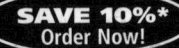
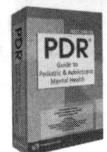
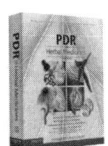
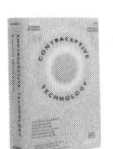
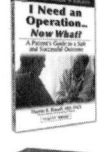
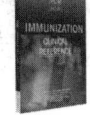
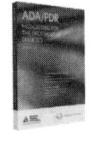
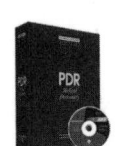
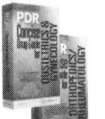
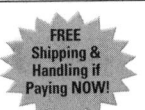

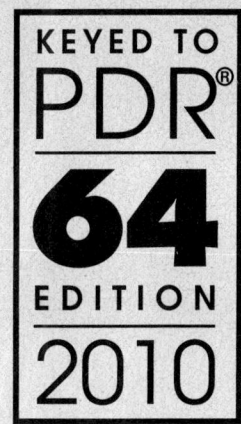

SLM 75.—
832008

PDR®

Guide to Drug Interactions, Side Effects, and Indications

ISBN: 978-1-56363-753-7

FOREWORD

Announcing PDR Network

Welcome to the 2010 edition of the *PDR® Guide to Drug Interactions, Side Effects, and Indications*. This year's Guide marks the introduction of the first national drug information and safety Alert service—**PDR Network**. This new service combines the expertise of PDR with the Health Care Notification Network (HCNN), the only network that delivers FDA-required drug Alerts and REMS programs to physicians and other prescribers online. PDR Network provides prescribers with a single, end-to-end drug information service, including:

- FDA-regulated drug labeling
- FDA-required drug Alerts
- Product-safety Alerts and recalls
- Information on the new FDA-required Risk Evaluation and Mitigation Strategies (REMS) program

By improving communication of important drug information and FDA safety Alerts, PDR Network's one-of-a-kind service will enhance patient safety, reduce medical liability, and ensure FDA compliance. For more information or to sign up for electronic Alerts, visit **www.PDRnet.com**.

About This Book

This edition of the *PDR Guide to Drug Interactions, Side Effects, and Indications* is cross-referenced with key facts from the 2010 editions of *Physicians' Desk Reference®* and *PDR® for Ophthalmic Medicines*, as well as updated labeling supplied by the manufacturer since the printing of the 2010 *PDR*. This unique handbook can help you to provide safe drug management. From its Indications Index, which permits you to instantly identify pharmaceutical alternatives for any given illness, to its Contraindications Index, which singles out products to avoid, this guide is designed to make safe, effective prescribing as fast, easy, and accurate as possible. Whether the challenge is detecting the source of an adverse reaction or avoiding a negative interaction, the *PDR Guide to Drug Interactions, Side Effects, and Indications* provides the tools you need to quickly find the answer. Here's a brief overview of the many features offered in the 2010 edition:

Interactions Index. This section includes an alphabetical listing of products followed by generic ingredients and dietary items that may cause an interaction as noted in the product's labeling. When applicable, specific brands that contain an interacting ingredient are also listed. A brief description of the interaction also appears. (Because product labeling varies in the scope of its interaction reporting, be sure to check the listing for each product in the patient's regimen.)

Food Interactions Cross-Reference. If you suspect an interaction with a specific dietary item, turn to this section. There you'll find potential drug/food and drug/alcohol interactions cross-referenced alphabetically by the name or type of food. Each entry includes a list of implicated drugs and a brief description of each interaction.

Side Effects Index. When a multidrug regimen masks the source of a side effect, this section can help provide the solution. Each entry includes an alphabetical list of the brands that have been associated with the problem. To help target the most likely offenders, incidence data are included whenever found in the official labeling.

Indications Index. If you need to locate an alternative to a medication—or simply want to review the full range of options for a particular diagnosis—turn to this part of the book. Here each indication is listed alphabetically, with a cross-reference to all brands approved for that purpose. For easy comparison, the listings include the generic name and manufacturer of each product. (Only FDA-regulated indications are referenced.)

Contraindications Index. When therapy is complicated by other medical conditions, this convenient index helps you to quickly eliminate contraindicated drugs from consideration. Here each contraindication is listed alphabetically, together with the drugs to avoid when the problem occurs.

The information in this edition of the *PDR Guide to Drug Interactions, Side Effects, and Indications* is based on FDA-regulated labeling found in the 2010 editions of *Physicians' Desk Reference* and *PDR for Ophthalmic Medicines*, or supplied by the manufacturer since the printing of the 2010 *PDR*. Please note that the entries in this Guide are derived directly from FDA-regulated prescribing information and only include products with labeling published by *PDR* or supplied to *PDR* by the manufacturer since the printing of the 2010 *PDR*. Note also that the publisher cannot guarantee that all entries are totally accurate or complete, nor is the publisher responsible for misuse of a product due to typographical error. Remember that important qualifications of the information listed in these indices may reside in the underlying text. Use this Guide as a convenient cross-reference, but consult the *PDR* or manufacturer when more detailed information is needed.

Web-Based Clinical Resources

PDR.net, a web portal designed specifically for healthcare professionals, provides a wealth of clinical information, including full FDA-regulated product labeling as well as concise drug information, disease monographs, patient education, clinical news, and conference information. PDR.net gives prescribers online access to authoritative, evidence-based information they need to support or confirm diagnosis and treatment decisions. PDR.net is also home to our **Clinical Resource Centers**, giving you the latest medical news and disease information all in one place. Online access is **free** for U.S.-based MDs, DOs, dentists, NPs, and PAs in full-time patient practice, as well as for medical students, residents, and other select prescribing allied health professionals. Register today at www.PDR.net.

Register for Product Safety Alerts at HCNN

Physicians and other prescribers may register to receive electronic Alerts online at **HCNN.net**, through participating medical societies and other HCNN partners, or by returning the qualification form distributed with physician copies of the 2010 *PDR*. Free to all licensed U.S. physicians and their staff, the HCNN is used exclusively for FDA-required product safety Alerts—not advertising or marketing—and fulfills FDA guidance for electronic delivery of Alerts.

Other Products from PDR

For those times when all you need is quick confirmation of a particular dosage, consult the 2010 **PDR® Pharmacopoeia Pocket Dosing Guide**. Only slightly larger than an index card and a half-inch thick, it fits easily into any pocket, and provides you with FDA-regulated dosing recommendations for more than 1,500 drugs.

Unlike other condensed drug references, the information is drawn exclusively from FDA-regulated drug labeling as published in *Physicians' Desk Reference* or supplied by the manufacturer.

To help you counsel patients who use over-the-counter supplements, the **PDR® for Nutritional Supplements, Second Edition** offers scientific consensus on hundreds of popular products, including amino acids, fatty acids, probiotics, phytoestrogens, phytosterols, over-the-counter hormones, and much more. Focused on the scientific evidence for each supplement's claims, this unique reference offers you a detailed, informed, and objective overview of a burgeoning area in the field of self-treatment.

For counseling patients who favor herbal remedies, the **PDR® for Herbal Medicines, Fourth Edition** provides you with science-based assessments of more than 700 botanicals. Indexed by scientific and common names (as well as Western, Asian, and homeopathic indications), this volume also includes a Side Effects Index, a Drug/Herb Interactions Guide, an Herb Identification Guide with nearly 400 color photos, and a Safety Guide that lists herbs to be avoided during pregnancy and those to be used only under professional supervision. Although botanical products are not officially regulated or monitored in the United States, *PDR for Herbal Medicines* provides you with authoritative information—the findings of the German Regulatory Authority's expert committee on herbal medicines, Commission E.

PDR prescribing information is also found in the **PDR® Electronic Library** on CD-ROM. This Windows® -compatible disc provides users with a complete database of *PDR* prescribing information, electronically searchable for instant retrieval. A standard subscription includes *PDR*'s sophisticated search software and an extensive file of chemical structures, illustrations, and full-color product photographs. For anyone who wants to run a fast double check on a proposed prescription, there's also the *PDR® Drug Interactions and Side Effects System*—sophisticated software capable of automatically screening a 20-drug regimen for conflicts, then proposing alternatives for any problematic medication. This unique decision-making tool comes free with the *PDR Electronic Library*.

For more information on these or any other members of the growing family of *PDR* products, please call, toll-free, 800-232-7379 or fax 201-722-2680, or visit *PDRbookstore.com*.

CONTENTS

SECTION 1

INTERACTIONS INDEX

Cataloged in this section are all interactions found during a review of product labeling as published by *Physicians' Desk Reference®* or supplied by the manufacturer since the printing of the 2010 *PDR*. The list is arranged alphabetically by brand or, when applicable, generic name.

Whenever appropriate, each brand-name heading is followed by a summary of the major pharmaceutical categories with which the product is said to interact. Beneath this summary is an alphabetical list of the compounds in these categories, each followed by a brief notation regarding the results of concurrent administration with the brand in question. After each notation is an alphabetical list of the brands with labeling published by *PDR* or supplied by the manufacturer since the printing

of the 2010 *PDR*. Page numbers refer to the 2010 editions of *Physicians' Desk Reference®* or *PDR® for Ophthalmic Medicines* (denoted with the ⊙ symbol).

Following the list of interacting drugs is a similar list of foods. Note that interactions with alcohol are listed here as well.

This index lists only interactions cited in FDA-regulated prescribing information as published by *PDR* or supplied by the manufacturer since the printing of the 2010 *PDR*. Because product labeling varies in the scope of its interaction reporting, you should check each product in the patient's regimen. Note also that cross-sensitivity reactions and effects on laboratory results are not included in the listings.

ACCOLATE TABLETS
(Zafirlukast) 3612
May interact with aspirin-acetylsalicylic acid, corticosteroids, cytochrome p450 2c9 substrates (selected), cytochrome p450 3a4 substrates (selected), dihydropyridine calcium channel blockers, erythromycin, oral anticoagulants, phenytoin, theophyllines, and certain other agents. Compounds in these categories include:

Acarbose (No formal drug-drug interaction studies with zafirlukast and other drugs known to be metabolized by the cytochrome P450 2C9 isoenzyme (eg, tolbutamide, phenytoin, carbamazepine) have been conducted; however, care should be exercised when zafirlukast is co-administered with these drugs).
No products indexed under this heading.

Alclometasone Dipropionate (In clinical trials, an increased proportion of zafirlukast patients over the age of 55 years reported infections as compared to placebo treated patients. A similar finding was not observed in other age groups studied. These infections were mostly mild or moderate in intensity and predominantly affected the respiratory tract. Infections occurred equally in both sexes, were dose-proportional to total milligrams of zafirlukast exposure, and were associated with co-administration of inhaled corticosteroids. The clinical significance of this finding is unknown).
No products indexed under this heading.

Alfentanil Hydrochloride (No formal drug-drug interaction studies between

zafirlukast and marketed drugs known to be metabolized by the P450 3A4 (CYP3A4) isoenzyme (eg, dihydropyridine calcium-channel blockers, cyclosporin, cisapride) have been conducted. As zafirlukast is known to be an inhibitor of CYP3A4 *in vitro*, it is reasonable to employ appropriate clinical monitoring when these drugs are co-administered with zafirlukast).
No products indexed under this heading.

Alprazolam (No formal drug-drug interaction studies between zafirlukast and marketed drugs known to be metabolized by the P450 3A4 (CYP3A4) isoenzyme (eg, dihydropyridine calcium-channel blockers, cyclosporin, cisapride) have been conducted. As zafirlukast is known to be an inhibitor of CYP3A4 *in vitro*, it is reasonable to employ appropriate clinical monitoring when these drugs are co-administered with zafirlukast).
No products indexed under this heading.

Amiodarone Hydrochloride (No formal drug-drug interaction studies between zafirlukast and marketed drugs known to be metabolized by the P450 3A4 (CYP3A4) isoenzyme (eg, dihydropyridine calcium-channel blockers, cyclosporin, cisapride) have been conducted. As zafirlukast is known to be an inhibitor of CYP3A4 *in vitro*, it is reasonable to employ appropriate clinical monitoring when zafirlukast is co-administered with zafirlukast).
No products indexed under this heading.

Amitriptyline Hydrochloride (No formal drug-drug interaction studies with zafirlukast and other drugs known to be metabolized by the cytochrome P450 2C9 isoenzyme (eg, tolbutamide, phenytoin, carbamazepine) have been conducted; however, care should be exercised when zafirlukast is co-administered with these drugs).
No products indexed under this heading.

Amlodipine Besylate (No formal drug-drug interaction studies between zafirlukast and marketed drugs known to be metabolized by the P450 3A4 (CYP3A4) isoenzyme (eg, dihydropyridine calcium-channel blockers, cyclosporin, cisapride) have been conducted. As zafirlukast is known to be an inhibitor of CYP3A4 *in vitro*, it is reasonable to employ appropriate clinical monitoring when these drugs are co-administered with zafirlukast). Products include:

Azor	1010
Exforge	2443
Exforge HCT	2449

Anisindione (Co-administration of multiple doses of zafirlukast (160 mg/day) to steady-state with a single 25 mg dose of warfarin (a substrate of CYP2C9) resulted in a significant increase in the mean AUC (+63%) and half-life (+36%) of S-warfarin. The mean prothrombin time increased by approximately 35%. The pharmacokinetics of zafirlukast were unaffected by co-administration with warfarin. Co-administration of zafirlukast with warfarin results in a clinically significant

increase in prothrombin time (PT). Patients on oral warfarin anticoagulant therapy and zafirlukast should have their prothrombin times monitored closely and anticoagulant dose adjusted accordingly).
No products indexed under this heading.

Aprepitant (No formal drug-drug interaction studies between zafirlukast and marketed drugs known to be metabolized by the P450 3A4 (CYP3A4) isoenzyme (eg, dihydropyridine calcium-channel blockers, cyclosporin, cisapride) have been conducted. As zafirlukast is known to be an inhibitor of CYP3A4 *in vitro*, it is reasonable to employ appropriate clinical monitoring when these drugs are co-administered with zafirlukast). Products include:

Emend	2124

Aspirin (Co-administration of zafirlukast (40 mg/day) with aspirin (650 mg four times daily) resulted in mean increased plasma concentrations of zafirlukast by approximately 45%). Products include:

Aggrenox	880
Bayer Aspirin	829
Percodan	1124
St. Joseph Aspirin	2045

Aspirin, Enteric Coated (Co-administration of zafirlukast (40 mg/day) with aspirin (650 mg four times daily) resulted in mean increased plasma concentrations of zafirlukast by approximately 45%).
No products indexed under this heading

Aspirin Buffered (Co-administration of zafirlukast (40 mg/day) with aspirin (650 mg four times daily) resulted in mean increased plasma concentrations of zafirlukast by approximately 45%).
No products indexed under this heading.

Astemizole (No formal drug-drug interaction studies between zafirlukast and marketed drugs known to be metabolized by the P450 3A4 (CYP3A4) isoenzyme (eg, dihydropyridine calcium-channel blockers, cyclosporin, cisapride) have been conducted. As zafirlukast is known to be an inhibitor of CYP3A4 *in vitro*, it is reasonable to employ appropriate clinical monitoring when these drugs are co-administered with zafirlukast).
No products indexed under this heading.

Atorvastatin Calcium (No formal drug-drug interaction studies between zafirlukast and marketed drugs known to be metabolized by the P450 3A4 (CYP3A4) isoenzyme (eg, dihydropyridine calcium-channel blockers, cyclosporin, cisapride) have been conducted. As zafirlukast is known to be an inhibitor of CYP3A4 *in vitro*, it is reasonable to employ appropriate clinical monitoring when these drugs are co-administered with zafirlukast). Products include:
Lipitor 2703

Beclomethasone Dipropionate (In clinical trials, an increased proportion of zafirlukast patients over the age of 55 years reported infections as compared to placebo treated patients. A similar finding was not observed in other age groups studied. These infections were mostly mild or moderate in intensity and predominantly affected the respiratory tract. Infections occurred equally in both sexes, were dose-proportional to total milligrams of zafirlukast exposure, and were associated with co-administration of inhaled corticosteroids. The clinical significance of this finding is unknown). Products include:
Qvar 3398

Beclomethasone Dipropionate Monohydrate (In clinical trials, an increased proportion of zafirlukast patients over the age of 55 years reported infections as compared to placebo treated patients. A similar finding was not observed in other age groups studied. These infections were mostly mild or moderate in intensity and predominantly affected the respiratory tract. Infections occurred equally in both sexes, were dose-proportional to total milligrams of zafirlukast exposure, and were associated with co-administration of inhaled corticosteroids. The clinical significance of this finding is unknown). Products include:
Beconase AQ 1386

Belladonna Ergotamine (No formal drug-drug interaction studies between zafirlukast and marketed drugs known to be metabolized by the P450 3A4 (CYP3A4) isoenzyme (eg, dihydropyridine calcium-channel blockers, cyclosporin, cisapride) have been conducted. As zafirlukast is known to be an inhibitor of CYP3A4 *in vitro*, it is reasonable to employ appropriate clinical monitoring when these drugs are co-administered with zafirlukast).
No products indexed under this heading.

Betamethasone (In clinical trials, an increased proportion of zafirlukast patients over the age of 55 years reported infections as compared to placebo treated patients. A similar finding was not observed in other age groups studied. These infections were mostly mild or moderate in intensity and predominantly affected the respiratory tract. Infections occurred equally in both sexes, were dose-proportional to total milligrams of zafirlukast exposure,

and were associated with co-administration of inhaled corticosteroids. The clinical significance of this finding is unknown).
No products indexed under this heading.

Betamethasone Acetate (In clinical trials, an increased proportion of zafirlukast patients over the age of 55 years reported infections as compared to placebo treated patients. A similar finding was not observed in other age groups studied. These infections were mostly mild or moderate in intensity and predominantly affected the respiratory tract. Infections occurred equally in both sexes, were dose-proportional to total milligrams of zafirlukast exposure, and were associated with co-administration of inhaled corticosteroids. The clinical significance of this finding is unknown).
No products indexed under this heading.

Betamethasone Benzoate (In clinical trials, an increased proportion of zafirlukast patients over the age of 55 years reported infections as compared to placebo treated patients. A similar finding was not observed in other age groups studied. These infections were mostly mild or moderate in intensity and predominantly affected the respiratory tract. Infections occurred equally in both sexes, were dose-proportional to total milligrams of zafirlukast exposure, and were associated with co-administration of inhaled corticosteroids. The clinical significance of this finding is unknown).
No products indexed under this heading.

Betamethasone Dipropionate (In clinical trials, an increased proportion of zafirlukast patients over the age of 55 years reported infections as compared to placebo treated patients. A similar finding was not observed in other age groups studied. These infections were mostly mild or moderate in intensity and predominantly affected the respiratory tract. Infections occurred equally in both sexes, were dose-proportional to total milligrams of zafirlukast exposure, and were associated with co-administration of inhaled corticosteroids. The clinical significance of this finding is unknown). Products include:
Diprolene Lotion 0.05% 3108
Diprolene Ointment 0.05% 3109
Diprolene AF Cream 0.05% 3107
Lotrisone 3163

Betamethasone Sodium Phosphate (In clinical trials, an increased proportion of zafirlukast patients over the age of 55 years reported infections as compared to placebo treated patients. A similar finding was not observed in other age groups studied. These infections were mostly mild or moderate in intensity and predominantly affected the respiratory tract. Infections occurred equally in both sexes, were dose-proportional to total milligrams of zafirlukast exposure, and were associated with co-administration of inhaled corticosteroids. The clinical significance of this finding is unknown).
No products indexed under this heading.

Betamethasone Valerate (In clinical trials, an increased proportion of zafirlukast patients over the age of 55 years reported infections as compared to placebo treated patients. A similar finding was not observed in other age groups studied. These infections were mostly mild or moderate in intensity and predominantly affected the respiratory tract. Infections occurred equally in both sexes, were dose-proportional to total milligrams of zafirlukast exposure, and were associated with co-administration of inhaled corticosteroids. The clinical significance of this finding is unknown). Products include:
Luxíq 3321

Budesonide (In clinical trials, an increased proportion of zafirlukast patients over the age of 55 years reported infections as compared to placebo treated patients. A similar finding was not observed in other age groups studied. These infections were mostly mild or moderate in intensity and predominantly affected the respiratory tract. Infections occurred equally in both sexes, were dose-proportional to total milligrams of zafirlukast exposure, and were associated with co-administration of inhaled corticosteroids. The clinical significance of this finding is unknown). Products include:
Pulmicort Flexhaler 714
Symbicort 80/4.5 720
Symbicort 160/4.5 720

Buspirone Hydrochloride (No formal drug-drug interaction studies between zafirlukast and marketed drugs known to be metabolized by the P450 3A4 (CYP3A4) isoenzyme (eg, dihydropyridine calcium-channel blockers, cyclosporin, cisapride) have been conducted. As zafirlukast is known to be an inhibitor of CYP3A4 *in vitro*, it is reasonable to employ appropriate clinical monitoring when these drugs are co-administered with zafirlukast).
No products indexed under this heading.

Busulfan (No formal drug-drug interaction studies between zafirlukast and marketed drugs known to be metabolized by the P450 3A4 (CYP3A4) isoenzyme (eg, dihydropyridine calcium-channel blockers, cyclosporin, cisapride) have been conducted. As zafirlukast is known to be an inhibitor of CYP3A4 *in vitro*, it is reasonable to employ appropriate clinical monitoring when these drugs are co-administered with zafirlukast). Products include:
Myleran 1581

Candesartan Cilexetil (No formal drug-drug interaction studies with zafirlukast and other drugs known to be metabolized by the cytochrome P450 2C9 isoenzyme (eg, tolbutamide, phenytoin, carbamazepine) have been conducted; however, care should be exercised when zafirlukast is co-administered with these drugs). Products include:
Atacand 697
Atacand HCT 700

Carbamazepine (No formal drug-drug interaction studies with zafirlukast and other drugs known to be metabolized by the cytochrome P450 2C9 isoenzyme (eg, tolbutamide, phenytoin, carbamazepine) have been conducted; however, care should be exercised when zafirlukast is co-administered with these drugs). Products include:
Carbatrol 3280
Equetro 3477

Carvedilol (No formal drug-drug interaction studies with zafirlukast and other drugs known to be metabolized by the cytochrome P450 2C9 isoenzyme (eg, tolbutamide, phenytoin, carbamazepine) have been conducted; however, care should be exercised when zafirlukast is co-administered with these drugs). Products include:
Coreg 1409

Celecoxib (No formal drug-drug interaction studies with zafirlukast and other drugs known to be metabolized by the cytochrome P450 2C9 isoenzyme (eg, tolbutamide, phenytoin, carbamazepine) have been conducted; however, care should be exercised when zafirlukast is co-administered with these drugs). Products include:
Celebrex 3272

Cerivastatin Sodium (No formal drug-drug interaction studies between zafirlukast and marketed drugs known to be metabolized by the P450 3A4 (CYP3A4) isoenzyme (eg, dihydropyri-

dine calcium-channel blockers, cyclosporin, cisapride) have been conducted. As zafirlukast is known to be an inhibitor of CYP3A4 *in vitro*, it is reasonable to employ appropriate clinical monitoring when these drugs are co-administered with zafirlukast).
No products indexed under this heading.

Chlorpheniramine (No formal drug-drug interaction studies between zafirlukast and marketed drugs known to be metabolized by the P450 3A4 (CYP3A4) isoenzyme (eg, dihydropyridine calcium-channel blockers, cyclosporin, cisapride) have been conducted. As zafirlukast is known to be an inhibitor of CYP3A4 *in vitro*, it is reasonable to employ appropriate clinical monitoring when these drugs are co-administered with zafirlukast).
No products indexed under this heading.

Chlorpheniramine Maleate (No formal drug-drug interaction studies between zafirlukast and marketed drugs known to be metabolized by the P450 3A4 (CYP3A4) isoenzyme (eg, dihydropyridine calcium-channel blockers, cyclosporin, cisapride) have been conducted. As zafirlukast is known to be an inhibitor of CYP3A4 *in vitro*, it is reasonable to employ appropriate clinical monitoring when these drugs are co-administered with zafirlukast).
No products indexed under this heading.

Chlorpheniramine Polistirex (No formal drug-drug interaction studies between zafirlukast and marketed drugs known to be metabolized by the P450 3A4 (CYP3A4) isoenzyme (eg, dihydropyridine calcium-channel blockers, cyclosporin, cisapride) have been conducted. As zafirlukast is known to be an inhibitor of CYP3A4 *in vitro*, it is reasonable to employ appropriate clinical monitoring when these drugs are co-administered with zafirlukast). Products include:
Tussionex 3443

Chlorpheniramine Tannate (No formal drug-drug interaction studies between zafirlukast and marketed drugs known to be metabolized by the P450 3A4 (CYP3A4) isoenzyme (eg, dihydropyridine calcium-channel blockers, cyclosporin, cisapride) have been conducted. As zafirlukast is known to be an inhibitor of CYP3A4 *in vitro*, it is reasonable to employ appropriate clinical monitoring when these drugs are co-administered with zafirlukast).
No products indexed under this heading.

Chlorpropamide (No formal drug-drug interaction studies with zafirlukast and other drugs known to be metabolized by the cytochrome P450 2C9 isoenzyme (eg, tolbutamide, phenytoin, carbamazepine) have been conducted; however, care should be exercised when zafirlukast is co-administered with these drugs).
No products indexed under this heading.

Ciclesonide (In clinical trials, an increased proportion of zafirlukast patients over the age of 55 years reported infections as compared to placebo treated patients. A similar finding was not observed in other age groups studied. These infections were mostly mild or moderate in intensity and predominantly affected the respiratory tract. Infections occurred equally in both sexes, were dose-proportional to total milligrams of zafirlukast exposure, and were associated with co-administration of inhaled corticosteroids. The clinical significance of this finding is unknown).
No products indexed under this heading.

Cisapride (No formal drug-drug interaction studies between zafirlukast and marketed drugs known to be metabolized by the P450 3A4 (CYP3A4) isoen-

zyme (eg, dihydropyridine calcium-channel blockers, cyclosporin, cisapride) have been conducted. As zafirlukast is known to be an inhibitor of CYP3A4 *in vitro*, it is reasonable to employ appropriate clinical monitoring when these drugs are co-administered with zafirlukast).
No products indexed under this heading.

Clarithromycin (No formal drug-drug interaction studies between zafirlukast and marketed drugs known to be metabolized by the P450 3A4 (CYP3A4) isoenzyme (eg, dihydropyridine calcium-channel blockers, cyclosporin, cisapride) have been conducted. As zafirlukast is known to be an inhibitor of CYP3A4 *in vitro*, it is reasonable to employ appropriate clinical monitoring when these drugs are co-administered with zafirlukast). Products include:
Biaxin/Biaxin XL 412

Clomipramine Hydrochloride (No formal drug-drug interaction studies with zafirlukast and other drugs known to be metabolized by the cytochrome P450 2C9 isoenzyme (eg, tolbutamide, phenytoin, carbamazepine) have been conducted; however, care should be exercised when zafirlukast is co-administered with these drugs).
No products indexed under this heading.

Cortisone Acetate (In clinical trials, an increased proportion of zafirlukast patients over the age of 55 years reported infections as compared to placebo treated patients. A similar finding was not observed in other age groups studied. These infections were mostly mild or moderate in intensity and predominantly affected the respiratory tract. Infections occurred equally in both sexes, were dose-proportional to total milligrams of zafirlukast exposure, and were associated with co-administration of inhaled corticosteroids. The clinical significance of this finding is unknown).
No products indexed under this heading.

Cyclosporine (No formal drug-drug interaction studies between zafirlukast and marketed drugs known to be metabolized by the P450 3A4 (CYP3A4) isoenzyme (eg, dihydropyridine calcium-channel blockers, cyclosporin, cisapride) have been conducted. As zafirlukast is known to be an inhibitor of CYP3A4 *in vitro*, it is reasonable to employ appropriate clinical monitoring when these drugs are co-administered with zafirlukast). Products include:
Gengraf 440
Neoral Oral Solution 2496
Neoral Capsules 2496
Restasis 605

Desogestrel (No formal drug-drug interaction studies with zafirlukast and other drugs known to be metabolized by the cytochrome P450 2C9 isoenzyme (eg, tolbutamide, phenytoin, carbamazepine) have been conducted; however, care should be exercised when zafirlukast is co-administered with these drugs).
No products indexed under this heading.

Desoximetasone (In clinical trials, an increased proportion of zafirlukast patients over the age of 55 years reported infections as compared to placebo treated patients. A similar finding was not observed in other age groups studied. These infections were mostly mild or moderate in intensity and predominantly affected the respiratory tract. Infections occurred equally in both sexes, were dose-proportional to total milligrams of zafirlukast exposure, and were associated with co-administration of inhaled corticosteroids. The clinical significance of this finding is unknown).
No products indexed under this heading.

Dexamethasone (In clinical trials, an increased proportion of zafirlukast patients over the age of 55 years reported infections as compared to placebo treated patients. A similar finding was not observed in other age groups studied. These infections were mostly mild or moderate in intensity and predominantly affected the respiratory tract. Infections occurred equally in both sexes, were dose-proportional to total milligrams of zafirlukast exposure, and were associated with co-administration of inhaled corticosteroids. The clinical significance of this finding is unknown). Products include:
Ciprodex 583
Ozurdex .... ⊙ 223
Tobramycin and Dexamethasone Ophthalmic Suspension .... ⊙ 251

Dexamethasone Acetate (In clinical trials, an increased proportion of zafirlukast patients over the age of 55 years reported infections as compared to placebo treated patients. A similar finding was not observed in other age groups studied. These infections were mostly mild or moderate in intensity and predominantly affected the respiratory tract. Infections occurred equally in both sexes, were dose-proportional to total milligrams of zafirlukast exposure, and were associated with co-administration of inhaled corticosteroids. The clinical significance of this finding is unknown).
No products indexed under this heading.

Dexamethasone Phosphate (In clinical trials, an increased proportion of zafirlukast patients over the age of 55 years reported infections as compared to placebo treated patients. A similar finding was not observed in other age groups studied. These infections were mostly mild or moderate in intensity and predominantly affected the respiratory tract. Infections occurred equally in both sexes, were dose-proportional to total milligrams of zafirlukast exposure, and were associated with co-administration of inhaled corticosteroids. The clinical significance of this finding is unknown).
No products indexed under this heading.

Dexamethasone Sodium (In clinical trials, an increased proportion of zafirlukast patients over the age of 55 years reported infections as compared to placebo treated patients. A similar finding was not observed in other age groups studied. These infections were mostly mild or moderate in intensity and predominantly affected the respiratory tract. Infections occurred equally in both sexes, were dose-proportional to total milligrams of zafirlukast exposure, and were associated with co-administration of inhaled corticosteroids. The clinical significance of this finding is unknown).
No products indexed under this heading.

Dexamethasone Sodium Phosphate (In clinical trials, an increased proportion of zafirlukast patients over the age of 55 years reported infections as compared to placebo treated patients. A similar finding was not observed in other age groups studied. These infections were mostly mild or moderate in intensity and predominantly affected the respiratory tract. Infections occurred equally in both sexes, were dose-proportional to total milligrams of zafirlukast exposure, and were associated with co-administration of inhaled corticosteroids. The clinical significance of this finding is unknown).
No products indexed under this heading.

Dexamethasone Sodium Phosphate Injection (In clinical trials, an increased proportion of zafirlukast patients over the age of 55 years reported infections as compared to placebo treated patients. A similar finding was not observed in other age groups studied. These infections were mostly mild or moderate in intensity and predominantly affected the respiratory tract. Infections occurred equally in both sexes, were dose-proportional to total milligrams of zafirlukast exposure, and were associated with co-administration of inhaled corticosteroids. The clinical significance of this finding is unknown).
No products indexed under this heading.

Dextromethorphan (No formal drug-drug interaction studies with zafirlukast and other drugs known to be metabolized by the cytochrome P450 2C9 isoenzyme (eg, tolbutamide, phenytoin, carbamazepine) have been conducted; however, care should be exercised when zafirlukast is co-administered with these drugs).
No products indexed under this heading.

Diazepam (No formal drug-drug interaction studies with zafirlukast and other drugs known to be metabolized by the cytochrome P450 2C9 isoenzyme (eg, tolbutamide, phenytoin, carbamazepine) have been conducted; however, care should be exercised when zafirlukast is co-administered with these drugs). Products include:
Valium Tablets 2880

Diclofenac Potassium (No formal drug-drug interaction studies with zafirlukast and other drugs known to be metabolized by the cytochrome P450 2C9 isoenzyme (eg, tolbutamide, phenytoin, carbamazepine) have been conducted; however, care should be exercised when zafirlukast is co-administered with these drugs).
No products indexed under this heading.

Diclofenac Sodium (No formal drug-drug interaction studies with zafirlukast and other drugs known to be metabolized by the cytochrome P450 2C9 isoenzyme (eg, tolbutamide, phenytoin, carbamazepine) have been conducted; however, care should be exercised when zafirlukast is co-administered with these drugs).
No products indexed under this heading.

Dicumarol (Co-administration of multiple doses of zafirlukast (160 mg/day) to steady-state with a single 25 mg dose of warfarin (a substrate of CYP2C9) resulted in a significant increase in the mean AUC (+63%) and half-life (+36%) of S-warfarin. The mean prothrombin time increased by approximately 35%. The pharmacokinetics of zafirlukast were unaffected by co-administration with warfarin. Co-administration of zafirlukast with warfarin results in a clinically significant increase in prothrombin time (PT). Patients on oral warfarin anticoagulant therapy and zafirlukast should have their prothrombin times monitored closely and anticoagulant dose adjusted accordingly).
No products indexed under this heading.

Diflorasone Diacetate (In clinical trials, an increased proportion of zafirlukast patients over the age of 55 years reported infections as compared to placebo treated patients. A similar finding was not observed in other age groups studied. These infections were mostly mild or moderate in intensity and predominantly affected the respiratory tract. Infections occurred equally in both sexes, were dose-proportional to total milligrams of zafirlukast exposure, and were associated with co-administration of inhaled corticosteroids. The clinical significance of this finding is unknown).
No products indexed under this heading.

Dihydroergotamine Mesylate (No formal drug-drug interaction studies between zafirlukast and marketed drugs known to be metabolized by the P450 3A4 (CYP3A4) isoenzyme (eg, dihydropyridine calcium-channel blockers, cyclosporin, cisapride) have been conducted. As zafirlukast is known to be an inhibitor of CYP3A4 *in vitro*, it is reasonable to employ appropriate clinical monitoring when these drugs are co-administered with zafirlukast).
No products indexed under this heading.

Diltiazem Hydrochloride (No formal drug-drug interaction studies between zafirlukast and marketed drugs known to be metabolized by the P450 3A4 (CYP3A4) isoenzyme (eg, dihydropyridine calcium-channel blockers, cyclosporin, cisapride) have been conducted. As zafirlukast is known to be an inhibitor of CYP3A4 *in vitro*, it is reasonable to employ appropriate clinical monitoring when these drugs are co-administered with zafirlukast). Products include:
Cardizem LA 423

Diltiazem Maleate (No formal drug-drug interaction studies between zafirlukast and marketed drugs known to be metabolized by the P450 3A4 (CYP3A4) isoenzyme (eg, dihydropyridine calcium-channel blockers, cyclosporin, cisapride) have been conducted. As zafirlukast is known to be an inhibitor of CYP3A4 *in vitro*, it is reasonable to employ appropriate clinical monitoring when these drugs are co-administered with zafirlukast).
No products indexed under this heading.

Disopyramide (No formal drug-drug interaction studies between zafirlukast and marketed drugs known to be metabolized by the P450 3A4 (CYP3A4) isoenzyme (eg, dihydropyridine calcium-channel blockers, cyclosporin, cisapride) have been conducted. As zafirlukast is known to be an inhibitor of CYP3A4 *in vitro*, it is reasonable to employ appropriate clinical monitoring when these drugs are co-administered with zafirlukast).
No products indexed under this heading.

Disopyramide Phosphate (No formal drug-drug interaction studies between zafirlukast and marketed drugs known to be metabolized by the P450 3A4 (CYP3A4) isoenzyme (eg, dihydropyridine calcium-channel blockers, cyclosporin, cisapride) have been conducted. As zafirlukast is known to be an inhibitor of CYP3A4 *in vitro*, it is reasonable to employ appropriate clinical monitoring when these drugs are co-administered with zafirlukast).
No products indexed under this heading.

Disulfiram (No formal drug-drug interaction studies between zafirlukast and marketed drugs known to be metabolized by the P450 3A4 (CYP3A4) isoenzyme (eg, dihydropyridine calcium-channel blockers, cyclosporin, cisapride) have been conducted. As zafirlukast is known to be an inhibitor of CYP3A4 *in vitro*, it is reasonable to employ appropriate clinical monitoring when these drugs are co-administered with zafirlukast).
No products indexed under this heading.

Doxorubicin Hydrochloride (No formal drug-drug interaction studies between zafirlukast and marketed drugs known to be metabolized by the P450 3A4 (CYP3A4) isoenzyme (eg, dihydropyridine calcium-channel blockers, cyclosporin, cisapride) have been conducted. As zafirlukast is known to be an inhibitor of CYP3A4 *in vitro*, it is reasonable to employ appropriate clinical monitoring when these drugs are co-administered with zafirlukast).
No products indexed under this heading.

IMPORTANT NOTE: Always consult each drug listing in the patient's regimen for possible interactions.

(⊙ Described in PDR® for Ophthalmic Medicines)

5 Interactions Index Accolate

metabolized by the cytochrome P450 2C9 isoenzyme (eg, tolbutamide, phenytoin, carbamazepine) have been conducted; however, care should be exercised when zafirlukast is co-administered with these drugs). Products include:
Prozac Weekly 1941
Prozac Pulvules 1941
Symbyax 1965

Flurbiprofen (No formal drug-drug interaction studies with zafirlukast and other drugs known to be metabolized by the cytochrome P450 2C9 isoenzyme (eg, tolbutamide, phenytoin, carbamazepine) have been conducted; however, care should be exercised when zafirlukast is co-administered with these drugs).
No products indexed under this heading.

Flurbiprofen Sodium (No formal drug-drug interaction studies with zafirlukast and other drugs known to be metabolized by the cytochrome P450 2C9 isoenzyme (eg, tolbutamide, phenytoin, carbamazepine) have been conducted; however, care should be exercised when zafirlukast is co-administered with these drugs).
No products indexed under this heading.

Fluticasone Furoate (In clinical trials, an increased proportion of zafirlukast patients over the age of 55 years reported infections as compared to placebo treated patients. A similar finding was not observed in other age groups studied. These infections were mostly mild or moderate in intensity and predominantly affected the respiratory tract. Infections occurred equally in both sexes, were dose-proportional to total milligrams of zafirlukast exposure, and were associated with co-administration of inhaled corticosteroids. The clinical significance of this finding is unknown). Products include:
Veramyst 1713

Fluticasone Propionate (In clinical trials, an increased proportion of zafirlukast patients over the age of 55 years reported infections as compared to placebo treated patients. A similar finding was not observed in other age groups studied. These infections were mostly mild or moderate in intensity and predominantly affected the respiratory tract. Infections occurred equally in both sexes, were dose-proportional to total milligrams of zafirlukast exposure, and were associated with co-administration of inhaled corticosteroids. The clinical significance of this finding is unknown). Products include:
Advair 100/50 1275
Advair 250/50 1275
Advair 500/50 1275
Advair HFA 45/21 1288
Advair HFA 115/21 1288
Advair HFA 230/21 1288
Flonase 1459
Flovent Diskus 1463
Flovent HFA 1470

Fluvastatin Sodium (No formal drug-drug interaction studies with zafirlukast and other drugs known to be metabolized by the cytochrome P450 2C9 isoenzyme (eg, tolbutamide, phenytoin, carbamazepine) have been conducted; however, care should be exercised when zafirlukast is co-administered with these drugs).
No products indexed under this heading.

Fosphenytoin (No formal drug-drug interaction studies with zafirlukast and other drugs known to be metabolized by the cytochrome P450 2C9 isoenzyme (eg, tolbutamide, phenytoin, carbamazepine) have been conducted; however, care should be exercised when zafirlukast is co-administered with these drugs).
No products indexed under this heading.

Fosphenytoin Sodium (No formal drug-drug interaction studies with zafirlukast and other drugs known to be metabolized by the cytochrome P450 2C9 isoenzyme (eg, tolbutamide, phenytoin, carbamazepine) have been conducted; however, care should be exercised when zafirlukast is co-administered with these drugs).
No products indexed under this heading.

Glimepiride (No formal drug-drug interaction studies with zafirlukast and other drugs known to be metabolized by the cytochrome P450 2C9 isoenzyme (eg, tolbutamide, phenytoin, carbamazepine) have been conducted; however, care should be exercised when zafirlukast is co-administered with these drugs). Products include:
Avandaryl 1356
Duetact 3354

Glipizide (No formal drug-drug interaction studies with zafirlukast and other drugs known to be metabolized by the cytochrome P450 2C9 isoenzyme (eg, tolbutamide, phenytoin, carbamazepine) have been conducted; however, care should be exercised when zafirlukast is co-administered with these drugs).
No products indexed under this heading.

Haloperidol (No formal drug-drug interaction studies between zafirlukast and marketed drugs known to be metabolized by the P450 3A4 (CYP3A4) isoenzyme (eg, dihydropyridine calcium-channel blockers, cyclosporin, cisapride) have been conducted. As zafirlukast is known to be an inhibitor of CYP3A4 *in vitro*, it is reasonable to employ appropriate clinical monitoring when these drugs are co-administered with zafirlukast).
No products indexed under this heading.

Haloperidol Decanoate (No formal drug-drug interaction studies between zafirlukast and marketed drugs known to be metabolized by the P450 3A4 (CYP3A4) isoenzyme (eg, dihydropyridine calcium-channel blockers, cyclosporin, cisapride) have been conducted. As zafirlukast is known to be an inhibitor of CYP3A4 *in vitro*, it is reasonable to employ appropriate clinical monitoring when these drugs are co-administered with zafirlukast).
No products indexed under this heading.

Haloperidol Lactate (No formal drug-drug interaction studies between zafirlukast and marketed drugs known to be metabolized by the P450 3A4 (CYP3A4) isoenzyme (eg, dihydropyridine calcium-channel blockers, cyclosporin, cisapride) have been conducted. As zafirlukast is known to be an inhibitor of CYP3A4 *in vitro*, it is reasonable to employ appropriate clinical monitoring when these drugs are co-administered with zafirlukast).
No products indexed under this heading.

Hydrocortisone (In clinical trials, an increased proportion of zafirlukast patients over the age of 55 years reported infections as compared to placebo treated patients. A similar finding was not observed in other age groups studied. These infections were mostly mild or moderate in intensity and predominantly affected the respiratory tract. Infections occurred equally in both sexes, were dose-proportional to total milligrams of zafirlukast exposure, and were associated with co-administration of inhaled corticosteroids. The clinical significance of this finding is unknown).
No products indexed under this heading.

Hydrocortisone (Alcohol) (In clinical trials, an increased proportion of zafirlukast patients over the age of 55 years reported infections as compared to placebo treated patients. A similar finding was not observed in other age groups studied. These infections were mostly mild or moderate in intensity and predominantly affected the respiratory tract. Infections occurred equally in both sexes, were dose-proportional to total milligrams of zafirlukast exposure, and were associated with co-administration of inhaled corticosteroids. The clinical significance of this finding is unknown).
No products indexed under this heading.

Hydrocortisone Acetate (In clinical trials, an increased proportion of zafirlukast patients over the age of 55 years reported infections as compared to placebo treated patients. A similar finding was not observed in other age groups studied. These infections were mostly mild or moderate in intensity and predominantly affected the respiratory tract. Infections occurred equally in both sexes, were dose-proportional to total milligrams of zafirlukast exposure, and were associated with co-administration of inhaled corticosteroids. The clinical significance of this finding is unknown).
No products indexed under this heading.

Hydrocortisone Butyrate (In clinical trials, an increased proportion of zafirlukast patients over the age of 55 years reported infections as compared to placebo treated patients. A similar finding was not observed in other age groups studied. These infections were mostly mild or moderate in intensity and predominantly affected the respiratory tract. Infections occurred equally in both sexes, were dose-proportional to total milligrams of zafirlukast exposure, and were associated with co-administration of inhaled corticosteroids. The clinical significance of this finding is unknown).
No products indexed under this heading.

Hydrocortisone Cypionate (In clinical trials, an increased proportion of zafirlukast patients over the age of 55 years reported infections as compared to placebo treated patients. A similar finding was not observed in other age groups studied. These infections were mostly mild or moderate in intensity and predominantly affected the respiratory tract. Infections occurred equally in both sexes, were dose-proportional to total milligrams of zafirlukast exposure, and were associated with co-administration of inhaled corticosteroids. The clinical significance of this finding is unknown).
No products indexed under this heading.

Hydrocortisone Hemisuccinate (In clinical trials, an increased proportion of zafirlukast patients over the age of 55 years reported infections as compared to placebo treated patients. A similar finding was not observed in other age groups studied. These infections were mostly mild or moderate in intensity and predominantly affected the respiratory tract. Infections occurred equally in both sexes, were dose-proportional to total milligrams of zafirlukast exposure, and were associated with co-administration of inhaled corticosteroids. The clinical significance of this finding is unknown).
No products indexed under this heading.

Hydrocortisone Probutate (In clinical trials, an increased proportion of zafirlukast patients over the age of 55 years reported infections as compared to placebo treated patients. A similar finding was not observed in other age groups studied. These infections were mostly mild or moderate in intensity and predominantly affected the respiratory tract. Infections occurred equally in both sexes, were dose-proportional to total milligrams of zafirlukast exposure, and were associated with co-administration of inhaled corticosteroids. The clinical significance of this finding is unknown).
No products indexed under this heading.

Hydrocortisone Sodium Phosphate (In clinical trials, an increased proportion of zafirlukast patients over the age of 55 years reported infections as compared to placebo treated patients. A similar finding was not observed in other age groups studied. These infections were mostly mild or moderate in intensity and predominantly affected the respiratory tract. Infections occurred equally in both sexes, were dose-proportional to total milligrams of zafirlukast exposure, and were associated with co-administration of inhaled corticosteroids. The clinical significance of this finding is unknown).
No products indexed under this heading.

Hydrocortisone Sodium Succinate (In clinical trials, an increased proportion of zafirlukast patients over the age of 55 years reported infections as compared to placebo treated patients. A similar finding was not observed in other age groups studied. These infections were mostly mild or moderate in intensity and predominantly affected the respiratory tract. Infections occurred equally in both sexes, were dose-proportional to total milligrams of zafirlukast exposure, and were associated with co-administration of inhaled corticosteroids. The clinical significance of this finding is unknown).
No products indexed under this heading.

Hydrocortisone Valerate (In clinical trials, an increased proportion of zafirlukast patients over the age of 55 years reported infections as compared to placebo treated patients. A similar finding was not observed in other age groups studied. These infections were mostly mild or moderate in intensity and predominantly affected the respiratory tract. Infections occurred equally in both sexes, were dose-proportional to total milligrams of zafirlukast exposure, and were associated with co-administration of inhaled corticosteroids. The clinical significance of this finding is unknown).
No products indexed under this heading.

Ibuprofen (No formal drug-drug interaction studies with zafirlukast and other drugs known to be metabolized by the cytochrome P450 2C9 isoenzyme (eg, tolbutamide, phenytoin, carbamazepine) have been conducted; however, care should be exercised when zafirlukast is co-administered with these drugs). Products include:
Motrin IB 2043
Children's Motrin 2044
Children's Motrin Non-Staining Dye-Free 2044
Infants' Motrin 2044
Infants' Motrin Dye-Free 2044
Junior Strength Motrin 2044
Vicoprofen 564

Imipramine Hydrochloride (No formal drug-drug interaction studies with zafirlukast and other drugs known to be metabolized by the cytochrome P450 2C9 isoenzyme (eg, tolbutamide, phenytoin, carbamazepine) have been conducted; however, care should be exercised when zafirlukast is co-administered with these drugs).
No products indexed under this heading.

Indinavir Sulfate (No formal drug-drug interaction studies between zafirlukast and marketed drugs known to be metabolized by the P450 3A4 (CYP3A4) isoenzyme (eg, dihydropyridine calcium-channel blockers, cyclosporin, cisapride) have been conducted. As zafirlukast is known to be an inhibitor of CYP3A4 *in vitro*, it is reasonable to employ appropriate clinical mon-

IMPORTANT NOTE: Always consult each drug listing in the patient's regimen for possible interactions.

itoring when these drugs are co-administered with zafirlukast). Products include:

Crixivan **2113**

Indomethacin (No formal drug-drug interaction studies with zafirlukast and other drugs known to be metabolized by the cytochrome P450 2C9 isoenzyme (eg, tolbutamide, phenytoin, carbamazepine) have been conducted; however, care should be exercised when zafirlukast is co-administered with these drugs). Products include:

Indocin **2167**

Indomethacin Sodium Trihydrate (No formal drug-drug interaction studies with zafirlukast and other drugs known to be metabolized by the cytochrome P450 2C9 isoenzyme (eg, tolbutamide, phenytoin, carbamazepine) have been conducted; however, care should be exercised when zafirlukast is co-administered with these drugs). Products include:

Indocin I.V. **2007**

Irbesartan (No formal drug-drug interaction studies with zafirlukast and other drugs known to be metabolized by the cytochrome P450 2C9 isoenzyme (eg, tolbutamide, phenytoin, carbamazepine) have been conducted; however, care should be exercised when zafirlukast is co-administered with these drugs). Products include:

Avalide **2956**
Avapro **2962**

Isradipine (No formal drug-drug interaction studies between zafirlukast and marketed drugs known to be metabolized by the P450 3A4 (CYP3A4) isoenzyme (eg, dihydropyridine calcium-channel blockers, cyclosporin, cisapride) have been conducted. As zafirlukast is known to be an inhibitor of CYP3A4 *in vitro*, it is reasonable to employ appropriate clinical monitoring when these drugs are co-administered with zafirlukast). Products include:

DynaCirc CR **1432**

Itraconazole (No formal drug-drug interaction studies between zafirlukast and marketed drugs known to be metabolized by the P450 3A4 (CYP3A4) isoenzyme (eg, dihydropyridine calcium-channel blockers, cyclosporin, cisapride) have been conducted. As zafirlukast is known to be an inhibitor of CYP3A4 *in vitro*, it is reasonable to employ appropriate clinical monitoring when these drugs are co-administered with zafirlukast).

No products indexed under this heading.

Ixabepilone (No formal drug-drug interaction studies between zafirlukast and marketed drugs known to be metabolized by the P450 3A4 (CYP3A4) isoenzyme (eg, dihydropyridine calcium-channel blockers, cyclosporin, cisapride) have been conducted. As zafirlukast is known to be an inhibitor of CYP3A4 *in vitro*, it is reasonable to employ appropriate clinical monitoring when these drugs are co-administered with zafirlukast).

No products indexed under this heading.

Ketoconazole (No formal drug-drug interaction studies between zafirlukast and marketed drugs known to be metabolized by the P450 3A4 (CYP3A4) isoenzyme (eg, dihydropyridine calcium-channel blockers, cyclosporin, cisapride) have been conducted. As zafirlukast is known to be an inhibitor of CYP3A4 *in vitro*, it is reasonable to employ appropriate clinical monitoring when these drugs are co-administered with zafirlukast). Products include:

Extina **3319**
Xolegel **3337**

Ketoprofen (No formal drug-drug interaction studies with zafirlukast and other drugs known to be metabolized by the cytochrome P450 2C9 isoenzyme (eg, tolbutamide, phenytoin, carbamazepine) have been conducted; however, care should be exercised when zafirlukast is co-administered with these drugs).

No products indexed under this heading.

Ketorolac Tromethamine (No formal drug-drug interaction studies with zafirlukast and other drugs known to be metabolized by the cytochrome P450 2C9 isoenzyme (eg, tolbutamide, phenytoin, carbamazepine) have been conducted; however, care should be exercised when zafirlukast is co-administered with these drugs). Products include:

Acuvail .... ⊙**209**

Lansoprazole (No formal drug-drug interaction studies with zafirlukast and other drugs known to be metabolized by the cytochrome P450 2C9 isoenzyme (eg, tolbutamide, phenytoin, carbamazepine) have been conducted; however, care should be exercised when zafirlukast is co-administered with these drugs).

No products indexed under this heading.

Levonorgestrel (No formal drug-drug interaction studies between zafirlukast and marketed drugs known to be metabolized by the P450 3A4 (CYP3A4) isoenzyme (eg, dihydropyridine calcium-channel blockers, cyclosporin, cisapride) have been conducted. As zafirlukast is known to be an inhibitor of CYP3A4 *in vitro*, it is reasonable to employ appropriate clinical monitoring when these drugs are co-administered with zafirlukast). Products include:

Climara Pro **847**
LoSeasonique **3407**
Lybrel **3514**
Mirena **854**
Plan B **3416**
Seasonique **3418**

Lidocaine (No formal drug-drug interaction studies between zafirlukast and marketed drugs known to be metabolized by the P450 3A4 (CYP3A4) isoenzyme (eg, dihydropyridine calcium-channel blockers, cyclosporin, cisapride) have been conducted. As zafirlukast is known to be an inhibitor of CYP3A4 *in vitro*, it is reasonable to employ appropriate clinical monitoring when these drugs are co-administered with zafirlukast). Products include:

Lidoderm **1107**

Lidocaine Hydrochloride (No formal drug-drug interaction studies between zafirlukast and marketed drugs known to be metabolized by the P450 3A4 (CYP3A4) isoenzyme (eg, dihydropyridine calcium-channel blockers, cyclosporin, cisapride) have been conducted. As zafirlukast is known to be an inhibitor of CYP3A4 *in vitro*, it is reasonable to employ appropriate clinical monitoring when these drugs are co-administered with zafirlukast).

No products indexed under this heading.

Losartan Potassium (No formal drug-drug interaction studies with zafirlukast and other drugs known to be metabolized by the cytochrome P450 2C9 isoenzyme (eg, tolbutamide, phenytoin, carbamazepine) have been conducted; however, care should be exercised when zafirlukast is co-administered with these drugs). Products include:

Cozaar **2106**
Hyzaar **2162**
Hyzaar 100-12.5 .... **2162**

Lovastatin (No formal drug-drug interaction studies between zafirlukast and marketed drugs known to be metabolized by the P450 3A4 (CYP3A4) isoenzyme (eg, dihydropyridine calcium-channel blockers, cyclosporin, cisapride) have been conducted. As zafirlukast is known to be an inhibitor of CYP3A4 *in vitro*, it is reasonable to employ appropriate clinical monitoring when these drugs are co-administered with zafirlukast). Products include:

Advicor **402**
Mevacor **2212**

Meclofenamate Sodium (No formal drug-drug interaction studies with zafirlukast and other drugs known to be metabolized by the cytochrome P450 2C9 isoenzyme (eg, tolbutamide, phenytoin, carbamazepine) have been conducted; however, care should be exercised when zafirlukast is co-administered with these drugs).

No products indexed under this heading.

Mefenamic Acid (No formal drug-drug interaction studies with zafirlukast and other drugs known to be metabolized by the cytochrome P450 2C9 isoenzyme (eg, tolbutamide, phenytoin, carbamazepine) have been conducted; however, care should be exercised when zafirlukast is co-administered with these drugs).

No products indexed under this heading.

Meloxicam (No formal drug-drug interaction studies with zafirlukast and other drugs known to be metabolized by the cytochrome P450 2C9 isoenzyme (eg, tolbutamide, phenytoin, carbamazepine) have been conducted; however, care should be exercised when zafirlukast is co-administered with these drugs).

No products indexed under this heading.

Mestranol (No formal drug-drug interaction studies between zafirlukast and marketed drugs known to be metabolized by the P450 3A4 (CYP3A4) isoenzyme (eg, dihydropyridine calcium-channel blockers, cyclosporin, cisapride) have been conducted. As zafirlukast is known to be an inhibitor of CYP3A4 *in vitro*, it is reasonable to employ appropriate clinical monitoring when these drugs are co-administered with zafirlukast).

No products indexed under this heading.

Metformin Hydrochloride (No formal drug-drug interaction studies with zafirlukast and other drugs known to be metabolized by the cytochrome P450 2C9 isoenzyme (eg, tolbutamide, phenytoin, carbamazepine) have been conducted; however, care should be exercised when zafirlukast is co-administered with these drugs). Products include:

ActoPlus **3338**
Avandamet **1345**
Janumet **2188**

Methadone Hydrochloride (No formal drug-drug interaction studies between zafirlukast and marketed drugs known to be metabolized by the P450 3A4 (CYP3A4) isoenzyme (eg, dihydropyridine calcium-channel blockers, cyclosporin, cisapride) have been conducted. As zafirlukast is known to be an inhibitor of CYP3A4 *in vitro*, it is reasonable to employ appropriate clinical monitoring when these drugs are co-administered with zafirlukast).

No products indexed under this heading.

Methylprednisolone (In clinical trials, an increased proportion of zafirlukast patients over the age of 55 years reported infections as compared to placebo treated patients. A similar finding was not observed in other age groups studied. These infections were mostly mild or moderate in intensity and predominantly affected the respiratory tract. Infections occurred equally in both sexes, were dose-proportional to total milligrams of zafirlukast exposure, and were associated with co-administration of inhaled corticosteroids. The clinical significance of this finding is unknown).

No products indexed under this heading.

Methylprednisolone Acetate (In clinical trials, an increased proportion of zafirlukast patients over the age of 55 years reported infections as compared to placebo treated patients. A similar finding was not observed in other age groups studied. These infections were mostly mild or moderate in intensity and predominantly affected the respiratory tract. Infections occurred equally in both sexes, were dose-proportional to total milligrams of zafirlukast exposure, and were associated with co-administration of inhaled corticosteroids. The clinical significance of this finding is unknown).

No products indexed under this heading.

Methylprednisolone Sodium Succinate (In clinical trials, an increased proportion of zafirlukast patients over the age of 55 years reported infections as compared to placebo treated patients. A similar finding was not observed in other age groups studied. These infections were mostly mild or moderate in intensity and predominantly affected the respiratory tract. Infections occurred equally in both sexes, were dose-proportional to total milligrams of zafirlukast exposure, and were associated with co-administration of inhaled corticosteroids. The clinical significance of this finding is unknown).

No products indexed under this heading.

Midazolam Hydrochloride (No formal drug-drug interaction studies between zafirlukast and marketed drugs known to be metabolized by the P450 3A4 (CYP3A4) isoenzyme (eg, dihydropyridine calcium-channel blockers, cyclosporin, cisapride) have been conducted. As zafirlukast is known to be an inhibitor of CYP3A4 *in vitro*, it is reasonable to employ appropriate clinical monitoring when these drugs are co-administered with zafirlukast).

No products indexed under this heading.

Miglitol (No formal drug-drug interaction studies with zafirlukast and other drugs known to be metabolized by the cytochrome P450 2C9 isoenzyme (eg, tolbutamide, phenytoin, carbamazepine) have been conducted; however, care should be exercised when zafirlukast is co-administered with these drugs).

No products indexed under this heading.

Mirtazapine (No formal drug-drug interaction studies with zafirlukast and other drugs known to be metabolized by the cytochrome P450 2C9 isoenzyme (eg, tolbutamide, phenytoin, carbamazepine) have been conducted; however, care should be exercised when zafirlukast is co-administered with these drugs). Products include:

Remeron Tablets **3214**
RemeronSolTab Tablets **3219**

Mometasone Furoate (In clinical trials, an increased proportion of zafirlukast patients over the age of 55 years reported infections as compared to placebo treated patients. A similar finding was not observed in other age groups studied. These infections were mostly mild or moderate in intensity and predominantly affected the respiratory tract. Infections occurred equally in both sexes, were dose-proportional to total milligrams of zafirlukast exposure, and were associated with co-administration of inhaled corticosteroids. The clinical significance of this finding is unknown). Products include:

Asmanex **3058**
Elocon Cream **3111**
Elocon Lotion **3112**
Elocon Ointment **3114**

7 **Interactions Index** **Accolate**

Mometasone Furoate Monohydrate (In clinical trials, an increased proportion of zafirlukast patients over the age of 55 years reported infections as compared to placebo treated patients. A similar finding was not observed in other age groups studied. These infections were mostly mild or moderate in intensity and predominantly affected the respiratory tract. Infections occurred equally in both sexes, were dose-proportional to total milligrams of zafirlukast exposure, and were associated with co-administration of inhaled corticosteroids. The clinical significance of this finding is unknown). Products include:

Nasonex 3166

Montelukast Sodium (No formal drug-drug interaction studies with zafirlukast and other drugs known to be metabolized by the cytochrome P450 2C9 isoenzyme (eg, tolbutamide, phenytoin, carbamazepine) have been conducted; however, care should be exercised when zafirlukast is co-administered with these drugs). Products include:

Singulair 2270

Nabumetone (No formal drug-drug interaction studies with zafirlukast and other drugs known to be metabolized by the cytochrome P450 2C9 isoenzyme (eg, tolbutamide, phenytoin, carbamazepine) have been conducted; however, care should be exercised when zafirlukast is co-administered with these drugs).

No products indexed under this heading.

Naproxen (No formal drug-drug interaction studies with zafirlukast and other drugs known to be metabolized by the cytochrome P450 2C9 isoenzyme (eg, tolbutamide, phenytoin, carbamazepine) have been conducted; however, care should be exercised when zafirlukast is co-administered with these drugs). Products include:

EC-Naprosyn 2850
Naprosyn 2850
Anaprox/Naprosyn 2850

Naproxen Sodium (No formal drug-drug interaction studies with zafirlukast and other drugs known to be metabolized by the cytochrome P450 2C9 isoenzyme (eg, tolbutamide, phenytoin, carbamazepine) have been conducted; however, care should be exercised when zafirlukast is co-administered with these drugs). Products include:

Anaprox 2850
Anaprox DS 2850
Treximet 1681

Nateglinide (No formal drug-drug interaction studies with zafirlukast and other drugs known to be metabolized by the cytochrome P450 2C9 isoenzyme (eg, tolbutamide, phenytoin, carbamazepine) have been conducted; however, care should be exercised when zafirlukast is co-administered with these drugs).

No products indexed under this heading.

Nefazodone Hydrochloride (No formal drug-drug interaction studies between zafirlukast and marketed drugs known to be metabolized by the P450 3A4 (CYP3A4) isoenzyme (eg, dihydropyridine calcium-channel blockers, cyclosporin, cisapride) have been conducted. As zafirlukast is known to be an inhibitor of CYP3A4 *in vitro*, it is reasonable to employ appropriate clinical monitoring when these drugs are co-administered with zafirlukast).

No products indexed under this heading.

Nelfinavir Mesylate (No formal drug-drug interaction studies between zafirlukast and marketed drugs known to be metabolized by the P450 3A4 (CYP3A4) isoenzyme (eg, dihydropyridine calcium-channel blockers, cyclosporin, cisapride) have been conducted. As zafirlukast is known to be an inhibitor of CYP3A4 *in vitro*, it is reasonable to employ appropriate clinical monitoring when these drugs are co-administered with zafirlukast).

No products indexed under this heading.

Nicardipine (No formal drug-drug interaction studies between zafirlukast and marketed drugs known to be metabolized by the P450 3A4 (CYP3A4) isoenzyme (eg, dihydropyridine calcium-channel blockers, cyclosporin, cisapride) have been conducted. As zafirlukast is known to be an inhibitor of CYP3A4 *in vitro*, it is reasonable to employ appropriate clinical monitoring when these drugs are co-administered with zafirlukast).

No products indexed under this heading.

Nicardipine Hydrochloride (No formal drug-drug interaction studies between zafirlukast and marketed drugs known to be metabolized by the P450 3A4 (CYP3A4) isoenzyme (eg, dihydropyridine calcium-channel blockers, cyclosporin, cisapride) have been conducted. As zafirlukast is known to be an inhibitor of CYP3A4 *in vitro*, it is reasonable to employ appropriate clinical monitoring when these drugs are co-administered with zafirlukast).

No products indexed under this heading.

Nifedipine (No formal drug-drug interaction studies with zafirlukast and other drugs known to be metabolized by the cytochrome P450 2C9 isoenzyme (eg, tolbutamide, phenytoin, carbamazepine) have been conducted; however, care should be exercised when zafirlukast is co-administered with these drugs).

No products indexed under this heading.

Nimodipine (No formal drug-drug interaction studies between zafirlukast and marketed drugs known to be metabolized by the P450 3A4 (CYP3A4) isoenzyme (eg, dihydropyridine calcium-channel blockers, cyclosporin, cisapride) have been conducted. As zafirlukast is known to be an inhibitor of CYP3A4 *in vitro*, it is reasonable to employ appropriate clinical monitoring when these drugs are co-administered with zafirlukast).

No products indexed under this heading.

Nisoldipine (No formal drug-drug interaction studies between zafirlukast and marketed drugs known to be metabolized by the P450 3A4 (CYP3A4) isoenzyme (eg, dihydropyridine calcium-channel blockers, cyclosporin, cisapride) have been conducted. As zafirlukast is known to be an inhibitor of CYP3A4 *in vitro*, it is reasonable to employ appropriate clinical monitoring when these drugs are co-administered with zafirlukast).

No products indexed under this heading.

Nitrendipine (No formal drug-drug interaction studies between zafirlukast and marketed drugs known to be metabolized by the P450 3A4 (CYP3A4) isoenzyme (eg, dihydropyridine calcium-channel blockers, cyclosporin, cisapride) have been conducted. As zafirlukast is known to be an inhibitor of CYP3A4 *in vitro*, it is reasonable to employ appropriate clinical monitoring when these drugs are co-administered with zafirlukast).

No products indexed under this heading.

Norethindrone (No formal drug-drug interaction studies between zafirlukast and marketed drugs known to be metabolized by the P450 3A4 (CYP3A4) isoenzyme (eg, dihydropyridine calcium-channel blockers, cyclosporin, cisapride) have been conducted. As zafirlukast is known to be an inhibitor of CYP3A4 *in vitro*, it is reasonable to employ appropriate clinical monitoring when these drugs are co-administered with zafirlukast). Products include:

Ortho Micronor 2660

Norethindrone Acetate (No formal drug-drug interaction studies between zafirlukast and marketed drugs known to be metabolized by the P450 3A4 (CYP3A4) isoenzyme (eg, dihydropyridine calcium-channel blockers, cyclosporin, cisapride) have been conducted. As zafirlukast is known to be an inhibitor of CYP3A4 *in vitro*, it is reasonable to employ appropriate clinical monitoring when these drugs are co-administered with zafirlukast). Products include:

Activella 2561

Norgestrel (No formal drug-drug interaction studies between zafirlukast and marketed drugs known to be metabolized by the P450 3A4 (CYP3A4) isoenzyme (eg, dihydropyridine calcium-channel blockers, cyclosporin, cisapride) have been conducted. As zafirlukast is known to be an inhibitor of CYP3A4 *in vitro*, it is reasonable to employ appropriate clinical monitoring when these drugs are co-administered with zafirlukast).

No products indexed under this heading.

Omeprazole (No formal drug-drug interaction studies with zafirlukast and other drugs known to be metabolized by the cytochrome P450 2C9 isoenzyme (eg, tolbutamide, phenytoin, carbamazepine) have been conducted; however, care should be exercised when zafirlukast is co-administered with these drugs).

No products indexed under this heading.

Ondansetron (No formal drug-drug interaction studies between zafirlukast and marketed drugs known to be metabolized by the P450 3A4 (CYP3A4) isoenzyme (eg, dihydropyridine calcium-channel blockers, cyclosporin, cisapride) have been conducted. As zafirlukast is known to be an inhibitor of CYP3A4 *in vitro*, it is reasonable to employ appropriate clinical monitoring when these drugs are co-administered with zafirlukast).

No products indexed under this heading.

Ondansetron Hydrochloride (No formal drug-drug interaction studies between zafirlukast and marketed drugs known to be metabolized by the P450 3A4 (CYP3A4) isoenzyme (eg, dihydropyridine calcium-channel blockers, cyclosporin, cisapride) have been conducted. As zafirlukast is known to be an inhibitor of CYP3A4 *in vitro*, it is reasonable to employ appropriate clinical monitoring when these drugs are co-administered with zafirlukast). Products include:

Zofran Injection 1750
Zofran 1756
Zofran ODT 1756

Oxaprozin (No formal drug-drug interaction studies with zafirlukast and other drugs known to be metabolized by the cytochrome P450 2C9 isoenzyme (eg, tolbutamide, phenytoin, carbamazepine) have been conducted; however, care should be exercised when zafirlukast is co-administered with these drugs).

No products indexed under this heading.

Paclitaxel (No formal drug-drug interaction studies between zafirlukast and marketed drugs known to be metabolized by the P450 3A4 (CYP3A4) isoenzyme (eg, dihydropyridine calcium-channel blockers, cyclosporin, cisapride) have been conducted. As zafirlukast is known to be an inhibitor of CYP3A4 *in vitro*, it is reasonable to employ appropriate clinical monitoring when these drugs are co-administered with zafirlukast).

No products indexed under this heading.

Phenylbutazone (No formal drug-drug interaction studies with zafirlukast and other drugs known to be metabolized by the cytochrome P450 2C9 isoenzyme (eg, tolbutamide, phenytoin, carbamazepine) have been conducted; however, care should be exercised when zafirlukast is co-administered with these drugs).

No products indexed under this heading.

Phenytoin (No formal drug-drug interaction studies with zafirlukast and other drugs known to be metabolized by the cytochrome P450 2C9 isoenzyme (eg, tolbutamide, phenytoin, carbamazepine) have been conducted; however, care should be exercised when zafirlukast is co-administered with these drugs).

No products indexed under this heading.

Phenytoin Sodium (No formal drug-drug interaction studies with zafirlukast and other drugs known to be metabolized by the cytochrome P450 2C9 isoenzyme (eg, tolbutamide, phenytoin, carbamazepine) have been conducted; however, care should be exercised when zafirlukast is co-administered with these drugs). Products include:

Phenytek Capsules 2380

Pimozide (No formal drug-drug interaction studies between zafirlukast and marketed drugs known to be metabolized by the P450 3A4 (CYP3A4) isoenzyme (eg, dihydropyridine calcium-channel blockers, cyclosporin, cisapride) have been conducted. As zafirlukast is known to be an inhibitor of CYP3A4 *in vitro*, it is reasonable to employ appropriate clinical monitoring when these drugs are co-administered with zafirlukast).

No products indexed under this heading.

Pioglitazone Hydrochloride (No formal drug-drug interaction studies with zafirlukast and other drugs known to be metabolized by the cytochrome P450 2C9 isoenzyme (eg, tolbutamide, phenytoin, carbamazepine) have been conducted; however, care should be exercised when zafirlukast is co-administered with these drugs). Products include:

ActoPlus 3338
Actos 3345
Duetact 3354

Piroxicam (No formal drug-drug interaction studies with zafirlukast and other drugs known to be metabolized by the cytochrome P450 2C9 isoenzyme (eg, tolbutamide, phenytoin, carbamazepine) have been conducted; however, care should be exercised when zafirlukast is co-administered with these drugs).

No products indexed under this heading.

Polyestradiol Phosphate (No formal drug-drug interaction studies between zafirlukast and marketed drugs known to be metabolized by the P450 3A4 (CYP3A4) isoenzyme (eg, dihydropyridine calcium-channel blockers, cyclosporin, cisapride) have been conducted. As zafirlukast is known to be an inhibitor of CYP3A4 *in vitro*, it is reasonable to employ appropriate clinical monitoring when these drugs are co-administered with zafirlukast).

No products indexed under this heading.

Prednisolone (In clinical trials, an increased proportion of zafirlukast patients over the age of 55 years reported infections as compared to placebo treated patients. A similar finding was not observed in other age groups studied. These infections were mostly mild or moderate in intensity and predominantly affected the respiratory tract. Infections occurred equally in both sexes, were dose-proportional to total milligrams of zafirlukast exposure, and were associated with co-

IMPORTANT NOTE: Always consult each drug listing in the patient's regimen for possible interactions.

administration of inhaled corticosteroids. The clinical significance of this finding is unknown).
No products indexed under this heading.

Prednisolone Acetate (In clinical trials, an increased proportion of zafirlukast patients over the age of 55 years reported infections as compared to placebo treated patients. A similar finding was not observed in other age groups studied. These infections were mostly mild or moderate in intensity and predominantly affected the respiratory tract. Infections occurred equally in both sexes, were dose-proportional to total milligrams of zafirlukast exposure, and were associated with co-administration of inhaled corticosteroids. The clinical significance of this finding is unknown). Products include:

Blephamide .... ⊙ **212**, ⊙ **214**
Pred Forte .... ⊙ **225**
Pred Mild .... ⊙ **230**
Pred-G .... ⊙ **226**, ⊙ **227**

Prednisolone Sodium Phosphate (In clinical trials, an increased proportion of zafirlukast patients over the age of 55 years reported infections as compared to placebo treated patients. A similar finding was not observed in other age groups studied. These infections were mostly mild or moderate in intensity and predominantly affected the respiratory tract. Infections occurred equally in both sexes, were dose-proportional to total milligrams of zafirlukast exposure, and were associated with co-administration of inhaled corticosteroids. The clinical significance of this finding is unknown).
No products indexed under this heading.

Prednisolone Tebutate (In clinical trials, an increased proportion of zafirlukast patients over the age of 55 years reported infections as compared to placebo treated patients. A similar finding was not observed in other age groups studied. These infections were mostly mild or moderate in intensity and predominantly affected the respiratory tract. Infections occurred equally in both sexes, were dose-proportional to total milligrams of zafirlukast exposure, and were associated with co-administration of inhaled corticosteroids. The clinical significance of this finding is unknown).
No products indexed under this heading.

Prednisone (In clinical trials, an increased proportion of zafirlukast patients over the age of 55 years reported infections as compared to placebo treated patients. A similar finding was not observed in other age groups studied. These infections were mostly mild or moderate in intensity and predominantly affected the respiratory tract. Infections occurred equally in both sexes, were dose-proportional to total milligrams of zafirlukast exposure, and were associated with co-administration of inhaled corticosteroids. The clinical significance of this finding is unknown).
No products indexed under this heading.

Prednisone sodium phosphate (In clinical trials, an increased proportion of zafirlukast patients over the age of 55 years reported infections as compared to placebo treated patients. A similar finding was not observed in other age groups studied. These infections were mostly mild or moderate in intensity and predominantly affected the respiratory tract. Infections occurred equally in both sexes, were dose-proportional to total milligrams of zafirlukast exposure, and were associated with co-administration of inhaled corticosteroids. The clinical significance of this finding is unknown).
No products indexed under this heading.

Quinidine Gluconate (No formal drug-drug interaction studies between zafirlukast and marketed drugs known to be metabolized by the P450 3A4 (CYP3A4) isoenzyme (eg, dihydropyridine calcium-channel blockers, cyclosporin, cisapride) have been conducted. As zafirlukast is known to be an inhibitor of CYP3A4 *in vitro*, it is reasonable to employ appropriate clinical monitoring when these drugs are co-administered with zafirlukast).
No products indexed under this heading.

Quinidine Polygalacturonate (No formal drug-drug interaction studies between zafirlukast and marketed drugs known to be metabolized by the P450 3A4 (CYP3A4) isoenzyme (eg, dihydropyridine calcium-channel blockers, cyclosporin, cisapride) have been conducted. As zafirlukast is known to be an inhibitor of CYP3A4 *in vitro*, it is reasonable to employ appropriate clinical monitoring when these drugs are co-administered with zafirlukast).
No products indexed under this heading.

Quinidine Sulfate (No formal drug-drug interaction studies between zafirlukast and marketed drugs known to be metabolized by the P450 3A4 (CYP3A4) isoenzyme (eg, dihydropyridine calcium-channel blockers, cyclosporin, cisapride) have been conducted. As zafirlukast is known to be an inhibitor of CYP3A4 *in vitro*, it is reasonable to employ appropriate clinical monitoring when these drugs are co-administered with zafirlukast).
No products indexed under this heading.

Repaglinide (No formal drug-drug interaction studies with zafirlukast and other drugs known to be metabolized by the cytochrome P450 2C9 isoenzyme (eg, tolbutamide, phenytoin, carbamazepine) have been conducted; however, care should be exercised when zafirlukast is co-administered with these drugs).
No products indexed under this heading.

Rifabutin (No formal drug-drug interaction studies between zafirlukast and marketed drugs known to be metabolized by the P450 3A4 (CYP3A4) isoenzyme (eg, dihydropyridine calcium-channel blockers, cyclosporin, cisapride) have been conducted. As zafirlukast is known to be an inhibitor of CYP3A4 *in vitro*, it is reasonable to employ appropriate clinical monitoring when these drugs are co-administered with zafirlukast).
No products indexed under this heading.

Ritonavir (No formal drug-drug interaction studies between zafirlukast and marketed drugs known to be metabolized by the P450 3A4 (CYP3A4) isoenzyme (eg, dihydropyridine calcium-channel blockers, cyclosporin, cisapride) have been conducted. As zafirlukast is known to be an inhibitor of CYP3A4 *in vitro*, it is reasonable to employ appropriate clinical monitoring when these drugs are co-administered with zafirlukast). Products include:

Kaletra **458**
Norvir **509**

Rofecoxib (No formal drug-drug interaction studies with zafirlukast and other drugs known to be metabolized by the cytochrome P450 2C9 isoenzyme (eg, tolbutamide, phenytoin, carbamazepine) have been conducted; however, care should be exercised when zafirlukast is co-administered with these drugs).
No products indexed under this heading.

Rosiglitazone Maleate (No formal drug-drug interaction studies with zafirlukast and other drugs known to be metabolized by the cytochrome P450 2C9 isoenzyme (eg, tolbutamide, phenytoin, carbamazepine) have been conducted; however, care should be exercised when zafirlukast is co-administered with these drugs). Products include:

Avandamet **1345**
Avandaryl **1356**
Avandia **1366**

Saquinavir (No formal drug-drug interaction studies between zafirlukast and marketed drugs known to be metabolized by the P450 3A4 (CYP3A4) isoenzyme (eg, dihydropyridine calcium-channel blockers, cyclosporin, cisapride) have been conducted. As zafirlukast is known to be an inhibitor of CYP3A4 *in vitro*, it is reasonable to employ appropriate clinical monitoring when these drugs are co-administered with zafirlukast).
No products indexed under this heading.

Saquinavir Mesylate (No formal drug-drug interaction studies between zafirlukast and marketed drugs known to be metabolized by the P450 3A4 (CYP3A4) isoenzyme (eg, dihydropyridine calcium-channel blockers, cyclosporin, cisapride) have been conducted. As zafirlukast is known to be an inhibitor of CYP3A4 *in vitro*, it is reasonable to employ appropriate clinical monitoring when these drugs are co-administered with zafirlukast).
No products indexed under this heading.

Sertraline Hydrochloride (No formal drug-drug interaction studies between zafirlukast and marketed drugs known to be metabolized by the P450 3A4 (CYP3A4) isoenzyme (eg, dihydropyridine calcium-channel blockers, cyclosporin, cisapride) have been conducted. As zafirlukast is known to be an inhibitor of CYP3A4 *in vitro*, it is reasonable to employ appropriate clinical monitoring when these drugs are co-administered with zafirlukast).
No products indexed under this heading.

Sildenafil Citrate (No formal drug-drug interaction studies with zafirlukast and other drugs known to be metabolized by the cytochrome P450 2C9 isoenzyme (eg, tolbutamide, phenytoin, carbamazepine) have been conducted; however, care should be exercised when zafirlukast is co-administered with these drugs).
No products indexed under this heading.

Simvastatin (No formal drug-drug interaction studies between zafirlukast and marketed drugs known to be metabolized by the P450 3A4 (CYP3A4) isoenzyme (eg, dihydropyridine calcium-channel blockers, cyclosporin, cisapride) have been conducted. As zafirlukast is known to be an inhibitor of CYP3A4 *in vitro*, it is reasonable to employ appropriate clinical monitoring when these drugs are co-administered with zafirlukast). Products include:

Simcor **524**
Vytorin 10/10 .... **2303, 3240**
Vytorin 10/20 .... **2303, 3240**
Vytorin 10/40 .... **2303, 3240**
Vytorin 10/80 .... **2303, 3240**
Zocor **2289**

Sirolimus (No formal drug-drug interaction studies between zafirlukast and marketed drugs known to be metabolized by the P450 3A4 (CYP3A4) isoenzyme (eg, dihydropyridine calcium-channel blockers, cyclosporin, cisapride) have been conducted. As zafirlukast is known to be an inhibitor of CYP3A4 *in vitro*, it is reasonable to employ appropriate clinical monitoring when these drugs are co-administered with zafirlukast). Products include:

Rapamune **3579**

Sulfamethoxazole (No formal drug-drug interaction studies with zafirlukast and other drugs known to be metabolized by the cytochrome P450 2C9 isoenzyme (eg, tolbutamide, phenytoin, carbamazepine) have been conducted; however, care should be exercised when zafirlukast is co-administered with these drugs).
No products indexed under this heading.

Sulindac (No formal drug-drug interaction studies with zafirlukast and other drugs known to be metabolized by the cytochrome P450 2C9 isoenzyme (eg, tolbutamide, phenytoin, carbamazepine) have been conducted; however, care should be exercised when zafirlukast is co-administered with these drugs). Products include:

Clinoril **2098**

Suprofen (No formal drug-drug interaction studies with zafirlukast and other drugs known to be metabolized by the cytochrome P450 2C9 isoenzyme (eg, tolbutamide, phenytoin, carbamazepine) have been conducted; however, care should be exercised when zafirlukast is co-administered with these drugs).
No products indexed under this heading.

Tacrolimus (No formal drug-drug interaction studies between zafirlukast and marketed drugs known to be metabolized by the P450 3A4 (CYP3A4) isoenzyme (eg, dihydropyridine calcium-channel blockers, cyclosporin, cisapride) have been conducted. As zafirlukast is known to be an inhibitor of CYP3A4 *in vitro*, it is reasonable to employ appropriate clinical monitoring when these drugs are co-administered with zafirlukast). Products include:

Prograf Capsules **677**
Prograf Injection **677**
Protopic **685**

Tadalafil (No formal drug-drug interaction studies between zafirlukast and marketed drugs known to be metabolized by the P450 3A4 (CYP3A4) isoenzyme (eg, dihydropyridine calcium-channel blockers, cyclosporin, cisapride) have been conducted. As zafirlukast is known to be an inhibitor of CYP3A4 *in vitro*, it is reasonable to employ appropriate clinical monitoring when these drugs are co-administered with zafirlukast). Products include:

Adcirca **3461**
Cialis **1861**

Tamoxifen Citrate (No formal drug-drug interaction studies with zafirlukast and other drugs known to be metabolized by the cytochrome P450 2C9 isoenzyme (eg, tolbutamide, phenytoin, carbamazepine) have been conducted; however, care should be exercised when zafirlukast is co-administered with these drugs).
No products indexed under this heading.

Telmisartan (No formal drug-drug interaction studies with zafirlukast and other drugs known to be metabolized by the cytochrome P450 2C9 isoenzyme (eg, tolbutamide, phenytoin, carbamazepine) have been conducted; however, care should be exercised when zafirlukast is co-administered with these drugs). Products include:

Micardis **887**
Micardis HCT **889**

Terfenadine (No formal drug-drug interaction studies between zafirlukast and marketed drugs known to be metabolized by the P450 3A4 (CYP3A4) isoenzyme (eg, dihydropyridine calcium-channel blockers, cyclosporin, cisapride) have been conducted. As zafirlukast is known to be an inhibitor of CYP3A4 *in vitro*, it is reasonable to employ appropriate clinical monitoring when these drugs are co-administered with zafirlukast).
No products indexed under this heading.

(⊙ Described in PDR® for Ophthalmic Medicines)

Theophylline (No formal drug-drug interaction studies between zafirlukast and marketed drugs known to be metabolized by the P450 3A4 (CYP3A4) isoenzyme (eg, dihydropyridine calcium-channel blockers, cyclosporin, cisapride) have been conducted. As zafirlukast is known to be an inhibitor of CYP3A4 *in vitro*, it is reasonable to employ appropriate clinical monitoring when these drugs are co-administered with zafirlukast).
No products indexed under this heading.

Theophylline Anhydrous (No formal drug-drug interaction studies between zafirlukast and marketed drugs known to be metabolized by the P450 3A4 (CYP3A4) isoenzyme (eg, dihydropyridine calcium-channel blockers, cyclosporin, cisapride) have been conducted. As zafirlukast is known to be an inhibitor of CYP3A4 *in vitro*, it is reasonable to employ appropriate clinical monitoring when these drugs are co-administered with zafirlukast). Products include:
Uniphyl 2817

Theophylline Calcium Salicylate (No formal drug-drug interaction studies between zafirlukast and marketed drugs known to be metabolized by the P450 3A4 (CYP3A4) isoenzyme (eg, dihydropyridine calcium-channel blockers, cyclosporin, cisapride) have been conducted. As zafirlukast is known to be an inhibitor of CYP3A4 *in vitro*, it is reasonable to employ appropriate clinical monitoring when these drugs are co-administered with zafirlukast).
No products indexed under this heading.

Theophylline Dihydroxypropyl (Glyceryl) (No formal drug-drug interaction studies between zafirlukast and marketed drugs known to be metabolized by the P450 3A4 (CYP3A4) isoenzyme (eg, dihydropyridine calcium-channel blockers, cyclosporin, cisapride) have been conducted. As zafirlukast is known to be an inhibitor of CYP3A4 *in vitro*, it is reasonable to employ appropriate clinical monitoring when these drugs are co-administered with zafirlukast).
No products indexed under this heading.

Theophylline Ethylenediamine (No formal drug-drug interaction studies between zafirlukast and marketed drugs known to be metabolized by the P450 3A4 (CYP3A4) isoenzyme (eg, dihydropyridine calcium-channel blockers, cyclosporin, cisapride) have been conducted. As zafirlukast is known to be an inhibitor of CYP3A4 *in vitro*, it is reasonable to employ appropriate clinical monitoring when these drugs are co-administered with zafirlukast).
No products indexed under this heading.

Theophylline Sodium Glycinate (No formal drug-drug interaction studies between zafirlukast and marketed drugs known to be metabolized by the P450 3A4 (CYP3A4) isoenzyme (eg, dihydropyridine calcium-channel blockers, cyclosporin, cisapride) have been conducted. As zafirlukast is known to be an inhibitor of CYP3A4 *in vitro*, it is reasonable to employ appropriate clinical monitoring when these drugs are co-administered with zafirlukast).
No products indexed under this heading.

Tiagabine Hydrochloride (No formal drug-drug interaction studies between zafirlukast and marketed drugs known to be metabolized by the P450 3A4 (CYP3A4) isoenzyme (eg, dihydropyridine calcium-channel blockers, cyclosporin, cisapride) have been conducted. As zafirlukast is known to be an inhibitor of CYP3A4 *in vitro*, it is reasonable to employ appropriate clinical monitoring when these drugs are co-administered with zafirlukast). Products include:
Gabitril 972

Tolazamide (No formal drug-drug interaction studies with zafirlukast and other drugs known to be metabolized by the cytochrome P450 2C9 isoenzyme (eg, tolbutamide, phenytoin, carbamazepine) have been conducted; however, care should be exercised when zafirlukast is co-administered with these drugs).
No products indexed under this heading.

Tolbutamide (No formal drug-drug interaction studies with zafirlukast and other drugs known to be metabolized by the cytochrome P450 2C9 isoenzyme (eg, tolbutamide, phenytoin, carbamazepine) have been conducted; however, care should be exercised when zafirlukast is co-administered with these drugs).
No products indexed under this heading.

Tolbutamide Sodium (No formal drug-drug interaction studies with zafirlukast and other drugs known to be metabolized by the cytochrome P450 2C9 isoenzyme (eg, tolbutamide, phenytoin, carbamazepine) have been conducted; however, care should be exercised when zafirlukast is co-administered with these drugs).
No products indexed under this heading.

Tolmetin Sodium (No formal drug-drug interaction studies with zafirlukast and other drugs known to be metabolized by the cytochrome P450 2C9 isoenzyme (eg, tolbutamide, phenytoin, carbamazepine) have been conducted; however, care should be exercised when zafirlukast is co-administered with these drugs).
No products indexed under this heading.

Tolterodine Tartrate (No formal drug-drug interaction studies between zafirlukast and marketed drugs known to be metabolized by the P450 3A4 (CYP3A4) isoenzyme (eg, dihydropyridine calcium-channel blockers, cyclosporin, cisapride) have been conducted. As zafirlukast is known to be an inhibitor of CYP3A4 *in vitro*, it is reasonable to employ appropriate clinical monitoring when these drugs are co-administered with zafirlukast).
No products indexed under this heading.

Torsemide (No formal drug-drug interaction studies with zafirlukast and other drugs known to be metabolized by the cytochrome P450 2C9 isoenzyme (eg, tolbutamide, phenytoin, carbamazepine) have been conducted; however, care should be exercised when zafirlukast is co-administered with these drugs).
No products indexed under this heading.

Trazodone Hydrochloride (No formal drug-drug interaction studies between zafirlukast and marketed drugs known to be metabolized by the P450 3A4 (CYP3A4) isoenzyme (eg, dihydropyridine calcium-channel blockers, cyclosporin, cisapride) have been conducted. As zafirlukast is known to be an inhibitor of CYP3A4 *in vitro*, it is reasonable to employ appropriate clinical monitoring when these drugs are co-administered with zafirlukast).
No products indexed under this heading.

Triamcinolone (In clinical trials, an increased proportion of zafirlukast patients over the age of 55 years reported infections as compared to placebo treated patients. A similar finding was not observed in other age groups studied. These infections were mostly mild or moderate in intensity and predominantly affected the respiratory tract. Infections occurred equally in both sexes, were dose-proportional to total milligrams of zafirlukast exposure, and were associated with co-administration of inhaled corticosteroids. The clinical significance of this finding is unknown).
No products indexed under this heading.

Triamcinolone Acetonide (In clinical trials, an increased proportion of zafirlukast patients over the age of 55 years reported infections as compared to placebo treated patients. A similar finding was not observed in other age groups studied. These infections were mostly mild or moderate in intensity and predominantly affected the respiratory tract. Infections occurred equally in both sexes, were dose-proportional to total milligrams of zafirlukast exposure, and were associated with co-administration of inhaled corticosteroids. The clinical significance of this finding is unknown). Products include:
Azmacort 408
Nasacort AQ 3019

Triamcinolone Diacetate (In clinical trials, an increased proportion of zafirlukast patients over the age of 55 years reported infections as compared to placebo treated patients. A similar finding was not observed in other age groups studied. These infections were mostly mild or moderate in intensity and predominantly affected the respiratory tract. Infections occurred equally in both sexes, were dose-proportional to total milligrams of zafirlukast exposure, and were associated with co-administration of inhaled corticosteroids. The clinical significance of this finding is unknown).
No products indexed under this heading.

Triamcinolone Hexacetonide (In clinical trials, an increased proportion of zafirlukast patients over the age of 55 years reported infections as compared to placebo treated patients. A similar finding was not observed in other age groups studied. These infections were mostly mild or moderate in intensity and predominantly affected the respiratory tract. Infections occurred equally in both sexes, were dose-proportional to total milligrams of zafirlukast exposure, and were associated with co-administration of inhaled corticosteroids. The clinical significance of this finding is unknown).
No products indexed under this heading.

Triazolam (No formal drug-drug interaction studies between zafirlukast and marketed drugs known to be metabolized by the P450 3A4 (CYP3A4) isoenzyme (eg, dihydropyridine calcium-channel blockers, cyclosporin, cisapride) have been conducted. As zafirlukast is known to be an inhibitor of CYP3A4 *in vitro*, it is reasonable to employ appropriate clinical monitoring when these drugs are co-administered with zafirlukast).
No products indexed under this heading.

Troglitazone (No formal drug-drug interaction studies with zafirlukast and other drugs known to be metabolized by the cytochrome P450 2C9 isoenzyme (eg, tolbutamide, phenytoin, carbamazepine) have been conducted; however, care should be exercised when zafirlukast is co-administered with these drugs).
No products indexed under this heading.

Valdecoxib (No formal drug-drug interaction studies with zafirlukast and other drugs known to be metabolized by the cytochrome P450 2C9 isoenzyme (eg, tolbutamide, phenytoin, carbamazepine) have been conducted; however, care should be exercised when zafirlukast is co-administered with these drugs).
No products indexed under this heading.

Valsartan (No formal drug-drug interaction studies with zafirlukast and other drugs known to be metabolized by the cytochrome P450 2C9 isoenzyme (eg, tolbutamide, phenytoin, carbamazepine) have been conducted; however, care should be exercised when zafirlukast is co-administered with these drugs). Products include:
Diovan 2413
Diovan HCT 2419
Exforge 2443
Exforge HCT 2449
Valturna 3637

Vardenafil Hydrochloride (No formal drug-drug interaction studies with zafirlukast and other drugs known to be metabolized by the cytochrome P450 2C9 isoenzyme (eg, tolbutamide, phenytoin, carbamazepine) have been conducted; however, care should be exercised when zafirlukast is co-administered with these drugs). Products include:
Levitra 3157

Verapamil Hydrochloride (No formal drug-drug interaction studies with zafirlukast and other drugs known to be metabolized by the cytochrome P450 2C9 isoenzyme (eg, tolbutamide, phenytoin, carbamazepine) have been conducted; however, care should be exercised when zafirlukast is co-administered with these drugs). Products include:
Tarka 534

Vinblastine Sulfate (No formal drug-drug interaction studies between zafirlukast and marketed drugs known to be metabolized by the P450 3A4 (CYP3A4) isoenzyme (eg, dihydropyridine calcium-channel blockers, cyclosporin, cisapride) have been conducted. As zafirlukast is known to be an inhibitor of CYP3A4 *in vitro*, it is reasonable to employ appropriate clinical monitoring when these drugs are co-administered with zafirlukast).
No products indexed under this heading.

Vincristine Sulfate (No formal drug-drug interaction studies between zafirlukast and marketed drugs known to be metabolized by the P450 3A4 (CYP3A4) isoenzyme (eg, dihydropyridine calcium-channel blockers, cyclosporin, cisapride) have been conducted. As zafirlukast is known to be an inhibitor of CYP3A4 *in vitro*, it is reasonable to employ appropriate clinical monitoring when these drugs are co-administered with zafirlukast).
No products indexed under this heading.

Voriconazole (No formal drug-drug interaction studies with zafirlukast and other drugs known to be metabolized by the cytochrome P450 2C9 isoenzyme (eg, tolbutamide, phenytoin, carbamazepine) have been conducted; however, care should be exercised when zafirlukast is co-administered with these drugs).
No products indexed under this heading.

Warfarin Sodium (Co-administration of multiple doses of zafirlukast (160 mg/day) to steady-state with a single 25 mg dose of warfarin (a substrate of CYP2C9) resulted in a significant increase in the mean AUC (+63%) and half-life (+36%) of S-warfarin. The mean prothrombin time increased by approximately 35%. The pharmacokinetics of zafirlukast were unaffected by co-administration with warfarin. Co-administration of zafirlukast with warfarin results in a clinically significant increase in prothrombin time (PT). Patients on oral warfarin anticoagulant therapy and zafirlukast should have their prothrombin times monitored closely and anticoagulant dose adjusted accordingly).
No products indexed under this heading.

Zileuton (No formal drug-drug interaction studies with zafirlukast and other drugs known to be metabolized by the cytochrome P450 2C9 isoenzyme (eg, tolbutamide, phenytoin, carbamazepine) have been conducted; however, care should be exercised when zafirlukast is co-administered with these drugs).
No products indexed under this heading.

IMPORTANT NOTE: Always consult each drug listing in the patient's regimen for possible interactions.

Food Interactions

Food, unspecified (The bioavailability of zafirlukast may be decreased when taken with food. Patients should be instructed to take zafirlukast at least 1 hour before or 2 hours after meals).

Meal, unspecified (The bioavailability of zafirlukast may be decreased when taken with food. Patients should be instructed to take zafirlukast at least 1 hour before or 2 hours after meals).

ACCUTANE CAPSULES

(Isotretinoin) 2832
May interact with corticosteroids, phenytoin, progestins, tetracyclines, and certain other agents. Compounds in these categories include:

Alclometasone Dipropionate (Systemic corticosteroids are known to cause osteoporosis; caution is advised if used concurrently because of potential interactive effect on bone loss between systemic corticosteroids and Accutane).
No products indexed under this heading.

Beclomethasone Dipropionate (Systemic corticosteroids are known to cause osteoporosis; caution is advised if used concurrently because of potential interactive effect on bone loss between systemic corticosteroids and Accutane). Products include:
Qvar 3398

Beclomethasone Dipropionate Monohydrate (Systemic corticosteroids are known to cause osteoporosis; caution is advised if used concurrently because of potential interactive effect on bone loss between systemic corticosteroids and Accutane). Products include:
Beconase AQ 1386

Betamethasone (Systemic corticosteroids are known to cause osteoporosis; caution is advised if used concurrently because of potential interactive effect on bone loss between systemic corticosteroids and Accutane).
No products indexed under this heading.

Betamethasone Acetate (Systemic corticosteroids are known to cause osteoporosis; caution is advised if used concurrently because of potential interactive effect on bone loss between systemic corticosteroids and Accutane).
No products indexed under this heading.

Betamethasone Benzoate (Systemic corticosteroids are known to cause osteoporosis; caution is advised if used concurrently because of potential interactive effect on bone loss between systemic corticosteroids and Accutane).
No products indexed under this heading.

Betamethasone Dipropionate (Systemic corticosteroids are known to cause osteoporosis; caution is advised if used concurrently because of potential interactive effect on bone loss between systemic corticosteroids and Accutane). Products include:
Diprolene Lotion 0.05% 3108
Diprolene Ointment 0.05% 3109
Diprolene AF Cream 0.05% 3107
Lotrisone 3163

Betamethasone Sodium Phosphate (Systemic corticosteroids are known to cause osteoporosis; caution is advised if used concurrently because of potential interactive effect on bone loss between systemic corticosteroids and Accutane).
No products indexed under this heading.

Betamethasone Valerate (Systemic corticosteroids are known to cause osteoporosis; caution is advised if used concurrently because of potential interactive effect on bone loss between systemic corticosteroids and Accutane).
Products include:

Luxiq 3321

Budesonide (Systemic corticosteroids are known to cause osteoporosis; caution is advised if used concurrently because of potential interactive effect on bone loss between systemic corticosteroids and Accutane). Products include:
Pulmicort Flexhaler 714
Symbicort 80/4.5 720
Symbicort 160/4.5 720

Ciclesonide (Systemic corticosteroids are known to cause osteoporosis; caution is advised if used concurrently because of potential interactive effect on bone loss between systemic corticosteroids and Accutane).
No products indexed under this heading.

Cortisone Acetate (Systemic corticosteroids are known to cause osteoporosis; caution is advised if used concurrently because of potential interactive effect on bone loss between systemic corticosteroids and Accutane).
No products indexed under this heading.

Demeclocycline Hydrochloride (Concomitant treatment with Accutane and tetracyclines should be avoided because Accutane is associated with a number of cases of pseudotumor cerebri, some of which involved concomitant use of tetracyclines).
No products indexed under this heading.

Desogestrel (Micro-dosed progesterone preparations ('minipills' that do not contain an estrogen) may be an inadequate method of contraception during isotretinoin therapy. Although other hormonal contraceptives are highly effective, there have been reports of pregnancy from female patients who have used combined oral contraceptives, as well as transdermal patch/injectable/ implantable/vaginal ring hormonal birth control products. These reports are more frequent for female patients who use only a single method of contraception. It is not known if hormonal contraceptives differ in their effectiveness when used with isotretinoin. Therefore, it is critically important for female patients of childbearing potential to select and commit to use 2 forms of effective contraception simultaneously, at least 1 of which must be a primary form).
No products indexed under this heading.

Desoximetasone (Systemic corticosteroids are known to cause osteoporosis; caution is advised if used concurrently because of potential interactive effect on bone loss between systemic corticosteroids and Accutane).
No products indexed under this heading.

Dexamethasone (Systemic corticosteroids are known to cause osteoporosis; caution is advised if used concurrently because of potential interactive effect on bone loss between systemic corticosteroids and Accutane).
Products include:
Ciprodex 583
Ozurdex .... ⊙ 223
Tobramycin and Dexamethasone
Ophthalmic Suspension .... ⊙ 251

Dexamethasone Acetate (Systemic corticosteroids are known to cause osteoporosis; caution is advised if used concurrently because of potential interactive effect on bone loss between systemic corticosteroids and Accutane).
No products indexed under this heading.

Dexamethasone Phosphate (Systemic corticosteroids are known to cause osteoporosis; caution is advised if used concurrently because of potential interactive effect on bone loss between systemic corticosteroids and Accutane).
No products indexed under this heading.

Dexamethasone Sodium (Systemic corticosteroids are known to cause osteoporosis; caution is advised if used concurrently because of potential interactive effect on bone loss between systemic corticosteroids and Accutane).
No products indexed under this heading.

Dexamethasone Sodium Phosphate (Systemic corticosteroids are known to cause osteoporosis; caution is advised if used concurrently because of potential interactive effect on bone loss between systemic corticosteroids and Accutane).
No products indexed under this heading.

Dexamethasone Sodium Phosphate Injection (Systemic corticosteroids are known to cause osteoporosis; caution is advised if used concurrently because of potential interactive effect on bone loss between systemic corticosteroids and Accutane).
No products indexed under this heading.

Diflorasone Diacetate (Systemic corticosteroids are known to cause osteoporosis; caution is advised if used concurrently because of potential interactive effect on bone loss between systemic corticosteroids and Accutane).
No products indexed under this heading.

Doxycycline (Concomitant treatment with Accutane and tetracyclines should be avoided because Accutane is associated with a number of cases of pseudotumor cerebri, some of which involved concomitant use of tetracyclines).
No products indexed under this heading.

Doxycycline Calcium (Concomitant treatment with Accutane and tetracyclines should be avoided because Accutane is associated with a number of cases of pseudotumor cerebri, some of which involved concomitant use of tetracyclines).
No products indexed under this heading.

Doxycycline Hyclate (Concomitant treatment with Accutane and tetracyclines should be avoided because Accutane is associated with a number of cases of pseudotumor cerebri, some of which involved concomitant use of tetracyclines).
No products indexed under this heading.

Doxycycline Monohydrate (Concomitant treatment with Accutane and tetracyclines should be avoided because Accutane is associated with a number of cases of pseudotumor cerebri, some of which involved concomitant use of tetracyclines).
No products indexed under this heading.

Fludrocortisone Acetate (Systemic corticosteroids are known to cause osteoporosis; caution is advised if used concurrently because of potential interactive effect on bone loss between systemic corticosteroids and Accutane).
No products indexed under this heading.

Flumethasone Pivalate (Systemic corticosteroids are known to cause osteoporosis; caution is advised if used concurrently because of potential interactive effect on bone loss between systemic corticosteroids and Accutane).
No products indexed under this heading.

Flunisolide Hemihydrate (Systemic corticosteroids are known to cause osteoporosis; caution is advised if used concurrently because of potential interactive effect on bone loss between systemic corticosteroids and Accutane).
No products indexed under this heading.

Fluticasone Furoate (Systemic corticosteroids are known to cause osteoporosis; caution is advised if used concurrently because of potential interactive effect on bone loss between systemic corticosteroids and Accutane).
Products include:
Veramyst 1713

Fluticasone Propionate (Systemic corticosteroids are known to cause osteoporosis; caution is advised if used concurrently because of potential interactive effect on bone loss between systemic corticosteroids and Accutane).
Products include:
Advair 100/50 1275
Advair 250/50 1275
Advair 500/50 1275
Advair HFA 45/21 1288
Advair HFA 115/21 1288
Advair HFA 230/21 1288
Flonase 1459
Flovent Diskus 1463
Flovent HFA 1470

Fosphenytoin (Phenytoin is known to cause osteomalacia; caution is advised if used concurrently because of potential interactive effect on bone loss between phenytoin and Accutane).
No products indexed under this heading.

Fosphenytoin Sodium (Phenytoin is known to cause osteomalacia; caution is advised if used concurrently because of potential interactive effect on bone loss between phenytoin and Accutane).
No products indexed under this heading.

Hydrocortisone (Systemic corticosteroids are known to cause osteoporosis; caution is advised if used concurrently because of potential interactive effect on bone loss between systemic corticosteroids and Accutane).
No products indexed under this heading.

Hydrocortisone (Alcohol) (Systemic corticosteroids are known to cause osteoporosis; caution is advised if used concurrently because of potential interactive effect on bone loss between systemic corticosteroids and Accutane).
No products indexed under this heading.

Hydrocortisone Acetate (Systemic corticosteroids are known to cause osteoporosis; caution is advised if used concurrently because of potential interactive effect on bone loss between systemic corticosteroids and Accutane).
No products indexed under this heading.

Hydrocortisone Butyrate (Systemic corticosteroids are known to cause osteoporosis; caution is advised if used concurrently because of potential interactive effect on bone loss between systemic corticosteroids and Accutane).
No products indexed under this heading.

Hydrocortisone Cypionate (Systemic corticosteroids are known to cause osteoporosis; caution is advised if used concurrently because of potential interactive effect on bone loss between systemic corticosteroids and Accutane).
No products indexed under this heading.

Hydrocortisone Hemisuccinate (Systemic corticosteroids are known to cause osteoporosis; caution is advised if used concurrently because of potential interactive effect on bone loss between systemic corticosteroids and Accutane).
No products indexed under this heading.

Hydrocortisone Probutate (Systemic corticosteroids are known to cause osteoporosis; caution is advised if used concurrently because of potential interactive effect on bone loss between systemic corticosteroids and Accutane).
No products indexed under this heading.

Hydrocortisone Sodium Phosphate (Systemic corticosteroids are known to cause osteoporosis; caution is advised if used concurrently because of potential interactive effect on bone loss between systemic corticosteroids and Accutane).
No products indexed under this heading.

(⊙ Described in PDR® for Ophthalmic Medicines)

Hydrocortisone Sodium Succinate (Systemic corticosteroids are known to cause osteoporosis; caution is advised if used concurrently because of potential interactive effect on bone loss between systemic corticosteroids and Accutane).
No products indexed under this heading.

Hydrocortisone Valerate (Systemic corticosteroids are known to cause osteoporosis; caution is advised if used concurrently because of potential interactive effect on bone loss between systemic corticosteroids and Accutane).
No products indexed under this heading.

Hypericum (Avoid St. John's Wort due to a possible interaction based on reports of breakthrough bleeding being reported on oral contraceptives shortly after starting St. John's Wort. Pregnancies have been reported by users of combined hormonal contraceptives who also used some form of St. John's Wort).
No products indexed under this heading.

Medroxyprogesterone Acetate (Micro-dosed progesterone preparations ('minipills' that do not contain an estrogen) may be an inadequate method of contraception during isotretinoin therapy. Although other hormonal contraceptives are highly effective, there have been reports of pregnancy from female patients who have used combined oral contraceptives, as well as transdermal patch/injectable/implantable/vaginal ring hormonal birth control products. These reports are more frequent for female patients who use only a single method of contraception. It is not known if hormonal contraceptives differ in their effectiveness when used with isotretinoin. Therefore, it is critically important for female patients of childbearing potential to select and commit to use 2 forms of effective contraception simultaneously, at least 1 of which must be a primary form). Products include:

Megestrol Acetate (Micro-dosed progesterone preparations ('minipills' that do not contain an estrogen) may be an inadequate method of contraception during isotretinoin therapy. Although other hormonal contraceptives are highly effective, there have been reports of pregnancy from female patients who have used combined oral contraceptives, as well as transdermal patch/injectable/implantable/vaginal ring hormonal birth control products. These reports are more frequent for female patients who use only a single method of contraception. It is not known if hormonal contraceptives differ in their effectiveness when used with isotretinoin. Therefore, it is critically important for female patients of childbearing potential to select and commit to use 2 forms of effective contraception simultaneously, at least 1 of which must be a primary form). Products include:

Methacycline Hydrochloride (Concomitant treatment with Accutane and tetracyclines should be avoided because Accutane is associated with a number of cases of pseudotumor cerebri, some of which involved concomitant use of tetracyclines).
No products indexed under this heading.

Methylprednisolone (Systemic corticosteroids are known to cause osteoporosis; caution is advised if used concurrently because of potential interactive effect on bone loss between systemic corticosteroids and Accutane).
No products indexed under this heading.

Methylprednisolone Acetate (Systemic corticosteroids are known to cause osteoporosis; caution is advised if used concurrently because of potential interactive effect on bone loss between systemic corticosteroids and Accutane).
No products indexed under this heading.

Methylprednisolone Sodium Succinate (Systemic corticosteroids are known to cause osteoporosis; caution is advised if used concurrently because of potential interactive effect on bone loss between systemic corticosteroids and Accutane).
No products indexed under this heading.

Minocycline Hydrochloride (Concomitant treatment with Accutane and tetracyclines should be avoided because Accutane is associated with a number of cases of pseudotumor cerebri, some of which involved concomitant use of tetracyclines). Products include:

Mometasone Furoate (Systemic corticosteroids are known to cause osteoporosis; caution is advised if used concurrently because of potential interactive effect on bone loss between systemic corticosteroids and Accutane). Products include:

Mometasone Furoate Monohydrate (Systemic corticosteroids are known to cause osteoporosis; caution is advised if used concurrently because of potential interactive effect on bone loss between systemic corticosteroids and Accutane). Products include:

Norethindrone (Microdosed progesterone preparations (minipills) may be an inadequate method of contraception during Accutane therapy). Products include:

Norethindrone Acetate (Micro-dosed progesterone preparations ('minipills' that do not contain an estrogen) may be an inadequate method of contraception during isotretinoin therapy. Although other hormonal contraceptives are highly effective, there have been reports of pregnancy from female patients who have used combined oral contraceptives, as well as transdermal patch/injectable/implantable/vaginal ring hormonal birth control products. These reports are more frequent for female patients who use only a single method of contraception. It is not known if hormonal contraceptives differ in their effectiveness when used with isotretinoin. Therefore, it is critically important for female patients of childbearing potential to select and commit to use 2 forms of effective contraception simultaneously, at least 1 of which must be a primary form). Products include:

Norgestimate (Micro-dosed progesterone preparations ('minipills' that do not contain an estrogen) may be an inadequate method of contraception during isotretinoin therapy. Although other hormonal contraceptives are highly effective, there have been reports of pregnancy from female patients who have used combined oral contraceptives, as well as transdermal patch/injectable/implantable/vaginal ring hormonal birth control products. These reports are more frequent for female patients who use only a single method of contraception. It is not known if hormonal contraceptives differ in their effectiveness when used with isotretinoin. Therefore, it is critically important for female patients of childbearing

potential to select and commit to use 2 forms of effective contraception simultaneously, at least 1 of which must be a primary form). Products include:

Oxytetracycline (Concomitant treatment with Accutane and tetracyclines should be avoided because Accutane is associated with a number of cases of pseudotumor cerebri, some of which involved concomitant use of tetracyclines).
No products indexed under this heading.

Oxytetracycline Hydrochloride (Concomitant treatment with Accutane and tetracyclines should be avoided because Accutane is associated with a number of cases of pseudotumor cerebri, some of which involved concomitant use of tetracyclines).
No products indexed under this heading.

Phenytoin (Phenytoin is known to cause osteomalacia; caution is advised if used concurrently because of potential interactive effect on bone loss between phenytoin and Accutane).
No products indexed under this heading.

Phenytoin Sodium (Phenytoin is known to cause osteomalacia; caution is advised if used concurrently because of potential interactive effect on bone loss between phenytoin and Accutane). Products include:

Prednisolone (Systemic corticosteroids are known to cause osteoporosis; caution is advised if used concurrently because of potential interactive effect on bone loss between systemic corticosteroids and Accutane).
No products indexed under this heading.

Prednisolone Acetate (Systemic corticosteroids are known to cause osteoporosis; caution is advised if used concurrently because of potential interactive effect on bone loss between systemic corticosteroids and Accutane). Products include:

Prednisolone Sodium Phosphate (Systemic corticosteroids are known to cause osteoporosis; caution is advised if used concurrently because of potential interactive effect on bone loss between systemic corticosteroids and Accutane).
No products indexed under this heading.

Prednisolone Tebutate (Systemic corticosteroids are known to cause osteoporosis; caution is advised if used concurrently because of potential interactive effect on bone loss between systemic corticosteroids and Accutane).
No products indexed under this heading.

Prednisone (Systemic corticosteroids are known to cause osteoporosis; caution is advised if used concurrently because of potential interactive effect on bone loss between systemic corticosteroids and Accutane).
No products indexed under this heading.

Prednisone sodium phosphate (Systemic corticosteroids are known to cause osteoporosis; caution is advised if used concurrently because of potential interactive effect on bone loss between systemic corticosteroids and Accutane).
No products indexed under this heading.

Tetracycline Hydrochloride (Concomitant treatment with Accutane and tetracyclines should be avoided because Accutane is associated with a number of cases of pseudotumor cerebri, some of which involved concomitant use of tetracyclines). Products include:

Tetracycline Phosphate Complex (Concomitant treatment with Accutane and tetracyclines should be avoided because Accutane is associated with a number of cases of pseudotumor cerebri, some of which involved concomitant use of tetracyclines).
No products indexed under this heading.

Triamcinolone (Systemic corticosteroids are known to cause osteoporosis; caution is advised if used concurrently because of potential interactive effect on bone loss between systemic corticosteroids and Accutane).
No products indexed under this heading.

Triamcinolone Acetonide (Systemic corticosteroids are known to cause osteoporosis; caution is advised if used concurrently because of potential interactive effect on bone loss between systemic corticosteroids and Accutane). Products include:

Triamcinolone Diacetate (Systemic corticosteroids are known to cause osteoporosis; caution is advised if used concurrently because of potential interactive effect on bone loss between systemic corticosteroids and Accutane).
No products indexed under this heading.

Triamcinolone Hexacetonide (Systemic corticosteroids are known to cause osteoporosis; caution is advised if used concurrently because of potential interactive effect on bone loss between systemic corticosteroids and Accutane).
No products indexed under this heading.

Vitamin A (Additive Vitamin A toxicity). Products include:

ACETADOTE INJECTION
None cited in PDR database.

ACIPHEX TABLETS
May interact with drugs whose absorption can be affected by the level of gastric acidity (selected), and certain other agents. Compounds in these categories include:

Amoxicillin (Combined administration consisting of rabeprazole, amoxicillin, and clarithromycin resulted in increases in plasma concentrations of rabeprazole and 14-hydroxyclarithromycin). Products include:

Amoxicillin Trihydrate (Combined administration consisting of rabeprazole, amoxicillin, and clarithromycin resulted in increases in plasma concentrations of rabeprazole and 14-hydroxyclarithromycin).
No products indexed under this heading.

Atazanavir (Co-administration of atazanavir with proton pump inhibitors is expected to substantially decrease atazanavir plasma concentrations and thereby reduce its therapeutic effect. Concomitant use of atazanavir and proton pump inhibitors is not recommended).
No products indexed under this heading.

Atazanavir Sulfate (Co-administration of atazanavir with proton pump inhibitors is expected to substantially decrease atazanavir plasma concentrations and thereby reduce its therapeutic effect. Concomitant use of atazanavir and proton pump inhibitors is not recommended).
No products indexed under this heading.

Clarithromycin (Combined administration consisting of rabeprazole, amoxicillin, and clarithromycin resulted in increases in plasma concentrations of rabeprazole and 14-hydroxyclarithromycin). Products include:
Biaxin/Biaxin XL ... 412

Cyclosporine (In vitro incubations employing human liver microsomes indicated that rabeprazole inhibited cyclosporine metabolism with an IC50 of 62 micromolar, a concentration that is over 50 times higher than the C_{max} in healthy volunteers following 14 days of dosing with 20 mg of rabeprazole). Products include:
Gengraf ... 440
Neoral Oral Solution ... 2496
Neoral Capsules ... 2496
Restasis ... 605

Dapsone (Rabeprazole produces sustained inhibition of gastric acid secretion. An interaction with compounds which are dependent on gastric pH for absorption may occur due to the magnitude of acid suppression observed with rabeprazole. Patients may need to be monitored when such drugs are taken concomitantly with rabeprazole). Products include:
Aczone ... 593
Dapsone ... 1819

Digoxin (Rabeprazole produces sustained inhibition of gastric acid secretion. An interaction with compounds which are dependent on gastric pH for absorption may occur due to the magnitude of acid suppression observed with rabeprazole. For example, in normal subjects, co-administration of rabeprazole 20 mg q.d. resulted in the AUC and C_{max} for digoxin of 19% and 29%, respectively. Therefore, patients may need to be monitored when digoxin is taken concomitantly with rabeprazole). Products include:
Lanoxin Injection ... 1546
Lanoxin Injection Pediatric ... 1549
Lanoxin Tablets ... 1553

Ketoconazole (Rabeprazole produces sustained inhibition of gastric acid secretion. An interaction with compounds which are dependent on gastric pH for absorption may occur due to the magnitude of acid suppression observed with rabeprazole. For example, in normal subjects, co-administration of rabeprazole 20 mg q.d. resulted in an approximately 30% decrease in the bioavailability of ketoconazole. Therefore, patients may need to be monitored when ketoconazole is taken concomitantly with rabeprazole). Products include:
Extina ... 3319
Xolegel ... 3337

Warfarin Sodium (There have been reports of increased INR and prothrombin time in patients receiving proton pump inhibitors, including rabeprazole, and warfarin concomitantly. Increases in INR and prothrombin time may lead to abnormal bleeding and even death).
No products indexed under this heading.

ACTIMMUNE

(Interferon Gamma-1B) ... 1810
May interact with agents associated with myelosuppression, drugs which undergo biotransformation by cytochrome p-450 mixed function oxidase. Compounds in these categories include:

Acarbose (Preclinical studies have demonstrated a decrease in hepatic microsomal cytochrome P-450 concentrations. This could potentially lead to a depression of the hepatic metabolism of certain drugs that utilize this degradative pathway).
No products indexed under this heading.

Acetaminophen (Preclinical studies have demonstrated a decrease in hepatic microsomal cytochrome P-450 concentrations. This could potentially lead to a depression of the hepatic metabolism of certain drugs that utilize this degradative pathway). Products include:
Percocet ... 1121
Tylenol ... 2049
Tylenol 8 Hour ... 2049
Extra Strength Tylenol Caplets, Cool Caplets, and EZ Tabs ... 2049
Extra Strength Tylenol Adult Rapid Blast Liquid ... 2049
Extra Strength Tylenol Rapid Release ... 2049
Tylenol with Codeine ... 2691
Tylenol Arthritis Pain Extended Release Geltabs/Caplets ... 2049
Children's Tylenol Suspension Liquid ... 2048
Children's Tylenol Meltaways ... 2048
Tylenol, Infants' Drops ... 2048
Junior Tylenol ... 2048
Vicodin ... 560
Vicodin ES ... 561
Vicodin HP ... 563
Zydone ... 1138

Alatrofloxacin Mesylate (Preclinical studies have demonstrated a decrease in hepatic microsomal cytochrome P-450 concentrations. This could potentially lead to a depression of the hepatic metabolism of certain drugs that utilize this degradative pathway).
No products indexed under this heading.

Alfentanil Hydrochloride (Preclinical studies have demonstrated a decrease in hepatic microsomal cytochrome P-450 concentrations. This could potentially lead to a depression of the hepatic metabolism of certain drugs that utilize this degradative pathway).
No products indexed under this heading.

Alprazolam (Preclinical studies have demonstrated a decrease in hepatic microsomal cytochrome P-450 concentrations. This could potentially lead to a depression of the hepatic metabolism of certain drugs that utilize this degradative pathway).
No products indexed under this heading.

Altretamine (Caution should be exercised when administering with other potentially myelosuppressive agents). Products include:
Hexalen ... 1066

Aminophylline (Preclinical studies have demonstrated a decrease in hepatic microsomal cytochrome P-450 concentrations. This could potentially lead to a depression of the hepatic metabolism of certain drugs that utilize this degradative pathway).
No products indexed under this heading.

Amiodarone Hydrochloride (Preclinical studies have demonstrated a decrease in hepatic microsomal cytochrome P-450 concentrations. This could potentially lead to a depression of the hepatic metabolism of certain drugs that utilize this degradative pathway).
No products indexed under this heading.

Amitriptyline Hydrochloride (Preclinical studies have demonstrated a decrease in hepatic microsomal cytochrome P-450 concentrations. This could potentially lead to a depression of the hepatic metabolism of certain drugs that utilize this degradative pathway).
No products indexed under this heading.

Amlodipine Besylate (Preclinical studies have demonstrated a decrease in hepatic microsomal cytochrome P-450 concentrations. This could potentially lead to a depression of the hepatic metabolism of certain drugs that utilize this degradative pathway). Products include:
Azor ... 1010
Exforge ... 2443
Exforge HCT ... 2449

Amoxapine (Preclinical studies have demonstrated a decrease in hepatic microsomal cytochrome P-450 concentrations. This could potentially lead to a depression of the hepatic metabolism of certain drugs that utilize this degradative pathway).
No products indexed under this heading.

Amphetamine Aspartate (Preclinical studies have demonstrated a decrease in hepatic microsomal cytochrome P-450 concentrations. This could potentially lead to a depression of the hepatic metabolism of certain drugs that utilize this degradative pathway).
No products indexed under this heading.

Amphetamine Aspartate Monohydrate (Preclinical studies have demonstrated a decrease in hepatic microsomal cytochrome P-450 concentrations. This could potentially lead to a depression of the hepatic metabolism of certain drugs that utilize this degradative pathway).
No products indexed under this heading.

Amphetamine Sulfate (Preclinical studies have demonstrated a decrease in hepatic microsomal cytochrome P-450 concentrations. This could potentially lead to a depression of the hepatic metabolism of certain drugs that utilize this degradative pathway).
No products indexed under this heading.

Anagrelide Hydrochloride (Preclinical studies have demonstrated a decrease in hepatic microsomal cytochrome P-450 concentrations. This could potentially lead to a depression of the hepatic metabolism of certain drugs that utilize this degradative pathway).
No products indexed under this heading.

Aprepitant (Preclinical studies have demonstrated a decrease in hepatic microsomal cytochrome P-450 concentrations. This could potentially lead to a depression of the hepatic metabolism of certain drugs that utilize this degradative pathway). Products include:
Emend ... 2124

Astemizole (Preclinical studies have demonstrated a decrease in hepatic microsomal cytochrome P-450 concentrations. This could potentially lead to a depression of the hepatic metabolism of certain drugs that utilize this degradative pathway).
No products indexed under this heading.

Atomoxetine Hydrochloride (Preclinical studies have demonstrated a decrease in hepatic microsomal cytochrome P-450 concentrations. This could potentially lead to a depression of the hepatic metabolism of certain drugs that utilize this degradative pathway). Products include:
Strattera ... 1957

Atorvastatin Calcium (Preclinical studies have demonstrated a decrease in hepatic microsomal cytochrome P-450 concentrations. This could potentially lead to a depression of the hepatic metabolism of certain drugs that utilize this degradative pathway). Products include:
Lipitor ... 2703

Belladonna Ergotamine (Preclinical studies have demonstrated a decrease in hepatic microsomal cytochrome P-450 concentrations. This could potentially lead to a depression of the hepatic metabolism of certain drugs that utilize this degradative pathway).
No products indexed under this heading.

Benzphetamine Hydrochloride (Preclinical studies have demonstrated a decrease in hepatic microsomal cytochrome P-450 concentrations. This could potentially lead to a depression of the hepatic metabolism of certain drugs that utilize this degradative pathway).
No products indexed under this heading.

Bisoprolol Fumarate (Preclinical studies have demonstrated a decrease in hepatic microsomal cytochrome P-450 concentrations. This could potentially lead to a depression of the hepatic metabolism of certain drugs that utilize this degradative pathway).
No products indexed under this heading.

Bromocriptine Mesylate (Preclinical studies have demonstrated a decrease in hepatic microsomal cytochrome P-450 concentrations. This could potentially lead to a depression of the hepatic metabolism of certain drugs that utilize this degradative pathway).
No products indexed under this heading.

Buspirone Hydrochloride (Preclinical studies have demonstrated a decrease in hepatic microsomal cytochrome P-450 concentrations. This could potentially lead to a depression of the hepatic metabolism of certain drugs that utilize this degradative pathway).
No products indexed under this heading.

Busulfan (Caution should be exercised when administering with other potentially myelosuppressive agents). Products include:
Myleran ... 1581

Caffeine (Preclinical studies have demonstrated a decrease in hepatic microsomal cytochrome P-450 concentrations. This could potentially lead to a depression of the hepatic metabolism of certain drugs that utilize this degradative pathway).
No products indexed under this heading.

Caffeine Anhydrous (Preclinical studies have demonstrated a decrease in hepatic microsomal cytochrome P-450 concentrations. This could potentially lead to a depression of the hepatic metabolism of certain drugs that utilize this degradative pathway).
No products indexed under this heading.

Caffeine Citrate (Preclinical studies have demonstrated a decrease in hepatic microsomal cytochrome P-450 concentrations. This could potentially lead to a depression of the hepatic metabolism of certain drugs that utilize this degradative pathway).
No products indexed under this heading.

Caffeine-containing medications (Preclinical studies have demonstrated a decrease in hepatic microsomal cytochrome P-450 concentrations. This could potentially lead to a depression of the hepatic metabolism of certain drugs that utilize this degradative pathway).
No products indexed under this heading.

Caffeine Sodium Benzoate (Preclinical studies have demonstrated a decrease in hepatic microsomal cytochrome P-450 concentrations. This could potentially lead to a depression of the hepatic metabolism of certain drugs that utilize this degradative pathway).
No products indexed under this heading.

Candesartan Cilexetil (Preclinical studies have demonstrated a decrease in hepatic microsomal cytochrome P-450 concentrations. This could potentially lead to a depression of the hepatic metabolism of certain drugs that utilize this degradative pathway). Products include:
Atacand ... 697
Atacand HCT ... 700

Captopril (Preclinical studies have demonstrated a decrease in hepatic microsomal cytochrome P-450 concentrations. This could potentially lead to a

depression of the hepatic metabolism of certain drugs that utilize this degradative pathway). Products include:
Captopril **2341**

Carbamazepine (Preclinical studies have demonstrated a decrease in hepatic microsomal cytochrome P-450 concentrations. This could potentially lead to a depression of the hepatic metabolism of certain drugs that utilize this degradative pathway). Products include:
Carbatrol **3280**
Equetro **3477**

Carisoprodol (Preclinical studies have demonstrated a decrease in hepatic microsomal cytochrome P-450 concentrations. This could potentially lead to a depression of the hepatic metabolism of certain drugs that utilize this degradative pathway).
No products indexed under this heading.

Carvedilol (Preclinical studies have demonstrated a decrease in hepatic microsomal cytochrome P-450 concentrations. This could potentially lead to a depression of the hepatic metabolism of certain drugs that utilize this degradative pathway). Products include:
Coreg **1409**

Celecoxib (Preclinical studies have demonstrated a decrease in hepatic microsomal cytochrome P-450 concentrations. This could potentially lead to a depression of the hepatic metabolism of certain drugs that utilize this degradative pathway). Products include:
Celebrex **3272**

Cerivastatin Sodium (Preclinical studies have demonstrated a decrease in hepatic microsomal cytochrome P-450 concentrations. This could potentially lead to a depression of the hepatic metabolism of certain drugs that utilize this degradative pathway).
No products indexed under this heading.

Cevimeline Hydrochloride (Preclinical studies have demonstrated a decrease in hepatic microsomal cytochrome P-450 concentrations. This could potentially lead to a depression of the hepatic metabolism of certain drugs that utilize this degradative pathway). Products include:
Evoxac **1027**

Chlorambucil (Caution should be exercised when administering with other potentially myelosuppressive agents). Products include:
Leukeran **1557**

Chloramphenicol (Caution should be exercised when administering with other potentially myelosuppressive agents).
No products indexed under this heading.

Chloramphenicol Palmitate (Caution should be exercised when administering with other potentially myelosuppressive agents).
No products indexed under this heading.

Chloramphenicol Sodium Succinate (Caution should be exercised when administering with other potentially myelosuppressive agents).
No products indexed under this heading.

Chlordiazepoxide (Preclinical studies have demonstrated a decrease in hepatic microsomal cytochrome P-450 concentrations. This could potentially lead to a depression of the hepatic metabolism of certain drugs that utilize this degradative pathway).
No products indexed under this heading.

Chlordiazepoxide Hydrochloride (Preclinical studies have demonstrated a decrease in hepatic microsomal cytochrome P-450 concentrations. This could potentially lead to a depression of the hepatic metabolism of certain drugs that utilize this degradative pathway).
No products indexed under this heading.

Chlorpheniramine (Preclinical studies have demonstrated a decrease in hepatic microsomal cytochrome P-450 concentrations. This could potentially lead to a depression of the hepatic metabolism of certain drugs that utilize this degradative pathway).
No products indexed under this heading.

Chlorpheniramine Maleate (Preclinical studies have demonstrated a decrease in hepatic microsomal cytochrome P-450 concentrations. This could potentially lead to a depression of the hepatic metabolism of certain drugs that utilize this degradative pathway).
No products indexed under this heading.

Chlorpheniramine Polistirex (Preclinical studies have demonstrated a decrease in hepatic microsomal cytochrome P-450 concentrations. This could potentially lead to a depression of the hepatic metabolism of certain drugs that utilize this degradative pathway).
Products include:
Tussionex **3443**

Chlorpheniramine Tannate (Preclinical studies have demonstrated a decrease in hepatic microsomal cytochrome P-450 concentrations. This could potentially lead to a depression of the hepatic metabolism of certain drugs that utilize this degradative pathway).
No products indexed under this heading.

Chlorpromazine (Preclinical studies have demonstrated a decrease in hepatic microsomal cytochrome P-450 concentrations. This could potentially lead to a depression of the hepatic metabolism of certain drugs that utilize this degradative pathway).
No products indexed under this heading.

Chlorpromazine Hydrochloride (Preclinical studies have demonstrated a decrease in hepatic microsomal cytochrome P-450 concentrations. This could potentially lead to a depression of the hepatic metabolism of certain drugs that utilize this degradative pathway).
No products indexed under this heading.

Chlorpropamide (Preclinical studies have demonstrated a decrease in hepatic microsomal cytochrome P-450 concentrations. This could potentially lead to a depression of the hepatic metabolism of certain drugs that utilize this degradative pathway).
No products indexed under this heading.

Cilostazol (Preclinical studies have demonstrated a decrease in hepatic microsomal cytochrome P-450 concentrations. This could potentially lead to a depression of the hepatic metabolism of certain drugs that utilize this degradative pathway).
No products indexed under this heading.

Cimetidine Hydrochloride (Preclinical studies have demonstrated a decrease in hepatic microsomal cytochrome P-450 concentrations. This could potentially lead to a depression of the hepatic metabolism of certain drugs that utilize this degradative pathway).
No products indexed under this heading.

Ciprofloxacin (Preclinical studies have demonstrated a decrease in hepatic microsomal cytochrome P-450 concentrations. This could potentially lead to a depression of the hepatic metabolism of certain drugs that utilize this degradative pathway). Products include:
Cipro I.V. **3082**
Cipro **3073**
Cipro XR **3091**
Ciprodex **583**

Ciprofloxacin Hydrochloride (Preclinical studies have demonstrated a decrease in hepatic microsomal cytochrome P-450 concentrations. This could potentially lead to a depression of

the hepatic metabolism of certain drugs that utilize this degradative pathway). Products include:
Cipro **3073**

Cisapride (Preclinical studies have demonstrated a decrease in hepatic microsomal cytochrome P-450 concentrations. This could potentially lead to a depression of the hepatic metabolism of certain drugs that utilize this degradative pathway).
No products indexed under this heading.

Citalopram Hydrobromide (Preclinical studies have demonstrated a decrease in hepatic microsomal cytochrome P-450 concentrations. This could potentially lead to a depression of the hepatic metabolism of certain drugs that utilize this degradative pathway). Products include:
Celexa **1153**

Cladribine (Caution should be exercised when administering with other potentially myelosuppressive agents). Products include:
Leustatin **946**

Clarithromycin (Preclinical studies have demonstrated a decrease in hepatic microsomal cytochrome P-450 concentrations. This could potentially lead to a depression of the hepatic metabolism of certain drugs that utilize this degradative pathway). Products include:
Biaxin/Biaxin XL **412**

Clomipramine Hydrochloride (Preclinical studies have demonstrated a decrease in hepatic microsomal cytochrome P-450 concentrations. This could potentially lead to a depression of the hepatic metabolism of certain drugs that utilize this degradative pathway).
No products indexed under this heading.

Clopidogrel Bisulfate (Preclinical studies have demonstrated a decrease in hepatic microsomal cytochrome P-450 concentrations. This could potentially lead to a depression of the hepatic metabolism of certain drugs that utilize this degradative pathway). Products include:
Plavix **3027**

Clopidogrel Hydrogen Sulfate (Preclinical studies have demonstrated a decrease in hepatic microsomal cytochrome P-450 concentrations. This could potentially lead to a depression of the hepatic metabolism of certain drugs that utilize this degradative pathway).
No products indexed under this heading.

Clozapine (Preclinical studies have demonstrated a decrease in hepatic microsomal cytochrome P-450 concentrations. This could potentially lead to a depression of the hepatic metabolism of certain drugs that utilize this degradative pathway).
No products indexed under this heading.

Codeine Phosphate (Preclinical studies have demonstrated a decrease in hepatic microsomal cytochrome P-450 concentrations. This could potentially lead to a depression of the hepatic metabolism of certain drugs that utilize this degradative pathway). Products include:
Tylenol with Codeine **2691**

Codeine Sulfate (Preclinical studies have demonstrated a decrease in hepatic microsomal cytochrome P-450 concentrations. This could potentially lead to a depression of the hepatic metabolism of certain drugs that utilize this degradative pathway).
No products indexed under this heading.

Cyclobenzaprine (Preclinical studies have demonstrated a decrease in hepatic microsomal cytochrome P-450 concentrations. This could potentially lead to a depression of the hepatic metabolism of certain drugs that utilize this degradative pathway).
No products indexed under this heading.

Cyclobenzaprine Hydrochloride (Preclinical studies have demonstrated a decrease in hepatic microsomal cytochrome P-450 concentrations. This could potentially lead to a depression of the hepatic metabolism of certain drugs that utilize this degradative pathway). Products include:
Amrix **964**

Cyclophosphamide (Preclinical studies have demonstrated a decrease in hepatic microsomal cytochrome P-450 concentrations. This could potentially lead to a depression of the hepatic metabolism of certain drugs that utilize this degradative pathway).
No products indexed under this heading.

Cyclosporine (Preclinical studies have demonstrated a decrease in hepatic microsomal cytochrome P-450 concentrations. This could potentially lead to a depression of the hepatic metabolism of certain drugs that utilize this degradative pathway). Products include:
Gengraf **440**
Neoral Oral Solution **2496**
Neoral Capsules **2496**
Restasis **605**

Daunorubicin Citrate Liposome (Caution should be exercised when administering with other potentially myelosuppressive agents).
No products indexed under this heading.

Daunorubicin Hydrochloride (Caution should be exercised when administering with other potentially myelosuppressive agents).
No products indexed under this heading.

Desipramine Hydrochloride (Preclinical studies have demonstrated a decrease in hepatic microsomal cytochrome P-450 concentrations. This could potentially lead to a depression of the hepatic metabolism of certain drugs that utilize this degradative pathway).
No products indexed under this heading.

Desogestrel (Preclinical studies have demonstrated a decrease in hepatic microsomal cytochrome P-450 concentrations. This could potentially lead to a depression of the hepatic metabolism of certain drugs that utilize this degradative pathway).
No products indexed under this heading.

Dexamethasone (Preclinical studies have demonstrated a decrease in hepatic microsomal cytochrome P-450 concentrations. This could potentially lead to a depression of the hepatic metabolism of certain drugs that utilize this degradative pathway). Products include:
Ciprodex **583**
Ozurdex .... ⊙**223**
Tobramycin and Dexamethasone Ophthalmic Suspension .... ⊙**251**

Dexamethasone Acetate (Preclinical studies have demonstrated a decrease in hepatic microsomal cytochrome P-450 concentrations. This could potentially lead to a depression of the hepatic metabolism of certain drugs that utilize this degradative pathway).
No products indexed under this heading.

Dexamethasone Phosphate (Preclinical studies have demonstrated a decrease in hepatic microsomal cytochrome P-450 concentrations. This could potentially lead to a depression of the hepatic metabolism of certain drugs that utilize this degradative pathway).
No products indexed under this heading.

IMPORTANT NOTE: Always consult each drug listing in the patient's regimen for possible interactions.

Dexamethasone Sodium (Preclinical studies have demonstrated a decrease in hepatic microsomal cytochrome P-450 concentrations. This could potentially lead to a depression of the hepatic metabolism of certain drugs that utilize this degradative pathway).
No products indexed under this heading.

Dexamethasone Sodium Phosphate (Preclinical studies have demonstrated a decrease in hepatic microsomal cytochrome P-450 concentrations. This could potentially lead to a depression of the hepatic metabolism of certain drugs that utilize this degradative pathway).
No products indexed under this heading.

Dexfenfluramine Hydrochloride (Preclinical studies have demonstrated a decrease in hepatic microsomal cytochrome P-450 concentrations. This could potentially lead to a depression of the hepatic metabolism of certain drugs that utilize this degradative pathway).
No products indexed under this heading.

Dexrazoxane (Caution should be exercised when administering with other potentially myelosuppressive agents).
No products indexed under this heading.

Dextromethorphan (Preclinical studies have demonstrated a decrease in hepatic microsomal cytochrome P-450 concentrations. This could potentially lead to a depression of the hepatic metabolism of certain drugs that utilize this degradative pathway).
No products indexed under this heading.

Dextromethorphan Hydrobromide (Preclinical studies have demonstrated a decrease in hepatic microsomal cytochrome P-450 concentrations. This could potentially lead to a depression of the hepatic metabolism of certain drugs that utilize this degradative pathway).
No products indexed under this heading.

Dextromethorphan Polistirex (Preclinical studies have demonstrated a decrease in hepatic microsomal cytochrome P-450 concentrations. This could potentially lead to a depression of the hepatic metabolism of certain drugs that utilize this degradative pathway).
No products indexed under this heading.

Diazepam (Preclinical studies have demonstrated a decrease in hepatic microsomal cytochrome P-450 concentrations. This could potentially lead to a depression of the hepatic metabolism of certain drugs that utilize this degradative pathway). Products include:
Valium Tablets 2880

Diclofenac Potassium (Preclinical studies have demonstrated a decrease in hepatic microsomal cytochrome P-450 concentrations. This could potentially lead to a depression of the hepatic metabolism of certain drugs that utilize this degradative pathway).
No products indexed under this heading.

Diclofenac Sodium (Preclinical studies have demonstrated a decrease in hepatic microsomal cytochrome P-450 concentrations. This could potentially lead to a depression of the hepatic metabolism of certain drugs that utilize this degradative pathway).
No products indexed under this heading.

Dihydroergotamine Mesylate (Preclinical studies have demonstrated a decrease in hepatic microsomal cytochrome P-450 concentrations. This could potentially lead to a depression of the hepatic metabolism of certain drugs that utilize this degradative pathway).
No products indexed under this heading.

Diltiazem Hydrochloride (Preclinical studies have demonstrated a decrease in hepatic microsomal cytochrome P-450 concentrations. This could potentially lead to a depression of the hepatic

metabolism of certain drugs that utilize this degradative pathway). Products include:
Cardizem LA 423

Diltiazem Maleate (Preclinical studies have demonstrated a decrease in hepatic microsomal cytochrome P-450 concentrations. This could potentially lead to a depression of the hepatic metabolism of certain drugs that utilize this degradative pathway).
No products indexed under this heading.

Disopyramide (Preclinical studies have demonstrated a decrease in hepatic microsomal cytochrome P-450 concentrations. This could potentially lead to a depression of the hepatic metabolism of certain drugs that utilize this degradative pathway).
No products indexed under this heading.

Disopyramide Phosphate (Preclinical studies have demonstrated a decrease in hepatic microsomal cytochrome P-450 concentrations. This could potentially lead to a depression of the hepatic metabolism of certain drugs that utilize this degradative pathway).
No products indexed under this heading.

Disulfiram (Preclinical studies have demonstrated a decrease in hepatic microsomal cytochrome P-450 concentrations. This could potentially lead to a depression of the hepatic metabolism of certain drugs that utilize this degradative pathway).
No products indexed under this heading.

Divalproex Sodium (Preclinical studies have demonstrated a decrease in hepatic microsomal cytochrome P-450 concentrations. This could potentially lead to a depression of the hepatic metabolism of certain drugs that utilize this degradative pathway). Products include:
Depakote ER 426

Docetaxel (Preclinical studies have demonstrated a decrease in hepatic microsomal cytochrome P-450 concentrations. This could potentially lead to a depression of the hepatic metabolism of certain drugs that utilize this degradative pathway). Products include:
Taxotere 3035

Dolasetron Mesylate (Preclinical studies have demonstrated a decrease in hepatic microsomal cytochrome P-450 concentrations. This could potentially lead to a depression of the hepatic metabolism of certain drugs that utilize this degradative pathway). Products include:
Anzemet Injection 2931
Anzemet Tablets 2934

Donepezil Hydrochloride (Preclinical studies have demonstrated a decrease in hepatic microsomal cytochrome P-450 concentrations. This could potentially lead to a depression of the hepatic metabolism of certain drugs that utilize this degradative pathway). Products include:
Aricept 1045
Aricept ODT 1045

Doxepin Hydrochloride (Preclinical studies have demonstrated a decrease in hepatic microsomal cytochrome P-450 concentrations. This could potentially lead to a depression of the hepatic metabolism of certain drugs that utilize this degradative pathway).
No products indexed under this heading.

Doxorubicin Hydrochloride (Caution should be exercised when administering with other potentially myelosuppressive agents).
No products indexed under this heading.

Doxorubicin Hydrochloride Liposome (Caution should be exercised when administering with other potentially myelosuppressive agents). Products include:

Doxil 939

Dronabinol (Preclinical studies have demonstrated a decrease in hepatic microsomal cytochrome P-450 concentrations. This could potentially lead to a depression of the hepatic metabolism of certain drugs that utilize this degradative pathway).
No products indexed under this heading.

Drugs that Undergo Biotransformation by Cytochrome P-450 Mixed Function Oxidase (Preclinical studies have demonstrated a decrease in hepatic microsomal cytochrome P-450 concentrations. This could potentially lead to a depression of the hepatic metabolism of certain drugs that utilize this degradative pathway).
No products indexed under this heading.

Dyphylline (Preclinical studies have demonstrated a decrease in hepatic microsomal cytochrome P-450 concentrations. This could potentially lead to a depression of the hepatic metabolism of certain drugs that utilize this degradative pathway).
No products indexed under this heading.

Encainide Hydrochloride (Preclinical studies have demonstrated a decrease in hepatic microsomal cytochrome P-450 concentrations. This could potentially lead to a depression of the hepatic metabolism of certain drugs that utilize this degradative pathway).
No products indexed under this heading.

Enoxacin (Preclinical studies have demonstrated a decrease in hepatic microsomal cytochrome P-450 concentrations. This could potentially lead to a depression of the hepatic metabolism of certain drugs that utilize this degradative pathway).
No products indexed under this heading.

Eprosartan Mesylate (Preclinical studies have demonstrated a decrease in hepatic microsomal cytochrome P-450 concentrations. This could potentially lead to a depression of the hepatic metabolism of certain drugs that utilize this degradative pathway). Products include:
Teveten 538
Teveten HCT 541

Ergotamine Tartrate (Preclinical studies have demonstrated a decrease in hepatic microsomal cytochrome P-450 concentrations. This could potentially lead to a depression of the hepatic metabolism of certain drugs that utilize this degradative pathway).
No products indexed under this heading.

Erythromycin (Preclinical studies have demonstrated a decrease in hepatic microsomal cytochrome P-450 concentrations. This could potentially lead to a depression of the hepatic metabolism of certain drugs that utilize this degradative pathway).
No products indexed under this heading.

Erythromycin Estolate (Preclinical studies have demonstrated a decrease in hepatic microsomal cytochrome P-450 concentrations. This could potentially lead to a depression of the hepatic metabolism of certain drugs that utilize this degradative pathway).
No products indexed under this heading.

Erythromycin Ethylsuccinate (Preclinical studies have demonstrated a decrease in hepatic microsomal cytochrome P-450 concentrations. This could potentially lead to a depression of the hepatic metabolism of certain drugs that utilize this degradative pathway). Products include:
E.E.S. 437
EryPed 435

Erythromycin Gluceptate (Preclinical studies have demonstrated a decrease in hepatic microsomal cytochrome P-450 concentrations. This could potentially lead to a depression of the hepatic metabolism of certain drugs that utilize this degradative pathway).
No products indexed under this heading.

Erythromycin Lactobionate (Preclinical studies have demonstrated a decrease in hepatic microsomal cytochrome P-450 concentrations. This could potentially lead to a depression of the hepatic metabolism of certain drugs that utilize this degradative pathway).
No products indexed under this heading.

Erythromycin Stearate (Preclinical studies have demonstrated a decrease in hepatic microsomal cytochrome P-450 concentrations. This could potentially lead to a depression of the hepatic metabolism of certain drugs that utilize this degradative pathway).
No products indexed under this heading.

Esomeprazole Magnesium (Preclinical studies have demonstrated a decrease in hepatic microsomal cytochrome P-450 concentrations. This could potentially lead to a depression of the hepatic metabolism of certain drugs that utilize this degradative pathway). Products include:
Nexium Capsules 704
Nexium Oral Suspension 704

Esomeprazole Sodium (Preclinical studies have demonstrated a decrease in hepatic microsomal cytochrome P-450 concentrations. This could potentially lead to a depression of the hepatic metabolism of certain drugs that utilize this degradative pathway). Products include:
Nexium I.V. 712

Estradiol (Preclinical studies have demonstrated a decrease in hepatic microsomal cytochrome P-450 concentrations. This could potentially lead to a depression of the hepatic metabolism of certain drugs that utilize this degradative pathway). Products include:
Activella 2561
Angeliq 831
Climara 841
Climara Pro 847
Divigel 3467
Estrasorb 1777
Vagifem 2589

Estradiol Benzoate (Preclinical studies have demonstrated a decrease in hepatic microsomal cytochrome P-450 concentrations. This could potentially lead to a depression of the hepatic metabolism of certain drugs that utilize this degradative pathway).
No products indexed under this heading.

Estradiol Cypionate (Preclinical studies have demonstrated a decrease in hepatic microsomal cytochrome P-450 concentrations. This could potentially lead to a depression of the hepatic metabolism of certain drugs that utilize this degradative pathway).
No products indexed under this heading.

Estradiol Valerate (Preclinical studies have demonstrated a decrease in hepatic microsomal cytochrome P-450 concentrations. This could potentially lead to a depression of the hepatic metabolism of certain drugs that utilize this degradative pathway).
No products indexed under this heading.

Estrogen (Preclinical studies have demonstrated a decrease in hepatic microsomal cytochrome P-450 concentrations. This could potentially lead to a depression of the hepatic metabolism of certain drugs that utilize this degradative pathway).
No products indexed under this heading.

Estrogens, Conjugated (Preclinical studies have demonstrated a decrease

(⊙ Described in PDR® for Ophthalmic Medicines)

in hepatic microsomal cytochrome P-450 concentrations. This could potentially lead to a depression of the hepatic metabolism of certain drugs that utilize this degradative pathway). Products include:

- Premarin Intravenous 3528
- Premarin Tablets 3533
- Premarin Vaginal Cream 3540
- Premphase 3549
- Prempro 3549

Estrogens, Conjugated, Synthetic A (Preclinical studies have demonstrated a decrease in hepatic microsomal cytochrome P-450 concentrations. This could potentially lead to a depression of the hepatic metabolism of certain drugs that utilize this degradative pathway).
No products indexed under this heading.

Estrogens, Esterified (Preclinical studies have demonstrated a decrease in hepatic microsomal cytochrome P-450 concentrations. This could potentially lead to a depression of the hepatic metabolism of certain drugs that utilize this degradative pathway).
No products indexed under this heading.

Ethinyl Estradiol (Preclinical studies have demonstrated a decrease in hepatic microsomal cytochrome P-450 concentrations. This could potentially lead to a depression of the hepatic metabolism of certain drugs that utilize this degradative pathway). Products include:

- LoSeasonique 3407
- Lybrel 3514
- NuvaRing 3181
- Ortho Evra 2648
- Ortho-Cyclen/Ortho Tri-Cyclen 2663
- Ortho Tri-Cyclen Lo Tablets 2673
- Seasonique 3418
- Yaz 864

Ethosuximide (Preclinical studies have demonstrated a decrease in hepatic microsomal cytochrome P-450 concentrations. This could potentially lead to a depression of the hepatic metabolism of certain drugs that utilize this degradative pathway).
No products indexed under this heading.

Ethotoin (Preclinical studies have demonstrated a decrease in hepatic microsomal cytochrome P-450 concentrations. This could potentially lead to a depression of the hepatic metabolism of certain drugs that utilize this degradative pathway).
No products indexed under this heading.

Ethynodiol Diacetate (Preclinical studies have demonstrated a decrease in hepatic microsomal cytochrome P-450 concentrations. This could potentially lead to a depression of the hepatic metabolism of certain drugs that utilize this degradative pathway).
No products indexed under this heading.

Etodolac (Preclinical studies have demonstrated a decrease in hepatic microsomal cytochrome P-450 concentrations. This could potentially lead to a depression of the hepatic metabolism of certain drugs that utilize this degradative pathway).
No products indexed under this heading.

Etoposide (Preclinical studies have demonstrated a decrease in hepatic microsomal cytochrome P-450 concentrations. This could potentially lead to a depression of the hepatic metabolism of certain drugs that utilize this degradative pathway).
No products indexed under this heading.

Etoposide Phosphate (Preclinical studies have demonstrated a decrease in hepatic microsomal cytochrome P-450 concentrations. This could potentially lead to a depression of the hepatic metabolism of certain drugs that utilize this degradative pathway).
No products indexed under this heading.

Felbamate (Preclinical studies have demonstrated a decrease in hepatic microsomal cytochrome P-450 concentrations. This could potentially lead to a depression of the hepatic metabolism of certain drugs that utilize this degradative pathway).
No products indexed under this heading.

Felodipine (Preclinical studies have demonstrated a decrease in hepatic microsomal cytochrome P-450 concentrations. This could potentially lead to a depression of the hepatic metabolism of certain drugs that utilize this degradative pathway).
No products indexed under this heading.

Fenoprofen Calcium (Preclinical studies have demonstrated a decrease in hepatic microsomal cytochrome P-450 concentrations. This could potentially lead to a depression of the hepatic metabolism of certain drugs that utilize this degradative pathway).
No products indexed under this heading.

Fentanyl (Preclinical studies have demonstrated a decrease in hepatic microsomal cytochrome P-450 concentrations. This could potentially lead to a depression of the hepatic metabolism of certain drugs that utilize this degradative pathway). Products include:

- Duragesic 2604
- Fentanyl Transdermal System 2346
- Onsolis 2054

Fentanyl Citrate (Preclinical studies have demonstrated a decrease in hepatic microsomal cytochrome P-450 concentrations. This could potentially lead to a depression of the hepatic metabolism of certain drugs that utilize this degradative pathway). Products include:

- Fentora 966

Flecainide Acetate (Preclinical studies have demonstrated a decrease in hepatic microsomal cytochrome P-450 concentrations. This could potentially lead to a depression of the hepatic metabolism of certain drugs that utilize this degradative pathway).
No products indexed under this heading.

Fludarabine Phosphate (Caution should be exercised when administering with other potentially myelosuppressive agents). Products include:

- Oforta 3023

Fluoxetine (Preclinical studies have demonstrated a decrease in hepatic microsomal cytochrome P-450 concentrations. This could potentially lead to a depression of the hepatic metabolism of certain drugs that utilize this degradative pathway).
No products indexed under this heading.

Fluoxetine Hydrochloride (Preclinical studies have demonstrated a decrease in hepatic microsomal cytochrome P-450 concentrations. This could potentially lead to a depression of the hepatic metabolism of certain drugs that utilize this degradative pathway). Products include:

- Prozac Weekly 1941
- Prozac Pulvules 1941
- Symbyax 1965

Fluphenazine Decanoate (Preclinical studies have demonstrated a decrease in hepatic microsomal cytochrome P-450 concentrations. This could potentially lead to a depression of the hepatic metabolism of certain drugs that utilize this degradative pathway).
No products indexed under this heading.

Fluphenazine Enanthate (Preclinical studies have demonstrated a decrease in hepatic microsomal cytochrome P-450 concentrations. This could potentially lead to a depression of the hepatic metabolism of certain drugs that utilize this degradative pathway).
No products indexed under this heading.

Fluphenazine Hydrochloride (Preclinical studies have demonstrated a decrease in hepatic microsomal cytochrome P-450 concentrations. This could potentially lead to a depression of the hepatic metabolism of certain drugs that utilize this degradative pathway).
No products indexed under this heading.

Flurbiprofen (Preclinical studies have demonstrated a decrease in hepatic microsomal cytochrome P-450 concentrations. This could potentially lead to a depression of the hepatic metabolism of certain drugs that utilize this degradative pathway).
No products indexed under this heading.

Flurbiprofen Sodium (Preclinical studies have demonstrated a decrease in hepatic microsomal cytochrome P-450 concentrations. This could potentially lead to a depression of the hepatic metabolism of certain drugs that utilize this degradative pathway).
No products indexed under this heading.

Flutamide (Preclinical studies have demonstrated a decrease in hepatic microsomal cytochrome P-450 concentrations. This could potentially lead to a depression of the hepatic metabolism of certain drugs that utilize this degradative pathway).
No products indexed under this heading.

Fluticasone Propionate (Preclinical studies have demonstrated a decrease in hepatic microsomal cytochrome P-450 concentrations. This could potentially lead to a depression of the hepatic metabolism of certain drugs that utilize this degradative pathway). Products include:

- Advair 100/50 1275
- Advair 250/50 1275
- Advair 500/50 1275
- Advair HFA 45/21 1288
- Advair HFA 115/21 1288
- Advair HFA 230/21 1288
- Flonase 1459
- Flovent Diskus 1463
- Flovent HFA 1470

Fluvastatin Sodium (Preclinical studies have demonstrated a decrease in hepatic microsomal cytochrome P-450 concentrations. This could potentially lead to a depression of the hepatic metabolism of certain drugs that utilize this degradative pathway).
No products indexed under this heading.

Fluvoxamine Maleate (Preclinical studies have demonstrated a decrease in hepatic microsomal cytochrome P-450 concentrations. This could potentially lead to a depression of the hepatic metabolism of certain drugs that utilize this degradative pathway).
No products indexed under this heading.

Formoterol Fumarate (Preclinical studies have demonstrated a decrease in hepatic microsomal cytochrome P-450 concentrations. This could potentially lead to a depression of the hepatic metabolism of certain drugs that utilize this degradative pathway). Products include:

- Foradil 3121
- Perforomist 3634

Fosphenytoin (Preclinical studies have demonstrated a decrease in hepatic microsomal cytochrome P-450 concentrations. This could potentially lead to a depression of the hepatic metabolism of certain drugs that utilize this degradative pathway).
No products indexed under this heading.

Fosphenytoin Sodium (Preclinical studies have demonstrated a decrease in hepatic microsomal cytochrome P-450 concentrations. This could potentially lead to a depression of the hepatic metabolism of certain drugs that utilize this degradative pathway).
No products indexed under this heading.

Gabapentin (Preclinical studies have demonstrated a decrease in hepatic microsomal cytochrome P-450 concentrations. This could potentially lead to a depression of the hepatic metabolism of certain drugs that utilize this degradative pathway).
No products indexed under this heading.

Galantamine Hydrobromide (Preclinical studies have demonstrated a decrease in hepatic microsomal cytochrome P-450 concentrations. This could potentially lead to a depression of the hepatic metabolism of certain drugs that utilize this degradative pathway).
No products indexed under this heading.

Gemcitabine Hydrochloride (Caution should be exercised when administering with other potentially myelosuppressive agents). Products include:

- Gemzar 1900

Gemtuzumab Ozogamicin (Caution should be exercised when administering with other potentially myelosuppressive agents). Products include:

- Mylotarg 3524

Glimepiride (Preclinical studies have demonstrated a decrease in hepatic microsomal cytochrome P-450 concentrations. This could potentially lead to a depression of the hepatic metabolism of certain drugs that utilize this degradative pathway). Products include:

- Avandaryl 1356
- Duetact 3354

Glipizide (Preclinical studies have demonstrated a decrease in hepatic microsomal cytochrome P-450 concentrations. This could potentially lead to a depression of the hepatic metabolism of certain drugs that utilize this degradative pathway).
No products indexed under this heading.

Glyburide (Preclinical studies have demonstrated a decrease in hepatic microsomal cytochrome P-450 concentrations. This could potentially lead to a depression of the hepatic metabolism of certain drugs that utilize this degradative pathway).
No products indexed under this heading.

Grepafloxacin Hydrochloride (Preclinical studies have demonstrated a decrease in hepatic microsomal cytochrome P-450 concentrations. This could potentially lead to a depression of the hepatic metabolism of certain drugs that utilize this degradative pathway).
No products indexed under this heading.

Haloperidol (Preclinical studies have demonstrated a decrease in hepatic microsomal cytochrome P-450 concentrations. This could potentially lead to a depression of the hepatic metabolism of certain drugs that utilize this degradative pathway).
No products indexed under this heading.

Haloperidol Decanoate (Preclinical studies have demonstrated a decrease in hepatic microsomal cytochrome P-450 concentrations. This could potentially lead to a depression of the hepatic metabolism of certain drugs that utilize this degradative pathway).
No products indexed under this heading.

Haloperidol Lactate (Preclinical studies have demonstrated a decrease in hepatic microsomal cytochrome P-450 concentrations. This could potentially lead to a depression of the hepatic metabolism of certain drugs that utilize this degradative pathway).
No products indexed under this heading.

Hexobarbital (Preclinical studies have demonstrated a decrease in hepatic microsomal cytochrome P-450 concentrations. This could potentially lead to a depression of the hepatic metabolism of certain drugs that utilize this degradative pathway).
No products indexed under this heading.

IMPORTANT NOTE: Always consult each drug listing in the patient's regimen for possible interactions.

Hydrocodone Bitartrate (Preclinical studies have demonstrated a decrease in hepatic microsomal cytochrome P-450 concentrations. This could potentially lead to a depression of the hepatic metabolism of certain drugs that utilize this degradative pathway). Products include:

Ibuprofen (Preclinical studies have demonstrated a decrease in hepatic microsomal cytochrome P-450 concentrations. This could potentially lead to a depression of the hepatic metabolism of certain drugs that utilize this degradative pathway). Products include:

Idarubicin Hydrochloride (Caution should be exercised when administering with other potentially myelosuppressive agents).
No products indexed under this heading.

Imipramine Hydrochloride (Preclinical studies have demonstrated a decrease in hepatic microsomal cytochrome P-450 concentrations. This could potentially lead to a depression of the hepatic metabolism of certain drugs that utilize this degradative pathway).
No products indexed under this heading.

Imipramine Pamoate (Preclinical studies have demonstrated a decrease in hepatic microsomal cytochrome P-450 concentrations. This could potentially lead to a depression of the hepatic metabolism of certain drugs that utilize this degradative pathway).
No products indexed under this heading.

Indinavir Sulfate (Preclinical studies have demonstrated a decrease in hepatic microsomal cytochrome P-450 concentrations. This could potentially lead to a depression of the hepatic metabolism of certain drugs that utilize this degradative pathway). Products include:

Indomethacin (Preclinical studies have demonstrated a decrease in hepatic microsomal cytochrome P-450 concentrations. This could potentially lead to a depression of the hepatic metabolism of certain drugs that utilize this degradative pathway). Products include:

Indomethacin Sodium Trihydrate (Preclinical studies have demonstrated a decrease in hepatic microsomal cytochrome P-450 concentrations. This could potentially lead to a depression of the hepatic metabolism of certain drugs that utilize this degradative pathway). Products include:

Indoramin Hydrochloride (Preclinical studies have demonstrated a decrease in hepatic microsomal cytochrome P-450 concentrations. This could potentially lead to a depression of the hepatic metabolism of certain drugs that utilize this degradative pathway).
No products indexed under this heading.

Interferon alfa-2a, Recombinant (Caution should be exercised when administering with other potentially myelosuppressive agents).
No products indexed under this heading.

Irbesartan (Preclinical studies have demonstrated a decrease in hepatic microsomal cytochrome P-450 concen-trations. This could potentially lead to a depression of the hepatic metabolism of certain drugs that utilize this degradative pathway). Products include:

Irinotecan Hydrochloride (Caution should be exercised when administering with other potentially myelosuppressive agents).
No products indexed under this heading.

Isotretinoin (Preclinical studies have demonstrated a decrease in hepatic microsomal cytochrome P-450 concen-trations. This could potentially lead to a depression of the hepatic metabolism of certain drugs that utilize this degradative pathway). Products include:

Isradipine (Preclinical studies have demonstrated a decrease in hepatic microsomal cytochrome P-450 concen-trations. This could potentially lead to a depression of the hepatic metabolism of certain drugs that utilize this degradative pathway). Products include:

Itraconazole (Preclinical studies have demonstrated a decrease in hepatic microsomal cytochrome P-450 concen-trations. This could potentially lead to a depression of the hepatic metabolism of certain drugs that utilize this degradative pathway).
No products indexed under this heading.

Ixabepilone (Preclinical studies have demonstrated a decrease in hepatic microsomal cytochrome P-450 concen-trations. This could potentially lead to a depression of the hepatic metabolism of certain drugs that utilize this degradative pathway).
No products indexed under this heading.

Ketoconazole (Preclinical studies have demonstrated a decrease in hepatic microsomal cytochrome P-450 concentrations. This could potentially lead to a depression of the hepatic metabolism of certain drugs that utilize this degradative pathway). Products include:

Ketoprofen (Preclinical studies have demonstrated a decrease in hepatic microsomal cytochrome P-450 concen-trations. This could potentially lead to a depression of the hepatic metabolism of certain drugs that utilize this degradative pathway).
No products indexed under this heading.

Ketorolac Tromethamine (Preclinical studies have demonstrated a decrease in hepatic microsomal cytochrome P-450 concentrations. This could potentially lead to a depression of the hepatic metabolism of certain drugs that utilize this degradative pathway). Products include:

Labetalol Hydrochloride (Preclinical studies have demonstrated a decrease in hepatic microsomal cytochrome P-450 concentrations. This could potentially lead to a depression of the hepatic metabolism of certain drugs that utilize this degradative pathway).
No products indexed under this heading.

Lamotrigine (Preclinical studies have demonstrated a decrease in hepatic microsomal cytochrome P-450 concen-trations. This could potentially lead to a depression of the hepatic metabolism of certain drugs that utilize this degra-dative pathway). Products include:

Lansoprazole (Preclinical studies have demonstrated a decrease in hepatic microsomal cytochrome P-450 concentrations. This could potentially lead to a depression of the hepatic metabolism of certain drugs that utilize this degradative pathway).
No products indexed under this heading.

Levetiracetam (Preclinical studies have demonstrated a decrease in hepatic microsomal cytochrome P-450 concentrations. This could potentially lead to a depression of the hepatic metabolism of certain drugs that utilize this degradative pathway). Products include:

Levobupivacaine Hydrochloride (Preclinical studies have demonstrated a decrease in hepatic microsomal cyto-chrome P-450 concentrations. This could potentially lead to a depression of the hepatic metabolism of certain drugs that utilize this degradative pathway).
No products indexed under this heading.

Levonorgestrel (Preclinical studies have demonstrated a decrease in hepatic microsomal cytochrome P-450 concentrations. This could potentially lead to a depression of the hepatic metabolism of certain drugs that utilize this degradative pathway). Products include:

Lidocaine (Preclinical studies have demonstrated a decrease in hepatic microsomal cytochrome P-450 concen-trations. This could potentially lead to a depression of the hepatic metabolism of certain drugs that utilize this degra-dative pathway). Products include:

Lidocaine Base (Preclinical studies have demonstrated a decrease in hepatic microsomal cytochrome P-450 concentrations. This could potentially lead to a depression of the hepatic metabolism of certain drugs that utilize this degradative pathway).
No products indexed under this heading.

Lidocaine Hydrochloride (Preclinical studies have demonstrated a decrease in hepatic microsomal cytochrome P-450 concentrations. This could poten-tially lead to a depression of the hepatic metabolism of certain drugs that utilize this degradative pathway).
No products indexed under this heading.

Lomefloxacin Hydrochloride (Pre-clinical studies have demonstrated a decrease in hepatic microsomal cytochrome P-450 concentrations. This could potentially lead to a depression of the hepatic metabolism of certain drugs that utilize this degradative pathway).
No products indexed under this heading.

Losartan Potassium (Preclinical stud-ies have demonstrated a decrease in hepatic microsomal cytochrome P-450 concentrations. This could potentially lead to a depression of the hepatic metabolism of certain drugs that utilize this degradative pathway). Products include:

Lovastatin (Preclinical studies have demonstrated a decrease in hepatic microsomal cytochrome P-450 concen-trations. This could potentially lead to a depression of the hepatic metabolism of certain drugs that utilize this degra-dative pathway). Products include:

Maprotiline Hydrochloride (Preclini-cal studies have demonstrated a decrease in hepatic microsomal cyto-chrome P-450 concentrations. This could potentially lead to a depression of the hepatic metabolism of certain drugs that utilize this degradative pathway).
No products indexed under this heading.

Meclofenamate Sodium (Preclinical studies have demonstrated a decrease in hepatic microsomal cytochrome P-450 concentrations. This could poten-tially lead to a depression of the hepatic metabolism of certain drugs that utilize this degradative pathway).
No products indexed under this heading.

Mefenamic Acid (Preclinical studies have demonstrated a decrease in hepatic microsomal cytochrome P-450 concentrations. This could potentially lead to a depression of the hepatic metabolism of certain drugs that utilize this degradative pathway).
No products indexed under this heading.

Meloxicam (Preclinical studies have demonstrated a decrease in hepatic microsomal cytochrome P-450 concentrations. This could potentially lead to a depression of the hepatic metabolism of certain drugs that utilize this degra-dative pathway).
No products indexed under this heading.

Melphalan Hydrochloride (Caution should be exercised when administering with other potentially myelosuppressive agents). Products include:

Meperidine Hydrochloride (Preclini-cal studies have demonstrated a decrease in hepatic microsomal cyto-chrome P-450 concentrations. This could potentially lead to a depression of the hepatic metabolism of certain drugs that utilize this degradative pathway).
No products indexed under this heading.

Mephenytoin (Preclinical studies have demonstrated a decrease in hepatic microsomal cytochrome P-450 concen-trations. This could potentially lead to a depression of the hepatic metabolism of certain drugs that utilize this degra-dative pathway).
No products indexed under this heading.

Mephobarbital (Preclinical studies have demonstrated a decrease in hepatic microsomal cytochrome P-450 concentrations. This could potentially lead to a depression of the hepatic metabolism of certain drugs that utilize this degradative pathway).
No products indexed under this heading.

Meprobamate (Preclinical studies have demonstrated a decrease in hepatic microsomal cytochrome P-450 concentrations. This could potentially lead to a depression of the hepatic metabolism of certain drugs that utilize this degradative pathway).
No products indexed under this heading.

Mercaptopurine (Caution should be exercised when administering with other potentially myelosuppressive agents).
No products indexed under this heading.

Mestranol (Preclinical studies have demonstrated a decrease in hepatic microsomal cytochrome P-450 concen-trations. This could potentially lead to a depression of the hepatic metabolism of certain drugs that utilize this degra-dative pathway).
No products indexed under this heading.

Metformin Hydrochloride (Preclini-cal studies have demonstrated a decrease in hepatic microsomal cyto-chrome P-450 concentrations. This could potentially lead to a depression of the hepatic metabolism of certain drugs that utilize this degradative pathway). Products include:

IMPORTANT NOTE: Always consult each drug listing in the patient's regimen for possible interactions.

Oxcarbazepine (Preclinical studies have demonstrated a decrease in hepatic microsomal cytochrome P-450 concentrations. This could potentially lead to a depression of the hepatic metabolism of certain drugs that utilize this degradative pathway).
No products indexed under this heading.

Oxycodone Hydrochloride (Preclinical studies have demonstrated a decrease in hepatic microsomal cytochrome P-450 concentrations. This could potentially lead to a depression of the hepatic metabolism of certain drugs that utilize this degradative pathway). Products include:
OxyContin 2807
Percocet 1121
Percodan 1124

Paclitaxel (Preclinical studies have demonstrated a decrease in hepatic microsomal cytochrome P-450 concentrations. This could potentially lead to a depression of the hepatic metabolism of certain drugs that utilize this degradative pathway).
No products indexed under this heading.

Pantoprazole Sodium (Preclinical studies have demonstrated a decrease in hepatic microsomal cytochrome P-450 concentrations. This could potentially lead to a depression of the hepatic metabolism of certain drugs that utilize this degradative pathway). Products include:
Protonix Tablets 3571
Protonix 3575

Paramethadione (Preclinical studies have demonstrated a decrease in hepatic microsomal cytochrome P-450 concentrations. This could potentially lead to a depression of the hepatic metabolism of certain drugs that utilize this degradative pathway).
No products indexed under this heading.

Paroxetine Hydrochloride (Preclinical studies have demonstrated a decrease in hepatic microsomal cytochrome P-450 concentrations. This could potentially lead to a depression of the hepatic metabolism of certain drugs that utilize this degradative pathway). Products include:
Paroxetine CR 2361
Paroxetine ER 2371
Paxil 1586
Paxil CR 1596

Pentamidine Isethionate (Preclinical studies have demonstrated a decrease in hepatic microsomal cytochrome P-450 concentrations. This could potentially lead to a depression of the hepatic metabolism of certain drugs that utilize this degradative pathway).
No products indexed under this heading.

Phenacemide (Preclinical studies have demonstrated a decrease in hepatic microsomal cytochrome P-450 concentrations. This could potentially lead to a depression of the hepatic metabolism of certain drugs that utilize this degradative pathway).
No products indexed under this heading.

Phenobarbital (Preclinical studies have demonstrated a decrease in hepatic microsomal cytochrome P-450 concentrations. This could potentially lead to a depression of the hepatic metabolism of certain drugs that utilize this degradative pathway). Products include:
Donnatal 2711

Phenobarbital Sodium (Preclinical studies have demonstrated a decrease in hepatic microsomal cytochrome P-450 concentrations. This could potentially lead to a depression of the hepatic metabolism of certain drugs that utilize this degradative pathway).
No products indexed under this heading.

Phensuximide (Preclinical studies have demonstrated a decrease in hepatic microsomal cytochrome P-450 concentrations. This could potentially lead to a depression of the hepatic metabolism of certain drugs that utilize this degradative pathway).
No products indexed under this heading.

Phenylbutazone (Preclinical studies have demonstrated a decrease in hepatic microsomal cytochrome P-450 concentrations. This could potentially lead to a depression of the hepatic metabolism of certain drugs that utilize this degradative pathway).
No products indexed under this heading.

Phenytoin (Preclinical studies have demonstrated a decrease in hepatic microsomal cytochrome P-450 concentrations. This could potentially lead to a depression of the hepatic metabolism of certain drugs that utilize this degradative pathway).
No products indexed under this heading.

Phenytoin Sodium (Preclinical studies have demonstrated a decrease in hepatic microsomal cytochrome P-450 concentrations. This could potentially lead to a depression of the hepatic metabolism of certain drugs that utilize this degradative pathway). Products include:
Phenytek Capsules 2380

Pimozide (Preclinical studies have demonstrated a decrease in hepatic microsomal cytochrome P-450 concentrations. This could potentially lead to a depression of the hepatic metabolism of certain drugs that utilize this degradative pathway).
No products indexed under this heading.

Pindolol (Preclinical studies have demonstrated a decrease in hepatic microsomal cytochrome P-450 concentrations. This could potentially lead to a depression of the hepatic metabolism of certain drugs that utilize this degradative pathway).
No products indexed under this heading.

Pioglitazone Hydrochloride (Preclinical studies have demonstrated a decrease in hepatic microsomal cytochrome P-450 concentrations. This could potentially lead to a depression of the hepatic metabolism of certain drugs that utilize this degradative pathway). Products include:
ActoPlus 3338
Actos 3345
Duetact 3354

Piroxicam (Preclinical studies have demonstrated a decrease in hepatic microsomal cytochrome P-450 concentrations. This could potentially lead to a depression of the hepatic metabolism of certain drugs that utilize this degradative pathway).
No products indexed under this heading.

Polyestradiol Phosphate (Preclinical studies have demonstrated a decrease in hepatic microsomal cytochrome P-450 concentrations. This could potentially lead to a depression of the hepatic metabolism of certain drugs that utilize this degradative pathway).
No products indexed under this heading.

Primidone (Preclinical studies have demonstrated a decrease in hepatic microsomal cytochrome P-450 concentrations. This could potentially lead to a depression of the hepatic metabolism of certain drugs that utilize this degradative pathway).
No products indexed under this heading.

Progesterone (Preclinical studies have demonstrated a decrease in hepatic microsomal cytochrome P-450 concentrations. This could potentially lead to a depression of the hepatic metabolism of certain drugs that utilize this degradative pathway). Products include:

Crinone 4% 996
Crinone 8% 996
Prometrium 3307

Proguanil Hydrochloride (Preclinical studies have demonstrated a decrease in hepatic microsomal cytochrome P-450 concentrations. This could potentially lead to a depression of the hepatic metabolism of certain drugs that utilize this degradative pathway). Products include:
Malarone Pediatric Tablets 1572
Malarone 1572

Propafenone Hydrochloride (Preclinical studies have demonstrated a decrease in hepatic microsomal cytochrome P-450 concentrations. This could potentially lead to a depression of the hepatic metabolism of certain drugs that utilize this degradative pathway). Products include:
Rythmol 1648
Rythmol SR 1652

Propoxyphene Hydrochloride (Preclinical studies have demonstrated a decrease in hepatic microsomal cytochrome P-450 concentrations. This could potentially lead to a depression of the hepatic metabolism of certain drugs that utilize this degradative pathway).
No products indexed under this heading.

Propoxyphene Napsylate (Preclinical studies have demonstrated a decrease in hepatic microsomal cytochrome P-450 concentrations. This could potentially lead to a depression of the hepatic metabolism of certain drugs that utilize this degradative pathway).
No products indexed under this heading.

Propranolol Hydrochloride (Preclinical studies have demonstrated a decrease in hepatic microsomal cytochrome P-450 concentrations. This could potentially lead to a depression of the hepatic metabolism of certain drugs that utilize this degradative pathway). Products include:
InnoPran XL 1517

Protriptyline Hydrochloride (Preclinical studies have demonstrated a decrease in hepatic microsomal cytochrome P-450 concentrations. This could potentially lead to a depression of the hepatic metabolism of certain drugs that utilize this degradative pathway).
No products indexed under this heading.

Quetiapine Fumarate (Preclinical studies have demonstrated a decrease in hepatic microsomal cytochrome P-450 concentrations. This could potentially lead to a depression of the hepatic metabolism of certain drugs that utilize this degradative pathway). Products include:
Seroquel 750
Seroquel XR 759

Quinidine Gluconate (Preclinical studies have demonstrated a decrease in hepatic microsomal cytochrome P-450 concentrations. This could potentially lead to a depression of the hepatic metabolism of certain drugs that utilize this degradative pathway).
No products indexed under this heading.

Quinidine Hydrochloride (Preclinical studies have demonstrated a decrease in hepatic microsomal cytochrome P-450 concentrations. This could potentially lead to a depression of the hepatic metabolism of certain drugs that utilize this degradative pathway).
No products indexed under this heading.

Quinidine Polygalacturonate (Preclinical studies have demonstrated a decrease in hepatic microsomal cytochrome P-450 concentrations. This could potentially lead to a depression of the hepatic metabolism of certain drugs that utilize this degradative pathway).
No products indexed under this heading.

Quinidine Sulfate (Preclinical studies have demonstrated a decrease in hepatic microsomal cytochrome P-450 concentrations. This could potentially lead to a depression of the hepatic metabolism of certain drugs that utilize this degradative pathway).
No products indexed under this heading.

Quinine (Preclinical studies have demonstrated a decrease in hepatic microsomal cytochrome P-450 concentrations. This could potentially lead to a depression of the hepatic metabolism of certain drugs that utilize this degradative pathway). Products include:
Hyland's Leg Cramps PM with Quinine 3315

Quinine Sulfate (Preclinical studies have demonstrated a decrease in hepatic microsomal cytochrome P-450 concentrations. This could potentially lead to a depression of the hepatic metabolism of certain drugs that utilize this degradative pathway).
No products indexed under this heading.

Rabeprazole Sodium (Preclinical studies have demonstrated a decrease in hepatic microsomal cytochrome P-450 concentrations. This could potentially lead to a depression of the hepatic metabolism of certain drugs that utilize this degradative pathway). Products include:
Aciphex 1035

Repaglinide (Preclinical studies have demonstrated a decrease in hepatic microsomal cytochrome P-450 concentrations. This could potentially lead to a depression of the hepatic metabolism of certain drugs that utilize this degradative pathway).
No products indexed under this heading.

Rifabutin (Preclinical studies have demonstrated a decrease in hepatic microsomal cytochrome P-450 concentrations. This could potentially lead to a depression of the hepatic metabolism of certain drugs that utilize this degradative pathway).
No products indexed under this heading.

Riluzole (Preclinical studies have demonstrated a decrease in hepatic microsomal cytochrome P-450 concentrations. This could potentially lead to a depression of the hepatic metabolism of certain drugs that utilize this degradative pathway). Products include:
Rilutek 3032

Risperidone (Preclinical studies have demonstrated a decrease in hepatic microsomal cytochrome P-450 concentrations. This could potentially lead to a depression of the hepatic metabolism of certain drugs that utilize this degradative pathway). Products include:
Risperdal Consta 2682

Ritonavir (Preclinical studies have demonstrated a decrease in hepatic microsomal cytochrome P-450 concentrations. This could potentially lead to a depression of the hepatic metabolism of certain drugs that utilize this degradative pathway). Products include:
Kaletra 458
Norvir 509

Rofecoxib (Preclinical studies have demonstrated a decrease in hepatic microsomal cytochrome P-450 concentrations. This could potentially lead to a depression of the hepatic metabolism of certain drugs that utilize this degradative pathway).
No products indexed under this heading.

Ropinirole Hydrochloride (Preclinical studies have demonstrated a decrease in hepatic microsomal cytochrome P-450 concentrations. This could potentially lead to a depression of the hepatic metabolism of certain drugs that utilize this degradative pathway). Products include:

(⊙ Described in PDR® for Ophthalmic Medicines)

IMPORTANT NOTE: Always consult each drug listing in the patient's regimen for possible interactions.

(⊙ Described in PDR® for Ophthalmic Medicines)

21 **Interactions Index** **Actonel**

Quinapril Hydrochloride (Post-marketing reports of orolingual angioedema associated with alteplase have primarily been in acute ischemic stroke patients receiving concomitant ACE inhibitors).
No products indexed under this heading.

Ramipril (Post-marketing reports of orolingual angioedema associated with alteplase have primarily been in acute ischemic stroke patients receiving concomitant ACE inhibitors).
No products indexed under this heading.

Spirapril Hydrochloride (Post-marketing reports of orolingual angioedema associated with alteplase have primarily been in acute ischemic stroke patients receiving concomitant ACE inhibitors).
No products indexed under this heading.

Ticlopidine Hydrochloride (Drugs that alter platelet function, such as ticlopidine, may increase the risk of bleeding if administered prior to or after alteplase therapy).
No products indexed under this heading.

Tirofiban Hydrochloride (Drugs that alter platelet function, such as tirofiban, may increase the risk of bleeding if administered prior to or after alteplase therapy).
No products indexed under this heading.

Trandolapril (Post-marketing reports of orolingual angioedema associated with alteplase have primarily been in acute ischemic stroke patients receiving concomitant ACE inhibitors).
Products include:
Mavik 489
Tarka 534

Warfarin Sodium (Co-administration increases the risk of bleeding).
No products indexed under this heading.

ACTIVE CALCIUM TABLETS

(Calcium Citrate, Vitamin D) 3476
None cited in PDR database.

ACTIVELLA TABLETS

(Estradiol, Norethindrone Acetate) 2561
May interact with thyroid preparations. Compounds in these categories include:

Levothyroxine Sodium (Estrogen administration leads to increased thyroid-binding globulin (TBG) levels. Patients with normal thyroid function can compensate for the increased TBG by making more thyroid hormone, thus maintaining free T4 and T3 serum concentrations in the normal range. Patients dependent on thyroid hormone replacement therapy who are also receiving estrogen may require increased doses of their thyroid replacement therapy. These patients should have their thyroid function monitored to maintain their free throid hormone levels in an acceptable range).
Products include:
Levoxyl Tablets 1843
Synthroid 529

Liothyronine Sodium (Estrogen administration leads to increased thyroid-binding globulin (TBG) levels. Patients with normal thyroid function can compensate for the increased TBG by making more thyroid hormone, thus maintaining free T4 and T3 serum concentrations in the normal range. Patients dependent on thyroid hormone replacement therapy who are also receiving estrogen may require increased doses of their thyroid replacement therapy. These patients should have their thyroid function monitored to maintain their free throid hormone levels in an acceptable range).
Products include:
Cytomel 1830

Liotrix (Estrogen administration leads to increased thyroid-binding globulin (TBG) levels. Patients with normal thyroid function can compensate for the increased TBG by making more thyroid hormone, thus maintaining free T4 and T3 serum concentrations in the normal range. Patients dependent on thyroid hormone replacement therapy who are also receiving estrogen may require increased doses of their thyroid replacement therapy. These patients should have their thyroid function monitored to maintain their free throid hormone levels in an acceptable range).
No products indexed under this heading.

Thyroglobulin (Estrogen administration leads to increased thyroid-binding globulin (TBG) levels. Patients with normal thyroid function can compensate for the increased TBG by making more thyroid hormone, thus maintaining free T4 and T3 serum concentrations in the normal range. Patients dependent on thyroid hormone replacement therapy who are also receiving estrogen may require increased doses of their thyroid replacement therapy. These patients should have their thyroid function monitored to maintain their free throid hormone levels in an acceptable range).
No products indexed under this heading.

Thyroid (Estrogen administration leads to increased thyroid-binding globulin (TBG) levels. Patients with normal thyroid function can compensate for the increased TBG by making more thyroid hormone, thus maintaining free T4 and T3 serum concentrations in the normal range. Patients dependent on thyroid hormone replacement therapy who are also receiving estrogen may require increased doses of their thyroid replacement therapy. These patients should have their thyroid function monitored to maintain their free throid hormone levels in an acceptable range).
Products include:
Naturethroid 2830

Thyroxine (Estrogen administration leads to increased thyroid-binding globulin (TBG) levels. Patients with normal thyroid function can compensate for the increased TBG by making more thyroid hormone, thus maintaining free T4 and T3 serum concentrations in the normal range. Patients dependent on thyroid hormone replacement therapy who are also receiving estrogen may require increased doses of their thyroid replacement therapy. These patients should have their thyroid function monitored to maintain their free throid hormone levels in an acceptable range).
No products indexed under this heading.

Thyroxine Sodium (Estrogen administration leads to increased thyroid-binding globulin (TBG) levels. Patients with normal thyroid function can compensate for the increased TBG by making more thyroid hormone, thus maintaining free T4 and T3 serum concentrations in the normal range. Patients dependent on thyroid hormone replacement therapy who are also receiving estrogen may require increased doses of their thyroid replacement therapy. These patients should have their thyroid function monitored to maintain their free throid hormone levels in an acceptable range).
No products indexed under this heading.

ACTONEL TABLETS

(Risedronate Sodium) 2779
May interact with antacids, antacids containing aluminum, calcium and magnesium, antineoplastics, calcium preparations, cations, corticosteroids, and certain other agents. Compounds in these categories include:

Alclometasone Dipropionate (Osteonecrosis of the jaw (ONJ) been reported in patients taking bisphosphonates, including risedronate. Known risk factors for osteonecrosis of the jaw include concomitant therapy (eg, corticosteroids)).
No products indexed under this heading.

Altretamine (Osteonecrosis of the jaw (ONJ) been reported in patients taking bisphosphonates, including risedronate. Known risk factors for osteonecrosis of the jaw include concomitant therapy (eg, chemotherapy)). Products include:
Hexalen 1066

Aluminum Acetate (Co-administration of risedronate and calcium, antacids, or oral medications containing divalent cations will interfere with the absorption of risedronate).
No products indexed under this heading.

Aluminum Carbonate (Co-administration of risedronate and calcium, antacids, or oral medications containing divalent cations will interfere with the absorption of risedronate).
No products indexed under this heading.

Aluminum Chlorhydroxide (Co-administration of risedronate and calcium, antacids, or oral medications containing divalent cations will interfere with the absorption of risedronate).
No products indexed under this heading.

Aluminum Chloride (Co-administration of risedronate and calcium, antacids, or oral medications containing divalent cations will interfere with the absorption of risedronate).
No products indexed under this heading.

Aluminum Chlorohydrate (Co-administration of risedronate and calcium, antacids, or oral medications containing divalent cations will interfere with the absorption of risedronate).
No products indexed under this heading.

Aluminum Glycinate (Co-administration of risedronate and calcium, antacids, or oral medications containing divalent cations will interfere with the absorption of risedronate).
No products indexed under this heading.

Aluminum Hydroxide (Co-administration of risedronate and calcium, antacids, or oral medications containing divalent cations will interfere with the absorption of risedronate).
No products indexed under this heading.

Aluminum Hydroxide Preparations (Co-administration of risedronate and calcium, antacids, or oral medications containing divalent cations will interfere with the absorption of risedronate).
No products indexed under this heading.

Aluminum Sulfate (Co-administration of risedronate and calcium, antacids, or oral medications containing divalent cations will interfere with the absorption of risedronate).
No products indexed under this heading.

Anastrozole (Osteonecrosis of the jaw (ONJ) been reported in patients taking bisphosphonates, including risedronate. Known risk factors for osteonecrosis of the jaw include concomitant therapy (eg, chemotherapy)).
No products indexed under this heading.

Asparaginase (Osteonecrosis of the jaw (ONJ) been reported in patients taking bisphosphonates, including risedronate. Known risk factors for osteonecrosis of the jaw include concomitant therapy (eg, chemotherapy)). Products include:
Elspar 2005, 2122

Beclomethasone Dipropionate (Osteonecrosis of the jaw (ONJ) been reported in patients taking bisphosphonates, including risedronate. Known risk factors for osteonecrosis of the jaw include concomitant therapy (eg, corticosteroids)). Products include:
Qvar 3398

Beclomethasone Dipropionate Monohydrate (Osteonecrosis of the jaw (ONJ) been reported in patients taking bisphosphonates, including risedronate. Known risk factors for osteonecrosis of the jaw include concomitant therapy (eg, corticosteroids)). Products include:
Beconase AQ 1386

Betamethasone (Osteonecrosis of the jaw (ONJ) been reported in patients taking bisphosphonates, including risedronate. Known risk factors for osteonecrosis of the jaw include concomitant therapy (eg, corticosteroids)).
No products indexed under this heading.

Betamethasone Acetate (Osteonecrosis of the jaw (ONJ) been reported in patients taking bisphosphonates, including risedronate. Known risk factors for osteonecrosis of the jaw include concomitant therapy (eg, corticosteroids)).
No products indexed under this heading.

Betamethasone Benzoate (Osteonecrosis of the jaw (ONJ) been reported in patients taking bisphosphonates, including risedronate. Known risk factors for osteonecrosis of the jaw include concomitant therapy (eg, corticosteroids)).
No products indexed under this heading.

Betamethasone Dipropionate (Osteonecrosis of the jaw (ONJ) been reported in patients taking bisphosphonates, including risedronate. Known risk factors for osteonecrosis of the jaw include concomitant therapy (eg, corticosteroids)). Products include:
Diprolene Lotion 0.05% 3108
Diprolene Ointment 0.05% 3109
Diprolene AF Cream 0.05% 3107
Lotrisone 3163

Betamethasone Sodium Phosphate (Osteonecrosis of the jaw (ONJ) been reported in patients taking bisphosphonates, including risedronate. Known risk factors for osteonecrosis of the jaw include concomitant therapy (eg, corticosteroids)).
No products indexed under this heading.

Betamethasone Valerate (Osteonecrosis of the jaw (ONJ) been reported in patients taking bisphosphonates, including risedronate. Known risk factors for osteonecrosis of the jaw include concomitant therapy (eg, corticosteroids)).
Products include:
Luxiq 3321

Bicalutamide (Osteonecrosis of the jaw (ONJ) been reported in patients taking bisphosphonates, including risedronate. Known risk factors for osteonecrosis of the jaw include concomitant therapy (eg, chemotherapy)).
No products indexed under this heading.

Bleomycin Sulfate (Osteonecrosis of the jaw (ONJ) been reported in patients taking bisphosphonates, including risedronate. Known risk factors for osteonecrosis of the jaw include concomitant therapy (eg, chemotherapy)).
No products indexed under this heading.

Budesonide (Osteonecrosis of the jaw (ONJ) been reported in patients taking bisphosphonates, including risedronate. Known risk factors for osteonecrosis of the jaw include concomitant therapy (eg, corticosteroids)). Products include:
Pulmicort Flexhaler 714
Symbicort 80/4.5 720
Symbicort 160/4.5 720

Busulfan (Osteonecrosis of the jaw (ONJ) been reported in patients taking bisphosphonates, including risedronate. Known risk factors for osteonecrosis of the jaw include concomitant therapy (eg, chemotherapy)). Products include:

IMPORTANT NOTE: Always consult each drug listing in the patient's regimen for possible interactions.

(⊙ Described in PDR® for Ophthalmic Medicines)

IMPORTANT NOTE: Always consult each drug listing in the patient's regimen for possible interactions.

Magnesium Sulfate (Co-administration of risedronate and calcium, antacids, or oral medications containing divalent cations will interfere with the absorption of risedronate).
No products indexed under this heading.

Magnesium Trisilicate (Co-administration of risedronate and calcium, antacids, or oral medications containing divalent cations will interfere with the absorption of risedronate).
No products indexed under this heading.

Mechlorethamine Hydrochloride (Osteonecrosis of the jaw (ONJ) been reported in patients taking bisphosphonates, including risedronate. Known risk factors for osteonecrosis of the jaw include concomitant therapy (eg, chemotherapy)). Products include:
Mustargen 2010

Megestrol Acetate (Osteonecrosis of the jaw (ONJ) been reported in patients taking bisphosphonates, including risedronate. Known risk factors for osteonecrosis of the jaw include concomitant therapy (eg, chemotherapy)). Products include:
Megace ES 2698

Melphalan (Osteonecrosis of the jaw (ONJ) been reported in patients taking bisphosphonates, including risedronate. Known risk factors for osteonecrosis of the jaw include concomitant therapy (eg, chemotherapy)). Products include:
Alkeran 1302

Mercaptopurine (Osteonecrosis of the jaw (ONJ) been reported in patients taking bisphosphonates, including risedronate. Known risk factors for osteonecrosis of the jaw include concomitant therapy (eg, chemotherapy)).
No products indexed under this heading.

Methotrexate (Osteonecrosis of the jaw (ONJ) been reported in patients taking bisphosphonates, including risedronate. Known risk factors for osteonecrosis of the jaw include concomitant therapy (eg, chemotherapy)).
No products indexed under this heading.

Methotrexate Sodium (Osteonecrosis of the jaw (ONJ) been reported in patients taking bisphosphonates, including risedronate. Known risk factors for osteonecrosis of the jaw include concomitant therapy (eg, chemotherapy)).
No products indexed under this heading.

Methylprednisolone (Osteonecrosis of the jaw (ONJ) been reported in patients taking bisphosphonates, including risedronate. Known risk factors for osteonecrosis of the jaw include concomitant therapy (eg, corticosteroids)).
No products indexed under this heading.

Methylprednisolone Acetate (Osteonecrosis of the jaw (ONJ) been reported in patients taking bisphosphonates, including risedronate. Known risk factors for osteonecrosis of the jaw include concomitant therapy (eg, corticosteroids)).
No products indexed under this heading.

Methylprednisolone Sodium Succinate (Osteonecrosis of the jaw (ONJ) been reported in patients taking bisphosphonates, including risedronate. Known risk factors for osteonecrosis of the jaw include concomitant therapy (eg, corticosteroids)).
No products indexed under this heading.

Mitomycin (Mitomycin-C) (Osteonecrosis of the jaw (ONJ) been reported in patients taking bisphosphonates, including risedronate. Known risk factors for osteonecrosis of the jaw include concomitant therapy (eg, chemotherapy)).
No products indexed under this heading.

Mitotane (Osteonecrosis of the jaw (ONJ) been reported in patients taking bisphosphonates, including risedronate. Known risk factors for osteonecrosis of the jaw include concomitant therapy (eg, chemotherapy)).
No products indexed under this heading.

Mitoxantrone Hydrochloride (Osteonecrosis of the jaw (ONJ) been reported in patients taking bisphosphonates, including risedronate. Known risk factors for osteonecrosis of the jaw include concomitant therapy (eg, chemotherapy)). Products include:
Novantrone 1088

Mometasone Furoate (Osteonecrosis of the jaw (ONJ) been reported in patients taking bisphosphonates, including risedronate. Known risk factors for osteonecrosis of the jaw include concomitant therapy (eg, corticosteroids)). Products include:
Asmanex 3058
Elocon Cream 3111
Elocon Lotion 3112
Elocon Ointment 3114

Mometasone Furoate Monohydrate (Osteonecrosis of the jaw (ONJ) been reported in patients taking bisphosphonates, including risedronate. Known risk factors for osteonecrosis of the jaw include concomitant therapy (eg, corticosteroids)). Products include:
Nasonex 3166

Oxaliplatin (Osteonecrosis of the jaw (ONJ) been reported in patients taking bisphosphonates, including risedronate. Known risk factors for osteonecrosis of the jaw include concomitant therapy (eg, chemotherapy)). Products include:
Eloxatin 2975

Paclitaxel (Osteonecrosis of the jaw (ONJ) been reported in patients taking bisphosphonates, including risedronate. Known risk factors for osteonecrosis of the jaw include concomitant therapy (eg, chemotherapy)).
No products indexed under this heading.

Prednisolone (Osteonecrosis of the jaw (ONJ) been reported in patients taking bisphosphonates, including risedronate. Known risk factors for osteonecrosis of the jaw include concomitant therapy (eg, corticosteroids)).
No products indexed under this heading.

Prednisolone Acetate (Osteonecrosis of the jaw (ONJ) been reported in patients taking bisphosphonates, including risedronate. Known risk factors for osteonecrosis of the jaw include concomitant therapy (eg, corticosteroids)). Products include:
Blephamide .... ⊙212, ⊙214
Pred Forte .... ⊙225
Pred Mild .... ⊙230
Pred-G .... ⊙226, ⊙227

Prednisolone Sodium Phosphate (Osteonecrosis of the jaw (ONJ) been reported in patients taking bisphosphonates, including risedronate. Known risk factors for osteonecrosis of the jaw include concomitant therapy (eg, corticosteroids)).
No products indexed under this heading.

Prednisolone Tebutate (Osteonecrosis of the jaw (ONJ) been reported in patients taking bisphosphonates, including risedronate. Known risk factors for osteonecrosis of the jaw include concomitant therapy (eg, corticosteroids)).
No products indexed under this heading.

Prednisone (Osteonecrosis of the jaw (ONJ) been reported in patients taking bisphosphonates, including risedronate. Known risk factors for osteonecrosis of the jaw include concomitant therapy (eg, corticosteroids)).
No products indexed under this heading.

Prednisone sodium phosphate (Osteonecrosis of the jaw (ONJ) been reported in patients taking bisphosphonates, including risedronate. Known risk factors for osteonecrosis of the jaw include concomitant therapy (eg, corticosteroids)).
No products indexed under this heading.

Procarbazine Hydrochloride (Osteonecrosis of the jaw (ONJ) been reported in patients taking bisphosphonates, including risedronate. Known risk factors for osteonecrosis of the jaw include concomitant therapy (eg, chemotherapy)).
No products indexed under this heading.

Selenium (Co-administration of risedronate and calcium, antacids, or oral medications containing divalent cations will interfere with the absorption of risedronate). Products include:
Cardio Basics 3455
Chelated Mineral 3476

Selenium Sulfide (Co-administration of risedronate and calcium, antacids, or oral medications containing divalent cations will interfere with the absorption of risedronate).
No products indexed under this heading.

Sodium Bicarbonate (Co-administration of risedronate and calcium, antacids, or oral medications containing divalent cations will interfere with the absorption of risedronate).
No products indexed under this heading.

Streptozocin (Osteonecrosis of the jaw (ONJ) been reported in patients taking bisphosphonates, including risedronate. Known risk factors for osteonecrosis of the jaw include concomitant therapy (eg, chemotherapy)).
No products indexed under this heading.

Tamoxifen Citrate (Osteonecrosis of the jaw (ONJ) been reported in patients taking bisphosphonates, including risedronate. Known risk factors for osteonecrosis of the jaw include concomitant therapy (eg, chemotherapy)).
No products indexed under this heading.

Teniposide (Osteonecrosis of the jaw (ONJ) been reported in patients taking bisphosphonates, including risedronate. Known risk factors for osteonecrosis of the jaw include concomitant therapy (eg, chemotherapy)).
No products indexed under this heading.

Thioguanine (Osteonecrosis of the jaw (ONJ) been reported in patients taking bisphosphonates, including risedronate. Known risk factors for osteonecrosis of the jaw include concomitant therapy (eg, chemotherapy)). Products include:
Tabloid 1664

Thiotepa (Osteonecrosis of the jaw (ONJ) been reported in patients taking bisphosphonates, including risedronate. Known risk factors for osteonecrosis of the jaw include concomitant therapy (eg, chemotherapy)).
No products indexed under this heading.

Topotecan Hydrochloride (Osteonecrosis of the jaw (ONJ) been reported in patients taking bisphosphonates, including risedronate. Known risk factors for osteonecrosis of the jaw include concomitant therapy (eg, chemotherapy)). Products include:
Hycamtin 1491
Hycamtin Capsules 1488

Toremifene Citrate (Osteonecrosis of the jaw (ONJ) been reported in patients taking bisphosphonates, including risedronate. Known risk factors for osteonecrosis of the jaw include concomitant therapy (eg, chemotherapy)).
No products indexed under this heading.

Triamcinolone (Osteonecrosis of the jaw (ONJ) been reported in patients taking bisphosphonates, including risedronate. Known risk factors for osteonecrosis of the jaw include concomitant therapy (eg, corticosteroids)).
No products indexed under this heading.

Triamcinolone Acetonide (Osteonecrosis of the jaw (ONJ) been reported in patients taking bisphosphonates, including risedronate. Known risk factors for osteonecrosis of the jaw include concomitant therapy (eg, corticosteroids)). Products include:
Azmacort 408
Nasacort AQ 3019

Triamcinolone Diacetate (Osteonecrosis of the jaw (ONJ) been reported in patients taking bisphosphonates, including risedronate. Known risk factors for osteonecrosis of the jaw include concomitant therapy (eg, corticosteroids)).
No products indexed under this heading.

Triamcinolone Hexacetonide (Osteonecrosis of the jaw (ONJ) been reported in patients taking bisphosphonates, including risedronate. Known risk factors for osteonecrosis of the jaw include concomitant therapy (eg, corticosteroids)).
No products indexed under this heading.

Valrubicin (Osteonecrosis of the jaw (ONJ) been reported in patients taking bisphosphonates, including risedronate. Known risk factors for osteonecrosis of the jaw include concomitant therapy (eg, chemotherapy)). Products include:
Valstar 1131

Vincristine Sulfate (Osteonecrosis of the jaw (ONJ) been reported in patients taking bisphosphonates, including risedronate. Known risk factors for osteonecrosis of the jaw include concomitant therapy (eg, chemotherapy)).
No products indexed under this heading.

Vinorelbine Tartrate (Osteonecrosis of the jaw (ONJ) been reported in patients taking bisphosphonates, including risedronate. Known risk factors for osteonecrosis of the jaw include concomitant therapy (eg, chemotherapy)).
No products indexed under this heading.

Zinc (Co-administration of risedronate and calcium, antacids, or oral medications containing divalent cations will interfere with the absorption of risedronate). Products include:
BoneMate Plus 3454
Cardio Basics 3455
Chelated Mineral 3476
CitraNatal 90 DHA Capsules 2332
CitraNatal Assure 2332
Heplive 607
Visutein 3456

Zinc Acetate (Co-administration of risedronate and calcium, antacids, or oral medications containing divalent cations will interfere with the absorption of risedronate).
No products indexed under this heading.

Zinc Bisglycinate (Co-administration of risedronate and calcium, antacids, or oral medications containing divalent cations will interfere with the absorption of risedronate).
No products indexed under this heading.

Zinc Chloride (Co-administration of risedronate and calcium, antacids, or oral medications containing divalent cations will interfere with the absorption of risedronate).
No products indexed under this heading.

Zinc Citrate (Co-administration of risedronate and calcium, antacids, or oral medications containing divalent cations will interfere with the absorption of risedronate). Products include:
Chelated Mineral 3476

(⊙ Described in PDR® for Ophthalmic Medicines)

Zinc-Containing Multivitamins (Co-administration of risedronate and calcium, antacids, or oral medications containing divalent cations will interfere with the absorption of risedronate).
No products indexed under this heading.

Zinc Gluconate (Co-administration of risedronate and calcium, antacids, or oral medications containing divalent cations will interfere with the absorption of risedronate).
No products indexed under this heading.

Zinc Oxide (Co-administration of risedronate and calcium, antacids, or oral medications containing divalent cations will interfere with the absorption of risedronate). Products include:
Bausch & Lomb Ocuvite Adult 50+ .... ⊙238
CitraNatal Rx 2332
Vusion Ointment 3335

Zinc Phenosulfonate (Co-administration of risedronate and calcium, antacids, or oral medications containing divalent cations will interfere with the absorption of risedronate).
No products indexed under this heading.

Zinc Sulfate (Co-administration of risedronate and calcium, antacids, or oral medications containing divalent cations will interfere with the absorption of risedronate). Products include:
Heplive 607
Zinc-220 606

Food Interactions

Food, unspecified (The extent of absorption of a 30 mg dose (three 10 mg tablets) when administered 0.5 hours before breakfast is reduced by 55% compared to dosing in the fasting state (no food or drink for 10 hours prior to or 4 hours after dosing). Dosing 1 hour prior to breakfast reduces the extent of absorption by 30% compared to dosing in the fasting state. Dosing either 0.5 hours prior to breakfast or 2 hours after dinner (evening meal) results in a similar extent of absorption. Residronate is effective when administered at least 30 minutes before breakfast).

Iron Amino Acid Chelate (Co-administration of risedronate and calcium, antacids, or oral medications containing divalent cations will interfere with the absorption of risedronate).

Meal, unspecified (The extent of absorption of a 30 mg dose (three 10 mg tablets) when administered 0.5 hours before breakfast is reduced by 55% compared to dosing in the fasting state (no food or drink for 10 hours prior to or 4 hours after dosing). Dosing 1 hour prior to breakfast reduces the extent of absorption by 30% compared to dosing in the fasting state. Dosing either 0.5 hours prior to breakfast or 2 hours after dinner (evening meal) results in a similar extent of absorption. Residronate is effective when administered at least 30 minutes before breakfast).

ACTOPLUS MET TABLETS
(Metformin Hydrochloride, Pioglitazone Hydrochloride) 3338
May interact with alcohols, beta-blockers, calcium channel blockers, cationic drugs that are eliminated by renal tubular, chloramphenicols, corticosteroids, cytochrome p450 2c8 inducers (selected), cytochrome p450 2c8 inhibitors (selected), cytochrome p450 3a4 substrates (selected), diuretics, estrogens, highly protein bound drugs (selected), insulin, oral contraceptives, oral hypoglycemic agents, phenothiazines, phenytoin, quinidine, radiographic iodinated contrast media, salicylates, sulfonamides, sulfonylureas, sympathomimetics, thiazides, thyroid preparations, and certain other agents. Compounds in these categories include:

Acarbose (Pioglitazone, like other thiazolidinediones, can cause fluid retention when used alone or in combination with other antihyperglycemic agents, including insulin. Fluid retention may lead to or exacerbate heart failure. In addition, patients receiving pioglitazone in combination with insulin or oral hypoglycemic agents may be at risk for hypoglycemia, and a reduction in the dose of the concomitant agent may be necessary).
No products indexed under this heading.

Acebutolol Hydrochloride (Hypoglycemia due to metformin may be difficult to recognize in the elderly and in people who are taking β-adrenergic blocking drugs).
No products indexed under this heading.

Albuterol (Certain drugs, including sympathomimetics, tend to produce hyperglycemia and may lead to loss of glycemic control. When such drugs are administered to a patient receiving ActoPlus Met, the patient should be closely observed to maintain adequate glycemic control).
No products indexed under this heading.

Albuterol Sulfate (Certain drugs, including sympathomimetics, tend to produce hyperglycemia and may lead to loss of glycemic control. When such drugs are administered to a patient receiving ActoPlus Met, the patient should be closely observed to maintain adequate glycemic control). Products include:
ProAir HFA 3393
Proventil HFA 3204
Ventolin HFA 1708

Alclometasone Dipropionate (Certain drugs, including corticosteroids, tend to produce hyperglycemia and may lead to loss of glycemic control. When such drugs are administered to a patient receiving ActoPlus Met, the patient should be closely observed to maintain adequate glycemic control).
No products indexed under this heading.

Alfentanil Hydrochloride (In vivo drug-drug interaction studies have suggested that pioglitazone may be a weak inducer of CYP450 isoform 3A4 substrate).
No products indexed under this heading.

Alprazolam (In vivo drug-drug interaction studies have suggested that pioglitazone may be a weak inducer of CYP450 isoform 3A4 substrate).
No products indexed under this heading.

Amiloride Hydrochloride (Cationic drugs (eg, amiloride, digoxin, morphine, procainamide, quinidine, quinine, ranitidine, triamterene, trimethoprim, and vancomycin) that are eliminated by renal tubular secretion theoretically have the potential for interaction with metformin by competing for common renal tubular transport systems. Careful patient monitoring and dose adjustment of ActoPlus Met and/or the interfering drug is recommended in patients who are taking cationic medications that are excreted via the proximal renal tubular secretory system).
No products indexed under this heading.

Amiodarone Hydrochloride (In vivo drug-drug interaction studies have suggested that pioglitazone may be a weak inducer of CYP450 isoform 3A4 substrate).
No products indexed under this heading.

Amitriptyline Hydrochloride (In vivo drug-drug interaction studies have suggested that pioglitazone may be a weak inducer of CYP450 isoform 3A4 substrate).
No products indexed under this heading.

Amlodipine Besylate (Certain drugs, including calcium channel blockers, tend to produce hyperglycemia and may lead to loss of glycemic control. When

such drugs are administered to a patient receiving ActoPlus Met, the patient should be closely observed to maintain adequate glycemic control).
Products include:
Azor 1010
Exforge 2443
Exforge HCT 2449

Anastrozole (An enzyme inhibitor of CYP2C8 (such as gemfibrozil) may significantly increase the AUC of pioglitazone. Therefore, if an inhibitor of CYP2C8 is started or stopped during treatment with pioglitazone, changes in diabetes treatment may be needed based on clinical response).
No products indexed under this heading.

Aprepitant (In vivo drug-drug interaction studies have suggested that pioglitazone may be a weak inducer of CYP450 isoform 3A4 substrate).
Products include:
Emend 2124

Aspirin (Metformin is negligibly bound to plasma proteins and is, therefore, less likely to interact with highly protein-bound drugs, such as salicylates).
Products include:
Aggrenox 880
Bayer Aspirin 829
Percodan 1124
St. Joseph Aspirin 2045

Aspirin, Enteric Coated (Metformin is negligibly bound to plasma proteins and is, therefore, less likely to interact with highly protein-bound drugs, such as salicylates).
No products indexed under this heading.

Aspirin Buffered (Metformin is negligibly bound to plasma proteins and is, therefore, less likely to interact with highly protein-bound drugs, such as salicylates).
No products indexed under this heading.

Astemizole (In vivo drug-drug interaction studies have suggested that pioglitazone may be a weak inducer of CYP450 isoform 3A4 substrate).
No products indexed under this heading.

Atenolol (Hypoglycemia due to metformin may be difficult to recognize in the elderly and in people who are taking β-adrenergic blocking drugs).
No products indexed under this heading.

Atorvastatin Calcium (Co-administration of pioglitazone for 7 days with atorvastatin calcium 80 mg once daily resulted in a ratio of least square mean (90% CI) values for unchanged pioglitazone of 0.69 (0.57-0.85) for C_{max}, 0.76 (0.65-0.88) for AUC and 0.96 (0.87-1.05) for C_{min}. For unchanged atorvastatin the ratio of least square mean (90% CI) values were 0.77 (0.66 - 0.90) for C_{max}, 0.86 (0.78-0.94) for AUC and 0.92 (0.82 - 1.02) for C_{min}). Products include:
Lipitor 2703

Atovaquone (Metformin is negligibly bound to plasma proteins and is, therefore, less likely to interact with highly protein-bound drugs, such as salicylates, sulfonamides, chloramphenicol and probenecid). Products include:
Malarone Pediatric Tablets 1572
Malarone 1572
Mepron Suspension 1576

Beclomethasone Dipropionate (Certain drugs, including corticosteroids, tend to produce hyperglycemia and may lead to loss of glycemic control. When such drugs are administered to a patient receiving ActoPlus Met, the patient should be closely observed to maintain adequate glycemic control).
Products include:
Qvar 3398

Beclomethasone Dipropionate Monohydrate (Certain drugs, including corticosteroids, tend to produce hyperglycemia and may lead to loss of

glycemic control. When such drugs are administered to a patient receiving ActoPlus Met, the patient should be closely observed to maintain adequate glycemic control). Products include:
Beconase AQ 1386

Belladonna Ergotamine (In vivo drug-drug interaction studies have suggested that pioglitazone may be a weak inducer of CYP450 isoform 3A4 substrate).
No products indexed under this heading.

Bendroflumethiazide (Certain drugs, including thiazide diuretics, tend to produce hyperglycemia and may lead to loss of glycemic control. When such drugs are administered to a patient receiving ActoPlus Met, the patient should be closely observed to maintain adequate glycemic control).
No products indexed under this heading.

Bepridil Hydrochloride (Certain drugs, including calcium channel blockers, tend to produce hyperglycemia and may lead to loss of glycemic control. When such drugs are administered to a patient receiving ActoPlus Met, the patient should be closely observed to maintain adequate glycemic control).
No products indexed under this heading.

Betamethasone (Certain drugs, including corticosteroids, tend to produce hyperglycemia and may lead to loss of glycemic control. When such drugs are administered to a patient receiving ActoPlus Met, the patient should be closely observed to maintain adequate glycemic control).
No products indexed under this heading.

Betamethasone Acetate (Certain drugs, including corticosteroids, tend to produce hyperglycemia and may lead to loss of glycemic control. When such drugs are administered to a patient receiving ActoPlus Met, the patient should be closely observed to maintain adequate glycemic control).
No products indexed under this heading.

Betamethasone Benzoate (Certain drugs, including corticosteroids, tend to produce hyperglycemia and may lead to loss of glycemic control. When such drugs are administered to a patient receiving ActoPlus Met, the patient should be closely observed to maintain adequate glycemic control).
No products indexed under this heading.

Betamethasone Dipropionate (Certain drugs, including corticosteroids, tend to produce hyperglycemia and may lead to loss of glycemic control. When such drugs are administered to a patient receiving ActoPlus Met, the patient should be closely observed to maintain adequate glycemic control). Products include:
Diprolene Lotion 0.05% 3108
Diprolene Ointment 0.05% 3109
Diprolene AF Cream 0.05% 3107
Lotrisone 3163

Betamethasone Sodium Phosphate (Certain drugs, including corticosteroids, tend to produce hyperglycemia and may lead to loss of glycemic control. When such drugs are administered to a patient receiving ActoPlus Met, the patient should be closely observed to maintain adequate glycemic control).
No products indexed under this heading.

Betamethasone Valerate (Certain drugs, including corticosteroids, tend to produce hyperglycemia and may lead to loss of glycemic control. When such drugs are administered to a patient receiving ActoPlus Met, the patient should be closely observed to maintain adequate glycemic control). Products include:
Luxíq 3321

IMPORTANT NOTE: Always consult each drug listing in the patient's regimen for possible interactions.

Betaxolol Hydrochloride (Hypoglycemia due to metformin may be difficult to recognize in the elderly and in people who are taking β-adrenergic blocking drugs).
No products indexed under this heading.

Bisoprolol Fumarate (Hypoglycemia due to metformin may be difficult to recognize in the elderly and in people who are taking β-adrenergic blocking drugs).
No products indexed under this heading.

Budesonide (Certain drugs, including corticosteroids, tend to produce hyperglycemia and may lead to loss of glycemic control. When such drugs are administered to a patient receiving ActoPlus Met, the patient should be closely observed to maintain adequate glycemic control). Products include:

Bumetanide (Certain drugs, including thiazides and other diuretics, tend to produce hyperglycemia and may lead to loss of glycemic control. When such drugs are administered to a patient receiving ActoPlus Met, the patient should be closely observed to maintain adequate glycemic control).
No products indexed under this heading.

Buspirone Hydrochloride (In vivo drug-drug interaction studies have suggested that pioglitazone may be a weak inducer of CYP450 isoform 3A4 substrate).
No products indexed under this heading.

Busulfan (In vivo drug-drug interaction studies have suggested that pioglitazone may be a weak inducer of CYP450 isoform 3A4 substrate). Products include:

Carbamazepine (An enzyme inducer of CYP2C8 (such as rifampin) may significantly decrease the AUC of pioglitazone. Therefore, if an inducer of CYP2C8 is started or stopped during treatment with pioglitazone, changes in diabetes treatment may be needed based on clinical response). Products include:

Carteolol Hydrochloride (Hypoglycemia due to metformin may be difficult to recognize in the elderly and in people who are taking β-adrenergic blocking drugs).
No products indexed under this heading.

Carvedilol (Hypoglycemia due to metformin may be difficult to recognize in the elderly and in people who are taking β-adrenergic blocking drugs). Products include:

Carvedilol Phosphate (Hypoglycemia due to metformin may be difficult to recognize in the elderly and in people who are taking β-adrenergic blocking drugs). Products include:

Cefonicid Sodium (Metformin is negligibly bound to plasma proteins and is, therefore, less likely to interact with highly protein-bound drugs, such as salicylates, sulfonamides, chloramphenicol and probenecid).
No products indexed under this heading.

Celecoxib (Metformin is negligibly bound to plasma proteins and is, therefore, less likely to interact with highly protein-bound drugs, such as salicylates, sulfonamides, chloramphenicol and probenecid). Products include:

Cerivastatin Sodium (In vivo drug-drug interaction studies have suggested that pioglitazone may be a weak inducer of CYP450 isoform 3A4 substrate).
No products indexed under this heading.

Chloramphenicol (Metformin is negligibly bound to plasma proteins and is, therefore, less likely to interact with highly protein-bound drugs, such as chloramphenicol).
No products indexed under this heading.

Chloramphenicol Palmitate (Metformin is negligibly bound to plasma proteins and is, therefore, less likely to interact with highly protein-bound drugs, such as chloramphenicol).
No products indexed under this heading.

Chloramphenicol Sodium Succinate (Metformin is negligibly bound to plasma proteins and is, therefore, less likely to interact with highly protein-bound drugs, such as chloramphenicol).
No products indexed under this heading.

Chlordiazepoxide (Metformin is negligibly bound to plasma proteins and is, therefore, less likely to interact with highly protein-bound drugs, such as salicylates, sulfonamides, chloramphenicol and probenecid).
No products indexed under this heading.

Chlordiazepoxide Hydrochloride (Metformin is negligibly bound to plasma proteins and is, therefore, less likely to interact with highly protein-bound drugs, such as salicylates, sulfonamides, chloramphenicol and probenecid).
No products indexed under this heading.

Chlorothiazide (Certain drugs, including thiazide diuretics, tend to produce hyperglycemia and may lead to loss of glycemic control. When such drugs are administered to a patient receiving ActoPlus Met, the patient should be closely observed to maintain adequate glycemic control).
No products indexed under this heading.

Chlorothiazide Sodium (Certain drugs, including thiazide diuretics, tend to produce hyperglycemia and may lead to loss of glycemic control. When such drugs are administered to a patient receiving ActoPlus Met, the patient should be closely observed to maintain adequate glycemic control). Products include:

Chlorotrianisene (Certain drugs, including estrogens, tend to produce hyperglycemia and may lead to loss of glycemic control. When such drugs are administered to a patient receiving ActoPlus Met, the patient should be closely observed to maintain adequate glycemic control).
No products indexed under this heading.

Chlorpheniramine (In vivo drug-drug interaction studies have suggested that pioglitazone may be a weak inducer of CYP450 isoform 3A4 substrate).
No products indexed under this heading.

Chlorpheniramine Maleate (In vivo drug-drug interaction studies have suggested that pioglitazone may be a weak inducer of CYP450 isoform 3A4 substrate).
No products indexed under this heading.

Chlorpheniramine Polistirex (In vivo drug-drug interaction studies have suggested that pioglitazone may be a weak inducer of CYP450 isoform 3A4 substrate). Products include:

Chlorpheniramine Tannate (In vivo drug-drug interaction studies have suggested that pioglitazone may be a weak inducer of CYP450 isoform 3A4 substrate).
No products indexed under this heading.

Chlorpromazine (Certain drugs, including phenothiazines, tend to produce hyperglycemia and may lead to loss of glycemic control. When such drugs are administered to a patient receiving ActoPlus Met, the patient should be closely observed to maintain adequate glycemic control).
No products indexed under this heading.

Chlorpromazine Hydrochloride (Certain drugs, including phenothiazines, tend to produce hyperglycemia and may lead to loss of glycemic control. When such drugs are administered to a patient receiving ActoPlus Met, the patient should be closely observed to maintain adequate glycemic control).
No products indexed under this heading.

Chlorpropamide (Pioglitazone, like other thiazolidinediones, can cause fluid retention when used alone or in combination with other antihyperglycemic agents, including insulin. Fluid retention may lead to or exacerbate heart failure. In addition, patients receiving pioglitazone in combination with insulin or oral hypoglycemic agents may be at risk for hypoglycemia, and a reduction in the dose of the concomitant agent may be necessary).
No products indexed under this heading.

Chlorthalidone (Certain drugs, including thiazides and other diuretics, tend to produce hyperglycemia and may lead to loss of glycemic control. When such drugs are administered to a patient receiving ActoPlus Met, the patient should be closely observed to maintain adequate glycemic control). Products include:

Choline Magnesium Trisalicylate (Metformin is negligibly bound to plasma proteins and is, therefore, less likely to interact with highly protein-bound drugs, such as salicylates).
No products indexed under this heading.

Ciclesonide (Certain drugs, including corticosteroids, tend to produce hyperglycemia and may lead to loss of glycemic control. When such drugs are administered to a patient receiving ActoPlus Met, the patient should be closely observed to maintain adequate glycemic control).
No products indexed under this heading.

Cimetidine (An interaction between metformin and oral cimetidine has been observed in normal healthy volunteers in both single- and multiple-dose, metformin-cimetidine drug interaction studies with a 60% increase in peak metformin plasma and whole blood concentrations and a 40% increase in plasma and whole blood metformin AUC. There was no change in elimination half-life in the single-dose study. Metformin had no effect on cimetidine pharmacokinetics).
No products indexed under this heading.

Cimetidine Hydrochloride (An interaction between metformin and oral cimetidine has been observed in normal healthy volunteers in both single- and multiple-dose, metformin-cimetidine drug interaction studies with a 60% increase in peak metformin plasma and whole blood concentrations and a 40% increase in plasma and whole blood metformin AUC. There was no change in elimination half-life in the single-dose study. Metformin had no effect on cimetidine pharmacokinetics).
No products indexed under this heading.

Cisapride (In vivo drug-drug interaction studies have suggested that pioglitazone may be a weak inducer of CYP450 isoform 3A4 substrate).
No products indexed under this heading.

Clarithromycin (In vivo drug-drug interaction studies have suggested that pioglitazone may be a weak inducer of CYP450 isoform 3A4 substrate). Products include:

Clomipramine Hydrochloride (Metformin is negligibly bound to plasma proteins and is, therefore, less likely to interact with highly protein-bound drugs, such as salicylates, sulfonamides, chloramphenicol and probenecid).
No products indexed under this heading.

Clozapine (Metformin is negligibly bound to plasma proteins and is, therefore, less likely to interact with highly protein-bound drugs, such as salicylates, sulfonamides, chloramphenicol and probenecid).
No products indexed under this heading.

Cortisone Acetate (Certain drugs, including corticosteroids, tend to produce hyperglycemia and may lead to loss of glycemic control. When such drugs are administered to a patient receiving ActoPlus Met, the patient should be closely observed to maintain adequate glycemic control).
No products indexed under this heading.

Cyclosporine (In vivo drug-drug interaction studies have suggested that pioglitazone may be a weak inducer of CYP450 isoform 3A4 substrate). Products include:

Desogestrel (Certain drugs, including oral contraceptives, tend to produce hyperglycemia and may lead to loss of glycemic control. When such drugs are administered to a patient receiving ActoPlus Met, the patient should be closely observed to maintain adequate glycemic control. Co-administration of pioglitazone (45 mg once daily) and an oral contraceptive (1 mg norethindrone plus 0.035 mg ethinyl estradiol once daily) for 21 days, resulted in 11% and 11-14% decrease in ethinyl estradiol AUC (0-24h) and C_{max} respectively. There were no significant changes in norethindrone AUC (0-24h) and C_{max}. In view of the high variability of ethinyl estradiol pharmacokinetics, the clinical significance of this finding is unknown).
No products indexed under this heading.

Desoximetasone (Certain drugs, including corticosteroids, tend to produce hyperglycemia and may lead to loss of glycemic control. When such drugs are administered to a patient receiving ActoPlus Met, the patient should be closely observed to maintain adequate glycemic control).
No products indexed under this heading.

Dexamethasone (Certain drugs, including corticosteroids, tend to produce hyperglycemia and may lead to loss of glycemic control. When such drugs are administered to a patient receiving ActoPlus Met, the patient should be closely observed to maintain adequate glycemic control). Products include:

Dexamethasone Acetate (Certain drugs, including corticosteroids, tend to produce hyperglycemia and may lead to loss of glycemic control. When such drugs are administered to a patient receiving ActoPlus Met, the patient should be closely observed to maintain adequate glycemic control).
No products indexed under this heading.

Dexamethasone Phosphate (Certain drugs, including corticosteroids, tend to produce hyperglycemia and may lead to loss of glycemic control. When such drugs are administered to a patient receiving ActoPlus Met, the patient should be closely observed to maintain adequate glycemic control).
No products indexed under this heading.

Dexamethasone Sodium (Certain drugs, including corticosteroids, tend to produce hyperglycemia and may lead to loss of glycemic control. When such drugs are administered to a patient receiving ActoPlus Met, the patient should be closely observed to maintain adequate glycemic control).
No products indexed under this heading.

Dexamethasone Sodium Phosphate (Certain drugs, including corticosteroids, tend to produce hyperglycemia and may lead to loss of glycemic control. When such drugs are administered to a patient receiving ActoPlus Met, the patient should be closely observed to maintain adequate glycemic control).
No products indexed under this heading.

Dexamethasone Sodium Phosphate Injection (Certain drugs, including corticosteroids, tend to produce hyperglycemia and may lead to loss of glycemic control. When such drugs are administered to a patient receiving ActoPlus Met, the patient should be closely observed to maintain adequate glycemic control).
No products indexed under this heading.

Diatrizoate Meglumine (Radiologic studies involving the use of intravascular iodinated contrast materials is contraindicated during therapy with Actoplus Met. Intravascular contrast studies with iodinated materials can lead to acute alteration of renal function and have been associated with lactic acidosis in patients receiving metformin. Therefore, in patients in whom any such study is planned, ActoPlus Met should be temporarily discontinued at the time of or prior to the procedure, and withheld for 48 hours subsequent to the procedure and reinstituted only after renal function has been re-evaluated and found to be normal).
No products indexed under this heading.

Diatrizoate Sodium (Radiologic studies involving the use of intravascular iodinated contrast materials is contraindicated during therapy with Actoplus Met. Intravascular contrast studies with iodinated materials can lead to acute alteration of renal function and have been associated with lactic acidosis in patients receiving metformin. Therefore, in patients in whom any such study is planned, ActoPlus Met should be temporarily discontinued at the time of or prior to the procedure, and withheld for 48 hours subsequent to the procedure and reinstituted only after renal function has been re-evaluated and found to be normal).
No products indexed under this heading.

Diazepam (In vivo drug-drug interaction studies have suggested that pioglitazone may be a weak inducer of CYP450 isoform 3A4 substrate). Products include:
Valium Tablets 2880

Diclofenac Potassium (Metformin is negligibly bound to plasma proteins and is, therefore, less likely to interact with highly protein-bound drugs, such as salicylates, sulfonamides, chloramphenicol and probenecid).
No products indexed under this heading.

Diclofenac Sodium (Metformin is negligibly bound to plasma proteins and is, therefore, less likely to interact with highly protein-bound drugs, such as salicylates, sulfonamides, chloramphenicol and probenecid).
No products indexed under this heading.

Dienestrol (Certain drugs, including estrogens, tend to produce hyperglycemia and may lead to loss of glycemic control. When such drugs are administered to a patient receiving ActoPlus Met, the patient should be closely observed to maintain adequate glycemic control).
No products indexed under this heading.

Diethylstilbestrol (Certain drugs, including estrogens, tend to produce hyperglycemia and may lead to loss of glycemic control. When such drugs are administered to a patient receiving ActoPlus Met, the patient should be closely observed to maintain adequate glycemic control).
No products indexed under this heading.

Diflorasone Diacetate (Certain drugs, including corticosteroids, tend to produce hyperglycemia and may lead to loss of glycemic control. When such drugs are administered to a patient receiving ActoPlus Met, the patient should be closely observed to maintain adequate glycemic control).
No products indexed under this heading.

Diflunisal (Metformin is negligibly bound to plasma proteins and is, therefore, less likely to interact with highly protein-bound drugs, such as salicylates).
No products indexed under this heading.

Digitalis Glycoside Preparations (Metformin is negligibly bound to plasma proteins and is, therefore, less likely to interact with highly protein-bound drugs, such as salicylates, sulfonamides, chloramphenicol and probenecid).
No products indexed under this heading.

Digitalis Lanata (Metformin is negligibly bound to plasma proteins and is, therefore, less likely to interact with highly protein-bound drugs, such as salicylates, sulfonamides, chloramphenicol and probenecid).
No products indexed under this heading.

Digitalis Purpurea (Metformin is negligibly bound to plasma proteins and is, therefore, less likely to interact with highly protein-bound drugs, such as salicylates, sulfonamides, chloramphenicol and probenecid).
No products indexed under this heading.

Digoxin (Cationic drugs (eg, amiloride, digoxin, morphine, procainamide, quinidine, quinine, ranitidine, triamterene, trimethoprim, and vancomycin) that are eliminated by renal tubular secretion theoretically have the potential for interaction with metformin by competing for common renal tubular transport systems. Careful patient monitoring and dose adjustment of ActoPlus Met and/or the interfering drug is recommended in patients who are taking cationic medications that are excreted via the proximal renal tubular secretory system). Products include:
Lanoxin Injection 1546
Lanoxin Injection Pediatric 1549
Lanoxin Tablets 1553

Dihydroergotamine Mesylate (In vivo drug-drug interaction studies have suggested that pioglitazone may be a weak inducer of CYP450 isoform 3A4 substrate).
No products indexed under this heading.

Diltiazem Hydrochloride (Certain drugs, including calcium channel blockers, tend to produce hyperglycemia and may lead to loss of glycemic control. When such drugs are administered to a

patient receiving ActoPlus Met, the patient should be closely observed to maintain adequate glycemic control). Products include:
Cardizem LA 423

Diltiazem Maleate (In vivo drug-drug interaction studies have suggested that pioglitazone may be a weak inducer of CYP450 isoform 3A4 substrate).
No products indexed under this heading.

Dipyridamole (Metformin is negligibly bound to plasma proteins and is, therefore, less likely to interact with highly protein-bound drugs, such as salicylates, sulfonamides, chloramphenicol and probenecid). Products include:
Aggrenox 880

Disopyramide (In vivo drug-drug interaction studies have suggested that pioglitazone may be a weak inducer of CYP450 isoform 3A4 substrate).
No products indexed under this heading.

Disopyramide Phosphate (In vivo drug-drug interaction studies have suggested that pioglitazone may be a weak inducer of CYP450 isoform 3A4 substrate).
No products indexed under this heading.

Disulfiram (In vivo drug-drug interaction studies have suggested that pioglitazone may be a weak inducer of CYP450 isoform 3A4 substrate).
No products indexed under this heading.

Dobutamine Hydrochloride (Certain drugs, including sympathomimetics, tend to produce hyperglycemia and may lead to loss of glycemic control. When such drugs are administered to a patient receiving ActoPlus Met, the patient should be closely observed to maintain adequate glycemic control).
No products indexed under this heading.

Dopamine Hydrochloride (Certain drugs, including sympathomimetics, tend to produce hyperglycemia and may lead to loss of glycemic control. When such drugs are administered to a patient receiving ActoPlus Met, the patient should be closely observed to maintain adequate glycemic control).
No products indexed under this heading.

Doxorubicin Hydrochloride (In vivo drug-drug interaction studies have suggested that pioglitazone may be a weak inducer of CYP450 isoform 3A4 substrate).
No products indexed under this heading.

Dronabinol (In vivo drug-drug interaction studies have suggested that pioglitazone may be a weak inducer of CYP450 isoform 3A4 substrate).
No products indexed under this heading.

Ephedrine Hydrochloride (Certain drugs, including sympathomimetics, tend to produce hyperglycemia and may lead to loss of glycemic control. When such drugs are administered to a patient receiving ActoPlus Met, the patient should be closely observed to maintain adequate glycemic control).
No products indexed under this heading.

Ephedrine Sulfate (Certain drugs, including sympathomimetics, tend to produce hyperglycemia and may lead to loss of glycemic control. When such drugs are administered to a patient receiving ActoPlus Met, the patient should be closely observed to maintain adequate glycemic control).
No products indexed under this heading.

Ephedrine Tannate (Certain drugs, including sympathomimetics, tend to produce hyperglycemia and may lead to loss of glycemic control. When such drugs are administered to a patient receiving ActoPlus Met, the patient should be closely observed to maintain adequate glycemic control).
No products indexed under this heading.

Epinephrine (Certain drugs, including sympathomimetics, tend to produce

hyperglycemia and may lead to loss of glycemic control. When such drugs are administered to a patient receiving ActoPlus Met, the patient should be closely observed to maintain adequate glycemic control). Products include:
EpiPen 3631
Twinject 3268

Epinephrine Bitartrate (Certain drugs, including sympathomimetics, tend to produce hyperglycemia and may lead to loss of glycemic control. When such drugs are administered to a patient receiving ActoPlus Met, the patient should be closely observed to maintain adequate glycemic control).
No products indexed under this heading.

Epinephrine Hydrochloride (Certain drugs, including sympathomimetics, tend to produce hyperglycemia and may lead to loss of glycemic control. When such drugs are administered to a patient receiving ActoPlus Met, the patient should be closely observed to maintain adequate glycemic control).
No products indexed under this heading.

Ergotamine Tartrate (In vivo drug-drug interaction studies have suggested that pioglitazone may be a weak inducer of CYP450 isoform 3A4 substrate).
No products indexed under this heading.

Erythromycin (In vivo drug-drug interaction studies have suggested that pioglitazone may be a weak inducer of CYP450 isoform 3A4 substrate).
No products indexed under this heading.

Erythromycin Estolate (In vivo drug-drug interaction studies have suggested that pioglitazone may be a weak inducer of CYP450 isoform 3A4 substrate).
No products indexed under this heading.

Erythromycin Ethylsuccinate (In vivo drug-drug interaction studies have suggested that pioglitazone may be a weak inducer of CYP450 isoform 3A4 substrate). Products include:
E.E.S. 437
EryPed 435

Erythromycin Gluceptate (In vivo drug-drug interaction studies have suggested that pioglitazone may be a weak inducer of CYP450 isoform 3A4 substrate).
No products indexed under this heading.

Erythromycin Lactobionate (In vivo drug-drug interaction studies have suggested that pioglitazone may be a weak inducer of CYP450 isoform 3A4 substrate).
No products indexed under this heading.

Erythromycin Stearate (In vivo drug-drug interaction studies have suggested that pioglitazone may be a weak inducer of CYP450 isoform 3A4 substrate).
No products indexed under this heading.

Esmolol Hydrochloride (Hypoglycemia due to metformin may be difficult to recognize in the elderly and in people who are taking β-adrenergic blocking drugs).
No products indexed under this heading.

Estradiol (Certain drugs, including estrogens, tend to produce hyperglycemia and may lead to loss of glycemic control. When such drugs are administered to a patient receiving ActoPlus Met, the patient should be closely observed to maintain adequate glycemic control). Products include:
Activella 2561
Angeliq 831
Climara 841
Climara Pro 847
Divigel 3467
Estrasorb 1777
Vagifem 2589

IMPORTANT NOTE: Always consult each drug listing in the patient's regimen for possible interactions.

ActoPlus **Interactions Index** 28

Estradiol Benzoate (*In vivo* drug-drug interaction studies have suggested that pioglitazone may be a weak inducer of CYP450 isoform 3A4 substrate).
No products indexed under this heading.

Estradiol Cypionate (*In vivo* drug-drug interaction studies have suggested that pioglitazone may be a weak inducer of CYP450 isoform 3A4 substrate).
No products indexed under this heading.

Estradiol Valerate (*In vivo* drug-drug interaction studies have suggested that pioglitazone may be a weak inducer of CYP450 isoform 3A4 substrate).
No products indexed under this heading.

Estrogens, Conjugated (Certain drugs, including estrogens, tend to produce hyperglycemia and may lead to loss of glycemic control. When such drugs are administered to a patient receiving ActoPlus Met, the patient should be closely observed to maintain adequate glycemic control). Products include:
Premarin Intravenous **3528**
Premarin Tablets **3533**
Premarin Vaginal Cream **3540**
Premphase **3549**
Prempro **3549**

Estrogens, Esterified (Certain drugs, including estrogens, tend to produce hyperglycemia and may lead to loss of glycemic control. When such drugs are administered to a patient receiving ActoPlus Met, the patient should be closely observed to maintain adequate glycemic control).
No products indexed under this heading.

Estropipate (Certain drugs, including estrogens, tend to produce hyperglycemia and may lead to loss of glycemic control. When such drugs are administered to a patient receiving ActoPlus Met, the patient should be closely observed to maintain adequate glycemic control).
No products indexed under this heading.

Ethacrynic Acid (Certain drugs, including thiazides and other diuretics, tend to produce hyperglycemia and may lead to loss of glycemic control. When such drugs are administered to a patient receiving ActoPlus Met, the patient should be closely observed to maintain adequate glycemic control).
No products indexed under this heading.

Ethanol (Alcohol is known to potentiate the effect of metformin on lactate metabolism. Patients, therefore, should be warned against excessive alcohol intake, acute or chronic, while receiving ActoPlus Met. In addition, hypoglycemia does not occur in patients receiving metformin alone under usual circumstances of use, but could occur when during concomitant use with ethanol).
No products indexed under this heading.

Ethinyl Estradiol (Co-administration of pioglitazone (45 mg once daily) and an oral contraceptive (1 mg norethindrone plus 0.035 mg ethinyl estradiol once daily) for 21 days, resulted in 11% and 11-14% decrease in ethinyl estradiol AUC (0-24h) and C_{max}, respectively. There were no significant changes in norethindrone AUC (0-24h) and C_{max}. In view of the high variability of ethinyl estradiol pharmacokinetics, the clinical significance of this finding is unknown). Products include:
LoSeasonique **3407**
Lybrel **3514**
NuvaRing **3181**
Ortho Evra **2648**
Ortho-Cyclen/Ortho Tri-Cyclen **2663**
Ortho Tri-Cyclen Lo Tablets **2673**
Seasonique **3418**
Yaz **864**

Ethiodized Oil (Radiologic studies involving the use of intravascular iodinated contrast materials is contraindicated during therapy with Actoplus Met. Intravascular contrast studies with iodinated materials can lead to acute alteration of renal function and have been associated with lactic acidosis in patients receiving metformin. Therefore, in patients in whom any such study is planned, ActoPlus Met should be temporarily discontinued at the time of or prior to the procedure, and withheld for 48 hours subsequent to the procedure and reinstituted only after renal function has been re-evaluated and found to be normal).
No products indexed under this heading.

Ethosuximide (*In vivo* drug-drug interaction studies have suggested that pioglitazone may be a weak inducer of CYP450 isoform 3A4 substrate).
No products indexed under this heading.

Ethyl Alcohol (Alcohol is known to potentiate the effect of metformin on lactate metabolism. Patients, therefore, should be warned against excessive alcohol intake, acute or chronic, while receiving ActoPlus Met. In addition, hypoglycemia does not occur in patients receiving metformin alone under usual circumstances of use, but could occur when during concomitant use with ethanol).
No products indexed under this heading.

Ethynodiol Diacetate (Certain drugs, including oral contraceptives, tend to produce hyperglycemia and may lead to loss of glycemic control. When such drugs are administered to a patient receiving ActoPlus Met, the patient should be closely observed to maintain adequate glycemic control. Co-administration of pioglitazone (45 mg once daily) and an oral contraceptive (1 mg norethindrone plus 0.035 mg ethinyl estradiol once daily) for 21 days, resulted in 11% and 11-14% decrease in ethinyl estradiol AUC (0-24h) and C_{max} respectively. There were no significant changes in norethindrone AUC (0-24h) and C_{max}. In view of the high variability of ethinyl estradiol pharmacokinetics, the clinical significance of this finding is unknown).
No products indexed under this heading.

Etoposide (*In vivo* drug-drug interaction studies have suggested that pioglitazone may be a weak inducer of CYP450 isoform 3A4 substrate).
No products indexed under this heading.

Etoposide Phosphate (*In vivo* drug-drug interaction studies have suggested that pioglitazone may be a weak inducer of CYP450 isoform 3A4 substrate).
No products indexed under this heading.

Felodipine (Certain drugs, including calcium channel blockers, tend to produce hyperglycemia and may lead to loss of glycemic control. When such drugs are administered to a patient receiving ActoPlus Met, the patient should be closely observed to maintain adequate glycemic control).
No products indexed under this heading.

Fenoprofen Calcium (Metformin is negligibly bound to plasma proteins and is, therefore, less likely to interact with highly protein-bound drugs, such as salicylates, sulfonamides, chloramphenicol and probenecid).
No products indexed under this heading.

Fentanyl (*In vivo* drug-drug interaction studies have suggested that pioglitazone may be a weak inducer of CYP450 isoform 3A4 substrate). Products include:
Duragesic **2604**
Fentanyl Transdermal System **2346**
Onsolis **2054**

Fentanyl Citrate (*In vivo* drug-drug interaction studies have suggested that pioglitazone may be a weak inducer of CYP450 isoform 3A4 substrate). Products include:
Fentora **966**

Fludrocortisone Acetate (Certain drugs, including corticosteroids, tend to produce hyperglycemia and may lead to loss of glycemic control. When such drugs are administered to a patient receiving ActoPlus Met, the patient should be closely observed to maintain adequate glycemic control).
No products indexed under this heading.

Flumethasone Pivalate (Certain drugs, including corticosteroids, tend to produce hyperglycemia and may lead to loss of glycemic control. When such drugs are administered to a patient receiving ActoPlus Met, the patient should be closely observed to maintain adequate glycemic control).
No products indexed under this heading.

Flunisolide Hemihydrate (Certain drugs, including corticosteroids, tend to produce hyperglycemia and may lead to loss of glycemic control. When such drugs are administered to a patient receiving ActoPlus Met, the patient should be closely observed to maintain adequate glycemic control).
No products indexed under this heading.

Fluphenazine Decanoate (Certain drugs, including phenothiazines, tend to produce hyperglycemia and may lead to loss of glycemic control. When such drugs are administered to a patient receiving ActoPlus Met, the patient should be closely observed to maintain adequate glycemic control).
No products indexed under this heading.

Fluphenazine Enanthate (Certain drugs, including phenothiazines, tend to produce hyperglycemia and may lead to loss of glycemic control. When such drugs are administered to a patient receiving ActoPlus Met, the patient should be closely observed to maintain adequate glycemic control).
No products indexed under this heading.

Fluphenazine Hydrochloride (Certain drugs, including phenothiazines, tend to produce hyperglycemia and may lead to loss of glycemic control. When such drugs are administered to a patient receiving ActoPlus Met, the patient should be closely observed to maintain adequate glycemic control).
No products indexed under this heading.

Flurazepam Hydrochloride (Metformin is negligibly bound to plasma proteins and is, therefore, less likely to interact with highly protein-bound drugs, such as salicylates, sulfonamides, chloramphenicol and probenecid).
No products indexed under this heading.

Flurbiprofen (Metformin is negligibly bound to plasma proteins and is, therefore, less likely to interact with highly protein-bound drugs, such as salicylates, sulfonamides, chloramphenicol and probenecid).
No products indexed under this heading.

Fluticasone Furoate (Certain drugs, including corticosteroids, tend to produce hyperglycemia and may lead to loss of glycemic control. When such drugs are administered to a patient receiving ActoPlus Met, the patient should be closely observed to maintain adequate glycemic control). Products include:
Veramyst **1713**

Fluticasone Propionate (Certain drugs, including corticosteroids, tend to produce hyperglycemia and may lead to loss of glycemic control. When such drugs are administered to a patient receiving ActoPlus Met, the patient should be closely observed to maintain adequate glycemic control). Products include:
Advair 100/50 ..... **1275**
Advair 250/50 ..... **1275**
Advair 500/50 ..... **1275**
Advair HFA 45/21 ..... **1288**
Advair HFA 115/21 ..... **1288**
Advair HFA 230/21 ..... **1288**
Flonase **1459**
Flovent Diskus **1463**
Flovent HFA **1470**

Fosphenytoin (Certain drugs, including phenytoin, tend to produce hyperglycemia and may lead to loss of glycemic control. When such drugs are administered to a patient receiving ActoPlus Met, the patient should be closely observed to maintain adequate glycemic control).
No products indexed under this heading.

Fosphenytoin Sodium (Certain drugs, including phenytoin, tend to produce hyperglycemia and may lead to loss of glycemic control. When such drugs are administered to a patient receiving ActoPlus Met, the patient should be closely observed to maintain adequate glycemic control).
No products indexed under this heading.

Furosemide (A single-dose, metformin-furosemide drug interaction study in healthy subjects demonstrated that pharmacokinetic parameters of both compounds were affected by co-administration. Furosemide increased the metformin plasma and blood C_{max} by 22% and blood AUC by 15%, without any significant change in metformin renal clearance. When administered with metformin, the C_{max} and AUC of furosemide were 31% and 12% smaller, respectively, than when administered alone and the terminal half-life was decreased by 31%,without any significant change in furosemide renal clearance. No information is available about the interaction of metformin and furosemide when co-administered chronically). Products include:
Furosemide **2354**

Gadopentetate Dimeglumine (Radiologic studies involving the use of intravascular iodinated contrast materials is contraindicated during therapy with Actoplus Met. Intravascular contrast studies with iodinated materials can lead to acute alteration of renal function and have been associated with lactic acidosis in patients receiving metformin. Therefore, in patients in whom any such study is planned, ActoPlus Met should be temporarily discontinued at the time of or prior to the procedure, and withheld for 48 hours subsequent to the procedure and reinstituted only after renal function has been re-evaluated and found to be normal).
No products indexed under this heading.

Gemfibrozil (Concomitant administration of gemfibrozil (oral 600 mg twice daily), an inhibitor of CYP2C8, with pioglitazone (oral 30 mg) in 10 healthy volunteers pre-treated for 2 days prior with gemfibrozil (oral 600 mg twice daily) resulted in pioglitazone exposure (AUC_{0-24}) being 226% of the pioglitazone exposure in the absence of gemfibrozil. If an inhibitor of CYP2C8 (such as gemfibrozil) is started or stopped during treatment with pioglitazone, changes in diabetes treatment may be needed based on clinical response).
No products indexed under this heading.

Glibenclamide (Pioglitazone, like other thiazolidinediones, can cause fluid retention when used alone or in combination with other antihyperglycemic agents, including insulin. Fluid retention may lead to or exacerbate heart failure. In addition, patients receiving pioglitazone in combination with insulin or oral hypoglycemic agents may be at risk for

29 **Interactions Index** **ActoPlus**

hypoglycemia, and a reduction in the dose of the concomitant agent may be necessary).
No products indexed under this heading.

Glimepiride (Pioglitazone, like other thiazolidinediones, can cause fluid retention when used alone or in combination with other antihyperglycemic agents, including insulin. Fluid retention may lead to or exacerbate heart failure. In addition, patients receiving pioglitazone in combination with insulin or oral hypoglycemic agents may be at risk for hypoglycemia, and a reduction in the dose of the concomitant agent may be necessary). Products include:
Avandaryl **1356**
Duetact **3354**

Glipizide (Pioglitazone, like other thiazolidinediones, can cause fluid retention when used alone or in combination with other antihyperglycemic agents, including insulin. Fluid retention may lead to or exacerbate heart failure. In addition, patients receiving pioglitazone in combination with insulin or oral hypoglycemic agents may be at risk for hypoglycemia, and a reduction in the dose of the concomitant agent may be necessary).
No products indexed under this heading.

Glyburide (Pioglitazone, like other thiazolidinediones, can cause fluid retention when used alone or in combination with other antihyperglycemic agents, including insulin. Fluid retention may lead to or exacerbate heart failure. In addition, patients receiving pioglitazone in combination with insulin or oral hypoglycemic agents may be at risk for hypoglycemia, and a reduction in the dose of the concomitant agent may be necessary).
No products indexed under this heading.

Haloperidol (*In vivo* drug-drug interaction studies have suggested that pioglitazone may be a weak inducer of CYP450 isoform 3A4 substrate).
No products indexed under this heading.

Haloperidol Decanoate (*In vivo* drug-drug interaction studies have suggested that pioglitazone may be a weak inducer of CYP450 isoform 3A4 substrate).
No products indexed under this heading.

Haloperidol Lactate (*In vivo* drug-drug interaction studies have suggested that pioglitazone may be a weak inducer of CYP450 isoform 3A4 substrate).
No products indexed under this heading.

Hydrochlorothiazide (Certain drugs, including thiazide diuretics, tend to produce hyperglycemia and may lead to loss of glycemic control. When such drugs are administered to a patient receiving ActoPlus Met, the patient should be closely observed to maintain adequate glycemic control). Products include:
Atacand HCT **700**
Avalide **2956**
Benicar HCT **1017**
Diovan HCT **2419**
Dyazide **1429**
Exforge HCT **2449**
Hyzaar **2162**
Hyzaar 100-12.5 .... **2162**
Micardis HCT **889**
Prinzide **2246**
Tekturna HCT **2541**
Teveten HCT **541**

Hydrocortisone (Certain drugs, including corticosteroids, tend to produce hyperglycemia and may lead to loss of glycemic control. When such drugs are administered to a patient receiving ActoPlus Met, the patient should be closely observed to maintain adequate glycemic control).
No products indexed under this heading.

Hydrocortisone (Alcohol) (Certain drugs, including corticosteroids, tend to produce hyperglycemia and may lead to loss of glycemic control. When such drugs are administered to a patient receiving ActoPlus Met, the patient should be closely observed to maintain adequate glycemic control).
No products indexed under this heading.

Hydrocortisone Acetate (Certain drugs, including corticosteroids, tend to produce hyperglycemia and may lead to loss of glycemic control. When such drugs are administered to a patient receiving ActoPlus Met, the patient should be closely observed to maintain adequate glycemic control).
No products indexed under this heading.

Hydrocortisone Butyrate (Certain drugs, including corticosteroids, tend to produce hyperglycemia and may lead to loss of glycemic control. When such drugs are administered to a patient receiving ActoPlus Met, the patient should be closely observed to maintain adequate glycemic control).
No products indexed under this heading.

Hydrocortisone Cypionate (Certain drugs, including corticosteroids, tend to produce hyperglycemia and may lead to loss of glycemic control. When such drugs are administered to a patient receiving ActoPlus Met, the patient should be closely observed to maintain adequate glycemic control).
No products indexed under this heading.

Hydrocortisone Hemisuccinate (Certain drugs, including corticosteroids, tend to produce hyperglycemia and may lead to loss of glycemic control. When such drugs are administered to a patient receiving ActoPlus Met, the patient should be closely observed to maintain adequate glycemic control).
No products indexed under this heading.

Hydrocortisone Probutate (Certain drugs, including corticosteroids, tend to produce hyperglycemia and may lead to loss of glycemic control. When such drugs are administered to a patient receiving ActoPlus Met, the patient should be closely observed to maintain adequate glycemic control).
No products indexed under this heading.

Hydrocortisone Sodium Phosphate (Certain drugs, including corticosteroids, tend to produce hyperglycemia and may lead to loss of glycemic control. When such drugs are administered to a patient receiving ActoPlus Met, the patient should be closely observed to maintain adequate glycemic control).
No products indexed under this heading.

Hydrocortisone Sodium Succinate (Certain drugs, including corticosteroids, tend to produce hyperglycemia and may lead to loss of glycemic control. When such drugs are administered to a patient receiving ActoPlus Met, the patient should be closely observed to maintain adequate glycemic control).
No products indexed under this heading.

Hydrocortisone Valerate (Certain drugs, including corticosteroids, tend to produce hyperglycemia and may lead to loss of glycemic control. When such drugs are administered to a patient receiving ActoPlus Met, the patient should be closely observed to maintain adequate glycemic control).
No products indexed under this heading.

Hydroflumethiazide (Certain drugs, including thiazide diuretics, tend to produce hyperglycemia and may lead to loss of glycemic control. When such drugs are administered to a patient receiving ActoPlus Met, the patient should be closely observed to maintain adequate glycemic control).
No products indexed under this heading.

Ibuprofen (Metformin is negligibly bound to plasma proteins and is, therefore, less likely to interact with highly protein-bound drugs, such as salicylates, sulfonamides, chloramphenicol and probenecid). Products include:
Motrin IB **2043**
Children's Motrin **2044**
Children's Motrin Non-Staining Dye-Free **2044**
Infants' Motrin **2044**
Infants' Motrin Dye-Free **2044**
Junior Strength Motrin **2044**
Vicoprofen **564**

Imipramine Hydrochloride (Metformin is negligibly bound to plasma proteins and is, therefore, less likely to interact with highly protein-bound drugs, such as salicylates, sulfonamides, chloramphenicol and probenecid).
No products indexed under this heading.

Imipramine Pamoate (Metformin is negligibly bound to plasma proteins and is, therefore, less likely to interact with highly protein-bound drugs, such as salicylates, sulfonamides, chloramphenicol and probenecid).
No products indexed under this heading.

Indapamide (Certain drugs, including thiazides and other diuretics, tend to produce hyperglycemia and may lead to loss of glycemic control. When such drugs are administered to a patient receiving ActoPlus Met, the patient should be closely observed to maintain adequate glycemic control). Products include:
Indapamide **2356**

Indinavir Sulfate (*In vivo* drug-drug interaction studies have suggested that pioglitazone may be a weak inducer of CYP450 isoform 3A4 substrate). Products include:
Crixivan **2113**

Indomethacin (Metformin is negligibly bound to plasma proteins and is, therefore, less likely to interact with highly protein-bound drugs, such as salicylates, sulfonamides, chloramphenicol and probenecid). Products include:
Indocin **2167**

Indomethacin Sodium Trihydrate (Metformin is negligibly bound to plasma proteins and is, therefore, less likely to interact with highly protein-bound drugs, such as salicylates, sulfonamides, chloramphenicol and probenecid). Products include:
Indocin I.V. **2007**

Insulin (Pioglitazone, like other thiazolidinediones, can cause fluid retention when used alone or in combination with other antihyperglycemic agents, including insulin. Fluid retention may lead to or exacerbate heart failure. In addition, patients receiving pioglitazone in combination with insulin or oral hypoglycemic agents may be at risk for hypoglycemia, and a reduction in the dose of the concomitant agent may be necessary. Hypoglycemia does not occur in patients receiving metformin alone under usual circumstances of use, but could occur when caloric intake is deficient, when strenuous exercise is not compensated by caloric supplementation, or during concomitant use with hypoglycemic agents (such as sulfonylureas or insulin) or ethanol).
No products indexed under this heading.

Insulin, Human, Zinc Suspension (Pioglitazone, like other thiazolidinediones, can cause fluid retention when used alone or in combination with other antihyperglycemic agents, including insulin. Fluid retention may lead to or exacerbate heart failure. In addition, patients receiving pioglitazone in combination with insulin or oral hypoglycemic agents may be at risk for hypoglycemia, and a reduction in the dose of the concomitant agent may be necessary. Hypoglycemia does not occur in patients receiving metformin alone under usual circumstances of use, but could occur when caloric intake is deficient, when strenuous exercise is not compensated by caloric supplementation, or during concomitant use with hypoglycemic agents (such as sulfonylureas or insulin) or ethanol).
No products indexed under this heading.

Insulin, Human (rDNA origin) (Pioglitazone, like other thiazolidinediones, can cause fluid retention when used alone or in combination with other antihyperglycemic agents, including insulin. Fluid retention may lead to or exacerbate heart failure. In addition, patients receiving pioglitazone in combination with insulin or oral hypoglycemic agents may be at risk for hypoglycemia, and a reduction in the dose of the concomitant agent may be necessary. Hypoglycemia does not occur in patients receiving metformin alone under usual circumstances of use, but could occur when caloric intake is deficient, when strenuous exercise is not compensated by caloric supplementation, or during concomitant use with hypoglycemic agents (such as sulfonylureas or insulin) or ethanol). Products include:
Exubera **2717**

Insulin, Human NPH (Pioglitazone, like other thiazolidinediones, can cause fluid retention when used alone or in combination with other antihyperglycemic agents, including insulin. Fluid retention may lead to or exacerbate heart failure. In addition, patients receiving pioglitazone in combination with insulin or oral hypoglycemic agents may be at risk for hypoglycemia, and a reduction in the dose of the concomitant agent may be necessary. Hypoglycemia does not occur in patients receiving metformin alone under usual circumstances of use, but could occur when caloric intake is deficient, when strenuous exercise is not compensated by caloric supplementation, or during concomitant use with hypoglycemic agents (such as sulfonylureas or insulin) or ethanol). Products include:
Humulin N Vial **1934**

Insulin, Human Regular (Pioglitazone, like other thiazolidinediones, can cause fluid retention when used alone or in combination with other antihyperglycemic agents, including insulin. Fluid retention may lead to or exacerbate heart failure. In addition, patients receiving pioglitazone in combination with insulin or oral hypoglycemic agents may be at risk for hypoglycemia, and a reduction in the dose of the concomitant agent may be necessary. Hypoglycemia does not occur in patients receiving metformin alone under usual circumstances of use, but could occur when caloric intake is deficient, when strenuous exercise is not compensated by caloric supplementation, or during concomitant use with hypoglycemic agents (such as sulfonylureas or insulin) or ethanol). Products include:
Humulin R **1937**
Humulin R (U-500) **1939**

Insulin, Human Regular and Human NPH Mixture (Pioglitazone, like other thiazolidinediones, can cause fluid retention when used alone or in combination with other antihyperglycemic agents, including insulin. Fluid retention may lead to or exacerbate heart failure. In addition, patients receiving pioglitazone in combination with insulin or oral hypoglycemic agents may be at risk for hypoglycemia, and a reduction in the dose of the concomitant agent may be necessary. Hypoglycemia does not occur in patients receiving metformin alone under usual circumstances of use, but could occur when caloric intake is deficient, when

IMPORTANT NOTE: Always consult each drug listing in the patient's regimen for possible interactions.

strenuous exercise is not compensated by caloric supplementation, or during concomitant use with hypoglycemic agents (such as sulfonylureas or insulin) or ethanol). Products include:

Humulin 50/50 1930
Humulin 70/30 Vial 1931

Insulin, NPH (Pioglitazone, like other thiazolidinediones, can cause fluid retention when used alone or in combination with other antihyperglycemic agents, including insulin. Fluid retention may lead to or exacerbate heart failure. In addition, patients receiving pioglitazone in combination with insulin or oral hypoglycemic agents may be at risk for hypoglycemia, and a reduction in the dose of the concomitant agent may be necessary. Hypoglycemia does not occur in patients receiving metformin alone under usual circumstances of use, but could occur when caloric intake is deficient, when strenuous exercise is not compensated by caloric supplementation, or during concomitant use with hypoglycemic agents (such as sulfonylureas or insulin) or ethanol).

No products indexed under this heading.

Insulin, Regular (Pioglitazone, like other thiazolidinediones, can cause fluid retention when used alone or in combination with other antihyperglycemic agents, including insulin. Fluid retention may lead to or exacerbate heart failure. In addition, patients receiving pioglitazone in combination with insulin or oral hypoglycemic agents may be at risk for hypoglycemia, and a reduction in the dose of the concomitant agent may be necessary. Hypoglycemia does not occur in patients receiving metformin alone under usual circumstances of use, but could occur when caloric intake is deficient, when strenuous exercise is not compensated by caloric supplementation, or during concomitant use with hypoglycemic agents (such as sulfonylureas or insulin) or ethanol).

No products indexed under this heading.

Insulin, Regular and NPH mixture (Pioglitazone, like other thiazolidinediones, can cause fluid retention when used alone or in combination with other antihyperglycemic agents, including insulin. Fluid retention may lead to or exacerbate heart failure. In addition, patients receiving pioglitazone in combination with insulin or oral hypoglycemic agents may be at risk for hypoglycemia, and a reduction in the dose of the concomitant agent may be necessary. Hypoglycemia does not occur in patients receiving metformin alone under usual circumstances of use, but could occur when caloric intake is deficient, when strenuous exercise is not compensated by caloric supplementation, or during concomitant use with hypoglycemic agents (such as sulfonylureas or insulin) or ethanol).

No products indexed under this heading.

Insulin, Zinc Crystals (Pioglitazone, like other thiazolidinediones, can cause fluid retention when used alone or in combination with other antihyperglycemic agents, including insulin. Fluid retention may lead to or exacerbate heart failure. In addition, patients receiving pioglitazone in combination with insulin or oral hypoglycemic agents may be at risk for hypoglycemia, and a reduction in the dose of the concomitant agent may be necessary. Hypoglycemia does not occur in patients receiving metformin alone under usual circumstances of use, but could occur when caloric intake is deficient, when strenuous exercise is not compensated by caloric supplementation, or during concomitant use with hypoglycemic agents (such as sulfonylureas or insulin) or ethanol).

No products indexed under this heading.

Insulin, Zinc Suspension (Pioglitazone, like other thiazolidinediones, can cause fluid retention when used alone or in combination with other antihyperglycemic agents, including insulin. Fluid retention may lead to or exacerbate heart failure. In addition, patients receiving pioglitazone in combination with insulin or oral hypoglycemic agents may be at risk for hypoglycemia, and a reduction in the dose of the concomitant agent may be necessary. Hypoglycemia does not occur in patients receiving metformin alone under usual circumstances of use, but could occur when caloric intake is deficient, when strenuous exercise is not compensated by caloric supplementation, or during concomitant use with hypoglycemic agents (such as sulfonylureas or insulin) or ethanol).

No products indexed under this heading.

Insulin Aspart (Pioglitazone, like other thiazolidinediones, can cause fluid retention when used alone or in combination with other antihyperglycemic agents, including insulin. Fluid retention may lead to or exacerbate heart failure. In addition, patients receiving pioglitazone in combination with insulin or oral hypoglycemic agents may be at risk for hypoglycemia, and a reduction in the dose of the concomitant agent may be necessary. Hypoglycemia does not occur in patients receiving metformin alone under usual circumstances of use, but could occur when caloric intake is deficient, when strenuous exercise is not compensated by caloric supplementation, or during concomitant use with hypoglycemic agents (such as sulfonylureas or insulin) or ethanol).

No products indexed under this heading.

Insulin Aspart, Human (Pioglitazone, like other thiazolidinediones, can cause fluid retention when used alone or in combination with other antihyperglycemic agents, including insulin. Fluid retention may lead to or exacerbate heart failure. In addition, patients receiving pioglitazone in combination with insulin or oral hypoglycemic agents may be at risk for hypoglycemia, and a reduction in the dose of the concomitant agent may be necessary. Hypoglycemia does not occur in patients receiving metformin alone under usual circumstances of use, but could occur when caloric intake is deficient, when strenuous exercise is not compensated by caloric supplementation, or during concomitant use with hypoglycemic agents (such as sulfonylureas or insulin) or ethanol). Products include:

NovoLog Mix 70/30 2581

Insulin Aspart, Human Regular (Pioglitazone, like other thiazolidinediones, can cause fluid retention when used alone or in combination with other antihyperglycemic agents, including insulin. Fluid retention may lead to or exacerbate heart failure. In addition, patients receiving pioglitazone in combination with insulin or oral hypoglycemic agents may be at risk for hypoglycemia, and a reduction in the dose of the concomitant agent may be necessary. Hypoglycemia does not occur in patients receiving metformin alone under usual circumstances of use, but could occur when caloric intake is deficient, when strenuous exercise is not compensated by caloric supplementation, or during concomitant use with hypoglycemic agents (such as sulfonylureas or insulin) or ethanol). Products include:

NovoLog 2575

Insulin Aspart Protamine, Human (Pioglitazone, like other thiazolidinediones, can cause fluid retention when used alone or in combination with other antihyperglycemic agents, including

insulin. Fluid retention may lead to or exacerbate heart failure. In addition, patients receiving pioglitazone in combination with insulin or oral hypoglycemic agents may be at risk for hypoglycemia, and a reduction in the dose of the concomitant agent may be necessary. Hypoglycemia does not occur in patients receiving metformin alone under usual circumstances of use, but could occur when caloric intake is deficient, when strenuous exercise is not compensated by caloric supplementation, or during concomitant use with hypoglycemic agents (such as sulfonylureas or insulin) or ethanol). Products include:

NovoLog Mix 70/30 2581

Insulin Detemir (rDNA Origin) (Pioglitazone, like other thiazolidinediones, can cause fluid retention when used alone or in combination with other antihyperglycemic agents, including insulin. Fluid retention may lead to or exacerbate heart failure. In addition, patients receiving pioglitazone in combination with insulin or oral hypoglycemic agents may be at risk for hypoglycemia, and a reduction in the dose of the concomitant agent may be necessary. Hypoglycemia does not occur in patients receiving metformin alone under usual circumstances of use, but could occur when caloric intake is deficient, when strenuous exercise is not compensated by caloric supplementation, or during concomitant use with hypoglycemic agents (such as sulfonylureas or insulin) or ethanol). Products include:

Levemir 2566

Insulin Glargine (Pioglitazone, like other thiazolidinediones, can cause fluid retention when used alone or in combination with other antihyperglycemic agents, including insulin. Fluid retention may lead to or exacerbate heart failure. In addition, patients receiving pioglitazone in combination with insulin or oral hypoglycemic agents may be at risk for hypoglycemia, and a reduction in the dose of the concomitant agent may be necessary. Hypoglycemia does not occur in patients receiving metformin alone under usual circumstances of use, but could occur when caloric intake is deficient, when strenuous exercise is not compensated by caloric supplementation, or during concomitant use with hypoglycemic agents (such as sulfonylureas or insulin) or ethanol). Products include:

Lantus 2996

Insulin Glulisine (Pioglitazone, like other thiazolidinediones, can cause fluid retention when used alone or in combination with other antihyperglycemic agents, including insulin. Fluid retention may lead to or exacerbate heart failure. In addition, patients receiving pioglitazone in combination with insulin or oral hypoglycemic agents may be at risk for hypoglycemia, and a reduction in the dose of the concomitant agent may be necessary. Hypoglycemia does not occur in patients receiving metformin alone under usual circumstances of use, but could occur when caloric intake is deficient, when strenuous exercise is not compensated by caloric supplementation, or during concomitant use with hypoglycemic agents (such as sulfonylureas or insulin) or ethanol). Products include:

Apidra 2937
Apidra SoloStar 2937

Insulin Lispro, Human (Pioglitazone, like other thiazolidinediones, can cause fluid retention when used alone or in combination with other antihyperglycemic agents, including insulin. Fluid retention may lead to or exacerbate heart failure. In addition, patients receiving pioglitazone in combination with

insulin or oral hypoglycemic agents may be at risk for hypoglycemia, and a reduction in the dose of the concomitant agent may be necessary. Hypoglycemia does not occur in patients receiving metformin alone under usual circumstances of use, but could occur when caloric intake is deficient, when strenuous exercise is not compensated by caloric supplementation, or during concomitant use with hypoglycemic agents (such as sulfonylureas or insulin) or ethanol). Products include:

Humalog 1910
Humalog Mix 1914
Humalog Mix75/25 1917

Insulin Lispro Protamine, Human (Pioglitazone, like other thiazolidinediones, can cause fluid retention when used alone or in combination with other antihyperglycemic agents, including insulin. Fluid retention may lead to or exacerbate heart failure. In addition, patients receiving pioglitazone in combination with insulin or oral hypoglycemic agents may be at risk for hypoglycemia, and a reduction in the dose of the concomitant agent may be necessary. Hypoglycemia does not occur in patients receiving metformin alone under usual circumstances of use, but could occur when caloric intake is deficient, when strenuous exercise is not compensated by caloric supplementation, or during concomitant use with hypoglycemic agents (such as sulfonylureas or insulin) or ethanol). Products include:

Humalog Mix 1914
Humalog Mix75/25 1917

Iodamide Meglumine (Radiologic studies involving the use of intravascular iodinated contrast materials is contraindicated during therapy with Actoplus Met. Intravascular contrast studies with iodinated materials can lead to acute alteration of renal function and have been associated with lactic acidosis in patients receiving metformin. Therefore, in patients in whom any such study is planned, ActoPlus Met should be temporarily discontinued at the time of or prior to the procedure, and withheld for 48 hours subsequent to the procedure and reinstituted only after renal function has been re-evaluated and found to be normal).

No products indexed under this heading.

Iohexol (Radiologic studies involving the use of intravascular iodinated contrast materials is contraindicated during therapy with Actoplus Met. Intravascular contrast studies with iodinated materials can lead to acute alteration of renal function and have been associated with lactic acidosis in patients receiving metformin. Therefore, in patients in whom any such study is planned, ActoPlus Met should be temporarily discontinued at the time of or prior to the procedure, and withheld for 48 hours subsequent to the procedure and reinstituted only after renal function has been re-evaluated and found to be normal).

No products indexed under this heading.

Iopamidol (Radiologic studies involving the use of intravascular iodinated contrast materials is contraindicated during therapy with Actoplus Met. Intravascular contrast studies with iodinated materials can lead to acute alteration of renal function and have been associated with lactic acidosis in patients receiving metformin. Therefore, in patients in whom any such study is planned, ActoPlus Met should be temporarily discontinued at the time of or prior to the procedure, and withheld for 48 hours subsequent to the procedure and reinstituted only after renal function has been re-evaluated and found to be normal).

No products indexed under this heading.

31 Interactions Index ActoPlus

Iopanoic Acid (Radiologic studies involving the use of intravascular iodinated contrast materials is contraindicated during therapy with Actoplus Met. Intravascular contrast studies with iodinated materials can lead to acute alteration of renal function and have been associated with lactic acidosis in patients receiving metformin. Therefore, in patients in whom any such study is planned, ActoPlus Met should be temporarily discontinued at the time of or prior to the procedure, and withheld for 48 hours subsequent to the procedure and reinstituted only after renal function has been re-evaluated and found to be normal).
No products indexed under this heading.

Iothalamate Meglumine (Radiologic studies involving the use of intravascular iodinated contrast materials is contraindicated during therapy with Actoplus Met. Intravascular contrast studies with iodinated materials can lead to acute alteration of renal function and have been associated with lactic acidosis in patients receiving metformin. Therefore, in patients in whom any such study is planned, ActoPlus Met should be temporarily discontinued at the time of or prior to the procedure, and withheld for 48 hours subsequent to the procedure and reinstituted only after renal function has been re-evaluated and found to be normal).
No products indexed under this heading.

Ioxaglate Meglumine (Radiologic studies involving the use of intravascular iodinated contrast materials is contraindicated during therapy with Actoplus Met. Intravascular contrast studies with iodinated materials can lead to acute alteration of renal function and have been associated with lactic acidosis in patients receiving metformin. Therefore, in patients in whom any such study is planned, ActoPlus Met should be temporarily discontinued at the time of or prior to the procedure, and withheld for 48 hours subsequent to the procedure and reinstituted only after renal function has been re-evaluated and found to be normal).
No products indexed under this heading.

Ioxaglate Sodium (Radiologic studies involving the use of intravascular iodinated contrast materials is contraindicated during therapy with Actoplus Met. Intravascular contrast studies with iodinated materials can lead to acute alteration of renal function and have been associated with lactic acidosis in patients receiving metformin. Therefore, in patients in whom any such study is planned, ActoPlus Met should be temporarily discontinued at the time of or prior to the procedure, and withheld for 48 hours subsequent to the procedure and reinstituted only after renal function has been re-evaluated and found to be normal).
No products indexed under this heading.

Isoniazid (Certain drugs, including isoniazid, tend to produce hyperglycemia and may lead to loss of glycemic control. When such drugs are administered to a patient receiving ActoPlus Met, the patient should be closely observed to maintain adequate glycemic control).
No products indexed under this heading.

Isoproterenol Hydrochloride (Certain drugs, including sympathomimetics, tend to produce hyperglycemia and may lead to loss of glycemic control. When such drugs are administered to a patient receiving ActoPlus Met, the patient should be closely observed to maintain adequate glycemic control).
No products indexed under this heading.

Isoproterenol Sulfate (Certain drugs, including sympathomimetics, tend to produce hyperglycemia and may lead to loss of glycemic control. When such drugs are administered to a patient receiving ActoPlus Met, the patient should be closely observed to maintain adequate glycemic control).
No products indexed under this heading.

Isradipine (Certain drugs, including calcium channel blockers, tend to produce hyperglycemia and may lead to loss of glycemic control. When such drugs are administered to a patient receiving ActoPlus Met, the patient should be closely observed to maintain adequate glycemic control). Products include:
DynaCirc CR 1432

Itraconazole (*In vivo* drug-drug interaction studies have suggested that pioglitazone may be a weak inducer of CYP450 isoform 3A4 substrate).
No products indexed under this heading.

Ixabepilone (*In vivo* drug-drug interaction studies have suggested that pioglitazone may be a weak inducer of CYP450 isoform 3A4 substrate).
No products indexed under this heading.

Ketoconazole (Co-administration of pioglitazone for 7 days with ketoconazole 200 mg administered twice daily resulted in a ratio of least square mean (90% CI) values for unchanged pioglitazone of 1.14 (1.06-1.23) for C_{max}, 1.34 (1.26-1.41) for AUC and 1.87 (1.71-2.04) for C_{min}). Products include:
Extina 3319
Xolegel 3337

Ketoprofen (Metformin is negligibly bound to plasma proteins and is, therefore, less likely to interact with highly protein-bound drugs, such as salicylates, sulfonamides, chloramphenicol and probenecid).
No products indexed under this heading.

Ketorolac Tromethamine (Metformin is negligibly bound to plasma proteins and is, therefore, less likely to interact with highly protein-bound drugs, such as salicylates, sulfonamides, chloramphenicol and probenecid). Products include:
Acuvail .... ⊙ 209

Labetalol Hydrochloride (Hypoglycemia due to metformin may be difficult to recognize in the elderly and in people who are taking β-adrenergic blocking drugs).
No products indexed under this heading.

Levalbuterol Hydrochloride (Certain drugs, including sympathomimetics, tend to produce hyperglycemia and may lead to loss of glycemic control. When such drugs are administered to a patient receiving ActoPlus Met, the patient should be closely observed to maintain adequate glycemic control).
No products indexed under this heading.

Levobunolol Hydrochloride (Hypoglycemia due to metformin may be difficult to recognize in the elderly and in people who are taking β-adrenergic blocking drugs).
No products indexed under this heading.

Levonorgestrel (Certain drugs, including oral contraceptives, tend to produce hyperglycemia and may lead to loss of glycemic control. When such drugs are administered to a patient receiving ActoPlus Met, the patient should be closely observed to maintain adequate glycemic control. Co-administration of pioglitazone (45 mg once daily) and an oral contraceptive (1 mg norethindrone plus 0.035 mg ethinyl estradiol once daily) for 21 days, resulted in 11% and 11-14% decrease in ethinyl estradiol AUC (0-24h) and C_{max} respectively. There were no significant changes in norethindrone AUC (0-24h) and C_{max}. In view of the high variability of ethinyl estradiol pharmacokinetics, the clinical significance of this finding is unknown). Products include:
Climara Pro 847
LoSeasonique 3407
Lybrel 3514
Mirena 854
Plan B 3416
Seasonique 3418

Levothyroxine Sodium (Certain drugs, including thyroid products, tend to produce hyperglycemia and may lead to loss of glycemic control. When such drugs are administered to a patient receiving ActoPlus Met, the patient should be closely observed to maintain adequate glycemic control). Products include:
Levoxyl Tablets 1843
Synthroid 529

Lidocaine (*In vivo* drug-drug interaction studies have suggested that pioglitazone may be a weak inducer of CYP450 isoform 3A4 substrate). Products include:
Lidoderm 1107

Lidocaine Hydrochloride (*In vivo* drug-drug interaction studies have suggested that pioglitazone may be a weak inducer of CYP450 isoform 3A4 substrate).
No products indexed under this heading.

Liothyronine Sodium (Certain drugs, including thyroid products, tend to produce hyperglycemia and may lead to loss of glycemic control. When such drugs are administered to a patient receiving ActoPlus Met, the patient should be closely observed to maintain adequate glycemic control). Products include:
Cytomel 1830

Liotrix (Certain drugs, including thyroid products, tend to produce hyperglycemia and may lead to loss of glycemic control. When such drugs are administered to a patient receiving ActoPlus Met, the patient should be closely observed to maintain adequate glycemic control).
No products indexed under this heading.

Lovastatin (*In vivo* drug-drug interaction studies have suggested that pioglitazone may be a weak inducer of CYP450 isoform 3A4 substrate). Products include:
Advicor 402
Mevacor 2212

Magnesium Salicylate (Metformin is negligibly bound to plasma proteins and is, therefore, less likely to interact with highly protein-bound drugs, such as salicylates).
No products indexed under this heading.

Meclofenamate Sodium (Metformin is negligibly bound to plasma proteins and is, therefore, less likely to interact with highly protein-bound drugs, such as salicylates, sulfonamides, chloramphenicol and probenecid).
No products indexed under this heading.

Mefenamic Acid (Metformin is negligibly bound to plasma proteins and is, therefore, less likely to interact with highly protein-bound drugs, such as salicylates, sulfonamides, chloramphenicol and probenecid).
No products indexed under this heading.

Mesoridazine Besylate (Certain drugs, including phenothiazines, tend to produce hyperglycemia and may lead to loss of glycemic control. When such drugs are administered to a patient receiving ActoPlus Met, the patient should be closely observed to maintain adequate glycemic control).
No products indexed under this heading.

Mestranol (Certain drugs, including oral contraceptives, tend to produce hyperglycemia and may lead to loss of glycemic control. When such drugs are administered to a patient receiving ActoPlus Met, the patient should be closely observed to maintain adequate glycemic control. Co-administration of pioglitazone (45 mg once daily) and an oral contraceptive (1 mg norethindrone plus 0.035 mg ethinyl estradiol once daily) for 21 days, resulted in 11% and 11-14% decrease in ethinyl estradiol AUC (0-24h) and C_{max} respectively. There were no significant changes in norethindrone AUC (0-24h) and C_{max}. In view of the high variability of ethinyl estradiol pharmacokinetics, the clinical significance of this finding is unknown).
No products indexed under this heading.

Metaproterenol Sulfate (Certain drugs, including sympathomimetics, tend to produce hyperglycemia and may lead to loss of glycemic control. When such drugs are administered to a patient receiving ActoPlus Met, the patient should be closely observed to maintain adequate glycemic control).
No products indexed under this heading.

Metaraminol Bitartrate (Certain drugs, including sympathomimetics, tend to produce hyperglycemia and may lead to loss of glycemic control. When such drugs are administered to a patient receiving ActoPlus Met, the patient should be closely observed to maintain adequate glycemic control).
No products indexed under this heading.

Methadone Hydrochloride (*In vivo* drug-drug interaction studies have suggested that pioglitazone may be a weak inducer of CYP450 isoform 3A4 substrate).
No products indexed under this heading.

Methotrimeprazine (Certain drugs, including phenothiazines, tend to produce hyperglycemia and may lead to loss of glycemic control. When such drugs are administered to a patient receiving ActoPlus Met, the patient should be closely observed to maintain adequate glycemic control).
No products indexed under this heading.

Methoxamine Hydrochloride (Certain drugs, including sympathomimetics, tend to produce hyperglycemia and may lead to loss of glycemic control. When such drugs are administered to a patient receiving ActoPlus Met, the patient should be closely observed to maintain adequate glycemic control).
No products indexed under this heading.

Methyclothiazide (Certain drugs, including thiazide diuretics, tend to produce hyperglycemia and may lead to loss of glycemic control. When such drugs are administered to a patient receiving ActoPlus Met, the patient should be closely observed to maintain adequate glycemic control).
No products indexed under this heading.

Methylprednisolone (Certain drugs, including corticosteroids, tend to produce hyperglycemia and may lead to loss of glycemic control. When such drugs are administered to a patient receiving ActoPlus Met, the patient should be closely observed to maintain adequate glycemic control).
No products indexed under this heading.

Methylprednisolone Acetate (Certain drugs, including corticosteroids, tend to produce hyperglycemia and may lead to loss of glycemic control. When such drugs are administered to a patient receiving ActoPlus Met, the patient should be closely observed to maintain adequate glycemic control).
No products indexed under this heading.

IMPORTANT NOTE: Always consult each drug listing in the patient's regimen for possible interactions.

Methylprednisolone Sodium Succinate (Certain drugs, including corticosteroids, tend to produce hyperglycemia and may lead to loss of glycemic control. When such drugs are administered to a patient receiving ActoPlus Met, the patient should be closely observed to maintain adequate glycemic control).
No products indexed under this heading.

Metipranolol Hydrochloride (Hypoglycemia due to metformin may be difficult to recognize in the elderly and in people who are taking β-adrenergic blocking drugs).
No products indexed under this heading.

Metolazone (Certain drugs, including thiazides and other diuretics, tend to produce hyperglycemia and may lead to loss of glycemic control. When such drugs are administered to a patient receiving ActoPlus Met, the patient should be closely observed to maintain adequate glycemic control).
No products indexed under this heading.

Metoprolol Succinate (Hypoglycemia due to metformin may be difficult to recognize in the elderly and in people who are taking β-adrenergic blocking drugs). Products include:
Toprol XL 732

Metoprolol Tartrate (Hypoglycemia due to metformin may be difficult to recognize in the elderly and in people who are taking β-adrenergic blocking drugs).
No products indexed under this heading.

Mibefradil Dihydrochloride (Certain drugs, including calcium channel blockers, tend to produce hyperglycemia and may lead to loss of glycemic control. When such drugs are administered to a patient receiving ActoPlus Met, the patient should be closely observed to maintain adequate glycemic control).
No products indexed under this heading.

Midazolam Hydrochloride (Administration of pioglitazone for 15 days followed by a single 7.5 mg dose of midazolam syrup resulted in a 26% reduction in midazolam C_{max} and AUC).
No products indexed under this heading.

Miglitol (Pioglitazone, like other thiazolidinediones, can cause fluid retention when used alone or in combination with other antihyperglycemic agents, including insulin. Fluid retention may lead to or exacerbate heart failure. In addition, patients receiving pioglitazone in combination with insulin or oral hypoglycemic agents may be at risk for hypoglycemia, and a reduction in the dose of the concomitant agent may be necessary).
No products indexed under this heading.

Mometasone Furoate (Certain drugs, including corticosteroids, tend to produce hyperglycemia and may lead to loss of glycemic control. When such drugs are administered to a patient receiving ActoPlus Met, the patient should be closely observed to maintain adequate glycemic control). Products include:
Asmanex 3058
Elocon Cream 3111
Elocon Lotion 3112
Elocon Ointment 3114

Mometasone Furoate Monohydrate (Certain drugs, including corticosteroids, tend to produce hyperglycemia and may lead to loss of glycemic control. When such drugs are administered to a patient receiving ActoPlus Met, the patient should be closely observed to maintain adequate glycemic control). Products include:
Nasonex 3166

Morphine Sulfate (Cationic drugs (eg, amiloride, digoxin, morphine, procainamide, quinidine, quinine, ranitidine, triamterene, trimethoprim, and vanco-

mycin) that are eliminated by renal tubular secretion theoretically have the potential for interaction with metformin by competing for common renal tubular transport systems. Careful patient monitoring and dose adjustment of ActoPlus Met and/or the interfering drug is recommended in patients who are taking cationic medications that are excreted via the proximal renal tubular secretory system). Products include:
Avinza 1822
Embeda 1831
MS Contin 2803

Nadolol (Hypoglycemia due to metformin may be difficult to recognize in the elderly and in people who are taking β-adrenergic blocking drugs). Products include:
Nadolol 2359

Naproxen (Metformin is negligibly bound to plasma proteins and is, therefore, less likely to interact with highly protein-bound drugs, such as salicylates, sulfonamides, chloramphenicol and probenecid). Products include:
EC-Naprosyn 2850
Naprosyn 2850
Anaprox/Naprosyn 2850

Naproxen Sodium (Metformin is negligibly bound to plasma proteins and is, therefore, less likely to interact with highly protein-bound drugs, such as salicylates, sulfonamides, chloramphenicol and probenecid). Products include:
Anaprox 2850
Anaprox DS 2850
Treximet 1681

Nateglinide (Pioglitazone, like other thiazolidinediones, can cause fluid retention when used alone or in combination with other antihyperglycemic agents, including insulin. Fluid retention may lead to or exacerbate heart failure. In addition, patients receiving pioglitazone in combination with insulin or oral hypoglycemic agents may be at risk for hypoglycemia, and a reduction in the dose of the concomitant agent may be necessary).
No products indexed under this heading.

Nebivolol (Hypoglycemia due to metformin may be difficult to recognize in the elderly and in people who are taking β-adrenergic blocking drugs). Products include:
Bystolic 1147

Nefazodone Hydrochloride (In vivo drug-drug interaction studies have suggested that pioglitazone may be a weak inducer of CYP450 isoform 3A4 substrate).
No products indexed under this heading.

Nelfinavir Mesylate (In vivo drug-drug interaction studies have suggested that pioglitazone may be a weak inducer of CYP450 isoform 3A4 substrate).
No products indexed under this heading.

Nicardipine (Certain drugs, including calcium channel blockers, tend to produce hyperglycemia and may lead to loss of glycemic control. When such drugs are administered to a patient receiving ActoPlus Met, the patient should be closely observed to maintain adequate glycemic control).
No products indexed under this heading.

Nicardipine Hydrochloride (Certain drugs, including calcium channel blockers, tend to produce hyperglycemia and may lead to loss of glycemic control. When such drugs are administered to a patient receiving ActoPlus Met, the patient should be closely observed to maintain adequate glycemic control).
No products indexed under this heading.

Nicotinic Acid (Certain drugs, including nicotinic acid, tend to produce hyperglycemia and may lead to loss of glycemic control. When such drugs are administered to a patient receiving ActoPlus Met, the patient should be closely observed to maintain adequate glycemic control).
No products indexed under this heading.

Nifedipine (A single-dose, metformin-nifedipine drug interaction study in normal healthy volunteers demonstrated that co-administration of nifedipine increased plasma metformin C_{max} and AUC by 20% and 9%, respectively, and increased the amount excreted in the urine. T_{max} and half-life were unaffected. Nifedipine appears to enhance the absorption of metformin. Metformin had minimal effects on nifedipine. In addition, co-administration of pioglitazone for 7 days with 30 mg nifedipine ER administered orally once daily for 4 days to male and female volunteers resulted in a ratio of least square mean (90% CI) values for unchanged nifedipine of 0.83 (0.73 - 0.95) for C_{max} and 0.88 (0.80 - 0.96) for AUC. In view of the high variability of nifedipine pharmacokinetics, the clinical significance of this finding is unknown).
No products indexed under this heading.

Nimodipine (Certain drugs, including calcium channel blockers, tend to produce hyperglycemia and may lead to loss of glycemic control. When such drugs are administered to a patient receiving ActoPlus Met, the patient should be closely observed to maintain adequate glycemic control).
No products indexed under this heading.

Nisoldipine (Certain drugs, including calcium channel blockers, tend to produce hyperglycemia and may lead to loss of glycemic control. When such drugs are administered to a patient receiving ActoPlus Met, the patient should be closely observed to maintain adequate glycemic control).
No products indexed under this heading.

Nitrendipine (In vivo drug-drug interaction studies have suggested that pioglitazone may be a weak inducer of CYP450 isoform 3A4 substrate).
No products indexed under this heading.

Norepinephrine Bitartrate (Certain drugs, including sympathomimetics, tend to produce hyperglycemia and may lead to loss of glycemic control. When such drugs are administered to a patient receiving ActoPlus Met, the patient should be closely observed to maintain adequate glycemic control).
No products indexed under this heading.

Norethindrone (Co-administration of pioglitazone (45 mg once daily) and an oral contraceptive (1 mg norethindrone plus 0.035 mg ethinyl estradiol once daily) for 21 days, resulted in 11% and 11-14% decrease in ethinyl estradiol AUC (0-24h) and C_{max}, respectively. There were no significant changes in norethindrone AUC (0-24h) and C_{max}. In view of the high variability of ethinyl estradiol pharmacokinetics, the clinical significance of this finding is unknown). Products include:
Ortho Micronor 2660

Norethindrone Acetate (In vivo drug-drug interaction studies have suggested that pioglitazone may be a weak inducer of CYP450 isoform 3A4 substrate). Products include:
Activella 2561

Norethynodrel (Certain drugs, including oral contraceptives, tend to produce hyperglycemia and may lead to loss of glycemic control. When such drugs are administered to a patient receiving ActoPlus Met, the patient should be closely observed to maintain adequate glycemic control. Co-administration of

pioglitazone (45 mg once daily) and an oral contraceptive (1 mg norethindrone plus 0.035 mg ethinyl estradiol once daily) for 21 days, resulted in 11% and 11-14% decrease in ethinyl estradiol AUC (0-24h) and C_{max} respectively. There were no significant changes in norethindrone AUC (0-24h) and C_{max}. In view of the high variability of ethinyl estradiol pharmacokinetics, the clinical significance of this finding is unknown).
No products indexed under this heading.

Norgestimate (Certain drugs, including oral contraceptives, tend to produce hyperglycemia and may lead to loss of glycemic control. When such drugs are administered to a patient receiving ActoPlus Met, the patient should be closely observed to maintain adequate glycemic control. Co-administration of pioglitazone (45 mg once daily) and an oral contraceptive (1 mg norethindrone plus 0.035 mg ethinyl estradiol once daily) for 21 days, resulted in 11% and 11-14% decrease in ethinyl estradiol AUC (0-24h) and C_{max} respectively. There were no significant changes in norethindrone AUC (0-24h) and C_{max}. In view of the high variability of ethinyl estradiol pharmacokinetics, the clinical significance of this finding is unknown). Products include:
Ortho-Cyclen/Ortho Tri-Cyclen 2663
Ortho Tri-Cyclen Lo Tablets 2673

Norgestrel (Certain drugs, including oral contraceptives, tend to produce hyperglycemia and may lead to loss of glycemic control. When such drugs are administered to a patient receiving ActoPlus Met, the patient should be closely observed to maintain adequate glycemic control. Co-administration of pioglitazone (45 mg once daily) and an oral contraceptive (1 mg norethindrone plus 0.035 mg ethinyl estradiol once daily) for 21 days, resulted in 11% and 11-14% decrease in ethinyl estradiol AUC (0-24h) and C_{max} respectively. There were no significant changes in norethindrone AUC (0-24h) and C_{max}. In view of the high variability of ethinyl estradiol pharmacokinetics, the clinical significance of this finding is unknown).
No products indexed under this heading.

Nortriptyline Hydrochloride (Metformin is negligibly bound to plasma proteins and is, therefore, less likely to interact with highly protein-bound drugs, such as salicylates, sulfonamides, chloramphenicol and probenecid).
No products indexed under this heading.

Omeprazole (An enzyme inhibitor of CYP2C8 (such as gemfibrozil) may significantly increase the AUC of pioglitazone. Therefore, if an inhibitor of CYP2C8 is started or stopped during treatment with pioglitazone, changes in diabetes treatment may be needed based on clinical response).
No products indexed under this heading.

Ondansetron (In vivo drug-drug interaction studies have suggested that pioglitazone may be a weak inducer of CYP450 isoform 3A4 substrate).
No products indexed under this heading.

Ondansetron Hydrochloride (In vivo drug-drug interaction studies have suggested that pioglitazone may be a weak inducer of CYP450 isoform 3A4 substrate). Products include:
Zofran Injection 1750
Zofran 1756
Zofran ODT 1756

Oxaprozin (Metformin is negligibly bound to plasma proteins and is, therefore, less likely to interact with highly protein-bound drugs, such as salicylates, sulfonamides, chloramphenicol and probenecid).
No products indexed under this heading.

Oxazepam (Metformin is negligibly bound to plasma proteins and is, therefore, less likely to interact with highly protein-bound drugs, such as salicylates, sulfonamides, chloramphenicol and probenecid).
No products indexed under this heading.

Paclitaxel (*In vivo* drug-drug interaction studies have suggested that pioglitazone may be a weak inducer of CYP450 isoform 3A4 substrate).
No products indexed under this heading.

Penbutolol Sulfate (Hypoglycemia due to metformin may be difficult to recognize in the elderly and in people who are taking β-adrenergic blocking drugs).
No products indexed under this heading.

Perphenazine (Certain drugs, including phenothiazines, tend to produce hyperglycemia and may lead to loss of glycemic control. When such drugs are administered to a patient receiving ActoPlus Met, the patient should be closely observed to maintain adequate glycemic control).
No products indexed under this heading.

Phenobarbital (An enzyme inducer of CYP2C8 (such as rifampin) may significantly decrease the AUC of pioglitazone. Therefore, if an inducer of CYP2C8 is started or stopped during treatment with pioglitazone, changes in diabetes treatment may be needed based on clinical response). Products include:
Donnatal 2711

Phenobarbital Sodium (An enzyme inducer of CYP2C8 (such as rifampin) may significantly decrease the AUC of pioglitazone. Therefore, if an inducer of CYP2C8 is started or stopped during treatment with pioglitazone, changes in diabetes treatment may be needed based on clinical response).
No products indexed under this heading.

Phenothiazine Derivatives (Certain drugs, including phenothiazines, tend to produce hyperglycemia and may lead to loss of glycemic control. When such drugs are administered to a patient receiving ActoPlus Met, the patient should be closely observed to maintain adequate glycemic control).
No products indexed under this heading.

Phenothiazines (Certain drugs, including phenothiazines, tend to produce hyperglycemia and may lead to loss of glycemic control. When such drugs are administered to a patient receiving ActoPlus Met, the patient should be closely observed to maintain adequate glycemic control).
No products indexed under this heading.

Phenylbutazone (Metformin is negligibly bound to plasma proteins and is, therefore, less likely to interact with highly protein-bound drugs, such as salicylates, sulfonamides, chloramphenicol and probenecid).
No products indexed under this heading.

Phenylephrine Bitartrate (Certain drugs, including sympathomimetics, tend to produce hyperglycemia and may lead to loss of glycemic control. When such drugs are administered to a patient receiving ActoPlus Met, the patient should be closely observed to maintain adequate glycemic control).
No products indexed under this heading.

Phenylephrine Hydrochloride (Certain drugs, including sympathomimetics, tend to produce hyperglycemia and may lead to loss of glycemic control. When such drugs are administered to a patient receiving ActoPlus Met, the patient should be closely observed to maintain adequate glycemic control).
Products include:
Sudafed PE Nasal Decongestant **2048**

Children's Sudafed PE Nasal
Decongestant.............................. 2047

Phenylephrine Tannate (Certain drugs, including sympathomimetics, tend to produce hyperglycemia and may lead to loss of glycemic control. When such drugs are administered to a patient receiving ActoPlus Met, the patient should be closely observed to maintain adequate glycemic control).
No products indexed under this heading.

Phenylpropanolamine Hydrochloride (Certain drugs, including sympathomimetics, tend to produce hyperglycemia and may lead to loss of glycemic control. When such drugs are administered to a patient receiving ActoPlus Met, the patient should be closely observed to maintain adequate glycemic control).
No products indexed under this heading.

Phenytoin (Certain drugs, including phenytoin, tend to produce hyperglycemia and may lead to loss of glycemic control. When such drugs are administered to a patient receiving ActoPlus Met, the patient should be closely observed to maintain adequate glycemic control).
No products indexed under this heading.

Phenytoin Sodium (Certain drugs, including phenytoin, tend to produce hyperglycemia and may lead to loss of glycemic control. When such drugs are administered to a patient receiving ActoPlus Met, the patient should be closely observed to maintain adequate glycemic control). Products include:
Phenytek Capsules 2380

Pimozide (*In vivo* drug-drug interaction studies have suggested that pioglitazone may be a weak inducer of CYP450 isoform 3A4 substrate).
No products indexed under this heading.

Pindolol (Hypoglycemia due to metformin may be difficult to recognize in the elderly and in people who are taking β-adrenergic blocking drugs).
No products indexed under this heading.

Pirbuterol Acetate (Certain drugs, including sympathomimetics, tend to produce hyperglycemia and may lead to loss of glycemic control. When such drugs are administered to a patient receiving ActoPlus Met, the patient should be closely observed to maintain adequate glycemic control). Products include:
Maxair Autohaler **1782**

Piroxicam (Metformin is negligibly bound to plasma proteins and is, therefore, less likely to interact with highly protein-bound drugs, such as salicylates, sulfonamides, chloramphenicol and probenecid).
No products indexed under this heading.

Polyestradiol Phosphate (Certain drugs, including estrogens, tend to produce hyperglycemia and may lead to loss of glycemic control. When such drugs are administered to a patient receiving ActoPlus Met, the patient should be closely observed to maintain adequate glycemic control).
No products indexed under this heading.

Polythiazide (Certain drugs, including thiazide diuretics, tend to produce hyperglycemia and may lead to loss of glycemic control. When such drugs are administered to a patient receiving ActoPlus Met, the patient should be closely observed to maintain adequate glycemic control).
No products indexed under this heading.

Prednisolone (Certain drugs, including corticosteroids, tend to produce hyperglycemia and may lead to loss of glycemic control. When such drugs are administered to a patient receiving ActoPlus Met, the patient should be closely observed to maintain adequate glycemic control).
No products indexed under this heading.

Prednisolone Acetate (Certain drugs, including corticosteroids, tend to produce hyperglycemia and may lead to loss of glycemic control. When such drugs are administered to a patient receiving ActoPlus Met, the patient should be closely observed to maintain adequate glycemic control). Products include:
Blephamide .... ⊙**212,** ⊙**214**
Pred Forte .... ⊙**225**
Pred Mild .... ⊙**230**
Pred-G .... ⊙**226,** ⊙**227**

Prednisolone Sodium Phosphate (Certain drugs, including corticosteroids, tend to produce hyperglycemia and may lead to loss of glycemic control. When such drugs are administered to a patient receiving ActoPlus Met, the patient should be closely observed to maintain adequate glycemic control).
No products indexed under this heading.

Prednisolone Tebutate (Certain drugs, including corticosteroids, tend to produce hyperglycemia and may lead to loss of glycemic control. When such drugs are administered to a patient receiving ActoPlus Met, the patient should be closely observed to maintain adequate glycemic control).
No products indexed under this heading.

Prednisone (Certain drugs, including corticosteroids, tend to produce hyperglycemia and may lead to loss of glycemic control. When such drugs are administered to a patient receiving ActoPlus Met, the patient should be closely observed to maintain adequate glycemic control).
No products indexed under this heading.

Prednisone sodium phosphate (Certain drugs, including corticosteroids, tend to produce hyperglycemia and may lead to loss of glycemic control. When such drugs are administered to a patient receiving ActoPlus Met, the patient should be closely observed to maintain adequate glycemic control).
No products indexed under this heading.

Primidone (An enzyme inducer of CYP2C8 (such as rifampin) may significantly decrease the AUC of pioglitazone. Therefore, if an inducer of CYP2C8 is started or stopped during treatment with pioglitazone, changes in diabetes treatment may be needed based on clinical response).
No products indexed under this heading.

Probenecid (Metformin is negligibly bound to plasma proteins and is therefore, less likely to interact with highly protein-bound drugs, such as probenecid).
No products indexed under this heading.

Procainamide (Cationic drugs (eg, amiloride, digoxin, morphine, procainamide, quinidine, quinine, ranitidine, triamterene, trimethoprim, and vancomycin) that are eliminated by renal tubular secretion theoretically have the potential for interaction with metformin by competing for common renal tubular transport systems. Careful patient monitoring and dose adjustment of ActoPlus Met and/or the interfering drug is recommended in patients who are taking cationic medications that are excreted via the proximal renal tubular secretory system).
No products indexed under this heading.

Procainamide Hydrochloride (Cationic drugs (eg, amiloride, digoxin, morphine, procainamide, quinidine, quinine, ranitidine, triamterene, trimethoprim, and vancomycin) that are eliminated by renal tubular secretion theoretically have the potential for interaction with metformin by competing for common renal tubular transport systems. Careful patient monitoring and dose adjustment of ActoPlus Met and/or the interfering drug is recommended in patients who are taking cationic medications that are excreted via the proximal renal tubular secretory system).
No products indexed under this heading.

Prochlorperazine (Certain drugs, including phenothiazines, tend to produce hyperglycemia and may lead to loss of glycemic control. When such drugs are administered to a patient receiving ActoPlus Met, the patient should be closely observed to maintain adequate glycemic control).
No products indexed under this heading.

Prochlorperazine Edisylate (Certain drugs, including phenothiazines, tend to produce hyperglycemia and may lead to loss of glycemic control. When such drugs are administered to a patient receiving ActoPlus Met, the patient should be closely observed to maintain adequate glycemic control).
No products indexed under this heading.

Prochlorperazine Maleate (Certain drugs, including phenothiazines, tend to produce hyperglycemia and may lead to loss of glycemic control. When such drugs are administered to a patient receiving ActoPlus Met, the patient should be closely observed to maintain adequate glycemic control).
No products indexed under this heading.

Promethazine (Certain drugs, including phenothiazines, tend to produce hyperglycemia and may lead to loss of glycemic control. When such drugs are administered to a patient receiving ActoPlus Met, the patient should be closely observed to maintain adequate glycemic control).
No products indexed under this heading.

Promethazine Hydrochloride (Certain drugs, including phenothiazines, tend to produce hyperglycemia and may lead to loss of glycemic control. When such drugs are administered to a patient receiving ActoPlus Met, the patient should be closely observed to maintain adequate glycemic control).
No products indexed under this heading.

Propranolol Hydrochloride (Metformin is negligibly bound to plasma proteins and is, therefore, less likely to interact with highly protein-bound drugs, such as salicylates, sulfonamides, chloramphenicol and probenecid). Products include:
InnoPran XL **1517**

Pseudoephedrine Hydrochloride (Certain drugs, including sympathomimetics, tend to produce hyperglycemia and may lead to loss of glycemic control. When such drugs are administered to a patient receiving ActoPlus Met, the patient should be closely observed to maintain adequate glycemic control).
Products include:
Allegra-D **2915**
Allegra-D 24 ....**2918**
Sudafed 12 Hour Nasal
   Decongestant Non-Drowsy **2048**
Sudafed 24 Hour **2048**
Sudafed Nasal Decongestant **2047**
Children's Sudafed Nasal
   Decongestant Liquid **2047**
Zyrtec-D Allergy & Congestion **2054**

Pseudoephedrine Sulfate (Certain drugs, including sympathomimetics, tend to produce hyperglycemia and may lead to loss of glycemic control. When such drugs are administered to a patient receiving ActoPlus Met, the

ActoPlus Interactions Index 34

patient should be closely observed to maintain adequate glycemic control). Products include:
Clarinex-D 12-Hour 3101
Clarinex-D 3104

Quercetin (An enzyme inhibitor of CYP2C8 (such as gemfibrozil) may significantly increase the AUC of pioglitazone. Therefore, if an inhibitor of CYP2C8 is started or stopped during treatment with pioglitazone, changes in diabetes treatment may be needed based on clinical response).
No products indexed under this heading.

Quinestrol (Certain drugs, including estrogens, tend to produce hyperglycemia and may lead to loss of glycemic control. When such drugs are administered to a patient receiving ActoPlus Met, the patient should be closely observed to maintain adequate glycemic control).
No products indexed under this heading.

Quinidine (Cationic drugs (eg, quinidine) that are eliminated by renal tubular secretion theoretically have the potential for interaction with metformin by competing for common renal tubular transport systems. Careful patient monitoring and dose adjustment of ActoPlus Met and/or the interfering drug is recommended in patients who are taking cationic medications that are excreted via the proximal renal tubular secretory system).
No products indexed under this heading.

Quinidine Gluconate (Cationic drugs (eg, quinidine) that are eliminated by renal tubular secretion theoretically have the potential for interaction with metformin by competing for common renal tubular transport systems. Careful patient monitoring and dose adjustment of ActoPlus Met and/or the interfering drug is recommended in patients who are taking cationic medications that are excreted via the proximal renal tubular secretory system).
No products indexed under this heading.

Quinidine Hydrochloride (Cationic drugs (eg, quinidine) that are eliminated by renal tubular secretion theoretically have the potential for interaction with metformin by competing for common renal tubular transport systems. Careful patient monitoring and dose adjustment of ActoPlus Met and/or the interfering drug is recommended in patients who are taking cationic medications that are excreted via the proximal renal tubular secretory system).
No products indexed under this heading.

Quinidine Polygalacturonate (Cationic drugs (eg, quinidine) that are eliminated by renal tubular secretion theoretically have the potential for interaction with metformin by competing for common renal tubular transport systems. Careful patient monitoring and dose adjustment of ActoPlus Met and/or the interfering drug is recommended in patients who are taking cationic medications that are excreted via the proximal renal tubular secretory system).
No products indexed under this heading.

Quinidine Sulfate (Cationic drugs (eg, quinidine) that are eliminated by renal tubular secretion theoretically have the potential for interaction with metformin by competing for common renal tubular transport systems. Careful patient monitoring and dose adjustment of ActoPlus Met and/or the interfering drug is recommended in patients who are taking cationic medications that are excreted via the proximal renal tubular secretory system).
No products indexed under this heading.

Quinine (Cationic drugs (eg, amiloride, digoxin, morphine, procainamide, quinidine, quinine, ranitidine, triamterene, trimethoprim, and vancomycin) that are eliminated by renal tubular secretion theoretically have the potential for interaction with metformin by competing for common renal tubular transport systems. Careful patient monitoring and dose adjustment of ActoPlus Met and/or the interfering drug is recommended in patients who are taking cationic medications that are excreted via the proximal renal tubular secretory system). Products include:
Hyland's Leg Cramps PM with Quinine......................... 3315

Quinine Sulfate (Cationic drugs (eg, amiloride, digoxin, morphine, procainamide, quinidine, quinine, ranitidine, triamterene, trimethoprim, and vancomycin) that are eliminated by renal tubular secretion theoretically have the potential for interaction with metformin by competing for common renal tubular transport systems. Careful patient monitoring and dose adjustment of ActoPlus Met and/or the interfering drug is recommended in patients who are taking cationic medications that are excreted via the proximal renal tubular secretory system).
No products indexed under this heading.

Ranitidine Bismuth Citrate (Cationic drugs (eg, amiloride, digoxin, morphine, procainamide, quinidine, quinine, ranitidine, triamterene, trimethoprim, and vancomycin) that are eliminated by renal tubular secretion theoretically have the potential for interaction with metformin by competing for common renal tubular transport systems. Careful patient monitoring and dose adjustment of ActoPlus Met and/or the interfering drug is recommended in patients who are taking cationic medications that are excreted via the proximal renal tubular secretory system).
No products indexed under this heading.

Ranitidine Hydrochloride (Cationic drugs (eg, amiloride, digoxin, morphine, procainamide, quinidine, quinine, ranitidine, triamterene, trimethoprim, and vancomycin) that are eliminated by renal tubular secretion theoretically have the potential for interaction with metformin by competing for common renal tubular transport systems. Careful patient monitoring and dose adjustment of ActoPlus Met and/or the interfering drug is recommended in patients who are taking cationic medications that are excreted via the proximal renal tubular secretory system). Products include:
Zantac 1737
Zantac Injection 1732
Zantac Pharmacy 1735

Repaglinide (Pioglitazone, like other thiazolidinediones, can cause fluid retention when used alone or in combination with other antihyperglycemic agents, including insulin. Fluid retention may lead to or exacerbate heart failure. In addition, patients receiving pioglitazone in combination with insulin or oral hypoglycemic agents may be at risk for hypoglycemia, and a reduction in the dose of the concomitant agent may be necessary).
No products indexed under this heading.

Rifabutin (An enzyme inducer of CYP2C8 (such as rifampin) may significantly decrease the AUC of pioglitazone. Therefore, if an inducer of CYP2C8 is started or stopped during treatment with pioglitazone, changes in diabetes treatment may be needed based on clinical response).
No products indexed under this heading.

Rifampin (Concomitant administration of rifampin (oral 600 mg once daily), an inducer of CYP2C8 with pioglitazone (oral 30 mg) in 10 healthy volunteers pre-treated for 5 days prior with rifampin (oral 600 mg once daily) resulted in a decrease in the AUC of pioglitazone by 54%. If an inducer of CYP2C8 (such as rifampin) is started or stopped during treatment with pioglitazone, changes in diabetes treatment may be needed based on clinical response).
No products indexed under this heading.

Ritonavir (*In vivo* drug-drug interaction studies have suggested that pioglitazone may be a weak inducer of CYP450 isoform 3A4 substrate). Products include:
Kaletra 458
Norvir 509

Rosiglitazone Maleate (Pioglitazone, like other thiazolidinediones, can cause fluid retention when used alone or in combination with other antihyperglycemic agents, including insulin. Fluid retention may lead to or exacerbate heart failure. In addition, patients receiving pioglitazone in combination with insulin or oral hypoglycemic agents may be at risk for hypoglycemia, and a reduction in the dose of the concomitant agent may be necessary). Products include:
Avandamet 1345
Avandaryl 1356
Avandia 1366

Salmeterol Xinafoate (Certain drugs, including sympathomimetics, tend to produce hyperglycemia and may lead to loss of glycemic control. When such drugs are administered to a patient receiving ActoPlus Met, the patient should be closely observed to maintain adequate glycemic control). Products include:
Advair 100/50 1275
Advair 250/50 1275
Advair 500/50 1275
Advair HFA 45/21 1288
Advair HFA 115/21 1288
Advair HFA 230/21 1288
Serevent Diskus 1656

Salsalate (Metformin is negligibly bound to plasma proteins and is, therefore, less likely to interact with highly protein-bound drugs, such as salicylates).
No products indexed under this heading.

Saquinavir (*In vivo* drug-drug interaction studies have suggested that pioglitazone may be a weak inducer of CYP450 isoform 3A4 substrate).
No products indexed under this heading.

Saquinavir Mesylate (*In vivo* drug-drug interaction studies have suggested that pioglitazone may be a weak inducer of CYP450 isoform 3A4 substrate).
No products indexed under this heading.

Sertraline Hydrochloride (*In vivo* drug-drug interaction studies have suggested that pioglitazone may be a weak inducer of CYP450 isoform 3A4 substrate).
No products indexed under this heading.

Sildenafil Citrate (*In vivo* drug-drug interaction studies have suggested that pioglitazone may be a weak inducer of CYP450 isoform 3A4 substrate).
No products indexed under this heading.

Simvastatin (*In vivo* drug-drug interaction studies have suggested that pioglitazone may be a weak inducer of CYP450 isoform 3A4 substrate). Products include:
Simcor 524
Vytorin 10/10 .... 2303, 3240
Vytorin 10/20 .... 2303, 3240
Vytorin 10/40 .... 2303, 3240
Vytorin 10/80 .... 2303, 3240
Zocor 2289

Sirolimus (*In vivo* drug-drug interaction studies have suggested that pioglitazone may be a weak inducer of CYP450 isoform 3A4 substrate). Products include:
Rapamune 3579

Sitagliptin Phosphate (Pioglitazone, like other thiazolidinediones, can cause fluid retention when used alone or in combination with other antihyperglycemic agents, including insulin. Fluid retention may lead to or exacerbate heart failure. In addition, patients receiving pioglitazone in combination with insulin or oral hypoglycemic agents may be at risk for hypoglycemia, and a reduction in the dose of the concomitant agent may be necessary). Products include:
Janumet 2188
Januvia 2196

Sotalol Hydrochloride (Hypoglycemia due to metformin may be difficult to recognize in the elderly and in people who are taking β-adrenergic blocking drugs).
No products indexed under this heading.

Spironolactone (Certain drugs, including thiazides and other diuretics, tend to produce hyperglycemia and may lead to loss of glycemic control. When such drugs are administered to a patient receiving ActoPlus Met, the patient should be closely observed to maintain adequate glycemic control).
No products indexed under this heading.

Sulfacytine (Metformin is negligibly bound to plasma proteins and is, therefore, less likely to interact with highly protein-bound drugs, such as sulfonamides).
No products indexed under this heading.

Sulfamethizole (Metformin is negligibly bound to plasma proteins and is, therefore, less likely to interact with highly protein-bound drugs, such as sulfonamides).
No products indexed under this heading.

Sulfamethoxazole (Metformin is negligibly bound to plasma proteins and is, therefore, less likely to interact with highly protein-bound drugs, such as sulfonamides).
No products indexed under this heading.

Sulfaphenazole (An enzyme inhibitor of CYP2C8 (such as gemfibrozil) may significantly increase the AUC of pioglitazone. Therefore, if an inhibitor of CYP2C8 is started or stopped during treatment with pioglitazone, changes in diabetes treatment may be needed based on clinical response).
No products indexed under this heading.

Sulfasalazine (Metformin is negligibly bound to plasma proteins and is, therefore, less likely to interact with highly protein-bound drugs, such as sulfonamides).
No products indexed under this heading.

Sulfinpyrazone (An enzyme inhibitor of CYP2C8 (such as gemfibrozil) may significantly increase the AUC of pioglitazone. Therefore, if an inhibitor of CYP2C8 is started or stopped during treatment with pioglitazone, changes in diabetes treatment may be needed based on clinical response).
No products indexed under this heading.

Sulfisoxazole Acetyl (Metformin is negligibly bound to plasma proteins and is, therefore, less likely to interact with highly protein-bound drugs, such as sulfonamides).
No products indexed under this heading.

Sulfisoxazole Diolamine (Metformin is negligibly bound to plasma proteins and is, therefore, less likely to interact with highly protein-bound drugs, such as sulfonamides).
No products indexed under this heading.

Sulindac (Metformin is negligibly bound to plasma proteins and is, therefore, less likely to interact with highly protein-bound drugs, such as salicylates, sulfonamides, chloramphenicol and probenecid). Products include:
Clinoril 2098

Tacrolimus (*In vivo* drug-drug interaction studies have suggested that piogli-

tazone may be a weak inducer of CYP450 isoform 3A4 substrate). Products include:

Prograf Capsules 677
Prograf Injection 677
Protopic 685

Tadalafil (*In vivo* drug-drug interaction studies have suggested that pioglitazone may be a weak inducer of CYP450 isoform 3A4 substrate). Products include:

Adcirca 3461
Cialis 1861

Tamoxifen Citrate (*In vivo* drug-drug interaction studies have suggested that pioglitazone may be a weak inducer of CYP450 isoform 3A4 substrate).
No products indexed under this heading.

Temazepam (Metformin is negligibly bound to plasma proteins and is, therefore, less likely to interact with highly protein-bound drugs, such as salicylates, sulfonamides, chloramphenicol and probenecid).
No products indexed under this heading.

Terbutaline Sulfate (Certain drugs, including sympathomimetics, tend to produce hyperglycemia and may lead to loss of glycemic control. When such drugs are administered to a patient receiving ActoPlus Met, the patient should be closely observed to maintain adequate glycemic control).
No products indexed under this heading.

Terfenadine (*In vivo* drug-drug interaction studies have suggested that pioglitazone may be a weak inducer of CYP450 isoform 3A4 substrate).
No products indexed under this heading.

Theophylline (*In vivo* drug-drug interaction studies have suggested that pioglitazone may be a weak inducer of CYP450 isoform 3A4 substrate).
No products indexed under this heading.

Theophylline Anhydrous (*In vivo* drug-drug interaction studies have suggested that pioglitazone may be a weak inducer of CYP450 isoform 3A4 substrate). Products include:

Uniphyl 2817

Theophylline Calcium Salicylate (*In vivo* drug-drug interaction studies have suggested that pioglitazone may be a weak inducer of CYP450 isoform 3A4 substrate).
No products indexed under this heading.

Theophylline Dihydroxypropyl (Glyceryl) (*In vivo* drug-drug interaction studies have suggested that pioglitazone may be a weak inducer of CYP450 isoform 3A4 substrate).
No products indexed under this heading.

Theophylline Ethylenediamine (*In vivo* drug-drug interaction studies have suggested that pioglitazone may be a weak inducer of CYP450 isoform 3A4 substrate).
No products indexed under this heading.

Theophylline Sodium Glycinate (*In vivo* drug-drug interaction studies have suggested that pioglitazone may be a weak inducer of CYP450 isoform 3A4 substrate).
No products indexed under this heading.

Thioridazine (Certain drugs, including phenothiazines, tend to produce hyperglycemia and may lead to loss of glycemic control. When such drugs are administered to a patient receiving ActoPlus Met, the patient should be closely observed to maintain adequate glycemic control).
No products indexed under this heading.

Thioridazine Hydrochloride (Certain drugs, including phenothiazines, tend to produce hyperglycemia and may lead to loss of glycemic control. When such drugs are administered to a patient receiving ActoPlus Met, the

patient should be closely observed to maintain adequate glycemic control). Products include:

Thioridazine Hydrochloride 2384

Thyroglobulin (Certain drugs, including thyroid products, tend to produce hyperglycemia and may lead to loss of glycemic control. When such drugs are administered to a patient receiving ActoPlus Met, the patient should be closely observed to maintain adequate glycemic control).
No products indexed under this heading.

Thyroid (Certain drugs, including thyroid products, tend to produce hyperglycemia and may lead to loss of glycemic control. When such drugs are administered to a patient receiving ActoPlus Met, the patient should be closely observed to maintain adequate glycemic control). Products include:

Naturethroid 2830

Thyroxine (Certain drugs, including thyroid products, tend to produce hyperglycemia and may lead to loss of glycemic control. When such drugs are administered to a patient receiving ActoPlus Met, the patient should be closely observed to maintain adequate glycemic control).
No products indexed under this heading.

Thyroxine Sodium (Certain drugs, including thyroid products, tend to produce hyperglycemia and may lead to loss of glycemic control. When such drugs are administered to a patient receiving ActoPlus Met, the patient should be closely observed to maintain adequate glycemic control).
No products indexed under this heading.

Tiagabine Hydrochloride (*In vivo* drug-drug interaction studies have suggested that pioglitazone may be a weak inducer of CYP450 isoform 3A4 substrate). Products include:

Gabitril 972

Timolol Hemihydrate (Hypoglycemia due to metformin may be difficult to recognize in the elderly and in people who are taking β-adrenergic blocking drugs). Products include:

Betimol 3490

Timolol Maleate (Hypoglycemia due to metformin may be difficult to recognize in the elderly and in people who are taking β-adrenergic blocking drugs). Products include:

Combigan 601
Dorzolamide
Hydrochloride/Timolol Maleate
Ophthalmic Solution ....⊙243
Timoptic in Ocudose ....⊙231

Tolazamide (Pioglitazone, like other thiazolidinediones, can cause fluid retention when used alone or in combination with other antihyperglycemic agents, including insulin. Fluid retention may lead to or exacerbate heart failure. In addition, patients receiving pioglitazone in combination with insulin or oral hypoglycemic agents may be at risk for hypoglycemia, and a reduction in the dose of the concomitant agent may be necessary).
No products indexed under this heading.

Tolbutamide (Pioglitazone, like other thiazolidinediones, can cause fluid retention when used alone or in combination with other antihyperglycemic agents, including insulin. Fluid retention may lead to or exacerbate heart failure. In addition, patients receiving pioglitazone in combination with insulin or oral hypoglycemic agents may be at risk for hypoglycemia, and a reduction in the dose of the concomitant agent may be necessary).
No products indexed under this heading.

Tolmetin Sodium (Metformin is negligibly bound to plasma proteins and is, therefore, less likely to interact with highly protein-bound drugs, such as salicylates, sulfonamides, chloramphenicol and probenecid).
No products indexed under this heading.

Tolterodine Tartrate (*In vivo* drug-drug interaction studies have suggested that pioglitazone may be a weak inducer of CYP450 isoform 3A4 substrate).
No products indexed under this heading.

Torsemide (Certain drugs, including thiazides and other diuretics, tend to produce hyperglycemia and may lead to loss of glycemic control. When such drugs are administered to a patient receiving ActoPlus Met, the patient should be closely observed to maintain adequate glycemic control).
No products indexed under this heading.

Trazodone Hydrochloride (*In vivo* drug-drug interaction studies have suggested that pioglitazone may be a weak inducer of CYP450 isoform 3A4 substrate).
No products indexed under this heading.

Triamcinolone (Certain drugs, including corticosteroids, tend to produce hyperglycemia and may lead to loss of glycemic control. When such drugs are administered to a patient receiving ActoPlus Met, the patient should be closely observed to maintain adequate glycemic control).
No products indexed under this heading.

Triamcinolone Acetonide (Certain drugs, including corticosteroids, tend to produce hyperglycemia and may lead to loss of glycemic control. When such drugs are administered to a patient receiving ActoPlus Met, the patient should be closely observed to maintain adequate glycemic control). Products include:

Azmacort 408
Nasacort AQ 3019

Triamcinolone Diacetate (Certain drugs, including corticosteroids, tend to produce hyperglycemia and may lead to loss of glycemic control. When such drugs are administered to a patient receiving ActoPlus Met, the patient should be closely observed to maintain adequate glycemic control).
No products indexed under this heading.

Triamcinolone Hexacetonide (Certain drugs, including corticosteroids, tend to produce hyperglycemia and may lead to loss of glycemic control. When such drugs are administered to a patient receiving ActoPlus Met, the patient should be closely observed to maintain adequate glycemic control).
No products indexed under this heading.

Triamterene (Cationic drugs (eg, amiloride, digoxin, morphine, procainamide, quinidine, quinine, ranitidine, triamterene, trimethoprim, and vancomycin) that are eliminated by renal tubular secretion theoretically have the potential for interaction with metformin by competing for common renal tubular transport systems. Careful patient monitoring and dose adjustment of ActoPlus Met and/or the interfering drug is recommended in patients who are taking cationic medications that are excreted via the proximal renal tubular secretory system). Products include:

Dyazide 1429
Dyrenium 3495

Triazolam (*In vivo* drug-drug interaction studies have suggested that pioglitazone may be a weak inducer of CYP450 isoform 3A4 substrate).
No products indexed under this heading.

Trifluoperazine Hydrochloride (Certain drugs, including phenothiazines, tend to produce hyperglycemia and may lead to loss of glycemic control. When such drugs are administered to a patient receiving ActoPlus Met, the patient should be closely observed to maintain adequate glycemic control).
No products indexed under this heading.

Trimethoprim (Cationic drugs (eg, amiloride, digoxin, morphine, procainamide, quinidine, quinine, ranitidine, triamterene, trimethoprim, and vancomycin) that are eliminated by renal tubular secretion theoretically have the potential for interaction with metformin by competing for common renal tubular transport systems. Careful patient monitoring and dose adjustment of ActoPlus Met and/or the interfering drug is recommended in patients who are taking cationic medications that are excreted via the proximal renal tubular secretory system).
No products indexed under this heading.

Trimethoprim Hydrochloride (Cationic drugs (eg, amiloride, digoxin, morphine, procainamide, quinidine, quinine, ranitidine, triamterene, trimethoprim, and vancomycin) that are eliminated by renal tubular secretion theoretically have the potential for interaction with metformin by competing for common renal tubular transport systems. Careful patient monitoring and dose adjustment of ActoPlus Met and/or the interfering drug is recommended in patients who are taking cationic medications that are excreted via the proximal renal tubular secretory system).
No products indexed under this heading.

Trimethoprim Sulfate (Cationic drugs (eg, amiloride, digoxin, morphine, procainamide, quinidine, quinine, ranitidine, triamterene, trimethoprim, and vancomycin) that are eliminated by renal tubular secretion theoretically have the potential for interaction with metformin by competing for common renal tubular transport systems. Careful patient monitoring and dose adjustment of ActoPlus Met and/or the interfering drug is recommended in patients who are taking cationic medications that are excreted via the proximal renal tubular secretory system).
No products indexed under this heading.

Trimipramine Maleate (Metformin is negligibly bound to plasma proteins and is, therefore, less likely to interact with highly protein-bound drugs, such as salicylates, sulfonamides, chloramphenicol and probenecid).
No products indexed under this heading.

Troglitazone (Pioglitazone, like other thiazolidinediones, can cause fluid retention when used alone or in combination with other antihyperglycemic agents, including insulin. Fluid retention may lead to or exacerbate heart failure. In addition, patients receiving pioglitazone in combination with insulin or oral hypoglycemic agents may be at risk for hypoglycemia, and a reduction in the dose of the concomitant agent may be necessary).
No products indexed under this heading.

Tyropanoate Sodium (Radiologic studies involving the use of intravascular iodinated contrast materials is contraindicated during therapy with Actoplus Met. Intravascular contrast studies with iodinated materials can lead to acute alteration of renal function and have been associated with lactic acidosis in patients receiving metformin. Therefore, in patients in whom any such study is planned, ActoPlus Met should be temporarily discontinued at the time of or prior to the procedure, and withheld for 48 hours subsequent

---

IMPORTANT NOTE: Always consult each drug listing in the patient's regimen for possible interactions.

to the procedure and reinstituted only after renal function has been re-evaluated and found to be normal).

No products indexed under this heading.

Vancomycin Hydrochloride (Cationic drugs (eg, amiloride, digoxin, morphine, procainamide, quinidine, quinine, ranitidine, triamterene, trimethoprim, and vancomycin) that are eliminated by renal tubular secretion theoretically have the potential for interaction with metformin by competing for common renal tubular transport systems. Careful patient monitoring and dose adjustment of ActoPlus Met and/or the interfering drug is recommended in patients who are taking cationic medications that are excreted via the proximal renal tubular secretory system).

No products indexed under this heading.

Vardenafil Hydrochloride (In vivo drug-drug interaction studies have suggested that pioglitazone may be a weak inducer of CYP450 isoform 3A4 substrate). Products include:

Levitra 3157

Verapamil Hydrochloride (Certain drugs, including calcium channel blockers, tend to produce hyperglycemia and may lead to loss of glycemic control. When such drugs are administered to a patient receiving ActoPlus Met, the patient should be closely observed to maintain adequate glycemic control). Products include:

Tarka 534

Vinblastine Sulfate (In vivo drug-drug interaction studies have suggested that pioglitazone may be a weak inducer of CYP450 isoform 3A4 substrate).

No products indexed under this heading.

Vincristine Sulfate (In vivo drug-drug interaction studies have suggested that pioglitazone may be a weak inducer of CYP450 isoform 3A4 substrate).

No products indexed under this heading.

Vitamin B12 (In controlled clinical trials of metformin at 29 weeks' duration, a decrease to subnormal levels of previously normal serum vitamin B_{12} levels, without clinical manifestations, was observed in approximately 7% of patients). Products include:

Animi-3 2711
Authia 3497
Bevitamel 3497
Cardio Basics 3455
Divista 3474
Ferralet 2333
Heplive 607
Nascobal 2700

Warfarin Sodium (In vivo drug-drug interaction studies have suggested that pioglitazone may be a weak inducer of CYP450 isoform 3A4 substrate).

No products indexed under this heading.

Food Interactions

Alcohol (Alcohol is known to potentiate the effect of metformin on lactate metabolism. Patients, therefore, should be warned against excessive alcohol intake, acute or chronic, while receiving ActoPlus Met. In addition, hypoglycemia does not occur in patients receiving metformin alone under usual circumstances of use, but could occur when during concomitant use with ethanol).

Beer, reduced-alcohol (Alcohol is known to potentiate the effect of metformin on lactate metabolism. Patients, therefore, should be warned against excessive alcohol intake, acute or chronic, while receiving ActoPlus Met. In addition, hypoglycemia does not occur in patients receiving metformin alone under usual circumstances of use, but could occur when during concomitant use with ethanol).

Beer, unspecified (Alcohol is known to potentiate the effect of metformin on lactate metabolism. Patients, therefore, should be warned against excessive alcohol intake, acute or chronic, while receiving ActoPlus Met. In addition, hypoglycemia does not occur in patients receiving metformin alone under usual circumstances of use, but could occur when during concomitant use with ethanol).

Food, unspecified (Administration of ActoPlus Met 15 mg/850 mg with food resulted in no change in overall exposure of pioglitazone. With metformin there was no change in AUC; however, mean peak serum concentration of metformin was decreased by 28% when administered with food. A delayed time to peak serum concentration was observed for both components (1.9 hours for pioglitazone and 0.8 hours for metformin) under fed conditions. These changes are not likely to be clinically significant).

Meal, unspecified (Administration of ActoPlus Met 15 mg/850 mg with food resulted in no change in overall exposure of pioglitazone. With metformin there was no change in AUC; however, mean peak serum concentration of metformin was decreased by 28% when administered with food. A delayed time to peak serum concentration was observed for both components (1.9 hours for pioglitazone and 0.8 hours for metformin) under fed conditions. These changes are not likely to be clinically significant).

Wine, Chianti (Alcohol is known to potentiate the effect of metformin on lactate metabolism. Patients, therefore, should be warned against excessive alcohol intake, acute or chronic, while receiving ActoPlus Met. In addition, hypoglycemia does not occur in patients receiving metformin alone under usual circumstances of use, but could occur when during concomitant use with ethanol).

Wine, Red (Alcohol is known to potentiate the effect of metformin on lactate metabolism. Patients, therefore, should be warned against excessive alcohol intake, acute or chronic, while receiving ActoPlus Met. In addition, hypoglycemia does not occur in patients receiving metformin alone under usual circumstances of use, but could occur when during concomitant use with ethanol).

Wine, unspecified (Alcohol is known to potentiate the effect of metformin on lactate metabolism. Patients, therefore, should be warned against excessive alcohol intake, acute or chronic, while receiving ActoPlus Met. In addition, hypoglycemia does not occur in patients receiving metformin alone under usual circumstances of use, but could occur when during concomitant use with ethanol).

Wine products (Alcohol is known to potentiate the effect of metformin on lactate metabolism. Patients, therefore, should be warned against excessive alcohol intake, acute or chronic, while receiving ActoPlus Met. In addition, hypoglycemia does not occur in patients receiving metformin alone under usual circumstances of use, but could occur when during concomitant use with ethanol).

ACTOS TABLETS

(Pioglitazone Hydrochloride) 3345

May interact with cytochrome p450 2c8 inducers (selected), cytochrome p450 2c8 inhibitors (selected), cytochrome p450 3a4 substrates (selected), insulin, oral contraceptives,

oral hypoglycemic agents, sulfonylureas, and certain other agents. Compounds in these categories include:

Acarbose (Patients receiving pioglitazone in combination with other oral hypoglycemic agents may be at risk for hypoglycemia, and a reduction in the dose of the concomitant agent may be necessary).

No products indexed under this heading.

Alfentanil Hydrochloride (In vivo drug-drug interaction studies have suggested that pioglitazone may be a weak inducer of CYP 450 isoform 3A4 substrate).

No products indexed under this heading.

Alprazolam (In vivo drug-drug interaction studies have suggested that pioglitazone may be a weak inducer of CYP 450 isoform 3A4 substrate).

No products indexed under this heading.

Amiodarone Hydrochloride (In vivo drug-drug interaction studies have suggested that pioglitazone may be a weak inducer of CYP 450 isoform 3A4 substrate).

No products indexed under this heading.

Amitriptyline Hydrochloride (In vivo drug-drug interaction studies have suggested that pioglitazone may be a weak inducer of CYP 450 isoform 3A4 substrate).

No products indexed under this heading.

Amlodipine Besylate (In vivo drug-drug interaction studies have suggested that pioglitazone may be a weak inducer of CYP 450 isoform 3A4 substrate). Products include:

Azor 1010
Exforge 2443
Exforge HCT 2449

Anastrozole (An enzyme inhibitor of CYP2C8 (such as gemfibrozil) may significantly increase the AUC of pioglitazone. Therefore, if an inhibitor of CYP2C8 is started or stopped during treatment with pioglitazone, changes in diabetes treatment may be needed based on clinical response).

No products indexed under this heading.

Aprepitant (In vivo drug-drug interaction studies have suggested that pioglitazone may be a weak inducer of CYP 450 isoform 3A4 substrate). Products include:

Emend 2124

Astemizole (In vivo drug-drug interaction studies have suggested that pioglitazone may be a weak inducer of CYP 450 isoform 3A4 substrate).

No products indexed under this heading.

Atorvastatin Calcium (Co-administration of pioglitazone hydrochloride for 7 days with atorvastatin calcium 80 mg once daily resulted in least square mean (90% CI) values for unchanged pioglitazone of 0.69 (0.57 - 0.85) for C_{max}, 0.76 (0.65 - 0.88) for AUC, and 0.96 (0.87 - 1.05) for C_{min}. For unchanged atorvastatin the least square mean (90% CI) values were 0.77 (0.66 - 0.90) for C_{max}, 0.86 (0.78 - 0.94) for AUC, and 0.92 (0.82 - 1.02) for C_{min}). Products include:

Lipitor 2703

Belladonna Ergotamine (In vivo drug-drug interaction studies have suggested that pioglitazone may be a weak inducer of CYP 450 isoform 3A4 substrate).

No products indexed under this heading.

Buspirone Hydrochloride (In vivo drug-drug interaction studies have suggested that pioglitazone may be a weak inducer of CYP 450 isoform 3A4 substrate).

No products indexed under this heading.

Busulfan (In vivo drug-drug interaction studies have suggested that pioglita-

zone may be a weak inducer of CYP 450 isoform 3A4 substrate). Products include:

Myleran 1581

Carbamazepine (An enzyme inducer of CYP2C8 (such as rifampin) may significantly decrease the AUC of pioglitazone. Therefore, if an inducer of CYP2C8 is started or stopped during treatment with pioglitazone, changes in diabetes treatment may be needed based on clinical response). Products include:

Carbatrol 3280
Equetro 3477

Cerivastatin Sodium (In vivo drug-drug interaction studies have suggested that pioglitazone may be a weak inducer of CYP 450 isoform 3A4 substrate).

No products indexed under this heading.

Chlorpheniramine (In vivo drug-drug interaction studies have suggested that pioglitazone may be a weak inducer of CYP 450 isoform 3A4 substrate).

No products indexed under this heading.

Chlorpheniramine Maleate (In vivo drug-drug interaction studies have suggested that pioglitazone may be a weak inducer of CYP 450 isoform 3A4 substrate).

No products indexed under this heading.

Chlorpheniramine Polistirex (In vivo drug-drug interaction studies have suggested that pioglitazone may be a weak inducer of CYP 450 isoform 3A4 substrate). Products include:

Tussionex 3443

Chlorpheniramine Tannate (In vivo drug-drug interaction studies have suggested that pioglitazone may be a weak inducer of CYP 450 isoform 3A4 substrate).

No products indexed under this heading.

Chlorpropamide (In controlled combination therapy studies with a sulfonylurea (taken along with pioglitazone), mild to moderate hypoglycemia, which appears to be dose related, was reported. In combination therapy studies, edema was reported for 7.2% of patients treated with pioglitazone and sulfonylureas compared to 2.1% of patients on sulfonylureas alone. In addition, in U.S. double-blind studies, anemia was reported in ≤ 2% of patients treated with pioglitazone plus sulfonylurea, metformin, or insulin. Also, patients receiving pioglitazone in combination with other oral hypoglycemic agents may be at risk for hypoglycemia, and a reduction in the dose of the concomitant agent may be necessary).

No products indexed under this heading.

Cimetidine (An enzyme inhibitor of CYP2C8 (such as gemfibrozil) may significantly increase the AUC of pioglitazone. Therefore, if an inhibitor of CYP2C8 is started or stopped during treatment with pioglitazone, changes in diabetes treatment may be needed based on clinical response).

No products indexed under this heading.

Cimetidine Hydrochloride (An enzyme inhibitor of CYP2C8 (such as gemfibrozil) may significantly increase the AUC of pioglitazone. Therefore, if an inhibitor of CYP2C8 is started or stopped during treatment with pioglitazone, changes in diabetes treatment may be needed based on clinical response).

No products indexed under this heading.

Cisapride (In vivo drug-drug interaction studies have suggested that pioglitazone may be a weak inducer of CYP 450 isoform 3A4 substrate).

No products indexed under this heading.

Clarithromycin (In vivo drug-drug interaction studies have suggested that

pioglitazone may be a weak inducer of CYP 450 isoform 3A4 substrate).
Products include:

Cyclosporine (*In vivo* drug-drug interaction studies have suggested that pioglitazone may be a weak inducer of CYP 450 isoform 3A4 substrate).
Products include:

Desogestrel (Co-administration of pioglitazone hydrochloride (45 mg once daily) and an oral contraceptive (1 mg norethindrone plus 0.035 mg ethinyl estradiol once daily) for 21 days, resulted in 11% and 11-14% decrease in ethinyl estradiol AUC (0-24h) and C_{max}, respectively. There were no significant changes in norethindrone AUC (0-24h) and C_{max}. In view of the high variability of ethinyl estradiol pharmacokinetics, the clinical significance of this finding is unknown).
No products indexed under this heading.

Diazepam (*In vivo* drug-drug interaction studies have suggested that pioglitazone may be a weak inducer of CYP 450 isoform 3A4 substrate). Products include:

Dihydroergotamine Mesylate (*In vivo* drug-drug interaction studies have suggested that pioglitazone may be a weak inducer of CYP 450 isoform 3A4 substrate).
No products indexed under this heading.

Diltiazem Hydrochloride (*In vivo* drug-drug interaction studies have suggested that pioglitazone may be a weak inducer of CYP 450 isoform 3A4 substrate). Products include:

Diltiazem Maleate (*In vivo* drug-drug interaction studies have suggested that pioglitazone may be a weak inducer of CYP 450 isoform 3A4 substrate).
No products indexed under this heading.

Disopyramide (*In vivo* drug-drug interaction studies have suggested that pioglitazone may be a weak inducer of CYP 450 isoform 3A4 substrate).
No products indexed under this heading.

Disopyramide Phosphate (*In vivo* drug-drug interaction studies have suggested that pioglitazone may be a weak inducer of CYP 450 isoform 3A4 substrate).
No products indexed under this heading.

Disulfiram (*In vivo* drug-drug interaction studies have suggested that pioglitazone may be a weak inducer of CYP 450 isoform 3A4 substrate).
No products indexed under this heading.

Doxorubicin Hydrochloride (*In vivo* drug-drug interaction studies have suggested that pioglitazone may be a weak inducer of CYP 450 isoform 3A4 substrate).
No products indexed under this heading.

Dronabinol (*In vivo* drug-drug interaction studies have suggested that pioglitazone may be a weak inducer of CYP 450 isoform 3A4 substrate).
No products indexed under this heading.

Ergotamine Tartrate (*In vivo* drug-drug interaction studies have suggested that pioglitazone may be a weak inducer of CYP 450 isoform 3A4 substrate).
No products indexed under this heading.

Erythromycin (*In vivo* drug-drug interaction studies have suggested that pioglitazone may be a weak inducer of CYP 450 isoform 3A4 substrate).
No products indexed under this heading.

Erythromycin Estolate (*In vivo* drug-drug interaction studies have suggested that pioglitazone may be a weak inducer of CYP 450 isoform 3A4 substrate).
No products indexed under this heading.

Erythromycin Ethylsuccinate (*In vivo* drug-drug interaction studies have suggested that pioglitazone may be a weak inducer of CYP 450 isoform 3A4 substrate). Products include:

Erythromycin Gluceptate (*In vivo* drug-drug interaction studies have suggested that pioglitazone may be a weak inducer of CYP 450 isoform 3A4 substrate).
No products indexed under this heading.

Erythromycin Lactobionate (*In vivo* drug-drug interaction studies have suggested that pioglitazone may be a weak inducer of CYP 450 isoform 3A4 substrate).
No products indexed under this heading.

Erythromycin Stearate (*In vivo* drug-drug interaction studies have suggested that pioglitazone may be a weak inducer of CYP 450 isoform 3A4 substrate).
No products indexed under this heading.

Estradiol (*In vivo* drug-drug interaction studies have suggested that pioglitazone may be a weak inducer of CYP 450 isoform 3A4 substrate). Products include:

Estradiol Benzoate (*In vivo* drug-drug interaction studies have suggested that pioglitazone may be a weak inducer of CYP 450 isoform 3A4 substrate).
No products indexed under this heading.

Estradiol Cypionate (*In vivo* drug-drug interaction studies have suggested that pioglitazone may be a weak inducer of CYP 450 isoform 3A4 substrate).
No products indexed under this heading.

Estradiol Valerate (*In vivo* drug-drug interaction studies have suggested that pioglitazone may be a weak inducer of CYP 450 isoform 3A4 substrate).
No products indexed under this heading.

Ethinyl Estradiol (Co-administration of pioglitazone hydrochloride (45 mg once daily) and an oral contraceptive (1 mg norethindrone plus 0.035 mg ethinyl estradiol once daily) for 21 days, resulted in 11% and 11-14% decrease in ethinyl estradiol AUC (0-24h) and C_{max}, respectively. In view of the high variability of ethinyl estradiol pharmacokinetics, the clinical significance of this finding is unknown). Products include:

Ethosuximide (*In vivo* drug-drug interaction studies have suggested that pioglitazone may be a weak inducer of CYP 450 isoform 3A4 substrate).
No products indexed under this heading.

Ethynodiol Diacetate (Co-administration of pioglitazone hydrochloride (45 mg once daily) and an oral contraceptive (1 mg norethindrone plus 0.035 mg ethinyl estradiol once daily) for 21 days, resulted in 11% and 11-14% decrease in ethinyl estradiol AUC (0-24h) and C_{max}, respectively.

There were no significant changes in norethindrone AUC (0-24h) and C_{max}. In view of the high variability of ethinyl estradiol pharmacokinetics, the clinical significance of this finding is unknown).
No products indexed under this heading.

Etoposide (*In vivo* drug-drug interaction studies have suggested that pioglitazone may be a weak inducer of CYP 450 isoform 3A4 substrate).
No products indexed under this heading.

Etoposide Phosphate (*In vivo* drug-drug interaction studies have suggested that pioglitazone may be a weak inducer of CYP 450 isoform 3A4 substrate).
No products indexed under this heading.

Felodipine (*In vivo* drug-drug interaction studies have suggested that pioglitazone may be a weak inducer of CYP 450 isoform 3A4 substrate).
No products indexed under this heading.

Fentanyl (*In vivo* drug-drug interaction studies have suggested that pioglitazone may be a weak inducer of CYP 450 isoform 3A4 substrate). Products include:

Fentanyl Citrate (*In vivo* drug-drug interaction studies have suggested that pioglitazone may be a weak inducer of CYP 450 isoform 3A4 substrate). Products include:

Gemfibrozil (Concomitant administration of gemfibrozil (oral 600 mg twice daily), an inhibitor of CYP2C8, with pioglitazone (oral 30 mg) in 10 healthy volunteers pre-treated for 2 days prior with gemfibrozil (oral 600 mg twice daily) resulted in pioglitazone exposure (AUC_{0-24}) being 226% of the pioglitazone exposure in the absence of gemfibrozil. An enzyme inhibitor of CYP2C8 (such as gemfibrozil) may significantly increase the AUC of pioglitazone. Therefore, if an inhibitor of CYP2C8 is started or stopped during treatment with pioglitazone, changes in diabetes treatment may be needed based on clinical response).
No products indexed under this heading.

Glibenclamide (Patients receiving pioglitazone in combination with other oral hypoglycemic agents may be at risk for hypoglycemia, and a reduction in the dose of the concomitant agent may be necessary).
No products indexed under this heading.

Glimepiride (In controlled combination therapy studies with a sulfonylurea (taken along with pioglitazone), mild to moderate hypoglycemia, which appears to be dose related, was reported. In combination therapy studies, edema was reported for 7.2% of patients treated with pioglitazone and sulfonylureas compared to 2.1% of patients on sulfonylureas alone. In addition, in U.S. double-blind studies, anemia was reported in ≤ 2% of patients treated with pioglitazone plus sulfonylurea, metformin, or insulin. Also, patients receiving pioglitazone in combination with other oral hypoglycemic agents may be at risk for hypoglycemia, and a reduction in the dose of the concomitant agent may be necessary). Products include:

Glipizide (In controlled combination therapy studies with a sulfonylurea (taken along with pioglitazone), mild to moderate hypoglycemia, which appears to be dose related, was reported. In combination therapy studies, edema was reported for 7.2% of patients treated with pioglitazone and sulfonylureas compared to 2.1% of patients on sulfo-

nylureas alone. In addition, in U.S. double-blind studies, anemia was reported in ≤ 2% of patients treated with pioglitazone plus sulfonylurea, metformin, or insulin. Also, patients receiving pioglitazone in combination with other oral hypoglycemic agents may be at risk for hypoglycemia, and a reduction in the dose of the concomitant agent may be necessary).
No products indexed under this heading.

Glyburide (In controlled combination therapy studies with a sulfonylurea (taken along with pioglitazone), mild to moderate hypoglycemia, which appears to be dose related, was reported. In combination therapy studies, edema was reported for 7.2% of patients treated with pioglitazone and sulfonylureas compared to 2.1% of patients on sulfonylureas alone. In addition, in U.S. double-blind studies, anemia was reported in ≤ 2% of patients treated with pioglitazone plus sulfonylurea, metformin, or insulin. Also, patients receiving pioglitazone in combination with other oral hypoglycemic agents may be at risk for hypoglycemia, and a reduction in the dose of the concomitant agent may be necessary).
No products indexed under this heading.

Haloperidol (*In vivo* drug-drug interaction studies have suggested that pioglitazone may be a weak inducer of CYP 450 isoform 3A4 substrate).
No products indexed under this heading.

Haloperidol Decanoate (*In vivo* drug-drug interaction studies have suggested that pioglitazone may be a weak inducer of CYP 450 isoform 3A4 substrate).
No products indexed under this heading.

Haloperidol Lactate (*In vivo* drug-drug interaction studies have suggested that pioglitazone may be a weak inducer of CYP 450 isoform 3A4 substrate).
No products indexed under this heading.

Indinavir Sulfate (*In vivo* drug-drug interaction studies have suggested that pioglitazone may be a weak inducer of CYP 450 isoform 3A4 substrate). Products include:

Insulin (Patients receiving pioglitazone in combination with insulin may be at risk for hypoglycemia, and a reduction in the dose of the concomitant agent may be necessary. There was an increase in the occurrence of edema in patients treated with pioglitazone and insulin compared to insulin alone. In addition, in U.S. double-blind studies, anemia was reported in ≤ 2% of patients treated with pioglitazone plus sulfonylurea, metformin, or insulin).
No products indexed under this heading.

Insulin, Human, Zinc Suspension (Patients receiving pioglitazone in combination with insulin may be at risk for hypoglycemia, and a reduction in the dose of the concomitant agent may be necessary. There was an increase in the occurrence of edema in patients treated with pioglitazone and insulin compared to insulin alone. In addition, in U.S. double-blind studies, anemia was reported in ≤ 2% of patients treated with pioglitazone plus sulfonylurea, metformin, or insulin).
No products indexed under this heading.

Insulin, Human (rDNA origin) (Patients receiving pioglitazone in combination with insulin may be at risk for hypoglycemia, and a reduction in the dose of the concomitant agent may be necessary. There was an increase in the occurrence of edema in patients treated with pioglitazone and insulin compared to insulin alone. In addition, in U.S. double-blind studies, anemia was

Actos Interactions Index 38

reported in ≤ 2% of patients treated with pioglitazone plus sulfonylurea, metformin, or insulin). Products include:
Exubera 2717

Insulin, Human NPH (Patients receiving pioglitazone in combination with insulin may be at risk for hypoglycemia, and a reduction in the dose of the concomitant agent may be necessary. There was an increase in the occurrence of edema in patients treated with pioglitazone and insulin compared to insulin alone. In addition, in U.S. double-blind studies, anemia was reported in ≤ 2% of patients treated with pioglitazone plus sulfonylurea, metformin, or insulin). Products include:
Humulin N Vial 1934

Insulin, Human Regular (Patients receiving pioglitazone in combination with insulin may be at risk for hypoglycemia, and a reduction in the dose of the concomitant agent may be necessary. There was an increase in the occurrence of edema in patients treated with pioglitazone and insulin compared to insulin alone. In addition, in U.S. double-blind studies, anemia was reported in ≤ 2% of patients treated with pioglitazone plus sulfonylurea, metformin, or insulin). Products include:
Humulin R 1937
Humulin R (U-500) 1939

Insulin, Human Regular and Human NPH Mixture (Patients receiving pioglitazone in combination with insulin may be at risk for hypoglycemia, and a reduction in the dose of the concomitant agent may be necessary. There was an increase in the occurrence of edema in patients treated with pioglitazone and insulin compared to insulin alone. In addition, in U.S. double-blind studies, anemia was reported in ≤ 2% of patients treated with pioglitazone plus sulfonylurea, metformin, or insulin). Products include:
Humulin 50/50 1930
Humulin 70/30 Vial 1931

Insulin, NPH (Patients receiving pioglitazone in combination with insulin may be at risk for hypoglycemia, and a reduction in the dose of the concomitant agent may be necessary. There was an increase in the occurrence of edema in patients treated with pioglitazone and insulin compared to insulin alone. In addition, in U.S. double-blind studies, anemia was reported in ≤ 2% of patients treated with pioglitazone plus sulfonylurea, metformin, or insulin).
No products indexed under this heading.

Insulin, Regular (Patients receiving pioglitazone in combination with insulin may be at risk for hypoglycemia, and a reduction in the dose of the concomitant agent may be necessary. There was an increase in the occurrence of edema in patients treated with pioglitazone and insulin compared to insulin alone. In addition, in U.S. double-blind studies, anemia was reported in ≤ 2% of patients treated with pioglitazone plus sulfonylurea, metformin, or insulin).
No products indexed under this heading.

Insulin, Regular and NPH mixture (Patients receiving pioglitazone in combination with insulin may be at risk for hypoglycemia, and a reduction in the dose of the concomitant agent may be necessary. There was an increase in the occurrence of edema in patients treated with pioglitazone and insulin compared to insulin alone. In addition, in U.S. double-blind studies, anemia was reported in ≤ 2% of patients treated with pioglitazone plus sulfonylurea, metformin, or insulin).
No products indexed under this heading.

Insulin, Zinc Crystals (Patients receiving pioglitazone in combination with insulin may be at risk for hypoglycemia, and a reduction in the dose of the concomitant agent may be necessary. There was an increase in the occurrence of edema in patients treated with pioglitazone and insulin compared to insulin alone. In addition, in U.S. double-blind studies, anemia was reported in ≤ 2% of patients treated with pioglitazone plus sulfonylurea, metformin, or insulin).
No products indexed under this heading.

Insulin, Zinc Suspension (Patients receiving pioglitazone in combination with insulin may be at risk for hypoglycemia, and a reduction in the dose of the concomitant agent may be necessary. There was an increase in the occurrence of edema in patients treated with pioglitazone and insulin compared to insulin alone. In addition, in U.S. double-blind studies, anemia was reported in ≤ 2% of patients treated with pioglitazone plus sulfonylurea, metformin, or insulin).
No products indexed under this heading.

Insulin Aspart (Patients receiving pioglitazone in combination with insulin may be at risk for hypoglycemia, and a reduction in the dose of the concomitant agent may be necessary. There was an increase in the occurrence of edema in patients treated with pioglitazone and insulin compared to insulin alone. In addition, in U.S. double-blind studies, anemia was reported in ≤ 2% of patients treated with pioglitazone plus sulfonylurea, metformin, or insulin).
No products indexed under this heading.

Insulin Aspart, Human (Patients receiving pioglitazone in combination with insulin may be at risk for hypoglycemia, and a reduction in the dose of the concomitant agent may be necessary. There was an increase in the occurrence of edema in patients treated with pioglitazone and insulin compared to insulin alone. In addition, in U.S. double-blind studies, anemia was reported in ≤ 2% of patients treated with pioglitazone plus sulfonylurea, metformin, or insulin). Products include:
NovoLog Mix 70/30 2581

Insulin Aspart, Human Regular (Patients receiving pioglitazone in combination with insulin may be at risk for hypoglycemia, and a reduction in the dose of the concomitant agent may be necessary. There was an increase in the occurrence of edema in patients treated with pioglitazone and insulin compared to insulin alone. In addition, in U.S. double-blind studies, anemia was reported in ≤ 2% of patients treated with pioglitazone plus sulfonylurea, metformin, or insulin). Products include:
NovoLog 2575

Insulin Aspart Protamine, Human (Patients receiving pioglitazone in combination with insulin may be at risk for hypoglycemia, and a reduction in the dose of the concomitant agent may be necessary. There was an increase in the occurrence of edema in patients treated with pioglitazone and insulin compared to insulin alone. In addition, in U.S. double-blind studies, anemia was reported in ≤ 2% of patients treated with pioglitazone plus sulfonylurea, metformin, or insulin). Products include:
NovoLog Mix 70/30 2581

Insulin Detemir (rDNA Origin) (Patients receiving pioglitazone in combination with insulin may be at risk for hypoglycemia, and a reduction in the dose of the concomitant agent may be necessary. There was an increase in the occurrence of edema in patients treated with pioglitazone and insulin compared to insulin alone. In addition, in U.S. double-blind studies, anemia was reported in ≤ 2% of patients treated with pioglitazone plus sulfonylurea, metformin, or insulin). Products include:
Levemir 2566

Insulin Glargine (Patients receiving pioglitazone in combination with insulin may be at risk for hypoglycemia, and a reduction in the dose of the concomitant agent may be necessary. There was an increase in the occurrence of edema in patients treated with pioglitazone and insulin compared to insulin alone. In addition, in U.S. double-blind studies, anemia was reported in ≤ 2% of patients treated with pioglitazone plus sulfonylurea, metformin, or insulin). Products include:
Lantus 2996

Insulin Glulisine (Patients receiving pioglitazone in combination with insulin may be at risk for hypoglycemia, and a reduction in the dose of the concomitant agent may be necessary. There was an increase in the occurrence of edema in patients treated with pioglitazone and insulin compared to insulin alone. In addition, in U.S. double-blind studies, anemia was reported in ≤ 2% of patients treated with pioglitazone plus sulfonylurea, metformin, or insulin). Products include:
Apidra 2937
Apidra SoloStar 2937

Insulin Lispro, Human (Patients receiving pioglitazone in combination with insulin may be at risk for hypoglycemia, and a reduction in the dose of the concomitant agent may be necessary. There was an increase in the occurrence of edema in patients treated with pioglitazone and insulin compared to insulin alone. In addition, in U.S. double-blind studies, anemia was reported in ≤ 2% of patients treated with pioglitazone plus sulfonylurea, metformin, or insulin). Products include:
Humalog 1910
Humalog Mix 1914
Humalog Mix75/25 1917

Insulin Lispro Protamine, Human (Patients receiving pioglitazone in combination with insulin may be at risk for hypoglycemia, and a reduction in the dose of the concomitant agent may be necessary. There was an increase in the occurrence of edema in patients treated with pioglitazone and insulin compared to insulin alone. In addition, in U.S. double-blind studies, anemia was reported in ≤ 2% of patients treated with pioglitazone plus sulfonylurea, metformin, or insulin). Products include:
Humalog Mix 1914
Humalog Mix75/25 1917

Isradipine (*In vivo* drug-drug interaction studies have suggested that pioglitazone may be a weak inducer of CYP 450 isoform 3A4 substrate). Products include:
DynaCirc CR 1432

Itraconazole (*In vivo* drug-drug interaction studies have suggested that pioglitazone may be a weak inducer of CYP 450 isoform 3A4 substrate).
No products indexed under this heading.

Ixabepilone (*In vivo* drug-drug interaction studies have suggested that pioglitazone may be a weak inducer of CYP 450 isoform 3A4 substrate).
No products indexed under this heading.

Ketoconazole (Co-administration of pioglitazone hydrochloride for 7 days with ketoconazole 200 mg administered twice daily resulted in least square mean (90% CI) values for unchanged pioglitazone of 1.14 (1.06 - 1.23) for C_{max}, 1.34 (1.26 - 1.41) for AUC, and 1.87 (1.71 - 2.04) for C_{min}). Products include:
Extina 3319
Xolegel 3337

Levonorgestrel (Co-administration of pioglitazone hydrochloride (45 mg once daily) and an oral contraceptive (1 mg norethindrone plus 0.035 mg ethinyl estradiol once daily) for 21 days, resulted in 11% and 11-14% decrease in ethinyl estradiol AUC (0-24h) and C_{max}, respectively. There were no significant changes in norethindrone AUC (0-24h) and C_{max}. In view of the high variability of ethinyl estradiol pharmacokinetics, the clinical significance of this finding is unknown). Products include:
Climara Pro 847
LoSeasonique 3407
Lybrel 3514
Mirena 854
Plan B 3416
Seasonique 3418

Lidocaine (*In vivo* drug-drug interaction studies have suggested that pioglitazone may be a weak inducer of CYP 450 isoform 3A4 substrate). Products include:
Lidoderm 1107

Lidocaine Hydrochloride (*In vivo* drug-drug interaction studies have suggested that pioglitazone may be a weak inducer of CYP 450 isoform 3A4 substrate).
No products indexed under this heading.

Lovastatin (*In vivo* drug-drug interaction studies have suggested that pioglitazone may be a weak inducer of CYP 450 isoform 3A4 substrate). Products include:
Advicor 402
Mevacor 2212

Mestranol (Co-administration of pioglitazone hydrochloride (45 mg once daily) and an oral contraceptive (1 mg norethindrone plus 0.035 mg ethinyl estradiol once daily) for 21 days, resulted in 11% and 11-14% decrease in ethinyl estradiol AUC (0-24h) and C_{max}, respectively. There were no significant changes in norethindrone AUC (0-24h) and C_{max}. In view of the high variability of ethinyl estradiol pharmacokinetics, the clinical significance of this finding is unknown).
No products indexed under this heading.

Metformin (In combination therapy studies with metformin (taken along with pioglitazone), edema was reported in 6% of patients on combination therapy compared to 2.5% of patients on metformin alone. In addition, in U.S. double-blind studies, anemia was reported in ≤ 2% of patients treated with pioglitazone plus sulfonylurea, metformin, or insulin. Also, patients receiving pioglitazone in combination with oral hypoglycemic agents may be at risk for hypoglycemia, and a reduction in the dose of the concomitant agent may be necessary).
No products indexed under this heading.

Metformin Hydrochloride (In combination therapy studies with metformin (taken along with pioglitazone), edema was reported in 6% of patients on combination therapy compared to 2.5% of patients on metformin alone. In addition, in U.S. double-blind studies, anemia was reported in ≤ 2% of patients treated with pioglitazone plus sulfonylurea, metformin, or insulin. Also, patients receiving pioglitazone in combination with oral hypoglycemic agents may be at risk for hypoglycemia, and a reduction in the dose of the concomitant agent may be necessary). Products include:
ActoPlus 3338
Avandamet 1345
Janumet 2188

Methadone Hydrochloride (*In vivo* drug-drug interaction studies have suggested that pioglitazone may be a weak inducer of CYP 450 isoform 3A4 substrate).
No products indexed under this heading.

Midazolam Hydrochloride (Administration of pioglitazone hydrochloride for 15 days followed by a single 7.5 mg of midazolam syrup resulted in a 26% reduction in midazolam C_{max} and AUC). No products indexed under this heading.

Miglitol (Patients receiving pioglitazone in combination with other oral hypoglycemic agents may be at risk for hypoglycemia, and a reduction in the dose of the concomitant agent may be necessary). No products indexed under this heading.

Nateglinide (Patients receiving pioglitazone in combination with other oral hypoglycemic agents may be at risk for hypoglycemia, and a reduction in the dose of the concomitant agent may be necessary). No products indexed under this heading.

Nefazodone Hydrochloride (In vivo drug-drug interaction studies have suggested that pioglitazone may be a weak inducer of CYP 450 isoform 3A4 substrate). No products indexed under this heading.

Nelfinavir Mesylate (In vivo drug-drug interaction studies have suggested that pioglitazone may be a weak inducer of CYP 450 isoform 3A4 substrate). No products indexed under this heading.

Nicardipine (An enzyme inhibitor of CYP2C8 (such as gemfibrozil) may significantly increase the AUC of pioglitazone. Therefore, if an inhibitor of CYP2C8 is started or stopped during treatment with pioglitazone, changes in diabetes treatment may be needed based on clinical response). No products indexed under this heading.

Nicardipine Hydrochloride (An enzyme inhibitor of CYP2C8 (such as gemfibrozil) may significantly increase the AUC of pioglitazone. Therefore, if an inhibitor of CYP2C8 is started or stopped during treatment with pioglitazone, changes in diabetes treatment may be needed based on clinical response). No products indexed under this heading.

Nifedipine (Co-administration of pioglitazone for 7 days with 30 mg nifedipine ER administered orally once daily for 4 days to male and female volunteers resulted in least square mean (90% CI) values for unchanged nifedipine of 0.83 (0.73 - 0.95) for C_{max} and 0.88 (0.80 - 0.96) for AUC. In view of the high variability of nifedipine pharmacokinetics, the clinical significance of this finding is unknown). No products indexed under this heading.

Nimodipine (In vivo drug-drug interaction studies have suggested that pioglitazone may be a weak inducer of CYP 450 isoform 3A4 substrate). No products indexed under this heading.

Nisoldipine (In vivo drug-drug interaction studies have suggested that pioglitazone may be a weak inducer of CYP 450 isoform 3A4 substrate). No products indexed under this heading.

Nitrendipine (In vivo drug-drug interaction studies have suggested that pioglitazone may be a weak inducer of CYP 450 isoform 3A4 substrate). No products indexed under this heading.

Norethindrone (Co-administration of pioglitazone hydrochloride (45 mg once daily) and an oral contraceptive (1 mg norethindrone plus 0.035 mg ethinyl estradiol once daily) for 21 days, resulted in 11% and 11-14% decrease in ethinyl estradiol AUC (0-24h) and C_{max}, respectively. There were no significant changes in norethindrone AUC (0-24h) and C_{max}. In view of the high variability of ethinyl estradiol pharmacokinetics, the clinical significance of this finding is unknown). Products include:

Norethindrone Acetate (In vivo drug-drug interaction studies have suggested that pioglitazone may be a weak inducer of CYP 450 isoform 3A4 substrate). Products include:

Norethynodrel (Co-administration of pioglitazone hydrochloride (45 mg once daily) and an oral contraceptive (1 mg norethindrone plus 0.035 mg ethinyl estradiol once daily) for 21 days, resulted in 11% and 11-14% decrease in ethinyl estradiol AUC (0-24h) and C_{max}, respectively. There were no significant changes in norethindrone AUC (0-24h) and C_{max}. In view of the high variability of ethinyl estradiol pharmacokinetics, the clinical significance of this finding is unknown). No products indexed under this heading.

Norgestimate (Co-administration of pioglitazone hydrochloride (45 mg once daily) and an oral contraceptive (1 mg norethindrone plus 0.035 mg ethinyl estradiol once daily) for 21 days, resulted in 11% and 11-14% decrease in ethinyl estradiol AUC (0-24h) and C_{max}, respectively. There were no significant changes in norethindrone AUC (0-24h) and C_{max}. In view of the high variability of ethinyl estradiol pharmacokinetics, the clinical significance of this finding is unknown). Products include:

Norgestrel (Co-administration of pioglitazone hydrochloride (45 mg once daily) and an oral contraceptive (1 mg norethindrone plus 0.035 mg ethinyl estradiol once daily) for 21 days, resulted in 11% and 11-14% decrease in ethinyl estradiol AUC (0-24h) and C_{max}, respectively. There were no significant changes in norethindrone AUC (0-24h) and C_{max}. In view of the high variability of ethinyl estradiol pharmacokinetics, the clinical significance of this finding is unknown). No products indexed under this heading.

Omeprazole (An enzyme inhibitor of CYP2C8 (such as gemfibrozil) may significantly increase the AUC of pioglitazone. Therefore, if an inhibitor of CYP2C8 is started or stopped during treatment with pioglitazone, changes in diabetes treatment may be needed based on clinical response). No products indexed under this heading.

Ondansetron (In vivo drug-drug interaction studies have suggested that pioglitazone may be a weak inducer of CYP 450 isoform 3A4 substrate). No products indexed under this heading.

Ondansetron Hydrochloride (In vivo drug-drug interaction studies have suggested that pioglitazone may be a weak inducer of CYP 450 isoform 3A4 substrate). Products include:

Paclitaxel (In vivo drug-drug interaction studies have suggested that pioglitazone may be a weak inducer of CYP 450 isoform 3A4 substrate). No products indexed under this heading.

Phenobarbital (An enzyme inducer of CYP2C8 (such as rifampin) may significantly decrease the AUC of pioglitazone. Therefore, if an inducer of CYP2C8 is started or stopped during treatment with pioglitazone, changes in diabetes treatment may be needed based on clinical response). Products include:

Phenobarbital Sodium (An enzyme inducer of CYP2C8 (such as rifampin) may significantly decrease the AUC of pioglitazone. Therefore, if an inducer of CYP2C8 is started or stopped during treatment with pioglitazone, changes in diabetes treatment may be needed based on clinical response). No products indexed under this heading.

Pimozide (In vivo drug-drug interaction studies have suggested that pioglitazone may be a weak inducer of CYP 450 isoform 3A4 substrate). No products indexed under this heading.

Polyestradiol Phosphate (In vivo drug-drug interaction studies have suggested that pioglitazone may be a weak inducer of CYP 450 isoform 3A4 substrate). No products indexed under this heading.

Primidone (An enzyme inducer of CYP2C8 (such as rifampin) may significantly decrease the AUC of pioglitazone. Therefore, if an inducer of CYP2C8 is started or stopped during treatment with pioglitazone, changes in diabetes treatment may be needed based on clinical response). No products indexed under this heading.

Quercetin (An enzyme inhibitor of CYP2C8 (such as gemfibrozil) may significantly increase the AUC of pioglitazone. Therefore, if an inhibitor of CYP2C8 is started or stopped during treatment with pioglitazone, changes in diabetes treatment may be needed based on clinical response). No products indexed under this heading.

Quinidine Gluconate (In vivo drug-drug interaction studies have suggested that pioglitazone may be a weak inducer of CYP 450 isoform 3A4 substrate). No products indexed under this heading.

Quinidine Polygalacturonate (In vivo drug-drug interaction studies have suggested that pioglitazone may be a weak inducer of CYP 450 isoform 3A4 substrate). No products indexed under this heading.

Quinidine Sulfate (In vivo drug-drug interaction studies have suggested that pioglitazone may be a weak inducer of CYP 450 isoform 3A4 substrate). No products indexed under this heading.

Repaglinide (Patients receiving pioglitazone in combination with other oral hypoglycemic agents may be at risk for hypoglycemia, and a reduction in the dose of the concomitant agent may be necessary). No products indexed under this heading.

Rifabutin (An enzyme inducer of CYP2C8 (such as rifampin) may significantly decrease the AUC of pioglitazone. Therefore, if an inducer of CYP2C8 is started or stopped during treatment with pioglitazone, changes in diabetes treatment may be needed based on clinical response). No products indexed under this heading.

Rifampin (Concomitant administration of rifampin (oral 600 mg twice daily), an inducer of CYP2C8, with pioglitazone (oral 30 mg) in 10 healthy volunteers pre-treated for 5 days prior with rifampin (oral 600 mg twice daily) resulted in a decrease in the AUC of pioglitazone by 54%. An enzyme inducer of CYP2C8 (such as rifampin) may significantly decrease the AUC of pioglitazone. Therefore, if an inducer of CYP2C8 is started or stopped during treatment with pioglitazone, changes in diabetes treatment may be needed based on clinical response). No products indexed under this heading.

Ritonavir (In vivo drug-drug interaction studies have suggested that pioglita-

zone may be a weak inducer of CYP 450 isoform 3A4 substrate). Products include:

Rosiglitazone Maleate (Patients receiving pioglitazone in combination with other oral hypoglycemic agents may be at risk for hypoglycemia, and a reduction in the dose of the concomitant agent may be necessary). Products include:

Saquinavir (In vivo drug-drug interaction studies have suggested that pioglitazone may be a weak inducer of CYP 450 isoform 3A4 substrate). No products indexed under this heading.

Saquinavir Mesylate (In vivo drug-drug interaction studies have suggested that pioglitazone may be a weak inducer of CYP 450 isoform 3A4 substrate). No products indexed under this heading.

Sertraline Hydrochloride (In vivo drug-drug interaction studies have suggested that pioglitazone may be a weak inducer of CYP 450 isoform 3A4 substrate). No products indexed under this heading.

Sildenafil Citrate (In vivo drug-drug interaction studies have suggested that pioglitazone may be a weak inducer of CYP 450 isoform 3A4 substrate). No products indexed under this heading.

Simvastatin (In vivo drug-drug interaction studies have suggested that pioglitazone may be a weak inducer of CYP 450 isoform 3A4 substrate). Products include:

Sirolimus (In vivo drug-drug interaction studies have suggested that pioglitazone may be a weak inducer of CYP 450 isoform 3A4 substrate). Products include:

Sitagliptin Phosphate (Patients receiving pioglitazone in combination with other oral hypoglycemic agents may be at risk for hypoglycemia, and a reduction in the dose of the concomitant agent may be necessary). Products include:

Sulfaphenazole (An enzyme inhibitor of CYP2C8 (such as gemfibrozil) may significantly increase the AUC of pioglitazone. Therefore, if an inhibitor of CYP2C8 is started or stopped during treatment with pioglitazone, changes in diabetes treatment may be needed based on clinical response). No products indexed under this heading.

Sulfinpyrazone (An enzyme inhibitor of CYP2C8 (such as gemfibrozil) may significantly increase the AUC of pioglitazone. Therefore, if an inhibitor of CYP2C8 is started or stopped during treatment with pioglitazone, changes in diabetes treatment may be needed based on clinical response). No products indexed under this heading.

Tacrolimus (In vivo drug-drug interaction studies have suggested that pioglitazone may be a weak inducer of CYP 450 isoform 3A4 substrate). Products include:

Tadalafil (In vivo drug-drug interaction studies have suggested that pioglita-

---

IMPORTANT NOTE: Always consult each drug listing in the patient's regimen for possible interactions.

zone may be a weak inducer of CYP 450 isoform 3A4 substrate). Products include:

Adcirca 3461
Cialis 1861

Tamoxifen Citrate (*In vivo* drug-drug interaction studies have suggested that pioglitazone may be a weak inducer of CYP 450 isoform 3A4 substrate).
No products indexed under this heading.

Terfenadine (*In vivo* drug-drug interaction studies have suggested that pioglitazone may be a weak inducer of CYP 450 isoform 3A4 substrate).
No products indexed under this heading.

Theophylline (*In vivo* drug-drug interaction studies have suggested that pioglitazone may be a weak inducer of CYP 450 isoform 3A4 substrate).
No products indexed under this heading.

Theophylline Anhydrous (*In vivo* drug-drug interaction studies have suggested that pioglitazone may be a weak inducer of CYP 450 isoform 3A4 substrate). Products include:

Uniphyl 2817

Theophylline Calcium Salicylate (*In vivo* drug-drug interaction studies have suggested that pioglitazone may be a weak inducer of CYP 450 isoform 3A4 substrate).
No products indexed under this heading.

Theophylline Dihydroxypropyl (Glyceryl) (*In vivo* drug-drug interaction studies have suggested that pioglitazone may be a weak inducer of CYP 450 isoform 3A4 substrate).
No products indexed under this heading.

Theophylline Ethylenediamine (*In vivo* drug-drug interaction studies have suggested that pioglitazone may be a weak inducer of CYP 450 isoform 3A4 substrate).
No products indexed under this heading.

Theophylline Sodium Glycinate (*In vivo* drug-drug interaction studies have suggested that pioglitazone may be a weak inducer of CYP 450 isoform 3A4 substrate).
No products indexed under this heading.

Tiagabine Hydrochloride (*In vivo* drug-drug interaction studies have suggested that pioglitazone may be a weak inducer of CYP 450 isoform 3A4 substrate). Products include:

Gabitril 972

Tolazamide (In controlled combination therapy studies with a sulfonylurea (taken along with pioglitazone), mild to moderate hypoglycemia, which appears to be dose related, was reported. In combination therapy studies, edema was reported for 7.2% of patients treated with pioglitazone and sulfonylureas compared to 2.1% of patients on sulfonylureas alone. In addition, in U.S. double-blind studies, anemia was reported in ≤ 2% of patients treated with pioglitazone plus sulfonylurea, metformin, or insulin. Also, patients receiving pioglitazone in combination with other oral hypoglycemic agents may be at risk for hypoglycemia, and a reduction in the dose of the concomitant agent may be necessary).
No products indexed under this heading.

Tolbutamide (In controlled combination therapy studies with a sulfonylurea (taken along with pioglitazone), mild to moderate hypoglycemia, which appears to be dose related, was reported. In combination therapy studies, edema was reported for 7.2% of patients treated with pioglitazone and sulfonylureas compared to 2.1% of patients on sulfonylureas alone. In addition, in U.S. double-blind studies, anemia was reported in ≤ 2% of patients treated with pioglitazone plus sulfonylurea, metformin, or insulin. Also, patients receiving pioglitazone in combination with other oral hypoglycemic agents may be at risk for hypoglycemia, and a reduction in the dose of the concomitant agent may be necessary).
No products indexed under this heading.

Tolterodine Tartrate (*In vivo* drug-drug interaction studies have suggested that pioglitazone may be a weak inducer of CYP 450 isoform 3A4 substrate).
No products indexed under this heading.

Trazodone Hydrochloride (*In vivo* drug-drug interaction studies have suggested that pioglitazone may be a weak inducer of CYP 450 isoform 3A4 substrate).
No products indexed under this heading.

Triazolam (*In vivo* drug-drug interaction studies have suggested that pioglitazone may be a weak inducer of CYP 450 isoform 3A4 substrate).
No products indexed under this heading.

Trimethoprim (An enzyme inhibitor of CYP2C8 (such as gemfibrozil) may significantly increase the AUC of pioglitazone. Therefore, if an inhibitor of CYP2C8 is started or stopped during treatment with pioglitazone, changes in diabetes treatment may be needed based on clinical response).
No products indexed under this heading.

Trimethoprim Hydrochloride (An enzyme inhibitor of CYP2C8 (such as gemfibrozil) may significantly increase the AUC of pioglitazone. Therefore, if an inhibitor of CYP2C8 is started or stopped during treatment with pioglitazone, changes in diabetes treatment may be needed based on clinical response).
No products indexed under this heading.

Trimethoprim Sulfate (An enzyme inhibitor of CYP2C8 (such as gemfibrozil) may significantly increase the AUC of pioglitazone. Therefore, if an inhibitor of CYP2C8 is started or stopped during treatment with pioglitazone, changes in diabetes treatment may be needed based on clinical response).
No products indexed under this heading.

Troglitazone (Patients receiving pioglitazone in combination with other oral hypoglycemic agents may be at risk for hypoglycemia, and a reduction in the dose of the concomitant agent may be necessary).
No products indexed under this heading.

Vardenafil Hydrochloride (*In vivo* drug-drug interaction studies have suggested that pioglitazone may be a weak inducer of CYP 450 isoform 3A4 substrate). Products include:

Levitra 3157

Verapamil Hydrochloride (*In vivo* drug-drug interaction studies have suggested that pioglitazone may be a weak inducer of CYP 450 isoform 3A4 substrate). Products include:

Tarka 534

Vinblastine Sulfate (*In vivo* drug-drug interaction studies have suggested that pioglitazone may be a weak inducer of CYP 450 isoform 3A4 substrate).
No products indexed under this heading.

Vincristine Sulfate (*In vivo* drug-drug interaction studies have suggested that pioglitazone may be a weak inducer of CYP 450 isoform 3A4 substrate).
No products indexed under this heading.

Warfarin Sodium (*In vivo* drug-drug interaction studies have suggested that pioglitazone may be a weak inducer of CYP 450 isoform 3A4 substrate).
No products indexed under this heading.

Food Interactions

Food, unspecified (Food slightly delays the time to peak serum concentration of pioglitazone to 3 to 4 hours, but does not alter the extent of absorption).

Meal, unspecified (Food slightly delays the time to peak serum concentration of pioglitazone to 3 to 4 hours, but does not alter the extent of absorption).

ACUVAIL OPHTHALMIC SOLUTION

(Ketorolac Tromethamine) .... ⊙209
May interact with anticoagulants, corticosteroids. Compounds in these categories include:

Alclometasone Dipropionate (Topical nonsteroidal anti-inflammatory drugs (NSAIDs) may slow or delay healing. Topical corticosteroids are also known to slow or delay healing. Concomitant use of topical NSAIDs and topical steroids may increase the potential for healing problems).
No products indexed under this heading.

Anisindione (It is recommended that ketorolac tromethamine ophthalmic solution be used with caution in patients who are receiving other medications which may prolong bleeding time).
No products indexed under this heading.

Ardeparin Sodium (It is recommended that ketorolac tromethamine ophthalmic solution be used with caution in patients who are receiving other medications which may prolong bleeding time).
No products indexed under this heading.

Beclomethasone Dipropionate (Topical nonsteroidal anti-inflammatory drugs (NSAIDs) may slow or delay healing. Topical corticosteroids are also known to slow or delay healing. Concomitant use of topical NSAIDs and topical steroids may increase the potential for healing problems). Products include:

Qvar 3398

Beclomethasone Dipropionate Monohydrate (Topical nonsteroidal anti-inflammatory drugs (NSAIDs) may slow or delay healing. Topical corticosteroids are also known to slow or delay healing. Concomitant use of topical NSAIDs and topical steroids may increase the potential for healing problems). Products include:

Beconase AQ 1386

Betamethasone (Topical nonsteroidal anti-inflammatory drugs (NSAIDs) may slow or delay healing. Topical corticosteroids are also known to slow or delay healing. Concomitant use of topical NSAIDs and topical steroids may increase the potential for healing problems).
No products indexed under this heading.

Betamethasone Acetate (Topical nonsteroidal anti-inflammatory drugs (NSAIDs) may slow or delay healing. Topical corticosteroids are also known to slow or delay healing. Concomitant use of topical NSAIDs and topical steroids may increase the potential for healing problems).
No products indexed under this heading.

Betamethasone Benzoate (Topical nonsteroidal anti-inflammatory drugs (NSAIDs) may slow or delay healing. Topical corticosteroids are also known to slow or delay healing. Concomitant use of topical NSAIDs and topical steroids may increase the potential for healing problems).
No products indexed under this heading.

Betamethasone Dipropionate (Topical nonsteroidal anti-inflammatory drugs (NSAIDs) may slow or delay healing. Topical corticosteroids are also known to slow or delay healing. Concomitant use of topical NSAIDs and topical steroids may increase the potential for healing problems). Products include:

Diprolene Lotion 0.05% 3108
Diprolene Ointment 0.05% 3109
Diprolene AF Cream 0.05% 3107
Lotrisone 3163

Betamethasone Sodium Phosphate (Topical nonsteroidal anti-inflammatory drugs (NSAIDs) may slow or delay healing. Topical corticosteroids are also known to slow or delay healing. Concomitant use of topical NSAIDs and topical steroids may increase the potential for healing problems).
No products indexed under this heading.

Betamethasone Valerate (Topical nonsteroidal anti-inflammatory drugs (NSAIDs) may slow or delay healing. Topical corticosteroids are also known to slow or delay healing. Concomitant use of topical NSAIDs and topical steroids may increase the potential for healing problems). Products include:

Luxíq 3321

Budesonide (Topical nonsteroidal anti-inflammatory drugs (NSAIDs) may slow or delay healing. Topical corticosteroids are also known to slow or delay healing. Concomitant use of topical NSAIDs and topical steroids may increase the potential for healing problems). Products include:

Pulmicort Flexhaler 714
Symbicort 80/4.5 720
Symbicort 160/4.5 720

Ciclesonide (Topical nonsteroidal anti-inflammatory drugs (NSAIDs) may slow or delay healing. Topical corticosteroids are also known to slow or delay healing. Concomitant use of topical NSAIDs and topical steroids may increase the potential for healing problems).
No products indexed under this heading.

Cortisone Acetate (Topical nonsteroidal anti-inflammatory drugs (NSAIDs) may slow or delay healing. Topical corticosteroids are also known to slow or delay healing. Concomitant use of topical NSAIDs and topical steroids may increase the potential for healing problems).
No products indexed under this heading.

Dalteparin Sodium (It is recommended that ketorolac tromethamine ophthalmic solution be used with caution in patients who are receiving other medications which may prolong bleeding time). Products include:

Fragmin 1058

Danaparoid Sodium (It is recommended that ketorolac tromethamine ophthalmic solution be used with caution in patients who are receiving other medications which may prolong bleeding time).
No products indexed under this heading.

Desoximetasone (Topical nonsteroidal anti-inflammatory drugs (NSAIDs) may slow or delay healing. Topical corticosteroids are also known to slow or delay healing. Concomitant use of topical NSAIDs and topical steroids may increase the potential for healing problems).
No products indexed under this heading.

Dexamethasone (Topical nonsteroidal anti-inflammatory drugs (NSAIDs) may slow or delay healing. Topical corticosteroids are also known to slow or delay healing. Concomitant use of topical NSAIDs and topical steroids may increase the potential for healing problems). Products include:

Ciprodex 583
Ozurdex .... ⊙223
Tobramycin and Dexamethasone Ophthalmic Suspension .... ⊙251

(⊙ Described in PDR® for Ophthalmic Medicines)

Dexamethasone Acetate (Topical nonsteroidal anti-inflammatory drugs (NSAIDs) may slow or delay healing. Topical corticosteroids are also known to slow or delay healing. Concomitant use of topical NSAIDs and topical steroids may increase the potential for healing problems).
    No products indexed under this heading.

Dexamethasone Phosphate (Topical nonsteroidal anti-inflammatory drugs (NSAIDs) may slow or delay healing. Topical corticosteroids are also known to slow or delay healing. Concomitant use of topical NSAIDs and topical steroids may increase the potential for healing problems).
    No products indexed under this heading.

Dexamethasone Sodium (Topical nonsteroidal anti-inflammatory drugs (NSAIDs) may slow or delay healing. Topical corticosteroids are also known to slow or delay healing. Concomitant use of topical NSAIDs and topical steroids may increase the potential for healing problems).
    No products indexed under this heading.

Dexamethasone Sodium Phosphate (Topical nonsteroidal anti-inflammatory drugs (NSAIDs) may slow or delay healing. Topical corticosteroids are also known to slow or delay healing. Concomitant use of topical NSAIDs and topical steroids may increase the potential for healing problems).
    No products indexed under this heading.

Dexamethasone Sodium Phosphate Injection (Topical nonsteroidal anti-inflammatory drugs (NSAIDs) may slow or delay healing. Topical corticosteroids are also known to slow or delay healing. Concomitant use of topical NSAIDs and topical steroids may increase the potential for healing problems).
    No products indexed under this heading.

Dicumarol (It is recommended that ketorolac tromethamine ophthalmic solution be used with caution in patients who are receiving other medications which may prolong bleeding time).
    No products indexed under this heading.

Diflorasone Diacetate (Topical nonsteroidal anti-inflammatory drugs (NSAIDs) may slow or delay healing. Topical corticosteroids are also known to slow or delay healing. Concomitant use of topical NSAIDs and topical steroids may increase the potential for healing problems).
    No products indexed under this heading.

Enoxaparin Sodium (It is recommended that ketorolac tromethamine ophthalmic solution be used with caution in patients who are receiving other medications which may prolong bleeding time). Products include:
    Lovenox 3005

Fludrocortisone Acetate (Topical nonsteroidal anti-inflammatory drugs (NSAIDs) may slow or delay healing. Topical corticosteroids are also known to slow or delay healing. Concomitant use of topical NSAIDs and topical steroids may increase the potential for healing problems).
    No products indexed under this heading.

Flumethasone Pivalate (Topical nonsteroidal anti-inflammatory drugs (NSAIDs) may slow or delay healing. Topical corticosteroids are also known to slow or delay healing. Concomitant use of topical NSAIDs and topical steroids may increase the potential for healing problems).
    No products indexed under this heading.

Flunisolide Hemihydrate (Topical nonsteroidal anti-inflammatory drugs (NSAIDs) may slow or delay healing. Topical corticosteroids are also known to slow or delay healing. Concomitant use of topical NSAIDs and topical steroids may increase the potential for healing problems).
    No products indexed under this heading.

Fluticasone Furoate (Topical nonsteroidal anti-inflammatory drugs (NSAIDs) may slow or delay healing. Topical corticosteroids are also known to slow or delay healing. Concomitant use of topical NSAIDs and topical steroids may increase the potential for healing problems). Products include:
    Veramyst 1713

Fluticasone Propionate (Topical nonsteroidal anti-inflammatory drugs (NSAIDs) may slow or delay healing. Topical corticosteroids are also known to slow or delay healing. Concomitant use of topical NSAIDs and topical steroids may increase the potential for healing problems). Products include:
    Advair 100/50 1275
    Advair 250/50 1275
    Advair 500/50 1275
    Advair HFA 45/21 1288
    Advair HFA 115/21 1288
    Advair HFA 230/21 1288
    Flonase 1459
    Flovent Diskus 1463
    Flovent HFA 1470

Fondaparinux Sodium (It is recommended that ketorolac tromethamine ophthalmic solution be used with caution in patients who are receiving other medications which may prolong bleeding time). Products include:
    Arixtra 1320

Heparin Calcium (It is recommended that ketorolac tromethamine ophthalmic solution be used with caution in patients who are receiving other medications which may prolong bleeding time).
    No products indexed under this heading.

Heparin Sodium (It is recommended that ketorolac tromethamine ophthalmic solution be used with caution in patients who are receiving other medications which may prolong bleeding time).
    No products indexed under this heading.

Hydrocortisone (Topical nonsteroidal anti-inflammatory drugs (NSAIDs) may slow or delay healing. Topical corticosteroids are also known to slow or delay healing. Concomitant use of topical NSAIDs and topical steroids may increase the potential for healing problems).
    No products indexed under this heading.

Hydrocortisone (Alcohol) (Topical nonsteroidal anti-inflammatory drugs (NSAIDs) may slow or delay healing. Topical corticosteroids are also known to slow or delay healing. Concomitant use of topical NSAIDs and topical steroids may increase the potential for healing problems).
    No products indexed under this heading.

Hydrocortisone Acetate (Topical nonsteroidal anti-inflammatory drugs (NSAIDs) may slow or delay healing. Topical corticosteroids are also known to slow or delay healing. Concomitant use of topical NSAIDs and topical steroids may increase the potential for healing problems).
    No products indexed under this heading.

Hydrocortisone Butyrate (Topical nonsteroidal anti-inflammatory drugs (NSAIDs) may slow or delay healing. Topical corticosteroids are also known to slow or delay healing. Concomitant use of topical NSAIDs and topical steroids may increase the potential for healing problems).
    No products indexed under this heading.

Hydrocortisone Cypionate (Topical nonsteroidal anti-inflammatory drugs (NSAIDs) may slow or delay healing. Topical corticosteroids are also known to slow or delay healing. Concomitant use of topical NSAIDs and topical steroids may increase the potential for healing problems).
    No products indexed under this heading.

Hydrocortisone Hemisuccinate (Topical nonsteroidal anti-inflammatory drugs (NSAIDs) may slow or delay healing. Topical corticosteroids are also known to slow or delay healing. Concomitant use of topical NSAIDs and topical steroids may increase the potential for healing problems).
    No products indexed under this heading.

Hydrocortisone Probutate (Topical nonsteroidal anti-inflammatory drugs (NSAIDs) may slow or delay healing. Topical corticosteroids are also known to slow or delay healing. Concomitant use of topical NSAIDs and topical steroids may increase the potential for healing problems).
    No products indexed under this heading.

Hydrocortisone Sodium Phosphate (Topical nonsteroidal anti-inflammatory drugs (NSAIDs) may slow or delay healing. Topical corticosteroids are also known to slow or delay healing. Concomitant use of topical NSAIDs and topical steroids may increase the potential for healing problems).
    No products indexed under this heading.

Hydrocortisone Sodium Succinate (Topical nonsteroidal anti-inflammatory drugs (NSAIDs) may slow or delay healing. Topical corticosteroids are also known to slow or delay healing. Concomitant use of topical NSAIDs and topical steroids may increase the potential for healing problems).
    No products indexed under this heading.

Hydrocortisone Valerate (Topical nonsteroidal anti-inflammatory drugs (NSAIDs) may slow or delay healing. Topical corticosteroids are also known to slow or delay healing. Concomitant use of topical NSAIDs and topical steroids may increase the potential for healing problems).
    No products indexed under this heading.

Low Molecular Weight Heparins (It is recommended that ketorolac tromethamine ophthalmic solution be used with caution in patients who are receiving other medications which may prolong bleeding time).
    No products indexed under this heading.

Methylprednisolone (Topical nonsteroidal anti-inflammatory drugs (NSAIDs) may slow or delay healing. Topical corticosteroids are also known to slow or delay healing. Concomitant use of topical NSAIDs and topical steroids may increase the potential for healing problems).
    No products indexed under this heading.

Methylprednisolone Acetate (Topical nonsteroidal anti-inflammatory drugs (NSAIDs) may slow or delay healing. Topical corticosteroids are also known to slow or delay healing. Concomitant use of topical NSAIDs and topical steroids may increase the potential for healing problems).
    No products indexed under this heading.

Methylprednisolone Sodium Succinate (Topical nonsteroidal anti-inflammatory drugs (NSAIDs) may slow or delay healing. Topical corticosteroids are also known to slow or delay healing. Concomitant use of topical NSAIDs and topical steroids may increase the potential for healing problems).
    No products indexed under this heading.

Mometasone Furoate (Topical nonsteroidal anti-inflammatory drugs (NSAIDs) may slow or delay healing.

Topical corticosteroids are also known to slow or delay healing. Concomitant use of topical NSAIDs and topical steroids may increase the potential for healing problems). Products include:
    Asmanex 3058
    Elocon Cream 3111
    Elocon Lotion 3112
    Elocon Ointment 3114

Mometasone Furoate Monohydrate (Topical nonsteroidal anti-inflammatory drugs (NSAIDs) may slow or delay healing. Topical corticosteroids are also known to slow or delay healing. Concomitant use of topical NSAIDs and topical steroids may increase the potential for healing problems). Products include:
    Nasonex 3166

Prednisolone (Topical nonsteroidal anti-inflammatory drugs (NSAIDs) may slow or delay healing. Topical corticosteroids are also known to slow or delay healing. Concomitant use of topical NSAIDs and topical steroids may increase the potential for healing problems).
    No products indexed under this heading.

Prednisolone Acetate (Topical nonsteroidal anti-inflammatory drugs (NSAIDs) may slow or delay healing. Topical corticosteroids are also known to slow or delay healing. Concomitant use of topical NSAIDs and topical steroids may increase the potential for healing problems). Products include:
    Blephamide .... ⊙212, ⊙214
    Pred Forte .... ⊙225
    Pred Mild .... ⊙230
    Pred-G .... ⊙226, ⊙227

Prednisolone Sodium Phosphate (Topical nonsteroidal anti-inflammatory drugs (NSAIDs) may slow or delay healing. Topical corticosteroids are also known to slow or delay healing. Concomitant use of topical NSAIDs and topical steroids may increase the potential for healing problems).
    No products indexed under this heading.

Prednisolone Tebutate (Topical nonsteroidal anti-inflammatory drugs (NSAIDs) may slow or delay healing. Topical corticosteroids are also known to slow or delay healing. Concomitant use of topical NSAIDs and topical steroids may increase the potential for healing problems).
    No products indexed under this heading.

Prednisone (Topical nonsteroidal anti-inflammatory drugs (NSAIDs) may slow or delay healing. Topical corticosteroids are also known to slow or delay healing. Concomitant use of topical NSAIDs and topical steroids may increase the potential for healing problems).
    No products indexed under this heading.

Prednisone sodium phosphate (Topical nonsteroidal anti-inflammatory drugs (NSAIDs) may slow or delay healing. Topical corticosteroids are also known to slow or delay healing. Concomitant use of topical NSAIDs and topical steroids may increase the potential for healing problems).
    No products indexed under this heading.

Tinzaparin Sodium (It is recommended that ketorolac tromethamine ophthalmic solution be used with caution in patients who are receiving other medications which may prolong bleeding time).
    No products indexed under this heading.

Triamcinolone (Topical nonsteroidal anti-inflammatory drugs (NSAIDs) may slow or delay healing. Topical corticosteroids are also known to slow or delay healing. Concomitant use of topical NSAIDs and topical steroids may increase the potential for healing problems).
    No products indexed under this heading.

IMPORTANT NOTE: Always consult each drug listing in the patient's regimen for possible interactions.

Acuvail Interactions Index 42

Triamcinolone Acetonide (Topical nonsteroidal anti-inflammatory drugs (NSAIDs) may slow or delay healing. Topical corticosteroids are also known to slow or delay healing. Concomitant use of topical NSAIDs and topical steroids may increase the potential for healing problems). Products include:
Azmacort 408
Nasacort AQ 3019

Triamcinolone Diacetate (Topical nonsteroidal anti-inflammatory drugs (NSAIDs) may slow or delay healing. Topical corticosteroids are also known to slow or delay healing. Concomitant use of topical NSAIDs and topical steroids may increase the potential for healing problems).
No products indexed under this heading.

Triamcinolone Hexacetonide (Topical nonsteroidal anti-inflammatory drugs (NSAIDs) may slow or delay healing. Topical corticosteroids are also known to slow or delay healing. Concomitant use of topical NSAIDs and topical steroids may increase the potential for healing problems).
No products indexed under this heading.

Warfarin Sodium (It is recommended that ketorolac tromethamine ophthalmic solution be used with caution in patients who are receiving other medications which may prolong bleeding time).
No products indexed under this heading.

ACZONE GEL 5%

(Dapsone) 593
May interact with anticonvulsants, antimalarials, and certain other agents. Compounds in these categories include:

Benzoyl Peroxide (Topical application of dapsone gel dapsone gel followed by benzoyl peroxide in subjects with acne vulgaris resulted in a temporary local yellow or orange discoloration of the skin and facial hair (reported 7 out of 95 subjects) with resolution in 4 to 57 days). Products include:
Benzaclin 2965
Brevoxyl 3316, 3317
Duac 3317

Carbamazepine (Concomitant administration may increase the formation of dapsone hydroxylamine, a metabolite of dapsone associated with hemolysis). Products include:
Carbatrol 3280
Equetro 3477

Chloroquine (Dapsone gel, 5% should not be used in patients who are taking antimalarial medications because of the potential for hemolytic reactions).
No products indexed under this heading.

Chloroquine Hydrochloride (Dapsone gel, 5% should not be used in patients who are taking antimalarial medications because of the potential for hemolytic reactions).
No products indexed under this heading.

Chloroquine Phosphate (Dapsone gel, 5% should not be used in patients who are taking antimalarial medications because of the potential for hemolytic reactions).
No products indexed under this heading.

Divalproex Sodium (Concomitant administration may increase the formation of dapsone hydroxylamine, a metabolite of dapsone associated with hemolysis). Products include:
Depakote ER 426

Ethosuximide (Concomitant administration may increase the formation of dapsone hydroxylamine, a metabolite of dapsone associated with hemolysis).
No products indexed under this heading.

Ethotoin (Concomitant administration may increase the formation of dapsone hydroxylamine, a metabolite of dapsone associated with hemolysis).
No products indexed under this heading.

Felbamate (Concomitant administration may increase the formation of dapsone hydroxylamine, a metabolite of dapsone associated with hemolysis).
No products indexed under this heading.

Fosphenytoin (Concomitant administration may increase the formation of dapsone hydroxylamine, a metabolite of dapsone associated with hemolysis).
No products indexed under this heading.

Fosphenytoin Sodium (Concomitant administration may increase the formation of dapsone hydroxylamine, a metabolite of dapsone associated with hemolysis).
No products indexed under this heading.

Gabapentin (Concomitant administration may increase the formation of dapsone hydroxylamine, a metabolite of dapsone associated with hemolysis).
No products indexed under this heading.

Hypericum (Certain concomitant medications such as St. John's wort, may increase the formation of dapsone hydroxylamine, a metabolite of dapsone associated with hemolysis).
No products indexed under this heading.

Lamotrigine (Concomitant administration may increase the formation of dapsone hydroxylamine, a metabolite of dapsone associated with hemolysis). Products include:
Lamictal 1522
Lamictal ODT 1522
Lamictal XR 1536

Levetiracetam (Concomitant administration may increase the formation of dapsone hydroxylamine, a metabolite of dapsone associated with hemolysis). Products include:
Keppra XR 3434

Mefloquine Hydrochloride (Dapsone gel, 5% should not be used in patients who are taking antimalarial medications because of the potential for hemolytic reactions).
No products indexed under this heading.

Mephenytoin (Concomitant administration may increase the formation of dapsone hydroxylamine, a metabolite of dapsone associated with hemolysis).
No products indexed under this heading.

Methsuximide (Concomitant administration may increase the formation of dapsone hydroxylamine, a metabolite of dapsone associated with hemolysis).
No products indexed under this heading.

Oxcarbazepine (Concomitant administration may increase the formation of dapsone hydroxylamine, a metabolite of dapsone associated with hemolysis).
No products indexed under this heading.

Paramethadione (Concomitant administration may increase the formation of dapsone hydroxylamine, a metabolite of dapsone associated with hemolysis).
No products indexed under this heading.

Phenacemide (Concomitant administration may increase the formation of dapsone hydroxylamine, a metabolite of dapsone associated with hemolysis).
No products indexed under this heading.

Phenobarbital (Concomitant administration may increase the formation of dapsone hydroxylamine, a metabolite of dapsone associated with hemolysis). Products include:
Donnatal 2711

Phenobarbital Sodium (Concomitant administration may increase the formation of dapsone hydroxylamine, a metabolite of dapsone associated with hemolysis).
No products indexed under this heading.

Phensuximide (Concomitant administration may increase the formation of dapsone hydroxylamine, a metabolite of dapsone associated with hemolysis).
No products indexed under this heading.

Phenytoin (Concomitant administration may increase the formation of dapsone hydroxylamine, a metabolite of dapsone associated with hemolysis).
No products indexed under this heading.

Phenytoin Sodium (Concomitant administration may increase the formation of dapsone hydroxylamine, a metabolite of dapsone associated with hemolysis). Products include:
Phenytek Capsules 2380

Primidone (Concomitant administration may increase the formation of dapsone hydroxylamine, a metabolite of dapsone associated with hemolysis).
No products indexed under this heading.

Pyrimethamine (With oral dapsone treatment, folic acid antagonists such as pyrimethamine have been noted to possibly increase the likelihood of hematologic reactions). Products include:
Daraprim 1423

Rifampin (Certain concomitant medications such as rifampin may increase the formation of dapson hydroxylamine, a metabolite of dapsone associated with hemolysis).
No products indexed under this heading.

Rufinamide (Concomitant administration may increase the formation of dapsone hydroxylamine, a metabolite of dapsone associated with hemolysis). Products include:
Banzel 1050

Sulfamethoxazole (A study evaluated the effect of the use of dapsone gel in combination with trimethoprim-sulfamethoxazole (TMP/SMX). During co-administration, system levels of TMP and SMX were essentially unchanged. However, levels of dapsone and its metabolites increased in the presence of TMP/SMX. Systemic exposure (AUC 0-24) of dapsone and N-acetyl-dapsone were increased by about 40% and 20%, respectively, in the presence of TMP/SMX. Systemic exposure (AUC 0-24) of dapsone hydroxylamine was more than doubled in the presence of TMP/SMX. Exposure from the proposed topical dose is about 1% of that from the 100 mg oral dose, even when co-administered with TMP/SMX. Use of dapsone gel with TMP/SMX may increase the likelihood of hemolysis in patients with G6PD deficiency).
No products indexed under this heading.

Tiagabine Hydrochloride (Concomitant administration may increase the formation of dapsone hydroxylamine, a metabolite of dapsone associated with hemolysis). Products include:
Gabitril 972

Topiramate (Concomitant administration may increase the formation of dapsone hydroxylamine, a metabolite of dapsone associated with hemolysis).
No products indexed under this heading.

Trimethadione (Concomitant administration may increase the formation of dapsone hydroxylamine, a metabolite of dapsone associated with hemolysis).
No products indexed under this heading.

Trimethoprim (A study evaluated the effect of the use of dapsone gel in combination with trimethoprim-sulfamethoxazole (TMP/SMX). During co-administration, system levels of TMP and SMX were essentially unchanged. However, levels of dapsone and its metabolites increased in the presence of TMP/SMX. Systemic exposure (AUC 0-24) of dapsone and N-acetyl-dapsone were increased by about 40% and 20%, respectively, in the presence of TMP/SMX. Systemic exposure (AUC 0-24) of dapsone hydroxylamine was more than doubled in the presence of TMP/SMX. Exposure from the proposed topical dose is about 1% of that from the 100 mg oral dose, even when co-administered with TMP/SMX. Use of dapsone gel with TMP/SMX may increase the likelihood of hemolysis in patients with G6PD deficiency).
No products indexed under this heading.

Trimethoprim Hydrochloride (A study evaluated the effect of the use of dapsone gel in combination with trimethoprim-sulfamethoxazole (TMP/SMX). During co-administration, system levels of TMP and SMX were essentially unchanged. However, levels of dapsone and its metabolites increased in the presence of TMP/SMX. Systemic exposure (AUC 0-24) of dapsone and N-acetyl-dapsone were increased by about 40% and 20%, respectively, in the presence of TMP/SMX. Systemic exposure (AUC 0-24) of dapsone hydroxylamine was more than doubled in the presence of TMP/SMX. Exposure from the proposed topical dose is about 1% of that from the 100 mg oral dose, even when co-administered with TMP/SMX. Use of dapsone gel with TMP/SMX may increase the likelihood of hemolysis in patients with G6PD deficiency).
No products indexed under this heading.

Trimethoprim Sulfate (A study evaluated the effect of the use of dapsone gel in combination with trimethoprim-sulfamethoxazole (TMP/SMX). During co-administration, system levels of TMP and SMX were essentially unchanged. However, levels of dapsone and its metabolites increased in the presence of TMP/SMX. Systemic exposure (AUC 0-24) of dapsone and N-acetyl-dapsone were increased by about 40% and 20%, respectively, in the presence of TMP/SMX. Systemic exposure (AUC 0-24) of dapsone hydroxylamine was more than doubled in the presence of TMP/SMX. Exposure from the proposed topical dose is about 1% of that from the 100 mg oral dose, even when co-administered with TMP/SMX. Use of dapsone gel with TMP/SMX may increase the likelihood of hemolysis in patients with G6PD deficiency).
No products indexed under this heading.

Valproate Sodium (Concomitant administration may increase the formation of dapsone hydroxylamine, a metabolite of dapsone associated with hemolysis).
No products indexed under this heading.

Valproic Acid (Concomitant administration may increase the formation of dapsone hydroxylamine, a metabolite of dapsone associated with hemolysis).
No products indexed under this heading.

Zonisamide (Concomitant administration may increase the formation of dapsone hydroxylamine, a metabolite of dapsone associated with hemolysis). Products include:
Zonegran 1081

ADCIRCA TABLETS

(Tadalafil) 3461
May interact with alcohols, alpha adrenergic blockers, angiotensin-II receptor antagonists, antacids, antihypertensives, cytochrome p450 3a inducers (selected), cytochrome p450 3a inhibitors (selected), erythromycin, nitrates and nitrites, PDE5 inhibitors, phenytoin, protease inhibitors, theophyllines, and certain other agents. Compounds in these categories include:

Acebutolol Hydrochloride (Clinical pharmacology studies were conducted to assess the effect of tadalafil on the potentiation of the blood-pressure-lowering effects of selected antihyper-

(⊙ Described in PDR® for Ophthalmic Medicines)

tensive medications (amlodipine, angiotensin II receptor blockers, bendroflumethiazide, enalapril, and metoprolol). Small reductions in blood pressure occurred following co-administration of tadalafil with these agents compared with placebo).

No products indexed under this heading.

Alfuzosin Hydrochloride (PDE5 inhibitors, including tadalafil, and α-adrenergic blocking agents are vasodilators with blood pressure-lowering effects. When vasodilators are used in combination, an additive effect on blood pressure may be anticipated. In some patients, concomitant use of these two drug classes can lower blood pressure significantly, which may lead to symptomatic hypotension (eg, fainting). Safety of combined use of PDE5 inhibitors and α-blockers may be affected by other variables, including intravascular volume depletion and use of other antihypertensive drugs). Products include:

Uroxatral **3050**

Aliskiren (Clinical pharmacology studies were conducted to assess the effect of tadalafil on the potentiation of the blood-pressure-lowering effects of selected antihypertensive medications (amlodipine, angiotensin II receptor blockers, bendroflumethiazide, enalapril, and metoprolol). Small reductions in blood pressure occurred following co-administration of tadalafil with these agents compared with placebo). Products include:

Tekturna **2538**
Tekturna HCT **2541**
Valturna **3637**

Allium sativum (For patients chronically taking potent inducers of CYP3A, avoid use of tadalafil. Rifampin (600 mg qd), a CYP3A inducer, reduced tadalafil 10 mg single dose exposure (AUC) by 88% and C_{max} by 46%. Bosentan (125 mg bid), a substrate of CYP2C9 and CYP3A and a moderate inducer of CYP3A, CYP2C9, and possibly CYP2C19, reduced tadalafil (40 mg qd) systemic exposure by 42% and C_{max} by 27% following multiple dose co-administration. Although specific interactions have not been studied, other CYP3A inducers would likely decrease tadalafil exposure).

No products indexed under this heading.

Aluminum Carbonate (Simultaneous administration of an antacid (magnesium hydroxide/aluminum hydroxide) and tadalafil (10 mg) reduced the apparent rate of absorption of tadalafil without altering exposure (AUC) to tadalafil).

No products indexed under this heading.

Aluminum Hydroxide (Simultaneous administration of an antacid (magnesium hydroxide/aluminum hydroxide) and tadalafil (10 mg) reduced the apparent rate of absorption of tadalafil without altering exposure (AUC) to tadalafil).

No products indexed under this heading.

Amiodarone Hydrochloride (Tadalafil is metabolized predominantly by CYP3A in the liver. In patients taking potent inhibitors of CYP3A, avoid use of tadalafil. Ketoconazole (400 mg qd), a selective and potent inhibitor of CYP3A, increased tadalafil 20 mg single dose exposure (AUC) by 312% and C_{max} by 22%. Ketoconazole (200 mg qd) increased tadalafil 10 mg single dose exposure (AUC) by 107% and C_{max} by 15%. Although specific interactions have not been studied, other CYP3A inhibitors would likely increase tadalafil exposure).

No products indexed under this heading.

Amlodipine Besylate (A study assessed the interaction between amlodipine (5 mg qd) and tadalafil 10 mg. There was no effect of tadalafil on amlodipine blood levels and no effect of amlodipine on tadalafil blood levels. The mean reduction in supine systolic/diastolic blood pressure because of tadalafil 10 mg in subjects taking amlodipine was 3/2 mm Hg, compared to placebo. In a similar study using tadalafil 20 mg, there were no clinically significant differences between tadalafil and placebo in subjects taking amlodipine). Products include:

Azor **1010**
Exforge **2443**
Exforge HCT **2449**

Amprenavir (Ritonavir (500 mg or 600 mg bid at steady state), an inhibitor of CYP3A, CYP2C9, CYP2C19, and CYP2D6, increased tadalafil 20 mg single dose exposure (AUC) by 32% with a 30% reduction in C_{max}. Ritonavir (200 mg bid), increased tadalafil 20 mg single dose exposure (AUC) by 124% with no change in C_{max}. Ritonavir inhibits and induces CYP3A, the enzyme involved in the metabolism of tadalafil in a time dependent manner. The results suggest the initial inhibitory effect of ritonavir on CYP3A may be mitigated by a more slowly evolving induction effect so that after about 1 week of ritonavir bid, the exposure of tadalafil is similiar in the presence of and absence of ritonavir. Although specific interactions have not been studied, other HIV protease inhibitors would likely increase tadalafil exposure).

No products indexed under this heading.

Amyl Nitrite (Concomitant use of tadalafil with organic nitrates is contraindicated. Tadalafil should not be used in patients who are using any form of organic nitrate, either regular or intermittently. Tadalafil potentiates the hypotensive effect of nitrates. In a patient who has taken tadalafil, where nitrate administration is deemed medically necessary in a life-threatening situation, at least 48 hours should elapse after the last dose of tadalafil before nitrate administration is considered. In such circumstances, nitrates should still only be administered under close medical supervision with appropriate hemodynamic monitoring).

No products indexed under this heading.

Apraclonidine Hydrochloride (PDE5 inhibitors, including tadalafil, and α-adrenergic blocking agents are vasodilators with blood pressure-lowering effects. When vasodilators are used in combination, an additive effect on blood pressure may be anticipated. In some patients, concomitant use of these two drug classes can lower blood pressure significantly, which may lead to symptomatic hypotension (eg, fainting). Safety of combined use of PDE5 inhibitors and α-blockers may be affected by other variables, including intravascular volume depletion and use of other antihypertensive drugs).

No products indexed under this heading.

Aprepitant (Tadalafil is metabolized predominantly by CYP3A in the liver. In patients taking potent inhibitors of CYP3A, avoid use of tadalafil. Ketoconazole (400 mg qd), a selective and potent inhibitor of CYP3A, increased tadalafil 20 mg single dose exposure (AUC) by 312% and C_{max} by 22%. Ketoconazole (200 mg qd) increased tadalafil 10 mg single dose exposure (AUC) by 107% and C_{max} by 15%. Although specific interactions have not been studied, other CYP3A inhibitors would likely increase tadalafil exposure). Products include:

Emend **2124**

Atazanavir (Ritonavir (500 mg or 600 mg bid at steady state), an inhibitor of CYP3A, CYP2C9, CYP2C19, and CYP2D6, increased tadalafil 20 mg single dose exposure (AUC) by 32% with a 30% reduction in C_{max}. Ritonavir (200 mg bid), increased tadalafil 20 mg single dose exposure (AUC) by 124% with no change in C_{max}. Ritonavir inhibits and induces CYP3A, the enzyme involved in the metabolism of tadalafil in a time dependent manner. The results suggest the initial inhibitory effect of ritonavir on CYP3A may be mitigated by a more slowly evolving induction effect so that after about 1 week of ritonavir bid, the exposure of tadalafil is similiar in the presence of and absence of ritonavir. Although specific interactions have not been studied, other HIV protease inhibitors would likely increase tadalafil exposure).

No products indexed under this heading.

Atazanavir Sulfate (Ritonavir (500 mg or 600 mg bid at steady state), an inhibitor of CYP3A, CYP2C9, CYP2C19, and CYP2D6, increased tadalafil 20 mg single dose exposure (AUC) by 32% with a 30% reduction in C_{max}. Ritonavir (200 mg bid), increased tadalafil 20 mg single dose exposure (AUC) by 124% with no change in C_{max}. Ritonavir inhibits and induces CYP3A, the enzyme involved in the metabolism of tadalafil in a time dependent manner. The results suggest the initial inhibitory effect of ritonavir on CYP3A may be mitigated by a more slowly evolving induction effect so that after about 1 week of ritonavir bid, the exposure of tadalafil is similiar in the presence of and absence of ritonavir. Although specific interactions have not been studied, other HIV protease inhibitors would likely increase tadalafil exposure).

No products indexed under this heading.

Atenolol (Clinical pharmacology studies were conducted to assess the effect of tadalafil on the potentiation of the blood-pressure-lowering effects of selected antihypertensive medications (amlodipine, angiotensin II receptor blockers, bendroflumethiazide, enalapril, and metoprolol). Small reductions in blood pressure occurred following co-administration of tadalafil with these agents compared with placebo).

No products indexed under this heading.

Benazepril Hydrochloride (Clinical pharmacology studies were conducted to assess the effect of tadalafil on the potentiation of the blood-pressure-lowering effects of selected antihypertensive medications (amlodipine, angiotensin II receptor blockers, bendroflumethiazide, enalapril, and metoprolol). Small reductions in blood pressure occurred following co-administration of tadalafil with these agents compared with placebo).

No products indexed under this heading.

Bendroflumethiazide (A study assessed the interaction between bendroflumethiazide (2.5 mg daily) and tadalafil 10 mg. Following dosing, the mean reduction in supine systolic/diastolic blood pressure because of tadalafil 10 mg in subjects taking bendroflumethiazide was 6/4 mm Hg, compared to placebo).

No products indexed under this heading.

Betaxolol Hydrochloride (Clinical pharmacology studies were conducted to assess the effect of tadalafil on the potentiation of the blood-pressure-lowering effects of selected antihypertensive medications (amlodipine, angiotensin II receptor blockers, bendroflumethiazide, enalapril, and metoprolol). Small reductions in blood pressure occurred following co-administration of tadalafil with these agents compared with placebo).

No products indexed under this heading.

Bisoprolol Fumarate (Clinical pharmacology studies were conducted to assess the effect of tadalafil on the potentiation of the blood-pressure-lowering effects of selected antihypertensive medications (amlodipine, angiotensin II receptor blockers, bendroflumethiazide, enalapril, and metoprolol). Small reductions in blood pressure occurred following co-administration of tadalafil with these agents compared with placebo).

No products indexed under this heading.

Bosentan (For patients chronically taking potent inducers of CYP3A, avoid use of tadalafil. Bosentan (125 mg bid), a substrate of CYP2C9 and CYP3A and a moderate inducer of CYP3A, CYP2C9, and possibly CYP2C19, reduced tadalafil (40 mg qd) systemic exposure by 42% and C_{max} by 27% following multiple dose co-administration). Products include:

Tracleer **573**

Calcium Carbonate (Simultaneous administration of an antacid (magnesium hydroxide/aluminum hydroxide) and tadalafil (10 mg) reduced the apparent rate of absorption of tadalafil without altering exposure (AUC) to tadalafil). Products include:

Chelated Mineral **3476**
Pepcid Complete **1822**
Extra Strength Rolaids Softchews Vanilla Creme **2045**

Candesartan Cilexetil (A study assessed the interaction between angiotensin II receptor blockers and tadalafil 20 mg. Subjects in the study were taking any marketed angiotensin II receptor blocker, either alone, as a component of a combination product, or as part of a multiple antihypertensive regimen. Following dosing, ambulatory measurements of blood pressure revealed differences between tadalafil and placebo of 8/4 mm Hg in systolic/diastolic blood pressure). Products include:

Atacand **697**
Atacand HCT **700**

Captopril (Clinical pharmacology studies were conducted to assess the effect of tadalafil on the potentiation of the blood-pressure-lowering effects of selected antihypertensive medications (amlodipine, angiotensin II receptor blockers, bendroflumethiazide, enalapril, and metoprolol). Small reductions in blood pressure occurred following co-administration of tadalafil with these agents compared with placebo). Products include:

Captopril **2341**

Carbamazepine (For patients chronically taking potent inducers of CYP3A, avoid use of tadalafil. Rifampin (600 mg qd), a CYP3A inducer, reduced tadalafil 10 mg single dose exposure (AUC) by 88% and C_{max} by 46%. Bosentan (125 mg bid), a substrate of CYP2C9 and CYP3A and a moderate inducer of CYP3A, CYP2C9, and possibly CYP2C19, reduced tadalafil (40 mg qd) systemic exposure by 42% and C_{max} by 27% following multiple dose co-administration. Although specific interactions have not been studied, other CYP3A inducers, such as carbamazepine, would likely decrease tadalafil exposure). Products include:

Carbatrol **3280**
Equetro **3477**

Carteolol Hydrochloride (Clinical pharmacology studies were conducted to assess the effect of tadalafil on the potentiation of the blood-pressure-lowering effects of selected antihypertensive medications (amlodipine, angiotensin II receptor blockers, bendroflumethiazide, enalapril, and metoprolol). Small reductions in blood pressure occurred following co-administration of tadalafil with these agents compared with placebo).

No products indexed under this heading.

IMPORTANT NOTE: Always consult each drug listing in the patient's regimen for possible interactions.

component of a combination product, or as part of a multiple antihypertensive regimen. Following dosing, ambulatory measurements of blood pressure revealed differences between tadalafil and placebo of 8/4 mm Hg in systolic/diastolic blood pressure). Products include:

Teveten **538**
Teveten HCT **541**

Erythrityl Tetranitrate (Concomitant use of tadalafil with organic nitrates is contraindicated. Tadalafil should not be used in patients who are using any form of organic nitrate, either regular or intermittently. Tadalafil potentiates the hypotensive effect of nitrates. In a patient who has taken tadalafil, where nitrate administration is deemed medically necessary in a life-threatening situation, at least 48 hours should elapse after the last dose of tadalafil before nitrate administration is considered. In such circumstances, nitrates should still only be administered under close medical supervision with appropriate hemodynamic monitoring).

No products indexed under this heading.

Erythromycin (Tadalafil is metabolized predominantly by CYP3A in the liver. In patients taking potent inhibitors of CYP3A, avoid use of tadalafil. Ketoconazole (400 mg qd), a selective and potent inhibitor of CYP3A, increased tadalafil 20 mg single dose exposure (AUC) by 312% and C_{max} by 22%. Ketoconazole (200 mg qd) increased tadalafil 10 mg single dose exposure (AUC) by 107% and C_{max} by 15%. Although specific interactions have not been studied, other CYP3A inhibitors, such as erythromycin, would likely increase tadalafil exposure).

No products indexed under this heading.

Erythromycin, Topical (Tadalafil is metabolized predominantly by CYP3A in the liver. In patients taking potent inhibitors of CYP3A, avoid use of tadalafil. Ketoconazole (400 mg qd), a selective and potent inhibitor of CYP3A, increased tadalafil 20 mg single dose exposure (AUC) by 312% and C_{max} by 22%. Ketoconazole (200 mg qd) increased tadalafil 10 mg single dose exposure (AUC) by 107% and C_{max} by 15%. Although specific interactions have not been studied, other CYP3A inhibitors, such as erythromycin, would likely increase tadalafil exposure).

No products indexed under this heading.

Erythromycin Estolate (Tadalafil is metabolized predominantly by CYP3A in the liver. In patients taking potent inhibitors of CYP3A, avoid use of tadalafil. Ketoconazole (400 mg qd), a selective and potent inhibitor of CYP3A, increased tadalafil 20 mg single dose exposure (AUC) by 312% and C_{max} by 22%. Ketoconazole (200 mg qd) increased tadalafil 10 mg single dose exposure (AUC) by 107% and C_{max} by 15%. Although specific interactions have not been studied, other CYP3A inhibitors, such as erythromycin, would likely increase tadalafil exposure).

No products indexed under this heading.

Erythromycin Ethylsuccinate (Tadalafil is metabolized predominantly by CYP3A in the liver. In patients taking potent inhibitors of CYP3A, avoid use of tadalafil. Ketoconazole (400 mg qd), a selective and potent inhibitor of CYP3A, increased tadalafil 20 mg single dose exposure (AUC) by 312% and C_{max} by 22%. Ketoconazole (200 mg qd) increased tadalafil 10 mg single dose exposure (AUC) by 107% and C_{max} by 15%. Although specific interactions have not been studied, other CYP3A inhibitors, such as erythromycin, would likely increase tadalafil exposure). Products include:

E.E.S. **437**
EryPed **435**

Erythromycin Gluceptate (Tadalafil is metabolized predominantly by CYP3A in the liver. In patients taking potent inhibitors of CYP3A, avoid use of tadalafil. Ketoconazole (400 mg qd), a selective and potent inhibitor of CYP3A, increased tadalafil 20 mg single dose exposure (AUC) by 312% and C_{max} by 22%. Ketoconazole (200 mg qd) increased tadalafil 10 mg single dose exposure (AUC) by 107% and C_{max} by 15%. Although specific interactions have not been studied, other CYP3A inhibitors, such as erythromycin, would likely increase tadalafil exposure).

No products indexed under this heading.

Erythromycin Lactobionate (Tadalafil is metabolized predominantly by CYP3A in the liver. In patients taking potent inhibitors of CYP3A, avoid use of tadalafil. Ketoconazole (400 mg qd), a selective and potent inhibitor of CYP3A, increased tadalafil 20 mg single dose exposure (AUC) by 312% and C_{max} by 22%. Ketoconazole (200 mg qd) increased tadalafil 10 mg single dose exposure (AUC) by 107% and C_{max} by 15%. Although specific interactions have not been studied, other CYP3A inhibitors, such as erythromycin, would likely increase tadalafil exposure).

No products indexed under this heading.

Erythromycin Stearate (Tadalafil is metabolized predominantly by CYP3A in the liver. In patients taking potent inhibitors of CYP3A, avoid use of tadalafil. Ketoconazole (400 mg qd), a selective and potent inhibitor of CYP3A, increased tadalafil 20 mg single dose exposure (AUC) by 312% and C_{max} by 22%. Ketoconazole (200 mg qd) increased tadalafil 10 mg single dose exposure (AUC) by 107% and C_{max} by 15%. Although specific interactions have not been studied, other CYP3A inhibitors, such as erythromycin, would likely increase tadalafil exposure).

No products indexed under this heading.

Esmolol Hydrochloride (Clinical pharmacology studies were conducted to assess the effect of tadalafil on the potentiation of the blood-pressure-lowering effects of selected antihypertensive medications (amlodipine, angiotensin II receptor blockers, bendroflumethiazide, enalapril, and metoprolol). Small reductions in blood pressure occurred following co-administration of tadalafil with these agents compared with placebo).

No products indexed under this heading.

Ethanol (Both alcohol and tadalafil, a PDE5 inhibitor, act as mild vasodilators. When mild vasodilators are taken in combination, blood pressure–lowering effects of each individual compound may be increased. Substantial consumption of alcohol (eg, 5 units or greater) in combination with tadalafil can increase the potential for orthostatic signs and symptoms, including increase in heart rate, decrease in standing blood pressure, dizziness, and headache).

No products indexed under this heading.

Ethinyl Estradiol (At steady-state, tadalafil (40 mg qd) increased ethinyl estradiol exposure (AUC) by 26% and C_{max} by 70% relative to oral contraceptive administered with placebo). Products include:

LoSeasonique **3407**
Lybrel **3514**
NuvaRing **3181**
Ortho Evra **2648**
Ortho-Cyclen/Ortho Tri-Cyclen **2663**
Ortho Tri-Cyclen Lo Tablets **2673**
Seasonique **3418**
Yaz **864**

Ethosuximide (For patients chronically taking potent inducers of CYP3A, avoid use of tadalafil. Rifampin (600 mg qd), a CYP3A inducer, reduced tadalafil 10 mg single dose exposure (AUC) by 88% and C_{max} by 46%. Bosentan (125 mg bid), a substrate of CYP2C9 and CYP3A and a moderate inducer of CYP3A, CYP2C9, and possibly CYP2C19, reduced tadalafil (40 mg qd) systemic exposure by 42% and C_{max} by 27% following multiple dose co-administration. Although specific interactions have not been studied, other CYP3A inducers would likely decrease tadalafil exposure).

No products indexed under this heading.

Ethyl Alcohol (Both alcohol and tadalafil, a PDE5 inhibitor, act as mild vasodilators. When mild vasodilators are taken in combination, blood pressure–lowering effects of each individual compound may be increased. Substantial consumption of alcohol (eg, 5 units or greater) in combination with tadalafil can increase the potential for orthostatic signs and symptoms, including increase in heart rate, decrease in standing blood pressure, dizziness, and headache).

No products indexed under this heading.

Felodipine (Clinical pharmacology studies were conducted to assess the effect of tadalafil on the potentiation of the blood-pressure-lowering effects of selected antihypertensive medications (amlodipine, angiotensin II receptor blockers, bendroflumethiazide, enalapril, and metoprolol). Small reductions in blood pressure occurred following co-administration of tadalafil with these agents compared with placebo).

No products indexed under this heading.

Fluconazole (Tadalafil is metabolized predominantly by CYP3A in the liver. In patients taking potent inhibitors of CYP3A, avoid use of tadalafil. Ketoconazole (400 mg qd), a selective and potent inhibitor of CYP3A, increased tadalafil 20 mg single dose exposure (AUC) by 312% and C_{max} by 22%. Ketoconazole (200 mg qd) increased tadalafil 10 mg single dose exposure (AUC) by 107% and C_{max} by 15%. Although specific interactions have not been studied, other CYP3A inhibitors would likely increase tadalafil exposure).

No products indexed under this heading.

Fluoxetine (Tadalafil is metabolized predominantly by CYP3A in the liver. In patients taking potent inhibitors of CYP3A, avoid use of tadalafil. Ketoconazole (400 mg qd), a selective and potent inhibitor of CYP3A, increased tadalafil 20 mg single dose exposure (AUC) by 312% and C_{max} by 22%. Ketoconazole (200 mg qd) increased tadalafil 10 mg single dose exposure (AUC) by 107% and C_{max} by 15%. Although specific interactions have not been studied, other CYP3A inhibitors would likely increase tadalafil exposure).

No products indexed under this heading.

Fluoxetine Hydrochloride (Tadalafil is metabolized predominantly by CYP3A in the liver. In patients taking potent inhibitors of CYP3A, avoid use of tadalafil. Ketoconazole (400 mg qd), a selective and potent inhibitor of CYP3A, increased tadalafil 20 mg single dose exposure (AUC) by 312% and C_{max} by 22%. Ketoconazole (200 mg qd) increased tadalafil 10 mg single dose exposure (AUC) by 107% and C_{max} by 15%. Although specific interactions have not been studied, other CYP3A inhibitors would likely increase tadalafil exposure). Products include:

Prozac Weekly **1941**
Prozac Pulvules **1941**
Symbyax **1965**

Fluvoxamine Maleate (Tadalafil is metabolized predominantly by CYP3A in the liver. In patients taking potent inhibitors of CYP3A, avoid use of tadalafil. Ketoconazole (400 mg qd), a selective and potent inhibitor of CYP3A, increased tadalafil 20 mg single dose exposure (AUC) by 312% and C_{max} by 22%. Ketoconazole (200 mg qd) increased tadalafil 10 mg single dose exposure (AUC) by 107% and C_{max} by 15%. Although specific interactions have not been studied, other CYP3A inhibitors would likely increase tadalafil exposure).

No products indexed under this heading.

Fosamprenavir Calcium (Ritonavir (500 mg or 600 mg bid at steady state), an inhibitor of CYP3A, CYP2C9, CYP2C19, and CYP2D6, increased tadalafil 20 mg single dose exposure (AUC) by 32% with a 30% reduction in C_{max}. Ritonavir (200 mg bid), increased tadalafil 20 mg single dose exposure (AUC) by 124% with no change in C_{max}. Ritonavir inhibits and induces CYP3A, the enzyme involved in the metabolism of tadalafil in a time dependent manner. The results suggest the initial inhibitory effect of ritonavir on CYP3A may be mitigated by a more slowly evolving induction effect so that after about 1 week of ritonavir bid, the exposure of tadalafil is similiar in the presence of and absence of ritonavir. Although specific interactions have not been studied, other HIV protease inhibitors would likely increase tadalafil exposure). Products include:

Lexiva Oral Suspension **1558**
Lexiva **1558**

Fosinopril Sodium (Clinical pharmacology studies were conducted to assess the effect of tadalafil on the potentiation of the blood-pressure-lowering effects of selected antihypertensive medications (amlodipine, angiotensin II receptor blockers, bendroflumethiazide, enalapril, and metoprolol). Small reductions in blood pressure occurred following co-administration of tadalafil with these agents compared with placebo).

No products indexed under this heading.

Fosphenytoin (For patients chronically taking potent inducers of CYP3A, avoid use of tadalafil. Rifampin (600 mg qd), a CYP3A inducer, reduced tadalafil 10 mg single dose exposure (AUC) by 88% and C_{max} by 46%. Bosentan (125 mg bid), a substrate of CYP2C9 and CYP3A and a moderate inducer of CYP3A, CYP2C9, and possibly CYP2C19, reduced tadalafil (40 mg qd) systemic exposure by 42% and C_{max} by 27% following multiple dose co-administration. Although specific interactions have not been studied, other CYP3A inducers, such as phenytoin, would likely decrease tadalafil exposure).

No products indexed under this heading.

Fosphenytoin Sodium (For patients chronically taking potent inducers of CYP3A, avoid use of tadalafil. Rifampin (600 mg qd), a CYP3A inducer, reduced tadalafil 10 mg single dose exposure (AUC) by 88% and C_{max} by 46%. Bosentan (125 mg bid), a substrate of CYP2C9 and CYP3A and a moderate inducer of CYP3A, CYP2C9, and possibly CYP2C19, reduced tadalafil (40 mg qd) systemic exposure by 42% and C_{max} by 27% following multiple dose co-administration. Although specific interactions have not been studied, other CYP3A inducers, such as phenytoin, would likely decrease tadalafil exposure).

No products indexed under this heading.

Furosemide (Clinical pharmacology studies were conducted to assess the effect of tadalafil on the potentiation of the blood-pressure-lowering effects of selected antihypertensive medications (amlodipine, angiotensin II receptor blockers, bendroflumethiazide, enalapril, and metoprolol). Small reductions

in blood pressure occurred following co-administration of tadalafil with these agents compared with placebo).
Products include:
Furosemide 2354

Glyceryl Trinitrate (Concomitant use of tadalafil with organic nitrates is contraindicated. Tadalafil should not be used in patients who are using any form of organic nitrate, either regular or intermittently. Tadalafil potentiates the hypotensive effect of nitrates. In a patient who has taken tadalafil, where nitrate administration is deemed medically necessary in a life-threatening situation, at least 48 hours should elapse after the last dose of tadalafil before nitrate administration is considered. In such circumstances, nitrates should still only be administered under close medical supervision with appropriate hemodynamic monitoring).
No products indexed under this heading.

Guanabenz Acetate (Clinical pharmacology studies were conducted to assess the effect of tadalafil on the potentiation of the blood-pressure-lowering effects of selected antihypertensive medications (amlodipine, angiotensin II receptor blockers, bendroflumethiazide, enalapril, and metoprolol). Small reductions in blood pressure occurred following co-administration of tadalafil with these agents compared with placebo).
No products indexed under this heading.

Guanethidine (Clinical pharmacology studies were conducted to assess the effect of tadalafil on the potentiation of the blood-pressure-lowering effects of selected antihypertensive medications (amlodipine, angiotensin II receptor blockers, bendroflumethiazide, enalapril, and metoprolol). Small reductions in blood pressure occurred following co-administration of tadalafil with these agents compared with placebo).
No products indexed under this heading.

Guanethidine Monosulfate (Clinical pharmacology studies were conducted to assess the effect of tadalafil on the potentiation of the blood-pressure-lowering effects of selected antihypertensive medications (amlodipine, angiotensin II receptor blockers, bendroflumethiazide, enalapril, and metoprolol). Small reductions in blood pressure occurred following co-administration of tadalafil with these agents compared with placebo).
No products indexed under this heading.

Guanethidine Sulfate (Clinical pharmacology studies were conducted to assess the effect of tadalafil on the potentiation of the blood-pressure-lowering effects of selected antihypertensive medications (amlodipine, angiotensin II receptor blockers, bendroflumethiazide, enalapril, and metoprolol). Small reductions in blood pressure occurred following co-administration of tadalafil with these agents compared with placebo).
No products indexed under this heading.

Hydralazine Hydrochloride (Clinical pharmacology studies were conducted to assess the effect of tadalafil on the potentiation of the blood-pressure-lowering effects of selected antihypertensive medications (amlodipine, angiotensin II receptor blockers, bendroflumethiazide, enalapril, and metoprolol). Small reductions in blood pressure occurred following co-administration of tadalafil with these agents compared with placebo).
No products indexed under this heading.

Hydrochlorothiazide (Clinical pharmacology studies were conducted to assess the effect of tadalafil on the potentiation of the blood-pressure-lowering effects of selected antihypertensive medications (amlodipine, angiotensin II receptor blockers, bendroflumethiazide, enalapril, and metoprolol). Small reductions in blood pressure occurred following co-administration of tadalafil with these agents compared with placebo).
Products include:
Atacand HCT 700
Avalide 2956
Benicar HCT 1017
Diovan HCT 2419
Dyazide 1429
Exforge HCT 2449
Hyzaar 2162
Hyzaar 100-12.5 2162
Micardis HCT 889
Prinzide 2246
Tekturna HCT 2541
Teveten HCT 541

Hydroflumethiazide (Clinical pharmacology studies were conducted to assess the effect of tadalafil on the potentiation of the blood-pressure-lowering effects of selected antihypertensive medications (amlodipine, angiotensin II receptor blockers, bendroflumethiazide, enalapril, and metoprolol). Small reductions in blood pressure occurred following co-administration of tadalafil with these agents compared with placebo).
No products indexed under this heading.

Indapamide (Clinical pharmacology studies were conducted to assess the effect of tadalafil on the potentiation of the blood-pressure-lowering effects of selected antihypertensive medications (amlodipine, angiotensin II receptor blockers, bendroflumethiazide, enalapril, and metoprolol). Small reductions in blood pressure occurred following co-administration of tadalafil with these agents compared with placebo).
Products include:
Indapamide 2356

Indinavir Sulfate (Ritonavir (500 mg or 600 mg bid at steady state), an inhibitor of CYP3A, CYP2C9, CYP2C19, and CYP2D6, increased tadalafil 20 mg single dose exposure (AUC) by 32% with a 30% reduction in C_{max}. Ritonavir (200 mg bid), increased tadalafil 20 mg single dose exposure (AUC) by 124% with no change in C_{max}. Ritonavir inhibits and induces CYP3A, the enzyme involved in the metabolism of tadalafil in a time dependent manner. The results suggest the initial inhibitory effect of ritonavir on CYP3A may be mitigated by a more slowly evolving induction effect so that after about 1 week of ritonavir bid, the exposure of tadalafil is similiar in the presence of and absence of ritonavir. Although specific interactions have not been studied, other HIV protease inhibitors would likely increase tadalafil exposure). Products include:
Crixivan 2113

Irbesartan (A study assessed the interaction between angiotensin II receptor blockers and tadalafil 20 mg. Subjects in the study were taking any marketed angiotensin II receptor blocker, either alone, as a component of a combination product, or as part of a multiple antihypertensive regimen. Following dosing, ambulatory measurements of blood pressure revealed differences between tadalafil and placebo of 8/4 mm Hg in systolic/diastolic blood pressure). Products include:
Avalide 2956
Avapro 2962

Isoniazid (Tadalafil is metabolized predominantly by CYP3A in the liver. In patients taking potent inhibitors of CYP3A, avoid use of tadalafil. Ketoconazole (400 mg qd), a selective and potent inhibitor of CYP3A, increased tadalafil 20 mg single dose exposure (AUC) by 312% and C_{max} by 22%. Ketoconazole (200 mg qd) increased tadalafil 10 mg single dose exposure (AUC) by 107% and C_{max} by 15%. Although specific interactions have not been studied, other CYP3A inhibitors would likely increase tadalafil exposure).
No products indexed under this heading.

Isosorbide Dinitrate (Concomitant use of tadalafil with organic nitrates is contraindicated. Tadalafil should not be used in patients who are using any form of organic nitrate, either regular or intermittently. Tadalafil potentiates the hypotensive effect of nitrates. In a patient who has taken tadalafil, where nitrate administration is deemed medically necessary in a life-threatening situation, at least 48 hours should elapse after the last dose of tadalafil before nitrate administration is considered. In such circumstances, nitrates should still only be administered under close medical supervision with appropriate hemodynamic monitoring).
No products indexed under this heading.

Isosorbide Mononitrate (Concomitant use of tadalafil with organic nitrates is contraindicated. Tadalafil should not be used in patients who are using any form of organic nitrate, either regular or intermittently. Tadalafil potentiates the hypotensive effect of nitrates. In a patient who has taken tadalafil, where nitrate administration is deemed medically necessary in a life-threatening situation, at least 48 hours should elapse after the last dose of tadalafil before nitrate administration is considered. In such circumstances, nitrates should still only be administered under close medical supervision with appropriate hemodynamic monitoring).
No products indexed under this heading.

Isradipine (Clinical pharmacology studies were conducted to assess the effect of tadalafil on the potentiation of the blood-pressure-lowering effects of selected antihypertensive medications (amlodipine, angiotensin II receptor blockers, bendroflumethiazide, enalapril, and metoprolol). Small reductions in blood pressure occurred following co-administration of tadalafil with these agents compared with placebo).
Products include:
DynaCirc CR 1432

Itraconazole (Tadalafil is metabolized predominantly by CYP3A in the liver. In patients taking potent inhibitors of CYP3A such as itraconazole, avoid use of tadalafil. Ketoconazole (400 mg qd), a selective and potent inhibitor of CYP3A, increased tadalafil 20 mg single dose exposure (AUC) by 312% and C_{max} by 22%. Ketoconazole (200 mg qd) increased tadalafil 10 mg single dose exposure (AUC) by 107% and C_{max} by 15%. Although specific interactions have not been studied, other CYP3A inhibitors, such as itraconazole, would likely increase tadalafil exposure).
No products indexed under this heading.

Ketoconazole (Tadalafil is metabolized predominantly by CYP3A in the liver. In patients taking potent inhibitors of CYP3A, such as ketoconazole, avoid use of tadalafil. Ketoconazole (400 mg qd), a selective and potent inhibitor of CYP3A, increased tadalafil 20 mg single dose exposure (AUC) by 312% and C_{max} by 22%. Ketoconazole (200 mg qd) increased tadalafil 10 mg single dose exposure (AUC) by 107% and C_{max} by 15%). Products include:
Extina 3319
Xolegel 3337

Labetalol Hydrochloride (Clinical pharmacology studies were conducted to assess the effect of tadalafil on the potentiation of the blood-pressure-lowering effects of selected antihypertensive medications (amlodipine, angiotensin II receptor blockers, bendroflumethiazide, enalapril, and metoprolol). Small reductions in blood pressure occurred following co-administration of tadalafil with these agents compared with placebo).
No products indexed under this heading.

Lisinopril (Clinical pharmacology studies were conducted to assess the effect of tadalafil on the potentiation of the blood-pressure-lowering effects of selected antihypertensive medications (amlodipine, angiotensin II receptor blockers, bendroflumethiazide, enalapril, and metoprolol). Small reductions in blood pressure occurred following co-administration of tadalafil with these agents compared with placebo).
Products include:
Prinivil 2241
Prinzide 2246

Lopinavir (Ritonavir (500 mg or 600 mg bid at steady state), an inhibitor of CYP3A, CYP2C9, CYP2C19, and CYP2D6, increased tadalafil 20 mg single dose exposure (AUC) by 32% with a 30% reduction in C_{max}. Ritonavir (200 mg bid), increased tadalafil 20 mg single dose exposure (AUC) by 124% with no change in C_{max}. Ritonavir inhibits and induces CYP3A, the enzyme involved in the metabolism of tadalafil in a time dependent manner. The results suggest the initial inhibitory effect of ritonavir on CYP3A may be mitigated by a more slowly evolving induction effect so that after about 1 week of ritonavir bid, the exposure of tadalafil is similiar in the presence of and absence of ritonavir. Although specific interactions have not been studied, other HIV protease inhibitors would likely increase tadalafil exposure). Products include:
Kaletra 458

Losartan Potassium (A study assessed the interaction between angiotensin II receptor blockers and tadalafil 20 mg. Subjects in the study were taking any marketed angiotensin II receptor blocker, either alone, as a component of a combination product, or as part of a multiple antihypertensive regimen. Following dosing, ambulatory measurements of blood pressure revealed differences between tadalafil and placebo of 8/4 mm Hg in systolic/diastolic blood pressure). Products include:
Cozaar 2106
Hyzaar 2162
Hyzaar 100-12.5 2162

Magaldrate (Simultaneous administration of an antacid (magnesium hydroxide/aluminum hydroxide) and tadalafil (10 mg) reduced the apparent rate of absorption of tadalafil without altering exposure (AUC) to tadalafil).
No products indexed under this heading.

Magnesium Carbonate (Simultaneous administration of an antacid (magnesium hydroxide/aluminum hydroxide) and tadalafil (10 mg) reduced the apparent rate of absorption of tadalafil without altering exposure (AUC) to tadalafil).
No products indexed under this heading.

Magnesium Hydroxide (Simultaneous administration of an antacid (magnesium hydroxide/aluminum hydroxide) and tadalafil (10 mg) reduced the apparent rate of absorption of tadalafil without altering exposure (AUC) to tadalafil). Products include:
Fleet Pedia-Lax Chewable Tablets 1144
Pepcid Complete 1822

Magnesium Oxide (Simultaneous administration of an antacid (magnesium hydroxide/aluminum hydroxide) and tadalafil (10 mg) reduced the apparent rate of absorption of tadalafil without altering exposure (AUC) to tadalafil).
Products include:
Beelith 873

Magnesium Trisilicate (Simultaneous administration of an antacid (magnesium hydroxide/aluminum hydroxide) and tadalafil (10 mg) reduced the apparent rate of absorption of tadalafil without altering exposure (AUC) to tadalafil).
No products indexed under this heading.

Mecamylamine Hydrochloride (Clinical pharmacology studies were conducted to assess the effect of tadalafil on the potentiation of the blood-pressure-lowering effects of selected antihypertensive medications (amlodipine, angiotensin II receptor blockers, bendroflumethiazide, enalapril, and metoprolol). Small reductions in blood pressure occurred following co-administration of tadalafil with these agents compared with placebo).
No products indexed under this heading.

Methyclothiazide (Clinical pharmacology studies were conducted to assess the effect of tadalafil on the potentiation of the blood-pressure-lowering effects of selected antihypertensive medications (amlodipine, angiotensin II receptor blockers, bendroflumethiazide, enalapril, and metoprolol). Small reductions in blood pressure occurred following co-administration of tadalafil with these agents compared with placebo).
No products indexed under this heading.

Methyldopa (Clinical pharmacology studies were conducted to assess the effect of tadalafil on the potentiation of the blood-pressure-lowering effects of selected antihypertensive medications (amlodipine, angiotensin II receptor blockers, bendroflumethiazide, enalapril, and metoprolol). Small reductions in blood pressure occurred following co-administration of tadalafil with these agents compared with placebo).
No products indexed under this heading.

Methyldopate Hydrochloride (Clinical pharmacology studies were conducted to assess the effect of tadalafil on the potentiation of the blood-pressure-lowering effects of selected antihypertensive medications (amlodipine, angiotensin II receptor blockers, bendroflumethiazide, enalapril, and metoprolol). Small reductions in blood pressure occurred following co-administration of tadalafil with these agents compared with placebo).
No products indexed under this heading.

Metolazone (Clinical pharmacology studies were conducted to assess the effect of tadalafil on the potentiation of the blood-pressure-lowering effects of selected antihypertensive medications (amlodipine, angiotensin II receptor blockers, bendroflumethiazide, enalapril, and metoprolol). Small reductions in blood pressure occurred following co-administration of tadalafil with these agents compared with placebo).
No products indexed under this heading.

Metoprolol Succinate (A study assessed the interaction between sustained-release metoprolol (25 to 200 mg daily) and tadalafil 10 mg. Following dosing, the mean reduction in supine systolic/diastolic blood pressure because of tadalafil 10 mg in subjects taking metoprolol was 5/3 mm Hg, compared to placebo). Products include:
Toprol XL 732

Metoprolol Tartrate (A study assessed the interaction between sustained-release metoprolol (25 to 200 mg daily) and tadalafil 10 mg. Following dosing, the mean reduction in supine systolic/diastolic blood pressure because of tadalafil 10 mg in subjects taking metoprolol was 5/3 mm Hg, compared to placebo).
No products indexed under this heading.

Metronidazole (Tadalafil is metabolized predominantly by CYP3A in the liver. In patients taking potent inhibitors of CYP3A, avoid use of tadalafil. Ketoconazole (400 mg qd), a selective and potent inhibitor of CYP3A, increased tadalafil 20 mg single dose exposure (AUC) by 312% and C_{max} by 22%. Ketoconazole (200 mg qd) increased tadalafil 10 mg single dose exposure (AUC) by 107% and C_{max} by 15%. Although specific interactions have not been studied, other CYP3A inhibitors would likely increase tadalafil exposure). Products include:
Pylera 793

Metronidazole Benzoate (Tadalafil is metabolized predominantly by CYP3A in the liver. In patients taking potent inhibitors of CYP3A, avoid use of tadalafil. Ketoconazole (400 mg qd), a selective and potent inhibitor of CYP3A, increased tadalafil 20 mg single dose exposure (AUC) by 312% and C_{max} by 22%. Ketoconazole (200 mg qd) increased tadalafil 10 mg single dose exposure (AUC) by 107% and C_{max} by 15%. Although specific interactions have not been studied, other CYP3A inhibitors would likely increase tadalafil exposure).
No products indexed under this heading.

Metronidazole Hydrochloride (Tadalafil is metabolized predominantly by CYP3A in the liver. In patients taking potent inhibitors of CYP3A, avoid use of tadalafil. Ketoconazole (400 mg qd), a selective and potent inhibitor of CYP3A, increased tadalafil 20 mg single dose exposure (AUC) by 312% and C_{max} by 22%. Ketoconazole (200 mg qd) increased tadalafil 10 mg single dose exposure (AUC) by 107% and C_{max} by 15%. Although specific interactions have not been studied, other CYP3A inhibitors would likely increase tadalafil exposure).
No products indexed under this heading.

Metyrosine (Clinical pharmacology studies were conducted to assess the effect of tadalafil on the potentiation of the blood-pressure-lowering effects of selected antihypertensive medications (amlodipine, angiotensin II receptor blockers, bendroflumethiazide, enalapril, and metoprolol). Small reductions in blood pressure occurred following co-administration of tadalafil with these agents compared with placebo).
No products indexed under this heading.

Mibefradil Dihydrochloride (Clinical pharmacology studies were conducted to assess the effect of tadalafil on the potentiation of the blood-pressure-lowering effects of selected antihypertensive medications (amlodipine, angiotensin II receptor blockers, bendroflumethiazide, enalapril, and metoprolol). Small reductions in blood pressure occurred following co-administration of tadalafil with these agents compared with placebo).
No products indexed under this heading.

Miconazole (Tadalafil is metabolized predominantly by CYP3A in the liver. In patients taking potent inhibitors of CYP3A, avoid use of tadalafil. Ketoconazole (400 mg qd), a selective and potent inhibitor of CYP3A, increased tadalafil 20 mg single dose exposure (AUC) by 312% and C_{max} by 22%. Ketoconazole (200 mg qd) increased tadalafil 10 mg single dose exposure (AUC) by 107% and C_{max} by 15%. Although specific interactions have not been studied, other CYP3A inhibitors would likely increase tadalafil exposure).
No products indexed under this heading.

Minoxidil (Clinical pharmacology studies were conducted to assess the effect of tadalafil on the potentiation of the blood-pressure-lowering effects of selected antihypertensive medications

(amlodipine, angiotensin II receptor blockers, bendroflumethiazide, enalapril, and metoprolol). Small reductions in blood pressure occurred following co-administration of tadalafil with these agents compared with placebo).
No products indexed under this heading.

Modafinil (For patients chronically taking potent inducers of CYP3A, avoid use of tadalafil. Rifampin (600 mg qd), a CYP3A inducer, reduced tadalafil 10 mg single dose exposure (AUC) by 88% and C_{max} by 46%. Bosentan (125 mg bid), a substrate of CYP2C9 and CYP3A and a moderate inducer of CYP3A, CYP2C9, and possibly CYP2C19, reduced tadalafil (40 mg qd) systemic exposure by 42% and C_{max} by 27% following multiple dose co-administration. Although specific interactions have not been studied, other CYP3A inducers would likely decrease tadalafil exposure). Products include:
Provigil 983

Moexipril Hydrochloride (Clinical pharmacology studies were conducted to assess the effect of tadalafil on the potentiation of the blood-pressure-lowering effects of selected antihypertensive medications (amlodipine, angiotensin II receptor blockers, bendroflumethiazide, enalapril, and metoprolol). Small reductions in blood pressure occurred following co-administration of tadalafil with these agents compared with placebo).
No products indexed under this heading.

Nadolol (Clinical pharmacology studies were conducted to assess the effect of tadalafil on the potentiation of the blood-pressure-lowering effects of selected antihypertensive medications (amlodipine, angiotensin II receptor blockers, bendroflumethiazide, enalapril, and metoprolol). Small reductions in blood pressure occurred following co-administration of tadalafil with these agents compared with placebo).
Products include:
Nadolol 2359

Nebivolol (Clinical pharmacology studies were conducted to assess the effect of tadalafil on the potentiation of the blood-pressure-lowering effects of selected antihypertensive medications (amlodipine, angiotensin II receptor blockers, bendroflumethiazide, enalapril, and metoprolol). Small reductions in blood pressure occurred following co-administration of tadalafil with these agents compared with placebo).
Products include:
Bystolic 1147

Nefazodone Hydrochloride (Tadalafil is metabolized predominantly by CYP3A in the liver. In patients taking potent inhibitors of CYP3A, avoid use of tadalafil. Ketoconazole (400 mg qd), a selective and potent inhibitor of CYP3A, increased tadalafil 20 mg single dose exposure (AUC) by 312% and C_{max} by 22%. Ketoconazole (200 mg qd) increased tadalafil 10 mg single dose exposure (AUC) by 107% and C_{max} by 15%. Although specific interactions have not been studied, other CYP3A inhibitors would likely increase tadalafil exposure).
No products indexed under this heading.

Nelfinavir Mesylate (Ritonavir (500 mg or 600 mg bid at steady state), an inhibitor of CYP3A, CYP2C9, CYP2C19, and CYP2D6, increased tadalafil 20 mg single dose exposure (AUC) by 32% with a 30% reduction in C_{max}. Ritonavir (200 mg bid), increased tadalafil 20 mg single dose exposure (AUC) by 124% with no change in C_{max}. Ritonavir inhibits and induces CYP3A, the enzyme involved in the metabolism of tadalafil in a time dependent manner. The results suggest the initial inhibitory effect of ritonavir on CYP3A may be

mitigated by a more slowly evolving induction effect so that after about 1 week of ritonavir bid, the exposure of tadalafil is similiar in the presence of and absence of ritonavir. Although specific interactions have not been studied, other HIV protease inhibitors would likely increase tadalafil exposure).
No products indexed under this heading.

Nevirapine (For patients chronically taking potent inducers of CYP3A, avoid use of tadalafil. Rifampin (600 mg qd), a CYP3A inducer, reduced tadalafil 10 mg single dose exposure (AUC) by 88% and C_{max} by 46%. Bosentan (125 mg bid), a substrate of CYP2C9 and CYP3A and a moderate inducer of CYP3A, CYP2C9, and possibly CYP2C19, reduced tadalafil (40 mg qd) systemic exposure by 42% and C_{max} by 27% following multiple dose co-administration. Although specific interactions have not been studied, other CYP3A inducers would likely decrease tadalafil exposure). Products include:
Viramune Oral Suspension 897
Viramune Tablets 897

Nicardipine Hydrochloride (Clinical pharmacology studies were conducted to assess the effect of tadalafil on the potentiation of the blood-pressure-lowering effects of selected antihypertensive medications (amlodipine, angiotensin II receptor blockers, bendroflumethiazide, enalapril, and metoprolol). Small reductions in blood pressure occurred following co-administration of tadalafil with these agents compared with placebo).
No products indexed under this heading.

Nifedipine (Clinical pharmacology studies were conducted to assess the effect of tadalafil on the potentiation of the blood-pressure-lowering effects of selected antihypertensive medications (amlodipine, angiotensin II receptor blockers, bendroflumethiazide, enalapril, and metoprolol). Small reductions in blood pressure occurred following co-administration of tadalafil with these agents compared with placebo).
No products indexed under this heading.

Nisoldipine (Clinical pharmacology studies were conducted to assess the effect of tadalafil on the potentiation of the blood-pressure-lowering effects of selected antihypertensive medications (amlodipine, angiotensin II receptor blockers, bendroflumethiazide, enalapril, and metoprolol). Small reductions in blood pressure occurred following co-administration of tadalafil with these agents compared with placebo).
No products indexed under this heading.

Nitrate & Nitrite Preparations (Concomitant use of tadalafil with organic nitrates is contraindicated. Tadalafil should not be used in patients who are using any form of organic nitrate, either regular or intermittently. Tadalafil potentiates the hypotensive effect of nitrates. In a patient who has taken tadalafil, where nitrate administration is deemed medically necessary in a life-threatening situation, at least 48 hours should elapse after the last dose of tadalafil before nitrate administration is considered. In such circumstances, nitrates should still only be administered under close medical supervision with appropriate hemodynamic monitoring).
No products indexed under this heading.

Nitrates, organic (Concomitant use of tadalafil with organic nitrates is contraindicated. Tadalafil should not be used in patients who are using any form of organic nitrate, either regular or intermittently. Tadalafil potentiates the hypotensive effect of nitrates. In a patient who has taken tadalafil, where nitrate administration is deemed medically necessary in a life-threatening situation, at least 48 hours should elapse after the

last dose of tadalafil before nitrate administration is considered. In such circumstances, nitrates should still only be administered under close medical supervision with appropriate hemodynamic monitoring).
No products indexed under this heading.

Nitrates and Nitrites (Concomitant use of tadalafil with organic nitrates is contraindicated. Tadalafil should not be used in patients who are using any form of organic nitrate, either regular or intermittently. Tadalafil potentiates the hypotensive effect of nitrates. In a patient who has taken tadalafil, where nitrate administration is deemed medically necessary in a life-threatening situation, at least 48 hours should elapse after the last dose of tadalafil before nitrate administration is considered. In such circumstances, nitrates should still only be administered under close medical supervision with appropriate hemodynamic monitoring).
No products indexed under this heading.

Nitroglycerin (Concomitant use of tadalafil with organic nitrates is contraindicated. Tadalafil should not be used in patients who are using any form of organic nitrate, either regular or intermittently. Tadalafil potentiates the hypotensive effect of nitrates. In a patient who has taken tadalafil, where nitrate administration is deemed medically necessary in a life-threatening situation, at least 48 hours should elapse after the last dose of tadalafil before nitrate administration is considered. In such circumstances, nitrates should still only be administered under close medical supervision with appropriate hemodynamic monitoring). Products include:
Nitro-Dur **3170**
Nitrolingual **3266**

Nitroglycerin, long-acting formulations (Concomitant use of tadalafil with organic nitrates is contraindicated. Tadalafil should not be used in patients who are using any form of organic nitrate, either regular or intermittently. Tadalafil potentiates the hypotensive effect of nitrates. In a patient who has taken tadalafil, where nitrate administration is deemed medically necessary in a life-threatening situation, at least 48 hours should elapse after the last dose of tadalafil before nitrate administration is considered. In such circumstances, nitrates should still only be administered under close medical supervision with appropriate hemodynamic monitoring).
No products indexed under this heading.

Nitroglycerin Intravenous (Concomitant use of tadalafil with organic nitrates is contraindicated. Tadalafil should not be used in patients who are using any form of organic nitrate, either regular or intermittently. Tadalafil potentiates the hypotensive effect of nitrates. In a patient who has taken tadalafil, where nitrate administration is deemed medically necessary in a life-threatening situation, at least 48 hours should elapse after the last dose of tadalafil before nitrate administration is considered. In such circumstances, nitrates should still only be administered under close medical supervision with appropriate hemodynamic monitoring).
No products indexed under this heading.

Norfloxacin (Tadalafil is metabolized predominantly by CYP3A in the liver. In patients taking potent inhibitors of CYP3A, avoid use of tadalafil. Ketoconazole (400 mg qd), a selective and potent inhibitor of CYP3A, increased tadalafil 20 mg single dose exposure (AUC) by 312% and C_{max} by 22%. Ketoconazole (200 mg qd) increased tadalafil 10 mg single dose exposure (AUC) by 107% and C_{max} by 15%. Although specific interactions have not been studied, other CYP3A inhibitors would likely increase tadalafil exposure). Products include:
Noroxin **2220**

Paroxetine Hydrochloride (Tadalafil is metabolized predominantly by CYP3A in the liver. In patients taking potent inhibitors of CYP3A, avoid use of tadalafil. Ketoconazole (400 mg qd), a selective and potent inhibitor of CYP3A, increased tadalafil 20 mg single dose exposure (AUC) by 312% and C_{max} by 22%. Ketoconazole (200 mg qd) increased tadalafil 10 mg single dose exposure (AUC) by 107% and C_{max} by 15%. Although specific interactions have not been studied, other CYP3A inhibitors would likely increase tadalafil exposure). Products include:
Paroxetine CR **2361**
Paroxetine ER **2371**
Paxil **1586**
Paxil CR **1596**

Penbutolol Sulfate (Clinical pharmacology studies were conducted to assess the effect of tadalafil on the potentiation of the blood-pressure-lowering effects of selected antihypertensive medications (amlodipine, angiotensin II receptor blockers, bendroflumethiazide, enalapril, and metoprolol). Small reductions in blood pressure occurred following co-administration of tadalafil with these agents compared with placebo).
No products indexed under this heading.

Pentaerythritol Tetranitrate (Concomitant use of tadalafil with organic nitrates is contraindicated. Tadalafil should not be used in patients who are using any form of organic nitrate, either regular or intermittently. Tadalafil potentiates the hypotensive effect of nitrates. In a patient who has taken tadalafil, where nitrate administration is deemed medically necessary in a life-threatening situation, at least 48 hours should elapse after the last dose of tadalafil before nitrate administration is considered. In such circumstances, nitrates should still only be administered under close medical supervision with appropriate hemodynamic monitoring).
No products indexed under this heading.

Perindopril Erbumine (Clinical pharmacology studies were conducted to assess the effect of tadalafil on the potentiation of the blood-pressure-lowering effects of selected antihypertensive medications (amlodipine, angiotensin II receptor blockers, bendroflumethiazide, enalapril, and metoprolol). Small reductions in blood pressure occurred following co-administration of tadalafil with these agents compared with placebo).
No products indexed under this heading.

Phenobarbital (For patients chronically taking potent inducers of CYP3A, avoid use of tadalafil. Rifampin (600 mg qd), a CYP3A inducer, reduced tadalafil 10 mg single dose exposure (AUC) by 88% and C_{max} by 46%. Bosentan (125 mg bid), a substrate of CYP2C9 and CYP3A and a moderate inducer of CYP3A, CYP2C9, and possibly CYP2C19, reduced tadalafil (40 mg qd) systemic exposure by 42% and C_{max} by 27% following multiple dose co-administration. Although specific interactions have not been studied, other CYP3A inducers, such as phenobarbital, would likely decrease tadalafil exposure). Products include:
Donnatal **2711**

Phenobarbital Sodium (For patients chronically taking potent inducers of CYP3A, avoid use of tadalafil. Rifampin (600 mg qd), a CYP3A inducer, reduced tadalafil 10 mg single dose exposure (AUC) by 88% and C_{max} by 46%. Bosentan (125 mg bid), a substrate of CYP2C9 and CYP3A and a moderate inducer of CYP3A, CYP2C9, and possibly CYP2C19, reduced tadalafil (40 mg qd) systemic exposure by 42% and C_{max} by 27% following multiple dose co-administration. Although specific interactions have not been studied, other CYP3A inducers, such as phenobarbital, would likely decrease tadalafil exposure).
No products indexed under this heading.

Phenoxybenzamine Hydrochloride (Clinical pharmacology studies were conducted to assess the effect of tadalafil on the potentiation of the blood-pressure-lowering effects of selected antihypertensive medications (amlodipine, angiotensin II receptor blockers, bendroflumethiazide, enalapril, and metoprolol). Small reductions in blood pressure occurred following co-administration of tadalafil with these agents compared with placebo). Products include:
Dibenzyline **3495**

Phentolamine Mesylate (Clinical pharmacology studies were conducted to assess the effect of tadalafil on the potentiation of the blood-pressure-lowering effects of selected antihypertensive medications (amlodipine, angiotensin II receptor blockers, bendroflumethiazide, enalapril, and metoprolol). Small reductions in blood pressure occurred following co-administration of tadalafil with these agents compared with placebo).
No products indexed under this heading.

Phenytoin (For patients chronically taking potent inducers of CYP3A, avoid use of tadalafil. Rifampin (600 mg qd), a CYP3A inducer, reduced tadalafil 10 mg single dose exposure (AUC) by 88% and C_{max} by 46%. Bosentan (125 mg bid), a substrate of CYP2C9 and CYP3A and a moderate inducer of CYP3A, CYP2C9, and possibly CYP2C19, reduced tadalafil (40 mg qd) systemic exposure by 42% and C_{max} by 27% following multiple dose co-administration. Although specific interactions have not been studied, other CYP3A inducers, such as phenytoin, would likely decrease tadalafil exposure).
No products indexed under this heading.

Phenytoin Sodium (For patients chronically taking potent inducers of CYP3A, avoid use of tadalafil. Rifampin (600 mg qd), a CYP3A inducer, reduced tadalafil 10 mg single dose exposure (AUC) by 88% and C_{max} by 46%. Bosentan (125 mg bid), a substrate of CYP2C9 and CYP3A and a moderate inducer of CYP3A, CYP2C9, and possibly CYP2C19, reduced tadalafil (40 mg qd) systemic exposure by 42% and C_{max} by 27% following multiple dose co-administration. Although specific interactions have not been studied, other CYP3A inducers, such as phenytoin, would likely decrease tadalafil exposure). Products include:
Phenytek Capsules **2380**

Pindolol (Clinical pharmacology studies were conducted to assess the effect of tadalafil on the potentiation of the blood-pressure-lowering effects of selected antihypertensive medications (amlodipine, angiotensin II receptor blockers, bendroflumethiazide, enalapril, and metoprolol). Small reductions in blood pressure occurred following co-administration of tadalafil with these agents compared with placebo).
No products indexed under this heading.

Polythiazide (Clinical pharmacology studies were conducted to assess the effect of tadalafil on the potentiation of the blood-pressure-lowering effects of selected antihypertensive medications (amlodipine, angiotensin II receptor blockers, bendroflumethiazide, enalapril, and metoprolol). Small reductions in blood pressure occurred following co-administration of tadalafil with these agents compared with placebo).
No products indexed under this heading.

Prazosin Hydrochloride (PDE5 inhibitors, including tadalafil, and α-adrenergic blocking agents are vasodilators with blood pressure-lowering effects. When vasodilators are used in combination, an additive effect on blood pressure may be anticipated. In some patients, concomitant use of these two drug classes can lower blood pressure significantly, which may lead to symptomatic hypotension (eg, fainting). Safety of combined use of PDE5 inhibitors and α-blockers may be affected by other variables, including intravascular volume depletion and use of other antihypertensive drugs).
No products indexed under this heading.

Propranolol Hydrochloride (Clinical pharmacology studies were conducted to assess the effect of tadalafil on the potentiation of the blood-pressure-lowering effects of selected antihypertensive medications (amlodipine, angiotensin II receptor blockers, bendroflumethiazide, enalapril, and metoprolol). Small reductions in blood pressure occurred following co-administration of tadalafil with these agents compared with placebo). Products include:
InnoPran XL **1517**

Quinapril Hydrochloride (Clinical pharmacology studies were conducted to assess the effect of tadalafil on the potentiation of the blood-pressure-lowering effects of selected antihypertensive medications (amlodipine, angiotensin II receptor blockers, bendroflumethiazide, enalapril, and metoprolol). Small reductions in blood pressure occurred following co-administration of tadalafil with these agents compared with placebo).
No products indexed under this heading.

Quinine (Tadalafil is metabolized predominantly by CYP3A in the liver. In patients taking potent inhibitors of CYP3A, avoid use of tadalafil. Ketoconazole (400 mg qd), a selective and potent inhibitor of CYP3A, increased tadalafil 20 mg single dose exposure (AUC) by 312% and C_{max} by 22%. Ketoconazole (200 mg qd) increased tadalafil 10 mg single dose exposure (AUC) by 107% and C_{max} by 15%. Although specific interactions have not been studied, other CYP3A inhibitors would likely increase tadalafil exposure). Products include:
Hyland's Leg Cramps PM with Quinine **3315**

Quinine Sulfate (Tadalafil is metabolized predominantly by CYP3A in the liver. In patients taking potent inhibitors of CYP3A, avoid use of tadalafil. Ketoconazole (400 mg qd), a selective and potent inhibitor of CYP3A, increased tadalafil 20 mg single dose exposure (AUC) by 312% and C_{max} by 22%. Ketoconazole (200 mg qd) increased tadalafil 10 mg single dose exposure (AUC) by 107% and C_{max} by 15%. Although specific interactions have not been studied, other CYP3A inhibitors would likely increase tadalafil exposure).
No products indexed under this heading.

Ramipril (Clinical pharmacology studies were conducted to assess the effect of tadalafil on the potentiation of the blood-pressure-lowering effects of selected antihypertensive medications (amlodipine, angiotensin II receptor blockers, bendroflumethiazide, enalapril, and metoprolol). Small reductions in blood pressure occurred following co-administration of tadalafil with these agents compared with placebo).
No products indexed under this heading.

Rauwolfia Serpentina (Clinical pharmacology studies were conducted to assess the effect of tadalafil on the potentiation of the blood-pressure-lowering effects of selected antihypertensive medications (amlodipine, angiotensin II receptor blockers, bendroflumethiazide, enalapril, and metoprolol). Small reductions in blood pressure occurred following co-administration of tadalafil with these agents compared with placebo).
No products indexed under this heading.

Rescinnamine (Clinical pharmacology studies were conducted to assess the effect of tadalafil on the potentiation of the blood-pressure-lowering effects of selected antihypertensive medications (amlodipine, angiotensin II receptor blockers, bendroflumethiazide, enalapril, and metoprolol). Small reductions in blood pressure occurred following co-administration of tadalafil with these agents compared with placebo).
No products indexed under this heading.

Reserpine (Clinical pharmacology studies were conducted to assess the effect of tadalafil on the potentiation of the blood-pressure-lowering effects of selected antihypertensive medications (amlodipine, angiotensin II receptor blockers, bendroflumethiazide, enalapril, and metoprolol). Small reductions in blood pressure occurred following co-administration of tadalafil with these agents compared with placebo).
No products indexed under this heading.

Rifabutin (For patients chronically taking potent inducers of CYP3A, avoid use of tadalafil. Rifampin (600 mg qd), a CYP3A inducer, reduced tadalafil 10 mg single dose exposure (AUC) by 88% and C_{max} by 46%. Bosentan (125 mg bid), a substrate of CYP2C9 and CYP3A and a moderate inducer of CYP3A, CYP2C9, and possibly CYP2C19, reduced tadalafil (40 mg qd) systemic exposure by 42% and C_{max} by 27% following multiple dose co-administration. Although specific interactions have not been studied, other CYP3A inducers would likely decrease tadalafil exposure).
No products indexed under this heading.

Rifampicin (For patients chronically taking potent inducers of CYP3A, avoid use of tadalafil. Rifampin (600 mg qd), a CYP3A inducer, reduced tadalafil 10 mg single dose exposure (AUC) by 88% and C_{max} by 46%. Bosentan (125 mg bid), a substrate of CYP2C9 and CYP3A and a moderate inducer of CYP3A, CYP2C9, and possibly CYP2C19, reduced tadalafil (40 mg qd) systemic exposure by 42% and C_{max} by 27% following multiple dose co-administration. Although specific interactions have not been studied, other CYP3A inducers would likely decrease tadalafil exposure).
No products indexed under this heading.

Rifampin (For patients chronically taking potent inducers of CYP3A, such as rifampin, avoid use of tadalafil. Rifampin (600 mg qd), a CYP3A inducer, reduced tadalafil 10 mg single dose exposure (AUC) by 88% and C_{max} by 46%, relative to the values for tadalafil 10 mg alone).
No products indexed under this heading.

Rifapentine (For patients chronically taking potent inducers of CYP3A, avoid use of tadalafil. Rifampin (600 mg qd), a CYP3A inducer, reduced tadalafil 10 mg single dose exposure (AUC) by 88% and C_{max} by 46%. Bosentan (125 mg bid), a substrate of CYP2C9 and CYP3A and a moderate inducer of CYP3A, CYP2C9, and possibly CYP2C19, reduced tadalafil (40 mg qd) systemic exposure by 42% and C_{max} by 27% following multiple dose co-administration. Although specific interactions have not been studied, other CYP3A inducers would likely decrease tadalafil exposure).
No products indexed under this heading.

Ritonavir (Ritonavir (500 mg or 600 mg bid at steady state), an inhibitor of CYP3A, CYP2C9, CYP2C19, and CYP2D6, increased tadalafil 20 mg single dose exposure (AUC) by 32% with a 30% reduction in C_{max}. Ritonavir (200 mg bid) increased tadalafil 20 mg single dose exposure (AUC) by 124% with no change in C_{max}. Ritonavir inhibits and induces CYP3A, the enzyme involved in the metabolism of tadalafil in a time dependent manner. The results suggest the initial inhibitory effect of ritonavir on CYP3A may be mitigated by a more slowly evolving induction effect so that after about 1 week of ritonavir bid, the exposure of tadalafil is similiar in the presence of and absence of ritonavir. Tadalafil should be avoided during the initiation of ritonavir. Tadalafil should be stopped at least 24 hours prior to starting ritonavir. After at least one week following the initiation of ritonavir, tadalafil can be resumed at 20 mg qd, and can be increased to 40 mg qd based upon individual tolerability. If receiving ritonavir for at least 1 week, start tadalafil at 20 mg qd. Increase the dose to 40 mg qd based on individual tolerability). Products include:
Kaletra **458**
Norvir **509**

Saquinavir (Ritonavir (500 mg or 600 mg bid at steady state), an inhibitor of CYP3A, CYP2C9, CYP2C19, and CYP2D6, increased tadalafil 20 mg single dose exposure (AUC) by 32% with a 30% reduction in C_{max}. Ritonavir (200 mg bid), increased tadalafil 20 mg single dose exposure (AUC) by 124% with no change in C_{max}. Ritonavir inhibits and induces CYP3A, the enzyme involved in the metabolism of tadalafil in a time dependent manner. The results suggest the initial inhibitory effect of ritonavir on CYP3A may be mitigated by a more slowly evolving induction effect so that after about 1 week of ritonavir bid, the exposure of tadalafil is similiar in the presence of and absence of ritonavir. Although specific interactions have not been studied, other HIV protease inhibitors would likely increase tadalafil exposure).
No products indexed under this heading.

Saquinavir Mesylate (Ritonavir (500 mg or 600 mg bid at steady state), an inhibitor of CYP3A, CYP2C9, CYP2C19, and CYP2D6, increased tadalafil 20 mg single dose exposure (AUC) by 32% with a 30% reduction in C_{max}. Ritonavir (200 mg bid), increased tadalafil 20 mg single dose exposure (AUC) by 124% with no change in C_{max}. Ritonavir inhibits and induces CYP3A, the enzyme involved in the metabolism of tadalafil in a time dependent manner. The results suggest the initial inhibitory effect of ritonavir on CYP3A may be mitigated by a more slowly evolving induction effect so that after about 1 week of ritonavir bid, the exposure of tadalafil is similiar in the presence of and absence of ritonavir. Although specific interactions have not been studied, other HIV protease inhibitors would likely increase tadalafil exposure).
No products indexed under this heading.

Sertraline Hydrochloride (Tadalafil is metabolized predominantly by CYP3A in the liver. In patients taking potent inhibitors of CYP3A, avoid use of tadalafil. Ketoconazole (400 mg qd), a selective and potent inhibitor of CYP3A, increased tadalafil 20 mg single dose exposure (AUC) by 312% and C_{max} by 22%. Ketoconazole (200 mg qd) increased tadalafil 10 mg single dose exposure (AUC) by 107% and C_{max} by 15%. Although specific interactions have not been studied, other CYP3A inhibitors would likely increase tadalafil exposure).
No products indexed under this heading.

Sildenafil Citrate (Tadalafil is also marketed as Cialis. The safety and efficacy of taking tadalafil together with Cialis or other PDE5 inhibitors have not been studied. Patients taking tadalafil should be informed not to take Cialis or other PDE5 inhibitors).
No products indexed under this heading.

Sodium Bicarbonate (Simultaneous administration of an antacid (magnesium hydroxide/aluminum hydroxide) and tadalafil (10 mg) reduced the apparent rate of absorption of tadalafil without altering exposure (AUC) to tadalafil).
No products indexed under this heading.

Sodium Nitroprusside (Clinical pharmacology studies were conducted to assess the effect of tadalafil on the potentiation of the blood-pressure-lowering effects of selected antihypertensive medications (amlodipine, angiotensin II receptor blockers, bendroflumethiazide, enalapril, and metoprolol). Small reductions in blood pressure occurred following co-administration of tadalafil with these agents compared with placebo).
No products indexed under this heading.

Sotalol Hydrochloride (Clinical pharmacology studies were conducted to assess the effect of tadalafil on the potentiation of the blood-pressure-lowering effects of selected antihypertensive medications (amlodipine, angiotensin II receptor blockers, bendroflumethiazide, enalapril, and metoprolol). Small reductions in blood pressure occurred following co-administration of tadalafil with these agents compared with placebo).
No products indexed under this heading.

Spirapril Hydrochloride (Clinical pharmacology studies were conducted to assess the effect of tadalafil on the potentiation of the blood-pressure-lowering effects of selected antihypertensive medications (amlodipine, angiotensin II receptor blockers, bendroflumethiazide, enalapril, and metoprolol). Small reductions in blood pressure occurred following co-administration of tadalafil with these agents compared with placebo).
No products indexed under this heading.

Tamsulosin Hydrochloride (PDE5 inhibitors, including tadalafil, and α-adrenergic blocking agents are vasodilators with blood pressure-lowering effects. When vasodilators are used in combination, an additive effect on blood pressure may be anticipated. In some patients, concomitant use of these two drug classes can lower blood pressure significantly, which may lead to symptomatic hypotension (eg, fainting). Safety of combined use of PDE5 inhibitors and α-blockers may be affected by other variables, including intravascular volume depletion and use of other antihypertensive drugs).
No products indexed under this heading.

Telmisartan (A study assessed the interaction between angiotensin II receptor blockers and tadalafil 20 mg. Subjects in the study were taking any marketed angiotensin II receptor blocker, either alone, as a component of a combination product, or as part of a multiple antihypertensive regimen. Following dosing, ambulatory measurements of blood pressure revealed differences between tadalafil and placebo of 8/4 mm Hg in systolic/diastolic blood pressure). Products include:
Micardis **887**
Micardis HCT **889**

Terazosin Hydrochloride (PDE5 inhibitors, including tadalafil, and α-adrenergic blocking agents are vasodilators with blood pressure-lowering effects. When vasodilators are used in combination, an additive effect on blood pressure may be anticipated. In some patients, concomitant use of these two drug classes can lower blood pressure significantly, which may lead to symptomatic hypotension (eg, fainting). Safety of combined use of PDE5 inhibitors and α-blockers may be affected by other variables, including intravascular volume depletion and use of other antihypertensive drugs).
No products indexed under this heading.

Theophylline (Tadalafil (10 mg qd) had no significant effect on the pharmacokinetics of theophylline. When tadalafil was administered to subjects taking theophylline, a small augmentation (3 beats per minute) of the increase in heart rate associated with theophylline was observed).
No products indexed under this heading.

Theophylline Anhydrous (Tadalafil (10 mg qd) had no significant effect on the pharmacokinetics of theophylline. When tadalafil was administered to subjects taking theophylline, a small augmentation (3 beats per minute) of the increase in heart rate associated with theophylline was observed). Products include:
Uniphyl **2817**

Theophylline Calcium Salicylate (Tadalafil (10 mg qd) had no significant effect on the pharmacokinetics of theophylline. When tadalafil was administered to subjects taking theophylline, a small augmentation (3 beats per minute) of the increase in heart rate associated with theophylline was observed).
No products indexed under this heading.

Theophylline Dihydroxypropyl (Glyceryl) (Tadalafil (10 mg qd) had no significant effect on the pharmacokinetics of theophylline. When tadalafil was administered to subjects taking theophylline, a small augmentation (3 beats per minute) of the increase in heart rate associated with theophylline was observed).
No products indexed under this heading.

Theophylline Ethylenediamine (Tadalafil (10 mg qd) had no significant effect on the pharmacokinetics of theophylline. When tadalafil was administered to subjects taking theophylline, a small augmentation (3 beats per minute) of the increase in heart rate associated with theophylline was observed).
No products indexed under this heading.

Theophylline Sodium Glycinate (Tadalafil (10 mg qd) had no significant effect on the pharmacokinetics of theophylline. When tadalafil was administered to subjects taking theophylline, a small augmentation (3 beats per minute) of the increase in heart rate associated with theophylline was observed).
No products indexed under this heading.

Timolol Maleate (Clinical pharmacology studies were conducted to assess the effect of tadalafil on the potentiation of the blood-pressure-lowering effects of selected antihypertensive medications (amlodipine, angiotensin II receptor blockers, bendroflumethiazide, enalapril, and metoprolol). Small reductions in blood pressure occurred following co-administration of tadalafil with these agents compared with placebo). Products include:
Combigan **601**
Dorzolamide Hydrochloride/Timolol Maleate Ophthalmic Solution .... ⊙**243**
Timoptic in Ocudose .... ⊙**231**

Tipranavir (Ritonavir (500 mg or 600 mg bid at steady state), an inhibitor of CYP3A, CYP2C9, CYP2C19, and CYP2D6, increased tadalafil 20 mg sin-

gle dose exposure (AUC) by 32% with a 30% reduction in C_{max}. Ritonavir (200 mg bid), increased tadalafil 20 mg single dose exposure (AUC) by 124% with no change in C_{max}. Ritonavir inhibits and induces CYP3A, the enzyme involved in the metabolism of tadalafil in a time dependent manner. The results suggest the initial inhibitory effect of ritonavir on CYP3A may be mitigated by a more slowly evolving induction effect so that after about 1 week of ritonavir bid, the exposure of tadalafil is similiar in the presence of and absence of ritonavir. Although specific interactions have not been studied, other HIV protease inhibitors would likely increase tadalafil exposure).
No products indexed under this heading.

Torsemide (Clinical pharmacology studies were conducted to assess the effect of tadalafil on the potentiation of the blood-pressure-lowering effects of selected antihypertensive medications (amlodipine, angiotensin II receptor blockers, bendroflumethiazide, enalapril, and metoprolol). Small reductions in blood pressure occurred following co-administration of tadalafil with these agents compared with placebo).
No products indexed under this heading.

Trandolapril (Clinical pharmacology studies were conducted to assess the effect of tadalafil on the potentiation of the blood-pressure-lowering effects of selected antihypertensive medications (amlodipine, angiotensin II receptor blockers, bendroflumethiazide, enalapril, and metoprolol). Small reductions in blood pressure occurred following co-administration of tadalafil with these agents compared with placebo).
Products include:
Mavik 489
Tarka 534

Trimethaphan Camsylate (Clinical pharmacology studies were conducted to assess the effect of tadalafil on the potentiation of the blood-pressure-lowering effects of selected antihypertensive medications (amlodipine, angiotensin II receptor blockers, bendroflumethiazide, enalapril, and metoprolol). Small reductions in blood pressure occurred following co-administration of tadalafil with these agents compared with placebo).
No products indexed under this heading.

Troleandomycin (Tadalafil is metabolized predominantly by CYP3A in the liver. In patients taking potent inhibitors of CYP3A, avoid use of tadalafil. Ketoconazole (400 mg qd), a selective and potent inhibitor of CYP3A, increased tadalafil 20 mg single dose exposure (AUC) by 312% and C_{max} by 22%. Ketoconazole (200 mg qd) increased tadalafil 10 mg single dose exposure (AUC) by 107% and C_{max} by 15%. Although specific interactions have not been studied, other CYP3A inhibitors would likely increase tadalafil exposure).
No products indexed under this heading.

Valsartan (A study assessed the interaction between angiotensin II receptor blockers and tadalafil 20 mg. Subjects in the study were taking any marketed angiotensin II receptor blocker, either alone, as a component of a combination product, or as part of a multiple antihypertensive regimen. Following dosing, ambulatory measurements of blood pressure revealed differences between tadalafil and placebo of 8/4 mm Hg in systolic/diastolic blood pressure).
Products include:
Diovan 2413
Diovan HCT 2419
Exforge 2443
Exforge HCT 2449
Valturna 3637

Vardenafil Hydrochloride (Tadalafil is also marketed as Cialis. The safety and efficacy of taking tadalafil together with Cialis or other PDE5 inhibitors have not been studied. Patients taking tadalafil should be informed not to take Cialis or other PDE5 inhibitors). Products include:
Levitra 3157

Venlafaxine Hydrochloride (Tadalafil is metabolized predominantly by CYP3A in the liver. In patients taking potent inhibitors of CYP3A, avoid use of tadalafil. Ketoconazole (400 mg qd), a selective and potent inhibitor of CYP3A, increased tadalafil 20 mg single dose exposure (AUC) by 312% and C_{max} by 22%. Ketoconazole (200 mg qd) increased tadalafil 10 mg single dose exposure (AUC) by 107% and C_{max} by 15%. Although specific interactions have not been studied, other CYP3A inhibitors would likely increase tadalafil exposure). Products include:
Effexor XR 3504
Venlafaxine Hydrochloride Tablets ... 2388

Verapamil Hydrochloride (Clinical pharmacology studies were conducted to assess the effect of tadalafil on the potentiation of the blood-pressure-lowering effects of selected antihypertensive medications (amlodipine, angiotensin II receptor blockers, bendroflumethiazide, enalapril, and metoprolol). Small reductions in blood pressure occurred following co-administration of tadalafil with these agents compared with placebo).
Products include:
Tarka 534

Voriconazole (Tadalafil is metabolized predominantly by CYP3A in the liver. In patients taking potent inhibitors of CYP3A, avoid use of tadalafil. Ketoconazole (400 mg qd), a selective and potent inhibitor of CYP3A, increased tadalafil 20 mg single dose exposure (AUC) by 312% and C_{max} by 22%. Ketoconazole (200 mg qd) increased tadalafil 10 mg single dose exposure (AUC) by 107% and C_{max} by 15%. Although specific interactions have not been studied, other CYP3A inhibitors would likely increase tadalafil exposure).
No products indexed under this heading.

Zafirlukast (Tadalafil is metabolized predominantly by CYP3A in the liver. In patients taking potent inhibitors of CYP3A, avoid use of tadalafil. Ketoconazole (400 mg qd), a selective and potent inhibitor of CYP3A, increased tadalafil 20 mg single dose exposure (AUC) by 312% and C_{max} by 22%. Ketoconazole (200 mg qd) increased tadalafil 10 mg single dose exposure (AUC) by 107% and C_{max} by 15%. Although specific interactions have not been studied, other CYP3A inhibitors would likely increase tadalafil exposure). Products include:
Accolate 3612

Zileuton (Tadalafil is metabolized predominantly by CYP3A in the liver. In patients taking potent inhibitors of CYP3A, avoid use of tadalafil. Ketoconazole (400 mg qd), a selective and potent inhibitor of CYP3A, increased tadalafil 20 mg single dose exposure (AUC) by 312% and C_{max} by 22%. Ketoconazole (200 mg qd) increased tadalafil 10 mg single dose exposure (AUC) by 107% and C_{max} by 15%. Although specific interactions have not been studied, other CYP3A inhibitors would likely increase tadalafil exposure).
No products indexed under this heading.

Food Interactions

Alcohol (Both alcohol and tadalafil, a PDE5 inhibitor, act as mild vasodilators. When mild vasodilators are taken in combination, blood pressure–lowering effects of each individual compound may be increased. Substantial consumption of alcohol (eg, 5 units or greater) in combination with tadalafil can increase the potential for orthostatic signs and symptoms, including increase in heart rate, decrease in standing blood pressure, dizziness, and headache).

Beer, reduced-alcohol (Both alcohol and tadalafil, a PDE5 inhibitor, act as mild vasodilators. When mild vasodilators are taken in combination, blood pressure–lowering effects of each individual compound may be increased. Substantial consumption of alcohol (eg, 5 units or greater) in combination with tadalafil can increase the potential for orthostatic signs and symptoms, including increase in heart rate, decrease in standing blood pressure, dizziness, and headache).

Beer, unspecified (Both alcohol and tadalafil, a PDE5 inhibitor, act as mild vasodilators. When mild vasodilators are taken in combination, blood pressure–lowering effects of each individual compound may be increased. Substantial consumption of alcohol (eg, 5 units or greater) in combination with tadalafil can increase the potential for orthostatic signs and symptoms, including increase in heart rate, decrease in standing blood pressure, dizziness, and headache).

Grapefruit (Tadalafil is metabolized predominantly by CYP3A in the liver. In patients taking potent inhibitors of CYP3A, avoid use of tadalafil. Ketoconazole (400 mg qd), a selective and potent inhibitor of CYP3A, increased tadalafil 20 mg single dose exposure (AUC) by 312% and C_{max} by 22%. Ketoconazole (200 mg qd) increased tadalafil 10 mg single dose exposure (AUC) by 107% and C_{max} by 15%. Although specific interactions have not been studied, other CYP3A inhibitors would likely increase tadalafil exposure).

Grapefruit Juice (Tadalafil is metabolized predominantly by CYP3A in the liver. In patients taking potent inhibitors of CYP3A, avoid use of tadalafil. Ketoconazole (400 mg qd), a selective and potent inhibitor of CYP3A, increased tadalafil 20 mg single dose exposure (AUC) by 312% and C_{max} by 22%. Ketoconazole (200 mg qd) increased tadalafil 10 mg single dose exposure (AUC) by 107% and C_{max} by 15%. Although specific interactions have not been studied, other CYP3A inhibitors, such as grapefruit juice, would likely increase tadalafil exposure).

Wine, Chianti (Both alcohol and tadalafil, a PDE5 inhibitor, act as mild vasodilators. When mild vasodilators are taken in combination, blood pressure–lowering effects of each individual compound may be increased. Substantial consumption of alcohol (eg, 5 units or greater) in combination with tadalafil can increase the potential for orthostatic signs and symptoms, including increase in heart rate, decrease in standing blood pressure, dizziness, and headache).

Wine, Red (Both alcohol and tadalafil, a PDE5 inhibitor, act as mild vasodilators. When mild vasodilators are taken in combination, blood pressure–lowering effects of each individual compound may be increased. Substantial consumption of alcohol (eg, 5 units or greater) in combination with tadalafil can increase the potential for orthostatic signs and symptoms, including increase in heart rate, decrease in standing blood pressure, dizziness, and headache).

Wine, unspecified (Both alcohol and tadalafil, a PDE5 inhibitor, act as mild vasodilators. When mild vasodilators are taken in combination, blood pressure–lowering effects of each individual compound may be increased. Substantial consumption of alcohol (eg, 5 units or greater) in combination with tadalafil can increase the potential for orthostatic signs and symptoms, including increase in heart rate, decrease in standing blood pressure, dizziness, and headache).

Wine products (Both alcohol and tadalafil, a PDE5 inhibitor, act as mild vasodilators. When mild vasodilators are taken in combination, blood pressure–lowering effects of each individual compound may be increased. Substantial consumption of alcohol (eg, 5 units or greater) in combination with tadalafil can increase the potential for orthostatic signs and symptoms, including increase in heart rate, decrease in standing blood pressure, dizziness, and headache).

ADENOCARD IV INJECTION

(Adenosine) 656
May interact with cardiac glycosides, xanthines, and certain other agents. Compounds in these categories include:

Aminophylline (The effects of adenosine are antagonized by co-administration with methylxanthines, such as theophylline; larger doses of adenosine may be required or adenosine may not be effective).
No products indexed under this heading.

Caffeine (The effects of adenosine are antagonized by co-administration with methylxanthines, such as caffeine; larger doses of adenosine may be required or adenosine may not be effective).
No products indexed under this heading.

Carbamazepine (Adenosine decreases the conduction through AV node, higher degrees of heart block may be produced in the presence of carbamazepine). Products include:
Carbatrol 3280
Equetro 3477

Deslanoside (The use of adenosine in patients receiving digitalis may be rarely associated with ventricular fibrillation).
No products indexed under this heading.

Digitalis Glycoside Preparations (The use of adenosine in patients receiving digitalis may be rarely associated with ventricular fibrillation).
No products indexed under this heading.

Digitalis Lanata (The use of adenosine in patients receiving digitalis may be rarely associated with ventricular fibrillation).
No products indexed under this heading.

Digitalis Purpurea (The use of adenosine in patients receiving digitalis may be rarely associated with ventricular fibrillation).
No products indexed under this heading.

Digitoxin (The use of adenosine in patients receiving digitalis may be rarely associated with ventricular fibrillation).
No products indexed under this heading.

Digoxin (The use of adenosine in patients receiving digitalis may be rarely associated with ventricular fibrillation).
Products include:
Lanoxin Injection 1546
Lanoxin Injection Pediatric 1549
Lanoxin Tablets 1553

Dipyridamole (Adenosine effects are potentiated by dipyridamole; smaller doses of adenosine may be effective with concurrent use). Products include:
Aggrenox 880

51 Interactions Index Adenoscan

Dyphylline (The effects of adenosine are antagonized by co-administration with methylxanthines, such as theophylline; larger doses of adenosine may be required or adenosine may not be effective).
No products indexed under this heading.

Theophylline (The effects of adenosine are antagonized by co-administration with methylxanthines, such as theophylline; larger doses of adenosine may be required or adenosine may not be effective).
No products indexed under this heading.

Theophylline Anhydrous (The effects of adenosine are antagonized by co-administration with methylxanthines, such as theophylline; larger doses of adenosine may be required or adenosine may not be effective). Products include:
Uniphyl 2817

Theophylline Calcium Salicylate (The effects of adenosine are antagonized by co-administration with methylxanthines, such as theophylline; larger doses of adenosine may be required or adenosine may not be effective).
No products indexed under this heading.

Theophylline Dihydroxypropyl (Glyceryl) (The effects of adenosine are antagonized by co-administration with methylxanthines, such as theophylline; larger doses of adenosine may be required or adenosine may not be effective).
No products indexed under this heading.

Theophylline Ethylenediamine (The effects of adenosine are antagonized by co-administration with methylxanthines, such as theophylline; larger doses of adenosine may be required or adenosine may not be effective).
No products indexed under this heading.

Theophylline Sodium Glycinate (The effects of adenosine are antagonized by co-administration with methylxanthines, such as theophylline; larger doses of adenosine may be required or adenosine may not be effective).
No products indexed under this heading.

Verapamil Hydrochloride (Digoxin and verapamil use may be rarely associated with ventricular fibrillation when combined with adenosine; potential for additive or synergistic depressant effects on the SA and AV nodes).
Products include:
Tarka 534

ADENOSCAN

(Adenosine) 657
May interact with adenosine receptor antagonists, beta-blockers, calcium channel blockers, cardiac glycosides, nucleoside transport inhibitors, xanthines. Compounds in these categories include:

Acebutolol Hydrochloride (Intravenous adenosine has been given with other cardioactive drugs (such as β-adrenergic blocking agents, cardiac glycosides, and calcium channel blockers) without apparent adverse interactions, but its effectiveness with these agents has not been systematically evaluated. Because of the potential for additive or synergistic depressant effects on the SA and AV nodes, however, adenosine should be used with caution in the presence of these agents).
No products indexed under this heading.

Aminophylline (The vasoactive effects of adenosine are inhibited by adenosine receptor antagonists, such as methylxanthines (eg, caffeine and theophylline). The safety and efficacy of adenosine in the presence of these agents has not been systematically evaluated).
No products indexed under this heading.

Amlodipine Besylate (Intravenous adenosine has been given with other cardioactive drugs (such as β-adrenergic blocking agents, cardiac glycosides, and calcium channel blockers) without apparent adverse interactions, but its effectiveness with these agents has not been systematically evaluated. Because of the potential for additive or synergistic depressant effects on the SA and AV nodes, however, adenosine should be used with caution in the presence of these agents).
Products include:
Azor 1010
Exforge 2443
Exforge HCT 2449

Atenolol (Intravenous adenosine has been given with other cardioactive drugs (such as β-adrenergic blocking agents, cardiac glycosides, and calcium channel blockers) without apparent adverse interactions, but its effectiveness with these agents has not been systematically evaluated. Because of the potential for additive or synergistic depressant effects on the SA and AV nodes, however, adenosine should be used with caution in the presence of these agents).
No products indexed under this heading.

Bepridil Hydrochloride (Intravenous adenosine has been given with other cardioactive drugs (such as β-adrenergic blocking agents, cardiac glycosides, and calcium channel blockers) without apparent adverse interactions, but its effectiveness with these agents has not been systematically evaluated. Because of the potential for additive or synergistic depressant effects on the SA and AV nodes, however, adenosine should be used with caution in the presence of these agents).
No products indexed under this heading.

Betaxolol Hydrochloride (Intravenous adenosine has been given with other cardioactive drugs (such as β-adrenergic blocking agents, cardiac glycosides, and calcium channel blockers) without apparent adverse interactions, but its effectiveness with these agents has not been systematically evaluated. Because of the potential for additive or synergistic depressant effects on the SA and AV nodes, however, adenosine should be used with caution in the presence of these agents).
No products indexed under this heading.

Bisoprolol Fumarate (Intravenous adenosine has been given with other cardioactive drugs (such as β-adrenergic blocking agents, cardiac glycosides, and calcium channel blockers) without apparent adverse interactions, but its effectiveness with these agents has not been systematically evaluated. Because of the potential for additive or synergistic depressant effects on the SA and AV nodes, however, adenosine should be used with caution in the presence of these agents).
No products indexed under this heading.

Caffeine (The vasoactive effects of adenosine are inhibited by adenosine receptor antagonists, such as methylxanthines (eg, caffeine and theophylline). The safety and efficacy of adenosine in the presence of these agents has not been systematically evaluated).
No products indexed under this heading.

Carteolol Hydrochloride (Intravenous adenosine has been given with other cardioactive drugs (such as β-adrenergic blocking agents, cardiac glycosides, and calcium channel blockers) without apparent adverse interactions, but its effectiveness with these agents has not been systematically evaluated. Because of the potential for additive or synergistic depressant effects on the SA and AV nodes, however, adenosine should be used with caution in the presence of these agents).
No products indexed under this heading.

Carvedilol (Intravenous adenosine has been given with other cardioactive drugs (such as β-adrenergic blocking agents, cardiac glycosides, and calcium channel blockers) without apparent adverse interactions, but its effectiveness with these agents has not been systematically evaluated. Because of the potential for additive or synergistic depressant effects on the SA and AV nodes, however, adenosine should be used with caution in the presence of these agents). Products include:
Coreg 1409

Carvedilol Phosphate (Intravenous adenosine has been given with other cardioactive drugs (such as β-adrenergic blocking agents, cardiac glycosides, and calcium channel blockers) without apparent adverse interactions, but its effectiveness with these agents has not been systematically evaluated. Because of the potential for additive or synergistic depressant effects on the SA and AV nodes, however, adenosine should be used with caution in the presence of these agents).
Products include:
Coreg CR 1416

Deslanoside (Intravenous adenosine has been given with other cardioactive drugs (such as β-adrenergic blocking agents, cardiac glycosides, and calcium channel blockers) without apparent adverse interactions, but its effectiveness with these agents has not been systematically evaluated. Because of the potential for additive or synergistic depressant effects on the SA and AV nodes, however, adenosine should be used with caution in the presence of these agents).
No products indexed under this heading.

Digitalis Glycoside Preparations (Intravenous adenosine has been given with other cardioactive drugs (such as β-adrenergic blocking agents, cardiac glycosides, and calcium channel blockers) without apparent adverse interactions, but its effectiveness with these agents has not been systematically evaluated. Because of the potential for additive or synergistic depressant effects on the SA and AV nodes, however, adenosine should be used with caution in the presence of these agents).
No products indexed under this heading.

Digitalis Lanata (Intravenous adenosine has been given with other cardioactive drugs (such as β-adrenergic blocking agents, cardiac glycosides, and calcium channel blockers) without apparent adverse interactions, but its effectiveness with these agents has not been systematically evaluated. Because of the potential for additive or synergistic depressant effects on the SA and AV nodes, however, adenosine should be used with caution in the presence of these agents).
No products indexed under this heading.

Digitalis Purpurea (Intravenous adenosine has been given with other cardioactive drugs (such as β-adrenergic blocking agents, cardiac glycosides, and calcium channel blockers) without apparent adverse interactions, but its effectiveness with these agents has not been systematically evaluated. Because of the potential for additive or synergistic depressant effects on the SA and AV nodes, however, adenosine should be used with caution in the presence of these agents).
No products indexed under this heading.

Digitoxin (Intravenous adenosine has been given with other cardioactive drugs (such as β-adrenergic blocking agents, cardiac glycosides, and calcium channel blockers) without apparent adverse interactions, but its effectiveness with these agents has not been systematically evaluated. Because of the potential for additive or synergistic depressant effects on the SA and AV nodes, however, adenosine should be used with caution in the presence of these agents).
No products indexed under this heading.

Digoxin (Intravenous adenosine has been given with other cardioactive drugs (such as β-adrenergic blocking agents, cardiac glycosides, and calcium channel blockers) without apparent adverse interactions, but its effectiveness with these agents has not been systematically evaluated. Because of the potential for additive or synergistic depressant effects on the SA and AV nodes, however, adenosine should be used with caution in the presence of these agents). Products include:
Lanoxin Injection 1546
Lanoxin Injection Pediatric 1549
Lanoxin Tablets 1553

Diltiazem Hydrochloride (Intravenous adenosine has been given with other cardioactive drugs (such as β-adrenergic blocking agents, cardiac glycosides, and calcium channel blockers) without apparent adverse interactions, but its effectiveness with these agents has not been systematically evaluated. Because of the potential for additive or synergistic depressant effects on the SA and AV nodes, however, adenosine should be used with caution in the presence of these agents).
Products include:
Cardizem LA 423

Dipyridamole (Vasoactive effects of adenosine are potentiated by nucleoside transport inhibitors, such as dipyridamole. The safety and efficacy of adenosine in the presence of dipyridamole has not been systematically evaluated). Products include:
Aggrenox 880

Dyphylline (The vasoactive effects of adenosine are inhibited by adenosine receptor antagonists, such as methylxanthines (eg, caffeine and theophylline). The safety and efficacy of adenosine in the presence of these agents has not been systematically evaluated).
No products indexed under this heading.

Esmolol Hydrochloride (Intravenous adenosine has been given with other cardioactive drugs (such as β-adrenergic blocking agents, cardiac glycosides, and calcium channel blockers) without apparent adverse interactions, but its effectiveness with these agents has not been systematically evaluated. Because of the potential for additive or synergistic depressant effects on the SA and AV nodes, however, adenosine should be used with caution in the presence of these agents).
No products indexed under this heading.

Felodipine (Intravenous adenosine has been given with other cardioactive drugs (such as β-adrenergic blocking agents, cardiac glycosides, and calcium channel blockers) without apparent adverse interactions, but its effectiveness with these agents has not been systematically evaluated. Because of the potential for additive or synergistic depressant effects on the SA and AV nodes, however, adenosine should be used with caution in the presence of these agents).
No products indexed under this heading.

Isradipine (Intravenous adenosine has been given with other cardioactive drugs (such as β-adrenergic blocking agents, cardiac glycosides, and calcium channel blockers) without apparent adverse interactions, but its effectiveness with these agents has not been

systematically evaluated. Because of the potential for additive or synergistic depressant effects on the SA and AV nodes, however, adenosine should be used with caution in the presence of these agents). Products include:
DynaCirc CR 1432

Labetalol Hydrochloride (Intravenous adenosine has been given with other cardioactive drugs (such as β-adrenergic blocking agents, cardiac glycosides, and calcium channel blockers) without apparent adverse interactions, but its effectiveness with these agents has not been systematically evaluated. Because of the potential for additive or synergistic depressant effects on the SA and AV nodes, however, adenosine should be used with caution in the presence of these agents).
No products indexed under this heading.

Levobunolol Hydrochloride (Intravenous adenosine has been given with other cardioactive drugs (such as β-adrenergic blocking agents, cardiac glycosides, and calcium channel blockers) without apparent adverse interactions, but its effectiveness with these agents has not been systematically evaluated. Because of the potential for additive or synergistic depressant effects on the SA and AV nodes, however, adenosine should be used with caution in the presence of these agents).
No products indexed under this heading.

Metipranolol Hydrochloride (Intravenous adenosine has been given with other cardioactive drugs (such as β-adrenergic blocking agents, cardiac glycosides, and calcium channel blockers) without apparent adverse interactions, but its effectiveness with these agents has not been systematically evaluated. Because of the potential for additive or synergistic depressant effects on the SA and AV nodes, however, adenosine should be used with caution in the presence of these agents).
No products indexed under this heading.

Metoprolol Succinate (Intravenous adenosine has been given with other cardioactive drugs (such as β-adrenergic blocking agents, cardiac glycosides, and calcium channel blockers) without apparent adverse interactions, but its effectiveness with these agents has not been systematically evaluated. Because of the potential for additive or synergistic depressant effects on the SA and AV nodes, however, adenosine should be used with caution in the presence of these agents). Products include:
Toprol XL 732

Metoprolol Tartrate (Intravenous adenosine has been given with other cardioactive drugs (such as β-adrenergic blocking agents, cardiac glycosides, and calcium channel blockers) without apparent adverse interactions, but its effectiveness with these agents has not been systematically evaluated. Because of the potential for additive or synergistic depressant effects on the SA and AV nodes, however, adenosine should be used with caution in the presence of these agents).
No products indexed under this heading.

Mibefradil Dihydrochloride (Intravenous adenosine has been given with other cardioactive drugs (such as β-adrenergic blocking agents, cardiac glycosides, and calcium channel blockers) without apparent adverse interactions, but its effectiveness with these agents has not been systematically evaluated. Because of the potential for additive or synergistic depressant effects on the SA and AV nodes, however, adenosine should be used with caution in the presence of these agents).
No products indexed under this heading.

Nadolol (Intravenous adenosine has been given with other cardioactive drugs (such as β-adrenergic blocking agents, cardiac glycosides, and calcium channel blockers) without apparent adverse interactions, but its effectiveness with these agents has not been systematically evaluated. Because of the potential for additive or synergistic depressant effects on the SA and AV nodes, however, adenosine should be used with caution in the presence of these agents). Products include:
Nadolol 2359

Nebivolol (Intravenous adenosine has been given with other cardioactive drugs (such as β-adrenergic blocking agents, cardiac glycosides, and calcium channel blockers) without apparent adverse interactions, but its effectiveness with these agents has not been systematically evaluated. Because of the potential for additive or synergistic depressant effects on the SA and AV nodes, however, adenosine should be used with caution in the presence of these agents). Products include:
Bystolic 1147

Nicardipine (Intravenous adenosine has been given with other cardioactive drugs (such as β-adrenergic blocking agents, cardiac glycosides, and calcium channel blockers) without apparent adverse interactions, but its effectiveness with these agents has not been systematically evaluated. Because of the potential for additive or synergistic depressant effects on the SA and AV nodes, however, adenosine should be used with caution in the presence of these agents).
No products indexed under this heading.

Nicardipine Hydrochloride (Intravenous adenosine has been given with other cardioactive drugs (such as β-adrenergic blocking agents, cardiac glycosides, and calcium channel blockers) without apparent adverse interactions, but its effectiveness with these agents has not been systematically evaluated. Because of the potential for additive or synergistic depressant effects on the SA and AV nodes, however, adenosine should be used with caution in the presence of these agents).
No products indexed under this heading.

Nifedipine (Intravenous adenosine has been given with other cardioactive drugs (such as β-adrenergic blocking agents, cardiac glycosides, and calcium channel blockers) without apparent adverse interactions, but its effectiveness with these agents has not been systematically evaluated. Because of the potential for additive or synergistic depressant effects on the SA and AV nodes, however, adenosine should be used with caution in the presence of these agents).
No products indexed under this heading.

Nimodipine (Intravenous adenosine has been given with other cardioactive drugs (such as β-adrenergic blocking agents, cardiac glycosides, and calcium channel blockers) without apparent adverse interactions, but its effectiveness with these agents has not been systematically evaluated. Because of the potential for additive or synergistic depressant effects on the SA and AV nodes, however, adenosine should be used with caution in the presence of these agents).
No products indexed under this heading.

Nisoldipine (Intravenous adenosine has been given with other cardioactive drugs (such as β-adrenergic blocking agents, cardiac glycosides, and calcium channel blockers) without apparent adverse interactions, but its effectiveness with these agents has not been systematically evaluated. Because of the potential for additive or synergistic

depressant effects on the SA and AV nodes, however, adenosine should be used with caution in the presence of these agents).
No products indexed under this heading.

Penbutolol Sulfate (Intravenous adenosine has been given with other cardioactive drugs (such as β-adrenergic blocking agents, cardiac glycosides, and calcium channel blockers) without apparent adverse interactions, but its effectiveness with these agents has not been systematically evaluated. Because of the potential for additive or synergistic depressant effects on the SA and AV nodes, however, adenosine should be used with caution in the presence of these agents).
No products indexed under this heading.

Pindolol (Intravenous adenosine has been given with other cardioactive drugs (such as β-adrenergic blocking agents, cardiac glycosides, and calcium channel blockers) without apparent adverse interactions, but its effectiveness with these agents has not been systematically evaluated. Because of the potential for additive or synergistic depressant effects on the SA and AV nodes, however, adenosine should be used with caution in the presence of these agents).
No products indexed under this heading.

Propranolol Hydrochloride (Intravenous adenosine has been given with other cardioactive drugs (such as β-adrenergic blocking agents, cardiac glycosides, and calcium channel blockers) without apparent adverse interactions, but its effectiveness with these agents has not been systematically evaluated. Because of the potential for additive or synergistic depressant effects on the SA and AV nodes, however, adenosine should be used with caution in the presence of these agents). Products include:
InnoPran XL 1517

Sotalol Hydrochloride (Intravenous adenosine has been given with other cardioactive drugs (such as β-adrenergic blocking agents, cardiac glycosides, and calcium channel blockers) without apparent adverse interactions, but its effectiveness with these agents has not been systematically evaluated. Because of the potential for additive or synergistic depressant effects on the SA and AV nodes, however, adenosine should be used with caution in the presence of these agents).
No products indexed under this heading.

Theophylline (The vasoactive effects of adenosine are inhibited by adenosine receptor antagonists, such as methylxanthines (eg, caffeine and theophylline). The safety and efficacy of adenosine in the presence of these agents has not been systematically evaluated).
No products indexed under this heading.

Theophylline Anhydrous (The vasoactive effects of adenosine are inhibited by adenosine receptor antagonists, such as methylxanthines (eg, caffeine and theophylline). The safety and efficacy of adenosine in the presence of these agents has not been systematically evaluated). Products include:
Uniphyl 2817

Theophylline Calcium Salicylate (The vasoactive effects of adenosine are inhibited by adenosine receptor antagonists, such as methylxanthines (eg, caffeine and theophylline). The safety and efficacy of adenosine in the presence of these agents has not been systematically evaluated).
No products indexed under this heading.

Theophylline Dihydroxypropyl (Glyceryl) (The vasoactive effects of adenosine are inhibited by adenosine receptor antagonists, such as methylxanthines (eg, caffeine and theophylline). The safety and efficacy of adenosine in the presence of these agents has not been systematically evaluated).
No products indexed under this heading.

Theophylline Ethylenediamine (The vasoactive effects of adenosine are inhibited by adenosine receptor antagonists, such as methylxanthines (eg, caffeine and theophylline). The safety and efficacy of adenosine in the presence of these agents has not been systematically evaluated).
No products indexed under this heading.

Theophylline Sodium Glycinate (The vasoactive effects of adenosine are inhibited by adenosine receptor antagonists, such as methylxanthines (eg, caffeine and theophylline). The safety and efficacy of adenosine in the presence of these agents has not been systematically evaluated).
No products indexed under this heading.

Timolol Hemihydrate (Intravenous adenosine has been given with other cardioactive drugs (such as β-adrenergic blocking agents, cardiac glycosides, and calcium channel blockers) without apparent adverse interactions, but its effectiveness with these agents has not been systematically evaluated. Because of the potential for additive or synergistic depressant effects on the SA and AV nodes, however, adenosine should be used with caution in the presence of these agents). Products include:
Betimol 3490

Timolol Maleate (Intravenous adenosine has been given with other cardioactive drugs (such as β-adrenergic blocking agents, cardiac glycosides, and calcium channel blockers) without apparent adverse interactions, but its effectiveness with these agents has not been systematically evaluated. Because of the potential for additive or synergistic depressant effects on the SA and AV nodes, however, adenosine should be used with caution in the presence of these agents). Products include:
Combigan 601
Dorzolamide
Hydrochloride/Timolol Maleate
Ophthalmic Solution .... ⊙243
Timoptic in Ocudose .... ⊙231

Verapamil Hydrochloride (Intravenous adenosine has been given with other cardioactive drugs (such as β-adrenergic blocking agents, cardiac glycosides, and calcium channel blockers) without apparent adverse interactions, but its effectiveness with these agents has not been systematically evaluated. Because of the potential for additive or synergistic depressant effects on the SA and AV nodes, however, adenosine should be used with caution in the presence of these agents). Products include:
Tarka 534

ADIPEX-P CAPSULES
(Phentermine Hydrochloride) 1178
See Adipex-P Tablets

ADIPEX-P TABLETS
(Phentermine Hydrochloride) 1178
May interact with alcohols, insulin, monoamine oxidase inhibitors, selective serotonin reuptake inhibitors, and certain other agents. Compounds in these categories include:

Citalopram Hydrobromide (The safety and efficacy of combination therapy with phentermine and any other drug products for weight loss, including selective serotonin reuptake inhibitors, have not been established; co-

administration of these products for weight loss is not recommended). Products include:

Dexfenfluramine Hydrochloride (Co-administration has resulted in primary pulmonary hypertension, a rare, frequently fatal disease of the lungs and serious regurgitant cardiac valvular disease).

No products indexed under this heading.

Escitalopram Oxalate (The safety and efficacy of combination therapy with phentermine and any other drug products for weight loss, including selective serotonin reuptake inhibitors, have not been established; co-administration of these products for weight loss is not recommended). Products include:

Ethanol (May result in adverse drug interaction).

No products indexed under this heading.

Ethyl Alcohol (May result in adverse drug interaction).

No products indexed under this heading.

Fenfluramine Hydrochloride (Co-administration has resulted in primary pulmonary hypertension, a rare, frequently fatal disease of the lungs and serious regurgitant cardiac valvular disease).

No products indexed under this heading.

Fluoxetine (The safety and efficacy of combination therapy with phentermine and any other drug products for weight loss, including selective serotonin reuptake inhibitors, have not been established; co-administration of these products for weight loss is not recommended).

No products indexed under this heading.

Fluoxetine Hydrochloride (The safety and efficacy of combination therapy with phentermine and any other drug products for weight loss, including selective serotonin reuptake inhibitors, have not been established; co-administration of these products for weight loss is not recommended). Products include:

Fluvoxamine (The safety and efficacy of combination therapy with phentermine and any other drug products for weight loss, including selective serotonin reuptake inhibitors, have not been established; co-administration of these products for weight loss is not recommended).

No products indexed under this heading.

Fluvoxamine Maleate (The safety and efficacy of combination therapy with phentermine and any other drug products for weight loss, including selective serotonin reuptake inhibitors, have not been established; co-administration of these products for weight loss is not recommended).

No products indexed under this heading.

Guanethidine Monosulfate (Decreased hypotensive effect of guanethidine).

No products indexed under this heading.

Insulin (Insulin requirement may be altered).

No products indexed under this heading.

Insulin, Human, Zinc Suspension (Insulin requirement may be altered).

No products indexed under this heading.

Insulin, Human (rDNA origin) (Insulin requirement may be altered). Products include:

Insulin, Human NPH (Insulin requirement may be altered). Products include:

Insulin, Human Regular (Insulin requirement may be altered). Products include:

Insulin, Human Regular and Human NPH Mixture (Insulin requirement may be altered). Products include:

Insulin, NPH (Insulin requirement may be altered).

No products indexed under this heading.

Insulin, Regular (Insulin requirement may be altered).

No products indexed under this heading.

Insulin, Regular and NPH mixture (Insulin requirement may be altered).

No products indexed under this heading.

Insulin, Zinc Crystals (Insulin requirement may be altered).

No products indexed under this heading.

Insulin, Zinc Suspension (Insulin requirement may be altered).

No products indexed under this heading.

Insulin Aspart (Insulin requirement may be altered).

No products indexed under this heading.

Insulin Aspart, Human (Insulin requirement may be altered). Products include:

Insulin Aspart, Human Regular (Insulin requirement may be altered). Products include:

Insulin Aspart Protamine, Human (Insulin requirement may be altered). Products include:

Insulin Detemir (rDNA Origin) (Insulin requirement may be altered). Products include:

Insulin Glargine (Insulin requirement may be altered). Products include:

Insulin Glulisine (Insulin requirement may be altered). Products include:

Insulin Lispro, Human (Insulin requirement may be altered). Products include:

Insulin Lispro Protamine, Human (Insulin requirement may be altered). Products include:

Isocarboxazid (Concurrent and/or sequential administration with MAO inhibitors may result in hypertensive crises; co-administration is contraindicated). Products include:

Moclobemide (Concurrent and/or sequential administration with MAO inhibitors may result in hypertensive crises; co-administration is contraindicated).

No products indexed under this heading.

Pargyline Hydrochloride (Concurrent and/or sequential administration with MAO inhibitors may result in hypertensive crises; co-administration is contraindicated).

No products indexed under this heading.

Paroxetine (The safety and efficacy of combination therapy with phentermine and any other drug products for weight loss, including selective serotonin reuptake inhibitors, have not been established; co-administration of these products for weight loss is not recommended).

No products indexed under this heading.

Paroxetine Hydrochloride (The safety and efficacy of combination therapy with phentermine and any other drug products for weight loss, including selective serotonin reuptake inhibitors, have not been established; co-administration of these products for weight loss is not recommended). Products include:

Paroxetine Mesylate (The safety and efficacy of combination therapy with phentermine and any other drug products for weight loss, including selective serotonin reuptake inhibitors, have not been established; co-administration of these products for weight loss is not recommended).

No products indexed under this heading.

Phenelzine Sulfate (Concurrent and/or sequential administration with MAO inhibitors may result in hypertensive crises; co-administration is contraindicated).

No products indexed under this heading.

Procarbazine Hydrochloride (Concurrent and/or sequential administration with MAO inhibitors may result in hypertensive crises; co-administration is contraindicated).

No products indexed under this heading.

Rasagiline Mesylate (Concurrent and/or sequential administration with MAO inhibitors may result in hypertensive crises; co-administration is contraindicated). Products include:

Selegiline (Concurrent and/or sequential administration with MAO inhibitors may result in hypertensive crises; co-administration is contraindicated). Products include:

Selegiline Hydrochloride (Concurrent and/or sequential administration with MAO inhibitors may result in hypertensive crises; co-administration is contraindicated). Products include:

Sertraline Hydrochloride (The safety and efficacy of combination therapy with phentermine and any other drug products for weight loss, including selective serotonin reuptake inhibitors, have not been established; co-administration of these products for weight loss is not recommended).

No products indexed under this heading.

Tranylcypromine Sulfate (Concurrent and/or sequential administration with MAO inhibitors may result in hypertensive crises; co-administration is contraindicated). Products include:

Food Interactions

Alcohol (May result in adverse drug interaction).

Beer, reduced-alcohol (May result in adverse drug interaction).

Beer, unspecified (May result in adverse drug interaction).

Wine, Chianti (May result in adverse drug interaction).

Wine, Red (May result in adverse drug interaction).

Wine, unspecified (May result in adverse drug interaction).

Wine products (May result in adverse drug interaction).

ADVAIR DISKUS 100/50

May interact with anticonvulsants, beta-blockers, corticosteroids, cytochrome p450 3a4 inhibitors (selected), cytochrome p450 3a4 inhibitors, potent (selected), loop diuretics, monoamine oxidase inhibitors, potassium-depleting diuretics, thiazides, tricyclic antidepressants, and certain other agents. Compounds in these categories include:

Acebutolol Hydrochloride (β-blockers not only block the pulmonary effect of β-agonists, such as salmeterol, a component of Advair Diskus, but may produce severe bronchospasm in patients with reversible obstructive airways disease. Therefore, patients with asthma and COPD should not normally be treated with β-blockers. However, under certain circumstances, there may be no acceptable alternatives to the use of β-adrenergic blocking agents for these patients; cardioselective β-blockers could be considered, although they should be administered with caution).

No products indexed under this heading.

Acetazolamide (Fluticasone propionate and salmeterol, the individual components of Advair Diskus, are substrates of CYP3A4. The use of strong CYP3A4 inhibitors with Advair Diskus is not recommended because increased corticosteroid and increased cardiovascular adverse effects may occur).

No products indexed under this heading.

Acetazolamide Sodium (Fluticasone propionate and salmeterol, the individual components of Advair Diskus, are substrates of CYP3A4. The use of strong CYP3A4 inhibitors with Advair Diskus is not recommended because increased corticosteroid and increased cardiovascular adverse effects may occur).

No products indexed under this heading.

Alclometasone Dipropionate (Decreases in bone mineral density (BMD) have been observed with long-term administration of products containing inhaled corticosteroids. Patients with major risk factors for decreased bone mineral content, such chronic use of drugs that can reduce bone mass (eg, oral corticosteroids) should be monitored and treated with established standards of care).

No products indexed under this heading.

Amiodarone Hydrochloride (Fluticasone propionate and salmeterol, the individual components of Advair Diskus, are substrates of CYP3A4. The use of strong CYP3A4 inhibitors with Advair Diskus is not recommended because increased corticosteroid and increased cardiovascular adverse effects may occur).

No products indexed under this heading.

Amitriptyline Hydrochloride (Advair Diskus should be administered with extreme caution to patients being treated with tricyclic antidepressants, or within 2 weeks of discontinuation of such agents, because the action of salmeterol, a component of Advair Diskus, on the vascular system may be potentiated by these agents).

No products indexed under this heading.

Amoxapine (Advair Diskus should be administered with extreme caution to patients being treated with tricyclic antidepressants, or within 2 weeks of discontinuation of such agents, because the action of salmeterol, a component of Advair Diskus, on the vascular system may be potentiated by these agents).

No products indexed under this heading.

IMPORTANT NOTE: Always consult each drug listing in the patient's regimen for possible interactions.

Clarithromycin (Fluticasone propionate and salmeterol, the individual components of Advair Diskus, are substrates of CYP3A4. The use of strong CYP3A4 inhibitors (eg, clarithromycin) with Advair Diskus is not recommended because increased systemic corticosteroid and increased cardiovascular adverse effects may occur). Products include:
Biaxin/Biaxin XL 412

Clomipramine Hydrochloride (Advair Diskus should be administered with extreme caution to patients being treated with tricyclic antidepressants, or within 2 weeks of discontinuation of such agents, because the action of salmeterol, a component of Advair Diskus, on the vascular system may be potentiated by these agents).
No products indexed under this heading.

Clotrimazole (Fluticasone propionate and salmeterol, the individual components of Advair Diskus, are substrates of CYP3A4. The use of strong CYP3A4 inhibitors with Advair Diskus is not recommended because increased corticosteroid and increased cardiovascular adverse effects may occur). Products include:
Lotrisone 3163

Conivaptan Hydrochloride (Fluticasone propionate and salmeterol, the individual components of Advair Diskus, are substrates of CYP3A4. The use of strong CYP3A4 inhibitors with Advair Diskus is not recommended because increased corticosteroid and increased cardiovascular adverse effects may occur). Products include:
Vaprisol 689

Cortisone Acetate (Decreases in bone mineral density (BMD) have been observed with long-term administration of products containing inhaled corticosteroids. Patients with major risk factors for decreased bone mineral content, such chronic use of drugs that can reduce bone mass (eg, oral corticosteroids) should be monitored and treated with established standards of care).
No products indexed under this heading.

Cyclosporine (Fluticasone propionate and salmeterol, the individual components of Advair Diskus, are substrates of CYP3A4. The use of strong CYP3A4 inhibitors with Advair Diskus is not recommended because increased corticosteroid and increased cardiovascular adverse effects may occur). Products include:
Gengraf 440
Neoral Oral Solution 2496
Neoral Capsules 2496
Restasis 605

Dalfopristin (Fluticasone propionate and salmeterol, the individual components of Advair Diskus, are substrates of CYP3A4. The use of strong CYP3A4 inhibitors with Advair Diskus is not recommended because increased corticosteroid and increased cardiovascular adverse effects may occur).
No products indexed under this heading.

Danazol (Fluticasone propionate and salmeterol, the individual components of Advair Diskus, are substrates of CYP3A4. The use of strong CYP3A4 inhibitors with Advair Diskus is not recommended because increased corticosteroid and increased cardiovascular adverse effects may occur).
No products indexed under this heading.

Darunavir (Fluticasone propionate and salmeterol, the individual components of Advair Diskus, are substrates of CYP3A4. The use of strong CYP3A4 inhibitors with Advair Diskus is not recommended because increased corticosteroid and increased cardiovascular adverse effects may occur).
No products indexed under this heading.

Dasatinib (Fluticasone propionate and salmeterol, the individual components of Advair Diskus, are substrates of CYP3A4. The use of strong CYP3A4 inhibitors with Advair Diskus is not recommended because increased corticosteroid and increased cardiovascular adverse effects may occur).
No products indexed under this heading.

Delavirdine Mesylate (Fluticasone propionate and salmeterol, the individual components of Advair Diskus, are substrates of CYP3A4. The use of strong CYP3A4 inhibitors with Advair Diskus is not recommended because increased corticosteroid and increased cardiovascular adverse effects may occur).
No products indexed under this heading.

Delavirine (Fluticasone propionate and salmeterol, the individual components of Advair Diskus, are substrates of CYP3A4. The use of strong CYP3A4 inhibitors with Advair Diskus is not recommended because increased corticosteroid and increased cardiovascular adverse effects may occur).
No products indexed under this heading.

Desipramine Hydrochloride (Advair Diskus should be administered with extreme caution to patients being treated with tricyclic antidepressants, or within 2 weeks of discontinuation of such agents, because the action of salmeterol, a component of Advair Diskus, on the vascular system may be potentiated by these agents).
No products indexed under this heading.

Desloratadine (Fluticasone propionate and salmeterol, the individual components of Advair Diskus, are substrates of CYP3A4. The use of strong CYP3A4 inhibitors with Advair Diskus is not recommended because increased corticosteroid and increased cardiovascular adverse effects may occur). Products include:
Clarinex Syrup 3098
Clarinex 3098
Clarinex Reditabs 3098
Clarinex-D 12-Hour 3101
Clarinex-D 3104

Desoximetasone (Decreases in bone mineral density (BMD) have been observed with long-term administration of products containing inhaled corticosteroids. Patients with major risk factors for decreased bone mineral content, such chronic use of drugs that can reduce bone mass (eg, oral corticosteroids) should be monitored and treated with established standards of care).
No products indexed under this heading.

Dexamethasone (Decreases in bone mineral density (BMD) have been observed with long-term administration of products containing inhaled corticosteroids. Patients with major risk factors for decreased bone mineral content, such chronic use of drugs that can reduce bone mass (eg, oral corticosteroids) should be monitored and treated with established standards of care). Products include:
Ciprodex 583
Ozurdex .... ⊙223
Tobramycin and Dexamethasone
Ophthalmic Suspension .... ⊙251

Dexamethasone Acetate (Decreases in bone mineral density (BMD) have been observed with long-term administration of products containing inhaled corticosteroids. Patients with major risk factors for decreased bone mineral content, such chronic use of drugs that can reduce bone mass (eg, oral corticosteroids) should be monitored and treated with established standards of care).
No products indexed under this heading.

Dexamethasone Phosphate (Decreases in bone mineral density (BMD) have been observed with long-term administration of products containing inhaled corticosteroids. Patients with major risk factors for decreased bone mineral content, such chronic use of drugs that can reduce bone mass (eg, oral corticosteroids) should be monitored and treated with established standards of care).
No products indexed under this heading.

Dexamethasone Sodium (Decreases in bone mineral density (BMD) have been observed with long-term administration of products containing inhaled corticosteroids. Patients with major risk factors for decreased bone mineral content, such chronic use of drugs that can reduce bone mass (eg, oral corticosteroids) should be monitored and treated with established standards of care).
No products indexed under this heading.

Dexamethasone Sodium Phosphate (Decreases in bone mineral density (BMD) have been observed with long-term administration of products containing inhaled corticosteroids. Patients with major risk factors for decreased bone mineral content, such chronic use of drugs that can reduce bone mass (eg, oral corticosteroids) should be monitored and treated with established standards of care).
No products indexed under this heading.

Dexamethasone Sodium Phosphate Injection (Decreases in bone mineral density (BMD) have been observed with long-term administration of products containing inhaled corticosteroids. Patients with major risk factors for decreased bone mineral content, such chronic use of drugs that can reduce bone mass (eg, oral corticosteroids) should be monitored and treated with established standards of care).
No products indexed under this heading.

Diflorasone Diacetate (Decreases in bone mineral density (BMD) have been observed with long-term administration of products containing inhaled corticosteroids. Patients with major risk factors for decreased bone mineral content, such chronic use of drugs that can reduce bone mass (eg, oral corticosteroids) should be monitored and treated with established standards of care).
No products indexed under this heading.

Diltiazem Hydrochloride (Fluticasone propionate and salmeterol, the individual components of Advair Diskus, are substrates of CYP3A4. The use of strong CYP3A4 inhibitors with Advair Diskus is not recommended because increased corticosteroid and increased cardiovascular adverse effects may occur). Products include:
Cardizem LA 423

Diltiazem Maleate (Fluticasone propionate and salmeterol, the individual components of Advair Diskus, are substrates of CYP3A4. The use of strong CYP3A4 inhibitors with Advair Diskus is not recommended because increased corticosteroid and increased cardiovascular adverse effects may occur).
No products indexed under this heading.

Divalproex Sodium (Decreases in bone mineral density (BMD) have been observed with long-term administration of products containing inhaled corticosteroids. Patients with major risk factors for decreased bone mineral content, such chronic use of drugs that can reduce bone mass (eg, anticonvulsants) should be monitored and treated with established standards of care). Products include:
Depakote ER 426

Doxepin Hydrochloride (Advair Diskus should be administered with extreme caution to patients being treated with tricyclic antidepressants, or within 2 weeks of discontinuation of such agents, because the action of salmeterol, a component of Advair Diskus, on the vascular system may be potentiated by these agents).
No products indexed under this heading.

Efavirenz (Fluticasone propionate and salmeterol, the individual components of Advair Diskus, are substrates of CYP3A4. The use of strong CYP3A4 inhibitors with Advair Diskus is not recommended because increased corticosteroid and increased cardiovascular adverse effects may occur). Products include:
Atripla 906

Erythromycin (Fluticasone propionate and salmeterol, the individual components of Advair Diskus, are substrates of CYP3A4. The use of strong CYP3A4 inhibitors with Advair Diskus is not recommended because increased corticosteroid and increased cardiovascular adverse effects may occur).
No products indexed under this heading.

Erythromycin Estolate (Fluticasone propionate and salmeterol, the individual components of Advair Diskus, are substrates of CYP3A4. The use of strong CYP3A4 inhibitors with Advair Diskus is not recommended because increased corticosteroid and increased cardiovascular adverse effects may occur).
No products indexed under this heading.

Erythromycin Ethylsuccinate (Fluticasone propionate and salmeterol, the individual components of Advair Diskus, are substrates of CYP3A4. The use of strong CYP3A4 inhibitors with Advair Diskus is not recommended because increased corticosteroid and increased cardiovascular adverse effects may occur). Products include:
E.E.S. 437
EryPed 435

Erythromycin Gluceptate (Fluticasone propionate and salmeterol, the individual components of Advair Diskus, are substrates of CYP3A4. The use of strong CYP3A4 inhibitors with Advair Diskus is not recommended because increased corticosteroid and increased cardiovascular adverse effects may occur).
No products indexed under this heading.

Erythromycin Lactobionate (Fluticasone propionate and salmeterol, the individual components of Advair Diskus, are substrates of CYP3A4. The use of strong CYP3A4 inhibitors with Advair Diskus is not recommended because increased corticosteroid and increased cardiovascular adverse effects may occur).
No products indexed under this heading.

Erythromycin Stearate (Fluticasone propionate and salmeterol, the individual components of Advair Diskus, are substrates of CYP3A4. The use of strong CYP3A4 inhibitors with Advair Diskus is not recommended because increased corticosteroid and increased cardiovascular adverse effects may occur).
No products indexed under this heading.

Esmolol Hydrochloride (β-blockers not only block the pulmonary effect of β-agonists, such as salmeterol, a component of Advair Diskus, but may produce severe bronchospasm in patients with reversible obstructive airways disease. Therefore, patients with asthma and COPD should not normally be treated with β-blockers. However, under certain circumstances, there may be no acceptable alternatives to the use of β-adrenergic blocking agents for these

---

IMPORTANT NOTE: Always consult each drug listing in the patient's regimen for possible interactions.

patients; cardioselective β-blockers could be considered, although they should be administered with caution).
No products indexed under this heading.

Esomeprazole Magnesium (Fluticasone propionate and salmeterol, the individual components of Advair Diskus, are substrates of CYP3A4. The use of strong CYP3A4 inhibitors with Advair Diskus is not recommended because increased corticosteroid and increased cardiovascular adverse effects may occur). Products include:

Esomeprazole Sodium (Fluticasone propionate and salmeterol, the individual components of Advair Diskus, are substrates of CYP3A4. The use of strong CYP3A4 inhibitors with Advair Diskus is not recommended because increased corticosteroid and increased cardiovascular adverse effects may occur). Products include:

Ethacrynic Acid (The ECG changes and/or hypokalemia that may result from the administration of nonpotassium-sparing diuretics (eg, loop diuretics) can be acutely worsened by β-agonists, especially when the recommended dose of the β-agonist is exceeded. Although the clinical relevance of these effects is not known, caution is advised in the co-administration of β-agonists with nonpotassium-sparing diuretics).
No products indexed under this heading.

Ethosuximide (Decreases in bone mineral density (BMD) have been observed with long-term administration of products containing inhaled corticosteroids. Patients with major risk factors for decreased bone mineral content, such chronic use of drugs that can reduce bone mass (eg, anticonvulsants) should be monitored and treated with established standards of care).
No products indexed under this heading.

Ethotoin (Decreases in bone mineral density (BMD) have been observed with long-term administration of products containing inhaled corticosteroids. Patients with major risk factors for decreased bone mineral content, such chronic use of drugs that can reduce bone mass (eg, anticonvulsants) should be monitored and treated with established standards of care).
No products indexed under this heading.

Felbamate (Decreases in bone mineral density (BMD) have been observed with long-term administration of products containing inhaled corticosteroids. Patients with major risk factors for decreased bone mineral content, such chronic use of drugs that can reduce bone mass (eg, anticonvulsants) should be monitored and treated with established standards of care).
No products indexed under this heading.

Fluconazole (Fluticasone propionate and salmeterol, the individual components of Advair Diskus, are substrates of CYP3A4. The use of strong CYP3A4 inhibitors with Advair Diskus is not recommended because increased corticosteroid and increased cardiovascular adverse effects may occur).
No products indexed under this heading.

Fludrocortisone Acetate (Decreases in bone mineral density (BMD) have been observed with long-term administration of products containing inhaled corticosteroids. Patients with major risk factors for decreased bone mineral content, such chronic use of drugs that can reduce bone mass (eg, oral corticosteroids) should be monitored and treated with established standards of care).
No products indexed under this heading.

Flumethasone Pivalate (Decreases in bone mineral density (BMD) have been observed with long-term administration of products containing inhaled corticosteroids. Patients with major risk factors for decreased bone mineral content, such chronic use of drugs that can reduce bone mass (eg, oral corticosteroids) should be monitored and treated with established standards of care).
No products indexed under this heading.

Flunisolide Hemihydrate (Decreases in bone mineral density (BMD) have been observed with long-term administration of products containing inhaled corticosteroids. Patients with major risk factors for decreased bone mineral content, such chronic use of drugs that can reduce bone mass (eg, oral corticosteroids) should be monitored and treated with established standards of care).
No products indexed under this heading.

Fluoxetine (Fluticasone propionate and salmeterol, the individual components of Advair Diskus, are substrates of CYP3A4. The use of strong CYP3A4 inhibitors with Advair Diskus is not recommended because increased corticosteroid and increased cardiovascular adverse effects may occur).
No products indexed under this heading.

Fluoxetine Hydrochloride (Fluticasone propionate and salmeterol, the individual components of Advair Diskus, are substrates of CYP3A4. The use of strong CYP3A4 inhibitors with Advair Diskus is not recommended because increased corticosteroid and increased cardiovascular adverse effects may occur). Products include:

Fluticasone Furoate (Decreases in bone mineral density (BMD) have been observed with long-term administration of products containing inhaled corticosteroids. Patients with major risk factors for decreased bone mineral content, such chronic use of drugs that can reduce bone mass (eg, oral corticosteroids) should be monitored and treated with established standards of care). Products include:

Fluvoxamine Maleate (Fluticasone propionate and salmeterol, the individual components of Advair Diskus, are substrates of CYP3A4. The use of strong CYP3A4 inhibitors with Advair Diskus is not recommended because increased corticosteroid and increased cardiovascular adverse effects may occur).
No products indexed under this heading.

Fosamprenavir Calcium (Fluticasone propionate and salmeterol, the individual components of Advair Diskus, are substrates of CYP3A4. The use of strong CYP3A4 inhibitors with Advair Diskus is not recommended because increased corticosteroid and increased cardiovascular adverse effects may occur). Products include:

Fosphenytoin (Decreases in bone mineral density (BMD) have been observed with long-term administration of products containing inhaled corticosteroids. Patients with major risk factors for decreased bone mineral content, such chronic use of drugs that can reduce bone mass (eg, anticonvulsants) should be monitored and treated with established standards of care).
No products indexed under this heading.

Fosphenytoin Sodium (Decreases in bone mineral density (BMD) have been observed with long-term administration of products containing inhaled corticosteroids. Patients with major risk factors for decreased bone mineral content, such chronic use of drugs that can reduce bone mass (eg, anticonvulsants) should be monitored and treated with established standards of care).
No products indexed under this heading.

Furosemide (The ECG changes and/or hypokalemia that may result from the administration of nonpotassium-sparing diuretics (eg, loop diuretics) can be acutely worsened by β-agonists, especially when the recommended dose of the β-agonist is exceeded. Although the clinical relevance of these effects is not known, caution is advised in the co-administration of β-agonists with nonpotassium-sparing diuretics). Products include:

Gabapentin (Decreases in bone mineral density (BMD) have been observed with long-term administration of products containing inhaled corticosteroids. Patients with major risk factors for decreased bone mineral content, such chronic use of drugs that can reduce bone mass (eg, anticonvulsants) should be monitored and treated with established standards of care).
No products indexed under this heading.

Hydrochlorothiazide (The ECG changes and/or hypokalemia that may result from the administration of nonpotassium-sparing diuretics (eg, thiazide diuretics) can be acutely worsened by β-agonists, especially when the recommended dose of the β-agonist is exceeded. Although the clinical relevance of these effects is not known, caution is advised in the co-administration of β-agonists with nonpotassium-sparing diuretics). Products include:

Hydrocortisone (Decreases in bone mineral density (BMD) have been observed with long-term administration of products containing inhaled corticosteroids. Patients with major risk factors for decreased bone mineral content, such chronic use of drugs that can reduce bone mass (eg, oral corticosteroids) should be monitored and treated with established standards of care).
No products indexed under this heading.

Hydrocortisone (Alcohol) (Decreases in bone mineral density (BMD) have been observed with long-term administration of products containing inhaled corticosteroids. Patients with major risk factors for decreased bone mineral content, such chronic use of drugs that can reduce bone mass (eg, oral corticosteroids) should be monitored and treated with established standards of care).
No products indexed under this heading.

Hydrocortisone Acetate (Decreases in bone mineral density (BMD) have been observed with long-term administration of products containing inhaled corticosteroids. Patients with major risk factors for decreased bone mineral content, such chronic use of drugs that can reduce bone mass (eg, oral corticosteroids) should be monitored and treated with established standards of care).
No products indexed under this heading.

Hydrocortisone Butyrate (Decreases in bone mineral density (BMD) have been observed with long-term administration of products containing inhaled corticosteroids. Patients with major risk factors for decreased bone mineral content, such chronic use of drugs that can reduce bone mass (eg, oral corticosteroids) should be monitored and treated with established standards of care).
No products indexed under this heading.

Hydrocortisone Cypionate (Decreases in bone mineral density (BMD) have been observed with long-term administration of products containing inhaled corticosteroids. Patients with major risk factors for decreased bone mineral content, such chronic use of drugs that can reduce bone mass (eg, oral corticosteroids) should be monitored and treated with established standards of care).
No products indexed under this heading.

Hydrocortisone Hemisuccinate (Decreases in bone mineral density (BMD) have been observed with long-term administration of products containing inhaled corticosteroids. Patients with major risk factors for decreased bone mineral content, such chronic use of drugs that can reduce bone mass (eg, oral corticosteroids) should be monitored and treated with established standards of care).
No products indexed under this heading.

Hydrocortisone Probutate (Decreases in bone mineral density (BMD) have been observed with long-term administration of products containing inhaled corticosteroids. Patients with major risk factors for decreased bone mineral content, such chronic use of drugs that can reduce bone mass (eg, oral corticosteroids) should be monitored and treated with established standards of care).
No products indexed under this heading.

Hydrocortisone Sodium Phosphate (Decreases in bone mineral density (BMD) have been observed with long-term administration of products containing inhaled corticosteroids. Patients with major risk factors for decreased bone mineral content, such chronic use of drugs that can reduce bone mass (eg, oral corticosteroids) should be monitored and treated with established standards of care).
No products indexed under this heading.

Hydrocortisone Sodium Succinate (Decreases in bone mineral density (BMD) have been observed with long-term administration of products containing inhaled corticosteroids. Patients with major risk factors for decreased bone mineral content, such chronic use of drugs that can reduce bone mass (eg, oral corticosteroids) should be monitored and treated with established standards of care).
No products indexed under this heading.

Hydrocortisone Valerate
(Decreases in bone mineral density (BMD) have been observed with long-term administration of products containing inhaled corticosteroids. Patients with major risk factors for decreased bone mineral content, such chronic use of drugs that can reduce bone mass (eg, oral corticosteroids) should be monitored and treated with established standards of care).
No products indexed under this heading.

Hydroflumethiazide (The ECG changes and/or hypokalemia that may result from the administration of nonpotassium-sparing diuretics (eg, thiazide diuretics) can be acutely worsened by β-agonists, especially when the recommended dose of the β-agonist is exceeded. Although the clinical relevance of these effects is not known, caution is advised in the co-administration of β-agonists with nonpotassium-sparing diuretics).
No products indexed under this heading.

Imatinib Mesylate (Fluticasone propionate and salmeterol, the individual components of Advair Diskus, are substrates of CYP3A4. The use of strong CYP3A4 inhibitors with Advair Diskus is not recommended because increased corticosteroid and increased cardiovascular adverse effects may occur). Products include:
Gleevec 2477

Imipramine Hydrochloride (Advair Diskus should be administered with extreme caution to patients being treated with tricyclic antidepressants, or within 2 weeks of discontinuation of such agents, because the action of salmeterol, a component of Advair Diskus, on the vascular system may be potentiated by these agents).
No products indexed under this heading.

Imipramine Pamoate (Advair Diskus should be administered with extreme caution to patients being treated with tricyclic antidepressants, or within 2 weeks of discontinuation of such agents, because the action of salmeterol, a component of Advair Diskus, on the vascular system may be potentiated by these agents).
No products indexed under this heading.

Indinavir Sulfate (Fluticasone propionate and salmeterol, the individual components of Advair Diskus, are substrates of CYP3A4. The use of strong CYP3A4 inhibitors (eg, indinavir) with Advair Diskus is not recommended because increased systemic corticosteroid and increased cardiovascular adverse effects may occur). Products include:
Crixivan 2113

Isocarboxazid (Advair Diskus should be administered with extreme caution to patients being treated with monoamine oxidase inhibitors, or within 2 weeks of discontinuation of such agents, because the action of salmeterol, a component of Advair Diskus, on the vascular system may be potentiated by these agents). Products include:
Marplan 3481

Isoniazid (Fluticasone propionate and salmeterol, the individual components of Advair Diskus, are substrates of CYP3A4. The use of strong CYP3A4 inhibitors with Advair Diskus is not recommended because increased corticosteroid and increased cardiovascular adverse effects may occur).
No products indexed under this heading.

Itraconazole (Fluticasone propionate and salmeterol, the individual components of Advair Diskus, are substrates of CYP3A4. The use of strong CYP3A4 inhibitors (eg, itraconazole) with Advair Diskus is not recommended because increased systemic corticosteroid and increased cardiovascular adverse effects may occur).
No products indexed under this heading.

Ketoconazole (Co-administration of orally inhaled fluticasone propionate (1,000 mcg) and ketoconazole (200 mg qd) resulted in increased plasma fluticasone propionate exposure and reduced plasma cortisol area under the curve (AUC), but had no effect on urinary excretion of cortisol. In addition, in a study in 20 healthy subjects, co-administration of inhaled salmeterol (50 mcg bid) and oral ketoconazole (400 mg qd) for 7 days resulted in greater systemic exposure to salmeterol (AUC increased 16-fold and C_{max} increased 1.4- fold). Three subjects were withdrawn due to β-agonist side effects (2 with prolonged QTc and 1 with palpitations and sinus tachycardia). Although there was no statistical effect on the mean QTc, co-administration of salmeterol and ketoconazole was associated with more frequent increases in QTc duration compared with salmeterol and placebo administration). Products include:
Extina 3319
Xolegel 3337

Labetalol Hydrochloride (β-blockers not only block the pulmonary effect of β-agonists, such as salmeterol, a component of Advair Diskus, but may produce severe bronchospasm in patients with reversible obstructive airways disease. Therefore, patients with asthma and COPD should not normally be treated with β-blockers. However, under certain circumstances, there may be no acceptable alternatives to the use of β-adrenergic blocking agents for these patients; cardioselective β-blockers could be considered, although they should be administered with caution).
No products indexed under this heading.

Lamotrigine (Decreases in bone mineral density (BMD) have been observed with long-term administration of products containing inhaled corticosteroids. Patients with major risk factors for decreased bone mineral content, such chronic use of drugs that can reduce bone mass (eg, anticonvulsants) should be monitored and treated with established standards of care). Products include:
Lamictal 1522
Lamictal ODT 1522
Lamictal XR 1536

Lapatinib (Fluticasone propionate and salmeterol, the individual components of Advair Diskus, are substrates of CYP3A4. The use of strong CYP3A4 inhibitors with Advair Diskus is not recommended because increased corticosteroid and increased cardiovascular adverse effects may occur). Products include:
Tykerb 1698

Levetiracetam (Decreases in bone mineral density (BMD) have been observed with long-term administration of products containing inhaled corticosteroids. Patients with major risk factors for decreased bone mineral content, such chronic use of drugs that can reduce bone mass (eg, anticonvulsants) should be monitored and treated with established standards of care). Products include:
Keppra XR 3434

Levobunolol Hydrochloride
(β-blockers not only block the pulmonary effect of β-agonists, such as salmeterol, a component of Advair Diskus, but may produce severe bronchospasm in patients with reversible obstructive airways disease. Therefore, patients with asthma and COPD should not normally be treated with β-blockers. However, under certain circumstances, there may be no acceptable alternatives to the use of β-adrenergic blocking agents for these patients; cardioselective β-blockers could be considered, although they should be administered with caution).
No products indexed under this heading.

Lopinavir (Fluticasone propionate and salmeterol, the individual components of Advair Diskus, are substrates of CYP3A4. The use of strong CYP3A4 inhibitors with Advair Diskus is not recommended because increased corticosteroid and increased cardiovascular adverse effects may occur). Products include:
Kaletra 458

Loratadine (Fluticasone propionate and salmeterol, the individual components of Advair Diskus, are substrates of CYP3A4. The use of strong CYP3A4 inhibitors with Advair Diskus is not recommended because increased corticosteroid and increased cardiovascular adverse effects may occur).
No products indexed under this heading.

Maprotiline Hydrochloride (Advair Diskus should be administered with extreme caution to patients being treated with tricyclic antidepressants, or within 2 weeks of discontinuation of such agents, because the action of salmeterol, a component of Advair Diskus, on the vascular system may be potentiated by these agents).
No products indexed under this heading.

Mephenytoin (Decreases in bone mineral density (BMD) have been observed with long-term administration of products containing inhaled corticosteroids. Patients with major risk factors for decreased bone mineral content, such chronic use of drugs that can reduce bone mass (eg, anticonvulsants) should be monitored and treated with established standards of care).
No products indexed under this heading.

Methsuximide (Decreases in bone mineral density (BMD) have been observed with long-term administration of products containing inhaled corticosteroids. Patients with major risk factors for decreased bone mineral content, such chronic use of drugs that can reduce bone mass (eg, anticonvulsants) should be monitored and treated with established standards of care).
No products indexed under this heading.

Methyclothiazide (The ECG changes and/or hypokalemia that may result from the administration of nonpotassium-sparing diuretics (eg, thiazide diuretics) can be acutely worsened by β-agonists, especially when the recommended dose of the β-agonist is exceeded. Although the clinical relevance of these effects is not known, caution is advised in the co-administration of β-agonists with nonpotassium-sparing diuretics).
No products indexed under this heading.

Methylprednisolone (Decreases in bone mineral density (BMD) have been observed with long-term administration of products containing inhaled corticosteroids. Patients with major risk factors for decreased bone mineral content, such chronic use of drugs that can reduce bone mass (eg, oral corticosteroids) should be monitored and treated with established standards of care).
No products indexed under this heading.

Methylprednisolone Acetate
(Decreases in bone mineral density (BMD) have been observed with long-term administration of products containing inhaled corticosteroids. Patients with major risk factors for decreased bone mineral content, such chronic use of drugs that can reduce bone mass (eg, oral corticosteroids) should be monitored and treated with established standards of care).
No products indexed under this heading.

Methylprednisolone Sodium Succinate (Decreases in bone mineral density (BMD) have been observed with long-term administration of products containing inhaled corticosteroids. Patients with major risk factors for decreased bone mineral content, such chronic use of drugs that can reduce bone mass (eg, oral corticosteroids) should be monitored and treated with established standards of care).
No products indexed under this heading.

Metipranolol Hydrochloride
(β-blockers not only block the pulmonary effect of β-agonists, such as salmeterol, a component of Advair Diskus, but may produce severe bronchospasm in patients with reversible obstructive airways disease. Therefore, patients with asthma and COPD should not normally be treated with β-blockers. However, under certain circumstances, there may be no acceptable alternatives to the use of β-adrenergic blocking agents for these patients; cardioselective β-blockers could be considered, although they should be administered with caution).
No products indexed under this heading.

Metoprolol Succinate (β-blockers not only block the pulmonary effect of β-agonists, such as salmeterol, a component of Advair Diskus, but may produce severe bronchospasm in patients with reversible obstructive airways disease. Therefore, patients with asthma and COPD should not normally be treated with β-blockers. However, under certain circumstances, there may be no acceptable alternatives to the use of β-adrenergic blocking agents for these patients; cardioselective β-blockers could be considered, although they should be administered with caution). Products include:
Toprol XL 732

Metoprolol Tartrate (β-blockers not only block the pulmonary effect of β-agonists, such as salmeterol, a component of Advair Diskus, but may produce severe bronchospasm in patients with reversible obstructive airways disease. Therefore, patients with asthma and COPD should not normally be treated with β-blockers. However, under certain circumstances, there may be no acceptable alternatives to the use of β-adrenergic blocking agents for these patients; cardioselective β-blockers could be considered, although they should be administered with caution).
No products indexed under this heading.

Metronidazole (Fluticasone propionate and salmeterol, the individual components of Advair Diskus, are substrates of CYP3A4. The use of strong CYP3A4 inhibitors with Advair Diskus is not recommended because increased corticosteroid and increased cardiovascular adverse effects may occur). Products include:
Pylera 793

IMPORTANT NOTE: Always consult each drug listing in the patient's regimen for possible interactions.

Advair **Interactions Index** 58

Metronidazole Benzoate (Fluticasone propionate and salmeterol, the individual components of Advair Diskus, are substrates of CYP3A4. The use of strong CYP3A4 inhibitors with Advair Diskus is not recommended because increased corticosteroid and increased cardiovascular adverse effects may occur).
No products indexed under this heading.

Metronidazole Hydrochloride (Fluticasone propionate and salmeterol, the individual components of Advair Diskus, are substrates of CYP3A4. The use of strong CYP3A4 inhibitors with Advair Diskus is not recommended because increased corticosteroid and increased cardiovascular adverse effects may occur).
No products indexed under this heading.

Metronidazole Sodium (Fluticasone propionate and salmeterol, the individual components of Advair Diskus, are substrates of CYP3A4. The use of strong CYP3A4 inhibitors with Advair Diskus is not recommended because increased corticosteroid and increased cardiovascular adverse effects may occur).
No products indexed under this heading.

Miconazole (Fluticasone propionate and salmeterol, the individual components of Advair Diskus, are substrates of CYP3A4. The use of strong CYP3A4 inhibitors with Advair Diskus is not recommended because increased corticosteroid and increased cardiovascular adverse effects may occur).
No products indexed under this heading.

Miconazole Nitrate (Fluticasone propionate and salmeterol, the individual components of Advair Diskus, are substrates of CYP3A4. The use of strong CYP3A4 inhibitors with Advair Diskus is not recommended because increased corticosteroid and increased cardiovascular adverse effects may occur). Products include:
Vusion Ointment **3335**

Mifepristone (Fluticasone propionate and salmeterol, the individual components of Advair Diskus, are substrates of CYP3A4. The use of strong CYP3A4 inhibitors with Advair Diskus is not recommended because increased corticosteroid and increased cardiovascular adverse effects may occur).
No products indexed under this heading.

Moclobemide (Advair Diskus should be administered with extreme caution to patients being treated with monoamine oxidase inhibitors, or within 2 weeks of discontinuation of such agents, because the action of salmeterol, a component of Advair Diskus, on the vascular system may be potentiated by these agents).
No products indexed under this heading.

Mometasone Furoate (Decreases in bone mineral density (BMD) have been observed with long-term administration of products containing inhaled corticosteroids. Patients with major risk factors for decreased bone mineral content, such chronic use of drugs that can reduce bone mass (eg, oral corticosteroids) should be monitored and treated with established standards of care). Products include:
Asmanex **3058**
Elocon Cream **3111**
Elocon Lotion **3112**
Elocon Ointment **3114**

Mometasone Furoate Monohydrate (Decreases in bone mineral density (BMD) have been observed with long-term administration of products containing inhaled corticosteroids. Patients with major risk factors for decreased bone mineral content, such chronic use of drugs that can reduce bone mass (eg, oral corticosteroids) should be monitored and treated with established standards of care). Products include:
Nasonex **3166**

Nadolol (β-blockers not only block the pulmonary effect of β-agonists, such as salmeterol, a component of Advair Diskus, but may produce severe bronchospasm in patients with reversible obstructive airways disease. Therefore, patients with asthma and COPD should not normally be treated with β-blockers. However, under certain circumstances, there may be no acceptable alternatives to the use of β-adrenergic blocking agents for these patients; cardioselective β-blockers could be considered, although they should be administered with caution). Products include:
Nadolol **2359**

Nebivolol (β-blockers not only block the pulmonary effect of β-agonists, such as salmeterol, a component of Advair Diskus, but may produce severe bronchospasm in patients with reversible obstructive airways disease. Therefore, patients with asthma and COPD should not normally be treated with β-blockers. However, under certain circumstances, there may be no acceptable alternatives to the use of β-adrenergic blocking agents for these patients; cardioselective β-blockers could be considered, although they should be administered with caution). Products include:
Bystolic **1147**

Nefazodone Hydrochloride (Fluticasone propionate and salmeterol, the individual components of Advair Diskus, are substrates of CYP3A4. The use of strong CYP3A4 inhibitors (eg, nefazodone) with Advair Diskus is not recommended because increased systemic corticosteroid and increased cardiovascular adverse effects may occur).
No products indexed under this heading.

Nelfinavir Mesylate (Fluticasone propionate and salmeterol, the individual components of Advair Diskus, are substrates of CYP3A4. The use of strong CYP3A4 inhibitors (eg, nelfinavir) with Advair Diskus is not recommended because increased systemic corticosteroid and increased cardiovascular adverse effects may occur).
No products indexed under this heading.

Nevirapine (Fluticasone propionate and salmeterol, the individual components of Advair Diskus, are substrates of CYP3A4. The use of strong CYP3A4 inhibitors with Advair Diskus is not recommended because increased corticosteroid and increased cardiovascular adverse effects may occur). Products include:
Viramune Oral Suspension **897**
Viramune Tablets **897**

Niacin (Fluticasone propionate and salmeterol, the individual components of Advair Diskus, are substrates of CYP3A4. The use of strong CYP3A4 inhibitors with Advair Diskus is not recommended because increased corticosteroid and increased cardiovascular adverse effects may occur). Products include:
Advicor **402**
Cardio Basics **3455**
Niaspan **497**
Simcor **524**

Niacinamide (Fluticasone propionate and salmeterol, the individual components of Advair Diskus, are substrates of CYP3A4. The use of strong CYP3A4 inhibitors with Advair Diskus is not recommended because increased corticosteroid and increased cardiovascular adverse effects may occur). Products include:
CitraNatal 90 DHA Capsules **2332**
CitraNatal Assure **2332**
CitraNatal Rx **2332**
Heplive **607**

Niacinamide Hydroiodide (Fluticasone propionate and salmeterol, the individual components of Advair Diskus, are substrates of CYP3A4. The use of strong CYP3A4 inhibitors with Advair Diskus is not recommended because increased corticosteroid and increased cardiovascular adverse effects may occur).
No products indexed under this heading.

Nicotinamide (Fluticasone propionate and salmeterol, the individual components of Advair Diskus, are substrates of CYP3A4. The use of strong CYP3A4 inhibitors with Advair Diskus is not recommended because increased corticosteroid and increased cardiovascular adverse effects may occur).
No products indexed under this heading.

Nifedipine (Fluticasone propionate and salmeterol, the individual components of Advair Diskus, are substrates of CYP3A4. The use of strong CYP3A4 inhibitors with Advair Diskus is not recommended because increased corticosteroid and increased cardiovascular adverse effects may occur).
No products indexed under this heading.

Norfloxacin (Fluticasone propionate and salmeterol, the individual components of Advair Diskus, are substrates of CYP3A4. The use of strong CYP3A4 inhibitors with Advair Diskus is not recommended because increased corticosteroid and increased cardiovascular adverse effects may occur). Products include:
Noroxin **2220**

Nortriptyline Hydrochloride (Advair Diskus should be administered with extreme caution to patients being treated with tricyclic antidepressants, or within 2 weeks of discontinuation of such agents, because the action of salmeterol, a component of Advair Diskus, on the vascular system may be potentiated by these agents).
No products indexed under this heading.

Omeprazole (Fluticasone propionate and salmeterol, the individual components of Advair Diskus, are substrates of CYP3A4. The use of strong CYP3A4 inhibitors with Advair Diskus is not recommended because increased corticosteroid and increased cardiovascular adverse effects may occur).
No products indexed under this heading.

Oxcarbazepine (Decreases in bone mineral density (BMD) have been observed with long-term administration of products containing inhaled corticosteroids. Patients with major risk factors for decreased bone mineral content, such chronic use of drugs that can reduce bone mass (eg, anticonvulsants) should be monitored and treated with established standards of care).
No products indexed under this heading.

Paramethadione (Decreases in bone mineral density (BMD) have been observed with long-term administration of products containing inhaled corticosteroids. Patients with major risk factors for decreased bone mineral content, such chronic use of drugs that can reduce bone mass (eg, anticonvulsants) should be monitored and treated with established standards of care).
No products indexed under this heading.

Pargyline Hydrochloride (Advair Diskus should be administered with extreme caution to patients being treated with monoamine oxidase inhibitors, or within 2 weeks of discontinuation of such agents, because the action of salmeterol, a component of Advair Diskus, on the vascular system may be potentiated by these agents).
No products indexed under this heading.

Paroxetine Hydrochloride (Fluticasone propionate and salmeterol, the individual components of Advair Diskus, are substrates of CYP3A4. The use of strong CYP3A4 inhibitors with Advair Diskus is not recommended because increased corticosteroid and increased cardiovascular adverse effects may occur). Products include:
Paroxetine CR **2361**
Paroxetine ER **2371**
Paxil **1586**
Paxil CR **1596**

Penbutolol Sulfate (β-blockers not only block the pulmonary effect of β-agonists, such as salmeterol, a component of Advair Diskus, but may produce severe bronchospasm in patients with reversible obstructive airways disease. Therefore, patients with asthma and COPD should not normally be treated with β-blockers. However, under certain circumstances, there may be no acceptable alternatives to the use of β-adrenergic blocking agents for these patients; cardioselective β-blockers could be considered, although they should be administered with caution).
No products indexed under this heading.

Phenacemide (Decreases in bone mineral density (BMD) have been observed with long-term administration of products containing inhaled corticosteroids. Patients with major risk factors for decreased bone mineral content, such chronic use of drugs that can reduce bone mass (eg, anticonvulsants) should be monitored and treated with established standards of care).
No products indexed under this heading.

Phenelzine Sulfate (Advair Diskus should be administered with extreme caution to patients being treated with monoamine oxidase inhibitors, or within 2 weeks of discontinuation of such agents, because the action of salmeterol, a component of Advair Diskus, on the vascular system may be potentiated by these agents).
No products indexed under this heading.

Phenobarbital (Decreases in bone mineral density (BMD) have been observed with long-term administration of products containing inhaled corticosteroids. Patients with major risk factors for decreased bone mineral content, such chronic use of drugs that can reduce bone mass (eg, anticonvulsants) should be monitored and treated with established standards of care). Products include:
Donnatal **2711**

Phenobarbital Sodium (Decreases in bone mineral density (BMD) have been observed with long-term administration of products containing inhaled corticosteroids. Patients with major risk factors for decreased bone mineral content, such chronic use of drugs that can reduce bone mass (eg, anticonvulsants) should be monitored and treated with established standards of care).
No products indexed under this heading.

Phensuximide (Decreases in bone mineral density (BMD) have been observed with long-term administration of products containing inhaled corticosteroids. Patients with major risk factors for decreased bone mineral content, such chronic use of drugs that can reduce bone mass (eg, anticonvulsants) should be monitored and treated with established standards of care).
No products indexed under this heading.

Phenytoin (Decreases in bone mineral density (BMD) have been observed with long-term administration of products containing inhaled corticosteroids. Patients with major risk factors for decreased bone mineral content, such chronic use of drugs that can reduce bone mass (eg, anticonvulsants) should be monitored and treated with established standards of care).
No products indexed under this heading.

Phenytoin Sodium (Decreases in bone mineral density (BMD) have been observed with long-term administration of products containing inhaled corticosteroids. Patients with major risk factors for decreased bone mineral content, such chronic use of drugs that can reduce bone mass (eg, anticonvulsants) should be monitored and treated with established standards of care).
Products include:
Phenytek Capsules 2380

Pindolol (β-blockers not only block the pulmonary effect of β-agonists, such as salmeterol, a component of Advair Diskus, but may produce severe bronchospasm in patients with reversible obstructive airways disease. Therefore, patients with asthma and COPD should not normally be treated with β-blockers. However, under certain circumstances, there may be no acceptable alternatives to the use of β-adrenergic blocking agents for these patients; cardioselective β-blockers could be considered, although they should be administered with caution).
No products indexed under this heading.

Polythiazide (The ECG changes and/or hypokalemia that may result from the administration of nonpotassium-sparing diuretics (eg, thiazide diuretics) can be acutely worsened by β-agonists, especially when the recommended dose of the β-agonist is exceeded. Although the clinical relevance of these effects is not known, caution is advised in the co-administration of β-agonists with nonpotassium-sparing diuretics).
No products indexed under this heading.

Posaconazole (Fluticasone propionate and salmeterol, the individual components of Advair Diskus, are substrates of CYP3A4. The use of strong CYP3A4 inhibitors with Advair Diskus is not recommended because increased corticosteroid and increased cardiovascular adverse effects may occur).
Products include:
Noxafil 3172

Prednisolone (Decreases in bone mineral density (BMD) have been observed with long-term administration of products containing inhaled corticosteroids. Patients with major risk factors for decreased bone mineral content, such chronic use of drugs that can reduce bone mass (eg, oral corticosteroids) should be monitored and treated with established standards of care).
No products indexed under this heading.

Prednisolone Acetate (Decreases in bone mineral density (BMD) have been observed with long-term administration of products containing inhaled corticosteroids. Patients with major risk factors for decreased bone mineral content, such chronic use of drugs that can reduce bone mass (eg, oral corticosteroids) should be monitored and treated with established standards of care).
Products include:
Blephamide .... ⊙212, ⊙214
Pred Forte .... ⊙225
Pred Mild .... ⊙230
Pred-G .... ⊙226, ⊙227

Prednisolone Sodium Phosphate (Decreases in bone mineral density (BMD) have been observed with long-term administration of products containing inhaled corticosteroids. Patients with major risk factors for decreased bone mineral content, such chronic use of drugs that can reduce bone mass (eg, oral corticosteroids) should be monitored and treated with established standards of care).
No products indexed under this heading.

Prednisolone Tebutate (Decreases in bone mineral density (BMD) have been observed with long-term administration of products containing inhaled corticosteroids. Patients with major risk factors for decreased bone mineral content, such chronic use of drugs that can reduce bone mass (eg, oral corticosteroids) should be monitored and treated with established standards of care).
No products indexed under this heading.

Prednisone (Decreases in bone mineral density (BMD) have been observed with long-term administration of products containing inhaled corticosteroids. Patients with major risk factors for decreased bone mineral content, such chronic use of drugs that can reduce bone mass (eg, oral corticosteroids) should be monitored and treated with established standards of care).
No products indexed under this heading.

Prednisone sodium phosphate (Decreases in bone mineral density (BMD) have been observed with long-term administration of products containing inhaled corticosteroids. Patients with major risk factors for decreased bone mineral content, such chronic use of drugs that can reduce bone mass (eg, oral corticosteroids) should be monitored and treated with established standards of care).
No products indexed under this heading.

Primidone (Decreases in bone mineral density (BMD) have been observed with long-term administration of products containing inhaled corticosteroids. Patients with major risk factors for decreased bone mineral content, such chronic use of drugs that can reduce bone mass (eg, anticonvulsants) should be monitored and treated with established standards of care).
No products indexed under this heading.

Procarbazine Hydrochloride (Advair Diskus should be administered with extreme caution to patients being treated with monoamine oxidase inhibitors, or within 2 weeks of discontinuation of such agents, because the action of salmeterol, a component of Advair Diskus, on the vascular system may be potentiated by these agents).
No products indexed under this heading.

Propoxyphene Hydrochloride (Fluticasone propionate and salmeterol, the individual components of Advair Diskus, are substrates of CYP3A4. The use of strong CYP3A4 inhibitors with Advair Diskus is not recommended because increased corticosteroid and increased cardiovascular adverse effects may occur).
No products indexed under this heading.

Propoxyphene Napsylate (Fluticasone propionate and salmeterol, the individual components of Advair Diskus, are substrates of CYP3A4. The use of strong CYP3A4 inhibitors with Advair Diskus is not recommended because increased corticosteroid and increased cardiovascular adverse effects may occur).
No products indexed under this heading.

Propranolol Hydrochloride (β-blockers not only block the pulmonary effect of β-agonists, such as salmeterol, a component of Advair Diskus, but may produce severe bronchospasm

in patients with reversible obstructive airways disease. Therefore, patients with asthma and COPD should not normally be treated with β-blockers. However, under certain circumstances, there may be no acceptable alternatives to the use of β-adrenergic blocking agents for these patients; cardioselective β-blockers could be considered, although they should be administered with caution). Products include:
InnoPran XL 1517

Protriptyline Hydrochloride (Advair Diskus should be administered with extreme caution to patients being treated with tricyclic antidepressants, or within 2 weeks of discontinuation of such agents, because the action of salmeterol, a component of Advair Diskus, on the vascular system may be potentiated by these agents).
No products indexed under this heading.

Quinidine (Fluticasone propionate and salmeterol, the individual components of Advair Diskus, are substrates of CYP3A4. The use of strong CYP3A4 inhibitors with Advair Diskus is not recommended because increased corticosteroid and increased cardiovascular adverse effects may occur).
No products indexed under this heading.

Quinidine Hydrochloride (Fluticasone propionate and salmeterol, the individual components of Advair Diskus, are substrates of CYP3A4. The use of strong CYP3A4 inhibitors with Advair Diskus is not recommended because increased corticosteroid and increased cardiovascular adverse effects may occur).
No products indexed under this heading.

Quinidine Polygalacturonate (Fluticasone propionate and salmeterol, the individual components of Advair Diskus, are substrates of CYP3A4. The use of strong CYP3A4 inhibitors with Advair Diskus is not recommended because increased corticosteroid and increased cardiovascular adverse effects may occur).
No products indexed under this heading.

Quinidine Sulfate (Fluticasone propionate and salmeterol, the individual components of Advair Diskus, are substrates of CYP3A4. The use of strong CYP3A4 inhibitors with Advair Diskus is not recommended because increased corticosteroid and increased cardiovascular adverse effects may occur).
No products indexed under this heading.

Quinine (Fluticasone propionate and salmeterol, the individual components of Advair Diskus, are substrates of CYP3A4. The use of strong CYP3A4 inhibitors with Advair Diskus is not recommended because increased corticosteroid and increased cardiovascular adverse effects may occur). Products include:
Hyland's Leg Cramps PM with Quinine 3315

Quinine Sulfate (Fluticasone propionate and salmeterol, the individual components of Advair Diskus, are substrates of CYP3A4. The use of strong CYP3A4 inhibitors with Advair Diskus is not recommended because increased corticosteroid and increased cardiovascular adverse effects may occur).
No products indexed under this heading.

Quinupristin (Fluticasone propionate and salmeterol, the individual components of Advair Diskus, are substrates of CYP3A4. The use of strong CYP3A4 inhibitors with Advair Diskus is not recommended because increased corticosteroid and increased cardiovascular adverse effects may occur).
No products indexed under this heading.

Ranitidine Bismuth Citrate (Fluticasone propionate and salmeterol, the individual components of Advair Diskus, are substrates of CYP3A4. The use of strong CYP3A4 inhibitors with Advair Diskus is not recommended because increased corticosteroid and increased cardiovascular adverse effects may occur).
No products indexed under this heading.

Ranitidine Hydrochloride (Fluticasone propionate and salmeterol, the individual components of Advair Diskus, are substrates of CYP3A4. The use of strong CYP3A4 inhibitors with Advair Diskus is not recommended because increased corticosteroid and increased cardiovascular adverse effects may occur). Products include:
Zantac 1737
Zantac Injection 1732
Zantac Pharmacy 1735

Rasagiline Mesylate (Advair Diskus should be administered with extreme caution to patients being treated with monoamine oxidase inhibitors, or within 2 weeks of discontinuation of such agents, because the action of salmeterol, a component of Advair Diskus, on the vascular system may be potentiated by these agents). Products include:
Azilect 3383

Ritonavir (Fluticasone propionate and salmeterol, the individual components of Advair Diskus, are substrates of CYP3A4. The use of strong CYP3A4 inhibitors (eg, ritonavir) with Advair Diskus is not recommended because increased systemic corticosteroid and increased cardiovascular adverse effects may occur. A study has shown that concomitant use with fluticasone propionate aqueous nasal spray with ritonavir, in healthy subjects, can result in significantly reduced serum cortisol concentrations. During postmarketing use, there have been reports of clinically significant drug interactions in patients receiving fluticasone propionate and ritonavir, resulting in systemic corticosteroid effects including Cushing syndrome and adrenal suppression). Products include:
Kaletra 458
Norvir 509

Rufinamide (Decreases in bone mineral density (BMD) have been observed with long-term administration of products containing inhaled corticosteroids. Patients with major risk factors for decreased bone mineral content, such chronic use of drugs that can reduce bone mass (eg, anticonvulsants) should be monitored and treated with established standards of care). Products include:
Banzel 1050

Saquinavir (Fluticasone propionate and salmeterol, the individual components of Advair Diskus are substrates of CYP3A4. The use of strong CYP3A4 inhibitors (eg, saquinavir) with Advair Diskus is not recommended because increased systemic corticosteroid and increased cardiovascular adverse effects may occur).
No products indexed under this heading.

Saquinavir Mesylate (Fluticasone propionate and salmeterol, the individual components of Advair Diskus are substrates of CYP3A4. The use of strong CYP3A4 inhibitors (eg, saquinavir) with Advair Diskus is not recommended because increased systemic corticosteroid and increased cardiovascular adverse effects may occur).
No products indexed under this heading.

Selegiline (Advair Diskus should be administered with extreme caution to patients being treated with monoamine oxidase inhibitors, or within 2 weeks of discontinuation of such agents, because the action of salmeterol, a

component of Advair Diskus, on the vascular system may be potentiated by these agents). Products include:

Emsam 3623

Selegiline Hydrochloride (Advair Diskus should be administered with extreme caution to patients being treated with monoamine oxidase inhibitors, or within 2 weeks of discontinuation of such agents, because the action of salmeterol, a component of Advair Diskus, on the vascular system may be potentiated by these agents). Products include:

Eldepryl 3312

Sertraline Hydrochloride (Fluticasone propionate and salmeterol, the individual components of Advair Diskus, are substrates of CYP3A4. The use of strong CYP3A4 inhibitors with Advair Diskus is not recommended because increased corticosteroid and increased cardiovascular adverse effects may occur).

No products indexed under this heading.

Sildenafil Citrate (Fluticasone propionate and salmeterol, the individual components of Advair Diskus, are substrates of CYP3A4. The use of strong CYP3A4 inhibitors with Advair Diskus is not recommended because increased corticosteroid and increased cardiovascular adverse effects may occur).

No products indexed under this heading.

Sotalol Hydrochloride (β-blockers not only block the pulmonary effect of β-agonists, such as salmeterol, a component of Advair Diskus, but may produce severe bronchospasm in patients with reversible obstructive airways disease. Therefore, patients with asthma and COPD should not normally be treated with β-blockers. However, under certain circumstances, there may be no acceptable alternatives to the use of β-adrenergic blocking agents for these patients; cardioselective β-blockers could be considered, although they should be administered with caution).

No products indexed under this heading.

Telithromycin (Fluticasone propionate and salmeterol, the individual components of Advair Diskus, are substrates of CYP3A4. The use of strong CYP3A4 inhibitors with Advair Diskus is not recommended because increased corticosteroid and increased cardiovascular adverse effects may occur). Products include:

Ketek 2991

Tiagabine Hydrochloride (Decreases in bone mineral density (BMD) have been observed with long-term administration of products containing inhaled corticosteroids. Patients with major risk factors for decreased bone mineral content, such chronic use of drugs that can reduce bone mass (eg, anticonvulsants) should be monitored and treated with established standards of care). Products include:

Gabitril 972

Timolol Hemihydrate (β-blockers not only block the pulmonary effect of β-agonists, such as salmeterol, a component of Advair Diskus, but may produce severe bronchospasm in patients with reversible obstructive airways disease. Therefore, patients with asthma and COPD should not normally be treated with β-blockers. However, under certain circumstances, there may be no acceptable alternatives to the use of β-adrenergic blocking agents for these patients; cardioselective β-blockers could be considered, although they should be administered with caution). Products include:

Betimol 3490

Timolol Maleate (β-blockers not only block the pulmonary effect of β-agonists, such as salmeterol, a com-

ponent of Advair Diskus, but may produce severe bronchospasm in patients with reversible obstructive airways disease. Therefore, patients with asthma and COPD should not normally be treated with β-blockers. However, under certain circumstances, there may be no acceptable alternatives to the use of β-adrenergic blocking agents for these patients; cardioselective β-blockers could be considered, although they should be administered with caution). Products include:

Combigan 601
Dorzolamide
Hydrochloride/Timolol Maleate
Ophthalmic Solution.................. ⊙ 243
Timoptic in Ocudose .... ⊙ 231

Tobacco (Decreases in bone mineral density (BMD) have been observed with long-term administration of products containing inhaled corticosteroids. Patients with major risk factors for decreased bone mineral content, such tobacco use, should be monitored and treated with established standards of care).

No products indexed under this heading.

Topiramate (Decreases in bone mineral density (BMD) have been observed with long-term administration of products containing inhaled corticosteroids. Patients with major risk factors for decreased bone mineral content, such chronic use of drugs that can reduce bone mass (eg, anticonvulsants) should be monitored and treated with established standards of care).

No products indexed under this heading.

Torsemide (The ECG changes and/or hypokalemia that may result from the administration of nonpotassium-sparing diuretics (eg, loop diuretics) can be acutely worsened by β-agonists, especially when the recommended dose of the β-agonist is exceeded. Although the clinical relevance of these effects is not known, caution is advised in the co-administration of β-agonists with nonpotassium-sparing diuretics).

No products indexed under this heading.

Tranylcypromine Sulfate (Advair Diskus should be administered with extreme caution to patients being treated with monoamine oxidase inhibitors, or within 2 weeks of discontinuation of such agents, because the action of salmeterol, a component of Advair Diskus, on the vascular system may be potentiated by these agents). Products include:

Parnate 1584

Triamcinolone (Decreases in bone mineral density (BMD) have been observed with long-term administration of products containing inhaled corticosteroids. Patients with major risk factors for decreased bone mineral content, such chronic use of drugs that can reduce bone mass (eg, oral corticosteroids) should be monitored and treated with established standards of care).

No products indexed under this heading.

Triamcinolone Acetonide (Decreases in bone mineral density (BMD) have been observed with long-term administration of products containing inhaled corticosteroids. Patients with major risk factors for decreased bone mineral content, such chronic use of drugs that can reduce bone mass (eg, oral corticosteroids) should be monitored and treated with established standards of care). Products include:

Azmacort 408
Nasacort AQ 3019

Triamcinolone Diacetate (Decreases in bone mineral density (BMD) have been observed with long-term administration of products containing inhaled corticosteroids. Patients with major risk factors for decreased bone mineral content, such chronic use of drugs that can reduce bone mass (eg, oral corticosteroids) should be monitored and treated with established standards of care).

No products indexed under this heading.

Triamcinolone Hexacetonide (Decreases in bone mineral density (BMD) have been observed with long-term administration of products containing inhaled corticosteroids. Patients with major risk factors for decreased bone mineral content, such chronic use of drugs that can reduce bone mass (eg, oral corticosteroids) should be monitored and treated with established standards of care).

No products indexed under this heading.

Trimethadione (Decreases in bone mineral density (BMD) have been observed with long-term administration of products containing inhaled corticosteroids. Patients with major risk factors for decreased bone mineral content, such chronic use of drugs that can reduce bone mass (eg, anticonvulsants) should be monitored and treated with established standards of care).

No products indexed under this heading.

Trimipramine Maleate (Advair Diskus should be administered with extreme caution to patients being treated with tricyclic antidepressants, or within 2 weeks of discontinuation of such agents, because the action of salmeterol, a component of Advair Diskus, on the vascular system may be potentiated by these agents).

No products indexed under this heading.

Troglitazone (Fluticasone propionate and salmeterol, the individual components of Advair Diskus, are substrates of CYP3A4. The use of strong CYP3A4 inhibitors with Advair Diskus is not recommended because increased corticosteroid and increased cardiovascular adverse effects may occur).

No products indexed under this heading.

Troleandomycin (Fluticasone propionate and salmeterol, the individual components of Advair Diskus, are substrates of CYP3A4. The use of strong CYP3A4 inhibitors with Advair Diskus is not recommended because increased corticosteroid and increased cardiovascular adverse effects may occur).

No products indexed under this heading.

Valproate Sodium (Decreases in bone mineral density (BMD) have been observed with long-term administration of products containing inhaled corticosteroids. Patients with major risk factors for decreased bone mineral content, such chronic use of drugs that can reduce bone mass (eg, anticonvulsants) should be monitored and treated with established standards of care).

No products indexed under this heading.

Valproic Acid (Decreases in bone mineral density (BMD) have been observed with long-term administration of products containing inhaled corticosteroids. Patients with major risk factors for decreased bone mineral content, such chronic use of drugs that can reduce bone mass (eg, anticonvulsants) should be monitored and treated with established standards of care).

No products indexed under this heading.

Vardenafil Hydrochloride (Fluticasone propionate and salmeterol, the individual components of Advair Diskus, are substrates of CYP3A4. The use of strong CYP3A4 inhibitors with Advair Diskus is not recommended because

increased corticosteroid and increased cardiovascular adverse effects may occur). Products include:

Levitra 3157

Verapamil Hydrochloride (Fluticasone propionate and salmeterol, the individual components of Advair Diskus, are substrates of CYP3A4. The use of strong CYP3A4 inhibitors with Advair Diskus is not recommended because increased corticosteroid and increased cardiovascular adverse effects may occur). Products include:

Tarka 534

Voriconazole (Fluticasone propionate and salmeterol, the individual components of Advair Diskus, are substrates of CYP3A4. The use of strong CYP3A4 inhibitors with Advair Diskus is not recommended because increased corticosteroid and increased cardiovascular adverse effects may occur).

No products indexed under this heading.

Zafirlukast (Fluticasone propionate and salmeterol, the individual components of Advair Diskus, are substrates of CYP3A4. The use of strong CYP3A4 inhibitors with Advair Diskus is not recommended because increased corticosteroid and increased cardiovascular adverse effects may occur). Products include:

Accolate 3612

Zileuton (Fluticasone propionate and salmeterol, the individual components of Advair Diskus, are substrates of CYP3A4. The use of strong CYP3A4 inhibitors with Advair Diskus is not recommended because increased corticosteroid and increased cardiovascular adverse effects may occur).

No products indexed under this heading.

Zonisamide (Decreases in bone mineral density (BMD) have been observed with long-term administration of products containing inhaled corticosteroids. Patients with major risk factors for decreased bone mineral content, such chronic use of drugs that can reduce bone mass (eg, anticonvulsants) should be monitored and treated with established standards of care). Products include:

Zonegran 1081

Food Interactions

Grapefruit (Fluticasone propionate and salmeterol, the individual components of Advair Diskus, are substrates of CYP3A4. The use of strong CYP3A4 inhibitors with Advair Diskus is not recommended because increased corticosteroid and increased cardiovascular adverse effects may occur).

Grapefruit Juice (Fluticasone propionate and salmeterol, the individual components of Advair Diskus, are substrates of CYP3A4. The use of strong CYP3A4 inhibitors with Advair Diskus is not recommended because increased corticosteroid and increased cardiovascular adverse effects may occur).

ADVAIR DISKUS 250/50
(Fluticasone Propionate, Salmeterol Xinafoate)... 1275
See Advair Diskus 100/50

ADVAIR DISKUS 500/50
(Fluticasone Propionate, Salmeterol Xinafoate)... 1275
See Advair Diskus 100/50

ADVAIR HFA 45/21 INHALATION AEROSOL
(Fluticasone Propionate, Salmeterol Xinafoate)... 1288
May interact with anticonvulsants, beta-blockers, beta2 agonists, corticosteroids, cytochrome p450 3a4 inhibitors (selected), cytochrome p450 3a4 inhibitors, potent (selected), erythromy-

cin, loop diuretics, monoamine oxidase inhibitors, nonpotassium-sparing diuretics, thiazides, tricyclic antidepressants, and certain other agents. Compounds in these categories include:

Acebutolol Hydrochloride (β-blockers not only block the pulmonary effect of β-agonists, such as salmeterol, a component of Advair HFA, but may produce severe bronchospasm in patients with asthma. Therefore, patients with asthma should not normally be treated with β-blockers. However, under certain circumstances, there may be no acceptable alternatives to the use of β-adrenergic blocking agents in patients with asthma. In this setting, cardioselective β-blockers could be considered, although they should be administered with caution).
No products indexed under this heading.

Acetazolamide (Both fluticasone propionate and salmeterol are substrates of CYP 3A4. There is a potential drug interaction with CYP 3A4 inhibitors).
No products indexed under this heading.

Acetazolamide Sodium (Both fluticasone propionate and salmeterol are substrates of CYP 3A4. There is a potential drug interaction with CYP 3A4 inhibitors).
No products indexed under this heading.

Albuterol (Patients who are receiving Advair HFA twice daily should not use additional salmeterol or other long-acting β-agonists (eg, formoterol) for prevention of exercise-induced bronchospasm (EIB) or the maintenance treatment of asthma. Additional benefit would not be gained from using supplemental salmeterol or formoterol for prevention of EIB since Advair HFA already contains an inhaled, long-acting β_2-agonist).
No products indexed under this heading.

Albuterol Sulfate (Patients who are receiving Advair HFA twice daily should not use additional salmeterol or other long-acting β-agonists (eg, formoterol) for prevention of exercise-induced bronchospasm (EIB) or the maintenance treatment of asthma. Additional benefit would not be gained from using supplemental salmeterol or formoterol for prevention of EIB since Advair HFA already contains an inhaled, long-acting β_2-agonist). Products include:
ProAir HFA **3393**
Proventil HFA **3204**
Ventolin HFA **1708**

Alclometasone Dipropionate (Long-term use of orally inhaled corticosteroids may affect normal bone metabolism, resulting in a loss of bone mineral density. In patients with major risk factors for decreased bone mineral content, such as chronic use of drugs that can reduce bone mass (eg, corticosteroids), Advair HFA may pose an additional risk).
No products indexed under this heading.

Amiodarone Hydrochloride (Both fluticasone propionate and salmeterol are substrates of CYP 3A4. There is a potential drug interaction with CYP 3A4 inhibitors).
No products indexed under this heading.

Amitriptyline Hydrochloride (Advair HFA should be administered with extreme caution to patients being treated with tricyclic antidepressants, or within 2 weeks of discontinuation of such agents, because the action of salmeterol, a component of Advair HFA, on the vascular system may be potentiated by these agents).
No products indexed under this heading.

Amoxapine (Advair HFA should be administered with extreme caution to patients being treated with tricyclic antidepressants, or within 2 weeks of discontinuation of such agents, because the action of salmeterol, a component of Advair HFA, on the vascular system may be potentiated by these agents).
No products indexed under this heading.

Amprenavir (Due to the potential increased risk of cardiovascular adverse events, the concomitant use of salmeterol with strong CYP3A4 inhibitors (eg, ketoconazole, ritonavir, atazanavir, clarithromycin, indinavir, itraconazole, nefazodone, nelfinavir, saquinavir, telithromycin) is not recommended).
No products indexed under this heading.

Anastrozole (Both fluticasone propionate and salmeterol are substrates of CYP 3A4. There is a potential drug interaction with CYP 3A4 inhibitors).
No products indexed under this heading.

Aprepitant (Both fluticasone propionate and salmeterol are substrates of CYP 3A4. There is a potential drug interaction with CYP 3A4 inhibitors).
Products include:
Emend **2124**

Atazanavir (Due to the potential increased risk of cardiovascular adverse events, the concomitant use of salmeterol with strong CYP3A4 inhibitors (eg, ketoconazole, ritonavir, atazanavir, clarithromycin, indinavir, itraconazole, nefazodone, nelfinavir, saquinavir, telithromycin) is not recommended).
No products indexed under this heading.

Atazanavir Sulfate (Due to the potential increased risk of cardiovascular adverse events, the concomitant use of salmeterol with strong CYP3A4 inhibitors (eg, ketoconazole, ritonavir, atazanavir, clarithromycin, indinavir, itraconazole, nefazodone, nelfinavir, saquinavir, telithromycin) is not recommended).
No products indexed under this heading.

Atenolol (β-blockers not only block the pulmonary effect of β-agonists, such as salmeterol, a component of Advair HFA, but may produce severe bronchospasm in patients with asthma. Therefore, patients with asthma should not normally be treated with β-blockers. However, under certain circumstances, there may be no acceptable alternatives to the use of β-adrenergic blocking agents in patients with asthma. In this setting, cardioselective β-blockers could be considered, although they should be administered with caution).
No products indexed under this heading.

Beclomethasone Dipropionate (Long-term use of orally inhaled corticosteroids may affect normal bone metabolism, resulting in a loss of bone mineral density. In patients with major risk factors for decreased bone mineral content, such as chronic use of drugs that can reduce bone mass (eg, corticosteroids), Advair HFA may pose an additional risk). Products include:
Qvar **3398**

Beclomethasone Dipropionate Monohydrate (Long-term use of orally inhaled corticosteroids may affect normal bone metabolism, resulting in a loss of bone mineral density. In patients with major risk factors for decreased bone mineral content, such as chronic use of drugs that can reduce bone mass (eg, corticosteroids), Advair HFA may pose an additional risk). Products include:
Beconase AQ **1386**

Bendroflumethiazide (The ECG changes and/or hypokalemia that may result from the administration of nonpotassium-sparing diuretics (such as loop or thiazide diuretics) can be acutely worsened by β-agonists, especially when the recommended dose of the β-agonist is exceeded. Although the clinical significance of these effects is not known, caution is advised in the co-administration of β-agonists with nonpotassium-sparing diuretics).
No products indexed under this heading.

Betamethasone (Long-term use of orally inhaled corticosteroids may affect normal bone metabolism, resulting in a loss of bone mineral density. In patients with major risk factors for decreased bone mineral content, such as chronic use of drugs that can reduce bone mass (eg, corticosteroids), Advair HFA may pose an additional risk).
No products indexed under this heading.

Betamethasone Acetate (Long-term use of orally inhaled corticosteroids may affect normal bone metabolism, resulting in a loss of bone mineral density. In patients with major risk factors for decreased bone mineral content, such as chronic use of drugs that can reduce bone mass (eg, corticosteroids), Advair HFA may pose an additional risk).
No products indexed under this heading.

Betamethasone Benzoate (Long-term use of orally inhaled corticosteroids may affect normal bone metabolism, resulting in a loss of bone mineral density. In patients with major risk factors for decreased bone mineral content, such as chronic use of drugs that can reduce bone mass (eg, corticosteroids), Advair HFA may pose an additional risk).
No products indexed under this heading.

Betamethasone Dipropionate (Long-term use of orally inhaled corticosteroids may affect normal bone metabolism, resulting in a loss of bone mineral density. In patients with major risk factors for decreased bone mineral content, such as chronic use of drugs that can reduce bone mass (eg, corticosteroids), Advair HFA may pose an additional risk). Products include:
Diprolene Lotion 0.05% **3108**
Diprolene Ointment 0.05% **3109**
Diprolene AF Cream 0.05% **3107**
Lotrisone **3163**

Betamethasone Sodium Phosphate (Long-term use of orally inhaled corticosteroids may affect normal bone metabolism, resulting in a loss of bone mineral density. In patients with major risk factors for decreased bone mineral content, such as chronic use of drugs that can reduce bone mass (eg, corticosteroids), Advair HFA may pose an additional risk).
No products indexed under this heading.

Betamethasone Valerate (Long-term use of orally inhaled corticosteroids may affect normal bone metabolism, resulting in a loss of bone mineral density. In patients with major risk factors for decreased bone mineral content, such as chronic use of drugs that can reduce bone mass (eg, corticosteroids), Advair HFA may pose an additional risk). Products include:
Luxíq **3321**

Betaxolol Hydrochloride (β-blockers not only block the pulmonary effect of β-agonists, such as salmeterol, a component of Advair HFA, but may produce severe bronchospasm in patients with asthma. Therefore, patients with asthma should not normally be treated with β-blockers. However, under certain circumstances, there may be no acceptable alternatives to the use of β-adrenergic blocking agents in patients with asthma. In this setting, cardioselective β-blockers could be considered, although they should be administered with caution).
No products indexed under this heading.

Bisoprolol Fumarate (β-blockers not only block the pulmonary effect of β-agonists, such as salmeterol, a component of Advair HFA, but may produce severe bronchospasm in patients with asthma. Therefore, patients with asthma should not normally be treated with β-blockers. However, under certain circumstances, there may be no acceptable alternatives to the use of β-adrenergic blocking agents in patients with asthma. In this setting, cardioselective β-blockers could be considered, although they should be administered with caution).
No products indexed under this heading.

Bitolterol Mesylate (Patients who are receiving Advair HFA twice daily should not use additional salmeterol or other long-acting β-agonists (eg, formoterol) for prevention of exercise-induced bronchospasm (EIB) or the maintenance treatment of asthma. Additional benefit would not be gained from using supplemental salmeterol or formoterol for prevention of EIB since Advair HFA already contains an inhaled, long-acting β_2-agonist).
No products indexed under this heading.

Budesonide (Long-term use of orally inhaled corticosteroids may affect normal bone metabolism, resulting in a loss of bone mineral density. In patients with major risk factors for decreased bone mineral content, such as chronic use of drugs that can reduce bone mass (eg, corticosteroids), Advair HFA may pose an additional risk). Products include:
Pulmicort Flexhaler **714**
Symbicort 80/4.5 .... **720**
Symbicort 160/4.5 .... **720**

Bumetanide (The ECG changes and/or hypokalemia that may result from the administration of nonpotassium-sparing diuretics (such as loop or thiazide diuretics) can be acutely worsened by β-agonists, especially when the recommended dose of the β-agonist is exceeded. Although the clinical significance of these effects is not known, caution is advised in the co-administration of β-agonists with nonpotassium-sparing diuretics).
No products indexed under this heading.

Carbamazepine (Long-term use of orally inhaled corticosteroids may affect normal bone metabolism, resulting in a loss of bone mineral density. In patients with major risk factors for decreased bone mineral content, such as chronic use of drugs that can reduce bone mass (eg, anticonvulsants), Advair HFA may pose an additional risk). Products include:
Carbatrol **3280**
Equetro **3477**

Carteolol Hydrochloride (β-blockers not only block the pulmonary effect of β-agonists, such as salmeterol, a component of Advair HFA, but may produce severe bronchospasm in patients with asthma. Therefore, patients with asthma should not normally be treated with β-blockers. However, under certain circumstances, there may be no acceptable alternatives to the use of β-adrenergic blocking agents in patients with asthma. In this setting, cardioselective β-blockers could be considered, although they should be administered with caution).
No products indexed under this heading.

Carvedilol (β-blockers not only block the pulmonary effect of β-agonists, such as salmeterol, a component of Advair HFA, but may produce severe bronchospasm in patients with asthma. Therefore, patients with asthma should not normally be treated with β-blockers. However, under certain circumstances, there may be no acceptable alternatives to the use of β-adrenergic blocking agents in patients with asthma. In this setting, cardioselective β-blockers

IMPORTANT NOTE: Always consult each drug listing in the patient's regimen for possible interactions.

Advair HFA Interactions Index 62

could be considered, although they should be administered with caution). Products include:
Coreg 1409

Carvedilol Phosphate (β-blockers not only block the pulmonary effect of β-agonists, such as salmeterol, a component of Advair HFA, but may produce severe bronchospasm in patients with asthma. Therefore, patients with asthma should not normally be treated with β-blockers. However, under certain circumstances, there may be no acceptable alternatives to the use of β-adrenergic blocking agents in patients with asthma. In this setting, cardioselective β-blockers could be considered, although they should be administered with caution). Products include:
Coreg CR 1416

Chlorothiazide (The ECG changes and/or hypokalemia that may result from the administration of nonpotassium-sparing diuretics (such as loop or thiazide diuretics) can be acutely worsened by β-agonists, especially when the recommended dose of the β-agonist is exceeded. Although the clinical significance of these effects is not known, caution is advised in the co-administration of β-agonists with nonpotassium-sparing diuretics).
No products indexed under this heading.

Chlorothiazide Sodium (The ECG changes and/or hypokalemia that may result from the administration of nonpotassium-sparing diuretics (such as loop or thiazide diuretics) can be acutely worsened by β-agonists, especially when the recommended dose of the β-agonist is exceeded. Although the clinical significance of these effects is not known, caution is advised in the co-administration of β-agonists with nonpotassium-sparing diuretics).
Products include:
Diuril Intravenous 2009

Ciclesonide (Long-term use of orally inhaled corticosteroids may affect normal bone metabolism, resulting in a loss of bone mineral density. In patients with major risk factors for decreased bone mineral content, such as chronic use of drugs that can reduce bone mass (eg, corticosteroids), Advair HFA may pose an additional risk).
No products indexed under this heading.

Cimetidine (Both fluticasone propionate and salmeterol are substrates of CYP 3A4. There is a potential drug interaction with CYP 3A4 inhibitors).
No products indexed under this heading.

Cimetidine Hydrochloride (Both fluticasone propionate and salmeterol are substrates of CYP 3A4. There is a potential drug interaction with CYP 3A4 inhibitors).
No products indexed under this heading.

Ciprofloxacin (Both fluticasone propionate and salmeterol are substrates of CYP 3A4. There is a potential drug interaction with CYP 3A4 inhibitors).
Products include:
Cipro I.V. 3082
Cipro 3073
Cipro XR 3091
Ciprodex 583

Clarithromycin (Due to the potential increased risk of cardiovascular adverse events, the concomitant use of salmeterol with strong CYP3A4 inhibitors (eg, ketoconazole, ritonavir, atazanavir, clarithromycin, indinavir, itraconazole, nefazodone, nelfinavir, saquinavir, telithromycin) is not recommended).
Products include:
Biaxin/Biaxin XL 412

Clomipramine Hydrochloride (Advair HFA should be administered with extreme caution to patients being treated with tricyclic antidepressants, or within 2 weeks of discontinuation of such agents, because the action of salmeterol, a component of Advair HFA, on the vascular system may be potentiated by these agents).
No products indexed under this heading.

Clotrimazole (Both fluticasone propionate and salmeterol are substrates of CYP 3A4. There is a potential drug interaction with CYP 3A4 inhibitors).
Products include:
Lotrisone 3163

Conivaptan Hydrochloride (Both fluticasone propionate and salmeterol are substrates of CYP 3A4. There is a potential drug interaction with CYP 3A4 inhibitors). Products include:
Vaprisol 689

Cortisone Acetate (Long-term use of orally inhaled corticosteroids may affect normal bone metabolism, resulting in a loss of bone mineral density. In patients with major risk factors for decreased bone mineral content, such as chronic use of drugs that can reduce bone mass (eg, corticosteroids), Advair HFA may pose an additional risk).
No products indexed under this heading.

Cyclosporine (Both fluticasone propionate and salmeterol are substrates of CYP 3A4. There is a potential drug interaction with CYP 3A4 inhibitors).
Products include:
Gengraf 440
Neoral Oral Solution 2496
Neoral Capsules 2496
Restasis 605

Dalfopristin (Both fluticasone propionate and salmeterol are substrates of CYP 3A4. There is a potential drug interaction with CYP 3A4 inhibitors).
No products indexed under this heading.

Danazol (Both fluticasone propionate and salmeterol are substrates of CYP 3A4. There is a potential drug interaction with CYP 3A4 inhibitors).
No products indexed under this heading.

Darunavir (Both fluticasone propionate and salmeterol are substrates of CYP 3A4. There is a potential drug interaction with CYP 3A4 inhibitors).
No products indexed under this heading.

Dasatinib (Both fluticasone propionate and salmeterol are substrates of CYP 3A4. There is a potential drug interaction with CYP 3A4 inhibitors).
No products indexed under this heading.

Delavirdine Mesylate (Due to the potential increased risk of cardiovascular adverse events, the concomitant use of salmeterol with strong CYP3A4 inhibitors (eg, ketoconazole, ritonavir, atazanavir, clarithromycin, indinavir, itraconazole, nefazodone, nelfinavir, saquinavir, telithromycin) is not recommended).
No products indexed under this heading.

Delavirine (Due to the potential increased risk of cardiovascular adverse events, the concomitant use of salmeterol with strong CYP3A4 inhibitors (eg, ketoconazole, ritonavir, atazanavir, clarithromycin, indinavir, itraconazole, nefazodone, nelfinavir, saquinavir, telithromycin) is not recommended).
No products indexed under this heading.

Desipramine Hydrochloride (Advair HFA should be administered with extreme caution to patients being treated with tricyclic antidepressants, or within 2 weeks of discontinuation of such agents, because the action of salmeterol, a component of Advair HFA, on the vascular system may be potentiated by these agents).
No products indexed under this heading.

Desloratadine (Both fluticasone propionate and salmeterol are substrates of CYP 3A4. There is a potential drug interaction with CYP 3A4 inhibitors).
Products include:
Clarinex Syrup 3098
Clarinex 3098
Clarinex Reditabs 3098
Clarinex-D 12-Hour 3101
Clarinex-D 3104

Desoximetasone (Long-term use of orally inhaled corticosteroids may affect normal bone metabolism, resulting in a loss of bone mineral density. In patients with major risk factors for decreased bone mineral content, such as chronic use of drugs that can reduce bone mass (eg, corticosteroids), Advair HFA may pose an additional risk).
No products indexed under this heading.

Dexamethasone (Long-term use of orally inhaled corticosteroids may affect normal bone metabolism, resulting in a loss of bone mineral density. In patients with major risk factors for decreased bone mineral content, such as chronic use of drugs that can reduce bone mass (eg, corticosteroids), Advair HFA may pose an additional risk). Products include:
Ciprodex 583
Ozurdex .... ⊙223
Tobramycin and Dexamethasone Ophthalmic Suspension .... ⊙251

Dexamethasone Acetate (Long-term use of orally inhaled corticosteroids may affect normal bone metabolism, resulting in a loss of bone mineral density. In patients with major risk factors for decreased bone mineral content, such as chronic use of drugs that can reduce bone mass (eg, corticosteroids), Advair HFA may pose an additional risk).
No products indexed under this heading.

Dexamethasone Phosphate (Long-term use of orally inhaled corticosteroids may affect normal bone metabolism, resulting in a loss of bone mineral density. In patients with major risk factors for decreased bone mineral content, such as chronic use of drugs that can reduce bone mass (eg, corticosteroids), Advair HFA may pose an additional risk).
No products indexed under this heading.

Dexamethasone Sodium (Long-term use of orally inhaled corticosteroids may affect normal bone metabolism, resulting in a loss of bone mineral density. In patients with major risk factors for decreased bone mineral content, such as chronic use of drugs that can reduce bone mass (eg, corticosteroids), Advair HFA may pose an additional risk).
No products indexed under this heading.

Dexamethasone Sodium Phosphate (Long-term use of orally inhaled corticosteroids may affect normal bone metabolism, resulting in a loss of bone mineral density. In patients with major risk factors for decreased bone mineral content, such as chronic use of drugs that can reduce bone mass (eg, corticosteroids), Advair HFA may pose an additional risk).
No products indexed under this heading.

Dexamethasone Sodium Phosphate Injection (Long-term use of orally inhaled corticosteroids may affect normal bone metabolism, resulting in a loss of bone mineral density. In patients with major risk factors for decreased bone mineral content, such as chronic use of drugs that can reduce bone mass (eg, corticosteroids), Advair HFA may pose an additional risk).
No products indexed under this heading.

Diflorasone Diacetate (Long-term use of orally inhaled corticosteroids may affect normal bone metabolism, resulting in a loss of bone mineral density. In patients with major risk factors for decreased bone mineral content, such as chronic use of drugs that can reduce bone mass (eg, corticosteroids), Advair HFA may pose an additional risk).
No products indexed under this heading.

Diltiazem Hydrochloride (Both fluticasone propionate and salmeterol are substrates of CYP 3A4. There is a potential drug interaction with CYP 3A4 inhibitors). Products include:
Cardizem LA 423

Diltiazem Maleate (Both fluticasone propionate and salmeterol are substrates of CYP 3A4. There is a potential drug interaction with CYP 3A4 inhibitors).
No products indexed under this heading.

Divalproex Sodium (Long-term use of orally inhaled corticosteroids may affect normal bone metabolism, resulting in a loss of bone mineral density. In patients with major risk factors for decreased bone mineral content, such as chronic use of drugs that can reduce bone mass (eg, anticonvulsants), Advair HFA may pose an additional risk).
Products include:
Depakote ER 426

Doxepin Hydrochloride (Advair HFA should be administered with extreme caution to patients being treated with tricyclic antidepressants, or within 2 weeks of discontinuation of such agents, because the action of salmeterol, a component of Advair HFA, on the vascular system may be potentiated by these agents).
No products indexed under this heading.

Efavirenz (Both fluticasone propionate and salmeterol are substrates of CYP 3A4. There is a potential drug interaction with CYP 3A4 inhibitors). Products include:
Atripla 906

Ephedrine Hydrochloride (Patients who are receiving Advair HFA twice daily should not use additional salmeterol or other long-acting β-agonists (eg, formoterol) for prevention of exercise-induced bronchospasm (EIB) or the maintenance treatment of asthma. Additional benefit would not be gained from using supplemental salmeterol or formoterol for prevention of EIB since Advair HFA already contains an inhaled, long-acting $β_2$-agonist).
No products indexed under this heading.

Ephedrine Sulfate (Patients who are receiving Advair HFA twice daily should not use additional salmeterol or other long-acting β-agonists (eg, formoterol) for prevention of exercise-induced bronchospasm (EIB) or the maintenance treatment of asthma. Additional benefit would not be gained from using supplemental salmeterol or formoterol for prevention of EIB since Advair HFA already contains an inhaled, long-acting $β_2$-agonist).
No products indexed under this heading.

Ephedrine Tannate (Patients who are receiving Advair HFA twice daily should not use additional salmeterol or other long-acting β-agonists (eg, formoterol) for prevention of exercise-induced bronchospasm (EIB) or the maintenance treatment of asthma. Additional benefit would not be gained from using supplemental salmeterol or formoterol for prevention of EIB since Advair HFA already contains an inhaled, long-acting $β_2$-agonist).
No products indexed under this heading.

Epinephrine (Patients who are receiving Advair HFA twice daily should not use additional salmeterol or other long-acting β-agonists (eg, formoterol) for

prevention of exercise-induced broncho-spasm (EIB) or the maintenance treatment of asthma. Additional benefit would not be gained from using supplemental salmeterol or formoterol for prevention of EIB since Advair HFA already contains an inhaled, long-acting β_2-agonist). Products include:

Epinephrine Hydrochloride (Patients who are receiving Advair HFA twice daily should not use additional salmeterol or other long-acting β-agonists (eg, formoterol) for prevention of exercise-induced bronchospasm (EIB) or the maintenance treatment of asthma. Additional benefit would not be gained from using supplemental salmeterol or formoterol for prevention of EIB since Advair HFA already contains an inhaled, long-acting β_2-agonist).
No products indexed under this heading.

Erythromycin (In a repeat-dose study in 13 healthy subjects, concomitant administration of erythromycin (a moderate CYP3A4 inhibitor) and salmeterol inhalation aerosol resulted in a 40% increase in salmeterol C_{max} at steady state, a 3.6-beat/min increase in heart rate, a 5.8-msec increase in QTc interval, and no change in plasma potassium).
No products indexed under this heading.

Erythromycin, Topical (In a repeat-dose study in 13 healthy subjects, concomitant administration of erythromycin (a moderate CYP3A4 inhibitor) and salmeterol inhalation aerosol resulted in a 40% increase in salmeterol C_{max} at steady state, a 3.6-beat/min increase in heart rate, a 5.8-msec increase in QTc interval, and no change in plasma potassium).
No products indexed under this heading.

Erythromycin Estolate (In a repeat-dose study in 13 healthy subjects, concomitant administration of erythromycin (a moderate CYP3A4 inhibitor) and salmeterol inhalation aerosol resulted in a 40% increase in salmeterol C_{max} at steady state, a 3.6-beat/min increase in heart rate, a 5.8-msec increase in QTc interval, and no change in plasma potassium).
No products indexed under this heading.

Erythromycin Ethylsuccinate (In a repeat-dose study in 13 healthy subjects, concomitant administration of erythromycin (a moderate CYP3A4 inhibitor) and salmeterol inhalation aerosol resulted in a 40% increase in salmeterol C_{max} at steady state, a 3.6-beat/min increase in heart rate, a 5.8-msec increase in QTc interval, and no change in plasma potassium). Products include:

Erythromycin Gluceptate (In a repeat-dose study in 13 healthy subjects, concomitant administration of erythromycin (a moderate CYP3A4 inhibitor) and salmeterol inhalation aerosol resulted in a 40% increase in salmeterol C_{max} at steady state, a 3.6-beat/min increase in QTc interval, and no change in plasma potassium).
No products indexed under this heading.

Erythromycin Lactobionate (In a repeat-dose study in 13 healthy subjects, concomitant administration of erythromycin (a moderate CYP3A4 inhibitor) and salmeterol inhalation aerosol resulted in a 40% increase in salmeterol C_{max} at steady state, a 3.6-beat/min increase in QTc interval, and no change in plasma potassium).
No products indexed under this heading.

Erythromycin Stearate (In a repeat-dose study in 13 healthy subjects, concomitant administration of erythromycin (a moderate CYP3A4 inhibitor) and salmeterol inhalation aerosol resulted in a 40% increase in salmeterol C_{max} at steady state, a 3.6-beat/min increase in heart rate, a 5.8-msec increase in QTc interval, and no change in plasma potassium).
No products indexed under this heading.

Esmolol Hydrochloride (β-blockers not only block the pulmonary effect of β-agonists, such as salmeterol, a component of Advair HFA, but may produce severe bronchospasm in patients with asthma. Therefore, patients with asthma should not normally be treated with β-blockers. However, under certain circumstances, there may be no acceptable alternatives to the use of β-adrenergic blocking agents in patients with asthma. In this setting, cardioselective β-blockers could be considered, although they should be administered with caution).
No products indexed under this heading.

Esomeprazole Magnesium (Both fluticasone propionate and salmeterol are substrates of CYP 3A4. There is a potential drug interaction with CYP 3A4 inhibitors). Products include:

Esomeprazole Sodium (Both fluticasone propionate and salmeterol are substrates of CYP 3A4. There is a potential drug interaction with CYP 3A4 inhibitors). Products include:

Ethacrynic Acid (The ECG changes and/or hypokalemia that may result from the administration of nonpotassium-sparing diuretics (such as loop or thiazide diuretics) can be acutely worsened by β-agonists, especially when the recommended dose of the β-agonist is exceeded. Although the clinical significance of these effects is not known, caution is advised in the co-administration of β-agonists with nonpotassium-sparing diuretics).
No products indexed under this heading.

Ethosuximide (Long-term use of orally inhaled corticosteroids may affect normal bone metabolism, resulting in a loss of bone mineral density. In patients with major risk factors for decreased bone mineral content, such as chronic use of drugs that can reduce bone mass (eg, anticonvulsants), Advair HFA may pose an additional risk).
No products indexed under this heading.

Ethotoin (Long-term use of orally inhaled corticosteroids may affect normal bone metabolism, resulting in a loss of bone mineral density. In patients with major risk factors for decreased bone mineral content, such as chronic use of drugs that can reduce bone mass (eg, anticonvulsants), Advair HFA may pose an additional risk).
No products indexed under this heading.

Felbamate (Long-term use of orally inhaled corticosteroids may affect normal bone metabolism, resulting in a loss of bone mineral density. In patients with major risk factors for decreased bone mineral content, such as chronic use of drugs that can reduce bone mass (eg, anticonvulsants), Advair HFA may pose an additional risk).
No products indexed under this heading.

Fluconazole (Both fluticasone propionate and salmeterol are substrates of CYP 3A4. There is a potential drug interaction with CYP 3A4 inhibitors).
No products indexed under this heading.

Fludrocortisone Acetate (Long-term use of orally inhaled corticosteroids may affect normal bone metabolism, resulting in a loss of bone mineral density. In patients with major risk factors for decreased bone mineral content, such as chronic use of drugs that can reduce bone mass (eg, corticosteroids), Advair HFA may pose an additional risk).
No products indexed under this heading.

Flumethasone Pivalate (Long-term use of orally inhaled corticosteroids may affect normal bone metabolism, resulting in a loss of bone mineral density. In patients with major risk factors for decreased bone mineral content, such as chronic use of drugs that can reduce bone mass (eg, corticosteroids), Advair HFA may pose an additional risk).
No products indexed under this heading.

Flunisolide Hemihydrate (Long-term use of orally inhaled corticosteroids may affect normal bone metabolism, resulting in a loss of bone mineral density. In patients with major risk factors for decreased bone mineral content, such as chronic use of drugs that can reduce bone mass (eg, corticosteroids), Advair HFA may pose an additional risk).
No products indexed under this heading.

Fluoxetine (Both fluticasone propionate and salmeterol are substrates of CYP 3A4. There is a potential drug interaction with CYP 3A4 inhibitors).
No products indexed under this heading.

Fluoxetine Hydrochloride (Both fluticasone propionate and salmeterol are substrates of CYP 3A4. There is a potential drug interaction with CYP 3A4 inhibitors). Products include:

Fluticasone Furoate (Long-term use of orally inhaled corticosteroids may affect normal bone metabolism, resulting in a loss of bone mineral density. In patients with major risk factors for decreased bone mineral content, such as chronic use of drugs that can reduce bone mass (eg, corticosteroids), Advair HFA may pose an additional risk). Products include:

Fluvoxamine Maleate (Both fluticasone and salmeterol are substrates of CYP 3A4. There is a potential drug interaction with CYP 3A4 inhibitors).
No products indexed under this heading.

Formoterol Fumarate (Patients who are receiving Advair HFA twice daily should not use additional salmeterol or other long-acting β-agonists (eg, formoterol) for prevention of exercise-induced bronchospasm (EIB) or the maintenance treatment of asthma. Additional benefit would not be gained from using supplemental salmeterol or formoterol for prevention of EIB since Advair HFA already contains an inhaled, long-acting β_2-agonist). Products include:

Formoterol fumarate dihydrate (Patients who are receiving Advair HFA twice daily should not use additional salmeterol or other long-acting β-agonists (eg, formoterol) for prevention of exercise-induced bronchospasm (EIB) or the maintenance treatment of asthma. Additional benefit would not be gained from using supplemental salmeterol or formoterol for prevention of EIB since Advair HFA already contains an inhaled, long-acting β_2-agonist). Products include:

Fosamprenavir Calcium (Due to the potential increased risk of cardiovascu-lar adverse events, the concomitant use of salmeterol with strong CYP3A4 inhibitors (eg, ketoconazole, ritonavir, atazanavir, clarithromycin, indinavir, itraconazole, nefazodone, nelfinavir, saquinavir, telithromycin) is not recommended). Products include:

Fosphenytoin (Long-term use of orally inhaled corticosteroids may affect normal bone metabolism, resulting in a loss of bone mineral density. In patients with major risk factors for decreased bone mineral content, such as chronic use of drugs that can reduce bone mass (eg, anticonvulsants), Advair HFA may pose an additional risk).
No products indexed under this heading.

Fosphenytoin Sodium (Long-term use of orally inhaled corticosteroids may affect normal bone metabolism, resulting in a loss of bone mineral density. In patients with major risk factors for decreased bone mineral content, such as chronic use of drugs that can reduce bone mass (eg, anticonvulsants), Advair HFA may pose an additional risk).
No products indexed under this heading.

Furosemide (The ECG changes and/or hypokalemia that may result from the administration of nonpotassium-sparing diuretics (such as loop or thiazide diuretics) can be acutely worsened by β-agonists, especially when the recommended dose of the β-agonist is exceeded. Although the clinical significance of these effects is not known, caution is advised in the co-administration of β-agonists with nonpotassium-sparing diuretics). Products include:

Gabapentin (Long-term use of orally inhaled corticosteroids may affect normal bone metabolism, resulting in a loss of bone mineral density. In patients with major risk factors for decreased bone mineral content, such as chronic use of drugs that can reduce bone mass (eg, anticonvulsants), Advair HFA may pose an additional risk).
No products indexed under this heading.

Hydrochlorothiazide (The ECG changes and/or hypokalemia that may result from the administration of nonpotassium-sparing diuretics (such as loop or thiazide diuretics) can be acutely worsened by β-agonists, especially when the recommended dose of the β-agonist is exceeded. Although the clinical significance of these effects is not known, caution is advised in the co-administration of β-agonists with nonpotassium-sparing diuretics). Products include:

Hydrocortisone (Long-term use of orally inhaled corticosteroids may affect normal bone metabolism, resulting in a loss of bone mineral density. In patients with major risk factors for decreased bone mineral content, such as chronic use of drugs that can reduce bone mass (eg, corticosteroids), Advair HFA may pose an additional risk).
No products indexed under this heading.

Hydrocortisone (Alcohol) (Long-term use of orally inhaled corticosteroids may affect normal bone metabolism, resulting in a loss of bone mineral density. In patients with major risk factors for decreased bone mineral content, such as chronic use of drugs that can reduce bone mass (eg, corticosteroids), Advair HFA may pose an additional risk).
No products indexed under this heading.

Hydrocortisone Acetate (Long-term use of orally inhaled corticosteroids may affect normal bone metabolism, resulting in a loss of bone mineral density. In patients with major risk factors for decreased bone mineral content, such as chronic use of drugs that can reduce bone mass (eg, corticosteroids), Advair HFA may pose an additional risk).
No products indexed under this heading.

Hydrocortisone Butyrate (Long-term use of orally inhaled corticosteroids may affect normal bone metabolism, resulting in a loss of bone mineral density. In patients with major risk factors for decreased bone mineral content, such as chronic use of drugs that can reduce bone mass (eg, corticosteroids), Advair HFA may pose an additional risk).
No products indexed under this heading.

Hydrocortisone Cypionate (Long-term use of orally inhaled corticosteroids may affect normal bone metabolism, resulting in a loss of bone mineral density. In patients with major risk factors for decreased bone mineral content, such as chronic use of drugs that can reduce bone mass (eg, corticosteroids), Advair HFA may pose an additional risk).
No products indexed under this heading.

Hydrocortisone Hemisuccinate (Long-term use of orally inhaled corticosteroids may affect normal bone metabolism, resulting in a loss of bone mineral density. In patients with major risk factors for decreased bone mineral content, such as chronic use of drugs that can reduce bone mass (eg, corticosteroids), Advair HFA may pose an additional risk).
No products indexed under this heading.

Hydrocortisone Probutate (Long-term use of orally inhaled corticosteroids may affect normal bone metabolism, resulting in a loss of bone mineral density. In patients with major risk factors for decreased bone mineral content, such as chronic use of drugs that can reduce bone mass (eg, corticosteroids), Advair HFA may pose an additional risk).
No products indexed under this heading.

Hydrocortisone Sodium Phosphate (Long-term use of orally inhaled corticosteroids may affect normal bone metabolism, resulting in a loss of bone mineral density. In patients with major risk factors for decreased bone mineral content, such as chronic use of drugs that can reduce bone mass (eg, corticosteroids), Advair HFA may pose an additional risk).
No products indexed under this heading.

Hydrocortisone Sodium Succinate (Long-term use of orally inhaled corticosteroids may affect normal bone metabolism, resulting in a loss of bone mineral density. In patients with major risk factors for decreased bone mineral content, such as chronic use of drugs that can reduce bone mass (eg, corticosteroids), Advair HFA may pose an additional risk).
No products indexed under this heading.

Hydrocortisone Valerate (Long-term use of orally inhaled corticosteroids may affect normal bone metabolism, resulting in a loss of bone mineral density. In patients with major risk factors for decreased bone mineral content, such as chronic use of drugs that can reduce bone mass (eg, corticosteroids), Advair HFA may pose an additional risk).
No products indexed under this heading.

Hydroflumethiazide (The ECG changes and/or hypokalemia that may result from the administration of nonpotassium-sparing diuretics (such as loop or thiazide diuretics) can be acutely worsened by β-agonists, especially when the recommended dose of the β-agonist is exceeded. Although the clinical significance of these effects is not known, caution is advised in the co-administration of β-agonists with nonpotassium-sparing diuretics).
No products indexed under this heading.

Imatinib Mesylate (Both fluticasone propionate and salmeterol are substrates of CYP 3A4. There is a potential drug interaction with CYP 3A4 inhibitors). Products include:
Gleevec 2477

Imipramine Hydrochloride (Advair HFA should be administered with extreme caution to patients being treated with tricyclic antidepressants, or within 2 weeks of discontinuation of such agents, because the action of salmeterol, a component of Advair HFA, on the vascular system may be potentiated by these agents).
No products indexed under this heading.

Imipramine Pamoate (Advair HFA should be administered with extreme caution to patients being treated with tricyclic antidepressants, or within 2 weeks of discontinuation of such agents, because the action of salmeterol, a component of Advair HFA, on the vascular system may be potentiated by these agents).
No products indexed under this heading.

Indinavir Sulfate (Due to the potential increased risk of cardiovascular adverse events, the concomitant use of salmeterol with strong CYP3A4 inhibitors (eg, ketoconazole, ritonavir, atazanavir, clarithromycin, indinavir, itraconazole, nefazodone, nelfinavir, saquinavir, telithromycin) is not recommended). Products include:
Crixivan 2113

Isocarboxazid (Advair HFA should be administered with extreme caution to patients being treated with monoamine oxidase inhibitors, or within 2 weeks of discontinuation of such agents, because the action of salmeterol, a component of Advair HFA, on the vascular system may be potentiated by these agents). Products include:
Marplan 3481

Isoetharine (Patients who are receiving Advair HFA twice daily should not use additional salmeterol or other long-acting β-agonists (eg, formoterol) for prevention of exercise-induced bronchospasm (EIB) or the maintenance treatment of asthma. Additional benefit would not be gained from using supplemental salmeterol or formoterol for prevention of EIB since Advair HFA already contains an inhaled, long-acting β_2-agonist).
No products indexed under this heading.

Isoniazid (Both fluticasone propionate and salmeterol are substrates of CYP 3A4. There is a potential drug interaction with CYP 3A4 inhibitors).
No products indexed under this heading.

Isoproterenol Hydrochloride (Patients who are receiving Advair HFA twice daily should not use additional salmeterol or other long-acting β-agonists (eg, formoterol) for prevention of exercise-induced bronchospasm (EIB) or the maintenance treatment of asthma. Additional benefit would not be gained from using supplemental salmeterol or formoterol for prevention of EIB since Advair HFA already contains an inhaled, long-acting β_2-agonist).
No products indexed under this heading.

Isoproterenol Sulfate (Patients who are receiving Advair HFA twice daily should not use additional salmeterol or other long-acting β-agonists (eg, formoterol) for prevention of exercise-induced bronchospasm (EIB) or the maintenance treatment of asthma. Additional benefit would not be gained from using supplemental salmeterol or formoterol for prevention of EIB since Advair HFA already contains an inhaled, long-acting β_2-agonist).
No products indexed under this heading.

Itraconazole (Due to the potential increased risk of cardiovascular adverse events, the concomitant use of salmeterol with strong CYP3A4 inhibitors (eg, ketoconazole, ritonavir, atazanavir, clarithromycin, indinavir, itraconazole, nefazodone, nelfinavir, saquinavir, telithromycin) is not recommended).
No products indexed under this heading.

Ketoconazole (In a placebo-controlled, crossover drug interaction study, co-administration of a single dose of orally inhaled fluticasone propionate (1,000 mcg) with multiple doses of ketoconazole (200 mg) to steady state resulted in increased systemic fluticasone propionate exposure, a reduction in plasma cortisol AUC, and no effect on urinary excretion of cortisol. In addition, in a drug interaction study, co-administration of inhaled salmeterol (50 mcg twice daily) and oral ketoconazole (400 mg once daily) for 7 days resulted in greater systemic exposure to salmeterol (AUC increased 16-fold and C_{max} increased 1.4-fold). Three subjects were withdrawn due to β-agonist side effects (2 with prolonged QTc and 1 with palpitations and sinus tachycardia). Although there was no statistical effect on the mean QTc, co-administration of salmeterol and ketoconazole was associated with more frequent increases in QTc duration compared with salmeterol and placebo administration. Due to the potential increased risk of cardiovascular adverse events, the concomitant use of salmeterol with strong CYP3A4 inhibitors (eg, ketoconazole) is not recommended). Products include:
Extina 3319
Xolegel 3337

Labetalol Hydrochloride (β-blockers not only block the pulmonary effect of β-agonists, such as salmeterol, a component of Advair HFA, but may produce severe bronchospasm in patients with asthma. Therefore, patients with asthma should not normally be treated with β-blockers. However, under certain circumstances, there may be no acceptable alternatives to the use of β-adrenergic blocking agents in patients with asthma. In this setting, cardioselective β-blockers could be considered, although they should be administered with caution).
No products indexed under this heading.

Lamotrigine (Long-term use of orally inhaled corticosteroids may affect normal bone metabolism, resulting in a loss of bone mineral density. In patients with major risk factors for decreased bone mineral content, such as chronic use of drugs that can reduce bone mass (eg, anticonvulsants), Advair HFA may pose an additional risk). Products include:
Lamictal 1522
Lamictal ODT 1522
Lamictal XR 1536

Lapatinib (Both fluticasone propionate and salmeterol are substrates of CYP 3A4. There is a potential drug interaction with CYP 3A4 inhibitors). Products include:
Tykerb 1698

Levalbuterol Hydrochloride (Patients who are receiving Advair HFA twice daily should not use additional salmeterol or other long-acting β-agonists (eg, formoterol) for prevention of exercise-induced bronchospasm (EIB) or the maintenance treatment of asthma. Additional benefit would not be gained from using supplemental salmeterol or formoterol for prevention of EIB since Advair HFA already contains an inhaled, long-acting β_2-agonist).
No products indexed under this heading.

Levetiracetam (Long-term use of orally inhaled corticosteroids may affect normal bone metabolism, resulting in a loss of bone mineral density. In patients with major risk factors for decreased bone mineral content, such as chronic use of drugs that can reduce bone mass (eg, anticonvulsants), Advair HFA may pose an additional risk). Products include:
Keppra XR 3434

Levobunolol Hydrochloride (β-blockers not only block the pulmonary effect of β-agonists, such as salmeterol, a component of Advair HFA, but may produce severe bronchospasm in patients with asthma. Therefore, patients with asthma should not normally be treated with β-blockers. However, under certain circumstances, there may be no acceptable alternatives to the use of β-adrenergic blocking agents in patients with asthma. In this setting, cardioselective β-blockers could be considered, although they should be administered with caution).
No products indexed under this heading.

Lopinavir (Due to the potential increased risk of cardiovascular adverse events, the concomitant use of salmeterol with strong CYP3A4 inhibitors (eg, ketoconazole, ritonavir, atazanavir, clarithromycin, indinavir, itraconazole, nefazodone, nelfinavir, saquinavir, telithromycin) is not recommended). Products include:
Kaletra 458

Loratadine (Both fluticasone propionate and salmeterol are substrates of CYP 3A4. There is a potential drug interaction with CYP 3A4 inhibitors).
No products indexed under this heading.

Maprotiline Hydrochloride (Advair HFA should be administered with extreme caution to patients being treated with tricyclic antidepressants, or within 2 weeks of discontinuation of such agents, because the action of salmeterol, a component of Advair HFA, on the vascular system may be potentiated by these agents).
No products indexed under this heading.

Mephenytoin (Long-term use of orally inhaled corticosteroids may affect normal bone metabolism, resulting in a loss of bone mineral density. In patients with major risk factors for decreased bone mineral content, such as chronic use of drugs that can reduce bone mass (eg, anticonvulsants), Advair HFA may pose an additional risk).
No products indexed under this heading.

Metaproterenol Sulfate (Patients who are receiving Advair HFA twice daily should not use additional salmeterol or other long-acting β-agonists (eg, formoterol) for prevention of exercise-induced bronchospasm (EIB) or the maintenance treatment of asthma. Additional benefit would not be gained from using supplemental salmeterol or for-

moterol for prevention of EIB since Advair HFA already contains an inhaled, long-acting β_2-agonist).
No products indexed under this heading.

Methsuximide (Long-term use of orally inhaled corticosteroids may affect normal bone metabolism, resulting in a loss of bone mineral density. In patients with major risk factors for decreased bone mineral content, such as chronic use of drugs that can reduce bone mass (eg, anticonvulsants), Advair HFA may pose an additional risk).
No products indexed under this heading.

Methyclothiazide (The ECG changes and/or hypokalemia that may result from the administration of nonpotassium-sparing diuretics (such as loop or thiazide diuretics) can be acutely worsened by β-agonists, especially when the recommended dose of the β-agonist is exceeded. Although the clinical significance of these effects is not known, caution is advised in the co-administration of β-agonists with nonpotassium-sparing diuretics).
No products indexed under this heading.

Methylprednisolone (Long-term use of orally inhaled corticosteroids may affect normal bone metabolism, resulting in a loss of bone mineral density. In patients with major risk factors for decreased bone mineral content, such as chronic use of drugs that can reduce bone mass (eg, corticosteroids), Advair HFA may pose an additional risk).
No products indexed under this heading.

Methylprednisolone Acetate (Long-term use of orally inhaled corticosteroids may affect normal bone metabolism, resulting in a loss of bone mineral density. In patients with major risk factors for decreased bone mineral content, such as chronic use of drugs that can reduce bone mass (eg, corticosteroids), Advair HFA may pose an additional risk).
No products indexed under this heading.

Methylprednisolone Sodium Succinate (Long-term use of orally inhaled corticosteroids may affect normal bone metabolism, resulting in a loss of bone mineral density. In patients with major risk factors for decreased bone mineral content, such as chronic use of drugs that can reduce bone mass (eg, corticosteroids), Advair HFA may pose an additional risk).
No products indexed under this heading.

Metipranolol Hydrochloride (β-blockers not only block the pulmonary effect of β-agonists, such as salmeterol, a component of Advair HFA, but may produce severe bronchospasm in patients with asthma. Therefore, patients with asthma should not normally be treated with β-blockers. However, under certain circumstances, there may be no acceptable alternatives to the use of β-adrenergic blocking agents in patients with asthma. In this setting, cardioselective β-blockers could be considered, although they should be administered with caution).
No products indexed under this heading.

Metoprolol Succinate (β-blockers not only block the pulmonary effect of β-agonists, such as salmeterol, a component of Advair HFA, but may produce severe bronchospasm in patients with asthma. Therefore, patients with asthma should not normally be treated with β-blockers. However, under certain circumstances, there may be no acceptable alternatives to the use of β-adrenergic blocking agents in patients with asthma. In this setting, cardioselective β-blockers could be considered, although they should be administered with caution). Products include:
Toprol XL 732

Metoprolol Tartrate (β-blockers not only block the pulmonary effect of β-agonists, such as salmeterol, a component of Advair HFA, but may produce severe bronchospasm in patients with asthma. Therefore, patients with asthma should not normally be treated with β-blockers. However, under certain circumstances, there may be no acceptable alternatives to the use of β-adrenergic blocking agents in patients with asthma. In this setting, cardioselective β-blockers could be considered, although they should be administered with caution).
No products indexed under this heading.

Metronidazole (Both fluticasone propionate and salmeterol are substrates of CYP 3A4. There is a potential drug interaction with CYP 3A4 inhibitors). Products include:
Pylera 793

Metronidazole Benzoate (Both fluticasone propionate and salmeterol are substrates of CYP 3A4. There is a potential drug interaction with CYP 3A4 inhibitors).
No products indexed under this heading.

Metronidazole Hydrochloride (Both fluticasone propionate and salmeterol are substrates of CYP 3A4. There is a potential drug interaction with CYP 3A4 inhibitors).
No products indexed under this heading.

Metronidazole Sodium (Both fluticasone propionate and salmeterol are substrates of CYP 3A4. There is a potential drug interaction with CYP 3A4 inhibitors).
No products indexed under this heading.

Miconazole (Both fluticasone propionate and salmeterol are substrates of CYP 3A4. There is a potential drug interaction with CYP 3A4 inhibitors).
No products indexed under this heading.

Miconazole Nitrate (Both fluticasone propionate and salmeterol are substrates of CYP 3A4. There is a potential drug interaction with CYP 3A4 inhibitors). Products include:
Vusion Ointment 3335

Mifepristone (Both fluticasone propionate and salmeterol are substrates of CYP 3A4. There is a potential drug interaction with CYP 3A4 inhibitors).
No products indexed under this heading.

Moclobemide (Advair HFA should be administered with extreme caution to patients being treated with monoamine oxidase inhibitors, or within 2 weeks of discontinuation of such agents, because the action of salmeterol, a component of Advair HFA, on the vascular system may be potentiated by these agents).
No products indexed under this heading.

Mometasone Furoate (Long-term use of orally inhaled corticosteroids may affect normal bone metabolism, resulting in a loss of bone mineral density. In patients with major risk factors for decreased bone mineral content, such as chronic use of drugs that can reduce bone mass (eg, corticosteroids), Advair HFA may pose an additional risk). Products include:
Asmanex 3058
Elocon Cream 3111
Elocon Lotion 3112
Elocon Ointment 3114

Mometasone Furoate Monohydrate (Long-term use of orally inhaled corticosteroids may affect normal bone metabolism, resulting in a loss of bone mineral density. In patients with major risk factors for decreased bone mineral content, such as chronic use of drugs that can reduce bone mass (eg, corticosteroids), Advair HFA may pose an additional risk). Products include:
Nasonex 3166

Nadolol (β-blockers not only block the pulmonary effect of β-agonists, such as salmeterol, a component of Advair HFA, but may produce severe bronchospasm in patients with asthma. Therefore, patients with asthma should not normally be treated with β-blockers. However, under certain circumstances, there may be no acceptable alternatives to the use of β-adrenergic blocking agents in patients with asthma. In this setting, cardioselective β-blockers could be considered, although they should be administered with caution). Products include:
Nadolol 2359

Nebivolol (β-blockers not only block the pulmonary effect of β-agonists, such as salmeterol, a component of Advair HFA, but may produce severe bronchospasm in patients with asthma. Therefore, patients with asthma should not normally be treated with β-blockers. However, under certain circumstances, there may be no acceptable alternatives to the use of β-adrenergic blocking agents in patients with asthma. In this setting, cardioselective β-blockers could be considered, although they should be administered with caution). Products include:
Bystolic 1147

Nefazodone Hydrochloride (Due to the potential increased risk of cardiovascular adverse events, the concomitant use of salmeterol with strong CYP3A4 inhibitors (eg, ketoconazole, ritonavir, atazanavir, clarithromycin, indinavir, itraconazole, nefazodone, nelfinavir, saquinavir, telithromycin) is not recommended).
No products indexed under this heading.

Nelfinavir Mesylate (Due to the potential increased risk of cardiovascular adverse events, the concomitant use of salmeterol with strong CYP3A4 inhibitors (eg, ketoconazole, ritonavir, atazanavir, clarithromycin, indinavir, itraconazole, nefazodone, nelfinavir, saquinavir, telithromycin) is not recommended).
No products indexed under this heading.

Nevirapine (Both fluticasone propionate and salmeterol are substrates of CYP 3A4. There is a potential drug interaction with CYP 3A4 inhibitors). Products include:
Viramune Oral Suspension 897
Viramune Tablets 897

Niacin (Both fluticasone propionate and salmeterol are substrates of CYP 3A4. There is a potential drug interaction with CYP 3A4 inhibitors). Products include:
Advicor 402
Cardio Basics 3455
Niaspan 497
Simcor 524

Niacinamide (Both fluticasone propionate and salmeterol are substrates of CYP 3A4. There is a potential drug interaction with CYP 3A4 inhibitors). Products include:
CitraNatal 90 DHA Capsules 2332
CitraNatal Assure 2332
CitraNatal Rx 2332
Heplive 607

Niacinamide Hydroiodide (Both fluticasone propionate and salmeterol are substrates of CYP 3A4. There is a potential drug interaction with CYP 3A4 inhibitors).
No products indexed under this heading.

Nicotinamide (Both fluticasone propionate and salmeterol are substrates of CYP 3A4. There is a potential drug interaction with CYP 3A4 inhibitors).
No products indexed under this heading.

Nifedipine (Both fluticasone propionate and salmeterol are substrates of CYP 3A4. There is a potential drug interaction with CYP 3A4 inhibitors).
No products indexed under this heading.

Norfloxacin (Both fluticasone propionate and salmeterol are substrates of CYP 3A4. There is a potential drug interaction with CYP 3A4 inhibitors). Products include:
Noroxin 2220

Nortriptyline Hydrochloride (Advair HFA should be administered with extreme caution to patients being treated with tricyclic antidepressants, or within 2 weeks of discontinuation of such agents, because the action of salmeterol, a component of Advair HFA, on the vascular system may be potentiated by these agents).
No products indexed under this heading.

Omeprazole (Both fluticasone propionate and salmeterol are substrates of CYP 3A4. There is a potential drug interaction with CYP 3A4 inhibitors).
No products indexed under this heading.

Oxcarbazepine (Long-term use of orally inhaled corticosteroids may affect normal bone metabolism, resulting in a loss of bone mineral density. In patients with major risk factors for decreased bone mineral content, such as chronic use of drugs that can reduce bone mass (eg, anticonvulsants), Advair HFA may pose an additional risk).
No products indexed under this heading.

Paramethadione (Long-term use of orally inhaled corticosteroids may affect normal bone metabolism, resulting in a loss of bone mineral density. In patients with major risk factors for decreased bone mineral content, such as chronic use of drugs that can reduce bone mass (eg, anticonvulsants), Advair HFA may pose an additional risk).
No products indexed under this heading.

Pargyline Hydrochloride (Advair HFA should be administered with extreme caution to patients being treated with monoamine oxidase inhibitors, or within 2 weeks of discontinuation of such agents, because the action of salmeterol, a component of Advair HFA, on the vascular system may be potentiated by these agents).
No products indexed under this heading.

Paroxetine Hydrochloride (Both fluticasone propionate and salmeterol are substrates of CYP 3A4. There is a potential drug interaction with CYP 3A4 inhibitors). Products include:
Paroxetine CR 2361
Paroxetine ER 2371
Paxil 1586
Paxil CR 1596

Penbutolol Sulfate (β-blockers not only block the pulmonary effect of β-agonists, such as salmeterol, a component of Advair HFA, but may produce severe bronchospasm in patients with asthma. Therefore, patients with asthma should not normally be treated with β-blockers. However, under certain circumstances, there may be no acceptable alternatives to the use of β-adrenergic blocking agents in patients with asthma. In this setting, cardioselective β-blockers could be considered, although they should be administered with caution).
No products indexed under this heading.

Phenacemide (Long-term use of orally inhaled corticosteroids may affect normal bone metabolism, resulting in a loss of bone mineral density. In patients with major risk factors for decreased bone mineral content, such as chronic use of drugs that can reduce bone mass (eg, anticonvulsants), Advair HFA may pose an additional risk).
No products indexed under this heading.

IMPORTANT NOTE: Always consult each drug listing in the patient's regimen for possible interactions.

Phenelzine Sulfate (Advair HFA should be administered with extreme caution to patients being treated with monoamine oxidase inhibitors, or within 2 weeks of discontinuation of such agents, because the action of salmeterol, a component of Advair HFA, on the vascular system may be potentiated by these agents).
No products indexed under this heading.

Phenobarbital (Long-term use of orally inhaled corticosteroids may affect normal bone metabolism, resulting in a loss of bone mineral density. In patients with major risk factors for decreased bone mineral content, such as chronic use of drugs that can reduce bone mass (eg, anticonvulsants), Advair HFA may pose an additional risk). Products include:
Donnatal **2711**

Phenobarbital Sodium (Long-term use of orally inhaled corticosteroids may affect normal bone metabolism, resulting in a loss of bone mineral density. In patients with major risk factors for decreased bone mineral content, such as chronic use of drugs that can reduce bone mass (eg, anticonvulsants), Advair HFA may pose an additional risk).
No products indexed under this heading.

Phensuximide (Long-term use of orally inhaled corticosteroids may affect normal bone metabolism, resulting in a loss of bone mineral density. In patients with major risk factors for decreased bone mineral content, such as chronic use of drugs that can reduce bone mass (eg, anticonvulsants), Advair HFA may pose an additional risk).
No products indexed under this heading.

Phenytoin (Long-term use of orally inhaled corticosteroids may affect normal bone metabolism, resulting in a loss of bone mineral density. In patients with major risk factors for decreased bone mineral content, such as chronic use of drugs that can reduce bone mass (eg, anticonvulsants), Advair HFA may pose an additional risk).
No products indexed under this heading.

Phenytoin Sodium (Long-term use of orally inhaled corticosteroids may affect normal bone metabolism, resulting in a loss of bone mineral density. In patients with major risk factors for decreased bone mineral content, such as chronic use of drugs that can reduce bone mass (eg, anticonvulsants), Advair HFA may pose an additional risk). Products include:
Phenytek Capsules **2380**

Pindolol (β-blockers not only block the pulmonary effect of β-agonists, such as salmeterol, a component of Advair HFA, but may produce severe bronchospasm in patients with asthma. Therefore, patients with asthma should not normally be treated with β-blockers. However, under certain circumstances, there may be no acceptable alternatives to the use of β-adrenergic blocking agents in patients with asthma. In this setting, cardioselective β-blockers could be considered, although they should be administered with caution).
No products indexed under this heading.

Pirbuterol Acetate (Patients who are receiving Advair HFA twice daily should not use additional salmeterol or other long-acting β-agonists (eg, formoterol) for prevention of exercise-induced bronchospasm (EIB) or the maintenance treatment of asthma. Additional benefit would not be gained from using supplemental salmeterol or formoterol for prevention of EIB since Advair HFA already contains an inhaled, long-acting β_2-agonist). Products include:
Maxair Autohaler **1782**

Polythiazide (The ECG changes and/or hypokalemia that may result from the administration of nonpotassium-sparing diuretics (such as loop or thiazide diuretics) can be acutely worsened by β-agonists, especially when the recommended dose of the β-agonist is exceeded. Although the clinical significance of these effects is not known, caution is advised in the co-administration of β-agonists with nonpotassium-sparing diuretics).
No products indexed under this heading.

Posaconazole (Both fluticasone propionate and salmeterol are substrates of CYP 3A4. There is a potential drug interaction with CYP 3A4 inhibitors). Products include:
Noxafil **3172**

Prednisolone (Long-term use of orally inhaled corticosteroids may affect normal bone metabolism, resulting in a loss of bone mineral density. In patients with major risk factors for decreased bone mineral content, such as chronic use of drugs that can reduce bone mass (eg, corticosteroids), Advair HFA may pose an additional risk).
No products indexed under this heading.

Prednisolone Acetate (Long-term use of orally inhaled corticosteroids may affect normal bone metabolism, resulting in a loss of bone mineral density. In patients with major risk factors for decreased bone mineral content, such as chronic use of drugs that can reduce bone mass (eg, corticosteroids), Advair HFA may pose an additional risk). Products include:
Blephamide .... ⊙**212**, ⊙**214**
Pred Forte .... ⊙**225**
Pred Mild .... ⊙**230**
Pred-G .... ⊙**226**, ⊙**227**

Prednisolone Sodium Phosphate (Long-term use of orally inhaled corticosteroids may affect normal bone metabolism, resulting in a loss of bone mineral density. In patients with major risk factors for decreased bone mineral content, such as chronic use of drugs that can reduce bone mass (eg, corticosteroids), Advair HFA may pose an additional risk).
No products indexed under this heading.

Prednisolone Tebutate (Long-term use of orally inhaled corticosteroids may affect normal bone metabolism, resulting in a loss of bone mineral density. In patients with major risk factors for decreased bone mineral content, such as chronic use of drugs that can reduce bone mass (eg, corticosteroids), Advair HFA may pose an additional risk).
No products indexed under this heading.

Prednisone (Long-term use of orally inhaled corticosteroids may affect normal bone metabolism, resulting in a loss of bone mineral density. In patients with major risk factors for decreased bone mineral content, such as chronic use of drugs that can reduce bone mass (eg, corticosteroids), Advair HFA may pose an additional risk).
No products indexed under this heading.

Prednisone sodium phosphate (Long-term use of orally inhaled corticosteroids may affect normal bone metabolism, resulting in a loss of bone mineral density. In patients with major risk factors for decreased bone mineral content, such as chronic use of drugs that can reduce bone mass (eg, corticosteroids), Advair HFA may pose an additional risk).
No products indexed under this heading.

Primidone (Long-term use of orally inhaled corticosteroids may affect normal bone metabolism, resulting in a loss of bone mineral density. In patients with major risk factors for decreased bone mineral content, such as chronic use of drugs that can reduce bone mass (eg, anticonvulsants), Advair HFA may pose an additional risk).
No products indexed under this heading.

Procarbazine Hydrochloride (Advair HFA should be administered with extreme caution to patients being treated with monoamine oxidase inhibitors, or within 2 weeks of discontinuation of such agents, because the action of salmeterol, a component of Advair HFA, on the vascular system may be potentiated by these agents).
No products indexed under this heading.

Propoxyphene Hydrochloride (Both fluticasone propionate and salmeterol are substrates of CYP 3A4. There is a potential drug interaction with CYP 3A4 inhibitors).
No products indexed under this heading.

Propoxyphene Napsylate (Both fluticasone propionate and salmeterol are substrates of CYP 3A4. There is a potential drug interaction with CYP 3A4 inhibitors).
No products indexed under this heading.

Propranolol Hydrochloride (β-blockers not only block the pulmonary effect of β-agonists, such as salmeterol, a component of Advair HFA, but may produce severe bronchospasm in patients with asthma. Therefore, patients with asthma should not normally be treated with β-blockers. However, under certain circumstances, there may be no acceptable alternatives to the use of β-adrenergic blocking agents in patients with asthma. In this setting, cardioselective β-blockers could be considered, although they should be administered with caution). Products include:
InnoPran XL **1517**

Protriptyline Hydrochloride (Advair HFA should be administered with extreme caution to patients being treated with tricyclic antidepressants, or within 2 weeks of discontinuation of such agents, because the action of salmeterol, a component of Advair HFA, on the vascular system may be potentiated by these agents).
No products indexed under this heading.

Quinidine (Both fluticasone propionate and salmeterol are substrates of CYP 3A4. There is a potential drug interaction with CYP 3A4 inhibitors).
No products indexed under this heading.

Quinidine Hydrochloride (Both fluticasone propionate and salmeterol are substrates of CYP 3A4. There is a potential drug interaction with CYP 3A4 inhibitors).
No products indexed under this heading.

Quinidine Polygalacturonate (Both fluticasone propionate and salmeterol are substrates of CYP 3A4. There is a potential drug interaction with CYP 3A4 inhibitors).
No products indexed under this heading.

Quinidine Sulfate (Both fluticasone propionate and salmeterol are substrates of CYP 3A4. There is a potential drug interaction with CYP 3A4 inhibitors).
No products indexed under this heading.

Quinine (Both fluticasone propionate and salmeterol are substrates of CYP 3A4. There is a potential drug interaction with CYP 3A4 inhibitors). Products include:
Hyland's Leg Cramps PM with Quinine **3315**

Quinine Sulfate (Both fluticasone propionate and salmeterol are substrates of CYP 3A4. There is a potential drug interaction with CYP 3A4 inhibitors).
No products indexed under this heading.

Quinupristin (Both fluticasone propionate and salmeterol are substrates of CYP 3A4. There is a potential drug interaction with CYP 3A4 inhibitors).
No products indexed under this heading.

Ranitidine Bismuth Citrate (Both fluticasone propionate and salmeterol are substrates of CYP 3A4. There is a potential drug interaction with CYP 3A4 inhibitors).
No products indexed under this heading.

Ranitidine Hydrochloride (Both fluticasone propionate and salmeterol are substrates of CYP 3A4. There is a potential drug interaction with CYP 3A4 inhibitors). Products include:
Zantac **1737**
Zantac Injection **1732**
Zantac Pharmacy **1735**

Rasagiline Mesylate (Advair HFA should be administered with extreme caution to patients being treated with monoamine oxidase inhibitors, or within 2 weeks of discontinuation of such agents, because the action of salmeterol, a component of Advair HFA, on the vascular system may be potentiated by these agents). Products include:
Azilect **3383**

Ritonavir (Co-administration of fluticasone propionate and the strong cytochrome P450 3A4 inhibitor ritonavir is not recommended. A drug interaction study with fluticasone propionate aqueous nasal spray in healthy subjects has shown that ritonavir can significantly increase plasma fluticasone propionate exposure (AUC), resulting in significantly reduced serum cortisol concentrations. During post-marketing use, there have been reports of clinically significant drug interactions in patients receiving fluticasone propionate and ritonavir, resulting in systemic corticosteroid effects including Cushing's syndrome and adrenal suppression. Therefore, co-administration of fluticasone propionate and ritonavir is not recommended unless the potential benefit to the patient outweighs the risk of systemic corticosteroid side effects). Products include:
Kaletra **458**
Norvir **509**

Rufinamide (Long-term use of orally inhaled corticosteroids may affect normal bone metabolism, resulting in a loss of bone mineral density. In patients with major risk factors for decreased bone mineral content, such as chronic use of drugs that can reduce bone mass (eg, anticonvulsants), Advair HFA may pose an additional risk). Products include:
Banzel **1050**

Saquinavir (Due to the potential increased risk of cardiovascular adverse events, the concomitant use of salmeterol with strong CYP3A4 inhibitors (eg, ketoconazole, ritonavir, atazanavir, clarithromycin, indinavir, itraconazole, nefazodone, nelfinavir, saquinavir, telithromycin) is not recommended).
No products indexed under this heading.

Saquinavir Mesylate (Due to the potential increased risk of cardiovascular adverse events, the concomitant use of salmeterol with strong CYP3A4 inhibitors (eg, ketoconazole, ritonavir, atazanavir, clarithromycin, indinavir, itraconazole, nefazodone, nelfinavir, saquinavir, telithromycin) is not recommended).
No products indexed under this heading.

Selegiline (Advair HFA should be administered with extreme caution to patients being treated with monoamine oxidase inhibitors, or within 2 weeks of

discontinuation of such agents, because the action of salmeterol, a component of Advair HFA, on the vascular system may be potentiated by these agents). Products include:

Selegiline Hydrochloride (Advair HFA should be administered with extreme caution to patients being treated with monoamine oxidase inhibitors, or within 2 weeks of discontinuation of such agents, because the action of salmeterol, a component of Advair HFA, on the vascular system may be potentiated by these agents). Products include:

Sertraline Hydrochloride (Both fluticasone propionate and salmeterol are substrates of CYP 3A4. There is a potential drug interaction with CYP 3A4 inhibitors).
No products indexed under this heading.

Sildenafil Citrate (Both fluticasone propionate and salmeterol are substrates of CYP 3A4. There is a potential drug interaction with CYP 3A4 inhibitors).
No products indexed under this heading.

Sotalol Hydrochloride (β-blockers not only block the pulmonary effect of β-agonists, such as salmeterol, a component of Advair HFA, but may produce severe bronchospasm in patients with asthma. Therefore, patients with asthma should not normally be treated with β-blockers. However, under certain circumstances, there may be no acceptable alternatives to the use of β-adrenergic blocking agents in patients with asthma. In this setting, cardioselective β-blockers could be considered, although they should be administered with caution).
No products indexed under this heading.

Telithromycin (Due to the potential increased risk of cardiovascular adverse events, the concomitant use of salmeterol with strong CYP3A4 inhibitors (eg, ketoconazole, ritonavir, atazanavir, clarithromycin, indinavir, itraconazole, nefazodone, nelfinavir, saquinavir, telithromycin) is not recommended). Products include:

Terbutaline Sulfate (Patients who are receiving Advair HFA twice daily should not use additional salmeterol or other long-acting β-agonists (eg, formoterol) for prevention of exercise-induced bronchospasm (EIB) or the maintenance treatment of asthma. Additional benefit would not be gained from using supplemental salmeterol or formoterol for prevention of EIB since Advair HFA already contains an inhaled, long-acting β₂-agonist).
No products indexed under this heading.

Tiagabine Hydrochloride (Long-term use of orally inhaled corticosteroids may affect normal bone metabolism, resulting in a loss of bone mineral density. In patients with major risk factors for decreased bone mineral content, such as chronic use of drugs that can reduce bone mass (eg, anticonvulsants), Advair HFA may pose an additional risk). Products include:

Timolol Hemihydrate (β-blockers not only block the pulmonary effect of β-agonists, such as salmeterol, a component of Advair HFA, but may produce severe bronchospasm in patients with asthma. Therefore, patients with asthma should not normally be treated with β-blockers. However, under certain circumstances, there may be no acceptable alternatives to the use of β-adrenergic blocking agents in patients with asthma. In this setting, cardioselec-

tive β-blockers could be considered, although they should be administered with caution). Products include:

Timolol Maleate (β-blockers not only block the pulmonary effect of β-agonists, such as salmeterol, a component of Advair HFA, but may produce severe bronchospasm in patients with asthma. Therefore, patients with asthma should not normally be treated with β-blockers. However, under certain circumstances, there may be no acceptable alternatives to the use of β-adrenergic blocking agents in patients with asthma. In this setting, cardioselective β-blockers could be considered, although they should be administered with caution). Products include:

Tobacco (Long-term use of orally inhaled corticosteroids may affect normal bone metabolism, resulting in a loss of bone mineral density. In patients with major risk factors for decreased bone mineral content, such as tobacco use, Advair HFA may pose an additional risk).
No products indexed under this heading.

Topiramate (Long-term use of orally inhaled corticosteroids may affect normal bone metabolism, resulting in a loss of bone mineral density. In patients with major risk factors for decreased bone mineral content, such as chronic use of drugs that can reduce bone mass (eg, anticonvulsants), Advair HFA may pose an additional risk).
No products indexed under this heading.

Torsemide (The ECG changes and/or hypokalemia that may result from the administration of nonpotassium-sparing diuretics (such as loop or thiazide diuretics) can be acutely worsened by β-agonists, especially when the recommended dose of the β-agonist is exceeded. Although the clinical significance of these effects is not known, caution is advised in the co-administration of β-agonists with nonpotassium-sparing diuretics).
No products indexed under this heading.

Tranylcypromine Sulfate (Advair HFA should be administered with extreme caution to patients being treated with monoamine oxidase inhibitors, or within 2 weeks of discontinuation of such agents, because the action of salmeterol, a component of Advair HFA, on the vascular system may be potentiated by these agents). Products include:

Triamcinolone (Long-term use of orally inhaled corticosteroids may affect normal bone metabolism, resulting in a loss of bone mineral density. In patients with major risk factors for decreased bone mineral content, such as chronic use of drugs that can reduce bone mass (eg, corticosteroids), Advair HFA may pose an additional risk).
No products indexed under this heading.

Triamcinolone Acetonide (Long-term use of orally inhaled corticosteroids may affect normal bone metabolism, resulting in a loss of bone mineral density. In patients with major risk factors for decreased bone mineral content, such as chronic use of drugs that can reduce bone mass (eg, corticosteroids), Advair HFA may pose an additional risk). Products include:

Triamcinolone Diacetate (Long-term use of orally inhaled corticosteroids may affect normal bone metabolism, resulting in a loss of bone mineral density. In patients with major risk factors for decreased bone mineral content, such as chronic use of drugs that can reduce bone mass (eg, corticosteroids), Advair HFA may pose an additional risk).
No products indexed under this heading.

Triamcinolone Hexacetonide (Long-term use of orally inhaled corticosteroids may affect normal bone metabolism, resulting in a loss of bone mineral density. In patients with major risk factors for decreased bone mineral content, such as chronic use of drugs that can reduce bone mass (eg, corticosteroids), Advair HFA may pose an additional risk).
No products indexed under this heading.

Trimethadione (Long-term use of orally inhaled corticosteroids may affect normal bone metabolism, resulting in a loss of bone mineral density. In patients with major risk factors for decreased bone mineral content, such as chronic use of drugs that can reduce bone mass (eg, anticonvulsants), Advair HFA may pose an additional risk).
No products indexed under this heading.

Trimipramine Maleate (Advair HFA should be administered with extreme caution to patients being treated with tricyclic antidepressants, or within 2 weeks of discontinuation of such agents, because the action of salmeterol, a component of Advair HFA, on the vascular system may be potentiated by these agents).
No products indexed under this heading.

Troglitazone (Both fluticasone propionate and salmeterol are substrates of CYP 3A4. There is a potential drug interaction with CYP 3A4 inhibitors).
No products indexed under this heading.

Troleandomycin (Due to the potential increased risk of cardiovascular adverse events, the concomitant use of salmeterol with strong CYP3A4 inhibitors (eg, ketoconazole, ritonavir, atazanavir, clarithromycin, indinavir, itraconazole, nefazodone, nelfinavir, saquinavir, telithromycin) is not recommended).
No products indexed under this heading.

Valproate Sodium (Long-term use of orally inhaled corticosteroids may affect normal bone metabolism, resulting in a loss of bone mineral density. In patients with major risk factors for decreased bone mineral content, such as chronic use of drugs that can reduce bone mass (eg, anticonvulsants), Advair HFA may pose an additional risk).
No products indexed under this heading.

Valproic Acid (Long-term use of orally inhaled corticosteroids may affect normal bone metabolism, resulting in a loss of bone mineral density. In patients with major risk factors for decreased bone mineral content, such as chronic use of drugs that can reduce bone mass (eg, anticonvulsants), Advair HFA may pose an additional risk).
No products indexed under this heading.

Vardenafil Hydrochloride (Both fluticasone propionate and salmeterol are substrates of CYP 3A4. There is a potential drug interaction with CYP 3A4 inhibitors). Products include:

Verapamil Hydrochloride (Both fluticasone propionate and salmeterol are substrates of CYP 3A4. There is a potential drug interaction with CYP 3A4 inhibitors). Products include:

Voriconazole (Due to the potential increased risk of cardiovascular adverse events, the concomitant use of salmeterol with strong CYP3A4 inhibitors (eg, ketoconazole, ritonavir, atazanavir, clarithromycin, indinavir, itraconazole, nefazodone, nelfinavir, saquinavir, telithromycin) is not recommended).
No products indexed under this heading.

Zafirlukast (Both fluticasone propionate and salmeterol are substrates of CYP 3A4. There is a potential drug interaction with CYP 3A4 inhibitors). Products include:

Zileuton (Both fluticasone propionate and salmeterol are substrates of CYP 3A4. There is a potential drug interaction with CYP 3A4 inhibitors).
No products indexed under this heading.

Zonisamide (Long-term use of orally inhaled corticosteroids may affect normal bone metabolism, resulting in a loss of bone mineral density. In patients with major risk factors for decreased bone mineral content, such as chronic use of drugs that can reduce bone mass (eg, anticonvulsants), Advair HFA may pose an additional risk). Products include:

Food Interactions

Grapefruit (Both fluticasone propionate and salmeterol are substrates of CYP 3A4. There is a potential drug interaction with CYP 3A4 inhibitors).

Grapefruit Juice (Both fluticasone propionate and salmeterol are substrates of CYP 3A4. There is a potential drug interaction with CYP 3A4 inhibitors).

ADVAIR HFA 115/21 INHALATION AEROSOL
See Advair HFA 45/21 Inhalation Aerosol

ADVAIR HFA 230/21 INHALATION AEROSOL
See Advair HFA 45/21 Inhalation Aerosol

ADVATE
None cited in PDR database.

ADVICOR TABLETS
May interact with alcohols, azole antifungals, beta-blockers, calcium channel blockers, cytochrome p450 3a4 inhibitors (selected), erythromycin, fibrates, nitrates and nitrites, oral anticoagulants, protease inhibitors, and certain other agents. Compounds in these categories include:

Acebutolol Hydrochloride (Co-administration of niacin with vasoactive drugs, such as adrenergic blocking agents, may result in postural hypotension, particularly in patients with unstable angina or acute phase of myocardial infarction).
No products indexed under this heading.

Acetazolamide (The risk of myopathy appears to be increased by high levels of HMG-CoA reductase inhibitory activity in plasma. Lovastatin is metabolized by the cytochrome P450 isoform 3A4. Certain drugs which share this metabolic pathway can raise the plasma levels of lovastatin and may increase the risk of myopathy).
No products indexed under this heading.

IMPORTANT NOTE: Always consult each drug listing in the patient's regimen for possible interactions.

Advicor Interactions Index 68

Acetazolamide Sodium (The risk of myopathy appears to be increased by high levels of HMG-CoA reductase inhibitory activity in plasma. Lovastatin is metabolized by the cytochrome P450 isoform 3A4. Certain drugs which share this metabolic pathway can raise the plasma levels of lovastatin and may increase the risk of myopathy).
No products indexed under this heading.

Amiodarone Hydrochloride (The risk of myopathy appears to be increased by high levels of HMG-CoA reductase inhibitory activity in plasma. Lovastatin is metabolized by the cytochrome P450 isoform 3A4. Certain drugs which share this metabolic pathway can raise the plasma levels of lovastatin and may increase the risk of myopathy).
No products indexed under this heading.

Amlodipine Besylate (Co-administration of niacin with vasoactive drugs, such as calcium channel blockers, may result in postural hypotension, particularly in patients with unstable angina or acute phase of myocardial infarction). Products include:
Azor 1010
Exforge 2443
Exforge HCT 2449

Amprenavir (Co-administration results in serious skeletal muscle disorders, such as rhabdomyolysis and myopathy).
No products indexed under this heading.

Amyl Nitrite (Co-administration of niacin with vasoactive drugs, such as nitrates, may result in postural hypotension, particularly in patients with unstable angina or acute phase of myocardial infarction).
No products indexed under this heading.

Anastrozole (The risk of myopathy appears to be increased by high levels of HMG-CoA reductase inhibitory activity in plasma. Lovastatin is metabolized by the cytochrome P450 isoform 3A4. Certain drugs which share this metabolic pathway can raise the plasma levels of lovastatin and may increase the risk of myopathy).
No products indexed under this heading.

Anisindione (Co-administration has resulted in increased bleeding and/or prothrombin time).
No products indexed under this heading.

Aprepitant (The risk of myopathy appears to be increased by high levels of HMG-CoA reductase inhibitory activity in plasma. Lovastatin is metabolized by the cytochrome P450 isoform 3A4. Certain drugs which share this metabolic pathway can raise the plasma levels of lovastatin and may increase the risk of myopathy). Products include:
Emend 2124

Aspirin (May decrease the metabolic clearance of niacin; the clinical relevance of this finding is unclear). Products include:
Aggrenox 880
Bayer Aspirin 829
Percodan 1124
St. Joseph Aspirin 2045

Atazanavir (Co-administration results in serious skeletal muscle disorders, such as rhabdomyolysis and myopathy).
No products indexed under this heading.

Atazanavir Sulfate (Co-administration results in serious skeletal muscle disorders, such as rhabdomyolysis and myopathy).
No products indexed under this heading.

Atenolol (Co-administration of niacin with vasoactive drugs, such as adrenergic blocking agents, may result in postural hypotension, particularly in patients with unstable angina or acute phase of myocardial infarction).
No products indexed under this heading.

Bepridil Hydrochloride (Co-administration of niacin with vasoactive drugs, such as calcium channel blockers, may result in postural hypotension, particularly in patients with unstable angina or acute phase of myocardial infarction).
No products indexed under this heading.

Betaxolol Hydrochloride (Co-administration of niacin with vasoactive drugs, such as adrenergic blocking agents, may result in postural hypotension, particularly in patients with unstable angina or acute phase of myocardial infarction).
No products indexed under this heading.

Bisoprolol Fumarate (Co-administration of niacin with vasoactive drugs, such as adrenergic blocking agents, may result in postural hypotension, particularly in patients with unstable angina or acute phase of myocardial infarction).
No products indexed under this heading.

Butoconazole Nitrate (Co-administration results in serious skeletal muscle disorders, such as rhabdomyolysis and myopathy).
No products indexed under this heading.

Carteolol Hydrochloride (Co-administration of niacin with vasoactive drugs, such as adrenergic blocking agents, may result in postural hypotension, particularly in patients with unstable angina or acute phase of myocardial infarction).
No products indexed under this heading.

Carvedilol (Co-administration of niacin with vasoactive drugs, such as adrenergic blocking agents, may result in postural hypotension, particularly in patients with unstable angina or acute phase of myocardial infarction). Products include:
Coreg 1409

Carvedilol Phosphate (Co-administration of niacin with vasoactive drugs, such as adrenergic blocking agents, may result in postural hypotension, particularly in patients with unstable angina or acute phase of myocardial infarction). Products include:
Coreg CR 1416

Cholestyramine (In-vitro study resulted in approximately 10% to 30% of available niacin bound to cholestyramine; 4 to 6 hours should elapse between ingestion of bile acid-binding resins and the administration of Advicor).
No products indexed under this heading.

Cimetidine (The risk of myopathy appears to be increased by high levels of HMG-CoA reductase inhibitory activity in plasma. Lovastatin is metabolized by the cytochrome P450 isoform 3A4. Certain drugs which share this metabolic pathway can raise the plasma levels of lovastatin and may increase the risk of myopathy).
No products indexed under this heading.

Cimetidine Hydrochloride (The risk of myopathy appears to be increased by high levels of HMG-CoA reductase inhibitory activity in plasma. Lovastatin is metabolized by the cytochrome P450 isoform 3A4. Certain drugs which share this metabolic pathway can raise the plasma levels of lovastatin and may increase the risk of myopathy).
No products indexed under this heading.

Ciprofloxacin (The risk of myopathy appears to be increased by high levels of HMG-CoA reductase inhibitory activity in plasma. Lovastatin is metabolized by the cytochrome P450 isoform 3A4. Certain drugs which share this metabolic pathway can raise the plasma levels of lovastatin and may increase the risk of myopathy). Products include:
Cipro I.V. 3082
Cipro 3073
Cipro XR 3091
Ciprodex 583

Clarithromycin (Co-administration results in serious skeletal muscle disorders, such as rhabdomyolysis and myopathy). Products include:
Biaxin/Biaxin XL 412

Clofibrate (The incidence and severity of myopathy are increased by co-administration of Advicor with drugs that cause myopathy when given alone, such as fibrates; combined use should be avoided).
No products indexed under this heading.

Clotrimazole (Co-administration results in serious skeletal muscle disorders, such as rhabdomyolysis and myopathy). Products include:
Lotrisone 3163

Colestipol Hydrochloride (In-vitro study resulted in approximately 90% of available niacin bound to colestipol; 4 to 6 hours should elapse between ingestion of bile acid-binding resins and the administration of Advicor).
No products indexed under this heading.

Conivaptan Hydrochloride (The risk of myopathy appears to be increased by high levels of HMG-CoA reductase inhibitory activity in plasma. Lovastatin is metabolized by the cytochrome P450 isoform 3A4. Certain drugs which share this metabolic pathway can raise the plasma levels of lovastatin and may increase the risk of myopathy). Products include:
Vaprisol 689

Cyclosporine (Co-administration results in serious skeletal muscle disorders, such as rhabdomyolysis and myopathy. Cyclosporine has been shown to increase the AUC of HMG-CoA reductase inhibitors). Products include:
Gengraf 440
Neoral Oral Solution 2496
Neoral Capsules 2496
Restasis 605

Dalfopristin (The risk of myopathy appears to be increased by high levels of HMG-CoA reductase inhibitory activity in plasma. Lovastatin is metabolized by the cytochrome P450 isoform 3A4. Certain drugs which share this metabolic pathway can raise the plasma levels of lovastatin and may increase the risk of myopathy).
No products indexed under this heading.

Danazol (Co-administration results in serious skeletal muscle disorders, such as rhabdomyolysis and myopathy).
No products indexed under this heading.

Darunavir (Co-administration results in serious skeletal muscle disorders, such as rhabdomyolysis and myopathy).
No products indexed under this heading.

Dasatinib (The risk of myopathy appears to be increased by high levels of HMG-CoA reductase inhibitory activity in plasma. Lovastatin is metabolized by the cytochrome P450 isoform 3A4. Certain drugs which share this metabolic pathway can raise the plasma levels of lovastatin and may increase the risk of myopathy).
No products indexed under this heading.

Delavirdine Mesylate (The risk of myopathy appears to be increased by high levels of HMG-CoA reductase inhibitory activity in plasma. Lovastatin is metabolized by the cytochrome P450 isoform 3A4. Certain drugs which share this metabolic pathway can raise the plasma levels of lovastatin and may increase the risk of myopathy).
No products indexed under this heading.

Delavirine (The risk of myopathy appears to be increased by high levels of HMG-CoA reductase inhibitory activity in plasma. Lovastatin is metabolized by the cytochrome P450 isoform 3A4. Certain drugs which share this metabolic pathway can raise the plasma levels of lovastatin and may increase the risk of myopathy).
No products indexed under this heading.

Desloratadine (The risk of myopathy appears to be increased by high levels of HMG-CoA reductase inhibitory activity in plasma. Lovastatin is metabolized by the cytochrome P450 isoform 3A4. Certain drugs which share this metabolic pathway can raise the plasma levels of lovastatin and may increase the risk of myopathy). Products include:
Clarinex Syrup 3098
Clarinex 3098
Clarinex Reditabs 3098
Clarinex-D 12-Hour 3101
Clarinex-D 3104

Dicumarol (Co-administration has resulted in increased bleeding and/or prothrombin time).
No products indexed under this heading.

Diltiazem Hydrochloride (Co-administration of niacin with vasoactive drugs, such as calcium channel blockers, may result in postural hypotension, particularly in patients with unstable angina or acute phase of myocardial infarction). Products include:
Cardizem LA 423

Diltiazem Maleate (The risk of myopathy appears to be increased by high levels of HMG-CoA reductase inhibitory activity in plasma. Lovastatin is metabolized by the cytochrome P450 isoform 3A4. Certain drugs which share this metabolic pathway can raise the plasma levels of lovastatin and may increase the risk of myopathy).
No products indexed under this heading.

Econazole Nitrate (Co-administration results in serious skeletal muscle disorders, such as rhabdomyolysis and myopathy).
No products indexed under this heading.

Efavirenz (The risk of myopathy appears to be increased by high levels of HMG-CoA reductase inhibitory activity in plasma. Lovastatin is metabolized by the cytochrome P450 isoform 3A4. Certain drugs which share this metabolic pathway can raise the plasma levels of lovastatin and may increase the risk of myopathy). Products include:
Atripla 906

Erythrityl Tetranitrate (Co-administration of niacin with vasoactive drugs, such as nitrates, may result in postural hypotension, particularly in patients with unstable angina or acute phase of myocardial infarction).
No products indexed under this heading.

Erythromycin (Co-administration results in serious skeletal muscle disorders, such as rhabdomyolysis and myopathy).
No products indexed under this heading.

Erythromycin, Topical (Co-administration results in serious skeletal muscle disorders, such as rhabdomyolysis and myopathy).
No products indexed under this heading.

Erythromycin Estolate (Co-administration results in serious skeletal muscle disorders, such as rhabdomyolysis and myopathy).
No products indexed under this heading.

Erythromycin Ethylsuccinate (Co-administration results in serious skeletal muscle disorders, such as rhabdomyolysis and myopathy). Products include:
E.E.S. 437
EryPed 435

(⊙ Described in PDR® for Ophthalmic Medicines)

69 Interactions Index Advicor

Erythromycin Gluceptate (Co-administration results in serious skeletal muscle disorders, such as rhabdomyolysis and myopathy).
No products indexed under this heading.

Erythromycin Lactobionate (Co-administration results in serious skeletal muscle disorders, such as rhabdomyolysis and myopathy).
No products indexed under this heading.

Erythromycin Stearate (Co-administration results in serious skeletal muscle disorders, such as rhabdomyolysis and myopathy).
No products indexed under this heading.

Esmolol Hydrochloride (Co-administration of niacin with vasoactive drugs, such as adrenergic blocking agents, may result in postural hypotension, particularly in patients with unstable angina or acute phase of myocardial infarction).
No products indexed under this heading.

Esomeprazole Magnesium (The risk of myopathy appears to be increased by high levels of HMG-CoA reductase inhibitory activity in plasma. Lovastatin is metabolized by the cytochrome P450 isoform 3A4. Certain drugs which share this metabolic pathway can raise the plasma levels of lovastatin and may increase the risk of myopathy). Products include:
Nexium Capsules 704
Nexium Oral Suspension 704

Esomeprazole Sodium (The risk of myopathy appears to be increased by high levels of HMG-CoA reductase inhibitory activity in plasma. Lovastatin is metabolized by the cytochrome P450 isoform 3A4. Certain drugs which share this metabolic pathway can raise the plasma levels of lovastatin and may increase the risk of myopathy). Products include:
Nexium I.V. 712

Ethanol (Concomitant alcohol may increase the flushing and its use should be avoided around the time of Advicor administration).
No products indexed under this heading.

Ethyl Alcohol (Concomitant alcohol may increase the flushing and its use should be avoided around the time of Advicor administration).
No products indexed under this heading.

Felodipine (Co-administration of niacin with vasoactive drugs, such as calcium channel blockers, may result in postural hypotension, particularly in patients with unstable angina or acute phase of myocardial infarction).
No products indexed under this heading.

Fenofibrate (The incidence and severity of myopathy are increased by co-administration of Advicor with drugs that cause myopathy when given alone, such as fibrates; combined use should be avoided). Products include:
Fenoglide 3263
Tricor 544
Trilipix 548

Fluconazole (Co-administration results in serious skeletal muscle disorders, such as rhabdomyolysis and myopathy).
No products indexed under this heading.

Fluoxetine (The risk of myopathy appears to be increased by high levels of HMG-CoA reductase inhibitory activity in plasma. Lovastatin is metabolized by the cytochrome P450 isoform 3A4. Certain drugs which share this metabolic pathway can raise the plasma levels of lovastatin and may increase the risk of myopathy).
No products indexed under this heading.

Fluoxetine Hydrochloride (The risk of myopathy appears to be increased by high levels of HMG-CoA reductase inhibitory activity in plasma. Lovastatin is metabolized by the cytochrome P450 isoform 3A4. Certain drugs which share this metabolic pathway can raise the plasma levels of lovastatin and may increase the risk of myopathy). Products include:
Prozac Weekly 1941
Prozac Pulvules 1941
Symbyax 1965

Fluvoxamine Maleate (The risk of myopathy appears to be increased by high levels of HMG-CoA reductase inhibitory activity in plasma. Lovastatin is metabolized by the cytochrome P450 isoform 3A4. Certain drugs which share this metabolic pathway can raise the plasma levels of lovastatin and may increase the risk of myopathy).
No products indexed under this heading.

Fosamprenavir Calcium (Co-administration results in serious skeletal muscle disorders, such as rhabdomyolysis and myopathy). Products include:
Lexiva Oral Suspension 1558
Lexiva 1558

Gemfibrozil (The incidence and severity of myopathy are increased by co-administration of Advicor with drugs that cause myopathy when given alone, such as fibrates; combined use should be avoided).
No products indexed under this heading.

Glyceryl Trinitrate (Co-administration of niacin with vasoactive drugs, such as nitrates, may result in postural hypotension, particularly in patients with unstable angina or acute phase of myocardial infarction).
No products indexed under this heading.

Imatinib Mesylate (The risk of myopathy appears to be increased by high levels of HMG-CoA reductase inhibitory activity in plasma. Lovastatin is metabolized by the cytochrome P450 isoform 3A4. Certain drugs which share this metabolic pathway can raise the plasma levels of lovastatin and may increase the risk of myopathy). Products include:
Gleevec 2477

Indinavir Sulfate (Co-administration results in serious skeletal muscle disorders, such as rhabdomyolysis and myopathy). Products include:
Crixivan 2113

Isoniazid (The risk of myopathy appears to be increased by high levels of HMG-CoA reductase inhibitory activity in plasma. Lovastatin is metabolized by the cytochrome P450 isoform 3A4. Certain drugs which share this metabolic pathway can raise the plasma levels of lovastatin and may increase the risk of myopathy).
No products indexed under this heading.

Isosorbide Dinitrate (Co-administration of niacin with vasoactive drugs, such as nitrates, may result in postural hypotension, particularly in patients with unstable angina or acute phase of myocardial infarction).
No products indexed under this heading.

Isosorbide Mononitrate (Co-administration of niacin with vasoactive drugs, such as nitrates, may result in postural hypotension, particularly in patients with unstable angina or acute phase of myocardial infarction).
No products indexed under this heading.

Isradipine (Co-administration of niacin with vasoactive drugs, such as calcium channel blockers, may result in postural hypotension, particularly in patients with unstable angina or acute phase of myocardial infarction). Products include:
DynaCirc CR 1432

Itraconazole (Co-administration results in serious skeletal muscle disorders, such as rhabdomyolysis and myopathy).
No products indexed under this heading.

Ketoconazole (Co-administration results in serious skeletal muscle disorders, such as rhabdomyolysis and myopathy). Products include:
Extina 3319
Xolegel 3337

Labetalol Hydrochloride (Co-administration of niacin with vasoactive drugs, such as adrenergic blocking agents, may result in postural hypotension, particularly in patients with unstable angina or acute phase of myocardial infarction).
No products indexed under this heading.

Lapatinib (The risk of myopathy appears to be increased by high levels of HMG-CoA reductase inhibitory activity in plasma. Lovastatin is metabolized by the cytochrome P450 isoform 3A4. Certain drugs which share this metabolic pathway can raise the plasma levels of lovastatin and may increase the risk of myopathy). Products include:
Tykerb 1698

Levobunolol Hydrochloride (Co-administration of niacin with vasoactive drugs, such as adrenergic blocking agents, may result in postural hypotension, particularly in patients with unstable angina or acute phase of myocardial infarction).
No products indexed under this heading.

Lopinavir (Co-administration results in serious skeletal muscle disorders, such as rhabdomyolysis and myopathy). Products include:
Kaletra 458

Loratadine (The risk of myopathy appears to be increased by high levels of HMG-CoA reductase inhibitory activity in plasma. Lovastatin is metabolized by the cytochrome P450 isoform 3A4. Certain drugs which share this metabolic pathway can raise the plasma levels of lovastatin and may increase the risk of myopathy).
No products indexed under this heading.

Metipranolol Hydrochloride (Co-administration of niacin with vasoactive drugs, such as adrenergic blocking agents, may result in postural hypotension, particularly in patients with unstable angina or acute phase of myocardial infarction).
No products indexed under this heading.

Metoprolol Succinate (Co-administration of niacin with vasoactive drugs, such as adrenergic blocking agents, may result in postural hypotension, particularly in patients with unstable angina or acute phase of myocardial infarction). Products include:
Toprol XL 732

Metoprolol Tartrate (Co-administration of niacin with vasoactive drugs, such as adrenergic blocking agents, may result in postural hypotension, particularly in patients with unstable angina or acute phase of myocardial infarction).
No products indexed under this heading.

Metronidazole (The risk of myopathy appears to be increased by high levels of HMG-CoA reductase inhibitory activity in plasma. Lovastatin is metabolized by the cytochrome P450 isoform 3A4. Certain drugs which share this metabolic pathway can raise the plasma levels of lovastatin and may increase the risk of myopathy). Products include:
Pylera 793

Metronidazole Benzoate (The risk of myopathy appears to be increased by high levels of HMG-CoA reductase inhibitory activity in plasma. Lovastatin is metabolized by the cytochrome P450 isoform 3A4. Certain drugs which share this metabolic pathway can raise the plasma levels of lovastatin and may increase the risk of myopathy).
No products indexed under this heading.

Metronidazole Hydrochloride (The risk of myopathy appears to be increased by high levels of HMG-CoA reductase inhibitory activity in plasma. Lovastatin is metabolized by the cytochrome P450 isoform 3A4. Certain drugs which share this metabolic pathway can raise the plasma levels of lovastatin and may increase the risk of myopathy).
No products indexed under this heading.

Metronidazole Sodium (The risk of myopathy appears to be increased by high levels of HMG-CoA reductase inhibitory activity in plasma. Lovastatin is metabolized by the cytochrome P450 isoform 3A4. Certain drugs which share this metabolic pathway can raise the plasma levels of lovastatin and may increase the risk of myopathy).
No products indexed under this heading.

Mibefradil Dihydrochloride (Co-administration of niacin with vasoactive drugs, such as calcium channel blockers, may result in postural hypotension, particularly in patients with unstable angina or acute phase of myocardial infarction).
No products indexed under this heading.

Miconazole (Co-administration results in serious skeletal muscle disorders, such as rhabdomyolysis and myopathy).
No products indexed under this heading.

Miconazole Nitrate (The risk of myopathy appears to be increased by high levels of HMG-CoA reductase inhibitory activity in plasma. Lovastatin is metabolized by the cytochrome P450 isoform 3A4. Certain drugs which share this metabolic pathway can raise the plasma levels of lovastatin and may increase the risk of myopathy). Products include:
Vusion Ointment 3335

Mifepristone (The risk of myopathy appears to be increased by high levels of HMG-CoA reductase inhibitory activity in plasma. Lovastatin is metabolized by the cytochrome P450 isoform 3A4. Certain drugs which share this metabolic pathway can raise the plasma levels of lovastatin and may increase the risk of myopathy).
No products indexed under this heading.

Nadolol (Co-administration of niacin with vasoactive drugs, such as adrenergic blocking agents, may result in postural hypotension, particularly in patients with unstable angina or acute phase of myocardial infarction). Products include:
Nadolol 2359

Nebivolol (Co-administration of niacin with vasoactive drugs, such as adrenergic blocking agents, may result in postural hypotension, particularly in patients with unstable angina or acute phase of myocardial infarction). Products include:
Bystolic 1147

Nefazodone Hydrochloride (Co-administration results in serious skeletal muscle disorders, such as rhabdomyolysis and myopathy).
No products indexed under this heading.

Nelfinavir Mesylate (Co-administration results in serious skeletal muscle disorders, such as rhabdomyolysis and myopathy).
No products indexed under this heading.

Nevirapine (The risk of myopathy appears to be increased by high levels of HMG-CoA reductase inhibitory activity in plasma. Lovastatin is metabolized by the cytochrome P450 isoform 3A4. Certain drugs which share this metabolic pathway can raise the plasma levels of lovastatin and may increase the risk of myopathy). Products include:
Viramune Oral Suspension 897
Viramune Tablets 897

IMPORTANT NOTE: Always consult each drug listing in the patient's regimen for possible interactions.

Advicor **Interactions Index** **70**

Niacinamide (The risk of myopathy appears to be increased by high levels of HMG-CoA reductase inhibitory activity in plasma. Lovastatin is metabolized by the cytochrome P450 isoform 3A4. Certain drugs which share this metabolic pathway can raise the plasma levels of lovastatin and may increase the risk of myopathy). Products include:
CitraNatal 90 DHA Capsules **2332**
CitraNatal Assure **2332**
CitraNatal Rx **2332**
Heplive **607**

Niacinamide Hydroiodide (The risk of myopathy appears to be increased by high levels of HMG-CoA reductase inhibitory activity in plasma. Lovastatin is metabolized by the cytochrome P450 isoform 3A4. Certain drugs which share this metabolic pathway can raise the plasma levels of lovastatin and may increase the risk of myopathy).
No products indexed under this heading.

Nicardipine (Co-administration of niacin with vasoactive drugs, such as calcium channel blockers, may result in postural hypotension, particularly in patients with unstable angina or acute phase of myocardial infarction).
No products indexed under this heading.

Nicardipine Hydrochloride (Co-administration of niacin with vasoactive drugs, such as calcium channel blockers, may result in postural hypotension, particularly in patients with unstable angina or acute phase of myocardial infarction).
No products indexed under this heading.

Nicotinamide (May potentiate the adverse effects of Advicor).
No products indexed under this heading.

Nifedipine (Co-administration of niacin with vasoactive drugs, such as calcium channel blockers, may result in postural hypotension, particularly in patients with unstable angina or acute phase of myocardial infarction).
No products indexed under this heading.

Nimodipine (Co-administration of niacin with vasoactive drugs, such as calcium channel blockers, may result in postural hypotension, particularly in patients with unstable angina or acute phase of myocardial infarction).
No products indexed under this heading.

Nisoldipine (Co-administration of niacin with vasoactive drugs, such as calcium channel blockers, may result in postural hypotension, particularly in patients with unstable angina or acute phase of myocardial infarction).
No products indexed under this heading.

Nitrate & Nitrite Preparations (Co-administration of niacin with vasoactive drugs, such as nitrates, may result in postural hypotension, particularly in patients with unstable angina or acute phase of myocardial infarction).
No products indexed under this heading.

Nitrates, organic (Co-administration of niacin with vasoactive drugs, such as nitrates, may result in postural hypotension, particularly in patients with unstable angina or acute phase of myocardial infarction).
No products indexed under this heading.

Nitrates and Nitrites (Co-administration of niacin with vasoactive drugs, such as nitrates, may result in postural hypotension, particularly in patients with unstable angina or acute phase of myocardial infarction).
No products indexed under this heading.

Nitroglycerin (Co-administration of niacin with vasoactive drugs, such as nitrates, may result in postural hypotension, particularly in patients with unstable angina or acute phase of myocardial infarction). Products include:
Nitro-Dur **3170**
Nitrolingual **3266**

Nitroglycerin, long-acting formulations (Co-administration of niacin with vasoactive drugs, such as nitrates, may result in postural hypotension, particularly in patients with unstable angina or acute phase of myocardial infarction).
No products indexed under this heading.

Nitroglycerin Intravenous (Co-administration of niacin with vasoactive drugs, such as nitrates, may result in postural hypotension, particularly in patients with unstable angina or acute phase of myocardial infarction).
No products indexed under this heading.

Norfloxacin (The risk of myopathy appears to be increased by high levels of HMG-CoA reductase inhibitory activity in plasma. Lovastatin is metabolized by the cytochrome P450 isoform 3A4. Certain drugs which share this metabolic pathway can raise the plasma levels of lovastatin and may increase the risk of myopathy). Products include:
Noroxin **2220**

Omeprazole (The risk of myopathy appears to be increased by high levels of HMG-CoA reductase inhibitory activity in plasma. Lovastatin is metabolized by the cytochrome P450 isoform 3A4. Certain drugs which share this metabolic pathway can raise the plasma levels of lovastatin and may increase the risk of myopathy).
No products indexed under this heading.

Oxiconazole Nitrate (Co-administration results in serious skeletal muscle disorders, such as rhabdomyolysis and myopathy).
No products indexed under this heading.

Paroxetine Hydrochloride (The risk of myopathy appears to be increased by high levels of HMG-CoA reductase inhibitory activity in plasma. Lovastatin is metabolized by the cytochrome P450 isoform 3A4. Certain drugs which share this metabolic pathway can raise the plasma levels of lovastatin and may increase the risk of myopathy).
Products include:
Paroxetine CR **2361**
Paroxetine ER **2371**
Paxil **1586**
Paxil CR **1596**

Penbutolol Sulfate (Co-administration of niacin with vasoactive drugs, such as adrenergic blocking agents, may result in postural hypotension, particularly in patients with unstable angina or acute phase of myocardial infarction).
No products indexed under this heading.

Pentaerythritol Tetranitrate (Co-administration of niacin with vasoactive drugs, such as nitrates, may result in postural hypotension, particularly in patients with unstable angina or acute phase of myocardial infarction).
No products indexed under this heading.

Pindolol (Co-administration of niacin with vasoactive drugs, such as adrenergic blocking agents, may result in postural hypotension, particularly in patients with unstable angina or acute phase of myocardial infarction).
No products indexed under this heading.

Posaconazole (Co-administration results in serious skeletal muscle disorders, such as rhabdomyolysis and myopathy). Products include:
Noxafil **3172**

Propoxyphene Hydrochloride (The risk of myopathy appears to be increased by high levels of HMG-CoA reductase inhibitory activity in plasma. Lovastatin is metabolized by the cytochrome P450 isoform 3A4. Certain drugs which share this metabolic pathway can raise the plasma levels of lovastatin and may increase the risk of myopathy).
No products indexed under this heading.

Propoxyphene Napsylate (The risk of myopathy appears to be increased by high levels of HMG-CoA reductase inhibitory activity in plasma. Lovastatin is metabolized by the cytochrome P450 isoform 3A4. Certain drugs which share this metabolic pathway can raise the plasma levels of lovastatin and may increase the risk of myopathy).
No products indexed under this heading.

Propranolol Hydrochloride (Co-administration of niacin with vasoactive drugs, such as adrenergic blocking agents, may result in postural hypotension, particularly in patients with unstable angina or acute phase of myocardial infarction). Products include:
InnoPran XL **1517**

Quinidine (The risk of myopathy appears to be increased by high levels of HMG-CoA reductase inhibitory activity in plasma. Lovastatin is metabolized by the cytochrome P450 isoform 3A4. Certain drugs which share this metabolic pathway can raise the plasma levels of lovastatin and may increase the risk of myopathy).
No products indexed under this heading.

Quinidine Hydrochloride (The risk of myopathy appears to be increased by high levels of HMG-CoA reductase inhibitory activity in plasma. Lovastatin is metabolized by the cytochrome P450 isoform 3A4. Certain drugs which share this metabolic pathway can raise the plasma levels of lovastatin and may increase the risk of myopathy).
No products indexed under this heading.

Quinidine Polygalacturonate (The risk of myopathy appears to be increased by high levels of HMG-CoA reductase inhibitory activity in plasma. Lovastatin is metabolized by the cytochrome P450 isoform 3A4. Certain drugs which share this metabolic pathway can raise the plasma levels of lovastatin and may increase the risk of myopathy).
No products indexed under this heading.

Quinidine Sulfate (The risk of myopathy appears to be increased by high levels of HMG-CoA reductase inhibitory activity in plasma. Lovastatin is metabolized by the cytochrome P450 isoform 3A4. Certain drugs which share this metabolic pathway can raise the plasma levels of lovastatin and may increase the risk of myopathy).
No products indexed under this heading.

Quinine (The risk of myopathy appears to be increased by high levels of HMG-CoA reductase inhibitory activity in plasma. Lovastatin is metabolized by the cytochrome P450 isoform 3A4. Certain drugs which share this metabolic pathway can raise the plasma levels of lovastatin and may increase the risk of myopathy). Products include:
Hyland's Leg Cramps PM with Quinine **3315**

Quinine Sulfate (The risk of myopathy appears to be increased by high levels of HMG-CoA reductase inhibitory activity in plasma. Lovastatin is metabolized by the cytochrome P450 isoform 3A4. Certain drugs which share this metabolic pathway can raise the plasma levels of lovastatin and may increase the risk of myopathy).
No products indexed under this heading.

Quinupristin (The risk of myopathy appears to be increased by high levels of HMG-CoA reductase inhibitory activity in plasma. Lovastatin is metabolized by the cytochrome P450 isoform 3A4. Certain drugs which share this metabolic pathway can raise the plasma levels of lovastatin and may increase the risk of myopathy).
No products indexed under this heading.

Ranitidine Bismuth Citrate (The risk of myopathy appears to be increased by high levels of HMG-CoA reductase inhibitory activity in plasma. Lovastatin is metabolized by the cytochrome P450 isoform 3A4. Certain drugs which share this metabolic pathway can raise the plasma levels of lovastatin and may increase the risk of myopathy).
No products indexed under this heading.

Ranitidine Hydrochloride (The risk of myopathy appears to be increased by high levels of HMG-CoA reductase inhibitory activity in plasma. Lovastatin is metabolized by the cytochrome P450 isoform 3A4. Certain drugs which share this metabolic pathway can raise the plasma levels of lovastatin and may increase the risk of myopathy).
Products include:
Zantac **1737**
Zantac Injection **1732**
Zantac Pharmacy **1735**

Ritonavir (Co-administration results in serious skeletal muscle disorders, such as rhabdomyolysis and myopathy).
Products include:
Kaletra **458**
Norvir **509**

Saquinavir (Co-administration results in serious skeletal muscle disorders, such as rhabdomyolysis and myopathy).
No products indexed under this heading.

Saquinavir Mesylate (Co-administration results in serious skeletal muscle disorders, such as rhabdomyolysis and myopathy).
No products indexed under this heading.

Sertaconazole Nitrate (Co-administration results in serious skeletal muscle disorders, such as rhabdomyolysis and myopathy).
No products indexed under this heading.

Sertraline Hydrochloride (The risk of myopathy appears to be increased by high levels of HMG-CoA reductase inhibitory activity in plasma. Lovastatin is metabolized by the cytochrome P450 isoform 3A4. Certain drugs which share this metabolic pathway can raise the plasma levels of lovastatin and may increase the risk of myopathy).
No products indexed under this heading.

Sildenafil Citrate (The risk of myopathy appears to be increased by high levels of HMG-CoA reductase inhibitory activity in plasma. Lovastatin is metabolized by the cytochrome P450 isoform 3A4. Certain drugs which share this metabolic pathway can raise the plasma levels of lovastatin and may increase the risk of myopathy).
No products indexed under this heading.

Sotalol Hydrochloride (Co-administration of niacin with vasoactive drugs, such as adrenergic blocking agents, may result in postural hypotension, particularly in patients with unstable angina or acute phase of myocardial infarction).
No products indexed under this heading.

Telithromycin (Co-administration results in serious skeletal muscle disorders, such as rhabdomyolysis and myopathy). Products include:
Ketek **2991**

Terconazole (Co-administration results in serious skeletal muscle disorders, such as rhabdomyolysis and myopathy).
No products indexed under this heading.

Timolol Hemihydrate (Co-administration of niacin with vasoactive drugs, such as adrenergic blocking agents, may result in postural hypotension, particularly in patients with unstable angina or acute phase of myocardial infarction). Products include:
Betimol **3490**

Timolol Maleate (Co-administration of niacin with vasoactive drugs, such as

(⊙ Described in PDR® for Ophthalmic Medicines)

adrenergic blocking agents, may result in postural hypotension, particularly in patients with unstable angina or acute phase of myocardial infarction).
Products include:
Combigan 601
Dorzolamide Hydrochloride/Timolol Maleate Ophthalmic Solution..................... ⊙243
Timoptic in Ocudose .... ⊙231

Tipranavir (Co-administration results in serious skeletal muscle disorders, such as rhabdomyolysis and myopathy).
No products indexed under this heading.

Troglitazone (The risk of myopathy appears to be increased by high levels of HMG-CoA reductase inhibitory activity in plasma. Lovastatin is metabolized by the cytochrome P450 isoform 3A4. Certain drugs which share this metabolic pathway can raise the plasma levels of lovastatin and may increase the risk of myopathy).
No products indexed under this heading.

Troleandomycin (The risk of myopathy appears to be increased by high levels of HMG-CoA reductase inhibitory activity in plasma. Lovastatin is metabolized by the cytochrome P450 isoform 3A4. Certain drugs which share this metabolic pathway can raise the plasma levels of lovastatin and may increase the risk of myopathy).
No products indexed under this heading.

Valproate Sodium (The risk of myopathy appears to be increased by high levels of HMG-CoA reductase inhibitory activity in plasma. Lovastatin is metabolized by the cytochrome P450 isoform 3A4. Certain drugs which share this metabolic pathway can raise the plasma levels of lovastatin and may increase the risk of myopathy).
No products indexed under this heading.

Vardenafil Hydrochloride (The risk of myopathy appears to be increased by high levels of HMG-CoA reductase inhibitory activity in plasma. Lovastatin is metabolized by the cytochrome P450 isoform 3A4. Certain drugs which share this metabolic pathway can raise the plasma levels of lovastatin and may increase the risk of myopathy).
Products include:
Levitra 3157

Verapamil Hydrochloride (Co-administration of niacin with vasoactive drugs, such as calcium channel blockers, may result in postural hypotension, particularly in patients with unstable angina or acute phase of myocardial infarction). Products include:
Tarka 534

Voriconazole (Co-administration results in serious skeletal muscle disorders, such as rhabdomyolysis and myopathy).
No products indexed under this heading.

Warfarin Sodium (Co-administration has resulted in increased bleeding and/or prothrombin time).
No products indexed under this heading.

Zafirlukast (The risk of myopathy appears to be increased by high levels of HMG-CoA reductase inhibitory activity in plasma. Lovastatin is metabolized by the cytochrome P450 isoform 3A4. Certain drugs which share this metabolic pathway can raise the plasma levels of lovastatin and may increase the risk of myopathy). Products include:
Accolate 3612

Zileuton (The risk of myopathy appears to be increased by high levels of HMG-CoA reductase inhibitory activity in plasma. Lovastatin is metabolized by the cytochrome P450 isoform 3A4. Certain drugs which share this metabolic pathway can raise the plasma levels of lovastatin and may increase the risk of myopathy).
No products indexed under this heading.

Food Interactions

Alcohol (Concomitant alcohol may increase the flushing and its use should be avoided around the time of Advicor administration).

Beer, reduced-alcohol (Concomitant alcohol may increase the flushing and its use should be avoided around the time of Advicor administration).

Beer, unspecified (Concomitant alcohol may increase the flushing and its use should be avoided around the time of Advicor administration).

Drinks, hot, unspecified (Concomitant hot drinks may increase the flushing and its use should be avoided around the time of Advicor administration).

Grapefruit (The risk of myopathy appears to be increased by high levels of HMG-CoA reductase inhibitory activity in plasma. Lovastatin is metabolized by the cytochrome P450 isoform 3A4. Certain drugs which share this metabolic pathway can raise the plasma levels of lovastatin and may increase the risk of myopathy).

Grapefruit Juice (Inhibits CYP3A4 and can increase the plasma concentration of lovastatin; concurrent use should be avoided).

Wine, Chianti (Concomitant alcohol may increase the flushing and its use should be avoided around the time of Advicor administration).

Wine, Red (Concomitant alcohol may increase the flushing and its use should be avoided around the time of Advicor administration).

Wine, unspecified (Concomitant alcohol may increase the flushing and its use should be avoided around the time of Advicor administration).

Wine products (Concomitant alcohol may increase the flushing and its use should be avoided around the time of Advicor administration).

AEROCHAMBER PLUS AND AEROCHAMBER PLUS WITH MASK

(Spacer, Inhalation) 1147
None cited in PDR database.

AFINITOR TABLETS

(Everolimus) 2398
May interact with cytochrome p450 3a4 inducers (selected), cytochrome p450 3a4 inhibitors (selected), cytochrome p450 3a4 inhibitors, potent (selected), dexamethasones, erythromycin, P-glycoprotein inhibitors, phenytoin, vaccines, live, and certain other agents. Compounds in these categories include:

Acetazolamide (Co-administration of everolimus with strong or moderate inhibitors of CYP3A4 (eg, ketoconazole, itraconazole, clarithromycin, atazanavir, nefazodone, saquinavir, telithromycin, ritonavir, amprenavir, indinavir, nelfinavir, delavirdine, fosamprenavir, voriconazole, aprepitant, erythromycin, fluconazole, grapefruit juice, verapamil or diltazem) should be avoided due to significant increase in exposure of everolimus).
No products indexed under this heading.

Acetazolamide Sodium (Co-administration of everolimus with strong or moderate inhibitors of CYP3A4 (eg, ketoconazole, itraconazole, clarithromycin, atazanavir, nefazodone, saquinavir, telithromycin, ritonavir, amprenavir, indinavir, nelfinavir, delavirdine, fosamprenavir, voriconazole, aprepitant, erythromycin, fluconazole, grapefruit juice, verapamil or diltazem) should be avoided due to significant increase in exposure of everolimus).
No products indexed under this heading.

Allium sativum (Co-administration of everolimus with strong CYP3A4 inducers (eg, dexamethasone, phenytoin, carbamazepine, rifampin, rifabutin, phenobarbital) should be avoided. If patients require co-administration of a strong CYP3A4 inducer, consider increasing the everolimus dose from 10 mg daily up to 20 mg daily (based on pharmacokinetic data), using 5 mg increments. This dose of everolimus is predicted to adjust the AUC to the range observed without inducers. However, there are no clinical data with this dose adjustment in patients receiving strong CYP3A4 inducers. If the strong inducer is discontinued, the everolimus dose should be returned to the dose used prior to initiation of the strong CYP3A4 inducer).
No products indexed under this heading.

Aminoglutethimide (Co-administration of everolimus with strong CYP3A4 inducers (eg, dexamethasone, phenytoin, carbamazepine, rifampin, rifabutin, phenobarbital) should be avoided. If patients require co-administration of a strong CYP3A4 inducer, consider increasing the everolimus dose from 10 mg daily up to 20 mg daily (based on pharmacokinetic data), using 5 mg increments. This dose of everolimus is predicted to adjust the AUC to the range observed without inducers. However, there are no clinical data with this dose adjustment in patients receiving strong CYP3A4 inducers. If the strong inducer is discontinued, the everolimus dose should be returned to the dose used prior to initiation of the strong CYP3A4 inducer).
No products indexed under this heading.

Amiodarone Hydrochloride (Co-administration of everolimus with strong or moderate inhibitors of CYP3A4 (eg, ketoconazole, itraconazole, clarithromycin, atazanavir, nefazodone, saquinavir, telithromycin, ritonavir, amprenavir, indinavir, nelfinavir, delavirdine, fosamprenavir, voriconazole, aprepitant, erythromycin, fluconazole, grapefruit juice, verapamil or diltazem) should be avoided due to significant increase in exposure of everolimus).
No products indexed under this heading.

Amlodipine Besylate (Co-administration of everolimus with P-glycoprotein (pgP) should be avoided due to significant increase in exposure of everolimus). Products include:
Azor 1010
Exforge 2443
Exforge HCT 2449

Amprenavir (Co-administration of everolimus with strong or moderate inhibitors of CYP3A4 (eg, ketoconazole, itraconazole, clarithromycin, atazanavir, nefazodone, saquinavir, telithromycin, ritonavir, amprenavir, indinavir, nelfinavir, delavirdine, fosamprenavir, voriconazole, aprepitant, erythromycin, fluconazole, grapefruit juice, verapamil or diltazem) should be avoided due to significant increase in exposure of everolimus).
No products indexed under this heading.

Anastrozole (Co-administration of everolimus with strong or moderate inhibitors of CYP3A4 (eg, ketoconazole, itraconazole, clarithromycin, atazanavir, nefazodone, saquinavir, telithromycin, ritonavir, amprenavir, indinavir, nelfinavir, delavirdine, fosamprenavir, voriconazole, aprepitant, erythromycin, fluconazole, grapefruit juice, verapamil or diltazem) should be avoided due to significant increase in exposure of everolimus).
No products indexed under this heading.

Aprepitant (Co-administration of everolimus with strong CYP3A4 inducers (eg, dexamethasone, phenytoin, carbamazepine, rifampin, rifabutin, phenobarbital) should be avoided. If patients require co-administration of a strong CYP3A4 inducer, consider increasing the everolimus dose from 10 mg daily up to 20 mg daily (based on pharmacokinetic data), using 5 mg increments. This dose of everolimus is predicted to adjust the AUC to the range observed without inducers. However, there are no clinical data with this dose adjustment in patients receiving strong CYP3A4 inducers. If the strong inducer is discontinued, the everolimus dose should be returned to the dose used prior to initiation of the strong CYP3A4 inducer). Products include:
Emend 2124

Atazanavir (Co-administration of everolimus with strong or moderate inhibitors of CYP3A4 (eg, ketoconazole, itraconazole, clarithromycin, atazanavir, nefazodone, saquinavir, telithromycin, ritonavir, amprenavir, indinavir, nelfinavir, delavirdine, fosamprenavir, voriconazole, aprepitant, erythromycin, fluconazole, grapefruit juice, verapamil or diltazem) should be avoided due to significant increase in exposure of everolimus).
No products indexed under this heading.

Atazanavir Sulfate (Co-administration of everolimus with strong or moderate inhibitors of CYP3A4 (eg, ketoconazole, itraconazole, clarithromycin, atazanavir, nefazodone, saquinavir, telithromycin, ritonavir, amprenavir, indinavir, nelfinavir, delavirdine, fosamprenavir, voriconazole, aprepitant, erythromycin, fluconazole, grapefruit juice, verapamil or diltazem) should be avoided due to significant increase in exposure of everolimus).
No products indexed under this heading.

Atenolol (Co-administration of everolimus with P-glycoprotein (pgP) should be avoided due to significant increase in exposure of everolimus).
No products indexed under this heading.

Atorvastatin Calcium (Co-administration of everolimus with P-glycoprotein (pgP) should be avoided due to significant increase in exposure of everolimus). Products include:
Lipitor 2703

Azithromycin Dihydrate (Co-administration of everolimus with P-glycoprotein (pgP) should be avoided due to significant increase in exposure of everolimus).
No products indexed under this heading.

BCG Vaccine (The use of live vaccines and close contact with those who have received live vaccines should be avoided during treatment with everolimus).
No products indexed under this heading.

Betamethasone (Co-administration of everolimus with strong CYP3A4 inducers (eg, dexamethasone, phenytoin, carbamazepine, rifampin, rifabutin, phenobarbital) should be avoided. If patients require co-administration of a strong CYP3A4 inducer, consider increasing the everolimus dose from 10 mg daily up to 20 mg daily (based on pharmacokinetic data), using 5 mg increments. This dose of everolimus is predicted to adjust the AUC to the range observed without inducers. However, there are no clinical data with this dose adjustment in patients receiving strong CYP3A4 inducers. If the strong inducer is discontinued, the everolimus dose should be returned to the dose used prior to initiation of the strong CYP3A4 inducer).
No products indexed under this heading.

Betamethasone Acetate (Co-administration of everolimus with strong CYP3A4 inducers (eg, dexamethasone, phenytoin, carbamazepine, rifampin, rifabutin, phenobarbital) should be

IMPORTANT NOTE: Always consult each drug listing in the patient's regimen for possible interactions.

avoided. If patients require co-administration of a strong CYP3A4 inducer, consider increasing the everolimus dose from 10 mg daily up to 20 mg daily (based on pharmacokinetic data), using 5 mg increments. This dose of everolimus is predicted to adjust the AUC to the range observed without inducers. However, there are no clinical data with this dose adjustment in patients receiving strong CYP3A4 inducers. If the strong inducer is discontinued, the everolimus dose should be returned to the dose used prior to initiation of the strong CYP3A4 inducer).
No products indexed under this heading.

Betamethasone Benzoate (Co-administration of everolimus with strong CYP3A4 inducers (eg, dexamethasone, phenytoin, carbamazepine, rifampin, rifabutin, phenobarbital) should be avoided. If patients require co-administration of a strong CYP3A4 inducer, consider increasing the everolimus dose from 10 mg daily up to 20 mg daily (based on pharmacokinetic data), using 5 mg increments. This dose of everolimus is predicted to adjust the AUC to the range observed without inducers. However, there are no clinical data with this dose adjustment in patients receiving strong CYP3A4 inducers. If the strong inducer is discontinued, the everolimus dose should be returned to the dose used prior to initiation of the strong CYP3A4 inducer).
No products indexed under this heading.

Betamethasone Dipropionate (Co-administration of everolimus with strong CYP3A4 inducers (eg, dexamethasone, phenytoin, carbamazepine, rifampin, rifabutin, phenobarbital) should be avoided. If patients require co-administration of a strong CYP3A4 inducer, consider increasing the everolimus dose from 10 mg daily up to 20 mg daily (based on pharmacokinetic data), using 5 mg increments. This dose of everolimus is predicted to adjust the AUC to the range observed without inducers. However, there are no clinical data with this dose adjustment in patients receiving strong CYP3A4 inducers. If the strong inducer is discontinued, the everolimus dose should be returned to the dose used prior to initiation of the strong CYP3A4 inducer). Products include:
Diprolene Lotion 0.05% 3108
Diprolene Ointment 0.05% 3109
Diprolene AF Cream 0.05% 3107
Lotrisone 3163

Betamethasone Sodium Phosphate (Co-administration of everolimus with strong CYP3A4 inducers (eg, dexamethasone, phenytoin, carbamazepine, rifampin, rifabutin, phenobarbital) should be avoided. If patients require co-administration of a strong CYP3A4 inducer, consider increasing the everolimus dose from 10 mg daily up to 20 mg daily (based on pharmacokinetic data), using 5 mg increments. This dose of everolimus is predicted to adjust the AUC to the range observed without inducers. However, there are no clinical data with this dose adjustment in patients receiving strong CYP3A4 inducers. If the strong inducer is discontinued, the everolimus dose should be returned to the dose used prior to initiation of the strong CYP3A4 inducer).
No products indexed under this heading.

Betamethasone Valerate (Co-administration of everolimus with strong CYP3A4 inducers (eg, dexamethasone, phenytoin, carbamazepine, rifampin, rifabutin, phenobarbital) should be avoided. If patients require co-administration of a strong CYP3A4 inducer, consider increasing the everolimus dose from 10 mg daily up to 20 mg daily (based on pharmacokinetic data), using 5 mg increments. This dose of everolimus is predicted to adjust the AUC to the range observed without inducers. However, there are no clinical data with this dose adjustment in patients receiving strong CYP3A4 inducers. If the strong inducer is discontinued, the everolimus dose should be returned to the dose used prior to initiation of the strong CYP3A4 inducer). Products include:
Luxíq 3321

Bosentan (Co-administration of everolimus with strong CYP3A4 inducers (eg, dexamethasone, phenytoin, carbamazepine, rifampin, rifabutin, phenobarbital) should be avoided. If patients require co-administration of a strong CYP3A4 inducer, consider increasing the everolimus dose from 10 mg daily up to 20 mg daily (based on pharmacokinetic data), using 5 mg increments. This dose of everolimus is predicted to adjust the AUC to the range observed without inducers. However, there are no clinical data with this dose adjustment in patients receiving strong CYP3A4 inducers. If the strong inducer is discontinued, the everolimus dose should be returned to the dose used prior to initiation of the strong CYP3A4 inducer). Products include:
Tracleer 573

Carbamazepine (Co-administration of everolimus with strong CYP3A4 inducers (eg, dexamethasone, phenytoin, carbamazepine, rifampin, rifabutin, phenobarbital) should be avoided. If patients require co-administration of a strong CYP3A4 inducer, consider increasing the everolimus dose from 10 mg daily up to 20 mg daily (based on pharmacokinetic data), using 5 mg increments. This dose of everolimus is predicted to adjust the AUC to the range observed without inducers. However, there are no clinical data with this dose adjustment in patients receiving strong CYP3A4 inducers. If the strong inducer is discontinued, the everolimus dose should be returned to the dose used prior to initiation of the strong CYP3A4 inducer). Products include:
Carbatrol 3280
Equetro 3477

Carvedilol (Co-administration of everolimus with P-glycoprotein (pgP) should be avoided due to significant increase in exposure of everolimus). Products include:
Coreg 1409

Carvedilol Phosphate (Co-administration of everolimus with P-glycoprotein (pgP) should be avoided due to significant increase in exposure of everolimus). Products include:
Coreg CR 1416

Cimetidine (Co-administration of everolimus with strong or moderate inhibitors of CYP3A4 (eg, ketoconazole, itraconazole, clarithromycin, atazanavir, nefazodone, saquinavir, telithromycin, ritonavir, amprenavir, indinavir, nelfinavir, delavirdine, fosamprenavir, voriconazole, aprepitant, erythromycin, fluconazole, grapefruit juice, verapamil or diltazem) should be avoided due to significant increase in exposure of everolimus).
No products indexed under this heading.

Cimetidine Hydrochloride (Co-administration of everolimus with strong or moderate inhibitors of CYP3A4 (eg, ketoconazole, itraconazole, clarithromycin, atazanavir, nefazodone, saquinavir, telithromycin, ritonavir, amprenavir, indinavir, nelfinavir, delavirdine, fosamprenavir, voriconazole, aprepitant, erythromycin, fluconazole, grapefruit juice, verapamil or diltazem) should be avoided due to significant increase in exposure of everolimus).
No products indexed under this heading.

Ciprofloxacin (Co-administration of everolimus with strong CYP3A4 inducers (eg, dexamethasone, phenytoin, carbamazepine, rifampin, rifabutin, phenobarbital) should be avoided. If patients require co-administration of a strong CYP3A4 inducer, consider increasing the everolimus dose from 10 mg daily up to 20 mg daily (based on pharmacokinetic data), using 5 mg increments. This dose of everolimus is predicted to adjust the AUC to the range observed without inducers. However, there are no clinical data with this dose adjustment in patients receiving strong CYP3A4 inducers. If the strong inducer is discontinued, the everolimus dose should be returned to the dose used prior to initiation of the strong CYP3A4 inducer). Products include:
Cipro I.V. 3082
Cipro 3073
Cipro XR 3091
Ciprodex 583

Ciprofloxacin Hydrochloride (Co-administration of everolimus with strong CYP3A4 inducers (eg, dexamethasone, phenytoin, carbamazepine, rifampin, rifabutin, phenobarbital) should be avoided. If patients require co-administration of a strong CYP3A4 inducer, consider increasing the everolimus dose from 10 mg daily up to 20 mg daily (based on pharmacokinetic data), using 5 mg increments. This dose of everolimus is predicted to adjust the AUC to the range observed without inducers. However, there are no clinical data with this dose adjustment in patients receiving strong CYP3A4 inducers. If the strong inducer is discontinued, the everolimus dose should be returned to the dose used prior to initiation of the strong CYP3A4 inducer). Products include:
Cipro 3073

Cisplatin (Co-administration of everolimus with strong CYP3A4 inducers (eg, dexamethasone, phenytoin, carbamazepine, rifampin, rifabutin, phenobarbital) should be avoided. If patients require co-administration of a strong CYP3A4 inducer, consider increasing the everolimus dose from 10 mg daily up to 20 mg daily (based on pharmacokinetic data), using 5 mg increments. This dose of everolimus is predicted to adjust the AUC to the range observed without inducers. However, there are no clinical data with this dose adjustment in patients receiving strong CYP3A4 inducers. If the strong inducer is discontinued, the everolimus dose should be returned to the dose used prior to initiation of the strong CYP3A4 inducer).
No products indexed under this heading.

Clarithromycin (Co-administration of everolimus with strong or moderate inhibitors of CYP3A4 (eg, ketoconazole, itraconazole, clarithromycin, atazanavir, nefazodone, saquinavir, telithromycin, ritonavir, amprenavir, indinavir, nelfinavir, delavirdine, fosamprenavir, voriconazole, aprepitant, erythromycin, fluconazole, grapefruit juice, verapamil or diltazem) should be avoided due to significant increase in exposure of everolimus). Products include:
Biaxin/Biaxin XL 412

Clotrimazole (Co-administration of everolimus with strong or moderate inhibitors of CYP3A4 (eg, ketoconazole, itraconazole, clarithromycin, atazanavir, nefazodone, saquinavir, telithromycin, ritonavir, amprenavir, indinavir, nelfinavir, delavirdine, fosamprenavir, voriconazole, aprepitant, erythromycin, fluconazole, grapefruit juice, verapamil or diltazem) should be avoided due to significant increase in exposure of everolimus). Products include:
Lotrisone 3163

Conivaptan Hydrochloride (Co-administration of everolimus with strong or moderate inhibitors of CYP3A4 (eg, ketoconazole, itraconazole, clarithromycin, atazanavir, nefazodone, saquinavir, telithromycin, ritonavir, amprenavir, indinavir, nelfinavir, delavirdine, fosamprenavir, voriconazole, aprepitant, erythromycin, fluconazole, grapefruit juice, verapamil or diltazem) should be avoided due to significant increase in exposure of everolimus). Products include:
Vaprisol 689

Cortisone Acetate (Co-administration of everolimus with strong CYP3A4 inducers (eg, dexamethasone, phenytoin, carbamazepine, rifampin, rifabutin, phenobarbital) should be avoided. If patients require co-administration of a strong CYP3A4 inducer, consider increasing the everolimus dose from 10 mg daily up to 20 mg daily (based on pharmacokinetic data), using 5 mg increments. This dose of everolimus is predicted to adjust the AUC to the range observed without inducers. However, there are no clinical data with this dose adjustment in patients receiving strong CYP3A4 inducers. If the strong inducer is discontinued, the everolimus dose should be returned to the dose used prior to initiation of the strong CYP3A4 inducer).
No products indexed under this heading.

Cyclosporine (Co-administration of everolimus with strong or moderate inhibitors of CYP3A4 (eg, ketoconazole, itraconazole, clarithromycin, atazanavir, nefazodone, saquinavir, telithromycin, ritonavir, amprenavir, indinavir, nelfinavir, delavirdine, fosamprenavir, voriconazole, aprepitant, erythromycin, fluconazole, grapefruit juice, verapamil or diltazem) should be avoided due to significant increase in exposure of everolimus). Products include:
Gengraf 440
Neoral Oral Solution 2496
Neoral Capsules 2496
Restasis 605

Dalfopristin (Co-administration of everolimus with strong or moderate inhibitors of CYP3A4 (eg, ketoconazole, itraconazole, clarithromycin, atazanavir, nefazodone, saquinavir, telithromycin, ritonavir, amprenavir, indinavir, nelfinavir, delavirdine, fosamprenavir, voriconazole, aprepitant, erythromycin, fluconazole, grapefruit juice, verapamil or diltazem) should be avoided due to significant increase in exposure of everolimus).
No products indexed under this heading.

Danazol (Co-administration of everolimus with strong or moderate inhibitors of CYP3A4 (eg, ketoconazole, itraconazole, clarithromycin, atazanavir, nefazodone, saquinavir, telithromycin, ritonavir, amprenavir, indinavir, nelfinavir, delavirdine, fosamprenavir, voriconazole, aprepitant, erythromycin, fluconazole, grapefruit juice, verapamil or diltazem) should be avoided due to significant increase in exposure of everolimus).
No products indexed under this heading.

Darunavir (Co-administration of everolimus with strong or moderate inhibitors of CYP3A4 (eg, ketoconazole, itraconazole, clarithromycin, atazanavir, nefazodone, saquinavir, telithromycin, ritonavir, amprenavir, indinavir, nelfinavir, delavirdine, fosamprenavir, voriconazole, aprepitant, erythromycin, fluconazole, grapefruit juice, verapamil or diltazem) should be avoided due to significant increase in exposure of everolimus).
No products indexed under this heading.

Dasatinib (Co-administration of everolimus with strong or moderate inhibitors of CYP3A4 (eg, ketoconazole, itracona-

zole, clarithromycin, atazanavir, nefazodone, saquinavir, telithromycin, ritonavir, amprenavir, indinavir, nelfinavir, delavirdine, fosamprenavir, voriconazole, aprepitant, erythromycin, fluconazole, grapefruit juice, verapamil or diltazem) should be avoided due to significant increase in exposure of everolimus).
No products indexed under this heading.

Delavirdine Mesylate (Co-administration of everolimus with strong or moderate inhibitors of CYP3A4 (eg, ketoconazole, itraconazole, clarithromycin, atazanavir, nefazodone, saquinavir, telithromycin, ritonavir, amprenavir, indinavir, nelfinavir, delavirdine, fosamprenavir, voriconazole, aprepitant, erythromycin, fluconazole, grapefruit juice, verapamil or diltazem) should be avoided due to significant increase in exposure of everolimus).
No products indexed under this heading.

Delavirine (Co-administration of everolimus with strong or moderate inhibitors of CYP3A4 (eg, ketoconazole, itraconazole, clarithromycin, atazanavir, nefazodone, saquinavir, telithromycin, ritonavir, amprenavir, indinavir, nelfinavir, delavirdine, fosamprenavir, voriconazole, aprepitant, erythromycin, fluconazole, grapefruit juice, verapamil or diltazem) should be avoided due to significant increase in exposure of everolimus).
No products indexed under this heading.

Desloratadine (Co-administration of everolimus with strong or moderate inhibitors of CYP3A4 (eg, ketoconazole, itraconazole, clarithromycin, atazanavir, nefazodone, saquinavir, telithromycin, ritonavir, amprenavir, indinavir, nelfinavir, delavirdine, fosamprenavir, voriconazole, aprepitant, erythromycin, fluconazole, grapefruit juice, verapamil or diltazem) should be avoided due to significant increase in exposure of everolimus). Products include:
Clarinex Syrup **3098**
Clarinex **3098**
Clarinex Reditabs **3098**
Clarinex-D 12-Hour **3101**
Clarinex-D **3104**

Dexamethasone (Co-administration of everolimus with strong CYP3A4 inducers (eg, dexamethasone) should be avoided. If patients require co-administration of a strong CYP3A4 inducer, consider increasing the everolimus dose from 10 mg daily up to 20 mg daily (based on pharmacokinetic data), using 5 mg increments. This dose of everolimus is predicted to adjust the AUC to the range observed without inducers. However, there are no clinical data with this dose adjustment in patients receiving strong CYP3A4 inducers. If the strong inducer is discontinued, the everolimus dose should be returned to the dose used prior to initiation of the strong CYP3A4 inducer). Products include:
Ciprodex **583**
Ozurdex .... ⊙ **223**
Tobramycin and Dexamethasone Ophthalmic Suspension .... ⊙ **251**

Dexamethasone Acetate (Co-administration of everolimus with strong CYP3A4 inducers (eg, dexamethasone) should be avoided. If patients require co-administration of a strong CYP3A4 inducer, consider increasing the everolimus dose from 10 mg daily up to 20 mg daily (based on pharmacokinetic data), using 5 mg increments. This dose of everolimus is predicted to adjust the AUC to the range observed without inducers. However, there are no clinical data with this dose adjustment in patients receiving strong CYP3A4 inducers. If the strong inducer is discontinued, the everolimus dose should be returned to the dose used prior to initiation of the strong CYP3A4 inducer).
No products indexed under this heading.

Dexamethasone Phosphate (Co-administration of everolimus with strong CYP3A4 inducers (eg, dexamethasone) should be avoided. If patients require co-administration of a strong CYP3A4 inducer, consider increasing the everolimus dose from 10 mg daily up to 20 mg daily (based on pharmacokinetic data), using 5 mg increments. This dose of everolimus is predicted to adjust the AUC to the range observed without inducers. However, there are no clinical data with this dose adjustment in patients receiving strong CYP3A4 inducers. If the strong inducer is discontinued, the everolimus dose should be returned to the dose used prior to initiation of the strong CYP3A4 inducer).
No products indexed under this heading.

Dexamethasone Sodium (Co-administration of everolimus with strong CYP3A4 inducers (eg, dexamethasone) should be avoided. If patients require co-administration of a strong CYP3A4 inducer, consider increasing the everolimus dose from 10 mg daily up to 20 mg daily (based on pharmacokinetic data), using 5 mg increments. This dose of everolimus is predicted to adjust the AUC to the range observed without inducers. However, there are no clinical data with this dose adjustment in patients receiving strong CYP3A4 inducers. If the strong inducer is discontinued, the everolimus dose should be returned to the dose used prior to initiation of the strong CYP3A4 inducer).
No products indexed under this heading.

Dexamethasone Sodium Phosphate (Co-administration of everolimus with strong CYP3A4 inducers (eg, dexamethasone) should be avoided. If patients require co-administration of a strong CYP3A4 inducer, consider increasing the everolimus dose from 10 mg daily up to 20 mg daily (based on pharmacokinetic data), using 5 mg increments. This dose of everolimus is predicted to adjust the AUC to the range observed without inducers. However, there are no clinical data with this dose adjustment in patients receiving strong CYP3A4 inducers. If the strong inducer is discontinued, the everolimus dose should be returned to the dose used prior to initiation of the strong CYP3A4 inducer).
No products indexed under this heading.

Dexamethasone Sodium Phosphate Injection (Co-administration of everolimus with strong CYP3A4 inducers (eg, dexamethasone) should be avoided. If patients require co-administration of a strong CYP3A4 inducer, consider increasing the everolimus dose from 10 mg daily up to 20 mg daily (based on pharmacokinetic data), using 5 mg increments. This dose of everolimus is predicted to adjust the AUC to the range observed without inducers. However, there are no clinical data with this dose adjustment in patients receiving strong CYP3A4 inducers. If the strong inducer is discontinued, the everolimus dose should be returned to the dose used prior to initiation of the strong CYP3A4 inducer).
No products indexed under this heading.

Digoxin (Co-administration of everolimus with P-glycoprotein (pgP) should be avoided due to significant increase in exposure of everolimus). Products include:
Lanoxin Injection **1546**
Lanoxin Injection Pediatric **1549**
Lanoxin Tablets **1553**

Diltiazem Hydrochloride (Co-administration of everolimus with strong or moderate inhibitors of CYP3A4 (eg, ketoconazole, itraconazole, clarithromycin, atazanavir, nefazodone, saquinavir, telithromycin, ritonavir, amprenavir, indinavir, nelfinavir, delavirdine, fosamprenavir, voriconazole, aprepitant, erythromycin, fluconazole, grapefruit juice, verapamil or diltazem) should be avoided due to significant increase in exposure of everolimus). Products include:
Cardizem LA **423**

Diltiazem Maleate (Co-administration of everolimus with strong or moderate inhibitors of CYP3A4 (eg, ketoconazole, itraconazole, clarithromycin, atazanavir, nefazodone, saquinavir, telithromycin, ritonavir, amprenavir, indinavir, nelfinavir, delavirdine, fosamprenavir, voriconazole, aprepitant, erythromycin, fluconazole, grapefruit juice, verapamil or diltazem) should be avoided due to significant increase in exposure of everolimus).
No products indexed under this heading.

Dirithromycin (Co-administration of everolimus with P-glycoprotein (pgP) should be avoided due to significant increase in exposure of everolimus).
No products indexed under this heading.

Doxorubicin Hydrochloride (Co-administration of everolimus with strong CYP3A4 inducers (eg, dexamethasone, phenytoin, carbamazepine, rifampin, rifabutin, phenobarbital) should be avoided. If patients require co-administration of a strong CYP3A4 inducer, consider increasing the everolimus dose from 10 mg daily up to 20 mg daily (based on pharmacokinetic data), using 5 mg increments. This dose of everolimus is predicted to adjust the AUC to the range observed without inducers. However, there are no clinical data with this dose adjustment in patients receiving strong CYP3A4 inducers. If the strong inducer is discontinued, the everolimus dose should be returned to the dose used prior to initiation of the strong CYP3A4 inducer).
No products indexed under this heading.

Efavirenz (Co-administration of everolimus with strong CYP3A4 inducers (eg, dexamethasone, phenytoin, carbamazepine, rifampin, rifabutin, phenobarbital) should be avoided. If patients require co-administration of a strong CYP3A4 inducer, consider increasing the everolimus dose from 10 mg daily up to 20 mg daily (based on pharmacokinetic data), using 5 mg increments. This dose of everolimus is predicted to adjust the AUC to the range observed without inducers. However, there are no clinical data with this dose adjustment in patients receiving strong CYP3A4 inducers. If the strong inducer is discontinued, the everolimus dose should be returned to the dose used prior to initiation of the strong CYP3A4 inducer). Products include:
Atripla **906**

Elacridar (Co-administration of everolimus with P-glycoprotein (pgP) should be avoided due to significant increase in exposure of everolimus).
No products indexed under this heading.

Erythromycin (Co-administration of everolimus with a moderate CYP3A4 inhibitor and a PgP inhibitor (eg, erythromycin) should be avoided. In healthy subjects, compared to everolimus treatment alone, there were significant increases in everolimus exposure when everolimus was co-administered with erythromycin. Everolimus C_{max} and AUC increased by 2.0- and 4.4-fold, respectively).
No products indexed under this heading.

Erythromycin, Topical (Co-administration of everolimus with a moderate CYP3A4 inhibitor and a PgP inhibitor (eg, erythromycin) should be avoided. In healthy subjects, compared to everolimus treatment alone, there were significant increases in everolimus exposure when everolimus was co-administered with erythromycin. Everolimus C_{max} and AUC increased by 2.0- and 4.4-fold, respectively).
No products indexed under this heading.

Erythromycin Estolate (Co-administration of everolimus with a moderate CYP3A4 inhibitor and a PgP inhibitor (eg, erythromycin) should be avoided. In healthy subjects, compared to everolimus treatment alone, there were significant increases in everolimus exposure when everolimus was co-administered with erythromycin. Everolimus C_{max} and AUC increased by 2.0- and 4.4-fold, respectively).
No products indexed under this heading.

Erythromycin Ethylsuccinate (Co-administration of everolimus with a moderate CYP3A4 inhibitor and a PgP inhibitor (eg, erythromycin) should be avoided. In healthy subjects, compared to everolimus treatment alone, there were significant increases in everolimus exposure when everolimus was co-administered with erythromycin. Everolimus C_{max} and AUC increased by 2.0- and 4.4-fold, respectively). Products include:
E.E.S. **437**
EryPed **435**

Erythromycin Gluceptate (Co-administration of everolimus with a moderate CYP3A4 inhibitor and a PgP inhibitor (eg, erythromycin) should be avoided. In healthy subjects, compared to everolimus treatment alone, there were significant increases in everolimus exposure when everolimus was co-administered with erythromycin. Everolimus C_{max} and AUC increased by 2.0- and 4.4-fold, respectively).
No products indexed under this heading.

Erythromycin Lactobionate (Co-administration of everolimus with a moderate CYP3A4 inhibitor and a PgP inhibitor (eg, erythromycin) should be avoided. In healthy subjects, compared to everolimus treatment alone, there were significant increases in everolimus exposure when everolimus was co-administered with erythromycin. Everolimus C_{max} and AUC increased by 2.0- and 4.4-fold, respectively).
No products indexed under this heading.

Erythromycin Stearate (Co-administration of everolimus with a moderate CYP3A4 inhibitor and a PgP inhibitor (eg, erythromycin) should be avoided. In healthy subjects, compared to everolimus treatment alone, there were significant increases in everolimus exposure when everolimus was co-administered with erythromycin. Everolimus C_{max} and AUC increased by 2.0- and 4.4-fold, respectively).
No products indexed under this heading.

Esomeprazole Magnesium (Co-administration of everolimus with strong or moderate inhibitors of CYP3A4 (eg, ketoconazole, itraconazole, clarithromycin, atazanavir, nefazodone, saquinavir, telithromycin, ritonavir, amprenavir, indinavir, nelfinavir, delavirdine, fosamprenavir, voriconazole, aprepitant, erythromycin, fluconazole, grapefruit juice, verapamil or diltazem) should be avoided due to significant increase in exposure of everolimus). Products include:
Nexium Capsules **704**
Nexium Oral Suspension **704**

Esomeprazole Sodium (Co-administration of everolimus with strong or moderate inhibitors of CYP3A4 (eg, ketoconazole, itraconazole, clarithromycin, atazanavir, nefazodone, saquinavir, telithromycin, ritonavir, amprenavir, indinavir, nelfinavir, delavirdine, fosamprenavir, voriconazole, aprepitant,

erythromycin, fluconazole, grapefruit juice, verapamil or diltazem) should be avoided due to significant increase in exposure of everolimus). Products include:

Nexium I.V. 712

Ethosuximide (Co-administration of everolimus with strong CYP3A4 inducers (eg, dexamethasone, phenytoin, carbamazepine, rifampin, rifabutin, phenobarbital) should be avoided. If patients require co-administration of a strong CYP3A4 inducer, consider increasing the everolimus dose from 10 mg daily up to 20 mg daily (based on pharmacokinetic data), using 5 mg increments. This dose of everolimus is predicted to adjust the AUC to the range observed without inducers. However, there are no clinical data with this dose adjustment in patients receiving strong CYP3A4 inducers. If the strong inducer is discontinued, the everolimus dose should be returned to the dose used prior to initiation of the strong CYP3A4 inducer).

No products indexed under this heading.

Fat (Based on data in healthy subjects taking 1 mg everolimus tablets, a high-fat meal reduced C_{max} and AUC by 60% and 16%, respectively. No data are available with everolimus 5 mg and 10 mg tablets).

No products indexed under this heading.

Felbamate (Co-administration of everolimus with strong CYP3A4 inducers (eg, dexamethasone, phenytoin, carbamazepine, rifampin, rifabutin, phenobarbital) should be avoided. If patients require co-administration of a strong CYP3A4 inducer, consider increasing the everolimus dose from 10 mg daily up to 20 mg daily (based on pharmacokinetic data), using 5 mg increments. This dose of everolimus is predicted to adjust the AUC to the range observed without inducers. However, there are no clinical data with this dose adjustment in patients receiving strong CYP3A4 inducers. If the strong inducer is discontinued, the everolimus dose should be returned to the dose used prior to initiation of the strong CYP3A4 inducer).

No products indexed under this heading.

Fluconazole (Co-administration of everolimus with strong or moderate inhibitors of CYP3A4 (eg, ketoconazole, itraconazole, clarithromycin, atazanavir, nefazodone, saquinavir, telithromycin, ritonavir, amprenavir, indinavir, nelfinavir, delavirdine, fosamprenavir, voriconazole, aprepitant, erythromycin, fluconazole, grapefruit juice, verapamil or diltazem) should be avoided due to significant increase in exposure of everolimus).

No products indexed under this heading.

Fludrocortisone Acetate (Co-administration of everolimus with strong CYP3A4 inducers (eg, dexamethasone, phenytoin, carbamazepine, rifampin, rifabutin, phenobarbital) should be avoided. If patients require co-administration of a strong CYP3A4 inducer, consider increasing the everolimus dose from 10 mg daily up to 20 mg daily (based on pharmacokinetic data), using 5 mg increments. This dose of everolimus is predicted to adjust the AUC to the range observed without inducers. However, there are no clinical data with this dose adjustment in patients receiving strong CYP3A4 inducers. If the strong inducer is discontinued, the everolimus dose should be returned to the dose used prior to initiation of the strong CYP3A4 inducer).

No products indexed under this heading.

Fluoxetine (Co-administration of everolimus with strong or moderate inhibitors of CYP3A4 (eg, ketoconazole, itraconazole, clarithromycin, atazanavir, nefazodone, saquinavir, telithromycin, ritonavir, amprenavir, indinavir, nelfinavir, delavirdine, fosamprenavir, voriconazole, aprepitant, erythromycin, fluconazole, grapefruit juice, verapamil or diltazem) should be avoided due to significant increase in exposure of everolimus).

No products indexed under this heading.

Fluoxetine Hydrochloride (Co-administration of everolimus with strong or moderate inhibitors of CYP3A4 (eg, ketoconazole, itraconazole, clarithromycin, atazanavir, nefazodone, saquinavir, telithromycin, ritonavir, amprenavir, indinavir, nelfinavir, delavirdine, fosamprenavir, voriconazole, aprepitant, erythromycin, fluconazole, grapefruit juice, verapamil or diltazem) should be avoided due to significant increase in exposure of everolimus). Products include:

Prozac Weekly 1941
Prozac Pulvules 1941
Symbyax 1965

Fluvoxamine Maleate (Co-administration of everolimus with strong or moderate inhibitors of CYP3A4 (eg, ketoconazole, itraconazole, clarithromycin, atazanavir, nefazodone, saquinavir, telithromycin, ritonavir, amprenavir, indinavir, nelfinavir, delavirdine, fosamprenavir, voriconazole, aprepitant, erythromycin, fluconazole, grapefruit juice, verapamil or diltazem) should be avoided due to significant increase in exposure of everolimus).

No products indexed under this heading.

Fosamprenavir Calcium (Co-administration of everolimus with strong or moderate inhibitors of CYP3A4 (eg, ketoconazole, itraconazole, clarithromycin, atazanavir, nefazodone, saquinavir, telithromycin, ritonavir, amprenavir, indinavir, nelfinavir, delavirdine, fosamprenavir, voriconazole, aprepitant, erythromycin, fluconazole, grapefruit juice, verapamil or diltazem) should be avoided due to significant increase in exposure of everolimus). Products include:

Lexiva Oral Suspension 1558
Lexiva 1558

Fosphenytoin (Co-administration of everolimus with strong CYP3A4 inducers (eg, phenytoin) should be avoided. If patients require co-administration of a strong CYP3A4 inducer, consider increasing the everolimus dose from 10 mg daily up to 20 mg daily (based on pharmacokinetic data), using 5 mg increments. This dose of everolimus is predicted to adjust the AUC to the range observed without inducers. However, there are no clinical data with this dose adjustment in patients receiving strong CYP3A4 inducers. If the strong inducer is discontinued, the everolimus dose should be returned to the dose used prior to initiation of the strong CYP3A4 inducer).

No products indexed under this heading.

Fosphenytoin Sodium (Co-administration of everolimus with strong CYP3A4 inducers (eg, phenytoin) should be avoided. If patients require co-administration of a strong CYP3A4 inducer, consider increasing the everolimus dose from 10 mg daily up to 20 mg daily (based on pharmacokinetic data), using 5 mg increments. This dose of everolimus is predicted to adjust the AUC to the range observed without inducers. However, there are no clinical data with this dose adjustment in patients receiving strong CYP3A4 inducers. If the strong inducer is discontinued, the everolimus dose should be returned to the dose used prior to initiation of the strong CYP3A4 inducer).

No products indexed under this heading.

Garlic Extract (Co-administration of everolimus with strong CYP3A4 inducers (eg, dexamethasone, phenytoin, carbamazepine, rifampin, rifabutin, phenobarbital) should be avoided. If patients require co-administration of a strong CYP3A4 inducer, consider increasing the everolimus dose from 10 mg daily up to 20 mg daily (based on pharmacokinetic data), using 5 mg increments. This dose of everolimus is predicted to adjust the AUC to the range observed without inducers. However, there are no clinical data with this dose adjustment in patients receiving strong CYP3A4 inducers. If the strong inducer is discontinued, the everolimus dose should be returned to the dose used prior to initiation of the strong CYP3A4 inducer).

No products indexed under this heading.

Garlic Oil (Co-administration of everolimus with strong CYP3A4 inducers (eg, dexamethasone, phenytoin, carbamazepine, rifampin, rifabutin, phenobarbital) should be avoided. If patients require co-administration of a strong CYP3A4 inducer, consider increasing the everolimus dose from 10 mg daily up to 20 mg daily (based on pharmacokinetic data), using 5 mg increments. This dose of everolimus is predicted to adjust the AUC to the range observed without inducers. However, there are no clinical data with this dose adjustment in patients receiving strong CYP3A4 inducers. If the strong inducer is discontinued, the everolimus dose should be returned to the dose used prior to initiation of the strong CYP3A4 inducer).

No products indexed under this heading.

Hydrocortisone (Co-administration of everolimus with strong CYP3A4 inducers (eg, dexamethasone, phenytoin, carbamazepine, rifampin, rifabutin, phenobarbital) should be avoided. If patients require co-administration of a strong CYP3A4 inducer, consider increasing the everolimus dose from 10 mg daily up to 20 mg daily (based on pharmacokinetic data), using 5 mg increments. This dose of everolimus is predicted to adjust the AUC to the range observed without inducers. However, there are no clinical data with this dose adjustment in patients receiving strong CYP3A4 inducers. If the strong inducer is discontinued, the everolimus dose should be returned to the dose used prior to initiation of the strong CYP3A4 inducer).

No products indexed under this heading.

Hydrocortisone (Alcohol) (Co-administration of everolimus with strong CYP3A4 inducers (eg, dexamethasone, phenytoin, carbamazepine, rifampin, rifabutin, phenobarbital) should be avoided. If patients require co-administration of a strong CYP3A4 inducer, consider increasing the everolimus dose from 10 mg daily up to 20 mg daily (based on pharmacokinetic data), using 5 mg increments. This dose of everolimus is predicted to adjust the AUC to the range observed without inducers. However, there are no clinical data with this dose adjustment in patients receiving strong CYP3A4 inducers. If the strong inducer is discontinued, the everolimus dose should be returned to the dose used prior to initiation of the strong CYP3A4 inducer).

No products indexed under this heading.

Hydrocortisone Acetate (Co-administration of everolimus with strong CYP3A4 inducers (eg, dexamethasone, phenytoin, carbamazepine, rifampin, rifabutin, phenobarbital) should be avoided. If patients require co-administration of a strong CYP3A4 inducer, consider increasing the everolimus dose from 10 mg daily up to 20 mg daily (based on pharmacokinetic data), using 5 mg increments. This dose of everolimus is predicted to adjust the AUC to the range observed without inducers. However, there are no clinical data with this dose adjustment in patients receiving strong CYP3A4 inducers. If the strong inducer is discontinued, the everolimus dose should be returned to the dose used prior to initiation of the strong CYP3A4 inducer).

No products indexed under this heading.

Hydrocortisone Butyrate (Co-administration of everolimus with strong CYP3A4 inducers (eg, dexamethasone, phenytoin, carbamazepine, rifampin, rifabutin, phenobarbital) should be avoided. If patients require co-administration of a strong CYP3A4 inducer, consider increasing the everolimus dose from 10 mg daily up to 20 mg daily (based on pharmacokinetic data), using 5 mg increments. This dose of everolimus is predicted to adjust the AUC to the range observed without inducers. However, there are no clinical data with this dose adjustment in patients receiving strong CYP3A4 inducers. If the strong inducer is discontinued, the everolimus dose should be returned to the dose used prior to initiation of the strong CYP3A4 inducer).

No products indexed under this heading.

Hydrocortisone Cypionate (Co-administration of everolimus with strong CYP3A4 inducers (eg, dexamethasone, phenytoin, carbamazepine, rifampin, rifabutin, phenobarbital) should be avoided. If patients require co-administration of a strong CYP3A4 inducer, consider increasing the everolimus dose from 10 mg daily up to 20 mg daily (based on pharmacokinetic data), using 5 mg increments. This dose of everolimus is predicted to adjust the AUC to the range observed without inducers. However, there are no clinical data with this dose adjustment in patients receiving strong CYP3A4 inducers. If the strong inducer is discontinued, the everolimus dose should be returned to the dose used prior to initiation of the strong CYP3A4 inducer).

No products indexed under this heading.

Hydrocortisone Hemisuccinate (Co-administration of everolimus with strong CYP3A4 inducers (eg, dexamethasone, phenytoin, carbamazepine, rifampin, rifabutin, phenobarbital) should be avoided. If patients require co-administration of a strong CYP3A4 inducer, consider increasing the everolimus dose from 10 mg daily up to 20 mg daily (based on pharmacokinetic data), using 5 mg increments. This dose of everolimus is predicted to adjust the AUC to the range observed without inducers. However, there are no clinical data with this dose adjustment in patients receiving strong CYP3A4 inducers. If the strong inducer is discontinued, the everolimus dose should be returned to the dose used prior to initiation of the strong CYP3A4 inducer).

No products indexed under this heading.

Hydrocortisone Probutate (Co-administration of everolimus with strong CYP3A4 inducers (eg, dexamethasone, phenytoin, carbamazepine, rifampin, rifabutin, phenobarbital) should be avoided. If patients require co-administration of a strong CYP3A4 inducer, consider increasing the everolimus dose from 10 mg daily up to 20 mg daily (based on pharmacokinetic data), using 5 mg increments. This dose of everolimus is predicted to adjust the AUC to the range observed without inducers. However, there are no clinical data with this dose adjustment in patients receiving strong CYP3A4 inducers. If the strong inducer is discontinued, the everolimus dose should be returned to the dose used prior to initiation of the strong CYP3A4 inducer).

No products indexed under this heading.

Hydrocortisone Sodium Phosphate (Co-administration of everolimus with strong CYP3A4 inducers (eg, dexamethasone, phenytoin, carbamazepine, rifampin, rifabutin, phenobarbital) should be avoided. If patients require co-administration of a strong CYP3A4 inducer, consider increasing the everolimus dose from 10 mg daily up to 20 mg daily (based on pharmacokinetic data), using 5 mg increments. This dose of everolimus is predicted to adjust the AUC to the range observed without inducers. However, there are no clinical data with this dose adjustment in patients receiving strong CYP3A4 inducers. If the strong inducer is discontinued, the everolimus dose should be returned to the dose used prior to initiation of the strong CYP3A4 inducer).
    No products indexed under this heading.

Hydrocortisone Sodium Succinate (Co-administration of everolimus with strong CYP3A4 inducers (eg, dexamethasone, phenytoin, carbamazepine, rifampin, rifabutin, phenobarbital) should be avoided. If patients require co-administration of a strong CYP3A4 inducer, consider increasing the everolimus dose from 10 mg daily up to 20 mg daily (based on pharmacokinetic data), using 5 mg increments. This dose of everolimus is predicted to adjust the AUC to the range observed without inducers. However, there are no clinical data with this dose adjustment in patients receiving strong CYP3A4 inducers. If the strong inducer is discontinued, the everolimus dose should be returned to the dose used prior to initiation of the strong CYP3A4 inducer).
    No products indexed under this heading.

Hydrocortisone Valerate (Co-administration of everolimus with strong CYP3A4 inducers (eg, dexamethasone, phenytoin, carbamazepine, rifampin, rifabutin, phenobarbital) should be avoided. If patients require co-administration of a strong CYP3A4 inducer, consider increasing the everolimus dose from 10 mg daily up to 20 mg daily (based on pharmacokinetic data), using 5 mg increments. This dose of everolimus is predicted to adjust the AUC to the range observed without inducers. However, there are no clinical data with this dose adjustment in patients receiving strong CYP3A4 inducers. If the strong inducer is discontinued, the everolimus dose should be returned to the dose used prior to initiation of the strong CYP3A4 inducer).
    No products indexed under this heading.

Hypericum (Co-administration of everolimus with strong CYP3A4 inducers (eg, dexamethasone, phenytoin, carbamazepine, rifampin, rifabutin, phenobarbital) should be avoided. If patients require co-administration of a strong CYP3A4 inducer, consider increasing the everolimus dose from 10 mg daily up to 20 mg daily (based on pharmacokinetic data), using 5 mg increments. This dose of everolimus is predicted to adjust the AUC to the range observed without inducers. However, there are no clinical data with this dose adjustment in patients receiving strong CYP3A4 inducers. If the strong inducer is discontinued, the everolimus dose should be returned to the dose used prior to initiation of the strong CYP3A4 inducer).
    No products indexed under this heading.

Hypericum Perforatum (Co-administration of everolimus with strong CYP3A4 inducers (eg, dexamethasone, phenytoin, carbamazepine, rifampin, rifabutin, phenobarbital) should be avoided. If patients require co-administration of a strong CYP3A4 inducer, consider increasing the everolimus dose from 10 mg daily up to

20 mg daily (based on pharmacokinetic data), using 5 mg increments. This dose of everolimus is predicted to adjust the AUC to the range observed without inducers. However, there are no clinical data with this dose adjustment in patients receiving strong CYP3A4 inducers. If the strong inducer is discontinued, the everolimus dose should be returned to the dose used prior to initiation of the strong CYP3A4 inducer).
Products include:
    Traumeel 1800

Imatinib Mesylate (Co-administration of everolimus with strong or moderate inhibitors of CYP3A4 (eg, ketoconazole, itraconazole, clarithromycin, atazanavir, nefazodone, saquinavir, telithromycin, ritonavir, amprenavir, indinavir, nelfinavir, delavirdine, fosamprenavir, voriconazole, aprepitant, erythromycin, fluconazole, grapefruit juice, verapamil or diltazem) should be avoided due to significant increase in exposure of everolimus). Products include:
    Gleevec 2477

Indinavir Sulfate (Co-administration of everolimus with strong or moderate inhibitors of CYP3A4 (eg, ketoconazole, itraconazole, clarithromycin, atazanavir, nefazodone, saquinavir, telithromycin, ritonavir, amprenavir, indinavir, nelfinavir, delavirdine, fosamprenavir, voriconazole, aprepitant, erythromycin, fluconazole, grapefruit juice, verapamil or diltazem) should be avoided due to significant increase in exposure of everolimus). Products include:
    Crixivan 2113

Influenza Vaccine, Live Attenuated (The use of live vaccines and close contact with those who have received live vaccines should be avoided during treatment with everolimus).
    No products indexed under this heading.

Influenza Virus Vaccine Live, Intranasal (The use of live vaccines and close contact with those who have received live vaccines should be avoided during treatment with everolimus). Products include:
    FluMist 2078

Isoniazid (Co-administration of everolimus with strong or moderate inhibitors of CYP3A4 (eg, ketoconazole, itraconazole, clarithromycin, atazanavir, nefazodone, saquinavir, telithromycin, ritonavir, amprenavir, indinavir, nelfinavir, delavirdine, fosamprenavir, voriconazole, aprepitant, erythromycin, fluconazole, grapefruit juice, verapamil or diltazem) should be avoided due to significant increase in exposure of everolimus).
    No products indexed under this heading.

Itraconazole (Co-administration of everolimus with strong or moderate inhibitors of CYP3A4 (eg, ketoconazole, itraconazole, clarithromycin, atazanavir, nefazodone, saquinavir, telithromycin, ritonavir, amprenavir, indinavir, nelfinavir, delavirdine, fosamprenavir, voriconazole, aprepitant, erythromycin, fluconazole, grapefruit juice, verapamil or diltazem) should be avoided due to significant increase in exposure of everolimus).
    No products indexed under this heading.

Ketoconazole (Co-administration of everolimus with a strong CYP3A4 inhibitor and a PgP inhibitor (eg, ketoconazole) should be avoided. In healthy subjects, compared to everolimus treatment alone there were significant increases in everolimus exposure when everolimus was co-administered with ketoconazole. Everolimus C_{max} and AUC increased by 3.9- and 15.0-fold, respectively). Products include:
    Extina 3319
    Xolegel 3337

Lapatinib (Co-administration of everolimus with strong or moderate inhibitors of CYP3A4 (eg, ketoconazole, itraconazole, clarithromycin, atazanavir, nefazodone, saquinavir, telithromycin, ritonavir, amprenavir, indinavir, nelfinavir, delavirdine, fosamprenavir, voriconazole, aprepitant, erythromycin, fluconazole, grapefruit juice, verapamil or diltazem) should be avoided due to significant increase in exposure of everolimus). Products include:
    Tykerb 1698

Lopinavir (Co-administration of everolimus with strong or moderate inhibitors of CYP3A4 (eg, ketoconazole, itraconazole, clarithromycin, atazanavir, nefazodone, saquinavir, telithromycin, ritonavir, amprenavir, indinavir, nelfinavir, delavirdine, fosamprenavir, voriconazole, aprepitant, erythromycin, fluconazole, grapefruit juice, verapamil or diltazem) should be avoided due to significant increase in exposure of everolimus). Products include:
    Kaletra 458

Loratadine (Co-administration of everolimus with strong or moderate inhibitors of CYP3A4 (eg, ketoconazole, itraconazole, clarithromycin, atazanavir, nefazodone, saquinavir, telithromycin, ritonavir, amprenavir, indinavir, nelfinavir, delavirdine, fosamprenavir, voriconazole, aprepitant, erythromycin, fluconazole, grapefruit juice, verapamil or diltazem) should be avoided due to significant increase in exposure of everolimus).
    No products indexed under this heading.

Measles, Mumps, Rubella and Varicella Virus Vaccine Live (The use of live vaccines and close contact with those who have received live vaccines should be avoided during treatment with everolimus). Products include:
    ProQuad 2254

Measles, Mumps & Rubella Virus Vaccine, Live (The use of live vaccines and close contact with those who have received live vaccines should be avoided during treatment with everolimus). Products include:
    M-M-R II 2203
    ProQuad 2254

Measles & Rubella Virus Vaccine Live (The use of live vaccines and close contact with those who have received live vaccines should be avoided during treatment with everolimus).
    No products indexed under this heading.

Measles Virus Vaccine Live (The use of live vaccines and close contact with those who have received live vaccines should be avoided during treatment with everolimus). Products include:
    Attenuvax 2086

Mephenytoin (Co-administration of everolimus with strong CYP3A4 inducers (eg, dexamethasone, phenytoin, carbamazepine, rifampin, rifabutin, phenobarbital) should be avoided. If patients require co-administration of a strong CYP3A4 inducer, consider increasing the everolimus dose from 10 mg daily up to 20 mg daily (based on pharmacokinetic data), using 5 mg increments. This dose of everolimus is predicted to adjust the AUC to the range observed without inducers. However, there are no clinical data with this dose adjustment in patients receiving strong CYP3A4 inducers. If the strong inducer is discontinued, the everolimus dose should be returned to the dose used prior to initiation of the strong CYP3A4 inducer).
    No products indexed under this heading.

Methsuximide (Co-administration of everolimus with strong CYP3A4 inducers (eg, dexamethasone, phenytoin,

carbamazepine, rifampin, rifabutin, phenobarbital) should be avoided. If patients require co-administration of a strong CYP3A4 inducer, consider increasing the everolimus dose from 10 mg daily up to 20 mg daily (based on pharmacokinetic data), using 5 mg increments. This dose of everolimus is predicted to adjust the AUC to the range observed without inducers. However, there are no clinical data with this dose adjustment in patients receiving strong CYP3A4 inducers. If the strong inducer is discontinued, the everolimus dose should be returned to the dose used prior to initiation of the strong CYP3A4 inducer).
    No products indexed under this heading.

Methylprednisolone (Co-administration of everolimus with strong CYP3A4 inducers (eg, dexamethasone, phenytoin, carbamazepine, rifampin, rifabutin, phenobarbital) should be avoided. If patients require co-administration of a strong CYP3A4 inducer, consider increasing the everolimus dose from 10 mg daily up to 20 mg daily (based on pharmacokinetic data), using 5 mg increments. This dose of everolimus is predicted to adjust the AUC to the range observed without inducers. However, there are no clinical data with this dose adjustment in patients receiving strong CYP3A4 inducers. If the strong inducer is discontinued, the everolimus dose should be returned to the dose used prior to initiation of the strong CYP3A4 inducer).
    No products indexed under this heading.

Methylprednisolone Acetate (Co-administration of everolimus with strong CYP3A4 inducers (eg, dexamethasone, phenytoin, carbamazepine, rifampin, rifabutin, phenobarbital) should be avoided. If patients require co-administration of a strong CYP3A4 inducer, consider increasing the everolimus dose from 10 mg daily up to 20 mg daily (based on pharmacokinetic data), using 5 mg increments. This dose of everolimus is predicted to adjust the AUC to the range observed without inducers. However, there are no clinical data with this dose adjustment in patients receiving strong CYP3A4 inducers. If the strong inducer is discontinued, the everolimus dose should be returned to the dose used prior to initiation of the strong CYP3A4 inducer).
    No products indexed under this heading.

Methylprednisolone Sodium Succinate (Co-administration of everolimus with strong CYP3A4 inducers (eg, dexamethasone, phenytoin, carbamazepine, rifampin, rifabutin, phenobarbital) should be avoided. If patients require co-administration of a strong CYP3A4 inducer, consider increasing the everolimus dose from 10 mg daily up to 20 mg daily (based on pharmacokinetic data), using 5 mg increments. This dose of everolimus is predicted to adjust the AUC to the range observed without inducers. However, there are no clinical data with this dose adjustment in patients receiving strong CYP3A4 inducers. If the strong inducer is discontinued, the everolimus dose should be returned to the dose used prior to initiation of the strong CYP3A4 inducer).
    No products indexed under this heading.

Metronidazole (Co-administration of everolimus with strong or moderate inhibitors of CYP3A4 (eg, ketoconazole, itraconazole, clarithromycin, atazanavir, nefazodone, saquinavir, telithromycin, ritonavir, amprenavir, indinavir, nelfinavir, delavirdine, fosamprenavir, voriconazole, aprepitant, erythromycin, fluconazole, grapefruit juice, verapamil or diltazem) should be avoided due to significant increase in exposure of everolimus). Products include:

Pylera 793

Metronidazole Benzoate (Co-administration of everolimus with strong or moderate inhibitors of CYP3A4 (eg, ketoconazole, itraconazole, clarithromycin, atazanavir, nefazodone, saquinavir, telithromycin, ritonavir, amprenavir, indinavir, nelfinavir, delavirdine, fosamprenavir, voriconazole, aprepitant, erythromycin, fluconazole, grapefruit juice, verapamil or diltazem) should be avoided due to significant increase in exposure of everolimus).
No products indexed under this heading.

Metronidazole Hydrochloride (Co-administration of everolimus with strong or moderate inhibitors of CYP3A4 (eg, ketoconazole, itraconazole, clarithromycin, atazanavir, nefazodone, saquinavir, telithromycin, ritonavir, amprenavir, indinavir, nelfinavir, delavirdine, fosamprenavir, voriconazole, aprepitant, erythromycin, fluconazole, grapefruit juice, verapamil or diltazem) should be avoided due to significant increase in exposure of everolimus).
No products indexed under this heading.

Metronidazole Sodium (Co-administration of everolimus with strong or moderate inhibitors of CYP3A4 (eg, ketoconazole, itraconazole, clarithromycin, atazanavir, nefazodone, saquinavir, telithromycin, ritonavir, amprenavir, indinavir, nelfinavir, delavirdine, fosamprenavir, voriconazole, aprepitant, erythromycin, fluconazole, grapefruit juice, verapamil or diltazem) should be avoided due to significant increase in exposure of everolimus).
No products indexed under this heading.

Mibefradil Dihydrochloride (Co-administration of everolimus with P-glycoprotein (pgP) should be avoided due to significant increase in exposure of everolimus).
No products indexed under this heading.

Miconazole (Co-administration of everolimus with strong or moderate inhibitors of CYP3A4 (eg, ketoconazole, itraconazole, clarithromycin, atazanavir, nefazodone, saquinavir, telithromycin, ritonavir, amprenavir, indinavir, nelfinavir, delavirdine, fosamprenavir, voriconazole, aprepitant, erythromycin, fluconazole, grapefruit juice, verapamil or diltazem) should be avoided due to significant increase in exposure of everolimus).
No products indexed under this heading.

Miconazole Nitrate (Co-administration of everolimus with strong or moderate inhibitors of CYP3A4 (eg, ketoconazole, itraconazole, clarithromycin, atazanavir, nefazodone, saquinavir, telithromycin, ritonavir, amprenavir, indinavir, nelfinavir, delavirdine, fosamprenavir, voriconazole, aprepitant, erythromycin, fluconazole, grapefruit juice, verapamil or diltazem) should be avoided due to significant increase in exposure of everolimus). Products include:
Vusion Ointment 3335

Mifepristone (Co-administration of everolimus with strong or moderate inhibitors of CYP3A4 (eg, ketoconazole, itraconazole, clarithromycin, atazanavir, nefazodone, saquinavir, telithromycin, ritonavir, amprenavir, indinavir, nelfinavir, delavirdine, fosamprenavir, voriconazole, aprepitant, erythromycin, fluconazole, grapefruit juice, verapamil or diltazem) should be avoided due to significant increase in exposure of everolimus).
No products indexed under this heading.

Modafinil (Co-administration of everolimus with strong CYP3A4 inducers (eg, dexamethasone, phenytoin, carbamazepine, rifampin, rifabutin, phenobarbital) should be avoided. If patients require co-administration of a strong CYP3A4 inducer, consider increasing the everolimus dose from 10 mg daily up to 20 mg daily (based on pharmacokinetic data), using 5 mg increments. This dose of everolimus is predicted to adjust the AUC to the range observed without inducers. However, there are no clinical data with this dose adjustment in patients receiving strong CYP3A4 inducers. If the strong inducer is discontinued, the everolimus dose should be returned to the dose used prior to initiation of the strong CYP3A4 inducer). Products include:
Provigil 983

Mumps Virus Vaccine, Live (The use of live vaccines and close contact with those who have received live vaccines should be avoided during treatment with everolimus). Products include:
Mumpsvax 2218

Nafcillin Sodium (Co-administration of everolimus with strong CYP3A4 inducers (eg, dexamethasone, phenytoin, carbamazepine, rifampin, rifabutin, phenobarbital) should be avoided. If patients require co-administration of a strong CYP3A4 inducer, consider increasing the everolimus dose from 10 mg daily up to 20 mg daily (based on pharmacokinetic data), using 5 mg increments. This dose of everolimus is predicted to adjust the AUC to the range observed without inducers. However, there are no clinical data with this dose adjustment in patients receiving strong CYP3A4 inducers. If the strong inducer is discontinued, the everolimus dose should be returned to the dose used prior to initiation of the strong CYP3A4 inducer).
No products indexed under this heading.

Nefazodone Hydrochloride (Co-administration of everolimus with strong or moderate inhibitors of CYP3A4 (eg, ketoconazole, itraconazole, clarithromycin, atazanavir, nefazodone, saquinavir, telithromycin, ritonavir, amprenavir, indinavir, nelfinavir, delavirdine, fosamprenavir, voriconazole, aprepitant, erythromycin, fluconazole, grapefruit juice, verapamil or diltazem) should be avoided due to significant increase in exposure of everolimus).
No products indexed under this heading.

Nelfinavir Mesylate (Co-administration of everolimus with strong or moderate inhibitors of CYP3A4 (eg, ketoconazole, itraconazole, clarithromycin, atazanavir, nefazodone, saquinavir, telithromycin, ritonavir, amprenavir, indinavir, nelfinavir, delavirdine, fosamprenavir, voriconazole, aprepitant, erythromycin, fluconazole, grapefruit juice, verapamil or diltazem) should be avoided due to significant increase in exposure of everolimus).
No products indexed under this heading.

Nevirapine (Co-administration of everolimus with strong CYP3A4 inducers (eg, dexamethasone, phenytoin, carbamazepine, rifampin, rifabutin, phenobarbital) should be avoided. If patients require co-administration of a strong CYP3A4 inducer, consider increasing the everolimus dose from 10 mg daily up to 20 mg daily (based on pharmacokinetic data), using 5 mg increments. This dose of everolimus is predicted to adjust the AUC to the range observed without inducers. However, there are no clinical data with this dose adjustment in patients receiving strong CYP3A4 inducers. If the strong inducer is discontinued, the everolimus dose should be returned to the dose used prior to initiation of the strong CYP3A4 inducer). Products include:
Viramune Oral Suspension 897
Viramune Tablets 897

Niacin (Co-administration of everolimus with strong or moderate inhibitors of CYP3A4 (eg, ketoconazole, itraconazole, clarithromycin, atazanavir, nefazodone, saquinavir, telithromycin, ritonavir, amprenavir, indinavir, nelfinavir, delavirdine, fosamprenavir, voriconazole, aprepitant, erythromycin, fluconazole, grapefruit juice, verapamil or diltazem) should be avoided due to significant increase in exposure of everolimus). Products include:
Advicor 402
Cardio Basics 3455
Niaspan 497
Simcor 524

Niacinamide (Co-administration of everolimus with strong or moderate inhibitors of CYP3A4 (eg, ketoconazole, itraconazole, clarithromycin, atazanavir, nefazodone, saquinavir, telithromycin, ritonavir, amprenavir, indinavir, nelfinavir, delavirdine, fosamprenavir, voriconazole, aprepitant, erythromycin, fluconazole, grapefruit juice, verapamil or diltazem) should be avoided due to significant increase in exposure of everolimus). Products include:
CitraNatal 90 DHA Capsules 2332
CitraNatal Assure 2332
CitraNatal Rx 2332
Heplive 607

Niacinamide Hydroiodide (Co-administration of everolimus with strong or moderate inhibitors of CYP3A4 (eg, ketoconazole, itraconazole, clarithromycin, atazanavir, nefazodone, saquinavir, telithromycin, ritonavir, amprenavir, indinavir, nelfinavir, delavirdine, fosamprenavir, voriconazole, aprepitant, erythromycin, fluconazole, grapefruit juice, verapamil or diltazem) should be avoided due to significant increase in exposure of everolimus).
No products indexed under this heading.

Nicotinamide (Co-administration of everolimus with strong or moderate inhibitors of CYP3A4 (eg, ketoconazole, itraconazole, clarithromycin, atazanavir, nefazodone, saquinavir, telithromycin, ritonavir, amprenavir, indinavir, nelfinavir, delavirdine, fosamprenavir, voriconazole, aprepitant, erythromycin, fluconazole, grapefruit juice, verapamil or diltazem) should be avoided due to significant increase in exposure of everolimus).
No products indexed under this heading.

Nifedipine (Co-administration of everolimus with strong or moderate inhibitors of CYP3A4 (eg, ketoconazole, itraconazole, clarithromycin, atazanavir, nefazodone, saquinavir, telithromycin, ritonavir, amprenavir, indinavir, nelfinavir, delavirdine, fosamprenavir, voriconazole, aprepitant, erythromycin, fluconazole, grapefruit juice, verapamil or diltazem) should be avoided due to significant increase in exposure of everolimus).
No products indexed under this heading.

Norfloxacin (Co-administration of everolimus with strong or moderate inhibitors of CYP3A4 (eg, ketoconazole, itraconazole, clarithromycin, atazanavir, nefazodone, saquinavir, telithromycin, ritonavir, amprenavir, indinavir, nelfinavir, delavirdine, fosamprenavir, voriconazole, aprepitant, erythromycin, fluconazole, grapefruit juice, verapamil or diltazem) should be avoided due to significant increase in exposure of everolimus). Products include:
Noroxin 2220

Omeprazole (Co-administration of everolimus with strong or moderate inhibitors of CYP3A4 (eg, ketoconazole, itraconazole, clarithromycin, atazanavir, nefazodone, saquinavir, telithromycin, ritonavir, amprenavir, indinavir, nelfinavir, delavirdine, fosamprenavir, voriconazole, aprepitant, erythromycin, fluconazole, grapefruit juice, verapamil or diltazem) should be avoided due to significant increase in exposure of everolimus).
No products indexed under this heading.

Oxcarbazepine (Co-administration of everolimus with strong CYP3A4 inducers (eg, dexamethasone, phenytoin, carbamazepine, rifampin, rifabutin, phenobarbital) should be avoided. If patients require co-administration of a strong CYP3A4 inducer, consider increasing the everolimus dose from 10 mg daily up to 20 mg daily (based on pharmacokinetic data), using 5 mg increments. This dose of everolimus is predicted to adjust the AUC to the range observed without inducers. However, there are no clinical data with this dose adjustment in patients receiving strong CYP3A4 inducers. If the strong inducer is discontinued, the everolimus dose should be returned to the dose used prior to initiation of the strong CYP3A4 inducer).
No products indexed under this heading.

Paroxetine Hydrochloride (Co-administration of everolimus with strong or moderate inhibitors of CYP3A4 (eg, ketoconazole, itraconazole, clarithromycin, atazanavir, nefazodone, saquinavir, telithromycin, ritonavir, amprenavir, indinavir, nelfinavir, delavirdine, fosamprenavir, voriconazole, aprepitant, erythromycin, fluconazole, grapefruit juice, verapamil or diltazem) should be avoided due to significant increase in exposure of everolimus). Products include:
Paroxetine CR 2361
Paroxetine ER 2371
Paxil 1586
Paxil CR 1596

Phenobarbital (Co-administration of everolimus with strong CYP3A4 inducers (eg, dexamethasone, phenytoin, carbamazepine, rifampin, rifabutin, phenobarbital) should be avoided. If patients require co-administration of a strong CYP3A4 inducer, consider increasing the everolimus dose from 10 mg daily up to 20 mg daily (based on pharmacokinetic data), using 5 mg increments. This dose of everolimus is predicted to adjust the AUC to the range observed without inducers. However, there are no clinical data with this dose adjustment in patients receiving strong CYP3A4 inducers. If the strong inducer is discontinued, the everolimus dose should be returned to the dose used prior to initiation of the strong CYP3A4 inducer). Products include:
Donnatal 2711

Phenobarbital Sodium (Co-administration of everolimus with strong CYP3A4 inducers (eg, dexamethasone, phenytoin, carbamazepine, rifampin, rifabutin, phenobarbital) should be avoided. If patients require co-administration of a strong CYP3A4 inducer, consider increasing the everolimus dose from 10 mg daily up to 20 mg daily (based on pharmacokinetic data), using 5 mg increments. This dose of everolimus is predicted to adjust the AUC to the range observed without inducers. However, there are no clinical data with this dose adjustment in patients receiving strong CYP3A4 inducers. If the strong inducer is discontinued, the everolimus dose should be returned to the dose used prior to initiation of the strong CYP3A4 inducer).
No products indexed under this heading.

Phenytoin (Co-administration of everolimus with strong CYP3A4 inducers (eg, phenytoin) should be avoided. If patients require co-administration of a strong CYP3A4 inducer, consider increasing the everolimus dose from 10 mg daily up to 20 mg daily (based on pharmacokinetic data), using 5 mg increments. This dose of everolimus is

predicted to adjust the AUC to the range observed without inducers. However, there are no clinical data with this dose adjustment in patients receiving strong CYP3A4 inducers. If the strong inducer is discontinued, the everolimus dose should be returned to the dose used prior to initiation of the strong CYP3A4 inducer).
No products indexed under this heading.

Phenytoin Sodium (Co-administration of everolimus with strong CYP3A4 inducers (eg, phenytoin) should be avoided. If patients require co-administration of a strong CYP3A4 inducer, consider increasing the everolimus dose from 10 mg daily up to 20 mg daily (based on pharmacokinetic data), using 5 mg increments. This dose of everolimus is predicted to adjust the AUC to the range observed without inducers. However, there are no clinical data with this dose adjustment in patients receiving strong CYP3A4 inducers. If the strong inducer is discontinued, the everolimus dose should be returned to the dose used prior to initiation of the strong CYP3A4 inducer). Products include:
Phenytek Capsules 2380

Poliovirus Vaccine, Live, Oral, Trivalent, Types 1,2,3 (Sabin) (The use of live vaccines and close contact with those who have received live vaccines should be avoided during treatment with everolimus).
No products indexed under this heading.

Posaconazole (Co-administration of everolimus with strong or moderate inhibitors of CYP3A4 (eg, ketoconazole, itraconazole, clarithromycin, atazanavir, nefazodone, saquinavir, telithromycin, ritonavir, amprenavir, indinavir, nelfinavir, delavirdine, fosamprenavir, voriconazole, aprepitant, erythromycin, fluconazole, grapefruit juice, verapamil or diltazem) should be avoided due to significant increase in exposure of everolimus). Products include:
Noxafil 3172

Prednisolone (Co-administration of everolimus with strong CYP3A4 inducers (eg, dexamethasone, phenytoin, carbamazepine, rifampin, rifabutin, phenobarbital) should be avoided. If patients require co-administration of a strong CYP3A4 inducer, consider increasing the everolimus dose from 10 mg daily up to 20 mg daily (based on pharmacokinetic data), using 5 mg increments. This dose of everolimus is predicted to adjust the AUC to the range observed without inducers. However, there are no clinical data with this dose adjustment in patients receiving strong CYP3A4 inducers. If the strong inducer is discontinued, the everolimus dose should be returned to the dose used prior to initiation of the strong CYP3A4 inducer).
No products indexed under this heading.

Prednisolone Acetate (Co-administration of everolimus with strong CYP3A4 inducers (eg, dexamethasone, phenytoin, carbamazepine, rifampin, rifabutin, phenobarbital) should be avoided. If patients require co-administration of a strong CYP3A4 inducer, consider increasing the everolimus dose from 10 mg daily up to 20 mg daily (based on pharmacokinetic data), using 5 mg increments. This dose of everolimus is predicted to adjust the AUC to the range observed without inducers. However, there are no clinical data with this dose adjustment in patients receiving strong CYP3A4 inducers. If the strong inducer is discontinued, the everolimus dose should be returned to the dose used prior to initiation of the strong CYP3A4 inducer). Products include:
Blephamide .... ⊙212, ⊙214
Pred Forte .... ⊙225
Pred Mild .... ⊙230
Pred-G .... ⊙226, ⊙227

Prednisolone Sodium Phosphate (Co-administration of everolimus with strong CYP3A4 inducers (eg, dexamethasone, phenytoin, carbamazepine, rifampin, rifabutin, phenobarbital) should be avoided. If patients require co-administration of a strong CYP3A4 inducer, consider increasing the everolimus dose from 10 mg daily up to 20 mg daily (based on pharmacokinetic data), using 5 mg increments. This dose of everolimus is predicted to adjust the AUC to the range observed without inducers. However, there are no clinical data with this dose adjustment in patients receiving strong CYP3A4 inducers. If the strong inducer is discontinued, the everolimus dose should be returned to the dose used prior to initiation of the strong CYP3A4 inducer).
No products indexed under this heading.

Prednisolone Tebutate (Co-administration of everolimus with strong CYP3A4 inducers (eg, dexamethasone, phenytoin, carbamazepine, rifampin, rifabutin, phenobarbital) should be avoided. If patients require co-administration of a strong CYP3A4 inducer, consider increasing the everolimus dose from 10 mg daily up to 20 mg daily (based on pharmacokinetic data), using 5 mg increments. This dose of everolimus is predicted to adjust the AUC to the range observed without inducers. However, there are no clinical data with this dose adjustment in patients receiving strong CYP3A4 inducers. If the strong inducer is discontinued, the everolimus dose should be returned to the dose used prior to initiation of the strong CYP3A4 inducer).
No products indexed under this heading.

Prednisone (Co-administration of everolimus with strong CYP3A4 inducers (eg, dexamethasone, phenytoin, carbamazepine, rifampin, rifabutin, phenobarbital) should be avoided. If patients require co-administration of a strong CYP3A4 inducer, consider increasing the everolimus dose from 10 mg daily up to 20 mg daily (based on pharmacokinetic data), using 5 mg increments. This dose of everolimus is predicted to adjust the AUC to the range observed without inducers. However, there are no clinical data with this dose adjustment in patients receiving strong CYP3A4 inducers. If the strong inducer is discontinued, the everolimus dose should be returned to the dose used prior to initiation of the strong CYP3A4 inducer).
No products indexed under this heading.

Prednisone sodium phosphate (Co-administration of everolimus with strong CYP3A4 inducers (eg, dexamethasone, phenytoin, carbamazepine, rifampin, rifabutin, phenobarbital) should be avoided. If patients require co-administration of a strong CYP3A4 inducer, consider increasing the everolimus dose from 10 mg daily up to 20 mg daily (based on pharmacokinetic data), using 5 mg increments. This dose of everolimus is predicted to adjust the AUC to the range observed without inducers. However, there are no clinical data with this dose adjustment in patients receiving strong CYP3A4 inducers. If the strong inducer is discontinued, the everolimus dose should be returned to the dose used prior to initiation of the strong CYP3A4 inducer).
No products indexed under this heading.

Primidone (Co-administration of everolimus with strong CYP3A4 inducers (eg, dexamethasone, phenytoin, carbamazepine, rifampin, rifabutin, phenobarbital) should be avoided. If patients require co-administration of a strong CYP3A4 inducer, consider increasing the everolimus dose from 10 mg daily up to 20 mg daily (based on pharmacokinetic data), using 5 mg increments. This dose of everolimus is predicted to adjust the AUC to the range observed without inducers. However, there are no clinical data with this dose adjustment in patients receiving strong CYP3A4 inducers. If the strong inducer is discontinued, the everolimus dose should be returned to the dose used prior to initiation of the strong CYP3A4 inducer).
No products indexed under this heading.

Propoxyphene Hydrochloride (Co-administration of everolimus with strong or moderate inhibitors of CYP3A4 (eg, ketoconazole, itraconazole, clarithromycin, atazanavir, nefazodone, saquinavir, telithromycin, ritonavir, amprenavir, indinavir, nelfinavir, delavirdine, fosamprenavir, voriconazole, aprepitant, erythromycin, fluconazole, grapefruit juice, verapamil or diltazem) should be avoided due to significant increase in exposure of everolimus).
No products indexed under this heading.

Propoxyphene Napsylate (Co-administration of everolimus with strong or moderate inhibitors of CYP3A4 (eg, ketoconazole, itraconazole, clarithromycin, atazanavir, nefazodone, saquinavir, telithromycin, ritonavir, amprenavir, indinavir, nelfinavir, delavirdine, fosamprenavir, voriconazole, aprepitant, erythromycin, fluconazole, grapefruit juice, verapamil or diltazem) should be avoided due to significant increase in exposure of everolimus).
No products indexed under this heading.

Quinidine (Co-administration of everolimus with strong or moderate inhibitors of CYP3A4 (eg, ketoconazole, itraconazole, clarithromycin, atazanavir, nefazodone, saquinavir, telithromycin, ritonavir, amprenavir, indinavir, nelfinavir, delavirdine, fosamprenavir, voriconazole, aprepitant, erythromycin, fluconazole, grapefruit juice, verapamil or diltazem) should be avoided due to significant increase in exposure of everolimus).
No products indexed under this heading.

Quinidine Gluconate (Co-administration of everolimus with P-glycoprotein (pgP) should be avoided due to significant increase in exposure of everolimus).
No products indexed under this heading.

Quinidine Hydrochloride (Co-administration of everolimus with strong or moderate inhibitors of CYP3A4 (eg, ketoconazole, itraconazole, clarithromycin, atazanavir, nefazodone, saquinavir, telithromycin, ritonavir, amprenavir, indinavir, nelfinavir, delavirdine, fosamprenavir, voriconazole, aprepitant, erythromycin, fluconazole, grapefruit juice, verapamil or diltazem) should be avoided due to significant increase in exposure of everolimus).
No products indexed under this heading.

Quinidine Polygalacturonate (Co-administration of everolimus with strong or moderate inhibitors of CYP3A4 (eg, ketoconazole, itraconazole, clarithromycin, atazanavir, nefazodone, saquinavir, telithromycin, ritonavir, amprenavir, indinavir, nelfinavir, delavirdine, fosamprenavir, voriconazole, aprepitant, erythromycin, fluconazole, grapefruit juice, verapamil or diltazem) should be avoided due to significant increase in exposure of everolimus).
No products indexed under this heading.

Quinidine Sulfate (Co-administration of everolimus with strong or moderate inhibitors of CYP3A4 (eg, ketoconazole, itraconazole, clarithromycin, atazanavir, nefazodone, saquinavir, telithromycin, ritonavir, amprenavir, indinavir, nelfinavir, delavirdine, fosamprenavir, voriconazole, aprepitant, erythromycin, fluconazole, grapefruit juice, verapamil or diltazem) should be avoided due to significant increase in exposure of everolimus).
No products indexed under this heading.

Quinine (Co-administration of everolimus with strong or moderate inhibitors of CYP3A4 (eg, ketoconazole, itraconazole, clarithromycin, atazanavir, nefazodone, saquinavir, telithromycin, ritonavir, amprenavir, indinavir, nelfinavir, delavirdine, fosamprenavir, voriconazole, aprepitant, erythromycin, fluconazole, grapefruit juice, verapamil or diltazem) should be avoided due to significant increase in exposure of everolimus). Products include:
Hyland's Leg Cramps PM with Quinine 3315

Quinine Sulfate (Co-administration of everolimus with strong or moderate inhibitors of CYP3A4 (eg, ketoconazole, itraconazole, clarithromycin, atazanavir, nefazodone, saquinavir, telithromycin, ritonavir, amprenavir, indinavir, nelfinavir, delavirdine, fosamprenavir, voriconazole, aprepitant, erythromycin, fluconazole, grapefruit juice, verapamil or diltazem) should be avoided due to significant increase in exposure of everolimus).
No products indexed under this heading.

Quinupristin (Co-administration of everolimus with strong or moderate inhibitors of CYP3A4 (eg, ketoconazole, itraconazole, clarithromycin, atazanavir, nefazodone, saquinavir, telithromycin, ritonavir, amprenavir, indinavir, nelfinavir, delavirdine, fosamprenavir, voriconazole, aprepitant, erythromycin, fluconazole, grapefruit juice, verapamil or diltazem) should be avoided due to significant increase in exposure of everolimus).
No products indexed under this heading.

Ranitidine Bismuth Citrate (Co-administration of everolimus with strong or moderate inhibitors of CYP3A4 (eg, ketoconazole, itraconazole, clarithromycin, atazanavir, nefazodone, saquinavir, telithromycin, ritonavir, amprenavir, indinavir, nelfinavir, delavirdine, fosamprenavir, voriconazole, aprepitant, erythromycin, fluconazole, grapefruit juice, verapamil or diltazem) should be avoided due to significant increase in exposure of everolimus).
No products indexed under this heading.

Ranitidine Hydrochloride (Co-administration of everolimus with strong or moderate inhibitors of CYP3A4 (eg, ketoconazole, itraconazole, clarithromycin, atazanavir, nefazodone, saquinavir, telithromycin, ritonavir, amprenavir, indinavir, nelfinavir, delavirdine, fosamprenavir, voriconazole, aprepitant, erythromycin, fluconazole, grapefruit juice, verapamil or diltazem) should be avoided due to significant increase in exposure of everolimus). Products include:
Zantac 1737
Zantac Injection 1732
Zantac Pharmacy 1735

Rifabutin (Co-administration of everolimus with strong CYP3A4 inducers (eg, dexamethasone, phenytoin, carbamazepine, rifampin, rifabutin, phenobarbital) should be avoided. If patients require co-administration of a strong CYP3A4 inducer, consider increasing the everolimus dose from 10 mg daily up to 20 mg daily (based on pharmacokinetic data), using 5 mg increments. This dose of everolimus is predicted to adjust the AUC to the range observed without inducers. However, there are no clinical data with this dose adjustment in patients receiving strong CYP3A4 inducers. If the strong inducer is discon-

tinued, the everolimus dose should be returned to the dose used prior to initiation of the strong CYP3A4 inducer).

No products indexed under this heading.

Rifampicin (Co-administration of everolimus with strong CYP3A4 inducers (eg, dexamethasone, phenytoin, carbamazepine, rifampin, rifabutin, phenobarbital) should be avoided. If patients require co-administration of a strong CYP3A4 inducer, consider increasing the everolimus dose from 10 mg daily up to 20 mg daily (based on pharmacokinetic data), using 5 mg increments. This dose of everolimus is predicted to adjust the AUC to the range observed without inducers. However, there are no clinical data with this dose adjustment in patients receiving strong CYP3A4 inducers. If the strong inducer is discontinued, the everolimus dose should be returned to the dose used prior to initiation of the strong CYP3A4 inducer).

No products indexed under this heading.

Rifampin (Co-administration of everolimus with rifampin should be avoided. In healthy subjects, co-administration of everolimus with rifampin decreased everolimus AUC and C_{max} by 64% and 58% respectively, compared to everolimus treatment alone. Consider a dose increase of everolimus when co-administered with strong inducers of CYP3A4 or PgP if alternative treatment cannot be administered).

No products indexed under this heading.

Rifapentine (Co-administration of everolimus with strong CYP3A4 inducers (eg, dexamethasone, phenytoin, carbamazepine, rifampin, rifabutin, phenobarbital) should be avoided. If patients require co-administration of a strong CYP3A4 inducer, consider increasing the everolimus dose from 10 mg daily up to 20 mg daily (based on pharmacokinetic data), using 5 mg increments. This dose of everolimus is predicted to adjust the AUC to the range observed without inducers. However, there are no clinical data with this dose adjustment in patients receiving strong CYP3A4 inducers. If the strong inducer is discontinued, the everolimus dose should be returned to the dose used prior to initiation of the strong CYP3A4 inducer).

No products indexed under this heading.

Ritonavir (Co-administration of everolimus with strong or moderate inhibitors of CYP3A4 (eg, ketoconazole, itraconazole, clarithromycin, atazanavir, nefazodone, saquinavir, telithromycin, ritonavir, amprenavir, indinavir, nelfinavir, delavirdine, fosamprenavir, voriconazole, aprepitant, erythromycin, fluconazole, grapefruit juice, verapamil or diltazem) should be avoided due to significant increase in exposure of everolimus). Products include:

Kaletra 458
Norvir 509

Rotavirus Vaccine, Live, Oral, Tetravalent (The use of live vaccines and close contact with those who have received live vaccines should be avoided during treatment with everolimus).

No products indexed under this heading.

Rubella & Mumps Virus Vaccine Live (The use of live vaccines and close contact with those who have received live vaccines should be avoided during treatment with everolimus).

No products indexed under this heading.

Rubella Virus Vaccine Live (The use of live vaccines and close contact with those who have received live vaccines should be avoided during treatment with everolimus). Products include:

Meruvax II 2210

Saquinavir (Co-administration of everolimus with strong or moderate inhibitors of CYP3A4 (eg, ketoconazole, itraconazole, clarithromycin, atazanavir, nefazodone, saquinavir, telithromycin, ritonavir, amprenavir, indinavir, nelfinavir, delavirdine, fosamprenavir, voriconazole, aprepitant, erythromycin, fluconazole, grapefruit juice, verapamil or diltazem) should be avoided due to significant increase in exposure of everolimus).

No products indexed under this heading.

Saquinavir Mesylate (Co-administration of everolimus with strong or moderate inhibitors of CYP3A4 (eg, ketoconazole, itraconazole, clarithromycin, atazanavir, nefazodone, saquinavir, telithromycin, ritonavir, amprenavir, indinavir, nelfinavir, delavirdine, fosamprenavir, voriconazole, aprepitant, erythromycin, fluconazole, grapefruit juice, verapamil or diltazem) should be avoided due to significant increase in exposure of everolimus).

No products indexed under this heading.

Sertraline Hydrochloride (Co-administration of everolimus with strong or moderate inhibitors of CYP3A4 (eg, ketoconazole, itraconazole, clarithromycin, atazanavir, nefazodone, saquinavir, telithromycin, ritonavir, amprenavir, indinavir, nelfinavir, delavirdine, fosamprenavir, voriconazole, aprepitant, erythromycin, fluconazole, grapefruit juice, verapamil or diltazem) should be avoided due to significant increase in exposure of everolimus).

No products indexed under this heading.

Sildenafil Citrate (Co-administration of everolimus with strong or moderate inhibitors of CYP3A4 (eg, ketoconazole, itraconazole, clarithromycin, atazanavir, nefazodone, saquinavir, telithromycin, ritonavir, amprenavir, indinavir, nelfinavir, delavirdine, fosamprenavir, voriconazole, aprepitant, erythromycin, fluconazole, grapefruit juice, verapamil or diltazem) should be avoided due to significant increase in exposure of everolimus).

No products indexed under this heading.

Smallpox Vaccine (The use of live vaccines and close contact with those who have received live vaccines should be avoided during treatment with everolimus).

No products indexed under this heading.

Sulfinpyrazone (Co-administration of everolimus with strong CYP3A4 inducers (eg, dexamethasone, phenytoin, carbamazepine, rifampin, rifabutin, phenobarbital) should be avoided. If patients require co-administration of a strong CYP3A4 inducer, consider increasing the everolimus dose from 10 mg daily up to 20 mg daily (based on pharmacokinetic data), using 5 mg increments. This dose of everolimus is predicted to adjust the AUC to the range observed without inducers. However, there are no clinical data with this dose adjustment in patients receiving strong CYP3A4 inducers. If the strong inducer is discontinued, the everolimus dose should be returned to the dose used prior to initiation of the strong CYP3A4 inducer).

No products indexed under this heading.

Tamoxifen Citrate (Co-administration of everolimus with P-glycoprotein (pgP) should be avoided due to significant increase in exposure of everolimus).

No products indexed under this heading.

Telithromycin (Co-administration of everolimus with strong or moderate inhibitors of CYP3A4 (eg, ketoconazole, itraconazole, clarithromycin, atazanavir, nefazodone, saquinavir, telithromycin, ritonavir, amprenavir, indinavir, nelfinavir, delavirdine, fosamprenavir, voriconazole, aprepitant, erythromycin,

fluconazole, grapefruit juice, verapamil or diltazem) should be avoided due to significant increase in exposure of everolimus). Products include:

Ketek 2991

Theophyllinate (Co-administration of everolimus with strong CYP3A4 inducers (eg, dexamethasone, phenytoin, carbamazepine, rifampin, rifabutin, phenobarbital) should be avoided. If patients require co-administration of a strong CYP3A4 inducer, consider increasing the everolimus dose from 10 mg daily up to 20 mg daily (based on pharmacokinetic data), using 5 mg increments. This dose of everolimus is predicted to adjust the AUC to the range observed without inducers. However, there are no clinical data with this dose adjustment in patients receiving strong CYP3A4 inducers. If the strong inducer is discontinued, the everolimus dose should be returned to the dose used prior to initiation of the strong CYP3A4 inducer).

No products indexed under this heading.

Theophylline (Co-administration of everolimus with strong CYP3A4 inducers (eg, dexamethasone, phenytoin, carbamazepine, rifampin, rifabutin, phenobarbital) should be avoided. If patients require co-administration of a strong CYP3A4 inducer, consider increasing the everolimus dose from 10 mg daily up to 20 mg daily (based on pharmacokinetic data), using 5 mg increments. This dose of everolimus is predicted to adjust the AUC to the range observed without inducers. However, there are no clinical data with this dose adjustment in patients receiving strong CYP3A4 inducers. If the strong inducer is discontinued, the everolimus dose should be returned to the dose used prior to initiation of the strong CYP3A4 inducer).

No products indexed under this heading.

Theophylline Anhydrous (Co-administration of everolimus with strong CYP3A4 inducers (eg, dexamethasone, phenytoin, carbamazepine, rifampin, rifabutin, phenobarbital) should be avoided. If patients require co-administration of a strong CYP3A4 inducer, consider increasing the everolimus dose from 10 mg daily up to 20 mg daily (based on pharmacokinetic data), using 5 mg increments. This dose of everolimus is predicted to adjust the AUC to the range observed without inducers. However, there are no clinical data with this dose adjustment in patients receiving strong CYP3A4 inducers. If the strong inducer is discontinued, the everolimus dose should be returned to the dose used prior to initiation of the strong CYP3A4 inducer). Products include:

Uniphyl 2817

Theophylline Calcium Salicylate (Co-administration of everolimus with strong CYP3A4 inducers (eg, dexamethasone, phenytoin, carbamazepine, rifampin, rifabutin, phenobarbital) should be avoided. If patients require co-administration of a strong CYP3A4 inducer, consider increasing the everolimus dose from 10 mg daily up to 20 mg daily (based on pharmacokinetic data), using 5 mg increments. This dose of everolimus is predicted to adjust the AUC to the range observed without inducers. However, there are no clinical data with this dose adjustment in patients receiving strong CYP3A4 inducers. If the strong inducer is discontinued, the everolimus dose should be returned to the dose used prior to initiation of the strong CYP3A4 inducer).

No products indexed under this heading.

Theophylline Dihydroxypropyl (Glyceryl) (Co-administration of everolimus with strong CYP3A4 induc-

ers (eg, dexamethasone, phenytoin, carbamazepine, rifampin, rifabutin, phenobarbital) should be avoided. If patients require co-administration of a strong CYP3A4 inducer, consider increasing the everolimus dose from 10 mg daily up to 20 mg daily (based on pharmacokinetic data), using 5 mg increments. This dose of everolimus is predicted to adjust the AUC to the range observed without inducers. However, there are no clinical data with this dose adjustment in patients receiving strong CYP3A4 inducers. If the strong inducer is discontinued, the everolimus dose should be returned to the dose used prior to initiation of the strong CYP3A4 inducer).

No products indexed under this heading.

Theophylline Ethylenediamine (Co-administration of everolimus with strong CYP3A4 inducers (eg, dexamethasone, phenytoin, carbamazepine, rifampin, rifabutin, phenobarbital) should be avoided. If patients require co-administration of a strong CYP3A4 inducer, consider increasing the everolimus dose from 10 mg daily up to 20 mg daily (based on pharmacokinetic data), using 5 mg increments. This dose of everolimus is predicted to adjust the AUC to the range observed without inducers. However, there are no clinical data with this dose adjustment in patients receiving strong CYP3A4 inducers. If the strong inducer is discontinued, the everolimus dose should be returned to the dose used prior to initiation of the strong CYP3A4 inducer).

No products indexed under this heading.

Theophylline Sodium Glycinate (Co-administration of everolimus with strong CYP3A4 inducers (eg, dexamethasone, phenytoin, carbamazepine, rifampin, rifabutin, phenobarbital) should be avoided. If patients require co-administration of a strong CYP3A4 inducer, consider increasing the everolimus dose from 10 mg daily up to 20 mg daily (based on pharmacokinetic data), using 5 mg increments. This dose of everolimus is predicted to adjust the AUC to the range observed without inducers. However, there are no clinical data with this dose adjustment in patients receiving strong CYP3A4 inducers. If the strong inducer is discontinued, the everolimus dose should be returned to the dose used prior to initiation of the strong CYP3A4 inducer).

No products indexed under this heading.

Triamcinolone (Co-administration of everolimus with strong CYP3A4 inducers (eg, dexamethasone, phenytoin, carbamazepine, rifampin, rifabutin, phenobarbital) should be avoided. If patients require co-administration of a strong CYP3A4 inducer, consider increasing the everolimus dose from 10 mg daily up to 20 mg daily (based on pharmacokinetic data), using 5 mg increments. This dose of everolimus is predicted to adjust the AUC to the range observed without inducers. However, there are no clinical data with this dose adjustment in patients receiving strong CYP3A4 inducers. If the strong inducer is discontinued, the everolimus dose should be returned to the dose used prior to initiation of the strong CYP3A4 inducer).

No products indexed under this heading.

Triamcinolone Acetonide (Co-administration of everolimus with strong CYP3A4 inducers (eg, dexamethasone, phenytoin, carbamazepine, rifampin, rifabutin, phenobarbital) should be avoided. If patients require co-administration of a strong CYP3A4 inducer, consider increasing the everolimus dose from 10 mg daily up to 20 mg daily (based on pharmacokinetic data), using 5 mg increments. This

dose of everolimus is predicted to adjust the AUC to the range observed without inducers. However, there are no clinical data with this dose adjustment in patients receiving strong CYP3A4 inducers. If the strong inducer is discontinued, the everolimus dose should be returned to the dose used prior to initiation of the strong CYP3A4 inducer). Products include:
Azmacort 408
Nasacort AQ 3019

Triamcinolone Diacetate (Co-administration of everolimus with strong CYP3A4 inducers (eg, dexamethasone, phenytoin, carbamazepine, rifampin, rifabutin, phenobarbital) should be avoided. If patients require co-administration of a strong CYP3A4 inducer, consider increasing the everolimus dose from 10 mg daily up to 20 mg daily (based on pharmacokinetic data), using 5 mg increments. This dose of everolimus is predicted to adjust the AUC to the range observed without inducers. However, there are no clinical data with this dose adjustment in patients receiving strong CYP3A4 inducers. If the strong inducer is discontinued, the everolimus dose should be returned to the dose used prior to initiation of the strong CYP3A4 inducer).
No products indexed under this heading.

Triamcinolone Hexacetonide (Co-administration of everolimus with strong CYP3A4 inducers (eg, dexamethasone, phenytoin, carbamazepine, rifampin, rifabutin, phenobarbital) should be avoided. If patients require co-administration of a strong CYP3A4 inducer, consider increasing the everolimus dose from 10 mg daily up to 20 mg daily (based on pharmacokinetic data), using 5 mg increments. This dose of everolimus is predicted to adjust the AUC to the range observed without inducers. However, there are no clinical data with this dose adjustment in patients receiving strong CYP3A4 inducers. If the strong inducer is discontinued, the everolimus dose should be returned to the dose used prior to initiation of the strong CYP3A4 inducer).
No products indexed under this heading.

Troglitazone (Co-administration of everolimus with strong CYP3A4 inducers (eg, dexamethasone, phenytoin, carbamazepine, rifampin, rifabutin, phenobarbital) should be avoided. If patients require co-administration of a strong CYP3A4 inducer, consider increasing the everolimus dose from 10 mg daily up to 20 mg daily (based on pharmacokinetic data), using 5 mg increments. This dose of everolimus is predicted to adjust the AUC to the range observed without inducers. However, there are no clinical data with this dose adjustment in patients receiving strong CYP3A4 inducers. If the strong inducer is discontinued, the everolimus dose should be returned to the dose used prior to initiation of the strong CYP3A4 inducer).
No products indexed under this heading.

Troleandomycin (Co-administration of everolimus with strong or moderate inhibitors of CYP3A4 (eg, ketoconazole, itraconazole, clarithromycin, atazanavir, nefazodone, saquinavir, telithromycin, ritonavir, amprenavir, indinavir, nelfinavir, delavirdine, fosamprenavir, voriconazole, aprepitant, erythromycin, fluconazole, grapefruit juice, verapamil or diltazem) should be avoided due to significant increase in exposure of everolimus).
No products indexed under this heading.

Typhoid Vaccine (The use of live vaccines and close contact with those who have received live vaccines should be avoided during treatment with everolimus).
No products indexed under this heading.

Valproate Sodium (Co-administration of everolimus with strong or moderate inhibitors of CYP3A4 (eg, ketoconazole, itraconazole, clarithromycin, atazanavir, nefazodone, saquinavir, telithromycin, ritonavir, amprenavir, indinavir, nelfinavir, delavirdine, fosamprenavir, voriconazole, aprepitant, erythromycin, fluconazole, grapefruit juice, verapamil or diltazem) should be avoided due to significant increase in exposure of everolimus).
No products indexed under this heading.

Vardenafil Hydrochloride (Co-administration of everolimus with strong or moderate inhibitors of CYP3A4 (eg, ketoconazole, itraconazole, clarithromycin, atazanavir, nefazodone, saquinavir, telithromycin, ritonavir, amprenavir, indinavir, nelfinavir, delavirdine, fosamprenavir, voriconazole, aprepitant, erythromycin, fluconazole, grapefruit juice, verapamil or diltazem) should be avoided due to significant increase in exposure of everolimus). Products include:
Levitra 3157

Varicella Virus Vaccine, Live (The use of live vaccines and close contact with those who have received live vaccines should be avoided during treatment with everolimus). Products include:
Varivax 2285

Verapamil Hydrochloride (Co-administration of everolimus with a moderate CYP3A4 inhibitor and a PgP inhibitor (eg, verapamil) should be avoided. In healthy subjects, compared to everolimus treatment alone there were significant increases in everolimus exposure when everolimus was co-administered with verapamil. Everolimus C_{max} and AUC increased by 2.3-and 3.5-fold, respectively). Products include:
Tarka 534

Voriconazole (Co-administration of everolimus with strong or moderate inhibitors of CYP3A4 (eg, ketoconazole, itraconazole, clarithromycin, atazanavir, nefazodone, saquinavir, telithromycin, ritonavir, amprenavir, indinavir, nelfinavir, delavirdine, fosamprenavir, voriconazole, aprepitant, erythromycin, fluconazole, grapefruit juice, verapamil or diltazem) should be avoided due to significant increase in exposure of everolimus).
No products indexed under this heading.

Yellow Fever Vaccine (The use of live vaccines and close contact with those who have received live vaccines should be avoided during treatment with everolimus).
No products indexed under this heading.

Zafirlukast (Co-administration of everolimus with strong or moderate inhibitors of CYP3A4 (eg, ketoconazole, itraconazole, clarithromycin, atazanavir, nefazodone, saquinavir, telithromycin, ritonavir, amprenavir, indinavir, nelfinavir, delavirdine, fosamprenavir, voriconazole, aprepitant, erythromycin, fluconazole, grapefruit juice, verapamil or diltazem) should be avoided due to significant increase in exposure of everolimus). Products include:
Accolate 3612

Zileuton (Co-administration of everolimus with strong or moderate inhibitors of CYP3A4 (eg, ketoconazole, itraconazole, clarithromycin, atazanavir, nefazodone, saquinavir, telithromycin, ritonavir, amprenavir, indinavir, nelfinavir, delavirdine, fosamprenavir, voriconazole, aprepitant, erythromycin, fluconazole, grapefruit juice, verapamil or diltazem) should be avoided due to significant increase in exposure of everolimus).
No products indexed under this heading.

Zoster Vaccine Live (The use of live vaccines and close contact with those who have received live vaccines should be avoided during treatment with everolimus). Products include:
Zostavax 2299

Food Interactions

Food, unspecified (Based on data in healthy subjects taking 1 mg everolimus tablets, a high-fat meal reduced C_{max} and AUC by 60% and 16%, respectively. No data are available with everolimus 5 mg and 10 mg tablets).

Grapefruit (Co-administration of everolimus with strong or moderate inhibitors of CYP3A4 (eg, ketoconazole, itraconazole, clarithromycin, atazanavir, nefazodone, saquinavir, telithromycin, ritonavir, amprenavir, indinavir, nelfinavir, delavirdine, fosamprenavir, voriconazole, aprepitant, erythromycin, fluconazole, grapefruit juice, verapamil or diltazem) should be avoided due to significant increase in exposure of everolimus).

Grapefruit Juice (Co-administration of everolimus with strong or moderate inhibitors of CYP3A4 (eg, ketoconazole, itraconazole, clarithromycin, atazanavir, nefazodone, saquinavir, telithromycin, ritonavir, amprenavir, indinavir, nelfinavir, delavirdine, fosamprenavir, voriconazole, aprepitant, erythromycin, fluconazole, grapefruit juice, verapamil or diltazem) should be avoided due to significant increase in exposure of everolimus).

Meal, unspecified (Based on data in healthy subjects taking 1 mg everolimus tablets, a high-fat meal reduced C_{max} and AUC by 60% and 16%, respectively. No data are available with everolimus 5 mg and 10 mg tablets).

AGGRENOX CAPSULES

(Aspirin, Dipyridamole) 880

May interact with ACE inhibitors, alcohols, anticholinesterase drugs, anticoagulants, beta-blockers, diuretics, nonsteroidal anti-inflammatory agents, oral hypoglycemic agents, phenytoin, valproate, and certain other agents. Compounds in these categories include:

Acarbose (Moderate doses of aspirin may increase the effectiveness of renal hypoglycemic drugs, leading to hypoglycemia).
No products indexed under this heading.

Acebutolol Hydrochloride (The hypertensive effects of beta-blockers may be diminished by the concomitant administration of aspirin due to inhibition of renal prostaglandins, leading to decreased renal blood flow and salt and fluid retention).
No products indexed under this heading.

Acetazolamide (Co-administration can lead to high serum concentrations of acetazolamide (and toxicity) due to competition at the renal tube for secretion).
No products indexed under this heading.

Acetazolamide Sodium (Co-administration can lead to high serum concentrations of acetazolamide (and toxicity) due to competition at the renal tube for secretion).
No products indexed under this heading.

Adenosine (Dipyridamole has been reported to increase the plasma levels and cardiovascular effects of adenosine). Products include:
Adenocard 656
Adenoscan 657

Amiloride Hydrochloride (The effectiveness of diuretics in patients with underlying renal or cardiovascular disease may be diminished by co-administration of aspirin due to inhibition of renal prostaglandins, leading to decreased renal blood flow and salt and fluid retention).
No products indexed under this heading.

Anisindione (Patients on anticoagulation therapy are at risk for bleeding).
No products indexed under this heading.

Ardeparin Sodium (Patients on anticoagulation therapy are at risk for bleeding).
No products indexed under this heading.

Atenolol (The hypertensive effects of beta-blockers may be diminished by the concomitant administration of aspirin due to inhibition of renal prostaglandins, leading to decreased renal blood flow and salt and fluid retention).
No products indexed under this heading.

Benazepril Hydrochloride (Co-administration can result in diminished hypotensive and hyponatremic effects of ACE inhibitors due to the effect of aspirin on the renin-angiotensin conversion pathway).
No products indexed under this heading.

Bendroflumethiazide (The effectiveness of diuretics in patients with underlying renal or cardiovascular disease may be diminished by co-administration of aspirin due to inhibition of renal prostaglandins, leading to decreased renal blood flow and salt and fluid retention).
No products indexed under this heading.

Betaxolol Hydrochloride (The hypertensive effects of beta-blockers may be diminished by the concomitant administration of aspirin due to inhibition of renal prostaglandins, leading to decreased renal blood flow and salt and fluid retention).
No products indexed under this heading.

Bisoprolol Fumarate (The hypertensive effects of beta-blockers may be diminished by the concomitant administration of aspirin due to inhibition of renal prostaglandins, leading to decreased renal blood flow and salt and fluid retention).
No products indexed under this heading.

Bumetanide (The effectiveness of diuretics in patients with underlying renal or cardiovascular disease may be diminished by co-administration of aspirin due to inhibition of renal prostaglandins, leading to decreased renal blood flow and salt and fluid retention).
No products indexed under this heading.

Captopril (Co-administration can result in diminished hypotensive and hyponatremic effects of ACE inhibitors due to the effect of aspirin on the renin-angiotensin conversion pathway). Products include:
Captopril 2341

Carteolol Hydrochloride (The hypertensive effects of beta-blockers may be diminished by the concomitant administration of aspirin due to inhibition of renal prostaglandins, leading to decreased renal blood flow and salt and fluid retention).
No products indexed under this heading.

Carvedilol (The hypertensive effects of beta-blockers may be diminished by the concomitant administration of aspirin due to inhibition of renal prostaglandins, leading to decreased renal blood flow and salt and fluid retention). Products include:
Coreg 1409

Carvedilol Phosphate (The hypertensive effects of beta-blockers may be diminished by the concomitant administration of aspirin due to inhibition of

renal prostaglandins, leading to decreased renal blood flow and salt and fluid retention). Products include:
Coreg CR 1416

Celecoxib (Co-administration of non-steroidal anti-inflammatory drugs with aspirin may increase bleeding or lead to decreased renal function). Products include:
Celebrex 3272

Chlorothiazide (The effectiveness of diuretics in patients with underlying renal or cardiovascular disease may be diminished by co-administration of aspirin due to inhibition of renal prostaglandins, leading to decreased renal blood flow and salt and fluid retention).
No products indexed under this heading.

Chlorothiazide Sodium (The effectiveness of diuretics in patients with underlying renal or cardiovascular disease may be diminished by co-administration of aspirin due to inhibition of renal prostaglandins, leading to decreased renal blood flow and salt and fluid retention). Products include:
Diuril Intravenous 2009

Chlorpropamide (Moderate doses of aspirin may increase the effectiveness of renal hypoglycemic drugs, leading to hypoglycemia).
No products indexed under this heading.

Chlorthalidone (The effectiveness of diuretics in patients with underlying renal or cardiovascular disease may be diminished by co-administration of aspirin due to inhibition of renal prostaglandins, leading to decreased renal blood flow and salt and fluid retention). Products include:
Clorpres 2344

Dalteparin Sodium (Patients on anticoagulation therapy are at risk for bleeding). Products include:
Fragmin 1058

Danaparoid Sodium (Patients on anticoagulation therapy are at risk for bleeding).
No products indexed under this heading.

Diclofenac Epolamine (Co-administration of non-steroidal anti-inflammatory drugs with aspirin may increase bleeding or lead to decreased renal function). Products include:
Flector 1839

Diclofenac Potassium (Co-administration of non-steroidal anti-inflammatory drugs with aspirin may increase bleeding or lead to decreased renal function).
No products indexed under this heading.

Diclofenac Sodium (Co-administration of non-steroidal anti-inflammatory drugs with aspirin may increase bleeding or lead to decreased renal function).
No products indexed under this heading.

Dicumarol (Patients on anticoagulation therapy are at risk for bleeding).
No products indexed under this heading.

Divalproex Sodium (Salicylic acid can displace protein-bound valproic acid leading to an increase in serum valproic acid levels). Products include:
Depakote ER 426

Donepezil Hydrochloride (Dipyridamole may counteract the anticholinesterase effect of cholinesterase inhibitors, thereby potentially aggravating myasthenia gravis). Products include:
Aricept 1045
Aricept ODT 1045

Edrophonium Chloride (Dipyridamole may counteract the anticholinesterase effect of cholinesterase inhibitors, thereby potentially aggravating myasthenia gravis).
No products indexed under this heading.

Enalapril Maleate (Co-administration can result in diminished hypotensive and hyponatremic effects of ACE inhibitors due to the effect of aspirin on the renin-angiotensin conversion pathway).
No products indexed under this heading.

Enalaprilat (Co-administration can result in diminished hypotensive and hyponatremic effects of ACE inhibitors due to the effect of aspirin on the renin-angiotensin conversion pathway).
No products indexed under this heading.

Enoxaparin Sodium (Patients on anticoagulation therapy are at risk for bleeding). Products include:
Lovenox 3005

Esmolol Hydrochloride (The hypertensive effects of beta-blockers may be diminished by the concomitant administration of aspirin due to inhibition of renal prostaglandins, leading to decreased renal blood flow and salt and fluid retention).
No products indexed under this heading.

Ethacrynic Acid (The effectiveness of diuretics in patients with underlying renal or cardiovascular disease may be diminished by co-administration of aspirin due to inhibition of renal prostaglandins, leading to decreased renal blood flow and salt and fluid retention).
No products indexed under this heading.

Ethanol (Patients who consume three or more alcoholic drinks every day should be counseled about the bleeding risks involved with chronic, heavy alcohol use while taking aspirin).
No products indexed under this heading.

Ethyl Alcohol (Patients who consume three or more alcoholic drinks every day should be counseled about the bleeding risks involved with chronic, heavy alcohol use while taking aspirin).
No products indexed under this heading.

Etodolac (Co-administration of non-steroidal anti-inflammatory drugs with aspirin may increase bleeding or lead to decreased renal function).
No products indexed under this heading.

Fenoprofen Calcium (Co-administration of non-steroidal anti-inflammatory drugs with aspirin may increase bleeding or lead to decreased renal function).
No products indexed under this heading.

Flurbiprofen (Co-administration of non-steroidal anti-inflammatory drugs with aspirin may increase bleeding or lead to decreased renal function).
No products indexed under this heading.

Fondaparinux Sodium (Patients on anticoagulation therapy are at risk for bleeding). Products include:
Arixtra 1320

Fosinopril Sodium (Co-administration can result in diminished hypotensive and hyponatremic effects of ACE inhibitors due to the effect of aspirin on the renin-angiotensin conversion pathway).
No products indexed under this heading.

Fosphenytoin (Salicylic acid can displace protein-bound phenytoin leading to a decrease in the total concentration of phenytoin).
No products indexed under this heading.

Fosphenytoin Sodium (Salicylic acid can displace protein-bound phenytoin leading to a decrease in the total concentration of phenytoin).
No products indexed under this heading.

Furosemide (The effectiveness of diuretics in patients with underlying renal or cardiovascular disease may be diminished by co-administration of aspirin due to inhibition of renal prostaglandins, leading to decreased renal blood flow and salt and fluid retention). Products include:
Furosemide 2354

Galantamine Hydrobromide (Dipyridamole may counteract the anticholinesterase effect of cholinesterase inhibitors, thereby potentially aggravating myasthenia gravis).
No products indexed under this heading.

Glibenclamide (Moderate doses of aspirin may increase the effectiveness of renal hypoglycemic drugs, leading to hypoglycemia).
No products indexed under this heading.

Glimepiride (Moderate doses of aspirin may increase the effectiveness of renal hypoglycemic drugs, leading to hypoglycemia). Products include:
Avandaryl 1356
Duetact 3354

Glipizide (Moderate doses of aspirin may increase the effectiveness of renal hypoglycemic drugs, leading to hypoglycemia).
No products indexed under this heading.

Glyburide (Moderate doses of aspirin may increase the effectiveness of renal hypoglycemic drugs, leading to hypoglycemia).
No products indexed under this heading.

Heparin Calcium (Patients on anticoagulation therapy are at risk for bleeding).
No products indexed under this heading.

Heparin Sodium (Aspirin can increase the anticoagulant activity of heparin, increasing bleeding risk).
No products indexed under this heading.

Hydrochlorothiazide (The effectiveness of diuretics in patients with underlying renal or cardiovascular disease may be diminished by co-administration of aspirin due to inhibition of renal prostaglandins, leading to decreased renal blood flow and salt and fluid retention). Products include:
Atacand HCT 700
Avalide 2956
Benicar HCT 1017
Diovan HCT 2419
Dyazide 1429
Exforge HCT 2449
Hyzaar 2162
Hyzaar 100-12.5 2162
Micardis HCT 889
Prinzide 2246
Tekturna HCT 2541
Teveten HCT 541

Hydroflumethiazide (The effectiveness of diuretics in patients with underlying renal or cardiovascular disease may be diminished by co-administration of aspirin due to inhibition of renal prostaglandins, leading to decreased renal blood flow and salt and fluid retention).
No products indexed under this heading.

Ibuprofen (Co-administration of non-steroidal anti-inflammatory drugs with aspirin may increase bleeding or lead to decreased renal function). Products include:
Motrin IB 2043
Children's Motrin 2044
Children's Motrin Non-Staining Dye-Free 2044
Infants' Motrin 2044
Infants' Motrin Dye-Free 2044
Junior Strength Motrin 2044
Vicoprofen 564

Indapamide (The effectiveness of diuretics in patients with underlying renal or cardiovascular disease may be diminished by co-administration of aspirin due to inhibition of renal prostaglandins, leading to decreased renal blood flow and salt and fluid retention). Products include:
Indapamide 2356

Indomethacin (Co-administration of non-steroidal anti-inflammatory drugs with aspirin may increase bleeding or lead to decreased renal function). Products include:
Indocin 2167

Indomethacin Sodium Trihydrate (Co-administration of non-steroidal anti-inflammatory drugs with aspirin may increase bleeding or lead to decreased renal function). Products include:
Indocin I.V. 2007

Ketoprofen (Co-administration of non-steroidal anti-inflammatory drugs with aspirin may increase bleeding or lead to decreased renal function).
No products indexed under this heading.

Ketorolac Tromethamine (Co-administration of non-steroidal anti-inflammatory drugs with aspirin may increase bleeding or lead to decreased renal function). Products include:
Acuvail .... ⊙209

Labetalol Hydrochloride (The hypertensive effects of beta-blockers may be diminished by the concomitant administration of aspirin due to inhibition of renal prostaglandins, leading to decreased renal blood flow and salt and fluid retention).
No products indexed under this heading.

Levobunolol Hydrochloride (The hypertensive effects of beta-blockers may be diminished by the concomitant administration of aspirin due to inhibition of renal prostaglandins, leading to decreased renal blood flow and salt and fluid retention).
No products indexed under this heading.

Lisinopril (Co-administration can result in diminished hypotensive and hyponatremic effects of ACE inhibitors due to the effect of aspirin on the renin-angiotensin conversion pathway). Products include:
Prinivil 2241
Prinzide 2246

Low Molecular Weight Heparins (Patients on anticoagulation therapy are at risk for bleeding).
No products indexed under this heading.

Meclofenamate Sodium (Co-administration of non-steroidal anti-inflammatory drugs with aspirin may increase bleeding or lead to decreased renal function).
No products indexed under this heading.

Mefenamic Acid (Co-administration of non-steroidal anti-inflammatory drugs with aspirin may increase bleeding or lead to decreased renal function).
No products indexed under this heading.

Meloxicam (Co-administration of non-steroidal anti-inflammatory drugs with aspirin may increase bleeding or lead to decreased renal function).
No products indexed under this heading.

Metformin Hydrochloride (Moderate doses of aspirin may increase the effectiveness of renal hypoglycemic drugs, leading to hypoglycemia). Products include:
ActoPlus 3338
Avandamet 1345
Janumet 2188

Methotrexate Sodium (Salicylic acid can inhibit renal clearance of methotrexate, leading to bone marrow toxicity, especially in the elderly or renal impaired).
No products indexed under this heading.

Methyclothiazide (The effectiveness of diuretics in patients with underlying renal or cardiovascular disease may be diminished by co-administration of aspirin due to inhibition of renal prostaglandins, leading to decreased renal blood flow and salt and fluid retention).
No products indexed under this heading.

Metipranolol Hydrochloride (The hypertensive effects of beta-blockers may be diminished by the concomitant administration of aspirin due to inhibition of renal prostaglandins, leading to decreased renal blood flow and salt and fluid retention).
No products indexed under this heading.

Metolazone (The effectiveness of diuretics in patients with underlying renal or cardiovascular disease may be diminished by co-administration of aspirin due to inhibition of renal prostaglandins, leading to decreased renal blood flow and salt and fluid retention).
No products indexed under this heading.

Metoprolol Succinate (The hypertensive effects of beta-blockers may be diminished by the concomitant administration of aspirin due to inhibition of renal prostaglandins, leading to decreased renal blood flow and salt and fluid retention). Products include:
Toprol XL 732

Metoprolol Tartrate (The hypertensive effects of beta-blockers may be diminished by the concomitant administration of aspirin due to inhibition of renal prostaglandins, leading to decreased renal blood flow and salt and fluid retention).
No products indexed under this heading.

Miglitol (Moderate doses of aspirin may increase the effectiveness of renal hypoglycemic drugs, leading to hypoglycemia).
No products indexed under this heading.

Moexipril Hydrochloride (Co-administration can result in diminished hypotensive and hyponatremic effects of ACE inhibitors due to the effect of aspirin on the renin-angiotensin conversion pathway).
No products indexed under this heading.

Nabumetone (Co-administration of non-steroidal anti-inflammatory drugs with aspirin may increase bleeding or lead to decreased renal function).
No products indexed under this heading.

Nadolol (The hypertensive effects of beta-blockers may be diminished by the concomitant administration of aspirin due to inhibition of renal prostaglandins, leading to decreased renal blood flow and salt and fluid retention). Products include:
Nadolol 2359

Naproxen (Co-administration of non-steroidal anti-inflammatory drugs with aspirin may increase bleeding or lead to decreased renal function). Products include:
EC-Naprosyn 2850
Naprosyn 2850
Anaprox/Naprosyn 2850

Naproxen Sodium (Co-administration of non-steroidal anti-inflammatory drugs with aspirin may increase bleeding or lead to decreased renal function). Products include:
Anaprox 2850
Anaprox DS 2850
Treximet 1681

Nateglinide (Moderate doses of aspirin may increase the effectiveness of renal hypoglycemic drugs, leading to hypoglycemia).
No products indexed under this heading.

Nebivolol (The hypertensive effects of beta-blockers may be diminished by the concomitant administration of aspirin due to inhibition of renal prostaglandins, leading to decreased renal blood flow and salt and fluid retention). Products include:
Bystolic 1147

Neostigmine Bromide (Dipyridamole may counteract the anticholinesterase effect of cholinesterase inhibitors, thereby potentially aggravating myasthenia gravis).
No products indexed under this heading.

Neostigmine Methylsulfate (Dipyridamole may counteract the anticholinesterase effect of cholinesterase inhibitors, thereby potentially aggravating myasthenia gravis).
No products indexed under this heading.

Oxaprozin (Co-administration of non-steroidal anti-inflammatory drugs with aspirin may increase bleeding or lead to decreased renal function).
No products indexed under this heading.

Penbutolol Sulfate (The hypertensive effects of beta-blockers may be diminished by the concomitant administration of aspirin due to inhibition of renal prostaglandins, leading to decreased renal blood flow and salt and fluid retention).
No products indexed under this heading.

Perindopril Erbumine (Co-administration can result in diminished hypotensive and hyponatremic effects of ACE inhibitors due to the effect of aspirin on the renin-angiotensin conversion pathway).
No products indexed under this heading.

Phenylbutazone (Co-administration of non-steroidal anti-inflammatory drugs with aspirin may increase bleeding or lead to decreased renal function).
No products indexed under this heading.

Phenytoin (Salicylic acid can displace protein-bound phenytoin leading to a decrease in the total concentration of phenytoin).
No products indexed under this heading.

Phenytoin Sodium (Salicylic acid can displace protein-bound phenytoin leading to a decrease in the total concentration of phenytoin). Products include:
Phenytek Capsules 2380

Pindolol (The hypertensive effects of beta-blockers may be diminished by the concomitant administration of aspirin due to inhibition of renal prostaglandins, leading to decreased renal blood flow and salt and fluid retention).
No products indexed under this heading.

Pioglitazone Hydrochloride (Moderate doses of aspirin may increase the effectiveness of renal hypoglycemic drugs, leading to hypoglycemia). Products include:
ActoPlus 3338
Actos 3345
Duetact 3354

Piroxicam (Co-administration of non-steroidal anti-inflammatory drugs with aspirin may increase bleeding or lead to decreased renal function).
No products indexed under this heading.

Polythiazide (The effectiveness of diuretics in patients with underlying renal or cardiovascular disease may be diminished by co-administration of aspirin due to inhibition of renal prostaglandins, leading to decreased renal blood flow and salt and fluid retention).
No products indexed under this heading.

Probenecid (Salicylates antagonize the uricosuric action of uricosuric agents, such as probenecid).
No products indexed under this heading.

Propranolol Hydrochloride (The hypertensive effects of beta-blockers may be diminished by the concomitant administration of aspirin due to inhibition of renal prostaglandins, leading to decreased renal blood flow and salt and fluid retention). Products include:
InnoPran XL 1517

Pyridostigmine Bromide (Dipyridamole may counteract the anticholinesterase effect of cholinesterase inhibitors, thereby potentially aggravating myasthenia gravis).
No products indexed under this heading.

Quinapril Hydrochloride (Co-administration can result in diminished hypotensive and hyponatremic effects of ACE inhibitors due to the effect of aspirin on the renin-angiotensin conversion pathway).
No products indexed under this heading.

Ramipril (Co-administration can result in diminished hypotensive and hyponatremic effects of ACE inhibitors due to the effect of aspirin on the renin-angiotensin conversion pathway).
No products indexed under this heading.

Repaglinide (Moderate doses of aspirin may increase the effectiveness of renal hypoglycemic drugs, leading to hypoglycemia).
No products indexed under this heading.

Rivastigmine Tartrate (Dipyridamole may counteract the anticholinesterase effect of cholinesterase inhibitors, thereby potentially aggravating myasthenia gravis). Products include:
Exelon 2432
Exelon Oral 2432
Exelon Patch 2437

Rofecoxib (Co-administration of non-steroidal anti-inflammatory drugs with aspirin may increase bleeding or lead to decreased renal function).
No products indexed under this heading.

Rosiglitazone Maleate (Moderate doses of aspirin may increase the effectiveness of renal hypoglycemic drugs, leading to hypoglycemia). Products include:
Avandamet 1345
Avandaryl 1356
Avandia 1366

Sitagliptin Phosphate (Moderate doses of aspirin may increase the effectiveness of renal hypoglycemic drugs, leading to hypoglycemia). Products include:
Janumet 2188
Januvia 2196

Sotalol Hydrochloride (The hypertensive effects of beta-blockers may be diminished by the concomitant administration of aspirin due to inhibition of renal prostaglandins, leading to decreased renal blood flow and salt and fluid retention).
No products indexed under this heading.

Spirapril Hydrochloride (Co-administration can result in diminished hypotensive and hyponatremic effects of ACE inhibitors due to the effect of aspirin on the renin-angiotensin conversion pathway).
No products indexed under this heading.

Spironolactone (The effectiveness of diuretics in patients with underlying renal or cardiovascular disease may be diminished by co-administration of aspirin due to inhibition of renal prostaglandins, leading to decreased renal blood flow and salt and fluid retention).
No products indexed under this heading.

Sulfinpyrazone (Salicylates antagonize the uricosuric action of uricosuric agents, such as sulfinpyrazone).
No products indexed under this heading.

Sulindac (Co-administration of non-steroidal anti-inflammatory drugs with aspirin may increase bleeding or lead to decreased renal function). Products include:
Clinoril 2098

Tacrine Hydrochloride (Dipyridamole may counteract the anticholinesterase effect of cholinesterase inhibitors, thereby potentially aggravating myasthenia gravis).
No products indexed under this heading.

Timolol Hemihydrate (The hypertensive effects of beta-blockers may be diminished by the concomitant administration of aspirin due to inhibition of renal prostaglandins, leading to decreased renal blood flow and salt and fluid retention). Products include:
Betimol 3490

Timolol Maleate (The hypertensive effects of beta-blockers may be diminished by the concomitant administration of aspirin due to inhibition of renal prostaglandins, leading to decreased renal blood flow and salt and fluid retention). Products include:
Combigan 601
Dorzolamide
Hydrochloride/Timolol Maleate
Ophthalmic Solution............. ⊙243
Timoptic in Ocudose .... ⊙231

Tinzaparin Sodium (Patients on anticoagulation therapy are at risk for bleeding).
No products indexed under this heading.

Tolazamide (Moderate doses of aspirin may increase the effectiveness of renal hypoglycemic drugs, leading to hypoglycemia).
No products indexed under this heading.

Tolbutamide (Moderate doses of aspirin may increase the effectiveness of renal hypoglycemic drugs, leading to hypoglycemia).
No products indexed under this heading.

Tolmetin Sodium (Co-administration of non-steroidal anti-inflammatory drugs with aspirin may increase bleeding or lead to decreased renal function).
No products indexed under this heading.

Torsemide (The effectiveness of diuretics in patients with underlying renal or cardiovascular disease may be diminished by co-administration of aspirin due to inhibition of renal prostaglandins, leading to decreased renal blood flow and salt and fluid retention).
No products indexed under this heading.

Trandolapril (Co-administration can result in diminished hypotensive and hyponatremic effects of ACE inhibitors due to the effect of aspirin on the renin-angiotensin conversion pathway). Products include:
Mavik 489
Tarka 534

Triamterene (The effectiveness of diuretics in patients with underlying renal or cardiovascular disease may be diminished by co-administration of aspirin due to inhibition of renal prostaglandins, leading to decreased renal blood flow and salt and fluid retention). Products include:
Dyazide 1429
Dyrenium 3495

Troglitazone (Moderate doses of aspirin may increase the effectiveness of renal hypoglycemic drugs, leading to hypoglycemia).
No products indexed under this heading.

Valdecoxib (Co-administration of non-steroidal anti-inflammatory drugs with aspirin may increase bleeding or lead to decreased renal function).
No products indexed under this heading.

Valproate Sodium (Salicylic acid can displace protein-bound valproic acid leading to an increase in serum valproic acid levels).
No products indexed under this heading.

Valproic Acid (Salicylic acid can displace protein-bound valproic acid leading to an increase in serum valproic acid levels).
No products indexed under this heading.

IMPORTANT NOTE: Always consult each drug listing in the patient's regimen for possible interactions.

Warfarin Sodium (Aspirin can displace warfarin from protein binding sites, leading to a prolongation of both the prothrombin time and the bleeding time).
No products indexed under this heading.

Food Interactions

Alcohol (Patients who consume three or more alcoholic drinks every day should be counseled about the bleeding risks involved with chronic, heavy alcohol use while taking aspirin).

Beer, reduced-alcohol (Patients who consume three or more alcoholic drinks every day should be counseled about the bleeding risks involved with chronic, heavy alcohol use while taking aspirin).

Beer, unspecified (Patients who consume three or more alcoholic drinks every day should be counseled about the bleeding risks involved with chronic, heavy alcohol use while taking aspirin).

Wine, Chianti (Patients who consume three or more alcoholic drinks every day should be counseled about the bleeding risks involved with chronic, heavy alcohol use while taking aspirin).

Wine, Red (Patients who consume three or more alcoholic drinks every day should be counseled about the bleeding risks involved with chronic, heavy alcohol use while taking aspirin).

Wine, unspecified (Patients who consume three or more alcoholic drinks every day should be counseled about the bleeding risks involved with chronic, heavy alcohol use while taking aspirin).

Wine products (Patients who consume three or more alcoholic drinks every day should be counseled about the bleeding risks involved with chronic, heavy alcohol use while taking aspirin).

ALAMAST OPHTHALMIC SOLUTION

(Pemirolast Potassium) 3490
None cited in PDR database.

ALBENZA TABLETS

(Albendazole) 1298
May interact with dexamethasones, theophyllines, and certain other agents. Compounds in these categories include:

Cimetidine (Albendazole sulfoxide concentrations in bile and cystic fluid were increased (about 2-fold) in hydatid cyst patients treated with cimetidine (10 mg/kg/day) (n = 7) compared with albendazole (20 mg/kg/day) alone (n = 12). Albendazole sulfoxide plasma concentrations were unchanged 4 hours after dosing).
No products indexed under this heading.

Cimetidine Hydrochloride (Albendazole sulfoxide concentrations in bile and cystic fluid were increased (about 2-fold) in hydatid cyst patients treated with cimetidine (10 mg/kg/day) (n = 7) compared with albendazole (20 mg/kg/day) alone (n = 12). Albendazole sulfoxide plasma concentrations were unchanged 4 hours after dosing).
No products indexed under this heading.

Dexamethasone (Steady-state trough concentrations of albendazole sulfoxide were about 56% higher when 8 mg dexamethasone was co-administered with each dose of albendazole (15 mg/kg/day) in 8 neurocysticercosis patients).
Products include:
Ciprodex **583**
Ozurdex .... ⊙ **223**
Tobramycin and Dexamethasone
  Ophthalmic Suspension .... ⊙ **251**

Dexamethasone Acetate (Steady-state trough concentrations of albendazole sulfoxide were about 56% higher when 8 mg dexamethasone was co-administered with each dose of albendazole (15 mg/kg/day) in 8 neurocysticercosis patients).
No products indexed under this heading.

Dexamethasone Phosphate (Steady-state trough concentrations of albendazole sulfoxide were about 56% higher when 8 mg dexamethasone was co-administered with each dose of albendazole (15 mg/kg/day) in 8 neurocysticercosis patients).
No products indexed under this heading.

Dexamethasone Sodium (Steady-state trough concentrations of albendazole sulfoxide were about 56% higher when 8 mg dexamethasone was co-administered with each dose of albendazole (15 mg/kg/day) in 8 neurocysticercosis patients).
No products indexed under this heading.

Dexamethasone Sodium Phosphate (Steady-state trough concentrations of albendazole sulfoxide were about 56% higher when 8 mg dexamethasone was co-administered with each dose of albendazole (15 mg/kg/day) in 8 neurocysticercosis patients).
No products indexed under this heading.

Dexamethasone Sodium Phosphate Injection (Steady-state trough concentrations of albendazole sulfoxide were about 56% higher when 8 mg dexamethasone was co-administered with each dose of albendazole (15 mg/kg/day) in 8 neurocysticercosis patients).
No products indexed under this heading.

Fat (Oral bioavailability appears to be enhanced when albendazole is co-administered with a fatty meal (estimated fat content 40 g) as evidenced by higher (up to 5-fold on average) plasma concentrations of albendazole sulfoxide as compared to the fasted state).
No products indexed under this heading.

Praziquantel (In the fed state, praziquantel (40 mg/kg) increased mean maximum plasma concentration and area under the curve of albendazole sulfoxide by about 50% in healthy subjects (n = 10) compared with a separate group of subjects (n = 6) given albendazole alone. Mean T_{max} and mean plasma elimination half-life of albendazole sulfoxide were unchanged. The pharmacokinetics of praziquantel were unchanged following co-administration with albendazole (400 mg)).
No products indexed under this heading.

Theophylline (Although single doses of albendazole have been shown not to inhibit theophylline metabolism, albendazole does induce cytochrome P450 1A in human hepatoma cells. Therefore, it is recommended that plasma concentrations of theophylline be monitored during and after treatment with albendazole).
No products indexed under this heading.

Theophylline Anhydrous (Although single doses of albendazole have been shown not to inhibit theophylline metabolism, albendazole does induce cytochrome P450 1A in human hepatoma cells. Therefore, it is recommended that plasma concentrations of theophylline be monitored during and after treatment with albendazole). Products include:
Uniphyl **2817**

Theophylline Calcium Salicylate (Although single doses of albendazole have been shown not to inhibit theophylline metabolism, albendazole does induce cytochrome P450 1A in human hepatoma cells. Therefore, it is recommended that plasma concentrations of theophylline be monitored during and after treatment with albendazole).
No products indexed under this heading.

Theophylline Dihydroxypropyl (Glyceryl) (Although single doses of albendazole have been shown not to inhibit theophylline metabolism, albendazole does induce cytochrome P450 1A in human hepatoma cells. Therefore, it is recommended that plasma concentrations of theophylline be monitored during and after treatment with albendazole).
No products indexed under this heading.

Theophylline Ethylenediamine (Although single doses of albendazole have been shown not to inhibit theophylline metabolism, albendazole does induce cytochrome P450 1A in human hepatoma cells. Therefore, it is recommended that plasma concentrations of theophylline be monitored during and after treatment with albendazole).
No products indexed under this heading.

Theophylline Sodium Glycinate (Although single doses of albendazole have been shown not to inhibit theophylline metabolism, albendazole does induce cytochrome P450 1A in human hepatoma cells. Therefore, it is recommended that plasma concentrations of theophylline be monitored during and after treatment with albendazole).
No products indexed under this heading.

Food Interactions

Food, unspecified (Oral bioavailability appears to be enhanced when albendazole is co-administered with a fatty meal (estimated fat content 40 g) as evidenced by higher (up to 5-fold on average) plasma concentrations of albendazole sulfoxide as compared to the fasted state).

Meal, unspecified (Oral bioavailability appears to be enhanced when albendazole is co-administered with a fatty meal (estimated fat content 40 g) as evidenced by higher (up to 5-fold on average) plasma concentrations of albendazole sulfoxide as compared to the fasted state).

ALBUTEIN 5% SOLUTION

(Albumin (human)) 1783
None cited in PDR database.

ALBUTEIN 25% SOLUTION

(Albumin (human)) 1784
None cited in PDR database.

ALDARA CREAM, 5%

(Imiquimod) 1771
None cited in PDR database.

ALFERON N INJECTION

(Interferon alfa-N3 (Human Leukocyte Derived)) 1801
None cited in PDR database.

ALIMTA FOR INJECTION

(Pemetrexed Disodium) 1850
May interact with nephrotoxic agents, non-steroidal anti-inflammatory agents, and certain other agents. Compounds in these categories include:

Abacavir Sulfate (Concomitant administration of nephrotoxic drugs could result in delayed clearance of pemetrexed). Products include:
Epzicom **1448**

Trizivir **1688**
Ziagen **1740**

Acyclovir (Concomitant administration of nephrotoxic drugs could result in delayed clearance of pemetrexed). Products include:
Zovirax **1760**

Acyclovir Sodium (Concomitant administration of nephrotoxic drugs could result in delayed clearance of pemetrexed).
No products indexed under this heading.

Alatrofloxacin Mesylate (Concomitant administration of nephrotoxic drugs could result in delayed clearance of pemetrexed).
No products indexed under this heading.

Aldesleukin (Concomitant administration of nephrotoxic drugs could result in delayed clearance of pemetrexed). Products include:
Proleukin **2504**

Amikacin Sulfate (Concomitant administration of nephrotoxic drugs could result in delayed clearance of pemetrexed).
No products indexed under this heading.

Amoxicillin (Concomitant administration of nephrotoxic drugs could result in delayed clearance of pemetrexed). Products include:
Amoxil Capsules **1311**
Amoxil Chewable Tablets **1311**
Amoxil **1311**
Amoxil Powder **1311**
Augmentin **1331**
Augmentin Tablets **1335**
Augmentin ES-600 .... **1338**
Augmentin XR **1342**
Moxatag **2321**

Amoxicillin Trihydrate (Concomitant administration of nephrotoxic drugs could result in delayed clearance of pemetrexed).
No products indexed under this heading.

Amphotericin B (Concomitant administration of nephrotoxic drugs could result in delayed clearance of pemetrexed).
No products indexed under this heading.

Amphotericin B, liposomal (Concomitant administration of nephrotoxic drugs could result in delayed clearance of pemetrexed). Products include:
AmBisome **659**

Amphotericin B Cholesteryl Sulfate (Concomitant administration of nephrotoxic drugs could result in delayed clearance of pemetrexed).
No products indexed under this heading.

Amphotericin B Lipid Complex (Concomitant administration of nephrotoxic drugs could result in delayed clearance of pemetrexed).
No products indexed under this heading.

Ampicillin (Concomitant administration of nephrotoxic drugs could result in delayed clearance of pemetrexed).
No products indexed under this heading.

Ampicillin Sodium (Concomitant administration of nephrotoxic drugs could result in delayed clearance of pemetrexed).
No products indexed under this heading.

Ampicillin Trihydrate (Concomitant administration of nephrotoxic drugs could result in delayed clearance of pemetrexed).
No products indexed under this heading.

Amprenavir (Concomitant administration of nephrotoxic drugs could result in delayed clearance of pemetrexed).
No products indexed under this heading.

Aspirin (Concomitant administration of nephrotoxic drugs could result in delayed clearance of pemetrexed). Products include:
Aggrenox **880**
Bayer Aspirin **829**

Atazanavir (Concomitant administration of nephrotoxic drugs could result in delayed clearance of pemetrexed).
No products indexed under this heading.

Atorvastatin Calcium (Concomitant administration of nephrotoxic drugs could result in delayed clearance of pemetrexed). Products include:

Azithromycin Dihydrate (Concomitant administration of nephrotoxic drugs could result in delayed clearance of pemetrexed).
No products indexed under this heading.

Azlocillin Sodium (Concomitant administration of nephrotoxic drugs could result in delayed clearance of pemetrexed).
No products indexed under this heading.

Aztreonam (Concomitant administration of nephrotoxic drugs could result in delayed clearance of pemetrexed).
No products indexed under this heading.

Bacampicillin Hydrochloride (Concomitant administration of nephrotoxic drugs could result in delayed clearance of pemetrexed).
No products indexed under this heading.

Bacitracin (Concomitant administration of nephrotoxic drugs could result in delayed clearance of pemetrexed).
No products indexed under this heading.

Bacitracin Zinc (Concomitant administration of nephrotoxic drugs could result in delayed clearance of pemetrexed).
No products indexed under this heading.

Balsalazide Disodium (Concomitant administration of nephrotoxic drugs could result in delayed clearance of pemetrexed).
No products indexed under this heading.

Benazepril Hydrochloride (Concomitant administration of nephrotoxic drugs could result in delayed clearance of pemetrexed).
No products indexed under this heading.

Bendroflumethiazide (Concomitant administration of nephrotoxic drugs could result in delayed clearance of pemetrexed).
No products indexed under this heading.

Caffeine (Concomitant administration of nephrotoxic drugs could result in delayed clearance of pemetrexed).
No products indexed under this heading.

Captopril (Concomitant administration of nephrotoxic drugs could result in delayed clearance of pemetrexed). Products include:

Carbenicillin Disodium (Concomitant administration of nephrotoxic drugs could result in delayed clearance of pemetrexed).
No products indexed under this heading.

Carbenicillin Indanyl Sodium (Concomitant administration of nephrotoxic drugs could result in delayed clearance of pemetrexed).
No products indexed under this heading.

Carboplatin (Concomitant administration of nephrotoxic drugs could result in delayed clearance of pemetrexed).
No products indexed under this heading.

Carmustine (BCNU) (Concomitant administration of nephrotoxic drugs could result in delayed clearance of pemetrexed).
No products indexed under this heading.

Cefaclor (Concomitant administration of nephrotoxic drugs could result in delayed clearance of pemetrexed).
No products indexed under this heading.

Cefadroxil (Concomitant administration of nephrotoxic drugs could result in delayed clearance of pemetrexed).
No products indexed under this heading.

Cefamandole Nafate (Concomitant administration of nephrotoxic drugs could result in delayed clearance of pemetrexed).
No products indexed under this heading.

Cefazolin Sodium (Concomitant administration of nephrotoxic drugs could result in delayed clearance of pemetrexed).
No products indexed under this heading.

Cefdinir (Concomitant administration of nephrotoxic drugs could result in delayed clearance of pemetrexed). Products include:

Cefepime Hydrochloride (Concomitant administration of nephrotoxic drugs could result in delayed clearance of pemetrexed).
No products indexed under this heading.

Cefixime (Concomitant administration of nephrotoxic drugs could result in delayed clearance of pemetrexed). Products include:

Cefmetazole Sodium (Concomitant administration of nephrotoxic drugs could result in delayed clearance of pemetrexed).
No products indexed under this heading.

Cefonicid Sodium (Concomitant administration of nephrotoxic drugs could result in delayed clearance of pemetrexed).
No products indexed under this heading.

Cefoperazone Sodium (Concomitant administration of nephrotoxic drugs could result in delayed clearance of pemetrexed).
No products indexed under this heading.

Ceforanide (Concomitant administration of nephrotoxic drugs could result in delayed clearance of pemetrexed).
No products indexed under this heading.

Cefotaxime Sodium (Concomitant administration of nephrotoxic drugs could result in delayed clearance of pemetrexed).
No products indexed under this heading.

Cefotetan (Concomitant administration of nephrotoxic drugs could result in delayed clearance of pemetrexed).
No products indexed under this heading.

Cefoxitin Sodium (Concomitant administration of nephrotoxic drugs could result in delayed clearance of pemetrexed).
No products indexed under this heading.

Cefpodoxime Proxetil (Concomitant administration of nephrotoxic drugs could result in delayed clearance of pemetrexed).
No products indexed under this heading.

Cefprozil (Concomitant administration of nephrotoxic drugs could result in delayed clearance of pemetrexed).
No products indexed under this heading.

Ceftazidime (Concomitant administration of nephrotoxic drugs could result in delayed clearance of pemetrexed). Products include:

Ceftizoxime Sodium (Concomitant administration of nephrotoxic drugs could result in delayed clearance of pemetrexed).
No products indexed under this heading.

Ceftriaxone Sodium (Concomitant administration of nephrotoxic drugs could result in delayed clearance of pemetrexed). Products include:

Cefuroxime Axetil (Concomitant administration of nephrotoxic drugs could result in delayed clearance of pemetrexed). Products include:

Cefuroxime Sodium (Concomitant administration of nephrotoxic drugs could result in delayed clearance of pemetrexed).
No products indexed under this heading.

Celecoxib (Patients with mild to moderate renal insufficiency should avoid taking NSAIDs with short elimination half-lives for a period of 2 days before, the day of, and 2 days following administration of pemetrexed. In the absence of data regarding potential interaction between pemetrexed and NSAIDs with longer half-lives, all patients taking these NSAIDs should interrupt dosing for at least 5 days before, the day of, and 2 days following pemetrexed administration. If concomitant administration of an NSAID is necessary, patients should be monitored closely for toxicity, especially myelosuppression, renal, and gastrointestinal toxicity). Products include:

Cephalexin (Concomitant administration of nephrotoxic drugs could result in delayed clearance of pemetrexed).
No products indexed under this heading.

Cephalothin Sodium (Concomitant administration of nephrotoxic drugs could result in delayed clearance of pemetrexed).
No products indexed under this heading.

Cephapirin Sodium (Concomitant administration of nephrotoxic drugs could result in delayed clearance of pemetrexed).
No products indexed under this heading.

Cephradine (Concomitant administration of nephrotoxic drugs could result in delayed clearance of pemetrexed).
No products indexed under this heading.

Cerivastatin Sodium (Concomitant administration of nephrotoxic drugs could result in delayed clearance of pemetrexed).
No products indexed under this heading.

Chlorothiazide (Concomitant administration of nephrotoxic drugs could result in delayed clearance of pemetrexed).
No products indexed under this heading.

Chlorothiazide Sodium (Concomitant administration of nephrotoxic drugs could result in delayed clearance of pemetrexed). Products include:

Chlorpropamide (Concomitant administration of nephrotoxic drugs could result in delayed clearance of pemetrexed).
No products indexed under this heading.

Cidofovir (Concomitant administration of nephrotoxic drugs could result in delayed clearance of pemetrexed).
No products indexed under this heading.

Cilastatin Sodium (Concomitant administration of nephrotoxic drugs could result in delayed clearance of pemetrexed). Products include:

Cimetidine (Concomitant administration of nephrotoxic drugs could result in delayed clearance of pemetrexed).
No products indexed under this heading.

Cimetidine Hydrochloride (Concomitant administration of nephrotoxic drugs could result in delayed clearance of pemetrexed).
No products indexed under this heading.

Cisplatin (Concomitant administration of nephrotoxic drugs could result in delayed clearance of pemetrexed).
No products indexed under this heading.

Cladribine (Concomitant administration of nephrotoxic drugs could result in delayed clearance of pemetrexed). Products include:

Clozapine (Concomitant administration of nephrotoxic drugs could result in delayed clearance of pemetrexed).
No products indexed under this heading.

Colistimethate Sodium (Concomitant administration of nephrotoxic drugs could result in delayed clearance of pemetrexed).
No products indexed under this heading.

Colistin Sulfate (Concomitant administration of nephrotoxic drugs could result in delayed clearance of pemetrexed).
No products indexed under this heading.

Cyclophosphamide (Concomitant administration of nephrotoxic drugs could result in delayed clearance of pemetrexed).
No products indexed under this heading.

Cyclosporine (Concomitant administration of nephrotoxic drugs could result in delayed clearance of pemetrexed). Products include:

Cytarabine (Concomitant administration of nephrotoxic drugs could result in delayed clearance of pemetrexed).
No products indexed under this heading.

Cytarabine Liposome (Concomitant administration of nephrotoxic drugs could result in delayed clearance of pemetrexed).
No products indexed under this heading.

Delavirdine Mesylate (Concomitant administration of nephrotoxic drugs could result in delayed clearance of pemetrexed).
No products indexed under this heading.

Diatrizoate Meglumine (Concomitant administration of nephrotoxic drugs could result in delayed clearance of pemetrexed).
No products indexed under this heading.

Diatrizoate Sodium (Concomitant administration of nephrotoxic drugs could result in delayed clearance of pemetrexed).
No products indexed under this heading.

Diclofenac Epolamine (Patients with mild to moderate renal insufficiency should avoid taking NSAIDs with short elimination half-lives for a period of 2 days before, the day of, and 2 days following administration of pemetrexed. In the absence of data regarding potential interaction between pemetrexed and NSAIDs with longer half-lives, all patients taking these NSAIDs should interrupt dosing for at least 5 days before, the day of, and 2 days following pemetrexed administration. If concomitant administration of an NSAID is necessary, patients should be monitored closely for toxicity, especially myelosuppression, renal, and gastrointestinal toxicity). Products include:

Diclofenac Potassium (Patients with mild to moderate renal insufficiency should avoid taking NSAIDs with short elimination half-lives for a period of 2 days before, the day of, and 2 days following administration of pemetrexed. In the absence of data regarding potential interaction between pemetrexed and NSAIDs with longer half-lives, all patients taking these NSAIDs should interrupt dosing for at least 5 days before, the day of, and 2 days following pemetrexed administration. If concomitant administration of an NSAID is necessary, patients should be monitored

closely for toxicity, especially myelosuppression, renal, and gastrointestinal toxicity).
No products indexed under this heading.

Diclofenac Sodium (Patients with mild to moderate renal insufficiency should avoid taking NSAIDs with short elimination half-lives for a period of 2 days before, the day of, and 2 days following administration of pemetrexed. In the absence of data regarding potential interaction between pemetrexed and NSAIDs with longer half-lives, all patients taking these NSAIDs should interrupt dosing for at least 5 days before, the day of, and 2 days following pemetrexed administration. If concomitant administration of an NSAID is necessary, patients should be monitored closely for toxicity, especially myelosuppression, renal, and gastrointestinal toxicity).
No products indexed under this heading.

Dicloxacillin Sodium (Concomitant administration of nephrotoxic drugs could result in delayed clearance of pemetrexed).
No products indexed under this heading.

Didanosine (Concomitant administration of nephrotoxic drugs could result in delayed clearance of pemetrexed).
No products indexed under this heading.

Efavirenz (Concomitant administration of nephrotoxic drugs could result in delayed clearance of pemetrexed). Products include:
Atripla **906**

Emtricitabine (Concomitant administration of nephrotoxic drugs could result in delayed clearance of pemetrexed). Products include:
Atripla **906**
Emtriva **1238**
Emtriva Oral Solution **1238**
Truvada **1258**

Enalapril Maleate (Concomitant administration of nephrotoxic drugs could result in delayed clearance of pemetrexed).
No products indexed under this heading.

Enalaprilat (Concomitant administration of nephrotoxic drugs could result in delayed clearance of pemetrexed).
No products indexed under this heading.

Enfuvirtide (Concomitant administration of nephrotoxic drugs could result in delayed clearance of pemetrexed).
No products indexed under this heading.

Ethiodized Oil (Concomitant administration of nephrotoxic drugs could result in delayed clearance of pemetrexed).
No products indexed under this heading.

Etodolac (Patients with mild to moderate renal insufficiency should avoid taking NSAIDs with short elimination half-lives for a period of 2 days before, the day of, and 2 days following administration of pemetrexed. In the absence of data regarding potential interaction between pemetrexed and NSAIDs with longer half-lives, all patients taking these NSAIDs should interrupt dosing for at least 5 days before, the day of, and 2 days following pemetrexed administration. If concomitant administration of an NSAID is necessary, patients should be monitored closely for toxicity, especially myelosuppression, renal, and gastrointestinal toxicity).
No products indexed under this heading.

Fenoprofen Calcium (Patients with mild to moderate renal insufficiency should avoid taking NSAIDs with short elimination half-lives for a period of 2 days before, the day of, and 2 days following administration of pemetrexed. In the absence of data regarding potential interaction between pemetrexed and NSAIDs with longer half-lives, all patients taking these NSAIDs should interrupt dosing for at least 5 days before, the day of, and 2 days following pemetrexed administration. If concomitant administration of an NSAID is necessary, patients should be monitored closely for toxicity, especially myelosuppression, renal, and gastrointestinal toxicity).
No products indexed under this heading.

Filgrastim (Concomitant administration of nephrotoxic drugs could result in delayed clearance of pemetrexed). Products include:
Neupogen **631**

Fluorouracil (Concomitant administration of nephrotoxic drugs could result in delayed clearance of pemetrexed). Products include:
Carac **2966**

Flurbiprofen (Patients with mild to moderate renal insufficiency should avoid taking NSAIDs with short elimination half-lives for a period of 2 days before, the day of, and 2 days following administration of pemetrexed. In the absence of data regarding potential interaction between pemetrexed and NSAIDs with longer half-lives, all patients taking these NSAIDs should interrupt dosing for at least 5 days before, the day of, and 2 days following pemetrexed administration. If concomitant administration of an NSAID is necessary, patients should be monitored closely for toxicity, especially myelosuppression, renal, and gastrointestinal toxicity).
No products indexed under this heading.

Fluvastatin Sodium (Concomitant administration of nephrotoxic drugs could result in delayed clearance of pemetrexed).
No products indexed under this heading.

Foscarnet Sodium (Concomitant administration of nephrotoxic drugs could result in delayed clearance of pemetrexed).
No products indexed under this heading.

Fosinopril Sodium (Concomitant administration of nephrotoxic drugs could result in delayed clearance of pemetrexed).
No products indexed under this heading.

Furosemide (Concomitant administration of nephrotoxic drugs could result in delayed clearance of pemetrexed). Products include:
Furosemide **2354**

Gadopentetate Dimeglumine (Concomitant administration of nephrotoxic drugs could result in delayed clearance of pemetrexed).
No products indexed under this heading.

Gentamicin (Concomitant administration of nephrotoxic drugs could result in delayed clearance of pemetrexed).
No products indexed under this heading.

Gentamicin Sulfate (Concomitant administration of nephrotoxic drugs could result in delayed clearance of pemetrexed). Products include:
Pred-G .... **⊙226, ⊙227**

Glipizide (Concomitant administration of nephrotoxic drugs could result in delayed clearance of pemetrexed).
No products indexed under this heading.

Globulin, Immune (Human) (Concomitant administration of nephrotoxic drugs could result in delayed clearance of pemetrexed). Products include:

Glyburide (Concomitant administration of nephrotoxic drugs could result in delayed clearance of pemetrexed).
No products indexed under this heading.

Gold Therapy (Concomitant administration of nephrotoxic drugs could result in delayed clearance of pemetrexed).
No products indexed under this heading.

HMG-CoA Reductase Inhibitors (Concomitant administration of nephrotoxic drugs could result in delayed clearance of pemetrexed).
No products indexed under this heading.

Hydrochlorothiazide (Concomitant administration of nephrotoxic drugs could result in delayed clearance of pemetrexed). Products include:
Atacand HCT **700**
Avalide **2956**
Benicar HCT **1017**
Diovan HCT **2419**
Dyazide **1429**
Exforge HCT **2449**
Hyzaar **2162**
Hyzaar 100-12.5 .... **2162**
Micardis HCT **889**
Prinzide **2246**
Tekturna HCT **2541**
Teveten HCT **541**

Hydroflumethiazide (Concomitant administration of nephrotoxic drugs could result in delayed clearance of pemetrexed).
No products indexed under this heading.

Ibuprofen (Although ibuprofen (400 mg four times a day) can decrease the clearance of pemetrexed, it can be administered with pemetrexed in patients with normal renal function (creatinine clearance ≥ 80 mL/min). Caution should be used when administering ibuprofen concurrently with pemetrexed to patients with mild to moderate renal insufficiency (creatinine clearance from 45 to 79 mL/min)). Products include:
Motrin IB **2043**
Children's Motrin **2044**
Children's Motrin Non-Staining Dye-Free **2044**
Infants' Motrin **2044**
Infants' Motrin Dye-Free **2044**
Junior Strength Motrin **2044**
Vicoprofen **564**

Idarubicin Hydrochloride (Concomitant administration of nephrotoxic drugs could result in delayed clearance of pemetrexed).
No products indexed under this heading.

Ifosfamide (Concomitant administration of nephrotoxic drugs could result in delayed clearance of pemetrexed).
No products indexed under this heading.

Imipenem (Concomitant administration of nephrotoxic drugs could result in delayed clearance of pemetrexed). Products include:
Primaxin I.M. **2232**
Primaxin I.V. **2235**

Immune Globulin Intravenous (Human) (Concomitant administration of nephrotoxic drugs could result in delayed clearance of pemetrexed). Products include:
Flebogamma 5% DIF **1794**
Gammagard **812, 815**
Gamunex **3374**

Indinavir Sulfate (Concomitant administration of nephrotoxic drugs could result in delayed clearance of pemetrexed). Products include:
Crixivan **2113**

Indomethacin (Patients with mild to moderate renal insufficiency should avoid taking NSAIDs with short elimination half-lives for a period of 2 days before, the day of, and 2 days following administration of pemetrexed. In the absence of data regarding potential interaction between pemetrexed and NSAIDs with longer half-lives, all patients taking these NSAIDs should interrupt dosing for at least 5 days before, the day of, and 2 days following pemetrexed administration. If concomitant administration of an NSAID is necessary, patients should be monitored closely for toxicity, especially myelosuppression, renal, and gastrointestinal toxicity). Products include:
Indocin **2167**

Indomethacin Sodium Trihydrate (Patients with mild to moderate renal insufficiency should avoid taking NSAIDs with short elimination half-lives for a period of 2 days before, the day of, and 2 days following administration of pemetrexed. In the absence of data regarding potential interaction between pemetrexed and NSAIDs with longer half-lives, all patients taking these NSAIDs should interrupt dosing for at least 5 days before, the day of, and 2 days following pemetrexed administration. If concomitant administration of an NSAID is necessary, patients should be monitored closely for toxicity, especially myelosuppression, renal, and gastrointestinal toxicity). Products include:
Indocin I.V. **2007**

Interferon Beta-1b (Concomitant administration of nephrotoxic drugs could result in delayed clearance of pemetrexed). Products include:
Betaseron **836**
Extavia **2459**

Interleuken-2 (Concomitant administration of nephrotoxic drugs could result in delayed clearance of pemetrexed).
No products indexed under this heading.

Iodamide Meglumine (Concomitant administration of nephrotoxic drugs could result in delayed clearance of pemetrexed).
No products indexed under this heading.

Iohexol (Concomitant administration of nephrotoxic drugs could result in delayed clearance of pemetrexed).
No products indexed under this heading.

Iopamidol (Concomitant administration of nephrotoxic drugs could result in delayed clearance of pemetrexed).
No products indexed under this heading.

Iopanoic Acid (Concomitant administration of nephrotoxic drugs could result in delayed clearance of pemetrexed).
No products indexed under this heading.

Iothalamate Meglumine (Concomitant administration of nephrotoxic drugs could result in delayed clearance of pemetrexed).
No products indexed under this heading.

Ioxaglate Meglumine (Concomitant administration of nephrotoxic drugs could result in delayed clearance of pemetrexed).
No products indexed under this heading.

Ioxaglate Sodium (Concomitant administration of nephrotoxic drugs could result in delayed clearance of pemetrexed).
No products indexed under this heading.

Kanamycin Sulfate (Concomitant administration of nephrotoxic drugs could result in delayed clearance of pemetrexed).
No products indexed under this heading.

Ketoprofen (Patients with mild to moderate renal insufficiency should avoid taking NSAIDs with short elimination half-lives for a period of 2 days before, the day of, and 2 days following administration of pemetrexed. In the absence of data regarding potential interaction between pemetrexed and NSAIDs with longer half-lives, all patients taking these NSAIDs should interrupt dosing for at least 5 days before, the day of, and 2 days following pemetrexed administration. If concomitant administration of an NSAID is necessary, patients should be monitored closely for toxicity, especially myelosuppression, renal, and gastrointestinal toxicity).
No products indexed under this heading.

Ketorolac Tromethamine (Patients with mild to moderate renal insufficiency should avoid taking NSAIDs with short elimination half-lives for a period of 2 days before, the day of, and 2 days

(⊙ Described in PDR® for Ophthalmic Medicines)

following administration of pemetrexed. In the absence of data regarding potential interaction between pemetrexed and NSAIDs with longer half-lives, all patients taking these NSAIDs should interrupt dosing for at least 5 days before, the day of, and 2 days following pemetrexed administration. If concomitant administration of an NSAID is necessary, patients should be monitored closely for toxicity, especially myelosuppression, renal, and gastrointestinal toxicity). Products include:
Acuvail .... ⊙209

Lamium album (Concomitant administration of nephrotoxic drugs could result in delayed clearance of pemetrexed).
No products indexed under this heading.

Lisinopril (Concomitant administration of nephrotoxic drugs could result in delayed clearance of pemetrexed). Products include:
Prinivil 2241
Prinzide 2246

Lithium (Concomitant administration of nephrotoxic drugs could result in delayed clearance of pemetrexed).
No products indexed under this heading.

Lithium Carbonate (Concomitant administration of nephrotoxic drugs could result in delayed clearance of pemetrexed).
No products indexed under this heading.

Lithium Citrate (Concomitant administration of nephrotoxic drugs could result in delayed clearance of pemetrexed).
No products indexed under this heading.

Lopinavir (Concomitant administration of nephrotoxic drugs could result in delayed clearance of pemetrexed). Products include:
Kaletra 458

Loracarbef (Concomitant administration of nephrotoxic drugs could result in delayed clearance of pemetrexed).
No products indexed under this heading.

Lovastatin (Concomitant administration of nephrotoxic drugs could result in delayed clearance of pemetrexed). Products include:
Advicor 402
Mevacor 2212

Meclofenamate Sodium (Patients with mild to moderate renal insufficiency should avoid taking NSAIDs with short elimination half-lives for a period of 2 days before, the day of, and 2 days following administration of pemetrexed. In the absence of data regarding potential interaction between pemetrexed and NSAIDs with longer half-lives, all patients taking these NSAIDs should interrupt dosing for at least 5 days before, the day of, and 2 days following pemetrexed administration. If concomitant administration of an NSAID is necessary, patients should be monitored closely for toxicity, especially myelosuppression, renal, and gastrointestinal toxicity).
No products indexed under this heading.

Mefenamic Acid (Patients with mild to moderate renal insufficiency should avoid taking NSAIDs with short elimination half-lives for a period of 2 days before, the day of, and 2 days following administration of pemetrexed. In the absence of data regarding potential interaction between pemetrexed and NSAIDs with longer half-lives, all patients taking these NSAIDs should interrupt dosing for at least 5 days before, the day of, and 2 days following pemetrexed administration. If concomitant administration of an NSAID is necessary, patients should be monitored closely for toxicity, especially myelosuppression, renal, and gastrointestinal toxicity).
No products indexed under this heading.

Meloxicam (Patients with mild to moderate renal insufficiency should avoid taking NSAIDs with short elimination half-lives for a period of 2 days before, the day of, and 2 days following administration of pemetrexed. In the absence of data regarding potential interaction between pemetrexed and NSAIDs with longer half-lives, all patients taking these NSAIDs should interrupt dosing for at least 5 days before, the day of, and 2 days following pemetrexed administration. If concomitant administration of an NSAID is necessary, patients should be monitored closely for toxicity, especially myelosuppression, renal, and gastrointestinal toxicity).
No products indexed under this heading.

Melphalan Hydrochloride (Concomitant administration of nephrotoxic drugs could result in delayed clearance of pemetrexed). Products include:
Alkeran for Injection 1300

Mesalamine (Concomitant administration of nephrotoxic drugs could result in delayed clearance of pemetrexed). Products include:
Apriso 2899
Asacol 2786
Asacol HD 2787
Canasa 782
Lialda 3295
Pentasa 3297

Methimazole (Concomitant administration of nephrotoxic drugs could result in delayed clearance of pemetrexed).
No products indexed under this heading.

Methotrexate (Concomitant administration of nephrotoxic drugs could result in delayed clearance of pemetrexed).
No products indexed under this heading.

Methotrexate Sodium (Concomitant administration of nephrotoxic drugs could result in delayed clearance of pemetrexed).
No products indexed under this heading.

Methyclothiazide (Concomitant administration of nephrotoxic drugs could result in delayed clearance of pemetrexed).
No products indexed under this heading.

Mezlocillin Sodium (Concomitant administration of nephrotoxic drugs could result in delayed clearance of pemetrexed).
No products indexed under this heading.

Minocycline Hydrochloride (Concomitant administration of nephrotoxic drugs could result in delayed clearance of pemetrexed). Products include:
Solodyn 2073

Mitomycin (Mitomycin-C) (Concomitant administration of nephrotoxic drugs could result in delayed clearance of pemetrexed).
No products indexed under this heading.

Moexipril Hydrochloride (Concomitant administration of nephrotoxic drugs could result in delayed clearance of pemetrexed).
No products indexed under this heading.

Muromonab-CD3 (Concomitant administration of nephrotoxic drugs could result in delayed clearance of pemetrexed). Products include:
Orthoclone OKT3 949

Nabumetone (Patients with mild to moderate renal insufficiency should avoid taking NSAIDs with short elimination half-lives for a period of 2 days before, the day of, and 2 days following administration of pemetrexed. In the absence of data regarding potential interaction between pemetrexed and NSAIDs with longer half-lives, all patients taking these NSAIDs should interrupt dosing for at least 5 days before, the day of, and 2 days following pemetrexed administration. If concomitant administration of an NSAID is necessary, patients should be monitored

closely for toxicity, especially myelosuppression, renal, and gastrointestinal toxicity).
No products indexed under this heading.

Nafcillin Sodium (Concomitant administration of nephrotoxic drugs could result in delayed clearance of pemetrexed).
No products indexed under this heading.

Naproxen (Patients with mild to moderate renal insufficiency should avoid taking NSAIDs with short elimination half-lives for a period of 2 days before, the day of, and 2 days following administration of pemetrexed. In the absence of data regarding potential interaction between pemetrexed and NSAIDs with longer half-lives, all patients taking these NSAIDs should interrupt dosing for at least 5 days before, the day of, and 2 days following pemetrexed administration. If concomitant administration of an NSAID is necessary, patients should be monitored closely for toxicity, especially myelosuppression, renal, and gastrointestinal toxicity). Products include:
EC-Naprosyn 2850
Naprosyn 2850
Anaprox/Naprosyn 2850

Naproxen Sodium (Patients with mild to moderate renal insufficiency should avoid taking NSAIDs with short elimination half-lives for a period of 2 days before, the day of, and 2 days following administration of pemetrexed. In the absence of data regarding potential interaction between pemetrexed and NSAIDs with longer half-lives, all patients taking these NSAIDs should interrupt dosing for at least 5 days before, the day of, and 2 days following pemetrexed administration. If concomitant administration of an NSAID is necessary, patients should be monitored closely for toxicity, especially myelosuppression, renal, and gastrointestinal toxicity). Products include:
Anaprox 2850
Anaprox DS 2850
Treximet 1681

Nelfinavir Mesylate (Concomitant administration of nephrotoxic drugs could result in delayed clearance of pemetrexed).
No products indexed under this heading.

Neomycin (Concomitant administration of nephrotoxic drugs could result in delayed clearance of pemetrexed).
No products indexed under this heading.

Neomycin, oral (Concomitant administration of nephrotoxic drugs could result in delayed clearance of pemetrexed).
No products indexed under this heading.

Neomycin Sulfate (Concomitant administration of nephrotoxic drugs could result in delayed clearance of pemetrexed).
No products indexed under this heading.

Nevirapine (Concomitant administration of nephrotoxic drugs could result in delayed clearance of pemetrexed). Products include:
Viramune Oral Suspension 897
Viramune Tablets 897

Norfloxacin (Concomitant administration of nephrotoxic drugs could result in delayed clearance of pemetrexed). Products include:
Noroxin 2220

Olsalazine Sodium (Concomitant administration of nephrotoxic drugs could result in delayed clearance of pemetrexed).
No products indexed under this heading.

Omeprazole (Concomitant administration of nephrotoxic drugs could result in delayed clearance of pemetrexed).
No products indexed under this heading.

Oxaprozin (Patients with mild to moderate renal insufficiency should avoid taking NSAIDs with short elimination half-lives for a period of 2 days before, the day of, and 2 days following administration of pemetrexed. In the absence of data regarding potential interaction between pemetrexed and NSAIDs with longer half-lives, all patients taking these NSAIDs should interrupt dosing for at least 5 days before, the day of, and 2 days following pemetrexed administration. If concomitant administration of an NSAID is necessary, patients should be monitored closely for toxicity, especially myelosuppression, renal, and gastrointestinal toxicity).
No products indexed under this heading.

Pamidronate Disodium (Concomitant administration of nephrotoxic drugs could result in delayed clearance of pemetrexed).
No products indexed under this heading.

Paroxetine Hydrochloride (Concomitant administration of nephrotoxic drugs could result in delayed clearance of pemetrexed). Products include:
Paroxetine CR 2361
Paroxetine ER 2371
Paxil 1586
Paxil CR 1596

Penicillamine (Concomitant administration of nephrotoxic drugs could result in delayed clearance of pemetrexed).
No products indexed under this heading.

Penicillin G Benzathine (Concomitant administration of nephrotoxic drugs could result in delayed clearance of pemetrexed). Products include:
Bicillin C-R Injectable Suspension 1826
Bicillin L-A 1828

Penicillin G Potassium (Concomitant administration of nephrotoxic drugs could result in delayed clearance of pemetrexed).
No products indexed under this heading.

Penicillin G Procaine (Concomitant administration of nephrotoxic drugs could result in delayed clearance of pemetrexed). Products include:
Bicillin C-R Injectable Suspension 1826
Bicillin L-A 1828

Penicillin G Sodium (Concomitant administration of nephrotoxic drugs could result in delayed clearance of pemetrexed).
No products indexed under this heading.

Penicillin V Potassium (Concomitant administration of nephrotoxic drugs could result in delayed clearance of pemetrexed).
No products indexed under this heading.

Pentamidine Isethionate (Concomitant administration of nephrotoxic drugs could result in delayed clearance of pemetrexed).
No products indexed under this heading.

Perindopril Erbumine (Concomitant administration of nephrotoxic drugs could result in delayed clearance of pemetrexed).
No products indexed under this heading.

Phenylbutazone (Patients with mild to moderate renal insufficiency should avoid taking NSAIDs with short elimination half-lives for a period of 2 days before, the day of, and 2 days following administration of pemetrexed. In the absence of data regarding potential interaction between pemetrexed and NSAIDs with longer half-lives, all patients taking these NSAIDs should interrupt dosing for at least 5 days before, the day of, and 2 days following pemetrexed administration. If concomitant administration of an NSAID is necessary, patients should be monitored closely for toxicity, especially myelosuppression, renal, and gastrointestinal toxicity).
No products indexed under this heading.

IMPORTANT NOTE: Always consult each drug listing in the patient's regimen for possible interactions.

Piroxicam (Patients with mild to moderate renal insufficiency should avoid taking NSAIDs with short elimination half-lives for a period of 2 days before, the day of, and 2 days following administration of pemetrexed. In the absence of data regarding potential interaction between pemetrexed and NSAIDs with longer half-lives, all patients taking these NSAIDs should interrupt dosing for at least 5 days before, the day of, and 2 days following pemetrexed administration. If concomitant administration of an NSAID is necessary, patients should be monitored closely for toxicity, especially myelosuppression, renal, and gastrointestinal toxicity).
No products indexed under this heading.

Plicamycin (Concomitant administration of nephrotoxic drugs could result in delayed clearance of pemetrexed).
No products indexed under this heading.

Polymyxin (Concomitant administration of nephrotoxic drugs could result in delayed clearance of pemetrexed).
No products indexed under this heading.

Polymyxin B Sulfate (Concomitant administration of nephrotoxic drugs could result in delayed clearance of pemetrexed).
No products indexed under this heading.

Polythiazide (Concomitant administration of nephrotoxic drugs could result in delayed clearance of pemetrexed).
No products indexed under this heading.

Pravastatin Sodium (Concomitant administration of nephrotoxic drugs could result in delayed clearance of pemetrexed).
No products indexed under this heading.

Probenecid (Concomitant administration of substances that are tubularly secreted (eg, probenecid) could potentially result in delayed clearance of pemetrexed).
No products indexed under this heading.

Quinapril Hydrochloride (Concomitant administration of nephrotoxic drugs could result in delayed clearance of pemetrexed).
No products indexed under this heading.

Rabeprazole Sodium (Concomitant administration of nephrotoxic drugs could result in delayed clearance of pemetrexed). Products include:
Aciphex 1035

Ramipril (Concomitant administration of nephrotoxic drugs could result in delayed clearance of pemetrexed).
No products indexed under this heading.

Rifampin (Concomitant administration of nephrotoxic drugs could result in delayed clearance of pemetrexed).
No products indexed under this heading.

Riluzole (Concomitant administration of nephrotoxic drugs could result in delayed clearance of pemetrexed). Products include:
Rilutek 3032

Ritonavir (Concomitant administration of nephrotoxic drugs could result in delayed clearance of pemetrexed). Products include:
Kaletra 458
Norvir 509

Rofecoxib (Patients with mild to moderate renal insufficiency should avoid taking NSAIDs with short elimination half-lives for a period of 2 days before, the day of, and 2 days following administration of pemetrexed. In the absence of data regarding potential interaction between pemetrexed and NSAIDs with longer half-lives, all patients taking these NSAIDs should interrupt dosing for at least 5 days before, the day of, and 2 days following pemetrexed administration. If concomitant administration of an NSAID is necessary,

patients should be monitored closely for toxicity, especially myelosuppression, renal, and gastrointestinal toxicity).
No products indexed under this heading.

Saquinavir (Concomitant administration of nephrotoxic drugs could result in delayed clearance of pemetrexed).
No products indexed under this heading.

Sibutramine Hydrochloride Monohydrate (Concomitant administration of nephrotoxic drugs could result in delayed clearance of pemetrexed). Products include:
Meridia 492

Simvastatin (Concomitant administration of nephrotoxic drugs could result in delayed clearance of pemetrexed). Products include:
Simcor 524
Vytorin 10/10 .... 2303, 3240
Vytorin 10/20 .... 2303, 3240
Vytorin 10/40 .... 2303, 3240
Vytorin 10/80 .... 2303, 3240
Zocor 2289

Spirapril Hydrochloride (Concomitant administration of nephrotoxic drugs could result in delayed clearance of pemetrexed).
No products indexed under this heading.

Stavudine (Concomitant administration of nephrotoxic drugs could result in delayed clearance of pemetrexed).
No products indexed under this heading.

Streptomycin Sulfate (Concomitant administration of nephrotoxic drugs could result in delayed clearance of pemetrexed).
No products indexed under this heading.

Streptozocin (Concomitant administration of nephrotoxic drugs could result in delayed clearance of pemetrexed).
No products indexed under this heading.

Sulfacytine (Concomitant administration of nephrotoxic drugs could result in delayed clearance of pemetrexed).
No products indexed under this heading.

Sulfamethizole (Concomitant administration of nephrotoxic drugs could result in delayed clearance of pemetrexed).
No products indexed under this heading.

Sulfamethoxazole (Concomitant administration of nephrotoxic drugs could result in delayed clearance of pemetrexed).
No products indexed under this heading.

Sulfasalazine (Concomitant administration of nephrotoxic drugs could result in delayed clearance of pemetrexed).
No products indexed under this heading.

Sulfinpyrazone (Concomitant administration of nephrotoxic drugs could result in delayed clearance of pemetrexed).
No products indexed under this heading.

Sulfisoxazole Acetyl (Concomitant administration of nephrotoxic drugs could result in delayed clearance of pemetrexed).
No products indexed under this heading.

Sulfisoxazole Diolamine (Concomitant administration of nephrotoxic drugs could result in delayed clearance of pemetrexed).
No products indexed under this heading.

Sulindac (Patients with mild to moderate renal insufficiency should avoid taking NSAIDs with short elimination half-lives for a period of 2 days before, the day of, and 2 days following administration of pemetrexed. In the absence of data regarding potential interaction between pemetrexed and NSAIDs with longer half-lives, all patients taking these NSAIDs should interrupt dosing for at least 5 days before, the day of, and 2 days following pemetrexed administration. If concomitant administration of an NSAID is necessary,

patients should be monitored closely for toxicity, especially myelosuppression, renal, and gastrointestinal toxicity). Products include:
Clinoril 2098

Tacrolimus (Concomitant administration of nephrotoxic drugs could result in delayed clearance of pemetrexed). Products include:
Prograf Capsules 677
Prograf Injection 677
Protopic 685

Tenofovir Disoproxil Fumarate (Concomitant administration of nephrotoxic drugs could result in delayed clearance of pemetrexed). Products include:
Atripla 906
Truvada 1258
Viread 1266

Thioguanine (Concomitant administration of nephrotoxic drugs could result in delayed clearance of pemetrexed). Products include:
Tabloid 1664

Ticarcillin Disodium (Concomitant administration of nephrotoxic drugs could result in delayed clearance of pemetrexed). Products include:
Timentin ADD-Vantage 1670
Timentin Galaxy 1674
Timentin 1666
Timentin Pharmacy 1678

Tobramycin (Concomitant administration of nephrotoxic drugs could result in delayed clearance of pemetrexed). Products include:
Tobi Nebulizer 2546
Tobramycin and Dexamethasone
  Ophthalmic Suspension .... ⊙ 251
Zylet .... ⊙ 252

Tobramycin Sulfate (Concomitant administration of nephrotoxic drugs could result in delayed clearance of pemetrexed).
No products indexed under this heading.

Tolazamide (Concomitant administration of nephrotoxic drugs could result in delayed clearance of pemetrexed).
No products indexed under this heading.

Tolbutamide (Concomitant administration of nephrotoxic drugs could result in delayed clearance of pemetrexed).
No products indexed under this heading.

Tolmetin Sodium (Patients with mild to moderate renal insufficiency should avoid taking NSAIDs with short elimination half-lives for a period of 2 days before, the day of, and 2 days following administration of pemetrexed. In the absence of data regarding potential interaction between pemetrexed and NSAIDs with longer half-lives, all patients taking these NSAIDs should interrupt dosing for at least 5 days before, the day of, and 2 days following pemetrexed administration. If concomitant administration of an NSAID is necessary, patients should be monitored closely for toxicity, especially myelosuppression, renal, and gastrointestinal toxicity).
No products indexed under this heading.

Trandolapril (Concomitant administration of nephrotoxic drugs could result in delayed clearance of pemetrexed). Products include:
Mavik 489
Tarka 534

Triamterene (Concomitant administration of nephrotoxic drugs could result in delayed clearance of pemetrexed). Products include:
Dyazide 1429
Dyrenium 3495

Trimethadione (Concomitant administration of nephrotoxic drugs could result in delayed clearance of pemetrexed).
No products indexed under this heading.

Trovafloxacin Mesylate (Concomitant administration of nephrotoxic drugs could result in delayed clearance of pemetrexed).
No products indexed under this heading.

Tyropanoate Sodium (Concomitant administration of nephrotoxic drugs could result in delayed clearance of pemetrexed).
No products indexed under this heading.

Valacyclovir Hydrochloride (Concomitant administration of nephrotoxic drugs could result in delayed clearance of pemetrexed). Products include:
Valtrex 1702

Valdecoxib (Patients with mild to moderate renal insufficiency should avoid taking NSAIDs with short elimination half-lives for a period of 2 days before, the day of, and 2 days following administration of pemetrexed. In the absence of data regarding potential interaction between pemetrexed and NSAIDs with longer half-lives, all patients taking these NSAIDs should interrupt dosing for at least 5 days before, the day of, and 2 days following pemetrexed administration. If concomitant administration of an NSAID is necessary, patients should be monitored closely for toxicity, especially myelosuppression, renal, and gastrointestinal toxicity).
No products indexed under this heading.

Vancomycin Hydrochloride (Concomitant administration of nephrotoxic drugs could result in delayed clearance of pemetrexed).
No products indexed under this heading.

Voriconazole (Concomitant administration of nephrotoxic drugs could result in delayed clearance of pemetrexed).
No products indexed under this heading.

Zalcitabine (Concomitant administration of nephrotoxic drugs could result in delayed clearance of pemetrexed).
No products indexed under this heading.

Zidovudine (Concomitant administration of nephrotoxic drugs could result in delayed clearance of pemetrexed). Products include:
Combivir 1404
Retrovir 1634
Retrovir IV 1640
Trizivir 1688

Zoledronic Acid (Concomitant administration of nephrotoxic drugs could result in delayed clearance of pemetrexed). Products include:
Reclast 2509
Zometa 2554

ALKERAN FOR INJECTION

(Melphalan Hydrochloride) 1300

Carmustine (BCNU) (IV melphalan may reduce the threshold for BCNU lung toxicity).
No products indexed under this heading.

Cisplatin (Cisplatin may affect melphalan kinetics by inducing renal dysfunction and subsequently altering melphalan clearance).
No products indexed under this heading.

Cyclosporine (The development of severe renal failure has been reported in patients treated with a single dose of IV melphalan followed by standard oral doses of cyclosporine). Products include:
Gengraf 440
Neoral Oral Solution 2496
Neoral Capsules 2496
Restasis 605

Nalidixic Acid (When nalidixic acid and IV melphalan are given simultaneously, the incidence of severe hemorrhagic necrotic enterocolitis has been reported to increase in pediatric patients).
No products indexed under this heading.

(⊙ Described in PDR® for Ophthalmic Medicines)

ALKERAN TABLETS

(Melphalan) 1302
None cited in PDR database.

ALLEGRA ODT ORALLY DISINTEGRATING TABLETS

(Fexofenadine Hydrochloride) 2911
May interact with antacids containing aluminum, calcium and magnesium, erythromycin, magnesium-containing antacids, and certain other agents. Compounds in these categories include:

Aluminum Carbonate (Administration of 120 mg fexofenadine hydrochloride within 15 minutes of an aluminum and magnesium containing antacid (Maalox) decreased fexofenadine AUC by 41% and C_{max} by 43%. Fexofenadine hydrochloride should not be taken closely in time with aluminum and magnesium containing antacids).
No products indexed under this heading.

Aluminum Hydroxide (Administration of 120 mg fexofenadine hydrochloride within 15 minutes of an aluminum and magnesium containing antacid (Maalox) decreased fexofenadine AUC by 41% and C_{max} by 43%. Fexofenadine hydrochloride should not be taken closely in time with aluminum and magnesium containing antacids).
No products indexed under this heading.

Calcium Carbonate (Administration of 120 mg fexofenadine hydrochloride within 15 minutes of an aluminum and magnesium containing antacid (Maalox) decreased fexofenadine AUC by 41% and C_{max} by 43%. Fexofenadine hydrochloride should not be taken closely in time with aluminum and magnesium containing antacids). Products include:
Chelated Mineral 3476
Pepcid Complete 1822
Extra Strength Rolaids Softchews
   Vanilla Creme 2045

Erythromycin (Co-administration of fexofenadine hydrochloride with erythromycin has led to increased plasma concentrations of fexofenadine).
No products indexed under this heading.

Erythromycin, Topical (Co-administration of fexofenadine hydrochloride with erythromycin has led to increased plasma concentrations of fexofenadine).
No products indexed under this heading.

Erythromycin Estolate (Co-administration of fexofenadine hydrochloride with erythromycin has led to increased plasma concentrations of fexofenadine).
No products indexed under this heading.

Erythromycin Ethylsuccinate (Co-administration of fexofenadine hydrochloride with erythromycin has led to increased plasma concentrations of fexofenadine). Products include:
E.E.S. 437
EryPed 435

Erythromycin Gluceptate (Co-administration of fexofenadine hydrochloride with erythromycin has led to increased plasma concentrations of fexofenadine).
No products indexed under this heading.

Erythromycin Lactobionate (Co-administration of fexofenadine hydrochloride with erythromycin has led to increased plasma concentrations of fexofenadine).
No products indexed under this heading.

Erythromycin Stearate (Co-administration of fexofenadine hydrochloride with erythromycin has led to increased plasma concentrations of fexofenadine).
No products indexed under this heading.

Fat (Administration of fexofenadine hydrochloride 30 mg with a high-fat meal decreased the AUC and C_{max} by approximately 40% and 60%, respectively, and a 2-hour delay in the time to peak exposure (T_{max}) was observed).
No products indexed under this heading.

Ketoconazole (Co-administration of fexofenadine hydrochloride with ketoconazole has led to increased plasma concentrations of fexofenadine).
Products include:
Extina 3319
Xolegel 3337

Magaldrate (Administration of 120 mg fexofenadine hydrochloride within 15 minutes of an aluminum and magnesium containing antacid (Maalox) decreased fexofenadine AUC by 41% and C_{max} by 43%. Fexofenadine hydrochloride should not be taken closely in time with aluminum and magnesium containing antacids).
No products indexed under this heading.

Magnesium Carbonate (Administration of 120 mg fexofenadine hydrochloride within 15 minutes of an aluminum and magnesium containing antacid (Maalox) decreased fexofenadine AUC by 41% and C_{max} by 43%. Fexofenadine hydrochloride should not be taken closely in time with aluminum and magnesium containing antacids).
No products indexed under this heading.

Magnesium Hydroxide (Administration of 120 mg fexofenadine hydrochloride within 15 minutes of an aluminum and magnesium containing antacid (Maalox) decreased fexofenadine AUC by 41% and C_{max} by 43%. Fexofenadine hydrochloride should not be taken closely in time with aluminum and magnesium containing antacids). Products include:
Fleet Pedia-Lax Chewable Tablets 1144
Pepcid Complete 1822

Magnesium Oxide (Administration of 120 mg fexofenadine hydrochloride within 15 minutes of an aluminum and magnesium containing antacid (Maalox) decreased fexofenadine AUC by 41% and C_{max} by 43%. Fexofenadine hydrochloride should not be taken closely in time with aluminum and magnesium containing antacids). Products include:
Beelith 873

Magnesium Trisilicate (Administration of 120 mg fexofenadine hydrochloride within 15 minutes of an aluminum and magnesium containing antacid (Maalox) decreased fexofenadine AUC by 41% and C_{max} by 43%. Fexofenadine hydrochloride should not be taken closely in time with aluminum and magnesium containing antacids).
No products indexed under this heading.

Food Interactions

Apple Juice (Fruit juices such as grapefruit, orange and apple may reduce the bioavailability and exposure of fexofenadine).

Food, unspecified (Administration of fexofenadine hydrochloride 30 mg with a high-fat meal decreased the AUC and C_{max} by approximately 40% and 60%, respectively, and a 2-hour delay in the time to peak exposure (T_{max}) was observed).

Fruit juices, unspecified (Fruit juices such as grapefruit, orange and apple may reduce the bioavailability and exposure of fexofenadine).

Grapefruit Juice (Fruit juices such as grapefruit, orange and apple may reduce the bioavailability and exposure of fexofenadine).

Meal, unspecified (Administration of fexofenadine hydrochloride 30 mg with a high-fat meal decreased the AUC and C_{max} by approximately 40% and 60%,

respectively, and a 2-hour delay in the time to peak exposure (T_{max}) was observed).

Orange Juice (Fruit juices such as grapefruit, orange and apple may reduce the bioavailability and exposure of fexofenadine).

ALLEGRA ORAL SOLUTION

(Fexofenadine Hydrochloride) 2911
See Allegra Tablets

ALLEGRA TABLETS

(Fexofenadine Hydrochloride) 2911
May interact with erythromycin, and certain other agents. Compounds in these categories include:

Aluminum Hydroxide (Administration of fexofenadine within 15 minutes of an aluminum and magnesium containing antacid decreased fexofenadine AUC by 41% and C_{max} by 43%; Allegra should not be taken closely in time with aluminum and magnesium containing antacids).
No products indexed under this heading.

Erythromycin (Co-administration with erythromycin has led to increased plasma levels of fexofenadine).
No products indexed under this heading.

Erythromycin, Topical (Co-administration with erythromycin has led to increased plasma levels of fexofenadine).
No products indexed under this heading.

Erythromycin Estolate (Co-administration with erythromycin has led to increased plasma levels of fexofenadine).
No products indexed under this heading.

Erythromycin Ethylsuccinate (Co-administration with erythromycin has led to increased plasma levels of fexofenadine). Products include:
E.E.S. 437
EryPed 435

Erythromycin Gluceptate (Co-administration with erythromycin has led to increased plasma levels of fexofenadine).
No products indexed under this heading.

Erythromycin Lactobionate (Co-administration with erythromycin has led to increased plasma levels of fexofenadine).
No products indexed under this heading.

Erythromycin Stearate (Co-administration with erythromycin has led to increased plasma levels of fexofenadine).
No products indexed under this heading.

Ketoconazole (Co-administration with ketoconazole as led to increased plasma levels of fexofenadine). Products include:
Extina 3319
Xolegel 3337

Magnesium Hydroxide (Administration of fexofenadine within 15 minutes of an aluminum and magnesium containing antacid decreased fexofenadine AUC by 41% and C_{max} by 43%; Allegra should not be taken closely in time with aluminum and magnesium containing antacids). Products include:
Fleet Pedia-Lax Chewable Tablets 1144
Pepcid Complete 1822

Food Interactions

Fruit juices, unspecified (Grapefruit, orange and apple may reduce the bioavailability and exposure of fexofenadine; it is recommended that fexofenadine should be taken with water).

ALLEGRA-D 12 HOUR EXTENDED-RELEASE TABLETS

(Fexofenadine Hydrochloride, Pseudoephedrine Hydrochloride)........... 2915
May interact with antacids, cardiac glycosides, erythromycin, monoamine oxidase inhibitors, sympathomimetics, and certain other agents. Compounds in these categories include:

Albuterol (Combined effects of pseudoephedrine with other sympathomimetics on cardiovascular system may be harmful to the patient).
No products indexed under this heading.

Albuterol Sulfate (Combined effects of pseudoephedrine with other sympathomimetics on cardiovascular system may be harmful to the patient).
Products include:
ProAir HFA 3393
Proventil HFA 3204
Ventolin HFA 1708

Aluminum Carbonate (Co-administration with fexofenadine HCL may decrease fexofenadine AUC by 41% and C_{max} by 43%).
No products indexed under this heading.

Aluminum Hydroxide (Co-administration with fexofenadine HCL may decrease fexofenadine AUC by 41% and C_{max} by 43%).
No products indexed under this heading.

Calcium Carbonate (Co-administration with fexofenadine HCL may decrease fexofenadine AUC by 41% and C_{max} by 43%). Products include:
Chelated Mineral 3476
Pepcid Complete 1822
Extra Strength Rolaids Softchews
   Vanilla Creme 2045

Deslanoside (Increased ectopic pacemaker activity can occur when pseudoephedrine is used concomitantly with digitalis).
No products indexed under this heading.

Digitalis Glycoside Preparations (Increased ectopic pacemaker activity can occur when pseudoephedrine is used concomitantly with digitalis).
No products indexed under this heading.

Digitalis Lanata (Increased ectopic pacemaker activity can occur when pseudoephedrine is used concomitantly with digitalis).
No products indexed under this heading.

Digitalis Purpurea (Increased ectopic pacemaker activity can occur when pseudoephedrine is used concomitantly with digitalis).
No products indexed under this heading.

Digitoxin (Increased ectopic pacemaker activity can occur when pseudoephedrine is used concomitantly with digitalis).
No products indexed under this heading.

Digoxin (Increased ectopic pacemaker activity can occur when pseudoephedrine is used concomitantly with digitalis). Products include:
Lanoxin Injection 1546
Lanoxin Injection Pediatric 1549
Lanoxin Tablets 1553

Dobutamine Hydrochloride (Combined effects of pseudoephedrine with other sympathomimetics on cardiovascular system may be harmful to the patient).
No products indexed under this heading.

Dopamine Hydrochloride (Combined effects of pseudoephedrine with other sympathomimetics on cardiovascular system may be harmful to the patient).
No products indexed under this heading.

IMPORTANT NOTE: Always consult each drug listing in the patient's regimen for possible interactions.

Ephedrine Hydrochloride (Combined effects of pseudoephedrine with other sympathomimetics on cardiovascular system may be harmful to the patient).
No products indexed under this heading.

Ephedrine Sulfate (Combined effects of pseudoephedrine with other sympathomimetics on cardiovascular system may be harmful to the patient).
No products indexed under this heading.

Ephedrine Tannate (Combined effects of pseudoephedrine with other sympathomimetics on cardiovascular system may be harmful to the patient).
No products indexed under this heading.

Epinephrine (Combined effects of pseudoephedrine with other sympathomimetics on cardiovascular system may be harmful to the patient).
Products include:
   EpiPen 3631
   Twinject 3268

Epinephrine Bitartrate (Combined effects of pseudoephedrine with other sympathomimetics on cardiovascular system may be harmful to the patient).
No products indexed under this heading.

Epinephrine Hydrochloride (Combined effects of pseudoephedrine with other sympathomimetics on cardiovascular system may be harmful to the patient).
No products indexed under this heading.

Erythromycin (Co-administration with erythromycin enhances fexofenadine gastrointestinal absorption thereby increasing plasma levels of fexofenadine; *in vivo* animal studies suggest that erythromycin may also decrease biliary excretion).
No products indexed under this heading.

Erythromycin, Topical (Co-administration with erythromycin enhances fexofenadine gastrointestinal absorption thereby increasing plasma levels of fexofenadine; *in vivo* animal studies suggest that erythromycin may also decrease biliary excretion).
No products indexed under this heading.

Erythromycin Estolate (Co-administration with erythromycin enhances fexofenadine gastrointestinal absorption thereby increasing plasma levels of fexofenadine; *in vivo* animal studies suggest that erythromycin may also decrease biliary excretion).
No products indexed under this heading.

Erythromycin Ethylsuccinate (Co-administration with erythromycin enhances fexofenadine gastrointestinal absorption thereby increasing plasma levels of fexofenadine; *in vivo* animal studies suggest that erythromycin may also decrease biliary excretion).
Products include:
   E.E.S. 437
   EryPed 435

Erythromycin Gluceptate (Co-administration with erythromycin enhances fexofenadine gastrointestinal absorption thereby increasing plasma levels of fexofenadine; *in vivo* animal studies suggest that erythromycin may also decrease biliary excretion).
No products indexed under this heading.

Erythromycin Lactobionate (Co-administration with erythromycin enhances fexofenadine gastrointestinal absorption thereby increasing plasma levels of fexofenadine; *in vivo* animal studies suggest that erythromycin may also decrease biliary excretion).
No products indexed under this heading.

Erythromycin Stearate (Co-administration with erythromycin enhances fexofenadine gastrointestinal absorption thereby increasing plasma levels of fexofenadine; *in vivo* animal studies suggest that erythromycin may also decrease biliary excretion).
No products indexed under this heading.

Isocarboxazid (Concurrent and/or sequential use with MAO inhibitors is contraindicated). Products include:
   Marplan 3481

Isoproterenol Hydrochloride (Combined effects of pseudoephedrine with other sympathomimetics on cardiovascular system may be harmful to the patient).
No products indexed under this heading.

Isoproterenol Sulfate (Combined effects of pseudoephedrine with other sympathomimetics on cardiovascular system may be harmful to the patient).
No products indexed under this heading.

Ketoconazole (Co-administration with ketoconazole enhances fexofenadine gastrointestinal absorption thereby increasing plasma levels of fexofenadine; *in vivo* animal studies suggest that ketoconazole may also decrease fexofenadine gastrointestinal secretion).
Products include:
   Extina 3319
   Xolegel 3337

Levalbuterol Hydrochloride (Combined effects of pseudoephedrine with other sympathomimetics on cardiovascular system may be harmful to the patient).
No products indexed under this heading.

Magaldrate (Co-administration with fexofenadine HCL may decrease fexofenadine AUC by 41% and C_{max} by 43%).
No products indexed under this heading.

Magnesium Carbonate (Co-administration with fexofenadine HCL may decrease fexofenadine AUC by 41% and C_{max} by 43%).
No products indexed under this heading.

Magnesium Hydroxide (Co-administration with fexofenadine HCL may decrease fexofenadine AUC by 41% and C_{max} by 43%). Products include:
   Fleet Pedia-Lax Chewable Tablets 1144
   Pepcid Complete 1822

Magnesium Oxide (Co-administration with fexofenadine HCL may decrease fexofenadine AUC by 41% and C_{max} by 43%). Products include:
   Beelith 873

Magnesium Trisilicate (Co-administration with fexofenadine HCL may decrease fexofenadine AUC by 41% and C_{max} by 43%).
No products indexed under this heading.

Mecamylamine Hydrochloride (Reduced antihypertensive effects).
No products indexed under this heading.

Metaproterenol Sulfate (Combined effects of pseudoephedrine with other sympathomimetics on cardiovascular system may be harmful to the patient).
No products indexed under this heading.

Metaraminol Bitartrate (Combined effects of pseudoephedrine with other sympathomimetics on cardiovascular system may be harmful to the patient).
No products indexed under this heading.

Methoxamine Hydrochloride (Combined effects of pseudoephedrine with other sympathomimetics on cardiovascular system may be harmful to the patient).
No products indexed under this heading.

Methyldopa (Reduced antihypertensive effects).
No products indexed under this heading.

Methyldopate Hydrochloride (Reduced antihypertensive effects).
No products indexed under this heading.

Moclobemide (Concurrent and/or sequential use with MAO inhibitors is contraindicated).
No products indexed under this heading.

Norepinephrine Bitartrate (Combined effects of pseudoephedrine with other sympathomimetics on cardiovascular system may be harmful to the patient).
No products indexed under this heading.

Pargyline Hydrochloride (Concurrent and/or sequential use with MAO inhibitors is contraindicated).
No products indexed under this heading.

Phenelzine Sulfate (Concurrent and/or sequential use with MAO inhibitors is contraindicated).
No products indexed under this heading.

Phenylephrine Bitartrate (Combined effects of pseudoephedrine with other sympathomimetics on cardiovascular system may be harmful to the patient).
No products indexed under this heading.

Phenylephrine Hydrochloride (Combined effects of pseudoephedrine with other sympathomimetics on cardiovascular system may be harmful to the patient). Products include:
   Sudafed PE Nasal Decongestant 2048
   Children's Sudafed PE Nasal Decongestant 2047

Phenylephrine Tannate (Combined effects of pseudoephedrine with other sympathomimetics on cardiovascular system may be harmful to the patient).
No products indexed under this heading.

Phenylpropanolamine Hydrochloride (Combined effects of pseudoephedrine with other sympathomimetics on cardiovascular system may be harmful to the patient).
No products indexed under this heading.

Pirbuterol Acetate (Combined effects of pseudoephedrine with other sympathomimetics on cardiovascular system may be harmful to the patient). Products include:
   Maxair Autohaler 1782

Procarbazine Hydrochloride (Concurrent and/or sequential use with MAO inhibitors is contraindicated).
No products indexed under this heading.

Pseudoephedrine Sulfate (Combined effects of pseudoephedrine with other sympathomimetics on cardiovascular system may be harmful to the patient). Products include:
   Clarinex-D 12-Hour 3101
   Clarinex-D 3104

Rasagiline Mesylate (Concurrent and/or sequential use with MAO inhibitors is contraindicated). Products include:
   Azilect 3383

Reserpine (Reduced antihypertensive effects).
No products indexed under this heading.

Salmeterol Xinafoate (Combined effects of pseudoephedrine with other sympathomimetics on cardiovascular system may be harmful to the patient). Products include:
   Advair 100/50 1275
   Advair 250/50 1275
   Advair 500/50 1275
   Advair HFA 45/21 1288
   Advair HFA 115/21 1288
   Advair HFA 230/21 1288
   Serevent Diskus 1656

Selegiline (Concurrent and/or sequential use with MAO inhibitors is contraindicated). Products include:
   Emsam 3623

Selegiline Hydrochloride (Concurrent and/or sequential use with MAO inhibitors is contraindicated). Products include:
   Eldepryl 3312

Sodium Bicarbonate (Co-administration with fexofenadine HCL may decrease fexofenadine AUC by 41% and C_{max} by 43%).
No products indexed under this heading.

Terbutaline Sulfate (Combined effects of pseudoephedrine with other sympathomimetics on cardiovascular system may be harmful to the patient).
No products indexed under this heading.

Tranylcypromine Sulfate (Concurrent and/or sequential use with MAO inhibitors is contraindicated). Products include:
   Parnate 1584

Food Interactions

Apple Juice (Co-administration with grapefruit, orange or apple juice will reduce the bioavailability and exposure or fexofenadine).

Diet, high-lipid (Co-administration with a high-fat meal decreased fexofenadine plasma concentrations C_{max} and AUC, and T_{max} was delayed by 50%; the rate of extent of pseudoephedrine absorption was not affected by food; administration of Allegra-D with food should be avoided).

Grapefruit Juice (Co-administration with grapefruit, orange or apple juice will reduce the bioavailability and exposure or fexofenadine).

Orange Juice (Co-administration with grapefruit, orange or apple juice will reduce the bioavailability and exposure or fexofenadine).

ALLEGRA-D 24 HOUR EXTENDED-RELEASE TABLETS
(Fexofenadine Hydrochloride, Pseudoephedrine Hydrochloride) 2918
See Allegra-D 12 Hour Extended-Release Tablets

ALOXI INJECTION
(Palonosetron Hydrochloride) 1042
None cited in PDR database.

ALPHAGAN P OPHTHALMIC SOLUTION
(Brimonidine Tartrate) 596
May interact with alcohols, anesthetics, antihypertensives, barbiturates, beta-blockers, cardiac glycosides, central nervous system depressants, hypnotics and sedatives, monoamine oxidase inhibitors, narcotic analgesics, tricyclic antidepressants. Compounds in these categories include:

Acebutolol Hydrochloride (Concurrent use of brimonidine, an alpha adrenergic agonist, with beta blockers (ophthalmic and systemic) may reduce pulse and blood pressure however, in clinical trials brimonidine did not have any significant effects on pulse and blood pressure).
No products indexed under this heading.

Alfentanil Hydrochloride (Possible additive or potentiating effect with CNS depressants).
No products indexed under this heading.

Aliskiren (Concurrent use of brimonidine, an alpha adrenergic agonist, with antihypertensives may reduce pulse and blood pressure, however, in clinical trials brimonidine did not have any significant effects on pulse and blood pressure). Products include:
   Tekturna 2538
   Tekturna HCT 2541
   Valturna 3637

89 Interactions Index Alphagan P

Alprazolam (Possible additive or potentiating effect with CNS depressants).
No products indexed under this heading.

Amitriptyline Hydrochloride (Tricyclic antidepressants have been reported to blunt the hypotensive effect of systemic clonidine, an alpha adrenergic agonist; it is not known whether the concurrent use of these agents with brimonidine can lead to interference in IOP-lowering effect; caution is advised).
No products indexed under this heading.

Amlodipine Besylate (Concurrent use of brimonidine, an alpha adrenergic agonist, with antihypertensives may reduce pulse and blood pressure, however, in clinical trials brimonidine did not have any significant effects on pulse and blood pressure). Products include:
Azor **1010**
Exforge **2443**
Exforge HCT **2449**

Amobarbital (Possible additive or potentiating effect with CNS depressants).
No products indexed under this heading.

Amobarbital Sodium (Possible additive or potentiating effect with CNS depressants).
No products indexed under this heading.

Amoxapine (Tricyclic antidepressants have been reported to blunt the hypotensive effect of systemic clonidine, an alpha adrenergic agonist; it is not known whether the concurrent use of these agents with brimonidine can lead to interference in IOP-lowering effect; caution is advised).
No products indexed under this heading.

Apomorphine (Possible additive or potentiating effect with CNS depressants).
No products indexed under this heading.

Apomorphine Hydrochloride (Possible additive or potentiating effect with CNS depressants).
No products indexed under this heading.

Aprobarbital (Possible additive or potentiating effect with CNS depressants).
No products indexed under this heading.

Articaine Hydrochloride (Possible additive or potentiating effect with CNS depressants).
No products indexed under this heading.

Atenolol (Concurrent use of brimonidine, an alpha adrenergic agonist, with beta blockers (ophthalmic and systemic) may reduce pulse and blood pressure, however, in clinical trials brimonidine did not have any significant effects on pulse and blood pressure).
No products indexed under this heading.

Benazepril Hydrochloride (Concurrent use of brimonidine, an alpha adrenergic agonist, with antihypertensives may reduce pulse and blood pressure, however, in clinical trials brimonidine did not have any significant effects on pulse and blood pressure).
No products indexed under this heading.

Bendroflumethiazide (Concurrent use of brimonidine, an alpha adrenergic agonist, with antihypertensives may reduce pulse and blood pressure, however, in clinical trials brimonidine did not have any significant effects on pulse and blood pressure).
No products indexed under this heading.

Benzocaine (Possible additive or potentiating effect with CNS depressants).
No products indexed under this heading.

Betaxolol Hydrochloride (Concurrent use of brimonidine, an alpha adrenergic agonist, with beta blockers (ophthalmic and systemic) may reduce pulse and blood pressure, however, in clinical trials brimonidine did not have any significant effects on pulse and blood pressure).
No products indexed under this heading.

Bisoprolol Fumarate (Concurrent use of brimonidine, an alpha adrenergic agonist, with beta blockers (ophthalmic and systemic) may reduce pulse and blood pressure, however, in clinical trials brimonidine did not have any significant effects on pulse and blood pressure).
No products indexed under this heading.

Bupivacaine Hydrochloride (Possible additive or potentiating effect with CNS depressants).
No products indexed under this heading.

Buprenorphine Hydrochloride (Possible additive or potentiating effect with CNS depressants).
No products indexed under this heading.

Buspirone Hydrochloride (Possible additive or potentiating effect with CNS depressants).
No products indexed under this heading.

Butabarbital (Possible additive or potentiating effect with CNS depressants).
No products indexed under this heading.

Butabarbital Sodium (Possible additive or potentiating effect with CNS depressants).
No products indexed under this heading.

Butalbital (Possible additive or potentiating effect with CNS depressants).
No products indexed under this heading.

Candesartan Cilexetil (Concurrent use of brimonidine, an alpha adrenergic agonist, with antihypertensives may reduce pulse and blood pressure, however, in clinical trials brimonidine did not have any significant effects on pulse and blood pressure). Products include:
Atacand **697**
Atacand HCT **700**

Captopril (Concurrent use of brimonidine, an alpha adrenergic agonist, with antihypertensives may reduce pulse and blood pressure, however, in clinical trials brimonidine did not have any significant effects on pulse and blood pressure). Products include:
Captopril **2341**

Carteolol Hydrochloride (Concurrent use of brimonidine, an alpha adrenergic agonist, with beta blockers (ophthalmic and systemic) may reduce pulse and blood pressure, however, in clinical trials brimonidine did not have any significant effects on pulse and blood pressure).
No products indexed under this heading.

Carvedilol (Concurrent use of brimonidine, an alpha adrenergic agonist, with beta blockers (ophthalmic and systemic) may reduce pulse and blood pressure, however, in clinical trials brimonidine did not have any significant effects on pulse and blood pressure). Products include:
Coreg **1409**

Carvedilol Phosphate (Concurrent use of brimonidine, an alpha adrenergic agonist, with beta blockers (ophthalmic and systemic) may reduce pulse and blood pressure, however, in clinical trials brimonidine did not have any significant effects on pulse and blood pressure). Products include:
Coreg CR **1416**

Chloral Hydrate (Possible additive or potentiating effect with CNS depressants).
No products indexed under this heading.

Chlordiazepoxide (Possible additive or potentiating effect with CNS depressants).
No products indexed under this heading.

Chlordiazepoxide Hydrochloride (Possible additive or potentiating effect with CNS depressants).
No products indexed under this heading.

Chloroprocaine Hydrochloride (Possible additive or potentiating effect with CNS depressants).
No products indexed under this heading.

Chlorothiazide (Concurrent use of brimonidine, an alpha adrenergic agonist, with antihypertensives may reduce pulse and blood pressure, however, in clinical trials brimonidine did not have any significant effects on pulse and blood pressure).
No products indexed under this heading.

Chlorothiazide Sodium (Concurrent use of brimonidine, an alpha adrenergic agonist, with antihypertensives may reduce pulse and blood pressure, however, in clinical trials brimonidine did not have any significant effects on pulse and blood pressure). Products include:
Diuril Intravenous **2009**

Chlorpromazine (Possible additive or potentiating effect with CNS depressants).
No products indexed under this heading.

Chlorpromazine Hydrochloride (Possible additive or potentiating effect with CNS depressants).
No products indexed under this heading.

Chlorprothixene (Possible additive or potentiating effect with CNS depressants).
No products indexed under this heading.

Chlorprothixene Hydrochloride (Possible additive or potentiating effect with CNS depressants).
No products indexed under this heading.

Chlorprothixene Lactate (Possible additive or potentiating effect with CNS depressants).
No products indexed under this heading.

Chlorthalidone (Concurrent use of brimonidine, an alpha adrenergic agonist, with antihypertensives may reduce pulse and blood pressure, however, in clinical trials brimonidine did not have any significant effects on pulse and blood pressure). Products include:
Clorpres **2344**

Clomipramine Hydrochloride (Tricyclic antidepressants have been reported to blunt the hypotensive effect of systemic clonidine, an alpha adrenergic agonist; it is not known whether the concurrent use of these agents with brimonidine can lead to interference in IOP-lowering effect; caution is advised).
No products indexed under this heading.

Clonazepam (Possible additive or potentiating effect with CNS depressants). Products include:
Klonopin **2855**

Clonidine (Concurrent use of brimonidine, an alpha adrenergic agonist, with antihypertensives may reduce pulse and blood pressure, however, in clinical trials brimonidine did not have any significant effects on pulse and blood pressure). Products include:
Catapres-TTS **884**

Clonidine Hydrochloride (Concurrent use of brimonidine, an alpha adrenergic agonist, with antihypertensives may reduce pulse and blood pressure, however, in clinical trials brimonidine did not have any significant effects on pulse and blood pressure). Products include:
Clorpres **2344**

Clorazepate Dipotassium (Possible additive or potentiating effect with CNS depressants).
No products indexed under this heading.

Clozapine (Possible additive or potentiating effect with CNS depressants).
No products indexed under this heading.

Cocaine Hydrochloride (Possible additive or potentiating effect with CNS depressants).
No products indexed under this heading.

Codeine Phosphate (Possible additive or potentiating effect with CNS depressants). Products include:
Tylenol with Codeine **2691**

Codeine Sulfate (Possible additive or potentiating effect with CNS depressants).
No products indexed under this heading.

Deserpidine (Concurrent use of brimonidine, an alpha adrenergic agonist, with antihypertensives may reduce pulse and blood pressure, however, in clinical trials brimonidine did not have any significant effects on pulse and blood pressure).
No products indexed under this heading.

Desflurane (Possible additive or potentiating effect with CNS depressants).
No products indexed under this heading.

Desipramine Hydrochloride (Tricyclic antidepressants have been reported to blunt the hypotensive effect of systemic clonidine, an alpha adrenergic agonist; it is not known whether the concurrent use of these agents with brimonidine can lead to interference in IOP-lowering effect; caution is advised).
No products indexed under this heading.

Deslanoside (Concurrent use of brimonidine, an alpha adrenergic agonist, with cardiac glycosides may reduce pulse and blood pressure, however, in clinical trials brimonidine did not have any significant effects on pulse and blood pressure).
No products indexed under this heading.

Dezocine (Possible additive or potentiating effect with CNS depressants).
No products indexed under this heading.

Diazepam (Possible additive or potentiating effect with CNS depressants). Products include:
Valium Tablets **2880**

Diazoxide (Concurrent use of brimonidine, an alpha adrenergic agonist, with antihypertensives may reduce pulse and blood pressure, however, in clinical trials brimonidine did not have any significant effects on pulse and blood pressure). Products include:
Proglycem **1179**
Proglycem Suspension **1179**

Dibucaine (Possible additive or potentiating effect with CNS depressants).
No products indexed under this heading.

Dibucaine Hydrochloride (Possible additive or potentiating effect with CNS depressants).
No products indexed under this heading.

Digitalis Glycoside Preparations (Concurrent use of brimonidine, an alpha adrenergic agonist, with cardiac glycosides may reduce pulse and blood pressure, however, in clinical trials brimonidine did not have any significant effects on pulse and blood pressure).
No products indexed under this heading.

Digitalis Lanata (Concurrent use of brimonidine, an alpha adrenergic agonist, with cardiac glycosides may reduce pulse and blood pressure, however, in clinical trials brimonidine did not have any significant effects on pulse and blood pressure).
No products indexed under this heading.

IMPORTANT NOTE: Always consult each drug listing in the patient's regimen for possible interactions.

Alphagan P Interactions Index 90

Digitalis Purpurea (Concurrent use of brimonidine, an alpha adrenergic agonist, with cardiac glycosides may reduce pulse and blood pressure, however, in clinical trials brimonidine did not have any significant effects on pulse and blood pressure).
No products indexed under this heading.

Digitoxin (Concurrent use of brimonidine, an alpha adrenergic agonist, with cardiac glycosides may reduce pulse and blood pressure, however, in clinical trials brimonidine did not have any significant effects on pulse and blood pressure).
No products indexed under this heading.

Digoxin (Concurrent use of brimonidine, an alpha adrenergic agonist, with cardiac glycosides may reduce pulse and blood pressure, however, in clinical trials brimonidine did not have any significant effects on pulse and blood pressure). Products include:
Lanoxin Injection **1546**
Lanoxin Injection Pediatric **1549**
Lanoxin Tablets **1553**

Dihydrocodeine Bitartrate (Possible additive or potentiating effect with CNS depressants).
No products indexed under this heading.

Dihydrocodeinone Bitartrate (Possible additive or potentiating effect with CNS depressants).
No products indexed under this heading.

Diltiazem Hydrochloride (Concurrent use of brimonidine, an alpha adrenergic agonist, with antihypertensives may reduce pulse and blood pressure, however, in clinical trials brimonidine did not have any significant effects on pulse and blood pressure). Products include:
Cardizem LA **423**

Diltiazem Maleate (Concurrent use of brimonidine, an alpha adrenergic agonist, with antihypertensives may reduce pulse and blood pressure, however, in clinical trials brimonidine did not have any significant effects on pulse and blood pressure).
No products indexed under this heading.

Doxazosin Mesylate (Concurrent use of brimonidine, an alpha adrenergic agonist, with antihypertensives may reduce pulse and blood pressure, however, in clinical trials brimonidine did not have any significant effects on pulse and blood pressure).
No products indexed under this heading.

Doxepin Hydrochloride (Tricyclic antidepressants have been reported to blunt the hypotensive effect of systemic clonidine, an alpha adrenergic agonist; it is not known whether the concurrent use of these agents with brimonidine can lead to interference in IOP-lowering effect; caution is advised).
No products indexed under this heading.

Droperidol (Possible additive or potentiating effect with CNS depressants).
No products indexed under this heading.

Enalapril Maleate (Concurrent use of brimonidine, an alpha adrenergic agonist, with antihypertensives may reduce pulse and blood pressure, however, in clinical trials brimonidine did not have any significant effects on pulse and blood pressure).
No products indexed under this heading.

Enalaprilat (Concurrent use of brimonidine, an alpha adrenergic agonist, with antihypertensives may reduce pulse and blood pressure, however, in clinical trials brimonidine did not have any significant effects on pulse and blood pressure).
No products indexed under this heading.

Enflurane (Possible additive or potentiating effect with CNS depressants).
No products indexed under this heading.

Eprosartan Mesylate (Concurrent use of brimonidine, an alpha adrenergic agonist, with antihypertensives may reduce pulse and blood pressure, however, in clinical trials brimonidine did not have any significant effects on pulse and blood pressure). Products include:
Teveten **538**
Teveten HCT **541**

Esmolol Hydrochloride (Concurrent use of brimonidine, an alpha adrenergic agonist, with beta blockers (ophthalmic and systemic) may reduce pulse and blood pressure, however, in clinical trials brimonidine did not have any significant effects on pulse and blood pressure).
No products indexed under this heading.

Estazolam (Possible additive or potentiating effect with CNS depressants).
No products indexed under this heading.

Ethanol (Possible additive or potentiating effect with CNS depressants).
No products indexed under this heading.

Ethchlorvynol (Possible additive or potentiating effect with CNS depressants).
No products indexed under this heading.

Ethinamate (Possible additive or potentiating effect with CNS depressants).
No products indexed under this heading.

Ethyl Alcohol (Possible additive or potentiating effect with CNS depressants).
No products indexed under this heading.

Etidocaine Hydrochloride (Possible additive or potentiating effect with CNS depressants).
No products indexed under this heading.

Felodipine (Concurrent use of brimonidine, an alpha adrenergic agonist, with antihypertensives may reduce pulse and blood pressure, however, in clinical trials brimonidine did not have any significant effects on pulse and blood pressure).
No products indexed under this heading.

Fentanyl (Possible additive or potentiating effect with CNS depressants). Products include:
Duragesic **2604**
Fentanyl Transdermal System **2346**
Onsolis **2054**

Fentanyl Citrate (Possible additive or potentiating effect with CNS depressants). Products include:
Fentora **966**

Fluphenazine Decanoate (Possible additive or potentiating effect with CNS depressants).
No products indexed under this heading.

Fluphenazine Enanthate (Possible additive or potentiating effect with CNS depressants).
No products indexed under this heading.

Fluphenazine Hydrochloride (Possible additive or potentiating effect with CNS depressants).
No products indexed under this heading.

Flurazepam Hydrochloride (Possible additive or potentiating effect with CNS depressants).
No products indexed under this heading.

Fosinopril Sodium (Concurrent use of brimonidine, an alpha adrenergic agonist, with antihypertensives may reduce pulse and blood pressure, however, in clinical trials brimonidine did not have any significant effects on pulse and blood pressure).
No products indexed under this heading.

Furosemide (Concurrent use of brimonidine, an alpha adrenergic agonist, with antihypertensives may reduce pulse and blood pressure, however, in clinical trials brimonidine did not have any significant effects on pulse and blood pressure). Products include:
Furosemide **2354**

Glutethimide (Possible additive or potentiating effect with CNS depressants).
No products indexed under this heading.

Guanabenz Acetate (Concurrent use of brimonidine, an alpha adrenergic agonist, with antihypertensives may reduce pulse and blood pressure, however, in clinical trials brimonidine did not have any significant effects on pulse and blood pressure).
No products indexed under this heading.

Guanethidine (Concurrent use of brimonidine, an alpha adrenergic agonist, with antihypertensives may reduce pulse and blood pressure, however, in clinical trials brimonidine did not have any significant effects on pulse and blood pressure).
No products indexed under this heading.

Guanethidine Monosulfate (Concurrent use of brimonidine, an alpha adrenergic agonist, with antihypertensives may reduce pulse and blood pressure, however, in clinical trials brimonidine did not have any significant effects on pulse and blood pressure).
No products indexed under this heading.

Guanethidine Sulfate (Concurrent use of brimonidine, an alpha adrenergic agonist, with antihypertensives may reduce pulse and blood pressure, however, in clinical trials brimonidine did not have any significant effects on pulse and blood pressure).
No products indexed under this heading.

Halazepam (Possible additive or potentiating effect with CNS depressants).
No products indexed under this heading.

Haloperidol (Possible additive or potentiating effect with CNS depressants).
No products indexed under this heading.

Haloperidol Decanoate (Possible additive or potentiating effect with CNS depressants).
No products indexed under this heading.

Haloperidol Lactate (Possible additive or potentiating effect with CNS depressants).
No products indexed under this heading.

Halothane (Possible additive or potentiating effect with CNS depressants).
No products indexed under this heading.

Hexobarbital (Possible additive or potentiating effect with CNS depressants).
No products indexed under this heading.

Hydralazine Hydrochloride (Concurrent use of brimonidine, an alpha adrenergic agonist, with antihypertensives may reduce pulse and blood pressure, however, in clinical trials brimonidine did not have any significant effects on pulse and blood pressure).
No products indexed under this heading.

Hydrochlorothiazide (Concurrent use of brimonidine, an alpha adrenergic agonist, with antihypertensives may reduce pulse and blood pressure, however, in clinical trials brimonidine did not have any significant effects on pulse and blood pressure). Products include:
Atacand HCT **700**
Avalide **2956**
Benicar HCT **1017**
Diovan HCT **2419**
Dyazide **1429**
Exforge HCT **2449**
Hyzaar **2162**
Hyzaar 100-12.5 .... **2162**
Micardis HCT **889**
Prinzide **2246**
Tekturna HCT **2541**
Teveten HCT **541**

Hydrocodone Bitartrate (Possible additive or potentiating effect with CNS depressants). Products include:
Vicodin **560**
Vicodin ES **561**
Vicodin HP **563**
Vicoprofen **564**
Zydone **1138**

Hydrocodone Polistirex (Possible additive or potentiating effect with CNS depressants). Products include:
Tussionex **3443**

Hydroflumethiazide (Concurrent use of brimonidine, an alpha adrenergic agonist, with antihypertensives may reduce pulse and blood pressure, however, in clinical trials brimonidine did not have any significant effects on pulse and blood pressure).
No products indexed under this heading.

Hydromorphone (Possible additive or potentiating effect with CNS depressants).
No products indexed under this heading.

Hydromorphone Hydrochloride (Possible additive or potentiating effect with CNS depressants). Products include:
Dilaudid Injection **2800**
Dilaudid Oral **2797**
Dilaudid Tablets **2797**
Dilaudid-HP **2800**

Hydroxyzine Hydrochloride (Possible additive or potentiating effect with CNS depressants).
No products indexed under this heading.

Imipramine Hydrochloride (Tricyclic antidepressants have been reported to blunt the hypotensive effect of systemic clonidine, an alpha adrenergic agonist; it is not known whether the concurrent use of these agents with brimonidine can lead to interference in IOP-lowering effect; caution is advised).
No products indexed under this heading.

Imipramine Pamoate (Tricyclic antidepressants have been reported to blunt the hypotensive effect of systemic clonidine, an alpha adrenergic agonist; it is not known whether the concurrent use of these agents with brimonidine can lead to interference in IOP-lowering effect; caution is advised).
No products indexed under this heading.

Indapamide (Concurrent use of brimonidine, an alpha adrenergic agonist, with antihypertensives may reduce pulse and blood pressure, however, in clinical trials brimonidine did not have any significant effects on pulse and blood pressure). Products include:
Indapamide **2356**

Irbesartan (Concurrent use of brimonidine, an alpha adrenergic agonist, with antihypertensives may reduce pulse and blood pressure, however, in clinical trials brimonidine did not have any significant effects on pulse and blood pressure). Products include:
Avalide **2956**
Avapro **2962**

Isocarboxazid (Concurrent use of brimonidine, an alpha adrenergic agonist, and MAO inhibitor is contraindicated). Products include:
Marplan **3481**

Isoflurane (Possible additive or potentiating effect with CNS depressants).
No products indexed under this heading.

Isradipine (Concurrent use of brimonidine, an alpha adrenergic agonist, with antihypertensives may reduce pulse and blood pressure, however, in clinical trials brimonidine did not have any significant effects on pulse and blood pressure). Products include:
DynaCirc CR **1432**

Ketamine Hydrochloride (Possible additive or potentiating effect with CNS depressants).
No products indexed under this heading.

91 Interactions Index Alphagan P

Labetalol Hydrochloride (Concurrent use of brimonidine, an alpha adrenergic agonist, with beta blockers (ophthalmic and systemic) may reduce pulse and blood pressure, however, in clinical trials brimonidine did not have any significant effects on pulse and blood pressure).
No products indexed under this heading.

Levobunolol Hydrochloride (Concurrent use of brimonidine, an alpha adrenergic agonist, with beta blockers (ophthalmic and systemic) may reduce pulse and blood pressure, however, in clinical trials brimonidine did not have any significant effects on pulse and blood pressure).
No products indexed under this heading.

Levobupivacaine Hydrochloride (Possible additive or potentiating effect with CNS depressants).
No products indexed under this heading.

Levomethadyl Acetate Hydrochloride (Possible additive or potentiating effect with CNS depressants).
No products indexed under this heading.

Levorphanol Tartrate (Possible additive or potentiating effect with CNS depressants).
No products indexed under this heading.

Lidocaine (Possible additive or potentiating effect with CNS depressants). Products include:
Lidoderm 1107

Lidocaine Base (Possible additive or potentiating effect with CNS depressants).
No products indexed under this heading.

Lidocaine Hydrochloride (Possible additive or potentiating effect with CNS depressants).
No products indexed under this heading.

Lisinopril (Concurrent use of brimonidine, an alpha adrenergic agonist, with antihypertensives may reduce pulse and blood pressure, however, in clinical trials brimonidine did not have any significant effects on pulse and blood pressure). Products include:
Prinivil 2241
Prinzide 2246

Lorazepam (Possible additive or potentiating effect with CNS depressants).
No products indexed under this heading.

Losartan Potassium (Concurrent use of brimonidine, an alpha adrenergic agonist, with antihypertensives may reduce pulse and blood pressure, however, in clinical trials brimonidine did not have any significant effects on pulse and blood pressure). Products include:
Cozaar 2106
Hyzaar 2162
Hyzaar 100-12.5 2162

Loxapine Hydrochloride (Possible additive or potentiating effect with CNS depressants).
No products indexed under this heading.

Loxapine Succinate (Possible additive or potentiating effect with CNS depressants).
No products indexed under this heading.

Maprotiline Hydrochloride (Tricyclic antidepressants have been reported to blunt the hypotensive effect of systemic clonidine, an alpha adrenergic agonist; it is not known whether the concurrent use of these agents with brimonidine can lead to interference in IOP-lowering effect; caution is advised).
No products indexed under this heading.

Mecamylamine Hydrochloride (Concurrent use of brimonidine, an alpha adrenergic agonist, with antihypertensives may reduce pulse and blood pressure, however, in clinical trials brimonidine did not have any significant effects on pulse and blood pressure).
No products indexed under this heading.

Meperidine Hydrochloride (Possible additive or potentiating effect with CNS depressants).
No products indexed under this heading.

Mephobarbital (Possible additive or potentiating effect with CNS depressants).
No products indexed under this heading.

Mepivacaine Hydrochloride (Possible additive or potentiating effect with CNS depressants).
No products indexed under this heading.

Meprobamate (Possible additive or potentiating effect with CNS depressants).
No products indexed under this heading.

Mesoridazine Besylate (Possible additive or potentiating effect with CNS depressants).
No products indexed under this heading.

Methadone Hydrochloride (Possible additive or potentiating effect with CNS depressants).
No products indexed under this heading.

Methohexital Sodium (Possible additive or potentiating effect with CNS depressants).
No products indexed under this heading.

Methotrimeprazine (Possible additive or potentiating effect with CNS depressants).
No products indexed under this heading.

Methoxyflurane (Possible additive or potentiating effect with CNS depressants).
No products indexed under this heading.

Methyclothiazide (Concurrent use of brimonidine, an alpha adrenergic agonist, with antihypertensives may reduce pulse and blood pressure, however, in clinical trials brimonidine did not have any significant effects on pulse and blood pressure).
No products indexed under this heading.

Methyldopa (Concurrent use of brimonidine, an alpha adrenergic agonist, with antihypertensives may reduce pulse and blood pressure, however, in clinical trials brimonidine did not have any significant effects on pulse and blood pressure).
No products indexed under this heading.

Methyldopate Hydrochloride (Concurrent use of brimonidine, an alpha adrenergic agonist, with antihypertensives may reduce pulse and blood pressure, however, in clinical trials brimonidine did not have any significant effects on pulse and blood pressure).
No products indexed under this heading.

Metipranolol Hydrochloride (Concurrent use of brimonidine, an alpha adrenergic agonist, with beta blockers (ophthalmic and systemic) may reduce pulse and blood pressure, however, in clinical trials brimonidine did not have any significant effects on pulse and blood pressure).
No products indexed under this heading.

Metolazone (Concurrent use of brimonidine, an alpha adrenergic agonist, with antihypertensives may reduce pulse and blood pressure, however, in clinical trials brimonidine did not have any significant effects on pulse and blood pressure).
No products indexed under this heading.

Metoprolol Succinate (Concurrent use of brimonidine, an alpha adrenergic agonist, with beta blockers (ophthalmic and systemic) may reduce pulse and blood pressure, however, in clinical trials brimonidine did not have any significant effects on pulse and blood pressure). Products include:
Toprol XL 732

Metoprolol Tartrate (Concurrent use of brimonidine, an alpha adrenergic agonist, with beta blockers (ophthalmic and systemic) may reduce pulse and blood pressure, however, in clinical trials brimonidine did not have any significant effects on pulse and blood pressure).
No products indexed under this heading.

Metyrosine (Concurrent use of brimonidine, an alpha adrenergic agonist, with antihypertensives may reduce pulse and blood pressure, however, in clinical trials brimonidine did not have any significant effects on pulse and blood pressure).
No products indexed under this heading.

Mibefradil Dihydrochloride (Concurrent use of brimonidine, an alpha adrenergic agonist, with antihypertensives may reduce pulse and blood pressure, however, in clinical trials brimonidine did not have any significant effects on pulse and blood pressure).
No products indexed under this heading.

Midazolam Hydrochloride (Possible additive or potentiating effect with CNS depressants).
No products indexed under this heading.

Minoxidil (Concurrent use of brimonidine, an alpha adrenergic agonist, with antihypertensives may reduce pulse and blood pressure, however, in clinical trials brimonidine did not have any significant effects on pulse and blood pressure).
No products indexed under this heading.

Moclobemide (Concurrent use of brimonidine, an alpha adrenergic agonist, and MAO inhibitor is contraindicated).
No products indexed under this heading.

Moexipril Hydrochloride (Concurrent use of brimonidine, an alpha adrenergic agonist, with antihypertensives may reduce pulse and blood pressure, however, in clinical trials brimonidine did not have any significant effects on pulse and blood pressure).
No products indexed under this heading.

Molindone Hydrochloride (Possible additive or potentiating effect with CNS depressants). Products include:
Moban 1108

Morphine Sulfate (Possible additive or potentiating effect with CNS depressants). Products include:
Avinza 1822
Embeda 1831
MS Contin 2803

Morphine Sulfate, Liposomal (Possible additive or potentiating effect with CNS depressants).
No products indexed under this heading.

Nadolol (Concurrent use of brimonidine, an alpha adrenergic agonist, with beta blockers (ophthalmic and systemic) may reduce pulse and blood pressure, however, in clinical trials brimonidine did not have any significant effects on pulse and blood pressure). Products include:
Nadolol 2359

Nebivolol (Concurrent use of brimonidine, an alpha adrenergic agonist, with beta blockers (ophthalmic and systemic) may reduce pulse and blood pressure, however, in clinical trials brimonidine did not have any significant effects on pulse and blood pressure). Products include:
Bystolic 1147

Nicardipine Hydrochloride (Concurrent use of brimonidine, an alpha adrenergic agonist, with antihypertensives may reduce pulse and blood pressure, however, in clinical trials brimonidine did not have any significant effects on pulse and blood pressure).
No products indexed under this heading.

Nifedipine (Concurrent use of brimonidine, an alpha adrenergic agonist, with antihypertensives may reduce pulse and blood pressure, however, in clinical trials brimonidine did not have any significant effects on pulse and blood pressure).
No products indexed under this heading.

Nisoldipine (Concurrent use of brimonidine, an alpha adrenergic agonist, with antihypertensives may reduce pulse and blood pressure, however, in clinical trials brimonidine did not have any significant effects on pulse and blood pressure).
No products indexed under this heading.

Nitroglycerin (Concurrent use of brimonidine, an alpha adrenergic agonist, with antihypertensives may reduce pulse and blood pressure, however, in clinical trials brimonidine did not have any significant effects on pulse and blood pressure). Products include:
Nitro-Dur 3170
Nitrolingual 3266

Nortriptyline Hydrochloride (Tricyclic antidepressants have been reported to blunt the hypotensive effect of systemic clonidine, an alpha adrenergic agonist; it is not known whether the concurrent use of these agents with brimonidine can lead to interference in IOP-lowering effect; caution is advised).
No products indexed under this heading.

Olanzapine (Possible additive or potentiating effect with CNS depressants). Products include:
Symbyax 1965
Zyprexa 1984
Zyprexa IntraMuscular 1984
Zyprexa ZYDIS 1984

Oxazepam (Possible additive or potentiating effect with CNS depressants).
No products indexed under this heading.

Oxycodone Hydrochloride (Possible additive or potentiating effect with CNS depressants). Products include:
OxyContin 2807
Percocet 1121
Percodan 1124

Oxycodone Terephthalate (Possible additive or potentiating effect with CNS depressants).
No products indexed under this heading.

Oxymorphone Hydrochloride (Possible additive or potentiating effect with CNS depressants). Products include:
Opana 1110
Opana ER 1114

Pargyline Hydrochloride (Concurrent use of brimonidine, an alpha adrenergic agonist, and MAO inhibitor is contraindicated).
No products indexed under this heading.

Penbutolol Sulfate (Concurrent use of brimonidine, an alpha adrenergic agonist, with beta blockers (ophthalmic and systemic) may reduce pulse and blood pressure, however, in clinical trials brimonidine did not have any significant effects on pulse and blood pressure).
No products indexed under this heading.

Pentobarbital (Possible additive or potentiating effect with CNS depressants).
No products indexed under this heading.

Pentobarbital Sodium (Possible additive or potentiating effect with CNS depressants). Products include:
Nembutal 2012

IMPORTANT NOTE: Always consult each drug listing in the patient's regimen for possible interactions.

(⊙ Described in PDR® for Ophthalmic Medicines)

Torsemide (Concurrent use of brimonidine, an alpha adrenergic agonist, with antihypertensives may reduce pulse and blood pressure, however, in clinical trials brimonidine did not have any significant effects on pulse and blood pressure).
No products indexed under this heading.

Trandolapril (Concurrent use of brimonidine, an alpha adrenergic agonist, with antihypertensives may reduce pulse and blood pressure, however, in clinical trials brimonidine did not have any significant effects on pulse and blood pressure). Products include:
Mavik 489
Tarka 534

Tranylcypromine Sulfate (Concurrent use of brimonidine, an alpha adrenergic agonist, and MAO inhibitor is contraindicated). Products include:
Parnate 1584

Triazolam (Possible additive or potentiating effect with CNS depressants).
No products indexed under this heading.

Trifluoperazine Hydrochloride (Possible additive or potentiating effect with CNS depressants).
No products indexed under this heading.

Trimethaphan Camsylate (Concurrent use of brimonidine, an alpha adrenergic agonist, with antihypertensives may reduce pulse and blood pressure, however, in clinical trials brimonidine did not have any significant effects on pulse and blood pressure).
No products indexed under this heading.

Trimipramine Maleate (Tricyclic antidepressants have been reported to blunt the hypotensive effect of systemic clonidine, an alpha adrenergic agonist; it is not known whether the concurrent use of these agents with brimonidine can lead to interference in IOP-lowering effect; caution is advised).
No products indexed under this heading.

Valsartan (Concurrent use of brimonidine, an alpha adrenergic agonist, with antihypertensives may reduce pulse and blood pressure, however, in clinical trials brimonidine did not have any significant effects on pulse and blood pressure). Products include:
Diovan 2413
Diovan HCT 2419
Exforge 2443
Exforge HCT 2449
Valturna 3637

Verapamil Hydrochloride (Concurrent use of brimonidine, an alpha adrenergic agonist, with antihypertensives may reduce pulse and blood pressure, however, in clinical trials brimonidine did not have any significant effects on pulse and blood pressure). Products include:
Tarka 534

Zaleplon (Possible additive or potentiating effect with CNS depressants).
No products indexed under this heading.

Ziprasidone Hydrochloride (Possible additive or potentiating effect with CNS depressants). Products include:
Geodon 2723

Zolpidem Tartrate (Possible additive or potentiating effect with CNS depressants). Products include:
Ambien 2920
Ambien CR 2925

Food Interactions
Alcohol (Possible additive or potentiating effect with CNS depressants).
Beer, reduced-alcohol (Possible additive or potentiating effect with CNS depressants).
Beer, unspecified (Possible additive or potentiating effect with CNS depressants).
Wine, Chianti (Possible additive or potentiating effect with CNS depressants).

Wine, Red (Possible additive or potentiating effect with CNS depressants).
Wine, unspecified (Possible additive or potentiating effect with CNS depressants).
Wine products (Possible additive or potentiating effect with CNS depressants).

ALPHANATE
(Antihemophilic Factor (Human), von Willebrand Factor (Human)) 1786
None cited in PDR database.

ALPHANINE SD
(Factor IX (Human)) 1791
None cited in PDR database.

ALREX OPHTHALMIC SUSPENSION 0.2%
(Loteprednol Etabonate) .... ⊙235
None cited in PDR database.

ALTABAX OINTMENT
(Retapamulin) 1304

Ketoconazole (Co-administration of oral ketoconazole 200 mg twice daily increased retapamulin geometric mean AUC_{0-24} and C_{max} by 81% after topical application of retapamulin ointment, 1% on the abraded skin of healthy adult males. Due to low systemic exposure to retapamulin following topical application in patients, dosage adjustments for retapamulin are unnecessary when co-administered with CYP3A4 inhibitors, such as ketoconazole) Products include:
Extina 3319
Xolegel 3337

AMBIEN TABLETS
(Zolpidem Tartrate) 2920
May interact with alcohols, central nervous system depressants, cytochrome p450 3a inhibitors (selected), and certain other agents. Compounds in these categories include:

Alfentanil Hydrochloride (Since the systematic evaluations of zolpidem in combination with other CNS-active drugs have been limited, careful consideration should be given to the pharmacology of any CNS-active drug to be used with zolpidem. Any drug with CNS-depressant effects could potentially enhance the CNS depressant effects of zolpidem. Dosage adjustments may be necessary when zolpidem is combined with other CNS depressant drugs).
No products indexed under this heading.

Alprazolam (Since the systematic evaluations of zolpidem in combination with other CNS-active drugs have been limited, careful consideration should be given to the pharmacology of any CNS-active drug to be used with zolpidem. Any drug with CNS-depressant effects could potentially enhance the CNS depressant effects of zolpidem. Dosage adjustments may be necessary when zolpidem is combined with other CNS depressant drugs).
No products indexed under this heading.

Amiodarone Hydrochloride (Some compounds known to inhibit CYP3A may increase exposure to zolpidem).
No products indexed under this heading.

Amobarbital (Since the systematic evaluations of zolpidem in combination with other CNS-active drugs have been limited, careful consideration should be given to the pharmacology of any CNS-active drug to be used with zolpidem. Any drug with CNS-depressant effects could potentially enhance the CNS depressant effects of zolpidem. Dosage adjustments may be necessary when zolpidem is combined with other CNS depressant drugs).
No products indexed under this heading.

Amobarbital Sodium (Since the systematic evaluations of zolpidem in combination with other CNS-active drugs have been limited, careful consideration should be given to the pharmacology of any CNS-active drug to be used with zolpidem. Any drug with CNS-depressant effects could potentially enhance the CNS depressant effects of zolpidem. Dosage adjustments may be necessary when zolpidem is combined with other CNS depressant drugs).
No products indexed under this heading.

Amprenavir (Some compounds known to inhibit CYP3A may increase exposure to zolpidem).
No products indexed under this heading.

Aprepitant (Some compounds known to inhibit CYP3A may increase exposure to zolpidem). Products include:
Emend 2124

Aprobarbital (Since the systematic evaluations of zolpidem in combination with other CNS-active drugs have been limited, careful consideration should be given to the pharmacology of any CNS-active drug to be used with zolpidem. Any drug with CNS-depressant effects could potentially enhance the CNS depressant effects of zolpidem. Dosage adjustments may be necessary when zolpidem is combined with other CNS depressant drugs).
No products indexed under this heading.

Buprenorphine Hydrochloride (Since the systematic evaluations of zolpidem in combination with other CNS-active drugs have been limited, careful consideration should be given to the pharmacology of any CNS-active drug to be used with zolpidem. Any drug with CNS-depressant effects could potentially enhance the CNS depressant effects of zolpidem. Dosage adjustments may be necessary when zolpidem is combined with other CNS depressant drugs).
No products indexed under this heading.

Buspirone Hydrochloride (Since the systematic evaluations of zolpidem in combination with other CNS-active drugs have been limited, careful consideration should be given to the pharmacology of any CNS-active drug to be used with zolpidem. Any drug with CNS-depressant effects could potentially enhance the CNS depressant effects of zolpidem. Dosage adjustments may be necessary when zolpidem is combined with other CNS depressant drugs).
No products indexed under this heading.

Butabarbital (Since the systematic evaluations of zolpidem in combination with other CNS-active drugs have been limited, careful consideration should be given to the pharmacology of any CNS-active drug to be used with zolpidem. Any drug with CNS-depressant effects could potentially enhance the CNS depressant effects of zolpidem. Dosage adjustments may be necessary when zolpidem is combined with other CNS depressant drugs).
No products indexed under this heading.

Butabarbital Sodium (Since the systematic evaluations of zolpidem in combination with other CNS-active drugs have been limited, careful consideration should be given to the pharmacology of any CNS-active drug to be used with zolpidem. Any drug with CNS-depressant effects could potentially enhance the CNS depressant effects of zolpidem. Dosage adjustments may be necessary when zolpidem is combined with other CNS depressant drugs).
No products indexed under this heading.

Butalbital (Since the systematic evaluations of zolpidem in combination with other CNS-active drugs have been limited, careful consideration should be given to the pharmacology of any CNS-

active drug to be used with zolpidem. Any drug with CNS-depressant effects could potentially enhance the CNS depressant effects of zolpidem. Dosage adjustments may be necessary when zolpidem is combined with other CNS depressant drugs).
No products indexed under this heading.

Chlordiazepoxide (Since the systematic evaluations of zolpidem in combination with other CNS-active drugs have been limited, careful consideration should be given to the pharmacology of any CNS-active drug to be used with zolpidem. Any drug with CNS-depressant effects could potentially enhance the CNS depressant effects of zolpidem. Dosage adjustments may be necessary when zolpidem is combined with other CNS depressant drugs).
No products indexed under this heading.

Chlordiazepoxide Hydrochloride (Since the systematic evaluations of zolpidem in combination with other CNS-active drugs have been limited, careful consideration should be given to the pharmacology of any CNS-active drug to be used with zolpidem. Any drug with CNS-depressant effects could potentially enhance the CNS depressant effects of zolpidem. Dosage adjustments may be necessary when zolpidem is combined with other CNS depressant drugs).
No products indexed under this heading.

Chlorpromazine (The systematic evaluations of zolpidem in combination with other CNS-active drugs has been limited. Zolpidem was evaluated in healthy subjects in a single dose interaction study. Chlorpromazine in combination with zolpidem produced no pharmacokinetic interaction, but there was an additive effect of decreased alertness and psychomotor performance).
No products indexed under this heading.

Chlorpromazine Hydrochloride (The systematic evaluations of zolpidem in combination with other CNS-active drugs has been limited. Zolpidem was evaluated in healthy subjects in a single dose interaction study. Chlorpromazine in combination with zolpidem produced no pharmacokinetic interaction, but there was an additive effect of decreased alertness and psychomotor performance).
No products indexed under this heading.

Chlorprothixene (Since the systematic evaluations of zolpidem in combination with other CNS-active drugs have been limited, careful consideration should be given to the pharmacology of any CNS-active drug to be used with zolpidem. Any drug with CNS-depressant effects could potentially enhance the CNS depressant effects of zolpidem. Dosage adjustments may be necessary when zolpidem is combined with other CNS depressant drugs).
No products indexed under this heading.

Chlorprothixene Hydrochloride (Since the systematic evaluations of zolpidem in combination with other CNS-active drugs have been limited, careful consideration should be given to the pharmacology of any CNS-active drug to be used with zolpidem. Any drug with CNS-depressant effects could potentially enhance the CNS depressant effects of zolpidem. Dosage adjustments may be necessary when zolpidem is combined with other CNS depressant drugs).
No products indexed under this heading.

Chlorprothixene Lactate (Since the systematic evaluations of zolpidem in combination with other CNS-active drugs have been limited, careful consideration should be given to the pharmacology of any CNS-active drug to be used with zolpidem. Any drug with CNS-

---

IMPORTANT NOTE: Always consult each drug listing in the patient's regimen for possible interactions.

depressant effects could potentially enhance the CNS depressant effects of zolpidem. Dosage adjustments may be necessary when zolpidem is combined with other CNS depressant drugs).
No products indexed under this heading.

Cimetidine (Some compounds known to inhibit CYP3A may increase exposure to zolpidem).
No products indexed under this heading.

Cimetidine Hydrochloride (Some compounds known to inhibit CYP3A may increase exposure to zolpidem).
No products indexed under this heading.

Ciprofloxacin (Some compounds known to inhibit CYP3A may increase exposure to zolpidem). Products include:
Cipro I.V. **3082**
Cipro **3073**
Cipro XR **3091**
Ciprodex **583**

Ciprofloxacin Hydrochloride (Some compounds known to inhibit CYP3A may increase exposure to zolpidem). Products include:
Cipro **3073**

Clarithromycin (Some compounds known to inhibit CYP3A may increase exposure to zolpidem). Products include:
Biaxin/Biaxin XL **412**

Clonazepam (Since the systematic evaluations of zolpidem in combination with other CNS-active drugs have been limited, careful consideration should be given to the pharmacology of any CNS-active drug to be used with zolpidem. Any drug with CNS-depressant effects could potentially enhance the CNS depressant effects of zolpidem. Dosage adjustments may be necessary when zolpidem is combined with other CNS depressant drugs). Products include:
Klonopin **2855**

Clorazepate Dipotassium (Since the systematic evaluations of zolpidem in combination with other CNS-active drugs have been limited, careful consideration should be given to the pharmacology of any CNS-active drug to be used with zolpidem. Any drug with CNS-depressant effects could potentially enhance the CNS depressant effects of zolpidem. Dosage adjustments may be necessary when zolpidem is combined with other CNS depressant drugs).
No products indexed under this heading.

Clozapine (Since the systematic evaluations of zolpidem in combination with other CNS-active drugs have been limited, careful consideration should be given to the pharmacology of any CNS-active drug to be used with zolpidem. Any drug with CNS-depressant effects could potentially enhance the CNS depressant effects of zolpidem. Dosage adjustments may be necessary when zolpidem is combined with other CNS depressant drugs).
No products indexed under this heading.

Codeine Phosphate (Since the systematic evaluations of zolpidem in combination with other CNS-active drugs have been limited, careful consideration should be given to the pharmacology of any CNS-active drug to be used with zolpidem. Any drug with CNS-depressant effects could potentially enhance the CNS depressant effects of zolpidem. Dosage adjustments may be necessary when zolpidem is combined with other CNS depressant drugs). Products include:
Tylenol with Codeine **2691**

Codeine Sulfate (Since the systematic evaluations of zolpidem in combination with other CNS-active drugs have been limited, careful consideration should be given to the pharmacology of any CNS-active drug to be used with zolpidem. Any drug with CNS-depressant effects could potentially enhance the CNS depressant effects of zolpidem. Dosage adjustments may be necessary when zolpidem is combined with other CNS depressant drugs).
No products indexed under this heading.

Cyclosporine (Some compounds known to inhibit CYP3A may increase exposure to zolpidem). Products include:
Gengraf **440**
Neoral Oral Solution **2496**
Neoral Capsules **2496**
Restasis **605**

Delavirdine Mesylate (Some compounds known to inhibit CYP3A may increase exposure to zolpidem).
No products indexed under this heading.

Desflurane (Since the systematic evaluations of zolpidem in combination with other CNS-active drugs have been limited, careful consideration should be given to the pharmacology of any CNS-active drug to be used with zolpidem. Any drug with CNS-depressant effects could potentially enhance the CNS depressant effects of zolpidem. Dosage adjustments may be necessary when zolpidem is combined with other CNS depressant drugs).
No products indexed under this heading.

Dezocine (Since the systematic evaluations of zolpidem in combination with other CNS-active drugs have been limited, careful consideration should be given to the pharmacology of any CNS-active drug to be used with zolpidem. Any drug with CNS-depressant effects could potentially enhance the CNS depressant effects of zolpidem. Dosage adjustments may be necessary when zolpidem is combined with other CNS depressant drugs).
No products indexed under this heading.

Diazepam (Since the systematic evaluations of zolpidem in combination with other CNS-active drugs have been limited, careful consideration should be given to the pharmacology of any CNS-active drug to be used with zolpidem. Any drug with CNS-depressant effects could potentially enhance the CNS depressant effects of zolpidem. Dosage adjustments may be necessary when zolpidem is combined with other CNS depressant drugs). Products include:
Valium Tablets **2880**

Diltiazem Hydrochloride (Some compounds known to inhibit CYP3A may increase exposure to zolpidem). Products include:
Cardizem LA **423**

Diltiazem Maleate (Some compounds known to inhibit CYP3A may increase exposure to zolpidem).
No products indexed under this heading.

Droperidol (Since the systematic evaluations of zolpidem in combination with other CNS-active drugs have been limited, careful consideration should be given to the pharmacology of any CNS-active drug to be used with zolpidem. Any drug with CNS-depressant effects could potentially enhance the CNS depressant effects of zolpidem. Dosage adjustments may be necessary when zolpidem is combined with other CNS depressant drugs).
No products indexed under this heading.

Efavirenz (Some compounds known to inhibit CYP3A may increase exposure to zolpidem). Products include:
Atripla **906**

Enflurane (Since the systematic evaluations of zolpidem in combination with other CNS-active drugs have been limited, careful consideration should be given to the pharmacology of any CNS-active drug to be used with zolpidem. Any drug with CNS-depressant effects could potentially enhance the CNS depressant effects of zolpidem. Dosage adjustments may be necessary when zolpidem is combined with other CNS depressant drugs).
No products indexed under this heading.

Erythromycin (Some compounds known to inhibit CYP3A may increase exposure to zolpidem).
No products indexed under this heading.

Estazolam (Since the systematic evaluations of zolpidem in combination with other CNS-active drugs have been limited, careful consideration should be given to the pharmacology of any CNS-active drug to be used with zolpidem. Any drug with CNS-depressant effects could potentially enhance the CNS depressant effects of zolpidem. Dosage adjustments may be necessary when zolpidem is combined with other CNS depressant drugs).
No products indexed under this heading.

Ethanol (Since the systematic evaluations of zolpidem in combination with other CNS-active drugs have been limited, careful consideration should be given to the pharmacology of any CNS-active drug to be used with zolpidem. Any drug with CNS-depressant effects could potentially enhance the CNS depressant effects of zolpidem. Dosage adjustments may be necessary when zolpidem is combined with other CNS depressant drugs).
No products indexed under this heading.

Ethchlorvynol (Since the systematic evaluations of zolpidem in combination with other CNS-active drugs have been limited, careful consideration should be given to the pharmacology of any CNS-active drug to be used with zolpidem. Any drug with CNS-depressant effects could potentially enhance the CNS depressant effects of zolpidem. Dosage adjustments may be necessary when zolpidem is combined with other CNS depressant drugs).
No products indexed under this heading.

Ethinamate (Since the systematic evaluations of zolpidem in combination with other CNS-active drugs have been limited, careful consideration should be given to the pharmacology of any CNS-active drug to be used with zolpidem. Any drug with CNS-depressant effects could potentially enhance the CNS depressant effects of zolpidem. Dosage adjustments may be necessary when zolpidem is combined with other CNS depressant drugs).
No products indexed under this heading.

Ethyl Alcohol (Since the systematic evaluations of zolpidem in combination with other CNS-active drugs have been limited, careful consideration should be given to the pharmacology of any CNS-active drug to be used with zolpidem. Any drug with CNS-depressant effects could potentially enhance the CNS depressant effects of zolpidem. Dosage adjustments may be necessary when zolpidem is combined with other CNS depressant drugs).
No products indexed under this heading.

Fentanyl (Since the systematic evaluations of zolpidem in combination with other CNS-active drugs have been limited, careful consideration should be given to the pharmacology of any CNS-active drug to be used with zolpidem. Any drug with CNS-depressant effects could potentially enhance the CNS depressant effects of zolpidem. Dosage adjustments may be necessary when zolpidem is combined with other CNS depressant drugs). Products include:
Duragesic **2604**
Fentanyl Transdermal System **2346**
Onsolis **2054**

Fentanyl Citrate (Since the systematic evaluations of zolpidem in combination with other CNS-active drugs have been limited, careful consideration should be given to the pharmacology of any CNS-active drug to be used with zolpidem. Any drug with CNS-depressant effects could potentially enhance the CNS depressant effects of zolpidem. Dosage adjustments may be necessary when zolpidem is combined with other CNS depressant drugs). Products include:
Fentora **966**

Fluconazole (Some compounds known to inhibit CYP3A may increase exposure to zolpidem).
No products indexed under this heading.

Fluoxetine (A single dose interaction study with zolpidem 10 mg and fluoxetine 20 mg at steady-state levels in male volunteers did not demonstrate any clinically significant pharmacokinetic or pharmacodynamic interactions. When multiple doses of zolpidem and fluoxetine at steady-state concentrations were evaluated in healthy females, the only significant change was a 17% increase in zolpidem half-life. There was no evidence of an additive effect in psychomotor performance).
No products indexed under this heading.

Fluoxetine Hydrochloride (A single dose interaction study with zolpidem 10 mg and fluoxetine 20 mg at steady-state levels in male volunteers did not demonstrate any clinically significant pharmacokinetic or pharmacodynamic interactions. When multiple doses of zolpidem and fluoxetine at steady-state concentrations were evaluated in healthy females, the only significant change was a 17% increase in zolpidem half-life. There was no evidence of an additive effect in psychomotor performance). Products include:
Prozac Weekly **1941**
Prozac Pulvules **1941**
Symbyax **1965**

Fluphenazine Decanoate (Since the systematic evaluations of zolpidem in combination with other CNS-active drugs have been limited, careful consideration should be given to the pharmacology of any CNS-active drug to be used with zolpidem. Any drug with CNS-depressant effects could potentially enhance the CNS depressant effects of zolpidem. Dosage adjustments may be necessary when zolpidem is combined with other CNS depressant drugs).
No products indexed under this heading.

Fluphenazine Enanthate (Since the systematic evaluations of zolpidem in combination with other CNS-active drugs have been limited, careful consideration should be given to the pharmacology of any CNS-active drug to be used with zolpidem. Any drug with CNS-depressant effects could potentially enhance the CNS depressant effects of zolpidem. Dosage adjustments may be necessary when zolpidem is combined with other CNS depressant drugs).
No products indexed under this heading.

Fluphenazine Hydrochloride (Since the systematic evaluations of zolpidem in combination with other CNS-active drugs have been limited, careful consideration should be given to the pharmacology of any CNS-active drug to be used with zolpidem. Any drug with CNS-depressant effects could potentially enhance the CNS depressant effects of zolpidem. Dosage adjustments may be necessary when zolpidem is combined with other CNS depressant drugs).
No products indexed under this heading.

Flurazepam Hydrochloride (Since the systematic evaluations of zolpidem in combination with other CNS-active drugs have been limited, careful consideration should be given to the pharmacology of any CNS-active drug to be used with zolpidem. Any drug with CNS-depressant effects could potentially enhance the CNS depressant effects of

95 **Interactions Index** **Ambien**

zolpidem. Dosage adjustments may be necessary when zolpidem is combined with other CNS depressant drugs).
No products indexed under this heading.

Fluvoxamine Maleate (Some compounds known to inhibit CYP3A may increase exposure to zolpidem).
No products indexed under this heading.

Glutethimide (Since the systematic evaluations of zolpidem in combination with other CNS-active drugs have been limited, careful consideration should be given to the pharmacology of any CNS-active drug to be used with zolpidem. Any drug with CNS-depressant effects could potentially enhance the CNS depressant effects of zolpidem. Dosage adjustments may be necessary when zolpidem is combined with other CNS depressant drugs).
No products indexed under this heading.

Halazepam (Since the systematic evaluations of zolpidem in combination with other CNS-active drugs have been limited, careful consideration should be given to the pharmacology of any CNS-active drug to be used with zolpidem. Any drug with CNS-depressant effects could potentially enhance the CNS depressant effects of zolpidem. Dosage adjustments may be necessary when zolpidem is combined with other CNS depressant drugs).
No products indexed under this heading.

Haloperidol (The systematic evaluations of zolpidem in combination with other CNS-active drugs has been limited. Zolpidem was evaluated in healthy subjects in a single dose interaction study. A study involving haloperidol and zolpidem revealed no effect of haloperidol on the pharmacokinetics or pharmacodynamics of zolpidem. The lack of drug interaction following single dose administration does not predict a lack of a drug interaction following chronic administration).
No products indexed under this heading.

Haloperidol Decanoate (The systematic evaluations of zolpidem in combination with other CNS-active drugs has been limited. Zolpidem was evaluated in healthy subjects in a single dose interaction study. A study involving haloperidol and zolpidem revealed no effect of haloperidol on the pharmacokinetics or pharmacodynamics of zolpidem. The lack of drug interaction following single dose administration does not predict a lack of a drug interaction following chronic administration).
No products indexed under this heading.

Haloperidol Lactate (The systematic evaluations of zolpidem in combination with other CNS-active drugs has been limited. Zolpidem was evaluated in healthy subjects in a single dose interaction study. A study involving haloperidol and zolpidem revealed no effect of haloperidol on the pharmacokinetics or pharmacodynamics of zolpidem. The lack of drug interaction following single dose administration does not predict a lack of a drug interaction following chronic administration).
No products indexed under this heading.

Hexobarbital (Since the systematic evaluations of zolpidem in combination with other CNS-active drugs have been limited, careful consideration should be given to the pharmacology of any CNS-active drug to be used with zolpidem. Any drug with CNS-depressant effects could potentially enhance the CNS depressant effects of zolpidem. Dosage adjustments may be necessary when zolpidem is combined with other CNS depressant drugs).
No products indexed under this heading.

Hydrocodone Bitartrate (Since the systematic evaluations of zolpidem in combination with other CNS-active drugs have been limited, careful consideration should be given to the pharmacology of any CNS-active drug to be used with zolpidem. Any drug with CNS-depressant effects could potentially enhance the CNS depressant effects of zolpidem. Dosage adjustments may be necessary when zolpidem is combined with other CNS depressant drugs). Products include:
Vicodin **560**
Vicodin ES **561**
Vicodin HP **563**
Vicoprofen **564**
Zydone **1138**

Hydrocodone Polistirex (Since the systematic evaluations of zolpidem in combination with other CNS-active drugs have been limited, careful consideration should be given to the pharmacology of any CNS-active drug to be used with zolpidem. Any drug with CNS-depressant effects could potentially enhance the CNS depressant effects of zolpidem. Dosage adjustments may be necessary when zolpidem is combined with other CNS depressant drugs). Products include:
Tussionex **3443**

Hydromorphone (Since the systematic evaluations of zolpidem in combination with other CNS-active drugs have been limited, careful consideration should be given to the pharmacology of any CNS-active drug to be used with zolpidem. Any drug with CNS-depressant effects could potentially enhance the CNS depressant effects of zolpidem. Dosage adjustments may be necessary when zolpidem is combined with other CNS depressant drugs).
No products indexed under this heading.

Hydromorphone Hydrochloride (Since the systematic evaluations of zolpidem in combination with other CNS-active drugs have been limited, careful consideration should be given to the pharmacology of any CNS-active drug to be used with zolpidem. Any drug with CNS-depressant effects could potentially enhance the CNS depressant effects of zolpidem. Dosage adjustments may be necessary when zolpidem is combined with other CNS depressant drugs). Products include:
Dilaudid Injection **2800**
Dilaudid Oral **2797**
Dilaudid Tablets **2797**
Dilaudid-HP **2800**

Hydroxyzine Hydrochloride (Since the systematic evaluations of zolpidem in combination with other CNS-active drugs have been limited, careful consideration should be given to the pharmacology of any CNS-active drug to be used with zolpidem. Any drug with CNS-depressant effects could potentially enhance the CNS depressant effects of zolpidem. Dosage adjustments may be necessary when zolpidem is combined with other CNS depressant drugs).
No products indexed under this heading.

Imipramine Hydrochloride (The systematic evaluations of zolpidem in combination with other CNS-active drugs has been limited. Zolpidem was evaluated in healthy subjects in a single dose interaction study. Imipramine in combination with zolpidem produced no pharmacokinetic interaction other than a 20% decrease in peak levels of imipramine, but there was an additive effect of decreased alertness).
No products indexed under this heading.

Imipramine Pamoate (The systematic evaluations of zolpidem in combination with other CNS-active drugs has been limited. Zolpidem was evaluated in healthy subjects in a single dose interaction study. Imipramine in combination with zolpidem produced no pharmacokinetic interaction other than a 20% decrease in peak levels of imipramine, but there was an additive effect of decreased alertness).
No products indexed under this heading.

Indinavir Sulfate (Some compounds known to inhibit CYP3A may increase exposure to zolpidem). Products include:
Crixivan **2113**

Isoflurane (Since the systematic evaluations of zolpidem in combination with other CNS-active drugs have been limited, careful consideration should be given to the pharmacology of any CNS-active drug to be used with zolpidem. Any drug with CNS-depressant effects could potentially enhance the CNS depressant effects of zolpidem. Dosage adjustments may be necessary when zolpidem is combined with other CNS depressant drugs).
No products indexed under this heading.

Isoniazid (Some compounds known to inhibit CYP3A may increase exposure to zolpidem).
No products indexed under this heading.

Itraconazole (A randomized, double-blind, crossover interaction study in ten healthy volunteers between itraconazole (200 mg QD for 4 days) and a single dose of zolpidem (10 mg) given 5 hours after the last dose of itraconazole resulted in a 34% increase in AUC of zolpidem. There were no significant pharmacodynamic effects of zolpidem on subjective drowsiness, postural sway, or psychomotor performance).
No products indexed under this heading.

Ketamine Hydrochloride (Since the systematic evaluations of zolpidem in combination with other CNS-active drugs have been limited, careful consideration should be given to the pharmacology of any CNS-active drug to be used with zolpidem. Any drug with CNS-depressant effects could potentially enhance the CNS depressant effects of zolpidem. Dosage adjustments may be necessary when zolpidem is combined with other CNS depressant drugs).
No products indexed under this heading.

Ketoconazole (A randomized, double-blind, crossover interaction study in 12 healthy subjects showed that coadministration of a single 5 mg dose of zolpidem with ketoconazole, a potent CYP3A4 inhibitor, given as 200 mg bid for two days increased C_{max} of zolpidem by a factor of 1.3 and increased the total AUC of zolpidem by a factor of 1.7 compared to zolpidem alone and prolonged the elimination half-life by approximately 30% along with an increase in the pharmacodynamic effects of zolpidem. Caution should be used when ketoconazole is given with zolpidem and consideration should be given to using a lower dose of zolpidem when ketoconazole and zolpidem are given together. Patients should be advised that the use of zolpidem with ketoconazole may enhance sedative effects). Products include:
Extina **3319**
Xolegel **3337**

Levomethadyl Acetate Hydrochloride (Since the systematic evaluations of zolpidem in combination with other CNS-active drugs have been limited, careful consideration should be given to the pharmacology of any CNS-active drug to be used with zolpidem. Any drug with CNS-depressant effects could potentially enhance the CNS depressant effects of zolpidem. Dosage adjustments may be necessary when zolpidem is combined with other CNS depressant drugs).
No products indexed under this heading.

Levorphanol Tartrate (Since the systematic evaluations of zolpidem in combination with other CNS-active drugs have been limited, careful consideration should be given to the pharmacology of any CNS-active drug to be used with zolpidem. Any drug with CNS-depressant effects could potentially enhance the CNS depressant effects of zolpidem. Dosage adjustments may be necessary when zolpidem is combined with other CNS depressant drugs).
No products indexed under this heading.

Lopinavir (Some compounds known to inhibit CYP3A may increase exposure to zolpidem). Products include:
Kaletra **458**

Lorazepam (Since the systematic evaluations of zolpidem in combination with other CNS-active drugs have been limited, careful consideration should be given to the pharmacology of any CNS-active drug to be used with zolpidem. Any drug with CNS-depressant effects could potentially enhance the CNS depressant effects of zolpidem. Dosage adjustments may be necessary when zolpidem is combined with other CNS depressant drugs).
No products indexed under this heading.

Loxapine Hydrochloride (Since the systematic evaluations of zolpidem in combination with other CNS-active drugs have been limited, careful consideration should be given to the pharmacology of any CNS-active drug to be used with zolpidem. Any drug with CNS-depressant effects could potentially enhance the CNS depressant effects of zolpidem. Dosage adjustments may be necessary when zolpidem is combined with other CNS depressant drugs).
No products indexed under this heading.

Loxapine Succinate (Since the systematic evaluations of zolpidem in combination with other CNS-active drugs have been limited, careful consideration should be given to the pharmacology of any CNS-active drug to be used with zolpidem. Any drug with CNS-depressant effects could potentially enhance the CNS depressant effects of zolpidem. Dosage adjustments may be necessary when zolpidem is combined with other CNS depressant drugs).
No products indexed under this heading.

Meperidine Hydrochloride (Since the systematic evaluations of zolpidem in combination with other CNS-active drugs have been limited, careful consideration should be given to the pharmacology of any CNS-active drug to be used with zolpidem. Any drug with CNS-depressant effects could potentially enhance the CNS depressant effects of zolpidem. Dosage adjustments may be necessary when zolpidem is combined with other CNS depressant drugs).
No products indexed under this heading.

Mephobarbital (Since the systematic evaluations of zolpidem in combination with other CNS-active drugs have been limited, careful consideration should be given to the pharmacology of any CNS-active drug to be used with zolpidem. Any drug with CNS-depressant effects could potentially enhance the CNS depressant effects of zolpidem. Dosage adjustments may be necessary when zolpidem is combined with other CNS depressant drugs).
No products indexed under this heading.

Meprobamate (Since the systematic evaluations of zolpidem in combination with other CNS-active drugs have been limited, careful consideration should be given to the pharmacology of any CNS-active drug to be used with zolpidem. Any drug with CNS-depressant effects could potentially enhance the CNS depressant effects of zolpidem. Dosage adjustments may be necessary when zolpidem is combined with other CNS depressant drugs).
No products indexed under this heading.

IMPORTANT NOTE: Always consult each drug listing in the patient's regimen for possible interactions.

Mesoridazine Besylate (Since the systematic evaluations of zolpidem in combination with other CNS-active drugs have been limited, careful consideration should be given to the pharmacology of any CNS-active drug to be used with zolpidem. Any drug with CNS-depressant effects could potentially enhance the CNS depressant effects of zolpidem. Dosage adjustments may be necessary when zolpidem is combined with other CNS depressant drugs).
    No products indexed under this heading.

Methadone Hydrochloride (Since the systematic evaluations of zolpidem in combination with other CNS-active drugs have been limited, careful consideration should be given to the pharmacology of any CNS-active drug to be used with zolpidem. Any drug with CNS-depressant effects could potentially enhance the CNS depressant effects of zolpidem. Dosage adjustments may be necessary when zolpidem is combined with other CNS depressant drugs).
    No products indexed under this heading.

Methohexital Sodium (Since the systematic evaluations of zolpidem in combination with other CNS-active drugs have been limited, careful consideration should be given to the pharmacology of any CNS-active drug to be used with zolpidem. Any drug with CNS-depressant effects could potentially enhance the CNS depressant effects of zolpidem. Dosage adjustments may be necessary when zolpidem is combined with other CNS depressant drugs).
    No products indexed under this heading.

Methotrimeprazine (Since the systematic evaluations of zolpidem in combination with other CNS-active drugs have been limited, careful consideration should be given to the pharmacology of any CNS-active drug to be used with zolpidem. Any drug with CNS-depressant effects could potentially enhance the CNS depressant effects of zolpidem. Dosage adjustments may be necessary when zolpidem is combined with other CNS depressant drugs).
    No products indexed under this heading.

Methoxyflurane (Since the systematic evaluations of zolpidem in combination with other CNS-active drugs have been limited, careful consideration should be given to the pharmacology of any CNS-active drug to be used with zolpidem. Any drug with CNS-depressant effects could potentially enhance the CNS depressant effects of zolpidem. Dosage adjustments may be necessary when zolpidem is combined with other CNS depressant drugs).
    No products indexed under this heading.

Metronidazole (Some compounds known to inhibit CYP3A may increase exposure to zolpidem). Products include:
    Pylera 793

Metronidazole Benzoate (Some compounds known to inhibit CYP3A may increase exposure to zolpidem).
    No products indexed under this heading.

Metronidazole Hydrochloride (Some compounds known to inhibit CYP3A may increase exposure to zolpidem).
    No products indexed under this heading.

Miconazole (Some compounds known to inhibit CYP3A may increase exposure to zolpidem).
    No products indexed under this heading.

Midazolam Hydrochloride (Since the systematic evaluations of zolpidem in combination with other CNS-active drugs have been limited, careful consideration should be given to the pharmacology of any CNS-active drug to be used with zolpidem. Any drug with CNS-depressant effects could potentially enhance the CNS depressant effects of

zolpidem. Dosage adjustments may be necessary when zolpidem is combined with other CNS depressant drugs).
    No products indexed under this heading.

Molindone Hydrochloride (Since the systematic evaluations of zolpidem in combination with other CNS-active drugs have been limited, careful consideration should be given to the pharmacology of any CNS-active drug to be used with zolpidem. Any drug with CNS-depressant effects could potentially enhance the CNS depressant effects of zolpidem. Dosage adjustments may be necessary when zolpidem is combined with other CNS depressant drugs).
Products include:
    Moban 1108

Morphine Sulfate (Since the systematic evaluations of zolpidem in combination with other CNS-active drugs have been limited, careful consideration should be given to the pharmacology of any CNS-active drug to be used with zolpidem. Any drug with CNS-depressant effects could potentially enhance the CNS depressant effects of zolpidem. Dosage adjustments may be necessary when zolpidem is combined with other CNS depressant drugs).
Products include:
    Avinza 1822
    Embeda 1831
    MS Contin 2803

Morphine Sulfate, Liposomal (Since the systematic evaluations of zolpidem in combination with other CNS-active drugs have been limited, careful consideration should be given to the pharmacology of any CNS-active drug to be used with zolpidem. Any drug with CNS-depressant effects could potentially enhance the CNS depressant effects of zolpidem. Dosage adjustments may be necessary when zolpidem is combined with other CNS depressant drugs).
    No products indexed under this heading.

Nefazodone Hydrochloride (Some compounds known to inhibit CYP3A may increase exposure to zolpidem).
    No products indexed under this heading.

Nelfinavir Mesylate (Some compounds known to inhibit CYP3A may increase exposure to zolpidem).
    No products indexed under this heading.

Nifedipine (Some compounds known to inhibit CYP3A may increase exposure to zolpidem).
    No products indexed under this heading.

Norfloxacin (Some compounds known to inhibit CYP3A may increase exposure to zolpidem). Products include:
    Noroxin 2220

Olanzapine (Since the systematic evaluations of zolpidem in combination with other CNS-active drugs have been limited, careful consideration should be given to the pharmacology of any CNS-active drug to be used with zolpidem. Any drug with CNS-depressant effects could potentially enhance the CNS depressant effects of zolpidem. Dosage adjustments may be necessary when zolpidem is combined with other CNS depressant drugs). Products include:
    Symbyax 1965
    Zyprexa 1984
    Zyprexa IntraMuscular 1984
    Zyprexa ZYDIS 1984

Oxazepam (Since the systematic evaluations of zolpidem in combination with other CNS-active drugs have been limited, careful consideration should be given to the pharmacology of any CNS-active drug to be used with zolpidem. Any drug with CNS-depressant effects could potentially enhance the CNS depressant effects of zolpidem. Dosage

adjustments may be necessary when zolpidem is combined with other CNS depressant drugs).
    No products indexed under this heading.

Oxycodone Hydrochloride (Since the systematic evaluations of zolpidem in combination with other CNS-active drugs have been limited, careful consideration should be given to the pharmacology of any CNS-active drug to be used with zolpidem. Any drug with CNS-depressant effects could potentially enhance the CNS depressant effects of zolpidem. Dosage adjustments may be necessary when zolpidem is combined with other CNS depressant drugs).
Products include:
    OxyContin 2807
    Percocet 1121
    Percodan 1124

Oxycodone Terephthalate (Since the systematic evaluations of zolpidem in combination with other CNS-active drugs have been limited, careful consideration should be given to the pharmacology of any CNS-active drug to be used with zolpidem. Any drug with CNS-depressant effects could potentially enhance the CNS depressant effects of zolpidem. Dosage adjustments may be necessary when zolpidem is combined with other CNS depressant drugs).
    No products indexed under this heading.

Oxymorphone Hydrochloride (Since the systematic evaluations of zolpidem in combination with other CNS-active drugs have been limited, careful consideration should be given to the pharmacology of any CNS-active drug to be used with zolpidem. Any drug with CNS-depressant effects could potentially enhance the CNS depressant effects of zolpidem. Dosage adjustments may be necessary when zolpidem is combined with other CNS depressant drugs). Products include:
    Opana 1110
    Opana ER 1114

Paroxetine Hydrochloride (Some compounds known to inhibit CYP3A may increase exposure to zolpidem).
Products include:
    Paroxetine CR 2361
    Paroxetine ER 2371
    Paxil 1586
    Paxil CR 1596

Pentobarbital (Since the systematic evaluations of zolpidem in combination with other CNS-active drugs have been limited, careful consideration should be given to the pharmacology of any CNS-active drug to be used with zolpidem. Any drug with CNS-depressant effects could potentially enhance the CNS depressant effects of zolpidem. Dosage adjustments may be necessary when zolpidem is combined with other CNS depressant drugs).
    No products indexed under this heading.

Pentobarbital Sodium (Since the systematic evaluations of zolpidem in combination with other CNS-active drugs have been limited, careful consideration should be given to the pharmacology of any CNS-active drug to be used with zolpidem. Any drug with CNS-depressant effects could potentially enhance the CNS depressant effects of zolpidem. Dosage adjustments may be necessary when zolpidem is combined with other CNS depressant drugs).
Products include:
    Nembutal 2012

Perphenazine (Since the systematic evaluations of zolpidem in combination with other CNS-active drugs have been limited, careful consideration should be given to the pharmacology of any CNS-active drug to be used with zolpidem. Any drug with CNS-depressant effects could potentially enhance the CNS depressant effects of zolpidem. Dosage

adjustments may be necessary when zolpidem is combined with other CNS depressant drugs).
    No products indexed under this heading.

Phenobarbital (Since the systematic evaluations of zolpidem in combination with other CNS-active drugs have been limited, careful consideration should be given to the pharmacology of any CNS-active drug to be used with zolpidem. Any drug with CNS-depressant effects could potentially enhance the CNS depressant effects of zolpidem. Dosage adjustments may be necessary when zolpidem is combined with other CNS depressant drugs). Products include:
    Donnatal 2711

Phenobarbital Sodium (Since the systematic evaluations of zolpidem in combination with other CNS-active drugs have been limited, careful consideration should be given to the pharmacology of any CNS-active drug to be used with zolpidem. Any drug with CNS-depressant effects could potentially enhance the CNS depressant effects of zolpidem. Dosage adjustments may be necessary when zolpidem is combined with other CNS depressant drugs).
    No products indexed under this heading.

Prazepam (Since the systematic evaluations of zolpidem in combination with other CNS-active drugs have been limited, careful consideration should be given to the pharmacology of any CNS-active drug to be used with zolpidem. Any drug with CNS-depressant effects could potentially enhance the CNS depressant effects of zolpidem. Dosage adjustments may be necessary when zolpidem is combined with other CNS depressant drugs).
    No products indexed under this heading.

Prochlorperazine (Since the systematic evaluations of zolpidem in combination with other CNS-active drugs have been limited, careful consideration should be given to the pharmacology of any CNS-active drug to be used with zolpidem. Any drug with CNS-depressant effects could potentially enhance the CNS depressant effects of zolpidem. Dosage adjustments may be necessary when zolpidem is combined with other CNS depressant drugs).
    No products indexed under this heading.

Prochlorperazine Edisylate (Since the systematic evaluations of zolpidem in combination with other CNS-active drugs have been limited, careful consideration should be given to the pharmacology of any CNS-active drug to be used with zolpidem. Any drug with CNS-depressant effects could potentially enhance the CNS depressant effects of zolpidem. Dosage adjustments may be necessary when zolpidem is combined with other CNS depressant drugs).
    No products indexed under this heading.

Prochlorperazine Maleate (Since the systematic evaluations of zolpidem in combination with other CNS-active drugs have been limited, careful consideration should be given to the pharmacology of any CNS-active drug to be used with zolpidem. Any drug with CNS-depressant effects could potentially enhance the CNS depressant effects of zolpidem. Dosage adjustments may be necessary when zolpidem is combined with other CNS depressant drugs).
    No products indexed under this heading.

Promethazine (Since the systematic evaluations of zolpidem in combination with other CNS-active drugs have been limited, careful consideration should be given to the pharmacology of any CNS-active drug to be used with zolpidem. Any drug with CNS-depressant effects could potentially enhance the CNS depressant effects of zolpidem. Dosage

adjustments may be necessary when zolpidem is combined with other CNS depressant drugs).
No products indexed under this heading.

Promethazine Hydrochloride (Since the systematic evaluations of zolpidem in combination with other CNS-active drugs have been limited, careful consideration should be given to the pharmacology of any CNS-active drug to be used with zolpidem. Any drug with CNS-depressant effects could potentially enhance the CNS depressant effects of zolpidem. Dosage adjustments may be necessary when zolpidem is combined with other CNS depressant drugs).
No products indexed under this heading.

Propofol (Since the systematic evaluations of zolpidem in combination with other CNS-active drugs have been limited, careful consideration should be given to the pharmacology of any CNS-active drug to be used with zolpidem. Any drug with CNS-depressant effects could potentially enhance the CNS depressant effects of zolpidem. Dosage adjustments may be necessary when zolpidem is combined with other CNS depressant drugs).
No products indexed under this heading.

Propoxyphene Hydrochloride (Since the systematic evaluations of zolpidem in combination with other CNS-active drugs have been limited, careful consideration should be given to the pharmacology of any CNS-active drug to be used with zolpidem. Any drug with CNS-depressant effects could potentially enhance the CNS depressant effects of zolpidem. Dosage adjustments may be necessary when zolpidem is combined with other CNS depressant drugs).
No products indexed under this heading.

Propoxyphene Napsylate (Since the systematic evaluations of zolpidem in combination with other CNS-active drugs have been limited, careful consideration should be given to the pharmacology of any CNS-active drug to be used with zolpidem. Any drug with CNS-depressant effects could potentially enhance the CNS depressant effects of zolpidem. Dosage adjustments may be necessary when zolpidem is combined with other CNS depressant drugs).
No products indexed under this heading.

Quazepam (Since the systematic evaluations of zolpidem in combination with other CNS-active drugs have been limited, careful consideration should be given to the pharmacology of any CNS-active drug to be used with zolpidem. Any drug with CNS-depressant effects could potentially enhance the CNS depressant effects of zolpidem. Dosage adjustments may be necessary when zolpidem is combined with other CNS depressant drugs).
No products indexed under this heading.

Quetiapine Fumarate (Since the systematic evaluations of zolpidem in combination with other CNS-active drugs have been limited, careful consideration should be given to the pharmacology of any CNS-active drug to be used with zolpidem. Any drug with CNS-depressant effects could potentially enhance the CNS depressant effects of zolpidem. Dosage adjustments may be necessary when zolpidem is combined with other CNS depressant drugs).
Products include:

Quinine (Some compounds known to inhibit CYP3A may increase exposure to zolpidem). Products include:

Quinine Sulfate (Some compounds known to inhibit CYP3A may increase exposure to zolpidem).
No products indexed under this heading.

Remifentanil Hydrochloride (Since the systematic evaluations of zolpidem in combination with other CNS-active drugs have been limited, careful consideration should be given to the pharmacology of any CNS-active drug to be used with zolpidem. Any drug with CNS-depressant effects could potentially enhance the CNS depressant effects of zolpidem. Dosage adjustments may be necessary when zolpidem is combined with other CNS depressant drugs).
No products indexed under this heading.

Rifampin (A randomized, placebo-controlled, crossover interaction study in eight healthy female subjects between five consecutive daily doses of rifampin (600 mg) and a single dose of zolpidem (20 mg) given 17 hours after the last dose of rifampin showed significant reductions of the AUC (-73%), C_{max} (-58) and T1/2 (-36) of zolpidem together with significant reductions in the pharmacodynamics of zolpidem).
No products indexed under this heading.

Risperidone (Since the systematic evaluations of zolpidem in combination with other CNS-active drugs have been limited, careful consideration should be given to the pharmacology of any CNS-active drug to be used with zolpidem. Any drug with CNS-depressant effects could potentially enhance the CNS depressant effects of zolpidem. Dosage adjustments may be necessary when zolpidem is combined with other CNS depressant drugs). Products include:

Ritonavir (Some compounds known to inhibit CYP3A may increase exposure to zolpidem). Products include:

Saquinavir (Some compounds known to inhibit CYP3A may increase exposure to zolpidem).
No products indexed under this heading.

Saquinavir Mesylate (Some compounds known to inhibit CYP3A may increase exposure to zolpidem).
No products indexed under this heading.

Secobarbital Sodium (Since the systematic evaluations of zolpidem in combination with other CNS-active drugs have been limited, careful consideration should be given to the pharmacology of any CNS-active drug to be used with zolpidem. Any drug with CNS-depressant effects could potentially enhance the CNS depressant effects of zolpidem. Dosage adjustments may be necessary when zolpidem is combined with other CNS depressant drugs).
No products indexed under this heading.

Sertraline Hydrochloride (Following five consecutive nightly doses of zolpidem 10 mg in the presence of sertaline 50 mg (17 consecutive daily doses, at 7:00 am, in healthy female volunteers), zolpidem C_{max} was significantly higher (43%) and T_{max} was significantly decreased (53%). Pharmacokinetics of sertraline and N-desmethylsertraline were unaffected by zolpidem).
No products indexed under this heading.

Sevoflurane (Since the systematic evaluations of zolpidem in combination with other CNS-active drugs have been limited, careful consideration should be given to the pharmacology of any CNS-active drug to be used with zolpidem. Any drug with CNS-depressant effects could potentially enhance the CNS depressant effects of zolpidem. Dosage adjustments may be necessary when zolpidem is combined with other CNS depressant drugs). Products include:

Sodium Butabarbital (Since the systematic evaluations of zolpidem in combination with other CNS-active drugs have been limited, careful consideration should be given to the pharmacology of any CNS-active drug to be used with zolpidem. Any drug with CNS-depressant effects could potentially enhance the CNS depressant effects of zolpidem. Dosage adjustments may be necessary when zolpidem is combined with other CNS depressant drugs).
No products indexed under this heading.

Sodium Oxybate (Since the systematic evaluations of zolpidem in combination with other CNS-active drugs have been limited, careful consideration should be given to the pharmacology of any CNS-active drug to be used with zolpidem. Any drug with CNS-depressant effects could potentially enhance the CNS depressant effects of zolpidem. Dosage adjustments may be necessary when zolpidem is combined with other CNS depressant drugs).
No products indexed under this heading.

Sodium Pentobarbital (Since the systematic evaluations of zolpidem in combination with other CNS-active drugs have been limited, careful consideration should be given to the pharmacology of any CNS-active drug to be used with zolpidem. Any drug with CNS-depressant effects could potentially enhance the CNS depressant effects of zolpidem. Dosage adjustments may be necessary when zolpidem is combined with other CNS depressant drugs).
No products indexed under this heading.

Sufentanil Citrate (Since the systematic evaluations of zolpidem in combination with other CNS-active drugs have been limited, careful consideration should be given to the pharmacology of any CNS-active drug to be used with zolpidem. Any drug with CNS-depressant effects could potentially enhance the CNS depressant effects of zolpidem. Dosage adjustments may be necessary when zolpidem is combined with other CNS depressant drugs).
No products indexed under this heading.

Talbutal (Since the systematic evaluations of zolpidem in combination with other CNS-active drugs have been limited, careful consideration should be given to the pharmacology of any CNS-active drug to be used with zolpidem. Any drug with CNS-depressant effects could potentially enhance the CNS depressant effects of zolpidem. Dosage adjustments may be necessary when zolpidem is combined with other CNS depressant drugs).
No products indexed under this heading.

Temazepam (Since the systematic evaluations of zolpidem in combination with other CNS-active drugs have been limited, careful consideration should be given to the pharmacology of any CNS-active drug to be used with zolpidem. Any drug with CNS-depressant effects could potentially enhance the CNS depressant effects of zolpidem. Dosage adjustments may be necessary when zolpidem is combined with other CNS depressant drugs).
No products indexed under this heading.

Thiamylal Sodium (Since the systematic evaluations of zolpidem in combination with other CNS-active drugs have been limited, careful consideration should be given to the pharmacology of any CNS-active drug to be used with zolpidem. Any drug with CNS-depressant effects could potentially enhance the CNS depressant effects of zolpidem. Dosage adjustments may be necessary when zolpidem is combined with other CNS depressant drugs).
No products indexed under this heading.

Thioridazine (Since the systematic evaluations of zolpidem in combination with other CNS-active drugs have been limited, careful consideration should be given to the pharmacology of any CNS-active drug to be used with zolpidem. Any drug with CNS-depressant effects could potentially enhance the CNS depressant effects of zolpidem. Dosage adjustments may be necessary when zolpidem is combined with other CNS depressant drugs).
No products indexed under this heading.

Thioridazine Hydrochloride (Since the systematic evaluations of zolpidem in combination with other CNS-active drugs have been limited, careful consideration should be given to the pharmacology of any CNS-active drug to be used with zolpidem. Any drug with CNS-depressant effects could potentially enhance the CNS depressant effects of zolpidem. Dosage adjustments may be necessary when zolpidem is combined with other CNS depressant drugs).
Products include:

Thiothixene (Since the systematic evaluations of zolpidem in combination with other CNS-active drugs have been limited, careful consideration should be given to the pharmacology of any CNS-active drug to be used with zolpidem. Any drug with CNS-depressant effects could potentially enhance the CNS depressant effects of zolpidem. Dosage adjustments may be necessary when zolpidem is combined with other CNS depressant drugs). Products include:

Thiothixene Hydrochloride (Since the systematic evaluations of zolpidem in combination with other CNS-active drugs have been limited, careful consideration should be given to the pharmacology of any CNS-active drug to be used with zolpidem. Any drug with CNS-depressant effects could potentially enhance the CNS depressant effects of zolpidem. Dosage adjustments may be necessary when zolpidem is combined with other CNS depressant drugs).
No products indexed under this heading.

Triazolam (Since the systematic evaluations of zolpidem in combination with other CNS-active drugs have been limited, careful consideration should be given to the pharmacology of any CNS-active drug to be used with zolpidem. Any drug with CNS-depressant effects could potentially enhance the CNS depressant effects of zolpidem. Dosage adjustments may be necessary when zolpidem is combined with other CNS depressant drugs).
No products indexed under this heading.

Trifluoperazine Hydrochloride (Since the systematic evaluations of zolpidem in combination with other CNS-active drugs have been limited, careful consideration should be given to the pharmacology of any CNS-active drug to be used with zolpidem. Any drug with CNS-depressant effects could potentially enhance the CNS depressant effects of zolpidem. Dosage adjustments may be necessary when zolpidem is combined with other CNS depressant drugs).
No products indexed under this heading.

Troleandomycin (Some compounds known to inhibit CYP3A may increase exposure to zolpidem).
No products indexed under this heading.

Venlafaxine Hydrochloride (Some compounds known to inhibit CYP3A may increase exposure to zolpidem). Products include:

IMPORTANT NOTE: Always consult each drug listing in the patient's regimen for possible interactions.

Verapamil Hydrochloride (Some compounds known to inhibit CYP3A may increase exposure to zolpidem). Products include:

Voriconazole (Some compounds known to inhibit CYP3A may increase exposure to zolpidem).
    No products indexed under this heading.

Zafirlukast (Some compounds known to inhibit CYP3A may increase exposure to zolpidem). Products include:

Zaleplon (Since the systematic evaluations of zolpidem in combination with other CNS-active drugs have been limited, careful consideration should be given to the pharmacology of any CNS-active drug to be used with zolpidem. Any drug with CNS-depressant effects could potentially enhance the CNS depressant effects of zolpidem. Dosage adjustments may be necessary when zolpidem is combined with other CNS depressant drugs).
    No products indexed under this heading.

Zileuton (Some compounds known to inhibit CYP3A may increase exposure to zolpidem).
    No products indexed under this heading.

Ziprasidone Hydrochloride (Since the systematic evaluations of zolpidem in combination with other CNS-active drugs have been limited, careful consideration should be given to the pharmacology of any CNS-active drug to be used with zolpidem. Any drug with CNS-depressant effects could potentially enhance the CNS depressant effects of zolpidem. Dosage adjustments may be necessary when zolpidem is combined with other CNS depressant drugs). Products include:

Food Interactions

Alcohol (Since the systematic evaluations of zolpidem in combination with other CNS-active drugs have been limited, careful consideration should be given to the pharmacology of any CNS-active drug to be used with zolpidem. Any drug with CNS-depressant effects could potentially enhance the CNS depressant effects of zolpidem. Dosage adjustments may be necessary when zolpidem is combined with other CNS depressant drugs).

Beer, reduced-alcohol (An additive effect on psychomotor performance between alcohol and zolpidem was demonstrated. Zolpidem should not be taken with alcohol.)

Beer, unspecified (An additive effect on psychomotor performance between alcohol and zolpidem was demonstrated. Zolpidem should not be taken with alcohol.)

Grapefruit (Some compounds known to inhibit CYP3A may increase exposure to zolpidem).

Grapefruit Juice (Some compounds known to inhibit CYP3A may increase exposure to zolpidem).

Meal, unspecified (The effect of zolpidem may be slowed by ingestion with or immediately after a meal).

Wine, Chianti (An additive effect on psychomotor performance between alcohol and zolpidem was demonstrated. Zolpidem should not be taken with alcohol.)

Wine, Red (An additive effect on psychomotor performance between alcohol and zolpidem was demonstrated. Zolpidem should not be taken with alcohol.)

Wine, unspecified (An additive effect on psychomotor performance between alcohol and zolpidem was demonstrated. Zolpidem should not be taken with alcohol.)

Wine products (An additive effect on psychomotor performance between alcohol and zolpidem was demonstrated. Zolpidem should not be taken with alcohol.)

AMBIEN CR TABLETS

(Zolpidem Tartrate) **2925**
May interact with alcohols, central nervous system depressants, central nervous system stimulants, cytochrome p450 3a inhibitors (selected), and certain other agents. Compounds in these categories include:

Alfentanil Hydrochloride (Any drug with CNS-depressant effects could potentially enhance the CNS-depressant effects of zolpidem tartrate. Dosage adjustments may be necessary when zolpidem tartrate is combined with other CNS depressant drugs).
    No products indexed under this heading.

Alprazolam (Any drug with CNS-depressant effects could potentially enhance the CNS-depressant effects of zolpidem tartrate. Dosage adjustments may be necessary when zolpidem tartrate is combined with other CNS depressant drugs).
    No products indexed under this heading.

Amiodarone Hydrochloride (Some compounds known to inhibit CYP3A4 may increase exposure to zolpidem tartrate).
    No products indexed under this heading.

Amobarbital (Any drug with CNS-depressant effects could potentially enhance the CNS-depressant effects of zolpidem tartrate. Dosage adjustments may be necessary when zolpidem tartrate is combined with other CNS depressant drugs).
    No products indexed under this heading.

Amobarbital Sodium (Any drug with CNS-depressant effects could potentially enhance the CNS-depressant effects of zolpidem tartrate. Dosage adjustments may be necessary when zolpidem tartrate is combined with other CNS depressant drugs).
    No products indexed under this heading.

Amphetamine Aspartate (The systematic evaluation of zolpidem tartrate in combination with other CNS-active drugs has been very limited. Therefore, careful consideration should be given to the pharmacology of any CNS-active drug to be used with zolpidem tartrate).
    No products indexed under this heading.

Amphetamine Aspartate Monohydrate (The systematic evaluation of zolpidem tartrate in combination with other CNS-active drugs has been very limited. Therefore, careful consideration should be given to the pharmacology of any CNS-active drug to be used with zolpidem tartrate).
    No products indexed under this heading.

Amphetamine Resins (The systematic evaluation of zolpidem tartrate in combination with other CNS-active drugs has been very limited. Therefore, careful consideration should be given to the pharmacology of any CNS-active drug to be used with zolpidem tartrate).
    No products indexed under this heading.

Amphetamine Sulfate (The systematic evaluation of zolpidem tartrate in combination with other CNS-active drugs has been very limited. Therefore, careful consideration should be given to the pharmacology of any CNS-active drug to be used with zolpidem tartrate).
    No products indexed under this heading.

Amprenavir (Some compounds known to inhibit CYP3A4 may increase exposure to zolpidem tartrate).
    No products indexed under this heading.

Aprepitant (Some compounds known to inhibit CYP3A4 may increase exposure to zolpidem tartrate). Products include:

Aprobarbital (Any drug with CNS-depressant effects could potentially enhance the CNS-depressant effects of zolpidem tartrate. Dosage adjustments may be necessary when zolpidem tartrate is combined with other CNS depressant drugs).
    No products indexed under this heading.

Buprenorphine Hydrochloride (Any drug with CNS-depressant effects could potentially enhance the CNS-depressant effects of zolpidem tartrate. Dosage adjustments may be necessary when zolpidem tartrate is combined with other CNS depressant drugs).
    No products indexed under this heading.

Buspirone Hydrochloride (Any drug with CNS-depressant effects could potentially enhance the CNS-depressant effects of zolpidem tartrate. Dosage adjustments may be necessary when zolpidem tartrate is combined with other CNS depressant drugs).
    No products indexed under this heading.

Butabarbital (Any drug with CNS-depressant effects could potentially enhance the CNS-depressant effects of zolpidem tartrate. Dosage adjustments may be necessary when zolpidem tartrate is combined with other CNS depressant drugs).
    No products indexed under this heading.

Butabarbital Sodium (Any drug with CNS-depressant effects could potentially enhance the CNS-depressant effects of zolpidem tartrate. Dosage adjustments may be necessary when zolpidem tartrate is combined with other CNS depressant drugs).
    No products indexed under this heading.

Butalbital (Any drug with CNS-depressant effects could potentially enhance the CNS-depressant effects of zolpidem tartrate. Dosage adjustments may be necessary when zolpidem tartrate is combined with other CNS depressant drugs).
    No products indexed under this heading.

Chlordiazepoxide (Any drug with CNS-depressant effects could potentially enhance the CNS-depressant effects of zolpidem tartrate. Dosage adjustments may be necessary when zolpidem tartrate is combined with other CNS depressant drugs).
    No products indexed under this heading.

Chlordiazepoxide Hydrochloride (Any drug with CNS-depressant effects could potentially enhance the CNS-depressant effects of zolpidem tartrate. Dosage adjustments may be necessary when zolpidem tartrate is combined with other CNS depressant drugs).
    No products indexed under this heading.

Chlorpromazine (Chlorpromazine in combination with zolpidem tartrate produced no pharmacokinetic interaction, but there was an additive effect of decreased alertness and psychomotor performance).
    No products indexed under this heading.

Chlorpromazine Hydrochloride (Chlorpromazine in combination with zolpidem tartrate produced no pharmacokinetic interaction, but there was an additive effect of decreased alertness and psychomotor performance).
    No products indexed under this heading.

Chlorprothixene (Any drug with CNS-depressant effects could potentially enhance the CNS-depressant effects of zolpidem tartrate. Dosage adjustments may be necessary when zolpidem tartrate is combined with other CNS depressant drugs).
    No products indexed under this heading.

Chlorprothixene Hydrochloride (Any drug with CNS-depressant effects could potentially enhance the CNS-depressant effects of zolpidem tartrate. Dosage adjustments may be necessary when zolpidem tartrate is combined with other CNS depressant drugs).
    No products indexed under this heading.

Chlorprothixene Lactate (Any drug with CNS-depressant effects could potentially enhance the CNS-depressant effects of zolpidem tartrate. Dosage adjustments may be necessary when zolpidem tartrate is combined with other CNS depressant drugs).
    No products indexed under this heading.

Cimetidine (Some compounds known to inhibit CYP3A4 may increase exposure to zolpidem tartrate).
    No products indexed under this heading.

Cimetidine Hydrochloride (Some compounds known to inhibit CYP3A4 may increase exposure to zolpidem tartrate).
    No products indexed under this heading.

Ciprofloxacin (Some compounds known to inhibit CYP3A4 may increase exposure to zolpidem tartrate). Products include:

Ciprofloxacin Hydrochloride (Some compounds known to inhibit CYP3A4 may increase exposure to zolpidem tartrate). Products include:

Clarithromycin (Some compounds known to inhibit CYP3A4 may increase exposure to zolpidem tartrate). Products include:

Clonazepam (Any drug with CNS-depressant effects could potentially enhance the CNS-depressant effects of zolpidem tartrate. Dosage adjustments may be necessary when zolpidem tartrate is combined with other CNS depressant drugs). Products include:

Clorazepate Dipotassium (Any drug with CNS-depressant effects could potentially enhance the CNS-depressant effects of zolpidem tartrate. Dosage adjustments may be necessary when zolpidem tartrate is combined with other CNS depressant drugs).
    No products indexed under this heading.

Clozapine (Any drug with CNS-depressant effects could potentially enhance the CNS-depressant effects of zolpidem tartrate. Dosage adjustments may be necessary when zolpidem tartrate is combined with other CNS depressant drugs).
    No products indexed under this heading.

Codeine Phosphate (Any drug with CNS-depressant effects could potentially enhance the CNS-depressant effects of zolpidem tartrate. Dosage adjustments may be necessary when zolpidem tartrate is combined with other CNS depressant drugs). Products include:

(⊙ Described in PDR® for Ophthalmic Medicines)

Codeine Sulfate (Any drug with CNS-depressant effects could potentially enhance the CNS-depressant effects of zolpidem tartrate. Dosage adjustments may be necessary when zolpidem tartrate is combined with other CNS depressant drugs).
　No products indexed under this heading.

Cyclosporine (Some compounds known to inhibit CYP3A4 may increase exposure to zolpidem tartrate). Products include:

Delavirdine Mesylate (Some compounds known to inhibit CYP3A4 may increase exposure to zolpidem tartrate).
　No products indexed under this heading.

Desflurane (Any drug with CNS-depressant effects could potentially enhance the CNS-depressant effects of zolpidem tartrate. Dosage adjustments may be necessary when zolpidem tartrate is combined with other CNS depressant drugs).
　No products indexed under this heading.

Dexmethylphenidate Hydrochloride (The systematic evaluation of zolpidem tartrate in combination with other CNS-active drugs has been very limited. Therefore, careful consideration should be given to the pharmacology of any CNS-active drug to be used with zolpidem tartrate). Products include:

Dextroamphetamine (The systematic evaluation of zolpidem tartrate in combination with other CNS-active drugs has been very limited. Therefore, careful consideration should be given to the pharmacology of any CNS-active drug to be used with zolpidem tartrate).
　No products indexed under this heading.

Dextroamphetamine Saccharate (The systematic evaluation of zolpidem tartrate in combination with other CNS-active drugs has been very limited. Therefore, careful consideration should be given to the pharmacology of any CNS-active drug to be used with zolpidem tartrate).
　No products indexed under this heading.

Dextroamphetamine Sulfate (The systematic evaluation of zolpidem tartrate in combination with other CNS-active drugs has been very limited. Therefore, careful consideration should be given to the pharmacology of any CNS-active drug to be used with zolpidem tartrate). Products include:

Dezocine (Any drug with CNS-depressant effects could potentially enhance the CNS-depressant effects of zolpidem tartrate. Dosage adjustments may be necessary when zolpidem tartrate is combined with other CNS depressant drugs).
　No products indexed under this heading.

Diazepam (Any drug with CNS-depressant effects could potentially enhance the CNS-depressant effects of zolpidem tartrate. Dosage adjustments may be necessary when zolpidem tartrate is combined with other CNS depressant drugs). Products include:

Diltiazem Hydrochloride (Some compounds known to inhibit CYP3A4 may increase exposure to zolpidem tartrate). Products include:

Diltiazem Maleate (Some compounds known to inhibit CYP3A4 may increase exposure to zolpidem tartrate).
　No products indexed under this heading.

Droperidol (Any drug with CNS-depressant effects could potentially enhance the CNS-depressant effects of zolpidem tartrate. Dosage adjustments may be necessary when zolpidem tartrate is combined with other CNS depressant drugs).
　No products indexed under this heading.

Efavirenz (Some compounds known to inhibit CYP3A4 may increase exposure to zolpidem tartrate). Products include:

Enflurane (Any drug with CNS-depressant effects could potentially enhance the CNS-depressant effects of zolpidem tartrate. Dosage adjustments may be necessary when zolpidem tartrate is combined with other CNS depressant drugs).
　No products indexed under this heading.

Erythromycin (Some compounds known to inhibit CYP3A4 may increase exposure to zolpidem tartrate).
　No products indexed under this heading.

Estazolam (Any drug with CNS-depressant effects could potentially enhance the CNS-depressant effects of zolpidem tartrate. Dosage adjustments may be necessary when zolpidem tartrate is combined with other CNS depressant drugs).
　No products indexed under this heading.

Ethanol (Any drug with CNS-depressant effects could potentially enhance the CNS-depressant effects of zolpidem tartrate. Dosage adjustments may be necessary when zolpidem tartrate is combined with other CNS depressant drugs).
　No products indexed under this heading.

Ethchlorvynol (Any drug with CNS-depressant effects could potentially enhance the CNS-depressant effects of zolpidem tartrate. Dosage adjustments may be necessary when zolpidem tartrate is combined with other CNS depressant drugs).
　No products indexed under this heading.

Ethinamate (Any drug with CNS-depressant effects could potentially enhance the CNS-depressant effects of zolpidem tartrate. Dosage adjustments may be necessary when zolpidem tartrate is combined with other CNS depressant drugs).
　No products indexed under this heading.

Ethyl Alcohol (Any drug with CNS-depressant effects could potentially enhance the CNS-depressant effects of zolpidem tartrate. Dosage adjustments may be necessary when zolpidem tartrate is combined with other CNS depressant drugs).
　No products indexed under this heading.

Fentanyl (Any drug with CNS-depressant effects could potentially enhance the CNS-depressant effects of zolpidem tartrate. Dosage adjustments may be necessary when zolpidem tartrate is combined with other CNS depressant drugs). Products include:

Fentanyl Citrate (Any drug with CNS-depressant effects could potentially enhance the CNS-depressant effects of zolpidem tartrate. Dosage adjustments may be necessary when zolpidem tartrate is combined with other CNS depressant drugs). Products include:

Fluconazole (Some compounds known to inhibit CYP3A4 may increase exposure to zolpidem tartrate).
　No products indexed under this heading.

Fluoxetine (A single-dose interaction study with zolpidem tartrate 10 mg and fluoxetine 20 mg at steady-state levels in male volunteers did not demonstrate any clinically significant pharmacokinet-

ic or pharmacodynamic interactions. When multiple doses of zolpidem tartrate and fluoxetine at steady-state concentrations were evaluated in healthy females, the only significant change was a 17% increase in the zolpidem tartrate half-life. There was no evidence of an additive effect in psychomotor performance).
　No products indexed under this heading.

Fluoxetine Hydrochloride (A single-dose interaction study with zolpidem tartrate 10 mg and fluoxetine 20 mg at steady-state levels in male volunteers did not demonstrate any clinically significant pharmacokinetic or pharmacodynamic interactions. When multiple doses of zolpidem tartrate and fluoxetine at steady-state concentrations were evaluated in healthy females, the only significant change was a 17% increase in the zolpidem tartrate half-life. There was no evidence of an additive effect in psychomotor performance). Products include:

Fluphenazine Decanoate (Any drug with CNS-depressant effects could potentially enhance the CNS-depressant effects of zolpidem tartrate. Dosage adjustments may be necessary when zolpidem tartrate is combined with other CNS depressant drugs).
　No products indexed under this heading.

Fluphenazine Enanthate (Any drug with CNS-depressant effects could potentially enhance the CNS-depressant effects of zolpidem tartrate. Dosage adjustments may be necessary when zolpidem tartrate is combined with other CNS depressant drugs).
　No products indexed under this heading.

Fluphenazine Hydrochloride (Any drug with CNS-depressant effects could potentially enhance the CNS-depressant effects of zolpidem tartrate. Dosage adjustments may be necessary when zolpidem tartrate is combined with other CNS depressant drugs).
　No products indexed under this heading.

Flurazepam Hydrochloride (Any drug with CNS-depressant effects could potentially enhance the CNS-depressant effects of zolpidem tartrate. Dosage adjustments may be necessary when zolpidem tartrate is combined with other CNS depressant drugs).
　No products indexed under this heading.

Fluvoxamine Maleate (Some compounds known to inhibit CYP3A4 may increase exposure to zolpidem tartrate).
　No products indexed under this heading.

Glutethimide (Any drug with CNS-depressant effects could potentially enhance the CNS-depressant effects of zolpidem tartrate. Dosage adjustments may be necessary when zolpidem tartrate is combined with other CNS depressant drugs).
　No products indexed under this heading.

Halazepam (Any drug with CNS-depressant effects could potentially enhance the CNS-depressant effects of zolpidem tartrate. Dosage adjustments may be necessary when zolpidem tartrate is combined with other CNS depressant drugs).
　No products indexed under this heading.

Haloperidol (A study involving haloperidol and zolpidem tartrate revealed no effect of haloperidol on the pharmacokinetics or pharmacodynamics of zolpidem tartrate. The lack of a drug interaction following a single-dose administration does not predict a lack following chronic administration).
　No products indexed under this heading.

Haloperidol Decanoate (A study involving haloperidol and zolpidem tartrate revealed no effect of haloperidol on the pharmacokinetics or pharmacodynamics of zolpidem tartrate. The lack of a drug interaction following a single-dose administration does not predict a lack following chronic administration).
　No products indexed under this heading.

Haloperidol Lactate (A study involving haloperidol and zolpidem tartrate revealed no effect of haloperidol on the pharmacokinetics or pharmacodynamics of zolpidem tartrate. The lack of a drug interaction following a single-dose administration does not predict a lack following chronic administration).
　No products indexed under this heading.

Hexobarbital (Any drug with CNS-depressant effects could potentially enhance the CNS-depressant effects of zolpidem tartrate. Dosage adjustments may be necessary when zolpidem tartrate is combined with other CNS depressant drugs).
　No products indexed under this heading.

Hydrocodone Bitartrate (Any drug with CNS-depressant effects could potentially enhance the CNS-depressant effects of zolpidem tartrate. Dosage adjustments may be necessary when zolpidem tartrate is combined with other CNS depressant drugs). Products include:

Hydrocodone Polistirex (Any drug with CNS-depressant effects could potentially enhance the CNS-depressant effects of zolpidem tartrate. Dosage adjustments may be necessary when zolpidem tartrate is combined with other CNS depressant drugs). Products include:

Hydromorphone (Any drug with CNS-depressant effects could potentially enhance the CNS-depressant effects of zolpidem tartrate. Dosage adjustments may be necessary when zolpidem tartrate is combined with other CNS depressant drugs).
　No products indexed under this heading.

Hydromorphone Hydrochloride (Any drug with CNS-depressant effects could potentially enhance the CNS-depressant effects of zolpidem tartrate. Dosage adjustments may be necessary when zolpidem tartrate is combined with other CNS depressant drugs). Products include:

Hydroxyamphetamine Hydrobromide (The systematic evaluation of zolpidem tartrate in combination with other CNS-active drugs has been very limited. Therefore, careful consideration should be given to the pharmacology of any CNS-active drug to be used with zolpidem tartrate).
　No products indexed under this heading.

Hydroxyzine Hydrochloride (Any drug with CNS-depressant effects could potentially enhance the CNS-depressant effects of zolpidem tartrate. Dosage adjustments may be necessary when zolpidem tartrate is combined with other CNS depressant drugs).
　No products indexed under this heading.

IMPORTANT NOTE: Always consult each drug listing in the patient's regimen for possible interactions.

Imipramine Hydrochloride (Imipramine in combination with zolpidem tartrate produced no pharmacokinetic interaction other than a 20% decrease in peak levels of imipramine, but there was an additive effect of decreased alertness).

No products indexed under this heading.

Imipramine Pamoate (Imipramine in combination with zolpidem tartrate produced no pharmacokinetic interaction other than a 20% decrease in peak levels of imipramine, but there was an additive effect of decreased alertness).

No products indexed under this heading.

Indinavir Sulfate (Some compounds known to inhibit CYP3A4 may increase exposure to zolpidem tartrate). Products include:

Isoflurane (Any drug with CNS-depressant effects could potentially enhance the CNS-depressant effects of zolpidem tartrate. Dosage adjustments may be necessary when zolpidem tartrate is combined with other CNS depressant drugs).

No products indexed under this heading.

Isoniazid (Some compounds known to inhibit CYP3A4 may increase exposure to zolpidem tartrate).

No products indexed under this heading.

Itraconazole (A randomized, double-blind, crossover interaction study in 10 healthy volunteers between itraconazole (200 mg once daily for 4 days) and a single dose of zolpidem tartrate (10 mg) given 5 hours after the last dose of itraconazole resulted in a 34% increase in AUC of zolpidem tartrate. There were no significant pharmacodynamic effects of zolpidem tartrate on subjective drowsiness, postural sway, or psychomotor performance).

No products indexed under this heading.

Ketamine Hydrochloride (Any drug with CNS-depressant effects could potentially enhance the CNS-depressant effects of zolpidem tartrate. Dosage adjustments may be necessary when zolpidem tartrate is combined with other CNS depressant drugs).

No products indexed under this heading.

Ketoconazole (A study in 12 healthy subjects showed that co-administration of a single 5 mg dose of immediate-release zolpidem tartrate with ketoconazole, a potent CYP3A4 inhibitor, given as 200 mg b.i.d. for 2 days increased C_{max} of zolpidem by a factor of 1.3 and increased the total AUC of zolpidem by a factor of 1.7 compared to zolpidem alone and prolonged the elimination T1/2 by approximately 30% along with an increase in the pharmacodynamic effects of zolpidem. Caution should be used when ketoconazole is given with zolpidem and consideration should be given to using a lower dose of zolpidem when ketoconazole and zolpidem are given together. Advise patients that the use of zolpidem tartrate extended release tablets with ketoconazole may enhance the sedative effects). Products include:

Levomethadyl Acetate Hydrochloride (Any drug with CNS-depressant effects could potentially enhance the CNS-depressant effects of zolpidem tartrate. Dosage adjustments may be necessary when zolpidem tartrate is combined with other CNS depressant drugs).

No products indexed under this heading.

Levorphanol Tartrate (Any drug with CNS-depressant effects could potentially enhance the CNS-depressant effects of zolpidem tartrate. Dosage adjustments may be necessary when zolpidem tartrate is combined with other CNS depressant drugs).

No products indexed under this heading.

Lisdexamfetamine Dimesylate (The systematic evaluation of zolpidem tartrate in combination with other CNS-active drugs has been very limited. Therefore, careful consideration should be given to the pharmacology of any CNS-active drug to be used with zolpidem tartrate). Products include:

Lopinavir (Some compounds known to inhibit CYP3A4 may increase exposure to zolpidem tartrate). Products include:

Lorazepam (Any drug with CNS-depressant effects could potentially enhance the CNS-depressant effects of zolpidem tartrate. Dosage adjustments may be necessary when zolpidem tartrate is combined with other CNS depressant drugs).

No products indexed under this heading.

Loxapine Hydrochloride (Any drug with CNS-depressant effects could potentially enhance the CNS-depressant effects of zolpidem tartrate. Dosage adjustments may be necessary when zolpidem tartrate is combined with other CNS depressant drugs).

No products indexed under this heading.

Loxapine Succinate (Any drug with CNS-depressant effects could potentially enhance the CNS-depressant effects of zolpidem tartrate. Dosage adjustments may be necessary when zolpidem tartrate is combined with other CNS depressant drugs).

No products indexed under this heading.

Meperidine Hydrochloride (Any drug with CNS-depressant effects could potentially enhance the CNS-depressant effects of zolpidem tartrate. Dosage adjustments may be necessary when zolpidem tartrate is combined with other CNS depressant drugs).

No products indexed under this heading.

Mephobarbital (Any drug with CNS-depressant effects could potentially enhance the CNS-depressant effects of zolpidem tartrate. Dosage adjustments may be necessary when zolpidem tartrate is combined with other CNS depressant drugs).

No products indexed under this heading.

Meprobamate (Any drug with CNS-depressant effects could potentially enhance the CNS-depressant effects of zolpidem tartrate. Dosage adjustments may be necessary when zolpidem tartrate is combined with other CNS depressant drugs).

No products indexed under this heading.

Mesoridazine Besylate (Any drug with CNS-depressant effects could potentially enhance the CNS-depressant effects of zolpidem tartrate. Dosage adjustments may be necessary when zolpidem tartrate is combined with other CNS depressant drugs).

No products indexed under this heading.

Methadone Hydrochloride (Any drug with CNS-depressant effects could potentially enhance the CNS-depressant effects of zolpidem tartrate. Dosage adjustments may be necessary when zolpidem tartrate is combined with other CNS depressant drugs).

No products indexed under this heading.

Methamphetamine Hydrochloride (The systematic evaluation of zolpidem tartrate in combination with other CNS-active drugs has been very limited. Therefore, careful consideration should be given to the pharmacology of any CNS-active drug to be used with zolpidem tartrate).

No products indexed under this heading.

Methohexital Sodium (Any drug with CNS-depressant effects could potentially enhance the CNS-depressant effects of zolpidem tartrate. Dosage adjustments may be necessary when zolpidem tartrate is combined with other CNS depressant drugs).

No products indexed under this heading.

Methotrimeprazine (Any drug with CNS-depressant effects could potentially enhance the CNS-depressant effects of zolpidem tartrate. Dosage adjustments may be necessary when zolpidem tartrate is combined with other CNS depressant drugs).

No products indexed under this heading.

Methoxyflurane (Any drug with CNS-depressant effects could potentially enhance the CNS-depressant effects of zolpidem tartrate. Dosage adjustments may be necessary when zolpidem tartrate is combined with other CNS depressant drugs).

No products indexed under this heading.

Methylphenidate (The systematic evaluation of zolpidem tartrate in combination with other CNS-active drugs has been very limited. Therefore, careful consideration should be given to the pharmacology of any CNS-active drug to be used with zolpidem tartrate). Products include:

Methylphenidate Hydrochloride (The systematic evaluation of zolpidem tartrate in combination with other CNS-active drugs has been very limited. Therefore, careful consideration should be given to the pharmacology of any CNS-active drug to be used with zolpidem tartrate). Products include:

Metronidazole (Some compounds known to inhibit CYP3A4 may increase exposure to zolpidem tartrate). Products include:

Metronidazole Benzoate (Some compounds known to inhibit CYP3A4 may increase exposure to zolpidem tartrate).

No products indexed under this heading.

Metronidazole Hydrochloride (Some compounds known to inhibit CYP3A4 may increase exposure to zolpidem tartrate).

No products indexed under this heading.

Miconazole (Some compounds known to inhibit CYP3A4 may increase exposure to zolpidem tartrate).

No products indexed under this heading.

Midazolam Hydrochloride (Any drug with CNS-depressant effects could potentially enhance the CNS-depressant effects of zolpidem tartrate. Dosage adjustments may be necessary when zolpidem tartrate is combined with other CNS depressant drugs).

No products indexed under this heading.

Molindone Hydrochloride (Any drug with CNS-depressant effects could potentially enhance the CNS-depressant effects of zolpidem tartrate. Dosage adjustments may be necessary when zolpidem tartrate is combined with other CNS depressant drugs). Products include:

Morphine Sulfate (Any drug with CNS-depressant effects could potentially enhance the CNS-depressant effects

of zolpidem tartrate. Dosage adjustments may be necessary when zolpidem tartrate is combined with other CNS depressant drugs). Products include:

Morphine Sulfate, Liposomal (Any drug with CNS-depressant effects could potentially enhance the CNS-depressant effects of zolpidem tartrate. Dosage adjustments may be necessary when zolpidem tartrate is combined with other CNS depressant drugs).

No products indexed under this heading.

Nefazodone Hydrochloride (Some compounds known to inhibit CYP3A4 may increase exposure to zolpidem tartrate).

No products indexed under this heading.

Nelfinavir Mesylate (Some compounds known to inhibit CYP3A4 may increase exposure to zolpidem tartrate).

No products indexed under this heading.

Nifedipine (Some compounds known to inhibit CYP3A4 may increase exposure to zolpidem tartrate).

No products indexed under this heading.

Norfloxacin (Some compounds known to inhibit CYP3A4 may increase exposure to zolpidem tartrate). Products include:

Olanzapine (Any drug with CNS-depressant effects could potentially enhance the CNS-depressant effects of zolpidem tartrate. Dosage adjustments may be necessary when zolpidem tartrate is combined with other CNS depressant drugs). Products include:

Oxazepam (Any drug with CNS-depressant effects could potentially enhance the CNS-depressant effects of zolpidem tartrate. Dosage adjustments may be necessary when zolpidem tartrate is combined with other CNS depressant drugs).

No products indexed under this heading.

Oxycodone Hydrochloride (Any drug with CNS-depressant effects could potentially enhance the CNS-depressant effects of zolpidem tartrate. Dosage adjustments may be necessary when zolpidem tartrate is combined with other CNS depressant drugs). Products include:

Oxycodone Terephthalate (Any drug with CNS-depressant effects could potentially enhance the CNS-depressant effects of zolpidem tartrate. Dosage adjustments may be necessary when zolpidem tartrate is combined with other CNS depressant drugs).

No products indexed under this heading.

Oxymorphone Hydrochloride (Any drug with CNS-depressant effects could potentially enhance the CNS-depressant effects of zolpidem tartrate. Dosage adjustments may be necessary when zolpidem tartrate is combined with other CNS depressant drugs). Products include:

Paroxetine Hydrochloride (Some compounds known to inhibit CYP3A4 may increase exposure to zolpidem tartrate). Products include:

Pemoline (The systematic evaluation of zolpidem tartrate in combination with other CNS-active drugs has been very limited. Therefore, careful consideration should be given to the pharmacology of any CNS-active drug to be used with zolpidem tartrate).
No products indexed under this heading.

Pentobarbital (Any drug with CNS-depressant effects could potentially enhance the CNS-depressant effects of zolpidem tartrate. Dosage adjustments may be necessary when zolpidem tartrate is combined with other CNS depressant drugs).
No products indexed under this heading.

Pentobarbital Sodium (Any drug with CNS-depressant effects could potentially enhance the CNS-depressant effects of zolpidem tartrate. Dosage adjustments may be necessary when zolpidem tartrate is combined with other CNS depressant drugs). Products include:
Nembutal 2012

Perphenazine (Any drug with CNS-depressant effects could potentially enhance the CNS-depressant effects of zolpidem tartrate. Dosage adjustments may be necessary when zolpidem tartrate is combined with other CNS depressant drugs).
No products indexed under this heading.

Phenobarbital (Any drug with CNS-depressant effects could potentially enhance the CNS-depressant effects of zolpidem tartrate. Dosage adjustments may be necessary when zolpidem tartrate is combined with other CNS depressant drugs). Products include:
Donnatal 2711

Phenobarbital Sodium (Any drug with CNS-depressant effects could potentially enhance the CNS-depressant effects of zolpidem tartrate. Dosage adjustments may be necessary when zolpidem tartrate is combined with other CNS depressant drugs).
No products indexed under this heading.

Prazepam (Any drug with CNS-depressant effects could potentially enhance the CNS-depressant effects of zolpidem tartrate. Dosage adjustments may be necessary when zolpidem tartrate is combined with other CNS depressant drugs).
No products indexed under this heading.

Prochlorperazine (Any drug with CNS-depressant effects could potentially enhance the CNS-depressant effects of zolpidem tartrate. Dosage adjustments may be necessary when zolpidem tartrate is combined with other CNS depressant drugs).
No products indexed under this heading.

Prochlorperazine Edisylate (Any drug with CNS-depressant effects could potentially enhance the CNS-depressant effects of zolpidem tartrate. Dosage adjustments may be necessary when zolpidem tartrate is combined with other CNS depressant drugs).
No products indexed under this heading.

Prochlorperazine Maleate (Any drug with CNS-depressant effects could potentially enhance the CNS-depressant effects of zolpidem tartrate. Dosage adjustments may be necessary when zolpidem tartrate is combined with other CNS depressant drugs).
No products indexed under this heading.

Promethazine (Any drug with CNS-depressant effects could potentially enhance the CNS-depressant effects of zolpidem tartrate. Dosage adjustments may be necessary when zolpidem tartrate is combined with other CNS depressant drugs).
No products indexed under this heading.

Promethazine Hydrochloride (Any drug with CNS-depressant effects could potentially enhance the CNS-depressant effects of zolpidem tartrate. Dosage adjustments may be necessary when zolpidem tartrate is combined with other CNS depressant drugs).
No products indexed under this heading.

Propofol (Any drug with CNS-depressant effects could potentially enhance the CNS-depressant effects of zolpidem tartrate. Dosage adjustments may be necessary when zolpidem tartrate is combined with other CNS depressant drugs).
No products indexed under this heading.

Propoxyphene Hydrochloride (Any drug with CNS-depressant effects could potentially enhance the CNS-depressant effects of zolpidem tartrate. Dosage adjustments may be necessary when zolpidem tartrate is combined with other CNS depressant drugs).
No products indexed under this heading.

Propoxyphene Napsylate (Any drug with CNS-depressant effects could potentially enhance the CNS-depressant effects of zolpidem tartrate. Dosage adjustments may be necessary when zolpidem tartrate is combined with other CNS depressant drugs).
No products indexed under this heading.

Quazepam (Any drug with CNS-depressant effects could potentially enhance the CNS-depressant effects of zolpidem tartrate. Dosage adjustments may be necessary when zolpidem tartrate is combined with other CNS depressant drugs).
No products indexed under this heading.

Quetiapine Fumarate (Any drug with CNS-depressant effects could potentially enhance the CNS-depressant effects of zolpidem tartrate. Dosage adjustments may be necessary when zolpidem tartrate is combined with other CNS depressant drugs). Products include:
Seroquel 750
Seroquel XR 759

Quinine (Some compounds known to inhibit CYP3A4 may increase exposure to zolpidem tartrate). Products include:
Hyland's Leg Cramps PM with Quinine 3315

Quinine Sulfate (Some compounds known to inhibit CYP3A4 may increase exposure to zolpidem tartrate).
No products indexed under this heading.

Remifentanil Hydrochloride (Any drug with CNS-depressant effects could potentially enhance the CNS-depressant effects of zolpidem tartrate. Dosage adjustments may be necessary when zolpidem tartrate is combined with other CNS depressant drugs).
No products indexed under this heading.

Rifampin (A randomized, placebo-controlled, crossover interaction study in 8 healthy female subjects between 5 consecutive daily doses of rifampin (600 mg) and a single dose of an immediate-release formulation of zolpidem tartrate (20 mg) given 17 hours after the last dose of rifampin showed significant reductions of the AUC (-73%), C_{max} (-58%), and T1/2 (-36%) of zolpidem tartrate together with significant reductions in the pharmacodynamic effects of zolpidem tartrate).
No products indexed under this heading.

Risperidone (Any drug with CNS-depressant effects could potentially enhance the CNS-depressant effects of zolpidem tartrate. Dosage adjustments may be necessary when zolpidem tartrate is combined with other CNS depressant drugs). Products include:
Risperdal Consta 2682

Ritonavir (Some compounds known to inhibit CYP3A4 may increase exposure to zolpidem tartrate). Products include:
Kaletra 458
Norvir 509

Saquinavir (Some compounds known to inhibit CYP3A4 may increase exposure to zolpidem tartrate).
No products indexed under this heading.

Saquinavir Mesylate (Some compounds known to inhibit CYP3A4 may increase exposure to zolpidem tartrate).
No products indexed under this heading.

Secobarbital Sodium (Any drug with CNS-depressant effects could potentially enhance the CNS-depressant effects of zolpidem tartrate. Dosage adjustments may be necessary when zolpidem tartrate is combined with other CNS depressant drugs).
No products indexed under this heading.

Sertraline Hydrochloride (Following five consecutive nightly doses of zolpidem tartrate 10 mg in the presence of sertraline 50 mg (17 consecutive daily doses, at 7:00 AM, in healthy female volunteers), zolpidem tartrate C_{max} was significantly higher (43%) and T_{max} was significantly decreased (53%). Pharmacokinetics of sertraline and N-desmethylsertraline were unaffected by zolpidem tartrate).
No products indexed under this heading.

Sevoflurane (Any drug with CNS-depressant effects could potentially enhance the CNS-depressant effects of zolpidem tartrate. Dosage adjustments may be necessary when zolpidem tartrate is combined with other CNS depressant drugs). Products include:
Ultane 554

Sodium Butabarbital (Any drug with CNS-depressant effects could potentially enhance the CNS-depressant effects of zolpidem tartrate. Dosage adjustments may be necessary when zolpidem tartrate is combined with other CNS depressant drugs).
No products indexed under this heading.

Sodium Oxybate (Any drug with CNS-depressant effects could potentially enhance the CNS-depressant effects of zolpidem tartrate. Dosage adjustments may be necessary when zolpidem tartrate is combined with other CNS depressant drugs).
No products indexed under this heading.

Sodium Pentobarbital (Any drug with CNS-depressant effects could potentially enhance the CNS-depressant effects of zolpidem tartrate. Dosage adjustments may be necessary when zolpidem tartrate is combined with other CNS depressant drugs).
No products indexed under this heading.

Sufentanil Citrate (Any drug with CNS-depressant effects could potentially enhance the CNS-depressant effects of zolpidem tartrate. Dosage adjustments may be necessary when zolpidem tartrate is combined with other CNS depressant drugs).
No products indexed under this heading.

Talbutal (Any drug with CNS-depressant effects could potentially enhance the CNS-depressant effects of zolpidem tartrate. Dosage adjustments may be necessary when zolpidem tartrate is combined with other CNS depressant drugs).
No products indexed under this heading.

Temazepam (Any drug with CNS-depressant effects could potentially enhance the CNS-depressant effects of zolpidem tartrate. Dosage adjustments may be necessary when zolpidem tartrate is combined with other CNS depressant drugs).
No products indexed under this heading.

Thiamylal Sodium (Any drug with CNS-depressant effects could potentially enhance the CNS-depressant effects of zolpidem tartrate. Dosage adjustments may be necessary when zolpidem tartrate is combined with other CNS depressant drugs).
No products indexed under this heading.

Thioridazine (Any drug with CNS-depressant effects could potentially enhance the CNS-depressant effects of zolpidem tartrate. Dosage adjustments may be necessary when zolpidem tartrate is combined with other CNS depressant drugs).
No products indexed under this heading.

Thioridazine Hydrochloride (Any drug with CNS-depressant effects could potentially enhance the CNS-depressant effects of zolpidem tartrate. Dosage adjustments may be necessary when zolpidem tartrate is combined with other CNS depressant drugs). Products include:
Thioridazine Hydrochloride 2384

Thiothixene (Any drug with CNS-depressant effects could potentially enhance the CNS-depressant effects of zolpidem tartrate. Dosage adjustments may be necessary when zolpidem tartrate is combined with other CNS depressant drugs). Products include:
Thiothixene 2386

Thiothixene Hydrochloride (Any drug with CNS-depressant effects could potentially enhance the CNS-depressant effects of zolpidem tartrate. Dosage adjustments may be necessary when zolpidem tartrate is combined with other CNS depressant drugs).
No products indexed under this heading.

Triazolam (Any drug with CNS-depressant effects could potentially enhance the CNS-depressant effects of zolpidem tartrate. Dosage adjustments may be necessary when zolpidem tartrate is combined with other CNS depressant drugs).
No products indexed under this heading.

Trifluoperazine Hydrochloride (Any drug with CNS-depressant effects could potentially enhance the CNS-depressant effects of zolpidem tartrate. Dosage adjustments may be necessary when zolpidem tartrate is combined with other CNS depressant drugs).
No products indexed under this heading.

Troleandomycin (Some compounds known to inhibit CYP3A4 may increase exposure to zolpidem tartrate).
No products indexed under this heading.

Venlafaxine Hydrochloride (Some compounds known to inhibit CYP3A4 may increase exposure to zolpidem tartrate). Products include:
Effexor XR 3504
Venlafaxine Hydrochloride Tablets ... 2388

Verapamil Hydrochloride (Some compounds known to inhibit CYP3A4 may increase exposure to zolpidem tartrate). Products include:
Tarka 534

Voriconazole (Some compounds known to inhibit CYP3A4 may increase exposure to zolpidem tartrate).
No products indexed under this heading.

Zafirlukast (Some compounds known to inhibit CYP3A4 may increase exposure to zolpidem tartrate). Products include:
Accolate 3612

Zaleplon (Any drug with CNS-depressant effects could potentially enhance the CNS-depressant effects of zolpidem tartrate. Dosage adjustments may be necessary when zolpidem tartrate is combined with other CNS depressant drugs).
No products indexed under this heading.

IMPORTANT NOTE: Always consult each drug listing in the patient's regimen for possible interactions.

(⊙ Described in PDR® for Ophthalmic Medicines)

IMPORTANT NOTE: Always consult each drug listing in the patient's regimen for possible interactions.

Ethynodiol Diacetate (Co-administration with oral contraceptives has resulted in reduced clearance by 32% and volume of distribution by 22%, producing slightly higher concentrations of naratriptan).
No products indexed under this heading.

Fluoxetine (Cases of life-threatening serotonin syndrome, including mental status changes, autonomic instability, neuromuscular aberrations, and/or GI symptoms, have been reported during combination use of selective serotonin reuptake inhibitors and triptans. If concomitant treatment with naratriptan and an SSRI is clinically warranted, careful observation of the patient is advised, particularly during treatment initiation and dose increases).
No products indexed under this heading.

Fluoxetine Hydrochloride (Cases of life-threatening serotonin syndrome, including mental status changes, autonomic instability, neuromuscular aberrations, and/or GI symptoms, have been reported during combination use of selective serotonin reuptake inhibitors and triptans. If concomitant treatment with naratriptan and an SSRI is clinically warranted, careful observation of the patient is advised, particularly during treatment initiation and dose increases).
Products include:
Prozac Weekly	1941
Prozac Pulvules	1941
Symbyax	1965

Fluvoxamine (Cases of life-threatening serotonin syndrome, including mental status changes, autonomic instability, neuromuscular aberrations, and/or GI symptoms, have been reported during combination use of selective serotonin reuptake inhibitors and triptans. If concomitant treatment with naratriptan and an SSRI is clinically warranted, careful observation of the patient is advised, particularly during treatment initiation and dose increases).
No products indexed under this heading.

Fluvoxamine Maleate (Cases of life-threatening serotonin syndrome, including mental status changes, autonomic instability, neuromuscular aberrations, and/or GI symptoms, have been reported during combination use of selective serotonin reuptake inhibitors and triptans. If concomitant treatment with naratriptan and an SSRI is clinically warranted, careful observation of the patient is advised, particularly during treatment initiation and dose increases).
No products indexed under this heading.

Frovatriptan Succinate (Co-administration with other 5-HT1 agonists within 24 hours of each other is contraindicated because of the vasospastic effects may be additive).
Products include:
Frova	1103

Levonorgestrel (Co-administration with oral contraceptives has resulted in reduced clearance by 32% and volume of distribution by 22%, producing slightly higher concentrations of naratriptan).
Products include:
Climara Pro	847
LoSeasonique	3407
Lybrel	3514
Mirena	854
Plan B	3416
Seasonique	3418

Mestranol (Co-administration with oral contraceptives has resulted in reduced clearance by 32% and volume of distribution by 22%, producing slightly higher concentrations of naratriptan).
No products indexed under this heading.

Methylergonovine Maleate (Ergot-containing drugs have been reported to cause prolonged vasospastic reactions; because there is a theoretical basis that these effects may be additive, use of ergot-type agents and naratriptan within 24 hours is contraindicated).
No products indexed under this heading.

Methysergide Maleate (Ergot-containing drugs have been reported to cause prolonged vasospastic reactions; because there is a theoretical basis that these effects may be additive, use of ergot-type agents and naratriptan within 24 hours is contraindicated).
No products indexed under this heading.

Nefazodone Hydrochloride (Cases of life-threatening serotonin syndrome, including mental status changes, autonomic instability, neuromuscular aberrations, and/or GI symptoms, have been reported during combination use of serotonin and norepinephrine reuptake inhibitors and triptans. If concomitant treatment with naratriptan and an SNRI is clinically warranted, careful observation of the patient is advised, particularly during treatment initiation and dose increases).
No products indexed under this heading.

Norethindrone (Co-administration with oral contraceptives has resulted in reduced clearance by 32% and volume of distribution by 22%, producing slightly higher concentrations of naratriptan).
Products include:
Ortho Micronor	2660

Norethynodrel (Co-administration with oral contraceptives has resulted in reduced clearance by 32% and volume of distribution by 22%, producing slightly higher concentrations of naratriptan).
No products indexed under this heading.

Norgestimate (Co-administration with oral contraceptives has resulted in reduced clearance by 32% and volume of distribution by 22%, producing slightly higher concentrations of naratriptan).
Products include:
Ortho-Cyclen/Ortho Tri-Cyclen	2663
Ortho Tri-Cyclen Lo Tablets	2673

Norgestrel (Co-administration with oral contraceptives has resulted in reduced clearance by 32% and volume of distribution by 22%, producing slightly higher concentrations of naratriptan).
No products indexed under this heading.

Paroxetine (Cases of life-threatening serotonin syndrome, including mental status changes, autonomic instability, neuromuscular aberrations, and/or GI symptoms, have been reported during combination use of selective serotonin reuptake inhibitors and triptans. If concomitant treatment with naratriptan and an SSRI is clinically warranted, careful observation of the patient is advised, particularly during treatment initiation and dose increases).
No products indexed under this heading.

Paroxetine Hydrochloride (Cases of life-threatening serotonin syndrome, including mental status changes, autonomic instability, neuromuscular aberrations, and/or GI symptoms, have been reported during combination use of selective serotonin reuptake inhibitors and triptans. If concomitant treatment with naratriptan and an SSRI is clinically warranted, careful observation of the patient is advised, particularly during treatment initiation and dose increases).
Products include:
Paroxetine CR	2361
Paroxetine ER	2371
Paxil	1586
Paxil CR	1596

Paroxetine Mesylate (Cases of life-threatening serotonin syndrome, including mental status changes, autonomic instability, neuromuscular aberrations, and/or GI symptoms, have been report-

ed during combination use of selective serotonin reuptake inhibitors and triptans. If concomitant treatment with naratriptan and an SSRI is clinically warranted, careful observation of the patient is advised, particularly during treatment initiation and dose increases).
No products indexed under this heading.

Rizatriptan Benzoate (Co-administration with other 5-HT1 agonists within 24 hours of each other is contraindicated because of the vasospastic effects may be additive).
Products include:
Maxalt	2206
Maxalt-MLT	2206

Sertraline Hydrochloride (Cases of life-threatening serotonin syndrome, including mental status changes, autonomic instability, neuromuscular aberrations, and/or GI symptoms, have been reported during combination use of selective serotonin reuptake inhibitors and triptans. If concomitant treatment with naratriptan and an SSRI is clinically warranted, careful observation of the patient is advised, particularly during treatment initiation and dose increases).
No products indexed under this heading.

Sumatriptan (Co-administration with other 5-HT1 agonists within 24 hours of each other is contraindicated because of the vasospastic effects may be additive). Products include:
Imitrex Nasal	1503

Sumatriptan Succinate (Co-administration with other 5-HT1 agonists within 24 hours of each other is contraindicated because of the vasospastic effects may be additive).
Products include:
Imitrex	1497
Imitrex Tablets	1508
Treximet	1681

Venlafaxine Hydrochloride (Cases of life-threatening serotonin syndrome, including mental status changes, autonomic instability, neuromuscular aberrations, and/or GI symptoms, have been reported during combination use of serotonin and norepinephrine reuptake inhibitors and triptans. If concomitant treatment with naratriptan and an SNRI is clinically warranted, careful observation of the patient is advised, particularly during treatment initiation and dose increases). Products include:
Effexor XR	3504
Venlafaxine Hydrochloride Tablets	2388

Zolmitriptan (Co-administration with other 5-HT1 agonists within 24 hours of each other is contraindicated because of the vasospastic effects may be additive). Products include:
Zomig Tablets	773
Zomig Nasal Spray	768
Zomig-ZMT Tablets	773

AMEVIVE
(Alefacept) 665
None cited in PDR database.

AMINOHIPPURATE SODIUM "PAH" INJECTION
(Aminohippurate Sodium) 2084
May interact with sulfonamides, and certain other agents. Compounds in these categories include:

Bendroflumethiazide (Co-administration with sulfonamides interfere with chemical color development essential to the analytical procedures).
No products indexed under this heading.

Chlorothiazide (Co-administration with sulfonamides interfere with chemical color development essential to the analytical procedures).
No products indexed under this heading.

Chlorothiazide Sodium (Co-administration with sulfonamides inter-

fere with chemical color development essential to the analytical procedures).
Products include:
Diuril Intravenous	2009

Chlorpropamide (Co-administration with sulfonamides interfere with chemical color development essential to the analytical procedures).
No products indexed under this heading.

Glipizide (Co-administration with sulfonamides interfere with chemical color development essential to the analytical procedures).
No products indexed under this heading.

Glyburide (Co-administration with sulfonamides interfere with chemical color development essential to the analytical procedures).
No products indexed under this heading.

Hydrochlorothiazide (Co-administration with sulfonamides interfere with chemical color development essential to the analytical procedures).
Products include:
Atacand HCT	700
Avalide	2956
Benicar HCT	1017
Diovan HCT	2419
Dyazide	1429
Exforge HCT	2449
Hyzaar	2162
Hyzaar 100-12.5	2162
Micardis HCT	889
Prinzide	2246
Tekturna HCT	2541
Teveten HCT	541

Hydroflumethiazide (Co-administration with sulfonamides interfere with chemical color development essential to the analytical procedures).
No products indexed under this heading.

Methyclothiazide (Co-administration with sulfonamides interfere with chemical color development essential to the analytical procedures).
No products indexed under this heading.

Polythiazide (Co-administration with sulfonamides interfere with chemical color development essential to the analytical procedures).
No products indexed under this heading.

Probenecid (Tubular secretion of PAH depressed).
No products indexed under this heading.

Procaine Hydrochloride (Renal clearance measurements impaired).
No products indexed under this heading.

Sulfacytine (Co-administration with sulfonamides interfere with chemical color development essential to the analytical procedures).
No products indexed under this heading.

Sulfamethizole (Co-administration with sulfonamides interfere with chemical color development essential to the analytical procedures).
No products indexed under this heading.

Sulfamethoxazole (Co-administration with sulfonamides interfere with chemical color development essential to the analytical procedures).
No products indexed under this heading.

Sulfasalazine (Co-administration with sulfonamides interfere with chemical color development essential to the analytical procedures).
No products indexed under this heading.

Sulfinpyrazone (Co-administration with sulfonamides interfere with chemical color development essential to the analytical procedures).
No products indexed under this heading.

Sulfisoxazole Acetyl (Co-administration with sulfonamides interfere with chemical color development essential to the analytical procedures).
No products indexed under this heading.

Sulfisoxazole Diolamine (Co-administration with sulfonamides interfere with chemical color development essential to the analytical procedures).
No products indexed under this heading.

Tolazamide (Co-administration with sulfonamides interfere with chemical color development essential to the analytical procedures).
No products indexed under this heading.

Tolbutamide (Co-administration with sulfonamides interfere with chemical color development essential to the analytical procedures).
No products indexed under this heading.

AMITIZA CAPSULES

(Lubiprostone) 3351
None cited in PDR database.

AMOXIL CAPSULES

(Amoxicillin) 1311
See Amoxil Tablets

AMOXIL CHEWABLE TABLETS

(Amoxicillin) 1311
See Amoxil Tablets

AMOXIL PEDIATRIC DROPS FOR ORAL SUSPENSION

(Amoxicillin) 1311
See Amoxil Tablets

AMOXIL POWDER FOR ORAL SUSPENSION

(Amoxicillin) 1311
See Amoxil Tablets

AMOXIL TABLETS

(Amoxicillin) 1311
May interact with macrolide antibiotics, oral anticoagulants, oral contraceptives, sulfonamides, tetracyclines, and certain other agents. Compounds in these categories include:

Anisindione (Abnormal prolongation of prothrombin time (increased international normalized ratio [INR]) has been reported rarely in patients receiving amoxicillin and oral anticoagulants. Appropriate monitoring should be undertaken when anticoagulants are prescribed concurrently. Adjustments in the dose of oral anticoagulants may be necessary to maintain the desired level of anticoagulation).
No products indexed under this heading.

Azithromycin Dihydrate (Macrolides may interfere with the bactericidal effects of penicillin. This has been demonstrated *in vitro*; however, the clinical significance of this interaction is not well documented).
No products indexed under this heading.

Bendroflumethiazide (Sulfonamides may interfere with the bactericidal effects of penicillin. This has been demonstrated *in vitro*; however, the clinical significance of this interaction is not well documented).
No products indexed under this heading.

Chloramphenicol (Chloramphenicol may interfere with the bactericidal effects of penicillin. This has been demonstrated *in vitro*; however, the clinical significance of this interaction is not well documented).
No products indexed under this heading.

Chloramphenicol Palmitate (Chloramphenicol may interfere with the bactericidal effects of penicillin. This has been demonstrated *in vitro*; however, the clinical significance of this interaction is not well documented).
No products indexed under this heading.

Chloramphenicol Sodium Succinate (Chloramphenicol may interfere with the bactericidal effects of penicillin. This has been demonstrated *in vitro*; however, the clinical significance of this interaction is not well documented).
No products indexed under this heading.

Chlorothiazide (Sulfonamides may interfere with the bactericidal effects of penicillin. This has been demonstrated *in vitro*; however, the clinical significance of this interaction is not well documented).
No products indexed under this heading.

Chlorothiazide Sodium (Sulfonamides may interfere with the bactericidal effects of penicillin. This has been demonstrated *in vitro*; however, the clinical significance of this interaction is not well documented). Products include:
Diuril Intravenous 2009

Chlorpropamide (Sulfonamides may interfere with the bactericidal effects of penicillin. This has been demonstrated *in vitro*; however, the clinical significance of this interaction is not well documented).
No products indexed under this heading.

Clarithromycin (Macrolides may interfere with the bactericidal effects of penicillin. This has been demonstrated *in vitro*; however, the clinical significance of this interaction is not well documented). Products include:
Biaxin/Biaxin XL 412

Demeclocycline Hydrochloride (Tetracyclines may interfere with the bactericidal effects of penicillin. This has been demonstrated *in vitro*; however, the clinical significance of this interaction is not well documented).
No products indexed under this heading.

Desogestrel (In common with other antibiotics, amoxicillin may affect the gut flora, leading to lower estrogen reabsorption and reduced efficacy of combined oral estrogen/progesterone contraceptives).
No products indexed under this heading.

Dicumarol (Abnormal prolongation of prothrombin time (increased international normalized ratio [INR]) has been reported rarely in patients receiving amoxicillin and oral anticoagulants. Appropriate monitoring should be undertaken when anticoagulants are prescribed concurrently. Adjustments in the dose of oral anticoagulants may be necessary to maintain the desired level of anticoagulation).
No products indexed under this heading.

Dirithromycin (Macrolides may interfere with the bactericidal effects of penicillin. This has been demonstrated *in vitro*; however, the clinical significance of this interaction is not well documented).
No products indexed under this heading.

Doxycycline (Tetracyclines may interfere with the bactericidal effects of penicillin. This has been demonstrated *in vitro*; however, the clinical significance of this interaction is not well documented).
No products indexed under this heading.

Doxycycline Calcium (Tetracyclines may interfere with the bactericidal effects of penicillin. This has been demonstrated *in vitro*; however, the clinical significance of this interaction is not well documented).
No products indexed under this heading.

Doxycycline Hyclate (Tetracyclines may interfere with the bactericidal effects of penicillin. This has been demonstrated *in vitro*; however, the clinical significance of this interaction is not well documented).
No products indexed under this heading.

Doxycycline Monohydrate (Tetracyclines may interfere with the bactericidal effects of penicillin. This has been demonstrated *in vitro*; however, the clinical significance of this interaction is not well documented).
No products indexed under this heading.

Erythromycin (Macrolides may interfere with the bactericidal effects of penicillin. This has been demonstrated *in vitro*; however, the clinical significance of this interaction is not well documented).
No products indexed under this heading.

Erythromycin Estolate (Macrolides may interfere with the bactericidal effects of penicillin. This has been demonstrated *in vitro*; however, the clinical significance of this interaction is not well documented).
No products indexed under this heading.

Erythromycin Ethylsuccinate (Macrolides may interfere with the bactericidal effects of penicillin. This has been demonstrated *in vitro*; however, the clinical significance of this interaction is not well documented). Products include:
E.E.S. 437
EryPed 435

Erythromycin Gluceptate (Macrolides may interfere with the bactericidal effects of penicillin. This has been demonstrated *in vitro*; however, the clinical significance of this interaction is not well documented).
No products indexed under this heading.

Erythromycin Stearate (Macrolides may interfere with the bactericidal effects of penicillin. This has been demonstrated *in vitro*; however, the clinical significance of this interaction is not well documented).
No products indexed under this heading.

Ethinyl Estradiol (In common with other antibiotics, amoxicillin may affect the gut flora, leading to lower estrogen reabsorption and reduced efficacy of combined oral estrogen/progesterone contraceptives). Products include:
LoSeasonique 3407
Lybrel 3514
NuvaRing 3181
Ortho Evra 2648
Ortho-Cyclen/Ortho Tri-Cyclen 2663
Ortho Tri-Cyclen Lo Tablets 2673
Seasonique 3418
Yaz 864

Ethynodiol Diacetate (In common with other antibiotics, amoxicillin may affect the gut flora, leading to lower estrogen reabsorption and reduced efficacy of combined oral estrogen/progesterone contraceptives).
No products indexed under this heading.

Glipizide (Sulfonamides may interfere with the bactericidal effects of penicillin. This has been demonstrated *in vitro*; however, the clinical significance of this interaction is not well documented).
No products indexed under this heading.

Glyburide (Sulfonamides may interfere with the bactericidal effects of penicillin. This has been demonstrated *in vitro*; however, the clinical significance of this interaction is not well documented).
No products indexed under this heading.

Hydrochlorothiazide (Sulfonamides may interfere with the bactericidal effects of penicillin. This has been demonstrated *in vitro*; however, the clinical significance of this interaction is not well documented). Products include:
Atacand HCT 700
Avalide 2956
Benicar HCT 1017
Diovan HCT 2419
Dyazide 1429
Exforge HCT 2449
Hyzaar 2162
Hyzaar 100-12.5 2162
Micardis HCT 889
Prinzide 2246
Tekturna HCT 2541
Teveten HCT 541

Hydroflumethiazide (Sulfonamides may interfere with the bactericidal effects of penicillin. This has been demonstrated *in vitro*; however, the clinical significance of this interaction is not well documented).
No products indexed under this heading.

Levonorgestrel (In common with other antibiotics, amoxicillin may affect the gut flora, leading to lower estrogen reabsorption and reduced efficacy of combined oral estrogen/progesterone contraceptives). Products include:
Climara Pro 847
LoSeasonique 3407
Lybrel 3514
Mirena 854
Plan B 3416
Seasonique 3418

Mestranol (In common with other antibiotics, amoxicillin may affect the gut flora, leading to lower estrogen reabsorption and reduced efficacy of combined oral estrogen/progesterone contraceptives).
No products indexed under this heading.

Methacycline Hydrochloride (Tetracyclines may interfere with the bactericidal effects of penicillin. This has been demonstrated *in vitro*; however, the clinical significance of this interaction is not well documented).
No products indexed under this heading.

Methyclothiazide (Sulfonamides may interfere with the bactericidal effects of penicillin. This has been demonstrated *in vitro*; however, the clinical significance of this interaction is not well documented).
No products indexed under this heading.

Minocycline Hydrochloride (Tetracyclines may interfere with the bactericidal effects of penicillin. This has been demonstrated *in vitro*; however, the clinical significance of this interaction is not well documented). Products include:
Solodyn 2073

Norethindrone (In common with other antibiotics, amoxicillin may affect the gut flora, leading to lower estrogen reabsorption and reduced efficacy of combined oral estrogen/progesterone contraceptives). Products include:
Ortho Micronor 2660

Norethynodrel (In common with other antibiotics, amoxicillin may affect the gut flora, leading to lower estrogen reabsorption and reduced efficacy of combined oral estrogen/progesterone contraceptives).
No products indexed under this heading.

Norgestimate (In common with other antibiotics, amoxicillin may affect the gut flora, leading to lower estrogen reabsorption and reduced efficacy of combined oral estrogen/progesterone contraceptives). Products include:
Ortho-Cyclen/Ortho Tri-Cyclen 2663
Ortho Tri-Cyclen Lo Tablets 2673

Norgestrel (In common with other antibiotics, amoxicillin may affect the gut flora, leading to lower estrogen reabsorption and reduced efficacy of combined oral estrogen/progesterone contraceptives).
No products indexed under this heading.

Oxytetracycline (Tetracyclines may interfere with the bactericidal effects of penicillin. This has been demonstrated *in vitro*; however, the clinical significance of this interaction is not well documented).
No products indexed under this heading.

107 Interactions Index Amrix

Oxytetracycline Hydrochloride (Tetracyclines may interfere with the bactericidal effects of penicillin. This has been demonstrated *in vitro*; however, the clinical significance of this interaction is not well documented).
No products indexed under this heading.

Polythiazide (Sulfonamides may interfere with the bactericidal effects of penicillin. This has been demonstrated *in vitro*; however, the clinical significance of this interaction is not well documented).
No products indexed under this heading.

Probenecid (Probenecid decreases the renal tubular secretion of amoxicillin. Concurrent of amoxicillin and probenecid may result in increased and prolonged blood levels of amoxicillin).
No products indexed under this heading.

Sulfacytine (Sulfonamides may interfere with the bactericidal effects of penicillin. This has been demonstrated *in vitro*; however, the clinical significance of this interaction is not well documented).
No products indexed under this heading.

Sulfamethizole (Sulfonamides may interfere with the bactericidal effects of penicillin. This has been demonstrated *in vitro*; however, the clinical significance of this interaction is not well documented).
No products indexed under this heading.

Sulfamethoxazole (May interfere with bactericidal effects of penicillin. This has been demonstrated *in vitro*; however, the clinical significance of the interaction is not well documented).
No products indexed under this heading.

Sulfasalazine (Sulfonamides may interfere with the bactericidal effects of penicillin. This has been demonstrated *in vitro*; however, the clinical significance of this interaction is not well documented).
No products indexed under this heading.

Sulfinpyrazone (Sulfonamides may interfere with the bactericidal effects of penicillin. This has been demonstrated *in vitro*; however, the clinical significance of this interaction is not well documented).
No products indexed under this heading.

Sulfisoxazole Acetyl (May interfere with bactericidal effects of penicillin. This has been demonstrated *in vitro*; however, the clinical significance of the interaction is not well documented).
No products indexed under this heading.

Sulfisoxazole Diolamine (Sulfonamides may interfere with the bactericidal effects of penicillin. This has been demonstrated *in vitro*; however, the clinical significance of this interaction is not well documented).
No products indexed under this heading.

Tetracycline Hydrochloride (Tetracyclines may interfere with the bactericidal effects of penicillin. This has been demonstrated *in vitro*; however, the clinical significance of this interaction is not well documented). Products include:
Pylera 793

Tetracycline Phosphate Complex (Tetracyclines may interfere with the bactericidal effects of penicillin. This has been demonstrated *in vitro*; however, the clinical significance of this interaction is not well documented).
No products indexed under this heading.

Tolazamide (Sulfonamides may interfere with the bactericidal effects of penicillin. This has been demonstrated *in vitro*; however, the clinical significance of this interaction is not well documented).
No products indexed under this heading.

Tolbutamide (Sulfonamides may interfere with the bactericidal effects of penicillin. This has been demonstrated *in vitro*; however, the clinical significance of this interaction is not well documented).
No products indexed under this heading.

Troleandomycin (Macrolides may interfere with the bactericidal effects of penicillin. This has been demonstrated *in vitro*; however, the clinical significance of this interaction is not well documented).
No products indexed under this heading.

Warfarin Sodium (Abnormal prolongation of prothrombin time (increased international normalized ratio [INR]) has been reported rarely in patients receiving amoxicillin and oral anticoagulants. Appropriate monitoring should be undertaken when anticoagulants are prescribed concurrently. Adjustments in the dose of oral anticoagulants may be necessary to maintain the desired level of anticoagulation).
No products indexed under this heading.

AMRIX CAPSULES

(Cyclobenzaprine Hydrochloride) 964
May interact with alcohols, barbiturates, central nervous system depressants, monoamine oxidase inhibitors, and certain other agents. Compounds in these categories include:

Alfentanil Hydrochloride (Concomitant use with cyclobenzaprine HCl may enhance the effects of CNS depressants).
No products indexed under this heading.

Alprazolam (Concomitant use with cyclobenzaprine HCl may enhance the effects of CNS depressants).
No products indexed under this heading.

Amobarbital (Concomitant use with cyclobenzaprine HCl may enhance the effects of barbiturates).
No products indexed under this heading.

Amobarbital Sodium (Concomitant use with cyclobenzaprine HCl may enhance the effects of barbiturates).
No products indexed under this heading.

Aprobarbital (Concomitant use with cyclobenzaprine HCl may enhance the effects of barbiturates).
No products indexed under this heading.

Buprenorphine Hydrochloride (Concomitant use with cyclobenzaprine HCl may enhance the effects of CNS depressants).
No products indexed under this heading.

Buspirone Hydrochloride (Concomitant use with cyclobenzaprine HCl may enhance the effects of CNS depressants).
No products indexed under this heading.

Butabarbital (Concomitant use with cyclobenzaprine HCl may enhance the effects of barbiturates).
No products indexed under this heading.

Butabarbital Sodium (Concomitant use with cyclobenzaprine HCl may enhance the effects of barbiturates).
No products indexed under this heading.

Butalbital (Concomitant use with cyclobenzaprine HCl may enhance the effects of barbiturates).
No products indexed under this heading.

Chlordiazepoxide (Concomitant use with cyclobenzaprine HCl may enhance the effects of CNS depressants).
No products indexed under this heading.

Chlordiazepoxide Hydrochloride (Concomitant use with cyclobenzaprine HCl may enhance the effects of CNS depressants).
No products indexed under this heading.

Chlorpromazine (Concomitant use with cyclobenzaprine HCl may enhance the effects of CNS depressants).
No products indexed under this heading.

Chlorpromazine Hydrochloride (Concomitant use with cyclobenzaprine HCl may enhance the effects of CNS depressants).
No products indexed under this heading.

Chlorprothixene (Concomitant use with cyclobenzaprine HCl may enhance the effects of CNS depressants).
No products indexed under this heading.

Chlorprothixene Hydrochloride (Concomitant use with cyclobenzaprine HCl may enhance the effects of CNS depressants).
No products indexed under this heading.

Chlorprothixene Lactate (Concomitant use with cyclobenzaprine HCl may enhance the effects of CNS depressants).
No products indexed under this heading.

Clonazepam (Concomitant use with cyclobenzaprine HCl may enhance the effects of CNS depressants). Products include:
Klonopin 2855

Clorazepate Dipotassium (Concomitant use with cyclobenzaprine HCl may enhance the effects of CNS depressants).
No products indexed under this heading.

Clozapine (Concomitant use with cyclobenzaprine HCl may enhance the effects of CNS depressants).
No products indexed under this heading.

Codeine Phosphate (Concomitant use with cyclobenzaprine HCl may enhance the effects of CNS depressants). Products include:
Tylenol with Codeine 2691

Codeine Sulfate (Concomitant use with cyclobenzaprine HCl may enhance the effects of CNS depressants).
No products indexed under this heading.

Desflurane (Concomitant use with cyclobenzaprine HCl may enhance the effects of CNS depressants).
No products indexed under this heading.

Dezocine (Concomitant use with cyclobenzaprine HCl may enhance the effects of CNS depressants).
No products indexed under this heading.

Diazepam (Concomitant use with cyclobenzaprine HCl may enhance the effects of CNS depressants). Products include:
Valium Tablets 2880

Droperidol (Concomitant use with cyclobenzaprine HCl may enhance the effects of CNS depressants).
No products indexed under this heading.

Enflurane (Concomitant use with cyclobenzaprine HCl may enhance the effects of CNS depressants).
No products indexed under this heading.

Estazolam (Concomitant use with cyclobenzaprine HCl may enhance the effects of CNS depressants).
No products indexed under this heading.

Ethanol (Concomitant use with cyclobenzaprine HCl may enhance the effects of CNS depressants).
No products indexed under this heading.

Ethchlorvynol (Concomitant use with cyclobenzaprine HCl may enhance the effects of CNS depressants).
No products indexed under this heading.

Ethinamate (Concomitant use with cyclobenzaprine HCl may enhance the effects of CNS depressants).
No products indexed under this heading.

Ethyl Alcohol (Concomitant use with cyclobenzaprine HCl may enhance the effects of CNS depressants).
No products indexed under this heading.

Fentanyl (Concomitant use with cyclobenzaprine HCl may enhance the effects of CNS depressants). Products include:
Duragesic 2604
Fentanyl Transdermal System 2346
Onsolis 2054

Fentanyl Citrate (Concomitant use with cyclobenzaprine HCl may enhance the effects of CNS depressants). Products include:
Fentora 966

Fluphenazine Decanoate (Concomitant use with cyclobenzaprine HCl may enhance the effects of CNS depressants).
No products indexed under this heading.

Fluphenazine Enanthate (Concomitant use with cyclobenzaprine HCl may enhance the effects of CNS depressants).
No products indexed under this heading.

Fluphenazine Hydrochloride (Concomitant use with cyclobenzaprine HCl may enhance the effects of CNS depressants).
No products indexed under this heading.

Flurazepam Hydrochloride (Concomitant use with cyclobenzaprine HCl may enhance the effects of CNS depressants).
No products indexed under this heading.

Glutethimide (Concomitant use with cyclobenzaprine HCl may enhance the effects of CNS depressants).
No products indexed under this heading.

Guanethidine (Tricyclic antidepressants may block the antihypertensive action of guanethidine and similarly acting compounds).
No products indexed under this heading.

Halazepam (Concomitant use with cyclobenzaprine HCl may enhance the effects of CNS depressants).
No products indexed under this heading.

Haloperidol (Concomitant use with cyclobenzaprine HCl may enhance the effects of CNS depressants).
No products indexed under this heading.

Haloperidol Decanoate (Concomitant use with cyclobenzaprine HCl may enhance the effects of CNS depressants).
No products indexed under this heading.

Haloperidol Lactate (Concomitant use with cyclobenzaprine HCl may enhance the effects of CNS depressants).
No products indexed under this heading.

Hexobarbital (Concomitant use with cyclobenzaprine HCl may enhance the effects of barbiturates).
No products indexed under this heading.

Hydrocodone Bitartrate (Concomitant use with cyclobenzaprine HCl may enhance the effects of CNS depressants). Products include:
Vicodin 560
Vicodin ES 561
Vicodin HP 563
Vicoprofen 564
Zydone 1138

Hydrocodone Polistirex (Concomitant use with cyclobenzaprine HCl may enhance the effects of CNS depressants). Products include:
Tussionex 3443

Hydromorphone (Concomitant use with cyclobenzaprine HCl may enhance the effects of CNS depressants).
No products indexed under this heading.

Hydromorphone Hydrochloride (Concomitant use with cyclobenzaprine HCl may enhance the effects of CNS depressants). Products include:
Dilaudid Injection 2800
Dilaudid Oral 2797
Dilaudid Tablets 2797
Dilaudid-HP 2800

IMPORTANT NOTE: Always consult each drug listing in the patient's regimen for possible interactions.

Amrix Interactions Index 108

Hydroxyzine Hydrochloride (Concomitant use with cyclobenzaprine HCl may enhance the effects of CNS depressants).
No products indexed under this heading.

Isocarboxazid (Cyclobenzaprine HCl may have life-threatening interactions with MAO inhibitors. Concomitant use of monoamine oxidase (MAO) inhibitors or within 14 days after their discontinuation is contraindicated). Products include:
Marplan 3481

Isoflurane (Concomitant use with cyclobenzaprine HCl may enhance the effects of CNS depressants).
No products indexed under this heading.

Ketamine Hydrochloride (Concomitant use with cyclobenzaprine HCl may enhance the effects of CNS depressants).
No products indexed under this heading.

Levomethadyl Acetate Hydrochloride (Concomitant use with cyclobenzaprine HCl may enhance the effects of CNS depressants).
No products indexed under this heading.

Levorphanol Tartrate (Concomitant use with cyclobenzaprine HCl may enhance the effects of CNS depressants).
No products indexed under this heading.

Lorazepam (Concomitant use with cyclobenzaprine HCl may enhance the effects of CNS depressants).
No products indexed under this heading.

Loxapine Hydrochloride (Concomitant use with cyclobenzaprine HCl may enhance the effects of CNS depressants).
No products indexed under this heading.

Loxapine Succinate (Concomitant use with cyclobenzaprine HCl may enhance the effects of CNS depressants).
No products indexed under this heading.

Meperidine Hydrochloride (Concomitant use with cyclobenzaprine HCl may enhance the effects of CNS depressants).
No products indexed under this heading.

Mephobarbital (Concomitant use with cyclobenzaprine HCl may enhance the effects of barbiturates).
No products indexed under this heading.

Meprobamate (Concomitant use with cyclobenzaprine HCl may enhance the effects of CNS depressants).
No products indexed under this heading.

Mesoridazine Besylate (Concomitant use with cyclobenzaprine HCl may enhance the effects of CNS depressants).
No products indexed under this heading.

Methadone Hydrochloride (Concomitant use with cyclobenzaprine HCl may enhance the effects of CNS depressants).
No products indexed under this heading.

Methohexital Sodium (Concomitant use with cyclobenzaprine HCl may enhance the effects of CNS depressants).
No products indexed under this heading.

Methotrimeprazine (Concomitant use with cyclobenzaprine HCl may enhance the effects of CNS depressants).
No products indexed under this heading.

Methoxyflurane (Concomitant use with cyclobenzaprine HCl may enhance the effects of CNS depressants).
No products indexed under this heading.

Midazolam Hydrochloride (Concomitant use with cyclobenzaprine HCl may enhance the effects of CNS depressants).
No products indexed under this heading.

Moclobemide (Cyclobenzaprine HCl may have life-threatening interactions with MAO inhibitors. Concomitant use of monoamine oxidase (MAO) inhibitors or within 14 days after their discontinuation is contraindicated).
No products indexed under this heading.

Molindone Hydrochloride (Concomitant use with cyclobenzaprine HCl may enhance the effects of CNS depressants). Products include:
Moban 1108

Morphine Sulfate (Concomitant use with cyclobenzaprine HCl may enhance the effects of CNS depressants). Products include:
Avinza 1822
Embeda 1831
MS Contin 2803

Morphine Sulfate, Liposomal (Concomitant use with cyclobenzaprine HCl may enhance the effects of CNS depressants).
No products indexed under this heading.

Olanzapine (Concomitant use with cyclobenzaprine HCl may enhance the effects of CNS depressants). Products include:
Symbyax 1965
Zyprexa 1984
Zyprexa IntraMuscular 1984
Zyprexa ZYDIS 1984

Oxazepam (Concomitant use with cyclobenzaprine HCl may enhance the effects of CNS depressants).
No products indexed under this heading.

Oxycodone Hydrochloride (Concomitant use with cyclobenzaprine HCl may enhance the effects of CNS depressants). Products include:
OxyContin 2807
Percocet 1121
Percodan 1124

Oxycodone Terephthalate (Concomitant use with cyclobenzaprine HCl may enhance the effects of CNS depressants).
No products indexed under this heading.

Oxymorphone Hydrochloride (Concomitant use with cyclobenzaprine HCl may enhance the effects of CNS depressants). Products include:
Opana 1110
Opana ER 1114

Pargyline Hydrochloride (Cyclobenzaprine HCl may have life-threatening interactions with MAO inhibitors. Concomitant use of monoamine oxidase (MAO) inhibitors or within 14 days after their discontinuation is contraindicated).
No products indexed under this heading.

Pentobarbital (Concomitant use with cyclobenzaprine HCl may enhance the effects of barbiturates).
No products indexed under this heading.

Pentobarbital Sodium (Concomitant use with cyclobenzaprine HCl may enhance the effects of barbiturates). Products include:
Nembutal 2012

Perphenazine (Concomitant use with cyclobenzaprine HCl may enhance the effects of CNS depressants).
No products indexed under this heading.

Phenelzine Sulfate (Cyclobenzaprine HCl may have life-threatening interactions with MAO inhibitors. Concomitant use of monoamine oxidase (MAO) inhibitors or within 14 days after their discontinuation is contraindicated).
No products indexed under this heading.

Phenobarbital (Concomitant use with cyclobenzaprine HCl may enhance the effects of barbiturates). Products include:
Donnatal 2711

Phenobarbital Sodium (Concomitant use with cyclobenzaprine HCl may enhance the effects of barbiturates).
No products indexed under this heading.

Prazepam (Concomitant use with cyclobenzaprine HCl may enhance the effects of CNS depressants).
No products indexed under this heading.

Procarbazine Hydrochloride (Cyclobenzaprine HCl may have life-threatening interactions with MAO inhibitors. Concomitant use of monoamine oxidase (MAO) inhibitors or within 14 days after their discontinuation is contraindicated).
No products indexed under this heading.

Prochlorperazine (Concomitant use with cyclobenzaprine HCl may enhance the effects of CNS depressants).
No products indexed under this heading.

Prochlorperazine Edisylate (Concomitant use with cyclobenzaprine HCl may enhance the effects of CNS depressants).
No products indexed under this heading.

Prochlorperazine Maleate (Concomitant use with cyclobenzaprine HCl may enhance the effects of CNS depressants).
No products indexed under this heading.

Promethazine (Concomitant use with cyclobenzaprine HCl may enhance the effects of CNS depressants).
No products indexed under this heading.

Promethazine Hydrochloride (Concomitant use with cyclobenzaprine HCl may enhance the effects of CNS depressants).
No products indexed under this heading.

Propofol (Concomitant use with cyclobenzaprine HCl may enhance the effects of CNS depressants).
No products indexed under this heading.

Propoxyphene Hydrochloride (Concomitant use with cyclobenzaprine HCl may enhance the effects of CNS depressants).
No products indexed under this heading.

Propoxyphene Napsylate (Concomitant use with cyclobenzaprine HCl may enhance the effects of CNS depressants).
No products indexed under this heading.

Quazepam (Concomitant use with cyclobenzaprine HCl may enhance the effects of CNS depressants).
No products indexed under this heading.

Quetiapine Fumarate (Concomitant use with cyclobenzaprine HCl may enhance the effects of CNS depressants). Products include:
Seroquel 750
Seroquel XR 759

Rasagiline Mesylate (Cyclobenzaprine HCl may have life-threatening interactions with MAO inhibitors. Concomitant use of monoamine oxidase (MAO) inhibitors or within 14 days after their discontinuation is contraindicated). Products include:
Azilect 3383

Remifentanil Hydrochloride (Concomitant use with cyclobenzaprine HCl may enhance the effects of CNS depressants).
No products indexed under this heading.

Risperidone (Concomitant use with cyclobenzaprine HCl may enhance the effects of CNS depressants). Products include:
Risperdal Consta 2682

Secobarbital Sodium (Concomitant use with cyclobenzaprine HCl may enhance the effects of barbiturates).
No products indexed under this heading.

Selegiline (Cyclobenzaprine HCl may have life-threatening interactions with MAO inhibitors. Concomitant use of monoamine oxidase (MAO) inhibitors or within 14 days after their discontinuation is contraindicated). Products include:
Emsam 3623

Selegiline Hydrochloride (Cyclobenzaprine HCl may have life-threatening interactions with MAO inhibitors. Concomitant use of monoamine oxidase (MAO) inhibitors or within 14 days after their discontinuation is contraindicated). Products include:
Eldepryl 3312

Sevoflurane (Concomitant use with cyclobenzaprine HCl may enhance the effects of CNS depressants). Products include:
Ultane 554

Sodium Butabarbital (Concomitant use with cyclobenzaprine HCl may enhance the effects of barbiturates).
No products indexed under this heading.

Sodium Oxybate (Concomitant use with cyclobenzaprine HCl may enhance the effects of CNS depressants).
No products indexed under this heading.

Sodium Pentobarbital (Concomitant use with cyclobenzaprine HCl may enhance the effects of barbiturates).
No products indexed under this heading.

Sufentanil Citrate (Concomitant use with cyclobenzaprine HCl may enhance the effects of CNS depressants).
No products indexed under this heading.

Talbutal (Concomitant use with cyclobenzaprine HCl may enhance the effects of CNS depressants).
No products indexed under this heading.

Temazepam (Concomitant use with cyclobenzaprine HCl may enhance the effects of CNS depressants).
No products indexed under this heading.

Thiamylal Sodium (Concomitant use with cyclobenzaprine HCl may enhance the effects of barbiturates).
No products indexed under this heading.

Thioridazine (Concomitant use with cyclobenzaprine HCl may enhance the effects of CNS depressants).
No products indexed under this heading.

Thioridazine Hydrochloride (Concomitant use with cyclobenzaprine HCl may enhance the effects of CNS depressants). Products include:
Thioridazine Hydrochloride 2384

Thiothixene (Concomitant use with cyclobenzaprine HCl may enhance the effects of CNS depressants). Products include:
Thiothixene 2386

Thiothixene Hydrochloride (Concomitant use with cyclobenzaprine HCl may enhance the effects of CNS depressants).
No products indexed under this heading.

Tramadol Hydrochloride (Tricyclic antidepressants may enhance the seizure risk in patients taking tramadol). Products include:
Ryzolt 2813
Ultram ER 2693

Tranylcypromine Sulfate (Cyclobenzaprine HCl may have life-threatening interactions with MAO inhibitors. Concomitant use of monoamine oxidase (MAO) inhibitors or within 14 days after their discontinuation is contraindicated). Products include:
Parnate 1584

Triazolam (Concomitant use with cyclobenzaprine HCl may enhance the effects of CNS depressants).
No products indexed under this heading.

Trifluoperazine Hydrochloride (Concomitant use with cyclobenzaprine HCl may enhance the effects of CNS depressants).
No products indexed under this heading.

Zaleplon (Concomitant use with cyclobenzaprine HCl may enhance the effects of CNS depressants).
No products indexed under this heading.

(⊙ Described in PDR® for Ophthalmic Medicines)

Ziprasidone Hydrochloride (Concomitant use with cyclobenzaprine HCl may enhance the effects of CNS depressants). Products include:
Geodon 2723

Zolpidem Tartrate (Concomitant use with cyclobenzaprine HCl may enhance the effects of CNS depressants). Products include:
Ambien 2920
Ambien CR 2925

Food Interactions

Alcohol (Concomitant use with cyclobenzaprine HCl may enhance the effects of CNS depressants).

Beer, reduced-alcohol (Concomitant use with cyclobenzaprine HCl may enhance the effects of alcohol).

Beer, unspecified (Concomitant use with cyclobenzaprine HCl may enhance the effects of alcohol).

Wine, Chianti (Concomitant use with cyclobenzaprine HCl may enhance the effects of alcohol).

Wine, Red (Concomitant use with cyclobenzaprine HCl may enhance the effects of alcohol).

Wine, unspecified (Concomitant use with cyclobenzaprine HCl may enhance the effects of alcohol).

Wine products (Concomitant use with cyclobenzaprine HCl may enhance the effects of alcohol).

ANAPROX TABLETS

(Naproxen Sodium) 2850
See EC-Naprosyn Delayed-Release Tablets

ANAPROX DS TABLETS

(Naproxen Sodium) 2850
See EC-Naprosyn Delayed-Release Tablets

ANDROGEL

(Testosterone) 3456
May interact with corticosteroids, insulin, oral anticoagulants, and certain other agents. Compounds in these categories include:

ACTH (The concurrent use of testosterone with ACTH or corticosteroids may result in increased fluid retention and should be monitored cautiously, particularly in patients with cardiac, renal, or hepatic disease).
No products indexed under this heading.

Alclometasone Dipropionate (The concurrent use of testosterone with ACTH or corticosteroids may result in increased fluid retention and should be monitored cautiously, particularly in patients with cardiac, renal, or hepatic disease).
No products indexed under this heading.

Anisindione (Changes in anticoagulant activity may be seen with androgens. More frequent monitoring of INR and prothrombin time are recommended in patients taking anticoagulants, especially at the initiation and termination of androgen therapy).
No products indexed under this heading.

Beclomethasone Dipropionate (The concurrent use of testosterone with ACTH or corticosteroids may result in increased fluid retention and should be monitored cautiously, particularly in patients with cardiac, renal, or hepatic disease). Products include:
Qvar 3398

Beclomethasone Dipropionate Monohydrate (The concurrent use of testosterone with ACTH or corticosteroids may result in increased fluid retention and should be monitored cautiously, particularly in patients with cardiac, renal, or hepatic disease). Products include:

Beconase AQ 1386

Betamethasone (The concurrent use of testosterone with ACTH or corticosteroids may result in increased fluid retention and should be monitored cautiously, particularly in patients with cardiac, renal, or hepatic disease).
No products indexed under this heading.

Betamethasone Acetate (The concurrent use of testosterone with ACTH or corticosteroids may result in increased fluid retention and should be monitored cautiously, particularly in patients with cardiac, renal, or hepatic disease).
No products indexed under this heading.

Betamethasone Benzoate (The concurrent use of testosterone with ACTH or corticosteroids may result in increased fluid retention and should be monitored cautiously, particularly in patients with cardiac, renal, or hepatic disease).
No products indexed under this heading.

Betamethasone Dipropionate (The concurrent use of testosterone with ACTH or corticosteroids may result in increased fluid retention and should be monitored cautiously, particularly in patients with cardiac, renal, or hepatic disease). Products include:
Diprolene Lotion 0.05% 3108
Diprolene Ointment 0.05% 3109
Diprolene AF Cream 0.05% 3107
Lotrisone 3163

Betamethasone Sodium Phosphate (The concurrent use of testosterone with ACTH or corticosteroids may result in increased fluid retention and should be monitored cautiously, particularly in patients with cardiac, renal, or hepatic disease).
No products indexed under this heading.

Betamethasone Valerate (The concurrent use of testosterone with ACTH or corticosteroids may result in increased fluid retention and should be monitored cautiously, particularly in patients with cardiac, renal, or hepatic disease). Products include:
Luxíq 3321

Budesonide (The concurrent use of testosterone with ACTH or corticosteroids may result in increased fluid retention and should be monitored cautiously, particularly in patients with cardiac, renal, or hepatic disease). Products include:
Pulmicort Flexhaler 714
Symbicort 80/4.5 720
Symbicort 160/4.5 720

Ciclesonide (The concurrent use of testosterone with ACTH or corticosteroids may result in increased fluid retention and should be monitored cautiously, particularly in patients with cardiac, renal, or hepatic disease).
No products indexed under this heading.

Cortisone Acetate (The concurrent use of testosterone with ACTH or corticosteroids may result in increased fluid retention and should be monitored cautiously, particularly in patients with cardiac, renal, or hepatic disease).
No products indexed under this heading.

Desoximetasone (The concurrent use of testosterone with ACTH or corticosteroids may result in increased fluid retention and should be monitored cautiously, particularly in patients with cardiac, renal, or hepatic disease).
No products indexed under this heading.

Dexamethasone (The concurrent use of testosterone with ACTH or corticosteroids may result in increased fluid retention and should be monitored cautiously, particularly in patients with cardiac, renal, or hepatic disease). Products include:
Ciprodex 583
Ozurdex .... ☉223

Tobramycin and Dexamethasone Ophthalmic Suspension .... ☉251

Dexamethasone Acetate (The concurrent use of testosterone with ACTH or corticosteroids may result in increased fluid retention and should be monitored cautiously, particularly in patients with cardiac, renal, or hepatic disease).
No products indexed under this heading.

Dexamethasone Phosphate (The concurrent use of testosterone with ACTH or corticosteroids may result in increased fluid retention and should be monitored cautiously, particularly in patients with cardiac, renal, or hepatic disease).
No products indexed under this heading.

Dexamethasone Sodium (The concurrent use of testosterone with ACTH or corticosteroids may result in increased fluid retention and should be monitored cautiously, particularly in patients with cardiac, renal, or hepatic disease).
No products indexed under this heading.

Dexamethasone Sodium Phosphate (The concurrent use of testosterone with ACTH or corticosteroids may result in increased fluid retention and should be monitored cautiously, particularly in patients with cardiac, renal, or hepatic disease).
No products indexed under this heading.

Dexamethasone Sodium Phosphate Injection (The concurrent use of testosterone with ACTH or corticosteroids may result in increased fluid retention and should be monitored cautiously, particularly in patients with cardiac, renal, or hepatic disease).
No products indexed under this heading.

Dicumarol (Changes in anticoagulant activity may be seen with androgens. More frequent monitoring of INR and prothrombin time are recommended in patients taking anticoagulants, especially at the initiation and termination of androgen therapy).
No products indexed under this heading.

Diflorasone Diacetate (The concurrent use of testosterone with ACTH or corticosteroids may result in increased fluid retention and should be monitored cautiously, particularly in patients with cardiac, renal, or hepatic disease).
No products indexed under this heading.

Fludrocortisone Acetate (The concurrent use of testosterone with ACTH or corticosteroids may result in increased fluid retention and should be monitored cautiously, particularly in patients with cardiac, renal, or hepatic disease).
No products indexed under this heading.

Flumethasone Pivalate (The concurrent use of testosterone with ACTH or corticosteroids may result in increased fluid retention and should be monitored cautiously, particularly in patients with cardiac, renal, or hepatic disease).
No products indexed under this heading.

Flunisolide Hemihydrate (The concurrent use of testosterone with ACTH or corticosteroids may result in increased fluid retention and should be monitored cautiously, particularly in patients with cardiac, renal, or hepatic disease).
No products indexed under this heading.

Fluticasone Furoate (The concurrent use of testosterone with ACTH or corticosteroids may result in increased fluid retention and should be monitored cautiously, particularly in patients with cardiac, renal, or hepatic disease). Products include:
Veramyst 1713

Fluticasone Propionate (The concurrent use of testosterone with ACTH or corticosteroids may result in increased

fluid retention and should be monitored cautiously, particularly in patients with cardiac, renal, or hepatic disease). Products include:
Advair 100/50 1275
Advair 250/50 1275
Advair 500/50 1275
Advair HFA 45/21 1288
Advair HFA 115/21 1288
Advair HFA 230/21 1288
Flonase 1459
Flovent Diskus 1463
Flovent HFA 1470

Hydrocortisone (The concurrent use of testosterone with ACTH or corticosteroids may result in increased fluid retention and should be monitored cautiously, particularly in patients with cardiac, renal, or hepatic disease).
No products indexed under this heading.

Hydrocortisone (Alcohol) (The concurrent use of testosterone with ACTH or corticosteroids may result in increased fluid retention and should be monitored cautiously, particularly in patients with cardiac, renal, or hepatic disease).
No products indexed under this heading.

Hydrocortisone Acetate (The concurrent use of testosterone with ACTH or corticosteroids may result in increased fluid retention and should be monitored cautiously, particularly in patients with cardiac, renal, or hepatic disease).
No products indexed under this heading.

Hydrocortisone Butyrate (The concurrent use of testosterone with ACTH or corticosteroids may result in increased fluid retention and should be monitored cautiously, particularly in patients with cardiac, renal, or hepatic disease).
No products indexed under this heading.

Hydrocortisone Cypionate (The concurrent use of testosterone with ACTH or corticosteroids may result in increased fluid retention and should be monitored cautiously, particularly in patients with cardiac, renal, or hepatic disease).
No products indexed under this heading.

Hydrocortisone Hemisuccinate (The concurrent use of testosterone with ACTH or corticosteroids may result in increased fluid retention and should be monitored cautiously, particularly in patients with cardiac, renal, or hepatic disease).
No products indexed under this heading.

Hydrocortisone Probutate (The concurrent use of testosterone with ACTH or corticosteroids may result in increased fluid retention and should be monitored cautiously, particularly in patients with cardiac, renal, or hepatic disease).
No products indexed under this heading.

Hydrocortisone Sodium Phosphate (The concurrent use of testosterone with ACTH or corticosteroids may result in increased fluid retention and should be monitored cautiously, particularly in patients with cardiac, renal, or hepatic disease).
No products indexed under this heading.

Hydrocortisone Sodium Succinate (The concurrent use of testosterone with ACTH or corticosteroids may result in increased fluid retention and should be monitored cautiously, particularly in patients with cardiac, renal, or hepatic disease).
No products indexed under this heading.

Hydrocortisone Valerate (The concurrent use of testosterone with ACTH or corticosteroids may result in increased fluid retention and should be monitored cautiously, particularly in patients with cardiac, renal, or hepatic disease).
No products indexed under this heading.

IMPORTANT NOTE: Always consult each drug listing in the patient's regimen for possible interactions.

Insulin (Changes in insulin sensitivity or glycemic control may occur in patients treated with androgens. In diabetic patients, the metabolic effects of androgens may decrease blood glucose and, therefore, insulin requirements).
No products indexed under this heading.

Insulin, Human, Zinc Suspension (Changes in insulin sensitivity or glycemic control may occur in patients treated with androgens. In diabetic patients, the metabolic effects of androgens may decrease blood glucose and, therefore, insulin requirements).
No products indexed under this heading.

Insulin, Human (rDNA origin) (Changes in insulin sensitivity or glycemic control may occur in patients treated with androgens. In diabetic patients, the metabolic effects of androgens may decrease blood glucose and, therefore, insulin requirements). Products include:
Exubera 2717

Insulin, Human NPH (Changes in insulin sensitivity or glycemic control may occur in patients treated with androgens. In diabetic patients, the metabolic effects of androgens may decrease blood glucose and, therefore, insulin requirements). Products include:
Humulin N Vial 1934

Insulin, Human Regular (Changes in insulin sensitivity or glycemic control may occur in patients treated with androgens. In diabetic patients, the metabolic effects of androgens may decrease blood glucose and, therefore, insulin requirements). Products include:
Humulin R 1937
Humulin R (U-500) 1939

Insulin, Human Regular and Human NPH Mixture (Changes in insulin sensitivity or glycemic control may occur in patients treated with androgens. In diabetic patients, the metabolic effects of androgens may decrease blood glucose and, therefore, insulin requirements). Products include:
Humulin 50/50 1930
Humulin 70/30 Vial 1931

Insulin, NPH (Changes in insulin sensitivity or glycemic control may occur in patients treated with androgens. In diabetic patients, the metabolic effects of androgens may decrease blood glucose and, therefore, insulin requirements).
No products indexed under this heading.

Insulin, Regular (Changes in insulin sensitivity or glycemic control may occur in patients treated with androgens. In diabetic patients, the metabolic effects of androgens may decrease blood glucose and, therefore, insulin requirements).
No products indexed under this heading.

Insulin, Regular and NPH mixture (Changes in insulin sensitivity or glycemic control may occur in patients treated with androgens. In diabetic patients, the metabolic effects of androgens may decrease blood glucose and, therefore, insulin requirements).
No products indexed under this heading.

Insulin, Zinc Crystals (Changes in insulin sensitivity or glycemic control may occur in patients treated with androgens. In diabetic patients, the metabolic effects of androgens may decrease blood glucose and, therefore, insulin requirements).
No products indexed under this heading.

Insulin, Zinc Suspension (Changes in insulin sensitivity or glycemic control may occur in patients treated with androgens. In diabetic patients, the metabolic effects of androgens may decrease blood glucose and, therefore, insulin requirements).
No products indexed under this heading.

Insulin Aspart (Changes in insulin sensitivity or glycemic control may occur in patients treated with androgens. In diabetic patients, the metabolic effects of androgens may decrease blood glucose and, therefore, insulin requirements).
No products indexed under this heading.

Insulin Aspart, Human (Changes in insulin sensitivity or glycemic control may occur in patients treated with androgens. In diabetic patients, the metabolic effects of androgens may decrease blood glucose and, therefore, insulin requirements). Products include:
NovoLog Mix 70/30 2581

Insulin Aspart, Human Regular (Changes in insulin sensitivity or glycemic control may occur in patients treated with androgens. In diabetic patients, the metabolic effects of androgens may decrease blood glucose and, therefore, insulin requirements). Products include:
NovoLog 2575

Insulin Aspart Protamine, Human (Changes in insulin sensitivity or glycemic control may occur in patients treated with androgens. In diabetic patients, the metabolic effects of androgens may decrease blood glucose and, therefore, insulin requirements). Products include:
NovoLog Mix 70/30 2581

Insulin Detemir (rDNA Origin) (Changes in insulin sensitivity or glycemic control may occur in patients treated with androgens. In diabetic patients, the metabolic effects of androgens may decrease blood glucose and, therefore, insulin requirements). Products include:
Levemir 2566

Insulin Glargine (Changes in insulin sensitivity or glycemic control may occur in patients treated with androgens. In diabetic patients, the metabolic effects of androgens may decrease blood glucose and, therefore, insulin requirements). Products include:
Lantus 2996

Insulin Glulisine (Changes in insulin sensitivity or glycemic control may occur in patients treated with androgens. In diabetic patients, the metabolic effects of androgens may decrease blood glucose and, therefore, insulin requirements). Products include:
Apidra 2937
Apidra SoloStar 2937

Insulin Lispro, Human (Changes in insulin sensitivity or glycemic control may occur in patients treated with androgens. In diabetic patients, the metabolic effects of androgens may decrease blood glucose and, therefore, insulin requirements). Products include:
Humalog 1910
Humalog Mix 1914
Humalog Mix75/25 1917

Insulin Lispro Protamine, Human (Changes in insulin sensitivity or glycemic control may occur in patients treated with androgens. In diabetic patients, the metabolic effects of androgens may decrease blood glucose and, therefore, insulin requirements). Products include:
Humalog Mix 1914
Humalog Mix75/25 1917

Methylprednisolone (The concurrent use of testosterone with ACTH or corticosteroids may result in increased fluid retention and should be monitored cautiously, particularly in patients with cardiac, renal, or hepatic disease).
No products indexed under this heading.

Methylprednisolone Acetate (The concurrent use of testosterone with ACTH or corticosteroids may result in increased fluid retention and should be monitored cautiously, particularly in patients with cardiac, renal, or hepatic disease).
No products indexed under this heading.

Methylprednisolone Sodium Succinate (The concurrent use of testosterone with ACTH or corticosteroids may result in increased fluid retention and should be monitored cautiously, particularly in patients with cardiac, renal, or hepatic disease).
No products indexed under this heading.

Mometasone Furoate (The concurrent use of testosterone with ACTH or corticosteroids may result in increased fluid retention and should be monitored cautiously, particularly in patients with cardiac, renal, or hepatic disease). Products include:
Asmanex 3058
Elocon Cream 3111
Elocon Lotion 3112
Elocon Ointment 3114

Mometasone Furoate Monohydrate (The concurrent use of testosterone with ACTH or corticosteroids may result in increased fluid retention and should be monitored cautiously, particularly in patients with cardiac, renal, or hepatic disease). Products include:
Nasonex 3166

Oxyphenbutazone (Co-administration of androgens and oxyphenbutazone may result in elevated serum levels of oxyphenbutazone).
No products indexed under this heading.

Prednisolone (The concurrent use of testosterone with ACTH or corticosteroids may result in increased fluid retention and should be monitored cautiously, particularly in patients with cardiac, renal, or hepatic disease).
No products indexed under this heading.

Prednisolone Acetate (The concurrent use of testosterone with ACTH or corticosteroids may result in increased fluid retention and should be monitored cautiously, particularly in patients with cardiac, renal, or hepatic disease). Products include:
Blephamide ....⊙212, ⊙214
Pred Forte ....⊙225
Pred Mild ....⊙230
Pred-G ....⊙226, ⊙227

Prednisolone Sodium Phosphate (The concurrent use of testosterone with ACTH or corticosteroids may result in increased fluid retention and should be monitored cautiously, particularly in patients with cardiac, renal, or hepatic disease).
No products indexed under this heading.

Prednisolone Tebutate (The concurrent use of testosterone with ACTH or corticosteroids may result in increased fluid retention and should be monitored cautiously, particularly in patients with cardiac, renal, or hepatic disease).
No products indexed under this heading.

Prednisone (The concurrent use of testosterone with ACTH or corticosteroids may result in increased fluid retention and should be monitored cautiously, particularly in patients with cardiac, renal, or hepatic disease).
No products indexed under this heading.

Prednisone sodium phosphate (The concurrent use of testosterone with ACTH or corticosteroids may result in increased fluid retention and should be monitored cautiously, particularly in patients with cardiac, renal, or hepatic disease).
No products indexed under this heading.

Propranolol Hydrochloride (Co-administration of injectable testosterone cypionate has resulted in an increased clearance of propranolol). Products include:
InnoPran XL 1517

Triamcinolone (The concurrent use of testosterone with ACTH or corticosteroids may result in increased fluid retention and should be monitored cautiously, particularly in patients with cardiac, renal, or hepatic disease).
No products indexed under this heading.

Triamcinolone Acetonide (The concurrent use of testosterone with ACTH or corticosteroids may result in increased fluid retention and should be monitored cautiously, particularly in patients with cardiac, renal, or hepatic disease). Products include:
Azmacort 408
Nasacort AQ 3019

Triamcinolone Diacetate (The concurrent use of testosterone with ACTH or corticosteroids may result in increased fluid retention and should be monitored cautiously, particularly in patients with cardiac, renal, or hepatic disease).
No products indexed under this heading.

Triamcinolone Hexacetonide (The concurrent use of testosterone with ACTH or corticosteroids may result in increased fluid retention and should be monitored cautiously, particularly in patients with cardiac, renal, or hepatic disease).
No products indexed under this heading.

Warfarin Sodium (Changes in anticoagulant activity may be seen with androgens. More frequent monitoring of INR and prothrombin time are recommended in patients taking anticoagulants, especially at the initiation and termination of androgen therapy).
No products indexed under this heading.

ANGELIQ TABLETS

(Drospirenone, Estradiol) 831
May interact with ACE inhibitors, angiotensin-II receptor antagonists, cytochrome p450 3a4 inducers (selected), cytochrome p450 3a4 inhibitors (selected), non-steroidal anti-inflammatory agents. Compounds in these categories include:

Acetazolamide (Inhibitors of CYP3A4 such as erythromycin, clarithromycin, ketoconazole, itraconazole, ritonavir and grapefruit juice may increase plasma concentrations of estrogens and may result in side effects).
No products indexed under this heading.

Acetazolamide Sodium (Inhibitors of CYP3A4 such as erythromycin, clarithromycin, ketoconazole, itraconazole, ritonavir and grapefruit juice may increase plasma concentrations of estrogens and may result in side effects).
No products indexed under this heading.

Allium sativum (Inducers of CYP3A4, such as St. John's Wort preparations (Hypericum perforatum), phenobarbital, carbamazepine, and rifampin, may reduce plasma concentrations of estrogens, possibly resulting in a decrease in therapeutic effects and/or changes in the uterine bleeding profile).
No products indexed under this heading.

Aminoglutethimide (Inducers of CYP3A4, such as St. John's Wort preparations (Hypericum perforatum), phenobarbital, carbamazepine, and rifampin, may reduce plasma concentrations of estrogens, possibly resulting in a decrease in therapeutic effects and/or changes in the uterine bleeding profile).
No products indexed under this heading.

Amiodarone Hydrochloride (Inhibitors of CYP3A4 such as erythromycin, clarithromycin, ketoconazole, itraconazole, ritonavir and grapefruit juice may increase plasma concentrations of estrogens and may result in side effects).
No products indexed under this heading.

Amprenavir (Inhibitors of CYP3A4 such as erythromycin, clarithromycin, ketoconazole, itraconazole, ritonavir and grapefruit juice may increase plasma concentrations of estrogens and may result in side effects).
No products indexed under this heading.

Anastrozole (Inhibitors of CYP3A4 such as erythromycin, clarithromycin, ketoconazole, itraconazole, ritonavir and grapefruit juice may increase plasma concentrations of estrogens and may result in side effects).
No products indexed under this heading.

Aprepitant (Inhibitors of CYP3A4 such as erythromycin, clarithromycin, ketoconazole, itraconazole, ritonavir and grapefruit juice may increase plasma concentrations of estrogens and may result in side effects). Products include:
Emend 2124

Atazanavir (Inhibitors of CYP3A4 such as erythromycin, clarithromycin, ketoconazole, itraconazole, ritonavir and grapefruit juice may increase plasma concentrations of estrogens and may result in side effects).
No products indexed under this heading.

Atazanavir Sulfate (Inhibitors of CYP3A4 such as erythromycin, clarithromycin, ketoconazole, itraconazole, ritonavir and grapefruit juice may increase plasma concentrations of estrogens and may result in side effects).
No products indexed under this heading.

Benazepril Hydrochloride (There is potential for an increase in serum potassium in women taking drospirenone with other drugs that may affect electrolytes).
No products indexed under this heading.

Betamethasone (Inducers of CYP3A4, such as St. John's Wort preparations (Hypericum perforatum), phenobarbital, carbamazepine, and rifampin, may reduce plasma concentrations of estrogens, possibly resulting in a decrease in therapeutic effects and/or changes in the uterine bleeding profile).
No products indexed under this heading.

Betamethasone Acetate (Inducers of CYP3A4, such as St. John's Wort preparations (Hypericum perforatum), phenobarbital, carbamazepine, and rifampin, may reduce plasma concentrations of estrogens, possibly resulting in a decrease in therapeutic effects and/or changes in the uterine bleeding profile).
No products indexed under this heading.

Betamethasone Benzoate (Inducers of CYP3A4, such as St. John's Wort preparations (Hypericum perforatum), phenobarbital, carbamazepine, and rifampin, may reduce plasma concentrations of estrogens, possibly resulting in a decrease in therapeutic effects and/or changes in the uterine bleeding profile).
No products indexed under this heading.

Betamethasone Dipropionate (Inducers of CYP3A4, such as St. John's Wort preparations (Hypericum perforatum), phenobarbital, carbamazepine, and rifampin, may reduce plasma concentrations of estrogens, possibly resulting in a decrease in therapeutic effects and/or changes in the uterine bleeding profile). Products include:
Diprolene Lotion 0.05% 3108
Diprolene Ointment 0.05% 3109
Diprolene AF Cream 0.05% 3107
Lotrisone 3163

Betamethasone Sodium Phosphate (Inducers of CYP3A4, such as St. John's Wort preparations (Hypericum perforatum), phenobarbital, carbamazepine, and rifampin, may reduce plasma concentrations of estrogens, possibly resulting in a decrease in therapeutic effects and/or changes in the uterine bleeding profile).
No products indexed under this heading.

Betamethasone Valerate (Inducers of CYP3A4, such as St. John's Wort preparations (Hypericum perforatum), phenobarbital, carbamazepine, and rifampin, may reduce plasma concentrations of estrogens, possibly resulting in a decrease in therapeutic effects and/or changes in the uterine bleeding profile). Products include:
Luxiq 3321

Bosentan (Inducers of CYP3A4, such as St. John's Wort preparations (Hypericum perforatum), phenobarbital, carbamazepine, and rifampin, may reduce plasma concentrations of estrogens, possibly resulting in a decrease in therapeutic effects and/or changes in the uterine bleeding profile). Products include:
Tracleer 573

Candesartan Cilexetil (There is potential for an increase in serum potassium in women taking drospirenone with other drugs that may affect electrolytes). Products include:
Atacand 697
Atacand HCT 700

Captopril (There is potential for an increase in serum potassium in women taking drospirenone with other drugs that may affect electrolytes). Products include:
Captopril 2341

Carbamazepine (Inducers of CYP3A4, such as St. John's Wort preparations (Hypericum perforatum), phenobarbital, carbamazepine, and rifampin, may reduce plasma concentrations of estrogens, possibly resulting in a decrease in therapeutic effects and/or changes in the uterine bleeding profile). Products include:
Carbatrol 3280
Equetro 3477

Celecoxib (There is potential for an increase in serum potassium in women taking drospirenone with other drugs that may affect electrolytes). Products include:
Celebrex 3272

Cimetidine (Inhibitors of CYP3A4 such as erythromycin, clarithromycin, ketoconazole, itraconazole, ritonavir and grapefruit juice may increase plasma concentrations of estrogens and may result in side effects).
No products indexed under this heading.

Cimetidine Hydrochloride (Inhibitors of CYP3A4 such as erythromycin, clarithromycin, ketoconazole, itraconazole, ritonavir and grapefruit juice may increase plasma concentrations of estrogens and may result in side effects).
No products indexed under this heading.

Ciprofloxacin (Inhibitors of CYP3A4 such as erythromycin, clarithromycin, ketoconazole, itraconazole, ritonavir and grapefruit juice may increase plasma concentrations of estrogens and may result in side effects). Products include:
Cipro I.V. 3082
Cipro 3073
Cipro XR 3091
Ciprodex 583

Ciprofloxacin Hydrochloride (Inducers of CYP3A4, such as St. John's Wort preparations (Hypericum perforatum), phenobarbital, carbamazepine, and rifampin, may reduce plasma concentrations of estrogens, possibly resulting

in a decrease in therapeutic effects and/or changes in the uterine bleeding profile). Products include:
Cipro 3073

Cisplatin (Inducers of CYP3A4, such as St. John's Wort preparations (Hypericum perforatum), phenobarbital, carbamazepine, and rifampin, may reduce plasma concentrations of estrogens, possibly resulting in a decrease in therapeutic effects and/or changes in the uterine bleeding profile).
No products indexed under this heading.

Clarithromycin (Inhibitors of CYP3A4 such as erythromycin, clarithromycin, ketoconazole, itraconazole, ritonavir and grapefruit juice may increase plasma concentrations of estrogens and may result in side effects). Products include:
Biaxin/Biaxin XL 412

Clotrimazole (Inhibitors of CYP3A4 such as erythromycin, clarithromycin, ketoconazole, itraconazole, ritonavir and grapefruit juice may increase plasma concentrations of estrogens and may result in side effects). Products include:
Lotrisone 3163

Conivaptan Hydrochloride (Inhibitors of CYP3A4 such as erythromycin, clarithromycin, ketoconazole, itraconazole, ritonavir and grapefruit juice may increase plasma concentrations of estrogens and may result in side effects). Products include:
Vaprisol 689

Cortisone Acetate (Inducers of CYP3A4, such as St. John's Wort preparations (Hypericum perforatum), phenobarbital, carbamazepine, and rifampin, may reduce plasma concentrations of estrogens, possibly resulting in a decrease in therapeutic effects and/or changes in the uterine bleeding profile).
No products indexed under this heading.

Cyclosporine (Inhibitors of CYP3A4 such as erythromycin, clarithromycin, ketoconazole, itraconazole, ritonavir and grapefruit juice may increase plasma concentrations of estrogens and may result in side effects). Products include:
Gengraf 440
Neoral Oral Solution 2496
Neoral Capsules 2496
Restasis 605

Dalfopristin (Inhibitors of CYP3A4 such as erythromycin, clarithromycin, ketoconazole, itraconazole, ritonavir and grapefruit juice may increase plasma concentrations of estrogens and may result in side effects).
No products indexed under this heading.

Danazol (Inhibitors of CYP3A4 such as erythromycin, clarithromycin, ketoconazole, itraconazole, ritonavir and grapefruit juice may increase plasma concentrations of estrogens and may result in side effects).
No products indexed under this heading.

Darunavir (Inhibitors of CYP3A4 such as erythromycin, clarithromycin, ketoconazole, itraconazole, ritonavir and grapefruit juice may increase plasma concentrations of estrogens and may result in side effects).
No products indexed under this heading.

Dasatinib (Inhibitors of CYP3A4 such as erythromycin, clarithromycin, ketoconazole, itraconazole, ritonavir and grapefruit juice may increase plasma concentrations of estrogens and may result in side effects).
No products indexed under this heading.

Delavirdine Mesylate (Inhibitors of CYP3A4 such as erythromycin, clarithromycin, ketoconazole, itraconazole, ritonavir and grapefruit juice may increase plasma concentrations of estrogens and may result in side effects).
No products indexed under this heading.

Delavirine (Inhibitors of CYP3A4 such as erythromycin, clarithromycin, ketoconazole, itraconazole, ritonavir and grapefruit juice may increase plasma concentrations of estrogens and may result in side effects).
No products indexed under this heading.

Desloratadine (Inhibitors of CYP3A4 such as erythromycin, clarithromycin, ketoconazole, itraconazole, ritonavir and grapefruit juice may increase plasma concentrations of estrogens and may result in side effects). Products include:
Clarinex Syrup 3098
Clarinex 3098
Clarinex Reditabs 3098
Clarinex-D 12-Hour 3101
Clarinex-D 3104

Dexamethasone (Inducers of CYP3A4, such as St. John's Wort preparations (Hypericum perforatum), phenobarbital, carbamazepine, and rifampin, may reduce plasma concentrations of estrogens, possibly resulting in a decrease in therapeutic effects and/or changes in the uterine bleeding profile). Products include:
Ciprodex 583
Ozurdex .... ⊙223
Tobramycin and Dexamethasone Ophthalmic Suspension .... ⊙251

Dexamethasone Acetate (Inducers of CYP3A4, such as St. John's Wort preparations (Hypericum perforatum), phenobarbital, carbamazepine, and rifampin, may reduce plasma concentrations of estrogens, possibly resulting in a decrease in therapeutic effects and/or changes in the uterine bleeding profile).
No products indexed under this heading.

Dexamethasone Phosphate (Inducers of CYP3A4, such as St. John's Wort preparations (Hypericum perforatum), phenobarbital, carbamazepine, and rifampin, may reduce plasma concentrations of estrogens, possibly resulting in a decrease in therapeutic effects and/or changes in the uterine bleeding profile).
No products indexed under this heading.

Dexamethasone Sodium (Inducers of CYP3A4, such as St. John's Wort preparations (Hypericum perforatum), phenobarbital, carbamazepine, and rifampin, may reduce plasma concentrations of estrogens, possibly resulting in a decrease in therapeutic effects and/or changes in the uterine bleeding profile).
No products indexed under this heading.

Dexamethasone Sodium Phosphate (Inducers of CYP3A4, such as St. John's Wort preparations (Hypericum perforatum), phenobarbital, carbamazepine, and rifampin, may reduce plasma concentrations of estrogens, possibly resulting in a decrease in therapeutic effects and/or changes in the uterine bleeding profile).
No products indexed under this heading.

Dexamethasone Sodium Phosphate Injection (Inducers of CYP3A4, such as St. John's Wort preparations (Hypericum perforatum), phenobarbital, carbamazepine, and rifampin, may reduce plasma concentrations of estrogens, possibly resulting in a decrease in therapeutic effects and/or changes in the uterine bleeding profile).
No products indexed under this heading.

Diclofenac Epolamine (There is potential for an increase in serum

Angeliq Interactions Index 112

potassium in women taking drospirenone with other drugs that may affect electrolytes). Products include:
Flector 1839

Diclofenac Potassium (There is potential for an increase in serum potassium in women taking drospirenone with other drugs that may affect electrolytes).
No products indexed under this heading.

Diclofenac Sodium (There is potential for an increase in serum potassium in women taking drospirenone with other drugs that may affect electrolytes).
No products indexed under this heading.

Diltiazem Hydrochloride (Inhibitors of CYP3A4 such as erythromycin, clarithromycin, ketoconazole, itraconazole, ritonavir and grapefruit juice may increase plasma concentrations of estrogens and may result in side effects). Products include:
Cardizem LA 423

Diltiazem Maleate (Inhibitors of CYP3A4 such as erythromycin, clarithromycin, ketoconazole, itraconazole, ritonavir and grapefruit juice may increase plasma concentrations of estrogens and may result in side effects).
No products indexed under this heading.

Doxorubicin Hydrochloride (Inducers of CYP3A4, such as St. John's Wort preparations (Hypericum perforatum), phenobarbital, carbamazepine, and rifampin, may reduce plasma concentrations of estrogens, possibly resulting in a decrease in therapeutic effects and/or changes in the uterine bleeding profile).
No products indexed under this heading.

Efavirenz (Inhibitors of CYP3A4 such as erythromycin, clarithromycin, ketoconazole, itraconazole, ritonavir and grapefruit juice may increase plasma concentrations of estrogens and may result in side effects). Products include:
Atripla 906

Enalapril Maleate (There is potential for an increase in serum potassium in women taking drospirenone with other drugs that may affect electrolytes).
No products indexed under this heading.

Enalaprilat (There is potential for an increase in serum potassium in women taking drospirenone with other drugs that may affect electrolytes).
No products indexed under this heading.

Eprosartan Mesylate (There is potential for an increase in serum potassium in women taking drospirenone with other drugs that may affect electrolytes). Products include:
Teveten 538
Teveten HCT 541

Erythromycin (Inhibitors of CYP3A4 such as erythromycin, clarithromycin, ketoconazole, itraconazole, ritonavir and grapefruit juice may increase plasma concentrations of estrogens and may result in side effects).
No products indexed under this heading.

Erythromycin Estolate (Inhibitors of CYP3A4 such as erythromycin, clarithromycin, ketoconazole, itraconazole, ritonavir and grapefruit juice may increase plasma concentrations of estrogens and may result in side effects).
No products indexed under this heading.

Erythromycin Ethylsuccinate (Inhibitors of CYP3A4 such as erythromycin, clarithromycin, ketoconazole, itraconazole, ritonavir and grapefruit juice may increase plasma concentrations of estrogens and may result in side effects). Products include:
E.E.S. 437
EryPed 435

Erythromycin Gluceptate (Inhibitors of CYP3A4 such as erythromycin, clarithromycin, ketoconazole, itraconazole, ritonavir and grapefruit juice may increase plasma concentrations of estrogens and may result in side effects).
No products indexed under this heading.

Erythromycin Lactobionate (Inhibitors of CYP3A4 such as erythromycin, clarithromycin, ketoconazole, itraconazole, ritonavir and grapefruit juice may increase plasma concentrations of estrogens and may result in side effects).
No products indexed under this heading.

Erythromycin Stearate (Inhibitors of CYP3A4 such as erythromycin, clarithromycin, ketoconazole, itraconazole, ritonavir and grapefruit juice may increase plasma concentrations of estrogens and may result in side effects).
No products indexed under this heading.

Esomeprazole Magnesium (Inhibitors of CYP3A4 such as erythromycin, clarithromycin, ketoconazole, itraconazole, ritonavir and grapefruit juice may increase plasma concentrations of estrogens and may result in side effects). Products include:
Nexium Capsules 704
Nexium Oral Suspension 704

Esomeprazole Sodium (Inhibitors of CYP3A4 such as erythromycin, clarithromycin, ketoconazole, itraconazole, ritonavir and grapefruit juice may increase plasma concentrations of estrogens and may result in side effects). Products include:
Nexium I.V. 712

Ethosuximide (Inducers of CYP3A4, such as St. John's Wort preparations (Hypericum perforatum), phenobarbital, carbamazepine, and rifampin, may reduce plasma concentrations of estrogens, possibly resulting in a decrease in therapeutic effects and/or changes in the uterine bleeding profile).
No products indexed under this heading.

Etodolac (There is potential for an increase in serum potassium in women taking drospirenone with other drugs that may affect electrolytes).
No products indexed under this heading.

Felbamate (Inducers of CYP3A4, such as St. John's Wort preparations (Hypericum perforatum), phenobarbital, carbamazepine, and rifampin, may reduce plasma concentrations of estrogens, possibly resulting in a decrease in therapeutic effects and/or changes in the uterine bleeding profile).
No products indexed under this heading.

Fenoprofen Calcium (There is potential for an increase in serum potassium in women taking drospirenone with other drugs that may affect electrolytes).
No products indexed under this heading.

Fluconazole (Inhibitors of CYP3A4 such as erythromycin, clarithromycin, ketoconazole, itraconazole, ritonavir and grapefruit juice may increase plasma concentrations of estrogens and may result in side effects).
No products indexed under this heading.

Fludrocortisone Acetate (Inducers of CYP3A4, such as St. John's Wort preparations (Hypericum perforatum), phenobarbital, carbamazepine, and rifampin, may reduce plasma concentrations of estrogens, possibly resulting in a decrease in therapeutic effects and/or changes in the uterine bleeding profile).
No products indexed under this heading.

Fluoxetine (Inhibitors of CYP3A4 such as erythromycin, clarithromycin, ketoconazole, itraconazole, ritonavir and grapefruit juice may increase plasma concentrations of estrogens and may result in side effects).
No products indexed under this heading.

Fluoxetine Hydrochloride (Inhibitors of CYP3A4 such as erythromycin, clarithromycin, ketoconazole, itraconazole, ritonavir and grapefruit juice may increase plasma concentrations of estrogens and may result in side effects). Products include:
Prozac Weekly 1941
Prozac Pulvules 1941
Symbyax 1965

Flurbiprofen (There is potential for an increase in serum potassium in women taking drospirenone with other drugs that may affect electrolytes).
No products indexed under this heading.

Fluvoxamine Maleate (Inhibitors of CYP3A4 such as erythromycin, clarithromycin, ketoconazole, itraconazole, ritonavir and grapefruit juice may increase plasma concentrations of estrogens and may result in side effects).
No products indexed under this heading.

Fosamprenavir Calcium (Inhibitors of CYP3A4 such as erythromycin, clarithromycin, ketoconazole, itraconazole, ritonavir and grapefruit juice may increase plasma concentrations of estrogens and may result in side effects). Products include:
Lexiva Oral Suspension 1558
Lexiva 1558

Fosinopril Sodium (There is potential for an increase in serum potassium in women taking drospirenone with other drugs that may affect electrolytes).
No products indexed under this heading.

Fosphenytoin Sodium (Inducers of CYP3A4, such as St. John's Wort preparations (Hypericum perforatum), phenobarbital, carbamazepine, and rifampin, may reduce plasma concentrations of estrogens, possibly resulting in a decrease in therapeutic effects and/or changes in the uterine bleeding profile).
No products indexed under this heading.

Garlic Extract (Inducers of CYP3A4, such as St. John's Wort preparations (Hypericum perforatum), phenobarbital, carbamazepine, and rifampin, may reduce plasma concentrations of estrogens, possibly resulting in a decrease in therapeutic effects and/or changes in the uterine bleeding profile).
No products indexed under this heading.

Garlic Oil (Inducers of CYP3A4, such as St. John's Wort preparations (Hypericum perforatum), phenobarbital, carbamazepine, and rifampin, may reduce plasma concentrations of estrogens, possibly resulting in a decrease in therapeutic effects and/or changes in the uterine bleeding profile).
No products indexed under this heading.

Hydrocortisone (Inducers of CYP3A4, such as St. John's Wort preparations (Hypericum perforatum), phenobarbital, carbamazepine, and rifampin, may reduce plasma concentrations of estrogens, possibly resulting in a decrease in therapeutic effects and/or changes in the uterine bleeding profile).
No products indexed under this heading.

Hydrocortisone (Alcohol) (Inducers of CYP3A4, such as St. John's Wort preparations (Hypericum perforatum), phenobarbital, carbamazepine, and rifampin, may reduce plasma concentrations of estrogens, possibly resulting in a decrease in therapeutic effects and/or changes in the uterine bleeding profile).
No products indexed under this heading.

Hydrocortisone Acetate (Inducers of CYP3A4, such as St. John's Wort preparations (Hypericum perforatum), phenobarbital, carbamazepine, and rifampin, may reduce plasma concentrations of estrogens, possibly resulting in a decrease in therapeutic effects and/or changes in the uterine bleeding profile).
No products indexed under this heading.

Hydrocortisone Butyrate (Inducers of CYP3A4, such as St. John's Wort preparations (Hypericum perforatum), phenobarbital, carbamazepine, and rifampin, may reduce plasma concentrations of estrogens, possibly resulting in a decrease in therapeutic effects and/or changes in the uterine bleeding profile).
No products indexed under this heading.

Hydrocortisone Cypionate (Inducers of CYP3A4, such as St. John's Wort preparations (Hypericum perforatum), phenobarbital, carbamazepine, and rifampin, may reduce plasma concentrations of estrogens, possibly resulting in a decrease in therapeutic effects and/or changes in the uterine bleeding profile).
No products indexed under this heading.

Hydrocortisone Hemisuccinate (Inducers of CYP3A4, such as St. John's Wort preparations (Hypericum perforatum), phenobarbital, carbamazepine, and rifampin, may reduce plasma concentrations of estrogens, possibly resulting in a decrease in therapeutic effects and/or changes in the uterine bleeding profile).
No products indexed under this heading.

Hydrocortisone Probutate (Inducers of CYP3A4, such as St. John's Wort preparations (Hypericum perforatum), phenobarbital, carbamazepine, and rifampin, may reduce plasma concentrations of estrogens, possibly resulting in a decrease in therapeutic effects and/or changes in the uterine bleeding profile).
No products indexed under this heading.

Hydrocortisone Sodium Phosphate (Inducers of CYP3A4, such as St. John's Wort preparations (Hypericum perforatum), phenobarbital, carbamazepine, and rifampin, may reduce plasma concentrations of estrogens, possibly resulting in a decrease in therapeutic effects and/or changes in the uterine bleeding profile).
No products indexed under this heading.

Hydrocortisone Sodium Succinate (Inducers of CYP3A4, such as St. John's Wort preparations (Hypericum perforatum), phenobarbital, carbamazepine, and rifampin, may reduce plasma concentrations of estrogens, possibly resulting in a decrease in therapeutic effects and/or changes in the uterine bleeding profile).
No products indexed under this heading.

Hydrocortisone Valerate (Inducers of CYP3A4, such as St. John's Wort preparations (Hypericum perforatum), phenobarbital, carbamazepine, and rifampin, may reduce plasma concentrations of estrogens, possibly resulting in a decrease in therapeutic effects and/or changes in the uterine bleeding profile).
No products indexed under this heading.

Hypericum (Inducers of CYP3A4, such as St. John's Wort preparations (Hypericum perforatum), phenobarbital, carbamazepine, and rifampin, may reduce plasma concentrations of estrogens, possibly resulting in a decrease in therapeutic effects and/or changes in the uterine bleeding profile).
No products indexed under this heading.

Hypericum Perforatum (Inducers of CYP3A4, such as St. John's Wort prepa-

rations (Hypericum perforatum), phenobarbital, carbamazepine, and rifampin, may reduce plasma concentrations of estrogens, possibly resulting in a decrease in therapeutic effects and/or changes in the uterine bleeding profile). Products include:

Traumeel 1800

Ibuprofen (There is potential for an increase in serum potassium in women taking drospirenone with other drugs that may affect electrolytes). Products include:

Motrin IB 2043
Children's Motrin 2044
Children's Motrin Non-Staining
   Dye-Free 2044
Infants' Motrin 2044
Infants' Motrin Dye-Free 2044
Junior Strength Motrin 2044
Vicoprofen 564

Imatinib Mesylate (Inhibitors of CYP3A4 such as erythromycin, clarithromycin, ketoconazole, itraconazole, ritonavir and grapefruit juice may increase plasma concentrations of estrogens and may result in side effects). Products include:

Gleevec 2477

Indinavir Sulfate (Inhibitors of CYP3A4 such as erythromycin, clarithromycin, ketoconazole, itraconazole, ritonavir and grapefruit juice may increase plasma concentrations of estrogens and may result in side effects). Products include:

Crixivan 2113

Indomethacin (There is potential for an increase in serum potassium in women taking drospirenone with other drugs that may affect electrolytes). Products include:

Indocin 2167

Indomethacin Sodium Trihydrate (There is potential for an increase in serum potassium in women taking drospirenone with other drugs that may affect electrolytes). Products include:

Indocin I.V. 2007

Irbesartan (There is potential for an increase in serum potassium in women taking drospirenone with other drugs that may affect electrolytes). Products include:

Avalide 2956
Avapro 2962

Isoniazid (Inhibitors of CYP3A4 such as erythromycin, clarithromycin, ketoconazole, itraconazole, ritonavir and grapefruit juice may increase plasma concentrations of estrogens and may result in side effects).

No products indexed under this heading.

Itraconazole (Inhibitors of CYP3A4 such as erythromycin, clarithromycin, ketoconazole, itraconazole, ritonavir and grapefruit juice may increase plasma concentrations of estrogens and may result in side effects).

No products indexed under this heading.

Ketoconazole (Inhibitors of CYP3A4 such as erythromycin, clarithromycin, ketoconazole, itraconazole, ritonavir and grapefruit juice may increase plasma concentrations of estrogens and may result in side effects). Products include:

Extina 3319
Xolegel 3337

Ketoprofen (There is potential for an increase in serum potassium in women taking drospirenone with other drugs that may affect electrolytes).

No products indexed under this heading.

Ketorolac Tromethamine (There is potential for an increase in serum potassium in women taking drospirenone with other drugs that may affect electrolytes). Products include:

Acuvail .... ⊙209

Lapatinib (Inhibitors of CYP3A4 such as erythromycin, clarithromycin, ketoconazole, itraconazole, ritonavir and grapefruit juice may increase plasma concentrations of estrogens and may result in side effects). Products include:

Tykerb 1698

Lisinopril (There is potential for an increase in serum potassium in women taking drospirenone with other drugs that may affect electrolytes). Products include:

Prinivil 2241
Prinzide 2246

Lopinavir (Inhibitors of CYP3A4 such as erythromycin, clarithromycin, ketoconazole, itraconazole, ritonavir and grapefruit juice may increase plasma concentrations of estrogens and may result in side effects). Products include:

Kaletra 458

Loratadine (Inhibitors of CYP3A4 such as erythromycin, clarithromycin, ketoconazole, itraconazole, ritonavir and grapefruit juice may increase plasma concentrations of estrogens and may result in side effects).

No products indexed under this heading.

Losartan Potassium (There is potential for an increase in serum potassium in women taking drospirenone with other drugs that may affect electrolytes). Products include:

Cozaar 2106
Hyzaar 2162
Hyzaar 100-12.5 2162

Meclofenamate Sodium (There is potential for an increase in serum potassium in women taking drospirenone with other drugs that may affect electrolytes).

No products indexed under this heading.

Mefenamic Acid (There is potential for an increase in serum potassium in women taking drospirenone with other drugs that may affect electrolytes).

No products indexed under this heading.

Meloxicam (There is potential for an increase in serum potassium in women taking drospirenone with other drugs that may affect electrolytes).

No products indexed under this heading.

Mephenytoin (Inducers of CYP3A4, such as St. John's Wort preparations (Hypericum perforatum), phenobarbital, carbamazepine, and rifampin, may reduce plasma concentrations of estrogens, possibly resulting in a decrease in therapeutic effects and/or changes in the uterine bleeding profile).

No products indexed under this heading.

Methsuximide (Inducers of CYP3A4, such as St. John's Wort preparations (Hypericum perforatum), phenobarbital, carbamazepine, and rifampin, may reduce plasma concentrations of estrogens, possibly resulting in a decrease in therapeutic effects and/or changes in the uterine bleeding profile).

No products indexed under this heading.

Methylprednisolone (Inducers of CYP3A4, such as St. John's Wort preparations (Hypericum perforatum), phenobarbital, carbamazepine, and rifampin, may reduce plasma concentrations of estrogens, possibly resulting in a decrease in therapeutic effects and/or changes in the uterine bleeding profile).

No products indexed under this heading.

Methylprednisolone Acetate (Inducers of CYP3A4, such as St. John's Wort preparations (Hypericum perforatum), phenobarbital, carbamazepine, and rifampin, may reduce plasma concentrations of estrogens, possibly resulting in a decrease in therapeutic effects and/or changes in the uterine bleeding profile).

No products indexed under this heading.

Methylprednisolone Sodium Succinate (Inducers of CYP3A4, such as St. John's Wort preparations (Hypericum perforatum), phenobarbital, carbamazepine, and rifampin, may reduce plasma concentrations of estrogens, possibly resulting in a decrease in therapeutic effects and/or changes in the uterine bleeding profile).

No products indexed under this heading.

Metronidazole (Inhibitors of CYP3A4 such as erythromycin, clarithromycin, ketoconazole, itraconazole, ritonavir and grapefruit juice may increase plasma concentrations of estrogens and may result in side effects). Products include:

Pylera 793

Metronidazole Benzoate (Inhibitors of CYP3A4 such as erythromycin, clarithromycin, ketoconazole, itraconazole, ritonavir and grapefruit juice may increase plasma concentrations of estrogens and may result in side effects).

No products indexed under this heading.

Metronidazole Hydrochloride (Inhibitors of CYP3A4 such as erythromycin, clarithromycin, ketoconazole, itraconazole, ritonavir and grapefruit juice may increase plasma concentrations of estrogens and may result in side effects).

No products indexed under this heading.

Metronidazole Sodium (Inhibitors of CYP3A4 such as erythromycin, clarithromycin, ketoconazole, itraconazole, ritonavir and grapefruit juice may increase plasma concentrations of estrogens and may result in side effects).

No products indexed under this heading.

Miconazole (Inhibitors of CYP3A4 such as erythromycin, clarithromycin, ketoconazole, itraconazole, ritonavir and grapefruit juice may increase plasma concentrations of estrogens and may result in side effects).

No products indexed under this heading.

Miconazole Nitrate (Inhibitors of CYP3A4 such as erythromycin, clarithromycin, ketoconazole, itraconazole, ritonavir and grapefruit juice may increase plasma concentrations of estrogens and may result in side effects). Products include:

Vusion Ointment 3335

Mifepristone (Inhibitors of CYP3A4 such as erythromycin, clarithromycin, ketoconazole, itraconazole, ritonavir and grapefruit juice may increase plasma concentrations of estrogens and may result in side effects).

No products indexed under this heading.

Modafinil (Inducers of CYP3A4, such as St. John's Wort preparations (Hypericum perforatum), phenobarbital, carbamazepine, and rifampin, may reduce plasma concentrations of estrogens, possibly resulting in a decrease in therapeutic effects and/or changes in the uterine bleeding profile). Products include:

Provigil 983

Moexipril Hydrochloride (There is potential for an increase in serum potassium in women taking drospirenone with other drugs that may affect electrolytes).

No products indexed under this heading.

Nabumetone (There is potential for an increase in serum potassium in women taking drospirenone with other drugs that may affect electrolytes).

No products indexed under this heading.

Nafcillin Sodium (Inducers of CYP3A4, such as St. John's Wort preparations (Hypericum perforatum), phenobarbital, carbamazepine, and rifampin, may reduce plasma concentrations of estrogens, possibly resulting in a decrease in therapeutic effects and/or changes in the uterine bleeding profile).

No products indexed under this heading.

Naproxen (There is potential for an increase in serum potassium in women taking drospirenone with other drugs that may affect electrolytes). Products include:

EC-Naprosyn 2850
Naprosyn 2850
Anaprox/Naprosyn 2850

Naproxen Sodium (There is potential for an increase in serum potassium in women taking drospirenone with other drugs that may affect electrolytes). Products include:

Anaprox 2850
Anaprox DS 2850
Treximet 1681

Nefazodone Hydrochloride (Inhibitors of CYP3A4 such as erythromycin, clarithromycin, ketoconazole, itraconazole, ritonavir and grapefruit juice may increase plasma concentrations of estrogens and may result in side effects).

No products indexed under this heading.

Nelfinavir Mesylate (Inhibitors of CYP3A4 such as erythromycin, clarithromycin, ketoconazole, itraconazole, ritonavir and grapefruit juice may increase plasma concentrations of estrogens and may result in side effects).

No products indexed under this heading.

Nevirapine (Inhibitors of CYP3A4 such as erythromycin, clarithromycin, ketoconazole, itraconazole, ritonavir and grapefruit juice may increase plasma concentrations of estrogens and may result in side effects). Products include:

Viramune Oral Suspension 897
Viramune Tablets 897

Niacin (Inhibitors of CYP3A4 such as erythromycin, clarithromycin, ketoconazole, itraconazole, ritonavir and grapefruit juice may increase plasma concentrations of estrogens and may result in side effects). Products include:

Advicor 402
Cardio Basics 3455
Niaspan 497
Simcor 524

Niacinamide (Inhibitors of CYP3A4 such as erythromycin, clarithromycin, ketoconazole, itraconazole, ritonavir and grapefruit juice may increase plasma concentrations of estrogens and may result in side effects). Products include:

CitraNatal 90 DHA Capsules 2332
CitraNatal Assure 2332
CitraNatal Rx 2332
Heplive 607

Niacinamide Hydroiodide (Inhibitors of CYP3A4 such as erythromycin, clarithromycin, ketoconazole, itraconazole, ritonavir and grapefruit juice may increase plasma concentrations of estrogens and may result in side effects).

No products indexed under this heading.

Nicotinamide (Inhibitors of CYP3A4 such as erythromycin, clarithromycin, ketoconazole, itraconazole, ritonavir and grapefruit juice may increase plasma concentrations of estrogens and may result in side effects).

No products indexed under this heading.

Nifedipine (Inhibitors of CYP3A4 such as erythromycin, clarithromycin, ketoconazole, itraconazole, ritonavir and grapefruit juice may increase plasma concentrations of estrogens and may result in side effects).

No products indexed under this heading.

IMPORTANT NOTE: Always consult each drug listing in the patient's regimen for possible interactions.

115 Interactions Index Anzemet

Sulfinpyrazone (Inducers of CYP3A4, such as St. John's Wort preparations (Hypericum perforatum), phenobarbital, carbamazepine, and rifampin, may reduce plasma concentrations of estrogens, possibly resulting in a decrease in therapeutic effects and/or changes in the uterine bleeding profile).
No products indexed under this heading.

Sulindac (There is potential for an increase in serum potassium in women taking drospirenone with other drugs that may affect electrolytes). Products include:
Clinoril 2098

Telithromycin (Inhibitors of CYP3A4 such as erythromycin, clarithromycin, ketoconazole, itraconazole, ritonavir and grapefruit juice may increase plasma concentrations of estrogens and may result in side effects). Products include:
Ketek 2991

Telmisartan (There is potential for an increase in serum potassium in women taking drospirenone with other drugs that may affect electrolytes). Products include:
Micardis 887
Micardis HCT 889

Theophyllinate (Inducers of CYP3A4, such as St. John's Wort preparations (Hypericum perforatum), phenobarbital, carbamazepine, and rifampin, may reduce plasma concentrations of estrogens, possibly resulting in a decrease in therapeutic effects and/or changes in the uterine bleeding profile).
No products indexed under this heading.

Theophylline (Inducers of CYP3A4, such as St. John's Wort preparations (Hypericum perforatum), phenobarbital, carbamazepine, and rifampin, may reduce plasma concentrations of estrogens, possibly resulting in a decrease in therapeutic effects and/or changes in the uterine bleeding profile).
No products indexed under this heading.

Theophylline Anhydrous (Inducers of CYP3A4, such as St. John's Wort preparations (Hypericum perforatum), phenobarbital, carbamazepine, and rifampin, may reduce plasma concentrations of estrogens, possibly resulting in a decrease in therapeutic effects and/or changes in the uterine bleeding profile). Products include:
Uniphyl 2817

Theophylline Calcium Salicylate (Inducers of CYP3A4, such as St. John's Wort preparations (Hypericum perforatum), phenobarbital, carbamazepine, and rifampin, may reduce plasma concentrations of estrogens, possibly resulting in a decrease in therapeutic effects and/or changes in the uterine bleeding profile).
No products indexed under this heading.

Theophylline Dihydroxypropyl (Glyceryl) (Inducers of CYP3A4, such as St. John's Wort preparations (Hypericum perforatum), phenobarbital, carbamazepine, and rifampin, may reduce plasma concentrations of estrogens, possibly resulting in a decrease in therapeutic effects and/or changes in the uterine bleeding profile).
No products indexed under this heading.

Theophylline Ethylenediamine (Inducers of CYP3A4, such as St. John's Wort preparations (Hypericum perforatum), phenobarbital, carbamazepine, and rifampin, may reduce plasma concentrations of estrogens, possibly resulting in a decrease in therapeutic effects and/or changes in the uterine bleeding profile).
No products indexed under this heading.

Theophylline Sodium Glycinate (Inducers of CYP3A4, such as St. John's Wort preparations (Hypericum perforatum), phenobarbital, carbamazepine, and rifampin, may reduce plasma concentrations of estrogens, possibly resulting in a decrease in therapeutic effects and/or changes in the uterine bleeding profile).
No products indexed under this heading.

Tolmetin Sodium (There is potential for an increase in serum potassium in women taking drospirenone with other drugs that may affect electrolytes).
No products indexed under this heading.

Trandolapril (There is potential for an increase in serum potassium in women taking drospirenone with other drugs that may affect electrolytes). Products include:
Mavik 489
Tarka 534

Triamcinolone (Inducers of CYP3A4, such as St. John's Wort preparations (Hypericum perforatum), phenobarbital, carbamazepine, and rifampin, may reduce plasma concentrations of estrogens, possibly resulting in a decrease in therapeutic effects and/or changes in the uterine bleeding profile).
No products indexed under this heading.

Triamcinolone Acetonide (Inducers of CYP3A4, such as St. John's Wort preparations (Hypericum perforatum), phenobarbital, carbamazepine, and rifampin, may reduce plasma concentrations of estrogens, possibly resulting in a decrease in therapeutic effects and/or changes in the uterine bleeding profile). Products include:
Azmacort 408
Nasacort AQ 3019

Triamcinolone Diacetate (Inducers of CYP3A4, such as St. John's Wort preparations (Hypericum perforatum), phenobarbital, carbamazepine, and rifampin, may reduce plasma concentrations of estrogens, possibly resulting in a decrease in therapeutic effects and/or changes in the uterine bleeding profile).
No products indexed under this heading.

Triamcinolone Hexacetonide (Inducers of CYP3A4, such as St. John's Wort preparations (Hypericum perforatum), phenobarbital, carbamazepine, and rifampin, may reduce plasma concentrations of estrogens, possibly resulting in a decrease in therapeutic effects and/or changes in the uterine bleeding profile).
No products indexed under this heading.

Troglitazone (Inhibitors of CYP3A4 such as erythromycin, clarithromycin, ketoconazole, itraconazole, ritonavir and grapefruit juice may increase plasma concentrations of estrogens and may result in side effects).
No products indexed under this heading.

Troleandomycin (Inhibitors of CYP3A4 such as erythromycin, clarithromycin, ketoconazole, itraconazole, ritonavir and grapefruit juice may increase plasma concentrations of estrogens and may result in side effects).
No products indexed under this heading.

Valdecoxib (There is potential for an increase in serum potassium in women taking drospirenone with other drugs that may affect electrolytes).
No products indexed under this heading.

Valproate Sodium (Inhibitors of CYP3A4 such as erythromycin, clarithromycin, ketoconazole, itraconazole, ritonavir and grapefruit juice may increase plasma concentrations of estrogens and may result in side effects).
No products indexed under this heading.

Valsartan (There is potential for an increase in serum potassium in women taking drospirenone with other drugs that may affect electrolytes). Products include:
Diovan 2413
Diovan HCT 2419
Exforge 2443
Exforge HCT 2449
Valturna 3637

Vardenafil Hydrochloride (Inhibitors of CYP3A4 such as erythromycin, clarithromycin, ketoconazole, itraconazole, ritonavir and grapefruit juice may increase plasma concentrations of estrogens and may result in side effects). Products include:
Levitra 3157

Verapamil Hydrochloride (Inhibitors of CYP3A4 such as erythromycin, clarithromycin, ketoconazole, itraconazole, ritonavir and grapefruit juice may increase plasma concentrations of estrogens and may result in side effects). Products include:
Tarka 534

Voriconazole (Inhibitors of CYP3A4 such as erythromycin, clarithromycin, ketoconazole, itraconazole, ritonavir and grapefruit juice may increase plasma concentrations of estrogens and may result in side effects).
No products indexed under this heading.

Zafirlukast (Inhibitors of CYP3A4 such as erythromycin, clarithromycin, ketoconazole, itraconazole, ritonavir and grapefruit juice may increase plasma concentrations of estrogens and may result in side effects). Products include:
Accolate 3612

Zileuton (Inhibitors of CYP3A4 such as erythromycin, clarithromycin, ketoconazole, itraconazole, ritonavir and grapefruit juice may increase plasma concentrations of estrogens and may result in side effects).
No products indexed under this heading.

Food Interactions

Grapefruit (Inhibitors of CYP3A4 such as erythromycin, clarithromycin, ketoconazole, itraconazole, ritonavir and grapefruit juice may increase plasma concentrations of estrogens and may result in side effects).

Grapefruit Juice (Inhibitors of CYP3A4 such as erythromycin, clarithromycin, ketoconazole, itraconazole, ritonavir and grapefruit juice may increase plasma concentrations of estrogens and may result in side effects).

ANGIOMAX FOR INJECTION

(Bivalirudin) 2061
May interact with glycoprotein (GP) IIb/IIIa inhibitors, thrombolytics, and certain other agents. Compounds in these categories include:

Abciximab (Co-administration was associated with increased risks of major bleeding events). Products include:
ReoPro 1952

Alteplase (Co-administration was associated with increased risks of major bleeding events). Products include:
Activase 1183
Cathflo 1192

Anistreplase (Co-administration was associated with increased risks of major bleeding events).
No products indexed under this heading.

Eptifibatide (Co-administration was associated with increased risks of major bleeding events). Products include:
Integrilin 3135

Heparin Sodium (Co-administration was associated with increased risks of major bleeding events).
No products indexed under this heading.

Reteplase (Co-administration was associated with increased risks of major bleeding events).
No products indexed under this heading.

Streptokinase (Co-administration was associated with increased risks of major bleeding events).
No products indexed under this heading.

Tirofiban Hydrochloride (Co-administration was associated with increased risks of major bleeding events).
No products indexed under this heading.

Urokinase (Co-administration was associated with increased risks of major bleeding events).
No products indexed under this heading.

Warfarin Sodium (Co-administration was associated with increased risks of major bleeding events).
No products indexed under this heading.

ANIMI-3 CAPSULES

(Docosahexaenoic Acid (DHA), Eicosapentaenoic Acid (EPA), Folic Acid, Omega-3 Acids, Phytosterols, Vitamin B12, Vitamin B6) 2711
None cited in PDR database.

ANTIVENIN (BLACK WIDOW SPIDER ANTIVENIN)

(Black Widow Spider Antivenin (Equine)) 2085
None cited in PDR database.

ANZEMET INJECTION

(Dolasetron Mesylate) 2931
See Anzemet Tablets

ANZEMET TABLETS

(Dolasetron Mesylate) 2934
May interact with anthracyclines, antiarrhythmics, diuretics, drugs that prolong the QT interval, and certain other agents. Compounds in these categories include:

Acebutolol Hydrochloride (Dolasetron should be administered with caution in patients who have or may develop prolongation of cardiac conduction intervals, particularly QTc. These include patients taking anti-arrhythmic drugs).
No products indexed under this heading.

Adenosine (Dolasetron should be administered with caution in patients who have or may develop prolongation of cardiac conduction intervals, particularly QTc. These include patients taking anti-arrhythmic drugs). Products include:
Adenocard 656
Adenoscan 657

Alprazolam (Dolasetron should be administered with caution in patients who have or may develop prolongation of cardiac conduction intervals, particularly QTc. These include patients taking drugs which lead to QT prolongation).
No products indexed under this heading.

Amiloride Hydrochloride (Dolasetron should be administered with caution in patients who have or may develop prolongation of cardiac conduction intervals, particularly QTc. These include patients taking diuretics with potential for inducing electrolyte abnormalities).
No products indexed under this heading.

IMPORTANT NOTE: Always consult each drug listing in the patient's regimen for possible interactions.

(⊙ Described in PDR® for Ophthalmic Medicines)

Fluphenazine Enanthate (Dolasetron should be administered with caution in patients who have or may develop prolongation of cardiac conduction intervals, particularly QTc. These include patients taking drugs which lead to QT prolongation).
No products indexed under this heading.

Fluphenazine Hydrochloride (Dolasetron should be administered with caution in patients who have or may develop prolongation of cardiac conduction intervals, particularly QTc. These include patients taking drugs which lead to QT prolongation).
No products indexed under this heading.

Furosemide (Dolasetron should be administered with caution in patients who have or may develop prolongation of cardiac conduction intervals, particularly QTc. These include patients taking diuretics with potential for inducing electrolyte abnormalities). Products include:
Furosemide 2354

Haloperidol (Dolasetron should be administered with caution in patients who have or may develop prolongation of cardiac conduction intervals, particularly QTc. These include patients taking drugs which lead to QT prolongation).
No products indexed under this heading.

Haloperidol Decanoate (Dolasetron should be administered with caution in patients who have or may develop prolongation of cardiac conduction intervals, particularly QTc. These include patients taking drugs which lead to QT prolongation).
No products indexed under this heading.

Haloperidol Lactate (Dolasetron should be administered with caution in patients who have or may develop prolongation of cardiac conduction intervals, particularly QTc. These include patients taking drugs which lead to QT prolongation).
No products indexed under this heading.

Hydrochlorothiazide (Dolasetron should be administered with caution in patients who have or may develop prolongation of cardiac conduction intervals, particularly QTc. These include patients taking diuretics with potential for inducing electrolyte abnormalities).
Products include:
Atacand HCT 700
Avalide 2956
Benicar HCT 1017
Diovan HCT 2419
Dyazide 1429
Exforge HCT 2449
Hyzaar 2162
Hyzaar 100-12.5 2162
Micardis HCT 889
Prinzide 2246
Tekturna HCT 2541
Teveten HCT 541

Hydroflumethiazide (Dolasetron should be administered with caution in patients who have or may develop prolongation of cardiac conduction intervals, particularly QTc. These include patients taking diuretics with potential for inducing electrolyte abnormalities).
No products indexed under this heading.

Hydroxyzine Hydrochloride (Dolasetron should be administered with caution in patients who have or may develop prolongation of cardiac conduction intervals, particularly QTc. These include patients taking drugs which lead to QT prolongation).
No products indexed under this heading.

Idarubicin Hydrochloride (Dolasetron should be administered with caution in patients who have or may develop prolongation of cardiac conduction intervals, particularly QTc. These include patients receiving cumulative high dose anthracycline therapy).
No products indexed under this heading.

Imipramine Hydrochloride (Dolasetron should be administered with caution in patients who have or may develop prolongation of cardiac conduction intervals, particularly QTc. These include patients taking drugs which lead to QT prolongation).
No products indexed under this heading.

Imipramine Pamoate (Dolasetron should be administered with caution in patients who have or may develop prolongation of cardiac conduction intervals, particularly QTc. These include patients taking drugs which lead to QT prolongation).
No products indexed under this heading.

Indapamide (Dolasetron should be administered with caution in patients who have or may develop prolongation of cardiac conduction intervals, particularly QTc. These include patients taking diuretics with potential for inducing electrolyte abnormalities). Products include:
Indapamide 2356

Isocarboxazid (Dolasetron should be administered with caution in patients who have or may develop prolongation of cardiac conduction intervals, particularly QTc. These include patients taking drugs which lead to QT prolongation). Products include:
Marplan 3481

Lidocaine (Dolasetron should be administered with caution in patients who have or may develop prolongation of cardiac conduction intervals, particularly QTc. These include patients taking drugs which lead to QT prolongation). Products include:
Lidoderm 1107

Lidocaine Hydrochloride (Dolasetron should be administered with caution in patients who have or may develop prolongation of cardiac conduction intervals, particularly QTc. These include patients taking anti-arrhythmic drugs).
No products indexed under this heading.

Lithium Carbonate (Dolasetron should be administered with caution in patients who have or may develop prolongation of cardiac conduction intervals, particularly QTc. These include patients taking drugs which lead to QT prolongation).
No products indexed under this heading.

Lithium Citrate (Dolasetron should be administered with caution in patients who have or may develop prolongation of cardiac conduction intervals, particularly QTc. These include patients taking drugs which lead to QT prolongation).
No products indexed under this heading.

Lorazepam (Dolasetron should be administered with caution in patients who have or may develop prolongation of cardiac conduction intervals, particularly QTc. These include patients taking drugs which lead to QT prolongation).
No products indexed under this heading.

Loxapine Hydrochloride (Dolasetron should be administered with caution in patients who have or may develop prolongation of cardiac conduction intervals, particularly QTc. These include patients taking drugs which lead to QT prolongation).
No products indexed under this heading.

Loxapine Succinate (Dolasetron should be administered with caution in patients who have or may develop prolongation of cardiac conduction intervals, particularly QTc. These include patients taking drugs which lead to QT prolongation).
No products indexed under this heading.

Maprotiline Hydrochloride (Dolasetron should be administered with caution in patients who have or may develop prolongation of cardiac conduction intervals, particularly QTc. These include patients taking drugs which lead to QT prolongation).
No products indexed under this heading.

Meprobamate (Dolasetron should be administered with caution in patients who have or may develop prolongation of cardiac conduction intervals, particularly QTc. These include patients taking drugs which lead to QT prolongation).
No products indexed under this heading.

Mesoridazine Besylate (Dolasetron should be administered with caution in patients who have or may develop prolongation of cardiac conduction intervals, particularly QTc. These include patients taking drugs which lead to QT prolongation).
No products indexed under this heading.

Methyclothiazide (Dolasetron should be administered with caution in patients who have or may develop prolongation of cardiac conduction intervals, particularly QTc. These include patients taking diuretics with potential for inducing electrolyte abnormalities).
No products indexed under this heading.

Metolazone (Dolasetron should be administered with caution in patients who have or may develop prolongation of cardiac conduction intervals, particularly QTc. These include patients taking diuretics with potential for inducing electrolyte abnormalities).
No products indexed under this heading.

Mexiletine Hydrochloride (Dolasetron should be administered with caution in patients who have or may develop prolongation of cardiac conduction intervals, particularly QTc. These include patients taking anti-arrhythmic drugs).
No products indexed under this heading.

Midazolam Hydrochloride (Dolasetron should be administered with caution in patients who have or may develop prolongation of cardiac conduction intervals, particularly QTc. These include patients taking drugs which lead to QT prolongation).
No products indexed under this heading.

Molindone Hydrochloride (Dolasetron should be administered with caution in patients who have or may develop prolongation of cardiac conduction intervals, particularly QTc. These include patients taking drugs which lead to QT prolongation). Products include:
Moban 1108

Moricizine Hydrochloride (Dolasetron should be administered with caution in patients who have or may develop prolongation of cardiac conduction intervals, particularly QTc. These include patients taking anti-arrhythmic drugs).
No products indexed under this heading.

Nortriptyline Hydrochloride (Dolasetron should be administered with caution in patients who have or may develop prolongation of cardiac conduction intervals, particularly QTc. These include patients taking drugs which lead to QT prolongation).
No products indexed under this heading.

Olanzapine (Dolasetron should be administered with caution in patients who have or may develop prolongation of cardiac conduction intervals, particularly QTc. These include patients taking drugs which lead to QT prolongation).
Products include:
Symbyax 1965
Zyprexa 1984
Zyprexa IntraMuscular 1984
Zyprexa ZYDIS 1984

Oxazepam (Dolasetron should be administered with caution in patients who have or may develop prolongation of cardiac conduction intervals, particularly QTc. These include patients taking drugs which lead to QT prolongation).
No products indexed under this heading.

Perphenazine (Dolasetron should be administered with caution in patients who have or may develop prolongation of cardiac conduction intervals, particularly QTc. These include patients taking drugs which lead to QT prolongation).
No products indexed under this heading.

Phenelzine Sulfate (Dolasetron should be administered with caution in patients who have or may develop prolongation of cardiac conduction intervals, particularly QTc. These include patients taking drugs which lead to QT prolongation).
No products indexed under this heading.

Polythiazide (Dolasetron should be administered with caution in patients who have or may develop prolongation of cardiac conduction intervals, particularly QTc. These include patients taking diuretics with potential for inducing electrolyte abnormalities).
No products indexed under this heading.

Prazepam (Dolasetron should be administered with caution in patients who have or may develop prolongation of cardiac conduction intervals, particularly QTc. These include patients taking drugs which lead to QT prolongation).
No products indexed under this heading.

Procainamide Hydrochloride (Dolasetron should be administered with caution in patients who have or may develop prolongation of cardiac conduction intervals, particularly QTc. These include patients taking anti-arrhythmic drugs).
No products indexed under this heading.

Prochlorperazine (Dolasetron should be administered with caution in patients who have or may develop prolongation of cardiac conduction intervals, particularly QTc. These include patients taking drugs which lead to QT prolongation).
No products indexed under this heading.

Promethazine Hydrochloride (Dolasetron should be administered with caution in patients who have or may develop prolongation of cardiac conduction intervals, particularly QTc. These include patients taking drugs which lead to QT prolongation).
No products indexed under this heading.

Propafenone Hydrochloride (Dolasetron should be administered with caution in patients who have or may develop prolongation of cardiac conduction intervals, particularly QTc. These include patients taking anti-arrhythmic drugs). Products include:
Rythmol 1648
Rythmol SR 1652

Propranolol Hydrochloride (Dolasetron should be administered with caution in patients who have or may develop prolongation of cardiac conduction intervals, particularly QTc. These include patients taking anti-arrhythmic drugs). Products include:
InnoPran XL 1517

Protriptyline Hydrochloride (Dolasetron should be administered with caution in patients who have or may develop prolongation of cardiac conduction intervals, particularly QTc. These include patients taking drugs which lead to QT prolongation).
No products indexed under this heading.

Quetiapine Fumarate (Dolasetron should be administered with caution in patients who have or may develop prolongation of cardiac conduction inter-

IMPORTANT NOTE: Always consult each drug listing in the patient's regimen for possible interactions.

(⊙ Described in PDR® for Ophthalmic Medicines)

Chlorpromazine (Phenothiazine derivatives may reduce the blood glucose-lowering effect of insulin).
　No products indexed under this heading.

Chlorpromazine Hydrochloride (Phenothiazine derivatives may reduce the blood glucose-lowering effect of insulin).
　No products indexed under this heading.

Chlorpropamide (Sulfonamide antibiotics may increase the blood glucose-lowering effect and susceptibility to hypoglycemia of insulin).
　No products indexed under this heading.

Chlorthalidone (Diuretics may reduce the blood glucose-lowering effect of insulin). Products include:

Choline Magnesium Trisalicylate (Salicylates may increase the blood glucose-lowering effect and susceptibility to hypoglycemia of insulin).
　No products indexed under this heading.

Ciclesonide (Corticosteroids may reduce the blood glucose-lowering effect of insulin).
　No products indexed under this heading.

Clofibrate (Fibrates may increase the blood glucose-lowering effect and susceptibility to hypoglycemia of insulin).
　No products indexed under this heading.

Clonidine (Clonidine may either potentiate or weaken the blood glucose-lowering effect of insulin and reduce or hide the signs of hypoglycemia). Products include:

Clonidine Hydrochloride (Clonidine may either potentiate or weaken the blood glucose-lowering effect of insulin and reduce or hide the signs of hypoglycemia). Products include:

Clozapine (Atypical antipsychotics may reduce the blood glucose-lowering effect of insulin).
　No products indexed under this heading.

Cortisone Acetate (Corticosteroids may reduce the blood glucose-lowering effect of insulin).
　No products indexed under this heading.

Danazol (Danazol may reduce the blood glucose-lowering effect of insulin).
　No products indexed under this heading.

Darunavir (Protease inhibitors may reduce the blood glucose-lowering effect of insulin).
　No products indexed under this heading.

Desogestrel (Progestogens may reduce the blood glucose-lowering effect of insulin).
　No products indexed under this heading.

Desoximetasone (Corticosteroids may reduce the blood glucose-lowering effect of insulin).
　No products indexed under this heading.

Dexamethasone (Corticosteroids may reduce the blood glucose-lowering effect of insulin). Products include:

Dexamethasone Acetate (Corticosteroids may reduce the blood glucose-lowering effect of insulin).
　No products indexed under this heading.

Dexamethasone Phosphate (Corticosteroids may reduce the blood glucose-lowering effect of insulin).
　No products indexed under this heading.

Dexamethasone Sodium (Corticosteroids may reduce the blood glucose-lowering effect of insulin).
　No products indexed under this heading.

Dexamethasone Sodium Phosphate (Corticosteroids may reduce the blood glucose-lowering effect of insulin).
　No products indexed under this heading.

Dexamethasone Sodium Phosphate Injection (Corticosteroids may reduce the blood glucose-lowering effect of insulin).
　No products indexed under this heading.

Dienestrol (Estrogens may reduce the blood glucose-lowering effect of insulin).
　No products indexed under this heading.

Diethylstilbestrol (Estrogens may reduce the blood glucose-lowering effect of insulin).
　No products indexed under this heading.

Diflorasone Diacetate (Corticosteroids may reduce the blood glucose-lowering effect of insulin).
　No products indexed under this heading.

Diflunisal (Salicylates may increase the blood glucose-lowering effect and susceptibility to hypoglycemia of insulin).
　No products indexed under this heading.

Disopyramide (Disopyramide may increase the blood glucose-lowering effect and susceptibility to hypoglycemia of insulin).
　No products indexed under this heading.

Disopyramide Phosphate (Disopyramide may increase the blood glucose-lowering effect and susceptibility to hypoglycemia of insulin).
　No products indexed under this heading.

Dobutamine Hydrochloride (Sympathomimetic agents may reduce the blood glucose-lowering effect of insulin).
　No products indexed under this heading.

Dopamine Hydrochloride (Sympathomimetic agents may reduce the blood glucose-lowering effect of insulin).
　No products indexed under this heading.

Enalapril Maleate (ACE inhibitors may increase the blood glucose-lowering effect and susceptibility to hypoglycemia of insulin).
　No products indexed under this heading.

Enalaprilat (ACE inhibitors may increase the blood glucose-lowering effect and susceptibility to hypoglycemia of insulin).
　No products indexed under this heading.

Ephedrine Hydrochloride (Sympathomimetic agents may reduce the blood glucose-lowering effect of insulin).
　No products indexed under this heading.

Ephedrine Sulfate (Sympathomimetic agents may reduce the blood glucose-lowering effect of insulin).
　No products indexed under this heading.

Ephedrine Tannate (Sympathomimetic agents may reduce the blood glucose-lowering effect of insulin).
　No products indexed under this heading.

Epinephrine (Sympathomimetic agents may reduce the blood glucose-lowering effect of insulin). Products include:

Epinephrine Bitartrate (Sympathomimetic agents may reduce the blood glucose-lowering effect of insulin).
　No products indexed under this heading.

Epinephrine Hydrochloride (Sympathomimetic agents may reduce the blood glucose-lowering effect of insulin).
　No products indexed under this heading.

Esmolol Hydrochloride (Beta-blockers may either potentiate or weaken the blood glucose-lowering effect of insulin and reduce or hide the signs of hypoglycemia).
　No products indexed under this heading.

Estradiol (Estrogens may reduce the blood glucose-lowering effect of insulin). Products include:

Estrogens, Conjugated (Estrogens may reduce the blood glucose-lowering effect of insulin). Products include:

Estrogens, Esterified (Estrogens may reduce the blood glucose-lowering effect of insulin).
　No products indexed under this heading.

Estropipate (Estrogens may reduce the blood glucose-lowering effect of insulin).
　No products indexed under this heading.

Ethacrynic Acid (Diuretics may reduce the blood glucose-lowering effect of insulin).
　No products indexed under this heading.

Ethanol (Alcohol may either potentiate or weaken the blood glucose-lowering effect of insulin).
　No products indexed under this heading.

Ethinyl Estradiol (Estrogens may reduce the blood glucose-lowering effect of insulin). Products include:

Ethyl Alcohol (Alcohol may either potentiate or weaken the blood glucose-lowering effect of insulin).
　No products indexed under this heading.

Ethynodiol Diacetate (Progestogens (eg, oral contraceptives) may reduce the blood glucose-lowering effect of insulin).
　No products indexed under this heading.

Fenofibrate (Fibrates may increase the blood glucose-lowering effect and susceptibility to hypoglycemia of insulin). Products include:

Fludrocortisone Acetate (Corticosteroids may reduce the blood glucose-lowering effect of insulin).
　No products indexed under this heading.

Flumethasone Pivalate (Corticosteroids may reduce the blood glucose-lowering effect of insulin).
　No products indexed under this heading.

Flunisolide Hemihydrate (Corticosteroids may reduce the blood glucose-lowering effect of insulin).
　No products indexed under this heading.

Fluoxetine (Fluoxetine may increase the blood glucose-lowering effect and susceptibility to hypoglycemia of insulin).
　No products indexed under this heading.

Fluoxetine Hydrochloride (Fluoxetine may increase the blood glucose-lowering effect and susceptibility to hypoglycemia of insulin). Products include:

Fluphenazine Decanoate (Phenothiazine derivatives may reduce the blood glucose-lowering effect of insulin).
　No products indexed under this heading.

Fluphenazine Enanthate (Phenothiazine derivatives may reduce the blood glucose-lowering effect of insulin).
　No products indexed under this heading.

Fluphenazine Hydrochloride (Phenothiazine derivatives may reduce the blood glucose-lowering effect of insulin).
　No products indexed under this heading.

Fluticasone Furoate (Corticosteroids may reduce the blood glucose-lowering effect of insulin). Products include:

Fluticasone Propionate (Corticosteroids may reduce the blood glucose-lowering effect of insulin). Products include:

Fosamprenavir Calcium (Protease inhibitors may reduce the blood glucose-lowering effect of insulin). Products include:

Fosinopril Sodium (ACE inhibitors may increase the blood glucose-lowering effect and susceptibility to hypoglycemia of insulin).
　No products indexed under this heading.

Furosemide (Diuretics may reduce the blood glucose-lowering effect of insulin). Products include:

Gemfibrozil (Fibrates may increase the blood glucose-lowering effect and susceptibility to hypoglycemia of insulin).
　No products indexed under this heading.

Glibenclamide (Oral antidiabetic products may increase the blood glucose-lowering effect and susceptibility to hypoglycemia of insulin).
　No products indexed under this heading.

Glimepiride (Oral antidiabetic products may increase the blood glucose-lowering effect and susceptibility to hypoglycemia of insulin). Products include:

Glipizide (Sulfonamide antibiotics may increase the blood glucose-lowering effect and susceptibility to hypoglycemia of insulin).
　No products indexed under this heading.

Glucagon (Glucagon may reduce the blood glucose-lowering effect of insulin). Products include:

Glyburide (Sulfonamide antibiotics may increase the blood glucose-lowering effect and susceptibility to hypoglycemia of insulin).
　No products indexed under this heading.

Guanethidine (Under the influence of sympatholytic medicinal products, such as guanethidine, the signs of hypoglycemia may be reduced or absent).
　No products indexed under this heading.

Guanethidine Monosulfate (Under the influence of sympatholytic medicinal products, such as guanethidine, the signs of hypoglycemia may be reduced or absent).
　No products indexed under this heading.

IMPORTANT NOTE: Always consult each drug listing in the patient's regimen for possible interactions.

Guanethidine Sulfate (Under the influence of sympatholytic medicinal products, such as guanethidine, the signs of hypoglycemia may be reduced or absent).
No products indexed under this heading.

Hydrochlorothiazide (Diuretics may reduce the blood glucose-lowering effect of insulin). Products include:

Atacand HCT	700
Avalide	2956
Benicar HCT	1017
Diovan HCT	2419
Dyazide	1429
Exforge HCT	2449
Hyzaar	2162
Hyzaar 100-12.5	2162
Micardis HCT	889
Prinzide	2246
Tekturna HCT	2541
Teveten HCT	541

Hydrocortisone (Corticosteroids may reduce the blood glucose-lowering effect of insulin).
No products indexed under this heading.

Hydrocortisone (Alcohol) (Corticosteroids may reduce the blood glucose-lowering effect of insulin).
No products indexed under this heading.

Hydrocortisone Acetate (Corticosteroids may reduce the blood glucose-lowering effect of insulin).
No products indexed under this heading.

Hydrocortisone Butyrate (Corticosteroids may reduce the blood glucose-lowering effect of insulin).
No products indexed under this heading.

Hydrocortisone Cypionate (Corticosteroids may reduce the blood glucose-lowering effect of insulin).
No products indexed under this heading.

Hydrocortisone Hemisuccinate (Corticosteroids may reduce the blood glucose-lowering effect of insulin).
No products indexed under this heading.

Hydrocortisone Probutate (Corticosteroids may reduce the blood glucose-lowering effect of insulin).
No products indexed under this heading.

Hydrocortisone Sodium Phosphate (Corticosteroids may reduce the blood glucose-lowering effect of insulin).
No products indexed under this heading.

Hydrocortisone Sodium Succinate (Corticosteroids may reduce the blood glucose-lowering effect of insulin).
No products indexed under this heading.

Hydrocortisone Valerate (Corticosteroids may reduce the blood glucose-lowering effect of insulin).
No products indexed under this heading.

Hydroflumethiazide (Diuretics may reduce the blood glucose-lowering effect of insulin).
No products indexed under this heading.

Indapamide (Diuretics may reduce the blood glucose-lowering effect of insulin). Products include:
Indapamide ... 2356

Indinavir Sulfate (Protease inhibitors may reduce the blood glucose-lowering effect of insulin). Products include:
Crixivan ... 2113

Isocarboxazid (MAO inhibitors may increase the blood glucose-lowering effect and susceptibility to hypoglycemia of insulin). Products include:
Marplan ... 3481

Isoniazid (Isoniazid may reduce the blood glucose-lowering effect of insulin).
No products indexed under this heading.

Isoproterenol Hydrochloride (Sympathomimetic agents may reduce the blood glucose-lowering effect of insulin).
No products indexed under this heading.

Isoproterenol Sulfate (Sympathomimetic agents may reduce the blood glucose-lowering effect of insulin).
No products indexed under this heading.

Labetalol Hydrochloride (Beta-blockers may either potentiate or weaken the blood glucose-lowering effect of insulin and reduce or hide the signs of hypoglycemia).
No products indexed under this heading.

Lanreotide (Somatostatin analogs may increase the blood glucose-lowering effect and susceptibility to hypoglycemia of insulin).
No products indexed under this heading.

Levalbuterol Hydrochloride (Sympathomimetic agents may reduce the blood glucose-lowering effect of insulin).
No products indexed under this heading.

Levobunolol Hydrochloride (Beta-blockers may either potentiate or weaken the blood glucose-lowering effect of insulin and reduce or hide the signs of hypoglycemia).
No products indexed under this heading.

Levonorgestrel (Progestogens (eg, oral contraceptives) may reduce the blood glucose-lowering effect of insulin). Products include:

Climara Pro	847
LoSeasonique	3407
Lybrel	3514
Mirena	854
Plan B	3416
Seasonique	3418

Levothyroxine Sodium (Thyroid hormones may reduce the blood glucose-lowering effect of insulin). Products include:

Levoxyl Tablets	1843
Synthroid	529

Liothyronine Sodium (Thyroid hormones may reduce the blood glucose-lowering effect of insulin). Products include:
Cytomel ... 1830

Liotrix (Thyroid hormones may reduce the blood glucose-lowering effect of insulin).
No products indexed under this heading.

Lisinopril (ACE inhibitors may increase the blood glucose-lowering effect and susceptibility to hypoglycemia of insulin). Products include:

Prinivil	2241
Prinzide	2246

Lithium (Lithium salts may either potentiate or weaken the blood-glucose-lowering effect of insulin).
No products indexed under this heading.

Lithium Carbonate (Lithium salts may either potentiate or weaken the blood-glucose-lowering effect of insulin).
No products indexed under this heading.

Lithium Citrate (Lithium salts may either potentiate or weaken the blood-glucose-lowering effect of insulin).
No products indexed under this heading.

Lopinavir (Protease inhibitors may reduce the blood glucose-lowering effect of insulin). Products include:
Kaletra ... 458

Magnesium Salicylate (Salicylates may increase the blood glucose-lowering effect and susceptibility to hypoglycemia of insulin).
No products indexed under this heading.

Medroxyprogesterone Acetate (Progestogens may reduce the blood glucose-lowering effect of insulin). Products include:

Premphase	3549
Prempro	3549

Megestrol Acetate (Progestogens may reduce the blood glucose-lowering effect of insulin). Products include:
Megace ES ... 2698

Mesoridazine Besylate (Phenothiazine derivatives may reduce the blood glucose-lowering effect of insulin).
No products indexed under this heading.

Mestranol (Progestogens (eg, oral contraceptives) may reduce the blood glucose-lowering effect of insulin).
No products indexed under this heading.

Metaproterenol Sulfate (Sympathomimetic agents may reduce the blood glucose-lowering effect of insulin).
No products indexed under this heading.

Metaraminol Bitartrate (Sympathomimetic agents may reduce the blood glucose-lowering effect of insulin).
No products indexed under this heading.

Metformin Hydrochloride (Oral antidiabetic products may increase the blood glucose-lowering effect and susceptibility to hypoglycemia of insulin). Products include:

ActoPlus	3338
Avandamet	1345
Janumet	2188

Methotrimeprazine (Phenothiazine derivatives may reduce the blood glucose-lowering effect of insulin).
No products indexed under this heading.

Methoxamine Hydrochloride (Sympathomimetic agents may reduce the blood glucose-lowering effect of insulin).
No products indexed under this heading.

Methyclothiazide (Diuretics may reduce the blood glucose-lowering effect of insulin).
No products indexed under this heading.

Methylprednisolone (Corticosteroids may reduce the blood glucose-lowering effect of insulin).
No products indexed under this heading.

Methylprednisolone Acetate (Corticosteroids may reduce the blood glucose-lowering effect of insulin).
No products indexed under this heading.

Methylprednisolone Sodium Succinate (Corticosteroids may reduce the blood glucose-lowering effect of insulin).
No products indexed under this heading.

Metipranolol Hydrochloride (Beta-blockers may either potentiate or weaken the blood glucose-lowering effect of insulin and reduce or hide the signs of hypoglycemia).
No products indexed under this heading.

Metolazone (Diuretics may reduce the blood glucose-lowering effect of insulin).
No products indexed under this heading.

Metoprolol Succinate (Beta-blockers may either potentiate or weaken the blood glucose-lowering effect of insulin and reduce or hide the signs of hypoglycemia). Products include:
Toprol XL ... 732

Metoprolol Tartrate (Beta-blockers may either potentiate or weaken the blood glucose-lowering effect of insulin and reduce or hide the signs of hypoglycemia).
No products indexed under this heading.

Miglitol (Oral antidiabetic products may increase the blood glucose-lowering effect and susceptibility to hypoglycemia of insulin).
No products indexed under this heading.

Moclobemide (MAO inhibitors may increase the blood glucose-lowering effect and susceptibility to hypoglycemia of insulin).
No products indexed under this heading.

Moexipril Hydrochloride (ACE inhibitors may increase the blood glucose-lowering effect and susceptibility to hypoglycemia of insulin).
No products indexed under this heading.

Mometasone Furoate (Corticosteroids may reduce the blood glucose-lowering effect of insulin). Products include:

Asmanex	3058
Elocon Cream	3111
Elocon Lotion	3112
Elocon Ointment	3114

Mometasone Furoate Monohydrate (Corticosteroids may reduce the blood glucose-lowering effect of insulin). Products include:
Nasonex ... 3166

Nadolol (Beta-blockers may either potentiate or weaken the blood glucose-lowering effect of insulin and reduce or hide the signs of hypoglycemia). Products include:
Nadolol ... 2359

Nateglinide (Oral antidiabetic products may increase the blood glucose-lowering effect and susceptibility to hypoglycemia of insulin).
No products indexed under this heading.

Nebivolol (Beta-blockers may either potentiate or weaken the blood glucose-lowering effect of insulin and reduce or hide the signs of hypoglycemia). Products include:
Bystolic ... 1147

Nelfinavir Mesylate (Protease inhibitors may reduce the blood glucose-lowering effect of insulin).
No products indexed under this heading.

Niacin (Niacin may reduce the blood glucose-lowering effect of insulin). Products include:

Advicor	402
Cardio Basics	3455
Niaspan	497
Simcor	524

Norepinephrine Bitartrate (Sympathomimetic agents may reduce the blood glucose-lowering effect of insulin).
No products indexed under this heading.

Norethindrone (Progestogens may reduce the blood glucose-lowering effect of insulin). Products include:
Ortho Micronor ... 2660

Norethindrone Acetate (Progestogens may reduce the blood glucose-lowering effect of insulin). Products include:
Activella ... 2561

Norethynodrel (Progestogens (eg, oral contraceptives) may reduce the blood glucose-lowering effect of insulin).
No products indexed under this heading.

Norgestimate (Progestogens may reduce the blood glucose-lowering effect of insulin). Products include:

Ortho-Cyclen/Ortho Tri-Cyclen	2663
Ortho Tri-Cyclen Lo Tablets	2673

Norgestrel (Progestogens (eg, oral contraceptives) may reduce the blood glucose-lowering effect of insulin).
No products indexed under this heading.

Octreotide Acetate (Somatostatin analogs may increase the blood glucose-lowering effect and susceptibility to hypoglycemia of insulin). Products include:

Sandostatin	2517
Sandostatin LAR	2519

Olanzapine (Atypical antipsychotics may reduce the blood glucose-lowering effect of insulin). Products include:

Symbyax	1965
Zyprexa	1984
Zyprexa IntraMuscular	1984
Zyprexa ZYDIS	1984

Pargyline Hydrochloride (MAO inhibitors may increase the blood glucose-lowering effect and susceptibility to hypoglycemia of insulin).
No products indexed under this heading.

121 **Interactions Index** **Apidra**

Penbutolol Sulfate (Beta-blockers may either potentiate or weaken the blood glucose-lowering effect of insulin and reduce or hide the signs of hypoglycemia).
No products indexed under this heading.

Pentamidine Isethionate (Pentamidine may cause hypoglycemia, which may sometimes be followed by hyperglycemia).
No products indexed under this heading.

Pentoxifylline (Pentoxifylline may increase the blood glucose-lowering effect and susceptibility to hypoglycemia of insulin).
No products indexed under this heading.

Perindopril Erbumine (ACE inhibitors may increase the blood glucose-lowering effect and susceptibility to hypoglycemia of insulin).
No products indexed under this heading.

Perphenazine (Phenothiazine derivatives may reduce the blood glucose-lowering effect of insulin).
No products indexed under this heading.

Phenelzine Sulfate (MAO inhibitors may increase the blood glucose-lowering effect and susceptibility to hypoglycemia of insulin).
No products indexed under this heading.

Phenothiazine Derivatives (Phenothiazine derivatives may reduce the blood glucose-lowering effect of insulin).
No products indexed under this heading.

Phenothiazines (Phenothiazine derivatives may reduce the blood glucose-lowering effect of insulin).
No products indexed under this heading.

Phenylephrine Bitartrate (Sympathomimetic agents may reduce the blood glucose-lowering effect of insulin).
No products indexed under this heading.

Phenylephrine Hydrochloride (Sympathomimetic agents may reduce the blood glucose-lowering effect of insulin). Products include:
- Sudafed PE Nasal Decongestant 2048
- Children's Sudafed PE Nasal Decongestant 2047

Phenylephrine Tannate (Sympathomimetic agents may reduce the blood glucose-lowering effect of insulin).
No products indexed under this heading.

Phenylpropanolamine Hydrochloride (Sympathomimetic agents may reduce the blood glucose-lowering effect of insulin).
No products indexed under this heading.

Pindolol (Beta-blockers may either potentiate or weaken the blood glucose-lowering effect of insulin and reduce or hide the signs of hypoglycemia).
No products indexed under this heading.

Pioglitazone Hydrochloride (Oral antidiabetic products may increase the blood glucose-lowering effect and susceptibility to hypoglycemia of insulin). Products include:
- ActoPlus 3338
- Actos 3345
- Duetact 3354

Pirbuterol Acetate (Sympathomimetic agents may reduce the blood glucose-lowering effect of insulin). Products include:
- Maxair Autohaler 1782

Polyestradiol Phosphate (Estrogens may reduce the blood glucose-lowering effect of insulin).
No products indexed under this heading.

Polythiazide (Diuretics may reduce the blood glucose-lowering effect of insulin).
No products indexed under this heading.

Pramlintide Acetate (Pramlintide may increase the blood glucose-lowering effect and susceptibility to hypoglycemia of insulin). Products include:
- Symlin 651
- SymlinPen 651

Prednisolone (Corticosteroids may reduce the blood glucose-lowering effect of insulin).
No products indexed under this heading.

Prednisolone Acetate (Corticosteroids may reduce the blood glucose-lowering effect of insulin). Products include:
- Blephamide ..... ⊙212, ⊙214
- Pred Forte ..... ⊙225
- Pred Mild ..... ⊙230
- Pred-G ..... ⊙226, ⊙227

Prednisolone Sodium Phosphate (Corticosteroids may reduce the blood glucose-lowering effect of insulin).
No products indexed under this heading.

Prednisolone Tebutate (Corticosteroids may reduce the blood glucose-lowering effect of insulin).
No products indexed under this heading.

Prednisone (Corticosteroids may reduce the blood glucose-lowering effect of insulin).
No products indexed under this heading.

Prednisone sodium phosphate (Corticosteroids may reduce the blood glucose-lowering effect of insulin).
No products indexed under this heading.

Procarbazine Hydrochloride (MAO inhibitors may increase the blood glucose-lowering effect and susceptibility to hypoglycemia of insulin).
No products indexed under this heading.

Prochlorperazine (Phenothiazine derivatives may reduce the blood glucose-lowering effect of insulin).
No products indexed under this heading.

Prochlorperazine Edisylate (Phenothiazine derivatives may reduce the blood glucose-lowering effect of insulin).
No products indexed under this heading.

Prochlorperazine Maleate (Phenothiazine derivatives may reduce the blood glucose-lowering effect of insulin).
No products indexed under this heading.

Promethazine (Phenothiazine derivatives may reduce the blood glucose-lowering effect of insulin).
No products indexed under this heading.

Promethazine Hydrochloride (Phenothiazine derivatives may reduce the blood glucose-lowering effect of insulin).
No products indexed under this heading.

Propoxyphene Hydrochloride (Propoxyphene may increase the blood glucose-lowering effect and susceptibility to hypoglycemia of insulin).
No products indexed under this heading.

Propoxyphene Napsylate (Propoxyphene may increase the blood glucose-lowering effect and susceptibility to hypoglycemia of insulin).
No products indexed under this heading.

Propranolol Hydrochloride (Beta-blockers may either potentiate or weaken the blood glucose-lowering effect of insulin and reduce or hide the signs of hypoglycemia). Products include:
- InnoPran XL 1517

Pseudoephedrine Hydrochloride (Sympathomimetic agents may reduce the blood glucose-lowering effect of insulin). Products include:
- Allegra-D 2915
- Allegra-D 24 2918
- Sudafed 12 Hour Nasal Decongestant Non-Drowsy 2048
- Sudafed 24 Hour 2048
- Sudafed Nasal Decongestant 2047
- Children's Sudafed Nasal Decongestant Liquid 2047
- Zyrtec-D Allergy & Congestion 2054

Pseudoephedrine Sulfate (Sympathomimetic agents may reduce the blood glucose-lowering effect of insulin). Products include:
- Clarinex-D 12-Hour 3101
- Clarinex-D 3104

Quetiapine Fumarate (Atypical antipsychotics may reduce the blood glucose-lowering effect of insulin). Products include:
- Seroquel 750
- Seroquel XR 759

Quinapril Hydrochloride (ACE inhibitors may increase the blood glucose-lowering effect and susceptibility to hypoglycemia of insulin).
No products indexed under this heading.

Quinestrol (Estrogens may reduce the blood glucose-lowering effect of insulin).
No products indexed under this heading.

Ramipril (ACE inhibitors may increase the blood glucose-lowering effect and susceptibility to hypoglycemia of insulin).
No products indexed under this heading.

Rasagiline Mesylate (MAO inhibitors may increase the blood glucose-lowering effect and susceptibility to hypoglycemia of insulin). Products include:
- Azilect 3383

Repaglinide (Oral antidiabetic products may increase the blood glucose-lowering effect and susceptibility to hypoglycemia of insulin).
No products indexed under this heading.

Reserpine (Under the influence of sympatholytic medicinal products, such as reserpine, the signs of hypoglycemia may be reduced or absent).
No products indexed under this heading.

Risperidone (Atypical antipsychotics may reduce the blood glucose-lowering effect of insulin). Products include:
- Risperdal Consta 2682

Ritonavir (Protease inhibitors may reduce the blood glucose-lowering effect of insulin). Products include:
- Kaletra 458
- Norvir 509

Rosiglitazone Maleate (Oral antidiabetic products may increase the blood glucose-lowering effect and susceptibility to hypoglycemia of insulin). Products include:
- Avandamet 1345
- Avandaryl 1356
- Avandia 1366

Salmeterol Xinafoate (Sympathomimetic agents may reduce the blood glucose-lowering effect of insulin). Products include:
- Advair 100/50 1275
- Advair 250/50 1275
- Advair 500/50 1275
- Advair HFA 45/21 1288
- Advair HFA 115/21 1288
- Advair HFA 230/21 1288
- Serevent Diskus 1656

Salsalate (Salicylates may increase the blood glucose-lowering effect and susceptibility to hypoglycemia of insulin).
No products indexed under this heading.

Saquinavir (Protease inhibitors may reduce the blood glucose-lowering effect of insulin).
No products indexed under this heading.

Saquinavir Mesylate (Protease inhibitors may reduce the blood glucose-lowering effect of insulin).
No products indexed under this heading.

Selegiline (MAO inhibitors may increase the blood glucose-lowering effect and susceptibility to hypoglycemia of insulin). Products include:
- Emsam 3623

Selegiline Hydrochloride (MAO inhibitors may increase the blood glucose-lowering effect and susceptibility to hypoglycemia of insulin). Products include:
- Eldepryl 3312

Sitagliptin Phosphate (Oral antidiabetic products may increase the blood glucose-lowering effect and susceptibility to hypoglycemia of insulin). Products include:
- Janumet 2188
- Januvia 2196

Somatropin (Somatropin may reduce the blood glucose-lowering effect of insulin). Products include:
- Nutropin 1204
- Nutropin AQ 1209
- Nutropin AQ NuSpin 1209
- Nutropin AQ Pen 1209
- Nutropin AQ Pen Cartridge 1209

Sotalol Hydrochloride (Beta-blockers may either potentiate or weaken the blood glucose-lowering effect of insulin and reduce or hide the signs of hypoglycemia).
No products indexed under this heading.

Spirapril Hydrochloride (ACE inhibitors may increase the blood glucose-lowering effect and susceptibility to hypoglycemia of insulin).
No products indexed under this heading.

Spironolactone (Diuretics may reduce the blood glucose-lowering effect of insulin).
No products indexed under this heading.

Sulfacytine (Sulfonamide antibiotics may increase the blood glucose-lowering effect and susceptibility to hypoglycemia of insulin).
No products indexed under this heading.

Sulfamethizole (Sulfonamide antibiotics may increase the blood glucose-lowering effect and susceptibility to hypoglycemia of insulin).
No products indexed under this heading.

Sulfamethoxazole (Sulfonamide antibiotics may increase the blood glucose-lowering effect and susceptibility to hypoglycemia of insulin).
No products indexed under this heading.

Sulfasalazine (Sulfonamide antibiotics may increase the blood glucose-lowering effect and susceptibility to hypoglycemia of insulin).
No products indexed under this heading.

Sulfinpyrazone (Sulfonamide antibiotics may increase the blood glucose-lowering effect and susceptibility to hypoglycemia of insulin).
No products indexed under this heading.

Sulfisoxazole Acetyl (Sulfonamide antibiotics may increase the blood glucose-lowering effect and susceptibility to hypoglycemia of insulin).
No products indexed under this heading.

Sulfisoxazole Diolamine (Sulfonamide antibiotics may increase the blood glucose-lowering effect and susceptibility to hypoglycemia of insulin).
No products indexed under this heading.

Terbutaline Sulfate (Sympathomimetic agents may reduce the blood glucose-lowering effect of insulin).
No products indexed under this heading.

Thioridazine (Phenothiazine derivatives may reduce the blood glucose-lowering effect of insulin).
No products indexed under this heading.

Thioridazine Hydrochloride (Phenothiazine derivatives may reduce the blood glucose-lowering effect of insulin). Products include:
- Thioridazine Hydrochloride 2384

Thyroglobulin (Thyroid hormones may reduce the blood glucose-lowering effect of insulin).
No products indexed under this heading.

IMPORTANT NOTE: Always consult each drug listing in the patient's regimen for possible interactions.

Thyroid (Thyroid hormones may reduce the blood glucose-lowering effect of insulin). Products include:
Naturethroid 2830

Thyroxine (Thyroid hormones may reduce the blood glucose-lowering effect of insulin).
No products indexed under this heading.

Thyroxine Sodium (Thyroid hormones may reduce the blood glucose-lowering effect of insulin).
No products indexed under this heading.

Timolol Hemihydrate (Beta-blockers may either potentiate or weaken the blood glucose-lowering effect of insulin and reduce or hide the signs of hypoglycemia). Products include:
Betimol 3490

Timolol Maleate (Beta-blockers may either potentiate or weaken the blood glucose-lowering effect of insulin and reduce or hide the signs of hypoglycemia). Products include:
Combigan 601
Dorzolamide Hydrochloride/Timolol Maleate Ophthalmic Solution .... ⊙243
Timoptic in Ocudose .... ⊙231

Tipranavir (Protease inhibitors may reduce the blood glucose-lowering effect of insulin).
No products indexed under this heading.

Tolazamide (Sulfonamide antibiotics may increase the blood glucose-lowering effect and susceptibility to hypoglycemia of insulin).
No products indexed under this heading.

Tolbutamide (Sulfonamide antibiotics may increase the blood glucose-lowering effect and susceptibility to hypoglycemia of insulin).
No products indexed under this heading.

Torsemide (Diuretics may reduce the blood glucose-lowering effect of insulin).
No products indexed under this heading.

Trandolapril (ACE inhibitors may increase the blood glucose-lowering effect and susceptibility to hypoglycemia of insulin). Products include:
Mavik 489
Tarka 534

Tranylcypromine Sulfate (MAO inhibitors may increase the blood glucose-lowering effect and susceptibility to hypoglycemia of insulin). Products include:
Parnate 1584

Triamcinolone (Corticosteroids may reduce the blood glucose-lowering effect of insulin).
No products indexed under this heading.

Triamcinolone Acetonide (Corticosteroids may reduce the blood glucose-lowering effect of insulin). Products include:
Azmacort 408
Nasacort AQ 3019

Triamcinolone Diacetate (Corticosteroids may reduce the blood glucose-lowering effect of insulin).
No products indexed under this heading.

Triamcinolone Hexacetonide (Corticosteroids may reduce the blood glucose-lowering effect of insulin).
No products indexed under this heading.

Triamterene (Diuretics may reduce the blood glucose-lowering effect of insulin). Products include:
Dyazide 1429
Dyrenium 3495

Trifluoperazine Hydrochloride (Phenothiazine derivatives may reduce the blood glucose-lowering effect of insulin).
No products indexed under this heading.

Troglitazone (Oral antidiabetic products may increase the blood glucose-lowering effect and susceptibility to hypoglycemia of insulin).
No products indexed under this heading.

Ziprasidone Hydrochloride (Atypical antipsychotics may reduce the blood glucose-lowering effect of insulin). Products include:
Geodon 2723

Ziprasidone Mesylate (Atypical antipsychotics may reduce the blood glucose-lowering effect of insulin). Products include:
Geodon 2723

Food Interactions

Alcohol (Alcohol may either potentiate or weaken the blood glucose-lowering effect of insulin).

Beer, reduced-alcohol (Alcohol may either potentiate or weaken the blood glucose-lowering effect of insulin).

Beer, unspecified (Alcohol may either potentiate or weaken the blood glucose-lowering effect of insulin).

Wine, Chianti (Alcohol may either potentiate or weaken the blood glucose-lowering effect of insulin).

Wine, Red (Alcohol may either potentiate or weaken the blood glucose-lowering effect of insulin).

Wine, unspecified (Alcohol may either potentiate or weaken the blood glucose-lowering effect of insulin).

Wine products (Alcohol may either potentiate or weaken the blood glucose-lowering effect of insulin).

APIDRA SOLOSTAR INJECTION

(Insulin Glulisine) 2937
See Apidra Injection

APLENZIN EXTENDED-RELEASE TABLETS

(Bupropion Hydrochloride) 2948

May interact with alcohols, anorexiants, antidepressant drugs, antipsychotic agents, benzodiazepines, beta-blockers, central nervous system stimulants, class IC antiarrhythmics, corticosteroids, cytochrome p450 2b6 inhibitors (selected), cytochrome p450 2b6 substrates (selected), cytochrome p450 2d6 substrates (selected), drugs which lower seizure threshold, haloperidols, hepatic microsomal enzyme inducers, hypnotics and sedatives, insulin, monoamine oxidase inhibitors, narcotic analgesics, oral hypoglycemic agents, phenytoin, theophyllines, and certain other agents. Compounds in these categories include:

Acarbose (Concomitant use of oral hypoglycemics with bupropion is associated with an increased seizure risk).
No products indexed under this heading.

Acebutolol Hydrochloride (Co-administration of bupropion with drugs that are metabolized by the CYP2D6 isoenzyme including beta-blockers (eg, metoprolol) should be approached with caution and should be initiated at the lower end of the dose range of the concomitant medication. If bupropion is added to the treatment regimen of a patient already receiving a drug metabolized by CYP2D6, the need to decrease the dose of the original medication should be considered, particularly for those concomitant medications with a narrow therapeutic index).
No products indexed under this heading.

Alclometasone Dipropionate (Concurrent administration of bupropion and agents that lower seizure threshold, such as systemic steroids, should be undertaken with extreme caution. Low initial dosing and gradual dose increases should be employed).
No products indexed under this heading.

Alfentanil Hydrochloride (Concomitant use of opiates, cocaine, or stimulants with bupropion is associated with an increased seizure risk).
No products indexed under this heading.

Allium sativum (Bupropion may be an inducer of drug-metabolizing enzymes in humans. In one study, following chronic administration of bupropion hydrochloride, 100 mg 3 times daily to 8 healthy male volunteers for 14 days, there was no evidence of induction of its own metabolism. Nevertheless, there may be the potential for clinically important alterations of blood levels of co-administered drugs).
No products indexed under this heading.

Alprazolam (Bupropion is contraindicated in patients undergoing abrupt discontinuation of benzodiazepine sedatives. Concomitant use of benzodiazepine sedatives with bupropion is associated with an increased seizure risk).
No products indexed under this heading.

Amantadine Hydrochloride (Limited clinical data suggest a higher incidence of adverse experiences in patients receiving bupropion concurrently with amantadine. Administration of bupropion tablets to patients receiving amantadine concurrently should be undertaken with caution, using small initial doses and gradual dose increases).
No products indexed under this heading.

Aminoglutethimide (Bupropion may be an inducer of drug-metabolizing enzymes in humans. In one study, following chronic administration of bupropion hydrochloride, 100 mg 3 times daily to 8 healthy male volunteers for 14 days, there was no evidence of induction of its own metabolism. Nevertheless, there may be the potential for clinically important alterations of blood levels of co-administered drugs).
No products indexed under this heading.

Amiodarone Hydrochloride (Because bupropion is extensively metabolized, the co-administration of other drugs may affect its clinical activity. *In vitro* studies indicate that bupropion is primarily metabolized to hydroxybupropion by the CYP2B6 isoenzyme. Therefore, the potential exists for a drug interaction between bupropion and drugs that are substrates or inhibitors of the CYP2B6 isoenzyme (eg, orphenadrine, thiotepa, and cyclophosphamide). In addition, *in vitro* studies suggest that paroxetine, sertraline, norfluoxetine, and fluvoxamine as well as nelfinavir, ritonavir, and efavirenz inhibit the hydroxylation of bupropion).
No products indexed under this heading.

Amitriptyline Hydrochloride (Concurrent administration of bupropion and agents that lower seizure threshold should be undertaken with extreme caution. Low initial dosing and gradual dose increases should be employed).
No products indexed under this heading.

Amlodipine Besylate (Because bupropion is extensively metabolized, the co-administration of other drugs may affect its clinical activity. *In vitro* studies indicate that bupropion is primarily metabolized to hydroxybupropion by the CYP2B6 isoenzyme. Therefore, the potential exists for a drug interaction between bupropion and drugs that are substrates or inhibitors of the CYP2B6 isoenzyme (eg, orphenadrine, thiotepa, and cyclophosphamide). In addition, *in vitro* studies suggest that paroxetine, sertraline, norfluoxetine, and fluvoxamine as well as nelfinavir, ritonavir, and efavirenz inhibit the hydroxylation of bupropion). Products include:
Azor 1010
Exforge 2443
Exforge HCT 2449

Amoxapine (Concurrent administration of bupropion and agents that lower seizure threshold should be undertaken with extreme caution. Low initial dosing and gradual dose increases should be employed).
No products indexed under this heading.

Amphetamine Aspartate (Concomitant use of opiates, cocaine, or stimulants with bupropion is associated with an increased seizure risk).
No products indexed under this heading.

Amphetamine Aspartate Monohydrate (Concomitant use of opiates, cocaine, or stimulants with bupropion is associated with an increased seizure risk).
No products indexed under this heading.

Amphetamine Resins (Concomitant use of opiates, cocaine, or stimulants with bupropion is associated with an increased seizure risk).
No products indexed under this heading.

Amphetamine Sulfate (Concomitant use of opiates, cocaine, or stimulants with bupropion is associated with an increased seizure risk).
No products indexed under this heading.

Apomorphine (Concomitant use of opiates, cocaine, or stimulants with bupropion is associated with an increased seizure risk).
No products indexed under this heading.

Apomorphine Hydrochloride (Concomitant use of opiates, cocaine, or stimulants with bupropion is associated with an increased seizure risk).
No products indexed under this heading.

Aprepitant (Bupropion may be an inducer of drug-metabolizing enzymes in humans. In one study, following chronic administration of bupropion hydrochloride, 100 mg 3 times daily to 8 healthy male volunteers for 14 days, there was no evidence of induction of its own metabolism. Nevertheless, there may be the potential for clinically important alterations of blood levels of co-administered drugs). Products include:
Emend 2124

Aripiprazole (Concurrent administration of bupropion and agents that lower seizure threshold, such as antipsychotics, should be undertaken with extreme caution. Low initial dosing and gradual dose increases should be employed. Co-administration of bupropion with drugs that are metabolized by the CYP2D6 isoenzyme including antipsychotics (eg, haloperidol, risperidone, thioridazine) should be approached with caution and should be initiated at the lower end of the dose range of the concomitant medication. If bupropion is added to the treatment regimen of a patient already receiving a drug metabolized by CYP2D6, the need to decrease the dose of the original medication should be considered, particularly for those concomitant medications with a narrow therapeutic index).
No products indexed under this heading.

Atenolol (Co-administration of bupropion with drugs that are metabolized by the CYP2D6 isoenzyme including beta-blockers (eg, metoprolol) should be approached with caution and should be initiated at the lower end of the dose range of the concomitant medication. If bupropion is added to the treatment regimen of a patient already receiving a drug metabolized by CYP2D6, the need

(⊙ Described in PDR® for Ophthalmic Medicines)

123 Interactions Index Aplenzin

to decrease the dose of the original medication should be considered, particularly for those concomitant medications with a narrow therapeutic index).
No products indexed under this heading.

Atomoxetine Hydrochloride (Co-administration of bupropion with drugs that are metabolized by the CYP2D6 isoenzyme should be approached with caution and should be initiated at the lower end of the dose range of the concomitant medication. If bupropion is added to the treatment regimen of a patient already receiving a drug metabolized by CYP2D6, the need to decrease the dose of the original medication should be considered, particularly for those concomitant medications with a narrow therapeutic index).
Products include:
Strattera 1957

Azelastine Hydrochloride (Because bupropion is extensively metabolized, the co-administration of other drugs may affect its clinical activity. *In vitro* studies indicate that bupropion is primarily metabolized to hydroxybupropion by the CYP2B6 isoenzyme. Therefore, the potential exists for a drug interaction between bupropion and drugs that are substrates or inhibitors of the CYP2B6 isoenzyme (eg, orphenadrine, thiotepa, and cyclophosphamide). In addition, *in vitro* studies suggest that paroxetine, sertraline, norfluoxetine, and fluvoxamine as well as nelfinavir, ritonavir, and efavirenz inhibit the hydroxylation of bupropion).
No products indexed under this heading.

Beclomethasone Dipropionate (Concurrent administration of bupropion and agents that lower seizure threshold, such as systemic steroids, should be undertaken with extreme caution. Low initial dosing and gradual dose increases should be employed).
Products include:
Qvar 3398

Beclomethasone Dipropionate Monohydrate (Concurrent administration of bupropion and agents that lower seizure threshold, such as systemic steroids, should be undertaken with extreme caution. Low initial dosing and gradual dose increases should be employed). Products include:
Beconase AQ 1386

Benzphetamine Hydrochloride (Concomitant use of anorectics with bupropion is associated with an increased seizure risk).
No products indexed under this heading.

Betamethasone (Concurrent administration of bupropion and agents that lower seizure threshold, such as systemic steroids, should be undertaken with extreme caution. Low initial dosing and gradual dose increases should be employed).
No products indexed under this heading.

Betamethasone Acetate (Concurrent administration of bupropion and agents that lower seizure threshold, such as systemic steroids, should be undertaken with extreme caution. Low initial dosing and gradual dose increases should be employed).
No products indexed under this heading.

Betamethasone Benzoate (Concurrent administration of bupropion and agents that lower seizure threshold, such as systemic steroids, should be undertaken with extreme caution. Low initial dosing and gradual dose increases should be employed).
No products indexed under this heading.

Betamethasone Dipropionate (Concurrent administration of bupropion and agents that lower seizure threshold, such as systemic steroids, should be undertaken with extreme caution. Low initial dosing and gradual dose increases should be employed).
Products include:
Diprolene Lotion 0.05% 3108
Diprolene Ointment 0.05% 3109
Diprolene AF Cream 0.05% 3107
Lotrisone 3163

Betamethasone Sodium Phosphate (Concurrent administration of bupropion and agents that lower seizure threshold, such as systemic steroids, should be undertaken with extreme caution. Low initial dosing and gradual dose increases should be employed).
No products indexed under this heading.

Betamethasone Valerate (Concurrent administration of bupropion and agents that lower seizure threshold, such as systemic steroids, should be undertaken with extreme caution. Low initial dosing and gradual dose increases should be employed).
Products include:
Luxíq 3321

Betaxolol Hydrochloride (Co-administration of bupropion with drugs that are metabolized by the CYP2D6 isoenzyme including beta-blockers (eg, metoprolol) should be approached with caution and should be initiated at the lower end of the dose range of the concomitant medication. If bupropion is added to the treatment regimen of a patient already receiving a drug metabolized by CYP2D6, the need to decrease the dose of the original medication should be considered, particularly for those concomitant medications with a narrow therapeutic index).
No products indexed under this heading.

Bisoprolol Fumarate (Co-administration of bupropion with drugs that are metabolized by the CYP2D6 isoenzyme should be approached with caution and should be initiated at the lower end of the dose range of the concomitant medication. If bupropion is added to the treatment regimen of a patient already receiving a drug metabolized by CYP2D6, the need to decrease the dose of the original medication should be considered, particularly for those concomitant medications with a narrow therapeutic index).
No products indexed under this heading.

Bosentan (Bupropion may be an inducer of drug-metabolizing enzymes in humans. In one study, following chronic administration of bupropion hydrochloride, 100 mg 3 times daily to 8 healthy male volunteers for 14 days, there was no evidence of induction of its own metabolism. Nevertheless, there may be the potential for clinically important alterations of blood levels of co-administered drugs). Products include:
Tracleer 573

Budesonide (Concurrent administration of bupropion and agents that lower seizure threshold, such as systemic steroids, should be undertaken with extreme caution. Low initial dosing and gradual dose increases should be employed). Products include:
Pulmicort Flexhaler 714
Symbicort 80/4.5 720
Symbicort 160/4.5 720

Buprenorphine Hydrochloride (Concomitant use of opiates, cocaine, or stimulants with bupropion is associated with an increased seizure risk).
No products indexed under this heading.

Bupropion (Bupropion is contraindicated in patients treated with Zyban (bupropion hydrochloride) Sustained-Release Tablets; Wellbutrin (bupropion hydrochloride immediate-release formulation); Wellbutrin SR (bupropion hydrochloride sustained-release formulation); Wellbutrin XL (bupropion hydrochloride extended-release formulation); or any other medications that contain bupropion because the incidence of seizure is dose dependent. Patients should be made aware that bupropion contains the same active ingredient found in Zyban, used as an aid to smoking cessation treatment. Bupropion should not be used in combination with Zyban or any other medications that contain bupropion).
No products indexed under this heading.

Butabarbital (Bupropion is containdicated in patients undergoing abrupt discontinuation of sedatives. Concomitant use of sedatives with bupropion is associated with an increased seizure risk).
No products indexed under this heading.

Butabarbital Sodium (Bupropion is containdicated in patients undergoing abrupt discontinuation of sedatives. Concomitant use of sedatives with bupropion is associated with an increased seizure risk).
No products indexed under this heading.

Butalbital (Bupropion is containdicated in patients undergoing abrupt discontinuation of sedatives. Concomitant use of sedatives with bupropion is associated with an increased seizure risk).
No products indexed under this heading.

Captopril (Co-administration of bupropion with drugs that are metabolized by the CYP2D6 isoenzyme should be approached with caution and should be initiated at the lower end of the dose range of the concomitant medication. If bupropion is added to the treatment regimen of a patient already receiving a drug metabolized by CYP2D6, the need to decrease the dose of the original medication should be considered, particularly for those concomitant medications with a narrow therapeutic index).
Products include:
Captopril 2341

Carbamazepine (Carbamazepine may induce the metabolism of bupropion). Products include:
Carbatrol 3280
Equetro 3477

Carteolol Hydrochloride (Co-administration of bupropion with drugs that are metabolized by the CYP2D6 isoenzyme including beta-blockers (eg, metoprolol) should be approached with caution and should be initiated at the lower end of the dose range of the concomitant medication. If bupropion is added to the treatment regimen of a patient already receiving a drug metabolized by CYP2D6, the need to decrease the dose of the original medication should be considered, particularly for those concomitant medications with a narrow therapeutic index).
No products indexed under this heading.

Carvedilol (Co-administration of bupropion with drugs that are metabolized by the CYP2D6 isoenzyme should be approached with caution and should be initiated at the lower end of the dose range of the concomitant medication. If bupropion is added to the treatment regimen of a patient already receiving a drug metabolized by CYP2D6, the need to decrease the dose of the original medication should be considered, particularly for those concomitant medications with a narrow therapeutic index).
Products include:
Coreg 1409

Carvedilol Phosphate (Co-administration of bupropion with drugs that are metabolized by the CYP2D6 isoenzyme including beta-blockers (eg, metoprolol) should be approached with caution and should be initiated at the lower end of the dose range of the concomitant medication. If bupropion is added to the treatment regimen of a patient already receiving a drug metabolized by CYP2D6, the need to decrease the dose of the original medication should be considered, particularly for those concomitant medications with a narrow therapeutic index).
Products include:
Coreg CR 1416

Cevimeline Hydrochloride (Co-administration of bupropion with drugs that are metabolized by the CYP2D6 isoenzyme should be approached with caution and should be initiated at the lower end of the dose range of the concomitant medication. If bupropion is added to the treatment regimen of a patient already receiving a drug metabolized by CYP2D6, the need to decrease the dose of the original medication should be considered, particularly for those concomitant medications with a narrow therapeutic index).
Products include:
Evoxac 1027

Chloral Hydrate (Bupropion is containdicated in patients undergoing abrupt discontinuation of sedatives. Concomitant use of sedatives with bupropion is associated with an increased seizure risk).
No products indexed under this heading.

Chlordiazepoxide (Bupropion is contraindicated in patients undergoing abrupt discontinuation of benzodiazepine sedatives. Concomitant use of benzodiazepine sedatives with bupropion is associated with an increased seizure risk).
No products indexed under this heading.

Chlordiazepoxide Hydrochloride (Bupropion is contraindicated in patients undergoing abrupt discontinuation of benzodiazepine sedatives. Concomitant use of benzodiazepine sedatives with bupropion is associated with an increased seizure risk).
No products indexed under this heading.

Chlorpromazine (Concurrent administration of bupropion and agents that lower seizure threshold should be undertaken with extreme caution. Low initial dosing and gradual dose increases should be employed).
No products indexed under this heading.

Chlorpromazine Hydrochloride (Concurrent administration of bupropion and agents that lower seizure threshold should be undertaken with extreme caution. Low initial dosing and gradual dose increases should be employed).
No products indexed under this heading.

Chlorpropamide (Concomitant use of oral hypoglycemics with bupropion is associated with an increased seizure risk).
No products indexed under this heading.

Chlorprothixene (Concurrent administration of bupropion and agents that lower seizure threshold, such as antipsychotics, should be undertaken with extreme caution. Low initial dosing and gradual dose increases should be employed. Co-administration of bupropion with drugs that are metabolized by the CYP2D6 isoenzyme including antipsychotics (eg, haloperidol, risperidone, thioridazine) should be approached with caution and should be initiated at the lower end of the dose range of the concomitant medication. If bupropion is added to the treatment regimen of a patient already receiving a drug metabolized by CYP2D6, the need to decrease the dose of the original medication should be considered, particularly for those concomitant medications with a narrow therapeutic index).
No products indexed under this heading.

Chlorprothixene Hydrochloride (Concurrent administration of bupropion and agents that lower seizure threshold, such as antipsychotics, should be undertaken with extreme caution. Low

IMPORTANT NOTE: Always consult each drug listing in the patient's regimen for possible interactions.

initial dosing and gradual dose increases should be employed. Co-administration of bupropion with drugs that are metabolized by the CYP2D6 isoenzyme including antipsychotics (eg, haloperidol, risperidone, thioridazine) should be approached with caution and should be initiated at the lower end of the dose range of the concomitant medication. If bupropion is added to the treatment regimen of a patient already receiving a drug metabolized by CYP2D6, the need to decrease the dose of the original medication should be considered, particularly for those concomitant medications with a narrow therapeutic index).

No products indexed under this heading.

Chlorprothixene Lactate (Concurrent administration of bupropion and agents that lower seizure threshold, such as antipsychotics, should be undertaken with extreme caution. Low initial dosing and gradual dose increases should be employed. Co-administration of bupropion with drugs that are metabolized by the CYP2D6 isoenzyme including antipsychotics (eg, haloperidol, risperidone, thioridazine) should be approached with caution and should be initiated at the lower end of the dose range of the concomitant medication. If bupropion is added to the treatment regimen of a patient already receiving a drug metabolized by CYP2D6, the need to decrease the dose of the original medication should be considered, particularly for those concomitant medications with a narrow therapeutic index).

No products indexed under this heading.

Ciclesonide (Concurrent administration of bupropion and agents that lower seizure threshold, such as systemic steroids, should be undertaken with extreme caution. Low initial dosing and gradual dose increases should be employed).

No products indexed under this heading.

Cimetidine (Effects of concomitant administration of cimetidine on the pharmacokinetics of bupropion and hydroxybupropion were unaffected. However, there were 16% and 32% increases in the AUC and C_{max}, respectively, of the combined moieties of threohydrobupropion and erythrohydrobupropion).

No products indexed under this heading.

Cimetidine Hydrochloride (Effects of concomitant administration of cimetidine on the pharmacokinetics of bupropion and hydroxybupropion were unaffected. However, there were 16% and 32% increases in the AUC and C_{max}, respectively, of the combined moieties of threohydrobupropion and erythrohydrobupropion).

No products indexed under this heading.

Ciprofloxacin (Bupropion may be an inducer of drug-metabolizing enzymes in humans. In one study, following chronic administration of bupropion hydrochloride, 100 mg 3 times daily to 8 healthy male volunteers for 14 days, there was no evidence of induction of its own metabolism. Nevertheless, there may be the potential for clinically important alterations of blood levels of co-administered drugs). Products include:

Cipro I.V. 3082
Cipro 3073
Cipro XR 3091
Ciprodex 583

Ciprofloxacin Hydrochloride (Bupropion may be an inducer of drug-metabolizing enzymes in humans. In one study, following chronic administration of bupropion hydrochloride, 100 mg 3 times daily to 8 healthy male volunteers for 14 days, there was no evidence of induction of its own metabolism. Nevertheless, there may be the

potential for clinically important alterations of blood levels of co-administered drugs). Products include:

Cipro 3073

Cisapride (Because bupropion is extensively metabolized, the co-administration of other drugs may affect its clinical activity. In vitro studies indicate that bupropion is primarily metabolized to hydroxybupropion by the CYP2B6 isoenzyme. Therefore, the potential exists for a drug interaction between bupropion and drugs that are substrates or inhibitors of the CYP2B6 isoenzyme (eg, orphenadrine, thiotepa, and cyclophosphamide). In addition, in vitro studies suggest that paroxetine, sertraline, norfluoxetine, and fluvoxamine as well as nelfinavir, ritonavir, and efavirenz inhibit the hydroxylation of bupropion).

No products indexed under this heading.

Cisplatin (Bupropion may be an inducer of drug-metabolizing enzymes in humans. In one study, following chronic administration of bupropion hydrochloride, 100 mg 3 times daily to 8 healthy male volunteers for 14 days, there was no evidence of induction of its own metabolism. Nevertheless, there may be the potential for clinically important alterations of blood levels of co-administered drugs).

No products indexed under this heading.

Citalopram Hydrobromide (Concurrent administration of bupropion and agents that lower seizure threshold, such as antidepressants, should be undertaken with extreme caution. Low initial dosing and gradual dose increases should be employed. Co-administration of bupropion with drugs that are metabolized by the CYP2D6 isoenzyme including antidepressants (eg, nortriptyline, imipramine, desipramine, paroxentine, fluoxetine, sertraline) should be approached with caution and should be initiated at the lower end of the dose range of the concomitant medication. If bupropion is added to the treatment regimen of a patient already receiving a drug metabolized by CYP2D6, the need to decrease the dose of the original medication should be considered, particularly for those concomitant medications with a narrow therapeutic index). Products include:

Celexa 1153

Clomipramine Hydrochloride (Concurrent administration of bupropion and agents that lower seizure threshold should be undertaken with extreme caution. Low initial dosing and gradual dose increases should be employed).

No products indexed under this heading.

Clorazepate Dipotassium (Bupropion is contraindicated in patients undergoing abrupt discontinuation of benzodiazepine sedatives. Concomitant use of benzodiazepine sedatives with bupropion is associated with an increased seizure risk).

No products indexed under this heading.

Clotrimazole (Because bupropion is extensively metabolized, the co-administration of other drugs may affect its clinical activity. In vitro studies indicate that bupropion is primarily metabolized to hydroxybupropion by the CYP2B6 isoenzyme. Therefore, the potential exists for a drug interaction between bupropion and drugs that are substrates or inhibitors of the CYP2B6 isoenzyme (eg, orphenadrine, thiotepa, and cyclophosphamide). In addition, in vitro studies suggest that paroxetine, sertraline, norfluoxetine, and fluvoxamine as well as nelfinavir, ritonavir, and efavirenz inhibit the hydroxylation of bupropion). Products include:

Lotrisone 3163

Clotrimazole, Topical (Because bupropion is extensively metabolized,

the co-administration of other drugs may affect its clinical activity. In vitro studies indicate that bupropion is primarily metabolized to hydroxybupropion by the CYP2B6 isoenzyme. Therefore, the potential exists for a drug interaction between bupropion and drugs that are substrates or inhibitors of the CYP2B6 isoenzyme (eg, orphenadrine, thiotepa, and cyclophosphamide). In addition, in vitro studies suggest that paroxetine, sertraline, norfluoxetine, and fluvoxamine as well as nelfinavir, ritonavir, and efavirenz inhibit the hydroxylation of bupropion).

No products indexed under this heading.

Clozapine (Concurrent administration of bupropion and agents that lower seizure threshold, such as antipsychotics, should be undertaken with extreme caution. Low initial dosing and gradual dose increases should be employed. Co-administration of bupropion with drugs that are metabolized by the CYP2D6 isoenzyme including antipsychotics (eg, haloperidol, risperidone, thioridazine) should be approached with caution and should be initiated at the lower end of the dose range of the concomitant medication. If bupropion is added to the treatment regimen of a patient already receiving a drug metabolized by CYP2D6, the need to decrease the dose of the original medication should be considered, particularly for those concomitant medications with a narrow therapeutic index).

No products indexed under this heading.

Cocaine Hydrochloride (Concomitant use of cocaine with bupropion is associated with an increased seizure risk).

No products indexed under this heading.

Codeine Phosphate (Concomitant use of opiates, cocaine, or stimulants with bupropion is associated with an increased seizure risk). Products include:

Tylenol with Codeine 2691

Codeine Sulfate (Concomitant use of opiates, cocaine, or stimulants with bupropion is associated with an increased seizure risk).

No products indexed under this heading.

Cortisone Acetate (Concurrent administration of bupropion and agents that lower seizure threshold, such as systemic steroids, should be undertaken with extreme caution. Low initial dosing and gradual dose increases should be employed).

No products indexed under this heading.

Cyclobenzaprine Hydrochloride (Co-administration of bupropion with drugs that are metabolized by the CYP2D6 isoenzyme should be approached with caution and should be initiated at the lower end of the dose range of the concomitant medication. If bupropion is added to the treatment regimen of a patient already receiving a drug metabolized by CYP2D6, the need to decrease the dose of the original medication should be considered, particularly for those concomitant medications with a narrow therapeutic index). Products include:

Amrix 964

Cyclophosphamide (Because bupropion is extensively metabolized, the co-administration of other drugs may affect its clinical activity. In vitro studies indicate that bupropion is primarily metabolized to hydroxybupropion by the CYP2B6 isoenzyme. Therefore, the potential exists for a drug interaction between bupropion and drugs that are substrates or inhibitors of the CYP2B6 isoenzyme (eg, orphenadrine, thiotepa, and cyclophosphamide). In addition, in vitro studies suggest that paroxetine, sertraline, norfluoxetine, and fluvoxam-

ine as well as nelfinavir, ritonavir, and efavirenz inhibit the hydroxylation of bupropion).

No products indexed under this heading.

Debrisoquine (Co-administration of bupropion with drugs that are metabolized by the CYP2D6 isoenzyme should be approached with caution and should be initiated at the lower end of the dose range of the concomitant medication. If bupropion is added to the treatment regimen of a patient already receiving a drug metabolized by CYP2D6, the need to decrease the dose of the original medication should be considered, particularly for those concomitant medications with a narrow therapeutic index).

No products indexed under this heading.

Desipramine Hydrochloride (Many drugs, including most antidepressants (SSRIs, many tricyclics), β-blockers, antiarrhythmics, and antipsychotics are metabolized by the CYP2D6 isoenzyme. Although bupropion is not metabolized by this isoenzyme, bupropion and hydroxybupropion are inhibitors of CYP2D6 isoenzyme in vitro. In a study of 15 male subjects (ages 19 to 35 years) who were extensive metabolizers of the CYP2D6 isoenzyme, daily doses of bupropion hydrochloride given as 150 mg twice daily followed by a single dose of 50 mg desipramine increased the C_{max}, AUC, and $t_{1/2}$ of desipramine by an average of approximately 2-, 5-, and 2-fold, respectively. The effect was present for at least 7 days after the last dose of bupropion. Concomitant use of bupropion with other drugs metabolized by CYP2D6 has not been formally studied).

No products indexed under this heading.

Desoximetasone (Concurrent administration of bupropion and agents that lower seizure threshold, such as systemic steroids, should be undertaken with extreme caution. Low initial dosing and gradual dose increases should be employed).

No products indexed under this heading.

Desvenlafaxine (Because bupropion is extensively metabolized, the co-administration of other drugs may affect its clinical activity. In vitro studies indicate that bupropion is primarily metabolized to hydroxybupropion by the CYP2B6 isoenzyme. Therefore, the potential exists for a drug interaction between bupropion and drugs that are substrates or inhibitors of the CYP2B6 isoenzyme (eg, orphenadrine, thiotepa, and cyclophosphamide). In addition, in vitro studies suggest that paroxetine, sertraline, norfluoxetine, and fluvoxamine as well as nelfinavir, ritonavir, and efavirenz inhibit the hydroxylation of bupropion).

No products indexed under this heading.

Desvenlafaxine Succinate (Because bupropion is extensively metabolized, the co-administration of other drugs may affect its clinical activity. In vitro studies indicate that bupropion is primarily metabolized to hydroxybupropion by the CYP2B6 isoenzyme. Therefore, the potential exists for a drug interaction between bupropion and drugs that are substrates or inhibitors of the CYP2B6 isoenzyme (eg, orphenadrine, thiotepa, and cyclophosphamide). In addition, in vitro studies suggest that paroxetine, sertraline, norfluoxetine, and fluvoxamine as well as nelfinavir, ritonavir, and efavirenz inhibit the hydroxylation of bupropion). Products include:

Pristiq 3564

Dexamethasone (Concurrent administration of bupropion and agents that lower seizure threshold, such as systemic steroids, should be undertaken

125 **Interactions Index** **Aplenzin**

with extreme caution. Low initial dosing and gradual dose increases should be employed). Products include:

Ciprodex 583
Ozurdex .... ⊙223
Tobramycin and Dexamethasone Ophthalmic Suspension .... ⊙251

Dexamethasone Acetate (Concurrent administration of bupropion and agents that lower seizure threshold, such as systemic steroids, should be undertaken with extreme caution. Low initial dosing and gradual dose increases should be employed).
No products indexed under this heading.

Dexamethasone Phosphate (Concurrent administration of bupropion and agents that lower seizure threshold, such as systemic steroids, should be undertaken with extreme caution. Low initial dosing and gradual dose increases should be employed).
No products indexed under this heading.

Dexamethasone Sodium (Concurrent administration of bupropion and agents that lower seizure threshold, such as systemic steroids, should be undertaken with extreme caution. Low initial dosing and gradual dose increases should be employed).
No products indexed under this heading.

Dexamethasone Sodium Phosphate (Concurrent administration of bupropion and agents that lower seizure threshold, such as systemic steroids, should be undertaken with extreme caution. Low initial dosing and gradual dose increases should be employed).
No products indexed under this heading.

Dexamethasone Sodium Phosphate Injection (Concurrent administration of bupropion and agents that lower seizure threshold, such as systemic steroids, should be undertaken with extreme caution. Low initial dosing and gradual dose increases should be employed).
No products indexed under this heading.

Dexfenfluramine Hydrochloride (Concomitant use of anorectics with bupropion is associated with an increased seizure risk).
No products indexed under this heading.

Dexmethylphenidate Hydrochloride (Concomitant use of opiates, cocaine, or stimulants with bupropion is associated with an increased seizure risk). Products include:

Focalin XR 2472

Dextroamphetamine (Concomitant use of opiates, cocaine, or stimulants with bupropion is associated with an increased seizure risk).
No products indexed under this heading.

Dextroamphetamine Saccharate (Concomitant use of opiates, cocaine, or stimulants with bupropion is associated with an increased seizure risk).
No products indexed under this heading.

Dextroamphetamine Sulfate (Concomitant use of opiates, cocaine, or stimulants with bupropion is associated with an increased seizure risk). Products include:

Dexedrine 1425

Dextromethorphan Hydrobromide (Co-administration of bupropion with drugs that are metabolized by the CYP2D6 isoenzyme should be approached with caution and should be initiated at the lower end of the dose range of the concomitant medication. If bupropion is added to the treatment regimen of a patient already receiving a drug metabolized by CYP2D6, the need to decrease the dose of the original medication should be considered, particularly for those concomitant medications with a narrow therapeutic index).
No products indexed under this heading.

Dextromethorphan Polistirex (Co-administration of bupropion with drugs that are metabolized by the CYP2D6 isoenzyme should be approached with caution and should be initiated at the lower end of the dose range of the concomitant medication. If bupropion is added to the treatment regimen of a patient already receiving a drug metabolized by CYP2D6, the need to decrease the dose of the original medication should be considered, particularly for those concomitant medications with a narrow therapeutic index).
No products indexed under this heading.

Dezocine (Concomitant use of opiates, cocaine, or stimulants with bupropion is associated with an increased seizure risk).
No products indexed under this heading.

Diazepam (Bupropion is contraindicated in patients undergoing abrupt discontinuation of benzodiazepine sedatives. Concomitant use of benzodiazepine sedatives with bupropion is associated with an increased seizure risk). Products include:

Valium Tablets 2880

Diclofenac Epolamine (Because bupropion is extensively metabolized, the co-administration of other drugs may affect its clinical activity. *In vitro* studies indicate that bupropion is primarily metabolized to hydroxybupropion by the CYP2B6 isoenzyme. Therefore, the potential exists for a drug interaction between bupropion and drugs that are substrates or inhibitors of the CYP2B6 isoenzyme (eg, orphenadrine, thiotepa, and cyclophosphamide). In addition, *in vitro* studies suggest that paroxetine, sertraline, norfluoxetine, and fluvoxamine as well as nelfinavir, ritonavir, and efavirenz inhibit the hydroxylation of bupropion). Products include:

Flector 1839

Diclofenac Potassium (Because bupropion is extensively metabolized, the co-administration of other drugs may affect its clinical activity. *In vitro* studies indicate that bupropion is primarily metabolized to hydroxybupropion by the CYP2B6 isoenzyme. Therefore, the potential exists for a drug interaction between bupropion and drugs that are substrates or inhibitors of the CYP2B6 isoenzyme (eg, orphenadrine, thiotepa, and cyclophosphamide). In addition, *in vitro* studies suggest that paroxetine, sertraline, norfluoxetine, and fluvoxamine as well as nelfinavir, ritonavir, and efavirenz inhibit the hydroxylation of bupropion).
No products indexed under this heading.

Diclofenac Sodium (Because bupropion is extensively metabolized, the co-administration of other drugs may affect its clinical activity. *In vitro* studies indicate that bupropion is primarily metabolized to hydroxybupropion by the CYP2B6 isoenzyme. Therefore, the potential exists for a drug interaction between bupropion and drugs that are substrates or inhibitors of the CYP2B6 isoenzyme (eg, orphenadrine, thiotepa, and cyclophosphamide). In addition, *in vitro* studies suggest that paroxetine, sertraline, norfluoxetine, and fluvoxamine as well as nelfinavir, ritonavir, and efavirenz inhibit the hydroxylation of bupropion).
No products indexed under this heading.

Diethylpropion Hydrochloride (Concomitant use of anorectics with bupropion is associated with an increased seizure risk).
No products indexed under this heading.

Diflorasone Diacetate (Concurrent administration of bupropion and agents that lower seizure threshold, such as systemic steroids, should be undertaken with extreme caution. Low initial dosing and gradual dose increases should be employed).
No products indexed under this heading.

Dihydrocodeine Bitartrate (Concomitant use of opiates, cocaine, or stimulants with bupropion is associated with an increased seizure risk).
No products indexed under this heading.

Dihydrocodeinone Bitartrate (Concomitant use of opiates, cocaine, or stimulants with bupropion is associated with an increased seizure risk).
No products indexed under this heading.

Diltiazem Hydrochloride (Bupropion may be an inducer of drug-metabolizing enzymes in humans. In one study, following chronic administration of bupropion hydrochloride, 100 mg 3 times daily to 8 healthy male volunteers for 14 days, there was no evidence of induction of its own metabolism. Nevertheless, there may be the potential for clinically important alterations of blood levels of co-administered drugs). Products include:

Cardizem LA 423

Diltiazem Maleate (Bupropion may be an inducer of drug-metabolizing enzymes in humans. In one study, following chronic administration of bupropion hydrochloride, 100 mg 3 times daily to 8 healthy male volunteers for 14 days, there was no evidence of induction of its own metabolism. Nevertheless, there may be the potential for clinically important alterations of blood levels of co-administered drugs).
No products indexed under this heading.

Disulfiram (Because bupropion is extensively metabolized, the co-administration of other drugs may affect its clinical activity. *In vitro* studies indicate that bupropion is primarily metabolized to hydroxybupropion by the CYP2B6 isoenzyme. Therefore, the potential exists for a drug interaction between bupropion and drugs that are substrates or inhibitors of the CYP2B6 isoenzyme (eg, orphenadrine, thiotepa, and cyclophosphamide). In addition, *in vitro* studies suggest that paroxetine, sertraline, norfluoxetine, and fluvoxamine as well as nelfinavir, ritonavir, and efavirenz inhibit the hydroxylation of bupropion).
No products indexed under this heading.

Divalproex Sodium (Because bupropion is extensively metabolized, the co-administration of other drugs may affect its clinical activity. *In vitro* studies indicate that bupropion is primarily metabolized to hydroxybupropion by the CYP2B6 isoenzyme. Therefore, the potential exists for a drug interaction between bupropion and drugs that are substrates or inhibitors of the CYP2B6 isoenzyme (eg, orphenadrine, thiotepa, and cyclophosphamide). In addition, *in vitro* studies suggest that paroxetine, sertraline, norfluoxetine, and fluvoxamine as well as nelfinavir, ritonavir, and efavirenz inhibit the hydroxylation of bupropion). Products include:

Depakote ER 426

Dolasetron Mesylate (Co-administration of bupropion with drugs that are metabolized by the CYP2D6 isoenzyme should be approached with caution and should be initiated at the lower end of the dose range of the concomitant medication. If bupropion is added to the treatment regimen of a patient already receiving a drug metabolized by CYP2D6, the need to decrease the dose of the original medication should be considered, particularly for those concomitant medications with a narrow therapeutic index). Products include:

Anzemet Injection 2931
Anzemet Tablets 2934

Donepezil Hydrochloride (Co-administration of bupropion with drugs that are metabolized by the CYP2D6 isoenzyme should be approached with caution and should be initiated at the lower end of the dose range of the concomitant medication. If bupropion is added to the treatment regimen of a patient already receiving a drug metabolized by CYP2D6, the need to decrease the dose of the original medication should be considered, particularly for those concomitant medications with a narrow therapeutic index). Products include:

Aricept 1045
Aricept ODT 1045

Doxepin Hydrochloride (Concurrent administration of bupropion and agents that lower seizure threshold should be undertaken with extreme caution. Low initial dosing and gradual dose increases should be employed).
No products indexed under this heading.

Doxorubicin Hydrochloride (Because bupropion is extensively metabolized, the co-administration of other drugs may affect its clinical activity. *In vitro* studies indicate that bupropion is primarily metabolized to hydroxybupropion by the CYP2B6 isoenzyme. Therefore, the potential exists for a drug interaction between bupropion and drugs that are substrates or inhibitors of the CYP2B6 isoenzyme (eg, orphenadrine, thiotepa, and cyclophosphamide). In addition, *in vitro* studies suggest that paroxetine, sertraline, norfluoxetine, and fluvoxamine as well as nelfinavir, ritonavir, and efavirenz inhibit the hydroxylation of bupropion).
No products indexed under this heading.

Doxorubicin Hydrochloride Liposome (Because bupropion is extensively metabolized, the co-administration of other drugs may affect its clinical activity. *In vitro* studies indicate that bupropion is primarily metabolized to hydroxybupropion by the CYP2B6 isoenzyme. Therefore, the potential exists for a drug interaction between bupropion and drugs that are substrates or inhibitors of the CYP2B6 isoenzyme (eg, orphenadrine, thiotepa, and cyclophosphamide). In addition, *in vitro* studies suggest that paroxetine, sertraline, norfluoxetine, and fluvoxamine as well as nelfinavir, ritonavir, and efavirenz inhibit the hydroxylation of bupropion). Products include:

Doxil 939

Efavirenz (There is a potential drug interaction between bupropion and drugs that are subtrates or inhibitors of the CYP2B6 isoenzyme. *In vitro* studies suggest that efavirenz inhibits the hydroxylation of bupropion). Products include:

Atripla 906

Encainide Hydrochloride (Co-administration of bupropion with drugs that are metabolized by the CYP2D6 isoenzyme should be approached with caution and should be initiated at the lower end of the dose range of the concomitant medication. If bupropion is added to the treatment regimen of a patient already receiving a drug metabolized by CYP2D6, the need to decrease the dose of the original medication should be considered, particularly for those concomitant medications with a narrow therapeutic index).
No products indexed under this heading.

Erythromycin (Because bupropion is extensively metabolized, the co-administration of other drugs may affect its clinical activity. *In vitro* studies

IMPORTANT NOTE: Always consult each drug listing in the patient's regimen for possible interactions.

indicate that bupropion is primarily metabolized to hydroxybupropion by the CYP2B6 isoenzyme. Therefore, the potential exists for a drug interaction between bupropion and drugs that are substrates or inhibitors of the CYP2B6 isoenzyme (eg, orphenadrine, thiotepa, and cyclophosphamide). In addition, *in vitro* studies suggest that paroxetine, sertraline, norfluoxetine, and fluvoxamine as well as nelfinavir, ritonavir, and efavirenz inhibit the hydroxylation of bupropion).

No products indexed under this heading.

Erythromycin, Topical (Because bupropion is extensively metabolized, the co-administration of other drugs may affect its clinical activity. *In vitro* studies indicate that bupropion is primarily metabolized to hydroxybupropion by the CYP2B6 isoenzyme. Therefore, the potential exists for a drug interaction between bupropion and drugs that are substrates or inhibitors of the CYP2B6 isoenzyme (eg, orphenadrine, thiotepa, and cyclophosphamide). In addition, *in vitro* studies suggest that paroxetine, sertraline, norfluoxetine, and fluvoxamine as well as nelfinavir, ritonavir, and efavirenz inhibit the hydroxylation of bupropion).

No products indexed under this heading.

Erythromycin Estolate (Because bupropion is extensively metabolized, the co-administration of other drugs may affect its clinical activity. *In vitro* studies indicate that bupropion is primarily metabolized to hydroxybupropion by the CYP2B6 isoenzyme. Therefore, the potential exists for a drug interaction between bupropion and drugs that are substrates or inhibitors of the CYP2B6 isoenzyme (eg, orphenadrine, thiotepa, and cyclophosphamide). In addition, *in vitro* studies suggest that paroxetine, sertraline, norfluoxetine, and fluvoxamine as well as nelfinavir, ritonavir, and efavirenz inhibit the hydroxylation of bupropion).

No products indexed under this heading.

Erythromycin Ethylsuccinate (Because bupropion is extensively metabolized, the co-administration of other drugs may affect its clinical activity. *In vitro* studies indicate that bupropion is primarily metabolized to hydroxybupropion by the CYP2B6 isoenzyme. Therefore, the potential exists for a drug interaction between bupropion and drugs that are substrates or inhibitors of the CYP2B6 isoenzyme (eg, orphenadrine, thiotepa, and cyclophosphamide). In addition, *in vitro* studies suggest that paroxetine, sertraline, norfluoxetine, and fluvoxamine as well as nelfinavir, ritonavir, and efavirenz inhibit the hydroxylation of bupropion). Products include:

E.E.S. **437**
EryPed **435**

Erythromycin Gluceptate (Because bupropion is extensively metabolized, the co-administration of other drugs may affect its clinical activity. *In vitro* studies indicate that bupropion is primarily metabolized to hydroxybupropion by the CYP2B6 isoenzyme. Therefore, the potential exists for a drug interaction between bupropion and drugs that are substrates or inhibitors of the CYP2B6 isoenzyme (eg, orphenadrine, thiotepa, and cyclophosphamide). In addition, *in vitro* studies suggest that paroxetine, sertraline, norfluoxetine, and fluvoxamine as well as nelfinavir, ritonavir, and efavirenz inhibit the hydroxylation of bupropion).

No products indexed under this heading.

Erythromycin Lactobionate (Because bupropion is extensively metabolized, the co-administration of other drugs may affect its clinical activity. *In vitro* studies indicate that bupropion is primarily metabolized to hydroxybupropion by the CYP2B6 isoenzyme. Therefore, the potential exists for a drug interaction between bupropion and drugs that are substrates or inhibitors of the CYP2B6 isoenzyme (eg, orphenadrine, thiotepa, and cyclophosphamide). In addition, *in vitro* studies suggest that paroxetine, sertraline, norfluoxetine, and fluvoxamine as well as nelfinavir, ritonavir, and efavirenz inhibit the hydroxylation of bupropion).

No products indexed under this heading.

Erythromycin Stearate (Because bupropion is extensively metabolized, the co-administration of other drugs may affect its clinical activity. *In vitro* studies indicate that bupropion is primarily metabolized to hydroxybupropion by the CYP2B6 isoenzyme. Therefore, the potential exists for a drug interaction between bupropion and drugs that are substrates or inhibitors of the CYP2B6 isoenzyme (eg, orphenadrine, thiotepa, and cyclophosphamide). In addition, *in vitro* studies suggest that paroxetine, sertraline, norfluoxetine, and fluvoxamine as well as nelfinavir, ritonavir, and efavirenz inhibit the hydroxylation of bupropion).

No products indexed under this heading.

Escitalopram Oxalate (Concurrent administration of bupropion and agents that lower seizure threshold, such as antidepressants, should be undertaken with extreme caution. Low initial dosing and gradual dose increases should be employed. Co-administration of bupropion with drugs that are metabolized by the CYP2D6 isoenzyme including antidepressants (eg, nortriptyline, imipramine, desipramine, paroxetine, fluoxetine, sertraline) should be approached with caution and should be initiated at the lower end of the dose range of the concomitant medication. If bupropion is added to the treatment regimen of a patient already receiving a drug metabolized by CYP2D6, the need to decrease the dose of the original medication should be considered, particularly for those concomitant medications with a narrow therapeutic index). Products include:

Lexapro Oral Suspension **1160**
Lexapro Tablets **1160**

Esmolol Hydrochloride (Co-administration of bupropion with drugs that are metabolized by the CYP2D6 isoenzyme including beta-blockers (eg, metoprolol) should be approached with caution and should be initiated at the lower end of the dose range of the concomitant medication. If bupropion is added to the treatment regimen of a patient already receiving a drug metabolized by CYP2D6, the need to decrease the dose of the original medication should be considered, particularly for those concomitant medications with a narrow therapeutic index).

No products indexed under this heading.

Esomeprazole Magnesium (Bupropion may be an inducer of drug-metabolizing enzymes in humans. In one study, following chronic administration of bupropion hydrochloride, 100 mg 3 times daily to 8 healthy male volunteers for 14 days, there was no evidence of induction of its own metabolism. Nevertheless, there may be the potential for clinically important alterations of blood levels of co-administered drugs). Products include:

Nexium Capsules **704**
Nexium Oral Suspension **704**

Esomeprazole Sodium (Bupropion may be an inducer of drug-metabolizing enzymes in humans. In one study, following chronic administration of bupropion hydrochloride, 100 mg 3 times daily to 8 healthy male volunteers for 14 days, there was no evidence of induction of its own metabolism. Nevertheless, there may be the potential for clinically important alterations of blood levels of co-administered drugs). Products include:

Nexium I.V. **712**

Estazolam (Bupropion is contraindicated in patients undergoing abrupt discontinuation of benzodiazepine sedatives. Concomitant use of benzodiazepine sedatives with bupropion is associated with an increased seizure risk).

No products indexed under this heading.

Estradiol (Because bupropion is extensively metabolized, the co-administration of other drugs may affect its clinical activity. *In vitro* studies indicate that bupropion is primarily metabolized to hydroxybupropion by the CYP2B6 isoenzyme. Therefore, the potential exists for a drug interaction between bupropion and drugs that are substrates or inhibitors of the CYP2B6 isoenzyme (eg, orphenadrine, thiotepa, and cyclophosphamide). In addition, *in vitro* studies suggest that paroxetine, sertraline, norfluoxetine, and fluvoxamine as well as nelfinavir, ritonavir, and efavirenz inhibit the hydroxylation of bupropion). Products include:

Activella **2561**
Angeliq **831**
Climara **841**
Climara Pro **847**
Divigel **3467**
Estrasorb **1777**
Vagifem **2589**

Estradiol Acetate (Because bupropion is extensively metabolized, the co-administration of other drugs may affect its clinical activity. *In vitro* studies indicate that bupropion is primarily metabolized to hydroxybupropion by the CYP2B6 isoenzyme. Therefore, the potential exists for a drug interaction between bupropion and drugs that are substrates or inhibitors of the CYP2B6 isoenzyme (eg, orphenadrine, thiotepa, and cyclophosphamide). In addition, *in vitro* studies suggest that paroxetine, sertraline, norfluoxetine, and fluvoxamine as well as nelfinavir, ritonavir, and efavirenz inhibit the hydroxylation of bupropion).

No products indexed under this heading.

Estradiol Benzoate (Because bupropion is extensively metabolized, the co-administration of other drugs may affect its clinical activity. *In vitro* studies indicate that bupropion is primarily metabolized to hydroxybupropion by the CYP2B6 isoenzyme. Therefore, the potential exists for a drug interaction between bupropion and drugs that are substrates or inhibitors of the CYP2B6 isoenzyme (eg, orphenadrine, thiotepa, and cyclophosphamide). In addition, *in vitro* studies suggest that paroxetine, sertraline, norfluoxetine, and fluvoxamine as well as nelfinavir, ritonavir, and efavirenz inhibit the hydroxylation of bupropion).

No products indexed under this heading.

Estradiol Cypionate (Because bupropion is extensively metabolized, the co-administration of other drugs may affect its clinical activity. *In vitro* studies indicate that bupropion is primarily metabolized to hydroxybupropion by the CYP2B6 isoenzyme. Therefore, the potential exists for a drug interaction between bupropion and drugs that are substrates or inhibitors of the CYP2B6 isoenzyme (eg, orphenadrine, thiotepa, and cyclophosphamide). In addition, *in vitro* studies suggest that paroxetine, sertraline, norfluoxetine, and fluvoxamine as well as nelfinavir, ritonavir, and efavirenz inhibit the hydroxylation of bupropion).

No products indexed under this heading.

Estradiol Valerate (Because bupropion is extensively metabolized, the co-administration of other drugs may affect its clinical activity. *In vitro* studies indicate that bupropion is primarily metabolized to hydroxybupropion by the CYP2B6 isoenzyme. Therefore, the potential exists for a drug interaction between bupropion and drugs that are substrates or inhibitors of the CYP2B6 isoenzyme (eg, orphenadrine, thiotepa, and cyclophosphamide). In addition, *in vitro* studies suggest that paroxetine, sertraline, norfluoxetine, and fluvoxamine as well as nelfinavir, ritonavir, and efavirenz inhibit the hydroxylation of bupropion).

No products indexed under this heading.

Estrogen (Because bupropion is extensively metabolized, the co-administration of other drugs may affect its clinical activity. *In vitro* studies indicate that bupropion is primarily metabolized to hydroxybupropion by the CYP2B6 isoenzyme. Therefore, the potential exists for a drug interaction between bupropion and drugs that are substrates or inhibitors of the CYP2B6 isoenzyme (eg, orphenadrine, thiotepa, and cyclophosphamide). In addition, *in vitro* studies suggest that paroxetine, sertraline, norfluoxetine, and fluvoxamine as well as nelfinavir, ritonavir, and efavirenz inhibit the hydroxylation of bupropion).

No products indexed under this heading.

Estrogens, Conjugated (Because bupropion is extensively metabolized, the co-administration of other drugs may affect its clinical activity. *In vitro* studies indicate that bupropion is primarily metabolized to hydroxybupropion by the CYP2B6 isoenzyme. Therefore, the potential exists for a drug interaction between bupropion and drugs that are substrates or inhibitors of the CYP2B6 isoenzyme (eg, orphenadrine, thiotepa, and cyclophosphamide). In addition, *in vitro* studies suggest that paroxetine, sertraline, norfluoxetine, and fluvoxamine as well as nelfinavir, ritonavir, and efavirenz inhibit the hydroxylation of bupropion). Products include:

Premarin Intravenous **3528**
Premarin Tablets **3533**
Premarin Vaginal Cream **3540**
Premphase **3549**
Prempro **3549**

Estrogens, Conjugated, Synthetic A (Because bupropion is extensively metabolized, the co-administration of other drugs may affect its clinical activity. *In vitro* studies indicate that bupropion is primarily metabolized to hydroxybupropion by the CYP2B6 isoenzyme. Therefore, the potential exists for a drug interaction between bupropion and drugs that are substrates or inhibitors of the CYP2B6 isoenzyme (eg, orphenadrine, thiotepa, and cyclophosphamide). In addition, *in vitro* studies suggest that paroxetine, sertraline, norfluoxetine, and fluvoxamine as well as nelfinavir, ritonavir, and efavirenz inhibit the hydroxylation of bupropion).

No products indexed under this heading.

Estrogens, Conjugated, Synthetic B (Because bupropion is extensively metabolized, the co-administration of other drugs may affect its clinical activity. *In vitro* studies indicate that bupropion is primarily metabolized to hydroxybupropion by the CYP2B6 isoenzyme. Therefore, the potential exists for a drug interaction between bupropion and drugs that are substrates or inhibitors of the CYP2B6 isoenzyme (eg, orphenadrine, thiotepa, and cyclophosphamide). In addition, *in vitro* studies suggest that paroxetine, sertraline, norfluoxetine, and fluvoxamine as well as nelfinavir, ritonavir, and efavirenz inhibit the hydroxylation of bupropion). Products include:

Enjuvia **3401**

Estrogens, Esterified (Because bupropion is extensively metabolized, the co-administration of other drugs may affect its clinical activity. *In vitro* studies indicate that bupropion is primarily metabolized to hydroxybupropion by the CYP2B6 isoenzyme. Therefore, the potential exists for a drug interaction between bupropion and drugs that are substrates or inhibitors of the CYP2B6 isoenzyme (eg, orphenadrine, thiotepa, and cyclophosphamide). In addition, *in vitro* studies suggest that paroxetine, sertraline, norfluoxetine, and fluvoxamine as well as nelfinavir, ritonavir, and efavirenz inhibit the hydroxylation of bupropion).
No products indexed under this heading.

Estrone (Because bupropion is extensively metabolized, the co-administration of other drugs may affect its clinical activity. *In vitro* studies indicate that bupropion is primarily metabolized to hydroxybupropion by the CYP2B6 isoenzyme. Therefore, the potential exists for a drug interaction between bupropion and drugs that are substrates or inhibitors of the CYP2B6 isoenzyme (eg, orphenadrine, thiotepa, and cyclophosphamide). In addition, *in vitro* studies suggest that paroxetine, sertraline, norfluoxetine, and fluvoxamine as well as nelfinavir, ritonavir, and efavirenz inhibit the hydroxylation of bupropion).
No products indexed under this heading.

Estropipate (Because bupropion is extensively metabolized, the co-administration of other drugs may affect its clinical activity. *In vitro* studies indicate that bupropion is primarily metabolized to hydroxybupropion by the CYP2B6 isoenzyme. Therefore, the potential exists for a drug interaction between bupropion and drugs that are substrates or inhibitors of the CYP2B6 isoenzyme (eg, orphenadrine, thiotepa, and cyclophosphamide). In addition, *in vitro* studies suggest that paroxetine, sertraline, norfluoxetine, and fluvoxamine as well as nelfinavir, ritonavir, and efavirenz inhibit the hydroxylation of bupropion).
No products indexed under this heading.

Ethanol (Bupropion is contraindicated in patients undergoing abrupt discontinuation of alcohol. Concomitant use of alcohol with bupropion is associated with an increased seizure risk. There have been rare reports of adverse neuropsychiatric events or reduced alcohol tolerance in patients who were drinking alcohol during treatment with bupropion. The consumption of alcohol during treatment with bupropion should be minimized or avoided).
No products indexed under this heading.

Ethchlorvynol (Bupropion is containdicated in patients undergoing abrupt discontinuation of sedatives. Concomitant use of sedatives with bupropion is associated with an increased seizure risk).
No products indexed under this heading.

Ethinamate (Bupropion is containdicated in patients undergoing abrupt discontinuation of sedatives. Concomitant use of sedatives with bupropion is associated with an increased seizure risk).
No products indexed under this heading.

Ethinyl Estradiol (Because bupropion is extensively metabolized, the co-administration of other drugs may affect its clinical activity. *In vitro* studies indicate that bupropion is primarily metabolized to hydroxybupropion by the CYP2B6 isoenzyme. Therefore, the potential exists for a drug interaction between bupropion and drugs that are substrates or inhibitors of the CYP2B6 isoenzyme (eg, orphenadrine, thiotepa, and cyclophosphamide). In addition, *in vitro* studies suggest that paroxetine, sertraline, norfluoxetine, and fluvoxamine as well as nelfinavir, ritonavir, and efavirenz inhibit the hydroxylation of bupropion). Products include:
LoSeasonique **3407**
Lybrel **3514**
NuvaRing **3181**
Ortho Evra **2648**
Ortho-Cyclen/Ortho Tri-Cyclen **2663**
Ortho Tri-Cyclen Lo Tablets **2673**
Seasonique **3418**
Yaz **864**

Ethosuximide (Bupropion may be an inducer of drug-metabolizing enzymes in humans. In one study, following chronic administration of bupropion hydrochloride, 100 mg 3 times daily to 8 healthy male volunteers for 14 days, there was no evidence of induction of its own metabolism. Nevertheless, there may be the potential for clinically important alterations of blood levels of co-administered drugs).
No products indexed under this heading.

Ethyl Alcohol (Bupropion is contraindicated in patients undergoing abrupt discontinuation of alcohol. Concomitant use of alcohol with bupropion is associated with an increased seizure risk. There have been rare reports of adverse neuropsychiatric events or reduced alcohol tolerance in patients who were drinking alcohol during treatment with bupropion. The consumption of alcohol during treatment with bupropion should be minimized or avoided).
No products indexed under this heading.

Felbamate (Bupropion may be an inducer of drug-metabolizing enzymes in humans. In one study, following chronic administration of bupropion hydrochloride, 100 mg 3 times daily to 8 healthy male volunteers for 14 days, there was no evidence of induction of its own metabolism. Nevertheless, there may be the potential for clinically important alterations of blood levels of co-administered drugs).
No products indexed under this heading.

Fenfluramine Hydrochloride (Concomitant use of anorectics with bupropion is associated with an increased seizure risk).
No products indexed under this heading.

Fentanyl (Concomitant use of opiates, cocaine, or stimulants with bupropion is associated with an increased seizure risk). Products include:
Duragesic **2604**
Fentanyl Transdermal System **2346**
Onsolis **2054**

Fentanyl Citrate (Concomitant use of opiates, cocaine, or stimulants with bupropion is associated with an increased seizure risk). Products include:
Fentora **966**

Flecainide Acetate (Co-administration of bupropion with drugs that are metabolized by the CYP2D6 isoenzyme should be approached with caution and should be initiated at the lower end of the dose range of the concomitant medication. If bupropion is added to the treatment regimen of a patient already receiving a drug metabolized by CYP2D6, the need to decrease the dose of the original medication should be considered, particularly for those concomitant medications with a narrow therapeutic index).
No products indexed under this heading.

Fludrocortisone Acetate (Concurrent administration of bupropion and agents that lower seizure threshold, such as systemic steroids, should be undertaken with extreme caution. Low initial dosing and gradual dose increases should be employed).
No products indexed under this heading.

Flumethasone Pivalate (Concurrent administration of bupropion and agents that lower seizure threshold, such as systemic steroids, should be undertaken with extreme caution. Low initial dosing and gradual dose increases should be employed).
No products indexed under this heading.

Flunisolide Hemihydrate (Concurrent administration of bupropion and agents that lower seizure threshold, such as systemic steroids, should be undertaken with extreme caution. Low initial dosing and gradual dose increases should be employed).
No products indexed under this heading.

Fluoxetine (Co-administration of bupropion with drugs that are metabolized by the CYP2D6 isoenzyme should be approached with caution and should be initiated at the lower end of the dose range of the concomitant medication. If bupropion is added to the treatment regimen of a patient already receiving a drug metabolized by CYP2D6, the need to decrease the dose of the original medication should be considered, particularly for those concomitant medications with a narrow therapeutic index).
No products indexed under this heading.

Fluoxetine Hydrochloride (Concurrent administration of bupropion and agents that lower seizure threshold should be undertaken with extreme caution. Low initial dosing and gradual dose increases should be employed). Products include:
Prozac Weekly **1941**
Prozac Pulvules **1941**
Symbyax **1965**

Fluphenazine Decanoate (Concurrent administration of bupropion and agents that lower seizure threshold should be undertaken with extreme caution. Low initial dosing and gradual dose increases should be employed).
No products indexed under this heading.

Fluphenazine Enanthate (Concurrent administration of bupropion and agents that lower seizure threshold should be undertaken with extreme caution. Low initial dosing and gradual dose increases should be employed).
No products indexed under this heading.

Fluphenazine Hydrochloride (Concurrent administration of bupropion and agents that lower seizure threshold should be undertaken with extreme caution. Low initial dosing and gradual dose increases should be employed).
No products indexed under this heading.

Flurazepam Hydrochloride (Bupropion is contraindicated in patients undergoing abrupt discontinuation of benzodiazepine sedatives. Concomitant use of benzodiazepine sedatives with bupropion is associated with an increased seizure risk).
No products indexed under this heading.

Fluticasone Furoate (Concurrent administration of bupropion and agents that lower seizure threshold, such as systemic steroids, should be undertaken with extreme caution. Low initial dosing and gradual dose increases should be employed). Products include:
Veramyst **1713**

Fluticasone Propionate (Concurrent administration of bupropion and agents that lower seizure threshold, such as systemic steroids, should be undertaken with extreme caution. Low initial dosing and gradual dose increases should be employed). Products include:
Advair 100/50 .... **1275**
Advair 250/50 .... **1275**
Advair 500/50 .... **1275**
Advair HFA 45/21 .... **1288**
Advair HFA 115/21 .... **1288**
Advair HFA 230/21 .... **1288**
Flonase **1459**
Flovent Diskus **1463**
Flovent HFA **1470**

Fluvoxamine (*In vitro* studies suggest that fluvoxamine inhibits the hydroxylation of bupropion and thus may increase bupropion activity).
No products indexed under this heading.

Fluvoxamine Maleate (*In vitro* studies suggest that fluvoxamine inhibits the hydroxylation of bupropion and thus may increase bupropion activity).
No products indexed under this heading.

Formoterol Fumarate (Co-administration of bupropion with drugs that are metabolized by the CYP2D6 isoenzyme should be approached with caution and should be initiated at the lower end of the dose range of the concomitant medication. If bupropion is added to the treatment regimen of a patient already receiving a drug metabolized by CYP2D6, the need to decrease the dose of the original medication should be considered, particularly for those concomitant medications with a narrow therapeutic index). Products include:
Foradil **3121**
Perforomist **3634**

Fosphenytoin (Phenytoin may induce the metabolism of bupropion).
No products indexed under this heading.

Fosphenytoin Sodium (Phenytoin may induce the metabolism of bupropion).
No products indexed under this heading.

Galantamine Hydrobromide (Co-administration of bupropion with drugs that are metabolized by the CYP2D6 isoenzyme should be approached with caution and should be initiated at the lower end of the dose range of the concomitant medication. If bupropion is added to the treatment regimen of a patient already receiving a drug metabolized by CYP2D6, the need to decrease the dose of the original medication should be considered, particularly for those concomitant medications with a narrow therapeutic index).
No products indexed under this heading.

Garlic Extract (Bupropion may be an inducer of drug-metabolizing enzymes in humans. In one study, following chronic administration of bupropion hydrochloride, 100 mg 3 times daily to 8 healthy male volunteers for 14 days, there was no evidence of induction of its own metabolism. Nevertheless, there may be the potential for clinically important alterations of blood levels of co-administered drugs).
No products indexed under this heading.

Garlic Oil (Bupropion may be an inducer of drug-metabolizing enzymes in humans. In one study, following chronic administration of bupropion hydrochloride, 100 mg 3 times daily to 8 healthy male volunteers for 14 days, there was no evidence of induction of its own metabolism. Nevertheless, there may be the potential for clinically important alterations of blood levels of co-administered drugs).
No products indexed under this heading.

Glibenclamide (Concomitant use of oral hypoglycemics with bupropion is associated with an increased seizure risk).
No products indexed under this heading.

IMPORTANT NOTE: Always consult each drug listing in the patient's regimen for possible interactions.

Glimepiride (Concomitant use of oral hypoglycemics with bupropion is associated with an increased seizure risk). Products include:

Glipizide (Concomitant use of oral hypoglycemics with bupropion is associated with an increased seizure risk).
No products indexed under this heading.

Glutethimide (Bupropion is contraindicated in patients undergoing abrupt discontinuation of sedatives. Concomitant use of sedatives with bupropion is associated with an increased seizure risk).
No products indexed under this heading.

Glyburide (Concomitant use of oral hypoglycemics with bupropion is associated with an increased seizure risk).
No products indexed under this heading.

Halazepam (Bupropion is contraindicated in patients undergoing abrupt discontinuation of benzodiazepine sedatives. Concomitant use of benzodiazepine sedatives with bupropion is associated with an increased seizure risk).
No products indexed under this heading.

Haloperidol (Concurrent administration of bupropion and agents that lower seizure threshold should be undertaken with extreme caution. Low initial dosing and gradual dose increases should be employed).
No products indexed under this heading.

Haloperidol Decanoate (Concurrent administration of bupropion and agents that lower seizure threshold should be undertaken with extreme caution. Low initial dosing and gradual dose increases should be employed).
No products indexed under this heading.

Haloperidol Lactate (Concurrent administration of bupropion and agents that lower seizure threshold, such as antipsychotics, should be undertaken with extreme caution. Low initial dosing and gradual dose increases should be employed. Co-administration of bupropion with drugs that are metabolized by the CYP2D6 isoenzyme including antipsychotics (eg, haloperidol, risperidone, thioridazine) should be approached with caution and should be initiated at the lower end of the dose range of the concomitant medication. If bupropion is added to the treatment regimen of a patient already receiving a drug metabolized by CYP2D6, the need to decrease the dose of the original medication should be considered, particularly for those concomitant medications with a narrow therapeutic index).
No products indexed under this heading.

Halothane (Because bupropion is extensively metabolized, the co-administration of other drugs may affect its clinical activity. *In vitro* studies indicate that bupropion is primarily metabolized to hydroxybupropion by the CYP2B6 isoenzyme. Therefore, the potential exists for a drug interaction between bupropion and drugs that are substrates or inhibitors of the CYP2B6 isoenzyme (eg, orphenadrine, thiotepa, and cyclophosphamide). In addition, *in vitro* studies suggest that paroxetine, sertraline, norfluoxetine, and fluvoxamine as well as nelfinavir, ritonavir, and efavirenz inhibit the hydroxylation of bupropion).
No products indexed under this heading.

Hepatic Enzyme-Inducing Agents (Bupropion may be an inducer of drug-metabolizing enzymes in humans. In one study, following chronic administration of bupropion hydrochloride, 100 mg 3 times daily to 8 healthy male volunteers for 14 days, there was no evidence of induction of its own metabolism. Nevertheless, there may be the

potential for clinically important alterations of blood levels of co-administered drugs).
No products indexed under this heading.

Hydrocodone Bitartrate (Concomitant use of opiates, cocaine, or stimulants with bupropion is associated with an increased seizure risk). Products include:

Hydrocodone Polistirex (Concomitant use of opiates, cocaine, or stimulants with bupropion is associated with an increased seizure risk). Products include:

Hydrocortisone (Concurrent administration of bupropion and agents that lower seizure threshold, such as systemic steroids, should be undertaken with extreme caution. Low initial dosing and gradual dose increases should be employed).
No products indexed under this heading.

Hydrocortisone (Alcohol) (Concurrent administration of bupropion and agents that lower seizure threshold, such as systemic steroids, should be undertaken with extreme caution. Low initial dosing and gradual dose increases should be employed).
No products indexed under this heading.

Hydrocortisone Acetate (Concurrent administration of bupropion and agents that lower seizure threshold, such as systemic steroids, should be undertaken with extreme caution. Low initial dosing and gradual dose increases should be employed).
No products indexed under this heading.

Hydrocortisone Butyrate (Concurrent administration of bupropion and agents that lower seizure threshold, such as systemic steroids, should be undertaken with extreme caution. Low initial dosing and gradual dose increases should be employed).
No products indexed under this heading.

Hydrocortisone Cypionate (Concurrent administration of bupropion and agents that lower seizure threshold, such as systemic steroids, should be undertaken with extreme caution. Low initial dosing and gradual dose increases should be employed).
No products indexed under this heading.

Hydrocortisone Hemisuccinate (Concurrent administration of bupropion and agents that lower seizure threshold, such as systemic steroids, should be undertaken with extreme caution. Low initial dosing and gradual dose increases should be employed).
No products indexed under this heading.

Hydrocortisone Probutate (Concurrent administration of bupropion and agents that lower seizure threshold, such as systemic steroids, should be undertaken with extreme caution. Low initial dosing and gradual dose increases should be employed).
No products indexed under this heading.

Hydrocortisone Sodium Phosphate (Concurrent administration of bupropion and agents that lower seizure threshold, such as systemic steroids, should be undertaken with extreme caution. Low initial dosing and gradual dose increases should be employed).
No products indexed under this heading.

Hydrocortisone Sodium Succinate (Concurrent administration of bupropion and agents that lower seizure threshold, such as systemic steroids, should be undertaken with extreme caution. Low initial dosing and gradual dose increases should be employed).
No products indexed under this heading.

Hydrocortisone Valerate (Concurrent administration of bupropion and agents that lower seizure threshold, such as systemic steroids, should be undertaken with extreme caution. Low initial dosing and gradual dose increases should be employed).
No products indexed under this heading.

Hydromorphone (Concomitant use of opiates, cocaine, or stimulants with bupropion is associated with an increased seizure risk).
No products indexed under this heading.

Hydromorphone Hydrochloride (Concomitant use of opiates, cocaine, or stimulants with bupropion is associated with an increased seizure risk). Products include:

Hydroxyamphetamine Hydrobromide (Concomitant use of opiates, cocaine, or stimulants with bupropion is associated with an increased seizure risk).
No products indexed under this heading.

Hypericum (Bupropion may be an inducer of drug-metabolizing enzymes in humans. In one study, following chronic administration of bupropion hydrochloride, 100 mg 3 times daily to 8 healthy male volunteers for 14 days, there was no evidence of induction of its own metabolism. Nevertheless, there may be the potential for clinically important alterations of blood levels of co-administered drugs).
No products indexed under this heading.

Hypericum Perforatum (Bupropion may be an inducer of drug-metabolizing enzymes in humans. In one study, following chronic administration of bupropion hydrochloride, 100 mg 3 times daily to 8 healthy male volunteers for 14 days, there was no evidence of induction of its own metabolism. Nevertheless, there may be the potential for clinically important alterations of blood levels of co-administered drugs). Products include:

Ifosfamide (Because bupropion is extensively metabolized, the co-administration of other drugs may affect its clinical activity. *In vitro* studies indicate that bupropion is primarily metabolized to hydroxybupropion by the CYP2B6 isoenzyme. Therefore, the potential exists for a drug interaction between bupropion and drugs that are substrates or inhibitors of the CYP2B6 isoenzyme (eg, orphenadrine, thiotepa, and cyclophosphamide). In addition, *in vitro* studies suggest that paroxetine, sertraline, norfluoxetine, and fluvoxamine as well as nelfinavir, ritonavir, and efavirenz inhibit the hydroxylation of bupropion).
No products indexed under this heading.

Imipramine Hydrochloride (Concurrent administration of bupropion and agents that lower seizure threshold should be undertaken with extreme caution. Low initial dosing and gradual dose increases should be employed).
No products indexed under this heading.

Imipramine Pamoate (Concurrent administration of bupropion and agents that lower seizure threshold should be undertaken with extreme caution. Low initial dosing and gradual dose increases should be employed).
No products indexed under this heading.

Indoramin Hydrochloride (Co-administration of bupropion with drugs that are metabolized by the CYP2D6 isoenzyme should be approached with caution and should be initiated at the lower end of the dose range of the concomitant medication. If bupropion is added to the treatment regimen of a patient already receiving a drug metabolized by CYP2D6, the need to decrease the dose of the original medication should be considered, particularly for those concomitant medications with a narrow therapeutic index).
No products indexed under this heading.

Insulin (Concomitant use of insulin with bupropion is associated with an increased seizure risk).
No products indexed under this heading.

Insulin, Human, Zinc Suspension (Concomitant use of insulin with bupropion is associated with an increased seizure risk).
No products indexed under this heading.

Insulin, Human (rDNA origin) (Concomitant use of insulin with bupropion is associated with an increased seizure risk). Products include:

Insulin, Human NPH (Concomitant use of insulin with bupropion is associated with an increased seizure risk). Products include:

Insulin, Human Regular (Concomitant use of insulin with bupropion is associated with an increased seizure risk). Products include:

Insulin, Human Regular and Human NPH Mixture (Concomitant use of insulin with bupropion is associated with an increased seizure risk). Products include:

Insulin, NPH (Concomitant use of insulin with bupropion is associated with an increased seizure risk).
No products indexed under this heading.

Insulin, Regular (Concomitant use of insulin with bupropion is associated with an increased seizure risk).
No products indexed under this heading.

Insulin, Regular and NPH mixture (Concomitant use of insulin with bupropion is associated with an increased seizure risk).
No products indexed under this heading.

Insulin, Zinc Crystals (Concomitant use of insulin with bupropion is associated with an increased seizure risk).
No products indexed under this heading.

Insulin, Zinc Suspension (Concomitant use of insulin with bupropion is associated with an increased seizure risk).
No products indexed under this heading.

Insulin Aspart (Concomitant use of insulin with bupropion is associated with an increased seizure risk).
No products indexed under this heading.

Insulin Aspart, Human (Concomitant use of insulin with bupropion is associated with an increased seizure risk). Products include:

Insulin Aspart, Human Regular (Concomitant use of insulin with bupropion is associated with an increased seizure risk). Products include:

129 Interactions Index Aplenzin

NovoLog 2575

Insulin Aspart Protamine, Human (Concomitant use of insulin with bupropion is associated with an increased seizure risk). Products include:
NovoLog Mix 70/30 2581

Insulin Detemir (rDNA Origin) (Concomitant use of insulin with bupropion is associated with an increased seizure risk). Products include:
Levemir 2566

Insulin Glargine (Concomitant use of insulin with bupropion is associated with an increased seizure risk). Products include:
Lantus 2996

Insulin Glulisine (Concomitant use of insulin with bupropion is associated with an increased seizure risk). Products include:
Apidra 2937
Apidra SoloStar 2937

Insulin Lispro, Human (Concomitant use of insulin with bupropion is associated with an increased seizure risk). Products include:
Humalog 1910
Humalog Mix 1914
Humalog Mix75/25 1917

Insulin Lispro Protamine, Human (Concomitant use of insulin with bupropion is associated with an increased seizure risk). Products include:
Humalog Mix 1914
Humalog Mix75/25 1917

Irinotecan Hydrochloride (Because bupropion is extensively metabolized, the co-administration of other drugs may affect its clinical activity. *In vitro* studies indicate that bupropion is primarily metabolized to hydroxybupropion by the CYP2B6 isoenzyme. Therefore, the potential exists for a drug interaction between bupropion and drugs that are substrates or inhibitors of the CYP2B6 isoenzyme (eg, orphenadrine, thiotepa, and cyclophosphamide). In addition, *in vitro* studies suggest that paroxetine, sertraline, norfluoxetine, and fluvoxamine as well as nelfinavir, ritonavir, and efavirenz inhibit the hydroxylation of bupropion).
No products indexed under this heading.

Isocarboxazid (Concurrent administration of bupropion and monoamine oxidase (MAO) inhibitors is contraindicated. At least 14 days should elapse between discontinuation of a MAO inhibitor and initiation of treatment with bupropion. MAO inhibitors increases bupropion toxicity). Products include:
Marplan 3481

Isoflurane (Because bupropion is extensively metabolized, the co-administration of other drugs may affect its clinical activity. *In vitro* studies indicate that bupropion is primarily metabolized to hydroxybupropion by the CYP2B6 isoenzyme. Therefore, the potential exists for a drug interaction between bupropion and drugs that are substrates or inhibitors of the CYP2B6 isoenzyme (eg, orphenadrine, thiotepa, and cyclophosphamide). In addition, *in vitro* studies suggest that paroxetine, sertraline, norfluoxetine, and fluvoxamine as well as nelfinavir, ritonavir, and efavirenz inhibit the hydroxylation of bupropion).
No products indexed under this heading.

Isotretinoin (Because bupropion is extensively metabolized, the co-administration of other drugs may affect its clinical activity. *In vitro* studies indicate that bupropion is primarily metabolized to hydroxybupropion by the CYP2B6 isoenzyme. Therefore, the potential exists for a drug interaction between bupropion and drugs that are substrates or inhibitors of the CYP2B6 isoenzyme (eg, orphenadrine, thiotepa, and cyclophosphamide). In addition, *in vitro* studies suggest that paroxetine, sertraline, norfluoxetine, and fluvoxamine as well as nelfinavir, ritonavir, and efavirenz inhibit the hydroxylation of bupropion). Products include:
Accutane 2832

Ketamine (Because bupropion is extensively metabolized, the co-administration of other drugs may affect its clinical activity. *In vitro* studies indicate that bupropion is primarily metabolized to hydroxybupropion by the CYP2B6 isoenzyme. Therefore, the potential exists for a drug interaction between bupropion and drugs that are substrates or inhibitors of the CYP2B6 isoenzyme (eg, orphenadrine, thiotepa, and cyclophosphamide). In addition, *in vitro* studies suggest that paroxetine, sertraline, norfluoxetine, and fluvoxamine as well as nelfinavir, ritonavir, and efavirenz inhibit the hydroxylation of bupropion).
No products indexed under this heading.

Ketamine Hydrochloride (Because bupropion is extensively metabolized, the co-administration of other drugs may affect its clinical activity. *In vitro* studies indicate that bupropion is primarily metabolized to hydroxybupropion by the CYP2B6 isoenzyme. Therefore, the potential exists for a drug interaction between bupropion and drugs that are substrates or inhibitors of the CYP2B6 isoenzyme (eg, orphenadrine, thiotepa, and cyclophosphamide). In addition, *in vitro* studies suggest that paroxetine, sertraline, norfluoxetine, and fluvoxamine as well as nelfinavir, ritonavir, and efavirenz inhibit the hydroxylation of bupropion).
No products indexed under this heading.

Ketoconazole (Because bupropion is extensively metabolized, the co-administration of other drugs may affect its clinical activity. *In vitro* studies indicate that bupropion is primarily metabolized to hydroxybupropion by the CYP2B6 isoenzyme. Therefore, the potential exists for a drug interaction between bupropion and drugs that are substrates or inhibitors of the CYP2B6 isoenzyme (eg, orphenadrine, thiotepa, and cyclophosphamide). In addition, *in vitro* studies suggest that paroxetine, sertraline, norfluoxetine, and fluvoxamine as well as nelfinavir, ritonavir, and efavirenz inhibit the hydroxylation of bupropion). Products include:
Extina 3319
Xolegel 3337

Labetalol Hydrochloride (Co-administration of bupropion with drugs that are metabolized by the CYP2D6 isoenzyme should be approached with caution and should be initiated at the lower end of the dose range of the concomitant medication. If bupropion is added to the treatment regimen of a patient already receiving a drug metabolized by CYP2D6, the need to decrease the dose of the original medication should be considered, particularly for those concomitant medications with a narrow therapeutic index).
No products indexed under this heading.

Lansoprazole (Bupropion may be an inducer of drug-metabolizing enzymes in humans. In one study, following chronic administration of bupropion hydrochloride, 100 mg 3 times daily to 8 healthy male volunteers for 14 days, there was no evidence of induction of its own metabolism. Nevertheless, there may be the potential for clinically important alterations of blood levels of co-administered drugs).
No products indexed under this heading.

Levobunolol Hydrochloride (Co-administration of bupropion with drugs that are metabolized by the CYP2D6 isoenzyme including beta-blockers (eg, metoprolol) should be approached with caution and should be initiated at the lower end of the dose range of the concomitant medication. If bupropion is added to the treatment regimen of a patient already receiving a drug metabolized by CYP2D6, the need to decrease the dose of the original medication should be considered, particularly for those concomitant medications with a narrow therapeutic index).
No products indexed under this heading.

Levodopa (Limited clinical data suggest a higher incidence of adverse experiences in patients receiving bupropion concurrently with levodopa. Administration of burpopion tablets to patients receiving levodopa concurrently should be undertaken with caution, using small initial doses and gradual dose increases). Products include:
Stalevo 2526

Levorphanol Tartrate (Concomitant use of opiates, cocaine, or stimulants with bupropion is associated with an increased seizure risk).
No products indexed under this heading.

Lidocaine (Co-administration of bupropion with drugs that are metabolized by the CYP2D6 isoenzyme should be approached with caution and should be initiated at the lower end of the dose range of the concomitant medication. If bupropion is added to the treatment regimen of a patient already receiving a drug metabolized by CYP2D6, the need to decrease the dose of the original medication should be considered, particularly for those concomitant medications with a narrow therapeutic index). Products include:
Lidoderm 1107

Lidocaine Base (Because bupropion is extensively metabolized, the co-administration of other drugs may affect its clinical activity. *In vitro* studies indicate that bupropion is primarily metabolized to hydroxybupropion by the CYP2B6 isoenzyme. Therefore, the potential exists for a drug interaction between bupropion and drugs that are substrates or inhibitors of the CYP2B6 isoenzyme (eg, orphenadrine, thiotepa, and cyclophosphamide). In addition, *in vitro* studies suggest that paroxetine, sertraline, norfluoxetine, and fluvoxamine as well as nelfinavir, ritonavir, and efavirenz inhibit the hydroxylation of bupropion).
No products indexed under this heading.

Lidocaine Hydrochloride (Co-administration of bupropion with drugs that are metabolized by the CYP2D6 isoenzyme should be approached with caution and should be initiated at the lower end of the dose range of the concomitant medication. If bupropion is added to the treatment regimen of a patient already receiving a drug metabolized by CYP2D6, the need to decrease the dose of the original medication should be considered, particularly for those concomitant medications with a narrow therapeutic index).
No products indexed under this heading.

Lisdexamfetamine Dimesylate (Concomitant use of opiates, cocaine, or stimulants with bupropion is associated with an increased seizure risk). Products include:
Vyvanse 3298

Lithium (Concurrent administration of bupropion and agents that lower seizure threshold, such as antipsychotics, should be undertaken with extreme caution. Low initial dosing and gradual dose increases should be employed. Co-administration of bupropion with drugs that are metabolized by the CYP2D6 isoenzyme including antipsychotics (eg, haloperidol, risperidone, thioridazine) should be approached with caution and should be initiated at the lower end of the dose range of the concomitant medication. If bupropion is added to the treatment regimen of a patient already receiving a drug metabolized by CYP2D6, the need to decrease the dose of the original medication should be considered, particularly for those concomitant medications with a narrow therapeutic index).
No products indexed under this heading.

Lithium Carbonate (Concurrent administration of bupropion and agents that lower seizure threshold, such as antipsychotics, should be undertaken with extreme caution. Low initial dosing and gradual dose increases should be employed. Co-administration of bupropion with drugs that are metabolized by the CYP2D6 isoenzyme including antipsychotics (eg, haloperidol, risperidone, thioridazine) should be approached with caution and should be initiated at the lower end of the dose range of the concomitant medication. If bupropion is added to the treatment regimen of a patient already receiving a drug metabolized by CYP2D6, the need to decrease the dose of the original medication should be considered, particularly for those concomitant medications with a narrow therapeutic index).
No products indexed under this heading.

Lithium Citrate (Concurrent administration of bupropion and agents that lower seizure threshold, such as antipsychotics, should be undertaken with extreme caution. Low initial dosing and gradual dose increases should be employed. Co-administration of bupropion with drugs that are metabolized by the CYP2D6 isoenzyme including antipsychotics (eg, haloperidol, risperidone, thioridazine) should be approached with caution and should be initiated at the lower end of the dose range of the concomitant medication. If bupropion is added to the treatment regimen of a patient already receiving a drug metabolized by CYP2D6, the need to decrease the dose of the original medication should be considered, particularly for those concomitant medications with a narrow therapeutic index).
No products indexed under this heading.

Lorazepam (Bupropion is contraindicated in patients undergoing abrupt discontinuation of benzodiazepine sedatives. Concomitant use of benzodiazepine sedatives with bupropion is associated with an increased seizure risk).
No products indexed under this heading.

Loxapine Hydrochloride (Concurrent administration of bupropion and agents that lower seizure threshold, such as antipsychotics, should be undertaken with extreme caution. Low initial dosing and gradual dose increases should be employed. Co-administration of bupropion with drugs that are metabolized by the CYP2D6 isoenzyme including antipsychotics (eg, haloperidol, risperidone, thioridazine) should be approached with caution and should be initiated at the lower end of the dose range of the concomitant medication. If bupropion is added to the treatment regimen of a patient already receiving a drug metabolized by CYP2D6, the need to decrease the dose of the original medication should be considered, particularly for those concomitant medications with a narrow therapeutic index).
No products indexed under this heading.

Loxapine Succinate (Concurrent administration of bupropion and agents that lower seizure threshold, such as antipsychotics, should be undertaken with extreme caution. Low initial dosing and gradual dose increases should be employed. Co-administration of bupropion with drugs that are metabolized by the CYP2D6 isoenzyme including antipsychotics (eg, haloperidol, risperidone,

IMPORTANT NOTE: Always consult each drug listing in the patient's regimen for possible interactions.

Aplenzin Interactions Index 130

thioridazine) should be approached with caution and should be initiated at the lower end of the dose range of the concomitant medication. If bupropion is added to the treatment regimen of a patient already receiving a drug metabolized by CYP2D6, the need to decrease the dose of the original medication should be considered, particularly for those concomitant medications with a narrow therapeutic index).
No products indexed under this heading.

Maprotiline Hydrochloride (Concurrent administration of bupropion and agents that lower seizure threshold should be undertaken with extreme caution. Low initial dosing and gradual dose increases should be employed).
No products indexed under this heading.

Mazindol (Concomitant use of anorectics with bupropion is associated with an increased seizure risk).
No products indexed under this heading.

Meperidine Hydrochloride (Concomitant use of opiates, cocaine, or stimulants with bupropion is associated with an increased seizure risk).
No products indexed under this heading.

Mephenytoin (Because bupropion is extensively metabolized, the co-administration of other drugs may affect its clinical activity. *In vitro* studies indicate that bupropion is primarily metabolized to hydroxybupropion by the CYP2B6 isoenzyme. Therefore, the potential exists for a drug interaction between bupropion and drugs that are substrates or inhibitors of the CYP2B6 isoenzyme (eg, orphenadrine, thiotepa, and cyclophosphamide). In addition, *in vitro* studies suggest that paroxetine, sertraline, norfluoxetine, and fluvoxamine as well as nelfinavir, ritonavir, and efavirenz inhibit the hydroxylation of bupropion).
No products indexed under this heading.

Mephobarbital (Because bupropion is extensively metabolized, the co-administration of other drugs may affect its clinical activity. *In vitro* studies indicate that bupropion is primarily metabolized to hydroxybupropion by the CYP2B6 isoenzyme. Therefore, the potential exists for a drug interaction between bupropion and drugs that are substrates or inhibitors of the CYP2B6 isoenzyme (eg, orphenadrine, thiotepa, and cyclophosphamide). In addition, *in vitro* studies suggest that paroxetine, sertraline, norfluoxetine, and fluvoxamine as well as nelfinavir, ritonavir, and efavirenz inhibit the hydroxylation of bupropion).
No products indexed under this heading.

Mesoridazine Besylate (Concurrent administration of bupropion and agents that lower seizure threshold should be undertaken with extreme caution. Low initial dosing and gradual dose increases should be employed).
No products indexed under this heading.

Metformin Hydrochloride (Concomitant use of oral hypoglycemics with bupropion is associated with an increased seizure risk). Products include:
ActoPlus **3338**
Avandamet **1345**
Janumet **2188**

Methadone Hydrochloride (Concomitant use of opiates, cocaine, or stimulants with bupropion is associated with an increased seizure risk).
No products indexed under this heading.

Methamphetamine Hydrochloride (Concomitant use of opiates, cocaine, or stimulants with bupropion is associated with an increased seizure risk).
No products indexed under this heading.

Methimazole (Because bupropion is extensively metabolized, the co-administration of other drugs may affect its clinical activity. *In vitro* studies indicate that bupropion is primarily metabolized to hydroxybupropion by the CYP2B6 isoenzyme. Therefore, the potential exists for a drug interaction between bupropion and drugs that are substrates or inhibitors of the CYP2B6 isoenzyme (eg, orphenadrine, thiotepa, and cyclophosphamide). In addition, *in vitro* studies suggest that paroxetine, sertraline, norfluoxetine, and fluvoxamine as well as nelfinavir, ritonavir, and efavirenz inhibit the hydroxylation of bupropion).
No products indexed under this heading.

Methotrimeprazine (Concurrent administration of bupropion and agents that lower seizure threshold, such as antipsychotics, should be undertaken with extreme caution. Low initial dosing and gradual dose increases should be employed. Co-administration of bupropion with drugs that are metabolized by the CYP2D6 isoenzyme including antipsychotics (eg, haloperidol, risperidone, thioridazine) should be approached with caution and should be initiated at the lower end of the dose range of the concomitant medication. If bupropion is added to the treatment regimen of a patient already receiving a drug metabolized by CYP2D6, the need to decrease the dose of the original medication should be considered, particularly for those concomitant medications with a narrow therapeutic index).
No products indexed under this heading.

Methoxyphenamine (Co-administration of bupropion with drugs that are metabolized by the CYP2D6 isoenzyme should be approached with caution and should be initiated at the lower end of the dose range of the concomitant medication. If bupropion is added to the treatment regimen of a patient already receiving a drug metabolized by CYP2D6, the need to decrease the dose of the original medication should be considered, particularly for those concomitant medications with a narrow therapeutic index).
No products indexed under this heading.

Methsuximide (Bupropion may be an inducer of drug-metabolizing enzymes in humans. In one study, following chronic administration of bupropion hydrochloride, 100 mg 3 times daily to 8 healthy male volunteers for 14 days, there was no evidence of induction of its own metabolism. Nevertheless, there may be the potential for clinically important alterations of blood levels of co-administered drugs).
No products indexed under this heading.

Methylphenidate (Concomitant use of opiates, cocaine, or stimulants with bupropion is associated with an increased seizure risk). Products include:
Daytrana **3283**

Methylphenidate Hydrochloride (Concomitant use of opiates, cocaine, or stimulants with bupropion is associated with an increased seizure risk). Products include:
Concerta **2598**
Metadate CD **3439**

Methylprednisolone (Concurrent administration of bupropion and agents that lower seizure threshold, such as systemic steroids, should be undertaken with extreme caution. Low initial dosing and gradual dose increases should be employed).
No products indexed under this heading.

Methylprednisolone Acetate (Concurrent administration of bupropion and agents that lower seizure threshold, such as systemic steroids, should be undertaken with extreme caution. Low initial dosing and gradual dose increases should be employed).
No products indexed under this heading.

Methylprednisolone Sodium Succinate (Concurrent administration of bupropion and agents that lower seizure threshold, such as systemic steroids, should be undertaken with extreme caution. Low initial dosing and gradual dose increases should be employed).
No products indexed under this heading.

Methyltestosterone (Because bupropion is extensively metabolized, the co-administration of other drugs may affect its clinical activity. *In vitro* studies indicate that bupropion is primarily metabolized to hydroxybupropion by the CYP2B6 isoenzyme. Therefore, the potential exists for a drug interaction between bupropion and drugs that are substrates or inhibitors of the CYP2B6 isoenzyme (eg, orphenadrine, thiotepa, and cyclophosphamide). In addition, *in vitro* studies suggest that paroxetine, sertraline, norfluoxetine, and fluvoxamine as well as nelfinavir, ritonavir, and efavirenz inhibit the hydroxylation of bupropion).
No products indexed under this heading.

Metipranolol Hydrochloride (Co-administration of bupropion with drugs that are metabolized by the CYP2D6 isoenzyme including beta-blockers (eg, metoprolol) should be approached with caution and should be initiated at the lower end of the dose range of the concomitant medication. If bupropion is added to the treatment regimen of a patient already receiving a drug metabolized by CYP2D6, the need to decrease the dose of the original medication should be considered, particularly for those concomitant medications with a narrow therapeutic index).
No products indexed under this heading.

Metoprolol Succinate (Co-administration of bupropion with drugs that are metabolized by the CYP2D6 isoenzyme should be approached with caution and should be initiated at the lower end of the dose range of the concomitant medication. If bupropion is added to the treatment regimen of a patient already receiving a drug metabolized by CYP2D6, the need to decrease the dose of the original medication should be considered, particularly for those concomitant medications with a narrow therapeutic index). Products include:
Toprol XL **732**

Metoprolol Tartrate (Co-administration of bupropion with drugs that are metabolized by the CYP2D6 isoenzyme should be approached with caution and should be initiated at the lower end of the dose range of the concomitant medication. If bupropion is added to the treatment regimen of a patient already receiving a drug metabolized by CYP2D6, the need to decrease the dose of the original medication should be considered, particularly for those concomitant medications with a narrow therapeutic index).
No products indexed under this heading.

Mexiletine Hydrochloride (Co-administration of bupropion with drugs that are metabolized by the CYP2D6 isoenzyme should be approached with caution and should be initiated at the lower end of the dose range of the concomitant medication. If bupropion is added to the treatment regimen of a patient already receiving a drug metabolized by CYP2D6, the need to decrease the dose of the original medication should be considered, particularly for those concomitant medications with a narrow therapeutic index).
No products indexed under this heading.

Miconazole (Because bupropion is extensively metabolized, the co-administration of other drugs may affect its clinical activity. *In vitro* studies indicate that bupropion is primarily metabolized to hydroxybupropion by the CYP2B6 isoenzyme. Therefore, the potential exists for a drug interaction between bupropion and drugs that are substrates or inhibitors of the CYP2B6 isoenzyme (eg, orphenadrine, thiotepa, and cyclophosphamide). In addition, *in vitro* studies suggest that paroxetine, sertraline, norfluoxetine, and fluvoxamine as well as nelfinavir, ritonavir, and efavirenz inhibit the hydroxylation of bupropion).
No products indexed under this heading.

Miconazole Nitrate (Because bupropion is extensively metabolized, the co-administration of other drugs may affect its clinical activity. *In vitro* studies indicate that bupropion is primarily metabolized to hydroxybupropion by the CYP2B6 isoenzyme. Therefore, the potential exists for a drug interaction between bupropion and drugs that are substrates or inhibitors of the CYP2B6 isoenzyme (eg, orphenadrine, thiotepa, and cyclophosphamide). In addition, *in vitro* studies suggest that paroxetine, sertraline, norfluoxetine, and fluvoxamine as well as nelfinavir, ritonavir, and efavirenz inhibit the hydroxylation of bupropion). Products include:
Vusion Ointment **3335**

Midazolam Hydrochloride (Bupropion is contraindicated in patients undergoing abrupt discontinuation of benzodiazepine sedatives. Concomitant use of benzodiazepine sedatives with bupropion is associated with an increased seizure risk).
No products indexed under this heading.

Miglitol (Concomitant use of oral hypoglycemics with bupropion is associated with an increased seizure risk).
No products indexed under this heading.

Mirtazapine (Concurrent administration of bupropion and agents that lower seizure threshold, such as antidepressants, should be undertaken with extreme caution. Low initial dosing and gradual dose increases should be employed. Co-administration of bupropion with drugs that are metabolized by the CYP2D6 isoenzyme including antidepressants (eg, nortriptyline, imipramine, desipramine, paroxentine, fluoxetine, sertraline) should be approached with caution and should be initiated at the lower end of the dose range of the concomitant medication. If bupropion is added to the treatment regimen of a patient already receiving a drug metabolized by CYP2D6, the need to decrease the dose of the original medication should be considered, particularly for those concomitant medications with a narrow therapeutic index). Products include:
Remeron Tablets **3214**
RemeronSolTab Tablets **3219**

Moclobemide (Concurrent administration of bupropion and monoamine oxidase (MAO) inhibitors is contraindicated. At least 14 days should elapse between discontinuation of a MAO inhibitor and initiation of treatment with bupropion. MAO inhibitors increases bupropion toxicity).
No products indexed under this heading.

Modafinil (Bupropion may be an inducer of drug-metabolizing enzymes in humans. In one study, following chronic administration of bupropion hydrochloride, 100 mg 3 times daily to 8 healthy male volunteers for 14 days, there was

131 **Interactions Index** **Aplenzin**

no evidence of induction of its own metabolism. Nevertheless, there may be the potential for clinically important alterations of blood levels of co-administered drugs). Products include:
Provigil ... 983

Molindone Hydrochloride (Concurrent administration of bupropion and agents that lower seizure threshold, such as antipsychotics, should be undertaken with extreme caution. Low initial dosing and gradual dose increases should be employed. Co-administration of bupropion with drugs that are metabolized by the CYP2D6 isoenzyme including antipsychotics (eg, haloperidol, risperidone, thioridazine) should be approached with caution and should be initiated at the lower end of the dose range of the concomitant medication. If bupropion is added to the treatment regimen of a patient already receiving a drug metabolized by CYP2D6, the need to decrease the dose of the original medication should be considered, particularly for those concomitant medications with a narrow therapeutic index). Products include:
Moban ... 1108

Mometasone Furoate (Concurrent administration of bupropion and agents that lower seizure threshold, such as systemic steroids, should be undertaken with extreme caution. Low initial dosing and gradual dose increases should be employed). Products include:
Asmanex ... 3058
Elocon Cream ... 3111
Elocon Lotion ... 3112
Elocon Ointment ... 3114

Mometasone Furoate Monohydrate (Concurrent administration of bupropion and agents that lower seizure threshold, such as systemic steroids, should be undertaken with extreme caution. Low initial dosing and gradual dose increases should be employed). Products include:
Nasonex ... 3166

Morphine Sulfate (Concomitant use of opiates, cocaine, or stimulants with bupropion is associated with an increased seizure risk). Products include:
Avinza ... 1822
Embeda ... 1831
MS Contin ... 2803

Morphine Sulfate, Liposomal (Concomitant use of opiates, cocaine, or stimulants with bupropion is associated with an increased seizure risk).
No products indexed under this heading.

Nadolol (Co-administration of bupropion with drugs that are metabolized by the CYP2D6 isoenzyme including beta-blockers (eg, metoprolol) should be approached with caution and should be initiated at the lower end of the dose range of the concomitant medication. If bupropion is added to the treatment regimen of a patient already receiving a drug metabolized by CYP2D6, the need to decrease the dose of the original medication should be considered, particularly for those concomitant medications with a narrow therapeutic index). Products include:
Nadolol ... 2359

Nafcillin Sodium (Bupropion may be an inducer of drug-metabolizing enzymes in humans. In one study, following chronic administration of bupropion hydrochloride, 100 mg 3 times daily to 8 healthy male volunteers for 14 days, there was no evidence of induction of its own metabolism. Nevertheless, there may be the potential for clinically important alterations of blood levels of co-administered drugs).
No products indexed under this heading.

Nateglinide (Concomitant use of oral hypoglycemics with bupropion is associated with an increased seizure risk).
No products indexed under this heading.

Nebivolol (Co-administration of bupropion with drugs that are metabolized by the CYP2D6 isoenzyme including beta-blockers (eg, metoprolol) should be approached with caution and should be initiated at the lower end of the dose range of the concomitant medication. If bupropion is added to the treatment regimen of a patient already receiving a drug metabolized by CYP2D6, the need to decrease the dose of the original medication should be considered, particularly for those concomitant medications with a narrow therapeutic index). Products include:
Bystolic ... 1147

Nefazodone Hydrochloride (Concurrent administration of bupropion and agents that lower seizure threshold, such as antidepressants, should be undertaken with extreme caution. Low initial dosing and gradual dose increases should be employed. Co-administration of bupropion with drugs that are metabolized by the CYP2D6 isoenzyme including antidepressants (eg, nortriptyline, imipramine, desipramine, paroxentine, fluoxetine, sertraline) should be approached with caution and should be initiated at the lower end of the dose range of the concomitant medication. If bupropion is added to the treatment regimen of a patient already receiving a drug metabolized by CYP2D6, the need to decrease the dose of the original medication should be considered, particularly for those concomitant medications with a narrow therapeutic index).
No products indexed under this heading.

Nelfinavir Mesylate (*In vitro* studies suggest that nelfinavir inhibits the hydroxylation of bupropion and thus may increase bupropion activity).
No products indexed under this heading.

Nevirapine (Because bupropion is extensively metabolized, the co-administration of other drugs may affect its clinical activity. *In vitro* studies indicate that bupropion is primarily metabolized to hydroxybupropion by the CYP2B6 isoenzyme. Therefore, the potential exists for a drug interaction between bupropion and drugs that are substrates or inhibitors of the CYP2B6 isoenzyme (eg, orphenadrine, thiotepa, and cyclophosphamide). In addition, *in vitro* studies suggest that paroxetine, sertraline, norfluoxetine, and fluvoxamine as well as nelfinavir, ritonavir, and efavirenz inhibit the hydroxylation of bupropion). Products include:
Viramune Oral Suspension ... 897
Viramune Tablets ... 897

Nicotine (In clinical practice, hypertension, in some cases severe, requiring acute treatment, has been reported in patients receiving bupropion alone and in combination with nicotine replacement therapy. These events have been observed in both patients with and without evidence of preexisting hypertension. Monitoring of blood pressure is recommended in patients who receive the combination of bupropion and nicotine replacement).
No products indexed under this heading.

Nicotine Polacrilex (Because bupropion is extensively metabolized, the co-administration of other drugs may affect its clinical activity. *In vitro* studies indicate that bupropion is primarily metabolized to hydroxybupropion by the CYP2B6 isoenzyme. Therefore, the potential exists for a drug interaction between bupropion and drugs that are substrates or inhibitors of the CYP2B6 isoenzyme (eg, orphenadrine, thiotepa, and cyclophosphamide). In addition, *in vitro* studies suggest that paroxetine, sertraline, norfluoxetine, and fluvoxamine as well as nelfinavir, ritonavir, and efavirenz inhibit the hydroxylation of bupropion).
No products indexed under this heading.

Nicotine Salicylate (Because bupropion is extensively metabolized, the co-administration of other drugs may affect its clinical activity. *In vitro* studies indicate that bupropion is primarily metabolized to hydroxybupropion by the CYP2B6 isoenzyme. Therefore, the potential exists for a drug interaction between bupropion and drugs that are substrates or inhibitors of the CYP2B6 isoenzyme (eg, orphenadrine, thiotepa, and cyclophosphamide). In addition, *in vitro* studies suggest that paroxetine, sertraline, norfluoxetine, and fluvoxamine as well as nelfinavir, ritonavir, and efavirenz inhibit the hydroxylation of bupropion).
No products indexed under this heading.

Nicotine Sulfate (Because bupropion is extensively metabolized, the co-administration of other drugs may affect its clinical activity. *In vitro* studies indicate that bupropion is primarily metabolized to hydroxybupropion by the CYP2B6 isoenzyme. Therefore, the potential exists for a drug interaction between bupropion and drugs that are substrates or inhibitors of the CYP2B6 isoenzyme (eg, orphenadrine, thiotepa, and cyclophosphamide). In addition, *in vitro* studies suggest that paroxetine, sertraline, norfluoxetine, and fluvoxamine as well as nelfinavir, ritonavir, and efavirenz inhibit the hydroxylation of bupropion).
No products indexed under this heading.

Norethindrone (Bupropion may be an inducer of drug-metabolizing enzymes in humans. In one study, following chronic administration of bupropion hydrochloride, 100 mg 3 times daily to 8 healthy male volunteers for 14 days, there was no evidence of induction of its own metabolism. Nevertheless, there may be the potential for clinically important alterations of blood levels of co-administered drugs). Products include:
Ortho Micronor ... 2660

Norethindrone Acetate (Bupropion may be an inducer of drug-metabolizing enzymes in humans. In one study, following chronic administration of bupropion hydrochloride, 100 mg 3 times daily to 8 healthy male volunteers for 14 days, there was no evidence of induction of its own metabolism. Nevertheless, there may be the potential for clinically important alterations of blood levels of co-administered drugs). Products include:
Activella ... 2561

Norfluoxetine (Because bupropion is extensively metabolized, the co-administration of other drugs may affect its clinical activity. *In vitro* studies indicate that bupropion is primarily metabolized to hydroxybupropion by the CYP2B6 isoenzyme. Therefore, the potential exists for a drug interaction between bupropion and drugs that are substrates or inhibitors of the CYP2B6 isoenzyme (eg, orphenadrine, thiotepa, and cyclophosphamide). In addition, *in vitro* studies suggest that paroxetine, sertraline, norfluoxetine, and fluvoxamine as well as nelfinavir, ritonavir, and efavirenz inhibit the hydroxylation of bupropion).
No products indexed under this heading.

Nortriptyline Hydrochloride (Concurrent administration of bupropion and agents that lower seizure threshold should be undertaken with extreme caution. Low initial dosing and gradual dose increases should be employed).
No products indexed under this heading.

Olanzapine (Concurrent administration of bupropion and agents that lower seizure threshold, such as antipsychotics, should be undertaken with extreme caution. Low initial dosing and gradual dose increases should be employed. Co-administration of bupropion with drugs that are metabolized by the CYP2D6 isoenzyme including antipsychotics (eg, haloperidol, risperidone, thioridazine) should be approached with caution and should be initiated at the lower end of the dose range of the concomitant medication. If bupropion is added to the treatment regimen of a patient already receiving a drug metabolized by CYP2D6, the need to decrease the dose of the original medication should be considered, particularly for those concomitant medications with a narrow therapeutic index). Products include:
Symbyax ... 1965
Zyprexa ... 1984
Zyprexa IntraMuscular ... 1984
Zyprexa ZYDIS ... 1984

Omeprazole (Co-administration of bupropion with drugs that are metabolized by the CYP2D6 isoenzyme should be approached with caution and should be initiated at the lower end of the dose range of the concomitant medication. If bupropion is added to the treatment regimen of a patient already receiving a drug metabolized by CYP2D6, the need to decrease the dose of the original medication should be considered, particularly for those concomitant medications with a narrow therapeutic index).
No products indexed under this heading.

Omeprazole Magnesium (Bupropion may be an inducer of drug-metabolizing enzymes in humans. In one study, following chronic administration of bupropion hydrochloride, 100 mg 3 times daily to 8 healthy male volunteers for 14 days, there was no evidence of induction of its own metabolism. Nevertheless, there may be the potential for clinically important alterations of blood levels of co-administered drugs).
No products indexed under this heading.

Ondansetron (Co-administration of bupropion with drugs that are metabolized by the CYP2D6 isoenzyme should be approached with caution and should be initiated at the lower end of the dose range of the concomitant medication. If bupropion is added to the treatment regimen of a patient already receiving a drug metabolized by CYP2D6, the need to decrease the dose of the original medication should be considered, particularly for those concomitant medications with a narrow therapeutic index).
No products indexed under this heading.

Ondansetron Hydrochloride (Co-administration of bupropion with drugs that are metabolized by the CYP2D6 isoenzyme should be approached with caution and should be initiated at the lower end of the dose range of the concomitant medication. If bupropion is added to the treatment regimen of a patient already receiving a drug metabolized by CYP2D6, the need to decrease the dose of the original medication should be considered, particularly for those concomitant medications with a narrow therapeutic index). Products include:
Zofran Injection ... 1750
Zofran ... 1756
Zofran ODT ... 1756

Orphenadrine Citrate (Because bupropion is extensively metabolized, the co-administration of other drugs may affect its clinical activity. *In vitro* studies indicate that bupropion is primarily metabolized to hydroxybupropion by the CYP2B6 isoenzyme. Therefore, the potential exists for a drug interaction between bupropion and drugs that

IMPORTANT NOTE: Always consult each drug listing in the patient's regimen for possible interactions.

are substrates or inhibitors of the CYP2B6 isoenzyme (eg, orphenadrine, thiotepa, and cyclophosphamide). In addition, *in vitro* studies suggest that paroxetine, sertraline, norfluoxetine, and fluvoxamine as well as nelfinavir, ritonavir, and efavirenz inhibit the hydroxylation of bupropion).
No products indexed under this heading.

Orphenadrine Hydrochloride (Because bupropion is extensively metabolized, the co-administration of other drugs may affect its clinical activity. *In vitro* studies indicate that bupropion is primarily metabolized to hydroxybupropion by the CYP2B6 isoenzyme. Therefore, the potential exists for a drug interaction between bupropion and drugs that are substrates or inhibitors of the CYP2B6 isoenzyme (eg, orphenadrine, thiotepa, and cyclophosphamide). In addition, *in vitro* studies suggest that paroxetine, sertraline, norfluoxetine, and fluvoxamine as well as nelfinavir, ritonavir, and efavirenz inhibit the hydroxylation of bupropion).
No products indexed under this heading.

Oxazepam (Bupropion is contraindicated in patients undergoing abrupt discontinuation of benzodiazepine sedatives. Concomitant use of benzodiazepine sedatives with bupropion is associated with an increased seizure risk).
No products indexed under this heading.

Oxcarbazepine (Bupropion may be an inducer of drug-metabolizing enzymes in humans. In one study, following chronic administration of bupropion hydrochloride, 100 mg 3 times daily to 8 healthy male volunteers for 14 days, there was no evidence of induction of its own metabolism. Nevertheless, there may be the potential for clinically important alterations of blood levels of co-administered drugs).
No products indexed under this heading.

Oxycodone Hydrochloride (Concomitant use of opiates, cocaine, or stimulants with bupropion is associated with an increased seizure risk).
Products include:
OxyContin **2807**
Percocet **1121**
Percodan **1124**

Oxycodone Terephthalate (Concomitant use of opiates, cocaine, or stimulants with bupropion is associated with an increased seizure risk).
No products indexed under this heading.

Oxymorphone Hydrochloride (Concomitant use of opiates, cocaine, or stimulants with bupropion is associated with an increased seizure risk).
Products include:
Opana **1110**
Opana ER **1114**

Paclitaxel (Co-administration of bupropion with drugs that are metabolized by the CYP2D6 isoenzyme should be approached with caution and should be initiated at the lower end of the dose range of the concomitant medication. If bupropion is added to the treatment regimen of a patient already receiving a drug metabolized by CYP2D6, the need to decrease the dose of the original medication should be considered, particularly for those concomitant medications with a narrow therapeutic index).
No products indexed under this heading.

Paliperidone (Concurrent administration of bupropion and agents that lower seizure threshold, such as antipsychotics, should be undertaken with extreme caution. Low initial dosing and gradual dose increases should be employed. Co-administration of bupropion with drugs that are metabolized by the CYP2D6 isoenzyme including antipsychotics (eg, haloperidol, risperidone, thioridazine) should be approached with caution and should be initiated at the lower end of the dose range of the concomitant medication. If bupropion is added to the treatment regimen of a patient already receiving a drug metabolized by CYP2D6, the need to decrease the dose of the original medication should be considered, particularly for those concomitant medications with a narrow therapeutic index).
Products include:
Invega **2613**
Invega Sustenna **2621**

Pargyline Hydrochloride (Concurrent administration of bupropion and monoamine oxidase (MAO) inhibitors is contraindicated. At least 14 days should elapse between discontinuation of a MAO inhibitor and initiation of treatment with bupropion. MAO inhibitors increases bupropion toxicity).
No products indexed under this heading.

Paroxetine (*In vitro* studies suggest that paroxetine inhibits the hydroxylation of bupropion and thus may increase bupropion activity).
No products indexed under this heading.

Paroxetine Hydrochloride (*In vitro* studies suggest that paroxetine inhibits the hydroxylation of bupropion and thus may increase bupropion activity).
Products include:
Paroxetine CR **2361**
Paroxetine ER **2371**
Paxil **1586**
Paxil CR **1596**

Paroxetine Mesylate (*In vitro* studies suggest that paroxetine inhibits the hydroxylation of bupropion and thus may increase bupropion activity).
No products indexed under this heading.

Pemoline (Concomitant use of opiates, cocaine, or stimulants with bupropion is associated with an increased seizure risk).
No products indexed under this heading.

Penbutolol Sulfate (Co-administration of bupropion with drugs that are metabolized by the CYP2D6 isoenzyme including beta-blockers (eg, metoprolol) should be approached with caution and should be initiated at the lower end of the dose range of the concomitant medication. If bupropion is added to the treatment regimen of a patient already receiving a drug metabolized by CYP2D6, the need to decrease the dose of the original medication should be considered, particularly for those concomitant medications with a narrow therapeutic index).
No products indexed under this heading.

Perphenazine (Concurrent administration of bupropion and agents that lower seizure threshold should be undertaken with extreme caution. Low initial dosing and gradual dose increases should be employed).
No products indexed under this heading.

Phendimetrazine Tartrate (Concomitant use of anorectics with bupropion is associated with an increased seizure risk).
No products indexed under this heading.

Phenelzine Sulfate (Concurrent and/or sequential use with MAO inhibitors is contraindicated; acute toxicity of bupropion is enhanced by phenelzine).
No products indexed under this heading.

Phenmetrazine Hydrochloride (Concomitant use of anorectics with bupropion is associated with an increased seizure risk).
No products indexed under this heading.

Phenobarbital (Phenobarbital may induce the metabolism of bupropion).
Products include:
Donnatal **2711**

Phenobarbital Sodium (Bupropion may be an inducer of drug-metabolizing enzymes in humans. In one study, following chronic administration of bupropion hydrochloride, 100 mg 3 times daily to 8 healthy male volunteers for 14 days, there was no evidence of induction of its own metabolism. Nevertheless, there may be the potential for clinically important alterations of blood levels of co-administered drugs).
No products indexed under this heading.

Phenylbutazone (Bupropion may be an inducer of drug-metabolizing enzymes in humans. In one study, following chronic administration of bupropion hydrochloride, 100 mg 3 times daily to 8 healthy male volunteers for 14 days, there was no evidence of induction of its own metabolism. Nevertheless, there may be the potential for clinically important alterations of blood levels of co-administered drugs).
No products indexed under this heading.

Phenytoin (Phenytoin may induce the metabolism of bupropion).
No products indexed under this heading.

Phenytoin Sodium (Phenytoin may induce the metabolism of bupropion).
Products include:
Phenytek Capsules **2380**

Pimozide (Concurrent administration of bupropion and agents that lower seizure threshold, such as antipsychotics, should be undertaken with extreme caution. Low initial dosing and gradual dose increases should be employed. Co-administration of bupropion with drugs that are metabolized by the CYP2D6 isoenzyme including antipsychotics (eg, haloperidol, risperidone, thioridazine) should be approached with caution and should be initiated at the lower end of the dose range of the concomitant medication. If bupropion is added to the treatment regimen of a patient already receiving a drug metabolized by CYP2D6, the need to decrease the dose of the original medication should be considered, particularly for those concomitant medications with a narrow therapeutic index).
No products indexed under this heading.

Pindolol (Co-administration of bupropion with drugs that are metabolized by the CYP2D6 isoenzyme should be approached with caution and should be initiated at the lower end of the dose range of the concomitant medication. If bupropion is added to the treatment regimen of a patient already receiving a drug metabolized by CYP2D6, the need to decrease the dose of the original medication should be considered, particularly for those concomitant medications with a narrow therapeutic index).
No products indexed under this heading.

Pioglitazone Hydrochloride (Concomitant use of oral hypoglycemics with bupropion is associated with an increased seizure risk). Products include:
ActoPlus **3338**
Actos **3345**
Duetact **3354**

Polyestradiol Phosphate (Because bupropion is extensively metabolized, the co-administration of other drugs may affect its clinical activity. *In vitro* studies indicate that bupropion is primarily metabolized to hydroxybupropion by the CYP2B6 isoenzyme. Therefore, the potential exists for a drug interaction between bupropion and drugs that are substrates or inhibitors of the CYP2B6 isoenzyme (eg, orphenadrine, thiotepa, and cyclophosphamide). In addition, *in vitro* studies suggest that paroxetine, sertraline, norfluoxetine, and fluvoxamine as well as nelfinavir, ritonavir, and efavirenz inhibit the hydroxylation of bupropion).
No products indexed under this heading.

Prazepam (Bupropion is contraindicated in patients undergoing abrupt discontinuation of benzodiazepine sedatives. Concomitant use of benzodiazepine sedatives with bupropion is associated with an increased seizure risk).
No products indexed under this heading.

Prednisolone (Concurrent administration of bupropion and agents that lower seizure threshold, such as systemic steroids, should be undertaken with extreme caution. Low initial dosing and gradual dose increases should be employed).
No products indexed under this heading.

Prednisolone Acetate (Concurrent administration of bupropion and agents that lower seizure threshold, such as systemic steroids, should be undertaken with extreme caution. Low initial dosing and gradual dose increases should be employed). Products include:
Blephamide .... ⊙**212**, ⊙**214**
Pred Forte .... ⊙**225**
Pred Mild .... ⊙**230**
Pred-G .... ⊙**226**, ⊙**227**

Prednisolone Sodium Phosphate (Concurrent administration of bupropion and agents that lower seizure threshold, such as systemic steroids, should be undertaken with extreme caution. Low initial dosing and gradual dose increases should be employed).
No products indexed under this heading.

Prednisolone Tebutate (Concurrent administration of bupropion and agents that lower seizure threshold, such as systemic steroids, should be undertaken with extreme caution. Low initial dosing and gradual dose increases should be employed).
No products indexed under this heading.

Prednisone (Concurrent administration of bupropion and agents that lower seizure threshold, such as systemic steroids, should be undertaken with extreme caution. Low initial dosing and gradual dose increases should be employed).
No products indexed under this heading.

Prednisone sodium phosphate (Concurrent administration of bupropion and agents that lower seizure threshold, such as systemic steroids, should be undertaken with extreme caution. Low initial dosing and gradual dose increases should be employed).
No products indexed under this heading.

Primidone (Bupropion may be an inducer of drug-metabolizing enzymes in humans. In one study, following chronic administration of bupropion hydrochloride, 100 mg 3 times daily to 8 healthy male volunteers for 14 days, there was no evidence of induction of its own metabolism. Nevertheless, there may be the potential for clinically important alterations of blood levels of co-administered drugs).
No products indexed under this heading.

Procarbazine Hydrochloride (Concurrent administration of bupropion and monoamine oxidase (MAO) inhibitors is contraindicated. At least 14 days should elapse between discontinuation of a MAO inhibitor and initiation of treatment with bupropion. MAO inhibitors increases bupropion toxicity).
No products indexed under this heading.

Prochlorperazine (Concurrent administration of bupropion and agents that lower seizure threshold should be undertaken with extreme caution. Low initial dosing and gradual dose increases should be employed).
No products indexed under this heading.

Promethazine (Because bupropion is extensively metabolized, the co-administration of other drugs may affect its clinical activity. *In vitro* studies indicate that bupropion is primarily

133 Interactions Index Aplenzin

metabolized to hydroxybupropion by the CYP2B6 isoenzyme. Therefore, the potential exists for a drug interaction between bupropion and drugs that are substrates or inhibitors of the CYP2B6 isoenzyme (eg, orphenadrine, thiotepa, and cyclophosphamide). In addition, *in vitro* studies suggest that paroxetine, sertraline, norfluoxetine, and fluvoxamine as well as nelfinavir, ritonavir, and efavirenz inhibit the hydroxylation of bupropion).
No products indexed under this heading.

Promethazine Hydrochloride (Concurrent administration of bupropion and agents that lower seizure threshold should be undertaken with extreme caution. Low initial dosing and gradual dose increases should be employed).
No products indexed under this heading.

Propafenone Hydrochloride (Co-administration of bupropion with drugs that are metabolized by the CYP2D6 isoenzyme should be approached with caution and should be initiated at the lower end of the dose range of the concomitant medication. If bupropion is added to the treatment regimen of a patient already receiving a drug metabolized by CYP2D6, the need to decrease the dose of the original medication should be considered, particularly for those concomitant medications with a narrow therapeutic index).
Products include:
Rythmol 1648
Rythmol SR 1652

Propofol (Bupropion is containdicated in patients undergoing abrupt discontinuation of sedatives. Concomitant use of sedatives with bupropion is associated with an increased seizure risk).
No products indexed under this heading.

Propoxyphene Hydrochloride (Concomitant use of opiates, cocaine, or stimulants with bupropion is associated with an increased seizure risk).
No products indexed under this heading.

Propoxyphene Napsylate (Concomitant use of opiates, cocaine, or stimulants with bupropion is associated with an increased seizure risk).
No products indexed under this heading.

Propranolol Hydrochloride (Co-administration of bupropion with drugs that are metabolized by the CYP2D6 isoenzyme should be approached with caution and should be initiated at the lower end of the dose range of the concomitant medication. If bupropion is added to the treatment regimen of a patient already receiving a drug metabolized by CYP2D6, the need to decrease the dose of the original medication should be considered, particularly for those concomitant medications with a narrow therapeutic index).
Products include:
InnoPran XL 1517

Protriptyline Hydrochloride (Concurrent administration of bupropion and agents that lower seizure threshold should be undertaken with extreme caution. Low initial dosing and gradual dose increases should be employed).
No products indexed under this heading.

Quazepam (Bupropion is contraindicated in patients undergoing abrupt discontinuation of benzodiazepine sedatives. Concomitant use of benzodiazepine sedatives with bupropion is associated with an increased seizure risk).
No products indexed under this heading.

Quetiapine Fumarate (Concurrent administration of bupropion and agents that lower seizure threshold, such as antipsychotics, should be undertaken with extreme caution. Low initial dosing and gradual dose increases should be employed. Co-administration of bupropion with drugs that are metabolized by the CYP2D6 isoenzyme including antipsychotics (eg, haloperidol, risperidone, thioridazine) should be approached with caution and should be initiated at the lower end of the dose range of the concomitant medication. If bupropion is added to the treatment regimen of a patient already receiving a drug metabolized by CYP2D6, the need to decrease the dose of the original medication should be considered, particularly for those concomitant medications with a narrow therapeutic index).
Products include:
Seroquel 750
Seroquel XR 759

Quinidine Gluconate (Co-administration of bupropion with drugs that are metabolized by the CYP2D6 isoenzyme should be approached with caution and should be initiated at the lower end of the dose range of the concomitant medication. If bupropion is added to the treatment regimen of a patient already receiving a drug metabolized by CYP2D6, the need to decrease the dose of the original medication should be considered, particularly for those concomitant medications with a narrow therapeutic index).
No products indexed under this heading.

Quinidine Hydrochloride (Co-administration of bupropion with drugs that are metabolized by the CYP2D6 isoenzyme should be approached with caution and should be initiated at the lower end of the dose range of the concomitant medication. If bupropion is added to the treatment regimen of a patient already receiving a drug metabolized by CYP2D6, the need to decrease the dose of the original medication should be considered, particularly for those concomitant medications with a narrow therapeutic index).
No products indexed under this heading.

Quinidine Polygalacturonate (Co-administration of bupropion with drugs that are metabolized by the CYP2D6 isoenzyme should be approached with caution and should be initiated at the lower end of the dose range of the concomitant medication. If bupropion is added to the treatment regimen of a patient already receiving a drug metabolized by CYP2D6, the need to decrease the dose of the original medication should be considered, particularly for those concomitant medications with a narrow therapeutic index).
No products indexed under this heading.

Quinidine Sulfate (Co-administration of bupropion with drugs that are metabolized by the CYP2D6 isoenzyme should be approached with caution and should be initiated at the lower end of the dose range of the concomitant medication. If bupropion is added to the treatment regimen of a patient already receiving a drug metabolized by CYP2D6, the need to decrease the dose of the original medication should be considered, particularly for those concomitant medications with a narrow therapeutic index).
No products indexed under this heading.

Ramelteon (Bupropion is containdicated in patients undergoing abrupt discontinuation of sedatives. Concomitant use of sedatives with bupropion is associated with an increased seizure risk). Products include:
Rozerem 3366

Rasagiline Mesylate (Concurrent administration of bupropion and monoamine oxidase (MAO) inhibitors is contraindicated. At least 14 days should elapse between discontinuation of a MAO inhibitor and initiation of treatment with bupropion. MAO inhibitors increases bupropion toxicity). Products include:
Azilect 3383

Remifentanil Hydrochloride (Concomitant use of opiates, cocaine, or stimulants with bupropion is associated with an increased seizure risk).
No products indexed under this heading.

Repaglinide (Concomitant use of oral hypoglycemics with bupropion is associated with an increased seizure risk).
No products indexed under this heading.

Rifabutin (Bupropion may be an inducer of drug-metabolizing enzymes in humans. In one study, following chronic administration of bupropion hydrochloride, 100 mg 3 times daily to 8 healthy male volunteers for 14 days, there was no evidence of induction of its own metabolism. Nevertheless, there may be the potential for clinically important alterations of blood levels of co-administered drugs).
No products indexed under this heading.

Rifampicin (Bupropion may be an inducer of drug-metabolizing enzymes in humans. In one study, following chronic administration of bupropion hydrochloride, 100 mg 3 times daily to 8 healthy male volunteers for 14 days, there was no evidence of induction of its own metabolism. Nevertheless, there may be the potential for clinically important alterations of blood levels of co-administered drugs).
No products indexed under this heading.

Rifampin (Bupropion may be an inducer of drug-metabolizing enzymes in humans. In one study, following chronic administration of bupropion hydrochloride, 100 mg 3 times daily to 8 healthy male volunteers for 14 days, there was no evidence of induction of its own metabolism. Nevertheless, there may be the potential for clinically important alterations of blood levels of co-administered drugs).
No products indexed under this heading.

Rifapentine (Bupropion may be an inducer of drug-metabolizing enzymes in humans. In one study, following chronic administration of bupropion hydrochloride, 100 mg 3 times daily to 8 healthy male volunteers for 14 days, there was no evidence of induction of its own metabolism. Nevertheless, there may be the potential for clinically important alterations of blood levels of co-administered drugs).
No products indexed under this heading.

Risperidone (Concurrent administration of bupropion and agents that lower seizure threshold, such as antipsychotics, should be undertaken with extreme caution. Low initial dosing and gradual dose increases should be employed. Co-administration of bupropion with drugs that are metabolized by the CYP2D6 isoenzyme including antipsychotics (eg, haloperidol, risperidone, thioridazine) should be approached with caution and should be initiated at the lower end of the dose range of the concomitant medication. If bupropion is added to the treatment regimen of a patient already receiving a drug metabolized by CYP2D6, the need to decrease the dose of the original medication should be considered, particularly for those concomitant medications with a narrow therapeutic index).
Products include:
Risperdal Consta 2682

Ritonavir (*In vitro* studies suggest that ritonavir inhibits the hydroxylation of bupropion and thus may increase bupropion activity). Products include:
Kaletra 458
Norvir 509

Ropivacaine Hydrochloride (Because bupropion is extensively metabolized, the co-administration of other drugs may affect its clinical activity. *In vitro* studies indicate that bupropion is primarily metabolized to hydroxybupropion by the CYP2B6 isoenzyme. Therefore, the potential exists for a drug interaction between bupropion and drugs that are substrates or inhibitors of the CYP2B6 isoenzyme (eg, orphenadrine, thiotepa, and cyclophosphamide). In addition, *in vitro* studies suggest that paroxetine, sertraline, norfluoxetine, and fluvoxamine as well as nelfinavir, ritonavir, and efavirenz inhibit the hydroxylation of bupropion).
No products indexed under this heading.

Rosiglitazone Maleate (Concomitant use of oral hypoglycemics with bupropion is associated with an increased seizure risk). Products include:
Avandamet 1345
Avandaryl 1356
Avandia 1366

Secobarbital Sodium (Bupropion is containdicated in patients undergoing abrupt discontinuation of sedatives. Concomitant use of sedatives with bupropion is associated with an increased seizure risk).
No products indexed under this heading.

Selegiline (Concurrent administration of bupropion and monoamine oxidase (MAO) inhibitors is contraindicated. At least 14 days should elapse between discontinuation of a MAO inhibitor and initiation of treatment with bupropion. MAO inhibitors increases bupropion toxicity). Products include:
Emsam 3623

Selegiline Hydrochloride (Concurrent administration of bupropion and monoamine oxidase (MAO) inhibitors is contraindicated. At least 14 days should elapse between discontinuation of a MAO inhibitor and initiation of treatment with bupropion. MAO inhibitors increases bupropion toxicity). Products include:
Eldepryl 3312

Sertraline Hydrochloride (*In vitro* studies suggest that sertraline inhibits the hydroxylation of bupropion and thus may increase bupropion activity).
No products indexed under this heading.

Sevoflurane (Because bupropion is extensively metabolized, the co-administration of other drugs may affect its clinical activity. *In vitro* studies indicate that bupropion is primarily metabolized to hydroxybupropion by the CYP2B6 isoenzyme. Therefore, the potential exists for a drug interaction between bupropion and drugs that are substrates or inhibitors of the CYP2B6 isoenzyme (eg, orphenadrine, thiotepa, and cyclophosphamide). In addition, *in vitro* studies suggest that paroxetine, sertraline, norfluoxetine, and fluvoxamine as well as nelfinavir, ritonavir, and efavirenz inhibit the hydroxylation of bupropion). Products include:
Ultane 554

Sibutramine Hydrochloride Monohydrate (Concomitant use of anorectics with bupropion is associated with an increased seizure risk). Products include:
Meridia 492

Sitagliptin Phosphate (Concomitant use of oral hypoglycemics with bupropion is associated with an increased seizure risk). Products include:
Janumet 2188
Januvia 2196

Sodium Butabarbital (Bupropion is containdicated in patients undergoing abrupt discontinuation of sedatives. Concomitant use of sedatives with bupropion is associated with an increased seizure risk).
No products indexed under this heading.

Sotalol Hydrochloride (Co-administration of bupropion with drugs that are metabolized by the CYP2D6 isoenzyme including beta-blockers (eg, metoprolol) should be approached with

IMPORTANT NOTE: Always consult each drug listing in the patient's regimen for possible interactions.

caution and should be initiated at the lower end of the dose range of the concomitant medication. If bupropion is added to the treatment regimen of a patient already receiving a drug metabolized by CYP2D6, the need to decrease the dose of the original medication should be considered, particularly for those concomitant medications with a narrow therapeutic index).
No products indexed under this heading.

Sufentanil Citrate (Concomitant use of opiates, cocaine, or stimulants with bupropion is associated with an increased seizure risk).
No products indexed under this heading.

Tamoxifen Citrate (Co-administration of bupropion with drugs that are metabolized by the CYP2D6 isoenzyme should be approached with caution and should be initiated at the lower end of the dose range of the concomitant medication. If bupropion is added to the treatment regimen of a patient already receiving a drug metabolized by CYP2D6, the need to decrease the dose of the original medication should be considered, particularly for those concomitant medications with a narrow therapeutic index).
No products indexed under this heading.

Temazepam (Bupropion is contraindicated in patients undergoing abrupt discontinuation of benzodiazepine sedatives. Concomitant use of benzodiazepine sedatives with bupropion is associated with an increased seizure risk).
No products indexed under this heading.

Teniposide (Co-administration of bupropion with drugs that are metabolized by the CYP2D6 isoenzyme should be approached with caution and should be initiated at the lower end of the dose range of the concomitant medication. If bupropion is added to the treatment regimen of a patient already receiving a drug metabolized by CYP2D6, the need to decrease the dose of the original medication should be considered, particularly for those concomitant medications with a narrow therapeutic index).
No products indexed under this heading.

Testosterone (Co-administration of bupropion with drugs that are metabolized by the CYP2D6 isoenzyme should be approached with caution and should be initiated at the lower end of the dose range of the concomitant medication. If bupropion is added to the treatment regimen of a patient already receiving a drug metabolized by CYP2D6, the need to decrease the dose of the original medication should be considered, particularly for those concomitant medications with a narrow therapeutic index).
Products include:
AndroGel 3456

Testosterone Cypionate (Co-administration of bupropion with drugs that are metabolized by the CYP2D6 isoenzyme should be approached with caution and should be initiated at the lower end of the dose range of the concomitant medication. If bupropion is added to the treatment regimen of a patient already receiving a drug metabolized by CYP2D6, the need to decrease the dose of the original medication should be considered, particularly for those concomitant medications with a narrow therapeutic index).
No products indexed under this heading.

Testosterone Enanthate (Co-administration of bupropion with drugs that are metabolized by the CYP2D6 isoenzyme should be approached with caution and should be initiated at the lower end of the dose range of the concomitant medication. If bupropion is added to the treatment regimen of a patient already receiving a drug metabolized by CYP2D6, the need to

decrease the dose of the original medication should be considered, particularly for those concomitant medications with a narrow therapeutic index).
Products include:
Delatestryl 1102

Testosterone Propionate (Co-administration of bupropion with drugs that are metabolized by the CYP2D6 isoenzyme should be approached with caution and should be initiated at the lower end of the dose range of the concomitant medication. If bupropion is added to the treatment regimen of a patient already receiving a drug metabolized by CYP2D6, the need to decrease the dose of the original medication should be considered, particularly for those concomitant medications with a narrow therapeutic index).
No products indexed under this heading.

Theophylline (Concurrent administration of bupropion agents that lower seizure threshold, such as theophylline, should be undertaken with extreme caution. Low initial dosing and gradual dose increases should be employed).
No products indexed under this heading.

Theophylline Anhydrous (Concurrent administration of bupropion agents that lower seizure threshold, such as theophylline, should be undertaken with extreme caution. Low initial dosing and gradual dose increases should be employed). Products include:
Uniphyl 2817

Theophylline Calcium Salicylate (Concurrent administration of bupropion agents that lower seizure threshold, such as theophylline, should be undertaken with extreme caution. Low initial dosing and gradual dose increases should be employed).
No products indexed under this heading.

Theophylline Dihydroxypropyl (Glyceryl) (Concurrent administration of bupropion agents that lower seizure threshold, such as theophylline, should be undertaken with extreme caution. Low initial dosing and gradual dose increases should be employed).
No products indexed under this heading.

Theophylline Ethylenediamine (Concurrent administration of bupropion agents that lower seizure threshold, such as theophylline, should be undertaken with extreme caution. Low initial dosing and gradual dose increases should be employed).
No products indexed under this heading.

Theophylline Sodium Glycinate (Concurrent administration of bupropion agents that lower seizure threshold, such as theophylline, should be undertaken with extreme caution. Low initial dosing and gradual dose increases should be employed).
No products indexed under this heading.

Thioridazine (Co-administration of bupropion with drugs that are metabolized by the CYP2D6 isoenzyme should be approached with caution and should be initiated at the lower end of the dose range of the concomitant medication. If bupropion is added to the treatment regimen of a patient already receiving a drug metabolized by CYP2D6, the need to decrease the dose of the original medication should be considered, particularly for those concomitant medications with a narrow therapeutic index).
No products indexed under this heading.

Thioridazine Hydrochloride (Co-administration of bupropion with drugs that are metabolized by the CYP2D6 isoenzyme, including thioridazine, should be approached with caution and should be initiated at the lower end of the dose range of the concomitant medication. If bupropion is added to the treatment regimen of a patient already receiving a drug metabolized by

CYP2D6, the need to decrease the dose of the original medication should be considered, particularly for those concomitant medications with a narrow therapeutic index). Products include:
Thioridazine Hydrochloride 2384

Thiotepa (Because bupropion is extensively metabolized, the co-administration of other drugs may affect its clinical activity. *In vitro* studies indicate that bupropion is primarily metabolized to hydroxybupropion by the CYP2B6 isoenzyme. Therefore, the potential exists for a drug interaction between bupropion and drugs that are substrates or inhibitors of the CYP2B6 isoenzyme (eg, orphenadrine, thiotepa, and cyclophosphamide). In addition, *in vitro* studies suggest that paroxetine, sertraline, norfluoxetine, and fluvoxamine as well as nelfinavir, ritonavir, and efavirenz inhibit the hydroxylation of bupropion).
No products indexed under this heading.

Thiothixene (Concurrent administration of bupropion and agents that lower seizure threshold, such as antipsychotics, should be undertaken with extreme caution. Low initial dosing and gradual dose increases should be employed. Co-administration of bupropion with drugs that are metabolized by the CYP2D6 isoenzyme including antipsychotics (eg, haloperidol, risperidone, thioridazine) should be approached with caution and should be initiated at the lower end of the dose range of the concomitant medication. If bupropion is added to the treatment regimen of a patient already receiving a drug metabolized by CYP2D6, the need to decrease the dose of the original medication should be considered, particularly for those concomitant medications with a narrow therapeutic index). Products include:
Thiothixene 2386

Timolol Hemihydrate (Co-administration of bupropion with drugs that are metabolized by the CYP2D6 isoenzyme including beta-blockers (eg, metoprolol) should be approached with caution and should be initiated at the lower end of the dose range of the concomitant medication. If bupropion is added to the treatment regimen of a patient already receiving a drug metabolized by CYP2D6, the need to decrease the dose of the original medication should be considered, particularly for those concomitant medications with a narrow therapeutic index). Products include:
Betimol 3490

Timolol Maleate (Co-administration of bupropion with drugs that are metabolized by the CYP2D6 isoenzyme should be approached with caution and should be initiated at the lower end of the dose range of the concomitant medication. If bupropion is added to the treatment regimen of a patient already receiving a drug metabolized by CYP2D6, the need to decrease the dose of the original medication should be considered, particularly for those concomitant medications with a narrow therapeutic index). Products include:
Combigan 601
Dorzolamide Hydrochloride/Timolol Maleate Ophthalmic Solution .... ⊙243
Timoptic in Ocudose .... ⊙231

Tobacco (Bupropion may be an inducer of drug-metabolizing enzymes in humans. In one study, following chronic administration of bupropion hydrochloride, 100 mg 3 times daily to 8 healthy male volunteers for 14 days, there was no evidence of induction of its own metabolism. Nevertheless, there may

be the potential for clinically important alterations of blood levels of co-administered drugs).
No products indexed under this heading.

Tolazamide (Concomitant use of oral hypoglycemics with bupropion is associated with an increased seizure risk).
No products indexed under this heading.

Tolbutamide (Concomitant use of oral hypoglycemics with bupropion is associated with an increased seizure risk).
No products indexed under this heading.

Tolterodine Tartrate (Co-administration of bupropion with drugs that are metabolized by the CYP2D6 isoenzyme should be approached with caution and should be initiated at the lower end of the dose range of the concomitant medication. If bupropion is added to the treatment regimen of a patient already receiving a drug metabolized by CYP2D6, the need to decrease the dose of the original medication should be considered, particularly for those concomitant medications with a narrow therapeutic index).
No products indexed under this heading.

Tramadol Hydrochloride (Co-administration of bupropion with drugs that are metabolized by the CYP2D6 isoenzyme should be approached with caution and should be initiated at the lower end of the dose range of the concomitant medication. If bupropion is added to the treatment regimen of a patient already receiving a drug metabolized by CYP2D6, the need to decrease the dose of the original medication should be considered, particularly for those concomitant medications with a narrow therapeutic index).
Products include:
Ryzolt 2813
Ultram ER 2693

Tranylcypromine Sulfate (Concurrent administration of bupropion and monoamine oxidase (MAO) inhibitors is contraindicated. At least 14 days should elapse between discontinuation of a MAO inhibitor and initiation of treatment with bupropion. MAO inhibitors increases bupropion toxicity). Products include:
Parnate 1584

Trazodone Hydrochloride (Concurrent administration of bupropion and agents that lower seizure threshold should be undertaken with extreme caution. Low initial dosing and gradual dose increases should be employed).
No products indexed under this heading.

Tretinoin (Because bupropion is extensively metabolized, the co-administration of other drugs may affect its clinical activity. *In vitro* studies indicate that bupropion is primarily metabolized to hydroxybupropion by the CYP2B6 isoenzyme. Therefore, the potential exists for a drug interaction between bupropion and drugs that are substrates or inhibitors of the CYP2B6 isoenzyme (eg, orphenadrine, thiotepa, and cyclophosphamide). In addition, *in vitro* studies suggest that paroxetine, sertraline, norfluoxetine, and fluvoxamine as well as nelfinavir, ritonavir, and efavirenz inhibit the hydroxylation of bupropion).
No products indexed under this heading.

Triamcinolone (Concurrent administration of bupropion and agents that lower seizure threshold, such as systemic steroids, should be undertaken with extreme caution. Low initial dosing and gradual dose increases should be employed).
No products indexed under this heading.

Triamcinolone Acetonide (Concurrent administration of bupropion and agents that lower seizure threshold, such as systemic steroids, should be undertaken with extreme caution. Low

(⊙ Described in PDR® for Ophthalmic Medicines)

initial dosing and gradual dose increases should be employed). Products include:
Azmacort 408
Nasacort AQ 3019

Triamcinolone Diacetate (Concurrent administration of bupropion and agents that lower seizure threshold, such as systemic steroids, should be undertaken with extreme caution. Low initial dosing and gradual dose increases should be employed).
No products indexed under this heading.

Triamcinolone Hexacetonide (Concurrent administration of bupropion and agents that lower seizure threshold, such as systemic steroids, should be undertaken with extreme caution. Low initial dosing and gradual dose increases should be employed).
No products indexed under this heading.

Triazolam (Bupropion is contraindicated in patients undergoing abrupt discontinuation of benzodiazepine sedatives. Concomitant use of benzodiazepine sedatives with bupropion is associated with an increased seizure risk).
No products indexed under this heading.

Trifluoperazine Hydrochloride (Concurrent administration of bupropion and agents that lower seizure threshold should be undertaken with extreme caution. Low initial dosing and gradual dose increases should be employed).
No products indexed under this heading.

Trimipramine Maleate (Concurrent administration of bupropion and agents that lower seizure threshold should be undertaken with extreme caution. Low initial dosing and gradual dose increases should be employed).
No products indexed under this heading.

Troglitazone (Concomitant use of oral hypoglycemics with bupropion is associated with an increased seizure risk).
No products indexed under this heading.

Valproate Sodium (Because bupropion is extensively metabolized, the co-administration of other drugs may affect its clinical activity. *In vitro* studies indicate that bupropion is primarily metabolized to hydroxybupropion by the CYP2B6 isoenzyme. Therefore, the potential exists for a drug interaction between bupropion and drugs that are substrates or inhibitors of the CYP2B6 isoenzyme (eg, orphenadrine, thiotepa, and cyclophosphamide). In addition, *in vitro* studies suggest that paroxetine, sertraline, norfluoxetine, and fluvoxamine as well as nelfinavir, ritonavir, and efavirenz inhibit the hydroxylation of bupropion).
No products indexed under this heading.

Valproic Acid (Because bupropion is extensively metabolized, the co-administration of other drugs may affect its clinical activity. *In vitro* studies indicate that bupropion is primarily metabolized to hydroxybupropion by the CYP2B6 isoenzyme. Therefore, the potential exists for a drug interaction between bupropion and drugs that are substrates or inhibitors of the CYP2B6 isoenzyme (eg, orphenadrine, thiotepa, and cyclophosphamide). In addition, *in vitro* studies suggest that paroxetine, sertraline, norfluoxetine, and fluvoxamine as well as nelfinavir, ritonavir, and efavirenz inhibit the hydroxylation of bupropion).
No products indexed under this heading.

Venlafaxine Hydrochloride (Concurrent administration of bupropion and agents that lower seizure threshold, such as antidepressants, should be undertaken with extreme caution. Low initial dosing and gradual dose increases should be employed. Co-administration of bupropion with drugs that are metabolized by the CYP2D6 isoenzyme including antidepressants (eg, nortriptyline, imipramine, desipramine, paroxetine, fluoxetine, sertraline) should be approached with caution and should be initiated at the lower end of the dose range of the concomitant medication. If bupropion is added to the treatment regimen of a patient already receiving a drug metabolized by CYP2D6, the need to decrease the dose of the original medication should be considered, particularly for those concomitant medications with a narrow therapeutic index). Products include:
Effexor XR 3504
Venlafaxine Hydrochloride Tablets ... 2388

Verapamil Hydrochloride (Because bupropion is extensively metabolized, the co-administration of other drugs may affect its clinical activity. *In vitro* studies indicate that bupropion is primarily metabolized to hydroxybupropion by the CYP2B6 isoenzyme. Therefore, the potential exists for a drug interaction between bupropion and drugs that are substrates or inhibitors of the CYP2B6 isoenzyme (eg, orphenadrine, thiotepa, and cyclophosphamide). In addition, *in vitro* studies suggest that paroxetine, sertraline, norfluoxetine, and fluvoxamine as well as nelfinavir, ritonavir, and efavirenz inhibit the hydroxylation of bupropion). Products include:
Tarka 534

Vinblastine Sulfate (Co-administration of bupropion with drugs that are metabolized by the CYP2D6 isoenzyme should be approached with caution and should be initiated at the lower end of the dose range of the concomitant medication. If bupropion is added to the treatment regimen of a patient already receiving a drug metabolized by CYP2D6, the need to decrease the dose of the original medication should be considered, particularly for those concomitant medications with a narrow therapeutic index).
No products indexed under this heading.

Warfarin Sodium (Altered PT and/or INR, infrequently associated with hemorrhagic or thrombotic complications, were observed when bupropion was co-administered with warfarin).
No products indexed under this heading.

Zaleplon (Bupropion is containdicated in patients undergoing abrupt discontinuation of sedatives. Concomitant use of sedatives with bupropion is associated with an increased seizure risk).
No products indexed under this heading.

Ziprasidone Hydrochloride (Concurrent administration of bupropion and agents that lower seizure threshold, such as antipsychotics, should be undertaken with extreme caution. Low initial dosing and gradual dose increases should be employed. Co-administration of bupropion with drugs that are metabolized by the CYP2D6 isoenzyme including antipsychotics (eg, haloperidol, risperidone, thioridazine) should be approached with caution and should be initiated at the lower end of the dose range of the concomitant medication. If bupropion is added to the treatment regimen of a patient already receiving a drug metabolized by CYP2D6, the need to decrease the dose of the original medication should be considered, particularly for those concomitant medications with a narrow therapeutic index). Products include:
Geodon 2723

Zolpidem Tartrate (Bupropion is containdicated in patients undergoing abrupt discontinuation of sedatives. Concomitant use of sedatives with bupropion is associated with an increased seizure risk). Products include:
Ambien 2920
Ambien CR 2925

Zonisamide (Co-administration of bupropion with drugs that are metabolized by the CYP2D6 isoenzyme should be approached with caution and should be initiated at the lower end of the dose range of the concomitant medication. If bupropion is added to the treatment regimen of a patient already receiving a drug metabolized by CYP2D6, the need to decrease the dose of the original medication should be considered, particularly for those concomitant medications with a narrow therapeutic index). Products include:
Zonegran 1081

Food Interactions

Alcohol (Bupropion is contraindicated in patients undergoing abrupt discontinuation of alcohol. Concomitant use of alcohol with bupropion is associated with an increased seizure risk. There have been rare reports of adverse neuropsychiatric events or reduced alcohol tolerance in patients who were drinking alcohol during treatment with bupropion. The consumption of alcohol during treatment with bupropion should be minimized or avoided).

Beer, reduced-alcohol (Bupropion is contraindicated in patients undergoing abrupt discontinuation of alcohol. Concomitant use of alcohol with bupropion is associated with an increased seizure risk. There have been rare reports of adverse neuropsychiatric events or reduced alcohol tolerance in patients who were drinking alcohol during treatment with bupropion. The consumption of alcohol during treatment with bupropion should be minimized or avoided).

Beer, unspecified (Bupropion is contraindicated in patients undergoing abrupt discontinuation of alcohol. Concomitant use of alcohol with bupropion is associated with an increased seizure risk. There have been rare reports of adverse neuropsychiatric events or reduced alcohol tolerance in patients who were drinking alcohol during treatment with bupropion. The consumption of alcohol during treatment with bupropion should be minimized or avoided).

Broccoli (Bupropion may be an inducer of drug-metabolizing enzymes in humans. In one study, following chronic administration of bupropion hydrochloride, 100 mg 3 times daily to 8 healthy male volunteers for 14 days, there was no evidence of induction of its own metabolism. Nevertheless, there may be the potential for clinically important alterations of blood levels of co-administered drugs).

Brussel Sprouts (Bupropion may be an inducer of drug-metabolizing enzymes in humans. In one study, following chronic administration of bupropion hydrochloride, 100 mg 3 times daily to 8 healthy male volunteers for 14 days, there was no evidence of induction of its own metabolism. Nevertheless, there may be the potential for clinically important alterations of blood levels of co-administered drugs).

Charbroiled Food (Bupropion may be an inducer of drug-metabolizing enzymes in humans. In one study, following chronic administration of bupropion hydrochloride, 100 mg 3 times daily to 8 healthy male volunteers for 14 days, there was no evidence of induction of its own metabolism. Nevertheless, there may be the potential for clinically important alterations of blood levels of co-administered drugs).

Wine, Chianti (Bupropion is contraindicated in patients undergoing abrupt discontinuation of alcohol. Concomitant use of alcohol with bupropion is associated with an increased seizure risk. There have been rare reports of adverse neuropsychiatric events or reduced alcohol tolerance in patients who were drinking alcohol during treatment with bupropion. The consumption of alcohol during treatment with bupropion should be minimized or avoided).

Wine, Red (Bupropion is contraindicated in patients undergoing abrupt discontinuation of alcohol. Concomitant use of alcohol with bupropion is associated with an increased seizure risk. There have been rare reports of adverse neuropsychiatric events or reduced alcohol tolerance in patients who were drinking alcohol during treatment with bupropion. The consumption of alcohol during treatment with bupropion should be minimized or avoided).

Wine, unspecified (Bupropion is contraindicated in patients undergoing abrupt discontinuation of alcohol. Concomitant use of alcohol with bupropion is associated with an increased seizure risk. There have been rare reports of adverse neuropsychiatric events or reduced alcohol tolerance in patients who were drinking alcohol during treatment with bupropion. The consumption of alcohol during treatment with bupropion should be minimized or avoided).

Wine products (Bupropion is contraindicated in patients undergoing abrupt discontinuation of alcohol. Concomitant use of alcohol with bupropion is associated with an increased seizure risk. There have been rare reports of adverse neuropsychiatric events or reduced alcohol tolerance in patients who were drinking alcohol during treatment with bupropion. The consumption of alcohol during treatment with bupropion should be minimized or avoided).

APPEAREX TABLETS

(Biotin) 2319
May interact with phenytoin, and certain other agents. Compounds in these categories include:

Antibiotics, unspecified (The use of antibiotics may reduce the contribution of biotin made by bacteria within the large intestine).
No products indexed under this heading.

Carbamazepine (May accelerate biotin metabolism, leading to a reduction in available biotin). Products include:
Carbatrol 3280
Equetro 3477

Fosphenytoin (May accelerate biotin metabolism, leading to a reduction in available biotin).
No products indexed under this heading.

Fosphenytoin Sodium (May accelerate biotin metabolism, leading to a reduction in available biotin).
No products indexed under this heading.

Phenobarbital (May accelerate biotin metabolism, leading to a reduction in available biotin). Products include:
Donnatal 2711

Phenytoin (May accelerate biotin metabolism, leading to a reduction in available biotin).
No products indexed under this heading.

Phenytoin Sodium (May accelerate biotin metabolism, leading to a reduction in available biotin). Products include:
Phenytek Capsules 2380

IMPORTANT NOTE: Always consult each drug listing in the patient's regimen for possible interactions.

Appearex | Interactions Index | 136

Primidone (May accelerate biotin metabolism, leading to a reduction in available biotin).
No products indexed under this heading.

APRISO CAPSULES

(Mesalamine) 2899
May interact with antacids, and certain other agents. Compounds in these categories include:

Aluminum Carbonate (Because the dissolution of the coating of the granules in mesalamine capsules depends on pH, mesalamine capsules should not be co-administered with antacids).
No products indexed under this heading.

Aluminum Hydroxide (Because the dissolution of the coating of the granules in mesalamine capsules depends on pH, mesalamine capsules should not be co-administered with antacids).
No products indexed under this heading.

Calcium Carbonate (Because the dissolution of the coating of the granules in mesalamine capsules depends on pH, mesalamine capsules should not be co-administered with antacids).
Products include:
Chelated Mineral 3476
Pepcid Complete 1822
Extra Strength Rolaids Softchews Vanilla Creme 2045

Fat (A high fat meal did not affect C_{max} for 5-ASA, but a 27% increase in the cumulative urinary excretion of 5-ASA was observed with a high fat meal. The overall extent of absorption of N-Ac-5-ASA was not affected by a high fat meal. As mesalamine and mesalamine granules in sachet were bioequivalent, mesalamine can be taken without regard to food).
No products indexed under this heading.

Magaldrate (Because the dissolution of the coating of the granules in mesalamine capsules depends on pH, mesalamine capsules should not be co-administered with antacids).
No products indexed under this heading.

Magnesium Carbonate (Because the dissolution of the coating of the granules in mesalamine capsules depends on pH, mesalamine capsules should not be co-administered with antacids).
No products indexed under this heading.

Magnesium Hydroxide (Because the dissolution of the coating of the granules in mesalamine capsules depends on pH, mesalamine capsules should not be co-administered with antacids).
Products include:
Fleet Pedia-Lax Chewable Tablets 1144
Pepcid Complete 1822

Magnesium Oxide (Because the dissolution of the coating of the granules in mesalamine capsules depends on pH, mesalamine capsules should not be co-administered with antacids).
Products include:
Beelith 873

Magnesium Trisilicate (Because the dissolution of the coating of the granules in mesalamine capsules depends on pH, mesalamine capsules should not be co-administered with antacids).
No products indexed under this heading.

Sodium Bicarbonate (Because the dissolution of the coating of the granules in mesalamine capsules depends on pH, mesalamine capsules should not be co-administered with antacids).
No products indexed under this heading.

Food Interactions

Food, unspecified (A high fat meal did not affect C_{max} for 5-ASA, but a 27% increase in the cumulative urinary excretion of 5-ASA was observed with a high fat meal. The overall extent of absorption of N-Ac-5-ASA was not affected by a high fat meal. As mesalamine and mesalamine granules in sachet were bioequivalent, mesalamine can be taken without regard to food).

Meal, unspecified (A high fat meal did not affect C_{max} for 5-ASA, but a 27% increase in the cumulative urinary excretion of 5-ASA was observed with a high fat meal. The overall extent of absorption of N-Ac-5-ASA was not affected by a high fat meal. As mesalamine and mesalamine granules in sachet were bioequivalent, mesalamine can be taken without regard to food).

ARALAST NP SOLVENT

(Alpha1-Proteinase Inhibitor (Human)) 806
None cited in PDR database.

ARANESP FOR INJECTION

(Darbepoetin Alfa) 607
None cited in PDR database.

ARCALYST FOR SUBCUTANEOUS INJECTION

(Rilonacept) 2824
May interact with drugs which undergo biotransformation by cytochrome p-450 mixed function oxidase, TNF antagonists, vaccines, live. Compounds in these categories include:

Acarbose (This is clinically relevant for CYP450 substrates with a narrow therapeutic index, where the dose is individually adjusted (eg, warfarin). Upon initiation of rilonacept, in patients being treated with these types of medicinal products, therapeutic monitoring of the effect or drug concentration should be performed and the individual dose of the medicinal product may need to be adjusted as needed).
No products indexed under this heading.

Acetaminophen (This is clinically relevant for CYP450 substrates with a narrow therapeutic index, where the dose is individually adjusted (eg, warfarin). Upon initiation of rilonacept, in patients being treated with these types of medicinal products, therapeutic monitoring of the effect or drug concentration should be performed and the individual dose of the medicinal product may need to be adjusted as needed). Products include:
Percocet 1121
Tylenol 2049
Tylenol 8 Hour 2049
Extra Strength Tylenol Caplets, Cool Caplets, and EZ Tabs 2049
Extra Strength Tylenol Adult Rapid Blast Liquid 2049
Extra Strength Tylenol Rapid Release 2049
Tylenol with Codeine 2691
Tylenol Arthritis Pain Extended Release Geltabs/Caplets 2049
Children's Tylenol Suspension Liquid 2048
Children's Tylenol Meltaways 2048
Tylenol, Infants' Drops 2048
Junior Tylenol 2048
Vicodin 560
Vicodin ES 561
Vicodin HP 563
Zydone 1138

Adalimumab (Concomitant administration of another drug that blocks IL-1 with a TNF-blocking agent in another patient population has been associated with an increased risk of serious infections and an increased risk of neutropenia. The concomitant administration of rilonacept with TNF-blocking agents may also result in similar toxicities and is not recommended). Products include:
Humira 448

Alatrofloxacin Mesylate (This is clinically relevant for CYP450 substrates with a narrow therapeutic index, where the dose is individually adjusted (eg, warfarin). Upon initiation of rilonacept, in patients being treated with these types of medicinal products, therapeutic monitoring of the effect or drug concentration should be performed and the individual dose of the medicinal product may need to be adjusted as needed).
No products indexed under this heading.

Alfentanil Hydrochloride (This is clinically relevant for CYP450 substrates with a narrow therapeutic index, where the dose is individually adjusted (eg, warfarin). Upon initiation of rilonacept, in patients being treated with these types of medicinal products, therapeutic monitoring of the effect or drug concentration should be performed and the individual dose of the medicinal product may need to be adjusted as needed).
No products indexed under this heading.

Alprazolam (This is clinically relevant for CYP450 substrates with a narrow therapeutic index, where the dose is individually adjusted (eg, warfarin). Upon initiation of rilonacept, in patients being treated with these types of medicinal products, therapeutic monitoring of the effect or drug concentration should be performed and the individual dose of the medicinal product may need to be adjusted as needed).
No products indexed under this heading.

Aminophylline (This is clinically relevant for CYP450 substrates with a narrow therapeutic index, where the dose is individually adjusted (eg, warfarin). Upon initiation of rilonacept, in patients being treated with these types of medicinal products, therapeutic monitoring of the effect or drug concentration should be performed and the individual dose of the medicinal product may need to be adjusted as needed).
No products indexed under this heading.

Amiodarone Hydrochloride (This is clinically relevant for CYP450 substrates with a narrow therapeutic index, where the dose is individually adjusted (eg, warfarin). Upon initiation of rilonacept, in patients being treated with these types of medicinal products, therapeutic monitoring of the effect or drug concentration should be performed and the individual dose of the medicinal product may need to be adjusted as needed).
No products indexed under this heading.

Amitriptyline Hydrochloride (This is clinically relevant for CYP450 substrates with a narrow therapeutic index, where the dose is individually adjusted (eg, warfarin). Upon initiation of rilonacept, in patients being treated with these types of medicinal products, therapeutic monitoring of the effect or drug concentration should be performed and the individual dose of the medicinal product may need to be adjusted as needed).
No products indexed under this heading.

Amlodipine Besylate (This is clinically relevant for CYP450 substrates with a narrow therapeutic index, where the dose is individually adjusted (eg, warfarin). Upon initiation of rilonacept, in patients being treated with these types of medicinal products, therapeutic monitoring of the effect or drug concentration should be performed and the individual dose of the medicinal product may need to be adjusted as needed).
Products include:
Azor 1010
Exforge 2443
Exforge HCT 2449

Amoxapine (This is clinically relevant for CYP450 substrates with a narrow therapeutic index, where the dose is individually adjusted (eg, warfarin). Upon initiation of rilonacept, in patients being treated with these types of medicinal products, therapeutic monitoring of the effect or drug concentration should be performed and the individual dose of the medicinal product may need to be adjusted as needed).
No products indexed under this heading.

Amphetamine Aspartate (This is clinically relevant for CYP450 substrates with a narrow therapeutic index, where the dose is individually adjusted (eg, warfarin). Upon initiation of rilonacept, in patients being treated with these types of medicinal products, therapeutic monitoring of the effect or drug concentration should be performed and the individual dose of the medicinal product may need to be adjusted as needed).
No products indexed under this heading.

Amphetamine Aspartate Monohydrate (This is clinically relevant for CYP450 substrates with a narrow therapeutic index, where the dose is individually adjusted (eg, warfarin). Upon initiation of rilonacept, in patients being treated with these types of medicinal products, therapeutic monitoring of the effect or drug concentration should be performed and the individual dose of the medicinal product may need to be adjusted as needed).
No products indexed under this heading.

Amphetamine Sulfate (This is clinically relevant for CYP450 substrates with a narrow therapeutic index, where the dose is individually adjusted (eg, warfarin). Upon initiation of rilonacept, in patients being treated with these types of medicinal products, therapeutic monitoring of the effect or drug concentration should be performed and the individual dose of the medicinal product may need to be adjusted as needed).
No products indexed under this heading.

Anagrelide Hydrochloride (This is clinically relevant for CYP450 substrates with a narrow therapeutic index, where the dose is individually adjusted (eg, warfarin). Upon initiation of rilonacept, in patients being treated with these types of medicinal products, therapeutic monitoring of the effect or drug concentration should be performed and the individual dose of the medicinal product may need to be adjusted as needed).
No products indexed under this heading.

Aprepitant (This is clinically relevant for CYP450 substrates with a narrow therapeutic index, where the dose is individually adjusted (eg, warfarin). Upon initiation of rilonacept, in patients being treated with these types of medicinal products, therapeutic monitoring of the effect or drug concentration should be performed and the individual dose of the medicinal product may need to be adjusted as needed). Products include:
Emend 2124

Astemizole (This is clinically relevant for CYP450 substrates with a narrow therapeutic index, where the dose is individually adjusted (eg, warfarin). Upon initiation of rilonacept, in patients being treated with these types of medicinal products, therapeutic monitoring of the effect or drug concentration should be performed and the individual dose of the medicinal product may need to be adjusted as needed).
No products indexed under this heading.

Atomoxetine Hydrochloride (This is clinically relevant for CYP450 substrates with a narrow therapeutic index, where the dose is individually adjusted (eg, warfarin). Upon initiation of rilonacept, in patients being treated with these types of medicinal products, therapeutic monitoring of the effect or drug concentration should be performed and

(⊙ Described in PDR® for Ophthalmic Medicines)

the individual dose of the medicinal product may need to be adjusted as needed). Products include:

Strattera **1957**

Atorvastatin Calcium (This is clinically relevant for CYP450 substrates with a narrow therapeutic index, where the dose is individually adjusted (eg, warfarin). Upon initiation of rilonacept, in patients being treated with these types of medicinal products, therapeutic monitoring of the effect or drug concentration should be performed and the individual dose of the medicinal product may need to be adjusted as needed). Products include:

Lipitor **2703**

BCG Vaccine (Since no data are available on either the efficacy of live vaccines or on the risks of secondary transmission of infection by live vaccines in patients receiving rilonacept, live vaccines should not be given concurrently with rilonacept. In addition, because rilonacept may interfere with normal immune response to new antigens, vaccinations may not be effective in patients receiving rilonacept. No data are available on the effectiveness of vaccination with inactivated (killed) antigens in patients receiving rilonacept).

No products indexed under this heading.

Belladonna Ergotamine (This is clinically relevant for CYP450 substrates with a narrow therapeutic index, where the dose is individually adjusted (eg, warfarin). Upon initiation of rilonacept, in patients being treated with these types of medicinal products, therapeutic monitoring of the effect or drug concentration should be performed and the individual dose of the medicinal product may need to be adjusted as needed).

No products indexed under this heading.

Benzphetamine Hydrochloride (This is clinically relevant for CYP450 substrates with a narrow therapeutic index, where the dose is individually adjusted (eg, warfarin). Upon initiation of rilonacept, in patients being treated with these types of medicinal products, therapeutic monitoring of the effect or drug concentration should be performed and the individual dose of the medicinal product may need to be adjusted as needed).

No products indexed under this heading.

Bisoprolol Fumarate (This is clinically relevant for CYP450 substrates with a narrow therapeutic index, where the dose is individually adjusted (eg, warfarin). Upon initiation of rilonacept, in patients being treated with these types of medicinal products, therapeutic monitoring of the effect or drug concentration should be performed and the individual dose of the medicinal product may need to be adjusted as needed).

No products indexed under this heading.

Bromocriptine Mesylate (This is clinically relevant for CYP450 substrates with a narrow therapeutic index, where the dose is individually adjusted (eg, warfarin). Upon initiation of rilonacept, in patients being treated with these types of medicinal products, therapeutic monitoring of the effect or drug concentration should be performed and the individual dose of the medicinal product may need to be adjusted as needed).

No products indexed under this heading.

Buspirone Hydrochloride (This is clinically relevant for CYP450 substrates with a narrow therapeutic index, where the dose is individually adjusted (eg, warfarin). Upon initiation of rilonacept, in patients being treated with these types of medicinal products, therapeutic monitoring of the effect or drug concentration should be performed and the individual dose of the medicinal product may need to be adjusted as needed).

No products indexed under this heading.

Busulfan (This is clinically relevant for CYP450 substrates with a narrow therapeutic index, where the dose is individually adjusted (eg, warfarin). Upon initiation of rilonacept, in patients being treated with these types of medicinal products, therapeutic monitoring of the effect or drug concentration should be performed and the individual dose of the medicinal product may need to be adjusted as needed). Products include:

Myleran **1581**

Caffeine (This is clinically relevant for CYP450 substrates with a narrow therapeutic index, where the dose is individually adjusted (eg, warfarin). Upon initiation of rilonacept, in patients being treated with these types of medicinal products, therapeutic monitoring of the effect or drug concentration should be performed and the individual dose of the medicinal product may need to be adjusted as needed).

No products indexed under this heading.

Caffeine Anhydrous (This is clinically relevant for CYP450 substrates with a narrow therapeutic index, where the dose is individually adjusted (eg, warfarin). Upon initiation of rilonacept, in patients being treated with these types of medicinal products, therapeutic monitoring of the effect or drug concentration should be performed and the individual dose of the medicinal product may need to be adjusted as needed).

No products indexed under this heading.

Caffeine Citrate (This is clinically relevant for CYP450 substrates with a narrow therapeutic index, where the dose is individually adjusted (eg, warfarin). Upon initiation of rilonacept, in patients being treated with these types of medicinal products, therapeutic monitoring of the effect or drug concentration should be performed and the individual dose of the medicinal product may need to be adjusted as needed).

No products indexed under this heading.

Caffeine-containing medications (This is clinically relevant for CYP450 substrates with a narrow therapeutic index, where the dose is individually adjusted (eg, warfarin). Upon initiation of rilonacept, in patients being treated with these types of medicinal products, therapeutic monitoring of the effect or drug concentration should be performed and the individual dose of the medicinal product may need to be adjusted as needed).

No products indexed under this heading.

Caffeine Sodium Benzoate (This is clinically relevant for CYP450 substrates with a narrow therapeutic index, where the dose is individually adjusted (eg, warfarin). Upon initiation of rilonacept, in patients being treated with these types of medicinal products, therapeutic monitoring of the effect or drug concentration should be performed and the individual dose of the medicinal product may need to be adjusted as needed).

No products indexed under this heading.

Candesartan Cilexetil (This is clinically relevant for CYP450 substrates with a narrow therapeutic index, where the dose is individually adjusted (eg, warfarin). Upon initiation of rilonacept, in patients being treated with these types of medicinal products, therapeutic monitoring of the effect or drug concentration should be performed and the individual dose of the medicinal product may need to be adjusted as needed). Products include:

Atacand **697**

Atacand HCT **700**

Captopril (This is clinically relevant for CYP450 substrates with a narrow therapeutic index, where the dose is individually adjusted (eg, warfarin). Upon initiation of rilonacept, in patients being treated with these types of medicinal products, therapeutic monitoring of the effect or drug concentration should be performed and the individual dose of the medicinal product may need to be adjusted as needed). Products include:

Captopril **2341**

Carbamazepine (This is clinically relevant for CYP450 substrates with a narrow therapeutic index, where the dose is individually adjusted (eg, warfarin). Upon initiation of rilonacept, in patients being treated with these types of medicinal products, therapeutic monitoring of the effect or drug concentration should be performed and the individual dose of the medicinal product may need to be adjusted as needed). Products include:

Carbatrol **3280**

Equetro **3477**

Carisoprodol (This is clinically relevant for CYP450 substrates with a narrow therapeutic index, where the dose is individually adjusted (eg, warfarin). Upon initiation of rilonacept, in patients being treated with these types of medicinal products, therapeutic monitoring of the effect or drug concentration should be performed and the individual dose of the medicinal product may need to be adjusted as needed).

No products indexed under this heading.

Carvedilol (This is clinically relevant for CYP450 substrates with a narrow therapeutic index, where the dose is individually adjusted (eg, warfarin). Upon initiation of rilonacept, in patients being treated with these types of medicinal products, therapeutic monitoring of the effect or drug concentration should be performed and the individual dose of the medicinal product may need to be adjusted as needed). Products include:

Coreg **1409**

Celecoxib (This is clinically relevant for CYP450 substrates with a narrow therapeutic index, where the dose is individually adjusted (eg, warfarin). Upon initiation of rilonacept, in patients being treated with these types of medicinal products, therapeutic monitoring of the effect or drug concentration should be performed and the individual dose of the medicinal product may need to be adjusted as needed). Products include:

Celebrex **3272**

Cerivastatin Sodium (This is clinically relevant for CYP450 substrates with a narrow therapeutic index, where the dose is individually adjusted (eg, warfarin). Upon initiation of rilonacept, in patients being treated with these types of medicinal products, therapeutic monitoring of the effect or drug concentration should be performed and the individual dose of the medicinal product may need to be adjusted as needed).

No products indexed under this heading.

Cevimeline Hydrochloride (This is clinically relevant for CYP450 substrates with a narrow therapeutic index, where the dose is individually adjusted (eg, warfarin). Upon initiation of rilonacept, in patients being treated with these types of medicinal products, therapeutic monitoring of the effect or drug concentration should be performed and the individual dose of the medicinal product may need to be adjusted as needed). Products include:

Evoxac **1027**

Chlordiazepoxide (This is clinically relevant for CYP450 substrates with a narrow therapeutic index, where the dose is individually adjusted (eg, warfarin). Upon initiation of rilonacept, in patients being treated with these types of medicinal products, therapeutic monitoring of the effect or drug concentration should be performed and the individual dose of the medicinal product may need to be adjusted as needed).

No products indexed under this heading.

Chlordiazepoxide Hydrochloride (This is clinically relevant for CYP450 substrates with a narrow therapeutic index, where the dose is individually adjusted (eg, warfarin). Upon initiation of rilonacept, in patients being treated with these types of medicinal products, therapeutic monitoring of the effect or drug concentration should be performed and the individual dose of the medicinal product may need to be adjusted as needed).

No products indexed under this heading.

Chlorpheniramine (This is clinically relevant for CYP450 substrates with a narrow therapeutic index, where the dose is individually adjusted (eg, warfarin). Upon initiation of rilonacept, in patients being treated with these types of medicinal products, therapeutic monitoring of the effect or drug concentration should be performed and the individual dose of the medicinal product may need to be adjusted as needed).

No products indexed under this heading.

Chlorpheniramine Maleate (This is clinically relevant for CYP450 substrates with a narrow therapeutic index, where the dose is individually adjusted (eg, warfarin). Upon initiation of rilonacept, in patients being treated with these types of medicinal products, therapeutic monitoring of the effect or drug concentration should be performed and the individual dose of the medicinal product may need to be adjusted as needed).

No products indexed under this heading.

Chlorpheniramine Polistirex (This is clinically relevant for CYP450 substrates with a narrow therapeutic index, where the dose is individually adjusted (eg, warfarin). Upon initiation of rilonacept, in patients being treated with these types of medicinal products, therapeutic monitoring of the effect or drug concentration should be performed and the individual dose of the medicinal product may need to be adjusted as needed). Products include:

Tussionex **3443**

Chlorpheniramine Tannate (This is clinically relevant for CYP450 substrates with a narrow therapeutic index, where the dose is individually adjusted (eg, warfarin). Upon initiation of rilonacept, in patients being treated with these types of medicinal products, therapeutic monitoring of the effect or drug concentration should be performed and the individual dose of the medicinal product may need to be adjusted as needed).

No products indexed under this heading.

Chlorpromazine (This is clinically relevant for CYP450 substrates with a narrow therapeutic index, where the dose is individually adjusted (eg, warfarin). Upon initiation of rilonacept, in patients being treated with these types of medicinal products, therapeutic monitoring of the effect or drug concentration should be performed and the individual dose of the medicinal product may need to be adjusted as needed).

No products indexed under this heading.

Chlorpromazine Hydrochloride (This is clinically relevant for CYP450 substrates with a narrow therapeutic index, where the dose is individually adjusted (eg, warfarin). Upon initiation of rilonacept, in patients being treated with these types of medicinal products, therapeutic monitoring of the effect or drug concentration should be per-

formed and the individual dose of the medicinal product may need to be adjusted as needed).
No products indexed under this heading.

Chlorpropamide (This is clinically relevant for CYP450 substrates with a narrow therapeutic index, where the dose is individually adjusted (eg, warfarin). Upon initiation of rilonacept, in patients being treated with these types of medicinal products, therapeutic monitoring of the effect or drug concentration should be performed and the individual dose of the medicinal product may need to be adjusted as needed).
No products indexed under this heading.

Cilostazol (This is clinically relevant for CYP450 substrates with a narrow therapeutic index, where the dose is individually adjusted (eg, warfarin). Upon initiation of rilonacept, in patients being treated with these types of medicinal products, therapeutic monitoring of the effect or drug concentration should be performed and the individual dose of the medicinal product may need to be adjusted as needed).
No products indexed under this heading.

Cimetidine Hydrochloride (This is clinically relevant for CYP450 substrates with a narrow therapeutic index, where the dose is individually adjusted (eg, warfarin). Upon initiation of rilonacept, in patients being treated with these types of medicinal products, therapeutic monitoring of the effect or drug concentration should be performed and the individual dose of the medicinal product may need to be adjusted as needed).
No products indexed under this heading.

Ciprofloxacin (This is clinically relevant for CYP450 substrates with a narrow therapeutic index, where the dose is individually adjusted (eg, warfarin). Upon initiation of rilonacept, in patients being treated with these types of medicinal products, therapeutic monitoring of the effect or drug concentration should be performed and the individual dose of the medicinal product may need to be adjusted as needed). Products include:
Cipro I.V. **3082**
Cipro **3073**
Cipro XR **3091**
Ciprodex **583**

Ciprofloxacin Hydrochloride (This is clinically relevant for CYP450 substrates with a narrow therapeutic index, where the dose is individually adjusted (eg, warfarin). Upon initiation of rilonacept, in patients being treated with these types of medicinal products, therapeutic monitoring of the effect or drug concentration should be performed and the individual dose of the medicinal product may need to be adjusted as needed). Products include:
Cipro **3073**

Cisapride (This is clinically relevant for CYP450 substrates with a narrow therapeutic index, where the dose is individually adjusted (eg, warfarin). Upon initiation of rilonacept, in patients being treated with these types of medicinal products, therapeutic monitoring of the effect or drug concentration should be performed and the individual dose of the medicinal product may need to be adjusted as needed).
No products indexed under this heading.

Citalopram Hydrobromide (This is clinically relevant for CYP450 substrates with a narrow therapeutic index, where the dose is individually adjusted (eg, warfarin). Upon initiation of rilonacept, in patients being treated with these types of medicinal products, therapeutic monitoring of the effect or drug concentration should be performed and the individual dose of the medicinal product may need to be adjusted as needed). Products include:
Celexa **1153**

Clarithromycin (This is clinically relevant for CYP450 substrates with a narrow therapeutic index, where the dose is individually adjusted (eg, warfarin). Upon initiation of rilonacept, in patients being treated with these types of medicinal products, therapeutic monitoring of the effect or drug concentration should be performed and the individual dose of the medicinal product may need to be adjusted as needed). Products include:
Biaxin/Biaxin XL **412**

Clomipramine Hydrochloride (This is clinically relevant for CYP450 substrates with a narrow therapeutic index, where the dose is individually adjusted (eg, warfarin). Upon initiation of rilonacept, in patients being treated with these types of medicinal products, therapeutic monitoring of the effect or drug concentration should be performed and the individual dose of the medicinal product may need to be adjusted as needed).
No products indexed under this heading.

Clopidogrel Bisulfate (This is clinically relevant for CYP450 substrates with a narrow therapeutic index, where the dose is individually adjusted (eg, warfarin). Upon initiation of rilonacept, in patients being treated with these types of medicinal products, therapeutic monitoring of the effect or drug concentration should be performed and the individual dose of the medicinal product may need to be adjusted as needed). Products include:
Plavix **3027**

Clopidogrel Hydrogen Sulfate (This is clinically relevant for CYP450 substrates with a narrow therapeutic index, where the dose is individually adjusted (eg, warfarin). Upon initiation of rilonacept, in patients being treated with these types of medicinal products, therapeutic monitoring of the effect or drug concentration should be performed and the individual dose of the medicinal product may need to be adjusted as needed).
No products indexed under this heading.

Clozapine (This is clinically relevant for CYP450 substrates with a narrow therapeutic index, where the dose is individually adjusted (eg, warfarin). Upon initiation of rilonacept, in patients being treated with these types of medicinal products, therapeutic monitoring of the effect or drug concentration should be performed and the individual dose of the medicinal product may need to be adjusted as needed).
No products indexed under this heading.

Codeine Phosphate (This is clinically relevant for CYP450 substrates with a narrow therapeutic index, where the dose is individually adjusted (eg, warfarin). Upon initiation of rilonacept, in patients being treated with these types of medicinal products, therapeutic monitoring of the effect or drug concentration should be performed and the individual dose of the medicinal product may need to be adjusted as needed). Products include:
Tylenol with Codeine **2691**

Codeine Sulfate (This is clinically relevant for CYP450 substrates with a narrow therapeutic index, where the dose is individually adjusted (eg, warfarin). Upon initiation of rilonacept, in patients being treated with these types of medicinal products, therapeutic monitoring of the effect or drug concentration should be performed and the individual dose of the medicinal product may need to be adjusted as needed).
No products indexed under this heading.

Cyclobenzaprine (This is clinically relevant for CYP450 substrates with a narrow therapeutic index, where the dose is individually adjusted (eg, warfarin). Upon initiation of rilonacept, in patients being treated with these types of medicinal products, therapeutic monitoring of the effect or drug concentration should be performed and the individual dose of the medicinal product may need to be adjusted as needed).
No products indexed under this heading.

Cyclobenzaprine Hydrochloride (This is clinically relevant for CYP450 substrates with a narrow therapeutic index, where the dose is individually adjusted (eg, warfarin). Upon initiation of rilonacept, in patients being treated with these types of medicinal products, therapeutic monitoring of the effect or drug concentration should be performed and the individual dose of the medicinal product may need to be adjusted as needed). Products include:
Amrix **964**

Cyclophosphamide (This is clinically relevant for CYP450 substrates with a narrow therapeutic index, where the dose is individually adjusted (eg, warfarin). Upon initiation of rilonacept, in patients being treated with these types of medicinal products, therapeutic monitoring of the effect or drug concentration should be performed and the individual dose of the medicinal product may need to be adjusted as needed).
No products indexed under this heading.

Cyclosporine (This is clinically relevant for CYP450 substrates with a narrow therapeutic index, where the dose is individually adjusted (eg, warfarin). Upon initiation of rilonacept, in patients being treated with these types of medicinal products, therapeutic monitoring of the effect or drug concentration should be performed and the individual dose of the medicinal product may need to be adjusted as needed). Products include:
Gengraf **440**
Neoral Oral Solution **2496**
Neoral Capsules **2496**
Restasis **605**

Desipramine Hydrochloride (This is clinically relevant for CYP450 substrates with a narrow therapeutic index, where the dose is individually adjusted (eg, warfarin). Upon initiation of rilonacept, in patients being treated with these types of medicinal products, therapeutic monitoring of the effect or drug concentration should be performed and the individual dose of the medicinal product may need to be adjusted as needed).
No products indexed under this heading.

Desogestrel (This is clinically relevant for CYP450 substrates with a narrow therapeutic index, where the dose is individually adjusted (eg, warfarin). Upon initiation of rilonacept, in patients being treated with these types of medicinal products, therapeutic monitoring of the effect or drug concentration should be performed and the individual dose of the medicinal product may need to be adjusted as needed).
No products indexed under this heading.

Dexamethasone (This is clinically relevant for CYP450 substrates with a narrow therapeutic index, where the dose is individually adjusted (eg, warfarin). Upon initiation of rilonacept, in patients being treated with these types of medicinal products, therapeutic monitoring of the effect or drug concentration should be performed and the individual dose of the medicinal product may need to be adjusted as needed). Products include:
Ciprodex **583**
Ozurdex .... ⊙**223**
Tobramycin and Dexamethasone Ophthalmic Suspension .... ⊙**251**

Dexamethasone Acetate (This is clinically relevant for CYP450 substrates with a narrow therapeutic index, where the dose is individually adjusted (eg, warfarin). Upon initiation of rilonacept, in patients being treated with these types of medicinal products, therapeutic monitoring of the effect or drug concentration should be performed and the individual dose of the medicinal product may need to be adjusted as needed).
No products indexed under this heading.

Dexamethasone Phosphate (This is clinically relevant for CYP450 substrates with a narrow therapeutic index, where the dose is individually adjusted (eg, warfarin). Upon initiation of rilonacept, in patients being treated with these types of medicinal products, therapeutic monitoring of the effect or drug concentration should be performed and the individual dose of the medicinal product may need to be adjusted as needed).
No products indexed under this heading.

Dexamethasone Sodium (This is clinically relevant for CYP450 substrates with a narrow therapeutic index, where the dose is individually adjusted (eg, warfarin). Upon initiation of rilonacept, in patients being treated with these types of medicinal products, therapeutic monitoring of the effect or drug concentration should be performed and the individual dose of the medicinal product may need to be adjusted as needed).
No products indexed under this heading.

Dexamethasone Sodium Phosphate (This is clinically relevant for CYP450 substrates with a narrow therapeutic index, where the dose is individually adjusted (eg, warfarin). Upon initiation of rilonacept, in patients being treated with these types of medicinal products, therapeutic monitoring of the effect or drug concentration should be performed and the individual dose of the medicinal product may need to be adjusted as needed).
No products indexed under this heading.

Dexfenfluramine Hydrochloride (This is clinically relevant for CYP450 substrates with a narrow therapeutic index, where the dose is individually adjusted (eg, warfarin). Upon initiation of rilonacept, in patients being treated with these types of medicinal products, therapeutic monitoring of the effect or drug concentration should be performed and the individual dose of the medicinal product may need to be adjusted as needed).
No products indexed under this heading.

Dextromethorphan (This is clinically relevant for CYP450 substrates with a narrow therapeutic index, where the dose is individually adjusted (eg, warfarin). Upon initiation of rilonacept, in patients being treated with these types of medicinal products, therapeutic monitoring of the effect or drug concentration should be performed and the individual dose of the medicinal product may need to be adjusted as needed).
No products indexed under this heading.

Dextromethorphan Hydrobromide (This is clinically relevant for CYP450 substrates with a narrow therapeutic index, where the dose is individually adjusted (eg, warfarin). Upon initiation of rilonacept, in patients being treated with these types of medicinal products, therapeutic monitoring of the effect or drug concentration should be performed and the individual dose of the medicinal product may need to be adjusted as needed).
No products indexed under this heading.

139 Interactions Index Arcalyst

Dextromethorphan Polistirex (This is clinically relevant for CYP450 substrates with a narrow therapeutic index, where the dose is individually adjusted (eg, warfarin). Upon initiation of rilonacept, in patients being treated with these types of medicinal products, therapeutic monitoring of the effect or drug concentration should be performed and the individual dose of the medicinal product may need to be adjusted as needed).
No products indexed under this heading.

Diazepam (This is clinically relevant for CYP450 substrates with a narrow therapeutic index, where the dose is individually adjusted (eg, warfarin). Upon initiation of rilonacept, in patients being treated with these types of medicinal products, therapeutic monitoring of the effect or drug concentration should be performed and the individual dose of the medicinal product may need to be adjusted as needed). Products include:
Valium Tablets 2880

Diclofenac Potassium (This is clinically relevant for CYP450 substrates with a narrow therapeutic index, where the dose is individually adjusted (eg, warfarin). Upon initiation of rilonacept, in patients being treated with these types of medicinal products, therapeutic monitoring of the effect or drug concentration should be performed and the individual dose of the medicinal product may need to be adjusted as needed).
No products indexed under this heading.

Diclofenac Sodium (This is clinically relevant for CYP450 substrates with a narrow therapeutic index, where the dose is individually adjusted (eg, warfarin). Upon initiation of rilonacept, in patients being treated with these types of medicinal products, therapeutic monitoring of the effect or drug concentration should be performed and the individual dose of the medicinal product may need to be adjusted as needed).
No products indexed under this heading.

Dihydroergotamine Mesylate (This is clinically relevant for CYP450 substrates with a narrow therapeutic index, where the dose is individually adjusted (eg, warfarin). Upon initiation of rilonacept, in patients being treated with these types of medicinal products, therapeutic monitoring of the effect or drug concentration should be performed and the individual dose of the medicinal product may need to be adjusted as needed).
No products indexed under this heading.

Diltiazem Hydrochloride (This is clinically relevant for CYP450 substrates with a narrow therapeutic index, where the dose is individually adjusted (eg, warfarin). Upon initiation of rilonacept, in patients being treated with these types of medicinal products, therapeutic monitoring of the effect or drug concentration should be performed and the individual dose of the medicinal product may need to be adjusted as needed). Products include:
Cardizem LA 423

Diltiazem Maleate (This is clinically relevant for CYP450 substrates with a narrow therapeutic index, where the dose is individually adjusted (eg, warfarin). Upon initiation of rilonacept, in patients being treated with these types of medicinal products, therapeutic monitoring of the effect or drug concentration should be performed and the individual dose of the medicinal product may need to be adjusted as needed).
No products indexed under this heading.

Disopyramide (This is clinically relevant for CYP450 substrates with a narrow therapeutic index, where the dose is individually adjusted (eg, warfarin). Upon initiation of rilonacept, in patients being treated with these types of medicinal products, therapeutic monitoring of the effect or drug concentration should be performed and the individual dose of the medicinal product may need to be adjusted as needed).
No products indexed under this heading.

Disopyramide Phosphate (This is clinically relevant for CYP450 substrates with a narrow therapeutic index, where the dose is individually adjusted (eg, warfarin). Upon initiation of rilonacept, in patients being treated with these types of medicinal products, therapeutic monitoring of the effect or drug concentration should be performed and the individual dose of the medicinal product may need to be adjusted as needed).
No products indexed under this heading.

Disulfiram (This is clinically relevant for CYP450 substrates with a narrow therapeutic index, where the dose is individually adjusted (eg, warfarin). Upon initiation of rilonacept, in patients being treated with these types of medicinal products, therapeutic monitoring of the effect or drug concentration should be performed and the individual dose of the medicinal product may need to be adjusted as needed).
No products indexed under this heading.

Divalproex Sodium (This is clinically relevant for CYP450 substrates with a narrow therapeutic index, where the dose is individually adjusted (eg, warfarin). Upon initiation of rilonacept, in patients being treated with these types of medicinal products, therapeutic monitoring of the effect or drug concentration should be performed and the individual dose of the medicinal product may need to be adjusted as needed). Products include:
Depakote ER 426

Docetaxel (This is clinically relevant for CYP450 substrates with a narrow therapeutic index, where the dose is individually adjusted (eg, warfarin). Upon initiation of rilonacept, in patients being treated with these types of medicinal products, therapeutic monitoring of the effect or drug concentration should be performed and the individual dose of the medicinal product may need to be adjusted as needed). Products include:
Taxotere 3035

Dolasetron Mesylate (This is clinically relevant for CYP450 substrates with a narrow therapeutic index, where the dose is individually adjusted (eg, warfarin). Upon initiation of rilonacept, in patients being treated with these types of medicinal products, therapeutic monitoring of the effect or drug concentration should be performed and the individual dose of the medicinal product may need to be adjusted as needed). Products include:
Anzemet Injection 2931
Anzemet Tablets 2934

Donepezil Hydrochloride (This is clinically relevant for CYP450 substrates with a narrow therapeutic index, where the dose is individually adjusted (eg, warfarin). Upon initiation of rilonacept, in patients being treated with these types of medicinal products, therapeutic monitoring of the effect or drug concentration should be performed and the individual dose of the medicinal product may need to be adjusted as needed). Products include:
Aricept 1045
Aricept ODT 1045

Doxepin Hydrochloride (This is clinically relevant for CYP450 substrates with a narrow therapeutic index, where the dose is individually adjusted (eg, warfarin). Upon initiation of rilonacept, in patients being treated with these types of medicinal products, therapeutic monitoring of the effect or drug concentration should be performed and the individual dose of the medicinal product may need to be adjusted as needed).
No products indexed under this heading.

Doxorubicin Hydrochloride (This is clinically relevant for CYP450 substrates with a narrow therapeutic index, where the dose is individually adjusted (eg, warfarin). Upon initiation of rilonacept, in patients being treated with these types of medicinal products, therapeutic monitoring of the effect or drug concentration should be performed and the individual dose of the medicinal product may need to be adjusted as needed).
No products indexed under this heading.

Dronabinol (This is clinically relevant for CYP450 substrates with a narrow therapeutic index, where the dose is individually adjusted (eg, warfarin). Upon initiation of rilonacept, in patients being treated with these types of medicinal products, therapeutic monitoring of the effect or drug concentration should be performed and the individual dose of the medicinal product may need to be adjusted as needed).
No products indexed under this heading.

Drugs that Undergo Biotransformation by Cytochrome P-450 Mixed Function Oxidase (This is clinically relevant for CYP450 substrates with a narrow therapeutic index, where the dose is individually adjusted (eg, warfarin). Upon initiation of rilonacept, in patients being treated with these types of medicinal products, therapeutic monitoring of the effect or drug concentration should be performed and the individual dose of the medicinal product may need to be adjusted as needed).
No products indexed under this heading.

Dyphylline (This is clinically relevant for CYP450 substrates with a narrow therapeutic index, where the dose is individually adjusted (eg, warfarin). Upon initiation of rilonacept, in patients being treated with these types of medicinal products, therapeutic monitoring of the effect or drug concentration should be performed and the individual dose of the medicinal product may need to be adjusted as needed).
No products indexed under this heading.

Encainide Hydrochloride (This is clinically relevant for CYP450 substrates with a narrow therapeutic index, where the dose is individually adjusted (eg, warfarin). Upon initiation of rilonacept, in patients being treated with these types of medicinal products, therapeutic monitoring of the effect or drug concentration should be performed and the individual dose of the medicinal product may need to be adjusted as needed).
No products indexed under this heading.

Enoxacin (This is clinically relevant for CYP450 substrates with a narrow therapeutic index, where the dose is individually adjusted (eg, warfarin). Upon initiation of rilonacept, in patients being treated with these types of medicinal products, therapeutic monitoring of the effect or drug concentration should be performed and the individual dose of the medicinal product may need to be adjusted as needed).
No products indexed under this heading.

Eprosartan Mesylate (This is clinically relevant for CYP450 substrates with a narrow therapeutic index, where the dose is individually adjusted (eg, warfarin). Upon initiation of rilonacept, in patients being treated with these types of medicinal products, therapeutic monitoring of the effect or drug concentration should be performed and the individual dose of the medicinal product may need to be adjusted as needed). Products include:
Teveten 538
Teveten HCT 541

Ergotamine Tartrate (This is clinically relevant for CYP450 substrates with a narrow therapeutic index, where the dose is individually adjusted (eg, warfarin). Upon initiation of rilonacept, in patients being treated with these types of medicinal products, therapeutic monitoring of the effect or drug concentration should be performed and the individual dose of the medicinal product may need to be adjusted as needed).
No products indexed under this heading.

Erythromycin (This is clinically relevant for CYP450 substrates with a narrow therapeutic index, where the dose is individually adjusted (eg, warfarin). Upon initiation of rilonacept, in patients being treated with these types of medicinal products, therapeutic monitoring of the effect or drug concentration should be performed and the individual dose of the medicinal product may need to be adjusted as needed).
No products indexed under this heading.

Erythromycin Estolate (This is clinically relevant for CYP450 substrates with a narrow therapeutic index, where the dose is individually adjusted (eg, warfarin). Upon initiation of rilonacept, in patients being treated with these types of medicinal products, therapeutic monitoring of the effect or drug concentration should be performed and the individual dose of the medicinal product may need to be adjusted as needed).
No products indexed under this heading.

Erythromycin Ethylsuccinate (This is clinically relevant for CYP450 substrates with a narrow therapeutic index, where the dose is individually adjusted (eg, warfarin). Upon initiation of rilonacept, in patients being treated with these types of medicinal products, therapeutic monitoring of the effect or drug concentration should be performed and the individual dose of the medicinal product may need to be adjusted as needed). Products include:
E.E.S. 437
EryPed 435

Erythromycin Gluceptate (This is clinically relevant for CYP450 substrates with a narrow therapeutic index, where the dose is individually adjusted (eg, warfarin). Upon initiation of rilonacept, in patients being treated with these types of medicinal products, therapeutic monitoring of the effect or drug concentration should be performed and the individual dose of the medicinal product may need to be adjusted as needed).
No products indexed under this heading.

Erythromycin Lactobionate (This is clinically relevant for CYP450 substrates with a narrow therapeutic index, where the dose is individually adjusted (eg, warfarin). Upon initiation of rilonacept, in patients being treated with these types of medicinal products, therapeutic monitoring of the effect or drug concentration should be performed and the individual dose of the medicinal product may need to be adjusted as needed).
No products indexed under this heading.

Erythromycin Stearate (This is clinically relevant for CYP450 substrates with a narrow therapeutic index, where the dose is individually adjusted (eg, warfarin). Upon initiation of rilonacept, in patients being treated with these types of medicinal products, therapeutic monitoring of the effect or drug concentration should be performed and the individual dose of the medicinal product may need to be adjusted as needed).
No products indexed under this heading.

IMPORTANT NOTE: Always consult each drug listing in the patient's regimen for possible interactions.

Esomeprazole Magnesium (This is clinically relevant for CYP450 substrates with a narrow therapeutic index, where the dose is individually adjusted (eg, warfarin). Upon initiation of rilonacept, in patients being treated with these types of medicinal products, therapeutic monitoring of the effect or drug concentration should be performed and the individual dose of the medicinal product may need to be adjusted as needed). Products include:

Nexium Capsules **704**
Nexium Oral Suspension **704**

Esomeprazole Sodium (This is clinically relevant for CYP450 substrates with a narrow therapeutic index, where the dose is individually adjusted (eg, warfarin). Upon initiation of rilonacept, in patients being treated with these types of medicinal products, therapeutic monitoring of the effect or drug concentration should be performed and the individual dose of the medicinal product may need to be adjusted as needed). Products include:

Nexium I.V. **712**

Estradiol (This is clinically relevant for CYP450 substrates with a narrow therapeutic index, where the dose is individually adjusted (eg, warfarin). Upon initiation of rilonacept, in patients being treated with these types of medicinal products, therapeutic monitoring of the effect or drug concentration should be performed and the individual dose of the medicinal product may need to be adjusted as needed). Products include:

Activella **2561**
Angeliq **831**
Climara **841**
Climara Pro **847**
Divigel **3467**
Estrasorb **1777**
Vagifem **2589**

Estradiol Benzoate (This is clinically relevant for CYP450 substrates with a narrow therapeutic index, where the dose is individually adjusted (eg, warfarin). Upon initiation of rilonacept, in patients being treated with these types of medicinal products, therapeutic monitoring of the effect or drug concentration should be performed and the individual dose of the medicinal product may need to be adjusted as needed).

No products indexed under this heading.

Estradiol Cypionate (This is clinically relevant for CYP450 substrates with a narrow therapeutic index, where the dose is individually adjusted (eg, warfarin). Upon initiation of rilonacept, in patients being treated with these types of medicinal products, therapeutic monitoring of the effect or drug concentration should be performed and the individual dose of the medicinal product may need to be adjusted as needed).

No products indexed under this heading.

Estradiol Valerate (This is clinically relevant for CYP450 substrates with a narrow therapeutic index, where the dose is individually adjusted (eg, warfarin). Upon initiation of rilonacept, in patients being treated with these types of medicinal products, therapeutic monitoring of the effect or drug concentration should be performed and the individual dose of the medicinal product may need to be adjusted as needed).

No products indexed under this heading.

Estrogen (This is clinically relevant for CYP450 substrates with a narrow therapeutic index, where the dose is individually adjusted (eg, warfarin). Upon initiation of rilonacept, in patients being treated with these types of medicinal products, therapeutic monitoring of the effect or drug concentration should be performed and the individual dose of the medicinal product may need to be adjusted as needed).

No products indexed under this heading.

Estrogens, Conjugated (This is clinically relevant for CYP450 substrates with a narrow therapeutic index, where the dose is individually adjusted (eg, warfarin). Upon initiation of rilonacept, in patients being treated with these types of medicinal products, therapeutic monitoring of the effect or drug concentration should be performed and the individual dose of the medicinal product may need to be adjusted as needed). Products include:

Premarin Intravenous **3528**
Premarin Tablets **3533**
Premarin Vaginal Cream **3540**
Premphase **3549**
Prempro **3549**

Estrogens, Conjugated, Synthetic A (This is clinically relevant for CYP450 substrates with a narrow therapeutic index, where the dose is individually adjusted (eg, warfarin). Upon initiation of rilonacept, in patients being treated with these types of medicinal products, therapeutic monitoring of the effect or drug concentration should be performed and the individual dose of the medicinal product may need to be adjusted as needed).

No products indexed under this heading.

Estrogens, Esterified (This is clinically relevant for CYP450 substrates with a narrow therapeutic index, where the dose is individually adjusted (eg, warfarin). Upon initiation of rilonacept, in patients being treated with these types of medicinal products, therapeutic monitoring of the effect or drug concentration should be performed and the individual dose of the medicinal product may need to be adjusted as needed).

No products indexed under this heading.

Etanercept (Concomitant administration of another drug that blocks IL-1 with a TNF-blocking agent in another patient population has been associated with an increased risk of serious infections and an increased risk of neutropenia. The concomitant administration of rilonacept with TNF-blocking agents may also result in similar toxicities and is not recommended). Products include:

Enbrel **613**

Ethinyl Estradiol (This is clinically relevant for CYP450 substrates with a narrow therapeutic index, where the dose is individually adjusted (eg, warfarin). Upon initiation of rilonacept, in patients being treated with these types of medicinal products, therapeutic monitoring of the effect or drug concentration should be performed and the individual dose of the medicinal product may need to be adjusted as needed). Products include:

LoSeasonique **3407**
Lybrel **3514**
NuvaRing **3181**
Ortho Evra **2648**
Ortho-Cyclen/Ortho Tri-Cyclen **2663**
Ortho Tri-Cyclen Lo Tablets **2673**
Seasonique **3418**
Yaz **864**

Ethosuximide (This is clinically relevant for CYP450 substrates with a narrow therapeutic index, where the dose is individually adjusted (eg, warfarin). Upon initiation of rilonacept, in patients being treated with these types of medicinal products, therapeutic monitoring of the effect or drug concentration should be performed and the individual dose of the medicinal product may need to be adjusted as needed).

No products indexed under this heading.

Ethotoin (This is clinically relevant for CYP450 substrates with a narrow therapeutic index, where the dose is individually adjusted (eg, warfarin). Upon initiation of rilonacept, in patients being treated with these types of medicinal products, therapeutic monitoring of the effect or drug concentration should be performed and the individual dose of the medicinal product may need to be adjusted as needed).

No products indexed under this heading.

Ethynodiol Diacetate (This is clinically relevant for CYP450 substrates with a narrow therapeutic index, where the dose is individually adjusted (eg, warfarin). Upon initiation of rilonacept, in patients being treated with these types of medicinal products, therapeutic monitoring of the effect or drug concentration should be performed and the individual dose of the medicinal product may need to be adjusted as needed).

No products indexed under this heading.

Etodolac (This is clinically relevant for CYP450 substrates with a narrow therapeutic index, where the dose is individually adjusted (eg, warfarin). Upon initiation of rilonacept, in patients being treated with these types of medicinal products, therapeutic monitoring of the effect or drug concentration should be performed and the individual dose of the medicinal product may need to be adjusted as needed).

No products indexed under this heading.

Etoposide (This is clinically relevant for CYP450 substrates with a narrow therapeutic index, where the dose is individually adjusted (eg, warfarin). Upon initiation of rilonacept, in patients being treated with these types of medicinal products, therapeutic monitoring of the effect or drug concentration should be performed and the individual dose of the medicinal product may need to be adjusted as needed).

No products indexed under this heading.

Etoposide Phosphate (This is clinically relevant for CYP450 substrates with a narrow therapeutic index, where the dose is individually adjusted (eg, warfarin). Upon initiation of rilonacept, in patients being treated with these types of medicinal products, therapeutic monitoring of the effect or drug concentration should be performed and the individual dose of the medicinal product may need to be adjusted as needed).

No products indexed under this heading.

Felbamate (This is clinically relevant for CYP450 substrates with a narrow therapeutic index, where the dose is individually adjusted (eg, warfarin). Upon initiation of rilonacept, in patients being treated with these types of medicinal products, therapeutic monitoring of the effect or drug concentration should be performed and the individual dose of the medicinal product may need to be adjusted as needed).

No products indexed under this heading.

Felodipine (This is clinically relevant for CYP450 substrates with a narrow therapeutic index, where the dose is individually adjusted (eg, warfarin). Upon initiation of rilonacept, in patients being treated with these types of medicinal products, therapeutic monitoring of the effect or drug concentration should be performed and the individual dose of the medicinal product may need to be adjusted as needed).

No products indexed under this heading.

Fenoprofen Calcium (This is clinically relevant for CYP450 substrates with a narrow therapeutic index, where the dose is individually adjusted (eg, warfarin). Upon initiation of rilonacept, in patients being treated with these types of medicinal products, therapeutic monitoring of the effect or drug concentration should be performed and the individual dose of the medicinal product may need to be adjusted as needed).

No products indexed under this heading.

Fentanyl (This is clinically relevant for CYP450 substrates with a narrow therapeutic index, where the dose is individually adjusted (eg, warfarin). Upon initiation of rilonacept, in patients being treated with these types of medicinal products, therapeutic monitoring of the effect or drug concentration should be performed and the individual dose of the medicinal product may need to be adjusted as needed). Products include:

Duragesic **2604**
Fentanyl Transdermal System **2346**
Onsolis **2054**

Fentanyl Citrate (This is clinically relevant for CYP450 substrates with a narrow therapeutic index, where the dose is individually adjusted (eg, warfarin). Upon initiation of rilonacept, in patients being treated with these types of medicinal products, therapeutic monitoring of the effect or drug concentration should be performed and the individual dose of the medicinal product may need to be adjusted as needed). Products include:

Fentora **966**

Flecainide Acetate (This is clinically relevant for CYP450 substrates with a narrow therapeutic index, where the dose is individually adjusted (eg, warfarin). Upon initiation of rilonacept, in patients being treated with these types of medicinal products, therapeutic monitoring of the effect or drug concentration should be performed and the individual dose of the medicinal product may need to be adjusted as needed).

No products indexed under this heading.

Fluoxetine (This is clinically relevant for CYP450 substrates with a narrow therapeutic index, where the dose is individually adjusted (eg, warfarin). Upon initiation of rilonacept, in patients being treated with these types of medicinal products, therapeutic monitoring of the effect or drug concentration should be performed and the individual dose of the medicinal product may need to be adjusted as needed).

No products indexed under this heading.

Fluoxetine Hydrochloride (This is clinically relevant for CYP450 substrates with a narrow therapeutic index, where the dose is individually adjusted (eg, warfarin). Upon initiation of rilonacept, in patients being treated with these types of medicinal products, therapeutic monitoring of the effect or drug concentration should be performed and the individual dose of the medicinal product may need to be adjusted as needed). Products include:

Prozac Weekly **1941**
Prozac Pulvules **1941**
Symbyax **1965**

Fluphenazine Decanoate (This is clinically relevant for CYP450 substrates with a narrow therapeutic index, where the dose is individually adjusted (eg, warfarin). Upon initiation of rilonacept, in patients being treated with these types of medicinal products, therapeutic monitoring of the effect or drug concentration should be performed and the individual dose of the medicinal product may need to be adjusted as needed).

No products indexed under this heading.

Fluphenazine Enanthate (This is clinically relevant for CYP450 substrates with a narrow therapeutic index, where the dose is individually adjusted (eg, warfarin). Upon initiation of rilonacept, in patients being treated with these types of medicinal products, therapeutic monitoring of the effect or drug concentration should be performed and the individual dose of the medicinal product may need to be adjusted as needed).

No products indexed under this heading.

Fluphenazine Hydrochloride (This is clinically relevant for CYP450 substrates with a narrow therapeutic index, where the dose is individually adjusted (eg, warfarin). Upon initiation of rilona-

cept, in patients being treated with these types of medicinal products, therapeutic monitoring of the effect or drug concentration should be performed and the individual dose of the medicinal product may need to be adjusted as needed).

No products indexed under this heading.

Flurbiprofen (This is clinically relevant for CYP450 substrates with a narrow therapeutic index, where the dose is individually adjusted (eg, warfarin). Upon initiation of rilonacept, in patients being treated with these types of medicinal products, therapeutic monitoring of the effect or drug concentration should be performed and the individual dose of the medicinal product may need to be adjusted as needed).

No products indexed under this heading.

Flurbiprofen Sodium (This is clinically relevant for CYP450 substrates with a narrow therapeutic index, where the dose is individually adjusted (eg, warfarin). Upon initiation of rilonacept, in patients being treated with these types of medicinal products, therapeutic monitoring of the effect or drug concentration should be performed and the individual dose of the medicinal product may need to be adjusted as needed).

No products indexed under this heading.

Flutamide (This is clinically relevant for CYP450 substrates with a narrow therapeutic index, where the dose is individually adjusted (eg, warfarin). Upon initiation of rilonacept, in patients being treated with these types of medicinal products, therapeutic monitoring of the effect or drug concentration should be performed and the individual dose of the medicinal product may need to be adjusted as needed).

No products indexed under this heading.

Fluticasone Propionate (This is clinically relevant for CYP450 substrates with a narrow therapeutic index, where the dose is individually adjusted (eg, warfarin). Upon initiation of rilonacept, in patients being treated with these types of medicinal products, therapeutic monitoring of the effect or drug concentration should be performed and the individual dose of the medicinal product may need to be adjusted as needed). Products include:

Advair 100/50 .... **1275**
Advair 250/50 .... **1275**
Advair 500/50 .... **1275**
Advair HFA 45/21 .... **1288**
Advair HFA 115/21 .... **1288**
Advair HFA 230/21 .... **1288**
Flonase **1459**
Flovent Diskus **1463**
Flovent HFA **1470**

Fluvastatin Sodium (This is clinically relevant for CYP450 substrates with a narrow therapeutic index, where the dose is individually adjusted (eg, warfarin). Upon initiation of rilonacept, in patients being treated with these types of medicinal products, therapeutic monitoring of the effect or drug concentration should be performed and the individual dose of the medicinal product may need to be adjusted as needed).

No products indexed under this heading.

Fluvoxamine Maleate (This is clinically relevant for CYP450 substrates with a narrow therapeutic index, where the dose is individually adjusted (eg, warfarin). Upon initiation of rilonacept, in patients being treated with these types of medicinal products, therapeutic monitoring of the effect or drug concentration should be performed and the individual dose of the medicinal product may need to be adjusted as needed).

No products indexed under this heading.

Formoterol Fumarate (This is clinically relevant for CYP450 substrates with a narrow therapeutic index, where the dose is individually adjusted (eg, warfarin). Upon initiation of rilonacept, in patients being treated with these types of medicinal products, therapeutic monitoring of the effect or drug concentration should be performed and the individual dose of the medicinal product may need to be adjusted as needed). Products include:

Foradil **3121**
Perforomist **3634**

Fosphenytoin (This is clinically relevant for CYP450 substrates with a narrow therapeutic index, where the dose is individually adjusted (eg, warfarin). Upon initiation of rilonacept, in patients being treated with these types of medicinal products, therapeutic monitoring of the effect or drug concentration should be performed and the individual dose of the medicinal product may need to be adjusted as needed).

No products indexed under this heading.

Fosphenytoin Sodium (This is clinically relevant for CYP450 substrates with a narrow therapeutic index, where the dose is individually adjusted (eg, warfarin). Upon initiation of rilonacept, in patients being treated with these types of medicinal products, therapeutic monitoring of the effect or drug concentration should be performed and the individual dose of the medicinal product may need to be adjusted as needed).

No products indexed under this heading.

Gabapentin (This is clinically relevant for CYP450 substrates with a narrow therapeutic index, where the dose is individually adjusted (eg, warfarin). Upon initiation of rilonacept, in patients being treated with these types of medicinal products, therapeutic monitoring of the effect or drug concentration should be performed and the individual dose of the medicinal product may need to be adjusted as needed).

No products indexed under this heading.

Galantamine Hydrobromide (This is clinically relevant for CYP450 substrates with a narrow therapeutic index, where the dose is individually adjusted (eg, warfarin). Upon initiation of rilonacept, in patients being treated with these types of medicinal products, therapeutic monitoring of the effect or drug concentration should be performed and the individual dose of the medicinal product may need to be adjusted as needed).

No products indexed under this heading.

Glimepiride (This is clinically relevant for CYP450 substrates with a narrow therapeutic index, where the dose is individually adjusted (eg, warfarin). Upon initiation of rilonacept, in patients being treated with these types of medicinal products, therapeutic monitoring of the effect or drug concentration should be performed and the individual dose of the medicinal product may need to be adjusted as needed). Products include:

Avandaryl **1356**
Duetact **3354**

Glipizide (This is clinically relevant for CYP450 substrates with a narrow therapeutic index, where the dose is individually adjusted (eg, warfarin). Upon initiation of rilonacept, in patients being treated with these types of medicinal products, therapeutic monitoring of the effect or drug concentration should be performed and the individual dose of the medicinal product may need to be adjusted as needed).

No products indexed under this heading.

Glyburide (This is clinically relevant for CYP450 substrates with a narrow therapeutic index, where the dose is individually adjusted (eg, warfarin). Upon initiation of rilonacept, in patients being treated with these types of medicinal products, therapeutic monitoring of the effect or drug concentration should be performed and the individual dose of the medicinal product may need to be adjusted as needed).

No products indexed under this heading.

Grepafloxacin Hydrochloride (This is clinically relevant for CYP450 substrates with a narrow therapeutic index, where the dose is individually adjusted (eg, warfarin). Upon initiation of rilonacept, in patients being treated with these types of medicinal products, therapeutic monitoring of the effect or drug concentration should be performed and the individual dose of the medicinal product may need to be adjusted as needed).

No products indexed under this heading.

Haloperidol (This is clinically relevant for CYP450 substrates with a narrow therapeutic index, where the dose is individually adjusted (eg, warfarin). Upon initiation of rilonacept, in patients being treated with these types of medicinal products, therapeutic monitoring of the effect or drug concentration should be performed and the individual dose of the medicinal product may need to be adjusted as needed).

No products indexed under this heading.

Haloperidol Decanoate (This is clinically relevant for CYP450 substrates with a narrow therapeutic index, where the dose is individually adjusted (eg, warfarin). Upon initiation of rilonacept, in patients being treated with these types of medicinal products, therapeutic monitoring of the effect or drug concentration should be performed and the individual dose of the medicinal product may need to be adjusted as needed).

No products indexed under this heading.

Haloperidol Lactate (This is clinically relevant for CYP450 substrates with a narrow therapeutic index, where the dose is individually adjusted (eg, warfarin). Upon initiation of rilonacept, in patients being treated with these types of medicinal products, therapeutic monitoring of the effect or drug concentration should be performed and the individual dose of the medicinal product may need to be adjusted as needed).

No products indexed under this heading.

Hexobarbital (This is clinically relevant for CYP450 substrates with a narrow therapeutic index, where the dose is individually adjusted (eg, warfarin). Upon initiation of rilonacept, in patients being treated with these types of medicinal products, therapeutic monitoring of the effect or drug concentration should be performed and the individual dose of the medicinal product may need to be adjusted as needed).

No products indexed under this heading.

Hydrocodone Bitartrate (This is clinically relevant for CYP450 substrates with a narrow therapeutic index, where the dose is individually adjusted (eg, warfarin). Upon initiation of rilonacept, in patients being treated with these types of medicinal products, therapeutic monitoring of the effect or drug concentration should be performed and the individual dose of the medicinal product may need to be adjusted as needed). Products include:

Vicodin **560**
Vicodin ES **561**
Vicodin HP **563**
Vicoprofen **564**
Zydone **1138**

Ibuprofen (This is clinically relevant for CYP450 substrates with a narrow therapeutic index, where the dose is individually adjusted (eg, warfarin). Upon initiation of rilonacept, in patients being treated with these types of medicinal products, therapeutic monitoring of the effect or drug concentration should be performed and the individual dose of the medicinal product may need to be adjusted as needed). Products include:

Motrin IB **2043**
Children's Motrin **2044**
Children's Motrin Non-Staining Dye-Free **2044**
Infants' Motrin **2044**
Infants' Motrin Dye-Free **2044**
Junior Strength Motrin **2044**
Vicoprofen **564**

Imipramine Hydrochloride (This is clinically relevant for CYP450 substrates with a narrow therapeutic index, where the dose is individually adjusted (eg, warfarin). Upon initiation of rilonacept, in patients being treated with these types of medicinal products, therapeutic monitoring of the effect or drug concentration should be performed and the individual dose of the medicinal product may need to be adjusted as needed).

No products indexed under this heading.

Imipramine Pamoate (This is clinically relevant for CYP450 substrates with a narrow therapeutic index, where the dose is individually adjusted (eg, warfarin). Upon initiation of rilonacept, in patients being treated with these types of medicinal products, therapeutic monitoring of the effect or drug concentration should be performed and the individual dose of the medicinal product may need to be adjusted as needed).

No products indexed under this heading.

Indinavir Sulfate (This is clinically relevant for CYP450 substrates with a narrow therapeutic index, where the dose is individually adjusted (eg, warfarin). Upon initiation of rilonacept, in patients being treated with these types of medicinal products, therapeutic monitoring of the effect or drug concentration should be performed and the individual dose of the medicinal product may need to be adjusted as needed). Products include:

Crixivan **2113**

Indomethacin (This is clinically relevant for CYP450 substrates with a narrow therapeutic index, where the dose is individually adjusted (eg, warfarin). Upon initiation of rilonacept, in patients being treated with these types of medicinal products, therapeutic monitoring of the effect or drug concentration should be performed and the individual dose of the medicinal product may need to be adjusted as needed). Products include:

Indocin **2167**

Indomethacin Sodium Trihydrate (This is clinically relevant for CYP450 substrates with a narrow therapeutic index, where the dose is individually adjusted (eg, warfarin). Upon initiation of rilonacept, in patients being treated with these types of medicinal products, therapeutic monitoring of the effect or drug concentration should be performed and the individual dose of the medicinal product may need to be adjusted as needed). Products include:

Indocin I.V. **2007**

Indoramin Hydrochloride (This is clinically relevant for CYP450 substrates with a narrow therapeutic index, where the dose is individually adjusted (eg, warfarin). Upon initiation of rilonacept, in patients being treated with these types of medicinal products, therapeutic monitoring of the effect or drug concentration should be performed and the individual dose of the medicinal product may need to be adjusted as needed).

No products indexed under this heading.

Infliximab (Concomitant administration of another drug that blocks IL-1 with a TNF-blocking agent in another patient population has been associated with an increased risk of serious infections and an increased risk of neutropenia. The concomitant administration of

143 **Interactions Index** **Arcalyst**

vaccination with inactivated (killed) antigens in patients receiving rilonacept). Products include:
Attenuvax 2086

Meclofenamate Sodium (This is clinically relevant for CYP450 substrates with a narrow therapeutic index, where the dose is individually adjusted (eg, warfarin). Upon initiation of rilonacept, in patients being treated with these types of medicinal products, therapeutic monitoring of the effect or drug concentration should be performed and the individual dose of the medicinal product may need to be adjusted as needed).
No products indexed under this heading.

Mefenamic Acid (This is clinically relevant for CYP450 substrates with a narrow therapeutic index, where the dose is individually adjusted (eg, warfarin). Upon initiation of rilonacept, in patients being treated with these types of medicinal products, therapeutic monitoring of the effect or drug concentration should be performed and the individual dose of the medicinal product may need to be adjusted as needed).
No products indexed under this heading.

Meloxicam (This is clinically relevant for CYP450 substrates with a narrow therapeutic index, where the dose is individually adjusted (eg, warfarin). Upon initiation of rilonacept, in patients being treated with these types of medicinal products, therapeutic monitoring of the effect or drug concentration should be performed and the individual dose of the medicinal product may need to be adjusted as needed).
No products indexed under this heading.

Meperidine Hydrochloride (This is clinically relevant for CYP450 substrates with a narrow therapeutic index, where the dose is individually adjusted (eg, warfarin). Upon initiation of rilonacept, in patients being treated with these types of medicinal products, therapeutic monitoring of the effect or drug concentration should be performed and the individual dose of the medicinal product may need to be adjusted as needed).
No products indexed under this heading.

Mephenytoin (This is clinically relevant for CYP450 substrates with a narrow therapeutic index, where the dose is individually adjusted (eg, warfarin). Upon initiation of rilonacept, in patients being treated with these types of medicinal products, therapeutic monitoring of the effect or drug concentration should be performed and the individual dose of the medicinal product may need to be adjusted as needed).
No products indexed under this heading.

Mephobarbital (This is clinically relevant for CYP450 substrates with a narrow therapeutic index, where the dose is individually adjusted (eg, warfarin). Upon initiation of rilonacept, in patients being treated with these types of medicinal products, therapeutic monitoring of the effect or drug concentration should be performed and the individual dose of the medicinal product may need to be adjusted as needed).
No products indexed under this heading.

Meprobamate (This is clinically relevant for CYP450 substrates with a narrow therapeutic index, where the dose is individually adjusted (eg, warfarin). Upon initiation of rilonacept, in patients being treated with these types of medicinal products, therapeutic monitoring of the effect or drug concentration should be performed and the individual dose of the medicinal product may need to be adjusted as needed).
No products indexed under this heading.

Mestranol (This is clinically relevant for CYP450 substrates with a narrow therapeutic index, where the dose is individually adjusted (eg, warfarin). Upon initiation of rilonacept, in patients being treated with these types of medicinal products, therapeutic monitoring of the effect or drug concentration should be performed and the individual dose of the medicinal product may need to be adjusted as needed).
No products indexed under this heading.

Metformin Hydrochloride (This is clinically relevant for CYP450 substrates with a narrow therapeutic index, where the dose is individually adjusted (eg, warfarin). Upon initiation of rilonacept, in patients being treated with these types of medicinal products, therapeutic monitoring of the effect or drug concentration should be performed and the individual dose of the medicinal product may need to be adjusted as needed). Products include:
ActoPlus 3338
Avandamet 1345
Janumet 2188

Methadone Hydrochloride (This is clinically relevant for CYP450 substrates with a narrow therapeutic index, where the dose is individually adjusted (eg, warfarin). Upon initiation of rilonacept, in patients being treated with these types of medicinal products, therapeutic monitoring of the effect or drug concentration should be performed and the individual dose of the medicinal product may need to be adjusted as needed).
No products indexed under this heading.

Methamphetamine Hydrochloride (This is clinically relevant for CYP450 substrates with a narrow therapeutic index, where the dose is individually adjusted (eg, warfarin). Upon initiation of rilonacept, in patients being treated with these types of medicinal products, therapeutic monitoring of the effect or drug concentration should be performed and the individual dose of the medicinal product may need to be adjusted as needed).
No products indexed under this heading.

Methsuximide (This is clinically relevant for CYP450 substrates with a narrow therapeutic index, where the dose is individually adjusted (eg, warfarin). Upon initiation of rilonacept, in patients being treated with these types of medicinal products, therapeutic monitoring of the effect or drug concentration should be performed and the individual dose of the medicinal product may need to be adjusted as needed).
No products indexed under this heading.

Metoprolol Succinate (This is clinically relevant for CYP450 substrates with a narrow therapeutic index, where the dose is individually adjusted (eg, warfarin). Upon initiation of rilonacept, in patients being treated with these types of medicinal products, therapeutic monitoring of the effect or drug concentration should be performed and the individual dose of the medicinal product may need to be adjusted as needed). Products include:
Toprol XL 732

Metoprolol Tartrate (This is clinically relevant for CYP450 substrates with a narrow therapeutic index, where the dose is individually adjusted (eg, warfarin). Upon initiation of rilonacept, in patients being treated with these types of medicinal products, therapeutic monitoring of the effect or drug concentration should be performed and the individual dose of the medicinal product may need to be adjusted as needed).
No products indexed under this heading.

Mexiletine Hydrochloride (This is clinically relevant for CYP450 substrates with a narrow therapeutic index, where the dose is individually adjusted (eg, warfarin). Upon initiation of rilonacept, in patients being treated with these types of medicinal products, therapeutic monitoring of the effect or drug concentration should be performed and the individual dose of the medicinal product may need to be adjusted as needed).
No products indexed under this heading.

Midazolam Hydrochloride (This is clinically relevant for CYP450 substrates with a narrow therapeutic index, where the dose is individually adjusted (eg, warfarin). Upon initiation of rilonacept, in patients being treated with these types of medicinal products, therapeutic monitoring of the effect or drug concentration should be performed and the individual dose of the medicinal product may need to be adjusted as needed).
No products indexed under this heading.

Miglitol (This is clinically relevant for CYP450 substrates with a narrow therapeutic index, where the dose is individually adjusted (eg, warfarin). Upon initiation of rilonacept, in patients being treated with these types of medicinal products, therapeutic monitoring of the effect or drug concentration should be performed and the individual dose of the medicinal product may need to be adjusted as needed).
No products indexed under this heading.

Mirtazapine (This is clinically relevant for CYP450 substrates with a narrow therapeutic index, where the dose is individually adjusted (eg, warfarin). Upon initiation of rilonacept, in patients being treated with these types of medicinal products, therapeutic monitoring of the effect or drug concentration should be performed and the individual dose of the medicinal product may need to be adjusted as needed). Products include:
Remeron Tablets 3214
RemeronSolTab Tablets 3219

Montelukast Sodium (This is clinically relevant for CYP450 substrates with a narrow therapeutic index, where the dose is individually adjusted (eg, warfarin). Upon initiation of rilonacept, in patients being treated with these types of medicinal products, therapeutic monitoring of the effect or drug concentration should be performed and the individual dose of the medicinal product may need to be adjusted as needed). Products include:
Singulair 2270

Morphine Sulfate (This is clinically relevant for CYP450 substrates with a narrow therapeutic index, where the dose is individually adjusted (eg, warfarin). Upon initiation of rilonacept, in patients being treated with these types of medicinal products, therapeutic monitoring of the effect or drug concentration should be performed and the individual dose of the medicinal product may need to be adjusted as needed). Products include:
Avinza 1822
Embeda 1831
MS Contin 2803

Moxifloxacin Hydrochloride (This is clinically relevant for CYP450 substrates with a narrow therapeutic index, where the dose is individually adjusted (eg, warfarin). Upon initiation of rilonacept, in patients being treated with these types of medicinal products, therapeutic monitoring of the effect or drug concentration should be performed and the individual dose of the medicinal product may need to be adjusted as needed). Products include:
Avelox 3064
Vigamox 589

Mumps Virus Vaccine, Live (Since no data are available on either the efficacy of live vaccines or on the risks of secondary transmission of infection by live vaccines in patients receiving rilonacept, live vaccines should not be given concurrently with rilonacept. In addition, because rilonacept may interfere with normal immune response to new antigens, vaccinations may not be effective in patients receiving rilonacept. No data are available on the effectiveness of vaccination with inactivated (killed) antigens in patients receiving rilonacept). Products include:
Mumpsvax 2218

Nabumetone (This is clinically relevant for CYP450 substrates with a narrow therapeutic index, where the dose is individually adjusted (eg, warfarin). Upon initiation of rilonacept, in patients being treated with these types of medicinal products, therapeutic monitoring of the effect or drug concentration should be performed and the individual dose of the medicinal product may need to be adjusted as needed).
No products indexed under this heading.

Nafcillin Sodium (This is clinically relevant for CYP450 substrates with a narrow therapeutic index, where the dose is individually adjusted (eg, warfarin). Upon initiation of rilonacept, in patients being treated with these types of medicinal products, therapeutic monitoring of the effect or drug concentration should be performed and the individual dose of the medicinal product may need to be adjusted as needed).
No products indexed under this heading.

Naproxen (This is clinically relevant for CYP450 substrates with a narrow therapeutic index, where the dose is individually adjusted (eg, warfarin). Upon initiation of rilonacept, in patients being treated with these types of medicinal products, therapeutic monitoring of the effect or drug concentration should be performed and the individual dose of the medicinal product may need to be adjusted as needed). Products include:
EC-Naprosyn 2850
Naprosyn 2850
Anaprox/Naprosyn 2850

Naproxen Sodium (This is clinically relevant for CYP450 substrates with a narrow therapeutic index, where the dose is individually adjusted (eg, warfarin). Upon initiation of rilonacept, in patients being treated with these types of medicinal products, therapeutic monitoring of the effect or drug concentration should be performed and the individual dose of the medicinal product may need to be adjusted as needed). Products include:
Anaprox 2850
Anaprox DS 2850
Treximet 1681

Nateglinide (This is clinically relevant for CYP450 substrates with a narrow therapeutic index, where the dose is individually adjusted (eg, warfarin). Upon initiation of rilonacept, in patients being treated with these types of medicinal products, therapeutic monitoring of the effect or drug concentration should be performed and the individual dose of the medicinal product may need to be adjusted as needed).
No products indexed under this heading.

Nefazodone Hydrochloride (This is clinically relevant for CYP450 substrates with a narrow therapeutic index, where the dose is individually adjusted (eg, warfarin). Upon initiation of rilonacept, in patients being treated with these types of medicinal products, therapeutic monitoring of the effect or drug concentration should be performed and the individual dose of the medicinal product may need to be adjusted as needed).
No products indexed under this heading.

Nelfinavir Mesylate (This is clinically relevant for CYP450 substrates with a

strates with a narrow therapeutic index, where the dose is individually adjusted (eg, warfarin). Upon initiation of rilonacept, in patients being treated with these types of medicinal products, therapeutic monitoring of the effect or drug concentration should be performed and the individual dose of the medicinal product may need to be adjusted as needed).
No products indexed under this heading.

Phenacemide (This is clinically relevant for CYP450 substrates with a narrow therapeutic index, where the dose is individually adjusted (eg, warfarin). Upon initiation of rilonacept, in patients being treated with these types of medicinal products, therapeutic monitoring of the effect or drug concentration should be performed and the individual dose of the medicinal product may need to be adjusted as needed).
No products indexed under this heading.

Phenobarbital (This is clinically relevant for CYP450 substrates with a narrow therapeutic index, where the dose is individually adjusted (eg, warfarin). Upon initiation of rilonacept, in patients being treated with these types of medicinal products, therapeutic monitoring of the effect or drug concentration should be performed and the individual dose of the medicinal product may need to be adjusted as needed). Products include:
Donnatal **2711**

Phenobarbital Sodium (This is clinically relevant for CYP450 substrates with a narrow therapeutic index, where the dose is individually adjusted (eg, warfarin). Upon initiation of rilonacept, in patients being treated with these types of medicinal products, therapeutic monitoring of the effect or drug concentration should be performed and the individual dose of the medicinal product may need to be adjusted as needed).
No products indexed under this heading.

Phensuximide (This is clinically relevant for CYP450 substrates with a narrow therapeutic index, where the dose is individually adjusted (eg, warfarin). Upon initiation of rilonacept, in patients being treated with these types of medicinal products, therapeutic monitoring of the effect or drug concentration should be performed and the individual dose of the medicinal product may need to be adjusted as needed).
No products indexed under this heading.

Phenylbutazone (This is clinically relevant for CYP450 substrates with a narrow therapeutic index, where the dose is individually adjusted (eg, warfarin). Upon initiation of rilonacept, in patients being treated with these types of medicinal products, therapeutic monitoring of the effect or drug concentration should be performed and the individual dose of the medicinal product may need to be adjusted as needed).
No products indexed under this heading.

Phenytoin (This is clinically relevant for CYP450 substrates with a narrow therapeutic index, where the dose is individually adjusted (eg, warfarin). Upon initiation of rilonacept, in patients being treated with these types of medicinal products, therapeutic monitoring of the effect or drug concentration should be performed and the individual dose of the medicinal product may need to be adjusted as needed).
No products indexed under this heading.

Phenytoin Sodium (This is clinically relevant for CYP450 substrates with a narrow therapeutic index, where the dose is individually adjusted (eg, warfarin). Upon initiation of rilonacept, in patients being treated with these types of medicinal products, therapeutic monitoring of the effect or drug concentration should be performed and the individual dose of the medicinal product may need to be adjusted as needed). Products include:
Phenytek Capsules **2380**

Pimozide (This is clinically relevant for CYP450 substrates with a narrow therapeutic index, where the dose is individually adjusted (eg, warfarin). Upon initiation of rilonacept, in patients being treated with these types of medicinal products, therapeutic monitoring of the effect or drug concentration should be performed and the individual dose of the medicinal product may need to be adjusted as needed).
No products indexed under this heading.

Pindolol (This is clinically relevant for CYP450 substrates with a narrow therapeutic index, where the dose is individually adjusted (eg, warfarin). Upon initiation of rilonacept, in patients being treated with these types of medicinal products, therapeutic monitoring of the effect or drug concentration should be performed and the individual dose of the medicinal product may need to be adjusted as needed).
No products indexed under this heading.

Pioglitazone Hydrochloride (This is clinically relevant for CYP450 substrates with a narrow therapeutic index, where the dose is individually adjusted (eg, warfarin). Upon initiation of rilonacept, in patients being treated with these types of medicinal products, therapeutic monitoring of the effect or drug concentration should be performed and the individual dose of the medicinal product may need to be adjusted as needed). Products include:
ActoPlus **3338**
Actos **3345**
Duetact **3354**

Piroxicam (This is clinically relevant for CYP450 substrates with a narrow therapeutic index, where the dose is individually adjusted (eg, warfarin). Upon initiation of rilonacept, in patients being treated with these types of medicinal products, therapeutic monitoring of the effect or drug concentration should be performed and the individual dose of the medicinal product may need to be adjusted as needed).
No products indexed under this heading.

Poliovirus Vaccine, Live, Oral, Trivalent, Types 1,2,3 (Sabin) (Since no data are available on either the efficacy of live vaccines or on the risks of secondary transmission of infection by live vaccines in patients receiving rilonacept, live vaccines should not be given concurrently with rilonacept. In addition, because rilonacept may interfere with normal immune response to new antigens, vaccinations may not be effective in patients receiving rilonacept. No data are available on the effectiveness of vaccination with inactivated (killed) antigens in patients receiving rilonacept).
No products indexed under this heading.

Polyestradiol Phosphate (This is clinically relevant for CYP450 substrates with a narrow therapeutic index, where the dose is individually adjusted (eg, warfarin). Upon initiation of rilonacept, in patients being treated with these types of medicinal products, therapeutic monitoring of the effect or drug concentration should be performed and the individual dose of the medicinal product may need to be adjusted as needed).
No products indexed under this heading.

Primidone (This is clinically relevant for CYP450 substrates with a narrow therapeutic index, where the dose is individually adjusted (eg, warfarin). Upon initiation of rilonacept, in patients being treated with these types of medicinal products, therapeutic monitoring of the effect or drug concentration should be performed and the individual dose of the medicinal product may need to be adjusted as needed).
No products indexed under this heading.

Progesterone (This is clinically relevant for CYP450 substrates with a narrow therapeutic index, where the dose is individually adjusted (eg, warfarin). Upon initiation of rilonacept, in patients being treated with these types of medicinal products, therapeutic monitoring of the effect or drug concentration should be performed and the individual dose of the medicinal product may need to be adjusted as needed). Products include:
Crinone 4% **996**
Crinone 8% **996**
Prometrium **3307**

Proguanil Hydrochloride (This is clinically relevant for CYP450 substrates with a narrow therapeutic index, where the dose is individually adjusted (eg, warfarin). Upon initiation of rilonacept, in patients being treated with these types of medicinal products, therapeutic monitoring of the effect or drug concentration should be performed and the individual dose of the medicinal product may need to be adjusted as needed). Products include:
Malarone Pediatric Tablets **1572**
Malarone **1572**

Propafenone Hydrochloride (This is clinically relevant for CYP450 substrates with a narrow therapeutic index, where the dose is individually adjusted (eg, warfarin). Upon initiation of rilonacept, in patients being treated with these types of medicinal products, therapeutic monitoring of the effect or drug concentration should be performed and the individual dose of the medicinal product may need to be adjusted as needed). Products include:
Rythmol **1648**
Rythmol SR **1652**

Propoxyphene Hydrochloride (This is clinically relevant for CYP450 substrates with a narrow therapeutic index, where the dose is individually adjusted (eg, warfarin). Upon initiation of rilonacept, in patients being treated with these types of medicinal products, therapeutic monitoring of the effect or drug concentration should be performed and the individual dose of the medicinal product may need to be adjusted as needed).
No products indexed under this heading.

Propoxyphene Napsylate (This is clinically relevant for CYP450 substrates with a narrow therapeutic index, where the dose is individually adjusted (eg, warfarin). Upon initiation of rilonacept, in patients being treated with these types of medicinal products, therapeutic monitoring of the effect or drug concentration should be performed and the individual dose of the medicinal product may need to be adjusted as needed).
No products indexed under this heading.

Propranolol Hydrochloride (This is clinically relevant for CYP450 substrates with a narrow therapeutic index, where the dose is individually adjusted (eg, warfarin). Upon initiation of rilonacept, in patients being treated with these types of medicinal products, therapeutic monitoring of the effect or drug concentration should be performed and the individual dose of the medicinal product may need to be adjusted as needed). Products include:
InnoPran XL **1517**

Protriptyline Hydrochloride (This is clinically relevant for CYP450 substrates with a narrow therapeutic index, where the dose is individually adjusted (eg, warfarin). Upon initiation of rilonacept, in patients being treated with these types of medicinal products, therapeutic monitoring of the effect or drug concentration should be performed and the individual dose of the medicinal product may need to be adjusted as needed).
No products indexed under this heading.

Quetiapine Fumarate (This is clinically relevant for CYP450 substrates with a narrow therapeutic index, where the dose is individually adjusted (eg, warfarin). Upon initiation of rilonacept, in patients being treated with these types of medicinal products, therapeutic monitoring of the effect or drug concentration should be performed and the individual dose of the medicinal product may need to be adjusted as needed). Products include:
Seroquel **750**
Seroquel XR **759**

Quinidine Gluconate (This is clinically relevant for CYP450 substrates with a narrow therapeutic index, where the dose is individually adjusted (eg, warfarin). Upon initiation of rilonacept, in patients being treated with these types of medicinal products, therapeutic monitoring of the effect or drug concentration should be performed and the individual dose of the medicinal product may need to be adjusted as needed).
No products indexed under this heading.

Quinidine Hydrochloride (This is clinically relevant for CYP450 substrates with a narrow therapeutic index, where the dose is individually adjusted (eg, warfarin). Upon initiation of rilonacept, in patients being treated with these types of medicinal products, therapeutic monitoring of the effect or drug concentration should be performed and the individual dose of the medicinal product may need to be adjusted as needed).
No products indexed under this heading.

Quinidine Polygalacturonate (This is clinically relevant for CYP450 substrates with a narrow therapeutic index, where the dose is individually adjusted (eg, warfarin). Upon initiation of rilonacept, in patients being treated with these types of medicinal products, therapeutic monitoring of the effect or drug concentration should be performed and the individual dose of the medicinal product may need to be adjusted as needed).
No products indexed under this heading.

Quinidine Sulfate (This is clinically relevant for CYP450 substrates with a narrow therapeutic index, where the dose is individually adjusted (eg, warfarin). Upon initiation of rilonacept, in patients being treated with these types of medicinal products, therapeutic monitoring of the effect or drug concentration should be performed and the individual dose of the medicinal product may need to be adjusted as needed).
No products indexed under this heading.

Quinine (This is clinically relevant for CYP450 substrates with a narrow therapeutic index, where the dose is individually adjusted (eg, warfarin). Upon initiation of rilonacept, in patients being treated with these types of medicinal products, therapeutic monitoring of the effect or drug concentration should be performed and the individual dose of the medicinal product may need to be adjusted as needed). Products include:
Hyland's Leg Cramps PM with Quinine **3315**

Quinine Sulfate (This is clinically relevant for CYP450 substrates with a narrow therapeutic index, where the dose is individually adjusted (eg, warfarin). Upon initiation of rilonacept, in patients being treated with these types of medicinal products, therapeutic monitoring of the effect or drug concentration should

be performed and the individual dose of the medicinal product may need to be adjusted as needed).

No products indexed under this heading.

Rabeprazole Sodium (This is clinically relevant for CYP450 substrates with a narrow therapeutic index, where the dose is individually adjusted (eg, warfarin). Upon initiation of rilonacept, in patients being treated with these types of medicinal products, therapeutic monitoring of the effect or drug concentration should be performed and the individual dose of the medicinal product may need to be adjusted as needed). Products include:

Aciphex 1035

Repaglinide (This is clinically relevant for CYP450 substrates with a narrow therapeutic index, where the dose is individually adjusted (eg, warfarin). Upon initiation of rilonacept, in patients being treated with these types of medicinal products, therapeutic monitoring of the effect or drug concentration should be performed and the individual dose of the medicinal product may need to be adjusted as needed).

No products indexed under this heading.

Rifabutin (This is clinically relevant for CYP450 substrates with a narrow therapeutic index, where the dose is individually adjusted (eg, warfarin). Upon initiation of rilonacept, in patients being treated with these types of medicinal products, therapeutic monitoring of the effect or drug concentration should be performed and the individual dose of the medicinal product may need to be adjusted as needed).

No products indexed under this heading.

Riluzole (This is clinically relevant for CYP450 substrates with a narrow therapeutic index, where the dose is individually adjusted (eg, warfarin). Upon initiation of rilonacept, in patients being treated with these types of medicinal products, therapeutic monitoring of the effect or drug concentration should be performed and the individual dose of the medicinal product may need to be adjusted as needed). Products include:

Rilutek 3032

Risperidone (This is clinically relevant for CYP450 substrates with a narrow therapeutic index, where the dose is individually adjusted (eg, warfarin). Upon initiation of rilonacept, in patients being treated with these types of medicinal products, therapeutic monitoring of the effect or drug concentration should be performed and the individual dose of the medicinal product may need to be adjusted as needed). Products include:

Risperdal Consta 2682

Ritonavir (This is clinically relevant for CYP450 substrates with a narrow therapeutic index, where the dose is individually adjusted (eg, warfarin). Upon initiation of rilonacept, in patients being treated with these types of medicinal products, therapeutic monitoring of the effect or drug concentration should be performed and the individual dose of the medicinal product may need to be adjusted as needed). Products include:

Kaletra 458
Norvir 509

Rofecoxib (This is clinically relevant for CYP450 substrates with a narrow therapeutic index, where the dose is individually adjusted (eg, warfarin). Upon initiation of rilonacept, in patients being treated with these types of medicinal products, therapeutic monitoring of the effect or drug concentration should be performed and the individual dose of the medicinal product may need to be adjusted as needed).

No products indexed under this heading.

Ropinirole Hydrochloride (This is clinically relevant for CYP450 sub-

strates with a narrow therapeutic index, where the dose is individually adjusted (eg, warfarin). Upon initiation of rilonacept, in patients being treated with these types of medicinal products, therapeutic monitoring of the effect or drug concentration should be performed and the individual dose of the medicinal product may need to be adjusted as needed). Products include:

Requip 1620
Requip XL 1628

Ropivacaine Hydrochloride (This is clinically relevant for CYP450 substrates with a narrow therapeutic index, where the dose is individually adjusted (eg, warfarin). Upon initiation of rilonacept, in patients being treated with these types of medicinal products, therapeutic monitoring of the effect or drug concentration should be performed and the individual dose of the medicinal product may need to be adjusted as needed).

No products indexed under this heading.

Rosiglitazone (This is clinically relevant for CYP450 substrates with a narrow therapeutic index, where the dose is individually adjusted (eg, warfarin). Upon initiation of rilonacept, in patients being treated with these types of medicinal products, therapeutic monitoring of the effect or drug concentration should be performed and the individual dose of the medicinal product may need to be adjusted as needed).

No products indexed under this heading.

Rosiglitazone Maleate (This is clinically relevant for CYP450 substrates with a narrow therapeutic index, where the dose is individually adjusted (eg, warfarin). Upon initiation of rilonacept, in patients being treated with these types of medicinal products, therapeutic monitoring of the effect or drug concentration should be performed and the individual dose of the medicinal product may need to be adjusted as needed). Products include:

Avandamet 1345
Avandaryl 1356
Avandia 1366

Rosiglitazone/Metformin (This is clinically relevant for CYP450 substrates with a narrow therapeutic index, where the dose is individually adjusted (eg, warfarin). Upon initiation of rilonacept, in patients being treated with these types of medicinal products, therapeutic monitoring of the effect or drug concentration should be performed and the individual dose of the medicinal product may need to be adjusted as needed).

No products indexed under this heading.

Rotavirus Vaccine, Live, Oral, Tetravalent (Since no data are available on either the efficacy of live vaccines or on the risks of secondary transmission of infection by live vaccines in patients receiving rilonacept, live vaccines should not be given concurrently with rilonacept. In addition, because rilonacept may interfere with normal immune response to new antigens, vaccinations may not be effective in patients receiving rilonacept. No data are available on the effectiveness of vaccination with inactivated (killed) antigens in patients receiving rilonacept).

No products indexed under this heading.

Rubella & Mumps Virus Vaccine Live (Since no data are available on either the efficacy of live vaccines or on the risks of secondary transmission of infection by live vaccines in patients receiving rilonacept, live vaccines should not be given concurrently with rilonacept. In addition, because rilonacept may interfere with normal immune response to new antigens, vaccinations may not be effective in patients receiving rilonacept. No data are available on

the effectiveness of vaccination with inactivated (killed) antigens in patients receiving rilonacept).

No products indexed under this heading.

Rubella Virus Vaccine Live (Since no data are available on either the efficacy of live vaccines or on the risks of secondary transmission of infection by live vaccines in patients receiving rilonacept, live vaccines should not be given concurrently with rilonacept. In addition, because rilonacept may interfere with normal immune response to new antigens, vaccinations may not be effective in patients receiving rilonacept. No data are available on the effectiveness of vaccination with inactivated (killed) antigens in patients receiving rilonacept). Products include:

Meruvax II 2210

Saquinavir (This is clinically relevant for CYP450 substrates with a narrow therapeutic index, where the dose is individually adjusted (eg, warfarin). Upon initiation of rilonacept, in patients being treated with these types of medicinal products, therapeutic monitoring of the effect or drug concentration should be performed and the individual dose of the medicinal product may need to be adjusted as needed).

No products indexed under this heading.

Saquinavir Mesylate (This is clinically relevant for CYP450 substrates with a narrow therapeutic index, where the dose is individually adjusted (eg, warfarin). Upon initiation of rilonacept, in patients being treated with these types of medicinal products, therapeutic monitoring of the effect or drug concentration should be performed and the individual dose of the medicinal product may need to be adjusted as needed).

No products indexed under this heading.

Sertraline Hydrochloride (This is clinically relevant for CYP450 substrates with a narrow therapeutic index, where the dose is individually adjusted (eg, warfarin). Upon initiation of rilonacept, in patients being treated with these types of medicinal products, therapeutic monitoring of the effect or drug concentration should be performed and the individual dose of the medicinal product may need to be adjusted as needed).

No products indexed under this heading.

Sildenafil Citrate (This is clinically relevant for CYP450 substrates with a narrow therapeutic index, where the dose is individually adjusted (eg, warfarin). Upon initiation of rilonacept, in patients being treated with these types of medicinal products, therapeutic monitoring of the effect or drug concentration should be performed and the individual dose of the medicinal product may need to be adjusted as needed).

No products indexed under this heading.

Simvastatin (This is clinically relevant for CYP450 substrates with a narrow therapeutic index, where the dose is individually adjusted (eg, warfarin). Upon initiation of rilonacept, in patients being treated with these types of medicinal products, therapeutic monitoring of the effect or drug concentration should be performed and the individual dose of the medicinal product may need to be adjusted as needed). Products include:

Simcor 524
Vytorin 10/10 .... 2303, 3240
Vytorin 10/20 .... 2303, 3240
Vytorin 10/40 .... 2303, 3240
Vytorin 10/80 .... 2303, 3240
Zocor 2289

Sirolimus (This is clinically relevant for CYP450 substrates with a narrow therapeutic index, where the dose is individually adjusted (eg, warfarin). Upon initiation of rilonacept, in patients being treated with these types of medicinal

products, therapeutic monitoring of the effect or drug concentration should be performed and the individual dose of the medicinal product may need to be adjusted as needed). Products include:

Rapamune 3579

Smallpox Vaccine (Since no data are available on either the efficacy of live vaccines or on the risks of secondary transmission of infection by live vaccines in patients receiving rilonacept, live vaccines should not be given concurrently with rilonacept. In addition, because rilonacept may interfere with normal immune response to new antigens, vaccinations may not be effective in patients receiving rilonacept. No data are available on the effectiveness of vaccination with inactivated (killed) antigens in patients receiving rilonacept).

No products indexed under this heading.

Sulfamethoxazole (This is clinically relevant for CYP450 substrates with a narrow therapeutic index, where the dose is individually adjusted (eg, warfarin). Upon initiation of rilonacept, in patients being treated with these types of medicinal products, therapeutic monitoring of the effect or drug concentration should be performed and the individual dose of the medicinal product may need to be adjusted as needed).

No products indexed under this heading.

Sulindac (This is clinically relevant for CYP450 substrates with a narrow therapeutic index, where the dose is individually adjusted (eg, warfarin). Upon initiation of rilonacept, in patients being treated with these types of medicinal products, therapeutic monitoring of the effect or drug concentration should be performed and the individual dose of the medicinal product may need to be adjusted as needed). Products include:

Clinoril 2098

Suprofen (This is clinically relevant for CYP450 substrates with a narrow therapeutic index, where the dose is individually adjusted (eg, warfarin). Upon initiation of rilonacept, in patients being treated with these types of medicinal products, therapeutic monitoring of the effect or drug concentration should be performed and the individual dose of the medicinal product may need to be adjusted as needed).

No products indexed under this heading.

Tacrine Hydrochloride (This is clinically relevant for CYP450 substrates with a narrow therapeutic index, where the dose is individually adjusted (eg, warfarin). Upon initiation of rilonacept, in patients being treated with these types of medicinal products, therapeutic monitoring of the effect or drug concentration should be performed and the individual dose of the medicinal product may need to be adjusted as needed).

No products indexed under this heading.

Tacrolimus (This is clinically relevant for CYP450 substrates with a narrow therapeutic index, where the dose is individually adjusted (eg, warfarin). Upon initiation of rilonacept, in patients being treated with these types of medicinal products, therapeutic monitoring of the effect or drug concentration should be performed and the individual dose of the medicinal product may need to be adjusted as needed). Products include:

Prograf Capsules 677
Prograf Injection 677
Protopic 685

Tadalafil (This is clinically relevant for CYP450 substrates with a narrow therapeutic index, where the dose is individually adjusted (eg, warfarin). Upon initiation of rilonacept, in patients being treated with these types of medicinal products, therapeutic monitoring of the effect or drug concentration should be performed and the individual dose of

the medicinal product may need to be adjusted as needed). Products include:

Adcirca 3461
Cialis 1861

Tamoxifen Citrate (This is clinically relevant for CYP450 substrates with a narrow therapeutic index, where the dose is individually adjusted (eg, warfarin). Upon initiation of rilonacept, in patients being treated with these types of medicinal products, therapeutic monitoring of the effect or drug concentration should be performed and the individual dose of the medicinal product may need to be adjusted as needed).

No products indexed under this heading.

Telmisartan (This is clinically relevant for CYP450 substrates with a narrow therapeutic index, where the dose is individually adjusted (eg, warfarin). Upon initiation of rilonacept, in patients being treated with these types of medicinal products, therapeutic monitoring of the effect or drug concentration should be performed and the individual dose of the medicinal product may need to be adjusted as needed). Products include:

Micardis 887
Micardis HCT 889

Teniposide (This is clinically relevant for CYP450 substrates with a narrow therapeutic index, where the dose is individually adjusted (eg, warfarin). Upon initiation of rilonacept, in patients being treated with these types of medicinal products, therapeutic monitoring of the effect or drug concentration should be performed and the individual dose of the medicinal product may need to be adjusted as needed).

No products indexed under this heading.

Terfenadine (This is clinically relevant for CYP450 substrates with a narrow therapeutic index, where the dose is individually adjusted (eg, warfarin). Upon initiation of rilonacept, in patients being treated with these types of medicinal products, therapeutic monitoring of the effect or drug concentration should be performed and the individual dose of the medicinal product may need to be adjusted as needed).

No products indexed under this heading.

Testosterone (This is clinically relevant for CYP450 substrates with a narrow therapeutic index, where the dose is individually adjusted (eg, warfarin). Upon initiation of rilonacept, in patients being treated with these types of medicinal products, therapeutic monitoring of the effect or drug concentration should be performed and the individual dose of the medicinal product may need to be adjusted as needed). Products include:

AndroGel 3456

Testosterone Cypionate (This is clinically relevant for CYP450 substrates with a narrow therapeutic index, where the dose is individually adjusted (eg, warfarin). Upon initiation of rilonacept, in patients being treated with these types of medicinal products, therapeutic monitoring of the effect or drug concentration should be performed and the individual dose of the medicinal product may need to be adjusted as needed).

No products indexed under this heading.

Testosterone Enanthate (This is clinically relevant for CYP450 substrates with a narrow therapeutic index, where the dose is individually adjusted (eg, warfarin). Upon initiation of rilonacept, in patients being treated with these types of medicinal products, therapeutic monitoring of the effect or drug concentration should be performed and the individual dose of the medicinal product may need to be adjusted as needed). Products include:

Delatestryl 1102

Testosterone Propionate (This is clinically relevant for CYP450 substrates with a narrow therapeutic index, where the dose is individually adjusted (eg, warfarin). Upon initiation of rilonacept, in patients being treated with these types of medicinal products, therapeutic monitoring of the effect or drug concentration should be performed and the individual dose of the medicinal product may need to be adjusted as needed).

No products indexed under this heading.

Theophylline (This is clinically relevant for CYP450 substrates with a narrow therapeutic index, where the dose is individually adjusted (eg, warfarin). Upon initiation of rilonacept, in patients being treated with these types of medicinal products, therapeutic monitoring of the effect or drug concentration should be performed and the individual dose of the medicinal product may need to be adjusted as needed).

No products indexed under this heading.

Theophylline Anhydrous (This is clinically relevant for CYP450 substrates with a narrow therapeutic index, where the dose is individually adjusted (eg, warfarin). Upon initiation of rilonacept, in patients being treated with these types of medicinal products, therapeutic monitoring of the effect or drug concentration should be performed and the individual dose of the medicinal product may need to be adjusted as needed). Products include:

Uniphyl 2817

Theophylline Calcium Salicylate (This is clinically relevant for CYP450 substrates with a narrow therapeutic index, where the dose is individually adjusted (eg, warfarin). Upon initiation of rilonacept, in patients being treated with these types of medicinal products, therapeutic monitoring of the effect or drug concentration should be performed and the individual dose of the medicinal product may need to be adjusted as needed).

No products indexed under this heading.

Theophylline Dihydroxypropyl (Glyceryl) (This is clinically relevant for CYP450 substrates with a narrow therapeutic index, where the dose is individually adjusted (eg, warfarin). Upon initiation of rilonacept, in patients being treated with these types of medicinal products, therapeutic monitoring of the effect or drug concentration should be performed and the individual dose of the medicinal product may need to be adjusted as needed).

No products indexed under this heading.

Theophylline Ethylenediamine (This is clinically relevant for CYP450 substrates with a narrow therapeutic index, where the dose is individually adjusted (eg, warfarin). Upon initiation of rilonacept, in patients being treated with these types of medicinal products, therapeutic monitoring of the effect or drug concentration should be performed and the individual dose of the medicinal product may need to be adjusted as needed).

No products indexed under this heading.

Theophylline Sodium Glycinate (This is clinically relevant for CYP450 substrates with a narrow therapeutic index, where the dose is individually adjusted (eg, warfarin). Upon initiation of rilonacept, in patients being treated with these types of medicinal products, therapeutic monitoring of the effect or drug concentration should be performed and the individual dose of the medicinal product may need to be adjusted as needed).

No products indexed under this heading.

Thioridazine (This is clinically relevant for CYP450 substrates with a narrow therapeutic index, where the dose is individually adjusted (eg, warfarin). Upon initiation of rilonacept, in patients being treated with these types of medicinal products, therapeutic monitoring of the effect or drug concentration should be performed and the individual dose of the medicinal product may need to be adjusted as needed).

No products indexed under this heading.

Thioridazine Hydrochloride (This is clinically relevant for CYP450 substrates with a narrow therapeutic index, where the dose is individually adjusted (eg, warfarin). Upon initiation of rilonacept, in patients being treated with these types of medicinal products, therapeutic monitoring of the effect or drug concentration should be performed and the individual dose of the medicinal product may need to be adjusted as needed). Products include:

Thioridazine Hydrochloride 2384

Tiagabine Hydrochloride (This is clinically relevant for CYP450 substrates with a narrow therapeutic index, where the dose is individually adjusted (eg, warfarin). Upon initiation of rilonacept, in patients being treated with these types of medicinal products, therapeutic monitoring of the effect or drug concentration should be performed and the individual dose of the medicinal product may need to be adjusted as needed). Products include:

Gabitril 972

Timolol Maleate (This is clinically relevant for CYP450 substrates with a narrow therapeutic index, where the dose is individually adjusted (eg, warfarin). Upon initiation of rilonacept, in patients being treated with these types of medicinal products, therapeutic monitoring of the effect or drug concentration should be performed and the individual dose of the medicinal product may need to be adjusted as needed). Products include:

Combigan 601
Dorzolamide Hydrochloride/Timolol Maleate Ophthalmic Solution .... ⊙243
Timoptic in Ocudose .... ⊙231

Tolazamide (This is clinically relevant for CYP450 substrates with a narrow therapeutic index, where the dose is individually adjusted (eg, warfarin). Upon initiation of rilonacept, in patients being treated with these types of medicinal products, therapeutic monitoring of the effect or drug concentration should be performed and the individual dose of the medicinal product may need to be adjusted as needed).

No products indexed under this heading.

Tolbutamide (This is clinically relevant for CYP450 substrates with a narrow therapeutic index, where the dose is individually adjusted (eg, warfarin). Upon initiation of rilonacept, in patients being treated with these types of medicinal products, therapeutic monitoring of the effect or drug concentration should be performed and the individual dose of the medicinal product may need to be adjusted as needed).

No products indexed under this heading.

Tolbutamide Sodium (This is clinically relevant for CYP450 substrates with a narrow therapeutic index, where the dose is individually adjusted (eg, warfarin). Upon initiation of rilonacept, in patients being treated with these types of medicinal products, therapeutic monitoring of the effect or drug concentration should be performed and the individual dose of the medicinal product may need to be adjusted as needed).

No products indexed under this heading.

Tolmetin Sodium (This is clinically relevant for CYP450 substrates with a narrow therapeutic index, where the dose is individually adjusted (eg, warfarin). Upon initiation of rilonacept, in patients being treated with these types of medicinal products, therapeutic monitoring of the effect or drug concentration should be performed and the individual dose of the medicinal product may need to be adjusted as needed).

No products indexed under this heading.

Tolterodine Tartrate (This is clinically relevant for CYP450 substrates with a narrow therapeutic index, where the dose is individually adjusted (eg, warfarin). Upon initiation of rilonacept, in patients being treated with these types of medicinal products, therapeutic monitoring of the effect or drug concentration should be performed and the individual dose of the medicinal product may need to be adjusted as needed).

No products indexed under this heading.

Topiramate (This is clinically relevant for CYP450 substrates with a narrow therapeutic index, where the dose is individually adjusted (eg, warfarin). Upon initiation of rilonacept, in patients being treated with these types of medicinal products, therapeutic monitoring of the effect or drug concentration should be performed and the individual dose of the medicinal product may need to be adjusted as needed).

No products indexed under this heading.

Torsemide (This is clinically relevant for CYP450 substrates with a narrow therapeutic index, where the dose is individually adjusted (eg, warfarin). Upon initiation of rilonacept, in patients being treated with these types of medicinal products, therapeutic monitoring of the effect or drug concentration should be performed and the individual dose of the medicinal product may need to be adjusted as needed).

No products indexed under this heading.

Tramadol Hydrochloride (This is clinically relevant for CYP450 substrates with a narrow therapeutic index, where the dose is individually adjusted (eg, warfarin). Upon initiation of rilonacept, in patients being treated with these types of medicinal products, therapeutic monitoring of the effect or drug concentration should be performed and the individual dose of the medicinal product may need to be adjusted as needed). Products include:

Ryzolt 2813
Ultram ER 2693

Trazodone Hydrochloride (This is clinically relevant for CYP450 substrates with a narrow therapeutic index, where the dose is individually adjusted (eg, warfarin). Upon initiation of rilonacept, in patients being treated with these types of medicinal products, therapeutic monitoring of the effect or drug concentration should be performed and the individual dose of the medicinal product may need to be adjusted as needed).

No products indexed under this heading.

Tretinoin (This is clinically relevant for CYP450 substrates with a narrow therapeutic index, where the dose is individually adjusted (eg, warfarin). Upon initiation of rilonacept, in patients being treated with these types of medicinal products, therapeutic monitoring of the effect or drug concentration should be performed and the individual dose of the medicinal product may need to be adjusted as needed).

No products indexed under this heading.

Triazolam (This is clinically relevant for CYP450 substrates with a narrow therapeutic index, where the dose is individually adjusted (eg, warfarin). Upon initiation of rilonacept, in patients being treated with these types of medicinal products, therapeutic monitoring of the effect or drug concentration should

be performed and the individual dose of the medicinal product may need to be adjusted as needed).

No products indexed under this heading.

Trimethadione (This is clinically relevant for CYP450 substrates with a narrow therapeutic index, where the dose is individually adjusted (eg, warfarin). Upon initiation of rilonacept, in patients being treated with these types of medicinal products, therapeutic monitoring of the effect or drug concentration should be performed and the individual dose of the medicinal product may need to be adjusted as needed).

No products indexed under this heading.

Trimethaphan Camsylate (This is clinically relevant for CYP450 substrates with a narrow therapeutic index, where the dose is individually adjusted (eg, warfarin). Upon initiation of rilonacept, in patients being treated with these types of medicinal products, therapeutic monitoring of the effect or drug concentration should be performed and the individual dose of the medicinal product may need to be adjusted as needed).

No products indexed under this heading.

Trimipramine Maleate (This is clinically relevant for CYP450 substrates with a narrow therapeutic index, where the dose is individually adjusted (eg, warfarin). Upon initiation of rilonacept, in patients being treated with these types of medicinal products, therapeutic monitoring of the effect or drug concentration should be performed and the individual dose of the medicinal product may need to be adjusted as needed).

No products indexed under this heading.

Troglitazone (This is clinically relevant for CYP450 substrates with a narrow therapeutic index, where the dose is individually adjusted (eg, warfarin). Upon initiation of rilonacept, in patients being treated with these types of medicinal products, therapeutic monitoring of the effect or drug concentration should be performed and the individual dose of the medicinal product may need to be adjusted as needed).

No products indexed under this heading.

Trovafloxacin Mesylate (This is clinically relevant for CYP450 substrates with a narrow therapeutic index, where the dose is individually adjusted (eg, warfarin). Upon initiation of rilonacept, in patients being treated with these types of medicinal products, therapeutic monitoring of the effect or drug concentration should be performed and the individual dose of the medicinal product may need to be adjusted as needed).

No products indexed under this heading.

Typhoid Vaccine (Since no data are available on either the efficacy of live vaccines or on the risks of secondary transmission of infection by live vaccines in patients receiving rilonacept, live vaccines should not be given concurrently with rilonacept. In addition, because rilonacept may interfere with normal immune response to new antigens, vaccinations may not be effective in patients receiving rilonacept. No data are available on the effectiveness of vaccination with inactivated (killed) antigens in patients receiving rilonacept).

No products indexed under this heading.

Valdecoxib (This is clinically relevant for CYP450 substrates with a narrow therapeutic index, where the dose is individually adjusted (eg, warfarin). Upon initiation of rilonacept, in patients being treated with these types of medicinal products, therapeutic monitoring of the effect or drug concentration should be performed and the individual dose of the medicinal product may need to be adjusted as needed).

No products indexed under this heading.

Valproate Sodium (This is clinically relevant for CYP450 substrates with a narrow therapeutic index, where the dose is individually adjusted (eg, warfarin). Upon initiation of rilonacept, in patients being treated with these types of medicinal products, therapeutic monitoring of the effect or drug concentration should be performed and the individual dose of the medicinal product may need to be adjusted as needed).

No products indexed under this heading.

Valproic Acid (This is clinically relevant for CYP450 substrates with a narrow therapeutic index, where the dose is individually adjusted (eg, warfarin). Upon initiation of rilonacept, in patients being treated with these types of medicinal products, therapeutic monitoring of the effect or drug concentration should be performed and the individual dose of the medicinal product may need to be adjusted as needed).

No products indexed under this heading.

Valsartan (This is clinically relevant for CYP450 substrates with a narrow therapeutic index, where the dose is individually adjusted (eg, warfarin). Upon initiation of rilonacept, in patients being treated with these types of medicinal products, therapeutic monitoring of the effect or drug concentration should be performed and the individual dose of the medicinal product may need to be adjusted as needed). Products include:

Diovan ... **2413**
Diovan HCT ... **2419**
Exforge ... **2443**
Exforge HCT ... **2449**
Valturna ... **3637**

Vardenafil Hydrochloride (This is clinically relevant for CYP450 substrates with a narrow therapeutic index, where the dose is individually adjusted (eg, warfarin). Upon initiation of rilonacept, in patients being treated with these types of medicinal products, therapeutic monitoring of the effect or drug concentration should be performed and the individual dose of the medicinal product may need to be adjusted as needed). Products include:

Levitra ... **3157**

Varicella Virus Vaccine, Live (Since no data are available on either the efficacy of live vaccines or on the risks of secondary transmission of infection by live vaccines in patients receiving rilonacept, live vaccines should not be given concurrently with rilonacept. In addition, because rilonacept may interfere with normal immune response to new antigens, vaccinations may not be effective in patients receiving rilonacept. No data are available on the effectiveness of vaccination with inactivated (killed) antigens in patients receiving rilonacept). Products include:

Varivax ... **2285**

Venlafaxine Hydrochloride (This is clinically relevant for CYP450 substrates with a narrow therapeutic index, where the dose is individually adjusted (eg, warfarin). Upon initiation of rilonacept, in patients being treated with these types of medicinal products, therapeutic monitoring of the effect or drug concentration should be performed and the individual dose of the medicinal product may need to be adjusted as needed). Products include:

Effexor XR ... **3504**
Venlafaxine Hydrochloride Tablets ... **2388**

Verapamil Hydrochloride (This is clinically relevant for CYP450 substrates with a narrow therapeutic index, where the dose is individually adjusted (eg, warfarin). Upon initiation of rilonacept, in patients being treated with these types of medicinal products, therapeutic monitoring of the effect or drug concentration should be performed and the individual dose of the medicinal product may need to be adjusted as needed). Products include:

Tarka ... **534**

Vinblastine Sulfate (This is clinically relevant for CYP450 substrates with a narrow therapeutic index, where the dose is individually adjusted (eg, warfarin). Upon initiation of rilonacept, in patients being treated with these types of medicinal products, therapeutic monitoring of the effect or drug concentration should be performed and the individual dose of the medicinal product may need to be adjusted as needed).

No products indexed under this heading.

Vincristine Sulfate (This is clinically relevant for CYP450 substrates with a narrow therapeutic index, where the dose is individually adjusted (eg, warfarin). Upon initiation of rilonacept, in patients being treated with these types of medicinal products, therapeutic monitoring of the effect or drug concentration should be performed and the individual dose of the medicinal product may need to be adjusted as needed).

No products indexed under this heading.

Vitamin A (This is clinically relevant for CYP450 substrates with a narrow therapeutic index, where the dose is individually adjusted (eg, warfarin). Upon initiation of rilonacept, in patients being treated with these types of medicinal products, therapeutic monitoring of the effect or drug concentration should be performed and the individual dose of the medicinal product may need to be adjusted as needed). Products include:

Cardio Basics ... **3455**
Heplive ... **607**
Norwegian Cod Liver Oil ... **919**

Vitamin A Acetate (This is clinically relevant for CYP450 substrates with a narrow therapeutic index, where the dose is individually adjusted (eg, warfarin). Upon initiation of rilonacept, in patients being treated with these types of medicinal products, therapeutic monitoring of the effect or drug concentration should be performed and the individual dose of the medicinal product may need to be adjusted as needed).

No products indexed under this heading.

Voriconazole (This is clinically relevant for CYP450 substrates with a narrow therapeutic index, where the dose is individually adjusted (eg, warfarin). Upon initiation of rilonacept, in patients being treated with these types of medicinal products, therapeutic monitoring of the effect or drug concentration should be performed and the individual dose of the medicinal product may need to be adjusted as needed).

No products indexed under this heading.

Warfarin Sodium (This is clinically relevant for CYP450 substrates with a narrow therapeutic index, where the dose is individually adjusted (eg, warfarin). Upon initiation of rilonacept, in patients being treated with these types of medicinal products, therapeutic monitoring of the effect or drug concentration should be performed and the individual dose of the medicinal product may need to be adjusted as needed).

No products indexed under this heading.

Yellow Fever Vaccine (Since no data are available on either the efficacy of live vaccines or on the risks of secondary transmission of infection by live vaccines in patients receiving rilonacept, live vaccines should not be given concurrently with rilonacept. In addition, because rilonacept may interfere with normal immune response to new antigens, vaccinations may not be effective in patients receiving rilonacept. No data are available on the effectiveness of vaccination with inactivated (killed) antigens in patients receiving rilonacept).

No products indexed under this heading.

Zafirlukast (This is clinically relevant for CYP450 substrates with a narrow therapeutic index, where the dose is individually adjusted (eg, warfarin). Upon initiation of rilonacept, in patients being treated with these types of medicinal products, therapeutic monitoring of the effect or drug concentration should be performed and the individual dose of the medicinal product may need to be adjusted as needed). Products include:

Accolate ... **3612**

Zileuton (This is clinically relevant for CYP450 substrates with a narrow therapeutic index, where the dose is individually adjusted (eg, warfarin). Upon initiation of rilonacept, in patients being treated with these types of medicinal products, therapeutic monitoring of the effect or drug concentration should be performed and the individual dose of the medicinal product may need to be adjusted as needed).

No products indexed under this heading.

Zolmitriptan (This is clinically relevant for CYP450 substrates with a narrow therapeutic index, where the dose is individually adjusted (eg, warfarin). Upon initiation of rilonacept, in patients being treated with these types of medicinal products, therapeutic monitoring of the effect or drug concentration should be performed and the individual dose of the medicinal product may need to be adjusted as needed). Products include:

Zomig Tablets ... **773**
Zomig Nasal Spray ... **768**
Zomig-ZMT Tablets ... **773**

Zonisamide (This is clinically relevant for CYP450 substrates with a narrow therapeutic index, where the dose is individually adjusted (eg, warfarin). Upon initiation of rilonacept, in patients being treated with these types of medicinal products, therapeutic monitoring of the effect or drug concentration should be performed and the individual dose of the medicinal product may need to be adjusted as needed). Products include:

Zonegran ... **1081**

Zopiclone (This is clinically relevant for CYP450 substrates with a narrow therapeutic index, where the dose is individually adjusted (eg, warfarin). Upon initiation of rilonacept, in patients being treated with these types of medicinal products, therapeutic monitoring of the effect or drug concentration should be performed and the individual dose of the medicinal product may need to be adjusted as needed).

No products indexed under this heading.

Zoster Vaccine Live (Since no data are available on either the efficacy of live vaccines or on the risks of secondary transmission of infection by live vaccines in patients receiving rilonacept, live vaccines should not be given concurrently with rilonacept. In addition, because rilonacept may interfere with normal immune response to new antigens, vaccinations may not be effective in patients receiving rilonacept. No data are available on the effectiveness of vaccination with inactivated (killed) antigens in patients receiving rilonacept). Products include:

Zostavax ... **2299**

Food Interactions

Beverages, caffeine-containing (This is clinically relevant for CYP450 substrates with a narrow therapeutic index, where the dose is individually adjusted (eg, warfarin). Upon initiation of rilonacept, in patients being treated with these types of medicinal products, therapeutic monitoring of the effect or drug concentration should be performed and the individual dose of the medicinal product may need to be adjusted as needed).

149 **Interactions Index** **Aricept**

Food, caffeine-containing (This is clinically relevant for CYP450 substrates with a narrow therapeutic index, where the dose is individually adjusted (eg, warfarin). Upon initiation of rilonacept, in patients being treated with these types of medicinal products, therapeutic monitoring of the effect or drug concentration should be performed and the individual dose of the medicinal product may need to be adjusted as needed).

ARGATROBAN INJECTION

(Argatroban) 1314
May interact with anticoagulants, thrombolytics, and certain other agents. Compounds in these categories include:

Alteplase (Co-administration with thrombolytic agents may increase the risk of bleeding). Products include:
Activase 1183
Cathflo 1192

Anisindione (Co-administration with other anticoagulants may increase the risk of bleeding).
No products indexed under this heading.

Anistreplase (Co-administration with thrombolytic agents may increase the risk of bleeding).
No products indexed under this heading.

Ardeparin Sodium (Co-administration with other anticoagulants may increase the risk of bleeding).
No products indexed under this heading.

Aspirin (Co-administration with antiplatelet agents, such as aspirin, may increase the risk of bleeding). Products include:
Aggrenox 880
Bayer Aspirin 829
Percodan 1124
St. Joseph Aspirin 2045

Bivalirudin (Co-administration with thrombolytic agents may increase the risk of bleeding). Products include:
Angiomax for Injection 2061

Clopidogrel Bisulfate (Co-administration with antiplatelet agents may increase the risk of bleeding). Products include:
Plavix 3027

Dalteparin Sodium (Co-administration with other anticoagulants may increase the risk of bleeding). Products include:
Fragmin 1058

Danaparoid Sodium (Co-administration with other anticoagulants may increase the risk of bleeding).
No products indexed under this heading.

Dicumarol (Co-administration with other anticoagulants may increase the risk of bleeding).
No products indexed under this heading.

Dipyridamole (Co-administration with antiplatelet agents may increase the risk of bleeding). Products include:
Aggrenox 880

Enoxaparin Sodium (Co-administration with other anticoagulants may increase the risk of bleeding). Products include:
Lovenox 3005

Fondaparinux Sodium (Co-administration with other anticoagulants may increase the risk of bleeding). Products include:
Arixtra 1320

Heparin Calcium (Co-administration with other anticoagulants may increase the risk of bleeding).
No products indexed under this heading.

Heparin Sodium (Co-administration with other anticoagulants may increase the risk of bleeding).
No products indexed under this heading.

Low Molecular Weight Heparins (Co-administration with other anticoagulants may increase the risk of bleeding).
No products indexed under this heading.

Reteplase (Co-administration with thrombolytic agents may increase the risk of bleeding).
No products indexed under this heading.

Streptokinase (Co-administration with thrombolytic agents may increase the risk of bleeding).
No products indexed under this heading.

Tinzaparin Sodium (Co-administration with other anticoagulants may increase the risk of bleeding).
No products indexed under this heading.

Urokinase (Co-administration with thrombolytic agents may increase the risk of bleeding).
No products indexed under this heading.

Warfarin Sodium (Co-administration with other anticoagulants may increase the risk of bleeding).
No products indexed under this heading.

ARICEPT TABLETS

(Donepezil Hydrochloride) 1045
May interact with anticholinergics, cytochrome p450 2d6 inducers (selected), cytochrome p450 3a4 inducers (selected), dexamethasones, non-steroidal anti-inflammatory agents, phenytoin, quinidine, and certain other agents. Compounds in these categories include:

Allium sativum (Inducers of CYP3A4 could increase the rate of elimination of donepezil).
No products indexed under this heading.

Aminoglutethimide (Inducers of CYP3A4 could increase the rate of elimination of donepezil).
No products indexed under this heading.

Aprepitant (Inducers of CYP3A4 could increase the rate of elimination of donepezil). Products include:
Emend 2124

Atropine Sulfate (Donepezil, a cholinesterase inhibitor, has the potential to interfere with the activity of anticholinergic medications). Products include:
Donnatal 2711

Belladonna Alkaloids (Donepezil, a cholinesterase inhibitor, has the potential to interfere with the activity of anticholinergic medications). Products include:
Hyland's Teething Tablets 3316

Benztropine Mesylate (Donepezil, a cholinesterase inhibitor, has the potential to interfere with the activity of anticholinergic medications).
No products indexed under this heading.

Betamethasone (Inducers of CYP3A4 could increase the rate of elimination of donepezil).
No products indexed under this heading.

Betamethasone Acetate (Inducers of CYP3A4 could increase the rate of elimination of donepezil).
No products indexed under this heading.

Betamethasone Benzoate (Inducers of CYP3A4 could increase the rate of elimination of donepezil).
No products indexed under this heading.

Betamethasone Dipropionate (Inducers of CYP3A4 could increase the rate of elimination of donepezil). Products include:
Diprolene Lotion 0.05% 3108
Diprolene Ointment 0.05% 3109
Diprolene AF Cream 0.05% 3107
Lotrisone 3163

Betamethasone Sodium Phosphate (Inducers of CYP3A4 could increase the rate of elimination of donepezil).
No products indexed under this heading.

Betamethasone Valerate (Inducers of CYP3A4 could increase the rate of elimination of donepezil). Products include:
Luxiq 3321

Bethanechol Chloride (Potential for synergistic effect).
No products indexed under this heading.

Biperiden Hydrochloride (Donepezil, a cholinesterase inhibitor, has the potential to interfere with the activity of anticholinergic medications).
No products indexed under this heading.

Bosentan (Inducers of CYP3A4 could increase the rate of elimination of donepezil). Products include:
Tracleer 573

Carbamazepine (Inducers of CYP2D6 and CYP3A4, such as carbamazepine, could increase the rate of elimination of donepezil). Products include:
Carbatrol 3280
Equetro 3477

Celecoxib (Cholinesterase inhibitors, such as donepezil, may be expected to increase gastric acid secretion due to increased cholinergic activity, therefore, patients on concurrent NSAID therapy should be monitored closely for increased risk of developing ulcers or symptoms of active or occult gastrointestinal bleeding). Products include:
Celebrex 3272

Ciprofloxacin (Inducers of CYP3A4 could increase the rate of elimination of donepezil). Products include:
Cipro I.V. 3082
Cipro 3073
Cipro XR 3091
Ciprodex 583

Ciprofloxacin Hydrochloride (Inducers of CYP3A4 could increase the rate of elimination of donepezil). Products include:
Cipro 3073

Cisplatin (Inducers of CYP3A4 could increase the rate of elimination of donepezil).
No products indexed under this heading.

Clidinium Bromide (Donepezil, a cholinesterase inhibitor, has the potential to interfere with the activity of anticholinergic medications).
No products indexed under this heading.

Cortisone Acetate (Inducers of CYP3A4 could increase the rate of elimination of donepezil).
No products indexed under this heading.

Dexamethasone (Inducers of CYP2D6 and CYP3A4, such as dexamethasone, could increase the rate of elimination of donepezil). Products include:
Ciprodex 583
Ozurdex .... ⊙ 223
Tobramycin and Dexamethasone Ophthalmic Suspension .... ⊙ 251

Dexamethasone Acetate (Inducers of CYP2D6 and CYP3A4, such as dexamethasone, could increase the rate of elimination of donepezil).
No products indexed under this heading.

Dexamethasone Phosphate (Inducers of CYP2D6 and CYP3A4, such as dexamethasone, could increase the rate of elimination of donepezil).
No products indexed under this heading.

Dexamethasone Sodium (Inducers of CYP2D6 and CYP3A4, such as dexamethasone, could increase the rate of elimination of donepezil).
No products indexed under this heading.

Dexamethasone Sodium Phosphate (Inducers of CYP2D6 and CYP3A4, such as dexamethasone, could increase the rate of elimination of donepezil).
No products indexed under this heading.

Dexamethasone Sodium Phosphate Injection (Inducers of CYP2D6 and CYP3A4, such as dexamethasone, could increase the rate of elimination of donepezil).
No products indexed under this heading.

Diclofenac Epolamine (Cholinesterase inhibitors, such as donepezil, may be expected to increase gastric acid secretion due to increased cholinergic activity, therefore, patients on concurrent NSAID therapy should be monitored closely for increased risk of developing ulcers or symptoms of active or occult gastrointestinal bleeding). Products include:
Flector 1839

Diclofenac Potassium (Cholinesterase inhibitors, such as donepezil, may be expected to increase gastric acid secretion due to increased cholinergic activity, therefore, patients on concurrent NSAID therapy should be monitored closely for increased risk of developing ulcers or symptoms of active or occult gastrointestinal bleeding).
No products indexed under this heading.

Diclofenac Sodium (Cholinesterase inhibitors, such as donepezil, may be expected to increase gastric acid secretion due to increased cholinergic activity, therefore, patients on concurrent NSAID therapy should be monitored closely for increased risk of developing ulcers or symptoms of active or occult gastrointestinal bleeding).
No products indexed under this heading.

Dicyclomine Hydrochloride (Donepezil, a cholinesterase inhibitor, has the potential to interfere with the activity of anticholinergic medications). Products include:
Bentyl Capsules 780
Bentyl Injection 780
Bentyl Syrup 780
Bentyl Tablets 780

Doxorubicin Hydrochloride (Inducers of CYP3A4 could increase the rate of elimination of donepezil).
No products indexed under this heading.

Efavirenz (Inducers of CYP3A4 could increase the rate of elimination of donepezil). Products include:
Atripla 906

Ethanol (Inducers of CYP2D6 could increase the rate of elimination of donepezil).
No products indexed under this heading.

Ethosuximide (Inducers of CYP3A4 could increase the rate of elimination of donepezil).
No products indexed under this heading.

Etodolac (Cholinesterase inhibitors, such as donepezil, may be expected to increase gastric acid secretion due to increased cholinergic activity, therefore, patients on concurrent NSAID therapy should be monitored closely for increased risk of developing ulcers or symptoms of active or occult gastrointestinal bleeding).
No products indexed under this heading.

Felbamate (Inducers of CYP3A4 could increase the rate of elimination of donepezil).
No products indexed under this heading.

Fenoprofen Calcium (Cholinesterase inhibitors, such as donepezil, may be expected to increase gastric acid secretion due to increased cholinergic activity, therefore, patients on concurrent NSAID therapy should be monitored closely for increased risk of developing ulcers or symptoms of active or occult gastrointestinal bleeding).
No products indexed under this heading.

Fludrocortisone Acetate (Inducers of CYP3A4 could increase the rate of elimination of donepezil).
No products indexed under this heading.

IMPORTANT NOTE: Always consult each drug listing in the patient's regimen for possible interactions.

151 Interactions Index Arixtra

Primidone (Inducers of CYP3A4 could increase the rate of elimination of donepezil).
No products indexed under this heading.

Procyclidine Hydrochloride (Donepezil, a cholinesterase inhibitor, has the potential to interfere with the activity of anticholinergic medications).
No products indexed under this heading.

Propantheline Bromide (Donepezil, a cholinesterase inhibitor, has the potential to interfere with the activity of anticholinergic medications).
No products indexed under this heading.

Quinidine (Inhibitors of CYP450, 2D6 and 3A4, such as quinidine, inhibit donepezil metabolism *in vitro*).
No products indexed under this heading.

Quinidine Gluconate (Inhibitors of CYP450, 2D6 and 3A4, such as quinidine, inhibit donepezil metabolism *in vitro*).
No products indexed under this heading.

Quinidine Hydrochloride (Inhibitors of CYP450, 2D6 and 3A4, such as quinidine, inhibit donepezil metabolism *in vitro*).
No products indexed under this heading.

Quinidine Polygalacturonate (Inhibitors of CYP450, 2D6 and 3A4, such as quinidine, inhibit donepezil metabolism *in vitro*).
No products indexed under this heading.

Quinidine Sulfate (Inhibitors of CYP450, 2D6 and 3A4, such as quinidine, inhibit donepezil metabolism *in vitro*).
No products indexed under this heading.

Rifabutin (Inducers of CYP3A4 could increase the rate of elimination of donepezil).
No products indexed under this heading.

Rifampicin (Inducers of CYP3A4 could increase the rate of elimination of donepezil).
No products indexed under this heading.

Rifampin (Inducers of CYP2D6 and CYP3A4, such as rifampin, could increase the rate of elimination of donepezil).
No products indexed under this heading.

Rifapentine (Inducers of CYP3A4 could increase the rate of elimination of donepezil).
No products indexed under this heading.

Ritonavir (Inducers of CYP2D6 could increase the rate of elimination of donepezil). Products include:
Kaletra 458
Norvir 509

Rofecoxib (Cholinesterase inhibitors, such as donepezil, may be expected to increase gastric acid secretion due to increased cholinergic activity, therefore, patients on concurrent NSAID therapy should be monitored closely for increased risk of developing ulcers or symptoms of active or occult gastrointestinal bleeding).
No products indexed under this heading.

Scopolamine (Donepezil, a cholinesterase inhibitor, has the potential to interfere with the activity of anticholinergic medications). Products include:
Transderm Scōp 2397

Scopolamine Hydrobromide (Donepezil, a cholinesterase inhibitor, has the potential to interfere with the activity of anticholinergic medications). Products include:
Donnatal 2711

Succinylcholine Chloride (Potential for synergistic effect).
No products indexed under this heading.

Sulfinpyrazone (Inducers of CYP3A4 could increase the rate of elimination of donepezil).
No products indexed under this heading.

Sulindac (Cholinesterase inhibitors, such as donepezil, may be expected to increase gastric acid secretion due to increased cholinergic activity, therefore, patients on concurrent NSAID therapy should be monitored closely for increased risk of developing ulcers or symptoms of active or occult gastrointestinal bleeding). Products include:
Clinoril 2098

Theophyllinate (Inducers of CYP3A4 could increase the rate of elimination of donepezil).
No products indexed under this heading.

Theophylline (Inducers of CYP3A4 could increase the rate of elimination of donepezil).
No products indexed under this heading.

Theophylline Anhydrous (Inducers of CYP3A4 could increase the rate of elimination of donepezil). Products include:
Uniphyl 2817

Theophylline Calcium Salicylate (Inducers of CYP3A4 could increase the rate of elimination of donepezil).
No products indexed under this heading.

Theophylline Dihydroxypropyl (Glyceryl) (Inducers of CYP3A4 could increase the rate of elimination of donepezil).
No products indexed under this heading.

Theophylline Ethylenediamine (Inducers of CYP3A4 could increase the rate of elimination of donepezil).
No products indexed under this heading.

Theophylline Sodium Glycinate (Inducers of CYP3A4 could increase the rate of elimination of donepezil).
No products indexed under this heading.

Tolmetin Sodium (Cholinesterase inhibitors, such as donepezil, may be expected to increase gastric acid secretion due to increased cholinergic activity, therefore, patients on concurrent NSAID therapy should be monitored closely for increased risk of developing ulcers or symptoms of active or occult gastrointestinal bleeding).
No products indexed under this heading.

Tolterodine Tartrate (Donepezil, a cholinesterase inhibitor, has the potential to interfere with the activity of anticholinergic medications).
No products indexed under this heading.

Triamcinolone (Inducers of CYP3A4 could increase the rate of elimination of donepezil).
No products indexed under this heading.

Triamcinolone Acetonide (Inducers of CYP3A4 could increase the rate of elimination of donepezil). Products include:
Azmacort 408
Nasacort AQ 3019

Triamcinolone Diacetate (Inducers of CYP3A4 could increase the rate of elimination of donepezil).
No products indexed under this heading.

Triamcinolone Hexacetonide (Inducers of CYP3A4 could increase the rate of elimination of donepezil).
No products indexed under this heading.

Tridihexethyl Chloride (Donepezil, a cholinesterase inhibitor, has the potential to interfere with the activity of anticholinergic medications).
No products indexed under this heading.

Trihexyphenidyl Hydrochloride (Donepezil, a cholinesterase inhibitor, has the potential to interfere with the activity of anticholinergic medications).
No products indexed under this heading.

Troglitazone (Inducers of CYP3A4 could increase the rate of elimination of donepezil).
No products indexed under this heading.

Valdecoxib (Cholinesterase inhibitors, such as donepezil, may be expected to increase gastric acid secretion due to increased cholinergic activity, therefore, patients on concurrent NSAID therapy should be monitored closely for increased risk of developing ulcers or symptoms of active or occult gastrointestinal bleeding).
No products indexed under this heading.

ARICEPT ODT TABLETS

(Donepezil Hydrochloride) 1045
See Aricept Tablets

ARIXTRA INJECTION

(Fondaparinux Sodium) 1320
May interact with anticoagulants, aspirin-acetylsalicylic acid, glycoprotein (GP) IIb/IIIa inhibitors, non-steroidal anti-inflammatory agents, oral anticoagulants, platelet inhibitors, spinal and peridural anesthetics. Compounds in these categories include:

Abciximab (Agents that may enhance the risk of hemorrhage should be discontinued prior to initiation of therapy with fondaparinux sodium. If co-administration is necessary, close monitoring may be appropriate). Products include:
ReoPro 1952

Anisindione (Agents that may enhance the risk of hemorrhage should be discontinued prior to initiation of therapy with fondaparinux sodium. If co-administration is necessary, close monitoring may be appropriate).
No products indexed under this heading.

Ardeparin Sodium (Agents that may enhance the risk of hemorrhage should be discontinued prior to initiation of therapy with fondaparinux sodium. If co-administration is necessary, close monitoring may be appropriate).
No products indexed under this heading.

Aspirin (Agents that may enhance the risk of hemorrhage should be discontinued prior to initiation of therapy with fondaparinux sodium. If co-administration is necessary, close monitoring may be appropriate). Products include:
Aggrenox 880
Bayer Aspirin 829
Percodan 1124
St. Joseph Aspirin 2045

Aspirin, Enteric Coated (Agents that may enhance the risk of hemorrhage should be discontinued prior to initiation of therapy with fondaparinux sodium. If co-administration is necessary, close monitoring may be appropriate).
No products indexed under this heading.

Aspirin Buffered (Agents that may enhance the risk of hemorrhage should be discontinued prior to initiation of therapy with fondaparinux sodium. If co-administration is necessary, close monitoring may be appropriate).
No products indexed under this heading.

Azlocillin Sodium (Agents that may enhance the risk of hemorrhage should be discontinued prior to initiation of therapy with fondaparinux sodium. If co-administration is necessary, close monitoring may be appropriate).
No products indexed under this heading.

Bupivacaine Hydrochloride (When neuraxial anesthesia (epidural/spinal anesthesia) is employed, patients anticoagulated or scheduled to be anticoagulated with fondaparinux sodium for prevention of thromboembolic complications are at risk of developing an epidural or spinal hematoma which can result in long-term or permanent paralysis).
No products indexed under this heading.

Carbenicillin Indanyl Sodium (Agents that may enhance the risk of hemorrhage should be discontinued prior to initiation of therapy with fondaparinux sodium. If co-administration is necessary, close monitoring may be appropriate).
No products indexed under this heading.

Celecoxib (Agents that may enhance the risk of hemorrhage should be discontinued prior to initiation of therapy with fondaparinux sodium. If co-administration is necessary, close monitoring may be appropriate). Products include:
Celebrex 3272

Choline Magnesium Trisalicylate (Agents that may enhance the risk of hemorrhage should be discontinued prior to initiation of therapy with fondaparinux sodium. If co-administration is necessary, close monitoring may be appropriate).
No products indexed under this heading.

Clopidogrel Bisulfate (Agents that may enhance the risk of hemorrhage should be discontinued prior to initiation of therapy with fondaparinux sodium. If co-administration is necessary, close monitoring may be appropriate). Products include:
Plavix 3027

Dalteparin Sodium (Agents that may enhance the risk of hemorrhage should be discontinued prior to initiation of therapy with fondaparinux sodium. If co-administration is necessary, close monitoring may be appropriate). Products include:
Fragmin 1058

Danaparoid Sodium (Agents that may enhance the risk of hemorrhage should be discontinued prior to initiation of therapy with fondaparinux sodium. If co-administration is necessary, close monitoring may be appropriate).
No products indexed under this heading.

Dextran (Agents that may enhance the risk of hemorrhage should be discontinued prior to initiation of therapy with fondaparinux sodium. If co-administration is necessary, close monitoring may be appropriate).
No products indexed under this heading.

Dextran 40 (Agents that may enhance the risk of hemorrhage should be discontinued prior to initiation of therapy with fondaparinux sodium. If co-administration is necessary, close monitoring may be appropriate).
No products indexed under this heading.

Dextran 70 (Agents that may enhance the risk of hemorrhage should be discontinued prior to initiation of therapy with fondaparinux sodium. If co-administration is necessary, close monitoring may be appropriate).
No products indexed under this heading.

Dextran I (Agents that may enhance the risk of hemorrhage should be discontinued prior to initiation of therapy with fondaparinux sodium. If co-administration is necessary, close monitoring may be appropriate).
No products indexed under this heading.

Dextrans (Low Molecular Weight) (Agents that may enhance the risk of hemorrhage should be discontinued prior to initiation of therapy with fondaparinux sodium. If co-administration is necessary, close monitoring may be appropriate).
No products indexed under this heading.

Diclofenac Epolamine (Agents that may enhance the risk of hemorrhage should be discontinued prior to initiation of therapy with fondaparinux sodium. If co-administration is necessary, close monitoring may be appropriate). Products include:

IMPORTANT NOTE: Always consult each drug listing in the patient's regimen for possible interactions.

Tinzaparin Sodium (Agents that may enhance the risk of hemorrhage should be discontinued prior to initiation of therapy with fondaparinux sodium. If co-administration is necessary, close monitoring may be appropriate).
No products indexed under this heading.

Tirofiban Hydrochloride (Agents that may enhance the risk of hemorrhage should be discontinued prior to initiation of therapy with fondaparinux sodium. If co-administration is necessary, close monitoring may be appropriate).
No products indexed under this heading.

Tolmetin Sodium (Agents that may enhance the risk of hemorrhage should be discontinued prior to initiation of therapy with fondaparinux sodium. If co-administration is necessary, close monitoring may be appropriate).
No products indexed under this heading.

Valdecoxib (Agents that may enhance the risk of hemorrhage should be discontinued prior to initiation of therapy with fondaparinux sodium. If co-administration is necessary, close monitoring may be appropriate).
No products indexed under this heading.

Warfarin Sodium (Agents that may enhance the risk of hemorrhage should be discontinued prior to initiation of therapy with fondaparinux sodium. If co-administration is necessary, close monitoring may be appropriate).
No products indexed under this heading.

AROMASIN TABLETS

(Exemestane) 2758
May interact with cytochrome p450 3a4 inducers (selected), estrogens, and certain other agents. Compounds in these categories include:

Allium sativum (Co-medications that induce CYP 3A4 (eg, rifampicin, phenytoin, carbamazepine, phenobarbital, or St. John's wort) may significantly decrease exposure to exemestane. Dose modification is recommended for patients who are also receiving a potent CYP 3A4 inducer).
No products indexed under this heading.

Aminoglutethimide (Co-medications that induce CYP 3A4 (eg, rifampicin, phenytoin, carbamazepine, phenobarbital, or St. John's wort) may significantly decrease exposure to exemestane. Dose modification is recommended for patients who are also receiving a potent CYP 3A4 inducer).
No products indexed under this heading.

Aprepitant (Co-medications that induce CYP 3A4 (eg, rifampicin, phenytoin, carbamazepine, phenobarbital, or St. John's wort) may significantly decrease exposure to exemestane. Dose modification is recommended for patients who are also receiving a potent CYP 3A4 inducer). Products include:
Emend 2124

Betamethasone (Co-medications that induce CYP 3A4 (eg, rifampicin, phenytoin, carbamazepine, phenobarbital, or St. John's wort) may significantly decrease exposure to exemestane. Dose modification is recommended for patients who are also receiving a potent CYP 3A4 inducer).
No products indexed under this heading.

Betamethasone Acetate (Co-medications that induce CYP 3A4 (eg, rifampicin, phenytoin, carbamazepine, phenobarbital, or St. John's wort) may significantly decrease exposure to exemestane. Dose modification is recommended for patients who are also receiving a potent CYP 3A4 inducer).
No products indexed under this heading.

Betamethasone Benzoate (Co-medications that induce CYP 3A4 (eg, rifampicin, phenytoin, carbamazepine, phenobarbital, or St. John's wort) may significantly decrease exposure to exemestane. Dose modification is recommended for patients who are also receiving a potent CYP 3A4 inducer).
No products indexed under this heading.

Betamethasone Dipropionate (Co-medications that induce CYP 3A4 (eg, rifampicin, phenytoin, carbamazepine, phenobarbital, or St. John's wort) may significantly decrease exposure to exemestane. Dose modification is recommended for patients who are also receiving a potent CYP 3A4 inducer). Products include:
Diprolene Lotion 0.05% 3108
Diprolene Ointment 0.05% 3109
Diprolene AF Cream 0.05% 3107
Lotrisone 3163

Betamethasone Sodium Phosphate (Co-medications that induce CYP 3A4 (eg, rifampicin, phenytoin, carbamazepine, phenobarbital, or St. John's wort) may significantly decrease exposure to exemestane. Dose modification is recommended for patients who are also receiving a potent CYP 3A4 inducer).
No products indexed under this heading.

Betamethasone Valerate (Co-medications that induce CYP 3A4 (eg, rifampicin, phenytoin, carbamazepine, phenobarbital, or St. John's wort) may significantly decrease exposure to exemestane. Dose modification is recommended for patients who are also receiving a potent CYP 3A4 inducer). Products include:
Luxiq 3321

Bosentan (Co-medications that induce CYP 3A4 (eg, rifampicin, phenytoin, carbamazepine, phenobarbital, or St. John's wort) may significantly decrease exposure to exemestane. Dose modification is recommended for patients who are also receiving a potent CYP 3A4 inducer). Products include:
Tracleer 573

Carbamazepine (Co-medications that induce CYP 3A4 (eg, rifampicin, phenytoin, carbamazepine, phenobarbital, or St. John's wort) may significantly decrease exposure to exemestane. Dose modification is recommended for patients who are also receiving a potent CYP 3A4 inducer). Products include:
Carbatrol 3280
Equetro 3477

Chlorotrianisene (Exemestane should not be co-administered with estrogen-containing agents, as these could interfere with its pharmacologic action).
No products indexed under this heading.

Ciprofloxacin (Co-medications that induce CYP 3A4 (eg, rifampicin, phenytoin, carbamazepine, phenobarbital, or St. John's wort) may significantly decrease exposure to exemestane. Dose modification is recommended for patients who are also receiving a potent CYP 3A4 inducer). Products include:
Cipro I.V. 3082
Cipro 3073
Cipro XR 3091
Ciprodex 583

Ciprofloxacin Hydrochloride (Co-medications that induce CYP 3A4 (eg, rifampicin, phenytoin, carbamazepine, phenobarbital, or St. John's wort) may significantly decrease exposure to exemestane. Dose modification is recommended for patients who are also receiving a potent CYP 3A4 inducer). Products include:
Cipro 3073

Cisplatin (Co-medications that induce CYP 3A4 (eg, rifampicin, phenytoin, carbamazepine, phenobarbital, or St. John's wort) may significantly decrease exposure to exemestane. Dose modification is recommended for patients who are also receiving a potent CYP 3A4 inducer).
No products indexed under this heading.

Cortisone Acetate (Co-medications that induce CYP 3A4 (eg, rifampicin, phenytoin, carbamazepine, phenobarbital, or St. John's wort) may significantly decrease exposure to exemestane. Dose modification is recommended for patients who are also receiving a potent CYP 3A4 inducer).
No products indexed under this heading.

Dexamethasone (Co-medications that induce CYP 3A4 (eg, rifampicin, phenytoin, carbamazepine, phenobarbital, or St. John's wort) may significantly decrease exposure to exemestane. Dose modification is recommended for patients who are also receiving a potent CYP 3A4 inducer). Products include:
Ciprodex 583
Ozurdex .... ⊙ 223
Tobramycin and Dexamethasone Ophthalmic Suspension .... ⊙ 251

Dexamethasone Acetate (Co-medications that induce CYP 3A4 (eg, rifampicin, phenytoin, carbamazepine, phenobarbital, or St. John's wort) may significantly decrease exposure to exemestane. Dose modification is recommended for patients who are also receiving a potent CYP 3A4 inducer).
No products indexed under this heading.

Dexamethasone Phosphate (Co-medications that induce CYP 3A4 (eg, rifampicin, phenytoin, carbamazepine, phenobarbital, or St. John's wort) may significantly decrease exposure to exemestane. Dose modification is recommended for patients who are also receiving a potent CYP 3A4 inducer).
No products indexed under this heading.

Dexamethasone Sodium (Co-medications that induce CYP 3A4 (eg, rifampicin, phenytoin, carbamazepine, phenobarbital, or St. John's wort) may significantly decrease exposure to exemestane. Dose modification is recommended for patients who are also receiving a potent CYP 3A4 inducer).
No products indexed under this heading.

Dexamethasone Sodium Phosphate (Co-medications that induce CYP 3A4 (eg, rifampicin, phenytoin, carbamazepine, phenobarbital, or St. John's wort) may significantly decrease exposure to exemestane. Dose modification is recommended for patients who are also receiving a potent CYP 3A4 inducer).
No products indexed under this heading.

Dexamethasone Sodium Phosphate Injection (Co-medications that induce CYP 3A4 (eg, rifampicin, phenytoin, carbamazepine, phenobarbital, or St. John's wort) may significantly decrease exposure to exemestane. Dose modification is recommended for patients who are also receiving a potent CYP 3A4 inducer).
No products indexed under this heading.

Dienestrol (Exemestane should not be co-administered with estrogen-containing agents, as these could interfere with its pharmacologic action).
No products indexed under this heading.

Diethylstilbestrol (Exemestane should not be co-administered with estrogen-containing agents, as these could interfere with its pharmacologic action).
No products indexed under this heading.

Doxorubicin Hydrochloride (Co-medications that induce CYP 3A4 (eg, rifampicin, phenytoin, carbamazepine, phenobarbital, or St. John's wort) may significantly decrease exposure to exemestane. Dose modification is recommended for patients who are also receiving a potent CYP 3A4 inducer).
No products indexed under this heading.

Efavirenz (Co-medications that induce CYP 3A4 (eg, rifampicin, phenytoin, carbamazepine, phenobarbital, or St. John's wort) may significantly decrease exposure to exemestane. Dose modification is recommended for patients who are also receiving a potent CYP 3A4 inducer). Products include:
Atripla 906

Estradiol (Exemestane should not be co-administered with estrogen-containing agents, as these could interfere with its pharmacologic action). Products include:
Activella 2561
Angeliq 831
Climara 841
Climara Pro 847
Divigel 3467
Estrasorb 1777
Vagifem 2589

Estrogens, Conjugated (Exemestane should not be co-administered with estrogen-containing agents, as these could interfere with its pharmacologic action). Products include:
Premarin Intravenous 3528
Premarin Tablets 3533
Premarin Vaginal Cream 3540
Premphase 3549
Prempro 3549

Estrogens, Esterified (Exemestane should not be co-administered with estrogen-containing agents, as these could interfere with its pharmacologic action).
No products indexed under this heading.

Estropipate (Exemestane should not be co-administered with estrogen-containing agents, as these could interfere with its pharmacologic action).
No products indexed under this heading.

Ethinyl Estradiol (Exemestane should not be co-administered with estrogen-containing agents, as these could interfere with its pharmacologic action). Products include:
LoSeasonique 3407
Lybrel 3514
NuvaRing 3181
Ortho Evra 2648
Ortho-Cyclen/Ortho Tri-Cyclen 2663
Ortho Tri-Cyclen Lo Tablets 2673
Seasonique 3418
Yaz 864

Ethosuximide (Co-medications that induce CYP 3A4 (eg, rifampicin, phenytoin, carbamazepine, phenobarbital, or St. John's wort) may significantly decrease exposure to exemestane. Dose modification is recommended for patients who are also receiving a potent CYP 3A4 inducer).
No products indexed under this heading.

Felbamate (Co-medications that induce CYP 3A4 (eg, rifampicin, phenytoin, carbamazepine, phenobarbital, or St. John's wort) may significantly decrease exposure to exemestane. Dose modification is recommended for patients who are also receiving a potent CYP 3A4 inducer).
No products indexed under this heading.

Fludrocortisone Acetate (Co-medications that induce CYP 3A4 (eg, rifampicin, phenytoin, carbamazepine, phenobarbital, or St. John's wort) may significantly decrease exposure to exemestane. Dose modification is recommended for patients who are also receiving a potent CYP 3A4 inducer).
No products indexed under this heading.

IMPORTANT NOTE: Always consult each drug listing in the patient's regimen for possible interactions.

Fosphenytoin Sodium (Co-medications that induce CYP 3A4 (eg, rifampicin, phenytoin, carbamazepine, phenobarbital, or St. John's wort) may significantly decrease exposure to exemestane. Dose modification is recommended for patients who are also receiving a potent CYP 3A4 inducer).
No products indexed under this heading.

Garlic Extract (Co-medications that induce CYP 3A4 (eg, rifampicin, phenytoin, carbamazepine, phenobarbital, or St. John's wort) may significantly decrease exposure to exemestane. Dose modification is recommended for patients who are also receiving a potent CYP 3A4 inducer).
No products indexed under this heading.

Garlic Oil (Co-medications that induce CYP 3A4 (eg, rifampicin, phenytoin, carbamazepine, phenobarbital, or St. John's wort) may significantly decrease exposure to exemestane. Dose modification is recommended for patients who are also receiving a potent CYP 3A4 inducer).
No products indexed under this heading.

Hydrocortisone (Co-medications that induce CYP 3A4 (eg, rifampicin, phenytoin, carbamazepine, phenobarbital, or St. John's wort) may significantly decrease exposure to exemestane. Dose modification is recommended for patients who are also receiving a potent CYP 3A4 inducer).
No products indexed under this heading.

Hydrocortisone (Alcohol) (Co-medications that induce CYP 3A4 (eg, rifampicin, phenytoin, carbamazepine, phenobarbital, or St. John's wort) may significantly decrease exposure to exemestane. Dose modification is recommended for patients who are also receiving a potent CYP 3A4 inducer).
No products indexed under this heading.

Hydrocortisone Acetate (Co-medications that induce CYP 3A4 (eg, rifampicin, phenytoin, carbamazepine, phenobarbital, or St. John's wort) may significantly decrease exposure to exemestane. Dose modification is recommended for patients who are also receiving a potent CYP 3A4 inducer).
No products indexed under this heading.

Hydrocortisone Butyrate (Co-medications that induce CYP 3A4 (eg, rifampicin, phenytoin, carbamazepine, phenobarbital, or St. John's wort) may significantly decrease exposure to exemestane. Dose modification is recommended for patients who are also receiving a potent CYP 3A4 inducer).
No products indexed under this heading.

Hydrocortisone Cypionate (Co-medications that induce CYP 3A4 (eg, rifampicin, phenytoin, carbamazepine, phenobarbital, or St. John's wort) may significantly decrease exposure to exemestane. Dose modification is recommended for patients who are also receiving a potent CYP 3A4 inducer).
No products indexed under this heading.

Hydrocortisone Hemisuccinate (Co-medications that induce CYP 3A4 (eg, rifampicin, phenytoin, carbamazepine, phenobarbital, or St. John's wort) may significantly decrease exposure to exemestane. Dose modification is recommended for patients who are also receiving a potent CYP 3A4 inducer).
No products indexed under this heading.

Hydrocortisone Probutate (Co-medications that induce CYP 3A4 (eg, rifampicin, phenytoin, carbamazepine, phenobarbital, or St. John's wort) may significantly decrease exposure to exemestane. Dose modification is recommended for patients who are also receiving a potent CYP 3A4 inducer).
No products indexed under this heading.

Hydrocortisone Sodium Phosphate (Co-medications that induce CYP 3A4 (eg, rifampicin, phenytoin, carbamazepine, phenobarbital, or St. John's wort) may significantly decrease exposure to exemestane. Dose modification is recommended for patients who are also receiving a potent CYP 3A4 inducer).
No products indexed under this heading.

Hydrocortisone Sodium Succinate (Co-medications that induce CYP 3A4 (eg, rifampicin, phenytoin, carbamazepine, phenobarbital, or St. John's wort) may significantly decrease exposure to exemestane. Dose modification is recommended for patients who are also receiving a potent CYP 3A4 inducer).
No products indexed under this heading.

Hydrocortisone Valerate (Co-medications that induce CYP 3A4 (eg, rifampicin, phenytoin, carbamazepine, phenobarbital, or St. John's wort) may significantly decrease exposure to exemestane. Dose modification is recommended for patients who are also receiving a potent CYP 3A4 inducer).
No products indexed under this heading.

Hypericum (Co-medications that induce CYP 3A4 (eg, rifampicin, phenytoin, carbamazepine, phenobarbital, or St. John's wort) may significantly decrease exposure to exemestane. Dose modification is recommended for patients who are also receiving a potent CYP 3A4 inducer).
No products indexed under this heading.

Hypericum Perforatum (Co-medications that induce CYP 3A4 (eg, rifampicin, phenytoin, carbamazepine, phenobarbital, or St. John's wort) may significantly decrease exposure to exemestane. Dose modification is recommended for patients who are also receiving a potent CYP 3A4 inducer). Products include:
Traumeel 1800

Mephenytoin (Co-medications that induce CYP 3A4 (eg, rifampicin, phenytoin, carbamazepine, phenobarbital, or St. John's wort) may significantly decrease exposure to exemestane. Dose modification is recommended for patients who are also receiving a potent CYP 3A4 inducer).
No products indexed under this heading.

Methsuximide (Co-medications that induce CYP 3A4 (eg, rifampicin, phenytoin, carbamazepine, phenobarbital, or St. John's wort) may significantly decrease exposure to exemestane. Dose modification is recommended for patients who are also receiving a potent CYP 3A4 inducer).
No products indexed under this heading.

Methylprednisolone (Co-medications that induce CYP 3A4 (eg, rifampicin, phenytoin, carbamazepine, phenobarbital, or St. John's wort) may significantly decrease exposure to exemestane. Dose modification is recommended for patients who are also receiving a potent CYP 3A4 inducer).
No products indexed under this heading.

Methylprednisolone Acetate (Co-medications that induce CYP 3A4 (eg, rifampicin, phenytoin, carbamazepine, phenobarbital, or St. John's wort) may significantly decrease exposure to exemestane. Dose modification is recommended for patients who are also receiving a potent CYP 3A4 inducer).
No products indexed under this heading.

Methylprednisolone Sodium Succinate (Co-medications that induce CYP 3A4 (eg, rifampicin, phenytoin, carbamazepine, phenobarbital, or St. John's wort) may significantly decrease exposure to exemestane. Dose modification is recommended for patients who are also receiving a potent CYP 3A4 inducer).
No products indexed under this heading.

Modafinil (Co-medications that induce CYP 3A4 (eg, rifampicin, phenytoin, carbamazepine, phenobarbital, or St. John's wort) may significantly decrease exposure to exemestane. Dose modification is recommended for patients who are also receiving a potent CYP 3A4 inducer). Products include:
Provigil 983

Nafcillin Sodium (Co-medications that induce CYP 3A4 (eg, rifampicin, phenytoin, carbamazepine, phenobarbital, or St. John's wort) may significantly decrease exposure to exemestane. Dose modification is recommended for patients who are also receiving a potent CYP 3A4 inducer).
No products indexed under this heading.

Nevirapine (Co-medications that induce CYP 3A4 (eg, rifampicin, phenytoin, carbamazepine, phenobarbital, or St. John's wort) may significantly decrease exposure to exemestane. Dose modification is recommended for patients who are also receiving a potent CYP 3A4 inducer). Products include:
Viramune Oral Suspension 897
Viramune Tablets 897

Oxcarbazepine (Co-medications that induce CYP 3A4 (eg, rifampicin, phenytoin, carbamazepine, phenobarbital, or St. John's wort) may significantly decrease exposure to exemestane. Dose modification is recommended for patients who are also receiving a potent CYP 3A4 inducer).
No products indexed under this heading.

Phenobarbital (Co-medications that induce CYP 3A4 (eg, rifampicin, phenytoin, carbamazepine, phenobarbital, or St. John's wort) may significantly decrease exposure to exemestane. Dose modification is recommended for patients who are also receiving a potent CYP 3A4 inducer). Products include:
Donnatal 2711

Phenobarbital Sodium (Co-medications that induce CYP 3A4 (eg, rifampicin, phenytoin, carbamazepine, phenobarbital, or St. John's wort) may significantly decrease exposure to exemestane. Dose modification is recommended for patients who are also receiving a potent CYP 3A4 inducer).
No products indexed under this heading.

Phenytoin (Co-medications that induce CYP 3A4 (eg, rifampicin, phenytoin, carbamazepine, phenobarbital, or St. John's wort) may significantly decrease exposure to exemestane. Dose modification is recommended for patients who are also receiving a potent CYP 3A4 inducer).
No products indexed under this heading.

Phenytoin Sodium (Co-medications that induce CYP 3A4 (eg, rifampicin, phenytoin, carbamazepine, phenobarbital, or St. John's wort) may significantly decrease exposure to exemestane. Dose modification is recommended for patients who are also receiving a potent CYP 3A4 inducer). Products include:
Phenytek Capsules 2380

Polyestradiol Phosphate (Exemestane should not be co-administered with estrogen-containing agents, as these could interfere with its pharmacologic action).
No products indexed under this heading.

Prednisolone (Co-medications that induce CYP 3A4 (eg, rifampicin, phenytoin, carbamazepine, phenobarbital, or St. John's wort) may significantly decrease exposure to exemestane. Dose modification is recommended for patients who are also receiving a potent CYP 3A4 inducer).
No products indexed under this heading.

Prednisolone Acetate (Co-medications that induce CYP 3A4 (eg, rifampicin, phenytoin, carbamazepine, phenobarbital, or St. John's wort) may significantly decrease exposure to exemestane. Dose modification is recommended for patients who are also receiving a potent CYP 3A4 inducer). Products include:
Blephamide .... ⊙212, ⊙214
Pred Forte .... ⊙225
Pred Mild .... ⊙230
Pred-G .... ⊙226, ⊙227

Prednisolone Sodium Phosphate (Co-medications that induce CYP 3A4 (eg, rifampicin, phenytoin, carbamazepine, phenobarbital, or St. John's wort) may significantly decrease exposure to exemestane. Dose modification is recommended for patients who are also receiving a potent CYP 3A4 inducer).
No products indexed under this heading.

Prednisolone Tebutate (Co-medications that induce CYP 3A4 (eg, rifampicin, phenytoin, carbamazepine, phenobarbital, or St. John's wort) may significantly decrease exposure to exemestane. Dose modification is recommended for patients who are also receiving a potent CYP 3A4 inducer).
No products indexed under this heading.

Prednisone (Co-medications that induce CYP 3A4 (eg, rifampicin, phenytoin, carbamazepine, phenobarbital, or St. John's wort) may significantly decrease exposure to exemestane. Dose modification is recommended for patients who are also receiving a potent CYP 3A4 inducer).
No products indexed under this heading.

Prednisone sodium phosphate (Co-medications that induce CYP 3A4 (eg, rifampicin, phenytoin, carbamazepine, phenobarbital, or St. John's wort) may significantly decrease exposure to exemestane. Dose modification is recommended for patients who are also receiving a potent CYP 3A4 inducer).
No products indexed under this heading.

Primidone (Co-medications that induce CYP 3A4 (eg, rifampicin, phenytoin, carbamazepine, phenobarbital, or St. John's wort) may significantly decrease exposure to exemestane. Dose modification is recommended for patients who are also receiving a potent CYP 3A4 inducer).
No products indexed under this heading.

Quinestrol (Exemestane should not be co-administered with estrogen-containing agents, as these could interfere with its pharmacologic action).
No products indexed under this heading.

Rifabutin (Co-medications that induce CYP 3A4 (eg, rifampicin, phenytoin, carbamazepine, phenobarbital, or St. John's wort) may significantly decrease exposure to exemestane. Dose modification is recommended for patients who are also receiving a potent CYP 3A4 inducer).
No products indexed under this heading.

Rifampicin (In a pharmacokinetic interaction study of 10 healthy postmenopausal volunteers pretreated with potent CYP 3A4 inducer rifampicin 600 mg daily for 14 days followed by a single dose of exemestane 25 mg, the mean plasma C_{max} and AUC of exemestane were decreased by 41% and 54%, respectively).
No products indexed under this heading.

(⊙ Described in PDR® for Ophthalmic Medicines)

Rifampin (Co-medications that induce CYP 3A4 (eg, rifampicin, phenytoin, carbamazepine, phenobarbital, or St. John's wort) may significantly decrease exposure to exemestane. Dose modification is recommended for patients who are also receiving a potent CYP 3A4 inducer).
No products indexed under this heading.

Rifapentine (Co-medications that induce CYP 3A4 (eg, rifampicin, phenytoin, carbamazepine, phenobarbital, or St. John's wort) may significantly decrease exposure to exemestane. Dose modification is recommended for patients who are also receiving a potent CYP 3A4 inducer).
No products indexed under this heading.

Sulfinpyrazone (Co-medications that induce CYP 3A4 (eg, rifampicin, phenytoin, carbamazepine, phenobarbital, or St. John's wort) may significantly decrease exposure to exemestane. Dose modification is recommended for patients who are also receiving a potent CYP 3A4 inducer).
No products indexed under this heading.

Theophyllinate (Co-medications that induce CYP 3A4 (eg, rifampicin, phenytoin, carbamazepine, phenobarbital, or St. John's wort) may significantly decrease exposure to exemestane. Dose modification is recommended for patients who are also receiving a potent CYP 3A4 inducer).
No products indexed under this heading.

Theophylline (Co-medications that induce CYP 3A4 (eg, rifampicin, phenytoin, carbamazepine, phenobarbital, or St. John's wort) may significantly decrease exposure to exemestane. Dose modification is recommended for patients who are also receiving a potent CYP 3A4 inducer).
No products indexed under this heading.

Theophylline Anhydrous (Co-medications that induce CYP 3A4 (eg, rifampicin, phenytoin, carbamazepine, phenobarbital, or St. John's wort) may significantly decrease exposure to exemestane. Dose modification is recommended for patients who are also receiving a potent CYP 3A4 inducer). Products include:
Uniphyl 2817

Theophylline Calcium Salicylate (Co-medications that induce CYP 3A4 (eg, rifampicin, phenytoin, carbamazepine, phenobarbital, or St. John's wort) may significantly decrease exposure to exemestane. Dose modification is recommended for patients who are also receiving a potent CYP 3A4 inducer).
No products indexed under this heading.

Theophylline Dihydroxypropyl (Glyceryl) (Co-medications that induce CYP 3A4 (eg, rifampicin, phenytoin, carbamazepine, phenobarbital, or St. John's wort) may significantly decrease exposure to exemestane. Dose modification is recommended for patients who are also receiving a potent CYP 3A4 inducer).
No products indexed under this heading.

Theophylline Ethylenediamine (Co-medications that induce CYP 3A4 (eg, rifampicin, phenytoin, carbamazepine, phenobarbital, or St. John's wort) may significantly decrease exposure to exemestane. Dose modification is recommended for patients who are also receiving a potent CYP 3A4 inducer).
No products indexed under this heading.

Theophylline Sodium Glycinate (Co-medications that induce CYP 3A4 (eg, rifampicin, phenytoin, carbamazepine, phenobarbital, or St. John's wort) may significantly decrease exposure to exemestane. Dose modification is recommended for patients who are also receiving a potent CYP 3A4 inducer).
No products indexed under this heading.

Triamcinolone (Co-medications that induce CYP 3A4 (eg, rifampicin, phenytoin, carbamazepine, phenobarbital, or St. John's wort) may significantly decrease exposure to exemestane. Dose modification is recommended for patients who are also receiving a potent CYP 3A4 inducer).
No products indexed under this heading.

Triamcinolone Acetonide (Co-medications that induce CYP 3A4 (eg, rifampicin, phenytoin, carbamazepine, phenobarbital, or St. John's wort) may significantly decrease exposure to exemestane. Dose modification is recommended for patients who are also receiving a potent CYP 3A4 inducer). Products include:
Azmacort 408
Nasacort AQ 3019

Triamcinolone Diacetate (Co-medications that induce CYP 3A4 (eg, rifampicin, phenytoin, carbamazepine, phenobarbital, or St. John's wort) may significantly decrease exposure to exemestane. Dose modification is recommended for patients who are also receiving a potent CYP 3A4 inducer).
No products indexed under this heading.

Triamcinolone Hexacetonide (Co-medications that induce CYP 3A4 (eg, rifampicin, phenytoin, carbamazepine, phenobarbital, or St. John's wort) may significantly decrease exposure to exemestane. Dose modification is recommended for patients who are also receiving a potent CYP 3A4 inducer).
No products indexed under this heading.

Troglitazone (Co-medications that induce CYP 3A4 (eg, rifampicin, phenytoin, carbamazepine, phenobarbital, or St. John's wort) may significantly decrease exposure to exemestane. Dose modification is recommended for patients who are also receiving a potent CYP 3A4 inducer).
No products indexed under this heading.

Food Interactions
Food, unspecified (Exemestane plasma levels increased by approximately 40% after a high-fat breakfast).
Meal, unspecified (Exemestane plasma levels increased by approximately 40% after a high-fat breakfast).

ARRANON INJECTION
(Nelarabine) 1327
Pentostatin (Co-administration of nelarabine with adenosine deaminase inhibitors, such as pentostatin, is not recommended).
No products indexed under this heading.

ASACOL DELAYED-RELEASE TABLETS
(Mesalamine) 2786
None cited in PDR database.

ASACOL HD DELAYED-RELEASE TABLETS
(Mesalamine) 2787
Fat (A high fat meal does not affect the extent of systemic exposure to mesalamine after single-dose administration of mesalamine, but mesalamine C_{max} decreases by 47% and t_{max} is delayed by 14 hours under fed conditions).
No products indexed under this heading.

Food Interactions
Food, unspecified (A high fat meal does not affect the extent of systemic exposure to mesalamine after single-dose administration of mesalamine, but mesalamine C_{max} decreases by 47% and t_{max} is delayed by 14 hours under fed conditions).

Meal, unspecified (A high fat meal does not affect the extent of systemic exposure to mesalamine after single-dose administration of mesalamine, but mesalamine C_{max} decreases by 47% and t_{max} is delayed by 14 hours under fed conditions).

ASMANEX TWISTHALER
(Mometasone Furoate) 3058
Ketoconazole (Ketoconazone, a strong inhibitor of cytochrome P4503A4, may increase plasma levels of mometasone furoate during concomitant dosing). Products include:
Extina 3319
Xolegel 3337

ATACAND TABLETS
(Candesartan Cilexetil) 697
May interact with lithium preparations. Compounds in these categories include:

Lithium (An increase in serum lithium concentration has been reported during concomitant administration of lithium with candesartan cilexetil, so careful monitoring of serum lithium levels is recommended during concomitant use).
No products indexed under this heading.

Lithium Carbonate (An increase in serum lithium concentration has been reported during concomitant administration of lithium with candesartan cilexetil, so careful monitoring of serum lithium levels is recommended during concomitant use).
No products indexed under this heading.

Lithium Citrate (An increase in serum lithium concentration has been reported during concomitant administration of lithium with candesartan cilexetil, so careful monitoring of serum lithium levels is recommended during concomitant use).
No products indexed under this heading.

ATACAND HCT 16-12.5 TABLETS
(Candesartan Cilexetil, Hydrochlorothiazide)............................ 700
May interact with alcohols, antihypertensives, barbiturates, corticosteroids, insulin, lithium preparations, narcotic analgesics, non-steroidal anti-inflammatory agents, nondepolarizing neuromuscular blocking agents, oral hypoglycemic agents, and certain other agents. Compounds in these categories include:

Acarbose (Hyperglycemia may occur with thiazide diuretics; dosage adjustment of the antidiabetic drugs may be required).
No products indexed under this heading.

Acebutolol Hydrochloride (Co-administration with other antihypertensive drugs may result in additive effect or potentiation of the antihypertensive effects with a potential for aggravation of orthostatic hypotension).
No products indexed under this heading.

ACTH (Co-administration with ACTH intensifies the electrolyte depletion, particularly hypokalemia).
No products indexed under this heading.

Alclometasone Dipropionate (Co-administration with corticosteroids intensifies the electrolyte depletion, particularly hypokalemia).
No products indexed under this heading.

Alfentanil Hydrochloride (Narcotics may aggravate hypotension produced by hydrochlorothiazide).
No products indexed under this heading.

Aliskiren (Co-administration with other antihypertensive drugs may result in additive effect or potentiation of the antihypertensive effects with a potential for aggravation of orthostatic hypotension). Products include:

Tekturna 2538
Tekturna HCT 2541
Valturna 3637

Amlodipine Besylate (Co-administration with other antihypertensive drugs may result in additive effect or potentiation of the antihypertensive effects with a potential for aggravation of orthostatic hypotension). Products include:
Azor 1010
Exforge 2443
Exforge HCT 2449

Amobarbital (Barbiturates may aggravate orthostatic hypotension produced by hydrochlorothiazide).
No products indexed under this heading.

Amobarbital Sodium (Barbiturates may aggravate orthostatic hypotension produced by hydrochlorothiazide).
No products indexed under this heading.

Apomorphine (Narcotics may aggravate hypotension produced by hydrochlorothiazide).
No products indexed under this heading.

Apomorphine Hydrochloride (Narcotics may aggravate hypotension produced by hydrochlorothiazide).
No products indexed under this heading.

Aprobarbital (Barbiturates may aggravate orthostatic hypotension produced by hydrochlorothiazide).
No products indexed under this heading.

Atenolol (Co-administration with other antihypertensive drugs may result in additive effect or potentiation of the antihypertensive effects with a potential for aggravation of orthostatic hypotension).
No products indexed under this heading.

Atracurium Besylate (Possible increased responsiveness to the muscle relaxant).
No products indexed under this heading.

Beclomethasone Dipropionate (Co-administration with corticosteroids intensifies the electrolyte depletion, particularly hypokalemia). Products include:
Qvar 3398

Beclomethasone Dipropionate Monohydrate (Co-administration with corticosteroids intensifies the electrolyte depletion, particularly hypokalemia). Products include:
Beconase AQ 1386

Benazepril Hydrochloride (Co-administration with other antihypertensive drugs may result in additive effect or potentiation of the antihypertensive effects with a potential for aggravation of orthostatic hypotension).
No products indexed under this heading.

Bendroflumethiazide (Co-administration with other antihypertensive drugs may result in additive effect or potentiation of the antihypertensive effects with a potential for aggravation of orthostatic hypotension).
No products indexed under this heading.

Betamethasone (Co-administration with corticosteroids intensifies the electrolyte depletion, particularly hypokalemia).
No products indexed under this heading.

Betamethasone Acetate (Co-administration with corticosteroids intensifies the electrolyte depletion, particularly hypokalemia).
No products indexed under this heading.

Betamethasone Benzoate (Co-administration with corticosteroids intensifies the electrolyte depletion, particularly hypokalemia).
No products indexed under this heading.

Betamethasone Dipropionate (Co-administration with corticosteroids intensifies the electrolyte depletion, particularly hypokalemia). Products include:
Diprolene Lotion 0.05% 3108

IMPORTANT NOTE: Always consult each drug listing in the patient's regimen for possible interactions.

(⊙ Described in PDR® for Ophthalmic Medicines)

Fludrocortisone Acetate (Co-administration with corticosteroids intensifies the electrolyte depletion, particularly hypokalemia).
No products indexed under this heading.

Flumethasone Pivalate (Co-administration with corticosteroids intensifies the electrolyte depletion, particularly hypokalemia).
No products indexed under this heading.

Flunisolide Hemihydrate (Co-administration with corticosteroids intensifies the electrolyte depletion, particularly hypokalemia).
No products indexed under this heading.

Flurbiprofen (Co-administration of non-steroidal anti-inflammatory agents can reduce the diuretic, natriuretic, and antihypertensive effects of thiazide diuretics).
No products indexed under this heading.

Fluticasone Furoate (Co-administration with corticosteroids intensifies the electrolyte depletion, particularly hypokalemia). Products include:
Veramyst 1713

Fluticasone Propionate (Co-administration with corticosteroids intensifies the electrolyte depletion, particularly hypokalemia). Products include:
Advair 100/50 1275
Advair 250/50 1275
Advair 500/50 1275
Advair HFA 45/21 1288
Advair HFA 115/21 1288
Advair HFA 230/21 1288
Flonase 1459
Flovent Diskus 1463
Flovent HFA 1470

Fosinopril Sodium (Co-administration with other antihypertensive drugs may result in additive effect or potentiation of the antihypertensive effects with a potential for aggravation of orthostatic hypotension).
No products indexed under this heading.

Furosemide (Co-administration with other antihypertensive drugs may result in additive effect or potentiation of the antihypertensive effects with a potential for aggravation of orthostatic hypotension). Products include:
Furosemide 2354

Gallamine (Possible increased responsiveness to the muscle relaxant).
No products indexed under this heading.

Gallamine Triethiodide (Possible increased responsiveness to the muscle relaxant).
No products indexed under this heading.

Glibenclamide (Hyperglycemia may occur with thiazide diuretics; dosage adjustment of the antidiabetic drugs may be required).
No products indexed under this heading.

Glimepiride (Hyperglycemia may occur with thiazide diuretics; dosage adjustment of the antidiabetic drugs may be required). Products include:
Avandaryl 1356
Duetact 3354

Glipizide (Hyperglycemia may occur with thiazide diuretics; dosage adjustment of the antidiabetic drugs may be required).
No products indexed under this heading.

Glyburide (Hyperglycemia may occur with thiazide diuretics; dosage adjustment of the antidiabetic drugs may be required).
No products indexed under this heading.

Guanabenz Acetate (Co-administration with other antihypertensive drugs may result in additive effect or potentiation of the antihypertensive effects with a potential for aggravation of orthostatic hypotension).
No products indexed under this heading.

Guanethidine (Co-administration with other antihypertensive drugs may result in additive effect or potentiation of the antihypertensive effects with a potential for aggravation of orthostatic hypotension).
No products indexed under this heading.

Guanethidine Monosulfate (Co-administration with other antihypertensive drugs may result in additive effect or potentiation of the antihypertensive effects with a potential for aggravation of orthostatic hypotension).
No products indexed under this heading.

Guanethidine Sulfate (Co-administration with other antihypertensive drugs may result in additive effect or potentiation of the antihypertensive effects with a potential for aggravation of orthostatic hypotension).
No products indexed under this heading.

Hexobarbital (Barbiturates may aggravate orthostatic hypotension produced by hydrochlorothiazide).
No products indexed under this heading.

Hydralazine Hydrochloride (Co-administration with other antihypertensive drugs may result in additive effect or potentiation of the antihypertensive effects with a potential for aggravation of orthostatic hypotension).
No products indexed under this heading.

Hydrocodone Bitartrate (Narcotics may aggravate hypotension produced by hydrochlorothiazide). Products include:
Vicodin 560
Vicodin ES 561
Vicodin HP 563
Vicoprofen 564
Zydone 1138

Hydrocodone Polistirex (Narcotics may aggravate hypotension produced by hydrochlorothiazide). Products include:
Tussionex 3443

Hydrocortisone (Co-administration with corticosteroids intensifies the electrolyte depletion, particularly hypokalemia).
No products indexed under this heading.

Hydrocortisone (Alcohol) (Co-administration with corticosteroids intensifies the electrolyte depletion, particularly hypokalemia).
No products indexed under this heading.

Hydrocortisone Acetate (Co-administration with corticosteroids intensifies the electrolyte depletion, particularly hypokalemia).
No products indexed under this heading.

Hydrocortisone Butyrate (Co-administration with corticosteroids intensifies the electrolyte depletion, particularly hypokalemia).
No products indexed under this heading.

Hydrocortisone Cypionate (Co-administration with corticosteroids intensifies the electrolyte depletion, particularly hypokalemia).
No products indexed under this heading.

Hydrocortisone Hemisuccinate (Co-administration with corticosteroids intensifies the electrolyte depletion, particularly hypokalemia).
No products indexed under this heading.

Hydrocortisone Probutate (Co-administration with corticosteroids intensifies the electrolyte depletion, particularly hypokalemia).
No products indexed under this heading.

Hydrocortisone Sodium Phosphate (Co-administration with corticosteroids intensifies the electrolyte depletion, particularly hypokalemia).
No products indexed under this heading.

Hydrocortisone Sodium Succinate (Co-administration with corticosteroids intensifies the electrolyte depletion, particularly hypokalemia).
No products indexed under this heading.

Hydrocortisone Valerate (Co-administration with corticosteroids intensifies the electrolyte depletion, particularly hypokalemia).
No products indexed under this heading.

Hydroflumethiazide (Co-administration with other antihypertensive drugs may result in additive effect or potentiation of the antihypertensive effects with a potential for aggravation of orthostatic hypotension).
No products indexed under this heading.

Hydromorphone (Narcotics may aggravate hypotension produced by hydrochlorothiazide).
No products indexed under this heading.

Hydromorphone Hydrochloride (Narcotics may aggravate hypotension produced by hydrochlorothiazide). Products include:
Dilaudid Injection 2800
Dilaudid Oral 2797
Dilaudid Tablets 2797
Dilaudid-HP 2800

Ibuprofen (Co-administration of non-steroidal anti-inflammatory agents can reduce the diuretic, natriuretic, and antihypertensive effects of thiazide diuretics). Products include:
Motrin IB 2043
Children's Motrin 2044
Children's Motrin Non-Staining Dye-Free 2044
Infants' Motrin 2044
Infants' Motrin Dye-Free 2044
Junior Strength Motrin 2044
Vicoprofen 564

Indapamide (Co-administration with other antihypertensive drugs may result in additive effect or potentiation of the antihypertensive effects with a potential for aggravation of orthostatic hypotension). Products include:
Indapamide 2356

Indomethacin (Co-administration of non-steroidal anti-inflammatory agents can reduce the diuretic, natriuretic, and antihypertensive effects of thiazide diuretics). Products include:
Indocin 2167

Indomethacin Sodium Trihydrate (Co-administration of non-steroidal anti-inflammatory agents can reduce the diuretic, natriuretic, and antihypertensive effects of thiazide diuretics). Products include:
Indocin I.V. 2007

Insulin (Hyperglycemia may occur with thiazide diuretics; dosage adjustment of the insulin may be required).
No products indexed under this heading.

Insulin, Human, Zinc Suspension (Hyperglycemia may occur with thiazide diuretics; dosage adjustment of the insulin may be required).
No products indexed under this heading.

Insulin, Human (rDNA origin) (Hyperglycemia may occur with thiazide diuretics; dosage adjustment of the insulin may be required). Products include:
Exubera 2717

Insulin, Human NPH (Hyperglycemia may occur with thiazide diuretics; dosage adjustment of the insulin may be required). Products include:
Humulin N Vial 1934

Insulin, Human Regular (Hyperglycemia may occur with thiazide diuretics; dosage adjustment of the insulin may be required). Products include:
Humulin R 1937
Humulin R (U-500) 1939

Insulin, Human Regular and Human NPH Mixture (Hyperglycemia

may occur with thiazide diuretics; dosage adjustment of the insulin may be required). Products include:
Humulin 50/50 1930
Humulin 70/30 Vial 1931

Insulin, NPH (Hyperglycemia may occur with thiazide diuretics; dosage adjustment of the insulin may be required).
No products indexed under this heading.

Insulin, Regular (Hyperglycemia may occur with thiazide diuretics; dosage adjustment of the insulin may be required).
No products indexed under this heading.

Insulin, Regular and NPH mixture (Hyperglycemia may occur with thiazide diuretics; dosage adjustment of the insulin may be required).
No products indexed under this heading.

Insulin, Zinc Crystals (Hyperglycemia may occur with thiazide diuretics; dosage adjustment of the insulin may be required).
No products indexed under this heading.

Insulin, Zinc Suspension (Hyperglycemia may occur with thiazide diuretics; dosage adjustment of the insulin may be required).
No products indexed under this heading.

Insulin Aspart (Hyperglycemia may occur with thiazide diuretics; dosage adjustment of the insulin may be required).
No products indexed under this heading.

Insulin Aspart, Human (Hyperglycemia may occur with thiazide diuretics; dosage adjustment of the insulin may be required). Products include:
NovoLog Mix 70/30 2581

Insulin Aspart, Human Regular (Hyperglycemia may occur with thiazide diuretics; dosage adjustment of the insulin may be required). Products include:
NovoLog 2575

Insulin Aspart Protamine, Human (Hyperglycemia may occur with thiazide diuretics; dosage adjustment of the insulin may be required). Products include:
NovoLog Mix 70/30 2581

Insulin Detemir (rDNA Origin) (Hyperglycemia may occur with thiazide diuretics; dosage adjustment of the insulin may be required). Products include:
Levemir 2566

Insulin Glargine (Hyperglycemia may occur with thiazide diuretics; dosage adjustment of the insulin may be required). Products include:
Lantus 2996

Insulin Glulisine (Hyperglycemia may occur with thiazide diuretics; dosage adjustment of the insulin may be required). Products include:
Apidra 2937
Apidra SoloStar 2937

Insulin Lispro, Human (Hyperglycemia may occur with thiazide diuretics; dosage adjustment of the insulin may be required). Products include:
Humalog 1910
Humalog Mix 1914
Humalog Mix 75/25 1917

Insulin Lispro Protamine, Human (Hyperglycemia may occur with thiazide diuretics; dosage adjustment of the insulin may be required). Products include:
Humalog Mix 1914
Humalog Mix 75/25 1917

Irbesartan (Co-administration with other antihypertensive drugs may result in additive effect or potentiation of the antihypertensive effects with a potential for aggravation of orthostatic hypotension). Products include:
Avalide 2956

IMPORTANT NOTE: Always consult each drug listing in the patient's regimen for possible interactions.

Avapro 2962

Isradipine (Co-administration with other antihypertensive drugs may result in additive effect or potentiation of the antihypertensive effects with a potential for aggravation of orthostatic hypotension). Products include:
DynaCirc CR 1432

Ketoprofen (Co-administration of non-steroidal anti-inflammatory agents can reduce the diuretic, natriuretic, and antihypertensive effects of thiazide diuretics).
No products indexed under this heading.

Ketorolac Tromethamine (Co-administration of non-steroidal anti-inflammatory agents can reduce the diuretic, natriuretic, and antihypertensive effects of thiazide diuretics). Products include:
Acuvail .... ⊙209

Labetalol Hydrochloride (Co-administration with other antihypertensive drugs may result in additive effect or potentiation of the antihypertensive effects with a potential for aggravation of orthostatic hypotension).
No products indexed under this heading.

Levorphanol Tartrate (Narcotics may aggravate hypotension produced by hydrochlorothiazide).
No products indexed under this heading.

Lisinopril (Co-administration with other antihypertensive drugs may result in additive effect or potentiation of the antihypertensive effects with a potential for aggravation of orthostatic hypotension). Products include:
Prinivil 2241
Prinzide 2246

Lithium (Hydrochlorothiazide reduces the renal clearance of lithium and can cause a high risk of lithium toxicity; in general, lithium should not be given with diuretics. An increase in serum lithium concentration has been reported during concomitant administration of lithium with candesartan cilexetil; careful monitoring of serum lithium levels is recommended during concomitant use).
No products indexed under this heading.

Lithium Carbonate (Hydrochlorothiazide reduces the renal clearance of lithium and can cause a high risk of lithium toxicity; in general, lithium should not be given with diuretics. An increase in serum lithium concentration has been reported during concomitant administration of lithium with candesartan cilexetil; careful monitoring of serum lithium levels is recommended during concomitant use).
No products indexed under this heading.

Lithium Citrate (Hydrochlorothiazide reduces the renal clearance of lithium and can cause a high risk of lithium toxicity; in general, lithium should not be given with diuretics. An increase in serum lithium concentration has been reported during concomitant administration of lithium with candesartan cilexetil; careful monitoring of serum lithium levels is recommended during concomitant use).
No products indexed under this heading.

Losartan Potassium (Co-administration with other antihypertensive drugs may result in additive effect or potentiation of the antihypertensive effects with a potential for aggravation of orthostatic hypotension). Products include:
Cozaar 2106
Hyzaar 2162
Hyzaar 100-12.5 2162

Mecamylamine Hydrochloride (Co-administration with other antihypertensive drugs may result in additive effect or potentiation of the antihypertensive effects with a potential for aggravation of orthostatic hypotension).
No products indexed under this heading.

Meclofenamate Sodium (Co-administration of non-steroidal anti-inflammatory agents can reduce the diuretic, natriuretic, and antihypertensive effects of thiazide diuretics).
No products indexed under this heading.

Mefenamic Acid (Co-administration of non-steroidal anti-inflammatory agents can reduce the diuretic, natriuretic, and antihypertensive effects of thiazide diuretics).
No products indexed under this heading.

Meloxicam (Co-administration of non-steroidal anti-inflammatory agents can reduce the diuretic, natriuretic, and antihypertensive effects of thiazide diuretics).
No products indexed under this heading.

Meperidine Hydrochloride (Narcotics may aggravate hypotension produced by hydrochlorothiazide).
No products indexed under this heading.

Mephobarbital (Barbiturates may aggravate orthostatic hypotension produced by hydrochlorothiazide).
No products indexed under this heading.

Metformin Hydrochloride (Hyperglycemia may occur with thiazide diuretics; dosage adjustment of the antidiabetic drugs may be required). Products include:
ActoPlus 3338
Avandamet 1345
Janumet 2188

Methadone Hydrochloride (Narcotics may aggravate hypotension produced by hydrochlorothiazide).
No products indexed under this heading.

Methyclothiazide (Co-administration with other antihypertensive drugs may result in additive effect or potentiation of the antihypertensive effects with a potential for aggravation of orthostatic hypotension).
No products indexed under this heading.

Methyldopa (Co-administration with other antihypertensive drugs may result in additive effect or potentiation of the antihypertensive effects with a potential for aggravation of orthostatic hypotension).
No products indexed under this heading.

Methyldopate Hydrochloride (Co-administration with other antihypertensive drugs may result in additive effect or potentiation of the antihypertensive effects with a potential for aggravation of orthostatic hypotension).
No products indexed under this heading.

Methylprednisolone (Co-administration with corticosteroids intensifies the electrolyte depletion, particularly hypokalemia).
No products indexed under this heading.

Methylprednisolone Acetate (Co-administration with corticosteroids intensifies the electrolyte depletion, particularly hypokalemia).
No products indexed under this heading.

Methylprednisolone Sodium Succinate (Co-administration with corticosteroids intensifies the electrolyte depletion, particularly hypokalemia).
No products indexed under this heading.

Metocurine Iodide (Possible increased responsiveness to the muscle relaxant).
No products indexed under this heading.

Metolazone (Co-administration with other antihypertensive drugs may result in additive effect or potentiation of the antihypertensive effects with a potential for aggravation of orthostatic hypotension).
No products indexed under this heading.

Metoprolol Succinate (Co-administration with other antihypertensive drugs may result in additive effect or potentiation of the antihypertensive effects with a potential for aggravation of orthostatic hypotension). Products include:
Toprol XL 732

Metoprolol Tartrate (Co-administration with other antihypertensive drugs may result in additive effect or potentiation of the antihypertensive effects with a potential for aggravation of orthostatic hypotension).
No products indexed under this heading.

Metyrosine (Co-administration with other antihypertensive drugs may result in additive effect or potentiation of the antihypertensive effects with a potential for aggravation of orthostatic hypotension).
No products indexed under this heading.

Mibefradil Dihydrochloride (Co-administration with other antihypertensive drugs may result in additive effect or potentiation of the antihypertensive effects with a potential for aggravation of orthostatic hypotension).
No products indexed under this heading.

Miglitol (Hyperglycemia may occur with thiazide diuretics; dosage adjustment of the antidiabetic drugs may be required).
No products indexed under this heading.

Minoxidil (Co-administration with other antihypertensive drugs may result in additive effect or potentiation of the antihypertensive effects with a potential for aggravation of orthostatic hypotension).
No products indexed under this heading.

Mivacurium Chloride (Possible increased responsiveness to the muscle relaxant).
No products indexed under this heading.

Moexipril Hydrochloride (Co-administration with other antihypertensive drugs may result in additive effect or potentiation of the antihypertensive effects with a potential for aggravation of orthostatic hypotension).
No products indexed under this heading.

Mometasone Furoate (Co-administration with corticosteroids intensifies the electrolyte depletion, particularly hypokalemia). Products include:
Asmanex 3058
Elocon Cream 3111
Elocon Lotion 3112
Elocon Ointment 3114

Mometasone Furoate Monohydrate (Co-administration with corticosteroids intensifies the electrolyte depletion, particularly hypokalemia). Products include:
Nasonex 3166

Morphine Sulfate (Narcotics may aggravate hypotension produced by hydrochlorothiazide). Products include:
Avinza 1822
Embeda 1831
MS Contin 2803

Morphine Sulfate, Liposomal (Narcotics may aggravate hypotension produced by hydrochlorothiazide).
No products indexed under this heading.

Nabumetone (Co-administration of non-steroidal anti-inflammatory agents can reduce the diuretic, natriuretic, and antihypertensive effects of thiazide diuretics).
No products indexed under this heading.

Nadolol (Co-administration with other antihypertensive drugs may result in additive effect or potentiation of the antihypertensive effects with a potential for aggravation of orthostatic hypotension). Products include:
Nadolol 2359

Naproxen (Co-administration of non-steroidal anti-inflammatory agents can reduce the diuretic, natriuretic, and antihypertensive effects of thiazide diuretics). Products include:
EC-Naprosyn 2850
Naprosyn 2850
Anaprox/Naprosyn 2850

Naproxen Sodium (Co-administration of non-steroidal anti-inflammatory agents can reduce the diuretic, natriuretic, and antihypertensive effects of thiazide diuretics). Products include:
Anaprox 2850
Anaprox DS 2850
Treximet 1681

Nateglinide (Hyperglycemia may occur with thiazide diuretics; dosage adjustment of the antidiabetic drugs may be required).
No products indexed under this heading.

Nebivolol (Co-administration with other antihypertensive drugs may result in additive effect or potentiation of the antihypertensive effects with a potential for aggravation of orthostatic hypotension). Products include:
Bystolic 1147

Nicardipine Hydrochloride (Co-administration with other antihypertensive drugs may result in additive effect or potentiation of the antihypertensive effects with a potential for aggravation of orthostatic hypotension).
No products indexed under this heading.

Nifedipine (Co-administration with other antihypertensive drugs may result in additive effect or potentiation of the antihypertensive effects with a potential for aggravation of orthostatic hypotension).
No products indexed under this heading.

Nisoldipine (Co-administration with other antihypertensive drugs may result in additive effect or potentiation of the antihypertensive effects with a potential for aggravation of orthostatic hypotension).
No products indexed under this heading.

Nitroglycerin (Co-administration with other antihypertensive drugs may result in additive effect or potentiation of the antihypertensive effects with a potential for aggravation of orthostatic hypotension). Products include:
Nitro-Dur 3170
Nitrolingual 3266

Norepinephrine Bitartrate (Possible decreased response to pressor amines).
No products indexed under this heading.

Oxaprozin (Co-administration of non-steroidal anti-inflammatory agents can reduce the diuretic, natriuretic, and antihypertensive effects of thiazide diuretics).
No products indexed under this heading.

Oxycodone Hydrochloride (Narcotics may aggravate hypotension produced by hydrochlorothiazide). Products include:
OxyContin 2807
Percocet 1121
Percodan 1124

Oxycodone Terephthalate (Narcotics may aggravate hypotension produced by hydrochlorothiazide).
No products indexed under this heading.

Oxymorphone Hydrochloride (Narcotics may aggravate hypotension produced by hydrochlorothiazide). Products include:
Opana 1110

(⊙ Described in PDR® for Ophthalmic Medicines)

IMPORTANT NOTE: Always consult each drug listing in the patient's regimen for possible interactions.

Tubocurarine Chloride (Possible increased responsiveness to the muscle relaxant).

No products indexed under this heading.

Valdecoxib (Co-administration of non-steroidal anti-inflammatory agents can reduce the diuretic, natriuretic, and anti-hypertensive effects of thiazide diuretics).

No products indexed under this heading.

Valsartan (Co-administration with other antihypertensive drugs may result in additive effect or potentiation of the antihypertensive effects with a potential for aggravation of orthostatic hypotension). Products include:

Diovan 2413
Diovan HCT 2419
Exforge 2443
Exforge HCT 2449
Valturna 3637

Vecuronium Bromide (Possible increased responsiveness to the muscle relaxant).

No products indexed under this heading.

Verapamil Hydrochloride (Co-administration with other antihypertensive drugs may result in additive effect or potentiation of the antihypertensive effects with a potential for aggravation of orthostatic hypotension). Products include:

Tarka 534

Food Interactions

Alcohol (May aggravate orthostatic hypotension produced by hydrochlorothiazide).

Beer, reduced-alcohol (May aggravate orthostatic hypotension produced by hydrochlorothiazide).

Beer, unspecified (May aggravate orthostatic hypotension produced by hydrochlorothiazide).

Wine, Chianti (May aggravate orthostatic hypotension produced by hydrochlorothiazide).

Wine, Red (May aggravate orthostatic hypotension produced by hydrochlorothiazide).

Wine, unspecified (May aggravate orthostatic hypotension produced by hydrochlorothiazide).

Wine products (May aggravate orthostatic hypotension produced by hydrochlorothiazide).

ATACAND HCT 32-12.5 TABLETS

(Candesartan Cilexetil,
Hydrochlorothiazide) 700
See Atacand HCT 16-12.5 Tablets

ATRIPLA TABLETS

(Efavirenz, Emtricitabine, Tenofovir
Disoproxil Fumarate) 906
May interact with cytochrome p450 2c19 substrates (selected), cytochrome p450 2c9 substrates (selected), cytochrome p450 3a4 inducers (selected), cytochrome p450 3a4 substrates (selected), nephrotoxic agents, and certain other agents. Compounds in these categories include:

Abacavir Sulfate (Renal impairment, including cases of acute renal failure and Fanconi syndrome (renal tubular injury with severe hypophosphatemia), has been reported in association with the use of tenofovir DF. The majority of these cases occurred in patients with underlying systemic or renal disease, or in patients taking nephrotoxic agents; however, some cases occured in patients without identified risk factors. Atripla should be avoided with concurrent or recent use of a nephrotoxic agent). Products include:

Epzicom 1448

Trizivir 1688
Ziagen 1740

Acarbose (In vitro studies have demonstrated that efavirenz inhibits CYP2C9 in the range of observed efavirenz plasma concentrations. Co-administration of efavirenz with drugs primarily metabolized by CYP2C9 may result in altered plasma concentrations of the co-administered drug. Therefore, appropriate dose adjustments may be necessary for these drugs).

No products indexed under this heading.

Acyclovir (Since emtricitabine and tenofovir are primarily eliminated by the kidneys, co-administration of ATRIPLA with drugs that reduce renal fuction or compete for active tubular secretion may increase serum concentrations of emtricitabine, tenofovir, and/or other renally eliminated drugs). Products include:

Zovirax 1760

Acyclovir Sodium (Since emtricitabine and tenofovir are primarily eliminated by the kidneys, co-administration of ATRIPLA with drugs that reduce renal fuction or compete for active tubular secretion may increase serum concentrations of emtricitabine, tenofovir, and/or other renally eliminated drugs).

No products indexed under this heading.

Adefovir dipivoxil (Since emtricitabine and tenofovir are primarily eliminated by the kidneys, co-administration of ATRIPLA with drugs that reduce renal fuction or compete for active tubular secretion may increase serum concentrations of emtricitabine, tenofovir, and/or other renally eliminated drugs). Products include:

Hepsera 1244

Alatrofloxacin Mesylate (Renal impairment, including cases of acute renal failure and Fanconi syndrome (renal tubular injury with severe hypophosphatemia), has been reported in association with the use of tenofovir DF. The majority of these cases occurred in patients with underlying systemic or renal disease, or in patients taking nephrotoxic agents; however, some cases occured in patients without identified risk factors. Atripla should be avoided with concurrent or recent use of a nephrotoxic agent).

No products indexed under this heading.

Aldesleukin (Renal impairment, including cases of acute renal failure and Fanconi syndrome (renal tubular injury with severe hypophosphatemia), has been reported in association with the use of tenofovir DF. The majority of these cases occurred in patients with underlying systemic or renal disease, or in patients taking nephrotoxic agents; however, some cases occured in patients without identified risk factors. Atripla should be avoided with concurrent or recent use of a nephrotoxic agent). Products include:

Proleukin 2504

Alfentanil Hydrochloride (Efavirenz has been shown in vivo to induce CYP3A4. Other compounds that are substrates of CYP3A4 may have decreased plasma concentrations when co-administered with efavirenz).

No products indexed under this heading.

Allium sativum (Drugs which induce CYP3A4 activity would be expected to increase the clearance of efavirenz resulting in lower plasma concentrations).

No products indexed under this heading.

Alprazolam (Efavirenz has been shown in vivo to induce CYP3A4. Other compounds that are substrates of CYP3A4 may have decreased plasma concentrations when co-administered with efavirenz).

No products indexed under this heading.

Amikacin Sulfate (Renal impairment, including cases of acute renal failure and Fanconi syndrome (renal tubular injury with severe hypophosphatemia), has been reported in association with the use of tenofovir DF. The majority of these cases occurred in patients with underlying systemic or renal disease, or in patients taking nephrotoxic agents; however, some cases occured in patients without identified risk factors. Atripla should be avoided with concurrent or recent use of a nephrotoxic agent).

No products indexed under this heading.

Aminoglutethimide (Drugs which induce CYP3A4 activity would be expected to increase the clearance of efavirenz resulting in lower plasma concentrations).

No products indexed under this heading.

Amiodarone Hydrochloride (Efavirenz has been shown in vivo to induce CYP3A4. Other compounds that are substrates of CYP3A4 may have decreased plasma concentrations when co-administered with efavirenz).

No products indexed under this heading.

Amitriptyline Hydrochloride (Efavirenz has been shown in vivo to induce CYP3A4. Other compounds that are substrates of CYP3A4 may have decreased plasma concentrations when co-administered with efavirenz).

No products indexed under this heading.

Amlodipine Besylate (Efavirenz has been shown in vivo to induce CYP3A4. Other compounds that are substrates of CYP3A4 may have decreased plasma concentrations when co-administered with efavirenz). Products include:

Azor 1010
Exforge 2443
Exforge HCT 2449

Amoxapine (In vitro studies have demonstrated that efavirenz inhibits CYP2C19 in the range of observed efavirenz plasma concentrations. Co-administration of efavirenz with drugs primarily metabolized by CYP2C19 may result in altered plasma concentrations of the co-administered drug. Therefore, appropriate dose adjustments may be necessary for these drugs).

No products indexed under this heading.

Amoxicillin (Renal impairment, including cases of acute renal failure and Fanconi syndrome (renal tubular injury with severe hypophosphatemia), has been reported in association with the use of tenofovir DF. The majority of these cases occurred in patients with underlying systemic or renal disease, or in patients taking nephrotoxic agents; however, some cases occured in patients without identified risk factors. Atripla should be avoided with concurrent or recent use of a nephrotoxic agent). Products include:

Amoxil Capsules 1311
Amoxil Chewable Tablets 1311
Amoxil 1311
Amoxil Powder 1311
Augmentin 1331
Augmentin Tablets 1335
Augmentin ES-600 1338
Augmentin XR 1342
Moxatag 2321

Amoxicillin Trihydrate (Renal impairment, including cases of acute renal failure and Fanconi syndrome (renal tubular injury with severe hypophosphatemia), has been reported in association with the use of tenofovir DF. The majority of these cases occurred in patients with underlying systemic or renal disease, or in patients taking nephrotoxic agents; however, some cases occured in patients without identi-

fied risk factors. Atripla should be avoided with concurrent or recent use of a nephrotoxic agent).

No products indexed under this heading.

Amphotericin B (Renal impairment, including cases of acute renal failure and Fanconi syndrome (renal tubular injury with severe hypophosphatemia), has been reported in association with the use of tenofovir DF. The majority of these cases occurred in patients with underlying systemic or renal disease, or in patients taking nephrotoxic agents; however, some cases occured in patients without identified risk factors. Atripla should be avoided with concurrent or recent use of a nephrotoxic agent).

No products indexed under this heading.

Amphotericin B, liposomal (Renal impairment, including cases of acute renal failure and Fanconi syndrome (renal tubular injury with severe hypophosphatemia), has been reported in association with the use of tenofovir DF. The majority of these cases occurred in patients with underlying systemic or renal disease, or in patients taking nephrotoxic agents; however, some cases occured in patients without identified risk factors. Atripla should be avoided with concurrent or recent use of a nephrotoxic agent). Products include:

AmBisome 659

Amphotericin B Cholesteryl Sulfate (Renal impairment, including cases of acute renal failure and Fanconi syndrome (renal tubular injury with severe hypophosphatemia), has been reported in association with the use of tenofovir DF. The majority of these cases occurred in patients with underlying systemic or renal disease, or in patients taking nephrotoxic agents; however, some cases occured in patients without identified risk factors. Atripla should be avoided with concurrent or recent use of a nephrotoxic agent).

No products indexed under this heading.

Amphotericin B Lipid Complex (Renal impairment, including cases of acute renal failure and Fanconi syndrome (renal tubular injury with severe hypophosphatemia), has been reported in association with the use of tenofovir DF. The majority of these cases occurred in patients with underlying systemic or renal disease, or in patients taking nephrotoxic agents; however, some cases occured in patients without identified risk factors. Atripla should be avoided with concurrent or recent use of a nephrotoxic agent).

No products indexed under this heading.

Ampicillin (Renal impairment, including cases of acute renal failure and Fanconi syndrome (renal tubular injury with severe hypophosphatemia), has been reported in association with the use of tenofovir DF. The majority of these cases occurred in patients with underlying systemic or renal disease, or in patients taking nephrotoxic agents; however, some cases occured in patients without identified risk factors. Atripla should be avoided with concurrent or recent use of a nephrotoxic agent).

No products indexed under this heading.

Ampicillin Sodium (Renal impairment, including cases of acute renal failure and Fanconi syndrome (renal tubular injury with severe hypophosphatemia), has been reported in association with the use of tenofovir DF. The majority of these cases occurred in patients with underlying systemic or renal disease, or in patients taking nephrotoxic agents; however, some cases occured in patients without identi-

161 Interactions Index Atripla

fied risk factors. Atripla should be avoided with concurrent or recent use of a nephrotoxic agent).
No products indexed under this heading.

Ampicillin Trihydrate (Renal impairment, including cases of acute renal failure and Fanconi syndrome (renal tubular injury with severe hypophosphatemia), has been reported in association with the use of tenofovir DF. The majority of these cases occurred in patients with underlying systemic or renal disease, or in patients taking nephrotoxic agents; however, some cases occured in patients without identified risk factors. Atripla should be avoided with concurrent or recent use of a nephrotoxic agent).
No products indexed under this heading.

Amprenavir (Efavirenz has the potential to decrease serum concentrations of amprenavir).
No products indexed under this heading.

Aprepitant (Efavirenz has been shown *in vivo* to induce CYP3A4. Other compounds that are substrates of CYP3A4 may have decreased plasma concentrations when co-administered with efavirenz). Products include:
Emend 2124

Aspirin (Renal impairment, including cases of acute renal failure and Fanconi syndrome (renal tubular injury with severe hypophosphatemia), has been reported in association with the use of tenofovir DF. The majority of these cases occurred in patients with underlying systemic or renal disease, or in patients taking nephrotoxic agents; however, some cases occured in patients without identified risk factors. Atripla should be avoided with concurrent or recent use of a nephrotoxic agent). Products include:
Aggrenox 880
Bayer Aspirin 829
Percodan 1124
St. Joseph Aspirin 2045

Astemizole (Due to the potential for serious and/or life-threatening reactions, such as cardiac arrhythmias with astemizole, concomitant use is contraindicated).
No products indexed under this heading.

Atazanavir (Atazanavir has been shown to increase tenofovir concentrations. The mechanism of this interaction is unknown. Higher tenofovir concentrations could potentiate tenofovir-associated adverse events, including renal disorders. Patients receiving either atazanavir with tenofovir DF should be monitored for tenofovir-associated adverse events. Atripla should be discontinued in patients who develop tenofovir-assocatied adverse events).
No products indexed under this heading.

Atorvastatin Calcium (Plasma concentrations of atorvastatin, pravastatin, and simvastatin decreased with efavirenz. Consult the complete prescribing information for the HMGCoA reductase inhibitor for guidance on individualizing the dose). Products include:
Lipitor 2703

Azithromycin Dihydrate (Renal impairment, including cases of acute renal failure and Fanconi syndrome (renal tubular injury with severe hypophosphatemia), has been reported in association with the use of tenofovir DF. The majority of these cases occurred in patients with underlying systemic or renal disease, or in patients taking nephrotoxic agents; however, some cases occured in patients without identified risk factors. Atripla should be avoided with concurrent or recent use of a nephrotoxic agent).
No products indexed under this heading.

Azlocillin Sodium (Renal impairment, including cases of acute renal failure and Fanconi syndrome (renal tubular injury with severe hypophosphatemia), has been reported in association with the use of tenofovir DF. The majority of these cases occurred in patients with underlying systemic or renal disease, or in patients taking nephrotoxic agents; however, some cases occured in patients without identified risk factors. Atripla should be avoided with concurrent or recent use of a nephrotoxic agent).
No products indexed under this heading.

Aztreonam (Renal impairment, including cases of acute renal failure and Fanconi syndrome (renal tubular injury with severe hypophosphatemia), has been reported in association with the use of tenofovir DF. The majority of these cases occurred in patients with underlying systemic or renal disease, or in patients taking nephrotoxic agents; however, some cases occured in patients without identified risk factors. Atripla should be avoided with concurrent or recent use of a nephrotoxic agent).
No products indexed under this heading.

Bacampicillin Hydrochloride (Renal impairment, including cases of acute renal failure and Fanconi syndrome (renal tubular injury with severe hypophosphatemia), has been reported in association with the use of tenofovir DF. The majority of these cases occurred in patients with underlying systemic or renal disease, or in patients taking nephrotoxic agents; however, some cases occured in patients without identified risk factors. Atripla should be avoided with concurrent or recent use of a nephrotoxic agent).
No products indexed under this heading.

Bacitracin (Renal impairment, including cases of acute renal failure and Fanconi syndrome (renal tubular injury with severe hypophosphatemia), has been reported in association with the use of tenofovir DF. The majority of these cases occurred in patients with underlying systemic or renal disease, or in patients taking nephrotoxic agents; however, some cases occured in patients without identified risk factors. Atripla should be avoided with concurrent or recent use of a nephrotoxic agent).
No products indexed under this heading.

Bacitracin Zinc (Renal impairment, including cases of acute renal failure and Fanconi syndrome (renal tubular injury with severe hypophosphatemia), has been reported in association with the use of tenofovir DF. The majority of these cases occurred in patients with underlying systemic or renal disease, or in patients taking nephrotoxic agents; however, some cases occured in patients without identified risk factors. Atripla should be avoided with concurrent or recent use of a nephrotoxic agent).
No products indexed under this heading.

Balsalazide Disodium (Renal impairment, including cases of acute renal failure and Fanconi syndrome (renal tubular injury with severe hypophosphatemia), has been reported in association with the use of tenofovir DF. The majority of these cases occurred in patients with underlying systemic or renal disease, or in patients taking nephrotoxic agents; however, some cases occured in patients without identified risk factors. Atripla should be avoided with concurrent or recent use of a nephrotoxic agent).
No products indexed under this heading.

Belladonna Ergotamine (Efavirenz has been shown *in vivo* to induce CYP3A4. Other compounds that are substrates of CYP3A4 may have decreased plasma concentrations when co-administered with efavirenz).
No products indexed under this heading.

Benazepril Hydrochloride (Renal impairment, including cases of acute renal failure and Fanconi syndrome (renal tubular injury with severe hypophosphatemia), has been reported in association with the use of tenofovir DF. The majority of these cases occurred in patients with underlying systemic or renal disease, or in patients taking nephrotoxic agents; however, some cases occured in patients without identified risk factors. Atripla should be avoided with concurrent or recent use of a nephrotoxic agent).
No products indexed under this heading.

Bendroflumethiazide (Renal impairment, including cases of acute renal failure and Fanconi syndrome (renal tubular injury with severe hypophosphatemia), has been reported in association with the use of tenofovir DF. The majority of these cases occurred in patients with underlying systemic or renal disease, or in patients taking nephrotoxic agents; however, some cases occured in patients without identified risk factors. Atripla should be avoided with concurrent or recent use of a nephrotoxic agent).
No products indexed under this heading.

Bepridil Hydrochloride (Due to the potential for serious and/or life threatening reactions, such as cardiac arrhythmias, concomitant use with bepridil is contraindicated).
No products indexed under this heading.

Betamethasone (Drugs which induce CYP3A4 activity would be expected to increase the clearance of efavirenz resulting in lower plasma concentrations).
No products indexed under this heading.

Betamethasone Acetate (Drugs which induce CYP3A4 activity would be expected to increase the clearance of efavirenz resulting in lower plasma concentrations).
No products indexed under this heading.

Betamethasone Benzoate (Drugs which induce CYP3A4 activity would be expected to increase the clearance of efavirenz resulting in lower plasma concentrations).
No products indexed under this heading.

Betamethasone Dipropionate (Drugs which induce CYP3A4 activity would be expected to increase the clearance of efavirenz resulting in lower plasma concentrations). Products include:
Diprolene Lotion 0.05% 3108
Diprolene Ointment 0.05% 3109
Diprolene AF Cream 0.05% 3107
Lotrisone 3163

Betamethasone Sodium Phosphate (Drugs which induce CYP3A4 activity would be expected to increase the clearance of efavirenz resulting in lower plasma concentrations).
No products indexed under this heading.

Betamethasone Valerate (Drugs which induce CYP3A4 activity would be expected to increase the clearance of efavirenz resulting in lower plasma concentrations). Products include:
Luxíq 3321

Bosentan (Drugs which induce CYP3A4 activity would be expected to increase the clearance of efavirenz resulting in lower plasma concentrations). Products include:
Tracleer 573

Buspirone Hydrochloride (Efavirenz has been shown *in vivo* to induce CYP3A4. Other compounds that are substrates of CYP3A4 may have decreased plasma concentrations when co-administered with efavirenz).
No products indexed under this heading.

Busulfan (Efavirenz has been shown *in vivo* to induce CYP3A4. Other compounds that are substrates of CYP3A4 may have decreased plasma concentrations when co-administered with efavirenz). Products include:
Myleran 1581

Caffeine (Renal impairment, including cases of acute renal failure and Fanconi syndrome (renal tubular injury with severe hypophosphatemia), has been reported in association with the use of tenofovir DF. The majority of these cases occurred in patients with underlying systemic or renal disease, or in patients taking nephrotoxic agents; however, some cases occured in patients without identified risk factors. Atripla should be avoided with concurrent or recent use of a nephrotoxic agent).
No products indexed under this heading.

Candesartan Cilexetil (In vitro studies have demonstrated that efavirenz inhibits CYP2C9 in the range of observed efavirenz plasma concentrations. Co-administration of efavirenz with drugs primarily metabolized by CYP2C9 may result in altered plasma concentrations of the co-administered drug. Therefore, appropriate dose adjustments may be necessary for these drugs). Products include:
Atacand 697
Atacand HCT 700

Captopril (Renal impairment, including cases of acute renal failure and Fanconi syndrome (renal tubular injury with severe hypophosphatemia), has been reported in association with the use of tenofovir DF. The majority of these cases occurred in patients with underlying systemic or renal disease, or in patients taking nephrotoxic agents; however, some cases occured in patients without identified risk factors. Atripla should be avoided with concurrent or recent use of a nephrotoxic agent). Products include:
Captopril 2341

Carbamazepine (Alternative anticonvulsant treatments should be used due to decreases in both carbamazepine and efavirenz concentrations). Products include:
Carbatrol 3280
Equetro 3477

Carbenicillin Disodium (Renal impairment, including cases of acute renal failure and Fanconi syndrome (renal tubular injury with severe hypophosphatemia), has been reported in association with the use of tenofovir DF. The majority of these cases occurred in patients with underlying systemic or renal disease, or in patients taking nephrotoxic agents; however, some cases occured in patients without identified risk factors. Atripla should be avoided with concurrent or recent use of a nephrotoxic agent).
No products indexed under this heading.

Carbenicillin Indanyl Sodium (Renal impairment, including cases of acute renal failure and Fanconi syndrome (renal tubular injury with severe hypophosphatemia), has been reported in association with the use of tenofovir DF. The majority of these cases occurred in patients with underlying systemic or renal disease, or in patients taking nephrotoxic agents; however, some cases occured in patients without

IMPORTANT NOTE: Always consult each drug listing in the patient's regimen for possible interactions.

identified risk factors. Atripla should be avoided with concurrent or recent use of a nephrotoxic agent).
No products indexed under this heading.

Carboplatin (Renal impairment, including cases of acute renal failure and Fanconi syndrome (renal tubular injury with severe hypophosphatemia), has been reported in association with the use of tenofovir DF. The majority of these cases occurred in patients with underlying systemic or renal disease, or in patients taking nephrotoxic agents; however, some cases occured in patients without identified risk factors. Atripla should be avoided with concurrent or recent use of a nephrotoxic agent).
No products indexed under this heading.

Carisoprodol (In vitro studies have demonstrated that efavirenz inhibits CYP2C19 in the range of observed efavirenz plasma concentrations. Co-administration of efavirenz with drugs primarily metabolized by CYP2C19 may result in altered plasma concentrations of the co-administered drug. Therefore, appropriate dose adjustments may be necessary for these drugs).
No products indexed under this heading.

Carmustine (BCNU) (Renal impairment, including cases of acute renal failure and Fanconi syndrome (renal tubular injury with severe hypophosphatemia), has been reported in association with the use of tenofovir DF. The majority of these cases occurred in patients with underlying systemic or renal disease, or in patients taking nephrotoxic agents; however, some cases occured in patients without identified risk factors. Atripla should be avoided with concurrent or recent use of a nephrotoxic agent).
No products indexed under this heading.

Carvedilol (In vitro studies have demonstrated that efavirenz inhibits CYP2C9 in the range of observed efavirenz plasma concentrations. Co-administration of efavirenz with drugs primarily metabolized by CYP2C9 may result in altered plasma concentrations of the co-administered drug. Therefore, appropriate dose adjustments may be necessary for these drugs). Products include:
Coreg 1409

Cefaclor (Renal impairment, including cases of acute renal failure and Fanconi syndrome (renal tubular injury with severe hypophosphatemia), has been reported in association with the use of tenofovir DF. The majority of these cases occurred in patients with underlying systemic or renal disease, or in patients taking nephrotoxic agents; however, some cases occured in patients without identified risk factors. Atripla should be avoided with concurrent or recent use of a nephrotoxic agent).
No products indexed under this heading.

Cefadroxil (Renal impairment, including cases of acute renal failure and Fanconi syndrome (renal tubular injury with severe hypophosphatemia), has been reported in association with the use of tenofovir DF. The majority of these cases occurred in patients with underlying systemic or renal disease, or in patients taking nephrotoxic agents; however, some cases occured in patients without identified risk factors. Atripla should be avoided with concurrent or recent use of a nephrotoxic agent).
No products indexed under this heading.

Cefamandole Nafate (Renal impairment, including cases of acute renal failure and Fanconi syndrome (renal tubular injury with severe hypophosphatemia), has been reported in associa-

tion with the use of tenofovir DF. The majority of these cases occurred in patients with underlying systemic or renal disease, or in patients taking nephrotoxic agents; however, some cases occured in patients without identified risk factors. Atripla should be avoided with concurrent or recent use of a nephrotoxic agent).
No products indexed under this heading.

Cefazolin Sodium (Renal impairment, including cases of acute renal failure and Fanconi syndrome (renal tubular injury with severe hypophosphatemia), has been reported in association with the use of tenofovir DF. The majority of these cases occurred in patients with underlying systemic or renal disease, or in patients taking nephrotoxic agents; however, some cases occured in patients without identified risk factors. Atripla should be avoided with concurrent or recent use of a nephrotoxic agent).
No products indexed under this heading.

Cefdinir (Renal impairment, including cases of acute renal failure and Fanconi syndrome (renal tubular injury with severe hypophosphatemia), has been reported in association with the use of tenofovir DF. The majority of these cases occurred in patients with underlying systemic or renal disease, or in patients taking nephrotoxic agents; however, some cases occured in patients without identified risk factors. Atripla should be avoided with concurrent or recent use of a nephrotoxic agent). Products include:
Omnicef Capsules 518
Omnicef Oral Suspension 518

Cefepime Hydrochloride (Renal impairment, including cases of acute renal failure and Fanconi syndrome (renal tubular injury with severe hypophosphatemia), has been reported in association with the use of tenofovir DF. The majority of these cases occurred in patients with underlying systemic or renal disease, or in patients taking nephrotoxic agents; however, some cases occured in patients without identified risk factors. Atripla should be avoided with concurrent or recent use of a nephrotoxic agent).
No products indexed under this heading.

Cefixime (Renal impairment, including cases of acute renal failure and Fanconi syndrome (renal tubular injury with severe hypophosphatemia), has been reported in association with the use of tenofovir DF. The majority of these cases occurred in patients with underlying systemic or renal disease, or in patients taking nephrotoxic agents; however, some cases occured in patients without identified risk factors. Atripla should be avoided with concurrent or recent use of a nephrotoxic agent). Products include:
Suprax for Oral Suspension 2038
Suprax Tablets 2038

Cefmetazole Sodium (Renal impairment, including cases of acute renal failure and Fanconi syndrome (renal tubular injury with severe hypophosphatemia), has been reported in association with the use of tenofovir DF. The majority of these cases occurred in patients with underlying systemic or renal disease, or in patients taking nephrotoxic agents; however, some cases occured in patients without identified risk factors. Atripla should be avoided with concurrent or recent use of a nephrotoxic agent).
No products indexed under this heading.

Cefonicid Sodium (Renal impairment, including cases of acute renal failure and Fanconi syndrome (renal tubular injury with severe hypophosphatemia), has been reported in association with the use of tenofovir DF. The majority of

these cases occurred in patients with underlying systemic or renal disease, or in patients taking nephrotoxic agents; however, some cases occured in patients without identified risk factors. Atripla should be avoided with concurrent or recent use of a nephrotoxic agent).
No products indexed under this heading.

Cefoperazone Sodium (Renal impairment, including cases of acute renal failure and Fanconi syndrome (renal tubular injury with severe hypophosphatemia), has been reported in association with the use of tenofovir DF. The majority of these cases occurred in patients with underlying systemic or renal disease, or in patients taking nephrotoxic agents; however, some cases occured in patients without identified risk factors. Atripla should be avoided with concurrent or recent use of a nephrotoxic agent).
No products indexed under this heading.

Ceforanide (Renal impairment, including cases of acute renal failure and Fanconi syndrome (renal tubular injury with severe hypophosphatemia), has been reported in association with the use of tenofovir DF. The majority of these cases occurred in patients with underlying systemic or renal disease, or in patients taking nephrotoxic agents; however, some cases occured in patients without identified risk factors. Atripla should be avoided with concurrent or recent use of a nephrotoxic agent).
No products indexed under this heading.

Cefotaxime Sodium (Renal impairment, including cases of acute renal failure and Fanconi syndrome (renal tubular injury with severe hypophosphatemia), has been reported in association with the use of tenofovir DF. The majority of these cases occurred in patients with underlying systemic or renal disease, or in patients taking nephrotoxic agents; however, some cases occured in patients without identified risk factors. Atripla should be avoided with concurrent or recent use of a nephrotoxic agent).
No products indexed under this heading.

Cefotetan (Renal impairment, including cases of acute renal failure and Fanconi syndrome (renal tubular injury with severe hypophosphatemia), has been reported in association with the use of tenofovir DF. The majority of these cases occurred in patients with underlying systemic or renal disease, or in patients taking nephrotoxic agents; however, some cases occured in patients without identified risk factors. Atripla should be avoided with concurrent or recent use of a nephrotoxic agent).
No products indexed under this heading.

Cefoxitin Sodium (Renal impairment, including cases of acute renal failure and Fanconi syndrome (renal tubular injury with severe hypophosphatemia), has been reported in association with the use of tenofovir DF. The majority of these cases occurred in patients with underlying systemic or renal disease, or in patients taking nephrotoxic agents; however, some cases occured in patients without identified risk factors. Atripla should be avoided with concurrent or recent use of a nephrotoxic agent).
No products indexed under this heading.

Cefpodoxime Proxetil (Renal impairment, including cases of acute renal failure and Fanconi syndrome (renal tubular injury with severe hypophosphatemia), has been reported in association with the use of tenofovir DF. The majority of these cases occurred in patients with underlying systemic or renal disease, or in patients taking

nephrotoxic agents; however, some cases occured in patients without identified risk factors. Atripla should be avoided with concurrent or recent use of a nephrotoxic agent).
No products indexed under this heading.

Cefprozil (Renal impairment, including cases of acute renal failure and Fanconi syndrome (renal tubular injury with severe hypophosphatemia), has been reported in association with the use of tenofovir DF. The majority of these cases occurred in patients with underlying systemic or renal disease, or in patients taking nephrotoxic agents; however, some cases occured in patients without identified risk factors. Atripla should be avoided with concurrent or recent use of a nephrotoxic agent).
No products indexed under this heading.

Ceftazidime (Renal impairment, including cases of acute renal failure and Fanconi syndrome (renal tubular injury with severe hypophosphatemia), has been reported in association with the use of tenofovir DF. The majority of these cases occurred in patients with underlying systemic or renal disease, or in patients taking nephrotoxic agents; however, some cases occured in patients without identified risk factors. Atripla should be avoided with concurrent or recent use of a nephrotoxic agent). Products include:
Fortaz 1481

Ceftizoxime Sodium (Renal impairment, including cases of acute renal failure and Fanconi syndrome (renal tubular injury with severe hypophosphatemia), has been reported in association with the use of tenofovir DF. The majority of these cases occurred in patients with underlying systemic or renal disease, or in patients taking nephrotoxic agents; however, some cases occured in patients without identified risk factors. Atripla should be avoided with concurrent or recent use of a nephrotoxic agent).
No products indexed under this heading.

Ceftriaxone Sodium (Renal impairment, including cases of acute renal failure and Fanconi syndrome (renal tubular injury with severe hypophosphatemia), has been reported in association with the use of tenofovir DF. The majority of these cases occurred in patients with underlying systemic or renal disease, or in patients taking nephrotoxic agents; however, some cases occured in patients without identified risk factors. Atripla should be avoided with concurrent or recent use of a nephrotoxic agent). Products include:
Rocephin 2859

Cefuroxime Axetil (Renal impairment, including cases of acute renal failure and Fanconi syndrome (renal tubular injury with severe hypophosphatemia), has been reported in association with the use of tenofovir DF. The majority of these cases occurred in patients with underlying systemic or renal disease, or in patients taking nephrotoxic agents; however, some cases occured in patients without identified risk factors. Atripla should be avoided with concurrent or recent use of a nephrotoxic agent). Products include:
Ceftin 1399

Cefuroxime Sodium (Renal impairment, including cases of acute renal failure and Fanconi syndrome (renal tubular injury with severe hypophosphatemia), has been reported in association with the use of tenofovir DF. The majority of these cases occurred in patients with underlying systemic or renal disease, or in patients taking nephrotoxic agents; however, some

(⊙ Described in PDR® for Ophthalmic Medicines)

cases occured in patients without identified risk factors. Atripla should be avoided with concurrent or recent use of a nephrotoxic agent).
No products indexed under this heading.

Celecoxib (Renal impairment, including cases of acute renal failure and Fanconi syndrome (renal tubular injury with severe hypophosphatemia), has been reported in association with the use of tenofovir DF. The majority of these cases occurred in patients with underlying systemic or renal disease, or in patients taking nephrotoxic agents; however, some cases occured in patients without identified risk factors. Atripla should be avoided with concurrent or recent use of a nephrotoxic agent). Products include:
Celebrex 3272

Cephalexin (Renal impairment, including cases of acute renal failure and Fanconi syndrome (renal tubular injury with severe hypophosphatemia), has been reported in association with the use of tenofovir DF. The majority of these cases occurred in patients with underlying systemic or renal disease, or in patients taking nephrotoxic agents; however, some cases occured in patients without identified risk factors. Atripla should be avoided with concurrent or recent use of a nephrotoxic agent).
No products indexed under this heading.

Cephalothin Sodium (Renal impairment, including cases of acute renal failure and Fanconi syndrome (renal tubular injury with severe hypophosphatemia), has been reported in association with the use of tenofovir DF. The majority of these cases occurred in patients with underlying systemic or renal disease, or in patients taking nephrotoxic agents; however, some cases occured in patients without identified risk factors. Atripla should be avoided with concurrent or recent use of a nephrotoxic agent).
No products indexed under this heading.

Cephapirin Sodium (Renal impairment, including cases of acute renal failure and Fanconi syndrome (renal tubular injury with severe hypophosphatemia), has been reported in association with the use of tenofovir DF. The majority of these cases occurred in patients with underlying systemic or renal disease, or in patients taking nephrotoxic agents; however, some cases occured in patients without identified risk factors. Atripla should be avoided with concurrent or recent use of a nephrotoxic agent).
No products indexed under this heading.

Cephradine (Renal impairment, including cases of acute renal failure and Fanconi syndrome (renal tubular injury with severe hypophosphatemia), has been reported in association with the use of tenofovir DF. The majority of these cases occurred in patients with underlying systemic or renal disease, or in patients taking nephrotoxic agents; however, some cases occured in patients without identified risk factors. Atripla should be avoided with concurrent or recent use of a nephrotoxic agent).
No products indexed under this heading.

Cerivastatin Sodium (Renal impairment, including cases of acute renal failure and Fanconi syndrome (renal tubular injury with severe hypophosphatemia), has been reported in association with the use of tenofovir DF. The majority of these cases occurred in patients with underlying systemic or renal disease, or in patients taking nephrotoxic agents; however, some cases occured in patients without identified risk factors. Atripla should be avoided with concurrent or recent use of a nephrotoxic agent).
No products indexed under this heading.

Chlorothiazide (Renal impairment, including cases of acute renal failure and Fanconi syndrome (renal tubular injury with severe hypophosphatemia), has been reported in association with the use of tenofovir DF. The majority of these cases occurred in patients with underlying systemic or renal disease, or in patients taking nephrotoxic agents; however, some cases occured in patients without identified risk factors. Atripla should be avoided with concurrent or recent use of a nephrotoxic agent).
No products indexed under this heading.

Chlorothiazide Sodium (Renal impairment, including cases of acute renal failure and Fanconi syndrome (renal tubular injury with severe hypophosphatemia), has been reported in association with the use of tenofovir DF. The majority of these cases occurred in patients with underlying systemic or renal disease, or in patients taking nephrotoxic agents; however, some cases occured in patients without identified risk factors. Atripla should be avoided with concurrent or recent use of a nephrotoxic agent). Products include:
Diuril Intravenous 2009

Chlorpheniramine (Efavirenz has been shown *in vivo* to induce CYP3A4. Other compounds that are substrates of CYP3A4 may have decreased plasma concentrations when co-administered with efavirenz).
No products indexed under this heading.

Chlorpheniramine Maleate (Efavirenz has been shown *in vivo* to induce CYP3A4. Other compounds that are substrates of CYP3A4 may have decreased plasma concentrations when co-administered with efavirenz).
No products indexed under this heading.

Chlorpheniramine Polistirex (Efavirenz has been shown *in vivo* to induce CYP3A4. Other compounds that are substrates of CYP3A4 may have decreased plasma concentrations when co-administered with efavirenz). Products include:
Tussionex 3443

Chlorpheniramine Tannate (Efavirenz has been shown *in vivo* to induce CYP3A4. Other compounds that are substrates of CYP3A4 may have decreased plasma concentrations when co-administered with efavirenz).
No products indexed under this heading.

Chlorpropamide (Renal impairment, including cases of acute renal failure and Fanconi syndrome (renal tubular injury with severe hypophosphatemia), has been reported in association with the use of tenofovir DF. The majority of these cases occurred in patients with underlying systemic or renal disease, or in patients taking nephrotoxic agents; however, some cases occured in patients without identified risk factors. Atripla should be avoided with concurrent or recent use of a nephrotoxic agent).
No products indexed under this heading.

Cidofovir (Since emtricitabine and tenofovir are primarily eliminated by the kidneys, co-administration of Atripla with drugs that reduce renal fuction or compete for active tubular secretion may increase serum concentrations of emtricitabine, tenofovir, and/or other renally eliminated drugs).
No products indexed under this heading.

Cilastatin Sodium (Renal impairment, including cases of acute renal failure and Fanconi syndrome (renal tubular injury with severe hypophosphatemia), has been reported in association with the use of tenofovir DF. The majority of these cases occurred in patients with underlying systemic or renal disease, or in patients taking nephrotoxic agents; however, some cases occured in patients without identified risk factors. Atripla should be avoided with concurrent or recent use of a nephrotoxic agent). Products include:
Primaxin I.M. 2232
Primaxin I.V. 2235

Cilostazol (In vitro studies have demonstrated that efavirenz inhibits CYP2C19 in the range of observed efavirenz plasma concentrations. Co-administration of efavirenz with drugs primarily metabolized by CYP2C19 may result in altered plasma concentrations of the co-administered drug. Therefore, appropriate dose adjustments may be necessary for these drugs).
No products indexed under this heading.

Cimetidine (Renal impairment, including cases of acute renal failure and Fanconi syndrome (renal tubular injury with severe hypophosphatemia), has been reported in association with the use of tenofovir DF. The majority of these cases occurred in patients with underlying systemic or renal disease, or in patients taking nephrotoxic agents; however, some cases occured in patients without identified risk factors. Atripla should be avoided with concurrent or recent use of a nephrotoxic agent).
No products indexed under this heading.

Cimetidine Hydrochloride (Renal impairment, including cases of acute renal failure and Fanconi syndrome (renal tubular injury with severe hypophosphatemia), has been reported in association with the use of tenofovir DF. The majority of these cases occurred in patients with underlying systemic or renal disease, or in patients taking nephrotoxic agents; however, some cases occured in patients without identified risk factors. Atripla should be avoided with concurrent or recent use of a nephrotoxic agent).
No products indexed under this heading.

Ciprofloxacin (Drugs which induce CYP3A4 activity would be expected to increase the clearance of efavirenz resulting in lower plasma concentrations). Products include:
Cipro I.V. 3082
Cipro 3073
Cipro XR 3091
Ciprodex 583

Ciprofloxacin Hydrochloride (Drugs which induce CYP3A4 activity would be expected to increase the clearance of efavirenz resulting in lower plasma concentrations). Products include:
Cipro 3073

Cisapride (Due to the potential for serious and/or life-threatening reactions, such as cardiac arrhythmias, concomitant use with cisapride is contraindicated).
No products indexed under this heading.

Cisplatin (Renal impairment, including cases of acute renal failure and Fanconi syndrome (renal tubular injury with severe hypophosphatemia), has been reported in association with the use of tenofovir DF. The majority of these cases occurred in patients with underlying systemic or renal disease, or in patients taking nephrotoxic agents; however, some cases occured in patients without identified risk factors. Atripla should be avoided with concurrent or recent use of a nephrotoxic agent).
No products indexed under this heading.

Citalopram Hydrobromide (In vitro studies have demonstrated that efavirenz inhibits CYP2C19 in the range of observed efavirenz plasma concentrations. Co-administration of efavirenz with drugs primarily metabolized by CYP2C19 may result in altered plasma concentrations of the co-administered drug. Therefore, appropriate dose adjustments may be necessary for these drugs). Products include:
Celexa 1153

Cladribine (Renal impairment, including cases of acute renal failure and Fanconi syndrome (renal tubular injury with severe hypophosphatemia), has been reported in association with the use of tenofovir DF. The majority of these cases occurred in patients with underlying systemic or renal disease, or in patients taking nephrotoxic agents; however, some cases occured in patients without identified risk factors. Atripla should be avoided with concurrent or recent use of a nephrotoxic agent). Products include:
Leustatin 946

Clarithromycin (In uninfected volunteers, 46% developed a rash while receiving efavirenz and clarithromycin. No dose adjustment of Atripla is recommended when given with clarithromycin. Alternatives to clarithromycin, such as azithromycin, should be considered. Other macrolide antibiotics, such as erythromycin, have not been studied in combination with Atripla). Products include:
Biaxin/Biaxin XL 412

Clomipramine Hydrochloride (In vitro studies have demonstrated that efavirenz inhibits CYP2C9 in the range of observed efavirenz plasma concentrations. Co-administration of efavirenz with drugs primarily metabolized by CYP2C9 may result in altered plasma concentrations of the co-administered drug. Therefore, appropriate dose adjustments may be necessary for these drugs).
No products indexed under this heading.

Clozapine (Renal impairment, including cases of acute renal failure and Fanconi syndrome (renal tubular injury with severc hypophosphatemia), has been reported in association with the use of tenofovir DF. The majority of these cases occurred in patients with underlying systemic or renal disease, or in patients taking nephrotoxic agents; however, some cases occured in patients without identified risk factors. Atripla should be avoided with concurrent or recent use of a nephrotoxic agent).
No products indexed under this heading.

Colistimethate Sodium (Renal impairment, including cases of acute renal failure and Fanconi syndrome (renal tubular injury with severe hypophosphatemia), has been reported in association with the use of tenofovir DF. The majority of these cases occurred in patients with underlying systemic or renal disease, or in patients taking nephrotoxic agents; however, some cases occured in patients without identified risk factors. Atripla should be avoided with concurrent or recent use of a nephrotoxic agent).
No products indexed under this heading.

Colistin Sulfate (Renal impairment, including cases of acute renal failure and Fanconi syndrome (renal tubular injury with severe hypophosphatemia), has been reported in association with the use of tenofovir DF. The majority of these cases occurred in patients with underlying systemic or renal disease, or in patients taking nephrotoxic agents; however, some cases occured in patients without identified risk factors. Atripla should be avoided with concurrent or recent use of a nephrotoxic agent).
No products indexed under this heading.

IMPORTANT NOTE: Always consult each drug listing in the patient's regimen for possible interactions.

Cortisone Acetate (Drugs which induce CYP3A4 activity would be expected to increase the clearance of efavirenz resulting in lower plasma concentrations).
No products indexed under this heading.

Cyclophosphamide (Renal impairment, including cases of acute renal failure and Fanconi syndrome (renal tubular injury with severe hypophosphatemia), has been reported in association with the use of tenofovir DF. The majority of these cases occurred in patients with underlying systemic or renal disease, or in patients taking nephrotoxic agents; however, some cases occured in patients without identified risk factors. Atripla should be avoided with concurrent or recent use of a nephrotoxic agent).
No products indexed under this heading.

Cyclosporine (Renal impairment, including cases of acute renal failure and Fanconi syndrome (renal tubular injury with severe hypophosphatemia), has been reported in association with the use of tenofovir DF. The majority of these cases occurred in patients with underlying systemic or renal disease, or in patients taking nephrotoxic agents; however, some cases occured in patients without identified risk factors. Atripla should be avoided with concurrent or recent use of a nephrotoxic agent). Products include:
Gengraf 440
Neoral Oral Solution 2496
Neoral Capsules 2496
Restasis 605

Cytarabine (Renal impairment, including cases of acute renal failure and Fanconi syndrome (renal tubular injury with severe hypophosphatemia), has been reported in association with the use of tenofovir DF. The majority of these cases occurred in patients with underlying systemic or renal disease, or in patients taking nephrotoxic agents; however, some cases occured in patients without identified risk factors. Atripla should be avoided with concurrent or recent use of a nephrotoxic agent).
No products indexed under this heading.

Cytarabine Liposome (Renal impairment, including cases of acute renal failure and Fanconi syndrome (renal tubular injury with severe hypophosphatemia), has been reported in association with the use of tenofovir DF. The majority of these cases occurred in patients with underlying systemic or renal disease, or in patients taking nephrotoxic agents; however, some cases occured in patients without identified risk factors. Atripla should be avoided with concurrent or recent use of a nephrotoxic agent).
No products indexed under this heading.

Delavirdine Mesylate (Renal impairment, including cases of acute renal failure and Fanconi syndrome (renal tubular injury with severe hypophosphatemia), has been reported in association with the use of tenofovir DF. The majority of these cases occurred in patients with underlying systemic or renal disease, or in patients taking nephrotoxic agents; however, some cases occured in patients without identified risk factors. Atripla should be avoided with concurrent or recent use of a nephrotoxic agent).
No products indexed under this heading.

Desipramine Hydrochloride (In vitro studies have demonstrated that efavirenz inhibits CYP2C19 in the range of observed efavirenz plasma concentrations. Co-administration of efavirenz with drugs primarily metabolized by CYP2C19 may result in altered plasma concentrations of the co-administered drug. Therefore, appropriate dose adjustments may be necessary for these drugs).
No products indexed under this heading.

Desogestrel (Efavirenz has been shown *in vivo* to induce CYP3A4. Other compounds that are substrates of CYP3A4 may have decreased plasma concentrations when co-administered with efavirenz).
No products indexed under this heading.

Dexamethasone (Drugs which induce CYP3A4 activity would be expected to increase the clearance of efavirenz resulting in lower plasma concentrations). Products include:
Ciprodex 583
Ozurdex .... ⊙223
Tobramycin and Dexamethasone Ophthalmic Suspension .... ⊙251

Dexamethasone Acetate (Drugs which induce CYP3A4 activity would be expected to increase the clearance of efavirenz resulting in lower plasma concentrations).
No products indexed under this heading.

Dexamethasone Phosphate (Drugs which induce CYP3A4 activity would be expected to increase the clearance of efavirenz resulting in lower plasma concentrations).
No products indexed under this heading.

Dexamethasone Sodium (Drugs which induce CYP3A4 activity would be expected to increase the clearance of efavirenz resulting in lower plasma concentrations).
No products indexed under this heading.

Dexamethasone Sodium Phosphate (Drugs which induce CYP3A4 activity would be expected to increase the clearance of efavirenz resulting in lower plasma concentrations).
No products indexed under this heading.

Dexamethasone Sodium Phosphate Injection (Drugs which induce CYP3A4 activity would be expected to increase the clearance of efavirenz resulting in lower plasma concentrations).
No products indexed under this heading.

Dextromethorphan (In vitro studies have demonstrated that efavirenz inhibits CYP2C9 in the range of observed efavirenz plasma concentrations. Co-administration of efavirenz with drugs primarily metabolized by CYP2C9 may result in altered plasma concentrations of the co-administered drug. Therefore, appropriate dose adjustments may be necessary for these drugs).
No products indexed under this heading.

Dextromethorphan Hydrobromide (In vitro studies have demonstrated that efavirenz inhibits CYP2C19 in the range of observed efavirenz plasma concentrations. Co-administration of efavirenz with drugs primarily metabolized by CYP2C19 may result in altered plasma concentrations of the co-administered drug. Therefore, appropriate dose adjustments may be necessary for these drugs).
No products indexed under this heading.

Diatrizoate Meglumine (Renal impairment, including cases of acute renal failure and Fanconi syndrome (renal tubular injury with severe hypophosphatemia), has been reported in association with the use of tenofovir DF. The majority of these cases occurred in patients with underlying systemic or renal disease, or in patients taking nephrotoxic agents; however, some cases occured in patients without identified risk factors. Atripla should be avoided with concurrent or recent use of a nephrotoxic agent).
No products indexed under this heading.

Diatrizoate Sodium (Renal impairment, including cases of acute renal failure and Fanconi syndrome (renal tubular injury with severe hypophosphatemia), has been reported in association with the use of tenofovir DF. The majority of these cases occurred in patients with underlying systemic or renal disease, or in patients taking nephrotoxic agents; however, some cases occured in patients without identified risk factors. Atripla should be avoided with concurrent or recent use of a nephrotoxic agent).
No products indexed under this heading.

Diazepam (Efavirenz has been shown *in vivo* to induce CYP3A4. Other compounds that are substrates of CYP3A4 may have decreased plasma concentrations when co-administered with efavirenz). Products include:
Valium Tablets 2880

Diclofenac Potassium (Renal impairment, including cases of acute renal failure and Fanconi syndrome (renal tubular injury with severe hypophosphatemia), has been reported in association with the use of tenofovir DF. The majority of these cases occurred in patients with underlying systemic or renal disease, or in patients taking nephrotoxic agents; however, some cases occured in patients without identified risk factors. Atripla should be avoided with concurrent or recent use of a nephrotoxic agent).
No products indexed under this heading.

Diclofenac Sodium (Renal impairment, including cases of acute renal failure and Fanconi syndrome (renal tubular injury with severe hypophosphatemia), has been reported in association with the use of tenofovir DF. The majority of these cases occurred in patients with underlying systemic or renal disease, or in patients taking nephrotoxic agents; however, some cases occured in patients without identified risk factors. Atripla should be avoided with concurrent or recent use of a nephrotoxic agent).
No products indexed under this heading.

Dicloxacillin Sodium (Renal impairment, including cases of acute renal failure and Fanconi syndrome (renal tubular injury with severe hypophosphatemia), has been reported in association with the use of tenofovir DF. The majority of these cases occurred in patients with underlying systemic or renal disease, or in patients taking nephrotoxic agents; however, some cases occured in patients without identified risk factors. Atripla should be avoided with concurrent or recent use of a nephrotoxic agent).
No products indexed under this heading.

Didanosine (Co-administration of tenofovir DF and didanosine should be undertaken with caution and patients receiving this combination should be monitored closely for didanosine-associated adverse events. Didanosine should be discontinued in patients who develop didanosine-associated adverse events).
No products indexed under this heading.

Dihydroergotamine Mesylate (Due to the potential for serious and/or life-threatening reactions, such as acute ergot toxicity characterized by peripheral vasospasm and ischemia of the extremities and other tissues, concomitant use with ergot derivatives is contraindicated).
No products indexed under this heading.

Diltiazem Hydrochloride (Efavirenz has been shown *in vivo* to induce CYP3A4. Other compounds that are substrates of CYP3A4 may have decreased plasma concentrations when co-administered with efavirenz). Products include:
Cardizem LA 423

Diltiazem Maleate (Efavirenz has been shown *in vivo* to induce CYP3A4. Other compounds that are substrates of CYP3A4 may have decreased plasma concentrations when co-administered with efavirenz).
No products indexed under this heading.

Disopyramide (Efavirenz has been shown *in vivo* to induce CYP3A4. Other compounds that are substrates of CYP3A4 may have decreased plasma concentrations when co-administered with efavirenz).
No products indexed under this heading.

Disopyramide Phosphate (Efavirenz has been shown *in vivo* to induce CYP3A4. Other compounds that are substrates of CYP3A4 may have decreased plasma concentrations when co-administered with efavirenz).
No products indexed under this heading.

Disulfiram (Efavirenz has been shown *in vivo* to induce CYP3A4. Other compounds that are substrates of CYP3A4 may have decreased plasma concentrations when co-administered with efavirenz).
No products indexed under this heading.

Divalproex Sodium (In vitro studies have demonstrated that efavirenz inhibits CYP2C19 in the range of observed efavirenz plasma concentrations. Co-administration of efavirenz with drugs primarily metabolized by CYP2C19 may result in altered plasma concentrations of the co-administered drug. Therefore, appropriate dose adjustments may be necessary for these drugs). Products include:
Depakote ER 426

Doxepin Hydrochloride (In vitro studies have demonstrated that efavirenz inhibits CYP2C19 in the range of observed efavirenz plasma concentrations. Co-administration of efavirenz with drugs primarily metabolized by CYP2C19 may result in altered plasma concentrations of the co-administered drug. Therefore, appropriate dose adjustments may be necessary for these drugs).
No products indexed under this heading.

Doxorubicin Hydrochloride (Efavirenz has been shown *in vivo* to induce CYP3A4. Other compounds that are substrates of CYP3A4 may have decreased plasma concentrations when co-administered with efavirenz).
No products indexed under this heading.

Dronabinol (Efavirenz has been shown *in vivo* to induce CYP3A4. Other compounds that are substrates of CYP3A4 may have decreased plasma concentrations when co-administered with efavirenz).
No products indexed under this heading.

Enalapril Maleate (Renal impairment, including cases of acute renal failure and Fanconi syndrome (renal tubular injury with severe hypophosphatemia), has been reported in association with the use of tenofovir DF. The majority of these cases occurred in patients with underlying systemic or renal disease, or in patients taking nephrotoxic agents; however, some cases occured in patients without identified risk factors. Atripla should be avoided with concurrent or recent use of a nephrotoxic agent).
No products indexed under this heading.

Enalaprilat (Renal impairment, including cases of acute renal failure and Fan-

coni syndrome (renal tubular injury with severe hypophosphatemia), has been reported in association with the use of tenofovir DF. The majority of these cases occurred in patients with underlying systemic or renal disease, or in patients taking nephrotoxic agents; however, some cases occured in patients without identified risk factors. Atripla should be avoided with concurrent or recent use of a nephrotoxic agent).
No products indexed under this heading.

Enfuvirtide (Renal impairment, including cases of acute renal failure and Fanconi syndrome (renal tubular injury with severe hypophosphatemia), has been reported in association with the use of tenofovir DF. The majority of these cases occurred in patients with underlying systemic or renal disease, or in patients taking nephrotoxic agents; however, some cases occured in patients without identified risk factors. Atripla should be avoided with concurrent or recent use of a nephrotoxic agent).
No products indexed under this heading.

Eprosartan Mesylate (In vitro studies have demonstrated that efavirenz inhibits CYP2C9 in the range of observed efavirenz plasma concentrations. Co-administration of efavirenz with drugs primarily metabolized by CYP2C9 may result in altered plasma concentrations of the co-administered drug. Therefore, appropriate dose adjustments may be necessary for these drugs). Products include:
Teveten 538
Teveten HCT 541

Ergonovine Maleate (Due to the potential for serious and/or life-threatening reactions, such as acute ergot toxicity characterized by peripheral vasospasm and ischemia of the extremities and other tissues, concomitant use with ergot derivatives is contraindicated).
No products indexed under this heading.

Ergotamine Tartrate (Due to the potential for serious and/or life-threatening reactions, such as acute ergot toxicity characterized by peripheral vasospasm and ischemia of the extremities and other tissues, concomitant use with ergot derivatives is contraindicated).
No products indexed under this heading.

Erythromycin (Efavirenz has been shown in vivo to induce CYP3A4. Other compounds that are substrates of CYP3A4 may have decreased plasma concentrations when co-administered with efavirenz).
No products indexed under this heading.

Erythromycin Estolate (Efavirenz has been shown in vivo to induce CYP3A4. Other compounds that are substrates of CYP3A4 may have decreased plasma concentrations when co-administered with efavirenz).
No products indexed under this heading.

Erythromycin Ethylsuccinate (Efavirenz has been shown in vivo to induce CYP3A4. Other compounds that are substrates of CYP3A4 may have decreased plasma concentrations when co-administered with efavirenz). Products include:
E.E.S. 437
EryPed 435

Erythromycin Gluceptate (Efavirenz has been shown in vivo to induce CYP3A4. Other compounds that are substrates of CYP3A4 may have decreased plasma concentrations when co-administered with efavirenz).
No products indexed under this heading.

Erythromycin Lactobionate (Efavirenz has been shown in vivo to induce CYP3A4. Other compounds that are substrates of CYP3A4 may have decreased plasma concentrations when co-administered with efavirenz).
No products indexed under this heading.

Erythromycin Stearate (Efavirenz has been shown in vivo to induce CYP3A4. Other compounds that are substrates of CYP3A4 may have decreased plasma concentrations when co-administered with efavirenz).
No products indexed under this heading.

Esomeprazole Magnesium (In vitro studies have demonstrated that efavirenz inhibits CYP2C19 in the range of observed efavirenz plasma concentrations. Co-administration of efavirenz with drugs primarily metabolized by CYP2C19 may result in altered plasma concentrations of the co-administered drug. Therefore, appropriate dose adjustments may be necessary for these drugs). Products include:
Nexium Capsules 704
Nexium Oral Suspension 704

Esomeprazole Sodium (In vitro studies have demonstrated that efavirenz inhibits CYP2C19 in the range of observed efavirenz plasma concentrations. Co-administration of efavirenz with drugs primarily metabolized by CYP2C19 may result in altered plasma concentrations of the co-administered drug. Therefore, appropriate dose adjustments may be necessary for these drugs). Products include:
Nexium I.V. 712

Estradiol (Efavirenz has been shown in vivo to induce CYP3A4. Other compounds that are substrates of CYP3A4 may have decreased plasma concentrations when co-administered with efavirenz). Products include:
Activella 2561
Angeliq 831
Climara 841
Climara Pro 847
Divigel 3467
Estrasorb 1777
Vagifem 2589

Estradiol Benzoate (Efavirenz has been shown in vivo to induce CYP3A4. Other compounds that are substrates of CYP3A4 may have decreased plasma concentrations when co-administered with efavirenz).
No products indexed under this heading.

Estradiol Cypionate (Efavirenz has been shown in vivo to induce CYP3A4. Other compounds that are substrates of CYP3A4 may have decreased plasma concentrations when co-administered with efavirenz).
No products indexed under this heading.

Estradiol Valerate (Efavirenz has been shown in vivo to induce CYP3A4. Other compounds that are substrates of CYP3A4 may have decreased plasma concentrations when co-administered with efavirenz).
No products indexed under this heading.

Ethinyl Estradiol (Because the potential interaction of efavirenz with oral contraceptives has not been fully characterized, a reliable method of barrier contraception should be used in addition to oral contraceptives). Products include:
LoSeasonique 3407
Lybrel 3514
NuvaRing 3181
Ortho Evra 2648
Ortho-Cyclen/Ortho Tri-Cyclen 2663
Ortho Tri-Cyclen Lo Tablets 2673
Seasonique 3418
Yaz 864

Ethiodized Oil (Renal impairment, including cases of acute renal failure and Fanconi syndrome (renal tubular

injury with severe hypophosphatemia), has been reported in association with the use of tenofovir DF. The majority of these cases occurred in patients with underlying systemic or renal disease, or in patients taking nephrotoxic agents; however, some cases occured in patients without identified risk factors. Atripla should be avoided with concurrent or recent use of a nephrotoxic agent).
No products indexed under this heading.

Ethosuximide (Efavirenz has been shown in vivo to induce CYP3A4. Other compounds that are substrates of CYP3A4 may have decreased plasma concentrations when co-administered with efavirenz).
No products indexed under this heading.

Ethotoin (In vitro studies have demonstrated that efavirenz inhibits CYP2C19 in the range of observed efavirenz plasma concentrations. Co-administration of efavirenz with drugs primarily metabolized by CYP2C19 may result in altered plasma concentrations of the co-administered drug. Therefore, appropriate dose adjustments may be necessary for these drugs).
No products indexed under this heading.

Ethynodiol Diacetate (Efavirenz has been shown in vivo to induce CYP3A4. Other compounds that are substrates of CYP3A4 may have decreased plasma concentrations when co-administered with efavirenz).
No products indexed under this heading.

Etodolac (Renal impairment, including cases of acute renal failure and Fanconi syndrome (renal tubular injury with severe hypophosphatemia), has been reported in association with the use of tenofovir DF. The majority of these cases occurred in patients with underlying systemic or renal disease, or in patients taking nephrotoxic agents; however, some cases occured in patients without identified risk factors. Atripla should be avoided with concurrent or recent use of a nephrotoxic agent).
No products indexed under this heading.

Etoposide (Efavirenz has been shown in vivo to induce CYP3A4. Other compounds that are substrates of CYP3A4 may have decreased plasma concentrations when co-administered with efavirenz).
No products indexed under this heading.

Etoposide Phosphate (Efavirenz has been shown in vivo to induce CYP3A4. Other compounds that are substrates of CYP3A4 may have decreased plasma concentrations when co-administered with efavirenz).
No products indexed under this heading.

Felbamate (Drugs which induce CYP3A4 activity would be expected to increase the clearance of efavirenz resulting in lower plasma concentrations).
No products indexed under this heading.

Felodipine (Efavirenz has been shown in vivo to induce CYP3A4. Other compounds that are substrates of CYP3A4 may have decreased plasma concentrations when co-administered with efavirenz).
No products indexed under this heading.

Fenoprofen Calcium (Renal impairment, including cases of acute renal failure and Fanconi syndrome (renal tubular injury with severe hypophosphatemia), has been reported in association with the use of tenofovir DF. The majority of these cases occurred in patients with underlying systemic or renal disease, or in patients taking nephrotoxic agents; however, some cases occured in patients without identi-

fied risk factors. Atripla should be avoided with concurrent or recent use of a nephrotoxic agent).
No products indexed under this heading.

Fentanyl (Efavirenz has been shown in vivo to induce CYP3A4. Other compounds that are substrates of CYP3A4 may have decreased plasma concentrations when co-administered with efavirenz). Products include:
Duragesic 2604
Fentanyl Transdermal System 2346
Onsolis 2054

Fentanyl Citrate (Efavirenz has been shown in vivo to induce CYP3A4. Other compounds that are substrates of CYP3A4 may have decreased plasma concentrations when co-administered with efavirenz). Products include:
Fentora 966

Filgrastim (Renal impairment, including cases of acute renal failure and Fanconi syndrome (renal tubular injury with severe hypophosphatemia), has been reported in association with the use of tenofovir DF. The majority of these cases occurred in patients with underlying systemic or renal disease, or in patients taking nephrotoxic agents; however, some cases occured in patients without identified risk factors. Atripla should be avoided with concurrent or recent use of a nephrotoxic agent). Products include:
Neupogen 631

Fludrocortisone Acetate (Drugs which induce CYP3A4 activity would be expected to increase the clearance of efavirenz resulting in lower plasma concentrations).
No products indexed under this heading.

Fluorouracil (Renal impairment, including cases of acute renal failure and Fanconi syndrome (renal tubular injury with severe hypophosphatemia), has been reported in association with the use of tenofovir DF. The majority of these cases occurred in patients with underlying systemic or renal disease, or in patients taking nephrotoxic agents; however, some cases occured in patients without identified risk factors. Atripla should be avoided with concurrent or recent use of a nephrotoxic agent). Products include:
Carac 2966

Fluoxetine Hydrochloride (In vitro studies have demonstrated that efavirenz inhibits CYP2C9 in the range of observed efavirenz plasma concentrations. Co-administration of efavirenz with drugs primarily metabolized by CYP2C9 may result in altered plasma concentrations of the co-administered drug. Therefore, appropriate dose adjustments may be necessary for these drugs). Products include:
Prozac Weekly 1941
Prozac Pulvules 1941
Symbyax 1965

Flurbiprofen (Renal impairment, including cases of acute renal failure and Fanconi syndrome (renal tubular injury with severe hypophosphatemia), has been reported in association with the use of tenofovir DF. The majority of these cases occurred in patients with underlying systemic or renal disease, or in patients taking nephrotoxic agents; however, some cases occured in patients without identified risk factors. Atripla should be avoided with concurrent or recent use of a nephrotoxic agent).
No products indexed under this heading.

IMPORTANT NOTE: Always consult each drug listing in the patient's regimen for possible interactions.

Flurbiprofen Sodium (In vitro studies have demonstrated that efavirenz inhibits CYP2C9 in the range of observed efavirenz plasma concentrations. Co-administration of efavirenz with drugs primarily metabolized by CYP2C9 may result in altered plasma concentrations of the co-administered drug. Therefore, appropriate dose adjustments may be necessary for these drugs).
No products indexed under this heading.

Fluvastatin Sodium (Renal impairment, including cases of acute renal failure and Fanconi syndrome (renal tubular injury with severe hypophosphatemia), has been reported in association with the use of tenofovir DF. The majority of these cases occurred in patients with underlying systemic or renal disease, or in patients taking nephrotoxic agents; however, some cases occured in patients without identified risk factors. Atripla should be avoided with concurrent or recent use of a nephrotoxic agent).
No products indexed under this heading.

Formoterol Fumarate (In vitro studies have demonstrated that efavirenz inhibits CYP2C19 in the range of observed efavirenz plasma concentrations. Co-administration of efavirenz with drugs primarily metabolized by CYP2C19 may result in altered plasma concentrations of the co-administered drug. Therefore, appropriate dose adjustments may be necessary for these drugs). Products include:
Foradil 3121
Perforomist 3634

Fosamprenavir Calcium (An additional 100 mg/day (300 mg total) of ritonavir is recommended when Atripla is administered with fosamprenavir/ritonavir once daily. No change in the ritonavir dose is required when Atripla is administered with fosamprenavir plus ritonavir twice daily). Products include:
Lexiva Oral Suspension 1558
Lexiva 1558

Foscarnet Sodium (Renal impairment, including cases of acute renal failure and Fanconi syndrome (renal tubular injury with severe hypophosphatemia), has been reported in association with the use of tenofovir DF. The majority of these cases occurred in patients with underlying systemic or renal disease, or in patients taking nephrotoxic agents; however, some cases occured in patients without identified risk factors. Atripla should be avoided with concurrent or recent use of a nephrotoxic agent).
No products indexed under this heading.

Fosinopril Sodium (Renal impairment, including cases of acute renal failure and Fanconi syndrome (renal tubular injury with severe hypophosphatemia), has been reported in association with the use of tenofovir DF. The majority of these cases occurred in patients with underlying systemic or renal disease, or in patients taking nephrotoxic agents; however, some cases occured in patients without identified risk factors. Atripla should be avoided with concurrent or recent use of a nephrotoxic agent).
No products indexed under this heading.

Fosphenytoin (In vitro studies have demonstrated that efavirenz inhibits CYP2C19 in the range of observed efavirenz plasma concentrations. Co-administration of efavirenz with drugs primarily metabolized by CYP2C19 may result in altered plasma concentrations of the co-administered drug. Therefore, appropriate dose adjustments may be necessary for these drugs).
No products indexed under this heading.

Fosphenytoin Sodium (Drugs which induce CYP3A4 activity would be expected to increase the clearance of efavirenz resulting in lower plasma concentrations).
No products indexed under this heading.

Furosemide (Renal impairment, including cases of acute renal failure and Fanconi syndrome (renal tubular injury with severe hypophosphatemia), has been reported in association with the use of tenofovir DF. The majority of these cases occurred in patients with underlying systemic or renal disease, or in patients taking nephrotoxic agents; however, some cases occured in patients without identified risk factors. Atripla should be avoided with concurrent or recent use of a nephrotoxic agent). Products include:
Furosemide 2354

Gabapentin (In vitro studies have demonstrated that efavirenz inhibits CYP2C19 in the range of observed efavirenz plasma concentrations. Co-administration of efavirenz with drugs primarily metabolized by CYP2C19 may result in altered plasma concentrations of the co-administered drug. Therefore, appropriate dose adjustments may be necessary for these drugs).
No products indexed under this heading.

Gadopentetate Dimeglumine (Renal impairment, including cases of acute renal failure and Fanconi syndrome (renal tubular injury with severe hypophosphatemia), has been reported in association with the use of tenofovir DF. The majority of these cases occurred in patients with underlying systemic or renal disease, or in patients taking nephrotoxic agents; however, some cases occured in patients without identified risk factors. Atripla should be avoided with concurrent or recent use of a nephrotoxic agent).
No products indexed under this heading.

Ganciclovir (Since emtricitabine and tenofovir are primarily eliminated by the kidneys, co-administration of Atripla with drugs that reduce renal fuction or compete for active tubular secretion may increase serum concentrations of emtricitabine, tenofovir, and/or other renally eliminated drugs).
No products indexed under this heading.

Ganciclovir Sodium (Since emtricitabine and tenofovir are primarily eliminated by the kidneys, co-administration of Atripla with drugs that reduce renal fuction or compete for active tubular secretion may increase serum concentrations of emtricitabine, tenofovir, and/or other renally eliminated drugs).
No products indexed under this heading.

Garlic Extract (Drugs which induce CYP3A4 activity would be expected to increase the clearance of efavirenz resulting in lower plasma concentrations).
No products indexed under this heading.

Garlic Oil (Drugs which induce CYP3A4 activity would be expected to increase the clearance of efavirenz resulting in lower plasma concentrations).
No products indexed under this heading.

Gentamicin (Renal impairment, including cases of acute renal failure and Fanconi syndrome (renal tubular injury with severe hypophosphatemia), has been reported in association with the use of tenofovir DF. The majority of these cases occurred in patients with underlying systemic or renal disease, or in patients taking nephrotoxic agents; however, some cases occured in patients without identified risk factors. Atripla should be avoided with concurrent or recent use of a nephrotoxic agent).
No products indexed under this heading.

Gentamicin Sulfate (Renal impairment, including cases of acute renal failure and Fanconi syndrome (renal tubular injury with severe hypophosphatemia), has been reported in association with the use of tenofovir DF. The majority of these cases occurred in patients with underlying systemic or renal disease, or in patients taking nephrotoxic agents; however, some cases occured in patients without identified risk factors. Atripla should be avoided with concurrent or recent use of a nephrotoxic agent). Products include:
Pred-G .... ⊙**226**, ⊙**227**

Glimepiride (In vitro studies have demonstrated that efavirenz inhibits CYP2C9 in the range of observed efavirenz plasma concentrations. Co-administration of efavirenz with drugs primarily metabolized by CYP2C9 may result in altered plasma concentrations of the co-administered drug. Therefore, appropriate dose adjustments may be necessary for these drugs). Products include:
Avandaryl **1356**
Duetact **3354**

Glipizide (Renal impairment, including cases of acute renal failure and Fanconi syndrome (renal tubular injury with severe hypophosphatemia), has been reported in association with the use of tenofovir DF. The majority of these cases occurred in patients with underlying systemic or renal disease, or in patients taking nephrotoxic agents; however, some cases occured in patients without identified risk factors. Atripla should be avoided with concurrent or recent use of a nephrotoxic agent).
No products indexed under this heading.

Globulin, Immune (Human) (Renal impairment, including cases of acute renal failure and Fanconi syndrome (renal tubular injury with severe hypophosphatemia), has been reported in association with the use of tenofovir DF. The majority of these cases occurred in patients with underlying systemic or renal disease, or in patients taking nephrotoxic agents; however, some cases occured in patients without identified risk factors. Atripla should be avoided with concurrent or recent use of a nephrotoxic agent). Products include:

Glyburide (Renal impairment, including cases of acute renal failure and Fanconi syndrome (renal tubular injury with severe hypophosphatemia), has been reported in association with the use of tenofovir DF. The majority of these cases occurred in patients with underlying systemic or renal disease, or in patients taking nephrotoxic agents; however, some cases occured in patients without identified risk factors. Atripla should be avoided with concurrent or recent use of a nephrotoxic agent).
No products indexed under this heading.

Gold Therapy (Renal impairment, including cases of acute renal failure and Fanconi syndrome (renal tubular injury with severe hypophosphatemia), has been reported in association with the use of tenofovir DF. The majority of these cases occurred in patients with underlying systemic or renal disease, or in patients taking nephrotoxic agents; however, some cases occured in patients without identified risk factors. Atripla should be avoided with concurrent or recent use of a nephrotoxic agent).
No products indexed under this heading.

Haloperidol (Efavirenz has been shown in vivo to induce CYP3A4. Other compounds that are substrates of CYP3A4 may have decreased plasma concentrations when co-administered with efavirenz).
No products indexed under this heading.

Haloperidol Decanoate (Efavirenz has been shown in vivo to induce CYP3A4. Other compounds that are substrates of CYP3A4 may have decreased plasma concentrations when co-administered with efavirenz).
No products indexed under this heading.

Haloperidol Lactate (Efavirenz has been shown in vivo to induce CYP3A4. Other compounds that are substrates of CYP3A4 may have decreased plasma concentrations when co-administered with efavirenz).
No products indexed under this heading.

HMG-CoA Reductase Inhibitors (Renal impairment, including cases of acute renal failure and Fanconi syndrome (renal tubular injury with severe hypophosphatemia), has been reported in association with the use of tenofovir DF. The majority of these cases occurred in patients with underlying systemic or renal disease, or in patients taking nephrotoxic agents; however, some cases occured in patients without identified risk factors. Atripla should be avoided with concurrent or recent use of a nephrotoxic agent).
No products indexed under this heading.

Hydrochlorothiazide (Renal impairment, including cases of acute renal failure and Fanconi syndrome (renal tubular injury with severe hypophosphatemia), has been reported in association with the use of tenofovir DF. The majority of these cases occurred in patients with underlying systemic or renal disease, or in patients taking nephrotoxic agents; however, some cases occured in patients without identified risk factors. Atripla should be avoided with concurrent or recent use of a nephrotoxic agent). Products include:
Atacand HCT **700**
Avalide **2956**
Benicar HCT **1017**
Diovan HCT **2419**
Dyazide **1429**
Exforge HCT **2449**
Hyzaar **2162**
Hyzaar 100-12.5 ....**2162**
Micardis HCT **889**
Prinzide **2246**
Tekturna HCT **2541**
Teveten HCT **541**

Hydrocortisone (Drugs which induce CYP3A4 activity would be expected to increase the clearance of efavirenz resulting in lower plasma concentrations).
No products indexed under this heading.

Hydrocortisone (Alcohol) (Drugs which induce CYP3A4 activity would be expected to increase the clearance of efavirenz resulting in lower plasma concentrations).
No products indexed under this heading.

Hydrocortisone Acetate (Drugs which induce CYP3A4 activity would be expected to increase the clearance of efavirenz resulting in lower plasma concentrations).
No products indexed under this heading.

Hydrocortisone Butyrate (Drugs which induce CYP3A4 activity would be expected to increase the clearance of efavirenz resulting in lower plasma concentrations).
No products indexed under this heading.

Hydrocortisone Cypionate (Drugs which induce CYP3A4 activity would be expected to increase the clearance of efavirenz resulting in lower plasma concentrations).
No products indexed under this heading.

Hydrocortisone Hemisuccinate (Drugs which induce CYP3A4 activity would be expected to increase the clearance of efavirenz resulting in lower plasma concentrations).
No products indexed under this heading.

Hydrocortisone Probutate (Drugs which induce CYP3A4 activity would be expected to increase the clearance of efavirenz resulting in lower plasma concentrations).
No products indexed under this heading.

Hydrocortisone Sodium Phosphate (Drugs which induce CYP3A4 activity would be expected to increase the clearance of efavirenz resulting in lower plasma concentrations).
No products indexed under this heading.

Hydrocortisone Sodium Succinate (Drugs which induce CYP3A4 activity would be expected to increase the clearance of efavirenz resulting in lower plasma concentrations).
No products indexed under this heading.

Hydrocortisone Valerate (Drugs which induce CYP3A4 activity would be expected to increase the clearance of efavirenz resulting in lower plasma concentrations).
No products indexed under this heading.

Hydroflumethiazide (Renal impairment, including cases of acute renal failure and Fanconi syndrome (renal tubular injury with severe hypophosphatemia), has been reported in association with the use of tenofovir DF. The majority of these cases occurred in patients with underlying systemic or renal disease, or in patients taking nephrotoxic agents; however, some cases occured in patients without identified risk factors. Atripla should be avoided with concurrent or recent use of a nephrotoxic agent).
No products indexed under this heading.

Hypericum (Drugs which induce CYP3A4 activity would be expected to increase the clearance of efavirenz resulting in lower plasma concentrations).
No products indexed under this heading.

Hypericum Perforatum (Hypericum perforatum is expected to substantially decrease plasma levels of efavirenz. It has not been studied in combination with efavirenz, but concomitant use is not recommended). Products include:
Traumeel 1800

Ibuprofen (Renal impairment, including cases of acute renal failure and Fanconi syndrome (renal tubular injury with severe hypophosphatemia), has been reported in association with the use of tenofovir DF. The majority of these cases occurred in patients with underlying systemic or renal disease, or in patients taking nephrotoxic agents; however, some cases occured in patients without identified risk factors. Atripla should be avoided with concurrent or recent use of a nephrotoxic agent). Products include:
Motrin IB 2043
Children's Motrin 2044
Children's Motrin Non-Staining
Dye-Free 2044
Infants' Motrin 2044
Infants' Motrin Dye-Free 2044
Junior Strength Motrin 2044
Vicoprofen 564

Idarubicin Hydrochloride (Renal impairment, including cases of acute renal failure and Fanconi syndrome (renal tubular injury with severe hypophosphatemia), has been reported in

association with the use of tenofovir DF. The majority of these cases occurred in patients with underlying systemic or renal disease, or in patients taking nephrotoxic agents; however, some cases occured in patients without identified risk factors. Atripla should be avoided with concurrent or recent use of a nephrotoxic agent).
No products indexed under this heading.

Ifosfamide (Renal impairment, including cases of acute renal failure and Fanconi syndrome (renal tubular injury with severe hypophosphatemia), has been reported in association with the use of tenofovir DF. The majority of these cases occurred in patients with underlying systemic or renal disease, or in patients taking nephrotoxic agents; however, some cases occured in patients without identified risk factors. Atripla should be avoided with concurrent or recent use of a nephrotoxic agent).
No products indexed under this heading.

Imipenem (Renal impairment, including cases of acute renal failure and Fanconi syndrome (renal tubular injury with severe hypophosphatemia), has been reported in association with the use of tenofovir DF. The majority of these cases occurred in patients with underlying systemic or renal disease, or in patients taking nephrotoxic agents; however, some cases occured in patients without identified risk factors. Atripla should be avoided with concurrent or recent use of a nephrotoxic agent). Products include:
Primaxin I.M. 2232
Primaxin I.V. 2235

Imipramine Hydrochloride (In vitro studies have demonstrated that efavirenz inhibits CYP2C9 in the range of observed efavirenz plasma concentrations. Co-administration of efavirenz with drugs primarily metabolized by CYP2C9 may result in altered plasma concentrations of the co-administered drug. Therefore, appropriate dose adjustments may be necessary for these drugs).
No products indexed under this heading.

Imipramine Pamoate (In vitro studies have demonstrated that efavirenz inhibits CYP2C19 in the range of observed efavirenz plasma concentrations. Co-administration of efavirenz with drugs primarily metabolized by CYP2C19 may result in altered plasma concentrations of the co-administered drug. Therefore, appropriate dose adjustments may be necessary for these drugs).
No products indexed under this heading.

Immune Globulin Intravenous (Human) (Renal impairment, including cases of acute renal failure and Fanconi syndrome (renal tubular injury with severe hypophosphatemia), has been reported in association with the use of tenofovir DF. The majority of these cases occurred in patients with underlying systemic or renal disease, or in patients taking nephrotoxic agents; however, some cases occured in patients without identified risk factors. Atripla should be avoided with concurrent or recent use of a nephrotoxic agent). Products include:
Flebogamma 5% DIF 1794
Gammagard 812, 815
Gamunex 3374

Indinavir Sulfate (The optimal dose of indinavir, when given in combination with efavirenz, is not known. Increasing the indinavir dose to 1000 mg every 8 hours does not compensate for the increased indinavir metabolism due to efavirenz). Products include:
Crixivan 2113

Indomethacin (Renal impairment, including cases of acute renal failure and Fanconi syndrome (renal tubular injury with severe hypophosphatemia), has been reported in association with the use of tenofovir DF. The majority of these cases occurred in patients with underlying systemic or renal disease, or in patients taking nephrotoxic agents; however, some cases occured in patients without identified risk factors. Atripla should be avoided with concurrent or recent use of a nephrotoxic agent). Products include:
Indocin 2167

Indomethacin Sodium Trihydrate (Renal impairment, including cases of acute renal failure and Fanconi syndrome (renal tubular injury with severe hypophosphatemia), has been reported in association with the use of tenofovir DF. The majority of these cases occurred in patients with underlying systemic or renal disease, or in patients taking nephrotoxic agents; however, some cases occured in patients without identified risk factors. Atripla should be avoided with concurrent or recent use of a nephrotoxic agent). Products include:
Indocin I.V. 2007

Interferon Beta-1b (Renal impairment, including cases of acute renal failure and Fanconi syndrome (renal tubular injury with severe hypophosphatemia), has been reported in association with the use of tenofovir DF. The majority of these cases occurred in patients with underlying systemic or renal disease, or in patients taking nephrotoxic agents; however, some cases occured in patients without identified risk factors. Atripla should be avoided with concurrent or recent use of a nephrotoxic agent). Products include:
Betaseron 836
Extavia 2459

Interleuken-2 (Renal impairment, including cases of acute renal failure and Fanconi syndrome (renal tubular injury with severe hypophosphatemia), has been reported in association with the use of tenofovir DF. The majority of these cases occurred in patients with underlying systemic or renal disease, or in patients taking nephrotoxic agents; however, some cases occured in patients without identified risk factors. Atripla should be avoided with concurrent or recent use of a nephrotoxic agent).
No products indexed under this heading.

Iodamide Meglumine (Renal impairment, including cases of acute renal failure and Fanconi syndrome (renal tubular injury with severe hypophosphatemia), has been reported in association with the use of tenofovir DF. The majority of these cases occurred in patients with underlying systemic or renal disease, or in patients taking nephrotoxic agents; however, some cases occured in patients without identified risk factors. Atripla should be avoided with concurrent or recent use of a nephrotoxic agent).
No products indexed under this heading.

Iohexol (Renal impairment, including cases of acute renal failure and Fanconi syndrome (renal tubular injury with severe hypophosphatemia), has been reported in association with the use of tenofovir DF. The majority of these cases occurred in patients with underlying systemic or renal disease, or in patients taking nephrotoxic agents; however, some cases occured in patients without identified risk factors. Atripla should be avoided with concurrent or recent use of a nephrotoxic agent).
No products indexed under this heading.

Iopamidol (Renal impairment, including cases of acute renal failure and Fanconi syndrome (renal tubular injury with severe hypophosphatemia), has been reported in association with the use of tenofovir DF. The majority of these cases occurred in patients with underlying systemic or renal disease, or in patients taking nephrotoxic agents; however, some cases occured in patients without identified risk factors. Atripla should be avoided with concurrent or recent use of a nephrotoxic agent).
No products indexed under this heading.

Iopanoic Acid (Renal impairment, including cases of acute renal failure and Fanconi syndrome (renal tubular injury with severe hypophosphatemia), has been reported in association with the use of tenofovir DF. The majority of these cases occurred in patients with underlying systemic or renal disease, or in patients taking nephrotoxic agents; however, some cases occured in patients without identified risk factors. Atripla should be avoided with concurrent or recent use of a nephrotoxic agent).
No products indexed under this heading.

Iothalamate Meglumine (Renal impairment, including cases of acute renal failure and Fanconi syndrome (renal tubular injury with severe hypophosphatemia), has been reported in association with the use of tenofovir DF. The majority of these cases occurred in patients with underlying systemic or renal disease, or in patients taking nephrotoxic agents; however, some cases occured in patients without identified risk factors. Atripla should be avoided with concurrent or recent use of a nephrotoxic agent).
No products indexed under this heading.

Ioxaglate Meglumine (Renal impairment, including cases of acute renal failure and Fanconi syndrome (renal tubular injury with severe hypophosphatemia), has been reported in association with the use of tenofovir DF. The majority of these cases occurred in patients with underlying systemic or renal disease, or in patients taking nephrotoxic agents; however, some cases occured in patients without identified risk factors. Atripla should be avoided with concurrent or recent use of a nephrotoxic agent).
No products indexed under this heading.

Ioxaglate Sodium (Renal impairment, including cases of acute renal failure and Fanconi syndrome (renal tubular injury with severe hypophosphatemia), has been reported in association with the use of tenofovir DF. The majority of these cases occurred in patients with underlying systemic or renal disease, or in patients taking nephrotoxic agents; however, some cases occured in patients without identified risk factors. Atripla should be avoided with concurrent or recent use of a nephrotoxic agent).
No products indexed under this heading.

Irbesartan (In vitro studies have demonstrated that efavirenz inhibits CYP2C9 in the range of observed efavirenz plasma concentrations. Co-administration of efavirenz with drugs primarily metabolized by CYP2C9 may result in altered plasma concentrations of the co-administered drug. Therefore, appropriate dose adjustments may be necessary for these drugs). Products include:
Avalide 2956
Avapro 2962

Isradipine (Efavirenz has been shown in vivo to induce CYP3A4. Other compounds that are substrates of CYP3A4

IMPORTANT NOTE: Always consult each drug listing in the patient's regimen for possible interactions.

may have decreased plasma concentrations when co-administered with efavirenz). Products include:
DynaCirc CR 1432

Itraconazole (Drug interaction studies with Atripla and these imidazole and triazole antifungals have not been conducted. Efavirenz has the potential to decrease plasma concentrations of itraconazole and ketoconazole).
No products indexed under this heading.

Ixabepilone (Efavirenz has been shown *in vivo* to induce CYP3A4. Other compounds that are substrates of CYP3A4 may have decreased plasma concentrations when co-administered with efavirenz).
No products indexed under this heading.

Kanamycin Sulfate (Renal impairment, including cases of acute renal failure and Fanconi syndrome (renal tubular injury with severe hypophosphatemia), has been reported in association with the use of tenofovir DF. The majority of these cases occurred in patients with underlying systemic or renal disease, or in patients taking nephrotoxic agents; however, some cases occured in patients without identified risk factors. Atripla should be avoided with concurrent or recent use of a nephrotoxic agent).
No products indexed under this heading.

Ketoconazole (Drug interaction studies with Atripla and these imidazole and triazole antifungals have not been conducted. Efavirenz has the potential to decrease plasma concentrations of itraconazole and ketoconazole). Products include:
Extina 3319
Xolegel 3337

Ketoprofen (Renal impairment, including cases of acute renal failure and Fanconi syndrome (renal tubular injury with severe hypophosphatemia), has been reported in association with the use of tenofovir DF. The majority of these cases occurred in patients with underlying systemic or renal disease, or in patients taking nephrotoxic agents; however, some cases occured in patients without identified risk factors. Atripla should be avoided with concurrent or recent use of a nephrotoxic agent).
No products indexed under this heading.

Ketorolac Tromethamine (Renal impairment, including cases of acute renal failure and Fanconi syndrome (renal tubular injury with severe hypophosphatemia), has been reported in association with the use of tenofovir DF. The majority of these cases occurred in patients with underlying systemic or renal disease, or in patients taking nephrotoxic agents; however, some cases occured in patients without identified risk factors. Atripla should be avoided with concurrent or recent use of a nephrotoxic agent). Products include:
Acuvail .... ⊙209

Lamium album (Renal impairment, including cases of acute renal failure and Fanconi syndrome (renal tubular injury with severe hypophosphatemia), has been reported in association with the use of tenofovir DF. The majority of these cases occurred in patients with underlying systemic or renal disease, or in patients taking nephrotoxic agents; however, some cases occured in patients without identified risk factors. Atripla should be avoided with concurrent or recent use of a nephrotoxic agent).
No products indexed under this heading.

Lamotrigine (In vitro studies have demonstrated that efavirenz inhibits CYP2C19 in the range of observed efavirenz plasma concentrations. Co-

administration of efavirenz with drugs primarily metabolized by CYP2C19 may result in altered plasma concentrations of the co-administered drug. Therefore, appropriate dose adjustments may be necessary for these drugs). Products include:
Lamictal 1522
Lamictal ODT 1522
Lamictal XR 1536

Lansoprazole (In vitro studies have demonstrated that efavirenz inhibits CYP2C9 in the range of observed efavirenz plasma concentrations. Co-administration of efavirenz with drugs primarily metabolized by CYP2C9 may result in altered plasma concentrations of the co-administered drug. Therefore, appropriate dose adjustments may be necessary for these drugs).
No products indexed under this heading.

Levetiracetam (In vitro studies have demonstrated that efavirenz inhibits CYP2C19 in the range of observed efavirenz plasma concentrations. Co-administration of efavirenz with drugs primarily metabolized by CYP2C19 may result in altered plasma concentrations of the co-administered drug. Therefore, appropriate dose adjustments may be necessary for these drugs). Products include:
Keppra XR 3434

Levonorgestrel (Efavirenz has been shown *in vivo* to induce CYP3A4. Other compounds that are substrates of CYP3A4 may have decreased plasma concentrations when co-administered with efavirenz). Products include:
Climara Pro 847
LoSeasonique 3407
Lybrel 3514
Mirena 854
Plan B 3416
Seasonique 3418

Lidocaine (Efavirenz has been shown *in vivo* to induce CYP3A4. Other compounds that are substrates of CYP3A4 may have decreased plasma concentrations when co-administered with efavirenz). Products include:
Lidoderm 1107

Lidocaine Hydrochloride (Efavirenz has been shown *in vivo* to induce CYP3A4. Other compounds that are substrates of CYP3A4 may have decreased plasma concentrations when co-administered with efavirenz).
No products indexed under this heading.

Lisinopril (Renal impairment, including cases of acute renal failure and Fanconi syndrome (renal tubular injury with severe hypophosphatemia), has been reported in association with the use of tenofovir DF. The majority of these cases occurred in patients with underlying systemic or renal disease, or in patients taking nephrotoxic agents; however, some cases occured in patients without identified risk factors. Atripla should be avoided with concurrent or recent use of a nephrotoxic agent). Products include:
Prinivil 2241
Prinzide 2246

Lithium (Renal impairment, including cases of acute renal failure and Fanconi syndrome (renal tubular injury with severe hypophosphatemia), has been reported in association with the use of tenofovir DF. The majority of these cases occurred in patients with underlying systemic or renal disease, or in patients taking nephrotoxic agents; however, some cases occured in patients without identified risk factors. Atripla should be avoided with concurrent or recent use of a nephrotoxic agent).
No products indexed under this heading.

Lithium Carbonate (Renal impairment, including cases of acute renal

failure and Fanconi syndrome (renal tubular injury with severe hypophosphatemia), has been reported in association with the use of tenofovir DF. The majority of these cases occurred in patients with underlying systemic or renal disease, or in patients taking nephrotoxic agents; however, some cases occured in patients without identified risk factors. Atripla should be avoided with concurrent or recent use of a nephrotoxic agent).
No products indexed under this heading.

Lithium Citrate (Renal impairment, including cases of acute renal failure and Fanconi syndrome (renal tubular injury with severe hypophosphatemia), has been reported in association with the use of tenofovir DF. The majority of these cases occurred in patients with underlying systemic or renal disease, or in patients taking nephrotoxic agents; however, some cases occured in patients without identified risk factors. Atripla should be avoided with concurrent or recent use of a nephrotoxic agent).
No products indexed under this heading.

Lopinavir (Kaletra has been shown to increase tenofovir concentrations. The mechanism of this interaction is unknown. Higher tenofovir concentrations could potentiate tenofovir-associated adverse events, including renal disorders. Patients receiving Kaletra with tenofovir DF should be monitored for tenofovir-associated adverse events. Atripla should be discontinued in patients who develop tenofovir-associated adverse events). Products include:
Kaletra 458

Loracarbef (Renal impairment, including cases of acute renal failure and Fanconi syndrome (renal tubular injury with severe hypophosphatemia), has been reported in association with the use of tenofovir DF. The majority of these cases occurred in patients with underlying systemic or renal disease, or in patients taking nephrotoxic agents; however, some cases occured in patients without identified risk factors. Atripla should be avoided with concurrent or recent use of a nephrotoxic agent).
No products indexed under this heading.

Losartan Potassium (In vitro studies have demonstrated that efavirenz inhibits CYP2C9 in the range of observed efavirenz plasma concentrations. Co-administration of efavirenz with drugs primarily metabolized by CYP2C9 may result in altered plasma concentrations of the co-administered drug. Therefore, appropriate dose adjustments may be necessary for these drugs). Products include:
Cozaar 2106
Hyzaar 2162
Hyzaar 100-12.5 2162

Lovastatin (Renal impairment, including cases of acute renal failure and Fanconi syndrome (renal tubular injury with severe hypophosphatemia), has been reported in association with the use of tenofovir DF. The majority of these cases occurred in patients with underlying systemic or renal disease, or in patients taking nephrotoxic agents; however, some cases occured in patients without identified risk factors. Atripla should be avoided with concurrent or recent use of a nephrotoxic agent). Products include:
Advicor 402
Mevacor 2212

Maprotiline Hydrochloride (In vitro studies have demonstrated that efavirenz inhibits CYP2C19 in the range of observed efavirenz plasma concentrations. Co-administration of efavirenz with drugs primarily metabolized by CYP2C19 may result in altered plasma concentrations of the co-administered drug. Therefore, appropriate dose adjustments may be necessary for these drugs).
No products indexed under this heading.

Meclofenamate Sodium (Renal impairment, including cases of acute renal failure and Fanconi syndrome (renal tubular injury with severe hypophosphatemia), has been reported in association with the use of tenofovir DF. The majority of these cases occurred in patients with underlying systemic or renal disease, or in patients taking nephrotoxic agents; however, some cases occured in patients without identified risk factors. Atripla should be avoided with concurrent or recent use of a nephrotoxic agent).
No products indexed under this heading.

Mefenamic Acid (Renal impairment, including cases of acute renal failure and Fanconi syndrome (renal tubular injury with severe hypophosphatemia), has been reported in association with the use of tenofovir DF. The majority of these cases occurred in patients with underlying systemic or renal disease, or in patients taking nephrotoxic agents; however, some cases occured in patients without identified risk factors. Atripla should be avoided with concurrent or recent use of a nephrotoxic agent).
No products indexed under this heading.

Meloxicam (Renal impairment, including cases of acute renal failure and Fanconi syndrome (renal tubular injury with severe hypophosphatemia), has been reported in association with the use of tenofovir DF. The majority of these cases occurred in patients with underlying systemic or renal disease, or in patients taking nephrotoxic agents; however, some cases occured in patients without identified risk factors. Atripla should be avoided with concurrent or recent use of a nephrotoxic agent).
No products indexed under this heading.

Melphalan Hydrochloride (Renal impairment, including cases of acute renal failure and Fanconi syndrome (renal tubular injury with severe hypophosphatemia), has been reported in association with the use of tenofovir DF. The majority of these cases occurred in patients with underlying systemic or renal disease, or in patients taking nephrotoxic agents; however, some cases occured in patients without identified risk factors. Atripla should be avoided with concurrent or recent use of a nephrotoxic agent). Products include:
Alkeran for Injection 1300

Mephenytoin (Drugs which induce CYP3A4 activity would be expected to increase the clearance of efavirenz resulting in lower plasma concentrations).
No products indexed under this heading.

Mephobarbital (In vitro studies have demonstrated that efavirenz inhibits CYP2C19 in the range of observed efavirenz plasma concentrations. Co-administration of efavirenz with drugs primarily metabolized by CYP2C19 may result in altered plasma concentrations of the co-administered drug. Therefore, appropriate dose adjustments may be necessary for these drugs).
No products indexed under this heading.

Meprobamate (In vitro studies have demonstrated that efavirenz inhibits CYP2C19 in the range of observed efavirenz plasma concentrations. Co-administration of efavirenz with drugs primarily metabolized by CYP2C19 may result in altered plasma concentrations of the co-administered drug. Therefore, appropriate dose adjustments may be necessary for these drugs).
No products indexed under this heading.

Mesalamine (Renal impairment, including cases of acute renal failure and Fanconi syndrome (renal tubular injury with severe hypophosphatemia), has been reported in association with the use of tenofovir DF. The majority of these cases occurred in patients with underlying systemic or renal disease, or in patients taking nephrotoxic agents; however, some cases occured in patients without identified risk factors. Atripla should be avoided with concurrent or recent use of a nephrotoxic agent). Products include:
Apriso **2899**
Asacol **2786**
Asacol HD **2787**
Canasa **782**
Lialda **3295**
Pentasa **3297**

Mestranol (Efavirenz has been shown *in vivo* to induce CYP3A4. Other compounds that are substrates of CYP3A4 may have decreased plasma concentrations when co-administered with efavirenz).
No products indexed under this heading.

Metformin Hydrochloride (In vitro studies have demonstrated that efavirenz inhibits CYP2C9 in the range of observed efavirenz plasma concentrations. Co-administration of efavirenz with drugs primarily metabolized by CYP2C9 may result in altered plasma concentrations of the co-administered drug. Therefore, appropriate dose adjustments may be necessary for these drugs). Products include:
ActoPlus **3338**
Avandamet **1345**
Janumet **2188**

Methadone Hydrochloride (Co-administration of efavirenz in HIV-infected individuals with a history of injection drug use resulted in decreased plasma levels of methadone and signs of opiate withdrawal. Methadone dose was increased by a mean of 22% to alleviate withdrawal symptoms. Patients should be monitored for signs of withdrawal and their methadone dose increased as required to alleviate withdrawal symptoms).
No products indexed under this heading.

Methimazole (Renal impairment, including cases of acute renal failure and Fanconi syndrome (renal tubular injury with severe hypophosphatemia), has been reported in association with the use of tenofovir DF. The majority of these cases occurred in patients with underlying systemic or renal disease, or in patients taking nephrotoxic agents; however, some cases occured in patients without identified risk factors. Atripla should be avoided with concurrent or recent use of a nephrotoxic agent).
No products indexed under this heading.

Methotrexate (Renal impairment, including cases of acute renal failure and Fanconi syndrome (renal tubular injury with severe hypophosphatemia), has been reported in association with the use of tenofovir DF. The majority of these cases occurred in patients with underlying systemic or renal disease, or in patients taking nephrotoxic agents; however, some cases occured in patients without identified risk factors. Atripla should be avoided with concurrent or recent use of a nephrotoxic agent).
No products indexed under this heading.

Methotrexate Sodium (Renal impairment, including cases of acute renal failure and Fanconi syndrome (renal tubular injury with severe hypophosphatemia), has been reported in association with the use of tenofovir DF. The majority of these cases occurred in patients with underlying systemic or renal disease, or in patients taking nephrotoxic agents; however, some cases occured in patients without identified risk factors. Atripla should be avoided with concurrent or recent use of a nephrotoxic agent).
No products indexed under this heading.

Methsuximide (Drugs which induce CYP3A4 activity would be expected to increase the clearance of efavirenz resulting in lower plasma concentrations).
No products indexed under this heading.

Methyclothiazide (Renal impairment, including cases of acute renal failure and Fanconi syndrome (renal tubular injury with severe hypophosphatemia), has been reported in association with the use of tenofovir DF. The majority of these cases occurred in patients with underlying systemic or renal disease, or in patients taking nephrotoxic agents; however, some cases occured in patients without identified risk factors. Atripla should be avoided with concurrent or recent use of a nephrotoxic agent).
No products indexed under this heading.

Methylergonovine Maleate (Due to the potential for serious and/or life-threatening reactions, such as acute ergot toxicity characterized by peripheral vasospasm and ischemia of the extremities and other tissues, concomitant use with ergot derivatives is contraindicated).
No products indexed under this heading.

Methylprednisolone (Drugs which induce CYP3A4 activity would be expected to increase the clearance of efavirenz resulting in lower plasma concentrations).
No products indexed under this heading.

Methylprednisolone Acetate (Drugs which induce CYP3A4 activity would be expected to increase the clearance of efavirenz resulting in lower plasma concentrations).
No products indexed under this heading.

Methylprednisolone Sodium Succinate (Drugs which induce CYP3A4 activity would be expected to increase the clearance of efavirenz resulting in lower plasma concentrations).
No products indexed under this heading.

Mezlocillin Sodium (Renal impairment, including cases of acute renal failure and Fanconi syndrome (renal tubular injury with severe hypophosphatemia), has been reported in association with the use of tenofovir DF. The majority of these cases occurred in patients with underlying systemic or renal disease, or in patients taking nephrotoxic agents; however, some cases occured in patients without identified risk factors. Atripla should be avoided with concurrent or recent use of a nephrotoxic agent).
No products indexed under this heading.

Midazolam Hydrochloride (Due to the potential for serious and/or life-threatening reactions, such as prolonged or increased sedation or respiratory depression, concomitant use with midazolam hydrochloride is contraindicated).
No products indexed under this heading.

Miglitol (In vitro studies have demonstrated that efavirenz inhibits CYP2C9 in the range of observed efavirenz plasma concentrations. Co-administration of efavirenz with drugs primarily metabolized by CYP2C9 may result in altered plasma concentrations of the co-administered drug. Therefore, appropriate dose adjustments may be necessary for these drugs).
No products indexed under this heading.

Minocycline Hydrochloride (Renal impairment, including cases of acute renal failure and Fanconi syndrome (renal tubular injury with severe hypophosphatemia), has been reported in association with the use of tenofovir DF. The majority of these cases occurred in patients with underlying systemic or renal disease, or in patients taking nephrotoxic agents; however, some cases occured in patients without identified risk factors. Atripla should be avoided with concurrent or recent use of a nephrotoxic agent). Products include:
Solodyn **2073**

Mirtazapine (In vitro studies have demonstrated that efavirenz inhibits CYP2C9 in the range of observed efavirenz plasma concentrations. Co-administration of efavirenz with drugs primarily metabolized by CYP2C9 may result in altered plasma concentrations of the co-administered drug. Therefore, appropriate dose adjustments may be necessary for these drugs). Products include:
Remeron Tablets **3214**
RemeronSolTab Tablets **3219**

Mitomycin (Mitomycin-C) (Renal impairment, including cases of acute renal failure and Fanconi syndrome (renal tubular injury with severe hypophosphatemia), has been reported in association with the use of tenofovir DF. The majority of these cases occurred in patients with underlying systemic or renal disease, or in patients taking nephrotoxic agents; however, some cases occured in patients without identified risk factors. Atripla should be avoided with concurrent or recent use of a nephrotoxic agent).
No products indexed under this heading.

Modafinil (Drugs which induce CYP3A4 activity would be expected to increase the clearance of efavirenz resulting in lower plasma concentrations). Products include:
Provigil **983**

Moexipril Hydrochloride (Renal impairment, including cases of acute renal failure and Fanconi syndrome (renal tubular injury with severe hypophosphatemia), has been reported in association with the use of tenofovir DF. The majority of these cases occurred in patients with underlying systemic or renal disease, or in patients taking nephrotoxic agents; however, some cases occured in patients without identified risk factors. Atripla should be avoided with concurrent or recent use of a nephrotoxic agent).
No products indexed under this heading.

Montelukast Sodium (In vitro studies have demonstrated that efavirenz inhibits CYP2C9 in the range of observed efavirenz plasma concentrations. Co-administration of efavirenz with drugs primarily metabolized by CYP2C9 may result in altered plasma concentrations of the co-administered drug. Therefore, appropriate dose adjustments may be necessary for these drugs). Products include:
Singulair **2270**

Muromonab-CD3 (Renal impairment, including cases of acute renal failure and Fanconi syndrome (renal tubular injury with severe hypophosphatemia), has been reported in association with the use of tenofovir DF. The majority of these cases occurred in patients with underlying systemic or renal disease, or in patients taking nephrotoxic agents; however, some cases occured in patients without identified risk factors. Atripla should be avoided with concurrent or recent use of a nephrotoxic agent). Products include:
Orthoclone OKT3 .... **949**

Nabumetone (Renal impairment, including cases of acute renal failure and Fanconi syndrome (renal tubular injury with severe hypophosphatemia), has been reported in association with the use of tenofovir DF. The majority of these cases occurred in patients with underlying systemic or renal disease, or in patients taking nephrotoxic agents; however, some cases occured in patients without identified risk factors. Atripla should be avoided with concurrent or recent use of a nephrotoxic agent).
No products indexed under this heading.

Nafcillin Sodium (Renal impairment, including cases of acute renal failure and Fanconi syndrome (renal tubular injury with severe hypophosphatemia), has been reported in association with the use of tenofovir DF. The majority of these cases occurred in patients with underlying systemic or renal disease, or in patients taking nephrotoxic agents; however, some cases occured in patients without identified risk factors. Atripla should be avoided with concurrent or recent use of a nephrotoxic agent).
No products indexed under this heading.

Naproxen (Renal impairment, including cases of acute renal failure and Fanconi syndrome (renal tubular injury with severe hypophosphatemia), has been reported in association with the use of tenofovir DF. The majority of these cases occurred in patients with underlying systemic or renal disease, or in patients taking nephrotoxic agents; however, some cases occured in patients without identified risk factors. Atripla should be avoided with concurrent or recent use of a nephrotoxic agent). Products include:
EC-Naprosyn **2850**
Naprosyn **2850**
Anaprox/Naprosyn **2850**

Naproxen Sodium (Renal impairment, including cases of acute renal failure and Fanconi syndrome (renal tubular injury with severe hypophosphatemia), has been reported in association with the use of tenofovir DF. The majority of these cases occurred in patients with underlying systemic or renal disease, or in patients taking nephrotoxic agents; however, some cases occured in patients without identified risk factors. Atripla should be avoided with concurrent or recent use of a nephrotoxic agent). Products include:
Anaprox **2850**
Anaprox DS **2850**
Treximet **1681**

Nateglinide (In vitro studies have demonstrated that efavirenz inhibits CYP2C9 in the range of observed efavirenz plasma concentrations. Co-administration of efavirenz with drugs primarily metabolized by CYP2C9 may result in altered plasma concentrations of the co-administered drug. Therefore, appropriate dose adjustments may be necessary for these drugs).
No products indexed under this heading.

Nefazodone Hydrochloride (Efavirenz has been shown *in vivo* to induce CYP3A4. Other compounds that are substrates of CYP3A4 may have decreased plasma concentrations when co-administered with efavirenz).
No products indexed under this heading.

fied risk factors. Atripla should be avoided with concurrent or recent use of a nephrotoxic agent).
No products indexed under this heading.

Penicillin G Procaine (Renal impairment, including cases of acute renal failure and Fanconi syndrome (renal tubular injury with severe hypophosphatemia), has been reported in association with the use of tenofovir DF. The majority of these cases occurred in patients with underlying systemic or renal disease, or in patients taking nephrotoxic agents; however, some cases occured in patients without identified risk factors. Atripla should be avoided with concurrent or recent use of a nephrotoxic agent). Products include:
Bicillin C-R Injectable Suspension 1826
Bicillin L-A 1828

Penicillin G Sodium (Renal impairment, including cases of acute renal failure and Fanconi syndrome (renal tubular injury with severe hypophosphatemia), has been reported in association with the use of tenofovir DF. The majority of these cases occurred in patients with underlying systemic or renal disease, or in patients taking nephrotoxic agents; however, some cases occured in patients without identified risk factors. Atripla should be avoided with concurrent or recent use of a nephrotoxic agent).
No products indexed under this heading.

Penicillin V Potassium (Renal impairment, including cases of acute renal failure and Fanconi syndrome (renal tubular injury with severe hypophosphatemia), has been reported in association with the use of tenofovir DF. The majority of these cases occurred in patients with underlying systemic or renal disease, or in patients taking nephrotoxic agents; however, some cases occured in patients without identified risk factors. Atripla should be avoided with concurrent or recent use of a nephrotoxic agent).
No products indexed under this heading.

Pentamidine Isethionate (Renal impairment, including cases of acute renal failure and Fanconi syndrome (renal tubular injury with severe hypophosphatemia), has been reported in association with the use of tenofovir DF. The majority of these cases occurred in patients with underlying systemic or renal disease, or in patients taking nephrotoxic agents; however, some cases occured in patients without identified risk factors. Atripla should be avoided with concurrent or recent use of a nephrotoxic agent).
No products indexed under this heading.

Perindopril Erbumine (Renal impairment, including cases of acute renal failure and Fanconi syndrome (renal tubular injury with severe hypophosphatemia), has been reported in association with the use of tenofovir DF. The majority of these cases occurred in patients with underlying systemic or renal disease, or in patients taking nephrotoxic agents; however, some cases occured in patients without identified risk factors. Atripla should be avoided with concurrent or recent use of a nephrotoxic agent).
No products indexed under this heading.

Phenacemide (In vitro studies have demonstrated that efavirenz inhibits CYP2C19 in the range of observed efavirenz plasma concentrations. Co-administration of efavirenz with drugs primarily metabolized by CYP2C19 may result in altered plasma concentrations of the co-administered drug. Therefore, appropriate dose adjustments may be necessary for these drugs).
No products indexed under this heading.

Phenobarbital (Potential for reduction in anticonvulsant and/or efavirenz plasma levels; periodic monitoring of anticonvulsant plasma levels should be conducted). Products include:
Donnatal 2711

Phenobarbital Sodium (Potential for reduction in anticonvulsant and/or efavirenz plasma levels; periodic monitoring of anticonvulsant plasma levels should be conducted).
No products indexed under this heading.

Phensuximide (In vitro studies have demonstrated that efavirenz inhibits CYP2C19 in the range of observed efavirenz plasma concentrations. Co-administration of efavirenz with drugs primarily metabolized by CYP2C19 may result in altered plasma concentrations of the co-administered drug. Therefore, appropriate dose adjustments may be necessary for these drugs).
No products indexed under this heading.

Phenylbutazone (Renal impairment, including cases of acute renal failure and Fanconi syndrome (renal tubular injury with severe hypophosphatemia), has been reported in association with the use of tenofovir DF. The majority of these cases occurred in patients with underlying systemic or renal disease, or in patients taking nephrotoxic agents; however, some cases occured in patients without identified risk factors. Atripla should be avoided with concurrent or recent use of a nephrotoxic agent).
No products indexed under this heading.

Phenytoin (Potential for reduction in anticonvulsant and/or efavirenz plasma levels; periodic monitoring of anticonvulsant plasma levels should be conducted).
No products indexed under this heading.

Phenytoin Sodium (Potential for reduction in anticonvulsant and/or efavirenz plasma levels; periodic monitoring of anticonvulsant plasma levels should be conducted). Products include:
Phenytek Capsules 2380

Pimozide (Due to the potential for serious and/or life threatening reactions, such as cardiac arrhythmias, concomitant use with pimozide is contraindicated).
No products indexed under this heading.

Pioglitazone Hydrochloride (In vitro studies have demonstrated that efavirenz inhibits CYP2C9 in the range of observed efavirenz plasma concentrations. Co-administration of efavirenz with drugs primarily metabolized by CYP2C9 may result in altered plasma concentrations of the co-administered drug. Therefore, appropriate dose adjustments may be necessary for these drugs). Products include:
ActoPlus 3338
Actos 3345
Duetact 3354

Piroxicam (Renal impairment, including cases of acute renal failure and Fanconi syndrome (renal tubular injury with severe hypophosphatemia), has been reported in association with the use of tenofovir DF. The majority of these cases occurred in patients with underlying systemic or renal disease, or in patients taking nephrotoxic agents; however, some cases occured in patients without identified risk factors. Atripla should be avoided with concurrent or recent use of a nephrotoxic agent).
No products indexed under this heading.

Plicamycin (Renal impairment, including cases of acute renal failure and Fanconi syndrome (renal tubular injury with severe hypophosphatemia), has been reported in association with the use of tenofovir DF. The majority of these cases occurred in patients with underlying systemic or renal disease, or in patients taking nephrotoxic agents; however, some cases occured in patients without identified risk factors. Atripla should be avoided with concurrent or recent use of a nephrotoxic agent).
No products indexed under this heading.

Polyestradiol Phosphate (Efavirenz has been shown *in vivo* to induce CYP3A4. Other compounds that are substrates of CYP3A4 may have decreased plasma concentrations when co-administered with efavirenz).
No products indexed under this heading.

Polymyxin (Renal impairment, including cases of acute renal failure and Fanconi syndrome (renal tubular injury with severe hypophosphatemia), has been reported in association with the use of tenofovir DF. The majority of these cases occurred in patients with underlying systemic or renal disease, or in patients taking nephrotoxic agents; however, some cases occured in patients without identified risk factors. Atripla should be avoided with concurrent or recent use of a nephrotoxic agent).
No products indexed under this heading.

Polymyxin B Sulfate (Renal impairment, including cases of acute renal failure and Fanconi syndrome (renal tubular injury with severe hypophosphatemia), has been reported in association with the use of tenofovir DF. The majority of these cases occurred in patients with underlying systemic or renal disease, or in patients taking nephrotoxic agents; however, some cases occured in patients without identified risk factors. Atripla should be avoided with concurrent or recent use of a nephrotoxic agent).
No products indexed under this heading.

Polythiazide (Renal impairment, including cases of acute renal failure and Fanconi syndrome (renal tubular injury with severe hypophosphatemia), has been reported in association with the use of tenofovir DF. The majority of these cases occurred in patients with underlying systemic or renal disease, or in patients taking nephrotoxic agents; however, some cases occured in patients without identified risk factors. Atripla should be avoided with concurrent or recent use of a nephrotoxic agent).
No products indexed under this heading.

Pravastatin Sodium (Plasma concentrations of atorvastatin, pravastatin, and simvastatin decreased with efavirenz. Consult the complete prescribing information for the HMGCoA reductase inhibitor for guidance on individualizing the dose).
No products indexed under this heading.

Prednisolone (Drugs which induce CYP3A4 activity would be expected to increase the clearance of efavirenz resulting in lower plasma concentrations).
No products indexed under this heading.

Prednisolone Acetate (Drugs which induce CYP3A4 activity would be expected to increase the clearance of efavirenz resulting in lower plasma concentrations). Products include:
Blephamide .... ⊙ 212, ⊙ 214
Pred Forte .... ⊙ 225
Pred Mild .... ⊙ 230
Pred-G .... ⊙ 226, ⊙ 227

Prednisolone Sodium Phosphate (Drugs which induce CYP3A4 activity would be expected to increase the clearance of efavirenz resulting in lower plasma concentrations).
No products indexed under this heading.

Prednisolone Tebutate (Drugs which induce CYP3A4 activity would be expected to increase the clearance of efavirenz resulting in lower plasma concentrations).
No products indexed under this heading.

Prednisone (Drugs which induce CYP3A4 activity would be expected to increase the clearance of efavirenz resulting in lower plasma concentrations).
No products indexed under this heading.

Prednisone sodium phosphate (Drugs which induce CYP3A4 activity would be expected to increase the clearance of efavirenz resulting in lower plasma concentrations).
No products indexed under this heading.

Primidone (Drugs which induce CYP3A4 activity would be expected to increase the clearance of efavirenz resulting in lower plasma concentrations).
No products indexed under this heading.

Progesterone (In vitro studies have demonstrated that efavirenz inhibits CYP2C19 in the range of observed efavirenz plasma concentrations. Co-administration of efavirenz with drugs primarily metabolized by CYP2C19 may result in altered plasma concentrations of the co-administered drug. Therefore, appropriate dose adjustments may be necessary for these drugs). Products include:
Crinone 4% 996
Crinone 8% 996
Prometrium 3307

Proguanil Hydrochloride (In vitro studies have demonstrated that efavirenz inhibits CYP2C19 in the range of observed efavirenz plasma concentrations. Co-administration of efavirenz with drugs primarily metabolized by CYP2C19 may result in altered plasma concentrations of the co-administered drug. Therefore, appropriate dose adjustments may be necessary for these drugs). Products include:
Malarone Pediatric Tablets 1572
Malarone 1572

Propranolol Hydrochloride (In vitro studies have demonstrated that efavirenz inhibits CYP2C19 in the range of observed efavirenz plasma concentrations. Co-administration of efavirenz with drugs primarily metabolized by CYP2C19 may result in altered plasma concentrations of the co-administered drug. Therefore, appropriate dose adjustments may be necessary for these drugs). Products include:
InnoPran XL 1517

Protriptyline Hydrochloride (In vitro studies have demonstrated that efavirenz inhibits CYP2C19 in the range of observed efavirenz plasma concentrations. Co-administration of efavirenz with drugs primarily metabolized by CYP2C19 may result in altered plasma concentrations of the co-administered drug. Therefore, appropriate dose adjustments may be necessary for these drugs).
No products indexed under this heading.

Quinapril Hydrochloride (Renal impairment, including cases of acute renal failure and Fanconi syndrome (renal tubular injury with severe hypophosphatemia), has been reported in association with the use of tenofovir DF. The majority of these cases occurred in patients with underlying systemic or renal disease, or in patients taking nephrotoxic agents; however, some cases occured in patients without identified risk factors. Atripla should be avoided with concurrent or recent use of a nephrotoxic agent).
No products indexed under this heading.

IMPORTANT NOTE: Always consult each drug listing in the patient's regimen for possible interactions.

Atripla Interactions Index 172

Quinidine Gluconate (Efavirenz has been shown *in vivo* to induce CYP3A4. Other compounds that are substrates of CYP3A4 may have decreased plasma concentrations when co-administered with efavirenz).
No products indexed under this heading.

Quinidine Polygalacturonate (Efavirenz has been shown *in vivo* to induce CYP3A4. Other compounds that are substrates of CYP3A4 may have decreased plasma concentrations when co-administered with efavirenz).
No products indexed under this heading.

Quinidine Sulfate (Efavirenz has been shown *in vivo* to induce CYP3A4. Other compounds that are substrates of CYP3A4 may have decreased plasma concentrations when co-administered with efavirenz).
No products indexed under this heading.

Rabeprazole Sodium (Renal impairment, including cases of acute renal failure and Fanconi syndrome (renal tubular injury with severe hypophosphatemia), has been reported in association with the use of tenofovir DF. The majority of these cases occurred in patients with underlying systemic or renal disease, or in patients taking nephrotoxic agents; however, some cases occured in patients without identified risk factors. Atripla should be avoided with concurrent or recent use of a nephrotoxic agent). Products include:
Aciphex 1035

Ramipril (Renal impairment, including cases of acute renal failure and Fanconi syndrome (renal tubular injury with severe hypophosphatemia), has been reported in association with the use of tenofovir DF. The majority of these cases occurred in patients with underlying systemic or renal disease, or in patients taking nephrotoxic agents; however, some cases occured in patients without identified risk factors. Atripla should be avoided with concurrent or recent use of a nephrotoxic agent).
No products indexed under this heading.

Repaglinide (In vitro studies have demonstrated that efavirenz inhibits CYP2C9 in the range of observed efavirenz plasma concentrations. Co-administration of efavirenz with drugs primarily metabolized by CYP2C9 may result in altered plasma concentrations of the co-administered drug. Therefore, appropriate dose adjustments may be necessary for these drugs).
No products indexed under this heading.

Rifabutin (Increase daily dose of rifabutin by 50%. Consider doubling the rifabutin dose regimens where rifabutin is given 2 or 3 times a week).
No products indexed under this heading.

Rifampicin (Drugs which induce CYP3A4 activity would be expected to increase the clearance of efavirenz resulting in lower plasma concentrations).
No products indexed under this heading.

Rifampin (Rifampin reduced plasma concentrations of efavirenz).
No products indexed under this heading.

Rifapentine (Drugs which induce CYP3A4 activity would be expected to increase the clearance of efavirenz resulting in lower plasma concentrations).
No products indexed under this heading.

Riluzole (Renal impairment, including cases of acute renal failure and Fanconi syndrome (renal tubular injury with severe hypophosphatemia), has been reported in association with the use of tenofovir DF. The majority of these cases occurred in patients with underlying systemic or renal disease, or in patients taking nephrotoxic agents; however, some cases occured in patients without identified risk factors. Atripla should be avoided with concurrent or recent use of a nephrotoxic agent). Products include:
Rilutek 3032

Ritonavir (Kaletra may increase tenofovir concentrations. The mechanism of this interaction is unknown. Higher tenofovir concentrations could potentiate tenofovir-associated adverse events. Patients receiving Kaletra with tenofovir DF should be monitored for tenofovir-associated adverse events. Atripla should be discontinued in patients who develop tenofovir-assocatied adverse events. When ritonavir 500 mg every 12 hours was co-administered with efavirenz 600 mg once daily, the combination was associated with a higher frequency of adverse clinical experiences (eg, dizziness, nausea, paresthesia) and lab abnormalities (elevated liver enzymes). Monitoring of liver enzymes is recommended when Atripla is used with ritonavir). Products include:
Kaletra 458
Norvir 509

Rofecoxib (Renal impairment, including cases of acute renal failure and Fanconi syndrome (renal tubular injury with severe hypophosphatemia), has been reported in association with the use of tenofovir DF. The majority of these cases occurred in patients with underlying systemic or renal disease, or in patients taking nephrotoxic agents; however, some cases occured in patients without identified risk factors. Atripla should be avoided with concurrent or recent use of a nephrotoxic agent).
No products indexed under this heading.

Rosiglitazone Maleate (In vitro studies have demonstrated that efavirenz inhibits CYP2C9 in the range of observed efavirenz plasma concentrations. Co-administration of efavirenz with drugs primarily metabolized by CYP2C9 may result in altered plasma concentrations of the co-administered drug. Therefore, appropriate dose adjustments may be necessary for these drugs). Products include:
Avandamet 1345
Avandaryl 1356
Avandia 1366

Saquinavir (Due to a decrease in its concentration, saquinavir should not be used as sole protease inhibitor in combination with Atripla).
No products indexed under this heading.

Saquinavir Mesylate (Due to a decrease in its concentration, saquinavir should not be used as sole protease inhibitor in combination with Atripla).
No products indexed under this heading.

Sertraline Hydrochloride (Increases in sertraline dose should be guided by clinical response).
No products indexed under this heading.

Sibutramine Hydrochloride Monohydrate (Renal impairment, including cases of acute renal failure and Fanconi syndrome (renal tubular injury with severe hypophosphatemia), has been reported in association with the use of tenofovir DF. The majority of these cases occurred in patients with underlying systemic or renal disease, or in patients taking nephrotoxic agents; however, some cases occured in patients without identified risk factors. Atripla should be avoided with concurrent or recent use of a nephrotoxic agent). Products include:
Meridia 492

Sildenafil Citrate (Efavirenz has been shown *in vivo* to induce CYP3A4. Other compounds that are substrates of CYP3A4 may have decreased plasma concentrations when co-administered with efavirenz).
No products indexed under this heading.

Simvastatin (Plasma concentrations of atorvastatin, pravastatin, and simvastatin decreased with efavirenz. Consult the complete prescribing information for the HMGCoA reductase inhibitor for guidance on individualizing the dose). Products include:
Simcor 524
Vytorin 10/10 .... 2303, 3240
Vytorin 10/20 .... 2303, 3240
Vytorin 10/40 .... 2303, 3240
Vytorin 10/80 .... 2303, 3240
Zocor 2289

Sirolimus (Efavirenz has been shown *in vivo* to induce CYP3A4. Other compounds that are substrates of CYP3A4 may have decreased plasma concentrations when co-administered with efavirenz). Products include:
Rapamune 3579

Spirapril Hydrochloride (Renal impairment, including cases of acute renal failure and Fanconi syndrome (renal tubular injury with severe hypophosphatemia), has been reported in association with the use of tenofovir DF. The majority of these cases occurred in patients with underlying systemic or renal disease, or in patients taking nephrotoxic agents; however, some cases occured in patients without identified risk factors. Atripla should be avoided with concurrent or recent use of a nephrotoxic agent).
No products indexed under this heading.

Stavudine (Renal impairment, including cases of acute renal failure and Fanconi syndrome (renal tubular injury with severe hypophosphatemia), has been reported in association with the use of tenofovir DF. The majority of these cases occurred in patients with underlying systemic or renal disease, or in patients taking nephrotoxic agents; however, some cases occured in patients without identified risk factors. Atripla should be avoided with concurrent or recent use of a nephrotoxic agent).
No products indexed under this heading.

Streptomycin Sulfate (Renal impairment, including cases of acute renal failure and Fanconi syndrome (renal tubular injury with severe hypophosphatemia), has been reported in association with the use of tenofovir DF. The majority of these cases occurred in patients with underlying systemic or renal disease, or in patients taking nephrotoxic agents; however, some cases occured in patients without identified risk factors. Atripla should be avoided with concurrent or recent use of a nephrotoxic agent).
No products indexed under this heading.

Streptozocin (Renal impairment, including cases of acute renal failure and Fanconi syndrome (renal tubular injury with severe hypophosphatemia), has been reported in association with the use of tenofovir DF. The majority of these cases occurred in patients with underlying systemic or renal disease, or in patients taking nephrotoxic agents; however, some cases occured in patients without identified risk factors. Atripla should be avoided with concurrent or recent use of a nephrotoxic agent).
No products indexed under this heading.

Sulfacytine (Renal impairment, including cases of acute renal failure and Fanconi syndrome (renal tubular injury with severe hypophosphatemia), has been reported in association with the use of tenofovir DF. The majority of these cases occurred in patients with underlying systemic or renal disease, or in patients taking nephrotoxic agents; however, some cases occured in patients without identified risk factors. Atripla should be avoided with concurrent or recent use of a nephrotoxic agent).
No products indexed under this heading.

Sulfamethizole (Renal impairment, including cases of acute renal failure and Fanconi syndrome (renal tubular injury with severe hypophosphatemia), has been reported in association with the use of tenofovir DF. The majority of these cases occurred in patients with underlying systemic or renal disease, or in patients taking nephrotoxic agents; however, some cases occured in patients without identified risk factors. Atripla should be avoided with concurrent or recent use of a nephrotoxic agent).
No products indexed under this heading.

Sulfamethoxazole (Renal impairment, including cases of acute renal failure and Fanconi syndrome (renal tubular injury with severe hypophosphatemia), has been reported in association with the use of tenofovir DF. The majority of these cases occurred in patients with underlying systemic or renal disease, or in patients taking nephrotoxic agents; however, some cases occured in patients without identified risk factors. Atripla should be avoided with concurrent or recent use of a nephrotoxic agent).
No products indexed under this heading.

Sulfasalazine (Renal impairment, including cases of acute renal failure and Fanconi syndrome (renal tubular injury with severe hypophosphatemia), has been reported in association with the use of tenofovir DF. The majority of these cases occurred in patients with underlying systemic or renal disease, or in patients taking nephrotoxic agents; however, some cases occured in patients without identified risk factors. Atripla should be avoided with concurrent or recent use of a nephrotoxic agent).
No products indexed under this heading.

Sulfinpyrazone (Renal impairment, including cases of acute renal failure and Fanconi syndrome (renal tubular injury with severe hypophosphatemia), has been reported in association with the use of tenofovir DF. The majority of these cases occurred in patients with underlying systemic or renal disease, or in patients taking nephrotoxic agents; however, some cases occured in patients without identified risk factors. Atripla should be avoided with concurrent or recent use of a nephrotoxic agent).
No products indexed under this heading.

Sulfisoxazole Acetyl (Renal impairment, including cases of acute renal failure and Fanconi syndrome (renal tubular injury with severe hypophosphatemia), has been reported in association with the use of tenofovir DF. The majority of these cases occurred in patients with underlying systemic or renal disease, or in patients taking nephrotoxic agents; however, some cases occured in patients without identified risk factors. Atripla should be avoided with concurrent or recent use of a nephrotoxic agent).
No products indexed under this heading.

Sulfisoxazole Diolamine (Renal impairment, including cases of acute renal failure and Fanconi syndrome (renal tubular injury with severe hypophosphatemia), has been reported in association with the use of tenofovir DF. The majority of these cases occurred in patients with underlying systemic or

renal disease, or in patients taking nephrotoxic agents; however, some cases occured in patients without identified risk factors. Atripla should be avoided with concurrent or recent use of a nephrotoxic agent).

No products indexed under this heading.

Sulindac (Renal impairment, including cases of acute renal failure and Fanconi syndrome (renal tubular injury with severe hypophosphatemia), has been reported in association with the use of tenofovir DF. The majority of these cases occurred in patients with underlying systemic or renal disease, or in patients taking nephrotoxic agents; however, some cases occured in patients without identified risk factors. Atripla should be avoided with concurrent or recent use of a nephrotoxic agent). Products include:
Clinoril 2098

Suprofen (In vitro studies have demonstrated that efavirenz inhibits CYP2C9 in the range of observed efavirenz plasma concentrations. Co-administration of efavirenz with drugs primarily metabolized by CYP2C9 may result in altered plasma concentrations of the co-administered drug. Therefore, appropriate dose adjustments may be necessary for these drugs).

No products indexed under this heading.

Tacrolimus (Renal impairment, including cases of acute renal failure and Fanconi syndrome (renal tubular injury with severe hypophosphatemia), has been reported in association with the use of tenofovir DF. The majority of these cases occurred in patients with underlying systemic or renal disease, or in patients taking nephrotoxic agents; however, some cases occured in patients without identified risk factors. Atripla should be avoided with concurrent or recent use of a nephrotoxic agent). Products include:
Prograf Capsules 677
Prograf Injection 677
Protopic 685

Tadalafil (Efavirenz has been shown *in vivo* to induce CYP3A4. Other compounds that are substrates of CYP3A4 may have decreased plasma concentrations when co-administered with efavirenz). Products include:
Adcirca 3461
Cialis 1861

Tamoxifen Citrate (Efavirenz has been shown *in vivo* to induce CYP3A4. Other compounds that are substrates of CYP3A4 may have decreased plasma concentrations when co-administered with efavirenz).

No products indexed under this heading.

Telmisartan (In vitro studies have demonstrated that efavirenz inhibits CYP2C9 in the range of observed efavirenz plasma concentrations. Co-administration of efavirenz with drugs primarily metabolized by CYP2C9 may result in altered plasma concentrations of the co-administered drug. Therefore, appropriate dose adjustments may be necessary for these drugs). Products include:
Micardis 887
Micardis HCT 889

Teniposide (In vitro studies have demonstrated that efavirenz inhibits CYP2C19 in the range of observed efavirenz plasma concentrations. Co-administration of efavirenz with drugs primarily metabolized by CYP2C19 may result in altered plasma concentrations of the co-administered drug. Therefore, appropriate dose adjustments may be necessary for these drugs).

No products indexed under this heading.

Terfenadine (Efavirenz has been shown *in vivo* to induce CYP3A4. Other compounds that are substrates of CYP3A4 may have decreased plasma concentrations when co-administered with efavirenz).

No products indexed under this heading.

Theophyllinate (Drugs which induce CYP3A4 activity would be expected to increase the clearance of efavirenz resulting in lower plasma concentrations).

No products indexed under this heading.

Theophylline (Efavirenz has been shown *in vivo* to induce CYP3A4. Other compounds that are substrates of CYP3A4 may have decreased plasma concentrations when co-administered with efavirenz).

No products indexed under this heading.

Theophylline Anhydrous (Efavirenz has been shown *in vivo* to induce CYP3A4. Other compounds that are substrates of CYP3A4 may have decreased plasma concentrations when co-administered with efavirenz). Products include:
Uniphyl 2817

Theophylline Calcium Salicylate (Efavirenz has been shown *in vivo* to induce CYP3A4. Other compounds that are substrates of CYP3A4 may have decreased plasma concentrations when co-administered with efavirenz).

No products indexed under this heading.

Theophylline Dihydroxypropyl (Glyceryl) (Efavirenz has been shown *in vivo* to induce CYP3A4. Other compounds that are substrates of CYP3A4 may have decreased plasma concentrations when co-administered with efavirenz).

No products indexed under this heading.

Theophylline Ethylenediamine (Efavirenz has been shown *in vivo* to induce CYP3A4. Other compounds that are substrates of CYP3A4 may have decreased plasma concentrations when co-administered with efavirenz).

No products indexed under this heading.

Theophylline Sodium Glycinate (Efavirenz has been shown *in vivo* to induce CYP3A4. Other compounds that are substrates of CYP3A4 may have decreased plasma concentrations when co-administered with efavirenz).

No products indexed under this heading.

Thioguanine (Renal impairment, including cases of acute renal failure and Fanconi syndrome (renal tubular injury with severe hypophosphatemia), has been reported in association with the use of tenofovir DF. The majority of these cases occurred in patients with underlying systemic or renal disease, or in patients taking nephrotoxic agents; however, some cases occured in patients without identified risk factors. Atripla should be avoided with concurrent or recent use of a nephrotoxic agent). Products include:
Tabloid 1664

Thioridazine (In vitro studies have demonstrated that efavirenz inhibits CYP2C19 in the range of observed efavirenz plasma concentrations. Co-administration of efavirenz with drugs primarily metabolized by CYP2C19 may result in altered plasma concentrations of the co-administered drug. Therefore, appropriate dose adjustments may be necessary for these drugs).

No products indexed under this heading.

Thioridazine Hydrochloride (In vitro studies have demonstrated that efavirenz inhibits CYP2C19 in the range of observed efavirenz plasma concentrations. Co-administration of efavirenz with drugs primarily metabolized by CYP2C19 may result in altered plasma concentrations of the co-administered

drug. Therefore, appropriate dose adjustments may be necessary for these drugs). Products include:
Thioridazine Hydrochloride 2384

Tiagabine Hydrochloride (Efavirenz has been shown *in vivo* to induce CYP3A4. Other compounds that are substrates of CYP3A4 may have decreased plasma concentrations when co-administered with efavirenz). Products include:
Gabitril 972

Ticarcillin Disodium (Renal impairment, including cases of acute renal failure and Fanconi syndrome (renal tubular injury with severe hypophosphatemia), has been reported in association with the use of tenofovir DF. The majority of these cases occurred in patients with underlying systemic or renal disease, or in patients taking nephrotoxic agents; however, some cases occured in patients without identified risk factors. Atripla should be avoided with concurrent or recent use of a nephrotoxic agent). Products include:
Timentin ADD-Vantage 1670
Timentin Galaxy 1674
Timentin 1666
Timentin Pharmacy 1678

Tobramycin (Renal impairment, including cases of acute renal failure and Fanconi syndrome (renal tubular injury with severe hypophosphatemia), has been reported in association with the use of tenofovir DF. The majority of these cases occurred in patients with underlying systemic or renal disease, or in patients taking nephrotoxic agents; however, some cases occured in patients without identified risk factors. Atripla should be avoided with concurrent or recent use of a nephrotoxic agent). Products include:
Tobi Nebulizer 2546
Tobramycin and Dexamethasone Ophthalmic Suspension ....⊙251
Zylet ....⊙252

Tobramycin Sulfate (Renal impairment, including cases of acute renal failure and Fanconi syndrome (renal tubular injury with severe hypophosphatemia), has been reported in association with the use of tenofovir DF. The majority of these cases occurred in patients with underlying systemic or renal disease, or in patients taking nephrotoxic agents; however, some cases occured in patients without identified risk factors. Atripla should be avoided with concurrent or recent use of a nephrotoxic agent).

No products indexed under this heading.

Tolazamide (Renal impairment, including cases of acute renal failure and Fanconi syndrome (renal tubular injury with severe hypophosphatemia), has been reported in association with the use of tenofovir DF. The majority of these cases occurred in patients with underlying systemic or renal disease, or in patients taking nephrotoxic agents; however, some cases occured in patients without identified risk factors. Atripla should be avoided with concurrent or recent use of a nephrotoxic agent).

No products indexed under this heading.

Tolbutamide (Renal impairment, including cases of acute renal failure and Fanconi syndrome (renal tubular injury with severe hypophosphatemia), has been reported in association with the use of tenofovir DF. The majority of these cases occurred in patients with underlying systemic or renal disease, or in patients taking nephrotoxic agents; however, some cases occured in patients without identified risk factors.

Atripla should be avoided with concurrent or recent use of a nephrotoxic agent).

No products indexed under this heading.

Tolbutamide Sodium (In vitro studies have demonstrated that efavirenz inhibits CYP2C9 in the range of observed efavirenz plasma concentrations. Co-administration of efavirenz with drugs primarily metabolized by CYP2C9 may result in altered plasma concentrations of the co-administered drug. Therefore, appropriate dose adjustments may be necessary for these drugs).

No products indexed under this heading.

Tolmetin Sodium (Renal impairment, including cases of acute renal failure and Fanconi syndrome (renal tubular injury with severe hypophosphatemia), has been reported in association with the use of tenofovir DF. The majority of these cases occurred in patients with underlying systemic or renal disease, or in patients taking nephrotoxic agents; however, some cases occured in patients without identified risk factors. Atripla should be avoided with concurrent or recent use of a nephrotoxic agent).

No products indexed under this heading.

Tolterodine Tartrate (Efavirenz has been shown *in vivo* to induce CYP3A4. Other compounds that are substrates of CYP3A4 may have decreased plasma concentrations when co-administered with efavirenz).

No products indexed under this heading.

Topiramate (In vitro studies have demonstrated that efavirenz inhibits CYP2C19 in the range of observed efavirenz plasma concentrations. Co-administration of efavirenz with drugs primarily metabolized by CYP2C19 may result in altered plasma concentrations of the co-administered drug. Therefore, appropriate dose adjustments may be necessary for these drugs).

No products indexed under this heading.

Torsemide (In vitro studies have demonstrated that efavirenz inhibits CYP2C9 in the range of observed efavirenz plasma concentrations. Co-administration of efavirenz with drugs primarily metabolized by CYP2C9 may result in altered plasma concentrations of the co-administered drug. Therefore, appropriate dose adjustments may be necessary for these drugs).

No products indexed under this heading.

Trandolapril (Renal impairment, including cases of acute renal failure and Fanconi syndrome (renal tubular injury with severe hypophosphatemia), has been reported in association with the use of tenofovir DF. The majority of these cases occurred in patients with underlying systemic or renal disease, or in patients taking nephrotoxic agents; however, some cases occured in patients without identified risk factors. Atripla should be avoided with concurrent or recent use of a nephrotoxic agent). Products include:
Mavik 489
Tarka 534

Trazodone Hydrochloride (Efavirenz has been shown *in vivo* to induce CYP3A4. Other compounds that are substrates of CYP3A4 may have decreased plasma concentrations when co-administered with efavirenz).

No products indexed under this heading.

Triamcinolone (Drugs which induce CYP3A4 activity would be expected to increase the clearance of efavirenz resulting in lower plasma concentrations).

No products indexed under this heading.

Triamcinolone Acetonide (Drugs which induce CYP3A4 activity would be

IMPORTANT NOTE: Always consult each drug listing in the patient's regimen for possible interactions.

Atripla Interactions Index 174

expected to increase the clearance of efavirenz resulting in lower plasma concentrations). Products include:
Azmacort 408
Nasacort AQ 3019

Triamcinolone Diacetate (Drugs which induce CYP3A4 activity would be expected to increase the clearance of efavirenz resulting in lower plasma concentrations).
No products indexed under this heading.

Triamcinolone Hexacetonide (Drugs which induce CYP3A4 activity would be expected to increase the clearance of efavirenz resulting in lower plasma concentrations).
No products indexed under this heading.

Triamterene (Renal impairment, including cases of acute renal failure and Fanconi syndrome (renal tubular injury with severe hypophosphatemia), has been reported in association with the use of tenofovir DF. The majority of these cases occurred in patients with underlying systemic or renal disease, or in patients taking nephrotoxic agents; however, some cases occured in patients without identified risk factors. Atripla should be avoided with concurrent or recent use of a nephrotoxic agent). Products include:
Dyazide 1429
Dyrenium 3495

Triazolam (Due to the potential for serious and/or life-threatening reactions, such as prolonged or increased sedation or respiratory depression, concomitant use with triazolam is contraindicated).
No products indexed under this heading.

Trimethadione (Renal impairment, including cases of acute renal failure and Fanconi syndrome (renal tubular injury with severe hypophosphatemia), has been reported in association with the use of tenofovir DF. The majority of these cases occurred in patients with underlying systemic or renal disease, or in patients taking nephrotoxic agents; however, some cases occured in patients without identified risk factors. Atripla should be avoided with concurrent or recent use of a nephrotoxic agent).
No products indexed under this heading.

Trimipramine Maleate (In vitro studies have demonstrated that efavirenz inhibits CYP2C19 in the range of observed efavirenz plasma concentrations. Co-administration of efavirenz with drugs primarily metabolized by CYP2C19 may result in altered plasma concentrations of the co-administered drug. Therefore, appropriate dose adjustments may be necessary for these drugs).
No products indexed under this heading.

Troglitazone (Drugs which induce CYP3A4 activity would be expected to increase the clearance of efavirenz resulting in lower plasma concentrations).
No products indexed under this heading.

Trovafloxacin Mesylate (Renal impairment, including cases of acute renal failure and Fanconi syndrome (renal tubular injury with severe hypophosphatemia), has been reported in association with the use of tenofovir DF. The majority of these cases occurred in patients with underlying systemic or renal disease, or in patients taking nephrotoxic agents; however, some cases occured in patients without identified risk factors. Atripla should be avoided with concurrent or recent use of a nephrotoxic agent).
No products indexed under this heading.

Tyropanoate Sodium (Renal impairment, including cases of acute renal failure and Fanconi syndrome (renal tubular injury with severe hypophosphatemia), has been reported in association with the use of tenofovir DF. The majority of these cases occurred in patients with underlying systemic or renal disease, or in patients taking nephrotoxic agents; however, some cases occured in patients without identified risk factors. Atripla should be avoided with concurrent or recent use of a nephrotoxic agent).
No products indexed under this heading.

Valacyclovir Hydrochloride (Since emtricitabine and tenofovir are primarily eliminated by the kidneys, co-administration of Atripla with drugs that reduce renal fuction or compete for active tubular secretion may increase serum concentrations of emtricitabine, tenofovir, and/or other renally eliminated drugs). Products include:
Valtrex 1702

Valdecoxib (Renal impairment, including cases of acute renal failure and Fanconi syndrome (renal tubular injury with severe hypophosphatemia), has been reported in association with the use of tenofovir DF. The majority of these cases occurred in patients with underlying systemic or renal disease, or in patients taking nephrotoxic agents; however, some cases occured in patients without identified risk factors. Atripla should be avoided with concurrent or recent use of a nephrotoxic agent).
No products indexed under this heading.

Valganciclovir Hydrochloride (Since emtricitabine and tenofovir are primarily eliminated by the kidneys, co-administration of Atripla with drugs that reduce renal fuction or compete for active tubular secretion may increase serum concentrations of emtricitabine, tenofovir, and/or other renally eliminated drugs). Products include:
Valcyte 2872

Valproate Sodium (In vitro studies have demonstrated that efavirenz inhibits CYP2C19 in the range of observed efavirenz plasma concentrations. Co-administration of efavirenz with drugs primarily metabolized by CYP2C19 may result in altered plasma concentrations of the co-administered drug. Therefore, appropriate dose adjustments may be necessary for these drugs).
No products indexed under this heading.

Valproic Acid (In vitro studies have demonstrated that efavirenz inhibits CYP2C19 in the range of observed efavirenz plasma concentrations. Co-administration of efavirenz with drugs primarily metabolized by CYP2C19 may result in altered plasma concentrations of the co-administered drug. Therefore, appropriate dose adjustments may be necessary for these drugs).
No products indexed under this heading.

Valsartan (In vitro studies have demonstrated that efavirenz inhibits CYP2C9 in the range of observed efavirenz plasma concentrations. Co-administration of efavirenz with drugs primarily metabolized by CYP2C9 may result in altered plasma concentrations of the co-administered drug. Therefore, appropriate dose adjustments may be necessary for these drugs). Products include:
Diovan 2413
Diovan HCT 2419
Exforge 2443
Exforge HCT 2449
Valturna 3637

Vancomycin Hydrochloride (Renal impairment, including cases of acute renal failure and Fanconi syndrome (renal tubular injury with severe hypophosphatemia), has been reported in association with the use of tenofovir DF. The majority of these cases occurred in patients with underlying systemic or renal disease, or in patients taking nephrotoxic agents; however, some cases occured in patients without identified risk factors. Atripla should be avoided with concurrent or recent use of a nephrotoxic agent).
No products indexed under this heading.

Vardenafil Hydrochloride (Efavirenz has been shown *in vivo* to induce CYP3A4. Other compounds that are substrates of CYP3A4 may have decreased plasma concentrations when co-administered with efavirenz). Products include:
Levitra 3157

Verapamil Hydrochloride (Efavirenz has been shown *in vivo* to induce CYP3A4. Other compounds that are substrates of CYP3A4 may have decreased plasma concentrations when co-administered with efavirenz). Products include:
Tarka 534

Vinblastine Sulfate (Efavirenz has been shown *in vivo* to induce CYP3A4. Other compounds that are substrates of CYP3A4 may have decreased plasma concentrations when co-administered with efavirenz).
No products indexed under this heading.

Vincristine Sulfate (Efavirenz has been shown *in vivo* to induce CYP3A4. Other compounds that are substrates of CYP3A4 may have decreased plasma concentrations when co-administered with efavirenz).
No products indexed under this heading.

Voriconazole (Efavirenz significantly decreases voriconazole plasma concentrations, and co-administration may decrease the therapeutic effectiveness of voriconazole. Also, voriconazole significantly increases efavirenz plasma concentrations, which may increase the risk of efavirenz-associated side effects. Concomitant use is contraindicated).
No products indexed under this heading.

Warfarin Sodium (Plasma concentrations and effects to warfarin sodium potentially increased or decreased by efavirenz).
No products indexed under this heading.

Zafirlukast (In vitro studies have demonstrated that efavirenz inhibits CYP2C9 in the range of observed efavirenz plasma concentrations. Co-administration of efavirenz with drugs primarily metabolized by CYP2C9 may result in altered plasma concentrations of the co-administered drug. Therefore, appropriate dose adjustments may be necessary for these drugs). Products include:
Accolate 3612

Zalcitabine (Renal impairment, including cases of acute renal failure and Fanconi syndrome (renal tubular injury with severe hypophosphatemia), has been reported in association with the use of tenofovir DF. The majority of these cases occurred in patients with underlying systemic or renal disease, or in patients taking nephrotoxic agents; however, some cases occured in patients without identified risk factors. Atripla should be avoided with concurrent or recent use of a nephrotoxic agent).
No products indexed under this heading.

Zidovudine (Renal impairment, including cases of acute renal failure and Fanconi syndrome (renal tubular injury with severe hypophosphatemia), has been reported in association with the use of tenofovir DF. The majority of these cases occurred in patients with underlying systemic or renal disease, or in patients taking nephrotoxic agents; however, some cases occured in patients without identified risk factors. Atripla should be avoided with concurrent or recent use of a nephrotoxic agent). Products include:
Combivir 1404
Retrovir 1634
Retrovir IV 1640
Trizivir 1688

Zileuton (In vitro studies have demonstrated that efavirenz inhibits CYP2C9 in the range of observed efavirenz plasma concentrations. Co-administration of efavirenz with drugs primarily metabolized by CYP2C9 may result in altered plasma concentrations of the co-administered drug. Therefore, appropriate dose adjustments may be necessary for these drugs).
No products indexed under this heading.

Zoledronic Acid (Renal impairment, including cases of acute renal failure and Fanconi syndrome (renal tubular injury with severe hypophosphatemia), has been reported in association with the use of tenofovir DF. The majority of these cases occurred in patients with underlying systemic or renal disease, or in patients taking nephrotoxic agents; however, some cases occured in patients without identified risk factors. Atripla should be avoided with concurrent or recent use of a nephrotoxic agent). Products include:
Reclast 2509
Zometa 2554

Zonisamide (In vitro studies have demonstrated that efavirenz inhibits CYP2C19 in the range of observed efavirenz plasma concentrations. Co-administration of efavirenz with drugs primarily metabolized by CYP2C19 may result in altered plasma concentrations of the co-administered drug. Therefore, appropriate dose adjustments may be necessary for these drugs). Products include:
Zonegran 1081

ATRYN LYOPHILIZED POWDER

(Antithrombin) 1998
May interact with anticoagulants, low molecular weight heparins, and certain other agents. Compounds in these categories include:

Anisindione (Concurrent administration of antithrombin with other anticoagulants that use antithrombin to exert their anticoagulant effect must be monitored clinically and biologically. The anticoagulant effect of drugs that use antithrombin to exert their anticoagulation may be altered when antithrombin is added or withdrawn. To avoid excessive or insufficient anticoagulation, regularly perform coagulation tests (aPTT, and where appropriate, anti-Factor Xa activity) suitable for the anticoagulant used, at close intervals, especially in the first hours following the start or withdrawal of antithrombin and monitor patients for bleeding or thrombosis).
No products indexed under this heading.

Ardeparin Sodium (Concurrent administration of antithrombin with other anticoagulants that use antithrombin to exert their anticoagulant effect must be monitored clinically and biologically. The anticoagulant effect of drugs that use antithrombin to exert their anticoagulation may be altered when antithrombin is added or withdrawn. To avoid excessive or insufficient anticoagulation, regularly perform coagulation tests (aPTT, and where appropriate, anti-Factor Xa activity) suitable for the anticoagulant used, at close intervals, especially in the first hours following the start or withdrawal of antithrombin and monitor patients for bleeding or thrombosis).
No products indexed under this heading.

Dalteparin Sodium (The anticoagulant effect of low molecular weight hep-

arin (LMWH) is enhanced by antithrombin. The half-life of antithrombin may be altered by concomitant treatment with these anticoagulants due to an altered antithrombin turnover. Thus, concurrent administration of antithrombin with low molecular weight heparin must be monitored clinically and biologically. To avoid excessive anticoagulation, regular coagulation tests (aPTT, and where appropriate, anti-Factor Xa activity) are to be performed at close intervals, with adjustment in dosage of the anticoagulant as necessary). Products include:
Fragmin 1058

Danaparoid Sodium (Concurrent administration of antithrombin with other anticoagulants that use antithrombin to exert their anticoagulant effect must be monitored clinically and biologically. The anticoagulant effect of drugs that use antithrombin to exert their anticoagulation may be altered when antithrombin is added or withdrawn. To avoid excessive or insufficient anticoagulation, regularly perform coagulation tests (aPTT, and where appropriate, anti-Factor Xa activity) suitable for the anticoagulant used, at close intervals, especially in the first hours following the start or withdrawal of antithrombin and monitor patients for bleeding or thrombosis).
No products indexed under this heading.

Dicumarol (Concurrent administration of antithrombin with other anticoagulants that use antithrombin to exert their anticoagulant effect must be monitored clinically and biologically. The anticoagulant effect of drugs that use antithrombin to exert their anticoagulation may be altered when antithrombin is added or withdrawn. To avoid excessive or insufficient anticoagulation, regularly perform coagulation tests (aPTT, and where appropriate, anti-Factor Xa activity) suitable for the anticoagulant used, at close intervals, especially in the first hours following the start or withdrawal of antithrombin and monitor patients for bleeding or thrombosis).
No products indexed under this heading.

Enoxaparin Sodium (The anticoagulant effect of low molecular weight heparin (LMWH) is enhanced by antithrombin. The half-life of antithrombin may be altered by concomitant treatment with these anticoagulants due to an altered antithrombin turnover. Thus, concurrent administration of antithrombin with low molecular weight heparin must be monitored clinically and biologically. To avoid excessive anticoagulation, regular coagulation tests (aPTT, and where appropriate, anti-Factor Xa activity) are to be performed at close intervals, with adjustment in dosage of the anticoagulant as necessary). Products include:
Lovenox 3005

Fondaparinux Sodium (Concurrent administration of antithrombin with other anticoagulants that use antithrombin to exert their anticoagulant effect must be monitored clinically and biologically. The anticoagulant effect of drugs that use antithrombin to exert their anticoagulation may be altered when antithrombin is added or withdrawn. To avoid excessive or insufficient anticoagulation, regularly perform coagulation tests (aPTT, and where appropriate, anti-Factor Xa activity) suitable for the anticoagulant used, at close intervals, especially in the first hours following the start or withdrawal of antithrombin and monitor patients for bleeding or thrombosis). Products include:
Arixtra 1320

Heparin (The anticoagulant effect of heparin is enhanced by antithrombin. The half-life of antithrombin may be altered by concomitant treatment with these anticoagulants due to an altered

antithrombin turnover. Thus, concurrent administration of antithrombin with heparin must be monitored clinically and biologically. To avoid excessive anticoagulation, regular coagulation tests (aPTT, and where appropriate, anti-Factor Xa activity) are to be performed at close intervals, with adjustment in dosage of the anticoagulant as necessary).
No products indexed under this heading.

Heparin Calcium (The anticoagulant effect of heparin is enhanced by antithrombin. The half-life of antithrombin may be altered by concomitant treatment with these anticoagulants due to an altered antithrombin turnover. Thus, concurrent administration of antithrombin with heparin must be monitored clinically and biologically. To avoid excessive anticoagulation, regular coagulation tests (aPTT, and where appropriate, anti-Factor Xa activity) are to be performed at close intervals, with adjustment in dosage of the anticoagulant as necessary).
No products indexed under this heading.

Heparin Sodium (The anticoagulant effect of heparin is enhanced by antithrombin. The half-life of antithrombin may be altered by concomitant treatment with these anticoagulants due to an altered antithrombin turnover. Thus, concurrent administration of antithrombin with heparin must be monitored clinically and biologically. To avoid excessive anticoagulation, regular coagulation tests (aPTT, and where appropriate, anti-Factor Xa activity) are to be performed at close intervals, with adjustment in dosage of the anticoagulant as necessary).
No products indexed under this heading.

Low Molecular Weight Heparins (Concurrent administration of antithrombin with other anticoagulants that use antithrombin to exert their anticoagulant effect must be monitored clinically and biologically. The anticoagulant effect of drugs that use antithrombin to exert their anticoagulation may be altered when antithrombin is added or withdrawn. To avoid excessive or insufficient anticoagulation, regularly perform coagulation tests (aPTT, and where appropriate, anti-Factor Xa activity) suitable for the anticoagulant used, at close intervals, especially in the first hours following the start or withdrawal of antithrombin and monitor patients for bleeding or thrombosis).
No products indexed under this heading.

Tinzaparin Sodium (The anticoagulant effect of low molecular weight heparin (LMWH) is enhanced by antithrombin. The half-life of antithrombin may be altered by concomitant treatment with these anticoagulants due to an altered antithrombin turnover. Thus, concurrent administration of antithrombin with low molecular weight heparin must be monitored clinically and biologically. To avoid excessive anticoagulation, regular coagulation tests (aPTT, and where appropriate, anti-Factor Xa activity) are to be performed at close intervals, with adjustment in dosage of the anticoagulant as necessary).
No products indexed under this heading.

Warfarin Sodium (Concurrent administration of antithrombin with other anticoagulants that use antithrombin to exert their anticoagulant effect must be monitored clinically and biologically. The anticoagulant effect of drugs that use antithrombin to exert their anticoagulation may be altered when antithrombin is added or withdrawn. To avoid excessive or insufficient anticoagulation, regularly perform coagulation tests (aPTT, and where appropriate, anti-Factor Xa activity) suitable for the anticoagulant used, at close intervals, especially in

the first hours following the start or withdrawal of antithrombin and monitor patients for bleeding or thrombosis).
No products indexed under this heading.

ATTENUVAX

(Measles Virus Vaccine Live) 2086
May interact with immunosuppressive agents. Compounds in these categories include:

Azathioprine (Concurrent use in individuals on immunosuppressive therapy is contraindicated).
No products indexed under this heading.

Basiliximab (Concurrent use in individuals on immunosuppressive therapy is contraindicated). Products include:
Simulect 2524

Cyclosporine (Concurrent use in individuals on immunosuppressive therapy is contraindicated). Products include:
Gengraf 440
Neoral Oral Solution 2496
Neoral Capsules 2496
Restasis 605

Muromonab-CD3 (Concurrent use in individuals on immunosuppressive therapy is contraindicated). Products include:
Orthoclone OKT3 949

Mycophenolate Mofetil (Concurrent use in individuals on immunosuppressive therapy is contraindicated).
No products indexed under this heading.

Rapamycin (Concurrent use in individuals on immunosuppressive therapy is contraindicated).
No products indexed under this heading.

Sirolimus (Concurrent use in individuals on immunosuppressive therapy is contraindicated). Products include:
Rapamune 3579

Tacrolimus (Concurrent use in individuals on immunosuppressive therapy is contraindicated). Products include:
Prograf Capsules 677
Prograf Injection 677
Protopic 685

AUGMENTIN CHEWABLE TABLETS

(Amoxicillin, Clavulanate Potassium) 1331
See Augmentin ES-600 Powder for Oral Suspension

AUGMENTIN POWDER FOR ORAL SUSPENSION

(Amoxicillin, Clavulanate Potassium) 1331
See Augmentin ES-600 Powder for Oral Suspension

AUGMENTIN TABLETS

(Amoxicillin, Clavulanate Potassium) 1335
See Augmentin ES-600 Powder for Oral Suspension

AUGMENTIN ES-600 POWDER FOR ORAL SUSPENSION

(Amoxicillin, Clavulanate Potassium) 1338
May interact with anticoagulants, oral contraceptives, and certain other agents. Compounds in these categories include:

Allopurinol (Co-administration of ampicillin with allopurinol substantially increases the incidence of rashes; there are no data with Augmentin and allopurinol administered concurrently).
No products indexed under this heading.

Anisindione (There have been reports of increased prothrombin time in patients receiving Augmentin and anticoagulant therapy concomitantly).
No products indexed under this heading.

Ardeparin Sodium (There have been reports of increased prothrombin time in patients receiving Augmentin and anticoagulant therapy concomitantly).
No products indexed under this heading.

Dalteparin Sodium (There have been reports of increased prothrombin time in patients receiving Augmentin and anticoagulant therapy concomitantly). Products include:
Fragmin 1058

Danaparoid Sodium (There have been reports of increased prothrombin time in patients receiving Augmentin and anticoagulant therapy concomitantly).
No products indexed under this heading.

Desogestrel (Potential for reduced efficacy of oral contraceptives).
No products indexed under this heading.

Dicumarol (There have been reports of increased prothrombin time in patients receiving Augmentin and anticoagulant therapy concomitantly).
No products indexed under this heading.

Enoxaparin Sodium (There have been reports of increased prothrombin time in patients receiving Augmentin and anticoagulant therapy concomitantly). Products include:
Lovenox 3005

Ethinyl Estradiol (Potential for reduced efficacy of oral contraceptives). Products include:
LoSeasonique 3407
Lybrel 3514
NuvaRing 3181
Ortho Evra 2648
Ortho-Cyclen/Ortho Tri-Cyclen 2663
Ortho Tri-Cyclen Lo Tablets 2673
Seasonique 3418
Yaz 864

Ethynodiol Diacetate (Potential for reduced efficacy of oral contraceptives).
No products indexed under this heading.

Fondaparinux Sodium (There have been reports of increased prothrombin time in patients receiving Augmentin and anticoagulant therapy concomitantly). Products include:
Arixtra 1320

Heparin Calcium (There have been reports of increased prothrombin time in patients receiving Augmentin and anticoagulant therapy concomitantly).
No products indexed under this heading.

Heparin Sodium (There have been reports of increased prothrombin time in patients receiving Augmentin and anticoagulant therapy concomitantly).
No products indexed under this heading.

Levonorgestrel (Potential for reduced efficacy of oral contraceptives). Products include:
Climara Pro 847
LoSeasonique 3407
Lybrel 3514
Mirena 854
Plan B 3416
Seasonique 3418

Low Molecular Weight Heparins (There have been reports of increased prothrombin time in patients receiving Augmentin and anticoagulant therapy concomitantly).
No products indexed under this heading.

Mestranol (Potential for reduced efficacy of oral contraceptives).
No products indexed under this heading.

Norethindrone (Potential for reduced efficacy of oral contraceptives). Products include:
Ortho Micronor 2660

Norethynodrel (Potential for reduced efficacy of oral contraceptives).
No products indexed under this heading.

Norgestimate (Potential for reduced efficacy of oral contraceptives). Products include:

Norgestrel (Potential for reduced efficacy of oral contraceptives).
No products indexed under this heading.

Probenecid (Decreases the renal tubular secretion of amoxicillin; concurrent use may result in increased and prolonged blood levels of amoxicillin; therefore, concomitant use is not recommended).
No products indexed under this heading.

Tinzaparin Sodium (There have been reports of increased prothrombin time in patients receiving Augmentin and anticoagulant therapy concomitantly).
No products indexed under this heading.

Warfarin Sodium (There have been reports of increased prothrombin time in patients receiving Augmentin and anticoagulant therapy concomitantly).
No products indexed under this heading.

AUGMENTIN XR EXTENDED RELEASE TABLETS

AUTHIA CREAM

AVALIDE FILM-COATED TABLETS

AVALIDE TABLETS

May interact with alcohols, antihypertensives, barbiturates, cardiac glycosides, corticosteroids, diuretics, insulin, lithium preparations, narcotic analgesics, non-steroidal anti-inflammatory agents, nondepolarizing neuromuscular blocking agents, oral hypoglycemic agents, vasopressors, and certain other agents. Compounds in these categories include:

Acarbose (Hyperglycemia may occur with thiazide diuretics. In diabetic patients, dosage adjustments of insulin or oral hypoglycemic agents may be required).
No products indexed under this heading.

Acebutolol Hydrochloride (Concomitant use of hydrochlorothiazide with other antihypertensive drugs may produce an additive effect or potentiation).
No products indexed under this heading.

ACTH (Concurrent use of hydrochlorothiazide with ACTH may cause intensified electrolyte depletion, particularly hypokalemia).
No products indexed under this heading.

Alclometasone Dipropionate (Concurrent use of hydrochlorothiazide with corticosteroids may cause intensified electrolyte depletion, particularly hypokalemia).
No products indexed under this heading.

Alfentanil Hydrochloride (Potentiation of orthostatic hypertension may occur during concomitant administration of hydrochlorothiazide with narcotics).
No products indexed under this heading.

Aliskiren (Concomitant use of hydrochlorothiazide with other antihypertensive drugs may produce an additive effect or potentiation). Products include:

Amiloride Hydrochloride (Initiation of antihypertensive therapy may cause symptomatic hypotension in patients with intravascular volume- or sodium-depletion, eg, in patients treated vigorously with diuretics).
No products indexed under this heading.

Amlodipine Besylate (Concomitant use of hydrochlorothiazide with other antihypertensive drugs may produce an additive effect or potentiation). Products include:

Amobarbital (Potentiation of orthostatic hypertension may occur during concomitant administration of hydrochlorothiazide with barbiturates).
No products indexed under this heading.

Amobarbital Sodium (Potentiation of orthostatic hypertension may occur during concomitant administration of hydrochlorothiazide with barbiturates).
No products indexed under this heading.

Apomorphine (Potentiation of orthostatic hypertension may occur during concomitant administration of hydrochlorothiazide with narcotics).
No products indexed under this heading.

Apomorphine Hydrochloride (Potentiation of orthostatic hypertension may occur during concomitant administration of hydrochlorothiazide with narcotics).
No products indexed under this heading.

Aprobarbital (Potentiation of orthostatic hypertension may occur during concomitant administration of hydrochlorothiazide with barbiturates).
No products indexed under this heading.

Atenolol (Concomitant use of hydrochlorothiazide with other antihypertensive drugs may produce an additive effect or potentiation).
No products indexed under this heading.

Atracurium Besylate (Hydrochlorothiazide may cause possible increased responsiveness to non-depolarizing skeletal muscle relaxants (eg, tubocurarine)).
No products indexed under this heading.

Beclomethasone Dipropionate (Concurrent use of hydrochlorothiazide with corticosteroids may cause intensified electrolyte depletion, particularly hypokalemia). Products include:

Beclomethasone Dipropionate Monohydrate (Concurrent use of hydrochlorothiazide with corticosteroids may cause intensified electrolyte depletion, particularly hypokalemia). Products include:

Benazepril Hydrochloride (Concomitant use of hydrochlorothiazide with other antihypertensive drugs may produce an additive effect or potentiation).
No products indexed under this heading.

Bendroflumethiazide (Concomitant use of hydrochlorothiazide with other antihypertensive drugs may produce an additive effect or potentiation).
No products indexed under this heading.

Betamethasone (Concurrent use of hydrochlorothiazide with corticosteroids may cause intensified electrolyte depletion, particularly hypokalemia).
No products indexed under this heading.

Betamethasone Acetate (Concurrent use of hydrochlorothiazide with corticosteroids may cause intensified electrolyte depletion, particularly hypokalemia).
No products indexed under this heading.

Betamethasone Benzoate (Concurrent use of hydrochlorothiazide with corticosteroids may cause intensified electrolyte depletion, particularly hypokalemia).
No products indexed under this heading.

Betamethasone Dipropionate (Concurrent use of hydrochlorothiazide with corticosteroids may cause intensified electrolyte depletion, particularly hypokalemia). Products include:

Betamethasone Sodium Phosphate (Concurrent use of hydrochlorothiazide with corticosteroids may cause intensified electrolyte depletion, particularly hypokalemia).
No products indexed under this heading.

Betamethasone Valerate (Concurrent use of hydrochlorothiazide with corticosteroids may cause intensified electrolyte depletion, particularly hypokalemia). Products include:

Betaxolol Hydrochloride (Concomitant use of hydrochlorothiazide with other antihypertensive drugs may produce an additive effect or potentiation).
No products indexed under this heading.

Bisoprolol Fumarate (Concomitant use of hydrochlorothiazide with other antihypertensive drugs may produce an additive effect or potentiation).
No products indexed under this heading.

Budesonide (Concurrent use of hydrochlorothiazide with corticosteroids may cause intensified electrolyte depletion, particularly hypokalemia). Products include:

Bumetanide (Initiation of antihypertensive therapy may cause symptomatic hypotension in patients with intravascular volume- or sodium-depletion, eg, in patients treated vigorously with diuretics).
No products indexed under this heading.

Buprenorphine Hydrochloride (Potentiation of orthostatic hypertension may occur during concomitant administration of hydrochlorothiazide with narcotics).
No products indexed under this heading.

Butabarbital (Potentiation of orthostatic hypertension may occur during concomitant administration of hydrochlorothiazide with barbiturates).
No products indexed under this heading.

Butabarbital Sodium (Potentiation of orthostatic hypertension may occur during concomitant administration of hydrochlorothiazide with barbiturates).
No products indexed under this heading.

Butalbital (Potentiation of orthostatic hypertension may occur during concomitant administration of hydrochlorothiazide with barbiturates).
No products indexed under this heading.

Candesartan Cilexetil (Concomitant use of hydrochlorothiazide with other antihypertensive drugs may produce an additive effect or potentiation). Products include:

Captopril (Concomitant use of hydrochlorothiazide with other antihypertensive drugs may produce an additive effect or potentiation). Products include:

Carteolol Hydrochloride (Concomitant use of hydrochlorothiazide with other antihypertensive drugs may produce an additive effect or potentiation).
No products indexed under this heading.

Carvedilol (Concomitant use of hydrochlorothiazide with other antihypertensive drugs may produce an additive effect or potentiation). Products include:

Carvedilol Phosphate (Concomitant use of hydrochlorothiazide with other antihypertensive drugs may produce an additive effect or potentiation). Products include:

Celecoxib (In some patients, the administration of a non-steroidal anti-inflammatory agent can reduce the diuretic, natriuretic, and antihypertensive effects of loop, potassium-sparing and thiazide diuretics. Therefore, when Avalide tablets and non-steroidal anti-inflammatory agents are used concomitantly, the patient should be observed closely to determine if the desired effect on the diuretic is obtained). Products include:

Chlorothiazide (Concomitant use of hydrochlorothiazide with other antihypertensive drugs may produce an additive effect or potentiation).
No products indexed under this heading.

Chlorothiazide Sodium (Concomitant use of hydrochlorothiazide with other antihypertensive drugs may produce an additive effect or potentiation). Products include:

Chlorpropamide (Hyperglycemia may occur with thiazide diuretics. In diabetic patients, dosage adjustments of insulin or oral hypoglycemic agents may be required).
No products indexed under this heading.

Chlorthalidone (Concomitant use of hydrochlorothiazide with other antihypertensive drugs may produce an additive effect or potentiation). Products include:

Cholestyramine (Absorption of hydrochlorothiazide is impaired in the presence of anionic exchange resins. Single doses of cholestyramine bind the hydrochlorothiazide and reduce its absorption from the gastrointestinal tract by up to 85%).
No products indexed under this heading.

Ciclesonide (Concurrent use of hydrochlorothiazide with corticosteroids may cause intensified electrolyte depletion, particularly hypokalemia).
No products indexed under this heading.

Cisatracurium Besylate (Hydrochlorothiazide may cause possible increased responsiveness to non-depolarizing skeletal muscle relaxants (eg, tubocurarine)). Products include:

Clonidine (Concomitant use of hydrochlorothiazide with other antihypertensive drugs may produce an additive effect or potentiation). Products include:

Clonidine Hydrochloride (Concomitant use of hydrochlorothiazide with other antihypertensive drugs may produce an additive effect or potentiation). Products include:

Codeine Phosphate (Potentiation of orthostatic hypertension may occur during concomitant administration of hydrochlorothiazide with narcotics). Products include:

177 Interactions Index Avalide

Codeine Sulfate (Potentiation of orthostatic hypertension may occur during concomitant administration of hydrochlorothiazide with narcotics).
No products indexed under this heading.

Colestipol (Absorption of hydrochlorothiazide is impaired in the presence of anionic exchange resins. Single doses of colestipol resins bind the hydrochlorothiazide and reduce its absorption from the gastrointestinal tract by up to 43%).
No products indexed under this heading.

Colestipol Hydrochloride (Absorption of hydrochlorothiazide is impaired in the presence of anionic exchange resins. Single doses of colestipol resins bind the hydrochlorothiazide and reduce its absorption from the gastrointestinal tract by up to 43%).
No products indexed under this heading.

Cortisone Acetate (Concurrent use of hydrochlorothiazide with corticosteroids may cause intensified electrolyte depletion, particularly hypokalemia).
No products indexed under this heading.

Deserpidine (Concomitant use of hydrochlorothiazide with other antihypertensive drugs may produce an additive effect or potentiation).
No products indexed under this heading.

Deslanoside (Hypokalemia may develop during therapy with Avalide. Hypokalemia may sensitize or exaggerate the response of the heart to the toxic effects of digitalis (eg, increased ventricular irritability)).
No products indexed under this heading.

Desoximetasone (Concurrent use of hydrochlorothiazide with corticosteroids may cause intensified electrolyte depletion, particularly hypokalemia).
No products indexed under this heading.

Dexamethasone (Concurrent use of hydrochlorothiazide with corticosteroids may cause intensified electrolyte depletion, particularly hypokalemia). Products include:
Ciprodex 583
Ozurdex .... ⊙ 223
Tobramycin and Dexamethasone Ophthalmic Suspension .... ⊙ 251

Dexamethasone Acetate (Concurrent use of hydrochlorothiazide with corticosteroids may cause intensified electrolyte depletion, particularly hypokalemia).
No products indexed under this heading.

Dexamethasone Phosphate (Concurrent use of hydrochlorothiazide with corticosteroids may cause intensified electrolyte depletion, particularly hypokalemia).
No products indexed under this heading.

Dexamethasone Sodium (Concurrent use of hydrochlorothiazide with corticosteroids may cause intensified electrolyte depletion, particularly hypokalemia).
No products indexed under this heading.

Dexamethasone Sodium Phosphate (Concurrent use of hydrochlorothiazide with corticosteroids may cause intensified electrolyte depletion, particularly hypokalemia).
No products indexed under this heading.

Dexamethasone Sodium Phosphate Injection (Concurrent use of hydrochlorothiazide with corticosteroids may cause intensified electrolyte depletion, particularly hypokalemia).
No products indexed under this heading.

Dezocine (Potentiation of orthostatic hypertension may occur during concomitant administration of hydrochlorothiazide with narcotics).
No products indexed under this heading.

Diazoxide (Concomitant use of hydrochlorothiazide with other antihypertensive drugs may produce an additive effect or potentiation). Products include:
Proglycem 1179
Proglycem Suspension 1179

Diclofenac Epolamine (In some patients, the administration of a non-steroidal anti-inflammatory agent can reduce the diuretic, natriuretic, and antihypertensive effects of loop, potassium-sparing and thiazide diuretics. Therefore, when Avalide tablets and non-steroidal anti-inflammatory agents are used concomitantly, the patient should be observed closely to determine if the desired effect on the diuretic is obtained). Products include:
Flector 1839

Diclofenac Potassium (In some patients, the administration of a non-steroidal anti-inflammatory agent can reduce the diuretic, natriuretic, and antihypertensive effects of loop, potassium-sparing and thiazide diuretics. Therefore, when Avalide tablets and non-steroidal anti-inflammatory agents are used concomitantly, the patient should be observed closely to determine if the desired effect on the diuretic is obtained).
No products indexed under this heading.

Diclofenac Sodium (In some patients, the administration of a non-steroidal anti-inflammatory agent can reduce the diuretic, natriuretic, and antihypertensive effects of loop, potassium-sparing and thiazide diuretics. Therefore, when Avalide tablets and non-steroidal anti-inflammatory agents are used concomitantly, the patient should be observed closely to determine if the desired effect on the diuretic is obtained).
No products indexed under this heading.

Diflorasone Diacetate (Concurrent use of hydrochlorothiazide with corticosteroids may cause intensified electrolyte depletion, particularly hypokalemia).
No products indexed under this heading.

Digitalis Glycoside Preparations (Hypokalemia may develop during therapy with Avalide. Hypokalemia may sensitize or exaggerate the response of the heart to the toxic effects of digitalis (eg, increased ventricular irritability)).
No products indexed under this heading.

Digitalis Lanata (Hypokalemia may develop during therapy with Avalide. Hypokalemia may sensitize or exaggerate the response of the heart to the toxic effects of digitalis (eg, increased ventricular irritability)).
No products indexed under this heading.

Digitalis Purpurea (Hypokalemia may develop during therapy with Avalide. Hypokalemia may sensitize or exaggerate the response of the heart to the toxic effects of digitalis (eg, increased ventricular irritability)).
No products indexed under this heading.

Digitoxin (Hypokalemia may develop during therapy with Avalide. Hypokalemia may sensitize or exaggerate the response of the heart to the toxic effects of digitalis (eg, increased ventricular irritability)).
No products indexed under this heading.

Digoxin (Hypokalemia may develop during therapy with Avalide. Hypokalemia may sensitize or exaggerate the response of the heart to the toxic effects of digitalis (eg, increased ventricular irritability)). Products include:
Lanoxin Injection 1546
Lanoxin Injection Pediatric 1549
Lanoxin Tablets 1553

Dihydrocodeine Bitartrate (Potentiation of orthostatic hypertension may occur during concomitant administration of hydrochlorothiazide with narcotics).
No products indexed under this heading.

Dihydrocodeinone Bitartrate (Potentiation of orthostatic hypertension may occur during concomitant administration of hydrochlorothiazide with narcotics).
No products indexed under this heading.

Diltiazem Hydrochloride (Concomitant use of hydrochlorothiazide with other antihypertensive drugs may produce an additive effect or potentiation). Products include:
Cardizem LA 423

Diltiazem Maleate (Concomitant use of hydrochlorothiazide with other antihypertensive drugs may produce an additive effect or potentiation).
No products indexed under this heading.

Dobutamine (Hydrochlorothiazide may cause possible decreased response to pressor amines (eg, norepinephrine), but this is not sufficient to preclude their use).
No products indexed under this heading.

Dobutamine Hydrochloride (Hydrochlorothiazide may cause possible decreased response to pressor amines (eg, norepinephrine), but this is not sufficient to preclude their use).
No products indexed under this heading.

Dopamine Hydrochloride (Hydrochlorothiazide may cause possible decreased response to pressor amines (eg, norepinephrine), but this is not sufficient to preclude their use).
No products indexed under this heading.

Doxacurium Chloride (Hydrochlorothiazide may cause possible increased responsiveness to non-depolarizing skeletal muscle relaxants (eg, tubocurarine)).
No products indexed under this heading.

Doxazosin Mesylate (Concomitant use of hydrochlorothiazide with other antihypertensive drugs may produce an additive effect or potentiation).
No products indexed under this heading.

d-Tubocurarine (Hydrochlorothiazide may cause possible increased responsiveness to non-depolarizing skeletal muscle relaxants (eg, tubocurarine)).
No products indexed under this heading.

Enalapril Maleate (Concomitant use of hydrochlorothiazide with other antihypertensive drugs may produce an additive effect or potentiation).
No products indexed under this heading.

Enalaprilat (Concomitant use of hydrochlorothiazide with other antihypertensive drugs may produce an additive effect or potentiation).
No products indexed under this heading.

Ephedrine Sulfate (Hydrochlorothiazide may cause possible decreased response to pressor amines (eg, norepinephrine), but this is not sufficient to preclude their use).
No products indexed under this heading.

Epinephrine Bitartrate (Hydrochlorothiazide may cause possible decreased response to pressor amines (eg, norepinephrine), but this is not sufficient to preclude their use).
No products indexed under this heading.

Epinephrine Hydrochloride (Hydrochlorothiazide may cause possible decreased response to pressor amines (eg, norepinephrine), but this is not sufficient to preclude their use).
No products indexed under this heading.

Eprosartan Mesylate (Concomitant use of hydrochlorothiazide with other antihypertensive drugs may produce an additive effect or potentiation). Products include:
Teveten 538
Teveten HCT 541

Esmolol Hydrochloride (Concomitant use of hydrochlorothiazide with other antihypertensive drugs may produce an additive effect or potentiation).
No products indexed under this heading.

Ethacrynic Acid (Initiation of antihypertensive therapy may cause symptomatic hypotension in patients with intravascular volume- or sodium-depletion, eg, in patients treated vigorously with diuretics).
No products indexed under this heading.

Ethanol (Potentiation of orthostatic hypertension may occur during concomitant administration of hydrochlorothiazide with alcohol).
No products indexed under this heading.

Ethyl Alcohol (Potentiation of orthostatic hypertension may occur during concomitant administration of hydrochlorothiazide with alcohol).
No products indexed under this heading.

Etodolac (In some patients, the administration of a non-steroidal anti-inflammatory agent can reduce the diuretic, natriuretic, and antihypertensive effects of loop, potassium-sparing and thiazide diuretics. Therefore, when Avalide tablets and non-steroidal anti-inflammatory agents are used concomitantly, the patient should be observed closely to determine if the desired effect on the diuretic is obtained).
No products indexed under this heading.

Felodipine (Concomitant use of hydrochlorothiazide with other antihypertensive drugs may produce an additive effect or potentiation).
No products indexed under this heading.

Fenoprofen Calcium (In some patients, the administration of a non-steroidal anti-inflammatory agent can reduce the diuretic, natriuretic, and antihypertensive effects of loop, potassium-sparing and thiazide diuretics. Therefore, when Avalide tablets and non-steroidal anti-inflammatory agents are used concomitantly, the patient should be observed closely to determine if the desired effect on the diuretic is obtained).
No products indexed under this heading.

Fentanyl (Potentiation of orthostatic hypertension may occur during concomitant administration of hydrochlorothiazide with narcotics). Products include:
Duragesic 2604
Fentanyl Transdermal System 2346
Onsolis 2054

Fentanyl Citrate (Potentiation of orthostatic hypertension may occur during concomitant administration of hydrochlorothiazide with narcotics). Products include:
Fentora 966

Fludrocortisone Acetate (Concurrent use of hydrochlorothiazide with corticosteroids may cause intensified electrolyte depletion, particularly hypokalemia).
No products indexed under this heading.

Flumethasone Pivalate (Concurrent use of hydrochlorothiazide with corticosteroids may cause intensified electrolyte depletion, particularly hypokalemia).
No products indexed under this heading.

Flunisolide Hemihydrate (Concurrent use of hydrochlorothiazide with corticosteroids may cause intensified electrolyte depletion, particularly hypokalemia).
No products indexed under this heading.

Flurbiprofen (In some patients, the administration of a non-steroidal anti-inflammatory agent can reduce the diuretic, natriuretic, and antihypertensive

patients, dosage adjustments of insulin or oral hypoglycemic agents may be required). Products include:

Insulin Glulisine (Hyperglycemia may occur with thiazide diuretics. In diabetic patients, dosage adjustments of insulin or oral hypoglycemic agents may be required). Products include:

Insulin Lispro, Human (Hyperglycemia may occur with thiazide diuretics. In diabetic patients, dosage adjustments of insulin or oral hypoglycemic agents may be required). Products include:

Insulin Lispro Protamine, Human (Hyperglycemia may occur with thiazide diuretics. In diabetic patients, dosage adjustments of insulin or oral hypoglycemic agents may be required). Products include:

Isoproterenol Hydrochloride (Hydrochlorothiazide may cause possible decreased response to pressor amines (eg, norepinephrine), but this is not sufficient to preclude their use).
No products indexed under this heading.

Isoproterenol Sulfate (Hydrochlorothiazide may cause possible decreased response to pressor amines (eg, norepinephrine), but this is not sufficient to preclude their use).
No products indexed under this heading.

Isradipine (Concomitant use of hydrochlorothiazide with other antihypertensive drugs may produce an additive effect or potentiation). Products include:

Ketoprofen (In some patients, the administration of a non-steroidal anti-inflammatory agent can reduce the diuretic, natriuretic, and antihypertensive effects of loop, potassium-sparing and thiazide diuretics. Therefore, when Avalide tablets and non-steroidal anti-inflammatory agents are used concomitantly, the patient should be observed closely to determine if the desired effect on the diuretic is obtained).
No products indexed under this heading.

Ketorolac Tromethamine (In some patients, the administration of a non-steroidal anti-inflammatory agent can reduce the diuretic, natriuretic, and antihypertensive effects of loop, potassium-sparing and thiazide diuretics. Therefore, when Avalide tablets and non-steroidal anti-inflammatory agents are used concomitantly, the patient should be observed closely to determine if the desired effect on the diuretic is obtained). Products include:

Labetalol Hydrochloride (Concomitant use of hydrochlorothiazide with other antihypertensive drugs may produce an additive effect or potentiation).
No products indexed under this heading.

Levorphanol Tartrate (Potentiation of orthostatic hypertension may occur during concomitant administration of hydrochlorothiazide with narcotics).
No products indexed under this heading.

Lisinopril (Concomitant use of hydrochlorothiazide with other antihypertensive drugs may produce an additive effect or potentiation). Products include:

Lithium (Lithium should not generally be given with diuretics, such as hydrochlorothiazide. Diuretic agents reduce the renal clearance of lithium and add a high risk of lithium toxicity).
No products indexed under this heading.

Lithium Carbonate (Lithium should not generally be given with diuretics, such as hydrochlorothiazide. Diuretic agents reduce the renal clearance of lithium and add a high risk of lithium toxicity).
No products indexed under this heading.

Lithium Citrate (Lithium should not generally be given with diuretics, such as hydrochlorothiazide. Diuretic agents reduce the renal clearance of lithium and add a high risk of lithium toxicity).
No products indexed under this heading.

Losartan Potassium (Concomitant use of hydrochlorothiazide with other antihypertensive drugs may produce an additive effect or potentiation). Products include:

Mecamylamine Hydrochloride (Concomitant use of hydrochlorothiazide with other antihypertensive drugs may produce an additive effect or potentiation).
No products indexed under this heading.

Meclofenamate Sodium (In some patients, the administration of a non-steroidal anti-inflammatory agent can reduce the diuretic, natriuretic, and antihypertensive effects of loop, potassium-sparing and thiazide diuretics. Therefore, when Avalide tablets and non-steroidal anti-inflammatory agents are used concomitantly, the patient should be observed closely to determine if the desired effect on the diuretic is obtained).
No products indexed under this heading.

Mefenamic Acid (In some patients, the administration of a non-steroidal anti-inflammatory agent can reduce the diuretic, natriuretic, and antihypertensive effects of loop, potassium-sparing and thiazide diuretics. Therefore, when Avalide tablets and non-steroidal anti-inflammatory agents are used concomitantly, the patient should be observed closely to determine if the desired effect on the diuretic is obtained).
No products indexed under this heading.

Meloxicam (In some patients, the administration of a non-steroidal anti-inflammatory agent can reduce the diuretic, natriuretic, and antihypertensive effects of loop, potassium-sparing and thiazide diuretics. Therefore, when Avalide tablets and non-steroidal anti-inflammatory agents are used concomitantly, the patient should be observed closely to determine if the desired effect on the diuretic is obtained).
No products indexed under this heading.

Meperidine Hydrochloride (Potentiation of orthostatic hypertension may occur during concomitant administration of hydrochlorothiazide with narcotics).
No products indexed under this heading.

Mephentermine Sulfate (Hydrochlorothiazide may cause possible decreased response to pressor amines (eg, norepinephrine), but this is not sufficient to preclude their use).
No products indexed under this heading.

Mephobarbital (Potentiation of orthostatic hypertension may occur during concomitant administration of hydrochlorothiazide with barbiturates).
No products indexed under this heading.

Metaraminol Bitartrate (Hydrochlorothiazide may cause possible decreased response to pressor amines (eg, norepinephrine), but this is not sufficient to preclude their use).
No products indexed under this heading.

Metformin Hydrochloride (Hyperglycemia may occur with thiazide diuretics. In diabetic patients, dosage adjustments of insulin or oral hypoglycemic agents may be required). Products include:

Methadone Hydrochloride (Potentiation of orthostatic hypertension may occur during concomitant administration of hydrochlorothiazide with narcotics).
No products indexed under this heading.

Methoxamine Hydrochloride (Hydrochlorothiazide may cause possible decreased response to pressor amines (eg, norepinephrine), but this is not sufficient to preclude their use).
No products indexed under this heading.

Methyclothiazide (Concomitant use of hydrochlorothiazide with other antihypertensive drugs may produce an additive effect or potentiation).
No products indexed under this heading.

Methyldopa (Concomitant use of hydrochlorothiazide with other antihypertensive drugs may produce an additive effect or potentiation).
No products indexed under this heading.

Methyldopate Hydrochloride (Concomitant use of hydrochlorothiazide with other antihypertensive drugs may produce an additive effect or potentiation).
No products indexed under this heading.

Methylprednisolone (Concurrent use of hydrochlorothiazide with corticosteroids may cause intensified electrolyte depletion, particularly hypokalemia).
No products indexed under this heading.

Methylprednisolone Acetate (Concurrent use of hydrochlorothiazide with corticosteroids may cause intensified electrolyte depletion, particularly hypokalemia).
No products indexed under this heading.

Methylprednisolone Sodium Succinate (Concurrent use of hydrochlorothiazide with corticosteroids may cause intensified electrolyte depletion, particularly hypokalemia).
No products indexed under this heading.

Metocurine Iodide (Hydrochlorothiazide may cause possible increased responsiveness to non-depolarizing skeletal muscle relaxants (eg, tubocurarine)).
No products indexed under this heading.

Metolazone (Concomitant use of hydrochlorothiazide with other antihypertensive drugs may produce an additive effect or potentiation).
No products indexed under this heading.

Metoprolol Succinate (Concomitant use of hydrochlorothiazide with other antihypertensive drugs may produce an additive effect or potentiation). Products include:

Metoprolol Tartrate (Concomitant use of hydrochlorothiazide with other antihypertensive drugs may produce an additive effect or potentiation).
No products indexed under this heading.

Metyrosine (Concomitant use of hydrochlorothiazide with other antihypertensive drugs may produce an additive effect or potentiation).
No products indexed under this heading.

Mibefradil Dihydrochloride (Concomitant use of hydrochlorothiazide with other antihypertensive drugs may produce an additive effect or potentiation).
No products indexed under this heading.

Miglitol (Hyperglycemia may occur with thiazide diuretics. In diabetic patients, dosage adjustments of insulin or oral hypoglycemic agents may be required).
No products indexed under this heading.

Minoxidil (Concomitant use of hydrochlorothiazide with other antihypertensive drugs may produce an additive effect or potentiation).
No products indexed under this heading.

Mivacurium Chloride (Hydrochlorothiazide may cause possible increased responsiveness to non-depolarizing skeletal muscle relaxants (eg, tubocurarine)).
No products indexed under this heading.

Moexipril Hydrochloride (Concomitant use of hydrochlorothiazide with other antihypertensive drugs may produce an additive effect or potentiation).
No products indexed under this heading.

Mometasone Furoate (Concurrent use of hydrochlorothiazide with corticosteroids may cause intensified electrolyte depletion, particularly hypokalemia). Products include:

Mometasone Furoate Monohydrate (Concurrent use of hydrochlorothiazide with corticosteroids may cause intensified electrolyte depletion, particularly hypokalemia). Products include:

Morphine Sulfate (Potentiation of orthostatic hypertension may occur during concomitant administration of hydrochlorothiazide with narcotics). Products include:

Morphine Sulfate, Liposomal (Potentiation of orthostatic hypertension may occur during concomitant administration of hydrochlorothiazide with narcotics).
No products indexed under this heading.

Nabumetone (In some patients, the administration of a non-steroidal anti-inflammatory agent can reduce the diuretic, natriuretic, and antihypertensive effects of loop, potassium-sparing and thiazide diuretics. Therefore, when Avalide tablets and non-steroidal anti-inflammatory agents are used concomitantly, the patient should be observed closely to determine if the desired effect on the diuretic is obtained).
No products indexed under this heading.

Nadolol (Concomitant use of hydrochlorothiazide with other antihypertensive drugs may produce an additive effect or potentiation). Products include:

Naproxen (In some patients, the administration of a non-steroidal anti-inflammatory agent can reduce the diuretic, natriuretic, and antihypertensive effects of loop, potassium-sparing and thiazide diuretics. Therefore, when Avalide tablets and non-steroidal anti-inflammatory agents are used concomitantly, the patient should be observed closely to determine if the desired effect on the diuretic is obtained). Products include:

IMPORTANT NOTE: Always consult each drug listing in the patient's regimen for possible interactions.

Sodium Pentobarbital (Potentiation of orthostatic hypertension may occur during concomitant administration of hydrochlorothiazide with barbiturates).
No products indexed under this heading.

Sotalol Hydrochloride (Concomitant use of hydrochlorothiazide with other antihypertensive drugs may produce an additive effect or potentiation).
No products indexed under this heading.

Spirapril Hydrochloride (Concomitant use of hydrochlorothiazide with other antihypertensive drugs may produce an additive effect or potentiation).
No products indexed under this heading.

Spironolactone (Initiation of antihypertensive therapy may cause symptomatic hypotension in patients with intravascular volume- or sodium-depletion, eg, in patients treated vigorously with diuretics).
No products indexed under this heading.

Sufentanil Citrate (Potentiation of orthostatic hypertension may occur during concomitant administration of hydrochlorothiazide with narcotics).
No products indexed under this heading.

Sulindac (In some patients, the administration of a non-steroidal anti-inflammatory agent can reduce the diuretic, natriuretic, and antihypertensive effects of loop, potassium-sparing and thiazide diuretics. Therefore, when Avalide tablets and non-steroidal anti-inflammatory agents are used concomitantly, the patient should be observed closely to determine if the desired effect on the diuretic is obtained). Products include:
Clinoril 2098

Telmisartan (Concomitant use of hydrochlorothiazide with other antihypertensive drugs may produce an additive effect or potentiation). Products include:
Micardis 887
Micardis HCT 889

Terazosin Hydrochloride (Concomitant use of hydrochlorothiazide with other antihypertensive drugs may produce an additive effect or potentiation).
No products indexed under this heading.

Thiamylal Sodium (Potentiation of orthostatic hypertension may occur during concomitant administration of hydrochlorothiazide with barbiturates).
No products indexed under this heading.

Timolol Maleate (Concomitant use of hydrochlorothiazide with other antihypertensive drugs may produce an additive effect or potentiation). Products include:
Combigan 601
Dorzolamide Hydrochloride/Timolol Maleate Ophthalmic Solution .... ⊙243
Timoptic in Ocudose .... ⊙231

Tolazamide (Hyperglycemia may occur with thiazide diuretics. In diabetic patients, dosage adjustments of insulin or oral hypoglycemic agents may be required).
No products indexed under this heading.

Tolbutamide (Hyperglycemia may occur with thiazide diuretics. In diabetic patients, dosage adjustments of insulin or oral hypoglycemic agents may be required).
No products indexed under this heading.

Tolmetin Sodium (In some patients, the administration of a non-steroidal anti-inflammatory agent can reduce the diuretic, natriuretic, and antihypertensive effects of loop, potassium-sparing and thiazide diuretics. Therefore, when Avalide tablets and non-steroidal anti-inflammatory agents are used concomitantly, the patient should be observed closely to determine if the desired effect on the diuretic is obtained).
No products indexed under this heading.

Torsemide (Concomitant use of hydrochlorothiazide with other antihypertensive drugs may produce an additive effect or potentiation).
No products indexed under this heading.

Trandolapril (Concomitant use of hydrochlorothiazide with other antihypertensive drugs may produce an additive effect or potentiation). Products include:
Mavik 489
Tarka 534

Triamcinolone (Concurrent use of hydrochlorothiazide with corticosteroids may cause intensified electrolyte depletion, particularly hypokalemia).
No products indexed under this heading.

Triamcinolone Acetonide (Concurrent use of hydrochlorothiazide with corticosteroids may cause intensified electrolyte depletion, particularly hypokalemia). Products include:
Azmacort 408
Nasacort AQ 3019

Triamcinolone Diacetate (Concurrent use of hydrochlorothiazide with corticosteroids may cause intensified electrolyte depletion, particularly hypokalemia).
No products indexed under this heading.

Triamcinolone Hexacetonide (Concurrent use of hydrochlorothiazide with corticosteroids may cause intensified electrolyte depletion, particularly hypokalemia).
No products indexed under this heading.

Triamterene (Initiation of antihypertensive therapy may cause symptomatic hypotension in patients with intravascular volume- or sodium-depletion, eg, in patients treated vigorously with diuretics). Products include:
Dyazide 1429
Dyrenium 3495

Trimethaphan Camsylate (Concomitant use of hydrochlorothiazide with other antihypertensive drugs may produce an additive effect or potentiation).
No products indexed under this heading.

Troglitazone (Hyperglycemia may occur with thiazide diuretics. In diabetic patients, dosage adjustments of insulin or oral hypoglycemic agents may be required).
No products indexed under this heading.

Tubocurarine Chloride (Hydrochlorothiazide may cause possible increased responsiveness to non-depolarizing skeletal muscle relaxants (eg, tubocurarine)).
No products indexed under this heading.

Valdecoxib (In some patients, the administration of a non-steroidal anti-inflammatory agent can reduce the diuretic, natriuretic, and antihypertensive effects of loop, potassium-sparing and thiazide diuretics. Therefore, when Avalide tablets and non-steroidal anti-inflammatory agents are used concomitantly, the patient should be observed closely to determine if the desired effect on the diuretic is obtained).
No products indexed under this heading.

Valsartan (Concomitant use of hydrochlorothiazide with other antihypertensive drugs may produce an additive effect or potentiation). Products include:
Diovan 2413
Diovan HCT 2419
Exforge 2443
Exforge HCT 2449
Valturna 3637

Vecuronium Bromide (Hydrochlorothiazide may cause possible increased responsiveness to non-depolarizing skeletal muscle relaxants (eg, tubocurarine)).
No products indexed under this heading.

Verapamil Hydrochloride (Concomitant use of hydrochlorothiazide with

other antihypertensive drugs may produce an additive effect or potentiation). Products include:
Tarka 534

Food Interactions

Alcohol (Potentiation of orthostatic hypertension may occur during concomitant administration of hydrochlorothiazide with alcohol).

Beer, reduced-alcohol (Potentiation of orthostatic hypertension may occur during concomitant administration of hydrochlorothiazide with alcohol).

Beer, unspecified (Potentiation of orthostatic hypertension may occur during concomitant administration of hydrochlorothiazide with alcohol).

Wine, Chianti (Potentiation of orthostatic hypertension may occur during concomitant administration of hydrochlorothiazide with alcohol).

Wine, Red (Potentiation of orthostatic hypertension may occur during concomitant administration of hydrochlorothiazide with alcohol).

Wine, unspecified (Potentiation of orthostatic hypertension may occur during concomitant administration of hydrochlorothiazide with alcohol).

Wine products (Potentiation of orthostatic hypertension may occur during concomitant administration of hydrochlorothiazide with alcohol).

AVANDAMET TABLETS

(Metformin Hydrochloride, Rosiglitazone Maleate) 1345
May interact with alcohols, calcium channel blockers, cationic drugs that are eliminated by renal tubular, corticosteroids, cytochrome p450 2c8 inducers (selected), cytochrome p450 2c8 inhibitors (selected), diuretics, estrogens, insulin, oral contraceptives, oral hypoglycemic agents, phenothiazines, phenytoin, quinidine, radiographic iodinated contrast media, sulfonylureas, sympathomimetics, thiazides, thyroid preparations, and certain other agents. Compounds in these categories include:

Acarbose (Patients receiving rosiglitazone in combination with other hypoglycemic agents may be at risk for hypoglycemia and a reduction in the dose of the concomitant agent may be necessary).
No products indexed under this heading.

Albuterol (Certain drugs, such as sympathomimetics, tend to produce hyperglycemia and may lead to loss of glycemic control).
No products indexed under this heading.

Albuterol Sulfate (Certain drugs, such as sympathomimetics, tend to produce hyperglycemia and may lead to loss of glycemic control). Products include:
ProAir HFA 3393
Proventil HFA 3204
Ventolin HFA 1708

Alclometasone Dipropionate (Certain drugs, such as corticosteroids, tend to produce hyperglycemia and may lead to loss of glycemic control).
No products indexed under this heading.

Amiloride Hydrochloride (Potential for loss of glycemic control; theoretical potential for interaction with metformin by competing for common renal tubular transport system).
No products indexed under this heading.

Amlodipine Besylate (Certain drugs, such as calcium channel blockers, tend to produce hyperglycemia and may lead to loss of glycemic control). Products include:
Azor 1010
Exforge 2443

Exforge HCT 2449

Anastrozole (An inhibitor of CYP2C8 may increase the AUC of rosiglitazone).
No products indexed under this heading.

Beclomethasone Dipropionate (Certain drugs, such as corticosteroids, tend to produce hyperglycemia and may lead to loss of glycemic control). Products include:
Qvar 3398

Beclomethasone Dipropionate Monohydrate (Certain drugs, such as corticosteroids, tend to produce hyperglycemia and may lead to loss of glycemic control). Products include:
Beconase AQ 1386

Bendroflumethiazide (Certain drugs, such as thiazides and other diuretics, tend to produce hyperglycemia and may lead to loss of glycemic control).
No products indexed under this heading.

Bepridil Hydrochloride (Certain drugs, such as calcium channel blockers, tend to produce hyperglycemia and may lead to loss of glycemic control).
No products indexed under this heading.

Betamethasone (Certain drugs, such as corticosteroids, tend to produce hyperglycemia and may lead to loss of glycemic control).
No products indexed under this heading.

Betamethasone Acetate (Certain drugs, such as corticosteroids, tend to produce hyperglycemia and may lead to loss of glycemic control).
No products indexed under this heading.

Betamethasone Benzoate (Certain drugs, such as corticosteroids, tend to produce hyperglycemia and may lead to loss of glycemic control).
No products indexed under this heading.

Betamethasone Dipropionate (Certain drugs, such as corticosteroids, tend to produce hyperglycemia and may lead to loss of glycemic control). Products include:
Diprolene Lotion 0.05% 3108
Diprolene Ointment 0.05% 3109
Diprolene AF Cream 0.05% 3107
Lotrisone 3163

Betamethasone Sodium Phosphate (Certain drugs, such as corticosteroids, tend to produce hyperglycemia and may lead to loss of glycemic control).
No products indexed under this heading.

Betamethasone Valerate (Certain drugs, such as corticosteroids, tend to produce hyperglycemia and may lead to loss of glycemic control). Products include:
Luxiq 3321

Budesonide (Certain drugs, such as corticosteroids, tend to produce hyperglycemia and may lead to loss of glycemic control). Products include:
Pulmicort Flexhaler 714
Symbicort 80/4.5 720
Symbicort 160/4.5 720

Bumetanide (Certain drugs, such as diuretics, tend to produce hyperglycemia and may lead to loss of glycemic control).
No products indexed under this heading.

Carbamazepine (An inducer of CYP2C8 may decrease the AUC of rosiglitazone). Products include:
Carbatrol 3280
Equetro 3477

Chlorothiazide (Certain drugs, such as thiazides and other diuretics, tend to produce hyperglycemia and may lead to loss of glycemic control).
No products indexed under this heading.

Chlorothiazide Sodium (Certain drugs, such as thiazides and other diuretics, tend to produce hyperglycemia and may lead to loss of glycemic control). Products include:

IMPORTANT NOTE: Always consult each drug listing in the patient's regimen for possible interactions.

Avandamet Interactions Index 182

Diuril Intravenous 2009

Chlorotrianisene (Certain drugs, such as estrogens, tend to produce hyperglycemia and may lead to loss of glycemic control).
No products indexed under this heading.

Chlorpromazine (Certain drugs, such as phenothiazines, tend to produce hyperglycemia and may lead to loss of glycemic control).
No products indexed under this heading.

Chlorpromazine Hydrochloride (Certain drugs, such as phenothiazines, tend to produce hyperglycemia and may lead to loss of glycemic control).
No products indexed under this heading.

Chlorpropamide (An increased incidence of heart failure has been observed when rosiglitazone was added to a sulfonylurea or to a sulfonylurea plus metformin).
No products indexed under this heading.

Chlorthalidone (Certain drugs, such as diuretics, tend to produce hyperglycemia and may lead to loss of glycemic control). Products include:
Clorpres 2344

Ciclesonide (Certain drugs, such as corticosteroids, tend to produce hyperglycemia and may lead to loss of glycemic control).
No products indexed under this heading.

Cimetidine (Co-administered with oral cimetidine may increase peak metformin plasma and whole blood concentrations by 60% and a 40% increase in plasma and whole blood metformin AUC).
No products indexed under this heading.

Cimetidine Hydrochloride (An inhibitor of CYP2C8 may increase the AUC of rosiglitazone).
No products indexed under this heading.

Cortisone Acetate (Certain drugs, such as corticosteroids, tend to produce hyperglycemia and may lead to loss of glycemic control).
No products indexed under this heading.

Desogestrel (Certain drugs, such as oral contraceptives, tend to produce hyperglycemia and may lead to loss of glycemic control).
No products indexed under this heading.

Desoximetasone (Certain drugs, such as corticosteroids, tend to produce hyperglycemia and may lead to loss of glycemic control).
No products indexed under this heading.

Dexamethasone (Certain drugs, such as corticosteroids, tend to produce hyperglycemia and may lead to loss of glycemic control). Products include:
Ciprodex 583
Ozurdex .... ⊙ 223
Tobramycin and Dexamethasone Ophthalmic Suspension .... ⊙ 251

Dexamethasone Acetate (Certain drugs, such as corticosteroids, tend to produce hyperglycemia and may lead to loss of glycemic control).
No products indexed under this heading.

Dexamethasone Phosphate (Certain drugs, such as corticosteroids, tend to produce hyperglycemia and may lead to loss of glycemic control).
No products indexed under this heading.

Dexamethasone Sodium (Certain drugs, such as corticosteroids, tend to produce hyperglycemia and may lead to loss of glycemic control).
No products indexed under this heading.

Dexamethasone Sodium Phosphate (Certain drugs, such as corticosteroids, tend to produce hyperglycemia and may lead to loss of glycemic control).
No products indexed under this heading.

Dexamethasone Sodium Phosphate Injection (Certain drugs, such as corticosteroids, tend to produce hyperglycemia and may lead to loss of glycemic control).
No products indexed under this heading.

Diatrizoate Meglumine (Potential for acute alteration of renal function; metformin should be temporarily withheld in patients undergoing radiologic studies involving parenteral iodinated contrast material).
No products indexed under this heading.

Diatrizoate Sodium (Potential for acute alteration of renal function; metformin should be temporarily withheld in patients undergoing radiologic studies involving parenteral iodinated contrast material).
No products indexed under this heading.

Dienestrol (Certain drugs, such as estrogens, tend to produce hyperglycemia and may lead to loss of glycemic control).
No products indexed under this heading.

Diethylstilbestrol (Certain drugs, such as estrogens, tend to produce hyperglycemia and may lead to loss of glycemic control).
No products indexed under this heading.

Diflorasone Diacetate (Certain drugs, such as corticosteroids, tend to produce hyperglycemia and may lead to loss of glycemic control).
No products indexed under this heading.

Digoxin (Theoretical potential for interaction with metformin by competing for common renal tubular transport system). Products include:
Lanoxin Injection 1546
Lanoxin Injection Pediatric 1549
Lanoxin Tablets 1553

Diltiazem Hydrochloride (Certain drugs, such as calcium channel blockers, tend to produce hyperglycemia and may lead to loss of glycemic control). Products include:
Cardizem LA 423

Dobutamine Hydrochloride (Certain drugs, such as sympathomimetics, tend to produce hyperglycemia and may lead to loss of glycemic control).
No products indexed under this heading.

Dopamine Hydrochloride (Certain drugs, such as sympathomimetics, tend to produce hyperglycemia and may lead to loss of glycemic control).
No products indexed under this heading.

Ephedrine Hydrochloride (Certain drugs, such as sympathomimetics, tend to produce hyperglycemia and may lead to loss of glycemic control).
No products indexed under this heading.

Ephedrine Sulfate (Certain drugs, such as sympathomimetics, tend to produce hyperglycemia and may lead to loss of glycemic control).
No products indexed under this heading.

Ephedrine Tannate (Certain drugs, such as sympathomimetics, tend to produce hyperglycemia and may lead to loss of glycemic control).
No products indexed under this heading.

Epinephrine (Certain drugs, such as sympathomimetics, tend to produce hyperglycemia and may lead to loss of glycemic control). Products include:
EpiPen 3631
Twinject 3268

Epinephrine Bitartrate (Certain drugs, such as sympathomimetics, tend to produce hyperglycemia and may lead to loss of glycemic control).
No products indexed under this heading.

Epinephrine Hydrochloride (Certain drugs, such as sympathomimetics, tend to produce hyperglycemia and may lead to loss of glycemic control).
No products indexed under this heading.

Estradiol (Certain drugs, such as estrogens, tend to produce hyperglycemia and may lead to loss of glycemic control). Products include:
Activella 2561
Angeliq 831
Climara 841
Climara Pro 847
Divigel 3467
Estrasorb 1777
Vagifem 2589

Estrogens, Conjugated (Certain drugs, such as estrogens, tend to produce hyperglycemia and may lead to loss of glycemic control). Products include:
Premarin Intravenous 3528
Premarin Tablets 3533
Premarin Vaginal Cream 3540
Premphase 3549
Prempro 3549

Estrogens, Esterified (Certain drugs, such as estrogens, tend to produce hyperglycemia and may lead to loss of glycemic control).
No products indexed under this heading.

Estropipate (Certain drugs, such as estrogens, tend to produce hyperglycemia and may lead to loss of glycemic control).
No products indexed under this heading.

Ethacrynic Acid (Certain drugs, such as diuretics, tend to produce hyperglycemia and may lead to loss of glycemic control).
No products indexed under this heading.

Ethanol (Alcohol potentiates the effect of metformin on lactate metabolism; patients should be warned against excessive alcohol intake, acute or chronic).
No products indexed under this heading.

Ethinyl Estradiol (Certain drugs, such as estrogens, tend to produce hyperglycemia and may lead to loss of glycemic control). Products include:
LoSeasonique 3407
Lybrel 3514
NuvaRing 3181
Ortho Evra 2648
Ortho-Cyclen/Ortho Tri-Cyclen 2663
Ortho Tri-Cyclen Lo Tablets 2673
Seasonique 3418
Yaz 864

Ethiodized Oil (Potential for acute alteration of renal function; metformin should be temporarily withheld in patients undergoing radiologic studies involving parenteral iodinated contrast material).
No products indexed under this heading.

Ethyl Alcohol (Alcohol potentiates the effect of metformin on lactate metabolism; patients should be warned against excessive alcohol intake, acute or chronic).
No products indexed under this heading.

Ethynodiol Diacetate (Certain drugs, such as oral contraceptives, tend to produce hyperglycemia and may lead to loss of glycemic control).
No products indexed under this heading.

Felodipine (Certain drugs, such as calcium channel blockers, tend to produce hyperglycemia and may lead to loss of glycemic control).
No products indexed under this heading.

Fludrocortisone Acetate (Certain drugs, such as corticosteroids, tend to produce hyperglycemia and may lead to loss of glycemic control).
No products indexed under this heading.

Flumethasone Pivalate (Certain drugs, such as corticosteroids, tend to produce hyperglycemia and may lead to loss of glycemic control).
No products indexed under this heading.

Flunisolide Hemihydrate (Certain drugs, such as corticosteroids, tend to produce hyperglycemia and may lead to loss of glycemic control).
No products indexed under this heading.

Fluphenazine Decanoate (Certain drugs, such as phenothiazines, tend to produce hyperglycemia and may lead to loss of glycemic control).
No products indexed under this heading.

Fluphenazine Enanthate (Certain drugs, such as phenothiazines, tend to produce hyperglycemia and may lead to loss of glycemic control).
No products indexed under this heading.

Fluphenazine Hydrochloride (Certain drugs, such as phenothiazines, tend to produce hyperglycemia and may lead to loss of glycemic control).
No products indexed under this heading.

Fluticasone Furoate (Certain drugs, such as corticosteroids, tend to produce hyperglycemia and may lead to loss of glycemic control). Products include:
Veramyst 1713

Fluticasone Propionate (Certain drugs, such as corticosteroids, tend to produce hyperglycemia and may lead to loss of glycemic control). Products include:
Advair 100/50 1275
Advair 250/50 1275
Advair 500/50 1275
Advair HFA 45/21 1288
Advair HFA 115/21 1288
Advair HFA 230/21 1288
Flonase 1459
Flovent Diskus 1463
Flovent HFA 1470

Fosphenytoin (Certain drugs, such as phenytoin, tend to produce hyperglycemia and may lead to loss of glycemic control).
No products indexed under this heading.

Fosphenytoin Sodium (Certain drugs, such as phenytoin, tend to produce hyperglycemia and may lead to loss of glycemic control).
No products indexed under this heading.

Furosemide (Increases metformin plasma and blood C_{max} by 22% and blood AUC by 15%; the C_{max} and AUC of furosemide were 31% and 12% smaller when co-administered; potential for loss of glycemic control). Products include:
Furosemide 2354

Gadopentetate Dimeglumine (Potential for acute alteration of renal function; metformin should be temporarily withheld in patients undergoing radiologic studies involving parenteral iodinated contrast material).
No products indexed under this heading.

Gemfibrozil (Concomitant administration of gemfibrozil (600 mg bid), an inhibitor of CYP2C8, and rosiglitazone (4 mg qd) for 7 days increased rosiglitazone AUC by 127%, compared to administration of rosiglitazone (4 mg qd) alone).
No products indexed under this heading.

Glibenclamide (Patients receiving rosiglitazone in combination with other hypoglycemic agents may be at risk for hypoglycemia and a reduction in the dose of the concomitant agent may be necessary).
No products indexed under this heading.

Glimepiride (An increased incidence of heart failure has been observed when rosiglitazone was added to a sulfonylurea or to a sulfonylurea plus metformin). Products include:
Avandaryl 1356
Duetact 3354

(⊙ Described in PDR® for Ophthalmic Medicines)

IMPORTANT NOTE: Always consult each drug listing in the patient's regimen for possible interactions.

(⊙ Described in PDR® for Ophthalmic Medicines)

Rifabutin (An inducer of CYP2C8 may decrease the AUC of rosiglitazone).
No products indexed under this heading.

Rifampin (Rifampin administration (600 mg qd) an inducer of CYP2C8, for 6 days is reported to decrease rosiglitazone AUC by 66%, compared to administration of rosiglitazone (8 mg) alone).
No products indexed under this heading.

Salmeterol Xinafoate (Certain drugs, such as sympathomimetics, tend to produce hyperglycemia and may lead to loss of glycemic control). Products include:

Sitagliptin Phosphate (Patients receiving rosiglitazone in combination with other hypoglycemic agents may be at risk for hypoglycemia and a reduction in the dose of the concomitant agent may be necessary). Products include:

Spironolactone (Certain drugs, such as diuretics, tend to produce hyperglycemia and may lead to loss of glycemic control).
No products indexed under this heading.

Sulfaphenazole (An inhibitor of CYP2C8 may increase the AUC of rosiglitazone).
No products indexed under this heading.

Sulfinpyrazone (An inhibitor of CYP2C8 may increase the AUC of rosiglitazone).
No products indexed under this heading.

Terbutaline Sulfate (Certain drugs, such as sympathomimetics, tend to produce hyperglycemia and may lead to loss of glycemic control).
No products indexed under this heading.

Thioridazine (Certain drugs, such as phenothiazines, tend to produce hyperglycemia and may lead to loss of glycemic control).
No products indexed under this heading.

Thioridazine Hydrochloride (Certain drugs, such as phenothiazines, tend to produce hyperglycemia and may lead to loss of glycemic control). Products include:

Thyroglobulin (Certain drugs, such as thyroid products, tend to produce hyperglycemia and may lead to loss of glycemic control).
No products indexed under this heading.

Thyroid (Certain drugs, such as thyroid products, tend to produce hyperglycemia and may lead to loss of glycemic control). Products include:

Thyroxine (Certain drugs, such as thyroid products, tend to produce hyperglycemia and may lead to loss of glycemic control).
No products indexed under this heading.

Thyroxine Sodium (Certain drugs, such as thyroid products, tend to produce hyperglycemia and may lead to loss of glycemic control).
No products indexed under this heading.

Tolazamide (An increased incidence of heart failure has been observed when rosiglitazone was added to a sulfonylurea or to a sulfonylurea plus metformin).
No products indexed under this heading.

Tolbutamide (An increased incidence of heart failure has been observed when rosiglitazone was added to a sulfonylurea or to a sulfonylurea plus metformin).
No products indexed under this heading.

Torsemide (Certain drugs, such as diuretics, tend to produce hyperglycemia and may lead to loss of glycemic control).
No products indexed under this heading.

Triamcinolone (Certain drugs, such as corticosteroids, tend to produce hyperglycemia and may lead to loss of glycemic control).
No products indexed under this heading.

Triamcinolone Acetonide (Certain drugs, such as corticosteroids, tend to produce hyperglycemia and may lead to loss of glycemic control). Products include:

Triamcinolone Diacetate (Certain drugs, such as corticosteroids, tend to produce hyperglycemia and may lead to loss of glycemic control).
No products indexed under this heading.

Triamcinolone Hexacetonide (Certain drugs, such as corticosteroids, tend to produce hyperglycemia and may lead to loss of glycemic control).
No products indexed under this heading.

Triamterene (Potential for loss of glycemic control; theoretical potential for interaction with metformin by competing for common renal tubular transport system). Products include:

Trifluoperazine Hydrochloride (Certain drugs, such as phenothiazines, tend to produce hyperglycemia and may lead to loss of glycemic control).
No products indexed under this heading.

Trimethoprim (Theoretical potential for interaction with metformin by competing for common renal tubular transport system).
No products indexed under this heading.

Trimethoprim Hydrochloride (An inhibitor of CYP2C8 may increase the AUC of rosiglitazone).
No products indexed under this heading.

Trimethoprim Sulfate (Theoretical potential for interaction with metformin by competing for common renal tubular transport system).
No products indexed under this heading.

Troglitazone (Patients receiving rosiglitazone in combination with other hypoglycemic agents may be at risk for hypoglycemia and a reduction in the dose of the concomitant agent may be necessary).
No products indexed under this heading.

Tyropanoate Sodium (Potential for acute alteration of renal function; metformin should be temporarily withheld in patients undergoing radiologic studies involving parenteral iodinated contrast material).
No products indexed under this heading.

Vancomycin Hydrochloride (Theoretical potential for interaction with metformin by competing for common renal tubular transport system).
No products indexed under this heading.

Verapamil Hydrochloride (Certain drugs, such as calcium channel blockers, tend to produce hyperglycemia and may lead to loss of glycemic control). Products include:

Food Interactions

Alcohol (Alcohol potentiates the effect of metformin on lactate metabolism; patients should be warned against excessive alcohol intake, acute or chronic).

Beer, reduced-alcohol (Alcohol potentiates the effect of metformin on lactate metabolism; patients should be warned against excessive alcohol intake, acute or chronic).

Beer, unspecified (Alcohol potentiates the effect of metformin on lactate metabolism; patients should be warned against excessive alcohol intake, acute or chronic).

Food, unspecified (Food decreases the extent and slightly delays the absorption of metformin).

Wine, Chianti (Alcohol potentiates the effect of metformin on lactate metabolism; patients should be warned against excessive alcohol intake, acute or chronic).

Wine, Red (Alcohol potentiates the effect of metformin on lactate metabolism; patients should be warned against excessive alcohol intake, acute or chronic).

Wine, unspecified (Alcohol potentiates the effect of metformin on lactate metabolism; patients should be warned against excessive alcohol intake, acute or chronic).

Wine products (Alcohol potentiates the effect of metformin on lactate metabolism; patients should be warned against excessive alcohol intake, acute or chronic).

AVANDARYL TABLETS

(Glimepiride, Rosiglitazone Maleate) 1356
May interact with beta-blockers, corticosteroids, cytochrome p450 2c8 inducers (selected), cytochrome p450 2c8 inhibitors (selected), diuretics, estrogens, insulin, monoamine oxidase inhibitors, non-steroidal anti-inflammatory agents, oral anticoagulants, oral contraceptives, phenothiazines, salicylates, sulfonamides, sympathomimetics, thiazides, thyroid preparations, and certain other agents. Compounds in these categories include:

Acebutolol Hydrochloride (May potentiate hypoglycemic action. Hypoglycemia may be difficult to recognize in patients taking β-blockers).
No products indexed under this heading.

Albuterol (Sympathomimetics tend to produce hyperglycemia and concurrent use may lead to loss of control).
No products indexed under this heading.

Albuterol Sulfate (Sympathomimetics tend to produce hyperglycemia and concurrent use may lead to loss of control). Products include:

Alclometasone Dipropionate (Corticosteroids tend to produce hyperglycemia and concurrent use may lead to loss of control).
No products indexed under this heading.

Amiloride Hydrochloride (Diuretics tend to produce hyperglycemia and concurrent use may lead to loss of control).
No products indexed under this heading.

Anastrozole (An inhibitor of CYP2C8 may decrease the AUC of rosiglitazone. Therefore, if an inducer of CYP2C8 is started or stopped during treatment with rosiglitazone, changes in diabetes treatment may be needed upon clinical response).
No products indexed under this heading.

Anisindione (May potentiate hypoglycemic action).
No products indexed under this heading.

Aspirin (Co-administration of aspirin (1 g tid) led to a 34% decrease in the mean glimepiride AUC and, therefore, a 34% increase in the mean CL/F. The mean C_{max} had a decrease of 4%. Blood glucose and serum C-peptide concentrations were unaffected and no hypoglycemic symptoms were reported). Products include:

Aspirin, Enteric Coated (Co-administration of aspirin (1 g tid) led to a 34% decrease in the mean glimepiride AUC and, therefore, a 34% increase in the mean CL/F. The mean C_{max} had a decrease of 4%. Blood glucose and serum C-peptide concentrations were unaffected and no hypoglycemic symptoms were reported).
No products indexed under this heading.

Aspirin Buffered (Co-administration of aspirin (1 g tid) led to a 34% decrease in the mean glimepiride AUC and, therefore, a 34% increase in the mean CL/F. The mean C_{max} had a decrease of 4%. Blood glucose and serum C-peptide concentrations were unaffected and no hypoglycemic symptoms were reported).
No products indexed under this heading.

Atenolol (May potentiate hypoglycemic action. Hypoglycemia may be difficult to recognize in patients taking β-blockers).
No products indexed under this heading.

Beclomethasone Dipropionate (Corticosteroids tend to produce hyperglycemia and concurrent use may lead to loss of control). Products include:

Beclomethasone Dipropionate Monohydrate (Corticosteroids tend to produce hyperglycemia and concurrent use may lead to loss of control). Products include:

Bendroflumethiazide (Diuretics tend to produce hyperglycemia and concurrent use may lead to loss of control).
No products indexed under this heading.

Betamethasone (Corticosteroids tend to produce hyperglycemia and concurrent use may lead to loss of control).
No products indexed under this heading.

Betamethasone Acetate (Corticosteroids tend to produce hyperglycemia and concurrent use may lead to loss of control).
No products indexed under this heading.

Betamethasone Benzoate (Corticosteroids tend to produce hyperglycemia and concurrent use may lead to loss of control).
No products indexed under this heading.

Betamethasone Dipropionate (Corticosteroids tend to produce hyperglycemia and concurrent use may lead to loss of control). Products include:

Betamethasone Sodium Phosphate (Corticosteroids tend to produce hyperglycemia and concurrent use may lead to loss of control).
No products indexed under this heading.

Betamethasone Valerate (Corticosteroids tend to produce hyperglycemia and concurrent use may lead to loss of control). Products include:

Betaxolol Hydrochloride (May potentiate hypoglycemic action. Hypoglycemia may be difficult to recognize in patients taking β-blockers).
No products indexed under this heading.

Bisoprolol Fumarate (May potentiate hypoglycemic action. Hypoglycemia may be difficult to recognize in patients taking β-blockers).
No products indexed under this heading.

Budesonide (Corticosteroids tend to produce hyperglycemia and concurrent use may lead to loss of control). Products include:

Pulmicort Flexhaler	714
Symbicort 80/4.5	720
Symbicort 160/4.5	720

Bumetanide (Diuretics tend to produce hyperglycemia and concurrent use may lead to loss of control).
No products indexed under this heading.

Carbamazepine (An inhibitor of CYP2C8 may decrease the AUC of rosiglitazone. Therefore, if an inducer of CYP2C8 is started or stopped during treatment with rosiglitazone, changes in diabetes treatment may be needed upon clinical response). Products include:

Carbatrol	3280
Equetro	3477

Carteolol Hydrochloride (May potentiate hypoglycemic action. Hypoglycemia may be difficult to recognize in patients taking β-blockers).
No products indexed under this heading.

Carvedilol (May potentiate hypoglycemic action. Hypoglycemia may be difficult to recognize in patients taking β-blockers). Products include:

Coreg	1409

Carvedilol Phosphate (May potentiate hypoglycemic action. Hypoglycemia may be difficult to recognize in patients taking β-blockers). Products include:

Coreg CR	1416

Celecoxib (May potentiate hypoglycemic action). Products include:

Celebrex	3272

Chloramphenicol (May potentiate hypoglycemic action).
No products indexed under this heading.

Chloramphenicol Palmitate (May potentiate hypoglycemic action).
No products indexed under this heading.

Chloramphenicol Sodium Succinate (May potentiate hypoglycemic action).
No products indexed under this heading.

Chlorothiazide (Diuretics tend to produce hyperglycemia and concurrent use may lead to loss of control).
No products indexed under this heading.

Chlorothiazide Sodium (Diuretics tend to produce hyperglycemia and concurrent use may lead to loss of control). Products include:

Diuril Intravenous	2009

Chlorotrianisene (Estrogens tend to produce hyperglycemia and concurrent use may lead to loss of control).
No products indexed under this heading.

Chlorpromazine (Phenothiazines tend to produce hyperglycemia and concurrent use may lead to loss of control).
No products indexed under this heading.

Chlorpromazine Hydrochloride (Phenothiazines tend to produce hyperglycemia and concurrent use may lead to loss of control).
No products indexed under this heading.

Chlorpropamide (May potentiate hypoglycemic action).
No products indexed under this heading.

Chlorthalidone (Diuretics tend to produce hyperglycemia and concurrent use may lead to loss of control). Products include:

Clorpres	2344

Choline Magnesium Trisalicylate (May potentiate hypoglycemic action; clinical trials data indicate no evidence of significant adverse interaction with concurrent use).
No products indexed under this heading.

Ciclesonide (Corticosteroids tend to produce hyperglycemia and concurrent use may lead to loss of control).
No products indexed under this heading.

Cimetidine (An inhibitor of CYP2C8 may decrease the AUC of rosiglitazone. Therefore, if an inducer of CYP2C8 is started or stopped during treatment with rosiglitazone, changes in diabetes treatment may be needed upon clinical response).
No products indexed under this heading.

Cimetidine Hydrochloride (An inhibitor of CYP2C8 may decrease the AUC of rosiglitazone. Therefore, if an inducer of CYP2C8 is started or stopped during treatment with rosiglitazone, changes in diabetes treatment may be needed upon clinical response).
No products indexed under this heading.

Cortisone Acetate (Corticosteroids tend to produce hyperglycemia and concurrent use may lead to loss of control).
No products indexed under this heading.

Desogestrel (Oral contraceptives tend to produce hyperglycemia and concurrent use may lead to loss of control).
No products indexed under this heading.

Desoximetasone (Corticosteroids tend to produce hyperglycemia and concurrent use may lead to loss of control).
No products indexed under this heading.

Dexamethasone (Corticosteroids tend to produce hyperglycemia and concurrent use may lead to loss of control). Products include:

Ciprodex	583
Ozurdex	⊙ 223
Tobramycin and Dexamethasone Ophthalmic Suspension	⊙ 251

Dexamethasone Acetate (Corticosteroids tend to produce hyperglycemia and concurrent use may lead to loss of control).
No products indexed under this heading.

Dexamethasone Phosphate (Corticosteroids tend to produce hyperglycemia and concurrent use may lead to loss of control).
No products indexed under this heading.

Dexamethasone Sodium (Corticosteroids tend to produce hyperglycemia and concurrent use may lead to loss of control).
No products indexed under this heading.

Dexamethasone Sodium Phosphate (Corticosteroids tend to produce hyperglycemia and concurrent use may lead to loss of control).
No products indexed under this heading.

Dexamethasone Sodium Phosphate Injection (Corticosteroids tend to produce hyperglycemia and concurrent use may lead to loss of control).
No products indexed under this heading.

Diclofenac Epolamine (May potentiate hypoglycemic action). Products include:

Flector	1839

Diclofenac Potassium (May potentiate hypoglycemic action).
No products indexed under this heading.

Diclofenac Sodium (May potentiate hypoglycemic action).
No products indexed under this heading.

Dicumarol (May potentiate hypoglycemic action).
No products indexed under this heading.

Dienestrol (Estrogens tend to produce hyperglycemia and concurrent use may lead to loss of control).
No products indexed under this heading.

Diethylstilbestrol (Estrogens tend to produce hyperglycemia and concurrent use may lead to loss of control).
No products indexed under this heading.

Diflorasone Diacetate (Corticosteroids tend to produce hyperglycemia and concurrent use may lead to loss of control).
No products indexed under this heading.

Diflunisal (May potentiate hypoglycemic action; clinical trials data indicate no evidence of significant adverse interaction with concurrent use).
No products indexed under this heading.

Dobutamine Hydrochloride (Sympathomimetics tend to produce hyperglycemia and concurrent use may lead to loss of control).
No products indexed under this heading.

Dopamine Hydrochloride (Sympathomimetics tend to produce hyperglycemia and concurrent use may lead to loss of control).
No products indexed under this heading.

Ephedrine Hydrochloride (Sympathomimetics tend to produce hyperglycemia and concurrent use may lead to loss of control).
No products indexed under this heading.

Ephedrine Sulfate (Sympathomimetics tend to produce hyperglycemia and concurrent use may lead to loss of control).
No products indexed under this heading.

Ephedrine Tannate (Sympathomimetics tend to produce hyperglycemia and concurrent use may lead to loss of control).
No products indexed under this heading.

Epinephrine (Sympathomimetics tend to produce hyperglycemia and concurrent use may lead to loss of control). Products include:

EpiPen	3631
Twinject	3268

Epinephrine Bitartrate (Sympathomimetics tend to produce hyperglycemia and concurrent use may lead to loss of control).
No products indexed under this heading.

Epinephrine Hydrochloride (Sympathomimetics tend to produce hyperglycemia and concurrent use may lead to loss of control).
No products indexed under this heading.

Esmolol Hydrochloride (May potentiate hypoglycemic action. Hypoglycemia may be difficult to recognize in patients taking β-blockers).
No products indexed under this heading.

Estradiol (Estrogens tend to produce hyperglycemia and concurrent use may lead to loss of control). Products include:

Activella	2561
Angeliq	831
Climara	841
Climara Pro	847
Divigel	3467
Estrasorb	1777
Vagifem	2589

Estrogens, Conjugated (Estrogens tend to produce hyperglycemia and concurrent use may lead to loss of control). Products include:

Premarin Intravenous	3528
Premarin Tablets	3533
Premarin Vaginal Cream	3540
Premphase	3549
Prempro	3549

Estrogens, Esterified (Estrogens tend to produce hyperglycemia and concurrent use may lead to loss of control).
No products indexed under this heading.

Estropipate (Estrogens tend to produce hyperglycemia and concurrent use may lead to loss of control).
No products indexed under this heading.

Ethacrynic Acid (Diuretics tend to produce hyperglycemia and concurrent use may lead to loss of control).
No products indexed under this heading.

Ethinyl Estradiol (Estrogens tend to produce hyperglycemia and concurrent use may lead to loss of control). Products include:

LoSeasonique	3407
Lybrel	3514
NuvaRing	3181
Ortho Evra	2648
Ortho-Cyclen/Ortho Tri-Cyclen	2663
Ortho Tri-Cyclen Lo Tablets	2673
Seasonique	3418
Yaz	864

Ethynodiol Diacetate (Oral contraceptives tend to produce hyperglycemia and concurrent use may lead to loss of control).
No products indexed under this heading.

Etodolac (May potentiate hypoglycemic action).
No products indexed under this heading.

Fenoprofen Calcium (May potentiate hypoglycemic action).
No products indexed under this heading.

Fludrocortisone Acetate (Corticosteroids tend to produce hyperglycemia and concurrent use may lead to loss of control).
No products indexed under this heading.

Flumethasone Pivalate (Corticosteroids tend to produce hyperglycemia and concurrent use may lead to loss of control).
No products indexed under this heading.

Flunisolide Hemihydrate (Corticosteroids tend to produce hyperglycemia and concurrent use may lead to loss of control).
No products indexed under this heading.

Fluphenazine Decanoate (Phenothiazines tend to produce hyperglycemia and concurrent use may lead to loss of control).
No products indexed under this heading.

Fluphenazine Enanthate (Phenothiazines tend to produce hyperglycemia and concurrent use may lead to loss of control).
No products indexed under this heading.

Fluphenazine Hydrochloride (Phenothiazines tend to produce hyperglycemia and concurrent use may lead to loss of control).
No products indexed under this heading.

Flurbiprofen (May potentiate hypoglycemic action).
No products indexed under this heading.

Fluticasone Furoate (Corticosteroids tend to produce hyperglycemia and concurrent use may lead to loss of control). Products include:

Veramyst	1713

Fluticasone Propionate (Corticosteroids tend to produce hyperglycemia and concurrent use may lead to loss of control). Products include:

Advair 100/50	1275
Advair 250/50	1275
Advair 500/50	1275
Advair HFA 45/21	1288
Advair HFA 115/21	1288
Advair HFA 230/21	1288
Flonase	1459
Flovent Diskus	1463
Flovent HFA	1470

Furosemide (Diuretics tend to produce hyperglycemia and concurrent use may lead to loss of control). Products include:

Furosemide	2354

Gemfibrozil (Concomitant administration of gemfibrozil (600 mg twice daily), an inhibitor of CYP2C8 and rosiglitazone (4 mg once daily) for 7 days increased rosiglitazone AUC by 127% compared to the administration of

rosiglitazone (4 mg once daily) alone. Given the potential for dose-related adverse events with rosiglitazone, a decrease in the dose of rosiglitazone may be needed when gemfibrozil is introduced.

No products indexed under this heading.

Glipizide (May potentiate hypoglycemic action).

No products indexed under this heading.

Glyburide (Rosiglitazone (2 mg twice daily) taken concomitantly with glyburide (3.75 to 10 mg/day) for 7 days did not alter the mean steady-state 24-hour plasma glucose concentrations in diabetic patients stabilized on glyburide therapy. Repeat doses of rosiglitazone (8 mg once daily) for 8 days in healthy adult Caucasian subjects caused a decrease in glyburide AUC (32%) and C_{max} (35%). In Japanese subjects, glyburide AUC (14%) and C_{max} (31%) slightly increased following co-administration of rosiglitazone).

No products indexed under this heading.

Hydrochlorothiazide (Diuretics tend to produce hyperglycemia and concurrent use may lead to loss of control). Products include:

Atacand HCT	700
Avalide	2956
Benicar HCT	1017
Diovan HCT	2419
Dyazide	1429
Exforge HCT	2449
Hyzaar	2162
Hyzaar 100-12.5	2162
Micardis HCT	889
Prinzide	2246
Tekturna HCT	2541
Teveten HCT	541

Hydrocortisone (Corticosteroids tend to produce hyperglycemia and concurrent use may lead to loss of control).

No products indexed under this heading.

Hydrocortisone (Alcohol) (Corticosteroids tend to produce hyperglycemia and concurrent use may lead to loss of control).

No products indexed under this heading.

Hydrocortisone Acetate (Corticosteroids tend to produce hyperglycemia and concurrent use may lead to loss of control).

No products indexed under this heading.

Hydrocortisone Butyrate (Corticosteroids tend to produce hyperglycemia and concurrent use may lead to loss of control).

No products indexed under this heading.

Hydrocortisone Cypionate (Corticosteroids tend to produce hyperglycemia and concurrent use may lead to loss of control).

No products indexed under this heading.

Hydrocortisone Hemisuccinate (Corticosteroids tend to produce hyperglycemia and concurrent use may lead to loss of control).

No products indexed under this heading.

Hydrocortisone Probutate (Corticosteroids tend to produce hyperglycemia and concurrent use may lead to loss of control).

No products indexed under this heading.

Hydrocortisone Sodium Phosphate (Corticosteroids tend to produce hyperglycemia and concurrent use may lead to loss of control).

No products indexed under this heading.

Hydrocortisone Sodium Succinate (Corticosteroids tend to produce hyperglycemia and concurrent use may lead to loss of control).

No products indexed under this heading.

Hydrocortisone Valerate (Corticosteroids tend to produce hyperglycemia and concurrent use may lead to loss of control).

No products indexed under this heading.

Hydroflumethiazide (Diuretics tend to produce hyperglycemia and concurrent use may lead to loss of control).

No products indexed under this heading.

Ibuprofen (May potentiate hypoglycemic action). Products include:

Motrin IB	2043
Children's Motrin	2044
Children's Motrin Non-Staining Dye-Free	2044
Infants' Motrin	2044
Infants' Motrin Dye-Free	2044
Junior Strength Motrin	2044
Vicoprofen	564

Indapamide (Diuretics tend to produce hyperglycemia and concurrent use may lead to loss of control). Products include:

Indapamide	2356

Indomethacin (May potentiate hypoglycemic action). Products include:

Indocin	2167

Indomethacin Sodium Trihydrate (May potentiate hypoglycemic action). Products include:

Indocin I.V.	2007

Insulin (Co-administration of glimepiride with insulin may increase the potential for hypoglycemia. Co-administration of rosiglitazone with insulin has resulted in increased incidence of cardiac failure and other cardiovascular adverse events).

No products indexed under this heading.

Insulin, Human, Zinc Suspension (Co-administration of glimepiride with insulin may increase the potential for hypoglycemia. Co-administration of rosiglitazone with insulin has resulted in increased incidence of cardiac failure and other cardiovascular adverse events).

No products indexed under this heading.

Insulin, Human (rDNA origin) (Co-administration of glimepiride with insulin may increase the potential for hypoglycemia. Co-administration of rosiglitazone with insulin has resulted in increased incidence of cardiac failure and other cardiovascular adverse events). Products include:

Exubera	2717

Insulin, Human NPH (Co-administration of glimepiride with insulin may increase the potential for hypoglycemia. Co-administration of rosiglitazone with insulin has resulted in increased incidence of cardiac failure and other cardiovascular adverse events). Products include:

Humulin N Vial	1934

Insulin, Human Regular (Co-administration of glimepiride with insulin may increase the potential for hypoglycemia. Co-administration of rosiglitazone with insulin has resulted in increased incidence of cardiac failure and other cardiovascular adverse events). Products include:

Humulin R	1937
Humulin R (U-500)	1939

Insulin, Human Regular and Human NPH Mixture (Co-administration of glimepiride with insulin may increase the potential for hypoglycemia. Co-administration of rosiglitazone with insulin has resulted in increased incidence of cardiac failure and other cardiovascular adverse events). Products include:

Humulin 50/50	1930
Humulin 70/30 Vial	1931

Insulin, NPH (Co-administration of glimepiride with insulin may increase the potential for hypoglycemia. Co-administration of rosiglitazone with insulin has resulted in increased incidence of cardiac failure and other cardiovascular adverse events).

No products indexed under this heading.

Insulin, Regular (Co-administration of glimepiride with insulin may increase the potential for hypoglycemia. Co-administration of rosiglitazone with insulin has resulted in increased incidence of cardiac failure and other cardiovascular adverse events).

No products indexed under this heading.

Insulin, Regular and NPH mixture (Co-administration of glimepiride with insulin may increase the potential for hypoglycemia. Co-administration of rosiglitazone with insulin has resulted in increased incidence of cardiac failure and other cardiovascular adverse events).

No products indexed under this heading.

Insulin, Zinc Crystals (Co-administration of glimepiride with insulin may increase the potential for hypoglycemia. Co-administration of rosiglitazone with insulin has resulted in increased incidence of cardiac failure and other cardiovascular adverse events).

No products indexed under this heading.

Insulin, Zinc Suspension (Co-administration of glimepiride with insulin may increase the potential for hypoglycemia. Co-administration of rosiglitazone with insulin has resulted in increased incidence of cardiac failure and other cardiovascular adverse events).

No products indexed under this heading.

Insulin Aspart (Co-administration of glimepiride with insulin may increase the potential for hypoglycemia. Co-administration of rosiglitazone with insulin has resulted in increased incidence of cardiac failure and other cardiovascular adverse events).

No products indexed under this heading.

Insulin Aspart, Human (Co-administration of glimepiride with insulin may increase the potential for hypoglycemia. Co-administration of rosiglitazone with insulin has resulted in increased incidence of cardiac failure and other cardiovascular adverse events). Products include:

NovoLog Mix 70/30	2581

Insulin Aspart, Human Regular (Co-administration of glimepiride with insulin may increase the potential for hypoglycemia. Co-administration of rosiglitazone with insulin has resulted in increased incidence of cardiac failure and other cardiovascular adverse events). Products include:

NovoLog	2575

Insulin Aspart Protamine, Human (Co-administration of glimepiride with insulin may increase the potential for hypoglycemia. Co-administration of rosiglitazone with insulin has resulted in increased incidence of cardiac failure and other cardiovascular adverse events). Products include:

NovoLog Mix 70/30	2581

Insulin Detemir (rDNA Origin) (Co-administration of glimepiride with insulin may increase the potential for hypoglycemia. Co-administration of rosiglitazone with insulin has resulted in increased incidence of cardiac failure and other cardiovascular adverse events). Products include:

Levemir	2566

Insulin Glargine (Co-administration of glimepiride with insulin may increase the potential for hypoglycemia. Co-administration of rosiglitazone with insulin has resulted in increased incidence of cardiac failure and other cardiovascular adverse events). Products include:

Lantus	2996

Insulin Glulisine (Co-administration of glimepiride with insulin may increase the potential for hypoglycemia. Co-administration of rosiglitazone with insulin has resulted in increased incidence of cardiac failure and other cardiovascular adverse events). Products include:

Apidra	2937
Apidra SoloStar	2937

Insulin Lispro, Human (Co-administration of glimepiride with insulin may increase the potential for hypoglycemia. Co-administration of rosiglitazone with insulin has resulted in increased incidence of cardiac failure and other cardiovascular adverse events). Products include:

Humalog	1910
Humalog Mix	1914
Humalog Mix75/25	1917

Insulin Lispro Protamine, Human (Co-administration of glimepiride with insulin may increase the potential for hypoglycemia. Co-administration of rosiglitazone with insulin has resulted in increased incidence of cardiac failure and other cardiovascular adverse events). Products include:

Humalog Mix	1914
Humalog Mix75/25	1917

Isocarboxazid (May potentiate hypoglycemic action). Products include:

Marplan	3481

Isoniazid (Isoniazid tends to produce hyperglycemia and concurrent use may lead to loss of control).

No products indexed under this heading.

Isoproterenol Hydrochloride (Sympathomimetics tend to produce hyperglycemia and concurrent use may lead to loss of control).

No products indexed under this heading.

Isoproterenol Sulfate (Sympathomimetics tend to produce hyperglycemia and concurrent use may lead to loss of control).

No products indexed under this heading.

Ketoprofen (May potentiate hypoglycemic action).

No products indexed under this heading.

Ketorolac Tromethamine (May potentiate hypoglycemic action). Products include:

Acuvail	⊙209

Labetalol Hydrochloride (May potentiate hypoglycemic action. Hypoglycemia may be difficult to recognize in patients taking β-blockers).

No products indexed under this heading.

Levalbuterol Hydrochloride (Sympathomimetics tend to produce hyperglycemia and concurrent use may lead to loss of control).

No products indexed under this heading.

Levobunolol Hydrochloride (May potentiate hypoglycemic action. Hypoglycemia may be difficult to recognize in patients taking β-blockers).

No products indexed under this heading.

Levonorgestrel (Oral contraceptives tend to produce hyperglycemia and concurrent use may lead to loss of control). Products include:

Climara Pro	847
LoSeasonique	3407
Lybrel	3514
Mirena	854
Plan B	3416
Seasonique	3418

Levothyroxine Sodium (Thyroid products tend to produce hyperglycemia and concurrent use may lead to loss of control). Products include:

Levoxyl Tablets	1843
Synthroid	529

Liothyronine Sodium (Thyroid products tend to produce hyperglycemia and concurrent use may lead to loss of control). Products include:

Cytomel	1830

Liotrix (Thyroid products tend to produce hyperglycemia and concurrent use may lead to loss of control).

No products indexed under this heading.

IMPORTANT NOTE: Always consult each drug listing in the patient's regimen for possible interactions.

Magnesium Salicylate (May potentiate hypoglycemic action; clinical trials data indicate no evidence of significant adverse interaction with concurrent use).
 No products indexed under this heading.

Meclofenamate Sodium (May potentiate hypoglycemic action).
 No products indexed under this heading.

Mefenamic Acid (May potentiate hypoglycemic action).
 No products indexed under this heading.

Meloxicam (May potentiate hypoglycemic action).
 No products indexed under this heading.

Mesoridazine Besylate (Phenothiazines tend to produce hyperglycemia and concurrent use may lead to loss of control).
 No products indexed under this heading.

Mestranol (Oral contraceptives tend to produce hyperglycemia and concurrent use may lead to loss of control).
 No products indexed under this heading.

Metaproterenol Sulfate (Sympathomimetics tend to produce hyperglycemia and concurrent use may lead to loss of control).
 No products indexed under this heading.

Metaraminol Bitartrate (Sympathomimetics tend to produce hyperglycemia and concurrent use may lead to loss of control).
 No products indexed under this heading.

Metformin Hydrochloride (Co-administration of glimepiride with metformin may increase the potential for hypoglycemia). Products include:
 ActoPlus 3338
 Avandamet 1345
 Janumet 2188

Methotrimeprazine (Phenothiazines tend to produce hyperglycemia and concurrent use may lead to loss of control).
 No products indexed under this heading.

Methoxamine Hydrochloride (Sympathomimetics tend to produce hyperglycemia and concurrent use may lead to loss of control).
 No products indexed under this heading.

Methyclothiazide (Diuretics tend to produce hyperglycemia and concurrent use may lead to loss of control).
 No products indexed under this heading.

Methylprednisolone (Corticosteroids tend to produce hyperglycemia and concurrent use may lead to loss of control).
 No products indexed under this heading.

Methylprednisolone Acetate (Corticosteroids tend to produce hyperglycemia and concurrent use may lead to loss of control).
 No products indexed under this heading.

Methylprednisolone Sodium Succinate (Corticosteroids tend to produce hyperglycemia and concurrent use may lead to loss of control).
 No products indexed under this heading.

Metipranolol Hydrochloride (May potentiate hypoglycemic action. Hypoglycemia may be difficult to recognize in patients taking β-blockers).
 No products indexed under this heading.

Metolazone (Diuretics tend to produce hyperglycemia and concurrent use may lead to loss of control).
 No products indexed under this heading.

Metoprolol Succinate (May potentiate hypoglycemic action. Hypoglycemia may be difficult to recognize in patients taking β-blockers). Products include:
 Toprol XL 732

Metoprolol Tartrate (May potentiate hypoglycemic action. Hypoglycemia may be difficult to recognize in patients taking β-blockers).
 No products indexed under this heading.

Miconazole (A potential interaction between oral miconazole and oral hypoglycemic agents leading to severe hypoglycemia has been reported).
 No products indexed under this heading.

Moclobemide (May potentiate hypoglycemic action).
 No products indexed under this heading.

Mometasone Furoate (Corticosteroids tend to produce hyperglycemia and concurrent use may lead to loss of control). Products include:
 Asmanex 3058
 Elocon Cream 3111
 Elocon Lotion 3112
 Elocon Ointment 3114

Mometasone Furoate Monohydrate (Corticosteroids tend to produce hyperglycemia and concurrent use may lead to loss of control). Products include:
 Nasonex 3166

Nabumetone (May potentiate hypoglycemic action).
 No products indexed under this heading.

Nadolol (May potentiate hypoglycemic action. Hypoglycemia may be difficult to recognize in patients taking β-blockers). Products include:
 Nadolol 2359

Naproxen (May potentiate hypoglycemic action). Products include:
 EC-Naprosyn 2850
 Naprosyn 2850
 Anaprox/Naprosyn 2850

Naproxen Sodium (May potentiate hypoglycemic action). Products include:
 Anaprox 2850
 Anaprox DS 2850
 Treximet 1681

Nebivolol (May potentiate hypoglycemic action. Hypoglycemia may be difficult to recognize in patients taking β-blockers). Products include:
 Bystolic 1147

Nicardipine (An inhibitor of CYP2C8 may decrease the AUC of rosiglitazone. Therefore, if an inducer of CYP2C8 is started or stopped during treatment with rosiglitazone, changes in diabetes treatment may be needed upon clinical response).
 No products indexed under this heading.

Nicardipine Hydrochloride (An inhibitor of CYP2C8 may decrease the AUC of rosiglitazone. Therefore, if an inducer of CYP2C8 is started or stopped during treatment with rosiglitazone, changes in diabetes treatment may be needed upon clinical response).
 No products indexed under this heading.

Nicotinic Acid (Nicotinic acid tends to produce hyperglycemia and concurrent use may lead to loss of control).
 No products indexed under this heading.

Norepinephrine Bitartrate (Sympathomimetics tend to produce hyperglycemia and concurrent use may lead to loss of control).
 No products indexed under this heading.

Norethindrone (Oral contraceptives tend to produce hyperglycemia and concurrent use may lead to loss of control). Products include:
 Ortho Micronor 2660

Norethynodrel (Oral contraceptives tend to produce hyperglycemia and concurrent use may lead to loss of control).
 No products indexed under this heading.

Norgestimate (Oral contraceptives tend to produce hyperglycemia and concurrent use may lead to loss of control). Products include:
 Ortho-Cyclen/Ortho Tri-Cyclen 2663
 Ortho Tri-Cyclen Lo Tablets 2673

Norgestrel (Oral contraceptives tend to produce hyperglycemia and concurrent use may lead to loss of control).
 No products indexed under this heading.

Omeprazole (An inhibitor of CYP2C8 may decrease the AUC of rosiglitazone. Therefore, if an inducer of CYP2C8 is started or stopped during treatment with rosiglitazone, changes in diabetes treatment may be needed upon clinical response).
 No products indexed under this heading.

Oxaprozin (May potentiate hypoglycemic action).
 No products indexed under this heading.

Pargyline Hydrochloride (May potentiate hypoglycemic action).
 No products indexed under this heading.

Penbutolol Sulfate (May potentiate hypoglycemic action. Hypoglycemia may be difficult to recognize in patients taking β-blockers).
 No products indexed under this heading.

Perphenazine (Phenothiazines tend to produce hyperglycemia and concurrent use may lead to loss of control).
 No products indexed under this heading.

Phenelzine Sulfate (May potentiate hypoglycemic action).
 No products indexed under this heading.

Phenobarbital (An inhibitor of CYP2C8 may decrease the AUC of rosiglitazone. Therefore, if an inducer of CYP2C8 is started or stopped during treatment with rosiglitazone, changes in diabetes treatment may be needed upon clinical response). Products include:
 Donnatal 2711

Phenobarbital Sodium (An inhibitor of CYP2C8 may decrease the AUC of rosiglitazone. Therefore, if an inducer of CYP2C8 is started or stopped during treatment with rosiglitazone, changes in diabetes treatment may be needed upon clinical response).
 No products indexed under this heading.

Phenothiazine Derivatives (Phenothiazines tend to produce hyperglycemia and concurrent use may lead to loss of control).
 No products indexed under this heading.

Phenothiazines (Phenothiazines tend to produce hyperglycemia and concurrent use may lead to loss of control).
 No products indexed under this heading.

Phenylbutazone (May potentiate hypoglycemic action).
 No products indexed under this heading.

Phenylephrine Bitartrate (Sympathomimetics tend to produce hyperglycemia and concurrent use may lead to loss of control).
 No products indexed under this heading.

Phenylephrine Hydrochloride (Sympathomimetics tend to produce hyperglycemia and concurrent use may lead to loss of control). Products include:
 Sudafed PE Nasal Decongestant 2048
 Children's Sudafed PE Nasal
  Decongestant 2047

Phenylephrine Tannate (Sympathomimetics tend to produce hyperglycemia and concurrent use may lead to loss of control).
 No products indexed under this heading.

Phenylpropanolamine Hydrochloride (Sympathomimetics tend to produce hyperglycemia and concurrent use may lead to loss of control).
 No products indexed under this heading.

Phenytoin (Phenytoin tends to produce hyperglycemia and concurrent use may lead to loss of control).
 No products indexed under this heading.

Phenytoin Sodium (Phenytoin tends to produce hyperglycemia and concurrent use may lead to loss of control). Products include:
 Phenytek Capsules 2380

Pindolol (May potentiate hypoglycemic action. Hypoglycemia may be difficult to recognize in patients taking β-blockers).
 No products indexed under this heading.

Pirbuterol Acetate (Sympathomimetics tend to produce hyperglycemia and concurrent use may lead to loss of control). Products include:
 Maxair Autohaler 1782

Piroxicam (May potentiate hypoglycemic action).
 No products indexed under this heading.

Polyestradiol Phosphate (Estrogens tend to produce hyperglycemia and concurrent use may lead to loss of control).
 No products indexed under this heading.

Polythiazide (Diuretics tend to produce hyperglycemia and concurrent use may lead to loss of control).
 No products indexed under this heading.

Prednisolone (Corticosteroids tend to produce hyperglycemia and concurrent use may lead to loss of control).
 No products indexed under this heading.

Prednisolone Acetate (Corticosteroids tend to produce hyperglycemia and concurrent use may lead to loss of control). Products include:
 Blephamide .... ⊙212, ⊙214
 Pred Forte .... ⊙225
 Pred Mild .... ⊙230
 Pred-G .... ⊙226, ⊙227

Prednisolone Sodium Phosphate (Corticosteroids tend to produce hyperglycemia and concurrent use may lead to loss of control).
 No products indexed under this heading.

Prednisolone Tebutate (Corticosteroids tend to produce hyperglycemia and concurrent use may lead to loss of control).
 No products indexed under this heading.

Prednisone (Corticosteroids tend to produce hyperglycemia and concurrent use may lead to loss of control).
 No products indexed under this heading.

Prednisone sodium phosphate (Corticosteroids tend to produce hyperglycemia and concurrent use may lead to loss of control).
 No products indexed under this heading.

Primidone (An inhibitor of CYP2C8 may decrease the AUC of rosiglitazone. Therefore, if an inducer of CYP2C8 is started or stopped during treatment with rosiglitazone, changes in diabetes treatment may be needed upon clinical response).
 No products indexed under this heading.

Probenecid (May potentiate hypoglycemic action).
 No products indexed under this heading.

Procarbazine Hydrochloride (May potentiate hypoglycemic action).
 No products indexed under this heading.

Prochlorperazine (Phenothiazines tend to produce hyperglycemia and concurrent use may lead to loss of control).
 No products indexed under this heading.

Prochlorperazine Edisylate (Phenothiazines tend to produce hyperglycemia and concurrent use may lead to loss of control).
 No products indexed under this heading.

Prochlorperazine Maleate (Phenothiazines tend to produce hyperglycemia and concurrent use may lead to loss of control).
 No products indexed under this heading.

Promethazine (Phenothiazines tend to produce hyperglycemia and concurrent use may lead to loss of control).
 No products indexed under this heading.

Promethazine Hydrochloride (Phenothiazines tend to produce hyperglycemia and concurrent use may lead to loss of control).
 No products indexed under this heading.

(⊙ Described in PDR® for Ophthalmic Medicines)

Propranolol Hydrochloride (Co-administration of propranolol (40 mg tid) and glimiperideincreases C_{max}, AUC, and $T_{1/2}$ of glimepiride by 23%, 22%, and 15%, respectively, and it decreased CL/F by 18%; no evidence of clinically significant adverse interactions). Products include:
InnoPran XL 1517

Pseudoephedrine Hydrochloride (Sympathomimetics tend to produce hyperglycemia and concurrent use may lead to loss of control). Products include:
Allegra-D 2915
Allegra-D 24 2918
Sudafed 12 Hour Nasal
Decongestant Non-Drowsy 2048
Sudafed 24 Hour 2048
Sudafed Nasal Decongestant 2047
Children's Sudafed Nasal
Decongestant Liquid 2047
Zyrtec-D Allergy & Congestion 2054

Pseudoephedrine Sulfate (Sympathomimetics tend to produce hyperglycemia and concurrent use may lead to loss of control). Products include:
Clarinex-D 12-Hour 3101
Clarinex-D 3104

Quercetin (An inhibitor of CYP2C8 may decrease the AUC of rosiglitazone. Therefore, if an inducer of CYP2C8 is started or stopped during treatment with rosiglitazone, changes in diabetes treatment may be needed upon clinical response).
No products indexed under this heading.

Quinestrol (Estrogens tend to produce hyperglycemia and concurrent use may lead to loss of control).
No products indexed under this heading.

Rasagiline Mesylate (May potentiate hypoglycemic action). Products include:
Azilect 3383

Rifabutin (An inhibitor of CYP2C8 may decrease the AUC of rosiglitazone. Therefore, if an inducer of CYP2C8 is started or stopped during treatment with rosiglitazone, changes in diabetes treatment may be needed upon clinical response).
No products indexed under this heading.

Rifampin (Rifampin administration (600 mg qd), an inducer of CYP2C8, for 6 days is reported to decrease rosiglitazone AUC by 66%, compared to the administration of rosiglitazone (8 mg) alone).
No products indexed under this heading.

Rofecoxib (May potentiate hypoglycemic action).
No products indexed under this heading.

Salmeterol Xinafoate (Sympathomimetics tend to produce hyperglycemia and concurrent use may lead to loss of control). Products include:
Advair 100/50 1275
Advair 250/50 1275
Advair 500/50 1275
Advair HFA 45/21 1288
Advair HFA 115/21 1288
Advair HFA 230/21 1288
Serevent Diskus 1656

Salsalate (May potentiate hypoglycemic action; clinical trials data indicate no evidence of significant adverse interaction with concurrent use).
No products indexed under this heading.

Selegiline (May potentiate hypoglycemic action). Products include:
Emsam 3623

Selegiline Hydrochloride (May potentiate hypoglycemic action). Products include:
Eldepryl 3312

Sotalol Hydrochloride (May potentiate hypoglycemic action. Hypoglycemia may be difficult to recognize in patients taking β-blockers).
No products indexed under this heading.

Spironolactone (Diuretics tend to produce hyperglycemia and concurrent use may lead to loss of control).
No products indexed under this heading.

Sulfacytine (May potentiate hypoglycemic action).
No products indexed under this heading.

Sulfamethizole (May potentiate hypoglycemic action).
No products indexed under this heading.

Sulfamethoxazole (May potentiate hypoglycemic action).
No products indexed under this heading.

Sulfaphenazole (An inhibitor of CYP2C8 may decrease the AUC of rosiglitazone. Therefore, if an inducer of CYP2C8 is started or stopped during treatment with rosiglitazone, changes in diabetes treatment may be needed upon clinical response).
No products indexed under this heading.

Sulfasalazine (May potentiate hypoglycemic action).
No products indexed under this heading.

Sulfinpyrazone (May potentiate hypoglycemic action).
No products indexed under this heading.

Sulfisoxazole Acetyl (May potentiate hypoglycemic action).
No products indexed under this heading.

Sulfisoxazole Diolamine (May potentiate hypoglycemic action).
No products indexed under this heading.

Sulindac (May potentiate hypoglycemic action). Products include:
Clinoril 2098

Terbutaline Sulfate (Sympathomimetics tend to produce hyperglycemia and concurrent use may lead to loss of control).
No products indexed under this heading.

Thioridazine (Phenothiazines tend to produce hyperglycemia and concurrent use may lead to loss of control).
No products indexed under this heading.

Thioridazine Hydrochloride (Phenothiazines tend to produce hyperglycemia and concurrent use may lead to loss of control). Products include:
Thioridazine Hydrochloride 2384

Thyroglobulin (Thyroid products tend to produce hyperglycemia and concurrent use may lead to loss of control).
No products indexed under this heading.

Thyroid (Thyroid products tend to produce hyperglycemia and concurrent use may lead to loss of control). Products include:
Naturethroid 2830

Thyroxine (Thyroid products tend to produce hyperglycemia and concurrent use may lead to loss of control).
No products indexed under this heading.

Thyroxine Sodium (Thyroid products tend to produce hyperglycemia and concurrent use may lead to loss of control).
No products indexed under this heading.

Timolol Hemihydrate (May potentiate hypoglycemic action. Hypoglycemia may be difficult to recognize in patients taking β-blockers). Products include:
Betimol 3490

Timolol Maleate (May potentiate hypoglycemic action. Hypoglycemia may be difficult to recognize in patients taking β-blockers). Products include:
Combigan 601
Dorzolamide
Hydrochloride/Timolol Maleate
Ophthalmic Solution .... ⊙243
Timoptic in Ocudose .... ⊙231

Tolazamide (May potentiate hypoglycemic action).
No products indexed under this heading.

Tolbutamide (May potentiate hypoglycemic action).
No products indexed under this heading.

Tolmetin Sodium (May potentiate hypoglycemic action).
No products indexed under this heading.

Torsemide (Diuretics tend to produce hyperglycemia and concurrent use may lead to loss of control).
No products indexed under this heading.

Tranylcypromine Sulfate (May potentiate hypoglycemic action). Products include:
Parnate 1584

Triamcinolone (Corticosteroids tend to produce hyperglycemia and concurrent use may lead to loss of control).
No products indexed under this heading.

Triamcinolone Acetonide (Corticosteroids tend to produce hyperglycemia and concurrent use may lead to loss of control). Products include:
Azmacort 408
Nasacort AQ 3019

Triamcinolone Diacetate (Corticosteroids tend to produce hyperglycemia and concurrent use may lead to loss of control).
No products indexed under this heading.

Triamcinolone Hexacetonide (Corticosteroids tend to produce hyperglycemia and concurrent use may lead to loss of control).
No products indexed under this heading.

Triamterene (Diuretics tend to produce hyperglycemia and concurrent use may lead to loss of control). Products include:
Dyazide 1429
Dyrenium 3495

Trifluoperazine Hydrochloride (Phenothiazines tend to produce hyperglycemia and concurrent use may lead to loss of control).
No products indexed under this heading.

Trimethoprim (An inhibitor of CYP2C8 may decrease the AUC of rosiglitazone. Therefore, if an inducer of CYP2C8 is started or stopped during treatment with rosiglitazone, changes in diabetes treatment may be needed upon clinical response).
No products indexed under this heading.

Trimethoprim Hydrochloride (An inhibitor of CYP2C8 may decrease the AUC of rosiglitazone. Therefore, if an inducer of CYP2C8 is started or stopped during treatment with rosiglitazone, changes in diabetes treatment may be needed upon clinical response).
No products indexed under this heading.

Trimethoprim Sulfate (An inhibitor of CYP2C8 may decrease the AUC of rosiglitazone. Therefore, if an inducer of CYP2C8 is started or stopped during treatment with rosiglitazone, changes in diabetes treatment may be needed upon clinical response).
No products indexed under this heading.

Valdecoxib (May potentiate hypoglycemic action).
No products indexed under this heading.

Warfarin Sodium (May potentiate hypoglycemic action).
No products indexed under this heading.

AVANDIA TABLETS
(Rosiglitazone Maleate) 1366
May interact with cytochrome p450 2c8 inducers (selected), cytochrome p450 2c8 inhibitors (selected), insulin, nitrates and nitrites, oral hypoglycemic agents, and certain other agents. Compounds in these categories include:

Acarbose (Patients receiving rosiglitazone in combination with other hypoglycemic agents may be at risk for hypoglycemic, and a reduction in the dose of the concomitant agent may be necessary).
No products indexed under this heading.

Amyl Nitrite (The use of rosiglitazone with nitrates is not recommended).
No products indexed under this heading.

Anastrozole (An inhibitor of CYP2C8 may increase the AUC of rosiglitazone. Therefore, if an inhibitor of CYP2C8 is started or stopped during treatment with rosiglitazone, changes in diabetes treatment may be needed based on clinical response).
No products indexed under this heading.

Carbamazepine (An inducer of CYP2C8 may decrease the AUC of rosiglitazone. Therefore, if an inducer of CYP2C8 is started or stopped during treatment with rosiglitazone, changes in diabetes treatment may be needed based on clinical response). Products include:
Carbatrol 3280
Equetro 3477

Chlorpropamide (Patients receiving rosiglitazone in combination with other hypoglycemic agents may be at risk for hypoglycemic, and a reduction in the dose of the concomitant agent may be necessary).
No products indexed under this heading.

Cimetidine (An inhibitor of CYP2C8 may increase the AUC of rosiglitazone. Therefore, if an inhibitor of CYP2C8 is started or stopped during treatment with rosiglitazone, changes in diabetes treatment may be needed based on clinical response).
No products indexed under this heading.

Cimetidine Hydrochloride (An inhibitor of CYP2C8 may increase the AUC of rosiglitazone. Therefore, if an inhibitor of CYP2C8 is started or stopped during treatment with rosiglitazone, changes in diabetes treatment may be needed based on clinical response).
No products indexed under this heading.

Erythrityl Tetranitrate (The use of rosiglitazone with nitrates is not recommended).
No products indexed under this heading.

Gemfibrozil (Concomitant administration of gemfibrozil (600 mg twice daily), an inhibitor of CYP2C8, and rosiglitazone (4 mg once daily) for 7 days increased rosiglitazone AUC by 127%, compared to the administration of rosiglitazone (4 mg once daily) alone. Given the potential for dose-related adverse events with rosiglitazone, a decrease in the dose of rosiglitazone may be needed when gemfibrozil is introduced).
No products indexed under this heading.

Glibenclamide (Patients receiving rosiglitazone in combination with other hypoglycemic agents may be at risk for hypoglycemic, and a reduction in the dose of the concomitant agent may be necessary).
No products indexed under this heading.

Glimepiride (Patients receiving rosiglitazone in combination with other hypoglycemic agents may be at risk for hypoglycemic, and a reduction in the dose of the concomitant agent may be necessary). Products include:
Avandaryl 1356
Duetact 3354

Glipizide (Patients receiving rosiglitazone in combination with other hypoglycemic agents may be at risk for hypoglycemic, and a reduction in the dose of the concomitant agent may be necessary).
No products indexed under this heading.

Glyburide (Rosiglitazone (2 mg twice daily) taken concomitantly with glyburide (3.75 to 10 mg/day) for 7 days did not alter the mean steady-state 24-hour plasma glucose concentrations in diabetic patients stabilized on glyburide therapy. Repeat doses of rosiglitazone (8 mg once daily) for 8 days in

healthy adult Caucasian subjects caused a decrease in glyburide AUC and C_{max} of approximately 30%. In Japanese subjects, glyburide AUC and C_{max} slightly increased following co-administration of rosiglitazone).

No products indexed under this heading.

Glyceryl Trinitrate (The use of rosiglitazone with nitrates is not recommended).

No products indexed under this heading.

Insulin (In studies in which rosiglitazone was added to insulin, rosiglitazone increased the risk of congestive heart failure and myocardial ischemia. Co-administration of rosiglitazone and insulin is not recommended).

No products indexed under this heading.

Insulin, Human, Zinc Suspension (In studies in which rosiglitazone was added to insulin, rosiglitazone increased the risk of congestive heart failure and myocardial ischemia. Co-administration of rosiglitazone and insulin is not recommended).

No products indexed under this heading.

Insulin, Human (rDNA origin) (In studies in which rosiglitazone was added to insulin, rosiglitazone increased the risk of congestive heart failure and myocardial ischemia. Co-administration of rosiglitazone and insulin is not recommended). Products include:

Insulin, Human NPH (In studies in which rosiglitazone was added to insulin, rosiglitazone increased the risk of congestive heart failure and myocardial ischemia. Co-administration of rosiglitazone and insulin is not recommended). Products include:

Insulin, Human Regular (In studies in which rosiglitazone was added to insulin, rosiglitazone increased the risk of congestive heart failure and myocardial ischemia. Co-administration of rosiglitazone and insulin is not recommended). Products include:

Insulin, Human Regular and Human NPH Mixture (In studies in which rosiglitazone was added to insulin, rosiglitazone increased the risk of congestive heart failure and myocardial ischemia. Co-administration of rosiglitazone and insulin is not recommended). Products include:

Insulin, NPH (In studies in which rosiglitazone was added to insulin, rosiglitazone increased the risk of congestive heart failure and myocardial ischemia. Co-administration of rosiglitazone and insulin is not recommended).

No products indexed under this heading.

Insulin, Regular (In studies in which rosiglitazone was added to insulin, rosiglitazone increased the risk of congestive heart failure and myocardial ischemia. Co-administration of rosiglitazone and insulin is not recommended).

No products indexed under this heading.

Insulin, Regular and NPH mixture (In studies in which rosiglitazone was added to insulin, rosiglitazone increased the risk of congestive heart failure and myocardial ischemia. Co-administration of rosiglitazone and insulin is not recommended).

No products indexed under this heading.

Insulin, Zinc Crystals (In studies in which rosiglitazone was added to insulin, rosiglitazone increased the risk of congestive heart failure and myocardial ischemia. Co-administration of rosiglitazone and insulin is not recommended).

No products indexed under this heading.

Insulin, Zinc Suspension (In studies in which rosiglitazone was added to insulin, rosiglitazone increased the risk of congestive heart failure and myocardial ischemia. Co-administration of rosiglitazone and insulin is not recommended).

No products indexed under this heading.

Insulin Aspart (In studies in which rosiglitazone was added to insulin, rosiglitazone increased the risk of congestive heart failure and myocardial ischemia. Co-administration of rosiglitazone and insulin is not recommended).

No products indexed under this heading.

Insulin Aspart, Human (In studies in which rosiglitazone was added to insulin, rosiglitazone increased the risk of congestive heart failure and myocardial ischemia. Co-administration of rosiglitazone and insulin is not recommended). Products include:

Insulin Aspart, Human Regular (In studies in which rosiglitazone was added to insulin, rosiglitazone increased the risk of congestive heart failure and myocardial ischemia. Co-administration of rosiglitazone and insulin is not recommended). Products include:

Insulin Aspart Protamine, Human (In studies in which rosiglitazone was added to insulin, rosiglitazone increased the risk of congestive heart failure and myocardial ischemia. Co-administration of rosiglitazone and insulin is not recommended). Products include:

Insulin Detemir (rDNA Origin) (In studies in which rosiglitazone was added to insulin, rosiglitazone increased the risk of congestive heart failure and myocardial ischemia. Co-administration of rosiglitazone and insulin is not recommended). Products include:

Insulin Glargine (In studies in which rosiglitazone was added to insulin, rosiglitazone increased the risk of congestive heart failure and myocardial ischemia. Co-administration of rosiglitazone and insulin is not recommended). Products include:

Insulin Glulisine (In studies in which rosiglitazone was added to insulin, rosiglitazone increased the risk of congestive heart failure and myocardial ischemia. Co-administration of rosiglitazone and insulin is not recommended). Products include:

Insulin Lispro, Human (In studies in which rosiglitazone was added to insulin, rosiglitazone increased the risk of congestive heart failure and myocardial ischemia. Co-administration of rosiglitazone and insulin is not recommended). Products include:

Insulin Lispro Protamine, Human (In studies in which rosiglitazone was added to insulin, rosiglitazone increased the risk of congestive heart failure and myocardial ischemia. Co-administration of rosiglitazone and insulin is not recommended). Products include:

Isosorbide Dinitrate (The use of rosiglitazone with nitrates is not recommended).

No products indexed under this heading.

Isosorbide Mononitrate (The use of rosiglitazone with nitrates is not recommended).

No products indexed under this heading.

Metformin Hydrochloride (Patients receiving rosiglitazone in combination with other hypoglycemic agents may be at risk for hypoglycemic, and a reduction in the dose of the concomitant agent may be necessary). Products include:

Miglitol (Patients receiving rosiglitazone in combination with other hypoglycemic agents may be at risk for hypoglycemic, and a reduction in the dose of the concomitant agent may be necessary).

No products indexed under this heading.

Nateglinide (Patients receiving rosiglitazone in combination with other hypoglycemic agents may be at risk for hypoglycemic, and a reduction in the dose of the concomitant agent may be necessary).

No products indexed under this heading.

Nicardipine (An inhibitor of CYP2C8 may increase the AUC of rosiglitazone. Therefore, if an inhibitor of CYP2C8 is started or stopped during treatment with rosiglitazone, changes in diabetes treatment may be needed based on clinical response).

No products indexed under this heading.

Nicardipine Hydrochloride (An inhibitor of CYP2C8 may increase the AUC of rosiglitazone. Therefore, if an inhibitor of CYP2C8 is started or stopped during treatment with rosiglitazone, changes in diabetes treatment may be needed based on clinical response).

No products indexed under this heading.

Nitrate & Nitrite Preparations (The use of rosiglitazone with nitrates is not recommended).

No products indexed under this heading.

Nitrates, organic (The use of rosiglitazone with nitrates is not recommended).

No products indexed under this heading.

Nitrates and Nitrites (The use of rosiglitazone with nitrates is not recommended).

No products indexed under this heading.

Nitroglycerin (The use of rosiglitazone with nitrates is not recommended). Products include:

Nitroglycerin, long-acting formulations (The use of rosiglitazone with nitrates is not recommended).

No products indexed under this heading.

Nitroglycerin Intravenous (The use of rosiglitazone with nitrates is not recommended).

No products indexed under this heading.

Omeprazole (An inhibitor of CYP2C8 may increase the AUC of rosiglitazone. Therefore, if an inhibitor of CYP2C8 is started or stopped during treatment with rosiglitazone, changes in diabetes treatment may be needed based on clinical response).

No products indexed under this heading.

Pentaerythritol Tetranitrate (The use of rosiglitazone with nitrates is not recommended).

No products indexed under this heading.

Phenobarbital (An inducer of CYP2C8 may decrease the AUC of rosiglitazone. Therefore, if an inducer of CYP2C8 is started or stopped during treatment with rosiglitazone, changes in diabetes treatment may be needed based on clinical response). Products include:

Phenobarbital Sodium (An inducer of CYP2C8 may decrease the AUC of rosiglitazone. Therefore, if an inducer of CYP2C8 is started or stopped during treatment with rosiglitazone, changes in diabetes treatment may be needed based on clinical response).

No products indexed under this heading.

Pioglitazone Hydrochloride (Patients receiving rosiglitazone in combination with other hypoglycemic agents may be at risk for hypoglycemic, and a reduction in the dose of the concomitant agent may be necessary). Products include:

Primidone (An inducer of CYP2C8 may decrease the AUC of rosiglitazone. Therefore, if an inducer of CYP2C8 is started or stopped during treatment with rosiglitazone, changes in diabetes treatment may be needed based on clinical response).

No products indexed under this heading.

Quercetin (An inhibitor of CYP2C8 may increase the AUC of rosiglitazone. Therefore, if an inhibitor of CYP2C8 is started or stopped during treatment with rosiglitazone, changes in diabetes treatment may be needed based on clinical response).

No products indexed under this heading.

Repaglinide (Patients receiving rosiglitazone in combination with other hypoglycemic agents may be at risk for hypoglycemic, and a reduction in the dose of the concomitant agent may be necessary).

No products indexed under this heading.

Rifabutin (An inducer of CYP2C8 may decrease the AUC of rosiglitazone. Therefore, if an inducer of CYP2C8 is started or stopped during treatment with rosiglitazone, changes in diabetes treatment may be needed based on clinical response).

No products indexed under this heading.

Rifampin (Rifampin administration (600 mg once a day), an inducer of CYP2C8, for 6 days is reported to decrease rosiglitazone AUC by 66%, compared to the administration of rosiglitazone (8 mg) alone).

No products indexed under this heading.

Sitagliptin Phosphate (Patients receiving rosiglitazone in combination with other hypoglycemic agents may be at risk for hypoglycemic, and a reduction in the dose of the concomitant agent may be necessary). Products include:

Sulfaphenazole (An inhibitor of CYP2C8 may increase the AUC of rosiglitazone. Therefore, if an inhibitor of CYP2C8 is started or stopped during treatment with rosiglitazone, changes in diabetes treatment may be needed based on clinical response).

No products indexed under this heading.

Sulfinpyrazone (An inhibitor of CYP2C8 may increase the AUC of rosiglitazone. Therefore, if an inhibitor of CYP2C8 is started or stopped during treatment with rosiglitazone, changes in diabetes treatment may be needed based on clinical response).

No products indexed under this heading.

Tolazamide (Patients receiving rosiglitazone in combination with other hypoglycemic agents may be at risk for hypoglycemic, and a reduction in the dose of the concomitant agent may be necessary).

No products indexed under this heading.

Tolbutamide (Patients receiving rosiglitazone in combination with other hypoglycemic agents may be at risk for hypoglycemic, and a reduction in the dose of the concomitant agent may be necessary).

No products indexed under this heading.

Trimethoprim (An inhibitor of CYP2C8 may increase the AUC of rosiglitazone. Therefore, if an inhibitor of CYP2C8 is started or stopped during treatment with rosiglitazone, changes in diabetes treatment may be needed based on clinical response).

No products indexed under this heading.

Trimethoprim Hydrochloride (An inhibitor of CYP2C8 may increase the AUC of rosiglitazone. Therefore, if an inhibitor of CYP2C8 is started or stopped during treatment with rosiglitazone, changes in diabetes treatment may be needed based on clinical response).

No products indexed under this heading.

Trimethoprim Sulfate (An inhibitor of CYP2C8 may increase the AUC of rosiglitazone. Therefore, if an inhibitor of CYP2C8 is started or stopped during treatment with rosiglitazone, changes in diabetes treatment may be needed based on clinical response).

No products indexed under this heading.

Troglitazone (Patients receiving rosiglitazone in combination with other hypoglycemic agents may be at risk for hypoglycemic, and a reduction in the dose of the concomitant agent may be necessary).

No products indexed under this heading.

AVAPRO TABLETS

(Irbesartan) 2962
None cited in PDR database.

AVASTIN IV

(Bevacizumab) 1187

Carboplatin (In a clinical study, based on limited data, there did not appear to be a difference in the mean exposure of either carboplatin or paclitaxel when each was administered alone or in combination with bevacizumab. However, 3 of the 8 patients receiving bevacizumab plus paclitaxel/carboplatin had substantially lower paclitaxel exposure after four cycles of treatment (at Day 63) than those at Day 0, while patients receiving paclitaxel/carboplatin without bevacizumab had a greater paclitaxel exposure at Day 63 than at Day 0).

No products indexed under this heading.

Paclitaxel (In a clinical study, based on limited data, there did not appear to be a difference in the mean exposure of either carboplatin or paclitaxel when each was administered alone or in combination with bevacizumab. However, 3 of the 8 patients receiving bevacizumab plus paclitaxel/carboplatin had substantially lower paclitaxel exposure after four cycles of treatment (at Day 63) than those at Day 0, while patients receiving paclitaxel/carboplatin without bevacizumab had a greater paclitaxel exposure at Day 63 than at Day 0).

No products indexed under this heading.

Paclitaxel, protein-bound (In a clinical study, based on limited data, there did not appear to be a difference in the mean exposure of either carboplatin or paclitaxel when each was administered alone or in combination with bevacizumab. However, 3 of the 8 patients receiving bevacizumab plus paclitaxel/carboplatin had substantially lower paclitaxel exposure after four cycles of treatment (at Day 63) than those at Day 0, while patients receiving paclitaxel/carboplatin without bevacizumab had a greater paclitaxel exposure at Day 63 than at Day 0).

No products indexed under this heading.

AVELOX I.V.

(Moxifloxacin Hydrochloride) 3064
See Avelox Tablets

AVELOX TABLETS

(Moxifloxacin Hydrochloride) 3064
May interact with antacids, antacids containing aluminum, calcium and magnesium, antipsychotic agents, cations, class 1A antiarrhythmics, class III antiarrhythmics, corticosteroids, erythromycin, iron containing oral preparations, iron salts, magnesium-containing antacids, non-steroidal anti-inflammatory agents, oral anticoagulants, quinidine, tricyclic antidepressants, zincs, and certain other agents. Compounds in these categories include:

Alclometasone Dipropionate (The risk of developing fluoroquinolone-associated tendinitis and tendon rupture is further increased in older patients usually over 60 years of age, in patients taking corticosteroid drugs, and in patients with kidney, heart or lung transplants).

No products indexed under this heading.

Aluminum Acetate (When moxifloxacin (single 400 mg tablet dose) was administered two hours before, concomitantly, or 4 hours after an aluminum/magnesium-containing antacid (900 mg aluminum hydroxide and 600 mg magnesium hydroxide as a single oral dose) to 12 healthy volunteers there, was a 26%, 60% and 23% reduction in the mean AUC of moxifloxacin, respectively. Moxifloxacin should be taken at least 4 hours before or 8 hours after metal cations).

No products indexed under this heading.

Aluminum Carbonate (When moxifloxacin (single 400 mg tablet dose) was administered two hours before, concomitantly, or 4 hours after an aluminum/magnesium-containing antacid (900 mg aluminum hydroxide and 600 mg magnesium hydroxide as a single oral dose) to 12 healthy volunteers, there was a 26%, 60%, and 23% reduction in the mean AUC of moxifloxacin, respectively. Moxifloxacin should be taken at least 4 hours before or 8 hours after antacids containing magnesium or aluminum).

No products indexed under this heading.

Aluminum Chlorhydroxide (When moxifloxacin (single 400 mg tablet dose) was administered two hours before, concomitantly, or 4 hours after an aluminum/magnesium-containing antacid (900 mg aluminum hydroxide and 600 mg magnesium hydroxide as a single oral dose) to 12 healthy volunteers there, was a 26%, 60% and 23% reduction in the mean AUC of moxifloxacin, respectively. Moxifloxacin should be taken at least 4 hours before or 8 hours after metal cations).

No products indexed under this heading.

Aluminum Chloride (When moxifloxacin (single 400 mg tablet dose) was administered two hours before, concomitantly, or 4 hours after an aluminum/magnesium-containing antacid (900 mg aluminum hydroxide and 600 mg magnesium hydroxide as a single oral dose) to 12 healthy volunteers there, was a 26%, 60% and 23% reduction in the mean AUC of moxifloxacin, respectively. Moxifloxacin should be taken at least 4 hours before or 8 hours after metal cations).

No products indexed under this heading.

Aluminum Chlorohydrate (When moxifloxacin (single 400 mg tablet dose) was administered two hours before, concomitantly, or 4 hours after an aluminum/magnesium-containing antacid (900 mg aluminum hydroxide and 600 mg magnesium hydroxide as a single oral dose) to 12 healthy volunteers there, was a 26%, 60% and 23%

reduction in the mean AUC of moxifloxacin, respectively. Moxifloxacin should be taken at least 4 hours before or 8 hours after metal cations).

No products indexed under this heading.

Aluminum Glycinate (When moxifloxacin (single 400 mg tablet dose) was administered two hours before, concomitantly, or 4 hours after an aluminum/magnesium-containing antacid (900 mg aluminum hydroxide and 600 mg magnesium hydroxide as a single oral dose) to 12 healthy volunteers there, was a 26%, 60% and 23% reduction in the mean AUC of moxifloxacin, respectively. Moxifloxacin should be taken at least 4 hours before or 8 hours after metal cations).

No products indexed under this heading.

Aluminum Hydroxide (When moxifloxacin (single 400 mg tablet dose) was administered two hours before, concomitantly, or 4 hours after an aluminum/magnesium-containing antacid (900 mg aluminum hydroxide and 600 mg magnesium hydroxide as a single oral dose) to 12 healthy volunteers, there was a 26%, 60%, and 23% reduction in the mean AUC of moxifloxacin, respectively. Moxifloxacin should be taken at least 4 hours before or 8 hours after antacids containing magnesium or aluminum).

No products indexed under this heading.

Aluminum Hydroxide Preparations (When moxifloxacin (single 400 mg tablet dose) was administered two hours before, concomitantly, or 4 hours after an aluminum/magnesium-containing antacid (900 mg aluminum hydroxide and 600 mg magnesium hydroxide as a single oral dose) to 12 healthy volunteers there, was a 26%, 60% and 23% reduction in the mean AUC of moxifloxacin, respectively. Moxifloxacin should be taken at least 4 hours before or 8 hours after metal cations).

No products indexed under this heading.

Aluminum Sulfate (When moxifloxacin (single 400 mg tablet dose) was administered two hours before, concomitantly, or 4 hours after an aluminum/magnesium-containing antacid (900 mg aluminum hydroxide and 600 mg magnesium hydroxide as a single oral dose) to 12 healthy volunteers there, was a 26%, 60% and 23% reduction in the mean AUC of moxifloxacin, respectively. Moxifloxacin should be taken at least 4 hours before or 8 hours after metal cations).

No products indexed under this heading.

Amiodarone Hydrochloride (Moxifloxacin has been shown to prolong the QT interval of the electrocardiogram in some patients. The drug should be avoided in patients receiving Class III antiarrhythmic agents, such as amiodarone, due to the lack of clinical experience with the drug in this patient population).

No products indexed under this heading.

Amitriptyline Hydrochloride (Moxifloxacin has been shown to prolong the QT interval of the electrocardiogram in some patients. Pharmacokinetic studies between moxifloxacin and other drugs that prolong the QT interval, such as tricyclic antidepressants, have not been performed. An additive effect of moxifloxacin and tricyclic antidepressants cannot be excluded, therefore, caution should be exercised when moxifloxacin is given concurrently with tricyclic antidepressants).

No products indexed under this heading.

Amoxapine (Moxifloxacin has been shown to prolong the QT interval of the electrocardiogram in some patients. Pharmacokinetic studies between moxifloxacin and other drugs that prolong

the QT interval, such as tricyclic antidepressants, have not been performed. An additive effect of moxifloxacin and tricyclic antidepressants cannot be excluded, therefore, caution should be exercised when moxifloxacin is given concurrently with tricyclic antidepressants).

No products indexed under this heading.

Anisindione (Quinolones, including moxifloxacin, have been reported to enhance the anticoagulant effects of warfarin or its derivatives in the patient population. In addition, infectious disease and its accompanying inflammatory process, age, and general status of the patient are risk factors for increased anticoagulant activity. Therefore, the prothrombin time, International Normalized Ratio (INR), or other suitable anticoagulation tests should be closely monitored if a quinolone is administered concomitantly with warfarin or its derivatives).

No products indexed under this heading.

Aripiprazole (Moxifloxacin has been shown to prolong the QT interval of the electrocardiogram in some patients. Pharmacokinetic studies between moxifloxacin and other drugs that prolong the QT interval, such as antipsychotics, has not been performed. An additive effect of moxifloxacin and antipsychotic phenthiazines cannot be excluded, therefore, caution should be exercised when moxifloxacin is given concurrently with antipsychotics).

No products indexed under this heading.

Atenolol (In a crossover study involving 24 healthy volunteers (12 male; 12 female), the mean atenolol AUC following a single oral dose of 50 mg atenolol with placebo was similar to that observed when atenolol was given concomitantly with a single 400 mg oral dose of moxifloxacin. The mean C_{max} of single dose atenolol decreased by about 10% following co-administration with a single dose of moxifloxacin).

No products indexed under this heading.

Beclomethasone Dipropionate (The risk of developing fluoroquinolone-associated tendinitis and tendon rupture is further increased in older patients usually over 60 years of age, in patients taking corticosteroid drugs, and in patients with kidney, heart or lung transplants). Products include:
Qvar 3398

Beclomethasone Dipropionate Monohydrate (The risk of developing fluoroquinolone-associated tendinitis and tendon rupture is further increased in older patients usually over 60 years of age, in patients taking corticosteroid drugs, and in patients with kidney, heart or lung transplants). Products include:
Beconase AQ 1386

Betamethasone (The risk of developing fluoroquinolone-associated tendinitis and tendon rupture is further increased in older patients usually over 60 years of age, in patients taking corticosteroid drugs, and in patients with kidney, heart or lung transplants).

No products indexed under this heading.

Betamethasone Acetate (The risk of developing fluoroquinolone-associated tendinitis and tendon rupture is further increased in older patients usually over 60 years of age, in patients taking corticosteroid drugs, and in patients with kidney, heart or lung transplants).

No products indexed under this heading.

IMPORTANT NOTE: Always consult each drug listing in the patient's regimen for possible interactions.

Avelox Interactions Index 192

Betamethasone Benzoate (The risk of developing fluoroquinolone-associated tendinitis and tendon rupture is further increased in older patients usually over 60 years of age, in patients taking corticosteroid drugs, and in patients with kidney, heart or lung transplants).
No products indexed under this heading.

Betamethasone Dipropionate (The risk of developing fluoroquinolone-associated tendinitis and tendon rupture is further increased in older patients usually over 60 years of age, in patients taking corticosteroid drugs, and in patients with kidney, heart or lung transplants). Products include:
Diprolene Lotion 0.05% 3108
Diprolene Ointment 0.05% 3109
Diprolene AF Cream 0.05% 3107
Lotrisone 3163

Betamethasone Sodium Phosphate (The risk of developing fluoroquinolone-associated tendinitis and tendon rupture is further increased in older patients usually over 60 years of age, in patients taking corticosteroid drugs, and in patients with kidney, heart or lung transplants).
No products indexed under this heading.

Betamethasone Valerate (The risk of developing fluoroquinolone-associated tendinitis and tendon rupture is further increased in older patients usually over 60 years of age, in patients taking corticosteroid drugs, and in patients with kidney, heart or lung transplants). Products include:
Luxiq 3321

Bretylium Tosylate (Moxifloxacin has been shown to prolong QT interval of the electrocardiogram in some patients. The drug should be avoided in patients receiving Class III antiarrhythmic agents, due to lack of clinical experience with the drug in these populations).
No products indexed under this heading.

Budesonide (The risk of developing fluoroquinolone-associated tendinitis and tendon rupture is further increased in older patients usually over 60 years of age, in patients taking corticosteroid drugs, and in patients with kidney, heart or lung transplants). Products include:
Pulmicort Flexhaler 714
Symbicort 80/4.5 720
Symbicort 160/4.5 720

Calcium (When moxifloxacin (single 400 mg tablet dose) was administered two hours before, concomitantly, or 4 hours after an aluminum/magnesium-containing antacid (900 mg aluminum hydroxide and 600 mg magnesium hydroxide as a single oral dose) to 12 healthy volunteers there, was a 26%, 60% and 23% reduction in the mean AUC of moxifloxacin, respectively. Moxifloxacin should be taken at least 4 hours before or 8 hours after metal cations). Products include:
BoneMate Plus 3454
Cardio Basics 3455
Chelated Mineral 3476
CitraNatal 90 DHA Capsules 2332
CitraNatal Harmony 2332

Calcium (Oyster Shell) (When moxifloxacin (single 400 mg tablet dose) was administered two hours before, concomitantly, or 4 hours after an aluminum/magnesium-containing antacid (900 mg aluminum hydroxide and 600 mg magnesium hydroxide as a single oral dose) to 12 healthy volunteers there, was a 26%, 60% and 23% reduction in the mean AUC of moxifloxacin, respectively. Moxifloxacin should be taken at least 4 hours before or 8 hours after metal cations).
No products indexed under this heading.

Calcium Acetate (When moxifloxacin (single 400 mg tablet dose) was administered two hours before, concomitantly, or 4 hours after an aluminum/magnesium-containing antacid (900 mg aluminum hydroxide and 600 mg magnesium hydroxide as a single oral dose) to 12 healthy volunteers there, was a 26%, 60% and 23% reduction in the mean AUC of moxifloxacin, respectively. Moxifloxacin should be taken at least 4 hours before or 8 hours after metal cations).
No products indexed under this heading.

Calcium Ascorbate (When moxifloxacin (single 400 mg tablet dose) was administered two hours before, concomitantly, or 4 hours after an aluminum/magnesium-containing antacid (900 mg aluminum hydroxide and 600 mg magnesium hydroxide as a single oral dose) to 12 healthy volunteers there, was a 26%, 60% and 23% reduction in the mean AUC of moxifloxacin, respectively. Moxifloxacin should be taken at least 4 hours before or 8 hours after metal cations). Products include:
Bio-C 3454
Procosa II 3476
Proflavanol 90 3476

Calcium Carbaspirin (When moxifloxacin (single 400 mg tablet dose) was administered two hours before, concomitantly, or 4 hours after an aluminum/magnesium-containing antacid (900 mg aluminum hydroxide and 600 mg magnesium hydroxide as a single oral dose) to 12 healthy volunteers there, was a 26%, 60% and 23% reduction in the mean AUC of moxifloxacin, respectively. Moxifloxacin should be taken at least 4 hours before or 8 hours after metal cations).
No products indexed under this heading.

Calcium Carbonate (When moxifloxacin (single 400 mg tablet dose) was administered two hours before, concomitantly, or 4 hours after an aluminum/magnesium-containing antacid (900 mg aluminum hydroxide and 600 mg magnesium hydroxide as a single oral dose) to 12 healthy volunteers, there was a 26%, 60%, and 23% reduction in the mean AUC of moxifloxacin, respectively. Moxifloxacin should be taken at least 4 hours before or 8 hours after antacids containing magnesium or aluminum). Products include:
Chelated Mineral 3476
Pepcid Complete 1822
Extra Strength Rolaids Softchews Vanilla Creme 2045

Calcium Carbonate, Precipitated (When moxifloxacin (single 400 mg tablet dose) was administered two hours before, concomitantly, or 4 hours after an aluminum/magnesium-containing antacid (900 mg aluminum hydroxide and 600 mg magnesium hydroxide as a single oral dose) to 12 healthy volunteers there, was a 26%, 60% and 23% reduction in the mean AUC of moxifloxacin, respectively. Moxifloxacin should be taken at least 4 hours before or 8 hours after metal cations).
No products indexed under this heading.

Calcium Caseinate (When moxifloxacin (single 400 mg tablet dose) was administered two hours before, concomitantly, or 4 hours after an aluminum/magnesium-containing antacid (900 mg aluminum hydroxide and 600 mg magnesium hydroxide as a single oral dose) to 12 healthy volunteers there, was a 26%, 60% and 23% reduction in the mean AUC of moxifloxacin, respectively. Moxifloxacin should be taken at least 4 hours before or 8 hours after metal cations).
No products indexed under this heading.

Calcium Chloride (When moxifloxacin (single 400 mg tablet dose) was administered two hours before, concomitantly, or 4 hours after an aluminum/magnesium-containing antacid (900 mg aluminum hydroxide and 600 mg magnesium hydroxide as a single oral dose) to 12 healthy volunteers there, was a 26%, 60% and 23% reduction in the mean AUC of moxifloxacin, respectively. Moxifloxacin should be taken at least 4 hours before or 8 hours after metal cations).
No products indexed under this heading.

Calcium Citrate (When moxifloxacin (single 400 mg tablet dose) was administered two hours before, concomitantly, or 4 hours after an aluminum/magnesium-containing antacid (900 mg aluminum hydroxide and 600 mg magnesium hydroxide as a single oral dose) to 12 healthy volunteers there, was a 26%, 60% and 23% reduction in the mean AUC of moxifloxacin, respectively. Moxifloxacin should be taken at least 4 hours before or 8 hours after metal cations). Products include:
Active Calcium 3476
Chelated Mineral 3476
CitraNatal 90 DHA Capsules 2332
CitraNatal Assure 2332
CitraNatal Harmony 2332
CitraNatal Rx 2332

Calcium Disodium Edetate (When moxifloxacin (single 400 mg tablet dose) was administered two hours before, concomitantly, or 4 hours after an aluminum/magnesium-containing antacid (900 mg aluminum hydroxide and 600 mg magnesium hydroxide as a single oral dose) to 12 healthy volunteers there, was a 26%, 60% and 23% reduction in the mean AUC of moxifloxacin, respectively. Moxifloxacin should be taken at least 4 hours before or 8 hours after metal cations).
No products indexed under this heading.

Calcium Glubionate (When moxifloxacin (single 400 mg tablet dose) was administered two hours before, concomitantly, or 4 hours after an aluminum/magnesium-containing antacid (900 mg aluminum hydroxide and 600 mg magnesium hydroxide as a single oral dose) to 12 healthy volunteers there, was a 26%, 60% and 23% reduction in the mean AUC of moxifloxacin, respectively. Moxifloxacin should be taken at least 4 hours before or 8 hours after metal cations).
No products indexed under this heading.

Calcium Gluconate (When moxifloxacin (single 400 mg tablet dose) was administered two hours before, concomitantly, or 4 hours after an aluminum/magnesium-containing antacid (900 mg aluminum hydroxide and 600 mg magnesium hydroxide as a single oral dose) to 12 healthy volunteers there, was a 26%, 60% and 23% reduction in the mean AUC of moxifloxacin, respectively. Moxifloxacin should be taken at least 4 hours before or 8 hours after metal cations).
No products indexed under this heading.

Calcium Glycerophosphate (When moxifloxacin (single 400 mg tablet dose) was administered two hours before, concomitantly, or 4 hours after an aluminum/magnesium-containing antacid (900 mg aluminum hydroxide and 600 mg magnesium hydroxide as a single oral dose) to 12 healthy volunteers there, was a 26%, 60% and 23% reduction in the mean AUC of moxifloxacin, respectively. Moxifloxacin should be taken at least 4 hours before or 8 hours after metal cations).
No products indexed under this heading.

Calcium Iodide (When moxifloxacin (single 400 mg tablet dose) was administered two hours before, concomitantly, or 4 hours after an aluminum/magnesium-containing antacid (900 mg aluminum hydroxide and 600 mg magnesium hydroxide as a single oral dose) to 12 healthy volunteers there, was a 26%, 60% and 23% reduction in the mean AUC of moxifloxacin, respectively. Moxifloxacin should be taken at least 4 hours before or 8 hours after metal cations).
No products indexed under this heading.

Calcium Lactate (When moxifloxacin (single 400 mg tablet dose) was administered two hours before, concomitantly, or 4 hours after an aluminum/magnesium-containing antacid (900 mg aluminum hydroxide and 600 mg magnesium hydroxide as a single oral dose) to 12 healthy volunteers there, was a 26%, 60% and 23% reduction in the mean AUC of moxifloxacin, respectively. Moxifloxacin should be taken at least 4 hours before or 8 hours after metal cations).
No products indexed under this heading.

Calcium Levulinate (When moxifloxacin (single 400 mg tablet dose) was administered two hours before, concomitantly, or 4 hours after an aluminum/magnesium-containing antacid (900 mg aluminum hydroxide and 600 mg magnesium hydroxide as a single oral dose) to 12 healthy volunteers there, was a 26%, 60% and 23% reduction in the mean AUC of moxifloxacin, respectively. Moxifloxacin should be taken at least 4 hours before or 8 hours after metal cations).
No products indexed under this heading.

Calcium Pantothenate (When moxifloxacin (single 400 mg tablet dose) was administered two hours before, concomitantly, or 4 hours after an aluminum/magnesium-containing antacid (900 mg aluminum hydroxide and 600 mg magnesium hydroxide as a single oral dose) to 12 healthy volunteers there, was a 26%, 60% and 23% reduction in the mean AUC of moxifloxacin, respectively. Moxifloxacin should be taken at least 4 hours before or 8 hours after metal cations). Products include:
Cardio Basics 3455

Calcium Phosphate (When moxifloxacin (single 400 mg tablet dose) was administered two hours before, concomitantly, or 4 hours after an aluminum/magnesium-containing antacid (900 mg aluminum hydroxide and 600 mg magnesium hydroxide as a single oral dose) to 12 healthy volunteers there, was a 26%, 60% and 23% reduction in the mean AUC of moxifloxacin, respectively. Moxifloxacin should be taken at least 4 hours before or 8 hours after metal cations).
No products indexed under this heading.

Calcium Phosphate, Dibasic (When moxifloxacin (single 400 mg tablet dose) was administered two hours before, concomitantly, or 4 hours after an aluminum/magnesium-containing antacid (900 mg aluminum hydroxide and 600 mg magnesium hydroxide as a single oral dose) to 12 healthy volunteers there, was a 26%, 60% and 23% reduction in the mean AUC of moxifloxacin, respectively. Moxifloxacin should be taken at least 4 hours before or 8 hours after metal cations).
No products indexed under this heading.

Calcium Phosphate, Tribasic (When moxifloxacin (single 400 mg tablet dose) was administered two hours before, concomitantly, or 4 hours after an aluminum/magnesium-containing antacid (900 mg aluminum hydroxide and 600 mg magnesium hydroxide as a single oral dose) to 12 healthy volunteers there, was a 26%, 60% and 23% reduction in the mean AUC of moxifloxacin, respectively. Moxifloxacin should be taken at least 4 hours before or 8 hours after metal cations).
No products indexed under this heading.

Calcium Phosphorus Preparations (When moxifloxacin (single 400 mg tablet dose) was administered two hours

before, concomitantly, or 4 hours after an aluminum/magnesium-containing antacid (900 mg aluminum hydroxide and 600 mg magnesium hydroxide as a single oral dose) to 12 healthy volunteers there, was a 26%, 60% and 23% reduction in the mean AUC of moxifloxacin, respectively. Moxifloxacin should be taken at least 4 hours before or 8 hours after metal cations).
No products indexed under this heading.

Calcium Polycarbophil (When moxifloxacin (single 400 mg tablet dose) was administered two hours before, concomitantly, or 4 hours after an aluminum/magnesium-containing antacid (900 mg aluminum hydroxide and 600 mg magnesium hydroxide as a single oral dose) to 12 healthy volunteers there, was a 26%, 60% and 23% reduction in the mean AUC of moxifloxacin, respectively. Moxifloxacin should be taken at least 4 hours before or 8 hours after metal cations).
No products indexed under this heading.

Calcium Salts (When moxifloxacin (single 400 mg tablet dose) was administered two hours before, concomitantly, or 4 hours after an aluminum/magnesium-containing antacid (900 mg aluminum hydroxide and 600 mg magnesium hydroxide as a single oral dose) to 12 healthy volunteers there, was a 26%, 60% and 23% reduction in the mean AUC of moxifloxacin, respectively. Moxifloxacin should be taken at least 4 hours before or 8 hours after metal cations).
No products indexed under this heading.

Calcium Sodium Alginate Fiber (When moxifloxacin (single 400 mg tablet dose) was administered two hours before, concomitantly, or 4 hours after an aluminum/magnesium-containing antacid (900 mg aluminum hydroxide and 600 mg magnesium hydroxide as a single oral dose) to 12 healthy volunteers there, was a 26%, 60% and 23% reduction in the mean AUC of moxifloxacin, respectively. Moxifloxacin should be taken at least 4 hours before or 8 hours after metal cations).
No products indexed under this heading.

Calcium Undecylenate (When moxifloxacin (single 400 mg tablet dose) was administered two hours before, concomitantly, or 4 hours after an aluminum/magnesium-containing antacid (900 mg aluminum hydroxide and 600 mg magnesium hydroxide as a single oral dose) to 12 healthy volunteers there, was a 26%, 60% and 23% reduction in the mean AUC of moxifloxacin, respectively. Moxifloxacin should be taken at least 4 hours before or 8 hours after metal cations).
No products indexed under this heading.

Celecoxib (Although not observed with moxifloxacin in preclinical and clinical trials, the concomitant administration of a nonsteriodal anti-inflammatory drug with a quinolone may increase the risks of CNS stimulation and convulsions). Products include:
Celebrex **3272**

Chlorpromazine (Moxifloxacin has been shown to prolong the QT interval of the electrocardiogram in some patients. Pharmacokinetic studies between moxifloxacin and other drugs that prolong the QT interval, such as antipsychotics, has not been performed. An additive effect of moxifloxacin and antipsychotic phenthiazines cannot be excluded, therefore, caution should be exercised when moxifloxacin is given concurrently with antipsychotics).
No products indexed under this heading.

Chlorpromazine Hydrochloride (Moxifloxacin has been shown to prolong the QT interval of the electrocardiogram in some patients. Pharmacokinetic studies between moxifloxacin and other drugs that prolong the QT interval, such as antipsychotics, has not been performed. An additive effect of moxifloxacin and antipsychotic phenthiazines cannot be excluded, therefore, caution should be exercised when moxifloxacin is given concurrently with antipsychotics).
No products indexed under this heading.

Chlorprothixene (Moxifloxacin has been shown to prolong the QT interval of the electrocardiogram in some patients. Pharmacokinetic studies between moxifloxacin and other drugs that prolong the QT interval, such as antipsychotics, has not been performed. An additive effect of moxifloxacin and antipsychotic phenthiazines cannot be excluded, therefore, caution should be exercised when moxifloxacin is given concurrently with antipsychotics).
No products indexed under this heading.

Chlorprothixene Hydrochloride (Moxifloxacin has been shown to prolong the QT interval of the electrocardiogram in some patients. Pharmacokinetic studies between moxifloxacin and other drugs that prolong the QT interval, such as antipsychotics, has not been performed. An additive effect of moxifloxacin and antipsychotic phenthiazines cannot be excluded, therefore, caution should be exercised when moxifloxacin is given concurrently with antipsychotics).
No products indexed under this heading.

Chlorprothixene Lactate (Moxifloxacin has been shown to prolong the QT interval of the electrocardiogram in some patients. Pharmacokinetic studies between moxifloxacin and other drugs that prolong the QT interval, such as antipsychotics, has not been performed. An additive effect of moxifloxacin and antipsychotic phenthiazines cannot be excluded, therefore, caution should be exercised when moxifloxacin is given concurrently with antipsychotics).
No products indexed under this heading.

Ciclesonide (The risk of developing fluoroquinolone-associated tendinitis and tendon rupture is further increased in older patients usually over 60 years of age, in patients taking corticosteroid drugs, and in patients with kidney, heart or lung transplants).
No products indexed under this heading.

Cisapride (Moxifloxacin has been shown to prolong the QT interval of the electrocardiogram in some patients. Pharmacokinetic studies between moxifloxacin and other drugs that prolong the QT interval, such as cisapride, has not been performed. An additive effect of moxifloxacin and cisapride cannot be excluded, therefore, caution should be exercised when moxifloxacin is given concurrently with cisapride).
No products indexed under this heading.

Clomipramine Hydrochloride (Moxifloxacin has been shown to prolong the QT interval of the electrocardiogram in some patients. Pharmacokinetic studies between moxifloxacin and other drugs that prolong the QT interval, such as tricyclic antidepressants, have not been performed. An additive effect of moxifloxacin and tricyclic antidepressants cannot be excluded, therefore, caution should be exercised when moxifloxacin is given concurrently with tricyclic antidepressants).
No products indexed under this heading.

Clozapine (Moxifloxacin has been shown to prolong the QT interval of the electrocardiogram in some patients. Pharmacokinetic studies between moxifloxacin and other drugs that prolong the QT interval, such as antipsychotics, has not been performed. An additive effect of moxifloxacin and antipsychotic phenthiazines cannot be excluded, therefore, caution should be exercised when moxifloxacin is given concurrently with antipsychotics).
No products indexed under this heading.

Cortisone Acetate (The risk of developing fluoroquinolone-associated tendinitis and tendon rupture is further increased in older patients usually over 60 years of age, in patients taking corticosteroid drugs, and in patients with kidney, heart or lung transplants).
No products indexed under this heading.

Desipramine Hydrochloride (Moxifloxacin has been shown to prolong the QT interval of the electrocardiogram in some patients. Pharmacokinetic studies between moxifloxacin and other drugs that prolong the QT interval, such as tricyclic antidepressants, have not been performed. An additive effect of moxifloxacin and tricyclic antidepressants cannot be excluded, therefore, caution should be exercised when moxifloxacin is given concurrently with tricyclic antidepressants).
No products indexed under this heading.

Desoximetasone (The risk of developing fluoroquinolone-associated tendinitis and tendon rupture is further increased in older patients usually over 60 years of age, in patients taking corticosteroid drugs, and in patients with kidney, heart or lung transplants).
No products indexed under this heading.

Dexamethasone (The risk of developing fluoroquinolone-associated tendinitis and tendon rupture is further increased in older patients usually over 60 years of age, in patients taking corticosteroid drugs, and in patients with kidney, heart or lung transplants). Products include:
Ciprodex **583**
Ozurdex .... ⊙ **223**
Tobramycin and Dexamethasone Ophthalmic Suspension .... ⊙ **251**

Dexamethasone Acetate (The risk of developing fluoroquinolone-associated tendinitis and tendon rupture is further increased in older patients usually over 60 years of age, in patients taking corticosteroid drugs, and in patients with kidney, heart or lung transplants).
No products indexed under this heading.

Dexamethasone Phosphate (The risk of developing fluoroquinolone-associated tendinitis and tendon rupture is further increased in older patients usually over 60 years of age, in patients taking corticosteroid drugs, and in patients with kidney, heart or lung transplants).
No products indexed under this heading.

Dexamethasone Sodium (The risk of developing fluoroquinolone-associated tendinitis and tendon rupture is further increased in older patients usually over 60 years of age, in patients taking corticosteroid drugs, and in patients with kidney, heart or lung transplants).
No products indexed under this heading.

Dexamethasone Sodium Phosphate (The risk of developing fluoroquinolone-associated tendinitis and tendon rupture is further increased in older patients usually over 60 years of age, in patients taking corticosteroid drugs, and in patients with kidney, heart or lung transplants).
No products indexed under this heading.

Dexamethasone Sodium Phosphate Injection (The risk of developing fluoroquinolone-associated tendinitis and tendon rupture is further increased in older patients usually over 60 years of age, in patients taking corticosteroid drugs, and in patients with kidney, heart or lung transplants).
No products indexed under this heading.

Diclofenac Epolamine (Although not observed with moxifloxacin in preclinical and clinical trials, the concomitant administration of a nonsteriodal anti-inflammatory drug with a quinolone may increase the risks of CNS stimulation and convulsions). Products include:
Flector **1839**

Diclofenac Potassium (Although not observed with moxifloxacin in preclinical and clinical trials, the concomitant administration of a nonsteriodal anti-inflammatory drug with a quinolone may increase the risks of CNS stimulation and convulsions).
No products indexed under this heading.

Diclofenac Sodium (Although not observed with moxifloxacin in preclinical and clinical trials, the concomitant administration of a nonsteriodal anti-inflammatory drug with a quinolone may increase the risks of CNS stimulation and convulsions).
No products indexed under this heading.

Dicumarol (Quinolones, including moxifloxacin, have been reported to enhance the anticoagulant effects of warfarin or its derivatives in the patient population. In addition, infectious disease and its accompanying inflammatory process, age, and general status of the patient are risk factors for increased anticoagulant activity. Therefore, the prothrombin time, International Normalized Ratio (INR), or other suitable anticoagulation tests should be closely monitored if a quinolone is administered concomitantly with warfarin or its derivatives).
No products indexed under this heading.

Didanosine (Oral administration of quinolones with formulations containing divalent and trivalent cations, such as didanosine, chewable/buffered tablets or the pediatric powder for oral solution, may substantially interfere with the absorption of quinolones, resulting in systemic concentrations considerably lower than desired. Therefore, moxifloxacin should be taken at least 4 hours before or 8 hours after didanosine).
No products indexed under this heading.

Diflorasone Diacetate (The risk of developing fluoroquinolone-associated tendinitis and tendon rupture is further increased in older patients usually over 60 years of age, in patients taking corticosteroid drugs, and in patients with kidney, heart or lung transplants).
No products indexed under this heading.

Digoxin (No significant effect of moxifloxacin (400 mg once daily for 2 days) on digoxin (0.6 mg as a single dose) AUC was detected in a study involving 12 healthy volunteers. The mean digoxin C_{max} increased by about 50% during the distrubution phase of digoxin. This transient increase in digoxin C_{max} is not viewed to be clinically significant. Moxifloxacin pharmacokinetics were similar in the presence or absence of digoxin. No dosage adjustment for moxifloxacin or digoxin is required when these drugs are administered concomitantly).
Products include:
Lanoxin Injection **1546**
Lanoxin Injection Pediatric **1549**
Lanoxin Tablets **1553**

IMPORTANT NOTE: Always consult each drug listing in the patient's regimen for possible interactions.

Disopyramide (Moxifloxacin has been shown to prolong the QT interval of the electrocardiogram in some patients. The drug should be avoided in patients receiving Class IA antiarrhythmic agents, due to the lack of clinical experience with the drug in these patient populations).
No products indexed under this heading.

Disopyramide Phosphate (Moxifloxacin has been shown to prolong the QT interval of the electrocardiogram in some patients. The drug should be avoided in patients receiving Class IA antiarrhythmic agents, due to the lack of clinical experience with the drug in these patient populations).
No products indexed under this heading.

Doxepin Hydrochloride (Moxifloxacin has been shown to prolong the QT interval of the electrocardiogram in some patients. Pharmacokinetic studies between moxifloxacin and other drugs that prolong the QT interval, such as tricyclic antidepressants, have not been performed. An additive effect of moxifloxacin and tricyclic antidepressants cannot be excluded, therefore, caution should be exercised when moxifloxacin is given concurrently with tricyclic antidepressants).
No products indexed under this heading.

Erythromycin (Moxifloxacin has been shown to prolong the QT interval of the electrocardiogram in some patients. Pharmacokinetic studies between moxifloxacin and other drugs that prolong the QT interval, such as erythromycin, has not been performed. An additive effect of moxifloxacin and erythromycin cannot be excluded, therefore, caution should be exercised when moxifloxacin is given concurrently with erythromycin).
No products indexed under this heading.

Erythromycin, Topical (Moxifloxacin has been shown to prolong the QT interval of the electrocardiogram in some patients. Pharmacokinetic studies between moxifloxacin and other drugs that prolong the QT interval, such as erythromycin, has not been performed. An additive effect of moxifloxacin and erythromycin cannot be excluded, therefore, caution should be exercised when moxifloxacin is given concurrently with erythromycin).
No products indexed under this heading.

Erythromycin Estolate (Moxifloxacin has been shown to prolong the QT interval of the electrocardiogram in some patients. Pharmacokinetic studies between moxifloxacin and other drugs that prolong the QT interval, such as erythromycin, has not been performed. An additive effect of moxifloxacin and erythromycin cannot be excluded, therefore, caution should be exercised when moxifloxacin is given concurrently with erythromycin).
No products indexed under this heading.

Erythromycin Ethylsuccinate (Moxifloxacin has been shown to prolong the QT interval of the electrocardiogram in some patients. Pharmacokinetic studies between moxifloxacin and other drugs that prolong the QT interval, such as erythromycin, has not been performed. An additive effect of moxifloxacin and erythromycin cannot be excluded, therefore, caution should be exercised when moxifloxacin is given concurrently with erythromycin). Products include:
E.E.S. **437**
EryPed **435**

Erythromycin Gluceptate (Moxifloxacin has been shown to prolong the QT interval of the electrocardiogram in some patients. Pharmacokinetic studies between moxifloxacin and other drugs that prolong the QT interval, such as erythromycin, has not been performed.

An additive effect of moxifloxacin and erythromycin cannot be excluded, therefore, caution should be exercised when moxifloxacin is given concurrently with erythromycin).
No products indexed under this heading.

Erythromycin Lactobionate (Moxifloxacin has been shown to prolong the QT interval of the electrocardiogram in some patients. Pharmacokinetic studies between moxifloxacin and other drugs that prolong the QT interval, such as erythromycin, has not been performed. An additive effect of moxifloxacin and erythromycin cannot be excluded, therefore, caution should be exercised when moxifloxacin is given concurrently with erythromycin).
No products indexed under this heading.

Erythromycin Stearate (Moxifloxacin has been shown to prolong the QT interval of the electrocardiogram in some patients. Pharmacokinetic studies between moxifloxacin and other drugs that prolong the QT interval, such as erythromycin, has not been performed. An additive effect of moxifloxacin and erythromycin cannot be excluded, therefore, caution should be exercised when moxifloxacin is given concurrently with erythromycin).
No products indexed under this heading.

Etodolac (Although not observed with moxifloxacin in preclinical and clinical trials, the concomitant administration of a nonsteriodal anti-inflammatory drug with a quinolone may increase the risks of CNS stimulation and convulsions).
No products indexed under this heading.

Fenoprofen Calcium (Although not observed with moxifloxacin in preclinical and clinical trials, the concomitant administration of a nonsteriodal anti-inflammatory drug with a quinolone may increase the risks of CNS stimulation and convulsions).
No products indexed under this heading.

Ferrous Fumarate (When moxifloxacin tablets were administered concomitantly with iron (ferrous sulfate 100 mg once daily for two days), the mean AUC and C_{max} of moxifloxacin was reduced by 39% and 59%, respectively. Moxifloxacin should only be taken more than 4 hours before or 8 hours after iron products). Products include:
PreNexa **3473**

Ferrous Gluconate (When moxifloxacin tablets were administered concomitantly with iron (ferrous sulfate 100 mg once daily for two days), the mean AUC and C_{max} of moxifloxacin was reduced by 39% and 59%, respectively. Moxifloxacin should only be taken more than 4 hours before or 8 hours after iron products). Products include:
CitraNatal Assure **2332**
CitraNatal Rx **2332**

Ferrous Sulfate (When moxifloxacin tablets were administered concomitantly with iron (ferrous sulfate 100 mg once daily for two days), the mean AUC and C_{max} of moxifloxacin was reduced by 39% and 59%, respectively. Moxifloxacin should only be taken more than 4 hours before or 8 hours after iron products).
No products indexed under this heading.

Fludrocortisone Acetate (The risk of developing fluoroquinolone-associated tendinitis and tendon rupture is further increased in older patients usually over 60 years of age, in patients taking corticosteroid drugs, and in patients with kidney, heart or lung transplants).
No products indexed under this heading.

Flumethasone Pivalate (The risk of developing fluoroquinolone-associated tendinitis and tendon rupture is further increased in older patients usually over 60 years of age, in patients taking corticosteroid drugs, and in patients with kidney, heart or lung transplants).
No products indexed under this heading.

Flunisolide Hemihydrate (The risk of developing fluoroquinolone-associated tendinitis and tendon rupture is further increased in older patients usually over 60 years of age, in patients taking corticosteroid drugs, and in patients with kidney, heart or lung transplants).
No products indexed under this heading.

Fluphenazine Decanoate (Moxifloxacin has been shown to prolong the QT interval of the electrocardiogram in some patients. Pharmacokinetic studies between moxifloxacin and other drugs that prolong the QT interval, such as antipsychotics, has not been performed. An additive effect of moxifloxacin and antipsychotic phenthiazines cannot be excluded, therefore, caution should be exercised when moxifloxacin is given concurrently with antipsychotics).
No products indexed under this heading.

Fluphenazine Enanthate (Moxifloxacin has been shown to prolong the QT interval of the electrocardiogram in some patients. Pharmacokinetic studies between moxifloxacin and other drugs that prolong the QT interval, such as antipsychotics, has not been performed. An additive effect of moxifloxacin and antipsychotic phenthiazines cannot be excluded, therefore, caution should be exercised when moxifloxacin is given concurrently with antipsychotics).
No products indexed under this heading.

Fluphenazine Hydrochloride (Moxifloxacin has been shown to prolong the QT interval of the electrocardiogram in some patients. Pharmacokinetic studies between moxifloxacin and other drugs that prolong the QT interval, such as antipsychotics, has not been performed. An additive effect of moxifloxacin and antipsychotic phenthiazines cannot be excluded, therefore, caution should be exercised when moxifloxacin is given concurrently with antipsychotics).
No products indexed under this heading.

Flurbiprofen (Although not observed with moxifloxacin in preclinical and clinical trials, the concomitant administration of a nonsteriodal anti-inflammatory drug with a quinolone may increase the risks of CNS stimulation and convulsions).
No products indexed under this heading.

Fluticasone Furoate (The risk of developing fluoroquinolone-associated tendinitis and tendon rupture is further increased in older patients usually over 60 years of age, in patients taking corticosteroid drugs, and in patients with kidney, heart or lung transplants). Products include:
Veramyst **1713**

Fluticasone Propionate (The risk of developing fluoroquinolone-associated tendinitis and tendon rupture is further increased in older patients usually over 60 years of age, in patients taking corticosteroid drugs, and in patients with kidney, heart or lung transplants). Products include:
Advair 100/50 .... **1275**
Advair 250/50 .... **1275**
Advair 500/50 .... **1275**
Advair HFA 45/21 .... **1288**
Advair HFA 115/21 .... **1288**
Advair HFA 230/21 .... **1288**
Flonase **1459**
Flovent Diskus **1463**

Flovent HFA **1470**

Glyburide (In diabetics, glyburide (2.5 mg once daily for two weeks pretreatment and for five days concurrently) mean AUC and C_{max} were 12% and 21% lower, respectively, when taken with moxifloxacin (400 mg once daily for five days) in comparison to placebo. Nonetheless, blood glucose levels were decreased slightly in patients taking glyburide and moxifloxacin in comparison to those taking glyburide alone, suggesting no interference by moxifloxacin on the activity of glyburide. These interaction results are not viewed as clinically significant).
No products indexed under this heading.

Haloperidol (Moxifloxacin has been shown to prolong the QT interval of the electrocardiogram in some patients. Pharmacokinetic studies between moxifloxacin and other drugs that prolong the QT interval, such as antipsychotics, has not been performed. An additive effect of moxifloxacin and antipsychotic phenthiazines cannot be excluded, therefore, caution should be exercised when moxifloxacin is given concurrently with antipsychotics).
No products indexed under this heading.

Haloperidol Decanoate (Moxifloxacin has been shown to prolong the QT interval of the electrocardiogram in some patients. Pharmacokinetic studies between moxifloxacin and other drugs that prolong the QT interval, such as antipsychotics, has not been performed. An additive effect of moxifloxacin and antipsychotic phenthiazines cannot be excluded, therefore, caution should be exercised when moxifloxacin is given concurrently with antipsychotics).
No products indexed under this heading.

Haloperidol Lactate (Moxifloxacin has been shown to prolong the QT interval of the electrocardiogram in some patients. Pharmacokinetic studies between moxifloxacin and other drugs that prolong the QT interval, such as antipsychotics, has not been performed. An additive effect of moxifloxacin and antipsychotic phenthiazines cannot be excluded, therefore, caution should be exercised when moxifloxacin is given concurrently with antipsychotics).
No products indexed under this heading.

Hydrocortisone (The risk of developing fluoroquinolone-associated tendinitis and tendon rupture is further increased in older patients usually over 60 years of age, in patients taking corticosteroid drugs, and in patients with kidney, heart or lung transplants).
No products indexed under this heading.

Hydrocortisone (Alcohol) (The risk of developing fluoroquinolone-associated tendinitis and tendon rupture is further increased in older patients usually over 60 years of age, in patients taking corticosteroid drugs, and in patients with kidney, heart or lung transplants).
No products indexed under this heading.

Hydrocortisone Acetate (The risk of developing fluoroquinolone-associated tendinitis and tendon rupture is further increased in older patients usually over 60 years of age, in patients taking corticosteroid drugs, and in patients with kidney, heart or lung transplants).
No products indexed under this heading.

Hydrocortisone Butyrate (The risk of developing fluoroquinolone-associated tendinitis and tendon rupture is further increased in older patients usually over 60 years of age, in patients taking corticosteroid drugs, and in patients with kidney, heart or lung transplants).
No products indexed under this heading.

(⊙ Described in PDR® for Ophthalmic Medicines)

Hydrocortisone Cypionate (The risk of developing fluoroquinolone-associated tendinitis and tendon rupture is further increased in older patients usually over 60 years of age, in patients taking corticosteroid drugs, and in patients with kidney, heart or lung transplants).
No products indexed under this heading.

Hydrocortisone Hemisuccinate (The risk of developing fluoroquinolone-associated tendinitis and tendon rupture is further increased in older patients usually over 60 years of age, in patients taking corticosteroid drugs, and in patients with kidney, heart or lung transplants).
No products indexed under this heading.

Hydrocortisone Probutate (The risk of developing fluoroquinolone-associated tendinitis and tendon rupture is further increased in older patients usually over 60 years of age, in patients taking corticosteroid drugs, and in patients with kidney, heart or lung transplants).
No products indexed under this heading.

Hydrocortisone Sodium Phosphate (The risk of developing fluoroquinolone-associated tendinitis and tendon rupture is further increased in older patients usually over 60 years of age, in patients taking corticosteroid drugs, and in patients with kidney, heart or lung transplants).
No products indexed under this heading.

Hydrocortisone Sodium Succinate (The risk of developing fluoroquinolone-associated tendinitis and tendon rupture is further increased in older patients usually over 60 years of age, in patients taking corticosteroid drugs, and in patients with kidney, heart or lung transplants).
No products indexed under this heading.

Hydrocortisone Valerate (The risk of developing fluoroquinolone-associated tendinitis and tendon rupture is further increased in older patients usually over 60 years of age, in patients taking corticosteroid drugs, and in patients with kidney, heart or lung transplants).
No products indexed under this heading.

Ibuprofen (Although not observed with moxifloxacin in preclinical and clinical trials, the concomitant administration of a nonsteriodal anti-inflammatory drug with a quinolone may increase the risks of CNS stimulation and convulsions). Products include:
Motrin IB 2043
Children's Motrin 2044
Children's Motrin Non-Staining Dye-Free 2044
Infants' Motrin 2044
Infants' Motrin Dye-Free 2044
Junior Strength Motrin 2044
Vicoprofen 564

Imipramine Hydrochloride (Moxifloxacin has been shown to prolong the QT interval of the electrocardiogram in some patients. Pharmacokinetic studies between moxifloxacin and other drugs that prolong the QT interval, such as tricyclic antidepressants, have not been performed. An additive effect of moxifloxacin and tricyclic antidepressants cannot be excluded, therefore, caution should be exercised when moxifloxacin is given concurrently with tricyclic antidepressants).
No products indexed under this heading.

Imipramine Pamoate (Moxifloxacin has been shown to prolong the QT interval of the electrocardiogram in some patients. Pharmacokinetic studies between moxifloxacin and other drugs that prolong the QT interval, such as tricyclic antidepressants, have not been performed. An additive effect of moxifloxacin and tricyclic antidepressants cannot be excluded, therefore, caution should be exercised when moxifloxacin is given concurrently with tricyclic antidepressants).
No products indexed under this heading.

Indomethacin (Although not observed with moxifloxacin in preclinical and clinical trials, the concomitant administration of a nonsteriodal anti-inflammatory drug with a quinolone may increase the risks of CNS stimulation and convulsions). Products include:
Indocin 2167

Indomethacin Sodium Trihydrate (Although not observed with moxifloxacin in preclinical and clinical trials, the concomitant administration of a nonsteriodal anti-inflammatory drug with a quinolone may increase the risks of CNS stimulation and convulsions). Products include:
Indocin I.V. 2007

Iron (When moxifloxacin tablets were administered concomitantly with iron (ferrous sulfate 100 mg once daily for two days), the mean AUC and C_{max} of moxifloxacin was reduced by 39% and 59%, respectively. Moxifloxacin should only be taken more than 4 hours before or 8 hours after iron products).
No products indexed under this heading.

Iron, Peptonized (When moxifloxacin tablets were administered concomitantly with iron (ferrous sulfate 100 mg once daily for two days), the mean AUC and C_{max} of moxifloxacin was reduced by 39% and 59%, respectively. Moxifloxacin should only be taken more than 4 hours before or 8 hours after iron products).
No products indexed under this heading.

Iron & Ammonium Citrate (When moxifloxacin (single 400 mg tablet dose) was administered two hours before, concomitantly, or 4 hours after an aluminum/magnesium-containing antacid (900 mg aluminum hydroxide and 600 mg magnesium hydroxide as a single oral dose) to 12 healthy volunteers there, was a 26%, 60% and 23% reduction in the mean AUC of moxifloxacin, respectively. Moxifloxacin should be taken at least 4 hours before or 8 hours after metal cations).
No products indexed under this heading.

Iron Cacodylate (When moxifloxacin tablets were administered concomitantly with iron (ferrous sulfate 100 mg once daily for two days), the mean AUC and C_{max} of moxifloxacin was reduced by 39% and 59%, respectively. Moxifloxacin should only be taken more than 4 hours before or 8 hours after iron products).
No products indexed under this heading.

Iron Carbonyl (When moxifloxacin tablets were administered concomitantly with iron (ferrous sulfate 100 mg once daily for two days), the mean AUC and C_{max} of moxifloxacin was reduced by 39% and 59%, respectively. Moxifloxacin should only be taken more than 4 hours before or 8 hours after iron products). Products include:
CitraNatal 90 DHA Capsules 2332
CitraNatal Assure 2332
CitraNatal Harmony 2332
CitraNatal Rx 2332
Ferralet 2333

Iron Dextran (When moxifloxacin tablets were administered concomitantly with iron (ferrous sulfate 100 mg once daily for two days), the mean AUC and C_{max} of moxifloxacin was reduced by 39% and 59%, respectively. Moxifloxacin should only be taken more than 4 hours before or 8 hours after iron products).
No products indexed under this heading.

Iron Polysaccharide Complex (When moxifloxacin tablets were administered concomitantly with iron (ferrous sulfate 100 mg once daily for two days), the mean AUC and C_{max} of moxifloxacin was reduced by 39% and 59%, respectively. Moxifloxacin should only be taken more than 4 hours before or 8 hours after iron products).
No products indexed under this heading.

Iron Sucrose (When moxifloxacin tablets were administered concomitantly with iron (ferrous sulfate 100 mg once daily for two days), the mean AUC and C_{max} of moxifloxacin was reduced by 39% and 59%, respectively. Moxifloxacin should only be taken more than 4 hours before or 8 hours after iron products).
No products indexed under this heading.

Iron Supplements (When moxifloxacin tablets were administered concomitantly with iron (ferrous sulfate 100 mg once daily for two days), the mean AUC and C_{max} of moxifloxacin was reduced by 39% and 59%, respectively. Moxifloxacin should only be taken more than 4 hours before or 8 hours after iron products).
No products indexed under this heading.

Ketoprofen (Although not observed with moxifloxacin in preclinical and clinical trials, the concomitant administration of a nonsteriodal anti-inflammatory drug with a quinolone may increase the risks of CNS stimulation and convulsions).
No products indexed under this heading.

Ketorolac Tromethamine (Although not observed with moxifloxacin in preclinical and clinical trials, the concomitant administration of a nonsteriodal anti-inflammatory drug with a quinolone may increase the risks of CNS stimulation and convulsions). Products include:
Acuvail .... ⊙ 209

Lithium (Moxifloxacin has been shown to prolong the QT interval of the electrocardiogram in some patients. Pharmacokinetic studies between moxifloxacin and other drugs that prolong the QT interval, such as antipsychotics, has not been performed. An additive effect of moxifloxacin and antipsychotic phenthiazines cannot be excluded, therefore, caution should be exercised when moxifloxacin is given concurrently with antipsychotics).
No products indexed under this heading.

Lithium Carbonate (Moxifloxacin has been shown to prolong the QT interval of the electrocardiogram in some patients. Pharmacokinetic studies between moxifloxacin and other drugs that prolong the QT interval, such as antipsychotics, has not been performed. An additive effect of moxifloxacin and antipsychotic phenthiazines cannot be excluded, therefore, caution should be exercised when moxifloxacin is given concurrently with antipsychotics).
No products indexed under this heading.

Lithium Citrate (Moxifloxacin has been shown to prolong the QT interval of the electrocardiogram in some patients. Pharmacokinetic studies between moxifloxacin and other drugs that prolong the QT interval, such as antipsychotics, has not been performed. An additive effect of moxifloxacin and antipsychotic phenthiazines cannot be excluded, therefore, caution should be exercised when moxifloxacin is given concurrently with antipsychotics).
No products indexed under this heading.

Loxapine Hydrochloride (Moxifloxacin has been shown to prolong the QT interval of the electrocardiogram in some patients. Pharmacokinetic studies between moxifloxacin and other drugs that prolong the QT interval, such as antipsychotics, has not been performed. An additive effect of moxifloxacin and antipsychotic phenthiazines cannot be excluded, therefore, caution should be exercised when moxifloxacin is given concurrently with antipsychotics).
No products indexed under this heading.

Loxapine Succinate (Moxifloxacin has been shown to prolong the QT interval of the electrocardiogram in some patients. Pharmacokinetic studies between moxifloxacin and other drugs that prolong the QT interval, such as antipsychotics, has not been performed. An additive effect of moxifloxacin and antipsychotic phenthiazines cannot be excluded, therefore, caution should be exercised when moxifloxacin is given concurrently with antipsychotics).
No products indexed under this heading.

Magaldrate (When moxifloxacin (single 400 mg tablet dose) was administered two hours before, concomitantly, or 4 hours after an aluminum/magnesium-containing antacid (900 mg aluminum hydroxide and 600 mg magnesium hydroxide as a single oral dose) to 12 healthy volunteers, there was a 26%, 60%, and 23% reduction in the mean AUC of moxifloxacin, respectively. Moxifloxacin should be taken at least 4 hours before or 8 hours after antacids containing magnesium or aluminum).
No products indexed under this heading.

Magnesium (When moxifloxacin (single 400 mg tablet dose) was administered two hours before, concomitantly, or 4 hours after an aluminum/magnesium-containing antacid (900 mg aluminum hydroxide and 600 mg magnesium hydroxide as a single oral dose) to 12 healthy volunteers there, was a 26%, 60% and 23% reduction in the mean AUC of moxifloxacin, respectively. Moxifloxacin should be taken at least 4 hours before or 8 hours after metal cations). Products include:
BoneMate Plus 3454
Cardio Basics 3455
Chelated Mineral 3476

Magnesium Aluminum Silicate (When moxifloxacin (single 400 mg tablet dose) was administered two hours before, concomitantly, or 4 hours after an aluminum/magnesium-containing antacid (900 mg aluminum hydroxide and 600 mg magnesium hydroxide as a single oral dose) to 12 healthy volunteers there, was a 26%, 60% and 23% reduction in the mean AUC of moxifloxacin, respectively. Moxifloxacin should be taken at least 4 hours before or 8 hours after metal cations).
No products indexed under this heading.

Magnesium Carbonate (When moxifloxacin (single 400 mg tablet dose) was administered two hours before, concomitantly, or 4 hours after an aluminum/magnesium-containing antacid (900 mg aluminum hydroxide and 600 mg magnesium hydroxide as a single oral dose) to 12 healthy volunteers, there was a 26%, 60%, and 23% reduction in the mean AUC of moxifloxacin, respectively. Moxifloxacin should be taken at least 4 hours before or 8 hours after antacids containing magnesium or aluminum).
No products indexed under this heading.

Magnesium Chloride (When moxifloxacin (single 400 mg tablet dose) was administered two hours before, concomitantly, or 4 hours after an aluminum/magnesium-containing antacid (900 mg aluminum hydroxide and 600 mg magnesium hydroxide as a single oral dose) to 12 healthy volunteers there, was a 26%, 60% and 23% reduction in the mean AUC of moxifloxa-

IMPORTANT NOTE: Always consult each drug listing in the patient's regimen for possible interactions.

Avelox **Interactions Index** **196**

cin, respectively. Moxifloxacin should be taken at least 4 hours before or 8 hours after metal cations).
No products indexed under this heading.

Magnesium Citrate (When moxifloxacin (single 400 mg tablet dose) was administered two hours before, concomitantly, or 4 hours after an aluminum/magnesium-containing antacid (900 mg aluminum hydroxide and 600 mg magnesium hydroxide as a single oral dose) to 12 healthy volunteers there, was a 26%, 60% and 23% reduction in the mean AUC of moxifloxacin, respectively. Moxifloxacin should be taken at least 4 hours before or 8 hours after metal cations). Products include:
Chelated Mineral 3476

Magnesium Gluconate (When moxifloxacin (single 400 mg tablet dose) was administered two hours before, concomitantly, or 4 hours after an aluminum/magnesium-containing antacid (900 mg aluminum hydroxide and 600 mg magnesium hydroxide as a single oral dose) to 12 healthy volunteers there, was a 26%, 60% and 23% reduction in the mean AUC of moxifloxacin, respectively. Moxifloxacin should be taken at least 4 hours before or 8 hours after metal cations).
No products indexed under this heading.

Magnesium Hydroxide (When moxifloxacin (single 400 mg tablet dose) was administered two hours before, concomitantly, or 4 hours after an aluminum/magnesium-containing antacid (900 mg aluminum hydroxide and 600 mg magnesium hydroxide as a single oral dose) to 12 healthy volunteers, there was a 26%, 60%, and 23% reduction in the mean AUC of moxifloxacin, respectively. Moxifloxacin should be taken at least 4 hours before or 8 hours after antacids containing magnesium or aluminum). Products include:
Fleet Pedia-Lax Chewable Tablets 1144
Pepcid Complete 1822

Magnesium Lactate (When moxifloxacin (single 400 mg tablet dose) was administered two hours before, concomitantly, or 4 hours after an aluminum/magnesium-containing antacid (900 mg aluminum hydroxide and 600 mg magnesium hydroxide as a single oral dose) to 12 healthy volunteers there, was a 26%, 60% and 23% reduction in the mean AUC of moxifloxacin, respectively. Moxifloxacin should be taken at least 4 hours before or 8 hours after metal cations).
No products indexed under this heading.

Magnesium Oxide (When moxifloxacin (single 400 mg tablet dose) was administered two hours before, concomitantly, or 4 hours after an aluminum/magnesium-containing antacid (900 mg aluminum hydroxide and 600 mg magnesium hydroxide as a single oral dose) to 12 healthy volunteers, there was a 26%, 60%, and 23% reduction in the mean AUC of moxifloxacin, respectively. Moxifloxacin should be taken at least 4 hours before or 8 hours after antacids containing magnesium or aluminum). Products include:
Beelith 873

Magnesium Salicylate (When moxifloxacin (single 400 mg tablet dose) was administered two hours before, concomitantly, or 4 hours after an aluminum/magnesium-containing antacid (900 mg aluminum hydroxide and 600 mg magnesium hydroxide as a single oral dose) to 12 healthy volunteers there, was a 26%, 60% and 23% reduction in the mean AUC of moxifloxacin, respectively. Moxifloxacin should be taken at least 4 hours before or 8 hours after metal cations).
No products indexed under this heading.

Magnesium Salicylate Tetrahydrate (When moxifloxacin (single 400 mg tablet dose) was administered two hours before, concomitantly, or 4 hours after an aluminum/magnesium-containing antacid (900 mg aluminum hydroxide and 600 mg magnesium hydroxide as a single oral dose) to 12 healthy volunteers there, was a 26%, 60% and 23% reduction in the mean AUC of moxifloxacin, respectively. Moxifloxacin should be taken at least 4 hours before or 8 hours after metal cations).
No products indexed under this heading.

Magnesium Salts (When moxifloxacin (single 400 mg tablet dose) was administered two hours before, concomitantly, or 4 hours after an aluminum/magnesium-containing antacid (900 mg aluminum hydroxide and 600 mg magnesium hydroxide as a single oral dose) to 12 healthy volunteers there, was a 26%, 60% and 23% reduction in the mean AUC of moxifloxacin, respectively. Moxifloxacin should be taken at least 4 hours before or 8 hours after metal cations).
No products indexed under this heading.

Magnesium Sulfate (When moxifloxacin (single 400 mg tablet dose) was administered two hours before, concomitantly, or 4 hours after an aluminum/magnesium-containing antacid (900 mg aluminum hydroxide and 600 mg magnesium hydroxide as a single oral dose) to 12 healthy volunteers there, was a 26%, 60% and 23% reduction in the mean AUC of moxifloxacin, respectively. Moxifloxacin should be taken at least 4 hours before or 8 hours after metal cations).
No products indexed under this heading.

Magnesium Trisilicate (When moxifloxacin (single 400 mg tablet dose) was administered two hours before, concomitantly, or 4 hours after an aluminum/magnesium-containing antacid (900 mg aluminum hydroxide and 600 mg magnesium hydroxide as a single oral dose) to 12 healthy volunteers, there was a 26%, 60%, and 23% reduction in the mean AUC of moxifloxacin, respectively. Moxifloxacin should be taken at least 4 hours before or 8 hours after antacids containing magnesium or aluminum).
No products indexed under this heading.

Maprotiline Hydrochloride (Moxifloxacin has been shown to prolong the QT interval of the electrocardiogram in some patients. Pharmacokinetic studies between moxifloxacin and other drugs that prolong the QT interval, such as tricyclic antidepressants, have not been performed. An additive effect of moxifloxacin and tricyclic antidepressants cannot be excluded, therefore, caution should be exercised when moxifloxacin is given concurrently with tricyclic antidepressants).
No products indexed under this heading.

Meclofenamate Sodium (Although not observed with moxifloxacin in preclinical and clinical trials, the concomitant administration of a nonsteriodal anti-inflammatory drug with a quinolone may increase the risks of CNS stimulation and convulsions).
No products indexed under this heading.

Mefenamic Acid (Although not observed with moxifloxacin in preclinical and clinical trials, the concomitant administration of a nonsteriodal anti-inflammatory drug with a quinolone may increase the risks of CNS stimulation and convulsions).
No products indexed under this heading.

Meloxicam (Although not observed with moxifloxacin in preclinical and clinical trials, the concomitant administration of a nonsteriodal anti-inflammatory drug with a quinolone may increase the risks of CNS stimulation and convulsions).
No products indexed under this heading.

Mesoridazine Besylate (Moxifloxacin has been shown to prolong the QT interval of the electrocardiogram in some patients. Pharmacokinetic studies between moxifloxacin and other drugs that prolong the QT interval, such as antipsychotics, has not been performed. An additive effect of moxifloxacin and antipsychotic phenthiazines cannot be excluded, therefore, caution should be exercised when moxifloxacin is given concurrently with antipsychotics).
No products indexed under this heading.

Methotrimeprazine (Moxifloxacin has been shown to prolong the QT interval of the electrocardiogram in some patients. Pharmacokinetic studies between moxifloxacin and other drugs that prolong the QT interval, such as antipsychotics, has not been performed. An additive effect of moxifloxacin and antipsychotic phenthiazines cannot be excluded, therefore, caution should be exercised when moxifloxacin is given concurrently with antipsychotics).
No products indexed under this heading.

Methylprednisolone (The risk of developing fluoroquinolone-associated tendinitis and tendon rupture is further increased in older patients usually over 60 years of age, in patients taking corticosteroid drugs, and in patients with kidney, heart or lung transplants).
No products indexed under this heading.

Methylprednisolone Acetate (The risk of developing fluoroquinolone-associated tendinitis and tendon rupture is further increased in older patients usually over 60 years of age, in patients taking corticosteroid drugs, and in patients with kidney, heart or lung transplants).
No products indexed under this heading.

Methylprednisolone Sodium Succinate (The risk of developing fluoroquinolone-associated tendinitis and tendon rupture is further increased in older patients usually over 60 years of age, in patients taking corticosteroid drugs, and in patients with kidney, heart or lung transplants).
No products indexed under this heading.

Molindone Hydrochloride (Moxifloxacin has been shown to prolong the QT interval of the electrocardiogram in some patients. Pharmacokinetic studies between moxifloxacin and other drugs that prolong the QT interval, such as antipsychotics, has not been performed. An additive effect of moxifloxacin and antipsychotic phenthiazines cannot be excluded, therefore, caution should be exercised when moxifloxacin is given concurrently with antipsychotics). Products include:
Moban 1108

Mometasone Furoate (The risk of developing fluoroquinolone-associated tendinitis and tendon rupture is further increased in older patients usually over 60 years of age, in patients taking corticosteroid drugs, and in patients with kidney, heart or lung transplants).
Products include:
Asmanex 3058
Elocon Cream 3111
Elocon Lotion 3112
Elocon Ointment 3114

Mometasone Furoate Monohydrate (The risk of developing fluoroquinolone-associated tendinitis and tendon rupture is further increased in older patients usually over 60 years of age, in patients taking corticosteroid drugs, and in patients with kidney, heart or lung transplants). Products include:
Nasonex 3166

Moricizine Hydrochloride (Moxifloxacin has been shown to prolong the QT interval of the electrocardiogram in some patients. The drug should be avoided in patients receiving Class IA antiarrhythmic agents, due to the lack of clinical experience with the drug in these patient populations).
No products indexed under this heading.

Nabumetone (Although not observed with moxifloxacin in preclinical and clinical trials, the concomitant administration of a nonsteriodal anti-inflammatory drug with a quinolone may increase the risks of CNS stimulation and convulsions).
No products indexed under this heading.

Naproxen (Although not observed with moxifloxacin in preclinical and clinical trials, the concomitant administration of a nonsteriodal anti-inflammatory drug with a quinolone may increase the risks of CNS stimulation and convulsions).
Products include:
EC-Naprosyn 2850
Naprosyn 2850
Anaprox/Naprosyn 2850

Naproxen Sodium (Although not observed with moxifloxacin in preclinical and clinical trials, the concomitant administration of a nonsteriodal anti-inflammatory drug with a quinolone may increase the risks of CNS stimulation and convulsions). Products include:
Anaprox 2850
Anaprox DS 2850
Treximet 1681

Nortriptyline Hydrochloride (Moxifloxacin has been shown to prolong the QT interval of the electrocardiogram in some patients. Pharmacokinetic studies between moxifloxacin and other drugs that prolong the QT interval, such as tricyclic antidepressants, have not been performed. An additive effect of moxifloxacin and tricyclic antidepressants cannot be excluded, therefore, caution should be exercised when moxifloxacin is given concurrently with tricyclic antidepressants).
No products indexed under this heading.

Olanzapine (Moxifloxacin has been shown to prolong the QT interval of the electrocardiogram in some patients. Pharmacokinetic studies between moxifloxacin and other drugs that prolong the QT interval, such as antipsychotics, has not been performed. An additive effect of moxifloxacin and antipsychotic phenthiazines cannot be excluded, therefore, caution should be exercised when moxifloxacin is given concurrently with antipsychotics). Products include:
Symbyax 1965
Zyprexa 1984
Zyprexa IntraMuscular 1984
Zyprexa ZYDIS 1984

Oxaprozin (Although not observed with moxifloxacin in preclinical and clinical trials, the concomitant administration of a nonsteriodal anti-inflammatory drug with a quinolone may increase the risks of CNS stimulation and convulsions).
No products indexed under this heading.

Paliperidone (Moxifloxacin has been shown to prolong the QT interval of the electrocardiogram in some patients. Pharmacokinetic studies between moxifloxacin and other drugs that prolong the QT interval, such as antipsychotics, has not been performed. An additive effect of moxifloxacin and antipsychotic phenthiazines cannot be excluded, therefore, caution should be exercised when moxifloxacin is given concurrently with antipsychotics). Products include:

197 **Interactions Index** **Avelox**

Invega 2613
Invega Sustenna 2621

Perphenazine (Moxifloxacin has been shown to prolong the QT interval of the electrocardiogram in some patients. Pharmacokinetic studies between moxifloxacin and other drugs that prolong the QT interval, such as antipsychotics, has not been performed. An additive effect of moxifloxacin and antipsychotic phenthiazines cannot be excluded, therefore, caution should be exercised when moxifloxacin is given concurrently with antipsychotics).
No products indexed under this heading.

Phenylbutazone (Although not observed with moxifloxacin in preclinical and clinical trials, the concomitant administration of a nonsteriodal anti-inflammatory drug with a quinolone may increase the risks of CNS stimulation and convulsions).
No products indexed under this heading.

Pimozide (Moxifloxacin has been shown to prolong the QT interval of the electrocardiogram in some patients. Pharmacokinetic studies between moxifloxacin and other drugs that prolong the QT interval, such as antipsychotics, has not been performed. An additive effect of moxifloxacin and antipsychotic phenthiazines cannot be excluded, therefore, caution should be exercised when moxifloxacin is given concurrently with antipsychotics).
No products indexed under this heading.

Piroxicam (Although not observed with moxifloxacin in preclinical and clinical trials, the concomitant administration of a nonsteriodal anti-inflammatory drug with a quinolone may increase the risks of CNS stimulation and convulsions).
No products indexed under this heading.

Polysaccharide Iron Complex (When moxifloxacin tablets were administered concomitantly with iron (ferrous sulfate 100 mg once daily for two days), the mean AUC and C_{max} of moxifloxacin was reduced by 39% and 59%, respectively. Moxifloxacin should only be taken more than 4 hours before or 8 hours after iron products). Products include:
Nu-Iron 150 2321

Prednisolone (The risk of developing fluoroquinolone-associated tendinitis and tendon rupture is further increased in older patients usually over 60 years of age, in patients taking corticosteroid drugs, and in patients with kidney, heart or lung transplants).
No products indexed under this heading.

Prednisolone Acetate (The risk of developing fluoroquinolone-associated tendinitis and tendon rupture is further increased in older patients usually over 60 years of age, in patients taking corticosteroid drugs, and in patients with kidney, heart or lung transplants).
Products include:
Blephamide .... ⊙ 212, ⊙ 214
Pred Forte .... ⊙ 225
Pred Mild .... ⊙ 230
Pred-G .... ⊙ 226, ⊙ 227

Prednisolone Sodium Phosphate (The risk of developing fluoroquinolone-associated tendinitis and tendon rupture is further increased in older patients usually over 60 years of age, in patients taking corticosteroid drugs, and in patients with kidney, heart or lung transplants).
No products indexed under this heading.

Prednisolone Tebutate (The risk of developing fluoroquinolone-associated tendinitis and tendon rupture is further increased in older patients usually over 60 years of age, in patients taking corticosteroid drugs, and in patients with kidney, heart or lung transplants).
No products indexed under this heading.

Prednisone (The risk of developing fluoroquinolone-associated tendinitis and tendon rupture is further increased in older patients usually over 60 years of age, in patients taking corticosteroid drugs, and in patients with kidney, heart or lung transplants).
No products indexed under this heading.

Prednisone sodium phosphate (The risk of developing fluoroquinolone-associated tendinitis and tendon rupture is further increased in older patients usually over 60 years of age, in patients taking corticosteroid drugs, and in patients with kidney, heart or lung transplants).
No products indexed under this heading.

Procainamide (Moxifloxacin has been shown to prolong the QT interval of the electrocardiogram in some patients. The drug should be avoided in patients receiving Class IA antiarrhythmic agents, such as procainamide, due to the lack of clinical experience with the drug in this patient population).
No products indexed under this heading.

Procainamide Hydrochloride (Moxifloxacin has been shown to prolong the QT interval of the electrocardiogram in some patients. The drug should be avoided in patients receiving Class IA antiarrhythmic agents, such as procainamide, due to the lack of clinical experience with the drug in this patient population).
No products indexed under this heading.

Prochlorperazine (Moxifloxacin has been shown to prolong the QT interval of the electrocardiogram in some patients. Pharmacokinetic studies between moxifloxacin and other drugs that prolong the QT interval, such as antipsychotics, has not been performed. An additive effect of moxifloxacin and antipsychotic phenthiazines cannot be excluded, therefore, caution should be exercised when moxifloxacin is given concurrently with antipsychotics).
No products indexed under this heading.

Protriptyline Hydrochloride (Moxifloxacin has been shown to prolong the QT interval of the electrocardiogram in some patients. Pharmacokinetic studies between moxifloxacin and other drugs that prolong the QT interval, such as tricyclic antidepressants, have not been performed. An additive effect of moxifloxacin and tricyclic antidepressants cannot be excluded, therefore, caution should be exercised when moxifloxacin is given concurrently with tricyclic antidepressants).
No products indexed under this heading.

Quetiapine Fumarate (Moxifloxacin has been shown to prolong the QT interval of the electrocardiogram in some patients. Pharmacokinetic studies between moxifloxacin and other drugs that prolong the QT interval, such as antipsychotics, has not been performed. An additive effect of moxifloxacin and antipsychotic phenthiazines cannot be excluded, therefore, caution should be exercised when moxifloxacin is given concurrently with antipsychotics). Products include:
Seroquel 750
Seroquel XR 759

Quinidine (Moxifloxacin has been shown to prolong the QT interval of the electrocardiogram in some patients. The drug should be avoided in patients receiving Class IA antiarrhythmic agents, due to the lack of clinical experience with the drug in these patient populations).
No products indexed under this heading.

Quinidine Gluconate (Moxifloxacin has been shown to prolong the QT interval of the electrocardiogram in some patients. The drug should be avoided in patients receiving Class IA antiarrhythmic agents, due to the lack of clinical experience with the drug in these patient populations).
No products indexed under this heading.

Quinidine Hydrochloride (Moxifloxacin has been shown to prolong the QT interval of the electrocardiogram in some patients. The drug should be avoided in patients receiving Class IA antiarrhythmic agents, due to the lack of clinical experience with the drug in these patient populations).
No products indexed under this heading.

Quinidine Polygalacturonate (Moxifloxacin has been shown to prolong the QT interval of the electrocardiogram in some patients. The drug should be avoided in patients receiving Class IA antiarrhythmic agents, due to the lack of clinical experience with the drug in these patient populations).
No products indexed under this heading.

Quinidine Sulfate (Moxifloxacin has been shown to prolong the QT interval of the electrocardiogram in some patients. The drug should be avoided in patients receiving Class IA antiarrhythmic agents, due to the lack of clinical experience with the drug in these patient populations).
No products indexed under this heading.

Risperidone (Moxifloxacin has been shown to prolong the QT interval of the electrocardiogram in some patients. Pharmacokinetic studies between moxifloxacin and other drugs that prolong the QT interval, such as antipsychotics, has not been performed. An additive effect of moxifloxacin and antipsychotic phenthiazines cannot be excluded, therefore, caution should be exercised when moxifloxacin is given concurrently with antipsychotics). Products include:
Risperdal Consta 2682

Rofecoxib (Although not observed with moxifloxacin in preclinical and clinical trials, the concomitant administration of a nonsteriodal anti-inflammatory drug with a quinolone may increase the risks of CNS stimulation and convulsions).
No products indexed under this heading.

Selenium (When moxifloxacin (single 400 mg tablet dose) was administered two hours before, concomitantly, or 4 hours after an aluminum/magnesium-containing antacid (900 mg aluminum hydroxide and 600 mg magnesium hydroxide as a single oral dose) to 12 healthy volunteers there, was a 26%, 60% and 23% reduction in the mean AUC of moxifloxacin, respectively. Moxifloxacin should be taken at least 4 hours before or 8 hours after metal cations). Products include:
Cardio Basics 3455
Chelated Mineral 3476

Selenium Sulfide (When moxifloxacin (single 400 mg tablet dose) was administered two hours before, concomitantly, or 4 hours after an aluminum/magnesium-containing antacid (900 mg aluminum hydroxide and 600 mg magnesium hydroxide as a single oral dose) to 12 healthy volunteers there, was a 26%, 60% and 23% reduction in the mean AUC of moxifloxacin, respectively. Moxifloxacin should be taken at least 4 hours before or 8 hours after metal cations).
No products indexed under this heading.

Sodium Bicarbonate (When moxifloxacin (single 400 mg tablet dose) was administered two hours before, concomitantly, or 4 hours after an aluminum/magnesium-containing antacid (900 mg aluminum hydroxide and 600 mg magnesium hydroxide as a single oral dose) to 12 healthy volunteers, there was a 26%, 60%, and 23% reduction in the mean AUC of moxifloxacin, respectively. Moxifloxacin should be taken at least 4 hours before or 8 hours after antacids).
No products indexed under this heading.

Sotalol Hydrochloride (Moxifloxacin has been shown to prolong the QT interval of the electrocardiogram in some patients. The drug should be avoided in patients receiving Class III antiarrhythmic agents, such as sotalol, due to the lack of clinical experience with the drug in this patient population).
No products indexed under this heading.

Sucralfate (Oral administration of quinolones with sucralfate may substantially interfere with the absorption of quinolones, resulting in systemic concentrations considerably lower than desired. Therefore, moxifloxacin should be taken at least 4 hours before or 8 hours after these agents). Products include:
Carafate Suspension 784
Carafate Tablets 785

Sulindac (Although not observed with moxifloxacin in preclinical and clinical trials, the concomitant administration of a nonsteriodal anti-inflammatory drug with a quinolone may increase the risks of CNS stimulation and convulsions). Products include:
Clinoril 2098

Thioridazine Hydrochloride (Moxifloxacin has been shown to prolong the QT interval of the electrocardiogram in some patients. Pharmacokinetic studies between moxifloxacin and other drugs that prolong the QT interval, such as antipsychotics, has not been performed. An additive effect of moxifloxacin and antipsychotic phenthiazines cannot be excluded, therefore, caution should be exercised when moxifloxacin is given concurrently with antipsychotics). Products include:
Thioridazine Hydrochloride 2384

Thiothixene (Moxifloxacin has been shown to prolong the QT interval of the electrocardiogram in some patients. Pharmacokinetic studies between moxifloxacin and other drugs that prolong the QT interval, such as antipsychotics, has not been performed. An additive effect of moxifloxacin and antipsychotic phenthiazines cannot be excluded, therefore, caution should be exercised when moxifloxacin is given concurrently with antipsychotics). Products include:
Thiothixene 2386

Tolmetin Sodium (Although not observed with moxifloxacin in preclinical and clinical trials, the concomitant administration of a nonsteriodal anti-inflammatory drug with a quinolone may increase the risks of CNS stimulation and convulsions).
No products indexed under this heading.

Triamcinolone (The risk of developing fluoroquinolone-associated tendinitis and tendon rupture is further increased in older patients usually over 60 years of age, in patients taking corticosteroid drugs, and in patients with kidney, heart or lung transplants).
No products indexed under this heading.

Triamcinolone Acetonide (The risk of developing fluoroquinolone-associated tendinitis and tendon rupture is further increased in older patients usually over 60 years of age, in patients taking corticosteroid drugs, and in patients with kidney, heart or lung transplants). Products include:
Azmacort 408
Nasacort AQ 3019

IMPORTANT NOTE: Always consult each drug listing in the patient's regimen for possible interactions.

Avelox Interactions Index 198

Triamcinolone Diacetate (The risk of developing fluoroquinolone-associated tendinitis and tendon rupture is further increased in older patients usually over 60 years of age, in patients taking corticosteroid drugs, and in patients with kidney, heart or lung transplants).
No products indexed under this heading.

Triamcinolone Hexacetonide (The risk of developing fluoroquinolone-associated tendinitis and tendon rupture is further increased in older patients usually over 60 years of age, in patients taking corticosteroid drugs, and in patients with kidney, heart or lung transplants).
No products indexed under this heading.

Trifluoperazine Hydrochloride (Moxifloxacin has been shown to prolong the QT interval of the electrocardiogram in some patients. Pharmacokinetic studies between moxifloxacin and other drugs that prolong the QT interval, such as antipsychotics, has not been performed. An additive effect of moxifloxacin and antipsychotic phenthiazines cannot be excluded, therefore, caution should be exercised when moxifloxacin is given concurrently with antipsychotics).
No products indexed under this heading.

Trimipramine Maleate (Moxifloxacin has been shown to prolong the QT interval of the electrocardiogram in some patients. Pharmacokinetic studies between moxifloxacin and other drugs that prolong the QT interval, such as tricyclic antidepressants, have not been performed. An additive effect of moxifloxacin and tricyclic antidepressants cannot be excluded, therefore, caution should be exercised when moxifloxacin is given concurrently with tricyclic antidepressants).
No products indexed under this heading.

Valdecoxib (Although not observed with moxifloxacin in preclinical and clinical trials, the concomitant administration of a nonsteriodal anti-inflammatory drug with a quinolone may increase the risks of CNS stimulation and convulsions).
No products indexed under this heading.

Vitamins with Iron (Quinolones form chelates with alkaline earth and transition metal cations. Oral administration of quinolones with multivitamins containing iron or zinc may substantially interfere with the absorption of quinolones, resulting in systemic concentrations considerably lower than desired. Therefore, moxifloxacin should be taken at least 4 hours before or 8 hours after these agents).
No products indexed under this heading.

Warfarin Sodium (Quinolones, including moxifloxacin, have been reported to enhance the anticoagulant effects of warfarin or its derivatives in the patient population. In addition, infectious disease and its accompanying inflammatory process, age, and general status of the patient are risk factors for increased anticoagulant activity. Therefore, the prothrombin time, International Normalized Ratio (INR), or other suitable anticoagulation tests should be closely monitored if a quinolone is administered concomitantly with warfarin or its derivatives).
No products indexed under this heading.

Zinc (Quinolones form chelates with alkaline earth and transition metal cations. Oral administration of quinolones with metal cations may substantially interfere with the absorption of quinolones, resulting in systemic concentrations considerably lower than desired. Therefore, moxifloxacin should be taken at least 4 hours before or 8 hours after metal cations such as zinc). Products include:
BoneMate Plus **3454**
Cardio Basics **3455**
Chelated Mineral **3476**
CitraNatal 90 DHA Capsules **2332**
CitraNatal Assure **2332**
Heplive **607**
Visutein **3456**

Zinc Acetate (Quinolones form chelates with alkaline earth and transition metal cations. Oral administration of quinolones with metal cations may substantially interfere with the absorption of quinolones, resulting in systemic concentrations considerably lower than desired. Therefore, moxifloxacin should be taken at least 4 hours before or 8 hours after metal cations, such as zinc).
No products indexed under this heading.

Zinc Bisglycinate (Quinolones form chelates with alkaline earth and transition metal cations. Oral administration of quinolones with metal cations may substantially interfere with the absorption of quinolones, resulting in systemic concentrations considerably lower than desired. Therefore, moxifloxacin should be taken at least 4 hours before or 8 hours after metal cations, such as zinc).
No products indexed under this heading.

Zinc Chloride (Quinolones form chelates with alkaline earth and transition metal cations. Oral administration of quinolones with metal cations may substantially interfere with the absorption of quinolones, resulting in systemic concentrations considerably lower than desired. Therefore, moxifloxacin should be taken at least 4 hours before or 8 hours after metal cations, such as zinc).
No products indexed under this heading.

Zinc Citrate (Quinolones form chelates with alkaline earth and transition metal cations. Oral administration of quinolones with metal cations may substantially interfere with the absorption of quinolones, resulting in systemic concentrations considerably lower than desired. Therefore, moxifloxacin should be taken at least 4 hours before or 8 hours after metal cations, such as zinc). Products include:
Chelated Mineral **3476**

Zinc-Containing Multivitamins (Quinolones form chelates with alkaline earth and transition metal cations. Oral administration of quinolones with multivitamins containing iron or zinc may substantially interfere with the absorption of quinolones, resulting in systemic concentrations considerably lower than desired. Therefore, moxifloxacin should be taken at least 4 hours before or 8 hours after these agents).
No products indexed under this heading.

Zinc Gluconate (Quinolones form chelates with alkaline earth and transition metal cations. Oral administration of quinolones with metal cations may substantially interfere with the absorption of quinolones, resulting in systemic concentrations considerably lower than desired. Therefore, moxifloxacin should be taken at least 4 hours before or 8 hours after metal cations, such as zinc).
No products indexed under this heading.

Zinc Oxide (Quinolones form chelates with alkaline earth and transition metal cations. Oral administration of quinolones with metal cations may substantially interfere with the absorption of quinolones, resulting in systemic concentrations considerably lower than desired. Therefore, moxifloxacin should be taken at least 4 hours before or 8 hours after metal cations, such as zinc). Products include:
Bausch & Lomb Ocuvite Adult 50+ .... ⊙238
CitraNatal Rx **2332**
Vusion Ointment **3335**

Zinc Phenosulfonate (Quinolones form chelates with alkaline earth and transition metal cations. Oral administration of quinolones with metal cations may substantially interfere with the absorption of quinolones, resulting in systemic concentrations considerably lower than desired. Therefore, moxifloxacin should be taken at least 4 hours before or 8 hours after metal cations, such as zinc).
No products indexed under this heading.

Zinc Pyrithione (Quinolones form chelates with alkaline earth and transition metal cations. Oral administration of quinolones with metal cations may substantially interfere with the absorption of quinolones, resulting in systemic concentrations considerably lower than desired. Therefore, moxifloxacin should be taken at least 4 hours before or 8 hours after metal cations, such as zinc).
No products indexed under this heading.

Zinc Sulfate (Quinolones form chelates with alkaline earth and transition metal cations. Oral administration of quinolones with metal cations may substantially interfere with the absorption of quinolones, resulting in systemic concentrations considerably lower than desired. Therefore, moxifloxacin should be taken at least 4 hours before or 8 hours after metal cations, such as zinc). Products include:
Heplive **607**
Zinc-220 .... **606**

Zinc Undecylenate (Quinolones form chelates with alkaline earth and transition metal cations. Oral administration of quinolones with metal cations may substantially interfere with the absorption of quinolones, resulting in systemic concentrations considerably lower than desired. Therefore, moxifloxacin should be taken at least 4 hours before or 8 hours after metal cations, such as zinc).
No products indexed under this heading.

Ziprasidone Hydrochloride (Moxifloxacin has been shown to prolong the QT interval of the electrocardiogram in some patients. Pharmacokinetic studies between moxifloxacin and other drugs that prolong the QT interval, such as antipsychotics, has not been performed. An additive effect of moxifloxacin and antipsychotic phenthiazines cannot be excluded, therefore, caution should be exercised when moxifloxacin is given concurrently with antipsychotics). Products include:
Geodon **2723**

Food Interactions

Iron Amino Acid Chelate (When moxifloxacin (single 400 mg tablet dose) was administered two hours before, concomitantly, or 4 hours after an aluminum/magnesium-containing antacid (900 mg aluminum hydroxide and 600 mg magnesium hydroxide as a single oral dose) to 12 healthy volunteers there, was a 26%, 60% and 23% reduction in the mean AUC of moxifloxacin, respectively. Moxifloxacin should be taken at least 4 hours before or 8 hours after metal cations).

AVINZA CAPSULES

(Morphine Sulfate) **1822**

May interact with alcohols, antiemetics, central nervous system depressants, general anesthetics, hypnotics and sedatives, mixed agonist/antagonist opioid analgesics, monoamine oxidase inhibitors, narcotic analgesics, phenothiazines, skeletal muscle relaxants, tranquilizers, and certain other agents. Compounds in these categories include:

Alfentanil Hydrochloride (The concurrent use of other central nervous system (CNS) depressants, including sedatives, hypnotics, general anesthetics, antiemetics, phenothiazines, or other tranquilizers or alcohol, increases the risk of respiratory depression, hypotension, profound sedation, or coma. Use with caution and in reduced dosages in patients taking these agents).
No products indexed under this heading.

Alprazolam (The concurrent use of other central nervous system (CNS) depressants, including sedatives, hypnotics, general anesthetics, antiemetics, phenothiazines, or other tranquilizers or alcohol, increases the risk of respiratory depression, hypotension, profound sedation, or coma. Use with caution and in reduced dosages in patients taking these agents).
No products indexed under this heading.

Amobarbital (The concurrent use of other central nervous system (CNS) depressants, including sedatives, hypnotics, general anesthetics, antiemetics, phenothiazines, or other tranquilizers or alcohol, increases the risk of respiratory depression, hypotension, profound sedation, or coma. Use with caution and in reduced dosages in patients taking these agents).
No products indexed under this heading.

Amobarbital Sodium (The concurrent use of other central nervous system (CNS) depressants, including sedatives, hypnotics, general anesthetics, antiemetics, phenothiazines, or other tranquilizers or alcohol, increases the risk of respiratory depression, hypotension, profound sedation, or coma. Use with caution and in reduced dosages in patients taking these agents).
No products indexed under this heading.

Apomorphine (Morphine may be expected to have additive effects when used in conjunction with other opioids or illicit drugs that cause central nervous system depression).
No products indexed under this heading.

Apomorphine Hydrochloride (Morphine may be expected to have additive effects when used in conjunction with other opioids or illicit drugs that cause central nervous system depression).
No products indexed under this heading.

Aprepitant (The concurrent use of other central nervous system (CNS) depressants, including antiemetics, increases the risk of respiratory depression, hypotension, profound sedation, or coma. Use with caution and in reduced dosages in patients taking these agents). Products include:
Emend **2124**

Aprobarbital (The concurrent use of other central nervous system (CNS) depressants, including sedatives, hypnotics, general anesthetics, antiemetics, phenothiazines, or other tranquilizers or alcohol, increases the risk of respiratory depression, hypotension, profound sedation, or coma. Use with caution and in reduced dosages in patients taking these agents).
No products indexed under this heading.

Atracurium Besylate (Morphine may enhance the neuromuscular blocking action of skeletal muscle relaxants and produce an increased degree of respiratory depression).
No products indexed under this heading.

Baclofen (Morphine may enhance the neuromuscular blocking action of skeletal muscle relaxants and produce an increased degree of respiratory depression).
No products indexed under this heading.

Buprenorphine Hydrochloride (Mixed agonist/antagonist analgesics (ie, pentazocine, nalbuphine and butorphanol) may reduce the analgesic effect and/or may precipitate withdrawal symptoms; mixed agonist/antagonist analgesics should not be administered to patients who have received or are receiving a course of therapy with pure opioid agonist analgesic).
No products indexed under this heading.

Buspirone Hydrochloride (The concurrent use of other central nervous system (CNS) depressants, including sedatives, hypnotics, general anesthetics, antiemetics, phenothiazines, or other tranquilizers or alcohol, increases the risk of respiratory depression, hypotension, profound sedation, or coma. Use with caution and in reduced dosages in patients taking these agents).
No products indexed under this heading.

Butabarbital (The concurrent use of other central nervous system (CNS) depressants, including sedatives, hypnotics, general anesthetics, antiemetics, phenothiazines, or other tranquilizers or alcohol, increases the risk of respiratory depression, hypotension, profound sedation, or coma. Use with caution and in reduced dosages in patients taking these agents).
No products indexed under this heading.

Butabarbital Sodium (The concurrent use of other central nervous system (CNS) depressants, including sedatives, hypnotics, general anesthetics, antiemetics, phenothiazines, or other tranquilizers or alcohol, increases the risk of respiratory depression, hypotension, profound sedation, or coma. Use with caution and in reduced dosages in patients taking these agents).
No products indexed under this heading.

Butalbital (The concurrent use of other central nervous system (CNS) depressants, including sedatives, hypnotics, general anesthetics, antiemetics, phenothiazines, or other tranquilizers or alcohol, increases the risk of respiratory depression, hypotension, profound sedation, or coma. Use with caution and in reduced dosages in patients taking these agents).
No products indexed under this heading.

Butorphanol Tartrate (Mixed agonist/antagonist analgesics (ie, pentazocine, nalbuphine and butorphanol) may reduce the analgesic effect and/or may precipitate withdrawal symptoms; mixed agonist/antagonist analgesics should not be administered to patients who have received or are receiving a course of therapy with pure opioid agonist analgesic).
No products indexed under this heading.

Carisoprodol (Morphine may enhance the neuromuscular blocking action of skeletal muscle relaxants and produce an increased degree of respiratory depression).
No products indexed under this heading.

Chloral Hydrate (The concurrent use of other central nervous system (CNS) depressants, including sedatives/hypnotics, increases the risk of respiratory depression, hypotension, profound sedation, or coma. Use with caution and in reduced dosages in patients taking these agents).
No products indexed under this heading.

Chlordiazepoxide (The concurrent use of other central nervous system (CNS) depressants, including sedatives, hypnotics, general anesthetics, antiemetics, phenothiazines, or other tranquilizers or alcohol, increases the risk of respiratory depression, hypotension, profound sedation, or coma. Use with caution and in reduced dosages in patients taking these agents).
No products indexed under this heading.

Chlordiazepoxide Hydrochloride (The concurrent use of other central nervous system (CNS) depressants, including sedatives, hypnotics, general anesthetics, antiemetics, phenothiazines, or other tranquilizers or alcohol, increases the risk of respiratory depression, hypotension, profound sedation, or coma. Use with caution and in reduced dosages in patients taking these agents).
No products indexed under this heading.

Chlorpromazine (The concurrent use of other central nervous system (CNS) depressants, including sedatives, hypnotics, general anesthetics, antiemetics, phenothiazines, or other tranquilizers or alcohol, increases the risk of respiratory depression, hypotension, profound sedation, or coma. Use with caution and in reduced dosages in patients taking these agents).
No products indexed under this heading.

Chlorpromazine Hydrochloride (The concurrent use of other central nervous system (CNS) depressants, including sedatives, hypnotics, general anesthetics, antiemetics, phenothiazines, or other tranquilizers or alcohol, increases the risk of respiratory depression, hypotension, profound sedation, or coma. Use with caution and in reduced dosages in patients taking these agents).
No products indexed under this heading.

Chlorprothixene (The concurrent use of other central nervous system (CNS) depressants, including sedatives, hypnotics, general anesthetics, antiemetics, phenothiazines, or other tranquilizers or alcohol, increases the risk of respiratory depression, hypotension, profound sedation, or coma. Use with caution and in reduced dosages in patients taking these agents).
No products indexed under this heading.

Chlorprothixene Hydrochloride (The concurrent use of other central nervous system (CNS) depressants, including sedatives, hypnotics, general anesthetics, antiemetics, phenothiazines, or other tranquilizers or alcohol, increases the risk of respiratory depression, hypotension, profound sedation, or coma. Use with caution and in reduced dosages in patients taking these agents).
No products indexed under this heading.

Chlorprothixene Lactate (The concurrent use of other central nervous system (CNS) depressants, including sedatives, hypnotics, general anesthetics, antiemetics, phenothiazines, or other tranquilizers or alcohol, increases the risk of respiratory depression, hypotension, profound sedation, or coma. Use with caution and in reduced dosages in patients taking these agents).
No products indexed under this heading.

Chlorzoxazone (Morphine may enhance the neuromuscular blocking action of skeletal muscle relaxants and produce an increased degree of respiratory depression).
No products indexed under this heading.

Cimetidine (Co-administration has been reported to precipitate apnea, confusion and muscle twitching in an isolated report. Patients should be monitored for increased respiratory and CNS depression when receiving cimetidine concomitantly with morphine).
No products indexed under this heading.

Cisatracurium Besylate (Morphine may enhance the neuromuscular blocking action of skeletal muscle relaxants and produce an increased degree of respiratory depression). Products include:
Nimbex 503

Clonazepam (The concurrent use of other central nervous system (CNS) depressants, including sedatives, hypnotics, general anesthetics, antiemetics, phenothiazines, or other tranquilizers or alcohol, increases the risk of respiratory depression, hypotension, profound sedation, or coma. Use with caution and in reduced dosages in patients taking these agents). Products include:
Klonopin 2855

Clorazepate Dipotassium (The concurrent use of other central nervous system (CNS) depressants, including sedatives, hypnotics, general anesthetics, antiemetics, phenothiazines, or other tranquilizers or alcohol, increases the risk of respiratory depression, hypotension, profound sedation, or coma. Use with caution and in reduced dosages in patients taking these agents).
No products indexed under this heading.

Clozapine (The concurrent use of other central nervous system (CNS) depressants, including sedatives, hypnotics, general anesthetics, antiemetics, phenothiazines, or other tranquilizers or alcohol, increases the risk of respiratory depression, hypotension, profound sedation, or coma. Use with caution and in reduced dosages in patients taking these agents).
No products indexed under this heading.

Codeine Phosphate (The concurrent use of other central nervous system (CNS) depressants, including sedatives, hypnotics, general anesthetics, antiemetics, phenothiazines, or other tranquilizers or alcohol, increases the risk of respiratory depression, hypotension, profound sedation, or coma. Use with caution and in reduced dosages in patients taking these agents). Products include:
Tylenol with Codeine 2691

Codeine Sulfate (The concurrent use of other central nervous system (CNS) depressants, including sedatives, hypnotics, general anesthetics, antiemetics, phenothiazines, or other tranquilizers or alcohol, increases the risk of respiratory depression, hypotension, profound sedation, or coma. Use with caution and in reduced dosages in patients taking these agents).
No products indexed under this heading.

Cyclobenzaprine Hydrochloride (Morphine may enhance the neuromuscular blocking action of skeletal muscle relaxants and produce an increased degree of respiratory depression). Products include:
Amrix 964

Dantrolene Sodium (Morphine may enhance the neuromuscular blocking action of skeletal muscle relaxants and produce an increased degree of respiratory depression).
No products indexed under this heading.

Desflurane (The concurrent use of other central nervous system (CNS) depressants, including sedatives, hypnotics, general anesthetics, antiemetics, phenothiazines, or other tranquilizers or alcohol, increases the risk of respiratory depression, hypotension, profound sedation, or coma. Use with caution and in reduced dosages in patients taking these agents).
No products indexed under this heading.

Dezocine (The concurrent use of other central nervous system (CNS) depressants, including sedatives, hypnotics, general anesthetics, antiemetics, phenothiazines, or other tranquilizers or alcohol, increases the risk of respiratory depression, hypotension, profound sedation, or coma. Use with caution and in reduced dosages in patients taking these agents).
No products indexed under this heading.

Diazepam (The concurrent use of other central nervous system (CNS) depressants, including sedatives, hypnotics, general anesthetics, antiemetics, phenothiazines, or other tranquilizers or alcohol, increases the risk of respiratory depression, hypotension, profound sedation, or coma. Use with caution and in reduced dosages in patients taking these agents). Products include:
Valium Tablets 2880

Dihydrocodeine Bitartrate (Morphine may be expected to have additive effects when used in conjunction with other opioids or illicit drugs that cause central nervous system depression).
No products indexed under this heading.

Dihydrocodeinone Bitartrate (Morphine may be expected to have additive effects when used in conjunction with other opioids or illicit drugs that cause central nervous system depression).
No products indexed under this heading.

Dimenhydrinate (The concurrent use of other central nervous system (CNS) depressants, including antiemetics, increases the risk of respiratory depression, hypotension, profound sedation, or coma. Use with caution and in reduced dosages in patients taking these agents).
No products indexed under this heading.

Diphenhydramine (The concurrent use of other central nervous system (CNS) depressants, including antiemetics, increases the risk of respiratory depression, hypotension, profound sedation, or coma. Use with caution and in reduced dosages in patients taking these agents).
No products indexed under this heading.

Diphenhydramine Hydrochloride (The concurrent use of other central nervous system (CNS) depressants, including antiemetics, increases the risk of respiratory depression, hypotension, profound sedation, or coma. Use with caution and in reduced dosages in patients taking these agents). Products include:
Benadryl Allergy Ultratab 2042
Children's Benadryl Allergy Liquid 2042

Dolasetron Mesylate (The concurrent use of other central nervous system (CNS) depressants, including antiemetics, increases the risk of respiratory depression, hypotension, profound sedation, or coma. Use with caution and in reduced dosages in patients taking these agents). Products include:
Anzemet Injection 2931
Anzemet Tablets 2934

Doxacurium Chloride (Morphine may enhance the neuromuscular blocking action of skeletal muscle relaxants and produce an increased degree of respiratory depression).
No products indexed under this heading.

Dronabinol (The concurrent use of other central nervous system (CNS) depressants, including antiemetics, increases the risk of respiratory depression, hypotension, profound sedation, or coma. Use with caution and in reduced dosages in patients taking these agents).
No products indexed under this heading.

Droperidol (The concurrent use of other central nervous system (CNS) depressants, including sedatives, hypnotics, general anesthetics, antiemetics, phenothiazines, or other tranquilizers or alcohol, increases the risk of respiratory depression, hypotension, profound sedation, or coma. Use with caution and in reduced dosages in patients taking these agents).
No products indexed under this heading.

IMPORTANT NOTE: Always consult each drug listing in the patient's regimen for possible interactions.

Avinza **Interactions Index** 200

d-Tubocurarine (Morphine may enhance the neuromuscular blocking action of skeletal muscle relaxants and produce an increased degree of respiratory depression).
No products indexed under this heading.

Enflurane (The concurrent use of other central nervous system (CNS) depressants, including sedatives, hypnotics, general anesthetics, antiemetics, phenothiazines, or other tranquilizers or alcohol, increases the risk of respiratory depression, hypotension, profound sedation, or coma. Use with caution and in reduced dosages in patients taking these agents).
No products indexed under this heading.

Estazolam (The concurrent use of other central nervous system (CNS) depressants, including sedatives, hypnotics, general anesthetics, antiemetics, phenothiazines, or other tranquilizers or alcohol, increases the risk of respiratory depression, hypotension, profound sedation, or coma. Use with caution and in reduced dosages in patients taking these agents).
No products indexed under this heading.

Ethanol (Patients must not consume alcoholic beverages, prescription or non-prescription medications containing alcohol while on morphine sulfate therapy. Consumption of alcohol while taking morphine sulfate may result in the rapid release and absorption of a potentially fatal dose of morphine).
No products indexed under this heading.

Ethchlorvynol (The concurrent use of other central nervous system (CNS) depressants, including sedatives, hypnotics, general anesthetics, antiemetics, phenothiazines, or other tranquilizers or alcohol, increases the risk of respiratory depression, hypotension, profound sedation, or coma. Use with caution and in reduced dosages in patients taking these agents).
No products indexed under this heading.

Ethinamate (The concurrent use of other central nervous system (CNS) depressants, including sedatives, hypnotics, general anesthetics, antiemetics, phenothiazines, or other tranquilizers or alcohol, increases the risk of respiratory depression, hypotension, profound sedation, or coma. Use with caution and in reduced dosages in patients taking these agents).
No products indexed under this heading.

Ethyl Alcohol (Patients must not consume alcoholic beverages, prescription or non-prescription medications containing alcohol while on morphine sulfate therapy. Consumption of alcohol while taking morphine sulfate may result in the rapid release and absorption of a potentially fatal dose of morphine).
No products indexed under this heading.

Fentanyl (The concurrent use of other central nervous system (CNS) depressants, including sedatives, hypnotics, general anesthetics, antiemetics, phenothiazines, or other tranquilizers or alcohol, increases the risk of respiratory depression, hypotension, profound sedation, or coma. Use with caution and in reduced dosages in patients taking these agents). Products include:
Duragesic **2604**
Fentanyl Transdermal System **2346**
Onsolis **2054**

Fentanyl Citrate (The concurrent use of other central nervous system (CNS) depressants, including sedatives, hypnotics, general anesthetics, antiemetics, phenothiazines, or other tranquilizers or alcohol, increases the risk of respiratory depression, hypotension, profound sedation, or coma. Use with caution and in reduced dosages in patients taking these agents). Products include:
Fentora **966**

Fluphenazine Decanoate (The concurrent use of other central nervous system (CNS) depressants, including sedatives, hypnotics, general anesthetics, antiemetics, phenothiazines, or other tranquilizers or alcohol, increases the risk of respiratory depression, hypotension, profound sedation, or coma. Use with caution and in reduced dosages in patients taking these agents).
No products indexed under this heading.

Fluphenazine Enanthate (The concurrent use of other central nervous system (CNS) depressants, including sedatives, hypnotics, general anesthetics, antiemetics, phenothiazines, or other tranquilizers or alcohol, increases the risk of respiratory depression, hypotension, profound sedation, or coma. Use with caution and in reduced dosages in patients taking these agents).
No products indexed under this heading.

Fluphenazine Hydrochloride (The concurrent use of other central nervous system (CNS) depressants, including sedatives, hypnotics, general anesthetics, antiemetics, phenothiazines, or other tranquilizers or alcohol, increases the risk of respiratory depression, hypotension, profound sedation, or coma. Use with caution and in reduced dosages in patients taking these agents).
No products indexed under this heading.

Flurazepam Hydrochloride (The concurrent use of other central nervous system (CNS) depressants, including sedatives, hypnotics, general anesthetics, antiemetics, phenothiazines, or other tranquilizers or alcohol, increases the risk of respiratory depression, hypotension, profound sedation, or coma. Use with caution and in reduced dosages in patients taking these agents).
No products indexed under this heading.

Gallamine (Morphine may enhance the neuromuscular blocking action of skeletal muscle relaxants and produce an increased degree of respiratory depression).
No products indexed under this heading.

Gallamine Triethiodide (Morphine may enhance the neuromuscular blocking action of skeletal muscle relaxants and produce an increased degree of respiratory depression).
No products indexed under this heading.

Glutethimide (The concurrent use of other central nervous system (CNS) depressants, including sedatives, hypnotics, general anesthetics, antiemetics, phenothiazines, or other tranquilizers or alcohol, increases the risk of respiratory depression, hypotension, profound sedation, or coma. Use with caution and in reduced dosages in patients taking these agents).
No products indexed under this heading.

Granisetron Hydrochloride (The concurrent use of other central nervous system (CNS) depressants, including antiemetics, increases the risk of respiratory depression, hypotension, profound sedation, or coma. Use with caution and in reduced dosages in patients taking these agents).
No products indexed under this heading.

Halazepam (The concurrent use of other central nervous system (CNS) depressants, including sedatives, hypnotics, general anesthetics, antiemetics, phenothiazines, or other tranquilizers or alcohol, increases the risk of respiratory depression, hypotension, profound sedation, or coma. Use with caution and in reduced dosages in patients taking these agents).
No products indexed under this heading.

Haloperidol (The concurrent use of other central nervous system (CNS) depressants, including sedatives, hypnotics, general anesthetics, antiemetics, phenothiazines, or other tranquilizers or alcohol, increases the risk of respiratory depression, hypotension, profound sedation, or coma. Use with caution and in reduced dosages in patients taking these agents).
No products indexed under this heading.

Haloperidol Decanoate (The concurrent use of other central nervous system (CNS) depressants, including sedatives, hypnotics, general anesthetics, antiemetics, phenothiazines, or other tranquilizers or alcohol, increases the risk of respiratory depression, hypotension, profound sedation, or coma. Use with caution and in reduced dosages in patients taking these agents).
No products indexed under this heading.

Haloperidol Lactate (The concurrent use of other central nervous system (CNS) depressants, including sedatives, hypnotics, general anesthetics, antiemetics, phenothiazines, or other tranquilizers or alcohol, increases the risk of respiratory depression, hypotension, profound sedation, or coma. Use with caution and in reduced dosages in patients taking these agents).
No products indexed under this heading.

Halothane (The concurrent use of other central nervous system (CNS) depressants, including general anesthetics, increases the risk of respiratory depression, hypotension, profound sedation, or coma. Use with caution and in reduced dosages in patients taking these agents).
No products indexed under this heading.

Hexobarbital (The concurrent use of other central nervous system (CNS) depressants, including sedatives, hypnotics, general anesthetics, antiemetics, phenothiazines, or other tranquilizers or alcohol, increases the risk of respiratory depression, hypotension, profound sedation, or coma. Use with caution and in reduced dosages in patients taking these agents).
No products indexed under this heading.

Hydrocodone Bitartrate (The concurrent use of other central nervous system (CNS) depressants, including sedatives, hypnotics, general anesthetics, antiemetics, phenothiazines, or other tranquilizers or alcohol, increases the risk of respiratory depression, hypotension, profound sedation, or coma. Use with caution and in reduced dosages in patients taking these agents). Products include:
Vicodin **560**
Vicodin ES **561**
Vicodin HP **563**
Vicoprofen **564**
Zydone **1138**

Hydrocodone Polistirex (The concurrent use of other central nervous system (CNS) depressants, including sedatives, hypnotics, general anesthetics, antiemetics, phenothiazines, or other tranquilizers or alcohol, increases the risk of respiratory depression, hypotension, profound sedation, or coma. Use with caution and in reduced dosages in patients taking these agents). Products include:
Tussionex **3443**

Hydromorphone (The concurrent use of other central nervous system (CNS) depressants, including sedatives, hypnotics, general anesthetics, antiemetics, phenothiazines, or other tranquilizers or alcohol, increases the risk of respiratory depression, hypotension, profound sedation, or coma. Use with caution and in reduced dosages in patients taking these agents).
No products indexed under this heading.

Hydromorphone Hydrochloride (The concurrent use of other central nervous system (CNS) depressants, including sedatives, hypnotics, general anesthetics, antiemetics, phenothiazines, or other tranquilizers or alcohol, increases the risk of respiratory depression, hypotension, profound sedation, or coma. Use with caution and in reduced dosages in patients taking these agents). Products include:
Dilaudid Injection **2800**
Dilaudid Oral **2797**
Dilaudid Tablets **2797**
Dilaudid-HP **2800**

Hydroxyzine Hydrochloride (The concurrent use of other central nervous system (CNS) depressants, including sedatives, hypnotics, general anesthetics, antiemetics, phenothiazines, or other tranquilizers or alcohol, increases the risk of respiratory depression, hypotension, profound sedation, or coma. Use with caution and in reduced dosages in patients taking these agents).
No products indexed under this heading.

Isocarboxazid (MAO inhibitors markedly potentiate the action of morphine; concurrent use should be avoided in patients taking MAOIs or within 14 days of stopping such treatment). Products include:
Marplan **3481**

Isoflurane (The concurrent use of other central nervous system (CNS) depressants, including sedatives, hypnotics, general anesthetics, antiemetics, phenothiazines, or other tranquilizers or alcohol, increases the risk of respiratory depression, hypotension, profound sedation, or coma. Use with caution and in reduced dosages in patients taking these agents).
No products indexed under this heading.

Ketamine Hydrochloride (The concurrent use of other central nervous system (CNS) depressants, including sedatives, hypnotics, general anesthetics, antiemetics, phenothiazines, or other tranquilizers or alcohol, increases the risk of respiratory depression, hypotension, profound sedation, or coma. Use with caution and in reduced dosages in patients taking these agents).
No products indexed under this heading.

Levomethadyl Acetate Hydrochloride (The concurrent use of other central nervous system (CNS) depressants, including sedatives, hypnotics, general anesthetics, antiemetics, phenothiazines, or other tranquilizers or alcohol, increases the risk of respiratory depression, hypotension, profound sedation, or coma. Use with caution and in reduced dosages in patients taking these agents).
No products indexed under this heading.

Levorphanol Tartrate (The concurrent use of other central nervous system (CNS) depressants, including sedatives, hypnotics, general anesthetics, antiemetics, phenothiazines, or other tranquilizers or alcohol, increases the risk of respiratory depression, hypotension, profound sedation, or coma. Use with caution and in reduced dosages in patients taking these agents).
No products indexed under this heading.

Lorazepam (The concurrent use of other central nervous system (CNS) depressants, including sedatives, hypnotics, general anesthetics, antiemetics, phenothiazines, or other tranquilizers or alcohol, increases the risk of respiratory depression, hypotension, profound sedation, or coma. Use with caution and in reduced dosages in patients taking these agents).
No products indexed under this heading.

(⊙ Described in PDR® for Ophthalmic Medicines)

201 **Interactions Index** **Avinza**

Loxapine Hydrochloride (The concurrent use of other central nervous system (CNS) depressants, including sedatives, hypnotics, general anesthetics, antiemetics, phenothiazines, or other tranquilizers or alcohol, increases the risk of respiratory depression, hypotension, profound sedation, or coma. Use with caution and in reduced dosages in patients taking these agents).
No products indexed under this heading.

Loxapine Succinate (The concurrent use of other central nervous system (CNS) depressants, including sedatives, hypnotics, general anesthetics, antiemetics, phenothiazines, or other tranquilizers or alcohol, increases the risk of respiratory depression, hypotension, profound sedation, or coma. Use with caution and in reduced dosages in patients taking these agents).
No products indexed under this heading.

Meclizine Hydrochloride (The concurrent use of other central nervous system (CNS) depressants, including antiemetics, increases the risk of respiratory depression, hypotension, profound sedation, or coma. Use with caution and in reduced dosages in patients taking these agents).
No products indexed under this heading.

Meperidine Hydrochloride (The concurrent use of other central nervous system (CNS) depressants, including sedatives, hypnotics, general anesthetics, antiemetics, phenothiazines, or other tranquilizers or alcohol, increases the risk of respiratory depression, hypotension, profound sedation, or coma. Use with caution and in reduced dosages in patients taking these agents).
No products indexed under this heading.

Mephobarbital (The concurrent use of other central nervous system (CNS) depressants, including sedatives, hypnotics, general anesthetics, antiemetics, phenothiazines, or other tranquilizers or alcohol, increases the risk of respiratory depression, hypotension, profound sedation, or coma. Use with caution and in reduced dosages in patients taking these agents).
No products indexed under this heading.

Meprobamate (The concurrent use of other central nervous system (CNS) depressants, including sedatives, hypnotics, general anesthetics, antiemetics, phenothiazines, or other tranquilizers or alcohol, increases the risk of respiratory depression, hypotension, profound sedation, or coma. Use with caution and in reduced dosages in patients taking these agents).
No products indexed under this heading.

Mesoridazine Besylate (The concurrent use of other central nervous system (CNS) depressants, including sedatives, hypnotics, general anesthetics, antiemetics, phenothiazines, or other tranquilizers or alcohol, increases the risk of respiratory depression, hypotension, profound sedation, or coma. Use with caution and in reduced dosages in patients taking these agents).
No products indexed under this heading.

Metaxalone (Morphine may enhance the neuromuscular blocking action of skeletal muscle relaxants and produce an increased degree of respiratory depression). Products include:
Skelaxin 1848

Methadone Hydrochloride (The concurrent use of other central nervous system (CNS) depressants, including sedatives, hypnotics, general anesthetics, antiemetics, phenothiazines, or other tranquilizers or alcohol, increases the risk of respiratory depression, hypotension, profound sedation, or coma. Use with caution and in reduced dosages in patients taking these agents).
No products indexed under this heading.

Methocarbamol (Morphine may enhance the neuromuscular blocking action of skeletal muscle relaxants and produce an increased degree of respiratory depression).
No products indexed under this heading.

Methohexital Sodium (The concurrent use of other central nervous system (CNS) depressants, including sedatives, hypnotics, general anesthetics, antiemetics, phenothiazines, or other tranquilizers or alcohol, increases the risk of respiratory depression, hypotension, profound sedation, or coma. Use with caution and in reduced dosages in patients taking these agents).
No products indexed under this heading.

Methotrimeprazine (The concurrent use of other central nervous system (CNS) depressants, including sedatives, hypnotics, general anesthetics, antiemetics, phenothiazines, or other tranquilizers or alcohol, increases the risk of respiratory depression, hypotension, profound sedation, or coma. Use with caution and in reduced dosages in patients taking these agents).
No products indexed under this heading.

Methoxyflurane (The concurrent use of other central nervous system (CNS) depressants, including sedatives, hypnotics, general anesthetics, antiemetics, phenothiazines, or other tranquilizers or alcohol, increases the risk of respiratory depression, hypotension, profound sedation, or coma. Use with caution and in reduced dosages in patients taking these agents).
No products indexed under this heading.

Metoclopramide Hydrochloride (The concurrent use of other central nervous system (CNS) depressants, including antiemetics, increases the risk of respiratory depression, hypotension, profound sedation, or coma. Use with caution and in reduced dosages in patients taking these agents). Products include:
Metozolv ODT 2901

Metocurine Iodide (Morphine may enhance the neuromuscular blocking action of skeletal muscle relaxants and produce an increased degree of respiratory depression).
No products indexed under this heading.

Midazolam Hydrochloride (The concurrent use of other central nervous system (CNS) depressants, including sedatives, hypnotics, general anesthetics, antiemetics, phenothiazines, or other tranquilizers or alcohol, increases the risk of respiratory depression, hypotension, profound sedation, or coma. Use with caution and in reduced dosages in patients taking these agents).
No products indexed under this heading.

Mivacurium Chloride (Morphine may enhance the neuromuscular blocking action of skeletal muscle relaxants and produce an increased degree of respiratory depression).
No products indexed under this heading.

Moclobemide (MAO inhibitors markedly potentiate the action of morphine; concurrent use should be avoided in patients taking MAOIs or within 14 days of stopping such treatment).
No products indexed under this heading.

Molindone Hydrochloride (The concurrent use of other central nervous system (CNS) depressants, including sedatives, hypnotics, general anesthetics, antiemetics, phenothiazines, or other tranquilizers or alcohol, increases the risk of respiratory depression, hypotension, profound sedation, or coma. Use with caution and in reduced dosages in patients taking these agents). Products include:
Moban 1108

Morphine Sulfate, Liposomal (The concurrent use of other central nervous system (CNS) depressants, including sedatives, hypnotics, general anesthetics, antiemetics, phenothiazines, or other tranquilizers or alcohol, increases the risk of respiratory depression, hypotension, profound sedation, or coma. Use with caution and in reduced dosages in patients taking these agents).
No products indexed under this heading.

Nabilone (The concurrent use of other central nervous system (CNS) depressants, including antiemetics, increases the risk of respiratory depression, hypotension, profound sedation, or coma. Use with caution and in reduced dosages in patients taking these agents).
No products indexed under this heading.

Nalbuphine Hydrochloride (Mixed agonist/antagonist analgesics (ie, pentazocine, nalbuphine and butorphanol) may reduce the analgesic effect and/or may precipitate withdrawal symptoms; mixed agonist/antagonist analgesics should not be administered to patients who have received or are receiving a course of therapy with pure opioid agonist analgesic).
No products indexed under this heading.

Nitrous Oxide (The concurrent use of other central nervous system (CNS) depressants, including general anesthetics, increases the risk of respiratory depression, hypotension, profound sedation, or coma. Use with caution and in reduced dosages in patients taking these agents).
No products indexed under this heading.

Olanzapine (The concurrent use of other central nervous system (CNS) depressants, including sedatives, hypnotics, general anesthetics, antiemetics, phenothiazines, or other tranquilizers or alcohol, increases the risk of respiratory depression, hypotension, profound sedation, or coma. Use with caution and in reduced dosages in patients taking these agents). Products include:
Symbyax 1965
Zyprexa 1984
Zyprexa IntraMuscular 1984
Zyprexa ZYDIS 1984

Ondansetron (The concurrent use of other central nervous system (CNS) depressants, including antiemetics, increases the risk of respiratory depression, hypotension, profound sedation, or coma. Use with caution and in reduced dosages in patients taking these agents).
No products indexed under this heading.

Ondansetron Hydrochloride (The concurrent use of other central nervous system (CNS) depressants, including antiemetics, increases the risk of respiratory depression, hypotension, profound sedation, or coma. Use with caution and in reduced dosages in patients taking these agents). Products include:
Zofran Injection 1750
Zofran 1756
Zofran ODT 1756

Orphenadrine Citrate (Morphine may enhance the neuromuscular blocking action of skeletal muscle relaxants and produce an increased degree of respiratory depression).
No products indexed under this heading.

Oxazepam (The concurrent use of other central nervous system (CNS) depressants, including sedatives, hypnotics, general anesthetics, antiemetics, phenothiazines, or other tranquilizers or alcohol, increases the risk of respiratory depression, hypotension, profound sedation, or coma. Use with caution and in reduced dosages in patients taking these agents).
No products indexed under this heading.

Oxycodone Hydrochloride (The concurrent use of other central nervous system (CNS) depressants, including sedatives, hypnotics, general anesthetics, antiemetics, phenothiazines, or other tranquilizers or alcohol, increases the risk of respiratory depression, hypotension, profound sedation, or coma. Use with caution and in reduced dosages in patients taking these agents). Products include:
OxyContin 2807
Percocet 1121
Percodan 1124

Oxycodone Terephthalate (The concurrent use of other central nervous system (CNS) depressants, including sedatives, hypnotics, general anesthetics, antiemetics, phenothiazines, or other tranquilizers or alcohol, increases the risk of respiratory depression, hypotension, profound sedation, or coma. Use with caution and in reduced dosages in patients taking these agents).
No products indexed under this heading.

Oxymorphone Hydrochloride (The concurrent use of other central nervous system (CNS) depressants, including sedatives, hypnotics, general anesthetics, antiemetics, phenothiazines, or other tranquilizers or alcohol, increases the risk of respiratory depression, hypotension, profound sedation, or coma. Use with caution and in reduced dosages in patients taking these agents). Products include:
Opana 1110
Opana ER 1114

Palonosetron Hydrochloride (The concurrent use of other central nervous system (CNS) depressants, including antiemetics, increases the risk of respiratory depression, hypotension, profound sedation, or coma. Use with caution and in reduced dosages in patients taking these agents). Products include:
Aloxi 1042

Pancuronium Bromide (Morphine may enhance the neuromuscular blocking action of skeletal muscle relaxants and produce an increased degree of respiratory depression).
No products indexed under this heading.

Pargyline Hydrochloride (MAO inhibitors markedly potentiate the action of morphine; concurrent use should be avoided in patients taking MAOIs or within 14 days of stopping such treatment).
No products indexed under this heading.

Pentazocine Hydrochloride (Mixed agonist/antagonist analgesics (ie, pentazocine, nalbuphine and butorphanol) may reduce the analgesic effect and/or may precipitate withdrawal symptoms; mixed agonist/antagonist analgesics should not be administered to patients who have received or are receiving a course of therapy with pure opioid agonist analgesic).
No products indexed under this heading.

Pentazocine Lactate (Mixed agonist/antagonist analgesics (ie, pentazocine, nalbuphine and butorphanol) may reduce the analgesic effect and/or may precipitate withdrawal symptoms; mixed agonist/antagonist analgesics should not be administered to patients who have received or are receiving a course of therapy with pure opioid agonist analgesic).
No products indexed under this heading.

Pentobarbital (The concurrent use of other central nervous system (CNS) depressants, including sedatives, hypnotics, general anesthetics, antiemetics, phenothiazines, or other tranquilizers or alcohol, increases the risk of respiratory depression, hypotension, profound sedation, or coma. Use with caution and in reduced dosages in patients taking these agents).
No products indexed under this heading.

IMPORTANT NOTE: Always consult each drug listing in the patient's regimen for possible interactions.

Avinza Interactions Index 202

Pentobarbital Sodium (The concurrent use of other central nervous system (CNS) depressants, including sedatives, hypnotics, general anesthetics, antiemetics, phenothiazines, or other tranquilizers or alcohol, increases the risk of respiratory depression, hypotension, profound sedation, or coma. Use with caution and in reduced dosages in patients taking these agents). Products include:
Nembutal 2012

Perphenazine (The concurrent use of other central nervous system (CNS) depressants, including sedatives, hypnotics, general anesthetics, antiemetics, phenothiazines, or other tranquilizers or alcohol, increases the risk of respiratory depression, hypotension, profound sedation, or coma. Use with caution and in reduced dosages in patients taking these agents).
No products indexed under this heading.

Phenelzine Sulfate (MAO inhibitors markedly potentiate the action of morphine; concurrent use should be avoided in patients taking MAOIs or within 14 days of stopping such treatment).
No products indexed under this heading.

Phenobarbital (The concurrent use of other central nervous system (CNS) depressants, including sedatives, hypnotics, general anesthetics, antiemetics, phenothiazines, or other tranquilizers or alcohol, increases the risk of respiratory depression, hypotension, profound sedation, or coma. Use with caution and in reduced dosages in patients taking these agents). Products include:
Donnatal 2711

Phenobarbital Sodium (The concurrent use of other central nervous system (CNS) depressants, including sedatives, hypnotics, general anesthetics, antiemetics, phenothiazines, or other tranquilizers or alcohol, increases the risk of respiratory depression, hypotension, profound sedation, or coma. Use with caution and in reduced dosages in patients taking these agents).
No products indexed under this heading.

Phenothiazine Derivatives (The concurrent use of other central nervous system (CNS) depressants, including phenothiazines, increases the risk of respiratory depression, hypotension, profound sedation, or coma. Use with caution and in reduced dosages in patients taking these agents).
No products indexed under this heading.

Phenothiazines (The concurrent use of other central nervous system (CNS) depressants, including phenothiazines, increases the risk of respiratory depression, hypotension, profound sedation, or coma. Use with caution and in reduced dosages in patients taking these agents).
No products indexed under this heading.

Pipecuronium Bromide (Morphine may enhance the neuromuscular blocking action of skeletal muscle relaxants and produce an increased degree of respiratory depression).
No products indexed under this heading.

Prazepam (The concurrent use of other central nervous system (CNS) depressants, including sedatives, hypnotics, general anesthetics, antiemetics, phenothiazines, or other tranquilizers or alcohol, increases the risk of respiratory depression, hypotension, profound sedation, or coma. Use with caution and in reduced dosages in patients taking these agents).
No products indexed under this heading.

Procarbazine Hydrochloride (MAO inhibitors markedly potentiate the action of morphine; concurrent use should be avoided in patients taking MAOIs or within 14 days of stopping such treatment).
No products indexed under this heading.

Prochlorperazine (The concurrent use of other central nervous system (CNS) depressants, including sedatives, hypnotics, general anesthetics, antiemetics, phenothiazines, or other tranquilizers or alcohol, increases the risk of respiratory depression, hypotension, profound sedation, or coma. Use with caution and in reduced dosages in patients taking these agents).
No products indexed under this heading.

Prochlorperazine Edisylate (The concurrent use of other central nervous system (CNS) depressants, including sedatives, hypnotics, general anesthetics, antiemetics, phenothiazines, or other tranquilizers or alcohol, increases the risk of respiratory depression, hypotension, profound sedation, or coma. Use with caution and in reduced dosages in patients taking these agents).
No products indexed under this heading.

Prochlorperazine Maleate (The concurrent use of other central nervous system (CNS) depressants, including sedatives, hypnotics, general anesthetics, antiemetics, phenothiazines, or other tranquilizers or alcohol, increases the risk of respiratory depression, hypotension, profound sedation, or coma. Use with caution and in reduced dosages in patients taking these agents).
No products indexed under this heading.

Promethazine (The concurrent use of other central nervous system (CNS) depressants, including sedatives, hypnotics, general anesthetics, antiemetics, phenothiazines, or other tranquilizers or alcohol, increases the risk of respiratory depression, hypotension, profound sedation, or coma. Use with caution and in reduced dosages in patients taking these agents).
No products indexed under this heading.

Promethazine Hydrochloride (The concurrent use of other central nervous system (CNS) depressants, including sedatives, hypnotics, general anesthetics, antiemetics, phenothiazines, or other tranquilizers or alcohol, increases the risk of respiratory depression, hypotension, profound sedation, or coma. Use with caution and in reduced dosages in patients taking these agents).
No products indexed under this heading.

Propofol (The concurrent use of other central nervous system (CNS) depressants, including sedatives, hypnotics, general anesthetics, antiemetics, phenothiazines, or other tranquilizers or alcohol, increases the risk of respiratory depression, hypotension, profound sedation, or coma. Use with caution and in reduced dosages in patients taking these agents).
No products indexed under this heading.

Propoxyphene Hydrochloride (The concurrent use of other central nervous system (CNS) depressants, including sedatives, hypnotics, general anesthetics, antiemetics, phenothiazines, or other tranquilizers or alcohol, increases the risk of respiratory depression, hypotension, profound sedation, or coma. Use with caution and in reduced dosages in patients taking these agents).
No products indexed under this heading.

Propoxyphene Napsylate (The concurrent use of other central nervous system (CNS) depressants, including sedatives, hypnotics, general anesthetics, antiemetics, phenothiazines, or other tranquilizers or alcohol, increases the risk of respiratory depression, hypotension, profound sedation, or coma. Use with caution and in reduced dosages in patients taking these agents).
No products indexed under this heading.

Quazepam (The concurrent use of other central nervous system (CNS) depressants, including sedatives, hypnotics, general anesthetics, antiemetics, phenothiazines, or other tranquilizers or alcohol, increases the risk of respiratory depression, hypotension, profound sedation, or coma. Use with caution and in reduced dosages in patients taking these agents).
No products indexed under this heading.

Quetiapine Fumarate (The concurrent use of other central nervous system (CNS) depressants, including sedatives, hypnotics, general anesthetics, antiemetics, phenothiazines, or other tranquilizers or alcohol, increases the risk of respiratory depression, hypotension, profound sedation, or coma. Use with caution and in reduced dosages in patients taking these agents). Products include:
Seroquel 750
Seroquel XR 759

Ramelteon (The concurrent use of other central nervous system (CNS) depressants, including sedatives/hypnotics, increases the risk of respiratory depression, hypotension, profound sedation, or coma. Use with caution and in reduced dosages in patients taking these agents). Products include:
Rozerem 3366

Rapacuronium Bromide (Morphine may enhance the neuromuscular blocking action of skeletal muscle relaxants and produce an increased degree of respiratory depression).
No products indexed under this heading.

Rasagiline Mesylate (MAO inhibitors markedly potentiate the action of morphine; concurrent use should be avoided in patients taking MAOIs or within 14 days of stopping such treatment). Products include:
Azilect 3383

Remifentanil Hydrochloride (The concurrent use of other central nervous system (CNS) depressants, including sedatives, hypnotics, general anesthetics, antiemetics, phenothiazines, or other tranquilizers or alcohol, increases the risk of respiratory depression, hypotension, profound sedation, or coma. Use with caution and in reduced dosages in patients taking these agents).
No products indexed under this heading.

Risperidone (The concurrent use of other central nervous system (CNS) depressants, including sedatives, hypnotics, general anesthetics, antiemetics, phenothiazines, or other tranquilizers or alcohol, increases the risk of respiratory depression, hypotension, profound sedation, or coma. Use with caution and in reduced dosages in patients taking these agents). Products include:
Risperdal Consta 2682

Rocuronium Bromide (Morphine may enhance the neuromuscular blocking action of skeletal muscle relaxants and produce an increased degree of respiratory depression). Products include:
Zemuron 3249

Scopolamine (The concurrent use of other central nervous system (CNS) depressants, including antiemetics, increases the risk of respiratory depression, hypotension, profound sedation, or coma. Use with caution and in reduced dosages in patients taking these agents). Products include:
Transderm Scōp 2397

Scopolamine Hydrobromide (The concurrent use of other central nervous system (CNS) depressants, including antiemetics, increases the risk of respiratory depression, hypotension, profound sedation, or coma. Use with caution and in reduced dosages in patients taking these agents). Products include:
Donnatal 2711

Secobarbital Sodium (The concurrent use of other central nervous system (CNS) depressants, including sedatives, hypnotics, general anesthetics, antiemetics, phenothiazines, or other tranquilizers or alcohol, increases the risk of respiratory depression, hypotension, profound sedation, or coma. Use with caution and in reduced dosages in patients taking these agents).
No products indexed under this heading.

Selegiline (MAO inhibitors markedly potentiate the action of morphine; concurrent use should be avoided in patients taking MAOIs or within 14 days of stopping such treatment). Products include:
Emsam 3623

Selegiline Hydrochloride (MAO inhibitors markedly potentiate the action of morphine; concurrent use should be avoided in patients taking MAOIs or within 14 days of stopping such treatment). Products include:
Eldepryl 3312

Sevoflurane (The concurrent use of other central nervous system (CNS) depressants, including sedatives, hypnotics, general anesthetics, antiemetics, phenothiazines, or other tranquilizers or alcohol, increases the risk of respiratory depression, hypotension, profound sedation, or coma. Use with caution and in reduced dosages in patients taking these agents). Products include:
Ultane 554

Sodium Butabarbital (The concurrent use of other central nervous system (CNS) depressants, including sedatives, hypnotics, general anesthetics, antiemetics, phenothiazines, or other tranquilizers or alcohol, increases the risk of respiratory depression, hypotension, profound sedation, or coma. Use with caution and in reduced dosages in patients taking these agents).
No products indexed under this heading.

Sodium Oxybate (The concurrent use of other central nervous system (CNS) depressants, including sedatives, hypnotics, general anesthetics, antiemetics, phenothiazines, or other tranquilizers or alcohol, increases the risk of respiratory depression, hypotension, profound sedation, or coma. Use with caution and in reduced dosages in patients taking these agents).
No products indexed under this heading.

Sodium Pentobarbital (The concurrent use of other central nervous system (CNS) depressants, including sedatives, hypnotics, general anesthetics, antiemetics, phenothiazines, or other tranquilizers or alcohol, increases the risk of respiratory depression, hypotension, profound sedation, or coma. Use with caution and in reduced dosages in patients taking these agents).
No products indexed under this heading.

Succinylcholine Chloride (Morphine may enhance the neuromuscular blocking action of skeletal muscle relaxants and produce an increased degree of respiratory depression).
No products indexed under this heading.

(⊙ Described in PDR® for Ophthalmic Medicines)

Sufentanil Citrate (The concurrent use of other central nervous system (CNS) depressants, including sedatives, hypnotics, general anesthetics, antiemetics, phenothiazines, or other tranquilizers or alcohol, increases the risk of respiratory depression, hypotension, profound sedation, or coma. Use with caution and in reduced dosages in patients taking these agents).
No products indexed under this heading.

Talbutal (The concurrent use of other central nervous system (CNS) depressants, including sedatives, hypnotics, general anesthetics, antiemetics, phenothiazines, or other tranquilizers or alcohol, increases the risk of respiratory depression, hypotension, profound sedation, or coma. Use with caution and in reduced dosages in patients taking these agents).
No products indexed under this heading.

Temazepam (The concurrent use of other central nervous system (CNS) depressants, including sedatives, hypnotics, general anesthetics, antiemetics, phenothiazines, or other tranquilizers or alcohol, increases the risk of respiratory depression, hypotension, profound sedation, or coma. Use with caution and in reduced dosages in patients taking these agents).
No products indexed under this heading.

Thiamylal Sodium (The concurrent use of other central nervous system (CNS) depressants, including sedatives, hypnotics, general anesthetics, antiemetics, phenothiazines, or other tranquilizers or alcohol, increases the risk of respiratory depression, hypotension, profound sedation, or coma. Use with caution and in reduced dosages in patients taking these agents).
No products indexed under this heading.

Thioridazine (The concurrent use of other central nervous system (CNS) depressants, including sedatives, hypnotics, general anesthetics, antiemetics, phenothiazines, or other tranquilizers or alcohol, increases the risk of respiratory depression, hypotension, profound sedation, or coma. Use with caution and in reduced dosages in patients taking these agents).
No products indexed under this heading.

Thioridazine Hydrochloride (The concurrent use of other central nervous system (CNS) depressants, including sedatives, hypnotics, general anesthetics, antiemetics, phenothiazines, or other tranquilizers or alcohol, increases the risk of respiratory depression, hypotension, profound sedation, or coma. Use with caution and in reduced dosages in patients taking these agents). Products include:
Thioridazine Hydrochloride 2384

Thiothixene (The concurrent use of other central nervous system (CNS) depressants, including sedatives, hypnotics, general anesthetics, antiemetics, phenothiazines, or other tranquilizers or alcohol, increases the risk of respiratory depression, hypotension, profound sedation, or coma. Use with caution and in reduced dosages in patients taking these agents). Products include:
Thiothixene 2386

Thiothixene Hydrochloride (The concurrent use of other central nervous system (CNS) depressants, including sedatives, hypnotics, general anesthetics, antiemetics, phenothiazines, or other tranquilizers or alcohol, increases the risk of respiratory depression, hypotension, profound sedation, or coma. Use with caution and in reduced dosages in patients taking these agents).
No products indexed under this heading.

Tizanidine (Morphine may enhance the neuromuscular blocking action of skeletal muscle relaxants and produce an increased degree of respiratory depression).
No products indexed under this heading.

Tizanidine Hydrochloride (Morphine may enhance the neuromuscular blocking action of skeletal muscle relaxants and produce an increased degree of respiratory depression).
No products indexed under this heading.

Tranylcypromine Sulfate (MAO inhibitors markedly potentiate the action of morphine; concurrent use should be avoided in patients taking MAOIs or within 14 days of stopping such treatment). Products include:
Parnate 1584

Triazolam (The concurrent use of other central nervous system (CNS) depressants, including sedatives, hypnotics, general anesthetics, antiemetics, phenothiazines, or other tranquilizers or alcohol, increases the risk of respiratory depression, hypotension, profound sedation, or coma. Use with caution and in reduced dosages in patients taking these agents).
No products indexed under this heading.

Trifluoperazine Hydrochloride (The concurrent use of other central nervous system (CNS) depressants, including sedatives, hypnotics, general anesthetics, antiemetics, phenothiazines, or other tranquilizers or alcohol, increases the risk of respiratory depression, hypotension, profound sedation, or coma. Use with caution and in reduced dosages in patients taking these agents).
No products indexed under this heading.

Trimethobenzamide Hydrochloride (The concurrent use of other central nervous system (CNS) depressants, including antiemetics, increases the risk of respiratory depression, hypotension, profound sedation, or coma. Use with caution and in reduced dosages in patients taking these agents).
No products indexed under this heading.

Tubocurarine Chloride (Morphine may enhance the neuromuscular blocking action of skeletal muscle relaxants and produce an increased degree of respiratory depression).
No products indexed under this heading.

Vecuronium Bromide (Morphine may enhance the neuromuscular blocking action of skeletal muscle relaxants and produce an increased degree of respiratory depression).
No products indexed under this heading.

Zaleplon (The concurrent use of other central nervous system (CNS) depressants, including sedatives, hypnotics, general anesthetics, antiemetics, phenothiazines, or other tranquilizers or alcohol, increases the risk of respiratory depression, hypotension, profound sedation, or coma. Use with caution and in reduced dosages in patients taking these agents).
No products indexed under this heading.

Ziprasidone Hydrochloride (The concurrent use of other central nervous system (CNS) depressants, including sedatives, hypnotics, general anesthetics, antiemetics, phenothiazines, or other tranquilizers or alcohol, increases the risk of respiratory depression, hypotension, profound sedation, or coma. Use with caution and in reduced dosages in patients taking these agents). Products include:
Geodon 2723

Zolpidem Tartrate (The concurrent use of other central nervous system (CNS) depressants, including sedatives, hypnotics, general anesthetics, antiemetics, phenothiazines, or other tranquilizers or alcohol, increases the risk of respiratory depression, hypotension, profound sedation, or coma. Use with caution and in reduced dosages in patients taking these agents). Products include:
Ambien 2920
Ambien CR 2925

Food Interactions

Alcohol (Patients must not consume alcoholic beverages, prescription or non-prescription medications containing alcohol while on morphine sulfate therapy. Consumption of alcohol while taking morphine sulfate may result in the rapid release and absorption of a potentially fatal dose of morphine).

Beer, reduced-alcohol (Patients must not consume alcoholic beverages, prescription or non-prescription medications containing alcohol while on morphine sulfate therapy. Consumption of alcohol while taking morphine sulfate may result in the rapid release and absorption of a potentially fatal dose of morphine).

Beer, unspecified (Patients must not consume alcoholic beverages, prescription or non-prescription medications containing alcohol while on morphine sulfate therapy. Consumption of alcohol while taking morphine sulfate may result in the rapid release and absorption of a potentially fatal dose of morphine).

Wine, Chianti (Patients must not consume alcoholic beverages, prescription or non-prescription medications containing alcohol while on morphine sulfate therapy. Consumption of alcohol while taking morphine sulfate may result in the rapid release and absorption of a potentially fatal dose of morphine).

Wine, Red (Patients must not consume alcoholic beverages, prescription or non-prescription medications containing alcohol while on morphine sulfate therapy. Consumption of alcohol while taking morphine sulfate may result in the rapid release and absorption of a potentially fatal dose of morphine).

Wine, unspecified (Patients must not consume alcoholic beverages, prescription or non-prescription medications containing alcohol while on morphine sulfate therapy. Consumption of alcohol while taking morphine sulfate may result in the rapid release and absorption of a potentially fatal dose of morphine).

Wine products (Patients must not consume alcoholic beverages, prescription or non-prescription medications containing alcohol while on morphine sulfate therapy. Consumption of alcohol while taking morphine sulfate may result in the rapid release and absorption of a potentially fatal dose of morphine).

AVODART SOFT GELATIN CAPSULES
(Dutasteride) 1375
May interact with cytochrome p450 3a4 inhibitors (selected), cytochrome p450 3a4 inhibitors, potent (selected), and certain other agents. Compounds in these categories include:

Acetazolamide (Based on *in vitro* data, blood concentrations of dutasteride may increase in the presence of inhibitors of CYP3A4/5).
No products indexed under this heading.

Acetazolamide Sodium (Based on *in vitro* data, blood concentrations of dutasteride may increase in the presence of inhibitors of CYP3A4/5).
No products indexed under this heading.

Amiodarone Hydrochloride (Based on *in vitro* data, blood concentrations of dutasteride may increase in the presence of inhibitors of CYP3A4/5).
No products indexed under this heading.

Amprenavir (Use caution when prescribing dutasteride to patients taking potent, chronic CYP3A4 enzyme inhibitors (eg, ritonavir)).
No products indexed under this heading.

Anastrozole (Based on *in vitro* data, blood concentrations of dutasteride may increase in the presence of inhibitors of CYP3A4/5).
No products indexed under this heading.

Aprepitant (Based on *in vitro* data, blood concentrations of dutasteride may increase in the presence of inhibitors of CYP3A4/5). Products include:
Emend 2124

Atazanavir (Use caution when prescribing dutasteride to patients taking potent, chronic CYP3A4 enzyme inhibitors (eg, ritonavir)).
No products indexed under this heading.

Atazanavir Sulfate (Use caution when prescribing dutasteride to patients taking potent, chronic CYP3A4 enzyme inhibitors (eg, ritonavir)).
No products indexed under this heading.

Cimetidine (Based on *in vitro* data, blood concentrations of dutasteride may increase in the presence of inhibitors of CYP3A4/5).
No products indexed under this heading.

Cimetidine Hydrochloride (Based on *in vitro* data, blood concentrations of dutasteride may increase in the presence of inhibitors of CYP3A4/5).
No products indexed under this heading.

Ciprofloxacin (Based on *in vitro* data, blood concentrations of dutasteride may increase in the presence of inhibitors of CYP3A4/5). Products include:
Cipro I.V. 3082
Cipro 3073
Cipro XR 3091
Ciprodex 583

Clarithromycin (Use caution when prescribing dutasteride to patients taking potent, chronic CYP3A4 enzyme inhibitors (eg, ritonavir)). Products include:
Biaxin/Biaxin XL 412

Clotrimazole (Based on *in vitro* data, blood concentrations of dutasteride may increase in the presence of inhibitors of CYP3A4/5). Products include:
Lotrisone 3163

Conivaptan Hydrochloride (Based on *in vitro* data, blood concentrations of dutasteride may increase in the presence of inhibitors of CYP3A4/5). Products include:
Vaprisol 689

Cyclosporine (Based on *in vitro* data, blood concentrations of dutasteride may increase in the presence of inhibitors of CYP3A4/5). Products include:
Gengraf 440
Neoral Oral Solution 2496
Neoral Capsules 2496
Restasis 605

Dalfopristin (Based on *in vitro* data, blood concentrations of dutasteride may increase in the presence of inhibitors of CYP3A4/5).
No products indexed under this heading.

Danazol (Based on *in vitro* data, blood concentrations of dutasteride may increase in the presence of inhibitors of CYP3A4/5).
No products indexed under this heading.

Darunavir (Based on *in vitro* data, blood concentrations of dutasteride may increase in the presence of inhibitors of CYP3A4/5).
No products indexed under this heading.

IMPORTANT NOTE: Always consult each drug listing in the patient's regimen for possible interactions.

(⊙ Described in PDR® for Ophthalmic Medicines)

Sertraline Hydrochloride (Based on *in vitro* data, blood concentrations of dutasteride may increase in the presence of inhibitors of CYP3A4/5).
No products indexed under this heading.

Sildenafil Citrate (Based on *in vitro* data, blood concentrations of dutasteride may increase in the presence of inhibitors of CYP3A4/5).
No products indexed under this heading.

Telithromycin (Use caution when prescribing dutasteride to patients taking potent, chronic CYP3A4 enzyme inhibitors (eg, ritonavir)). Products include:
Ketek 2991

Troglitazone (Based on *in vitro* data, blood concentrations of dutasteride may increase in the presence of inhibitors of CYP3A4/5).
No products indexed under this heading.

Troleandomycin (Use caution when prescribing dutasteride to patients taking potent, chronic CYP3A4 enzyme inhibitors (eg, ritonavir)).
No products indexed under this heading.

Valproate Sodium (Based on *in vitro* data, blood concentrations of dutasteride may increase in the presence of inhibitors of CYP3A4/5).
No products indexed under this heading.

Vardenafil Hydrochloride (Based on *in vitro* data, blood concentrations of dutasteride may increase in the presence of inhibitors of CYP3A4/5).
Products include:
Levitra 3157

Verapamil Hydrochloride (Co-administration of verapamil decreases dutasteride clearance and leads to increased exposure to dutasteride. The change in dutasteride exposure is not considered to be clinically significant. No dose adjustment is recommended). Products include:
Tarka 534

Voriconazole (Use caution when prescribing dutasteride to patients taking potent, chronic CYP3A4 enzyme inhibitors (eg, ritonavir)).
No products indexed under this heading.

Zafirlukast (Based on *in vitro* data, blood concentrations of dutasteride may increase in the presence of inhibitors of CYP3A4/5). Products include:
Accolate 3612

Zileuton (Based on *in vitro* data, blood concentrations of dutasteride may increase in the presence of inhibitors of CYP3A4/5).
No products indexed under this heading.

Food Interactions

Food, unspecified (When the drug is administered with food, the maximum serum concentrations were reduced by 10% to 15%. This reduction is of no clinical significance).

Grapefruit (Based on *in vitro* data, blood concentrations of dutasteride may increase in the presence of inhibitors of CYP3A4/5).

Grapefruit Juice (Based on *in vitro* data, blood concentrations of dutasteride may increase in the presence of inhibitors of CYP3A4/5).

Meal, unspecified (When the drug is administered with food, the maximum serum concentrations were reduced by 10% to 15%. This reduction is of no clinical significance).

AXERT TABLETS

(Almotriptan Malate) 2593
May interact with 5HT1-receptor agonists, cytochrome p450 3a4 inhibitors, potent (selected), ergot-containing drugs, selective serotonin reuptake inhibitors, serotonin and norepinephrine reuptake inhibitors, triptans, and certain other agents. Compounds in these categories include:

Amprenavir (Co-administration of almotriptan and oral ketoconazole, a potent CYP3A4 inhibitor, resulted in an approximately 60% increase in exposure of almotriptan. Increased exposures to almotriptan may be expected when almotriptan is used concomitantly with other potent CYP3A4 inhibitors. In patients concomitantly using potent CYP3A4 inhibitors, the recommended starting dose of almotriptan is 6.25 mg. The maximum daily dose should not exceed 12.5 mg within a 24-hour period. Concomitant use of almotriptan and potent CYP3A4 inhibitors should be avoided in patients with renal or hepatic impairment).
No products indexed under this heading.

Atazanavir (Co-administration of almotriptan and oral ketoconazole, a potent CYP3A4 inhibitor, resulted in an approximately 60% increase in exposure of almotriptan. Increased exposures to almotriptan may be expected when almotriptan is used concomitantly with other potent CYP3A4 inhibitors. In patients concomitantly using potent CYP3A4 inhibitors, the recommended starting dose of almotriptan is 6.25 mg. The maximum daily dose should not exceed 12.5 mg within a 24-hour period. Concomitant use of almotriptan and potent CYP3A4 inhibitors should be avoided in patients with renal or hepatic impairment).
No products indexed under this heading.

Atazanavir Sulfate (Co-administration of almotriptan and oral ketoconazole, a potent CYP3A4 inhibitor, resulted in an approximately 60% increase in exposure of almotriptan. Increased exposures to almotriptan may be expected when almotriptan is used concomitantly with other potent CYP3A4 inhibitors. In patients concomitantly using potent CYP3A4 inhibitors, the recommended starting dose of almotriptan is 6.25 mg. The maximum daily dose should not exceed 12.5 mg within a 24-hour period. Concomitant use of almotriptan and potent CYP3A4 inhibitors should be avoided in patients with renal or hepatic impairment).
No products indexed under this heading.

Citalopram Hydrobromide (Cases of life-threatening serotonin syndrome have been reported during combined use of selective serotonin reuptake inhibitors (SSRIs) and triptans. If concomitant treatment with almotriptan and an SSRI (eg, citalopram) is clinically warranted, careful observation of the patient is advised, particularly during treatment initiation and dose increases). Products include:
Celexa 1153

Clarithromycin (Co-administration of almotriptan and oral ketoconazole, a potent CYP3A4 inhibitor, resulted in an approximately 60% increase in exposure of almotriptan. Increased exposures to almotriptan may be expected when almotriptan is used concomitantly with other potent CYP3A4 inhibitors. In patients concomitantly using potent CYP3A4 inhibitors, the recommended starting dose of almotriptan is 6.25 mg. The maximum daily dose should not exceed 12.5 mg within a 24-hour period. Concomitant use of almotriptan and potent CYP3A4 inhibitors should be avoided in patients with renal or hepatic impairment). Products include:
Biaxin/Biaxin XL 412

Delavirdine Mesylate (Co-administration of almotriptan and oral ketoconazole, a potent CYP3A4 inhibitor, resulted in an approximately 60% increase in exposure of almotriptan. Increased exposures to almotriptan may be expected when almotriptan is used concomitantly with other potent CYP3A4 inhibitors. In patients concomi-

tantly using potent CYP3A4 inhibitors, the recommended starting dose of almotriptan is 6.25 mg. The maximum daily dose should not exceed 12.5 mg within a 24-hour period. Concomitant use of almotriptan and potent CYP3A4 inhibitors should be avoided in patients with renal or hepatic impairment).
No products indexed under this heading.

Delavirine (Co-administration of almotriptan and oral ketoconazole, a potent CYP3A4 inhibitor, resulted in an approximately 60% increase in exposure of almotriptan. Increased exposures to almotriptan may be expected when almotriptan is used concomitantly with other potent CYP3A4 inhibitors. In patients concomitantly using potent CYP3A4 inhibitors, the recommended starting dose of almotriptan is 6.25 mg. The maximum daily dose should not exceed 12.5 mg within a 24-hour period. Concomitant use of almotriptan and potent CYP3A4 inhibitors should be avoided in patients with renal or hepatic impairment).
No products indexed under this heading.

Desvenlafaxine Succinate (Cases of life-threatening serotonin syndrome have been reported during combined use of selective serotonin norepinephrine reuptake inhibitors (SNRIs) and triptans. If concomitant treatment with almotriptan and an SNRI is clinically warranted, careful observation of the patient is advised, particularly during treatment initiation and dose increases). Products include:
Pristiq 3564

Dihydroergotamine Mesylate (Ergot-containing drugs have been reported to cause prolonged vasospastic reactions. Because in theory vasospastic effects may be additive, concomitant use of ergotamine containing or ergot type medications (eg, dihydroergotamine) and almotriptan within 24 hours of each other is contraindicated).
No products indexed under this heading.

Duloxetine Hydrochloride (Cases of life-threatening serotonin syndrome have been reported during combined use of selective serotonin norepinephrine reuptake inhibitors (SNRIs) and triptans. If concomitant treatment with almotriptan and an SNRI (eg, duloxetine) is clinically warranted, careful observation of the patient is advised, particularly during treatment initiation and dose increases). Products include:
Cymbalta 1871

Eletriptan Hydrobromide (Concomitant use of other 5-HT1 agonists (eg, triptans) within 24 hours of treatment with almotriptan is contraindicated).
No products indexed under this heading.

Ergonovine Maleate (Ergot-containing drugs have been reported to cause prolonged vasospastic reactions. Because in theory vasospastic effects may be additive, concomitant use of ergotamine containing or ergot type medications and almotriptan within 24 hours of each other is contraindicated).
No products indexed under this heading.

Ergotamine Tartrate (Ergot-containing drugs have been reported to cause prolonged vasospastic reactions. Because in theory vasospastic effects may be additive, concomitant use of ergotamine containing or ergot type medications (eg, ergotamine tartrate) and almotriptan within 24 hours of each other is contraindicated).
No products indexed under this heading.

Escitalopram Oxalate (Cases of life-threatening serotonin syndrome have been reported during combined use of selective serotonin reuptake inhibitors (SSRIs) and triptans. If concomitant treatment with almotriptan and an SSRI (eg, escitalopram) is clinically

warranted, careful observation of the patient is advised, particularly during treatment initiation and dose increases). Products include:
Lexapro Oral Suspension 1160
Lexapro Tablets 1160

Fluoxetine (Cases of life-threatening serotonin syndrome have been reported during combined use of selective serotonin reuptake inhibitors (SSRIs) and triptans. If concomitant treatment with almotriptan and an SSRI (eg, fluoxetine) is clinically warranted, careful observation of the patient is advised, particularly during treatment initiation and dose increases. In addition, co-administration of almotriptan and fluoxetine (60 mg qd for 8 days), a potent inhibitor of CYP2D6, had no effect on almotriptan clearance, but maximal concentrations of almotriptan were increased 18%. This difference is not clinically significant).
No products indexed under this heading.

Fluoxetine Hydrochloride (Cases of life-threatening serotonin syndrome have been reported during combined use of selective serotonin reuptake inhibitors (SSRIs) and triptans. If concomitant treatment with almotriptan and an SSRI (eg, fluoxetine) is clinically warranted, careful observation of the patient is advised, particularly during treatment initiation and dose increases. In addition, co-administration of almotriptan and fluoxetine (60 mg qd for 8 days), a potent inhibitor of CYP2D6, had no effect on almotriptan clearance, but maximal concentrations of almotriptan were increased 18%. This difference is not clinically significant). Products include:
Prozac Weekly 1941
Prozac Pulvules 1941
Symbyax 1965

Fluvoxamine (Cases of life-threatening serotonin syndrome have been reported during combined use of selective serotonin reuptake inhibitors (SSRIs) and triptans. If concomitant treatment with almotriptan and an SSRI (eg, fluvoxamine) is clinically warranted, careful observation of the patient is advised, particularly during treatment initiation and dose increases).
No products indexed under this heading.

Fluvoxamine Maleate (Cases of life-threatening serotonin syndrome have been reported during combined use of selective serotonin reuptake inhibitors (SSRIs) and triptans. If concomitant treatment with almotriptan and an SSRI (eg, fluvoxamine) is clinically warranted, careful observation of the patient is advised, particularly during treatment initiation and dose increases).
No products indexed under this heading.

Fosamprenavir Calcium (Co-administration of almotriptan and oral ketoconazole, a potent CYP3A4 inhibitor, resulted in an approximately 60% increase in exposure of almotriptan. Increased exposures to almotriptan may be expected when almotriptan is used concomitantly with other potent CYP3A4 inhibitors. In patients concomitantly using potent CYP3A4 inhibitors, the recommended starting dose of almotriptan is 6.25 mg. The maximum daily dose should not exceed 12.5 mg within a 24-hour period. Concomitant use of almotriptan and potent CYP3A4 inhibitors should be avoided in patients with renal or hepatic impairment).
Products include:
Lexiva Oral Suspension 1558
Lexiva 1558

Frovatriptan Succinate (Concomitant use of other 5-HT1 agonists (eg, triptans) within 24 hours of treatment with almotriptan is contraindicated).
Products include:

IMPORTANT NOTE: Always consult each drug listing in the patient's regimen for possible interactions.

Aspirin Buffered (In patients given very high doses (3,900 mg) of aspirin daily, increases in serum salicylate levels were seen when nizatidine, 150 mg b.i.d., were administered concurrently). No products indexed under this heading.

AZASITE OPHTHALMIC DROPS

(Azithromycin) 1806
None cited in PDR database.

AZILECT TABLETS

(Rasagiline Mesylate) 3383
May interact with cytochrome p450 1a2 inhibitors (selected), monoamine oxidase inhibitors, nonselective MAO inhibitors, selective serotonin reuptake inhibitors, serotonin and norepinephrine reuptake inhibitors, sympathomimetics, tricyclic antidepressants, and certain other agents. Compounds in these categories include:

Alatrofloxacin Mesylate (Rasagiline plasma concentrations may increase up to 2 fold in patients using concomitant CYP1A2 inhibitors). No products indexed under this heading.

Albuterol (Severe hypertensive reactions have followed the administration of sympathomimetics and non-selective MAO inhibitors and concomitant use is contraindicated). No products indexed under this heading.

Albuterol Sulfate (Severe hypertensive reactions have followed the administration of sympathomimetics and non-selective MAO inhibitors and concomitant use is contraindicated). Products include:
ProAir HFA 3393
Proventil HFA 3204
Ventolin HFA 1708

Amiodarone Hydrochloride (Rasagiline plasma concentrations may increase up to 2 fold in patients using concomitant CYP1A2 inhibitors). No products indexed under this heading.

Amitriptyline Hydrochloride (Severe CNS toxicity associated with hyperpyrexia and death has been reported with the combination of tricyclic antidepressants (TCAs) and non-selective MAOIs or selective MAO-B inhibitors. Because the mechanisms of these reactions are not fully understood, the combination of rasagiline with TCAs should be avoided. At least 14 days should elapse between discontinuation of rasagiline and initiation of treatment with a TCA). No products indexed under this heading.

Amoxapine (Severe CNS toxicity associated with hyperpyrexia and death has been reported with the combination of tricyclic antidepressants (TCAs) and non-selective MAOIs or selective MAO-B inhibitors. Because the mechanisms of these reactions are not fully understood, the combination of rasagiline with TCAs should be avoided. At least 14 days should elapse between discontinuation of rasagiline and initiation of treatment with a TCA). No products indexed under this heading.

Anastrozole (Rasagiline plasma concentrations may increase up to 2 fold in patients using concomitant CYP1A2 inhibitors). No products indexed under this heading.

Cimetidine (Rasagiline plasma concentrations may increase up to 2 fold in patients using concomitant CYP1A2 inhibitors). No products indexed under this heading.

Cimetidine Hydrochloride (Rasagiline plasma concentrations may increase up to 2 fold in patients using concomitant CYP1A2 inhibitors). No products indexed under this heading.

Ciprofloxacin (Rasagiline plasma concentrations may increase up to 2 fold in patients using concomitant ciprofloxacin). Products include:
Cipro I.V. 3082
Cipro 3073
Cipro XR 3091
Ciprodex 583

Ciprofloxacin Hydrochloride (Rasagiline plasma concentrations may increase up to 2 fold in patients using concomitant ciprofloxacin). Products include:
Cipro 3073

Citalopram Hydrobromide (Severe CNS toxicity associated with hyperpyrexia and death has been reported with the combination of selective serotonin reuptake inhibitors (SSRIs) and non-selective MAOIs or selective MAO-B inhibitors. Because the mechanisms of these reactions are not fully understood, the combination of rasagiline with SSRI antidepressants should be avoided. At least 14 days should elapse between discontinuation of rasagiline and initiation of treatment with a SSRI antidepressant. Because of the long half lives offluoxetine and its active metabolite, at least five weeks (perhaps longer, especially if fluoxetine has been prescribed chronically and/or at higher doses) should elapse between discontinuation of fluoxetine and inititation of rasagiline). Products include:
Celexa 1153

Clarithromycin (Rasagiline plasma concentrations may increase up to 2 fold in patients using concomitant CYP1A2 inhibitors). Products include:
Biaxin/Biaxin XL 412

Clomipramine Hydrochloride (Severe CNS toxicity associated with hyperpyrexia and death has been reported with the combination of tricyclic antidepressants (TCAs) and non-selective MAOIs or selective MAO-B inhibitors. Because the mechanisms of these reactions are not fully understood, the combination of rasagiline with TCAs should be avoided. At least 14 days should elapse between discontinuation of rasagiline and initiation of treatment with a TCA). No products indexed under this heading.

Cyclobenzaprine (Rasagiline is contraindicated for use with cyclobenzaprine). No products indexed under this heading.

Cyclobenzaprine Hydrochloride (Rasagiline is contraindicated for use with cyclobenzaprine). Products include:
Amrix 964

Desipramine Hydrochloride (Severe CNS toxicity associated with hyperpyrexia and death has been reported with the combination of tricyclic antidepressants (TCAs) and non-selective MAOIs or selective MAO-B inhibitors. Because the mechanisms of these reactions are not fully understood, the combination of rasagiline with TCAs should be avoided. At least 14 days should elapse between discontinuation of rasagiline and initiation of treatment with a TCA). No products indexed under this heading.

Desogestrel (Rasagiline plasma concentrations may increase up to 2 fold in patients using concomitant CYP1A2 inhibitors). No products indexed under this heading.

Desvenlafaxine Succinate (Severe CNS toxicity associated with hyperpyrexia and death has been reported with the combination of serotonin-norepinephrine reuptake inhibitors (SNRIs) and non-selective MAOIs or selective MAO-B inhibitors. Furthermore, because the mechanisms of these reactions are not fully under-

stood, it seems prudent, in general, to avoid the combination of rasagiline with SNRI antidepressants. At least 14 days should elapse between discontinuation of rasagiline and initiation of treatment with a SNRI antidepressant). Products include:
Pristiq 3564

Dextromethorphan (The combination of MAO inhibitors and dextromethorphan has been reported to cause brief episodes of psychosis or bizarre behavior and concomitant use is contraindicated). No products indexed under this heading.

Dextromethorphan Hydrobromide (The combination of MAO inhibitors and dextromethorphan has been reported to cause brief episodes of psychosis or bizarre behavior and concomitant use is contraindicated). No products indexed under this heading.

Dextromethorphan Polistirex (The combination of MAO inhibitors and dextromethorphan has been reported to cause brief episodes of psychosis or bizarre behavior and concomitant use is contraindicated). No products indexed under this heading.

Dobutamine Hydrochloride (Severe hypertensive reactions have followed the administration of sympathomimetics and non-selective MAO inhibitors and concomitant use is contraindicated). No products indexed under this heading.

Dopamine Hydrochloride (Severe hypertensive reactions have followed the administration of sympathomimetics and non-selective MAO inhibitors and concomitant use is contraindicated). No products indexed under this heading.

Doxepin Hydrochloride (Severe CNS toxicity associated with hyperpyrexia and death has been reported with the combination of tricyclic antidepressants (TCAs) and non-selective MAOIs or selective MAO-B inhibitors. Because the mechanisms of these reactions are not fully understood, the combination of rasagiline with TCAs should be avoided. At least 14 days should elapse between discontinuation of rasagiline and initiation of treatment with a TCA). No products indexed under this heading.

Duloxetine Hydrochloride (Severe CNS toxicity associated with hyperpyrexia and death has been reported with the combination of serotonin-norepinephrine reuptake inhibitors (SNRIs) and non-selective MAOIs or selective MAO-B inhibitors. Furthermore, because the mechanisms of these reactions are not fully understood, it seems prudent, in general, to avoid the combination of rasagiline with SNRI antidepressants. At least 14 days should elapse between discontinuation of rasagiline and initiation of treatment with a SNRI antidepressant). Products include:
Cymbalta 1871

Enoxacin (Rasagiline plasma concentrations may increase up to 2 fold in patients using concomitant CYP1A2 inhibitors). No products indexed under this heading.

Ephedrine Hydrochloride (Severe hypertensive reactions have followed the administration of sympathomimetics and non-selective MAO inhibitors and concomitant use is contraindicated). No products indexed under this heading.

Ephedrine Sulfate (Severe hypertensive reactions have followed the administration of sympathomimetics and non-selective MAO inhibitors and concomitant use is contraindicated). No products indexed under this heading.

Ephedrine Tannate (Severe hypertensive reactions have followed the administration of sympathomimetics and non-selective MAO inhibitors and concomitant use is contraindicated). No products indexed under this heading.

Epinephrine (Severe hypertensive reactions have followed the administration of sympathomimetics and non-selective MAO inhibitors and concomitant use is contraindicated). Products include:
EpiPen 3631
Twinject 3268

Epinephrine Bitartrate (Severe hypertensive reactions have followed the administration of sympathomimetics and non-selective MAO inhibitors and concomitant use is contraindicated). No products indexed under this heading.

Epinephrine Hydrochloride (Severe hypertensive reactions have followed the administration of sympathomimetics and non-selective MAO inhibitors and concomitant use is contraindicated). No products indexed under this heading.

Escitalopram Oxalate (Severe CNS toxicity associated with hyperpyrexia and death has been reported with the combination of selective serotonin reuptake inhibitors (SSRIs) and non-selective MAOIs or selective MAO-B inhibitors. Because the mechanisms of these reactions are not fully understood, the combination of rasagiline with SSRI antidepressants should be avoided. At least 14 days should elapse between discontinuation of rasagiline and initiation of treatment with a SSRI antidepressant. Because of the long half lives offluoxetine and its active metabolite, at least five weeks (perhaps longer, especially if fluoxetine has been prescribed chronically and/or at higher doses) should elapse between discontinuation of fluoxetine and inititation of rasagiline). Products include:
Lexapro Oral Suspension 1160
Lexapro Tablets 1160

Esomeprazole Magnesium (Rasagiline plasma concentrations may increase up to 2 fold in patients using concomitant CYP1A2 inhibitors). Products include:
Nexium Capsules 704
Nexium Oral Suspension 704

Esomeprazole Sodium (Rasagiline plasma concentrations may increase up to 2 fold in patients using concomitant CYP1A2 inhibitors). Products include:
Nexium I.V. 712

Ethinyl Estradiol (Rasagiline plasma concentrations may increase up to 2 fold in patients using concomitant CYP1A2 inhibitors). Products include:
LoSeasonique 3407
Lybrel 3514
NuvaRing 3181
Ortho Evra 2648
Ortho-Cyclen/Ortho Tri-Cyclen 2663
Ortho Tri-Cyclen Lo Tablets 2673
Seasonique 3418
Yaz 864

Fluoxetine (Severe CNS toxicity associated with hyperpyrexia and death has been reported with the combination of selective serotonin reuptake inhibitors (SSRIs) and non-selective MAOIs or selective MAO-B inhibitors. Because the mechanisms of these reactions are not fully understood, the combination of rasagiline with SSRI antidepressants should be avoided. At least 14 days should elapse between discontinuation of rasagiline and initiation of treatment with a SSRI antidepressant. Because of the long half lives offluoxetine and its active metabolite, at least five weeks (perhaps longer, especially if fluoxetine has been prescribed chronically and/or

IMPORTANT NOTE: Always consult each drug listing in the patient's regimen for possible interactions.

Azilect Interactions Index 208

at higher doses) should elapse between discontinuation of fluoxetine and inititation of rasagiline).
No products indexed under this heading.

Fluoxetine Hydrochloride (Severe CNS toxicity associated with hyperpyrexia and death has been reported with the combination of selective serotonin reuptake inhibitors (SSRIs) and non-selective MAOIs or selective MAO-B inhibitors. Because the mechanisms of these reactions are not fully understood, the combination of rasagiline with SSRI antidepressants should be avoided. At least 14 days should elapse between discontinuation of rasagiline and initiation of treatment with a SSRI antidepressant. Because of the long half lives offluoxetine and its active metabolite, at least five weeks (perhaps longer, especially if fluoxetine has been prescribed chronically and/or at higher doses) should elapse between discontinuation of fluoxetine and inititation of rasagiline). Products include:
Prozac Weekly 1941
Prozac Pulvules 1941
Symbyax 1965

Fluvoxamine (Severe CNS toxicity associated with hyperpyrexia and death has been reported with the combination of selective serotonin reuptake inhibitors (SSRIs) and non-selective MAOIs or selective MAO-B inhibitors. Because the mechanisms of these reactions are not fully understood, the combination of rasagiline with SSRI antidepressants should be avoided. At least 14 days should elapse between discontinuation of rasagiline and initiation of treatment with a SSRI antidepressant. Because of the long half lives offluoxetine and its active metabolite, at least five weeks (perhaps longer, especially if fluoxetine has been prescribed chronically and/or at higher doses) should elapse between discontinuation of fluoxetine and inititation of rasagiline).
No products indexed under this heading.

Fluvoxamine Maleate (Severe CNS toxicity associated with hyperpyrexia and death has been reported with the combination of selective serotonin reuptake inhibitors (SSRIs) and non-selective MAOIs or selective MAO-B inhibitors. Because the mechanisms of these reactions are not fully understood, the combination of rasagiline with SSRI antidepressants should be avoided. At least 14 days should elapse between discontinuation of rasagiline and initiation of treatment with a SSRI antidepressant. Because of the long half lives offluoxetine and its active metabolite, at least five weeks (perhaps longer, especially if fluoxetine has been prescribed chronically and/or at higher doses) should elapse between discontinuation of fluoxetine and inititation of rasagiline).
No products indexed under this heading.

Gatifloxacin (Rasagiline plasma concentrations may increase up to 2 fold in patients using concomitant CYP1A2 inhibitors).
No products indexed under this heading.

Gemifloxacin Mesylate (Rasagiline plasma concentrations may increase up to 2 fold in patients using concomitant CYP1A2 inhibitors).
No products indexed under this heading.

Grepafloxacin Hydrochloride (Rasagiline plasma concentrations may increase up to 2 fold in patients using concomitant CYP1A2 inhibitors).
No products indexed under this heading.

Hypericum (Rasagiline is contraindicated for use with St. John's wort).
No products indexed under this heading.

Hypericum Perforatum (Rasagiline is contraindicated for use with St. John's wort). Products include:
Traumeel 1800

Imipramine Hydrochloride (Severe CNS toxicity associated with hyperpyrexia and death has been reported with the combination of tricyclic antidepressants (TCAs) and non-selective MAOIs or selective MAO-B inhibitors. Because the mechanisms of these reactions are not fully understood, the combination of rasagiline with TCAs should be avoided. At least 14 days should elapse between discontinuation of rasagiline and initiation of treatment with a TCA).
No products indexed under this heading.

Imipramine Pamoate (Severe CNS toxicity associated with hyperpyrexia and death has been reported with the combination of tricyclic antidepressants (TCAs) and non-selective MAOIs or selective MAO-B inhibitors. Because the mechanisms of these reactions are not fully understood, the combination of rasagiline with TCAs should be avoided. At least 14 days should elapse between discontinuation of rasagiline and initiation of treatment with a TCA).
No products indexed under this heading.

Isocarboxazid (Rasagiline should not be administered along with other MAO inhibitors because of the increased risk of non-selective MAO inhibition that may lead to a hypertensive crisis. At least 14 days should elapse between discontinuation of rasagiline and initiation of treatment with MAO inhibitors).
Products include:
Marplan 3481

Isoniazid (Rasagiline plasma concentrations may increase up to 2 fold in patients using concomitant CYP1A2 inhibitors).
No products indexed under this heading.

Isoproterenol Hydrochloride (Severe hypertensive reactions have followed the administration of sympathomimetics and non-selective MAO inhibitors and concomitant use is contraindicated).
No products indexed under this heading.

Isoproterenol Sulfate (Severe hypertensive reactions have followed the administration of sympathomimetics and non-selective MAO inhibitors and concomitant use is contraindicated).
No products indexed under this heading.

Ketoconazole (Rasagiline plasma concentrations may increase up to 2 fold in patients using concomitant CYP1A2 inhibitors). Products include:
Extina 3319
Xolegel 3337

Levalbuterol Hydrochloride (Severe hypertensive reactions have followed the administration of sympathomimetics and non-selective MAO inhibitors and concomitant use is contraindicated).
No products indexed under this heading.

Levofloxacin (Rasagiline plasma concentrations may increase up to 2 fold in patients using concomitant CYP1A2 inhibitors). Products include:
Iquix 3492
Levaquin 2629
Levaquin in 5% Dextrose 2629
Quixin 3493

Levonorgestrel (Rasagiline plasma concentrations may increase up to 2 fold in patients using concomitant CYP1A2 inhibitors). Products include:
Climara Pro 847
LoSeasonique 3407
Lybrel 3514
Mirena 854
Plan B 3416
Seasonique 3418

Lomefloxacin Hydrochloride (Rasagiline plasma concentrations may increase up to 2 fold in patients using concomitant CYP1A2 inhibitors).
No products indexed under this heading.

Maprotiline Hydrochloride (Severe CNS toxicity associated with hyperpyrexia and death has been reported with the combination of tricyclic antidepressants (TCAs) and non-selective MAOIs or selective MAO-B inhibitors. Because the mechanisms of these reactions are not fully understood, the combination of rasagiline with TCAs should be avoided. At least 14 days should elapse between discontinuation of rasagiline and initiation of treatment with a TCA).
No products indexed under this heading.

Meperidine Hydrochloride (Serious, sometimes fatal reactions have been precipitated with concomitant use of meperidine and MAO inhibitors and concomitant use is contraindicated).
No products indexed under this heading.

Mestranol (Rasagiline plasma concentrations may increase up to 2 fold in patients using concomitant CYP1A2 inhibitors).
No products indexed under this heading.

Metaproterenol Sulfate (Severe hypertensive reactions have followed the administration of sympathomimetics and non-selective MAO inhibitors and concomitant use is contraindicated).
No products indexed under this heading.

Metaraminol Bitartrate (Severe hypertensive reactions have followed the administration of sympathomimetics and non-selective MAO inhibitors and concomitant use is contraindicated).
No products indexed under this heading.

Methadone Hydrochloride (Serious, sometimes fatal reactions have been precipitated with concomitant use of methadone and MAO inhibitors and concomitant use is contraindicated).
No products indexed under this heading.

Methoxamine Hydrochloride (Severe hypertensive reactions have followed the administration of sympathomimetics and non-selective MAO inhibitors and concomitant use is contraindicated).
No products indexed under this heading.

Methoxsalen (Rasagiline plasma concentrations may increase up to 2 fold in patients using concomitant CYP1A2 inhibitors).
No products indexed under this heading.

Mexiletine Hydrochloride (Rasagiline plasma concentrations may increase up to 2 fold in patients using concomitant CYP1A2 inhibitors).
No products indexed under this heading.

Mibefradil Dihydrochloride (Rasagiline plasma concentrations may increase up to 2 fold in patients using concomitant CYP1A2 inhibitors).
No products indexed under this heading.

Mirtazapine (Rasagiline is contraindicated for use with mirtazapine).
Products include:
Remeron Tablets 3214
RemeronSolTab Tablets 3219

Moclobemide (Rasagiline should not be administered along with other MAO inhibitors because of the increased risk of non-selective MAO inhibition that may lead to a hypertensive crisis. At least 14 days should elapse between discontinuation of rasagiline and initiation of treatment with MAO inhibitors).
No products indexed under this heading.

Moxifloxacin Hydrochloride (Rasagiline plasma concentrations may increase up to 2 fold in patients using concomitant CYP1A2 inhibitors).
Products include:
Avelox 3064
Vigamox 589

Nalidixic Acid (Rasagiline plasma concentrations may increase up to 2 fold in patients using concomitant CYP1A2 inhibitors).
No products indexed under this heading.

Nefazodone Hydrochloride (Severe CNS toxicity associated with hyperpyrexia and death has been reported with the combination of serotonin-norepinephrine reuptake inhibitors (SNRIs) and non-selective MAOIs or selective MAO-B inhibitors. Furthermore, because the mechanisms of these reactions are not fully understood, it seems prudent, in general, to avoid the combination of rasagiline with SNRI antidepressants. At least 14 days should elapse between discontinuation of rasagiline and initiation of treatment with a SNRI antidepressant).
No products indexed under this heading.

Norepinephrine Bitartrate (Severe hypertensive reactions have followed the administration of sympathomimetics and non-selective MAO inhibitors and concomitant use is contraindicated).
No products indexed under this heading.

Norethindrone (Rasagiline plasma concentrations may increase up to 2 fold in patients using concomitant CYP1A2 inhibitors). Products include:
Ortho Micronor 2660

Norethindrone Acetate (Rasagiline plasma concentrations may increase up to 2 fold in patients using concomitant CYP1A2 inhibitors). Products include:
Activella 2561

Norfloxacin (Rasagiline plasma concentrations may increase up to 2 fold in patients using concomitant CYP1A2 inhibitors). Products include:
Noroxin 2220

Norgestrel (Rasagiline plasma concentrations may increase up to 2 fold in patients using concomitant CYP1A2 inhibitors).
No products indexed under this heading.

Nortriptyline Hydrochloride (Severe CNS toxicity associated with hyperpyrexia and death has been reported with the combination of tricyclic antidepressants (TCAs) and non-selective MAOIs or selective MAO-B inhibitors. Because the mechanisms of these reactions are not fully understood, the combination of rasagiline with TCAs should be avoided. At least 14 days should elapse between discontinuation of rasagiline and initiation of treatment with a TCA).
No products indexed under this heading.

Ofloxacin (Rasagiline plasma concentrations may increase up to 2 fold in patients using concomitant CYP1A2 inhibitors).
No products indexed under this heading.

Omeprazole (Rasagiline plasma concentrations may increase up to 2 fold in patients using concomitant CYP1A2 inhibitors).
No products indexed under this heading.

Omeprazole Magnesium (Rasagiline plasma concentrations may increase up to 2 fold in patients using concomitant CYP1A2 inhibitors).
No products indexed under this heading.

Pargyline Hydrochloride (Rasagiline should not be administered along with other MAO inhibitors because of the increased risk of non-selective MAO inhibition that may lead to a hypertensive crisis. At least 14 days should elapse between discontinuation of rasagiline and initiation of treatment with MAO inhibitors).
No products indexed under this heading.

Paroxetine (Severe CNS toxicity associated with hyperpyrexia and death has been reported with the combination of selective serotonin reuptake inhibitors (SSRIs) and non-selective MAOIs or selective MAO-B inhibitors. Because the mechanisms of these reactions are not fully understood, the combination of rasagiline with SSRI antidepressants should be avoided. At least 14 days

(⊙ Described in PDR® for Ophthalmic Medicines)

should elapse between discontinuation of rasagiline and initiation of treatment with a SSRI antidepressant. Because of the long half lives offluoxetine and its active metabolite, at least five weeks (perhaps longer, especially if fluoxetine has been prescribed chronically and/or at higher doses) should elapse between discontinuation of fluoxetine and initiation of rasagiline).
No products indexed under this heading.

Paroxetine Hydrochloride (Severe CNS toxicity associated with hyperpyrexia and death has been reported with the combination of selective serotonin reuptake inhibitors (SSRIs) and non-selective MAOIs or selective MAO-B inhibitors. Because the mechanisms of these reactions are not fully understood, the combination of rasagiline with SSRI antidepressants should be avoided. At least 14 days should elapse between discontinuation of rasagiline and initiation of treatment with a SSRI antidepressant. Because of the long half lives offluoxetine and its active metabolite, at least five weeks (perhaps longer, especially if fluoxetine has been prescribed chronically and/or at higher doses) should elapse between discontinuation of fluoxetine and inititation of rasagiline). Products include:

Paroxetine Mesylate (Severe CNS toxicity associated with hyperpyrexia and death has been reported with the combination of selective serotonin reuptake inhibitors (SSRIs) and non-selective MAOIs or selective MAO-B inhibitors. Because the mechanisms of these reactions are not fully understood, the combination of rasagiline with SSRI antidepressants should be avoided. At least 14 days should elapse between discontinuation of rasagiline and initiation of treatment with a SSRI antidepressant. Because of the long half lives offluoxetine and its active metabolite, at least five weeks (perhaps longer, especially if fluoxetine has been prescribed chronically and/or at higher doses) should elapse between discontinuation of fluoxetine and inititation of rasagiline).
No products indexed under this heading.

Phenelzine Sulfate (Rasagiline should not be administered along with other MAO inhibitors because of the increased risk of non-selective MAO inhibition that may lead to a hypertensive crisis. At least 14 days should elapse between discontinuation of rasagiline and initiation of treatment with MAO inhibitors).
No products indexed under this heading.

Phenylephrine Bitartrate (Severe hypertensive reactions have followed the administration of sympathomimetics and non-selective MAO inhibitors and concomitant use is contraindicated).
No products indexed under this heading.

Phenylephrine Hydrochloride (Severe hypertensive reactions have followed the administration of sympathomimetics and non-selective MAO inhibitors and concomitant use is contraindicated). Products include:

Phenylephrine Tannate (Severe hypertensive reactions have followed the administration of sympathomimetics and non-selective MAO inhibitors and concomitant use is contraindicated).
No products indexed under this heading.

Phenylpropanolamine Hydrochloride (Severe hypertensive reactions have followed the administration of sympathomimetics and non-selective MAO inhibitors and concomitant use is contraindicated).
No products indexed under this heading.

Pirbuterol Acetate (Severe hypertensive reactions have followed the administration of sympathomimetics and non-selective MAO inhibitors and concomitant use is contraindicated). Products include:

Procarbazine Hydrochloride (Rasagiline should not be administered along with other MAO inhibitors because of the increased risk of non-selective MAO inhibition that may lead to a hypertensive crisis. At least 14 days should elapse between discontinuation of rasagiline and initiation of treatment with MAO inhibitors).
No products indexed under this heading.

Protriptyline Hydrochloride (Severe CNS toxicity associated with hyperpyrexia and death has been reported with the combination of tricyclic antidepressants (TCAs) and non-selective MAOIs or selective MAO-B inhibitors. Because the mechanisms of these reactions are not fully understood, the combination of rasagiline with TCAs should be avoided. At least 14 days should elapse between discontinuation of rasagiline and initiation of treatment with a TCA).
No products indexed under this heading.

Pseudoephedrine Hydrochloride (Severe hypertensive reactions have followed the administration of sympathomimetics and non-selective MAO inhibitors and concomitant use is contraindicated). Products include:

Pseudoephedrine Sulfate (Severe hypertensive reactions have followed the administration of sympathomimetics and non-selective MAO inhibitors and concomitant use is contraindicated). Products include:

Ranitidine Bismuth Citrate (Rasagiline plasma concentrations may increase up to 2 fold in patients using concomitant CYP1A2 inhibitors).
No products indexed under this heading.

Ranitidine Hydrochloride (Rasagiline plasma concentrations may increase up to 2 fold in patients using concomitant CYP1A2 inhibitors). Products include:

Ritonavir (Rasagiline plasma concentrations may increase up to 2 fold in patients using concomitant CYP1A2 inhibitors). Products include:

Salmeterol Xinafoate (Severe hypertensive reactions have followed the administration of sympathomimetics and non-selective MAO inhibitors and concomitant use is contraindicated). Products include:

Selegiline (Rasagiline should not be administered along with other MAO inhibitors because of the increased risk of non-selective MAO inhibition that may lead to a hypertensive crisis. At least 14 days should elapse between discontinuation of rasagiline and initiation of treatment with MAO inhibitors). Products include:

Selegiline Hydrochloride (Rasagiline should not be administered along with other MAO inhibitors because of the increased risk of non-selective MAO inhibition that may lead to a hypertensive crisis. At least 14 days should elapse between discontinuation of rasagiline and initiation of treatment with MAO inhibitors). Products include:

Sertraline Hydrochloride (Severe CNS toxicity associated with hyperpyrexia and death has been reported with the combination of selective serotonin reuptake inhibitors (SSRIs) and non-selective MAOIs or selective MAO-B inhibitors. Because the mechanisms of these reactions are not fully understood, the combination of rasagiline with SSRI antidepressants should be avoided. At least 14 days should elapse between discontinuation of rasagiline and initiation of treatment with a SSRI antidepressant. Because of the long half lives offluoxetine and its active metabolite, at least five weeks (perhaps longer, especially if fluoxetine has been prescribed chronically and/or at higher doses) should elapse between discontinuation of fluoxetine and inititation of rasagiline).
No products indexed under this heading.

Sildenafil Citrate (Rasagiline plasma concentrations may increase up to 2 fold in patients using concomitant CYP1A2 inhibitors).
No products indexed under this heading.

Sparfloxacin (Rasagiline plasma concentrations may increase up to 2 fold in patients using concomitant CYP1A2 inhibitors).
No products indexed under this heading.

Tacrine Hydrochloride (Rasagiline plasma concentrations may increase up to 2 fold in patients using concomitant CYP1A2 inhibitors).
No products indexed under this heading.

Terbutaline Sulfate (Severe hypertensive reactions have followed the administration of sympathomimetics and non-selective MAO inhibitors and concomitant use is contraindicated).
No products indexed under this heading.

Ticlopidine Hydrochloride (Rasagiline plasma concentrations may increase up to 2 fold in patients using concomitant CYP1A2 inhibitors).
No products indexed under this heading.

Tramadol Hydrochloride (Serious, sometimes fatal reactions have been precipitated with concomitant use of tramadol and MAO inhibitors and concomitant use is contraindicated). Products include:

Tranylcypromine Sulfate (Rasagiline should not be administered along with other MAO inhibitors because of the increased risk of non-selective MAO inhibition that may lead to a hypertensive crisis. At least 14 days should elapse between discontinuation of rasagiline and initiation of treatment with MAO inhibitors). Products include:

Trimipramine Maleate (Severe CNS toxicity associated with hyperpyrexia and death has been reported with the combination of tricyclic antidepressants (TCAs) and non-selective MAOIs or selective MAO-B inhibitors. Because the

mechanisms of these reactions are not fully understood, the combination of rasagiline with TCAs should be avoided. At least 14 days should elapse between discontinuation of rasagiline and initiation of treatment with a TCA).
No products indexed under this heading.

Troleandomycin (Rasagiline plasma concentrations may increase up to 2 fold in patients using concomitant CYP1A2 inhibitors).
No products indexed under this heading.

Trovafloxacin Mesylate (Rasagiline plasma concentrations may increase up to 2 fold in patients using concomitant CYP1A2 inhibitors).
No products indexed under this heading.

Vardenafil Hydrochloride (Rasagiline plasma concentrations may increase up to 2 fold in patients using concomitant CYP1A2 inhibitors). Products include:

Venlafaxine Hydrochloride (Severe CNS toxicity associated with hyperpyrexia and death has been reported with the combination of serotonin-norepinephrine reuptake inhibitors (SNRIs) and non-selective MAOIs or selective MAO-B inhibitors. Furthermore, because the mechanisms of these reactions are not fully understood, it seems prudent, in general, to avoid the combination of rasagiline with SNRI antidepressants. At least 14 days should elapse between discontinuation of rasagiline and initiation of treatment with a SNRI antidepressant). Products include:

Zileuton (Rasagiline plasma concentrations may increase up to 2 fold in patients using concomitant CYP1A2 inhibitors).
No products indexed under this heading.

Food Interactions

Beverages with high tyramine (Severe hypertensive reactions have followed the administration of tyramine rich beverages and non-selective MAO inhibitors).

Food high in tyramine (Severe hypertensive reactions have followed the administration of tyramine rich foods and non-selective MAO inhibitors).

Grapefruit (Rasagiline plasma concentrations may increase up to 2 fold in patients using concomitant CYP1A2 inhibitors).

Grapefruit Juice (Rasagiline plasma concentrations may increase up to 2 fold in patients using concomitant CYP1A2 inhibitors).

AZMACORT INHALATION AEROSOL

(Triamcinolone Acetonide) 408

Prednisone (Potential for increased likelihood of HPA suppression).
No products indexed under this heading.

AZOPT OPHTHALMIC SUSPENSION

(Brinzolamide) ....○201
None cited in PDR database.

AZOR TABLETS

(Amlodipine Besylate, Olmesartan Medoxomil).. 1010
None cited in PDR database.

BACTROBAN CREAM

(Mupirocin Calcium) 1383
None cited in PDR database.

BACTROBAN NASAL

(Mupirocin Calcium) 1384
None cited in PDR database.

IMPORTANT NOTE: Always consult each drug listing in the patient's regimen for possible interactions.

Bactroban Ointment Interactions Index 210

BACTROBAN OINTMENT

(Mupirocin) 1385
None cited in PDR database.

BANZEL TABLETS

(Rufinamide) 1050
May interact with cytochrome p450 3a4 substrates (selected), oral contraceptives, phenytoin, and certain other agents. Compounds in these categories include:

Alfentanil Hydrochloride (Rufinamide is a weak inducer of the CYP3A4 enzyme and can decrease exposure of drugs that are substrates of CYP3A4).
No products indexed under this heading.

Alprazolam (Rufinamide is a weak inducer of the CYP3A4 enzyme and can decrease exposure of drugs that are substrates of CYP3A4).
No products indexed under this heading.

Amiodarone Hydrochloride (Rufinamide is a weak inducer of the CYP3A4 enzyme and can decrease exposure of drugs that are substrates of CYP3A4).
No products indexed under this heading.

Amitriptyline Hydrochloride (Rufinamide is a weak inducer of the CYP3A4 enzyme and can decrease exposure of drugs that are substrates of CYP3A4).
No products indexed under this heading.

Amlodipine Besylate (Rufinamide is a weak inducer of the CYP3A4 enzyme and can decrease exposure of drugs that are substrates of CYP3A4).
Products include:
Azor 1010
Exforge 2443
Exforge HCT 2449

Aprepitant (Rufinamide is a weak inducer of the CYP3A4 enzyme and can decrease exposure of drugs that are substrates of CYP3A4). Products include:
Emend 2124

Astemizole (Rufinamide is a weak inducer of the CYP3A4 enzyme and can decrease exposure of drugs that are substrates of CYP3A4).
No products indexed under this heading.

Atorvastatin Calcium (Rufinamide is a weak inducer of the CYP3A4 enzyme and can decrease exposure of drugs that are substrates of CYP3A4).
Products include:
Lipitor 2703

Belladonna Ergotamine (Rufinamide is a weak inducer of the CYP3A4 enzyme and can decrease exposure of drugs that are substrates of CYP3A4).
No products indexed under this heading.

Buspirone Hydrochloride (Rufinamide is a weak inducer of the CYP3A4 enzyme and can decrease exposure of drugs that are substrates of CYP3A4).
No products indexed under this heading.

Busulfan (Rufinamide is a weak inducer of the CYP3A4 enzyme and can decrease exposure of drugs that are substrates of CYP3A4). Products include:
Myleran 1581

Carbamazepine (Co-administration of carbamazepine and rufinamide led to a decrease of plasma concentration by 7% to 13% and a decrease plasma concentration of rufinamide by 19 to 26% dependent on dose of carbamazepine).
Products include:
Carbatrol 3280
Equetro 3477

Cerivastatin Sodium (Rufinamide is a weak inducer of the CYP3A4 enzyme and can decrease exposure of drugs that are substrates of CYP3A4).
No products indexed under this heading.

Chlorpheniramine (Rufinamide is a weak inducer of the CYP3A4 enzyme and can decrease exposure of drugs that are substrates of CYP3A4).
No products indexed under this heading.

Chlorpheniramine Maleate (Rufinamide is a weak inducer of the CYP3A4 enzyme and can decrease exposure of drugs that are substrates of CYP3A4).
No products indexed under this heading.

Chlorpheniramine Polistirex (Rufinamide is a weak inducer of the CYP3A4 enzyme and can decrease exposure of drugs that are substrates of CYP3A4). Products include:
Tussionex 3443

Chlorpheniramine Tannate (Rufinamide is a weak inducer of the CYP3A4 enzyme and can decrease exposure of drugs that are substrates of CYP3A4).
No products indexed under this heading.

Chlorzoxazone (Drugs that are substrates of CYP 2E1 (eg, chlorzoxazone) may have increased plasma levels in the presence of rufinamide, but this has not been studied).
No products indexed under this heading.

Cisapride (Rufinamide is a weak inducer of the CYP3A4 enzyme and can decrease exposure of drugs that are substrates of CYP3A4).
No products indexed under this heading.

Clarithromycin (Rufinamide is a weak inducer of the CYP3A4 enzyme and can decrease exposure of drugs that are substrates of CYP3A4). Products include:
Biaxin/Biaxin XL 412

Cyclosporine (Rufinamide is a weak inducer of the CYP3A4 enzyme and can decrease exposure of drugs that are substrates of CYP3A4). Products include:
Gengraf 440
Neoral Oral Solution 2496
Neoral Capsules 2496
Restasis 605

Desogestrel (Co-administration of rufinamide (800 mg BID for 14 days) and Ortho-Novum 1/35® resulted in a mean decrease in the ethinyl estradiol AUC0-24 of 22% and C_{max} by 18% and norethindrone AUC_{0-24} by 14% and C_{max} by 18%, respectively. The clinical significance of this decrease is unknown. Female patients of childbearing age should be warned that the concurrent use of rufinamide with hormonal contraceptives may render this method of contraception less effective. Additional non-hormonal forms of contraception are recommended when using rufinamide).
No products indexed under this heading.

Diazepam (Rufinamide is a weak inducer of the CYP3A4 enzyme and can decrease exposure of drugs that are substrates of CYP3A4). Products include:
Valium Tablets 2880

Dihydroergotamine Mesylate (Rufinamide is a weak inducer of the CYP3A4 enzyme and can decrease exposure of drugs that are substrates of CYP3A4).
No products indexed under this heading.

Diltiazem Hydrochloride (Rufinamide is a weak inducer of the CYP3A4 enzyme and can decrease exposure of drugs that are substrates of CYP3A4).
Products include:
Cardizem LA 423

Diltiazem Maleate (Rufinamide is a weak inducer of the CYP3A4 enzyme and can decrease exposure of drugs that are substrates of CYP3A4).
No products indexed under this heading.

Disopyramide (Rufinamide is a weak inducer of the CYP3A4 enzyme and can decrease exposure of drugs that are substrates of CYP3A4).
No products indexed under this heading.

Disopyramide Phosphate (Rufinamide is a weak inducer of the CYP3A4 enzyme and can decrease exposure of drugs that are substrates of CYP3A4).
No products indexed under this heading.

Disulfiram (Rufinamide is a weak inducer of the CYP3A4 enzyme and can decrease exposure of drugs that are substrates of CYP3A4).
No products indexed under this heading.

Doxorubicin Hydrochloride (Rufinamide is a weak inducer of the CYP3A4 enzyme and can decrease exposure of drugs that are substrates of CYP3A4).
No products indexed under this heading.

Dronabinol (Rufinamide is a weak inducer of the CYP3A4 enzyme and can decrease exposure of drugs that are substrates of CYP3A4).
No products indexed under this heading.

Ergotamine Tartrate (Rufinamide is a weak inducer of the CYP3A4 enzyme and can decrease exposure of drugs that are substrates of CYP3A4).
No products indexed under this heading.

Erythromycin (Rufinamide is a weak inducer of the CYP3A4 enzyme and can decrease exposure of drugs that are substrates of CYP3A4).
No products indexed under this heading.

Erythromycin Estolate (Rufinamide is a weak inducer of the CYP3A4 enzyme and can decrease exposure of drugs that are substrates of CYP3A4).
No products indexed under this heading.

Erythromycin Ethylsuccinate (Rufinamide is a weak inducer of the CYP3A4 enzyme and can decrease exposure of drugs that are substrates of CYP3A4). Products include:
E.E.S. 437
EryPed 435

Erythromycin Gluceptate (Rufinamide is a weak inducer of the CYP3A4 enzyme and can decrease exposure of drugs that are substrates of CYP3A4).
No products indexed under this heading.

Erythromycin Lactobionate (Rufinamide is a weak inducer of the CYP3A4 enzyme and can decrease exposure of drugs that are substrates of CYP3A4).
No products indexed under this heading.

Erythromycin Stearate (Rufinamide is a weak inducer of the CYP3A4 enzyme and can decrease exposure of drugs that are substrates of CYP3A4).
No products indexed under this heading.

Estradiol (Rufinamide is a weak inducer of the CYP3A4 enzyme and can decrease exposure of drugs that are substrates of CYP3A4). Products include:
Activella 2561
Angeliq 831
Climara 841
Climara Pro 847
Divigel 3467
Estrasorb 1777
Vagifem 2589

Estradiol Benzoate (Rufinamide is a weak inducer of the CYP3A4 enzyme and can decrease exposure of drugs that are substrates of CYP3A4).
No products indexed under this heading.

Estradiol Cypionate (Rufinamide is a weak inducer of the CYP3A4 enzyme and can decrease exposure of drugs that are substrates of CYP3A4).
No products indexed under this heading.

Estradiol Valerate (Rufinamide is a weak inducer of the CYP3A4 enzyme and can decrease exposure of drugs that are substrates of CYP3A4).
No products indexed under this heading.

Ethinyl Estradiol (Co-administration of rufinamide (800 mg BID for 14 days) and Ortho-Novum 1/35® resulted in a mean decrease in the ethinyl estradiol AUC0-24 of 22% and C_{max} by 18% and norethindrone AUC_{0-24} by 14% and C_{max} by 18%, respectively. The clinical significance of this decrease is unknown. Female patients of childbearing age should be warned that the concurrent use of rufinamide with hormonal contraceptives may render this method of contraception less effective. Additional non-hormonal forms of contraception are recommended when using rufinamide). Products include:
LoSeasonique 3407
Lybrel 3514
NuvaRing 3181
Ortho Evra 2648
Ortho-Cyclen/Ortho Tri-Cyclen 2663
Ortho Tri-Cyclen Lo Tablets 2673
Seasonique 3418
Yaz 864

Ethosuximide (Rufinamide is a weak inducer of the CYP3A4 enzyme and can decrease exposure of drugs that are substrates of CYP3A4).
No products indexed under this heading.

Ethynodiol Diacetate (Co-administration of rufinamide (800 mg BID for 14 days) and Ortho-Novum 1/35® resulted in a mean decrease in the ethinyl estradiol AUC0-24 of 22% and C_{max} by 18% and norethindrone AUC_{0-24} by 14% and C_{max} by 18%, respectively. The clinical significance of this decrease is unknown. Female patients of childbearing age should be warned that the concurrent use of rufinamide with hormonal contraceptives may render this method of contraception less effective. Additional non-hormonal forms of contraception are recommended when using rufinamide).
No products indexed under this heading.

Etoposide (Rufinamide is a weak inducer of the CYP3A4 enzyme and can decrease exposure of drugs that are substrates of CYP3A4).
No products indexed under this heading.

Etoposide Phosphate (Rufinamide is a weak inducer of the CYP3A4 enzyme and can decrease exposure of drugs that are substrates of CYP3A4).
No products indexed under this heading.

Felodipine (Rufinamide is a weak inducer of the CYP3A4 enzyme and can decrease exposure of drugs that are substrates of CYP3A4).
No products indexed under this heading.

Fentanyl (Rufinamide is a weak inducer of the CYP3A4 enzyme and can decrease exposure of drugs that are substrates of CYP3A4). Products include:
Duragesic 2604
Fentanyl Transdermal System 2346
Onsolis 2054

Fentanyl Citrate (Rufinamide is a weak inducer of the CYP3A4 enzyme and can decrease exposure of drugs that are substrates of CYP3A4).
Products include:
Fentora 966

Fosphenytoin (The decrease in clearance of phenytoin estimated at typical levels of rufinamide (Cavss 15 ug/mL) is predicted to increase plasma levels of phenytoin by 7% to 21%. The concentration of rufinamide with antiepileptic drugs is predicted to decrease by 25% to 46% independent of dose or concentration of phenytoin).
No products indexed under this heading.

(⊙ Described in PDR® for Ophthalmic Medicines)

Fosphenytoin Sodium (The decrease in clearance of phenytoin estimated at typical levels of rufinamide (Cavss 15 ug/mL) is predicted to increase plasma levels of phenytoin by 7% to 21%. The concentration of rufinamide with antiepileptic drugs is predicted to decrease by 25% to 46% independent of dose or concentration of phenytoin).
No products indexed under this heading.

Haloperidol (Rufinamide is a weak inducer of the CYP3A4 enzyme and can decrease exposure of drugs that are substrates of CYP3A4).
No products indexed under this heading.

Haloperidol Decanoate (Rufinamide is a weak inducer of the CYP3A4 enzyme and can decrease exposure of drugs that are substrates of CYP3A4).
No products indexed under this heading.

Haloperidol Lactate (Rufinamide is a weak inducer of the CYP3A4 enzyme and can decrease exposure of drugs that are substrates of CYP3A4).
No products indexed under this heading.

Indinavir Sulfate (Rufinamide is a weak inducer of the CYP3A4 enzyme and can decrease exposure of drugs that are substrates of CYP3A4).
Products include:

Isradipine (Rufinamide is a weak inducer of the CYP3A4 enzyme and can decrease exposure of drugs that are substrates of CYP3A4). Products include:

Itraconazole (Rufinamide is a weak inducer of the CYP3A4 enzyme and can decrease exposure of drugs that are substrates of CYP3A4).
No products indexed under this heading.

Ixabepilone (Rufinamide is a weak inducer of the CYP3A4 enzyme and can decrease exposure of drugs that are substrates of CYP3A4).
No products indexed under this heading.

Ketoconazole (Rufinamide is a weak inducer of the CYP3A4 enzyme and can decrease exposure of drugs that are substrates of CYP3A4). Products include:

Lamotrigine (The plasma levels of lamotrigine is predicted to decrease by 7% to 13% with rufinamide). Products include:

Levonorgestrel (Co-administration of rufinamide (800 mg BID for 14 days) and Ortho-Novum 1/35® resulted in a mean decrease in the ethinyl estradiol AUC0-24 of 22% and C_{max} by 18% and norethindrone AUC_{0-24} by 14% and C_{max} by 18%, respectively. The clinical significance of this decrease is unknown. Female patients of childbearing age should be warned that the concurrent use of rufinamide with hormonal contraceptives may render this method of contraception less effective. Additional non-hormonal forms of contraception are recommended when using rufinamide). Products include:

Lidocaine (Rufinamide is a weak inducer of the CYP3A4 enzyme and can decrease exposure of drugs that are substrates of CYP3A4). Products include:

Lidocaine Hydrochloride (Rufinamide is a weak inducer of the CYP3A4 enzyme and can decrease exposure of drugs that are substrates of CYP3A4).
No products indexed under this heading.

Lovastatin (Rufinamide is a weak inducer of the CYP3A4 enzyme and can decrease exposure of drugs that are substrates of CYP3A4). Products include:

Mestranol (Co-administration of rufinamide (800 mg BID for 14 days) and Ortho-Novum 1/35® resulted in a mean decrease in the ethinyl estradiol AUC0-24 of 22% and C_{max} by 18% and norethindrone AUC_{0-24} by 14% and C_{max} by 18%, respectively. The clinical significance of this decrease is unknown. Female patients of childbearing age should be warned that the concurrent use of rufinamide with hormonal contraceptives may render this method of contraception less effective. Additional non-hormonal forms of contraception are recommended when using rufinamide).
No products indexed under this heading.

Methadone Hydrochloride (Rufinamide is a weak inducer of the CYP3A4 enzyme and can decrease exposure of drugs that are substrates of CYP3A4).
No products indexed under this heading.

Midazolam Hydrochloride (Rufinamide is a weak inducer of the CYP3A4 enzyme and can decrease exposure of drugs that are substrates of CYP3A4).
No products indexed under this heading.

Nefazodone Hydrochloride (Rufinamide is a weak inducer of the CYP3A4 enzyme and can decrease exposure of drugs that are substrates of CYP3A4).
No products indexed under this heading.

Nelfinavir Mesylate (Rufinamide is a weak inducer of the CYP3A4 enzyme and can decrease exposure of drugs that are substrates of CYP3A4).
No products indexed under this heading.

Nicardipine (Rufinamide is a weak inducer of the CYP3A4 enzyme and can decrease exposure of drugs that are substrates of CYP3A4).
No products indexed under this heading.

Nicardipine Hydrochloride (Rufinamide is a weak inducer of the CYP3A4 enzyme and can decrease exposure of drugs that are substrates of CYP3A4).
No products indexed under this heading.

Nifedipine (Rufinamide is a weak inducer of the CYP3A4 enzyme and can decrease exposure of drugs that are substrates of CYP3A4).
No products indexed under this heading.

Nimodipine (Rufinamide is a weak inducer of the CYP3A4 enzyme and can decrease exposure of drugs that are substrates of CYP3A4).
No products indexed under this heading.

Nisoldipine (Rufinamide is a weak inducer of the CYP3A4 enzyme and can decrease exposure of drugs that are substrates of CYP3A4).
No products indexed under this heading.

Nitrendipine (Rufinamide is a weak inducer of the CYP3A4 enzyme and can decrease exposure of drugs that are substrates of CYP3A4).
No products indexed under this heading.

Norethindrone (Co-administration of rufinamide (800 mg BID for 14 days) and Ortho-Novum 1/35® resulted in a mean decrease in the ethinyl estradiol AUC0-24 of 22% and C_{max} by 18% and norethindrone AUC_{0-24} by 14% and C_{max} by 18%, respectively. The clinical significance of this decrease is unknown. Female patients of childbearing age should be warned that the con-

current use of rufinamide with hormonal contraceptives may render this method of contraception less effective. Additional non-hormonal forms of contraception are recommended when using rufinamide). Products include:

Norethindrone Acetate (Rufinamide is a weak inducer of the CYP3A4 enzyme and can decrease exposure of drugs that are substrates of CYP3A4). Products include:

Norethynodrel (Co-administration of rufinamide (800 mg BID for 14 days) and Ortho-Novum 1/35® resulted in a mean decrease in the ethinyl estradiol AUC0-24 of 22% and C_{max} by 18% and norethindrone AUC_{0-24} by 14% and C_{max} by 18%, respectively. The clinical significance of this decrease is unknown. Female patients of childbearing age should be warned that the concurrent use of rufinamide with hormonal contraceptives may render this method of contraception less effective. Additional non-hormonal forms of contraception are recommended when using rufinamide).
No products indexed under this heading.

Norgestimate (Co-administration of rufinamide (800 mg BID for 14 days) and Ortho-Novum 1/35® resulted in a mean decrease in the ethinyl estradiol AUC0-24 of 22% and C_{max} by 18% and norethindrone AUC_{0-24} by 14% and C_{max} by 18%, respectively. The clinical significance of this decrease is unknown. Female patients of childbearing age should be warned that the concurrent use of rufinamide with hormonal contraceptives may render this method of contraception less effective. Additional non-hormonal forms of contraception are recommended when using rufinamide). Products include:

Norgestrel (Co-administration of rufinamide (800 mg BID for 14 days) and Ortho-Novum 1/35® resulted in a mean decrease in the ethinyl estradiol AUC0-24 of 22% and C_{max} by 18% and norethindrone AUC_{0-24} by 14% and C_{max} by 18%, respectively. The clinical significance of this decrease is unknown. Female patients of childbearing age should be warned that the concurrent use of rufinamide with hormonal contraceptives may render this method of contraception less effective. Additional non-hormonal forms of contraception are recommended when using rufinamide).
No products indexed under this heading.

Ondansetron (Rufinamide is a weak inducer of the CYP3A4 enzyme and can decrease exposure of drugs that are substrates of CYP3A4).
No products indexed under this heading.

Ondansetron Hydrochloride (Rufinamide is a weak inducer of the CYP3A4 enzyme and can decrease exposure of drugs that are substrates of CYP3A4). Products include:

Paclitaxel (Rufinamide is a weak inducer of the CYP3A4 enzyme and can decrease exposure of drugs that are substrates of CYP3A4).
No products indexed under this heading.

Phenobarbital (Co-administration of phenobarbital and rufinamide led to an increase of plasma concentration by 8% to 13% and a decrease plasma concentration of rufinamide by 25% to 46% independent on dose or concentration of phenobarbital). Products include:

Phenytoin (The decrease in clearance of phenytoin estimated at typical levels of rufinamide (Cavss 15 ug/mL) is predicted to increase plasma levels of phenytoin by 7% to 21%. The concentration of rufinamide with antiepileptic drugs is predicted to decrease by 25% to 46% independent of dose or concentration of phenytoin).
No products indexed under this heading.

Phenytoin Sodium (The decrease in clearance of phenytoin estimated at typical levels of rufinamide (Cavss 15 ug/mL) is predicted to increase plasma levels of phenytoin by 7% to 21%. The concentration of rufinamide with antiepileptic drugs is predicted to decrease by 25% to 46% independent of dose or concentration of phenytoin). Products include:

Pimozide (Rufinamide is a weak inducer of the CYP3A4 enzyme and can decrease exposure of drugs that are substrates of CYP3A4).
No products indexed under this heading.

Polyestradiol Phosphate (Rufinamide is a weak inducer of the CYP3A4 enzyme and can decrease exposure of drugs that are substrates of CYP3A4).
No products indexed under this heading.

Primidone (Co-administration of primidone and rufinamide led to a decrease of plasma concentration by 25% to 46% of primidone).
No products indexed under this heading.

Quinidine Gluconate (Rufinamide is a weak inducer of the CYP3A4 enzyme and can decrease exposure of drugs that are substrates of CYP3A4).
No products indexed under this heading.

Quinidine Polygalacturonate (Rufinamide is a weak inducer of the CYP3A4 enzyme and can decrease exposure of drugs that are substrates of CYP3A4).
No products indexed under this heading.

Quinidine Sulfate (Rufinamide is a weak inducer of the CYP3A4 enzyme and can decrease exposure of drugs that are substrates of CYP3A4).
No products indexed under this heading.

Rifabutin (Rufinamide is a weak inducer of the CYP3A4 enzyme and can decrease exposure of drugs that are substrates of CYP3A4).
No products indexed under this heading.

Ritonavir (Rufinamide is a weak inducer of the CYP3A4 enzyme and can decrease exposure of drugs that are substrates of CYP3A4). Products include:

Saquinavir (Rufinamide is a weak inducer of the CYP3A4 enzyme and can decrease exposure of drugs that are substrates of CYP3A4).
No products indexed under this heading.

Saquinavir Mesylate (Rufinamide is a weak inducer of the CYP3A4 enzyme and can decrease exposure of drugs that are substrates of CYP3A4).
No products indexed under this heading.

Sertraline Hydrochloride (Rufinamide is a weak inducer of the CYP3A4 enzyme and can decrease exposure of drugs that are substrates of CYP3A4).
No products indexed under this heading.

Sildenafil Citrate (Rufinamide is a weak inducer of the CYP3A4 enzyme and can decrease exposure of drugs that are substrates of CYP3A4).
No products indexed under this heading.

Simvastatin (Rufinamide is a weak inducer of the CYP3A4 enzyme and can decrease exposure of drugs that are substrates of CYP3A4). Products include:

IMPORTANT NOTE: Always consult each drug listing in the patient's regimen for possible interactions.

Simcor **524**
Vytorin 10/10 .... **2303, 3240**
Vytorin 10/20 .... **2303, 3240**
Vytorin 10/40 .... **2303, 3240**
Vytorin 10/80 .... **2303, 3240**
Zocor **2289**

Sirolimus (Rufinamide is a weak inducer of the CYP3A4 enzyme and can decrease exposure of drugs that are substrates of CYP3A4). Products include:
Rapamune **3579**

Tacrolimus (Rufinamide is a weak inducer of the CYP3A4 enzyme and can decrease exposure of drugs that are substrates of CYP3A4). Products include:
Prograf Capsules **677**
Prograf Injection **677**
Protopic **685**

Tadalafil (Rufinamide is a weak inducer of the CYP3A4 enzyme and can decrease exposure of drugs that are substrates of CYP3A4). Products include:
Adcirca **3461**
Cialis **1861**

Tamoxifen Citrate (Rufinamide is a weak inducer of the CYP3A4 enzyme and can decrease exposure of drugs that are substrates of CYP3A4).
No products indexed under this heading.

Terfenadine (Rufinamide is a weak inducer of the CYP3A4 enzyme and can decrease exposure of drugs that are substrates of CYP3A4).
No products indexed under this heading.

Theophylline (Rufinamide is a weak inducer of the CYP3A4 enzyme and can decrease exposure of drugs that are substrates of CYP3A4).
No products indexed under this heading.

Theophylline Anhydrous (Rufinamide is a weak inducer of the CYP3A4 enzyme and can decrease exposure of drugs that are substrates of CYP3A4). Products include:
Uniphyl **2817**

Theophylline Calcium Salicylate (Rufinamide is a weak inducer of the CYP3A4 enzyme and can decrease exposure of drugs that are substrates of CYP3A4).
No products indexed under this heading.

Theophylline Dihydroxypropyl (Glyceryl) (Rufinamide is a weak inducer of the CYP3A4 enzyme and can decrease exposure of drugs that are substrates of CYP3A4).
No products indexed under this heading.

Theophylline Ethylenediamine (Rufinamide is a weak inducer of the CYP3A4 enzyme and can decrease exposure of drugs that are substrates of CYP3A4).
No products indexed under this heading.

Theophylline Sodium Glycinate (Rufinamide is a weak inducer of the CYP3A4 enzyme and can decrease exposure of drugs that are substrates of CYP3A4).
No products indexed under this heading.

Tiagabine Hydrochloride (Rufinamide is a weak inducer of the CYP3A4 enzyme and can decrease exposure of drugs that are substrates of CYP3A4). Products include:
Gabitril **972**

Tolterodine Tartrate (Rufinamide is a weak inducer of the CYP3A4 enzyme and can decrease exposure of drugs that are substrates of CYP3A4).
No products indexed under this heading.

Trazodone Hydrochloride (Rufinamide is a weak inducer of the CYP3A4 enzyme and can decrease exposure of drugs that are substrates of CYP3A4).
No products indexed under this heading.

Triazolam (Co-administration and pretreatment with rufinamide (400 mg bid) resulted in a 37% decrease in AUC and a 23% decrease in C_{max} of triazolam, a CYP3A4 substrate).
No products indexed under this heading.

Valproate Sodium (Based on a population pharmacokinetic analysis, rufinamide clearance was decreased by valproate. In children, valproate administration may lead to elevated levels of rufinamide by up to 70%. Patients stabilized on rufinamide before being prescribed valproate should begin valproate therapy at a low dose, and titrate to a clinically effective dose. Similarly, patients on valproate should begin at a rufinamide dose lower than 400 mg).
No products indexed under this heading.

Vardenafil Hydrochloride (Rufinamide is a weak inducer of the CYP3A4 enzyme and can decrease exposure of drugs that are substrates of CYP3A4). Products include:
Levitra **3157**

Verapamil Hydrochloride (Rufinamide is a weak inducer of the CYP3A4 enzyme and can decrease exposure of drugs that are substrates of CYP3A4). Products include:
Tarka **534**

Vinblastine Sulfate (Rufinamide is a weak inducer of the CYP3A4 enzyme and can decrease exposure of drugs that are substrates of CYP3A4).
No products indexed under this heading.

Vincristine Sulfate (Rufinamide is a weak inducer of the CYP3A4 enzyme and can decrease exposure of drugs that are substrates of CYP3A4).
No products indexed under this heading.

Warfarin Sodium (Rufinamide is a weak inducer of the CYP3A4 enzyme and can decrease exposure of drugs that are substrates of CYP3A4).
No products indexed under this heading.

Food Interactions

Food, unspecified (Food increased the extent of absorption of rufinamide in healthy volunteers by 34% and increased peak exposure by 56% after a single dose of 400 mg, although the T_{max} was not elevated. Clinical trials were performed under fed conditions and dosing is recommended with food).

BAUSCH & LOMB OCUVITE ADULT 50+ VITAMIN AND MINERAL SUPPLEMENT

(Copper, Lutein, Omega-3 Acids, Vitamin C, Vitamin E, Vitamins with Minerals, Zinc Oxide) .... ⊙**238**
None cited in PDR database.

BAUSCH & LOMB PRESERVISION AREDS TABLETS

(Vitamins with Minerals) .... ⊙**238**
None cited in PDR database.

BAUSCH & LOMB ALAWAY EYE DROPS

(Ketotifen Fumarate) .... ⊙**237**
None cited in PDR database.

BAUSCH & LOMB OCUVITE LUTEIN VITAMIN AND MINERAL SUPPLEMENT

(Lutein, Vitamins with Minerals) .... ⊙**239**
None cited in PDR database.

BAUSCH & LOMB PRESERVISION AREDS SOFTGELS

(Vitamins with Minerals) .... ⊙**239**
None cited in PDR database.

BAUSCH & LOMB PRESERVISION LUTEIN SOFTGELS

(Lutein, Vitamins with Minerals) .... ⊙**237**
None cited in PDR database.

BAYER ASPIRIN

(Aspirin) **829**
May interact with ACE inhibitors, anticoagulants, beta-blockers, diuretics, nonsteroidal anti-inflammatory agents, oral hypoglycemic agents, phenytoin, valproate, and certain other agents. Compounds in these categories include:

Acarbose (Moderate doses of aspirin may increase the effectiveness of oral hypoglycemic drugs, leading to hypoglycemia).
No products indexed under this heading.

Acebutolol Hydrochloride (The hypotensive effects of beta blockers may be diminished by the concomitant administration of aspirin due to inhibition of renal prostaglandins, leading to decreased renal blood flow, and salt and fluid retention).
No products indexed under this heading.

Acetazolamide (Concurrent use of aspirin and acetazolamide can lead to high serum concentrations of acetazolamide (and toxicity) due to competition at the renal tubule for secretion).
No products indexed under this heading.

Acetazolamide Sodium (Concurrent use of aspirin and acetazolamide can lead to high serum concentrations of acetazolamide (and toxicity) due to competition at the renal tubule for secretion).
No products indexed under this heading.

Amiloride Hydrochloride (The effectiveness of diuretics in patients with underlying renal or cardiovascular disease may be diminished by the concomitant administration of aspirin due to inhibition of renal prostaglandins, leading to decreased renal blood flow, and salt and fluidretention).
No products indexed under this heading.

Anisindione (Patients on anticoagulation therapy are at increased risk for bleeding because of drug-drug interactions and the effect on platelets. Aspirin can displace warfarin from protein binding sites, leading to prolongation of both the prothrombin time and bleeding time. Aspirin can increase the anticoagulant activity of heparin, increasing bleeding risk).
No products indexed under this heading.

Ardeparin Sodium (Patients on anticoagulation therapy are at increased risk for bleeding because of drug-drug interactions and the effect on platelets. Aspirin can displace warfarin from protein binding sites, leading to prolongation of both the prothrombin time and bleeding time. Aspirin can increase the anticoagulant activity of heparin, increasing bleeding risk).
No products indexed under this heading.

Atenolol (The hypotensive effects of beta blockers may be diminished by the concomitant administration of aspirin due to inhibition of renal prostaglandins, leading to decreased renal blood flow, and salt and fluid retention).
No products indexed under this heading.

Benazepril Hydrochloride (The hyponatremic and hypotensive effects of ACE inhibitors may be diminished by the concomitant administration of aspirin due to its indirect effect on the renin-angiotensin conversion pathway).
No products indexed under this heading.

Bendroflumethiazide (The effectiveness of diuretics in patients with underlying renal or cardiovascular disease may be diminished by the concomitant administration of aspirin due to inhibition of renal prostaglandins, leading to decreased renal blood flow, and salt and fluid retention).
No products indexed under this heading.

Betaxolol Hydrochloride (The hypotensive effects of beta blockers may be diminished by the concomitant administration of aspirin due to inhibition of renal prostaglandins, leading to decreased renal blood flow, and salt and fluid retention).
No products indexed under this heading.

Bisoprolol Fumarate (The hypotensive effects of beta blockers may be diminished by the concomitant administration of aspirin due to inhibition of renal prostaglandins, leading to decreased renal blood flow, and salt and fluid retention).
No products indexed under this heading.

Bumetanide (The effectiveness of diuretics in patients with underlying renal or cardiovascular disease may be diminished by the concomitant administration of aspirin due to inhibition of renal prostaglandins, leading to decreased renal blood flow, and salt and fluidretention).
No products indexed under this heading.

Captopril (The hyponatremic and hypotensive effects of ACE inhibitors may be diminished by the concomitant administration of aspirin due to its indirect effect on the renin-angiotensin conversion pathway). Products include:
Captopril **2341**

Carteolol Hydrochloride (The hypotensive effects of beta blockers may be diminished by the concomitant administration of aspirin due to inhibition of renal prostaglandins, leading to decreased renal blood flow, and salt and fluid retention).
No products indexed under this heading.

Carvedilol (The hypotensive effects of beta blockers may be diminished by the concomitant administration of aspirin due to inhibition of renal prostaglandins, leading to decreased renal blood flow, and salt and fluid retention). Products include:
Coreg **1409**

Carvedilol Phosphate (The hypotensive effects of beta blockers may be diminished by the concomitant administration of aspirin due to inhibition of renal prostaglandins, leading to decreased renal blood flow, and salt and fluid retention). Products include:
Coreg CR **1416**

Celecoxib (The concurrent use of aspirin with other NSAIDs should be avoided because this may increase bleeding or lead to decreased renal function). Products include:
Celebrex **3272**

Chlorothiazide (The effectiveness of diuretics in patients with underlying renal or cardiovascular disease may be diminished by the concomitant administration of aspirin due to inhibition of renal prostaglandins, leading to decreased renal blood flow, and salt and fluidretention).
No products indexed under this heading.

Chlorothiazide Sodium (The effectiveness of diuretics in patients with underlying renal or cardiovascular disease may be diminished by the concomitant administration of aspirin due to inhibition of renal prostaglandins, leading to decreased renal blood flow, and salt and fluidretention). Products include:
Diuril Intravenous **2009**

(⊙ Described in PDR® for Ophthalmic Medicines)

Chlorpropamide (Moderate doses of aspirin may increase the effectiveness of oral hypoglycemic drugs, leading to hypoglycemia).
No products indexed under this heading.

Chlorthalidone (The effectiveness of diuretics in patients with underlying renal or cardiovascular disease may be diminished by the concomitant administration of aspirin due to inhibition of renal prostaglandins, leading to decreased renal blood flow, and salt and fluidretention). Products include:
Clorpres 2344

Dalteparin Sodium (Patients on anticoagulation therapy are at increased risk for bleeding because of drug-drug interactions and the effect on platelets. Aspirin can displace warfarin from protein binding sites, leading to prolongation of both the prothrombin time and bleeding time. Aspirin can increase the anticoagulant activity of heparin, increasing bleeding risk). Products include:
Fragmin 1058

Danaparoid Sodium (Patients on anticoagulation therapy are at increased risk for bleeding because of drug-drug interactions and the effect on platelets. Aspirin can displace warfarin from protein binding sites, leading to prolongation of both the prothrombin time and bleeding time. Aspirin can increase the anticoagulant activity of heparin, increasing bleeding risk).
No products indexed under this heading.

Diclofenac Epolamine (The concurrent use of aspirin with other NSAIDs should be avoided because this may increase bleeding or lead to decreased renal function). Products include:
Flector 1839

Diclofenac Potassium (The concurrent use of aspirin with other NSAIDs should be avoided because this may increase bleeding or lead to decreased renal function).
No products indexed under this heading.

Diclofenac Sodium (The concurrent use of aspirin with other NSAIDs should be avoided because this may increase bleeding or lead to decreased renal function).
No products indexed under this heading.

Dicumarol (Patients on anticoagulation therapy are at increased risk for bleeding because of drug-drug interactions and the effect on platelets. Aspirin can displace warfarin from protein binding sites, leading to prolongation of both the prothrombin time and bleeding time. Aspirin can increase the anticoagulant activity of heparin, increasing bleeding risk).
No products indexed under this heading.

Divalproex Sodium (Salicylate can displace protein-bound valproic acid, leading to an increase in serum valproic acid levels). Products include:
Depakote ER 426

Enalapril Maleate (The hyponatremic and hypotensive effects of ACE inhibitors may be diminished by the concomitant administration of aspirin due to its indirect effect on the renin-angiotensin conversion pathway).
No products indexed under this heading.

Enalaprilat (The hyponatremic and hypotensive effects of ACE inhibitors may be diminished by the concomitant administration of aspirin due to its indirect effect on the renin-angiotensin conversion pathway).
No products indexed under this heading.

Enoxaparin Sodium (Patients on anticoagulation therapy are at increased risk for bleeding because of drug-drug interactions and the effect on platelets. Aspirin can displace warfarin from protein binding sites, leading to prolonga-

tion of both the prothrombin time and bleeding time. Aspirin can increase the anticoagulant activity of heparin, increasing bleeding risk). Products include:
Lovenox 3005

Esmolol Hydrochloride (The hypotensive effects of beta blockers may be diminished by the concomitant administration of aspirin due to inhibition of renal prostaglandins, leading to decreased renal blood flow, and salt and fluid retention).
No products indexed under this heading.

Ethacrynic Acid (The effectiveness of diuretics in patients with underlying renal or cardiovascular disease may be diminished by the concomitant administration of aspirin due to inhibition of renal prostaglandins, leading to decreased renal blood flow, and salt and fluidretention).
No products indexed under this heading.

Etodolac (The concurrent use of aspirin with other NSAIDs should be avoided because this may increase bleeding or lead to decreased renal function).
No products indexed under this heading.

Fenoprofen Calcium (The concurrent use of aspirin with other NSAIDs should be avoided because this may increase bleeding or lead to decreased renal function).
No products indexed under this heading.

Flurbiprofen (The concurrent use of aspirin with other NSAIDs should be avoided because this may increase bleeding or lead to decreased renal function).
No products indexed under this heading.

Fondaparinux Sodium (Patients on anticoagulation therapy are at increased risk for bleeding because of drug-drug interactions and the effect on platelets. Aspirin can displace warfarin from protein binding sites, leading to prolongation of both the prothrombin time and bleeding time. Aspirin can increase the anticoagulant activity of heparin, increasing bleeding risk). Products include:
Arixtra 1320

Fosinopril Sodium (The hyponatremic and hypotensive effects of ACE inhibitors may be diminished by the concomitant administration of aspirin due to its indirect effect on the renin-angiotensin conversion pathway).
No products indexed under this heading.

Fosphenytoin (Salicylate can displace protein-bound phenytoin, leading to a decrease in the total concentration of phenytoin).
No products indexed under this heading.

Fosphenytoin Sodium (Salicylate can displace protein-bound phenytoin, leading to a decrease in the total concentration of phenytoin).
No products indexed under this heading.

Furosemide (The effectiveness of diuretics in patients with underlying renal or cardiovascular disease may be diminished by the concomitant administration of aspirin due to inhibition of renal prostaglandins, leading to decreased renal blood flow, and salt and fluidretention). Products include:
Furosemide 2354

Glibenclamide (Moderate doses of aspirin may increase the effectiveness of oral hypoglycemic drugs, leading to hypoglycemia).
No products indexed under this heading.

Glimepiride (Moderate doses of aspirin may increase the effectiveness of oral hypoglycemic drugs, leading to hypoglycemia). Products include:
Avandaryl 1356
Duetact 3354

Glipizide (Moderate doses of aspirin may increase the effectiveness of oral hypoglycemic drugs, leading to hypoglycemia).
No products indexed under this heading.

Glyburide (Moderate doses of aspirin may increase the effectiveness of oral hypoglycemic drugs, leading to hypoglycemia).
No products indexed under this heading.

Heparin Calcium (Patients on anticoagulation therapy are at increased risk for bleeding because of drug-drug interactions and the effect on platelets. Aspirin can displace warfarin from protein binding sites, leading to prolongation of both the prothrombin time and bleeding time. Aspirin can increase the anticoagulant activity of heparin, increasing bleeding risk).
No products indexed under this heading.

Heparin Sodium (Patients on anticoagulation therapy are at increased risk for bleeding because of drug-drug interactions and the effect on platelets. Aspirin can displace warfarin from protein binding sites, leading to prolongation of both the prothrombin time and bleeding time. Aspirin can increase the anticoagulant activity of heparin, increasing bleeding risk).
No products indexed under this heading.

Hydrochlorothiazide (The effectiveness of diuretics in patients with underlying renal or cardiovascular disease may be diminished by the concomitant administration of aspirin due to inhibition of renal prostaglandins, leading to decreased renal blood flow, and salt and fluidretention). Products include:
Atacand HCT 700
Avalide 2956
Benicar HCT 1017
Diovan HCT 2419
Dyazide 1429
Exforge HCT 2449
Hyzaar 2162
Hyzaar 100-12.5 2162
Micardis HCT 889
Prinzide 2246
Tekturna HCT 2541
Teveten HCT 541

Hydroflumethiazide (The effectiveness of diuretics in patients with underlying renal or cardiovascular disease may be diminished by the concomitant administration of aspirin due to inhibition of renal prostaglandins, leading to decreased renal blood flow, and salt and fluidretention).
No products indexed under this heading.

Ibuprofen (The concurrent use of aspirin with other NSAIDs should be avoided because this may increase bleeding or lead to decreased renal function). Products include:
Motrin IB 2043
Children's Motrin 2044
Children's Motrin Non-Staining Dye-Free 2044
Infants' Motrin 2044
Infants' Motrin Dye-Free 2044
Junior Strength Motrin 2044
Vicoprofen 564

Indapamide (The effectiveness of diuretics in patients with underlying renal or cardiovascular disease may be diminished by the concomitant administration of aspirin due to inhibition of renal prostaglandins, leading to decreased renal blood flow, and salt and fluidretention). Products include:
Indapamide 2356

Indomethacin (The concurrent use of aspirin with other NSAIDs should be avoided because this may increase bleeding or lead to decreased renal function). Products include:
Indocin 2167

Indomethacin Sodium Trihydrate (The concurrent use of aspirin with other NSAIDs should be avoided because

this may increase bleeding or lead to decreased renal function). Products include:
Indocin I.V. 2007

Ketoprofen (The concurrent use of aspirin with other NSAIDs should be avoided because this may increase bleeding or lead to decreased renal function).
No products indexed under this heading.

Ketorolac Tromethamine (The concurrent use of aspirin with other NSAIDs should be avoided because this may increase bleeding or lead to decreased renal function). Products include:
Acuvail .... ⊙209

Labetalol Hydrochloride (The hypotensive effects of beta blockers may be diminished by the concomitant administration of aspirin due to inhibition of renal prostaglandins, leading to decreased renal blood flow, and salt and fluid retention).
No products indexed under this heading.

Levobunolol Hydrochloride (The hypotensive effects of beta blockers may be diminished by the concomitant administration of aspirin due to inhibition of renal prostaglandins, leading to decreased renal blood flow, and salt and fluid retention).
No products indexed under this heading.

Lisinopril (The hyponatremic and hypotensive effects of ACE inhibitors may be diminished by the concomitant administration of aspirin due to its indirect effect on the renin-angiotensin conversion pathway). Products include:
Prinivil 2241
Prinzide 2246

Low Molecular Weight Heparins (Patients on anticoagulation therapy are at increased risk for bleeding because of drug-drug interactions and the effect on platelets. Aspirin can displace warfarin from protein binding sites, leading to prolongation of both the prothrombin time and bleeding time. Aspirin can increase the anticoagulant activity of heparin, increasing bleeding risk).
No products indexed under this heading.

Meclofenamate Sodium (The concurrent use of aspirin with other NSAIDs should be avoided because this may increase bleeding or lead to decreased renal function).
No products indexed under this heading.

Mefenamic Acid (The concurrent use of aspirin with other NSAIDs should be avoided because this may increase bleeding or lead to decreased renal function).
No products indexed under this heading.

Meloxicam (The concurrent use of aspirin with other NSAIDs should be avoided because this may increase bleeding or lead to decreased renal function).
No products indexed under this heading.

Metformin Hydrochloride (Moderate doses of aspirin may increase the effectiveness of oral hypoglycemic drugs, leading to hypoglycemia). Products include:
ActoPlus 3338
Avandamet 1345
Janumet 2188

Methotrexate (Salicylate can inhibit renal clearance of methotrexate, leading to bone marrow toxicity, especially in the elderly or renal-impaired).
No products indexed under this heading.

Methotrexate Sodium (Salicylate can inhibit renal clearance of methotrexate, leading to bone marrow toxicity, especially in the elderly or renal-impaired).
No products indexed under this heading.

IMPORTANT NOTE: Always consult each drug listing in the patient's regimen for possible interactions.

Methyclothiazide (The effectiveness of diuretics in patients with underlying renal or cardiovascular disease may be diminished by the concomitant administration of aspirin due to inhibition of renal prostaglandins, leading to decreased renal blood flow, and salt and fluidretention).
　　No products indexed under this heading.

Metipranolol Hydrochloride (The hypotensive effects of beta blockers may be diminished by the concomitant administration of aspirin due to inhibition of renal prostaglandins, leading to decreased renal blood flow, and salt and fluid retention).
　　No products indexed under this heading.

Metolazone (The effectiveness of diuretics in patients with underlying renal or cardiovascular disease may be diminished by the concomitant administration of aspirin due to inhibition of renal prostaglandins, leading to decreased renal blood flow, and salt and fluidretention).
　　No products indexed under this heading.

Metoprolol Succinate (The hypotensive effects of beta blockers may be diminished by the concomitant administration of aspirin due to inhibition of renal prostaglandins, leading to decreased renal blood flow, and salt and fluid retention). Products include:

Metoprolol Tartrate (The hypotensive effects of beta blockers may be diminished by the concomitant administration of aspirin due to inhibition of renal prostaglandins, leading to decreased renal blood flow, and salt and fluid retention).
　　No products indexed under this heading.

Miglitol (Moderate doses of aspirin may increase the effectiveness of oral hypoglycemic drugs, leading to hypoglycemia).
　　No products indexed under this heading.

Moexipril Hydrochloride (The hyponatremic and hypotensive effects of ACE inhibitors may be diminished by the concomitant administration of aspirin due to its indirect effect on the renin-angiotensin conversion pathway).
　　No products indexed under this heading.

Nabumetone (The concurrent use of aspirin with other NSAIDs should be avoided because this may increase bleeding or lead to decreased renal function).
　　No products indexed under this heading.

Nadolol (The hypotensive effects of beta blockers may be diminished by the concomitant administration of aspirin due to inhibition of renal prostaglandins, leading to decreased renal blood flow, and salt and fluid retention). Products include:

Naproxen (The concurrent use of aspirin with other NSAIDs should be avoided because this may increase bleeding or lead to decreased renal function). Products include:

Naproxen Sodium (The concurrent use of aspirin with other NSAIDs should be avoided because this may increase bleeding or lead to decreased renal function). Products include:

Nateglinide (Moderate doses of aspirin may increase the effectiveness of oral hypoglycemic drugs, leading to hypoglycemia).
　　No products indexed under this heading.

Nebivolol (The hypotensive effects of beta blockers may be diminished by the

concomitant administration of aspirin due to inhibition of renal prostaglandins, leading to decreased renal blood flow, and salt and fluid retention). Products include:

Oxaprozin (The concurrent use of aspirin with other NSAIDs should be avoided because this may increase bleeding or lead to decreased renal function).
　　No products indexed under this heading.

Penbutolol Sulfate (The hypotensive effects of beta blockers may be diminished by the concomitant administration of aspirin due to inhibition of renal prostaglandins, leading to decreased renal blood flow, and salt and fluid retention).
　　No products indexed under this heading.

Perindopril Erbumine (The hyponatremic and hypotensive effects of ACE inhibitors may be diminished by the concomitant administration of aspirin due to its indirect effect on the renin-angiotensin conversion pathway).
　　No products indexed under this heading.

Phenylbutazone (The concurrent use of aspirin with other NSAIDs should be avoided because this may increase bleeding or lead to decreased renal function).
　　No products indexed under this heading.

Phenytoin (Salicylate can displace protein-bound phenytoin, leading to a decrease in the total concentration of phenytoin).
　　No products indexed under this heading.

Phenytoin Sodium (Salicylate can displace protein-bound phenytoin, leading to a decrease in the total concentration of phenytoin). Products include:

Pindolol (The hypotensive effects of beta blockers may be diminished by the concomitant administration of aspirin due to inhibition of renal prostaglandins, leading to decreased renal blood flow, and salt and fluid retention).
　　No products indexed under this heading.

Pioglitazone Hydrochloride (Moderate doses of aspirin may increase the effectiveness of oral hypoglycemic drugs, leading to hypoglycemia). Products include:

Piroxicam (The concurrent use of aspirin with other NSAIDs should be avoided because this may increase bleeding or lead to decreased renal function).
　　No products indexed under this heading.

Polythiazide (The effectiveness of diuretics in patients with underlying renal or cardiovascular disease may be diminished by the concomitant administration of aspirin due to inhibition of renal prostaglandins, leading to decreased renal blood flow, and salt and fluidretention).
　　No products indexed under this heading.

Probenecid (Salicylates antagonize the uricosuric action of uricouric agents).
　　No products indexed under this heading.

Propranolol Hydrochloride (The hypotensive effects of beta blockers may be diminished by the concomitant administration of aspirin due to inhibition of renal prostaglandins, leading to decreased renal blood flow, and salt and fluid retention). Products include:

Quinapril Hydrochloride (The hyponatremic and hypotensive effects of ACE inhibitors may be diminished by the concomitant administration of aspirin due to its indirect effect on the renin-angiotensin conversion pathway).
　　No products indexed under this heading.

Ramipril (The hyponatremic and hypotensive effects of ACE inhibitors may be diminished by the concomitant administration of aspirin due to its indirect effect on the renin-angiotensin conversion pathway).
　　No products indexed under this heading.

Repaglinide (Moderate doses of aspirin may increase the effectiveness of oral hypoglycemic drugs, leading to hypoglycemia).
　　No products indexed under this heading.

Rofecoxib (The concurrent use of aspirin with other NSAIDs should be avoided because this may increase bleeding or lead to decreased renal function).
　　No products indexed under this heading.

Rosiglitazone Maleate (Moderate doses of aspirin may increase the effectiveness of oral hypoglycemic drugs, leading to hypoglycemia). Products include:

Sitagliptin Phosphate (Moderate doses of aspirin may increase the effectiveness of oral hypoglycemic drugs, leading to hypoglycemia). Products include:

Sotalol Hydrochloride (The hypotensive effects of beta blockers may be diminished by the concomitant administration of aspirin due to inhibition of renal prostaglandins, leading to decreased renal blood flow, and salt and fluid retention).
　　No products indexed under this heading.

Spirapril Hydrochloride (The hyponatremic and hypotensive effects of ACE inhibitors may be diminished by the concomitant administration of aspirin due to its indirect effect on the renin-angiotensin conversion pathway).
　　No products indexed under this heading.

Spironolactone (The effectiveness of diuretics in patients with underlying renal or cardiovascular disease may be diminished by the concomitant administration of aspirin due to inhibition of renal prostaglandins, leading to decreased renal blood flow, and salt and fluidretention).
　　No products indexed under this heading.

Sulfinpyrazone (Salicylates antagonize the uricosuric action of uricouric agents).
　　No products indexed under this heading.

Sulindac (The concurrent use of aspirin with other NSAIDs should be avoided because this may increase bleeding or lead to decreased renal function). Products include:

Timolol Hemihydrate (The hypotensive effects of beta blockers may be diminished by the concomitant administration of aspirin due to inhibition of renal prostaglandins, leading to decreased renal blood flow, and salt and fluid retention). Products include:

Timolol Maleate (The hypotensive effects of beta blockers may be diminished by the concomitant administration of aspirin due to inhibition of renal prostaglandins, leading to decreased renal blood flow, and salt and fluid retention). Products include:

Tinzaparin Sodium (Patients on anticoagulation therapy are at increased risk for bleeding because of drug-drug interactions and the effect on platelets. Aspirin can displace warfarin from protein binding sites, leading to prolongation of both the prothrombin time and bleeding time. Aspirin can increase the anticoagulant activity of heparin, increasing bleeding risk).
　　No products indexed under this heading.

Tolazamide (Moderate doses of aspirin may increase the effectiveness of oral hypoglycemic drugs, leading to hypoglycemia).
　　No products indexed under this heading.

Tolbutamide (Moderate doses of aspirin may increase the effectiveness of oral hypoglycemic drugs, leading to hypoglycemia).
　　No products indexed under this heading.

Tolmetin Sodium (The concurrent use of aspirin with other NSAIDs should be avoided because this may increase bleeding or lead to decreased renal function).
　　No products indexed under this heading.

Torsemide (The effectiveness of diuretics in patients with underlying renal or cardiovascular disease may be diminished by the concomitant administration of aspirin due to inhibition of renal prostaglandins, leading to decreased renal blood flow, and salt and fluidretention).
　　No products indexed under this heading.

Trandolapril (The hyponatremic and hypotensive effects of ACE inhibitors may be diminished by the concomitant administration of aspirin due to its indirect effect on the renin-angiotensin conversion pathway). Products include:

Triamterene (The effectiveness of diuretics in patients with underlying renal or cardiovascular disease may be diminished by the concomitant administration of aspirin due to inhibition of renal prostaglandins, leading to decreased renal blood flow, and salt and fluidretention). Products include:

Troglitazone (Moderate doses of aspirin may increase the effectiveness of oral hypoglycemic drugs, leading to hypoglycemia).
　　No products indexed under this heading.

Valdecoxib (The concurrent use of aspirin with other NSAIDs should be avoided because this may increase bleeding or lead to decreased renal function).
　　No products indexed under this heading.

Valproate Sodium (Salicylate can displace protein-bound valproic acid, leading to an increase in serum valproic acid levels).
　　No products indexed under this heading.

Valproic Acid (Salicylate can displace protein-bound valproic acid, leading to an increase in serum valproic acid levels).
　　No products indexed under this heading.

Warfarin Sodium (Patients on anticoagulation therapy are at increased risk for bleeding because of drug-drug interactions and the effect on platelets. Aspirin can displace warfarin from protein binding sites, leading to prolongation of both the prothrombin time and bleeding time. Aspirin can increase the anticoagulant activity of heparin, increasing bleeding risk).
　　No products indexed under this heading.

BECONASE AQ NASAL SPRAY

(Beclomethasone Dipropionate · Monohydrate) 1386
None cited in PDR database.

BEELITH TABLETS

(Magnesium Oxide, Vitamin B6) 873

Prescription Drugs, unspecified (Concurrent use should be avoided).
No products indexed under this heading.

BENADRYL ALLERGY ULTRATAB TABLETS

(Diphenhydramine Hydrochloride) 2042
May interact with alcohols, hypnotics and sedatives, tranquilizers. Compounds in these categories include:

Alprazolam (Concurrent use may increase drowsiness effect).
No products indexed under this heading.

Buspirone Hydrochloride (Concurrent use may increase drowsiness effect).
No products indexed under this heading.

Butabarbital (Concurrent use may increase drowsiness effect).
No products indexed under this heading.

Butabarbital Sodium (Concurrent use may increase drowsiness effect).
No products indexed under this heading.

Butalbital (Concurrent use may increase drowsiness effect).
No products indexed under this heading.

Chloral Hydrate (Concurrent use may increase drowsiness effect).
No products indexed under this heading.

Chlordiazepoxide (Concurrent use may increase drowsiness effect).
No products indexed under this heading.

Chlordiazepoxide Hydrochloride (Concurrent use may increase drowsiness effect).
No products indexed under this heading.

Chlorpromazine (Concurrent use may increase drowsiness effect).
No products indexed under this heading.

Chlorpromazine Hydrochloride (Concurrent use may increase drowsiness effect).
No products indexed under this heading.

Chlorprothixene (Concurrent use may increase drowsiness effect).
No products indexed under this heading.

Chlorprothixene Hydrochloride (Concurrent use may increase drowsiness effect).
No products indexed under this heading.

Chlorprothixene Lactate (Concurrent use may increase drowsiness effect).
No products indexed under this heading.

Clorazepate Dipotassium (Concurrent use may increase drowsiness effect).
No products indexed under this heading.

Diazepam (Concurrent use may increase drowsiness effect). Products include:
Valium Tablets 2880

Droperidol (Concurrent use may increase drowsiness effect).
No products indexed under this heading.

Estazolam (Concurrent use may increase drowsiness effect).
No products indexed under this heading.

Ethanol (Increases drowsiness effect; avoid concomitant use).
No products indexed under this heading.

Ethchlorvynol (Concurrent use may increase drowsiness effect).
No products indexed under this heading.

Ethinamate (Concurrent use may increase drowsiness effect).
No products indexed under this heading.

Ethyl Alcohol (Increases drowsiness effect; avoid concomitant use).
No products indexed under this heading.

Fluphenazine Decanoate (Concurrent use may increase drowsiness effect).
No products indexed under this heading.

Fluphenazine Enanthate (Concurrent use may increase drowsiness effect).
No products indexed under this heading.

Fluphenazine Hydrochloride (Concurrent use may increase drowsiness effect).
No products indexed under this heading.

Flurazepam Hydrochloride (Concurrent use may increase drowsiness effect).
No products indexed under this heading.

Glutethimide (Concurrent use may increase drowsiness effect).
No products indexed under this heading.

Haloperidol (Concurrent use may increase drowsiness effect).
No products indexed under this heading.

Haloperidol Decanoate (Concurrent use may increase drowsiness effect).
No products indexed under this heading.

Hydroxyzine Hydrochloride (Concurrent use may increase drowsiness effect).
No products indexed under this heading.

Lorazepam (Concurrent use may increase drowsiness effect).
No products indexed under this heading.

Loxapine Hydrochloride (Concurrent use may increase drowsiness effect).
No products indexed under this heading.

Loxapine Succinate (Concurrent use may increase drowsiness effect).
No products indexed under this heading.

Meprobamate (Concurrent use may increase drowsiness effect).
No products indexed under this heading.

Mesoridazine Besylate (Concurrent use may increase drowsiness effect).
No products indexed under this heading.

Midazolam Hydrochloride (Concurrent use may increase drowsiness effect).
No products indexed under this heading.

Molindone Hydrochloride (Concurrent use may increase drowsiness effect). Products include:
Moban 1108

Oxazepam (Concurrent use may increase drowsiness effect).
No products indexed under this heading.

Perphenazine (Concurrent use may increase drowsiness effect).
No products indexed under this heading.

Prazepam (Concurrent use may increase drowsiness effect).
No products indexed under this heading.

Prochlorperazine (Concurrent use may increase drowsiness effect).
No products indexed under this heading.

Promethazine Hydrochloride (Concurrent use may increase drowsiness effect).
No products indexed under this heading.

Propofol (Concurrent use may increase drowsiness effect).
No products indexed under this heading.

Quazepam (Concurrent use may increase drowsiness effect).
No products indexed under this heading.

Ramelteon (Concurrent use may increase drowsiness effect). Products include:
Rozerem 3366

Secobarbital Sodium (Concurrent use may increase drowsiness effect).
No products indexed under this heading.

Sodium Butabarbital (Concurrent use may increase drowsiness effect).
No products indexed under this heading.

Temazepam (Concurrent use may increase drowsiness effect).
No products indexed under this heading.

Thioridazine Hydrochloride (Concurrent use may increase drowsiness effect). Products include:
Thioridazine Hydrochloride 2384

Thiothixene (Concurrent use may increase drowsiness effect). Products include:
Thiothixene 2386

Triazolam (Concurrent use may increase drowsiness effect).
No products indexed under this heading.

Trifluoperazine Hydrochloride (Concurrent use may increase drowsiness effect).
No products indexed under this heading.

Zaleplon (Concurrent use may increase drowsiness effect).
No products indexed under this heading.

Zolpidem Tartrate (Concurrent use may increase drowsiness effect). Products include:
Ambien 2920
Ambien CR 2925

Food Interactions

Alcohol (Increases drowsiness effect; avoid concomitant use).

Beer, reduced-alcohol (Increases drowsiness effect; avoid concomitant use).

Beer, unspecified (Increases drowsiness effect; avoid concomitant use).

Wine, Chianti (Increases drowsiness effect; avoid concomitant use).

Wine, Red (Increases drowsiness effect; avoid concomitant use).

Wine, unspecified (Increases drowsiness effect; avoid concomitant use).

Wine products (Increases drowsiness effect; avoid concomitant use).

CHILDREN'S BENADRYL ALLERGY LIQUID

(Diphenhydramine Hydrochloride) 2042
May interact with hypnotics and sedatives, tranquilizers. Compounds in these categories include:

Alprazolam (Concurrent use may increase drowsiness effect).
No products indexed under this heading.

Buspirone Hydrochloride (Concurrent use may increase drowsiness effect).
No products indexed under this heading.

Butabarbital (Concurrent use may increase drowsiness effect).
No products indexed under this heading.

Butabarbital Sodium (Concurrent use may increase drowsiness effect).
No products indexed under this heading.

Butalbital (Concurrent use may increase drowsiness effect).
No products indexed under this heading.

Chloral Hydrate (Concurrent use may increase drowsiness effect).
No products indexed under this heading.

Chlordiazepoxide (Concurrent use may increase drowsiness effect).
No products indexed under this heading.

Chlordiazepoxide Hydrochloride (Concurrent use may increase drowsiness effect).
No products indexed under this heading.

Chlorpromazine (Concurrent use may increase drowsiness effect).
No products indexed under this heading.

Chlorpromazine Hydrochloride (Concurrent use may increase drowsiness effect).
No products indexed under this heading.

Chlorprothixene (Concurrent use may increase drowsiness effect).
No products indexed under this heading.

Chlorprothixene Hydrochloride (Concurrent use may increase drowsiness effect).
No products indexed under this heading.

Chlorprothixene Lactate (Concurrent use may increase drowsiness effect).
No products indexed under this heading.

Clorazepate Dipotassium (Concurrent use may increase drowsiness effect).
No products indexed under this heading.

Diazepam (Concurrent use may increase drowsiness effect). Products include:
Valium Tablets 2880

Droperidol (Concurrent use may increase drowsiness effect).
No products indexed under this heading.

Estazolam (Concurrent use may increase drowsiness effect).
No products indexed under this heading.

Ethchlorvynol (Concurrent use may increase drowsiness effect).
No products indexed under this heading.

Ethinamate (Concurrent use may increase drowsiness effect).
No products indexed under this heading.

Fluphenazine Decanoate (Concurrent use may increase drowsiness effect).
No products indexed under this heading.

Fluphenazine Enanthate (Concurrent use may increase drowsiness effect).
No products indexed under this heading.

Fluphenazine Hydrochloride (Concurrent use may increase drowsiness effect).
No products indexed under this heading.

Flurazepam Hydrochloride (Concurrent use may increase drowsiness effect).
No products indexed under this heading.

Glutethimide (Concurrent use may increase drowsiness effect).
No products indexed under this heading.

Haloperidol (Concurrent use may increase drowsiness effect).
No products indexed under this heading.

Haloperidol Decanoate (Concurrent use may increase drowsiness effect).
No products indexed under this heading.

Hydroxyzine Hydrochloride (Concurrent use may increase drowsiness effect).
No products indexed under this heading.

Lorazepam (Concurrent use may increase drowsiness effect).
No products indexed under this heading.

Loxapine Hydrochloride (Concurrent use may increase drowsiness effect).
No products indexed under this heading.

Loxapine Succinate (Concurrent use may increase drowsiness effect).
No products indexed under this heading.

Meprobamate (Concurrent use may increase drowsiness effect).
No products indexed under this heading.

Mesoridazine Besylate (Concurrent use may increase drowsiness effect).
No products indexed under this heading.

Midazolam Hydrochloride (Concurrent use may increase drowsiness effect).
No products indexed under this heading.

Molindone Hydrochloride (Concurrent use may increase drowsiness effect). Products include:

IMPORTANT NOTE: Always consult each drug listing in the patient's regimen for possible interactions.

Moban 1108

Oxazepam (Concurrent use may increase drowsiness effect).
No products indexed under this heading.

Perphenazine (Concurrent use may increase drowsiness effect).
No products indexed under this heading.

Prazepam (Concurrent use may increase drowsiness effect).
No products indexed under this heading.

Prochlorperazine (Concurrent use may increase drowsiness effect).
No products indexed under this heading.

Promethazine Hydrochloride (Concurrent use may increase drowsiness effect).
No products indexed under this heading.

Propofol (Concurrent use may increase drowsiness effect).
No products indexed under this heading.

Quazepam (Concurrent use may increase drowsiness effect).
No products indexed under this heading.

Ramelteon (Concurrent use may increase drowsiness effect). Products include:
Rozerem 3366

Secobarbital Sodium (Concurrent use may increase drowsiness effect).
No products indexed under this heading.

Sodium Butabarbital (Concurrent use may increase drowsiness effect).
No products indexed under this heading.

Temazepam (Concurrent use may increase drowsiness effect).
No products indexed under this heading.

Thioridazine Hydrochloride (Concurrent use may increase drowsiness effect). Products include:
Thioridazine Hydrochloride 2384

Thiothixene (Concurrent use may increase drowsiness effect). Products include:
Thiothixene 2386

Triazolam (Concurrent use may increase drowsiness effect).
No products indexed under this heading.

Trifluoperazine Hydrochloride (Concurrent use may increase drowsiness effect).
No products indexed under this heading.

Zaleplon (Concurrent use may increase drowsiness effect).
No products indexed under this heading.

Zolpidem Tartrate (Concurrent use may increase drowsiness effect). Products include:
Ambien 2920
Ambien CR 2925

BENEFIX VIALS
(Antihemophilic Factor (Recombinant)) 3497
None cited in PDR database.

BENICAR TABLETS
(Olmesartan Medoxomil) 1015
None cited in PDR database.

BENICAR HCT TABLETS
(Hydrochlorothiazide, Olmesartan Medoxomil) 1017
May interact with alcohols, angiotensin-II receptor antagonists, antihypertensives, barbiturates, corticosteroids, curariform skeletal muscle relaxants, insulin, lithium preparations, narcotic analgesics, non-steroidal anti-inflammatory agents, oral hypoglycemic agents, vasopressors, and certain other agents. Compounds in these categories include:

Acarbose (Co-administration may require a dosage adjustment of the antidiabetic drug).
No products indexed under this heading.

Acebutolol Hydrochloride (Co-administration could have additive effect or potentiation).
No products indexed under this heading.

ACTH (Co-administration could cause intensified electrolyte depletion, particularly hypokalemia).
No products indexed under this heading.

Alclometasone Dipropionate (Co-administration could cause intensified electrolyte depletion, particularly hypokalemia).
No products indexed under this heading.

Alfentanil Hydrochloride (Concurrent administration could cause potentiation of orthostatic hypotension).
No products indexed under this heading.

Aliskiren (Co-administration could have additive effect or potentiation). Products include:
Tekturna 2538
Tekturna HCT 2541
Valturna 3637

Amlodipine Besylate (Co-administration could have additive effect or potentiation). Products include:
Azor 1010
Exforge 2443
Exforge HCT 2449

Amobarbital (Concurrent administration could cause potentiation of orthostatic hypotension).
No products indexed under this heading.

Amobarbital Sodium (Concurrent administration could cause potentiation of orthostatic hypotension).
No products indexed under this heading.

Apomorphine (Concurrent administration could cause potentiation of orthostatic hypotension).
No products indexed under this heading.

Apomorphine Hydrochloride (Concurrent administration could cause potentiation of orthostatic hypotension).
No products indexed under this heading.

Aprobarbital (Concurrent administration could cause potentiation of orthostatic hypotension).
No products indexed under this heading.

Atenolol (Co-administration could have additive effect or potentiation).
No products indexed under this heading.

Atracurium Besylate (Co-administration could cause possible increased responsiveness to the muscle relaxant).
No products indexed under this heading.

Beclomethasone Dipropionate (Co-administration could cause intensified electrolyte depletion, particularly hypokalemia). Products include:
Qvar 3398

Beclomethasone Dipropionate Monohydrate (Co-administration could cause intensified electrolyte depletion, particularly hypokalemia). Products include:
Beconase AQ 1386

Benazepril Hydrochloride (Co-administration could have additive effect or potentiation).
No products indexed under this heading.

Bendroflumethiazide (Co-administration could have additive effect or potentiation).
No products indexed under this heading.

Betamethasone (Co-administration could cause intensified electrolyte depletion, particularly hypokalemia).
No products indexed under this heading.

Betamethasone Acetate (Co-administration could cause intensified electrolyte depletion, particularly hypokalemia).
No products indexed under this heading.

Betamethasone Benzoate (Co-administration could cause intensified electrolyte depletion, particularly hypokalemia).
No products indexed under this heading.

Betamethasone Dipropionate (Co-administration could cause intensified electrolyte depletion, particularly hypokalemia). Products include:
Diprolene Lotion 0.05% 3108
Diprolene Ointment 0.05% 3109
Diprolene AF Cream 0.05% 3107
Lotrisone 3163

Betamethasone Sodium Phosphate (Co-administration could cause intensified electrolyte depletion, particularly hypokalemia).
No products indexed under this heading.

Betamethasone Valerate (Co-administration could cause intensified electrolyte depletion, particularly hypokalemia). Products include:
Luxíq 3321

Betaxolol Hydrochloride (Co-administration could have additive effect or potentiation).
No products indexed under this heading.

Bisoprolol Fumarate (Co-administration could have additive effect or potentiation).
No products indexed under this heading.

Budesonide (Co-administration could cause intensified electrolyte depletion, particularly hypokalemia). Products include:
Pulmicort Flexhaler 714
Symbicort 80/4.5 720
Symbicort 160/4.5 720

Buprenorphine Hydrochloride (Concurrent administration could cause potentiation of orthostatic hypotension).
No products indexed under this heading.

Butabarbital (Concurrent administration could cause potentiation of orthostatic hypotension).
No products indexed under this heading.

Butabarbital Sodium (Concurrent administration could cause potentiation of orthostatic hypotension).
No products indexed under this heading.

Butalbital (Concurrent administration could cause potentiation of orthostatic hypotension).
No products indexed under this heading.

Candesartan Cilexetil (Co-administration could have additive effect or potentiation). Products include:
Atacand 697
Atacand HCT 700

Captopril (Co-administration could have additive effect or potentiation). Products include:
Captopril 2341

Carteolol Hydrochloride (Co-administration could have additive effect or potentiation).
No products indexed under this heading.

Carvedilol (Co-administration could have additive effect or potentiation). Products include:
Coreg 1409

Carvedilol Phosphate (Co-administration could have additive effect or potentiation). Products include:
Coreg CR 1416

Celecoxib (In some patients the administration of a non-steroidal anti-inflammatory agent can reduce the diuretic, natriuretic and antihypertensive effects of loop, potassium-sparing and thiazide diuretics). Products include:
Celebrex 3272

Chlorothiazide (Co-administration could have additive effect or potentiation).
No products indexed under this heading.

Chlorothiazide Sodium (Co-administration could have additive effect or potentiation). Products include:
Diuril Intravenous 2009

Chlorpropamide (Co-administration may require a dosage adjustment of the antidiabetic drug).
No products indexed under this heading.

Chlorthalidone (Co-administration could have additive effect or potentiation). Products include:
Clorpres 2344

Cholestyramine (Absorption of hydrochlorothiazide is impaired in the presence of anionic exchange resins; single doses of cholestyramine bind the hydrochlorothiazide and reduce its absorption from the gastrointestinal tract by 85%).
No products indexed under this heading.

Ciclesonide (Co-administration could cause intensified electrolyte depletion, particularly hypokalemia).
No products indexed under this heading.

Cisatracurium Besylate (Co-administration could cause possible increased responsiveness to the muscle relaxant). Products include:
Nimbex 503

Clonidine (Co-administration could have additive effect or potentiation). Products include:
Catapres-TTS 884

Clonidine Hydrochloride (Co-administration could have additive effect or potentiation). Products include:
Clorpres 2344

Codeine Phosphate (Concurrent administration could cause potentiation of orthostatic hypotension). Products include:
Tylenol with Codeine 2691

Codeine Sulfate (Concurrent administration could cause potentiation of orthostatic hypotension).
No products indexed under this heading.

Colestipol (Absorption of hydrochlorothiazide is impaired in the presence of anionic exchange resins; single doses of colestipol bind the hydrochlorothiazide and reduce its absorption from the gastrointestinal tract by 43%).
No products indexed under this heading.

Colestipol Hydrochloride (Absorption of hydrochlorothiazide is impaired in the presence of anionic exchange resins; single doses of colestipol bind the hydrochlorothiazide and reduce its absorption from the gastrointestinal tract by 43%).
No products indexed under this heading.

Cortisone Acetate (Co-administration could cause intensified electrolyte depletion, particularly hypokalemia).
No products indexed under this heading.

Deserpidine (Co-administration could have additive effect or potentiation).
No products indexed under this heading.

Desoximetasone (Co-administration could cause intensified electrolyte depletion, particularly hypokalemia).
No products indexed under this heading.

Dexamethasone (Co-administration could cause intensified electrolyte depletion, particularly hypokalemia). Products include:
Ciprodex 583
Ozurdex .... ⊙ 223
Tobramycin and Dexamethasone Ophthalmic Suspension .... ⊙ 251

Dexamethasone Acetate (Co-administration could cause intensified electrolyte depletion, particularly hypokalemia).
No products indexed under this heading.

Dexamethasone Phosphate (Co-administration could cause intensified electrolyte depletion, particularly hypokalemia).
No products indexed under this heading.

Dexamethasone Sodium (Co-administration could cause intensified electrolyte depletion, particularly hypokalemia).
No products indexed under this heading.

Dexamethasone Sodium Phosphate (Co-administration could cause intensified electrolyte depletion, particularly hypokalemia).
No products indexed under this heading.

Dexamethasone Sodium Phosphate Injection (Co-administration could cause intensified electrolyte depletion, particularly hypokalemia).
No products indexed under this heading.

Dezocine (Concurrent administration could cause potentiation of orthostatic hypotension).
No products indexed under this heading.

Diazoxide (Co-administration could have additive effect or potentiation). Products include:
Proglycem 1179
Proglycem Suspension 1179

Diclofenac Epolamine (In some patients the administration of a non-steroidal anti-inflammatory agent can reduce the diuretic, natriuretic and antihypertensive effects of loop, potassium-sparing and thiazide diuretics). Products include:
Flector 1839

Diclofenac Potassium (In some patients the administration of a non-steroidal anti-inflammatory agent can reduce the diuretic, natriuretic and antihypertensive effects of loop, potassium-sparing and thiazide diuretics).
No products indexed under this heading.

Diclofenac Sodium (In some patients the administration of a non-steroidal anti-inflammatory agent can reduce the diuretic, natriuretic and antihypertensive effects of loop, potassium-sparing and thiazide diuretics).
No products indexed under this heading.

Diflorasone Diacetate (Co-administration could cause intensified electrolyte depletion, particularly hypokalemia).
No products indexed under this heading.

Dihydrocodeine Bitartrate (Concurrent administration could cause potentiation of orthostatic hypotension).
No products indexed under this heading.

Dihydrocodeinone Bitartrate (Concurrent administration could cause potentiation of orthostatic hypotension).
No products indexed under this heading.

Diltiazem Hydrochloride (Co-administration could have additive effect or potentiation). Products include:
Cardizem LA 423

Diltiazem Maleate (Co-administration could have additive effect or potentiation).
No products indexed under this heading.

Dobutamine (Co-administration could cause possible decreased response to pressor amines but not sufficient to preclude their use).
No products indexed under this heading.

Dobutamine Hydrochloride (Co-administration could cause possible decreased response to pressor amines but not sufficient to preclude their use).
No products indexed under this heading.

Dopamine Hydrochloride (Co-administration could cause possible decreased response to pressor amines but not sufficient to preclude their use).
No products indexed under this heading.

Doxacurium Chloride (Co-administration could cause possible increased responsiveness to the muscle relaxant).
No products indexed under this heading.

Doxazosin Mesylate (Co-administration could have additive effect or potentiation).
No products indexed under this heading.

d-Tubocurarine (Co-administration could cause possible increased responsiveness to the muscle relaxant).
No products indexed under this heading.

Enalapril Maleate (Co-administration could have additive effect or potentiation).
No products indexed under this heading.

Enalaprilat (Co-administration could have additive effect or potentiation).
No products indexed under this heading.

Ephedrine Sulfate (Co-administration could cause possible decreased response to pressor amines but not sufficient to preclude their use).
No products indexed under this heading.

Epinephrine Bitartrate (Co-administration could cause possible decreased response to pressor amines but not sufficient to preclude their use).
No products indexed under this heading.

Epinephrine Hydrochloride (Co-administration could cause possible decreased response to pressor amines but not sufficient to preclude their use).
No products indexed under this heading.

Eprosartan Mesylate (Co-administration could have additive effect or potentiation). Products include:
Teveten 538
Teveten HCT 541

Esmolol Hydrochloride (Co-administration could have additive effect or potentiation).
No products indexed under this heading.

Ethanol (Concurrent administration could cause potentiation of orthostatic hypotension).
No products indexed under this heading.

Ethyl Alcohol (Concurrent administration could cause potentiation of orthostatic hypotension).
No products indexed under this heading.

Etodolac (In some patients the administration of a non-steroidal anti-inflammatory agent can reduce the diuretic, natriuretic and antihypertensive effects of loop, potassium-sparing and thiazide diuretics).
No products indexed under this heading.

Felodipine (Co-administration could have additive effect or potentiation).
No products indexed under this heading.

Fenoprofen Calcium (In some patients the administration of a non-steroidal anti-inflammatory agent can reduce the diuretic, natriuretic and antihypertensive effects of loop, potassium-sparing and thiazide diuretics).
No products indexed under this heading.

Fentanyl (Concurrent administration could cause potentiation of orthostatic hypotension). Products include:
Duragesic 2604
Fentanyl Transdermal System 2346
Onsolis 2054

Fentanyl Citrate (Concurrent administration could cause potentiation of orthostatic hypotension). Products include:
Fentora 966

Fludrocortisone Acetate (Co-administration could cause intensified electrolyte depletion, particularly hypokalemia).
No products indexed under this heading.

Flumethasone Pivalate (Co-administration could cause intensified electrolyte depletion, particularly hypokalemia).
No products indexed under this heading.

Flunisolide Hemihydrate (Co-administration could cause intensified electrolyte depletion, particularly hypokalemia).
No products indexed under this heading.

Flurbiprofen (In some patients the administration of a non-steroidal anti-inflammatory agent can reduce the diuretic, natriuretic and antihypertensive effects of loop, potassium-sparing and thiazide diuretics).
No products indexed under this heading.

Fluticasone Furoate (Co-administration could cause intensified electrolyte depletion, particularly hypokalemia). Products include:
Veramyst 1713

Fluticasone Propionate (Co-administration could cause intensified electrolyte depletion, particularly hypokalemia). Products include:
Advair 100/50 1275
Advair 250/50 1275
Advair 500/50 1275
Advair HFA 45/21 1288
Advair HFA 115/21 1288
Advair HFA 230/21 1288
Flonase 1459
Flovent Diskus 1463
Flovent HFA 1470

Fosinopril Sodium (Co-administration could have additive effect or potentiation).
No products indexed under this heading.

Furosemide (Co-administration could have additive effect or potentiation). Products include:
Furosemide 2354

Gallamine (Co-administration could cause possible increased responsiveness to the muscle relaxant).
No products indexed under this heading.

Gallamine Triethiodide (Co-administration could cause possible increased responsiveness to the muscle relaxant).
No products indexed under this heading.

Glibenclamide (Co-administration may require a dosage adjustment of the antidiabetic drug).
No products indexed under this heading.

Glimepiride (Co-administration may require a dosage adjustment of the antidiabetic drug). Products include:
Avandaryl 1356
Duetact 3354

Glipizide (Co-administration may require a dosage adjustment of the antidiabetic drug).
No products indexed under this heading.

Glyburide (Co-administration may require a dosage adjustment of the antidiabetic drug).
No products indexed under this heading.

Guanabenz Acetate (Co-administration could have additive effect or potentiation).
No products indexed under this heading.

Guanethidine (Co-administration could have additive effect or potentiation).
No products indexed under this heading.

Guanethidine Monosulfate (Co-administration could have additive effect or potentiation).
No products indexed under this heading.

Guanethidine Sulfate (Co-administration could have additive effect or potentiation).
No products indexed under this heading.

Hexobarbital (Concurrent administration could cause potentiation of orthostatic hypotension).
No products indexed under this heading.

Hydralazine Hydrochloride (Co-administration could have additive effect or potentiation).
No products indexed under this heading.

Hydrocodone Bitartrate (Concurrent administration could cause potentiation of orthostatic hypotension). Products include:
Vicodin 560
Vicodin ES 561
Vicodin HP 563
Vicoprofen 564
Zydone 1138

Hydrocodone Polistirex (Concurrent administration could cause potentiation of orthostatic hypotension). Products include:
Tussionex 3443

Hydrocortisone (Co-administration could cause intensified electrolyte depletion, particularly hypokalemia).
No products indexed under this heading.

Hydrocortisone (Alcohol) (Co-administration could cause intensified electrolyte depletion, particularly hypokalemia).
No products indexed under this heading.

Hydrocortisone Acetate (Co-administration could cause intensified electrolyte depletion, particularly hypokalemia).
No products indexed under this heading.

Hydrocortisone Butyrate (Co-administration could cause intensified electrolyte depletion, particularly hypokalemia).
No products indexed under this heading.

Hydrocortisone Cypionate (Co-administration could cause intensified electrolyte depletion, particularly hypokalemia).
No products indexed under this heading.

Hydrocortisone Hemisuccinate (Co-administration could cause intensified electrolyte depletion, particularly hypokalemia).
No products indexed under this heading.

Hydrocortisone Probutate (Co-administration could cause intensified electrolyte depletion, particularly hypokalemia).
No products indexed under this heading.

Hydrocortisone Sodium Phosphate (Co-administration could cause intensified electrolyte depletion, particularly hypokalemia).
No products indexed under this heading.

Hydrocortisone Sodium Succinate (Co-administration could cause intensified electrolyte depletion, particularly hypokalemia).
No products indexed under this heading.

Hydrocortisone Valerate (Co-administration could cause intensified electrolyte depletion, particularly hypokalemia).
No products indexed under this heading.

Hydroflumethiazide (Co-administration could have additive effect or potentiation).
No products indexed under this heading.

Hydromorphone (Concurrent administration could cause potentiation of orthostatic hypotension).
No products indexed under this heading.

Hydromorphone Hydrochloride (Concurrent administration could cause potentiation of orthostatic hypotension). Products include:
Dilaudid Injection 2800
Dilaudid Oral 2797
Dilaudid Tablets 2797
Dilaudid-HP 2800

Ibuprofen (In some patients the administration of a non-steroidal anti-inflammatory agent can reduce the diuretic, natriuretic and antihypertensive effects of loop, potassium-sparing and thiazide diuretics). Products include:

IMPORTANT NOTE: Always consult each drug listing in the patient's regimen for possible interactions.

Indapamide (Co-administration could have additive effect or potentiation). Products include:

Indomethacin (In some patients the administration of a non-steroidal anti-inflammatory agent can reduce the diuretic, natriuretic and antihypertensive effects of loop, potassium-sparing and thiazide diuretics). Products include:

Indomethacin Sodium Trihydrate (In some patients the administration of a non-steroidal anti-inflammatory agent can reduce the diuretic, natriuretic and antihypertensive effects of loop, potassium-sparing and thiazide diuretics). Products include:

Insulin (Co-administration may require a dosage adjustment of the antidiabetic drug).
  No products indexed under this heading.

Insulin, Human, Zinc Suspension (Co-administration may require a dosage adjustment of the antidiabetic drug).
  No products indexed under this heading.

Insulin, Human (rDNA origin) (Co-administration may require a dosage adjustment of the antidiabetic drug). Products include:

Insulin, Human NPH (Co-administration may require a dosage adjustment of the antidiabetic drug). Products include:

Insulin, Human Regular (Co-administration may require a dosage adjustment of the antidiabetic drug). Products include:

Insulin, Human Regular and Human NPH Mixture (Co-administration may require a dosage adjustment of the antidiabetic drug). Products include:

Insulin, NPH (Co-administration may require a dosage adjustment of the antidiabetic drug).
  No products indexed under this heading.

Insulin, Regular (Co-administration may require a dosage adjustment of the antidiabetic drug).
  No products indexed under this heading.

Insulin, Regular and NPH mixture (Co-administration may require a dosage adjustment of the antidiabetic drug).
  No products indexed under this heading.

Insulin, Zinc Crystals (Co-administration may require a dosage adjustment of the antidiabetic drug).
  No products indexed under this heading.

Insulin, Zinc Suspension (Co-administration may require a dosage adjustment of the antidiabetic drug).
  No products indexed under this heading.

Insulin Aspart (Co-administration may require a dosage adjustment of the antidiabetic drug).
  No products indexed under this heading.

Insulin Aspart, Human (Co-administration may require a dosage adjustment of the antidiabetic drug). Products include:

Insulin Aspart, Human Regular (Co-administration may require a dosage adjustment of the antidiabetic drug). Products include:

Insulin Aspart Protamine, Human (Co-administration may require a dosage adjustment of the antidiabetic drug). Products include:

Insulin Detemir (rDNA Origin) (Co-administration may require a dosage adjustment of the antidiabetic drug). Products include:

Insulin Glargine (Co-administration may require a dosage adjustment of the antidiabetic drug). Products include:

Insulin Glulisine (Co-administration may require a dosage adjustment of the antidiabetic drug). Products include:

Insulin Lispro, Human (Co-administration may require a dosage adjustment of the antidiabetic drug). Products include:

Insulin Lispro Protamine, Human (Co-administration may require a dosage adjustment of the antidiabetic drug). Products include:

Irbesartan (Co-administration could have additive effect or potentiation). Products include:

Isoproterenol Hydrochloride (Co-administration could cause possible decreased response to pressor amines but not sufficient to preclude their use).
  No products indexed under this heading.

Isoproterenol Sulfate (Co-administration could cause possible decreased response to pressor amines but not sufficient to preclude their use).
  No products indexed under this heading.

Isradipine (Co-administration could have additive effect or potentiation). Products include:

Ketoprofen (In some patients the administration of a non-steroidal anti-inflammatory agent can reduce the diuretic, natriuretic and antihypertensive effects of loop, potassium-sparing and thiazide diuretics).
  No products indexed under this heading.

Ketorolac Tromethamine (In some patients the administration of a non-steroidal anti-inflammatory agent can reduce the diuretic, natriuretic and antihypertensive effects of loop, potassium-sparing and thiazide diuretics). Products include:

Labetalol Hydrochloride (Co-administration could have additive effect or potentiation).
  No products indexed under this heading.

Levorphanol Tartrate (Concurrent administration could cause potentiation of orthostatic hypotension).
  No products indexed under this heading.

Lisinopril (Co-administration could have additive effect or potentiation). Products include:

Lithium (Lithium should not generally be given with diuretics; diuretic agents reduce the renal clearance of lithium and add a high risk of lithium toxicity).
  No products indexed under this heading.

Lithium Carbonate (Lithium should not generally be given with diuretics; diuretic agents reduce the renal clearance of lithium and add a high risk of lithium toxicity).
  No products indexed under this heading.

Lithium Citrate (Lithium should not generally be given with diuretics; diuretic agents reduce the renal clearance of lithium and add a high risk of lithium toxicity).
  No products indexed under this heading.

Losartan Potassium (Co-administration could have additive effect or potentiation). Products include:

Mecamylamine Hydrochloride (Co-administration could have additive effect or potentiation).
  No products indexed under this heading.

Meclofenamate Sodium (In some patients the administration of a non-steroidal anti-inflammatory agent can reduce the diuretic, natriuretic and antihypertensive effects of loop, potassium-sparing and thiazide diuretics).
  No products indexed under this heading.

Mefenamic Acid (In some patients the administration of a non-steroidal anti-inflammatory agent can reduce the diuretic, natriuretic and antihypertensive effects of loop, potassium-sparing and thiazide diuretics).
  No products indexed under this heading.

Meloxicam (In some patients the administration of a non-steroidal anti-inflammatory agent can reduce the diuretic, natriuretic and antihypertensive effects of loop, potassium-sparing and thiazide diuretics).
  No products indexed under this heading.

Meperidine Hydrochloride (Concurrent administration could cause potentiation of orthostatic hypotension).
  No products indexed under this heading.

Mephentermine Sulfate (Co-administration could cause possible decreased response to pressor amines but not sufficient to preclude their use).
  No products indexed under this heading.

Mephobarbital (Concurrent administration could cause potentiation of orthostatic hypotension).
  No products indexed under this heading.

Metaraminol Bitartrate (Co-administration could cause possible decreased response to pressor amines but not sufficient to preclude their use).
  No products indexed under this heading.

Metformin Hydrochloride (Co-administration may require a dosage adjustment of the antidiabetic drug). Products include:

Methadone Hydrochloride (Concurrent administration could cause potentiation of orthostatic hypotension).
  No products indexed under this heading.

Methoxamine Hydrochloride (Co-administration could cause possible decreased response to pressor amines but not sufficient to preclude their use).
  No products indexed under this heading.

Methyclothiazide (Co-administration could have additive effect or potentiation).
  No products indexed under this heading.

Methyldopa (Co-administration could have additive effect or potentiation).
  No products indexed under this heading.

Methyldopate Hydrochloride (Co-administration could have additive effect or potentiation).
  No products indexed under this heading.

Methylprednisolone (Co-administration could cause intensified electrolyte depletion, particularly hypokalemia).
  No products indexed under this heading.

Methylprednisolone Acetate (Co-administration could cause intensified electrolyte depletion, particularly hypokalemia).
  No products indexed under this heading.

Methylprednisolone Sodium Succinate (Co-administration could cause intensified electrolyte depletion, particularly hypokalemia).
  No products indexed under this heading.

Metocurine Iodide (Co-administration could cause possible increased responsiveness to the muscle relaxant).
  No products indexed under this heading.

Metolazone (Co-administration could have additive effect or potentiation).
  No products indexed under this heading.

Metoprolol Succinate (Co-administration could have additive effect or potentiation). Products include:

Metoprolol Tartrate (Co-administration could have additive effect or potentiation).
  No products indexed under this heading.

Metyrosine (Co-administration could have additive effect or potentiation).
  No products indexed under this heading.

Mibefradil Dihydrochloride (Co-administration could have additive effect or potentiation).
  No products indexed under this heading.

Miglitol (Co-administration may require a dosage adjustment of the antidiabetic drug).
  No products indexed under this heading.

Minoxidil (Co-administration could have additive effect or potentiation).
  No products indexed under this heading.

Mivacurium Chloride (Co-administration could cause possible increased responsiveness to the muscle relaxant).
  No products indexed under this heading.

Moexipril Hydrochloride (Co-administration could have additive effect or potentiation).
  No products indexed under this heading.

Mometasone Furoate (Co-administration could cause intensified electrolyte depletion, particularly hypokalemia). Products include:

Mometasone Furoate Monohydrate (Co-administration could cause intensified electrolyte depletion, particularly hypokalemia). Products include:

Morphine Sulfate (Concurrent administration could cause potentiation of orthostatic hypotension). Products include:

Morphine Sulfate, Liposomal (Concurrent administration could cause potentiation of orthostatic hypotension).
  No products indexed under this heading.

Nabumetone (In some patients the administration of a non-steroidal anti-inflammatory agent can reduce the diuretic, natriuretic and antihypertensive effects of loop, potassium-sparing and thiazide diuretics).
  No products indexed under this heading.

Nadolol (Co-administration could have additive effect or potentiation). Products include:

219 Interactions Index Benicar HCT

Nadolol ... 2359

Naproxen (In some patients the administration of a non-steroidal anti-inflammatory agent can reduce the diuretic, natriuretic and antihypertensive effects of loop, potassium-sparing and thiazide diuretics). Products include:
EC-Naprosyn ... 2850
Naprosyn ... 2850
Anaprox/Naprosyn ... 2850

Naproxen Sodium (In some patients the administration of a non-steroidal anti-inflammatory agent can reduce the diuretic, natriuretic and antihypertensive effects of loop, potassium-sparing and thiazide diuretics). Products include:
Anaprox ... 2850
Anaprox DS ... 2850
Treximet ... 1681

Nateglinide (Co-administration may require a dosage adjustment of the antidiabetic drug).
No products indexed under this heading.

Nebivolol (Co-administration could have additive effect or potentiation). Products include:
Bystolic ... 1147

Nicardipine Hydrochloride (Co-administration could have additive effect or potentiation).
No products indexed under this heading.

Nifedipine (Co-administration could have additive effect or potentiation).
No products indexed under this heading.

Nisoldipine (Co-administration could have additive effect or potentiation).
No products indexed under this heading.

Nitroglycerin (Co-administration could have additive effect or potentiation). Products include:
Nitro-Dur ... 3170
Nitrolingual ... 3266

Norepinephrine Bitartrate (Co-administration could cause possible decreased response to pressor amines but not sufficient to preclude their use).
No products indexed under this heading.

Oxaprozin (In some patients the administration of a non-steroidal anti-inflammatory agent can reduce the diuretic, natriuretic and antihypertensive effects of loop, potassium-sparing and thiazide diuretics).
No products indexed under this heading.

Oxycodone Hydrochloride (Concurrent administration could cause potentiation of orthostatic hypotension). Products include:
OxyContin ... 2807
Percocet ... 1121
Percodan ... 1124

Oxycodone Terephthalate (Concurrent administration could cause potentiation of orthostatic hypotension).
No products indexed under this heading.

Oxymorphone Hydrochloride (Concurrent administration could cause potentiation of orthostatic hypotension). Products include:
Opana ... 1110
Opana ER ... 1114

Pancuronium Bromide (Co-administration could cause possible increased responsiveness to the muscle relaxant).
No products indexed under this heading.

Penbutolol Sulfate (Co-administration could have additive effect or potentiation).
No products indexed under this heading.

Pentobarbital (Concurrent administration could cause potentiation of orthostatic hypotension).
No products indexed under this heading.

Pentobarbital Sodium (Concurrent administration could cause potentiation of orthostatic hypotension). Products include:
Nembutal ... 2012

Perindopril Erbumine (Co-administration could have additive effect or potentiation).
No products indexed under this heading.

Phenobarbital (Concurrent administration could cause potentiation of orthostatic hypotension). Products include:
Donnatal ... 2711

Phenobarbital Sodium (Concurrent administration could cause potentiation of orthostatic hypotension).
No products indexed under this heading.

Phenoxybenzamine Hydrochloride (Co-administration could have additive effect or potentiation). Products include:
Dibenzyline ... 3495

Phentolamine Mesylate (Co-administration could have additive effect or potentiation).
No products indexed under this heading.

Phenylbutazone (In some patients the administration of a non-steroidal anti-inflammatory agent can reduce the diuretic, natriuretic and antihypertensive effects of loop, potassium-sparing and thiazide diuretics).
No products indexed under this heading.

Phenylephrine Hydrochloride (Co-administration could cause possible decreased response to pressor amines but not sufficient to preclude their use). Products include:
Sudafed PE Nasal Decongestant ... 2048
Children's Sudafed PE Nasal Decongestant ... 2047

Pindolol (Co-administration could have additive effect or potentiation).
No products indexed under this heading.

Pioglitazone Hydrochloride (Co-administration may require a dosage adjustment of the antidiabetic drug). Products include:
ActoPlus ... 3338
Actos ... 3345
Duetact ... 3354

Pipecuronium Bromide (Co-administration could cause possible increased responsiveness to the muscle relaxant).
No products indexed under this heading.

Piroxicam (In some patients the administration of a non-steroidal anti-inflammatory agent can reduce the diuretic, natriuretic and antihypertensive effects of loop, potassium-sparing and thiazide diuretics).
No products indexed under this heading.

Polythiazide (Co-administration could have additive effect or potentiation).
No products indexed under this heading.

Prazosin Hydrochloride (Co-administration could have additive effect or potentiation).
No products indexed under this heading.

Prednisolone (Co-administration could cause intensified electrolyte depletion, particularly hypokalemia).
No products indexed under this heading.

Prednisolone Acetate (Co-administration could cause intensified electrolyte depletion, particularly hypokalemia). Products include:
Blephamide ... ⊙212, ⊙214
Pred Forte ... ⊙225
Pred Mild ... ⊙230
Pred-G ... ⊙226, ⊙227

Prednisolone Sodium Phosphate (Co-administration could cause intensified electrolyte depletion, particularly hypokalemia).
No products indexed under this heading.

Prednisolone Tebutate (Co-administration could cause intensified electrolyte depletion, particularly hypokalemia).
No products indexed under this heading.

Prednisone (Co-administration could cause intensified electrolyte depletion, particularly hypokalemia).
No products indexed under this heading.

Prednisone sodium phosphate (Co-administration could cause intensified electrolyte depletion, particularly hypokalemia).
No products indexed under this heading.

Propoxyphene Hydrochloride (Concurrent administration could cause potentiation of orthostatic hypotension).
No products indexed under this heading.

Propoxyphene Napsylate (Concurrent administration could cause potentiation of orthostatic hypotension).
No products indexed under this heading.

Propranolol Hydrochloride (Co-administration could have additive effect or potentiation). Products include:
InnoPran XL ... 1517

Quinapril Hydrochloride (Co-administration could have additive effect or potentiation).
No products indexed under this heading.

Ramipril (Co-administration could have additive effect or potentiation).
No products indexed under this heading.

Rapacuronium Bromide (Co-administration could cause possible increased responsiveness to the muscle relaxant).
No products indexed under this heading.

Rauwolfia Serpentina (Co-administration could have additive effect or potentiation).
No products indexed under this heading.

Remifentanil Hydrochloride (Concurrent administration could cause potentiation of orthostatic hypotension).
No products indexed under this heading.

Repaglinide (Co-administration may require a dosage adjustment of the antidiabetic drug).
No products indexed under this heading.

Rescinnamine (Co-administration could have additive effect or potentiation).
No products indexed under this heading.

Reserpine (Co-administration could have additive effect or potentiation).
No products indexed under this heading.

Rocuronium Bromide (Co-administration could cause possible increased responsiveness to the muscle relaxant). Products include:
Zemuron ... 3249

Rofecoxib (In some patients the administration of a non-steroidal anti-inflammatory agent can reduce the diuretic, natriuretic and antihypertensive effects of loop, potassium-sparing and thiazide diuretics).
No products indexed under this heading.

Rosiglitazone Maleate (Co-administration may require a dosage adjustment of the antidiabetic drug). Products include:
Avandamet ... 1345
Avandaryl ... 1356
Avandia ... 1366

Secobarbital Sodium (Concurrent administration could cause potentiation of orthostatic hypotension).
No products indexed under this heading.

Sitagliptin Phosphate (Co-administration may require a dosage adjustment of the antidiabetic drug). Products include:
Janumet ... 2188
Januvia ... 2196

Sodium Butabarbital (Concurrent administration could cause potentiation of orthostatic hypotension).
No products indexed under this heading.

Sodium Nitroprusside (Co-administration could have additive effect or potentiation).
No products indexed under this heading.

Sodium Pentobarbital (Concurrent administration could cause potentiation of orthostatic hypotension).
No products indexed under this heading.

Sotalol Hydrochloride (Co-administration could have additive effect or potentiation).
No products indexed under this heading.

Spirapril Hydrochloride (Co-administration could have additive effect or potentiation).
No products indexed under this heading.

Sufentanil Citrate (Concurrent administration could cause potentiation of orthostatic hypotension).
No products indexed under this heading.

Sulindac (In some patients the administration of a non-steroidal anti-inflammatory agent can reduce the diuretic, natriuretic and antihypertensive effects of loop, potassium-sparing and thiazide diuretics). Products include:
Clinoril ... 2098

Telmisartan (Co-administration could have additive effect or potentiation). Products include:
Micardis ... 887
Micardis HCT ... 889

Terazosin Hydrochloride (Co-administration could have additive effect or potentiation).
No products indexed under this heading.

Thiamylal Sodium (Concurrent administration could cause potentiation of orthostatic hypotension).
No products indexed under this heading.

Timolol Maleate (Co-administration could have additive effect or potentiation). Products include:
Combigan ... 601
Dorzolamide Hydrochloride/Timolol Maleate Ophthalmic Solution ... ⊙243
Timoptic in Ocudose ... ⊙231

Tolazamide (Co-administration may require a dosage adjustment of the antidiabetic drug).
No products indexed under this heading.

Tolbutamide (Co-administration may require a dosage adjustment of the antidiabetic drug).
No products indexed under this heading.

Tolmetin Sodium (In some patients the administration of a non-steroidal anti-inflammatory agent can reduce the diuretic, natriuretic and antihypertensive effects of loop, potassium-sparing and thiazide diuretics).
No products indexed under this heading.

Torsemide (Co-administration could have additive effect or potentiation).
No products indexed under this heading.

Trandolapril (Co-administration could have additive effect or potentiation). Products include:
Mavik ... 489
Tarka ... 534

Triamcinolone (Co-administration could cause intensified electrolyte depletion, particularly hypokalemia).
No products indexed under this heading.

Triamcinolone Acetonide (Co-administration could cause intensified electrolyte depletion, particularly hypokalemia). Products include:
Azmacort ... 408
Nasacort AQ ... 3019

Triamcinolone Diacetate (Co-administration could cause intensified electrolyte depletion, particularly hypokalemia).
No products indexed under this heading.

IMPORTANT NOTE: Always consult each drug listing in the patient's regimen for possible interactions.

Benicar HCT Interactions Index 220

Triamcinolone Hexacetonide (Co-administration could cause intensified electrolyte depletion, particularly hypokalemia).
No products indexed under this heading.

Trimethaphan Camsylate (Co-administration could have additive effect or potentiation).
No products indexed under this heading.

Troglitazone (Co-administration may require a dosage adjustment of the antidiabetic drug).
No products indexed under this heading.

Tubocurarine Chloride (Co-administration could cause possible increased responsiveness to the muscle relaxant).
No products indexed under this heading.

Valdecoxib (In some patients the administration of a non-steroidal anti-inflammatory agent can reduce the diuretic, natriuretic and antihypertensive effects of loop, potassium-sparing and thiazide diuretics).
No products indexed under this heading.

Valsartan (Co-administration could have additive effect or potentiation). Products include:
Diovan ... **2413**
Diovan HCT ... **2419**
Exforge ... **2443**
Exforge HCT ... **2449**
Valturna ... **3637**

Vecuronium Bromide (Co-administration could cause possible increased responsiveness to the muscle relaxant).
No products indexed under this heading.

Verapamil Hydrochloride (Co-administration could have additive effect or potentiation). Products include:
Tarka ... **534**

Food Interactions

Alcohol (Concurrent administration could cause potentiation of orthostatic hypotension).

Beer, reduced-alcohol (Concurrent administration could cause potentiation of orthostatic hypotension).

Beer, unspecified (Concurrent administration could cause potentiation of orthostatic hypotension).

Wine, Chianti (Concurrent administration could cause potentiation of orthostatic hypotension).

Wine, Red (Concurrent administration could cause potentiation of orthostatic hypotension).

Wine, unspecified (Concurrent administration could cause potentiation of orthostatic hypotension).

Wine products (Concurrent administration could cause potentiation of orthostatic hypotension).

BENTYL CAPSULES
(Dicyclomine Hydrochloride) ... **780**
See Bentyl Tablets

BENTYL INJECTION
(Dicyclomine Hydrochloride) ... **780**
See Bentyl Tablets

BENTYL SYRUP
(Dicyclomine Hydrochloride) ... **780**
See Bentyl Tablets

BENTYL TABLETS
(Dicyclomine Hydrochloride) ... **780**
May interact with agents used to treat achlorhydria and/or to test gastric secretion, antacids, antiglaucoma agents, antihistamines, antipsychotic agents, benzodiazepines, corticosteroids, monoamine oxidase inhibitors, narcotic analgesics, nitrates and nitrites, sympathomimetics, tricyclic antidepressants, type 1 antiarrhythmic drugs, and certain other agents. Compounds in these categories include:

Acetazolamide (Anticholinergics antagonize the effects of antiglaucoma agents).
No products indexed under this heading.

Acetylcholine Chloride (Anticholinergics antagonize the effects of antiglaucoma agents).
No products indexed under this heading.

Acrivastine (Antihistamines may increase certain actions or side effects of anticholinergic agents).
No products indexed under this heading.

Albuterol (Sympathomimetic agents may increase certain actions or side effects of anticholinergic agents).
No products indexed under this heading.

Albuterol Sulfate (Sympathomimetic agents may increase certain actions or side effects of anticholinergic agents). Products include:
ProAir HFA ... **3393**
Proventil HFA ... **3204**
Ventolin HFA ... **1708**

Alclometasone Dipropionate (Anticholinergic drugs in the presence of increased intraocular pressure may be hazardous when taken concurrently with agents such as corticosteroids).
No products indexed under this heading.

Alfentanil Hydrochloride (Narcotic analgesics may increase certain actions or side effects of anticholinergic agents).
No products indexed under this heading.

Alprazolam (Benzodiazepines may increase certain actions or side effects of anticholinergic agents).
No products indexed under this heading.

Aluminum Carbonate (Antacids may interfere with the absorption of anticholinergic agents; therefore, simultaneous use of these drugs should be avoided).
No products indexed under this heading.

Aluminum Hydroxide (Antacids may interfere with the absorption of anticholinergic agents; therefore, simultaneous use of these drugs should be avoided).
No products indexed under this heading.

Amantadine Hydrochloride (Amantadine may increase certain actions or side effects of anticholinergic agents).
No products indexed under this heading.

Amitriptyline Hydrochloride (Tricyclic antidepressants may increase certain actions or side effects of anticholinergic agents).
No products indexed under this heading.

Amoxapine (Tricyclic antidepressants may increase certain actions or side effects of anticholinergic agents).
No products indexed under this heading.

Amyl Nitrite (Nitrates and nitrites may increase certain actions or side effects of anticholinergic agents).
No products indexed under this heading.

Apomorphine (Narcotic analgesics may increase certain actions or side effects of anticholinergic agents).
No products indexed under this heading.

Apomorphine Hydrochloride (Narcotic analgesics may increase certain actions or side effects of anticholinergic agents).
No products indexed under this heading.

Aripiprazole (Antipsychotic agents may increase certain actions or side effects of anticholinergic agents).
No products indexed under this heading.

Astemizole (Antihistamines may increase certain actions or side effects of anticholinergic agents).
No products indexed under this heading.

Azatadine Maleate (Antihistamines may increase certain actions or side effects of anticholinergic agents).
No products indexed under this heading.

Beclomethasone Dipropionate (Anticholinergic drugs in the presence of increased intraocular pressure may be hazardous when taken concurrently with agents such as corticosteroids). Products include:
Qvar ... **3398**

Beclomethasone Dipropionate Monohydrate (Anticholinergic drugs in the presence of increased intraocular pressure may be hazardous when taken concurrently with agents such as corticosteroids). Products include:
Beconase AQ ... **1386**

Betamethasone (Anticholinergic drugs in the presence of increased intraocular pressure may be hazardous when taken concurrently with agents such as corticosteroids).
No products indexed under this heading.

Betamethasone Acetate (Anticholinergic drugs in the presence of increased intraocular pressure may be hazardous when taken concurrently with agents such as corticosteroids).
No products indexed under this heading.

Betamethasone Benzoate (Anticholinergic drugs in the presence of increased intraocular pressure may be hazardous when taken concurrently with agents such as corticosteroids).
No products indexed under this heading.

Betamethasone Dipropionate (Anticholinergic drugs in the presence of increased intraocular pressure may be hazardous when taken concurrently with agents such as corticosteroids). Products include:
Diprolene Lotion 0.05% ... **3108**
Diprolene Ointment 0.05% ... **3109**
Diprolene AF Cream 0.05% ... **3107**
Lotrisone ... **3163**

Betamethasone Sodium Phosphate (Anticholinergic drugs in the presence of increased intraocular pressure may be hazardous when taken concurrently with agents such as corticosteroids).
No products indexed under this heading.

Betamethasone Valerate (Anticholinergic drugs in the presence of increased intraocular pressure may be hazardous when taken concurrently with agents such as corticosteroids). Products include:
Luxiq ... **3321**

Betaxolol Hydrochloride (Anticholinergics antagonize the effects of antiglaucoma agents).
No products indexed under this heading.

Bromodiphenhydramine Hydrochloride (Antihistamines may increase certain actions or side effects of anticholinergic agents).
No products indexed under this heading.

Brompheniramine Maleate (Antihistamines may increase certain actions or side effects of anticholinergic agents).
No products indexed under this heading.

Budesonide (Anticholinergic drugs in the presence of increased intraocular pressure may be hazardous when taken concurrently with agents such as corticosteroids). Products include:
Pulmicort Flexhaler ... **714**
Symbicort 80/4.5 ... **720**
Symbicort 160/4.5 ... **720**

Buprenorphine Hydrochloride (Narcotic analgesics may increase certain actions or side effects of anticholinergic agents).
No products indexed under this heading.

Calcium Carbonate (Antacids may interfere with the absorption of anticholinergic agents; therefore, simultaneous use of these drugs should be avoided). Products include:
Chelated Mineral ... **3476**
Pepcid Complete ... **1822**
Extra Strength Rolaids Softchews Vanilla Creme ... **2045**

Carbachol (Anticholinergics antagonize the effects of antiglaucoma agents).
No products indexed under this heading.

Cetirizine Hydrochloride (Antihistamines may increase certain actions or side effects of anticholinergic agents). Products include:
Zyrtec Allergy ... **2052**
Children's Zyrtec Allergy Syrup ... **2053**
Children's Zyrtec Allergy ... **2053**
Children's Zyrtec Hives Relief ... **2053**
Zyrtec-D Allergy & Congestion ... **2054**

Chlordiazepoxide (Benzodiazepines may increase certain actions or side effects of anticholinergic agents).
No products indexed under this heading.

Chlordiazepoxide Hydrochloride (Benzodiazepines may increase certain actions or side effects of anticholinergic agents).
No products indexed under this heading.

Chlorpheniramine Maleate (Antihistamines may increase certain actions or side effects of anticholinergic agents).
No products indexed under this heading.

Chlorpheniramine Polistirex (Antihistamines may increase certain actions or side effects of anticholinergic agents). Products include:
Tussionex ... **3443**

Chlorpheniramine Tannate (Antihistamines may increase certain actions or side effects of anticholinergic agents).
No products indexed under this heading.

Chlorpromazine (Antipsychotic agents may increase certain actions or side effects of anticholinergic agents).
No products indexed under this heading.

Chlorpromazine Hydrochloride (Antipsychotic agents may increase certain actions or side effects of anticholinergic agents).
No products indexed under this heading.

Chlorprothixene (Antipsychotic agents may increase certain actions or side effects of anticholinergic agents).
No products indexed under this heading.

Chlorprothixene Hydrochloride (Antipsychotic agents may increase certain actions or side effects of anticholinergic agents).
No products indexed under this heading.

Chlorprothixene Lactate (Antipsychotic agents may increase certain actions or side effects of anticholinergic agents).
No products indexed under this heading.

Ciclesonide (Anticholinergic drugs in the presence of increased intraocular pressure may be hazardous when taken concurrently with agents such as corticosteroids).
No products indexed under this heading.

Cisapride (Anticholinergic drugs may antagonize the effects of drugs that alter gastrointestinal motility).
No products indexed under this heading.

Clemastine Fumarate (Antihistamines may increase certain actions or side effects of anticholinergic agents).
No products indexed under this heading.

Clomipramine Hydrochloride (Tricyclic antidepressants may increase certain actions or side effects of anticholinergic agents).
No products indexed under this heading.

Clorazepate Dipotassium (Benzodiazepines may increase certain actions or side effects of anticholinergic agents).
No products indexed under this heading.

221 **Interactions Index** **Bentyl**

Clozapine (Antipsychotic agents may increase certain actions or side effects of anticholinergic agents).
No products indexed under this heading.

Codeine Phosphate (Narcotic analgesics may increase certain actions or side effects of anticholinergic agents). Products include:
Tylenol with Codeine **2691**

Codeine Sulfate (Narcotic analgesics may increase certain actions or side effects of anticholinergic agents).
No products indexed under this heading.

Cortisone Acetate (Anticholinergic drugs in the presence of increased intraocular pressure may be hazardous when taken concurrently with agents such as corticosteroids).
No products indexed under this heading.

Cyproheptadine Hydrochloride (Antihistamines may increase certain actions or side effects of anticholinergic agents).
No products indexed under this heading.

Demecarium Bromide (Anticholinergics antagonize the effects of antiglaucoma agents).
No products indexed under this heading.

Desipramine Hydrochloride (Tricyclic antidepressants may increase certain actions or side effects of anticholinergic agents).
No products indexed under this heading.

Desoximetasone (Anticholinergic drugs in the presence of increased intraocular pressure may be hazardous when taken concurrently with agents such as corticosteroids).
No products indexed under this heading.

Dexamethasone (Anticholinergic drugs in the presence of increased intraocular pressure may be hazardous when taken concurrently with agents such as corticosteroids). Products include:
Ciprodex **583**
Ozurdex .... ⊙ **223**
Tobramycin and Dexamethasone Ophthalmic Suspension .... ⊙ **251**

Dexamethasone Acetate (Anticholinergic drugs in the presence of increased intraocular pressure may be hazardous when taken concurrently with agents such as corticosteroids).
No products indexed under this heading.

Dexamethasone Phosphate (Anticholinergic drugs in the presence of increased intraocular pressure may be hazardous when taken concurrently with agents such as corticosteroids).
No products indexed under this heading.

Dexamethasone Sodium (Anticholinergic drugs in the presence of increased intraocular pressure may be hazardous when taken concurrently with agents such as corticosteroids).
No products indexed under this heading.

Dexamethasone Sodium Phosphate (Anticholinergic drugs in the presence of increased intraocular pressure may be hazardous when taken concurrently with agents such as corticosteroids).
No products indexed under this heading.

Dexamethasone Sodium Phosphate Injection (Anticholinergic drugs in the presence of increased intraocular pressure may be hazardous when taken concurrently with agents such as corticosteroids).
No products indexed under this heading.

Dexchlorpheniramine Maleate (Antihistamines may increase certain actions or side effects of anticholinergic agents).
No products indexed under this heading.

Dexpanthenol (Anticholinergic drugs may antagonize the effects of drugs that alter gastrointestinal motility).
No products indexed under this heading.

Dezocine (Narcotic analgesics may increase certain actions or side effects of anticholinergic agents).
No products indexed under this heading.

Diazepam (Benzodiazepines may increase certain actions or side effects of anticholinergic agents). Products include:
Valium Tablets **2880**

Dichlorphenamide (Anticholinergics antagonize the effects of antiglaucoma agents).
No products indexed under this heading.

Diflorasone Diacetate (Anticholinergic drugs in the presence of increased intraocular pressure may be hazardous when taken concurrently with agents such as corticosteroids).
No products indexed under this heading.

Digoxin (Anticholinergic agents may affect gastrointestinal absorption of various drugs, such as slowly dissolving dosage forms of digoxin; increased serum digoxin concentrations may result). Products include:
Lanoxin Injection **1546**
Lanoxin Injection Pediatric **1549**
Lanoxin Tablets **1553**

Dihydrocodeine Bitartrate (Narcotic analgesics may increase certain actions or side effects of anticholinergic agents).
No products indexed under this heading.

Dihydrocodeinone Bitartrate (Narcotic analgesics may increase certain actions or side effects of anticholinergic agents).
No products indexed under this heading.

Diphenhydramine Hydrochloride (Antihistamines may increase certain actions or side effects of anticholinergic agents). Products include:
Benadryl Allergy Ultratab **2042**
Children's Benadryl Allergy Liquid **2042**

Diphenylpyraline Hydrochloride (Antihistamines may increase certain actions or side effects of anticholinergic agents).
No products indexed under this heading.

Dipivefrin Hydrochloride (Anticholinergics antagonize the effects of antiglaucoma agents).
No products indexed under this heading.

Disopyramide Phosphate (Class I antiarrhythmic agents may increase certain actions or side effects of anticholinergic agents).
No products indexed under this heading.

Dobutamine Hydrochloride (Sympathomimetic agents may increase certain actions or side effects of anticholinergic agents).
No products indexed under this heading.

Dopamine Hydrochloride (Sympathomimetic agents may increase certain actions or side effects of anticholinergic agents).
No products indexed under this heading.

Doxepin Hydrochloride (Tricyclic antidepressants may increase certain actions or side effects of anticholinergic agents).
No products indexed under this heading.

Echothiophate Iodide (Anticholinergics antagonize the effects of antiglaucoma agents).
No products indexed under this heading.

Ephedrine Hydrochloride (Sympathomimetic agents may increase certain actions or side effects of anticholinergic agents).
No products indexed under this heading.

Ephedrine Sulfate (Sympathomimetic agents may increase certain actions or side effects of anticholinergic agents).
No products indexed under this heading.

Ephedrine Tannate (Sympathomimetic agents may increase certain actions or side effects of anticholinergic agents).
No products indexed under this heading.

Epinephrine (Sympathomimetic agents may increase certain actions or side effects of anticholinergic agents). Products include:
EpiPen **3631**
Twinject **3268**

Epinephrine Bitartrate (Sympathomimetic agents may increase certain actions or side effects of anticholinergic agents).
No products indexed under this heading.

Epinephrine Hydrochloride (Sympathomimetic agents may increase certain actions or side effects of anticholinergic agents).
No products indexed under this heading.

Epinephryl Borate (Anticholinergics antagonize the effects of antiglaucoma agents).
No products indexed under this heading.

Erythrityl Tetranitrate (Nitrates and nitrites may increase certain actions or side effects of anticholinergic agents).
No products indexed under this heading.

Estazolam (Benzodiazepines may increase certain actions or side effects of anticholinergic agents).
No products indexed under this heading.

Fentanyl (Narcotic analgesics may increase certain actions or side effects of anticholinergic agents). Products include:
Duragesic **2604**
Fentanyl Transdermal System **2346**
Onsolis **2054**

Fentanyl Citrate (Narcotic analgesics may increase certain actions or side effects of anticholinergic agents). Products include:
Fentora **966**

Fexofenadine Hydrochloride (Antihistamines may increase certain actions or side effects of anticholinergic agents). Products include:
Allegra ODT **2911**
Allegra Oral Solution **2911**
Allegra **2911**
Allegra-D **2915**
Allegra-D 24 .... **2918**

Fludrocortisone Acetate (Anticholinergic drugs in the presence of increased intraocular pressure may be hazardous when taken concurrently with agents such as corticosteroids).
No products indexed under this heading.

Flumethasone Pivalate (Anticholinergic drugs in the presence of increased intraocular pressure may be hazardous when taken concurrently with agents such as corticosteroids).
No products indexed under this heading.

Flunisolide Hemihydrate (Anticholinergic drugs in the presence of increased intraocular pressure may be hazardous when taken concurrently with agents such as corticosteroids).
No products indexed under this heading.

Fluphenazine Decanoate (Antipsychotic agents may increase certain actions or side effects of anticholinergic agents).
No products indexed under this heading.

Fluphenazine Enanthate (Antipsychotic agents may increase certain actions or side effects of anticholinergic agents).
No products indexed under this heading.

Fluphenazine Hydrochloride (Antipsychotic agents may increase certain actions or side effects of anticholinergic agents).
No products indexed under this heading.

Flurazepam Hydrochloride (Benzodiazepines may increase certain actions or side effects of anticholinergic agents).
No products indexed under this heading.

Fluticasone Furoate (Anticholinergic drugs in the presence of increased intraocular pressure may be hazardous when taken concurrently with agents such as corticosteroids). Products include:
Veramyst **1713**

Fluticasone Propionate (Anticholinergic drugs in the presence of increased intraocular pressure may be hazardous when taken concurrently with agents such as corticosteroids). Products include:
Advair 100/50 .... **1275**
Advair 250/50 .... **1275**
Advair 500/50 .... **1275**
Advair HFA 45/21 .... **1288**
Advair HFA 115/21 .... **1288**
Advair HFA 230/21 .... **1288**
Flonase **1459**
Flovent Diskus **1463**
Flovent HFA **1470**

Glutamic Acid Hydrochloride (The inhibiting effects of anticholinergic drugs on gastric hydrochloric acid secretion are antagonized by agents used to treat achlorhydria and those used to test gastric secretion).
No products indexed under this heading.

Glyceryl Trinitrate (Nitrates and nitrites may increase certain actions or side effects of anticholinergic agents).
No products indexed under this heading.

Halazepam (Benzodiazepines may increase certain actions or side effects of anticholinergic agents).
No products indexed under this heading.

Haloperidol (Antipsychotic agents may increase certain actions or side effects of anticholinergic agents).
No products indexed under this heading.

Haloperidol Decanoate (Antipsychotic agents may increase certain actions or side effects of anticholinergic agents).
No products indexed under this heading.

Haloperidol Lactate (Antipsychotic agents may increase certain actions or side effects of anticholinergic agents).
No products indexed under this heading.

Hydrocodone Bitartrate (Narcotic analgesics may increase certain actions or side effects of anticholinergic agents). Products include:
Vicodin **560**
Vicodin ES **561**
Vicodin HP **563**
Vicoprofen **564**
Zydone **1138**

Hydrocodone Polistirex (Narcotic analgesics may increase certain actions or side effects of anticholinergic agents). Products include:
Tussionex **3443**

Hydrocortisone (Anticholinergic drugs in the presence of increased intraocular pressure may be hazardous when taken concurrently with agents such as corticosteroids).
No products indexed under this heading.

Hydrocortisone (Alcohol) (Anticholinergic drugs in the presence of increased intraocular pressure may be hazardous when taken concurrently with agents such as corticosteroids).
No products indexed under this heading.

Hydrocortisone Acetate (Anticholinergic drugs in the presence of increased intraocular pressure may be hazardous when taken concurrently with agents such as corticosteroids).
No products indexed under this heading.

IMPORTANT NOTE: Always consult each drug listing in the patient's regimen for possible interactions.

Bentyl Interactions Index 222

Hydrocortisone Butyrate (Anticholinergic drugs in the presence of increased intraocular pressure may be hazardous when taken concurrently with agents such as corticosteroids).
No products indexed under this heading.

Hydrocortisone Cypionate (Anticholinergic drugs in the presence of increased intraocular pressure may be hazardous when taken concurrently with agents such as corticosteroids).
No products indexed under this heading.

Hydrocortisone Hemisuccinate (Anticholinergic drugs in the presence of increased intraocular pressure may be hazardous when taken concurrently with agents such as corticosteroids).
No products indexed under this heading.

Hydrocortisone Probutate (Anticholinergic drugs in the presence of increased intraocular pressure may be hazardous when taken concurrently with agents such as corticosteroids).
No products indexed under this heading.

Hydrocortisone Sodium Phosphate (Anticholinergic drugs in the presence of increased intraocular pressure may be hazardous when taken concurrently with agents such as corticosteroids).
No products indexed under this heading.

Hydrocortisone Sodium Succinate (Anticholinergic drugs in the presence of increased intraocular pressure may be hazardous when taken concurrently with agents such as corticosteroids).
No products indexed under this heading.

Hydrocortisone Valerate (Anticholinergic drugs in the presence of increased intraocular pressure may be hazardous when taken concurrently with agents such as corticosteroids).
No products indexed under this heading.

Hydromorphone (Narcotic analgesics may increase certain actions or side effects of anticholinergic agents).
No products indexed under this heading.

Hydromorphone Hydrochloride (Narcotic analgesics may increase certain actions or side effects of anticholinergic agents). Products include:
Dilaudid Injection **2800**
Dilaudid Oral **2797**
Dilaudid Tablets **2797**
Dilaudid-HP **2800**

Imipramine Hydrochloride (Tricyclic antidepressants may increase certain actions or side effects of anticholinergic agents).
No products indexed under this heading.

Imipramine Pamoate (Tricyclic antidepressants may increase certain actions or side effects of anticholinergic agents).
No products indexed under this heading.

Isocarboxazid (MAO inhibitors may increase certain actions or side effects of anticholinergic agents). Products include:
Marplan **3481**

Isoflurophate (Anticholinergics antagonize the effects of antiglaucoma agents).
No products indexed under this heading.

Isoproterenol Hydrochloride (Sympathomimetic agents may increase certain actions or side effects of anticholinergic agents).
No products indexed under this heading.

Isoproterenol Sulfate (Sympathomimetic agents may increase certain actions or side effects of anticholinergic agents).
No products indexed under this heading.

Isosorbide Dinitrate (Nitrates and nitrites may increase certain actions or side effects of anticholinergic agents).
No products indexed under this heading.

Isosorbide Mononitrate (Nitrates and nitrites may increase certain actions or side effects of anticholinergic agents).
No products indexed under this heading.

Levalbuterol Hydrochloride (Sympathomimetic agents may increase certain actions or side effects of anticholinergic agents).
No products indexed under this heading.

Levobunolol Hydrochloride (Anticholinergics antagonize the effects of antiglaucoma agents).
No products indexed under this heading.

Levorphanol Tartrate (Narcotic analgesics may increase certain actions or side effects of anticholinergic agents).
No products indexed under this heading.

Lithium (Antipsychotic agents may increase certain actions or side effects of anticholinergic agents).
No products indexed under this heading.

Lithium Carbonate (Antipsychotic agents may increase certain actions or side effects of anticholinergic agents).
No products indexed under this heading.

Lithium Citrate (Antipsychotic agents may increase certain actions or side effects of anticholinergic agents).
No products indexed under this heading.

Loratadine (Antihistamines may increase certain actions or side effects of anticholinergic agents).
No products indexed under this heading.

Lorazepam (Benzodiazepines may increase certain actions or side effects of anticholinergic agents).
No products indexed under this heading.

Loxapine Hydrochloride (Antipsychotic agents may increase certain actions or side effects of anticholinergic agents).
No products indexed under this heading.

Loxapine Succinate (Antipsychotic agents may increase certain actions or side effects of anticholinergic agents).
No products indexed under this heading.

Magaldrate (Antacids may interfere with the absorption of anticholinergic agents; therefore, simultaneous use of these drugs should be avoided).
No products indexed under this heading.

Magnesium Carbonate (Antacids may interfere with the absorption of anticholinergic agents; therefore, simultaneous use of these drugs should be avoided).
No products indexed under this heading.

Magnesium Hydroxide (Antacids may interfere with the absorption of anticholinergic agents; therefore, simultaneous use of these drugs should be avoided). Products include:
Fleet Pedia-Lax Chewable Tablets **1144**
Pepcid Complete **1822**

Magnesium Oxide (Antacids may interfere with the absorption of anticholinergic agents; therefore, simultaneous use of these drugs should be avoided). Products include:
Beelith **873**

Magnesium Trisilicate (Antacids may interfere with the absorption of anticholinergic agents; therefore, simultaneous use of these drugs should be avoided).
No products indexed under this heading.

Maprotiline Hydrochloride (Tricyclic antidepressants may increase certain actions or side effects of anticholinergic agents).
No products indexed under this heading.

Meperidine Hydrochloride (Narcotic analgesics may increase certain actions or side effects of anticholinergic agents).
No products indexed under this heading.

Mesoridazine Besylate (Antipsychotic agents may increase certain actions or side effects of anticholinergic agents).
No products indexed under this heading.

Metaproterenol Sulfate (Sympathomimetic agents may increase certain actions or side effects of anticholinergic agents).
No products indexed under this heading.

Metaraminol Bitartrate (Sympathomimetic agents may increase certain actions or side effects of anticholinergic agents).
No products indexed under this heading.

Methadone Hydrochloride (Narcotic analgesics may increase certain actions or side effects of anticholinergic agents).
No products indexed under this heading.

Methazolamide (Anticholinergics antagonize the effects of antiglaucoma agents).
No products indexed under this heading.

Methdilazine Hydrochloride (Antihistamines may increase certain actions or side effects of anticholinergic agents).
No products indexed under this heading.

Methotrimeprazine (Antipsychotic agents may increase certain actions or side effects of anticholinergic agents).
No products indexed under this heading.

Methoxamine Hydrochloride (Sympathomimetic agents may increase certain actions or side effects of anticholinergic agents).
No products indexed under this heading.

Methylprednisolone (Anticholinergic drugs in the presence of increased intraocular pressure may be hazardous when taken concurrently with agents such as corticosteroids).
No products indexed under this heading.

Methylprednisolone Acetate (Anticholinergic drugs in the presence of increased intraocular pressure may be hazardous when taken concurrently with agents such as corticosteroids).
No products indexed under this heading.

Methylprednisolone Sodium Succinate (Anticholinergic drugs in the presence of increased intraocular pressure may be hazardous when taken concurrently with agents such as corticosteroids).
No products indexed under this heading.

Metoclopramide Hydrochloride (Anticholinergic drugs may antagonize the effects of drugs that alter gastrointestinal motility). Products include:
Metozolv ODT **2901**

Midazolam Hydrochloride (Benzodiazepines may increase certain actions or side effects of anticholinergic agents).
No products indexed under this heading.

Moclobemide (MAO inhibitors may increase certain actions or side effects of anticholinergic agents).
No products indexed under this heading.

Molindone Hydrochloride (Antipsychotic agents may increase certain actions or side effects of anticholinergic agents). Products include:
Moban **1108**

Mometasone Furoate (Anticholinergic drugs in the presence of increased intraocular pressure may be hazardous when taken concurrently with agents such as corticosteroids). Products include:
Asmanex **3058**
Elocon Cream **3111**
Elocon Lotion **3112**
Elocon Ointment **3114**

Mometasone Furoate Monohydrate (Anticholinergic drugs in the presence of increased intraocular pressure may be hazardous when taken concurrently with agents such as corticosteroids). Products include:
Nasonex **3166**

Moricizine Hydrochloride (Class I antiarrhythmic agents may increase certain actions or side effects of anticholinergic agents).
No products indexed under this heading.

Morphine Sulfate (Narcotic analgesics may increase certain actions or side effects of anticholinergic agents). Products include:
Avinza **1822**
Embeda **1831**
MS Contin **2803**

Morphine Sulfate, Liposomal (Narcotic analgesics may increase certain actions or side effects of anticholinergic agents).
No products indexed under this heading.

Nitrate & Nitrite Preparations (Nitrates and nitrites may increase certain actions or side effects of anticholinergic agents).
No products indexed under this heading.

Nitrates, organic (Nitrates and nitrites may increase certain actions or side effects of anticholinergic agents).
No products indexed under this heading.

Nitrates and Nitrites (Nitrates and nitrites may increase certain actions or side effects of anticholinergic agents).
No products indexed under this heading.

Nitroglycerin (Nitrates and nitrites may increase certain actions or side effects of anticholinergic agents). Products include:
Nitro-Dur **3170**
Nitrolingual **3266**

Nitroglycerin, long-acting formulations (Nitrates and nitrites may increase certain actions or side effects of anticholinergic agents).
No products indexed under this heading.

Nitroglycerin Intravenous (Nitrates and nitrites may increase certain actions or side effects of anticholinergic agents).
No products indexed under this heading.

Norepinephrine Bitartrate (Sympathomimetic agents may increase certain actions or side effects of anticholinergic agents).
No products indexed under this heading.

Nortriptyline Hydrochloride (Tricyclic antidepressants may increase certain actions or side effects of anticholinergic agents).
No products indexed under this heading.

Olanzapine (Antipsychotic agents may increase certain actions or side effects of anticholinergic agents). Products include:
Symbyax **1965**
Zyprexa **1984**
Zyprexa IntraMuscular **1984**
Zyprexa ZYDIS **1984**

Oxazepam (Benzodiazepines may increase certain actions or side effects of anticholinergic agents).
No products indexed under this heading.

Oxycodone Hydrochloride (Narcotic analgesics may increase certain actions or side effects of anticholinergic agents). Products include:
OxyContin **2807**
Percocet **1121**
Percodan **1124**

Oxycodone Terephthalate (Narcotic analgesics may increase certain actions or side effects of anticholinergic agents).
No products indexed under this heading.

Oxymorphone Hydrochloride (Narcotic analgesics may increase certain actions or side effects of anticholinergic agents). Products include:
Opana **1110**

(⊙ Described in PDR® for Ophthalmic Medicines)

Opana ER 1114

Paliperidone (Antipsychotic agents may increase certain actions or side effects of anticholinergic agents). Products include:
  Invega 2613
  Invega Sustenna 2621

Pargyline Hydrochloride (MAO inhibitors may increase certain actions or side effects of anticholinergic agents).
  No products indexed under this heading.

Pentaerythritol Tetranitrate (Nitrates and nitrites may increase certain actions or side effects of anticholinergic agents).
  No products indexed under this heading.

Pentagastrin (The inhibiting effects of anticholinergic drugs on gastric hydrochloric acid secretion are antagonized by agents used to treat achlorhydria and those used to test gastric secretion).
  No products indexed under this heading.

Perphenazine (Antipsychotic agents may increase certain actions or side effects of anticholinergic agents).
  No products indexed under this heading.

Phenelzine Sulfate (MAO inhibitors may increase certain actions or side effects of anticholinergic agents).
  No products indexed under this heading.

Phenylephrine Bitartrate (Sympathomimetic agents may increase certain actions or side effects of anticholinergic agents).
  No products indexed under this heading.

Phenylephrine Hydrochloride (Sympathomimetic agents may increase certain actions or side effects of anticholinergic agents). Products include:
  Sudafed PE Nasal Decongestant 2048
  Children's Sudafed PE Nasal Decongestant 2047

Phenylephrine Tannate (Sympathomimetic agents may increase certain actions or side effects of anticholinergic agents).
  No products indexed under this heading.

Phenylpropanolamine Hydrochloride (Sympathomimetic agents may increase certain actions or side effects of anticholinergic agents).
  No products indexed under this heading.

Pilocarpine (Anticholinergics antagonize the effects of antiglaucoma agents).
  No products indexed under this heading.

Pilocarpine Hydrochloride (Anticholinergics antagonize the effects of antiglaucoma agents). Products include:
  Salagen 1072

Pimozide (Antipsychotic agents may increase certain actions or side effects of anticholinergic agents).
  No products indexed under this heading.

Pirbuterol Acetate (Sympathomimetic agents may increase certain actions or side effects of anticholinergic agents). Products include:
  Maxair Autohaler 1782

Prazepam (Benzodiazepines may increase certain actions or side effects of anticholinergic agents).
  No products indexed under this heading.

Prednisolone (Anticholinergic drugs in the presence of increased intraocular pressure may be hazardous when taken concurrently with agents such as corticosteroids).
  No products indexed under this heading.

Prednisolone Acetate (Anticholinergic drugs in the presence of increased intraocular pressure may be hazardous when taken concurrently with agents such as corticosteroids). Products include:
  Blephamide .... ⊙212, ⊙214

Pred Forte .... ⊙225
Pred Mild .... ⊙230
Pred-G .... ⊙226, ⊙227

Prednisolone Sodium Phosphate (Anticholinergic drugs in the presence of increased intraocular pressure may be hazardous when taken concurrently with agents such as corticosteroids).
  No products indexed under this heading.

Prednisolone Tebutate (Anticholinergic drugs in the presence of increased intraocular pressure may be hazardous when taken concurrently with agents such as corticosteroids).
  No products indexed under this heading.

Prednisone (Anticholinergic drugs in the presence of increased intraocular pressure may be hazardous when taken concurrently with agents such as corticosteroids).
  No products indexed under this heading.

Prednisone sodium phosphate (Anticholinergic drugs in the presence of increased intraocular pressure may be hazardous when taken concurrently with agents such as corticosteroids).
  No products indexed under this heading.

Procainamide Hydrochloride (Class I antiarrhythmic agents may increase certain actions or side effects of anticholinergic agents).
  No products indexed under this heading.

Procarbazine Hydrochloride (MAO inhibitors may increase certain actions or side effects of anticholinergic agents).
  No products indexed under this heading.

Prochlorperazine (Antipsychotic agents may increase certain actions or side effects of anticholinergic agents).
  No products indexed under this heading.

Promethazine Hydrochloride (Antihistamines may increase certain actions or side effects of anticholinergic agents).
  No products indexed under this heading.

Propafenone Hydrochloride (Class I antiarrhythmic agents may increase certain actions or side effects of anticholinergic agents). Products include:
  Rythmol 1648
  Rythmol SR 1652

Propoxyphene Hydrochloride (Narcotic analgesics may increase certain actions or side effects of anticholinergic agents).
  No products indexed under this heading.

Propoxyphene Napsylate (Narcotic analgesics may increase certain actions or side effects of anticholinergic agents).
  No products indexed under this heading.

Protriptyline Hydrochloride (Tricyclic antidepressants may increase certain actions or side effects of anticholinergic agents).
  No products indexed under this heading.

Pseudoephedrine Hydrochloride (Sympathomimetic agents may increase certain actions or side effects of anticholinergic agents). Products include:
  Allegra-D 2915
  Allegra-D 24 2918
  Sudafed 12 Hour Nasal Decongestant Non-Drowsy 2048
  Sudafed 24 Hour 2048
  Sudafed Nasal Decongestant 2047
  Children's Sudafed Nasal Decongestant Liquid 2047
  Zyrtec-D Allergy & Congestion 2054

Pseudoephedrine Sulfate (Sympathomimetic agents may increase certain actions or side effects of anticholinergic agents). Products include:
  Clarinex-D 12-Hour 3101
  Clarinex-D 3104

Pyrilamine Maleate (Antihistamines may increase certain actions or side effects of anticholinergic agents).
  No products indexed under this heading.

Pyrilamine Tannate (Antihistamines may increase certain actions or side effects of anticholinergic agents).
  No products indexed under this heading.

Quazepam (Benzodiazepines may increase certain actions or side effects of anticholinergic agents).
  No products indexed under this heading.

Quetiapine Fumarate (Antipsychotic agents may increase certain actions or side effects of anticholinergic agents). Products include:
  Seroquel 750
  Seroquel XR 759

Quinidine Gluconate (Class I antiarrhythmic agents may increase certain actions or side effects of anticholinergic agents).
  No products indexed under this heading.

Quinidine Polygalacturonate (Class I antiarrhythmic agents may increase certain actions or side effects of anticholinergic agents).
  No products indexed under this heading.

Quinidine Sulfate (Class I antiarrhythmic agents may increase certain actions or side effects of anticholinergic agents).
  No products indexed under this heading.

Rasagiline Mesylate (MAO inhibitors may increase certain actions or side effects of anticholinergic agents). Products include:
  Azilect 3383

Remifentanil Hydrochloride (Narcotic analgesics may increase certain actions or side effects of anticholinergic agents).
  No products indexed under this heading.

Risperidone (Antipsychotic agents may increase certain actions or side effects of anticholinergic agents). Products include:
  Risperdal Consta 2682

Salmeterol Xinafoate (Sympathomimetic agents may increase certain actions or side effects of anticholinergic agents). Products include:
  Advair 100/50 1275
  Advair 250/50 1275
  Advair 500/50 1275
  Advair HFA 45/21 1288
  Advair HFA 115/21 1288
  Advair HFA 230/21 1288
  Serevent Diskus 1656

Selegiline (MAO inhibitors may increase certain actions or side effects of anticholinergic agents). Products include:
  Emsam 3623

Selegiline Hydrochloride (MAO inhibitors may increase certain actions or side effects of anticholinergic agents). Products include:
  Eldepryl 3312

Sodium Bicarbonate (Antacids may interfere with the absorption of anticholinergic agents; therefore, simultaneous use of these drugs should be avoided).
  No products indexed under this heading.

Sufentanil Citrate (Narcotic analgesics may increase certain actions or side effects of anticholinergic agents).
  No products indexed under this heading.

Temazepam (Benzodiazepines may increase certain actions or side effects of anticholinergic agents).
  No products indexed under this heading.

Terbutaline Sulfate (Sympathomimetic agents may increase certain actions or side effects of anticholinergic agents).
  No products indexed under this heading.

Terfenadine (Antihistamines may increase certain actions or side effects of anticholinergic agents).
  No products indexed under this heading.

Thioridazine Hydrochloride (Antipsychotic agents may increase certain actions or side effects of anticholinergic agents). Products include:
  Thioridazine Hydrochloride 2384

Thiothixene (Antipsychotic agents may increase certain actions or side effects of anticholinergic agents). Products include:
  Thiothixene 2386

Timolol Maleate (Anticholinergics antagonize the effects of antiglaucoma agents). Products include:
  Combigan 601
  Dorzolamide Hydrochloride/Timolol Maleate Ophthalmic Solution........ ⊙243
  Timoptic in Ocudose .... ⊙231

Tranylcypromine Sulfate (MAO inhibitors may increase certain actions or side effects of anticholinergic agents). Products include:
  Parnate 1584

Triamcinolone (Anticholinergic drugs in the presence of increased intraocular pressure may be hazardous when taken concurrently with agents such as corticosteroids).
  No products indexed under this heading.

Triamcinolone Acetonide (Anticholinergic drugs in the presence of increased intraocular pressure may be hazardous when taken concurrently with agents such as corticosteroids). Products include:
  Azmacort 408
  Nasacort AQ 3019

Triamcinolone Diacetate (Anticholinergic drugs in the presence of increased intraocular pressure may be hazardous when taken concurrently with agents such as corticosteroids).
  No products indexed under this heading.

Triamcinolone Hexacetonide (Anticholinergic drugs in the presence of increased intraocular pressure may be hazardous when taken concurrently with agents such as corticosteroids).
  No products indexed under this heading.

Triazolam (Benzodiazepines may increase certain actions or side effects of anticholinergic agents).
  No products indexed under this heading.

Trifluoperazine Hydrochloride (Antipsychotic agents may increase certain actions or side effects of anticholinergic agents).
  No products indexed under this heading.

Trimeprazine Tartrate (Antihistamines may increase certain actions or side effects of anticholinergic agents).
  No products indexed under this heading.

Trimipramine Maleate (Tricyclic antidepressants may increase certain actions or side effects of anticholinergic agents).
  No products indexed under this heading.

Tripelennamine Hydrochloride (Antihistamines may increase certain actions or side effects of anticholinergic agents).
  No products indexed under this heading.

Triprolidine Hydrochloride (Antihistamines may increase certain actions or side effects of anticholinergic agents).
  No products indexed under this heading.

Ziprasidone Hydrochloride (Antipsychotic agents may increase certain actions or side effects of anticholinergic agents). Products include:
  Geodon 2723

BENZACLIN TOPICAL GEL

(Benzoyl Peroxide, Clindamycin Phosphate) 2965
May interact with antidiarrheals, drugs

affecting gastrointestinal motility, erythromycin, narcotic analgesics, peeling/desquamating agents, and certain other agents. Compounds in these categories include:

Acitretin (Concomitant topical acne therapy should be used with caution because a possible cumulative irritancy may occur, especially with the use of peeling, desquamating or abrasive agents). Products include:
Soriatane 3326

Adapalene (Concomitant topical acne therapy should be used with caution because a possible cumulative irritancy may occur, especially with the use of peeling, desquamating or abrasive agents).
No products indexed under this heading.

Albuterol (Diarrhea, bloody diarrhea, and colitis (including pseudomembranous colitis) have been reported with the use of topical and systemic clindamycin. Antiperistaltic agents may prolong and/or worsen the condition).
No products indexed under this heading.

Albuterol Sulfate (Diarrhea, bloody diarrhea, and colitis (including pseudomembranous colitis) have been reported with the use of topical and systemic clindamycin. Antiperistaltic agents may prolong and/or worsen the condition). Products include:
ProAir HFA 3393
Proventil HFA 3204
Ventolin HFA 1708

Alfentanil Hydrochloride (Diarrhea, bloody diarrhea, and colitis (including pseudomembranous colitis) have been reported with the use of topical and systemic clindamycin. Antiperistaltic agents, such as opiates and diphenoxylate, with atropine may prolong and/or worsen the condition).
No products indexed under this heading.

Alosetron Hydrochloride (Diarrhea, bloody diarrhea, and colitis (including pseudomembranous colitis) have been reported with the use of topical and systemic clindamycin. Antiperistaltic agents may prolong and/or worsen the condition).
No products indexed under this heading.

Amitriptyline Hydrochloride (Diarrhea, bloody diarrhea, and colitis (including pseudomembranous colitis) have been reported with the use of topical and systemic clindamycin. Antiperistaltic agents may prolong and/or worsen the condition).
No products indexed under this heading.

Amlodipine Besylate (Diarrhea, bloody diarrhea, and colitis (including pseudomembranous colitis) have been reported with the use of topical and systemic clindamycin. Antiperistaltic agents may prolong and/or worsen the condition). Products include:
Azor 1010
Exforge 2443
Exforge HCT 2449

Amoxapine (Diarrhea, bloody diarrhea, and colitis (including pseudomembranous colitis) have been reported with the use of topical and systemic clindamycin. Antiperistaltic agents may prolong and/or worsen the condition).
No products indexed under this heading.

Apomorphine (Diarrhea, bloody diarrhea, and colitis (including pseudomembranous colitis) have been reported with the use of topical and systemic clindamycin. Antiperistaltic agents, such as opiates and diphenoxylate, with atropine may prolong and/or worsen the condition).
No products indexed under this heading.

Apomorphine Hydrochloride (Diarrhea, bloody diarrhea, and colitis (including pseudomembranous colitis) have been reported with the use of topical and systemic clindamycin. Antiperistaltic agents, such as opiates and diphenoxylate, with atropine may prolong and/or worsen the condition).
No products indexed under this heading.

Astemizole (Diarrhea, bloody diarrhea, and colitis (including pseudomembranous colitis) have been reported with the use of topical and systemic clindamycin. Antiperistaltic agents may prolong and/or worsen the condition).
No products indexed under this heading.

Atropine Sulfate (Diarrhea, bloody diarrhea, and colitis (including pseudomembranous colitis) have been reported with the use of topical and systemic clindamycin. Antiperistaltic agents, such as opiates and diphenoxylate, with atropine may prolong and/or worsen the condition). Products include:
Donnatal 2711

Azatadine Maleate (Diarrhea, bloody diarrhea, and colitis (including pseudomembranous colitis) have been reported with the use of topical and systemic clindamycin. Antiperistaltic agents may prolong and/or worsen the condition).
No products indexed under this heading.

Azelaic Acid (Concomitant topical acne therapy should be used with caution because a possible cumulative irritancy may occur, especially with the use of peeling, desquamating or abrasive agents). Products include:
Finacea 1808

Belladonna Alkaloids (Diarrhea, bloody diarrhea, and colitis (including pseudomembranous colitis) have been reported with the use of topical and systemic clindamycin. Antiperistaltic agents may prolong and/or worsen the condition). Products include:
Hyland's Teething Tablets 3316

Benztropine Mesylate (Diarrhea, bloody diarrhea, and colitis (including pseudomembranous colitis) have been reported with the use of topical and systemic clindamycin. Antiperistaltic agents may prolong and/or worsen the condition).
No products indexed under this heading.

Bepridil Hydrochloride (Diarrhea, bloody diarrhea, and colitis (including pseudomembranous colitis) have been reported with the use of topical and systemic clindamycin. Antiperistaltic agents may prolong and/or worsen the condition).
No products indexed under this heading.

Bethanechol Chloride (Diarrhea, bloody diarrhea, and colitis (including pseudomembranous colitis) have been reported with the use of topical and systemic clindamycin. Antiperistaltic agents may prolong and/or worsen the condition).
No products indexed under this heading.

Biperiden Hydrochloride (Diarrhea, bloody diarrhea, and colitis (including pseudomembranous colitis) have been reported with the use of topical and systemic clindamycin. Antiperistaltic agents may prolong and/or worsen the condition).
No products indexed under this heading.

Bismuth Subsalicylate (Diarrhea, bloody diarrhea, and colitis (including pseudomembranous colitis) have been reported with the use of topical and systemic clindamycin. Antiperistaltic agents may prolong and/or worsen the condition).
No products indexed under this heading.

Bitolterol Mesylate (Diarrhea, bloody diarrhea, and colitis (including pseudomembranous colitis) have been reported with the use of topical and systemic clindamycin. Antiperistaltic agents may prolong and/or worsen the condition).
No products indexed under this heading.

Bromocriptine Mesylate (Diarrhea, bloody diarrhea, and colitis (including pseudomembranous colitis) have been reported with the use of topical and systemic clindamycin. Antiperistaltic agents may prolong and/or worsen the condition).
No products indexed under this heading.

Bromodiphenhydramine Hydrochloride (Diarrhea, bloody diarrhea, and colitis (including pseudomembranous colitis) have been reported with the use of topical and systemic clindamycin. Antiperistaltic agents may prolong and/or worsen the condition).
No products indexed under this heading.

Brompheniramine Maleate (Diarrhea, bloody diarrhea, and colitis (including pseudomembranous colitis) have been reported with the use of topical and systemic clindamycin. Antiperistaltic agents may prolong and/or worsen the condition).
No products indexed under this heading.

Buprenorphine Hydrochloride (Diarrhea, bloody diarrhea, and colitis (including pseudomembranous colitis) have been reported with the use of topical and systemic clindamycin. Antiperistaltic agents, such as opiates and diphenoxylate, with atropine may prolong and/or worsen the condition).
No products indexed under this heading.

Calcipotriene (Concomitant topical acne therapy should be used with caution because a possible cumulative irritancy may occur, especially with the use of peeling, desquamating or abrasive agents).
No products indexed under this heading.

Cevimeline Hydrochloride (Diarrhea, bloody diarrhea, and colitis (including pseudomembranous colitis) have been reported with the use of topical and systemic clindamycin. Antiperistaltic agents may prolong and/or worsen the condition). Products include:
Evoxac 1027

Chlorpheniramine Maleate (Diarrhea, bloody diarrhea, and colitis (including pseudomembranous colitis) have been reported with the use of topical and systemic clindamycin. Antiperistaltic agents may prolong and/or worsen the condition).
No products indexed under this heading.

Chlorpheniramine Polistirex (Diarrhea, bloody diarrhea, and colitis (including pseudomembranous colitis) have been reported with the use of topical and systemic clindamycin. Antiperistaltic agents may prolong and/or worsen the condition). Products include:
Tussionex 3443

Chlorpheniramine Tannate (Diarrhea, bloody diarrhea, and colitis (including pseudomembranous colitis) have been reported with the use of topical and systemic clindamycin. Antiperistaltic agents may prolong and/or worsen the condition).
No products indexed under this heading.

Cisapride (Diarrhea, bloody diarrhea, and colitis (including pseudomembranous colitis) have been reported with the use of topical and systemic clindamycin. Antiperistaltic agents may prolong and/or worsen the condition).
No products indexed under this heading.

Clemastine Fumarate (Diarrhea, bloody diarrhea, and colitis (including pseudomembranous colitis) have been reported with the use of topical and systemic clindamycin. Antiperistaltic agents may prolong and/or worsen the condition).
No products indexed under this heading.

Clidinium Bromide (Diarrhea, bloody diarrhea, and colitis (including pseudomembranous colitis) have been reported with the use of topical and systemic clindamycin. Antiperistaltic agents may prolong and/or worsen the condition).
No products indexed under this heading.

Clindamycin, Topical (Concomitant topical acne therapy should be used with caution because a possible cumulative irritancy may occur, especially with the use of peeling, desquamating or abrasive agents).
No products indexed under this heading.

Clomipramine Hydrochloride (Diarrhea, bloody diarrhea, and colitis (including pseudomembranous colitis) have been reported with the use of topical and systemic clindamycin. Antiperistaltic agents may prolong and/or worsen the condition).
No products indexed under this heading.

Clotrimazole, Topical (Concomitant topical acne therapy should be used with caution because a possible cumulative irritancy may occur, especially with the use of peeling, desquamating or abrasive agents).
No products indexed under this heading.

Coal Tar (Concomitant topical acne therapy should be used with caution because a possible cumulative irritancy may occur, especially with the use of peeling, desquamating or abrasive agents).
No products indexed under this heading.

Codeine Phosphate (Diarrhea, bloody diarrhea, and colitis (including pseudomembranous colitis) have been reported with the use of topical and systemic clindamycin. Antiperistaltic agents, such as opiates and diphenoxylate, with atropine may prolong and/or worsen the condition). Products include:
Tylenol with Codeine 2691

Codeine Sulfate (Diarrhea, bloody diarrhea, and colitis (including pseudomembranous colitis) have been reported with the use of topical and systemic clindamycin. Antiperistaltic agents, such as opiates and diphenoxylate, with atropine may prolong and/or worsen the condition).
No products indexed under this heading.

Concomitant Topical Acne Therapy (Concomitant topical acne therapy should be used with caution because a possible cumulative irritancy effect may occur, especially with the use of peeling, desquamating, or abrasive agents).
No products indexed under this heading.

Cyproheptadine Hydrochloride (Diarrhea, bloody diarrhea, and colitis (including pseudomembranous colitis) have been reported with the use of topical and systemic clindamycin. Antiperistaltic agents may prolong and/or worsen the condition).
No products indexed under this heading.

Desipramine Hydrochloride (Diarrhea, bloody diarrhea, and colitis (including pseudomembranous colitis) have been reported with the use of topical and systemic clindamycin. Antiperistaltic agents may prolong and/or worsen the condition).
No products indexed under this heading.

IMPORTANT NOTE: Always consult each drug listing in the patient's regimen for possible interactions.

systemic clindamycin. Antiperistaltic agents may prolong and/or worsen the condition). Products include:
Donnatal 2711

Imipramine Hydrochloride (Diarrhea, bloody diarrhea, and colitis (including pseudomembranous colitis) have been reported with the use of topical and systemic clindamycin. Antiperistaltic agents may prolong and/or worsen the condition).
No products indexed under this heading.

Imipramine Pamoate (Diarrhea, bloody diarrhea, and colitis (including pseudomembranous colitis) have been reported with the use of topical and systemic clindamycin. Antiperistaltic agents may prolong and/or worsen the condition).
No products indexed under this heading.

Ipratropium Bromide (Diarrhea, bloody diarrhea, and colitis (including pseudomembranous colitis) have been reported with the use of topical and systemic clindamycin. Antiperistaltic agents may prolong and/or worsen the condition).
No products indexed under this heading.

Isoetharine (Diarrhea, bloody diarrhea, and colitis (including pseudomembranous colitis) have been reported with the use of topical and systemic clindamycin. Antiperistaltic agents may prolong and/or worsen the condition).
No products indexed under this heading.

Isoproterenol Hydrochloride (Diarrhea, bloody diarrhea, and colitis (including pseudomembranous colitis) have been reported with the use of topical and systemic clindamycin. Antiperistaltic agents may prolong and/or worsen the condition).
No products indexed under this heading.

Isoproterenol Sulfate (Diarrhea, bloody diarrhea, and colitis (including pseudomembranous colitis) have been reported with the use of topical and systemic clindamycin. Antiperistaltic agents may prolong and/or worsen the condition).
No products indexed under this heading.

Isotretinoin (Concomitant topical acne therapy should be used with caution because a possible cumulative irritancy may occur, especially with the use of peeling, desquamating or abrasive agents). Products include:
Accutane 2832

Isradipine (Diarrhea, bloody diarrhea, and colitis (including pseudomembranous colitis) have been reported with the use of topical and systemic clindamycin. Antiperistaltic agents may prolong and/or worsen the condition). Products include:
DynaCirc CR 1432

Kaolin (Diarrhea, bloody diarrhea, and colitis (including pseudomembranous colitis) have been reported with the use of topical and systemic clindamycin. Antiperistaltic agents may prolong and/or worsen the condition).
No products indexed under this heading.

Levalbuterol Hydrochloride (Diarrhea, bloody diarrhea, and colitis (including pseudomembranous colitis) have been reported with the use of topical and systemic clindamycin. Antiperistaltic agents may prolong and/or worsen the condition).
No products indexed under this heading.

Levorphanol Tartrate (Diarrhea, bloody diarrhea, and colitis (including pseudomembranous colitis) have been reported with the use of topical and systemic clindamycin. Antiperistaltic agents, such as opiates and diphenoxylate, with atropine may prolong and/or worsen the condition).
No products indexed under this heading.

Loperamide Hydrochloride (Diarrhea, bloody diarrhea, and colitis (including pseudomembranous colitis) have been reported with the use of topical and systemic clindamycin. Antiperistaltic agents may prolong and/or worsen the condition). Products include:
Imodium A-D 2042
Imodium Multi-Symptom Relief 2043

Maprotiline Hydrochloride (Diarrhea, bloody diarrhea, and colitis (including pseudomembranous colitis) have been reported with the use of topical and systemic clindamycin. Antiperistaltic agents may prolong and/or worsen the condition).
No products indexed under this heading.

Mepenzolate Bromide (Diarrhea, bloody diarrhea, and colitis (including pseudomembranous colitis) have been reported with the use of topical and systemic clindamycin. Antiperistaltic agents may prolong and/or worsen the condition).
No products indexed under this heading.

Meperidine Hydrochloride (Diarrhea, bloody diarrhea, and colitis (including pseudomembranous colitis) have been reported with the use of topical and systemic clindamycin. Antiperistaltic agents, such as opiates and diphenoxylate, with atropine may prolong and/or worsen the condition).
No products indexed under this heading.

Mequinol (Concomitant topical acne therapy should be used with caution because a possible cumulative irritancy may occur, especially with the use of peeling, desquamating or abrasive agents).
No products indexed under this heading.

Metaproterenol Sulfate (Diarrhea, bloody diarrhea, and colitis (including pseudomembranous colitis) have been reported with the use of topical and systemic clindamycin. Antiperistaltic agents may prolong and/or worsen the condition).
No products indexed under this heading.

Methadone Hydrochloride (Diarrhea, bloody diarrhea, and colitis (including pseudomembranous colitis) have been reported with the use of topical and systemic clindamycin. Antiperistaltic agents, such as opiates and diphenoxylate, with atropine may prolong and/or worsen the condition).
No products indexed under this heading.

Methdilazine Hydrochloride (Diarrhea, bloody diarrhea, and colitis (including pseudomembranous colitis) have been reported with the use of topical and systemic clindamycin. Antiperistaltic agents may prolong and/or worsen the condition).
No products indexed under this heading.

Metoclopramide Hydrochloride (Diarrhea, bloody diarrhea, and colitis (including pseudomembranous colitis) have been reported with the use of topical and systemic clindamycin. Antiperistaltic agents may prolong and/or worsen the condition). Products include:
Metozolv ODT 2901

Mibefradil Dihydrochloride (Diarrhea, bloody diarrhea, and colitis (including pseudomembranous colitis) have been reported with the use of topical and systemic clindamycin. Antiperistaltic agents may prolong and/or worsen the condition).
No products indexed under this heading.

Morphine Sulfate (Diarrhea, bloody diarrhea, and colitis (including pseudomembranous colitis) have been reported with the use of topical and systemic clindamycin. Antiperistaltic agents, such as opiates and diphenoxylate, with atropine may prolong and/or worsen the condition). Products include:
Avinza 1822
Embeda 1831
MS Contin 2803

Morphine Sulfate, Liposomal (Diarrhea, bloody diarrhea, and colitis (including pseudomembranous colitis) have been reported with the use of topical and systemic clindamycin. Antiperistaltic agents, such as opiates and diphenoxylate, with atropine may prolong and/or worsen the condition).
No products indexed under this heading.

Neostigmine Bromide (Diarrhea, bloody diarrhea, and colitis (including pseudomembranous colitis) have been reported with the use of topical and systemic clindamycin. Antiperistaltic agents may prolong and/or worsen the condition).
No products indexed under this heading.

Neostigmine Methylsulfate (Diarrhea, bloody diarrhea, and colitis (including pseudomembranous colitis) have been reported with the use of topical and systemic clindamycin. Antiperistaltic agents may prolong and/or worsen the condition).
No products indexed under this heading.

Nicardipine Hydrochloride (Diarrhea, bloody diarrhea, and colitis (including pseudomembranous colitis) have been reported with the use of topical and systemic clindamycin. Antiperistaltic agents may prolong and/or worsen the condition).
No products indexed under this heading.

Nifedipine (Diarrhea, bloody diarrhea, and colitis (including pseudomembranous colitis) have been reported with the use of topical and systemic clindamycin. Antiperistaltic agents may prolong and/or worsen the condition).
No products indexed under this heading.

Nimodipine (Diarrhea, bloody diarrhea, and colitis (including pseudomembranous colitis) have been reported with the use of topical and systemic clindamycin. Antiperistaltic agents may prolong and/or worsen the condition).
No products indexed under this heading.

Nisoldipine (Diarrhea, bloody diarrhea, and colitis (including pseudomembranous colitis) have been reported with the use of topical and systemic clindamycin. Antiperistaltic agents may prolong and/or worsen the condition).
No products indexed under this heading.

Nitazoxanide (Diarrhea, bloody diarrhea, and colitis (including pseudomembranous colitis) have been reported with the use of topical and systemic clindamycin. Antiperistaltic agents may prolong and/or worsen the condition).
No products indexed under this heading.

Nortriptyline Hydrochloride (Diarrhea, bloody diarrhea, and colitis (including pseudomembranous colitis) have been reported with the use of topical and systemic clindamycin. Antiperistaltic agents may prolong and/or worsen the condition).
No products indexed under this heading.

Octreotide Acetate (Diarrhea, bloody diarrhea, and colitis (including pseudomembranous colitis) have been reported with the use of topical and systemic clindamycin. Antiperistaltic agents may prolong and/or worsen the condition). Products include:
Sandostatin 2517
Sandostatin LAR 2519

Oxybutynin Chloride (Diarrhea, bloody diarrhea, and colitis (including pseudomembranous colitis) have been reported with the use of topical and systemic clindamycin. Antiperistaltic agents may prolong and/or worsen the condition).
No products indexed under this heading.

Oxycodone Hydrochloride (Diarrhea, bloody diarrhea, and colitis (including pseudomembranous colitis) have been reported with the use of topical and systemic clindamycin. Antiperistaltic agents, such as opiates and diphenoxylate, with atropine may prolong and/or worsen the condition). Products include:
OxyContin 2807
Percocet 1121
Percodan 1124

Oxycodone Terephthalate (Diarrhea, bloody diarrhea, and colitis (including pseudomembranous colitis) have been reported with the use of topical and systemic clindamycin. Antiperistaltic agents, such as opiates and diphenoxylate, with atropine may prolong and/or worsen the condition).
No products indexed under this heading.

Oxymorphone Hydrochloride (Diarrhea, bloody diarrhea, and colitis (including pseudomembranous colitis) have been reported with the use of topical and systemic clindamycin. Antiperistaltic agents, such as opiates and diphenoxylate, with atropine may prolong and/or worsen the condition). Products include:
Opana 1110
Opana ER 1114

Oxyphenonium Bromide (Diarrhea, bloody diarrhea, and colitis (including pseudomembranous colitis) have been reported with the use of topical and systemic clindamycin. Antiperistaltic agents may prolong and/or worsen the condition).
No products indexed under this heading.

Pectin (Diarrhea, bloody diarrhea, and colitis (including pseudomembranous colitis) have been reported with the use of topical and systemic clindamycin. Antiperistaltic agents may prolong and/or worsen the condition).
No products indexed under this heading.

Pergolide Mesylate (Diarrhea, bloody diarrhea, and colitis (including pseudomembranous colitis) have been reported with the use of topical and systemic clindamycin. Antiperistaltic agents may prolong and/or worsen the condition).
No products indexed under this heading.

Pirbuterol Acetate (Diarrhea, bloody diarrhea, and colitis (including pseudomembranous colitis) have been reported with the use of topical and systemic clindamycin. Antiperistaltic agents may prolong and/or worsen the condition). Products include:
Maxair Autohaler 1782

Podofilox (Concomitant topical acne therapy should be used with caution because a possible cumulative irritancy may occur, especially with the use of peeling, desquamating or abrasive agents).
No products indexed under this heading.

Pramipexole Dihydrochloride (Diarrhea, bloody diarrhea, and colitis (including pseudomembranous colitis) have been reported with the use of topical and systemic clindamycin. Antiperistaltic agents may prolong and/or worsen the condition).
No products indexed under this heading.

Procainamide Hydrochloride (Diarrhea, bloody diarrhea, and colitis (including pseudomembranous colitis) have been reported with the use of topical and systemic clindamycin. Antiperistaltic agents may prolong and/or worsen the condition).
No products indexed under this heading.

Procyclidine Hydrochloride (Diarrhea, bloody diarrhea, and colitis (including pseudomembranous colitis) have been reported with the use of topical and systemic clindamycin. Antiperistaltic agents may prolong and/or worsen the condition).
No products indexed under this heading.

Promethazine Hydrochloride (Diarrhea, bloody diarrhea, and colitis (including pseudomembranous colitis) have been reported with the use of topical and systemic clindamycin. Antiperistaltic agents may prolong and/or worsen the condition).
No products indexed under this heading.

Propantheline Bromide (Diarrhea, bloody diarrhea, and colitis (including pseudomembranous colitis) have been reported with the use of topical and systemic clindamycin. Antiperistaltic agents may prolong and/or worsen the condition).
No products indexed under this heading.

Propoxyphene Hydrochloride (Diarrhea, bloody diarrhea, and colitis (including pseudomembranous colitis) have been reported with the use of topical and systemic clindamycin. Antiperistaltic agents, such as opiates and diphenoxylate, with atropine may prolong and/or worsen the condition).
No products indexed under this heading.

Propoxyphene Napsylate (Diarrhea, bloody diarrhea, and colitis (including pseudomembranous colitis) have been reported with the use of topical and systemic clindamycin. Antiperistaltic agents, such as opiates and diphenoxylate, with atropine may prolong and/or worsen the condition).
No products indexed under this heading.

Protriptyline Hydrochloride (Diarrhea, bloody diarrhea, and colitis (including pseudomembranous colitis) have been reported with the use of topical and systemic clindamycin. Antiperistaltic agents may prolong and/or worsen the condition).
No products indexed under this heading.

Pyridostigmine Bromide (Diarrhea, bloody diarrhea, and colitis (including pseudomembranous colitis) have been reported with the use of topical and systemic clindamycin. Antiperistaltic agents may prolong and/or worsen the condition).
No products indexed under this heading.

Pyrilamine Maleate (Diarrhea, bloody diarrhea, and colitis (including pseudomembranous colitis) have been reported with the use of topical and systemic clindamycin. Antiperistaltic agents may prolong and/or worsen the condition).
No products indexed under this heading.

Pyrilamine Tannate (Diarrhea, bloody diarrhea, and colitis (including pseudomembranous colitis) have been reported with the use of topical and systemic clindamycin. Antiperistaltic agents may prolong and/or worsen the condition).
No products indexed under this heading.

Quinidine Gluconate (Diarrhea, bloody diarrhea, and colitis (including pseudomembranous colitis) have been reported with the use of topical and systemic clindamycin. Antiperistaltic agents may prolong and/or worsen the condition).
No products indexed under this heading.

Quinidine Polygalacturonate (Diarrhea, bloody diarrhea, and colitis (including pseudomembranous colitis) have been reported with the use of topical and systemic clindamycin. Antiperistaltic agents may prolong and/or worsen the condition).
No products indexed under this heading.

Quinidine Sulfate (Diarrhea, bloody diarrhea, and colitis (including pseudomembranous colitis) have been reported with the use of topical and systemic clindamycin. Antiperistaltic agents may prolong and/or worsen the condition).
No products indexed under this heading.

Remifentanil Hydrochloride (Diarrhea, bloody diarrhea, and colitis (including pseudomembranous colitis) have been reported with the use of topical and systemic clindamycin. Antiperistaltic agents, such as opiates and diphenoxylate, with atropine may prolong and/or worsen the condition).
No products indexed under this heading.

Rifaximin (Diarrhea, bloody diarrhea, and colitis (including pseudomembranous colitis) have been reported with the use of topical and systemic clindamycin. Antiperistaltic agents may prolong and/or worsen the condition). Products include:
Xifaxan **2909**

Rivastigmine Tartrate (Diarrhea, bloody diarrhea, and colitis (including pseudomembranous colitis) have been reported with the use of topical and systemic clindamycin. Antiperistaltic agents may prolong and/or worsen the condition). Products include:
Exelon **2432**
Exelon Oral **2432**
Exelon Patch **2437**

Ropinirole Hydrochloride (Diarrhea, bloody diarrhea, and colitis (including pseudomembranous colitis) have been reported with the use of topical and systemic clindamycin. Antiperistaltic agents may prolong and/or worsen the condition). Products include:
Requip **1620**
Requip XL **1628**

Salicylic Acid (Concomitant topical acne therapy should be used with caution because a possible cumulative irritancy may occur, especially with the use of peeling, desquamating or abrasive agents).
No products indexed under this heading.

Salmeterol Xinafoate (Diarrhea, bloody diarrhea, and colitis (including pseudomembranous colitis) have been reported with the use of topical and systemic clindamycin. Antiperistaltic agents may prolong and/or worsen the condition). Products include:
Advair 100/50 .... **1275**
Advair 250/50 .... **1275**
Advair 500/50 .... **1275**
Advair HFA 45/21 .... **1288**
Advair HFA 115/21 .... **1288**
Advair HFA 230/21 .... **1288**
Serevent Diskus **1656**

Scopolamine (Diarrhea, bloody diarrhea, and colitis (including pseudomembranous colitis) have been reported with the use of topical and systemic clindamycin. Antiperistaltic agents may prolong and/or worsen the condition). Products include:
Transderm Scōp **2397**

Scopolamine Hydrobromide (Diarrhea, bloody diarrhea, and colitis (including pseudomembranous colitis) have been reported with the use of topical and systemic clindamycin. Antiperistaltic agents may prolong and/or worsen the condition). Products include:
Donnatal **2711**

Sucralfate (Diarrhea, bloody diarrhea, and colitis (including pseudomembranous colitis) have been reported with the use of topical and systemic clindamycin. Antiperistaltic agents may prolong and/or worsen the condition). Products include:
Carafate Suspension **784**
Carafate Tablets **785**

Sufentanil Citrate (Diarrhea, bloody diarrhea, and colitis (including pseudomembranous colitis) have been reported with the use of topical and systemic clindamycin. Antiperistaltic agents, such as opiates and diphenoxylate, with atropine may prolong and/or worsen the condition).
No products indexed under this heading.

Sulfur Preparations (Concomitant topical acne therapy should be used with caution because a possible cumulative irritancy may occur, especially with the use of peeling, desquamating or abrasive agents).
No products indexed under this heading.

Tacrine Hydrochloride (Diarrhea, bloody diarrhea, and colitis (including pseudomembranous colitis) have been reported with the use of topical and systemic clindamycin. Antiperistaltic agents may prolong and/or worsen the condition).
No products indexed under this heading.

Tazarotene (Concomitant topical acne therapy should be used with caution because a possible cumulative irritancy may occur, especially with the use of peeling, desquamating or abrasive agents).
No products indexed under this heading.

Terbutaline Sulfate (Diarrhea, bloody diarrhea, and colitis (including pseudomembranous colitis) have been reported with the use of topical and systemic clindamycin. Antiperistaltic agents may prolong and/or worsen the condition).
No products indexed under this heading.

Tolterodine Tartrate (Diarrhea, bloody diarrhea, and colitis (including pseudomembranous colitis) have been reported with the use of topical and systemic clindamycin. Antiperistaltic agents may prolong and/or worsen the condition).
No products indexed under this heading.

Tretinoin (Concomitant topical acne therapy should be used with caution because a possible cumulative irritancy may occur, especially with the use of peeling, desquamating or abrasive agents).
No products indexed under this heading.

Tridihexethyl Chloride (Diarrhea, bloody diarrhea, and colitis (including pseudomembranous colitis) have been reported with the use of topical and systemic clindamycin. Antiperistaltic agents may prolong and/or worsen the condition).
No products indexed under this heading.

Trihexyphenidyl Hydrochloride (Diarrhea, bloody diarrhea, and colitis (including pseudomembranous colitis) have been reported with the use of topical and systemic clindamycin. Antiperistaltic agents may prolong and/or worsen the condition).
No products indexed under this heading.

Trimeprazine Tartrate (Diarrhea, bloody diarrhea, and colitis (including pseudomembranous colitis) have been reported with the use of topical and systemic clindamycin. Antiperistaltic agents may prolong and/or worsen the condition).
No products indexed under this heading.

Trimipramine Maleate (Diarrhea, bloody diarrhea, and colitis (including pseudomembranous colitis) have been reported with the use of topical and systemic clindamycin. Antiperistaltic agents may prolong and/or worsen the condition).
No products indexed under this heading.

Tripelennamine Hydrochloride (Diarrhea, bloody diarrhea, and colitis (including pseudomembranous colitis) have been reported with the use of topical and systemic clindamycin. Antiperistaltic agents may prolong and/or worsen the condition).
No products indexed under this heading.

Triprolidine Hydrochloride (Diarrhea, bloody diarrhea, and colitis (including pseudomembranous colitis) have been reported with the use of topical and systemic clindamycin. Antiperistaltic agents may prolong and/or worsen the condition).
No products indexed under this heading.

Verapamil Hydrochloride (Diarrhea, bloody diarrhea, and colitis (including pseudomembranous colitis) have been reported with the use of topical and systemic clindamycin. Antiperistaltic agents may prolong and/or worsen the condition). Products include:
Tarka **534**

Zalcitabine (Concomitant topical acne therapy should be used with caution because a possible cumulative irritancy may occur, especially with the use of peeling, desquamating or abrasive agents).
No products indexed under this heading.

BESIVANCE OPHTHALMIC SUSPENSION

(Besifloxacin) **3621**
None cited in PDR database.

BETADINE 5% OPHTHALMIC SOLUTION

(Povidone Iodine) .... ⊙**202**
None cited in PDR database.

BETASERON FOR SC INJECTION

(Interferon Beta-1b) **836**
None cited in PDR database.

BETIMOL OPHTHALMIC SOLUTION

(Timolol Hemihydrate) **3490**
May interact with beta-blockers, calcium channel blockers, cardiac glycosides, and certain other agents. Compounds in these categories include:

Acebutolol Hydrochloride (Concurrent use with systemic beta blockers may result in additive effect either on the intraocular pressure or the known systemic effect of beta blockade).
No products indexed under this heading.

Amlodipine Besylate (Possible atrioventricular conduction disturbances, left ventricular failure, and hypotension). Products include:
Azor **1010**
Exforge **2443**
Exforge HCT **2449**

Atenolol (Concurrent use with systemic beta blockers may result in additive effect either on the intraocular pressure or the known systemic effect of beta blockade).
No products indexed under this heading.

Bepridil Hydrochloride (Possible atrioventricular conduction disturbances, left ventricular failure, and hypotension).
No products indexed under this heading.

Betaxolol Hydrochloride (Concurrent use with systemic beta blockers may result in additive effect either on the intraocular pressure or the known systemic effect of beta blockade).
No products indexed under this heading.

Bisoprolol Fumarate (Concurrent use with systemic beta blockers may result in additive effect either on the intraocular pressure or the known systemic effect of beta blockade).
No products indexed under this heading.

Carteolol Hydrochloride (Concurrent use with systemic beta blockers may result in additive effect either on the intraocular pressure or the known systemic effect of beta blockade).
No products indexed under this heading.

Carvedilol (Concurrent use with systemic beta blockers may result in addi-

IMPORTANT NOTE: Always consult each drug listing in the patient's regimen for possible interactions.

(☉ Described in PDR® for Ophthalmic Medicines)

Diclofenac Potassium (Due to the frequent occurrence of severe and prolonged thrombocytopenia, the potential benefits of medications that interfere with platelet function and/or anticoagulation should be weighed against the potential increased risk of bleeding and hemorrhage).
No products indexed under this heading.

Diclofenac Sodium (Due to the frequent occurrence of severe and prolonged thrombocytopenia, the potential benefits of medications that interfere with platelet function and/or anticoagulation should be weighed against the potential increased risk of bleeding and hemorrhage).
No products indexed under this heading.

Dicumarol (Due to the frequent occurrence of severe and prolonged thrombocytopenia, the potential benefits of medications that interfere with platelet function and/or anticoagulation should be weighed against the potential increased risk of bleeding and hemorrhage).
No products indexed under this heading.

Diflunisal (Due to the frequent occurrence of severe and prolonged thrombocytopenia, the potential benefits of medications that interfere with platelet function and/or anticoagulation should be weighed against the potential increased risk of bleeding and hemorrhage).
No products indexed under this heading.

Dipyridamole (Due to the frequent occurrence of severe and prolonged thrombocytopenia, the potential benefits of medications that interfere with platelet function and/or anticoagulation should be weighed against the potential increased risk of bleeding and hemorrhage). Products include:

Enoxaparin Sodium (Due to the frequent occurrence of severe and prolonged thrombocytopenia, the potential benefits of medications that interfere with platelet function and/or anticoagulation should be weighed against the potential increased risk of bleeding and hemorrhage). Products include:

Eptifibatide (Due to the frequent occurrence of severe and prolonged thrombocytopenia, the potential benefits of medications that interfere with platelet function and/or anticoagulation should be weighed against the potential increased risk of bleeding and hemorrhage). Products include:

Fenoprofen Calcium (Due to the frequent occurrence of severe and prolonged thrombocytopenia, the potential benefits of medications that interfere with platelet function and/or anticoagulation should be weighed against the potential increased risk of bleeding and hemorrhage).
No products indexed under this heading.

Flurbiprofen (Due to the frequent occurrence of severe and prolonged thrombocytopenia, the potential benefits of medications that interfere with platelet function and/or anticoagulation should be weighed against the potential increased risk of bleeding and hemorrhage).
No products indexed under this heading.

Fondaparinux Sodium (Due to the frequent occurrence of severe and prolonged thrombocytopenia, the potential benefits of medications that interfere with platelet function and/or anticoagulation should be weighed against the potential increased risk of bleeding and hemorrhage). Products include:

Heparin Calcium (Due to the frequent occurrence of severe and prolonged thrombocytopenia, the potential benefits of medications that interfere with platelet function and/or anticoagulation should be weighed against the potential increased risk of bleeding and hemorrhage).
No products indexed under this heading.

Heparin Sodium (Due to the frequent occurrence of severe and prolonged thrombocytopenia, the potential benefits of medications that interfere with platelet function and/or anticoagulation should be weighed against the potential increased risk of bleeding and hemorrhage).
No products indexed under this heading.

Hydroxychloroquine Sulfate (Due to the frequent occurrence of severe and prolonged thrombocytopenia, the potential benefits of medications that interfere with platelet function and/or anticoagulation should be weighed against the potential increased risk of bleeding and hemorrhage).
No products indexed under this heading.

Ibuprofen (Due to the frequent occurrence of severe and prolonged thrombocytopenia, the potential benefits of medications that interfere with platelet function and/or anticoagulation should be weighed against the potential increased risk of bleeding and hemorrhage). Products include:

Indomethacin (Due to the frequent occurrence of severe and prolonged thrombocytopenia, the potential benefits of medications that interfere with platelet function and/or anticoagulation should be weighed against the potential increased risk of bleeding and hemorrhage). Products include:

Indomethacin Sodium Trihydrate (Due to the frequent occurrence of severe and prolonged thrombocytopenia, the potential benefits of medications that interfere with platelet function and/or anticoagulation should be weighed against the potential increased risk of bleeding and hemorrhage). Products include:

Ketoprofen (Due to the frequent occurrence of severe and prolonged thrombocytopenia, the potential benefits of medications that interfere with platelet function and/or anticoagulation should be weighed against the potential increased risk of bleeding and hemorrhage).
No products indexed under this heading.

Low Molecular Weight Heparins (Due to the frequent occurrence of severe and prolonged thrombocytopenia, the potential benefits of medications that interfere with platelet function and/or anticoagulation should be weighed against the potential increased risk of bleeding and hemorrhage).
No products indexed under this heading.

Magnesium Salicylate (Due to the frequent occurrence of severe and prolonged thrombocytopenia, the potential benefits of medications that interfere with platelet function and/or anticoagulation should be weighed against the potential increased risk of bleeding and hemorrhage).
No products indexed under this heading.

Meclofenamate Sodium (Due to the frequent occurrence of severe and prolonged thrombocytopenia, the potential benefits of medications that interfere with platelet function and/or anticoagulation should be weighed against the potential increased risk of bleeding and hemorrhage).
No products indexed under this heading.

Mefenamic Acid (Due to the frequent occurrence of severe and prolonged thrombocytopenia, the potential benefits of medications that interfere with platelet function and/or anticoagulation should be weighed against the potential increased risk of bleeding and hemorrhage).
No products indexed under this heading.

Mezlocillin Sodium (Due to the frequent occurrence of severe and prolonged thrombocytopenia, the potential benefits of medications that interfere with platelet function and/or anticoagulation should be weighed against the potential increased risk of bleeding and hemorrhage).
No products indexed under this heading.

Nafcillin Sodium (Due to the frequent occurrence of severe and prolonged thrombocytopenia, the potential benefits of medications that interfere with platelet function and/or anticoagulation should be weighed against the potential increased risk of bleeding and hemorrhage).
No products indexed under this heading.

Naproxen (Due to the frequent occurrence of severe and prolonged thrombocytopenia, the potential benefits of medications that interfere with platelet function and/or anticoagulation should be weighed against the potential increased risk of bleeding and hemorrhage). Products include:

Naproxen Sodium (Due to the frequent occurrence of severe and prolonged thrombocytopenia, the potential benefits of medications that interfere with platelet function and/or anticoagulation should be weighed against the potential increased risk of bleeding and hemorrhage). Products include:

Penicillin G Benzathine (Due to the frequent occurrence of severe and prolonged thrombocytopenia, the potential benefits of medications that interfere with platelet function and/or anticoagulation should be weighed against the potential increased risk of bleeding and hemorrhage). Products include:

Penicillin G Procaine (Due to the frequent occurrence of severe and prolonged thrombocytopenia, the potential benefits of medications that interfere with platelet function and/or anticoagulation should be weighed against the potential increased risk of bleeding and hemorrhage). Products include:

Phenylbutazone (Due to the frequent occurrence of severe and prolonged thrombocytopenia, the potential benefits of medications that interfere with platelet function and/or anticoagulation should be weighed against the potential increased risk of bleeding and hemorrhage).
No products indexed under this heading.

Piroxicam (Due to the frequent occurrence of severe and prolonged thrombocytopenia, the potential benefits of medications that interfere with platelet function and/or anticoagulation should be weighed against the potential increased risk of bleeding and hemorrhage).
No products indexed under this heading.

Salsalate (Due to the frequent occurrence of severe and prolonged thrombocytopenia, the potential benefits of medications that interfere with platelet function and/or anticoagulation should be weighed against the potential increased risk of bleeding and hemorrhage).
No products indexed under this heading.

Sulindac (Due to the frequent occurrence of severe and prolonged thrombocytopenia, the potential benefits of medications that interfere with platelet function and/or anticoagulation should be weighed against the potential increased risk of bleeding and hemorrhage). Products include:

Ticarcillin Disodium (Due to the frequent occurrence of severe and prolonged thrombocytopenia, the potential benefits of medications that interfere with platelet function and/or anticoagulation should be weighed against the potential increased risk of bleeding and hemorrhage). Products include:

Ticlopidine Hydrochloride (Due to the frequent occurrence of severe and prolonged thrombocytopenia, the potential benefits of medications that interfere with platelet function and/or anticoagulation should be weighed against the potential increased risk of bleeding and hemorrhage).
No products indexed under this heading.

Tinzaparin Sodium (Due to the frequent occurrence of severe and prolonged thrombocytopenia, the potential benefits of medications that interfere with platelet function and/or anticoagulation should be weighed against the potential increased risk of bleeding and hemorrhage).
No products indexed under this heading.

Tirofiban Hydrochloride (Due to the frequent occurrence of severe and prolonged thrombocytopenia, the potential benefits of medications that interfere with platelet function and/or anticoagulation should be weighed against the potential increased risk of bleeding and hemorrhage).
No products indexed under this heading.

Tolmetin Sodium (Due to the frequent occurrence of severe and prolonged thrombocytopenia, the potential benefits of medications that interfere with platelet function and/or anticoagulation should be weighed against the potential increased risk of bleeding and hemorrhage).
No products indexed under this heading.

Warfarin Sodium (Due to the frequent occurrence of severe and prolonged thrombocytopenia, the potential benefits of medications that interfere with platelet function and/or anticoagulation should be weighed against the potential increased risk of bleeding and hemorrhage).
No products indexed under this heading.

BIAXIN FILMTAB TABLETS

(Clarithromycin) **412**
May interact with cytochrome p450 3a substrates (selected), cytochrome p450 inducers (selected), HMG-CoA reductase inhibitors, insulin, methylpredni-

---

IMPORTANT NOTE: Always consult each drug listing in the patient's regimen for possible interactions.

solone, oral anticoagulants, oral hypoglycemic agents, phenytoin, quinidine, theophyllines, triazolobenzodiazepines, valproate, and certain other agents. Compounds in these categories include:

Acarbose (There have been rare reports of hypoglycemia, some of which have occurred in patients taking oral hypoglycemic agents).
No products indexed under this heading.

Alfentanil Hydrochloride (Co-administration of clarithromycin, known to inhibit CYP3A, and a drug primarily metabolized by CYP3A may be associated with elevations in drug concentrations that could increase or prolong both therapeutic and adverse effects of the concomitant drug. There have been spontaneous or published reports of CYP3A based interactions of erythromycin and/or clarithromycin with alfentanil).
No products indexed under this heading.

Allium cepa (Strong inducers of the cytochrome P450 metabolism system such as efavirenz, nevirapine, rifampicin, rifabutin, and rifapentine may accelerate the metabolism of clarithromycin and thus lower the plasma levels of clarithromycin, while increasing those of 14-OH-clarithromycin, a metabolite that is also microbiologically active. Since the microbiological activities of clarithromycin and 14-OH-clarithromycin are different for different bacteria, the intended therapeutic effect could be impaired during concomitant administration of clarithromycin and enzyme inducers). Products include:
Hyland's Cold 'N Cough 3314
Mederma 2319
Mederma for Kids 2319

Allium sativum (Strong inducers of the cytochrome P450 metabolism system such as efavirenz, nevirapine, rifampicin, rifabutin, and rifapentine may accelerate the metabolism of clarithromycin and thus lower the plasma levels of clarithromycin, while increasing those of 14-OH-clarithromycin, a metabolite that is also microbiologically active. Since the microbiological activities of clarithromycin and 14-OH-clarithromycin are different for different bacteria, the intended therapeutic effect could be impaired during concomitant administration of clarithromycin and enzyme inducers).
No products indexed under this heading.

Allium schoenoprasum (Strong inducers of the cytochrome P450 metabolism system such as efavirenz, nevirapine, rifampicin, rifabutin, and rifapentine may accelerate the metabolism of clarithromycin and thus lower the plasma levels of clarithromycin, while increasing those of 14-OH-clarithromycin, a metabolite that is also microbiologically active. Since the microbiological activities of clarithromycin and 14-OH-clarithromycin are different for different bacteria, the intended therapeutic effect could be impaired during concomitant administration of clarithromycin and enzyme inducers).
No products indexed under this heading.

Allium ursinum (Strong inducers of the cytochrome P450 metabolism system such as efavirenz, nevirapine, rifampicin, rifabutin, and rifapentine may accelerate the metabolism of clarithromycin and thus lower the plasma levels of clarithromycin, while increasing those of 14-OH-clarithromycin, a metabolite that is also microbiologically active. Since the microbiological activities of clarithromycin and 14-OH-clarithromycin are different for different bacteria, the intended therapeutic effect could be

impaired during concomitant administration of clarithromycin and enzyme inducers).
No products indexed under this heading.

Alprazolam (Co-administration of erythromycin or clarithromycin and a drug primarily metabolized by CYP3A may be associated with elevation in drug concentrations that could increase or prolong both the therapeutic and adverse effects of the concomitant drug).
No products indexed under this heading.

Aminoglutethimide (Strong inducers of the cytochrome P450 metabolism system such as efavirenz, nevirapine, rifampicin, rifabutin, and rifapentine may accelerate the metabolism of clarithromycin and thus lower the plasma levels of clarithromycin, while increasing those of 14-OH-clarithromycin, a metabolite that is also microbiologically active. Since the microbiological activities of clarithromycin and 14-OH-clarithromycin are different for different bacteria, the intended therapeutic effect could be impaired during concomitant administration of clarithromycin and enzyme inducers).
No products indexed under this heading.

Aminophylline (Co-administration of erythromycin or clarithromycin and a drug primarily metabolized by CYP3A may be associated with elevation in drug concentrations that could increase or prolong both the therapeutic and adverse effects of the concomitant drug).
No products indexed under this heading.

Amitriptyline Hydrochloride (Co-administration of erythromycin or clarithromycin and a drug primarily metabolized by CYP3A may be associated with elevation in drug concentrations that could increase or prolong both the therapeutic and adverse effects of the concomitant drug).
No products indexed under this heading.

Amlodipine Besylate (Co-administration of erythromycin or clarithromycin and a drug primarily metabolized by CYP3A may be associated with elevation in drug concentrations that could increase or prolong both the therapeutic and adverse effects of the concomitant drug).
Products include:
Azor 1010
Exforge 2443
Exforge HCT 2449

Anisindione (Spontaneous reports in the post-marketing period suggest that concomitant administration of clarithromycin and oral anticoagulants may potentiate the effects of the oral anticoagulants. Prothrombin times should be carefully monitored while patients are receiving clarithromycin and oral anticoagulants simultaneously).
No products indexed under this heading.

Aprepitant (Co-administration of erythromycin or clarithromycin and a drug primarily metabolized by CYP3A may be associated with elevation in drug concentrations that could increase or prolong both the therapeutic and adverse effects of the concomitant drug).
Products include:
Emend 2124

Astemizole (Concomitant administration of clarithromycin with astemizole is contraindicated. There have been post-marketing reports of drug interactions when clarithromycin and/or erythromycin are co-administered with astemizole, resulting in cardiac arrhythmias (QT prolongation, ventricular tachycardia, ventricular fibrillation, and torsades de pointes) most likely due to inhibition of

metabolism of these drugs by erythromycin and clarithromycin. Fatalities have been reported).
No products indexed under this heading.

Atazanavir (Co-administration of clarithromycin (500 mg twice daily) with atazanavir (400 mg once daily) resulted in a 2-fold increase in exposure to clarithromycin and a 70% decrease in exposure to 14-OH-clarithromycin, with a 28% increase in the AUC of atazanavir).
No products indexed under this heading.

Atazanavir Sulfate (Co-administration of clarithromycin (500 mg twice daily) with atazanavir (400 mg once daily) resulted in a 2-fold increase in exposure to clarithromycin and a 70% decrease in exposure to 14-OH-clarithromycin, with a 28% increase in the AUC of atazanavir).
No products indexed under this heading.

Atorvastatin Calcium (As with other macrolides, clarithromycin has been reported to increase concentrations of HMG-CoA reductase inhibitors (eg, lovastatin, simvastatin). Rare reports of rhabdomyolysis have been reported in patients taking these drugs concomitantly). Products include:
Lipitor 2703

Betamethasone (Strong inducers of the cytochrome P450 metabolism system such as efavirenz, nevirapine, rifampicin, rifabutin, and rifapentine may accelerate the metabolism of clarithromycin and thus lower the plasma levels of clarithromycin, while increasing those of 14-OH-clarithromycin, a metabolite that is also microbiologically active. Since the microbiological activities of clarithromycin and 14-OH-clarithromycin are different for different bacteria, the intended therapeutic effect could be impaired during concomitant administration of clarithromycin and enzyme inducers).
No products indexed under this heading.

Betamethasone Acetate (Strong inducers of the cytochrome P450 metabolism system such as efavirenz, nevirapine, rifampicin, rifabutin, and rifapentine may accelerate the metabolism of clarithromycin and thus lower the plasma levels of clarithromycin, while increasing those of 14-OH-clarithromycin, a metabolite that is also microbiologically active. Since the microbiological activities of clarithromycin and 14-OH-clarithromycin are different for different bacteria, the intended therapeutic effect could be impaired during concomitant administration of clarithromycin and enzyme inducers).
No products indexed under this heading.

Betamethasone Benzoate (Strong inducers of the cytochrome P450 metabolism system such as efavirenz, nevirapine, rifampicin, rifabutin, and rifapentine may accelerate the metabolism of clarithromycin and thus lower the plasma levels of clarithromycin, while increasing those of 14-OH-clarithromycin, a metabolite that is also microbiologically active. Since the microbiological activities of clarithromycin and 14-OH-clarithromycin are different for different bacteria, the intended therapeutic effect could be impaired during concomitant administration of clarithromycin and enzyme inducers).
No products indexed under this heading.

Betamethasone Dipropionate (Strong inducers of the cytochrome P450 metabolism system such as efavirenz, nevirapine, rifampicin, rifabutin, and rifapentine may accelerate the metabolism of clarithromycin and thus lower the plasma levels of clarithromycin, while increasing those of 14-OH-clarithromycin, a metabolite that is also microbiologically active. Since the

microbiological activities of clarithromycin and 14-OH-clarithromycin are different for different bacteria, the intended therapeutic effect could be impaired during concomitant administration of clarithromycin and enzyme inducers).
Products include:
Diprolene Lotion 0.05% 3108
Diprolene Ointment 0.05% 3109
Diprolene AF Cream 0.05% 3107
Lotrisone 3163

Betamethasone Sodium Phosphate (Strong inducers of the cytochrome P450 metabolism system such as efavirenz, nevirapine, rifampicin, rifabutin, and rifapentine may accelerate the metabolism of clarithromycin and thus lower the plasma levels of clarithromycin, while increasing those of 14-OH-clarithromycin, a metabolite that is also microbiologically active. Since the microbiological activities of clarithromycin and 14-OH-clarithromycin are different for different bacteria, the intended therapeutic effect could be impaired during concomitant administration of clarithromycin and enzyme inducers).
No products indexed under this heading.

Betamethasone Valerate (Strong inducers of the cytochrome P450 metabolism system such as efavirenz, nevirapine, rifampicin, rifabutin, and rifapentine may accelerate the metabolism of clarithromycin and thus lower the plasma levels of clarithromycin, while increasing those of 14-OH-clarithromycin, a metabolite that is also microbiologically active. Since the microbiological activities of clarithromycin and 14-OH-clarithromycin are different for different bacteria, the intended therapeutic effect could be impaired during concomitant administration of clarithromycin and enzyme inducers).
Products include:
Luxíq 3321

Bosentan (Strong inducers of the cytochrome P450 metabolism system such as efavirenz, nevirapine, rifampicin, rifabutin, and rifapentine may accelerate the metabolism of clarithromycin and thus lower the plasma levels of clarithromycin, while increasing those of 14-OH-clarithromycin, a metabolite that is also microbiologically active. Since the microbiological activities of clarithromycin and 14-OH-clarithromycin are different for different bacteria, the intended therapeutic effect could be impaired during concomitant administration of clarithromycin and enzyme inducers). Products include:
Tracleer 573

Bromocriptine Mesylate (Co-administration of clarithromycin, known to inhibit CYP3A, and a drug primarily metabolized by CYP3A may be associated with elevations in drug concentrations that could increase or prolong both therapeutic and adverse effects of the concomitant drug. There have been spontaneous or published reports of CYP3A based interactions of erythromycin and/or clarithromycin with bromocriptine).
No products indexed under this heading.

Buspirone Hydrochloride (Co-administration of erythromycin or clarithromycin and a drug primarily metabolized by CYP3A may be associated with elevation in drug concentrations that could increase or prolong both the therapeutic and adverse effects of the concomitant drug).
No products indexed under this heading.

Busulfan (Co-administration of erythromycin or clarithromycin and a drug primarily metabolized by CYP3A may be associated with elevation in drug concentrations that could increase or pro-

long both the therapeutic and adverse effects of the concomitant drug). Products include:
Myleran 1581

Carbamazepine (Concomitant administration of single doses of clarithromycin and carbamazepine has been shown to result in increased plasma concentrations of carbamazepine. Blood level monitoring of carbamazepine may be considered). Products include:
Carbatrol 3280
Equetro 3477

Cerivastatin Sodium (As with other macrolides, clarithromycin has been reported to increase concentrations of HMG-CoA reductase inhibitors (eg, lovastatin, simvastatin). Rare reports of rhabdomyolysis have been reported in patients taking these drugs concomitantly).
No products indexed under this heading.

Chlorpheniramine (Co-administration of erythromycin or clarithromycin and a drug primarily metabolized by CYP3A may be associated with elevation in drug concentrations that could increase or prolong both the therapeutic and adverse effects of the concomitant drug).
No products indexed under this heading.

Chlorpheniramine Maleate (Co-administration of erythromycin or clarithromycin and a drug primarily metabolized by CYP3A may be associated with elevation in drug concentrations that could increase or prolong both the therapeutic and adverse effects of the concomitant drug).
No products indexed under this heading.

Chlorpheniramine Polistirex (Co-administration of erythromycin or clarithromycin and a drug primarily metabolized by CYP3A may be associated with elevation in drug concentrations that could increase or prolong both the therapeutic and adverse effects of the concomitant drug). Products include:
Tussionex 3443

Chlorpheniramine Tannate (Co-administration of erythromycin or clarithromycin and a drug primarily metabolized by CYP3A may be associated with elevation in drug concentrations that could increase or prolong both the therapeutic and adverse effects of the concomitant drug).
No products indexed under this heading.

Chlorpropamide (There have been rare reports of hypoglycemia, some of which have occurred in patients taking oral hypoglycemic agents).
No products indexed under this heading.

Cilostazol (Co-administration of clarithromycin, known to inhibit CYP3A, and a drug primarily metabolized by CYP3A may be associated with elevations in drug concentrations that could increase or prolong both therapeutic and adverse effects of the concomitant drug. There have been spontaneous or published reports of CYP3A based interactions of erythromycin and/or clarithromycin with cilostazol).
No products indexed under this heading.

Ciprofloxacin (Strong inducers of the cytochrome P450 metabolism system such as efavirenz, nevirapine, rifampicin, rifabutin, and rifapentine may accelerate the metabolism of clarithromycin and thus lower the plasma levels of clarithromycin, while increasing those of 14-OH-clarithromycin, a metabolite that is also microbiologically active. Since the microbiological activities of clarithromycin and 14-OH-clarithromycin are different for different bacteria, the intended therapeutic effect could be impaired during concomitant administration of clarithromycin and enzyme inducers). Products include:
Cipro I.V. 3082
Cipro 3073
Cipro XR 3091
Ciprodex 583

Ciprofloxacin Hydrochloride (Strong inducers of the cytochrome P450 metabolism system such as efavirenz, nevirapine, rifampicin, rifabutin, and rifapentine may accelerate the metabolism of clarithromycin and thus lower the plasma levels of clarithromycin, while increasing those of 14-OH-clarithromycin, a metabolite that is also microbiologically active. Since the microbiological activities of clarithromycin and 14-OH-clarithromycin are different for different bacteria, the intended therapeutic effect could be impaired during concomitant administration of clarithromycin and enzyme inducers). Products include:
Cipro 3073

Cisapride (Concomitant administration of clarithromycin with cisapride is contraindicated. There have been post-marketing reports of drug interactions when clarithromycin and/or erythromycin are co-administered with cisapride, resulting in cardiac arrhythmias (QT prolongation, ventricular tachycardia, ventricular fibrillation, and torsades de pointes) most likely due to inhibition of metabolism of these drugs by erythromycin and clarithromycin. Fatalities have been reported).
No products indexed under this heading.

Cisplatin (Strong inducers of the cytochrome P450 metabolism system such as efavirenz, nevirapine, rifampicin, rifabutin, and rifapentine may accelerate the metabolism of clarithromycin and thus lower the plasma levels of clarithromycin, while increasing those of 14-OH-clarithromycin, a metabolite that is also microbiologically active. Since the microbiological activities of clarithromycin and 14-OH-clarithromycin are different for different bacteria, the intended therapeutic effect could be impaired during concomitant administration of clarithromycin and enzyme inducers).
No products indexed under this heading.

Citalopram Hydrobromide (Strong inducers of the cytochrome P450 metabolism system such as efavirenz, nevirapine, rifampicin, rifabutin, and rifapentine may accelerate the metabolism of clarithromycin and thus lower the plasma levels of clarithromycin, while increasing those of 14-OH-clarithromycin, a metabolite that is also microbiologically active. Since the microbiological activities of clarithromycin and 14-OH-clarithromycin are different for different bacteria, the intended therapeutic effect could be impaired during concomitant administration of clarithromycin and enzyme inducers). Products include:
Celexa 1153

Colchicine (When clarithromycin and colchicine are administered together, inhibition of Pgp and/or CYP3A by clarithromycin may lead to increased exposure to colchicine. Patients should be monitored for clinical symptoms of colchicine toxicity).
No products indexed under this heading.

Cortisone Acetate (Strong inducers of the cytochrome P450 metabolism system such as efavirenz, nevirapine, rifampicin, rifabutin, and rifapentine may accelerate the metabolism of clarithromycin and thus lower the plasma levels of clarithromycin, while increasing those of 14-OH-clarithromycin, a metabolite that is also microbiologically active. Since the microbiological activities of clarithromycin and 14-OH-clarithromycin are different for different bacteria, the intended therapeutic effect could be impaired during concomitant administration of clarithromycin and enzyme inducers).
No products indexed under this heading.

Cyclosporine (Co-administration of clarithromycin, known to inhibit CYP3A, and a drug primarily metabolized by CYP3A may be associated with elevations in drug concentrations that could increase or prolong both therapeutic and adverse effects of the concomitant drug. There have been spontaneous or published reports of CYP3A based interactions of erythromycin and/or clarithromycin with cyclosporine). Products include:
Gengraf 440
Neoral Oral Solution 2496
Neoral Capsules 2496
Restasis 605

Desogestrel (Co-administration of erythromycin or clarithromycin and a drug primarily metabolized by CYP3A may be associated with elevation in drug concentrations that could increase or prolong both the therapeutic and adverse effects of the concomitant drug).
No products indexed under this heading.

Dexamethasone (Co-administration of erythromycin or clarithromycin and a drug primarily metabolized by CYP3A may be associated with elevation in drug concentrations that could increase or prolong both the therapeutic and adverse effects of the concomitant drug). Products include:
Ciprodex 583
Ozurdex ..... ⊙223
Tobramycin and Dexamethasone Ophthalmic Suspension ..... ⊙251

Dexamethasone Acetate (Co-administration of erythromycin or clarithromycin and a drug primarily metabolized by CYP3A may be associated with elevation in drug concentrations that could increase or prolong both the therapeutic and adverse effects of the concomitant drug).
No products indexed under this heading.

Dexamethasone Phosphate (Co-administration of erythromycin or clarithromycin and a drug primarily metabolized by CYP3A may be associated with elevation in drug concentrations that could increase or prolong both the therapeutic and adverse effects of the concomitant drug).
No products indexed under this heading.

Dexamethasone Sodium (Co-administration of erythromycin or clarithromycin and a drug primarily metabolized by CYP3A may be associated with elevation in drug concentrations that could increase or prolong both the therapeutic and adverse effects of the concomitant drug).
No products indexed under this heading.

Dexamethasone Sodium Phosphate (Co-administration of erythromycin or clarithromycin and a drug primarily metabolized by CYP3A may be associated with elevation in drug concentrations that could increase or prolong both the therapeutic and adverse effects of the concomitant drug).
No products indexed under this heading.

Dexamethasone Sodium Phosphate Injection (Strong inducers of the cytochrome P450 metabolism system such as efavirenz, nevirapine, rifampicin, rifabutin, and rifapentine may accelerate the metabolism of clarithromycin and thus lower the plasma levels of clarithromycin, while increasing those of 14-OH-clarithromycin, a metabolite that is also microbiologically active. Since the microbiological activities of clarithromycin and 14-OH-clarithromycin are different for different bacteria, the intended therapeutic effect could be impaired during concomitant administration of clarithromycin and enzyme inducers).
No products indexed under this heading.

Diazepam (Co-administration of erythromycin or clarithromycin and a drug primarily metabolized by CYP3A may be associated with elevation in drug concentrations that could increase or prolong both the therapeutic and adverse effects of the concomitant drug). Products include:
Valium Tablets 2880

Dicumarol (Spontaneous reports in the post-marketing period suggest that concomitant administration of clarithromycin and oral anticoagulants may potentiate the effects of the oral anticoagulants. Prothrombin times should be carefully monitored while patients are receiving clarithromycin and oral anticoagulants simultaneously).
No products indexed under this heading.

Digoxin (When clarithromycin and digoxin are administered together, inhibition of Pgp by clarithromycin may lead to increased exposure to digoxin. Elevated digoxin serum concentrations in patients receiving clarithromycin and digoxin concomitantly have also been reported in post-marketing surveillance. Some patients have shown clinical signs consistent with digoxin toxicity, including potentially fatal arrhythmias. Serum digoxin concentrations should be carefully monitored while patients are receiving digoxin and clarithromycin simultaneously). Products include:
Lanoxin Injection 1546
Lanoxin Injection Pediatric 1549
Lanoxin Tablets 1553

Dihydroergotamine Mesylate (Post-marketing reports indicate that co-administration of clarithromycin with dihydroergotamine has been associated with acute ergot toxicity characterized by vasospasm and ischemia of the extremities and other tissues including the central nervous system. Concomitant administration of clarithromycin with ergotamine or dihydroergotamine is contraindicated).
No products indexed under this heading.

Diltiazem Hydrochloride (Co-administration of erythromycin or clarithromycin and a drug primarily metabolized by CYP3A may be associated with elevation in drug concentrations that could increase or prolong both the therapeutic and adverse effects of the concomitant drug). Products include:
Cardizem LA 423

Diltiazem Maleate (Co-administration of erythromycin or clarithromycin and a drug primarily metabolized by CYP3A may be associated with elevation in drug concentrations that could increase or prolong both the therapeutic and adverse effects of the concomitant drug).
No products indexed under this heading.

Disopyramide (There have been post-marketing reports of torsades de pointes occurring with concurrent use of clarithromycin and disopyramide. Electrocardiograms should be monitored for QTc prolongation during co-administration of clarithromycin with these drugs. Serum concentrations of these medications should also be monitored).
No products indexed under this heading.

IMPORTANT NOTE: Always consult each drug listing in the patient's regimen for possible interactions.

Biaxin **Interactions Index** 232

Disopyramide Phosphate (There have been post-marketing reports of torsades de pointes occurring with concurrent use of clarithromycin and disopyramide. Electrocardiograms should be monitored for QTc prolongation during co-administration of clarithromycin with these drugs. Serum concentrations of these medications should also be monitored).
No products indexed under this heading.

Divalproex Sodium (Co-administration of clarithromycin, known to inhibit CYP3A, and a drug primarily metabolized by CYP3A may be associated with elevations in drug concentrations that could increase or prolong both therapeutic and adverse effects of the concomitant drug. There have been reports of interactions of erythromycin or clarithromycin with drugs not thought to be metabolized by CYP3A, including valproate). Products include:
Depakote ER **426**

Doxorubicin Hydrochloride (Co-administration of erythromycin or clarithromycin and a drug primarily metabolized by CYP3A may be associated with elevation in drug concentrations that could increase or prolong both the therapeutic and adverse effects of the concomitant drug).
No products indexed under this heading.

Dronabinol (Co-administration of erythromycin or clarithromycin and a drug primarily metabolized by CYP3A may be associated with elevation in drug concentrations that could increase or prolong both the therapeutic and adverse effects of the concomitant drug).
No products indexed under this heading.

Dyphylline (Co-administration of erythromycin or clarithromycin and a drug primarily metabolized by CYP3A may be associated with elevation in drug concentrations that could increase or prolong both the therapeutic and adverse effects of the concomitant drug).
No products indexed under this heading.

Efavirenz (Strong inducers of the cytochrome P450 metabolism system such as efavirenz may accelerate the metabolism of clarithromycin and thus lower the plasma levels of clarithromycin, while increasing those of 14-OH-clarithromycin, a metabolite that is also microbiologically active. Since the microbiological activities of clarithromycin and 14-OH-clarithromycin are different for different bacteria, the intended therapeutic effect could be impaired during concomitant administration of clarithromycin and enzyme inducers). Products include:
Atripla **906**

Ergotamine Tartrate (Post-marketing reports indicate that co-administration of clarithromycin with ergotamine has been associated with acute ergot toxicity characterized by vasospasm and ischemia of the extremities and other tissues including the central nervous system. Concomitant administration of clarithromycin with ergotamine is contraindicated).
No products indexed under this heading.

Erythromycin (Co-administration of erythromycin or clarithromycin and a drug primarily metabolized by CYP3A may be associated with elevation in drug concentrations that could increase or prolong both the therapeutic and adverse effects of the concomitant drug).
No products indexed under this heading.

Erythromycin, Topical (Strong inducers of the cytochrome P450 metabolism system such as efavirenz, nevirapine, rifampicin, rifabutin, and rifapentine may accelerate the metabolism of clarithromycin and thus lower the plasma levels of clarithromycin, while increasing those of 14-OH-clarithromycin, a metabolite that is also microbiologically active. Since the microbiological activities of clarithromycin and 14-OH-clarithromycin are different for different bacteria, the intended therapeutic effect could be impaired during concomitant administration of clarithromycin and enzyme inducers).
No products indexed under this heading.

Erythromycin Estolate (Co-administration of erythromycin or clarithromycin and a drug primarily metabolized by CYP3A may be associated with elevation in drug concentrations that could increase or prolong both the therapeutic and adverse effects of the concomitant drug).
No products indexed under this heading.

Erythromycin Ethylsuccinate (Co-administration of erythromycin or clarithromycin and a drug primarily metabolized by CYP3A may be associated with elevation in drug concentrations that could increase or prolong both the therapeutic and adverse effects of the concomitant drug). Products include:
E.E.S. **437**
EryPed **435**

Erythromycin Gluceptate (Co-administration of erythromycin or clarithromycin and a drug primarily metabolized by CYP3A may be associated with elevation in drug concentrations that could increase or prolong both the therapeutic and adverse effects of the concomitant drug).
No products indexed under this heading.

Erythromycin Lactobionate (Co-administration of erythromycin or clarithromycin and a drug primarily metabolized by CYP3A may be associated with elevation in drug concentrations that could increase or prolong both the therapeutic and adverse effects of the concomitant drug).
No products indexed under this heading.

Erythromycin Stearate (Co-administration of erythromycin or clarithromycin and a drug primarily metabolized by CYP3A may be associated with elevation in drug concentrations that could increase or prolong both the therapeutic and adverse effects of the concomitant drug).
No products indexed under this heading.

Escitalopram Oxalate (Strong inducers of the cytochrome P450 metabolism system such as efavirenz, nevirapine, rifampicin, rifabutin, and rifapentine may accelerate the metabolism of clarithromycin and thus lower the plasma levels of clarithromycin, while increasing those of 14-OH-clarithromycin, a metabolite that is also microbiologically active. Since the microbiological activities of clarithromycin and 14-OH-clarithromycin are different for different bacteria, the intended therapeutic effect could be impaired during concomitant administration of clarithromycin and enzyme inducers). Products include:
Lexapro Oral Suspension **1160**
Lexapro Tablets **1160**

Esomeprazole Magnesium (Strong inducers of the cytochrome P450 metabolism system such as efavirenz, nevirapine, rifampicin, rifabutin, and rifapentine may accelerate the metabolism of clarithromycin and thus lower the plasma levels of clarithromycin, while increasing those of 14-OH-clarithromycin, a metabolite that is also microbiologically active. Since the microbiological activities of clarithromycin and 14-OH-clarithromycin are different for different bacteria, the intended therapeutic effect could be impaired during concomitant administration of clarithromycin and enzyme inducers). Products include:
Nexium Capsules **704**
Nexium Oral Suspension **704**

Esomeprazole Sodium (Strong inducers of the cytochrome P450 metabolism system such as efavirenz, nevirapine, rifampicin, rifabutin, and rifapentine may accelerate the metabolism of clarithromycin and thus lower the plasma levels of clarithromycin, while increasing those of 14-OH-clarithromycin, a metabolite that is also microbiologically active. Since the microbiological activities of clarithromycin and 14-OH-clarithromycin are different for different bacteria, the intended therapeutic effect could be impaired during concomitant administration of clarithromycin and enzyme inducers). Products include:
Nexium I.V. **712**

Estrogen (Co-administration of erythromycin or clarithromycin and a drug primarily metabolized by CYP3A may be associated with elevation in drug concentrations that could increase or prolong both the therapeutic and adverse effects of the concomitant drug).
No products indexed under this heading.

Estrogens, Conjugated (Co-administration of erythromycin or clarithromycin and a drug primarily metabolized by CYP3A may be associated with elevation in drug concentrations that could increase or prolong both the therapeutic and adverse effects of the concomitant drug). Products include:
Premarin Intravenous **3528**
Premarin Tablets **3533**
Premarin Vaginal Cream **3540**
Premphase **3549**
Prempro **3549**

Estrogens, Conjugated, Synthetic A (Co-administration of erythromycin or clarithromycin and a drug primarily metabolized by CYP3A may be associated with elevation in drug concentrations that could increase or prolong both the therapeutic and adverse effects of the concomitant drug).
No products indexed under this heading.

Estrogens, Esterified (Co-administration of erythromycin or clarithromycin and a drug primarily metabolized by CYP3A may be associated with elevation in drug concentrations that could increase or prolong both the therapeutic and adverse effects of the concomitant drug).
No products indexed under this heading.

Ethanol (Strong inducers of the cytochrome P450 metabolism system such as efavirenz, nevirapine, rifampicin, rifabutin, and rifapentine may accelerate the metabolism of clarithromycin and thus lower the plasma levels of clarithromycin, while increasing those of 14-OH-clarithromycin, a metabolite that is also microbiologically active. Since the microbiological activities of clarithromycin and 14-OH-clarithromycin are different for different bacteria, the intended therapeutic effect could be impaired during concomitant administration of clarithromycin and enzyme inducers).
No products indexed under this heading.

Ethinyl Estradiol (Co-administration of erythromycin or clarithromycin and a drug primarily metabolized by CYP3A may be associated with elevation in drug concentrations that could increase or prolong both the therapeutic and adverse effects of the concomitant drug). Products include:
LoSeasonique **3407**
Lybrel **3514**
NuvaRing **3181**
Ortho Evra **2648**
Ortho-Cyclen/Ortho Tri-Cyclen **2663**
Ortho Tri-Cyclen Lo Tablets **2673**
Seasonique **3418**
Yaz **864**

Ethosuximide (Co-administration of erythromycin or clarithromycin and a drug primarily metabolized by CYP3A may be associated with elevation in drug concentrations that could increase or prolong both the therapeutic and adverse effects of the concomitant drug).
No products indexed under this heading.

Ethynodiol Diacetate (Co-administration of erythromycin or clarithromycin and a drug primarily metabolized by CYP3A may be associated with elevation in drug concentrations that could increase or prolong both the therapeutic and adverse effects of the concomitant drug).
No products indexed under this heading.

Etoposide (Co-administration of erythromycin or clarithromycin and a drug primarily metabolized by CYP3A may be associated with elevation in drug concentrations that could increase or prolong both the therapeutic and adverse effects of the concomitant drug).
No products indexed under this heading.

Etoposide Phosphate (Co-administration of erythromycin or clarithromycin and a drug primarily metabolized by CYP3A may be associated with elevation in drug concentrations that could increase or prolong both the therapeutic and adverse effects of the concomitant drug).
No products indexed under this heading.

Felbamate (Strong inducers of the cytochrome P450 metabolism system such as efavirenz, nevirapine, rifampicin, rifabutin, and rifapentine may accelerate the metabolism of clarithromycin and thus lower the plasma levels of clarithromycin, while increasing those of 14-OH-clarithromycin, a metabolite that is also microbiologically active. Since the microbiological activities of clarithromycin and 14-OH-clarithromycin are different for different bacteria, the intended therapeutic effect could be impaired during concomitant administration of clarithromycin and enzyme inducers).
No products indexed under this heading.

Felodipine (Co-administration of erythromycin or clarithromycin and a drug primarily metabolized by CYP3A may be associated with elevation in drug concentrations that could increase or prolong both the therapeutic and adverse effects of the concomitant drug).
No products indexed under this heading.

Fentanyl (Co-administration of erythromycin or clarithromycin and a drug primarily metabolized by CYP3A may be associated with elevation in drug concentrations that could increase or prolong both the therapeutic and adverse effects of the concomitant drug). Products include:
Duragesic **2604**
Fentanyl Transdermal System **2346**
Onsolis **2054**

Fentanyl Citrate (Co-administration of erythromycin or clarithromycin and a drug primarily metabolized by CYP3A may be associated with elevation in drug concentrations that could increase or prolong both the therapeutic and adverse effects of the concomitant drug). Products include:
Fentora **966**

Fluconazole (Concomitant administration of fluconazole 200 mg daily and clarithromycin 500 mg twice daily to 21 healthy volunteers led to increases in the mean steady-state clarithromycin C_{min} and AUC of 33% and 18%, respectively).
No products indexed under this heading.

Fludrocortisone Acetate (Strong inducers of the cytochrome P450 metabolism system such as efavirenz, nevirapine, rifampicin, rifabutin, and rifapentine may accelerate the metabolism of clarithromycin and thus lower the plasma levels of clarithromycin, while increasing those of 14-OH-clarithromycin, a metabolite that is also microbiologically active. Since the microbiological activities of clarithromycin and 14-OH-clarithromycin are different for different bacteria, the intended therapeutic effect could be impaired during concomitant administration of clarithromycin and enzyme inducers).
No products indexed under this heading.

Fluvastatin Sodium (As with other macrolides, clarithromycin has been reported to increase concentrations of HMG-CoA reductase inhibitors (eg, lovastatin, simvastatin). Rare reports of rhabdomyolysis have been reported in patients taking these drugs concomitantly).
No products indexed under this heading.

Fluvoxamine (Strong inducers of the cytochrome P450 metabolism system such as efavirenz, nevirapine, rifampicin, rifabutin, and rifapentine may accelerate the metabolism of clarithromycin and thus lower the plasma levels of clarithromycin, while increasing those of 14-OH-clarithromycin, a metabolite that is also microbiologically active. Since the microbiological activities of clarithromycin and 14-OH-clarithromycin are different for different bacteria, the intended therapeutic effect could be impaired during concomitant administration of clarithromycin and enzyme inducers).
No products indexed under this heading.

Fluvoxamine Maleate (Strong inducers of the cytochrome P450 metabolism system such as efavirenz, nevirapine, rifampicin, rifabutin, and rifapentine may accelerate the metabolism of clarithromycin and thus lower the plasma levels of clarithromycin, while increasing those of 14-OH-clarithromycin, a metabolite that is also microbiologically active. Since the microbiological activities of clarithromycin and 14-OH-clarithromycin are different for different bacteria, the intended therapeutic effect could be impaired during concomitant administration of clarithromycin and enzyme inducers).
No products indexed under this heading.

Fosphenytoin (Co-administration of clarithromycin, known to inhibit CYP3A, and a drug primarily metabolized by CYP3A may be associated with elevations in drug concentrations that could increase or prolong both therapeutic and adverse effects of the concomitant drug. There have been reports of interactions of erythromycin or clarithromycin with drugs not thought to be metabolized by CYP3A, including phenytoin).
No products indexed under this heading.

Fosphenytoin Sodium (Co-administration of clarithromycin, known to inhibit CYP3A, and a drug primarily metabolized by CYP3A may be associated with elevations in drug concentrations that could increase or prolong both therapeutic and adverse effects of the concomitant drug. There have been reports of interactions of erythromycin or clarithromycin with drugs not thought to be metabolized by CYP3A, including phenytoin).
No products indexed under this heading.

Garlic Extract (Strong inducers of the cytochrome P450 metabolism system such as efavirenz, nevirapine, rifampicin, rifabutin, and rifapentine may accelerate the metabolism of clarithromycin and thus lower the plasma levels of clarithromycin, while increasing those of 14-OH-clarithromycin, a metabolite that is also microbiologically active. Since the microbiological activities of clarithromycin and 14-OH-clarithromycin are different for different bacteria, the intended therapeutic effect could be impaired during concomitant administration of clarithromycin and enzyme inducers).
No products indexed under this heading.

Garlic Oil (Strong inducers of the cytochrome P450 metabolism system such as efavirenz, nevirapine, rifampicin, rifabutin, and rifapentine may accelerate the metabolism of clarithromycin and thus lower the plasma levels of clarithromycin, while increasing those of 14-OH-clarithromycin, a metabolite that is also microbiologically active. Since the microbiological activities of clarithromycin and 14-OH-clarithromycin are different for different bacteria, the intended therapeutic effect could be impaired during concomitant administration of clarithromycin and enzyme inducers).
No products indexed under this heading.

Glibenclamide (There have been rare reports of hypoglycemia, some of which have occurred in patients taking oral hypoglycemic agents).
No products indexed under this heading.

Glimepiride (There have been rare reports of hypoglycemia, some of which have occurred in patients taking oral hypoglycemic agents). Products include:
Avandaryl **1356**
Duetact **3354**

Glipizide (There have been rare reports of hypoglycemia, some of which have occurred in patients taking oral hypoglycemic agents).
No products indexed under this heading.

Glyburide (There have been rare reports of hypoglycemia, some of which have occurred in patients taking oral hypoglycemic agents).
No products indexed under this heading.

Haloperidol (Co-administration of erythromycin or clarithromycin and a drug primarily metabolized by CYP3A may be associated with elevation in drug concentrations that could increase or prolong both the therapeutic and adverse effects of the concomitant drug).
No products indexed under this heading.

Haloperidol Decanoate (Co-administration of erythromycin or clarithromycin and a drug primarily metabolized by CYP3A may be associated with elevation in drug concentrations that could increase or prolong both the therapeutic and adverse effects of the concomitant drug).
No products indexed under this heading.

Hexobarbital (Concurrent use of erythromycin and/or clarithromycin in patients receiving drugs metabolized by the cytochrome P450 system may be associated with elevation in serum levels of hexobarbital).
No products indexed under this heading.

Hydrocortisone (Strong inducers of the cytochrome P450 metabolism system such as efavirenz, nevirapine, rifampicin, rifabutin, and rifapentine may accelerate the metabolism of clarithromycin and thus lower the plasma levels of clarithromycin, while increasing those of 14-OH-clarithromycin, a metabolite that is also microbiologically active. Since the microbiological activities of clarithromycin and 14-OH-clarithromycin are different for different bacteria, the intended therapeutic effect could be impaired during concomitant administration of clarithromycin and enzyme inducers).
No products indexed under this heading.

Hydrocortisone (Alcohol) (Strong inducers of the cytochrome P450 metabolism system such as efavirenz, nevirapine, rifampicin, rifabutin, and rifapentine may accelerate the metabolism of clarithromycin and thus lower the plasma levels of clarithromycin, while increasing those of 14-OH-clarithromycin, a metabolite that is also microbiologically active. Since the microbiological activities of clarithromycin and 14-OH-clarithromycin are different for different bacteria, the intended therapeutic effect could be impaired during concomitant administration of clarithromycin and enzyme inducers).
No products indexed under this heading.

Hydrocortisone Acetate (Strong inducers of the cytochrome P450 metabolism system such as efavirenz, nevirapine, rifampicin, rifabutin, and rifapentine may accelerate the metabolism of clarithromycin and thus lower the plasma levels of clarithromycin, while increasing those of 14-OH-clarithromycin, a metabolite that is also microbiologically active. Since the microbiological activities of clarithromycin and 14-OH-clarithromycin are different for different bacteria, the intended therapeutic effect could be impaired during concomitant administration of clarithromycin and enzyme inducers).
No products indexed under this heading.

Hydrocortisone Butyrate (Strong inducers of the cytochrome P450 metabolism system such as efavirenz, nevirapine, rifampicin, rifabutin, and rifapentine may accelerate the metabolism of clarithromycin and thus lower the plasma levels of clarithromycin, while increasing those of 14-OH-clarithromycin, a metabolite that is also microbiologically active. Since the microbiological activities of clarithromycin and 14-OH-clarithromycin are different for different bacteria, the intended therapeutic effect could be impaired during concomitant administration of clarithromycin and enzyme inducers).
No products indexed under this heading.

Hydrocortisone Cypionate (Strong inducers of the cytochrome P450 metabolism system such as efavirenz, nevirapine, rifampicin, rifabutin, and rifapentine may accelerate the metabolism of clarithromycin and thus lower the plasma levels of clarithromycin, while increasing those of 14-OH-clarithromycin, a metabolite that is also microbiologically active. Since the microbiological activities of clarithromycin and 14-OH-clarithromycin are different for different bacteria, the intended therapeutic effect could be impaired during concomitant administration of clarithromycin and enzyme inducers).
No products indexed under this heading.

Hydrocortisone Hemisuccinate (Strong inducers of the cytochrome P450 metabolism system such as efavirenz, nevirapine, rifampicin, rifabutin, and rifapentine may accelerate the metabolism of clarithromycin and thus lower the plasma levels of clarithromycin, while increasing those of 14-OH-clarithromycin, a metabolite that is also microbiologically active. Since the microbiological activities of clarithromycin and 14-OH-clarithromycin are different for different bacteria, the intended therapeutic effect could be impaired during concomitant administration of clarithromycin and enzyme inducers).
No products indexed under this heading.

Hydrocortisone Probutate (Strong inducers of the cytochrome P450 metabolism system such as efavirenz, nevirapine, rifampicin, rifabutin, and rifapentine may accelerate the metabolism of clarithromycin and thus lower the plasma levels of clarithromycin, while increasing those of 14-OH-clarithromycin, a metabolite that is also microbiologically active. Since the microbiological activities of clarithromycin and 14-OH-clarithromycin are different for different bacteria, the intended therapeutic effect could be impaired during concomitant administration of clarithromycin and enzyme inducers).
No products indexed under this heading.

Hydrocortisone Sodium Phosphate (Strong inducers of the cytochrome P450 metabolism system such as efavirenz, nevirapine, rifampicin, rifabutin, and rifapentine may accelerate the metabolism of clarithromycin and thus lower the plasma levels of clarithromycin, while increasing those of 14-OH-clarithromycin, a metabolite that is also microbiologically active. Since the microbiological activities of clarithromycin and 14-OH-clarithromycin are different for different bacteria, the intended therapeutic effect could be impaired during concomitant administration of clarithromycin and enzyme inducers).
No products indexed under this heading.

Hydrocortisone Sodium Succinate (Strong inducers of the cytochrome P450 metabolism system such as efavirenz, nevirapine, rifampicin, rifabutin, and rifapentine may accelerate the metabolism of clarithromycin and thus lower the plasma levels of clarithromycin, while increasing those of 14-OH-clarithromycin, a metabolite that is also microbiologically active. Since the microbiological activities of clarithromycin and 14-OH-clarithromycin are different for different bacteria, the intended therapeutic effect could be impaired during concomitant administration of clarithromycin and enzyme inducers).
No products indexed under this heading.

Hydrocortisone Valerate (Strong inducers of the cytochrome P450 metabolism system such as efavirenz, nevirapine, rifampicin, rifabutin, and rifapentine may accelerate the metabolism of clarithromycin and thus lower the plasma levels of clarithromycin, while increasing those of 14-OH-clarithromycin, a metabolite that is also microbiologically active. Since the microbiological activities of clarithromycin and 14-OH-clarithromycin are different for different bacteria, the intended therapeutic effect could be impaired during concomitant administration of clarithromycin and enzyme inducers).
No products indexed under this heading.

Hypericum (Strong inducers of the cytochrome P450 metabolism system such as efavirenz, nevirapine, rifampicin, rifabutin, and rifapentine may accelerate the metabolism of clarithromycin and thus lower the plasma levels of clarithromycin, while increasing those of 14-OH-clarithromycin, a metabolite that is also microbiologically active. Since the microbiological activities of clarithromycin and 14-OH-clarithromycin are different for different bacteria, the intended therapeutic effect could be impaired during concomitant administration of clarithromycin and enzyme inducers).
No products indexed under this heading.

Hypericum Perforatum (Strong inducers of the cytochrome P450 metabolism system such as efavirenz, nevirapine, rifampicin, rifabutin, and rifapentine may accelerate the metabolism of clarithromycin and thus lower the plasma levels of clarithromycin, while increasing those of 14-OH-clarithromycin, a metabolite that is also microbiologically active. Since the microbiological activities of clarithromycin and 14-OH-clarithromycin are different for different bacteria, the intended therapeutic effect could be impaired during concomitant administration of clarithromycin and enzyme inducers). Products include:

IMPORTANT NOTE: Always consult each drug listing in the patient's regimen for possible interactions.

(⊙ Described in PDR® for Ophthalmic Medicines)

is also microbiologically active. Since the microbiological activities of clarithromycin and 14-OH-clarithromycin are different for different bacteria, the intended therapeutic effect could be impaired during concomitant administration of clarithromycin and enzyme inducers). Products include:
Provigil 983

Nafcillin Sodium (Strong inducers of the cytochrome P450 metabolism system such as efavirenz, nevirapine, rifampicin, rifabutin, and rifapentine may accelerate the metabolism of clarithromycin and thus lower the plasma levels of clarithromycin, while increasing those of 14-OH-clarithromycin, a metabolite that is also microbiologically active. Since the microbiological activities of clarithromycin and 14-OH-clarithromycin are different for different bacteria, the intended therapeutic effect could be impaired during concomitant administration of clarithromycin and enzyme inducers).
No products indexed under this heading.

Nateglinide (There have been rare reports of hypoglycemia, some of which have occurred in patients taking oral hypoglycemic agents).
No products indexed under this heading.

Nefazodone Hydrochloride (Co-administration of erythromycin or clarithromycin and a drug primarily metabolized by CYP3A may be associated with elevation in drug concentrations that could increase or prolong both the therapeutic and adverse effects of the concomitant drug).
No products indexed under this heading.

Nelfinavir Mesylate (Co-administration of erythromycin or clarithromycin and a drug primarily metabolized by CYP3A may be associated with elevation in drug concentrations that could increase or prolong both the therapeutic and adverse effects of the concomitant drug).
No products indexed under this heading.

Nevirapine (Strong inducers of the cytochrome P450 metabolism system such as nevirapine may accelerate the metabolism of clarithromycin and thus lower the plasma levels of clarithromycin, while increasing those of 14-OH-clarithromycin, a metabolite that is also microbiologically active. Since the microbiological activities of clarithromycin and 14-OH-clarithromycin are different for different bacteria, the intended therapeutic effect could be impaired during concomitant administration of clarithromycin and enzyme inducers). Products include:
Viramune Oral Suspension 897
Viramune Tablets 897

Nicardipine (Co-administration of erythromycin or clarithromycin and a drug primarily metabolized by CYP3A may be associated with elevation in drug concentrations that could increase or prolong both the therapeutic and adverse effects of the concomitant drug).
No products indexed under this heading.

Nicardipine Hydrochloride (Co-administration of erythromycin or clarithromycin and a drug primarily metabolized by CYP3A may be associated with elevation in drug concentrations that could increase or prolong both the therapeutic and adverse effects of the concomitant drug).
No products indexed under this heading.

Nicotine (Strong inducers of the cytochrome P450 metabolism system such as efavirenz, nevirapine, rifampicin, rifabutin, and rifapentine may accelerate the metabolism of clarithromycin and thus lower the plasma levels of clarithromycin, while increasing those of 14-OH-clarithromycin, a metabolite that

is also microbiologically active. Since the microbiological activities of clarithromycin and 14-OH-clarithromycin are different for different bacteria, the intended therapeutic effect could be impaired during concomitant administration of clarithromycin and enzyme inducers).
No products indexed under this heading.

Nicotine Polacrilex (Strong inducers of the cytochrome P450 metabolism system such as efavirenz, nevirapine, rifampicin, rifabutin, and rifapentine may accelerate the metabolism of clarithromycin and thus lower the plasma levels of clarithromycin, while increasing those of 14-OH-clarithromycin, a metabolite that is also microbiologically active. Since the microbiological activities of clarithromycin and 14-OH-clarithromycin are different for different bacteria, the intended therapeutic effect could be impaired during concomitant administration of clarithromycin and enzyme inducers).
No products indexed under this heading.

Nicotine Salicylate (Strong inducers of the cytochrome P450 metabolism system such as efavirenz, nevirapine, rifampicin, rifabutin, and rifapentine may accelerate the metabolism of clarithromycin and thus lower the plasma levels of clarithromycin, while increasing those of 14-OH-clarithromycin, a metabolite that is also microbiologically active. Since the microbiological activities of clarithromycin and 14-OH-clarithromycin are different for different bacteria, the intended therapeutic effect could be impaired during concomitant administration of clarithromycin and enzyme inducers).
No products indexed under this heading.

Nicotine Sulfate (Strong inducers of the cytochrome P450 metabolism system such as efavirenz, nevirapine, rifampicin, rifabutin, and rifapentine may accelerate the metabolism of clarithromycin and thus lower the plasma levels of clarithromycin, while increasing those of 14-OH-clarithromycin, a metabolite that is also microbiologically active. Since the microbiological activities of clarithromycin and 14-OH-clarithromycin are different for different bacteria, the intended therapeutic effect could be impaired during concomitant administration of clarithromycin and enzyme inducers).
No products indexed under this heading.

Nifedipine (Co-administration of erythromycin or clarithromycin and a drug primarily metabolized by CYP3A may be associated with elevation in drug concentrations that could increase or prolong both the therapeutic and adverse effects of the concomitant drug).
No products indexed under this heading.

Nimodipine (Co-administration of erythromycin or clarithromycin and a drug primarily metabolized by CYP3A may be associated with elevation in drug concentrations that could increase or prolong both the therapeutic and adverse effects of the concomitant drug).
No products indexed under this heading.

Nisoldipine (Co-administration of erythromycin or clarithromycin and a drug primarily metabolized by CYP3A may be associated with elevation in drug concentrations that could increase or prolong both the therapeutic and adverse effects of the concomitant drug).
No products indexed under this heading.

Norethindrone (Co-administration of erythromycin or clarithromycin and a drug primarily metabolized by CYP3A may be associated with elevation in drug concentrations that could increase

or prolong both the therapeutic and adverse effects of the concomitant drug). Products include:
Ortho Micronor 2660

Norethindrone Acetate (Strong inducers of the cytochrome P450 metabolism system such as efavirenz, nevirapine, rifampicin, rifabutin, and rifapentine may accelerate the metabolism of clarithromycin and thus lower the plasma levels of clarithromycin, while increasing those of 14-OH-clarithromycin, a metabolite that is also microbiologically active. Since the microbiological activities of clarithromycin and 14-OH-clarithromycin are different for different bacteria, the intended therapeutic effect could be impaired during concomitant administration of clarithromycin and enzyme inducers). Products include:
Activella 2561

Norgestrel (Co-administration of erythromycin or clarithromycin and a drug primarily metabolized by CYP3A may be associated with elevation in drug concentrations that could increase or prolong both the therapeutic and adverse effects of the concomitant drug).
No products indexed under this heading.

Omeprazole (Clarithromycin 500 mg every 8 hours was given in combination with omeprazole 40 mg daily to healthy adult subjects. The steady-state plasma concentrations of omeprazole were increased (C_{max}, AUC_{0-24}, and $t_{1/2}$ increases of 30%, 89%, and 34%, respectively), by the concomitant administration of clarithromycin. The mean 24-hour gastric pH value was 5.2 when omeprazole was administered alone and 5.7 when co-administered with clarithromycin).
No products indexed under this heading.

Omeprazole Magnesium (Strong inducers of the cytochrome P450 metabolism system such as efavirenz, nevirapine, rifampicin, rifabutin, and rifapentine may accelerate the metabolism of clarithromycin and thus lower the plasma levels of clarithromycin, while increasing those of 14-OH-clarithromycin, a metabolite that is also microbiologically active. Since the microbiological activities of clarithromycin and 14-OH-clarithromycin are different for different bacteria, the intended therapeutic effect could be impaired during concomitant administration of clarithromycin and enzyme inducers).
No products indexed under this heading.

Ondansetron Hydrochloride (Co-administration of erythromycin or clarithromycin and a drug primarily metabolized by CYP3A may be associated with elevation in drug concentrations that could increase or prolong both the therapeutic and adverse effects of the concomitant drug). Products include:
Zofran Injection 1750
Zofran 1756
Zofran ODT 1756

Oxcarbazepine (Strong inducers of the cytochrome P450 metabolism system such as efavirenz, nevirapine, rifampicin, rifabutin, and rifapentine may accelerate the metabolism of clarithromycin and thus lower the plasma levels of clarithromycin, while increasing those of 14-OH-clarithromycin, a metabolite that is also microbiologically active. Since the microbiological activities of clarithromycin and 14-OH-clarithromycin are different for different bacteria, the intended therapeutic effect could be impaired during concomitant administration of clarithromycin and enzyme inducers).
No products indexed under this heading.

Paclitaxel (Co-administration of erythromycin or clarithromycin and a drug primarily metabolized by CYP3A may be associated with elevation in drug concentrations that could increase or prolong both the therapeutic and adverse effects of the concomitant drug).
No products indexed under this heading.

Phenobarbital (Strong inducers of the cytochrome P450 metabolism system such as efavirenz, nevirapine, rifampicin, rifabutin, and rifapentine may accelerate the metabolism of clarithromycin and thus lower the plasma levels of clarithromycin, while increasing those of 14-OH-clarithromycin, a metabolite that is also microbiologically active. Since the microbiological activities of clarithromycin and 14-OH-clarithromycin are different for different bacteria, the intended therapeutic effect could be impaired during concomitant administration of clarithromycin and enzyme inducers). Products include:
Donnatal 2711

Phenobarbital Sodium (Strong inducers of the cytochrome P450 metabolism system such as efavirenz, nevirapine, rifampicin, rifabutin, and rifapentine may accelerate the metabolism of clarithromycin and thus lower the plasma levels of clarithromycin, while increasing those of 14-OH-clarithromycin, a metabolite that is also microbiologically active. Since the microbiological activities of clarithromycin and 14-OH-clarithromycin are different for different bacteria, the intended therapeutic effect could be impaired during concomitant administration of clarithromycin and enzyme inducers).
No products indexed under this heading.

Phenytoin (Co-administration of clarithromycin, known to inhibit CYP3A, and a drug primarily metabolized by CYP3A may be associated with elevations in drug concentrations that could increase or prolong both therapeutic and adverse effects of the concomitant drug. There have been reports of interactions of erythromycin or clarithromycin with drugs not thought to be metabolized by CYP3A, including phenytoin).
No products indexed under this heading.

Phenytoin Sodium (Co-administration of clarithromycin, known to inhibit CYP3A, and a drug primarily metabolized by CYP3A may be associated with elevations in drug concentrations that could increase or prolong both therapeutic and adverse effects of the concomitant drug. There have been reports of interactions of erythromycin or clarithromycin with drugs not thought to be metabolized by CYP3A, including phenytoin). Products include:
Phenytek Capsules 2380

Pimozide (Concurrent use of erythromycin and/or clarithromycin in patients receiving pimozide has been reported to result in rare cases of cardiovascular adverse events including prolonged QT interval, ventricular tachycardia, ventricular fibrillation, torsade de pointes, and death; co-administration is contraindicated).
No products indexed under this heading.

Pioglitazone Hydrochloride (There have been rare reports of hypoglycemia, some of which have occurred in patients taking oral hypoglycemic agents). Products include:
ActoPlus 3338
Actos 3345
Duetact 3354

Pravastatin Sodium (As with other macrolides, clarithromycin has been reported to increase concentrations of HMG-CoA reductase inhibitors (eg, lovastatin, simvastatin). Rare reports of rhabdomyolysis have been reported in patients taking these drugs concomitantly).
No products indexed under this heading.

Prednisolone (Strong inducers of the cytochrome P450 metabolism system such as efavirenz, nevirapine, rifampicin, rifabutin, and rifapentine may accelerate the metabolism of clarithromycin and thus lower the plasma levels of clarithromycin, while increasing those of 14-OH-clarithromycin, a metabolite that is also microbiologically active. Since the microbiological activities of clarithromycin and 14-OH-clarithromycin are different for different bacteria, the intended therapeutic effect could be impaired during concomitant administration of clarithromycin and enzyme inducers).
No products indexed under this heading.

Prednisolone Acetate (Strong inducers of the cytochrome P450 metabolism system such as efavirenz, nevirapine, rifampicin, rifabutin, and rifapentine may accelerate the metabolism of clarithromycin and thus lower the plasma levels of clarithromycin, while increasing those of 14-OH-clarithromycin, a metabolite that is also microbiologically active. Since the microbiological activities of clarithromycin and 14-OH-clarithromycin are different for different bacteria, the intended therapeutic effect could be impaired during concomitant administration of clarithromycin and enzyme inducers). Products include:
Blephamide .... ⊙ **212**, ⊙ **214**
Pred Forte .... ⊙ **225**
Pred Mild .... ⊙ **230**
Pred-G .... ⊙ **226**, ⊙ **227**

Prednisolone Sodium Phosphate (Strong inducers of the cytochrome P450 metabolism system such as efavirenz, nevirapine, rifampicin, rifabutin, and rifapentine may accelerate the metabolism of clarithromycin and thus lower the plasma levels of clarithromycin, while increasing those of 14-OH-clarithromycin, a metabolite that is also microbiologically active. Since the microbiological activities of clarithromycin and 14-OH-clarithromycin are different for different bacteria, the intended therapeutic effect could be impaired during concomitant administration of clarithromycin and enzyme inducers).
No products indexed under this heading.

Prednisolone Tebutate (Strong inducers of the cytochrome P450 metabolism system such as efavirenz, nevirapine, rifampicin, rifabutin, and rifapentine may accelerate the metabolism of clarithromycin and thus lower the plasma levels of clarithromycin, while increasing those of 14-OH-clarithromycin, a metabolite that is also microbiologically active. Since the microbiological activities of clarithromycin and 14-OH-clarithromycin are different for different bacteria, the intended therapeutic effect could be impaired during concomitant administration of clarithromycin and enzyme inducers).
No products indexed under this heading.

Prednisone (Strong inducers of the cytochrome P450 metabolism system such as efavirenz, nevirapine, rifampicin, rifabutin, and rifapentine may accelerate the metabolism of clarithromycin and thus lower the plasma levels of clarithromycin, while increasing those of 14-OH-clarithromycin, a metabolite that is also microbiologically active. Since the microbiological activities of clarithromycin and 14-OH-clarithromycin are different for different bacteria, the intended therapeutic effect could be impaired during concomitant administration of clarithromycin and enzyme inducers).
No products indexed under this heading.

Prednisone sodium phosphate (Strong inducers of the cytochrome P450 metabolism system such as efavirenz, nevirapine, rifampicin, rifabutin, and rifapentine may accelerate the metabolism of clarithromycin and thus lower the plasma levels of clarithromycin, while increasing those of 14-OH-clarithromycin, a metabolite that is also microbiologically active. Since the microbiological activities of clarithromycin and 14-OH-clarithromycin are different for different bacteria, the intended therapeutic effect could be impaired during concomitant administration of clarithromycin and enzyme inducers).
No products indexed under this heading.

Primidone (Strong inducers of the cytochrome P450 metabolism system such as efavirenz, nevirapine, rifampicin, rifabutin, and rifapentine may accelerate the metabolism of clarithromycin and thus lower the plasma levels of clarithromycin, while increasing those of 14-OH-clarithromycin, a metabolite that is also microbiologically active. Since the microbiological activities of clarithromycin and 14-OH-clarithromycin are different for different bacteria, the intended therapeutic effect could be impaired during concomitant administration of clarithromycin and enzyme inducers).
No products indexed under this heading.

Quinidine (There have been post-marketing reports of torsades de pointes occurring with concurrent use of clarithromycin and quinidine. Electrocardiograms should be monitored for QTc prolongation during co-administration of clarithromycin with quinidine. Serum concentrations of these medications should also be monitored).
No products indexed under this heading.

Quinidine Gluconate (There have been post-marketing reports of torsades de pointes occurring with concurrent use of clarithromycin and quinidine. Electrocardiograms should be monitored for QTc prolongation during co-administration of clarithromycin with quinidine. Serum concentrations of these medications should also be monitored).
No products indexed under this heading.

Quinidine Hydrochloride (There have been post-marketing reports of torsades de pointes occurring with concurrent use of clarithromycin and quinidine. Electrocardiograms should be monitored for QTc prolongation during co-administration of clarithromycin with quinidine. Serum concentrations of these medications should also be monitored).
No products indexed under this heading.

Quinidine Polygalacturonate (There have been post-marketing reports of torsades de pointes occurring with concurrent use of clarithromycin and quinidine. Electrocardiograms should be monitored for QTc prolongation during co-administration of clarithromycin with quinidine. Serum concentrations of these medications should also be monitored).
No products indexed under this heading.

Quinidine Sulfate (There have been post-marketing reports of torsades de pointes occurring with concurrent use of clarithromycin and quinidine. Electrocardiograms should be monitored for QTc prolongation during co-administration of clarithromycin with quinidine. Serum concentrations of these medications should also be monitored).
No products indexed under this heading.

Quinine (Co-administration of erythromycin or clarithromycin and a drug primarily metabolized by CYP3A may be associated with elevation in drug concentrations that could increase or prolong both the therapeutic and adverse effects of the concomitant drug). Products include:
Hyland's Leg Cramps PM with Quinine **3315**

Quinine Sulfate (Co-administration of erythromycin or clarithromycin and a drug primarily metabolized by CYP3A may be associated with elevation in drug concentrations that could increase or prolong both the therapeutic and adverse effects of the concomitant drug).
No products indexed under this heading.

Ranitidine Bismuth Citrate (Co-administration of clarithromycin with ranitidine bismuth citrate resulted in increased plasma ranitidine concentrations (57%), increased plasma bismuth trough concentrations (48%), and increased 14- hydroxy-clarithromycin plasma concentrations (31%). Clarithromycin in combination with ranitidine bismuth citrate therapy is not recommended in patients with creatinine clearance less than 25 mL/min and in patients with history of acute acute porphyria).
No products indexed under this heading.

Repaglinide (There have been rare reports of hypoglycemia, some of which have occurred in patients taking oral hypoglycemic agents).
No products indexed under this heading.

Rifabutin (Co-administration of clarithromycin, known to inhibit CYP3A, and a drug primarily metabolized by CYP3A may be associated with elevations in drug concentrations that could increase or prolong both therapeutic and adverse effects of the concomitant drug. There have been spontaneous or published reports of CYP3A based interactions of erythromycin and/or clarithromycin with rifabutin).
No products indexed under this heading.

Rifampicin (Strong inducers of the cytochrome P450 metabolism system such as rifampicin may accelerate the metabolism of clarithromycin and thus lower the plasma levels of clarithromycin, while increasing those of 14-OH-clarithromycin, a metabolite that is also microbiologically active. Since the microbiological activities of clarithromycin and 14-OH-clarithromycin are different for different bacteria, the intended therapeutic effect could be impaired during concomitant administration of clarithromycin and enzyme inducers).
No products indexed under this heading.

Rifampin (Strong inducers of the cytochrome P450 metabolism system such as efavirenz, nevirapine, rifampicin, rifabutin, and rifapentine may accelerate the metabolism of clarithromycin and thus lower the plasma levels of clarithromycin, while increasing those of 14-OH-clarithromycin, a metabolite that is also microbiologically active. Since the microbiological activities of clarithromycin and 14-OH-clarithromycin are different for different bacteria, the intended therapeutic effect could be impaired during concomitant administration of clarithromycin and enzyme inducers).
No products indexed under this heading.

Rifapentine (Strong inducers of the cytochrome P450 metabolism system such as rifapentine may accelerate the metabolism of clarithromycin and thus lower the plasma levels of clarithromycin, while increasing those of 14-OH-clarithromycin, a metabolite that is also microbiologically active. Since the microbiological activities of clarithromycin and 14-OH-clarithromycin are different for different bacteria, the intended therapeutic effect could be impaired during concomitant administration of clarithromycin and enzyme inducers).
No products indexed under this heading.

Ritonavir (Concomitant administration of clarithromycin and ritonavir (n = 22) resulted in a 77% increase in clarithromycin AUC and a 100% decrease in the AUC of 14-OH clarithromycin. Clarithromycin may be administered without dosage adjustment to patients with normal renal function taking ritonavir. However, for patients with renal impairment, dosage adjustments should be considered). Products include:
Kaletra **458**
Norvir **509**

Rosiglitazone Maleate (There have been rare reports of hypoglycemia, some of which have occurred in patients taking oral hypoglycemic agents). Products include:
Avandamet **1345**
Avandaryl **1356**
Avandia **1366**

Rosuvastatin Calcium (As with other macrolides, clarithromycin has been reported to increase concentrations of HMG-CoA reductase inhibitors (eg, lovastatin, simvastatin). Rare reports of rhabdomyolysis have been reported in patients taking these drugs concomitantly). Products include:
Crestor **736**

Saquinavir (Concomitant administration of clarithromycin (500 mg bid) and saquinavir (soft gelatin capsules, 1200 mg tid) to 12 healthy volunteers resulted in steady-state AUC and C_{max} values of saquinavir which were 177% and 187% higher than those seen with saquinavir alone. Clarithromycin AUC and C_{max} values were approximately 40% higher than those seen with clarithromycin alone).
No products indexed under this heading.

Saquinavir Mesylate (Co-administration of erythromycin or clarithromycin and a drug primarily metabolized by CYP3A may be associated with elevation in drug concentrations that could increase or prolong both the therapeutic and adverse effects of the concomitant drug).
No products indexed under this heading.

Secobarbital Sodium (Strong inducers of the cytochrome P450 metabolism system such as efavirenz, nevirapine, rifampicin, rifabutin, and rifapentine may accelerate the metabolism of clarithromycin and thus lower the plasma levels of clarithromycin, while increasing those of 14-OH-clarithromycin, a metabolite that is also microbiologically active. Since the microbiological activities of clarithromycin and 14-OH-clarithromycin are different for different bacteria, the intended therapeutic effect could be impaired during concomitant administration of clarithromycin and enzyme inducers).
No products indexed under this heading.

(⊙ Described in PDR® for Ophthalmic Medicines)

237 Interactions Index Biaxin

Sertraline Hydrochloride (Co-administration of erythromycin or clarithromycin and a drug primarily metabolized by CYP3A may be associated with elevation in drug concentrations that could increase or prolong both the therapeutic and adverse effects of the concomitant drug).
No products indexed under this heading.

Sildenafil Citrate (Co-administration of clarithromycin with sildenafil would likely result in increased phosphodiesterase inhibitor exposure. Reduction of sildenafil dosage should be considered when sildenafil is co-administered with clarithromycin).
No products indexed under this heading.

Simvastatin (As with other macrolides, clarithromycin has been reported to increase concentrations of HMG-CoA reductase inhibitors (eg, lovastatin, simvastatin). Rare reports of rhabdomyolysis have been reported in patients taking these drugs concomitantly). Products include:
Simcor 524
Vytorin 10/10 .... 2303, 3240
Vytorin 10/20 .... 2303, 3240
Vytorin 10/40 .... 2303, 3240
Vytorin 10/80 .... 2303, 3240
Zocor 2289

Sirolimus (Co-administration of erythromycin or clarithromycin and a drug primarily metabolized by CYP3A may be associated with elevation in drug concentrations that could increase or prolong both the therapeutic and adverse effects of the concomitant drug). Products include:
Rapamune 3579

Sitagliptin Phosphate (There have been rare reports of hypoglycemia, some of which have occurred in patients taking oral hypoglycemic agents). Products include:
Janumet 2188
Januvia 2196

Sulfinpyrazone (Strong inducers of the cytochrome P450 metabolism system such as efavirenz, nevirapine, rifampicin, rifabutin, and rifapentine may accelerate the metabolism of clarithromycin and thus lower the plasma levels of clarithromycin, while increasing those of 14-OH-clarithromycin, a metabolite that is also microbiologically active. Since the microbiological activities of clarithromycin and 14-OH-clarithromycin are different for different bacteria, the intended therapeutic effect could be impaired during concomitant administration of clarithromycin and enzyme inducers).
No products indexed under this heading.

Tacrolimus (Co-administration of clarithromycin, known to inhibit CYP3A, and a drug primarily metabolized by CYP3A may be associated with elevations in drug concentrations that could increase or prolong both therapeutic and adverse effects of the concomitant drug. There have been spontaneous or published reports of CYP3A based interactions of erythromycin and/or clarithromycin with tacrolimus). Products include:
Prograf Capsules 677
Prograf Injection 677
Protopic 685

Tadalafil (Co-administration of clarithromycin with tadalafil would likely result in increased phosphodiesterase inhibitor exposure. Reduction of tadalafil dosage should be considered when tadalafil is co-administered with clarithromycin). Products include:
Adcirca 3461
Cialis 1861

Tamoxifen Citrate (Co-administration of erythromycin or clarithromycin and a drug primarily metabolized by CYP3A may be associated with elevation in drug concentrations that could increase or prolong both the therapeutic and adverse effects of the concomitant drug).
No products indexed under this heading.

Terfenadine (Concomitant administration of clarithromycin with terfenadine is contraindicated. There have been postmarketing reports of drug interactions when clarithromycin and/or erythromycin are co-administered with terfenadine, resulting in cardiac arrhythmias (QT prolongation, ventricular tachycardia, ventricular fibrillation, and torsades de pointes) most likely due to inhibition of metabolism of terfenadine by erythromycin and clarithromycin).
No products indexed under this heading.

Testosterone (Co-administration of erythromycin or clarithromycin and a drug primarily metabolized by CYP3A may be associated with elevation in drug concentrations that could increase or prolong both the therapeutic and adverse effects of the concomitant drug). Products include:
AndroGel 3456

Testosterone Cypionate (Co-administration of erythromycin or clarithromycin and a drug primarily metabolized by CYP3A may be associated with elevation in drug concentrations that could increase or prolong both the therapeutic and adverse effects of the concomitant drug).
No products indexed under this heading.

Testosterone Enanthate (Co-administration of erythromycin or clarithromycin and a drug primarily metabolized by CYP3A may be associated with elevation in drug concentrations that could increase or prolong both the therapeutic and adverse effects of the concomitant drug). Products include:
Delatestryl 1102

Testosterone Propionate (Co-administration of erythromycin or clarithromycin and a drug primarily metabolized by CYP3A may be associated with elevation in drug concentrations that could increase or prolong both the therapeutic and adverse effects of the concomitant drug).
No products indexed under this heading.

Theophyllinate (Strong inducers of the cytochrome P450 metabolism system such as efavirenz, nevirapine, rifampicin, rifabutin, and rifapentine may accelerate the metabolism of clarithromycin and thus lower the plasma levels of clarithromycin, while increasing those of 14-OH-clarithromycin, a metabolite that is also microbiologically active. Since the microbiological activities of clarithromycin and 14-OH-clarithromycin are different for different bacteria, the intended therapeutic effect could be impaired during concomitant administration of clarithromycin and enzyme inducers).
No products indexed under this heading.

Theophylline (Clarithromycin use in patients who are receiving theophylline may be associated with an increase of serum theophylline concentrations. Monitoring of serum theophylline concentrations should be considered for patients receiving high doses of theophylline or with baseline concentrations in the upper therapeutic range).
No products indexed under this heading.

Theophylline Anhydrous (Clarithromycin use in patients who are receiving theophylline may be associated with an increase of serum theophylline concentrations. Monitoring of serum theophylline concentrations should be considered for patients receiving high doses of theophylline or with baseline concentrations in the upper therapeutic range). Products include:
Uniphyl 2817

Theophylline Calcium Salicylate (Clarithromycin use in patients who are receiving theophylline may be associated with an increase of serum theophylline concentrations. Monitoring of serum theophylline concentrations should be considered for patients receiving high doses of theophylline or with baseline concentrations in the upper therapeutic range).
No products indexed under this heading.

Theophylline Dihydroxypropyl (Glyceryl) (Clarithromycin use in patients who are receiving theophylline may be associated with an increase of serum theophylline concentrations. Monitoring of serum theophylline concentrations should be considered for patients receiving high doses of theophylline or with baseline concentrations in the upper therapeutic range).
No products indexed under this heading.

Theophylline Ethylenediamine (Clarithromycin use in patients who are receiving theophylline may be associated with an increase of serum theophylline concentrations. Monitoring of serum theophylline concentrations should be considered for patients receiving high doses of theophylline or with baseline concentrations in the upper therapeutic range).
No products indexed under this heading.

Theophylline Sodium Glycinate (Clarithromycin use in patients who are receiving theophylline may be associated with an increase of serum theophylline concentrations. Monitoring of serum theophylline concentrations should be considered for patients receiving high doses of theophylline or with baseline concentrations in the upper therapeutic range).
No products indexed under this heading.

Tiagabine Hydrochloride (Co-administration of erythromycin or clarithromycin and a drug primarily metabolized by CYP3A may be associated with elevation in drug concentrations that could increase or prolong both the therapeutic and adverse effects of the concomitant drug). Products include:
Gabitril 972

Tobacco (Strong inducers of the cytochrome P450 metabolism system such as efavirenz, nevirapine, rifampicin, rifabutin, and rifapentine may accelerate the metabolism of clarithromycin and thus lower the plasma levels of clarithromycin, while increasing those of 14-OH-clarithromycin, a metabolite that is also microbiologically active. Since the microbiological activities of clarithromycin and 14-OH-clarithromycin are different for different bacteria, the intended therapeutic effect could be impaired during concomitant administration of clarithromycin and enzyme inducers).
No products indexed under this heading.

Tolazamide (There have been rare reports of hypoglycemia, some of which have occurred in patients taking oral hypoglycemic agents).
No products indexed under this heading.

Tolbutamide (There have been rare reports of hypoglycemia, some of which have occurred in patients taking oral hypoglycemic agents).
No products indexed under this heading.

Tolterodine Tartrate (Inhibition of CYP3A results in significantly higher serum concentrations of tolterodine. A reduction in tolterodine dosage may be necessary in the presence of CYP3A inhibitors, such as clarithromycin in the CYP2D6 poor metabolizer population).
No products indexed under this heading.

Trazodone Hydrochloride (Co-administration of erythromycin or clarithromycin and a drug primarily metabolized by CYP3A may be associated with elevation in drug concentrations that could increase or prolong both the therapeutic and adverse effects of the concomitant drug).
No products indexed under this heading.

Triamcinolone (Strong inducers of the cytochrome P450 metabolism system such as efavirenz, nevirapine, rifampicin, rifabutin, and rifapentine may accelerate the metabolism of clarithromycin and thus lower the plasma levels of clarithromycin, while increasing those of 14-OH-clarithromycin, a metabolite that is also microbiologically active. Since the microbiological activities of clarithromycin and 14-OH-clarithromycin are different for different bacteria, the intended therapeutic effect could be impaired during concomitant administration of clarithromycin and enzyme inducers).
No products indexed under this heading.

Triamcinolone Acetonide (Strong inducers of the cytochrome P450 metabolism system such as efavirenz, nevirapine, rifampicin, rifabutin, and rifapentine may accelerate the metabolism of clarithromycin and thus lower the plasma levels of clarithromycin, while increasing those of 14-OH-clarithromycin, a metabolite that is also microbiologically active. Since the microbiological activities of clarithromycin and 14-OH-clarithromycin are different for different bacteria, the intended therapeutic effect could be impaired during concomitant administration of clarithromycin and enzyme inducers). Products include:
Azmacort 408
Nasacort AQ 3019

Triamcinolone Diacetate (Strong inducers of the cytochrome P450 metabolism system such as efavirenz, nevirapine, rifampicin, rifabutin, and rifapentine may accelerate the metabolism of clarithromycin and thus lower the plasma levels of clarithromycin, while increasing those of 14-OH-clarithromycin, a metabolite that is also microbiologically active. Since the microbiological activities of clarithromycin and 14-OH-clarithromycin are different for different bacteria, the intended therapeutic effect could be impaired during concomitant administration of clarithromycin and enzyme inducers).
No products indexed under this heading.

Triamcinolone Hexacetonide (Strong inducers of the cytochrome P450 metabolism system such as efavirenz, nevirapine, rifampicin, rifabutin, and rifapentine may accelerate the metabolism of clarithromycin and thus lower the plasma levels of clarithromycin, while increasing those of 14-OH-clarithromycin, a metabolite that is also microbiologically active. Since the microbiological activities of clarithromycin and 14-OH-clarithromycin are different for different bacteria, the intended therapeutic effect could be impaired during concomitant administration of clarithromycin and enzyme inducers).
No products indexed under this heading.

IMPORTANT NOTE: Always consult each drug listing in the patient's regimen for possible interactions.

Triazolam (Erthromycin has been reported to decrease the clearance of triazolam and thus may increase it pharmacologic effects. There have been post-marketing reports of drug interactions and CNS effects (eg, somnolence, confusion) with the concomitant use of clarithromycin and triazolam).
No products indexed under this heading.

Troglitazone (There have been rare reports of hypoglycemia, some of which have occurred in patients taking oral hypoglycemic agents).
No products indexed under this heading.

Valproate Sodium (Co-administration of clarithromycin, known to inhibit CYP3A, and a drug primarily metabolized by CYP3A may be associated with elevations in drug concentrations that could increase or prolong both therapeutic and adverse effects of the concomitant drug. There have been reports of interactions of erythromycin or clarithromycin with drugs not thought to be metabolized by CYP3A, including valproate).
No products indexed under this heading.

Valproic Acid (Co-administration of clarithromycin, known to inhibit CYP3A, and a drug primarily metabolized by CYP3A may be associated with elevations in drug concentrations that could increase or prolong both therapeutic and adverse effects of the concomitant drug. There have been reports of interactions of erythromycin or clarithromycin with drugs not thought to be metabolized by CYP3A, including valproate).
No products indexed under this heading.

Vardenafil Hydrochloride (Co-administration of clarithromycin with vardenafil would likely result in increased phosphodiesterase inhibitor exposure. Reduction of vardenafil dosage should be considered when vardenafil is co-administered with clarithromycin). Products include:
Levitra 3157

Venlafaxine Hydrochloride (Co-administration of erythromycin or clarithromycin and a drug primarily metabolized by CYP3A may be associated with elevation in drug concentrations that could increase or prolong both the therapeutic and adverse effects of the concomitant drug). Products include:
Effexor XR 3504
Venlafaxine Hydrochloride Tablets ... 2388

Verapamil Hydrochloride (Hypotension, bradyarrhythmias, and lactic acidosis have been observed in patients receiving concurrent verapamil, belonging to the calcium channel blockers drug class). Products include:
Tarka 534

Vinblastine Sulfate (Co-administration of clarithromycin, known to inhibit CYP3A, and a drug primarily metabolized by CYP3A may be associated with elevations in drug concentrations that could increase or prolong both therapeutic and adverse effects of the concomitant drug. There have been spontaneous or published reports of CYP3A based interactions of erythromycin and/or clarithromycin with vinblastine).
No products indexed under this heading.

Vincristine Sulfate (Co-administration of erythromycin or clarithromycin and a drug primarily metabolized by CYP3A may be associated with elevation in drug concentrations that could increase or prolong both the therapeutic and adverse effects of the concomitant drug).
No products indexed under this heading.

Warfarin Sodium (Spontaneous reports in the post-marketing period suggest that concomitant administration of clarithromycin and oral anticoagulants may potentiate the effects of the oral anticoagulants. Prothrombin times should be carefully monitored while patients are receiving clarithromycin and oral anticoagulants simultaneously).
No products indexed under this heading.

Zidovudine (Simultaneous oral administration of clarithromycin and zidovudine to HIV-infected adult patients may result in decreased steady-state zidovudine concentrations. Because clarithromycin appears to interfere with absorption of simultaneously administered oral zidovudine, this interaction can be largely avoided by staggering the doses of clarithromycin and zidovudine).
Products include:
Combivir 1404
Retrovir 1634
Retrovir IV 1640
Trizivir 1688

Food Interactions

Broccoli (Strong inducers of the cytochrome P450 metabolism system such as efavirenz, nevirapine, rifampicin, rifabutin, and rifapentine may accelerate the metabolism of clarithromycin and thus lower the plasma levels of clarithromycin, while increasing those of 14-OH-clarithromycin, a metabolite that is also microbiologically active. Since the microbiological activities of clarithromycin and 14-OH-clarithromycin are different for different bacteria, the intended therapeutic effect could be impaired during concomitant administration of clarithromycin and enzyme inducers).

Brussel Sprouts (Strong inducers of the cytochrome P450 metabolism system such as efavirenz, nevirapine, rifampicin, rifabutin, and rifapentine may accelerate the metabolism of clarithromycin and thus lower the plasma levels of clarithromycin, while increasing those of 14-OH-clarithromycin, a metabolite that is also microbiologically active. Since the microbiological activities of clarithromycin and 14-OH-clarithromycin are different for different bacteria, the intended therapeutic effect could be impaired during concomitant administration of clarithromycin and enzyme inducers).

Charbroiled Food (Strong inducers of the cytochrome P450 metabolism system such as efavirenz, nevirapine, rifampicin, rifabutin, and rifapentine may accelerate the metabolism of clarithromycin and thus lower the plasma levels of clarithromycin, while increasing those of 14-OH-clarithromycin, a metabolite that is also microbiologically active. Since the microbiological activities of clarithromycin and 14-OH-clarithromycin are different for different bacteria, the intended therapeutic effect could be impaired during concomitant administration of clarithromycin and enzyme inducers).

Food, unspecified (For a single 500 mg dose of clarithromycin, food slightly delays the onset of clarithromycin absorption, increasing the peak time from approximately 2 to 2.5 hours. Food also increases the clarithromycin peak plasma concentration by about 24%, but does not affect the extent of clarithromycin bioavailability).

Meal, unspecified (For a single 500 mg dose of clarithromycin, food slightly delays the onset of clarithromycin absorption, increasing the peak time from approximately 2 to 2.5 hours. Food

also increases the clarithromycin peak plasma concentration by about 24%, but does not affect the extent of clarithromycin bioavailability).

BIAXIN GRANULES
(Clarithromycin) 412
See Biaxin Filmtab Tablets

BIAXIN XL FILMTAB TABLETS
(Clarithromycin) 412
See Biaxin Filmtab Tablets

BICILLIN C-R INJECTABLE SUSPENSION
(Penicillin G Benzathine, Penicillin G Procaine)....................................... 1826
May interact with bacteriostatic antibiotics, parenteral tetracyclines, tetracyclines, and certain other agents. Compounds in these categories include:

Chloramphenicol (A bacteriostatic antibiotic may antagonize the bactericidal effect of penicillin, and concurrent use of these drugs should be avoided).
No products indexed under this heading.

Chloramphenicol Palmitate (A bacteriostatic antibiotic may antagonize the bactericidal effect of penicillin, and concurrent use of these drugs should be avoided).
No products indexed under this heading.

Chloramphenicol Sodium Succinate (A bacteriostatic antibiotic may antagonize the bactericidal effect of penicillin, and concurrent use of these drugs should be avoided).
No products indexed under this heading.

Demeclocycline Hydrochloride (A bacteriostatic antibiotic may antagonize the bactericidal effect of penicillin, and concurrent use of these drugs should be avoided).
No products indexed under this heading.

Doxycycline (A bacteriostatic antibiotic may antagonize the bactericidal effect of penicillin, and concurrent use of these drugs should be avoided).
No products indexed under this heading.

Doxycycline Calcium (A bacteriostatic antibiotic may antagonize the bactericidal effect of penicillin, and concurrent use of these drugs should be avoided).
No products indexed under this heading.

Doxycycline Hyclate (A bacteriostatic antibiotic may antagonize the bactericidal effect of penicillin, and concurrent use of these drugs should be avoided).
No products indexed under this heading.

Doxycycline Monohydrate (A bacteriostatic antibiotic may antagonize the bactericidal effect of penicillin, and concurrent use of these drugs should be avoided).
No products indexed under this heading.

Erythromycin (A bacteriostatic antibiotic may antagonize the bactericidal effect of penicillin, and concurrent use of these drugs should be avoided).
No products indexed under this heading.

Erythromycin Estolate (A bacteriostatic antibiotic may antagonize the bactericidal effect of penicillin, and concurrent use of these drugs should be avoided).
No products indexed under this heading.

Erythromycin Ethylsuccinate (A bacteriostatic antibiotic may antagonize the bactericidal effect of penicillin, and concurrent use of these drugs should be avoided). Products include:
E.E.S. 437
EryPed 435

Erythromycin Gluceptate (A bacteriostatic antibiotic may antagonize the bactericidal effect of penicillin, and concurrent use of these drugs should be avoided).
No products indexed under this heading.

Erythromycin Stearate (A bacteriostatic antibiotic may antagonize the bactericidal effect of penicillin, and concurrent use of these drugs should be avoided).
No products indexed under this heading.

Methacycline Hydrochloride (A bacteriostatic antibiotic may antagonize the bactericidal effect of penicillin, and concurrent use of these drugs should be avoided).
No products indexed under this heading.

Minocycline Hydrochloride (A bacteriostatic antibiotic may antagonize the bactericidal effect of penicillin, and concurrent use of these drugs should be avoided). Products include:
Solodyn 2073

Oxytetracycline (A bacteriostatic antibiotic may antagonize the bactericidal effect of penicillin, and concurrent use of these drugs should be avoided).
No products indexed under this heading.

Oxytetracycline Hydrochloride (A bacteriostatic antibiotic may antagonize the bactericidal effect of penicillin, and concurrent use of these drugs should be avoided).
No products indexed under this heading.

Probenecid (Concurrent administration of penicillin and probenecid increases and prolongs serum penicillin levels by decreasing the apparent volume of distribution and slowing the rate of excretion by competitively inhibiting renal tubular secretion of penicillin).
No products indexed under this heading.

Sulfamethizole (A bacteriostatic antibiotic may antagonize the bactericidal effect of penicillin, and concurrent use of these drugs should be avoided).
No products indexed under this heading.

Sulfamethoxazole (A bacteriostatic antibiotic may antagonize the bactericidal effect of penicillin, and concurrent use of these drugs should be avoided).
No products indexed under this heading.

Sulfisoxazole Acetyl (A bacteriostatic antibiotic may antagonize the bactericidal effect of penicillin, and concurrent use of these drugs should be avoided).
No products indexed under this heading.

Tetracycline Hydrochloride (A bacteriostatic antibiotic may antagonize the bactericidal effect of penicillin, and concurrent use of these drugs should be avoided). Products include:
Pylera 793

Tetracycline Phosphate Complex (A bacteriostatic antibiotic may antagonize the bactericidal effect of penicillin, and concurrent use of these drugs should be avoided).
No products indexed under this heading.

BICILLIN L-A INJECTION
(Penicillin G Benzathine, Penicillin G Procaine)....................................... 1828
May interact with bacteriostatic antibiotics, parenteral tetracyclines, tetracyclines, and certain other agents. Compounds in these categories include:

Chloramphenicol (A bacteriostatic antibiotic may antagonize the bactericidal effect of penicillin, and concurrent use of these drugs should be avoided).
No products indexed under this heading.

Chloramphenicol Palmitate (A bacteriostatic antibiotic may antagonize the bactericidal effect of penicillin, and concurrent use of these drugs should be avoided).
No products indexed under this heading.

Chloramphenicol Sodium Succinate (A bacteriostatic antibiotic may antagonize the bactericidal effect of penicillin, and concurrent use of these drugs should be avoided).
No products indexed under this heading.

Demeclocycline Hydrochloride (A bacteriostatic antibiotic may antagonize the bactericidal effect of penicillin, and concurrent use of these drugs should be avoided).
No products indexed under this heading.

Doxycycline (A bacteriostatic antibiotic may antagonize the bactericidal effect of penicillin, and concurrent use of these drugs should be avoided).
No products indexed under this heading.

Doxycycline Calcium (A bacteriostatic antibiotic may antagonize the bactericidal effect of penicillin, and concurrent use of these drugs should be avoided).
No products indexed under this heading.

Doxycycline Hyclate (A bacteriostatic antibiotic may antagonize the bactericidal effect of penicillin, and concurrent use of these drugs should be avoided).
No products indexed under this heading.

Doxycycline Monohydrate (A bacteriostatic antibiotic may antagonize the bactericidal effect of penicillin, and concurrent use of these drugs should be avoided).
No products indexed under this heading.

Erythromycin (A bacteriostatic antibiotic may antagonize the bactericidal effect of penicillin, and concurrent use of these drugs should be avoided).
No products indexed under this heading.

Erythromycin Estolate (A bacteriostatic antibiotic may antagonize the bactericidal effect of penicillin, and concurrent use of these drugs should be avoided).
No products indexed under this heading.

Erythromycin Ethylsuccinate (A bacteriostatic antibiotic may antagonize the bactericidal effect of penicillin, and concurrent use of these drugs should be avoided). Products include:
E.E.S. 437
EryPed 435

Erythromycin Gluceptate (A bacteriostatic antibiotic may antagonize the bactericidal effect of penicillin, and concurrent use of these drugs should be avoided).
No products indexed under this heading.

Erythromycin Stearate (A bacteriostatic antibiotic may antagonize the bactericidal effect of penicillin, and concurrent use of these drugs should be avoided).
No products indexed under this heading.

Methacycline Hydrochloride (A bacteriostatic antibiotic may antagonize the bactericidal effect of penicillin, and concurrent use of these drugs should be avoided).
No products indexed under this heading.

Minocycline Hydrochloride (A bacteriostatic antibiotic may antagonize the bactericidal effect of penicillin, and concurrent use of these drugs should be avoided). Products include:
Solodyn 2073

Oxytetracycline (A bacteriostatic antibiotic may antagonize the bactericidal effect of penicillin, and concurrent use of these drugs should be avoided).
No products indexed under this heading.

Oxytetracycline Hydrochloride (A bacteriostatic antibiotic may antagonize the bactericidal effect of penicillin, and concurrent use of these drugs should be avoided).
No products indexed under this heading.

Probenecid (Concurrent administration of penicillin and probenecid increases and prolongs serum penicillin levels by decreasing the apparent volume of distribution and slowing the rate of excretion by competitively inhibiting renal tubular secretion of penicillin).
No products indexed under this heading.

Sulfamethizole (A bacteriostatic antibiotic may antagonize the bactericidal effect of penicillin, and concurrent use of these drugs should be avoided).
No products indexed under this heading.

Sulfamethoxazole (A bacteriostatic antibiotic may antagonize the bactericidal effect of penicillin, and concurrent use of these drugs should be avoided).
No products indexed under this heading.

Sulfisoxazole Acetyl (A bacteriostatic antibiotic may antagonize the bactericidal effect of penicillin, and concurrent use of these drugs should be avoided).
No products indexed under this heading.

Tetracycline Hydrochloride (A bacteriostatic antibiotic may antagonize the bactericidal effect of penicillin, and concurrent use of these drugs should be avoided). Products include:
Pylera 793

Tetracycline Phosphate Complex (A bacteriostatic antibiotic may antagonize the bactericidal effect of penicillin, and concurrent use of these drugs should be avoided).
No products indexed under this heading.

BIO-C TABLETS
(Bioflavonoids, Calcium Ascorbate, Vitamin C) 3454
None cited in PDR database.

BIOS LIFE C ADVANCED FIBER AND NUTRIENT DRINK
(Dietary Supplement, Fiber, Fiber Supplement, Phytosterols, Policosanol, Vitamins with Minerals) 3454
None cited in PDR database.

BIOS LIFE SLIM ADVANCED FIBER AND NUTRIENT DRINK
(Fiber, Fiber Supplement, Multivitamins with Minerals, Vitamins with Minerals) 3454
None cited in PDR database.

BLEPH-10 OPHTHALMIC SOLUTION 10%
(Sulfacetamide Sodium) .... ☉211
May interact with silver preparations. Compounds in these categories include:

Silver Acetate (Incompatible).
No products indexed under this heading.

Silver Nitrate (Incompatible).
No products indexed under this heading.

Silver Sulfadiazine (Incompatible).
No products indexed under this heading.

BLEPHAMIDE OPHTHALMIC OINTMENT
(Prednisolone Acetate, Sulfacetamide Sodium) .... ☉214
None cited in PDR database.

BLEPHAMIDE OPHTHALMIC SUSPENSION
(Prednisolone Acetate, Sulfacetamide Sodium) .... ☉212
None cited in PDR database.

BONEMATE PLUS ADVANCED BONE HEALTH FORMULA
(Boron, Calcium, Copper, Magnesium, Manganese, Vitamin C, Vitamin D, Vitamin K, Vitamins with Minerals, Zinc)............................. 3454
None cited in PDR database. (None cited in PDR database).

BONIVA INJECTION
(Ibandronate Sodium) 2840
None cited in PDR database.

BONIVA TABLETS
(Ibandronate Sodium) 2844
May interact with antacids, antacids containing aluminum, calcium and magnesium, aspirin-acetylsalicylic acid, calcium preparations, cations, iron containing oral preparations, iron salts, magnesium salts, magnesium-containing antacids, non-steroidal anti-inflammatory agents, and certain other agents. Compounds in these categories include:

Aluminum Acetate (Products containing calcium and other multivalent cations (such as aluminum, magnesium, iron) are likely to interfere with absorption of ibandronate sodium. Ibandronate sodium should be taken at least 60 minutes before any oral medications, including medications containing multivalent cations (such as antacids, supplements or vitamins)).
No products indexed under this heading.

Aluminum Carbonate (Products containing calcium and other multivalent cations (such as aluminum, magnesium, iron) are likely to interfere with absorption of ibandronate sodium. Ibandronate sodium should be taken at least 60 minutes before any oral medications, including medications containing multivalent cations (such as antacids, supplements or vitamins)).
No products indexed under this heading.

Aluminum Chlorhydroxide (Products containing calcium and other multivalent cations (such as aluminum, magnesium, iron) are likely to interfere with absorption of ibandronate sodium. Ibandronate sodium should be taken at least 60 minutes before any oral medications, including medications containing multivalent cations (such as antacids, supplements or vitamins)).
No products indexed under this heading.

Aluminum Chloride (Products containing calcium and other multivalent cations (such as aluminum, magnesium, iron) are likely to interfere with absorption of ibandronate sodium. Ibandronate sodium should be taken at least 60 minutes before any oral medications, including medications containing multivalent cations (such as antacids, supplements or vitamins)).
No products indexed under this heading.

Aluminum Chlorohydrate (Products containing calcium and other multivalent cations (such as aluminum, magnesium, iron) are likely to interfere with absorption of ibandronate sodium. Ibandronate sodium should be taken at least 60 minutes before any oral medications, including medications containing multivalent cations (such as antacids, supplements or vitamins)).
No products indexed under this heading.

Aluminum Glycinate (Products containing calcium and other multivalent cations (such as aluminum, magnesium, iron) are likely to interfere with absorption of ibandronate sodium. Ibandronate sodium should be taken at least 60 minutes before any oral medications, including medications containing multivalent cations (such as antacids, supplements or vitamins)).
No products indexed under this heading.

Aluminum Hydroxide (Products containing calcium and other multivalent cations (such as aluminum, magnesium, iron) are likely to interfere with absorption of ibandronate sodium. Ibandronate sodium should be taken at least 60 minutes before any oral medications, including medications containing multivalent cations (such as antacids, supplements or vitamins)).
No products indexed under this heading.

Aluminum Hydroxide Preparations (Products containing calcium and other multivalent cations (such as aluminum, magnesium, iron) are likely to interfere with absorption of ibandronate sodium. Ibandronate sodium should be taken at least 60 minutes before any oral medications, including medications containing multivalent cations (such as antacids, supplements or vitamins)).
No products indexed under this heading.

Aluminum Sulfate (Products containing calcium and other multivalent cations (such as aluminum, magnesium, iron) are likely to interfere with absorption of ibandronate sodium. Ibandronate sodium should be taken at least 60 minutes before any oral medications, including medications containing multivalent cations (such as antacids, supplements or vitamins)).
No products indexed under this heading.

Aspirin (Since aspirin and bisphosphonates are associated with gastrointestinal irritation, caution should be exercised in the concomitant use of aspirin products with ibandronate sodium). Products include:
Aggrenox 880
Bayer Aspirin 829
Percodan 1124
St. Joseph Aspirin 2045

Aspirin, Enteric Coated (Since aspirin and bisphosphonates are associated with gastrointestinal irritation, caution should be exercised in the concomitant use of aspirin products with ibandronate sodium).
No products indexed under this heading.

Aspirin Buffered (Since aspirin and bisphosphonates are associated with gastrointestinal irritation, caution should be exercised in the concomitant use of aspirin products with ibandronate sodium).
No products indexed under this heading.

Calcium (Products containing calcium and other multivalent cations (such as aluminum, magnesium, iron) are likely to interfere with absorption of ibandronate sodium. Ibandronate sodium should be taken at least 60 minutes before any oral medications, including medications containing multivalent cations (such as antacids, supplements or vitamins)). Products include:
BoneMate Plus 3454
Cardio Basics 3455
Chelated Mineral 3476
CitraNatal 90 DHA Capsules 2332
CitraNatal Harmony 2332

Calcium (Oyster Shell) (Products containing calcium and other multivalent cations (such as aluminum, magnesium, iron) are likely to interfere with absorption of ibandronate sodium. Ibandronate sodium should be taken at least 60 minutes before any oral medications, including medications containing multivalent cations (such as antacids, supplements or vitamins)).
No products indexed under this heading.

IMPORTANT NOTE: Always consult each drug listing in the patient's regimen for possible interactions.

Calcium Acetate (Products containing calcium and other multivalent cations (such as aluminum, magnesium, iron) are likely to interfere with absorption of ibandronate sodium. Ibandronate sodium should be taken at least 60 minutes before any oral medications, including medications containing multivalent cations (such as antacids, supplements or vitamins)).
No products indexed under this heading.

Calcium Ascorbate (Products containing calcium and other multivalent cations (such as aluminum, magnesium, iron) are likely to interfere with absorption of ibandronate sodium. Ibandronate sodium should be taken at least 60 minutes before any oral medications, including medications containing multivalent cations (such as antacids, supplements or vitamins)). Products include:
Bio-C 3454
Procosa II 3476
Proflavanol 90 3476

Calcium Carbaspirin (Products containing calcium and other multivalent cations (such as aluminum, magnesium, iron) are likely to interfere with absorption of ibandronate sodium. Ibandronate sodium should be taken at least 60 minutes before any oral medications, including medications containing multivalent cations (such as antacids, supplements or vitamins)).
No products indexed under this heading.

Calcium Carbonate (Products containing calcium and other multivalent cations (such as aluminum, magnesium, iron) are likely to interfere with absorption of ibandronate sodium. Ibandronate sodium should be taken at least 60 minutes before any oral medications, including medications containing multivalent cations (such as antacids, supplements or vitamins)). Products include:
Chelated Mineral 3476
Pepcid Complete 1822
Extra Strength Rolaids Softchews Vanilla Creme 2045

Calcium Carbonate, Precipitated (Products containing calcium and other multivalent cations (such as aluminum, magnesium, iron) are likely to interfere with absorption of ibandronate sodium. Ibandronate sodium should be taken at least 60 minutes before any oral medications, including medications containing multivalent cations (such as antacids, supplements or vitamins)).
No products indexed under this heading.

Calcium Caseinate (Products containing calcium and other multivalent cations (such as aluminum, magnesium, iron) are likely to interfere with absorption of ibandronate sodium. Ibandronate sodium should be taken at least 60 minutes before any oral medications, including medications containing multivalent cations (such as antacids, supplements or vitamins)).
No products indexed under this heading.

Calcium Chloride (Products containing calcium and other multivalent cations (such as aluminum, magnesium, iron) are likely to interfere with absorption of ibandronate sodium. Ibandronate sodium should be taken at least 60 minutes before any oral medications, including medications containing multivalent cations (such as antacids, supplements or vitamins)).
No products indexed under this heading.

Calcium Citrate (Products containing calcium and other multivalent cations (such as aluminum, magnesium, iron) are likely to interfere with absorption of ibandronate sodium. Ibandronate sodium should be taken at least 60 minutes before any oral medications, including medications containing multivalent cations (such as antacids, supplements or vitamins)). Products include:
Active Calcium 3476
Chelated Mineral 3476
CitraNatal 90 DHA Capsules 2332
CitraNatal Assure 2332
CitraNatal Harmony 2332
CitraNatal Rx 2332

Calcium Disodium Edetate (Products containing calcium and other multivalent cations (such as aluminum, magnesium, iron) are likely to interfere with absorption of ibandronate sodium. Ibandronate sodium should be taken at least 60 minutes before any oral medications, including medications containing multivalent cations (such as antacids, supplements or vitamins)).
No products indexed under this heading.

Calcium Glubionate (Products containing calcium and other multivalent cations (such as aluminum, magnesium, iron) are likely to interfere with absorption of ibandronate sodium. Ibandronate sodium should be taken at least 60 minutes before any oral medications, including medications containing multivalent cations (such as antacids, supplements or vitamins)).
No products indexed under this heading.

Calcium Gluconate (Products containing calcium and other multivalent cations (such as aluminum, magnesium, iron) are likely to interfere with absorption of ibandronate sodium. Ibandronate sodium should be taken at least 60 minutes before any oral medications, including medications containing multivalent cations (such as antacids, supplements or vitamins)).
No products indexed under this heading.

Calcium Glycerophosphate (Products containing calcium and other multivalent cations (such as aluminum, magnesium, iron) are likely to interfere with absorption of ibandronate sodium. Ibandronate sodium should be taken at least 60 minutes before any oral medications, including medications containing multivalent cations (such as antacids, supplements or vitamins)).
No products indexed under this heading.

Calcium Iodide (Products containing calcium and other multivalent cations (such as aluminum, magnesium, iron) are likely to interfere with absorption of ibandronate sodium. Ibandronate sodium should be taken at least 60 minutes before any oral medications, including medications containing multivalent cations (such as antacids, supplements or vitamins)).
No products indexed under this heading.

Calcium Lactate (Products containing calcium and other multivalent cations (such as aluminum, magnesium, iron) are likely to interfere with absorption of ibandronate sodium. Ibandronate sodium should be taken at least 60 minutes before any oral medications, including medications containing multivalent cations (such as antacids, supplements or vitamins)).
No products indexed under this heading.

Calcium Levulinate (Products containing calcium and other multivalent cations (such as aluminum, magnesium, iron) are likely to interfere with absorption of ibandronate sodium. Ibandronate sodium should be taken at least 60 minutes before any oral medications, including medications containing multivalent cations (such as antacids, supplements or vitamins)).
No products indexed under this heading.

Calcium Pantothenate (Products containing calcium and other multivalent cations (such as aluminum, magnesium, iron) are likely to interfere with absorption of ibandronate sodium. Ibandronate sodium should be taken at least 60 minutes before any oral medications, including medications containing multivalent cations (such as antacids, supplements or vitamins)). Products include:
Cardio Basics 3455

Calcium Phosphate (Products containing calcium and other multivalent cations (such as aluminum, magnesium, iron) are likely to interfere with absorption of ibandronate sodium. Ibandronate sodium should be taken at least 60 minutes before any oral medications, including medications containing multivalent cations (such as antacids, supplements or vitamins)).
No products indexed under this heading.

Calcium Phosphate, Dibasic (Products containing calcium and other multivalent cations (such as aluminum, magnesium, iron) are likely to interfere with absorption of ibandronate sodium. Ibandronate sodium should be taken at least 60 minutes before any oral medications, including medications containing multivalent cations (such as antacids, supplements or vitamins)).
No products indexed under this heading.

Calcium Phosphate, Tribasic (Products containing calcium and other multivalent cations (such as aluminum, magnesium, iron) are likely to interfere with absorption of ibandronate sodium. Ibandronate sodium should be taken at least 60 minutes before any oral medications, including medications containing multivalent cations (such as antacids, supplements or vitamins)).
No products indexed under this heading.

Calcium Phosphorus Preparations (Products containing calcium and other multivalent cations (such as aluminum, magnesium, iron) are likely to interfere with absorption of ibandronate sodium. Ibandronate sodium should be taken at least 60 minutes before any oral medications, including medications containing multivalent cations (such as antacids, supplements or vitamins)).
No products indexed under this heading.

Calcium Polycarbophil (Products containing calcium and other multivalent cations (such as aluminum, magnesium, iron) are likely to interfere with absorption of ibandronate sodium. Ibandronate sodium should be taken at least 60 minutes before any oral medications, including medications containing multivalent cations (such as antacids, supplements or vitamins)).
No products indexed under this heading.

Calcium Salts (Products containing calcium and other multivalent cations (such as aluminum, magnesium, iron) are likely to interfere with absorption of ibandronate sodium. Ibandronate sodium should be taken at least 60 minutes before any oral medications, including medications containing multivalent cations (such as antacids, supplements or vitamins)).
No products indexed under this heading.

Calcium Sodium Alginate Fiber (Products containing calcium and other multivalent cations (such as aluminum, magnesium, iron) are likely to interfere with absorption of ibandronate sodium. Ibandronate sodium should be taken at least 60 minutes before any oral medications, including medications containing multivalent cations (such as antacids, supplements or vitamins)).
No products indexed under this heading.

Calcium Undecylenate (Products containing calcium and other multivalent cations (such as aluminum, magnesium, iron) are likely to interfere with absorption of ibandronate sodium. Ibandronate sodium should be taken at least 60 minutes before any oral medications, including medications containing multivalent cations (such as antacids, supplements or vitamins)).
No products indexed under this heading.

Celecoxib (Since NSAIDs and bisphosphonates are associated with gastrointestinal irritation, caution should be exercised in the concomitant use of NSAIDs with ibandronate sodium). Products include:
Celebrex 3272

Diclofenac Epolamine (Since NSAIDs and bisphosphonates are associated with gastrointestinal irritation, caution should be exercised in the concomitant use of NSAIDs with ibandronate sodium). Products include:
Flector 1839

Diclofenac Potassium (Since NSAIDs and bisphosphonates are associated with gastrointestinal irritation, caution should be exercised in the concomitant use of NSAIDs with ibandronate sodium).
No products indexed under this heading.

Diclofenac Sodium (Since NSAIDs and bisphosphonates are associated with gastrointestinal irritation, caution should be exercised in the concomitant use of NSAIDs with ibandronate sodium).
No products indexed under this heading.

Dietary Supplement (Products containing calcium and other multivalent cations (such as aluminum, magnesium, iron) are likely to interfere with absorption of ibandronate sodium. Ibandronate sodium should be taken at least 60 minutes before any oralmedications, including medications containing multivalent cations (such as antacids, supplements or vitamins)). Products include:
Bios Life C 3454
Hyland's Sniffles 'N Sneezes 4 Kids 3315
Immunizen 3455
Mega Antioxidant 3476
Sen-Sei-Ro Liquid 1849
Sen-Sei-Ro Powder 1849

Drugs, Oral, unspecified (Patients should wait at least 60 minutes after dosing before taking any other oral medications).
No products indexed under this heading.

Etodolac (Since NSAIDs and bisphosphonates are associated with gastrointestinal irritation, caution should be exercised in the concomitant use of NSAIDs with ibandronate sodium).
No products indexed under this heading.

Fenoprofen Calcium (Since NSAIDs and bisphosphonates are associated with gastrointestinal irritation, caution should be exercised in the concomitant use of NSAIDs with ibandronate sodium).
No products indexed under this heading.

Ferrous Fumarate (Products containing calcium and other multivalent cations (such as aluminum, magnesium, iron) are likely to interfere with absorption of ibandronate sodium. Ibandronate sodium should be taken at least 60 minutes before any oral medications, including medications containing multivalent cations (such as antacids, supplements or vitamins)). Products include:
PreNexa 3473

Ferrous Gluconate (Products containing calcium and other multivalent cations (such as aluminum, magnesium, iron) are likely to interfere with absorption of ibandronate sodium. Ibandronate

241 **Interactions Index** **Boniva**

sodium should be taken at least 60 minutes before any oral medications, including medications containing multivalent cations (such as antacids, supplements or vitamins)). Products include:

CitraNatal Assure 2332
CitraNatal Rx 2332

Ferrous Sulfate (Products containing calcium and other multivalent cations (such as aluminum, magnesium, iron) are likely to interfere with absorption of ibandronate sodium. Ibandronate sodium should be taken at least 60 minutes before any oral medications, including medications containing multivalent cations (such as antacids, supplements or vitamins)).
No products indexed under this heading.

Flurbiprofen (Since NSAIDs and bisphosphonates are associated with gastrointestinal irritation, caution should be exercised in the concomitant use of NSAIDs with ibandronate sodium).
No products indexed under this heading.

Ibuprofen (Since NSAIDs and bisphosphonates are associated with gastrointestinal irritation, caution should be exercised in the concomitant use of NSAIDs with ibandronate sodium). Products include:

Motrin IB 2043
Children's Motrin 2044
Children's Motrin Non-Staining Dye-Free 2044
Infants' Motrin 2044
Infants' Motrin Dye-Free 2044
Junior Strength Motrin 2044
Vicoprofen 564

Indomethacin (Since NSAIDs and bisphosphonates are associated with gastrointestinal irritation, caution should be exercised in the concomitant use of NSAIDs with ibandronate sodium). Products include:

Indocin 2167

Indomethacin Sodium Trihydrate (Since NSAIDs and bisphosphonates are associated with gastrointestinal irritation, caution should be exercised in the concomitant use of NSAIDs with ibandronate sodium). Products include:

Indocin I.V. 2007

Iron (Products containing calcium and other multivalent cations (such as aluminum, magnesium, iron) are likely to interfere with absorption of ibandronate sodium. Ibandronate sodium should be taken at least 60 minutes before any oral medications, including medications containing multivalent cations (such as antacids, supplements or vitamins)).
No products indexed under this heading.

Iron, Peptonized (Products containing calcium and other multivalent cations (such as aluminum, magnesium, iron) are likely to interfere with absorption of ibandronate sodium. Ibandronate sodium should be taken at least 60 minutes before any oral medications, including medications containing multivalent cations (such as antacids, supplements or vitamins)).
No products indexed under this heading.

Iron & Ammonium Citrate (Products containing calcium and other multivalent cations (such as aluminum, magnesium, iron) are likely to interfere with absorption of ibandronate sodium. Ibandronate sodium should be taken at least 60 minutes before any oral medications, including medications containing multivalent cations (such as antacids, supplements or vitamins)).
No products indexed under this heading.

Iron Cacodylate (Products containing calcium and other multivalent cations (such as aluminum, magnesium, iron) are likely to interfere with absorption of ibandronate sodium. Ibandronate sodium should be taken at least 60 minutes before any oral medications, including medications containing multivalent cations (such as antacids, supplements or vitamins)).
No products indexed under this heading.

Iron Carbonyl (Products containing calcium and other multivalent cations (such as aluminum, magnesium, iron) are likely to interfere with absorption of ibandronate sodium. Ibandronate sodium should be taken at least 60 minutes before any oral medications, including medications containing multivalent cations (such as antacids, supplements or vitamins)). Products include:

CitraNatal 90 DHA Capsules 2332
CitraNatal Assure 2332
CitraNatal Harmony 2332
CitraNatal Rx 2332
Ferralet 2333

Iron Dextran (Products containing calcium and other multivalent cations (such as aluminum, magnesium, iron) are likely to interfere with absorption of ibandronate sodium. Ibandronate sodium should be taken at least 60 minutes before any oral medications, including medications containing multivalent cations (such as antacids, supplements or vitamins)).
No products indexed under this heading.

Iron Polysaccharide Complex (Products containing calcium and other multivalent cations (such as aluminum, magnesium, iron) are likely to interfere with absorption of ibandronate sodium. Ibandronate sodium should be taken at least 60 minutes before any oral medications, including medications containing multivalent cations (such as antacids, supplements or vitamins)).
No products indexed under this heading.

Iron Sucrose (Products containing calcium and other multivalent cations (such as aluminum, magnesium, iron) are likely to interfere with absorption of ibandronate sodium. Ibandronate sodium should be taken at least 60 minutes before any oral medications, including medications containing multivalent cations (such as antacids, supplements or vitamins)).
No products indexed under this heading.

Iron Supplements (Products containing calcium and other multivalent cations (such as aluminum, magnesium, iron) are likely to interfere with absorption of ibandronate sodium. Ibandronate sodium should be taken at least 60 minutes before any oral medications, including medications containing multivalent cations (such as antacids, supplements or vitamins)).
No products indexed under this heading.

Ketoprofen (Since NSAIDs and bisphosphonates are associated with gastrointestinal irritation, caution should be exercised in the concomitant use of NSAIDs with ibandronate sodium).
No products indexed under this heading.

Ketorolac Tromethamine (Since NSAIDs and bisphosphonates are associated with gastrointestinal irritation, caution should be exercised in the concomitant use of NSAIDs with ibandronate sodium). Products include:

Acuvail .... ⊙209

Magaldrate (Products containing calcium and other multivalent cations (such as aluminum, magnesium, iron) are likely to interfere with absorption of ibandronate sodium. Ibandronate sodium should be taken at least 60 minutes before any oral medications, including medications containing multivalent cations (such as antacids, supplements or vitamins)).
No products indexed under this heading.

Magnesium (Products containing calcium and other multivalent cations (such as aluminum, magnesium, iron) are likely to interfere with absorption of ibandronate sodium. Ibandronate sodium should be taken at least 60 minutes before any oral medications, including medications containing multivalent cations (such as antacids, supplements or vitamins)). Products include:

BoneMate Plus 3454
Cardio Basics 3455
Chelated Mineral 3476

Magnesium Aluminum Silicate (Products containing calcium and other multivalent cations (such as aluminum, magnesium, iron) are likely to interfere with absorption of ibandronate sodium. Ibandronate sodium should be taken at least 60 minutes before any oral medications, including medications containing multivalent cations (such as antacids, supplements or vitamins)).
No products indexed under this heading.

Magnesium Carbonate (Products containing calcium and other multivalent cations (such as aluminum, magnesium, iron) are likely to interfere with absorption of ibandronate sodium. Ibandronate sodium should be taken at least 60 minutes before any oral medications, including medications containing multivalent cations (such as antacids, supplements or vitamins)).
No products indexed under this heading.

Magnesium Chloride (Products containing calcium and other multivalent cations (such as aluminum, magnesium, iron) are likely to interfere with absorption of ibandronate sodium. Ibandronate sodium should be taken at least 60 minutes before any oral medications, including medications containing multivalent cations (such as antacids, supplements or vitamins)).
No products indexed under this heading.

Magnesium Citrate (Products containing calcium and other multivalent cations (such as aluminum, magnesium, iron) are likely to interfere with absorption of ibandronate sodium. Ibandronate sodium should be taken at least 60 minutes before any oral medications, including medications containing multivalent cations (such as antacids, supplements or vitamins)). Products include:

Chelated Mineral 3476

Magnesium Gluconate (Products containing calcium and other multivalent cations (such as aluminum, magnesium, iron) are likely to interfere with absorption of ibandronate sodium. Ibandronate sodium should be taken at least 60 minutes before any oral medications, including medications containing multivalent cations (such as antacids, supplements or vitamins)).
No products indexed under this heading.

Magnesium Hydroxide (Products containing calcium and other multivalent cations (such as aluminum, magnesium, iron) are likely to interfere with absorption of ibandronate sodium. Ibandronate sodium should be taken at least 60 minutes before any oral medications, including medications containing multivalent cations (such as antacids, supplements or vitamins)). Products include:

Fleet Pedia-Lax Chewable Tablets 1144
Pepcid Complete 1822

Magnesium Lactate (Products containing calcium and other multivalent cations (such as aluminum, magnesium, iron) are likely to interfere with absorption of ibandronate sodium. Ibandronate sodium should be taken at least 60 minutes before any oral medications, including medications containing multivalent cations (such as antacids, supplements or vitamins)).
No products indexed under this heading.

Magnesium Oxide (Products containing calcium and other multivalent cations (such as aluminum, magnesium, iron) are likely to interfere with absorption of ibandronate sodium. Ibandronate sodium should be taken at least 60 minutes before any oral medications, including medications containing multivalent cations (such as antacids, supplements or vitamins)). Products include:

Beelith 873

Magnesium Salicylate (Products containing calcium and other multivalent cations (such as aluminum, magnesium, iron) are likely to interfere with absorption of ibandronate sodium. Ibandronate sodium should be taken at least 60 minutes before any oral medications, including medications containing multivalent cations (such as antacids, supplements or vitamins)).
No products indexed under this heading.

Magnesium Salicylate Tetrahydrate (Products containing calcium and other multivalent cations (such as aluminum, magnesium, iron) are likely to interfere with absorption of ibandronate sodium. Ibandronate sodium should be taken at least 60 minutes before any oral medications, including medications containing multivalent cations (such as antacids, supplements or vitamins)).
No products indexed under this heading.

Magnesium Salts (Products containing calcium and other multivalent cations (such as aluminum, magnesium, iron) are likely to interfere with absorption of ibandronate sodium. Ibandronate sodium should be taken at least 60 minutes before any oral medications, including medications containing multivalent cations (such as antacids, supplements or vitamins)).
No products indexed under this heading.

Magnesium Sulfate (Products containing calcium and other multivalent cations (such as aluminum, magnesium, iron) are likely to interfere with absorption of ibandronate sodium. Ibandronate sodium should be taken at least 60 minutes before any oral medications, including medications containing multivalent cations (such as antacids, supplements or vitamins)).
No products indexed under this heading.

Magnesium Trisilicate (Products containing calcium and other multivalent cations (such as aluminum, magnesium, iron) are likely to interfere with absorption of ibandronate sodium. Ibandronate sodium should be taken at least 60 minutes before any oral medications, including medications containing multivalent cations (such as antacids, supplements or vitamins)).
No products indexed under this heading.

Meclofenamate Sodium (Since NSAIDs and bisphosphonates are associated with gastrointestinal irritation, caution should be exercised in the concomitant use of NSAIDs with ibandronate sodium).
No products indexed under this heading.

Mefenamic Acid (Since NSAIDs and bisphosphonates are associated with gastrointestinal irritation, caution should be exercised in the concomitant use of NSAIDs with ibandronate sodium).
No products indexed under this heading.

IMPORTANT NOTE: Always consult each drug listing in the patient's regimen for possible interactions.

Meloxicam (Since NSAIDs and bisphosphonates are associated with gastrointestinal irritation, caution should be exercised in the concomitant use of NSAIDs with ibandronate sodium).
No products indexed under this heading.

Multivitamins (Products containing calcium and other multivalent cations (such as aluminum, magnesium, iron) are likely to interfere with absorption of ibandronate sodium. Ibandronate sodium should be taken at least 60 minutes before any oral medications containing multivalent cations (including vitamins)).
No products indexed under this heading.

Multivitamins with Minerals (Products containing calcium and other multivalent cations (such as aluminum, magnesium, iron) are likely to interfere with absorption of ibandronate sodium. Ibandronate sodium should be taken at least 60 minutes before any oral medications containing multivalent cations (including vitamins)). Products include:
Bios Life Slim 3454

Nabumetone (Since NSAIDs and bisphosphonates are associated with gastrointestinal irritation, caution should be exercised in the concomitant use of NSAIDs with ibandronate sodium).
No products indexed under this heading.

Naproxen (Since NSAIDs and bisphosphonates are associated with gastrointestinal irritation, caution should be exercised in the concomitant use of NSAIDs with ibandronate sodium). Products include:
EC-Naprosyn 2850
Naprosyn 2850
Anaprox/Naprosyn 2850

Naproxen Sodium (Since NSAIDs and bisphosphonates are associated with gastrointestinal irritation, caution should be exercised in the concomitant use of NSAIDs with ibandronate sodium). Products include:
Anaprox 2850
Anaprox DS 2850
Treximet 1681

Oral Medications, unspecified (Patients should wait at least 60 minutes after dosing before taking any other oral medications).
No products indexed under this heading.

Oxaprozin (Since NSAIDs and bisphosphonates are associated with gastrointestinal irritation, caution should be exercised in the concomitant use of NSAIDs with ibandronate sodium).
No products indexed under this heading.

Phenylbutazone (Since NSAIDs and bisphosphonates are associated with gastrointestinal irritation, caution should be exercised in the concomitant use of NSAIDs with ibandronate sodium).
No products indexed under this heading.

Piroxicam (Since NSAIDs and bisphosphonates are associated with gastrointestinal irritation, caution should be exercised in the concomitant use of NSAIDs with ibandronate sodium).
No products indexed under this heading.

Polysaccharide Iron Complex (Products containing calcium and other multivalent cations (such as aluminum, magnesium, iron) are likely to interfere with absorption of ibandronate sodium. Ibandronate sodium should be taken at least 60 minutes before any oral medications, including medications containing multivalent cations (such as antacids, supplements or vitamins)). Products include:
Nu-Iron 150 2321

Ranitidine Bismuth Citrate (In healthy volunteers, co-administration with ranitidine resulted in a 20% increased bioavailability of ibandronate, which was not considered to be clinically relevant).
No products indexed under this heading.

Ranitidine Hydrochloride (In healthy volunteers, co-administration with ranitidine resulted in a 20% increased bioavailability of ibandronate, which was not considered to be clinically relevant). Products include:
Zantac 1737
Zantac Injection 1732
Zantac Pharmacy 1735

Rofecoxib (Since NSAIDs and bisphosphonates are associated with gastrointestinal irritation, caution should be exercised in the concomitant use of NSAIDs with ibandronate sodium).
No products indexed under this heading.

Selenium (Products containing calcium and other multivalent cations (such as aluminum, magnesium, iron) are likely to interfere with absorption of ibandronate sodium. Ibandronate sodium should be taken at least 60 minutes before any oral medications, including medications containing multivalent cations (such as antacids, supplements or vitamins)). Products include:
Cardio Basics 3455
Chelated Mineral 3476

Selenium Sulfide (Products containing calcium and other multivalent cations (such as aluminum, magnesium, iron) are likely to interfere with absorption of ibandronate sodium. Ibandronate sodium should be taken at least 60 minutes before any oral medications, including medications containing multivalent cations (such as antacids, supplements or vitamins)).
No products indexed under this heading.

Sodium Bicarbonate (Products containing calcium and other multivalent cations (such as aluminum, magnesium, iron) are likely to interfere with absorption of ibandronate sodium. Ibandronate sodium should be taken at least 60 minutes before any oral medications, including medications containing multivalent cations (such as antacids, supplements or vitamins)).
No products indexed under this heading.

Sulindac (Since NSAIDs and bisphosphonates are associated with gastrointestinal irritation, caution should be exercised in the concomitant use of NSAIDs with ibandronate sodium). Products include:
Clinoril 2098

Tolmetin Sodium (Since NSAIDs and bisphosphonates are associated with gastrointestinal irritation, caution should be exercised in the concomitant use of NSAIDs with ibandronate sodium).
No products indexed under this heading.

Valdecoxib (Since NSAIDs and bisphosphonates are associated with gastrointestinal irritation, caution should be exercised in the concomitant use of NSAIDs with ibandronate sodium).
No products indexed under this heading.

Vitamins, Multiple (Products containing calcium and other multivalent cations (such as aluminum, magnesium, iron) are likely to interfere with absorption of ibandronate sodium. Ibandronate sodium should be taken at least 60 minutes before any oral medications, including medications containing multivalent cations (such as antacids, supplements or vitamins)). Products include:
Mega Antioxidant 3476

Vitamins, Supplement (Products containing calcium and other multivalent cations (such as aluminum, magnesium, iron) are likely to interfere with absorption of ibandronate sodium. Ibandronate sodium should be taken at least 60 minutes before any oral medications, including medications containing multivalent cations (such as antacids, supplements or vitamins)).
No products indexed under this heading.

Zinc (Products containing calcium and other multivalent cations (such as aluminum, magnesium, iron) are likely to interfere with absorption of ibandronate sodium. Ibandronate sodium should be taken at least 60 minutes before any oral medications, including medications containing multivalent cations (such as antacids, supplements or vitamins)). Products include:
BoneMate Plus 3454
Cardio Basics 3455
Chelated Mineral 3476
CitraNatal 90 DHA Capsules 2332
CitraNatal Assure 2332
Heplive 607
Visutein 3456

Zinc Acetate (Products containing calcium and other multivalent cations (such as aluminum, magnesium, iron) are likely to interfere with absorption of ibandronate sodium. Ibandronate sodium should be taken at least 60 minutes before any oral medications, including medications containing multivalent cations (such as antacids, supplements or vitamins)).
No products indexed under this heading.

Zinc Bisglycinate (Products containing calcium and other multivalent cations (such as aluminum, magnesium, iron) are likely to interfere with absorption of ibandronate sodium. Ibandronate sodium should be taken at least 60 minutes before any oral medications, including medications containing multivalent cations (such as antacids, supplements or vitamins)).
No products indexed under this heading.

Zinc Chloride (Products containing calcium and other multivalent cations (such as aluminum, magnesium, iron) are likely to interfere with absorption of ibandronate sodium. Ibandronate sodium should be taken at least 60 minutes before any oral medications, including medications containing multivalent cations (such as antacids, supplements or vitamins)).
No products indexed under this heading.

Zinc Citrate (Products containing calcium and other multivalent cations (such as aluminum, magnesium, iron) are likely to interfere with absorption of ibandronate sodium. Ibandronate sodium should be taken at least 60 minutes before any oral medications, including medications containing multivalent cations (such as antacids, supplements or vitamins)). Products include:
Chelated Mineral 3476

Zinc-Containing Multivitamins (Products containing calcium and other multivalent cations (such as aluminum, magnesium, iron) are likely to interfere with absorption of ibandronate sodium. Ibandronate sodium should be taken at least 60 minutes before any oral medications, including medications containing multivalent cations (such as antacids, supplements or vitamins)).
No products indexed under this heading.

Zinc Gluconate (Products containing calcium and other multivalent cations (such as aluminum, magnesium, iron) are likely to interfere with absorption of ibandronate sodium. Ibandronate sodium should be taken at least 60 minutes before any oral medications, including medications containing multivalent cations (such as antacids, supplements or vitamins)).
No products indexed under this heading.

Zinc Oxide (Products containing calcium and other multivalent cations (such as aluminum, magnesium, iron) are likely to interfere with absorption of ibandronate sodium. Ibandronate sodium should be taken at least 60 minutes before any oral medications, including medications containing multivalent cations (such as antacids, supplements or vitamins)). Products include:

Bausch & Lomb Ocuvite Adult
50+ .... ⊙238
CitraNatal Rx 2332
Vusion Ointment 3335

Zinc Phenosulfonate (Products containing calcium and other multivalent cations (such as aluminum, magnesium, iron) are likely to interfere with absorption of ibandronate sodium. Ibandronate sodium should be taken at least 60 minutes before any oral medications, including medications containing multivalent cations (such as antacids, supplements or vitamins)).
No products indexed under this heading.

Zinc Sulfate (Products containing calcium and other multivalent cations (such as aluminum, magnesium, iron) are likely to interfere with absorption of ibandronate sodium. Ibandronate sodium should be taken at least 60 minutes before any oral medications, including medications containing multivalent cations (such as antacids, supplements or vitamins)). Products include:
Heplive 607
Zinc-220 606

Food Interactions

Dairy products (Milk is likely to interfere with absorption of ibandronate. Ibandronate should be taken at least 60 minutes before the first food or drink (other than water) of the day).

Food, unspecified (The oral bioavailability of ibandronate is reduced by about 90% when ibandronate is administered concomitantly with a standard breakfast in comparison with bioavailability observed in fasted subjects. There is no meaningful reduction in bioavailability when ibandronate is taken at least 60 minutes before a meal. However, both bioavailability and the effect on bone mineral density (BMD) are reduced when food or beverages are taken less than 60 minutes following an ibandronate dose).

Iron Amino Acid Chelate (Products containing calcium and other multivalent cations (such as aluminum, magnesium, iron) are likely to interfere with absorption of ibandronate sodium. Ibandronate sodium should be taken at least 60 minutes before any oral medications, including medications containing multivalent cations (such as antacids, supplements or vitamins)).

Meal, unspecified (The oral bioavailability of ibandronate is reduced by about 90% when ibandronate is administered concomitantly with a standard breakfast in comparison with bioavailability observed in fasted subjects. There is no meaningful reduction in bioavailability when ibandronate is taken at least 60 minutes before a meal. However, both bioavailability and the effect on bone mineral density (BMD) are reduced when food or beverages are taken less than 60 minutes following an ibandronate dose).

BOOSTRIX VACCINE
(Diphtheria & Tetanus Toxoids and Acellular Pertussis Vaccine Adsorbed) 1395
May interact with alkylating agents, antimetabolites, corticosteroids, cytotoxic drugs, immunosuppressive agents, and certain other agents. Compounds in these categories include:

Alclometasone Dipropionate (Immunosuppressive therapies, including corticosteroids (used in greater than physiological doses), may reduce the immune response to Boostrix).
No products indexed under this heading.

243 **Interactions Index** **Boostrix**

Azathioprine (Immunosuppressive therapies may reduce the immune response to Boostrix).
No products indexed under this heading.

Basiliximab (Immunosuppressive therapies may reduce the immune response to Boostrix). Products include:
Simulect **2524**

Beclomethasone Dipropionate (Immunosuppressive therapies, including corticosteroids (used in greater than physiological doses), may reduce the immune response to Boostrix).
Products include:
Qvar **3398**

Beclomethasone Dipropionate Monohydrate (Immunosuppressive therapies, including corticosteroids (used in greater than physiological doses), may reduce the immune response to Boostrix). Products include:
Beconase AQ **1386**

Betamethasone (Immunosuppressive therapies, including corticosteroids (used in greater than physiological doses), may reduce the immune response to Boostrix).
No products indexed under this heading.

Betamethasone Acetate (Immunosuppressive therapies, including corticosteroids (used in greater than physiological doses), may reduce the immune response to Boostrix).
No products indexed under this heading.

Betamethasone Benzoate (Immunosuppressive therapies, including corticosteroids (used in greater than physiological doses), may reduce the immune response to Boostrix).
No products indexed under this heading.

Betamethasone Dipropionate (Immunosuppressive therapies, including corticosteroids (used in greater than physiological doses), may reduce the immune response to Boostrix).
Products include:
Diprolene Lotion 0.05% **3108**
Diprolene Ointment 0.05% **3109**
Diprolene AF Cream 0.05% **3107**
Lotrisone **3163**

Betamethasone Sodium Phosphate (Immunosuppressive therapies, including corticosteroids (used in greater than physiological doses), may reduce the immune response to Boostrix).
No products indexed under this heading.

Betamethasone Valerate (Immunosuppressive therapies, including corticosteroids (used in greater than physiological doses), may reduce the immune response to Boostrix). Products include:
Luxíq **3321**

Bleomycin Sulfate (Immunosuppressive therapies, including cytotoxic drugs, may reduce the immune response to Boostrix).
No products indexed under this heading.

Budesonide (Immunosuppressive therapies, including corticosteroids (used in greater than physiological doses), may reduce the immune response to Boostrix). Products include:
Pulmicort Flexhaler **714**
Symbicort 80/4.5 .... **720**
Symbicort 160/4.5 .... **720**

Busulfan (Immunosuppressive therapies, including alkylating agents, may reduce the immune response to Boostrix). Products include:
Myleran **1581**

Capecitabine (Immunosuppressive therapies, including antimetabolites, may reduce the immune response to Boostrix). Products include:
Xeloda **2882**

Carmustine (BCNU) (Immunosuppressive therapies, including alkylating agents, may reduce the immune response to Boostrix).
No products indexed under this heading.

Chlorambucil (Immunosuppressive therapies, including alkylating agents, may reduce the immune response to Boostrix). Products include:
Leukeran **1557**

Ciclesonide (Immunosuppressive therapies, including corticosteroids (used in greater than physiological doses), may reduce the immune response to Boostrix).
No products indexed under this heading.

Cladribine (Immunosuppressive therapies, including antimetabolites, may reduce the immune response to Boostrix). Products include:
Leustatin **946**

Cortisone Acetate (Immunosuppressive therapies, including corticosteroids (used in greater than physiological doses), may reduce the immune response to Boostrix).
No products indexed under this heading.

Cyclophosphamide (Immunosuppressive therapies, including alkylating agents, may reduce the immune response to Boostrix).
No products indexed under this heading.

Cyclosporine (Immunosuppressive therapies may reduce the immune response to Boostrix). Products include:
Gengraf **440**
Neoral Oral Solution **2496**
Neoral Capsules **2496**
Restasis **605**

Cytarabine (Immunosuppressive therapies, including antimetabolites, may reduce the immune response to Boostrix).
No products indexed under this heading.

Dacarbazine (Immunosuppressive therapies, including alkylating agents, may reduce the immune response to Boostrix).
No products indexed under this heading.

Daunorubicin Hydrochloride (Immunosuppressive therapies, including cytotoxic drugs, may reduce the immune response to Boostrix).
No products indexed under this heading.

Desoximetasone (Immunosuppressive therapies, including corticosteroids (used in greater than physiological doses), may reduce the immune response to Boostrix).
No products indexed under this heading.

Dexamethasone (Immunosuppressive therapies, including corticosteroids (used in greater than physiological doses), may reduce the immune response to Boostrix). Products include:
Ciprodex **583**
Ozurdex .... ⊙ **223**
Tobramycin and Dexamethasone Ophthalmic Suspension .... ⊙ **251**

Dexamethasone Acetate (Immunosuppressive therapies, including corticosteroids (used in greater than physiological doses), may reduce the immune response to Boostrix).
No products indexed under this heading.

Dexamethasone Phosphate (Immunosuppressive therapies, including corticosteroids (used in greater than physiological doses), may reduce the immune response to Boostrix).
No products indexed under this heading.

Dexamethasone Sodium (Immunosuppressive therapies, including corticosteroids (used in greater than physiological doses), may reduce the immune response to Boostrix).
No products indexed under this heading.

Dexamethasone Sodium Phosphate (Immunosuppressive therapies, including corticosteroids (used in greater than physiological doses), may reduce the immune response to Boostrix).
No products indexed under this heading.

Dexamethasone Sodium Phosphate Injection (Immunosuppressive therapies, including corticosteroids (used in greater than physiological doses), may reduce the immune response to Boostrix).
No products indexed under this heading.

Diflorasone Diacetate (Immunosuppressive therapies, including corticosteroids (used in greater than physiological doses), may reduce the immune response to Boostrix).
No products indexed under this heading.

Doxorubicin Hydrochloride (Immunosuppressive therapies, including cytotoxic drugs, may reduce the immune response to Boostrix).
No products indexed under this heading.

Epirubicin Hydrochloride (Immunosuppressive therapies, including cytotoxic drugs, may reduce the immune response to Boostrix).
No products indexed under this heading.

Floxuridine (Immunosuppressive therapies, including antimetabolites, may reduce the immune response to Boostrix).
No products indexed under this heading.

Fludarabine Phosphate (Immunosuppressive therapies, including antimetabolites, may reduce the immune response to Boostrix). Products include:
Oforta **3023**

Fludrocortisone Acetate (Immunosuppressive therapies, including corticosteroids (used in greater than physiological doses), may reduce the immune response to Boostrix).
No products indexed under this heading.

Flumethasone Pivalate (Immunosuppressive therapies, including corticosteroids (used in greater than physiological doses), may reduce the immune response to Boostrix).
No products indexed under this heading.

Flunisolide Hemihydrate (Immunosuppressive therapies, including corticosteroids (used in greater than physiological doses), may reduce the immune response to Boostrix).
No products indexed under this heading.

Fluorouracil (Immunosuppressive therapies, including antimetabolites, may reduce the immune response to Boostrix). Products include:
Carac **2966**

Fluticasone Furoate (Immunosuppressive therapies, including corticosteroids (used in greater than physiological doses), may reduce the immune response to Boostrix). Products include:
Veramyst **1713**

Fluticasone Propionate (Immunosuppressive therapies, including corticosteroids (used in greater than physiological doses), may reduce the immune response to Boostrix). Products include:
Advair 100/50 .... **1275**
Advair 250/50 .... **1275**
Advair 500/50 .... **1275**
Advair HFA 45/21 .... **1288**
Advair HFA 115/21 .... **1288**
Advair HFA 230/21 .... **1288**
Flonase **1459**
Flovent Diskus **1463**
Flovent HFA **1470**

Gemcitabine Hydrochloride (Immunosuppressive therapies, including antimetabolites, may reduce the immune response to Boostrix). Products include:
Gemzar **1900**

Hydrocortisone (Immunosuppressive therapies, including corticosteroids (used in greater than physiological doses), may reduce the immune response to Boostrix).
No products indexed under this heading.

Hydrocortisone (Alcohol) (Immunosuppressive therapies, including corticosteroids (used in greater than physiological doses), may reduce the immune response to Boostrix).
No products indexed under this heading.

Hydrocortisone Acetate (Immunosuppressive therapies, including corticosteroids (used in greater than physiological doses), may reduce the immune response to Boostrix).
No products indexed under this heading.

Hydrocortisone Butyrate (Immunosuppressive therapies, including corticosteroids (used in greater than physiological doses), may reduce the immune response to Boostrix).
No products indexed under this heading.

Hydrocortisone Cypionate (Immunosuppressive therapies, including corticosteroids (used in greater than physiological doses), may reduce the immune response to Boostrix).
No products indexed under this heading.

Hydrocortisone Hemisuccinate (Immunosuppressive therapies, including corticosteroids (used in greater than physiological doses), may reduce the immune response to Boostrix).
No products indexed under this heading.

Hydrocortisone Probutate (Immunosuppressive therapies, including corticosteroids (used in greater than physiological doses), may reduce the immune response to Boostrix).
No products indexed under this heading.

Hydrocortisone Sodium Phosphate (Immunosuppressive therapies, including corticosteroids (used in greater than physiological doses), may reduce the immune response to Boostrix).
No products indexed under this heading.

Hydrocortisone Sodium Succinate (Immunosuppressive therapies, including corticosteroids (used in greater than physiological doses), may reduce the immune response to Boostrix).
No products indexed under this heading.

Hydrocortisone Valerate (Immunosuppressive therapies, including corticosteroids (used in greater than physiological doses), may reduce the immune response to Boostrix).
No products indexed under this heading.

Hydroxyurea (Immunosuppressive therapies, including cytotoxic drugs, may reduce the immune response to Boostrix).
No products indexed under this heading.

Influenza Virus Vaccine (Boostrix was administered concomitantly with influenza virus vaccine in a clinical study. Lower geometric mean antibody concentrations (GMCs) for antibodies to the pertussis antigens filamentous hemagglutinin (FHA) and pertactin were observed when Boostrix was administered concomitantly with influenza virus vaccine as compared with Boostrix alone). Products include:
Fluarix **1476**
Flulaval **1479**

Lomustine (CCNU) (Immunosuppressive therapies, including alkylating agents, may reduce the immune response to Boostrix).
No products indexed under this heading.

Mechlorethamine Hydrochloride (Immunosuppressive therapies, including alkylating agents, may reduce the immune response to Boostrix).
Products include:

IMPORTANT NOTE: Always consult each drug listing in the patient's regimen for possible interactions.

(⊙ Described in PDR® for Ophthalmic Medicines)

Pancuronium Bromide (Co-administration of onabotulinumtoxinA and aminoglycosides or other agents interfering with neuromuscular transmission (eg, curare-like compounds) should only be performed with caution as the effect of the toxin may be potentiated).
No products indexed under this heading.

Pipecuronium Bromide (Co-administration of onabotulinumtoxinA and aminoglycosides or other agents interfering with neuromuscular transmission (eg, curare-like compounds) should only be performed with caution as the effect of the toxin may be potentiated).
No products indexed under this heading.

Rapacuronium Bromide (Co-administration of onabotulinumtoxinA and aminoglycosides or other agents interfering with neuromuscular transmission (eg, curare-like compounds) should only be performed with caution as the effect of the toxin may be potentiated).
No products indexed under this heading.

Rocuronium Bromide (Co-administration of onabotulinumtoxinA and aminoglycosides or other agents interfering with neuromuscular transmission (eg, curare-like compounds) should only be performed with caution as the effect of the toxin may be potentiated). Products include:
Zemuron 3249

Streptomycin Sulfate (Co-administration of onabotulinumtoxinA and aminoglycosides or other agents interfering with neuromuscular transmission (eg, curare-like compounds) should only be performed with caution as the effect of the toxin may be potentiated).
No products indexed under this heading.

Succinylcholine Chloride (Co-administration of onabotulinumtoxinA and aminoglycosides or other agents interfering with neuromuscular transmission (eg, curare-like compounds) should only be performed with caution as the effect of the toxin may be potentiated).
No products indexed under this heading.

Tobramycin (Co-administration of onabotulinumtoxinA and aminoglycosides or other agents interfering with neuromuscular transmission (eg, curare-like compounds) should only be performed with caution as the effect of the toxin may be potentiated). Products include:
Tobi Nebulizer 2546
Tobramycin and Dexamethasone Ophthalmic Suspension .... ⊙251
Zylet .... ⊙252

Tobramycin Sulfate (Co-administration of onabotulinumtoxinA and aminoglycosides or other agents interfering with neuromuscular transmission (eg, curare-like compounds) should only be performed with caution as the effect of the toxin may be potentiated).
No products indexed under this heading.

Tubocurarine Chloride (Co-administration of onabotulinumtoxinA and aminoglycosides or other agents interfering with neuromuscular transmission (eg, curare-like compounds) should only be performed with caution as the effect of the toxin may be potentiated).
No products indexed under this heading.

Vecuronium Bromide (Co-administration of onabotulinumtoxinA and aminoglycosides or other agents interfering with neuromuscular transmission (eg, curare-like compounds) should only be performed with caution as the effect of the toxin may be potentiated).
No products indexed under this heading.

BREVOXYL-4 CREAMY WASH
(Benzoyl Peroxide) 3317
None cited in PDR database.

BREVOXYL-4 GEL
(Benzoyl Peroxide) 3316
None cited in PDR database.

BREVOXYL-8 CREAMY WASH
(Benzoyl Peroxide) 3317
None cited in PDR database.

BREVOXYL-8 GEL
(Benzoyl Peroxide) 3316
None cited in PDR database.

BYETTA INJECTION
(Exenatide) 648
May interact with bacteriostatic antibiotics, beta-lactams antibiotics, fluoroquinolone antibiotics, macrolide antibiotics, oral contraceptives, penicillins, tetracyclines, and certain other agents. Compounds in these categories include:

Acetaminophen (When 1000 mg acetaminophen exlixir was given with 10 mcg of exenatide (0 hours) and 1 hour, 2 hours, and 4 hours after exenatide, acetaminophen AUCs were decreased by 21%, 23%, 24%, and 14%, respectively; C_{max} was decreased by 37%, 56%, 54%, and 41%, respectively; T_{max} was increased from 0.6 hour in the control period to 0.9 hour, 4.2 hours, 3.3 hours, and 1.6 hours, respectively. Acetaminohpen AUC, C_{max} and T_{max} were not significantly changed when acetaminophen was given 1 hour before exenatide). Products include:
Percocet 1121
Tylenol 2049
Tylenol 8 Hour 2049
Extra Strength Tylenol Caplets, Cool Caplets, and EZ Tabs 2049
Extra Strength Tylenol Adult Rapid Blast Liquid 2049
Extra Strength Tylenol Rapid Release 2049
Tylenol with Codeine 2691
Tylenol Arthritis Pain Extended Release Geltabs/Caplets 2049
Children's Tylenol Suspension Liquid 2048
Chlidren's Tylenol Meltaways 2048
Tylenol, Infants' Drops 2048
Junior Tylenol 2048
Vicodin 560
Vicodin ES 561
Vicodin HP 563
Zydone 1138

Alatrofloxacin Mesylate (The effect of exenatide to slow gastric emptying may reduce the extent and rate of absorption of orally administered drugs. Exenatide should be used with caution in patients receiving oral medications that require rapid gastrointestinal absorption. For oral medications that are dependent on threshold concentrations for efficacy, such as antibiotics, patients should be advised to take those drugs at least 1 hr before exenatide injection. If such drugs are to be administered with food, patients should be advised to take them with a meal or snack when exenatide is not administered).
No products indexed under this heading.

Amoxicillin (The effect of exenatide to slow gastric emptying may reduce the extent and rate of absorption of orally administered drugs. Exenatide should be used with caution in patients receiving oral medications that require rapid gastrointestinal absorption. For oral medications that are dependent on threshold concentrations for efficacy, such as antibiotics, patients should be advised to take those drugs at least 1 hr before exenatide injection. If such drugs are to be administered with food, patients should be advised to take them with a meal or snack when exenatide is not administered). Products include:
Amoxil Capsules 1311
Amoxil Chewable Tablets 1311
Amoxil 1311
Amoxil Powder 1311
Augmentin 1331
Augmentin Tablets 1335
Augmentin ES-600 1338
Augmentin XR 1342
Moxatag 2321

Amoxicillin Trihydrate (The effect of exenatide to slow gastric emptying may reduce the extent and rate of absorption of orally administered drugs. Exenatide should be used with caution in patients receiving oral medications that require rapid gastrointestinal absorption. For oral medications that are dependent on threshold concentrations for efficacy, such as antibiotics, patients should be advised to take those drugs at least 1 hr before exenatide injection. If such drugs are to be administered with food, patients should be advised to take them with a meal or snack when exenatide is not administered).
No products indexed under this heading.

Ampicillin (The effect of exenatide to slow gastric emptying may reduce the extent and rate of absorption of orally administered drugs. Exenatide should be used with caution in patients receiving oral medications that require rapid gastrointestinal absorption. For oral medications that are dependent on threshold concentrations for efficacy, such as antibiotics, patients should be advised to take those drugs at least 1 hr before exenatide injection. If such drugs are to be administered with food, patients should be advised to take them with a meal or snack when exenatide is not administered).
No products indexed under this heading.

Ampicillin Sodium (The effect of exenatide to slow gastric emptying may reduce the extent and rate of absorption of orally administered drugs. Exenatide should be used with caution in patients receiving oral medications that require rapid gastrointestinal absorption. For oral medications that are dependent on threshold concentrations for efficacy, such as antibiotics, patients should be advised to take those drugs at least 1 hr before exenatide injection. If such drugs are to be administered with food, patients should be advised to take them with a meal or snack when exenatide is not administered).
No products indexed under this heading.

Ampicillin Trihydrate (The effect of exenatide to slow gastric emptying may reduce the extent and rate of absorption of orally administered drugs. Exenatide should be used with caution in patients receiving oral medications that require rapid gastrointestinal absorption. For oral medications that are dependent on threshold concentrations for efficacy, such as antibiotics, patients should be advised to take those drugs at least 1 hr before exenatide injection. If such drugs are to be administered with food, patients should be advised to take them with a meal or snack when exenatide is not administered).
No products indexed under this heading.

Azithromycin Dihydrate (The effect of exenatide to slow gastric emptying may reduce the extent and rate of absorption of orally administered drugs. Exenatide should be used with caution in patients receiving oral medications that require rapid gastrointestinal absorption. For oral medications that are dependent on threshold concentrations for efficacy, such as antibiotics, patients should be advised to take those drugs at least 1 hr before exenatide injection. If such drugs are to be administered with food, patients should be advised to take them with a meal or snack when exenatide is not administered).
No products indexed under this heading.

Azlocillin Sodium (The effect of exenatide to slow gastric emptying may reduce the extent and rate of absorption of orally administered drugs. Exenatide should be used with caution in patients receiving oral medications that require rapid gastrointestinal absorption. For oral medications that are dependent on threshold concentrations for efficacy, such as antibiotics, patients should be advised to take those drugs at least 1 hr before exenatide injection. If such drugs are to be administered with food, patients should be advised to take them with a meal or snack when exenatide is not administered).
No products indexed under this heading.

Aztreonam (The effect of exenatide to slow gastric emptying may reduce the extent and rate of absorption of orally administered drugs. Exenatide should be used with caution in patients receiving oral medications that require rapid gastrointestinal absorption. For oral medications that are dependent on threshold concentrations for efficacy, such as antibiotics, patients should be advised to take those drugs at least 1 hr before exenatide injection. If such drugs are to be administered with food, patients should be advised to take them with a meal or snack when exenatide is not administered).
No products indexed under this heading.

Bacampicillin Hydrochloride (The effect of exenatide to slow gastric emptying may reduce the extent and rate of absorption of orally administered drugs. Exenatide should be used with caution in patients receiving oral medications that require rapid gastrointestinal absorption. For oral medications that are dependent on threshold concentrations for efficacy, such as antibiotics, patients should be advised to take those drugs at least 1 hr before exenatide injection. If such drugs are to be administered with food, patients should be advised to take them with a meal or snack when exenatide is not administered).
No products indexed under this heading.

Carbenicillin Disodium (The effect of exenatide to slow gastric emptying may reduce the extent and rate of absorption of orally administered drugs. Exenatide should be used with caution in patients receiving oral medications that require rapid gastrointestinal absorption. For oral medications that are dependent on threshold concentrations for efficacy, such as antibiotics, patients should be advised to take those drugs at least 1 hr before exenatide injection. If such drugs are to be administered with food, patients should be advised to take them with a meal or snack when exenatide is not administered).
No products indexed under this heading.

Carbenicillin Indanyl Sodium (The effect of exenatide to slow gastric emptying may reduce the extent and rate of absorption of orally administered drugs. Exenatide should be used with caution in patients receiving oral medications that require rapid gastrointestinal absorption. For oral medications that are dependent on threshold concentrations for efficacy, such as antibiotics, patients should be advised to take those drugs at least 1 hr before exenatide injection. If such drugs are to be administered with food, patients should be advised to take them with a meal or snack when exenatide is not administered).
No products indexed under this heading.

IMPORTANT NOTE: Always consult each drug listing in the patient's regimen for possible interactions.

Cefaclor (The effect of exenatide to slow gastric emptying may reduce the extent and rate of absorption of orally administered drugs. Exenatide should be used with caution in patients receiving oral medications that require rapid gastrointestinal absorption. For oral medications that are dependent on threshold concentrations for efficacy, such as antibiotics, patients should be advised to take those drugs at least 1 hr before exenatide injection. If such drugs are to be administered with food, patients should be advised to take them with a meal or snack when exenatide is not administered).
No products indexed under this heading.

Cefadroxil (The effect of exenatide to slow gastric emptying may reduce the extent and rate of absorption of orally administered drugs. Exenatide should be used with caution in patients receiving oral medications that require rapid gastrointestinal absorption. For oral medications that are dependent on threshold concentrations for efficacy, such as antibiotics, patients should be advised to take those drugs at least 1 hr before exenatide injection. If such drugs are to be administered with food, patients should be advised to take them with a meal or snack when exenatide is not administered).
No products indexed under this heading.

Cefamandole Nafate (The effect of exenatide to slow gastric emptying may reduce the extent and rate of absorption of orally administered drugs. Exenatide should be used with caution in patients receiving oral medications that require rapid gastrointestinal absorption. For oral medications that are dependent on threshold concentrations for efficacy, such as antibiotics, patients should be advised to take those drugs at least 1 hr before exenatide injection. If such drugs are to be administered with food, patients should be advised to take them with a meal or snack when exenatide is not administered).
No products indexed under this heading.

Cefazolin Sodium (The effect of exenatide to slow gastric emptying may reduce the extent and rate of absorption of orally administered drugs. Exenatide should be used with caution in patients receiving oral medications that require rapid gastrointestinal absorption. For oral medications that are dependent on threshold concentrations for efficacy, such as antibiotics, patients should be advised to take those drugs at least 1 hr before exenatide injection. If such drugs are to be administered with food, patients should be advised to take them with a meal or snack when exenatide is not administered).
No products indexed under this heading.

Cefixime (The effect of exenatide to slow gastric emptying may reduce the extent and rate of absorption of orally administered drugs. Exenatide should be used with caution in patients receiving oral medications that require rapid gastrointestinal absorption. For oral medications that are dependent on threshold concentrations for efficacy, such as antibiotics, patients should be advised to take those drugs at least 1 hr before exenatide injection. If such drugs are to be administered with food, patients should be advised to take them with a meal or snack when exenatide is not administered). Products include:
Suprax for Oral Suspension 2038
Suprax Tablets 2038

Cefmetazole Sodium (The effect of exenatide to slow gastric emptying may reduce the extent and rate of absorption of orally administered drugs. Exenatide should be used with caution

in patients receiving oral medications that require rapid gastrointestinal absorption. For oral medications that are dependent on threshold concentrations for efficacy, such as antibiotics, patients should be advised to take those drugs at least 1 hr before exenatide injection. If such drugs are to be administered with food, patients should be advised to take them with a meal or snack when exenatide is not administered).
No products indexed under this heading.

Cefonicid Sodium (The effect of exenatide to slow gastric emptying may reduce the extent and rate of absorption of orally administered drugs. Exenatide should be used with caution in patients receiving oral medications that require rapid gastrointestinal absorption. For oral medications that are dependent on threshold concentrations for efficacy, such as antibiotics, patients should be advised to take those drugs at least 1 hr before exenatide injection. If such drugs are to be administered with food, patients should be advised to take them with a meal or snack when exenatide is not administered).
No products indexed under this heading.

Cefoperazone Sodium (The effect of exenatide to slow gastric emptying may reduce the extent and rate of absorption of orally administered drugs. Exenatide should be used with caution in patients receiving oral medications that require rapid gastrointestinal absorption. For oral medications that are dependent on threshold concentrations for efficacy, such as antibiotics, patients should be advised to take those drugs at least 1 hr before exenatide injection. If such drugs are to be administered with food, patients should be advised to take them with a meal or snack when exenatide is not administered).
No products indexed under this heading.

Ceforanide (The effect of exenatide to slow gastric emptying may reduce the extent and rate of absorption of orally administered drugs. Exenatide should be used with caution in patients receiving oral medications that require rapid gastrointestinal absorption. For oral medications that are dependent on threshold concentrations for efficacy, such as antibiotics, patients should be advised to take those drugs at least 1 hr before exenatide injection. If such drugs are to be administered with food, patients should be advised to take them with a meal or snack when exenatide is not administered).
No products indexed under this heading.

Cefotaxime Sodium (The effect of exenatide to slow gastric emptying may reduce the extent and rate of absorption of orally administered drugs. Exenatide should be used with caution in patients receiving oral medications that require rapid gastrointestinal absorption. For oral medications that are dependent on threshold concentrations for efficacy, such as antibiotics, patients should be advised to take those drugs at least 1 hr before exenatide injection. If such drugs are to be administered with food, patients should be advised to take them with a meal or snack when exenatide is not administered).
No products indexed under this heading.

Cefotetan (The effect of exenatide to slow gastric emptying may reduce the extent and rate of absorption of orally administered drugs. Exenatide should be used with caution in patients receiving oral medications that require rapid gastrointestinal absorption. For oral medications that are dependent on threshold concentrations for efficacy,

such as antibiotics, patients should be advised to take those drugs at least 1 hr before exenatide injection. If such drugs are to be administered with food, patients should be advised to take them with a meal or snack when exenatide is not administered).
No products indexed under this heading.

Cefoxitin Sodium (The effect of exenatide to slow gastric emptying may reduce the extent and rate of absorption of orally administered drugs. Exenatide should be used with caution in patients receiving oral medications that require rapid gastrointestinal absorption. For oral medications that are dependent on threshold concentrations for efficacy, such as antibiotics, patients should be advised to take those drugs at least 1 hr before exenatide injection. If such drugs are to be administered with food, patients should be advised to take them with a meal or snack when exenatide is not administered).
No products indexed under this heading.

Cefpodoxime Proxetil (The effect of exenatide to slow gastric emptying may reduce the extent and rate of absorption of orally administered drugs. Exenatide should be used with caution in patients receiving oral medications that require rapid gastrointestinal absorption. For oral medications that are dependent on threshold concentrations for efficacy, such as antibiotics, patients should be advised to take those drugs at least 1 hr before exenatide injection. If such drugs are to be administered with food, patients should be advised to take them with a meal or snack when exenatide is not administered).
No products indexed under this heading.

Cefprozil (The effect of exenatide to slow gastric emptying may reduce the extent and rate of absorption of orally administered drugs. Exenatide should be used with caution in patients receiving oral medications that require rapid gastrointestinal absorption. For oral medications that are dependent on threshold concentrations for efficacy, such as antibiotics, patients should be advised to take those drugs at least 1 hr before exenatide injection. If such drugs are to be administered with food, patients should be advised to take them with a meal or snack when exenatide is not administered).
No products indexed under this heading.

Ceftazidime (The effect of exenatide to slow gastric emptying may reduce the extent and rate of absorption of orally administered drugs. Exenatide should be used with caution in patients receiving oral medications that require rapid gastrointestinal absorption. For oral medications that are dependent on threshold concentrations for efficacy, such as antibiotics, patients should be advised to take those drugs at least 1 hr before exenatide injection. If such drugs are to be administered with food, patients should be advised to take them with a meal or snack when exenatide is not administered). Products include:
Fortaz 1481

Ceftizoxime Sodium (The effect of exenatide to slow gastric emptying may reduce the extent and rate of absorption of orally administered drugs. Exenatide should be used with caution in patients receiving oral medications that require rapid gastrointestinal absorption. For oral medications that are dependent on threshold concentrations for efficacy, such as antibiotics, patients should be advised to take those drugs at least 1 hr before exenatide injection. If such drugs are to be administered with food, patients

should be advised to take them with a meal or snack when exenatide is not administered).
No products indexed under this heading.

Ceftriaxone Sodium (The effect of exenatide to slow gastric emptying may reduce the extent and rate of absorption of orally administered drugs. Exenatide should be used with caution in patients receiving oral medications that require rapid gastrointestinal absorption. For oral medications that are dependent on threshold concentrations for efficacy, such as antibiotics, patients should be advised to take those drugs at least 1 hr before exenatide injection. If such drugs are to be administered with food, patients should be advised to take them with a meal or snack when exenatide is not administered). Products include:
Rocephin 2859

Cefuroxime Axetil (The effect of exenatide to slow gastric emptying may reduce the extent and rate of absorption of orally administered drugs. Exenatide should be used with caution in patients receiving oral medications that require rapid gastrointestinal absorption. For oral medications that are dependent on threshold concentrations for efficacy, such as antibiotics, patients should be advised to take those drugs at least 1 hr before exenatide injection. If such drugs are to be administered with food, patients should be advised to take them with a meal or snack when exenatide is not administered). Products include:
Ceftin 1399

Cefuroxime Sodium (The effect of exenatide to slow gastric emptying may reduce the extent and rate of absorption of orally administered drugs. Exenatide should be used with caution in patients receiving oral medications that require rapid gastrointestinal absorption. For oral medications that are dependent on threshold concentrations for efficacy, such as antibiotics, patients should be advised to take those drugs at least 1 hr before exenatide injection. If such drugs are to be administered with food, patients should be advised to take them with a meal or snack when exenatide is not administered).
No products indexed under this heading.

Cephalexin (The effect of exenatide to slow gastric emptying may reduce the extent and rate of absorption of orally administered drugs. Exenatide should be used with caution in patients receiving oral medications that require rapid gastrointestinal absorption. For oral medications that are dependent on threshold concentrations for efficacy, such as antibiotics, patients should be advised to take those drugs at least 1 hr before exenatide injection. If such drugs are to be administered with food, patients should be advised to take them with a meal or snack when exenatide is not administered).
No products indexed under this heading.

Cephalothin Sodium (The effect of exenatide to slow gastric emptying may reduce the extent and rate of absorption of orally administered drugs. Exenatide should be used with caution in patients receiving oral medications that require rapid gastrointestinal absorption. For oral medications that are dependent on threshold concentrations for efficacy, such as antibiotics, patients should be advised to take those drugs at least 1 hr before exenatide injection. If such drugs are to be administered with food, patients should be advised to take them with a meal or snack when exenatide is not administered).
No products indexed under this heading.

Cephapirin Sodium (The effect of exenatide to slow gastric emptying may reduce the extent and rate of absorption of orally administered drugs. Exenatide should be used with caution in patients receiving oral medications that require rapid gastrointestinal absorption. For oral medications that are dependent on threshold concentrations for efficacy, such as antibiotics, patients should be advised to take those drugs at least 1 hr before exenatide injection. If such drugs are to be administered with food, patients should be advised to take them with a meal or snack when exenatide is not administered).
No products indexed under this heading.

Cephradine (The effect of exenatide to slow gastric emptying may reduce the extent and rate of absorption of orally administered drugs. Exenatide should be used with caution in patients receiving oral medications that require rapid gastrointestinal absorption. For oral medications that are dependent on threshold concentrations for efficacy, such as antibiotics, patients should be advised to take those drugs at least 1 hr before exenatide injection. If such drugs are to be administered with food, patients should be advised to take them with a meal or snack when exenatide is not administered).
No products indexed under this heading.

Chloramphenicol (The effect of exenatide to slow gastric emptying may reduce the extent and rate of absorption of orally administered drugs. Exenatide should be used with caution in patients receiving oral medications that require rapid gastrointestinal absorption. For oral medications that are dependent on threshold concentrations for efficacy, such as antibiotics, patients should be advised to take those drugs at least 1 hr before exenatide injection. If such drugs are to be administered with food, patients should be advised to take them with a meal or snack when exenatide is not administered).
No products indexed under this heading.

Chloramphenicol Palmitate (The effect of exenatide to slow gastric emptying may reduce the extent and rate of absorption of orally administered drugs. Exenatide should be used with caution in patients receiving oral medications that require rapid gastrointestinal absorption. For oral medications that are dependent on threshold concentrations for efficacy, such as antibiotics, patients should be advised to take those drugs at least 1 hr before exenatide injection. If such drugs are to be administered with food, patients should be advised to take them with a meal or snack when exenatide is not administered).
No products indexed under this heading.

Chloramphenicol Sodium Succinate (The effect of exenatide to slow gastric emptying may reduce the extent and rate of absorption of orally administered drugs. Exenatide should be used with caution in patients receiving oral medications that require rapid gastrointestinal absorption. For oral medications that are dependent on threshold concentrations for efficacy, such as antibiotics, patients should be advised to take those drugs at least 1 hr before exenatide injection. If such drugs are to be administered with food, patients should be advised to take them with a meal or snack when exenatide is not administered).
No products indexed under this heading.

Cilastatin Sodium (The effect of exenatide to slow gastric emptying may reduce the extent and rate of absorption of orally administered drugs.

Exenatide should be used with caution in patients receiving oral medications that require rapid gastrointestinal absorption. For oral medications that are dependent on threshold concentrations for efficacy, such as antibiotics, patients should be advised to take those drugs at least 1 hr before exenatide injection. If such drugs are to be administered with food, patients should be advised to take them with a meal or snack when exenatide is not administered). Products include:
    Primaxin I.M. 2232
    Primaxin I.V. 2235

Ciprofloxacin (The effect of exenatide to slow gastric emptying may reduce the extent and rate of absorption of orally administered drugs. Exenatide should be used with caution in patients receiving oral medications that require rapid gastrointestinal absorption. For oral medications that are dependent on threshold concentrations for efficacy, such as antibiotics, patients should be advised to take those drugs at least 1 hr before exenatide injection. If such drugs are to be administered with food, patients should be advised to take them with a meal or snack when exenatide is not administered). Products include:
    Cipro I.V. 3082
    Cipro 3073
    Cipro XR 3091
    Ciprodex 583

Ciprofloxacin Hydrochloride (The effect of exenatide to slow gastric emptying may reduce the extent and rate of absorption of orally administered drugs. Exenatide should be used with caution in patients receiving oral medications that require rapid gastrointestinal absorption. For oral medications that are dependent on threshold concentrations for efficacy, such as antibiotics, patients should be advised to take those drugs at least 1 hr before exenatide injection. If such drugs are to be administered with food, patients should be advised to take them with a meal or snack when exenatide is not administered). Products include:
    Cipro 3073

Clarithromycin (The effect of exenatide to slow gastric emptying may reduce the extent and rate of absorption of orally administered drugs. Exenatide should be used with caution in patients receiving oral medications that require rapid gastrointestinal absorption. For oral medications that are dependent on threshold concentrations for efficacy, such as antibiotics, patients should be advised to take those drugs at least 1 hr before exenatide injection. If such drugs are to be administered with food, patients should be advised to take them with a meal or snack when exenatide is not administered). Products include:
    Biaxin/Biaxin XL 412

Cloxacillin (The effect of exenatide to slow gastric emptying may reduce the extent and rate of absorption of orally administered drugs. Exenatide should be used with caution in patients receiving oral medications that require rapid gastrointestinal absorption. For oral medications that are dependent on threshold concentrations for efficacy, such as antibiotics, patients should be advised to take those drugs at least 1 hr before exenatide injection. If such drugs are to be administered with food, patients should be advised to take them with a meal or snack when exenatide is not administered).
No products indexed under this heading.

Cloxacillin Sodium (The effect of exenatide to slow gastric emptying may reduce the extent and rate of absorption of orally administered drugs.
Exenatide should be used with caution

in patients receiving oral medications that require rapid gastrointestinal absorption. For oral medications that are dependent on threshold concentrations for efficacy, such as antibiotics, patients should be advised to take those drugs at least 1 hr before exenatide injection. If such drugs are to be administered with food, patients should be advised to take them with a meal or snack when exenatide is not administered).
No products indexed under this heading.

Cloxacillin Sodium Monohydrate (The effect of exenatide to slow gastric emptying may reduce the extent and rate of absorption of orally administered drugs. Exenatide should be used with caution in patients receiving oral medications that require rapid gastrointestinal absorption. For oral medications that are dependent on threshold concentrations for efficacy, such as antibiotics, patients should be advised to take those drugs at least 1 hr before exenatide injection. If such drugs are to be administered with food, patients should be advised to take them with a meal or snack when exenatide is not administered).
No products indexed under this heading.

Demeclocycline Hydrochloride (The effect of exenatide to slow gastric emptying may reduce the extent and rate of absorption of orally administered drugs. Exenatide should be used with caution in patients receiving oral medications that require rapid gastrointestinal absorption. For oral medications that are dependent on threshold concentrations for efficacy, such as antibiotics, patients should be advised to take those drugs at least 1 hr before exenatide injection. If such drugs are to be administered with food, patients should be advised to take them with a meal or snack when exenatide is not administered).
No products indexed under this heading.

Desogestrel (The effect of exenatide to slow gastric emptying may reduce the extent and rate of absorption of orally administered drugs. Exenatide should be used with caution in patients receiving oral medications that require rapid gastrointestinal absorption. For oral medications that are dependent on threshold concentrations for efficacy, such as contraceptives, patients should be advised to take those drugs at least 1 hr before exenatide injection. If such drugs are to be administered with food, patients should be advised to take them with a meal or snack when exenatide is not administered).
No products indexed under this heading.

Dicloxacillin (The effect of exenatide to slow gastric emptying may reduce the extent and rate of absorption of orally administered drugs. Exenatide should be used with caution in patients receiving oral medications that require rapid gastrointestinal absorption. For oral medications that are dependent on threshold concentrations for efficacy, such as antibiotics, patients should be advised to take those drugs at least 1 hr before exenatide injection. If such drugs are to be administered with food, patients should be advised to take them with a meal or snack when exenatide is not administered).
No products indexed under this heading.

Dicloxacillin Sodium (The effect of exenatide to slow gastric emptying may reduce the extent and rate of absorption of orally administered drugs. Exenatide should be used with caution in patients receiving oral medications that require rapid gastrointestinal absorption. For oral medications that are dependent on threshold concentrations for efficacy, such as antibiotics,

patients should be advised to take those drugs at least 1 hr before exenatide injection. If such drugs are to be administered with food, patients should be advised to take them with a meal or snack when exenatide is not administered).
No products indexed under this heading.

Digoxin (Co-administration of repeated doses of exenatide (10 mcg BID) decreased the C_{max} of oral digoxin (0.25 mg QD) by 17% and delayed the T_{max} by approximately 2.5 hours; however, the overall steady-state pharmacokinetic exposure (AUC) was not changed). Products include:
    Lanoxin Injection 1546
    Lanoxin Injection Pediatric 1549
    Lanoxin Tablets 1553

Dirithromycin (The effect of exenatide to slow gastric emptying may reduce the extent and rate of absorption of orally administered drugs. Exenatide should be used with caution in patients receiving oral medications that require rapid gastrointestinal absorption. For oral medications that are dependent on threshold concentrations for efficacy, such as antibiotics, patients should be advised to take those drugs at least 1 hr before exenatide injection. If such drugs are to be administered with food, patients should be advised to take them with a meal or snack when exenatide is not administered).
No products indexed under this heading.

Disodium Carbenicillin (The effect of exenatide to slow gastric emptying may reduce the extent and rate of absorption of orally administered drugs. Exenatide should be used with caution in patients receiving oral medications that require rapid gastrointestinal absorption. For oral medications that are dependent on threshold concentrations for efficacy, such as antibiotics, patients should be advised to take those drugs at least 1 hr before exenatide injection. If such drugs are to be administered with food, patients should be advised to take them with a meal or snack when exenatide is not administered).
No products indexed under this heading.

Doxycycline (The effect of exenatide to slow gastric emptying may reduce the extent and rate of absorption of orally administered drugs. Exenatide should be used with caution in patients receiving oral medications that require rapid gastrointestinal absorption. For oral medications that are dependent on threshold concentrations for efficacy, such as antibiotics, patients should be advised to take those drugs at least 1 hr before exenatide injection. If such drugs are to be administered with food, patients should be advised to take them with a meal or snack when exenatide is not administered).
No products indexed under this heading.

Doxycycline Calcium (The effect of exenatide to slow gastric emptying may reduce the extent and rate of absorption of orally administered drugs. Exenatide should be used with caution in patients receiving oral medications that require rapid gastrointestinal absorption. For oral medications that are dependent on threshold concentrations for efficacy, such as antibiotics, patients should be advised to take those drugs at least 1 hr before exenatide injection. If such drugs are to be administered with food, patients should be advised to take them with a meal or snack when exenatide is not administered).
No products indexed under this heading.

Doxycycline Hyclate (The effect of exenatide to slow gastric emptying may reduce the extent and rate of absorp-

tion of orally administered drugs. Exenatide should be used with caution in patients receiving oral medications that require rapid gastrointestinal absorption. For oral medications that are dependent on threshold concentrations for efficacy, such as antibiotics, patients should be advised to take those drugs at least 1 hr before exenatide injection. If such drugs are to be administered with food, patients should be advised to take them with a meal or snack when exenatide is not administered).

No products indexed under this heading.

Doxycycline Monohydrate (The effect of exenatide to slow gastric emptying may reduce the extent and rate of absorption of orally administered drugs. Exenatide should be used with caution in patients receiving oral medications that require rapid gastrointestinal absorption. For oral medications that are dependent on threshold concentrations for efficacy, such as antibiotics, patients should be advised to take those drugs at least 1 hr before exenatide injection. If such drugs are to be administered with food, patients should be advised to take them with a meal or snack when exenatide is not administered).

No products indexed under this heading.

Enoxacin (The effect of exenatide to slow gastric emptying may reduce the extent and rate of absorption of orally administered drugs. Exenatide should be used with caution in patients receiving oral medications that require rapid gastrointestinal absorption. For oral medications that are dependent on threshold concentrations for efficacy, such as antibiotics, patients should be advised to take those drugs at least 1 hr before exenatide injection. If such drugs are to be administered with food, patients should be advised to take them with a meal or snack when exenatide is not administered).

No products indexed under this heading.

Erythromycin (The effect of exenatide to slow gastric emptying may reduce the extent and rate of absorption of orally administered drugs. Exenatide should be used with caution in patients receiving oral medications that require rapid gastrointestinal absorption. For oral medications that are dependent on threshold concentrations for efficacy, such as antibiotics, patients should be advised to take those drugs at least 1 hr before exenatide injection. If such drugs are to be administered with food, patients should be advised to take them with a meal or snack when exenatide is not administered).

No products indexed under this heading.

Erythromycin Estolate (The effect of exenatide to slow gastric emptying may reduce the extent and rate of absorption of orally administered drugs. Exenatide should be used with caution in patients receiving oral medications that require rapid gastrointestinal absorption. For oral medications that are dependent on threshold concentrations for efficacy, such as antibiotics, patients should be advised to take those drugs at least 1 hr before exenatide injection. If such drugs are to be administered with food, patients should be advised to take them with a meal or snack when exenatide is not administered).

No products indexed under this heading.

Erythromycin Ethylsuccinate (The effect of exenatide to slow gastric emptying may reduce the extent and rate of absorption of orally administered drugs. Exenatide should be used with caution in patients receiving oral medications that require rapid gastrointestinal absorption. For oral medications that are dependent on threshold concentrations for efficacy, such as antibiotics, patients should be advised to take those drugs at least 1 hr before exenatide injection. If such drugs are to be administered with food, patients should be advised to take them with a meal or snack when exenatide is not administered). Products include:

E.E.S. **437**
EryPed **435**

Erythromycin Gluceptate (The effect of exenatide to slow gastric emptying may reduce the extent and rate of absorption of orally administered drugs. Exenatide should be used with caution in patients receiving oral medications that require rapid gastrointestinal absorption. For oral medications that are dependent on threshold concentrations for efficacy, such as antibiotics, patients should be advised to take those drugs at least 1 hr before exenatide injection. If such drugs are to be administered with food, patients should be advised to take them with a meal or snack when exenatide is not administered).

No products indexed under this heading.

Erythromycin Stearate (The effect of exenatide to slow gastric emptying may reduce the extent and rate of absorption of orally administered drugs. Exenatide should be used with caution in patients receiving oral medications that require rapid gastrointestinal absorption. For oral medications that are dependent on threshold concentrations for efficacy, such as antibiotics, patients should be advised to take those drugs at least 1 hr before exenatide injection. If such drugs are to be administered with food, patients should be advised to take them with a meal or snack when exenatide is not administered).

No products indexed under this heading.

Ethinyl Estradiol (The effect of exenatide to slow gastric emptying may reduce the extent and rate of absorption of orally administered drugs. Exenatide should be used with caution in patients receiving oral medications that require rapid gastrointestinal absorption. For oral medications that are dependent on threshold concentrations for efficacy, such as contraceptives, patients should be advised to take those drugs at least 1 hr before exenatide injection. If such drugs are to be administered with food, patients should be advised to take them with a meal or snack when exenatide is not administered). Products include:

LoSeasonique **3407**
Lybrel **3514**
NuvaRing **3181**
Ortho Evra **2648**
Ortho-Cyclen/Ortho Tri-Cyclen **2663**
Ortho Tri-Cyclen Lo Tablets **2673**
Seasonique **3418**
Yaz **864**

Ethynodiol Diacetate (The effect of exenatide to slow gastric emptying may reduce the extent and rate of absorption of orally administered drugs. Exenatide should be used with caution in patients receiving oral medications that require rapid gastrointestinal absorption. For oral medications that are dependent on threshold concentrations for efficacy, such as contraceptives, patients should be advised to take those drugs at least 1 hr before exenatide injection. If such drugs are to be administered with food, patients should be advised to take them with a meal or snack when exenatide is not administered).

No products indexed under this heading.

Gatifloxacin (The effect of exenatide to slow gastric emptying may reduce the extent and rate of absorption of orally administered drugs. Exenatide should be used with caution in patients receiving oral medications that require rapid gastrointestinal absorption. For oral medications that are dependent on threshold concentrations for efficacy, such as antibiotics, patients should be advised to take those drugs at least 1 hr before exenatide injection. If such drugs are to be administered with food, patients should be advised to take them with a meal or snack when exenatide is not administered).

No products indexed under this heading.

Grepafloxacin Hydrochloride (The effect of exenatide to slow gastric emptying may reduce the extent and rate of absorption of orally administered drugs. Exenatide should be used with caution in patients receiving oral medications that require rapid gastrointestinal absorption. For oral medications that are dependent on threshold concentrations for efficacy, such as antibiotics, patients should be advised to take those drugs at least 1 hr before exenatide injection. If such drugs are to be administered with food, patients should be advised to take them with a meal or snack when exenatide is not administered).

No products indexed under this heading.

Imipenem (The effect of exenatide to slow gastric emptying may reduce the extent and rate of absorption of orally administered drugs. Exenatide should be used with caution in patients receiving oral medications that require rapid gastrointestinal absorption. For oral medications that are dependent on threshold concentrations for efficacy, such as antibiotics, patients should be advised to take those drugs at least 1 hr before exenatide injection. If such drugs are to be administered with food, patients should be advised to take them with a meal or snack when exenatide is not administered). Products include:

Primaxin I.M. **2232**
Primaxin I.V. **2235**

Levofloxacin (The effect of exenatide to slow gastric emptying may reduce the extent and rate of absorption of orally administered drugs. Exenatide should be used with caution in patients receiving oral medications that require rapid gastrointestinal absorption. For oral medications that are dependent on threshold concentrations for efficacy, such as antibiotics, patients should be advised to take those drugs at least 1 hr before exenatide injection. If such drugs are to be administered with food, patients should be advised to take them with a meal or snack when exenatide is not administered). Products include:

Iquix **3492**
Levaquin **2629**
Levaquin in 5% Dextrose **2629**
Quixin **3493**

Levonorgestrel (The effect of exenatide to slow gastric emptying may reduce the extent and rate of absorption of orally administered drugs. Exenatide should be used with caution in patients receiving oral medications that require rapid gastrointestinal absorption. For oral medications that are dependent on threshold concentrations for efficacy, such as contraceptives, patients should be advised to take those drugs at least 1 hr before exenatide injection. If such drugs are to be administered with food, patients should be advised to take them with a meal or snack when exenatide is not administered). Products include:

Climara Pro **847**
LoSeasonique **3407**
Lybrel **3514**
Mirena **854**
Plan B **3416**
Seasonique **3418**

Lisinopril (Lisinopril steady-state T_{max} was delayed 2 hours). Products include:

Prinivil **2241**
Prinzide **2246**

Lomefloxacin Hydrochloride (The effect of exenatide to slow gastric emptying may reduce the extent and rate of absorption of orally administered drugs. Exenatide should be used with caution in patients receiving oral medications that require rapid gastrointestinal absorption. For oral medications that are dependent on threshold concentrations for efficacy, such as antibiotics, patients should be advised to take those drugs at least 1 hr before exenatide injection. If such drugs are to be administered with food, patients should be advised to take them with a meal or snack when exenatide is not administered).

No products indexed under this heading.

Loracarbef (The effect of exenatide to slow gastric emptying may reduce the extent and rate of absorption of orally administered drugs. Exenatide should be used with caution in patients receiving oral medications that require rapid gastrointestinal absorption. For oral medications that are dependent on threshold concentrations for efficacy, such as antibiotics, patients should be advised to take those drugs at least 1 hr before exenatide injection. If such drugs are to be administered with food, patients should be advised to take them with a meal or snack when exenatide is not administered).

No products indexed under this heading.

Lovastatin (Lovastatin AUC and C_{max} were decreased approximately 40% and 28%, respectively, and T_{max} was delayed about 4 hours when exenatide was administered concomitantly with a single dose of lovastatin (40 mg) compared with lovastatin administered alone. In the30-week controlled clinical trials of exenatide, the use of exenatide in patients already receiving HMG CoA reductase inhibitors was not associated with consistent changes in lipid profiles compared to baseline). Products include:

Advicor **402**
Mevacor **2212**

Mestranol (The effect of exenatide to slow gastric emptying may reduce the extent and rate of absorption of orally administered drugs. Exenatide should be used with caution in patients receiving oral medications that require rapid gastrointestinal absorption. For oral medications that are dependent on threshold concentrations for efficacy, such as contraceptives, patients should be advised to take those drugs at least 1 hr before exenatide injection. If such drugs are to be administered with food, patients should be advised to take them with a meal or snack when exenatide is not administered).

No products indexed under this heading.

Methacycline Hydrochloride (The effect of exenatide to slow gastric emptying may reduce the extent and rate of absorption of orally administered drugs. Exenatide should be used with caution in patients receiving oral medications that require rapid gastrointestinal absorption. For oral medications that are dependent on threshold concentrations for efficacy, such as antibiotics, patients should be advised to take those drugs at least 1 hr before exenatide injection. If such drugs are to be administered with food, patients should be advised to take them with a meal or snack when exenatide is not administered).

No products indexed under this heading.

Methicillin Sodium (The effect of exenatide to slow gastric emptying may reduce the extent and rate of absorp-

249 Interactions Index Byetta

tion of orally administered drugs. Exenatide should be used with caution in patients receiving oral medications that require rapid gastrointestinal absorption. For oral medications that are dependent on threshold concentrations for efficacy, such as antibiotics, patients should be advised to take those drugs at least 1 hr before exenatide injection. If such drugs are to be administered with food, patients should be advised to take them with a meal or snack when exenatide is not administered).
No products indexed under this heading.

Mezlocillin Sodium (The effect of exenatide to slow gastric emptying may reduce the extent and rate of absorption of orally administered drugs. Exenatide should be used with caution in patients receiving oral medications that require rapid gastrointestinal absorption. For oral medications that are dependent on threshold concentrations for efficacy, such as antibiotics, patients should be advised to take those drugs at least 1 hr before exenatide injection. If such drugs are to be administered with food, patients should be advised to take them with a meal or snack when exenatide is not administered).
No products indexed under this heading.

Minocycline Hydrochloride (The effect of exenatide to slow gastric emptying may reduce the extent and rate of absorption of orally administered drugs. Exenatide should be used with caution in patients receiving oral medications that require rapid gastrointestinal absorption. For oral medications that are dependent on threshold concentrations for efficacy, such as antibiotics, patients should be advised to take those drugs at least 1 hr before exenatide injection. If such drugs are to be administered with food, patients should be advised to take them with a meal or snack when exenatide is not administered). Products include:
Solodyn 2073

Moxifloxacin Hydrochloride (The effect of exenatide to slow gastric emptying may reduce the extent and rate of absorption of orally administered drugs. Exenatide should be used with caution in patients receiving oral medications that require rapid gastrointestinal absorption. For oral medications that are dependent on threshold concentrations for efficacy, such as antibiotics, patients should be advised to take those drugs at least 1 hr before exenatide injection. If such drugs are to be administered with food, patients should be advised to take them with a meal or snack when exenatide is not administered). Products include:
Avelox 3064
Vigamox 589

Nafcillin Sodium (The effect of exenatide to slow gastric emptying may reduce the extent and rate of absorption of orally administered drugs. Exenatide should be used with caution in patients receiving oral medications that require rapid gastrointestinal absorption. For oral medications that are dependent on threshold concentrations for efficacy, such as antibiotics, patients should be advised to take those drugs at least 1 hr before exenatide injection. If such drugs are to be administered with food, patients should be advised to take them with a meal or snack when exenatide is not administered).
No products indexed under this heading.

Norethindrone (The effect of exenatide to slow gastric emptying may reduce the extent and rate of absorption of orally administered drugs. Exenatide should be used with caution in patients receiving oral medications that require rapid gastrointestinal absorption. For oral medications that are dependent on threshold concentrations for efficacy, such as contraceptives, patients should be advised to take those drugs at least 1 hr before exenatide injection. If such drugs are to be administered with food, patients should be advised to take them with a meal or snack when exenatide is not administered). Products include:
Ortho Micronor 2660

Norethynodrel (The effect of exenatide to slow gastric emptying may reduce the extent and rate of absorption of orally administered drugs. Exenatide should be used with caution in patients receiving oral medications that require rapid gastrointestinal absorption. For oral medications that are dependent on threshold concentrations for efficacy, such as contraceptives, patients should be advised to take those drugs at least 1 hr before exenatide injection. If such drugs are to be administered with food, patients should be advised to take them with a meal or snack when exenatide is not administered).
No products indexed under this heading.

Norfloxacin (The effect of exenatide to slow gastric emptying may reduce the extent and rate of absorption of orally administered drugs. Exenatide should be used with caution in patients receiving oral medications that require rapid gastrointestinal absorption. For oral medications that are dependent on threshold concentrations for efficacy, such as antibiotics, patients should be advised to take those drugs at least 1 hr before exenatide injection. If such drugs are to be administered with food, patients should be advised to take them with a meal or snack when exenatide is not administered). Products include:
Noroxin 2220

Norgestimate (The effect of exenatide to slow gastric emptying may reduce the extent and rate of absorption of orally administered drugs. Exenatide should be used with caution in patients receiving oral medications that require rapid gastrointestinal absorption. For oral medications that are dependent on threshold concentrations for efficacy, such as contraceptives, patients should be advised to take those drugs at least 1 hr before exenatide injection. If such drugs are to be administered with food, patients should be advised to take them with a meal or snack when exenatide is not administered). Products include:
Ortho-Cyclen/Ortho Tri-Cyclen 2663
Ortho Tri-Cyclen Lo Tablets 2673

Norgestrel (The effect of exenatide to slow gastric emptying may reduce the extent and rate of absorption of orally administered drugs. Exenatide should be used with caution in patients receiving oral medications that require rapid gastrointestinal absorption. For oral medications that are dependent on threshold concentrations for efficacy, such as contraceptives, patients should be advised to take those drugs at least 1 hr before exenatide injection. If such drugs are to be administered with food, patients should be advised to take them with a meal or snack when exenatide is not administered).
No products indexed under this heading.

Ofloxacin (The effect of exenatide to slow gastric emptying may reduce the extent and rate of absorption of orally administered drugs. Exenatide should be used with caution in patients receiving oral medications that require rapid gastrointestinal absorption. For oral medications that are dependent on threshold concentrations for efficacy, such as antibiotics, patients should be advised to take those drugs at least 1 hr before exenatide injection. If such drugs are to be administered with food, patients should be advised to take them with a meal or snack when exenatide is not administered).
No products indexed under this heading.

Oral Medications, unspecified (The effect of exenatide to slow gastric emptying may reduce the extent and rate of absorption of orally administered drugs. Exenatide should be used with caution in patients receiving oral medications that require rapid gastrointestinal absorption).
No products indexed under this heading.

Oxacillin (The effect of exenatide to slow gastric emptying may reduce the extent and rate of absorption of orally administered drugs. Exenatide should be used with caution in patients receiving oral medications that require rapid gastrointestinal absorption. For oral medications that are dependent on threshold concentrations for efficacy, such as antibiotics, patients should be advised to take those drugs at least 1 hr before exenatide injection. If such drugs are to be administered with food, patients should be advised to take them with a meal or snack when exenatide is not administered).
No products indexed under this heading.

Oxacillin Sodium (The effect of exenatide to slow gastric emptying may reduce the extent and rate of absorption of orally administered drugs. Exenatide should be used with caution in patients receiving oral medications that require rapid gastrointestinal absorption. For oral medications that are dependent on threshold concentrations for efficacy, such as antibiotics, patients should be advised to take those drugs at least 1 hr before exenatide injection. If such drugs are to be administered with food, patients should be advised to take them with a meal or snack when exenatide is not administered).
No products indexed under this heading.

Oxytetracycline (The effect of exenatide to slow gastric emptying may reduce the extent and rate of absorption of orally administered drugs. Exenatide should be used with caution in patients receiving oral medications that require rapid gastrointestinal absorption. For oral medications that are dependent on threshold concentrations for efficacy, such as antibiotics, patients should be advised to take those drugs at least 1 hr before exenatide injection. If such drugs are to be administered with food, patients should be advised to take them with a meal or snack when exenatide is not administered).
No products indexed under this heading.

Oxytetracycline Hydrochloride (The effect of exenatide to slow gastric emptying may reduce the extent and rate of absorption of orally administered drugs. Exenatide should be used with caution in patients receiving oral medications that require rapid gastrointestinal absorption. For oral medications that are dependent on threshold concentrations for efficacy, such as antibiotics, patients should be advised to take those drugs at least 1 hr before exenatide injection. If such drugs are to be administered with food, patients should be advised to take them with a meal or snack when exenatide is not administered).
No products indexed under this heading.

Penicillin, Potassium Phenoxymethyl (The effect of exenatide to slow gastric emptying may reduce the extent and rate of absorption of orally administered drugs. Exenatide should be used with caution in patients receiving oral medications that require rapid gastrointestinal absorption. For oral medications that are dependent on threshold concentrations for efficacy, such as antibiotics, patients should be advised to take those drugs at least 1 hr before exenatide injection. If such drugs are to be administered with food, patients should be advised to take them with a meal or snack when exenatide is not administered).
No products indexed under this heading.

Penicillin G Benzathine (The effect of exenatide to slow gastric emptying may reduce the extent and rate of absorption of orally administered drugs. Exenatide should be used with caution in patients receiving oral medications that require rapid gastrointestinal absorption. For oral medications that are dependent on threshold concentrations for efficacy, such as antibiotics, patients should be advised to take those drugs at least 1 hr before exenatide injection. If such drugs are to be administered with food, patients should be advised to take them with a meal or snack when exenatide is not administered). Products include:
Bicillin C-R Injectable Suspension 1826
Bicillin L-A 1828

Penicillin G Dibenzylethyenediamine (The effect of exenatide to slow gastric emptying may reduce the extent and rate of absorption of orally administered drugs. Exenatide should be used with caution in patients receiving oral medications that require rapid gastrointestinal absorption. For oral medications that are dependent on threshold concentrations for efficacy, such as antibiotics, patients should be advised to take those drugs at least 1 hr before exenatide injection. If such drugs are to be administered with food, patients should be advised to take them with a meal or snack when exenatide is not administered).
No products indexed under this heading.

Penicillin G Potassium (The effect of exenatide to slow gastric emptying may reduce the extent and rate of absorption of orally administered drugs. Exenatide should be used with caution in patients receiving oral medications that require rapid gastrointestinal absorption. For oral medications that are dependent on threshold concentrations for efficacy, such as antibiotics, patients should be advised to take those drugs at least 1 hr before exenatide injection. If such drugs are to be administered with food, patients should be advised to take them with a meal or snack when exenatide is not administered).
No products indexed under this heading.

Penicillin G Procaine (The effect of exenatide to slow gastric emptying may reduce the extent and rate of absorption of orally administered drugs. Exenatide should be used with caution in patients receiving oral medications that require rapid gastrointestinal absorption. For oral medications that are dependent on threshold concentrations for efficacy, such as antibiotics, patients should be advised to take those drugs at least 1 hr before exenatide injection. If such drugs are to be administered with food, patients should be advised to take them with a meal or snack when exenatide is not administered). Products include:
Bicillin C-R Injectable Suspension 1826
Bicillin L-A 1828

Penicillin G Sodium (The effect of exenatide to slow gastric emptying may reduce the extent and rate of absorption of orally administered drugs. Exenatide should be used with caution in patients receiving oral medications

that require rapid gastrointestinal absorption. For oral medications that are dependent on threshold concentrations for efficacy, such as antibiotics, patients should be advised to take those drugs at least 1 hr before exenatide injection. If such drugs are to be administered with food, patients should be advised to take them with a meal or snack when exenatide is not administered).

No products indexed under this heading.

Penicillin V (The effect of exenatide to slow gastric emptying may reduce the extent and rate of absorption of orally administered drugs. Exenatide should be used with caution in patients receiving oral medications that require rapid gastrointestinal absorption. For oral medications that are dependent on threshold concentrations for efficacy, such as antibiotics, patients should be advised to take those drugs at least 1 hr before exenatide injection. If such drugs are to be administered with food, patients should be advised to take them with a meal or snack when exenatide is not administered).

No products indexed under this heading.

Penicillin V Potassium (The effect of exenatide to slow gastric emptying may reduce the extent and rate of absorption of orally administered drugs. Exenatide should be used with caution in patients receiving oral medications that require rapid gastrointestinal absorption. For oral medications that are dependent on threshold concentrations for efficacy, such as antibiotics, patients should be advised to take those drugs at least 1 hr before exenatide injection. If such drugs are to be administered with food, patients should be advised to take them with a meal or snack when exenatide is not administered).

No products indexed under this heading.

Penicillins (The effect of exenatide to slow gastric emptying may reduce the extent and rate of absorption of orally administered drugs. Exenatide should be used with caution in patients receiving oral medications that require rapid gastrointestinal absorption. For oral medications that are dependent on threshold concentrations for efficacy, such as antibiotics, patients should be advised to take those drugs at least 1 hr before exenatide injection. If such drugs are to be administered with food, patients should be advised to take them with a meal or snack when exenatide is not administered).

No products indexed under this heading.

Piperacillin Sodium (The effect of exenatide to slow gastric emptying may reduce the extent and rate of absorption of orally administered drugs. Exenatide should be used with caution in patients receiving oral medications that require rapid gastrointestinal absorption. For oral medications that are dependent on threshold concentrations for efficacy, such as antibiotics, patients should be advised to take those drugs at least 1 hr before exenatide injection. If such drugs are to be administered with food, patients should be advised to take them with a meal or snack when exenatide is not administered). Products include:

Zosyn **3607**

Sodium Cloxacillin Monohydrate (The effect of exenatide to slow gastric emptying may reduce the extent and rate of absorption of orally administered drugs. Exenatide should be used with caution in patients receiving oral medications that require rapid gastrointestinal absorption. For oral medications that are dependent on threshold concentrations for efficacy, such as antibiotics, patients should be advised to take those drugs at least 1 hr before exenatide injection. If such drugs are to be administered with food, patients should be advised to take them with a meal or snack when exenatide is not administered).

No products indexed under this heading.

Sulfamethizole (The effect of exenatide to slow gastric emptying may reduce the extent and rate of absorption of orally administered drugs. Exenatide should be used with caution in patients receiving oral medications that require rapid gastrointestinal absorption. For oral medications that are dependent on threshold concentrations for efficacy, such as antibiotics, patients should be advised to take those drugs at least 1 hr before exenatide injection. If such drugs are to be administered with food, patients should be advised to take them with a meal or snack when exenatide is not administered).

No products indexed under this heading.

Sulfamethoxazole (The effect of exenatide to slow gastric emptying may reduce the extent and rate of absorption of orally administered drugs. Exenatide should be used with caution in patients receiving oral medications that require rapid gastrointestinal absorption. For oral medications that are dependent on threshold concentrations for efficacy, such as antibiotics, patients should be advised to take those drugs at least 1 hr before exenatide injection. If such drugs are to be administered with food, patients should be advised to take them with a meal or snack when exenatide is not administered).

No products indexed under this heading.

Sulfisoxazole Acetyl (The effect of exenatide to slow gastric emptying may reduce the extent and rate of absorption of orally administered drugs. Exenatide should be used with caution in patients receiving oral medications that require rapid gastrointestinal absorption. For oral medications that are dependent on threshold concentrations for efficacy, such as antibiotics, patients should be advised to take those drugs at least 1 hr before exenatide injection. If such drugs are to be administered with food, patients should be advised to take them with a meal or snack when exenatide is not administered).

No products indexed under this heading.

Tetracycline Hydrochloride (The effect of exenatide to slow gastric emptying may reduce the extent and rate of absorption of orally administered drugs. Exenatide should be used with caution in patients receiving oral medications that require rapid gastrointestinal absorption. For oral medications that are dependent on threshold concentrations for efficacy, such as antibiotics, patients should be advised to take those drugs at least 1 hr before exenatide injection. If such drugs are to be administered with food, patients should be advised to take them with a meal or snack when exenatide is not administered). Products include:

Pylera **793**

Tetracycline Phosphate Complex (The effect of exenatide to slow gastric emptying may reduce the extent and rate of absorption of orally administered drugs. Exenatide should be used with caution in patients receiving oral medications that require rapid gastrointestinal absorption. For oral medications that are dependent on threshold concentrations for efficacy, such as antibiotics, patients should be advised to take those drugs at least 1 hr before exenatide injection. If such drugs are to be administered with food, patients should be advised to take them with a meal or snack when exenatide is not administered).

No products indexed under this heading.

Ticarcillin Disodium (The effect of exenatide to slow gastric emptying may reduce the extent and rate of absorption of orally administered drugs. Exenatide should be used with caution in patients receiving oral medications that require rapid gastrointestinal absorption. For oral medications that are dependent on threshold concentrations for efficacy, such as antibiotics, patients should be advised to take those drugs at least 1 hr before exenatide injection. If such drugs are to be administered with food, patients should be advised to take them with a meal or snack when exenatide is not administered). Products include:

Timentin ADD-Vantage **1670**
Timentin Galaxy **1674**
Timentin **1666**
Timentin Pharmacy **1678**

Troleandomycin (The effect of exenatide to slow gastric emptying may reduce the extent and rate of absorption of orally administered drugs. Exenatide should be used with caution in patients receiving oral medications that require rapid gastrointestinal absorption. For oral medications that are dependent on threshold concentrations for efficacy, such as antibiotics, patients should be advised to take those drugs at least 1 hr before exenatide injection. If such drugs are to be administered with food, patients should be advised to take them with a meal or snack when exenatide is not administered).

No products indexed under this heading.

Trovafloxacin Mesylate (The effect of exenatide to slow gastric emptying may reduce the extent and rate of absorption of orally administered drugs. Exenatide should be used with caution in patients receiving oral medications that require rapid gastrointestinal absorption. For oral medications that are dependent on threshold concentrations for efficacy, such as antibiotics, patients should be advised to take those drugs at least 1 hr before exenatide injection. If such drugs are to be administered with food, patients should be advised to take them with a meal or snack when exenatide is not administered).

No products indexed under this heading.

Warfarin Sodium (In a controlled clinical pharmacology study in healthy volunteers, a delay in warfarin T_{max} of about 2 hours was observed when warfarin was administered 30 min after exenatide. No clinically relevant effects on C_{max} or AUC were observed. However, since market introduction there have been some spontaneously cases reported of increased INR with concomitant use of warfarin and exenatide, sometimes associated with bleeding).

No products indexed under this heading.

BYSTOLIC TABLETS

(Nebivolol) **1147**

May interact with antiarrhythmics, calcium channel blockers, cardiac glycosides, catecholamine-depleting drugs, cytochrome p450 2d6 inducers (selected), cytochrome p450 2d6 inhibitors (selected), insulin, oral hypoglycemic agents, and certain other agents. Compounds in these categories include:

Acarbose (Beta-blockers may mask some of the manifestations of hypoglycemia, particularly tachycardia. Nonselective beta-blockers may potentiate insulin-induced hypoglycemia and delay recovery of serum glucose levels. It is not known whether nebivolol has these effects. Patients subject to spontaneous hypoglycemia, or diabetic patients receiving insulin or oral hypoglycemic agents, should be advised about these possibilities and nebivolol should be used with caution).

No products indexed under this heading.

Acebutolol Hydrochloride (Nebivolol should be used with care when myocardial depressants or inhibitors of AV-conduction, such as antiarrhythmic agents, such as disopyramide, are used concurrently).

No products indexed under this heading.

Adenosine (Nebivolol should be used with care when myocardial depressants or inhibitors of AV-conduction, such as antiarrhythmic agents, such as disopyramide, are used concurrently). Products include:

Adenocard **656**
Adenoscan **657**

Amiodarone Hydrochloride (Nebivolol should be used with care when myocardial depressants or inhibitors of AV-conduction, such as antiarrhythmic agents, such as disopyramide, are used concurrently).

No products indexed under this heading.

Amitriptyline Hydrochloride (Drugs that inhibit CYP2D6 can be expected to increase plasma levels of nebivolol. When nebivolol is co-administered with an inhibitor of CYP2D6, patients should be closely monitored and the nebivolol dose adjusted according to blood pressure response. Use caution when nebivolol is co-administered with CYP2D6 inhibitors).

No products indexed under this heading.

Amlodipine Besylate (Because of significant negative inotropic and chronotropic effects in patients treated with beta-blockers and calcium channel blockers of the verapamil and diltiazem type, caution should be used in patients treated concomitantly with these agents and ECGand blood pressure should be monitored. Nebivolol should be used with care when myocardial depressants or inhibitors of AV-conduction, such as certain calcium antagonists (particularly of the phenylalkylamine [verapamil] and benzothiazepine [diltiazem] classes)). Products include:

Azor **1010**
Exforge **2443**
Exforge HCT **2449**

Amoxapine (Drugs that inhibit CYP2D6 can be expected to increase plasma levels of nebivolol. When nebivolol is co-administered with an inhibitor of CYP2D6, patients should be closely monitored and the nebivolol dose adjusted according to blood pressure response. Use caution when nebivolol is co-administered with CYP2D6 inhibitors).

No products indexed under this heading.

Bepridil Hydrochloride (Because of significant negative inotropic and chronotropic effects in patients treated with beta-blockers and calcium channel blockers of the verapamil and diltiazem type, caution should be used in patients treated concomitantly with these agents and ECGand blood pressure should be monitored. Nebivolol should be used with care when myocardial depressants or inhibitors of AV-conduction, such as certain calcium antagonists (particularly of the phenylalkylamine [verapamil] and benzothiazepine [diltiazem] classes)).

No products indexed under this heading.

Bretylium Tosylate (Nebivolol should be used with care when myocardial depressants or inhibitors of AV-conduction, such as antiarrhythmic agents, such as disopyramide, are used concurrently).

No products indexed under this heading.

Bupropion Hydrochloride (Drugs that inhibit CYP2D6 can be expected to increase plasma levels of nebivolol. When nebivolol is co-administered with an inhibitor of CYP2D6, patients should be closely monitored and the nebivolol dose adjusted according to blood pressure response. Use caution when nebivolol is co-administered with CYP2D6 inhibitors). Products include:

Carbamazepine (When nebivolol is co-administered with an inducer of CYP2D6, patients should be closely monitored and the nebivolol dose adjusted according to blood pressure response). Products include:

Celecoxib (Drugs that inhibit CYP2D6 can be expected to increase plasma levels of nebivolol. When nebivolol is co-administered with an inhibitor of CYP2D6, patients should be closely monitored and the nebivolol dose adjusted according to blood pressure response. Use caution when nebivolol is co-administered with CYP2D6 inhibitors). Products include:

Chloroquine (Drugs that inhibit CYP2D6 can be expected to increase plasma levels of nebivolol. When nebivolol is co-administered with an inhibitor of CYP2D6, patients should be closely monitored and the nebivolol dose adjusted according to blood pressure response. Use caution when nebivolol is co-administered with CYP2D6 inhibitors).
No products indexed under this heading.

Chloroquine Hydrochloride (Drugs that inhibit CYP2D6 can be expected to increase plasma levels of nebivolol. When nebivolol is co-administered with an inhibitor of CYP2D6, patients should be closely monitored and the nebivolol dose adjusted according to blood pressure response. Use caution when nebivolol is co-administered with CYP2D6 inhibitors).
No products indexed under this heading.

Chloroquine Phosphate (Drugs that inhibit CYP2D6 can be expected to increase plasma levels of nebivolol. When nebivolol is co-administered with an inhibitor of CYP2D6, patients should be closely monitored and the nebivolol dose adjusted according to blood pressure response. Use caution when nebivolol is co-administered with CYP2D6 inhibitors).
No products indexed under this heading.

Chlorpheniramine (Drugs that inhibit CYP2D6 can be expected to increase plasma levels of nebivolol. When nebivolol is co-administered with an inhibitor of CYP2D6, patients should be closely monitored and the nebivolol dose adjusted according to blood pressure response. Use caution when nebivolol is co-administered with CYP2D6 inhibitors).
No products indexed under this heading.

Chlorpheniramine Maleate (Drugs that inhibit CYP2D6 can be expected to increase plasma levels of nebivolol. When nebivolol is co-administered with an inhibitor of CYP2D6, patients should be closely monitored and the nebivolol dose adjusted according to blood pressure response. Use caution when nebivolol is co-administered with CYP2D6 inhibitors).
No products indexed under this heading.

Chlorpheniramine Polistirex (Drugs that inhibit CYP2D6 can be expected to increase plasma levels of nebivolol. When nebivolol is co-administered with

an inhibitor of CYP2D6, patients should be closely monitored and the nebivolol dose adjusted according to blood pressure response. Use caution when nebivolol is co-administered with CYP2D6 inhibitors). Products include:

Chlorpheniramine Tannate (Drugs that inhibit CYP2D6 can be expected to increase plasma levels of nebivolol. When nebivolol is co-administered with an inhibitor of CYP2D6, patients should be closely monitored and the nebivolol dose adjusted according to blood pressure response. Use caution when nebivolol is co-administered with CYP2D6 inhibitors).
No products indexed under this heading.

Chlorpropamide (Beta-blockers may mask some of the manifestations of hypoglycemia, particularly tachycardia. Nonselective beta-blockers may potentiate insulin-induced hypoglycemia and delay recovery of serum glucose levels. It is not known whether nebivolol has these effects. Patients subject to spontaneous hypoglycemia, or diabetic patients receiving insulin or oral hypoglycemic agents, should be advised about these possibilities and nebivolol should be used with caution).
No products indexed under this heading.

Cimetidine (Drugs that inhibit CYP2D6 can be expected to increase plasma levels of nebivolol. When nebivolol is co-administered with an inhibitor of CYP2D6, patients should be closely monitored and the nebivolol dose adjusted according to blood pressure response. Use caution when nebivolol is co-administered with CYP2D6 inhibitors).
No products indexed under this heading.

Cimetidine Hydrochloride (Drugs that inhibit CYP2D6 can be expected to increase plasma levels of nebivolol. When nebivolol is co-administered with an inhibitor of CYP2D6, patients should be closely monitored and the nebivolol dose adjusted according to blood pressure response. Use caution when nebivolol is co-administered with CYP2D6 inhibitors).
No products indexed under this heading.

Citalopram Hydrobromide (Drugs that inhibit CYP2D6 can be expected to increase plasma levels of nebivolol. When nebivolol is co-administered with an inhibitor of CYP2D6, patients should be closely monitored and the nebivolol dose adjusted according to blood pressure response. Use caution when nebivolol is co-administered with CYP2D6 inhibitors). Products include:

Clomipramine Hydrochloride (Drugs that inhibit CYP2D6 can be expected to increase plasma levels of nebivolol. When nebivolol is co-administered with an inhibitor of CYP2D6, patients should be closely monitored and the nebivolol dose adjusted according to blood pressure response. Use caution when nebivolol is co-administered with CYP2D6 inhibitors).
No products indexed under this heading.

Clonidine (In patients who are receiving nebivolol and clonidine, nebivolol should be discontinued for several days before the gradual tapering of clonidine). Products include:

Cocaine Hydrochloride (Drugs that inhibit CYP2D6 can be expected to increase plasma levels of nebivolol. When nebivolol is co-administered with an inhibitor of CYP2D6, patients should be closely monitored and the nebivolol dose adjusted according to blood pressure response. Use caution when nebivolol is co-administered with CYP2D6 inhibitors).
No products indexed under this heading.

Deserpidine (Patients receiving catecholamine-depleting drugs, such as reserpine or guanethidine, should be closely monitored, because the added beta-blocking action of nebivolol may produce excessive reduction of sympathetic activity).
No products indexed under this heading.

Desipramine Hydrochloride (Drugs that inhibit CYP2D6 can be expected to increase plasma levels of nebivolol. When nebivolol is co-administered with an inhibitor of CYP2D6, patients should be closely monitored and the nebivolol dose adjusted according to blood pressure response. Use caution when nebivolol is co-administered with CYP2D6 inhibitors).
No products indexed under this heading.

Deslanoside (Both digitalis glycosides and beta-blockers slow atrioventricular conduction and decrease heart rate. Concomitant use can increase the risk of bradycardia).
No products indexed under this heading.

Digitalis Glycoside Preparations (Both digitalis glycosides and beta-blockers slow atrioventricular conduction and decrease heart rate. Concomitant use can increase the risk of bradycardia).
No products indexed under this heading.

Digitalis Lanata (Both digitalis glycosides and beta-blockers slow atrioventricular conduction and decrease heart rate. Concomitant use can increase the risk of bradycardia).
No products indexed under this heading.

Digitalis Purpurea (Both digitalis glycosides and beta-blockers slow atrioventricular conduction and decrease heart rate. Concomitant use can increase the risk of bradycardia).
No products indexed under this heading.

Digitoxin (Both digitalis glycosides and beta-blockers slow atrioventricular conduction and decrease heart rate. Concomitant use can increase the risk of bradycardia).
No products indexed under this heading.

Digoxin (Both digitalis glycosides and beta-blockers slow atrioventricular conduction and decrease heart rate. Concomitant use can increase the risk of bradycardia). Products include:

Diltiazem Hydrochloride (Because of significant negative inotropic and chronotropic effects in patients treated with beta-blockers and calcium channel blockers of the verapamil and diltiazem type, caution should be used in patients treated concomitantly with these agents and ECGand blood pressure should be monitored. Nebivolol should be used with care when myocardial depressants or inhibitors of AV-conduction, such as certain calcium antagonists (particularly of the phenylalkylamine [verapamil] and benzothiazepine [diltiazem] classes)). Products include:

Diphenhydramine (Drugs that inhibit CYP2D6 can be expected to increase plasma levels of nebivolol. When nebivolol is co-administered with an inhibitor of CYP2D6, patients should be closely monitored and the nebivolol dose adjusted according to blood pressure response. Use caution when nebivolol is co-administered with CYP2D6 inhibitors).
No products indexed under this heading.

Diphenhydramine Hydrochloride (Drugs that inhibit CYP2D6 can be expected to increase plasma levels of nebivolol. When nebivolol is co-administered with an inhibitor of CYP2D6, patients should be closely monitored and the nebivolol dose adjusted according to blood pressure response. Use caution when nebivolol is co-administered with CYP2D6 inhibitors). Products include:

Disopyramide Phosphate (Nebivolol should be used with care when myocardial depressants or inhibitors of AV-conduction, such as antiarrhythmic agents, such as disopyramide, are used concurrently).
No products indexed under this heading.

Dofetilide (Nebivolol should be used with care when myocardial depressants or inhibitors of AV-conduction, such as antiarrhythmic agents, such as disopyramide, are used concurrently).
No products indexed under this heading.

Doxepin Hydrochloride (Drugs that inhibit CYP2D6 can be expected to increase plasma levels of nebivolol. When nebivolol is co-administered with an inhibitor of CYP2D6, patients should be closely monitored and the nebivolol dose adjusted according to blood pressure response. Use caution when nebivolol is co-administered with CYP2D6 inhibitors).
No products indexed under this heading.

Escitalopram Oxalate (Drugs that inhibit CYP2D6 can be expected to increase plasma levels of nebivolol. When nebivolol is co-administered with an inhibitor of CYP2D6, patients should be closely monitored and the nebivolol dose adjusted according to blood pressure response. Use caution when nebivolol is co-administered with CYP2D6 inhibitors). Products include:

Ethanol (When nebivolol is co-administered with an inducer of CYP2D6, patients should be closely monitored and the nebivolol dose adjusted according to blood pressure response).
No products indexed under this heading.

Felodipine (Because of significant negative inotropic and chronotropic effects in patients treated with beta-blockers and calcium channel blockers of the verapamil and diltiazem type, caution should be used in patients treated concomitantly with these agents and ECGand blood pressure should be monitored. Nebivolol should be used with care when myocardial depressants or inhibitors of AV-conduction, such as certain calcium antagonists (particularly of the phenylalkylamine [verapamil] and benzothiazepine [diltiazem] classes)).
No products indexed under this heading.

Flecainide Acetate (Nebivolol should be used with care when myocardial depressants or inhibitors of AV-conduction, such as antiarrhythmic agents, such as disopyramide, are used concurrently).
No products indexed under this heading.

Fluoxetine (Drugs that inhibit CYP2D6 can be expected to increase plasma levels of nebivolol. When nebivolol is co-administered with an inhibitor of CYP2D6, patients should be closely monitored and the nebivolol dose adjusted according to blood pressure response. Use caution when nebivolol is co-administered with CYP2D6 inhibitors).
No products indexed under this heading.

Fluoxetine Hydrochloride (Drugs that inhibit CYP2D6 can be expected to increase plasma levels of nebivolol. When nebivolol is co-administered with an inhibitor of CYP2D6, patients should be closely monitored and the nebivolol dose adjusted according to blood pressure response. Use caution when nebivolol is co-administered with CYP2D6 inhibitors). Products include:
Prozac Weekly **1941**
Prozac Pulvules **1941**
Symbyax **1965**

Fluphenazine Decanoate (Drugs that inhibit CYP2D6 can be expected to increase plasma levels of nebivolol. When nebivolol is co-administered with an inhibitor of CYP2D6, patients should be closely monitored and the nebivolol dose adjusted according to blood pressure response. Use caution when nebivolol is co-administered with CYP2D6 inhibitors).
No products indexed under this heading.

Fluphenazine Enanthate (Drugs that inhibit CYP2D6 can be expected to increase plasma levels of nebivolol. When nebivolol is co-administered with an inhibitor of CYP2D6, patients should be closely monitored and the nebivolol dose adjusted according to blood pressure response. Use caution when nebivolol is co-administered with CYP2D6 inhibitors).
No products indexed under this heading.

Fluphenazine Hydrochloride (Drugs that inhibit CYP2D6 can be expected to increase plasma levels of nebivolol. When nebivolol is co-administered with an inhibitor of CYP2D6, patients should be closely monitored and the nebivolol dose adjusted according to blood pressure response. Use caution when nebivolol is co-administered with CYP2D6 inhibitors).
No products indexed under this heading.

Fluvoxamine Maleate (Drugs that inhibit CYP2D6 can be expected to increase plasma levels of nebivolol. When nebivolol is co-administered with an inhibitor of CYP2D6, patients should be closely monitored and the nebivolol dose adjusted according to blood pressure response. Use caution when nebivolol is co-administered with CYP2D6 inhibitors).
No products indexed under this heading.

Glibenclamide (Beta-blockers may mask some of the manifestations of hypoglycemia, particularly tachycardia. Nonselective beta-blockers may potentiate insulin-induced hypoglycemia and delay recovery of serum glucose levels. It is not known whether nebivolol has these effects. Patients subject to spontaneous hypoglycemia, or diabetic patients receiving insulin or oral hypoglycemic agents, should be advised about these possibilities and nebivolol should be used with caution).
No products indexed under this heading.

Glimepiride (Beta-blockers may mask some of the manifestations of hypoglycemia, particularly tachycardia. Nonselective beta-blockers may potentiate insulin-induced hypoglycemia and delay recovery of serum glucose levels. It is not known whether nebivolol has these effects. Patients subject to spontaneous hypoglycemia, or diabetic patients receiving insulin or oral hypoglycemic agents, should be advised about these possibilities and nebivolol should be used with caution). Products include:
Avandaryl **1356**
Duetact **3354**

Glipizide (Beta-blockers may mask some of the manifestations of hypoglycemia, particularly tachycardia. Nonselective beta-blockers may potentiate insulin-induced hypoglycemia and delay recovery of serum glucose levels. It is not known whether nebivolol has these effects. Patients subject to spontaneous hypoglycemia, or diabetic patients receiving insulin or oral hypoglycemic agents, should be advised about these possibilities and nebivolol should be used with caution).
No products indexed under this heading.

Glyburide (Beta-blockers may mask some of the manifestations of hypoglycemia, particularly tachycardia. Nonselective beta-blockers may potentiate insulin-induced hypoglycemia and delay recovery of serum glucose levels. It is not known whether nebivolol has these effects. Patients subject to spontaneous hypoglycemia, or diabetic patients receiving insulin or oral hypoglycemic agents, should be advised about these possibilities and nebivolol should be used with caution).
No products indexed under this heading.

Guanethidine (Patients receiving catecholamine-depleting drugs, such as reserpine or guanethidine, should be closely monitored, because the added beta-blocking action of nebivolol may produce excessive reduction of sympathetic activity).
No products indexed under this heading.

Guanethidine Monosulfate (Patients receiving catecholamine-depleting drugs, such as reserpine or guanethidine, should be closely monitored, because the added beta-blocking action of nebivolol may produce excessive reduction of sympathetic activity).
No products indexed under this heading.

Guanethidine Sulfate (Patients receiving catecholamine-depleting drugs, such as reserpine or guanethidine, should be closely monitored, because the added beta-blocking action of nebivolol may produce excessive reduction of sympathetic activity).
No products indexed under this heading.

Halofantrine Hydrochloride (Drugs that inhibit CYP2D6 can be expected to increase plasma levels of nebivolol. When nebivolol is co-administered with an inhibitor of CYP2D6, patients should be closely monitored and the nebivolol dose adjusted according to blood pressure response. Use caution when nebivolol is co-administered with CYP2D6 inhibitors).
No products indexed under this heading.

Haloperidol (Drugs that inhibit CYP2D6 can be expected to increase plasma levels of nebivolol. When nebivolol is co-administered with an inhibitor of CYP2D6, patients should be closely monitored and the nebivolol dose adjusted according to blood pressure response. Use caution when nebivolol is co-administered with CYP2D6 inhibitors).
No products indexed under this heading.

Haloperidol Decanoate (Drugs that inhibit CYP2D6 can be expected to increase plasma levels of nebivolol. When nebivolol is co-administered with an inhibitor of CYP2D6, patients should be closely monitored and the nebivolol dose adjusted according to blood pressure response. Use caution when nebivolol is co-administered with CYP2D6 inhibitors).
No products indexed under this heading.

Haloperidol Lactate (Drugs that inhibit CYP2D6 can be expected to increase plasma levels of nebivolol. When nebivolol is co-administered with an inhibitor of CYP2D6, patients should be closely monitored and the nebivolol dose adjusted according to blood pressure response. Use caution when nebivolol is co-administered with CYP2D6 inhibitors).
No products indexed under this heading.

Hydroxychloroquine Sulfate (Drugs that inhibit CYP2D6 can be expected to increase plasma levels of nebivolol. When nebivolol is co-administered with an inhibitor of CYP2D6, patients should be closely monitored and the nebivolol dose adjusted according to blood pressure response. Use caution when nebivolol is co-administered with CYP2D6 inhibitors).
No products indexed under this heading.

Hypericum (When nebivolol is co-administered with an inducer of CYP2D6, patients should be closely monitored and the nebivolol dose adjusted according to blood pressure response).
No products indexed under this heading.

Hypericum Perforatum (When nebivolol is co-administered with an inducer of CYP2D6, patients should be closely monitored and the nebivolol dose adjusted according to blood pressure response). Products include:
Traumeel **1800**

Imatinib Mesylate (Drugs that inhibit CYP2D6 can be expected to increase plasma levels of nebivolol. When nebivolol is co-administered with an inhibitor of CYP2D6, patients should be closely monitored and the nebivolol dose adjusted according to blood pressure response. Use caution when nebivolol is co-administered with CYP2D6 inhibitors). Products include:
Gleevec **2477**

Imipramine Hydrochloride (Drugs that inhibit CYP2D6 can be expected to increase plasma levels of nebivolol. When nebivolol is co-administered with an inhibitor of CYP2D6, patients should be closely monitored and the nebivolol dose adjusted according to blood pressure response. Use caution when nebivolol is co-administered with CYP2D6 inhibitors).
No products indexed under this heading.

Imipramine Pamoate (Drugs that inhibit CYP2D6 can be expected to increase plasma levels of nebivolol. When nebivolol is co-administered with an inhibitor of CYP2D6, patients should be closely monitored and the nebivolol dose adjusted according to blood pressure response. Use caution when nebivolol is co-administered with CYP2D6 inhibitors).
No products indexed under this heading.

Insulin (Beta-blockers may mask some of the manifestations of hypoglycemia, partiuclarly tachycardia. Nonselective beta-blockers may potentiate insulin-induced hypoglycemia and delay recovery of serum glucose levels. It is not known whether nebivolol has these effects. Patients subject to spontaneous hypoglycemia, or diabetic patients receiving insulin or oral hypoglycemic agents, should be advised about these possibilities and nebivolol should be used with caution).
No products indexed under this heading.

Insulin, Human, Zinc Suspension (Beta-blockers may mask some of the manifestations of hypoglycemia, partiuclarly tachycardia. Nonselective beta-blockers may potentiate insulin-induced hypoglycemia and delay recovery of serum glucose levels. It is not known whether nebivolol has these effects. Patients subject to spontaneous hypoglycemia, or diabetic patients receiving insulin or oral hypoglycemic agents, should be advised about these possibilities and nebivolol should be used with caution).
No products indexed under this heading.

Insulin, Human (rDNA origin) (Beta-blockers may mask some of the manifestations of hypoglycemia, partiuclarly tachycardia. Nonselective beta-blockers may potentiate insulin-induced hypoglycemia and delay recovery of serum glucose levels. It is not known whether nebivolol has these effects. Patients subject to spontaneous hypoglycemia, or diabetic patients receiving insulin or oral hypoglycemic agents, should be advised about these possibilities and nebivolol should be used with caution). Products include:
Exubera **2717**

Insulin, Human NPH (Beta-blockers may mask some of the manifestations of hypoglycemia, partiuclarly tachycardia. Nonselective beta-blockers may potentiate insulin-induced hypoglycemia and delay recovery of serum glucose levels. It is not known whether nebivolol has these effects. Patients subject to spontaneous hypoglycemia, or diabetic patients receiving insulin or oral hypoglycemic agents, should be advised about these possibilities and nebivolol should be used with caution). Products include:
Humulin N Vial **1934**

Insulin, Human Regular (Beta-blockers may mask some of the manifestations of hypoglycemia, partiuclarly tachycardia. Nonselective beta-blockers may potentiate insulin-induced hypoglycemia and delay recovery of serum glucose levels. It is not known whether nebivolol has these effects. Patients subject to spontaneous hypoglycemia, or diabetic patients receiving insulin or oral hypoglycemic agents, should be advised about these possibilities and nebivolol should be used with caution). Products include:
Humulin R **1937**
Humulin R (U-500) **1939**

Insulin, Human Regular and Human NPH Mixture (Beta-blockers may mask some of the manifestations of hypoglycemia, partiuclarly tachycardia. Nonselective beta-blockers may potentiate insulin-induced hypoglycemia and delay recovery of serum glucose levels. It is not known whether nebivolol has these effects. Patients subject to spontaneous hypoglycemia, or diabetic patients receiving insulin or oral hypoglycemic agents, should be advised about these possibilities and nebivolol should be used with caution). Products include:
Humulin 50/50 .... **1930**
Humulin 70/30 Vial **1931**

Insulin, NPH (Beta-blockers may mask some of the manifestations of hypoglycemia, partiuclarly tachycardia. Nonselective beta-blockers may potentiate insulin-induced hypoglycemia and delay recovery of serum glucose levels. It is not known whether nebivolol has these effects. Patients subject to spontaneous hypoglycemia, or diabetic patients receiving insulin or oral hypoglycemic agents, should be advised about these possibilities and nebivolol should be used with caution).
No products indexed under this heading.

Insulin, Regular (Beta-blockers may mask some of the manifestations of hypoglycemia, particularly tachycardia. Nonselective beta-blockers may potentiate insulin-induced hypoglycemia and delay recovery of serum glucose levels. It is not known whether nebivolol has these effects. Patients subject to spontaneous hypoglycemia, or diabetic patients receiving insulin or oral hypo-

253 **Interactions Index** **Bystolic**

glycemic agents, should be advised about these possibilities and nebivolol should be used with caution).
No products indexed under this heading.

Insulin, Regular and NPH mixture (Beta-blockers may mask some of the manifestations of hypoglycemia, partiuclarly tachycardia. Nonselective beta-blockers may potentiate insulin-induced hypoglycemia and delay recovery of serum glucose levels. It is not known whether nebivolol has these effects. Patients subject to spontaneous hypoglycemia, or diabetic patients receiving insulin or oral hypoglycemic agents, should be advised about these possibilities and nebivolol should be used with caution).
No products indexed under this heading.

Insulin, Zinc Crystals (Beta-blockers may mask some of the manifestations of hypoglycemia, partiuclarly tachycardia. Nonselective beta-blockers may potentiate insulin-induced hypoglycemia and delay recovery of serum glucose levels. It is not known whether nebivolol has these effects. Patients subject to spontaneous hypoglycemia, or diabetic patients receiving insulin or oral hypoglycemic agents, should be advised about these possibilities and nebivolol should be used with caution).
No products indexed under this heading.

Insulin, Zinc Suspension (Beta-blockers may mask some of the manifestations of hypoglycemia, partiuclarly tachycardia. Nonselective beta-blockers may potentiate insulin-induced hypoglycemia and delay recovery of serum glucose levels. It is not known whether nebivolol has these effects. Patients subject to spontaneous hypoglycemia, or diabetic patients receiving insulin or oral hypoglycemic agents, should be advised about these possibilities and nebivolol should be used with caution).
No products indexed under this heading.

Insulin Aspart (Beta-blockers may mask some of the manifestations of hypoglycemia, partiuclarly tachycardia. Nonselective beta-blockers may potentiate insulin-induced hypoglycemia and delay recovery of serum glucose levels. It is not known whether nebivolol has these effects. Patients subject to spontaneous hypoglycemia, or diabetic patients receiving insulin or oral hypoglycemic agents, should be advised about these possibilities and nebivolol should be used with caution).
No products indexed under this heading.

Insulin Aspart, Human (Beta-blockers may mask some of the manifestations of hypoglycemia, partiuclarly tachycardia. Nonselective beta-blockers may potentiate insulin-induced hypoglycemia and delay recovery of serum glucose levels. It is not known whether nebivolol has these effects. Patients subject to spontaneous hypoglycemia, or diabetic patients receiving insulin or oral hypoglycemic agents, should be advised about these possibilities and nebivolol should be used with caution). Products include:
NovoLog Mix 70/30 2581

Insulin Aspart, Human Regular (Beta-blockers may mask some of the manifestations of hypoglycemia, partiuclarly tachycardia. Nonselective beta-blockers may potentiate insulin-induced hypoglycemia and delay recovery of serum glucose levels. It is not known whether nebivolol has these effects. Patients subject to spontaneous hypoglycemia, or diabetic patients receiving insulin or oral hypoglycemic agents, should be advised about these possibilities and nebivolol should be used with caution). Products include:
NovoLog 2575

Insulin Aspart Protamine, Human (Beta-blockers may mask some of the manifestations of hypoglycemia, partiuclarly tachycardia. Nonselective beta-blockers may potentiate insulin-induced hypoglycemia and delay recovery of serum glucose levels. It is not known whether nebivolol has these effects. Patients subject to spontaneous hypoglycemia, or diabetic patients receiving insulin or oral hypoglycemic agents, should be advised about these possibilities and nebivolol should be used with caution). Products include:
NovoLog Mix 70/30 2581

Insulin Detemir (rDNA Origin) (Beta-blockers may mask some of the manifestations of hypoglycemia, partiuclarly tachycardia. Nonselective beta-blockers may potentiate insulin-induced hypoglycemia and delay recovery of serum glucose levels. It is not known whether nebivolol has these effects. Patients subject to spontaneous hypoglycemia, or diabetic patients receiving insulin or oral hypoglycemic agents, should be advised about these possibilities and nebivolol should be used with caution). Products include:
Levemir 2566

Insulin Glargine (Beta-blockers may mask some of the manifestations of hypoglycemia, partiuclarly tachycardia. Nonselective beta-blockers may potentiate insulin-induced hypoglycemia and delay recovery of serum glucose levels. It is not known whether nebivolol has these effects. Patients subject to spontaneous hypoglycemia, or diabetic patients receiving insulin or oral hypoglycemic agents, should be advised about these possibilities and nebivolol should be used with caution). Products include:
Lantus 2996

Insulin Glulisine (Beta-blockers may mask some of the manifestations of hypoglycemia, partiuclarly tachycardia. Nonselective beta-blockers may potentiate insulin-induced hypoglycemia and delay recovery of serum glucose levels. It is not known whether nebivolol has these effects. Patients subject to spontaneous hypoglycemia, or diabetic patients receiving insulin or oral hypoglycemic agents, should be advised about these possibilities and nebivolol should be used with caution). Products include:
Apidra 2937
Apidra SoloStar 2937

Insulin Lispro, Human (Beta-blockers may mask some of the manifestations of hypoglycemia, partiuclarly tachycardia. Nonselective beta-blockers may potentiate insulin-induced hypoglycemia and delay recovery of serum glucose levels. It is not known whether nebivolol has these effects. Patients subject to spontaneous hypoglycemia, or diabetic patients receiving insulin or oral hypoglycemic agents, should be advised about these possibilities and nebivolol should be used with caution). Products include:
Humalog 1910
Humalog Mix 1914
Humalog Mix75/25 1917

Insulin Lispro Protamine, Human (Beta-blockers may mask some of the manifestations of hypoglycemia, partiuclarly tachycardia. Nonselective beta-blockers may potentiate insulin-induced hypoglycemia and delay recovery of serum glucose levels. It is not known whether nebivolol has these effects. Patients subject to spontaneous hypoglycemia, or diabetic patients receiving insulin or oral hypoglycemic agents, should be advised about these possibilities and nebivolol should be used with caution). Products include:
Humalog Mix 1914
Humalog Mix75/25 1917

Isradipine (Because of significant negative inotropic and chronotropic effects in patients treated with beta-blockers and calcium channel blockers of the verapamil and diltiazem type, caution should be used in patients treated concomitantly with these agents and ECGand blood pressure should be monitored. Nebivolol should be used with care when myocardial depressants or inhibitors of AV-conduction, such as certain calcium antagonists (particularly of the phenylalkylamine [verapamil] and benzothiazepine [diltiazem] classes)). Products include:
DynaCirc CR 1432

Lidocaine Hydrochloride (Nebivolol should be used with care when myocardial depressants or inhibitors of AV-conduction, such as antiarrhythmic agents, such as disopyramide, are used concurrently).
No products indexed under this heading.

Maprotiline Hydrochloride (Drugs that inhibit CYP2D6 can be expected to increase plasma levels of nebivolol. When nebivolol is co-administered with an inhibitor of CYP2D6, patients should be closely monitored and the nebivolol dose adjusted according to blood pressure response. Use caution when nebivolol is co-administered with CYP2D6 inhibitors).
No products indexed under this heading.

Metformin Hydrochloride (Beta-blockers may mask some of the manifestations of hypoglycemia, particularly tachycardia. Nonselective beta-blockers may potentiate insulin-induced hypoglycemia and delay recovery of serum glucose levels. It is not known whether nebivolol has these effects. Patients subject to spontaneous hypoglycemia, or diabetic patients receiving insulin or oral hypoglycemic agents, should be advised about these possibilities and nebivolol should be used with caution). Products include:
ActoPlus 3338
Avandamet 1345
Janumet 2188

Methadone Hydrochloride (Drugs that inhibit CYP2D6 can be expected to increase plasma levels of nebivolol. When nebivolol is co-administered with an inhibitor of CYP2D6, patients should be closely monitored and the nebivolol dose adjusted according to blood pressure response. Use caution when nebivolol is co-administered with CYP2D6 inhibitors).
No products indexed under this heading.

Mexiletine Hydrochloride (Nebivolol should be used with care when myocardial depressants or inhibitors of AV-conduction, such as antiarrhythmic agents, such as disopyramide, are used concurrently).
No products indexed under this heading.

Mibefradil Dihydrochloride (Because of significant negative inotropic and chronotropic effects in patients treated with beta-blockers and calcium channel blockers of the verapamil and diltiazem type, caution should be used in patients treated concomitantly with these agents and ECGand blood pressure should be monitored. Nebivolol should be used with care when myocardial depressants or inhibitors of AV-conduction, such as certain calcium antagonists (particularly of the phenylalkylamine [verapamil] and benzothiazepine [diltiazem] classes)).
No products indexed under this heading.

Miglitol (Beta-blockers may mask some of the manifestations of hypoglycemia, particularly tachycardia. Nonselective beta-blockers may potentiate insulin-induced hypoglycemia and delay recovery of serum glucose levels. It is not known whether nebivolol has these effects. Patients subject to spontaneous hypoglycemia, or diabetic patients receiving insulin or oral hypoglycemic agents, should be advised about these possibilities and nebivolol should be used with caution).
No products indexed under this heading.

Moclobemide (Drugs that inhibit CYP2D6 can be expected to increase plasma levels of nebivolol. When nebivolol is co-administered with an inhibitor of CYP2D6, patients should be closely monitored and the nebivolol dose adjusted according to blood pressure response. Use caution when nebivolol is co-administered with CYP2D6 inhibitors).
No products indexed under this heading.

Moricizine Hydrochloride (Nebivolol should be used with care when myocardial depressants or inhibitors of AV-conduction, such as antiarrhythmic agents, such as disopyramide, are used concurrently).
No products indexed under this heading.

Nateglinide (Beta-blockers may mask some of the manifestations of hypoglycemia, particularly tachycardia. Nonselective beta-blockers may potentiate insulin-induced hypoglycemia and delay recovery of serum glucose levels. It is not known whether nebivolol has these effects. Patients subject to spontaneous hypoglycemia, or diabetic patients receiving insulin or oral hypoglycemic agents, should be advised about these possibilities and nebivolol should be used with caution).
No products indexed under this heading.

Nicardipine (Because of significant negative inotropic and chronotropic effects in patients treated with beta-blockers and calcium channel blockers of the verapamil and diltiazem type, caution should be used in patients treated concomitantly with these agents and ECGand blood pressure should be monitored. Nebivolol should be used with care when myocardial depressants or inhibitors of AV-conduction, such as certain calcium antagonists (particularly of the phenylalkylamine [verapamil] and benzothiazepine [diltiazem] classes)).
No products indexed under this heading.

Nicardipine Hydrochloride (Because of significant negative inotropic and chronotropic effects in patients treated with beta-blockers and calcium channel blockers of the verapamil and diltiazem type, caution should be used in patients treated concomitantly with these agents and ECGand blood pressure should be monitored. Nebivolol should be used with care when myocardial depressants or inhibitors of AV-conduction, such as certain calcium antagonists (particularly of the phenylalkylamine [verapamil] and benzothiazepine [diltiazem] classes)).
No products indexed under this heading.

Nifedipine (Because of significant negative inotropic and chronotropic effects in patients treated with beta-blockers and calcium channel blockers of the verapamil and diltiazem type, caution should be used in patients treated concomitantly with these agents and ECGand blood pressure should be monitored. Nebivolol should be used with care when myocardial depressants or inhibitors of AV-conduction, such as certain calcium antagonists (particularly of the phenylalkylamine [verapamil] and benzothiazepine [diltiazem] classes)).
No products indexed under this heading.

Nimodipine (Because of significant negative inotropic and chronotropic effects in patients treated with beta-blockers and calcium channel blockers of the verapamil and diltiazem type, caution should be used in patients treat-

IMPORTANT NOTE: Always consult each drug listing in the patient's regimen for possible interactions.

Bystolic Interactions Index 254

ed concomitantly with these agents and ECGand blood pressure should be monitored. Nebivolol should be used with care when myocardial depressants or inhibitors of AV-conduction, such as certain calcium antagonists (particularly of the phenylalkylamine [verapamil] and benzothiazepine [diltiazem] classes)).
No products indexed under this heading.

Nisoldipine (Because of significant negative inotropic and chronotropic effects in patients treated with beta-blockers and calcium channel blockers of the verapamil and diltiazem type, caution should be used in patients treated concomitantly with these agents and ECGand blood pressure should be monitored. Nebivolol should be used with care when myocardial depressants or inhibitors of AV-conduction, such as certain calcium antagonists (particularly of the phenylalkylamine [verapamil] and benzothiazepine [diltiazem] classes)).
No products indexed under this heading.

Nortriptyline Hydrochloride (Drugs that inhibit CYP2D6 can be expected to increase plasma levels of nebivolol. When nebivolol is co-administered with an inhibitor of CYP2D6, patients should be closely monitored and the nebivolol dose adjusted according to blood pressure response. Use caution when nebivolol is co-administered with CYP2D6 inhibitors).
No products indexed under this heading.

Paroxetine Hydrochloride (Drugs that inhibit CYP2D6 can be expected to increase plasma levels of nebivolol. When nebivolol is co-administered with an inhibitor of CYP2D6, patients should be closely monitored and the nebivolol dose adjusted according to blood pressure response. Use caution when nebivolol is co-administered with CYP2D6 inhibitors). Products include:
Paroxetine CR ... **2361**
Paroxetine ER ... **2371**
Paxil ... **1586**
Paxil CR ... **1596**

Perphenazine (Drugs that inhibit CYP2D6 can be expected to increase plasma levels of nebivolol. When nebivolol is co-administered with an inhibitor of CYP2D6, patients should be closely monitored and the nebivolol dose adjusted according to blood pressure response. Use caution when nebivolol is co-administered with CYP2D6 inhibitors).
No products indexed under this heading.

Phenobarbital (When nebivolol is co-administered with an inducer of CYP2D6, patients should be closely monitored and the nebivolol dose adjusted according to blood pressure response). Products include:
Donnatal ... **2711**

Phenobarbital Sodium (When nebivolol is co-administered with an inducer of CYP2D6, patients should be closely monitored and the nebivolol dose adjusted according to blood pressure response).
No products indexed under this heading.

Phenytoin (When nebivolol is co-administered with an inducer of CYP2D6, patients should be closely monitored and the nebivolol dose adjusted according to blood pressure response).
No products indexed under this heading.

Phenytoin Sodium (When nebivolol is co-administered with an inducer of CYP2D6, patients should be closely monitored and the nebivolol dose adjusted according to blood pressure response). Products include:
Phenytek Capsules ... **2380**

Pioglitazone Hydrochloride (Beta-blockers may mask some of the manifestations of hypoglycemia, particularly tachycardia. Nonselective beta-blockers may potentiate insulin-induced hypoglycemia and delay recovery of serum glucose levels. It is not known whether nebivolol has these effects. Patients subject to spontaneous hypoglycemia, or diabetic patients receiving insulin or oral hypoglycemic agents, should be advised about these possibilities and nebivolol should be used with caution). Products include:
ActoPlus ... **3338**
Actos ... **3345**
Duetact ... **3354**

Primidone (When nebivolol is co-administered with an inducer of CYP2D6, patients should be closely monitored and the nebivolol dose adjusted according to blood pressure response).
No products indexed under this heading.

Procainamide Hydrochloride (Nebivolol should be used with care when myocardial depressants or inhibitors of AV-conduction, such as antiarrhythmic agents, such as disopyramide, are used concurrently).
No products indexed under this heading.

Propafenone Hydrochloride (Nebivolol should be used with care when myocardial depressants or inhibitors of AV-conduction, such as antiarrhythmic agents, such as disopyramide, are used concurrently). Products include:
Rythmol ... **1648**
Rythmol SR ... **1652**

Propoxyphene Hydrochloride (Drugs that inhibit CYP2D6 can be expected to increase plasma levels of nebivolol. When nebivolol is co-administered with an inhibitor of CYP2D6, patients should be closely monitored and the nebivolol dose adjusted according to blood pressure response. Use caution when nebivolol is co-administered with CYP2D6 inhibitors).
No products indexed under this heading.

Propoxyphene Napsylate (Drugs that inhibit CYP2D6 can be expected to increase plasma levels of nebivolol. When nebivolol is co-administered with an inhibitor of CYP2D6, patients should be closely monitored and the nebivolol dose adjusted according to blood pressure response. Use caution when nebivolol is co-administered with CYP2D6 inhibitors).
No products indexed under this heading.

Propranolol Hydrochloride (Nebivolol should be used with care when myocardial depressants or inhibitors of AV-conduction, such as antiarrhythmic agents, such as disopyramide, are used concurrently). Products include:
InnoPran XL ... **1517**

Protriptyline Hydrochloride (Drugs that inhibit CYP2D6 can be expected to increase plasma levels of nebivolol. When nebivolol is co-administered with an inhibitor of CYP2D6, patients should be closely monitored and the nebivolol dose adjusted according to blood pressure response. Use caution when nebivolol is co-administered with CYP2D6 inhibitors).
No products indexed under this heading.

Quinacrine Hydrochloride (Drugs that inhibit CYP2D6 can be expected to increase plasma levels of nebivolol. When nebivolol is co-administered with an inhibitor of CYP2D6, patients should be closely monitored and the nebivolol dose adjusted according to blood pressure response. Use caution when nebivolol is co-administered with CYP2D6 inhibitors).
No products indexed under this heading.

Quinidine (Drugs that inhibit CYP2D6 can be expected to increase plasma levels of nebivolol. When nebivolol is co-administered with an inhibitor of CYP2D6, patients should be closely monitored and the nebivolol dose adjusted according to blood pressure response. Use caution when nebivolol is co-administered with CYP2D6 inhibitors).
No products indexed under this heading.

Quinidine Gluconate (Nebivolol should be used with care when myocardial depressants or inhibitors of AV-conduction, such as antiarrhythmic agents, such as disopyramide, are used concurrently).
No products indexed under this heading.

Quinidine Hydrochloride (Drugs that inhibit CYP2D6 can be expected to increase plasma levels of nebivolol. When nebivolol is co-administered with an inhibitor of CYP2D6, patients should be closely monitored and the nebivolol dose adjusted according to blood pressure response. Use caution when nebivolol is co-administered with CYP2D6 inhibitors).
No products indexed under this heading.

Quinidine Polygalacturonate (Nebivolol should be used with care when myocardial depressants or inhibitors of AV-conduction, such as antiarrhythmic agents, such as disopyramide, are used concurrently).
No products indexed under this heading.

Quinidine Sulfate (Nebivolol should be used with care when myocardial depressants or inhibitors of AV-conduction, such as antiarrhythmic agents, such as disopyramide, are used concurrently).
No products indexed under this heading.

Ranitidine Bismuth Citrate (Drugs that inhibit CYP2D6 can be expected to increase plasma levels of nebivolol. When nebivolol is co-administered with an inhibitor of CYP2D6, patients should be closely monitored and the nebivolol dose adjusted according to blood pressure response. Use caution when nebivolol is co-administered with CYP2D6 inhibitors).
No products indexed under this heading.

Ranitidine Hydrochloride (Drugs that inhibit CYP2D6 can be expected to increase plasma levels of nebivolol. When nebivolol is co-administered with an inhibitor of CYP2D6, patients should be closely monitored and the nebivolol dose adjusted according to blood pressure response. Use caution when nebivolol is co-administered with CYP2D6 inhibitors). Products include:
Zantac ... **1737**
Zantac Injection ... **1732**
Zantac Pharmacy ... **1735**

Rauwolfia Serpentina (Patients receiving catecholamine-depleting drugs, such as reserpine or guanethidine, should be closely monitored, because the added beta-blocking action of nebivolol may produce excessive reduction of sympathetic activity).
No products indexed under this heading.

Repaglinide (Beta-blockers may mask some of the manifestations of hypoglycemia, particularly tachycardia. Nonselective beta-blockers may potentiate insulin-induced hypoglycemia and delay recovery of serum glucose levels. It is not known whether nebivolol has these effects. Patients subject to spontaneous hypoglycemia, or diabetic patients receiving insulin or oral hypoglycemic agents, should be advised about these possibilities and nebivolol should be used with caution).
No products indexed under this heading.

Rescinnamine (Patients receiving catecholamine-depleting drugs, such as reserpine or guanethidine, should be closely monitored, because the added beta-blocking action of nebivolol may produce excessive reduction of sympathetic activity).
No products indexed under this heading.

Reserpine (Patients receiving catecholamine-depleting drugs, such as reserpine or guanethidine, should be closely monitored, because the added beta-blocking action of nebivolol may produce excessive reduction of sympathetic activity).
No products indexed under this heading.

Rifampin (When nebivolol is co-administered with an inducer of CYP2D6, patients should be closely monitored and the nebivolol dose adjusted according to blood pressure response).
No products indexed under this heading.

Ritonavir (Drugs that inhibit CYP2D6 can be expected to increase plasma levels of nebivolol. When nebivolol is co-administered with an inhibitor of CYP2D6, patients should be closely monitored and the nebivolol dose adjusted according to blood pressure response. Use caution when nebivolol is co-administered with CYP2D6 inhibitors). Products include:
Kaletra ... **458**
Norvir ... **509**

Rosiglitazone Maleate (Beta-blockers may mask some of the manifestations of hypoglycemia, particularly tachycardia. Nonselective beta-blockers may potentiate insulin-induced hypoglycemia and delay recovery of serum glucose levels. It is not known whether nebivolol has these effects. Patients subject to spontaneous hypoglycemia, or diabetic patients receiving insulin or oral hypoglycemic agents, should be advised about these possibilities and nebivolol should be used with caution). Products include:
Avandamet ... **1345**
Avandaryl ... **1356**
Avandia ... **1366**

Sertraline Hydrochloride (Drugs that inhibit CYP2D6 can be expected to increase plasma levels of nebivolol. When nebivolol is co-administered with an inhibitor of CYP2D6, patients should be closely monitored and the nebivolol dose adjusted according to blood pressure response. Use caution when nebivolol is co-administered with CYP2D6 inhibitors).
No products indexed under this heading.

Sildenafil Citrate (The co-administration of nebivolol and sildenafil decreased AUC and C_{max} of sildenafil by 21 and 23%, respectively. The effect on the C_{max} and AUC for d-nebivolol was also small (less than 20%). The effect on vital signs (eg, pulse and blood pressure) was approximately the sum of the effects of sildenafil and nebivolol).
No products indexed under this heading.

Sitagliptin Phosphate (Beta-blockers may mask some of the manifestations of hypoglycemia, particularly tachycardia. Nonselective beta-blockers may potentiate insulin-induced hypoglycemia and delay recovery of serum glucose levels. It is not known whether nebivolol has these effects. Patients subject to spontaneous hypoglycemia, or diabetic patients receiving insulin or oral hypoglycemic agents, should be advised about these possibilities and nebivolol should be used with caution). Products include:
Janumet ... **2188**
Januvia ... **2196**

(⊙ Described in PDR® for Ophthalmic Medicines)

255 Interactions Index Campral

Sotalol Hydrochloride (Nebivolol should be used with care when myocardial depressants or inhibitors of AV-conduction, such as antiarrhythmic agents, such as disopyramide, are used concurrently).
No products indexed under this heading.

Terbinafine Hydrochloride (Drugs that inhibit CYP2D6 can be expected to increase plasma levels of nebivolol. When nebivolol is co-administered with an inhibitor of CYP2D6, patients should be closely monitored and the nebivolol dose adjusted according to blood pressure response. Use caution when nebivolol is co-administered with CYP2D6 inhibitors).
No products indexed under this heading.

Thioridazine Hydrochloride (Drugs that inhibit CYP2D6 can be expected to increase plasma levels of nebivolol. When nebivolol is co-administered with an inhibitor of CYP2D6, patients should be closely monitored and the nebivolol dose adjusted according to blood pressure response. Use caution when nebivolol is co-administered with CYP2D6 inhibitors). Products include:
Thioridazine Hydrochloride 2384

Tocainide Hydrochloride (Nebivolol should be used with care when myocardial depressants or inhibitors of AV-conduction, such as antiarrhythmic agents, such as disopyramide, are used concurrently).
No products indexed under this heading.

Tolazamide (Beta-blockers may mask some of the manifestations of hypoglycemia, particularly tachycardia. Nonselective beta-blockers may potentiate insulin-induced hypoglycemia and delay recovery of serum glucose levels. It is not known whether nebivolol has these effects. Patients subject to spontaneous hypoglycemia, or diabetic patients receiving insulin or oral hypoglycemic agents, should be advised about these possibilities and nebivolol should be used with caution).
No products indexed under this heading.

Tolbutamide (Beta-blockers may mask some of the manifestations of hypoglycemia, particularly tachycardia. Nonselective beta-blockers may potentiate insulin-induced hypoglycemia and delay recovery of serum glucose levels. It is not known whether nebivolol has these effects. Patients subject to spontaneous hypoglycemia, or diabetic patients receiving insulin or oral hypoglycemic agents, should be advised about these possibilities and nebivolol should be used with caution).
No products indexed under this heading.

Trimipramine Maleate (Drugs that inhibit CYP2D6 can be expected to increase plasma levels of nebivolol. When nebivolol is co-administered with an inhibitor of CYP2D6, patients should be closely monitored and the nebivolol dose adjusted according to blood pressure response. Use caution when nebivolol is co-administered with CYP2D6 inhibitors).
No products indexed under this heading.

Troglitazone (Beta-blockers may mask some of the manifestations of hypoglycemia, particularly tachycardia. Nonselective beta-blockers may potentiate insulin-induced hypoglycemia and delay recovery of serum glucose levels. It is not known whether nebivolol has these effects. Patients subject to spontaneous hypoglycemia, or diabetic patients receiving insulin or oral hypoglycemic agents, should be advised about these possibilities and nebivolol should be used with caution).
No products indexed under this heading.

Vardenafil Hydrochloride (Drugs that inhibit CYP2D6 can be expected to increase plasma levels of nebivolol. When nebivolol is co-administered with an inhibitor of CYP2D6, patients should be closely monitored and the nebivolol dose adjusted according to blood pressure response. Use caution when nebivolol is co-administered with CYP2D6 inhibitors). Products include:
Levitra 3157

Verapamil Hydrochloride (Because of significant negative inotropic and chronotropic effects in patients treated with beta-blockers and calcium channel blockers of the verapamil and diltiazem type, caution should be used in patients treated concomitantly with these agents and ECGand blood pressure should be monitored. Nebivolol should be used with care when myocardial depressants or inhibitors of AV-conduction, such as certain calcium antagonists (particularly of the phenylalkylamine [verapamil] and benzothiazepine [diltiazem] classes)). Products include:
Tarka 534

CALCIJEX INJECTION

(Calcitriol) 422

Magnesium Carbonate (Co-administration with magnesium-containing antacids may lead to the development of hypermagnesemia; concurrent use should be avoided).
No products indexed under this heading.

Magnesium Hydroxide (Co-administration with magnesium-containing antacids may lead to the development of hypermagnesemia; concurrent use should be avoided). Products include:
Fleet Pedia-Lax Chewable Tablets 1144
Pepcid Complete 1822

Vitamin D (Since calcitriol is the most potent metabolite of vitamin D available, vitamin D and its derivatives should be withheld during treatment). Products include:
Active Calcium 3476
BoneMate Plus 3454
Cardio Basics 3455
Norwegian Cod Liver Oil 919

CAMPRAL TABLETS

(Acamprosate Calcium) 1150
May interact with antidepressant drugs, and certain other agents. Compounds in these categories include:

Amitriptyline Hydrochloride (Patients taking acaprosate calcium concomitantly with antidepressants more commonly reported both weight gain and weight loss, compared with patients taking either medication alone).
No products indexed under this heading.

Amoxapine (Patients taking acaprosate calcium concomitantly with antidepressants more commonly reported both weight gain and weight loss, compared with patients taking either medication alone).
No products indexed under this heading.

Bupropion Hydrochloride (Patients taking acaprosate calcium concomitantly with antidepressants more commonly reported both weight gain and weight loss, compared with patients taking either medication alone). Products include:
Aplenzin 2948
Wellbutrin 1719
Wellbutrin SR 1725
Zyban 1762

Citalopram Hydrobromide (Patients taking acaprosate calcium concomitantly with antidepressants more commonly reported both weight gain and weight loss, compared with patients taking either medication alone). Products include:
Celexa 1153

Desipramine Hydrochloride (Patients taking acaprosate calcium concomitantly with antidepressants more commonly reported both weight gain and weight loss, compared with patients taking either medication alone).
No products indexed under this heading.

Doxepin Hydrochloride (Patients taking acaprosate calcium concomitantly with antidepressants more commonly reported both weight gain and weight loss, compared with patients taking either medication alone).
No products indexed under this heading.

Escitalopram Oxalate (Patients taking acaprosate calcium concomitantly with antidepressants more commonly reported both weight gain and weight loss, compared with patients taking either medication alone). Products include:
Lexapro Oral Suspension 1160
Lexapro Tablets 1160

Fluoxetine Hydrochloride (Patients taking acaprosate calcium concomitantly with antidepressants more commonly reported both weight gain and weight loss, compared with patients taking either medication alone). Products include:
Prozac Weekly 1941
Prozac Pulvules 1941
Symbyax 1965

Fluvoxamine (Patients taking acaprosate calcium concomitantly with antidepressants more commonly reported both weight gain and weight loss, compared with patients taking either medication alone).
No products indexed under this heading.

Fluvoxamine Maleate (Patients taking acaprosate calcium concomitantly with antidepressants more commonly reported both weight gain and weight loss, compared with patients taking either medication alone).
No products indexed under this heading.

Imipramine Hydrochloride (Patients taking acaprosate calcium concomitantly with antidepressants more commonly reported both weight gain and weight loss, compared with patients taking either medication alone).
No products indexed under this heading.

Imipramine Pamoate (Patients taking acaprosate calcium concomitantly with antidepressants more commonly reported both weight gain and weight loss, compared with patients taking either medication alone).
No products indexed under this heading.

Isocarboxazid (Patients taking acaprosate calcium concomitantly with antidepressants more commonly reported both weight gain and weight loss, compared with patients taking either medication alone). Products include:
Marplan 3481

Maprotiline Hydrochloride (Patients taking acaprosate calcium concomitantly with antidepressants more commonly reported both weight gain and weight loss, compared with patients taking either medication alone).
No products indexed under this heading.

Mirtazapine (Patients taking acaprosate calcium concomitantly with antidepressants more commonly reported both weight gain and weight loss, compared with patients taking either medication alone). Products include:
Remeron Tablets 3214
RemeronSolTab Tablets 3219

Naltrexone Hydrochloride (Co-administration of naltrexone with acamprosate calcium produced a 25% increase in AUC and a 33% increase in the C_{max} of acamprosate. No adjustment of dosage is recommended in such patients). Products include:
Embeda 1831

Nefazodone Hydrochloride (Patients taking acaprosate calcium concomitantly with antidepressants more commonly reported both weight gain and weight loss, compared with patients taking either medication alone).
No products indexed under this heading.

Nortriptyline Hydrochloride (Patients taking acaprosate calcium concomitantly with antidepressants more commonly reported both weight gain and weight loss, compared with patients taking either medication alone).
No products indexed under this heading.

Paroxetine (Patients taking acaprosate calcium concomitantly with antidepressants more commonly reported both weight gain and weight loss, compared with patients taking either medication alone).
No products indexed under this heading.

Paroxetine Hydrochloride (Patients taking acaprosate calcium concomitantly with antidepressants more commonly reported both weight gain and weight loss, compared with patients taking either medication alone). Products include:
Paroxetine CR 2361
Paroxetine ER 2371
Paxil 1586
Paxil CR 1596

Paroxetine Mesylate (Patients taking acaprosate calcium concomitantly with antidepressants more commonly reported both weight gain and weight loss, compared with patients taking either medication alone).
No products indexed under this heading.

Phenelzine Sulfate (Patients taking acaprosate calcium concomitantly with antidepressants more commonly reported both weight gain and weight loss, compared with patients taking either medication alone).
No products indexed under this heading.

Protriptyline Hydrochloride (Patients taking acaprosate calcium concomitantly with antidepressants more commonly reported both weight gain and weight loss, compared with patients taking either medication alone).
No products indexed under this heading.

Selegiline (Patients taking acaprosate calcium concomitantly with antidepressants more commonly reported both weight gain and weight loss, compared with patients taking either medication alone). Products include:
Emsam 3623

Selegiline Hydrochloride (Patients taking acaprosate calcium concomitantly with antidepressants more commonly reported both weight gain and weight loss, compared with patients taking either medication alone). Products include:
Eldepryl 3312

Sertraline Hydrochloride (Patients taking acaprosate calcium concomitantly with antidepressants more commonly reported both weight gain and weight loss, compared with patients taking either medication alone).
No products indexed under this heading.

Tranylcypromine Sulfate (Patients taking acaprosate calcium concomitantly with antidepressants more commonly reported both weight gain and weight loss, compared with patients taking either medication alone). Products include:
Parnate 1584

Trazodone Hydrochloride (Patients taking acaprosate calcium concomitantly with antidepressants more commonly reported both weight gain and weight loss, compared with patients taking either medication alone).
No products indexed under this heading.

IMPORTANT NOTE: Always consult each drug listing in the patient's regimen for possible interactions.

(☉ Described in PDR® for Ophthalmic Medicines)

CAPTOPRIL TABLETS

(Captopril) 2341
May interact with agents causing renin release, beta-blockers, diuretics, ganglionic blocking agents, inhibitors of endogenous prostaglandin synthesis, lithium preparations, nitrates and nitrites, non-steroidal anti-inflammatory agents, peripheral adrenergic blockers, potassium preparations, potassium sparing diuretics, thiazides, vasodilators, and certain other agents. Compounds in these categories include:

Acebutolol Hydrochloride (Less than additive antihypertensive effect).
No products indexed under this heading.

Alfuzosin Hydrochloride (Use with caution). Products include:
Uroxatral 3050

Amiloride Hydrochloride (Hypotension; increased serum potassium).
No products indexed under this heading.

Amyl Nitrite (Discontinue before starting captopril; if resumed administer at lower dosage).
No products indexed under this heading.

Aspirin (Antihypertensive effects of captopril reduced). Products include:
Aggrenox 880
Bayer Aspirin 829
Percodan 1124
St. Joseph Aspirin 2045

Atenolol (Less than additive antihypertensive effect).
No products indexed under this heading.

Bendroflumethiazide (Captopril's effect will be augmented).
No products indexed under this heading.

Betaxolol Hydrochloride (Less than additive antihypertensive effect).
No products indexed under this heading.

Bisabolol (Use with caution).
No products indexed under this heading.

Bisoprolol Fumarate (Less than additive antihypertensive effect).
No products indexed under this heading.

Bumetanide (Captopril's effect will be augmented; hypotension).
No products indexed under this heading.

Carteolol Hydrochloride (Less than additive antihypertensive effect).
No products indexed under this heading.

Carvedilol (Less than additive antihypertensive effect). Products include:
Coreg 1409

Carvedilol Phosphate (Less than additive antihypertensive effect). Products include:
Coreg CR 1416

Celecoxib (Antihypertensive effects of captopril reduced). Products include:
Celebrex 3272

Chlorothiazide (Captopril's effect will be augmented).
No products indexed under this heading.

Chlorothiazide Sodium (Captopril's effect will be augmented). Products include:
Diuril Intravenous 2009

Chlorthalidone (Captopril's effect will be augmented; hypotension; increased serum potassium). Products include:
Clorpres 2344

Diazoxide (Drugs having vasodilator activity should, if possible, be discontinued before starting captopril). Products include:
Proglycem 1179
Proglycem Suspension 1179

Diclofenac Epolamine (Antihypertensive effects of captopril reduced). Products include:
Flector 1839

Diclofenac Potassium (Antihypertensive effects of captopril reduced).
No products indexed under this heading.

Diclofenac Sodium (Antihypertensive effects of captopril reduced).
No products indexed under this heading.

Doxazosin Mesylate (Use with caution).
No products indexed under this heading.

Epoprostenol Sodium (Drugs having vasodilator activity should, if possible, be discontinued before starting captopril). Products include:
Flolan 1453

Erythrityl Tetranitrate (Discontinue before starting captopril; if resumed administer at lower dosage).
No products indexed under this heading.

Esmolol Hydrochloride (Less than additive antihypertensive effect).
No products indexed under this heading.

Ethacrynic Acid (Captopril's effect will be augmented; hypotension).
No products indexed under this heading.

Ethaverine Hydrochloride (Drugs having vasodilator activity should, if possible, be discontinued before starting captopril).
No products indexed under this heading.

Etodolac (Antihypertensive effects of captopril reduced).
No products indexed under this heading.

Fenoprofen Calcium (Antihypertensive effects of captopril reduced).
No products indexed under this heading.

Flurbiprofen (Antihypertensive effects of captopril reduced).
No products indexed under this heading.

Furosemide (Captopril's effect will be augmented; hypotension). Products include:
Furosemide 2354

Glyceryl Trinitrate (Discontinue before starting captopril; if resumed administer at lower dosage).
No products indexed under this heading.

Hydralazine Hydrochloride (Drugs having vasodilator activity should, if possible, be discontinued before starting captopril).
No products indexed under this heading.

Hydrochlorothiazide (Captopril's effect will be augmented). Products include:
Atacand HCT 700
Avalide 2956
Benicar HCT 1017
Diovan HCT 2419
Dyazide 1429
Exforge HCT 2449
Hyzaar 2162
Hyzaar 100-12.5 2162
Micardis HCT 889
Prinzide 2246
Tekturna HCT 2541
Teveten HCT 541

Hydroflumethiazide (Captopril's effect will be augmented).
No products indexed under this heading.

Ibuprofen (Antihypertensive effects of captopril reduced). Products include:
Motrin IB 2043
Children's Motrin 2044
Children's Motrin Non-Staining
Dye-Free 2044
Infants' Motrin 2044
Infants' Motrin Dye-Free 2044
Junior Strength Motrin 2044
Vicoprofen 564

Indapamide (Captopril's effect will be augmented; hypotension). Products include:
Indapamide 2356

Indomethacin (Antihypertensive effects of captopril reduced). Products include:
Indocin 2167

Indomethacin Sodium Trihydrate (Antihypertensive effects of captopril reduced). Products include:
Indocin I.V. 2007

Isosorbide Dinitrate (Discontinue before starting captopril; if resumed administer at lower dosage).
No products indexed under this heading.

Isosorbide Mononitrate (Discontinue before starting captopril; if resumed administer at lower dosage).
No products indexed under this heading.

Isoxsuprine Hydrochloride (Drugs having vasodilator activity should, if possible, be discontinued before starting captopril).
No products indexed under this heading.

Ketoprofen (Antihypertensive effects of captopril reduced).
No products indexed under this heading.

Ketorolac Tromethamine (Antihypertensive effects of captopril reduced). Products include:
Acuvail .... ☉209

Labetalol Hydrochloride (Less than additive antihypertensive effect).
No products indexed under this heading.

Levobetaxolol Hydrochloride (Use with caution).
No products indexed under this heading.

Levobunolol Hydrochloride (Less than additive antihypertensive effect).
No products indexed under this heading.

Lithium (Increased serum lithium levels and symptoms of lithium toxicity).
No products indexed under this heading.

Lithium Carbonate (Increased serum lithium levels and symptoms of lithium toxicity).
No products indexed under this heading.

Lithium Citrate (Increased serum lithium levels and symptoms of lithium toxicity).
No products indexed under this heading.

Mecamylamine Hydrochloride (Use with caution).
No products indexed under this heading.

Meclofenamate Sodium (Antihypertensive effects of captopril reduced).
No products indexed under this heading.

Mefenamic Acid (Antihypertensive effects of captopril reduced).
No products indexed under this heading.

Meloxicam (Antihypertensive effects of captopril reduced).
No products indexed under this heading.

Methyclothiazide (Captopril's effect will be augmented).
No products indexed under this heading.

Metipranolol (Use with caution). Products include:
Optipranolol .... ☉249

Metipranolol Hydrochloride (Less than additive antihypertensive effect).
No products indexed under this heading.

Metolazone (Captopril's effect will be augmented; hypotension).
No products indexed under this heading.

Metoprolol Succinate (Less than additive antihypertensive effect). Products include:
Toprol XL 732

Metoprolol Tartrate (Less than additive antihypertensive effect).
No products indexed under this heading.

Minoxidil (Drugs having vasodilator activity should, if possible, be discontinued before starting captopril).
No products indexed under this heading.

Nabumetone (Antihypertensive effects of captopril reduced).
No products indexed under this heading.

Nadolol (Less than additive antihypertensive effect). Products include:
Nadolol 2359

Naproxen (Antihypertensive effects of captopril reduced). Products include:
EC-Naprosyn 2850
Naprosyn 2850

Anaprox/Naprosyn 2850

Naproxen Sodium (Antihypertensive effects of captopril reduced). Products include:
Anaprox 2850
Anaprox DS 2850
Treximet 1681

Nebivolol (Less than additive antihypertensive effect). Products include:
Bystolic 1147

Nitrate & Nitrite Preparations (Discontinue before starting captopril; if resumed administer at lower dosage).
No products indexed under this heading.

Nitrates, organic (Discontinue before starting captopril; if resumed administer at lower dosage).
No products indexed under this heading.

Nitrates and Nitrites (Discontinue before starting captopril; if resumed administer at lower dosage).
No products indexed under this heading.

Nitroglycerin (Discontinue before starting captopril; if resumed administer at lower dosage). Products include:
Nitro-Dur 3170
Nitrolingual 3266

Nitroglycerin, long-acting formulations (Discontinue before starting captopril; if resumed administer at lower dosage).
No products indexed under this heading.

Nitroglycerin Intravenous (Discontinue before starting captopril; if resumed administer at lower dosage).
No products indexed under this heading.

Oxaprozin (Antihypertensive effects of captopril reduced).
No products indexed under this heading.

Papaverine (Drugs having vasodilator activity should, if possible, be discontinued before starting captopril).
No products indexed under this heading.

Papaverine Hydrochloride (Drugs having vasodilator activity should, if possible, be discontinued before starting captopril).
No products indexed under this heading.

Penbutolol Sulfate (Less than additive antihypertensive effect).
No products indexed under this heading.

Pentaerythritol Tetranitrate (Discontinue before starting captopril; if resumed administer at lower dosage).
No products indexed under this heading.

Phenylbutazone (Antihypertensive effects of captopril reduced).
No products indexed under this heading.

Pindolol (Less than additive antihypertensive effect).
No products indexed under this heading.

Piroxicam (Antihypertensive effects of captopril reduced).
No products indexed under this heading.

Polythiazide (Captopril's effect will be augmented).
No products indexed under this heading.

Potassium Acid Phosphate (Potential for significant increase in serum potassium). Products include:
K-Phos Original 874

Potassium Bicarbonate (Potential for significant increase in serum potassium).
No products indexed under this heading.

Potassium Chloride (Potential for significant increase in serum potassium). Products include:
MoviPrep Oral Solution 2905

Potassium Citrate (Potential for significant increase in serum potassium). Products include:
Urocit-K 2333

Potassium Gluconate (Potential for significant increase in serum potassium).
No products indexed under this heading.

IMPORTANT NOTE: Always consult each drug listing in the patient's regimen for possible interactions.

Potassium Phosphate (Potential for significant increase in serum potassium). Products include:
K-Phos Neutral 873

Prazosin Hydrochloride (Use with caution).
No products indexed under this heading.

Propranolol (Use with caution).
No products indexed under this heading.

Propranolol Hydrochloride (Less than additive antihypertensive effect). Products include:
InnoPran XL 1517

Rofecoxib (Antihypertensive effects of captopril reduced).
No products indexed under this heading.

Sotalol Hydrochloride (Less than additive antihypertensive effect).
No products indexed under this heading.

Spironolactone (Captopril's effect will be augmented; hypotension; increased serum potassium).
No products indexed under this heading.

Sulindac (Antihypertensive effects of captopril reduced). Products include:
Clinoril 2098

Terazosin Hydrochloride (Use with caution).
No products indexed under this heading.

Timolol Hemihydrate (Less than additive antihypertensive effect). Products include:
Betimol 3490

Timolol Maleate (Less than additive antihypertensive effect). Products include:
Combigan 601
Dorzolamide Hydrochloride/Timolol Maleate Ophthalmic Solution .... ⊙243
Timoptic in Ocudose .... ⊙231

Tolazoline Hydrochloride (Drugs having vasodilator activity should, if possible, be discontinued before starting captopril).
No products indexed under this heading.

Tolmetin Sodium (Antihypertensive effects of captopril reduced).
No products indexed under this heading.

Torsemide (Captopril's effect will be augmented; hypotension).
No products indexed under this heading.

Triamterene (Captopril's effect will be augmented; hypotension; increased serum potassium). Products include:
Dyazide 1429
Dyrenium 3495

Trimethaphan Camsylate (Use with caution).
No products indexed under this heading.

Valdecoxib (Antihypertensive effects of captopril reduced).
No products indexed under this heading.

Food Interactions

Alcohol (Drugs having vasodilator activity should, if possible, be discontinued before starting captopril).

Food, unspecified (Reduces absorption by about 30% to 40%; should be given one hour before meals).

CARAC CREAM 0.5%
(Fluorouracil) 2966
None cited in PDR database.

CARAFATE SUSPENSION
(Sucralfate) 784
May interact with fluoroquinolone antibiotics, quinidine, xanthines, and certain other agents. Compounds in these categories include:

Alatrofloxacin Mesylate (Potential for reduced extent of absorption (bioavailability) with concomitant oral administration; dosing the concomitant medication 2 hours before sucralfate eliminates the interaction).
No products indexed under this heading.

Aluminum Carbonate (Simultaneous administration within one-half hour before or after sucralfate should be avoided; may increase the total body burden of aluminum).
No products indexed under this heading.

Aluminum Hydroxide (Simultaneous administration within one-half hour before or after sucralfate should be avoided; may increase the total body burden of aluminum).
No products indexed under this heading.

Aminophylline (Simultaneous administration results in reduced oral absorption of theophylline).
No products indexed under this heading.

Cimetidine (Simultaneous administration results in reduced oral absorption of oral cimetidine; dosing the concomitant medication 2 hours before sucralfate eliminates the interaction).
No products indexed under this heading.

Cimetidine Hydrochloride (Simultaneous administration results in reduced oral absorption of oral cimetidine; dosing the concomitant medication 2 hours before sucralfate eliminates the interaction).
No products indexed under this heading.

Ciprofloxacin (Potential for reduced extent of absorption (bioavailability) with concomitant oral administration; dosing the concomitant medication 2 hours before sucralfate eliminates the interaction). Products include:
Cipro I.V. 3082
Cipro 3073
Cipro XR 3091
Ciprodex 583

Ciprofloxacin Hydrochloride (Potential for reduced extent of absorption (bioavailability) with concomitant oral administration; dosing the concomitant medication 2 hours before sucralfate eliminates the interaction). Products include:
Cipro 3073

Digoxin (Simultaneous administration results in reduced oral absorption of oral digoxin; dosing the concomitant medication 2 hours before sucralfate eliminates the interaction). Products include:
Lanoxin Injection 1546
Lanoxin Injection Pediatric 1549
Lanoxin Tablets 1553

Dyphylline (Simultaneous administration results in reduced oral absorption of theophylline).
No products indexed under this heading.

Enoxacin (Potential for reduced extent of absorption (bioavailability) with concomitant oral administration; dosing the concomitant medication 2 hours before sucralfate eliminates the interaction).
No products indexed under this heading.

Gatifloxacin (Potential for reduced extent of absorption (bioavailability) with concomitant oral administration; dosing the concomitant medication 2 hours before sucralfate eliminates the interaction).
No products indexed under this heading.

Grepafloxacin Hydrochloride (Potential for reduced extent of absorption (bioavailability) with concomitant oral administration; dosing the concomitant medication 2 hours before sucralfate eliminates the interaction).
No products indexed under this heading.

Ketoconazole (Simultaneous administration results in reduced oral absorption of oral ketoconazole). Products include:

Extina 3319
Xolegel 3337

Levofloxacin (Potential for reduced extent of absorption (bioavailability) with concomitant oral administration; dosing the concomitant medication 2 hours before sucralfate eliminates the interaction). Products include:
Iquix 3492
Levaquin 2629
Levaquin in 5% Dextrose 2629
Quixin 3493

Levothyroxine Sodium (Potential for reduced extent of absorption (bioavailability) with concomitant oral administration). Products include:
Levoxyl Tablets 1843
Synthroid 529

Lomefloxacin Hydrochloride (Potential for reduced extent of absorption (bioavailability) with concomitant oral administration; dosing the concomitant medication 2 hours before sucralfate eliminates the interaction).
No products indexed under this heading.

Magnesium Hydroxide (Simultaneous administration within one-half hour before or after sucralfate should be avoided; may increase the total body burden of aluminum). Products include:
Fleet Pedia-Lax Chewable Tablets 1144
Pepcid Complete 1822

Magnesium Oxide (Simultaneous administration within one-half hour before or after sucralfate should be avoided; may increase the total body burden of aluminum). Products include:
Beelith 873

Moxifloxacin Hydrochloride (Potential for reduced extent of absorption (bioavailability) with concomitant oral administration; dosing the concomitant medication 2 hours before sucralfate eliminates the interaction). Products include:
Avelox 3064
Vigamox 589

Norfloxacin (Potential for reduced extent of absorption (bioavailability) with concomitant oral administration; dosing the concomitant medication 2 hours before sucralfate eliminates the interaction). Products include:
Noroxin 2220

Ofloxacin (Potential for reduced extent of absorption (bioavailability) with concomitant oral administration; dosing the concomitant medication 2 hours before sucralfate eliminates the interaction).
No products indexed under this heading.

Phenytoin (Simultaneous administration results in reduced oral absorption of oral phenytoin).
No products indexed under this heading.

Phenytoin Sodium (Simultaneous administration results in reduced oral absorption of oral phenytoin). Products include:
Phenytek Capsules 2380

Quinidine (Potential for reduced extent of absorption (bioavailability) with concomitant oral administration).
No products indexed under this heading.

Quinidine Gluconate (Potential for reduced extent of absorption (bioavailability) with concomitant oral administration).
No products indexed under this heading.

Quinidine Hydrochloride (Potential for reduced extent of absorption (bioavailability) with concomitant oral administration).
No products indexed under this heading.

Quinidine Polygalacturonate (Potential for reduced extent of absorption (bioavailability) with concomitant oral administration).
No products indexed under this heading.

Quinidine Sulfate (Potential for reduced extent of absorption (bioavailability) with concomitant oral administration).
No products indexed under this heading.

Ranitidine Hydrochloride (Simultaneous administration results in reduced oral absorption of oral ranitidine; dosing the concomitant medication 2 hours before sucralfate eliminates the interaction). Products include:
Zantac 1737
Zantac Injection 1732
Zantac Pharmacy 1735

Tetracycline Hydrochloride (Simultaneous administration results in reduced oral absorption of oral tetracycline). Products include:
Pylera 793

Theophylline (Simultaneous administration results in reduced oral absorption of theophylline).
No products indexed under this heading.

Theophylline Anhydrous (Simultaneous administration results in reduced oral absorption of theophylline). Products include:
Uniphyl 2817

Theophylline Calcium Salicylate (Simultaneous administration results in reduced oral absorption of theophylline).
No products indexed under this heading.

Theophylline Dihydroxypropyl (Glyceryl) (Simultaneous administration results in reduced oral absorption of theophylline).
No products indexed under this heading.

Theophylline Ethylenediamine (Simultaneous administration results in reduced oral absorption of theophylline).
No products indexed under this heading.

Theophylline Sodium Glycinate (Simultaneous administration results in reduced oral absorption of theophylline).
No products indexed under this heading.

Trovafloxacin Mesylate (Potential for reduced extent of absorption (bioavailability) with concomitant oral administration; dosing the concomitant medication 2 hours before sucralfate eliminates the interaction).
No products indexed under this heading.

Warfarin Sodium (Subtherapeutic prothrombin times with concomitant warfarin and sucralfate have been reported in spontaneous and published reports; clinical studies have demonstrated no changes in the prothrombin time with the addition of sucralfate to chronic warfarin therapy).
No products indexed under this heading.

CARAFATE TABLETS
(Sucralfate) 785
May interact with fluoroquinolone antibiotics, quinidine, xanthines, and certain other agents. Compounds in these categories include:

Alatrofloxacin Mesylate (Potential for reduced extent of absorption (bioavailability) with concomitant oral administration; dosing the concomitant medication 2 hours before sucralfate eliminates the interaction).
No products indexed under this heading.

Aluminum Carbonate (Simultaneous administration within one-half hour before or after sucralfate should be avoided; may increase the total body burden of aluminum).
No products indexed under this heading.

Aluminum Hydroxide (Simultaneous administration within one-half hour before or after sucralfate should be avoided; may increase the total body burden of aluminum).
No products indexed under this heading.

(⊙ Described in PDR® for Ophthalmic Medicines)

259 Interactions Index Carbatrol

Aminophylline (Simultaneous administration results in reduced oral absorption of theophylline).
No products indexed under this heading.

Cimetidine (Simultaneous administration results in reduced oral absorption of oral cimetidine; dosing the concomitant medication 2 hours before sucralfate eliminates the interaction).
No products indexed under this heading.

Cimetidine Hydrochloride (Simultaneous administration results in reduced oral absorption of oral cimetidine; dosing the concomitant medication 2 hours before sucralfate eliminates the interaction).
No products indexed under this heading.

Ciprofloxacin (Potential for reduced extent of absorption (bioavailability) with concomitant oral administration; dosing the concomitant medication 2 hours before sucralfate eliminates the interaction). Products include:
Cipro I.V. 3082
Cipro 3073
Cipro XR 3091
Ciprodex 583

Ciprofloxacin Hydrochloride (Potential for reduced extent of absorption (bioavailability) with concomitant oral administration; dosing the concomitant medication 2 hours before sucralfate eliminates the interaction). Products include:
Cipro 3073

Digoxin (Simultaneous administration results in reduced oral absorption of oral digoxin; dosing the concomitant medication 2 hours before sucralfate eliminates the interaction). Products include:
Lanoxin Injection 1546
Lanoxin Injection Pediatric 1549
Lanoxin Tablets 1553

Dyphylline (Simultaneous administration results in reduced oral absorption of theophylline).
No products indexed under this heading.

Enoxacin (Potential for reduced extent of absorption (bioavailability) with concomitant oral administration; dosing the concomitant medication 2 hours before sucralfate eliminates the interaction).
No products indexed under this heading.

Gatifloxacin (Potential for reduced extent of absorption (bioavailability) with concomitant oral administration; dosing the concomitant medication 2 hours before sucralfate eliminates the interaction).
No products indexed under this heading.

Grepafloxacin Hydrochloride (Potential for reduced extent of absorption (bioavailability) with concomitant oral administration; dosing the concomitant medication 2 hours before sucralfate eliminates the interaction).
No products indexed under this heading.

Ketoconazole (Simultaneous administration results in reduced oral absorption of oral ketoconazole). Products include:
Extina 3319
Xolegel 3337

Levofloxacin (Potential for reduced extent of absorption (bioavailability) with concomitant oral administration; dosing the concomitant medication 2 hours before sucralfate eliminates the interaction). Products include:
Iquix 3492
Levaquin 2629
Levaquin in 5% Dextrose 2629
Quixin 3493

Levothyroxine Sodium (Potential for reduced extent of absorption (bioavailability) with concomitant oral administration). Products include:
Levoxyl Tablets 1843
Synthroid 529

Lomefloxacin Hydrochloride (Potential for reduced extent of absorption (bioavailability) with concomitant oral administration; dosing the concomitant medication 2 hours before sucralfate eliminates the interaction).
No products indexed under this heading.

Magnesium Hydroxide (Simultaneous administration within one-half hour before or after sucralfate should be avoided; may increase the total body burden of aluminum). Products include:
Fleet Pedia-Lax Chewable Tablets 1144
Pepcid Complete 1822

Magnesium Oxide (Simultaneous administration within one-half hour before or after sucralfate should be avoided; may increase the total body burden of aluminum). Products include:
Beelith 873

Moxifloxacin Hydrochloride (Potential for reduced extent of absorption (bioavailability) with concomitant oral administration; dosing the concomitant medication 2 hours before sucralfate eliminates the interaction). Products include:
Avelox 3064
Vigamox 589

Norfloxacin (Potential for reduced extent of absorption (bioavailability) with concomitant oral administration; dosing the concomitant medication 2 hours before sucralfate eliminates the interaction). Products include:
Noroxin 2220

Ofloxacin (Potential for reduced extent of absorption (bioavailability) with concomitant oral administration; dosing the concomitant medication 2 hours before sucralfate eliminates the interaction).
No products indexed under this heading.

Phenytoin (Simultaneous administration results in reduced oral absorption of oral phenytoin).
No products indexed under this heading.

Phenytoin Sodium (Simultaneous administration results in reduced oral absorption of oral phenytoin). Products include:
Phenytek Capsules 2380

Quinidine (Potential for reduced extent of absorption (bioavailability) with concomitant oral administration).
No products indexed under this heading.

Quinidine Gluconate (Potential for reduced extent of absorption (bioavailability) with concomitant oral administration).
No products indexed under this heading.

Quinidine Hydrochloride (Potential for reduced extent of absorption (bioavailability) with concomitant oral administration).
No products indexed under this heading.

Quinidine Polygalacturonate (Potential for reduced extent of absorption (bioavailability) with concomitant oral administration).
No products indexed under this heading.

Quinidine Sulfate (Potential for reduced extent of absorption (bioavailability) with concomitant oral administration).
No products indexed under this heading.

Ranitidine Hydrochloride (Simultaneous administration results in reduced oral absorption of oral ranitidine; dosing the concomitant medication 2 hours before sucralfate eliminates the interaction). Products include:
Zantac 1737
Zantac Injection 1732
Zantac Pharmacy 1735

Tetracycline Hydrochloride (Simultaneous administration results in reduced oral absorption of oral tetracycline). Products include:
Pylera 793

Theophylline (Simultaneous administration results in reduced oral absorption of theophylline).
No products indexed under this heading.

Theophylline Anhydrous (Simultaneous administration results in reduced oral absorption of theophylline). Products include:
Uniphyl 2817

Theophylline Calcium Salicylate (Simultaneous administration results in reduced oral absorption of theophylline).
No products indexed under this heading.

Theophylline Dihydroxypropyl (Glyceryl) (Simultaneous administration results in reduced oral absorption of theophylline).
No products indexed under this heading.

Theophylline Ethylenediamine (Simultaneous administration results in reduced oral absorption of theophylline).
No products indexed under this heading.

Theophylline Sodium Glycinate (Simultaneous administration results in reduced oral absorption of theophylline).
No products indexed under this heading.

Trovafloxacin Mesylate (Potential for reduced extent of absorption (bioavailability) with concomitant oral administration; dosing the concomitant medication 2 hours before sucralfate eliminates the interaction).
No products indexed under this heading.

Warfarin Sodium (Subtherapeutic prothrombin times with concomitant warfarin and sucralfate have been reported in spontaneous and published reports; clinical studies have demonstrated no changes in the prothrombin time with the addition of sucralfate to chronic warfarin therapy).
No products indexed under this heading.

CARBATROL CAPSULES

(Carbamazepine) 3280
May interact with alcohols, antimalarials, aspirin and acetaminophen containing products, azole antifungals, centrally-acting drugs, cytochrome p450 1a2 substrates (selected), cytochrome p450 3a4 inducers (selected), cytochrome p450 3a4 inhibitors (selected), cytochrome p450 3a4 substrates (selected), erythromycin, glucocorticoids, haloperidols, lithium preparations, monoamine oxidase inhibitors, oral contraceptives, phenytoin, protease inhibitors, theophyllines, valproate, and certain other agents. Compounds in these categories include:

Acetaminophen (Carbamazepine is known to induce CYP1A2 and CYP3A4. Therefore, the potential exists for interaction between carbamazepine and any agent metabolized by one (or more) of these enzymes. Agents that are metabolized by CYP1A2 and CYP3A4 may have decreased plasma levels when administered concomitantly with carbamazepine. Thus, if a patient has been titrated to a stable dosage on one of the agents in these categories, and then begins a course of treatment with carbamazepine, it is reasonable to expect that a dose increase for the concomitant agent may be necessary). Products include:
Percocet 1121
Tylenol 2049
Tylenol 8 Hour 2049
Extra Strength Tylenol Caplets, Cool Caplets, and EZ Tabs 2049
Extra Strength Tylenol Adult Rapid Blast Liquid 2049
Extra Strength Tylenol Rapid Release 2049
Tylenol with Codeine 2691
Tylenol Arthritis Pain Extended Release Geltabs/Caplets 2049
Children's Tylenol Suspension Liquid 2048
Children's Tylenol Meltaways 2048
Tylenol, Infants' Drops 2048
Junior Tylenol 2048
Vicodin 560
Vicodin ES 561
Vicodin HP 563
Zydone 1138

Acetazolamide (Carbamazepine is metabolized mainly by CYP3A4, the active carbamazepine 10,11-epoxide, which is futher metabolized to the trans-diol by epoxide hydrolase. Therefore, the potential exists for interaction between carbamazepine and any agent that inhibits CYP3A4 and/or epoxide hydrolase. Agents that are CYP3A4 inhibitors may increase the plasma levels of carbamazepine. Thus, if a patient has been titrated to a stable dosage of carbamazepine, and then begins a course of treatment with a CYP3A4 or epoxide hydrolase inhibitor, it is reasonable to expect that a dose reduction for carbamazepine may be necessary).
No products indexed under this heading.

Acetazolamide Sodium (Carbamazepine is metabolized mainly by CYP3A4, the active carbamazepine 10,11-epoxide, which is futher metabolized to the trans-diol by epoxide hydrolase. Therefore, the potential exists for interaction between carbamazepine and any agent that inhibits CYP3A4 and/or epoxide hydrolase. Agents that are CYP3A4 inhibitors may increase the plasma levels of carbamazepine. Thus, if a patient has been titrated to a stable dosage of carbamazepine, and then begins a course of treatment with a CYP3A4 or epoxide hydrolase inhibitor, it is reasonable to expect that a dose reduction for carbamazepine may be necessary).
No products indexed under this heading.

Alatrofloxacin Mesylate (Carbamazepine is known to induce CYP1A2 and CYP3A4. Therefore, the potential exists for interaction between carbamazepine and any agent metabolized by one (or more) of these enzymes. Agents that are metabolized by CYP1A2 and CYP3A4 may have decreased plasma levels when administered concomitantly with carbamazepine. Thus, if a patient has been titrated to a stable dosage on one of the agents in these categories, and then begins a course of treatment with carbamazepine, it is reasonable to expect that a dose increase for the concomitant agent may be necessary).
No products indexed under this heading.

Alfentanil Hydrochloride (Carbamazepine is known to induce CYP1A2 and CYP3A4. Therefore, the potential exists for interaction between carbamazepine and any agent metabolized by one (or more) of these enzymes. Agents that are metabolized by CYP1A2 and CYP3A4 may have decreased plasma levels when administered concomitantly with carbamazepine. Thus, if a patient has been titrated to a stable dosage on one of the agents in these categories, and then begins a course of treatment with carbamazepine, it is reasonable to expect that a dose increase for the concomitant agent may be necessary).
No products indexed under this heading.

Allium sativum (Carbamazepine is metabolized by CYP3A4. Therefore, the potential exists for interaction between carbamazepine and any agent that induces CYP3A4. Agents that are CYP3A4 inducers may decrease plasma levels of carbamazepine. Thus, if a patient has been titrated to a stable dosage on carbamazepine, and then begins a course of treatment with

IMPORTANT NOTE: Always consult each drug listing in the patient's regimen for possible interactions.

CYP3A4 inducers, it is reasonable to expect that a dose increase for carbamazepine may be necessary).
No products indexed under this heading.

Alprazolam (Carbamazepine is known to induce CYP1A2 and CYP3A4. Therefore, the potential exists for interaction between carbamazepine and any agent metabolized by one (or more) of these enzymes. Agents that are metabolized by CYP1A2 and CYP3A4 may have decreased plasma levels when administered concomitantly with carbamazepine. Thus, if a patient has been titrated to a stable dosage on one of the agents in these categories, and then begins a course of treatment with carbamazepine, it is reasonable to expect that a dose increase for the concomitant agent may be necessary).
No products indexed under this heading.

Aminoglutethimide (Carbamazepine is metabolized by CYP3A4. Therefore, the potential exists for interaction between carbamazepine and any agent that induces CYP3A4. Agents that are CYP3A4 inducers may decrease plasma levels of carbamazepine. Thus, if a patient has been titrated to a stable dosage on carbamazepine, and then begins a course of treatment with CYP3A4 inducers, it is reasonable to expect that a dose increase for carbamazepine may be necessary).
No products indexed under this heading.

Aminophylline (Carbamazepine is known to induce CYP1A2 and CYP3A4. Therefore, the potential exists for interaction between carbamazepine and any agent metabolized by one (or more) of these enzymes. Agents that are metabolized by CYP1A2 and CYP3A4 may have decreased plasma levels when administered concomitantly with carbamazepine. Thus, if a patient has been titrated to a stable dosage on one of the agents in these categories, and then begins a course of treatment with carbamazepine, it is reasonable to expect that a dose increase for the concomitant agent may be necessary).
No products indexed under this heading.

Amiodarone Hydrochloride (Carbamazepine is metabolized mainly by CYP3A4, the active carbamazepine 10,11-epoxide, which is futher metabolized to the trans-diol by epoxide hydrolase. Therefore, the potential exists for interaction between carbamazepine and any agent that inhibits CYP3A4 and/or epoxide hydrolase. Agents that are CYP3A4 inhibitors may increase the plasma levels of carbamazepine. Thus, if a patient has been titrated to a stable dosage of carbamazepine, and then begins a course of treatment with a CYP3A4 or epoxide hydrolase inhibitor, it is reasonable to expect that a dose reduction for carbamazepine may be necessary).
No products indexed under this heading.

Amitriptyline Hydrochloride (Carbamazepine is known to induce CYP1A2 and CYP3A4. Therefore, the potential exists for interaction between carbamazepine and any agent metabolized by one (or more) of these enzymes. Agents that are metabolized by CYP1A2 and CYP3A4 may have decreased plasma levels when administered concomitantly with carbamazepine. Thus, if a patient has been titrated to a stable dosage on one of the agents in these categories, and then begins a course of treatment with carbamazepine, it is reasonable to expect that a dose increase for the concomitant agent may be necessary).
No products indexed under this heading.

Amlodipine Besylate (Carbamazepine is known to induce CYP1A2 and CYP3A4. Therefore, the potential exists for interaction between carbamazepine and any agent metabolized by one (or

more) of these enzymes. Agents that are metabolized by CYP1A2 and CYP3A4 may have decreased plasma levels when administered concomitantly with carbamazepine. Thus, if a patient has been titrated to a stable dosage on one of the agents in these categories, and then begins a course of treatment with carbamazepine, it is reasonable to expect that a dose increase for the concomitant agent may be necessary).
Products include:

Azor	1010
Exforge	2443
Exforge HCT	2449

Amoxapine (Carbamazepine is known to induce CYP1A2 and CYP3A4. Therefore, the potential exists for interaction between carbamazepine and any agent metabolized by one (or more) of these enzymes. Agents that are metabolized by CYP1A2 and CYP3A4 may have decreased plasma levels when administered concomitantly with carbamazepine. Thus, if a patient has been titrated to a stable dosage on one of the agents in these categories, and then begins a course of treatment with carbamazepine, it is reasonable to expect that a dose increase for the concomitant agent may be necessary).
No products indexed under this heading.

Amphetamine Aspartate (Because of its primary CNS effect, caution should be used when carbamazepine is taken with other centrally acting drugs).
No products indexed under this heading.

Amphetamine Aspartate Monohydrate (Because of its primary CNS effect, caution should be used when carbamazepine is taken with other centrally acting drugs).
No products indexed under this heading.

Amphetamine Resins (Because of its primary CNS effect, caution should be used when carbamazepine is taken with other centrally acting drugs).
No products indexed under this heading.

Amphetamine Sulfate (Because of its primary CNS effect, caution should be used when carbamazepine is taken with other centrally acting drugs).
No products indexed under this heading.

Amprenavir (Carbamazepine is metabolized mainly by CYP3A4, the active carbamazepine 10,11-epoxide, which is futher metabolized to the trans-diol by epoxide hydrolase. Therefore, the potential exists for interaction between carbamazepine and any agent that inhibits CYP3A4 and/or epoxide hydrolase. Agents that are CYP3A4 inhibitors may increase the plasma levels of carbamazepine. Thus, if a patient has been titrated to a stable dosage of carbamazepine, and then begins a course of treatment with a CYP3A4 or epoxide hydrolase inhibitor, it is reasonable to expect that a dose reduction for carbamazepine may be necessary).
No products indexed under this heading.

Anagrelide Hydrochloride (Carbamazepine is known to induce CYP1A2 and CYP3A4. Therefore, the potential exists for interaction between carbamazepine and any agent metabolized by one (or more) of these enzymes. Agents that are metabolized by CYP1A2 and CYP3A4 may have decreased plasma levels when administered concomitantly with carbamazepine. Thus, if a patient has been titrated to a stable dosage on one of the agents in these categories, and then begins a course of treatment with carbamazepine, it is reasonable to expect that a dose increase for the concomitant agent may be necessary).
No products indexed under this heading.

Anastrozole (Carbamazepine is metabolized mainly by CYP3A4, the active carbamazepine 10,11-epoxide, which is futher metabolized to the trans-

diol by epoxide hydrolase. Therefore, the potential exists for interaction between carbamazepine and any agent that inhibits CYP3A4 and/or epoxide hydrolase. Agents that are CYP3A4 inhibitors may increase the plasma levels of carbamazepine. Thus, if a patient has been titrated to a stable dosage of carbamazepine, and then begins a course of treatment with a CYP3A4 or epoxide hydrolase inhibitor, it is reasonable to expect that a dose reduction for carbamazepine may be necessary).
No products indexed under this heading.

Aprepitant (Carbamazepine is metabolized mainly by CYP3A4, the active carbamazepine 10,11-epoxide, which is futher metabolized to the trans-diol by epoxide hydrolase. Therefore, the potential exists for interaction between carbamazepine and any agent that inhibits CYP3A4 and/or epoxide hydrolase. Agents that are CYP3A4 inhibitors may increase the plasma levels of carbamazepine. Thus, if a patient has been titrated to a stable dosage of carbamazepine, and then begins a course of treatment with a CYP3A4 or epoxide hydrolase inhibitor, it is reasonable to expect that a dose reduction for carbamazepine may be necessary).
Products include:

Emend	2124

Aprobarbital (Because of its primary CNS effect, caution should be used when carbamazepine is taken with other centrally acting drugs).
No products indexed under this heading.

Aspirin (Carbamazepine is known to induce CYP1A2 and CYP3A4. Therefore, the potential exists for interaction between carbamazepine and any agent metabolized by one (or more) of these enzymes. Agents that are metabolized by CYP1A2 and CYP3A4 may have decreased plasma levels when administered concomitantly with carbamazepine. Thus, if a patient has been titrated to a stable dosage on one of the agents in these categories, and then begins a course of treatment with carbamazepine, it is reasonable to expect that a dose increase for the concomitant agent may be necessary). Products include:

Aggrenox	880
Bayer Aspirin	829
Percodan	1124
St. Joseph Aspirin	2045

Astemizole (Carbamazepine is known to induce CYP1A2 and CYP3A4. Therefore, the potential exists for interaction between carbamazepine and any agent metabolized by one (or more) of these enzymes. Agents that are metabolized by CYP1A2 and CYP3A4 may have decreased plasma levels when administered concomitantly with carbamazepine. Thus, if a patient has been titrated to a stable dosage on one of the agents in these categories, and then begins a course of treatment with carbamazepine, it is reasonable to expect that a dose increase for the concomitant agent may be necessary).
No products indexed under this heading.

Atazanavir (Carbamazepine is metabolized mainly by CYP3A4, the active carbamazepine 10,11-epoxide, which is futher metabolized to the trans-diol by epoxide hydrolase. Therefore, the potential exists for interaction between carbamazepine and any agent that inhibits CYP3A4 and/or epoxide hydrolase. Agents that are CYP3A4 inhibitors may increase the plasma levels of carbamazepine. Thus, if a patient has been titrated to a stable dosage of carbamazepine, and then begins a course of treatment with a CYP3A4 or epoxide

hydrolase inhibitor, it is reasonable to expect that a dose reduction for carbamazepine may be necessary).
No products indexed under this heading.

Atazanavir Sulfate (Carbamazepine is metabolized mainly by CYP3A4, the active carbamazepine 10,11-epoxide, which is futher metabolized to the trans-diol by epoxide hydrolase. Therefore, the potential exists for interaction between carbamazepine and any agent that inhibits CYP3A4 and/or epoxide hydrolase. Agents that are CYP3A4 inhibitors may increase the plasma levels of carbamazepine. Thus, if a patient has been titrated to a stable dosage of carbamazepine, and then begins a course of treatment with a CYP3A4 or epoxide hydrolase inhibitor, it is reasonable to expect that a dose reduction for carbamazepine may be necessary).
No products indexed under this heading.

Atorvastatin Calcium (Carbamazepine is known to induce CYP1A2 and CYP3A4. Therefore, the potential exists for interaction between carbamazepine and any agent metabolized by one (or more) of these enzymes. Agents that are metabolized by CYP1A2 and CYP3A4 may have decreased plasma levels when administered concomitantly with carbamazepine. Thus, if a patient has been titrated to a stable dosage on one of the agents in these categories, and then begins a course of treatment with carbamazepine, it is reasonable to expect that a dose increase for the concomitant agent may be necessary).
Products include:

Lipitor	2703

Belladonna Ergotamine (Carbamazepine is known to induce CYP1A2 and CYP3A4. Therefore, the potential exists for interaction between carbamazepine and any agent metabolized by one (or more) of these enzymes. Agents that are metabolized by CYP1A2 and CYP3A4 may have decreased plasma levels when administered concomitantly with carbamazepine. Thus, if a patient has been titrated to a stable dosage on one of the agents in these categories, and then begins a course of treatment with carbamazepine, it is reasonable to expect that a dose increase for the concomitant agent may be necessary).
No products indexed under this heading.

Betamethasone (Carbamazepine is metabolized by CYP3A4. Therefore, the potential exists for interaction between carbamazepine and any agent that induces CYP3A4. Agents that are CYP3A4 inducers may decrease plasma levels of carbamazepine. Thus, if a patient has been titrated to a stable dosage on carbamazepine, and then begins a course of treatment with CYP3A4 inducers, it is reasonable to expect that a dose increase for carbamazepine may be necessary).
No products indexed under this heading.

Betamethasone Acetate (Carbamazepine is metabolized by CYP3A4. Therefore, the potential exists for interaction between carbamazepine and any agent that induces CYP3A4. Agents that are CYP3A4 inducers may decrease plasma levels of carbamazepine. Thus, if a patient has been titrated to a stable dosage on carbamazepine, and then begins a course of treatment with CYP3A4 inducers, it is reasonable to expect that a dose increase for carbamazepine may be necessary).
No products indexed under this heading.

Betamethasone Benzoate (Carbamazepine is metabolized by CYP3A4. Therefore, the potential exists for interaction between carbamazepine and any agent that induces CYP3A4. Agents that are CYP3A4 inducers may decrease plasma levels of carbamazepine. Thus, if a patient has been titrated to a stable

dosage on carbamazepine, and then begins a course of treatment with CYP3A4 inducers, it is reasonable to expect that a dose increase for carbamazepine may be necessary).
No products indexed under this heading.

Betamethasone Dipropionate (Carbamazepine is metabolized by CYP3A4. Therefore, the potential exists for interaction between carbamazepine and any agent that induces CYP3A4. Agents that are CYP3A4 inducers may decrease plasma levels of carbamazepine. Thus, if a patient has been titrated to a stable dosage on carbamazepine, and then begins a course of treatment with CYP3A4 inducers, it is reasonable to expect that a dose increase for carbamazepine may be necessary). Products include:
Diprolene Lotion 0.05% 3108
Diprolene Ointment 0.05% 3109
Diprolene AF Cream 0.05% 3107
Lotrisone 3163

Betamethasone Sodium Phosphate (Carbamazepine is metabolized by CYP3A4. Therefore, the potential exists for interaction between carbamazepine and any agent that induces CYP3A4. Agents that are CYP3A4 inducers may decrease plasma levels of carbamazepine. Thus, if a patient has been titrated to a stable dosage on carbamazepine, and then begins a course of treatment with CYP3A4 inducers, it is reasonable to expect that a dose increase for carbamazepine may be necessary).
No products indexed under this heading.

Betamethasone Valerate (Carbamazepine is metabolized by CYP3A4. Therefore, the potential exists for interaction between carbamazepine and any agent that induces CYP3A4. Agents that are CYP3A4 inducers may decrease plasma levels of carbamazepine. Thus, if a patient has been titrated to a stable dosage on carbamazepine, and then begins a course of treatment with CYP3A4 inducers, it is reasonable to expect that a dose increase for carbamazepine may be necessary). Products include:
Luxíq 3321

Bosentan (Carbamazepine is metabolized by CYP3A4. Therefore, the potential exists for interaction between carbamazepine and any agent that induces CYP3A4. Agents that are CYP3A4 inducers may decrease plasma levels of carbamazepine. Thus, if a patient has been titrated to a stable dosage on carbamazepine, and then begins a course of treatment with CYP3A4 inducers, it is reasonable to expect that a dose increase for carbamazepine may be necessary). Products include:
Tracleer 573

Budesonide (Carbamazepine is known to induce CYP1A2 and CYP3A4. Therefore, the potential exists for interaction between carbamazepine and any agent metabolized by one (or more) of these enzymes. Agents that are metabolized by CYP1A2 and CYP3A4 may have decreased plasma levels when administered concomitantly with carbamazepine. Thus, if a patient has been titrated to a stable dosage on one of the agents in these categories, and then begins a course of treatment with carbamazepine, it is reasonable to expect that a dose increase for the concomitant agent may be necessary). Products include:
Pulmicort Flexhaler 714
Symbicort 80/4.5 720
Symbicort 160/4.5 720

Buprenorphine Hydrochloride (Because of its primary CNS effect, caution should be used when carbamazepine is taken with other centrally acting drugs).
No products indexed under this heading.

Buspirone Hydrochloride (Carbamazepine is known to induce CYP1A2 and CYP3A4. Therefore, the potential exists for interaction between carbamazepine and any agent metabolized by one (or more) of these enzymes. Agents that are metabolized by CYP1A2 and CYP3A4 may have decreased plasma levels when administered concomitantly with carbamazepine. Thus, if a patient has been titrated to a stable dosage on one of the agents in these categories, and then begins a course of treatment with carbamazepine, it is reasonable to expect that a dose increase for the concomitant agent may be necessary).
No products indexed under this heading.

Busulfan (Carbamazepine is known to induce CYP1A2 and CYP3A4. Therefore, the potential exists for interaction between carbamazepine and any agent metabolized by one (or more) of these enzymes. Agents that are metabolized by CYP1A2 and CYP3A4 may have decreased plasma levels when administered concomitantly with carbamazepine. Thus, if a patient has been titrated to a stable dosage on one of the agents in these categories, and then begins a course of treatment with carbamazepine, it is reasonable to expect that a dose increase for the concomitant agent may be necessary). Products include:
Myleran 1581

Butabarbital (Because of its primary CNS effect, caution should be used when carbamazepine is taken with other centrally acting drugs).
No products indexed under this heading.

Butalbital (Because of its primary CNS effect, caution should be used when carbamazepine is taken with other centrally acting drugs).
No products indexed under this heading.

Butoconazole Nitrate (Carbamazepine is metabolized mainly by CYP3A4, the active carbamazepine 10,11-epoxide, which is futher metabolized to the trans-diol by epoxide hydrolase. Therefore, the potential exists for interaction between carbamazepine and any agent that inhibits CYP3A4 and/or epoxide hydrolase. Agents that are CYP3A4 inhibitors may increase the plasma levels of carbamazepine. Thus, if a patient has been titrated to a stable dosage of carbamazepine, and then begins a course of treatment with a CYP3A4 or epoxide hydrolase inhibitor, it is reasonable to expect that a dose reduction for carbamazepine may be necessary).
No products indexed under this heading.

Caffeine (Carbamazepine is known to induce CYP1A2 and CYP3A4. Therefore, the potential exists for interaction between carbamazepine and any agent metabolized by one (or more) of these enzymes. Agents that are metabolized by CYP1A2 and CYP3A4 may have decreased plasma levels when administered concomitantly with carbamazepine. Thus, if a patient has been titrated to a stable dosage on one of the agents in these categories, and then begins a course of treatment with carbamazepine, it is reasonable to expect that a dose increase for the concomitant agent may be necessary).
No products indexed under this heading.

Caffeine Anhydrous (Carbamazepine is known to induce CYP1A2 and CYP3A4. Therefore, the potential exists for interaction between carbamazepine and any agent metabolized by one (or more) of these enzymes. Agents that are metabolized by CYP1A2 and CYP3A4 may have decreased plasma levels when administered concomitantly with carbamazepine. Thus, if a patient has been titrated to a stable dosage on one of the agents in these categories, and then begins a course of treatment with carbamazepine, it is reasonable to expect that a dose increase for the concomitant agent may be necessary).
No products indexed under this heading.

Caffeine Citrate (Carbamazepine is known to induce CYP1A2 and CYP3A4. Therefore, the potential exists for interaction between carbamazepine and any agent metabolized by one (or more) of these enzymes. Agents that are metabolized by CYP1A2 and CYP3A4 may have decreased plasma levels when administered concomitantly with carbamazepine. Thus, if a patient has been titrated to a stable dosage on one of the agents in these categories, and then begins a course of treatment with carbamazepine, it is reasonable to expect that a dose increase for the concomitant agent may be necessary).
No products indexed under this heading.

Caffeine-containing medications (Carbamazepine is known to induce CYP1A2 and CYP3A4. Therefore, the potential exists for interaction between carbamazepine and any agent metabolized by one (or more) of these enzymes. Agents that are metabolized by CYP1A2 and CYP3A4 may have decreased plasma levels when administered concomitantly with carbamazepine. Thus, if a patient has been titrated to a stable dosage on one of the agents in these categories, and then begins a course of treatment with carbamazepine, it is reasonable to expect that a dose increase for the concomitant agent may be necessary).
No products indexed under this heading.

Caffeine Sodium Benzoate (Carbamazepine is known to induce CYP1A2 and CYP3A4. Therefore, the potential exists for interaction between carbamazepine and any agent metabolized by one (or more) of these enzymes. Agents that are metabolized by CYP1A2 and CYP3A4 may have decreased plasma levels when administered concomitantly with carbamazepine. Thus, if a patient has been titrated to a stable dosage on one of the agents in these categories, and then begins a course of treatment with carbamazepine, it is reasonable to expect that a dose increase for the concomitant agent may be necessary).
No products indexed under this heading.

Cerivastatin Sodium (Carbamazepine is known to induce CYP1A2 and CYP3A4. Therefore, the potential exists for interaction between carbamazepine and any agent metabolized by one (or more) of these enzymes. Agents that are metabolized by CYP1A2 and CYP3A4 may have decreased plasma levels when administered concomitantly with carbamazepine. Thus, if a patient has been titrated to a stable dosage on one of the agents in these categories, and then begins a course of treatment with carbamazepine, it is reasonable to expect that a dose increase for the concomitant agent may be necessary).
No products indexed under this heading.

Chlordiazepoxide (Carbamazepine is known to induce CYP1A2 and CYP3A4. Therefore, the potential exists for interaction between carbamazepine and any agent metabolized by one (or more) of these enzymes. Agents that are metabolized by CYP1A2 and CYP3A4 may have decreased plasma levels when administered concomitantly with carbamazepine. Thus, if a patient has been titrated to a stable dosage on one of the agents in these categories, and then begins a course of treatment with carbamazepine, it is reasonable to expect that a dose increase for the concomitant agent may be necessary).
No products indexed under this heading.

Chlordiazepoxide Hydrochloride (Carbamazepine is known to induce CYP1A2 and CYP3A4. Therefore, the potential exists for interaction between carbamazepine and any agent metabolized by one (or more) of these enzymes. Agents that are metabolized by CYP1A2 and CYP3A4 may have decreased plasma levels when administered concomitantly with carbamazepine. Thus, if a patient has been titrated to a stable dosage on one of the agents in these categories, and then begins a course of treatment with carbamazepine, it is reasonable to expect that a dose increase for the concomitant agent may be necessary).
No products indexed under this heading.

Chloroquine (Anti-malarial drugs, such as chloroquine and mefloquine, may antagonize the activity of carbamazepine).
No products indexed under this heading.

Chloroquine Hydrochloride (Anti-malarial drugs, such as chloroquine and mefloquine, may antagonize the activity of carbamazepine).
No products indexed under this heading.

Chloroquine Phosphate (Anti-malarial drugs, such as chloroquine and mefloquine, may antagonize the activity of carbamazepine).
No products indexed under this heading.

Chlorpheniramine (Carbamazepine is known to induce CYP1A2 and CYP3A4. Therefore, the potential exists for interaction between carbamazepine and any agent metabolized by one (or more) of these enzymes. Agents that are metabolized by CYP1A2 and CYP3A4 may have decreased plasma levels when administered concomitantly with carbamazepine. Thus, if a patient has been titrated to a stable dosage on one of the agents in these categories, and then begins a course of treatment with carbamazepine, it is reasonable to expect that a dose increase for the concomitant agent may be necessary).
No products indexed under this heading.

Chlorpheniramine Maleate (Carbamazepine is known to induce CYP1A2 and CYP3A4. Therefore, the potential exists for interaction between carbamazepine and any agent metabolized by one (or more) of these enzymes. Agents that are metabolized by CYP1A2 and CYP3A4 may have decreased plasma levels when administered concomitantly with carbamazepine. Thus, if a patient has been titrated to a stable dosage on one of the agents in these categories, and then begins a course of treatment with carbamazepine, it is reasonable to expect that a dose increase for the concomitant agent may be necessary).
No products indexed under this heading.

Chlorpheniramine Polistirex (Carbamazepine is known to induce CYP1A2 and CYP3A4. Therefore, the potential exists for interaction between carbamazepine and any agent metabolized by one (or more) of these enzymes. Agents that are metabolized by CYP1A2 and CYP3A4 may have decreased plasma levels when administered concomitantly with carbamazepine. Thus, if a patient has been titrated to a stable dosage on one of the agents in these categories, and then begins a course of treatment with carbamazepine, it is reasonable to expect that a dose increase for the concomitant agent may be necessary). Products include:
Tussionex 3443

Chlorpheniramine Tannate (Carbamazepine is known to induce CYP1A2

IMPORTANT NOTE: Always consult each drug listing in the patient's regimen for possible interactions.

Carbatrol
Interactions Index
262

and CYP3A4. Therefore, the potential exists for interaction between carbamazepine and any agent metabolized by one (or more) of these enzymes. Agents that are metabolized by CYP1A2 and CYP3A4 may have decreased plasma levels when administered concomitantly with carbamazepine. Thus, if a patient has been titrated to a stable dosage on one of the agents in these categories, and then begins a course of treatment with carbamazepine, it is reasonable to expect that a dose increase for the concomitant agent may be necessary).
No products indexed under this heading.

Chlorpromazine (Because of its primary CNS effect, caution should be used when carbamazepine is taken with other centrally acting drugs).
No products indexed under this heading.

Chlorpromazine Hydrochloride (Because of its primary CNS effect, caution should be used when carbamazepine is taken with other centrally acting drugs).
No products indexed under this heading.

Chlorprothixene (Because of its primary CNS effect, caution should be used when carbamazepine is taken with other centrally acting drugs).
No products indexed under this heading.

Chlorprothixene Hydrochloride (Because of its primary CNS effect, caution should be used when carbamazepine is taken with other centrally acting drugs).
No products indexed under this heading.

Chlorprothixene Lactate (Because of its primary CNS effect, caution should be used when carbamazepine is taken with other centrally acting drugs).
No products indexed under this heading.

Cimetidine (Carbamazepine is metabolized mainly by CYP3A4, the active carbamazepine 10,11-epoxide, which is futher metabolized to the trans-diol by epoxide hydrolase. Therefore, the potential exists for interaction between carbamazepine and any agent that inhibits CYP3A4 and/or epoxide hydrolase. Agents that are CYP3A4 inhibitors may increase the plasma levels of carbamazepine. Thus, if a patient has been titrated to a stable dosage of carbamazepine, and then begins a course of treatment with a CYP3A4 or epoxide hydrolase inhibitor, it is reasonable to expect that a dose reduction for carbamazepine may be necessary).
No products indexed under this heading.

Cimetidine Hydrochloride (Carbamazepine is metabolized mainly by CYP3A4, the active carbamazepine 10,11-epoxide, which is futher metabolized to the trans-diol by epoxide hydrolase. Therefore, the potential exists for interaction between carbamazepine and any agent that inhibits CYP3A4 and/or epoxide hydrolase. Agents that are CYP3A4 inhibitors may increase the plasma levels of carbamazepine. Thus, if a patient has been titrated to a stable dosage of carbamazepine, and then begins a course of treatment with a CYP3A4 or epoxide hydrolase inhibitor, it is reasonable to expect that a dose reduction for carbamazepine may be necessary).
No products indexed under this heading.

Ciprofloxacin (Carbamazepine is metabolized mainly by CYP3A4, the active carbamazepine 10,11-epoxide, which is futher metabolized to the trans-diol by epoxide hydrolase. Therefore, the potential exists for interaction between carbamazepine and any agent that inhibits CYP3A4 and/or epoxide hydrolase. Agents that are CYP3A4 inhibitors may increase the plasma levels of carbamazepine. Thus, if a patient has been titrated to a stable dosage of carbamazepine, and then begins a course of treatment with a CYP3A4 or epoxide hydrolase inhibitor, it is reasonable to expect that a dose reduction for carbamazepine may be necessary). Products include:
Cipro I.V. 3082
Cipro 3073
Cipro XR 3091
Ciprodex 583

Ciprofloxacin Hydrochloride (Carbamazepine is metabolized by CYP3A4. Therefore, the potential exists for interaction between carbamazepine and any agent that induces CYP3A4. Agents that are CYP3A4 inducers may decrease plasma levels of carbamazepine. Thus, if a patient has been titrated to a stable dosage on carbamazepine, and then begins a course of treatment with CYP3A4 inducers, it is reasonable to expect that a dose increase for carbamazepine may be necessary). Products include:
Cipro 3073

Cisapride (Carbamazepine is known to induce CYP1A2 and CYP3A4. Therefore, the potential exists for interaction between carbamazepine and any agent metabolized by one (or more) of these enzymes. Agents that are metabolized by CYP1A2 and CYP3A4 may have decreased plasma levels when administered concomitantly with carbamazepine. Thus, if a patient has been titrated to a stable dosage on one of the agents in these categories, and then begins a course of treatment with carbamazepine, it is reasonable to expect that a dose increase for the concomitant agent may be necessary).
No products indexed under this heading.

Cisplatin (Carbamazepine is metabolized by CYP3A4. Therefore, the potential exists for interaction between carbamazepine and any agent that induces CYP3A4. Agents that are CYP3A4 inducers may decrease plasma levels of carbamazepine. Thus, if a patient has been titrated to a stable dosage on carbamazepine, and then begins a course of treatment with CYP3A4 inducers, it is reasonable to expect that a dose increase for carbamazepine may be necessary).
No products indexed under this heading.

Clarithromycin (Carbamazepine is metabolized mainly by CYP3A4, the active carbamazepine 10,11-epoxide, which is futher metabolized to the trans-diol by epoxide hydrolase. Therefore, the potential exists for interaction between carbamazepine and any agent that inhibits CYP3A4 and/or epoxide hydrolase. Agents that are CYP3A4 inhibitors may increase the plasma levels of carbamazepine. Thus, if a patient has been titrated to a stable dosage of carbamazepine, and then begins a course of treatment with a CYP3A4 or epoxide hydrolase inhibitor, it is reasonable to expect that a dose reduction for carbamazepine may be necessary). Products include:
Biaxin/Biaxin XL 412

Clomipramine Hydrochloride (Carbamazepine increases the plasma levels of clomipramine HCl).
No products indexed under this heading.

Clopidogrel Bisulfate (Carbamazepine is known to induce CYP1A2 and CYP3A4. Therefore, the potential exists for interaction between carbamazepine and any agent metabolized by one (or more) of these enzymes. Agents that are metabolized by CYP1A2 and CYP3A4 may have decreased plasma levels when administered concomitantly with carbamazepine. Thus, if a patient has been titrated to a stable dosage on one of the agents in these categories, and then begins a course of treatment with carbamazepine, it is reasonable to expect that a dose increase for the concomitant agent may be necessary). Products include:
Plavix 3027

Clorazepate Dipotassium (Because of its primary CNS effect, caution should be used when carbamazepine is taken with other centrally acting drugs).
No products indexed under this heading.

Clotrimazole (Carbamazepine is metabolized mainly by CYP3A4, the active carbamazepine 10,11-epoxide, which is futher metabolized to the trans-diol by epoxide hydrolase. Therefore, the potential exists for interaction between carbamazepine and any agent that inhibits CYP3A4 and/or epoxide hydrolase. Agents that are CYP3A4 inhibitors may increase the plasma levels of carbamazepine. Thus, if a patient has been titrated to a stable dosage of carbamazepine, and then begins a course of treatment with a CYP3A4 or epoxide hydrolase inhibitor, it is reasonable to expect that a dose reduction for carbamazepine may be necessary). Products include:
Lotrisone 3163

Clozapine (Carbamazepine is known to induce CYP1A2 and CYP3A4. Therefore, the potential exists for interaction between carbamazepine and any agent metabolized by one (or more) of these enzymes. Agents that are metabolized by CYP1A2 and CYP3A4 may have decreased plasma levels when administered concomitantly with carbamazepine. Thus, if a patient has been titrated to a stable dosage on one of the agents in these categories, and then begins a course of treatment with carbamazepine, it is reasonable to expect that a dose increase for the concomitant agent may be necessary).
No products indexed under this heading.

Codeine Phosphate (Because of its primary CNS effect, caution should be used when carbamazepine is taken with other centrally acting drugs). Products include:
Tylenol with Codeine 2691

Codeine Sulfate (Because of its primary CNS effect, caution should be used when carbamazepine is taken with other centrally acting drugs).
No products indexed under this heading.

Conivaptan Hydrochloride (Carbamazepine is metabolized mainly by CYP3A4, the active carbamazepine 10,11-epoxide, which is futher metabolized to the trans-diol by epoxide hydrolase. Therefore, the potential exists for interaction between carbamazepine and any agent that inhibits CYP3A4 and/or epoxide hydrolase. Agents that are CYP3A4 inhibitors may increase the plasma levels of carbamazepine. Thus, if a patient has been titrated to a stable dosage of carbamazepine, and then begins a course of treatment with a CYP3A4 or epoxide hydrolase inhibitor, it is reasonable to expect that a dose reduction for carbamazepine may be necessary). Products include:
Vaprisol 689

Cortisone Acetate (Carbamazepine is metabolized by CYP3A4. Therefore, the potential exists for interaction between carbamazepine and any agent that induces CYP3A4. Agents that are CYP3A4 inducers may decrease plasma levels of carbamazepine. Thus, if a patient has been titrated to a stable dosage on carbamazepine, and then begins a course of treatment with CYP3A4 inducers, it is reasonable to expect that a dose increase for carbamazepine may be necessary).
No products indexed under this heading.

Cyclobenzaprine (Carbamazepine is known to induce CYP1A2 and CYP3A4. Therefore, the potential exists for interaction between carbamazepine and any agent metabolized by one (or more) of these enzymes. Agents that are metabolized by CYP1A2 and CYP3A4 may have decreased plasma levels when administered concomitantly with carbamazepine. Thus, if a patient has been titrated to a stable dosage on one of the agents in these categories, and then begins a course of treatment with carbamazepine, it is reasonable to expect that a dose increase for the concomitant agent may be necessary).
No products indexed under this heading.

Cyclobenzaprine Hydrochloride (Carbamazepine is known to induce CYP1A2 and CYP3A4. Therefore, the potential exists for interaction between carbamazepine and any agent metabolized by one (or more) of these enzymes. Agents that are metabolized by CYP1A2 and CYP3A4 may have decreased plasma levels when administered concomitantly with carbamazepine. Thus, if a patient has been titrated to a stable dosage on one of the agents in these categories, and then begins a course of treatment with carbamazepine, it is reasonable to expect that a dose increase for the concomitant agent may be necessary). Products include:
Amrix 964

Cyclosporine (Carbamazepine is metabolized mainly by CYP3A4, the active carbamazepine 10,11-epoxide, which is futher metabolized to the trans-diol by epoxide hydrolase. Therefore, the potential exists for interaction between carbamazepine and any agent that inhibits CYP3A4 and/or epoxide hydrolase. Agents that are CYP3A4 inhibitors may increase the plasma levels of carbamazepine. Thus, if a patient has been titrated to a stable dosage of carbamazepine, and then begins a course of treatment with a CYP3A4 or epoxide hydrolase inhibitor, it is reasonable to expect that a dose reduction for carbamazepine may be necessary). Products include:
Gengraf 440
Neoral Oral Solution 2496
Neoral Capsules 2496
Restasis 605

Dalfopristin (Carbamazepine is metabolized mainly by CYP3A4, the active carbamazepine 10,11-epoxide, which is futher metabolized to the trans-diol by epoxide hydrolase. Therefore, the potential exists for interaction between carbamazepine and any agent that inhibits CYP3A4 and/or epoxide hydrolase. Agents that are CYP3A4 inhibitors may increase the plasma levels of carbamazepine. Thus, if a patient has been titrated to a stable dosage of carbamazepine, and then begins a course of treatment with a CYP3A4 or epoxide hydrolase inhibitor, it is reasonable to expect that a dose reduction for carbamazepine may be necessary).
No products indexed under this heading.

Danazol (Carbamazepine is metabolized mainly by CYP3A4, the active carbamazepine 10,11-epoxide, which is futher metabolized to the trans-diol by epoxide hydrolase. Therefore, the potential exists for interaction between carbamazepine and any agent that inhibits CYP3A4 and/or epoxide hydrolase. Agents that are CYP3A4 inhibitors may increase the plasma levels of carbamazepine. Thus, if a patient has been titrated to a stable dosage of carbamazepine, and then begins a course of treatment with a CYP3A4 or epoxide hydrolase inhibitor, it is reasonable to expect that a dose reduction for carbamazepine may be necessary).
No products indexed under this heading.

Darunavir (Carbamazepine is metabolized mainly by CYP3A4, the active car-

bamazepine 10,11-epoxide, which is futher metabolized to the trans-diol by epoxide hydrolase. Therefore, the potential exists for interaction between carbamazepine and any agent that inhibits CYP3A4 and/or epoxide hydrolase. Agents that are CYP3A4 inhibitors may increase the plasma levels of carbamazepine. Thus, if a patient has been titrated to a stable dosage of carbamazepine, and then begins a course of treatment with a CYP3A4 or epoxide hydrolase inhibitor, it is reasonable to expect that a dose reduction for carbamazepine may be necessary).
No products indexed under this heading.

Dasatinib (Carbamazepine is metabolized mainly by CYP3A4, the active carbamazepine 10,11-epoxide, which is futher metabolized to the trans-diol by epoxide hydrolase. Therefore, the potential exists for interaction between carbamazepine and any agent that inhibits CYP3A4 and/or epoxide hydrolase. Agents that are CYP3A4 inhibitors may increase the plasma levels of carbamazepine. Thus, if a patient has been titrated to a stable dosage of carbamazepine, and then begins a course of treatment with a CYP3A4 or epoxide hydrolase inhibitor, it is reasonable to expect that a dose reduction for carbamazepine may be necessary).
No products indexed under this heading.

Delavirdine Mesylate (Co-administration of carbamazepine and delavirdine may lead to loss of virologic response and possible resistance to rescriptor or to the class of non-nucleoside reverse transcriptasee inhibitors).
No products indexed under this heading.

Delavirine (Carbamazepine is metabolized mainly by CYP3A4, the active carbamazepine 10,11-epoxide, which is futher metabolized to the trans-diol by epoxide hydrolase. Therefore, the potential exists for interaction between carbamazepine and any agent that inhibits CYP3A4 and/or epoxide hydrolase. Agents that are CYP3A4 inhibitors may increase the plasma levels of carbamazepine. Thus, if a patient has been titrated to a stable dosage of carbamazepine, and then begins a course of treatment with a CYP3A4 or epoxide hydrolase inhibitor, it is reasonable to expect that a dose reduction for carbamazepine may be necessary).
No products indexed under this heading.

Desflurane (Because of its primary CNS effect, caution should be used when carbamazepine is taken with other centrally acting drugs).
No products indexed under this heading.

Desipramine Hydrochloride (Carbamazepine is known to induce CYP1A2 and CYP3A4. Therefore, the potential exists for interaction between carbamazepine and any agent metabolized by one (or more) of these enzymes. Agents that are metabolized by CYP1A2 and CYP3A4 may have decreased plasma levels when administered concomitantly with carbamazepine. Thus, if a patient has been titrated to a stable dosage on one of the agents in these categories, and then begins a course of treatment with carbamazepine, it is reasonable to expect that a dose increase for the concomitant agent may be necessary).
No products indexed under this heading.

Desloratadine (Carbamazepine is metabolized mainly by CYP3A4, the active carbamazepine 10,11-epoxide, which is futher metabolized to the trans-diol by epoxide hydrolase. Therefore, the potential exists for interaction between carbamazepine and any agent that inhibits CYP3A4 and/or epoxide hydrolase. Agents that are CYP3A4 inhibitors may increase the plasma levels of carbamazepine. Thus, if a patient has been titrated to a stable dosage of carbamazepine, and then begins a course of treatment with a CYP3A4 or epoxide hydrolase inhibitor, it is reasonable to expect that a dose reduction for carbamazepine may be necessary).
Products include:
Clarinex Syrup **3098**
Clarinex **3098**
Clarinex Reditabs **3098**
Clarinex-D 12-Hour **3101**
Clarinex-D **3104**

Desogestrel (Carbamazepine is known to induce CYP1A2 and CYP3A4. Therefore, the potential exists for interaction between carbamazepine and any agent metabolized by one (or more) of these enzymes. Agents that are metabolized by CYP1A2 or CYP3A4 may have decreased plasma levels when administered concomitantly with carbamazepine. Breakthrough bleeding has been reported among patients receiving concomitant oral contraceptives and their reliability may be adversely affected).
No products indexed under this heading.

Dexamethasone (Carbamazepine is metabolized by CYP3A4. Therefore, the potential exists for interaction between carbamazepine and any agent that induces CYP3A4. Agents that are CYP3A4 inducers may decrease plasma levels of carbamazepine. Thus, if a patient has been titrated to a stable dosage on carbamazepine, and then begins a course of treatment with CYP3A4 inducers, it is reasonable to expect that a dose increase for carbamazepine may be necessary). Products include:
Ciprodex **583**
Ozurdex .... ⊙**223**
Tobramycin and Dexamethasone Ophthalmic Suspension .... ⊙**251**

Dexamethasone Acetate (Carbamazepine is metabolized by CYP3A4. Therefore, the potential exists for interaction between carbamazepine and any agent that induces CYP3A4. Agents that are CYP3A4 inducers may decrease plasma levels of carbamazepine. Thus, if a patient has been titrated to a stable dosage on carbamazepine, and then begins a course of treatment with CYP3A4 inducers, it is reasonable to expect that a dose increase for carbamazepine may be necessary).
No products indexed under this heading.

Dexamethasone Phosphate (Carbamazepine is metabolized by CYP3A4. Therefore, the potential exists for interaction between carbamazepine and any agent that induces CYP3A4. Agents that are CYP3A4 inducers may decrease plasma levels of carbamazepine. Thus, if a patient has been titrated to a stable dosage on carbamazepine, and then begins a course of treatment with CYP3A4 inducers, it is reasonable to expect that a dose increase for carbamazepine may be necessary).
No products indexed under this heading.

Dexamethasone Sodium (Carbamazepine is metabolized by CYP3A4. Therefore, the potential exists for interaction between carbamazepine and any agent that induces CYP3A4. Agents that are CYP3A4 inducers may decrease plasma levels of carbamazepine. Thus, if a patient has been titrated to a stable dosage on carbamazepine, and then begins a course of treatment with CYP3A4 inducers, it is reasonable to expect that a dose increase for carbamazepine may be necessary).
No products indexed under this heading.

Dexamethasone Sodium Phosphate (Carbamazepine is metabolized by CYP3A4. Therefore, the potential exists for interaction between carbamazepine and any agent that induces CYP3A4. Agents that are CYP3A4 inducers may decrease plasma levels of carbamazepine. Thus, if a patient has been titrated to a stable dosage on carbamazepine, and then begins a course of treatment with CYP3A4 inducers, it is reasonable to expect that a dose increase for carbamazepine may be necessary).
No products indexed under this heading.

Dexamethasone Sodium Phosphate Injection (Carbamazepine is metabolized by CYP3A4. Therefore, the potential exists for interaction between carbamazepine and any agent that induces CYP3A4. Agents that are CYP3A4 inducers may decrease plasma levels of carbamazepine. Thus, if a patient has been titrated to a stable dosage on carbamazepine, and then begins a course of treatment with CYP3A4 inducers, it is reasonable to expect that a dose increase for carbamazepine may be necessary).
No products indexed under this heading.

Dexmethylphenidate Hydrochloride (Because of its primary CNS effect, caution should be used when carbamazepine is taken with other centrally acting drugs). Products include:
Focalin XR **2472**

Dextroamphetamine (Because of its primary CNS effect, caution should be used when carbamazepine is taken with other centrally acting drugs).
No products indexed under this heading.

Dextroamphetamine Saccharate (Because of its primary CNS effect, caution should be used when carbamazepine is taken with other centrally acting drugs).
No products indexed under this heading.

Dextroamphetamine Sulfate (Because of its primary CNS effect, caution should be used when carbamazepine is taken with other centrally acting drugs). Products include:
Dexedrine **1425**

Dezocine (Because of its primary CNS effect, caution should be used when carbamazepine is taken with other centrally acting drugs).
No products indexed under this heading.

Diazepam (Carbamazepine is known to induce CYP1A2 and CYP3A4. Therefore, the potential exists for interaction between carbamazepine and any agent metabolized by one (or more) of these enzymes. Agents that are metabolized by CYP1A2 and CYP3A4 may have decreased plasma levels when administered concomitantly with carbamazepine. Thus, if a patient has been titrated to a stable dosage on one of the agents in these categories, and then begins a course of treatment with carbamazepine, it is reasonable to expect that a dose increase for the concomitant agent may be necessary). Products include:
Valium Tablets **2880**

Dihydroergotamine Mesylate (Carbamazepine is known to induce CYP1A2 and CYP3A4. Therefore, the potential exists for interaction between carbamazepine and any agent metabolized by one (or more) of these enzymes. Agents that are metabolized by CYP1A2 and CYP3A4 may have decreased plasma levels when administered concomitantly with carbamazepine. Thus, if a patient has been titrated to a stable dosage on one of the agents in these categories, and then begins a course of treatment with carbamazepine, it is reasonable to expect that a dose increase for the concomitant agent may be necessary).
No products indexed under this heading.

Diltiazem Hydrochloride (Carbamazepine is metabolized mainly by CYP3A4, the active carbamazepine 10,11-epoxide, which is futher metabolized to the trans-diol by epoxide hydrolase. Therefore, the potential exists for interaction between carbamazepine and any agent that inhibits CYP3A4 and/or epoxide hydrolase. Agents that are CYP3A4 inhibitors may increase the plasma levels of carbamazepine. Thus, if a patient has been titrated to a stable dosage of carbamazepine, and then begins a course of treatment with a CYP3A4 or epoxide hydrolase inhibitor, it is reasonable to expect that a dose reduction for carbamazepine may be necessary). Products include:
Cardizem LA **423**

Diltiazem Maleate (Carbamazepine is metabolized mainly by CYP3A4, the active carbamazepine 10,11-epoxide, which is futher metabolized to the trans-diol by epoxide hydrolase. Therefore, the potential exists for interaction between carbamazepine and any agent that inhibits CYP3A4 and/or epoxide hydrolase. Agents that are CYP3A4 inhibitors may increase the plasma levels of carbamazepine. Thus, if a patient has been titrated to a stable dosage of carbamazepine, and then begins a course of treatment with a CYP3A4 or epoxide hydrolase inhibitor, it is reasonable to expect that a dose reduction for carbamazepine may be necessary).
No products indexed under this heading.

Disopyramide (Carbamazepine is known to induce CYP1A2 and CYP3A4. Therefore, the potential exists for interaction between carbamazepine and any agent metabolized by one (or more) of these enzymes. Agents that are metabolized by CYP1A2 and CYP3A4 may have decreased plasma levels when administered concomitantly with carbamazepine. Thus, if a patient has been titrated to a stable dosage on one of the agents in these categories, and then begins a course of treatment with carbamazepine, it is reasonable to expect that a dose increase for the concomitant agent may be necessary).
No products indexed under this heading.

Disopyramide Phosphate (Carbamazepine is known to induce CYP1A2 and CYP3A4. Therefore, the potential exists for interaction between carbamazepine and any agent metabolized by one (or more) of these enzymes. Agents that are metabolized by CYP1A2 and CYP3A4 may have decreased plasma levels when administered concomitantly with carbamazepine. Thus, if a patient has been titrated to a stable dosage on one of the agents in these categories, and then begins a course of treatment with carbamazepine, it is reasonable to expect that a dose increase for the concomitant agent may be necessary).
No products indexed under this heading.

Disulfiram (Carbamazepine is known to induce CYP1A2 and CYP3A4. Therefore, the potential exists for interaction between carbamazepine and any agent metabolized by one (or more) of these enzymes. Agents that are metabolized by CYP1A2 and CYP3A4 may have decreased plasma levels when administered concomitantly with carbamazepine. Thus, if a patient has been titrated to a stable dosage on one of the agents in these categories, and then begins a course of treatment with carbamazepine, it is reasonable to expect that a dose increase for the concomitant agent may be necessary).
No products indexed under this heading.

Divalproex Sodium (Carbamazepine is metabolized mainly by CYP3A4 the active carbamazepine 10,11-epoxide, which is futher metabolized to the trans-diol by epoxide hydrolase. Therefore, the potential exists for interaction between carbamazepine and any agent that inhibits CYP3A4 and/or epoxide hydrolase. Agents that are CYP3A4 inhibitors may increase the plasma levels of carbamazepine. Also inhibits

Carbatrol Interactions Index 264

epoxide hydroxylase, resulting in increased levels of the active metabolite carbamazepine-10,11-epoxide. Thus, if a patient has been titrated to a stable dosage of carbamazepine, and then begins a course of treatment with a CYP3A4 or epoxide hydrolase inhibitor, it is reasonable to expect that a dose reduction for carbamazepine may be necessary). Products include:

Depakote ER 426

Doxepin Hydrochloride (Carbamazepine is known to induce CYP1A2 and CYP3A4. Therefore, the potential exists for interaction between carbamazepine and any agent metabolized by one (or more) of these enzymes. Agents that are metabolized by CYP1A2 and CYP3A4 may have decreased plasma levels when administered concomitantly with carbamazepine. Thus, if a patient has been titrated to a stable dosage on one of the agents in these categories, and then begins a course of treatment with carbamazepine, it is reasonable to expect that a dose increase for the concomitant agent may be necessary).

No products indexed under this heading.

Doxorubicin Hydrochloride (Carbamazepine is metabolized by CYP3A4. Therefore, the potential exists for interaction between carbamazepine and any agent that induces CYP3A4. Agents that are CYP3A4 inducers may decrease plasma levels of carbamazepine. Thus, if a patient has been titrated to a stable dosage on carbamazepine, and then begins a course of treatment with CYP3A4 inducers, it is reasonable to expect that a dose increase for carbamazepine may be necessary).

No products indexed under this heading.

Dronabinol (Carbamazepine is known to induce CYP1A2 and CYP3A4. Therefore, the potential exists for interaction between carbamazepine and any agent metabolized by one (or more) of these enzymes. Agents that are metabolized by CYP1A2 and CYP3A4 may have decreased plasma levels when administered concomitantly with carbamazepine. Thus, if a patient has been titrated to a stable dosage on one of the agents in these categories, and then begins a course of treatment with carbamazepine, it is reasonable to expect that a dose increase for the concomitant agent may be necessary).

No products indexed under this heading.

Droperidol (Because of its primary CNS effect, caution should be used when carbamazepine is taken with other centrally acting drugs).

No products indexed under this heading.

Econazole Nitrate (Carbamazepine is metabolized mainly by CYP3A4, the active carbamazepine 10,11-epoxide, which is futher metabolized to the trans-diol by epoxide hydrolase. Therefore, the potential exists for interaction between carbamazepine and any agent that inhibits CYP3A4 and/or epoxide hydrolase. Agents that are CYP3A4 inhibitors may increase the plasma levels of carbamazepine. Thus, if a patient has been titrated to a stable dosage of carbamazepine, and then begins a course of treatment with a CYP3A4 or epoxide hydrolase inhibitor, it is reasonable to expect that a dose reduction for carbamazepine may be necessary).

No products indexed under this heading.

Efavirenz (Carbamazepine is metabolized mainly by CYP3A4, the active carbamazepine 10,11-epoxide, which is futher metabolized to the trans-diol by epoxide hydrolase. Therefore, the potential exists for interaction between carbamazepine and any agent that inhibits CYP3A4 and/or epoxide hydrolase. Agents that are CYP3A4 inhibitors may increase the plasma levels of carbamazepine. Thus, if a patient has been titrated to a stable dosage of carbamazepine, and then begins a course of treatment with a CYP3A4 or epoxide hydrolase inhibitor, it is reasonable to expect that a dose reduction for carbamazepine may be necessary). Products include:

Atripla 906

Enflurane (Because of its primary CNS effect, caution should be used when carbamazepine is taken with other centrally acting drugs).

No products indexed under this heading.

Enoxacin (Carbamazepine is known to induce CYP1A2 and CYP3A4. Therefore, the potential exists for interaction between carbamazepine and any agent metabolized by one (or more) of these enzymes. Agents that are metabolized by CYP1A2 and CYP3A4 may have decreased plasma levels when administered concomitantly with carbamazepine. Thus, if a patient has been titrated to a stable dosage on one of the agents in these categories, and then begins a course of treatment with carbamazepine, it is reasonable to expect that a dose increase for the concomitant agent may be necessary).

No products indexed under this heading.

Ergotamine Tartrate (Carbamazepine is known to induce CYP1A2 and CYP3A4. Therefore, the potential exists for interaction between carbamazepine and any agent metabolized by one (or more) of these enzymes. Agents that are metabolized by CYP1A2 and CYP3A4 may have decreased plasma levels when administered concomitantly with carbamazepine. Thus, if a patient has been titrated to a stable dosage on one of the agents in these categories, and then begins a course of treatment with carbamazepine, it is reasonable to expect that a dose increase for the concomitant agent may be necessary).

No products indexed under this heading.

Erythromycin (Carbamazepine is metabolized mainly by CYP3A4, the active carbamazepine 10,11-epoxide, which is futher metabolized to the trans-diol by epoxide hydrolase. Therefore, the potential exists for interaction between carbamazepine and any agent that inhibits CYP3A4 and/or epoxide hydrolase. Agents that are CYP3A4 inhibitors may increase the plasma levels of carbamazepine. Thus, if a patient has been titrated to a stable dosage of carbamazepine, and then begins a course of treatment with a CYP3A4 or epoxide hydrolase inhibitor, it is reasonable to expect that a dose reduction for carbamazepine may be necessary).

No products indexed under this heading.

Erythromycin, Topical (Carbamazepine is metabolized mainly by CYP3A4, the active carbamazepine 10,11-epoxide, which is futher metabolized to the trans-diol by epoxide hydrolase. Therefore, the potential exists for interaction between carbamazepine and any agent that inhibits CYP3A4 and/or epoxide hydrolase. Agents that are CYP3A4 inhibitors may increase the plasma levels of carbamazepine. Also inhibits epoxide hydroxylase, resulting in increased levels of the active metabolite carbamazepine-10,11-epoxide. Thus, if a patient has been titrated to a stable dosage of carbamazepine, and then begins a course of treatment with a CYP3A4 or epoxide hydrolase inhibitor, it is reasonable to expect that a dose reduction for carbamazepine may be necessary).

No products indexed under this heading.

Erythromycin Estolate (Carbamazepine is metabolized mainly by CYP3A4, the active carbamazepine 10,11-epoxide, which is futher metabolized to the trans-diol by epoxide hydrolase. Therefore, the potential exists for interaction between carbamazepine and any agent that inhibits CYP3A4 and/or epoxide hydrolase. Agents that are CYP3A4 inhibitors may increase the plasma levels of carbamazepine. Thus, if a patient has been titrated to a stable dosage of carbamazepine, and then begins a course of treatment with a CYP3A4 or epoxide hydrolase inhibitor, it is reasonable to expect that a dose reduction for carbamazepine may be necessary).

No products indexed under this heading.

Erythromycin Ethylsuccinate (Carbamazepine is metabolized mainly by CYP3A4, the active carbamazepine 10,11-epoxide, which is futher metabolized to the trans-diol by epoxide hydrolase. Therefore, the potential exists for interaction between carbamazepine and any agent that inhibits CYP3A4 and/or epoxide hydrolase. Agents that are CYP3A4 inhibitors may increase the plasma levels of carbamazepine. Thus, if a patient has been titrated to a stable dosage of carbamazepine, and then begins a course of treatment with a CYP3A4 or epoxide hydrolase inhibitor, it is reasonable to expect that a dose reduction for carbamazepine may be necessary). Products include:

E.E.S. 437
EryPed 435

Erythromycin Gluceptate (Carbamazepine is metabolized mainly by CYP3A4, the active carbamazepine 10,11-epoxide, which is futher metabolized to the trans-diol by epoxide hydrolase. Therefore, the potential exists for interaction between carbamazepine and any agent that inhibits CYP3A4 and/or epoxide hydrolase. Agents that are CYP3A4 inhibitors may increase the plasma levels of carbamazepine. Thus, if a patient has been titrated to a stable dosage of carbamazepine, and then begins a course of treatment with a CYP3A4 or epoxide hydrolase inhibitor, it is reasonable to expect that a dose reduction for carbamazepine may be necessary).

No products indexed under this heading.

Erythromycin Lactobionate (Carbamazepine is metabolized mainly by CYP3A4, the active carbamazepine 10,11-epoxide, which is futher metabolized to the trans-diol by epoxide hydrolase. Therefore, the potential exists for interaction between carbamazepine and any agent that inhibits CYP3A4 and/or epoxide hydrolase. Agents that are CYP3A4 inhibitors may increase the plasma levels of carbamazepine. Thus, if a patient has been titrated to a stable dosage of carbamazepine, and then begins a course of treatment with a CYP3A4 or epoxide hydrolase inhibitor, it is reasonable to expect that a dose reduction for carbamazepine may be necessary).

No products indexed under this heading.

Erythromycin Stearate (Carbamazepine is metabolized mainly by CYP3A4, the active carbamazepine 10,11-epoxide, which is futher metabolized to the trans-diol by epoxide hydrolase. Therefore, the potential exists for interaction between carbamazepine and any agent that inhibits CYP3A4 and/or epoxide hydrolase. Agents that are CYP3A4 inhibitors may increase the plasma levels of carbamazepine. Thus, if a patient has been titrated to a stable dosage of carbamazepine, and then begins a course of treatment with a CYP3A4 or epoxide hydrolase inhibitor, it is reasonable to expect that a dose reduction for carbamazepine may be necessary).

No products indexed under this heading.

Esomeprazole Magnesium (Carbamazepine is metabolized mainly by CYP3A4, the active carbamazepine 10,11-epoxide, which is futher metabolized to the trans-diol by epoxide hydrolase. Therefore, the potential exists for interaction between carbamazepine and any agent that inhibits CYP3A4 and/or epoxide hydrolase. Agents that are CYP3A4 inhibitors may increase the plasma levels of carbamazepine. Thus, if a patient has been titrated to a stable dosage of carbamazepine, and then begins a course of treatment with a CYP3A4 or epoxide hydrolase inhibitor, it is reasonable to expect that a dose reduction for carbamazepine may be necessary). Products include:

Nexium Capsules 704
Nexium Oral Suspension 704

Esomeprazole Sodium (Carbamazepine is metabolized mainly by CYP3A4, the active carbamazepine 10,11-epoxide, which is futher metabolized to the trans-diol by epoxide hydrolase. Therefore, the potential exists for interaction between carbamazepine and any agent that inhibits CYP3A4 and/or epoxide hydrolase. Agents that are CYP3A4 inhibitors may increase the plasma levels of carbamazepine. Thus, if a patient has been titrated to a stable dosage of carbamazepine, and then begins a course of treatment with a CYP3A4 or epoxide hydrolase inhibitor, it is reasonable to expect that a dose reduction for carbamazepine may be necessary). Products include:

Nexium I.V. 712

Estazolam (Because of its primary CNS effect, caution should be used when carbamazepine is taken with other centrally acting drugs).

No products indexed under this heading.

Estradiol (Carbamazepine is known to induce CYP1A2 and CYP3A4. Therefore, the potential exists for interaction between carbamazepine and any agent metabolized by one (or more) of these enzymes. Agents that are metabolized by CYP1A2 and CYP3A4 may have decreased plasma levels when administered concomitantly with carbamazepine. Thus, if a patient has been titrated to a stable dosage on one of the agents in these categories, and then begins a course of treatment with carbamazepine, it is reasonable to expect that a dose increase for the concomitant agent may be necessary). Products include:

Activella 2561
Angeliq 831
Climara 841
Climara Pro 847
Divigel 3467
Estrasorb 1777
Vagifem 2589

Estradiol Benzoate (Carbamazepine is known to induce CYP1A2 and CYP3A4. Therefore, the potential exists for interaction between carbamazepine and any agent metabolized by one (or more) of these enzymes. Agents that are metabolized by CYP1A2 and CYP3A4 may have decreased plasma levels when administered concomitantly with carbamazepine. Thus, if a patient has been titrated to a stable dosage on one of the agents in these categories, and then begins a course of treatment with carbamazepine, it is reasonable to expect that a dose increase for the concomitant agent may be necessary).

No products indexed under this heading.

Estradiol Cypionate (Carbamazepine is known to induce CYP1A2 and CYP3A4. Therefore, the potential exists for interaction between carbamazepine and any agent metabolized by one (or more) of these enzymes. Agents that are metabolized by CYP1A2 and CYP3A4 may have decreased plasma levels when administered concomitantly with carbamazepine. Thus, if a patient has been titrated to a stable dosage on

one of the agents in these categories, and then begins a course of treatment with carbamazepine, it is reasonable to expect that a dose increase for the concomitant agent may be necessary).
No products indexed under this heading.

Estradiol Valerate (Carbamazepine is known to induce CYP1A2 and CYP3A4. Therefore, the potential exists for interaction between carbamazepine and any agent metabolized by one (or more) of these enzymes. Agents that are metabolized by CYP1A2 and CYP3A4 may have decreased plasma levels when administered concomitantly with carbamazepine. Thus, if a patient has been titrated to a stable dosage on one of the agents in these categories, and then begins a course of treatment with carbamazepine, it is reasonable to expect that a dose increase for the concomitant agent may be necessary).
No products indexed under this heading.

Ethanol (Because of its primary CNS effect, caution should be used when carbamazepine is taken with alcohol).
No products indexed under this heading.

Ethchlorvynol (Because of its primary CNS effect, caution should be used when carbamazepine is taken with other centrally acting drugs).
No products indexed under this heading.

Ethinamate (Because of its primary CNS effect, caution should be used when carbamazepine is taken with other centrally acting drugs).
No products indexed under this heading.

Ethinyl Estradiol (Carbamazepine is known to induce CYP1A2 and CYP3A4. Therefore, the potential exists for interaction between carbamazepine and any agent metabolized by one (or more) of these enzymes. Agents that are metabolized by CYP1A2 or CYP3A4 may have decreased plasma levels when administered concomitantly with carbamazepine. Breakthrough bleeding has been reported among patients receiving concomitant oral contraceptives and their reliability may be adversely affected).
Products include:
LoSeasonique **3407**
Lybrel **3514**
NuvaRing **3181**
Ortho Evra **2648**
Ortho-Cyclen/Ortho Tri-Cyclen **2663**
Ortho Tri-Cyclen Lo Tablets **2673**
Seasonique **3418**
Yaz **864**

Ethosuximide (Carbamazepine is metabolized by CYP3A4. Therefore, the potential exists for interaction between carbamazepine and any agent that induces CYP3A4. Agents that are CYP3A4 inducers may decrease plasma levels of carbamazepine. Thus, if a patient has been titrated to a stable dosage on carbamazepine, and then begins a course of treatment with CYP3A4 inducers, it is reasonable to expect that a dose increase for carbamazepine may be necessary).
No products indexed under this heading.

Ethyl Alcohol (Because of its primary CNS effect, caution should be used when carbamazepine is taken with alcohol).
No products indexed under this heading.

Ethynodiol Diacetate (Carbamazepine is known to induce CYP1A2 and CYP3A4. Therefore, the potential exists for interaction between carbamazepine and any agent metabolized by one (or more) of these enzymes. Agents that are metabolized by CYP1A2 or CYP3A4 may have decreased plasma levels when administered concomitantly with carbamazepine. Breakthrough bleeding has been reported among patients receiving concomitant oral contraceptives and their reliability may be adversely affected).
No products indexed under this heading.

Etoposide (Carbamazepine is known to induce CYP1A2 and CYP3A4. Therefore, the potential exists for interaction between carbamazepine and any agent metabolized by one (or more) of these enzymes. Agents that are metabolized by CYP1A2 and CYP3A4 may have decreased plasma levels when administered concomitantly with carbamazepine. Thus, if a patient has been titrated to a stable dosage on one of the agents in these categories, and then begins a course of treatment with carbamazepine, it is reasonable to expect that a dose increase for the concomitant agent may be necessary).
No products indexed under this heading.

Etoposide Phosphate (Carbamazepine is known to induce CYP1A2 and CYP3A4. Therefore, the potential exists for interaction between carbamazepine and any agent metabolized by one (or more) of these enzymes. Agents that are metabolized by CYP1A2 and CYP3A4 may have decreased plasma levels when administered concomitantly with carbamazepine. Thus, if a patient has been titrated to a stable dosage on one of the agents in these categories, and then begins a course of treatment with carbamazepine, it is reasonable to expect that a dose increase for the concomitant agent may be necessary).
No products indexed under this heading.

Fat (A high fat meal diet increased the rate of absorption of a single 400 mg dose (mean T_{max} was reduced from 24 hours, in the fasting state, to 14 hours and C_{max} increased from 3.2 to 4.3 μg/mL) but not the extent (AUC) of absorption. The elimination half-life remains unchanged between fed and fasting state. The multiple dose study conducted in the fed state showed that the steady-state C_{max} values were within the therapeutic concentration range. The pharmacokinetic profile of extended-release carbamazepine was similar when given by sprinkling the beads over applesauce compared to the intact capsule administered in the fasted state).
No products indexed under this heading.

Felbamate (Carbamazepine is metabolized by CYP3A4. Therefore, the potential exists for interaction between carbamazepine and any agent that induces CYP3A4. Agents that are CYP3A4 inducers may decrease plasma levels of carbamazepine. Thus, if a patient has been titrated to a stable dosage on carbamazepine, and then begins a course of treatment with CYP3A4 inducers, it is reasonable to expect that a dose increase for carbamazepine may be necessary).
No products indexed under this heading.

Felodipine (Carbamazepine is known to induce CYP1A2 and CYP3A4. Therefore, the potential exists for interaction between carbamazepine and any agent metabolized by one (or more) of these enzymes. Agents that are metabolized by CYP1A2 and CYP3A4 may have decreased plasma levels when administered concomitantly with carbamazepine. Thus, if a patient has been titrated to a stable dosage on one of the agents in these categories, and then begins a course of treatment with carbamazepine, it is reasonable to expect that a dose increase for the concomitant agent may be necessary).
No products indexed under this heading.

Fentanyl (Carbamazepine is known to induce CYP1A2 and CYP3A4. Therefore, the potential exists for interaction between carbamazepine and any agent metabolized by one (or more) of these enzymes. Agents that are metabolized by CYP1A2 and CYP3A4 may have decreased plasma levels when administered concomitantly with carbamazepine. Thus, if a patient has been titrated to a stable dosage on one of the agents in these categories, and then begins a course of treatment with carbamazepine, it is reasonable to expect that a dose increase for the concomitant agent may be necessary). Products include:
Duragesic **2604**
Fentanyl Transdermal System **2346**
Onsolis **2054**

Fentanyl Citrate (Carbamazepine is known to induce CYP1A2 and CYP3A4. Therefore, the potential exists for interaction between carbamazepine and any agent metabolized by one (or more) of these enzymes. Agents that are metabolized by CYP1A2 and CYP3A4 may have decreased plasma levels when administered concomitantly with carbamazepine. Thus, if a patient has been titrated to a stable dosage on one of the agents in these categories, and then begins a course of treatment with carbamazepine, it is reasonable to expect that a dose increase for the concomitant agent may be necessary).
Products include:
Fentora **966**

Fluconazole (Carbamazepine is metabolized mainly by CYP3A4, the active carbamazepine 10,11-epoxide, which is futher metabolized to the trans-diol by epoxide hydrolase. Therefore, the potential exists for interaction between carbamazepine and any agent that inhibits CYP3A4 and/or epoxide hydrolase. Agents that are CYP3A4 inhibitors may increase the plasma levels of carbamazepine. Thus, if a patient has been titrated to a stable dosage of carbamazepine, and then begins a course of treatment with a CYP3A4 or epoxide hydrolase inhibitor, it is reasonable to expect that a dose reduction for carbamazepine may be necessary).
No products indexed under this heading.

Fludrocortisone Acetate (Carbamazepine is metabolized by CYP3A4. Therefore, the potential exists for interaction between carbamazepine and any agent that induces CYP3A4. Agents that are CYP3A4 inducers may decrease plasma levels of carbamazepine. Thus, if a patient has been titrated to a stable dosage on carbamazepine, and then begins a course of treatment with CYP3A4 inducers, it is reasonable to expect that a dose increase for carbamazepine may be necessary).
No products indexed under this heading.

Fluoxetine (Carbamazepine is metabolized mainly by CYP3A4, the active carbamazepine 10,11-epoxide, which is futher metabolized to the trans-diol by epoxide hydrolase. Therefore, the potential exists for interaction between carbamazepine and any agent that inhibits CYP3A4 and/or epoxide hydrolase. Agents that are CYP3A4 inhibitors may increase the plasma levels of carbamazepine. Thus, if a patient has been titrated to a stable dosage of carbamazepine, and then begins a course of treatment with a CYP3A4 or epoxide hydrolase inhibitor, it is reasonable to expect that a dose reduction for carbamazepine may be necessary).
No products indexed under this heading.

Fluoxetine Hydrochloride (Carbamazepine is metabolized mainly by CYP3A4, the active carbamazepine 10,11-epoxide, which is futher metabolized to the trans-diol by epoxide hydrolase. Therefore, the potential exists for interaction between carbamazepine and any agent that inhibits CYP3A4 and/or epoxide hydrolase. Agents that are CYP3A4 inhibitors may increase the plasma levels of carbamazepine. Thus, if a patient has been titrated to a stable dosage of carbamazepine, and then begins a course of treatment with a CYP3A4 or epoxide hydrolase inhibitor, it is reasonable to expect that a dose reduction for carbamazepine may be necessary). Products include:
Prozac Weekly **1941**
Prozac Pulvules **1941**
Symbyax **1965**

Fluphenazine Decanoate (Because of its primary CNS effect, caution should be used when carbamazepine is taken with other centrally acting drugs).
No products indexed under this heading.

Fluphenazine Enanthate (Because of its primary CNS effect, caution should be used when carbamazepine is taken with other centrally acting drugs).
No products indexed under this heading.

Fluphenazine Hydrochloride (Because of its primary CNS effect, caution should be used when carbamazepine is taken with other centrally acting drugs).
No products indexed under this heading.

Flurazepam Hydrochloride (Because of its primary CNS effect, caution should be used when carbamazepine is taken with other centrally acting drugs).
No products indexed under this heading.

Flutamide (Carbamazepine is known to induce CYP1A2 and CYP3A4. Therefore, the potential exists for interaction between carbamazepine and any agent metabolized by one (or more) of these enzymes. Agents that are metabolized by CYP1A2 and CYP3A4 may have decreased plasma levels when administered concomitantly with carbamazepine. Thus, if a patient has been titrated to a stable dosage on one of the agents in these categories, and then begins a course of treatment with carbamazepine, it is reasonable to expect that a dose increase for the concomitant agent may be necessary).
No products indexed under this heading.

Fluticasone Propionate (Carbamazepine is known to induce CYP1A2 and CYP3A4. Therefore, the potential exists for interaction between carbamazepine and any agent metabolized by one (or more) of these enzymes. Agents that are metabolized by CYP1A2 and CYP3A4 may have decreased plasma levels when administered concomitantly with carbamazepine. Thus, if a patient has been titrated to a stable dosage on one of the agents in these categories, and then begins a course of treatment with carbamazepine, it is reasonable to expect that a dose increase for the concomitant agent may be necessary).
Products include:
Advair 100/50 .... **1275**
Advair 250/50 .... **1275**
Advair 500/50 .... **1275**
Advair HFA 45/21 .... **1288**
Advair HFA 115/21 .... **1288**
Advair HFA 230/21 .... **1288**
Flonase **1459**
Flovent Diskus **1463**
Flovent HFA **1470**

Fluvoxamine Maleate (Carbamazepine is metabolized mainly by CYP3A4, the active carbamazepine 10,11-epoxide, which is futher metabolized to the trans-diol by epoxide hydrolase. Therefore, the potential exists for interaction between carbamazepine and any agent that inhibits CYP3A4 and/or epoxide hydrolase. Agents that are CYP3A4 inhibitors may increase the plasma levels of carbamazepine. Thus, if a patient has been titrated to a stable dosage of carbamazepine, and then begins a course of treatment with a CYP3A4 or epoxide hydrolase inhibitor,

Carbatrol Interactions Index 266

it is reasonable to expect that a dose reduction for carbamazepine may be necessary).
No products indexed under this heading.

Fosamprenavir Calcium (Carbamazepine is metabolized mainly by CYP3A4, the active carbamazepine 10,11-epoxide, which is futher metabolized to the trans-diol by epoxide hydrolase. Therefore, the potential exists for interaction between carbamazepine and any agent that inhibits CYP3A4 and/or epoxide hydrolase. Agents that are CYP3A4 inhibitors may increase the plasma levels of carbamazepine. Thus, if a patient has been titrated to a stable dosage of carbamazepine, and then begins a course of treatment with a CYP3A4 or epoxide hydrolase inhibitor, it is reasonable to expect that a dose reduction for carbamazepine may be necessary). Products include:
Lexiva Oral Suspension 1558
Lexiva 1558

Fosphenytoin (Carbamazepine is metabolized by CYP3A4. Therefore, the potential exists for interaction between carbamazepine and any agent that induces CYP3A4. Agents that are CYP3A4 inducers may decrease plasma levels of carbamazepine. Thus, if a patient has been titrated to a stable dosage on carbamazepine, and then begins a course of treatment with a CYP3A4 inducers, it is reasonable to expect that a dose increase for carbamazepine may be necessary. Carbamazepine may increase the plasma levels of phenytoin; careful monitoring of phenytoin plasma levels following comedication with carbamazepine is advised).
No products indexed under this heading.

Fosphenytoin Sodium (Carbamazepine is metabolized by CYP3A4. Therefore, the potential exists for interaction between carbamazepine and any agent that induces CYP3A4. Agents that are CYP3A4 inducers may decrease plasma levels of carbamazepine. Thus, if a patient has been titrated to a stable dosage on carbamazepine, and then begins a course of treatment with a CYP3A4 inducers, it is reasonable to expect that a dose increase for carbamazepine may be necessary. Carbamazepine may increase the plasma levels of phenytoin; careful monitoring of phenytoin plasma levels following comedication with carbamazepine is advised).
No products indexed under this heading.

Garlic Extract (Carbamazepine is metabolized by CYP3A4. Therefore, the potential exists for interaction between carbamazepine and any agent that induces CYP3A4. Agents that are CYP3A4 inducers may decrease plasma levels of carbamazepine. Thus, if a patient has been titrated to a stable dosage on carbamazepine, and then begins a course of treatment with CYP3A4 inducers, it is reasonable to expect that a dose increase for carbamazepine may be necessary).
No products indexed under this heading.

Garlic Oil (Carbamazepine is metabolized by CYP3A4. Therefore, the potential exists for interaction between carbamazepine and any agent that induces CYP3A4. Agents that are CYP3A4 inducers may decrease plasma levels of carbamazepine. Thus, if a patient has been titrated to a stable dosage on carbamazepine, and then begins a course of treatment with CYP3A4 inducers, it is reasonable to expect that a dose increase for carbamazepine may be necessary).
No products indexed under this heading.

Glutethimide (Because of its primary CNS effect, caution should be used when carbamazepine is taken with other centrally acting drugs).
No products indexed under this heading.

Grepafloxacin Hydrochloride (Carbamazepine is known to induce CYP1A2 and CYP3A4. Therefore, the potential exists for interaction between carbamazepine and any agent metabolized by one (or more) of these enzymes. Agents that are metabolized by CYP1A2 and CYP3A4 may have decreased plasma levels when administered concomitantly with carbamazepine. Thus, if a patient has been titrated to a stable dosage on one of the agents in these categories, and then begins a course of treatment with carbamazepine, it is reasonable to expect that a dose increase for the concomitant agent may be necessary).
No products indexed under this heading.

Haloperidol (Carbamazepine is known to induce CYP1A2 and CYP3A4. Therefore, the potential exists for interaction between carbamazepine and any agent metabolized by one (or more) of these enzymes. Agents that are metabolized by CYP1A2 and CYP3A4 may have decreased plasma levels when administered concomitantly with carbamazepine. Thus, if a patient has been titrated to a stable dosage on one of the agents in these categories, and then begins a course of treatment with carbamazepine, it is reasonable to expect that a dose increase for the concomitant agent may be necessary).
No products indexed under this heading.

Haloperidol Decanoate (Carbamazepine is known to induce CYP1A2 and CYP3A4. Therefore, the potential exists for interaction between carbamazepine and any agent metabolized by one (or more) of these enzymes. Agents that are metabolized by CYP1A2 and CYP3A4 may have decreased plasma levels when administered concomitantly with carbamazepine. Thus, if a patient has been titrated to a stable dosage on one of the agents in these categories, and then begins a course of treatment with carbamazepine, it is reasonable to expect that a dose increase for the concomitant agent may be necessary).
No products indexed under this heading.

Haloperidol Lactate (Carbamazepine is known to induce CYP1A2 and CYP3A4. Therefore, the potential exists for interaction between carbamazepine and any agent metabolized by one (or more) of these enzymes. Agents that are metabolized by CYP1A2 and CYP3A4 may have decreased plasma levels when administered concomitantly with carbamazepine. Thus, if a patient has been titrated to a stable dosage on one of the agents in these categories, and then begins a course of treatment with carbamazepine, it is reasonable to expect that a dose increase for the concomitant agent may be necessary).
No products indexed under this heading.

Hydrocodone Bitartrate (Because of its primary CNS effect, caution should be used when carbamazepine is taken with other centrally acting drugs). Products include:
Vicodin 560
Vicodin ES 561
Vicodin HP 563
Vicoprofen 564
Zydone 1138

Hydrocodone Polistirex (Because of its primary CNS effect, caution should be used when carbamazepine is taken with other centrally acting drugs). Products include:
Tussionex 3443

Hydrocortisone (Carbamazepine is metabolized by CYP3A4. Therefore, the potential exists for interaction between carbamazepine and any agent that induces CYP3A4. Agents that are CYP3A4 inducers may decrease plasma levels of carbamazepine. Thus, if a patient has been titrated to a stable dosage on carbamazepine, and then begins a course of treatment with CYP3A4 inducers, it is reasonable to expect that a dose increase for carbamazepine may be necessary).
No products indexed under this heading.

Hydrocortisone (Alcohol) (Carbamazepine is metabolized by CYP3A4. Therefore, the potential exists for interaction between carbamazepine and any agent that induces CYP3A4. Agents that are CYP3A4 inducers may decrease plasma levels of carbamazepine. Thus, if a patient has been titrated to a stable dosage on carbamazepine, and then begins a course of treatment with CYP3A4 inducers, it is reasonable to expect that a dose increase for carbamazepine may be necessary).
No products indexed under this heading.

Hydrocortisone Acetate (Carbamazepine is metabolized by CYP3A4. Therefore, the potential exists for interaction between carbamazepine and any agent that induces CYP3A4. Agents that are CYP3A4 inducers may decrease plasma levels of carbamazepine. Thus, if a patient has been titrated to a stable dosage on carbamazepine, and then begins a course of treatment with CYP3A4 inducers, it is reasonable to expect that a dose increase for carbamazepine may be necessary).
No products indexed under this heading.

Hydrocortisone Butyrate (Carbamazepine is metabolized by CYP3A4. Therefore, the potential exists for interaction between carbamazepine and any agent that induces CYP3A4. Agents that are CYP3A4 inducers may decrease plasma levels of carbamazepine. Thus, if a patient has been titrated to a stable dosage on carbamazepine, and then begins a course of treatment with CYP3A4 inducers, it is reasonable to expect that a dose increase for carbamazepine may be necessary).
No products indexed under this heading.

Hydrocortisone Cypionate (Carbamazepine is metabolized by CYP3A4. Therefore, the potential exists for interaction between carbamazepine and any agent that induces CYP3A4. Agents that are CYP3A4 inducers may decrease plasma levels of carbamazepine. Thus, if a patient has been titrated to a stable dosage on carbamazepine, and then begins a course of treatment with CYP3A4 inducers, it is reasonable to expect that a dose increase for carbamazepine may be necessary).
No products indexed under this heading.

Hydrocortisone Hemisuccinate (Carbamazepine is metabolized by CYP3A4. Therefore, the potential exists for interaction between carbamazepine and any agent that induces CYP3A4. Agents that are CYP3A4 inducers may decrease plasma levels of carbamazepine. Thus, if a patient has been titrated to a stable dosage on carbamazepine, and then begins a course of treatment with CYP3A4 inducers, it is reasonable to expect that a dose increase for carbamazepine may be necessary).
No products indexed under this heading.

Hydrocortisone Probutate (Carbamazepine is metabolized by CYP3A4. Therefore, the potential exists for interaction between carbamazepine and any agent that induces CYP3A4. Agents that are CYP3A4 inducers may decrease plasma levels of carbamazepine. Thus, if a patient has been titrated to a stable dosage on carbamazepine, and then begins a course of treatment with CYP3A4 inducers, it is reasonable to expect that a dose increase for carbamazepine may be necessary).
No products indexed under this heading.

Hydrocortisone Sodium Phosphate (Carbamazepine is metabolized by CYP3A4. Therefore, the potential exists for interaction between carbamazepine and any agent that induces CYP3A4. Agents that are CYP3A4 inducers may decrease plasma levels of carbamazepine. Thus, if a patient has been titrated to a stable dosage on carbamazepine, and then begins a course of treatment with CYP3A4 inducers, it is reasonable to expect that a dose increase for carbamazepine may be necessary).
No products indexed under this heading.

Hydrocortisone Sodium Succinate (Carbamazepine is metabolized by CYP3A4. Therefore, the potential exists for interaction between carbamazepine and any agent that induces CYP3A4. Agents that are CYP3A4 inducers may decrease plasma levels of carbamazepine. Thus, if a patient has been titrated to a stable dosage on carbamazepine, and then begins a course of treatment with CYP3A4 inducers, it is reasonable to expect that a dose increase for carbamazepine may be necessary).
No products indexed under this heading.

Hydrocortisone Valerate (Carbamazepine is metabolized by CYP3A4. Therefore, the potential exists for interaction between carbamazepine and any agent that induces CYP3A4. Agents that are CYP3A4 inducers may decrease plasma levels of carbamazepine. Thus, if a patient has been titrated to a stable dosage on carbamazepine, and then begins a course of treatment with CYP3A4 inducers, it is reasonable to expect that a dose increase for carbamazepine may be necessary).
No products indexed under this heading.

Hydromorphone Hydrochloride (Because of its primary CNS effect, caution should be used when carbamazepine is taken with other centrally acting drugs). Products include:
Dilaudid Injection 2800
Dilaudid Oral 2797
Dilaudid Tablets 2797
Dilaudid-HP 2800

Hydroxyamphetamine Hydrobromide (Because of its primary CNS effect, caution should be used when carbamazepine is taken with other centrally acting drugs).
No products indexed under this heading.

Hydroxyzine Hydrochloride (Because of its primary CNS effect, caution should be used when carbamazepine is taken with other centrally acting drugs).
No products indexed under this heading.

Hypericum (Carbamazepine is metabolized by CYP3A4. Therefore, the potential exists for interaction between carbamazepine and any agent that induces CYP3A4. Agents that are CYP3A4 inducers may decrease plasma levels of carbamazepine. Thus, if a patient has been titrated to a stable dosage on carbamazepine, and then begins a course of treatment with CYP3A4 inducers, it is reasonable to expect that a dose increase for carbamazepine may be necessary).
No products indexed under this heading.

Hypericum Perforatum (Carbamazepine is metabolized by CYP3A4. Therefore, the potential exists for interaction between carbamazepine and any agent that induces CYP3A4. Agents that are CYP3A4 inducers may decrease plasma levels of carbamazepine. Thus, if a patient has been titrated to a stable dosage on carbamazepine, and then begins a course of treatment with

267 Interactions Index Carbatrol

CYP3A4 inducers, it is reasonable to expect that a dose increase for carbamazepine may be necessary). Products include:
Traumeel 1800

Imatinib Mesylate (Carbamazepine is metabolized mainly by CYP3A4, the active carbamazepine 10,11-epoxide, which is futher metabolized to the trans-diol by epoxide hydrolase. Therefore, the potential exists for interaction between carbamazepine and any agent that inhibits CYP3A4 and/or epoxide hydrolase. Agents that are CYP3A4 inhibitors may increase the plasma levels of carbamazepine. Thus, if a patient has been titrated to a stable dosage of carbamazepine, and then begins a course of treatment with a CYP3A4 or epoxide hydrolase inhibitor, it is reasonable to expect that a dose reduction for carbamazepine may be necessary). Products include:
Gleevec 2477

Imipramine Hydrochloride (Carbamazepine is known to induce CYP1A2 and CYP3A4. Therefore, the potential exists for interaction between carbamazepine and any agent metabolized by one (or more) of these enzymes. Agents that are metabolized by CYP1A2 and CYP3A4 may have decreased plasma levels when administered concomitantly with carbamazepine. Thus, if a patient has been titrated to a stable dosage on one of the agents in these categories, and then begins a course of treatment with carbamazepine, it is reasonable to expect that a dose increase for the concomitant agent may be necessary).
No products indexed under this heading.

Imipramine Pamoate (Carbamazepine is known to induce CYP1A2 and CYP3A4. Therefore, the potential exists for interaction between carbamazepine and any agent metabolized by one (or more) of these enzymes. Agents that are metabolized by CYP1A2 and CYP3A4 may have decreased plasma levels when administered concomitantly with carbamazepine. Thus, if a patient has been titrated to a stable dosage on one of the agents in these categories, and then begins a course of treatment with carbamazepine, it is reasonable to expect that a dose increase for the concomitant agent may be necessary).
No products indexed under this heading.

Indinavir Sulfate (Carbamazepine is metabolized mainly by CYP3A4, the active carbamazepine 10,11-epoxide, which is futher metabolized to the trans-diol by epoxide hydrolase. Therefore, the potential exists for interaction between carbamazepine and any agent that inhibits CYP3A4 and/or epoxide hydrolase. Agents that are CYP3A4 inhibitors may increase the plasma levels of carbamazepine. Thus, if a patient has been titrated to a stable dosage of carbamazepine, and then begins a course of treatment with a CYP3A4 or epoxide hydrolase inhibitor, it is reasonable to expect that a dose reduction for carbamazepine may be necessary). Products include:
Crixivan 2113

Isocarboxazid (Co-administration of carbamazepine with monoamine oxidase inhibitors is contraindicated, therefore, not recommended. Before administration of carbamazepine, MAO inhibitors should be discontinued for a minimum of 14 days, or longer if the clinical situation permits). Products include:
Marplan 3481

Isoflurane (Because of its primary CNS effect, caution should be used when carbamazepine is taken with other centrally acting drugs).
No products indexed under this heading.

Isoniazid (Carbamazepine is metabolized mainly by CYP3A4, the active carbamazepine 10,11-epoxide, which is futher metabolized to the trans-diol by epoxide hydrolase. Therefore, the potential exists for interaction between carbamazepine and any agent that inhibits CYP3A4 and/or epoxide hydrolase. Agents that are CYP3A4 inhibitors may increase the plasma levels of carbamazepine. Thus, if a patient has been titrated to a stable dosage of carbamazepine, and then begins a course of treatment with a CYP3A4 or epoxide hydrolase inhibitor, it is reasonable to expect that a dose reduction for carbamazepine may be necessary).
No products indexed under this heading.

Isradipine (Carbamazepine is known to induce CYP1A2 and CYP3A4. Therefore, the potential exists for interaction between carbamazepine and any agent metabolized by one (or more) of these enzymes. Agents that are metabolized by CYP1A2 and CYP3A4 may have decreased plasma levels when administered concomitantly with carbamazepine. Thus, if a patient has been titrated to a stable dosage on one of the agents in these categories, and then begins a course of treatment with carbamazepine, it is reasonable to expect that a dose increase for the concomitant agent may be necessary). Products include:
DynaCirc CR 1432

Itraconazole (Carbamazepine is metabolized mainly by CYP3A4, the active carbamazepine 10,11-epoxide, which is futher metabolized to the trans-diol by epoxide hydrolase. Therefore, the potential exists for interaction between carbamazepine and any agent that inhibits CYP3A4 and/or epoxide hydrolase. Agents that are CYP3A4 inhibitors may increase the plasma levels of carbamazepine. Thus, if a patient has been titrated to a stable dosage of carbamazepine, and then begins a course of treatment with a CYP3A4 or epoxide hydrolase inhibitor, it is reasonable to expect that a dose reduction for carbamazepine may be necessary).
No products indexed under this heading.

Ixabepilone (Carbamazepine is known to induce CYP1A2 and CYP3A4. Therefore, the potential exists for interaction between carbamazepine and any agent metabolized by one (or more) of these enzymes. Agents that are metabolized by CYP1A2 and CYP3A4 may have decreased plasma levels when administered concomitantly with carbamazepine. Thus, if a patient has been titrated to a stable dosage on one of the agents in these categories, and then begins a course of treatment with carbamazepine, it is reasonable to expect that a dose increase for the concomitant agent may be necessary).
No products indexed under this heading.

Ketamine Hydrochloride (Because of its primary CNS effect, caution should be used when carbamazepine is taken with other centrally acting drugs).
No products indexed under this heading.

Ketoconazole (Carbamazepine is metabolized mainly by CYP3A4, the active carbamazepine 10,11-epoxide, which is futher metabolized to the trans-diol by epoxide hydrolase. Therefore, the potential exists for interaction between carbamazepine and any agent that inhibits CYP3A4 and/or epoxide hydrolase. Agents that are CYP3A4 inhibitors may increase the plasma levels of carbamazepine. Thus, if a patient has been titrated to a stable dosage of carbamazepine, and then begins a course of treatment with a CYP3A4 or epoxide hydrolase inhibitor, it is reasonable to expect that a dose reduction for carbamazepine may be necessary). Products include:
Extina 3319
Xolegel 3337

Lapatinib (Carbamazepine is metabolized mainly by CYP3A4, the active carbamazepine 10,11-epoxide, which is futher metabolized to the trans-diol by epoxide hydrolase. Therefore, the potential exists for interaction between carbamazepine and any agent that inhibits CYP3A4 and/or epoxide hydrolase. Agents that are CYP3A4 inhibitors may increase the plasma levels of carbamazepine. Thus, if a patient has been titrated to a stable dosage of carbamazepine, and then begins a course of treatment with a CYP3A4 or epoxide hydrolase inhibitor, it is reasonable to expect that a dose reduction for carbamazepine may be necessary). Products include:
Tykerb 1698

Levobupivacaine Hydrochloride (Carbamazepine is known to induce CYP1A2 and CYP3A4. Therefore, the potential exists for interaction between carbamazepine and any agent metabolized by one (or more) of these enzymes. Agents that are metabolized by CYP1A2 and CYP3A4 may have decreased plasma levels when administered concomitantly with carbamazepine. Thus, if a patient has been titrated to a stable dosage on one of the agents in these categories, and then begins a course of treatment with carbamazepine, it is reasonable to expect that a dose increase for the concomitant agent may be necessary).
No products indexed under this heading.

Levomethadyl Acetate Hydrochloride (Because of its primary CNS effect, caution should be used when carbamazepine is taken with other centrally acting drugs).
No products indexed under this heading.

Levonorgestrel (Carbamazepine is known to induce CYP1A2 and CYP3A4. Therefore, the potential exists for interaction between carbamazepine and any agent metabolized by one (or more) of these enzymes. Agents that are metabolized by CYP1A2 or CYP3A4 may have decreased plasma levels when administered concomitantly with carbamazepine. Breakthrough bleeding has been reported among patients receiving concomitant oral contraceptives and their reliability may be adversely affected). Products include:
Climara Pro 847
LoSeasonique 3407
Lybrel 3514
Mirena 854
Plan B 3416
Seasonique 3418

Levorphanol Tartrate (Because of its primary CNS effect, caution should be used when carbamazepine is taken with other centrally acting drugs).
No products indexed under this heading.

Lidocaine (Carbamazepine is known to induce CYP1A2 and CYP3A4. Therefore, the potential exists for interaction between carbamazepine and any agent metabolized by one (or more) of these enzymes. Agents that are metabolized by CYP1A2 and CYP3A4 may have decreased plasma levels when administered concomitantly with carbamazepine. Thus, if a patient has been titrated to a stable dosage on one of the agents in these categories, and then begins a course of treatment with carbamazepine, it is reasonable to expect that a dose increase for the concomitant agent may be necessary). Products include:
Lidoderm 1107

Lidocaine Hydrochloride (Carbamazepine is known to induce CYP1A2 and CYP3A4. Therefore, the potential exists for interaction between carbamazepine and any agent metabolized by one (or more) of these enzymes. Agents that are metabolized by CYP1A2 and CYP3A4 may have decreased plasma levels when administered concomitantly with carbamazepine. Thus, if a patient has been titrated to a stable dosage on one of the agents in these categories, and then begins a course of treatment with carbamazepine, it is reasonable to expect that a dose increase for the concomitant agent may be necessary).
No products indexed under this heading.

Lisdexamfetamine Dimesylate (Because of its primary CNS effect, caution should be used when carbamazepine is taken with other centrally acting drugs). Products include:
Vyvanse 3298

Lithium (Concomitant administration of carbamazepine and lithium may increase the risk of neurotoxic side effects).
No products indexed under this heading.

Lithium Carbonate (Concomitant administration of carbamazepine and lithium may increase the risk of neurotoxic side effects).
No products indexed under this heading.

Lithium Citrate (Concomitant administration of carbamazepine and lithium may increase the risk of neurotoxic side effects).
No products indexed under this heading.

Lomefloxacin Hydrochloride (Carbamazepine is known to induce CYP1A2 and CYP3A4. Therefore, the potential exists for interaction between carbamazepine and any agent metabolized by one (or more) of these enzymes. Agents that are metabolized by CYP1A2 and CYP3A4 may have decreased plasma levels when administered concomitantly with carbamazepine. Thus, if a patient has been titrated to a stable dosage on one of the agents in these categories, and then begins a course of treatment with carbamazepine, it is reasonable to expect that a dose increase for the concomitant agent may be necessary).
No products indexed under this heading.

Lopinavir (Carbamazepine is metabolized mainly by CYP3A4, the active carbamazepine 10,11-epoxide, which is futher metabolized to the trans-diol by epoxide hydrolase. Therefore, the potential exists for interaction between carbamazepine and any agent that inhibits CYP3A4 and/or epoxide hydrolase. Agents that are CYP3A4 inhibitors may increase the plasma levels of carbamazepine. Thus, if a patient has been titrated to a stable dosage of carbamazepine, and then begins a course of treatment with a CYP3A4 or epoxide hydrolase inhibitor, it is reasonable to expect that a dose reduction for carbamazepine may be necessary). Products include:
Kaletra 458

Loratadine (Carbamazepine is metabolized mainly by CYP3A4, the active carbamazepine 10,11-epoxide, which is futher metabolized to the trans-diol by epoxide hydrolase. Therefore, the potential exists for interaction between carbamazepine and any agent that inhibits CYP3A4 and/or epoxide hydrolase. Agents that are CYP3A4 inhibitors may increase the plasma levels of carbamazepine. Thus, if a patient has been titrated to a stable dosage of carbamazepine, and then begins a course of treatment with a CYP3A4 or epoxide hydrolase inhibitor, it is reasonable to expect that a dose reduction for carbamazepine may be necessary).
No products indexed under this heading.

IMPORTANT NOTE: Always consult each drug listing in the patient's regimen for possible interactions.

Carbatrol Interactions Index 268

Lorazepam (Because of its primary CNS effect, caution should be used when carbamazepine is taken with other centrally acting drugs).
No products indexed under this heading.

Lovastatin (Carbamazepine is known to induce CYP1A2 and CYP3A4. Therefore, the potential exists for interaction between carbamazepine and any agent metabolized by one (or more) of these enzymes. Agents that are metabolized by CYP1A2 and CYP3A4 may have decreased plasma levels when administered concomitantly with carbamazepine. Thus, if a patient has been titrated to a stable dosage on one of the agents in these categories, and then begins a course of treatment with carbamazepine, it is reasonable to expect that a dose increase for the concomitant agent may be necessary). Products include:
Advicor 402
Mevacor 2212

Loxapine Hydrochloride (Because of its primary CNS effect, caution should be used when carbamazepine is taken with other centrally acting drugs).
No products indexed under this heading.

Loxapine Succinate (Because of its primary CNS effect, caution should be used when carbamazepine is taken with other centrally acting drugs).
No products indexed under this heading.

Maprotiline Hydrochloride (Carbamazepine is known to induce CYP1A2 and CYP3A4. Therefore, the potential exists for interaction between carbamazepine and any agent metabolized by one (or more) of these enzymes. Agents that are metabolized by CYP1A2 and CYP3A4 may have decreased plasma levels when administered concomitantly with carbamazepine. Thus, if a patient has been titrated to a stable dosage on one of the agents in these categories, and then begins a course of treatment with carbamazepine, it is reasonable to expect that a dose increase for the concomitant agent may be necessary).
No products indexed under this heading.

Mefloquine Hydrochloride (Antimalarial drugs, such as chloroquine and mefloquine, may antagonize the activity of carbamazepine).
No products indexed under this heading.

Meperidine Hydrochloride (Because of its primary CNS effect, caution should be used when carbamazepine is taken with other centrally acting drugs).
No products indexed under this heading.

Mephenytoin (Carbamazepine is metabolized by CYP3A4. Therefore, the potential exists for interaction between carbamazepine and any agent that induces CYP3A4. Agents that are CYP3A4 inducers may decrease plasma levels of carbamazepine. Thus, if a patient has been titrated to a stable dosage on carbamazepine, and then begins a course of treatment with CYP3A4 inducers, it is reasonable to expect that a dose increase for carbamazepine may be necessary).
No products indexed under this heading.

Mephobarbital (Because of its primary CNS effect, caution should be used when carbamazepine is taken with other centrally acting drugs).
No products indexed under this heading.

Meprobamate (Because of its primary CNS effect, caution should be used when carbamazepine is taken with other centrally acting drugs).
No products indexed under this heading.

Mesoridazine Besylate (Because of its primary CNS effect, caution should be used when carbamazepine is taken with other centrally acting drugs).
No products indexed under this heading.

Mestranol (Carbamazepine is known to induce CYP1A2 and CYP3A4. Therefore, the potential exists for interaction between carbamazepine and any agent metabolized by one (or more) of these enzymes. Agents that are metabolized by CYP1A2 or CYP3A4 may have decreased plasma levels when administered concomitantly with carbamazepine. Breakthrough bleeding has been reported among patients receiving concomitant oral contraceptives and their reliability may be adversely affected).
No products indexed under this heading.

Methadone Hydrochloride (Carbamazepine is known to induce CYP1A2 and CYP3A4. Therefore, the potential exists for interaction between carbamazepine and any agent metabolized by one (or more) of these enzymes. Agents that are metabolized by CYP1A2 and CYP3A4 may have decreased plasma levels when administered concomitantly with carbamazepine. Thus, if a patient has been titrated to a stable dosage on one of the agents in these categories, and then begins a course of treatment with carbamazepine, it is reasonable to expect that a dose increase for the concomitant agent may be necessary).
No products indexed under this heading.

Methamphetamine Hydrochloride (Because of its primary CNS effect, caution should be used when carbamazepine is taken with other centrally acting drugs).
No products indexed under this heading.

Methohexital Sodium (Because of its primary CNS effect, caution should be used when carbamazepine is taken with other centrally acting drugs).
No products indexed under this heading.

Methotrimeprazine (Because of its primary CNS effect, caution should be used when carbamazepine is taken with other centrally acting drugs).
No products indexed under this heading.

Methoxyflurane (Because of its primary CNS effect, caution should be used when carbamazepine is taken with other centrally acting drugs).
No products indexed under this heading.

Methsuximide (Carbamazepine is metabolized by CYP3A4. Therefore, the potential exists for interaction between carbamazepine and any agent that induces CYP3A4. Agents that are CYP3A4 inducers may decrease plasma levels of carbamazepine. Thus, if a patient has been titrated to a stable dosage on carbamazepine, and then begins a course of treatment with CYP3A4 inducers, it is reasonable to expect that a dose increase for carbamazepine may be necessary).
No products indexed under this heading.

Methylphenidate (Because of its primary CNS effect, caution should be used when carbamazepine is taken with other centrally acting drugs). Products include:
Daytrana 3283

Methylphenidate Hydrochloride (Because of its primary CNS effect, caution should be used when carbamazepine is taken with other centrally acting drugs). Products include:
Concerta 2598
Metadate CD 3439

Methylprednisolone (Carbamazepine is metabolized by CYP3A4. Therefore, the potential exists for interaction between carbamazepine and any agent that induces CYP3A4. Agents that are CYP3A4 inducers may decrease plasma levels of carbamazepine. Thus, if a patient has been titrated to a stable dosage on carbamazepine, and then begins a course of treatment with CYP3A4 inducers, it is reasonable to expect that a dose increase for carbamazepine may be necessary).
No products indexed under this heading.

Methylprednisolone Acetate (Carbamazepine is metabolized by CYP3A4. Therefore, the potential exists for interaction between carbamazepine and any agent that induces CYP3A4. Agents that are CYP3A4 inducers may decrease plasma levels of carbamazepine. Thus, if a patient has been titrated to a stable dosage on carbamazepine, and then begins a course of treatment with CYP3A4 inducers, it is reasonable to expect that a dose increase for carbamazepine may be necessary).
No products indexed under this heading.

Methylprednisolone Sodium Succinate (Carbamazepine is metabolized by CYP3A4. Therefore, the potential exists for interaction between carbamazepine and any agent that induces CYP3A4. Agents that are CYP3A4 inducers may decrease plasma levels of carbamazepine. Thus, if a patient has been titrated to a stable dosage on carbamazepine, and then begins a course of treatment with CYP3A4 inducers, it is reasonable to expect that a dose increase for carbamazepine may be necessary).
No products indexed under this heading.

Metronidazole (Carbamazepine is metabolized mainly by CYP3A4, the active carbamazepine 10,11-epoxide, which is futher metabolized to the trans-diol by epoxide hydrolase. Therefore, the potential exists for interaction between carbamazepine and any agent that inhibits CYP3A4 and/or epoxide hydrolase. Agents that are CYP3A4 inhibitors may increase the plasma levels of carbamazepine. Thus, if a patient has been titrated to a stable dosage of carbamazepine, and then begins a course of treatment with a CYP3A4 or epoxide hydrolase inhibitor, it is reasonable to expect that a dose reduction for carbamazepine may be necessary). Products include:
Pylera 793

Metronidazole Benzoate (Carbamazepine is metabolized mainly by CYP3A4, the active carbamazepine 10,11-epoxide, which is futher metabolized to the trans-diol by epoxide hydrolase. Therefore, the potential exists for interaction between carbamazepine and any agent that inhibits CYP3A4 and/or epoxide hydrolase. Agents that are CYP3A4 inhibitors may increase the plasma levels of carbamazepine. Thus, if a patient has been titrated to a stable dosage of carbamazepine, and then begins a course of treatment with a CYP3A4 or epoxide hydrolase inhibitor, it is reasonable to expect that a dose reduction for carbamazepine may be necessary).
No products indexed under this heading.

Metronidazole Hydrochloride (Carbamazepine is metabolized mainly by CYP3A4, the active carbamazepine 10,11-epoxide, which is futher metabolized to the trans-diol by epoxide hydrolase. Therefore, the potential exists for interaction between carbamazepine and any agent that inhibits CYP3A4 and/or epoxide hydrolase. Agents that are CYP3A4 inhibitors may increase the plasma levels of carbamazepine. Thus, if a patient has been titrated to a stable dosage of carbamazepine, and then begins a course of treatment with a CYP3A4 or epoxide hydrolase inhibitor, it is reasonable to expect that a dose reduction for carbamazepine may be necessary).
No products indexed under this heading.

Metronidazole Sodium (Carbamazepine is metabolized mainly by CYP3A4, the active carbamazepine 10,11-epoxide, which is futher metabolized to the trans-diol by epoxide hydrolase. Therefore, the potential exists for interaction between carbamazepine and any agent that inhibits CYP3A4 and/or epoxide hydrolase. Agents that are CYP3A4 inhibitors may increase the plasma levels of carbamazepine. Thus, if a patient has been titrated to a stable dosage of carbamazepine, and then begins a course of treatment with a CYP3A4 or epoxide hydrolase inhibitor, it is reasonable to expect that a dose reduction for carbamazepine may be necessary).
No products indexed under this heading.

Mexiletine Hydrochloride (Carbamazepine is known to induce CYP1A2 and CYP3A4. Therefore, the potential exists for interaction between carbamazepine and any agent metabolized by one (or more) of these enzymes. Agents that are metabolized by CYP1A2 and CYP3A4 may have decreased plasma levels when administered concomitantly with carbamazepine. Thus, if a patient has been titrated to a stable dosage on one of the agents in these categories, and then begins a course of treatment with carbamazepine, it is reasonable to expect that a dose increase for the concomitant agent may be necessary).
No products indexed under this heading.

Miconazole (Carbamazepine is metabolized mainly by CYP3A4, the active carbamazepine 10,11-epoxide, which is futher metabolized to the trans-diol by epoxide hydrolase. Therefore, the potential exists for interaction between carbamazepine and any agent that inhibits CYP3A4 and/or epoxide hydrolase. Agents that are CYP3A4 inhibitors may increase the plasma levels of carbamazepine. Thus, if a patient has been titrated to a stable dosage of carbamazepine, and then begins a course of treatment with a CYP3A4 or epoxide hydrolase inhibitor, it is reasonable to expect that a dose reduction for carbamazepine may be necessary).
No products indexed under this heading.

Miconazole Nitrate (Carbamazepine is metabolized mainly by CYP3A4, the active carbamazepine 10,11-epoxide, which is futher metabolized to the trans-diol by epoxide hydrolase. Therefore, the potential exists for interaction between carbamazepine and any agent that inhibits CYP3A4 and/or epoxide hydrolase. Agents that are CYP3A4 inhibitors may increase the plasma levels of carbamazepine. Thus, if a patient has been titrated to a stable dosage of carbamazepine, and then begins a course of treatment with a CYP3A4 or epoxide hydrolase inhibitor, it is reasonable to expect that a dose reduction for carbamazepine may be necessary). Products include:
Vusion Ointment 3335

Midazolam Hydrochloride (Carbamazepine is known to induce CYP1A2 and CYP3A4. Therefore, the potential exists for interaction between carbamazepine and any agent metabolized by one (or more) of these enzymes. Agents that are metabolized by CYP1A2 and CYP3A4 may have decreased plasma levels when administered concomitantly with carbamazepine. Thus, if a patient has been titrated to a stable dosage on one of the agents in these categories, and then begins a course of treatment with carbamazepine, it is reasonable to expect that a dose increase for the concomitant agent may be necessary).
No products indexed under this heading.

Mifepristone (Carbamazepine is metabolized mainly by CYP3A4, the active carbamazepine 10,11-epoxide, which is futher metabolized to the trans-diol by epoxide hydrolase. Therefore, the potential exists for interaction

269 **Interactions Index** **Carbatrol**

between carbamazepine and any agent that inhibits CYP3A4 and/or epoxide hydrolase. Agents that are CYP3A4 inhibitors may increase the plasma levels of carbamazepine. Thus, if a patient has been titrated to a stable dosage of carbamazepine, and then begins a course of treatment with a CYP3A4 or epoxide hydrolase inhibitor, it is reasonable to expect that a dose reduction for carbamazepine may be necessary).
No products indexed under this heading.

Mirtazapine (Carbamazepine is known to induce CYP1A2 and CYP3A4. Therefore, the potential exists for interaction between carbamazepine and any agent metabolized by one (or more) of these enzymes. Agents that are metabolized by CYP1A2 and CYP3A4 may have decreased plasma levels when administered concomitantly with carbamazepine. Thus, if a patient has been titrated to a stable dosage on one of the agents in these categories, and then begins a course of treatment with carbamazepine, it is reasonable to expect that a dose increase for the concomitant agent may be necessary). Products include:
Remeron Tablets 3214
RemeronSolTab Tablets 3219

Moclobemide (Co-administration of carbamazepine with monoamine oxidase inhibitors is contraindicated, therefore, not recommended. Before administration of carbamazepine, MAO inhibitors should be discontinued for a minimum of 14 days, or longer if the clinical situation permits).
No products indexed under this heading.

Modafinil (Carbamazepine is metabolized by CYP3A4. Therefore, the potential exists for interaction between carbamazepine and any agent that induces CYP3A4. Agents that are CYP3A4 inducers may decrease plasma levels of carbamazepine. Thus, if a patient has been titrated to a stable dosage on carbamazepine, and then begins a course of treatment with CYP3A4 inducers, it is reasonable to expect that a dose increase for carbamazepine may be necessary). Products include:
Provigil 983

Molindone Hydrochloride (Because of its primary CNS effect, caution should be used when carbamazepine is taken with other centrally acting drugs). Products include:
Moban 1108

Morphine Sulfate (Because of its primary CNS effect, caution should be used when carbamazepine is taken with other centrally acting drugs). Products include:
Avinza 1822
Embeda 1831
MS Contin 2803

Moxifloxacin Hydrochloride (Carbamazepine is known to induce CYP1A2 and CYP3A4. Therefore, the potential exists for interaction between carbamazepine and any agent metabolized by one (or more) of these enzymes. Agents that are metabolized by CYP1A2 and CYP3A4 may have decreased plasma levels when administered concomitantly with carbamazepine. Thus, if a patient has been titrated to a stable dosage on one of the agents in these categories, and then begins a course of treatment with carbamazepine, it is reasonable to expect that a dose increase for the concomitant agent may be necessary). Products include:
Avelox 3064
Vigamox 589

Nafcillin Sodium (Carbamazepine is metabolized by CYP3A4. Therefore, the potential exists for interaction between carbamazepine and any agent that induces CYP3A4. Agents that are CYP3A4 inducers may decrease plasma levels of carbamazepine. Thus, if a patient has been titrated to a stable dosage on carbamazepine, and then begins a course of treatment with CYP3A4 inducers, it is reasonable to expect that a dose increase for carbamazepine may be necessary).
No products indexed under this heading.

Naproxen (Carbamazepine is known to induce CYP1A2 and CYP3A4. Therefore, the potential exists for interaction between carbamazepine and any agent metabolized by one (or more) of these enzymes. Agents that are metabolized by CYP1A2 and CYP3A4 may have decreased plasma levels when administered concomitantly with carbamazepine. Thus, if a patient has been titrated to a stable dosage on one of the agents in these categories, and then begins a course of treatment with carbamazepine, it is reasonable to expect that a dose increase for the concomitant agent may be necessary). Products include:
EC-Naprosyn 2850
Naprosyn 2850
Anaprox/Naprosyn 2850

Naproxen Sodium (Carbamazepine is known to induce CYP1A2 and CYP3A4. Therefore, the potential exists for interaction between carbamazepine and any agent metabolized by one (or more) of these enzymes. Agents that are metabolized by CYP1A2 and CYP3A4 may have decreased plasma levels when administered concomitantly with carbamazepine. Thus, if a patient has been titrated to a stable dosage on one of the agents in these categories, and then begins a course of treatment with carbamazepine, it is reasonable to expect that a dose increase for the concomitant agent may be necessary). Products include:
Anaprox 2850
Anaprox DS 2850
Treximet 1681

Nefazodone Hydrochloride (Carbamazepine is metabolized mainly by CYP3A4, the active carbamazepine 10,11-epoxide, which is futher metabolized to the trans-diol by epoxide hydrolase. Therefore, the potential exists for interaction between carbamazepine and any agent that inhibits CYP3A4 and/or epoxide hydrolase. Agents that are CYP3A4 inhibitors may increase the plasma levels of carbamazepine. Thus, if a patient has been titrated to a stable dosage of carbamazepine, and then begins a course of treatment with a CYP3A4 or epoxide hydrolase inhibitor, it is reasonable to expect that a dose reduction for carbamazepine may be necessary).
No products indexed under this heading.

Nelfinavir Mesylate (Carbamazepine is metabolized mainly by CYP3A4, the active carbamazepine 10,11-epoxide, which is futher metabolized to the trans-diol by epoxide hydrolase. Therefore, the potential exists for interaction between carbamazepine and any agent that inhibits CYP3A4 and/or epoxide hydrolase. Agents that are CYP3A4 inhibitors may increase the plasma levels of carbamazepine. Thus, if a patient has been titrated to a stable dosage of carbamazepine, and then begins a course of treatment with a CYP3A4 or epoxide hydrolase inhibitor, it is reasonable to expect that a dose reduction for carbamazepine may be necessary).
No products indexed under this heading.

Nevirapine (Carbamazepine is metabolized mainly by CYP3A4, the active carbamazepine 10,11-epoxide, which is futher metabolized to the trans-diol by epoxide hydrolase. Therefore, the potential exists for interaction between carbamazepine and any agent that inhibits CYP3A4 and/or epoxide hydrolase. Agents that are CYP3A4 inhibitors may increase the plasma levels of carbamazepine. Thus, if a patient has been titrated to a stable dosage of carbamazepine, and then begins a course of treatment with a CYP3A4 or epoxide hydrolase inhibitor, it is reasonable to expect that a dose reduction for carbamazepine may be necessary). Products include:
Viramune Oral Suspension 897
Viramune Tablets 897

Niacin (Carbamazepine is metabolized mainly by CYP3A4, the active carbamazepine 10,11-epoxide, which is futher metabolized to the trans-diol by epoxide hydrolase. Therefore, the potential exists for interaction between carbamazepine and any agent that inhibits CYP3A4 and/or epoxide hydrolase. Agents that are CYP3A4 inhibitors may increase the plasma levels of carbamazepine. Thus, if a patient has been titrated to a stable dosage of carbamazepine, and then begins a course of treatment with a CYP3A4 or epoxide hydrolase inhibitor, it is reasonable to expect that a dose reduction for carbamazepine may be necessary). Products include:
Advicor 402
Cardio Basics 3455
Niaspan 497
Simcor 524

Niacinamide (Carbamazepine is metabolized mainly by CYP3A4, the active carbamazepine 10,11-epoxide, which is futher metabolized to the trans-diol by epoxide hydrolase. Therefore, the potential exists for interaction between carbamazepine and any agent that inhibits CYP3A4 and/or epoxide hydrolase. Agents that are CYP3A4 inhibitors may increase the plasma levels of carbamazepine. Thus, if a patient has been titrated to a stable dosage of carbamazepine, and then begins a course of treatment with a CYP3A4 or epoxide hydrolase inhibitor, it is reasonable to expect that a dose reduction for carbamazepine may be necessary). Products include:
CitraNatal 90 DHA Capsules 2332
CitraNatal Assure 2332
CitraNatal Rx 2332
Heplive 607

Niacinamide Hydroiodide (Carbamazepine is metabolized mainly by CYP3A4, the active carbamazepine 10,11-epoxide, which is futher metabolized to the trans-diol by epoxide hydrolase. Therefore, the potential exists for interaction between carbamazepine and any agent that inhibits CYP3A4 and/or epoxide hydrolase. Agents that are CYP3A4 inhibitors may increase the plasma levels of carbamazepine. Thus, if a patient has been titrated to a stable dosage of carbamazepine, and then begins a course of treatment with a CYP3A4 or epoxide hydrolase inhibitor, it is reasonable to expect that a dose reduction for carbamazepine may be necessary).
No products indexed under this heading.

Nicardipine (Carbamazepine is known to induce CYP1A2 and CYP3A4. Therefore, the potential exists for interaction between carbamazepine and any agent metabolized by one (or more) of these enzymes. Agents that are metabolized by CYP1A2 and CYP3A4 may have decreased plasma levels when administered concomitantly with carbamazepine. Thus, if a patient has been titrated to a stable dosage on one of the agents in these categories, and then begins a course of treatment with carbamazepine, it is reasonable to expect that a dose increase for the concomitant agent may be necessary).
No products indexed under this heading.

Nicardipine Hydrochloride (Carbamazepine is known to induce CYP1A2 and CYP3A4. Therefore, the potential exists for interaction between carbamazepine and any agent metabolized by one (or more) of these enzymes. Agents that are metabolized by CYP1A2 and CYP3A4 may have decreased plasma levels when administered concomitantly with carbamazepine. Thus, if a patient has been titrated to a stable dosage on one of the agents in these categories, and then begins a course of treatment with carbamazepine, it is reasonable to expect that a dose increase for the concomitant agent may be necessary).
No products indexed under this heading.

Nicotinamide (Carbamazepine is metabolized mainly by CYP3A4, the active carbamazepine 10,11-epoxide, which is futher metabolized to the trans-diol by epoxide hydrolase. Therefore, the potential exists for interaction between carbamazepine and any agent that inhibits CYP3A4 and/or epoxide hydrolase. Agents that are CYP3A4 inhibitors may increase the plasma levels of carbamazepine. Thus, if a patient has been titrated to a stable dosage of carbamazepine, and then begins a course of treatment with a CYP3A4 or epoxide hydrolase inhibitor, it is reasonable to expect that a dose reduction for carbamazepine may be necessary).
No products indexed under this heading.

Nicotine Polacrilex (Carbamazepine is known to induce CYP1A2 and CYP3A4. Therefore, the potential exists for interaction between carbamazepine and any agent metabolized by one (or more) of these enzymes. Agents that are metabolized by CYP1A2 and CYP3A4 may have decreased plasma levels when administered concomitantly with carbamazepine. Thus, if a patient has been titrated to a stable dosage on one of the agents in these categories, and then begins a course of treatment with carbamazepine, it is reasonable to expect that a dose increase for the concomitant agent may be necessary).
No products indexed under this heading.

Nicotine Salicylate (Carbamazepine is known to induce CYP1A2 and CYP3A4. Therefore, the potential exists for interaction between carbamazepine and any agent metabolized by one (or more) of these enzymes. Agents that are metabolized by CYP1A2 and CYP3A4 may have decreased plasma levels when administered concomitantly with carbamazepine. Thus, if a patient has been titrated to a stable dosage on one of the agents in these categories, and then begins a course of treatment with carbamazepine, it is reasonable to expect that a dose increase for the concomitant agent may be necessary).
No products indexed under this heading.

Nicotine Sulfate (Carbamazepine is known to induce CYP1A2 and CYP3A4. Therefore, the potential exists for interaction between carbamazepine and any agent metabolized by one (or more) of these enzymes. Agents that are metabolized by CYP1A2 and CYP3A4 may have decreased plasma levels when administered concomitantly with carbamazepine. Thus, if a patient has been titrated to a stable dosage on one of the agents in these categories, and then begins a course of treatment with carbamazepine, it is reasonable to expect that a dose increase for the concomitant agent may be necessary).
No products indexed under this heading.

Nifedipine (Carbamazepine is metabolized mainly by CYP3A4, the active carbamazepine 10,11-epoxide, which is futher metabolized to the trans-diol by epoxide hydrolase. Therefore, the potential exists for interaction between carbamazepine and any agent that

IMPORTANT NOTE: Always consult each drug listing in the patient's regimen for possible interactions.

inhibits CYP3A4 and/or epoxide hydrolase. Agents that are CYP3A4 inhibitors may increase the plasma levels of carbamazepine. Thus, if a patient has been titrated to a stable dosage of carbamazepine, and then begins a course of treatment with a CYP3A4 or epoxide hydrolase inhibitor, it is reasonable to expect that a dose reduction for carbamazepine may be necessary).
No products indexed under this heading.

Nimodipine (Carbamazepine is known to induce CYP1A2 and CYP3A4. Therefore, the potential exists for interaction between carbamazepine and any agent metabolized by one (or more) of these enzymes. Agents that are metabolized by CYP1A2 and CYP3A4 may have decreased plasma levels when administered concomitantly with carbamazepine. Thus, if a patient has been titrated to a stable dosage on one of the agents in these categories, and then begins a course of treatment with carbamazepine, it is reasonable to expect that a dose increase for the concomitant agent may be necessary).
No products indexed under this heading.

Nisoldipine (Carbamazepine is known to induce CYP1A2 and CYP3A4. Therefore, the potential exists for interaction between carbamazepine and any agent metabolized by one (or more) of these enzymes. Agents that are metabolized by CYP1A2 and CYP3A4 may have decreased plasma levels when administered concomitantly with carbamazepine. Thus, if a patient has been titrated to a stable dosage on one of the agents in these categories, and then begins a course of treatment with carbamazepine, it is reasonable to expect that a dose increase for the concomitant agent may be necessary).
No products indexed under this heading.

Nitrendipine (Carbamazepine is known to induce CYP1A2 and CYP3A4. Therefore, the potential exists for interaction between carbamazepine and any agent metabolized by one (or more) of these enzymes. Agents that are metabolized by CYP1A2 and CYP3A4 may have decreased plasma levels when administered concomitantly with carbamazepine. Thus, if a patient has been titrated to a stable dosage on one of the agents in these categories, and then begins a course of treatment with carbamazepine, it is reasonable to expect that a dose increase for the concomitant agent may be necessary).
No products indexed under this heading.

Norethindrone (Carbamazepine is known to induce CYP1A2 and CYP3A4. Therefore, the potential exists for interaction between carbamazepine and any agent metabolized by one (or more) of these enzymes. Agents that are metabolized by CYP1A2 or CYP3A4 may have decreased plasma levels when administered concomitantly with carbamazepine. Breakthrough bleeding has been reported among patients receiving concomitant oral contraceptives and their reliability may be adversely affected). Products include:
Ortho Micronor **2660**

Norethindrone Acetate (Carbamazepine is known to induce CYP1A2 and CYP3A4. Therefore, the potential exists for interaction between carbamazepine and any agent metabolized by one (or more) of these enzymes. Agents that are metabolized by CYP1A2 and CYP3A4 may have decreased plasma levels when administered concomitantly with carbamazepine. Thus, if a patient has been titrated to a stable dosage on one of the agents in these categories, and then begins a course of treatment with carbamazepine, it is reasonable to expect that a dose increase for the concomitant agent may be necessary). Products include:
Activella **2561**

Norethynodrel (Carbamazepine is known to induce CYP1A2 and CYP3A4. Therefore, the potential exists for interaction between carbamazepine and any agent metabolized by one (or more) of these enzymes. Agents that are metabolized by CYP1A2 or CYP3A4 may have decreased plasma levels when administered concomitantly with carbamazepine. Breakthrough bleeding has been reported among patients receiving concomitant oral contraceptives and their reliability may be adversely affected).
No products indexed under this heading.

Norfloxacin (Carbamazepine is metabolized mainly by CYP3A4, the active carbamazepine 10,11-epoxide, which is futher metabolized to the trans-diol by epoxide hydrolase. Therefore, the potential exists for interaction between carbamazepine and any agent that inhibits CYP3A4 and/or epoxide hydrolase. Agents that are CYP3A4 inhibitors may increase the plasma levels of carbamazepine. Thus, if a patient has been titrated to a stable dosage of carbamazepine, and then begins a course of treatment with a CYP3A4 or epoxide hydrolase inhibitor, it is reasonable to expect that a dose reduction for carbamazepine may be necessary). Products include:
Noroxin **2220**

Norgestimate (Carbamazepine is known to induce CYP1A2 and CYP3A4. Therefore, the potential exists for interaction between carbamazepine and any agent metabolized by one (or more) of these enzymes. Agents that are metabolized by CYP1A2 or CYP3A4 may have decreased plasma levels when administered concomitantly with carbamazepine. Breakthrough bleeding has been reported among patients receiving concomitant oral contraceptives and their reliability may be adversely affected). Products include:
Ortho-Cyclen/Ortho Tri-Cyclen **2663**
Ortho Tri-Cyclen Lo Tablets **2673**

Norgestrel (Carbamazepine is known to induce CYP1A2 and CYP3A4. Therefore, the potential exists for interaction between carbamazepine and any agent metabolized by one (or more) of these enzymes. Agents that are metabolized by CYP1A2 or CYP3A4 may have decreased plasma levels when administered concomitantly with carbamazepine. Breakthrough bleeding has been reported among patients receiving concomitant oral contraceptives and their reliability may be adversely affected).
No products indexed under this heading.

Nortriptyline Hydrochloride (Carbamazepine is known to induce CYP1A2 and CYP3A4. Therefore, the potential exists for interaction between carbamazepine and any agent metabolized by one (or more) of these enzymes. Agents that are metabolized by CYP1A2 and CYP3A4 may have decreased plasma levels when administered concomitantly with carbamazepine. Thus, if a patient has been titrated to a stable dosage on one of the agents in these categories, and then begins a course of treatment with carbamazepine, it is reasonable to expect that a dose increase for the concomitant agent may be necessary).
No products indexed under this heading.

Ofloxacin (Carbamazepine is known to induce CYP1A2 and CYP3A4. Therefore, the potential exists for interaction between carbamazepine and any agent metabolized by one (or more) of these enzymes. Agents that are metabolized by CYP1A2 and CYP3A4 may have decreased plasma levels when administered concomitantly with carbamazepine. Thus, if a patient has been titrated to a stable dosage on one of the agents in these categories, and then begins a course of treatment with carbamazepine, it is reasonable to expect that a dose increase for the concomitant agent may be necessary).
No products indexed under this heading.

Olanzapine (Carbamazepine is known to induce CYP1A2 and CYP3A4. Therefore, the potential exists for interaction between carbamazepine and any agent metabolized by one (or more) of these enzymes. Agents that are metabolized by CYP1A2 and CYP3A4 may have decreased plasma levels when administered concomitantly with carbamazepine. Thus, if a patient has been titrated to a stable dosage on one of the agents in these categories, and then begins a course of treatment with carbamazepine, it is reasonable to expect that a dose increase for the concomitant agent may be necessary). Products include:
Symbyax **1965**
Zyprexa **1984**
Zyprexa IntraMuscular **1984**
Zyprexa ZYDIS **1984**

Omeprazole (Carbamazepine is metabolized mainly by CYP3A4, the active carbamazepine 10,11-epoxide, which is futher metabolized to the trans-diol by epoxide hydrolase. Therefore, the potential exists for interaction between carbamazepine and any agent that inhibits CYP3A4 and/or epoxide hydrolase. Agents that are CYP3A4 inhibitors may increase the plasma levels of carbamazepine. Thus, if a patient has been titrated to a stable dosage of carbamazepine, and then begins a course of treatment with a CYP3A4 or epoxide hydrolase inhibitor, it is reasonable to expect that a dose reduction for carbamazepine may be necessary).
No products indexed under this heading.

Ondansetron (Carbamazepine is known to induce CYP1A2 and CYP3A4. Therefore, the potential exists for interaction between carbamazepine and any agent metabolized by one (or more) of these enzymes. Agents that are metabolized by CYP1A2 and CYP3A4 may have decreased plasma levels when administered concomitantly with carbamazepine. Thus, if a patient has been titrated to a stable dosage on one of the agents in these categories, and then begins a course of treatment with carbamazepine, it is reasonable to expect that a dose increase for the concomitant agent may be necessary).
No products indexed under this heading.

Ondansetron Hydrochloride (Carbamazepine is known to induce CYP1A2 and CYP3A4. Therefore, the potential exists for interaction between carbamazepine and any agent metabolized by one (or more) of these enzymes. Agents that are metabolized by CYP1A2 and CYP3A4 may have decreased plasma levels when administered concomitantly with carbamazepine. Thus, if a patient has been titrated to a stable dosage on one of the agents in these categories, and then begins a course of treatment with carbamazepine, it is reasonable to expect that a dose increase for the concomitant agent may be necessary). Products include:
Zofran Injection **1750**
Zofran **1756**
Zofran ODT **1756**

Oxazepam (Because of its primary CNS effect, caution should be used when carbamazepine is taken with other centrally acting drugs).
No products indexed under this heading.

Oxcarbazepine (Carbamazepine is metabolized by CYP3A4. Therefore, the potential exists for interaction between carbamazepine and any agent that induces CYP3A4. Agents that are CYP3A4 inducers may decrease plasma levels of carbamazepine. Thus, if a patient has been titrated to a stable dosage on carbamazepine, and then begins a course of treatment with CYP3A4 inducers, it is reasonable to expect that a dose increase for carbamazepine may be necessary).
No products indexed under this heading.

Oxiconazole Nitrate (Carbamazepine is metabolized mainly by CYP3A4, the active carbamazepine 10,11-epoxide, which is futher metabolized to the trans-diol by epoxide hydrolase. Therefore, the potential exists for interaction between carbamazepine and any agent that inhibits CYP3A4 and/or epoxide hydrolase. Agents that are CYP3A4 inhibitors may increase the plasma levels of carbamazepine. Thus, if a patient has been titrated to a stable dosage of carbamazepine, and then begins a course of treatment with a CYP3A4 or epoxide hydrolase inhibitor, it is reasonable to expect that a dose reduction for carbamazepine may be necessary).
No products indexed under this heading.

Oxycodone Hydrochloride (Because of its primary CNS effect, caution should be used when carbamazepine is taken with other centrally acting drugs). Products include:
OxyContin **2807**
Percocet **1121**
Percodan **1124**

Paclitaxel (Carbamazepine is known to induce CYP1A2 and CYP3A4. Therefore, the potential exists for interaction between carbamazepine and any agent metabolized by one (or more) of these enzymes. Agents that are metabolized by CYP1A2 and CYP3A4 may have decreased plasma levels when administered concomitantly with carbamazepine. Thus, if a patient has been titrated to a stable dosage on one of the agents in these categories, and then begins a course of treatment with carbamazepine, it is reasonable to expect that a dose increase for the concomitant agent may be necessary).
No products indexed under this heading.

Pargyline Hydrochloride (Coadministration of carbamazepine with monoamine oxidase inhibitors is contraindicated, therefore, not recommended. Before administration of carbamazepine, MAO inhibitors should be discontinued for a minimum of 14 days, or longer if the clinical situation permits).
No products indexed under this heading.

Paroxetine Hydrochloride (Carbamazepine is metabolized mainly by CYP3A4, the active carbamazepine 10,11-epoxide, which is futher metabolized to the trans-diol by epoxide hydrolase. Therefore, the potential exists for interaction between carbamazepine and any agent that inhibits CYP3A4 and/or epoxide hydrolase. Agents that are CYP3A4 inhibitors may increase the plasma levels of carbamazepine. Thus, if a patient has been titrated to a stable dosage of carbamazepine, and then begins a course of treatment with a CYP3A4 or epoxide hydrolase inhibitor, it is reasonable to expect that a dose reduction for carbamazepine may be necessary). Products include:
Paroxetine CR **2361**
Paroxetine ER **2371**
Paxil **1586**
Paxil CR **1596**

Pemoline (Because of its primary CNS effect, caution should be used when carbamazepine is taken with other centrally acting drugs).
No products indexed under this heading.

Pentobarbital Sodium (Because of its primary CNS effect, caution should

be used when carbamazepine is taken with other centrally acting drugs). Products include:
Nembutal 2012

Perphenazine (Because of its primary CNS effect, caution should be used when carbamazepine is taken with other centrally acting drugs).
No products indexed under this heading.

Phenelzine Sulfate (Co-administration of carbamazepine with monoamine oxidase inhibitors is contra-indicated, therefore, not recommended. Before administration of carbamaze-pine, MAO inhibitors should be discon-tinued for a minimum of 14 days, or longer if the clinical situation permits).
No products indexed under this heading.

Phenobarbital (Carbamazepine is metabolized by CYP3A4. Therefore, the potential exists for interaction between carbamazepine and any agent that induces CYP3A4. Agents that are CYP3A4 inducers may decrease plasma levels of carbamazepine. Thus, if a patient has been titrated to a stable dosage on carbamazepine, and then begins a course of treatment with CYP3A4 inducers, it is reasonable to expect that a dose increase for carbam-azepine may be necessary). Products include:
Donnatal 2711

Phenobarbital Sodium (Carbamaze-pine is metabolized by CYP3A4. There-fore, the potential exists for interaction between carbamazepine and any agent that induces CYP3A4. Agents that are CYP3A4 inducers may decrease plasma levels of carbamazepine. Thus, if a patient has been titrated to a stable dosage on carbamazepine, and then begins a course of treatment with CYP3A4 inducers, it is reasonable to expect that a dose increase for carbam-azepine may be necessary).
No products indexed under this heading.

Phenytoin (Carbamazepine is metabo-lized by CYP3A4. Therefore, the poten-tial exists for interaction between car-bamazepine and any agent that induces CYP3A4. Agents that are CYP3A4 inducers may decrease plasma levels of carbamazepine. Thus, if a patient has been titrated to a stable dosage on car-bamazepine, and then begins a course of treatment with a CYP3A4 inducers, it is reasonable to expect that a dose increase for carbamazepine may be necessary. Carbamazepine may increase the plasma levels of phenytoin; careful monitoring of phenytoin plasma levels following co-medication with car-bamazepine is advised).
No products indexed under this heading.

Phenytoin Sodium (Carbamazepine is metabolized by CYP3A4. Therefore, the potential exists for interaction between carbamazepine and any agent that induces CYP3A4. Agents that are CYP3A4 inducers may decrease plasma levels of carbamazepine. Thus, if a patient has been titrated to a stable dosage on carbamazepine, and then begins a course of treatment with a CYP3A4 inducers, it is reasonable to expect that a dose increase for carbam-azepine may be necessary. Carbamaze-pine may increase the plasma levels of phenytoin; careful monitoring of pheny-toin plasma levels following co-medication with carbamazepine is advised). Products include:
Phenytek Capsules 2380

Pimozide (Carbamazepine is known to induce CYP1A2 and CYP3A4. There-fore, the potential exists for interaction between carbamazepine and any agent metabolized by one (or more) of these enzymes. Agents that are metabolized by CYP1A2 and CYP3A4 may have decreased plasma levels when adminis-tered concomitantly with carbamaze-

pine. Thus, if a patient has been titrated to a stable dosage on one of the agents in these categories, and then begins a course of treatment with carbamaze-pine, it is reasonable to expect that a dose increase for the concomitant agent may be necessary).
No products indexed under this heading.

Polyestradiol Phosphate (Carbam-azepine is known to induce CYP1A2 and CYP3A4. Therefore, the potential exists for interaction between carbamazepine and any agent metabolized by one (or more) of these enzymes. Agents that are metabolized by CYP1A2 and CYP3A4 may have decreased plasma levels when administered concomitantly with carbamazepine. Thus, if a patient has been titrated to a stable dosage on one of the agents in these categories, and then begins a course of treatment with carbamazepine, it is reasonable to expect that a dose increase for the con-comitant agent may be necessary).
No products indexed under this heading.

Posaconazole (Carbamazepine is metabolized mainly by CYP3A4, the active carbamazepine 10,11-epoxide, which is futher metabolized to the trans-diol by epoxide hydrolase. Therefore, the potential exists for interaction between carbamazepine and any agent that inhibits CYP3A4 and/or epoxide hydrolase. Agents that are CYP3A4 inhibitors may increase the plasma lev-els of carbamazepine. Thus, if a patient has been titrated to a stable dosage of carbamazepine, and then begins a course of treatment with a CYP3A4 or epoxide hydrolase inhibitor, it is reason-able to expect that a dose reduction for carbamazepine may be necessary).
Products include:
Noxafil 3172

Prazepam (Because of its primary CNS effect, caution should be used when carbamazepine is taken with other centrally acting drugs).
No products indexed under this heading.

Prednisolone (Carbamazepine is metabolized by CYP3A4. Therefore, the potential exists for interaction between carbamazepine and any agent that induces CYP3A4. Agents that are CYP3A4 inducers may decrease plasma levels of carbamazepine. Thus, if a patient has been titrated to a stable dosage on carbamazepine, and then begins a course of treatment with CYP3A4 inducers, it is reasonable to expect that a dose increase for carbam-azepine may be necessary).
No products indexed under this heading.

Prednisolone Acetate (Carbamaze-pine is metabolized by CYP3A4. There-fore, the potential exists for interaction between carbamazepine and any agent that induces CYP3A4. Agents that are CYP3A4 inducers may decrease plasma levels of carbamazepine. Thus, if a patient has been titrated to a stable dosage on carbamazepine, and then begins a course of treatment with CYP3A4 inducers, it is reasonable to expect that a dose increase for carbam-azepine may be necessary). Products include:
Blephamide .... ⊙**212**, ⊙**214**
Pred Forte .... ⊙**225**
Pred Mild .... ⊙**230**
Pred-G .... ⊙**226**, ⊙**227**

Prednisolone Sodium Phosphate (Carbamazepine is metabolized by CYP3A4. Therefore, the potential exists for interaction between carbamazepine and any agent that induces CYP3A4. Agents that are CYP3A4 inducers may decrease plasma levels of carbamaze-pine. Thus, if a patient has been titrated to a stable dosage on carbamazepine, and then begins a course of treatment

with CYP3A4 inducers, it is reasonable to expect that a dose increase for car-bamazepine may be necessary).
No products indexed under this heading.

Prednisolone Tebutate (Carbamaze-pine is metabolized by CYP3A4. There-fore, the potential exists for interaction between carbamazepine and any agent that induces CYP3A4. Agents that are CYP3A4 inducers may decrease plasma levels of carbamazepine. Thus, if a patient has been titrated to a stable dosage on carbamazepine, and then begins a course of treatment with CYP3A4 inducers, it is reasonable to expect that a dose increase for carbam-azepine may be necessary).
No products indexed under this heading.

Prednisone (Carbamazepine is metab-olized by CYP3A4. Therefore, the poten-tial exists for interaction between car-bamazepine and any agent that induces CYP3A4. Agents that are CYP3A4 inducers may decrease plasma levels of carbamazepine. Thus, if a patient has been titrated to a stable dosage on car-bamazepine, and then begins a course of treatment with CYP3A4 inducers, it is reasonable to expect that a dose increase for carbamazepine may be necessary).
No products indexed under this heading.

Prednisone sodium phosphate (Carbamazepine is metabolized by CYP3A4. Therefore, the potential exists for interaction between carbamazepine and any agent that induces CYP3A4. Agents that are CYP3A4 inducers may decrease plasma levels of carbamaze-pine. Thus, if a patient has been titrated to a stable dosage on carbamazepine, and then begins a course of treatment with CYP3A4 inducers, it is reasonable to expect that a dose increase for car-bamazepine may be necessary).
No products indexed under this heading.

Primidone (Carbamazepine increases the plasma levels of primidone).
No products indexed under this heading.

Procarbazine Hydrochloride (Co-administration of carbamazepine with monoamine oxidase inhibitors is contra-indicated, therefore, not recommended. Before administration of carbamaze-pine, MAO inhibitors should be discon-tinued for a minimum of 14 days, or longer if the clinical situation permits).
No products indexed under this heading.

Prochlorperazine (Because of its primary CNS effect, caution should be used when carbamazepine is taken with other centrally acting drugs).
No products indexed under this heading.

Promethazine Hydrochloride (Because of its primary CNS effect, caution should be used when carbamaz-epine is taken with other centrally act-ing drugs).
No products indexed under this heading.

Propafenone Hydrochloride (Car-bamazepine is known to induce CYP1A2 and CYP3A4. Therefore, the potential exists for interaction between carbam-azepine and any agent metabolized by one (or more) of these enzymes. Agents that are metabolized by CYP1A2 and CYP3A4 may have decreased plasma levels when administered concomitantly with carbamazepine. Thus, if a patient has been titrated to a stable dosage on one of the agents in these categories, and then begins a course of treatment with carbamazepine, it is reasonable to expect that a dose increase for the con-comitant agent may be necessary). Products include:
Rythmol 1648
Rythmol SR 1652

Propofol (Because of its primary CNS effect, caution should be used when carbamazepine is taken with other cen-trally acting drugs).
No products indexed under this heading.

Propoxyphene Hydrochloride (Car-bamazepine is metabolized mainly by CYP3A4, the active carbamazepine 10,11-epoxide, which is futher metabo-lized to the trans-diol by epoxide hydro-lase. Therefore, the potential exists for interaction between carbamazepine and any agent that inhibits CYP3A4 and/or epoxide hydrolase. Agents that are CYP3A4 inhibitors may increase the plasma levels of carbamazepine. Thus, if a patient has been titrated to a stable dosage of carbamazepine, and then begins a course of treatment with a CYP3A4 or epoxide hydrolase inhibitor, it is reasonable to expect that a dose reduction for carbamazepine may be necessary).
No products indexed under this heading.

Propoxyphene Napsylate (Carbam-azepine is metabolized mainly by CYP3A4, the active carbamazepine 10,11-epoxide, which is futher metabo-lized to the trans-diol by epoxide hydro-lase. Therefore, the potential exists for interaction between carbamazepine and any agent that inhibits CYP3A4 and/or epoxide hydrolase. Agents that are CYP3A4 inhibitors may increase the plasma levels of carbamazepine. Thus, if a patient has been titrated to a stable dosage of carbamazepine, and then begins a course of treatment with a CYP3A4 or epoxide hydrolase inhibitor, it is reasonable to expect that a dose reduction for carbamazepine may be necessary).
No products indexed under this heading.

Propranolol Hydrochloride (Car-bamazepine is known to induce CYP1A2 and CYP3A4. Therefore, the potential exists for interaction between carbam-azepine and any agent metabolized by one (or more) of these enzymes. Agents that are metabolized by CYP1A2 and CYP3A4 may have decreased plasma levels when administered concomitantly with carbamazepine. Thus, if a patient has been titrated to a stable dosage on one of the agents in these categories, and then begins a course of treatment with carbamazepine, it is reasonable to expect that a dose increase for the con-comitant agent may be necessary). Products include:
InnoPran XL 1517

Protriptyline Hydrochloride (Car-bamazepine is known to induce CYP1A2 and CYP3A4. Therefore, the potential exists for interaction between carbam-azepine and any agent metabolized by one (or more) of these enzymes. Agents that are metabolized by CYP1A2 and CYP3A4 may have decreased plasma levels when administered concomitantly with carbamazepine. Thus, if a patient has been titrated to a stable dosage on one of the agents in these categories, and then begins a course of treatment with carbamazepine, it is reasonable to expect that a dose increase for the con-comitant agent may be necessary).
No products indexed under this heading.

Pyrimethamine (Anti-malarial drugs, such as chloroquine and mefloquine, may antagonize the activity of carbam-azepine). Products include:
Daraprim 1423

Quazepam (Because of its primary CNS effect, caution should be used when carbamazepine is taken with other centrally acting drugs).
No products indexed under this heading.

Quetiapine Fumarate (Because of its primary CNS effect, caution should

---

IMPORTANT NOTE: Always consult each drug listing in the patient's regimen for possible interactions.

be used when carbamazepine is taken with other centrally acting drugs). Products include:

Seroquel 750
Seroquel XR 759

Quinidine (Carbamazepine is metabolized mainly by CYP3A4, the active carbamazepine 10,11-epoxide, which is futher metabolized to the trans-diol by epoxide hydrolase. Therefore, the potential exists for interaction between carbamazepine and any agent that inhibits CYP3A4 and/or epoxide hydrolase. Agents that are CYP3A4 inhibitors may increase the plasma levels of carbamazepine. Thus, if a patient has been titrated to a stable dosage of carbamazepine, and then begins a course of treatment with a CYP3A4 or epoxide hydrolase inhibitor, it is reasonable to expect that a dose reduction for carbamazepine may be necessary).
No products indexed under this heading.

Quinidine Gluconate (Carbamazepine is known to induce CYP1A2 and CYP3A4. Therefore, the potential exists for interaction between carbamazepine and any agent metabolized by one (or more) of these enzymes. Agents that are metabolized by CYP1A2 and CYP3A4 may have decreased plasma levels when administered concomitantly with carbamazepine. Thus, if a patient has been titrated to a stable dosage on one of the agents in these categories, and then begins a course of treatment with carbamazepine, it is reasonable to expect that a dose increase for the concomitant agent may be necessary).
No products indexed under this heading.

Quinidine Hydrochloride (Carbamazepine is metabolized mainly by CYP3A4, the active carbamazepine 10,11-epoxide, which is futher metabolized to the trans-diol by epoxide hydrolase. Therefore, the potential exists for interaction between carbamazepine and any agent that inhibits CYP3A4 and/or epoxide hydrolase. Agents that are CYP3A4 inhibitors may increase the plasma levels of carbamazepine. Thus, if a patient has been titrated to a stable dosage of carbamazepine, and then begins a course of treatment with a CYP3A4 or epoxide hydrolase inhibitor, it is reasonable to expect that a dose reduction for carbamazepine may be necessary).
No products indexed under this heading.

Quinidine Polygalacturonate (Carbamazepine is metabolized mainly by CYP3A4, the active carbamazepine 10,11-epoxide, which is futher metabolized to the trans-diol by epoxide hydrolase. Therefore, the potential exists for interaction between carbamazepine and any agent that inhibits CYP3A4 and/or epoxide hydrolase. Agents that are CYP3A4 inhibitors may increase the plasma levels of carbamazepine. Thus, if a patient has been titrated to a stable dosage of carbamazepine, and then begins a course of treatment with a CYP3A4 or epoxide hydrolase inhibitor, it is reasonable to expect that a dose reduction for carbamazepine may be necessary).
No products indexed under this heading.

Quinidine Sulfate (Carbamazepine is metabolized mainly by CYP3A4, the active carbamazepine 10,11-epoxide, which is futher metabolized to the trans-diol by epoxide hydrolase. Therefore, the potential exists for interaction between carbamazepine and any agent that inhibits CYP3A4 and/or epoxide hydrolase. Agents that are CYP3A4 inhibitors may increase the plasma levels of carbamazepine. Thus, if a patient has been titrated to a stable dosage of carbamazepine, and then begins a course of treatment with a CYP3A4 or epoxide hydrolase inhibitor, it is reasonable to expect that a dose reduction for carbamazepine may be necessary).
No products indexed under this heading.

Quinine (Carbamazepine is metabolized mainly by CYP3A4, the active carbamazepine 10,11-epoxide, which is futher metabolized to the trans-diol by epoxide hydrolase. Therefore, the potential exists for interaction between carbamazepine and any agent that inhibits CYP3A4 and/or epoxide hydrolase. Agents that are CYP3A4 inhibitors may increase the plasma levels of carbamazepine. Thus, if a patient has been titrated to a stable dosage of carbamazepine, and then begins a course of treatment with a CYP3A4 or epoxide hydrolase inhibitor, it is reasonable to expect that a dose reduction for carbamazepine may be necessary). Products include:

Hyland's Leg Cramps PM with Quinine 3315

Quinine Sulfate (Carbamazepine is metabolized mainly by CYP3A4, the active carbamazepine 10,11-epoxide, which is futher metabolized to the trans-diol by epoxide hydrolase. Therefore, the potential exists for interaction between carbamazepine and any agent that inhibits CYP3A4 and/or epoxide hydrolase. Agents that are CYP3A4 inhibitors may increase the plasma levels of carbamazepine. Thus, if a patient has been titrated to a stable dosage of carbamazepine, and then begins a course of treatment with a CYP3A4 or epoxide hydrolase inhibitor, it is reasonable to expect that a dose reduction for carbamazepine may be necessary).
No products indexed under this heading.

Quinupristin (Carbamazepine is metabolized mainly by CYP3A4, the active carbamazepine 10,11-epoxide, which is futher metabolized to the trans-diol by epoxide hydrolase. Therefore, the potential exists for interaction between carbamazepine and any agent that inhibits CYP3A4 and/or epoxide hydrolase. Agents that are CYP3A4 inhibitors may increase the plasma levels of carbamazepine. Thus, if a patient has been titrated to a stable dosage of carbamazepine, and then begins a course of treatment with a CYP3A4 or epoxide hydrolase inhibitor, it is reasonable to expect that a dose reduction for carbamazepine may be necessary).
No products indexed under this heading.

Ranitidine Bismuth Citrate (Carbamazepine is metabolized mainly by CYP3A4, the active carbamazepine 10,11-epoxide, which is futher metabolized to the trans-diol by epoxide hydrolase. Therefore, the potential exists for interaction between carbamazepine and any agent that inhibits CYP3A4 and/or epoxide hydrolase. Agents that are CYP3A4 inhibitors may increase the plasma levels of carbamazepine. Thus, if a patient has been titrated to a stable dosage of carbamazepine, and then begins a course of treatment with a CYP3A4 or epoxide hydrolase inhibitor, it is reasonable to expect that a dose reduction for carbamazepine may be necessary).
No products indexed under this heading.

Ranitidine Hydrochloride (Carbamazepine is metabolized mainly by CYP3A4, the active carbamazepine 10,11-epoxide, which is futher metabolized to the trans-diol by epoxide hydrolase. Therefore, the potential exists for interaction between carbamazepine and any agent that inhibits CYP3A4 and/or epoxide hydrolase. Agents that are CYP3A4 inhibitors may increase the plasma levels of carbamazepine. Thus, if a patient has been titrated to a stable dosage of carbamazepine, and then begins a course of treatment with a CYP3A4 or epoxide hydrolase inhibitor, it is reasonable to expect that a dose reduction for carbamazepine may be necessary). Products include:

Zantac 1737
Zantac Injection 1732
Zantac Pharmacy 1735

Rasagiline Mesylate (Co-administration of carbamazepine with monoamine oxidase inhibitors is contraindicated, therefore, not recommended. Before administration of carbamazepine, MAO inhibitors should be discontinued for a minimum of 14 days, or longer if the clinical situation permits). Products include:

Azilect 3383

Remifentanil Hydrochloride (Because of its primary CNS effect, caution should be used when carbamazepine is taken with other centrally acting drugs).
No products indexed under this heading.

Rifabutin (Carbamazepine is metabolized by CYP3A4. Therefore, the potential exists for interaction between carbamazepine and any agent that induces CYP3A4. Agents that are CYP3A4 inducers may decrease plasma levels of carbamazepine. Thus, if a patient has been titrated to a stable dosage on carbamazepine, and then begins a course of treatment with CYP3A4 inducers, it is reasonable to expect that a dose increase for carbamazepine may be necessary).
No products indexed under this heading.

Rifampicin (Carbamazepine is metabolized by CYP3A4. Therefore, the potential exists for interaction between carbamazepine and any agent that induces CYP3A4. Agents that are CYP3A4 inducers may decrease plasma levels of carbamazepine. Thus, if a patient has been titrated to a stable dosage on carbamazepine, and then begins a course of treatment with CYP3A4 inducers, it is reasonable to expect that a dose increase for carbamazepine may be necessary).
No products indexed under this heading.

Rifampin (Carbamazepine is metabolized by CYP3A4. Therefore, the potential exists for interaction between carbamazepine and any agent that induces CYP3A4. Agents that are CYP3A4 inducers may decrease plasma levels of carbamazepine. Thus, if a patient has been titrated to a stable dosage on carbamazepine, and then begins a course of treatment with CYP3A4 inducers, it is reasonable to expect that a dose increase for carbamazepine may be necessary).
No products indexed under this heading.

Rifapentine (Carbamazepine is metabolized by CYP3A4. Therefore, the potential exists for interaction between carbamazepine and any agent that induces CYP3A4. Agents that are CYP3A4 inducers may decrease plasma levels of carbamazepine. Thus, if a patient has been titrated to a stable dosage on carbamazepine, and then begins a course of treatment with CYP3A4 inducers, it is reasonable to expect that a dose increase for carbamazepine may be necessary).
No products indexed under this heading.

Riluzole (Carbamazepine is known to induce CYP1A2 and CYP3A4. Therefore, the potential exists for interaction between carbamazepine and any agent metabolized by one (or more) of these enzymes. Agents that are metabolized by CYP1A2 and CYP3A4 may have decreased plasma levels when administered concomitantly with carbamazepine. Thus, if a patient has been titrated to a stable dosage on one of the agents in these categories, and then begins a course of treatment with carbamazepine, it is reasonable to expect that a dose increase for the concomitant agent may be necessary). Products include:

Rilutek 3032

Risperidone (Because of its primary CNS effect, caution should be used when carbamazepine is taken with other centrally acting drugs). Products include:

Risperdal Consta 2682

Ritonavir (Carbamazepine is metabolized mainly by CYP3A4, the active carbamazepine 10,11-epoxide, which is futher metabolized to the trans-diol by epoxide hydrolase. Therefore, the potential exists for interaction between carbamazepine and any agent that inhibits CYP3A4 and/or epoxide hydrolase. Agents that are CYP3A4 inhibitors may increase the plasma levels of carbamazepine. Thus, if a patient has been titrated to a stable dosage of carbamazepine, and then begins a course of treatment with a CYP3A4 or epoxide hydrolase inhibitor, it is reasonable to expect that a dose reduction for carbamazepine may be necessary). Products include:

Kaletra 458
Norvir 509

Ropinirole Hydrochloride (Carbamazepine is known to induce CYP1A2 and CYP3A4. Therefore, the potential exists for interaction between carbamazepine and any agent metabolized by one (or more) of these enzymes. Agents that are metabolized by CYP1A2 and CYP3A4 may have decreased plasma levels when administered concomitantly with carbamazepine. Thus, if a patient has been titrated to a stable dosage on one of the agents in these categories, and then begins a course of treatment with carbamazepine, it is reasonable to expect that a dose increase for the concomitant agent may be necessary). Products include:

Requip 1620
Requip XL 1628

Ropivacaine Hydrochloride (Carbamazepine is known to induce CYP1A2 and CYP3A4. Therefore, the potential exists for interaction between carbamazepine and any agent metabolized by one (or more) of these enzymes. Agents that are metabolized by CYP1A2 and CYP3A4 may have decreased plasma levels when administered concomitantly with carbamazepine. Thus, if a patient has been titrated to a stable dosage on one of the agents in these categories, and then begins a course of treatment with carbamazepine, it is reasonable to expect that a dose increase for the concomitant agent may be necessary).
No products indexed under this heading.

Saquinavir (Carbamazepine is metabolized mainly by CYP3A4, the active carbamazepine 10,11-epoxide, which is futher metabolized to the trans-diol by epoxide hydrolase. Therefore, the potential exists for interaction between carbamazepine and any agent that inhibits CYP3A4 and/or epoxide hydrolase. Agents that are CYP3A4 inhibitors may increase the plasma levels of carbamazepine. Thus, if a patient has been titrated to a stable dosage of carbamazepine, and then begins a course of treatment with a CYP3A4 or epoxide hydrolase inhibitor, it is reasonable to expect that a dose reduction for carbamazepine may be necessary).
No products indexed under this heading.

Saquinavir Mesylate (Carbamazepine is metabolized mainly by CYP3A4, the active carbamazepine 10,11-epoxide, which is futher metabolized to the trans-diol by epoxide hydrolase. Therefore, the potential exists for interaction between carbamazepine and any agent that inhibits CYP3A4 and/or

epoxide hydrolase. Agents that are CYP3A4 inhibitors may increase the plasma levels of carbamazepine. Thus, if a patient has been titrated to a stable dosage of carbamazepine, and then begins a course of treatment with a CYP3A4 or epoxide hydrolase inhibitor, it is reasonable to expect that a dose reduction for carbamazepine may be necessary).

No products indexed under this heading.

Secobarbital Sodium (Because of its primary CNS effect, caution should be used when carbamazepine is taken with other centrally acting drugs).

No products indexed under this heading.

Selegiline (Co-administration of carbamazepine with monoamine oxidase inhibitors is contraindicated, therefore, not recommended. Before administration of carbamazepine, MAO inhibitors should be discontinued for a minimum of 14 days, or longer if the clinical situation permits). Products include:

Emsam 3623

Selegiline Hydrochloride (Co-administration of carbamazepine with monoamine oxidase inhibitors is contraindicated, therefore, not recommended. Before administration of carbamazepine, MAO inhibitors should be discontinued for a minimum of 14 days, or longer if the clinical situation permits). Products include:

Eldepryl 3312

Sertaconazole Nitrate (Carbamazepine is metabolized mainly by CYP3A4, the active carbamazepine 10,11-epoxide, which is futher metabolized to the trans-diol by epoxide hydrolase. Therefore, the potential exists for interaction between carbamazepine and any agent that inhibits CYP3A4 and/or epoxide hydrolase. Agents that are CYP3A4 inhibitors may increase the plasma levels of carbamazepine. Thus, if a patient has been titrated to a stable dosage of carbamazepine, and then begins a course of treatment with a CYP3A4 or epoxide hydrolase inhibitor, it is reasonable to expect that a dose reduction for carbamazepine may be necessary).

No products indexed under this heading.

Sertraline Hydrochloride (Carbamazepine is metabolized mainly by CYP3A4, the active carbamazepine 10,11-epoxide, which is futher metabolized to the trans-diol by epoxide hydrolase. Therefore, the potential exists for interaction between carbamazepine and any agent that inhibits CYP3A4 and/or epoxide hydrolase. Agents that are CYP3A4 inhibitors may increase the plasma levels of carbamazepine. Thus, if a patient has been titrated to a stable dosage of carbamazepine, and then begins a course of treatment with a CYP3A4 or epoxide hydrolase inhibitor, it is reasonable to expect that a dose reduction for carbamazepine may be necessary).

No products indexed under this heading.

Sevoflurane (Because of its primary CNS effect, caution should be used when carbamazepine is taken with other centrally acting drugs). Products include:

Ultane 554

Sildenafil Citrate (Carbamazepine is metabolized mainly by CYP3A4, the active carbamazepine 10,11-epoxide, which is futher metabolized to the trans-diol by epoxide hydrolase. Therefore, the potential exists for interaction between carbamazepine and any agent that inhibits CYP3A4 and/or epoxide hydrolase. Agents that are CYP3A4 inhibitors may increase the plasma levels of carbamazepine. Thus, if a patient has been titrated to a stable dosage of carbamazepine, and then begins a course of treatment with a CYP3A4 or epoxide hydrolase inhibitor, it is reasonable to expect that a dose reduction for carbamazepine may be necessary).

No products indexed under this heading.

Simvastatin (Carbamazepine is known to induce CYP1A2 and CYP3A4. Therefore, the potential exists for interaction between carbamazepine and any agent metabolized by one (or more) of these enzymes. Agents that are metabolized by CYP1A2 and CYP3A4 may have decreased plasma levels when administered concomitantly with carbamazepine. Thus, if a patient has been titrated to a stable dosage on one of the agents in these categories, and then begins a course of treatment with carbamazepine, it is reasonable to expect that a dose increase for the concomitant agent may be necessary). Products include:

Simcor 524
Vytorin 10/10 .... 2303, 3240
Vytorin 10/20 .... 2303, 3240
Vytorin 10/40 .... 2303, 3240
Vytorin 10/80 .... 2303, 3240
Zocor 2289

Sirolimus (Carbamazepine is known to induce CYP1A2 and CYP3A4. Therefore, the potential exists for interaction between carbamazepine and any agent metabolized by one (or more) of these enzymes. Agents that are metabolized by CYP1A2 and CYP3A4 may have decreased plasma levels when administered concomitantly with carbamazepine. Thus, if a patient has been titrated to a stable dosage on one of the agents in these categories, and then begins a course of treatment with carbamazepine, it is reasonable to expect that a dose increase for the concomitant agent may be necessary). Products include:

Rapamune 3579

Sodium Oxybate (Because of its primary CNS effect, caution should be used when carbamazepine is taken with other centrally acting drugs).

No products indexed under this heading.

Sufentanil Citrate (Because of its primary CNS effect, caution should be used when carbamazepine is taken with other centrally acting drugs).

No products indexed under this heading.

Sulfinpyrazone (Carbamazepine is metabolized by CYP3A4. Therefore, the potential exists for interaction between carbamazepine and any agent that induces CYP3A4. Agents that are CYP3A4 inducers may decrease plasma levels of carbamazepine. Thus, if a patient has been titrated to a stable dosage on carbamazepine, and then begins a course of treatment with CYP3A4 inducers, it is reasonable to expect that a dose increase for carbamazepine may be necessary).

No products indexed under this heading.

Tacrine Hydrochloride (Carbamazepine is known to induce CYP1A2 and CYP3A4. Therefore, the potential exists for interaction between carbamazepine and any agent metabolized by one (or more) of these enzymes. Agents that are metabolized by CYP1A2 and CYP3A4 may have decreased plasma levels when administered concomitantly with carbamazepine. Thus, if a patient has been titrated to a stable dosage on one of the agents in these categories, and then begins a course of treatment with carbamazepine, it is reasonable to expect that a dose increase for the concomitant agent may be necessary).

No products indexed under this heading.

Tacrolimus (Carbamazepine is known to induce CYP1A2 and CYP3A4. Therefore, the potential exists for interaction between carbamazepine and any agent metabolized by one (or more) of these enzymes. Agents that are metabolized by CYP1A2 and CYP3A4 may have decreased plasma levels when administered concomitantly with carbamazepine. Thus, if a patient has been titrated to a stable dosage on one of the agents in these categories, and then begins a course of treatment with carbamazepine, it is reasonable to expect that a dose increase for the concomitant agent may be necessary). Products include:

Prograf Capsules 677
Prograf Injection 677
Protopic 685

Tadalafil (Carbamazepine is known to induce CYP1A2 and CYP3A4. Therefore, the potential exists for interaction between carbamazepine and any agent metabolized by one (or more) of these enzymes. Agents that are metabolized by CYP1A2 and CYP3A4 may have decreased plasma levels when administered concomitantly with carbamazepine. Thus, if a patient has been titrated to a stable dosage on one of the agents in these categories, and then begins a course of treatment with carbamazepine, it is reasonable to expect that a dose increase for the concomitant agent may be necessary). Products include:

Adcirca 3461
Cialis 1861

Tamoxifen Citrate (Carbamazepine is known to induce CYP1A2 and CYP3A4. Therefore, the potential exists for interaction between carbamazepine and any agent metabolized by one (or more) of these enzymes. Agents that are metabolized by CYP1A2 and CYP3A4 may have decreased plasma levels when administered concomitantly with carbamazepine. Thus, if a patient has been titrated to a stable dosage on one of the agents in these categories, and then begins a course of treatment with carbamazepine, it is reasonable to expect that a dose increase for the concomitant agent may be necessary).

No products indexed under this heading.

Telithromycin (Carbamazepine is metabolized mainly by CYP3A4, the active carbamazepine 10,11-epoxide, which is futher metabolized to the trans-diol by epoxide hydrolase. Therefore, the potential exists for interaction between carbamazepine and any agent that inhibits CYP3A4 and/or epoxide hydrolase. Agents that are CYP3A4 inhibitors may increase the plasma levels of carbamazepine. Thus, if a patient has been titrated to a stable dosage of carbamazepine, and then begins a course of treatment with a CYP3A4 or epoxide hydrolase inhibitor, it is reasonable to expect that a dose reduction for carbamazepine may be necessary). Products include:

Ketek 2991

Temazepam (Because of its primary CNS effect, caution should be used when carbamazepine is taken with other centrally acting drugs).

No products indexed under this heading.

Terconazole (Carbamazepine is metabolized mainly by CYP3A4, the active carbamazepine 10,11-epoxide, which is futher metabolized to the trans-diol by epoxide hydrolase. Therefore, the potential exists for interaction between carbamazepine and any agent that inhibits CYP3A4 and/or epoxide hydrolase. Agents that are CYP3A4 inhibitors may increase the plasma levels of carbamazepine. Thus, if a patient has been titrated to a stable dosage of carbamazepine, and then begins a course of treatment with a CYP3A4 or epoxide hydrolase inhibitor, it is reasonable to expect that a dose reduction for carbamazepine may be necessary).

No products indexed under this heading.

Terfenadine (Carbamazepine is known to induce CYP1A2 and CYP3A4. Therefore, the potential exists for interaction between carbamazepine and any agent metabolized by one (or more) of these enzymes. Agents that are metabolized by CYP1A2 and CYP3A4 may have decreased plasma levels when administered concomitantly with carbamazepine. Thus, if a patient has been titrated to a stable dosage on one of the agents in these categories, and then begins a course of treatment with carbamazepine, it is reasonable to expect that a dose increase for the concomitant agent may be necessary).

No products indexed under this heading.

Theobromine (Carbamazepine is known to induce CYP1A2 and CYP3A4. Therefore, the potential exists for interaction between carbamazepine and any agent metabolized by one (or more) of these enzymes. Agents that are metabolized by CYP1A2 and CYP3A4 may have decreased plasma levels when administered concomitantly with carbamazepine. Thus, if a patient has been titrated to a stable dosage on one of the agents in these categories, and then begins a course of treatment with carbamazepine, it is reasonable to expect that a dose increase for the concomitant agent may be necessary).

No products indexed under this heading.

Theophyllinate (Carbamazepine is metabolized by CYP3A4. Therefore, the potential exists for interaction between carbamazepine and any agent that induces CYP3A4. Agents that are CYP3A4 inducers may decrease plasma levels of carbamazepine. Thus, if a patient has been titrated to a stable dosage on carbamazepine, and then begins a course of treatment with CYP3A4 inducers, it is reasonable to expect that a dose increase for carbamazepine may be necessary).

No products indexed under this heading.

Theophylline (Carbamazepine is metabolized by CYP3A4. Therefore, the potential exists for interaction between carbamazepine and any agent that induces CYP3A4. Agents that are CYP3A4 inducers may decrease plasma levels of carbamazepine. Thus, if a patient has been titrated to a stable dosage on carbamazepine, and then begins a course of treatment with CYP3A4 inducers, it is reasonable to expect that a dose increase for carbamazepine may be necessary).

No products indexed under this heading.

Theophylline Anhydrous (Carbamazepine is metabolized by CYP3A4. Therefore, the potential exists for interaction between carbamazepine and any agent that induces CYP3A4. Agents that are CYP3A4 inducers may decrease plasma levels of carbamazepine. Thus, if a patient has been titrated to a stable dosage on carbamazepine, and then begins a course of treatment with CYP3A4 inducers, it is reasonable to expect that a dose increase for carbamazepine may be necessary). Products include:

Uniphyl 2817

Theophylline Calcium Salicylate (Carbamazepine is metabolized by CYP3A4. Therefore, the potential exists for interaction between carbamazepine and any agent that induces CYP3A4. Agents that are CYP3A4 inducers may decrease plasma levels of carbamazepine. Thus, if a patient has been titrated to a stable dosage on carbamazepine, and then begins a course of treatment with CYP3A4 inducers, it is reasonable to expect that a dose increase for carbamazepine may be necessary).

No products indexed under this heading.

Theophylline Dihydroxypropyl (Glyceryl) (Carbamazepine is metabo-

Carbatrol Interactions Index 274

lized by CYP3A4. Therefore, the potential exists for interaction between carbamazepine and any agent that induces CYP3A4. Agents that are CYP3A4 inducers may decrease plasma levels of carbamazepine. Thus, if a patient has been titrated to a stable dosage on carbamazepine, and then begins a course of treatment with CYP3A4 inducers, it is reasonable to expect that a dose increase for carbamazepine may be necessary).
No products indexed under this heading.

Theophylline Ethylenediamine (Carbamazepine is metabolized by CYP3A4. Therefore, the potential exists for interaction between carbamazepine and any agent that induces CYP3A4. Agents that are CYP3A4 inducers may decrease plasma levels of carbamazepine. Thus, if a patient has been titrated to a stable dosage on carbamazepine, and then begins a course of treatment with CYP3A4 inducers, it is reasonable to expect that a dose increase for carbamazepine may be necessary).
No products indexed under this heading.

Theophylline Sodium Glycinate (Carbamazepine is metabolized by CYP3A4. Therefore, the potential exists for interaction between carbamazepine and any agent that induces CYP3A4. Agents that are CYP3A4 inducers may decrease plasma levels of carbamazepine. Thus, if a patient has been titrated to a stable dosage on carbamazepine, and then begins a course of treatment with CYP3A4 inducers, it is reasonable to expect that a dose increase for carbamazepine may be necessary).
No products indexed under this heading.

Thiamylal Sodium (Because of its primary CNS effect, caution should be used when carbamazepine is taken with other centrally acting drugs).
No products indexed under this heading.

Thioridazine Hydrochloride (Because of its primary CNS effect, caution should be used when carbamazepine is taken with other centrally acting drugs). Products include:
Thioridazine Hydrochloride 2384

Thiothixene (Because of its primary CNS effect, caution should be used when carbamazepine is taken with other centrally acting drugs). Products include:
Thiothixene 2386

Tiagabine Hydrochloride (Carbamazepine is known to induce CYP1A2 and CYP3A4. Therefore, the potential exists for interaction between carbamazepine and any agent metabolized by one (or more) of these enzymes. Agents that are metabolized by CYP1A2 and CYP3A4 may have decreased plasma levels when administered concomitantly with carbamazepine. Thus, if a patient has been titrated to a stable dosage on one of the agents in these categories, and then begins a course of treatment with carbamazepine, it is reasonable to expect that a dose increase for the concomitant agent may be necessary). Products include:
Gabitril 972

Tipranavir (Carbamazepine is metabolized mainly by CYP3A4, the active carbamazepine 10,11-epoxide, which is futher metabolized to the trans-diol by epoxide hydrolase. Therefore, the potential exists for interaction between carbamazepine and any agent that inhibits CYP3A4 and/or epoxide hydrolase. Agents that are CYP3A4 inhibitors may increase the plasma levels of carbamazepine. Thus, if a patient has been titrated to a stable dosage of carbamazepine, and then begins a course of treatment with a CYP3A4 or epoxide hydrolase inhibitor, it is reasonable to expect that a dose reduction for carbamazepine may be necessary).
No products indexed under this heading.

Tizanidine (Carbamazepine is known to induce CYP1A2 and CYP3A4. Therefore, the potential exists for interaction between carbamazepine and any agent metabolized by one (or more) of these enzymes. Agents that are metabolized by CYP1A2 and CYP3A4 may have decreased plasma levels when administered concomitantly with carbamazepine. Thus, if a patient has been titrated to a stable dosage on one of the agents in these categories, and then begins a course of treatment with carbamazepine, it is reasonable to expect that a dose increase for the concomitant agent may be necessary).
No products indexed under this heading.

Tizanidine Hydrochloride (Carbamazepine is known to induce CYP1A2 and CYP3A4. Therefore, the potential exists for interaction between carbamazepine and any agent metabolized by one (or more) of these enzymes. Agents that are metabolized by CYP1A2 and CYP3A4 may have decreased plasma levels when administered concomitantly with carbamazepine. Thus, if a patient has been titrated to a stable dosage on one of the agents in these categories, and then begins a course of treatment with carbamazepine, it is reasonable to expect that a dose increase for the concomitant agent may be necessary).
No products indexed under this heading.

Tolterodine Tartrate (Carbamazepine is known to induce CYP1A2 and CYP3A4. Therefore, the potential exists for interaction between carbamazepine and any agent metabolized by one (or more) of these enzymes. Agents that are metabolized by CYP1A2 and CYP3A4 may have decreased plasma levels when administered concomitantly with carbamazepine. Thus, if a patient has been titrated to a stable dosage on one of the agents in these categories, and then begins a course of treatment with carbamazepine, it is reasonable to expect that a dose increase for the concomitant agent may be necessary).
No products indexed under this heading.

Tranylcypromine Sulfate (Coadministration of carbamazepine with monoamine oxidase inhibitors is contraindicated, therefore, not recommended. Before administration of carbamazepine, MAO inhibitors should be discontinued for a minimum of 14 days, or longer if the clinical situation permits). Products include:
Parnate 1584

Trazodone Hydrochloride (Carbamazepine is known to induce CYP1A2 and CYP3A4. Therefore, the potential exists for interaction between carbamazepine and any agent metabolized by one (or more) of these enzymes. Agents that are metabolized by CYP1A2 and CYP3A4 may have decreased plasma levels when administered concomitantly with carbamazepine. Thus, if a patient has been titrated to a stable dosage on one of the agents in these categories, and then begins a course of treatment with carbamazepine, it is reasonable to expect that a dose increase for the concomitant agent may be necessary).
No products indexed under this heading.

Triamcinolone (Carbamazepine is metabolized by CYP3A4. Therefore, the potential exists for interaction between carbamazepine and any agent that induces CYP3A4. Agents that are CYP3A4 inducers may decrease plasma levels of carbamazepine. Thus, if a patient has been titrated to a stable dosage on carbamazepine, and then begins a course of treatment with CYP3A4 inducers, it is reasonable to expect that a dose increase for carbamazepine may be necessary).
No products indexed under this heading.

Triamcinolone Acetonide (Carbamazepine is metabolized by CYP3A4. Therefore, the potential exists for interaction between carbamazepine and any agent that induces CYP3A4. Agents that are CYP3A4 inducers may decrease plasma levels of carbamazepine. Thus, if a patient has been titrated to a stable dosage on carbamazepine, and then begins a course of treatment with CYP3A4 inducers, it is reasonable to expect that a dose increase for carbamazepine may be necessary). Products include:
Azmacort 408
Nasacort AQ 3019

Triamcinolone Diacetate (Carbamazepine is metabolized by CYP3A4. Therefore, the potential exists for interaction between carbamazepine and any agent that induces CYP3A4. Agents that are CYP3A4 inducers may decrease plasma levels of carbamazepine. Thus, if a patient has been titrated to a stable dosage on carbamazepine, and then begins a course of treatment with CYP3A4 inducers, it is reasonable to expect that a dose increase for carbamazepine may be necessary).
No products indexed under this heading.

Triamcinolone Hexacetonide (Carbamazepine is metabolized by CYP3A4. Therefore, the potential exists for interaction between carbamazepine and any agent that induces CYP3A4. Agents that are CYP3A4 inducers may decrease plasma levels of carbamazepine. Thus, if a patient has been titrated to a stable dosage on carbamazepine, and then begins a course of treatment with CYP3A4 inducers, it is reasonable to expect that a dose increase for carbamazepine may be necessary).
No products indexed under this heading.

Triazolam (Carbamazepine is known to induce CYP1A2 and CYP3A4. Therefore, the potential exists for interaction between carbamazepine and any agent metabolized by one (or more) of these enzymes. Agents that are metabolized by CYP1A2 and CYP3A4 may have decreased plasma levels when administered concomitantly with carbamazepine. Thus, if a patient has been titrated to a stable dosage on one of the agents in these categories, and then begins a course of treatment with carbamazepine, it is reasonable to expect that a dose increase for the concomitant agent may be necessary).
No products indexed under this heading.

Trifluoperazine Hydrochloride (Because of its primary CNS effect, caution should be used when carbamazepine is taken with other centrally acting drugs).
No products indexed under this heading.

Trimethaphan Camsylate (Carbamazepine is known to induce CYP1A2 and CYP3A4. Therefore, the potential exists for interaction between carbamazepine and any agent metabolized by one (or more) of these enzymes. Agents that are metabolized by CYP1A2 and CYP3A4 may have decreased plasma levels when administered concomitantly with carbamazepine. Thus, if a patient has been titrated to a stable dosage on one of the agents in these categories, and then begins a course of treatment with carbamazepine, it is reasonable to expect that a dose increase for the concomitant agent may be necessary).
No products indexed under this heading.

Trimipramine Maleate (Carbamazepine is known to induce CYP1A2 and CYP3A4. Therefore, the potential exists for interaction between carbamazepine and any agent metabolized by one (or more) of these enzymes. Agents that are metabolized by CYP1A2 and CYP3A4 may have decreased plasma levels when administered concomitantly with carbamazepine. Thus, if a patient has been titrated to a stable dosage on one of the agents in these categories, and then begins a course of treatment with carbamazepine, it is reasonable to expect that a dose increase for the concomitant agent may be necessary).
No products indexed under this heading.

Troglitazone (Carbamazepine is metabolized mainly by CYP3A4, the active carbamazepine 10,11-epoxide, which is futher metabolized to the trans-diol by epoxide hydrolase. Therefore, the potential exists for interaction between carbamazepine and any agent that inhibits CYP3A4 and/or epoxide hydrolase. Agents that are CYP3A4 inhibitors may increase the plasma levels of carbamazepine. Thus, if a patient has been titrated to a stable dosage of carbamazepine, and then begins a course of treatment with a CYP3A4 or epoxide hydrolase inhibitor, it is reasonable to expect that a dose reduction for carbamazepine may be necessary).
No products indexed under this heading.

Troleandomycin (Carbamazepine is metabolized mainly by CYP3A4, the active carbamazepine 10,11-epoxide, which is futher metabolized to the trans-diol by epoxide hydrolase. Therefore, the potential exists for interaction between carbamazepine and any agent that inhibits CYP3A4 and/or epoxide hydrolase. Agents that are CYP3A4 inhibitors may increase the plasma levels of carbamazepine. Thus, if a patient has been titrated to a stable dosage of carbamazepine, and then begins a course of treatment with a CYP3A4 or epoxide hydrolase inhibitor, it is reasonable to expect that a dose reduction for carbamazepine may be necessary).
No products indexed under this heading.

Trovafloxacin Mesylate (Carbamazepine is known to induce CYP1A2 and CYP3A4. Therefore, the potential exists for interaction between carbamazepine and any agent metabolized by one (or more) of these enzymes. Agents that are metabolized by CYP1A2 and CYP3A4 may have decreased plasma levels when administered concomitantly with carbamazepine. Thus, if a patient has been titrated to a stable dosage on one of the agents in these categories, and then begins a course of treatment with carbamazepine, it is reasonable to expect that a dose increase for the concomitant agent may be necessary).
No products indexed under this heading.

Valproate Sodium (Carbamazepine is metabolized mainly by CYP3A4, the active carbamazepine 10,11-epoxide, which is futher metabolized to the trans-diol by epoxide hydrolase. Therefore, the potential exists for interaction between carbamazepine and any agent that inhibits CYP3A4 and/or epoxide hydrolase. Agents that are CYP3A4 inhibitors may increase the plasma levels of carbamazepine. Thus, if a patient has been titrated to a stable dosage of carbamazepine, and then begins a course of treatment with a CYP3A4 or epoxide hydrolase inhibitor, it is reasonable to expect that a dose reduction for carbamazepine may be necessary).
No products indexed under this heading.

Valproic Acid (Carbamazepine is metabolized mainly by CYP3A4 the active carbamazepine 10,11-epoxide, which is futher metabolized to the trans-diol by epoxide hydrolase. Therefore, the potential exists for interaction between carbamazepine and any agent that inhibits CYP3A4 and/or epoxide hydrolase. Agents that are CYP3A4

inhibitors may increase the plasma levels of carbamazepine. Also inhibits epoxide hydroxylase, resulting in increased levels of the active metabolite carbamazepine-10,11-epoxide. Thus, if a patient has been titrated to a stable dosage of carbamazepine, and then begins a course of treatment with a CYP3A4 or epoxide hydrolase inhibitor, it is reasonable to expect that a dose reduction for carbamazepine may be necessary).
No products indexed under this heading.

Vardenafil Hydrochloride (Carbamazepine is metabolized mainly by CYP3A4, the active carbamazepine 10,11-epoxide, which is futher metabolized to the trans-diol by epoxide hydrolase. Therefore, the potential exists for interaction between carbamazepine and any agent that inhibits CYP3A4 and/or epoxide hydrolase. Agents that are CYP3A4 inhibitors may increase the plasma levels of carbamazepine. Thus, if a patient has been titrated to a stable dosage of carbamazepine, and then begins a course of treatment with a CYP3A4 or epoxide hydrolase inhibitor, it is reasonable to expect that a dose reduction for carbamazepine may be necessary). Products include:
Levitra 3157

Verapamil Hydrochloride (Carbamazepine is metabolized mainly by CYP3A4, the active carbamazepine 10,11-epoxide, which is futher metabolized to the trans-diol by epoxide hydrolase. Therefore, the potential exists for interaction between carbamazepine and any agent that inhibits CYP3A4 and/or epoxide hydrolase. Agents that are CYP3A4 inhibitors may increase the plasma levels of carbamazepine. Thus, if a patient has been titrated to a stable dosage of carbamazepine, and then begins a course of treatment with a CYP3A4 or epoxide hydrolase inhibitor, it is reasonable to expect that a dose reduction for carbamazepine may be necessary). Products include:
Tarka 534

Vinblastine Sulfate (Carbamazepine is known to induce CYP1A2 and CYP3A4. Therefore, the potential exists for interaction between carbamazepine and any agent metabolized by one (or more) of these enzymes. Agents that are metabolized by CYP1A2 and CYP3A4 may have decreased plasma levels when administered concomitantly with carbamazepine. Thus, if a patient has been titrated to a stable dosage on one of the agents in these categories, and then begins a course of treatment with carbamazepine, it is reasonable to expect that a dose increase for the concomitant agent may be necessary).
No products indexed under this heading.

Vincristine Sulfate (Carbamazepine is known to induce CYP1A2 and CYP3A4. Therefore, the potential exists for interaction between carbamazepine and any agent metabolized by one (or more) of these enzymes. Agents that are metabolized by CYP1A2 and CYP3A4 may have decreased plasma levels when administered concomitantly with carbamazepine. Thus, if a patient has been titrated to a stable dosage on one of the agents in these categories, and then begins a course of treatment with carbamazepine, it is reasonable to expect that a dose increase for the concomitant agent may be necessary).
No products indexed under this heading.

Voriconazole (Carbamazepine is metabolized mainly by CYP3A4, the active carbamazepine 10,11-epoxide, which is futher metabolized to the trans-diol by epoxide hydrolase. Therefore, the potential exists for interaction between carbamazepine and any agent that inhibits CYP3A4 and/or epoxide hydrolase. Agents that are CYP3A4 inhibitors may increase the plasma levels of carbamazepine. Thus, if a patient has been titrated to a stable dosage of carbamazepine, and then begins a course of treatment with a CYP3A4 or epoxide hydrolase inhibitor, it is reasonable to expect that a dose reduction for carbamazepine may be necessary).
No products indexed under this heading.

Warfarin Sodium (Carbamazepine is known to induce CYP1A2 and CYP3A4. Therefore, the potential exists for interaction between carbamazepine and any agent metabolized by one (or more) of these enzymes. Agents that are metabolized by CYP1A2 or CYP3A4 may have decreased plasma levels when administered concomitantly with carbamazepine. Thus, if a patient has been titrated to a stable dosage on one of the agents in these categories, and then begins a course of treatment with carbamazepine, it is reasonable to expect that a dose increase for the concomitant agent may be necessary. Therefore, warfarin's anticoagulant effect may be reduced in the presence of carbamazepine and dosage adjustment may be necessary).
No products indexed under this heading.

Zafirlukast (Carbamazepine is metabolized mainly by CYP3A4, the active carbamazepine 10,11-epoxide, which is futher metabolized to the trans-diol by epoxide hydrolase. Therefore, the potential exists for interaction between carbamazepine and any agent that inhibits CYP3A4 and/or epoxide hydrolase. Agents that are CYP3A4 inhibitors may increase the plasma levels of carbamazepine. Thus, if a patient has been titrated to a stable dosage of carbamazepine, and then begins a course of treatment with a CYP3A4 or epoxide hydrolase inhibitor, it is reasonable to expect that a dose reduction for carbamazepine may be necessary). Products include:
Accolate 3612

Zaleplon (Because of its primary CNS effect, caution should be used when carbamazepine is taken with other centrally acting drugs).
No products indexed under this heading.

Zileuton (Carbamazepine is metabolized mainly by CYP3A4, the active carbamazepine 10,11-epoxide, which is futher metabolized to the trans-diol by epoxide hydrolase. Therefore, the potential exists for interaction between carbamazepine and any agent that inhibits CYP3A4 and/or epoxide hydrolase. Agents that are CYP3A4 inhibitors may increase the plasma levels of carbamazepine. Thus, if a patient has been titrated to a stable dosage of carbamazepine, and then begins a course of treatment with a CYP3A4 or epoxide hydrolase inhibitor, it is reasonable to expect that a dose reduction for carbamazepine may be necessary).
No products indexed under this heading.

Ziprasidone Hydrochloride (Because of its primary CNS effect, caution should be used when carbamazepine is taken with other centrally acting drugs). Products include:
Geodon 2723

Zolmitriptan (Carbamazepine is known to induce CYP1A2 and CYP3A4. Therefore, the potential exists for interaction between carbamazepine and any agent metabolized by one (or more) of these enzymes. Agents that are metabolized by CYP1A2 and CYP3A4 may have decreased plasma levels when administered concomitantly with carbamazepine. Thus, if a patient has been titrated to a stable dosage on one of the agents in these categories, and then begins a course of treatment with carbamazepine, it is reasonable to expect that a dose increase for the concomitant agent may be necessary). Products include:
Zomig Tablets 773
Zomig Nasal Spray 768
Zomig-ZMT Tablets 773

Zolpidem Tartrate (Because of its primary CNS effect, caution should be used when carbamazepine is taken with other centrally acting drugs). Products include:
Ambien 2920
Ambien CR 2925

Food Interactions

Alcohol (Because of its primary CNS effect, caution should be used when carbamazepine is taken with alcohol).

Beer, reduced-alcohol (Because of its primary CNS effect, caution should be used when carbamazepine is taken with alcohol).

Beer, unspecified (Because of its primary CNS effect, caution should be used when carbamazepine is taken with alcohol).

Food, caffeine-containing (Carbamazepine is known to induce CYP1A2 and CYP3A4. Therefore, the potential exists for interaction between carbamazepine and any agent metabolized by one (or more) of these enzymes. Agents that are metabolized by CYP1A2 and CYP3A4 may have decreased plasma levels when administered concomitantly with carbamazepine. Thus, if a patient has been titrated to a stable dosage on one of the agents in these categories, and then begins a course of treatment with carbamazepine, it is reasonable to expect that a dose increase for the concomitant agent may be necessary).

Food, unspecified (A high fat meal diet increased the rate of absorption of a single 400 mg dose (mean T_{max} was reduced from 24 hours, in the fasting state, to 14 hours and C_{max} increased from 3.2 to 4.3 μg/mL) but not the extent (AUC) of absorption. The elimination half-life remains unchanged between fed and fasting state. The multiple dose study conducted in the fed state showed that the steady-state C_{max} values were within the therapeutic concentration range. The pharmacokinetic profile of extended-release carbamazepine was similar when given by sprinkling the beads over applesauce compared to the intact capsule administered in the fasted state).

Grapefruit (Carbamazepine is metabolized mainly by CYP3A4, the active carbamazepine 10,11-epoxide, which is futher metabolized to the trans-diol by epoxide hydrolase. Therefore, the potential exists for interaction between carbamazepine and any agent that inhibits CYP3A4 and/or epoxide hydrolase. Agents that are CYP3A4 inhibitors may increase the plasma levels of carbamazepine. Thus, if a patient has been titrated to a stable dosage of carbamazepine, and then begins a course of treatment with a CYP3A4 or epoxide hydrolase inhibitor, it is reasonable to expect that a dose reduction for carbamazepine may be necessary).

Grapefruit Juice (Carbamazepine is metabolized mainly by CYP3A4, the active carbamazepine 10,11-epoxide, which is futher metabolized to the trans-diol by epoxide hydrolase. Therefore, the potential exists for interaction between carbamazepine and any agent that inhibits CYP3A4 and/or epoxide hydrolase. Agents that are CYP3A4 inhibitors may increase the plasma levels of carbamazepine. Thus, if a patient has been titrated to a stable dosage of carbamazepine, and then begins a course of treatment with a CYP3A4 or epoxide hydrolase inhibitor, it is reasonable to expect that a dose reduction for carbamazepine may be necessary).

Meal, unspecified (A high fat meal diet increased the rate of absorption of a single 400 mg dose (mean T_{max} was reduced from 24 hours, in the fasting state, to 14 hours and C_{max} increased from 3.2 to 4.3 μg/mL) but not the extent (AUC) of absorption. The elimination half-life remains unchanged between fed and fasting state. The multiple dose study conducted in the fed state showed that the steady-state C_{max} values were within the therapeutic concentration range. The pharmacokinetic profile of extended-release carbamazepine was similar when given by sprinkling the beads over applesauce compared to the intact capsule administered in the fasted state).

Wine, Chianti (Because of its primary CNS effect, caution should be used when carbamazepine is taken with alcohol).

Wine, Red (Because of its primary CNS effect, caution should be used when carbamazepine is taken with alcohol).

Wine, unspecified (Because of its primary CNS effect, caution should be used when carbamazepine is taken with alcohol).

Wine products (Because of its primary CNS effect, caution should be used when carbamazepine is taken with alcohol).

CARDIO BASICS TABLETS

(Amino Acid Preparations, Beta-Carotene, Biotin, Calcium, Calcium Pantothenate, Cholecalciferol, Chromium, Coenzyme Q-10, Copper, L-Cysteine, D-Alpha Tocopherol, Folate, Inositol, L-Arginine, Levocarnitine, L-Proline, L-Lysine, Magnesium, Manganese, Maritime Pine Extract, Molybdenum, Niacin, Phosphorus, Potassium, Selenium, Sodium, Vitamin A, Vitamin B1, Vitamin B12, Vitamin B2, Vitamin B6, Vitamin C, Vitamin D, Vitamin E, Vitamins with Minerals, Zinc) 3455
None cited in PDR database.

CARDIOESSENTIALS CAPSULES

(Coenzyme Q-10, Levocarnitine, Taurine) 3455
None cited in PDR database.

CARDIZEM LA EXTENDED RELEASE TABLETS

(Diltiazem Hydrochloride) 423
May interact with anesthetics, antihypertensives, benzodiazepines, beta-blockers, cardiac glycosides, cytochrome p450 3a4 inducers (selected), cytochrome p450 3a4 inhibitors (selected), cytochrome p450 3a4 substrates (selected), quinidine, and certain other agents. Compounds in these categories include:

Acebutolol Hydrochloride (Pharmacologic studies indicate that there may be additive effects in prolonging A-V conduction when using beta-blockers or digitalis concomitantly with diltiazem).
No products indexed under this heading.

Acetazolamide (Diltiazem is both a substrate and an inhibitor of the CYP3A4 enzyme system. Other drugs that are specific substrates, inhibitors, or inducers of this enzyme system may have a significant impact on the efficacy and side effect profile of diltiazem).
No products indexed under this heading.

IMPORTANT NOTE: Always consult each drug listing in the patient's regimen for possible interactions.

Acetazolamide Sodium (Diltiazem is both a substrate and an inhibitor of the CYP3A4 enzyme system. Other drugs that are specific substrates, inhibitors, or inducers of this enzyme system may have a significant impact on the efficacy and side effect profile of diltiazem).
No products indexed under this heading.

Alfentanil Hydrochloride (The depression of cardiac contractility, conductivity, and automaticity, as well as the vascular dilation associated with anesthetics, may be potentiated by calcium channel blockers).
No products indexed under this heading.

Aliskiren (Diltiazem has an additive effect when used with other antihypertensive agents. Therefore, the dosage of diltiazem or concomitant antihypertensives may need to be adjusted when adding one to the other). Products include:
Tekturna 2538
Tekturna HCT 2541
Valturna 3637

Allium sativum (Diltiazem is both a substrate and an inhibitor of the CYP3A4 enzyme system. Other drugs that are specific substrates, inhibitors, or inducers of this enzyme system may have a significant impact on the efficacy and side effect profile of diltiazem).
No products indexed under this heading.

Alprazolam (Studies showed that diltiazem increased the AUC of midazolam and triazolam by 3- to 4-fold and the C_{max} by 2-fold, compared to placebo. The elimination half-life of midazolam and triazolam also increased during co-administration with diltiazem).
No products indexed under this heading.

Aminoglutethimide (Diltiazem is both a substrate and an inhibitor of the CYP3A4 enzyme system. Other drugs that are specific substrates, inhibitors, or inducers of this enzyme system may have a significant impact on the efficacy and side effect profile of diltiazem).
No products indexed under this heading.

Amiodarone Hydrochloride (Patients taking other drugs that are substrates of CYP450, especially patients with renal and/or hepatic impairment, may require dosage adjustment when starting or stopping concomitantly administered diltiazem in order to maintain optimum therapeutic blood levels).
No products indexed under this heading.

Amitriptyline Hydrochloride (Patients taking other drugs that are substrates of CYP450, especially patients with renal and/or hepatic impairment, may require dosage adjustment when starting or stopping concomitantly administered diltiazem in order to maintain optimum therapeutic blood levels).
No products indexed under this heading.

Amlodipine Besylate (Diltiazem has an additive effect when used with other antihypertensive agents. Therefore, the dosage of diltiazem or concomitant antihypertensives may need to be adjusted when adding one to the other). Products include:
Azor 1010
Exforge 2443
Exforge HCT 2449

Amprenavir (Diltiazem is both a substrate and an inhibitor of the CYP3A4 enzyme system. Other drugs that are specific substrates, inhibitors, or inducers of this enzyme system may have a significant impact on the efficacy and side effect profile of diltiazem).
No products indexed under this heading.

Anastrozole (Diltiazem is both a substrate and an inhibitor of the CYP3A4 enzyme system. Other drugs that are specific substrates, inhibitors, or inducers of this enzyme system may have a significant impact on the efficacy and side effect profile of diltiazem).
No products indexed under this heading.

Aprepitant (Patients taking other drugs that are substrates of CYP450, especially patients with renal and/or hepatic impairment, may require dosage adjustment when starting or stopping concomitantly administered diltiazem in order to maintain optimum therapeutic blood levels). Products include:
Emend 2124

Articaine Hydrochloride (The depression of cardiac contractility, conductivity, and automaticity, as well as the vascular dilation associated with anesthetics, may be potentiated by calcium channel blockers).
No products indexed under this heading.

Astemizole (Patients taking other drugs that are substrates of CYP450, especially patients with renal and/or hepatic impairment, may require dosage adjustment when starting or stopping concomitantly administered diltiazem in order to maintain optimum therapeutic blood levels).
No products indexed under this heading.

Atazanavir (Diltiazem is both a substrate and an inhibitor of the CYP3A4 enzyme system. Other drugs that are specific substrates, inhibitors, or inducers of this enzyme system may have a significant impact on the efficacy and side effect profile of diltiazem).
No products indexed under this heading.

Atazanavir Sulfate (Diltiazem is both a substrate and an inhibitor of the CYP3A4 enzyme system. Other drugs that are specific substrates, inhibitors, or inducers of this enzyme system may have a significant impact on the efficacy and side effect profile of diltiazem).
No products indexed under this heading.

Atenolol (Pharmacologic studies indicate that there may be additive effects in prolonging A-V conduction when using beta-blockers or digitalis concomitantly with diltiazem).
No products indexed under this heading.

Atorvastatin Calcium (Patients taking other drugs that are substrates of CYP450, especially patients with renal and/or hepatic impairment, may require dosage adjustment when starting or stopping concomitantly administered diltiazem in order to maintain optimum therapeutic blood levels). Products include:
Lipitor 2703

Belladonna Ergotamine (Patients taking other drugs that are substrates of CYP450, especially patients with renal and/or hepatic impairment, may require dosage adjustment when starting or stopping concomitantly administered diltiazem in order to maintain optimum therapeutic blood levels).
No products indexed under this heading.

Benazepril Hydrochloride (Diltiazem has an additive effect when used with other antihypertensive agents. Therefore, the dosage of diltiazem or concomitant antihypertensives may need to be adjusted when adding one to the other).
No products indexed under this heading.

Bendroflumethiazide (Diltiazem has an additive effect when used with other antihypertensive agents. Therefore, the dosage of diltiazem or concomitant antihypertensives may need to be adjusted when adding one to the other).
No products indexed under this heading.

Benzocaine (The depression of cardiac contractility, conductivity, and automaticity, as well as the vascular dilation associated with anesthetics, may be potentiated by calcium channel blockers).
No products indexed under this heading.

Betamethasone (Diltiazem is both a substrate and an inhibitor of the CYP3A4 enzyme system. Other drugs that are specific substrates, inhibitors, or inducers of this enzyme system may have a significant impact on the efficacy and side effect profile of diltiazem).
No products indexed under this heading.

Betamethasone Acetate (Diltiazem is both a substrate and an inhibitor of the CYP3A4 enzyme system. Other drugs that are specific substrates, inhibitors, or inducers of this enzyme system may have a significant impact on the efficacy and side effect profile of diltiazem).
No products indexed under this heading.

Betamethasone Benzoate (Diltiazem is both a substrate and an inhibitor of the CYP3A4 enzyme system. Other drugs that are specific substrates, inhibitors, or inducers of this enzyme system may have a significant impact on the efficacy and side effect profile of diltiazem).
No products indexed under this heading.

Betamethasone Dipropionate (Diltiazem is both a substrate and an inhibitor of the CYP3A4 enzyme system. Other drugs that are specific substrates, inhibitors, or inducers of this enzyme system may have a significant impact on the efficacy and side effect profile of diltiazem). Products include:
Diprolene Lotion 0.05% 3108
Diprolene Ointment 0.05% 3109
Diprolene AF Cream 0.05% 3107
Lotrisone 3163

Betamethasone Sodium Phosphate (Diltiazem is both a substrate and an inhibitor of the CYP3A4 enzyme system. Other drugs that are specific substrates, inhibitors, or inducers of this enzyme system may have a significant impact on the efficacy and side effect profile of diltiazem).
No products indexed under this heading.

Betamethasone Valerate (Diltiazem is both a substrate and an inhibitor of the CYP3A4 enzyme system. Other drugs that are specific substrates, inhibitors, or inducers of this enzyme system may have a significant impact on the efficacy and side effect profile of diltiazem). Products include:
Luxíq 3321

Betaxolol Hydrochloride (Pharmacologic studies indicate that there may be additive effects in prolonging A-V conduction when using beta-blockers or digitalis concomitantly with diltiazem).
No products indexed under this heading.

Bisoprolol Fumarate (Pharmacologic studies indicate that there may be additive effects in prolonging A-V conduction when using beta-blockers or digitalis concomitantly with diltiazem).
No products indexed under this heading.

Bosentan (Diltiazem is both a substrate and an inhibitor of the CYP3A4 enzyme system. Other drugs that are specific substrates, inhibitors, or inducers of this enzyme system may have a significant impact on the efficacy and side effect profile of diltiazem). Products include:
Tracleer 573

Bupivacaine Hydrochloride (The depression of cardiac contractility, conductivity, and automaticity, as well as the vascular dilation associated with anesthetics, may be potentiated by calcium channel blockers).
No products indexed under this heading.

Buspirone Hydrochloride (Studies showed that diltiazem increased the AUC of buspirone by 5.5 fold and the C_{max} by 4.1 fold. Enhanced effects of buspirone may be possible).
No products indexed under this heading.

Busulfan (Patients taking other drugs that are substrates of CYP450, especially patients with renal and/or hepatic impairment, may require dosage adjustment when starting or stopping concomitantly administered diltiazem in order to maintain optimum therapeutic blood levels). Products include:
Myleran 1581

Candesartan Cilexetil (Diltiazem has an additive effect when used with other antihypertensive agents. Therefore, the dosage of diltiazem or concomitant antihypertensives may need to be adjusted when adding one to the other). Products include:
Atacand 697
Atacand HCT 700

Captopril (Diltiazem has an additive effect when used with other antihypertensive agents. Therefore, the dosage of diltiazem or concomitant antihypertensives may need to be adjusted when adding one to the other). Products include:
Captopril 2341

Carbamazepine (Concomitant administration of diltiazem with carbamazepine has been reported to result in elevated serum levels of carbamazepine (40% to 72% increase), resulting in toxicity in some cases). Products include:
Carbatrol 3280
Equetro 3477

Carteolol Hydrochloride (Pharmacologic studies indicate that there may be additive effects in prolonging A-V conduction when using beta-blockers or digitalis concomitantly with diltiazem).
No products indexed under this heading.

Carvedilol (Pharmacologic studies indicate that there may be additive effects in prolonging A-V conduction when using beta-blockers or digitalis concomitantly with diltiazem). Products include:
Coreg 1409

Carvedilol Phosphate (Pharmacologic studies indicate that there may be additive effects in prolonging A-V conduction when using beta-blockers or digitalis concomitantly with diltiazem). Products include:
Coreg CR 1416

Cerivastatin Sodium (Patients taking other drugs that are substrates of CYP450, especially patients with renal and/or hepatic impairment, may require dosage adjustment when starting or stopping concomitantly administered diltiazem in order to maintain optimum therapeutic blood levels).
No products indexed under this heading.

Chlordiazepoxide (Studies showed that diltiazem increased the AUC of midazolam and triazolam by 3- to 4-fold and the C_{max} by 2-fold, compared to placebo. The elimination half-life of midazolam and triazolam also increased during co-administration with diltiazem).
No products indexed under this heading.

Chlordiazepoxide Hydrochloride (Studies showed that diltiazem increased the AUC of midazolam and triazolam by 3- to 4-fold and the C_{max} by 2-fold, compared to placebo. The elimination half-life of midazolam and triazolam also increased during co-administration with diltiazem).
No products indexed under this heading.

(⊙ Described in PDR® for Ophthalmic Medicines)

Chloroprocaine Hydrochloride
(The depression of cardiac contractility, conductivity, and automaticity, as well as the vascular dilation associated with anesthetics, may be potentiated by calcium channel blockers).
No products indexed under this heading.

Chlorothiazide (Diltiazem has an additive effect when used with other antihypertensive agents. Therefore, the dosage of diltiazem or concomitant antihypertensives may need to be adjusted when adding one to the other).
No products indexed under this heading.

Chlorothiazide Sodium (Diltiazem has an additive effect when used with other antihypertensive agents. Therefore, the dosage of diltiazem or concomitant antihypertensives may need to be adjusted when adding one to the other). Products include:
Diuril Intravenous 2009

Chlorpheniramine (Patients taking other drugs that are substrates of CYP450, especially patients with renal and/or hepatic impairment, may require dosage adjustment when starting or stopping concomitantly administered diltiazem in order to maintain optimum therapeutic blood levels).
No products indexed under this heading.

Chlorpheniramine Maleate
(Patients taking other drugs that are substrates of CYP450, especially patients with renal and/or hepatic impairment, may require dosage adjustment when starting or stopping concomitantly administered diltiazem in order to maintain optimum therapeutic blood levels).
No products indexed under this heading.

Chlorpheniramine Polistirex
(Patients taking other drugs that are substrates of CYP450, especially patients with renal and/or hepatic impairment, may require dosage adjustment when starting or stopping concomitantly administered diltiazem in order to maintain optimum therapeutic blood levels). Products include:
Tussionex 3443

Chlorpheniramine Tannate
(Patients taking other drugs that are substrates of CYP450, especially patients with renal and/or hepatic impairment, may require dosage adjustment when starting or stopping concomitantly administered diltiazem in order to maintain optimum therapeutic blood levels).
No products indexed under this heading.

Chlorthalidone (Diltiazem has an additive effect when used with other antihypertensive agents. Therefore, the dosage of diltiazem or concomitant antihypertensives may need to be adjusted when adding one to the other). Products include:
Clorpres 2344

Cimetidine (A study in six healthy volunteers has shown a significant increase in peak diltiazem plasma levels (58%) and AUC (53%) after a 1-week course of cimetidine at 1200 mg per day and a single dose of diltiazem 60 mg).
No products indexed under this heading.

Cimetidine Hydrochloride (A study in six healthy volunteers has shown a significant increase in peak diltiazem plasma levels (58%) and AUC (53%) after a 1-week course of cimetidine at 1200 mg per day and a single dose of diltiazem 60 mg).
No products indexed under this heading.

Ciprofloxacin (Diltiazem is both a substrate and an inhibitor of the CYP3A4 enzyme system. Other drugs that are specific substrates, inhibitors, or inducers of this enzyme system may have a

significant impact on the efficacy and side effect profile of diltiazem).
Products include:
Cipro I.V. 3082
Cipro 3073
Cipro XR 3091
Ciprodex 583

Ciprofloxacin Hydrochloride (Diltiazem is both a substrate and an inhibitor of the CYP3A4 enzyme system. Other drugs that are specific substrates, inhibitors, or inducers of this enzyme system may have a significant impact on the efficacy and side effect profile of diltiazem). Products include:
Cipro 3073

Cisapride (Patients taking other drugs that are substrates of CYP450, especially patients with renal and/or hepatic impairment, may require dosage adjustment when starting or stopping concomitantly administered diltiazem in order to maintain optimum therapeutic blood levels).
No products indexed under this heading.

Cisplatin (Diltiazem is both a substrate and an inhibitor of the CYP3A4 enzyme system. Other drugs that are specific substrates, inhibitors, or inducers of this enzyme system may have a significant impact on the efficacy and side effect profile of diltiazem).
No products indexed under this heading.

Clarithromycin (Patients taking other drugs that are substrates of CYP450, especially patients with renal and/or hepatic impairment, may require dosage adjustment when starting or stopping concomitantly administered diltiazem in order to maintain optimum therapeutic blood levels). Products include:
Biaxin/Biaxin XL 412

Clonidine (Diltiazem has an additive effect when used with other antihypertensive agents. Therefore, the dosage of diltiazem or concomitant antihypertensives may need to be adjusted when adding one to the other). Products include:
Catapres-TTS 884

Clonidine Hydrochloride (Diltiazem has an additive effect when used with other antihypertensive agents. Therefore, the dosage of diltiazem or concomitant antihypertensives may need to be adjusted when adding one to the other). Products include:
Clorpres 2344

Clorazepate Dipotassium (Studies showed that diltiazem increased the AUC of midazolam and triazolam by 3- to 4-fold and the C_{max} by 2-fold, compared to placebo. The elimination half-life of midazolam and triazolam also increased during co-administration with diltiazem).
No products indexed under this heading.

Clotrimazole (Diltiazem is both a substrate and an inhibitor of the CYP3A4 enzyme system. Other drugs that are specific substrates, inhibitors, or inducers of this enzyme system may have a significant impact on the efficacy and side effect profile of diltiazem). Products include:
Lotrisone 3163

Cocaine Hydrochloride (The depression of cardiac contractility, conductivity, and automaticity, as well as the vascular dilation associated with anesthetics, may be potentiated by calcium channel blockers).
No products indexed under this heading.

Conivaptan Hydrochloride (Diltiazem is both a substrate and an inhibitor of the CYP3A4 enzyme system. Other drugs that are specific substrates, inhibitors, or inducers of this enzyme system may have a significant impact on the efficacy and side effect profile of diltiazem). Products include:

Vaprisol 689

Cortisone Acetate (Diltiazem is both a substrate and an inhibitor of the CYP3A4 enzyme system. Other drugs that are specific substrates, inhibitors, or inducers of this enzyme system may have a significant impact on the efficacy and side effect profile of diltiazem).
No products indexed under this heading.

Cyclosporine (In renal and cardiac transplant recipients, a reduction of cyclosporine dose ranging from 15% to 48% was necessary to maintain cyclosporine trough concentrations similar to those seen prior to the addition of diltiazem. If these agents are to be administered concurrently, cyclosporine concentrations should be monitored, especially when diltiazem therapy is initiated, adjusted or discontinued). Products include:
Gengraf 440
Neoral Oral Solution 2496
Neoral Capsules 2496
Restasis 605

Dalfopristin (Diltiazem is both a substrate and an inhibitor of the CYP3A4 enzyme system. Other drugs that are specific substrates, inhibitors, or inducers of this enzyme system may have a significant impact on the efficacy and side effect profile of diltiazem).
No products indexed under this heading.

Danazol (Diltiazem is both a substrate and an inhibitor of the CYP3A4 enzyme system. Other drugs that are specific substrates, inhibitors, or inducers of this enzyme system may have a significant impact on the efficacy and side effect profile of diltiazem).
No products indexed under this heading.

Darunavir (Diltiazem is both a substrate and an inhibitor of the CYP3A4 enzyme system. Other drugs that are specific substrates, inhibitors, or inducers of this enzyme system may have a significant impact on the efficacy and side effect profile of diltiazem).
No products indexed under this heading.

Dasatinib (Diltiazem is both a substrate and an inhibitor of the CYP3A4 enzyme system. Other drugs that are specific substrates, inhibitors, or inducers of this enzyme system may have a significant impact on the efficacy and side effect profile of diltiazem).
No products indexed under this heading.

Delavirdine Mesylate (Diltiazem is both a substrate and an inhibitor of the CYP3A4 enzyme system. Other drugs that are specific substrates, inhibitors, or inducers of this enzyme system may have a significant impact on the efficacy and side effect profile of diltiazem).
No products indexed under this heading.

Delavirine (Diltiazem is both a substrate and an inhibitor of the CYP3A4 enzyme system. Other drugs that are specific substrates, inhibitors, or inducers of this enzyme system may have a significant impact on the efficacy and side effect profile of diltiazem).
No products indexed under this heading.

Deserpidine (Diltiazem has an additive effect when used with other antihypertensive agents. Therefore, the dosage of diltiazem or concomitant antihypertensives may need to be adjusted when adding one to the other).
No products indexed under this heading.

Deslanoside (Pharmacologic studies indicate that there may be additive effects in prolonging A-V conduction when using beta-blockers or digitalis concomitantly with diltiazem).
No products indexed under this heading.

Desloratadine (Diltiazem is both a substrate and an inhibitor of the CYP3A4 enzyme system. Other drugs that are specific substrates, inhibitors, or inducers of this enzyme system may

have a significant impact on the efficacy and side effect profile of diltiazem).
Products include:
Clarinex Syrup 3098
Clarinex 3098
Clarinex Reditabs 3098
Clarinex-D 12-Hour 3101
Clarinex-D 3104

Desogestrel (Patients taking other drugs that are substrates of CYP450, especially patients with renal and/or hepatic impairment, may require dosage adjustment when starting or stopping concomitantly administered diltiazem in order to maintain optimum therapeutic blood levels).
No products indexed under this heading.

Dexamethasone (Diltiazem is both a substrate and an inhibitor of the CYP3A4 enzyme system. Other drugs that are specific substrates, inhibitors, or inducers of this enzyme system may have a significant impact on the efficacy and side effect profile of diltiazem). Products include:
Ciprodex 583
Ozurdex .... ⊙223
Tobramycin and Dexamethasone Ophthalmic Suspension .... ⊙251

Dexamethasone Acetate (Diltiazem is both a substrate and an inhibitor of the CYP3A4 enzyme system. Other drugs that are specific substrates, inhibitors, or inducers of this enzyme system may have a significant impact on the efficacy and side effect profile of diltiazem).
No products indexed under this heading.

Dexamethasone Phosphate (Diltiazem is both a substrate and an inhibitor of the CYP3A4 enzyme system. Other drugs that are specific substrates, inhibitors, or inducers of this enzyme system may have a significant impact on the efficacy and side effect profile of diltiazem).
No products indexed under this heading.

Dexamethasone Sodium (Diltiazem is both a substrate and an inhibitor of the CYP3A4 enzyme system. Other drugs that are specific substrates, inhibitors, or inducers of this enzyme system may have a significant impact on the efficacy and side effect profile of diltiazem).
No products indexed under this heading.

Dexamethasone Sodium Phosphate (Diltiazem is both a substrate and an inhibitor of the CYP3A4 enzyme system. Other drugs that are specific substrates, inhibitors, or inducers of this enzyme system may have a significant impact on the efficacy and side effect profile of diltiazem).
No products indexed under this heading.

Dexamethasone Sodium Phosphate Injection (Diltiazem is both a substrate and an inhibitor of the CYP3A4 enzyme system. Other drugs that are specific substrates, inhibitors, or inducers of this enzyme system may have a significant impact on the efficacy and side effect profile of diltiazem).
No products indexed under this heading.

Diazepam (Studies showed that diltiazem increased the AUC of midazolam and triazolam by 3- to 4-fold and the C_{max} by 2-fold, compared to placebo. The elimination half-life of midazolam and triazolam also increased during co-administration with diltiazem). Products include:
Valium Tablets 2880

Diazoxide (Diltiazem has an additive effect when used with other antihypertensive agents. Therefore, the dosage of diltiazem or concomitant antihypertensives may need to be adjusted when adding one to the other). Products include:
Proglycem 1179

IMPORTANT NOTE: Always consult each drug listing in the patient's regimen for possible interactions.

Cardizem Interactions Index 278

Proglycem Suspension 1179

Dibucaine (The depression of cardiac contractility, conductivity, and automaticity, as well as the vascular dilation associated with anesthetics, may be potentiated by calcium channel blockers).
No products indexed under this heading.

Dibucaine Hydrochloride (The depression of cardiac contractility, conductivity, and automaticity, as well as the vascular dilation associated with anesthetics, may be potentiated by calcium channel blockers).
No products indexed under this heading.

Digitalis Glycoside Preparations (Pharmacologic studies indicate that there may be additive effects in prolonging A-V conduction when using beta-blockers or digitalis concomitantly with diltiazem).
No products indexed under this heading.

Digitalis Lanata (Pharmacologic studies indicate that there may be additive effects in prolonging A-V conduction when using beta-blockers or digitalis concomitantly with diltiazem).
No products indexed under this heading.

Digitalis Purpurea (Pharmacologic studies indicate that there may be additive effects in prolonging A-V conduction when using beta-blockers or digitalis concomitantly with diltiazem).
No products indexed under this heading.

Digitoxin (Pharmacologic studies indicate that there may be additive effects in prolonging A-V conduction when using beta-blockers or digitalis concomitantly with diltiazem).
No products indexed under this heading.

Digoxin (Pharmacologic studies indicate that there may be additive effects in prolonging A-V conduction when using beta-blockers or digitalis concomitantly with diltiazem). Products include:
Lanoxin Injection 1546
Lanoxin Injection Pediatric 1549
Lanoxin Tablets 1553

Dihydroergotamine Mesylate (Patients taking other drugs that are substrates of CYP450, especially patients with renal and/or hepatic impairment, may require dosage adjustment when starting or stopping concomitantly administered diltiazem in order to maintain optimum therapeutic blood levels).
No products indexed under this heading.

Diltiazem Maleate (Diltiazem has an additive effect when used with other antihypertensive agents. Therefore, the dosage of diltiazem or concomitant antihypertensives may need to be adjusted when adding one to the other).
No products indexed under this heading.

Disopyramide (Patients taking other drugs that are substrates of CYP450, especially patients with renal and/or hepatic impairment, may require dosage adjustment when starting or stopping concomitantly administered diltiazem in order to maintain optimum therapeutic blood levels).
No products indexed under this heading.

Disopyramide Phosphate (Patients taking other drugs that are substrates of CYP450, especially patients with renal and/or hepatic impairment, may require dosage adjustment when starting or stopping concomitantly administered diltiazem in order to maintain optimum therapeutic blood levels).
No products indexed under this heading.

Disulfiram (Patients taking other drugs that are substrates of CYP450, especially patients with renal and/or hepatic impairment, may require dosage adjustment when starting or stopping concomitantly administered diltiazem in order to maintain optimum therapeutic blood levels).
No products indexed under this heading.

Doxazosin Mesylate (Diltiazem has an additive effect when used with other antihypertensive agents. Therefore, the dosage of diltiazem or concomitant antihypertensives may need to be adjusted when adding one to the other).
No products indexed under this heading.

Doxorubicin Hydrochloride (Patients taking other drugs that are substrates of CYP450, especially patients with renal and/or hepatic impairment, may require dosage adjustment when starting or stopping concomitantly administered diltiazem in order to maintain optimum therapeutic blood levels).
No products indexed under this heading.

Dronabinol (Patients taking other drugs that are substrates of CYP450, especially patients with renal and/or hepatic impairment, may require dosage adjustment when starting or stopping concomitantly administered diltiazem in order to maintain optimum therapeutic blood levels).
No products indexed under this heading.

Efavirenz (Diltiazem is both a substrate and an inhibitor of the CYP3A4 enzyme system. Other drugs that are specific substrates, inhibitors, or inducers of this enzyme system may have a significant impact on the efficacy and side effect profile of diltiazem). Products include:
Atripla 906

Enalapril Maleate (Diltiazem has an additive effect when used with other antihypertensive agents. Therefore, the dosage of diltiazem or concomitant antihypertensives may need to be adjusted when adding one to the other).
No products indexed under this heading.

Enalaprilat (Diltiazem has an additive effect when used with other antihypertensive agents. Therefore, the dosage of diltiazem or concomitant antihypertensives may need to be adjusted when adding one to the other).
No products indexed under this heading.

Enflurane (The depression of cardiac contractility, conductivity, and automaticity, as well as the vascular dilation associated with anesthetics, may be potentiated by calcium channel blockers).
No products indexed under this heading.

Eprosartan Mesylate (Diltiazem has an additive effect when used with other antihypertensive agents. Therefore, the dosage of diltiazem or concomitant antihypertensives may need to be adjusted when adding one to the other). Products include:
Teveten 538
Teveten HCT 541

Ergotamine Tartrate (Patients taking other drugs that are substrates of CYP450, especially patients with renal and/or hepatic impairment, may require dosage adjustment when starting or stopping concomitantly administered diltiazem in order to maintain optimum therapeutic blood levels).
No products indexed under this heading.

Erythromycin (Patients taking other drugs that are substrates of CYP450, especially patients with renal and/or hepatic impairment, may require dosage adjustment when starting or stopping concomitantly administered diltiazem in order to maintain optimum therapeutic blood levels).
No products indexed under this heading.

Erythromycin Estolate (Patients taking other drugs that are substrates of CYP450, especially patients with renal and/or hepatic impairment, may require dosage adjustment when starting or stopping concomitantly administered diltiazem in order to maintain optimum therapeutic blood levels).
No products indexed under this heading.

Erythromycin Ethylsuccinate (Patients taking other drugs that are substrates of CYP450, especially patients with renal and/or hepatic impairment, may require dosage adjustment when starting or stopping concomitantly administered diltiazem in order to maintain optimum therapeutic blood levels). Products include:
E.E.S. 437
EryPed 435

Erythromycin Gluceptate (Patients taking other drugs that are substrates of CYP450, especially patients with renal and/or hepatic impairment, may require dosage adjustment when starting or stopping concomitantly administered diltiazem in order to maintain optimum therapeutic blood levels).
No products indexed under this heading.

Erythromycin Lactobionate (Patients taking other drugs that are substrates of CYP450, especially patients with renal and/or hepatic impairment, may require dosage adjustment when starting or stopping concomitantly administered diltiazem in order to maintain optimum therapeutic blood levels).
No products indexed under this heading.

Erythromycin Stearate (Patients taking other drugs that are substrates of CYP450, especially patients with renal and/or hepatic impairment, may require dosage adjustment when starting or stopping concomitantly administered diltiazem in order to maintain optimum therapeutic blood levels).
No products indexed under this heading.

Esmolol Hydrochloride (Pharmacologic studies indicate that there may be additive effects in prolonging A-V conduction when using beta-blockers or digitalis concomitantly with diltiazem).
No products indexed under this heading.

Esomeprazole Magnesium (Diltiazem is both a substrate and an inhibitor of the CYP3A4 enzyme system. Other drugs that are specific substrates, inhibitors, or inducers of this enzyme system may have a significant impact on the efficacy and side effect profile of diltiazem). Products include:
Nexium Capsules 704
Nexium Oral Suspension 704

Esomeprazole Sodium (Diltiazem is both a substrate and an inhibitor of the CYP3A4 enzyme system. Other drugs that are specific substrates, inhibitors, or inducers of this enzyme system may have a significant impact on the efficacy and side effect profile of diltiazem). Products include:
Nexium I.V. 712

Estazolam (Studies showed that diltiazem increased the AUC of midazolam and triazolam by 3- to 4-fold and the C_{max} by 2-fold, compared to placebo. The elimination half-life of midazolam and triazolam also increased during co-administration with diltiazem).
No products indexed under this heading.

Estradiol (Patients taking other drugs that are substrates of CYP450, especially patients with renal and/or hepatic impairment, may require dosage adjustment when starting or stopping concomitantly administered diltiazem in order to maintain optimum therapeutic blood levels). Products include:
Activella 2561
Angeliq 831
Climara 841
Climara Pro 847
Divigel 3467
Estrasorb 1777
Vagifem 2589

Estradiol Benzoate (Patients taking other drugs that are substrates of CYP450, especially patients with renal and/or hepatic impairment, may require dosage adjustment when starting or stopping concomitantly administered diltiazem in order to maintain optimum therapeutic blood levels).
No products indexed under this heading.

Estradiol Cypionate (Patients taking other drugs that are substrates of CYP450, especially patients with renal and/or hepatic impairment, may require dosage adjustment when starting or stopping concomitantly administered diltiazem in order to maintain optimum therapeutic blood levels).
No products indexed under this heading.

Estradiol Valerate (Patients taking other drugs that are substrates of CYP450, especially patients with renal and/or hepatic impairment, may require dosage adjustment when starting or stopping concomitantly administered diltiazem in order to maintain optimum therapeutic blood levels).
No products indexed under this heading.

Ethinyl Estradiol (Patients taking other drugs that are substrates of CYP450, especially patients with renal and/or hepatic impairment, may require dosage adjustment when starting or stopping concomitantly administered diltiazem in order to maintain optimum therapeutic blood levels). Products include:
LoSeasonique 3407
Lybrel 3514
NuvaRing 3181
Ortho Evra 2648
Ortho-Cyclen/Ortho Tri-Cyclen 2663
Ortho Tri-Cyclen Lo Tablets 2673
Seasonique 3418
Yaz 864

Ethosuximide (Patients taking other drugs that are substrates of CYP450, especially patients with renal and/or hepatic impairment, may require dosage adjustment when starting or stopping concomitantly administered diltiazem in order to maintain optimum therapeutic blood levels).
No products indexed under this heading.

Ethynodiol Diacetate (Patients taking other drugs that are substrates of CYP450, especially patients with renal and/or hepatic impairment, may require dosage adjustment when starting or stopping concomitantly administered diltiazem in order to maintain optimum therapeutic blood levels).
No products indexed under this heading.

Etidocaine Hydrochloride (The depression of cardiac contractility, conductivity, and automaticity, as well as the vascular dilation associated with anesthetics, may be potentiated by calcium channel blockers).
No products indexed under this heading.

Etoposide (Patients taking other drugs that are substrates of CYP450, especially patients with renal and/or hepatic impairment, may require dosage adjustment when starting or stopping concomitantly administered diltiazem in order to maintain optimum therapeutic blood levels).
No products indexed under this heading.

Etoposide Phosphate (Patients taking other drugs that are substrates of CYP450, especially patients with renal and/or hepatic impairment, may require dosage adjustment when starting or stopping concomitantly administered diltiazem in order to maintain optimum therapeutic blood levels).
No products indexed under this heading.

(⊙ Described in PDR® for Ophthalmic Medicines)

Felbamate (Diltiazem is both a substrate and an inhibitor of the CYP3A4 enzyme system. Other drugs that are specific substrates, inhibitors, or inducers of this enzyme system may have a significant impact on the efficacy and side effect profile of diltiazem).
No products indexed under this heading.

Felodipine (Diltiazem has an additive effect when used with other antihypertensive agents. Therefore, the dosage of diltiazem or concomitant antihypertensives may need to be adjusted when adding one to the other).
No products indexed under this heading.

Fentanyl (Patients taking other drugs that are substrates of CYP450, especially patients with renal and/or hepatic impairment, may require dosage adjustment when starting or stopping concomitantly administered diltiazem in order to maintain optimum therapeutic blood levels). Products include:

Duragesic 2604

Fentanyl Transdermal System 2346

Onsolis 2054

Fentanyl Citrate (The depression of cardiac contractility, conductivity, and automaticity, as well as the vascular dilation associated with anesthetics, may be potentiated by calcium channel blockers). Products include:

Fentora 966

Fluconazole (Diltiazem is both a substrate and an inhibitor of the CYP3A4 enzyme system. Other drugs that are specific substrates, inhibitors, or inducers of this enzyme system may have a significant impact on the efficacy and side effect profile of diltiazem).
No products indexed under this heading.

Fludrocortisone Acetate (Diltiazem is both a substrate and an inhibitor of the CYP3A4 enzyme system. Other drugs that are specific substrates, inhibitors, or inducers of this enzyme system may have a significant impact on the efficacy and side effect profile of diltiazem).
No products indexed under this heading.

Fluoxetine (Diltiazem is both a substrate and an inhibitor of the CYP3A4 enzyme system. Other drugs that are specific substrates, inhibitors, or inducers of this enzyme system may have a significant impact on the efficacy and side effect profile of diltiazem).
No products indexed under this heading.

Fluoxetine Hydrochloride (Diltiazem is both a substrate and an inhibitor of the CYP3A4 enzyme system. Other drugs that are specific substrates, inhibitors, or inducers of this enzyme system may have a significant impact on the efficacy and side effect profile of diltiazem). Products include:

Prozac Weekly 1941

Prozac Pulvules 1941

Symbyax 1965

Flurazepam Hydrochloride (Studies showed that diltiazem increased the AUC of midazolam and triazolam by 3- to 4-fold and the C_{max} by 2-fold, compared to placebo. The elimination half-life of midazolam and triazolam also increased during co-administration with diltiazem).
No products indexed under this heading.

Fluvoxamine Maleate (Diltiazem is both a substrate and an inhibitor of the CYP3A4 enzyme system. Other drugs that are specific substrates, inhibitors, or inducers of this enzyme system may have a significant impact on the efficacy and side effect profile of diltiazem).
No products indexed under this heading.

Fosamprenavir Calcium (Diltiazem is both a substrate and an inhibitor of the CYP3A4 enzyme system. Other drugs that are specific substrates, inhibitors, or inducers of this enzyme system may have a significant impact on the efficacy and side effect profile of diltiazem). Products include:

Lexiva Oral Suspension 1558

Lexiva 1558

Fosinopril Sodium (Diltiazem has an additive effect when used with other antihypertensive agents. Therefore, the dosage of diltiazem or concomitant antihypertensives may need to be adjusted when adding one to the other).
No products indexed under this heading.

Fosphenytoin Sodium (Diltiazem is both a substrate and an inhibitor of the CYP3A4 enzyme system. Other drugs that are specific substrates, inhibitors, or inducers of this enzyme system may have a significant impact on the efficacy and side effect profile of diltiazem).
No products indexed under this heading.

Furosemide (Diltiazem has an additive effect when used with other antihypertensive agents. Therefore, the dosage of diltiazem or concomitant antihypertensives may need to be adjusted when adding one to the other). Products include:

Furosemide 2354

Garlic Extract (Diltiazem is both a substrate and an inhibitor of the CYP3A4 enzyme system. Other drugs that are specific substrates, inhibitors, or inducers of this enzyme system may have a significant impact on the efficacy and side effect profile of diltiazem).
No products indexed under this heading.

Garlic Oil (Diltiazem is both a substrate and an inhibitor of the CYP3A4 enzyme system. Other drugs that are specific substrates, inhibitors, or inducers of this enzyme system may have a significant impact on the efficacy and side effect profile of diltiazem).
No products indexed under this heading.

Guanabenz Acetate (Diltiazem has an additive effect when used with other antihypertensive agents. Therefore, the dosage of diltiazem or concomitant antihypertensives may need to be adjusted when adding one to the other).
No products indexed under this heading.

Guanethidine (Diltiazem has an additive effect when used with other antihypertensive agents. Therefore, the dosage of diltiazem or concomitant antihypertensives may need to be adjusted when adding one to the other).
No products indexed under this heading.

Guanethidine Monosulfate (Diltiazem has an additive effect when used with other antihypertensive agents. Therefore, the dosage of diltiazem or concomitant antihypertensives may need to be adjusted when adding one to the other).
No products indexed under this heading.

Guanethidine Sulfate (Diltiazem has an additive effect when used with other antihypertensive agents. Therefore, the dosage of diltiazem or concomitant antihypertensives may need to be adjusted when adding one to the other).
No products indexed under this heading.

Halazepam (Studies showed that diltiazem increased the AUC of midazolam and triazolam by 3- to 4-fold and the C_{max} by 2-fold, compared to placebo. The elimination half-life of midazolam and triazolam also increased during co-administration with diltiazem).
No products indexed under this heading.

Haloperidol (Patients taking other drugs that are substrates of CYP450, especially patients with renal and/or hepatic impairment, may require dosage adjustment when starting or stopping concomitantly administered diltiazem in order to maintain optimum therapeutic blood levels).
No products indexed under this heading.

Haloperidol Decanoate (Patients taking other drugs that are substrates of CYP450, especially patients with renal and/or hepatic impairment, may require dosage adjustment when starting or stopping concomitantly administered diltiazem in order to maintain optimum therapeutic blood levels).
No products indexed under this heading.

Haloperidol Lactate (Patients taking other drugs that are substrates of CYP450, especially patients with renal and/or hepatic impairment, may require dosage adjustment when starting or stopping concomitantly administered diltiazem in order to maintain optimum therapeutic blood levels).
No products indexed under this heading.

Halothane (The depression of cardiac contractility, conductivity, and automaticity, as well as the vascular dilation associated with anesthetics, may be potentiated by calcium channel blockers).
No products indexed under this heading.

Hydralazine Hydrochloride (Diltiazem has an additive effect when used with other antihypertensive agents. Therefore, the dosage of diltiazem or concomitant antihypertensives may need to be adjusted when adding one to the other).
No products indexed under this heading.

Hydrochlorothiazide (Diltiazem has an additive effect when used with other antihypertensive agents. Therefore, the dosage of diltiazem or concomitant antihypertensives may need to be adjusted when adding one to the other). Products include:

Atacand HCT 700

Avalide 2956

Benicar HCT 1017

Diovan HCT 2419

Dyazide 1429

Exforge HCT 2449

Hyzaar 2162

Hyzaar 100-12.5 2162

Micardis HCT 889

Prinzide 2246

Tekturna HCT 2541

Teveten HCT 541

Hydrocortisone (Diltiazem is both a substrate and an inhibitor of the CYP3A4 enzyme system. Other drugs that are specific substrates, inhibitors, or inducers of this enzyme system may have a significant impact on the efficacy and side effect profile of diltiazem).
No products indexed under this heading.

Hydrocortisone (Alcohol) (Diltiazem is both a substrate and an inhibitor of the CYP3A4 enzyme system. Other drugs that are specific substrates, inhibitors, or inducers of this enzyme system may have a significant impact on the efficacy and side effect profile of diltiazem).
No products indexed under this heading.

Hydrocortisone Acetate (Diltiazem is both a substrate and an inhibitor of the CYP3A4 enzyme system. Other drugs that are specific substrates, inhibitors, or inducers of this enzyme system may have a significant impact on the efficacy and side effect profile of diltiazem).
No products indexed under this heading.

Hydrocortisone Butyrate (Diltiazem is both a substrate and an inhibitor of the CYP3A4 enzyme system. Other drugs that are specific substrates, inhibitors, or inducers of this enzyme system may have a significant impact on the efficacy and side effect profile of diltiazem).
No products indexed under this heading.

Hydrocortisone Cypionate (Diltiazem is both a substrate and an inhibitor of the CYP3A4 enzyme system. Other drugs that are specific substrates, inhibitors, or inducers of this enzyme system may have a significant impact on the efficacy and side effect profile of diltiazem).
No products indexed under this heading.

Hydrocortisone Hemisuccinate (Diltiazem is both a substrate and an inhibitor of the CYP3A4 enzyme system. Other drugs that are specific substrates, inhibitors, or inducers of this enzyme system may have a significant impact on the efficacy and side effect profile of diltiazem).
No products indexed under this heading.

Hydrocortisone Probutate (Diltiazem is both a substrate and an inhibitor of the CYP3A4 enzyme system. Other drugs that are specific substrates, inhibitors, or inducers of this enzyme system may have a significant impact on the efficacy and side effect profile of diltiazem).
No products indexed under this heading.

Hydrocortisone Sodium Phosphate (Diltiazem is both a substrate and an inhibitor of the CYP3A4 enzyme system. Other drugs that are specific substrates, inhibitors, or inducers of this enzyme system may have a significant impact on the efficacy and side effect profile of diltiazem).
No products indexed under this heading.

Hydrocortisone Sodium Succinate (Diltiazem is both a substrate and an inhibitor of the CYP3A4 enzyme system. Other drugs that are specific substrates, inhibitors, or inducers of this enzyme system may have a significant impact on the efficacy and side effect profile of diltiazem).
No products indexed under this heading.

Hydrocortisone Valerate (Diltiazem is both a substrate and an inhibitor of the CYP3A4 enzyme system. Other drugs that are specific substrates, inhibitors, or inducers of this enzyme system may have a significant impact on the efficacy and side effect profile of diltiazem).
No products indexed under this heading.

Hydroflumethiazide (Diltiazem has an additive effect when used with other antihypertensive agents. Therefore, the dosage of diltiazem or concomitant antihypertensives may need to be adjusted when adding one to the other).
No products indexed under this heading.

Hypericum (Diltiazem is both a substrate and an inhibitor of the CYP3A4 enzyme system. Other drugs that are specific substrates, inhibitors, or inducers of this enzyme system may have a significant impact on the efficacy and side effect profile of diltiazem).
No products indexed under this heading.

Hypericum Perforatum (Diltiazem is both a substrate and an inhibitor of the CYP3A4 enzyme system. Other drugs that are specific substrates, inhibitors, or inducers of this enzyme system may have a significant impact on the efficacy and side effect profile of diltiazem). Products include:

Traumeel 1800

Imatinib Mesylate (Diltiazem is both a substrate and an inhibitor of the CYP3A4 enzyme system. Other drugs that are specific substrates, inhibitors, or inducers of this enzyme system may have a significant impact on the efficacy and side effect profile of diltiazem). Products include:

Gleevec 2477

Indapamide (Diltiazem has an additive effect when used with other antihypertensive agents. Therefore, the dosage of diltiazem or concomitant antihyper-

tensives may need to be adjusted when adding one to the other). Products include:

Indinavir Sulfate (Patients taking other drugs that are substrates of CYP450, especially patients with renal and/or hepatic impairment, may require dosage adjustment when starting or stopping concomitantly administered diltiazem in order to maintain optimum therapeutic blood levels). Products include:

Irbesartan (Diltiazem has an additive effect when used with other antihypertensive agents. Therefore, the dosage of diltiazem or concomitant antihypertensives may need to be adjusted when adding one to the other). Products include:

Isoflurane (The depression of cardiac contractility, conductivity, and automaticity, as well as the vascular dilation associated with anesthetics, may be potentiated by calcium channel blockers).

No products indexed under this heading.

Isoniazid (Diltiazem is both a substrate and an inhibitor of the CYP3A4 enzyme system. Other drugs that are specific substrates, inhibitors, or inducers of this enzyme system may have a significant impact on the efficacy and side effect profile of diltiazem).

No products indexed under this heading.

Isradipine (Diltiazem has an additive effect when used with other antihypertensive agents. Therefore, the dosage of diltiazem or concomitant antihypertensives may need to be adjusted when adding one to the other). Products include:

Itraconazole (Patients taking other drugs that are substrates of CYP450, especially patients with renal and/or hepatic impairment, may require dosage adjustment when starting or stopping concomitantly administered diltiazem in order to maintain optimum therapeutic blood levels).

No products indexed under this heading.

Ixabepilone (Patients taking other drugs that are substrates of CYP450, especially patients with renal and/or hepatic impairment, may require dosage adjustment when starting or stopping concomitantly administered diltiazem in order to maintain optimum therapeutic blood levels).

No products indexed under this heading.

Ketamine Hydrochloride (The depression of cardiac contractility, conductivity, and automaticity, as well as the vascular dilation associated with anesthetics, may be potentiated by calcium channel blockers).

No products indexed under this heading.

Ketoconazole (Patients taking other drugs that are substrates of CYP450, especially patients with renal and/or hepatic impairment, may require dosage adjustment when starting or stopping concomitantly administered diltiazem in order to maintain optimum therapeutic blood levels). Products include:

Labetalol Hydrochloride (Pharmacologic studies indicate that there may be additive effects in prolonging A-V conduction when using beta-blockers or digitalis concomitantly with diltiazem).

No products indexed under this heading.

Lapatinib (Diltiazem is both a substrate and an inhibitor of the CYP3A4 enzyme system. Other drugs that are

specific substrates, inhibitors, or inducers of this enzyme system may have a significant impact on the efficacy and side effect profile of diltiazem). Products include:

Levobunolol Hydrochloride (Pharmacologic studies indicate that there may be additive effects in prolonging A-V conduction when using beta-blockers or digitalis concomitantly with diltiazem).

No products indexed under this heading.

Levobupivacaine Hydrochloride (The depression of cardiac contractility, conductivity, and automaticity, as well as the vascular dilation associated with anesthetics, may be potentiated by calcium channel blockers).

No products indexed under this heading.

Levonorgestrel (Patients taking other drugs that are substrates of CYP450, especially patients with renal and/or hepatic impairment, may require dosage adjustment when starting or stopping concomitantly administered diltiazem in order to maintain optimum therapeutic blood levels). Products include:

Lidocaine (The depression of cardiac contractility, conductivity, and automaticity, as well as the vascular dilation associated with anesthetics, may be potentiated by calcium channel blockers). Products include:

Lidocaine Base (The depression of cardiac contractility, conductivity, and automaticity, as well as the vascular dilation associated with anesthetics, may be potentiated by calcium channel blockers).

No products indexed under this heading.

Lidocaine Hydrochloride (The depression of cardiac contractility, conductivity, and automaticity, as well as the vascular dilation associated with anesthetics, may be potentiated by calcium channel blockers).

No products indexed under this heading.

Lisinopril (Diltiazem has an additive effect when used with other antihypertensive agents. Therefore, the dosage of diltiazem or concomitant antihypertensives may need to be adjusted when adding one to the other). Products include:

Lopinavir (Diltiazem is both a substrate and an inhibitor of the CYP3A4 enzyme system. Other drugs that are specific substrates, inhibitors, or inducers of this enzyme system may have a significant impact on the efficacy and side effect profile of diltiazem). Products include:

Loratadine (Diltiazem is both a substrate and an inhibitor of the CYP3A4 enzyme system. Other drugs that are specific substrates, inhibitors, or inducers of this enzyme system may have a significant impact on the efficacy and side effect profile of diltiazem).

No products indexed under this heading.

Lorazepam (Studies showed that diltiazem increased the AUC of midazolam and triazolam by 3- to 4-fold and the C_{max} by 2-fold, compared to placebo. The elimination half-life of midazolam and triazolam also increased during co-administration with diltiazem).

No products indexed under this heading.

Losartan Potassium (Diltiazem has an additive effect when used with other

antihypertensive agents. Therefore, the dosage of diltiazem or concomitant antihypertensives may need to be adjusted when adding one to the other). Products include:

Lovastatin (In a ten-subject study, co-administration of diltiazem (120 mg bid diltiazem SR) with lovastatin resulted in a 3-4 times increase in mean lovastatin AUC and C_{max} versus lovastatin alone). Products include:

Mecamylamine Hydrochloride (Diltiazem has an additive effect when used with other antihypertensive agents. Therefore, the dosage of diltiazem or concomitant antihypertensives may need to be adjusted when adding one to the other).

No products indexed under this heading.

Mephenytoin (Diltiazem is both a substrate and an inhibitor of the CYP3A4 enzyme system. Other drugs that are specific substrates, inhibitors, or inducers of this enzyme system may have a significant impact on the efficacy and side effect profile of diltiazem).

No products indexed under this heading.

Mepivacaine Hydrochloride (The depression of cardiac contractility, conductivity, and automaticity, as well as the vascular dilation associated with anesthetics, may be potentiated by calcium channel blockers).

No products indexed under this heading.

Mestranol (Patients taking other drugs that are substrates of CYP450, especially patients with renal and/or hepatic impairment, may require dosage adjustment when starting or stopping concomitantly administered diltiazem in order to maintain optimum therapeutic blood levels).

No products indexed under this heading.

Methadone Hydrochloride (Patients taking other drugs that are substrates of CYP450, especially patients with renal and/or hepatic impairment, may require dosage adjustment when starting or stopping concomitantly administered diltiazem in order to maintain optimum therapeutic blood levels).

No products indexed under this heading.

Methohexital Sodium (The depression of cardiac contractility, conductivity, and automaticity, as well as the vascular dilation associated with anesthetics, may be potentiated by calcium channel blockers).

No products indexed under this heading.

Methsuximide (Diltiazem is both a substrate and an inhibitor of the CYP3A4 enzyme system. Other drugs that are specific substrates, inhibitors, or inducers of this enzyme system may have a significant impact on the efficacy and side effect profile of diltiazem).

No products indexed under this heading.

Methyclothiazide (Diltiazem has an additive effect when used with other antihypertensive agents. Therefore, the dosage of diltiazem or concomitant antihypertensives may need to be adjusted when adding one to the other).

No products indexed under this heading.

Methyldopa (Diltiazem has an additive effect when used with other antihypertensive agents. Therefore, the dosage of diltiazem or concomitant antihypertensives may need to be adjusted when adding one to the other).

No products indexed under this heading.

Methyldopate Hydrochloride (Diltiazem has an additive effect when used with other antihypertensive agents. Therefore, the dosage of diltiazem or concomitant antihypertensives may need to be adjusted when adding one to the other).

No products indexed under this heading.

Methylprednisolone (Diltiazem is both a substrate and an inhibitor of the CYP3A4 enzyme system. Other drugs that are specific substrates, inhibitors, or inducers of this enzyme system may have a significant impact on the efficacy and side effect profile of diltiazem).

No products indexed under this heading.

Methylprednisolone Acetate (Diltiazem is both a substrate and an inhibitor of the CYP3A4 enzyme system. Other drugs that are specific substrates, inhibitors, or inducers of this enzyme system may have a significant impact on the efficacy and side effect profile of diltiazem).

No products indexed under this heading.

Methylprednisolone Sodium Succinate (Diltiazem is both a substrate and an inhibitor of the CYP3A4 enzyme system. Other drugs that are specific substrates, inhibitors, or inducers of this enzyme system may have a significant impact on the efficacy and side effect profile of diltiazem).

No products indexed under this heading.

Metipranolol Hydrochloride (Pharmacologic studies indicate that there may be additive effects in prolonging A-V conduction when using beta-blockers or digitalis concomitantly with diltiazem).

No products indexed under this heading.

Metolazone (Diltiazem has an additive effect when used with other antihypertensive agents. Therefore, the dosage of diltiazem or concomitant antihypertensives may need to be adjusted when adding one to the other).

No products indexed under this heading.

Metoprolol Succinate (Pharmacologic studies indicate that there may be additive effects in prolonging A-V conduction when using beta-blockers or digitalis concomitantly with diltiazem). Products include:

Metoprolol Tartrate (Pharmacologic studies indicate that there may be additive effects in prolonging A-V conduction when using beta-blockers or digitalis concomitantly with diltiazem).

No products indexed under this heading.

Metronidazole (Diltiazem is both a substrate and an inhibitor of the CYP3A4 enzyme system. Other drugs that are specific substrates, inhibitors, or inducers of this enzyme system may have a significant impact on the efficacy and side effect profile of diltiazem). Products include:

Metronidazole Benzoate (Diltiazem is both a substrate and an inhibitor of the CYP3A4 enzyme system. Other drugs that are specific substrates, inhibitors, or inducers of this enzyme system may have a significant impact on the efficacy and side effect profile of diltiazem).

No products indexed under this heading.

Metronidazole Hydrochloride (Diltiazem is both a substrate and an inhibitor of the CYP3A4 enzyme system. Other drugs that are specific substrates, inhibitors, or inducers of this enzyme system may have a significant impact on the efficacy and side effect profile of diltiazem).

No products indexed under this heading.

Metronidazole Sodium (Diltiazem is both a substrate and an inhibitor of the CYP3A4 enzyme system. Other drugs that are specific substrates, inhibitors, or inducers of this enzyme system may have a significant impact on the efficacy and side effect profile of diltiazem).
No products indexed under this heading.

Metyrosine (Diltiazem has an additive effect when used with other antihypertensive agents. Therefore, the dosage of diltiazem or concomitant antihypertensives may need to be adjusted when adding one to the other).
No products indexed under this heading.

Mibefradil Dihydrochloride (Diltiazem has an additive effect when used with other antihypertensive agents. Therefore, the dosage of diltiazem or concomitant antihypertensives may need to be adjusted when adding one to the other).
No products indexed under this heading.

Miconazole (Diltiazem is both a substrate and an inhibitor of the CYP3A4 enzyme system. Other drugs that are specific substrates, inhibitors, or inducers of this enzyme system may have a significant impact on the efficacy and side effect profile of diltiazem).
No products indexed under this heading.

Miconazole Nitrate (Diltiazem is both a substrate and an inhibitor of the CYP3A4 enzyme system. Other drugs that are specific substrates, inhibitors, or inducers of this enzyme system may have a significant impact on the efficacy and side effect profile of diltiazem).
Products include:
Vusion Ointment 3335

Midazolam Hydrochloride (The depression of cardiac contractility, conductivity, and automaticity, as well as the vascular dilation associated with anesthetics, may be potentiated by calcium channel blockers).
No products indexed under this heading.

Mifepristone (Diltiazem is both a substrate and an inhibitor of the CYP3A4 enzyme system. Other drugs that are specific substrates, inhibitors, or inducers of this enzyme system may have a significant impact on the efficacy and side effect profile of diltiazem).
No products indexed under this heading.

Minoxidil (Diltiazem has an additive effect when used with other antihypertensive agents. Therefore, the dosage of diltiazem or concomitant antihypertensives may need to be adjusted when adding one to the other).
No products indexed under this heading.

Modafinil (Diltiazem is both a substrate and an inhibitor of the CYP3A4 enzyme system. Other drugs that are specific substrates, inhibitors, or inducers of this enzyme system may have a significant impact on the efficacy and side effect profile of diltiazem).
Products include:
Provigil 983

Moexipril Hydrochloride (Diltiazem has an additive effect when used with other antihypertensive agents. Therefore, the dosage of diltiazem or concomitant antihypertensives may need to be adjusted when adding one to the other).
No products indexed under this heading.

Nadolol (Pharmacologic studies indicate that there may be additive effects in prolonging A-V conduction when using beta-blockers or digitalis concomitantly with diltiazem). Products include:
Nadolol 2359

Nafcillin Sodium (Diltiazem is both a substrate and an inhibitor of the CYP3A4 enzyme system. Other drugs that are specific substrates, inhibitors, or inducers of this enzyme system may have a significant impact on the efficacy and side effect profile of diltiazem).
No products indexed under this heading.

Nebivolol (Pharmacologic studies indicate that there may be additive effects in prolonging A-V conduction when using beta-blockers or digitalis concomitantly with diltiazem). Products include:
Bystolic 1147

Nefazodone Hydrochloride (Patients taking other drugs that are substrates of CYP450, especially patients with renal and/or hepatic impairment, may require dosage adjustment when starting or stopping concomitantly administered diltiazem in order to maintain optimum therapeutic blood levels).
No products indexed under this heading.

Nelfinavir Mesylate (Patients taking other drugs that are substrates of CYP450, especially patients with renal and/or hepatic impairment, may require dosage adjustment when starting or stopping concomitantly administered diltiazem in order to maintain optimum therapeutic blood levels).
No products indexed under this heading.

Nevirapine (Diltiazem is both a substrate and an inhibitor of the CYP3A4 enzyme system. Other drugs that are specific substrates, inhibitors, or inducers of this enzyme system may have a significant impact on the efficacy and side effect profile of diltiazem).
Products include:
Viramune Oral Suspension 897
Viramune Tablets 897

Niacin (Diltiazem is both a substrate and an inhibitor of the CYP3A4 enzyme system. Other drugs that are specific substrates, inhibitors, or inducers of this enzyme system may have a significant impact on the efficacy and side effect profile of diltiazem). Products include:
Advicor 402
Cardio Basics 3455
Niaspan 497
Simcor 524

Niacinamide (Diltiazem is both a substrate and an inhibitor of the CYP3A4 enzyme system. Other drugs that are specific substrates, inhibitors, or inducers of this enzyme system may have a significant impact on the efficacy and side effect profile of diltiazem).
Products include:
CitraNatal 90 DHA Capsules 2332
CitraNatal Assure 2332
CitraNatal Rx 2332
Heplive 607

Niacinamide Hydroiodide (Diltiazem is both a substrate and an inhibitor of the CYP3A4 enzyme system. Other drugs that are specific substrates, inhibitors, or inducers of this enzyme system may have a significant impact on the efficacy and side effect profile of diltiazem).
No products indexed under this heading.

Nicardipine (Patients taking other drugs that are substrates of CYP450, especially patients with renal and/or hepatic impairment, may require dosage adjustment when starting or stopping concomitantly administered diltiazem in order to maintain optimum therapeutic blood levels).
No products indexed under this heading.

Nicardipine Hydrochloride (Diltiazem has an additive effect when used with other antihypertensive agents. Therefore, the dosage of diltiazem or concomitant antihypertensives may need to be adjusted when adding one to the other).
No products indexed under this heading.

Nicotinamide (Diltiazem is both a substrate and an inhibitor of the CYP3A4 enzyme system. Other drugs that are specific substrates, inhibitors, or inducers of this enzyme system may have a significant impact on the efficacy and side effect profile of diltiazem).
No products indexed under this heading.

Nifedipine (Diltiazem has an additive effect when used with other antihypertensive agents. Therefore, the dosage of diltiazem or concomitant antihypertensives may need to be adjusted when adding one to the other).
No products indexed under this heading.

Nimodipine (Patients taking other drugs that are substrates of CYP450, especially patients with renal and/or hepatic impairment, may require dosage adjustment when starting or stopping concomitantly administered diltiazem in order to maintain optimum therapeutic blood levels).
No products indexed under this heading.

Nisoldipine (Diltiazem has an additive effect when used with other antihypertensive agents. Therefore, the dosage of diltiazem or concomitant antihypertensives may need to be adjusted when adding one to the other).
No products indexed under this heading.

Nitrendipine (Patients taking other drugs that are substrates of CYP450, especially patients with renal and/or hepatic impairment, may require dosage adjustment when starting or stopping concomitantly administered diltiazem in order to maintain optimum therapeutic blood levels).
No products indexed under this heading.

Nitroglycerin (Diltiazem has an additive effect when used with other antihypertensive agents. Therefore, the dosage of diltiazem or concomitant antihypertensives may need to be adjusted when adding one to the other).
Products include:
Nitro-Dur 3170
Nitrolingual 3266

Norethindrone (Patients taking other drugs that are substrates of CYP450, especially patients with renal and/or hepatic impairment, may require dosage adjustment when starting or stopping concomitantly administered diltiazem in order to maintain optimum therapeutic blood levels). Products include:
Ortho Micronor 2660

Norethindrone Acetate (Patients taking other drugs that are substrates of CYP450, especially patients with renal and/or hepatic impairment, may require dosage adjustment when starting or stopping concomitantly administered diltiazem in order to maintain optimum therapeutic blood levels).
Products include:
Activella 2561

Norfloxacin (Diltiazem is both a substrate and an inhibitor of the CYP3A4 enzyme system. Other drugs that are specific substrates, inhibitors, or inducers of this enzyme system may have a significant impact on the efficacy and side effect profile of diltiazem).
Products include:
Noroxin 2220

Norgestrel (Patients taking other drugs that are substrates of CYP450, especially patients with renal and/or hepatic impairment, may require dosage adjustment when starting or stopping concomitantly administered diltiazem in order to maintain optimum therapeutic blood levels).
No products indexed under this heading.

Omeprazole (Diltiazem is both a substrate and an inhibitor of the CYP3A4 enzyme system. Other drugs that are specific substrates, inhibitors, or inducers of this enzyme system may have a significant impact on the efficacy and side effect profile of diltiazem).
No products indexed under this heading.

Ondansetron (Patients taking other drugs that are substrates of CYP450, especially patients with renal and/or hepatic impairment, may require dosage adjustment when starting or stopping concomitantly administered diltiazem in order to maintain optimum therapeutic blood levels).
No products indexed under this heading.

Ondansetron Hydrochloride (Patients taking other drugs that are substrates of CYP450, especially patients with renal and/or hepatic impairment, may require dosage adjustment when starting or stopping concomitantly administered diltiazem in order to maintain optimum therapeutic blood levels). Products include:
Zofran Injection 1750
Zofran 1756
Zofran ODT 1756

Oxazepam (Studies showed that diltiazem increased the AUC of midazolam and triazolam by 3- to 4-fold and the C_{max} by 2-fold, compared to placebo. The elimination half-life of midazolam and triazolam also increased during co-administration with diltiazem).
No products indexed under this heading.

Oxcarbazepine (Diltiazem is both a substrate and an inhibitor of the CYP3A4 enzyme system. Other drugs that are specific substrates, inhibitors, or inducers of this enzyme system may have a significant impact on the efficacy and side effect profile of diltiazem).
No products indexed under this heading.

Paclitaxel (Patients taking other drugs that are substrates of CYP450, especially patients with renal and/or hepatic impairment, may require dosage adjustment when starting or stopping concomitantly administered diltiazem in order to maintain optimum therapeutic blood levels).
No products indexed under this heading.

Paroxetine Hydrochloride (Diltiazem is both a substrate and an inhibitor of the CYP3A4 enzyme system. Other drugs that are specific substrates, inhibitors, or inducers of this enzyme system may have a significant impact on the efficacy and side effect profile of diltiazem). Products include:
Paroxetine CR 2361
Paroxetine ER 2371
Paxil 1586
Paxil CR 1596

Penbutolol Sulfate (Pharmacologic studies indicate that there may be additive effects in prolonging A-V conduction when using beta-blockers or digitalis concomitantly with diltiazem).
No products indexed under this heading.

Perindopril Erbumine (Diltiazem has an additive effect when used with other antihypertensive agents. Therefore, the dosage of diltiazem or concomitant antihypertensives may need to be adjusted when adding one to the other).
No products indexed under this heading.

Phenobarbital (Diltiazem is both a substrate and an inhibitor of the CYP3A4 enzyme system. Other drugs

IMPORTANT NOTE: Always consult each drug listing in the patient's regimen for possible interactions.

that are specific substrates, inhibitors, or inducers of this enzyme system may have a significant impact on the efficacy and side effect profile of diltiazem). Products include:
Donnatal 2711

Phenobarbital Sodium (Diltiazem is both a substrate and an inhibitor of the CYP3A4 enzyme system. Other drugs that are specific substrates, inhibitors, or inducers of this enzyme system may have a significant impact on the efficacy and side effect profile of diltiazem).
No products indexed under this heading.

Phenoxybenzamine Hydrochloride (Diltiazem has an additive effect when used with other antihypertensive agents. Therefore, the dosage of diltiazem or concomitant antihypertensives may need to be adjusted when adding one to the other). Products include:
Dibenzyline 3495

Phentolamine Mesylate (Diltiazem has an additive effect when used with other antihypertensive agents. Therefore, the dosage of diltiazem or concomitant antihypertensives may need to be adjusted when adding one to the other).
No products indexed under this heading.

Phenytoin (Diltiazem is both a substrate and an inhibitor of the CYP3A4 enzyme system. Other drugs that are specific substrates, inhibitors, or inducers of this enzyme system may have a significant impact on the efficacy and side effect profile of diltiazem).
No products indexed under this heading.

Phenytoin Sodium (Diltiazem is both a substrate and an inhibitor of the CYP3A4 enzyme system. Other drugs that are specific substrates, inhibitors, or inducers of this enzyme system may have a significant impact on the efficacy and side effect profile of diltiazem). Products include:
Phenytek Capsules 2380

Pimozide (Patients taking other drugs that are substrates of CYP450, especially patients with renal and/or hepatic impairment, may require dosage adjustment when starting or stopping concomitantly administered diltiazem in order to maintain optimum therapeutic blood levels).
No products indexed under this heading.

Pindolol (Pharmacologic studies indicate that there may be additive effects in prolonging A-V conduction when using beta-blockers or digitalis concomitantly with diltiazem).
No products indexed under this heading.

Polyestradiol Phosphate (Patients taking other drugs that are substrates of CYP450, especially patients with renal and/or hepatic impairment, may require dosage adjustment when starting or stopping concomitantly administered diltiazem in order to maintain optimum therapeutic blood levels).
No products indexed under this heading.

Polythiazide (Diltiazem has an additive effect when used with other antihypertensive agents. Therefore, the dosage of diltiazem or concomitant antihypertensives may need to be adjusted when adding one to the other).
No products indexed under this heading.

Posaconazole (Diltiazem is both a substrate and an inhibitor of the CYP3A4 enzyme system. Other drugs that are specific substrates, inhibitors, or inducers of this enzyme system may have a significant impact on the efficacy and side effect profile of diltiazem). Products include:
Noxafil 3172

Prazepam (Studies showed that diltiazem increased the AUC of midazolam and triazolam by 3- to 4-fold and the C_{max} by 2-fold, compared to placebo. The elimination half-life of midazolam and triazolam also increased during co-administration with diltiazem).
No products indexed under this heading.

Prazosin Hydrochloride (Diltiazem has an additive effect when used with other antihypertensive agents. Therefore, the dosage of diltiazem or concomitant antihypertensives may need to be adjusted when adding one to the other).
No products indexed under this heading.

Prednisolone (Diltiazem is both a substrate and an inhibitor of the CYP3A4 enzyme system. Other drugs that are specific substrates, inhibitors, or inducers of this enzyme system may have a significant impact on the efficacy and side effect profile of diltiazem).
No products indexed under this heading.

Prednisolone Acetate (Diltiazem is both a substrate and an inhibitor of the CYP3A4 enzyme system. Other drugs that are specific substrates, inhibitors, or inducers of this enzyme system may have a significant impact on the efficacy and side effect profile of diltiazem). Products include:
Blephamide .... ⊙ 212, ⊙ 214
Pred Forte .... ⊙ 225
Pred Mild .... ⊙ 230
Pred-G .... ⊙ 226, ⊙ 227

Prednisolone Sodium Phosphate (Diltiazem is both a substrate and an inhibitor of the CYP3A4 enzyme system. Other drugs that are specific substrates, inhibitors, or inducers of this enzyme system may have a significant impact on the efficacy and side effect profile of diltiazem).
No products indexed under this heading.

Prednisolone Tebutate (Diltiazem is both a substrate and an inhibitor of the CYP3A4 enzyme system. Other drugs that are specific substrates, inhibitors, or inducers of this enzyme system may have a significant impact on the efficacy and side effect profile of diltiazem).
No products indexed under this heading.

Prednisone (Diltiazem is both a substrate and an inhibitor of the CYP3A4 enzyme system. Other drugs that are specific substrates, inhibitors, or inducers of this enzyme system may have a significant impact on the efficacy and side effect profile of diltiazem).
No products indexed under this heading.

Prednisone sodium phosphate (Diltiazem is both a substrate and an inhibitor of the CYP3A4 enzyme system. Other drugs that are specific substrates, inhibitors, or inducers of this enzyme system may have a significant impact on the efficacy and side effect profile of diltiazem).
No products indexed under this heading.

Prilocaine (The depression of cardiac contractility, conductivity, and automaticity, as well as the vascular dilation associated with anesthetics, may be potentiated by calcium channel blockers).
No products indexed under this heading.

Prilocaine Hydrochloride (The depression of cardiac contractility, conductivity, and automaticity, as well as the vascular dilation associated with anesthetics, may be potentiated by calcium channel blockers).
No products indexed under this heading.

Primidone (Diltiazem is both a substrate and an inhibitor of the CYP3A4 enzyme system. Other drugs that are specific substrates, inhibitors, or inducers of this enzyme system may have a significant impact on the efficacy and side effect profile of diltiazem).
No products indexed under this heading.

Procaine (The depression of cardiac contractility, conductivity, and automaticity, as well as the vascular dilation associated with anesthetics, may be potentiated by calcium channel blockers).
No products indexed under this heading.

Procaine Hydrochloride (The depression of cardiac contractility, conductivity, and automaticity, as well as the vascular dilation associated with anesthetics, may be potentiated by calcium channel blockers).
No products indexed under this heading.

Proparacaine Hydrochloride (The depression of cardiac contractility, conductivity, and automaticity, as well as the vascular dilation associated with anesthetics, may be potentiated by calcium channel blockers).
No products indexed under this heading.

Propofol (The depression of cardiac contractility, conductivity, and automaticity, as well as the vascular dilation associated with anesthetics, may be potentiated by calcium channel blockers).
No products indexed under this heading.

Propoxyphene Hydrochloride (Diltiazem is both a substrate and an inhibitor of the CYP3A4 enzyme system. Other drugs that are specific substrates, inhibitors, or inducers of this enzyme system may have a significant impact on the efficacy and side effect profile of diltiazem).
No products indexed under this heading.

Propoxyphene Napsylate (Diltiazem is both a substrate and an inhibitor of the CYP3A4 enzyme system. Other drugs that are specific substrates, inhibitors, or inducers of this enzyme system may have a significant impact on the efficacy and side effect profile of diltiazem).
No products indexed under this heading.

Propranolol Hydrochloride (Pharmacologic studies indicate that there may be additive effects in prolonging A-V conduction when using beta-blockers or digitalis concomitantly with diltiazem). Products include:
InnoPran XL 1517

Quazepam (Studies showed that diltiazem increased the AUC of midazolam and triazolam by 3- to 4-fold and the C_{max} by 2-fold, compared to placebo. The elimination half-life of midazolam and triazolam also increased during co-administration with diltiazem).
No products indexed under this heading.

Quinapril Hydrochloride (Diltiazem has an additive effect when used with other antihypertensive agents. Therefore, the dosage of diltiazem or concomitant antihypertensives may need to be adjusted when adding one to the other).
No products indexed under this heading.

Quinidine (Diltiazem significantly increases the AUC of quinidine by 51%, t1/2 by 36%, and decreases it Cloral by 33%. Monitoring for quinidine adverse effects may be warranted and the dose adjusted accordingly).
No products indexed under this heading.

Quinidine Gluconate (Diltiazem significantly increases the AUC of quinidine by 51%, t1/2 by 36%, and decreases it Cloral by 33%. Monitoring for quinidine adverse effects may be warranted and the dose adjusted accordingly).
No products indexed under this heading.

Quinidine Hydrochloride (Diltiazem significantly increases the AUC of quinidine by 51%, t1/2 by 36%, and decreases it Cloral by 33%. Monitoring for quinidine adverse effects may be warranted and the dose adjusted accordingly).
No products indexed under this heading.

Quinidine Polygalacturonate (Diltiazem significantly increases the AUC of quinidine by 51%, t1/2 by 36%, and decreases it Cloral by 33%. Monitoring for quinidine adverse effects may be warranted and the dose adjusted accordingly).
No products indexed under this heading.

Quinidine Sulfate (Diltiazem significantly increases the AUC of quinidine by 51%, t1/2 by 36%, and decreases it Cloral by 33%. Monitoring for quinidine adverse effects may be warranted and the dose adjusted accordingly).
No products indexed under this heading.

Quinine (Diltiazem is both a substrate and an inhibitor of the CYP3A4 enzyme system. Other drugs that are specific substrates, inhibitors, or inducers of this enzyme system may have a significant impact on the efficacy and side effect profile of diltiazem). Products include:
Hyland's Leg Cramps PM with Quinine 3315

Quinine Sulfate (Diltiazem is both a substrate and an inhibitor of the CYP3A4 enzyme system. Other drugs that are specific substrates, inhibitors, or inducers of this enzyme system may have a significant impact on the efficacy and side effect profile of diltiazem).
No products indexed under this heading.

Quinupristin (Diltiazem is both a substrate and an inhibitor of the CYP3A4 enzyme system. Other drugs that are specific substrates, inhibitors, or inducers of this enzyme system may have a significant impact on the efficacy and side effect profile of diltiazem).
No products indexed under this heading.

Ramipril (Diltiazem has an additive effect when used with other antihypertensive agents. Therefore, the dosage of diltiazem or concomitant antihypertensives may need to be adjusted when adding one to the other).
No products indexed under this heading.

Ranitidine Bismuth Citrate (Diltiazem is both a substrate and an inhibitor of the CYP3A4 enzyme system. Other drugs that are specific substrates, inhibitors, or inducers of this enzyme system may have a significant impact on the efficacy and side effect profile of diltiazem).
No products indexed under this heading.

Ranitidine Hydrochloride (Diltiazem is both a substrate and an inhibitor of the CYP3A4 enzyme system. Other drugs that are specific substrates, inhibitors, or inducers of this enzyme system may have a significant impact on the efficacy and side effect profile of diltiazem). Products include:
Zantac 1737
Zantac Injection 1732
Zantac Pharmacy 1735

Rauwolfia Serpentina (Diltiazem has an additive effect when used with other antihypertensive agents. Therefore, the dosage of diltiazem or concomitant antihypertensives may need to be adjusted when adding one to the other).
No products indexed under this heading.

Remifentanil Hydrochloride (The depression of cardiac contractility, conductivity, and automaticity, as well as the vascular dilation associated with anesthetics, may be potentiated by calcium channel blockers).
No products indexed under this heading.

Rescinnamine (Diltiazem has an additive effect when used with other antihypertensive agents. Therefore, the dosage of diltiazem or concomitant antihypertensives may need to be adjusted when adding one to the other).
No products indexed under this heading.

Reserpine (Diltiazem has an additive effect when used with other antihypertensive agents. Therefore, the dosage of diltiazem or concomitant antihypertensives may need to be adjusted when adding one to the other).
No products indexed under this heading.

Rifabutin (Patients taking other drugs that are substrates of CYP450, especially patients with renal and/or hepatic impairment, may require dosage adjustment when starting or stopping concomitantly administered diltiazem in order to maintain optimum therapeutic blood levels).
No products indexed under this heading.

Rifampicin (Diltiazem is both a substrate and an inhibitor of the CYP3A4 enzyme system. Other drugs that are specific substrates, inhibitors, or inducers of this enzyme system may have a significant impact on the efficacy and side effect profile of diltiazem).
No products indexed under this heading.

Rifampin (Co-administration of rifampin with diltiazem lowered the diltiazem plasma concentrations to undetectable levels. Co-administration of diltiazem with rifampin or any known CYP3A4 inducer should be avoided when possible and alternative therapy considered).
No products indexed under this heading.

Rifapentine (Diltiazem is both a substrate and an inhibitor of the CYP3A4 enzyme system. Other drugs that are specific substrates, inhibitors, or inducers of this enzyme system may have a significant impact on the efficacy and side effect profile of diltiazem).
No products indexed under this heading.

Ritonavir (Patients taking other drugs that are substrates of CYP450, especially patients with renal and/or hepatic impairment, may require dosage adjustment when starting or stopping concomitantly administered diltiazem in order to maintain optimum therapeutic blood levels). Products include:
Kaletra **458**
Norvir **509**

Ropivacaine Hydrochloride (The depression of cardiac contractility, conductivity, and automaticity, as well as the vascular dilation associated with anesthetics, may be potentiated by calcium channel blockers).
No products indexed under this heading.

Saquinavir (Patients taking other drugs that are substrates of CYP450, especially patients with renal and/or hepatic impairment, may require dosage adjustment when starting or stopping concomitantly administered diltiazem in order to maintain optimum therapeutic blood levels).
No products indexed under this heading.

Saquinavir Mesylate (Patients taking other drugs that are substrates of CYP450, especially patients with renal and/or hepatic impairment, may require dosage adjustment when starting or stopping concomitantly administered diltiazem in order to maintain optimum therapeutic blood levels).
No products indexed under this heading.

Sertraline Hydrochloride (Patients taking other drugs that are substrates of CYP450, especially patients with renal and/or hepatic impairment, may require dosage adjustment when starting or stopping concomitantly administered diltiazem in order to maintain optimum therapeutic blood levels).
No products indexed under this heading.

Sildenafil Citrate (Patients taking other drugs that are substrates of CYP450, especially patients with renal and/or hepatic impairment, may require dosage adjustment when starting or stopping concomitantly administered diltiazem in order to maintain optimum therapeutic blood levels).
No products indexed under this heading.

Simvastatin (Patients taking other drugs that are substrates of CYP450, especially patients with renal and/or hepatic impairment, may require dosage adjustment when starting or stopping concomitantly administered diltiazem in order to maintain optimum therapeutic blood levels). Products include:
Simcor **524**
Vytorin 10/10 .... **2303, 3240**
Vytorin 10/20 .... **2303, 3240**
Vytorin 10/40 .... **2303, 3240**
Vytorin 10/80 .... **2303, 3240**
Zocor **2289**

Sirolimus (Patients taking other drugs that are substrates of CYP450, especially patients with renal and/or hepatic impairment, may require dosage adjustment when starting or stopping concomitantly administered diltiazem in order to maintain optimum therapeutic blood levels). Products include:
Rapamune **3579**

Sodium Nitroprusside (Diltiazem has an additive effect when used with other antihypertensive agents. Therefore, the dosage of diltiazem or concomitant antihypertensives may need to be adjusted when adding one to the other).
No products indexed under this heading.

Sotalol Hydrochloride (Pharmacologic studies indicate that there may be additive effects in prolonging A-V conduction when using beta-blockers or digitalis concomitantly with diltiazem).
No products indexed under this heading.

Spirapril Hydrochloride (Diltiazem has an additive effect when used with other antihypertensive agents. Therefore, the dosage of diltiazem or concomitant antihypertensives may need to be adjusted when adding one to the other).
No products indexed under this heading.

Sufentanil Citrate (The depression of cardiac contractility, conductivity, and automaticity, as well as the vascular dilation associated with anesthetics, may be potentiated by calcium channel blockers).
No products indexed under this heading.

Sulfinpyrazone (Diltiazem is both a substrate and an inhibitor of the CYP3A4 enzyme system. Other drugs that are specific substrates, inhibitors, or inducers of this enzyme system may have a significant impact on the efficacy and side effect profile of diltiazem).
No products indexed under this heading.

Tacrolimus (Patients taking other drugs that are substrates of CYP450, especially patients with renal and/or hepatic impairment, may require dosage adjustment when starting or stopping concomitantly administered diltiazem in order to maintain optimum therapeutic blood levels). Products include:
Prograf Capsules **677**
Prograf Injection **677**
Protopic **685**

Tadalafil (Patients taking other drugs that are substrates of CYP450, especially patients with renal and/or hepatic impairment, may require dosage adjustment when starting or stopping concomitantly administered diltiazem in order to maintain optimum therapeutic blood levels). Products include:
Adcirca **3461**
Cialis **1861**

Tamoxifen Citrate (Patients taking other drugs that are substrates of CYP450, especially patients with renal and/or hepatic impairment, may require dosage adjustment when starting or stopping concomitantly administered diltiazem in order to maintain optimum therapeutic blood levels).
No products indexed under this heading.

Telithromycin (Diltiazem is both a substrate and an inhibitor of the CYP3A4 enzyme system. Other drugs that are specific substrates, inhibitors, or inducers of this enzyme system may have a significant impact on the efficacy and side effect profile of diltiazem). Products include:
Ketek **2991**

Telmisartan (Diltiazem has an additive effect when used with other antihypertensive agents. Therefore, the dosage of diltiazem or concomitant antihypertensives may need to be adjusted when adding one to the other). Products include:
Micardis **887**
Micardis HCT **889**

Temazepam (Studies showed that diltiazem increased the AUC of midazolam and triazolam by 3- to 4-fold and the C_{max} by 2-fold, compared to placebo. The elimination half-life of midazolam and triazolam also increased during co-administration with diltiazem).
No products indexed under this heading.

Terazosin Hydrochloride (Diltiazem has an additive effect when used with other antihypertensive agents. Therefore, the dosage of diltiazem or concomitant antihypertensives may need to be adjusted when adding one to the other).
No products indexed under this heading.

Terfenadine (Patients taking other drugs that are substrates of CYP450, especially patients with renal and/or hepatic impairment, may require dosage adjustment when starting or stopping concomitantly administered diltiazem in order to maintain optimum therapeutic blood levels).
No products indexed under this heading.

Tetracaine (The depression of cardiac contractility, conductivity, and automaticity, as well as the vascular dilation associated with anesthetics, may be potentiated by calcium channel blockers).
No products indexed under this heading.

Tetracaine Hydrochloride (The depression of cardiac contractility, conductivity, and automaticity, as well as the vascular dilation associated with anesthetics, may be potentiated by calcium channel blockers).
No products indexed under this heading.

Theophyllinate (Diltiazem is both a substrate and an inhibitor of the CYP3A4 enzyme system. Other drugs that are specific substrates, inhibitors, or inducers of this enzyme system may have a significant impact on the efficacy and side effect profile of diltiazem).
No products indexed under this heading.

Theophylline (Patients taking other drugs that are substrates of CYP450, especially patients with renal and/or hepatic impairment, may require dosage adjustment when starting or stopping concomitantly administered diltiazem in order to maintain optimum therapeutic blood levels).
No products indexed under this heading.

Theophylline Anhydrous (Patients taking other drugs that are substrates of CYP450, especially patients with renal and/or hepatic impairment, may require dosage adjustment when starting or stopping concomitantly administered diltiazem in order to maintain optimum therapeutic blood levels). Products include:
Uniphyl **2817**

Theophylline Calcium Salicylate (Patients taking other drugs that are substrates of CYP450, especially patients with renal and/or hepatic impairment, may require dosage adjustment when starting or stopping concomitantly administered diltiazem in order to maintain optimum therapeutic blood levels).
No products indexed under this heading.

Theophylline Dihydroxypropyl (Glyceryl) (Patients taking other drugs that are substrates of CYP450, especially patients with renal and/or hepatic impairment, may require dosage adjustment when starting or stopping concomitantly administered diltiazem in order to maintain optimum therapeutic blood levels).
No products indexed under this heading.

Theophylline Ethylenediamine (Patients taking other drugs that are substrates of CYP450, especially patients with renal and/or hepatic impairment, may require dosage adjustment when starting or stopping concomitantly administered diltiazem in order to maintain optimum therapeutic blood levels).
No products indexed under this heading.

Theophylline Sodium Glycinate (Patients taking other drugs that are substrates of CYP450, especially patients with renal and/or hepatic impairment, may require dosage adjustment when starting or stopping concomitantly administered diltiazem in order to maintain optimum therapeutic blood levels).
No products indexed under this heading.

Thiamylal Sodium (The depression of cardiac contractility, conductivity, and automaticity, as well as the vascular dilation associated with anesthetics, may be potentiated by calcium channel blockers).
No products indexed under this heading.

Tiagabine Hydrochloride (Patients taking other drugs that are substrates of CYP450, especially patients with renal and/or hepatic impairment, may require dosage adjustment when starting or stopping concomitantly administered diltiazem in order to maintain optimum therapeutic blood levels). Products include:
Gabitril **972**

Timolol Hemihydrate (Pharmacologic studies indicate that there may be additive effects in prolonging A-V conduction when using beta-blockers or digitalis concomitantly with diltiazem). Products include:
Betimol **3490**

Timolol Maleate (Pharmacologic studies indicate that there may be additive effects in prolonging A-V conduction when using beta-blockers or digitalis concomitantly with diltiazem). Products include:
Combigan **601**
Dorzolamide Hydrochloride/Timolol Maleate Ophthalmic Solution .... ⊙ **243**
Timoptic in Ocudose .... ⊙ **231**

Tolterodine Tartrate (Patients taking other drugs that are substrates of CYP450, especially patients with renal and/or hepatic impairment, may require dosage adjustment when starting or stopping concomitantly administered diltiazem in order to maintain optimum therapeutic blood levels).
No products indexed under this heading.

Torsemide (Diltiazem has an additive effect when used with other antihypertensive agents. Therefore, the dosage of diltiazem or concomitant antihypertensives may need to be adjusted when adding one to the other).
No products indexed under this heading.

IMPORTANT NOTE: Always consult each drug listing in the patient's regimen for possible interactions.

Food Interactions

CATAPRES-TTS

(⊙ Described in PDR® for Ophthalmic Medicines)

Desipramine Hydrochloride (If a patient receiving clonidine is also taking tricyclic antidepressants, the hypotensive effect of clonidine may be reduced, necessitating an increase in the clonidine dose).
No products indexed under this heading.

Deslanoside (Due to a potential for additive effects, such as bradycardia and AV block, caution is warranted in patients receiving clonidine concomitantly with agents known to affect sinus node function or AV nodal conduction (eg, digitalis, calcium channel blockers and β-blockers). Cases of sinus bradycardia and atrioventricular block have been reported, both with and without the use of concomitant digitalis).
No products indexed under this heading.

Digitalis Glycoside Preparations (Due to a potential for additive effects, such as bradycardia and AV block, caution is warranted in patients receiving clonidine concomitantly with agents known to affect sinus node function or AV nodal conduction (eg, digitalis, calcium channel blockers and β-blockers). Cases of sinus bradycardia and atrioventricular block have been reported, both with and without the use of concomitant digitalis).
No products indexed under this heading.

Digitalis Lanata (Due to a potential for additive effects, such as bradycardia and AV block, caution is warranted in patients receiving clonidine concomitantly with agents known to affect sinus node function or AV nodal conduction (eg, digitalis, calcium channel blockers and β-blockers). Cases of sinus bradycardia and atrioventricular block have been reported, both with and without the use of concomitant digitalis).
No products indexed under this heading.

Digitalis Purpurea (Due to a potential for additive effects, such as bradycardia and AV block, caution is warranted in patients receiving clonidine concomitantly with agents known to affect sinus node function or AV nodal conduction (eg, digitalis, calcium channel blockers and β-blockers). Cases of sinus bradycardia and atrioventricular block have been reported, both with and without the use of concomitant digitalis).
No products indexed under this heading.

Digitoxin (Due to a potential for additive effects, such as bradycardia and AV block, caution is warranted in patients receiving clonidine concomitantly with agents known to affect sinus node function or AV nodal conduction (eg, digitalis, calcium channel blockers and β-blockers). Cases of sinus bradycardia and atrioventricular block have been reported, both with and without the use of concomitant digitalis).
No products indexed under this heading.

Digoxin (Due to a potential for additive effects, such as bradycardia and AV block, caution is warranted in patients receiving clonidine concomitantly with agents known to affect sinus node function or AV nodal conduction (eg, digitalis, calcium channel blockers and β-blockers). Cases of sinus bradycardia and atrioventricular block have been reported, both with and without the use of concomitant digitalis). Products include:
Lanoxin Injection 1546
Lanoxin Injection Pediatric 1549
Lanoxin Tablets 1553

Diltiazem Hydrochloride (Due to a potential for additive effects, such as bradycardia and AV block, caution is warranted in patients receiving clonidine concomitantly with agents known to affect sinus node function or AV nodal conduction (eg, digitalis, calcium channel blockers and β-blockers)). Products include:
Cardizem LA 423

Doxepin Hydrochloride (If a patient receiving clonidine is also taking tricyclic antidepressants, the hypotensive effect of clonidine may be reduced, necessitating an increase in the clonidine dose).
No products indexed under this heading.

Enflurane (Due to a potential for additive effects, such as bradycardia and AV block, caution is warranted in patients receiving clonidine concomitantly with agents known to affect sinus node function or AV nodal conduction (eg, digitalis, calcium channel blockers and β-blockers)).
No products indexed under this heading.

Esmolol Hydrochloride (Due to a potential for additive effects, such as bradycardia and AV block, caution is warranted in patients receiving clonidine concomitantly with agents known to affect sinus node function or AV nodal conduction (eg, digitalis, calcium channel blockers and β-blockers)).
No products indexed under this heading.

Estazolam (Clonidine may potentiate the CNS-depressive effects of alcohol, barbiturates or other sedating drugs).
No products indexed under this heading.

Ethanol (Clonidine may potentiate the CNS-depressive effects of alcohol, barbiturates or other sedating drugs).
No products indexed under this heading.

Ethchlorvynol (Clonidine may potentiate the CNS-depressive effects of alcohol, barbiturates or other sedating drugs).
No products indexed under this heading.

Ethinamate (Clonidine may potentiate the CNS-depressive effects of alcohol, barbiturates or other sedating drugs).
No products indexed under this heading.

Ethyl Alcohol (Clonidine may potentiate the CNS-depressive effects of alcohol, barbiturates or other sedating drugs).
No products indexed under this heading.

Felodipine (Due to a potential for additive effects, such as bradycardia and AV block, caution is warranted in patients receiving clonidine concomitantly with agents known to affect sinus node function or AV nodal conduction (eg, digitalis, calcium channel blockers and β-blockers)).
No products indexed under this heading.

Fentanyl Citrate (Due to a potential for additive effects, such as bradycardia and AV block, caution is warranted in patients receiving clonidine concomitantly with agents known to affect sinus node function or AV nodal conduction (eg, digitalis, calcium channel blockers and β-blockers)). Products include:
Fentora 966

Flurazepam Hydrochloride (Clonidine may potentiate the CNS-depressive effects of alcohol, barbiturates or other sedating drugs).
No products indexed under this heading.

Glutethimide (Clonidine may potentiate the CNS-depressive effects of alcohol, barbiturates or other sedating drugs).
No products indexed under this heading.

Halothane (Due to a potential for additive effects, such as bradycardia and AV block, caution is warranted in patients receiving clonidine concomitantly with agents known to affect sinus node function or AV nodal conduction (eg, digitalis, calcium channel blockers and β-blockers)).
No products indexed under this heading.

Hexobarbital (Clonidine may potentiate the CNS-depressive effects of alcohol, barbiturates or other sedating drugs).
No products indexed under this heading.

Imipramine Hydrochloride (If a patient receiving clonidine is also taking tricyclic antidepressants, the hypotensive effect of clonidine may be reduced, necessitating an increase in the clonidine dose).
No products indexed under this heading.

Imipramine Pamoate (If a patient receiving clonidine is also taking tricyclic antidepressants, the hypotensive effect of clonidine may be reduced, necessitating an increase in the clonidine dose).
No products indexed under this heading.

Isoflurane (Due to a potential for additive effects, such as bradycardia and AV block, caution is warranted in patients receiving clonidine concomitantly with agents known to affect sinus node function or AV nodal conduction (eg, digitalis, calcium channel blockers and β-blockers)).
No products indexed under this heading.

Isradipine (Due to a potential for additive effects, such as bradycardia and AV block, caution is warranted in patients receiving clonidine concomitantly with agents known to affect sinus node function or AV nodal conduction (eg, digitalis, calcium channel blockers and β-blockers)). Products include:
DynaCirc CR 1432

Ketamine Hydrochloride (Due to a potential for additive effects, such as bradycardia and AV block, caution is warranted in patients receiving clonidine concomitantly with agents known to affect sinus node function or AV nodal conduction (eg, digitalis, calcium channel blockers and β-blockers)).
No products indexed under this heading.

Labetalol Hydrochloride (Due to a potential for additive effects, such as bradycardia and AV block, caution is warranted in patients receiving clonidine concomitantly with agents known to affect sinus node function or AV nodal conduction (eg, digitalis, calcium channel blockers and β-blockers)).
No products indexed under this heading.

Levobunolol Hydrochloride (Due to a potential for additive effects, such as bradycardia and AV block, caution is warranted in patients receiving clonidine concomitantly with agents known to affect sinus node function or AV nodal conduction (eg, digitalis, calcium channel blockers and β-blockers)).
No products indexed under this heading.

Lorazepam (Clonidine may potentiate the CNS-depressive effects of alcohol, barbiturates or other sedating drugs).
No products indexed under this heading.

Maprotiline Hydrochloride (If a patient receiving clonidine is also taking tricyclic antidepressants, the hypotensive effect of clonidine may be reduced, necessitating an increase in the clonidine dose).
No products indexed under this heading.

Mephobarbital (Clonidine may potentiate the CNS-depressive effects of alcohol, barbiturates or other sedating drugs).
No products indexed under this heading.

Methohexital Sodium (Due to a potential for additive effects, such as bradycardia and AV block, caution is warranted in patients receiving clonidine concomitantly with agents known to affect sinus node function or AV nodal conduction (eg, digitalis, calcium channel blockers and β-blockers)).
No products indexed under this heading.

Methylphenidate (Serious adverse events, including death, have been reported in concomitant use with methylphenidate, although no causality for the combination has been established. The safety of using clonidine in combination with methylphenidate has not been systematically evaluated). Products include:
Daytrana 3283

Methylphenidate Hydrochloride (Serious adverse events, including death, have been reported in concomitant use with methylphenidate, although no causality for the combination has been established. The safety of using clonidine in combination with methylphenidate has not been systematically evaluated). Products include:
Concerta 2598
Metadate CD 3439

Metipranolol Hydrochloride (Due to a potential for additive effects, such as bradycardia and AV block, caution is warranted in patients receiving clonidine concomitantly with agents known to affect sinus node function or AV nodal conduction (eg, digitalis, calcium channel blockers and β-blockers)).
No products indexed under this heading.

Metoprolol Succinate (Due to a potential for additive effects, such as bradycardia and AV block, caution is warranted in patients receiving clonidine concomitantly with agents known to affect sinus node function or AV nodal conduction (eg, digitalis, calcium channel blockers and β-blockers)). Products include:
Toprol XL 732

Metoprolol Tartrate (Due to a potential for additive effects, such as bradycardia and AV block, caution is warranted in patients receiving clonidine concomitantly with agents known to affect sinus node function or AV nodal conduction (eg, digitalis, calcium channel blockers and β-blockers)).
No products indexed under this heading.

Mibefradil Dihydrochloride (Due to a potential for additive effects, such as bradycardia and AV block, caution is warranted in patients receiving clonidine concomitantly with agents known to affect sinus node function or AV nodal conduction (eg, digitalis, calcium channel blockers and β-blockers)).
No products indexed under this heading.

Midazolam Hydrochloride (Clonidine may potentiate the CNS-depressive effects of alcohol, barbiturates or other sedating drugs).
No products indexed under this heading.

Nadolol (Due to a potential for additive effects, such as bradycardia and AV block, caution is warranted in patients receiving clonidine concomitantly with agents known to affect sinus node function or AV nodal conduction (eg, digitalis, calcium channel blockers and β-blockers)). Products include:
Nadolol 2359

Nebivolol (Due to a potential for additive effects, such as bradycardia and AV block, caution is warranted in patients receiving clonidine concomitantly with agents known to affect sinus node function or AV nodal conduction (eg, digitalis, calcium channel blockers and β-blockers)). Products include:
Bystolic 1147

Nicardipine (Due to a potential for additive effects, such as bradycardia and AV block, caution is warranted in patients receiving clonidine concomitantly with agents known to affect sinus node function or AV nodal conduction (eg, digitalis, calcium channel blockers and β-blockers)).
No products indexed under this heading.

IMPORTANT NOTE: Always consult each drug listing in the patient's regimen for possible interactions.

Nicardipine Hydrochloride (Due to a potential for additive effects, such as bradycardia and AV block, caution is warranted in patients receiving clonidine concomitantly with agents known to affect sinus node function or AV nodal conduction (eg, digitalis, calcium channel blockers and β-blockers)).
No products indexed under this heading.

Nifedipine (Due to a potential for additive effects, such as bradycardia and AV block, caution is warranted in patients receiving clonidine concomitantly with agents known to affect sinus node function or AV nodal conduction (eg, digitalis, calcium channel blockers and β-blockers)).
No products indexed under this heading.

Nimodipine (Due to a potential for additive effects, such as bradycardia and AV block, caution is warranted in patients receiving clonidine concomitantly with agents known to affect sinus node function or AV nodal conduction (eg, digitalis, calcium channel blockers and β-blockers)).
No products indexed under this heading.

Nisoldipine (Due to a potential for additive effects, such as bradycardia and AV block, caution is warranted in patients receiving clonidine concomitantly with agents known to affect sinus node function or AV nodal conduction (eg, digitalis, calcium channel blockers and β-blockers)).
No products indexed under this heading.

Nortriptyline Hydrochloride (If a patient receiving clonidine is also taking tricyclic antidepressants, the hypotensive effect of clonidine may be reduced, necessitating an increase in the clonidine dose).
No products indexed under this heading.

Penbutolol Sulfate (Due to a potential for additive effects, such as bradycardia and AV block, caution is warranted in patients receiving clonidine concomitantly with agents known to affect sinus node function or AV nodal conduction (eg, digitalis, calcium channel blockers and β-blockers)).
No products indexed under this heading.

Pentobarbital (Clonidine may potentiate the CNS-depressive effects of alcohol, barbiturates or other sedating drugs).
No products indexed under this heading.

Pentobarbital Sodium (Clonidine may potentiate the CNS-depressive effects of alcohol, barbiturates or other sedating drugs). Products include:
Nembutal 2012

Phenobarbital (Clonidine may potentiate the CNS-depressive effects of alcohol, barbiturates or other sedating drugs). Products include:
Donnatal 2711

Phenobarbital Sodium (Clonidine may potentiate the CNS-depressive effects of alcohol, barbiturates or other sedating drugs).
No products indexed under this heading.

Pindolol (Due to a potential for additive effects, such as bradycardia and AV block, caution is warranted in patients receiving clonidine concomitantly with agents known to affect sinus node function or AV nodal conduction (eg, digitalis, calcium channel blockers and β-blockers)).
No products indexed under this heading.

Propofol (Clonidine may potentiate the CNS-depressive effects of alcohol, barbiturates or other sedating drugs).
No products indexed under this heading.

Propranolol Hydrochloride (Due to a potential for additive effects, such as bradycardia and AV block, caution is warranted in patients receiving clonidine concomitantly with agents known to affect sinus node function or AV nodal

conduction (eg, digitalis, calcium channel blockers and β-blockers)). Products include:
InnoPran XL 1517

Protriptyline Hydrochloride (If a patient receiving clonidine is also taking tricyclic antidepressants, the hypotensive effect of clonidine may be reduced, necessitating an increase in the clonidine dose).
No products indexed under this heading.

Quazepam (Clonidine may potentiate the CNS-depressive effects of alcohol, barbiturates or other sedating drugs).
No products indexed under this heading.

Ramelteon (Clonidine may potentiate the CNS-depressive effects of alcohol, barbiturates or other sedating drugs). Products include:
Rozerem 3366

Secobarbital Sodium (Clonidine may potentiate the CNS-depressive effects of alcohol, barbiturates or other sedating drugs).
No products indexed under this heading.

Sodium Butabarbital (Clonidine may potentiate the CNS-depressive effects of alcohol, barbiturates or other sedating drugs).
No products indexed under this heading.

Sodium Pentobarbital (Clonidine may potentiate the CNS-depressive effects of alcohol, barbiturates or other sedating drugs).
No products indexed under this heading.

Sotalol Hydrochloride (Due to a potential for additive effects, such as bradycardia and AV block, caution is warranted in patients receiving clonidine concomitantly with agents known to affect sinus node function or AV nodal conduction (eg, digitalis, calcium channel blockers and β-blockers)).
No products indexed under this heading.

Sufentanil Citrate (Due to a potential for additive effects, such as bradycardia and AV block, caution is warranted in patients receiving clonidine concomitantly with agents known to affect sinus node function or AV nodal conduction (eg, digitalis, calcium channel blockers and β-blockers)).
No products indexed under this heading.

Temazepam (Clonidine may potentiate the CNS-depressive effects of alcohol, barbiturates or other sedating drugs).
No products indexed under this heading.

Thiamylal Sodium (Clonidine may potentiate the CNS-depressive effects of alcohol, barbiturates or other sedating drugs).
No products indexed under this heading.

Timolol Hemihydrate (Due to a potential for additive effects, such as bradycardia and AV block, caution is warranted in patients receiving clonidine concomitantly with agents known to affect sinus node function or AV nodal conduction (eg, digitalis, calcium channel blockers and β-blockers)). Products include:
Betimol 3490

Timolol Maleate (Due to a potential for additive effects, such as bradycardia and AV block, caution is warranted in patients receiving clonidine concomitantly with agents known to affect sinus node function or AV nodal conduction (eg, digitalis, calcium channel blockers and β-blockers)). Products include:
Combigan 601
Dorzolamide
Hydrochloride/Timolol Maleate
Ophthalmic Solution .... ⊙243
Timoptic in Ocudose .... ⊙231

Triazolam (Clonidine may potentiate the CNS-depressive effects of alcohol, barbiturates or other sedating drugs).
No products indexed under this heading.

Trimipramine Maleate (If a patient receiving clonidine is also taking tricyclic antidepressants, the hypotensive effect of clonidine may be reduced, necessitating an increase in the clonidine dose).
No products indexed under this heading.

Verapamil Hydrochloride (Due to a potential for additive effects, such as bradycardia and AV block, caution is warranted in patients receiving clonidine concomitantly with agents known to affect sinus node function or AV nodal conduction (eg, digitalis, calcium channel blockers and β-blockers)). Products include:
Tarka 534

Zaleplon (Clonidine may potentiate the CNS-depressive effects of alcohol, barbiturates or other sedating drugs).
No products indexed under this heading.

Zolpidem Tartrate (Clonidine may potentiate the CNS-depressive effects of alcohol, barbiturates or other sedating drugs). Products include:
Ambien 2920
Ambien CR 2925

Food Interactions

Alcohol (Clonidine may potentiate the CNS-depressive effects of alcohol, barbiturates or other sedating drugs).

Beer, reduced-alcohol (Clonidine may potentiate the CNS-depressive effects of alcohol, barbiturates or other sedating drugs).

Beer, unspecified (Clonidine may potentiate the CNS-depressive effects of alcohol, barbiturates or other sedating drugs).

Wine, Chianti (Clonidine may potentiate the CNS-depressive effects of alcohol, barbiturates or other sedating drugs).

Wine, Red (Clonidine may potentiate the CNS-depressive effects of alcohol, barbiturates or other sedating drugs).

Wine, unspecified (Clonidine may potentiate the CNS-depressive effects of alcohol, barbiturates or other sedating drugs).

Wine products (Clonidine may potentiate the CNS-depressive effects of alcohol, barbiturates or other sedating drugs).

CATHFLO ACTIVASE
(Alteplase) 1192
See Activase I.V.

CEFTIN FOR ORAL SUSPENSION
(Cefuroxime Axetil) 1399
See Ceftin Tablets

CEFTIN TABLETS
(Cefuroxime Axetil) 1399
May interact with drugs that reduce gastric acidity, oral anticoagulants, and certain other agents. Compounds in these categories include:

Aluminum Carbonate (Drugs that reduce gastric acidity may result in a lower bioavailability of Ceftin compared with that of fasting state and tend to cancel the effect of postprandial absorption).
No products indexed under this heading.

Aluminum Hydroxide (Drugs that reduce gastric acidity may result in a lower bioavailability of Ceftin compared with that of fasting state and tend to cancel the effect of postprandial absorption).
No products indexed under this heading.

Anisindione (Cephalosporins may be associated with a fall in prothrombin activity; those at risk include patients previously stabilized on anticoagulant therapy).
No products indexed under this heading.

Cimetidine (Drugs that reduce gastric acidity may result in a lower bioavailability of Ceftin compared with that of fasting state and tend to cancel the effect of postprandial absorption).
No products indexed under this heading.

Cimetidine Hydrochloride (Drugs that reduce gastric acidity may result in a lower bioavailability of Ceftin compared with that of fasting state and tend to cancel the effect of postprandial absorption).
No products indexed under this heading.

Dicumarol (Cephalosporins may be associated with a fall in prothrombin activity; those at risk include patients previously stabilized on anticoagulant therapy).
No products indexed under this heading.

Esomeprazole Magnesium (Drugs that reduce gastric acidity may result in a lower bioavailability of Ceftin compared with that of fasting state and tend to cancel the effect of postprandial absorption). Products include:
Nexium Capsules 704
Nexium Oral Suspension 704

Famotidine (Drugs that reduce gastric acidity may result in a lower bioavailability of Ceftin compared with that of fasting state and tend to cancel the effect of postprandial absorption). Products include:
Pepcid 2227
Original Strength Pepcid AC
Gelcaps 1821
Original Strength Pepcid AC 1821
Maximum Strength Pepcid AC 1821
Pepcid Complete 1822

Lansoprazole (Drugs that reduce gastric acidity may result in a lower bioavailability of Ceftin compared with that of fasting state and tend to cancel the effect of postprandial absorption).
No products indexed under this heading.

Magnesium Hydroxide (Drugs that reduce gastric acidity may result in a lower bioavailability of Ceftin compared with that of fasting state and tend to cancel the effect of postprandial absorption). Products include:
Fleet Pedia-Lax Chewable Tablets 1144
Pepcid Complete 1822

Nizatidine (Drugs that reduce gastric acidity may result in a lower bioavailability of Ceftin compared with that of fasting state and tend to cancel the effect of postprandial absorption). Products include:
Axid 1381

Omeprazole (Drugs that reduce gastric acidity may result in a lower bioavailability of Ceftin compared with that of fasting state and tend to cancel the effect of postprandial absorption).
No products indexed under this heading.

Probenecid (Increases serum concentration of cefuroxime).
No products indexed under this heading.

Rabeprazole Sodium (Drugs that reduce gastric acidity may result in a lower bioavailability of Ceftin compared with that of fasting state and tend to cancel the effect of postprandial absorption). Products include:
Aciphex 1035

Ranitidine Hydrochloride (Drugs that reduce gastric acidity may result in a lower bioavailability of Ceftin compared with that of fasting state and tend to cancel the effect of postprandial absorption). Products include:
Zantac 1737
Zantac Injection 1732

(⊙ Described in PDR® for Ophthalmic Medicines)

Zantac Pharmacy 1735

Warfarin Sodium (Cephalosporins may be associated with a fall in prothrombin activity; those at risk include patients previously stabilized on anticoagulant therapy).
No products indexed under this heading.

Food Interactions

Food, unspecified (Absorption is greater when taken after food).

CELEBREX CAPSULES

(Celecoxib) 3272
May interact with ACE inhibitors, alcohols, angiotensin-II receptor antagonists, antacids containing aluminum, calcium and magnesium, anticoagulants, aspirin-acetylsalicylic acid, corticosteroids, cytochrome p450 2c9 inhibitors (selected), cytochrome p450 2d6 substrates (selected), diuretics, lithium preparations, loop diuretics, non-steroidal anti-inflammatory agents, oral anticoagulants, thiazides, and certain other agents. Compounds in these categories include:

Alclometasone Dipropionate (Other factors that increase the risk of GI bleeding in patients treated with NSAIDs include concomitant use of oral corticosteroids. Most spontaneous reports of fatal GI events are in elderly or debilitated patients and therefore special care should be taken in treating this population).
No products indexed under this heading.

Aluminum Carbonate (Co-administration of celecoxib with aluminum- and magnesium-containing antacids resulted in a reduction in plasma celecoxib concentrations with a decrease of 37% in C_{max} and 10% in AUC. Higher doses (400 mg twice daily) should be administered with food to improve absorption).
No products indexed under this heading.

Aluminum Hydroxide (Co-administration of celecoxib with aluminum- and magnesium-containing antacids resulted in a reduction in plasma celecoxib concentrations with a decrease of 37% in C_{max} and 10% in AUC. Higher doses (400 mg twice daily) should be administered with food to improve absorption).
No products indexed under this heading.

Amiloride Hydrochloride (Renal toxicity has also been seen in patients in whom renal prostaglandins have a compensatory role in the maintenance of renal perfusion. In these patients, administration of an NSAID may cause a dose-dependent reduction in prostaglandin formation and, secondarily, in renal blood flow, which may precipitate overt renal decompensation. Patients at greatest risk of this reaction are those with impaired renal function, heart failure, liver dysfunction, and those taking diuretics).
No products indexed under this heading.

Amiodarone Hydrochloride (Celecoxib metabolism is predominantly mediated via cytochrome P450 (CYP) 2C9 in the liver. Co-administration of celecoxib with drugs that are known to inhibit CYP2C9 should be done with caution. Significant interactions may occur when celecoxib is administered together with drugs that inhibit CYP2C9).
No products indexed under this heading.

Amitriptyline Hydrochloride (In vitro studies indicate that celecoxib, although not a substrate, is an inhibitor of CYP2D6. Therefore, there is a potential for an in vivo drug interaction with drugs that are metabolized by CYP2D6).
No products indexed under this heading.

Amphetamine Aspartate (In vitro studies indicate that celecoxib, although not a substrate, is an inhibitor of CYP2D6. Therefore, there is a potential for an in vivo drug interaction with drugs that are metabolized by CYP2D6).
No products indexed under this heading.

Amphetamine Aspartate Monohydrate (In vitro studies indicate that celecoxib, although not a substrate, is an inhibitor of CYP2D6. Therefore, there is a potential for an in vivo drug interaction with drugs that are metabolized by CYP2D6).
No products indexed under this heading.

Amphetamine Sulfate (In vitro studies indicate that celecoxib, although not a substrate, is an inhibitor of CYP2D6. Therefore, there is a potential for an in vivo drug interaction with drugs that are metabolized by CYP2D6).
No products indexed under this heading.

Anastrozole (Celecoxib metabolism is predominantly mediated via cytochrome P450 (CYP) 2C9 in the liver. Co-administration of celecoxib with drugs that are known to inhibit CYP2C9 should be done with caution. Significant interactions may occur when celecoxib is administered together with drugs that inhibit CYP2C9).
No products indexed under this heading.

Anisindione (Anticoagulant activity should be monitored, particularly in the first few days, after initiating or changing celecoxib therapy in patients receiving warfarin or similar agents, since these patients are at an increased risk of bleeding complications. In post-marketing experience, serious bleeding events, some of which were fatal, have been reported, predominantly in the elderly, in association with increases in prothrombin time in patients receiving celecoxib concurrently with warfarin).
No products indexed under this heading.

Ardeparin Sodium (Other factors that increase the risk of GI bleeding in patients treated with NSAIDs include concomitant use of anticoagulants. Most spontaneous reports of fatal GI events are in elderly or debilitated patients and therefore special care should be taken in treating this population).
No products indexed under this heading.

Aspirin (Celecoxib can be used with low-dose aspirin. However, concomitant administration of aspirin with celecoxib increases the rate of GI ulceration or other complications, compared to use of celecoxib alone. Because of its lack of platelet effects, celecoxib is not a substitute for aspirin for cardiovascular prophylaxis). Products include:
Aggrenox 880
Bayer Aspirin 829
Percodan 1124
St. Joseph Aspirin 2045

Aspirin, Enteric Coated (Celecoxib can be used with low-dose aspirin. However, concomitant administration of aspirin with celecoxib increases the rate of GI ulceration or other complications, compared to use of celecoxib alone. Because of its lack of platelet effects, celecoxib is not a substitute for aspirin for cardiovascular prophylaxis).
No products indexed under this heading.

Aspirin Buffered (Celecoxib can be used with low-dose aspirin. However, concomitant administration of aspirin with celecoxib increases the rate of GI ulceration or other complications, compared to use of celecoxib alone. Because of its lack of platelet effects, celecoxib is not a substitute for aspirin for cardiovascular prophylaxis).
No products indexed under this heading.

Atomoxetine Hydrochloride (In vitro studies indicate that celecoxib, although

not a substrate, is an inhibitor of CYP2D6. Therefore, there is a potential for an in vivo drug interaction with drugs that are metabolized by CYP2D6). Products include:
Strattera 1957

Beclomethasone Dipropionate (Other factors that increase the risk of GI bleeding in patients treated with NSAIDs include concomitant use of oral corticosteroids. Most spontaneous reports of fatal GI events are in elderly or debilitated patients and therefore special care should be taken in treating this population). Products include:
Qvar 3398

Beclomethasone Dipropionate Monohydrate (Other factors that increase the risk of GI bleeding in patients treated with NSAIDs include concomitant use of oral corticosteroids. Most spontaneous reports of fatal GI events are in elderly or debilitated patients and therefore special care should be taken in treating this population). Products include:
Beconase AQ 1386

Benazepril Hydrochloride (Reports suggest that NSAIDs may diminish the antihypertensive effect of Angiotensin Converting Enzyme (ACE) inhibitors. This interaction should be given consideration in patients taking celecoxib concomitantly with ACE inhibitors).
No products indexed under this heading.

Bendroflumethiazide (Patients taking thiazides may have impaired response to these therapies when taking NSAIDs. NSAIDs, including celecoxib, should be used with caution in patients with hypertension. Blood pressure should be monitored closely during the initiation of therapy with celecoxib and throughout the course of therapy).
No products indexed under this heading.

Betamethasone (Other factors that increase the risk of GI bleeding in patients treated with NSAIDs include concomitant use of oral corticosteroids. Most spontaneous reports of fatal GI events are in elderly or debilitated patients and therefore special care should be taken in treating this population).
No products indexed under this heading.

Betamethasone Acetate (Other factors that increase the risk of GI bleeding in patients treated with NSAIDs include concomitant use of oral corticosteroids. Most spontaneous reports of fatal GI events are in elderly or debilitated patients and therefore special care should be taken in treating this population).
No products indexed under this heading.

Betamethasone Benzoate (Other factors that increase the risk of GI bleeding in patients treated with NSAIDs include concomitant use of oral corticosteroids. Most spontaneous reports of fatal GI events are in elderly or debilitated patients and therefore special care should be taken in treating this population).
No products indexed under this heading.

Betamethasone Dipropionate (Other factors that increase the risk of GI bleeding in patients treated with NSAIDs include concomitant use of oral corticosteroids. Most spontaneous reports of fatal GI events are in elderly or debilitated patients and therefore special care should be taken in treating this population). Products include:
Diprolene Lotion 0.05% 3108
Diprolene Ointment 0.05% 3109
Diprolene AF Cream 0.05% 3107
Lotrisone 3163

Betamethasone Sodium Phosphate (Other factors that increase the risk of GI bleeding in patients treated with NSAIDs include concomitant use of oral corticosteroids. Most spontaneous reports of fatal GI events are in elderly or debilitated patients and therefore special care should be taken in treating this population).
No products indexed under this heading.

Betamethasone Valerate (Other factors that increase the risk of GI bleeding in patients treated with NSAIDs include concomitant use of oral corticosteroids. Most spontaneous reports of fatal GI events are in elderly or debilitated patients and therefore special care should be taken in treating this population). Products include:
Luxíq 3321

Bisoprolol Fumarate (In vitro studies indicate that celecoxib, although not a substrate, is an inhibitor of CYP2D6. Therefore, there is a potential for an in vivo drug interaction with drugs that are metabolized by CYP2D6).
No products indexed under this heading.

Budesonide (Other factors that increase the risk of GI bleeding in patients treated with NSAIDs include concomitant use of oral corticosteroids. Most spontaneous reports of fatal GI events are in elderly or debilitated patients and therefore special care should be taken in treating this population). Products include:
Pulmicort Flexhaler 714
Symbicort 80/4.5 720
Symbicort 160/4.5 720

Bumetanide (Patients taking thiazides or loop diuretics may have impaired response to these therapies when taking NSAIDs. NSAIDs, including celecoxib, should be used with caution in patients with hypertension. Blood pressure should be monitored closely during the initiation of therapy with celecoxib and throughout the course of therapy).
No products indexed under this heading.

Calcium Carbonate (Co-administration of celecoxib with aluminum- and magnesium-containing antacids resulted in a reduction in plasma celecoxib concentrations with a decrease of 37% in C_{max} and 10% in AUC. Higher doses (400 mg twice daily) should be administered with food to improve absorption). Products include:
Chelated Mineral 3476
Pepcid Complete 1822
Extra Strength Rolaids Softchews Vanilla Creme 2045

Candesartan Cilexetil (Reports suggest that NSAIDs may diminish the antihypertensive effect of angiotensin II antagonists. This interaction should be given consideration in patients taking celecoxib concomitantly with angiotensin II antagonists. Patients are at greater risk of renal toxicity when taking angiotensin II receptor antagonists with NSAIDs). Products include:
Atacand 697
Atacand HCT 700

Captopril (Reports suggest that NSAIDs may diminish the antihypertensive effect of Angiotensin Converting Enzyme (ACE) inhibitors. This interaction should be given consideration in patients taking celecoxib concomitantly with ACE inhibitors). Products include:
Captopril 2341

Carvedilol (In vitro studies indicate that celecoxib, although not a substrate, is an inhibitor of CYP2D6. Therefore, there is a potential for an in vivo drug interaction with drugs that are metabolized by CYP2D6). Products include:
Coreg 1409

Cevimeline Hydrochloride (In vitro studies indicate that celecoxib, although

---

IMPORTANT NOTE: Always consult each drug listing in the patient's regimen for possible interactions.

not a substrate, is an inhibitor of CYP2D6. Therefore, there is a potential for an *in vivo* drug interaction with drugs that are metabolized by CYP2D6). Products include:

Evoxac 1027

Chloramphenicol (Celecoxib metabolism is predominantly mediated via cytochrome P450 (CYP) 2C9 in the liver. Co-administration of celecoxib with drugs that are known to inhibit CYP2C9 should be done with caution. Significant interactions may occur when celecoxib is administered together with drugs that inhibit CYP2C9).

No products indexed under this heading.

Chloramphenicol Palmitate (Celecoxib metabolism is predominantly mediated via cytochrome P450 (CYP) 2C9 in the liver. Co-administration of celecoxib with drugs that are known to inhibit CYP2C9 should be done with caution. Significant interactions may occur when celecoxib is administered together with drugs that inhibit CYP2C9).

No products indexed under this heading.

Chloramphenicol Sodium Succinate (Celecoxib metabolism is predominantly mediated via cytochrome P450 (CYP) 2C9 in the liver. Co-administration of celecoxib with drugs that are known to inhibit CYP2C9 should be done with caution. Significant interactions may occur when celecoxib is administered together with drugs that inhibit CYP2C9).

No products indexed under this heading.

Chlorothiazide (Patients taking thiazides may have impaired response to these therapies when taking NSAIDs. NSAIDs, including celecoxib, should be used with caution in patients with hypertension. Blood pressure should be monitored closely during the initiation of therapy with celecoxib and throughout the course of therapy).

No products indexed under this heading.

Chlorothiazide Sodium (Patients taking thiazides may have impaired response to these therapies when taking NSAIDs. NSAIDs, including celecoxib, should be used with caution in patients with hypertension. Blood pressure should be monitored closely during the initiation of therapy with celecoxib and throughout the course of therapy). Products include:

Diuril Intravenous 2009

Chlorpromazine (*In vitro* studies indicate that celecoxib, although not a substrate, is an inhibitor of CYP2D6. Therefore, there is a potential for an *in vivo* drug interaction with drugs that are metabolized by CYP2D6).

No products indexed under this heading.

Chlorpromazine Hydrochloride (*In vitro* studies indicate that celecoxib, although not a substrate, is an inhibitor of CYP2D6. Therefore, there is a potential for an *in vivo* drug interaction with drugs that are metabolized by CYP2D6).

No products indexed under this heading.

Chlorpropamide (Celecoxib metabolism is predominantly mediated via cytochrome P450 (CYP) 2C9 in the liver. Co-administration of celecoxib with drugs that are known to inhibit CYP2C9 should be done with caution. Significant interactions may occur when celecoxib is administered together with drugs that inhibit CYP2C9).

No products indexed under this heading.

Chlorthalidone (Renal toxicity has also been seen in patients in whom renal prostaglandins have a compensatory role in the maintenance of renal perfusion. In these patients, administration of an NSAID may cause a dose-dependent reduction in prostaglandin formation and, secondarily, in renal

blood flow, which may precipitate overt renal decompensation. Patients at greatest risk of this reaction are those with impaired renal function, heart failure, liver dysfunction, and those taking diuretics). Products include:

Clorpres 2344

Ciclesonide (Other factors that increase the risk of GI bleeding in patients treated with NSAIDs include concomitant use of oral corticosteroids. Most spontaneous reports of fatal GI events are in elderly or debilitated patients and therefore special care should be taken in treating this population).

No products indexed under this heading.

Cimetidine (Celecoxib metabolism is predominantly mediated via cytochrome P450 (CYP) 2C9 in the liver. Co-administration of celecoxib with drugs that are known to inhibit CYP2C9 should be done with caution. Significant interactions may occur when celecoxib is administered together with drugs that inhibit CYP2C9).

No products indexed under this heading.

Cimetidine Hydrochloride (Celecoxib metabolism is predominantly mediated via cytochrome P450 (CYP) 2C9 in the liver. Co-administration of celecoxib with drugs that are known to inhibit CYP2C9 should be done with caution. Significant interactions may occur when celecoxib is administered together with drugs that inhibit CYP2C9).

No products indexed under this heading.

Clomipramine Hydrochloride (*In vitro* studies indicate that celecoxib, although not a substrate, is an inhibitor of CYP2D6. Therefore, there is a potential for an *in vivo* drug interaction with drugs that are metabolized by CYP2D6).

No products indexed under this heading.

Clopidogrel Bisulfate (Celecoxib metabolism is predominantly mediated via cytochrome P450 (CYP) 2C9 in the liver. Co-administration of celecoxib with drugs that are known to inhibit CYP2C9 should be done with caution. Significant interactions may occur when celecoxib is administered together with drugs that inhibit CYP2C9). Products include:

Plavix 3027

Clopidogrel Hydrogen Sulfate (Celecoxib metabolism is predominantly mediated via cytochrome P450 (CYP) 2C9 in the liver. Co-administration of celecoxib with drugs that are known to inhibit CYP2C9 should be done with caution. Significant interactions may occur when celecoxib is administered together with drugs that inhibit CYP2C9).

No products indexed under this heading.

Clotrimazole (Celecoxib metabolism is predominantly mediated via cytochrome P450 (CYP) 2C9 in the liver. Co-administration of celecoxib with drugs that are known to inhibit CYP2C9 should be done with caution. Significant interactions may occur when celecoxib is administered together with drugs that inhibit CYP2C9). Products include:

Lotrisone 3163

Clozapine (*In vitro* studies indicate that celecoxib, although not a substrate, is an inhibitor of CYP2D6. Therefore, there is a potential for an *in vivo* drug interaction with drugs that are metabolized by CYP2D6).

No products indexed under this heading.

Codeine Phosphate (*In vitro* studies indicate that celecoxib, although not a substrate, is an inhibitor of CYP2D6. Therefore, there is a potential for an *in vivo* drug interaction with drugs that are metabolized by CYP2D6). Products include:

Tylenol with Codeine 2691

Codeine Sulfate (*In vitro* studies indicate that celecoxib, although not a substrate, is an inhibitor of CYP2D6. Therefore, there is a potential for an *in vivo* drug interaction with drugs that are metabolized by CYP2D6).

No products indexed under this heading.

Cortisone Acetate (Other factors that increase the risk of GI bleeding in patients treated with NSAIDs include concomitant use of oral corticosteroids. Most spontaneous reports of fatal GI events are in elderly or debilitated patients and therefore special care should be taken in treating this population).

No products indexed under this heading.

Cyclobenzaprine Hydrochloride (*In vitro* studies indicate that celecoxib, although not a substrate, is an inhibitor of CYP2D6. Therefore, there is a potential for an *in vivo* drug interaction with drugs that are metabolized by CYP2D6). Products include:

Amrix 964

Dalteparin Sodium (Other factors that increase the risk of GI bleeding in patients treated with NSAIDs include concomitant use of anticoagulants. Most spontaneous reports of fatal GI events are in elderly or debilitated patients and therefore special care should be taken in treating this population). Products include:

Fragmin 1058

Danaparoid Sodium (Other factors that increase the risk of GI bleeding in patients treated with NSAIDs include concomitant use of anticoagulants. Most spontaneous reports of fatal GI events are in elderly or debilitated patients and therefore special care should be taken in treating this population).

No products indexed under this heading.

Debrisoquine (*In vitro* studies indicate that celecoxib, although not a substrate, is an inhibitor of CYP2D6. Therefore, there is a potential for an *in vivo* drug interaction with drugs that are metabolized by CYP2D6).

No products indexed under this heading.

Desipramine Hydrochloride (*In vitro* studies indicate that celecoxib, although not a substrate, is an inhibitor of CYP2D6. Therefore, there is a potential for an *in vivo* drug interaction with drugs that are metabolized by CYP2D6).

No products indexed under this heading.

Desoximetasone (Other factors that increase the risk of GI bleeding in patients treated with NSAIDs include concomitant use of oral corticosteroids. Most spontaneous reports of fatal GI events are in elderly or debilitated patients and therefore special care should be taken in treating this population).

No products indexed under this heading.

Dexamethasone (Other factors that increase the risk of GI bleeding in patients treated with NSAIDs include concomitant use of oral corticosteroids. Most spontaneous reports of fatal GI events are in elderly or debilitated patients and therefore special care should be taken in treating this population). Products include:

Ciprodex 583
Ozurdex .... ⊙ 223
Tobramycin and Dexamethasone Ophthalmic Suspension .... ⊙ 251

Dexamethasone Acetate (Other factors that increase the risk of GI bleeding in patients treated with NSAIDs include concomitant use of oral corticosteroids. Most spontaneous reports of fatal GI events are in elderly or debilitated patients and therefore special care should be taken in treating this population).

No products indexed under this heading.

Dexamethasone Phosphate (Other factors that increase the risk of GI bleeding in patients treated with NSAIDs include concomitant use of oral corticosteroids. Most spontaneous reports of fatal GI events are in elderly or debilitated patients and therefore special care should be taken in treating this population).

No products indexed under this heading.

Dexamethasone Sodium (Other factors that increase the risk of GI bleeding in patients treated with NSAIDs include concomitant use of oral corticosteroids. Most spontaneous reports of fatal GI events are in elderly or debilitated patients and therefore special care should be taken in treating this population).

No products indexed under this heading.

Dexamethasone Sodium Phosphate (Other factors that increase the risk of GI bleeding in patients treated with NSAIDs include concomitant use of oral corticosteroids. Most spontaneous reports of fatal GI events are in elderly or debilitated patients and therefore special care should be taken in treating this population).

No products indexed under this heading.

Dexamethasone Sodium Phosphate Injection (Other factors that increase the risk of GI bleeding in patients treated with NSAIDs include concomitant use of oral corticosteroids. Most spontaneous reports of fatal GI events are in elderly or debilitated patients and therefore special care should be taken in treating this population).

No products indexed under this heading.

Dexfenfluramine Hydrochloride (*In vitro* studies indicate that celecoxib, although not a substrate, is an inhibitor of CYP2D6. Therefore, there is a potential for an *in vivo* drug interaction with drugs that are metabolized by CYP2D6).

No products indexed under this heading.

Dextromethorphan Hydrobromide (*In vitro* studies indicate that celecoxib, although not a substrate, is an inhibitor of CYP2D6. Therefore, there is a potential for an *in vivo* drug interaction with drugs that are metabolized by CYP2D6).

No products indexed under this heading.

Dextromethorphan Polistirex (*In vitro* studies indicate that celecoxib, although not a substrate, is an inhibitor of CYP2D6. Therefore, there is a potential for an *in vivo* drug interaction with drugs that are metabolized by CYP2D6).

No products indexed under this heading.

Diclofenac Epolamine (The concomitant use of celecoxib with any dose of a non-aspirin NSAID should be avoided due to the potential for increased risk of adverse reactions. Other factors that increase the risk of GI bleeding in patients treated with NSAIDs include concomitant use of longer duration of NSAID therapy. Most spontaneous reports of fatal GI events are in elderly or debilitated patients and therefore special care should be taken in treating this population). Products include:

Flector 1839

Diclofenac Potassium (The concomitant use of celecoxib with any dose of a non-aspirin NSAID should be avoided

289 Interactions Index Celebrex

due to the potential for increased risk of adverse reactions. Other factors that increase the risk of GI bleeding in patients treated with NSAIDs include concomitant use of longer duration of NSAID therapy. Most spontaneous reports of fatal GI events are in elderly or debilitated patients and therefore special care should be taken in treating this population).
No products indexed under this heading.

Diclofenac Sodium (The concomitant use of celecoxib with any dose of a non-aspirin NSAID should be avoided due to the potential for increased risk of adverse reactions. Other factors that increase the risk of GI bleeding in patients treated with NSAIDs include concomitant use of longer duration of NSAID therapy. Most spontaneous reports of fatal GI events are in elderly or debilitated patients and therefore special care should be taken in treating this population).
No products indexed under this heading.

Dicumarol (Anticoagulant activity should be monitored, particularly in the first few days, after initiating or changing celecoxib therapy in patients receiving warfarin or similar agents, since these patients are at an increased risk of bleeding complications. In postmarketing experience, serious bleeding events, some of which were fatal, have been reported, predominantly in the elderly, in association with increases in prothrombin time in patients receiving celecoxib concurrently with warfarin).
No products indexed under this heading.

Diflorasone Diacetate (Other factors that increase the risk of GI bleeding in patients treated with NSAIDs include concomitant use of oral corticosteroids. Most spontaneous reports of fatal GI events are in elderly or debilitated patients and therefore special care should be taken in treating this population).
No products indexed under this heading.

Disulfiram (Celecoxib metabolism is predominantly mediated via cytochrome P450 (CYP) 2C9 in the liver. Co-administration of celecoxib with drugs that are known to inhibit CYP2C9 should be done with caution. Significant interactions may occur when celecoxib is administered together with drugs that inhibit CYP2C9).
No products indexed under this heading.

Dolasetron Mesylate (*In vitro* studies indicate that celecoxib, although not a substrate, is an inhibitor of CYP2D6. Therefore, there is a potential for an *in vivo* drug interaction with drugs that are metabolized by CYP2D6). Products include:
Anzemet Injection **2931**
Anzemet Tablets **2934**

Donepezil Hydrochloride (*In vitro* studies indicate that celecoxib, although not a substrate, is an inhibitor of CYP2D6. Therefore, there is a potential for an *in vivo* drug interaction with drugs that are metabolized by CYP2D6). Products include:
Aricept **1045**
Aricept ODT **1045**

Doxepin Hydrochloride (*In vitro* studies indicate that celecoxib, although not a substrate, is an inhibitor of CYP2D6. Therefore, there is a potential for an *in vivo* drug interaction with drugs that are metabolized by CYP2D6).
No products indexed under this heading.

Efavirenz (Celecoxib metabolism is predominantly mediated via cytochrome P450 (CYP) 2C9 in the liver. Co-administration of celecoxib with drugs that are known to inhibit CYP2C9 should be done with caution. Significant interactions may occur when celecoxib is administered together with drugs that inhibit CYP2C9). Products include:
Atripla **906**

Enalapril Maleate (Reports suggest that NSAIDs may diminish the antihypertensive effect of Angiotensin Converting Enzyme (ACE) inhibitors. This interaction should be given consideration in patients taking celecoxib concomitantly with ACE inhibitors).
No products indexed under this heading.

Enalaprilat (Reports suggest that NSAIDs may diminish the antihypertensive effect of Angiotensin Converting Enzyme (ACE) inhibitors. This interaction should be given consideration in patients taking celecoxib concomitantly with ACE inhibitors).
No products indexed under this heading.

Encainide Hydrochloride (*In vitro* studies indicate that celecoxib, although not a substrate, is an inhibitor of CYP2D6. Therefore, there is a potential for an *in vivo* drug interaction with drugs that are metabolized by CYP2D6).
No products indexed under this heading.

Enoxaparin Sodium (Other factors that increase the risk of GI bleeding in patients treated with NSAIDs include concomitant use of anticoagulants. Most spontaneous reports of fatal GI events are in elderly or debilitated patients and therefore special care should be taken in treating this population). Products include:
Lovenox **3005**

Eprosartan Mesylate (Reports suggest that NSAIDs may diminish the antihypertensive effect of angiotensin II antagonists. This interaction should be given consideration in patients taking celecoxib concomitantly with angiotensin II antagonists. Patients are at greater risk of renal toxicity when taking angiotensin II receptor antagonists with NSAIDs). Products include:
Teveten **538**
Teveten HCT **541**

Ethacrynic Acid (Patients taking thiazides or loop diuretics may have impaired response to these therapies when taking NSAIDs. NSAIDs, including celecoxib, should be used with caution in patients with hypertension. Blood pressure should be monitored closely during the initiation of therapy with celecoxib and throughout the course of therapy).
No products indexed under this heading.

Ethanol (Other factors that increase the risk of GI bleeding in patients treated with NSAIDs include concomitant use of alcohol. Most spontaneous reports of fatal GI events are in elderly or debilitated patients and therefore special care should be taken in treating this population).
No products indexed under this heading.

Ethyl Alcohol (Other factors that increase the risk of GI bleeding in patients treated with NSAIDs include concomitant use of alcohol. Most spontaneous reports of fatal GI events are in elderly or debilitated patients and therefore special care should be taken in treating this population).
No products indexed under this heading.

Etodolac (The concomitant use of celecoxib with any dose of a non-aspirin NSAID should be avoided due to the potential for increased risk of adverse reactions. Other factors that increase the risk of GI bleeding in patients treated with NSAIDs include concomitant use of longer duration of NSAID therapy. Most spontaneous reports of fatal GI events are in elderly or debilitated patients and therefore special care should be taken in treating this population).
No products indexed under this heading.

Fat (When celecoxib capsules were taken with a high fat meal, peak plasma levels were delayed for about 1 to 2 hours with an increase in total absorption (AUC) of 10% to 20%. Under fasting conditions, at doses above 200 mg, there is less than a proportional increase in C_{max} and AUC, which is thought to be due to the low solubility of the drug in aqueous media. Celecoxib, at doses up to 200 mg twice daily, can be administered without regard to timing of meals. Higher doses (400 mg twice daily) should be administered with food to improve absorption).
No products indexed under this heading.

Fenofibrate (Celecoxib metabolism is predominantly mediated via cytochrome P450 (CYP) 2C9 in the liver. Co-administration of celecoxib with drugs that are known to inhibit CYP2C9 should be done with caution. Significant interactions may occur when celecoxib is administered together with drugs that inhibit CYP2C9). Products include:
Fenoglide **3263**
Tricor **544**
Trilipix **548**

Fenoprofen Calcium (The concomitant use of celecoxib with any dose of a non-aspirin NSAID should be avoided due to the potential for increased risk of adverse reactions. Other factors that increase the risk of GI bleeding in patients treated with NSAIDs include concomitant use of longer duration of NSAID therapy. Most spontaneous reports of fatal GI events are in elderly or debilitated patients and therefore special care should be taken in treating this population).
No products indexed under this heading.

Fentanyl (*In vitro* studies indicate that celecoxib, although not a substrate, is an inhibitor of CYP2D6. Therefore, there is a potential for an *in vivo* drug interaction with drugs that are metabolized by CYP2D6). Products include:
Duragesic **2604**
Fentanyl Transdermal System **2346**
Onsolis **2054**

Fentanyl Citrate (*In vitro* studies indicate that celecoxib, although not a substrate, is an inhibitor of CYP2D6. Therefore, there is a potential for an *in vivo* drug interaction with drugs that are metabolized by CYP2D6). Products include:
Fentora **966**

Flecainide Acetate (*In vitro* studies indicate that celecoxib, although not a substrate, is an inhibitor of CYP2D6. Therefore, there is a potential for an *in vivo* drug interaction with drugs that are metabolized by CYP2D6).
No products indexed under this heading.

Fluconazole (Concomitant administration of fluconazole at 200 mg once daily resulted in a two-fold increase in celecoxib plasma concentration. This increase is due to the inhibition of celecoxib metabolism via P450 2C9 by fluconazole. Celecoxib should be introduced at the lowest recommended dose in patients receiving fluconazole).
No products indexed under this heading.

Fludrocortisone Acetate (Other factors that increase the risk of GI bleeding in patients treated with NSAIDs include concomitant use of oral corticosteroids. Most spontaneous reports of fatal GI events are in elderly or debilitated patients and therefore special care should be taken in treating this population).
No products indexed under this heading.

Flumethasone Pivalate (Other factors that increase the risk of GI bleeding in patients treated with NSAIDs include concomitant use of oral corticosteroids. Most spontaneous reports of fatal GI events are in elderly or debilitated patients and therefore special care should be taken in treating this population).
No products indexed under this heading.

Flunisolide Hemihydrate (Other factors that increase the risk of GI bleeding in patients treated with NSAIDs include concomitant use of oral corticosteroids. Most spontaneous reports of fatal GI events are in elderly or debilitated patients and therefore special care should be taken in treating this population).
No products indexed under this heading.

Fluorouracil (Celecoxib metabolism is predominantly mediated via cytochrome P450 (CYP) 2C9 in the liver. Co-administration of celecoxib with drugs that are known to inhibit CYP2C9 should be done with caution. Significant interactions may occur when celecoxib is administered together with drugs that inhibit CYP2C9). Products include:
Carac **2966**

Fluoxetine (*In vitro* studies indicate that celecoxib, although not a substrate, is an inhibitor of CYP2D6. Therefore, there is a potential for an *in vivo* drug interaction with drugs that are metabolized by CYP2D6).
No products indexed under this heading.

Fluoxetine Hydrochloride (Celecoxib metabolism is predominantly mediated via cytochrome P450 (CYP) 2C9 in the liver. Co-administration of celecoxib with drugs that are known to inhibit CYP2C9 should be done with caution. Significant interactions may occur when celecoxib is administered together with drugs that inhibit CYP2C9). Products include:
Prozac Weekly **1941**
Prozac Pulvules **1941**
Symbyax **1965**

Fluphenazine Decanoate (*In vitro* studies indicate that celecoxib, although not a substrate, is an inhibitor of CYP2D6. Therefore, there is a potential for an *in vivo* drug interaction with drugs that are metabolized by CYP2D6).
No products indexed under this heading.

Fluphenazine Enanthate (*In vitro* studies indicate that celecoxib, although not a substrate, is an inhibitor of CYP2D6. Therefore, there is a potential for an *in vivo* drug interaction with drugs that are metabolized by CYP2D6).
No products indexed under this heading.

Fluphenazine Hydrochloride (*In vitro* studies indicate that celecoxib, although not a substrate, is an inhibitor of CYP2D6. Therefore, there is a potential for an *in vivo* drug interaction with drugs that are metabolized by CYP2D6).
No products indexed under this heading.

Flurbiprofen (The concomitant use of celecoxib with any dose of a non-aspirin NSAID should be avoided due to the potential for increased risk of adverse reactions. Other factors that increase the risk of GI bleeding in patients treated with NSAIDs include concomitant use of longer duration of NSAID therapy. Most spontaneous reports of fatal GI events are in elderly or debilitated patients and therefore special care should be taken in treating this population).
No products indexed under this heading.

IMPORTANT NOTE: Always consult each drug listing in the patient's regimen for possible interactions.

Flurbiprofen Sodium (Celecoxib metabolism is predominantly mediated via cytochrome P450 (CYP) 2C9 in the liver. Co-administration of celecoxib with drugs that are known to inhibit CYP2C9 should be done with caution. Significant interactions may occur when celecoxib is administered together with drugs that inhibit CYP2C9).
No products indexed under this heading.

Fluticasone Furoate (Other factors that increase the risk of GI bleeding in patients treated with NSAIDs include concomitant use of oral corticosteroids. Most spontaneous reports of fatal GI events are in elderly or debilitated patients and therefore special care should be taken in treating this population). Products include:

Fluticasone Propionate (Other factors that increase the risk of GI bleeding in patients treated with NSAIDs include concomitant use of oral corticosteroids. Most spontaneous reports of fatal GI events are in elderly or debilitated patients and therefore special care should be taken in treating this population). Products include:

Fluvastatin Sodium (Celecoxib metabolism is predominantly mediated via cytochrome P450 (CYP) 2C9 in the liver. Co-administration of celecoxib with drugs that are known to inhibit CYP2C9 should be done with caution. Significant interactions may occur when celecoxib is administered together with drugs that inhibit CYP2C9).
No products indexed under this heading.

Fluvoxamine Maleate (Celecoxib metabolism is predominantly mediated via cytochrome P450 (CYP) 2C9 in the liver. Co-administration of celecoxib with drugs that are known to inhibit CYP2C9 should be done with caution. Significant interactions may occur when celecoxib is administered together with drugs that inhibit CYP2C9).
No products indexed under this heading.

Fondaparinux Sodium (Other factors that increase the risk of GI bleeding in patients treated with NSAIDs include concomitant use of anticoagulants. Most spontaneous reports of fatal GI events are in elderly or debilitated patients and therefore special care should be taken in treating this population). Products include:

Formoterol Fumarate (In vitro studies indicate that celecoxib, although not a substrate, is an inhibitor of CYP2D6. Therefore, there is a potential for an in vivo drug interaction with drugs that are metabolized by CYP2D6). Products include:

Fosinopril Sodium (Reports suggest that NSAIDs may diminish the antihypertensive effect of Angiotensin Converting Enzyme (ACE) inhibitors. This interaction should be given consideration in patients taking celecoxib concomitantly with ACE inhibitors).
No products indexed under this heading.

Furosemide (Clinical studies, as well as post-marketing observations, have shown that NSAIDs can reduce the natriuretic effect of furosemide and thiazides in some patients. This response

has been attributed to inhibition of renal prostaglandin synthesis). Products include:

Galantamine Hydrobromide (In vitro studies indicate that celecoxib, although not a substrate, is an inhibitor of CYP2D6. Therefore, there is a potential for an in vivo drug interaction with drugs that are metabolized by CYP2D6).
No products indexed under this heading.

Gemfibrozil (Celecoxib metabolism is predominantly mediated via cytochrome P450 (CYP) 2C9 in the liver. Co-administration of celecoxib with drugs that are known to inhibit CYP2C9 should be done with caution. Significant interactions may occur when celecoxib is administered together with drugs that inhibit CYP2C9).
No products indexed under this heading.

Glipizide (Celecoxib metabolism is predominantly mediated via cytochrome P450 (CYP) 2C9 in the liver. Co-administration of celecoxib with drugs that are known to inhibit CYP2C9 should be done with caution. Significant interactions may occur when celecoxib is administered together with drugs that inhibit CYP2C9).
No products indexed under this heading.

Glyburide (Celecoxib metabolism is predominantly mediated via cytochrome P450 (CYP) 2C9 in the liver. Co-administration of celecoxib with drugs that are known to inhibit CYP2C9 should be done with caution. Significant interactions may occur when celecoxib is administered together with drugs that inhibit CYP2C9).
No products indexed under this heading.

Haloperidol (In vitro studies indicate that celecoxib, although not a substrate, is an inhibitor of CYP2D6. Therefore, there is a potential for an in vivo drug interaction with drugs that are metabolized by CYP2D6).
No products indexed under this heading.

Haloperidol Decanoate (In vitro studies indicate that celecoxib, although not a substrate, is an inhibitor of CYP2D6. Therefore, there is a potential for an in vivo drug interaction with drugs that are metabolized by CYP2D6).
No products indexed under this heading.

Heparin Calcium (Other factors that increase the risk of GI bleeding in patients treated with NSAIDs include concomitant use of anticoagulants. Most spontaneous reports of fatal GI events are in elderly or debilitated patients and therefore special care should be taken in treating this population).
No products indexed under this heading.

Heparin Sodium (Other factors that increase the risk of GI bleeding in patients treated with NSAIDs include concomitant use of anticoagulants. Most spontaneous reports of fatal GI events are in elderly or debilitated patients and therefore special care should be taken in treating this population).
No products indexed under this heading.

Hydrochlorothiazide (Patients taking thiazides may have impaired response to these therapies when taking NSAIDs. NSAIDs, including celecoxib, should be used with caution in patients with hypertension. Blood pressure should be monitored closely during the initiation of therapy with celecoxib and throughout the course of therapy). Products include:

Hydrochlorothiazide Hydrochloride (Celecoxib metabolism is predominantly mediated via cytochrome (CYP) 2C9 in the liver. Co-administration of celecoxib with drugs that are known to inhibit CYP2C9 should be done with caution. Significant interactions may occur when celecoxib is administered together with drugs that inhibit CYP2C9).
No products indexed under this heading.

Hydrocodone Bitartrate (In vitro studies indicate that celecoxib, although not a substrate, is an inhibitor of CYP2D6. Therefore, there is a potential for an in vivo drug interaction with drugs that are metabolized by CYP2D6). Products include:

Hydrocortisone (Other factors that increase the risk of GI bleeding in patients treated with NSAIDs include concomitant use of oral corticosteroids. Most spontaneous reports of fatal GI events are in elderly or debilitated patients and therefore special care should be taken in treating this population).
No products indexed under this heading.

Hydrocortisone (Alcohol) (Other factors that increase the risk of GI bleeding in patients treated with NSAIDs include concomitant use of oral corticosteroids. Most spontaneous reports of fatal GI events are in elderly or debilitated patients and therefore special care should be taken in treating this population).
No products indexed under this heading.

Hydrocortisone Acetate (Other factors that increase the risk of GI bleeding in patients treated with NSAIDs include concomitant use of oral corticosteroids. Most spontaneous reports of fatal GI events are in elderly or debilitated patients and therefore special care should be taken in treating this population).
No products indexed under this heading.

Hydrocortisone Butyrate (Other factors that increase the risk of GI bleeding in patients treated with NSAIDs include concomitant use of oral corticosteroids. Most spontaneous reports of fatal GI events are in elderly or debilitated patients and therefore special care should be taken in treating this population).
No products indexed under this heading.

Hydrocortisone Cypionate (Other factors that increase the risk of GI bleeding in patients treated with NSAIDs include concomitant use of oral corticosteroids. Most spontaneous reports of fatal GI events are in elderly or debilitated patients and therefore special care should be taken in treating this population).
No products indexed under this heading.

Hydrocortisone Hemisuccinate (Other factors that increase the risk of GI bleeding in patients treated with NSAIDs include concomitant use of oral corticosteroids. Most spontaneous reports of fatal GI events are in elderly or debilitated patients and therefore special care should be taken in treating this population).
No products indexed under this heading.

Hydrocortisone Probutate (Other factors that increase the risk of GI bleeding in patients treated with NSAIDs include concomitant use of oral corticosteroids. Most spontaneous reports of fatal GI events are in elderly or debilitated patients and therefore special care should be taken in treating this population).
No products indexed under this heading.

Hydrocortisone Sodium Phosphate (Other factors that increase the risk of GI bleeding in patients treated with NSAIDs include concomitant use of oral corticosteroids. Most spontaneous reports of fatal GI events are in elderly or debilitated patients and therefore special care should be taken in treating this population).
No products indexed under this heading.

Hydrocortisone Sodium Succinate (Other factors that increase the risk of GI bleeding in patients treated with NSAIDs include concomitant use of oral corticosteroids. Most spontaneous reports of fatal GI events are in elderly or debilitated patients and therefore special care should be taken in treating this population).
No products indexed under this heading.

Hydrocortisone Valerate (Other factors that increase the risk of GI bleeding in patients treated with NSAIDs include concomitant use of oral corticosteroids. Most spontaneous reports of fatal GI events are in elderly or debilitated patients and therefore special care should be taken in treating this population).
No products indexed under this heading.

Hydroflumethiazide (Patients taking thiazides may have impaired response to these therapies when taking NSAIDs. NSAIDs, including celecoxib, should be used with caution in patients with hypertension. Blood pressure should be monitored closely during the initiation of therapy with celecoxib and throughout the course of therapy).
No products indexed under this heading.

Ibuprofen (The concomitant use of celecoxib with any dose of a non-aspirin NSAID should be avoided due to the potential for increased risk of adverse reactions. Other factors that increase the risk of GI bleeding in patients treated with NSAIDs include concomitant use of longer duration of NSAID therapy. Most spontaneous reports of fatal GI events are in elderly or debilitated patients and therefore special care should be taken in treating this population). Products include:

Imatinib Mesylate (Celecoxib metabolism is predominantly mediated via cytochrome P450 (CYP) 2C9 in the liver. Co-administration of celecoxib with drugs that are known to inhibit CYP2C9 should be done with caution. Significant interactions may occur when celecoxib is administered together with drugs that inhibit CYP2C9). Products include:

Imipramine Hydrochloride (In vitro studies indicate that celecoxib, although not a substrate, is an inhibitor of CYP2D6. Therefore, there is a potential for an in vivo drug interaction with drugs that are metabolized by CYP2D6).
No products indexed under this heading.

Imipramine Pamoate (*In vitro* studies indicate that celecoxib, although not a substrate, is an inhibitor of CYP2D6. Therefore, there is a potential for an *in vivo* drug interaction with drugs that are metabolized by CYP2D6).
No products indexed under this heading.

Indapamide (Renal toxicity has also been seen in patients in whom renal prostaglandins have a compensatory role in the maintenance of renal perfusion. In these patients, administration of an NSAID may cause a dose-dependent reduction in prostaglandin formation and, secondarily, in renal blood flow, which may precipitate overt renal decompensation. Patients at greatest risk of this reaction are those with impaired renal function, heart failure, liver dysfunction, and those taking diuretics). Products include:
Indapamide 2356

Indomethacin (The concomitant use of celecoxib with any dose of a non-aspirin NSAID should be avoided due to the potential for increased risk of adverse reactions. Other factors that increase the risk of GI bleeding in patients treated with NSAIDs include concomitant use of longer duration of NSAID therapy. Most spontaneous reports of fatal GI events are in elderly or debilitated patients and therefore special care should be taken in treating this population). Products include:
Indocin 2167

Indomethacin Sodium Trihydrate (The concomitant use of celecoxib with any dose of a non-aspirin NSAID should be avoided due to the potential for increased risk of adverse reactions. Other factors that increase the risk of GI bleeding in patients treated with NSAIDs include concomitant use of longer duration of NSAID therapy. Most spontaneous reports of fatal GI events are in elderly or debilitated patients and therefore special care should be taken in treating this population). Products include:
Indocin I.V. 2007

Indoramin Hydrochloride (*In vitro* studies indicate that celecoxib, although not a substrate, is an inhibitor of CYP2D6. Therefore, there is a potential for an *in vivo* drug interaction with drugs that are metabolized by CYP2D6).
No products indexed under this heading.

Irbesartan (Reports suggest that NSAIDs may diminish the antihypertensive effect of angiotensin II antagonists. This interaction should be given consideration in patients taking celecoxib concomitantly with angiotensin II antagonists. Patients are at greater risk of renal toxicity when taking angiotensin II receptor antagonists with NSAIDs). Products include:
Avalide 2956
Avapro 2962

Isoniazid (Celecoxib metabolism is predominantly mediated via cytochrome P450 (CYP) 2C9 in the liver. Co-administration of celecoxib with drugs that are known to inhibit CYP2C9 should be done with caution. Significant interactions may occur when celecoxib is administered together with drugs that inhibit CYP2C9).
No products indexed under this heading.

Itraconazole (Celecoxib metabolism is predominantly mediated via cytochrome P450 (CYP) 2C9 in the liver. Co-administration of celecoxib with drugs that are known to inhibit CYP2C9 should be done with caution. Significant interactions may occur when celecoxib is administered together with drugs that inhibit CYP2C9).
No products indexed under this heading.

Ketoconazole (Celecoxib metabolism is predominantly mediated via cytochrome P450 (CYP) 2C9 in the liver. Co-administration of celecoxib with drugs that are known to inhibit CYP2C9 should be done with caution. Significant interactions may occur when celecoxib is administered together with drugs that inhibit CYP2C9). Products include:
Extina 3319
Xolegel 3337

Ketoprofen (The concomitant use of celecoxib with any dose of a non-aspirin NSAID should be avoided due to the potential for increased risk of adverse reactions. Other factors that increase the risk of GI bleeding in patients treated with NSAIDs include concomitant use of longer duration of NSAID therapy. Most spontaneous reports of fatal GI events are in elderly or debilitated patients and therefore special care should be taken in treating this population).
No products indexed under this heading.

Ketorolac Tromethamine (The concomitant use of celecoxib with any dose of a non-aspirin NSAID should be avoided due to the potential for increased risk of adverse reactions. Other factors that increase the risk of GI bleeding in patients treated with NSAIDs include concomitant use of longer duration of NSAID therapy. Most spontaneous reports of fatal GI events are in elderly or debilitated patients and therefore special care should be taken in treating this population). Products include:
Acuvail .... ⊙ 209

Labetalol Hydrochloride (*In vitro* studies indicate that celecoxib, although not a substrate, is an inhibitor of CYP2D6. Therefore, there is a potential for an *in vivo* drug interaction with drugs that are metabolized by CYP2D6).
No products indexed under this heading.

Leflunomide (Celecoxib metabolism is predominantly mediated via cytochrome P450 (CYP) 2C9 in the liver. Co-administration of celecoxib with drugs that are known to inhibit CYP2C9 should be done with caution. Significant interactions may occur when celecoxib is administered together with drugs that inhibit CYP2C9).
No products indexed under this heading.

Lidocaine (*In vitro* studies indicate that celecoxib, although not a substrate, is an inhibitor of CYP2D6. Therefore, there is a potential for an *in vivo* drug interaction with drugs that are metabolized by CYP2D6). Products include:
Lidoderm 1107

Lidocaine Hydrochloride (*In vitro* studies indicate that celecoxib, although not a substrate, is an inhibitor of CYP2D6. Therefore, there is a potential for an *in vivo* drug interaction with drugs that are metabolized by CYP2D6).
No products indexed under this heading.

Lisinopril (Reports suggest that NSAIDs may diminish the antihypertensive effect of Angiotensin Converting Enzyme (ACE) inhibitors. This interaction should be given consideration in patients taking celecoxib concomitantly with ACE inhibitors). Products include:
Prinivil 2241
Prinzide 2246

Lithium (In a study conducted in healthy subjects, mean steady-state lithium plasma levels increased approximately 17% in subjects receiving lithium 450 mg twice daily with celecoxib 200 mg twice daily as compared to subjects receiving lithium alone. Patients on lithium treatment should be closely monitored when celecoxib is introduced or withdrawn).
No products indexed under this heading.

Lithium Carbonate (In a study conducted in healthy subjects, mean steady-state lithium plasma levels increased approximately 17% in subjects receiving lithium 450 mg twice daily with celecoxib 200 mg twice daily as compared to subjects receiving lithium alone. Patients on lithium treatment should be closely monitored when celecoxib is introduced or withdrawn).
No products indexed under this heading.

Lithium Citrate (In a study conducted in healthy subjects, mean steady-state lithium plasma levels increased approximately 17% in subjects receiving lithium 450 mg twice daily with celecoxib 200 mg twice daily as compared to subjects receiving lithium alone. Patients on lithium treatment should be closely monitored when celecoxib is introduced or withdrawn).
No products indexed under this heading.

Losartan Potassium (Reports suggest that NSAIDs may diminish the antihypertensive effect of angiotensin II antagonists. This interaction should be given consideration in patients taking celecoxib concomitantly with angiotensin II antagonists. Patients are at greater risk of renal toxicity when taking angiotensin II receptor antagonists with NSAIDs). Products include:
Cozaar 2106
Hyzaar 2162
Hyzaar 100-12.5 2162

Lovastatin (Celecoxib metabolism is predominantly mediated via cytochrome P450 (CYP) 2C9 in the liver. Co-administration of celecoxib with drugs that are known to inhibit CYP2C9 should be done with caution. Significant interactions may occur when celecoxib is administered together with drugs that inhibit CYP2C9). Products include:
Advicor 402
Mevacor 2212

Low Molecular Weight Heparins (Other factors that increase the risk of GI bleeding in patients treated with NSAIDs include concomitant use of anticoagulants. Most spontaneous reports of fatal GI events are in elderly or debilitated patients and therefore special care should be taken in treating this population).
No products indexed under this heading.

Magaldrate (Co-administration of celecoxib with aluminum- and magnesium-containing antacids resulted in a reduction in plasma celecoxib concentrations with a decrease of 37% in C_{max} and 10% in AUC. Higher doses (400 mg twice daily) should be administered with food to improve absorption).
No products indexed under this heading.

Magnesium Carbonate (Co-administration of celecoxib with aluminum- and magnesium-containing antacids resulted in a reduction in plasma celecoxib concentrations with a decrease of 37% in C_{max} and 10% in AUC. Higher doses (400 mg twice daily) should be administered with food to improve absorption).
No products indexed under this heading.

Magnesium Hydroxide (Co-administration of celecoxib with aluminum- and magnesium-containing antacids resulted in a reduction in plasma celecoxib concentrations with a decrease of 37% in C_{max} and 10% in AUC. Higher doses (400 mg twice daily) should be administered with food to improve absorption). Products include:
Fleet Pedia-Lax Chewable Tablets 1144
Pepcid Complete 1822

Magnesium Oxide (Co-administration of celecoxib with aluminum- and magnesium-containing antacids resulted in a reduction in plasma celecoxib concentrations with a decrease of 37% in C_{max} and 10% in AUC. Higher doses (400 mg twice daily) should be administered with food to improve absorption). Products include:
Beelith 873

Magnesium Trisilicate (Co-administration of celecoxib with aluminum- and magnesium-containing antacids resulted in a reduction in plasma celecoxib concentrations with a decrease of 37% in C_{max} and 10% in AUC. Higher doses (400 mg twice daily) should be administered with food to improve absorption).
No products indexed under this heading.

Maprotiline Hydrochloride (*In vitro* studies indicate that celecoxib, although not a substrate, is an inhibitor of CYP2D6. Therefore, there is a potential for an *in vivo* drug interaction with drugs that are metabolized by CYP2D6).
No products indexed under this heading.

Meclofenamate Sodium (The concomitant use of celecoxib with any dose of a non-aspirin NSAID should be avoided due to the potential for increased risk of adverse reactions. Other factors that increase the risk of GI bleeding in patients treated with NSAIDs include concomitant use of longer duration of NSAID therapy. Most spontaneous reports of fatal GI events are in elderly or debilitated patients and therefore special care should be taken in treating this population).
No products indexed under this heading.

Mefenamic Acid (The concomitant use of celecoxib with any dose of a non-aspirin NSAID should be avoided due to the potential for increased risk of adverse reactions. Other factors that increase the risk of GI bleeding in patients treated with NSAIDs include concomitant use of longer duration of NSAID therapy. Most spontaneous reports of fatal GI events are in elderly or debilitated patients and therefore special care should be taken in treating this population).
No products indexed under this heading.

Meloxicam (The concomitant use of celecoxib with any dose of a non-aspirin NSAID should be avoided due to the potential for increased risk of adverse reactions. Other factors that increase the risk of GI bleeding in patients treated with NSAIDs include concomitant use of longer duration of NSAID therapy. Most spontaneous reports of fatal GI events are in elderly or debilitated patients and therefore special care should be taken in treating this population).
No products indexed under this heading.

Meperidine Hydrochloride (*In vitro* studies indicate that celecoxib, although not a substrate, is an inhibitor of CYP2D6. Therefore, there is a potential for an *in vivo* drug interaction with drugs that are metabolized by CYP2D6).
No products indexed under this heading.

Methadone Hydrochloride (*In vitro* studies indicate that celecoxib, although not a substrate, is an inhibitor of CYP2D6. Therefore, there is a potential for an *in vivo* drug interaction with drugs that are metabolized by CYP2D6).
No products indexed under this heading.

Methamphetamine Hydrochloride (*In vitro* studies indicate that celecoxib, although not a substrate, is an inhibitor of CYP2D6. Therefore, there is a potential for an *in vivo* drug interaction with drugs that are metabolized by CYP2D6).
No products indexed under this heading.

IMPORTANT NOTE: Always consult each drug listing in the patient's regimen for possible interactions.

inhibit CYP2C9 should be done with caution. Significant interactions may occur when celecoxib is administered together with drugs that inhibit CYP2C9). Products include:

Paroxetine CR **2361**
Paroxetine ER **2371**
Paxil **1586**
Paxil CR **1596**

Perindopril Erbumine (Reports suggest that NSAIDs may diminish the antihypertensive effect of Angiotensin Converting Enzyme (ACE) inhibitors. This interaction should be given consideration in patients taking celecoxib concomitantly with ACE inhibitors).
No products indexed under this heading.

Phenylbutazone (The concomitant use of celecoxib with any dose of a non-aspirin NSAID should be avoided due to the potential for increased risk of adverse reactions. Other factors that increase the risk of GI bleeding in patients treated with NSAIDs include concomitant use of longer duration of NSAID therapy. Most spontaneous reports of fatal GI events are in elderly or debilitated patients and therefore special care should be taken in treating this population).
No products indexed under this heading.

Pindolol (*In vitro* studies indicate that celecoxib, although not a substrate, is an inhibitor of CYP2D6. Therefore, there is a potential for an *in vivo* drug interaction with drugs that are metabolized by CYP2D6).
No products indexed under this heading.

Piroxicam (The concomitant use of celecoxib with any dose of a non-aspirin NSAID should be avoided due to the potential for increased risk of adverse reactions. Other factors that increase the risk of GI bleeding in patients treated with NSAIDs include concomitant use of longer duration of NSAID therapy. Most spontaneous reports of fatal GI events are in elderly or debilitated patients and therefore special care should be taken in treating this population).
No products indexed under this heading.

Polythiazide (Patients taking thiazides may have impaired response to these therapies when taking NSAIDs. NSAIDs, including celecoxib, should be used with caution in patients with hypertension. Blood pressure should be monitored closely during the initiation of therapy with celecoxib and throughout the course of therapy).
No products indexed under this heading.

Prednisolone (Other factors that increase the risk of GI bleeding in patients treated with NSAIDs include concomitant use of oral corticosteroids. Most spontaneous reports of fatal GI events are in elderly or debilitated patients and therefore special care should be taken in treating this population).
No products indexed under this heading.

Prednisolone Acetate (Other factors that increase the risk of GI bleeding in patients treated with NSAIDs include concomitant use of oral corticosteroids. Most spontaneous reports of fatal GI events are in elderly or debilitated patients and therefore special care should be taken in treating this population). Products include:

Blephamide .... ⊙**212**, ⊙**214**
Pred Forte .... ⊙**225**
Pred Mild .... ⊙**230**
Pred-G .... ⊙**226**, ⊙**227**

Prednisolone Sodium Phosphate (Other factors that increase the risk of GI bleeding in patients treated with NSAIDs include concomitant use of oral corticosteroids. Most spontaneous reports of fatal GI events are in elderly or debilitated patients and therefore special care should be taken in treating this population).
No products indexed under this heading.

Prednisolone Tebutate (Other factors that increase the risk of GI bleeding in patients treated with NSAIDs include concomitant use of oral corticosteroids. Most spontaneous reports of fatal GI events are in elderly or debilitated patients and therefore special care should be taken in treating this population).
No products indexed under this heading.

Prednisone (Other factors that increase the risk of GI bleeding in patients treated with NSAIDs include concomitant use of oral corticosteroids. Most spontaneous reports of fatal GI events are in elderly or debilitated patients and therefore special care should be taken in treating this population).
No products indexed under this heading.

Prednisone sodium phosphate (Other factors that increase the risk of GI bleeding in patients treated with NSAIDs include concomitant use of oral corticosteroids. Most spontaneous reports of fatal GI events are in elderly or debilitated patients and therefore special care should be taken in treating this population).
No products indexed under this heading.

Propafenone Hydrochloride (*In vitro* studies indicate that celecoxib, although not a substrate, is an inhibitor of CYP2D6. Therefore, there is a potential for an *in vivo* drug interaction with drugs that are metabolized by CYP2D6). Products include:

Rythmol **1648**
Rythmol SR **1652**

Propoxyphene Hydrochloride (*In vitro* studies indicate that celecoxib, although not a substrate, is an inhibitor of CYP2D6. Therefore, there is a potential for an *in vivo* drug interaction with drugs that are metabolized by CYP2D6).
No products indexed under this heading.

Propoxyphene Napsylate (*In vitro* studies indicate that celecoxib, although not a substrate, is an inhibitor of CYP2D6. Therefore, there is a potential for an *in vivo* drug interaction with drugs that are metabolized by CYP2D6).
No products indexed under this heading.

Propranolol Hydrochloride (*In vitro* studies indicate that celecoxib, although not a substrate, is an inhibitor of CYP2D6. Therefore, there is a potential for an *in vivo* drug interaction with drugs that are metabolized by CYP2D6). Products include:

InnoPran XL **1517**

Quetiapine Fumarate (*In vitro* studies indicate that celecoxib, although not a substrate, is an inhibitor of CYP2D6. Therefore, there is a potential for an *in vivo* drug interaction with drugs that are metabolized by CYP2D6). Products include:

Seroquel **750**
Seroquel XR **759**

Quinapril Hydrochloride (Reports suggest that NSAIDs may diminish the antihypertensive effect of Angiotensin Converting Enzyme (ACE) inhibitors. This interaction should be given consideration in patients taking celecoxib concomitantly with ACE inhibitors).
No products indexed under this heading.

Quinidine Gluconate (*In vitro* studies indicate that celecoxib, although not a substrate, is an inhibitor of CYP2D6. Therefore, there is a potential for an *in vivo* drug interaction with drugs that are metabolized by CYP2D6).
No products indexed under this heading.

Quinidine Hydrochloride (*In vitro* studies indicate that celecoxib, although not a substrate, is an inhibitor of CYP2D6. Therefore, there is a potential for an *in vivo* drug interaction with drugs that are metabolized by CYP2D6).
No products indexed under this heading.

Quinidine Polygalacturonate (*In vitro* studies indicate that celecoxib, although not a substrate, is an inhibitor of CYP2D6. Therefore, there is a potential for an *in vivo* drug interaction with drugs that are metabolized by CYP2D6).
No products indexed under this heading.

Quinidine Sulfate (*In vitro* studies indicate that celecoxib, although not a substrate, is an inhibitor of CYP2D6. Therefore, there is a potential for an *in vivo* drug interaction with drugs that are metabolized by CYP2D6).
No products indexed under this heading.

Ramipril (Reports suggest that NSAIDs may diminish the antihypertensive effect of Angiotensin Converting Enzyme (ACE) inhibitors. This interaction should be given consideration in patients taking celecoxib concomitantly with ACE inhibitors).
No products indexed under this heading.

Risperidone (*In vitro* studies indicate that celecoxib, although not a substrate, is an inhibitor of CYP2D6. Therefore, there is a potential for an *in vivo* drug interaction with drugs that are metabolized by CYP2D6). Products include:

Risperdal Consta **2682**

Ritonavir (Celecoxib metabolism is predominantly mediated via cytochrome P450 (CYP) 2C9 in the liver. Co-administration of celecoxib with drugs that are known to inhibit CYP2C9 should be done with caution. Significant interactions may occur when celecoxib is administered together with drugs that inhibit CYP2C9). Products include:

Kaletra **458**
Norvir **509**

Rofecoxib (The concomitant use of celecoxib with any dose of a non-aspirin NSAID should be avoided due to the potential for increased risk of adverse reactions. Other factors that increase the risk of GI bleeding in patients treated with NSAIDs include concomitant use of longer duration of NSAID therapy. Most spontaneous reports of fatal GI events are in elderly or debilitated patients and therefore special care should be taken in treating this population).
No products indexed under this heading.

Sertraline Hydrochloride (Celecoxib metabolism is predominantly mediated via cytochrome P450 (CYP) 2C9 in the liver. Co-administration of celecoxib with drugs that are known to inhibit CYP2C9 should be done with caution. Significant interactions may occur when celecoxib is administered together with drugs that inhibit CYP2C9).
No products indexed under this heading.

Sildenafil Citrate (Celecoxib metabolism is predominantly mediated via cytochrome P450 (CYP) 2C9 in the liver. Co-administration of celecoxib with drugs that are known to inhibit CYP2C9 should be done with caution. Significant interactions may occur when celecoxib is administered together with drugs that inhibit CYP2C9).
No products indexed under this heading.

Spirapril Hydrochloride (Reports suggest that NSAIDs may diminish the antihypertensive effect of Angiotensin Converting Enzyme (ACE) inhibitors. This interaction should be given consideration in patients taking celecoxib concomitantly with ACE inhibitors).
No products indexed under this heading.

Spironolactone (Renal toxicity has also been seen in patients in whom renal prostaglandins have a compensatory role in the maintenance of renal perfusion. In these patients, administration of an NSAID may cause a dose-dependent reduction in prostaglandin formation and, secondarily, in renal blood flow, which may precipitate overt renal decompensation. Patients at greatest risk of this reaction are those with impaired renal function, heart failure, liver dysfunction, and those taking diuretics).
No products indexed under this heading.

Sulfacytine (Celecoxib metabolism is predominantly mediated via cytochrome P450 (CYP) 2C9 in the liver. Co-administration of celecoxib with drugs that are known to inhibit CYP2C9 should be done with caution. Significant interactions may occur when celecoxib is administered together with drugs that inhibit CYP2C9).
No products indexed under this heading.

Sulfamethizole (Celecoxib metabolism is predominantly mediated via cytochrome P450 (CYP) 2C9 in the liver. Co-administration of celecoxib with drugs that are known to inhibit CYP2C9 should be done with caution. Significant interactions may occur when celecoxib is administered together with drugs that inhibit CYP2C9).
No products indexed under this heading.

Sulfamethoxazole (Celecoxib metabolism is predominantly mediated via cytochrome P450 (CYP) 2C9 in the liver. Co-administration of celecoxib with drugs that are known to inhibit CYP2C9 should be done with caution. Significant interactions may occur when celecoxib is administered together with drugs that inhibit CYP2C9).
No products indexed under this heading.

Sulfasalazine (Celecoxib metabolism is predominantly mediated via cytochrome P450 (CYP) 2C9 in the liver. Co-administration of celecoxib with drugs that are known to inhibit CYP2C9 should be done with caution. Significant interactions may occur when celecoxib is administered together with drugs that inhibit CYP2C9).
No products indexed under this heading.

Sulfinpyrazone (Celecoxib metabolism is predominantly mediated via cytochrome P450 (CYP) 2C9 in the liver. Co-administration of celecoxib with drugs that are known to inhibit CYP2C9 should be done with caution. Significant interactions may occur when celecoxib is administered together with drugs that inhibit CYP2C9).
No products indexed under this heading.

Sulfisoxazole Acetyl (Celecoxib metabolism is predominantly mediated via cytochrome P450 (CYP) 2C9 in the liver. Co-administration of celecoxib with drugs that are known to inhibit CYP2C9 should be done with caution. Significant interactions may occur when celecoxib is administered together with drugs that inhibit CYP2C9).
No products indexed under this heading.

Sulfisoxazole Diolamine (Celecoxib metabolism is predominantly mediated via cytochrome P450 (CYP) 2C9 in the liver. Co-administration of celecoxib with drugs that are known to inhibit CYP2C9 should be done with caution. Significant interactions may occur when celecoxib is administered together with drugs that inhibit CYP2C9).
No products indexed under this heading.

Sulindac (The concomitant use of celecoxib with any dose of a non-aspirin NSAID should be avoided due to the potential for increased risk of adverse reactions. Other factors that increase the risk of GI bleeding in patients treated with NSAIDs include concomitant use of longer duration of NSAID therapy. Most spontaneous reports of fatal GI events are in elderly or debilitated patients and therefore special care should be taken in treating this population). Products include:
Clinoril 2098

Tamoxifen Citrate (In vitro studies indicate that celecoxib, although not a substrate, is an inhibitor of CYP2D6. Therefore, there is a potential for an in vivo drug interaction with drugs that are metabolized by CYP2D6).
No products indexed under this heading.

Telmisartan (Reports suggest that NSAIDs may diminish the antihypertensive effect of angiotensin II antagonists. This interaction should be given consideration in patients taking celecoxib concomitantly with angiotensin II antagonists. Patients are at greater risk of renal toxicity when taking angiotensin II receptor antagonists with NSAIDs). Products include:
Micardis 887
Micardis HCT 889

Teniposide (In vitro studies indicate that celecoxib, although not a substrate, is an inhibitor of CYP2D6. Therefore, there is a potential for an in vivo drug interaction with drugs that are metabolized by CYP2D6).
No products indexed under this heading.

Terconazole (Celecoxib metabolism is predominantly mediated via cytochrome P450 (CYP) 2C9 in the liver. Co-administration of celecoxib with drugs that are known to inhibit CYP2C9 should be done with caution. Significant interactions may occur when celecoxib is administered together with drugs that inhibit CYP2C9).
No products indexed under this heading.

Testosterone (In vitro studies indicate that celecoxib, although not a substrate, is an inhibitor of CYP2D6. Therefore, there is a potential for an in vivo drug interaction with drugs that are metabolized by CYP2D6). Products include:
AndroGel 3456

Testosterone Cypionate (In vitro studies indicate that celecoxib, although not a substrate, is an inhibitor of CYP2D6. Therefore, there is a potential for an in vivo drug interaction with drugs that are metabolized by CYP2D6).
No products indexed under this heading.

Testosterone Enanthate (In vitro studies indicate that celecoxib, although not a substrate, is an inhibitor of CYP2D6. Therefore, there is a potential for an in vivo drug interaction with drugs that are metabolized by CYP2D6). Products include:
Delatestryl 1102

Testosterone Propionate (In vitro studies indicate that celecoxib, although not a substrate, is an inhibitor of CYP2D6. Therefore, there is a potential for an in vivo drug interaction with drugs that are metabolized by CYP2D6).
No products indexed under this heading.

Thioridazine (In vitro studies indicate that celecoxib, although not a substrate, is an inhibitor of CYP2D6. Therefore, there is a potential for an in vivo drug interaction with drugs that are metabolized by CYP2D6).
No products indexed under this heading.

Thioridazine Hydrochloride (In vitro studies indicate that celecoxib, although not a substrate, is an inhibitor of CYP2D6. Therefore, there is a potential for an in vivo drug interaction with drugs that are metabolized by CYP2D6). Products include:
Thioridazine Hydrochloride 2384

Ticlopidine Hydrochloride (Celecoxib metabolism is predominantly mediated via cytochrome P450 (CYP) 2C9 in the liver. Co-administration of celecoxib with drugs that are known to inhibit CYP2C9 should be done with caution. Significant interactions may occur when celecoxib is administered together with drugs that inhibit CYP2C9).
No products indexed under this heading.

Timolol Maleate (In vitro studies indicate that celecoxib, although not a substrate, is an inhibitor of CYP2D6. Therefore, there is a potential for an in vivo drug interaction with drugs that are metabolized by CYP2D6). Products include:
Combigan 601
Dorzolamide
Hydrochloride/Timolol Maleate
Ophthalmic Solution .... ⊙243
Timoptic in Ocudose .... ⊙231

Tinzaparin Sodium (Other factors that increase the risk of GI bleeding in patients treated with NSAIDs include concomitant use of anticoagulants. Most spontaneous reports of fatal GI events are in elderly or debilitated patients and therefore special care should be taken in treating this population).
No products indexed under this heading.

Tobacco (Other factors that increase the risk of GI bleeding in patients treated with NSAIDs include concomitant use of tobacco. Most spontaneous reports of fatal GI events are in elderly or debilitated patients and therefore special care should be taken in treating this population).
No products indexed under this heading.

Tolazamide (Celecoxib metabolism is predominantly mediated via cytochrome P450 (CYP) 2C9 in the liver. Co-administration of celecoxib with drugs that are known to inhibit CYP2C9 should be done with caution. Significant interactions may occur when celecoxib is administered together with drugs that inhibit CYP2C9).
No products indexed under this heading.

Tolbutamide (Celecoxib metabolism is predominantly mediated via cytochrome P450 (CYP) 2C9 in the liver. Co-administration of celecoxib with drugs that are known to inhibit CYP2C9 should be done with caution. Significant interactions may occur when celecoxib is administered together with drugs that inhibit CYP2C9).
No products indexed under this heading.

Tolbutamide Sodium (Celecoxib metabolism is predominantly mediated via cytochrome P450 (CYP) 2C9 in the liver. Co-administration of celecoxib with drugs that are known to inhibit CYP2C9 should be done with caution. Significant interactions may occur when celecoxib is administered together with drugs that inhibit CYP2C9).
No products indexed under this heading.

Tolmetin Sodium (The concomitant use of celecoxib with any dose of a non-aspirin NSAID should be avoided due to the potential for increased risk of adverse reactions. Other factors that increase the risk of GI bleeding in patients treated with NSAIDs include concomitant use of longer duration of NSAID therapy. Most spontaneous reports of fatal GI events are in elderly or debilitated patients and therefore special care should be taken in treating this population).
No products indexed under this heading.

Tolterodine Tartrate (In vitro studies indicate that celecoxib, although not a substrate, is an inhibitor of CYP2D6. Therefore, there is a potential for an in vivo drug interaction with drugs that are metabolized by CYP2D6).
No products indexed under this heading.

Torsemide (Patients taking thiazides or loop diuretics may have impaired response to these therapies when taking NSAIDs. NSAIDs, including celecoxib, should be used with caution in patients with hypertension. Blood pressure should be monitored closely during the initiation of therapy with celecoxib and throughout the course of therapy).
No products indexed under this heading.

Tramadol Hydrochloride (In vitro studies indicate that celecoxib, although not a substrate, is an inhibitor of CYP2D6. Therefore, there is a potential for an in vivo drug interaction with drugs that are metabolized by CYP2D6). Products include:
Ryzolt 2813
Ultram ER 2693

Trandolapril (Reports suggest that NSAIDs may diminish the antihypertensive effect of Angiotensin Converting Enzyme (ACE) inhibitors. This interaction should be given consideration in patients taking celecoxib concomitantly with ACE inhibitors). Products include:
Mavik 489
Tarka 534

Trazodone Hydrochloride (In vitro studies indicate that celecoxib, although not a substrate, is an inhibitor of CYP2D6. Therefore, there is a potential for an in vivo drug interaction with drugs that are metabolized by CYP2D6).
No products indexed under this heading.

Triamcinolone (Other factors that increase the risk of GI bleeding in patients treated with NSAIDs include concomitant use of oral corticosteroids. Most spontaneous reports of fatal GI events are in elderly or debilitated patients and therefore special care should be taken in treating this population).
No products indexed under this heading.

Triamcinolone Acetonide (Other factors that increase the risk of GI bleeding in patients treated with NSAIDs include concomitant use of oral corticosteroids. Most spontaneous reports of fatal GI events are in elderly or debilitated patients and therefore special care should be taken in treating this population). Products include:
Azmacort 408
Nasacort AQ 3019

Triamcinolone Diacetate (Other factors that increase the risk of GI bleeding in patients treated with NSAIDs include concomitant use of oral corticosteroids. Most spontaneous reports of fatal GI events are in elderly or debilitated patients and therefore special care should be taken in treating this population).
No products indexed under this heading.

Triamcinolone Hexacetonide (Other factors that increase the risk of GI bleeding in patients treated with NSAIDs include concomitant use of oral corticosteroids. Most spontaneous reports of fatal GI events are in elderly or debilitated patients and therefore special care should be taken in treating this population).
No products indexed under this heading.

Triamterene (Renal toxicity has also been seen in patients in whom renal prostaglandins have a compensatory role in the maintenance of renal perfusion. In these patients, administration of an NSAID may cause a dose-dependent reduction in prostaglandin formation and, secondarily, in renal blood flow, which may precipitate overt renal decompensation. Patients at greatest risk of this reaction are those with impaired renal function, heart failure, liver dysfunction, and those taking diuretics). Products include:
Dyazide 1429
Dyrenium 3495

Triazolam (In vitro studies indicate that celecoxib, although not a substrate, is an inhibitor of CYP2D6. Therefore, there is a potential for an in vivo drug interaction with drugs that are metabolized by CYP2D6).
No products indexed under this heading.

Trimipramine Maleate (In vitro studies indicate that celecoxib, although not a substrate, is an inhibitor of CYP2D6. Therefore, there is a potential for an in vivo drug interaction with drugs that are metabolized by CYP2D6).
No products indexed under this heading.

Troglitazone (Celecoxib metabolism is predominantly mediated via cytochrome P450 (CYP) 2C9 in the liver. Co-administration of celecoxib with drugs that are known to inhibit CYP2C9 should be done with caution. Significant interactions may occur when celecoxib is administered together with drugs that inhibit CYP2C9).
No products indexed under this heading.

Valdecoxib (The concomitant use of celecoxib with any dose of a non-aspirin NSAID should be avoided due to the potential for increased risk of adverse reactions. Other factors that increase the risk of GI bleeding in patients treated with NSAIDs include concomitant use of longer duration of NSAID therapy. Most spontaneous reports of fatal GI events are in elderly or debilitated patients and therefore special care should be taken in treating this population).
No products indexed under this heading.

Valsartan (Reports suggest that NSAIDs may diminish the antihypertensive effect of angiotensin II antagonists. This interaction should be given consideration in patients taking celecoxib concomitantly with angiotensin II antagonists. Patients are at greater risk of renal toxicity when taking angiotensin II receptor antagonists with NSAIDs). Products include:
Diovan 2413
Diovan HCT 2419
Exforge 2443
Exforge HCT 2449
Valturna 3637

Vardenafil Hydrochloride (Celecoxib metabolism is predominantly mediated via cytochrome P450 (CYP) 2C9 in the liver. Co-administration of celecoxib with drugs that are known to inhibit CYP2C9 should be done with caution. Significant interactions may occur when celecoxib is administered together with drugs that inhibit CYP2C9). Products include:
Levitra 3157

Venlafaxine Hydrochloride (In vitro studies indicate that celecoxib, although

not a substrate, is an inhibitor of CYP2D6. Therefore, there is a potential for an *in vivo* drug interaction with drugs that are metabolized by CYP2D6). Products include:
Effexor XR **3504**
Venlafaxine Hydrochloride Tablets ... **2388**

Vinblastine Sulfate (*In vitro* studies indicate that celecoxib, although not a substrate, is an inhibitor of CYP2D6. Therefore, there is a potential for an *in vivo* drug interaction with drugs that are metabolized by CYP2D6).
No products indexed under this heading.

Voriconazole (Celecoxib metabolism is predominantly mediated via cytochrome P450 (CYP) 2C9 in the liver. Co-administration of celecoxib with drugs that are known to inhibit CYP2C9 should be done with caution. Significant interactions may occur when celecoxib is administered together with drugs that inhibit CYP2C9).
No products indexed under this heading.

Warfarin Sodium (Anticoagulant activity should be monitored, particularly in the first few days, after initiating or changing celecoxib therapy in patients receiving warfarin or similar agents, since these patients are at an increased risk of bleeding complications. The effect of celecoxib on the anticoagulant effect of warfarin was studied in a group of healthy subjects receiving daily 2-5 mg doses of warfarin. In these subjects, celecoxib did not alter the anticoagulant effect of warfarin as determined by prothrombin time. However, in postmarketing experience, serious bleeding events, some of which were fatal, have been reported, predominantly in the elderly, in association with increases in prothrombin time in patients receiving celecoxib concurrently with warfarin).
No products indexed under this heading.

Zafirlukast (Celecoxib metabolism is predominantly mediated via cytochrome P450 (CYP) 2C9 in the liver. Co-administration of celecoxib with drugs that are known to inhibit CYP2C9 should be done with caution. Significant interactions may occur when celecoxib is administered together with drugs that inhibit CYP2C9). Products include:
Accolate **3612**

Zonisamide (*In vitro* studies indicate that celecoxib, although not a substrate, is an inhibitor of CYP2D6. Therefore, there is a potential for an *in vivo* drug interaction with drugs that are metabolized by CYP2D6). Products include:
Zonegran **1081**

Food Interactions

Alcohol (Other factors that increase the risk of GI bleeding in patients treated with NSAIDs include concomitant use of alcohol. Most spontaneous reports of fatal GI events are in elderly or debilitated patients and therefore special care should be taken in treating this population).

Beer, reduced-alcohol (Other factors that increase the risk of GI bleeding in patients treated with NSAIDs include concomitant use of alcohol. Most spontaneous reports of fatal GI events are in elderly or debilitated patients and therefore special care should be taken in treating this population).

Beer, unspecified (Other factors that increase the risk of GI bleeding in patients treated with NSAIDs include concomitant use of alcohol. Most spontaneous reports of fatal GI events are in elderly or debilitated patients and therefore special care should be taken in treating this population).

Food, unspecified (When celecoxib capsules were taken with a high fat meal, peak plasma levels were delayed for about 1 to 2 hours with an increase in total absorption (AUC) of 10% to 20%. Under fasting conditions, at doses above 200 mg, there is less than a proportional increase in C_{max} and AUC, which is thought to be due to the low solubility of the drug in aqueous media. Celecoxib, at doses up to 200 mg twice daily, can be administered without regard to timing of meals. Higher doses (400 mg twice daily) should be administered with food to improve absorption).

Meal, unspecified (When celecoxib capsules were taken with a high fat meal, peak plasma levels were delayed for about 1 to 2 hours with an increase in total absorption (AUC) of 10% to 20%. Under fasting conditions, at doses above 200 mg, there is less than a proportional increase in C_{max} and AUC, which is thought to be due to the low solubility of the drug in aqueous media. Celecoxib, at doses up to 200 mg twice daily, can be administered without regard to timing of meals. Higher doses (400 mg twice daily) should be administered with food to improve absorption).

Wine, Chianti (Other factors that increase the risk of GI bleeding in patients treated with NSAIDs include concomitant use of alcohol. Most spontaneous reports of fatal GI events are in elderly or debilitated patients and therefore special care should be taken in treating this population).

Wine, Red (Other factors that increase the risk of GI bleeding in patients treated with NSAIDs include concomitant use of alcohol. Most spontaneous reports of fatal GI events are in elderly or debilitated patients and therefore special care should be taken in treating this population).

Wine, unspecified (Other factors that increase the risk of GI bleeding in patients treated with NSAIDs include concomitant use of alcohol. Most spontaneous reports of fatal GI events are in elderly or debilitated patients and therefore special care should be taken in treating this population).

Wine products (Other factors that increase the risk of GI bleeding in patients treated with NSAIDs include concomitant use of alcohol. Most spontaneous reports of fatal GI events are in elderly or debilitated patients and therefore special care should be taken in treating this population).

CELEXA ORAL SOLUTION

(Citalopram Hydrobromide) **1153**
See See Celexa Tablets

CELEXA TABLETS

(Citalopram Hydrobromide) **1153**
May interact with alcohols, anticoagulants, antipsychotic agents, aspirin-acetylsalicylic acid, central nervous system depressants, central nervous system stimulants, cytochrome p450 2c19 inhibitors (selected), cytochrome p450 3a4 inhibitors (selected), cytochrome p450 3a4 inhibitors, potent (selected), diuretics, dopamine antagonists, lithium preparations, macrolide antibiotics, monoamine oxidase inhibitors, non-steroidal anti-inflammatory agents, serotonin and norepinephrine reuptake inhibitors, serotoninergic agents, tricyclic antidepressants, triptans, and certain other agents. Compounds in these categories include:

Acetazolamide (*In vitro* studies indicated that CYP3A4 and CYP2C19 are the primary enzymes involved in the metabolism of citalopram. However, co-administration of citalopram (40 mg) and ketoconazole (200 mg), a potent inhibitor of CYP3A4, did not significantly affect the pharmacokinetics of citalopram. Because citalopram is metabolized by multiple enzyme systems, inhibition of a single enzyme may not appreciably decrease citalopram clearance).
No products indexed under this heading.

Acetazolamide Sodium (*In vitro* studies indicated that CYP3A4 and CYP2C19 are the primary enzymes involved in the metabolism of citalopram. However, co-administration of citalopram (40 mg) and ketoconazole (200 mg), a potent inhibitor of CYP3A4, did not significantly affect the pharmacokinetics of citalopram. Because citalopram is metabolized by multiple enzyme systems, inhibition of a single enzyme may not appreciably decrease citalopram clearance).
No products indexed under this heading.

Alfentanil Hydrochloride (Given the primary CNS effects of citalopram, caution should be used when it is taken in combination with other centrally acting drugs).
No products indexed under this heading.

Almotriptan Malate (The development of potentially life threatening serotonin syndrome or Neuroleptic Malignant syndrome (NMS)-like reactions have been reported with citalopram alone, but particularly with concomitant use of serotonergic drugs including triptans. Serotonin syndrome, in its most severe form can resemble neuroleptic malignant syndrome. Patients should be monitored for the emergence of serotonin syndrome or NMS-like signs and symptoms. If concomitant treatment of citalopram with a triptan is clinically warranted, careful observation of the patient is advised, particularly during treatment initiation and dose increases). Products include:
Axert **2593**

Alprazolam (Given the primary CNS effects of citalopram, caution should be used when it is taken in combination with other centrally acting drugs).
No products indexed under this heading.

Amiloride Hydrochloride (Hyponatremia may occur as a result of treatment with SSRIs including citalopram. Patients taking diuretics may be at greater risk. Discontinuation of citalopram should be considered in patients with symptomatic hyponatremia and appropriate medical intervention should be instituted).
No products indexed under this heading.

Amiodarone Hydrochloride (*In vitro* studies indicated that CYP3A4 and CYP2C19 are the primary enzymes involved in the metabolism of citalopram. However, co-administration of citalopram (40 mg) and ketoconazole (200 mg), a potent inhibitor of CYP3A4, did not significantly affect the pharmacokinetics of citalopram. Because citalopram is metabolized by multiple enzyme systems, inhibition of a single enzyme may not appreciably decrease citalopram clearance).
No products indexed under this heading.

Amitriptyline Hydrochloride (Co-administration of imipramine with citalopram has resulted in a 50% increase in active metabolite, desipramine concentration. The clinical significance of this finding is unknown. Caution is indicated if tricyclic antidepressants are co-administered with citalopram).
No products indexed under this heading.

Amobarbital (Given the primary CNS effects of citalopram, caution should be used when it is taken in combination with other centrally acting drugs).
No products indexed under this heading.

Amobarbital Sodium (Given the primary CNS effects of citalopram, caution should be used when it is taken in combination with other centrally acting drugs).
No products indexed under this heading.

Amoxapine (Co-administration of imipramine with citalopram has resulted in a 50% increase in active metabolite, desipramine concentration. The clinical significance of this finding is unknown. Caution is indicated if tricyclic antidepressants are co-administered with citalopram).
No products indexed under this heading.

Amphetamine Aspartate (Given the primary CNS effects of citalopram, caution should be used when it is taken in combination with other centrally acting drugs).
No products indexed under this heading.

Amphetamine Aspartate Monohydrate (Given the primary CNS effects of citalopram, caution should be used when it is taken in combination with other centrally acting drugs).
No products indexed under this heading.

Amphetamine Resins (Given the primary CNS effects of citalopram, caution should be used when it is taken in combination with other centrally acting drugs).
No products indexed under this heading.

Amphetamine Sulfate (Given the primary CNS effects of citalopram, caution should be used when it is taken in combination with other centrally acting drugs).
No products indexed under this heading.

Amprenavir (*In vitro* studies indicated that CYP3A4 and CYP2C19 are the primary enzymes involved in the metabolism of citalopram. However, co-administration of citalopram (40 mg) and ketoconazole (200 mg), a potent inhibitor of CYP3A4, did not significantly affect the pharmacokinetics of citalopram. Because citalopram is metabolized by multiple enzyme systems, inhibition of a single enzyme may not appreciably decrease citalopram clearance).
No products indexed under this heading.

Anastrozole (*In vitro* studies indicated that CYP3A4 and CYP2C19 are the primary enzymes involved in the metabolism of citalopram. However, co-administration of citalopram (40 mg) and ketoconazole (200 mg), a potent inhibitor of CYP3A4, did not significantly affect the pharmacokinetics of citalopram. Because citalopram is metabolized by multiple enzyme systems, inhibition of a single enzyme may not appreciably decrease citalopram clearance).
No products indexed under this heading.

Anisindione (Citalopram may increase the risk of bleeding events. Concomitant use of anticoagulants may add to the risk. Case reports and studies have demonstrated an association between use of drugs that interfere with serotonin reuptake and the occurrence of gastrointestinal bleeding. Patients should be cautioned about the risk of bleeding associated with the concomitant use of citalopram and drugs affecting coagulation).
No products indexed under this heading.

Aprepitant (*In vitro* studies indicated that CYP3A4 and CYP2C19 are the primary enzymes involved in the metabolism of citalopram. However, co-administration of citalopram (40 mg) and ketoconazole (200 mg), a potent inhibitor of CYP3A4, did not significantly affect the pharmacokinetics of citalopram. Because citalopram is metabolized by multiple enzyme systems, inhi-

IMPORTANT NOTE: Always consult each drug listing in the patient's regimen for possible interactions.

bition of a single enzyme may not appreciably decrease citalopram clearance). Products include:
Emend 2124

Aprobarbital (Given the primary CNS effects of citalopram, caution should be used when it is taken in combination with other centrally acting drugs).
No products indexed under this heading.

Ardeparin Sodium (Citalopram may increase the risk of bleeding events. Concomitant use of anticoagulants may add to the risk. Case reports and studies have demonstrated an association between use of drugs that interfere with serotonin reuptake and the occurrence of gastrointestinal bleeding. Patients should be cautioned about the risk of bleeding associated with the concomitant use of citalopram and drugs affecting coagulation).
No products indexed under this heading.

Aripiprazole (The development of a potentially life threatening serotonin syndrome or Neuroleptic Malignant Syndrome (NMS)-like reactions have been reported with citalopram alone, and with concomitant use of antipsychotics. Serotonin syndrome, in its most severe form can resemble neuroleptic malignant syndrome. Patients should be monitored for the emergence of serotonin syndrome or NMS-like signs and symptoms. Treatment with citalopram and any antipsychotics should be discontinued immediately if the above events occur and supportive symptomatic treatment should be initiated).
No products indexed under this heading.

Aspirin (Citalopram may increase the risk of bleeding events. Concomitant use of aspirin may add to the risk. Case reports and studies have demonstrated an association between use of drugs that interfere with serotonin reuptake and the occurrence of gastrointestinal bleeding. Patients should be cautioned about the risk of bleeding associated with the concomitant use of citalopram and aspirin). Products include:
Aggrenox 880
Bayer Aspirin 829
Percodan 1124
St. Joseph Aspirin 2045

Aspirin, Enteric Coated (Citalopram may increase the risk of bleeding events. Concomitant use of aspirin may add to the risk. Case reports and studies have demonstrated an association between use of drugs that interfere with serotonin reuptake and the occurrence of gastrointestinal bleeding. Patients should be cautioned about the risk of bleeding associated with the concomitant use of citalopram and aspirin).
No products indexed under this heading.

Aspirin Buffered (Citalopram may increase the risk of bleeding events. Concomitant use of aspirin may add to the risk. Case reports and studies have demonstrated an association between use of drugs that interfere with serotonin reuptake and the occurrence of gastrointestinal bleeding. Patients should be cautioned about the risk of bleeding associated with the concomitant use of citalopram and aspirin).
No products indexed under this heading.

Atazanavir (In vitro studies indicated that CYP3A4 and CYP2C19 are the primary enzymes involved in the metabolism of citalopram. However, co-administration of citalopram (40 mg) and ketoconazole (200 mg), a potent inhibitor of CYP3A4, did not significantly affect the pharmacokinetics of citalopram. Because citalopram is metabolized by multiple enzyme systems, inhibition of a single enzyme may not appreciably decrease citalopram clearance).
No products indexed under this heading.

Atazanavir Sulfate (In vitro studies indicated that CYP3A4 and CYP2C19 are the primary enzymes involved in the metabolism of citalopram. However, co-administration of citalopram (40 mg) and ketoconazole (200 mg), a potent inhibitor of CYP3A4, did not significantly affect the pharmacokinetics of citalopram. Because citalopram is metabolized by multiple enzyme systems, inhibition of a single enzyme may not appreciably decrease citalopram clearance).
No products indexed under this heading.

Azithromycin Dihydrate (Since CYP3A4 and 2C19 are the primary enzymes involved in the metabolism of citalopram, it is expected that potent inhibitors of 3A4 (eg, macrolide antibiotics) might decrease the clearance of citalopram. However, co-administration of citalopram and the potent 3A4 inhibitor ketoconazole did not significantly affect the pharmacokinetics of citalopram. Because citalopram is metabolized by multiple enzyme systems, inhibition of a single enzyme system may not appreciably decrease citalopram clearance).
No products indexed under this heading.

Bendroflumethiazide (Hyponatremia may occur as a result of treatment with SSRIs including citalopram. Patients taking diuretics may be at greater risk. Discontinuation of citalopram should be considered in patients with symptomatic hyponatremia and appropriate medical intervention should be instituted).
No products indexed under this heading.

Bumetanide (Hyponatremia may occur as a result of treatment with SSRIs including citalopram. Patients taking diuretics may be at greater risk. Discontinuation of citalopram should be considered in patients with symptomatic hyponatremia and appropriate medical intervention should be instituted).
No products indexed under this heading.

Buprenorphine Hydrochloride (Given the primary CNS effects of citalopram, caution should be used when it is taken in combination with other centrally acting drugs).
No products indexed under this heading.

Buspirone Hydrochloride (Given the primary CNS effects of citalopram, caution should be used when it is taken in combination with other centrally acting drugs).
No products indexed under this heading.

Butabarbital (Given the primary CNS effects of citalopram, caution should be used when it is taken in combination with other centrally acting drugs).
No products indexed under this heading.

Butabarbital Sodium (Given the primary CNS effects of citalopram, caution should be used when it is taken in combination with other centrally acting drugs).
No products indexed under this heading.

Butalbital (Given the primary CNS effects of citalopram, caution should be used when it is taken in combination with other centrally acting drugs).
No products indexed under this heading.

Carbamazepine (Combined administration of citalopram (40 mg/day for 14 days) and carbamazepine (titrated to 400 mg/day for 35 days) did not significantly affect the pharmacokinetics of carbamazepine, a CYP3A4 substrate. Although trough citalopram plasma levels were unaffected, given the enzyme inducing properties of carbamazepine, the possibility that carbamazepine might increase the clearance of citalopram should be considered if these two drugs are co-administered). Products include:
Carbatrol 3280

Equetro 3477

Celecoxib (Citalopram may increase the risk of bleeding events. Concomitant use of NSAIDs may add to the risk. Case reports and epidemiological studies have demonstrated an association between use of drugs that interfere with serotonin reuptake and the occurrence of gastrointestinal bleeding. Bleeding events related to SSRIs use have ranged from ecchymoses, hematomas, epitaxis, and petechiae to life-threatening hemorrhages. Patients should be cautioned about the risk of bleeding associated with the concomitant use of citalopram and NSAIDs). Products include:
Celebrex 3272

Chlordiazepoxide (Given the primary CNS effects of citalopram, caution should be used when it is taken in combination with other centrally acting drugs).
No products indexed under this heading.

Chlordiazepoxide Hydrochloride (Given the primary CNS effects of citalopram, caution should be used when it is taken in combination with other centrally acting drugs).
No products indexed under this heading.

Chlorothiazide (Hyponatremia may occur as a result of treatment with SSRIs including citalopram. Patients taking diuretics may be at greater risk. Discontinuation of citalopram should be considered in patients with symptomatic hyponatremia and appropriate medical intervention should be instituted).
No products indexed under this heading.

Chlorothiazide Sodium (Hyponatremia may occur as a result of treatment with SSRIs including citalopram. Patients taking diuretics may be at greater risk. Discontinuation of citalopram should be considered in patients with symptomatic hyponatremia and appropriate medical intervention should be instituted). Products include:
Diuril Intravenous 2009

Chlorpromazine (The development of a potentially life threatening serotonin syndrome or Neuroleptic Malignant Syndrome (NMS)-like reactions have been reported with citalopram alone, and with concomitant use of antipsychotics. Serotonin syndrome, in its most severe form can resemble neuroleptic malignant syndrome. Patients should be monitored for the emergence of serotonin syndrome or NMS-like signs and symptoms. Treatment with citalopram and any antipsychotics should be discontinued immediately if the above events occur and supportive symptomatic treatment should be initiated).
No products indexed under this heading.

Chlorpromazine Hydrochloride (The development of a potentially life threatening serotonin syndrome or Neuroleptic Malignant Syndrome (NMS)-like reactions have been reported with citalopram alone, and with concomitant use of antipsychotics. Serotonin syndrome, in its most severe form can resemble neuroleptic malignant syndrome. Patients should be monitored for the emergence of serotonin syndrome or NMS-like signs and symptoms. Treatment with citalopram and any antipsychotics should be discontinued immediately if the above events occur and supportive symptomatic treatment should be initiated).
No products indexed under this heading.

Chlorprothixene (The development of a potentially life threatening serotonin syndrome or Neuroleptic Malignant Syndrome (NMS)-like reactions have been reported with citalopram alone, and with concomitant use of antipsychotics. Serotonin syndrome, in its most severe form can resemble neuroleptic malig-

nant syndrome. Patients should be monitored for the emergence of serotonin syndrome or NMS-like signs and symptoms. Treatment with citalopram and any antipsychotics should be discontinued immediately if the above events occur and supportive symptomatic treatment should be initiated).
No products indexed under this heading.

Chlorprothixene Hydrochloride (The development of a potentially life threatening serotonin syndrome or Neuroleptic Malignant Syndrome (NMS)-like reactions have been reported with citalopram alone, and with concomitant use of antipsychotics. Serotonin syndrome, in its most severe form can resemble neuroleptic malignant syndrome. Patients should be monitored for the emergence of serotonin syndrome or NMS-like signs and symptoms. Treatment with citalopram and any antipsychotics should be discontinued immediately if the above events occur and supportive symptomatic treatment should be initiated).
No products indexed under this heading.

Chlorprothixene Lactate (The development of a potentially life threatening serotonin syndrome or Neuroleptic Malignant Syndrome (NMS)-like reactions have been reported with citalopram alone, and with concomitant use of antipsychotics. Serotonin syndrome, in its most severe form can resemble neuroleptic malignant syndrome. Patients should be monitored for the emergence of serotonin syndrome or NMS-like signs and symptoms. Treatment with citalopram and any antipsychotics should be discontinued immediately if the above events occur and supportive symptomatic treatment should be initiated).
No products indexed under this heading.

Chlorthalidone (Hyponatremia may occur as a result of treatment with SSRIs including citalopram. Patients taking diuretics may be at greater risk. Discontinuation of citalopram should be considered in patients with symptomatic hyponatremia and appropriate medical intervention should be instituted). Products include:
Clorpres 2344

Cimetidine (In subjects who had received 21 days of 40mg/day of citalopram, combined administration of 400 mg/day cimetidine for 8 days resulted in an increase in citalopram AUC and C_{max} by 43% and 39% respectively. The clinical significance of these findings is unknown).
No products indexed under this heading.

Cimetidine Hydrochloride (In subjects who had received 21 days of 40mg/day of citalopram, combined administration of 400 mg/day cimetidine for 8 days resulted in an increase in citalopram AUC and C_{max} by 43% and 39% respectively. The clinical significance of these findings is unknown).
No products indexed under this heading.

Ciprofloxacin (In vitro studies indicated that CYP3A4 and CYP2C19 are the primary enzymes involved in the metabolism of citalopram. However, co-administration of citalopram (40 mg) and ketoconazole (200 mg), a potent inhibitor of CYP3A4, did not significantly affect the pharmacokinetics of citalopram. Because citalopram is metabolized by multiple enzyme systems, inhibition of a single enzyme may not appreciably decrease citalopram clearance). Products include:
Cipro I.V. 3082
Cipro 3073
Cipro XR 3091
Ciprodex 583

Clarithromycin (Since CYP3A4 and 2C19 are the primary enzymes involved

in the metabolism of citalopram, it is expected that potent inhibitors of 3A4 (eg, macrolide antibiotics) might decrease the clearance of citalopram. However, co-administration of citalopram and the potent 3A4 inhibitor ketoconazole did not significantly affect the pharmacokinetics of citalopram. Because citalopram is metabolized by multiple enzyme systems, inhibition of a single enzyme system may not appreciably decrease citalopram clearance). Products include:

Biaxin/Biaxin XL 412

Clomipramine Hydrochloride (Co-administration of imipramine with citalopram has resulted in a 50% increase in active metabolite, desipramine concentration. The clinical significance of this finding is unknown. Caution is indicated if tricyclic antidepressants are co-administered with citalopram).

No products indexed under this heading.

Clonazepam (Given the primary CNS effects of citalopram, caution should be used when it is taken in combination with other centrally acting drugs). Products include:

Klonopin 2855

Clorazepate Dipotassium (Given the primary CNS effects of citalopram, caution should be used when it is taken in combination with other centrally acting drugs).

No products indexed under this heading.

Clotrimazole (In vitro studies indicated that CYP3A4 and CYP2C19 are the primary enzymes involved in the metabolism of citalopram. However, co-administration of citalopram (40 mg) and ketoconazole (200 mg), a potent inhibitor of CYP3A4, did not significantly affect the pharmacokinetics of citalopram. Because citalopram is metabolized by multiple enzyme systems, inhibition of a single enzyme may not appreciably decrease citalopram clearance). Products include:

Lotrisone 3163

Clozapine (The development of a potentially life threatening serotonin syndrome or Neuroleptic Malignant Syndrome (NMS)-like reactions have been reported with citalopram alone, and with concomitant use of antipsychotics. Serotonin syndrome, in its most severe form can resemble neuroleptic malignant syndrome. Patients should be monitored for the emergence of serotonin syndrome or NMS-like signs and symptoms. Treatment with citalopram and any antipsychotics should be discontinued immediately if the above events occur and supportive symptomatic treatment should be initiated).

No products indexed under this heading.

Codeine Phosphate (Given the primary CNS effects of citalopram, caution should be used when it is taken in combination with other centrally acting drugs). Products include:

Tylenol with Codeine 2691

Codeine Sulfate (Given the primary CNS effects of citalopram, caution should be used when it is taken in combination with other centrally acting drugs).

No products indexed under this heading.

Conivaptan Hydrochloride (In vitro studies indicated that CYP3A4 and CYP2C19 are the primary enzymes involved in the metabolism of citalopram. However, co-administration of citalopram (40 mg) and ketoconazole (200 mg), a potent inhibitor of CYP3A4, did not significantly affect the pharmacokinetics of citalopram. Because citalopram is metabolized by multiple enzyme systems, inhibition of a single enzyme may not appreciably decrease citalopram clearance). Products include:

Vaprisol 689

Cyclosporine (In vitro studies indicated that CYP3A4 and CYP2C19 are the primary enzymes involved in the metabolism of citalopram. However, co-administration of citalopram (40 mg) and ketoconazole (200 mg), a potent inhibitor of CYP3A4, did not significantly affect the pharmacokinetics of citalopram. Because citalopram is metabolized by multiple enzyme systems, inhibition of a single enzyme may not appreciably decrease citalopram clearance). Products include:

Gengraf 440
Neoral Oral Solution 2496
Neoral Capsules 2496
Restasis 605

Dalfopristin (In vitro studies indicated that CYP3A4 and CYP2C19 are the primary enzymes involved in the metabolism of citalopram. However, co-administration of citalopram (40 mg) and ketoconazole (200 mg), a potent inhibitor of CYP3A4, did not significantly affect the pharmacokinetics of citalopram. Because citalopram is metabolized by multiple enzyme systems, inhibition of a single enzyme may not appreciably decrease citalopram clearance).

No products indexed under this heading.

Dalteparin Sodium (Citalopram may increase the risk of bleeding events. Concomitant use of anticoagulants may add to the risk. Case reports and studies have demonstrated an association between use of drugs that interfere with serotonin reuptake and the occurrence of gastrointestinal bleeding. Patients should be cautioned about the risk of bleeding associated with the concomitant use of citalopram and drugs affecting coagulation). Products include:

Fragmin 1058

Danaparoid Sodium (Citalopram may increase the risk of bleeding events. Concomitant use of anticoagulants may add to the risk. Case reports and studies have demonstrated an association between use of drugs that interfere with serotonin reuptake and the occurrence of gastrointestinal bleeding. Patients should be cautioned about the risk of bleeding associated with the concomitant use of citalopram and drugs affecting coagulation).

No products indexed under this heading.

Danazol (In vitro studies indicated that CYP3A4 and CYP2C19 are the primary enzymes involved in the metabolism of citalopram. However, co-administration of citalopram (40 mg) and ketoconazole (200 mg), a potent inhibitor of CYP3A4, did not significantly affect the pharmacokinetics of citalopram. Because citalopram is metabolized by multiple enzyme systems, inhibition of a single enzyme may not appreciably decrease citalopram clearance).

No products indexed under this heading.

Darunavir (In vitro studies indicated that CYP3A4 and CYP2C19 are the primary enzymes involved in the metabolism of citalopram. However, co-administration of citalopram (40 mg) and ketoconazole (200 mg), a potent inhibitor of CYP3A4, did not significantly affect the pharmacokinetics of citalopram. Because citalopram is metabolized by multiple enzyme systems, inhibition of a single enzyme may not appreciably decrease citalopram clearance).

No products indexed under this heading.

Dasatinib (In vitro studies indicated that CYP3A4 and CYP2C19 are the primary enzymes involved in the metabolism of citalopram. However, co-administration of citalopram (40 mg) and ketoconazole (200 mg), a potent inhibitor of CYP3A4, did not significantly affect the pharmacokinetics of citalo-

pram. Because citalopram is metabolized by multiple enzyme systems, inhibition of a single enzyme may not appreciably decrease citalopram clearance).

No products indexed under this heading.

Delavirdine Mesylate (Since CYP3A4 and 2C19 are the primary enzymes involved in the metabolism of citalopram, it is expected that potent inhibitors of CYP219 (eg, omeprazole) might decrease the clearance of citalopram. However, co-administration of citalopram and the potent CYP3A4 inhibitor did not significantly affect the pharmacokinetics of citalopram. Because citalopram is metabolized by multiple enzyme systems, inhibition of a single enzyme system may not appreciably decrease citalopram clearance).

No products indexed under this heading.

Delavirine (In vitro studies indicated that CYP3A4 and CYP2C19 are the primary enzymes involved in the metabolism of citalopram. However, co-administration of citalopram (40 mg) and ketoconazole (200 mg), a potent inhibitor of CYP3A4, did not significantly affect the pharmacokinetics of citalopram. Because citalopram is metabolized by multiple enzyme systems, inhibition of a single enzyme may not appreciably decrease citalopram clearance).

No products indexed under this heading.

Desflurane (Given the primary CNS effects of citalopram, caution should be used when it is taken in combination with other centrally acting drugs).

No products indexed under this heading.

Desipramine Hydrochloride (Co-administration of imipramine with citalopram has resulted in a 50% increase in active metabolite, desipramine concentration. The clinical significance of this finding is unknown. Caution is indicated if tricyclic antidepressants are co-administered with citalopram).

No products indexed under this heading.

Desloratadine (In vitro studies indicated that CYP3A4 and CYP2C19 are the primary enzymes involved in the metabolism of citalopram. However, co-administration of citalopram (40 mg) and ketoconazole (200 mg), a potent inhibitor of CYP3A4, did not significantly affect the pharmacokinetics of citalopram. Because citalopram is metabolized by multiple enzyme systems, inhibition of a single enzyme may not appreciably decrease citalopram clearance). Products include:

Clarinex Syrup 3098
Clarinex 3098
Clarinex Reditabs 3098
Clarinex-D 12-Hour 3101
Clarinex-D 3104

Desogestrel (Since CYP3A4 and 2C19 are the primary enzymes involved in the metabolism of citalopram, it is expected that potent inhibitors of CYP219 (eg, omeprazole) might decrease the clearance of citalopram. However, co-administration of citalopram and the potent CYP3A4 inhibitor did not significantly affect the pharmacokinetics of citalopram. Because citalopram is metabolized by multiple enzyme systems, inhibition of a single enzyme system may not appreciably decrease citalopram clearance).

No products indexed under this heading.

Desvenlafaxine Succinate (The development of potentially life threatening serotonin syndrome or Neuroleptic Malignant Syndrome (NMS)-like reactions have been reported with citalopram alone, but particularly with concomitant use of serotonergic drugs. The concomitant use of citalopram with SNRIs is not recommended). Products include:

Pristiq 3564

Dexmethylphenidate Hydrochloride (Given the primary CNS effects of citalopram, caution should be used when it is taken in combination with other centrally acting drugs). Products include:

Focalin XR 2472

Dextroamphetamine (Given the primary CNS effects of citalopram, caution should be used when it is taken in combination with other centrally acting drugs).

No products indexed under this heading.

Dextroamphetamine Saccharate (Given the primary CNS effects of citalopram, caution should be used when it is taken in combination with other centrally acting drugs).

No products indexed under this heading.

Dextroamphetamine Sulfate (Given the primary CNS effects of citalopram, caution should be used when it is taken in combination with other centrally acting drugs). Products include:

Dexedrine 1425

Dezocine (Given the primary CNS effects of citalopram, caution should be used when it is taken in combination with other centrally acting drugs).

No products indexed under this heading.

Diazepam (Given the primary CNS effects of citalopram, caution should be used when it is taken in combination with other centrally acting drugs). Products include:

Valium Tablets 2880

Diclofenac Epolamine (Citalopram may increase the risk of bleeding events. Concomitant use of NSAIDs may add to the risk. Case reports and epidemiological studies have demonstrated an association between use of drugs that interfere with serotonin reuptake and the occurrence of gastrointestinal bleeding. Bleeding events related to SSRIs use have ranged from ecchymoses, hematomas, epitaxis, and petechiae to life-threatening hemorrhages. Patients should be cautioned about the risk of bleeding associated with the concomitant use of citalopram and NSAIDs). Products include:

Flector 1839

Diclofenac Potassium (Citalopram may increase the risk of bleeding events. Concomitant use of NSAIDs may add to the risk. Case reports and epidemiological studies have demonstrated an association between use of drugs that interfere with serotonin reuptake and the occurrence of gastrointestinal bleeding. Bleeding events related to SSRIs use have ranged from ecchymoses, hematomas, epitaxis, and petechiae to life-threatening hemorrhages. Patients should be cautioned about the risk of bleeding associated with the concomitant use of citalopram and NSAIDs).

No products indexed under this heading.

Diclofenac Sodium (Citalopram may increase the risk of bleeding events. Concomitant use of NSAIDs may add to the risk. Case reports and epidemiological studies have demonstrated an association between use of drugs that interfere with serotonin reuptake and the occurrence of gastrointestinal bleeding. Bleeding events related to SSRIs use have ranged from ecchymoses, hematomas, epitaxis, and petechiae to life-threatening hemorrhages. Patients should be cautioned about the risk of bleeding associated with the concomitant use of citalopram and NSAIDs).

No products indexed under this heading.

Dicumarol (Citalopram may increase the risk of bleeding events. Concomitant use of anticoagulants may add to the risk. Case reports and studies have demonstrated an association between

---

IMPORTANT NOTE: Always consult each drug listing in the patient's regimen for possible interactions.

use of drugs that interfere with serotonin reuptake and the occurrence of gastrointestinal bleeding. Patients should be cautioned about the risk of bleeding associated with the concomitant use of citalopram and drugs affecting coagulation).

No products indexed under this heading.

Diltiazem Hydrochloride (*In vitro* studies indicated that CYP3A4 and CYP2C19 are the primary enzymes involved in the metabolism of citalopram. However, co-administration of citalopram (40 mg) and ketoconazole (200 mg), a potent inhibitor of CYP3A4, did not significantly affect the pharmacokinetics of citalopram. Because citalopram is metabolized by multiple enzyme systems, inhibition of a single enzyme may not appreciably decrease citalopram clearance). Products include:

Cardizem LA 423

Diltiazem Maleate (*In vitro* studies indicated that CYP3A4 and CYP2C19 are the primary enzymes involved in the metabolism of citalopram. However, co-administration of citalopram (40 mg) and ketoconazole (200 mg), a potent inhibitor of CYP3A4, did not significantly affect the pharmacokinetics of citalopram. Because citalopram is metabolized by multiple enzyme systems, inhibition of a single enzyme may not appreciably decrease citalopram clearance).

No products indexed under this heading.

Dirithromycin (Since CYP3A4 and 2C19 are the primary enzymes involved in the metabolism of citalopram, it is expected that potent inhibitors of 3A4 (eg, macrolide antibiotics) might decrease the clearance of citalopram. However, co-administration of citalopram and the potent 3A4 inhibitor ketoconazole did not significantly affect the pharmacokinetics of citalopram. Because citalopram is metabolized by multiple enzyme systems, inhibition of a single enzyme system may not appreciably decrease citalopram clearance).

No products indexed under this heading.

Doxepin Hydrochloride (Co-administration of imipramine with citalopram has resulted in a 50% increase in active metabolite, desipramine concentration. The clinical significance of this finding is unknown. Caution is indicated if tricyclic antidepressants are co-administered with citalopram).

No products indexed under this heading.

Droperidol (Given the primary CNS effects of citalopram, caution should be used when it is taken in combination with other centrally acting drugs).

No products indexed under this heading.

Duloxetine Hydrochloride (The development of potentially life threatening serotonin syndrome or Neuroleptic Malignant Syndrome (NMS)-like reactions have been reported with citalopram alone, but particularly with concomitant use of serotonergic drugs. The concomitant use of citalopram with SNRIs is not recommended). Products include:

Cymbalta 1871

Efavirenz (Since CYP3A4 and 2C19 are the primary enzymes involved in the metabolism of citalopram, it is expected that potent inhibitors of CYP219 (eg, omeprazole) might decrease the clearance of citalopram. However, co-administration of citalopram and the potent CYP3A4 inhibitor did not significantly affect the pharmacokinetics of citalopram. Because citalopram is metabolized by multiple enzyme systems, inhibition of a single enzyme system may not appreciably decrease citalopram clearance). Products include:

Atripla 906

Eletriptan Hydrobromide (The development of potentially life threatening serotonin syndrome or Neuroleptic Malignant syndrome (NMS)-like reactions have been reported with citalopram alone, but particularly with concomitant use of serotonergic drugs including triptans. Serotonin syndrome, in its most severe form can resemble neuroleptic malignant syndrome. Patients should be monitored for the emergence of serotonin syndrome or NMS-like signs and symptoms. If concomitant treatment of citalopram with a triptan is clinically warranted, careful observation of the patient is advised, particularly during treatment initiation and dose increases).

No products indexed under this heading.

Enflurane (Given the primary CNS effects of citalopram, caution should be used when it is taken in combination with other centrally acting drugs).

No products indexed under this heading.

Enoxaparin Sodium (Citalopram may increase the risk of bleeding events. Concomitant use of anticoagulants may add to the risk. Case reports and studies have demonstrated an association between use of drugs that interfere with serotonin reuptake and the occurrence of gastrointestinal bleeding. Patients should be cautioned about the risk of bleeding associated with the concomitant use of citalopram and drugs affecting coagulation). Products include:

Lovenox 3005

Erythromycin (Since CYP3A4 and 2C19 are the primary enzymes involved in the metabolism of citalopram, it is expected that potent inhibitors of 3A4 (eg, macrolide antibiotics) might decrease the clearance of citalopram. However, co-administration of citalopram and the potent 3A4 inhibitor ketoconazole did not significantly affect the pharmacokinetics of citalopram. Because citalopram is metabolized by multiple enzyme systems, inhibition of a single enzyme system may not appreciably decrease citalopram clearance).

No products indexed under this heading.

Erythromycin Estolate (Since CYP3A4 and 2C19 are the primary enzymes involved in the metabolism of citalopram, it is expected that potent inhibitors of 3A4 (eg, macrolide antibiotics) might decrease the clearance of citalopram. However, co-administration of citalopram and the potent 3A4 inhibitor ketoconazole did not significantly affect the pharmacokinetics of citalopram. Because citalopram is metabolized by multiple enzyme systems, inhibition of a single enzyme system may not appreciably decrease citalopram clearance).

No products indexed under this heading.

Erythromycin Ethylsuccinate (Since CYP3A4 and 2C19 are the primary enzymes involved in the metabolism of citalopram, it is expected that potent inhibitors of 3A4 (eg, macrolide antibiotics) might decrease the clearance of citalopram. However, co-administration of citalopram and the potent 3A4 inhibitor ketoconazole did not significantly affect the pharmacokinetics of citalopram. Because citalopram is metabolized by multiple enzyme systems, inhibition of a single enzyme system may not appreciably decrease citalopram clearance). Products include:

E.E.S. 437

EryPed 435

Erythromycin Gluceptate (Since CYP3A4 and 2C19 are the primary enzymes involved in the metabolism of citalopram, it is expected that potent inhibitors of 3A4 (eg, macrolide antibiotics) might decrease the clearance of citalopram. However, co-administration of citalopram and the potent 3A4 inhibitor ketoconazole did not significantly affect the pharmacokinetics of citalopram. Because citalopram is metabolized by multiple enzyme systems, inhibition of a single enzyme system may not appreciably decrease citalopram clearance).

No products indexed under this heading.

Erythromycin Lactobionate (*In vitro* studies indicated that CYP3A4 and CYP2C19 are the primary enzymes involved in the metabolism of citalopram. However, co-administration of citalopram (40 mg) and ketoconazole (200 mg), a potent inhibitor of CYP3A4, did not significantly affect the pharmacokinetics of citalopram. Because citalopram is metabolized by multiple enzyme systems, inhibition of a single enzyme may not appreciably decrease citalopram clearance).

No products indexed under this heading.

Erythromycin Stearate (Since CYP3A4 and 2C19 are the primary enzymes involved in the metabolism of citalopram, it is expected that potent inhibitors of 3A4 (eg, macrolide antibiotics) might decrease the clearance of citalopram. However, co-administration of citalopram and the potent 3A4 inhibitor ketoconazole did not significantly affect the pharmacokinetics of citalopram. Because citalopram is metabolized by multiple enzyme systems, inhibition of a single enzyme system may not appreciably decrease citalopram clearance).

No products indexed under this heading.

Escitalopram Oxalate (The development of potentially life threatening serotonin syndrome or Neuroleptic Malignant Syndrome (NMS)-like reactions have been reported with citalopram alone, but particularly with concomitant use of serotonergic drugs. Serotonin syndrome, in its most severe form, can resemble neuroleptic malignant syndrome. Patients should be monitored for the emergence of serotonin syndrome or NMS-like signs and symptoms. Treatment with citalopram and any concomitant serotonergic agent should be discontinued immediately if the above events occur and supportive treatment should be initiated). Products include:

Lexapro Oral Suspension 1160

Lexapro Tablets 1160

Esomeprazole Magnesium (*In vitro* studies indicated that CYP3A4 and CYP2C19 are the primary enzymes involved in the metabolism of citalopram. However, co-administration of citalopram (40 mg) and ketoconazole (200 mg), a potent inhibitor of CYP3A4, did not significantly affect the pharmacokinetics of citalopram. Because citalopram is metabolized by multiple enzyme systems, inhibition of a single enzyme may not appreciably decrease citalopram clearance). Products include:

Nexium Capsules 704

Nexium Oral Suspension 704

Esomeprazole Sodium (*In vitro* studies indicated that CYP3A4 and CYP2C19 are the primary enzymes involved in the metabolism of citalopram. However, co-administration of citalopram (40 mg) and ketoconazole (200 mg), a potent inhibitor of CYP3A4, did not significantly affect the pharmacokinetics of citalopram. Because citalopram is metabolized by multiple enzyme systems, inhibition of a single enzyme may not appreciably decrease citalopram clearance). Products include:

Nexium I.V. 712

Estazolam (Given the primary CNS effects of citalopram, caution should be used when it is taken in combination with other centrally acting drugs).

No products indexed under this heading.

Ethacrynic Acid (Hyponatremia may occur as a result of treatment with SSRIs including citalopram. Patients taking diuretics may be at greater risk. Discontinuation of citalopram should be considered in patients with symptomatic hyponatremia and appropriate medical intervention should be instituted).

No products indexed under this heading.

Ethanol (Although citalopram did not potentiate cognitive and motor effects of alcohol, as with other psychotropic medications, the use of alcohol by depressed patients taking citalopram is not recommended).

No products indexed under this heading.

Ethchlorvynol (Given the primary CNS effects of citalopram, caution should be used when it is taken in combination with other centrally acting drugs).

No products indexed under this heading.

Ethinamate (Given the primary CNS effects of citalopram, caution should be used when it is taken in combination with other centrally acting drugs).

No products indexed under this heading.

Ethinyl Estradiol (Since CYP3A4 and 2C19 are the primary enzymes involved in the metabolism of citalopram, it is expected that potent inhibitors of CYP219 (eg, omeprazole) might decrease the clearance of citalopram. However, co-administration of citalopram and the potent CYP3A4 inhibitor did not significantly affect the pharmacokinetics of citalopram. Because citalopram is metabolized by multiple enzyme systems, inhibition of a single enzyme system may not appreciably decrease citalopram clearance). Products include:

LoSeasonique 3407

Lybrel 3514

NuvaRing 3181

Ortho Evra 2648

Ortho-Cyclen/Ortho Tri-Cyclen 2663

Ortho Tri-Cyclen Lo Tablets 2673

Seasonique 3418

Yaz 864

Ethyl Alcohol (Although citalopram did not potentiate cognitive and motor effects of alcohol, as with other psychotropic medications, the use of alcohol by depressed patients taking citalopram is not recommended).

No products indexed under this heading.

Ethynodiol Diacetate (Since CYP3A4 and 2C19 are the primary enzymes involved in the metabolism of citalopram, it is expected that potent inhibitors of CYP219 (eg, omeprazole) might decrease the clearance of citalopram. However, co-administration of citalopram and the potent CYP3A4 inhibitor did not significantly affect the pharmacokinetics of citalopram. Because citalopram is metabolized by multiple enzyme systems, inhibition of a single enzyme system may not appreciably decrease citalopram clearance).

No products indexed under this heading.

Etodolac (Citalopram may increase the risk of bleeding events. Concomitant use of NSAIDs may add to the risk. Case reports and epidemiological studies have demonstrated an association between use of drugs that interfere with serotonin reuptake and the occurrence of gastrointestinal bleeding. Bleeding events related to SSRIs use have ranged from ecchymoses, hematomas, epitaxis, and petechiae to life-threatening hemorrhages. Patients should be cautioned about the risk of bleeding associated with the concomitant use of citalopram and NSAIDs).

No products indexed under this heading.

Felbamate (Since CYP3A4 and 2C19 are the primary enzymes involved in the metabolism of citalopram, it is expected that potent inhibitors of CYP219 (eg, omeprazole) might decrease the clearance of citalopram. However, co-administration of citalopram and the potent CYP3A4 inhibitor did not significantly affect the pharmacokinetics of citalopram. Because citalopram is metabolized by multiple enzyme systems, inhibition of a single enzyme system may not appreciably decrease citalopram clearance).
No products indexed under this heading.

Fenoprofen Calcium (Citalopram may increase the risk of bleeding events. Concomitant use of NSAIDs may add to the risk. Case reports and epidemiological studies have demonstrated an association between use of drugs that interfere with serotonin reuptake and the occurrence of gastrointestinal bleeding. Bleeding events related to SSRIs use have ranged from ecchymoses, hematomas, epitaxis, and petechiae to life-threatening hemorrhages. Patients should be cautioned about the risk of bleeding associated with the concomitant use of citalopram and NSAIDs).
No products indexed under this heading.

Fentanyl (Given the primary CNS effects of citalopram, caution should be used when it is taken in combination with other centrally acting drugs).
Products include:
Duragesic 2604
Fentanyl Transdermal System 2346
Onsolis 2054

Fentanyl Citrate (Given the primary CNS effects of citalopram, caution should be used when it is taken in combination with other centrally acting drugs). Products include:
Fentora 966

Fluconazole (*In vitro* studies indicated that CYP3A4 and CYP2C19 are the primary enzymes involved in the metabolism of citalopram. However, co-administration of citalopram (40 mg) and ketoconazole (200 mg), a potent inhibitor of CYP3A4, did not significantly affect the pharmacokinetics of citalopram. Because citalopram is metabolized by multiple enzyme systems, inhibition of a single enzyme may not appreciably decrease citalopram clearance).
No products indexed under this heading.

Fluoxetine (Since CYP3A4 and 2C19 are the primary enzymes involved in the metabolism of citalopram, it is expected that potent inhibitors of CYP219 (eg, omeprazole) might decrease the clearance of citalopram. However, co-administration of citalopram and the potent CYP3A4 inhibitor did not significantly affect the pharmacokinetics of citalopram. Because citalopram is metabolized by multiple enzyme systems, inhibition of a single enzyme system may not appreciably decrease citalopram clearance).
No products indexed under this heading.

Fluoxetine Hydrochloride (The development of potentially life threatening serotonin syndrome or Neuroleptic Malignant Syndrome (NMS)-like reactions have been reported with citalopram alone, but particularly with concomitant use of serotonergic drugs. Serotonin syndrome, in its most severe form, can resemble neuroleptic malignant syndrome. Patients should be monitored for the emergence of serotonin syndrome or NMS-like signs and symptoms. Treatment with citalopram and any concomitant serotonergic agent should be discontinued immediately if the above events occur and supportive treatment should be initiated). Products include:
Prozac Weekly 1941
Prozac Pulvules 1941
Symbyax 1965

Fluphenazine Decanoate (The development of a potentially life threatening serotonin syndrome or Neuroleptic Malignant Syndrome (NMS)-like reactions have been reported with citalopram alone, and with concomitant use of antipsychotics. Serotonin syndrome, in its most severe form can resemble neuroleptic malignant syndrome. Patients should be monitored for the emergence of serotonin syndrome or NMS-like signs and symptoms. Treatment with citalopram and any antipsychotics should be discontinued immediately if the above events occur and supportive symptomatic treatment should be initiated).
No products indexed under this heading.

Fluphenazine Enanthate (The development of a potentially life threatening serotonin syndrome or Neuroleptic Malignant Syndrome (NMS)-like reactions have been reported with citalopram alone, and with concomitant use of antipsychotics. Serotonin syndrome, in its most severe form can resemble neuroleptic malignant syndrome. Patients should be monitored for the emergence of serotonin syndrome or NMS-like signs and symptoms. Treatment with citalopram and any antipsychotics should be discontinued immediately if the above events occur and supportive symptomatic treatment should be initiated).
No products indexed under this heading.

Fluphenazine Hydrochloride (The development of a potentially life threatening serotonin syndrome or Neuroleptic Malignant Syndrome (NMS)-like reactions have been reported with citalopram alone, and with concomitant use of antipsychotics. Serotonin syndrome, in its most severe form can resemble neuroleptic malignant syndrome. Patients should be monitored for the emergence of serotonin syndrome or NMS-like signs and symptoms. Treatment with citalopram and any antipsychotics should be discontinued immediately if the above events occur and supportive symptomatic treatment should be initiated).
No products indexed under this heading.

Flurazepam Hydrochloride (Given the primary CNS effects of citalopram, caution should be used when it is taken in combination with other centrally acting drugs).
No products indexed under this heading.

Flurbiprofen (Citalopram may increase the risk of bleeding events. Concomitant use of NSAIDs may add to the risk. Case reports and epidemiological studies have demonstrated an association between use of drugs that interfere with serotonin reuptake and the occurrence of gastrointestinal bleeding. Bleeding events related to SSRIs use have ranged from ecchymoses, hematomas, epitaxis, and petechiae to life-threatening hemorrhages. Patients should be cautioned about the risk of bleeding associated with the concomitant use of citalopram and NSAIDs).
No products indexed under this heading.

Fluvastatin Sodium (Since CYP3A4 and 2C19 are the primary enzymes involved in the metabolism of citalopram, it is expected that potent inhibitors of CYP219 (eg, omeprazole) might decrease the clearance of citalopram. However, co-administration of citalopram and the potent CYP3A4 inhibitor did not significantly affect the pharmacokinetics of citalopram. Because citalopram is metabolized by multiple enzyme systems, inhibition of a single enzyme system may not appreciably decrease citalopram clearance).
No products indexed under this heading.

Fluvoxamine (Since CYP3A4 and 2C19 are the primary enzymes involved in the metabolism of citalopram, it is expected that potent inhibitors of CYP219 (eg, omeprazole) might decrease the clearance of citalopram. However, co-administration of citalopram and the potent CYP3A4 inhibitor did not significantly affect the pharmacokinetics of citalopram. Because citalopram is metabolized by multiple enzyme systems, inhibition of a single enzyme system may not appreciably decrease citalopram clearance).
No products indexed under this heading.

Fluvoxamine Maleate (The development of potentially life threatening serotonin syndrome or Neuroleptic Malignant Syndrome (NMS)-like reactions have been reported with citalopram alone, but particularly with concomitant use of serotonergic drugs. Serotonin syndrome, in its most severe form, can resemble neuroleptic malignant syndrome. Patients should be monitored for the emergence of serotonin syndrome or NMS-like signs and symptoms. Treatment with citalopram and any concomitant serotonergic agent should be discontinued immediately if the above events occur and supportive treatment should be initiated).
No products indexed under this heading.

Fondaparinux Sodium (Citalopram may increase the risk of bleeding events. Concomitant use of anticoagulants may add to the risk. Case reports and studies have demonstrated an association between use of drugs that interfere with serotonin reuptake and the occurrence of gastrointestinal bleeding. Patients should be cautioned about the risk of bleeding associated with the concomitant use of citalopram and drugs affecting coagulation).
Products include:
Arixtra 1320

Fosamprenavir Calcium (*In vitro* studies indicated that CYP3A4 and CYP2C19 are the primary enzymes involved in the metabolism of citalopram. However, co-administration of citalopram (40 mg) and ketoconazole (200 mg), a potent inhibitor of CYP3A4, did not significantly affect the pharmacokinetics of citalopram. Because citalopram is metabolized by multiple enzyme systems, inhibition of a single enzyme may not appreciably decrease citalopram clearance). Products include:
Lexiva Oral Suspension 1558
Lexiva 1558

Frovatriptan Succinate (The development of a potentially life threatening serotonin syndrome or Neuroleptic Malignant syndrome (NMS)-like reactions have been reported with citalopram alone, but particularly with concomitant use of serotonergic drugs including triptans. Serotonin syndrome, in its most severe form can resemble neuroleptic malignant syndrome. Patients should be monitored for the emergence of serotonin syndrome or NMS-like signs and symptoms. If concomitant treatment of citalopram with a triptan is clinically warranted, careful observation of the patient is advised, particularly during treatment initiation and dose increases). Products include:
Frova 1103

Furosemide (Hyponatremia may occur as a result of treatment with SSRIs including citalopram. Patients taking diuretics may be at greater risk. Discontinuation of citalopram should be considered in patients with symptomatic hyponatremia and appropriate medical intervention should be instituted). Products include:
Furosemide 2354

Glutethimide (Given the primary CNS effects of citalopram, caution should be used when it is taken in combination with other centrally acting drugs).
No products indexed under this heading.

Halazepam (Given the primary CNS effects of citalopram, caution should be used when it is taken in combination with other centrally acting drugs).
No products indexed under this heading.

Haloperidol (The development of a potentially life threatening serotonin syndrome or Neuroleptic Malignant Syndrome (NMS)-like reactions have been reported with citalopram alone, and with concomitant use of antipsychotics. Serotonin syndrome, in its most severe form can resemble neuroleptic malignant syndrome. Patients should be monitored for the emergence of serotonin syndrome or NMS-like signs and symptoms. Treatment with citalopram and any antipsychotics should be discontinued immediately if the above events occur and supportive symptomatic treatment should be initiated).
No products indexed under this heading.

Haloperidol Decanoate (The development of a potentially life threatening serotonin syndrome or Neuroleptic Malignant Syndrome (NMS)-like reactions have been reported with citalopram alone, and with concomitant use of antipsychotics. Serotonin syndrome, in its most severe form can resemble neuroleptic malignant syndrome. Patients should be monitored for the emergence of serotonin syndrome or NMS-like signs and symptoms. Treatment with citalopram and any antipsychotics should be discontinued immediately if the above events occur and supportive symptomatic treatment should be initiated).
No products indexed under this heading.

Haloperidol Lactate (The development of a potentially life threatening serotonin syndrome or Neuroleptic Malignant Syndrome (NMS)-like reactions have been reported with citalopram alone, and with concomitant use of antipsychotics. Serotonin syndrome, in its most severe form can resemble neuroleptic malignant syndrome. Patients should be monitored for the emergence of serotonin syndrome or NMS-like signs and symptoms. Treatment with citalopram and any antipsychotics should be discontinued immediately if the above events occur and supportive symptomatic treatment should be initiated).
No products indexed under this heading.

Heparin Calcium (Citalopram may increase the risk of bleeding events. Concomitant use of anticoagulants may add to the risk. Case reports and studies have demonstrated an association between use of drugs that interfere with serotonin reuptake and the occurrence of gastrointestinal bleeding. Patients should be cautioned about the risk of bleeding associated with the concomitant use of citalopram and drugs affecting coagulation).
No products indexed under this heading.

Heparin Sodium (Citalopram may increase the risk of bleeding events. Concomitant use of anticoagulants may add to the risk. Case reports and studies have demonstrated an association between use of drugs that interfere with serotonin reuptake and the occurrence of gastrointestinal bleeding. Patients should be cautioned about the risk of bleeding associated with the concomitant use of citalopram and drugs affecting coagulation).
No products indexed under this heading.

IMPORTANT NOTE: Always consult each drug listing in the patient's regimen for possible interactions.

Hexobarbital (Given the primary CNS effects of citalopram, caution should be used when it is taken in combination with other centrally acting drugs).

No products indexed under this heading.

Hydrochlorothiazide (Hyponatremia may occur as a result of treatment with SSRIs including citalopram. Patients taking diuretics may be at greater risk. Discontinuation of citalopram should be considered in patients with symptomatic hyponatremia and appropriate medical intervention should be instituted). Products include:

Atacand HCT	700
Avalide	2956
Benicar HCT	1017
Diovan HCT	2419
Dyazide	1429
Exforge HCT	2449
Hyzaar	2162
Hyzaar 100-12.5	2162
Micardis HCT	889
Prinzide	2246
Tekturna HCT	2541
Teveten HCT	541

Hydrocodone Bitartrate (Given the primary CNS effects of citalopram, caution should be used when it is taken in combination with other centrally acting drugs). Products include:

Vicodin	560
Vicodin ES	561
Vicodin HP	563
Vicoprofen	564
Zydone	1138

Hydrocodone Polistirex (Given the primary CNS effects of citalopram, caution should be used when it is taken in combination with other centrally acting drugs). Products include:

Tussionex	3443

Hydroflumethiazide (Hyponatremia may occur as a result of treatment with SSRIs including citalopram. Patients taking diuretics may be at greater risk. Discontinuation of citalopram should be considered in patients with symptomatic hyponatremia and appropriate medical intervention should be instituted).

No products indexed under this heading.

Hydromorphone (Given the primary CNS effects of citalopram, caution should be used when it is taken in combination with other centrally acting drugs).

No products indexed under this heading.

Hydromorphone Hydrochloride (Given the primary CNS effects of citalopram, caution should be used when it is taken in combination with other centrally acting drugs). Products include:

Dilaudid Injection	2800
Dilaudid Oral	2797
Dilaudid Tablets	2797
Dilaudid-HP	2800

Hydroxyamphetamine Hydrobromide (Given the primary CNS effects of citalopram, caution should be used when it is taken in combination with other centrally acting drugs).

No products indexed under this heading.

Hydroxyzine Hydrochloride (Given the primary CNS effects of citalopram, caution should be used when it is taken in combination with other centrally acting drugs).

No products indexed under this heading.

Hypericum (Based on the mechanism of action of SSRIs, including citalopram, and the potential for serotonin syndrome, caution is advised when citalopram is co-administered with other drugs that may affect the serotonergic neurotransmitter systems such as St. John's Wort).

No products indexed under this heading.

Ibuprofen (Citalopram may increase the risk of bleeding events. Concomitant use of NSAIDs may add to the risk. Case reports and epidemiological studies have demonstrated an association

between use of drugs that interfere with serotonin reuptake and the occurrence of gastrointestinal bleeding. Bleeding events related to SSRIs use have ranged from ecchymoses, hematomas, epitaxis, and petechiae to life-threatening hemorrhages. Patients should be cautioned about the risk of bleeding associated with the concomitant use of citalopram and NSAIDs). Products include:

Motrin IB	2043
Children's Motrin	2044
Children's Motrin Non-Staining Dye-Free	2044
Infants' Motrin	2044
Infants' Motrin Dye-Free	2044
Junior Strength Motrin	2044
Vicoprofen	564

Imatinib Mesylate (*In vitro* studies indicated that CYP3A4 and CYP2C19 are the primary enzymes involved in the metabolism of citalopram. However, co-administration of citalopram (40 mg) and ketoconazole (200 mg), a potent inhibitor of CYP3A4, did not significantly affect the pharmacokinetics of citalopram. Because citalopram is metabolized by multiple enzyme systems, inhibition of a single enzyme may not appreciably decrease citalopram clearance). Products include:

Gleevec	2477

Imipramine Hydrochloride (Co-administration of imipramine with citalopram has resulted in a 50% increase in active metabolite, desipramine concentration. The clinical significance of this finding is unknown. Caution is indicated if tricyclic antidepressants are co-administered with citalopram).

No products indexed under this heading.

Imipramine Pamoate (Co-administration of imipramine with citalopram has resulted in a 50% increase in active metabolite, desipramine concentration. The clinical significance of this finding is unknown. Caution is indicated if tricyclic antidepressants are co-administered with citalopram).

No products indexed under this heading.

Indapamide (Hyponatremia may occur as a result of treatment with SSRIs including citalopram. Patients taking diuretics may be at greater risk. Discontinuation of citalopram should be considered in patients with symptomatic hyponatremia and appropriate medical intervention should be instituted). Products include:

Indapamide	2356

Indinavir Sulfate (*In vitro* studies indicated that CYP3A4 and CYP2C19 are the primary enzymes involved in the metabolism of citalopram. However, co-administration of citalopram (40 mg) and ketoconazole (200 mg), a potent inhibitor of CYP3A4, did not significantly affect the pharmacokinetics of citalopram. Because citalopram is metabolized by multiple enzyme systems, inhibition of a single enzyme may not appreciably decrease citalopram clearance). Products include:

Crixivan	2113

Indomethacin (Citalopram may increase the risk of bleeding events. Concomitant use of NSAIDs may add to the risk. Case reports and epidemiological studies have demonstrated an association between use of drugs that interfere with serotonin reuptake and the occurrence of gastrointestinal bleeding. Bleeding events related to SSRIs use have ranged from ecchymoses, hematomas, epitaxis, and petechiae to life-threatening hemorrhages. Patients should be cautioned about the risk of bleeding associated with the concomitant use of citalopram and NSAIDs). Products include:

Indocin	2167

Indomethacin Sodium Trihydrate (Citalopram may increase the risk of bleeding events. Concomitant use of NSAIDs may add to the risk. Case reports and epidemiological studies have demonstrated an association between use of drugs that interfere with serotonin reuptake and the occurrence of gastrointestinal bleeding. Bleeding events related to SSRIs use have ranged from ecchymoses, hematomas, epitaxis, and petechiae to life-threatening hemorrhages. Patients should be cautioned about the risk of bleeding associated with the concomitant use of citalopram and NSAIDs). Products include:

Indocin I.V.	2007

Isocarboxazid (The concomitant use of citalopram with MAO inhibitors is contraindicated. In patients receiving serotonin reuptake inhibitors (SSRIs) in combination with an MAO inhibitor, there have been reports of serious, sometimes fatal reactions. These reactions have also been reported in patients who have recently discontinued SSRI treatment and have been started on an MAO inhibitor. Some cases presented with features resembling neuroleptic malignant syndrome. In addition, there is data to indicate that SSRIs and MAO inhibitors may act synergistically to elevate blood pressure and evoke behavioral excitation. Therefore, it is recommended that citalopram should not be used in combination with an MAO inhibitor, or within 14 days of discontinuing treatment with an MAO inhibitor. Similarly, at least 14 days should be allowed after stopping citalopram before starting an MAO inhibitor). Products include:

Marplan	3481

Isoflurane (Given the primary CNS effects of citalopram, caution should be used when it is taken in combination with other centrally acting drugs).

No products indexed under this heading.

Isoniazid (Since CYP3A4 and 2C19 are the primary enzymes involved in the metabolism of citalopram, it is expected that potent inhibitors of CYP219 (eg, omeprazole) might decrease the clearance of citalopram. However, co-administration of citalopram and the potent CYP3A4 inhibitor did not significantly affect the pharmacokinetics of citalopram. Because citalopram is metabolized by multiple enzyme systems, inhibition of a single enzyme system may not appreciably decrease citalopram clearance).

No products indexed under this heading.

Itraconazole (Co-administration with potent inhibitors of CYP3A4, such as itraconazole, may decrease the clearance of citalopram).

No products indexed under this heading.

Ketamine Hydrochloride (Given the primary CNS effects of citalopram, caution should be used when it is taken in combination with other centrally acting drugs).

No products indexed under this heading.

Ketoconazole (Co-administration resulted in decreased C_{max} and AUC of ketoconazole by 21% and 10% respectively, and did not significantly affect the pharmacokinetics of citalopram). Products include:

Extina	3319
Xolegel	3337

Ketoprofen (Citalopram may increase the risk of bleeding events. Concomitant use of NSAIDs may add to the risk. Case reports and epidemiological studies have demonstrated an association between use of drugs that interfere with serotonin reuptake and the occurrence of gastrointestinal bleeding. Bleeding events related to SSRIs use have ranged from ecchymoses, hematomas, epitaxis, and petechiae to life-

threatening hemorrhages. Patients should be cautioned about the risk of bleeding associated with the concomitant use of citalopram and NSAIDs).

No products indexed under this heading.

Ketorolac Tromethamine (Citalopram may increase the risk of bleeding events. Concomitant use of NSAIDs may add to the risk. Case reports and epidemiological studies have demonstrated an association between use of drugs that interfere with serotonin reuptake and the occurrence of gastrointestinal bleeding. Bleeding events related to SSRIs use have ranged from ecchymoses, hematomas, epitaxis, and petechiae to life-threatening hemorrhages. Patients should be cautioned about the risk of bleeding associated with the concomitant use of citalopram and NSAIDs). Products include:

Acuvail	⊙209

Lansoprazole (Since CYP3A4 and 2C19 are the primary enzymes involved in the metabolism of citalopram, it is expected that potent inhibitors of CYP219 (eg, omeprazole) might decrease the clearance of citalopram. However, co-administration of citalopram and the potent CYP3A4 inhibitor did not significantly affect the pharmacokinetics of citalopram. Because citalopram is metabolized by multiple enzyme systems, inhibition of a single enzyme system may not appreciably decrease citalopram clearance).

No products indexed under this heading.

Lapatinib (*In vitro* studies indicated that CYP3A4 and CYP2C19 are the primary enzymes involved in the metabolism of citalopram. However, co-administration of citalopram (40 mg) and ketoconazole (200 mg), a potent inhibitor of CYP3A4, did not significantly affect the pharmacokinetics of citalopram. Because citalopram is metabolized by multiple enzyme systems, inhibition of a single enzyme may not appreciably decrease citalopram clearance). Products include:

Tykerb	1698

Letrozole (Since CYP3A4 and 2C19 are the primary enzymes involved in the metabolism of citalopram, it is expected that potent inhibitors of CYP219 (eg, omeprazole) might decrease the clearance of citalopram. However, co-administration of citalopram and the potent CYP3A4 inhibitor did not significantly affect the pharmacokinetics of citalopram. Because citalopram is metabolized by multiple enzyme systems, inhibition of a single enzyme system may not appreciably decrease citalopram clearance). Products include:

Femara	2466

Levomethadyl Acetate Hydrochloride (Given the primary CNS effects of citalopram, caution should be used when it is taken in combination with other centrally acting drugs).

No products indexed under this heading.

Levonorgestrel (Since CYP3A4 and 2C19 are the primary enzymes involved in the metabolism of citalopram, it is expected that potent inhibitors of CYP219 (eg, omeprazole) might decrease the clearance of citalopram. However, co-administration of citalopram and the potent CYP3A4 inhibitor did not significantly affect the pharmacokinetics of citalopram. Because citalopram is metabolized by multiple enzyme systems, inhibition of a single enzyme system may not appreciably decrease citalopram clearance). Products include:

Climara Pro	847
LoSeasonique	3407
Lybrel	3514
Mirena	854

Plan B 3416
Seasonique 3418

Levorphanol Tartrate (Given the primary CNS effects of citalopram, caution should be used when it is taken in combination with other centrally acting drugs).
No products indexed under this heading.

Linezolid (Based on the mechanism of action of SSRIs, including citalopram, and the potential for serotonin syndrome, caution is advised when citalopram is co-administered with other drugs that may affect the serotonergic neurotransmitter systems, such as linezolid). Products include:
Zyvox 2769

Lisdexamfetamine Dimesylate (Given the primary CNS effects of citalopram, caution should be used when it is taken in combination with other centrally acting drugs). Products include:
Vyvanse 3298

Lithium (The development of a potentially life threatening serotonin syndrome or Neuroleptic Malignant Syndrome (NMS)-like reactions have been reported with citalopram alone, and with concomitant use of antipsychotics. Serotonin syndrome, in its most severe form can resemble neuroleptic malignant syndrome. Patients should be monitored for the emergence of serotonin syndrome or NMS-like signs and symptoms. Treatment with citalopram and any antipsychotics should be discontinued immediately if the above events occur and supportive symptomatic treatment should be initiated).
No products indexed under this heading.

Lithium Carbonate (The development of a potentially life threatening serotonin syndrome or Neuroleptic Malignant Syndrome (NMS)-like reactions have been reported with citalopram alone, and with concomitant use of antipsychotics. Serotonin syndrome, in its most severe form can resemble neuroleptic malignant syndrome. Patients should be monitored for the emergence of serotonin syndrome or NMS-like signs and symptoms. Treatment with citalopram and any antipsychotics should be discontinued immediately if the above events occur and supportive symptomatic treatment should be initiated).
No products indexed under this heading.

Lithium Citrate (The development of a potentially life threatening serotonin syndrome or Neuroleptic Malignant Syndrome (NMS)-like reactions have been reported with citalopram alone, and with concomitant use of antipsychotics. Serotonin syndrome, in its most severe form can resemble neuroleptic malignant syndrome. Patients should be monitored for the emergence of serotonin syndrome or NMS-like signs and symptoms. Treatment with citalopram and any antipsychotics should be discontinued immediately if the above events occur and supportive symptomatic treatment should be initiated).
No products indexed under this heading.

Lopinavir (*In vitro* studies indicated that CYP3A4 and CYP2C19 are the primary enzymes involved in the metabolism of citalopram. However, co-administration of citalopram (40 mg) and ketoconazole (200 mg), a potent inhibitor of CYP3A4, did not significantly affect the pharmacokinetics of citalopram. Because citalopram is metabolized by multiple enzyme systems, inhibition of a single enzyme may not appreciably decrease citalopram clearance). Products include:
Kaletra 458

Loratadine (*In vitro* studies indicated that CYP3A4 and CYP2C19 are the primary enzymes involved in the metabolism of citalopram. However, co-administration of citalopram (40 mg) and ketoconazole (200 mg), a potent inhibitor of CYP3A4, did not significantly affect the pharmacokinetics of citalopram. Because citalopram is metabolized by multiple enzyme systems, inhibition of a single enzyme may not appreciably decrease citalopram clearance).
No products indexed under this heading.

Lorazepam (Given the primary CNS effects of citalopram, caution should be used when it is taken in combination with other centrally acting drugs).
No products indexed under this heading.

Low Molecular Weight Heparins (Citalopram may increase the risk of bleeding events. Concomitant use of anticoagulants may add to the risk. Case reports and studies have demonstrated an association between use of drugs that interfere with serotonin reuptake and the occurrence of gastrointestinal bleeding. Patients should be cautioned about the risk of bleeding associated with the concomitant use of citalopram and drugs affecting coagulation).
No products indexed under this heading.

Loxapine Hydrochloride (The development of a potentially life threatening serotonin syndrome or Neuroleptic Malignant Syndrome (NMS)-like reactions have been reported with citalopram alone, and with concomitant use of antipsychotics. Serotonin syndrome, in its most severe form can resemble neuroleptic malignant syndrome. Patients should be monitored for the emergence of serotonin syndrome or NMS-like signs and symptoms. Treatment with citalopram and any antipsychotics should be discontinued immediately if the above events occur and supportive symptomatic treatment should be initiated).
No products indexed under this heading.

Loxapine Succinate (The development of a potentially life threatening serotonin syndrome or Neuroleptic Malignant Syndrome (NMS)-like reactions have been reported with citalopram alone, and with concomitant use of antipsychotics. Serotonin syndrome, in its most severe form can resemble neuroleptic malignant syndrome. Patients should be monitored for the emergence of serotonin syndrome or NMS-like signs and symptoms. Treatment with citalopram and any antipsychotics should be discontinued immediately if the above events occur and supportive symptomatic treatment should be initiated).
No products indexed under this heading.

Maprotiline Hydrochloride (Co-administration of imipramine with citalopram has resulted in a 50% increase in active metabolite, desipramine concentration. The clinical significance of this finding is unknown. Caution is indicated if tricyclic antidepressants are co-administered with citalopram).
No products indexed under this heading.

Meclofenamate Sodium (Citalopram may increase the risk of bleeding events. Concomitant use of NSAIDs may add to the risk. Case reports and epidemiological studies have demonstrated an association between use of drugs that interfere with serotonin reuptake and the occurrence of gastrointestinal bleeding. Bleeding events related to SSRIs use have ranged from ecchymoses, hematomas, epitaxis, and petechiae to life-threatening hemorrhages. Patients should be cautioned about the risk of bleeding associated with the concomitant use of citalopram and NSAIDs).
No products indexed under this heading.

Mefenamic Acid (Citalopram may increase the risk of bleeding events. Concomitant use of NSAIDs may add to the risk. Case reports and epidemiological studies have demonstrated an association between use of drugs that interfere with serotonin reuptake and the occurrence of gastrointestinal bleeding. Bleeding events related to SSRIs use have ranged from ecchymoses, hematomas, epitaxis, and petechiae to life-threatening hemorrhages. Patients should be cautioned about the risk of bleeding associated with the concomitant use of citalopram and NSAIDs).
No products indexed under this heading.

Meloxicam (Citalopram may increase the risk of bleeding events. Concomitant use of NSAIDs may add to the risk. Case reports and epidemiological studies have demonstrated an association between use of drugs that interfere with serotonin reuptake and the occurrence of gastrointestinal bleeding. Bleeding events related to SSRIs use have ranged from ecchymoses, hematomas, epitaxis, and petechiae to life-threatening hemorrhages. Patients should be cautioned about the risk of bleeding associated with the concomitant use of citalopram and NSAIDs).
No products indexed under this heading.

Meperidine Hydrochloride (Given the primary CNS effects of citalopram, caution should be used when it is taken in combination with other centrally acting drugs).
No products indexed under this heading.

Mephobarbital (Given the primary CNS effects of citalopram, caution should be used when it is taken in combination with other centrally acting drugs).
No products indexed under this heading.

Meprobamate (Given the primary CNS effects of citalopram, caution should be used when it is taken in combination with other centrally acting drugs).
No products indexed under this heading.

Mesoridazine Besylate (The development of a potentially life threatening serotonin syndrome or Neuroleptic Malignant Syndrome (NMS)-like reactions have been reported with citalopram alone, and with concomitant use of antipsychotics. Serotonin syndrome, in its most severe form can resemble neuroleptic malignant syndrome. Patients should be monitored for the emergence of serotonin syndrome or NMS-like signs and symptoms. Treatment with citalopram and any antipsychotics should be discontinued immediately if the above events occur and supportive symptomatic treatment should be initiated).
No products indexed under this heading.

Mestranol (Since CYP3A4 and 2C19 are the primary enzymes involved in the metabolism of citalopram, it is expected that potent inhibitors of CYP219 (eg, omeprazole) might decrease the clearance of citalopram. However, co-administration of citalopram and the potent CYP3A4 inhibitor did not significantly affect the pharmacokinetics of citalopram. Because citalopram is metabolized by multiple enzyme systems, inhibition of a single enzyme system may not appreciably decrease citalopram clearance).
No products indexed under this heading.

Methadone Hydrochloride (Given the primary CNS effects of citalopram, caution should be used when it is taken in combination with other centrally acting drugs).
No products indexed under this heading.

Methamphetamine Hydrochloride (Given the primary CNS effects of citalopram, caution should be used when it is taken in combination with other centrally acting drugs).
No products indexed under this heading.

Methohexital Sodium (Given the primary CNS effects of citalopram, caution should be used when it is taken in combination with other centrally acting drugs).
No products indexed under this heading.

Methotrimeprazine (The development of a potentially life threatening serotonin syndrome or Neuroleptic Malignant Syndrome (NMS)-like reactions have been reported with citalopram alone, and with concomitant use of antipsychotics. Serotonin syndrome, in its most severe form can resemble neuroleptic malignant syndrome. Patients should be monitored for the emergence of serotonin syndrome or NMS-like signs and symptoms. Treatment with citalopram and any antipsychotics should be discontinued immediately if the above events occur and supportive symptomatic treatment should be initiated).
No products indexed under this heading.

Methoxyflurane (Given the primary CNS effects of citalopram, caution should be used when it is taken in combination with other centrally acting drugs).
No products indexed under this heading.

Methyclothiazide (Hyponatremia may occur as a result of treatment with SSRIs including citalopram. Patients taking diuretics may be at greater risk. Discontinuation of citalopram should be considered in patients with symptomatic hyponatremia and appropriate medical intervention should be instituted).
No products indexed under this heading.

Methylphenidate (Given the primary CNS effects of citalopram, caution should be used when it is taken in combination with other centrally acting drugs). Products include:
Daytrana 3283

Methylphenidate Hydrochloride (Given the primary CNS effects of citalopram, caution should be used when it is taken in combination with other centrally acting drugs). Products include:
Concerta 2598
Metadate CD 3439

Metoclopramide Hydrochloride (The development of a potentially life threatening serotonin syndrome or Neuroleptic Malignant Syndrome (NMS)-like reactions have been reported with citalopram alone, and with concomitant use of dopamine antagonists. Serotonin syndrome, in its most severe form can resemble neuroleptic malignant syndrome. Patients should be monitored for the emergence of serotonin syndrome or NMS-like signs and symptoms. Treatment with citalopram and any concomitant antidopaminergic agent should be discontinued immediately if the above events occur and supportive symptomatic treatment should be initiated). Products include:
Metozolv ODT 2901

Metolazone (Hyponatremia may occur as a result of treatment with SSRIs including citalopram. Patients taking diuretics may be at greater risk. Discontinuation of citalopram should be considered in patients with symptomatic hyponatremia and appropriate medical intervention should be instituted).
No products indexed under this heading.

Metoprolol Succinate (Co-administration has resulted in a two-fold increase in the plasma levels of metoprolol; increased plasma levels of metoprolol have been associated with decreased cardioselectivity; no clinically

IMPORTANT NOTE: Always consult each drug listing in the patient's regimen for possible interactions.

Celexa **Interactions Index** 302

significant effects on the blood pressure or heart rate have been reported with concurrent use). Products include:
Toprol XL 732

Metoprolol Tartrate (Co-administration has resulted in a two-fold increase in the plasma levels of metoprolol; increased plasma levels of metoprolol have been associated with decreased cardioselectivity; no clinically significant effects on the blood pressure or heart rate have been reported with concurrent use).
No products indexed under this heading.

Metronidazole (*In vitro* studies indicated that CYP3A4 and CYP2C19 are the primary enzymes involved in the metabolism of citalopram. However, co-administration of citalopram (40 mg) and ketoconazole (200 mg), a potent inhibitor of CYP3A4, did not significantly affect the pharmacokinetics of citalopram. Because citalopram is metabolized by multiple enzyme systems, inhibition of a single enzyme may not appreciably decrease citalopram clearance). Products include:
Pylera 793

Metronidazole Benzoate (*In vitro* studies indicated that CYP3A4 and CYP2C19 are the primary enzymes involved in the metabolism of citalopram. However, co-administration of citalopram (40 mg) and ketoconazole (200 mg), a potent inhibitor of CYP3A4, did not significantly affect the pharmacokinetics of citalopram. Because citalopram is metabolized by multiple enzyme systems, inhibition of a single enzyme may not appreciably decrease citalopram clearance).
No products indexed under this heading.

Metronidazole Hydrochloride (*In vitro* studies indicated that CYP3A4 and CYP2C19 are the primary enzymes involved in the metabolism of citalopram. However, co-administration of citalopram (40 mg) and ketoconazole (200 mg), a potent inhibitor of CYP3A4, did not significantly affect the pharmacokinetics of citalopram. Because citalopram is metabolized by multiple enzyme systems, inhibition of a single enzyme may not appreciably decrease citalopram clearance).
No products indexed under this heading.

Metronidazole Sodium (*In vitro* studies indicated that CYP3A4 and CYP2C19 are the primary enzymes involved in the metabolism of citalopram. However, co-administration of citalopram (40 mg) and ketoconazole (200 mg), a potent inhibitor of CYP3A4, did not significantly affect the pharmacokinetics of citalopram. Because citalopram is metabolized by multiple enzyme systems, inhibition of a single enzyme may not appreciably decrease citalopram clearance).
No products indexed under this heading.

Miconazole (*In vitro* studies indicated that CYP3A4 and CYP2C19 are the primary enzymes involved in the metabolism of citalopram. However, co-administration of citalopram (40 mg) and ketoconazole (200 mg), a potent inhibitor of CYP3A4, did not significantly affect the pharmacokinetics of citalopram. Because citalopram is metabolized by multiple enzyme systems, inhibition of a single enzyme may not appreciably decrease citalopram clearance).
No products indexed under this heading.

Miconazole Nitrate (*In vitro* studies indicated that CYP3A4 and CYP2C19 are the primary enzymes involved in the metabolism of citalopram. However, co-administration of citalopram (40 mg) and ketoconazole (200 mg), a potent inhibitor of CYP3A4, did not significantly affect the pharmacokinetics of citalopram. Because citalopram is metabolized by multiple enzyme systems, inhibition of a single enzyme may not appreciably decrease citalopram clearance). Products include:
Vusion Ointment 3335

Midazolam Hydrochloride (Given the primary CNS effects of citalopram, caution should be used when it is taken in combination with other centrally acting drugs).
No products indexed under this heading.

Mifepristone (*In vitro* studies indicated that CYP3A4 and CYP2C19 are the primary enzymes involved in the metabolism of citalopram. However, co-administration of citalopram (40 mg) and ketoconazole (200 mg), a potent inhibitor of CYP3A4, did not significantly affect the pharmacokinetics of citalopram. Because citalopram is metabolized by multiple enzyme systems, inhibition of a single enzyme may not appreciably decrease citalopram clearance).
No products indexed under this heading.

Moclobemide (The concomitant use of citalopram with MAO inhibitors is contraindicated. In patients receiving serotonin reuptake inhibitors (SSRIs) in combination with an MAO inhibitor, there have been reports of serious, sometimes fatal reactions. These reactions have also been reported in patients who have recently discontinued SSRI treatment and have been started on an MAO inhibitor. Some cases presented with features resembling neuroleptic malignant syndrome. In addition, there is data to indicate that SSRIs and MAO inhibitors may act synergistically to elevate blood pressure and evoke behavioral excitation. Therefore, it is recommended that citalopram should not be used in combination with an MAO inhibitor, or within 14 days of discontinuing treatment with an MAO inhibitor. Similarly, at least 14 days should be allowed after stopping citalopram before starting an MAO inhibitor).
No products indexed under this heading.

Modafinil (Since CYP3A4 and 2C19 are the primary enzymes involved in the metabolism of citalopram, it is expected that potent inhibitors of CYP219 (eg, omeprazole) might decrease the clearance of citalopram. However, co-administration of citalopram and the potent CYP3A4 inhibitor did not significantly affect the pharmacokinetics of citalopram. Because citalopram is metabolized by multiple enzyme systems, inhibition of a single enzyme system may not appreciably decrease citalopram clearance). Products include:
Provigil 983

Molindone Hydrochloride (The development of a potentially life threatening serotonin syndrome or Neuroleptic Malignant Syndrome (NMS)-like reactions have been reported with citalopram alone, and with concomitant use of antipsychotics. Serotonin syndrome, in its most severe form can resemble neuroleptic malignant syndrome. Patients should be monitored for the emergence of serotonin syndrome or NMS-like signs and symptoms. Treatment with citalopram and any antipsychotics should be discontinued immediately if the above events occur and supportive symptomatic treatment should be initiated). Products include:
Moban 1108

Morphine Sulfate (Given the primary CNS effects of citalopram, caution should be used when it is taken in combination with other centrally acting drugs). Products include:
Avinza 1822
Embeda 1831
MS Contin 2803

Morphine Sulfate, Liposomal (Given the primary CNS effects of citalopram, caution should be used when it is taken in combination with other centrally acting drugs).
No products indexed under this heading.

Nabumetone (Citalopram may increase the risk of bleeding events. Concomitant use of NSAIDs may add to the risk. Case reports and epidemiological studies have demonstrated an association between use of drugs that interfere with serotonin reuptake and the occurrence of gastrointestinal bleeding. Bleeding events related to SSRIs use have ranged from ecchymoses, hematomas, epitaxis, and petechiae to life-threatening hemorrhages. Patients should be cautioned about the risk of bleeding associated with the concomitant use of citalopram and NSAIDs).
No products indexed under this heading.

Naproxen (Citalopram may increase the risk of bleeding events. Concomitant use of NSAIDs may add to the risk. Case reports and epidemiological studies have demonstrated an association between use of drugs that interfere with serotonin reuptake and the occurrence of gastrointestinal bleeding. Bleeding events related to SSRIs use have ranged from ecchymoses, hematomas, epitaxis, and petechiae to life-threatening hemorrhages. Patients should be cautioned about the risk of bleeding associated with the concomitant use of citalopram and NSAIDs). Products include:
EC-Naprosyn 2850
Naprosyn 2850
Anaprox/Naprosyn 2850

Naproxen Sodium (Citalopram may increase the risk of bleeding events. Concomitant use of NSAIDs may add to the risk. Case reports and epidemiological studies have demonstrated an association between use of drugs that interfere with serotonin reuptake and the occurrence of gastrointestinal bleeding. Bleeding events related to SSRIs use have ranged from ecchymoses, hematomas, epitaxis, and petechiae to life-threatening hemorrhages. Patients should be cautioned about the risk of bleeding associated with the concomitant use of citalopram and NSAIDs). Products include:
Anaprox 2850
Anaprox DS 2850
Treximet 1681

Naratriptan Hydrochloride (The development of potentially life threatening serotonin syndrome or Neuroleptic Malignant syndrome (NMS)-like reactions have been reported with citalopram alone, but particularly with concomitant use of serotonergic drugs including triptans. Serotonin syndrome, in its most severe form can resemble neuroleptic malignant syndrome. Patients should be monitored for the emergence of serotonin syndrome or NMS-like signs and symptoms. If concomitant treatment of citalopram with a triptan is clinically warranted, careful observation of the patient is advised, particularly during treatment initiation and dose increases). Products include:
Amerge 1306

Nefazodone Hydrochloride (The development of potentially life threatening serotonin syndrome or Neuroleptic Malignant Syndrome (NMS)-like reactions have been reported with citalopram alone, but particularly with concomitant use of serotonergic drugs. The concomitant use of citalopram with SNRIs is not recommended).
No products indexed under this heading.

Nelfinavir Mesylate (*In vitro* studies indicated that CYP3A4 and CYP2C19 are the primary enzymes involved in the metabolism of citalopram. However, co-administration of citalopram (40 mg) and ketoconazole (200 mg), a potent inhibitor of CYP3A4, did not significantly affect the pharmacokinetics of citalopram. Because citalopram is metabolized by multiple enzyme systems, inhibition of a single enzyme may not appreciably decrease citalopram clearance).
No products indexed under this heading.

Nevirapine (*In vitro* studies indicated that CYP3A4 and CYP2C19 are the primary enzymes involved in the metabolism of citalopram. However, co-administration of citalopram (40 mg) and ketoconazole (200 mg), a potent inhibitor of CYP3A4, did not significantly affect the pharmacokinetics of citalopram. Because citalopram is metabolized by multiple enzyme systems, inhibition of a single enzyme may not appreciably decrease citalopram clearance). Products include:
Viramune Oral Suspension 897
Viramune Tablets 897

Niacin (*In vitro* studies indicated that CYP3A4 and CYP2C19 are the primary enzymes involved in the metabolism of citalopram. However, co-administration of citalopram (40 mg) and ketoconazole (200 mg), a potent inhibitor of CYP3A4, did not significantly affect the pharmacokinetics of citalopram. Because citalopram is metabolized by multiple enzyme systems, inhibition of a single enzyme may not appreciably decrease citalopram clearance). Products include:
Advicor 402
Cardio Basics 3455
Niaspan 497
Simcor 524

Niacinamide (*In vitro* studies indicated that CYP3A4 and CYP2C19 are the primary enzymes involved in the metabolism of citalopram. However, co-administration of citalopram (40 mg) and ketoconazole (200 mg), a potent inhibitor of CYP3A4, did not significantly affect the pharmacokinetics of citalopram. Because citalopram is metabolized by multiple enzyme systems, inhibition of a single enzyme may not appreciably decrease citalopram clearance). Products include:
CitraNatal 90 DHA Capsules 2332
CitraNatal Assure 2332
CitraNatal Rx 2332
Heplive 607

Niacinamide Hydroiodide (*In vitro* studies indicated that CYP3A4 and CYP2C19 are the primary enzymes involved in the metabolism of citalopram. However, co-administration of citalopram (40 mg) and ketoconazole (200 mg), a potent inhibitor of CYP3A4, did not significantly affect the pharmacokinetics of citalopram. Because citalopram is metabolized by multiple enzyme systems, inhibition of a single enzyme may not appreciably decrease citalopram clearance).
No products indexed under this heading.

Nicotinamide (*In vitro* studies indicated that CYP3A4 and CYP2C19 are the primary enzymes involved in the metabolism of citalopram. However, co-administration of citalopram (40 mg) and ketoconazole (200 mg), a potent inhibitor of CYP3A4, did not significantly affect the pharmacokinetics of citalopram. Because citalopram is metabolized by multiple enzyme systems, inhibition of a single enzyme may not appreciably decrease citalopram clearance).
No products indexed under this heading.

Nifedipine (*In vitro* studies indicated that CYP3A4 and CYP2C19 are the primary enzymes involved in the metabolism of citalopram. However, co-

administration of citalopram (40 mg) and ketoconazole (200 mg), a potent inhibitor of CYP3A4, did not significantly affect the pharmacokinetics of citalopram. Because citalopram is metabolized by multiple enzyme systems, inhibition of a single enzyme may not appreciably decrease citalopram clearance).

No products indexed under this heading.

Norethindrone (Since CYP3A4 and 2C19 are the primary enzymes involved in the metabolism of citalopram, it is expected that potent inhibitors of CYP219 (eg, omeprazole) might decrease the clearance of citalopram. However, co-administration of citalopram and the potent CYP3A4 inhibitor did not significantly affect the pharmacokinetics of citalopram. Because citalopram is metabolized by multiple enzyme systems, inhibition of a single enzyme system may not appreciably decrease citalopram clearance). Products include:

Ortho Micronor 2660

Norethynodrel (Since CYP3A4 and 2C19 are the primary enzymes involved in the metabolism of citalopram, it is expected that potent inhibitors of CYP219 (eg, omeprazole) might decrease the clearance of citalopram. However, co-administration of citalopram and the potent CYP3A4 inhibitor did not significantly affect the pharmacokinetics of citalopram. Because citalopram is metabolized by multiple enzyme systems, inhibition of a single enzyme system may not appreciably decrease citalopram clearance).

No products indexed under this heading.

Norfloxacin (*In vitro* studies indicated that CYP3A4 and CYP2C19 are the primary enzymes involved in the metabolism of citalopram. However, co-administration of citalopram (40 mg) and ketoconazole (200 mg), a potent inhibitor of CYP3A4, did not significantly affect the pharmacokinetics of citalopram. Because citalopram is metabolized by multiple enzyme systems, inhibition of a single enzyme may not appreciably decrease citalopram clearance). Products include:

Noroxin 2220

Norgestimate (Since CYP3A4 and 2C19 are the primary enzymes involved in the metabolism of citalopram, it is expected that potent inhibitors of CYP219 (eg, omeprazole) might decrease the clearance of citalopram. However, co-administration of citalopram and the potent CYP3A4 inhibitor did not significantly affect the pharmacokinetics of citalopram. Because citalopram is metabolized by multiple enzyme systems, inhibition of a single enzyme system may not appreciably decrease citalopram clearance). Products include:

Ortho-Cyclen/Ortho Tri-Cyclen 2663
Ortho Tri-Cyclen Lo Tablets 2673

Norgestrel (Since CYP3A4 and 2C19 are the primary enzymes involved in the metabolism of citalopram, it is expected that potent inhibitors of CYP219 (eg, omeprazole) might decrease the clearance of citalopram. However, co-administration of citalopram and the potent CYP3A4 inhibitor did not significantly affect the pharmacokinetics of citalopram. Because citalopram is metabolized by multiple enzyme systems, inhibition of a single enzyme system may not appreciably decrease citalopram clearance).

No products indexed under this heading.

Nortriptyline Hydrochloride (Co-administration of imipramine with citalopram has resulted in a 50% increase in active metabolite, desipramine concentration. The clinical significance of this finding is unknown. Caution is indicated if tricyclic antidepressants are co-administered with citalopram).

No products indexed under this heading.

Olanzapine (The development of a potentially life threatening serotonin syndrome or Neuroleptic Malignant Syndrome (NMS)-like reactions have been reported with citalopram alone, and with concomitant use of antipsychotics. Serotonin syndrome, in its most severe form can resemble neuroleptic malignant syndrome. Patients should be monitored for the emergence of serotonin syndrome or NMS-like signs and symptoms. Treatment with citalopram and any antipsychotics should be discontinued immediately if the above events occur and supportive symptomatic treatment should be initiated). Products include:

Symbyax 1965
Zyprexa 1984
Zyprexa IntraMuscular 1984
Zyprexa ZYDIS 1984

Omeprazole (Since CYP3A4 and 2C19 are the primary enzymes involved in the metabolism of citalopram, it is expected that potent inhibitors of CYP219 (eg, omeprazole) might decrease the clearance of citalopram. However, co-administration of citalopram and the potent CYP3A4 inhibitor did not significantly affect the pharmacokinetics of citalopram. Because citalopram is metabolized by multiple enzyme systems, inhibition of a single enzyme system may not appreciably decrease citalopram clearance).

No products indexed under this heading.

Oxaprozin (Citalopram may increase the risk of bleeding events. Concomitant use of NSAIDs may add to the risk. Case reports and epidemiological studies have demonstrated an association between use of drugs that interfere with serotonin reuptake and the occurrence of gastrointestinal bleeding. Bleeding events related to SSRIs use have ranged from ecchymoses, hematomas, epitaxis, and petechiae to life-threatening hemorrhages. Patients should be cautioned about the risk of bleeding associated with the concomitant use of citalopram and NSAIDs).

No products indexed under this heading.

Oxazepam (Given the primary CNS effects of citalopram, caution should be used when it is taken in combination with other centrally acting drugs).

No products indexed under this heading.

Oxcarbazepine (Since CYP3A4 and 2C19 are the primary enzymes involved in the metabolism of citalopram, it is expected that potent inhibitors of CYP219 (eg, omeprazole) might decrease the clearance of citalopram. However, co-administration of citalopram and the potent CYP3A4 inhibitor did not significantly affect the pharmacokinetics of citalopram. Because citalopram is metabolized by multiple enzyme systems, inhibition of a single enzyme system may not appreciably decrease citalopram clearance).

No products indexed under this heading.

Oxycodone Hydrochloride (Given the primary CNS effects of citalopram, caution should be used when it is taken in combination with other centrally acting drugs). Products include:

OxyContin 2807
Percocet 1121
Percodan 1124

Oxycodone Terephthalate (Given the primary CNS effects of citalopram, caution should be used when it is taken in combination with other centrally acting drugs).

No products indexed under this heading.

Oxymorphone Hydrochloride (Given the primary CNS effects of citalopram, caution should be used when it is taken in combination with other centrally acting drugs). Products include:

Opana 1110
Opana ER 1114

Paliperidone (The development of a potentially life threatening serotonin syndrome or Neuroleptic Malignant Syndrome (NMS)-like reactions have been reported with citalopram alone, and with concomitant use of antipsychotics. Serotonin syndrome, in its most severe form can resemble neuroleptic malignant syndrome. Patients should be monitored for the emergence of serotonin syndrome or NMS-like signs and symptoms. Treatment with citalopram and any antipsychotics should be discontinued immediately if the above events occur and supportive symptomatic treatment should be initiated). Products include:

Invega 2613
Invega Sustenna 2621

Pargyline Hydrochloride (The concomitant use of citalopram with MAO inhibitors is contraindicated. In patients receiving serotonin reuptake inhibitors (SSRIs) in combination with an MAO inhibitor, there have been reports of serious, sometimes fatal reactions. These reactions have also been reported in patients who have recently discontinued SSRI treatment and have been started on an MAO inhibitor. Some cases presented with features resembling neuroleptic malignant syndrome. In addition, there is data to indicate that SSRIs and MAO inhibitors may act synergistically to elevate blood pressure and evoke behavioral excitation. Therefore, it is recommended that citalopram should not be used in combination with an MAO inhibitor, or within 14 days of discontinuing treatment with an MAO inhibitor. Similarly, at least 14 days should be allowed after stopping citalopram before starting an MAO inhibitor).

No products indexed under this heading.

Paroxetine Hydrochloride (The development of potentially life threatening serotonin syndrome or Neuroleptic Malignant Syndrome (NMS)-like reactions have been reported with citalopram alone, but particularly with concomitant use of serotonergic drugs. Serotonin syndrome, in its most severe form, can resemble neuroleptic malignant syndrome. Patients should be monitored for the emergence of serotonin syndrome or NMS-like signs and symptoms. Treatment with citalopram and any concomitant serotonergic agent should be discontinued immediately if the above events occur and supportive treatment should be initiated). Products include:

Paroxetine CR 2361
Paroxetine ER 2371
Paxil 1586
Paxil CR 1596

Pemoline (Given the primary CNS effects of citalopram, caution should be used when it is taken in combination with other centrally acting drugs).

No products indexed under this heading.

Pentobarbital (Given the primary CNS effects of citalopram, caution should be used when it is taken in combination with other centrally acting drugs).

No products indexed under this heading.

Pentobarbital Sodium (Given the primary CNS effects of citalopram, cau-

tion should be used when it is taken in combination with other centrally acting drugs). Products include:

Nembutal 2012

Perphenazine (The development of a potentially life threatening serotonin syndrome or Neuroleptic Malignant Syndrome (NMS)-like reactions have been reported with citalopram alone, and with concomitant use of antipsychotics. Serotonin syndrome, in its most severe form can resemble neuroleptic malignant syndrome. Patients should be monitored for the emergence of serotonin syndrome or NMS-like signs and symptoms. Treatment with citalopram and any antipsychotics should be discontinued immediately if the above events occur and supportive symptomatic treatment should be initiated).

No products indexed under this heading.

Phenelzine Sulfate (The concomitant use of citalopram with MAO inhibitors is contraindicated. In patients receiving serotonin reuptake inhibitors (SSRIs) in combination with an MAO inhibitor, there have been reports of serious, sometimes fatal reactions. These reactions have also been reported in patients who have recently discontinued SSRI treatment and have been started on an MAO inhibitor. Some cases presented with features resembling neuroleptic malignant syndrome. In addition, there is data to indicate that SSRIs and MAO inhibitors may act synergistically to elevate blood pressure and evoke behavioral excitation. Therefore, it is recommended that citalopram should not be used in combination with an MAO inhibitor, or within 14 days of discontinuing treatment with an MAO inhibitor. Similarly, at least 14 days should be allowed after stopping citalopram before starting an MAO inhibitor).

No products indexed under this heading.

Phenobarbital (Given the primary CNS effects of citalopram, caution should be used when it is taken in combination with other centrally acting drugs). Products include:

Donnatal 2711

Phenobarbital Sodium (Given the primary CNS effects of citalopram, caution should be used when it is taken in combination with other centrally acting drugs).

No products indexed under this heading.

Phenylbutazone (Citalopram may increase the risk of bleeding events. Concomitant use of NSAIDs may add to the risk. Case reports and epidemiological studies have demonstrated an association between use of drugs that interfere with serotonin reuptake and the occurrence of gastrointestinal bleeding. Bleeding events related to SSRIs use have ranged from ecchymoses, hematomas, epitaxis, and petechiae to life-threatening hemorrhages. Patients should be cautioned about the risk of bleeding associated with the concomitant use of citalopram and NSAIDs).

No products indexed under this heading.

Pimozide (Concomitant use of pimozide is contraindicated. In a controlled study, a single dose of pimozide 2 mg co-administered with citalopram 40 mg given once daily for 11 days was associated with a mean increase in QTc values of approximately 10 msec compared to pimozide given alone).

No products indexed under this heading.

Piroxicam (Citalopram may increase the risk of bleeding events. Concomitant use of NSAIDs may add to the risk. Case reports and epidemiological studies have demonstrated an association between use of drugs that interfere with serotonin reuptake and the occurrence of gastrointestinal bleeding. Bleeding events related to SSRIs use have ranged from ecchymoses, hematomas,

---

IMPORTANT NOTE: Always consult each drug listing in the patient's regimen for possible interactions.

epitaxis, and petechiae to life-threatening hemorrhages. Patients should be cautioned about the risk of bleeding associated with the concomitant use of citalopram and NSAIDs). No products indexed under this heading.

Polythiazide (Hyponatremia may occur as a result of treatment with SSRIs including citalopram. Patients taking diuretics may be at greater risk. Discontinuation of citalopram should be considered in patients with symptomatic hyponatremia and appropriate medical intervention should be instituted). No products indexed under this heading.

Posaconazole (In vitro studies indicated that CYP3A4 and CYP2C19 are the primary enzymes involved in the metabolism of citalopram. However, co-administration of citalopram (40 mg) and ketoconazole (200 mg), a potent inhibitor of CYP3A4, did not significantly affect the pharmacokinetics of citalopram. Because citalopram is metabolized by multiple enzyme systems, inhibition of a single enzyme may not appreciably decrease citalopram clearance). Products include:
Noxafil 3172

Prazepam (Given the primary CNS effects of citalopram, caution should be used when it is taken in combination with other centrally acting drugs). No products indexed under this heading.

Procarbazine Hydrochloride (The concomitant use of citalopram with MAO inhibitors is contraindicated. In patients receiving serotonin reuptake inhibitors (SSRIs) in combination with an MAO inhibitor, there have been reports of serious, sometimes fatal reactions. These reactions have also been reported in patients who have recently discontinued SSRI treatment and have been started on an MAO inhibitor. Some cases presented with features resembling neuroleptic malignant syndrome. In addition, there is data to indicate that SSRIs and MAO inhibitors may act synergistically to elevate blood pressure and evoke behavioral excitation. Therefore, it is recommended that citalopram should not be used in combination with an MAO inhibitor, or within 14 days of discontinuing treatment with an MAO inhibitor. Similarly, at least 14 days should be allowed after stopping citalopram before starting an MAO inhibitor). No products indexed under this heading.

Prochlorperazine (The development of a potentially life threatening serotonin syndrome or Neuroleptic Malignant Syndrome (NMS)-like reactions have been reported with citalopram alone, and with concomitant use of antipsychotics. Serotonin syndrome, in its most severe form can resemble neuroleptic malignant syndrome. Patients should be monitored for the emergence of serotonin syndrome or NMS-like signs and symptoms. Treatment with citalopram and any antipsychotics should be discontinued immediately if the above events occur and supportive symptomatic treatment should be initiated). No products indexed under this heading.

Prochlorperazine Edisylate (Given the primary CNS effects of citalopram, caution should be used when it is taken in combination with other centrally acting drugs). No products indexed under this heading.

Prochlorperazine Maleate (Given the primary CNS effects of citalopram, caution should be used when it is taken in combination with other centrally acting drugs). No products indexed under this heading.

Promethazine (The development of a potentially life threatening serotonin syndrome or Neuroleptic Malignant Syndrome (NMS)-like reactions have been

reported with citalopram alone, and with concomitant use of dopamine antagonists. Serotonin syndrome, in its most severe form can resemble neuroleptic malignant syndrome. Patients should be monitored for the emergence of serotonin syndrome or NMS-like signs and symptoms. Treatment with citalopram and any concomitant antidopaminergic agent should be discontinued immediately if the above events occur and supportive symptomatic treatment should be initiated). No products indexed under this heading.

Promethazine Hydrochloride (The development of a potentially life threatening serotonin syndrome or Neuroleptic Malignant Syndrome (NMS)-like reactions have been reported with citalopram alone, and with concomitant use of dopamine antagonists. Serotonin syndrome, in its most severe form can resemble neuroleptic malignant syndrome. Patients should be monitored for the emergence of serotonin syndrome or NMS-like signs and symptoms. Treatment with citalopram and any concomitant antidopaminergic agent should be discontinued immediately if the above events occur and supportive symptomatic treatment should be initiated). No products indexed under this heading.

Propofol (Given the primary CNS effects of citalopram, caution should be used when it is taken in combination with other centrally acting drugs). No products indexed under this heading.

Propoxyphene Hydrochloride (Given the primary CNS effects of citalopram, caution should be used when it is taken in combination with other centrally acting drugs). No products indexed under this heading.

Propoxyphene Napsylate (Given the primary CNS effects of citalopram, caution should be used when it is taken in combination with other centrally acting drugs). No products indexed under this heading.

Protriptyline Hydrochloride (Co-administration of imipramine with citalopram has resulted in a 50% increase in active metabolite, desipramine concentration. The clinical significance of this finding is unknown. Caution is indicated if tricyclic antidepressants are co-administered with citalopram). No products indexed under this heading.

Quazepam (Given the primary CNS effects of citalopram, caution should be used when it is taken in combination with other centrally acting drugs). No products indexed under this heading.

Quetiapine Fumarate (The development of a potentially life threatening serotonin syndrome or Neuroleptic Malignant Syndrome (NMS)-like reactions have been reported with citalopram alone, and with concomitant use of antipsychotics. Serotonin syndrome, in its most severe form can resemble neuroleptic malignant syndrome. Patients should be monitored for the emergence of serotonin syndrome or NMS-like signs and symptoms. Treatment with citalopram and any antipsychotics should be discontinued immediately if the above events occur and supportive symptomatic treatment should be initiated). Products include:
Seroquel 750
Seroquel XR 759

Quinidine (Since CYP3A4 and 2C19 are the primary enzymes involved in the metabolism of citalopram, it is expected that potent inhibitors of CYP219 (eg, omeprazole) might decrease the clearance of citalopram. However, co-administration of citalopram and the potent CYP3A4 inhibitor did not significantly affect the pharma-

cokinetics of citalopram. Because citalopram is metabolized by multiple enzyme systems, inhibition of a single enzyme system may not appreciably decrease citalopram clearance). No products indexed under this heading.

Quinidine Gluconate (Since CYP3A4 and 2C19 are the primary enzymes involved in the metabolism of citalopram, it is expected that potent inhibitors of CYP219 (eg, omeprazole) might decrease the clearance of citalopram. However, co-administration of citalopram and the potent CYP3A4 inhibitor did not significantly affect the pharmacokinetics of citalopram. Because citalopram is metabolized by multiple enzyme systems, inhibition of a single enzyme system may not appreciably decrease citalopram clearance). No products indexed under this heading.

Quinidine Hydrochloride (Since CYP3A4 and 2C19 are the primary enzymes involved in the metabolism of citalopram, it is expected that potent inhibitors of CYP219 (eg, omeprazole) might decrease the clearance of citalopram. However, co-administration of citalopram and the potent CYP3A4 inhibitor did not significantly affect the pharmacokinetics of citalopram. Because citalopram is metabolized by multiple enzyme systems, inhibition of a single enzyme system may not appreciably decrease citalopram clearance). No products indexed under this heading.

Quinidine Polygalacturonate (Since CYP3A4 and 2C19 are the primary enzymes involved in the metabolism of citalopram, it is expected that potent inhibitors of CYP219 (eg, omeprazole) might decrease the clearance of citalopram. However, co-administration of citalopram and the potent CYP3A4 inhibitor did not significantly affect the pharmacokinetics of citalopram. Because citalopram is metabolized by multiple enzyme systems, inhibition of a single enzyme system may not appreciably decrease citalopram clearance). No products indexed under this heading.

Quinidine Sulfate (Since CYP3A4 and 2C19 are the primary enzymes involved in the metabolism of citalopram, it is expected that potent inhibitors of CYP219 (eg, omeprazole) might decrease the clearance of citalopram. However, co-administration of citalopram and the potent CYP3A4 inhibitor did not significantly affect the pharmacokinetics of citalopram. Because citalopram is metabolized by multiple enzyme systems, inhibition of a single enzyme system may not appreciably decrease citalopram clearance). No products indexed under this heading.

Quinine (In vitro studies indicated that CYP3A4 and CYP2C19 are the primary enzymes involved in the metabolism of citalopram. However, co-administration of citalopram (40 mg) and ketoconazole (200 mg), a potent inhibitor of CYP3A4, did not significantly affect the pharmacokinetics of citalopram. Because citalopram is metabolized by multiple enzyme systems, inhibition of a single enzyme may not appreciably decrease citalopram clearance). Products include:
Hyland's Leg Cramps PM with Quinine 3315

Quinine Sulfate (In vitro studies indicated that CYP3A4 and CYP2C19 are the primary enzymes involved in the metabolism of citalopram. However, co-administration of citalopram (40 mg) and ketoconazole (200 mg), a potent inhibitor of CYP3A4, did not significantly affect the pharmacokinetics of citalopram. Because citalopram is metabolized by multiple enzyme systems, inhi-

bition of a single enzyme may not appreciably decrease citalopram clearance). No products indexed under this heading.

Quinupristin (In vitro studies indicated that CYP3A4 and CYP2C19 are the primary enzymes involved in the metabolism of citalopram. However, co-administration of citalopram (40 mg) and ketoconazole (200 mg), a potent inhibitor of CYP3A4, did not significantly affect the pharmacokinetics of citalopram. Because citalopram is metabolized by multiple enzyme systems, inhibition of a single enzyme may not appreciably decrease citalopram clearance). No products indexed under this heading.

Ranitidine Bismuth Citrate (In vitro studies indicated that CYP3A4 and CYP2C19 are the primary enzymes involved in the metabolism of citalopram. However, co-administration of citalopram (40 mg) and ketoconazole (200 mg), a potent inhibitor of CYP3A4, did not significantly affect the pharmacokinetics of citalopram. Because citalopram is metabolized by multiple enzyme systems, inhibition of a single enzyme may not appreciably decrease citalopram clearance). No products indexed under this heading.

Ranitidine Hydrochloride (In vitro studies indicated that CYP3A4 and CYP2C19 are the primary enzymes involved in the metabolism of citalopram. However, co-administration of citalopram (40 mg) and ketoconazole (200 mg), a potent inhibitor of CYP3A4, did not significantly affect the pharmacokinetics of citalopram. Because citalopram is metabolized by multiple enzyme systems, inhibition of a single enzyme may not appreciably decrease citalopram clearance). Products include:
Zantac 1737
Zantac Injection 1732
Zantac Pharmacy 1735

Rasagiline Mesylate (The concomitant use of citalopram with MAO inhibitors is contraindicated. In patients receiving serotonin reuptake inhibitors (SSRIs) in combination with an MAO inhibitor, there have been reports of serious, sometimes fatal reactions. These reactions have also been reported in patients who have recently discontinued SSRI treatment and have been started on an MAO inhibitor. Some cases presented with features resembling neuroleptic malignant syndrome. In addition, there is data to indicate that SSRIs and MAO inhibitors may act synergistically to elevate blood pressure and evoke behavioral excitation. Therefore, it is recommended that citalopram should not be used in combination with an MAO inhibitor, or within 14 days of discontinuing treatment with an MAO inhibitor. Similarly, at least 14 days should be allowed after stopping citalopram before starting an MAO inhibitor). Products include:
Azilect 3383

Remifentanil Hydrochloride (Given the primary CNS effects of citalopram, caution should be used when it is taken in combination with other centrally acting drugs). No products indexed under this heading.

Risperidone (The development of a potentially life threatening serotonin syndrome or Neuroleptic Malignant Syndrome (NMS)-like reactions have been reported with citalopram alone, and with concomitant use of antipsychotics. Serotonin syndrome, in its most severe form can resemble neuroleptic malignant syndrome. Patients should be monitored for the emergence of serotonin syndrome or NMS-like signs and symptoms. Treatment with citalopram and

305 Interactions Index Celexa

any antipsychotics should be discontinued immediately if the above events occur and supportive symptomatic treatment should be initiated). Products include:

Risperdal Consta 2682

Ritonavir (Since CYP3A4 and 2C19 are the primary enzymes involved in the metabolism of citalopram, it is expected that potent inhibitors of CYP219 (eg, omeprazole) might decrease the clearance of citalopram. However, co-administration of citalopram and the potent CYP3A4 inhibitor did not significantly affect the pharmacokinetics of citalopram. Because citalopram is metabolized by multiple enzyme systems, inhibition of a single enzyme system may not appreciably decrease citalopram clearance). Products include:

Kaletra 458
Norvir 509

Rizatriptan Benzoate (The development of potentially life threatening serotonin syndrome or Neuroleptic Malignant syndrome (NMS)-like reactions have been reported with citalopram alone, but particularly with concomitant use of serotonergic drugs including triptans. Serotonin syndrome, in its most severe form can resemble neuroleptic malignant syndrome. Patients should be monitored for the emergence of serotonin syndrome or NMS-like signs and symptoms. If concomitant treatment of citalopram with a triptan is clinically warranted, careful observation of the patient is advised, particularly during treatment initiation and dose increases). Products include:

Maxalt 2206
Maxalt-MLT 2206

Rofecoxib (Citalopram may increase the risk of bleeding events. Concomitant use of NSAIDs may add to the risk. Case reports and epidemiological studies have demonstrated an association between use of drugs that interfere with serotonin reuptake and the occurrence of gastrointestinal bleeding. Bleeding events related to SSRIs use have ranged from ecchymoses, hematomas, epitaxis, and petechiae to life-threatening hemorrhages. Patients should be cautioned about the risk of bleeding associated with the concomitant use of citalopram and NSAIDs).
No products indexed under this heading.

Saquinavir (*In vitro* studies indicated that CYP3A4 and CYP2C19 are the primary enzymes involved in the metabolism of citalopram. However, co-administration of citalopram (40 mg) and ketoconazole (200 mg), a potent inhibitor of CYP3A4, did not significantly affect the pharmacokinetics of citalopram. Because citalopram is metabolized by multiple enzyme systems, inhibition of a single enzyme may not appreciably decrease citalopram clearance).
No products indexed under this heading.

Saquinavir Mesylate (*In vitro* studies indicated that CYP3A4 and CYP2C19 are the primary enzymes involved in the metabolism of citalopram. However, co-administration of citalopram (40 mg) and ketoconazole (200 mg), a potent inhibitor of CYP3A4, did not significantly affect the pharmacokinetics of citalopram. Because citalopram is metabolized by multiple enzyme systems, inhibition of a single enzyme may not appreciably decrease citalopram clearance).
No products indexed under this heading.

Secobarbital Sodium (Given the primary CNS effects of citalopram, caution should be used when it is taken in combination with other centrally acting drugs).
No products indexed under this heading.

Selegiline (The concomitant use of citalopram with MAO inhibitors is contraindicated. In patients receiving serotonin reuptake inhibitors (SSRIs) in combination with an MAO inhibitor, there have been reports of serious, sometimes fatal reactions. These reactions have also been reported in patients who have recently discontinued SSRI treatment and have been started on an MAO inhibitor. Some cases presented with features resembling neuroleptic malignant syndrome. In addition, there is data to indicate that SSRIs and MAO inhibitors may act synergistically to elevate blood pressure and evoke behavioral excitation. Therefore, it is recommended that citalopram should not be used in combination with an MAO inhibitor, or within 14 days of discontinuing treatment with an MAO inhibitor. Similarly, at least 14 days should be allowed after stopping citalopram before starting an MAO inhibitor). Products include:

Emsam 3623

Selegiline Hydrochloride (The concomitant use of citalopram with MAO inhibitors is contraindicated. In patients receiving serotonin reuptake inhibitors (SSRIs) in combination with an MAO inhibitor, there have been reports of serious, sometimes fatal reactions. These reactions have also been reported in patients who have recently discontinued SSRI treatment and have been started on an MAO inhibitor. Some cases presented with features resembling neuroleptic malignant syndrome. In addition, there is data to indicate that SSRIs and MAO inhibitors may act synergistically to elevate blood pressure and evoke behavioral excitation. Therefore, it is recommended that citalopram should not be used in combination with an MAO inhibitor, or within 14 days of discontinuing treatment with an MAO inhibitor. Similarly, at least 14 days should be allowed after stopping citalopram before starting an MAO inhibitor). Products include:

Eldepryl 3312

Sertraline Hydrochloride (The development of potentially life threatening serotonin syndrome or Neuroleptic Malignant Syndrome (NMS)-like reactions have been reported with citalopram alone, but particularly with concomitant use of serotonergic drugs. Serotonin syndrome, in its most severe form, can resemble neuroleptic malignant syndrome. Patients should be monitored for the emergence of serotonin syndrome or NMS-like signs and symptoms. Treatment with citalopram and any concomitant serotonergic agent should be discontinued immediately if the above events occur and supportive treatment should be initiated).
No products indexed under this heading.

Sevoflurane (Given the primary CNS effects of citalopram, caution should be used when it is taken in combination with other centrally acting drugs). Products include:

Ultane 554

Sildenafil Citrate (Since CYP3A4 and 2C19 are the primary enzymes involved in the metabolism of citalopram, it is expected that potent inhibitors of CYP219 (eg, omeprazole) might decrease the clearance of citalopram. However, co-administration of citalopram and the potent CYP3A4 inhibitor did not significantly affect the pharmacokinetics of citalopram. Because citalopram is metabolized by multiple enzyme systems, inhibition of a single enzyme system may not appreciably decrease citalopram clearance).
No products indexed under this heading.

Sodium Butabarbital (Given the primary CNS effects of citalopram, caution should be used when it is taken in combination with other centrally acting drugs).
No products indexed under this heading.

Sodium Oxybate (Given the primary CNS effects of citalopram, caution should be used when it is taken in combination with other centrally acting drugs).
No products indexed under this heading.

Sodium Pentobarbital (Given the primary CNS effects of citalopram, caution should be used when it is taken in combination with other centrally acting drugs).
No products indexed under this heading.

Spironolactone (Hyponatremia may occur as a result of treatment with SSRIs including citalopram. Patients taking diuretics may be at greater risk. Discontinuation of citalopram should be considered in patients with symptomatic hyponatremia and appropriate medical intervention should be instituted).
No products indexed under this heading.

Sufentanil Citrate (Given the primary CNS effects of citalopram, caution should be used when it is taken in combination with other centrally acting drugs).
No products indexed under this heading.

Sulfaphenazole (Since CYP3A4 and 2C19 are the primary enzymes involved in the metabolism of citalopram, it is expected that potent inhibitors of CYP219 (eg, omeprazole) might decrease the clearance of citalopram. However, co-administration of citalopram and the potent CYP3A4 inhibitor did not significantly affect the pharmacokinetics of citalopram. Because citalopram is metabolized by multiple enzyme systems, inhibition of a single enzyme system may not appreciably decrease citalopram clearance).
No products indexed under this heading.

Sulindac (Citalopram may increase the risk of bleeding events. Concomitant use of NSAIDs may add to the risk. Case reports and epidemiological studies have demonstrated an association between use of drugs that interfere with serotonin reuptake and the occurrence of gastrointestinal bleeding. Bleeding events related to SSRIs use have ranged from ecchymoses, hematomas, epitaxis, and petechiae to life-threatening hemorrhages. Patients should be cautioned about the risk of bleeding associated with the concomitant use of citalopram and NSAIDs). Products include:

Clinoril 2098

Sumatriptan (There have been rare post-marketing reports describing patients with weakness, hyperreflexia, and incoordination following the use of a SSRI and sumatriptan. If concomitant treatment with sumatriptan and citalopram is clinically warranted, appropriate observation of the patient is advised). Products include:

Imitrex Nasal 1503

Sumatriptan Succinate (There have been rare post-marketing reports describing patients with weakness, hyperreflexia, and incoordination following the use of a SSRI and sumatriptan. If concomitant treatment with sumatriptan and citalopram is clinically warranted, appropriate observation of the patient is advised). Products include:

Imitrex 1497
Imitrex Tablets 1508
Treximet 1681

Talbutal (Given the primary CNS effects of citalopram, caution should be used when it is taken in combination with other centrally acting drugs).
No products indexed under this heading.

Telithromycin (*In vitro* studies indicated that CYP3A4 and CYP2C19 are the primary enzymes involved in the metabolism of citalopram. However, co-administration of citalopram (40 mg) and ketoconazole (200 mg), a potent inhibitor of CYP3A4, did not significantly affect the pharmacokinetics of citalopram. Because citalopram is metabolized by multiple enzyme systems, inhibition of a single enzyme may not appreciably decrease citalopram clearance). Products include:

Ketek 2991

Telmisartan (Since CYP3A4 and 2C19 are the primary enzymes involved in the metabolism of citalopram, it is expected that potent inhibitors of CYP219 (eg, omeprazole) might decrease the clearance of citalopram. However, co-administration of citalopram and the potent CYP3A4 inhibitor did not significantly affect the pharmacokinetics of citalopram. Because citalopram is metabolized by multiple enzyme systems, inhibition of a single enzyme system may not appreciably decrease citalopram clearance). Products include:

Micardis 887
Micardis HCT 889

Temazepam (Given the primary CNS effects of citalopram, caution should be used when it is taken in combination with other centrally acting drugs).
No products indexed under this heading.

Thiamylal Sodium (Given the primary CNS effects of citalopram, caution should be used when it is taken in combination with other centrally acting drugs).
No products indexed under this heading.

Thioridazine (Given the primary CNS effects of citalopram, caution should be used when it is taken in combination with other centrally acting drugs).
No products indexed under this heading.

Thioridazine Hydrochloride (The development of a potentially life threatening serotonin syndrome or Neuroleptic Malignant Syndrome (NMS)-like reactions have been reported with citalopram alone, and with concomitant use of antipsychotics. Serotonin syndrome, in its most severe form can resemble neuroleptic malignant syndrome. Patients should be monitored for the emergence of serotonin syndrome or NMS-like signs and symptoms. Treatment with citalopram and any antipsychotics should be discontinued immediately if the above events occur and supportive symptomatic treatment should be initiated). Products include:

Thioridazine Hydrochloride 2384

Thiothixene (The development of a potentially life threatening serotonin syndrome or Neuroleptic Malignant Syndrome (NMS)-like reactions have been reported with citalopram alone, and with concomitant use of antipsychotics. Serotonin syndrome, in its most severe form can resemble neuroleptic malignant syndrome. Patients should be monitored for the emergence of serotonin syndrome or NMS-like signs and symptoms. Treatment with citalopram and any antipsychotics should be discontinued immediately if the above events occur and supportive symptomatic treatment should be initiated). Products include:

Thiothixene 2386

Thiothixene Hydrochloride (Given the primary CNS effects of citalopram, caution should be used when it is taken in combination with other centrally acting drugs).
No products indexed under this heading.

Ticlopidine Hydrochloride (Since CYP3A4 and 2C19 are the primary

enzymes involved in the metabolism of citalopram, it is expected that potent inhibitors of CYP219 (eg, omeprazole) might decrease the clearance of citalopram. However, co-administration of citalopram and the potent CYP3A4 inhibitor did not significantly affect the pharmacokinetics of citalopram. Because citalopram is metabolized by multiple enzyme systems, inhibition of a single enzyme system may not appreciably decrease citalopram clearance).

No products indexed under this heading.

Tinzaparin Sodium (Citalopram may increase the risk of bleeding events. Concomitant use of anticoagulants may add to the risk. Case reports and studies have demonstrated an association between use of drugs that interfere with serotonin reuptake and the occurrence of gastrointestinal bleeding. Patients should be cautioned about the risk of bleeding associated with the concomitant use of citalopram and drugs affecting coagulation).

No products indexed under this heading.

Tolbutamide (Since CYP3A4 and 2C19 are the primary enzymes involved in the metabolism of citalopram, it is expected that potent inhibitors of CYP219 (eg, omeprazole) might decrease the clearance of citalopram. However, co-administration of citalopram and the potent CYP3A4 inhibitor did not significantly affect the pharmacokinetics of citalopram. Because citalopram is metabolized by multiple enzyme systems, inhibition of a single enzyme system may not appreciably decrease citalopram clearance).

No products indexed under this heading.

Tolbutamide Sodium (Since CYP3A4 and 2C19 are the primary enzymes involved in the metabolism of citalopram, it is expected that potent inhibitors of CYP219 (eg, omeprazole) might decrease the clearance of citalopram. However, co-administration of citalopram and the potent CYP3A4 inhibitor did not significantly affect the pharmacokinetics of citalopram. Because citalopram is metabolized by multiple enzyme systems, inhibition of a single enzyme system may not appreciably decrease citalopram clearance).

No products indexed under this heading.

Tolmetin Sodium (Citalopram may increase the risk of bleeding events. Concomitant use of NSAIDs may add to the risk. Case reports and epidemiological studies have demonstrated an association between use of drugs that interfere with serotonin reuptake and the occurrence of gastrointestinal bleeding. Bleeding events related to SSRIs use have ranged from ecchymoses, hematomas, epitaxis, and petechiae to life-threatening hemorrhages. Patients should be cautioned about the risk of bleeding associated with the concomitant use of citalopram and NSAIDs).

No products indexed under this heading.

Topiramate (Since CYP3A4 and 2C19 are the primary enzymes involved in the metabolism of citalopram, it is expected that potent inhibitors of CYP219 (eg, omeprazole) might decrease the clearance of citalopram. However, co-administration of citalopram and the potent CYP3A4 inhibitor did not significantly affect the pharmacokinetics of citalopram. Because citalopram is metabolized by multiple enzyme systems, inhibition of a single enzyme system may not appreciably decrease citalopram clearance).

No products indexed under this heading.

Torsemide (Hyponatremia may occur as a result of treatment with SSRIs including citalopram. Patients taking diuretics may be at greater risk. Discontinuation of citalopram should be considered in patients with symptomatic hyponatremia and appropriate medical intervention should be instituted).

No products indexed under this heading.

Tramadol Hydrochloride (Based on the mechanism of action of SSRIs, including citalopram, and the potential for serotonin syndrome, caution is advised when citalopram is co-administered with other drugs that may affect the serotonergic neurotransmitter systems, such as tramadol). Products include:

Ryzolt 2813
Ultram ER 2693

Tranylcypromine Sulfate (The concomitant use of citalopram with MAO inhibitors is contraindicated. In patients receiving serotonin reuptake inhibitors (SSRIs) in combination with an MAO inhibitor, there have been reports of serious, sometimes fatal reactions. These reactions have also been reported in patients who have recently discontinued SSRI treatment and have been started on an MAO inhibitor. Some cases presented with features resembling neuroleptic malignant syndrome. In addition, there is data to indicate that SSRIs and MAO inhibitors may act synergistically to elevate blood pressure and evoke behavioral excitation. Therefore, it is recommended that citalopram should not be used in combination with an MAO inhibitor, or within 14 days of discontinuing treatment with an MAO inhibitor. Similarly, at least 14 days should be allowed after stopping citalopram before starting an MAO inhibitor). Products include:

Parnate 1584

Triamterene (Hyponatremia may occur as a result of treatment with SSRIs including citalopram. Patients taking diuretics may be at greater risk. Discontinuation of citalopram should be considered in patients with symptomatic hyponatremia and appropriate medical intervention should be instituted). Products include:

Dyazide 1429
Dyrenium 3495

Triazolam (Given the primary CNS effects of citalopram, caution should be used when it is taken in combination with other centrally acting drugs).

No products indexed under this heading.

Trifluoperazine Hydrochloride (The development of a potentially life threatening serotonin syndrome or Neuroleptic Malignant Syndrome (NMS)-like reactions have been reported with citalopram alone, and with concomitant use of antipsychotics. Serotonin syndrome, in its most severe form can resemble neuroleptic malignant syndrome. Patients should be monitored for the emergence of serotonin syndrome or NMS-like signs and symptoms. Treatment with citalopram and any antipsychotics should be discontinued immediately if the above events occur and supportive symptomatic treatment should be initiated).

No products indexed under this heading.

Trimipramine Maleate (Co-administration of imipramine with citalopram has resulted in a 50% increase in active metabolite, desipramine concentration. The clinical significance of this finding is unknown. Caution is indicated if tricyclic antidepressants are co-administered with citalopram).

No products indexed under this heading.

Troglitazone (In vitro studies indicated that CYP3A4 and CYP2C19 are the primary enzymes involved in the metabolism of citalopram. However, co-

administration of citalopram (40 mg) and ketoconazole (200 mg), a potent inhibitor of CYP3A4, did not significantly affect the pharmacokinetics of citalopram. Because citalopram is metabolized by multiple enzyme systems, inhibition of a single enzyme may not appreciably decrease citalopram clearance).

No products indexed under this heading.

Troleandomycin (Since CYP3A4 and 2C19 are the primary enzymes involved in the metabolism of citalopram, it is expected that potent inhibitors of 3A4 (eg, macrolide antibiotics) might decrease the clearance of citalopram. However, co-administration of citalopram and the potent 3A4 inhibitor ketoconazole did not significantly affect the pharmacokinetics of citalopram. Because citalopram is metabolized by multiple enzyme systems, inhibition of a single enzyme system may not appreciably decrease citalopram clearance).

No products indexed under this heading.

Tryptophan (The concomitant use of citalopram with serotonin precursors such as tryptophan is not recommended).

No products indexed under this heading.

Valdecoxib (Citalopram may increase the risk of bleeding events. Concomitant use of NSAIDs may add to the risk. Case reports and epidemiological studies have demonstrated an association between use of drugs that interfere with serotonin reuptake and the occurrence of gastrointestinal bleeding. Bleeding events related to SSRIs use have ranged from ecchymoses, hematomas, epitaxis, and petechiae to life-threatening hemorrhages. Patients should be cautioned about the risk of bleeding associated with the concomitant use of citalopram and NSAIDs).

No products indexed under this heading.

Valproate Sodium (In vitro studies indicated that CYP3A4 and CYP2C19 are the primary enzymes involved in the metabolism of citalopram. However, co-administration of citalopram (40 mg) and ketoconazole (200 mg), a potent inhibitor of CYP3A4, did not significantly affect the pharmacokinetics of citalopram. Because citalopram is metabolized by multiple enzyme systems, inhibition of a single enzyme may not appreciably decrease citalopram clearance).

No products indexed under this heading.

Vardenafil Hydrochloride (Since CYP3A4 and 2C19 are the primary enzymes involved in the metabolism of citalopram, it is expected that potent inhibitors of CYP219 (eg, omeprazole) might decrease the clearance of citalopram. However, co-administration of citalopram and the potent CYP3A4 inhibitor did not significantly affect the pharmacokinetics of citalopram. Because citalopram is metabolized by multiple enzyme systems, inhibition of a single enzyme system may not appreciably decrease citalopram clearance). Products include:

Levitra 3157

Venlafaxine Hydrochloride (The development of potentially life threatening serotonin syndrome or Neuroleptic Malignant Syndrome (NMS)-like reactions have been reported with citalopram alone, but particularly with concomitant use of serotonergic drugs. The concomitant use of citalopram with SNRIs is not recommended). Products include:

Effexor XR 3504
Venlafaxine Hydrochloride Tablets ... 2388

Verapamil Hydrochloride (In vitro studies indicated that CYP3A4 and CYP2C19 are the primary enzymes involved in the metabolism of citalo-

pram. However, co-administration of citalopram (40 mg) and ketoconazole (200 mg), a potent inhibitor of CYP3A4, did not significantly affect the pharmacokinetics of citalopram. Because citalopram is metabolized by multiple enzyme systems, inhibition of a single enzyme may not appreciably decrease citalopram clearance). Products include:

Tarka 534

Voriconazole (Since CYP3A4 and 2C19 are the primary enzymes involved in the metabolism of citalopram, it is expected that potent inhibitors of CYP219 (eg, omeprazole) might decrease the clearance of citalopram. However, co-administration of citalopram and the potent CYP3A4 inhibitor did not significantly affect the pharmacokinetics of citalopram. Because citalopram is metabolized by multiple enzyme systems, inhibition of a single enzyme system may not appreciably decrease citalopram clearance).

No products indexed under this heading.

Warfarin Sodium (Altered anticoagulant effects, including increased bleeding have been reported when SSRIs are co-administered with warfarin. Patients receiving warfarin therapy should be carefully monitored when citalopram is initiated or discontinued).

No products indexed under this heading.

Zafirlukast (In vitro studies indicated that CYP3A4 and CYP2C19 are the primary enzymes involved in the metabolism of citalopram. However, co-administration of citalopram (40 mg) and ketoconazole (200 mg), a potent inhibitor of CYP3A4, did not significantly affect the pharmacokinetics of citalopram. Because citalopram is metabolized by multiple enzyme systems, inhibition of a single enzyme may not appreciably decrease citalopram clearance). Products include:

Accolate 3612

Zaleplon (Given the primary CNS effects of citalopram, caution should be used when it is taken in combination with other centrally acting drugs).

No products indexed under this heading.

Zileuton (In vitro studies indicated that CYP3A4 and CYP2C19 are the primary enzymes involved in the metabolism of citalopram. However, co-administration of citalopram (40 mg) and ketoconazole (200 mg), a potent inhibitor of CYP3A4, did not significantly affect the pharmacokinetics of citalopram. Because citalopram is metabolized by multiple enzyme systems, inhibition of a single enzyme may not appreciably decrease citalopram clearance).

No products indexed under this heading.

Ziprasidone Hydrochloride (The development of a potentially life threatening serotonin syndrome or Neuroleptic Malignant Syndrome (NMS)-like reactions have been reported with citalopram alone, and with concomitant use of antipsychotics. Serotonin syndrome, in its most severe form can resemble neuroleptic malignant syndrome. Patients should be monitored for the emergence of serotonin syndrome or NMS-like signs and symptoms. Treatment with citalopram and any antipsychotics should be discontinued immediately if the above events occur and supportive symptomatic treatment should be initiated). Products include:

Geodon 2723

Zolmitriptan (The development of potentially life threatening serotonin syndrome or Neuroleptic Malignant syndrome (NMS)-like reactions have been reported with citalopram alone, but particularly with concomitant use of serotonergic drugs including triptans. Serotonin syndrome, in its most severe form

can resemble neuroleptic malignant syndrome. Patients should be monitored for the emergence of serotonin syndrome or NMS-like signs and symptoms. If concomitant treatment of citalopram with a triptan is clinically warranted, careful observation of the patient is advised, particularly during treatment initiation and dose increases). Products include:

Zomig Tablets 773
Zomig Nasal Spray 768
Zomig-ZMT Tablets 773

Zolpidem Tartrate (Given the primary CNS effects of citalopram, caution should be used when it is taken in combination with other centrally acting drugs). Products include:

Ambien 2920
Ambien CR 2925

Food Interactions

Alcohol (Although citalopram did not potentiate cognitive and motor effects of alcohol, as with other psychotropic medications, the use of alcohol by depressed patients taking citalopram is not recommended).

Beer, reduced-alcohol (Although citalopram did not potentiate cognitive and motor effects of alcohol, as with other psychotropic medications, the use of alcohol by depressed patients taking citalopram is not recommended).

Beer, unspecified (Although citalopram did not potentiate cognitive and motor effects of alcohol, as with other psychotropic medications, the use of alcohol by depressed patients taking citalopram is not recommended).

Grapefruit (*In vitro* studies indicated that CYP3A4 and CYP2C19 are the primary enzymes involved in the metabolism of citalopram. However, co-administration of citalopram (40 mg) and ketoconazole (200 mg), a potent inhibitor of CYP3A4, did not significantly affect the pharmacokinetics of citalopram. Because citalopram is metabolized by multiple enzyme systems, inhibition of a single enzyme may not appreciably decrease citalopram clearance).

Grapefruit Juice (*In vitro* studies indicated that CYP3A4 and CYP2C19 are the primary enzymes involved in the metabolism of citalopram. However, co-administration of citalopram (40 mg) and ketoconazole (200 mg), a potent inhibitor of CYP3A4, did not significantly affect the pharmacokinetics of citalopram. Because citalopram is metabolized by multiple enzyme systems, inhibition of a single enzyme may not appreciably decrease citalopram clearance).

Wine, Chianti (Although citalopram did not potentiate cognitive and motor effects of alcohol, as with other psychotropic medications, the use of alcohol by depressed patients taking citalopram is not recommended).

Wine, Red (Although citalopram did not potentiate cognitive and motor effects of alcohol, as with other psychotropic medications, the use of alcohol by depressed patients taking citalopram is not recommended).

Wine, unspecified (Although citalopram did not potentiate cognitive and motor effects of alcohol, as with other psychotropic medications, the use of alcohol by depressed patients taking citalopram is not recommended).

Wine products (Although citalopram did not potentiate cognitive and motor effects of alcohol, as with other psychotropic medications, the use of alcohol by depressed patients taking citalopram is not recommended).

CERVIDIL VAGINAL INSERT

(Dinoprostone) 1159

May interact with oxytocic drugs, and certain other agents. Compounds in these categories include:

Dihydroergotamine Mesylate (Dinoprostone is contraindicated in patients already receiving intravenous oxytocic drugs. Cervidil may augment the activity of oxytocic agents and their concomitant use is not recommended. A dosing interval of at least 30 minutes is recommended for the sequential use of oxytocin following the removal of the dinoprostone vaginal insert. Since prostaglandins potentiate the effect of oxytocin, dinoprostone must be removed before oxytocin administration is initiated and the patient's uterine activity carefully monitored for uterine hyperstimulation).
No products indexed under this heading.

Ergonovine Maleate (Dinoprostone is contraindicated in patients already receiving intravenous oxytocic drugs. Cervidil may augment the activity of oxytocic agents and their concomitant use is not recommended. A dosing interval of at least 30 minutes is recommended for the sequential use of oxytocin following the removal of the dinoprostone vaginal insert. Since prostaglandins potentiate the effect of oxytocin, dinoprostone must be removed before oxytocin administration is initiated and the patient's uterine activity carefully monitored for uterine hyperstimulation).
No products indexed under this heading.

Ergotamine Tartrate (Dinoprostone is contraindicated in patients already receiving intravenous oxytocic drugs. Cervidil may augment the activity of oxytocic agents and their concomitant use is not recommended. A dosing interval of at least 30 minutes is recommended for the sequential use of oxytocin following the removal of the dinoprostone vaginal insert. Since prostaglandins potentiate the effect of oxytocin, dinoprostone must be removed before oxytocin administration is initiated and the patient's uterine activity carefully monitored for uterine hyperstimulation).
No products indexed under this heading.

Methylergonovine Maleate (Dinoprostone is contraindicated in patients already receiving intravenous oxytocic drugs. Cervidil may augment the activity of oxytocic agents and their concomitant use is not recommended. A dosing interval of at least 30 minutes is recommended for the sequential use of oxytocin following the removal of the dinoprostone vaginal insert. Since prostaglandins potentiate the effect of oxytocin, dinoprostone must be removed before oxytocin administration is initiated and the patient's uterine activity carefully monitored for uterine hyperstimulation).
No products indexed under this heading.

Methysergide Maleate (Dinoprostone is contraindicated in patients already receiving intravenous oxytocic drugs. Cervidil may augment the activity of oxytocic agents and their concomitant use is not recommended. A dosing interval of at least 30 minutes is recommended for the sequential use of oxytocin following the removal of the dinoprostone vaginal insert. Since prostaglandins potentiate the effect of oxytocin, dinoprostone must be removed before oxytocin administration is initiated and the patient's uterine activity carefully monitored for uterine hyperstimulation).
No products indexed under this heading.

Oxytocin (Dinoprostone is contraindicated in patients already receiving intravenous oxytocic drugs. Cervidil may augment the activity of oxytocic agents and their concomitant use is not recommended. A dosing interval of at least 30 minutes is recommended for the sequential use of oxytocin following the removal of the dinoprostone vaginal insert. Since prostaglandins potentiate the effect of oxytocin, dinoprostone must be removed before oxytocin administration is initiated and the patient's uterine activity carefully monitored for uterine hyperstimulation).
No products indexed under this heading.

Oxytocin (Injection) (Dinoprostone is contraindicated in patients already receiving intravenous oxytocic drugs. Cervidil may augment the activity of oxytocic agents and their concomitant use is not recommended. A dosing interval of at least 30 minutes is recommended for the sequential use of oxytocin following the removal of the dinoprostone vaginal insert. Since prostaglandins potentiate the effect of oxytocin, dinoprostone must be removed before oxytocin administration is initiated and the patient's uterine activity carefully monitored for uterine hyperstimulation).
No products indexed under this heading.

CHANTIX TABLETS

(Varenicline Tartrate) 2712

May interact with nicotines, and certain other agents. Compounds in these categories include:

Bupropion (Varenicline (1 mg BID) did not alter the steady-state pharmacokinetics of bupropion (150 mg BID) in 46 smokers. The safety of the combination of bupropion and varenicline has not been established).
No products indexed under this heading.

Bupropion Hydrochloride (Varenicline (1 mg BID) did not alter the steady-state pharmacokinetics of bupropion (150 mg BID) in 46 smokers. The safety of the combination of bupropion and varenicline has not been established). Products include:

Aplenzin 2948
Wellbutrin 1719
Wellbutrin SR 1725
Zyban 1762

Cimetidine (Co-administration of an OCT2 inhibitor, cimetidine (300 mg QID), with varenicline (2 mg single dose) to 12 smokers increased the systemic exposure of varenicline by 29% (90% CI: 21.5%, 36.9%) due to a reduction in varenicline renal clearance).
No products indexed under this heading.

Cimetidine Hydrochloride (Co-administration of an OCT2 inhibitor, cimetidine (300 mg QID), with varenicline (2 mg single dose) to 12 smokers increased the systemic exposure of varenicline by 29% (90% CI: 21.5%, 36.9%) due to a reduction in varenicline renal clearance).
No products indexed under this heading.

Nicotine (Although co-administration of varenicline (1 mg BID) and transdermal nicotine (21 mg/day) for up to 12 days did not affect nicotine pharmacokinetics, the incidence of nausea, headache, vomiting, dizziness, dyspepsia and fatigue was greater for the combination than for Nicotine Replacement Therapy (NRT) alone. In this study, 8 of 22 (36%) subjects treated with the combination of varenicline and NRT prematurely discontinued treatment due to adverse events, compared to 1 of 17 (6%) of subjects treated with NRT and placebo).
No products indexed under this heading.

Nicotine Polacrilex (Although co-administration of varenicline (1 mg BID) and transdermal nicotine (21 mg/day) for up to 12 days did not affect nicotine pharmacokinetics, the incidence of nausea, headache, vomiting, dizziness, dyspepsia and fatigue was greater for the combination than for Nicotine Replacement Therapy (NRT) alone. In this study, 8 of 22 (36%) subjects treated with the combination of varenicline and NRT prematurely discontinued treatment due to adverse events, compared to 1 of 17 (6%) of subjects treated with NRT and placebo).
No products indexed under this heading.

Nicotine Salicylate (Although co-administration of varenicline (1 mg BID) and transdermal nicotine (21 mg/day) for up to 12 days did not affect nicotine pharmacokinetics, the incidence of nausea, headache, vomiting, dizziness, dyspepsia and fatigue was greater for the combination than for Nicotine Replacement Therapy (NRT) alone. In this study, 8 of 22 (36%) subjects treated with the combination of varenicline and NRT prematurely discontinued treatment due to adverse events, compared to 1 of 17 (6%) of subjects treated with NRT and placebo).
No products indexed under this heading.

Nicotine Sulfate (Although co-administration of varenicline (1 mg BID) and transdermal nicotine (21 mg/day) for up to 12 days did not affect nicotine pharmacokinetics, the incidence of nausea, headache, vomiting, dizziness, dyspepsia and fatigue was greater for the combination than for Nicotine Replacement Therapy (NRT) alone. In this study, 8 of 22 (36%) subjects treated with the combination of varenicline and NRT prematurely discontinued treatment due to adverse events, compared to 1 of 17 (6%) of subjects treated with NRT and placebo).
No products indexed under this heading.

CHELATED MINERAL TABLETS

(Boron, Calcium, Calcium Carbonate, Calcium Citrate, Chromium, Chromium Picolinate, Chromium Polynicotinate, Copper, Iodine, Magnesium, Magnesium Citrate, Manganese, Minerals, Molybdenum, Potassium Iodide, Selenium, Silicone, Vanadium, Zinc, Zinc Citrate) 3476
None cited in PDR database.

CHEMET CAPSULES

(Succimer) 2001

Calcium Disodium Edetate (Concomitant administration of succimer with other chelation therapy, such as $CaNa_2EDTA$, is not recommended).
No products indexed under this heading.

CIALIS TABLETS

(Tadalafil) 1861

May interact with alcohols, alpha adrenergic blockers, angiotensin-II receptor antagonists, antacids, antacids containing aluminum, calcium and magnesium, antihypertensives, cytochrome p450 3a4 inducers (selected), cytochrome p450 3a4 inhibitors (selected), cytochrome p450 3a4 inhibitors, potent (selected), erythromycin, magnesium-containing antacids, nitrates and nitrites, phenytoin, protease inhibitors, theophyllines, and certain other agents. Compounds in these categories include:

Acebutolol Hydrochloride (PDE5 inhibitors, including tadalafil, are mild systemic vasodilators. Clinical pharma-

IMPORTANT NOTE: Always consult each drug listing in the patient's regimen for possible interactions.

cology studies were conducted to assess the effect of tadalafil on the potentiation of the blood-pressure-lowering effects of selected antihypertensive medications (amlodipine, angiotesin II receptor blockers, bendrofluazide, enalapril, and metoprolol). Small reductions in blood pressure occurred following co-administration of tadalafil with these agents compared to placebo).

No products indexed under this heading.

Acetazolamide (Tadalafil is a substrate of and predominantly metabolized by CYP3A4. Studies have shown that drugs that inhibit CYP3A4 can increase tadalafil exposure. When tadalafil is used on an as-needed basis, patients taking concomitant potent inhibitors of CYP3A4, such as ketoconazole or ritonavir, the maximum recommended dose of tadalafil is 10 mg, not to exceed once every 72 hours. When tadalafil is used in a once-daily regimen, patients taking concomitant potent inhibitors of CYP3A4, such as ketoconazole or ritonavir, the dose should not exceed 2.5 mg).

No products indexed under this heading.

Acetazolamide Sodium (Tadalafil is a substrate of and predominantly metabolized by CYP3A4. Studies have shown that drugs that inhibit CYP3A4 can increase tadalafil exposure. When tadalafil is used on an as-needed basis, patients taking concomitant potent inhibitors of CYP3A4, such as ketoconazole or ritonavir, the maximum recommended dose of tadalafil is 10 mg, not to exceed once every 72 hours. When tadalafil is used in a once-daily regimen, patients taking concomitant potent inhibitors of CYP3A4, such as ketoconazole or ritonavir, the dose should not exceed 2.5 mg).

No products indexed under this heading.

Alfuzosin Hydrochloride (Caution is advised when PDE5 inhibitors are co-administered with α-blockers. Tadalafil and α-adrenergic blocking agents are both vasodilators with blood-pressure lowering effects. When vasodilators are used in combination, an additive effect on blood pressure may be anticipated. In some patients, concomitant use of these two drug classes can lower blood presure significantly, which may lead to symptomatic hypotension (eg, fainting). When tadalafil is co-administered with an α-blocker, patients should be stable on α-blocker therapy prior to initiating treatment with tadalafil, and tadalafil should be administered at the lowest recommended dose). Products include:

Aliskiren (PDE5 inhibitors, including tadalafil, are mild systemic vasodilators. Clinical pharmacology studies were conducted to assess the effect of tadalafil on the potentiation of the blood-pressure-lowering effects of selected antihypertensive medications (amlodipine, angiotesin II receptor blockers, bendrofluazide, enalapril, and metoprolol). Small reductions in blood pressure occurred following co-administration of tadalafil with these agents compared to placebo). Products include:

Allium sativum (Studies have shown that drugs that induce CYP3A4 can decrease tadalafil exposure. Rifampin (600 mg daily), a CYP3A4 inducer, reduced tadalafil 10 mg single-dose exposure (AUC) by 88% and C_{max} by 46%, relative to the values for tadalafil 10 mg alone. Although specific interactions have not been studied, other CYP3A4 inducers, such as carbamazepine, phenytoin, and phenobarbital,

would likely decrease tadalafil exposure. No dose adjustment is warranted. The reduced exposure of tadalafil with the co-administration of rifampin or other CYP3A4 inducers can be anticipated to decrease the efficacy of tadalafil for once daily use; the magnitude of decreased efficacy is unknown).

No products indexed under this heading.

Aluminum Carbonate (Simultaneous administration of an antacid (magnesium hydroxide/aluminum hydroxide) and tadalafil reduced the apparent rate of absorption of tadalafil without altering exposure (AUC) to tadalafil).

No products indexed under this heading.

Aluminum Hydroxide (Simultaneous administration of an antacid (magnesium hydroxide/aluminum hydroxide) and tadalafil reduced the apparent rate of absorption of tadalafil without altering exposure (AUC) to tadalafil).

No products indexed under this heading.

Aminoglutethimide (Studies have shown that drugs that induce CYP3A4 can decrease tadalafil exposure. Rifampin (600 mg daily), a CYP3A4 inducer, reduced tadalafil 10 mg single-dose exposure (AUC) by 88% and C_{max} by 46%, relative to the values for tadalafil 10 mg alone. Although specific interactions have not been studied, other CYP3A4 inducers, such as carbamazepine, phenytoin, and phenobarbital, would likely decrease tadalafil exposure. No dose adjustment is warranted. The reduced exposure of tadalafil with the co-administration of rifampin or other CYP3A4 inducers can be anticipated to decrease the efficacy of tadalafil for once daily use; the magnitude of decreased efficacy is unknown).

No products indexed under this heading.

Amiodarone Hydrochloride (Tadalafil is a substrate of and predominantly metabolized by CYP3A4. Studies have shown that drugs that inhibit CYP3A4 can increase tadalafil exposure. When tadalafil is used on an as-needed basis, patients taking concomitant potent inhibitors of CYP3A4, such as ketoconazole or ritonavir, the maximum recommended dose of tadalafil is 10 mg, not to exceed once every 72 hours. When tadalafil is used in a once-daily regimen, patients taking concomitant potent inhibitors of CYP3A4, such as ketoconazole or ritonavir, the dose should not exceed 2.5 mg).

No products indexed under this heading.

Amlodipine Besylate (A study was conducted to assess the interaction of amlodipine (5 mg daily) and tadalafil 10 mg. There was no effect of tadalafil on amlodipine blood levels and no effect of amlodipine on tadalafil blood levels. The mean reduction in supine systolic/diastolic blood pressure due to tadalafil 10 mg in subjects taking amlodipine was 3/2 mm Hg, compared to placebo. In a similar study using tadalafil 20 mg, there were no clinically significant differences between tadalafil and placebo in subjects taking amlodipine). Products include:

Amprenavir (Ritonavir (500 mg or 600 mg b.i.d. at steady state), an inhibitor of CYP3A4, CYP2C9, CYP2C19, and CYP2D6, increased tadalafil 20 mg single-dose exposure (AUC) by 32% with a 30% reduction in C_{max}, relative to the values for tadalafil 20 mg alone. Ritonavir (200 mg b.i.d.), increased tadalafil 20 mg single-dose exposure (AUC) by 124% with no change in C_{max}, relative to the values for tadalafil 20 mg alone. Although specific interactions

have not been studied, other HIV protease inhibitors would likely increase tadalafil exposure).

No products indexed under this heading.

Amyl Nitrite (Administration of tadalafil to patients using any form of organic nitrate, either regularly and/or intermittently, is contraindicated. In clinical pharmacology studies, tadalafil was shown to potentiate the hypotensive effects of nitrates. In a patient who has taken tadalafil, where nitrate administration is deemed medically necessary in a life threatening situation, at least 48 hours should elapse after the last dose of tadalafil before nitrate administration is considered. In such circumstances, nitrates should still only be administered under close medical supervision with appropriate hemodynamic monitoring).

No products indexed under this heading.

Anastrozole (Tadalafil is a substrate of and predominantly metabolized by CYP3A4. Studies have shown that drugs that inhibit CYP3A4 can increase tadalafil exposure. When tadalafil is used on an as-needed basis, patients taking concomitant potent inhibitors of CYP3A4, such as ketoconazole or ritonavir, the maximum recommended dose of tadalafil is 10 mg, not to exceed once every 72 hours. When tadalafil is used in a once-daily regimen, patients taking concomitant potent inhibitors of CYP3A4, such as ketoconazole or ritonavir, the dose should not exceed 2.5 mg).

No products indexed under this heading.

Apraclonidine Hydrochloride (Caution is advised when PDE5 inhibitors are co-administered with α-blockers. Tadalafil and α-adrenergic blocking agents are both vasodilators with blood-pressure lowering effects. When vasodilators are used in combination, an additive effect on blood pressure may be anticipated. In some patients, concomitant use of these two drug classes can lower blood presure significantly, which may lead to symptomatic hypotension (eg, fainting). When tadalafil is co-administered with an α-blocker, patients should be stable on α-blocker therapy prior to initiating treatment with tadalafil, and tadalafil should be administered at the lowest recommended dose).

No products indexed under this heading.

Aprepitant (Tadalafil is a substrate of and predominantly metabolized by CYP3A4. Studies have shown that drugs that inhibit CYP3A4 can increase tadalafil exposure. When tadalafil is used on an as-needed basis, patients taking concomitant potent inhibitors of CYP3A4, such as ketoconazole or ritonavir, the maximum recommended dose of tadalafil is 10 mg, not to exceed once every 72 hours. When tadalafil is used in a once-daily regimen, patients taking concomitant potent inhibitors of CYP3A4, such as ketoconazole or ritonavir, the dose should not exceed 2.5 mg). Products include:

Atazanavir (Ritonavir (500 mg or 600 mg b.i.d. at steady state), an inhibitor of CYP3A4, CYP2C9, CYP2C19, and CYP2D6, increased tadalafil 20 mg single-dose exposure (AUC) by 32% with a 30% reduction in C_{max}, relative to the values for tadalafil 20 mg alone. Ritonavir (200 mg b.i.d.), increased tadalafil 20 mg single-dose exposure (AUC) by 124% with no change in C_{max}, relative to the values for tadalafil 20 mg alone. Although specific interactions have not been studied, other HIV protease inhibitors would likely increase tadalafil exposure).

No products indexed under this heading.

Atazanavir Sulfate (Ritonavir (500 mg or 600 mg b.i.d. at steady state), an inhibitor of CYP3A4, CYP2C9,

CYP2C19, and CYP2D6, increased tadalafil 20 mg single-dose exposure (AUC) by 32% with a 30% reduction in C_{max}, relative to the values for tadalafil 20 mg alone. Ritonavir (200 mg b.i.d.), increased tadalafil 20 mg single-dose exposure (AUC) by 124% with no change in C_{max}, relative to the values for tadalafil 20 mg alone. Although specific interactions have not been studied, other HIV protease inhibitors would likely increase tadalafil exposure).

No products indexed under this heading.

Atenolol (PDE5 inhibitors, including tadalafil, are mild systemic vasodilators. Clinical pharmacology studies were conducted to assess the effect of tadalafil on the potentiation of the blood-pressure-lowering effects of selected antihypertensive medications (amlodipine, angiotesin II receptor blockers, bendrofluazide, enalapril, and metoprolol). Small reductions in blood pressure occurred following co-administration of tadalafil with these agents compared to placebo).

No products indexed under this heading.

Benazepril Hydrochloride (PDE5 inhibitors, including tadalafil, are mild systemic vasodilators. Clinical pharmacology studies were conducted to assess the effect of tadalafil on the potentiation of the blood-pressure-lowering effects of selected antihypertensive medications (amlodipine, angiotesin II receptor blockers, bendrofluazide, enalapril, and metoprolol). Small reductions in blood pressure occurred following co-administration of tadalafil with these agents compared to placebo).

No products indexed under this heading.

Bendrofluazide (A study was conducted to assess the interaction of bendrofluazide (2.5 mg daily) and tadalafil 10 mg. Following dosing, the mean reduction in supine systolic/diastolic blood pressure due to tadalafil 10 mg in subjects taking bendrofluazide was 6/4 mm Hg, compared to placebo).

No products indexed under this heading.

Bendroflumethiazide (PDE5 inhibitors, including tadalafil, are mild systemic vasodilators. Clinical pharmacology studies were conducted to assess the effect of tadalafil on the potentiation of the blood-pressure-lowering effects of selected antihypertensive medications (amlodipine, angiotesin II receptor blockers, bendrofluazide, enalapril, and metoprolol). Small reductions in blood pressure occurred following co-administration of tadalafil with these agents compared to placebo).

No products indexed under this heading.

Betamethasone (Studies have shown that drugs that induce CYP3A4 can decrease tadalafil exposure. Rifampin (600 mg daily), a CYP3A4 inducer, reduced tadalafil 10 mg single-dose exposure (AUC) by 88% and C_{max} by 46%, relative to the values for tadalafil 10 mg alone. Although specific interactions have not been studied, other CYP3A4 inducers, such as carbamazepine, phenytoin, and phenobarbital, would likely decrease tadalafil exposure. No dose adjustment is warranted. The reduced exposure of tadalafil with the co-administration of rifampin or other CYP3A4 inducers can be anticipated to decrease the efficacy of tadalafil for once daily use; the magnitude of decreased efficacy is unknown).

No products indexed under this heading.

Betamethasone Acetate (Studies have shown that drugs that induce CYP3A4 can decrease tadalafil exposure. Rifampin (600 mg daily), a CYP3A4 inducer, reduced tadalafil 10 mg single-dose exposure (AUC) by 88% and C_{max} by 46%, relative to the values for tadalafil 10 mg alone.

Although specific interactions have not been studied, other CYP3A4 inducers, such as carbamazepine, phenytoin, and phenobarbital, would likely decrease tadalafil exposure. No dose adjustment is warranted. The reduced exposure of tadalafil with the co-administration of rifampin or other CYP3A4 inducers can be anticipated to decrease the efficacy of tadalafil for once daily use; the magnitude of decreased efficacy is unknown).
No products indexed under this heading.

Betamethasone Benzoate (Studies have shown that drugs that induce CYP3A4 can decrease tadalafil exposure. Rifampin (600 mg daily), a CYP3A4 inducer, reduced tadalafil 10 mg single-dose exposure (AUC) by 88% and C_{max} by 46%, relative to the values for tadalafil 10 mg alone. Although specific interactions have not been studied, other CYP3A4 inducers, such as carbamazepine, phenytoin, and phenobarbital, would likely decrease tadalafil exposure. No dose adjustment is warranted. The reduced exposure of tadalafil with the co-administration of rifampin or other CYP3A4 inducers can be anticipated to decrease the efficacy of tadalafil for once daily use; the magnitude of decreased efficacy is unknown).
No products indexed under this heading.

Betamethasone Dipropionate (Studies have shown that drugs that induce CYP3A4 can decrease tadalafil exposure. Rifampin (600 mg daily), a CYP3A4 inducer, reduced tadalafil 10 mg single-dose exposure (AUC) by 88% and C_{max} by 46%, relative to the values for tadalafil 10 mg alone. Although specific interactions have not been studied, other CYP3A4 inducers, such as carbamazepine, phenytoin, and phenobarbital, would likely decrease tadalafil exposure. No dose adjustment is warranted. The reduced exposure of tadalafil with the co-administration of rifampin or other CYP3A4 inducers can be anticipated to decrease the efficacy of tadalafil for once daily use; the magnitude of decreased efficacy is unknown). Products include:
Diprolene Lotion 0.05% 3108
Diprolene Ointment 0.05% 3109
Diprolene AF Cream 0.05% 3107
Lotrisone 3163

Betamethasone Sodium Phosphate (Studies have shown that drugs that induce CYP3A4 can decrease tadalafil exposure. Rifampin (600 mg daily), a CYP3A4 inducer, reduced tadalafil 10 mg single-dose exposure (AUC) by 88% and C_{max} by 46%, relative to the values for tadalafil 10 mg alone. Although specific interactions have not been studied, other CYP3A4 inducers, such as carbamazepine, phenytoin, and phenobarbital, would likely decrease tadalafil exposure. No dose adjustment is warranted. The reduced exposure of tadalafil with the co-administration of rifampin or other CYP3A4 inducers can be anticipated to decrease the efficacy of tadalafil for once daily use; the magnitude of decreased efficacy is unknown).
No products indexed under this heading.

Betamethasone Valerate (Studies have shown that drugs that induce CYP3A4 can decrease tadalafil exposure. Rifampin (600 mg daily), a CYP3A4 inducer, reduced tadalafil 10 mg single-dose exposure (AUC) by 88% and C_{max} by 46%, relative to the values for tadalafil 10 mg alone. Although specific interactions have not been studied, other CYP3A4 inducers, such as carbamazepine, phenytoin, and phenobarbital, would likely decrease tadalafil exposure. No dose adjustment is warranted. The reduced exposure of tadalafil with the co-administration of rifampin or other CYP3A4 inducers can be anticipated to decrease the efficacy of tadalafil for once daily use; the magnitude of decreased efficacy is unknown). Products include:
Luxíq 3321

Betaxolol Hydrochloride (PDE5 inhibitors, including tadalafil, are mild systemic vasodilators. Clinical pharmacology studies were conducted to assess the effect of tadalafil on the potentiation of the blood-pressure-lowering effects of selected antihypertensive medications (amlodipine, angiotesin II receptor blockers, bendrofluazide, enalapril, and metoprolol). Small reductions in blood pressure occurred following co-administration of tadalafil with these agents compared to placebo).
No products indexed under this heading.

Bisoprolol Fumarate (PDE5 inhibitors, including tadalafil, are mild systemic vasodilators. Clinical pharmacology studies were conducted to assess the effect of tadalafil on the potentiation of the blood-pressure-lowering effects of selected antihypertensive medications (amlodipine, angiotesin II receptor blockers, bendrofluazide, enalapril, and metoprolol). Small reductions in blood pressure occurred following co-administration of tadalafil with these agents compared to placebo).
No products indexed under this heading.

Bosentan (Studies have shown that drugs that induce CYP3A4 can decrease tadalafil exposure. Rifampin (600 mg daily), a CYP3A4 inducer, reduced tadalafil 10 mg single-dose exposure (AUC) by 88% and C_{max} by 46%, relative to the values for tadalafil 10 mg alone. Although specific interactions have not been studied, other CYP3A4 inducers, such as carbamazepine, phenytoin, and phenobarbital, would likely decrease tadalafil exposure. No dose adjustment is warranted. The reduced exposure of tadalafil with the co-administration of rifampin or other CYP3A4 inducers can be anticipated to decrease the efficacy of tadalafil for once daily use; the magnitude of decreased efficacy is unknown). Products include:
Tracleer 573

Calcium Carbonate (Simultaneous administration of an antacid (magnesium hydroxide/aluminum hydroxide) and tadalafil reduced the apparent rate of absorption of tadalafil without altering exposure (AUC) to tadalafil). Products include:
Chelated Mineral 3476
Pepcid Complete 1822
Extra Strength Rolaids Softchews Vanilla Creme 2045

Candesartan Cilexetil (A study was conducted to assess the interaction of angiotensin II receptor blockers and tadalafil 20 mg. Subjects in the study were taking any marketed angiotensin II receptor blocker, either alone, as a component of a combination product, or as part of a multiple antihypertensive regimen. Following dosing, ambulatory measurements of blood pressure revealed differences between tadalafil and placebo of 8/4 mm Hg in systolic/diastolic blood pressure). Products include:
Atacand 697
Atacand HCT 700

Captopril (PDE5 inhibitors, including tadalafil, are mild systemic vasodilators. Clinical pharmacology studies were conducted to assess the effect of tadalafil on the potentiation of the blood-pressure-lowering effects of selected antihypertensive medications (amlodipine, angiotesin II receptor blockers, bendrofluazide, enalapril, and metoprolol). Small reductions in blood pressure occurred following co-administration of tadalafil with these agents compared to placebo). Products include:
Captopril 2341

Carbamazepine (Studies have shown that drugs that induce CYP3A4 can decrease tadalafil exposure. Rifampin (600 mg daily), a CYP3A4 inducer, reduced tadalafil 10 mg single-dose exposure (AUC) by 88% and C_{max} by 46%, relative to the values for tadalafil 10 mg alone. Although specific interactions have not been studied, other CYP3A4 inducers, such as carbamazepine, phenytoin, and phenobarbital, would likely decrease tadalafil exposure. No dose adjustment is warranted. The reduced exposure of tadalafil with the co-administration of CYP3A4 inducers can be anticipated to decrease the efficacy of tadalafil for once daily use; the magnitude of decreased efficacy is unknown). Products include:
Carbatrol 3280
Equetro 3477

Carteolol Hydrochloride (PDE5 inhibitors, including tadalafil, are mild systemic vasodilators. Clinical pharmacology studies were conducted to assess the effect of tadalafil on the potentiation of the blood-pressure-lowering effects of selected antihypertensive medications (amlodipine, angiotesin II receptor blockers, bendrofluazide, enalapril, and metoprolol). Small reductions in blood pressure occurred following co-administration of tadalafil with these agents compared to placebo).
No products indexed under this heading.

Carvedilol (PDE5 inhibitors, including tadalafil, are mild systemic vasodilators. Clinical pharmacology studies were conducted to assess the effect of tadalafil on the potentiation of the blood-pressure-lowering effects of selected antihypertensive medications (amlodipine, angiotesin II receptor blockers, bendrofluazide, enalapril, and metoprolol). Small reductions in blood pressure occurred following co-administration of tadalafil with these agents compared to placebo). Products include:
Coreg 1409

Carvedilol Phosphate (PDE5 inhibitors, including tadalafil, are mild systemic vasodilators. Clinical pharmacology studies were conducted to assess the effect of tadalafil on the potentiation of the blood-pressure-lowering effects of selected antihypertensive medications (amlodipine, angiotesin II receptor blockers, bendrofluazide, enalapril, and metoprolol). Small reductions in blood pressure occurred following co-administration of tadalafil with these agents compared to placebo). Products include:
Coreg CR 1416

Chlorothiazide (PDE5 inhibitors, including tadalafil, are mild systemic vasodilators. Clinical pharmacology studies were conducted to assess the effect of tadalafil on the potentiation of the blood-pressure-lowering effects of selected antihypertensive medications (amlodipine, angiotesin II receptor blockers, bendrofluazide, enalapril, and metoprolol). Small reductions in blood pressure occurred following co-administration of tadalafil with these agents compared to placebo).
No products indexed under this heading.

Chlorothiazide Sodium (PDE5 inhibitors, including tadalafil, are mild systemic vasodilators. Clinical pharmacology studies were conducted to assess the effect of tadalafil on the potentiation of the blood-pressure-lowering effects of selected antihypertensive medications (amlodipine, angiotesin II receptor blockers, bendrofluazide, enalapril, and metoprolol). Small reductions in blood pressure occurred following co-administration of tadalafil with these agents compared to placebo). Products include:
Diuril Intravenous 2009

Chlorthalidone (PDE5 inhibitors, including tadalafil, are mild systemic vasodilators. Clinical pharmacology studies were conducted to assess the effect of tadalafil on the potentiation of the blood-pressure-lowering effects of selected antihypertensive medications (amlodipine, angiotesin II receptor blockers, bendrofluazide, enalapril, and metoprolol). Small reductions in blood pressure occurred following co-administration of tadalafil with these agents compared to placebo). Products include:
Clorpres 2344

Cimetidine (Tadalafil is a substrate of and predominantly metabolized by CYP3A4. Studies have shown that drugs that inhibit CYP3A4 can increase tadalafil exposure. When tadalafil is used on an as-needed basis, patients taking concomitant potent inhibitors of CYP3A4, such as ketoconazole or ritonavir, the maximum recommended dose of tadalafil is 10 mg, not to exceed once every 72 hours. When tadalafil is used in a once-daily regimen, patients taking concomitant potent inhibitors of CYP3A4, such as ketoconazole or ritonavir, the dose should not exceed 2.5 mg).
No products indexed under this heading.

Cimetidine Hydrochloride (Tadalafil is a substrate of and predominantly metabolized by CYP3A4. Studies have shown that drugs that inhibit CYP3A4 can increase tadalafil exposure. When tadalafil is used on an as-needed basis, patients taking concomitant potent inhibitors of CYP3A4, such as ketoconazole or ritonavir, the maximum recommended dose of tadalafil is 10 mg, not to exceed once every 72 hours. When tadalafil is used in a once-daily regimen, patients taking concomitant potent inhibitors of CYP3A4, such as ketoconazole or ritonavir, the dose should not exceed 2.5 mg).
No products indexed under this heading.

Ciprofloxacin (Tadalafil is a substrate of and predominantly metabolized by CYP3A4. Studies have shown that drugs that inhibit CYP3A4 can increase tadalafil exposure. When tadalafil is used on an as-needed basis, patients taking concomitant potent inhibitors of CYP3A4, such as ketoconazole or ritonavir, the maximum recommended dose of tadalafil is 10 mg, not to exceed once every 72 hours. When tadalafil is used in a once-daily regimen, patients taking concomitant potent inhibitors of CYP3A4, such as ketoconazole or ritonavir, the dose should not exceed 2.5 mg). Products include:
Cipro I.V. 3082
Cipro 3073
Cipro XR 3091
Ciprodex 583

Ciprofloxacin Hydrochloride (Studies have shown that drugs that induce CYP3A4 can decrease tadalafil exposure. Rifampin (600 mg daily), a CYP3A4 inducer, reduced tadalafil 10 mg single-dose exposure (AUC) by 88% and C_{max} by 46%, relative to the values for tadalafil 10 mg alone. Although specific interactions have not been studied, other CYP3A4 inducers, such as carbamazepine, phenytoin, and phenobarbital, would likely decrease tadalafil exposure. No dose adjustment is warranted. The reduced exposure of tadalafil with the co-administration of rifampin or other CYP3A4 inducers can be anticipated to decrease the efficacy

IMPORTANT NOTE: Always consult each drug listing in the patient's regimen for possible interactions.

Cialis Interactions Index 310

of tadalafil for once daily use; the magnitude of decreased efficacy is unknown). Products include:
Cipro 3073

Cisplatin (Studies have shown that drugs that induce CYP3A4 can decrease tadalafil exposure. Rifampin (600 mg daily), a CYP3A4 inducer, reduced tadalafil 10 mg single-dose exposure (AUC) by 88% and C_{max} by 46%, relative to the values for tadalafil 10 mg alone. Although specific interactions have not been studied, other CYP3A4 inducers, such as carbamazepine, phenytoin, and phenobarbital, would likely decrease tadalafil exposure. No dose adjustment is warranted. The reduced exposure of tadalafil with the co-administration of rifampin or other CYP3A4 inducers can be anticipated to decrease the efficacy of tadalafil for once daily use; the magnitude of decreased efficacy is unknown).
No products indexed under this heading.

Clarithromycin (Tadalafil is a substrate of and metabolized predominantly by CYP3A4. Studies have shown that drugs that inhibit CYP3A4 can increase tadalafil exposure. When tadalafil is used on an as-needed basis, patients taking concomitant potent inhibitors of CYP3A4, such as ketoconazole or ritonavir, the maximum recommended dose of tadalafil is 10 mg, not to exceed once every 72 hours. When tadalafil is used in a once-daily regimen, patients taking concomitant potent inhibitors of CYP3A4, such as ketoconazole or ritonavir, the dose should not exceed 2.5 mg). Products include:
Biaxin/Biaxin XL 412

Clonidine (Caution is advised when PDE5 inhibitors are co-administered with α-blockers. Tadalafil and α-adrenergic blocking agents are both vasodilators with blood-pressure lowering effects. When vasodilators are used in combination, an additive effect on blood pressure may be anticipated. In some patients, concomitant use of these two drug classes can lower blood presure significantly, which may lead to symptomatic hypotension (eg, fainting). When tadalafil is co-administered with an α-blocker, patients should be stable on α-blocker therapy prior to initiating treatment with tadalafil, and tadalafil should be administered at the lowest recommended dose). Products include:
Catapres-TTS 884

Clonidine Hydrochloride (Caution is advised when PDE5 inhibitors are co-administered with α-blockers. Tadalafil and α-adrenergic blocking agents are both vasodilators with blood-pressure lowering effects. When vasodilators are used in combination, an additive effect on blood pressure may be anticipated. In some patients, concomitant use of these two drug classes can lower blood presure significantly, which may lead to symptomatic hypotension (eg, fainting). When tadalafil is co-administered with an α-blocker, patients should be stable on α-blocker therapy prior to initiating treatment with tadalafil, and tadalafil should be administered at the lowest recommended dose). Products include:
Clorpres 2344

Clotrimazole (Tadalafil is a substrate of and predominantly metabolized by CYP3A4. Studies have shown that drugs that inhibit CYP3A4 can increase tadalafil exposure. When tadalafil is used on an as-needed basis, patients taking concomitant potent inhibitors of CYP3A4, such as ketoconazole or ritonavir, the maximum recommended dose of tadalafil is 10 mg, not to exceed once every 72 hours. When tadalafil is used in a once-daily regimen, patients taking concomitant potent inhibitors of CYP3A4, such as ketoconazole or ritonavir, the dose should not exceed 2.5 mg). Products include:
Lotrisone 3163

Conivaptan Hydrochloride (Tadalafil is a substrate of and predominantly metabolized by CYP3A4. Studies have shown that drugs that inhibit CYP3A4 can increase tadalafil exposure. When tadalafil is used on an as-needed basis, patients taking concomitant potent inhibitors of CYP3A4, such as ketoconazole or ritonavir, the maximum recommended dose of tadalafil is 10 mg, not to exceed once every 72 hours. When tadalafil is used in a once-daily regimen, patients taking concomitant potent inhibitors of CYP3A4, such as ketoconazole or ritonavir, the dose should not exceed 2.5 mg). Products include:
Vaprisol 689

Cortisone Acetate (Studies have shown that drugs that induce CYP3A4 can decrease tadalafil exposure. Rifampin (600 mg daily), a CYP3A4 inducer, reduced tadalafil 10 mg single-dose exposure (AUC) by 88% and C_{max} by 46%, relative to the values for tadalafil 10 mg alone. Although specific interactions have not been studied, other CYP3A4 inducers, such as carbamazepine, phenytoin, and phenobarbital, would likely decrease tadalafil exposure. No dose adjustment is warranted. The reduced exposure of tadalafil with the co-administration of rifampin or other CYP3A4 inducers can be anticipated to decrease the efficacy of tadalafil for once daily use; the magnitude of decreased efficacy is unknown).
No products indexed under this heading.

Cyclosporine (Tadalafil is a substrate of and predominantly metabolized by CYP3A4. Studies have shown that drugs that inhibit CYP3A4 can increase tadalafil exposure. When tadalafil is used on an as-needed basis, patients taking concomitant potent inhibitors of CYP3A4, such as ketoconazole or ritonavir, the maximum recommended dose of tadalafil is 10 mg, not to exceed once every 72 hours. When tadalafil is used in a once-daily regimen, patients taking concomitant potent inhibitors of CYP3A4, such as ketoconazole or ritonavir, the dose should not exceed 2.5 mg). Products include:
Gengraf 440
Neoral Oral Solution 2496
Neoral Capsules 2496
Restasis 605

Dalfopristin (Tadalafil is a substrate of and predominantly metabolized by CYP3A4. Studies have shown that drugs that inhibit CYP3A4 can increase tadalafil exposure. When tadalafil is used on an as-needed basis, patients taking concomitant potent inhibitors of CYP3A4, such as ketoconazole or ritonavir, the maximum recommended dose of tadalafil is 10 mg, not to exceed once every 72 hours. When tadalafil is used in a once-daily regimen, patients taking concomitant potent inhibitors of CYP3A4, such as ketoconazole or ritonavir, the dose should not exceed 2.5 mg).
No products indexed under this heading.

Danazol (Tadalafil is a substrate of and predominantly metabolized by CYP3A4. Studies have shown that drugs that inhibit CYP3A4 can increase tadalafil exposure. When tadalafil is used on an as-needed basis, patients taking concomitant potent inhibitors of CYP3A4, such as ketoconazole or ritonavir, the maximum recommended dose of tadalafil is 10 mg, not to exceed once every 72 hours. When tadalafil is used in a once-daily regimen, patients taking concomitant potent inhibitors of CYP3A4, such as ketoconazole or ritonavir, the dose should not exceed 2.5 mg).
No products indexed under this heading.

Darunavir (Ritonavir (500 mg or 600 mg b.i.d. at steady state), an inhibitor of CYP3A4, CYP2C9, CYP2C19, and CYP2D6, increased tadalafil 20 mg single-dose exposure (AUC) by 32% with a 30% reduction in C_{max}, relative to the values for tadalafil 20 mg alone. Ritonavir (200 mg b.i.d.), increased tadalafil 20 mg single-dose exposure (AUC) by 124% with no change in C_{max}, relative to the values for tadalafil 20 mg alone. Although specific interactions have not been studied, other HIV protease inhibitors would likely increase tadalafil exposure).
No products indexed under this heading.

Dasatinib (Tadalafil is a substrate of and predominantly metabolized by CYP3A4. Studies have shown that drugs that inhibit CYP3A4 can increase tadalafil exposure. When tadalafil is used on an as-needed basis, patients taking concomitant potent inhibitors of CYP3A4, such as ketoconazole or ritonavir, the maximum recommended dose of tadalafil is 10 mg, not to exceed once every 72 hours. When tadalafil is used in a once-daily regimen, patients taking concomitant potent inhibitors of CYP3A4, such as ketoconazole or ritonavir, the dose should not exceed 2.5 mg).
No products indexed under this heading.

Delavirdine Mesylate (Tadalafil is a substrate of and metabolized predominantly by CYP3A4. Studies have shown that drugs that inhibit CYP3A4 can increase tadalafil exposure. When tadalafil is used on an as-needed basis, patients taking concomitant potent inhibitors of CYP3A4, such as ketoconazole or ritonavir, the maximum recommended dose of tadalafil is 10 mg, not to exceed once every 72 hours. When tadalafil is used in a once-daily regimen, patients taking concomitant potent inhibitors of CYP3A4, such as ketoconazole or ritonavir, the dose should not exceed 2.5 mg).
No products indexed under this heading.

Delavirine (Tadalafil is a substrate of and metabolized predominantly by CYP3A4. Studies have shown that drugs that inhibit CYP3A4 can increase tadalafil exposure. When tadalafil is used on an as-needed basis, patients taking concomitant potent inhibitors of CYP3A4, such as ketoconazole or ritonavir, the maximum recommended dose of tadalafil is 10 mg, not to exceed once every 72 hours. When tadalafil is used in a once-daily regimen, patients taking concomitant potent inhibitors of CYP3A4, such as ketoconazole or ritonavir, the dose should not exceed 2.5 mg).
No products indexed under this heading.

Deserpidine (PDE5 inhibitors, including tadalafil, are mild systemic vasodilators. Clinical pharmacology studies were conducted to assess the effect of tadalafil on the potentiation of the blood-pressure-lowering effects of selected antihypertensive medications (amlodipine, angiotesin II receptor blockers, bendrofluazide, enalapril, and metoprolol). Small reductions in blood pressure occurred following co-administration of tadalafil with these agents compared to placebo).
No products indexed under this heading.

Desloratadine (Tadalafil is a substrate of and predominantly metabolized by CYP3A4. Studies have shown that drugs that inhibit CYP3A4 can increase tadalafil exposure. When tadalafil is used on an as-needed basis, patients taking concomitant potent inhibitors of CYP3A4, such as ketoconazole or ritonavir, the maximum recommended dose of tadalafil is 10 mg, not to exceed once every 72 hours. When tadalafil is used in a once-daily regimen, patients taking concomitant potent inhibitors of CYP3A4, such as ketoconazole or ritonavir, the dose should not exceed 2.5 mg). Products include:
Clarinex Syrup 3098
Clarinex 3098
Clarinex Reditabs 3098
Clarinex-D 12-Hour 3101
Clarinex-D 3104

Dexamethasone (Studies have shown that drugs that induce CYP3A4 can decrease tadalafil exposure. Rifampin (600 mg daily), a CYP3A4 inducer, reduced tadalafil 10 mg single-dose exposure (AUC) by 88% and C_{max} by 46%, relative to the values for tadalafil 10 mg alone. Although specific interactions have not been studied, other CYP3A4 inducers, such as carbamazepine, phenytoin, and phenobarbital, would likely decrease tadalafil exposure. No dose adjustment is warranted. The reduced exposure of tadalafil with the co-administration of rifampin or other CYP3A4 inducers can be anticipated to decrease the efficacy of tadalafil for once daily use; the magnitude of decreased efficacy is unknown). Products include:
Ciprodex 583
Ozurdex .... ⊙223
Tobramycin and Dexamethasone Ophthalmic Suspension .... ⊙251

Dexamethasone Acetate (Studies have shown that drugs that induce CYP3A4 can decrease tadalafil exposure. Rifampin (600 mg daily), a CYP3A4 inducer, reduced tadalafil 10 mg single-dose exposure (AUC) by 88% and C_{max} by 46%, relative to the values for tadalafil 10 mg alone. Although specific interactions have not been studied, other CYP3A4 inducers, such as carbamazepine, phenytoin, and phenobarbital, would likely decrease tadalafil exposure. No dose adjustment is warranted. The reduced exposure of tadalafil with the co-administration of rifampin or other CYP3A4 inducers can be anticipated to decrease the efficacy of tadalafil for once daily use; the magnitude of decreased efficacy is unknown).
No products indexed under this heading.

Dexamethasone Phosphate (Studies have shown that drugs that induce CYP3A4 can decrease tadalafil exposure. Rifampin (600 mg daily), a CYP3A4 inducer, reduced tadalafil 10 mg single-dose exposure (AUC) by 88% and C_{max} by 46%, relative to the values for tadalafil 10 mg alone. Although specific interactions have not been studied, other CYP3A4 inducers, such as carbamazepine, phenytoin, and phenobarbital, would likely decrease tadalafil exposure. No dose adjustment is warranted. The reduced exposure of tadalafil with the co-administration of rifampin or other CYP3A4 inducers can be anticipated to decrease the efficacy of tadalafil for once daily use; the magnitude of decreased efficacy is unknown).
No products indexed under this heading.

Dexamethasone Sodium (Studies have shown that drugs that induce CYP3A4 can decrease tadalafil exposure. Rifampin (600 mg daily), a CYP3A4 inducer, reduced tadalafil 10 mg single-dose exposure (AUC) by 88% and C_{max} by 46%, relative to the values for tadalafil 10 mg alone. Although specific interactions have not been studied, other CYP3A4 inducers, such as carbamazepine, phenytoin, and phenobarbital, would likely decrease tadalafil exposure. No dose adjustment is warranted. The reduced exposure of tadalafil with the co-administration of

311 Interactions Index Cialis

rifampin or other CYP3A4 inducers can be anticipated to decrease the efficacy of tadalafil for once daily use; the magnitude of decreased efficacy is unknown).
No products indexed under this heading.

Dexamethasone Sodium Phosphate (Studies have shown that drugs that induce CYP3A4 can decrease tadalafil exposure. Rifampin (600 mg daily), a CYP3A4 inducer, reduced tadalafil 10 mg single-dose exposure (AUC) by 88% and C_{max} by 46%, relative to the values for tadalafil 10 mg alone. Although specific interactions have not been studied, other CYP3A4 inducers, such as carbamazepine, phenytoin, and phenobarbital, would likely decrease tadalafil exposure. No dose adjustment is warranted. The reduced exposure of tadalafil with the co-administration of rifampin or other CYP3A4 inducers can be anticipated to decrease the efficacy of tadalafil for once daily use; the magnitude of decreased efficacy is unknown).
No products indexed under this heading.

Dexamethasone Sodium Phosphate Injection (Studies have shown that drugs that induce CYP3A4 can decrease tadalafil exposure. Rifampin (600 mg daily), a CYP3A4 inducer, reduced tadalafil 10 mg single-dose exposure (AUC) by 88% and C_{max} by 46%, relative to the values for tadalafil 10 mg alone. Although specific interactions have not been studied, other CYP3A4 inducers, such as carbamazepine, phenytoin, and phenobarbital, would likely decrease tadalafil exposure. No dose adjustment is warranted. The reduced exposure of tadalafil with the co-administration of rifampin or other CYP3A4 inducers can be anticipated to decrease the efficacy of tadalafil for once daily use; the magnitude of decreased efficacy is unknown).
No products indexed under this heading.

Diazoxide (PDE5 inhibitors, including tadalafil, are mild systemic vasodilators. Clinical pharmacology studies were conducted to assess the effect of tadalafil on the potentiation of the blood-pressure-lowering effects of selected antihypertensive medications (amlodipine, angiotesin II receptor blockers, bendrofluazide, enalapril, and metoprolol). Small reductions in blood pressure occurred following co-administration of tadalafil with these agents compared to placebo). Products include:
Proglycem 1179
Proglycem Suspension 1179

Diltiazem Hydrochloride (PDE5 inhibitors, including tadalafil, are mild systemic vasodilators. Clinical pharmacology studies were conducted to assess the effect of tadalafil on the potentiation of the blood-pressure-lowering effects of selected antihypertensive medications (amlodipine, angiotesin II receptor blockers, bendrofluazide, enalapril, and metoprolol). Small reductions in blood pressure occurred following co-administration of tadalafil with these agents compared to placebo). Products include:
Cardizem LA 423

Diltiazem Maleate (PDE5 inhibitors, including tadalafil, are mild systemic vasodilators. Clinical pharmacology studies were conducted to assess the effect of tadalafil on the potentiation of the blood-pressure-lowering effects of selected antihypertensive medications (amlodipine, angiotesin II receptor blockers, bendrofluazide, enalapril, and metoprolol). Small reductions in blood pressure occurred following co-administration of tadalafil with these agents compared to placebo).
No products indexed under this heading.

Doxazosin Mesylate (Caution is advised when PDE5 inhibitors are co-administered with α-blockers. Tadalafil and α-adrenergic blocking agents are both vasodilators with blood-pressure lowering effects. When vasodilators are used in combination, an additive effect on blood pressure may be anticipated. In some patients, concomitant use of these two drug classes can lower blood presure significantly, which may lead to symptomatic hypotension (eg, fainting). When tadalafil is co-administered with an α-blocker, patients should be stable on α-blocker therapy prior to initiating treatment with tadalafil, and tadalafil should be administered at the lowest recommended dose).
No products indexed under this heading.

Doxorubicin Hydrochloride (Studies have shown that drugs that induce CYP3A4 can decrease tadalafil exposure. Rifampin (600 mg daily), a CYP3A4 inducer, reduced tadalafil 10 mg single-dose exposure (AUC) by 88% and C_{max} by 46%, relative to the values for tadalafil 10 mg alone. Although specific interactions have not been studied, other CYP3A4 inducers, such as carbamazepine, phenytoin, and phenobarbital, would likely decrease tadalafil exposure. No dose adjustment is warranted. The reduced exposure of tadalafil with the co-administration of rifampin or other CYP3A4 inducers can be anticipated to decrease the efficacy of tadalafil for once daily use; the magnitude of decreased efficacy is unknown).
No products indexed under this heading.

Efavirenz (Tadalafil is a substrate of and predominantly metabolized by CYP3A4. Studies have shown that drugs that inhibit CYP3A4 can increase tadalafil exposure. When tadalafil is used on an as-needed basis, patients taking concomitant potent inhibitors of CYP3A4, such as ketoconazole or ritonavir, the maximum recommended dose of tadalafil is 10 mg, not to exceed once every 72 hours. When tadalafil is used in a once-daily regimen, patients taking concomitant potent inhibitors of CYP3A4, such as ketoconazole or ritonavir, the dose should not exceed 2.5 mg). Products include:
Atripla 906

Enalapril Maleate (A study was conducted to assess the interaction of enalapril (10 to 20 mg daily) and tadalafil 10 mg. Following dosing, the mean reduction in supine systolic/diastolic blood pressure due to tadalafil 10 mg in subjects taking enalapril was 4/1 mm Hg, compared to placebo).
No products indexed under this heading.

Enalaprilat (A study was conducted to assess the interaction of enalapril (10 to 20 mg daily) and tadalafil 10 mg. Following dosing, the mean reduction in supine systolic/diastolic blood pressure due to tadalafil 10 mg in subjects taking enalapril was 4/1 mm Hg, compared to placebo).
No products indexed under this heading.

Eprosartan Mesylate (A study was conducted to assess the interaction of angiotensin II receptor blockers and tadalafil 20 mg. Subjects in the study were taking any marketed angiotensin II receptor blocker, either alone, as a component of a combination product, or as part of a multiple antihypertensive regimen. Following dosing, ambulatory measurements of blood pressure revealed differences between tadalafil and placebo of 8/4 mm Hg in systolic/diastolic blood pressure). Products include:
Teveten 538
Teveten HCT 541

Erythrityl Tetranitrate (Administration of tadalafil to patients using any form of organic nitrate, either regularly and/or intermittently, is contraindicated. In clinical pharmacology studies, tadalafil was shown to potentiate the hypotensive effects of nitrates. In a patient who has taken tadalafil, where nitrate administration is deemed medically necessary in a life threatening situation, at least 48 hours should elapse after the last dose of tadalafil before nitrate administration is considered. In such circumstances, nitrates should still only be administered under close medical supervision with appropriate hemodynamic monitoring).
No products indexed under this heading.

Erythromycin (CYP3A4 inhibitors such as erythromycin may likely increase tadalafil exposure).
No products indexed under this heading.

Erythromycin, Topical (CYP3A4 inhibitors such as erythromycin may likely increase tadalafil exposure).
No products indexed under this heading.

Erythromycin Estolate (CYP3A4 inhibitors such as erythromycin may likely increase tadalafil exposure).
No products indexed under this heading.

Erythromycin Ethylsuccinate (CYP3A4 inhibitors such as erythromycin may likely increase tadalafil exposure). Products include:
E.E.S. 437
EryPed 435

Erythromycin Gluceptate (CYP3A4 inhibitors such as erythromycin may likely increase tadalafil exposure).
No products indexed under this heading.

Erythromycin Lactobionate (CYP3A4 inhibitors such as erythromycin may likely increase tadalafil exposure).
No products indexed under this heading.

Erythromycin Stearate (CYP3A4 inhibitors such as erythromycin may likely increase tadalafil exposure).
No products indexed under this heading.

Esmolol Hydrochloride (PDE5 inhibitors, including tadalafil, are mild systemic vasodilators. Clinical pharmacology studies were conducted to assess the effect of tadalafil on the potentiation of the blood-pressure-lowering effects of selected antihypertensive medications (amlodipine, angiotesin II receptor blockers, bendrofluazide, enalapril, and metoprolol). Small reductions in blood pressure occurred following co-administration of tadalafil with these agents compared to placebo).
No products indexed under this heading.

Esomeprazole Magnesium (Tadalafil is a substrate of and predominantly metabolized by CYP3A4. Studies have shown that drugs that inhibit CYP3A4 can increase tadalafil exposure. When tadalafil is used on an as-needed basis, patients taking concomitant potent inhibitors of CYP3A4, such as ketoconazole or ritonavir, the maximum recommended dose of tadalafil is 10 mg, not to exceed once every 72 hours. When tadalafil is used in a once-daily regimen, patients taking concomitant potent inhibitors of CYP3A4, such as ketoconazole or ritonavir, the dose should not exceed 2.5 mg). Products include:
Nexium Capsules 704
Nexium Oral Suspension 704

Esomeprazole Sodium (Tadalafil is a substrate of and predominantly metabolized by CYP3A4. Studies have shown that drugs that inhibit CYP3A4 can increase tadalafil exposure. When tadalafil is used on an as-needed basis, patients taking concomitant potent inhibitors of CYP3A4, such as ketoconazole or ritonavir, the maximum recommended dose of tadalafil is 10 mg, not to exceed once every 72 hours. When tadalafil is used in a once-daily regimen, patients taking concomitant potent inhibitors of CYP3A4, such as ketoconazole or ritonavir, the dose should not exceed 2.5 mg). Products include:
Nexium I.V. 712

Ethanol (Both alcohol and tadalafil act as mild vasodilators. When mild vasodilators are taken in combination, blood-pressure-lowering effects of each individual compound may be increased. Substantial consumption of alcohol (eg, 5 units or greater) in combination with tadalafil can increase the potential for orthostatic signs and symptoms, including increase in heart rate, decrease in standing blood pressure, dizziness, and headache).
No products indexed under this heading.

Ethosuximide (Studies have shown that drugs that induce CYP3A4 can decrease tadalafil exposure. Rifampin (600 mg daily), a CYP3A4 inducer, reduced tadalafil 10 mg single-dose exposure (AUC) by 88% and C_{max} by 46%, relative to the values for tadalafil 10 mg alone. Although specific interactions have not been studied, other CYP3A4 inducers, such as carbamazepine, phenytoin, and phenobarbital, would likely decrease tadalafil exposure. No dose adjustment is warranted. The reduced exposure of tadalafil with the co-administration of rifampin or other CYP3A4 inducers can be anticipated to decrease the efficacy of tadalafil for once daily use; the magnitude of decreased efficacy is unknown).
No products indexed under this heading.

Ethyl Alcohol (Both alcohol and tadalafil act as mild vasodilators. When mild vasodilators are taken in combination, blood-pressure-lowering effects of each individual compound may be increased. Substantial consumption of alcohol (eg, 5 units or greater) in combination with tadalafil can increase the potential for orthostatic signs and symptoms, including increase in heart rate, decrease in standing blood pressure, dizziness, and headache).
No products indexed under this heading.

Felbamate (Studies have shown that drugs that induce CYP3A4 can decrease tadalafil exposure. Rifampin (600 mg daily), a CYP3A4 inducer, reduced tadalafil 10 mg single-dose exposure (AUC) by 88% and C_{max} by 46%, relative to the values for tadalafil 10 mg alone. Although specific interactions have not been studied, other CYP3A4 inducers, such as carbamazepine, phenytoin, and phenobarbital, would likely decrease tadalafil exposure. No dose adjustment is warranted. The reduced exposure of tadalafil with the co-administration of rifampin or other CYP3A4 inducers can be anticipated to decrease the efficacy of tadalafil for once daily use; the magnitude of decreased efficacy is unknown).
No products indexed under this heading.

Felodipine (PDE5 inhibitors, including tadalafil, are mild systemic vasodilators. Clinical pharmacology studies were conducted to assess the effect of tadalafil on the potentiation of the blood-pressure-lowering effects of selected antihypertensive medications (amlodipine, angiotesin II receptor blockers, bendrofluazide, enalapril, and metoprolol). Small reductions in blood pressure occurred following co-administration of tadalafil with these agents compared to placebo).
No products indexed under this heading.

Fluconazole (Tadalafil is a substrate of and predominantly metabolized by CYP3A4. Studies have shown that drugs that inhibit CYP3A4 can increase

IMPORTANT NOTE: Always consult each drug listing in the patient's regimen for possible interactions.

tadalafil exposure. When tadalafil is used on an as-needed basis, patients taking concomitant potent inhibitors of CYP3A4, such as ketoconazole or ritonavir, the maximum recommended dose of tadalafil is 10 mg, not to exceed once every 72 hours. When tadalafil is used in a once-daily regimen, patients taking concomitant potent inhibitors of CYP3A4, such as ketoconazole or ritonavir, the dose should not exceed 2.5 mg).
No products indexed under this heading.

Fludrocortisone Acetate (Studies have shown that drugs that induce CYP3A4 can decrease tadalafil exposure. Rifampin (600 mg daily), a CYP3A4 inducer, reduced tadalafil 10 mg single-dose exposure (AUC) by 88% and C_{max} by 46%, relative to the values for tadalafil 10 mg alone. Although specific interactions have not been studied, other CYP3A4 inducers, such as carbamazepine, phenytoin, and phenobarbital, would likely decrease tadalafil exposure. No dose adjustment is warranted. The reduced exposure of tadalafil with the co-administration of rifampin or other CYP3A4 inducers can be anticipated to decrease the efficacy of tadalafil for once daily use; the magnitude of decreased efficacy is unknown).
No products indexed under this heading.

Fluoxetine (Tadalafil is a substrate of and predominantly metabolized by CYP3A4. Studies have shown that drugs that inhibit CYP3A4 can increase tadalafil exposure. When tadalafil is used on an as-needed basis, patients taking concomitant potent inhibitors of CYP3A4, such as ketoconazole or ritonavir, the maximum recommended dose of tadalafil is 10 mg, not to exceed once every 72 hours. When tadalafil is used in a once-daily regimen, patients taking concomitant potent inhibitors of CYP3A4, such as ketoconazole or ritonavir, the dose should not exceed 2.5 mg).
No products indexed under this heading.

Fluoxetine Hydrochloride (Tadalafil is a substrate of and predominantly metabolized by CYP3A4. Studies have shown that drugs that inhibit CYP3A4 can increase tadalafil exposure. When tadalafil is used on an as-needed basis, patients taking concomitant potent inhibitors of CYP3A4, such as ketoconazole or ritonavir, the maximum recommended dose of tadalafil is 10 mg, not to exceed once every 72 hours. When tadalafil is used in a once-daily regimen, patients taking concomitant potent inhibitors of CYP3A4, such as ketoconazole or ritonavir, the dose should not exceed 2.5 mg). Products include:

Prozac Weekly **1941**
Prozac Pulvules **1941**
Symbyax **1965**

Fluvoxamine Maleate (Tadalafil is a substrate of and predominantly metabolized by CYP3A4. Studies have shown that drugs that inhibit CYP3A4 can increase tadalafil exposure. When tadalafil is used on an as-needed basis, patients taking concomitant potent inhibitors of CYP3A4, such as ketoconazole or ritonavir, the maximum recommended dose of tadalafil is 10 mg, not to exceed once every 72 hours. When tadalafil is used in a once-daily regimen, patients taking concomitant potent inhibitors of CYP3A4, such as ketoconazole or ritonavir, the dose should not exceed 2.5 mg).
No products indexed under this heading.

Fosamprenavir Calcium (Ritonavir (500 mg or 600 mg b.i.d. at steady state), an inhibitor of CYP3A4, CYP2C9, CYP2C19, and CYP2D6, increased tadalafil 20 mg single-dose exposure (AUC) by 32% with a 30% reduction in C_{max}, relative to the values for tadalafil 20 mg alone. Ritonavir (200 mg b.i.d.), increased tadalafil 20 mg single-dose exposure (AUC) by 124% with no change in C_{max}, relative to the values for tadalafil 20 mg alone. Although specific interactions have not been studied, other HIV protease inhibitors would likely increase tadalafil exposure). Products include:

Lexiva Oral Suspension **1558**
Lexiva **1558**

Fosinopril Sodium (PDE5 inhibitors, including tadalafil, are mild systemic vasodilators. Clinical pharmacology studies were conducted to assess the effect of tadalafil on the potentiation of the blood-pressure-lowering effects of selected antihypertensive medications (amlodipine, angiotesin II receptor blockers, bendrofluazide, enalapril, and metoprolol). Small reductions in blood pressure occurred following co-administration of tadalafil with these agents compared to placebo).
No products indexed under this heading.

Fosphenytoin (Studies have shown that drugs that induce CYP3A4 can decrease tadalafil exposure. Rifampin (600 mg daily), a CYP3A4 inducer, reduced tadalafil 10 mg single-dose exposure (AUC) by 88% and C_{max} by 46%, relative to the values for tadalafil 10 mg alone. Although specific interactions have not been studied, other CYP3A4 inducers, such as phenytoin would likely decrease tadalafil exposure. No dose adjustment is warranted. The reduced exposure of tadalafil with the co-administration of CYP3A4 inducers can be anticipated to decrease the efficacy of tadalafil for once daily use; the magnitude of decreased efficacy is unknown).
No products indexed under this heading.

Fosphenytoin Sodium (Studies have shown that drugs that induce CYP3A4 can decrease tadalafil exposure. Rifampin (600 mg daily), a CYP3A4 inducer, reduced tadalafil 10 mg single-dose exposure (AUC) by 88% and C_{max} by 46%, relative to the values for tadalafil 10 mg alone. Although specific interactions have not been studied, other CYP3A4 inducers, such as phenytoin would likely decrease tadalafil exposure. No dose adjustment is warranted. The reduced exposure of tadalafil with the co-administration of CYP3A4 inducers can be anticipated to decrease the efficacy of tadalafil for once daily use; the magnitude of decreased efficacy is unknown).
No products indexed under this heading.

Furosemide (PDE5 inhibitors, including tadalafil, are mild systemic vasodilators. Clinical pharmacology studies were conducted to assess the effect of tadalafil on the potentiation of the blood-pressure-lowering effects of selected antihypertensive medications (amlodipine, angiotesin II receptor blockers, bendrofluazide, enalapril, and metoprolol). Small reductions in blood pressure occurred following co-administration of tadalafil with these agents compared to placebo). Products include:

Furosemide **2354**

Garlic Extract (Studies have shown that drugs that induce CYP3A4 can decrease tadalafil exposure. Rifampin (600 mg daily), a CYP3A4 inducer, reduced tadalafil 10 mg single-dose exposure (AUC) by 88% and C_{max} by 46%, relative to the values for tadalafil 10 mg alone. Although specific interactions have not been studied, other CYP3A4 inducers, such as carbamazepine, phenytoin, and phenobarbital, would likely decrease tadalafil exposure. No dose adjustment is warranted. The reduced exposure of tadalafil with the co-administration of rifampin or other CYP3A4 inducers can be anticipated to decrease the efficacy of tadalafil for once daily use; the magnitude of decreased efficacy is unknown).
No products indexed under this heading.

Garlic Oil (Studies have shown that drugs that induce CYP3A4 can decrease tadalafil exposure. Rifampin (600 mg daily), a CYP3A4 inducer, reduced tadalafil 10 mg single-dose exposure (AUC) by 88% and C_{max} by 46%, relative to the values for tadalafil 10 mg alone. Although specific interactions have not been studied, other CYP3A4 inducers, such as carbamazepine, phenytoin, and phenobarbital, would likely decrease tadalafil exposure. No dose adjustment is warranted. The reduced exposure of tadalafil with the co-administration of rifampin or other CYP3A4 inducers can be anticipated to decrease the efficacy of tadalafil for once daily use; the magnitude of decreased efficacy is unknown).
No products indexed under this heading.

Glyceryl Trinitrate (Administration of tadalafil to patients using any form of organic nitrate, either regularly and/or intermittently, is contraindicated. In clinical pharmacology studies, tadalafil was shown to potentiate the hypotensive effects of nitrates. In a patient who has taken tadalafil, where nitrate administration is deemed medically necessary in a life threatening situation, at least 48 hours should elapse after the last dose of tadalafil before nitrate administration is considered. In such circumstances, nitrates should still only be administered under close medical supervision with appropriate hemodynamic monitoring).
No products indexed under this heading.

Guanabenz Acetate (PDE5 inhibitors, including tadalafil, are mild systemic vasodilators. Clinical pharmacology studies were conducted to assess the effect of tadalafil on the potentiation of the blood-pressure-lowering effects of selected antihypertensive medications (amlodipine, angiotesin II receptor blockers, bendrofluazide, enalapril, and metoprolol). Small reductions in blood pressure occurred following co-administration of tadalafil with these agents compared to placebo).
No products indexed under this heading.

Guanethidine (PDE5 inhibitors, including tadalafil, are mild systemic vasodilators. Clinical pharmacology studies were conducted to assess the effect of tadalafil on the potentiation of the blood-pressure-lowering effects of selected antihypertensive medications (amlodipine, angiotesin II receptor blockers, bendrofluazide, enalapril, and metoprolol). Small reductions in blood pressure occurred following co-administration of tadalafil with these agents compared to placebo).
No products indexed under this heading.

Guanethidine Monosulfate (PDE5 inhibitors, including tadalafil, are mild systemic vasodilators. Clinical pharmacology studies were conducted to assess the effect of tadalafil on the potentiation of the blood-pressure-lowering effects of selected antihypertensive medications (amlodipine, angiotesin II receptor blockers, bendrofluazide, enalapril, and metoprolol). Small reductions in blood pressure occurred following co-administration of tadalafil with these agents compared to placebo).
No products indexed under this heading.

Guanethidine Sulfate (PDE5 inhibitors, including tadalafil, are mild systemic vasodilators. Clinical pharmacology studies were conducted to assess the effect of tadalafil on the potentiation of the blood-pressure-lowering effects of selected antihypertensive medications (amlodipine, angiotesin II receptor blockers, bendrofluazide, enalapril, and metoprolol). Small reductions in blood pressure occurred following co-administration of tadalafil with these agents compared to placebo).
No products indexed under this heading.

Hydralazine Hydrochloride (PDE5 inhibitors, including tadalafil, are mild systemic vasodilators. Clinical pharmacology studies were conducted to assess the effect of tadalafil on the potentiation of the blood-pressure-lowering effects of selected antihypertensive medications (amlodipine, angiotesin II receptor blockers, bendrofluazide, enalapril, and metoprolol). Small reductions in blood pressure occurred following co-administration of tadalafil with these agents compared to placebo).
No products indexed under this heading.

Hydrochlorothiazide (PDE5 inhibitors, including tadalafil, are mild systemic vasodilators. Clinical pharmacology studies were conducted to assess the effect of tadalafil on the potentiation of the blood-pressure-lowering effects of selected antihypertensive medications (amlodipine, angiotesin II receptor blockers, bendrofluazide, enalapril, and metoprolol). Small reductions in blood pressure occurred following co-administration of tadalafil with these agents compared to placebo). Products include:

Atacand HCT **700**
Avalide **2956**
Benicar HCT **1017**
Diovan HCT **2419**
Dyazide **1429**
Exforge HCT **2449**
Hyzaar **2162**
Hyzaar 100-12.5 .... **2162**
Micardis HCT **889**
Prinzide **2246**
Tekturna HCT **2541**
Teveten HCT **541**

Hydrocortisone (Studies have shown that drugs that induce CYP3A4 can decrease tadalafil exposure. Rifampin (600 mg daily), a CYP3A4 inducer, reduced tadalafil 10 mg single-dose exposure (AUC) by 88% and C_{max} by 46%, relative to the values for tadalafil 10 mg alone. Although specific interactions have not been studied, other CYP3A4 inducers, such as carbamazepine, phenytoin, and phenobarbital, would likely decrease tadalafil exposure. No dose adjustment is warranted. The reduced exposure of tadalafil with the co-administration of rifampin or other CYP3A4 inducers can be anticipated to decrease the efficacy of tadalafil for once daily use; the magnitude of decreased efficacy is unknown).
No products indexed under this heading.

Hydrocortisone (Alcohol) (Studies have shown that drugs that induce CYP3A4 can decrease tadalafil exposure. Rifampin (600 mg daily), a CYP3A4 inducer, reduced tadalafil 10 mg single-dose exposure (AUC) by 88% and C_{max} by 46%, relative to the values for tadalafil 10 mg alone. Although specific interactions have not been studied, other CYP3A4 inducers, such as carbamazepine, phenytoin, and phenobarbital, would likely decrease tadalafil exposure. No dose adjustment is warranted. The reduced exposure of tadalafil with the co-administration of rifampin or other CYP3A4 inducers can be anticipated to decrease the efficacy of tadalafil for once daily use; the magnitude of decreased efficacy is unknown).
No products indexed under this heading.

Hydrocortisone Acetate (Studies have shown that drugs that induce CYP3A4 can decrease tadalafil exposure. Rifampin (600 mg daily), a

CYP3A4 inducer, reduced tadalafil 10 mg single-dose exposure (AUC) by 88% and C_{max} by 46%, relative to the values for tadalafil 10 mg alone. Although specific interactions have not been studied, other CYP3A4 inducers, such as carbamazepine, phenytoin, and phenobarbital, would likely decrease tadalafil exposure. No dose adjustment is warranted. The reduced exposure of tadalafil with the co-administration of rifampin or other CYP3A4 inducers can be anticipated to decrease the efficacy of tadalafil for once daily use; the magnitude of decreased efficacy is unknown).

No products indexed under this heading.

Hydrocortisone Butyrate (Studies have shown that drugs that induce CYP3A4 can decrease tadalafil exposure. Rifampin (600 mg daily), a CYP3A4 inducer, reduced tadalafil 10 mg single-dose exposure (AUC) by 88% and C_{max} by 46%, relative to the values for tadalafil 10 mg alone. Although specific interactions have not been studied, other CYP3A4 inducers, such as carbamazepine, phenytoin, and phenobarbital, would likely decrease tadalafil exposure. No dose adjustment is warranted. The reduced exposure of tadalafil with the co-administration of rifampin or other CYP3A4 inducers can be anticipated to decrease the efficacy of tadalafil for once daily use; the magnitude of decreased efficacy is unknown).

No products indexed under this heading.

Hydrocortisone Cypionate (Studies have shown that drugs that induce CYP3A4 can decrease tadalafil exposure. Rifampin (600 mg daily), a CYP3A4 inducer, reduced tadalafil 10 mg single-dose exposure (AUC) by 88% and C_{max} by 46%, relative to the values for tadalafil 10 mg alone. Although specific interactions have not been studied, other CYP3A4 inducers, such as carbamazepine, phenytoin, and phenobarbital, would likely decrease tadalafil exposure. No dose adjustment is warranted. The reduced exposure of tadalafil with the co-administration of rifampin or other CYP3A4 inducers can be anticipated to decrease the efficacy of tadalafil for once daily use; the magnitude of decreased efficacy is unknown).

No products indexed under this heading.

Hydrocortisone Hemisuccinate (Studies have shown that drugs that induce CYP3A4 can decrease tadalafil exposure. Rifampin (600 mg daily), a CYP3A4 inducer, reduced tadalafil 10 mg single-dose exposure (AUC) by 88% and C_{max} by 46%, relative to the values for tadalafil 10 mg alone. Although specific interactions have not been studied, other CYP3A4 inducers, such as carbamazepine, phenytoin, and phenobarbital, would likely decrease tadalafil exposure. No dose adjustment is warranted. The reduced exposure of tadalafil with the co-administration of rifampin or other CYP3A4 inducers can be anticipated to decrease the efficacy of tadalafil for once daily use; the magnitude of decreased efficacy is unknown).

No products indexed under this heading.

Hydrocortisone Probutate (Studies have shown that drugs that induce CYP3A4 can decrease tadalafil exposure. Rifampin (600 mg daily), a CYP3A4 inducer, reduced tadalafil 10 mg single-dose exposure (AUC) by 88% and C_{max} by 46%, relative to the values for tadalafil 10 mg alone. Although specific interactions have not been studied, other CYP3A4 inducers, such as carbamazepine, phenytoin, and phenobarbital, would likely decrease tadalafil exposure. No dose adjustment

is warranted. The reduced exposure of tadalafil with the co-administration of rifampin or other CYP3A4 inducers can be anticipated to decrease the efficacy of tadalafil for once daily use; the magnitude of decreased efficacy is unknown).

No products indexed under this heading.

Hydrocortisone Sodium Phosphate (Studies have shown that drugs that induce CYP3A4 can decrease tadalafil exposure. Rifampin (600 mg daily), a CYP3A4 inducer, reduced tadalafil 10 mg single-dose exposure (AUC) by 88% and C_{max} by 46%, relative to the values for tadalafil 10 mg alone. Although specific interactions have not been studied, other CYP3A4 inducers, such as carbamazepine, phenytoin, and phenobarbital, would likely decrease tadalafil exposure. No dose adjustment is warranted. The reduced exposure of tadalafil with the co-administration of rifampin or other CYP3A4 inducers can be anticipated to decrease the efficacy of tadalafil for once daily use; the magnitude of decreased efficacy is unknown).

No products indexed under this heading.

Hydrocortisone Sodium Succinate (Studies have shown that drugs that induce CYP3A4 can decrease tadalafil exposure. Rifampin (600 mg daily), a CYP3A4 inducer, reduced tadalafil 10 mg single-dose exposure (AUC) by 88% and C_{max} by 46%, relative to the values for tadalafil 10 mg alone. Although specific interactions have not been studied, other CYP3A4 inducers, such as carbamazepine, phenytoin, and phenobarbital, would likely decrease tadalafil exposure. No dose adjustment is warranted. The reduced exposure of tadalafil with the co-administration of rifampin or other CYP3A4 inducers can be anticipated to decrease the efficacy of tadalafil for once daily use; the magnitude of decreased efficacy is unknown).

No products indexed under this heading.

Hydrocortisone Valerate (Studies have shown that drugs that induce CYP3A4 can decrease tadalafil exposure. Rifampin (600 mg daily), a CYP3A4 inducer, reduced tadalafil 10 mg single-dose exposure (AUC) by 88% and C_{max} by 46%, relative to the values for tadalafil 10 mg alone. Although specific interactions have not been studied, other CYP3A4 inducers, such as carbamazepine, phenytoin, and phenobarbital, would likely decrease tadalafil exposure. No dose adjustment is warranted. The reduced exposure of tadalafil with the co-administration of rifampin or other CYP3A4 inducers can be anticipated to decrease the efficacy of tadalafil for once daily use; the magnitude of decreased efficacy is unknown).

No products indexed under this heading.

Hydroflumethiazide (PDE5 inhibitors, including tadalafil, are mild systemic vasodilators. Clinical pharmacology studies were conducted to assess the effect of tadalafil on the potentiation of the blood-pressure-lowering effects of selected antihypertensive medications (amlodipine, angiotesin II receptor blockers, bendrofluazide, enalapril, and metoprolol). Small reductions in blood pressure occurred following co-administration of tadalafil with these agents compared to placebo).

No products indexed under this heading.

Hypericum (Studies have shown that drugs that induce CYP3A4 can decrease tadalafil exposure. Rifampin (600 mg daily), a CYP3A4 inducer, reduced tadalafil 10 mg single-dose exposure (AUC) by 88% and C_{max} by 46%, relative to the values for tadalafil 10 mg alone. Although specific interac-

tions have not been studied, other CYP3A4 inducers, such as carbamazepine, phenytoin, and phenobarbital, would likely decrease tadalafil exposure. No dose adjustment is warranted. The reduced exposure of tadalafil with the co-administration of rifampin or other CYP3A4 inducers can be anticipated to decrease the efficacy of tadalafil for once daily use; the magnitude of decreased efficacy is unknown).

No products indexed under this heading.

Hypericum Perforatum (Studies have shown that drugs that induce CYP3A4 can decrease tadalafil exposure. Rifampin (600 mg daily), a CYP3A4 inducer, reduced tadalafil 10 mg single-dose exposure (AUC) by 88% and C_{max} by 46%, relative to the values for tadalafil 10 mg alone. Although specific interactions have not been studied, other CYP3A4 inducers, such as carbamazepine, phenytoin, and phenobarbital, would likely decrease tadalafil exposure. No dose adjustment is warranted. The reduced exposure of tadalafil with the co-administration of rifampin or other CYP3A4 inducers can be anticipated to decrease the efficacy of tadalafil for once daily use; the magnitude of decreased efficacy is unknown). Products include:

Traumeel 1800

Imatinib Mesylate (Tadalafil is a substrate of and predominantly metabolized by CYP3A4. Studies have shown that drugs that inhibit CYP3A4 can increase tadalafil exposure. When tadalafil is used on an as-needed basis, patients taking concomitant potent inhibitors of CYP3A4, such as ketoconazole or ritonavir, the maximum recommended dose of tadalafil is 10 mg, not to exceed once every 72 hours. When tadalafil is used in a once-daily regimen, patients taking concomitant potent inhibitors of CYP3A4, such as ketoconazole or ritonavir, the dose should not exceed 2.5 mg). Products include:

Gleevec 2477

Indapamide (PDE5 inhibitors, including tadalafil, are mild systemic vasodilators. Clinical pharmacology studies were conducted to assess the effect of tadalafil on the potentiation of the blood-pressure-lowering effects of selected antihypertensive medications (amlodipine, angiotesin II receptor blockers, bendrofluazide, enalapril, and metoprolol). Small reductions in blood pressure occurred following co-administration of tadalafil with these agents compared to placebo). Products include:

Indapamide 2356

Indinavir Sulfate (Ritonavir (500 mg or 600 mg b.i.d. at steady state), an inhibitor of CYP3A4, CYP2C9, CYP2C19, and CYP2D6, increased tadalafil 20 mg single-dose exposure (AUC) by 32% with a 30% reduction in C_{max}, relative to the values for tadalafil 20 mg alone. Ritonavir (200 mg b.i.d.), increased tadalafil 20 mg single-dose exposure (AUC) by 124% with no change in C_{max}, relative to the values for tadalafil 20 mg alone. Although specific interactions have not been studied, other HIV protease inhibitors would likely increase tadalafil exposure). Products include:

Crixivan 2113

Irbesartan (A study was conducted to assess the interaction of angiotensin II receptor blockers and tadalafil 20 mg. Subjects in the study were taking any marketed angiotensin II receptor blocker, either alone, as a component of a combination product, or as part of a multiple antihypertensive regimen. Following dosing, ambulatory measurements of blood pressure revealed differ-

ences between tadalafil and placebo of 8/4 mm Hg in systolic/diastolic blood pressure). Products include:

Avalide 2956
Avapro 2962

Isoniazid (Tadalafil is a substrate of and predominantly metabolized by CYP3A4. Studies have shown that drugs that inhibit CYP3A4 can increase tadalafil exposure. When tadalafil is used on an as-needed basis, patients taking concomitant potent inhibitors of CYP3A4, such as ketoconazole or ritonavir, the maximum recommended dose of tadalafil is 10 mg, not to exceed once every 72 hours. When tadalafil is used in a once-daily regimen, patients taking concomitant potent inhibitors of CYP3A4, such as ketoconazole or ritonavir, the dose should not exceed 2.5 mg).

No products indexed under this heading.

Isosorbide Dinitrate (Administration of tadalafil to patients using any form of organic nitrate, either regularly and/or intermittently, is contraindicated. In clinical pharmacology studies, tadalafil was shown to potentiate the hypotensive effects of nitrates. In a patient who has taken tadalafil, where nitrate administration is deemed medically necessary in a life threatening situation, at least 48 hours should elapse after the last dose of tadalafil before nitrate administration is considered. In such circumstances, nitrates should still only be administered under close medical supervision with appropriate hemodynamic monitoring).

No products indexed under this heading.

Isosorbide Mononitrate (Administration of tadalafil to patients using any form of organic nitrate, either regularly and/or intermittently, is contraindicated. In clinical pharmacology studies, tadalafil was shown to potentiate the hypotensive effects of nitrates. In a patient who has taken tadalafil, where nitrate administration is deemed medically necessary in a life threatening situation, at least 48 hours should elapse after the last dose of tadalafil before nitrate administration is considered. In such circumstances, nitrates should still only be administered under close medical supervision with appropriate hemodynamic monitoring).

No products indexed under this heading.

Isradipine (PDE5 inhibitors, including tadalafil, are mild systemic vasodilators. Clinical pharmacology studies were conducted to assess the effect of tadalafil on the potentiation of the blood-pressure-lowering effects of selected antihypertensive medications (amlodipine, angiotesin II receptor blockers, bendrofluazide, enalapril, and metoprolol). Small reductions in blood pressure occurred following co-administration of tadalafil with these agents compared to placebo). Products include:

DynaCirc CR 1432

Itraconazole (Tadalafil is metabolized predominantly by CYP3A4. CYP3A4 inhibitors, such as itraconazole, may likely increase tadalafil exposure. The dose of tadalafil should be limited to 10 mg no more than once every 72 hours in patients taking potent inhibitors of CYP3A4 such as itraconazole. In patients taking potent inhibitors of CYP3A4 and tadalafil for once daily use, the dose of tadalafil should not exceed 2.5 mg).

No products indexed under this heading.

Ketoconazole (Ketoconazole (400 mg daily), a selective and potent inhibitor of CYP3A4, increased tadalafil 20 mg single-dose exposure (AUC) by 312% and C_{max} by 22%, relative to the values for tadalafil 20 mg alone. Ketoconazole (200 mg daily) increased tadalafil 10 mg single-dose exposure (AUC)

by 107% and C_{max} by 15%, relative to the values for tadalafil 10 mg alone. For patients taking potent inhibitors of CYP3A4, such as ketoconazole, and are using tadalafil on an as needed basis, the dose of tadalafil should be limited to 10 mg no more than once every 72 hours. For once-daily use, the dose of tadalafil should not exceed 2.5 mg). Products include:

Extina 3319
Xolegel 3337

Labetalol Hydrochloride (PDE5 inhibitors, including tadalafil, are mild systemic vasodilators. Clinical pharmacology studies were conducted to assess the effect of tadalafil on the potentiation of the blood-pressure-lowering effects of selected antihypertensive medications (amlodipine, angiotesin II receptor blockers, bendrofluazide, enalapril, and metoprolol). Small reductions in blood pressure occurred following co-administration of tadalafil with these agents compared to placebo).

No products indexed under this heading.

Lapatinib (Tadalafil is a substrate of and predominantly metabolized by CYP3A4. Studies have shown that drugs that inhibit CYP3A4 can increase tadalafil exposure. When tadalafil is used on an as-needed basis, patients taking concomitant potent inhibitors of CYP3A4, such as ketoconazole or ritonavir, the maximum recommended dose of tadalafil is 10 mg, not to exceed once every 72 hours. When tadalafil is used in a once-daily regimen, patients taking concomitant potent inhibitors of CYP3A4, such as ketoconazole or ritonavir, the dose should not exceed 2.5 mg). Products include:

Tykerb 1698

Lisinopril (PDE5 inhibitors, including tadalafil, are mild systemic vasodilators. Clinical pharmacology studies were conducted to assess the effect of tadalafil on the potentiation of the blood-pressure-lowering effects of selected antihypertensive medications (amlodipine, angiotesin II receptor blockers, bendrofluazide, enalapril, and metoprolol). Small reductions in blood pressure occurred following co-administration of tadalafil with these agents compared to placebo). Products include:

Prinivil 2241
Prinzide 2246

Lopinavir (Ritonavir (500 mg or 600 mg b.i.d. at steady state), an inhibitor of CYP3A4, CYP2C9, CYP2C19, and CYP2D6, increased tadalafil 20 mg single-dose exposure (AUC) by 32% with a 30% reduction in C_{max}, relative to the values for tadalafil 20 mg alone. Ritonavir (200 mg b.i.d.), increased tadalafil 20 mg single-dose exposure (AUC) by 124% with no change in C_{max}, relative to the values for tadalafil 20 mg alone. Although specific interactions have not been studied, other HIV protease inhibitors would likely increase tadalafil exposure). Products include:

Kaletra 458

Loratadine (Tadalafil is a substrate of and predominantly metabolized by CYP3A4. Studies have shown that drugs that inhibit CYP3A4 can increase tadalafil exposure. When tadalafil is used on an as-needed basis, patients taking concomitant potent inhibitors of CYP3A4, such as ketoconazole or ritonavir, the maximum recommended dose of tadalafil is 10 mg, not to exceed once every 72 hours. When tadalafil is used in a once-daily regimen, patients taking concomitant potent inhibitors of CYP3A4, such as ketoconazole or ritonavir, the dose should not exceed 2.5 mg).

No products indexed under this heading.

Losartan Potassium (A study was conducted to assess the interaction of angiotensin II receptor blockers and tadalafil 20 mg. Subjects in the study were taking any marketed angiotensin II receptor blocker, either alone, as a component of a combination product, or as part of a multiple antihypertensive regimen. Following dosing, ambulatory measurements of blood pressure revealed differences between tadalafil and placebo of 8/4 mm Hg in systolic/diastolic blood pressure). Products include:

Cozaar 2106
Hyzaar 2162
Hyzaar 100-12.5 2162

Magaldrate (Simultaneous administration of an antacid (magnesium hydroxide/aluminum hydroxide) and tadalafil reduced the apparent rate of absorption of tadalafil without altering exposure (AUC) to tadalafil).

No products indexed under this heading.

Magnesium Carbonate (Simultaneous administration of an antacid (magnesium hydroxide/aluminum hydroxide) and tadalafil reduced the apparent rate of absorption of tadalafil without altering exposure (AUC) to tadalafil).

No products indexed under this heading.

Magnesium Hydroxide (Simultaneous administration of an antacid (magnesium hydroxide/aluminum hydroxide) and tadalafil reduced the apparent rate of absorption of tadalafil without altering exposure (AUC) to tadalafil). Products include:

Fleet Pedia-Lax Chewable Tablets 1144
Pepcid Complete 1822

Magnesium Oxide (Simultaneous administration of an antacid (magnesium hydroxide/aluminum hydroxide) and tadalafil reduced the apparent rate of absorption of tadalafil without altering exposure (AUC) to tadalafil). Products include:

Beelith 873

Magnesium Trisilicate (Simultaneous administration of an antacid (magnesium hydroxide/aluminum hydroxide) and tadalafil reduced the apparent rate of absorption of tadalafil without altering exposure (AUC) to tadalafil).

No products indexed under this heading.

Mecamylamine Hydrochloride (PDE5 inhibitors, including tadalafil, are mild systemic vasodilators. Clinical pharmacology studies were conducted to assess the effect of tadalafil on the potentiation of the blood-pressure-lowering effects of selected antihypertensive medications (amlodipine, angiotesin II receptor blockers, bendrofluazide, enalapril, and metoprolol). Small reductions in blood pressure occurred following co-administration of tadalafil with these agents compared to placebo).

No products indexed under this heading.

Mephenytoin (Studies have shown that drugs that induce CYP3A4 can decrease tadalafil exposure. Rifampin (600 mg daily), a CYP3A4 inducer, reduced tadalafil 10 mg single-dose exposure (AUC) by 88% and C_{max} by 46%, relative to the values for tadalafil 10 mg alone. Although specific interactions have not been studied, other CYP3A4 inducers, such as carbamazepine, phenytoin, and phenobarbital, would likely decrease tadalafil exposure. No dose adjustment is warranted. The reduced exposure of tadalafil with the co-administration of rifampin or other CYP3A4 inducers can be anticipated to decrease the efficacy of tadalafil for once daily use; the magnitude of decreased efficacy is unknown).

No products indexed under this heading.

Methsuximide (Studies have shown that drugs that induce CYP3A4 can decrease tadalafil exposure. Rifampin (600 mg daily), a CYP3A4 inducer, reduced tadalafil 10 mg single-dose exposure (AUC) by 88% and C_{max} by 46%, relative to the values for tadalafil 10 mg alone. Although specific interactions have not been studied, other CYP3A4 inducers, such as carbamazepine, phenytoin, and phenobarbital, would likely decrease tadalafil exposure. No dose adjustment is warranted. The reduced exposure of tadalafil with the co-administration of rifampin or other CYP3A4 inducers can be anticipated to decrease the efficacy of tadalafil for once daily use; the magnitude of decreased efficacy is unknown).

No products indexed under this heading.

Methyclothiazide (PDE5 inhibitors, including tadalafil, are mild systemic vasodilators. Clinical pharmacology studies were conducted to assess the effect of tadalafil on the potentiation of the blood-pressure-lowering effects of selected antihypertensive medications (amlodipine, angiotesin II receptor blockers, bendrofluazide, enalapril, and metoprolol). Small reductions in blood pressure occurred following co-administration of tadalafil with these agents compared to placebo).

No products indexed under this heading.

Methyldopa (PDE5 inhibitors, including tadalafil, are mild systemic vasodilators. Clinical pharmacology studies were conducted to assess the effect of tadalafil on the potentiation of the blood-pressure-lowering effects of selected antihypertensive medications (amlodipine, angiotesin II receptor blockers, bendrofluazide, enalapril, and metoprolol). Small reductions in blood pressure occurred following co-administration of tadalafil with these agents compared to placebo).

No products indexed under this heading.

Methyldopate Hydrochloride (PDE5 inhibitors, including tadalafil, are mild systemic vasodilators. Clinical pharmacology studies were conducted to assess the effect of tadalafil on the potentiation of the blood-pressure-lowering effects of selected antihypertensive medications (amlodipine, angiotesin II receptor blockers, bendrofluazide, enalapril, and metoprolol). Small reductions in blood pressure occurred following co-administration of tadalafil with these agents compared to placebo).

No products indexed under this heading.

Methylprednisolone (Studies have shown that drugs that induce CYP3A4 can decrease tadalafil exposure. Rifampin (600 mg daily), a CYP3A4 inducer, reduced tadalafil 10 mg single-dose exposure (AUC) by 88% and C_{max} by 46%, relative to the values for tadalafil 10 mg alone. Although specific interactions have not been studied, other CYP3A4 inducers, such as carbamazepine, phenytoin, and phenobarbital, would likely decrease tadalafil exposure. No dose adjustment is warranted. The reduced exposure of tadalafil with the co-administration of rifampin or other CYP3A4 inducers can be anticipated to decrease the efficacy of tadalafil for once daily use; the magnitude of decreased efficacy is unknown).

No products indexed under this heading.

Methylprednisolone Acetate (Studies have shown that drugs that induce CYP3A4 can decrease tadalafil exposure. Rifampin (600 mg daily), a CYP3A4 inducer, reduced tadalafil 10 mg single-dose exposure (AUC) by 88% and C_{max} by 46%, relative to the values for tadalafil 10 mg alone. Although specific interactions have not been studied, other CYP3A4 inducers, such as carbamazepine, phenytoin, and phenobarbital, would likely decrease tadalafil exposure. No dose adjustment is warranted. The reduced exposure of tadalafil with the co-administration of rifampin or other CYP3A4 inducers can be anticipated to decrease the efficacy of tadalafil for once daily use; the magnitude of decreased efficacy is unknown).

No products indexed under this heading.

Methylprednisolone Sodium Succinate (Studies have shown that drugs that induce CYP3A4 can decrease tadalafil exposure. Rifampin (600 mg daily), a CYP3A4 inducer, reduced tadalafil 10 mg single-dose exposure (AUC) by 88% and C_{max} by 46%, relative to the values for tadalafil 10 mg alone. Although specific interactions have not been studied, other CYP3A4 inducers, such as carbamazepine, phenytoin, and phenobarbital, would likely decrease tadalafil exposure. No dose adjustment is warranted. The reduced exposure of tadalafil with the co-administration of rifampin or other CYP3A4 inducers can be anticipated to decrease the efficacy of tadalafil for once daily use; the magnitude of decreased efficacy is unknown).

No products indexed under this heading.

Metolazone (PDE5 inhibitors, including tadalafil, are mild systemic vasodilators. Clinical pharmacology studies were conducted to assess the effect of tadalafil on the potentiation of the blood-pressure-lowering effects of selected antihypertensive medications (amlodipine, angiotesin II receptor blockers, bendrofluazide, enalapril, and metoprolol). Small reductions in blood pressure occurred following co-administration of tadalafil with these agents compared to placebo).

No products indexed under this heading.

Metoprolol Succinate (A study was conducted to assess the interaction of sustained-release metoprolol (25 to 200 mg daily) and tadalafil 10 mg. Following dosing, the mean reduction in supine systolic/diastolic blood pressure due to tadalafil 10 mg in subjects taking metoprolol was 5/3 mm Hg, compared to placebo). Products include:

Toprol XL 732

Metoprolol Tartrate (A study was conducted to assess the interaction of sustained-release metoprolol (25 to 200 mg daily) and tadalafil 10 mg. Following dosing, the mean reduction in supine systolic/diastolic blood pressure due to tadalafil 10 mg in subjects taking metoprolol was 5/3 mm Hg, compared to placebo).

No products indexed under this heading.

Metronidazole (Tadalafil is a substrate of and predominantly metabolized by CYP3A4. Studies have shown that drugs that inhibit CYP3A4 can increase tadalafil exposure. When tadalafil is used on an as-needed basis, patients taking concomitant potent inhibitors of CYP3A4, such as ketoconazole or ritonavir, the maximum recommended dose of tadalafil is 10 mg, not to exceed once every 72 hours. When tadalafil is used in a once-daily regimen, patients taking concomitant potent inhibitors of CYP3A4, such as ketoconazole or ritonavir, the dose should not exceed 2.5 mg). Products include:

Pylera 793

Metronidazole Benzoate (Tadalafil is a substrate of and predominantly metabolized by CYP3A4. Studies have shown that drugs that inhibit CYP3A4 can increase tadalafil exposure. When tadalafil is used on an as-needed basis, patients taking concomitant potent inhibitors of CYP3A4, such as ketoconazole or ritonavir, the maximum recommended dose of tadalafil is 10 mg, not

315 Interactions Index Cialis

to exceed once every 72 hours. When tadalafil is used in a once-daily regimen, patients taking concomitant potent inhibitors of CYP3A4, such as ketoconazole or ritonavir, the dose should not exceed 2.5 mg).
No products indexed under this heading.

Metronidazole Hydrochloride (Tadalafil is a substrate of and predominantly metabolized by CYP3A4. Studies have shown that drugs that inhibit CYP3A4 can increase tadalafil exposure. When tadalafil is used on an as-needed basis, patients taking concomitant potent inhibitors of CYP3A4, such as ketoconazole or ritonavir, the maximum recommended dose of tadalafil is 10 mg, not to exceed once every 72 hours. When tadalafil is used in a once-daily regimen, patients taking concomitant potent inhibitors of CYP3A4, such as ketoconazole or ritonavir, the dose should not exceed 2.5 mg).
No products indexed under this heading.

Metronidazole Sodium (Tadalafil is a substrate of and predominantly metabolized by CYP3A4. Studies have shown that drugs that inhibit CYP3A4 can increase tadalafil exposure. When tadalafil is used on an as-needed basis, patients taking concomitant potent inhibitors of CYP3A4, such as ketoconazole or ritonavir, the maximum recommended dose of tadalafil is 10 mg, not to exceed once every 72 hours. When tadalafil is used in a once-daily regimen, patients taking concomitant potent inhibitors of CYP3A4, such as ketoconazole or ritonavir, the dose should not exceed 2.5 mg).
No products indexed under this heading.

Metyrosine (PDE5 inhibitors, including tadalafil, are mild systemic vasodilators. Clinical pharmacology studies were conducted to assess the effect of tadalafil on the potentiation of the blood-pressure-lowering effects of selected antihypertensive medications (amlodipine, angiotesin II receptor blockers, bendrofluazide, enalapril, and metoprolol). Small reductions in blood pressure occurred following co-administration of tadalafil with these agents compared to placebo).
No products indexed under this heading.

Mibefradil Dihydrochloride (PDE5 inhibitors, including tadalafil, are mild systemic vasodilators. Clinical pharmacology studies were conducted to assess the effect of tadalafil on the potentiation of the blood-pressure-lowering effects of selected antihypertensive medications (amlodipine, angiotesin II receptor blockers, bendrofluazide, enalapril, and metoprolol). Small reductions in blood pressure occurred following co-administration of tadalafil with these agents compared to placebo).
No products indexed under this heading.

Miconazole (Tadalafil is a substrate of and predominantly metabolized by CYP3A4. Studies have shown that drugs that inhibit CYP3A4 can increase tadalafil exposure. When tadalafil is used on an as-needed basis, patients taking concomitant potent inhibitors of CYP3A4, such as ketoconazole or ritonavir, the maximum recommended dose of tadalafil is 10 mg, not to exceed once every 72 hours. When tadalafil is used in a once-daily regimen, patients taking concomitant potent inhibitors of CYP3A4, such as ketoconazole or ritonavir, the dose should not exceed 2.5 mg).
No products indexed under this heading.

Miconazole Nitrate (Tadalafil is a substrate of and predominantly metabolized by CYP3A4. Studies have shown that drugs that inhibit CYP3A4 can increase tadalafil exposure. When tadalafil is used on an as-needed basis, patients taking concomitant potent inhibitors of CYP3A4, such as ketoconazole or ritonavir, the maximum recommended dose of tadalafil is 10 mg, not to exceed once every 72 hours. When tadalafil is used in a once-daily regimen, patients taking concomitant potent inhibitors of CYP3A4, such as ketoconazole or ritonavir, the dose should not exceed 2.5 mg). Products include:
Vusion Ointment 3335

Mifepristone (Tadalafil is a substrate of and predominantly metabolized by CYP3A4. Studies have shown that drugs that inhibit CYP3A4 can increase tadalafil exposure. When tadalafil is used on an as-needed basis, patients taking concomitant potent inhibitors of CYP3A4, such as ketoconazole or ritonavir, the maximum recommended dose of tadalafil is 10 mg, not to exceed once every 72 hours. When tadalafil is used in a once-daily regimen, patients taking concomitant potent inhibitors of CYP3A4, such as ketoconazole or ritonavir, the dose should not exceed 2.5 mg).
No products indexed under this heading.

Minoxidil (PDE5 inhibitors, including tadalafil, are mild systemic vasodilators. Clinical pharmacology studies were conducted to assess the effect of tadalafil on the potentiation of the blood-pressure-lowering effects of selected antihypertensive medications (amlodipine, angiotesin II receptor blockers, bendrofluazide, enalapril, and metoprolol). Small reductions in blood pressure occurred following co-administration of tadalafil with these agents compared to placebo).
No products indexed under this heading.

Modafinil (Studies have shown that drugs that induce CYP3A4 can decrease tadalafil exposure. Rifampin (600 mg daily), a CYP3A4 inducer, reduced tadalafil 10 mg single-dose exposure (AUC) by 88% and C_{max} by 46%, relative to the values for tadalafil 10 mg alone. Although specific interactions have not been studied, other CYP3A4 inducers, such as carbamazepine, phenytoin, and phenobarbital, would likely decrease tadalafil exposure. No dose adjustment is warranted. The reduced exposure of tadalafil with the co-administration of rifampin or other CYP3A4 inducers can be anticipated to decrease the efficacy of tadalafil for once daily use; the magnitude of decreased efficacy is unknown). Products include:
Provigil 983

Moexipril Hydrochloride (PDE5 inhibitors, including tadalafil, are mild systemic vasodilators. Clinical pharmacology studies were conducted to assess the effect of tadalafil on the potentiation of the blood-pressure-lowering effects of selected antihypertensive medications (amlodipine, angiotesin II receptor blockers, bendrofluazide, enalapril, and metoprolol). Small reductions in blood pressure occurred following co-administration of tadalafil with these agents compared to placebo).
No products indexed under this heading.

Nadolol (PDE5 inhibitors, including tadalafil, are mild systemic vasodilators. Clinical pharmacology studies were conducted to assess the effect of tadalafil on the potentiation of the blood-pressure-lowering effects of selected antihypertensive medications (amlodipine, angiotesin II receptor blockers, bendrofluazide, enalapril, and metoprolol). Small reductions in blood pressure occurred following co-administration of tadalafil with these agents compared to placebo). Products include:
Nadolol 2359

Nafcillin Sodium (Studies have shown that drugs that induce CYP3A4 can decrease tadalafil exposure. Rifampin (600 mg daily), a CYP3A4 inducer, reduced tadalafil 10 mg single-dose exposure (AUC) by 88% and C_{max} by 46%, relative to the values for tadalafil 10 mg alone. Although specific interactions have not been studied, other CYP3A4 inducers, such as carbamazepine, phenytoin, and phenobarbital, would likely decrease tadalafil exposure. No dose adjustment is warranted. The reduced exposure of tadalafil with the co-administration of rifampin or other CYP3A4 inducers can be anticipated to decrease the efficacy of tadalafil for once daily use; the magnitude of decreased efficacy is unknown).
No products indexed under this heading.

Nebivolol (PDE5 inhibitors, including tadalafil, are mild systemic vasodilators. Clinical pharmacology studies were conducted to assess the effect of tadalafil on the potentiation of the blood-pressure-lowering effects of selected antihypertensive medications (amlodipine, angiotesin II receptor blockers, bendrofluazide, enalapril, and metoprolol). Small reductions in blood pressure occurred following co-administration of tadalafil with these agents compared to placebo). Products include:
Bystolic 1147

Nefazodone Hydrochloride (Tadalafil is a substrate of and metabolized predominantly by CYP3A4. Studies have shown that drugs that inhibit CYP3A4 can increase tadalafil exposure. When tadalafil is used on an as-needed basis, patients taking concomitant potent inhibitors of CYP3A4, such as ketoconazole or ritonavir, the maximum recommended dose of tadalafil is 10 mg, not to exceed once every 72 hours. When tadalafil is used in a once-daily regimen, patients taking concomitant potent inhibitors of CYP3A4, such as ketoconazole or ritonavir, the dose should not exceed 2.5 mg).
No products indexed under this heading.

Nelfinavir Mesylate (Ritonavir (500 mg or 600 mg b.i.d. at steady state), an inhibitor of CYP3A4, CYP2C9, CYP2C19, and CYP2D6, increased tadalafil 20 mg single-dose exposure (AUC) by 32% with a 30% reduction in C_{max}, relative to the values for tadalafil 20 mg alone. Ritonavir (200 mg b.i.d.), increased tadalafil 20 mg single-dose exposure (AUC) by 124% with no change in C_{max}, relative to the values for tadalafil 20 mg alone. Although specific interactions have not been studied, other HIV protease inhibitors would likely increase tadalafil exposure).
No products indexed under this heading.

Nevirapine (Tadalafil is a substrate of and predominantly metabolized by CYP3A4. Studies have shown that drugs that inhibit CYP3A4 can increase tadalafil exposure. When tadalafil is used on an as-needed basis, patients taking concomitant potent inhibitors of CYP3A4, such as ketoconazole or ritonavir, the maximum recommended dose of tadalafil is 10 mg, not to exceed once every 72 hours. When tadalafil is used in a once-daily regimen, patients taking concomitant potent inhibitors of CYP3A4, such as ketoconazole or ritonavir, the dose should not exceed 2.5 mg). Products include:
Viramune Oral Suspension 897
Viramune Tablets 897

Niacin (Tadalafil is a substrate of and predominantly metabolized by CYP3A4. Studies have shown that drugs that inhibit CYP3A4 can increase tadalafil exposure. When tadalafil is used on an as-needed basis, patients taking concomitant potent inhibitors of CYP3A4, such as ketoconazole or ritonavir, the maximum recommended dose of tadalafil is 10 mg, not to exceed once every 72 hours. When tadalafil is used in a once-daily regimen, patients taking concomitant potent inhibitors of CYP3A4, such as ketoconazole or ritonavir, the dose should not exceed 2.5 mg). Products include:
Advicor 402
Cardio Basics 3455
Niaspan 497
Simcor 524

Niacinamide (Tadalafil is a substrate of and predominantly metabolized by CYP3A4. Studies have shown that drugs that inhibit CYP3A4 can increase tadalafil exposure. When tadalafil is used on an as-needed basis, patients taking concomitant potent inhibitors of CYP3A4, such as ketoconazole or ritonavir, the maximum recommended dose of tadalafil is 10 mg, not to exceed once every 72 hours. When tadalafil is used in a once-daily regimen, patients taking concomitant potent inhibitors of CYP3A4, such as ketoconazole or ritonavir, the dose should not exceed 2.5 mg). Products include:
CitraNatal 90 DHA Capsules 2332
CitraNatal Assure 2332
CitraNatal Rx 2332
Heplive 607

Niacinamide Hydroiodide (Tadalafil is a substrate of and predominantly metabolized by CYP3A4. Studies have shown that drugs that inhibit CYP3A4 can increase tadalafil exposure. When tadalafil is used on an as-needed basis, patients taking concomitant potent inhibitors of CYP3A4, such as ketoconazole or ritonavir, the maximum recommended dose of tadalafil is 10 mg, not to exceed once every 72 hours. When tadalafil is used in a once-daily regimen, patients taking concomitant potent inhibitors of CYP3A4, such as ketoconazole or ritonavir, the dose should not exceed 2.5 mg).
No products indexed under this heading.

Nicardipine Hydrochloride (PDE5 inhibitors, including tadalafil, are mild systemic vasodilators. Clinical pharmacology studies were conducted to assess the effect of tadalafil on the potentiation of the blood-pressure-lowering effects of selected antihypertensive medications (amlodipine, angiotesin II receptor blockers, bendrofluazide, enalapril, and metoprolol). Small reductions in blood pressure occurred following co-administration of tadalafil with these agents compared to placebo).
No products indexed under this heading.

Nicotinamide (Tadalafil is a substrate of and predominantly metabolized by CYP3A4. Studies have shown that drugs that inhibit CYP3A4 can increase tadalafil exposure. When tadalafil is used on an as-needed basis, patients taking concomitant potent inhibitors of CYP3A4, such as ketoconazole or ritonavir, the maximum recommended dose of tadalafil is 10 mg, not to exceed once every 72 hours. When tadalafil is used in a once-daily regimen, patients taking concomitant potent inhibitors of CYP3A4, such as ketoconazole or ritonavir, the dose should not exceed 2.5 mg).
No products indexed under this heading.

Nifedipine (PDE5 inhibitors, including tadalafil, are mild systemic vasodilators. Clinical pharmacology studies were conducted to assess the effect of tadalafil on the potentiation of the blood-pressure-lowering effects of selected antihypertensive medications (amlodipine, angiotesin II receptor blockers, bendrofluazide, enalapril, and metoprolol). Small reductions in blood pres-

IMPORTANT NOTE: Always consult each drug listing in the patient's regimen for possible interactions.

sure occurred following co-administration of tadalafil with these agents compared to placebo).

No products indexed under this heading.

Nisoldipine (PDE5 inhibitors, including tadalafil, are mild systemic vasodilators. Clinical pharmacology studies were conducted to assess the effect of tadalafil on the potentiation of the blood-pressure-lowering effects of selected antihypertensive medications (amlodipine, angiotesin II receptor blockers, bendrofluazide, enalapril, and metoprolol). Small reductions in blood pressure occurred following co-administration of tadalafil with these agents compared to placebo).

No products indexed under this heading.

Nitrate & Nitrite Preparations (Administration of tadalafil to patients using any form of organic nitrate, either regularly and/or intermittently, is contraindicated. In clinical pharmacology studies, tadalafil was shown to potentiate the hypotensive effects of nitrates. In a patient who has taken tadalafil, where nitrate administration is deemed medically necessary in a life threatening situation, at least 48 hours should elapse after the last dose of tadalafil before nitrate administration is considered. In such circumstances, nitrates should still only be administered under close medical supervision with appropriate hemodynamic monitoring).

No products indexed under this heading.

Nitrates, organic (Administration of tadalafil to patients using any form of organic nitrate, either regularly and/or intermittently, is contraindicated. In clinical pharmacology studies, tadalafil was shown to potentiate the hypotensive effects of nitrates. In a patient who has taken tadalafil, where nitrate administration is deemed medically necessary in a life threatening situation, at least 48 hours should elapse after the last dose of tadalafil before nitrate administration is considered. In such circumstances, nitrates should still only be administered under close medical supervision with appropriate hemodynamic monitoring).

No products indexed under this heading.

Nitrates and Nitrites (Administration of tadalafil to patients using any form of organic nitrate, either regularly and/or intermittently, is contraindicated. In clinical pharmacology studies, tadalafil was shown to potentiate the hypotensive effects of nitrates. In a patient who has taken tadalafil, where nitrate administration is deemed medically necessary in a life threatening situation, at least 48 hours should elapse after the last dose of tadalafil before nitrate administration is considered. In such circumstances, nitrates should still only be administered under close medical supervision with appropriate hemodynamic monitoring).

No products indexed under this heading.

Nitroglycerin (Administration of tadalafil to patients using any form of organic nitrate, either regularly and/or intermittently, is contraindicated. In clinical pharmacology studies, tadalafil was shown to potentiate the hypotensive effects of nitrates. In a patient who has taken tadalafil, where nitrate administration is deemed medically necessary in a life threatening situation, at least 48 hours should elapse after the last dose of tadalafil before nitrate administration is considered. In such circumstances, nitrates should still only be administered under close medical supervision with appropriate hemodynamic monitoring). Products include:

Nitro-Dur 3170
Nitrolingual 3266

Nitroglycerin, long-acting formulations (Administration of tadalafil to patients using any form of organic nitrate, either regularly and/or intermit-

tently, is contraindicated. In clinical pharmacology studies, tadalafil was shown to potentiate the hypotensive effects of nitrates. In a patient who has taken tadalafil, where nitrate administration is deemed medically necessary in a life threatening situation, at least 48 hours should elapse after the last dose of tadalafil before nitrate administration is considered. In such circumstances, nitrates should still only be administered under close medical supervision with appropriate hemodynamic monitoring).

No products indexed under this heading.

Nitroglycerin Intravenous (Administration of tadalafil to patients using any form of organic nitrate, either regularly and/or intermittently, is contraindicated. In clinical pharmacology studies, tadalafil was shown to potentiate the hypotensive effects of nitrates. In a patient who has taken tadalafil, where nitrate administration is deemed medically necessary in a life threatening situation, at least 48 hours should elapse after the last dose of tadalafil before nitrate administration is considered. In such circumstances, nitrates should still only be administered under close medical supervision with appropriate hemodynamic monitoring).

No products indexed under this heading.

Norfloxacin (Tadalafil is a substrate of and predominantly metabolized by CYP3A4. Studies have shown that drugs that inhibit CYP3A4 can increase tadalafil exposure. When tadalafil is used on an as-needed basis, patients taking concomitant potent inhibitors of CYP3A4, such as ketoconazole or ritonavir, the maximum recommended dose of tadalafil is 10 mg, not to exceed once every 72 hours. When tadalafil is used in a once-daily regimen, patients taking concomitant potent inhibitors of CYP3A4, such as ketoconazole or ritonavir, the dose should not exceed 2.5 mg). Products include:

Noroxin 2220

Omeprazole (Tadalafil is a substrate of and predominantly metabolized by CYP3A4. Studies have shown that drugs that inhibit CYP3A4 can increase tadalafil exposure. When tadalafil is used on an as-needed basis, patients taking concomitant potent inhibitors of CYP3A4, such as ketoconazole or ritonavir, the maximum recommended dose of tadalafil is 10 mg, not to exceed once every 72 hours. When tadalafil is used in a once-daily regimen, patients taking concomitant potent inhibitors of CYP3A4, such as ketoconazole or ritonavir, the dose should not exceed 2.5 mg).

No products indexed under this heading.

Oxcarbazepine (Studies have shown that drugs that induce CYP3A4 can decrease tadalafil exposure. Rifampin (600 mg daily), a CYP3A4 inducer, reduced tadalafil 10 mg single-dose exposure (AUC) by 88% and C_{max} by 46%, relative to the values for tadalafil 10 mg alone. Although specific interactions have not been studied, other CYP3A4 inducers, such as carbamazepine, phenytoin, and phenobarbital, would likely decrease tadalafil exposure. No dose adjustment is warranted. The reduced exposure of tadalafil with the co-administration of rifampin or other CYP3A4 inducers can be anticipated to decrease the efficacy of tadalafil for once daily use; the magnitude of decreased efficacy is unknown).

No products indexed under this heading.

Paroxetine Hydrochloride (Tadalafil is a substrate of and predominantly metabolized by CYP3A4. Studies have shown that drugs that inhibit CYP3A4 can increase tadalafil exposure. When tadalafil is used on an as-needed basis, patients taking concomitant potent

inhibitors of CYP3A4, such as ketoconazole or ritonavir, the maximum recommended dose of tadalafil is 10 mg, not to exceed once every 72 hours. When tadalafil is used in a once-daily regimen, patients taking concomitant potent inhibitors of CYP3A4, such as ketoconazole or ritonavir, the dose should not exceed 2.5 mg). Products include:

Paroxetine CR 2361
Paroxetine ER 2371
Paxil 1586
Paxil CR 1596

Penbutolol Sulfate (PDE5 inhibitors, including tadalafil, are mild systemic vasodilators. Clinical pharmacology studies were conducted to assess the effect of tadalafil on the potentiation of the blood-pressure-lowering effects of selected antihypertensive medications (amlodipine, angiotesin II receptor blockers, bendrofluazide, enalapril, and metoprolol). Small reductions in blood pressure occurred following co-administration of tadalafil with these agents compared to placebo).

No products indexed under this heading.

Pentaerythritol Tetranitrate (Administration of tadalafil to patients using any form of organic nitrate, either regularly and/or intermittently, is contraindicated. In clinical pharmacology studies, tadalafil was shown to potentiate the hypotensive effects of nitrates. In a patient who has taken tadalafil, where nitrate administration is deemed medically necessary in a life threatening situation, at least 48 hours should elapse after the last dose of tadalafil before nitrate administration is considered. In such circumstances, nitrates should still only be administered under close medical supervision with appropriate hemodynamic monitoring).

No products indexed under this heading.

Perindopril Erbumine (PDE5 inhibitors, including tadalafil, are mild systemic vasodilators. Clinical pharmacology studies were conducted to assess the effect of tadalafil on the potentiation of the blood-pressure-lowering effects of selected antihypertensive medications (amlodipine, angiotesin II receptor blockers, bendrofluazide, enalapril, and metoprolol). Small reductions in blood pressure occurred following co-administration of tadalafil with these agents compared to placebo).

No products indexed under this heading.

Phenobarbital (Studies have shown that drugs that induce CYP3A4 can decrease tadalafil exposure. Rifampin (600 mg daily), a CYP3A4 inducer, reduced tadalafil 10 mg single-dose exposure (AUC) by 88% and C_{max} by 46%, relative to the values for tadalafil 10 mg alone. Although specific interactions have not been studied, other CYP3A4 inducers, such as phenobarbital, would likely decrease tadalafil exposure. No dose adjustment is warranted. The reduced exposure of tadalafil with the co-administration of CYP3A4 inducers can be anticipated to decrease the efficacy of tadalafil for once daily use; the magnitude of decreased efficacy is unknown). Products include:

Donnatal 2711

Phenobarbital Sodium (Studies have shown that drugs that induce CYP3A4 can decrease tadalafil exposure. Rifampin (600 mg daily), a CYP3A4 inducer, reduced tadalafil 10 mg single-dose exposure (AUC) by 88% and C_{max} by 46%, relative to the values for tadalafil 10 mg alone. Although specific interactions have not been studied, other CYP3A4 inducers, such as phenobarbital, would likely decrease tadalafil exposure. No dose adjustment is warranted. The reduced exposure of tadalafil with the co-administration of CYP3A4 inducers can be anticipated to decrease the

efficacy of tadalafil for once daily use; the magnitude of decreased efficacy is unknown).

No products indexed under this heading.

Phenoxybenzamine Hydrochloride (PDE5 inhibitors, including tadalafil, are mild systemic vasodilators. Clinical pharmacology studies were conducted to assess the effect of tadalafil on the potentiation of the blood-pressure-lowering effects of selected antihypertensive medications (amlodipine, angiotesin II receptor blockers, bendrofluazide, enalapril, and metoprolol). Small reductions in blood pressure occurred following co-administration of tadalafil with these agents compared to placebo). Products include:

Dibenzyline 3495

Phentolamine Mesylate (PDE5 inhibitors, including tadalafil, are mild systemic vasodilators. Clinical pharmacology studies were conducted to assess the effect of tadalafil on the potentiation of the blood-pressure-lowering effects of selected antihypertensive medications (amlodipine, angiotesin II receptor blockers, bendrofluazide, enalapril, and metoprolol). Small reductions in blood pressure occurred following co-administration of tadalafil with these agents compared to placebo).

No products indexed under this heading.

Phenytoin (Studies have shown that drugs that induce CYP3A4 can decrease tadalafil exposure. Rifampin (600 mg daily), a CYP3A4 inducer, reduced tadalafil 10 mg single-dose exposure (AUC) by 88% and C_{max} by 46%, relative to the values for tadalafil 10 mg alone. Although specific interactions have not been studied, other CYP3A4 inducers, such as phenytoin would likely decrease tadalafil exposure. No dose adjustment is warranted. The reduced exposure of tadalafil with the co-administration of CYP3A4 inducers can be anticipated to decrease the efficacy of tadalafil for once daily use; the magnitude of decreased efficacy is unknown).

No products indexed under this heading.

Phenytoin Sodium (Studies have shown that drugs that induce CYP3A4 can decrease tadalafil exposure. Rifampin (600 mg daily), a CYP3A4 inducer, reduced tadalafil 10 mg single-dose exposure (AUC) by 88% and C_{max} by 46%, relative to the values for tadalafil 10 mg alone. Although specific interactions have not been studied, other CYP3A4 inducers, such as phenytoin would likely decrease tadalafil exposure. No dose adjustment is warranted. The reduced exposure of tadalafil with the co-administration of CYP3A4 inducers can be anticipated to decrease the efficacy of tadalafil for once daily use; the magnitude of decreased efficacy is unknown). Products include:

Phenytek Capsules 2380

Pindolol (PDE5 inhibitors, including tadalafil, are mild systemic vasodilators. Clinical pharmacology studies were conducted to assess the effect of tadalafil on the potentiation of the blood-pressure-lowering effects of selected antihypertensive medications (amlodipine, angiotesin II receptor blockers, bendrofluazide, enalapril, and metoprolol). Small reductions in blood pressure occurred following co-administration of tadalafil with these agents compared to placebo).

No products indexed under this heading.

Polythiazide (PDE5 inhibitors, including tadalafil, are mild systemic vasodilators. Clinical pharmacology studies were conducted to assess the effect of tadalafil on the potentiation of the blood-pressure-lowering effects of selected

antihypertensive medications (amlodipine, angiotesin II receptor blockers, bendrofluazide, enalapril, and metoprolol). Small reductions in blood pressure occurred following co-administration of tadalafil with these agents compared to placebo).
No products indexed under this heading.

Posaconazole (Tadalafil is a substrate of and predominantly metabolized by CYP3A4. Studies have shown that drugs that inhibit CYP3A4 can increase tadalafil exposure. When tadalafil is used on an as-needed basis, patients taking concomitant potent inhibitors of CYP3A4, such as ketoconazole or ritonavir, the maximum recommended dose of tadalafil is 10 mg, not to exceed once every 72 hours. When tadalafil is used in a once-daily regimen, patients taking concomitant potent inhibitors of CYP3A4, such as ketoconazole or ritonavir, the dose should not exceed 2.5 mg). Products include:
Noxafil 3172

Prazosin Hydrochloride (Caution is advised when PDE5 inhibitors are co-administered with α-blockers. Tadalafil and α-adrenergic blocking agents are both vasodilators with blood-pressure lowering effects. When vasodilators are used in combination, an additive effect on blood pressure may be anticipated. In some patients, concomitant use of these two drug classes can lower blood presure significantly, which may lead to symptomatic hypotension (eg, fainting). When tadalafil is co-administered with an α-blocker, patients should be stable on α-blocker therapy prior to initiating treatment with tadalafil, and tadalafil should be administered at the lowest recommended dose).
No products indexed under this heading.

Prednisolone (Studies have shown that drugs that induce CYP3A4 can decrease tadalafil exposure. Rifampin (600 mg daily), a CYP3A4 inducer, reduced tadalafil 10 mg single-dose exposure (AUC) by 88% and C_{max} by 46%, relative to the values for tadalafil 10 mg alone. Although specific interactions have not been studied, other CYP3A4 inducers, such as carbamazepine, phenytoin, and phenobarbital, would likely decrease tadalafil exposure. No dose adjustment is warranted. The reduced exposure of tadalafil with the co-administration of rifampin or other CYP3A4 inducers can be anticipated to decrease the efficacy of tadalafil for once daily use; the magnitude of decreased efficacy is unknown).
No products indexed under this heading.

Prednisolone Acetate (Studies have shown that drugs that induce CYP3A4 can decrease tadalafil exposure. Rifampin (600 mg daily) a CYP3A4 inducer, reduced tadalafil 10 mg single-dose exposure (AUC) by 88% and C_{max} by 46%, relative to the values for tadalafil 10 mg alone. Although specific interactions have not been studied, other CYP3A4 inducers, such as carbamazepine, phenytoin, and phenobarbital, would likely decrease tadalafil exposure. No dose adjustment is warranted. The reduced exposure of tadalafil with the co-administration of rifampin or other CYP3A4 inducers can be anticipated to decrease the efficacy of tadalafil for once daily use; the magnitude of decreased efficacy is unknown). Products include:
Blephamide .... ⊙212, ⊙214
Pred Forte .... ⊙225
Pred Mild .... ⊙230
Pred-G .... ⊙226, ⊙227

Prednisolone Sodium Phosphate (Studies have shown that drugs that induce CYP3A4 can decrease tadalafil exposure. Rifampin (600 mg daily), a CYP3A4 inducer, reduced tadalafil

10 mg single-dose exposure (AUC) by 88% and C_{max} by 46%, relative to the values for tadalafil 10 mg alone. Although specific interactions have not been studied, other CYP3A4 inducers, such as carbamazepine, phenytoin, and phenobarbital, would likely decrease tadalafil exposure. No dose adjustment is warranted. The reduced exposure of tadalafil with the co-administration of rifampin or other CYP3A4 inducers can be anticipated to decrease the efficacy of tadalafil for once daily use; the magnitude of decreased efficacy is unknown).
No products indexed under this heading.

Prednisolone Tebutate (Studies have shown that drugs that induce CYP3A4 can decrease tadalafil exposure. Rifampin (600 mg daily), a CYP3A4 inducer, reduced tadalafil 10 mg single-dose exposure (AUC) by 88% and C_{max} by 46%, relative to the values for tadalafil 10 mg alone. Although specific interactions have not been studied, other CYP3A4 inducers, such as carbamazepine, phenytoin, and phenobarbital, would likely decrease tadalafil exposure. No dose adjustment is warranted. The reduced exposure of tadalafil with the co-administration of rifampin or other CYP3A4 inducers can be anticipated to decrease the efficacy of tadalafil for once daily use; the magnitude of decreased efficacy is unknown).
No products indexed under this heading.

Prednisone (Studies have shown that drugs that induce CYP3A4 can decrease tadalafil exposure. Rifampin (600 mg daily), a CYP3A4 inducer, reduced tadalafil 10 mg single-dose exposure (AUC) by 88% and C_{max} by 46%, relative to the values for tadalafil 10 mg alone. Although specific interactions have not been studied, other CYP3A4 inducers, such as carbamazepine, phenytoin, and phenobarbital, would likely decrease tadalafil exposure. No dose adjustment is warranted. The reduced exposure of tadalafil with the co-administration of rifampin or other CYP3A4 inducers can be anticipated to decrease the efficacy of tadalafil for once daily use; the magnitude of decreased efficacy is unknown).
No products indexed under this heading.

Prednisone sodium phosphate (Studies have shown that drugs that induce CYP3A4 can decrease tadalafil exposure. Rifampin (600 mg daily), a CYP3A4 inducer, reduced tadalafil 10 mg single-dose exposure (AUC) by 88% and C_{max} by 46%, relative to the values for tadalafil 10 mg alone. Although specific interactions have not been studied, other CYP3A4 inducers, such as carbamazepine, phenytoin, and phenobarbital, would likely decrease tadalafil exposure. No dose adjustment is warranted. The reduced exposure of tadalafil with the co-administration of rifampin or other CYP3A4 inducers can be anticipated to decrease the efficacy of tadalafil for once daily use; the magnitude of decreased efficacy is unknown).
No products indexed under this heading.

Primidone (Studies have shown that drugs that induce CYP3A4 can decrease tadalafil exposure. Rifampin (600 mg daily), a CYP3A4 inducer, reduced tadalafil 10 mg single-dose exposure (AUC) by 88% and C_{max} by 46%, relative to the values for tadalafil 10 mg alone. Although specific interactions have not been studied, other CYP3A4 inducers, such as carbamazepine, phenytoin, and phenobarbital, would likely decrease tadalafil exposure. No dose adjustment is warranted. The reduced exposure of tadalafil with the co-administration of rifampin or oth-

er CYP3A4 inducers can be anticipated to decrease the efficacy of tadalafil for once daily use; the magnitude of decreased efficacy is unknown).
No products indexed under this heading.

Propoxyphene Hydrochloride (Tadalafil is a substrate of and predominantly metabolized by CYP3A4. Studies have shown that drugs that inhibit CYP3A4 can increase tadalafil exposure. When tadalafil is used on an as-needed basis, patients taking concomitant potent inhibitors of CYP3A4, such as ketoconazole or ritonavir, the maximum recommended dose of tadalafil is 10 mg, not to exceed once every 72 hours. When tadalafil is used in a once-daily regimen, patients taking concomitant potent inhibitors of CYP3A4, such as ketoconazole or ritonavir, the dose should not exceed 2.5 mg).
No products indexed under this heading.

Propoxyphene Napsylate (Tadalafil is a substrate of and predominantly metabolized by CYP3A4. Studies have shown that drugs that inhibit CYP3A4 can increase tadalafil exposure. When tadalafil is used on an as-needed basis, patients taking concomitant potent inhibitors of CYP3A4, such as ketoconazole or ritonavir, the maximum recommended dose of tadalafil is 10 mg, not to exceed once every 72 hours. When tadalafil is used in a once-daily regimen, patients taking concomitant potent inhibitors of CYP3A4, such as ketoconazole or ritonavir, the dose should not exceed 2.5 mg).
No products indexed under this heading.

Propranolol Hydrochloride (PDE5 inhibitors, including tadalafil, are mild systemic vasodilators. Clinical pharmacology studies were conducted to assess the effect of tadalafil on the potentiation of the blood-pressure-lowering effects of selected antihypertensive medications (amlodipine, angiotesin II receptor blockers, bendrofluazide, enalapril, and metoprolol). Small reductions in blood pressure occurred following co-administration of tadalafil with these agents compared to placebo). Products include:
InnoPran XL 1517

Quinapril Hydrochloride (PDE5 inhibitors, including tadalafil, are mild systemic vasodilators. Clinical pharmacology studies were conducted to assess the effect of tadalafil on the potentiation of the blood-pressure-lowering effects of selected antihypertensive medications (amlodipine, angiotesin II receptor blockers, bendrofluazide, enalapril, and metoprolol). Small reductions in blood pressure occurred following co-administration of tadalafil with these agents compared to placebo).
No products indexed under this heading.

Quinidine (Tadalafil is a substrate of and predominantly metabolized by CYP3A4. Studies have shown that drugs that inhibit CYP3A4 can increase tadalafil exposure. When tadalafil is used on an as-needed basis, patients taking concomitant potent inhibitors of CYP3A4, such as ketoconazole or ritonavir, the maximum recommended dose of tadalafil is 10 mg, not to exceed once every 72 hours. When tadalafil is used in a once-daily regimen, patients taking concomitant potent inhibitors of CYP3A4, such as ketoconazole or ritonavir, the dose should not exceed 2.5 mg).
No products indexed under this heading.

Quinidine Hydrochloride (Tadalafil is a substrate of and predominantly metabolized by CYP3A4. Studies have shown that drugs that inhibit CYP3A4 can increase tadalafil exposure. When tadalafil is used on an as-needed basis,

patients taking concomitant potent inhibitors of CYP3A4, such as ketoconazole or ritonavir, the maximum recommended dose of tadalafil is 10 mg, not to exceed once every 72 hours. When tadalafil is used in a once-daily regimen, patients taking concomitant potent inhibitors of CYP3A4, such as ketoconazole or ritonavir, the dose should not exceed 2.5 mg).
No products indexed under this heading.

Quinidine Polygalacturonate (Tadalafil is a substrate of and predominantly metabolized by CYP3A4. Studies have shown that drugs that inhibit CYP3A4 can increase tadalafil exposure. When tadalafil is used on an as-needed basis, patients taking concomitant potent inhibitors of CYP3A4, such as ketoconazole or ritonavir, the maximum recommended dose of tadalafil is 10 mg, not to exceed once every 72 hours. When tadalafil is used in a once-daily regimen, patients taking concomitant potent inhibitors of CYP3A4, such as ketoconazole or ritonavir, the dose should not exceed 2.5 mg).
No products indexed under this heading.

Quinidine Sulfate (Tadalafil is a substrate of and predominantly metabolized by CYP3A4. Studies have shown that drugs that inhibit CYP3A4 can increase tadalafil exposure. When tadalafil is used on an as-needed basis, patients taking concomitant potent inhibitors of CYP3A4, such as ketoconazole or ritonavir, the maximum recommended dose of tadalafil is 10 mg, not to exceed once every 72 hours. When tadalafil is used in a once-daily regimen, patients taking concomitant potent inhibitors of CYP3A4, such as ketoconazole or ritonavir, the dose should not exceed 2.5 mg).
No products indexed under this heading.

Quinine (Tadalafil is a substrate of and predominantly metabolized by CYP3A4. Studies have shown that drugs that inhibit CYP3A4 can increase tadalafil exposure. When tadalafil is used on an as-needed basis, patients taking concomitant potent inhibitors of CYP3A4, such as ketoconazole or ritonavir, the maximum recommended dose of tadalafil is 10 mg, not to exceed once every 72 hours. When tadalafil is used in a once-daily regimen, patients taking concomitant potent inhibitors of CYP3A4, such as ketoconazole or ritonavir, the dose should not exceed 2.5 mg). Products include:
Hyland's Leg Cramps PM with
    Quinine 3315

Quinine Sulfate (Tadalafil is a substrate of and predominantly metabolized by CYP3A4. Studies have shown that drugs that inhibit CYP3A4 can increase tadalafil exposure. When tadalafil is used on an as-needed basis, patients taking concomitant potent inhibitors of CYP3A4, such as ketoconazole or ritonavir, the maximum recommended dose of tadalafil is 10 mg, not to exceed once every 72 hours. When tadalafil is used in a once-daily regimen, patients taking concomitant potent inhibitors of CYP3A4, such as ketoconazole or ritonavir, the dose should not exceed 2.5 mg).
No products indexed under this heading.

Quinupristin (Tadalafil is a substrate of and predominantly metabolized by CYP3A4. Studies have shown that drugs that inhibit CYP3A4 can increase tadalafil exposure. When tadalafil is used on an as-needed basis, patients taking concomitant potent inhibitors of CYP3A4, such as ketoconazole or ritonavir, the maximum recommended dose of tadalafil is 10 mg, not to exceed once every 72 hours. When tadalafil is used in a once-daily regimen, patients taking concomitant potent

---

IMPORTANT NOTE: Always consult each drug listing in the patient's regimen for possible interactions.

inhibitors of CYP3A4, such as ketoconazole or ritonavir, the dose should not exceed 2.5 mg).
No products indexed under this heading.

Ramipril (PDE5 inhibitors, including tadalafil, are mild systemic vasodilators. Clinical pharmacology studies were conducted to assess the effect of tadalafil on the potentiation of the blood-pressure-lowering effects of selected antihypertensive medications (amlodipine, angiotesin II receptor blockers, bendrofluazide, enalapril, and metoprolol). Small reductions in blood pressure occurred following co-administration of tadalafil with these agents compared to placebo).
No products indexed under this heading.

Ranitidine Bismuth Citrate (Tadalafil is a substrate of and predominantly metabolized by CYP3A4. Studies have shown that drugs that inhibit CYP3A4 can increase tadalafil exposure. When tadalafil is used on an as-needed basis, patients taking concomitant potent inhibitors of CYP3A4, such as ketoconazole or ritonavir, the maximum recommended dose of tadalafil is 10 mg, not to exceed once every 72 hours. When tadalafil is used in a once-daily regimen, patients taking concomitant potent inhibitors of CYP3A4, such as ketoconazole or ritonavir, the dose should not exceed 2.5 mg).
No products indexed under this heading.

Ranitidine Hydrochloride (Tadalafil is a substrate of and predominantly metabolized by CYP3A4. Studies have shown that drugs that inhibit CYP3A4 can increase tadalafil exposure. When tadalafil is used on an as-needed basis, patients taking concomitant potent inhibitors of CYP3A4, such as ketoconazole or ritonavir, the maximum recommended dose of tadalafil is 10 mg, not to exceed once every 72 hours. When tadalafil is used in a once-daily regimen, patients taking concomitant potent inhibitors of CYP3A4, such as ketoconazole or ritonavir, the dose should not exceed 2.5 mg). Products include:
Zantac **1737**
Zantac Injection **1732**
Zantac Pharmacy **1735**

Rauwolfia Serpentina (PDE5 inhibitors, including tadalafil, are mild systemic vasodilators. Clinical pharmacology studies were conducted to assess the effect of tadalafil on the potentiation of the blood-pressure-lowering effects of selected antihypertensive medications (amlodipine, angiotesin II receptor blockers, bendrofluazide, enalapril, and metoprolol). Small reductions in blood pressure occurred following co-administration of tadalafil with these agents compared to placebo).
No products indexed under this heading.

Rescinnamine (PDE5 inhibitors, including tadalafil, are mild systemic vasodilators. Clinical pharmacology studies were conducted to assess the effect of tadalafil on the potentiation of the blood-pressure-lowering effects of selected antihypertensive medications (amlodipine, angiotesin II receptor blockers, bendrofluazide, enalapril, and metoprolol). Small reductions in blood pressure occurred following co-administration of tadalafil with these agents compared to placebo).
No products indexed under this heading.

Reserpine (PDE5 inhibitors, including tadalafil, are mild systemic vasodilators. Clinical pharmacology studies were conducted to assess the effect of tadalafil on the potentiation of the blood-pressure-lowering effects of selected antihypertensive medications (amlodipine, angiotesin II receptor blockers, bendrofluazide, enalapril, and metoprolol). Small reductions in blood pressure occurred following co-administration of tadalafil with these agents compared to placebo).
No products indexed under this heading.

Rifabutin (Studies have shown that drugs that induce CYP3A4 can decrease tadalafil exposure. Rifampin (600 mg daily), a CYP3A4 inducer, reduced tadalafil 10 mg single-dose exposure (AUC) by 88% and C_{max} by 46%, relative to the values for tadalafil 10 mg alone. Although specific interactions have not been studied, other CYP3A4 inducers, such as carbamazepine, phenytoin, and phenobarbital, would likely decrease tadalafil exposure. No dose adjustment is warranted. The reduced exposure of tadalafil with the co-administration of rifampin or other CYP3A4 inducers can be anticipated to decrease the efficacy of tadalafil for once daily use; the magnitude of decreased efficacy is unknown).
No products indexed under this heading.

Rifampicin (Studies have shown that drugs that induce CYP3A4 can decrease tadalafil exposure. Rifampin (600 mg daily), a CYP3A4 inducer, reduced tadalafil 10 mg single-dose exposure (AUC) by 88% and C_{max} by 46%, relative to the values for tadalafil 10 mg alone. Although specific interactions have not been studied, other CYP3A4 inducers, such as carbamazepine, phenytoin, and phenobarbital, would likely decrease tadalafil exposure. No dose adjustment is warranted. The reduced exposure of tadalafil with the co-administration of rifampin or other CYP3A4 inducers can be anticipated to decrease the efficacy of tadalafil for once daily use; the magnitude of decreased efficacy is unknown).
No products indexed under this heading.

Rifampin (Studies have shown that drugs that induce CYP3A4 can decrease tadalafil exposure. Rifampin (600 mg daily), a CYP3A4 inducer, reduced tadalafil 10 mg single-dose exposure (AUC) by 88% and C_{max} by 46%, relative to the values for tadalafil 10 mg alone. No dose adjustment is warranted. The reduced exposure of tadalafil with the co-administration of rifampin can be anticipated to decrease the efficacy of tadalafil for once daily use; the magnitude of decreased efficacy is unknown).
No products indexed under this heading.

Rifapentine (Studies have shown that drugs that induce CYP3A4 can decrease tadalafil exposure. Rifampin (600 mg daily), a CYP3A4 inducer, reduced tadalafil 10 mg single-dose exposure (AUC) by 88% and C_{max} by 46%, relative to the values for tadalafil 10 mg alone. Although specific interactions have not been studied, other CYP3A4 inducers, such as carbamazepine, phenytoin, and phenobarbital, would likely decrease tadalafil exposure. No dose adjustment is warranted. The reduced exposure of tadalafil with the co-administration of rifampin or other CYP3A4 inducers can be anticipated to decrease the efficacy of tadalafil for once daily use; the magnitude of decreased efficacy is unknown).
No products indexed under this heading.

Ritonavir (Ritonavir (500 mg or 600 mg b.i.d. at steady state), an inhibitor of CYP3A4, CYP2C9, CYP2C19, and CYP2D6, increased tadalafil 20 mg single-dose exposure (AUC) by 32% with a 30% reduction in C_{max}, relative to the values for tadalafil 20 mg alone. Ritonavir (200 mg b.i.d.), increased tadalafil 20 mg single-dose exposure (AUC) by 124% with no change in C_{max}, relative to the values for tadalafil 20 mg alone. For patients taking potent inhibitors of CYP3A4, such as ritonavir, and are using tadalafil on an as needed basis, the dose of tadalafil should be limited to 10 mg no more than once every 72 hours. For once-daily use, the dose of tadalafil should not exceed 2.5 mg). Products include:
Kaletra **458**
Norvir **509**

Saquinavir (Ritonavir (500 mg or 600 mg b.i.d. at steady state), an inhibitor of CYP3A4, CYP2C9, CYP2C19, and CYP2D6, increased tadalafil 20 mg single-dose exposure (AUC) by 32% with a 30% reduction in C_{max}, relative to the values for tadalafil 20 mg alone. Ritonavir (200 mg b.i.d.), increased tadalafil 20 mg single-dose exposure (AUC) by 124% with no change in C_{max}, relative to the values for tadalafil 20 mg alone. Although specific interactions have not been studied, other HIV protease inhibitors would likely increase tadalafil exposure).
No products indexed under this heading.

Saquinavir Mesylate (Ritonavir (500 mg or 600 mg b.i.d. at steady state), an inhibitor of CYP3A4, CYP2C9, CYP2C19, and CYP2D6, increased tadalafil 20 mg single-dose exposure (AUC) by 32% with a 30% reduction in C_{max}, relative to the values for tadalafil 20 mg alone. Ritonavir (200 mg b.i.d.), increased tadalafil 20 mg single-dose exposure (AUC) by 124% with no change in C_{max}, relative to the values for tadalafil 20 mg alone. Although specific interactions have not been studied, other HIV protease inhibitors would likely increase tadalafil exposure).
No products indexed under this heading.

Sertraline Hydrochloride (Tadalafil is a substrate of and predominantly metabolized by CYP3A4. Studies have shown that drugs that inhibit CYP3A4 can increase tadalafil exposure. When tadalafil is used on an as-needed basis, patients taking concomitant potent inhibitors of CYP3A4, such as ketoconazole or ritonavir, the maximum recommended dose of tadalafil is 10 mg, not to exceed once every 72 hours. When tadalafil is used in a once-daily regimen, patients taking concomitant potent inhibitors of CYP3A4, such as ketoconazole or ritonavir, the dose should not exceed 2.5 mg).
No products indexed under this heading.

Sildenafil Citrate (Tadalafil is a substrate of and predominantly metabolized by CYP3A4. Studies have shown that drugs that inhibit CYP3A4 can increase tadalafil exposure. When tadalafil is used on an as-needed basis, patients taking concomitant potent inhibitors of CYP3A4, such as ketoconazole or ritonavir, the maximum recommended dose of tadalafil is 10 mg, not to exceed once every 72 hours. When tadalafil is used in a once-daily regimen, patients taking concomitant potent inhibitors of CYP3A4, such as ketoconazole or ritonavir, the dose should not exceed 2.5 mg).
No products indexed under this heading.

Sodium Bicarbonate (Simultaneous administration of an antacid (magnesium hydroxide/aluminum hydroxide) and tadalafil reduced the apparent rate of absorption of tadalafil without altering exposure (AUC) to tadalafil).
No products indexed under this heading.

Sodium Nitroprusside (PDE5 inhibitors, including tadalafil, are mild systemic vasodilators. Clinical pharmacology studies were conducted to assess the effect of tadalafil on the potentiation of the blood-pressure-lowering effects of selected antihypertensive medications (amlodipine, angiotesin II receptor blockers, bendrofluazide, enalapril, and metoprolol). Small reductions in blood pressure occurred following co-administration of tadalafil with these agents compared to placebo).
No products indexed under this heading.

Sotalol Hydrochloride (PDE5 inhibitors, including tadalafil, are mild systemic vasodilators. Clinical pharmacology studies were conducted to assess the effect of tadalafil on the potentiation of the blood-pressure-lowering effects of selected antihypertensive medications (amlodipine, angiotesin II receptor blockers, bendrofluazide, enalapril, and metoprolol). Small reductions in blood pressure occurred following co-administration of tadalafil with these agents compared to placebo).
No products indexed under this heading.

Spirapril Hydrochloride (PDE5 inhibitors, including tadalafil, are mild systemic vasodilators. Clinical pharmacology studies were conducted to assess the effect of tadalafil on the potentiation of the blood-pressure-lowering effects of selected antihypertensive medications (amlodipine, angiotesin II receptor blockers, bendrofluazide, enalapril, and metoprolol). Small reductions in blood pressure occurred following co-administration of tadalafil with these agents compared to placebo).
No products indexed under this heading.

Sulfinpyrazone (Studies have shown that drugs that induce CYP3A4 can decrease tadalafil exposure. Rifampin (600 mg daily), a CYP3A4 inducer, reduced tadalafil 10 mg single-dose exposure (AUC) by 88% and C_{max} by 46%, relative to the values for tadalafil 10 mg alone. Although specific interactions have not been studied, other CYP3A4 inducers, such as carbamazepine, phenytoin, and phenobarbital, would likely decrease tadalafil exposure. No dose adjustment is warranted. The reduced exposure of tadalafil with the co-administration of rifampin or other CYP3A4 inducers can be anticipated to decrease the efficacy of tadalafil for once daily use; the magnitude of decreased efficacy is unknown).
No products indexed under this heading.

Tamsulosin Hydrochloride (Caution is advised when PDE5 inhibitors are co-administered with α-blockers. Tadalafil and α-adrenergic blocking agents are both vasodilators with blood-pressure lowering effects. When vasodilators are used in combination, an additive effect on blood pressure may be anticipated. In some patients, concomitant use of these two drug classes can lower blood presure significantly, which may lead to symptomatic hypotension (eg, fainting). When tadalafil is co-administered with an α-blocker, patients should be stable on α-blocker therapy prior to initiating treatment with tadalafil, and tadalafil should be administered at the lowest recommended dose).
No products indexed under this heading.

Telithromycin (Tadalafil is a substrate of and metabolized predominantly by CYP3A4. Studies have shown that drugs that inhibit CYP3A4 can increase tadalafil exposure. When tadalafil is used on an as-needed basis, patients taking concomitant potent inhibitors of CYP3A4, such as ketoconazole or ritonavir, the maximum recommended dose of tadalafil is 10 mg, not to exceed once every 72 hours. When tadalafil is used in a once-daily regimen, patients taking concomitant potent inhibitors of CYP3A4, such as ketoconazole or ritonavir, the dose should not exceed 2.5 mg). Products include:
Ketek **2991**

Telmisartan (A study was conducted to assess the interaction of angiotensin II receptor blockers and tadalafil 20 mg. Subjects in the study were taking any

marketed angiotensin II receptor blocker, either alone, as a component of a combination product, or as part of a multiple antihypertensive regimen. Following dosing, ambulatory measurements of blood pressure revealed differences between tadalafil and placebo of 8/4 mm Hg in systolic/diastolic blood pressure). Products include:

Micardis **887**
Micardis HCT **889**

Terazosin Hydrochloride (Caution is advised when PDE5 inhibitors are co-administered with α-blockers. Tadalafil and α-adrenergic blocking agents are both vasodilators with blood-pressure lowering effects. When vasodilators are used in combination, an additive effect on blood pressure may be anticipated. In some patients, concomitant use of these two drug classes can lower blood presure significantly, which may lead to symptomatic hypotension (e.g., fainting). When tadalafil is co-administered with an α-blocker, patients should be stable on α-blocker therapy prior to initiating treatment with tadalafil, and tadalafil should be administered at the lowest recommended dose).

No products indexed under this heading.

Theophyllinate (Studies have shown that drugs that induce CYP3A4 can decrease tadalafil exposure. Rifampin (600 mg daily), a CYP3A4 inducer, reduced tadalafil 10 mg single-dose exposure (AUC) by 88% and C_{max} by 46%, relative to the values for tadalafil 10 mg alone. Although specific interactions have not been studied, other CYP3A4 inducers, such as carbamazepine, phenytoin, and phenobarbital, would likely decrease tadalafil exposure. No dose adjustment is warranted. The reduced exposure of tadalafil with the co-administration of rifampin or other CYP3A4 inducers can be anticipated to decrease the efficacy of tadalafil for once daily use; the magnitude of decreased efficacy is unknown).

No products indexed under this heading.

Theophylline (Tadalafil had no significant effect on the pharmacokinetics of theophylline. When tadalafil was administered to subjects taking theophylline, a small augmentation (3 beats per minute) of the increase in heart rate associated with theophylline was observed).

No products indexed under this heading.

Theophylline Anhydrous (Tadalafil had no significant effect on the pharmacokinetics of theophylline. When tadalafil was administered to subjects taking theophylline, a small augmentation (3 beats per minute) of the increase in heart rate associated with theophylline was observed). Products include:

Uniphyl **2817**

Theophylline Calcium Salicylate (Tadalafil had no significant effect on the pharmacokinetics of theophylline. When tadalafil was administered to subjects taking theophylline, a small augmentation (3 beats per minute) of the increase in heart rate associated with theophylline was observed).

No products indexed under this heading.

Theophylline Dihydroxypropyl (Glyceryl) (Tadalafil had no significant effect on the pharmacokinetics of theophylline. When tadalafil was administered to subjects taking theophylline, a small augmentation (3 beats per minute) of the increase in heart rate associated with theophylline was observed).

No products indexed under this heading.

Theophylline Ethylenediamine (Tadalafil had no significant effect on the pharmacokinetics of theophylline. When tadalafil was administered to subjects taking theophylline, a small augmentation (3 beats per minute) of the increase in heart rate associated with theophylline was observed).

No products indexed under this heading.

Theophylline Sodium Glycinate (Tadalafil had no significant effect on the pharmacokinetics of theophylline. When tadalafil was administered to subjects taking theophylline, a small augmentation (3 beats per minute) of the increase in heart rate associated with theophylline was observed).

No products indexed under this heading.

Timolol Maleate (PDE5 inhibitors, including tadalafil, are mild systemic vasodilators. Clinical pharmacology studies were conducted to assess the effect of tadalafil on the potentiation of the blood-pressure-lowering effects of selected antihypertensive medications (amlodipine, angiotesin II receptor blockers, bendrofluazide, enalapril, and metoprolol). Small reductions in blood pressure occurred following co-administration of tadalafil with these agents compared to placebo). Products include:

Combigan **601**
Dorzolamide Hydrochloride/Timolol Maleate Ophthalmic Solution .... ⊙**243**
Timoptic in Ocudose .... ⊙**231**

Tipranavir (Ritonavir (500 mg or 600 mg b.i.d. at steady state), an inhibitor of CYP3A4, CYP2C9, CYP2C19, and CYP2D6, increased tadalafil 20 mg single-dose exposure (AUC) by 32% with a 30% reduction in C_{max}, relative to the values for tadalafil 20 mg alone. Ritonavir (200 mg b.i.d.), increased tadalafil 20 mg single-dose exposure (AUC) by 124% with no change in C_{max}, relative to the values for tadalafil 20 mg alone. Although specific interactions have not been studied, other HIV protease inhibitors would likely increase tadalafil exposure).

No products indexed under this heading.

Torsemide (PDE5 inhibitors, including tadalafil, are mild systemic vasodilators. Clinical pharmacology studies were conducted to assess the effect of tadalafil on the potentiation of the blood-pressure-lowering effects of selected antihypertensive medications (amlodipine, angiotesin II receptor blockers, bendrofluazide, enalapril, and metoprolol). Small reductions in blood pressure occurred following co-administration of tadalafil with these agents compared to placebo).

No products indexed under this heading.

Trandolapril (PDE5 inhibitors, including tadalafil, are mild systemic vasodilators. Clinical pharmacology studies were conducted to assess the effect of tadalafil on the potentiation of the blood-pressure-lowering effects of selected antihypertensive medications (amlodipine, angiotesin II receptor blockers, bendrofluazide, enalapril, and metoprolol). Small reductions in blood pressure occurred following co-administration of tadalafil with these agents compared to placebo). Products include:

Mavik **489**
Tarka **534**

Triamcinolone (Studies have shown that drugs that induce CYP3A4 can decrease tadalafil exposure. Rifampin (600 mg daily), a CYP3A4 inducer, reduced tadalafil 10 mg single-dose exposure (AUC) by 88% and C_{max} by 46%, relative to the values for tadalafil 10 mg alone. Although specific interactions have not been studied, other CYP3A4 inducers, such as carbamazepine, phenytoin, and phenobarbital, would likely decrease tadalafil exposure. No dose adjustment is warranted. The reduced exposure of tadalafil with the co-administration of rifampin or other CYP3A4 inducers can be anticipated to decrease the efficacy of tadalafil for once daily use; the magnitude of decreased efficacy is unknown).

No products indexed under this heading.

Triamcinolone Acetonide (Studies have shown that drugs that induce CYP3A4 can decrease tadalafil exposure. Rifampin (600 mg daily), a CYP3A4 inducer, reduced tadalafil 10 mg single-dose exposure (AUC) by 88% and C_{max} by 46%, relative to the values for tadalafil 10 mg alone. Although specific interactions have not been studied, other CYP3A4 inducers, such as carbamazepine, phenytoin, and phenobarbital, would likely decrease tadalafil exposure. No dose adjustment is warranted. The reduced exposure of tadalafil with the co-administration of rifampin or other CYP3A4 inducers can be anticipated to decrease the efficacy of tadalafil for once daily use; the magnitude of decreased efficacy is unknown). Products include:

Azmacort **408**
Nasacort AQ **3019**

Triamcinolone Diacetate (Studies have shown that drugs that induce CYP3A4 can decrease tadalafil exposure. Rifampin (600 mg daily), a CYP3A4 inducer, reduced tadalafil 10 mg single-dose exposure (AUC) by 88% and C_{max} by 46%, relative to the values for tadalafil 10 mg alone. Although specific interactions have not been studied, other CYP3A4 inducers, such as carbamazepine, phenytoin, and phenobarbital, would likely decrease tadalafil exposure. No dose adjustment is warranted. The reduced exposure of tadalafil with the co-administration of rifampin or other CYP3A4 inducers can be anticipated to decrease the efficacy of tadalafil for once daily use; the magnitude of decreased efficacy is unknown).

No products indexed under this heading.

Triamcinolone Hexacetonide (Studies have shown that drugs that induce CYP3A4 can decrease tadalafil exposure. Rifampin (600 mg daily), a CYP3A4 inducer, reduced tadalafil 10 mg single-dose exposure (AUC) by 88% and C_{max} by 46%, relative to the values for tadalafil 10 mg alone. Although specific interactions have not been studied, other CYP3A4 inducers, such as carbamazepine, phenytoin, and phenobarbital, would likely decrease tadalafil exposure. No dose adjustment is warranted. The reduced exposure of tadalafil with the co-administration of rifampin or other CYP3A4 inducers can be anticipated to decrease the efficacy of tadalafil for once daily use; the magnitude of decreased efficacy is unknown).

No products indexed under this heading.

Trimethaphan Camsylate (PDE5 inhibitors, including tadalafil, are mild systemic vasodilators. Clinical pharmacology studies were conducted to assess the effect of tadalafil on the potentiation of the blood-pressure-lowering effects of selected antihypertensive medications (amlodipine, angiotesin II receptor blockers, bendrofluazide, enalapril, and metoprolol). Small reductions in blood pressure occurred following co-administration of tadalafil with these agents compared to placebo).

No products indexed under this heading.

Troglitazone (Tadalafil is a substrate of and predominantly metabolized by CYP3A4. Studies have shown that drugs that inhibit CYP3A4 can increase tadalafil exposure. When tadalafil is used on an as-needed basis, patients taking concomitant potent inhibitors of CYP3A4, such as ketoconazole or ritonavir, the maximum recommended dose of tadalafil is 10 mg, not to exceed once every 72 hours. When tadalafil is used in a once-daily regimen, patients taking concomitant potent inhibitors of CYP3A4, such as ketoconazole or ritonavir, the dose should not exceed 2.5 mg).

No products indexed under this heading.

Troleandomycin (Tadalafil is a substrate of and metabolized predominantly by CYP3A4. Studies have shown that drugs that inhibit CYP3A4 can increase tadalafil exposure. When tadalafil is used on an as-needed basis, patients taking concomitant potent inhibitors of CYP3A4, such as ketoconazole or ritonavir, the maximum recommended dose of tadalafil is 10 mg, not to exceed once every 72 hours. When tadalafil is used in a once-daily regimen, patients taking concomitant potent inhibitors of CYP3A4, such as ketoconazole or ritonavir, the dose should not exceed 2.5 mg).

No products indexed under this heading.

Valproate Sodium (Tadalafil is a substrate of and predominantly metabolized by CYP3A4. Studies have shown that drugs that inhibit CYP3A4 can increase tadalafil exposure. When tadalafil is used on an as-needed basis, patients taking concomitant potent inhibitors of CYP3A4, such as ketoconazole or ritonavir, the maximum recommended dose of tadalafil is 10 mg, not to exceed once every 72 hours. When tadalafil is used in a once-daily regimen, patients taking concomitant potent inhibitors of CYP3A4, such as ketoconazole or ritonavir, the dose should not exceed 2.5 mg).

No products indexed under this heading.

Valsartan (A study was conducted to assess the interaction of angiotensin II receptor blockers and tadalafil 20 mg. Subjects in the study were taking any marketed angiotensin II receptor blocker, either alone, as a component of a combination product, or as part of a multiple antihypertensive regimen. Following dosing, ambulatory measurements of blood pressure revealed differences between tadalafil and placebo of 8/4 mm Hg in systolic/diastolic blood pressure). Products include:

Diovan **2413**
Diovan HCT **2419**
Exforge **2443**
Exforge HCT **2449**
Valturna **3637**

Vardenafil Hydrochloride (Tadalafil is a substrate of and predominantly metabolized by CYP3A4. Studies have shown that drugs that inhibit CYP3A4 can increase tadalafil exposure. When tadalafil is used on an as-needed basis, patients taking concomitant potent inhibitors of CYP3A4, such as ketoconazole or ritonavir, the maximum recommended dose of tadalafil is 10 mg, not to exceed once every 72 hours. When tadalafil is used in a once-daily regimen, patients taking concomitant potent inhibitors of CYP3A4, such as ketoconazole or ritonavir, the dose should not exceed 2.5 mg). Products include:

Levitra **3157**

Verapamil Hydrochloride (PDE5 inhibitors, including tadalafil, are mild systemic vasodilators. Clinical pharmacology studies were conducted to assess the effect of tadalafil on the potentiation of the blood-pressure-lowering effects of selected antihypertensive medications (amlodipine, angiotesin II receptor blockers, bendrofluazide, enalapril, and metoprolol). Small reductions in blood pres-

IMPORTANT NOTE: Always consult each drug listing in the patient's regimen for possible interactions.

Cialis Interactions Index 320

sure occurred following co-administration of tadalafil with these agents compared to placebo). Products include:
Tarka 534

Voriconazole (Tadalafil is a substrate of and metabolized predominantly by CYP3A4. Studies have shown that drugs that inhibit CYP3A4 can increase tadalafil exposure. When tadalafil is used on an as-needed basis, patients taking concomitant potent inhibitors of CYP3A4, such as ketoconazole or ritonavir, the maximum recommended dose of tadalafil is 10 mg, not to exceed once every 72 hours. When tadalafil is used in a once-daily regimen, patients taking concomitant potent inhibitors of CYP3A4, such as ketoconazole or ritonavir, the dose should not exceed 2.5 mg).
No products indexed under this heading.

Zafirlukast (Tadalafil is a substrate of and predominantly metabolized by CYP3A4. Studies have shown that drugs that inhibit CYP3A4 can increase tadalafil exposure. When tadalafil is used on an as-needed basis, patients taking concomitant potent inhibitors of CYP3A4, such as ketoconazole or ritonavir, the maximum recommended dose of tadalafil is 10 mg, not to exceed once every 72 hours. When tadalafil is used in a once-daily regimen, patients taking concomitant potent inhibitors of CYP3A4, such as ketoconazole or ritonavir, the dose should not exceed 2.5 mg). Products include:
Accolate 3612

Zileuton (Tadalafil is a substrate of and predominantly metabolized by CYP3A4. Studies have shown that drugs that inhibit CYP3A4 can increase tadalafil exposure. When tadalafil is used on an as-needed basis, patients taking concomitant potent inhibitors of CYP3A4, such as ketoconazole or ritonavir, the maximum recommended dose of tadalafil is 10 mg, not to exceed once every 72 hours. When tadalafil is used in a once-daily regimen, patients taking concomitant potent inhibitors of CYP3A4, such as ketoconazole or ritonavir, the dose should not exceed 2.5 mg).
No products indexed under this heading.

Food Interactions

Alcohol (Both alcohol and tadalafil act as mild vasodilators. When mild vasodilators are taken in combination, blood-pressure-lowering effects of each individual compound may be increased. Substantial consumption of alcohol (eg, 5 units or greater) in combination with tadalafil can increase the potential for orthostatic signs and symptoms, including increase in heart rate, decrease in standing blood pressure, dizziness, and headache).

Beer, reduced-alcohol (Both alcohol and tadalafil act as mild vasodilators. When mild vasodilators are taken in combination, blood-pressure-lowering effects of each individual compound may be increased. Substantial consumption of alcohol (eg, 5 units or greater) in combination with tadalafil can increase the potential for orthostatic signs and symptoms, including increase in heart rate, decrease in standing blood pressure, dizziness, and headache).

Beer, unspecified (Both alcohol and tadalafil act as mild vasodilators. When mild vasodilators are taken in combination, blood-pressure-lowering effects of each individual compound may be increased. Substantial consumption of alcohol (eg, 5 units or greater) in combination with tadalafil can increase the potential for orthostatic signs and symptoms, including increase in heart rate, decrease in standing blood pressure, dizziness, and headache).

Grapefruit (Tadalafil is a substrate of and predominantly metabolized by CYP3A4. Studies have shown that drugs that inhibit CYP3A4 can increase tadalafil exposure. When tadalafil is used on an as-needed basis, patients taking concomitant potent inhibitors of CYP3A4, such as ketoconazole or ritonavir, the maximum recommended dose of tadalafil is 10 mg, not to exceed once every 72 hours. When tadalafil is used in a once-daily regimen, patients taking concomitant potent inhibitors of CYP3A4, such as ketoconazole or ritonavir, the dose should not exceed 2.5 mg).

Grapefruit Juice (CYP3A4 inhibitors, such as grapefruit juice, may likely increase tadalafil exposure).

Wine, Chianti (Both alcohol and tadalafil act as mild vasodilators. When mild vasodilators are taken in combination, blood-pressure-lowering effects of each individual compound may be increased. Substantial consumption of alcohol (eg, 5 units or greater) in combination with tadalafil can increase the potential for orthostatic signs and symptoms, including increase in heart rate, decrease in standing blood pressure, dizziness, and headache).

Wine, Red (Both alcohol and tadalafil act as mild vasodilators. When mild vasodilators are taken in combination, blood-pressure-lowering effects of each individual compound may be increased. Substantial consumption of alcohol (eg, 5 units or greater) in combination with tadalafil can increase the potential for orthostatic signs and symptoms, including increase in heart rate, decrease in standing blood pressure, dizziness, and headache).

Wine, unspecified (Both alcohol and tadalafil act as mild vasodilators. When mild vasodilators are taken in combination, blood-pressure-lowering effects of each individual compound may be increased. Substantial consumption of alcohol (eg, 5 units or greater) in combination with tadalafil can increase the potential for orthostatic signs and symptoms, including increase in heart rate, decrease in standing blood pressure, dizziness, and headache).

Wine products (Both alcohol and tadalafil act as mild vasodilators. When mild vasodilators are taken in combination, blood-pressure-lowering effects of each individual compound may be increased. Substantial consumption of alcohol (eg, 5 units or greater) in combination with tadalafil can increase the potential for orthostatic signs and symptoms, including increase in heart rate, decrease in standing blood pressure, dizziness, and headache).

CIMZIA

(Certolizumab pegol) 3426
May interact with corticosteroids, immunosuppressive agents, non-steroidal anti-inflammatory agents, vaccines, live, and certain other agents. Compounds in these categories include:

Abatacept (An increased risk of serious infections has been seen in clinical studies of other TNF-blocking agents used in combination with anakinra or abatacept, with no added benefit. Formal drug interaction studies have not been performed with rituximab or natalizumab. Because of the nature of the adverse events seen with these combinations with TNF blocker therapy, similar toxicities may also result from the use of certolizumab in these combinations. There is not enough information to assess the safety and efficacy of such combination therapy. Therefore, the use of certolizumab in combination with anakinra, abatacept, rituximab, or natalizumab is not recommended).
No products indexed under this heading.

Alclometasone Dipropionate (Patients treated with certolizumab are at increased risk for developing serious infections that may lead to hospitalization or death. Most patients who developed these infections were taking concomitant immunosuppressants such as methotrexate or corticosteroids. Hypertensive adverse reactions were observed more frequently in patients receiving certolizumab than in controls. These adverse reactions occurred more frequently among patients with a baseline history of hypertension and among patients receiving concomitant corticosteroids and non-steroidal anti-inflammatory drugs).
No products indexed under this heading.

Anakinra (An increased risk of serious infections has been seen in clinical studies of other TNF-blocking agents used in combination with anakinra or abatacept, with no added benefit. Formal drug interaction studies have not been performed with rituximab or natalizumab. Because of the nature of the adverse events seen with these combinations with TNF blocker therapy, similar toxicities may also result from the use of certolizumab in these combinations. There is not enough information to assess the safety and efficacy of such combination therapy. Therefore, the use of certolizumab in combination with anakinra, abatacept, rituximab, or natalizumab is not recommended). Products include:
Kineret 877

Azathioprine (Patients treated with certolizumab are at increased risk for developing serious infections that may lead to hospitalization or death. Most patients who developed these infections were taking concomitant immunosuppressants such as methotrexate or corticosteroids).
No products indexed under this heading.

Basiliximab (Patients treated with certolizumab are at increased risk for developing serious infections that may lead to hospitalization or death. Most patients who developed these infections were taking concomitant immunosuppressants such as methotrexate or corticosteroids). Products include:
Simulect 2524

BCG Vaccine (No data is available on the response to vaccinations or the secondary transmission of infection by live vaccines in patients receiving certolizumab pegol. Do not administer live vaccines or attenuated vaccines concurrently with certolizumab pegol).
No products indexed under this heading.

Beclomethasone Dipropionate (Patients treated with certolizumab are at increased risk for developing serious infections that may lead to hospitalization or death. Most patients who developed these infections were taking concomitant immunosuppressants such as methotrexate or corticosteroids. Hypertensive adverse reactions were observed more frequently in patients receiving certolizumab than in controls. These adverse reactions occurred more frequently among patients with a baseline history of hypertension and among patients receiving concomitant corticosteroids and non-steroidal anti-inflammatory drugs). Products include:
Qvar 3398

Beclomethasone Dipropionate Monohydrate (Patients treated with certolizumab are at increased risk for developing serious infections that may lead to hospitalization or death. Most patients who developed these infections were taking concomitant immunosuppressants such as methotrexate or corticosteroids. Hypertensive adverse reactions were observed more frequently in patients receiving certolizumab than in controls. These adverse reactions occurred more frequently among patients with a baseline history of hypertension and among patients receiving concomitant corticosteroids and non-steroidal anti-inflammatory drugs).
Products include:
Beconase AQ 1386

Betamethasone (Patients treated with certolizumab are at increased risk for developing serious infections that may lead to hospitalization or death. Most patients who developed these infections were taking concomitant immunosuppressants such as methotrexate or corticosteroids. Hypertensive adverse reactions were observed more frequently in patients receiving certolizumab than in controls. These adverse reactions occurred more frequently among patients with a baseline history of hypertension and among patients receiving concomitant corticosteroids and non-steroidal anti-inflammatory drugs).
No products indexed under this heading.

Betamethasone Acetate (Patients treated with certolizumab are at increased risk for developing serious infections that may lead to hospitalization or death. Most patients who developed these infections were taking concomitant immunosuppressants such as methotrexate or corticosteroids. Hypertensive adverse reactions were observed more frequently in patients receiving certolizumab than in controls. These adverse reactions occurred more frequently among patients with a baseline history of hypertension and among patients receiving concomitant corticosteroids and non-steroidal anti-inflammatory drugs).
No products indexed under this heading.

Betamethasone Benzoate (Patients treated with certolizumab are at increased risk for developing serious infections that may lead to hospitalization or death. Most patients who developed these infections were taking concomitant immunosuppressants such as methotrexate or corticosteroids. Hypertensive adverse reactions were observed more frequently in patients receiving certolizumab than in controls. These adverse reactions occurred more frequently among patients with a baseline history of hypertension and among patients receiving concomitant corticosteroids and non-steroidal anti-inflammatory drugs).
No products indexed under this heading.

Betamethasone Dipropionate (Patients treated with certolizumab are at increased risk for developing serious infections that may lead to hospitalization or death. Most patients who developed these infections were taking concomitant immunosuppressants such as methotrexate or corticosteroids. Hypertensive adverse reactions were observed more frequently in patients receiving certolizumab than in controls. These adverse reactions occurred more frequently among patients with a baseline history of hypertension and among patients receiving concomitant corticosteroids and non-steroidal anti-inflammatory drugs). Products include:
Diprolene Lotion 0.05% 3108
Diprolene Ointment 0.05% 3109
Diprolene AF Cream 0.05% 3107
Lotrisone 3163

Betamethasone Sodium Phosphate (Patients treated with certolizumab are at increased risk for develop-

ing serious infections that may lead to hospitalization or death. Most patients who developed these infections were taking concomitant immunosuppressants such as methotrexate or corticosteroids. Hypertensive adverse reactions were observed more frequently in patients receiving certolizumab than in controls. These adverse reactions occurred more frequently among patients with a baseline history of hypertension and among patients receiving concomitant corticosteroids and non-steroidal anti-inflammatory drugs).

No products indexed under this heading.

Betamethasone Valerate (Patients treated with certolizumab are at increased risk for developing serious infections that may lead to hospitalization or death. Most patients who developed these infections were taking concomitant immunosuppressants such as methotrexate or corticosteroids. Hypertensive adverse reactions were observed more frequently in patients receiving certolizumab than in controls. These adverse reactions occurred more frequently among patients with a baseline history of hypertension and among patients receiving concomitant corticosteroids and non-steroidal anti-inflammatory drugs). Products include:
Luxiq 3321

Budesonide (Patients treated with certolizumab are at increased risk for developing serious infections that may lead to hospitalization or death. Most patients who developed these infections were taking concomitant immunosuppressants such as methotrexate or corticosteroids. Hypertensive adverse reactions were observed more frequently in patients receiving certolizumab than in controls. These adverse reactions occurred more frequently among patients with a baseline history of hypertension and among patients receiving concomitant corticosteroids and non-steroidal anti-inflammatory drugs). Products include:
Pulmicort Flexhaler 714
Symbicort 80/4.5 720
Symbicort 160/4.5 720

Celecoxib (Hypertensive adverse reactions were observed more frequently in patients receiving certolizumab than in controls. These adverse reactions occurred more frequently among patients with a baseline history of hypertension and among patients receiving concomitant corticosteroids and non-steroidal anti-inflammatory drugs). Products include:
Celebrex 3272

Ciclesonide (Patients treated with certolizumab are at increased risk for developing serious infections that may lead to hospitalization or death. Most patients who developed these infections were taking concomitant immunosuppressants such as methotrexate or corticosteroids. Hypertensive adverse reactions were observed more frequently in patients receiving certolizumab than in controls. These adverse reactions occurred more frequently among patients with a baseline history of hypertension and among patients receiving concomitant corticosteroids and non-steroidal anti-inflammatory drugs).

No products indexed under this heading.

Cortisone Acetate (Patients treated with certolizumab are at increased risk for developing serious infections that may lead to hospitalization or death. Most patients who developed these infections were taking concomitant immunosuppressants such as methotrexate or corticosteroids. Hypertensive adverse reactions were observed more frequently in patients receiving certolizumab than in controls. These adverse reactions occurred more frequently

among patients with a baseline history of hypertension and among patients receiving concomitant corticosteroids and non-steroidal anti-inflammatory drugs).

No products indexed under this heading.

Cyclosporine (Patients treated with certolizumab are at increased risk for developing serious infections that may lead to hospitalization or death. Most patients who developed these infections were taking concomitant immunosuppressants such as methotrexate or corticosteroids). Products include:
Gengraf 440
Neoral Oral Solution 2496
Neoral Capsules 2496
Restasis 605

Desoximetasone (Patients treated with certolizumab are at increased risk for developing serious infections that may lead to hospitalization or death. Most patients who developed these infections were taking concomitant immunosuppressants such as methotrexate or corticosteroids. Hypertensive adverse reactions were observed more frequently in patients receiving certolizumab than in controls. These adverse reactions occurred more frequently among patients with a baseline history of hypertension and among patients receiving concomitant corticosteroids and non-steroidal anti-inflammatory drugs).

No products indexed under this heading.

Dexamethasone (Patients treated with certolizumab are at increased risk for developing serious infections that may lead to hospitalization or death. Most patients who developed these infections were taking concomitant immunosuppressants such as methotrexate or corticosteroids. Hypertensive adverse reactions were observed more frequently in patients receiving certolizumab than in controls. These adverse reactions occurred more frequently among patients with a baseline history of hypertension and among patients receiving concomitant corticosteroids and non-steroidal anti-inflammatory drugs). Products include:
Ciprodex 583
Ozurdex .... ⊙223
Tobramycin and Dexamethasone Ophthalmic Suspension .... ⊙251

Dexamethasone Acetate (Patients treated with certolizumab are at increased risk for developing serious infections that may lead to hospitalization or death. Most patients who developed these infections were taking concomitant immunosuppressants such as methotrexate or corticosteroids. Hypertensive adverse reactions were observed more frequently in patients receiving certolizumab than in controls. These adverse reactions occurred more frequently among patients with a baseline history of hypertension and among patients receiving concomitant corticosteroids and non-steroidal anti-inflammatory drugs).

No products indexed under this heading.

Dexamethasone Phosphate (Patients treated with certolizumab are at increased risk for developing serious infections that may lead to hospitalization or death. Most patients who developed these infections were taking concomitant immunosuppressants such as methotrexate or corticosteroids. Hypertensive adverse reactions were observed more frequently in patients receiving certolizumab than in controls. These adverse reactions occurred more frequently among patients with a baseline history of hypertension and among patients receiving concomitant corticosteroids and non-steroidal anti-inflammatory drugs).

No products indexed under this heading.

Dexamethasone Sodium (Patients treated with certolizumab are at increased risk for developing serious infections that may lead to hospitalization or death. Most patients who developed these infections were taking concomitant immunosuppressants such as methotrexate or corticosteroids. Hypertensive adverse reactions were observed more frequently in patients receiving certolizumab than in controls. These adverse reactions occurred more frequently among patients with a baseline history of hypertension and among patients receiving concomitant corticosteroids and non-steroidal anti-inflammatory drugs).

No products indexed under this heading.

Dexamethasone Sodium Phosphate (Patients treated with certolizumab are at increased risk for developing serious infections that may lead to hospitalization or death. Most patients who developed these infections were taking concomitant immunosuppressants such as methotrexate or corticosteroids. Hypertensive adverse reactions were observed more frequently in patients receiving certolizumab than in controls. These adverse reactions occurred more frequently among patients with a baseline history of hypertension and among patients receiving concomitant corticosteroids and non-steroidal anti-inflammatory drugs).

No products indexed under this heading.

Dexamethasone Sodium Phosphate Injection (Patients treated with certolizumab are at increased risk for developing serious infections that may lead to hospitalization or death. Most patients who developed these infections were taking concomitant immunosuppressants such as methotrexate or corticosteroids. Hypertensive adverse reactions were observed more frequently in patients receiving certolizumab than in controls. These adverse reactions occurred more frequently among patients with a baseline history of hypertension and among patients receiving concomitant corticosteroids and non-steroidal anti-inflammatory drugs).

No products indexed under this heading.

Diclofenac Epolamine (Hypertensive adverse reactions were observed more frequently in patients receiving certolizumab than in controls. These adverse reactions occurred more frequently among patients with a baseline history of hypertension and among patients receiving concomitant corticosteroids and non-steroidal anti-inflammatory drugs). Products include:
Flector 1839

Diclofenac Potassium (Hypertensive adverse reactions were observed more frequently in patients receiving certolizumab than in controls. These adverse reactions occurred more frequently among patients with a baseline history of hypertension and among patients receiving concomitant corticosteroids and non-steroidal anti-inflammatory drugs).

No products indexed under this heading.

Diclofenac Sodium (Hypertensive adverse reactions were observed more frequently in patients receiving certolizumab than in controls. These adverse reactions occurred more frequently among patients with a baseline history of hypertension and among patients receiving concomitant corticosteroids and non-steroidal anti-inflammatory drugs).

No products indexed under this heading.

Diflorasone Diacetate (Patients treated with certolizumab are at increased risk for developing serious infections that may lead to hospitalization or death. Most patients who developed these infections were taking con-

comitant immunosuppressants such as methotrexate or corticosteroids. Hypertensive adverse reactions were observed more frequently in patients receiving certolizumab than in controls. These adverse reactions occurred more frequently among patients with a baseline history of hypertension and among patients receiving concomitant corticosteroids and non-steroidal anti-inflammatory drugs).

No products indexed under this heading.

Etodolac (Hypertensive adverse reactions were observed more frequently in patients receiving certolizumab than in controls. These adverse reactions occurred more frequently among patients with a baseline history of hypertension and among patients receiving concomitant corticosteroids and non-steroidal anti-inflammatory drugs).

No products indexed under this heading.

Fenoprofen Calcium (Hypertensive adverse reactions were observed more frequently in patients receiving certolizumab than in controls. These adverse reactions occurred more frequently among patients with a baseline history of hypertension and among patients receiving concomitant corticosteroids and non-steroidal anti-inflammatory drugs).

No products indexed under this heading.

Fludrocortisone Acetate (Patients treated with certolizumab are at increased risk for developing serious infections that may lead to hospitalization or death. Most patients who developed these infections were taking concomitant immunosuppressants such as methotrexate or corticosteroids. Hypertensive adverse reactions were observed more frequently in patients receiving certolizumab than in controls. These adverse reactions occurred more frequently among patients with a baseline history of hypertension and among patients receiving concomitant corticosteroids and non-steroidal anti-inflammatory drugs).

No products indexed under this heading.

Flumethasone Pivalate (Patients treated with certolizumab are at increased risk for developing serious infections that may lead to hospitalization or death. Most patients who developed these infections were taking concomitant immunosuppressants such as methotrexate or corticosteroids. Hypertensive adverse reactions were observed more frequently in patients receiving certolizumab than in controls. These adverse reactions occurred more frequently among patients with a baseline history of hypertension and among patients receiving concomitant corticosteroids and non-steroidal anti-inflammatory drugs).

No products indexed under this heading.

Flunisolide Hemihydrate (Patients treated with certolizumab are at increased risk for developing serious infections that may lead to hospitalization or death. Most patients who developed these infections were taking concomitant immunosuppressants such as methotrexate or corticosteroids. Hypertensive adverse reactions were observed more frequently in patients receiving certolizumab than in controls. These adverse reactions occurred more frequently among patients with a baseline history of hypertension and among patients receiving concomitant corticosteroids and non-steroidal anti-inflammatory drugs).

No products indexed under this heading.

IMPORTANT NOTE: Always consult each drug listing in the patient's regimen for possible interactions.

Flurbiprofen (Hypertensive adverse reactions were observed more frequently in patients receiving certolizumab than in controls. These adverse reactions occurred more frequently among patients with a baseline history of hypertension and among patients receiving concomitant corticosteroids and non-steroidal anti-inflammatory drugs).

No products indexed under this heading.

Fluticasone Furoate (Patients treated with certolizumab are at increased risk for developing serious infections that may lead to hospitalization or death. Most patients who developed these infections were taking concomitant immunosuppressants such as methotrexate or corticosteroids. Hypertensive adverse reactions were observed more frequently in patients receiving certolizumab than in controls. These adverse reactions occurred more frequently among patients with a baseline history of hypertension and among patients receiving concomitant corticosteroids and non-steroidal anti-inflammatory drugs). Products include:

Veramyst 1713

Fluticasone Propionate (Patients treated with certolizumab are at increased risk for developing serious infections that may lead to hospitalization or death. Most patients who developed these infections were taking concomitant immunosuppressants such as methotrexate or corticosteroids. Hypertensive adverse reactions were observed more frequently in patients receiving certolizumab than in controls. These adverse reactions occurred more frequently among patients with a baseline history of hypertension and among patients receiving concomitant corticosteroids and non-steroidal anti-inflammatory drugs). Products include:

Advair 100/50 1275
Advair 250/50 1275
Advair 500/50 1275
Advair HFA 45/21 1288
Advair HFA 115/21 1288
Advair HFA 230/21 1288
Flonase 1459
Flovent Diskus 1463
Flovent HFA 1470

Hydrocortisone (Patients treated with certolizumab are at increased risk for developing serious infections that may lead to hospitalization or death. Most patients who developed these infections were taking concomitant immunosuppressants such as methotrexate or corticosteroids. Hypertensive adverse reactions were observed more frequently in patients receiving certolizumab than in controls. These adverse reactions occurred more frequently among patients with a baseline history of hypertension and among patients receiving concomitant corticosteroids and non-steroidal anti-inflammatory drugs).

No products indexed under this heading.

Hydrocortisone (Alcohol) (Patients treated with certolizumab are at increased risk for developing serious infections that may lead to hospitalization or death. Most patients who developed these infections were taking concomitant immunosuppressants such as methotrexate or corticosteroids. Hypertensive adverse reactions were observed more frequently in patients receiving certolizumab than in controls. These adverse reactions occurred more frequently among patients with a baseline history of hypertension and among patients receiving concomitant corticosteroids and non-steroidal anti-inflammatory drugs).

No products indexed under this heading.

Hydrocortisone Acetate (Patients treated with certolizumab are at increased risk for developing serious infections that may lead to hospitaliza-

tion or death. Most patients who developed these infections were taking concomitant immunosuppressants such as methotrexate or corticosteroids. Hypertensive adverse reactions were observed more frequently in patients receiving certolizumab than in controls. These adverse reactions occurred more frequently among patients with a baseline history of hypertension and among patients receiving concomitant corticosteroids and non-steroidal anti-inflammatory drugs).

No products indexed under this heading.

Hydrocortisone Butyrate (Patients treated with certolizumab are at increased risk for developing serious infections that may lead to hospitalization or death. Most patients who developed these infections were taking concomitant immunosuppressants such as methotrexate or corticosteroids. Hypertensive adverse reactions were observed more frequently in patients receiving certolizumab than in controls. These adverse reactions occurred more frequently among patients with a baseline history of hypertension and among patients receiving concomitant corticosteroids and non-steroidal anti-inflammatory drugs).

No products indexed under this heading.

Hydrocortisone Cypionate (Patients treated with certolizumab are at increased risk for developing serious infections that may lead to hospitalization or death. Most patients who developed these infections were taking concomitant immunosuppressants such as methotrexate or corticosteroids. Hypertensive adverse reactions were observed more frequently in patients receiving certolizumab than in controls. These adverse reactions occurred more frequently among patients with a baseline history of hypertension and among patients receiving concomitant corticosteroids and non-steroidal anti-inflammatory drugs).

No products indexed under this heading.

Hydrocortisone Hemisuccinate (Patients treated with certolizumab are at increased risk for developing serious infections that may lead to hospitalization or death. Most patients who developed these infections were taking concomitant immunosuppressants such as methotrexate or corticosteroids. Hypertensive adverse reactions were observed more frequently in patients receiving certolizumab than in controls. These adverse reactions occurred more frequently among patients with a baseline history of hypertension and among patients receiving concomitant corticosteroids and non-steroidal anti-inflammatory drugs).

No products indexed under this heading.

Hydrocortisone Probutate (Patients treated with certolizumab are at increased risk for developing serious infections that may lead to hospitalization or death. Most patients who developed these infections were taking concomitant immunosuppressants such as methotrexate or corticosteroids. Hypertensive adverse reactions were observed more frequently in patients receiving certolizumab than in controls. These adverse reactions occurred more frequently among patients with a baseline history of hypertension and among patients receiving concomitant corticosteroids and non-steroidal anti-inflammatory drugs).

No products indexed under this heading.

Hydrocortisone Sodium Phosphate (Patients treated with certolizumab are at increased risk for developing serious infections that may lead to hospitalization or death. Most patients who developed these infections were taking concomitant immunosuppres-

sants such as methotrexate or corticosteroids. Hypertensive adverse reactions were observed more frequently in patients receiving certolizumab than in controls. These adverse reactions occurred more frequently among patients with a baseline history of hypertension and among patients receiving concomitant corticosteroids and non-steroidal anti-inflammatory drugs).

No products indexed under this heading.

Hydrocortisone Sodium Succinate (Patients treated with certolizumab are at increased risk for developing serious infections that may lead to hospitalization or death. Most patients who developed these infections were taking concomitant immunosuppressants such as methotrexate or corticosteroids. Hypertensive adverse reactions were observed more frequently in patients receiving certolizumab than in controls. These adverse reactions occurred more frequently among patients with a baseline history of hypertension and among patients receiving concomitant corticosteroids and non-steroidal anti-inflammatory drugs).

No products indexed under this heading.

Hydrocortisone Valerate (Patients treated with certolizumab are at increased risk for developing serious infections that may lead to hospitalization or death. Most patients who developed these infections were taking concomitant immunosuppressants such as methotrexate or corticosteroids. Hypertensive adverse reactions were observed more frequently in patients receiving certolizumab than in controls. These adverse reactions occurred more frequently among patients with a baseline history of hypertension and among patients receiving concomitant corticosteroids and non-steroidal anti-inflammatory drugs).

No products indexed under this heading.

Ibuprofen (Hypertensive adverse reactions were observed more frequently in patients receiving certolizumab than in controls. These adverse reactions occurred more frequently among patients with a baseline history of hypertension and among patients receiving concomitant corticosteroids and non-steroidal anti-inflammatory drugs). Products include:

Motrin IB 2043
Children's Motrin 2044
Children's Motrin Non-Staining
   Dye-Free 2044
Infants' Motrin 2044
Infants' Motrin Dye-Free 2044
Junior Strength Motrin 2044
Vicoprofen 564

Indomethacin (Hypertensive adverse reactions were observed more frequently in patients receiving certolizumab than in controls. These adverse reactions occurred more frequently among patients with a baseline history of hypertension and among patients receiving concomitant corticosteroids and non-steroidal anti-inflammatory drugs). Products include:

Indocin 2167

Indomethacin Sodium Trihydrate (Hypertensive adverse reactions were observed more frequently in patients receiving certolizumab than in controls. These adverse reactions occurred more frequently among patients with a baseline history of hypertension and among patients receiving concomitant corticosteroids and non-steroidal anti-inflammatory drugs). Products include:

Indocin I.V. 2007

Influenza Vaccine, Live Attenuated (No data is available on the response to vaccinations or the secondary transmission of infection by live vaccines in patients receiving certolizumab pegol. Do not administer live vaccines or attenuated vaccines concurrently with certolizumab pegol).

No products indexed under this heading.

Influenza Virus Vaccine Live, Intranasal (No data is available on the response to vaccinations or the secondary transmission of infection by live vaccines in patients receiving certolizumab pegol. Do not administer live vaccines or attenuated vaccines concurrently with certolizumab pegol). Products include:

FluMist 2078

Ketoprofen (Hypertensive adverse reactions were observed more frequently in patients receiving certolizumab than in controls. These adverse reactions occurred more frequently among patients with a baseline history of hypertension and among patients receiving concomitant corticosteroids and non-steroidal anti-inflammatory drugs).

No products indexed under this heading.

Ketorolac Tromethamine (Hypertensive adverse reactions were observed more frequently in patients receiving certolizumab than in controls. These adverse reactions occurred more frequently among patients with a baseline history of hypertension and among patients receiving concomitant corticosteroids and non-steroidal anti-inflammatory drugs). Products include:

Acuvail .... ⊙ 209

Measles, Mumps, Rubella and Varicella Virus Vaccine Live (No data is available on the response to vaccinations or the secondary transmission of infection by live vaccines in patients receiving certolizumab pegol. Do not administer live vaccines or attenuated vaccines concurrently with certolizumab pegol). Products include:

ProQuad 2254

Measles, Mumps & Rubella Virus Vaccine, Live (No data is available on the response to vaccinations or the secondary transmission of infection by live vaccines in patients receiving certolizumab pegol. Do not administer live vaccines or attenuated vaccines concurrently with certolizumab pegol). Products include:

M-M-R II 2203
ProQuad 2254

Measles & Rubella Virus Vaccine Live (No data is available on the response to vaccinations or the secondary transmission of infection by live vaccines in patients receiving certolizumab pegol. Do not administer live vaccines or attenuated vaccines concurrently with certolizumab pegol).

No products indexed under this heading.

Measles Virus Vaccine Live (No data is available on the response to vaccinations or the secondary transmission of infection by live vaccines in patients receiving certolizumab pegol. Do not administer live vaccines or attenuated vaccines concurrently with certolizumab pegol). Products include:

Attenuvax 2086

Meclofenamate Sodium (Hypertensive adverse reactions were observed more frequently in patients receiving certolizumab than in controls. These adverse reactions occurred more frequently among patients with a baseline history of hypertension and among patients receiving concomitant corticosteroids and non-steroidal anti-inflammatory drugs).

No products indexed under this heading.

Mefenamic Acid (Hypertensive adverse reactions were observed more frequently in patients receiving certolizumab than in controls. These adverse reactions occurred more frequently among patients with a baseline history of hypertension and among patients receiving concomitant corticosteroids and non-steroidal anti-inflammatory drugs).
No products indexed under this heading.

Meloxicam (Hypertensive adverse reactions were observed more frequently in patients receiving certolizumab than in controls. These adverse reactions occurred more frequently among patients with a baseline history of hypertension and among patients receiving concomitant corticosteroids and non-steroidal anti-inflammatory drugs).
No products indexed under this heading.

Methotrexate (Patients treated with certolizumab are at increased risk for developing serious infections that may lead to hospitalization or death. Most patients who developed these infections were taking concomitant immunosuppressants such as methotrexate or corticosteroids).
No products indexed under this heading.

Methotrexate Sodium (Patients treated with certolizumab are at increased risk for developing serious infections that may lead to hospitalization or death. Most patients who developed these infections were taking concomitant immunosuppressants such as methotrexate or corticosteroids).
No products indexed under this heading.

Methylprednisolone (Patients treated with certolizumab are at increased risk for developing serious infections that may lead to hospitalization or death. Most patients who developed these infections were taking concomitant immunosuppressants such as methotrexate or corticosteroids. Hypertensive adverse reactions were observed more frequently in patients receiving certolizumab than in controls. These adverse reactions occurred more frequently among patients with a baseline history of hypertension and among patients receiving concomitant corticosteroids and non-steroidal anti-inflammatory drugs).
No products indexed under this heading.

Methylprednisolone Acetate (Patients treated with certolizumab are at increased risk for developing serious infections that may lead to hospitalization or death. Most patients who developed these infections were taking concomitant immunosuppressants such as methotrexate or corticosteroids. Hypertensive adverse reactions were observed more frequently in patients receiving certolizumab than in controls. These adverse reactions occurred more frequently among patients with a baseline history of hypertension and among patients receiving concomitant corticosteroids and non-steroidal anti-inflammatory drugs).
No products indexed under this heading.

Methylprednisolone Sodium Succinate (Patients treated with certolizumab are at increased risk for developing serious infections that may lead to hospitalization or death. Most patients who developed these infections were taking concomitant immunosuppressants such as methotrexate or corticosteroids. Hypertensive adverse reactions were observed more frequently in patients receiving certolizumab than in controls. These adverse reactions occurred more frequently among patients with a baseline history of hypertension and among patients receiving concomitant corticosteroids and non-steroidal anti-inflammatory drugs).
No products indexed under this heading.

Mometasone Furoate (Patients treated with certolizumab are at increased risk for developing serious infections that may lead to hospitalization or death. Most patients who developed these infections were taking concomitant immunosuppressants such as methotrexate or corticosteroids. Hypertensive adverse reactions were observed more frequently in patients receiving certolizumab than in controls. These adverse reactions occurred more frequently among patients with a baseline history of hypertension and among patients receiving concomitant corticosteroids and non-steroidal anti-inflammatory drugs). Products include:
Asmanex **3058**
Elocon Cream **3111**
Elocon Lotion **3112**
Elocon Ointment **3114**

Mometasone Furoate Monohydrate (Patients treated with certolizumab are at increased risk for developing serious infections that may lead to hospitalization or death. Most patients who developed these infections were taking concomitant immunosuppressants such as methotrexate or corticosteroids. Hypertensive adverse reactions were observed more frequently in patients receiving certolizumab than in controls. These adverse reactions occurred more frequently among patients with a baseline history of hypertension and among patients receiving concomitant corticosteroids and non-steroidal anti-inflammatory drugs). Products include:
Nasonex **3166**

Mumps Virus Vaccine, Live (No data is available on the response to vaccinations or the secondary transmission of infection by live vaccines in patients receiving certolizumab pegol. Do not administer live vaccines or attenuated vaccines concurrently with certolizumab pegol). Products include:
Mumpsvax **2218**

Muromonab-CD3 (Patients treated with certolizumab are at increased risk for developing serious infections that may lead to hospitalization or death. Most patients who developed these infections were taking concomitant immunosuppressants such as methotrexate or corticosteroids). Products include:
Orthoclone OKT3 .... **949**

Mycophenolate Mofetil (Patients treated with certolizumab are at increased risk for developing serious infections that may lead to hospitalization or death. Most patients who developed these infections were taking concomitant immunosuppressants such as methotrexate or corticosteroids).
No products indexed under this heading.

Nabumetone (Hypertensive adverse reactions were observed more frequently in patients receiving certolizumab than in controls. These adverse reactions occurred more frequently among patients with a baseline history of hypertension and among patients receiving concomitant corticosteroids and non-steroidal anti-inflammatory drugs).
No products indexed under this heading.

Naproxen (Hypertensive adverse reactions were observed more frequently in patients receiving certolizumab than in controls. These adverse reactions occurred more frequently among patients with a baseline history of hypertension and among patients receiving concomitant corticosteroids and non-steroidal anti-inflammatory drugs). Products include:
EC-Naprosyn **2850**
Naprosyn **2850**
Anaprox/Naprosyn **2850**

Naproxen Sodium (Hypertensive adverse reactions were observed more frequently in patients receiving certolizumab than in controls. These adverse reactions occurred more frequently among patients with a baseline history of hypertension and among patients receiving concomitant corticosteroids and non-steroidal anti-inflammatory drugs). Products include:
Anaprox **2850**
Anaprox DS **2850**
Treximet **1681**

Natalizumab (An increased risk of serious infections has been seen in clinical studies of other TNF-blocking agents used in combination with anakinra or abatacept, with no added benefit. Formal drug interaction studies have not been performed with rituximab or natalizumab. Because of the nature of the adverse events seen with these combinations with TNF blocker therapy, similar toxicities may also result from the use of certolizumab in these combinations. There is not enough information to assess the safety and efficacy of such combination therapy. Therefore, the use of certolizumab in combination with anakinra, abatacept, rituximab, or natalizumab is not recommended).
No products indexed under this heading.

Oxaprozin (Hypertensive adverse reactions were observed more frequently in patients receiving certolizumab than in controls. These adverse reactions occurred more frequently among patients with a baseline history of hypertension and among patients receiving concomitant corticosteroids and non-steroidal anti-inflammatory drugs).
No products indexed under this heading.

Phenylbutazone (Hypertensive adverse reactions were observed more frequently in patients receiving certolizumab than in controls. These adverse reactions occurred more frequently among patients with a baseline history of hypertension and among patients receiving concomitant corticosteroids and non-steroidal anti-inflammatory drugs).
No products indexed under this heading.

Piroxicam (Hypertensive adverse reactions were observed more frequently in patients receiving certolizumab than in controls. These adverse reactions occurred more frequently among patients with a baseline history of hypertension and among patients receiving concomitant corticosteroids and non-steroidal anti-inflammatory drugs).
No products indexed under this heading.

Poliovirus Vaccine, Live, Oral, Trivalent, Types 1,2,3 (Sabin) (No data is available on the response to vaccinations or the secondary transmission of infection by live vaccines in patients receiving certolizumab pegol. Do not administer live vaccines or attenuated vaccines concurrently with certolizumab pegol).
No products indexed under this heading.

Prednisolone (Patients treated with certolizumab are at increased risk for developing serious infections that may lead to hospitalization or death. Most patients who developed these infections were taking concomitant immunosuppressants such as methotrexate or corticosteroids. Hypertensive adverse reactions were observed more frequently in patients receiving certolizumab than in controls. These adverse reactions occurred more frequently among patients with a baseline history of hypertension and among patients receiving concomitant corticosteroids and non-steroidal anti-inflammatory drugs).
No products indexed under this heading.

Prednisolone Acetate (Patients treated with certolizumab are at increased risk for developing serious infections that may lead to hospitalization or death. Most patients who developed these infections were taking concomitant immunosuppressants such as methotrexate or corticosteroids. Hypertensive adverse reactions were observed more frequently in patients receiving certolizumab than in controls. These adverse reactions occurred more frequently among patients with a baseline history of hypertension and among patients receiving concomitant corticosteroids and non-steroidal anti-inflammatory drugs). Products include:
Blephamide .... ⊙**212**, ⊙**214**
Pred Forte .... ⊙**225**
Pred Mild .... ⊙**230**
Pred-G .... ⊙**226**, ⊙**227**

Prednisolone Sodium Phosphate (Patients treated with certolizumab are at increased risk for developing serious infections that may lead to hospitalization or death. Most patients who developed these infections were taking concomitant immunosuppressants such as methotrexate or corticosteroids. Hypertensive adverse reactions were observed more frequently in patients receiving certolizumab than in controls. These adverse reactions occurred more frequently among patients with a baseline history of hypertension and among patients receiving concomitant corticosteroids and non-steroidal anti-inflammatory drugs).
No products indexed under this heading.

Prednisolone Tebutate (Patients treated with certolizumab are at increased risk for developing serious infections that may lead to hospitalization or death. Most patients who developed these infections were taking concomitant immunosuppressants such as methotrexate or corticosteroids. Hypertensive adverse reactions were observed more frequently in patients receiving certolizumab than in controls. These adverse reactions occurred more frequently among patients with a baseline history of hypertension and among patients receiving concomitant corticosteroids and non-steroidal anti-inflammatory drugs).
No products indexed under this heading.

Prednisone (Patients treated with certolizumab are at increased risk for developing serious infections that may lead to hospitalization or death. Most patients who developed these infections were taking concomitant immunosuppressants such as methotrexate or corticosteroids. Hypertensive adverse reactions were observed more frequently in patients receiving certolizumab than in controls. These adverse reactions occurred more frequently among patients with a baseline history of hypertension and among patients receiving concomitant corticosteroids and non-steroidal anti-inflammatory drugs).
No products indexed under this heading.

Prednisone sodium phosphate (Patients treated with certolizumab are at increased risk for developing serious infections that may lead to hospitalization or death. Most patients who developed these infections were taking concomitant immunosuppressants such as methotrexate or corticosteroids. Hypertensive adverse reactions were observed more frequently in patients receiving certolizumab than in controls. These adverse reactions occurred more frequently among patients with a baseline history of hypertension and among patients receiving concomitant corticosteroids and non-steroidal anti-inflammatory drugs).
No products indexed under this heading.

IMPORTANT NOTE: Always consult each drug listing in the patient's regimen for possible interactions.

Aluminum Hydroxide (Concurrent administration of ciprofloxacin with multivalent cation-containing products, such as magnesium/aluminum antacids, may substantially decrease its absorption, resulting in serum and urine levels considerably lower than desired. Ciprofloxacin may be taken two hours before or six hours after taking magnesium or aluminum containing antacids. Concurrent administration of antacids containing magnesium hydroxide or aluminum hydroxide may reduce the bioavailability of ciprofloxacin by as much as 90%).
No products indexed under this heading.

Aluminum Hydroxide Preparations (Concurrent administration of ciprofloxacin with multivalent cation-containing products may substantially decrease its absorption, resulting in serum and urine levels considerably lower than desired).
No products indexed under this heading.

Aluminum Sulfate (Concurrent administration of ciprofloxacin with multivalent cation-containing products may substantially decrease its absorption, resulting in serum and urine levels considerably lower than desired).
No products indexed under this heading.

Aminophylline (Ciprofloxacin is an inhibitor of the hepatic CYP1A2 enzyme pathway. Co-administration of ciprofloxacin and other drugs primarily metabolized by CYP1A2, such as methylxanthines, results in increased plasma concentrations of co-administered drug and could lead to clinically significant pharmacodynamic side effects of the co-administered drug).
No products indexed under this heading.

Amiodarone Hydrochloride (In general, elderly patients may be more susceptible to drug-associated effects on the QT interval. Therefore, precautions should be taken when using ciprofloxacin with concomitant drugs that can result in prolongation of the QT interval).
No products indexed under this heading.

Amitriptyline Hydrochloride (In general, elderly patients may be more susceptible to drug-associated effects on the QT interval. Therefore, precautions should be taken when using ciprofloxacin with concomitant drugs that can result in prolongation of the QT interval).
No products indexed under this heading.

Amoxapine (In general, elderly patients may be more susceptible to drug-associated effects on the QT interval. Therefore, precautions should be taken when using ciprofloxacin with concomitant drugs that can result in prolongation of the QT interval).
No products indexed under this heading.

Anagrelide Hydrochloride (Ciprofloxacin is an inhibitor of the hepatic CYP1A2 enzyme pathway. Co-administration of ciprofloxacin and other drugs primarily metabolized by CYP1A2 results in increased plasma concentrations of the co-administered drug and could lead to clinically significant pharmacodynamic side effects of the co-administered drug).
No products indexed under this heading.

Anisindione (Ciprofloxacin has been reported to enhance the effects of the oral anticoagulant warfarin or its derivatives. When these products are administered concomitantly, prothrombin time or other suitable coagulant tests should be closely monitored).
No products indexed under this heading.

Astemizole (In general, elderly patients may be more susceptible to drug-associated effects on the QT interval. Therefore, precautions should be taken when using ciprofloxacin with concomitant drugs that can result in prolongation of the QT interval).
No products indexed under this heading.

Beclomethasone Dipropionate (Fluoroquinolones, including ciprofloxacin, are associated with an increased risk of tendinitis and tendon rupture in all ages. This adverse reaction most frequently involves the Achilles tendon, and rupture of the Achilles tendon may require surgical repair. Tendinitis and tendon rupture in the rotator cuff (the shoulder), the hand, the biceps, the thumb, and other tendon sites have also been reported. The risk of developing fluoroquinolone-associated tendinitis and tendon rupture is further increased in older patients usually over 60 years of age, in patients taking corticosteroid drugs, and in patients with kidney, heart or lung transplants). Products include:
Qvar 3398

Beclomethasone Dipropionate Monohydrate (Fluoroquinolones, including ciprofloxacin, are associated with an increased risk of tendinitis and tendon rupture in all ages. This adverse reaction most frequently involves the Achilles tendon, and rupture of the Achilles tendon may require surgical repair. Tendinitis and tendon rupture in the rotator cuff (the shoulder), the hand, the biceps, the thumb, and other tendon sites have also been reported. The risk of developing fluoroquinolone-associated tendinitis and tendon rupture is further increased in older patients usually over 60 years of age, in patients taking corticosteroid drugs, and in patients with kidney, heart or lung transplants). Products include:
Beconase AQ 1386

Betamethasone (Fluoroquinolones, including ciprofloxacin, are associated with an increased risk of tendinitis and tendon rupture in all ages. This adverse reaction most frequently involves the Achilles tendon, and rupture of the Achilles tendon may require surgical repair. Tendinitis and tendon rupture in the rotator cuff (the shoulder), the hand, the biceps, the thumb, and other tendon sites have also been reported. The risk of developing fluoroquinolone-associated tendinitis and tendon rupture is further increased in older patients usually over 60 years of age, in patients taking corticosteroid drugs, and in patients with kidney, heart or lung transplants).
No products indexed under this heading.

Betamethasone Acetate (Fluoroquinolones, including ciprofloxacin, are associated with an increased risk of tendinitis and tendon rupture in all ages. This adverse reaction most frequently involves the Achilles tendon, and rupture of the Achilles tendon may require surgical repair. Tendinitis and tendon rupture in the rotator cuff (the shoulder), the hand, the biceps, the thumb, and other tendon sites have also been reported. The risk of developing fluoroquinolone-associated tendinitis and tendon rupture is further increased in older patients usually over 60 years of age, in patients taking corticosteroid drugs, and in patients with kidney, heart or lung transplants).
No products indexed under this heading.

Betamethasone Benzoate (Fluoroquinolones, including ciprofloxacin, are associated with an increased risk of tendinitis and tendon rupture in all ages. This adverse reaction most frequently involves the Achilles tendon, and rupture of the Achilles tendon may require surgical repair. Tendinitis and tendon rupture in the rotator cuff (the shoulder), the hand, the biceps, the thumb, and other tendon sites have also been reported. The risk of developing fluoroquinolone-associated tendinitis and tendon rupture is further increased in older patients usually over 60 years

of age, in patients taking corticosteroid drugs, and in patients with kidney, heart or lung transplants).
No products indexed under this heading.

Betamethasone Dipropionate (Fluoroquinolones, including ciprofloxacin, are associated with an increased risk of tendinitis and tendon rupture in all ages. This adverse reaction most frequently involves the Achilles tendon, and rupture of the Achilles tendon may require surgical repair. Tendinitis and tendon rupture in the rotator cuff (the shoulder), the hand, the biceps, the thumb, and other tendon sites have also been reported. The risk of developing fluoroquinolone-associated tendinitis and tendon rupture is further increased in older patients usually over 60 years of age, in patients taking corticosteroid drugs, and in patients with kidney, heart or lung transplants). Products include:
Diprolene Lotion 0.05% 3108
Diprolene Ointment 0.05% 3109
Diprolene AF Cream 0.05% 3107
Lotrisone 3163

Betamethasone Sodium Phosphate (Fluoroquinolones, including ciprofloxacin, are associated with an increased risk of tendinitis and tendon rupture in all ages. This adverse reaction most frequently involves the Achilles tendon, and rupture of the Achilles tendon may require surgical repair. Tendinitis and tendon rupture in the rotator cuff (the shoulder), the hand, the biceps, the thumb, and other tendon sites have also been reported. The risk of developing fluoroquinolone-associated tendinitis and tendon rupture is further increased in older patients usually over 60 years of age, in patients taking corticosteroid drugs, and in patients with kidney, heart or lung transplants).
No products indexed under this heading.

Betamethasone Valerate (Fluoroquinolones, including ciprofloxacin, are associated with an increased risk of tendinitis and tendon rupture in all ages. This adverse reaction most frequently involves the Achilles tendon, and rupture of the Achilles tendon may require surgical repair. Tendinitis and tendon rupture in the rotator cuff (the shoulder), the hand, the biceps, the thumb, and other tendon sites have also been reported. The risk of developing fluoroquinolone-associated tendinitis and tendon rupture is further increased in older patients usually over 60 years of age, in patients taking corticosteroid drugs, and in patients with kidney, heart or lung transplants). Products include:
Luxiq 3321

Bretylium Tosylate (In general, elderly patients may be more susceptible to drug-associated effects on the QT interval. Therefore, precautions should be taken when using ciprofloxacin with concomitant drugs that can result in prolongation of the QT interval).
No products indexed under this heading.

Budesonide (Fluoroquinolones, including ciprofloxacin, are associated with an increased risk of tendinitis and tendon rupture in all ages. This adverse reaction most frequently involves the Achilles tendon, and rupture of the Achilles tendon may require surgical repair. Tendinitis and tendon rupture in the rotator cuff (the shoulder), the hand, the biceps, the thumb, and other tendon sites have also been reported. The risk of developing fluoroquinolone-associated tendinitis and tendon rupture is further increased in older patients usually over 60 years of age, in patients taking corticosteroid drugs, and in patients with kidney, heart or lung transplants). Products include:
Pulmicort Flexhaler 714
Symbicort 80/4.5 720

Symbicort 160/4.5 720

Buspirone Hydrochloride (In general, elderly patients may be more susceptible to drug-associated effects on the QT interval. Therefore, precautions should be taken when using ciprofloxacin with concomitant drugs that can result in prolongation of the QT interval).
No products indexed under this heading.

Caffeine (Ciprofloxacin is an inhibitor of the hepatic CYP1A2 enzyme pathway. Co-administration of ciprofloxacin and other drugs primarily metabolized by CYP1A2 results in increased plasma concentrations of the co-administered drug and could lead to clinically significant pharmacodynamic side effects of the co-administered drug).
No products indexed under this heading.

Caffeine Anhydrous (Ciprofloxacin is an inhibitor of the hepatic CYP1A2 enzyme pathway. Co-administration of ciprofloxacin and other drugs primarily metabolized by CYP1A2 results in increased plasma concentrations of the co-administered drug and could lead to clinically significant pharmacodynamic side effects of the co-administered drug).
No products indexed under this heading.

Caffeine Citrate (Ciprofloxacin is an inhibitor of the hepatic CYP1A2 enzyme pathway. Co-administration of ciprofloxacin and other drugs primarily metabolized by CYP1A2 results in increased plasma concentrations of the co-administered drug and could lead to clinically significant pharmacodynamic side effects of the co-administered drug).
No products indexed under this heading.

Caffeine-containing medications (Ciprofloxacin is an inhibitor of the hepatic CYP1A2 enzyme pathway. Co-administration of ciprofloxacin and other drugs primarily metabolized by CYP1A2 results in increased plasma concentrations of the co-administered drug and could lead to clinically significant pharmacodynamic side effects of the co-administered drug).
No products indexed under this heading.

Caffeine Sodium Benzoate (Ciprofloxacin is an inhibitor of the hepatic CYP1A2 enzyme pathway. Co-administration of ciprofloxacin and other drugs primarily metabolized by CYP1A2 results in increased plasma concentrations of the co-administered drug and could lead to clinically significant pharmacodynamic side effects of the co-administered drug).
No products indexed under this heading.

Calcium (Concurrent administration of ciprofloxacin with multivalent cation-containing products may substantially decrease its absorption, resulting in serum and urine levels considerably lower than desired). Products include:
BoneMate Plus 3454
Cardio Basics 3455
Chelated Mineral 3476
CitraNatal 90 DHA Capsules 2332
CitraNatal Harmony 2332

Calcium (Oyster Shell) (Concurrent administration of ciprofloxacin with multivalent cation-containing products may substantially decrease its absorption, resulting in serum and urine levels considerably lower than desired).
No products indexed under this heading.

Calcium Acetate (Concurrent administration of ciprofloxacin with multivalent cation-containing products may substantially decrease its absorption, resulting in serum and urine levels considerably lower than desired).
No products indexed under this heading.

Calcium Ascorbate (Concurrent administration of ciprofloxacin with multivalent cation-containing products may

---

IMPORTANT NOTE: Always consult each drug listing in the patient's regimen for possible interactions.

Cipro I.V. Interactions Index 326

substantially decrease its absorption, resulting in serum and urine levels considerably lower than desired). Products include:
Bio-C ... 3454
Procosa II ... 3476
Proflavanol 90 ... 3476

Calcium Carbaspirin (Concurrent administration of ciprofloxacin with multivalent cation-containing products may substantially decrease its absorption, resulting in serum and urine levels considerably lower than desired).
No products indexed under this heading.

Calcium Carbonate (Concurrent administration of ciprofloxacin with multivalent cation-containing products, such as magnesium/aluminum antacids, may substantially decrease its absorption, resulting in serum and urine levels considerably lower than desired. Ciprofloxacin may be taken two hours before or six hours after taking magnesium or aluminum containing antacids. Concurrent administration of antacids containing magnesium hydroxide or aluminum hydroxide may reduce the bioavailability of ciprofloxacin by as much as 90%). Products include:
Chelated Mineral ... 3476
Pepcid Complete ... 1822
Extra Strength Rolaids Softchews Vanilla Creme ... 2045

Calcium Carbonate, Precipitated (Concurrent administration of ciprofloxacin with multivalent cation-containing products may substantially decrease its absorption, resulting in serum and urine levels considerably lower than desired).
No products indexed under this heading.

Calcium Caseinate (Concurrent administration of ciprofloxacin with multivalent cation-containing products may substantially decrease its absorption, resulting in serum and urine levels considerably lower than desired).
No products indexed under this heading.

Calcium Chloride (Concurrent administration of ciprofloxacin with products containing calcium may substantially decrease its absorption, resulting in serum and urine levels considerably lower than desired. Ciprofloxacin should be administered at least 2 hours before or 6 hours after products containing calcium).
No products indexed under this heading.

Calcium Citrate (Concurrent administration of ciprofloxacin with products containing calcium may substantially decrease its absorption, resulting in serum and urine levels considerably lower than desired. Ciprofloxacin should be administered at least 2 hours before or 6 hours after products containing calcium). Products include:
Active Calcium ... 3476
Chelated Mineral ... 3476
CitraNatal 90 DHA Capsules ... 2332
CitraNatal Assure ... 2332
CitraNatal Harmony ... 2332
CitraNatal Rx ... 2332

Calcium Disodium Edetate (Concurrent administration of ciprofloxacin with multivalent cation-containing products may substantially decrease its absorption, resulting in serum and urine levels considerably lower than desired).
No products indexed under this heading.

Calcium Glubionate (Concurrent administration of ciprofloxacin with products containing calcium may substantially decrease its absorption, resulting in serum and urine levels considerably lower than desired. Ciprofloxacin should be administered at least 2 hours before or 6 hours after products containing calcium).
No products indexed under this heading.

Calcium Gluconate (Concurrent administration of ciprofloxacin with multivalent cation-containing products may substantially decrease its absorption, resulting in serum and urine levels considerably lower than desired).
No products indexed under this heading.

Calcium Glycerophosphate (Concurrent administration of ciprofloxacin with multivalent cation-containing products may substantially decrease its absorption, resulting in serum and urine levels considerably lower than desired).
No products indexed under this heading.

Calcium Iodide (Concurrent administration of ciprofloxacin with multivalent cation-containing products may substantially decrease its absorption, resulting in serum and urine levels considerably lower than desired).
No products indexed under this heading.

Calcium Lactate (Concurrent administration of ciprofloxacin with multivalent cation-containing products may substantially decrease its absorption, resulting in serum and urine levels considerably lower than desired).
No products indexed under this heading.

Calcium Levulinate (Concurrent administration of ciprofloxacin with multivalent cation-containing products may substantially decrease its absorption, resulting in serum and urine levels considerably lower than desired).
No products indexed under this heading.

Calcium Pantothenate (Concurrent administration of ciprofloxacin with multivalent cation-containing products may substantially decrease its absorption, resulting in serum and urine levels considerably lower than desired). Products include:
Cardio Basics ... 3455

Calcium Phosphate (Concurrent administration of ciprofloxacin with multivalent cation-containing products may substantially decrease its absorption, resulting in serum and urine levels considerably lower than desired).
No products indexed under this heading.

Calcium Phosphate, Dibasic (Concurrent administration of ciprofloxacin with multivalent cation-containing products may substantially decrease its absorption, resulting in serum and urine levels considerably lower than desired).
No products indexed under this heading.

Calcium Phosphate, Tribasic (Concurrent administration of ciprofloxacin with multivalent cation-containing products may substantially decrease its absorption, resulting in serum and urine levels considerably lower than desired).
No products indexed under this heading.

Calcium Phosphorus Preparations (Concurrent administration of ciprofloxacin with multivalent cation-containing products may substantially decrease its absorption, resulting in serum and urine levels considerably lower than desired).
No products indexed under this heading.

Calcium Polycarbophil (Concurrent administration of ciprofloxacin with multivalent cation-containing products may substantially decrease its absorption, resulting in serum and urine levels considerably lower than desired).
No products indexed under this heading.

Calcium Salts (Concurrent administration of ciprofloxacin with multivalent cation-containing products may substantially decrease its absorption, resulting in serum and urine levels considerably lower than desired).
No products indexed under this heading.

Calcium Sodium Alginate Fiber (Concurrent administration of ciprofloxacin with multivalent cation-containing products may substantially decrease its absorption, resulting in serum and urine levels considerably lower than desired).
No products indexed under this heading.

Calcium Undecylenate (Concurrent administration of ciprofloxacin with multivalent cation-containing products may substantially decrease its absorption, resulting in serum and urine levels considerably lower than desired).
No products indexed under this heading.

Celecoxib (Non-steroidal anti-inflammatory drugs in combination of very high doses of quinolones have been shown to provoke convulsions in pre-clinical studies). Products include:
Celebrex ... 3272

Chlordiazepoxide (In general, elderly patients may be more susceptible to drug-associated effects on the QT interval. Therefore, precautions should be taken when using ciprofloxacin with concomitant drugs that can result in prolongation of the QT interval).
No products indexed under this heading.

Chlordiazepoxide Hydrochloride (In general, elderly patients may be more susceptible to drug-associated effects on the QT interval. Therefore, precautions should be taken when using ciprofloxacin with concomitant drugs that can result in prolongation of the QT interval).
No products indexed under this heading.

Chlorpromazine (In general, elderly patients may be more susceptible to drug-associated effects on the QT interval. Therefore, precautions should be taken when using ciprofloxacin with concomitant drugs that can result in prolongation of the QT interval).
No products indexed under this heading.

Chlorpromazine Hydrochloride (In general, elderly patients may be more susceptible to drug-associated effects on the QT interval. Therefore, precautions should be taken when using ciprofloxacin with concomitant drugs that can result in prolongation of the QT interval).
No products indexed under this heading.

Chlorprothixene (In general, elderly patients may be more susceptible to drug-associated effects on the QT interval. Therefore, precautions should be taken when using ciprofloxacin with concomitant drugs that can result in prolongation of the QT interval).
No products indexed under this heading.

Chlorprothixene Hydrochloride (In general, elderly patients may be more susceptible to drug-associated effects on the QT interval. Therefore, precautions should be taken when using ciprofloxacin with concomitant drugs that can result in prolongation of the QT interval).
No products indexed under this heading.

Ciclesonide (Fluoroquinolones, including ciprofloxacin, are associated with an increased risk of tendinitis and tendon rupture in all ages. This adverse reaction most frequently involves the Achilles tendon, and rupture of the Achilles tendon may require surgical repair. Tendinitis and tendon rupture in the rotator cuff (the shoulder), the hand, the biceps, the thumb, and other tendon sites have also been reported. The risk of developing fluoroquinolone-associated tendinitis and tendon rupture is further increased in older patients usually over 60 years of age, in patients taking corticosteroid drugs, and in patients with kidney, heart or lung transplants).
No products indexed under this heading.

Cimetidine Hydrochloride (Ciprofloxacin is an inhibitor of the hepatic CYP1A2 enzyme pathway. Co-administration of ciprofloxacin and other drugs primarily metabolized by CYP1A2 results in increased plasma concentrations of the co-administered drug and could lead to clinically significant pharmacodynamic side effects of the co-administered drug).
No products indexed under this heading.

Ciprofloxacin Hydrochloride (Ciprofloxacin is an inhibitor of the hepatic CYP1A2 enzyme pathway. Co-administration of ciprofloxacin and other drugs primarily metabolized by CYP1A2 results in increased plasma concentrations of the co-administered drug and could lead to clinically significant pharmacodynamic side effects of the co-administered drug). Products include:
Cipro ... 3073

Clomipramine Hydrochloride (In general, elderly patients may be more susceptible to drug-associated effects on the QT interval. Therefore, precautions should be taken when using ciprofloxacin with concomitant drugs that can result in prolongation of the QT interval).
No products indexed under this heading.

Clopidogrel Bisulfate (Ciprofloxacin is an inhibitor of the hepatic CYP1A2 enzyme pathway. Co-administration of ciprofloxacin and other drugs primarily metabolized by CYP1A2 results in increased plasma concentrations of the co-administered drug and could lead to clinically significant pharmacodynamic side effects of the co-administered drug). Products include:
Plavix ... 3027

Clorazepate Dipotassium (In general, elderly patients may be more susceptible to drug-associated effects on the QT interval. Therefore, precautions should be taken when using ciprofloxacin with concomitant drugs that can result in prolongation of the QT interval).
No products indexed under this heading.

Clozapine (In general, elderly patients may be more susceptible to drug-associated effects on the QT interval. Therefore, precautions should be taken when using ciprofloxacin with concomitant drugs that can result in prolongation of the QT interval).
No products indexed under this heading.

Cortisone Acetate (Fluoroquinolones, including ciprofloxacin, are associated with an increased risk of tendinitis and tendon rupture in all ages. This adverse reaction most frequently involves the Achilles tendon, and rupture of the Achilles tendon may require surgical repair. Tendinitis and tendon rupture in the rotator cuff (the shoulder), the hand, the biceps, the thumb, and other tendon sites have also been reported. The risk of developing fluoroquinolone-associated tendinitis and tendon rupture is further increased in older patients usually over 60 years of age, in patients taking corticosteroid drugs, and in patients with kidney, heart or lung transplants).
No products indexed under this heading.

Cyclobenzaprine (Ciprofloxacin is an inhibitor of the hepatic CYP1A2 enzyme pathway. Co-administration of ciprofloxacin and other drugs primarily metabolized by CYP1A2 results in increased plasma concentrations of the co-administered drug and could lead to clinically significant pharmacodynamic side effects of the co-administered drug).
No products indexed under this heading.

Cyclobenzaprine Hydrochloride (Ciprofloxacin is an inhibitor of the hepatic CYP1A2 enzyme pathway. Co-administration of ciprofloxacin and oth-

er drugs primarily metabolized by CYP1A2 results in increased plasma concentrations of the co-administered drug and could lead to clinically significant pharmacodynamic side effects of the co-administered drug). Products include:

Cyclosporine (Ciprofloxacin has been associated with transient elevations in serum creatinine in patients receiving cyclosporine concomitantly). Products include:

Desipramine Hydrochloride (In general, elderly patients may be more susceptible to drug-associated effects on the QT interval. Therefore, precautions should be taken when using ciprofloxacin with concomitant drugs that can result in prolongation of the QT interval).
No products indexed under this heading.

Desoximetasone (Fluoroquinolones, including ciprofloxacin, are associated with an increased risk of tendinitis and tendon rupture in all ages. This adverse reaction most frequently involves the Achilles tendon, and rupture of the Achilles tendon may require surgical repair. Tendinitis and tendon rupture in the rotator cuff (the shoulder), the hand, the biceps, the thumb, and other tendon sites have also been reported. The risk of developing fluoroquinolone-associated tendinitis and tendon rupture is further increased in older patients usually over 60 years of age, in patients taking corticosteroid drugs, and in patients with kidney, heart or lung transplants).
No products indexed under this heading.

Dexamethasone (Fluoroquinolones, including ciprofloxacin, are associated with an increased risk of tendinitis and tendon rupture in all ages. This adverse reaction most frequently involves the Achilles tendon, and rupture of the Achilles tendon may require surgical repair. Tendinitis and tendon rupture in the rotator cuff (the shoulder), the hand, the biceps, the thumb, and other tendon sites have also been reported. The risk of developing fluoroquinolone-associated tendinitis and tendon rupture is further increased in older patients usually over 60 years of age, in patients taking corticosteroid drugs, and in patients with kidney, heart or lung transplants). Products include:

Dexamethasone Acetate (Fluoroquinolones, including ciprofloxacin, are associated with an increased risk of tendinitis and tendon rupture in all ages. This adverse reaction most frequently involves the Achilles tendon, and rupture of the Achilles tendon may require surgical repair. Tendinitis and tendon rupture in the rotator cuff (the shoulder), the hand, the biceps, the thumb, and other tendon sites have also been reported. The risk of developing fluoroquinolone-associated tendinitis and tendon rupture is further increased in older patients usually over 60 years of age, in patients taking corticosteroid drugs, and in patients with kidney, heart or lung transplants).
No products indexed under this heading.

Dexamethasone Phosphate (Fluoroquinolones, including ciprofloxacin, are associated with an increased risk of tendinitis and tendon rupture in all ages. This adverse reaction most frequently involves the Achilles tendon, and rupture of the Achilles tendon may require surgical repair. Tendinitis and tendon

rupture in the rotator cuff (the shoulder), the hand, the biceps, the thumb, and other tendon sites have also been reported. The risk of developing fluoroquinolone-associated tendinitis and tendon rupture is further increased in older patients usually over 60 years of age, in patients taking corticosteroid drugs, and in patients with kidney, heart or lung transplants).
No products indexed under this heading.

Dexamethasone Sodium (Fluoroquinolones, including ciprofloxacin, are associated with an increased risk of tendinitis and tendon rupture in all ages. This adverse reaction most frequently involves the Achilles tendon, and rupture of the Achilles tendon may require surgical repair. Tendinitis and tendon rupture in the rotator cuff (the shoulder), the hand, the biceps, the thumb, and other tendon sites have also been reported. The risk of developing fluoroquinolone-associated tendinitis and tendon rupture is further increased in older patients usually over 60 years of age, in patients taking corticosteroid drugs, and in patients with kidney, heart or lung transplants).
No products indexed under this heading.

Dexamethasone Sodium Phosphate (Fluoroquinolones, including ciprofloxacin, are associated with an increased risk of tendinitis and tendon rupture in all ages. This adverse reaction most frequently involves the Achilles tendon, and rupture of the Achilles tendon may require surgical repair. Tendinitis and tendon rupture in the rotator cuff (the shoulder), the hand, the biceps, the thumb, and other tendon sites have also been reported. The risk of developing fluoroquinolone-associated tendinitis and tendon rupture is further increased in older patients usually over 60 years of age, in patients taking corticosteroid drugs, and in patients with kidney, heart or lung transplants).
No products indexed under this heading.

Dexamethasone Sodium Phosphate Injection (Fluoroquinolones, including ciprofloxacin, are associated with an increased risk of tendinitis and tendon rupture in all ages. This adverse reaction most frequently involves the Achilles tendon, and rupture of the Achilles tendon may require surgical repair. Tendinitis and tendon rupture in the rotator cuff (the shoulder), the hand, the biceps, the thumb, and other tendon sites have also been reported. The risk of developing fluoroquinolone-associated tendinitis and tendon rupture is further increased in older patients usually over 60 years of age, in patients taking corticosteroid drugs, and in patients with kidney, heart or lung transplants).
No products indexed under this heading.

Diazepam (In general, elderly patients may be more susceptible to drug-associated effects on the QT interval. Therefore, precautions should be taken when using ciprofloxacin with concomitant drugs that can result in prolongation of the QT interval). Products include:

Diclofenac Epolamine (Non-steroidal anti-inflammatory drugs in combination of very high doses of quinolones have been shown to provoke convulsions in pre-clinical studies). Products include:

Diclofenac Potassium (Non-steroidal anti-inflammatory drugs in combination of very high doses of quinolones have been shown to provoke convulsions in pre-clinical studies).
No products indexed under this heading.

Diclofenac Sodium (Non-steroidal anti-inflammatory drugs in combination of very high doses of quinolones have been shown to provoke convulsions in pre-clinical studies).
No products indexed under this heading.

Dicumarol (Ciprofloxacin has been reported to enhance the effects of the oral anticoagulant warfarin or its derivatives. When these products are administered concomitantly, prothrombin time or other suitable coagulant tests should be closely monitored).
No products indexed under this heading.

Didanosine (Concurrent administration of ciprofloxacin with multivalent cation-containing products, such as didanosine, chewable/buffered tablets or pediatric powder, may substantially decrease its absorption, resulting in serum and urine levels considerably lower than desired. Ciprofloxacin should be administered at least 2 hours before or 6 hours after didanosine chewable/buffered tablets or pediatric powder for oral solution).
No products indexed under this heading.

Diflorasone Diacetate (Fluoroquinolones, including ciprofloxacin, are associated with an increased risk of tendinitis and tendon rupture in all ages. This adverse reaction most frequently involves the Achilles tendon, and rupture of the Achilles tendon may require surgical repair. Tendinitis and tendon rupture in the rotator cuff (the shoulder), the hand, the biceps, the thumb, and other tendon sites have also been reported. The risk of developing fluoroquinolone-associated tendinitis and tendon rupture is further increased in older patients usually over 60 years of age, in patients taking corticosteroid drugs, and in patients with kidney, heart or lung transplants).
No products indexed under this heading.

Diltiazem Hydrochloride (Ciprofloxacin is an inhibitor of the hepatic CYP1A2 enzyme pathway. Co-administration of ciprofloxacin and other drugs primarily metabolized by CYP1A2 results in increased plasma concentrations of the co-administered drug and could lead to clinically significant pharmacodynamic side effects of the co-administered drug). Products include:

Diltiazem Maleate (Ciprofloxacin is an inhibitor of the hepatic CYP1A2 enzyme pathway. Co-administration of ciprofloxacin and other drugs primarily metabolized by CYP1A2 results in increased plasma concentrations of the co-administered drug and could lead to clinically significant pharmacodynamic side effects of the co-administered drug).
No products indexed under this heading.

Disopyramide (In general, elderly patients may be more susceptible to drug-associated effects on the QT interval. Therefore, precautions should be taken when using ciprofloxacin with concomitant drugs that can result in prolongation of the QT interval).
No products indexed under this heading.

Disopyramide Phosphate (In general, elderly patients may be more susceptible to drug-associated effects on the QT interval. Therefore, precautions should be taken when using ciprofloxacin with concomitant drugs that can result in prolongation of the QT interval).
No products indexed under this heading.

Dofetilide (In general, elderly patients may be more susceptible to drug-associated effects on the QT interval. Therefore, precautions should be taken when using ciprofloxacin with concomitant drugs that can result in prolongation of the QT interval).
No products indexed under this heading.

Doxepin Hydrochloride (In general, elderly patients may be more susceptible to drug-associated effects on the QT interval. Therefore, precautions should be taken when using ciprofloxacin with concomitant drugs that can result in prolongation of the QT interval).
No products indexed under this heading.

Droperidol (In general, elderly patients may be more susceptible to drug-associated effects on the QT interval. Therefore, precautions should be taken when using ciprofloxacin with concomitant drugs that can result in prolongation of the QT interval).
No products indexed under this heading.

Dyphylline (Ciprofloxacin is an inhibitor of the hepatic CYP1A2 enzyme pathway. Co-administration of ciprofloxacin and other drugs primarily metabolized by CYP1A2, such as methylxanthines, results in increased plasma concentrations of co-administered drug and could lead to clinically significant pharmacodynamic side effects of the co-administered drug).
No products indexed under this heading.

Enoxacin (Ciprofloxacin is an inhibitor of the hepatic CYP1A2 enzyme pathway. Co-administration of ciprofloxacin and other drugs primarily metabolized by CYP1A2 results in increased plasma concentrations of the co-administered drug and could lead to clinically significant pharmacodynamic side effects of the co-administered drug).
No products indexed under this heading.

Erythromycin (In general, elderly patients may be more susceptible to drug-associated effects on the QT interval. Therefore, precautions should be taken when using ciprofloxacin with concomitant drugs that can result in prolongation of the QT interval).
No products indexed under this heading.

Erythromycin Estolate (In general, elderly patients may be more susceptible to drug-associated effects on the QT interval. Therefore, precautions should be taken when using ciprofloxacin with concomitant drugs that can result in prolongation of the QT interval).
No products indexed under this heading.

Erythromycin Ethylsuccinate (In general, elderly patients may be more susceptible to drug-associated effects on the QT interval. Therefore, precautions should be taken when using ciprofloxacin with concomitant drugs that can result in prolongation of the QT interval). Products include:

Erythromycin Gluceptate (In general, elderly patients may be more susceptible to drug-associated effects on the QT interval. Therefore, precautions should be taken when using ciprofloxacin with concomitant drugs that can result in prolongation of the QT interval).
No products indexed under this heading.

Erythromycin Lactobionate (In general, elderly patients may be more susceptible to drug-associated effects on the QT interval. Therefore, precautions should be taken when using ciprofloxacin with concomitant drugs that can result in prolongation of the QT interval).
No products indexed under this heading.

Erythromycin Stearate (In general, elderly patients may be more susceptible to drug-associated effects on the QT interval. Therefore, precautions should be taken when using ciprofloxacin with concomitant drugs that can result in prolongation of the QT interval).
No products indexed under this heading.

Estradiol (Ciprofloxacin is an inhibitor of the hepatic CYP1A2 enzyme pathway. Co-administration of ciprofloxacin and other drugs primarily metabolized

IMPORTANT NOTE: Always consult each drug listing in the patient's regimen for possible interactions.

Cipro I.V. Interactions Index 328

by CYP1A2 results in increased plasma concentrations of the co-administered drug and could lead to clinically significant pharmacodynamic side effects of the co-administered drug). Products include:
Activella 2561
Angeliq 831
Climara 841
Climara Pro 847
Divigel 3467
Estrasorb 1777
Vagifem 2589

Estradiol Benzoate (Ciprofloxacin is an inhibitor of the hepatic CYP1A2 enzyme pathway. Co-administration of ciprofloxacin and other drugs primarily metabolized by CYP1A2 results in increased plasma concentrations of the co-administered drug and could lead to clinically significant pharmacodynamic side effects of the co-administered drug).
No products indexed under this heading.

Estradiol Cypionate (Ciprofloxacin is an inhibitor of the hepatic CYP1A2 enzyme pathway. Co-administration of ciprofloxacin and other drugs primarily metabolized by CYP1A2 results in increased plasma concentrations of the co-administered drug and could lead to clinically significant pharmacodynamic side effects of the co-administered drug).
No products indexed under this heading.

Etodolac (Non-steroidal anti-inflammatory drugs in combination of very high doses of quinolones have been shown to provoke convulsions in pre-clinical studies).
No products indexed under this heading.

Fenoprofen Calcium (Non-steroidal anti-inflammatory drugs in combination of very high doses of quinolones have been shown to provoke convulsions in pre-clinical studies).
No products indexed under this heading.

Ferrous Fumarate (Concurrent administration of ciprofloxacin with products containing iron may substantially decrease its absorption, resulting in serum and urine levels considerably lower than desired. Ciprofloxacin should be administered at least 2 hours before or 6 hours after products containing iron). Products include:
PreNexa 3473

Ferrous Gluconate (Concurrent administration of ciprofloxacin with products containing iron may substantially decrease its absorption, resulting in serum and urine levels considerably lower than desired. Ciprofloxacin should be administered at least 2 hours before or 6 hours after products containing iron). Products include:
CitraNatal Assure 2332
CitraNatal Rx 2332

Ferrous Sulfate (Concurrent administration of ciprofloxacin with products containing iron may substantially decrease its absorption, resulting in serum and urine levels considerably lower than desired. Ciprofloxacin should be administered at least 2 hours before or 6 hours after products containing iron).
No products indexed under this heading.

Flecainide Acetate (In general, elderly patients may be more susceptible to drug-associated effects on the QT interval. Therefore, precautions should be taken when using ciprofloxacin with concomitant drugs that can result in prolongation of the QT interval).
No products indexed under this heading.

Fludrocortisone Acetate (Fluoroquinolones, including ciprofloxacin, are associated with an increased risk of tendinitis and tendon rupture in all ages. This adverse reaction most frequently involves the Achilles tendon, and rupture of the Achilles tendon may require surgical repair. Tendinitis and tendon rupture in the rotator cuff (the shoulder), the hand, the biceps, the thumb, and other tendon sites have also been reported. The risk of developing fluoroquinolone-associated tendinitis and tendon rupture is further increased in older patients usually over 60 years of age, in patients taking corticosteroid drugs, and in patients with kidney, heart or lung transplants).
No products indexed under this heading.

Flumethasone Pivalate (Fluoroquinolones, including ciprofloxacin, are associated with an increased risk of tendinitis and tendon rupture in all ages. This adverse reaction most frequently involves the Achilles tendon, and rupture of the Achilles tendon may require surgical repair. Tendinitis and tendon rupture in the rotator cuff (the shoulder), the hand, the biceps, the thumb, and other tendon sites have also been reported. The risk of developing fluoroquinolone-associated tendinitis and tendon rupture is further increased in older patients usually over 60 years of age, in patients taking corticosteroid drugs, and in patients with kidney, heart or lung transplants).
No products indexed under this heading.

Flunisolide Hemihydrate (Fluoroquinolones, including ciprofloxacin, are associated with an increased risk of tendinitis and tendon rupture in all ages. This adverse reaction most frequently involves the Achilles tendon, and rupture of the Achilles tendon may require surgical repair. Tendinitis and tendon rupture in the rotator cuff (the shoulder), the hand, the biceps, the thumb, and other tendon sites have also been reported. The risk of developing fluoroquinolone-associated tendinitis and tendon rupture is further increased in older patients usually over 60 years of age, in patients taking corticosteroid drugs, and in patients with kidney, heart or lung transplants).
No products indexed under this heading.

Fluphenazine Decanoate (In general, elderly patients may be more susceptible to drug-associated effects on the QT interval. Therefore, precautions should be taken when using ciprofloxacin with concomitant drugs that can result in prolongation of the QT interval).
No products indexed under this heading.

Fluphenazine Enanthate (In general, elderly patients may be more susceptible to drug-associated effects on the QT interval. Therefore, precautions should be taken when using ciprofloxacin with concomitant drugs that can result in prolongation of the QT interval).
No products indexed under this heading.

Fluphenazine Hydrochloride (In general, elderly patients may be more susceptible to drug-associated effects on the QT interval. Therefore, precautions should be taken when using ciprofloxacin with concomitant drugs that can result in prolongation of the QT interval).
No products indexed under this heading.

Flurbiprofen (Non-steroidal anti-inflammatory drugs in combination of very high doses of quinolones have been shown to provoke convulsions in pre-clinical studies).
No products indexed under this heading.

Flutamide (Ciprofloxacin is an inhibitor of the hepatic CYP1A2 enzyme pathway. Co-administration of ciprofloxacin and other drugs primarily metabolized by CYP1A2 results in increased plasma concentrations of the co-administered drug and could lead to clinically significant pharmacodynamic side effects of the co-administered drug).
No products indexed under this heading.

Fluticasone Furoate (Fluoroquinolones, including ciprofloxacin, are associated with an increased risk of tendinitis and tendon rupture in all ages. This adverse reaction most frequently involves the Achilles tendon, and rupture of the Achilles tendon may require surgical repair. Tendinitis and tendon rupture in the rotator cuff (the shoulder), the hand, the biceps, the thumb, and other tendon sites have also been reported. The risk of developing fluoroquinolone-associated tendinitis and tendon rupture is further increased in older patients usually over 60 years of age, in patients taking corticosteroid drugs, and in patients with kidney, heart or lung transplants). Products include:
Veramyst 1713

Fluticasone Propionate (Fluoroquinolones, including ciprofloxacin, are associated with an increased risk of tendinitis and tendon rupture in all ages. This adverse reaction most frequently involves the Achilles tendon, and rupture of the Achilles tendon may require surgical repair. Tendinitis and tendon rupture in the rotator cuff (the shoulder), the hand, the biceps, the thumb, and other tendon sites have also been reported. The risk of developing fluoroquinolone-associated tendinitis and tendon rupture is further increased in older patients usually over 60 years of age, in patients taking corticosteroid drugs, and in patients with kidney, heart or lung transplants). Products include:
Advair 100/50 1275
Advair 250/50 1275
Advair 500/50 1275
Advair HFA 45/21 1288
Advair HFA 115/21 1288
Advair HFA 230/21 1288
Flonase 1459
Flovent Diskus 1463
Flovent HFA 1470

Fluvoxamine Maleate (Ciprofloxacin is an inhibitor of the hepatic CYP1A2 enzyme pathway. Co-administration of ciprofloxacin and other drugs primarily metabolized by CYP1A2 results in increased plasma concentrations of the co-administered drug and could lead to clinically significant pharmacodynamic side effects of the co-administered drug).
No products indexed under this heading.

Fosphenytoin (Altered serum levels of phenytoin (increased and decreased) have been reported in patients receiving concomitant ciprofloxacin).
No products indexed under this heading.

Fosphenytoin Sodium (Altered serum levels of phenytoin (increased and decreased) have been reported in patients receiving concomitant ciprofloxacin).
No products indexed under this heading.

Glyburide (The concomitant administration of ciprofloxacin with the sulfonylurea glyburide has, on rare occasions, resulted in severe hypoglycemia).
No products indexed under this heading.

Grepafloxacin Hydrochloride (Ciprofloxacin is an inhibitor of the hepatic CYP1A2 enzyme pathway. Co-administration of ciprofloxacin and other drugs primarily metabolized by CYP1A2 results in increased plasma concentrations of the co-administered drug and could lead to clinically significant pharmacodynamic side effects of the co-administered drug).
No products indexed under this heading.

Haloperidol (In general, elderly patients may be more susceptible to drug-associated effects on the QT interval. Therefore, precautions should be taken when using ciprofloxacin with concomitant drugs that can result in prolongation of the QT interval).
No products indexed under this heading.

Haloperidol Decanoate (In general, elderly patients may be more susceptible to drug-associated effects on the QT interval. Therefore, precautions should be taken when using ciprofloxacin with concomitant drugs that can result in prolongation of the QT interval).
No products indexed under this heading.

Haloperidol Lactate (In general, elderly patients may be more susceptible to drug-associated effects on the QT interval. Therefore, precautions should be taken when using ciprofloxacin with concomitant drugs that can result in prolongation of the QT interval).
No products indexed under this heading.

Hydrocortisone (Fluoroquinolones, including ciprofloxacin, are associated with an increased risk of tendinitis and tendon rupture in all ages. This adverse reaction most frequently involves the Achilles tendon, and rupture of the Achilles tendon may require surgical repair. Tendinitis and tendon rupture in the rotator cuff (the shoulder), the hand, the biceps, the thumb, and other tendon sites have also been reported. The risk of developing fluoroquinolone-associated tendinitis and tendon rupture is further increased in older patients usually over 60 years of age, in patients taking corticosteroid drugs, and in patients with kidney, heart or lung transplants).
No products indexed under this heading.

Hydrocortisone (Alcohol) (Fluoroquinolones, including ciprofloxacin, are associated with an increased risk of tendinitis and tendon rupture in all ages. This adverse reaction most frequently involves the Achilles tendon, and rupture of the Achilles tendon may require surgical repair. Tendinitis and tendon rupture in the rotator cuff (the shoulder), the hand, the biceps, the thumb, and other tendon sites have also been reported. The risk of developing fluoroquinolone-associated tendinitis and tendon rupture is further increased in older patients usually over 60 years of age, in patients taking corticosteroid drugs, and in patients with kidney, heart or lung transplants).
No products indexed under this heading.

Hydrocortisone Acetate (Fluoroquinolones, including ciprofloxacin, are associated with an increased risk of tendinitis and tendon rupture in all ages. This adverse reaction most frequently involves the Achilles tendon, and rupture of the Achilles tendon may require surgical repair. Tendinitis and tendon rupture in the rotator cuff (the shoulder), the hand, the biceps, the thumb, and other tendon sites have also been reported. The risk of developing fluoroquinolone-associated tendinitis and tendon rupture is further increased in older patients usually over 60 years of age, in patients taking corticosteroid drugs, and in patients with kidney, heart or lung transplants).
No products indexed under this heading.

Hydrocortisone Butyrate (Fluoroquinolones, including ciprofloxacin, are associated with an increased risk of tendinitis and tendon rupture in all ages. This adverse reaction most frequently involves the Achilles tendon, and rupture of the Achilles tendon may require surgical repair. Tendinitis and tendon rupture in the rotator cuff (the shoulder), the hand, the biceps, the thumb, and other tendon sites have also been reported. The risk of developing fluoroquinolone-associated tendinitis and tendon rupture is further increased in older patients usually over 60 years of age, in patients taking corticosteroid drugs, and in patients with kidney, heart or lung transplants).
No products indexed under this heading.

Hydrocortisone Cypionate (Fluoroquinolones, including ciprofloxacin, are associated with an increased risk of tendinitis and tendon rupture in all ages. This adverse reaction most frequently involves the Achilles tendon, and rupture of the Achilles tendon may require surgical repair. Tendinitis and tendon rupture in the rotator cuff (the shoulder), the hand, the biceps, the thumb, and other tendon sites have also been reported. The risk of developing fluoroquinolone-associated tendinitis and tendon rupture is further increased in older patients usually over 60 years of age, in patients taking corticosteroid drugs, and in patients with kidney, heart or lung transplants).
No products indexed under this heading.

Hydrocortisone Hemisuccinate (Fluoroquinolones, including ciprofloxacin, are associated with an increased risk of tendinitis and tendon rupture in all ages. This adverse reaction most frequently involves the Achilles tendon, and rupture of the Achilles tendon may require surgical repair. Tendinitis and tendon rupture in the rotator cuff (the shoulder), the hand, the biceps, the thumb, and other tendon sites have also been reported. The risk of developing fluoroquinolone-associated tendinitis and tendon rupture is further increased in older patients usually over 60 years of age, in patients taking corticosteroid drugs, and in patients with kidney, heart or lung transplants).
No products indexed under this heading.

Hydrocortisone Probutate (Fluoroquinolones, including ciprofloxacin, are associated with an increased risk of tendinitis and tendon rupture in all ages. This adverse reaction most frequently involves the Achilles tendon, and rupture of the Achilles tendon may require surgical repair. Tendinitis and tendon rupture in the rotator cuff (the shoulder), the hand, the biceps, the thumb, and other tendon sites have also been reported. The risk of developing fluoroquinolone-associated tendinitis and tendon rupture is further increased in older patients usually over 60 years of age, in patients taking corticosteroid drugs, and in patients with kidney, heart or lung transplants).
No products indexed under this heading.

Hydrocortisone Sodium Phosphate (Fluoroquinolones, including ciprofloxacin, are associated with an increased risk of tendinitis and tendon rupture in all ages. This adverse reaction most frequently involves the Achilles tendon, and rupture of the Achilles tendon may require surgical repair. Tendinitis and tendon rupture in the rotator cuff (the shoulder), the hand, the biceps, the thumb, and other tendon sites have also been reported. The risk of developing fluoroquinolone-associated tendinitis and tendon rupture is further increased in older patients usually over 60 years of age, in patients taking corticosteroid drugs, and in patients with kidney, heart or lung transplants).
No products indexed under this heading.

Hydrocortisone Sodium Succinate (Fluoroquinolones, including ciprofloxacin, are associated with an increased risk of tendinitis and tendon rupture in all ages. This adverse reaction most frequently involves the Achilles tendon, and rupture of the Achilles tendon may require surgical repair. Tendinitis and tendon rupture in the rotator cuff (the shoulder), the hand, the biceps, the thumb, and other tendon sites have also been reported. The risk of developing fluoroquinolone-associated tendinitis and tendon rupture is further increased in older patients usually over 60 years

of age, in patients taking corticosteroid drugs, and in patients with kidney, heart or lung transplants).
No products indexed under this heading.

Hydrocortisone Valerate (Fluoroquinolones, including ciprofloxacin, are associated with an increased risk of tendinitis and tendon rupture in all ages. This adverse reaction most frequently involves the Achilles tendon, and rupture of the Achilles tendon may require surgical repair. Tendinitis and tendon rupture in the rotator cuff (the shoulder), the hand, the biceps, the thumb, and other tendon sites have also been reported. The risk of developing fluoroquinolone-associated tendinitis and tendon rupture is further increased in older patients usually over 60 years of age, in patients taking corticosteroid drugs, and in patients with kidney, heart or lung transplants).
No products indexed under this heading.

Hydroxyzine Hydrochloride (In general, elderly patients may be more susceptible to drug-associated effects on the QT interval. Therefore, precautions should be taken when using ciprofloxacin with concomitant drugs that can result in prolongation of the QT interval).
No products indexed under this heading.

Ibuprofen (Non-steroidal anti-inflammatory drugs in combination of very high doses of quinolones have been shown to provoke convulsions in pre-clinical studies). Products include:

Imipramine Hydrochloride (In general, elderly patients may be more susceptible to drug-associated effects on the QT interval. Therefore, precautions should be taken when using ciprofloxacin with concomitant drugs that can result in prolongation of the QT interval).
No products indexed under this heading.

Imipramine Pamoate (In general, elderly patients may be more susceptible to drug-associated effects on the QT interval. Therefore, precautions should be taken when using ciprofloxacin with concomitant drugs that can result in prolongation of the QT interval).
No products indexed under this heading.

Indomethacin (Non-steroidal anti-inflammatory drugs in combination of very high doses of quinolones have been shown to provoke convulsions in pre-clinical studies). Products include:

Indomethacin Sodium Trihydrate (Non-steroidal anti-inflammatory drugs in combination of very high doses of quinolones have been shown to provoke convulsions in pre-clinical studies). Products include:

Iron (Concurrent administration of ciprofloxacin with products containing iron may substantially decrease its absorption, resulting in serum and urine levels considerably lower than desired. Ciprofloxacin should be administered at least 2 hours before or 6 hours after products containing iron).
No products indexed under this heading.

Iron, Peptonized (Concurrent administration of ciprofloxacin with multivalent cation-containing products may substantially decrease its absorption, resulting in serum and urine levels considerably lower than desired).
No products indexed under this heading.

Iron & Ammonium Citrate (Concurrent administration of ciprofloxacin with multivalent cation-containing products may substantially decrease its absorption, resulting in serum and urine levels considerably lower than desired).
No products indexed under this heading.

Iron Cacodylate (Concurrent administration of ciprofloxacin with multivalent cation-containing products may substantially decrease its absorption, resulting in serum and urine levels considerably lower than desired).
No products indexed under this heading.

Iron Carbonyl (Concurrent administration of ciprofloxacin with multivalent cation-containing products may substantially decrease its absorption, resulting in serum and urine levels considerably lower than desired). Products include:

Iron Supplements (Concurrent administration of ciprofloxacin with multivalent cation-containing products may substantially decrease its absorption, resulting in serum and urine levels considerably lower than desired).
No products indexed under this heading.

Isocarboxazid (In general, elderly patients may be more susceptible to drug-associated effects on the QT interval. Therefore, precautions should be taken when using ciprofloxacin with concomitant drugs that can result in prolongation of the QT interval). Products include:

Ketoprofen (Non-steroidal anti-inflammatory drugs in combination of very high doses of quinolones have been shown to provoke convulsions in pre-clinical studies).
No products indexed under this heading.

Ketorolac Tromethamine (Non-steroidal anti-inflammatory drugs in combination of very high doses of quinolones have been shown to provoke convulsions in pre-clinical studies). Products include:

Levobupivacaine Hydrochloride (Ciprofloxacin is an inhibitor of the hepatic CYP1A2 enzyme pathway. Co-administration of ciprofloxacin and other drugs primarily metabolized by CYP1A2 results in increased plasma concentrations of the co-administered drug and could lead to clinically significant pharmacodynamic side effects of the co-administered drug).
No products indexed under this heading.

Lidocaine (In general, elderly patients may be more susceptible to drug-associated effects on the QT interval. Therefore, precautions should be taken when using ciprofloxacin with concomitant drugs that can result in prolongation of the QT interval). Products include:

Lidocaine Hydrochloride (In general, elderly patients may be more susceptible to drug-associated effects on the QT interval. Therefore, precautions should be taken when using ciprofloxacin with concomitant drugs that can result in prolongation of the QT interval).
No products indexed under this heading.

Lithium Carbonate (In general, elderly patients may be more susceptible to drug-associated effects on the QT interval. Therefore, precautions should be taken when using ciprofloxacin with concomitant drugs that can result in prolongation of the QT interval).
No products indexed under this heading.

Lithium Citrate (In general, elderly patients may be more susceptible to drug-associated effects on the QT interval. Therefore, precautions should be taken when using ciprofloxacin with concomitant drugs that can result in prolongation of the QT interval).
No products indexed under this heading.

Lomefloxacin Hydrochloride (Ciprofloxacin is an inhibitor of the hepatic CYP1A2 enzyme pathway. Co-administration of ciprofloxacin and other drugs primarily metabolized by CYP1A2 results in increased plasma concentrations of the co-administered drug and could lead to clinically significant pharmacodynamic side effects of the co-administered drug).
No products indexed under this heading.

Lorazepam (In general, elderly patients may be more susceptible to drug-associated effects on the QT interval. Therefore, precautions should be taken when using ciprofloxacin with concomitant drugs that can result in prolongation of the QT interval).
No products indexed under this heading.

Loxapine Hydrochloride (In general, elderly patients may be more susceptible to drug-associated effects on the QT interval. Therefore, precautions should be taken when using ciprofloxacin with concomitant drugs that can result in prolongation of the QT interval).
No products indexed under this heading.

Loxapine Succinate (In general, elderly patients may be more susceptible to drug-associated effects on the QT interval. Therefore, precautions should be taken when using ciprofloxacin with concomitant drugs that can result in prolongation of the QT interval).
No products indexed under this heading.

Magaldrate (Concurrent administration of ciprofloxacin with multivalent cation-containing products, such as magnesium/aluminum antacids, may substantially decrease its absorption, resulting in serum and urine levels considerably lower than desired. Ciprofloxacin may be taken two hours before or six hours after taking magnesium or aluminum containing antacids. Concurrent administration of antacids containing magnesium hydroxide or aluminum hydroxide may reduce the bioavailability of ciprofloxacin by as much as 90%).
No products indexed under this heading.

Magnesium (Concurrent administration of ciprofloxacin with multivalent cation-containing products may substantially decrease its absorption, resulting in serum and urine levels considerably lower than desired). Products include:

Magnesium Aluminum Silicate (Concurrent administration of ciprofloxacin with multivalent cation-containing products may substantially decrease its absorption, resulting in serum and urine levels considerably lower than desired).
No products indexed under this heading.

Magnesium Carbonate (Concurrent administration of ciprofloxacin with multivalent cation-containing products, such as magnesium/aluminum antacids, may substantially decrease its absorption, resulting in serum and urine levels considerably lower than desired. Ciprofloxacin may be taken two hours before or six hours after taking magnesium or aluminum containing antacids. Concurrent administration of antacids containing magnesium hydroxide or aluminum hydroxide may reduce the bioavailability of ciprofloxacin by as much as 90%).
No products indexed under this heading.

IMPORTANT NOTE: Always consult each drug listing in the patient's regimen for possible interactions.

Cipro I.V. Interactions Index 330

Magnesium Chloride (Concurrent administration of ciprofloxacin with multivalent cation-containing products may substantially decrease its absorption, resulting in serum and urine levels considerably lower than desired).
No products indexed under this heading.

Magnesium Citrate (Concurrent administration of ciprofloxacin with multivalent cation-containing products may substantially decrease its absorption, resulting in serum and urine levels considerably lower than desired). Products include:
Chelated Mineral 3476

Magnesium Gluconate (Concurrent administration of ciprofloxacin with multivalent cation-containing products may substantially decrease its absorption, resulting in serum and urine levels considerably lower than desired).
No products indexed under this heading.

Magnesium Hydroxide (Concurrent administration of ciprofloxacin with multivalent cation-containing products, such as magnesium/aluminum antacids, may substantially decrease its absorption, resulting in serum and urine levels considerably lower than desired. Ciprofloxacin may be taken two hours before or six hours after taking magnesium or aluminum containing antacids. Concurrent administration of antacids containing magnesium hydroxide or aluminum hydroxide may reduce the bioavailability of ciprofloxacin by as much as 90%). Products include:
Fleet Pedia-Lax Chewable Tablets 1144
Pepcid Complete 1822

Magnesium Lactate (Concurrent administration of ciprofloxacin with multivalent cation-containing products may substantially decrease its absorption, resulting in serum and urine levels considerably lower than desired).
No products indexed under this heading.

Magnesium Oxide (Concurrent administration of ciprofloxacin with multivalent cation-containing products, such as magnesium/aluminum antacids, may substantially decrease its absorption, resulting in serum and urine levels considerably lower than desired. Ciprofloxacin may be taken two hours before or six hours after taking magnesium or aluminum containing antacids. Concurrent administration of antacids containing magnesium hydroxide or aluminum hydroxide may reduce the bioavailability of ciprofloxacin by as much as 90%). Products include:
Beelith 873

Magnesium Salicylate (Concurrent administration of ciprofloxacin with multivalent cation-containing products may substantially decrease its absorption, resulting in serum and urine levels considerably lower than desired).
No products indexed under this heading.

Magnesium Salicylate Tetrahydrate (Concurrent administration of ciprofloxacin with multivalent cation-containing products may substantially decrease its absorption, resulting in serum and urine levels considerably lower than desired).
No products indexed under this heading.

Magnesium Salts (Concurrent administration of ciprofloxacin with multivalent cation-containing products may substantially decrease its absorption, resulting in serum and urine levels considerably lower than desired).
No products indexed under this heading.

Magnesium Sulfate (Concurrent administration of ciprofloxacin with multivalent cation-containing products may substantially decrease its absorption, resulting in serum and urine levels considerably lower than desired).
No products indexed under this heading.

Magnesium Trisilicate (Concurrent administration of ciprofloxacin with multivalent cation-containing products, such as magnesium/aluminum antacids, may substantially decrease its absorption, resulting in serum and urine levels considerably lower than desired. Ciprofloxacin may be taken two hours before or six hours after taking magnesium or aluminum containing antacids. Concurrent administration of antacids containing magnesium hydroxide or aluminum hydroxide may reduce the bioavailability of ciprofloxacin by as much as 90%).
No products indexed under this heading.

Maprotiline Hydrochloride (In general, elderly patients may be more susceptible to drug-associated effects on the QT interval. Therefore, precautions should be taken when using ciprofloxacin with concomitant drugs that can result in prolongation of the QT interval).
No products indexed under this heading.

Meclofenamate Sodium (Non-steroidal anti-inflammatory drugs in combination of very high doses of quinolones have been shown to provoke convulsions in pre-clinical studies).
No products indexed under this heading.

Mefenamic Acid (Non-steroidal anti-inflammatory drugs in combination of very high doses of quinolones have been shown to provoke convulsions in pre-clinical studies).
No products indexed under this heading.

Meloxicam (Non-steroidal anti-inflammatory drugs in combination of very high doses of quinolones have been shown to provoke convulsions in pre-clinical studies).
No products indexed under this heading.

Meprobamate (In general, elderly patients may be more susceptible to drug-associated effects on the QT interval. Therefore, precautions should be taken when using ciprofloxacin with concomitant drugs that can result in prolongation of the QT interval).
No products indexed under this heading.

Mesoridazine Besylate (In general, elderly patients may be more susceptible to drug-associated effects on the QT interval. Therefore, precautions should be taken when using ciprofloxacin with concomitant drugs that can result in prolongation of the QT interval).
No products indexed under this heading.

Methadone Hydrochloride (Ciprofloxacin is an inhibitor of the hepatic CYP1A2 enzyme pathway. Co-administration of ciprofloxacin and other drugs primarily metabolized by CYP1A2 results in increased plasma concentrations of the co-administered drug and could lead to clinically significant pharmacodynamic side effects of the co-administered drug).
No products indexed under this heading.

Methotrexate (Renal tubular transport of methotrexate may be inhibited by concomitant administration of ciprofloxacin, potentially leading to increased plasma levels of methotrexate. This might increase the risk of methotrexate associated toxic reactions. Therefore, patients under methotrexate therapy should be carefully monitored when concomitant ciprofloxacin therapy is indicated).
No products indexed under this heading.

Methotrexate Sodium (Renal tubular transport of methotrexate may be inhibited by concomitant administration of ciprofloxacin, potentially leading to increased plasma levels of methotrexate. This might increase the risk of methotrexate associated toxic reactions. Therefore, patients under methotrexate therapy should be carefully monitored when concomitant ciprofloxacin therapy is indicated).
No products indexed under this heading.

Methylprednisolone (Fluoroquinolones, including ciprofloxacin, are associated with an increased risk of tendinitis and tendon rupture in all ages. This adverse reaction most frequently involves the Achilles tendon, and rupture of the Achilles tendon may require surgical repair. Tendinitis and tendon rupture in the rotator cuff (the shoulder), the hand, the biceps, the thumb, and other tendon sites have also been reported. The risk of developing fluoroquinolone-associated tendinitis and tendon rupture is further increased in older patients usually over 60 years of age, in patients taking corticosteroid drugs, and in patients with kidney, heart or lung transplants).
No products indexed under this heading.

Methylprednisolone Acetate (Fluoroquinolones, including ciprofloxacin, are associated with an increased risk of tendinitis and tendon rupture in all ages. This adverse reaction most frequently involves the Achilles tendon, and rupture of the Achilles tendon may require surgical repair. Tendinitis and tendon rupture in the rotator cuff (the shoulder), the hand, the biceps, the thumb, and other tendon sites have also been reported. The risk of developing fluoroquinolone-associated tendinitis and tendon rupture is further increased in older patients usually over 60 years of age, in patients taking corticosteroid drugs, and in patients with kidney, heart or lung transplants).
No products indexed under this heading.

Methylprednisolone Sodium Succinate (Fluoroquinolones, including ciprofloxacin, are associated with an increased risk of tendinitis and tendon rupture in all ages. This adverse reaction most frequently involves the Achilles tendon, and rupture of the Achilles tendon may require surgical repair. Tendinitis and tendon rupture in the rotator cuff (the shoulder), the hand, the biceps, the thumb, and other tendon sites have also been reported. The risk of developing fluoroquinolone-associated tendinitis and tendon rupture is further increased in older patients usually over 60 years of age, in patients taking corticosteroid drugs, and in patients with kidney, heart or lung transplants).
No products indexed under this heading.

Metoclopramide Hydrochloride (Metoclopramide significantly accelerates the absorption of oral ciprofloxacin, resulting in shorter time to reach maximum plasma concentrations. No significant effect was observed on the bioavailability of ciprofloxacin). Products include:
Metozolv ODT 2901

Mexiletine Hydrochloride (In general, elderly patients may be more susceptible to drug-associated effects on the QT interval. Therefore, precautions should be taken when using ciprofloxacin with concomitant drugs that can result in prolongation of the QT interval).
No products indexed under this heading.

Midazolam Hydrochloride (In general, elderly patients may be more susceptible to drug-associated effects on the QT interval. Therefore, precautions should be taken when using ciprofloxacin with concomitant drugs that can result in prolongation of the QT interval).
No products indexed under this heading.

Mirtazapine (Ciprofloxacin is an inhibitor of the hepatic CYP1A2 enzyme pathway. Co-administration of ciprofloxacin and other drugs primarily metabolized by CYP1A2 results in increased plasma concentrations of the co-administered drug and could lead to clinically significant pharmacodynamic side effects of the co-administered drug). Products include:
Remeron Tablets 3214
RemeronSolTab Tablets 3219

Molindone Hydrochloride (In general, elderly patients may be more susceptible to drug-associated effects on the QT interval. Therefore, precautions should be taken when using ciprofloxacin with concomitant drugs that can result in prolongation of the QT interval). Products include:
Moban 1108

Mometasone Furoate (Fluoroquinolones, including ciprofloxacin, are associated with an increased risk of tendinitis and tendon rupture in all ages. This adverse reaction most frequently involves the Achilles tendon, and rupture of the Achilles tendon may require surgical repair. Tendinitis and tendon rupture in the rotator cuff (the shoulder), the hand, the biceps, the thumb, and other tendon sites have also been reported. The risk of developing fluoroquinolone-associated tendinitis and tendon rupture is further increased in older patients usually over 60 years of age, in patients taking corticosteroid drugs, and in patients with kidney, heart or lung transplants). Products include:
Asmanex 3058
Elocon Cream 3111
Elocon Lotion 3112
Elocon Ointment 3114

Mometasone Furoate Monohydrate (Fluoroquinolones, including ciprofloxacin, are associated with an increased risk of tendinitis and tendon rupture in all ages. This adverse reaction most frequently involves the Achilles tendon, and rupture of the Achilles tendon may require surgical repair. Tendinitis and tendon rupture in the rotator cuff (the shoulder), the hand, the biceps, the thumb, and other tendon sites have also been reported. The risk of developing fluoroquinolone-associated tendinitis and tendon rupture is further increased in older patients usually over 60 years of age, in patients taking corticosteroid drugs, and in patients with kidney, heart or lung transplants). Products include:
Nasonex 3166

Moricizine Hydrochloride (In general, eldery patients may be more susceptible to drug-associated effects on the QT interval. Therefore, precautions should be taken when using ciprofloxacin with concomitant drugs that can result in prolongation of the QT interval (eg, class IA antiarrhythmics)).
No products indexed under this heading.

Moxifloxacin Hydrochloride (Ciprofloxacin is an inhibitor of the hepatic CYP1A2 enzyme pathway. Co-administration of ciprofloxacin and other drugs primarily metabolized by CYP1A2 results in increased plasma concentrations of the co-administered drug and could lead to clinically significant pharmacodynamic side effects of the co-administered drug). Products include:
Avelox 3064
Vigamox 589

Nabumetone (Non-steroidal anti-inflammatory drugs in combination of very high doses of quinolones have been shown to provoke convulsions in pre-clinical studies).
No products indexed under this heading.

Nafcillin Sodium (Ciprofloxacin is an inhibitor of the hepatic CYP1A2 enzyme pathway. Co-administration of ciprofloxacin and other drugs primarily metabolized by CYP1A2 results in increased plasma concentrations of the co-administered drug and could lead to clinically significant pharmacodynamic side effects of the co-administered drug).
No products indexed under this heading.

(⊙ Described in PDR® for Ophthalmic Medicines)

Naproxen (Non-steroidal anti-inflammatory drugs in combination of very high doses of quinolones have been shown to provoke convulsions in preclinical studies). Products include:

Naproxen Sodium (Non-steroidal anti-inflammatory drugs in combination of very high doses of quinolones have been shown to provoke convulsions in pre-clinical studies). Products include:

Nicotine Polacrilex (Ciprofloxacin is an inhibitor of the hepatic CYP1A2 enzyme pathway. Co-administration of ciprofloxacin and other drugs primarily metabolized by CYP1A2 results in increased plasma concentrations of the co-administered drug and could lead to clinically significant pharmacodynamic side effects of the co-administered drug).
No products indexed under this heading.

Nicotine Salicylate (Ciprofloxacin is an inhibitor of the hepatic CYP1A2 enzyme pathway. Co-administration of ciprofloxacin and other drugs primarily metabolized by CYP1A2 results in increased plasma concentrations of the co-administered drug and could lead to clinically significant pharmacodynamic side effects of the co-administered drug).
No products indexed under this heading.

Nicotine Sulfate (Ciprofloxacin is an inhibitor of the hepatic CYP1A2 enzyme pathway. Co-administration of ciprofloxacin and other drugs primarily metabolized by CYP1A2 results in increased plasma concentrations of the co-administered drug and could lead to clinically significant pharmacodynamic side effects of the co-administered drug).
No products indexed under this heading.

Norethindrone Acetate (Ciprofloxacin is an inhibitor of the hepatic CYP1A2 enzyme pathway. Co-administration of ciprofloxacin and other drugs primarily metabolized by CYP1A2 results in increased plasma concentrations of the co-administered drug and could lead to clinically significant pharmacodynamic side effects of the co-administered drug). Products include:

Norfloxacin (Ciprofloxacin is an inhibitor of the hepatic CYP1A2 enzyme pathway. Co-administration of ciprofloxacin and other drugs primarily metabolized by CYP1A2 results in increased plasma concentrations of the co-administered drug and could lead to clinically significant pharmacodynamic side effects of the co-administered drug). Products include:

Nortriptyline Hydrochloride (In general, elderly patients may be more susceptible to drug-associated effects on the QT interval. Therefore, precautions should be taken when using ciprofloxacin with concomitant drugs that can result in prolongation of the QT interval).
No products indexed under this heading.

Ofloxacin (Ciprofloxacin is an inhibitor of the hepatic CYP1A2 enzyme pathway. Co-administration of ciprofloxacin and other drugs primarily metabolized by CYP1A2 results in increased plasma concentrations of the co-administered drug and could lead to clinically significant pharmacodynamic side effects of the co-administered drug).
No products indexed under this heading.

Olanzapine (In general, elderly patients may be more susceptible to drug-associated effects on the QT inter-

val. Therefore, precautions should be taken when using ciprofloxacin with concomitant drugs that can result in prolongation of the QT interval). Products include:

Ondansetron (Ciprofloxacin is an inhibitor of the hepatic CYP1A2 enzyme pathway. Co-administration of ciprofloxacin and other drugs primarily metabolized by CYP1A2 results in increased plasma concentrations of the co-administered drug and could lead to clinically significant pharmacodynamic side effects of the co-administered drug).
No products indexed under this heading.

Ondansetron Hydrochloride (Ciprofloxacin is an inhibitor of the hepatic CYP1A2 enzyme pathway. Co-administration of ciprofloxacin and other drugs primarily metabolized by CYP1A2 results in increased plasma concentrations of the co-administered drug and could lead to clinically significant pharmacodynamic side effects of the co-administered drug). Products include:

Oxaprozin (Non-steroidal anti-inflammatory drugs in combination of very high doses of quinolones have been shown to provoke convulsions in pre-clinical studies).
No products indexed under this heading.

Oxazepam (In general, elderly patients may be more susceptible to drug-associated effects on the QT interval. Therefore, precautions should be taken when using ciprofloxacin with concomitant drugs that can result in prolongation of the QT interval).
No products indexed under this heading.

Perphenazine (In general, elderly patients may be more susceptible to drug-associated effects on the QT interval. Therefore, precautions should be taken when using ciprofloxacin with concomitant drugs that can result in prolongation of the QT interval).
No products indexed under this heading.

Phenelzine Sulfate (In general, elderly patients may be more susceptible to drug-associated effects on the QT interval. Therefore, precautions should be taken when using ciprofloxacin with concomitant drugs that can result in prolongation of the QT interval).
No products indexed under this heading.

Phenobarbital (Ciprofloxacin is an inhibitor of the hepatic CYP1A2 enzyme pathway. Co-administration of ciprofloxacin and other drugs primarily metabolized by CYP1A2 results in increased plasma concentrations of the co-administered drug and could lead to clinically significant pharmacodynamic side effects of the co-administered drug). Products include:

Phenobarbital Sodium (Ciprofloxacin is an inhibitor of the hepatic CYP1A2 enzyme pathway. Co-administration of ciprofloxacin and other drugs primarily metabolized by CYP1A2 results in increased plasma concentrations of the co-administered drug and could lead to clinically significant pharmacodynamic side effects of the co-administered drug).
No products indexed under this heading.

Phenylbutazone (Non-steroidal anti-inflammatory drugs in combination of very high doses of quinolones have been shown to provoke convulsions in pre-clinical studies).
No products indexed under this heading.

Phenytoin (Altered serum levels of phenytoin (increased and decreased) have been reported in patients receiving concomitant ciprofloxacin).
No products indexed under this heading.

Phenytoin Sodium (Altered serum levels of phenytoin (increased and decreased) have been reported in patients receiving concomitant ciprofloxacin). Products include:

Piroxicam (Non-steroidal anti-inflammatory drugs in combination of very high doses of quinolones have been shown to provoke convulsions in pre-clinical studies).
No products indexed under this heading.

Polysaccharide Iron Complex (Concurrent administration of ciprofloxacin with products containing iron may substantially decrease its absorption, resulting in serum and urine levels considerably lower than desired. Ciprofloxacin should be administered at least 2 hours before or 6 hours after products containing iron). Products include:

Prazepam (In general, elderly patients may be more susceptible to drug-associated effects on the QT interval. Therefore, precautions should be taken when using ciprofloxacin with concomitant drugs that can result in prolongation of the QT interval).
No products indexed under this heading.

Prednisolone (Fluoroquinolones, including ciprofloxacin, are associated with an increased risk of tendinitis and tendon rupture in all ages. This adverse reaction most frequently involves the Achilles tendon, and rupture of the Achilles tendon may require surgical repair. Tendinitis and tendon rupture in the rotator cuff (the shoulder), the hand, the biceps, the thumb, and other tendon sites have also been reported. The risk of developing fluoroquinolone-associated tendinitis and tendon rupture is further increased in older patients usually over 60 years of age, in patients taking corticosteroid drugs, and in patients with kidney, heart or lung transplants).
No products indexed under this heading.

Prednisolone Acetate (Fluoroquinolones, including ciprofloxacin, are associated with an increased risk of tendinitis and tendon rupture in all ages. This adverse reaction most frequently involves the Achilles tendon, and rupture of the Achilles tendon may require surgical repair. Tendinitis and tendon rupture in the rotator cuff (the shoulder), the hand, the biceps, the thumb, and other tendon sites have also been reported. The risk of developing fluoroquinolone-associated tendinitis and tendon rupture is further increased in older patients usually over 60 years of age, in patients taking corticosteroid drugs, and in patients with kidney, heart or lung transplants). Products include:

Prednisolone Sodium Phosphate (Fluoroquinolones, including ciprofloxacin, are associated with an increased risk of tendinitis and tendon rupture in all ages. This adverse reaction most frequently involves the Achilles tendon, and rupture of the Achilles tendon may require surgical repair. Tendinitis and tendon rupture in the rotator cuff (the shoulder), the hand, the biceps, the thumb, and other tendon sites have also been reported. The risk of developing fluoroquinolone-associated tendinitis and tendon rupture is further increased in older patients usually over 60 years

of age, in patients taking corticosteroid drugs, and in patients with kidney, heart or lung transplants).
No products indexed under this heading.

Prednisolone Tebutate (Fluoroquinolones, including ciprofloxacin, are associated with an increased risk of tendinitis and tendon rupture in all ages. This adverse reaction most frequently involves the Achilles tendon, and rupture of the Achilles tendon may require surgical repair. Tendinitis and tendon rupture in the rotator cuff (the shoulder), the hand, the biceps, the thumb, and other tendon sites have also been reported. The risk of developing fluoroquinolone-associated tendinitis and tendon rupture is further increased in older patients usually over 60 years of age, in patients taking corticosteroid drugs, and in patients with kidney, heart or lung transplants).
No products indexed under this heading.

Prednisone (Fluoroquinolones, including ciprofloxacin, are associated with an increased risk of tendinitis and tendon rupture in all ages. This adverse reaction most frequently involves the Achilles tendon, and rupture of the Achilles tendon may require surgical repair. Tendinitis and tendon rupture in the rotator cuff (the shoulder), the hand, the biceps, the thumb, and other tendon sites have also been reported. The risk of developing fluoroquinolone-associated tendinitis and tendon rupture is further increased in older patients usually over 60 years of age, in patients taking corticosteroid drugs, and in patients with kidney, heart or lung transplants).
No products indexed under this heading.

Prednisone sodium phosphate (Fluoroquinolones, including ciprofloxacin, are associated with an increased risk of tendinitis and tendon rupture in all ages. This adverse reaction most frequently involves the Achilles tendon, and rupture of the Achilles tendon may require surgical repair. Tendinitis and tendon rupture in the rotator cuff (the shoulder), the hand, the biceps, the thumb, and other tendon sites have also been reported. The risk of developing fluoroquinolone-associated tendinitis and tendon rupture is further increased in older patients usually over 60 years of age, in patients taking corticosteroid drugs, and in patients with kidney, heart or lung transplants).
No products indexed under this heading.

Probenecid (Probenecid interferes with renal tubular secretion of ciprofloxacin and produces an increase in the level of ciprofloxacin in the serum. This should be considered if patients are receiving both drugs concomitantly).
No products indexed under this heading.

Procainamide (In general, eldery patients may be more susceptible to drug-associated effects on the QT interval. Therefore, precautions should be taken when using ciprofloxacin with concomitant drugs that can result in prolongation of the QT interval (eg, class IA antiarrhythmics)).
No products indexed under this heading.

Procainamide Hydrochloride (In general, elderly patients may be more susceptible to drug-associated effects on the QT interval. Therefore, precautions should be taken when using ciprofloxacin with concomitant drugs that can result in prolongation of the QT interval).
No products indexed under this heading.

Prochlorperazine (In general, elderly patients may be more susceptible to drug-associated effects on the QT interval. Therefore, precautions should be taken when using ciprofloxacin with concomitant drugs that can result in prolongation of the QT interval).
No products indexed under this heading.

IMPORTANT NOTE: Always consult each drug listing in the patient's regimen for possible interactions.

Promethazine Hydrochloride (In general, elderly patients may be more susceptible to drug-associated effects on the QT interval. Therefore, precautions should be taken when using ciprofloxacin with concomitant drugs that can result in prolongation of the QT interval).
No products indexed under this heading.

Propafenone Hydrochloride (In general, elderly patients may be more susceptible to drug-associated effects on the QT interval. Therefore, precautions should be taken when using ciprofloxacin with concomitant drugs that can result in prolongation of the QT interval). Products include:

Propranolol Hydrochloride (Ciprofloxacin is an inhibitor of the hepatic CYP1A2 enzyme pathway. Co-administration of ciprofloxacin and other drugs primarily metabolized by CYP1A2 results in increased plasma concentrations of the co-administered drug and could lead to clinically significant pharmacodynamic side effects of the co-administered drug). Products include:

Protriptyline Hydrochloride (In general, elderly patients may be more susceptible to drug-associated effects on the QT interval. Therefore, precautions should be taken when using ciprofloxacin with concomitant drugs that can result in prolongation of the QT interval).
No products indexed under this heading.

Quetiapine Fumarate (In general, elderly patients may be more susceptible to drug-associated effects on the QT interval. Therefore, precautions should be taken when using ciprofloxacin with concomitant drugs that can result in prolongation of the QT interval). Products include:

Quinidine (In general, elderly patients may be more susceptible to drug-associated effects on the QT interval. Therefore, precautions should be taken when using ciprofloxacin with concomitant drugs that can result in prolongation of the QT interval).
No products indexed under this heading.

Quinidine Gluconate (In general, elderly patients may be more susceptible to drug-associated effects on the QT interval. Therefore, precautions should be taken when using ciprofloxacin with concomitant drugs that can result in prolongation of the QT interval).
No products indexed under this heading.

Quinidine Hydrochloride (In general, elderly patients may be more susceptible to drug-associated effects on the QT interval. Therefore, precautions should be taken when using ciprofloxacin with concomitant drugs that can result in prolongation of the QT interval).
No products indexed under this heading.

Quinidine Polygalacturonate (In general, elderly patients may be more susceptible to drug-associated effects on the QT interval. Therefore, precautions should be taken when using ciprofloxacin with concomitant drugs that can result in prolongation of the QT interval).
No products indexed under this heading.

Quinidine Sulfate (In general, elderly patients may be more susceptible to drug-associated effects on the QT interval. Therefore, precautions should be taken when using ciprofloxacin with concomitant drugs that can result in prolongation of the QT interval).
No products indexed under this heading.

Riluzole (Ciprofloxacin is an inhibitor of the hepatic CYP1A2 enzyme pathway. Co-administration of ciprofloxacin and

other drugs primarily metabolized by CYP1A2 results in increased plasma concentrations of the co-administered drug and could lead to clinically significant pharmacodynamic side effects of the co-administered drug). Products include:

Risperidone (In general, elderly patients may be more susceptible to drug-associated effects on the QT interval. Therefore, precautions should be taken when using ciprofloxacin with concomitant drugs that can result in prolongation of the QT interval). Products include:

Ritonavir (Ciprofloxacin is an inhibitor of the hepatic CYP1A2 enzyme pathway. Co-administration of ciprofloxacin and other drugs primarily metabolized by CYP1A2 results in increased plasma concentrations of the co-administered drug and could lead to clinically significant pharmacodynamic side effects of the co-administered drug). Products include:

Rofecoxib (Non-steroidal anti-inflammatory drugs in combination of very high doses of quinolones have been shown to provoke convulsions in pre-clinical studies).
No products indexed under this heading.

Ropinirole Hydrochloride (Ciprofloxacin is an inhibitor of the hepatic CYP1A2 enzyme pathway. Co-administration of ciprofloxacin and other drugs primarily metabolized by CYP1A2 results in increased plasma concentrations of the co-administered drug and could lead to clinically significant pharmacodynamic side effects of the co-administered drug). Products include:

Ropivacaine Hydrochloride (Ciprofloxacin is an inhibitor of the hepatic CYP1A2 enzyme pathway. Co-administration of ciprofloxacin and other drugs primarily metabolized by CYP1A2 results in increased plasma concentrations of the co-administered drug and could lead to clinically significant pharmacodynamic side effects of the co-administered drug).
No products indexed under this heading.

Selenium (Concurrent administration of ciprofloxacin with multivalent cation-containing products may substantially decrease its absorption, resulting in serum and urine levels considerably lower than desired). Products include:

Selenium Sulfide (Concurrent administration of ciprofloxacin with multivalent cation-containing products may substantially decrease its absorption, resulting in serum and urine levels considerably lower than desired).
No products indexed under this heading.

Sotalol Hydrochloride (In general, elderly patients may be more susceptible to drug-associated effects on the QT interval. Therefore, precautions should be taken when using ciprofloxacin with concomitant drugs that can result in prolongation of the QT interval (eg, class III antiarrhythmics)).
No products indexed under this heading.

Sucralfate (Concurrent administration of ciprofloxacin with multivalent cation-containing products, such as sucralfate, may substantially decrease its absorption, resulting in serum and urine levels considerably lower than desired. Ciprofloxacin should be administered at least 2 hours before or 6 hours after sucralfate). Products include:

Sulindac (Non-steroidal anti-inflammatory drugs in combination of very high doses of quinolones have been shown to provoke convulsions in pre-clinical studies). Products include:

Tacrine Hydrochloride (Ciprofloxacin is an inhibitor of the hepatic CYP1A2 enzyme pathway. Co-administration of ciprofloxacin and other drugs primarily metabolized by CYP1A2 results in increased plasma concentrations of the co-administered drug and could lead to clinically significant pharmacodynamic side effects of the co-administered drug).
No products indexed under this heading.

Tamoxifen Citrate (Ciprofloxacin is an inhibitor of the hepatic CYP1A2 enzyme pathway. Co-administration of ciprofloxacin and other drugs primarily metabolized by CYP1A2 results in increased plasma concentrations of the co-administered drug and could lead to clinically significant pharmacodynamic side effects of the co-administered drug).
No products indexed under this heading.

Theobromine (Ciprofloxacin is an inhibitor of the hepatic CYP1A2 enzyme pathway. Co-administration of ciprofloxacin and other drugs primarily metabolized by CYP1A2 results in increased plasma concentrations of the co-administered drug and could lead to clinically significant pharmacodynamic side effects of the co-administered drug).
No products indexed under this heading.

Theophylline (Ciprofloxacin is an inhibitor of the hepatic CYP1A2 enzyme pathway. Co-administration of ciprofloxacin and other drugs primarily metabolized by CYP1A2 (eg, theophylline, methylxanthines, tizanidine) results in increased plasma concentrations of the co-administered drug and could lead to clinically significant pharmacodynamic side effects of the co-administered drug. Concurrent administration may lead to elevated serum concentrations of theophylline and prolongation of its elimination half-life. Serious and fatal reactions have been reported in patients receiving concurrent administration of ciprofloxacin and theophylline. These reactions have included cardiac arrest, seizures, status epilepticus, and respiratory failure. Although similar serious adverse effects have been reported in patients receiving theophylline alone, the possibility that these reactions may be potentiated by ciprofloxacin cannot be eliminated. If concomitant use cannot be avoided, serum levels of theophylline should be monitored and dosage adjustments made as appropriate).
No products indexed under this heading.

Theophylline Anhydrous (Ciprofloxacin is an inhibitor of the hepatic CYP1A2 enzyme pathway. Co-administration of ciprofloxacin and other drugs primarily metabolized by CYP1A2 (eg, theophylline, methylxanthines, tizanidine) results in increased plasma concentrations of the co-administered drug and could lead to clinically significant pharmacodynamic side effects of the co-administered drug. Concurrent administration may lead to elevated serum concentrations of theophylline and prolongation of its elimination half-life. Serious and fatal reactions have been reported in patients receiving concurrent administration of ciprofloxacin and theophylline. These reactions have included cardiac arrest, seizures, status epilepticus, and respiratory failure. Although similar serious adverse effects have been reported in patients receiving theophylline alone, the possibility that these reactions may

be potentiated by ciprofloxacin cannot be eliminated. If concomitant use cannot be avoided, serum levels of theophylline should be monitored and dosage adjustments made as appropriate). Products include:

Theophylline Calcium Salicylate (Ciprofloxacin is an inhibitor of the hepatic CYP1A2 enzyme pathway. Co-administration of ciprofloxacin and other drugs primarily metabolized by CYP1A2 (eg, theophylline, methylxanthines, tizanidine) results in increased plasma concentrations of the co-administered drug and could lead to clinically significant pharmacodynamic side effects of the co-administered drug. Concurrent administration may lead to elevated serum concentrations of theophylline and prolongation of its elimination half-life. Serious and fatal reactions have been reported in patients receiving concurrent administration of ciprofloxacin and theophylline. These reactions have included cardiac arrest, seizures, status epilepticus, and respiratory failure. Although similar serious adverse effects have been reported in patients receiving theophylline alone, the possibility that these reactions may be potentiated by ciprofloxacin cannot be eliminated. If concomitant use cannot be avoided, serum levels of theophylline should be monitored and dosage adjustments made as appropriate).
No products indexed under this heading.

Theophylline Dihydroxypropyl (Glyceryl) (Ciprofloxacin is an inhibitor of the hepatic CYP1A2 enzyme pathway. Co-administration of ciprofloxacin and other drugs primarily metabolized by CYP1A2 (eg, theophylline, methylxanthines, tizanidine) results in increased plasma concentrations of the co-administered drug and could lead to clinically significant pharmacodynamic side effects of the co-administered drug. Concurrent administration may lead to elevated serum concentrations of theophylline and prolongation of its elimination half-life. Serious and fatal reactions have been reported in patients receiving concurrent administration of ciprofloxacin and theophylline. These reactions have included cardiac arrest, seizures, status epilepticus, and respiratory failure. Although similar serious adverse effects have been reported in patients receiving theophylline alone, the possibility that these reactions may be potentiated by ciprofloxacin cannot be eliminated. If concomitant use cannot be avoided, serum levels of theophylline should be monitored and dosage adjustments made as appropriate).
No products indexed under this heading.

Theophylline Ethylenediamine (Ciprofloxacin is an inhibitor of the hepatic CYP1A2 enzyme pathway. Co-administration of ciprofloxacin and other drugs primarily metabolized by CYP1A2 (eg, theophylline, methylxanthines, tizanidine) results in increased plasma concentrations of the co-administered drug and could lead to clinically significant pharmacodynamic side effects of the co-administered drug. Concurrent administration may lead to elevated serum concentrations of theophylline and prolongation of its elimination half-life. Serious and fatal reactions have been reported in patients receiving concurrent administration of ciprofloxacin and theophylline. These reactions have included cardiac arrest, seizures, status epilepticus, and respiratory failure. Although similar serious adverse effects have been reported in patients receiving theophylline alone, the possibility that these reactions may be potentiated by ciprofloxacin cannot be eliminated. If concomitant use cannot be avoided, serum levels of theo-

phylline should be monitored and dosage adjustments made as appropriate).
No products indexed under this heading.

Theophylline Sodium Glycinate (Ciprofloxacin is an inhibitor of the hepatic CYP1A2 enzyme pathway. Co-administration of ciprofloxacin and other drugs primarily metabolized by CYP1A2 (eg, theophylline, methylxanthines, tizanidine) results in increased plasma concentrations of the co-administered drug and could lead to clinically significant pharmacodynamic side effects of the co-administered drug. Concurrent administration may lead to elevated serum concentrations of theophylline and prolongation of its elimination half-life. Serious and fatal reactions have been reported in patients receiving concurrent administration of ciprofloxacin and theophylline. These reactions have included cardiac arrest, seizures, status epilepticus, and respiratory failure. Although similar serious adverse effects have been reported in patients receiving theophylline alone, the possibility that these reactions may be potentiated by ciprofloxacin cannot be eliminated. If concomitant use cannot be avoided, serum levels of theophylline should be monitored and dosage adjustments made as appropriate).
No products indexed under this heading.

Thioridazine Hydrochloride (In general, elderly patients may be more susceptible to drug-associated effects on the QT interval. Therefore, precautions should be taken when using ciprofloxacin with concomitant drugs that can result in prolongation of the QT interval). Products include:
Thioridazine Hydrochloride 2384

Thiothixene (In general, elderly patients may be more susceptible to drug-associated effects on the QT interval. Therefore, precautions should be taken when using ciprofloxacin with concomitant drugs that can result in prolongation of the QT interval). Products include:
Thiothixene 2386

Tizanidine (Concomitant administration of tizanidine and ciprofloxacin is contraindicated. In a pharmacokinetic study, systemic exposure of tizanidine (4 mg single dose) was significantly increased (C_{max} 7-fold, AUC 10-fold) when the drug was given concomitantly with ciprofloxacin (500 mg b.i.d. for 3 days). The hypotensive and sedative effects of tizanidine were also potentiated).
No products indexed under this heading.

Tizanidine Hydrochloride (Concomitant administration of tizanidine and ciprofloxacin is contraindicated. In a pharmacokinetic study, systemic exposure of tizanidine (4 mg single dose) was significantly increased (C_{max} 7-fold, AUC 10-fold) when the drug was given concomitantly with ciprofloxacin (500 mg b.i.d. for 3 days). The hypotensive and sedative effects of tizanidine were also potentiated).
No products indexed under this heading.

Tocainide Hydrochloride (In general, elderly patients may be more susceptible to drug-associated effects on the QT interval. Therefore, precautions should be taken when using ciprofloxacin with concomitant drugs that can result in prolongation of the QT interval).
No products indexed under this heading.

Tolmetin Sodium (Non-steroidal anti-inflammatory drugs in combination of very high doses of quinolones have been shown to provoke convulsions in pre-clinical studies).
No products indexed under this heading.

Tranylcypromine Sulfate (In general, elderly patients may be more susceptible to drug-associated effects on

the QT interval. Therefore, precautions should be taken when using ciprofloxacin with concomitant drugs that can result in prolongation of the QT interval). Products include:
Parnate 1584

Triamcinolone (Fluoroquinolones, including ciprofloxacin, are associated with an increased risk of tendinitis and tendon rupture in all ages. This adverse reaction most frequently involves the Achilles tendon, and rupture of the Achilles tendon may require surgical repair. Tendinitis and tendon rupture in the rotator cuff (the shoulder), the hand, the biceps, the thumb, and other tendon sites have also been reported. The risk of developing fluoroquinolone-associated tendinitis and tendon rupture is further increased in older patients usually over 60 years of age, in patients taking corticosteroid drugs, and in patients with kidney, heart or lung transplants).
No products indexed under this heading.

Triamcinolone Acetonide (Fluoroquinolones, including ciprofloxacin, are associated with an increased risk of tendinitis and tendon rupture in all ages. This adverse reaction most frequently involves the Achilles tendon, and rupture of the Achilles tendon may require surgical repair. Tendinitis and tendon rupture in the rotator cuff (the shoulder), the hand, the biceps, the thumb, and other tendon sites have also been reported. The risk of developing fluoroquinolone-associated tendinitis and tendon rupture is further increased in older patients usually over 60 years of age, in patients taking corticosteroid drugs, and in patients with kidney, heart or lung transplants). Products include:
Azmacort 408
Nasacort AQ 3019

Triamcinolone Diacetate (Fluoroquinolones, including ciprofloxacin, are associated with an increased risk of tendinitis and tendon rupture in all ages. This adverse reaction most frequently involves the Achilles tendon, and rupture of the Achilles tendon may require surgical repair. Tendinitis and tendon rupture in the rotator cuff (the shoulder), the hand, the biceps, the thumb, and other tendon sites have also been reported. The risk of developing fluoroquinolone-associated tendinitis and tendon rupture is further increased in older patients usually over 60 years of age, in patients taking corticosteroid drugs, and in patients with kidney, heart or lung transplants).
No products indexed under this heading.

Triamcinolone Hexacetonide (Fluoroquinolones, including ciprofloxacin, are associated with an increased risk of tendinitis and tendon rupture in all ages. This adverse reaction most frequently involves the Achilles tendon, and rupture of the Achilles tendon may require surgical repair. Tendinitis and tendon rupture in the rotator cuff (the shoulder), the hand, the biceps, the thumb, and other tendon sites have also been reported. The risk of developing fluoroquinolone-associated tendinitis and tendon rupture is further increased in older patients usually over 60 years of age, in patients taking corticosteroid drugs, and in patients with kidney, heart or lung transplants).
No products indexed under this heading.

Trifluoperazine Hydrochloride (In general, elderly patients may be more susceptible to drug-associated effects on the QT interval. Therefore, precautions should be taken when using ciprofloxacin with concomitant drugs that can result in prolongation of the QT interval).
No products indexed under this heading.

Trimethaphan Camsylate (Ciprofloxacin is an inhibitor of the hepatic CYP1A2 enzyme pathway. Co-administration of ciprofloxacin and other drugs primarily metabolized by CYP1A2 results in increased plasma concentrations of the co-administered drug and could lead to clinically significant pharmacodynamic side effects of the co-administered drug).
No products indexed under this heading.

Trimipramine Maleate (In general, elderly patients may be more susceptible to drug-associated effects on the QT interval. Therefore, precautions should be taken when using ciprofloxacin with concomitant drugs that can result in prolongation of the QT interval).
No products indexed under this heading.

Trovafloxacin Mesylate (Ciprofloxacin is an inhibitor of the hepatic CYP1A2 enzyme pathway. Co-administration of ciprofloxacin and other drugs primarily metabolized by CYP1A2 results in increased plasma concentrations of the co-administered drug and could lead to clinically significant pharmacodynamic side effects of the co-administered drug).
No products indexed under this heading.

Valdecoxib (Non-steroidal anti-inflammatory drugs in combination of very high doses of quinolones have been shown to provoke convulsions in pre-clinical studies).
No products indexed under this heading.

Verapamil Hydrochloride (Ciprofloxacin is an inhibitor of the hepatic CYP1A2 enzyme pathway. Co-administration of ciprofloxacin and other drugs primarily metabolized by CYP1A2 results in increased plasma concentrations of the co-administered drug and could lead to clinically significant pharmacodynamic side effects of the co-administered drug). Products include:
Tarka 534

Warfarin Sodium (Ciprofloxacin has been reported to enhance the effects of the oral anticoagulant warfarin or its derivatives. When these products are administered concomitantly, prothrombin time or other suitable coagulant tests should be closely monitored).
No products indexed under this heading.

Zileuton (Ciprofloxacin is an inhibitor of the hepatic CYP1A2 enzyme pathway. Co-administration of ciprofloxacin and other drugs primarily metabolized by CYP1A2 results in increased plasma concentrations of the co-administered drug and could lead to clinically significant pharmacodynamic side effects of the co-administered drug).
No products indexed under this heading.

Zinc (Concurrent administration of ciprofloxacin with products containing zinc may substantially decrease its absorption, resulting in serum and urine levels considerably lower than desired. Ciprofloxacin should be administered at least 2 hours before or 6 hours after products containing zinc). Products include:
BoneMate Plus 3454
Cardio Basics 3455
Chelated Mineral 3476
CitraNatal 90 DHA Capsules 2332
CitraNatal Assure 2332
Heplive 607
Visutein 3456

Zinc Acetate (Concurrent administration of ciprofloxacin with multivalent cation-containing products may substantially decrease its absorption, resulting in serum and urine levels considerably lower than desired).
No products indexed under this heading.

Zinc Bisglycinate (Concurrent administration of ciprofloxacin with multivalent cation-containing products may substantially decrease its absorption, resulting in serum and urine levels considerably lower than desired).
No products indexed under this heading.

Zinc Chloride (Concurrent administration of ciprofloxacin with multivalent cation-containing products may substantially decrease its absorption, resulting in serum and urine levels considerably lower than desired).
No products indexed under this heading.

Zinc Citrate (Concurrent administration of ciprofloxacin with multivalent cation-containing products may substantially decrease its absorption, resulting in serum and urine levels considerably lower than desired). Products include:
Chelated Mineral 3476

Zinc-Containing Multivitamins (Concurrent administration of ciprofloxacin with multivalent cation-containing products may substantially decrease its absorption, resulting in serum and urine levels considerably lower than desired).
No products indexed under this heading.

Zinc Gluconate (Concurrent administration of ciprofloxacin with multivalent cation-containing products may substantially decrease its absorption, resulting in serum and urine levels considerably lower than desired).
No products indexed under this heading.

Zinc Oxide (Concurrent administration of ciprofloxacin with multivalent cation-containing products may substantially decrease its absorption, resulting in serum and urine levels considerably lower than desired). Products include:
Bausch & Lomb Ocuvite Adult
50+ .... ⊙238
CitraNatal Rx 2332
Vusion Ointment 3335

Zinc Phenosulfonate (Concurrent administration of ciprofloxacin with multivalent cation-containing products may substantially decrease its absorption, resulting in serum and urine levels considerably lower than desired).
No products indexed under this heading.

Zinc Sulfate (Concurrent administration of ciprofloxacin with multivalent cation-containing products may substantially decrease its absorption, resulting in serum and urine levels considerably lower than desired). Products include:
Heplive 607
Zinc-220 606

Ziprasidone Hydrochloride (In general, elderly patients may be more susceptible to drug-associated effects on the QT interval. Therefore, precautions should be taken when using ciprofloxacin with concomitant drugs that can result in prolongation of the QT interval). Products include:
Geodon 2723

Zolmitriptan (Ciprofloxacin is an inhibitor of the hepatic CYP1A2 enzyme pathway. Co-administration of ciprofloxacin and other drugs primarily metabolized by CYP1A2 results in increased plasma concentrations of the co-administered drug and could lead to clinically significant pharmacodynamic side effects of the co-administered drug). Products include:
Zomig Tablets 773
Zomig Nasal Spray 768
Zomig-ZMT Tablets 773

Food Interactions
Beverages, caffeine-containing (Ciprofloxacin has been shown to interfere with the metabolism of caffeine. This may lead to reduced clearance of caffeine and a prolongation of its serum half-life and inhibits the formation of

paraxanthine after caffeine administration).

Dairy products (Ciprofloxacin should not be taken with dairy products (like milk or yogurt) alone since absorption of ciprofloxacin may be significantly reduced; however, ciprofloxacin may be taken with a meal that contains these products).

Food, caffeine-containing (Ciprofloxacin is an inhibitor of the hepatic CYP1A2 enzyme pathway. Co-administration of ciprofloxacin and other drugs primarily metabolized by CYP1A2 results in increased plasma concentrations of the co-administered drug and could lead to clinically significant pharmacodynamic side effects of the co-administered drug).

Food, unspecified (When ciprofloxacin tablets are given concomitantly with food, there is a delay in the absorption of the drug, resulting in peak concentrations that occur closer to 2 hours after dosing rather than 1 hour, whereas there is no delay observed when ciprofloxacin suspension is given with food. The overall absorption of ciprofloxacin tablets or ciprofloxacin suspension, however, is not substantially affected. The pharmacokinetics of ciprofloxacin given as the suspension are also not affected by food).

Fruit juices, unspecified (Ciprofloxacin should not be taken with calcium-fortified juices alone since absorption of ciprofloxacin may be significantly reduced; however, ciprofloxacin may be taken with a meal that contains these products).

Iron Amino Acid Chelate (Concurrent administration of ciprofloxacin with multivalent cation-containing products may substantially decrease its absorption, resulting in serum and urine levels considerably lower than desired).

Meal, unspecified (When ciprofloxacin tablets are given concomitantly with food, there is a delay in the absorption of the drug, resulting in peak concentrations that occur closer to 2 hours after dosing rather than 1 hour, whereas there is no delay observed when ciprofloxacin suspension is given with food. The overall absorption of ciprofloxacin tablets or ciprofloxacin suspension, however, is not substantially affected. The pharmacokinetics of ciprofloxacin given as the suspension are also not affected by food).

CIPRO ORAL SUSPENSION

(Ciprofloxacin) 3073

See Cipro Tablets

CIPRO TABLETS

(Ciprofloxacin Hydrochloride) 3073

May interact with antacids containing aluminum, calcium and magnesium, caffeines, calcium preparations, cations, class I antiarrhythmics, class III antiarrhythmics, corticosteroids, cytochrome p450 1a2 substrates (selected), drugs that prolong the QT interval, iron containing oral preparations, non-steroidal anti-inflammatory agents, oral anticoagulants, phenytoin, theophyllines, xanthines, and certain other agents. Compounds in these categories include:

Acetaminophen (Ciprofloxacin is an inhibitor of the hepatic CYP1A2 enzyme pathway. Co-administration of ciprofloxacin and other drugs primarily metabolized by CYP1A2 results in increased plasma concentrations of the co-administered drug and could lead to clinically significant pharmacodynamic side effects of the co-administered drug). Products include:

Percocet 1121
Tylenol 2049
Tylenol 8 Hour 2049
Extra Strength Tylenol Caplets, Cool Caplets, and EZ Tabs 2049
Extra Strength Tylenol Adult Rapid Blast Liquid 2049
Extra Strength Tylenol Rapid Release 2049
Tylenol with Codeine 2691
Tylenol Arthritis Pain Extended Release Geltabs/Caplets 2049
Children's Tylenol Suspension Liquid 2048
Chlidren's Tylenol Meltaways 2048
Tylenol, Infants' Drops 2048
Junior Tylenol 2048
Vicodin 560
Vicodin ES 561
Vicodin HP 563
Zydone 1138

Alatrofloxacin Mesylate (Ciprofloxacin is an inhibitor of the hepatic CYP1A2 enzyme pathway. Co-administration of ciprofloxacin and other drugs primarily metabolized by CYP1A2 results in increased plasma concentrations of the co-administered drug and could lead to clinically significant pharmacodynamic side effects of the co-administered drug).
No products indexed under this heading.

Alclometasone Dipropionate (Fluoroquinolones including ciprofloxacin are associated with an increased risk of tendinitis and tendon rupture in all ages. This adverse reaction most frequently involves the Achilles tendon, and rupture of the Achilles tendon may require surgical repair. Tendinitis and tendon rupture in the rotator cuff (the shoulder), the hand, the biceps, the thumb, and other tendon sites have also been reported. The risk of developing fluoroquinolone-associated tendinitis and tendon rupture is further increased in older patients usually over 60 years of age, in patients taking corticosteroid drugs, and in patients with kidney, heart or lung transplants).
No products indexed under this heading.

Alprazolam (In general, elderly patients may be more susceptible to drug-associated effects on the QT interval. Therefore, precautions should be taken when using ciprofloxacin with concomitant drugs that can result in prolongation of the QT interval).
No products indexed under this heading.

Aluminum Acetate (Concurrent administration of ciprofloxacin with multivalent cation-containing products may substantially decrease its absorption, resulting in serum and urine levels considerably lower than desired).
No products indexed under this heading.

Aluminum Carbonate (Concurrent administration of ciprofloxacin with multivalent cation-containing products, such as magnesium/aluminum antacids, may substantially decrease its absorption, resulting in serum and urine levels considerably lower than desired. Ciprofloxacin may be taken two hours before or six hours after taking magnesium or aluminum containing antacids. Concurrent administration of antacids containing magnesium hydroxide or aluminum hydroxide may reduce the bioavailability of ciprofloxacin by as much as 90%).
No products indexed under this heading.

Aluminum Chlorhydroxide (Concurrent administration of ciprofloxacin with multivalent cation-containing products may substantially decrease its absorption, resulting in serum and urine levels considerably lower than desired).
No products indexed under this heading.

Aluminum Chloride (Concurrent administration of ciprofloxacin with multivalent cation-containing products may substantially decrease its absorption, resulting in serum and urine levels considerably lower than desired).
No products indexed under this heading.

Aluminum Chlorohydrate (Concurrent administration of ciprofloxacin with multivalent cation-containing products may substantially decrease its absorption, resulting in serum and urine levels considerably lower than desired).
No products indexed under this heading.

Aluminum Glycinate (Concurrent administration of ciprofloxacin with multivalent cation-containing products may substantially decrease its absorption, resulting in serum and urine levels considerably lower than desired).
No products indexed under this heading.

Aluminum Hydroxide (Concurrent administration of ciprofloxacin with multivalent cation-containing products, such as magnesium/aluminum antacids, may substantially decrease its absorption, resulting in serum and urine levels considerably lower than desired. Ciprofloxacin may be taken two hours before or six hours after taking magnesium or aluminum containing antacids. Concurrent administration of antacids containing magnesium hydroxide or aluminum hydroxide may reduce the bioavailability of ciprofloxacin by as much as 90%).
No products indexed under this heading.

Aluminum Hydroxide Preparations (Concurrent administration of ciprofloxacin with multivalent cation-containing products may substantially decrease its absorption, resulting in serum and urine levels considerably lower than desired).
No products indexed under this heading.

Aluminum Sulfate (Concurrent administration of ciprofloxacin with multivalent cation-containing products may substantially decrease its absorption, resulting in serum and urine levels considerably lower than desired).
No products indexed under this heading.

Aminophylline (Ciprofloxacin is an inhibitor of the hepatic CYP1A2 enzyme pathway. Co-administration of ciprofloxacin and other drugs primarily metabolized by CYP1A2, such as methylxanthines, results in increased plasma concentrations of co-administered drug and could lead to clinically significant pharmacodynamic side effects of the co-administered drug).
No products indexed under this heading.

Amiodarone Hydrochloride (In general, elderly patients may be more susceptible to drug-associated effects on the QT interval. Therefore, precautions should be taken when using ciprofloxacin with concomitant drugs that can result in prolongation of the QT interval).
No products indexed under this heading.

Amitriptyline Hydrochloride (In general, elderly patients may be more susceptible to drug-associated effects on the QT interval. Therefore, precautions should be taken when using ciprofloxacin with concomitant drugs that can result in prolongation of the QT interval).
No products indexed under this heading.

Amoxapine (In general, elderly patients may be more susceptible to drug-associated effects on the QT interval. Therefore, precautions should be taken when using ciprofloxacin with concomitant drugs that can result in prolongation of the QT interval).
No products indexed under this heading.

Anagrelide Hydrochloride (Ciprofloxacin is an inhibitor of the hepatic CYP1A2 enzyme pathway. Co-administration of ciprofloxacin and other drugs primarily metabolized by CYP1A2 results in increased plasma concentrations of the co-administered drug and could lead to clinically significant pharmacodynamic side effects of the co-administered drug).
No products indexed under this heading.

Anisindione (Ciprofloxacin has been reported to enhance the effects of the oral anticoagulant warfarin or its derivatives. When these products are administered concomitantly, prothrombin time or other suitable coagulant tests should be closely monitored).
No products indexed under this heading.

Astemizole (In general, elderly patients may be more susceptible to drug-associated effects on the QT interval. Therefore, precautions should be taken when using ciprofloxacin with concomitant drugs that can result in prolongation of the QT interval).
No products indexed under this heading.

Beclomethasone Dipropionate (Fluoroquinolones including ciprofloxacin are associated with an increased risk of tendinitis and tendon rupture in all ages. This adverse reaction most frequently involves the Achilles tendon, and rupture of the Achilles tendon may require surgical repair. Tendinitis and tendon rupture in the rotator cuff (the shoulder), the hand, the biceps, the thumb, and other tendon sites have also been reported. The risk of developing fluoroquinolone-associated tendinitis and tendon rupture is further increased in older patients usually over 60 years of age, in patients taking corticosteroid drugs, and in patients with kidney, heart or lung transplants). Products include:
Qvar 3398

Beclomethasone Dipropionate Monohydrate (Fluoroquinolones including ciprofloxacin are associated with an increased risk of tendinitis and tendon rupture in all ages. This adverse reaction most frequently involves the Achilles tendon, and rupture of the Achilles tendon may require surgical repair. Tendinitis and tendon rupture in the rotator cuff (the shoulder), the hand, the biceps, the thumb, and other tendon sites have also been reported. The risk of developing fluoroquinolone-associated tendinitis and tendon rupture is further increased in older patients usually over 60 years of age, in patients taking corticosteroid drugs, and in patients with kidney, heart or lung transplants). Products include:
Beconase AQ 1386

Betamethasone (Fluoroquinolones including ciprofloxacin are associated with an increased risk of tendinitis and tendon rupture in all ages. This adverse reaction most frequently involves the Achilles tendon, and rupture of the Achilles tendon may require surgical repair. Tendinitis and tendon rupture in the rotator cuff (the shoulder), the hand, the biceps, the thumb, and other tendon sites have also been reported. The risk of developing fluoroquinolone-associated tendinitis and tendon rupture is further increased in older patients usually over 60 years of age, in patients taking corticosteroid drugs, and in patients with kidney, heart or lung transplants).
No products indexed under this heading.

Betamethasone Acetate (Fluoroquinolones including ciprofloxacin are associated with an increased risk of tendinitis and tendon rupture in all ages. This adverse reaction most frequently involves the Achilles tendon, and rupture of the Achilles tendon may require surgical repair. Tendinitis and tendon

rupture in the rotator cuff (the shoulder), the hand, the biceps, the thumb, and other tendon sites have also been reported. The risk of developing fluoroquinolone-associated tendinitis and tendon rupture is further increased in older patients usually over 60 years of age, in patients taking corticosteroid drugs, and in patients with kidney, heart or lung transplants).

No products indexed under this heading.

Betamethasone Benzoate (Fluoroquinolones including ciprofloxacin are associated with an increased risk of tendinitis and tendon rupture in all ages. This adverse reaction most frequently involves the Achilles tendon, and rupture of the Achilles tendon may require surgical repair. Tendinitis and tendon rupture in the rotator cuff (the shoulder), the hand, the biceps, the thumb, and other tendon sites have also been reported. The risk of developing fluoroquinolone-associated tendinitis and tendon rupture is further increased in older patients usually over 60 years of age, in patients taking corticosteroid drugs, and in patients with kidney, heart or lung transplants).

No products indexed under this heading.

Betamethasone Dipropionate (Fluoroquinolones including ciprofloxacin are associated with an increased risk of tendinitis and tendon rupture in all ages. This adverse reaction most frequently involves the Achilles tendon, and rupture of the Achilles tendon may require surgical repair. Tendinitis and tendon rupture in the rotator cuff (the shoulder), the hand, the biceps, the thumb, and other tendon sites have also been reported. The risk of developing fluoroquinolone-associated tendinitis and tendon rupture is further increased in older patients usually over 60 years of age, in patients taking corticosteroid drugs, and in patients with kidney, heart or lung transplants). Products include:

Betamethasone Sodium Phosphate (Fluoroquinolones including ciprofloxacin are associated with an increased risk of tendinitis and tendon rupture in all ages. This adverse reaction most frequently involves the Achilles tendon, and rupture of the Achilles tendon may require surgical repair. Tendinitis and tendon rupture in the rotator cuff (the shoulder), the hand, the biceps, the thumb, and other tendon sites have also been reported. The risk of developing fluoroquinolone-associated tendinitis and tendon rupture is further increased in older patients usually over 60 years of age, in patients taking corticosteroid drugs, and in patients with kidney, heart or lung transplants).

No products indexed under this heading.

Betamethasone Valerate (Fluoroquinolones including ciprofloxacin are associated with an increased risk of tendinitis and tendon rupture in all ages. This adverse reaction most frequently involves the Achilles tendon, and rupture of the Achilles tendon may require surgical repair. Tendinitis and tendon rupture in the rotator cuff (the shoulder), the hand, the biceps, the thumb, and other tendon sites have also been reported. The risk of developing fluoroquinolone-associated tendinitis and tendon rupture is further increased in older patients usually over 60 years of age, in patients taking corticosteroid drugs, and in patients with kidney, heart or lung transplants). Products include:

Bretylium Tosylate (In general, elderly patients may be more susceptible to drug-associated effects on the QT interval. Therefore, precautions should be taken when using ciprofloxacin with concomitant drugs that can result in prolongation of the QT interval).

No products indexed under this heading.

Budesonide (Fluoroquinolones including ciprofloxacin are associated with an increased risk of tendinitis and tendon rupture in all ages. This adverse reaction most frequently involves the Achilles tendon, and rupture of the Achilles tendon may require surgical repair. Tendinitis and tendon rupture in the rotator cuff (the shoulder), the hand, the biceps, the thumb, and other tendon sites have also been reported. The risk of developing fluoroquinolone-associated tendinitis and tendon rupture is further increased in older patients usually over 60 years of age, in patients taking corticosteroid drugs, and in patients with kidney, heart or lung transplants). Products include:

Buspirone Hydrochloride (In general, elderly patients may be more susceptible to drug-associated effects on the QT interval. Therefore, precautions should be taken when using ciprofloxacin with concomitant drugs that can result in prolongation of the QT interval).

No products indexed under this heading.

Caffeine (Ciprofloxacin is an inhibitor of the hepatic CYP1A2 enzyme pathway. Co-administration of ciprofloxacin and other drugs primarily metabolized by CYP1A2 results in increased plasma concentrations of the co-administered drug and could lead to clinically significant pharmacodynamic side effects of the co-administered drug).

No products indexed under this heading.

Caffeine Anhydrous (Ciprofloxacin is an inhibitor of the hepatic CYP1A2 enzyme pathway. Co-administration of ciprofloxacin and other drugs primarily metabolized by CYP1A2 results in increased plasma concentrations of the co-administered drug and could lead to clinically significant pharmacodynamic side effects of the co-administered drug).

No products indexed under this heading.

Caffeine Citrate (Ciprofloxacin is an inhibitor of the hepatic CYP1A2 enzyme pathway. Co-administration of ciprofloxacin and other drugs primarily metabolized by CYP1A2 results in increased plasma concentrations of the co-administered drug and could lead to clinically significant pharmacodynamic side effects of the co-administered drug).

No products indexed under this heading.

Caffeine-containing medications (Ciprofloxacin is an inhibitor of the hepatic CYP1A2 enzyme pathway. Co-administration of ciprofloxacin and other drugs primarily metabolized by CYP1A2 results in increased plasma concentrations of the co-administered drug and could lead to clinically significant pharmacodynamic side effects of the co-administered drug).

No products indexed under this heading.

Caffeine Sodium Benzoate (Ciprofloxacin is an inhibitor of the hepatic CYP1A2 enzyme pathway. Co-administration of ciprofloxacin and other drugs primarily metabolized by CYP1A2 results in increased plasma concentrations of the co-administered drug and could lead to clinically significant pharmacodynamic side effects of the co-administered drug).

No products indexed under this heading.

Calcium (Concurrent administration of ciprofloxacin with multivalent cation-containing products may substantially decrease its absorption, resulting in serum and urine levels considerably lower than desired. Products include:

Calcium (Oyster Shell) (Concurrent administration of ciprofloxacin with multivalent cation-containing products may substantially decrease its absorption, resulting in serum and urine levels considerably lower than desired).

No products indexed under this heading.

Calcium Acetate (Concurrent administration of ciprofloxacin with multivalent cation-containing products may substantially decrease its absorption, resulting in serum and urine levels considerably lower than desired).

No products indexed under this heading.

Calcium Ascorbate (Concurrent administration of ciprofloxacin with multivalent cation-containing products may substantially decrease its absorption, resulting in serum and urine levels considerably lower than desired). Products include:

Calcium Carbaspirin (Concurrent administration of ciprofloxacin with multivalent cation-containing products may substantially decrease its absorption, resulting in serum and urine levels considerably lower than desired).

No products indexed under this heading.

Calcium Carbonate (Concurrent administration of ciprofloxacin with multivalent cation-containing products, such as magnesium/aluminum antacids, may substantially decrease its absorption, resulting in serum and urine levels considerably lower than desired. Ciprofloxacin may be taken two hours before or six hours after taking magnesium or aluminum containing antacids. Concurrent administration of antacids containing magnesium hydroxide or aluminum hydroxide may reduce the bioavailability of ciprofloxacin by as much as 90%). Products include:

Calcium Carbonate, Precipitated (Concurrent administration of ciprofloxacin with multivalent cation-containing products may substantially decrease its absorption, resulting in serum and urine levels considerably lower than desired).

No products indexed under this heading.

Calcium Caseinate (Concurrent administration of ciprofloxacin with multivalent cation-containing products may substantially decrease its absorption, resulting in serum and urine levels considerably lower than desired).

No products indexed under this heading.

Calcium Chloride (Concurrent administration of ciprofloxacin with products containing calcium may substantially decrease its absorption, resulting in serum and urine levels considerably lower than desired. Ciprofloxacin should be administered at least 2 hours before or 6 hours after products containing calcium).

No products indexed under this heading.

Calcium Citrate (Concurrent administration of ciprofloxacin with products containing calcium may substantially decrease its absorption, resulting in serum and urine levels considerably lower than desired. Ciprofloxacin should

be administered at least 2 hours before or 6 hours after products containing calcium). Products include:

Calcium Disodium Edetate (Concurrent administration of ciprofloxacin with multivalent cation-containing products may substantially decrease its absorption, resulting in serum and urine levels considerably lower than desired).

No products indexed under this heading.

Calcium Glubionate (Concurrent administration of ciprofloxacin with products containing calcium may substantially decrease its absorption, resulting in serum and urine levels considerably lower than desired. Ciprofloxacin should be administered at least 2 hours before or 6 hours after products containing calcium).

No products indexed under this heading.

Calcium Gluconate (Concurrent administration of ciprofloxacin with multivalent cation-containing products may substantially decrease its absorption, resulting in serum and urine levels considerably lower than desired).

No products indexed under this heading.

Calcium Glycerophosphate (Concurrent administration of ciprofloxacin with multivalent cation-containing products may substantially decrease its absorption, resulting in serum and urine levels considerably lower than desired).

No products indexed under this heading.

Calcium Iodide (Concurrent administration of ciprofloxacin with multivalent cation-containing products may substantially decrease its absorption, resulting in serum and urine levels considerably lower than desired).

No products indexed under this heading.

Calcium Lactate (Concurrent administration of ciprofloxacin with multivalent cation-containing products may substantially decrease its absorption, resulting in serum and urine levels considerably lower than desired).

No products indexed under this heading.

Calcium Levulinate (Concurrent administration of ciprofloxacin with multivalent cation-containing products may substantially decrease its absorption, resulting in serum and urine levels considerably lower than desired).

No products indexed under this heading.

Calcium Pantothenate (Concurrent administration of ciprofloxacin with multivalent cation-containing products may substantially decrease its absorption, resulting in serum and urine levels considerably lower than desired). Products include:

Calcium Phosphate (Concurrent administration of ciprofloxacin with multivalent cation-containing products may substantially decrease its absorption, resulting in serum and urine levels considerably lower than desired).

No products indexed under this heading.

Calcium Phosphate, Dibasic (Concurrent administration of ciprofloxacin with multivalent cation-containing products may substantially decrease its absorption, resulting in serum and urine levels considerably lower than desired).

No products indexed under this heading.

Calcium Phosphate, Tribasic (Concurrent administration of ciprofloxacin with multivalent cation-containing products may substantially decrease its absorption, resulting in serum and urine levels considerably lower than desired).

No products indexed under this heading.

IMPORTANT NOTE: Always consult each drug listing in the patient's regimen for possible interactions.

Cipro Tablets Interactions Index 336

Calcium Phosphorus Preparations (Concurrent administration of ciprofloxacin with multivalent cation-containing products may substantially decrease its absorption, resulting in serum and urine levels considerably lower than desired).
No products indexed under this heading.

Calcium Polycarbophil (Concurrent administration of ciprofloxacin with multivalent cation-containing products may substantially decrease its absorption, resulting in serum and urine levels considerably lower than desired).
No products indexed under this heading.

Calcium Salts (Concurrent administration of ciprofloxacin with multivalent cation-containing products may substantially decrease its absorption, resulting in serum and urine levels considerably lower than desired).
No products indexed under this heading.

Calcium Sodium Alginate Fiber (Concurrent administration of ciprofloxacin with multivalent cation-containing products may substantially decrease its absorption, resulting in serum and urine levels considerably lower than desired).
No products indexed under this heading.

Calcium Undecylenate (Concurrent administration of ciprofloxacin with multivalent cation-containing products may substantially decrease its absorption, resulting in serum and urine levels considerably lower than desired).
No products indexed under this heading.

Celecoxib (Non-steroidal anti-inflammatory drugs in combination of very high doses of quinolones have been shown to provoke convulsions in pre-clinical studies). Products include:
Celebrex 3272

Chlordiazepoxide (In general, elderly patients may be more susceptible to drug-associated effects on the QT interval. Therefore, precautions should be taken when using ciprofloxacin with concomitant drugs that can result in prolongation of the QT interval).
No products indexed under this heading.

Chlordiazepoxide Hydrochloride (In general, elderly patients may be more susceptible to drug-associated effects on the QT interval. Therefore, precautions should be taken when using ciprofloxacin with concomitant drugs that can result in prolongation of the QT interval).
No products indexed under this heading.

Chlorpromazine (In general, elderly patients may be more susceptible to drug-associated effects on the QT interval. Therefore, precautions should be taken when using ciprofloxacin with concomitant drugs that can result in prolongation of the QT interval).
No products indexed under this heading.

Chlorpromazine Hydrochloride (In general, elderly patients may be more susceptible to drug-associated effects on the QT interval. Therefore, precautions should be taken when using ciprofloxacin with concomitant drugs that can result in prolongation of the QT interval).
No products indexed under this heading.

Chlorprothixene (In general, elderly patients may be more susceptible to drug-associated effects on the QT interval. Therefore, precautions should be taken when using ciprofloxacin with concomitant drugs that can result in prolongation of the QT interval).
No products indexed under this heading.

Chlorprothixene Hydrochloride (In general, elderly patients may be more susceptible to drug-associated effects on the QT interval. Therefore, precautions should be taken when using ciprofloxacin with concomitant drugs that can result in prolongation of the QT interval).
No products indexed under this heading.

Ciclesonide (Fluoroquinolones including ciprofloxacin are associated with an increased risk of tendinitis and tendon rupture in all ages. This adverse reaction most frequently involves the Achilles tendon, and rupture of the Achilles tendon may require surgical repair. Tendinitis and tendon rupture in the rotator cuff (the shoulder), the hand, the biceps, the thumb, and other tendon sites have also been reported. The risk of developing fluoroquinolone-associated tendinitis and tendon rupture is further increased in older patients usually over 60 years of age, in patients taking corticosteroid drugs, and in patients with kidney, heart or lung transplants).
No products indexed under this heading.

Cimetidine Hydrochloride (Ciprofloxacin is an inhibitor of the hepatic CYP1A2 enzyme pathway. Co-administration of ciprofloxacin and other drugs primarily metabolized by CYP1A2 results in increased plasma concentrations of the co-administered drug and could lead to clinically significant pharmacodynamic side effects of the co-administered drug).
No products indexed under this heading.

Ciprofloxacin (Ciprofloxacin is an inhibitor of the hepatic CYP1A2 enzyme pathway. Co-administration of ciprofloxacin and other drugs primarily metabolized by CYP1A2 results in increased plasma concentrations of the co-administered drug and could lead to clinically significant pharmacodynamic side effects of the co-administered drug). Products include:
Cipro I.V. 3082
Cipro 3073
Cipro XR 3091
Ciprodex 583

Clomipramine Hydrochloride (In general, elderly patients may be more susceptible to drug-associated effects on the QT interval. Therefore, precautions should be taken when using ciprofloxacin with concomitant drugs that can result in prolongation of the QT interval).
No products indexed under this heading.

Clopidogrel Bisulfate (Ciprofloxacin is an inhibitor of the hepatic CYP1A2 enzyme pathway. Co-administration of ciprofloxacin and other drugs primarily metabolized by CYP1A2 results in increased plasma concentrations of the co-administered drug and could lead to clinically significant pharmacodynamic side effects of the co-administered drug). Products include:
Plavix 3027

Clorazepate Dipotassium (In general, elderly patients may be more susceptible to drug-associated effects on the QT interval. Therefore, precautions should be taken when using ciprofloxacin with concomitant drugs that can result in prolongation of the QT interval).
No products indexed under this heading.

Clozapine (In general, elderly patients may be more susceptible to drug-associated effects on the QT interval. Therefore, precautions should be taken when using ciprofloxacin with concomitant drugs that can result in prolongation of the QT interval).
No products indexed under this heading.

Cortisone Acetate (Fluoroquinolones including ciprofloxacin are associated with an increased risk of tendinitis and tendon rupture in all ages. This adverse reaction most frequently involves the Achilles tendon, and rupture of the Achilles tendon may require surgical repair. Tendinitis and tendon rupture in the rotator cuff (the shoulder), the hand, the biceps, the thumb, and other tendon sites have also been reported. The risk of developing fluoroquinolone-associated tendinitis and tendon rupture is further increased in older patients usually over 60 years of age, in patients taking corticosteroid drugs, and in patients with kidney, heart or lung transplants).
No products indexed under this heading.

Cyclobenzaprine (Ciprofloxacin is an inhibitor of the hepatic CYP1A2 enzyme pathway. Co-administration of ciprofloxacin and other drugs primarily metabolized by CYP1A2 results in increased plasma concentrations of the co-administered drug and could lead to clinically significant pharmacodynamic side effects of the co-administered drug).
No products indexed under this heading.

Cyclobenzaprine Hydrochloride (Ciprofloxacin is an inhibitor of the hepatic CYP1A2 enzyme pathway. Co-administration of ciprofloxacin and other drugs primarily metabolized by CYP1A2 results in increased plasma concentrations of the co-administered drug and could lead to clinically significant pharmacodynamic side effects of the co-administered drug). Products include:
Amrix 964

Cyclosporine (Ciprofloxacin has been associated with transient elevations in serum creatinine in patients receiving cyclosporine concomitantly). Products include:
Gengraf 440
Neoral Oral Solution 2496
Neoral Capsules 2496
Restasis 605

Desipramine Hydrochloride (In general, elderly patients may be more susceptible to drug-associated effects on the QT interval. Therefore, precautions should be taken when using ciprofloxacin with concomitant drugs that can result in prolongation of the QT interval).
No products indexed under this heading.

Desoximetasone (Fluoroquinolones including ciprofloxacin are associated with an increased risk of tendinitis and tendon rupture in all ages. This adverse reaction most frequently involves the Achilles tendon, and rupture of the Achilles tendon may require surgical repair. Tendinitis and tendon rupture in the rotator cuff (the shoulder), the hand, the biceps, the thumb, and other tendon sites have also been reported. The risk of developing fluoroquinolone-associated tendinitis and tendon rupture is further increased in older patients usually over 60 years of age, in patients taking corticosteroid drugs, and in patients with kidney, heart or lung transplants).
No products indexed under this heading.

Dexamethasone (Fluoroquinolones including ciprofloxacin are associated with an increased risk of tendinitis and tendon rupture in all ages. This adverse reaction most frequently involves the Achilles tendon, and rupture of the Achilles tendon may require surgical repair. Tendinitis and tendon rupture in the rotator cuff (the shoulder), the hand, the biceps, the thumb, and other tendon sites have also been reported. The risk of developing fluoroquinolone-associated tendinitis and tendon rupture is further increased in older patients usually over 60 years of age, in patients taking corticosteroid drugs, and in patients with kidney, heart or lung transplants). Products include:
Ciprodex 583
Ozurdex .... ⊙ 223
Tobramycin and Dexamethasone Ophthalmic Suspension .... ⊙ 251

Dexamethasone Acetate (Fluoroquinolones including ciprofloxacin are associated with an increased risk of tendinitis and tendon rupture in all ages. This adverse reaction most frequently involves the Achilles tendon, and rupture of the Achilles tendon may require surgical repair. Tendinitis and tendon rupture in the rotator cuff (the shoulder), the hand, the biceps, the thumb, and other tendon sites have also been reported. The risk of developing fluoroquinolone-associated tendinitis and tendon rupture is further increased in older patients usually over 60 years of age, in patients taking corticosteroid drugs, and in patients with kidney, heart or lung transplants).
No products indexed under this heading.

Dexamethasone Phosphate (Fluoroquinolones including ciprofloxacin are associated with an increased risk of tendinitis and tendon rupture in all ages. This adverse reaction most frequently involves the Achilles tendon, and rupture of the Achilles tendon may require surgical repair. Tendinitis and tendon rupture in the rotator cuff (the shoulder), the hand, the biceps, the thumb, and other tendon sites have also been reported. The risk of developing fluoroquinolone-associated tendinitis and tendon rupture is further increased in older patients usually over 60 years of age, in patients taking corticosteroid drugs, and in patients with kidney, heart or lung transplants).
No products indexed under this heading.

Dexamethasone Sodium (Fluoroquinolones including ciprofloxacin are associated with an increased risk of tendinitis and tendon rupture in all ages. This adverse reaction most frequently involves the Achilles tendon, and rupture of the Achilles tendon may require surgical repair. Tendinitis and tendon rupture in the rotator cuff (the shoulder), the hand, the biceps, the thumb, and other tendon sites have also been reported. The risk of developing fluoroquinolone-associated tendinitis and tendon rupture is further increased in older patients usually over 60 years of age, in patients taking corticosteroid drugs, and in patients with kidney, heart or lung transplants).
No products indexed under this heading.

Dexamethasone Sodium Phosphate (Fluoroquinolones including ciprofloxacin are associated with an increased risk of tendinitis and tendon rupture in all ages. This adverse reaction most frequently involves the Achilles tendon, and rupture of the Achilles tendon may require surgical repair. Tendinitis and tendon rupture in the rotator cuff (the shoulder), the hand, the biceps, the thumb, and other tendon sites have also been reported. The risk of developing fluoroquinolone-associated tendinitis and tendon rupture is further increased in older patients usually over 60 years of age, in patients taking corticosteroid drugs, and in patients with kidney, heart or lung transplants).
No products indexed under this heading.

Dexamethasone Sodium Phosphate Injection (Fluoroquinolones including ciprofloxacin are associated with an increased risk of tendinitis and tendon rupture in all ages. This adverse reaction most frequently involves the Achilles tendon, and rupture of the Achilles tendon may require surgical repair. Tendinitis and tendon rupture in the rotator cuff (the shoulder), the hand, the biceps, the thumb, and other tendon sites have also been reported. The risk of developing fluoroquinolone-associated tendinitis and tendon rupture is further increased in older patients usually over 60 years of age, in patients taking corticosteroid drugs, and in patients with kidney, heart or lung transplants).
No products indexed under this heading.

Diazepam (In general, elderly patients may be more susceptible to drug-

337 Interactions Index Cipro Tablets

associated effects on the QT interval. Therefore, precautions should be taken when using ciprofloxacin with concomitant drugs that can result in prolongation of the QT interval). Products include:
Valium Tablets 2880

Diclofenac Epolamine (Non-steroidal anti-inflammatory drugs in combination of very high doses of quinolones have been shown to provoke convulsions in pre-clinical studies). Products include:
Flector 1839

Diclofenac Potassium (Non-steroidal anti-inflammatory drugs in combination of very high doses of quinolones have been shown to provoke convulsions in pre-clinical studies).
No products indexed under this heading.

Diclofenac Sodium (Non-steroidal anti-inflammatory drugs in combination of very high doses of quinolones have been shown to provoke convulsions in pre-clinical studies).
No products indexed under this heading.

Dicumarol (Ciprofloxacin has been reported to enhance the effects of the oral anticoagulant warfarin or its derivatives. When these products are administered concomitantly, prothrombin time or other suitable coagulant tests should be closely monitored).
No products indexed under this heading.

Didanosine (Concurrent administration of ciprofloxacin with multivalent cation-containing products, such as didanosine chewable/buffered tablets or pediatric powder, may substantially decrease its absorption, resulting in serum and urine levels considerably lower than desired. Ciprofloxacin should be administered at least 2 hours before or 6 hours after didanosine chewable/buffered tablets or pediatric powder for oral solution).
No products indexed under this heading.

Diflorasone Diacetate (Fluoroquinolones including ciprofloxacin are associated with an increased risk of tendinitis and tendon rupture in all ages. This adverse reaction most frequently involves the Achilles tendon, and rupture of the Achilles tendon may require surgical repair. Tendinitis and tendon rupture in the rotator cuff (the shoulder), the hand, the biceps, the thumb, and other tendon sites have also been reported. The risk of developing fluoroquinolone-associated tendinitis and tendon rupture is further increased in older patients usually over 60 years of age, in patients taking corticosteroid drugs, and in patients with kidney, heart or lung transplants).
No products indexed under this heading.

Diltiazem Hydrochloride (Ciprofloxacin is an inhibitor of the hepatic CYP1A2 enzyme pathway. Co-administration of ciprofloxacin and other drugs primarily metabolized by CYP1A2 results in increased plasma concentrations of the co-administered drug and could lead to clinically significant pharmacodynamic side effects of the co-administered drug). Products include:
Cardizem LA 423

Diltiazem Maleate (Ciprofloxacin is an inhibitor of the hepatic CYP1A2 enzyme pathway. Co-administration of ciprofloxacin and other drugs primarily metabolized by CYP1A2 results in increased plasma concentrations of the co-administered drug and could lead to clinically significant pharmacodynamic side effects of the co-administered drug).
No products indexed under this heading.

Disopyramide (In general, elderly patients may be more susceptible to drug-associated effects on the QT interval. Therefore, precautions should be taken when using ciprofloxacin with concomitant drugs that can result in prolongation of the QT interval).
No products indexed under this heading.

Disopyramide Phosphate (In general, elderly patients may be more susceptible to drug-associated effects on the QT interval. Therefore, precautions should be taken when using ciprofloxacin with concomitant drugs that can result in prolongation of the QT interval).
No products indexed under this heading.

Dofetilide (In general, elderly patients may be more susceptible to drug-associated effects on the QT interval. Therefore, precautions should be taken when using ciprofloxacin with concomitant drugs that can result in prolongation of the QT interval).
No products indexed under this heading.

Doxepin Hydrochloride (In general, elderly patients may be more susceptible to drug-associated effects on the QT interval. Therefore, precautions should be taken when using ciprofloxacin with concomitant drugs that can result in prolongation of the QT interval).
No products indexed under this heading.

Droperidol (In general, elderly patients may be more susceptible to drug-associated effects on the QT interval. Therefore, precautions should be taken when using ciprofloxacin with concomitant drugs that can result in prolongation of the QT interval).
No products indexed under this heading.

Dyphylline (Ciprofloxacin is an inhibitor of the hepatic CYP1A2 enzyme pathway. Co-administration of ciprofloxacin and other drugs primarily metabolized by CYP1A2, such as methylxanthines, results in increased plasma concentrations of co-administered drug and could lead to clinically significant pharmacodynamic side effects of the co-administered drug).
No products indexed under this heading.

Enoxacin (Ciprofloxacin is an inhibitor of the hepatic CYP1A2 enzyme pathway. Co-administration of ciprofloxacin and other drugs primarily metabolized by CYP1A2 results in increased plasma concentrations of the co-administered drug and could lead to clinically significant pharmacodynamic side effects of the co-administered drug).
No products indexed under this heading.

Erythromycin (In general, elderly patients may be more susceptible to drug-associated effects on the QT interval. Therefore, precautions should be taken when using ciprofloxacin with concomitant drugs that can result in prolongation of the QT interval).
No products indexed under this heading.

Erythromycin Estolate (In general, elderly patients may be more susceptible to drug-associated effects on the QT interval. Therefore, precautions should be taken when using ciprofloxacin with concomitant drugs that can result in prolongation of the QT interval).
No products indexed under this heading.

Erythromycin Ethylsuccinate (In general, elderly patients may be more susceptible to drug-associated effects on the QT interval. Therefore, precautions should be taken when using ciprofloxacin with concomitant drugs that can result in prolongation of the QT interval). Products include:
E.E.S. 437
EryPed 435

Erythromycin Gluceptate (In general, elderly patients may be more susceptible to drug-associated effects on the QT interval. Therefore, precautions should be taken when using ciprofloxacin with concomitant drugs that can result in prolongation of the QT interval).
No products indexed under this heading.

Erythromycin Lactobionate (In general, elderly patients may be more susceptible to drug-associated effects on the QT interval. Therefore, precautions should be taken when using ciprofloxacin with concomitant drugs that can result in prolongation of the QT interval).
No products indexed under this heading.

Erythromycin Stearate (In general, elderly patients may be more susceptible to drug-associated effects on the QT interval. Therefore, precautions should be taken when using ciprofloxacin with concomitant drugs that can result in prolongation of the QT interval).
No products indexed under this heading.

Estradiol (Ciprofloxacin is an inhibitor of the hepatic CYP1A2 enzyme pathway. Co-administration of ciprofloxacin and other drugs primarily metabolized by CYP1A2 results in increased plasma concentrations of the co-administered drug and could lead to clinically significant pharmacodynamic side effects of the co-administered drug). Products include:
Activella 2561
Angeliq 831
Climara 841
Climara Pro 847
Divigel 3467
Estrasorb 1777
Vagifem 2589

Estradiol Benzoate (Ciprofloxacin is an inhibitor of the hepatic CYP1A2 enzyme pathway. Co-administration of ciprofloxacin and other drugs primarily metabolized by CYP1A2 results in increased plasma concentrations of the co-administered drug and could lead to clinically significant pharmacodynamic side effects of the co-administered drug).
No products indexed under this heading.

Estradiol Cypionate (Ciprofloxacin is an inhibitor of the hepatic CYP1A2 enzyme pathway. Co-administration of ciprofloxacin and other drugs primarily metabolized by CYP1A2 results in increased plasma concentrations of the co-administered drug and could lead to clinically significant pharmacodynamic side effects of the co-administered drug).
No products indexed under this heading.

Etodolac (Non-steroidal anti-inflammatory drugs in combination of very high doses of quinolones have been shown to provoke convulsions in pre-clinical studies).
No products indexed under this heading.

Fenoprofen Calcium (Non-steroidal anti-inflammatory drugs in combination of very high doses of quinolones have been shown to provoke convulsions in pre-clinical studies).
No products indexed under this heading.

Ferrous Fumarate (Concurrent administration of ciprofloxacin with products containing iron may substantially decrease its absorption, resulting in serum and urine levels considerably lower than desired. Ciprofloxacin should be administered at least 2 hours before or 6 hours after products containing iron). Products include:
PreNexa 3473

Ferrous Gluconate (Concurrent administration of ciprofloxacin with products containing iron may substantially decrease its absorption, resulting in serum and urine levels considerably lower than desired. Ciprofloxacin should be administered at least 2 hours before or 6 hours after products containing iron). Products include:
CitraNatal Assure 2332
CitraNatal Rx 2332

Ferrous Sulfate (Concurrent administration of ciprofloxacin with products containing iron may substantially decrease its absorption, resulting in serum and urine levels considerably lower than desired. Ciprofloxacin should be administered at least 2 hours before or 6 hours after products containing iron).
No products indexed under this heading.

Flecainide Acetate (In general, elderly patients may be more susceptible to drug-associated effects on the QT interval. Therefore, precautions should be taken when using ciprofloxacin with concomitant drugs that can result in prolongation of the QT interval).
No products indexed under this heading.

Fludrocortisone Acetate (Fluoroquinolones including ciprofloxacin are associated with an increased risk of tendinitis and tendon rupture in all ages. This adverse reaction most frequently involves the Achilles tendon, and rupture of the Achilles tendon may require surgical repair. Tendinitis and tendon rupture in the rotator cuff (the shoulder), the hand, the biceps, the thumb, and other tendon sites have also been reported. The risk of developing fluoroquinolone-associated tendinitis and tendon rupture is further increased in older patients usually over 60 years of age, in patients taking corticosteroid drugs, and in patients with kidney, heart or lung transplants).
No products indexed under this heading.

Flumethasone Pivalate (Fluoroquinolones including ciprofloxacin are associated with an increased risk of tendinitis and tendon rupture in all ages. This adverse reaction most frequently involves the Achilles tendon, and rupture of the Achilles tendon may require surgical repair. Tendinitis and tendon rupture in the rotator cuff (the shoulder), the hand, the biceps, the thumb, and other tendon sites have also been reported. The risk of developing fluoroquinolone-associated tendinitis and tendon rupture is further increased in older patients usually over 60 years of age, in patients taking corticosteroid drugs, and in patients with kidney, heart or lung transplants).
No products indexed under this heading.

Flunisolide Hemihydrate (Fluoroquinolones including ciprofloxacin are associated with an increased risk of tendinitis and tendon rupture in all ages. This adverse reaction most frequently involves the Achilles tendon, and rupture of the Achilles tendon may require surgical repair. Tendinitis and tendon rupture in the rotator cuff (the shoulder), the hand, the biceps, the thumb, and other tendon sites have also been reported. The risk of developing fluoroquinolone-associated tendinitis and tendon rupture is further increased in older patients usually over 60 years of age, in patients taking corticosteroid drugs, and in patients with kidney, heart or lung transplants).
No products indexed under this heading.

Fluphenazine Decanoate (In general, elderly patients may be more susceptible to drug-associated effects on the QT interval. Therefore, precautions should be taken when using ciprofloxacin with concomitant drugs that can result in prolongation of the QT interval).
No products indexed under this heading.

IMPORTANT NOTE: Always consult each drug listing in the patient's regimen for possible interactions.

Fluphenazine Enanthate (In general, elderly patients may be more susceptible to drug-associated effects on the QT interval. Therefore, precautions should be taken when using ciprofloxacin with concomitant drugs that can result in prolongation of the QT interval).
No products indexed under this heading.

Fluphenazine Hydrochloride (In general, elderly patients may be more susceptible to drug-associated effects on the QT interval. Therefore, precautions should be taken when using ciprofloxacin with concomitant drugs that can result in prolongation of the QT interval).
No products indexed under this heading.

Flurbiprofen (Non-steroidal anti-inflammatory drugs in combination of very high doses of quinolones have been shown to provoke convulsions in preclinical studies).
No products indexed under this heading.

Flutamide (Ciprofloxacin is an inhibitor of the hepatic CYP1A2 enzyme pathway. Co-administration of ciprofloxacin and other drugs primarily metabolized by CYP1A2 results in increased plasma concentrations of the co-administered drug and could lead to clinically significant pharmacodynamic side effects of the co-administered drug).
No products indexed under this heading.

Fluticasone Furoate (Fluoroquinolones including ciprofloxacin are associated with an increased risk of tendinitis and tendon rupture in all ages. This adverse reaction most frequently involves the Achilles tendon, and rupture of the Achilles tendon may require surgical repair. Tendinitis and tendon rupture in the rotator cuff (the shoulder), the hand, the biceps, the thumb, and other tendon sites have also been reported. The risk of developing fluoroquinolone-associated tendinitis and tendon rupture is further increased in older patients usually over 60 years of age, in patients taking corticosteroid drugs, and in patients with kidney, heart or lung transplants). Products include:
Veramyst ... **1713**

Fluticasone Propionate (Fluoroquinolones including ciprofloxacin are associated with an increased risk of tendinitis and tendon rupture in all ages. This adverse reaction most frequently involves the Achilles tendon, and rupture of the Achilles tendon may require surgical repair. Tendinitis and tendon rupture in the rotator cuff (the shoulder), the hand, the biceps, the thumb, and other tendon sites have also been reported. The risk of developing fluoroquinolone-associated tendinitis and tendon rupture is further increased in older patients usually over 60 years of age, in patients taking corticosteroid drugs, and in patients with kidney, heart or lung transplants). Products include:
Advair 100/50 ... **1275**
Advair 250/50 ... **1275**
Advair 500/50 ... **1275**
Advair HFA 45/21 ... **1288**
Advair HFA 115/21 ... **1288**
Advair HFA 230/21 ... **1288**
Flonase ... **1459**
Flovent Diskus ... **1463**
Flovent HFA ... **1470**

Fluvoxamine Maleate (Ciprofloxacin is an inhibitor of the hepatic CYP1A2 enzyme pathway. Co-administration of ciprofloxacin and other drugs primarily metabolized by CYP1A2 results in increased plasma concentrations of the co-administered drug and could lead to clinically significant pharmacodynamic side effects of the co-administered drug).
No products indexed under this heading.

Fosphenytoin (Altered serum levels of phenytoin (increased and decreased) have been reported in patients receiving concomitant ciprofloxacin).
No products indexed under this heading.

Fosphenytoin Sodium (Altered serum levels of phenytoin (increased and decreased) have been reported in patients receiving concomitant ciprofloxacin).
No products indexed under this heading.

Glyburide (The concomitant administration of ciprofloxacin with the sulfonylurea glyburide has, on rare occasions, resulted in severe hypoglycemia).
No products indexed under this heading.

Grepafloxacin Hydrochloride (Ciprofloxacin is an inhibitor of the hepatic CYP1A2 enzyme pathway. Co-administration of ciprofloxacin and other drugs primarily metabolized by CYP1A2 results in increased plasma concentrations of the co-administered drug and could lead to clinically significant pharmacodynamic side effects of the co-administered drug).
No products indexed under this heading.

Haloperidol (In general, elderly patients may be more susceptible to drug-associated effects on the QT interval. Therefore, precautions should be taken when using ciprofloxacin with concomitant drugs that can result in prolongation of the QT interval).
No products indexed under this heading.

Haloperidol Decanoate (In general, elderly patients may be more susceptible to drug-associated effects on the QT interval. Therefore, precautions should be taken when using ciprofloxacin with concomitant drugs that can result in prolongation of the QT interval).
No products indexed under this heading.

Haloperidol Lactate (In general, elderly patients may be more susceptible to drug-associated effects on the QT interval. Therefore, precautions should be taken when using ciprofloxacin with concomitant drugs that can result in prolongation of the QT interval).
No products indexed under this heading.

Hydrocortisone (Fluoroquinolones including ciprofloxacin are associated with an increased risk of tendinitis and tendon rupture in all ages. This adverse reaction most frequently involves the Achilles tendon, and rupture of the Achilles tendon may require surgical repair. Tendinitis and tendon rupture in the rotator cuff (the shoulder), the hand, the biceps, the thumb, and other tendon sites have also been reported. The risk of developing fluoroquinolone-associated tendinitis and tendon rupture is further increased in older patients usually over 60 years of age, in patients taking corticosteroid drugs, and in patients with kidney, heart or lung transplants).
No products indexed under this heading.

Hydrocortisone (Alcohol) (Fluoroquinolones including ciprofloxacin are associated with an increased risk of tendinitis and tendon rupture in all ages. This adverse reaction most frequently involves the Achilles tendon, and rupture of the Achilles tendon may require surgical repair. Tendinitis and tendon rupture in the rotator cuff (the shoulder), the hand, the biceps, the thumb, and other tendon sites have also been reported. The risk of developing fluoroquinolone-associated tendinitis and tendon rupture is further increased in older patients usually over 60 years of age, in patients taking corticosteroid drugs, and in patients with kidney, heart or lung transplants).
No products indexed under this heading.

Hydrocortisone Acetate (Fluoroquinolones including ciprofloxacin are associated with an increased risk of tendinitis and tendon rupture in all ages. This adverse reaction most frequently involves the Achilles tendon, and rupture of the Achilles tendon may require surgical repair. Tendinitis and tendon rupture in the rotator cuff (the shoulder), the hand, the biceps, the thumb, and other tendon sites have also been reported. The risk of developing fluoroquinolone-associated tendinitis and tendon rupture is further increased in older patients usually over 60 years of age, in patients taking corticosteroid drugs, and in patients with kidney, heart or lung transplants).
No products indexed under this heading.

Hydrocortisone Butyrate (Fluoroquinolones including ciprofloxacin are associated with an increased risk of tendinitis and tendon rupture in all ages. This adverse reaction most frequently involves the Achilles tendon, and rupture of the Achilles tendon may require surgical repair. Tendinitis and tendon rupture in the rotator cuff (the shoulder), the hand, the biceps, the thumb, and other tendon sites have also been reported. The risk of developing fluoroquinolone-associated tendinitis and tendon rupture is further increased in older patients usually over 60 years of age, in patients taking corticosteroid drugs, and in patients with kidney, heart or lung transplants).
No products indexed under this heading.

Hydrocortisone Cypionate (Fluoroquinolones including ciprofloxacin are associated with an increased risk of tendinitis and tendon rupture in all ages. This adverse reaction most frequently involves the Achilles tendon, and rupture of the Achilles tendon may require surgical repair. Tendinitis and tendon rupture in the rotator cuff (the shoulder), the hand, the biceps, the thumb, and other tendon sites have also been reported. The risk of developing fluoroquinolone-associated tendinitis and tendon rupture is further increased in older patients usually over 60 years of age, in patients taking corticosteroid drugs, and in patients with kidney, heart or lung transplants).
No products indexed under this heading.

Hydrocortisone Hemisuccinate (Fluoroquinolones including ciprofloxacin are associated with an increased risk of tendinitis and tendon rupture in all ages. This adverse reaction most frequently involves the Achilles tendon, and rupture of the Achilles tendon may require surgical repair. Tendinitis and tendon rupture in the rotator cuff (the shoulder), the hand, the biceps, the thumb, and other tendon sites have also been reported. The risk of developing fluoroquinolone-associated tendinitis and tendon rupture is further increased in older patients usually over 60 years of age, in patients taking corticosteroid drugs, and in patients with kidney, heart or lung transplants).
No products indexed under this heading.

Hydrocortisone Probutate (Fluoroquinolones including ciprofloxacin are associated with an increased risk of tendinitis and tendon rupture in all ages. This adverse reaction most frequently involves the Achilles tendon, and rupture of the Achilles tendon may require surgical repair. Tendinitis and tendon rupture in the rotator cuff (the shoulder), the hand, the biceps, the thumb, and other tendon sites have also been reported. The risk of developing fluoroquinolone-associated tendinitis and tendon rupture is further increased in older patients usually over 60 years of age, in patients taking corticosteroid drugs, and in patients with kidney, heart or lung transplants).
No products indexed under this heading.

Hydrocortisone Sodium Phosphate (Fluoroquinolones including ciprofloxacin are associated with an increased risk of tendinitis and tendon rupture in all ages. This adverse reaction most frequently involves the Achilles tendon, and rupture of the Achilles tendon may require surgical repair. Tendinitis and tendon rupture in the rotator cuff (the shoulder), the hand, the biceps, the thumb, and other tendon sites have also been reported. The risk of developing fluoroquinolone-associated tendinitis and tendon rupture is further increased in older patients usually over 60 years of age, in patients taking corticosteroid drugs, and in patients with kidney, heart or lung transplants).
No products indexed under this heading.

Hydrocortisone Sodium Succinate (Fluoroquinolones including ciprofloxacin are associated with an increased risk of tendinitis and tendon rupture in all ages. This adverse reaction most frequently involves the Achilles tendon, and rupture of the Achilles tendon may require surgical repair. Tendinitis and tendon rupture in the rotator cuff (the shoulder), the hand, the biceps, the thumb, and other tendon sites have also been reported. The risk of developing fluoroquinolone-associated tendinitis and tendon rupture is further increased in older patients usually over 60 years of age, in patients taking corticosteroid drugs, and in patients with kidney, heart or lung transplants).
No products indexed under this heading.

Hydrocortisone Valerate (Fluoroquinolones including ciprofloxacin are associated with an increased risk of tendinitis and tendon rupture in all ages. This adverse reaction most frequently involves the Achilles tendon, and rupture of the Achilles tendon may require surgical repair. Tendinitis and tendon rupture in the rotator cuff (the shoulder), the hand, the biceps, the thumb, and other tendon sites have also been reported. The risk of developing fluoroquinolone-associated tendinitis and tendon rupture is further increased in older patients usually over 60 years of age, in patients taking corticosteroid drugs, and in patients with kidney, heart or lung transplants).
No products indexed under this heading.

Hydroxyzine Hydrochloride (In general, elderly patients may be more susceptible to drug-associated effects on the QT interval. Therefore, precautions should be taken when using ciprofloxacin with concomitant drugs that can result in prolongation of the QT interval).
No products indexed under this heading.

Ibuprofen (Non-steroidal anti-inflammatory drugs in combination of very high doses of quinolones have been shown to provoke convulsions in pre-clinical studies). Products include:
Motrin IB ... **2043**
Children's Motrin ... **2044**
Children's Motrin Non-Staining Dye-Free ... **2044**
Infants' Motrin ... **2044**
Infants' Motrin Dye-Free ... **2044**
Junior Strength Motrin ... **2044**
Vicoprofen ... **564**

Imipramine Hydrochloride (In general, elderly patients may be more susceptible to drug-associated effects on the QT interval. Therefore, precautions should be taken when using ciprofloxacin with concomitant drugs that can result in prolongation of the QT interval).
No products indexed under this heading.

Imipramine Pamoate (In general, elderly patients may be more susceptible to drug-associated effects on the QT interval. Therefore, precautions should be taken when using ciprofloxacin with concomitant drugs that can result in prolongation of the QT interval).
No products indexed under this heading.

Indomethacin (Non-steroidal anti-inflammatory drugs in combination of very high doses of quinolones have been shown to provoke convulsions in pre-clinical studies). Products include:
Indocin 2167

Indomethacin Sodium Trihydrate (Non-steroidal anti-inflammatory drugs in combination of very high doses of quinolones have been shown to provoke convulsions in pre-clinical studies). Products include:
Indocin I.V. 2007

Iron (Concurrent administration of ciprofloxacin with products containing iron may substantially decrease its absorption, resulting in serum and urine levels considerably lower than desired. Ciprofloxacin should be administered at least 2 hours before or 6 hours after products containing iron).
No products indexed under this heading.

Iron, Peptonized (Concurrent administration of ciprofloxacin with multivalent cation-containing products may substantially decrease its absorption, resulting in serum and urine levels considerably lower than desired).
No products indexed under this heading.

Iron & Ammonium Citrate (Concurrent administration of ciprofloxacin with multivalent cation-containing products may substantially decrease its absorption, resulting in serum and urine levels considerably lower than desired).
No products indexed under this heading.

Iron Cacodylate (Concurrent administration of ciprofloxacin with multivalent cation-containing products may substantially decrease its absorption, resulting in serum and urine levels considerably lower than desired).
No products indexed under this heading.

Iron Carbonyl (Concurrent administration of ciprofloxacin with multivalent cation-containing products may substantially decrease its absorption, resulting in serum and urine levels considerably lower than desired). Products include:
CitraNatal 90 DHA Capsules 2332
CitraNatal Assure 2332
CitraNatal Harmony 2332
CitraNatal Rx 2332
Ferralet 2333

Iron Supplements (Concurrent administration of ciprofloxacin with multivalent cation-containing products may substantially decrease its absorption, resulting in serum and urine levels considerably lower than desired).
No products indexed under this heading.

Isocarboxazid (In general, elderly patients may be more susceptible to drug-associated effects on the QT interval. Therefore, precautions should be taken when using ciprofloxacin with concomitant drugs that can result in prolongation of the QT interval). Products include:
Marplan 3481

Ketoprofen (Non-steroidal anti-inflammatory drugs in combination of very high doses of quinolones have been shown to provoke convulsions in pre-clinical studies).
No products indexed under this heading.

Ketorolac Tromethamine (Non-steroidal anti-inflammatory drugs in combination of very high doses of quinolones have been shown to provoke convulsions in pre-clinical studies). Products include:

Acuvail .... ⊙209

Levobupivacaine Hydrochloride (Ciprofloxacin is an inhibitor of the hepatic CYP1A2 enzyme pathway. Co-administration of ciprofloxacin and other drugs primarily metabolized by CYP1A2 results in increased plasma concentrations of the co-administered drug and could lead to clinically significant pharmacodynamic side effects of the co-administered drug).
No products indexed under this heading.

Lidocaine (In general, elderly patients may be more susceptible to drug-associated effects on the QT interval. Therefore, precautions should be taken when using ciprofloxacin with concomitant drugs that can result in prolongation of the QT interval). Products include:
Lidoderm 1107

Lidocaine Hydrochloride (In general, elderly patients may be more susceptible to drug-associated effects on the QT interval. Therefore, precautions should be taken when using ciprofloxacin with concomitant drugs that can result in prolongation of the QT interval).
No products indexed under this heading.

Lithium Carbonate (In general, elderly patients may be more susceptible to drug-associated effects on the QT interval. Therefore, precautions should be taken when using ciprofloxacin with concomitant drugs that can result in prolongation of the QT interval).
No products indexed under this heading.

Lithium Citrate (In general, elderly patients may be more susceptible to drug-associated effects on the QT interval. Therefore, precautions should be taken when using ciprofloxacin with concomitant drugs that can result in prolongation of the QT interval).
No products indexed under this heading.

Lomefloxacin Hydrochloride (Ciprofloxacin is an inhibitor of the hepatic CYP1A2 enzyme pathway. Co-administration of ciprofloxacin and other drugs primarily metabolized by CYP1A2 results in increased plasma concentrations of the co-administered drug and could lead to clinically significant pharmacodynamic side effects of the co-administered drug).
No products indexed under this heading.

Lorazepam (In general, elderly patients may be more susceptible to drug-associated effects on the QT interval. Therefore, precautions should be taken when using ciprofloxacin with concomitant drugs that can result in prolongation of the QT interval).
No products indexed under this heading.

Loxapine Hydrochloride (In general, elderly patients may be more susceptible to drug-associated effects on the QT interval. Therefore, precautions should be taken when using ciprofloxacin with concomitant drugs that can result in prolongation of the QT interval).
No products indexed under this heading.

Loxapine Succinate (In general, elderly patients may be more susceptible to drug-associated effects on the QT interval. Therefore, precautions should be taken when using ciprofloxacin with concomitant drugs that can result in prolongation of the QT interval).
No products indexed under this heading.

Magaldrate (Concurrent administration of ciprofloxacin with multivalent cation-containing products, such as magnesium/aluminum antacids, may substantially decrease its absorption, resulting in serum and urine levels considerably lower than desired. Ciprofloxacin may be taken two hours before or six hours after taking magnesium or aluminum containing antacids. Concurrent administration of antacids contain-

ing magnesium hydroxide or aluminum hydroxide may reduce the bioavailability of ciprofloxacin by as much as 90%).
No products indexed under this heading.

Magnesium (Concurrent administration of ciprofloxacin with multivalent cation-containing products may substantially decrease its absorption, resulting in serum and urine levels considerably lower than desired). Products include:
BoneMate Plus 3454
Cardio Basics 3455
Chelated Mineral 3476

Magnesium Aluminum Silicate (Concurrent administration of ciprofloxacin with multivalent cation-containing products may substantially decrease its absorption, resulting in serum and urine levels considerably lower than desired).
No products indexed under this heading.

Magnesium Carbonate (Concurrent administration of ciprofloxacin with multivalent cation-containing products, such as magnesium/aluminum antacids, may substantially decrease its absorption, resulting in serum and urine levels considerably lower than desired. Ciprofloxacin may be taken two hours before or six hours after taking magnesium or aluminum containing antacids. Concurrent administration of antacids containing magnesium hydroxide or aluminum hydroxide may reduce the bioavailability of ciprofloxacin by as much as 90%).
No products indexed under this heading.

Magnesium Chloride (Concurrent administration of ciprofloxacin with multivalent cation-containing products may substantially decrease its absorption, resulting in serum and urine levels considerably lower than desired).
No products indexed under this heading.

Magnesium Citrate (Concurrent administration of ciprofloxacin with multivalent cation-containing products may substantially decrease its absorption, resulting in serum and urine levels considerably lower than desired). Products include:
Chelated Mineral 3476

Magnesium Gluconate (Concurrent administration of ciprofloxacin with multivalent cation-containing products may substantially decrease its absorption, resulting in serum and urine levels considerably lower than desired).
No products indexed under this heading.

Magnesium Hydroxide (Concurrent administration of ciprofloxacin with multivalent cation-containing products, such as magnesium/aluminum antacids, may substantially decrease its absorption, resulting in serum and urine levels considerably lower than desired. Ciprofloxacin may be taken two hours before or six hours after taking magnesium or aluminum containing antacids. Concurrent administration of antacids containing magnesium hydroxide or aluminum hydroxide may reduce the bioavailability of ciprofloxacin by as much as 90%). Products include:
Fleet Pedia-Lax Chewable Tablets 1144
Pepcid Complete 1822

Magnesium Lactate (Concurrent administration of ciprofloxacin with multivalent cation-containing products may substantially decrease its absorption, resulting in serum and urine levels considerably lower than desired).
No products indexed under this heading.

Magnesium Oxide (Concurrent administration of ciprofloxacin with multivalent cation-containing products, such as magnesium/aluminum antacids, may substantially decrease its absorption, resulting in serum and urine levels considerably lower than desired. Ciprofloxacin may be taken two hours before or six hours after taking magnesium or aluminum containing antacids. Concur-

rent administration of antacids containing magnesium hydroxide or aluminum hydroxide may reduce the bioavailability of ciprofloxacin by as much as 90%). Products include:
Beelith 873

Magnesium Salicylate (Concurrent administration of ciprofloxacin with multivalent cation-containing products may substantially decrease its absorption, resulting in serum and urine levels considerably lower than desired).
No products indexed under this heading.

Magnesium Salicylate Tetrahydrate (Concurrent administration of ciprofloxacin with multivalent cation-containing products may substantially decrease its absorption, resulting in serum and urine levels considerably lower than desired).
No products indexed under this heading.

Magnesium Salts (Concurrent administration of ciprofloxacin with multivalent cation-containing products may substantially decrease its absorption, resulting in serum and urine levels considerably lower than desired).
No products indexed under this heading.

Magnesium Sulfate (Concurrent administration of ciprofloxacin with multivalent cation-containing products may substantially decrease its absorption, resulting in serum and urine levels considerably lower than desired).
No products indexed under this heading.

Magnesium Trisilicate (Concurrent administration of ciprofloxacin with multivalent cation-containing products, such as magnesium/aluminum antacids, may substantially decrease its absorption, resulting in serum and urine levels considerably lower than desired. Ciprofloxacin may be taken two hours before or six hours after taking magnesium or aluminum containing antacids. Concurrent administration of antacids containing magnesium hydroxide or aluminum hydroxide may reduce the bioavailability of ciprofloxacin by as much as 90%).
No products indexed under this heading.

Maprotiline Hydrochloride (In general, elderly patients may be more susceptible to drug-associated effects on the QT interval. Therefore, precautions should be taken when using ciprofloxacin with concomitant drugs that can result in prolongation of the QT interval).
No products indexed under this heading.

Meclofenamate Sodium (Non-steroidal anti-inflammatory drugs in combination of very high doses of quinolones have been shown to provoke convulsions in pre-clinical studies).
No products indexed under this heading.

Mefenamic Acid (Non-steroidal anti-inflammatory drugs in combination of very high doses of quinolones have been shown to provoke convulsions in pre-clinical studies).
No products indexed under this heading.

Meloxicam (Non-steroidal anti-inflammatory drugs in combination of very high doses of quinolones have been shown to provoke convulsions in pre-clinical studies).
No products indexed under this heading.

Meprobamate (In general, elderly patients may be more susceptible to drug-associated effects on the QT interval. Therefore, precautions should be taken when using ciprofloxacin with concomitant drugs that can result in prolongation of the QT interval).
No products indexed under this heading.

IMPORTANT NOTE: Always consult each drug listing in the patient's regimen for possible interactions.

(⊙ Described in PDR® for Ophthalmic Medicines)

Perphenazine (In general, elderly patients may be more susceptible to drug-associated effects on the QT interval. Therefore, precautions should be taken when using ciprofloxacin with concomitant drugs that can result in prolongation of the QT interval).
No products indexed under this heading.

Phenelzine Sulfate (In general, elderly patients may be more susceptible to drug-associated effects on the QT interval. Therefore, precautions should be taken when using ciprofloxacin with concomitant drugs that can result in prolongation of the QT interval).
No products indexed under this heading.

Phenobarbital (Ciprofloxacin is an inhibitor of the hepatic CYP1A2 enzyme pathway. Co-administration of ciprofloxacin and other drugs primarily metabolized by CYP1A2 results in increased plasma concentrations of the co-administered drug and could lead to clinically significant pharmacodynamic side effects of the co-administered drug). Products include:
Donnatal 2711

Phenobarbital Sodium (Ciprofloxacin is an inhibitor of the hepatic CYP1A2 enzyme pathway. Co-administration of ciprofloxacin and other drugs primarily metabolized by CYP1A2 results in increased plasma concentrations of the co-administered drug and could lead to clinically significant pharmacodynamic side effects of the co-administered drug).
No products indexed under this heading.

Phenylbutazone (Non-steroidal anti-inflammatory drugs in combination of very high doses of quinolones have been shown to provoke convulsions in pre-clinical studies).
No products indexed under this heading.

Phenytoin (Altered serum levels of phenytoin (increased and decreased) have been reported in patients receiving concomitant ciprofloxacin).
No products indexed under this heading.

Phenytoin Sodium (Altered serum levels of phenytoin (increased and decreased) have been reported in patients receiving concomitant ciprofloxacin). Products include:
Phenytek Capsules 2380

Piroxicam (Non-steroidal anti-inflammatory drugs in combination of very high doses of quinolones have been shown to provoke convulsions in pre-clinical studies).
No products indexed under this heading.

Polysaccharide Iron Complex (Concurrent administration of ciprofloxacin with products containing iron may substantially decrease its absorption, resulting in serum and urine levels considerably lower than desired. Ciprofloxacin should be administered at least 2 hours before or 6 hours after products containing iron). Products include:
Nu-Iron 150 2321

Prazepam (In general, elderly patients may be more susceptible to drug-associated effects on the QT interval. Therefore, precautions should be taken when using ciprofloxacin with concomitant drugs that can result in prolongation of the QT interval).
No products indexed under this heading.

Prednisolone (Fluoroquinolones including ciprofloxacin are associated with an increased risk of tendinitis and tendon rupture in all ages. This adverse reaction most frequently involves the Achilles tendon, and rupture of the Achilles tendon may require surgical repair. Tendinitis and tendon rupture in the rotator cuff (the shoulder), the hand, the biceps, the thumb, and other tendon sites have also been reported. The risk of developing fluoroquinolone-associated tendinitis and tendon rupture

is further increased in older patients usually over 60 years of age, in patients taking corticosteroid drugs, and in patients with kidney, heart or lung transplants).
No products indexed under this heading.

Prednisolone Acetate (Fluoroquinolones including ciprofloxacin are associated with an increased risk of tendinitis and tendon rupture in all ages. This adverse reaction most frequently involves the Achilles tendon, and rupture of the Achilles tendon may require surgical repair. Tendinitis and tendon rupture in the rotator cuff (the shoulder), the hand, the biceps, the thumb, and other tendon sites have also been reported. The risk of developing fluoroquinolone-associated tendinitis and tendon rupture is further increased in older patients usually over 60 years of age, in patients taking corticosteroid drugs, and in patients with kidney, heart or lung transplants). Products include:
Blephamide .... ⊙212, ⊙214
Pred Forte ....⊙225
Pred Mild ....⊙230
Pred-G ....⊙226, ⊙227

Prednisolone Sodium Phosphate (Fluoroquinolones including ciprofloxacin are associated with an increased risk of tendinitis and tendon rupture in all ages. This adverse reaction most frequently involves the Achilles tendon, and rupture of the Achilles tendon may require surgical repair. Tendinitis and tendon rupture in the rotator cuff (the shoulder), the hand, the biceps, the thumb, and other tendon sites have also been reported. The risk of developing fluoroquinolone-associated tendinitis and tendon rupture is further increased in older patients usually over 60 years of age, in patients taking corticosteroid drugs, and in patients with kidney, heart or lung transplants).
No products indexed under this heading.

Prednisolone Tebutate (Fluoroquinolones including ciprofloxacin are associated with an increased risk of tendinitis and tendon rupture in all ages. This adverse reaction most frequently involves the Achilles tendon, and rupture of the Achilles tendon may require surgical repair. Tendinitis and tendon rupture in the rotator cuff (the shoulder), the hand, the biceps, the thumb, and other tendon sites have also been reported. The risk of developing fluoroquinolone-associated tendinitis and tendon rupture is further increased in older patients usually over 60 years of age, in patients taking corticosteroid drugs, and in patients with kidney, heart or lung transplants).
No products indexed under this heading.

Prednisone (Fluoroquinolones including ciprofloxacin are associated with an increased risk of tendinitis and tendon rupture in all ages. This adverse reaction most frequently involves the Achilles tendon, and rupture of the Achilles tendon may require surgical repair. Tendinitis and tendon rupture in the rotator cuff (the shoulder), the hand, the biceps, the thumb, and other tendon sites have also been reported. The risk of developing fluoroquinolone-associated tendinitis and tendon rupture is further increased in older patients usually over 60 years of age, in patients taking corticosteroid drugs, and in patients with kidney, heart or lung transplants).
No products indexed under this heading.

Prednisone sodium phosphate (Fluoroquinolones including ciprofloxacin are associated with an increased risk of tendinitis and tendon rupture in all ages. This adverse reaction most frequently involves the Achilles tendon, and rupture of the Achilles tendon may require surgical repair. Tendinitis and

tendon rupture in the rotator cuff (the shoulder), the hand, the biceps, the thumb, and other tendon sites have also been reported. The risk of developing fluoroquinolone-associated tendinitis and tendon rupture is further increased in older patients usually over 60 years of age, in patients taking corticosteroid drugs, and in patients with kidney, heart or lung transplants).
No products indexed under this heading.

Probenecid (Probenecid interferes with renal tubular secretion of ciprofloxacin and produces an increase in the level of ciprofloxacin in the serum. This should be considered if patients are receiving both drugs concomitantly).
No products indexed under this heading.

Procainamide (In general, eldery patients may be more susceptible to drug-associated effects on the QT interval. Therefore, precautions should be taken when using ciprofloxacin with concomitant drugs that can result in prolongation of the QT interval (eg, class IA antiarrhythmics)).
No products indexed under this heading.

Procainamide Hydrochloride (In general, elderly patients may be more susceptible to drug-associated effects on the QT interval. Therefore, precautions should be taken when using ciprofloxacin with concomitant drugs that can result in prolongation of the QT interval).
No products indexed under this heading.

Prochlorperazine (In general, elderly patients may be more susceptible to drug-associated effects on the QT interval. Therefore, precautions should be taken when using ciprofloxacin with concomitant drugs that can result in prolongation of the QT interval).
No products indexed under this heading.

Promethazine Hydrochloride (In general, elderly patients may be more susceptible to drug-associated effects on the QT interval. Therefore, precautions should be taken when using ciprofloxacin with concomitant drugs that can result in prolongation of the QT interval).
No products indexed under this heading.

Propafenone Hydrochloride (In general, elderly patients may be more susceptible to drug-associated effects on the QT interval. Therefore, precautions should be taken when using ciprofloxacin with concomitant drugs that can result in prolongation of the QT interval). Products include:
Rythmol 1648
Rythmol SR 1652

Propranolol Hydrochloride (Ciprofloxacin is an inhibitor of the hepatic CYP1A2 enzyme pathway. Co-administration of ciprofloxacin and other drugs primarily metabolized by CYP1A2 results in increased plasma concentrations of the co-administered drug and could lead to clinically significant pharmacodynamic side effects of the co-administered drug). Products include:
InnoPran XL 1517

Protriptyline Hydrochloride (In general, elderly patients may be more susceptible to drug-associated effects on the QT interval. Therefore, precautions should be taken when using ciprofloxacin with concomitant drugs that can result in prolongation of the QT interval).
No products indexed under this heading.

Quetiapine Fumarate (In general, elderly patients may be more susceptible to drug-associated effects on the QT interval. Therefore, precautions should be taken when using ciprofloxacin with concomitant drugs that can result in prolongation of the QT interval). Products include:
Seroquel 750
Seroquel XR 759

Quinidine (In general, elderly patients may be more susceptible to drug-associated effects on the QT interval. Therefore, precautions should be taken when using ciprofloxacin with concomitant drugs that can result in prolongation of the QT interval).
No products indexed under this heading.

Quinidine Gluconate (In general, elderly patients may be more susceptible to drug-associated effects on the QT interval. Therefore, precautions should be taken when using ciprofloxacin with concomitant drugs that can result in prolongation of the QT interval).
No products indexed under this heading.

Quinidine Hydrochloride (In general, elderly patients may be more susceptible to drug-associated effects on the QT interval. Therefore, precautions should be taken when using ciprofloxacin with concomitant drugs that can result in prolongation of the QT interval).
No products indexed under this heading.

Quinidine Polygalacturonate (In general, elderly patients may be more susceptible to drug-associated effects on the QT interval. Therefore, precautions should be taken when using ciprofloxacin with concomitant drugs that can result in prolongation of the QT interval).
No products indexed under this heading.

Quinidine Sulfate (In general, elderly patients may be more susceptible to drug-associated effects on the QT interval. Therefore, precautions should be taken when using ciprofloxacin with concomitant drugs that can result in prolongation of the QT interval).
No products indexed under this heading.

Riluzole (Ciprofloxacin is an inhibitor of the hepatic CYP1A2 enzyme pathway. Co-administration of ciprofloxacin and other drugs primarily metabolized by CYP1A2 results in increased plasma concentrations of the co-administered drug and could lead to clinically significant pharmacodynamic side effects of the co-administered drug). Products include:
Rilutek 3032

Risperidone (In general, elderly patients may be more susceptible to drug-associated effects on the QT interval. Therefore, precautions should be taken when using ciprofloxacin with concomitant drugs that can result in prolongation of the QT interval). Products include:
Risperdal Consta 2682

Ritonavir (Ciprofloxacin is an inhibitor of the hepatic CYP1A2 enzyme pathway. Co-administration of ciprofloxacin and other drugs primarily metabolized by CYP1A2 results in increased plasma concentrations of the co-administered drug and could lead to clinically significant pharmacodynamic side effects of the co-administered drug). Products include:
Kaletra 458
Norvir 509

Rofecoxib (Non-steroidal anti-inflammatory drugs in combination of very high doses of quinolones have been shown to provoke convulsions in pre-clinical studies).
No products indexed under this heading.

Ropinirole Hydrochloride (Ciprofloxacin is an inhibitor of the hepatic CYP1A2 enzyme pathway. Co-administration of ciprofloxacin and other drugs primarily metabolized by CYP1A2 results in increased plasma concentrations of the co-administered drug and could lead to clinically significant pharmacodynamic side effects of the co-administered drug). Products include:
Requip 1620
Requip XL 1628

IMPORTANT NOTE: Always consult each drug listing in the patient's regimen for possible interactions.

Ropivacaine Hydrochloride (Ciprofloxacin is an inhibitor of the hepatic CYP1A2 enzyme pathway. Co-administration of ciprofloxacin and other drugs primarily metabolized by CYP1A2 results in increased plasma concentrations of the co-administered drug and could lead to clinically significant pharmacodynamic side effects of the co-administered drug).
No products indexed under this heading.

Selenium (Concurrent administration of ciprofloxacin with multivalent cation-containing products may substantially decrease its absorption, resulting in serum and urine levels considerably lower than desired. Products include:
Cardio Basics 3455
Chelated Mineral 3476

Selenium Sulfide (Concurrent administration of ciprofloxacin with multivalent cation-containing products may substantially decrease its absorption, resulting in serum and urine levels considerably lower than desired).
No products indexed under this heading.

Sotalol Hydrochloride (In general, elderly patients may be more susceptible to drug-associated effects on the QT interval. Therefore, precautions should be taken when using ciprofloxacin with concomitant drugs that can result in prolongation of the QT interval (eg, class III antiarrhythmics)).
No products indexed under this heading.

Sucralfate (Concurrent administration of ciprofloxacin with multivalent cation-containing products, such as sucralfate, may substantially decrease its absorption, resulting in serum and urine levels considerably lower than desired. Ciprofloxacin should be administered at least 2 hours before or 6 hours after sucralfate). Products include:
Carafate Suspension 784
Carafate Tablets 785

Sulindac (Non-steroidal anti-inflammatory drugs in combination of very high doses of quinolones have been shown to provoke convulsions in pre-clinical studies). Products include:
Clinoril 2098

Tacrine Hydrochloride (Ciprofloxacin is an inhibitor of the hepatic CYP1A2 enzyme pathway. Co-administration of ciprofloxacin and other drugs primarily metabolized by CYP1A2 results in increased plasma concentrations of the co-administered drug and could lead to clinically significant pharmacodynamic side effects of the co-administered drug).
No products indexed under this heading.

Tamoxifen Citrate (Ciprofloxacin is an inhibitor of the hepatic CYP1A2 enzyme pathway. Co-administration of ciprofloxacin and other drugs primarily metabolized by CYP1A2 results in increased plasma concentrations of the co-administered drug and could lead to clinically significant pharmacodynamic side effects of the co-administered drug).
No products indexed under this heading.

Theobromine (Ciprofloxacin is an inhibitor of the hepatic CYP1A2 enzyme pathway. Co-administration of ciprofloxacin and other drugs primarily metabolized by CYP1A2 results in increased plasma concentrations of the co-administered drug and could lead to clinically significant pharmacodynamic side effects of the co-administered drug).
No products indexed under this heading.

Theophylline (Ciprofloxacin is an inhibitor of the hepatic CYP1A2 enzyme pathway. Co-administration of ciprofloxacin and other drugs primarily metabolized by CYP1A2 (eg, theophylline, methylxanthines, tizanidine) results in increased plasma concentrations of the co-administered drug and could lead to clinically significant pharmacodynamic side effects of the co-administered drug. Concurrent administration may lead to elevated serum concentrations of theophylline and prolongation of its elimination half-life. Serious and fatal reactions have been reported in patients receiving concurrent administration of ciprofloxacin and theophylline. These reactions have included cardiac arrest, seizures, status epilepticus, and respiratory failure. Although similar serious adverse effects have been reported in patients receiving theophylline alone, the possibility that these reactions may be potentiated by ciprofloxacin cannot be eliminated. If concomitant use cannot be avoided, serum levels of theophylline should be monitored and dosage adjustments made as appropriate).
No products indexed under this heading.

Theophylline Anhydrous (Ciprofloxacin is an inhibitor of the hepatic CYP1A2 enzyme pathway. Co-administration of ciprofloxacin and other drugs primarily metabolized by CYP1A2 (eg, theophylline, methylxanthines, tizanidine) results in increased plasma concentrations of the co-administered drug and could lead to clinically significant pharmacodynamic side effects of the co-administered drug. Concurrent administration may lead to elevated serum concentrations of theophylline and prolongation of its elimination half-life. Serious and fatal reactions have been reported in patients receiving concurrent administration of ciprofloxacin and theophylline. These reactions have included cardiac arrest, seizures, status epilepticus, and respiratory failure. Although similar serious adverse effects have been reported in patients receiving theophylline alone, the possibility that these reactions may be potentiated by ciprofloxacin cannot be eliminated. If concomitant use cannot be avoided, serum levels of theophylline should be monitored and dosage adjustments made as appropriate). Products include:
Uniphyl 2817

Theophylline Calcium Salicylate (Ciprofloxacin is an inhibitor of the hepatic CYP1A2 enzyme pathway. Co-administration of ciprofloxacin and other drugs primarily metabolized by CYP1A2 (eg, theophylline, methylxanthines, tizanidine) results in increased plasma concentrations of the co-administered drug and could lead to clinically significant pharmacodynamic side effects of the co-administered drug. Concurrent administration may lead to elevated serum concentrations of theophylline and prolongation of its elimination half-life. Serious and fatal reactions have been reported in patients receiving concurrent administration of ciprofloxacin and theophylline. These reactions have included cardiac arrest, seizures, status epilepticus, and respiratory failure. Although similar serious adverse effects have been reported in patients receiving theophylline alone, the possibility that these reactions may be potentiated by ciprofloxacin cannot be eliminated. If concomitant use cannot be avoided, serum levels of theophylline should be monitored and dosage adjustments made as appropriate).
No products indexed under this heading.

Theophylline Dihydroxypropyl (Glyceryl) (Ciprofloxacin is an inhibitor of the hepatic CYP1A2 enzyme pathway. Co-administration of ciprofloxacin and other drugs primarily metabolized by CYP1A2 (eg, theophylline, methylxanthines, tizanidine) results in increased plasma concentrations of the co-administered drug and could lead to clinically significant pharmacodynamic side effects of the co-administered drug. Concurrent administration may

lead to elevated serum concentrations of theophylline and prolongation of its elimination half-life. Serious and fatal reactions have been reported in patients receiving concurrent administration of ciprofloxacin and theophylline. These reactions have included cardiac arrest, seizures, status epilepticus, and respiratory failure. Although similar serious adverse effects have been reported in patients receiving theophylline alone, the possibility that these reactions may be potentiated by ciprofloxacin cannot be eliminated. If concomitant use cannot be avoided, serum levels of theophylline should be monitored and dosage adjustments made as appropriate).
No products indexed under this heading.

Theophylline Ethylenediamine (Ciprofloxacin is an inhibitor of the hepatic CYP1A2 enzyme pathway. Co-administration of ciprofloxacin and other drugs primarily metabolized by CYP1A2 (eg, theophylline, methylxanthines, tizanidine) results in increased plasma concentrations of the co-administered drug and could lead to clinically significant pharmacodynamic side effects of the co-administered drug. Concurrent administration may lead to elevated serum concentrations of theophylline and prolongation of its elimination half-life. Serious and fatal reactions have been reported in patients receiving concurrent administration of ciprofloxacin and theophylline. These reactions have included cardiac arrest, seizures, status epilepticus, and respiratory failure. Although similar serious adverse effects have been reported in patients receiving theophylline alone, the possibility that these reactions may be potentiated by ciprofloxacin cannot be eliminated. If concomitant use cannot be avoided, serum levels of theophylline should be monitored and dosage adjustments made as appropriate).
No products indexed under this heading.

Theophylline Sodium Glycinate (Ciprofloxacin is an inhibitor of the hepatic CYP1A2 enzyme pathway. Co-administration of ciprofloxacin and other drugs primarily metabolized by CYP1A2 (eg, theophylline, methylxanthines, tizanidine) results in increased plasma concentrations of the co-administered drug and could lead to clinically significant pharmacodynamic side effects of the co-administered drug. Concurrent administration may lead to elevated serum concentrations of theophylline and prolongation of its elimination half-life. Serious and fatal reactions have been reported in patients receiving concurrent administration of ciprofloxacin and theophylline. These reactions have included cardiac arrest, seizures, status epilepticus, and respiratory failure. Although similar serious adverse effects have been reported in patients receiving theophylline alone, the possibility that these reactions may be potentiated by ciprofloxacin cannot be eliminated. If concomitant use cannot be avoided, serum levels of theophylline should be monitored and dosage adjustments made as appropriate).
No products indexed under this heading.

Thioridazine Hydrochloride (In general, elderly patients may be more susceptible to drug-associated effects on the QT interval. Therefore, precautions should be taken when using ciprofloxacin with concomitant drugs that can result in prolongation of the QT interval). Products include:
Thioridazine Hydrochloride 2384

Thiothixene (In general, elderly patients may be more susceptible to drug-associated effects on the QT interval. Therefore, precautions should be taken when using ciprofloxacin with con-

comitant drugs that can result in prolongation of the QT interval). Products include:
Thiothixene 2386

Tizanidine (Concomitant administration of tizanidine and ciprofloxacin is contraindicated. In a pharmacokinetic study, systemic exposure of tizanidine (4 mg single dose) was significantly increased (C_{max} 7-fold, AUC 10-fold) when the drug was given concomitantly with ciprofloxacin (500 mg b.i.d. for 3 days). The hypotensive and sedative effects of tizanidine were also potentiated).
No products indexed under this heading.

Tizanidine Hydrochloride (Concomitant administration of tizanidine and ciprofloxacin is contraindicated. In a pharmacokinetic study, systemic exposure of tizanidine (4 mg single dose) was significantly increased (C_{max} 7-fold, AUC 10-fold) when the drug was given concomitantly with ciprofloxacin (500 mg b.i.d. for 3 days). The hypotensive and sedative effects of tizanidine were also potentiated).
No products indexed under this heading.

Tocainide Hydrochloride (In general, elderly patients may be more susceptible to drug-associated effects on the QT interval. Therefore, precautions should be taken when using ciprofloxacin with concomitant drugs that can result in prolongation of the QT interval).
No products indexed under this heading.

Tolmetin Sodium (Non-steroidal anti-inflammatory drugs in combination of very high doses of quinolones have been shown to provoke convulsions in pre-clinical studies).
No products indexed under this heading.

Tranylcypromine Sulfate (In general, elderly patients may be more susceptible to drug-associated effects on the QT interval. Therefore, precautions should be taken when using ciprofloxacin with concomitant drugs that can result in prolongation of the QT interval). Products include:
Parnate 1584

Triamcinolone (Fluoroquinolones including ciprofloxacin are associated with an increased risk of tendinitis and tendon rupture in all ages. This adverse reaction most frequently involves the Achilles tendon, and rupture of the Achilles tendon may require surgical repair. Tendinitis and tendon rupture in the rotator cuff (the shoulder), the hand, the biceps, the thumb, and other tendon sites have also been reported. The risk of developing fluoroquinolone-associated tendinitis and tendon rupture is further increased in older patients usually over 60 years of age, in patients taking corticosteroid drugs, and in patients with kidney, heart or lung transplants).
No products indexed under this heading.

Triamcinolone Acetonide (Fluoroquinolones including ciprofloxacin are associated with an increased risk of tendinitis and tendon rupture in all ages. This adverse reaction most frequently involves the Achilles tendon, and rupture of the Achilles tendon may require surgical repair. Tendinitis and tendon rupture in the rotator cuff (the shoulder), the hand, the biceps, the thumb, and other tendon sites have also been reported. The risk of developing fluoroquinolone-associated tendinitis and tendon rupture is further increased in older patients usually over 60 years of age, in patients taking corticosteroid drugs, and in patients with kidney, heart or lung transplants). Products include:
Azmacort 408
Nasacort AQ 3019

Triamcinolone Diacetate (Fluoroquinolones including ciprofloxacin are

associated with an increased risk of tendinitis and tendon rupture in all ages. This adverse reaction most frequently involves the Achilles tendon, and rupture of the Achilles tendon may require surgical repair. Tendinitis and tendon rupture in the rotator cuff (the shoulder), the hand, the biceps, the thumb, and other tendon sites have also been reported. The risk of developing fluoroquinolone-associated tendinitis and tendon rupture is further increased in older patients usually over 60 years of age, in patients taking corticosteroid drugs, and in patients with kidney, heart or lung transplants).

No products indexed under this heading.

Triamcinolone Hexacetonide (Fluoroquinolones including ciprofloxacin are associated with an increased risk of tendinitis and tendon rupture in all ages. This adverse reaction most frequently involves the Achilles tendon, and rupture of the Achilles tendon may require surgical repair. Tendinitis and tendon rupture in the rotator cuff (the shoulder), the hand, the biceps, the thumb, and other tendon sites have also been reported. The risk of developing fluoroquinolone-associated tendinitis and tendon rupture is further increased in older patients usually over 60 years of age, in patients taking corticosteroid drugs, and in patients with kidney, heart or lung transplants).

No products indexed under this heading.

Trifluoperazine Hydrochloride (In general, elderly patients may be more susceptible to drug-associated effects on the QT interval. Therefore, precautions should be taken when using ciprofloxacin with concomitant drugs that can result in prolongation of the QT interval).

No products indexed under this heading.

Trimethaphan Camsylate (Ciprofloxacin is an inhibitor of the hepatic CYP1A2 enzyme pathway. Co-administration of ciprofloxacin and other drugs primarily metabolized by CYP1A2 results in increased plasma concentrations of the co-administered drug and could lead to clinically significant pharmacodynamic side effects of the co-administered drug).

No products indexed under this heading.

Trimipramine Maleate (In general, elderly patients may be more susceptible to drug-associated effects on the QT interval. Therefore, precautions should be taken when using ciprofloxacin with concomitant drugs that can result in prolongation of the QT interval).

No products indexed under this heading.

Trovafloxacin Mesylate (Ciprofloxacin is an inhibitor of the hepatic CYP1A2 enzyme pathway. Co-administration of ciprofloxacin and other drugs primarily metabolized by CYP1A2 results in increased plasma concentrations of the co-administered drug and could lead to clinically significant pharmacodynamic side effects of the co-administered drug).

No products indexed under this heading.

Valdecoxib (Non-steroidal anti-inflammatory drugs in combination of very high doses of quinolones have been shown to provoke convulsions in preclinical studies).

No products indexed under this heading.

Verapamil Hydrochloride (Ciprofloxacin is an inhibitor of the hepatic CYP1A2 enzyme pathway. Co-administration of ciprofloxacin and other drugs primarily metabolized by CYP1A2 results in increased plasma concentrations of the co-administered drug and could lead to clinically significant pharmacodynamic side effects of the co-administered drug). Products include:

Warfarin Sodium (Ciprofloxacin has been reported to enhance the effects of the oral anticoagulant warfarin or its derivatives. When these products are administered concomitantly, prothrombin time or other suitable coagulant tests should be closely monitored).

No products indexed under this heading.

Zileuton (Ciprofloxacin is an inhibitor of the hepatic CYP1A2 enzyme pathway. Co-administration of ciprofloxacin and other drugs primarily metabolized by CYP1A2 results in increased plasma concentrations of the co-administered drug and could lead to clinically significant pharmacodynamic side effects of the co-administered drug).

No products indexed under this heading.

Zinc (Concurrent administration of ciprofloxacin with products containing zinc may substantially decrease its absorption, resulting in serum and urine levels considerably lower than desired. Ciprofloxacin should be administered at least 2 hours before or 6 hours after products containing zinc). Products include:

Zinc Acetate (Concurrent administration of ciprofloxacin with multivalent cation-containing products may substantially decrease its absorption, resulting in serum and urine levels considerably lower than desired).

No products indexed under this heading.

Zinc Bisglycinate (Concurrent administration of ciprofloxacin with multivalent cation-containing products may substantially decrease its absorption, resulting in serum and urine levels considerably lower than desired).

No products indexed under this heading.

Zinc Chloride (Concurrent administration of ciprofloxacin with multivalent cation-containing products may substantially decrease its absorption, resulting in serum and urine levels considerably lower than desired).

No products indexed under this heading.

Zinc Citrate (Concurrent administration of ciprofloxacin with multivalent cation-containing products may substantially decrease its absorption, resulting in serum and urine levels considerably lower than desired). Products include:

Zinc-Containing Multivitamins (Concurrent administration of ciprofloxacin with multivalent cation-containing products may substantially decrease its absorption, resulting in serum and urine levels considerably lower than desired).

No products indexed under this heading.

Zinc Gluconate (Concurrent administration of ciprofloxacin with multivalent cation-containing products may substantially decrease its absorption, resulting in serum and urine levels considerably lower than desired).

No products indexed under this heading.

Zinc Oxide (Concurrent administration of ciprofloxacin with multivalent cation-containing products may substantially decrease its absorption, resulting in serum and urine levels considerably lower than desired). Products include:

Zinc Phenosulfonate (Concurrent administration of ciprofloxacin with multivalent cation-containing products may substantially decrease its absorption, resulting in serum and urine levels considerably lower than desired).

No products indexed under this heading.

Zinc Sulfate (Concurrent administration of ciprofloxacin with multivalent cation-containing products may substantially decrease its absorption, resulting in serum and urine levels considerably lower than desired). Products include:

Ziprasidone Hydrochloride (In general, elderly patients may be more susceptible to drug-associated effects on the QT interval. Therefore, precautions should be taken when using ciprofloxacin with concomitant drugs that can result in prolongation of the QT interval). Products include:

Zolmitriptan (Ciprofloxacin is an inhibitor of the hepatic CYP1A2 enzyme pathway. Co-administration of ciprofloxacin and other drugs primarily metabolized by CYP1A2 results in increased plasma concentrations of the co-administered drug and could lead to clinically significant pharmacodynamic side effects of the co-administered drug). Products include:

Food Interactions

Beverages, caffeine-containing (Ciprofloxacin has been shown to interfere with the metabolism of caffeine. This may lead to reduced clearance of caffeine and a prolongation of its serum half-life and inhibits the formation of paraxanthine after caffeine administration).

Dairy products (Ciprofloxacin should not be taken with dairy products (like milk or yogurt) alone since absorption of ciprofloxacin may be significantly reduced; however, ciprofloxacin may be taken with a meal that contains these products).

Food, caffeine-containing (Ciprofloxacin is an inhibitor of the hepatic CYP1A2 enzyme pathway. Co-administration of ciprofloxacin and other drugs primarily metabolized by CYP1A2 results in increased plasma concentrations of the co-administered drug and could lead to clinically significant pharmacodynamic side effects of the co-administered drug).

Food, unspecified (When ciprofloxacin tablets are given concomitantly with food, there is a delay in the absorption of the drug, resulting in peak concentrations that occur closer to 2 hours after dosing rather than 1 hour, whereas there is no delay observed when ciprofloxacin suspension is given with food. The overall absorption of ciprofloxacin tablets or ciprofloxacin suspension, however, is not substantially affected. The pharmacokinetics of ciprofloxacin given as the suspension are also not affected by food).

Fruit juices, unspecified (Ciprofloxacin should not be taken with calcium-fortified juices alone since absorption of ciprofloxacin may be significantly reduced; however, ciprofloxacin may be taken with a meal that contains these products).

Iron Amino Acid Chelate (Concurrent administration of ciprofloxacin with multivalent cation-containing products may substantially decrease its absorption,

resulting in serum and urine levels considerably lower than desired).

Meal, unspecified (When ciprofloxacin tablets are given concomitantly with food, there is a delay in the absorption of the drug, and there is a delay in peak concentrations that occur closer to 2 hours after dosing rather than 1 hour, whereas there is no delay observed when ciprofloxacin suspension is given with food. The overall absorption of ciprofloxacin tablets or ciprofloxacin suspension, however, is not substantially affected. The pharmacokinetics of ciprofloxacin given as the suspension are also not affected by food).

CIPRO XR TABLETS

May interact with antacids containing aluminum, calcium and magnesium, caffeines, cations, class 1A antiarrhythmics, class III antiarrhythmics, corticosteroids, cytochrome p450 1a2 substrates (selected), non-steroidal anti-inflammatory agents, oral anticoagulants, phenytoin, theophyllines, xanthines, and certain other agents. Compounds in these categories include:

Acetaminophen (Ciprofloxacin is an inhibitor of the hepatic CYP1A2 enzyme pathway. Co-administration of ciprofloxacin and other drugs primarily metabolized by CYP1A2 results in increased plasma concentrations of the co-administered drug and could lead to clinically significant pharmacodynamic side effects of the co-administered drug). Products include:

Alatrofloxacin Mesylate (Ciprofloxacin is an inhibitor of the hepatic CYP1A2 enzyme pathway. Co-administration of ciprofloxacin and other drugs primarily metabolized by CYP1A2 results in increased plasma concentrations of the co-administered drug and could lead to clinically significant pharmacodynamic side effects of the co-administered drug).

No products indexed under this heading.

Alclometasone Dipropionate (Fluoroquinolones, including ciprofloxacin, are associated with an increased risk of tendinitis and tendon rupture in all ages. The risk is further increased in older patients usually over 60 years of age, in patients taking corticosteroid drugs, and in kidney, heart and lung transplant recipients).

No products indexed under this heading.

Aluminum Acetate (Concurrent administration of ciprofloxacin with multivalent cation-containing products may substantially interfere with the absorption of ciprofloxacin, resulting in serum and urine levels considerably lower than desired. Ciprofloxacin extended release tablets should be administered at least 2 hours before or 6 hours after metal cations).

No products indexed under this heading.

IMPORTANT NOTE: Always consult each drug listing in the patient's regimen for possible interactions.

Aluminum Carbonate (Concurrent administration of ciprofloxacin with multivalent cation-containing products may substantially interfere with the absorption of ciprofloxacin, resulting in serum and urine levels considerably lower than desired. Ciprofloxacin extended release tablets should be administered at least 2 hours before or 6 hours after metal cations).

No products indexed under this heading.

Aluminum Chlorhydroxide (Concurrent administration of ciprofloxacin with multivalent cation-containing products may substantially interfere with the absorption of ciprofloxacin, resulting in serum and urine levels considerably lower than desired. Ciprofloxacin extended release tablets should be administered at least 2 hours before or 6 hours after metal cations).

No products indexed under this heading.

Aluminum Chloride (Concurrent administration of ciprofloxacin with multivalent cation-containing products may substantially interfere with the absorption of ciprofloxacin, resulting in serum and urine levels considerably lower than desired. Ciprofloxacin extended release tablets should be administered at least 2 hours before or 6 hours after metal cations).

No products indexed under this heading.

Aluminum Chlorohydrate (Concurrent administration of ciprofloxacin with multivalent cation-containing products may substantially interfere with the absorption of ciprofloxacin, resulting in serum and urine levels considerably lower than desired. Ciprofloxacin extended release tablets should be administered at least 2 hours before or 6 hours after metal cations).

No products indexed under this heading.

Aluminum Glycinate (Concurrent administration of ciprofloxacin with multivalent cation-containing products may substantially interfere with the absorption of ciprofloxacin, resulting in serum and urine levels considerably lower than desired. Ciprofloxacin extended release tablets should be administered at least 2 hours before or 6 hours after metal cations).

No products indexed under this heading.

Aluminum Hydroxide (Concurrent administration of ciprofloxacin with multivalent cation-containing products may substantially interfere with the absorption of ciprofloxacin, resulting in serum and urine levels considerably lower than desired. Ciprofloxacin extended release tablets should be administered at least 2 hours before or 6 hours after metal cations).

No products indexed under this heading.

Aluminum Hydroxide Preparations (Concurrent administration of ciprofloxacin with multivalent cation-containing products may substantially interfere with the absorption of ciprofloxacin, resulting in serum and urine levels considerably lower than desired. Ciprofloxacin extended release tablets should be administered at least 2 hours before or 6 hours after metal cations).

No products indexed under this heading.

Aluminum Sulfate (Concurrent administration of ciprofloxacin with multivalent cation-containing products may substantially interfere with the absorption of ciprofloxacin, resulting in serum and urine levels considerably lower than desired. Ciprofloxacin extended release tablets should be administered at least 2 hours before or 6 hours after metal cations).

No products indexed under this heading.

Aminophylline (Ciprofloxacin is an inhibitor of the hepatic CYP1A2 enzyme pathway. Co-administration of ciprofloxacin and other drugs primarily metabolized by CYP1A2 (eg, methylxanthines) results in increased plasma concentrations of the co-administered drug and could lead to clinically significant pharmacodynamic side effects of the co-administered drug).

No products indexed under this heading.

Amiodarone Hydrochloride (Precaution should be taken when using ciprofloxacin with drugs that can result in prolongation of the QT interval, such as class III antiarrhythmics).

No products indexed under this heading.

Amitriptyline Hydrochloride (Ciprofloxacin is an inhibitor of the hepatic CYP1A2 enzyme pathway. Co-administration of ciprofloxacin and other drugs primarily metabolized by CYP1A2 results in increased plasma concentrations of the co-administered drug and could lead to clinically significant pharmacodynamic side effects of the co-administered drug).

No products indexed under this heading.

Amoxapine (Ciprofloxacin is an inhibitor of the hepatic CYP1A2 enzyme pathway. Co-administration of ciprofloxacin and other drugs primarily metabolized by CYP1A2 results in increased plasma concentrations of the co-administered drug and could lead to clinically significant pharmacodynamic side effects of the co-administered drug).

No products indexed under this heading.

Anagrelide Hydrochloride (Ciprofloxacin is an inhibitor of the hepatic CYP1A2 enzyme pathway. Co-administration of ciprofloxacin and other drugs primarily metabolized by CYP1A2 results in increased plasma concentrations of the co-administered drug and could lead to clinically significant pharmacodynamic side effects of the co-administered drug).

No products indexed under this heading.

Anisindione (Ciprofloxacin has been reported to enhance the effects of the oral anticoagulant warfarin or its derivatives. When these products are administered concomitantly, prothrombin time or other suitable coagulation tests should be closely monitored).

No products indexed under this heading.

Beclomethasone Dipropionate (Fluoroquinolones, including ciprofloxacin, are associated with an increased risk of tendinitis and tendon rupture in all ages. The risk is further increased in older patients usually over 60 years of age, in patients taking corticosteroid drugs, and in kidney, heart and lung transplant recipients). Products include:

Qvar **3398**

Beclomethasone Dipropionate Monohydrate (Fluoroquinolones, including ciprofloxacin, are associated with an increased risk of tendinitis and tendon rupture in all ages. The risk is further increased in older patients usually over 60 years of age, in patients taking corticosteroid drugs, and in kidney, heart and lung transplant recipients). Products include:

Beconase AQ **1386**

Betamethasone (Fluoroquinolones, including ciprofloxacin, are associated with an increased risk of tendinitis and tendon rupture in all ages. The risk is further increased in older patients usually over 60 years of age, in patients taking corticosteroid drugs, and in kidney, heart and lung transplant recipients).

No products indexed under this heading.

Betamethasone Acetate (Fluoroquinolones, including ciprofloxacin, are associated with an increased risk of tendinitis and tendon rupture in all ages. The risk is further increased in older patients usually over 60 years of age, in patients taking corticosteroid drugs, and in kidney, heart and lung transplant recipients).

No products indexed under this heading.

Betamethasone Benzoate (Fluoroquinolones, including ciprofloxacin, are associated with an increased risk of tendinitis and tendon rupture in all ages. The risk is further increased in older patients usually over 60 years of age, in patients taking corticosteroid drugs, and in kidney, heart and lung transplant recipients).

No products indexed under this heading.

Betamethasone Dipropionate (Fluoroquinolones, including ciprofloxacin, are associated with an increased risk of tendinitis and tendon rupture in all ages. The risk is further increased in older patients usually over 60 years of age, in patients taking corticosteroid drugs, and in kidney, heart and lung transplant recipients). Products include:

Diprolene Lotion 0.05% **3108**
Diprolene Ointment 0.05% **3109**
Diprolene AF Cream 0.05% **3107**
Lotrisone **3163**

Betamethasone Sodium Phosphate (Fluoroquinolones, including ciprofloxacin, are associated with an increased risk of tendinitis and tendon rupture in all ages. The risk is further increased in older patients usually over 60 years of age, in patients taking corticosteroid drugs, and in kidney, heart and lung transplant recipients).

No products indexed under this heading.

Betamethasone Valerate (Fluoroquinolones, including ciprofloxacin, are associated with an increased risk of tendinitis and tendon rupture in all ages. The risk is further increased in older patients usually over 60 years of age, in patients taking corticosteroid drugs, and in kidney, heart and lung transplant recipients). Products include:

Luxíq **3321**

Bretylium Tosylate (Precaution should be taken when using ciprofloxacin with drugs that can result in prolongation of the QT interval, such as class III antiarrhythmics).

No products indexed under this heading.

Budesonide (Fluoroquinolones, including ciprofloxacin, are associated with an increased risk of tendinitis and tendon rupture in all ages. The risk is further increased in older patients usually over 60 years of age, in patients taking corticosteroid drugs, and in kidney, heart and lung transplant recipients). Products include:

Pulmicort Flexhaler **714**
Symbicort 80/4.5 .... **720**
Symbicort 160/4.5 .... **720**

Caffeine (Ciprofloxacin has been shown to interfere with the metabolism of caffeine. This may lead to reduced clearance of caffeine and a prolongation of its serum half-life and inhibit the formation of paraxanthine after caffeine administration).

No products indexed under this heading.

Caffeine Anhydrous (Ciprofloxacin has been shown to interfere with the metabolism of caffeine. This may lead to reduced clearance of caffeine and a prolongation of its serum half-life and inhibit the formation of paraxanthine after caffeine administration).

No products indexed under this heading.

Caffeine Citrate (Ciprofloxacin has been shown to interfere with the metabolism of caffeine. This may lead to reduced clearance of caffeine and a prolongation of its serum half-life and inhibit the formation of paraxanthine after caffeine administration).

No products indexed under this heading.

Caffeine-containing medications (Ciprofloxacin has been shown to interfere with the metabolism of caffeine. This may lead to reduced clearance of caffeine and a prolongation of its serum half-life and inhibit the formation of paraxanthine after caffeine administration).

No products indexed under this heading.

Caffeine Sodium Benzoate (Ciprofloxacin has been shown to interfere with the metabolism of caffeine. This may lead to reduced clearance of caffeine and a prolongation of its serum half-life and inhibit the formation of paraxanthine after caffeine administration).

No products indexed under this heading.

Calcium (Concurrent administration of ciprofloxacin with multivalent cation-containing products may substantially interfere with the absorption of ciprofloxacin, resulting in serum and urine levels considerably lower than desired. Ciprofloxacin extended release tablets should be administered at least 2 hours before or 6 hours after metal cations). Products include:

BoneMate Plus **3454**
Cardio Basics **3455**
Chelated Mineral **3476**
CitraNatal 90 DHA Capsules **2332**
CitraNatal Harmony **2332**

Calcium (Oyster Shell) (Concurrent administration of ciprofloxacin with multivalent cation-containing products may substantially interfere with the absorption of ciprofloxacin, resulting in serum and urine levels considerably lower than desired. Ciprofloxacin extended release tablets should be administered at least 2 hours before or 6 hours after metal cations).

No products indexed under this heading.

Calcium Acetate (Concurrent administration of ciprofloxacin with multivalent cation-containing products may substantially interfere with the absorption of ciprofloxacin, resulting in serum and urine levels considerably lower than desired. Ciprofloxacin extended release tablets should be administered at least 2 hours before or 6 hours after metal cations).

No products indexed under this heading.

Calcium Ascorbate (Concurrent administration of ciprofloxacin with multivalent cation-containing products may substantially interfere with the absorption of ciprofloxacin, resulting in serum and urine levels considerably lower than desired. Ciprofloxacin extended release tablets should be administered at least 2 hours before or 6 hours after metal cations). Products include:

Bio-C **3454**
Procosa II **3476**
Proflavanol 90 .... **3476**

Calcium Carbaspirin (Concurrent administration of ciprofloxacin with multivalent cation-containing products may substantially interfere with the absorption of ciprofloxacin, resulting in serum and urine levels considerably lower than desired. Ciprofloxacin extended release tablets should be administered at least 2 hours before or 6 hours after metal cations).

No products indexed under this heading.

Calcium Carbonate (Concurrent administration of ciprofloxacin with multivalent cation-containing products may substantially interfere with the absorption of ciprofloxacin, resulting in serum and urine levels considerably lower than

345 Interactions Index Cipro XR

desired. Ciprofloxacin extended release tablets should be administered at least 2 hours before or 6 hours after metal cations). Products include:
Chelated Mineral 3476
Pepcid Complete 1822
Extra Strength Rolaids Softchews Vanilla Creme 2045

Calcium Carbonate, Precipitated (Concurrent administration of ciprofloxacin with multivalent cation-containing products may substantially interfere with the absorption of ciprofloxacin, resulting in serum and urine levels considerably lower than desired. Ciprofloxacin extended release tablets should be administered at least 2 hours before or 6 hours after metal cations).
No products indexed under this heading.

Calcium Caseinate (Concurrent administration of ciprofloxacin with multivalent cation-containing products may substantially interfere with the absorption of ciprofloxacin, resulting in serum and urine levels considerably lower than desired. Ciprofloxacin extended release tablets should be administered at least 2 hours before or 6 hours after metal cations).
No products indexed under this heading.

Calcium Chloride (Concurrent administration of ciprofloxacin with multivalent cation-containing products may substantially interfere with the absorption of ciprofloxacin, resulting in serum and urine levels considerably lower than desired. Ciprofloxacin extended release tablets should be administered at least 2 hours before or 6 hours after metal cations).
No products indexed under this heading.

Calcium Citrate (Concurrent administration of ciprofloxacin with multivalent cation-containing products may substantially interfere with the absorption of ciprofloxacin, resulting in serum and urine levels considerably lower than desired. Ciprofloxacin extended release tablets should be administered at least 2 hours before or 6 hours after metal cations). Products include:
Active Calcium 3476
Chelated Mineral 3476
CitraNatal 90 DHA Capsules 2332
CitraNatal Assure 2332
CitraNatal Harmony 2332
CitraNatal Rx 2332

Calcium Disodium Edetate (Concurrent administration of ciprofloxacin with multivalent cation-containing products may substantially interfere with the absorption of ciprofloxacin, resulting in serum and urine levels considerably lower than desired. Ciprofloxacin extended release tablets should be administered at least 2 hours before or 6 hours after metal cations).
No products indexed under this heading.

Calcium Glubionate (Concurrent administration of ciprofloxacin with multivalent cation-containing products may substantially interfere with the absorption of ciprofloxacin, resulting in serum and urine levels considerably lower than desired. Ciprofloxacin extended release tablets should be administered at least 2 hours before or 6 hours after metal cations).
No products indexed under this heading.

Calcium Gluconate (Concurrent administration of ciprofloxacin with multivalent cation-containing products may substantially interfere with the absorption of ciprofloxacin, resulting in serum and urine levels considerably lower than desired. Ciprofloxacin extended release tablets should be administered at least 2 hours before or 6 hours after metal cations).
No products indexed under this heading.

Calcium Glycerophosphate (Concurrent administration of ciprofloxacin with multivalent cation-containing products may substantially interfere with the absorption of ciprofloxacin, resulting in serum and urine levels considerably lower than desired. Ciprofloxacin extended release tablets should be administered at least 2 hours before or 6 hours after metal cations).
No products indexed under this heading.

Calcium Iodide (Concurrent administration of ciprofloxacin with multivalent cation-containing products may substantially interfere with the absorption of ciprofloxacin, resulting in serum and urine levels considerably lower than desired. Ciprofloxacin extended release tablets should be administered at least 2 hours before or 6 hours after metal cations).
No products indexed under this heading.

Calcium Lactate (Concurrent administration of ciprofloxacin with multivalent cation-containing products may substantially interfere with the absorption of ciprofloxacin, resulting in serum and urine levels considerably lower than desired. Ciprofloxacin extended release tablets should be administered at least 2 hours before or 6 hours after metal cations).
No products indexed under this heading.

Calcium Levulinate (Concurrent administration of ciprofloxacin with multivalent cation-containing products may substantially interfere with the absorption of ciprofloxacin, resulting in serum and urine levels considerably lower than desired. Ciprofloxacin extended release tablets should be administered at least 2 hours before or 6 hours after metal cations).
No products indexed under this heading.

Calcium Pantothenate (Concurrent administration of ciprofloxacin with multivalent cation-containing products may substantially interfere with the absorption of ciprofloxacin, resulting in serum and urine levels considerably lower than desired. Ciprofloxacin extended release tablets should be administered at least 2 hours before or 6 hours after metal cations). Products include:
Cardio Basics 3455

Calcium Phosphate (Concurrent administration of ciprofloxacin with multivalent cation-containing products may substantially interfere with the absorption of ciprofloxacin, resulting in serum and urine levels considerably lower than desired. Ciprofloxacin extended release tablets should be administered at least 2 hours before or 6 hours after metal cations).
No products indexed under this heading.

Calcium Phosphate, Dibasic (Concurrent administration of ciprofloxacin with multivalent cation-containing products may substantially interfere with the absorption of ciprofloxacin, resulting in serum and urine levels considerably lower than desired. Ciprofloxacin extended release tablets should be administered at least 2 hours before or 6 hours after metal cations).
No products indexed under this heading.

Calcium Phosphate, Tribasic (Concurrent administration of ciprofloxacin with multivalent cation-containing products may substantially interfere with the absorption of ciprofloxacin, resulting in serum and urine levels considerably lower than desired. Ciprofloxacin extended release tablets should be administered at least 2 hours before or 6 hours after metal cations).
No products indexed under this heading.

Calcium Phosphorus Preparations (Concurrent administration of ciprofloxacin with multivalent cation-containing products may substantially interfere with the absorption of ciprofloxacin, resulting in serum and urine levels considerably lower than desired. Ciprofloxacin extended release tablets should be administered at least 2 hours before or 6 hours after metal cations).
No products indexed under this heading.

Calcium Polycarbophil (Concurrent administration of ciprofloxacin with multivalent cation-containing products may substantially interfere with the absorption of ciprofloxacin, resulting in serum and urine levels considerably lower than desired. Ciprofloxacin extended release tablets should be administered at least 2 hours before or 6 hours after metal cations).
No products indexed under this heading.

Calcium Salts (Concurrent administration of ciprofloxacin with multivalent cation-containing products may substantially interfere with the absorption of ciprofloxacin, resulting in serum and urine levels considerably lower than desired. Ciprofloxacin extended release tablets should be administered at least 2 hours before or 6 hours after metal cations).
No products indexed under this heading.

Calcium Sodium Alginate Fiber (Concurrent administration of ciprofloxacin with multivalent cation-containing products may substantially interfere with the absorption of ciprofloxacin, resulting in serum and urine levels considerably lower than desired. Ciprofloxacin extended release tablets should be administered at least 2 hours before or 6 hours after metal cations).
No products indexed under this heading.

Calcium Undecylenate (Concurrent administration of ciprofloxacin with multivalent cation-containing products may substantially interfere with the absorption of ciprofloxacin, resulting in serum and urine levels considerably lower than desired. Ciprofloxacin extended release tablets should be administered at least 2 hours before or 6 hours after metal cations).
No products indexed under this heading.

Celecoxib (Non-steroidal anti-inflammatory drugs (but not acetyl salicylic acid) in combination of very high doses of quinolones have been shown to provoke convulsions in pre-clinical studies). Products include:
Celebrex 3272

Chlordiazepoxide (Ciprofloxacin is an inhibitor of the hepatic CYP1A2 enzyme pathway. Co-administration of ciprofloxacin and other drugs primarily metabolized by CYP1A2 results in increased plasma concentrations of the co-administered drug and could lead to clinically significant pharmacodynamic side effects of the co-administered drug).
No products indexed under this heading.

Chlordiazepoxide Hydrochloride (Ciprofloxacin is an inhibitor of the hepatic CYP1A2 enzyme pathway. Co-administration of ciprofloxacin and other drugs primarily metabolized by CYP1A2 results in increased plasma concentrations of the co-administered drug and could lead to clinically significant pharmacodynamic side effects of the co-administered drug).
No products indexed under this heading.

Ciclesonide (Fluoroquinolones, including ciprofloxacin, are associated with an increased risk of tendinitis and tendon rupture in all ages. The risk is further increased in older patients usually over 60 years of age, in patients taking corticosteroid drugs, and in kidney, heart and lung transplant recipients).
No products indexed under this heading.

Cimetidine Hydrochloride (Ciprofloxacin is an inhibitor of the hepatic CYP1A2 enzyme pathway. Co-administration of ciprofloxacin and other drugs primarily metabolized by CYP1A2 results in increased plasma concentrations of the co-administered drug and could lead to clinically significant pharmacodynamic side effects of the co-administered drug).
No products indexed under this heading.

Ciprofloxacin Hydrochloride (Ciprofloxacin is an inhibitor of the hepatic CYP1A2 enzyme pathway. Co-administration of ciprofloxacin and other drugs primarily metabolized by CYP1A2 results in increased plasma concentrations of the co-administered drug and could lead to clinically significant pharmacodynamic side effects of the co-administered drug). Products include:
Cipro 3073

Clomipramine Hydrochloride (Ciprofloxacin is an inhibitor of the hepatic CYP1A2 enzyme pathway. Co-administration of ciprofloxacin and other drugs primarily metabolized by CYP1A2 results in increased plasma concentrations of the co-administered drug and could lead to clinically significant pharmacodynamic side effects of the co-administered drug).
No products indexed under this heading.

Clopidogrel Bisulfate (Ciprofloxacin is an inhibitor of the hepatic CYP1A2 enzyme pathway. Co-administration of ciprofloxacin and other drugs primarily metabolized by CYP1A2 results in increased plasma concentrations of the co-administered drug and could lead to clinically significant pharmacodynamic side effects of the co-administered drug). Products include:
Plavix 3027

Clozapine (Ciprofloxacin is an inhibitor of the hepatic CYP1A2 enzyme pathway. Co-administration of ciprofloxacin and other drugs primarily metabolized by CYP1A2 results in increased plasma concentrations of the co-administered drug and could lead to clinically significant pharmacodynamic side effects of the co-administered drug).
No products indexed under this heading.

Cortisone Acetate (Fluoroquinolones, including ciprofloxacin, are associated with an increased risk of tendinitis and tendon rupture in all ages. The risk is further increased in older patients usually over 60 years of age, in patients taking corticosteroid drugs, and in kidney, heart and lung transplant recipients).
No products indexed under this heading.

Cyclobenzaprine (Ciprofloxacin is an inhibitor of the hepatic CYP1A2 enzyme pathway. Co-administration of ciprofloxacin and other drugs primarily metabolized by CYP1A2 results in increased plasma concentrations of the co-administered drug and could lead to clinically significant pharmacodynamic side effects of the co-administered drug).
No products indexed under this heading.

Cyclobenzaprine Hydrochloride (Ciprofloxacin is an inhibitor of the hepatic CYP1A2 enzyme pathway. Co-administration of ciprofloxacin and other drugs primarily metabolized by CYP1A2 results in increased plasma concentrations of the co-administered drug and could lead to clinically signifi-

cant pharmacodynamic side effects of the co-administered drug). Products include:

Cyclosporine (Quinolones, including ciprofloxacin, have been associated with transient elevations in serum creatinine in patients receiving cyclosporine concomitantly). Products include:

Desipramine Hydrochloride (Ciprofloxacin is an inhibitor of the hepatic CYP1A2 enzyme pathway. Co-administration of ciprofloxacin and other drugs primarily metabolized by CYP1A2 results in increased plasma concentrations of the co-administered drug and could lead to clinically significant pharmacodynamic side effects of the co-administered drug).
No products indexed under this heading.

Desoximetasone (Fluoroquinolones, including ciprofloxacin, are associated with an increased risk of tendinitis and tendon rupture in all ages. The risk is further increased in older patients usually over 60 years of age, in patients taking corticosteroid drugs, and in kidney, heart and lung transplant recipients).
No products indexed under this heading.

Dexamethasone (Fluoroquinolones, including ciprofloxacin, are associated with an increased risk of tendinitis and tendon rupture in all ages. The risk is further increased in older patients usually over 60 years of age, in patients taking corticosteroid drugs, and in kidney, heart and lung transplant recipients). Products include:

Dexamethasone Acetate (Fluoroquinolones, including ciprofloxacin, are associated with an increased risk of tendinitis and tendon rupture in all ages. The risk is further increased in older patients usually over 60 years of age, in patients taking corticosteroid drugs, and in kidney, heart and lung transplant recipients).
No products indexed under this heading.

Dexamethasone Phosphate (Fluoroquinolones, including ciprofloxacin, are associated with an increased risk of tendinitis and tendon rupture in all ages. The risk is further increased in older patients usually over 60 years of age, in patients taking corticosteroid drugs, and in kidney, heart and lung transplant recipients).
No products indexed under this heading.

Dexamethasone Sodium (Fluoroquinolones, including ciprofloxacin, are associated with an increased risk of tendinitis and tendon rupture in all ages. The risk is further increased in older patients usually over 60 years of age, in patients taking corticosteroid drugs, and in kidney, heart and lung transplant recipients).
No products indexed under this heading.

Dexamethasone Sodium Phosphate (Fluoroquinolones, including ciprofloxacin, are associated with an increased risk of tendinitis and tendon rupture in all ages. The risk is further increased in older patients usually over 60 years of age, in patients taking corticosteroid drugs, and in kidney, heart and lung transplant recipients).
No products indexed under this heading.

Dexamethasone Sodium Phosphate Injection (Fluoroquinolones, including ciprofloxacin, are associated with an increased risk of tendinitis and tendon rupture in all ages. The risk is further increased in older patients usually over 60 years of age, in patients taking corticosteroid drugs, and in kidney, heart and lung transplant recipients).
No products indexed under this heading.

Diazepam (Ciprofloxacin is an inhibitor of the hepatic CYP1A2 enzyme pathway. Co-administration of ciprofloxacin and other drugs primarily metabolized by CYP1A2 results in increased plasma concentrations of the co-administered drug and could lead to clinically significant pharmacodynamic side effects of the co-administered drug). Products include:

Diclofenac Epolamine (Non-steroidal anti-inflammatory drugs (but not acetyl salicylic acid) in combination of very high doses of quinolones have been shown to provoke convulsions in pre-clinical studies). Products include:

Diclofenac Potassium (Non-steroidal anti-inflammatory drugs (but not acetyl salicylic acid) in combination of very high doses of quinolones have been shown to provoke convulsions in pre-clinical studies).
No products indexed under this heading.

Diclofenac Sodium (Non-steroidal anti-inflammatory drugs (but not acetyl salicylic acid) in combination of very high doses of quinolones have been shown to provoke convulsions in pre-clinical studies).
No products indexed under this heading.

Dicumarol (Ciprofloxacin has been reported to enhance the effects of the oral anticoagulant warfarin or its derivatives. When these products are administered concomitantly, prothrombin time or other suitable coagulation tests should be closely monitored).
No products indexed under this heading.

Didanosine (Concurrent administration of ciprofloxacin with multivalent cation-containing products, such as didanosine chewable/buffered tablets or pediatric powder, may substantially interfere with the absorption of ciprofloxacin, resulting in serum and urine levels considerably lower than desired. Ciprofloxacin extended release tablets should be administered at least 2 hours before or 6 hours after didanosine).
No products indexed under this heading.

Diflorasone Diacetate (Fluoroquinolones, including ciprofloxacin, are associated with an increased risk of tendinitis and tendon rupture in all ages. The risk is further increased in older patients usually over 60 years of age, in patients taking corticosteroid drugs, and in kidney, heart and lung transplant recipients).
No products indexed under this heading.

Diltiazem Hydrochloride (Ciprofloxacin is an inhibitor of the hepatic CYP1A2 enzyme pathway. Co-administration of ciprofloxacin and other drugs primarily metabolized by CYP1A2 results in increased plasma concentrations of the co-administered drug and could lead to clinically significant pharmacodynamic side effects of the co-administered drug). Products include:

Diltiazem Maleate (Ciprofloxacin is an inhibitor of the hepatic CYP1A2 enzyme pathway. Co-administration of ciprofloxacin and other drugs primarily metabolized by CYP1A2 results in increased plasma concentrations of the co-administered drug and could lead to clinically significant pharmacodynamic side effects of the co-administered drug).
No products indexed under this heading.

Disopyramide (Precaution should be taken when using ciprofloxacin with drugs that can result in prolongation of the QT interval, such as class IA antiarrhythmics).
No products indexed under this heading.

Disopyramide Phosphate (Precaution should be taken when using ciprofloxacin with drugs that can result in prolongation of the QT interval, such as class IA antiarrhythmics).
No products indexed under this heading.

Doxepin Hydrochloride (Ciprofloxacin is an inhibitor of the hepatic CYP1A2 enzyme pathway. Co-administration of ciprofloxacin and other drugs primarily metabolized by CYP1A2 results in increased plasma concentrations of the co-administered drug and could lead to clinically significant pharmacodynamic side effects of the co-administered drug).
No products indexed under this heading.

Dyphylline (Ciprofloxacin is an inhibitor of the hepatic CYP1A2 enzyme pathway. Co-administration of ciprofloxacin and other drugs primarily metabolized by CYP1A2 (eg, methylxanthines) results in increased plasma concentrations of the co-administered drug and could lead to clinically significant pharmacodynamic side effects of the co-administered drug).
No products indexed under this heading.

Enoxacin (Ciprofloxacin is an inhibitor of the hepatic CYP1A2 enzyme pathway. Co-administration of ciprofloxacin and other drugs primarily metabolized by CYP1A2 results in increased plasma concentrations of the co-administered drug and could lead to clinically significant pharmacodynamic side effects of the co-administered drug).
No products indexed under this heading.

Erythromycin (Ciprofloxacin is an inhibitor of the hepatic CYP1A2 enzyme pathway. Co-administration of ciprofloxacin and other drugs primarily metabolized by CYP1A2 results in increased plasma concentrations of the co-administered drug and could lead to clinically significant pharmacodynamic side effects of the co-administered drug).
No products indexed under this heading.

Erythromycin Estolate (Ciprofloxacin is an inhibitor of the hepatic CYP1A2 enzyme pathway. Co-administration of ciprofloxacin and other drugs primarily metabolized by CYP1A2 results in increased plasma concentrations of the co-administered drug and could lead to clinically significant pharmacodynamic side effects of the co-administered drug).
No products indexed under this heading.

Erythromycin Ethylsuccinate (Ciprofloxacin is an inhibitor of the hepatic CYP1A2 enzyme pathway. Co-administration of ciprofloxacin and other drugs primarily metabolized by CYP1A2 results in increased plasma concentrations of the co-administered drug and could lead to clinically significant pharmacodynamic side effects of the co-administered drug). Products include:

Erythromycin Glucceptate (Ciprofloxacin is an inhibitor of the hepatic CYP1A2 enzyme pathway. Co-administration of ciprofloxacin and other drugs primarily metabolized by CYP1A2 results in increased plasma concentrations of the co-administered drug and could lead to clinically significant pharmacodynamic side effects of the co-administered drug).
No products indexed under this heading.

Erythromycin Lactobionate (Ciprofloxacin is an inhibitor of the hepatic CYP1A2 enzyme pathway. Co-administration of ciprofloxacin and other drugs primarily metabolized by CYP1A2 results in increased plasma concentrations of the co-administered drug and could lead to clinically significant pharmacodynamic side effects of the co-administered drug).
No products indexed under this heading.

Erythromycin Stearate (Ciprofloxacin is an inhibitor of the hepatic CYP1A2 enzyme pathway. Co-administration of ciprofloxacin and other drugs primarily metabolized by CYP1A2 results in increased plasma concentrations of the co-administered drug and could lead to clinically significant pharmacodynamic side effects of the co-administered drug).
No products indexed under this heading.

Estradiol (Ciprofloxacin is an inhibitor of the hepatic CYP1A2 enzyme pathway. Co-administration of ciprofloxacin and other drugs primarily metabolized by CYP1A2 results in increased plasma concentrations of the co-administered drug and could lead to clinically significant pharmacodynamic side effects of the co-administered drug). Products include:

Estradiol Benzoate (Ciprofloxacin is an inhibitor of the hepatic CYP1A2 enzyme pathway. Co-administration of ciprofloxacin and other drugs primarily metabolized by CYP1A2 results in increased plasma concentrations of the co-administered drug and could lead to clinically significant pharmacodynamic side effects of the co-administered drug).
No products indexed under this heading.

Estradiol Cypionate (Ciprofloxacin is an inhibitor of the hepatic CYP1A2 enzyme pathway. Co-administration of ciprofloxacin and other drugs primarily metabolized by CYP1A2 results in increased plasma concentrations of the co-administered drug and could lead to clinically significant pharmacodynamic side effects of the co-administered drug).
No products indexed under this heading.

Etodolac (Non-steroidal anti-inflammatory drugs (but not acetyl salicylic acid) in combination of very high doses of quinolones have been shown to provoke convulsions in pre-clinical studies).
No products indexed under this heading.

Fenoprofen Calcium (Non-steroidal anti-inflammatory drugs (but not acetyl salicylic acid) in combination of very high doses of quinolones have been shown to provoke convulsions in pre-clinical studies).
No products indexed under this heading.

Ferrous Fumarate (Concurrent administration of ciprofloxacin with multivalent cation-containing products may substantially interfere with the absorption of ciprofloxacin, resulting in serum and urine levels considerably lower than desired. Ciprofloxacin extended release

tablets should be administered at least 2 hours before or 6 hours after metal cations). Products include:

PreNexa 3473

Ferrous Gluconate (Concurrent administration of ciprofloxacin with multivalent cation-containing products may substantially interfere with the absorption of ciprofloxacin, resulting in serum and urine levels considerably lower than desired. Ciprofloxacin extended release tablets should be administered at least 2 hours before or 6 hours after metal cations). Products include:

CitraNatal Assure 2332
CitraNatal Rx 2332

Ferrous Sulfate (Concurrent administration of ciprofloxacin with multivalent cation-containing products may substantially interfere with the absorption of ciprofloxacin, resulting in serum and urine levels considerably lower than desired. Ciprofloxacin extended release tablets should be administered at least 2 hours before or 6 hours after metal cations).

No products indexed under this heading.

Fludrocortisone Acetate (Fluoroquinolones, including ciprofloxacin, are associated with an increased risk of tendinitis and tendon rupture in all ages. The risk is further increased in older patients usually over 60 years of age, in patients taking corticosteroid drugs, and in kidney, heart and lung transplant recipients).

No products indexed under this heading.

Flumethasone Pivalate (Fluoroquinolones, including ciprofloxacin, are associated with an increased risk of tendinitis and tendon rupture in all ages. The risk is further increased in older patients usually over 60 years of age, in patients taking corticosteroid drugs, and in kidney, heart and lung transplant recipients).

No products indexed under this heading.

Flunisolide Hemihydrate (Fluoroquinolones, including ciprofloxacin, are associated with an increased risk of tendinitis and tendon rupture in all ages. The risk is further increased in older patients usually over 60 years of age, in patients taking corticosteroid drugs, and in kidney, heart and lung transplant recipients).

No products indexed under this heading.

Flurbiprofen (Non-steroidal anti-inflammatory drugs (but not acetyl salicylic acid) in combination of very high doses of quinolones have been shown to provoke convulsions in pre-clinical studies).

No products indexed under this heading.

Flutamide (Ciprofloxacin is an inhibitor of the hepatic CYP1A2 enzyme pathway. Co-administration of ciprofloxacin and other drugs primarily metabolized by CYP1A2 results in increased plasma concentrations of the co-administered drug and could lead to clinically significant pharmacodynamic side effects of the co-administered drug).

No products indexed under this heading.

Fluticasone Furoate (Fluoroquinolones, including ciprofloxacin, are associated with an increased risk of tendinitis and tendon rupture in all ages. The risk is further increased in older patients usually over 60 years of age, in patients taking corticosteroid drugs, and in kidney, heart and lung transplant recipients). Products include:

Veramyst 1713

Fluticasone Propionate (Fluoroquinolones, including ciprofloxacin, are associated with an increased risk of tendinitis and tendon rupture in all ages. The risk is further increased in older patients usually over 60 years of age, in patients taking corticosteroid drugs, and in kidney, heart and lung transplant recipients). Products include:

Advair 100/50 1275
Advair 250/50 1275
Advair 500/50 1275
Advair HFA 45/21 1288
Advair HFA 115/21 1288
Advair HFA 230/21 1288
Flonase 1459
Flovent Diskus 1463
Flovent HFA 1470

Fluvoxamine Maleate (Ciprofloxacin is an inhibitor of the hepatic CYP1A2 enzyme pathway. Co-administration of ciprofloxacin and other drugs primarily metabolized by CYP1A2 results in increased plasma concentrations of the co-administered drug and could lead to clinically significant pharmacodynamic side effects of the co-administered drug).

No products indexed under this heading.

Fosphenytoin (Altered serum levels of phenytoin (increased and decreased) have been reported in patients receiving concomitant ciprofloxacin).

No products indexed under this heading.

Fosphenytoin Sodium (Altered serum levels of phenytoin (increased and decreased) have been reported in patients receiving concomitant ciprofloxacin).

No products indexed under this heading.

Glyburide (The concomitant administration of ciprofloxacin with the sulfonylurea glyburide has, on rare occasions, resulted in severe hypoglycemia).

No products indexed under this heading.

Grepafloxacin Hydrochloride (Ciprofloxacin is an inhibitor of the hepatic CYP1A2 enzyme pathway. Co-administration of ciprofloxacin and other drugs primarily metabolized by CYP1A2 results in increased plasma concentrations of the co-administered drug and could lead to clinically significant pharmacodynamic side effects of the co-administered drug).

No products indexed under this heading.

Haloperidol (Ciprofloxacin is an inhibitor of the hepatic CYP1A2 enzyme pathway. Co-administration of ciprofloxacin and other drugs primarily metabolized by CYP1A2 results in increased plasma concentrations of the co-administered drug and could lead to clinically significant pharmacodynamic side effects of the co-administered drug).

No products indexed under this heading.

Haloperidol Decanoate (Ciprofloxacin is an inhibitor of the hepatic CYP1A2 enzyme pathway. Co-administration of ciprofloxacin and other drugs primarily metabolized by CYP1A2 results in increased plasma concentrations of the co-administered drug and could lead to clinically significant pharmacodynamic side effects of the co-administered drug).

No products indexed under this heading.

Haloperidol Lactate (Ciprofloxacin is an inhibitor of the hepatic CYP1A2 enzyme pathway. Co-administration of ciprofloxacin and other drugs primarily metabolized by CYP1A2 results in increased plasma concentrations of the co-administered drug and could lead to clinically significant pharmacodynamic side effects of the co-administered drug).

No products indexed under this heading.

Hydrocortisone (Fluoroquinolones, including ciprofloxacin, are associated with an increased risk of tendinitis and tendon rupture in all ages. The risk is further increased in older patients usually over 60 years of age, in patients taking corticosteroid drugs, and in kidney, heart and lung transplant recipients).

No products indexed under this heading.

Hydrocortisone (Alcohol) (Fluoroquinolones, including ciprofloxacin, are associated with an increased risk of tendinitis and tendon rupture in all ages. The risk is further increased in older patients usually over 60 years of age, in patients taking corticosteroid drugs, and in kidney, heart and lung transplant recipients).

No products indexed under this heading.

Hydrocortisone Acetate (Fluoroquinolones, including ciprofloxacin, are associated with an increased risk of tendinitis and tendon rupture in all ages. The risk is further increased in older patients usually over 60 years of age, in patients taking corticosteroid drugs, and in kidney, heart and lung transplant recipients).

No products indexed under this heading.

Hydrocortisone Butyrate (Fluoroquinolones, including ciprofloxacin, are associated with an increased risk of tendinitis and tendon rupture in all ages. The risk is further increased in older patients usually over 60 years of age, in patients taking corticosteroid drugs, and in kidney, heart and lung transplant recipients).

No products indexed under this heading.

Hydrocortisone Cypionate (Fluoroquinolones, including ciprofloxacin, are associated with an increased risk of tendinitis and tendon rupture in all ages. The risk is further increased in older patients usually over 60 years of age, in patients taking corticosteroid drugs, and in kidney, heart and lung transplant recipients).

No products indexed under this heading.

Hydrocortisone Hemisuccinate (Fluoroquinolones, including ciprofloxacin, are associated with an increased risk of tendinitis and tendon rupture in all ages. The risk is further increased in older patients usually over 60 years of age, in patients taking corticosteroid drugs, and in kidney, heart and lung transplant recipients).

No products indexed under this heading.

Hydrocortisone Probutate (Fluoroquinolones, including ciprofloxacin, are associated with an increased risk of tendinitis and tendon rupture in all ages. The risk is further increased in older patients usually over 60 years of age, in patients taking corticosteroid drugs, and in kidney, heart and lung transplant recipients).

No products indexed under this heading.

Hydrocortisone Sodium Phosphate (Fluoroquinolones, including ciprofloxacin, are associated with an increased risk of tendinitis and tendon rupture in all ages. The risk is further increased in older patients usually over 60 years of age, in patients taking corticosteroid drugs, and in kidney, heart and lung transplant recipients).

No products indexed under this heading.

Hydrocortisone Sodium Succinate (Fluoroquinolones, including ciprofloxacin, are associated with an increased risk of tendinitis and tendon rupture in all ages. The risk is further increased in older patients usually over 60 years of age, in patients taking corticosteroid drugs, and in kidney, heart and lung transplant recipients).

No products indexed under this heading.

Hydrocortisone Valerate (Fluoroquinolones, including ciprofloxacin, are associated with an increased risk of tendinitis and tendon rupture in all ages. The risk is further increased in older patients usually over 60 years of age, in patients taking corticosteroid drugs, and in kidney, heart and lung transplant recipients).

No products indexed under this heading.

Ibuprofen (Non-steroidal anti-inflammatory drugs (but not acetyl salicylic acid) in combination of very high doses of quinolones have been shown to provoke convulsions in pre-clinical studies). Products include:

Motrin IB 2043
Children's Motrin 2044
Children's Motrin Non-Staining Dye-Free 2044
Infants' Motrin 2044
Infants' Motrin Dye-Free 2044
Junior Strength Motrin 2044
Vicoprofen 564

Imipramine Hydrochloride (Ciprofloxacin is an inhibitor of the hepatic CYP1A2 enzyme pathway. Co-administration of ciprofloxacin and other drugs primarily metabolized by CYP1A2 results in increased plasma concentrations of the co-administered drug and could lead to clinically significant pharmacodynamic side effects of the co-administered drug).

No products indexed under this heading.

Imipramine Pamoate (Ciprofloxacin is an inhibitor of the hepatic CYP1A2 enzyme pathway. Co-administration of ciprofloxacin and other drugs primarily metabolized by CYP1A2 results in increased plasma concentrations of the co-administered drug and could lead to clinically significant pharmacodynamic side effects of the co-administered drug).

No products indexed under this heading.

Indomethacin (Non-steroidal anti-inflammatory drugs (but not acetyl salicylic acid) in combination of very high doses of quinolones have been shown to provoke convulsions in pre-clinical studies). Products include:

Indocin 2167

Indomethacin Sodium Trihydrate (Non-steroidal anti-inflammatory drugs (but not acetyl salicylic acid) in combination of very high doses of quinolones have been shown to provoke convulsions in pre-clinical studies). Products include:

Indocin I.V. 2007

Iron (Concurrent administration of ciprofloxacin with multivalent cation-containing products may substantially interfere with the absorption of ciprofloxacin, resulting in serum and urine levels considerably lower than desired. Ciprofloxacin extended release tablets should be administered at least 2 hours before or 6 hours after metal cations).

No products indexed under this heading.

Iron, Peptonized (Concurrent administration of ciprofloxacin with multivalent cation-containing products may substantially interfere with the absorption of ciprofloxacin, resulting in serum and urine levels considerably lower than desired. Ciprofloxacin extended release tablets should be administered at least 2 hours before or 6 hours after metal cations).

No products indexed under this heading.

Iron & Ammonium Citrate (Concurrent administration of ciprofloxacin with multivalent cation-containing products may substantially interfere with the absorption of ciprofloxacin, resulting in serum and urine levels considerably lower than desired. Ciprofloxacin extended release tablets should be administered at least 2 hours before or 6 hours after metal cations).

No products indexed under this heading.

Iron Cacodylate (Concurrent administration of ciprofloxacin with multivalent cation-containing products may substantially interfere with the absorption of ciprofloxacin, resulting in serum and urine levels considerably lower than desired. Ciprofloxacin extended release tablets should be administered at least 2 hours before or 6 hours after metal cations).

No products indexed under this heading.

IMPORTANT NOTE: Always consult each drug listing in the patient's regimen for possible interactions.

Iron Carbonyl (Concurrent administration of ciprofloxacin with multivalent cation-containing products may substantially interfere with the absorption of ciprofloxacin, resulting in serum and urine levels considerably lower than desired. Ciprofloxacin extended release tablets should be administered at least 2 hours before or 6 hours after metal cations). Products include:

Iron Supplements (Concurrent administration of ciprofloxacin with multivalent cation-containing products may substantially interfere with the absorption of ciprofloxacin, resulting in serum and urine levels considerably lower than desired. Ciprofloxacin extended release tablets should be administered at least 2 hours before or 6 hours after metal cations).

No products indexed under this heading.

Ketoprofen (Non-steroidal anti-inflammatory drugs (but not acetyl salicylic acid) in combination of very high doses of quinolones have been shown to provoke convulsions in pre-clinical studies).

No products indexed under this heading.

Ketorolac Tromethamine (Non-steroidal anti-inflammatory drugs (but not acetyl salicylic acid) in combination of very high doses of quinolones have been shown to provoke convulsions in pre-clinical studies). Products include:

Levobupivacaine Hydrochloride (Ciprofloxacin is an inhibitor of the hepatic CYP1A2 enzyme pathway. Co-administration of ciprofloxacin and other drugs primarily metabolized by CYP1A2 results in increased plasma concentrations of the co-administered drug and could lead to clinically significant pharmacodynamic side effects of the co-administered drug).

No products indexed under this heading.

Lomefloxacin Hydrochloride (Ciprofloxacin is an inhibitor of the hepatic CYP1A2 enzyme pathway. Co-administration of ciprofloxacin and other drugs primarily metabolized by CYP1A2 results in increased plasma concentrations of the co-administered drug and could lead to clinically significant pharmacodynamic side effects of the co-administered drug).

No products indexed under this heading.

Magaldrate (When ciprofloxacin extended release tablets, given as a single 1000 mg dose, were administered 2 hours before or 4 hours after a magnesium/aluminum-containing antacid (900 mg aluminum hydroxide and 600 mg magnesium hydroxide as a single oral dose) to 18 healthy volunteers, there was a 4% and 19% reduction, respectively, in the mean C_{max} of ciprofloxacin. The reduction in the mean AUC was 24% and 26%, respectively. Ciprofloxacin extended release tablets should be administered at least 2 hours before or 6 hours after antacids containing magnesium or aluminum).

No products indexed under this heading.

Magnesium (Concurrent administration of ciprofloxacin with multivalent cation-containing products may substantially interfere with the absorption of ciprofloxacin, resulting in serum and urine levels considerably lower than desired. Ciprofloxacin extended release tablets should be administered at least 2 hours before or 6 hours after metal cations). Products include:

Magnesium Aluminum Silicate (Concurrent administration of ciprofloxacin with multivalent cation-containing products may substantially interfere with the absorption of ciprofloxacin, resulting in serum and urine levels considerably lower than desired. Ciprofloxacin extended release tablets should be administered at least 2 hours before or 6 hours after metal cations).

No products indexed under this heading.

Magnesium Carbonate (Concurrent administration of ciprofloxacin with multivalent cation-containing products may substantially interfere with the absorption of ciprofloxacin, resulting in serum and urine levels considerably lower than desired. Ciprofloxacin extended release tablets should be administered at least 2 hours before or 6 hours after metal cations).

No products indexed under this heading.

Magnesium Chloride (Concurrent administration of ciprofloxacin with multivalent cation-containing products may substantially interfere with the absorption of ciprofloxacin, resulting in serum and urine levels considerably lower than desired. Ciprofloxacin extended release tablets should be administered at least 2 hours before or 6 hours after metal cations).

No products indexed under this heading.

Magnesium Citrate (Concurrent administration of ciprofloxacin with multivalent cation-containing products may substantially interfere with the absorption of ciprofloxacin, resulting in serum and urine levels considerably lower than desired. Ciprofloxacin extended release tablets should be administered at least 2 hours before or 6 hours after metal cations). Products include:

Magnesium Gluconate (Concurrent administration of ciprofloxacin with multivalent cation-containing products may substantially interfere with the absorption of ciprofloxacin, resulting in serum and urine levels considerably lower than desired. Ciprofloxacin extended release tablets should be administered at least 2 hours before or 6 hours after metal cations).

No products indexed under this heading.

Magnesium Hydroxide (Concurrent administration of ciprofloxacin with multivalent cation-containing products may substantially interfere with the absorption of ciprofloxacin, resulting in serum and urine levels considerably lower than desired. Ciprofloxacin extended release tablets should be administered at least 2 hours before or 6 hours after metal cations). Products include:

Magnesium Lactate (Concurrent administration of ciprofloxacin with multivalent cation-containing products may substantially interfere with the absorption of ciprofloxacin, resulting in serum and urine levels considerably lower than desired. Ciprofloxacin extended release tablets should be administered at least 2 hours before or 6 hours after metal cations).

No products indexed under this heading.

Magnesium Oxide (Concurrent administration of ciprofloxacin with multivalent cation-containing products may substantially interfere with the absorption of ciprofloxacin, resulting in serum and urine levels considerably lower than desired. Ciprofloxacin extended release tablets should be administered at least 2 hours before or 6 hours after metal cations). Products include:

Magnesium Salicylate (Concurrent administration of ciprofloxacin with multivalent cation-containing products may substantially interfere with the absorption of ciprofloxacin, resulting in serum and urine levels considerably lower than desired. Ciprofloxacin extended release tablets should be administered at least 2 hours before or 6 hours after metal cations).

No products indexed under this heading.

Magnesium Salicylate Tetrahydrate (Concurrent administration of ciprofloxacin with multivalent cation-containing products may substantially interfere with the absorption of ciprofloxacin, resulting in serum and urine levels considerably lower than desired. Ciprofloxacin extended release tablets should be administered at least 2 hours before or 6 hours after metal cations).

No products indexed under this heading.

Magnesium Salts (Concurrent administration of ciprofloxacin with multivalent cation-containing products may substantially interfere with the absorption of ciprofloxacin, resulting in serum and urine levels considerably lower than desired. Ciprofloxacin extended release tablets should be administered at least 2 hours before or 6 hours after metal cations).

No products indexed under this heading.

Magnesium Sulfate (Concurrent administration of ciprofloxacin with multivalent cation-containing products may substantially interfere with the absorption of ciprofloxacin, resulting in serum and urine levels considerably lower than desired. Ciprofloxacin extended release tablets should be administered at least 2 hours before or 6 hours after metal cations).

No products indexed under this heading.

Magnesium Trisilicate (Concurrent administration of ciprofloxacin with multivalent cation-containing products may substantially interfere with the absorption of ciprofloxacin, resulting in serum and urine levels considerably lower than desired. Ciprofloxacin extended release tablets should be administered at least 2 hours before or 6 hours after metal cations).

No products indexed under this heading.

Maprotiline Hydrochloride (Ciprofloxacin is an inhibitor of the hepatic CYP1A2 enzyme pathway. Co-administration of ciprofloxacin and other drugs primarily metabolized by CYP1A2 results in increased plasma concentrations of the co-administered drug and could lead to clinically significant pharmacodynamic side effects of the co-administered drug).

No products indexed under this heading.

Meclofenamate Sodium (Non-steroidal anti-inflammatory drugs (but not acetyl salicylic acid) in combination of very high doses of quinolones have been shown to provoke convulsions in pre-clinical studies).

No products indexed under this heading.

Mefenamic Acid (Non-steroidal anti-inflammatory drugs (but not acetyl salicylic acid) in combination of very high doses of quinolones have been shown to provoke convulsions in pre-clinical studies).

No products indexed under this heading.

Meloxicam (Non-steroidal anti-inflammatory drugs (but not acetyl salicylic acid) in combination of very high doses of quinolones have been shown to provoke convulsions in pre-clinical studies).

No products indexed under this heading.

Methadone Hydrochloride (Ciprofloxacin is an inhibitor of the hepatic CYP1A2 enzyme pathway. Co-administration of ciprofloxacin and other drugs primarily metabolized by CYP1A2 results in increased plasma concentrations of the co-administered drug and could lead to clinically significant pharmacodynamic side effects of the co-administered drug).

No products indexed under this heading.

Methotrexate (Renal tubular transport of methotrexate may be inhibited by concomitant administration of ciprofloxacin, potentially leading to increased plasma levels of methotrexate. This might increase the risk of methotrexate associated toxic reactions. Therefore, patients under methotrexate therapy should be carefully monitored when concomitant ciprofloxacin therapy is indicated).

No products indexed under this heading.

Methotrexate Sodium (Renal tubular transport of methotrexate may be inhibited by concomitant administration of ciprofloxacin, potentially leading to increased plasma levels of methotrexate. This might increase the risk of methotrexate associated toxic reactions. Therefore, patients under methotrexate therapy should be carefully monitored when concomitant ciprofloxacin therapy is indicated).

No products indexed under this heading.

Methylprednisolone (Fluoroquinolones, including ciprofloxacin, are associated with an increased risk of tendinitis and tendon rupture in all ages. The risk is further increased in older patients usually over 60 years of age, in patients taking corticosteroid drugs, and in kidney, heart and lung transplant recipients).

No products indexed under this heading.

Methylprednisolone Acetate (Fluoroquinolones, including ciprofloxacin, are associated with an increased risk of tendinitis and tendon rupture in all ages. The risk is further increased in older patients usually over 60 years of age, in patients taking corticosteroid drugs, and in kidney, heart and lung transplant recipients).

No products indexed under this heading.

Methylprednisolone Sodium Succinate (Fluoroquinolones, including ciprofloxacin, are associated with an increased risk of tendinitis and tendon rupture in all ages. The risk is further increased in older patients usually over 60 years of age, in patients taking corticosteroid drugs, and in kidney, heart and lung transplant recipients).

No products indexed under this heading.

Metoclopramide Hydrochloride (Metoclopramide significantly accelerates the absorption of oral ciprofloxacin, resulting in a shorter time to reach maximum plasma concentrations. No significant effect was observed on the bioavailability of ciprofloxacin). Products include:

Mexiletine Hydrochloride (Ciprofloxacin is an inhibitor of the hepatic CYP1A2 enzyme pathway. Co-administration of ciprofloxacin and other drugs primarily metabolized by CYP1A2 results in increased plasma concentrations of the co-administered drug and could lead to clinically significant pharmacodynamic side effects of the co-administered drug).

No products indexed under this heading.

Mirtazapine (Ciprofloxacin is an inhibitor of the hepatic CYP1A2 enzyme pathway. Co-administration of ciprofloxacin and other drugs primarily metabolized by CYP1A2 results in increased plasma concentrations of the co-administered drug and could lead to clinically signifi-

IMPORTANT NOTE: Always consult each drug listing in the patient's regimen for possible interactions.

Propafenone Hydrochloride (Ciprofloxacin is an inhibitor of the hepatic CYP1A2 enzyme pathway. Co-administration of ciprofloxacin and other drugs primarily metabolized by CYP1A2 results in increased plasma concentrations of the co-administered drug and could lead to clinically significant pharmacodynamic side effects of the co-administered drug). Products include:

Rythmol **1648**
Rythmol SR **1652**

Propranolol Hydrochloride (Ciprofloxacin is an inhibitor of the hepatic CYP1A2 enzyme pathway. Co-administration of ciprofloxacin and other drugs primarily metabolized by CYP1A2 results in increased plasma concentrations of the co-administered drug and could lead to clinically significant pharmacodynamic side effects of the co-administered drug). Products include:

InnoPran XL **1517**

Protriptyline Hydrochloride (Ciprofloxacin is an inhibitor of the hepatic CYP1A2 enzyme pathway. Co-administration of ciprofloxacin and other drugs primarily metabolized by CYP1A2 results in increased plasma concentrations of the co-administered drug and could lead to clinically significant pharmacodynamic side effects of the co-administered drug).
No products indexed under this heading.

Quinidine (Precaution should be taken when using ciprofloxacin with drugs that can result in prolongation of the QT interval, such as class IA antiarrhythmics).
No products indexed under this heading.

Quinidine Gluconate (Precaution should be taken when using ciprofloxacin with drugs that can result in prolongation of the QT interval, such as class IA antiarrhythmics).
No products indexed under this heading.

Quinidine Hydrochloride (Precaution should be taken when using ciprofloxacin with drugs that can result in prolongation of the QT interval, such as class IA antiarrhythmics).
No products indexed under this heading.

Quinidine Polygalacturonate (Precaution should be taken when using ciprofloxacin with drugs that can result in prolongation of the QT interval, such as class IA antiarrhythmics).
No products indexed under this heading.

Quinidine Sulfate (Precaution should be taken when using ciprofloxacin with drugs that can result in prolongation of the QT interval, such as class IA antiarrhythmics).
No products indexed under this heading.

Riluzole (Ciprofloxacin is an inhibitor of the hepatic CYP1A2 enzyme pathway. Co-administration of ciprofloxacin and other drugs primarily metabolized by CYP1A2 results in increased plasma concentrations of the co-administered drug and could lead to clinically significant pharmacodynamic side effects of the co-administered drug). Products include:

Rilutek **3032**

Ritonavir (Ciprofloxacin is an inhibitor of the hepatic CYP1A2 enzyme pathway. Co-administration of ciprofloxacin and other drugs primarily metabolized by CYP1A2 results in increased plasma concentrations of the co-administered drug and could lead to clinically significant pharmacodynamic side effects of the co-administered drug). Products include:

Kaletra **458**
Norvir **509**

Rofecoxib (Non-steroidal anti-inflammatory drugs (but not acetyl salicylic acid) in combination of very high doses of quinolones have been shown to provoke convulsions in pre-clinical studies).
No products indexed under this heading.

Ropinirole Hydrochloride (Ciprofloxacin is an inhibitor of the hepatic CYP1A2 enzyme pathway. Co-administration of ciprofloxacin and other drugs primarily metabolized by CYP1A2 results in increased plasma concentrations of the co-administered drug and could lead to clinically significant pharmacodynamic side effects of the co-administered drug). Products include:

Requip **1620**
Requip XL **1628**

Ropivacaine Hydrochloride (Ciprofloxacin is an inhibitor of the hepatic CYP1A2 enzyme pathway. Co-administration of ciprofloxacin and other drugs primarily metabolized by CYP1A2 results in increased plasma concentrations of the co-administered drug and could lead to clinically significant pharmacodynamic side effects of the co-administered drug).
No products indexed under this heading.

Selenium (Concurrent administration of ciprofloxacin with multivalent cation-containing products may substantially interfere with the absorption of ciprofloxacin, resulting in serum and urine levels considerably lower than desired. Ciprofloxacin extended release tablets should be administered at least 2 hours before or 6 hours after metal cations). Products include:

Cardio Basics **3455**
Chelated Mineral **3476**

Selenium Sulfide (Concurrent administration of ciprofloxacin with multivalent cation-containing products may substantially interfere with the absorption of ciprofloxacin, resulting in serum and urine levels considerably lower than desired. Ciprofloxacin extended release tablets should be administered at least 2 hours before or 6 hours after metal cations).
No products indexed under this heading.

Sotalol Hydrochloride (Precaution should be taken when using ciprofloxacin with drugs that can result in prolongation of the QT interval, such as class III antiarrhythmics).
No products indexed under this heading.

Sucralfate (Concurrent administration of quinolone, including ciprofloxacin, with sucralfate may substantially interfere with the absorption of quinolone, resulting in serum and urine levels considerably lower than desired. Ciprofloxacin should be administered at least 2 hours before or 6 hours after sucralfate is given). Products include:

Carafate Suspension **784**
Carafate Tablets **785**

Sulindac (Non-steroidal anti-inflammatory drugs (but not acetyl salicylic acid) in combination of very high doses of quinolones have been shown to provoke convulsions in pre-clinical studies). Products include:

Clinoril **2098**

Tacrine Hydrochloride (Ciprofloxacin is an inhibitor of the hepatic CYP1A2 enzyme pathway. Co-administration of ciprofloxacin and other drugs primarily metabolized by CYP1A2 results in increased plasma concentrations of the co-administered drug and could lead to clinically significant pharmacodynamic side effects of the co-administered drug).
No products indexed under this heading.

Tamoxifen Citrate (Ciprofloxacin is an inhibitor of the hepatic CYP1A2 enzyme pathway. Co-administration of ciprofloxacin and other drugs primarily metabolized by CYP1A2 results in increased plasma concentrations of the co-administered drug and could lead to clinically significant pharmacodynamic side effects of the co-administered drug).
No products indexed under this heading.

Theobromine (Ciprofloxacin is an inhibitor of the hepatic CYP1A2 enzyme pathway. Co-administration of ciprofloxacin and other drugs primarily metabolized by CYP1A2 results in increased plasma concentrations of the co-administered drug and could lead to clinically significant pharmacodynamic side effects of the co-administered drug).
No products indexed under this heading.

Theophylline (Ciprofloxacin is an inhibitor of the hepatic CYP1A2 enzyme pathway. Co-administration of ciprofloxacin and other drugs primarily metabolized by CYP1A2 results in increased plasma concentrations of the co-administered drug and could lead to clinically significant pharmacodynamic side effects of the co-administered drug and prolongation of its elimination half-life. This may result in increased risk of theophylline-related adverse reactions. If concomitant use cannot be avoided, serum levels of theophylline should be monitored and dosage adjustments made as appropriate. Serious and fatal reactions have been reported in patients receiving concurrent administration of ciprofloxacin and theophylline).
No products indexed under this heading.

Theophylline Anhydrous (Ciprofloxacin is an inhibitor of the hepatic CYP1A2 enzyme pathway. Co-administration of ciprofloxacin and other drugs primarily metabolized by CYP1A2 results in increased plasma concentrations of the co-administered drug and could lead to clinically significant pharmacodynamic side effects of the co-administered drug and prolongation of its elimination half-life. This may result in increased risk of theophylline-related adverse reactions. If concomitant use cannot be avoided, serum levels of theophylline should be monitored and dosage adjustments made as appropriate. Serious and fatal reactions have been reported in patients receiving concurrent administration of ciprofloxacin and theophylline). Products include:

Uniphyl **2817**

Theophylline Calcium Salicylate (Ciprofloxacin is an inhibitor of the hepatic CYP1A2 enzyme pathway. Co-administration of ciprofloxacin and other drugs primarily metabolized by CYP1A2 results in increased plasma concentrations of the co-administered drug and could lead to clinically significant pharmacodynamic side effects of the co-administered drug and prolongation of its elimination half-life. This may result in increased risk of theophylline-related adverse reactions. If concomitant use cannot be avoided, serum levels of theophylline should be monitored and dosage adjustments made as appropriate. Serious and fatal reactions have been reported in patients receiving concurrent administration of ciprofloxacin and theophylline).
No products indexed under this heading.

Theophylline Dihydroxypropyl (Glyceryl) (Ciprofloxacin is an inhibitor of the hepatic CYP1A2 enzyme pathway. Co-administration of ciprofloxacin and other drugs primarily metabolized by CYP1A2 results in increased plasma concentrations of the co-administered drug and could lead to clinically significant pharmacodynamic side effects of the co-administered drug and prolongation of its elimination half-life. This may result in increased risk of theophylline-related adverse reactions. If concomitant use cannot be avoided, serum levels of theophylline should be monitored and dosage adjustments made as appropriate. Serious and fatal reactions have been reported in patients receiving concurrent administration of ciprofloxacin and theophylline).
No products indexed under this heading.

Theophylline Ethylenediamine (Ciprofloxacin is an inhibitor of the hepatic CYP1A2 enzyme pathway. Co-administration of ciprofloxacin and other drugs primarily metabolized by CYP1A2 results in increased plasma concentrations of the co-administered drug and could lead to clinically significant pharmacodynamic side effects of the co-administered drug and prolongation of its elimination half-life. This may result in increased risk of theophylline-related adverse reactions. If concomitant use cannot be avoided, serum levels of theophylline should be monitored and dosage adjustments made as appropriate. Serious and fatal reactions have been reported in patients receiving concurrent administration of ciprofloxacin and theophylline).
No products indexed under this heading.

Theophylline Sodium Glycinate (Ciprofloxacin is an inhibitor of the hepatic CYP1A2 enzyme pathway. Co-administration of ciprofloxacin and other drugs primarily metabolized by CYP1A2 results in increased plasma concentrations of the co-administered drug and could lead to clinically significant pharmacodynamic side effects of the co-administered drug and prolongation of its elimination half-life. This may result in increased risk of theophylline-related adverse reactions. If concomitant use cannot be avoided, serum levels of theophylline should be monitored and dosage adjustments made as appropriate. Serious and fatal reactions have been reported in patients receiving concurrent administration of ciprofloxacin and theophylline).
No products indexed under this heading.

Tizanidine (Concomitant administration of tizanidine and ciprofloxacin is contraindicated. Systemic exposure of tizanidine was significantly increased (C_{max} 7-fold, AUC 10-fold) when the drug was given concomitantly with ciprofloxacin. The hypotensive and sedative effects of tizanidine were also potentiated).
No products indexed under this heading.

Tizanidine Hydrochloride (Concomitant administration of tizanidine and ciprofloxacin is contraindicated. Systemic exposure of tizanidine was significantly increased (C_{max} 7-fold, AUC 10-fold) when the drug was given concomitantly with ciprofloxacin. The hypotensive and sedative effects of tizanidine were also potentiated).
No products indexed under this heading.

Tolmetin Sodium (Non-steroidal anti-inflammatory drugs (but not acetyl salicylic acid) in combination of very high doses of quinolones have been shown to provoke convulsions in pre-clinical studies).
No products indexed under this heading.

Triamcinolone (Fluoroquinolones, including ciprofloxacin, are associated with an increased risk of tendinitis and tendon rupture in all ages. The risk is further increased in older patients usually over 60 years of age, in patients taking corticosteroid drugs, and in kidney, heart and lung transplant recipients).
No products indexed under this heading.

Triamcinolone Acetonide (Fluoroquinolones, including ciprofloxacin, are

associated with an increased risk of tendinitis and tendon rupture in all ages. The risk is further increased in older patients usually over 60 years of age, in patients taking corticosteroid drugs, and in kidney, heart and lung transplant recipients). Products include:

Triamcinolone Diacetate (Fluoroquinolones, including ciprofloxacin, are associated with an increased risk of tendinitis and tendon rupture in all ages. The risk is further increased in older patients usually over 60 years of age, in patients taking corticosteroid drugs, and in kidney, heart and lung transplant recipients).
No products indexed under this heading.

Triamcinolone Hexacetonide (Fluoroquinolones, including ciprofloxacin, are associated with an increased risk of tendinitis and tendon rupture in all ages. The risk is further increased in older patients usually over 60 years of age, in patients taking corticosteroid drugs, and in kidney, heart and lung transplant recipients).
No products indexed under this heading.

Trimethaphan Camsylate (Ciprofloxacin is an inhibitor of the hepatic CYP1A2 enzyme pathway. Co-administration of ciprofloxacin and other drugs primarily metabolized by CYP1A2 results in increased plasma concentrations of the co-administered drug and could lead to clinically significant pharmacodynamic side effects of the co-administered drug).
No products indexed under this heading.

Trimipramine Maleate (Ciprofloxacin is an inhibitor of the hepatic CYP1A2 enzyme pathway. Co-administration of ciprofloxacin and other drugs primarily metabolized by CYP1A2 results in increased plasma concentrations of the co-administered drug and could lead to clinically significant pharmacodynamic side effects of the co-administered drug).
No products indexed under this heading.

Trovafloxacin Mesylate (Ciprofloxacin is an inhibitor of the hepatic CYP1A2 enzyme pathway. Co-administration of ciprofloxacin and other drugs primarily metabolized by CYP1A2 results in increased plasma concentrations of the co-administered drug and could lead to clinically significant pharmacodynamic side effects of the co-administered drug).
No products indexed under this heading.

Valdecoxib (Non-steroidal anti-inflammatory drugs (but not acetyl salicylic acid) in combination with very high doses of quinolones have been shown to provoke convulsions in pre-clinical studies).
No products indexed under this heading.

Verapamil Hydrochloride (Ciprofloxacin is an inhibitor of the hepatic CYP1A2 enzyme pathway. Co-administration of ciprofloxacin and other drugs primarily metabolized by CYP1A2 results in increased plasma concentrations of the co-administered drug and could lead to clinically significant pharmacodynamic side effects of the co-administered drug). Products include:

Warfarin Sodium (Ciprofloxacin has been reported to enhance the effects of the oral anticoagulant warfarin or its derivatives. When these products are administered concomitantly, prothrombin time or other suitable coagulation tests should be closely monitored).
No products indexed under this heading.

Zileuton (Ciprofloxacin is an inhibitor of the hepatic CYP1A2 enzyme pathway. Co-administration of ciprofloxacin and other drugs primarily metabolized by CYP1A2 results in increased plasma concentrations of the co-administered drug and could lead to clinically significant pharmacodynamic side effects of the co-administered drug).
No products indexed under this heading.

Zinc (Concurrent administration of ciprofloxacin with multivalent cation-containing products may substantially interfere with the absorption of ciprofloxacin, resulting in serum and urine levels considerably lower than desired. Ciprofloxacin extended release tablets should be administered at least 2 hours before or 6 hours after metal cations). Products include:

Zinc Acetate (Concurrent administration of ciprofloxacin with multivalent cation-containing products may substantially interfere with the absorption of ciprofloxacin, resulting in serum and urine levels considerably lower than desired. Ciprofloxacin extended release tablets should be administered at least 2 hours before or 6 hours after metal cations).
No products indexed under this heading.

Zinc Bisglycinate (Concurrent administration of ciprofloxacin with multivalent cation-containing products may substantially interfere with the absorption of ciprofloxacin, resulting in serum and urine levels considerably lower than desired. Ciprofloxacin extended release tablets should be administered at least 2 hours before or 6 hours after metal cations).
No products indexed under this heading.

Zinc Chloride (Concurrent administration of ciprofloxacin with multivalent cation-containing products may substantially interfere with the absorption of ciprofloxacin, resulting in serum and urine levels considerably lower than desired. Ciprofloxacin extended release tablets should be administered at least 2 hours before or 6 hours after metal cations).
No products indexed under this heading.

Zinc Citrate (Concurrent administration of ciprofloxacin with multivalent cation-containing products may substantially interfere with the absorption of ciprofloxacin, resulting in serum and urine levels considerably lower than desired. Ciprofloxacin extended release tablets should be administered at least 2 hours before or 6 hours after metal cations). Products include:

Zinc-Containing Multivitamins (Concurrent administration of ciprofloxacin with multivalent cation-containing products may substantially interfere with the absorption of ciprofloxacin, resulting in serum and urine levels considerably lower than desired. Ciprofloxacin extended release tablets should be administered at least 2 hours before or 6 hours after metal cations).
No products indexed under this heading.

Zinc Gluconate (Concurrent administration of ciprofloxacin with multivalent cation-containing products may substantially interfere with the absorption of ciprofloxacin, resulting in serum and urine levels considerably lower than desired. Ciprofloxacin extended release tablets should be administered at least 2 hours before or 6 hours after metal cations).
No products indexed under this heading.

Zinc Oxide (Concurrent administration of ciprofloxacin with multivalent cation-containing products may substantially interfere with the absorption of ciprofloxacin, resulting in serum and urine levels considerably lower than desired. Ciprofloxacin extended release tablets should be administered at least 2 hours before or 6 hours after metal cations). Products include:

Zinc Phenosulfonate (Concurrent administration of ciprofloxacin with multivalent cation-containing products may substantially interfere with the absorption of ciprofloxacin, resulting in serum and urine levels considerably lower than desired. Ciprofloxacin extended release tablets should be administered at least 2 hours before or 6 hours after metal cations).
No products indexed under this heading.

Zinc Sulfate (Concurrent administration of ciprofloxacin with multivalent cation-containing products may substantially interfere with the absorption of ciprofloxacin, resulting in serum and urine levels considerably lower than desired. Ciprofloxacin extended release tablets should be administered at least 2 hours before or 6 hours after metal cations). Products include:

Zolmitriptan (Ciprofloxacin is an inhibitor of the hepatic CYP1A2 enzyme pathway. Co-administration of ciprofloxacin and other drugs primarily metabolized by CYP1A2 results in increased plasma concentrations of the co-administered drug and could lead to clinically significant pharmacodynamic side effects of the co-administered drug). Products include:

Food Interactions

Beverages, caffeine-containing (Ciprofloxacin has been shown to interfere with the metabolism of caffeine. This may lead to reduced clearance of caffeine and a prolongation of its serum half-life and inhibit the formation of paraxanthine after caffeine administration).

Food, caffeine-containing (Ciprofloxacin has been shown to interfere with the metabolism of caffeine. This may lead to reduced clearance of caffeine and a prolongation of its serum half-life and inhibit the formation of paraxanthine after caffeine administration).

Food, calcium-rich (Concomitant administration of ciprofloxacin with milk products (dairy products) or calcium-fortified juices alone should be avoided since decreased absorption is possible).

Iron Amino Acid Chelate (Concurrent administration of ciprofloxacin with multivalent cation-containing products may substantially interfere with the absorption of ciprofloxacin, resulting in serum and urine levels considerably lower than desired. Ciprofloxacin extended release tablets should be administered at least 2 hours before or 6 hours after metal cations).

CIPRODEX OTIC SUSPENSION

(Ciprofloxacin, Dexamethasone) 583
None cited in PDR database.

CITRANATAL 90 DHA

(Calcium, Calcium Citrate, Copper, Docosahexaenoic Acid (DHA), Docusate Sodium, Eicosapentaenoic Acid (EPA), Folic Acid, Iodine, Iron Carbonyl, Niacinamide, Vitamin B1, Vitamin B2, Vitamin B6, Vitamin C, Vitamin D3, Vitamin E, Zinc) 2332
May interact with anticoagulants. Compounds in these categories include:

Anisindione (Ingestion of more than 3 grams of omega-3 fatty acids per day has shown to have potential antithrombotic effects including increased bleeding time and INR. Administration of omega-3 fatty acids should be avoided in patients on anticoagulants).
No products indexed under this heading.

Ardeparin Sodium (Ingestion of more than 3 grams of omega-3 fatty acids per day has shown to have potential antithrombotic effects including increased bleeding time and INR. Administration of omega-3 fatty acids should be avoided in patients on anticoagulants).
No products indexed under this heading.

Dalteparin Sodium (Ingestion of more than 3 grams of omega-3 fatty acids per day has shown to have potential antithrombotic effects including increased bleeding time and INR. Administration of omega-3 fatty acids should be avoided in patients on anticoagulants). Products include:

Danaparoid Sodium (Ingestion of more than 3 grams of omega-3 fatty acids per day has shown to have potential antithrombotic effects including increased bleeding time and INR. Administration of omega-3 fatty acids should be avoided in patients on anticoagulants).
No products indexed under this heading.

Dicumarol (Ingestion of more than 3 grams of omega-3 fatty acids per day has shown to have potential antithrombotic effects including increased bleeding time and INR. Administration of omega-3 fatty acids should be avoided in patients on anticoagulants).
No products indexed under this heading.

Enoxaparin Sodium (Ingestion of more than 3 grams of omega-3 fatty acids per day has shown to have potential antithrombotic effects including increased bleeding time and INR. Administration of omega-3 fatty acids should be avoided in patients on anticoagulants). Products include:

Fondaparinux Sodium (Ingestion of more than 3 grams of omega-3 fatty acids per day has shown to have potential antithrombotic effects including increased bleeding time and INR. Administration of omega-3 fatty acids should be avoided in patients on anticoagulants). Products include:

Heparin Calcium (Ingestion of more than 3 grams of omega-3 fatty acids per day has shown to have potential antithrombotic effects including increased bleeding time and INR. Administration of omega-3 fatty acids should be avoided in patients on anticoagulants).
No products indexed under this heading.

Heparin Sodium (Ingestion of more than 3 grams of omega-3 fatty acids per day has shown to have potential antithrombotic effects including increased bleeding time and INR. Administration of omega-3 fatty acids should be avoided in patients on anticoagulants).
No products indexed under this heading.

IMPORTANT NOTE: Always consult each drug listing in the patient's regimen for possible interactions.

Low Molecular Weight Heparins
(Ingestion of more than 3 grams of omega-3 fatty acids per day has shown to have potential antithrombotic effects including increased bleeding time and INR. Administration of omega-3 fatty acids should be avoided in patients on anticoagulants).
No products indexed under this heading.

Tinzaparin Sodium (Ingestion of more than 3 grams of omega-3 fatty acids per day has shown to have potential antithrombotic effects including increased bleeding time and INR. Administration of omega-3 fatty acids should be avoided in patients on anticoagulants).
No products indexed under this heading.

Warfarin Sodium (Ingestion of more than 3 grams of omega-3 fatty acids per day has shown to have potential antithrombotic effects including increased bleeding time and INR. Administration of omega-3 fatty acids should be avoided in patients on anticoagulants).
No products indexed under this heading.

CITRANATAL ASSURE

(Calcium Citrate, Copper, Docosahexaenoic Acid (DHA), Docusate Sodium, Eicosapentaenoic Acid (EPA), Ferrous Gluconate, Folic Acid, Iodine, Iron Carbonyl, Niacinamide, Vitamin B1, Vitamin B2, Vitamin B6, Vitamin C, Vitamin D3, Vitamin E, Zinc) 2332
May interact with anticoagulants. Compounds in these categories include:

Anisindione (Ingestion of more than 3 grams of omega-3 fatty acids per day has shown to have potential antithrombotic effects including increased bleeding time and INR. Administration of omega-3 fatty acids should be avoided in patients on anticoagulants).
No products indexed under this heading.

Ardeparin Sodium (Ingestion of more than 3 grams of omega-3 fatty acids per day has shown to have potential antithrombotic effects including increased bleeding time and INR. Administration of omega-3 fatty acids should be avoided in patients on anticoagulants).
No products indexed under this heading.

Dalteparin Sodium (Ingestion of more than 3 grams of omega-3 fatty acids per day has shown to have potential antithrombotic effects including increased bleeding time and INR. Administration of omega-3 fatty acids should be avoided in patients on anticoagulants). Products include:
Fragmin 1058

Danaparoid Sodium (Ingestion of more than 3 grams of omega-3 fatty acids per day has shown to have potential antithrombotic effects including increased bleeding time and INR. Administration of omega-3 fatty acids should be avoided in patients on anticoagulants).
No products indexed under this heading.

Dicumarol (Ingestion of more than 3 grams of omega-3 fatty acids per day has shown to have potential antithrombotic effects including increased bleeding time and INR. Administration of omega-3 fatty acids should be avoided in patients on anticoagulants).
No products indexed under this heading.

Enoxaparin Sodium (Ingestion of more than 3 grams of omega-3 fatty acids per day has shown to have potential antithrombotic effects including increased bleeding time and INR. Administration of omega-3 fatty acids should be avoided in patients on anticoagulants). Products include:

Lovenox 3005

Fondaparinux Sodium (Ingestion of more than 3 grams of omega-3 fatty acids per day has shown to have potential antithrombotic effects including increased bleeding time and INR. Administration of omega-3 fatty acids should be avoided in patients on anticoagulants). Products include:
Arixtra 1320

Heparin Calcium (Ingestion of more than 3 grams of omega-3 fatty acids per day has shown to have potential antithrombotic effects including increased bleeding time and INR. Administration of omega-3 fatty acids should be avoided in patients on anticoagulants).
No products indexed under this heading.

Heparin Sodium (Ingestion of more than 3 grams of omega-3 fatty acids per day has shown to have potential antithrombotic effects including increased bleeding time and INR. Administration of omega-3 fatty acids should be avoided in patients on anticoagulants).
No products indexed under this heading.

Low Molecular Weight Heparins
(Ingestion of more than 3 grams of omega-3 fatty acids per day has shown to have potential antithrombotic effects including increased bleeding time and INR. Administration of omega-3 fatty acids should be avoided in patients on anticoagulants).
No products indexed under this heading.

Tinzaparin Sodium (Ingestion of more than 3 grams of omega-3 fatty acids per day has shown to have potential antithrombotic effects including increased bleeding time and INR. Administration of omega-3 fatty acids should be avoided in patients on anticoagulants).
No products indexed under this heading.

Warfarin Sodium (Ingestion of more than 3 grams of omega-3 fatty acids per day has shown to have potential antithrombotic effects including increased bleeding time and INR. Administration of omega-3 fatty acids should be avoided in patients on anticoagulants).
No products indexed under this heading.

CITRANATAL HARMONY CAPSULES

(Calcium, Calcium Citrate, Docosahexaenoic Acid (DHA), Docusate Sodium, Folic Acid, Iron Carbonyl, Vitamin B6, Vitamin D3, Vitamin E) 2332
May interact with anticoagulants. Compounds in these categories include:

Anisindione (Ingestion of more than 3 grams of omega-3 fatty acids per day has been shown to have potential antithrombotic effects, including an increased bleeding time and INR. Administration of omega-3 fatty acids should be avoided in patients on anticoagulants).
No products indexed under this heading.

Ardeparin Sodium (Ingestion of more than 3 grams of omega-3 fatty acids per day has been shown to have potential antithrombotic effects, including an increased bleeding time and INR. Administration of omega-3 fatty acids should be avoided in patients on anticoagulants).
No products indexed under this heading.

Dalteparin Sodium (Ingestion of more than 3 grams of omega-3 fatty acids per day has been shown to have potential antithrombotic effects, including an increased bleeding time and INR. Administration of omega-3 fatty acids should be avoided in patients on anticoagulants). Products include:

Fragmin 1058

Danaparoid Sodium (Ingestion of more than 3 grams of omega-3 fatty acids per day has been shown to have potential antithrombotic effects, including an increased bleeding time and INR. Administration of omega-3 fatty acids should be avoided in patients on anticoagulants).
No products indexed under this heading.

Dicumarol (Ingestion of more than 3 grams of omega-3 fatty acids per day has been shown to have potential antithrombotic effects, including an increased bleeding time and INR. Administration of omega-3 fatty acids should be avoided in patients on anticoagulants).
No products indexed under this heading.

Enoxaparin Sodium (Ingestion of more than 3 grams of omega-3 fatty acids per day has been shown to have potential antithrombotic effects, including an increased bleeding time and INR. Administration of omega-3 fatty acids should be avoided in patients on anticoagulants). Products include:
Lovenox 3005

Fondaparinux Sodium (Ingestion of more than 3 grams of omega-3 fatty acids per day has been shown to have potential antithrombotic effects, including an increased bleeding time and INR. Administration of omega-3 fatty acids should be avoided in patients on anticoagulants). Products include:
Arixtra 1320

Heparin Calcium (Ingestion of more than 3 grams of omega-3 fatty acids per day has been shown to have potential antithrombotic effects, including an increased bleeding time and INR. Administration of omega-3 fatty acids should be avoided in patients on anticoagulants).
No products indexed under this heading.

Heparin Sodium (Ingestion of more than 3 grams of omega-3 fatty acids per day has been shown to have potential antithrombotic effects, including an increased bleeding time and INR. Administration of omega-3 fatty acids should be avoided in patients on anticoagulants).
No products indexed under this heading.

Low Molecular Weight Heparins
(Ingestion of more than 3 grams of omega-3 fatty acids per day has been shown to have potential antithrombotic effects, including an increased bleeding time and INR. Administration of omega-3 fatty acids should be avoided in patients on anticoagulants).
No products indexed under this heading.

Tinzaparin Sodium (Ingestion of more than 3 grams of omega-3 fatty acids per day has been shown to have potential antithrombotic effects, including an increased bleeding time and INR. Administration of omega-3 fatty acids should be avoided in patients on anticoagulants).
No products indexed under this heading.

Warfarin Sodium (Ingestion of more than 3 grams of omega-3 fatty acids per day has been shown to have potential antithrombotic effects, including an increased bleeding time and INR. Administration of omega-3 fatty acids should be avoided in patients on anticoagulants).
No products indexed under this heading.

CITRANATAL RX TABLETS

(Calcium Citrate, Cholecalciferol, Cupric Oxide, Docusate Sodium, Ferrous Gluconate, Folic Acid, Iron Carbonyl, Niacinamide, Potassium Iodide, Vitamin B1, Vitamin B2, Vitamin B6, Vitamin C, Vitamin E, Zinc Oxide) 2332
None cited in PDR database.

CLARINEX SYRUP

(Desloratadine) 3098
See Clarinex Tablets

CLARINEX TABLETS

(Desloratadine) 3098
May interact with erythromycin, and certain other agents. Compounds in these categories include:

Azithromycin Dihydrate (Co-administration resulted in increased C_{max} and AUC of desloratadine by 15% and 5% respectively; C_{max} and AUC of 3-hydroxydesloratadine increased by 15% and 4% respectively; there were no clinically relevant changes in the safety profile of desloratadine).
No products indexed under this heading.

Cimetidine (Co-administration resulted in increased C_{max} and AUC of desloratadine by 12% and 19% respectively; C_{max} and AUC of 3-hydroxydesloratadine decreased by 11% and 3% respectively; there were no clinically relevant changes in the safety profile of desloratadine).
No products indexed under this heading.

Cimetidine Hydrochloride (Co-administration resulted in increased C_{max} and AUC of desloratadine by 12% and 19% respectively; C_{max} and AUC of 3-hydroxydesloratadine decreased by 11% and 3% respectively; there were no clinically relevant changes in the safety profile of desloratadine).
No products indexed under this heading.

Erythromycin (Co-administration resulted in increased C_{max} and AUC of desloratadine by 24% and 14% respectively; C_{max} and AUC of 3-hydroxydesloratadine increased by 43% and 40% respectively; there were no clinically relevant changes in the safety profile of desloratadine).
No products indexed under this heading.

Erythromycin, Topical (Co-administration resulted in increased C_{max} and AUC of desloratadine by 24% and 14% respectively; C_{max} and AUC of 3-hydroxydesloratadine increased by 43% and 40% respectively; there were no clinically relevant changes in the safety profile of desloratadine).
No products indexed under this heading.

Erythromycin Estolate (Co-administration resulted in increased C_{max} and AUC of desloratadine by 24% and 14% respectively; C_{max} and AUC of 3-hydroxydesloratadine increased by 43% and 40% respectively; there were no clinically relevant changes in the safety profile of desloratadine).
No products indexed under this heading.

Erythromycin Ethylsuccinate (Co-administration resulted in increased C_{max} and AUC of desloratadine by 24% and 14% respectively; C_{max} and AUC of 3-hydroxydesloratadine increased by 43% and 40% respectively; there were no clinically relevant changes in the safety profile of desloratadine).
Products include:
E.E.S. 437
EryPed 435

Erythromycin Gluceptate (Co-administration resulted in increased C_{max} and AUC of desloratadine by 24% and 14% respectively; C_{max} and AUC of 3-hydroxydesloratadine increased by 43% and 40% respectively; there were no clinically relevant changes in the safety profile of desloratadine).
No products indexed under this heading.

(⊙ Described in PDR® for Ophthalmic Medicines)

Erythromycin Lactobionate (Co-administration resulted in increased C_{max} and AUC of desloratadine by 24% and 14% respectively; C_{max} and AUC of 3-hydroxydesloratadine increased by 43% and 40% respectively; there were no clinically relevant changes in the safety profile of desloratadine).
No products indexed under this heading.

Erythromycin Stearate (Co-administration resulted in increased C_{max} and AUC of desloratadine by 24% and 14% respectively; C_{max} and AUC of 3-hydroxydesloratadine increased by 43% and 40% respectively; there were no clinically relevant changes in the safety profile of desloratadine).
No products indexed under this heading.

Fluoxetine Hydrochloride (Co-administration resulted in increased C_{max} of desloratadine by 15%; C_{max} and AUC of 3-hydroxydesloratadine increased by 17% and 13% respectively; there were no clinically relevant changes in the safety profile of desloratadine). Products include:
Prozac Weekly 1941
Prozac Pulvules 1941
Symbyax 1965

Ketoconazole (Co-administration resulted in increased C_{max} and AUC of desloratadine by 45% and 39% respectively; C_{max} and AUC of 3-hydroxydesloratadine increased by 43% and 72% respectively; there were no clinically relevant changes in the safety profile of desloratadine).
Products include:
Extina 3319
Xolegel 3337

CLARINEX REDITABS TABLETS

(Desloratadine) 3098
See Clarinex Tablets

CLARINEX-D 12-HOUR EXTENDED-RELEASE TABLETS

(Desloratadine, Pseudoephedrine Sulfate) 3101
May interact with beta-blockers, cardiac glycosides, erythromycin, monoamine oxidase inhibitors, veratrum alkaloids, and certain other agents. Compounds in these categories include:

Acebutolol Hydrochloride (The antihypertensive effects of beta-adrenergic blocking agents, methyldopa, mecamylamine, reserpine, and veratrum alkaloids may be reduced by sympathomimetics).
No products indexed under this heading.

Atenolol (The antihypertensive effects of beta-adrenergic blocking agents, methyldopa, mecamylamine, reserpine, and veratrum alkaloids may be reduced by sympathomimetics).
No products indexed under this heading.

Azithromycin (Although increased plasma concentrations (C_{max} and AUC 0-24 hours) of desloratadine and/or 3-hydroxyloratadine were observed, there were no clinically relevant changes in the safety profile of desloratadine, as assessed by electrocardiographic parameters(including the corrected QT interval), clinical lab tests, vital signs, and adverse events). Products include:
AzaSite 1806

Azithromycin Dihydrate (Although increased plasma concentrations (C_{max} and AUC 0-24 hours) of desloratadine and/or 3-hydroxyloratadine were observed, there were no clinically relevant changes in the safety profile of desloratadine, as assessed by electrocardiographic parameters (including the corrected QT interval), clinical lab tests, vital signs, and adverse events).
No products indexed under this heading.

Betaxolol Hydrochloride (The antihypertensive effects of beta-adrenergic blocking agents, methyldopa, mecamylamine, reserpine, and veratrum alkaloids may be reduced by sympathomimetics).
No products indexed under this heading.

Bisoprolol Fumarate (The antihypertensive effects of beta-adrenergic blocking agents, methyldopa, mecamylamine, reserpine, and veratrum alkaloids may be reduced by sympathomimetics).
No products indexed under this heading.

Carteolol Hydrochloride (The antihypertensive effects of beta-adrenergic blocking agents, methyldopa, mecamylamine, reserpine, and veratrum alkaloids may be reduced by sympathomimetics).
No products indexed under this heading.

Carvedilol (The antihypertensive effects of beta-adrenergic blocking agents, methyldopa, mecamylamine, reserpine, and veratrum alkaloids may be reduced by sympathomimetics).
Products include:
Coreg 1409

Carvedilol Phosphate (The antihypertensive effects of beta-adrenergic blocking agents, methyldopa, mecamylamine, reserpine, and veratrum alkaloids may be reduced by sympathomimetics). Products include:
Coreg CR 1416

Cimetidine (Although increased plasma concentrations (C_{max} and AUC 0-24 hours) of desloratadine and/or 3-hydroxyloratadine were observed, there were no clinically relevant changes in the safety profile of desloratadine, as assessed by electrocardiographic parameters (including the corrected QT interval), clinical lab tests, vital signs, and adverse events).
No products indexed under this heading.

Cimetidine Hydrochloride (Although increased plasma concentrations (C_{max} and AUC 0-24 hours) of desloratadine and/or 3-hydroxyloratadine were observed, there were no clinically relevant changes in the safety profile of desloratadine, as assessed by electrocardiographic parameters (including the corrected QT interval), clinical lab tests, vital signs, and adverse events).
No products indexed under this heading.

Cryptenamine Preparations (The antihypertensive effects of beta-adrenergic blocking agents, methyldopa, mecamylamine, reserpine, and veratrum alkaloids may be reduced by sympathomimetics).
No products indexed under this heading.

Deslanoside (Increased ectopic pacemaker activity can occur when pseudoephedrine is used concomitantly with digitalis).
No products indexed under this heading.

Digitalis Glycoside Preparations (Increased ectopic pacemaker activity can occur when pseudoephedrine is used concomitantly with digitalis).
No products indexed under this heading.

Digitalis Lanata (Increased ectopic pacemaker activity can occur when pseudoephedrine is used concomitantly with digitalis).
No products indexed under this heading.

Digitalis Purpurea (Increased ectopic pacemaker activity can occur when pseudoephedrine is used concomitantly with digitalis).
No products indexed under this heading.

Digitoxin (Increased ectopic pacemaker activity can occur when pseudoephedrine is used concomitantly with digitalis).
No products indexed under this heading.

Digoxin (Increased ectopic pacemaker activity can occur when pseudoephedrine is used concomitantly with digitalis). Products include:
Lanoxin Injection 1546
Lanoxin Injection Pediatric 1549
Lanoxin Tablets 1553

Erythromycin (Although increased plasma concentrations (C_{max} and AUC 0-24 hours) of desloratadine and/or 3-hydroxydesloratadine were observed, there were no clinically relevant changes in the safety profile of desloratadine, as were assessed by electrocardiographic parameters (including the corrected QT interval), clinical lab tests, vital signs, and adverse events).
No products indexed under this heading.

Erythromycin, Topical (Although increased plasma concentrations (C_{max} and AUC 0-24 hours) of desloratadine and/or 3-hydroxydesloratadine were observed, there were no clinically relevant changes in the safety profile of desloratadine, as were assessed by electrocardiographic parameters (including the corrected QT interval), clinical lab tests, vital signs, and adverse events).
No products indexed under this heading.

Erythromycin Estolate (Although increased plasma concentrations (C_{max} and AUC 0-24 hours) of desloratadine and/or 3-hydroxydesloratadine were observed, there were no clinically relevant changes in the safety profile of desloratadine, as were assessed by electrocardiographic parameters (including the corrected QT interval), clinical lab tests, vital signs, and adverse events).
No products indexed under this heading.

Erythromycin Ethylsuccinate (Although increased plasma concentrations (C_{max} and AUC 0-24 hours) of desloratadine and/or 3-hydroxydesloratadine were observed, there were no clinically relevant changes in the safety profile of desloratadine, as were assessed by electrocardiographic parameters (including the corrected QT interval), clinical lab tests, vital signs, and adverse events).
Products include:
E.E.S. 437
EryPed 435

Erythromycin Gluceptate (Although increased plasma concentrations (C_{max} and AUC 0-24 hours) of desloratadine and/or 3-hydroxydesloratadine were observed, there were no clinically relevant changes in the safety profile of desloratadine, as were assessed by electrocardiographic parameters (including the corrected QT interval), clinical lab tests, vital signs, and adverse events).
No products indexed under this heading.

Erythromycin Lactobionate (Although increased plasma concentrations (C_{max} and AUC 0-24 hours) of desloratadine and/or 3-hydroxydesloratadine were observed, there were no clinically relevant changes in the safety profile of desloratadine, as were assessed by electrocardiographic parameters (including the corrected QT interval), clinical lab tests, vital signs, and adverse events).
No products indexed under this heading.

Erythromycin Stearate (Although increased plasma concentrations (C_{max} and AUC 0-24 hours) of desloratadine and/or 3-hydroxydesloratadine were observed, there were no clinically relevant changes in the safety profile of desloratadine, as were assessed by electrocardiographic parameters (including the corrected QT interval), clinical lab tests, vital signs, and adverse events).
No products indexed under this heading.

Esmolol Hydrochloride (The antihypertensive effects of beta-adrenergic blocking agents, methyldopa, mecamylamine, reserpine, and veratrum alkaloids may be reduced by sympathomimetics).
No products indexed under this heading.

Fluoxetine (Although increased plasma concentrations (C_{max} and/or AUC 0-24 hours) of desloratadine and/or 3-hydroxyloratadine were observed, there were no clinically relevant changes in the safety profile of desloratadine, as assessed by electrocardiographic parameters (including the corrected QT interval), clinical lab tests, vital signs, and adverse events).
No products indexed under this heading.

Fluoxetine Hydrochloride (Although increased plasma concentrations (C_{max} and AUC 0-24 hours) of desloratadine and/or 3-hydroxyloratadine were observed, there were no clinically relevant changes in the safety profile of desloratadine, as assessed by electrocardiographic parameters (including the corrected QT interval), clinical lab tests, vital signs, and adverse events).
Products include:
Prozac Weekly 1941
Prozac Pulvules 1941
Symbyax 1965

Isocarboxazid (Due to the pseudoephedrine component, concomitant use with monoamine oxidase inhibitors (MAOIs) or within 14 days after stopping treatment with MAOIs is contraindicated). Products include:
Marplan 3481

Ketoconazole (Although increased plasma concentrations (C_{max} and AUC 0-24 hours) of desloratadine and/or 3-hydroxyloratadine were observed, there were no clinically relevant changes in the safety profile of desloratadine, as assessed by electrocardiographic parameters (including the corrected QT interval), clinical lab tests, vital signs, and adverse events). Products include:
Extina 3319
Xolegel 3337

Labetalol Hydrochloride (The antihypertensive effects of beta-adrenergic blocking agents, methyldopa, mecamylamine, reserpine, and veratrum alkaloids may be reduced by sympathomimetics).
No products indexed under this heading.

Levobunolol Hydrochloride (The antihypertensive effects of beta-adrenergic blocking agents, methyldopa, mecamylamine, reserpine, and veratrum alkaloids may be reduced by sympathomimetics).
No products indexed under this heading.

Mecamylamine Hydrochloride (The antihypertensive effects of beta-adrenergic blocking agents, methyldopa, mecamylamine, reserpine, and veratrum alkaloids may be reduced by sympathomimetics).
No products indexed under this heading.

Methyldopa (The antihypertensive effects of beta-adrenergic blocking agents, methyldopa, mecamylamine, reserpine, and veratrum alkaloids may be reduced by sympathomimetics).
No products indexed under this heading.

Methyldopate Hydrochloride (The antihypertensive effects of beta-adrenergic blocking agents, methyldopa, mecamylamine, reserpine, and veratrum alkaloids may be reduced by sympathomimetics).
No products indexed under this heading.

Metipranolol Hydrochloride (The antihypertensive effects of beta-adrenergic blocking agents, methyldopa, mecamylamine, reserpine, and veratrum alkaloids may be reduced by sympathomimetics).
No products indexed under this heading.

IMPORTANT NOTE: Always consult each drug listing in the patient's regimen for possible interactions.

Clarinex-D Interactions Index 354

Metoprolol Succinate (The antihypertensive effects of beta-adrenergic blocking agents, methyldopa, mecamylamine, reserpine, and veratrum alkaloids may be reduced by sympathomimetics). Products include:

Toprol XL 732

Metoprolol Tartrate (The antihypertensive effects of beta-adrenergic blocking agents, methyldopa, mecamylamine, reserpine, and veratrum alkaloids may be reduced by sympathomimetics).

No products indexed under this heading.

Moclobemide (Due to the pseudoephedrine component, concomitant use with monoamine oxidase inhibitors (MAOIs) or within 14 days after stopping treatment with MAOIs is contraindicated).

No products indexed under this heading.

Nadolol (The antihypertensive effects of beta-adrenergic blocking agents, methyldopa, mecamylamine, reserpine, and veratrum alkaloids may be reduced by sympathomimetics). Products include:

Nadolol 2359

Nebivolol (The antihypertensive effects of beta-adrenergic blocking agents, methyldopa, mecamylamine, reserpine, and veratrum alkaloids may be reduced by sympathomimetics). Products include:

Bystolic 1147

Pargyline Hydrochloride (Due to the pseudoephedrine component, concomitant use with monoamine oxidase inhibitors (MAOIs) or within 14 days after stopping treatment with MAOIs is contraindicated).

No products indexed under this heading.

Penbutolol Sulfate (The antihypertensive effects of beta-adrenergic blocking agents, methyldopa, mecamylamine, reserpine, and veratrum alkaloids may be reduced by sympathomimetics).

No products indexed under this heading.

Phenelzine Sulfate (Due to the pseudoephedrine component, concomitant use with monoamine oxidase inhibitors (MAOIs) or within 14 days after stopping treatment with MAOIs is contraindicated).

No products indexed under this heading.

Pindolol (The antihypertensive effects of beta-adrenergic blocking agents, methyldopa, mecamylamine, reserpine, and veratrum alkaloids may be reduced by sympathomimetics).

No products indexed under this heading.

Procarbazine Hydrochloride (Due to the pseudoephedrine component, concomitant use with monoamine oxidase inhibitors (MAOIs) or within 14 days after stopping treatment with MAOIs is contraindicated).

No products indexed under this heading.

Propranolol Hydrochloride (The antihypertensive effects of beta-adrenergic blocking agents, methyldopa, mecamylamine, reserpine, and veratrum alkaloids may be reduced by sympathomimetics). Products include:

InnoPran XL 1517

Rasagiline Mesylate (Due to the pseudoephedrine component, concomitant use with monoamine oxidase inhibitors (MAOIs) or within 14 days after stopping treatment with MAOIs is contraindicated). Products include:

Azilect 3383

Selegiline (Due to the pseudoephedrine component, concomitant use with monoamine oxidase inhibitors (MAOIs) or within 14 days after stopping treatment with MAOIs is contraindicated). Products include:

Emsam 3623

Selegiline Hydrochloride (Due to the pseudoephedrine component, concomitant use with monoamine oxidase inhibitors (MAOIs) or within 14 days after stopping treatment with MAOIs is contraindicated). Products include:

Eldepryl 3312

Sotalol Hydrochloride (The antihypertensive effects of beta-adrenergic blocking agents, methyldopa, mecamylamine, reserpine, and veratrum alkaloids may be reduced by sympathomimetics).

No products indexed under this heading.

Timolol Hemihydrate (The antihypertensive effects of beta-adrenergic blocking agents, methyldopa, mecamylamine, reserpine, and veratrum alkaloids may be reduced by sympathomimetics). Products include:

Betimol 3490

Timolol Maleate (The antihypertensive effects of beta-adrenergic blocking agents, methyldopa, mecamylamine, reserpine, and veratrum alkaloids may be reduced by sympathomimetics). Products include:

Combigan 601

Dorzolamide Hydrochloride/Timolol Maleate Ophthalmic Solution .... ⊙243

Timoptic in Ocudose .... ⊙231

Tranylcypromine Sulfate (Due to the pseudoephedrine component, concomitant use with monoamine oxidase inhibitors (MAOIs) or within 14 days after stopping treatment with MAOIs is contraindicated). Products include:

Parnate 1584

CLARINEX-D 24-HOUR EXTENDED-RELEASE TABLETS

(Desloratadine, Pseudoephedrine Sulfate) 3104

May interact with beta-blockers, cardiac glycosides, monoamine oxidase inhibitors, veratrum alkaloids, and certain other agents. Compounds in these categories include:

Acebutolol Hydrochloride (The antihypertensive effects of beta-adrenergic blocking agents may be reduced by sympathomimetics).

No products indexed under this heading.

Atenolol (The antihypertensive effects of beta-adrenergic blocking agents may be reduced by sympathomimetics).

No products indexed under this heading.

Betaxolol Hydrochloride (The antihypertensive effects of beta-adrenergic blocking agents may be reduced by sympathomimetics).

No products indexed under this heading.

Bisoprolol Fumarate (The antihypertensive effects of beta-adrenergic blocking agents may be reduced by sympathomimetics).

No products indexed under this heading.

Carteolol Hydrochloride (The antihypertensive effects of beta-adrenergic blocking agents may be reduced by sympathomimetics).

No products indexed under this heading.

Carvedilol (The antihypertensive effects of beta-adrenergic blocking agents may be reduced by sympathomimetics). Products include:

Coreg 1409

Carvedilol Phosphate (The antihypertensive effects of beta-adrenergic blocking agents may be reduced by sympathomimetics). Products include:

Coreg CR 1416

Cryptenamine Preparations (The antihypertensive effects of veratrum alkaloids may be reduced by sympathomimetics).

No products indexed under this heading.

Deslanoside (Increased ectopic pacemaker activity can occur when pseudoephedrine is used concomitantly with digitalis).

No products indexed under this heading.

Digitalis Glycoside Preparations (Increased ectopic pacemaker activity can occur when pseudoephedrine is used concomitantly with digitalis).

No products indexed under this heading.

Digitalis Lanata (Increased ectopic pacemaker activity can occur when pseudoephedrine is used concomitantly with digitalis).

No products indexed under this heading.

Digitalis Purpurea (Increased ectopic pacemaker activity can occur when pseudoephedrine is used concomitantly with digitalis).

No products indexed under this heading.

Digitoxin (Increased ectopic pacemaker activity can occur when pseudoephedrine is used concomitantly with digitalis).

No products indexed under this heading.

Digoxin (Increased ectopic pacemaker activity can occur when pseudoephedrine is used concomitantly with digitalis). Products include:

Lanoxin Injection 1546

Lanoxin Injection Pediatric 1549

Lanoxin Tablets 1553

Esmolol Hydrochloride (The antihypertensive effects of beta-adrenergic blocking agents may be reduced by sympathomimetics).

No products indexed under this heading.

Isocarboxazid (Due to the pseudoephedrine component, Clarinex-D 24 Hour extended-release tablets should not be used by patients taking monoamine oxidase inhibitors or within 14 days after stopping such treatment). Products include:

Marplan 3481

Labetalol Hydrochloride (The antihypertensive effects of beta-adrenergic blocking agents may be reduced by sympathomimetics).

No products indexed under this heading.

Levobunolol Hydrochloride (The antihypertensive effects of beta-adrenergic blocking agents may be reduced by sympathomimetics).

No products indexed under this heading.

Mecamylamine Hydrochloride (The antihypertensive effects of mecamylamine may be reduced by sympathomimetics).

No products indexed under this heading.

Methyldopa (The antihypertensive effects of methyldopa may be reduced by sympathomimetics).

No products indexed under this heading.

Methyldopate Hydrochloride (The antihypertensive effects of methyldopa may be reduced by sympathomimetics).

No products indexed under this heading.

Metipranolol Hydrochloride (The antihypertensive effects of beta-adrenergic blocking agents may be reduced by sympathomimetics).

No products indexed under this heading.

Metoprolol Succinate (The antihypertensive effects of beta-adrenergic blocking agents may be reduced by sympathomimetics). Products include:

Toprol XL 732

Metoprolol Tartrate (The antihypertensive effects of beta-adrenergic blocking agents may be reduced by sympathomimetics).

No products indexed under this heading.

Moclobemide (Due to the pseudoephedrine component, Clarinex-D 24 Hour extended-release tablets should not be used by patients taking monoamine oxidase inhibitors or within 14 days after stopping such treatment).

No products indexed under this heading.

Nadolol (The antihypertensive effects of beta-adrenergic blocking agents may be reduced by sympathomimetics). Products include:

Nadolol 2359

Nebivolol (The antihypertensive effects of beta-adrenergic blocking agents may be reduced by sympathomimetics). Products include:

Bystolic 1147

Pargyline Hydrochloride (Due to the pseudoephedrine component, Clarinex-D 24 Hour extended-release tablets should not be used by patients taking monoamine oxidase inhibitors or within 14 days after stopping such treatment).

No products indexed under this heading.

Penbutolol Sulfate (The antihypertensive effects of beta-adrenergic blocking agents may be reduced by sympathomimetics).

No products indexed under this heading.

Phenelzine Sulfate (Due to the pseudoephedrine component, Clarinex-D 24 Hour extended-release tablets should not be used by patients taking monoamine oxidase inhibitors or within 14 days after stopping such treatment).

No products indexed under this heading.

Pindolol (The antihypertensive effects of beta-adrenergic blocking agents may be reduced by sympathomimetics).

No products indexed under this heading.

Procarbazine Hydrochloride (Due to the pseudoephedrine component, Clarinex-D 24 Hour extended-release tablets should not be used by patients taking monoamine oxidase inhibitors or within 14 days after stopping such treatment).

No products indexed under this heading.

Propranolol Hydrochloride (The antihypertensive effects of beta-adrenergic blocking agents may be reduced by sympathomimetics). Products include:

InnoPran XL 1517

Rasagiline Mesylate (Due to the pseudoephedrine component, Clarinex-D 24 Hour extended-release tablets should not be used by patients taking monoamine oxidase inhibitors or within 14 days after stopping such treatment). Products include:

Azilect 3383

Reserpine (The antihypertensive effects of reserpine may be reduced by sympathomimetics).

No products indexed under this heading.

Selegiline (Due to the pseudoephedrine component, Clarinex-D 24 Hour extended-release tablets should not be used by patients taking monoamine oxidase inhibitors or within 14 days after stopping such treatment). Products include:

Emsam 3623

Selegiline Hydrochloride (Due to the pseudoephedrine component, Clarinex-D 24 Hour extended-release tablets should not be used by patients taking monoamine oxidase inhibitors or within 14 days after stopping such treatment). Products include:

Eldepryl 3312

Sotalol Hydrochloride (The antihypertensive effects of beta-adrenergic blocking agents may be reduced by sympathomimetics).

No products indexed under this heading.

(⊙ Described in PDR® for Ophthalmic Medicines)

355 **Interactions Index** **Climara**

Timolol Hemihydrate (The antihypertensive effects of beta-adrenergic blocking agents may be reduced by sympathomimetics). Products include:
Betimol 3490

Timolol Maleate (The antihypertensive effects of beta-adrenergic blocking agents may be reduced by sympathomimetics). Products include:
Combigan 601
Dorzolamide Hydrochloride/Timolol Maleate Ophthalmic Solution .... ⊙243
Timoptic in Ocudose .... ⊙231

Tranylcypromine Sulfate (Due to the pseudoephedrine component, Clarinex-D 24 Hour extended-release tablets should not be used by patients taking monoamine oxidase inhibitors or within 14 days after stopping such treatment). Products include:
Parnate 1584

CLEVIPREX
(Clevidipine Butyrate) 2064
None cited in PDR database.

CLIMARA TRANSDERMAL SYSTEM
(Estradiol) 841
May interact with cytochrome p450 3a4 inducers (selected), cytochrome p450 3a4 inhibitors (selected), erythromycin, thyroid preparations, and certain other agents. Compounds in these categories include:

Acetazolamide (Inhibitors of CYP3A4 may increase plasma concentrations of estrogens and may result in side effects).
No products indexed under this heading.

Acetazolamide Sodium (Inhibitors of CYP3A4 may increase plasma concentrations of estrogens and may result in side effects).
No products indexed under this heading.

Allium sativum (Inducers of CYP3A4 may reduce plasma concentrations of estrogens, possibly resulting in a decrease in therapeutic effects and/or changes in the uterine bleeding profile).
No products indexed under this heading.

Aminoglutethimide (Inducers of CYP3A4 may reduce plasma concentrations of estrogens, possibly resulting in a decrease in therapeutic effects and/or changes in the uterine bleeding profile).
No products indexed under this heading.

Amiodarone Hydrochloride (Inhibitors of CYP3A4 may increase plasma concentrations of estrogens and may result in side effects).
No products indexed under this heading.

Amprenavir (Inhibitors of CYP3A4 may increase plasma concentrations of estrogens and may result in side effects).
No products indexed under this heading.

Anastrozole (Inhibitors of CYP3A4 may increase plasma concentrations of estrogens and may result in side effects).
No products indexed under this heading.

Aprepitant (Inhibitors of CYP3A4 may increase plasma concentrations of estrogens and may result in side effects). Products include:
Emend 2124

Atazanavir (Inhibitors of CYP3A4 may increase plasma concentrations of estrogens and may result in side effects).
No products indexed under this heading.

Atazanavir Sulfate (Inhibitors of CYP3A4 may increase plasma concentrations of estrogens and may result in side effects).
No products indexed under this heading.

Betamethasone (Inducers of CYP3A4 may reduce plasma concentrations of estrogens, possibly resulting in a decrease in therapeutic effects and/or changes in the uterine bleeding profile).
No products indexed under this heading.

Betamethasone Acetate (Inducers of CYP3A4 may reduce plasma concentrations of estrogens, possibly resulting in a decrease in therapeutic effects and/or changes in the uterine bleeding profile).
No products indexed under this heading.

Betamethasone Benzoate (Inducers of CYP3A4 may reduce plasma concentrations of estrogens, possibly resulting in a decrease in therapeutic effects and/or changes in the uterine bleeding profile).
No products indexed under this heading.

Betamethasone Dipropionate (Inducers of CYP3A4 may reduce plasma concentrations of estrogens, possibly resulting in a decrease in therapeutic effects and/or changes in the uterine bleeding profile). Products include:
Diprolene Lotion 0.05% 3108
Diprolene Ointment 0.05% 3109
Diprolene AF Cream 0.05% 3107
Lotrisone 3163

Betamethasone Sodium Phosphate (Inducers of CYP3A4 may reduce plasma concentrations of estrogens, possibly resulting in a decrease in therapeutic effects and/or changes in the uterine bleeding profile).
No products indexed under this heading.

Betamethasone Valerate (Inducers of CYP3A4 may reduce plasma concentrations of estrogens, possibly resulting in a decrease in therapeutic effects and/or changes in the uterine bleeding profile). Products include:
Luxiq 3321

Bosentan (Inducers of CYP3A4 may reduce plasma concentrations of estrogens, possibly resulting in a decrease in therapeutic effects and/or changes in the uterine bleeding profile). Products include:
Tracleer 573

Carbamazepine (Inducers of CYP3A4, such as carbamazepine, may reduce plasma concentrations of estrogens, possibly resulting in a decrease in therapeutic effects and/or changes in uterine bleeding profile). Products include:
Carbatrol 3280
Equetro 3477

Cimetidine (Inhibitors of CYP3A4 may increase plasma concentrations of estrogens and may result in side effects).
No products indexed under this heading.

Cimetidine Hydrochloride (Inhibitors of CYP3A4 may increase plasma concentrations of estrogens and may result in side effects).
No products indexed under this heading.

Ciprofloxacin (Inhibitors of CYP3A4 may increase plasma concentrations of estrogens and may result in side effects). Products include:
Cipro I.V. 3082
Cipro 3073
Cipro XR 3091
Ciprodex 583

Ciprofloxacin Hydrochloride (Inducers of CYP3A4 may reduce plasma concentrations of estrogens, possibly resulting in a decrease in therapeutic effects and/or changes in the uterine bleeding profile). Products include:
Cipro 3073

Cisplatin (Inducers of CYP3A4 may reduce plasma concentrations of estrogens, possibly resulting in a decrease in therapeutic effects and/or changes in the uterine bleeding profile).
No products indexed under this heading.

Clarithromycin (Inhibitors of CYP3A4, such as clarithromycin, may increase plasma concentrations of estrogens and may result in side effects). Products include:
Biaxin/Biaxin XL 412

Clotrimazole (Inhibitors of CYP3A4 may increase plasma concentrations of estrogens and may result in side effects). Products include:
Lotrisone 3163

Conivaptan Hydrochloride (Inhibitors of CYP3A4 may increase plasma concentrations of estrogens and may result in side effects). Products include:
Vaprisol 689

Cortisone Acetate (Inducers of CYP3A4 may reduce plasma concentrations of estrogens, possibly resulting in a decrease in therapeutic effects and/or changes in the uterine bleeding profile).
No products indexed under this heading.

Cyclosporine (Inhibitors of CYP3A4 may increase plasma concentrations of estrogens and may result in side effects). Products include:
Gengraf 440
Neoral Oral Solution 2496
Neoral Capsules 2496
Restasis 605

Dalfopristin (Inhibitors of CYP3A4 may increase plasma concentrations of estrogens and may result in side effects).
No products indexed under this heading.

Danazol (Inhibitors of CYP3A4 may increase plasma concentrations of estrogens and may result in side effects).
No products indexed under this heading.

Darunavir (Inhibitors of CYP3A4 may increase plasma concentrations of estrogens and may result in side effects).
No products indexed under this heading.

Dasatinib (Inhibitors of CYP3A4 may increase plasma concentrations of estrogens and may result in side effects).
No products indexed under this heading.

Delavirdine Mesylate (Inhibitors of CYP3A4 may increase plasma concentrations of estrogens and may result in side effects).
No products indexed under this heading.

Delavirine (Inhibitors of CYP3A4 may increase plasma concentrations of estrogens and may result in side effects).
No products indexed under this heading.

Desloratadine (Inhibitors of CYP3A4 may increase plasma concentrations of estrogens and may result in side effects). Products include:
Clarinex Syrup 3098
Clarinex 3098
Clarinex Reditabs 3098
Clarinex-D 12-Hour 3101
Clarinex-D 3104

Dexamethasone (Inducers of CYP3A4 may reduce plasma concentrations of estrogens, possibly resulting in a decrease in therapeutic effects and/or changes in the uterine bleeding profile). Products include:
Ciprodex 583
Ozurdex .... ⊙223
Tobramycin and Dexamethasone Ophthalmic Suspension .... ⊙251

Dexamethasone Acetate (Inducers of CYP3A4 may reduce plasma concentrations of estrogens, possibly resulting in a decrease in therapeutic effects and/or changes in the uterine bleeding profile).
No products indexed under this heading.

Dexamethasone Phosphate (Inducers of CYP3A4 may reduce plasma concentrations of estrogens, possibly resulting in a decrease in therapeutic effects and/or changes in the uterine bleeding profile).
No products indexed under this heading.

Dexamethasone Sodium (Inducers of CYP3A4 may reduce plasma concentrations of estrogens, possibly resulting in a decrease in therapeutic effects and/or changes in the uterine bleeding profile).
No products indexed under this heading.

Dexamethasone Sodium Phosphate (Inducers of CYP3A4 may reduce plasma concentrations of estrogens, possibly resulting in a decrease in therapeutic effects and/or changes in the uterine bleeding profile).
No products indexed under this heading.

Dexamethasone Sodium Phosphate Injection (Inducers of CYP3A4 may reduce plasma concentrations of estrogens, possibly resulting in a decrease in therapeutic effects and/or changes in the uterine bleeding profile).
No products indexed under this heading.

Diltiazem Hydrochloride (Inhibitors of CYP3A4 may increase plasma concentrations of estrogens and may result in side effects). Products include:
Cardizem LA 423

Diltiazem Maleate (Inhibitors of CYP3A4 may increase plasma concentrations of estrogens and may result in side effects).
No products indexed under this heading.

Doxorubicin Hydrochloride (Inducers of CYP3A4 may reduce plasma concentrations of estrogens, possibly resulting in a decrease in therapeutic effects and/or changes in the uterine bleeding profile).
No products indexed under this heading.

Efavirenz (Inhibitors of CYP3A4 may increase plasma concentrations of estrogens and may result in side effects). Products include:
Atripla 906

Erythromycin (Inhibitors of CYP3A4, such as erythromycin, may increase plasma concentrations of estrogens and may result in side effects).
No products indexed under this heading.

Erythromycin, Topical (Inhibitors of CYP3A4, such as erythromycin, may increase plasma concentrations of estrogens and may result in side effects).
No products indexed under this heading.

Erythromycin Estolate (Inhibitors of CYP3A4, such as erythromycin, may increase plasma concentrations of estrogens and may result in side effects).
No products indexed under this heading.

Erythromycin Ethylsuccinate (Inhibitors of CYP3A4, such as erythromycin, may increase plasma concentrations of estrogens and may result in side effects). Products include:
E.E.S. 437
EryPed 435

Erythromycin Gluceptate (Inhibitors of CYP3A4, such as erythromycin, may increase plasma concentrations of estrogens and may result in side effects).
No products indexed under this heading.

IMPORTANT NOTE: Always consult each drug listing in the patient's regimen for possible interactions.

Erythromycin Lactobionate (Inhibitors of CYP3A4, such as erythromycin, may increase plasma concentrations of estrogens and may result in side effects).
No products indexed under this heading.

Erythromycin Stearate (Inhibitors of CYP3A4, such as erythromycin, may increase plasma concentrations of estrogens and may result in side effects).
No products indexed under this heading.

Esomeprazole Magnesium (Inhibitors of CYP3A4 may increase plasma concentrations of estrogens and may result in side effects). Products include:

Esomeprazole Sodium (Inhibitors of CYP3A4 may increase plasma concentrations of estrogens and may result in side effects). Products include:

Ethosuximide (Inducers of CYP3A4 may reduce plasma concentrations of estrogens, possibly resulting in a decrease in therapeutic effects and/or changes in the uterine bleeding profile).
No products indexed under this heading.

Felbamate (Inducers of CYP3A4 may reduce plasma concentrations of estrogens, possibly resulting in a decrease in therapeutic effects and/or changes in the uterine bleeding profile).
No products indexed under this heading.

Fluconazole (Inhibitors of CYP3A4 may increase plasma concentrations of estrogens and may result in side effects).
No products indexed under this heading.

Fludrocortisone Acetate (Inducers of CYP3A4 may reduce plasma concentrations of estrogens, possibly resulting in a decrease in therapeutic effects and/or changes in the uterine bleeding profile).
No products indexed under this heading.

Fluoxetine (Inhibitors of CYP3A4 may increase plasma concentrations of estrogens and may result in side effects).
No products indexed under this heading.

Fluoxetine Hydrochloride (Inhibitors of CYP3A4 may increase plasma concentrations of estrogens and may result in side effects). Products include:

Fluvoxamine Maleate (Inhibitors of CYP3A4 may increase plasma concentrations of estrogens and may result in side effects).
No products indexed under this heading.

Fosamprenavir Calcium (Inhibitors of CYP3A4 may increase plasma concentrations of estrogens and may result in side effects). Products include:

Fosphenytoin Sodium (Inducers of CYP3A4 may reduce plasma concentrations of estrogens, possibly resulting in a decrease in therapeutic effects and/or changes in the uterine bleeding profile).
No products indexed under this heading.

Garlic Extract (Inducers of CYP3A4 may reduce plasma concentrations of estrogens, possibly resulting in a decrease in therapeutic effects and/or changes in the uterine bleeding profile).
No products indexed under this heading.

Garlic Oil (Inducers of CYP3A4 may reduce plasma concentrations of estrogens, possibly resulting in a decrease in therapeutic effects and/or changes in the uterine bleeding profile).
No products indexed under this heading.

Hydrocortisone (Inducers of CYP3A4 may reduce plasma concentrations of estrogens, possibly resulting in a decrease in therapeutic effects and/or changes in the uterine bleeding profile).
No products indexed under this heading.

Hydrocortisone (Alcohol) (Inducers of CYP3A4 may reduce plasma concentrations of estrogens, possibly resulting in a decrease in therapeutic effects and/or changes in the uterine bleeding profile).
No products indexed under this heading.

Hydrocortisone Acetate (Inducers of CYP3A4 may reduce plasma concentrations of estrogens, possibly resulting in a decrease in therapeutic effects and/or changes in the uterine bleeding profile).
No products indexed under this heading.

Hydrocortisone Butyrate (Inducers of CYP3A4 may reduce plasma concentrations of estrogens, possibly resulting in a decrease in therapeutic effects and/or changes in the uterine bleeding profile).
No products indexed under this heading.

Hydrocortisone Cypionate (Inducers of CYP3A4 may reduce plasma concentrations of estrogens, possibly resulting in a decrease in therapeutic effects and/or changes in the uterine bleeding profile).
No products indexed under this heading.

Hydrocortisone Hemisuccinate (Inducers of CYP3A4 may reduce plasma concentrations of estrogens, possibly resulting in a decrease in therapeutic effects and/or changes in the uterine bleeding profile).
No products indexed under this heading.

Hydrocortisone Probutate (Inducers of CYP3A4 may reduce plasma concentrations of estrogens, possibly resulting in a decrease in therapeutic effects and/or changes in the uterine bleeding profile).
No products indexed under this heading.

Hydrocortisone Sodium Phosphate (Inducers of CYP3A4 may reduce plasma concentrations of estrogens, possibly resulting in a decrease in therapeutic effects and/or changes in the uterine bleeding profile).
No products indexed under this heading.

Hydrocortisone Sodium Succinate (Inducers of CYP3A4 may reduce plasma concentrations of estrogens, possibly resulting in a decrease in therapeutic effects and/or changes in the uterine bleeding profile).
No products indexed under this heading.

Hydrocortisone Valerate (Inducers of CYP3A4 may reduce plasma concentrations of estrogens, possibly resulting in a decrease in therapeutic effects and/or changes in the uterine bleeding profile).
No products indexed under this heading.

Hypericum (Inducers of CYP3A4 may reduce plasma concentrations of estrogens, possibly resulting in a decrease in therapeutic effects and/or changes in the uterine bleeding profile).
No products indexed under this heading.

Hypericum Perforatum (Inducers of CYP3A4, such as St. John's Wort preparations (hypericum perforatum), may reduce plasma concentrations of estrogens, possibly resulting in a decrease in therapeutic effects and/or changes in uterine bleeding profile). Products include:

Imatinib Mesylate (Inhibitors of CYP3A4 may increase plasma concentrations of estrogens and may result in side effects). Products include:

Indinavir Sulfate (Inhibitors of CYP3A4 may increase plasma concentrations of estrogens and may result in side effects). Products include:

Isoniazid (Inhibitors of CYP3A4 may increase plasma concentrations of estrogens and may result in side effects).
No products indexed under this heading.

Itraconazole (Inhibitors of CYP3A4, such as itraconazole, may increase plasma concentrations of estrogens and may result in side effects).
No products indexed under this heading.

Ketoconazole (Inhibitors of CYP3A4, such as ketoconazole, may increase plasma concentrations of estrogens and may result in side effects). Products include:

Lapatinib (Inhibitors of CYP3A4 may increase plasma concentrations of estrogens and may result in side effects). Products include:

Levothyroxine Sodium (Estrogen administration leads to increased thyroid-binding globulin (TBG) levels. Patients dependent on thyroid hormone replacement therapy who are also receiving estrogens may require increased doses of their thyroid replacement therapy. These patients should have their thyroid function monitored in order to maintain their free thyroid hormone levels in an acceptable range). Products include:

Liothyronine Sodium (Estrogen administration leads to increased thyroid-binding globulin (TBG) levels. Patients dependent on thyroid hormone replacement therapy who are also receiving estrogens may require increased doses of their thyroid replacement therapy. These patients should have their thyroid function monitored in order to maintain their free thyroid hormone levels in an acceptable range). Products include:

Liotrix (Estrogen administration leads to increased thyroid-binding globulin (TBG) levels. Patients dependent on thyroid hormone replacement therapy who are also receiving estrogens may require increased doses of their thyroid replacement therapy. These patients should have their thyroid function monitored in order to maintain their free thyroid hormone levels in an acceptable range).
No products indexed under this heading.

Lopinavir (Inhibitors of CYP3A4 may increase plasma concentrations of estrogens and may result in side effects). Products include:

Loratadine (Inhibitors of CYP3A4 may increase plasma concentrations of estrogens and may result in side effects).
No products indexed under this heading.

Mephenytoin (Inducers of CYP3A4 may reduce plasma concentrations of estrogens, possibly resulting in a decrease in therapeutic effects and/or changes in the uterine bleeding profile).
No products indexed under this heading.

Methsuximide (Inducers of CYP3A4 may reduce plasma concentrations of estrogens, possibly resulting in a decrease in therapeutic effects and/or changes in the uterine bleeding profile).
No products indexed under this heading.

Methylprednisolone (Inducers of CYP3A4 may reduce plasma concentrations of estrogens, possibly resulting in a decrease in therapeutic effects and/or changes in the uterine bleeding profile).
No products indexed under this heading.

Methylprednisolone Acetate (Inducers of CYP3A4 may reduce plasma concentrations of estrogens, possibly resulting in a decrease in therapeutic effects and/or changes in the uterine bleeding profile).
No products indexed under this heading.

Methylprednisolone Sodium Succinate (Inducers of CYP3A4 may reduce plasma concentrations of estrogens, possibly resulting in a decrease in therapeutic effects and/or changes in the uterine bleeding profile).
No products indexed under this heading.

Metronidazole (Inhibitors of CYP3A4 may increase plasma concentrations of estrogens and may result in side effects). Products include:

Metronidazole Benzoate (Inhibitors of CYP3A4 may increase plasma concentrations of estrogens and may result in side effects).
No products indexed under this heading.

Metronidazole Hydrochloride (Inhibitors of CYP3A4 may increase plasma concentrations of estrogens and may result in side effects).
No products indexed under this heading.

Metronidazole Sodium (Inhibitors of CYP3A4 may increase plasma concentrations of estrogens and may result in side effects).
No products indexed under this heading.

Miconazole (Inhibitors of CYP3A4 may increase plasma concentrations of estrogens and may result in side effects).
No products indexed under this heading.

Miconazole Nitrate (Inhibitors of CYP3A4 may increase plasma concentrations of estrogens and may result in side effects). Products include:

Mifepristone (Inhibitors of CYP3A4 may increase plasma concentrations of estrogens and may result in side effects).
No products indexed under this heading.

Modafinil (Inducers of CYP3A4 may reduce plasma concentrations of estrogens, possibly resulting in a decrease in therapeutic effects and/or changes in the uterine bleeding profile). Products include:

Nafcillin Sodium (Inducers of CYP3A4 may reduce plasma concentrations of estrogens, possibly resulting in a decrease in therapeutic effects and/or changes in the uterine bleeding profile).
No products indexed under this heading.

Nefazodone Hydrochloride (Inhibitors of CYP3A4 may increase plasma concentrations of estrogens and may result in side effects).
No products indexed under this heading.

Nelfinavir Mesylate (Inhibitors of CYP3A4 may increase plasma concentrations of estrogens and may result in side effects).
No products indexed under this heading.

Nevirapine (Inhibitors of CYP3A4 may increase plasma concentrations of estrogens and may result in side effects). Products include:

Niacin (Inhibitors of CYP3A4 may increase plasma concentrations of estrogens and may result in side effects). Products include:

IMPORTANT NOTE: Always consult each drug listing in the patient's regimen for possible interactions.

Triamcinolone (Inducers of CYP3A4 may reduce plasma concentrations of estrogens, possibly resulting in a decrease in therapeutic effects and/or changes in the uterine bleeding profile).
No products indexed under this heading.

Triamcinolone Acetonide (Inducers of CYP3A4 may reduce plasma concentrations of estrogens, possibly resulting in a decrease in therapeutic effects and/or changes in the uterine bleeding profile). Products include:

Triamcinolone Diacetate (Inducers of CYP3A4 may reduce plasma concentrations of estrogens, possibly resulting in a decrease in therapeutic effects and/or changes in the uterine bleeding profile).
No products indexed under this heading.

Triamcinolone Hexacetonide (Inducers of CYP3A4 may reduce plasma concentrations of estrogens, possibly resulting in a decrease in therapeutic effects and/or changes in the uterine bleeding profile).
No products indexed under this heading.

Troglitazone (Inhibitors of CYP3A4 may increase plasma concentrations of estrogens and may result in side effects).
No products indexed under this heading.

Troleandomycin (Inhibitors of CYP3A4 may increase plasma concentrations of estrogens and may result in side effects).
No products indexed under this heading.

Valproate Sodium (Inhibitors of CYP3A4 may increase plasma concentrations of estrogens and may result in side effects).
No products indexed under this heading.

Vardenafil Hydrochloride (Inhibitors of CYP3A4 may increase plasma concentrations of estrogens and may result in side effects). Products include:

Verapamil Hydrochloride (Inhibitors of CYP3A4 may increase plasma concentrations of estrogens and may result in side effects). Products include:

Voriconazole (Inhibitors of CYP3A4 may increase plasma concentrations of estrogens and may result in side effects).
No products indexed under this heading.

Zafirlukast (Inhibitors of CYP3A4 may increase plasma concentrations of estrogens and may result in side effects). Products include:

Zileuton (Inhibitors of CYP3A4 may increase plasma concentrations of estrogens and may result in side effects).
No products indexed under this heading.

Food Interactions

Grapefruit (Inhibitors of CYP3A4 may increase plasma concentrations of estrogens and may result in side effects).

Grapefruit Juice (Inhibitors of CYP3A4, such as grapefruit juice, may increase plasma concentrations of estrogens and may result in side effects).

CLIMARA PRO TRANSDERMAL SYSTEM

(Estradiol, Levonorgestrel) 847
May interact with cytochrome p450 2c18 inhibitors (selected), cytochrome p450 2c19 inducers (selected), cytochrome p450 2c19 inhibitors (selected), cytochrome p450 2c8 inducers (selected), cytochrome p450 2c8 inhibitors (selected), cytochrome p450 2c9 inducers (selected), cytochrome p450 2c9 inhibitors (selected), cytochrome p450 3a4 inducers (selected), cytochrome p450 3a4 inhibitors (selected). Compounds in these categories include:

Acetazolamide (Inhibitors of CYP3A4 such as erythromycin, clarithromycin, ketoconazole, itraconazole, ritonavir and grapefruit juice may increase plasma concentrations of estrogens and may result in side effects).
No products indexed under this heading.

Acetazolamide Sodium (Inhibitors of CYP3A4 such as erythromycin, clarithromycin, ketoconazole, itraconazole, ritonavir and grapefruit juice may increase plasma concentrations of estrogens and may result in side effects).
No products indexed under this heading.

Allium sativum (Inducers of CYP3A4 may reduce plasma concentrations of estrogens, possibly resulting in a decrease in therapeutic effects and/or changes in the uterine bleeding profile).
No products indexed under this heading.

Aminoglutethimide (Inducers of CYP3A4 may reduce plasma concentrations of estrogens, possibly resulting in a decrease in therapeutic effects and/or changes in the uterine bleeding profile).
No products indexed under this heading.

Amiodarone Hydrochloride (Inhibitors of CYP3A4 such as erythromycin, clarithromycin, ketoconazole, itraconazole, ritonavir and grapefruit juice may increase plasma concentrations of estrogens and may result in side effects).
No products indexed under this heading.

Amprenavir (Inhibitors of CYP3A4 such as erythromycin, clarithromycin, ketoconazole, itraconazole, ritonavir and grapefruit juice may increase plasma concentrations of estrogens and may result in side effects).
No products indexed under this heading.

Anastrozole (Inhibitors of CYP3A4 such as erythromycin, clarithromycin, ketoconazole, itraconazole, ritonavir and grapefruit juice may increase plasma concentrations of estrogens and may result in side effects).
No products indexed under this heading.

Aprepitant (Inducers of CYP3A4 may reduce plasma concentrations of estrogens, possibly resulting in a decrease in therapeutic effects and/or changes in the uterine bleeding profile). Products include:

Atazanavir (Inhibitors of CYP3A4 such as erythromycin, clarithromycin, ketoconazole, itraconazole, ritonavir and grapefruit juice may increase plasma concentrations of estrogens and may result in side effects).
No products indexed under this heading.

Atazanavir Sulfate (Inhibitors of CYP3A4 such as erythromycin, clarithromycin, ketoconazole, itraconazole, ritonavir and grapefruit juice may increase plasma concentrations of estrogens and may result in side effects).
No products indexed under this heading.

Bendroflumethiazide (Based on in-vitro and in-vivo studies, it can be assumed that CYP3A, CYP2E and CYP2C are involved in the metabolism of levonorgestrel. Likewise, inducers or inhibitors of these enzymes may either, respectively, decrease the therapeutic effects or result in side effects).
No products indexed under this heading.

Betamethasone (Inducers of CYP3A4 may reduce plasma concentrations of estrogens, possibly resulting in a decrease in therapeutic effects and/or changes in the uterine bleeding profile).
No products indexed under this heading.

Betamethasone Acetate (Inducers of CYP3A4 may reduce plasma concentrations of estrogens, possibly resulting in a decrease in therapeutic effects and/or changes in the uterine bleeding profile).
No products indexed under this heading.

Betamethasone Benzoate (Inducers of CYP3A4 may reduce plasma concentrations of estrogens, possibly resulting in a decrease in therapeutic effects and/or changes in the uterine bleeding profile).
No products indexed under this heading.

Betamethasone Dipropionate (Inducers of CYP3A4 may reduce plasma concentrations of estrogens, possibly resulting in a decrease in therapeutic effects and/or changes in the uterine bleeding profile). Products include:

Betamethasone Sodium Phosphate (Inducers of CYP3A4 may reduce plasma concentrations of estrogens, possibly resulting in a decrease in therapeutic effects and/or changes in the uterine bleeding profile).
No products indexed under this heading.

Betamethasone Valerate (Inducers of CYP3A4 may reduce plasma concentrations of estrogens, possibly resulting in a decrease in therapeutic effects and/or changes in the uterine bleeding profile). Products include:

Bosentan (Inducers of CYP3A4 may reduce plasma concentrations of estrogens, possibly resulting in a decrease in therapeutic effects and/or changes in the uterine bleeding profile). Products include:

Carbamazepine (Inducers of CYP3A4 may reduce plasma concentrations of estrogens, possibly resulting in a decrease in therapeutic effects and/or changes in the uterine bleeding profile). Products include:

Chloramphenicol (Based on in-vitro and in-vivo studies, it can be assumed that CYP3A, CYP2E and CYP2C are involved in the metabolism of levonorgestrel. Likewise, inducers or inhibitors of these enzymes may either, respectively, decrease the therapeutic effects or result in side effects).
No products indexed under this heading.

Chloramphenicol Palmitate (Based on in-vitro and in-vivo studies, it can be assumed that CYP3A, CYP2E and CYP2C are involved in the metabolism of levonorgestrel. Likewise, inducers or inhibitors of these enzymes may either, respectively, decrease the therapeutic effects or result in side effects).
No products indexed under this heading.

Chloramphenicol Sodium Succinate (Based on in-vitro and in-vivo studies, it can be assumed that CYP3A, CYP2E and CYP2C are involved in the metabolism of levonorgestrel. Likewise, inducers or inhibitors of these enzymes may either, respectively, decrease the therapeutic effects or result in side effects).
No products indexed under this heading.

Chlorothiazide (Based on in-vitro and in-vivo studies, it can be assumed that CYP3A, CYP2E and CYP2C are involved in the metabolism of levonorgestrel. Likewise, inducers or inhibitors of these enzymes may either, respectively, decrease the therapeutic effects or result in side effects).
No products indexed under this heading.

Chlorothiazide Sodium (Based on in-vitro and in-vivo studies, it can be assumed that CYP3A, CYP2E and CYP2C are involved in the metabolism of levonorgestrel. Likewise, inducers or inhibitors of these enzymes may either, respectively, decrease the therapeutic effects or result in side effects).
Products include:

Chlorpropamide (Based on in-vitro and in-vivo studies, it can be assumed that CYP3A, CYP2E and CYP2C are involved in the metabolism of levonorgestrel. Likewise, inducers or inhibitors of these enzymes may either, respectively, decrease the therapeutic effects or result in side effects).
No products indexed under this heading.

Cimetidine (Inhibitors of CYP3A4 such as erythromycin, clarithromycin, ketoconazole, itraconazole, ritonavir and grapefruit juice may increase plasma concentrations of estrogens and may result in side effects).
No products indexed under this heading.

Cimetidine Hydrochloride (Inhibitors of CYP3A4 such as erythromycin, clarithromycin, ketoconazole, itraconazole, ritonavir and grapefruit juice may increase plasma concentrations of estrogens and may result in side effects).
No products indexed under this heading.

Ciprofloxacin (Inducers of CYP3A4 may reduce plasma concentrations of estrogens, possibly resulting in a decrease in therapeutic effects and/or changes in the uterine bleeding profile). Products include:

Ciprofloxacin Hydrochloride (Inducers of CYP3A4 may reduce plasma concentrations of estrogens, possibly resulting in a decrease in therapeutic effects and/or changes in the uterine bleeding profile). Products include:

Cisplatin (Inducers of CYP3A4 may reduce plasma concentrations of estrogens, possibly resulting in a decrease in therapeutic effects and/or changes in the uterine bleeding profile).
No products indexed under this heading.

Citalopram Hydrobromide (Based on in-vitro and in-vivo studies, it can be assumed that CYP3A, CYP2E and CYP2C are involved in the metabolism of levonorgestrel. Likewise, inducers or inhibitors of these enzymes may either, respectively, decrease the therapeutic effects or result in side effects).
Products include:

Clarithromycin (Inhibitors of CYP3A4 such as erythromycin, clarithromycin, ketoconazole, itraconazole, ritonavir and grapefruit juice may increase plasma concentrations of estrogens and may result in side effects). Products include:

Clopidogrel Bisulfate (Based on in-vitro and in-vivo studies, it can be assumed that CYP3A, CYP2E and CYP2C are involved in the metabolism of levonorgestrel. Likewise, inducers or inhibitors of these enzymes may either, respectively, decrease the therapeutic effects or result in side effects).
Products include:

Clopidogrel Hydrogen Sulfate (Based on in-vitro and in-vivo studies, it can be assumed that CYP3A, CYP2E and CYP2C are involved in the metabolism of levonorgestrel. Likewise, inducers or inhibitors of these enzymes may either, respectively, decrease the therapeutic effects or resultin side effects). No products indexed under this heading.

Clotrimazole (Inhibitors of CYP3A4 such as erythromycin, clarithromycin, ketoconazole, itraconazole, ritonavir and grapefruit juice may increase plasma concentrations of estrogens and may result in side effects). Products include:

Conivaptan Hydrochloride (Inhibitors of CYP3A4 such as erythromycin, clarithromycin, ketoconazole, itraconazole, ritonavir and grapefruit juice may increase plasma concentrations of estrogens and may result in side effects). Products include:

Cortisone Acetate (Inducers of CYP3A4 may reduce plasma concentrations of estrogens, possibly resulting in a decrease in therapeutic effects and/or changes in the uterine bleeding profile). No products indexed under this heading.

Cyclosporine (Inhibitors of CYP3A4 such as erythromycin, clarithromycin, ketoconazole, itraconazole, ritonavir and grapefruit juice may increase plasma concentrations of estrogens and may result in side effects). Products include:

Dalfopristin (Inhibitors of CYP3A4 such as erythromycin, clarithromycin, ketoconazole, itraconazole, ritonavir and grapefruit juice may increase plasma concentrations of estrogens and may result in side effects). No products indexed under this heading.

Danazol (Inhibitors of CYP3A4 such as erythromycin, clarithromycin, ketoconazole, itraconazole, ritonavir and grapefruit juice may increase plasma concentrations of estrogens and may result in side effects). No products indexed under this heading.

Darunavir (Inhibitors of CYP3A4 such as erythromycin, clarithromycin, ketoconazole, itraconazole, ritonavir and grapefruit juice may increase plasma concentrations of estrogens and may result in side effects). No products indexed under this heading.

Dasatinib (Inhibitors of CYP3A4 such as erythromycin, clarithromycin, ketoconazole, itraconazole, ritonavir and grapefruit juice may increase plasma concentrations of estrogens and may result in side effects). No products indexed under this heading.

Delavirdine Mesylate (Inhibitors of CYP3A4 such as erythromycin, clarithromycin, ketoconazole, itraconazole, ritonavir and grapefruit juice may increase plasma concentrations of estrogens and may result in side effects). No products indexed under this heading.

Delavirine (Inhibitors of CYP3A4 such as erythromycin, clarithromycin, ketoconazole, itraconazole, ritonavir and grapefruit juice may increase plasma concentrations of estrogens and may result in side effects). No products indexed under this heading.

Desloratadine (Inhibitors of CYP3A4 such as erythromycin, clarithromycin, ketoconazole, itraconazole, ritonavir and grapefruit juice may increase plas-

ma concentrations of estrogens and may result in side effects). Products include:

Desogestrel (Based on in-vitro and in-vivo studies, it can be assumed that CYP3A, CYP2E and CYP2C are involved in the metabolism of levonorgestrel. Likewise, inducers or inhibitors of these enzymes may either, respectively, decrease the therapeutic effects or resultin side effects). No products indexed under this heading.

Dexamethasone (Inducers of CYP3A4 may reduce plasma concentrations of estrogens, possibly resulting in a decrease in therapeutic effects and/or changes in the uterine bleeding profile). Products include:

Dexamethasone Acetate (Inducers of CYP3A4 may reduce plasma concentrations of estrogens, possibly resulting in a decrease in therapeutic effects and/or changes in the uterine bleeding profile). No products indexed under this heading.

Dexamethasone Phosphate (Inducers of CYP3A4 may reduce plasma concentrations of estrogens, possibly resulting in a decrease in therapeutic effects and/or changes in the uterine bleeding profile). No products indexed under this heading.

Dexamethasone Sodium (Inducers of CYP3A4 may reduce plasma concentrations of estrogens, possibly resulting in a decrease in therapeutic effects and/or changes in the uterine bleeding profile). No products indexed under this heading.

Dexamethasone Sodium Phosphate (Inducers of CYP3A4 may reduce plasma concentrations of estrogens, possibly resulting in a decrease in therapeutic effects and/or changes in the uterine bleeding profile). No products indexed under this heading.

Dexamethasone Sodium Phosphate Injection (Inducers of CYP3A4 may reduce plasma concentrations of estrogens, possibly resulting in a decrease in therapeutic effects and/or changes in the uterine bleeding profile). No products indexed under this heading.

Diclofenac Epolamine (Based on in-vitro and in-vivo studies, it can be assumed that CYP3A, CYP2E and CYP2C are involved in the metabolism of levonorgestrel. Likewise, inducers or inhibitors of these enzymes may either, respectively, decrease the therapeutic effects or resultin side effects). Products include:

Diclofenac Potassium (Based on in-vitro and in-vivo studies, it can be assumed that CYP3A, CYP2E and CYP2C are involved in the metabolism of levonorgestrel. Likewise, inducers or inhibitors of these enzymes may either, respectively, decrease the therapeutic effects or resultin side effects). No products indexed under this heading.

Diclofenac Sodium (Based on in-vitro and in-vivo studies, it can be assumed that CYP3A, CYP2E and CYP2C are involved in the metabolism of levonorgestrel. Likewise, inducers or inhibitors of these enzymes may either, respectively, decrease the therapeutic effects or resultin side effects). No products indexed under this heading.

Diltiazem Hydrochloride (Inhibitors of CYP3A4 such as erythromycin, clarithromycin, ketoconazole, itraconazole, ritonavir and grapefruit juice may increase plasma concentrations of estrogens and may result in side effects). Products include:

Diltiazem Maleate (Inhibitors of CYP3A4 such as erythromycin, clarithromycin, ketoconazole, itraconazole, ritonavir and grapefruit juice may increase plasma concentrations of estrogens and may result in side effects). No products indexed under this heading.

Disulfiram (Based on in-vitro and in-vivo studies, it can be assumed that CYP3A, CYP2E and CYP2C are involved in the metabolism of levonorgestrel. Likewise, inducers or inhibitors of these enzymes may either, respectively, decrease the therapeutic effects or resultin side effects). No products indexed under this heading.

Doxorubicin Hydrochloride (Inducers of CYP3A4 may reduce plasma concentrations of estrogens, possibly resulting in a decrease in therapeutic effects and/or changes in the uterine bleeding profile). No products indexed under this heading.

Efavirenz (Inducers of CYP3A4 may reduce plasma concentrations of estrogens, possibly resulting in a decrease in therapeutic effects and/or changes in the uterine bleeding profile). Products include:

Erythromycin (Inhibitors of CYP3A4 such as erythromycin, clarithromycin, ketoconazole, itraconazole, ritonavir and grapefruit juice may increase plasma concentrations of estrogens and may result in side effects). No products indexed under this heading.

Erythromycin Estolate (Inhibitors of CYP3A4 such as erythromycin, clarithromycin, ketoconazole, itraconazole, ritonavir and grapefruit juice may increase plasma concentrations of estrogens and may result in side effects). No products indexed under this heading.

Erythromycin Ethylsuccinate (Inhibitors of CYP3A4 such as erythromycin, clarithromycin, ketoconazole, itraconazole, ritonavir and grapefruit juice may increase plasma concentrations of estrogens and may result in side effects). Products include:

Erythromycin Gluceptate (Inhibitors of CYP3A4 such as erythromycin, clarithromycin, ketoconazole, itraconazole, ritonavir and grapefruit juice may increase plasma concentrations of estrogens and may result in side effects). No products indexed under this heading.

Erythromycin Lactobionate (Inhibitors of CYP3A4 such as erythromycin, clarithromycin, ketoconazole, itraconazole, ritonavir and grapefruit juice may increase plasma concentrations of estrogens and may result in side effects). No products indexed under this heading.

Erythromycin Stearate (Inhibitors of CYP3A4 such as erythromycin, clarithromycin, ketoconazole, itraconazole, ritonavir and grapefruit juice may increase plasma concentrations of estrogens and may result in side effects). No products indexed under this heading.

Esomeprazole Magnesium (Inhibitors of CYP3A4 such as erythromycin, clarithromycin, ketoconazole, itraconazole, ritonavir and grapefruit juice may

increase plasma concentrations of estrogens and may result in side effects). Products include:

Esomeprazole Sodium (Inhibitors of CYP3A4 such as erythromycin, clarithromycin, ketoconazole, itraconazole, ritonavir and grapefruit juice may increase plasma concentrations of estrogens and may result in side effects). Products include:

Ethinyl Estradiol (Based on in-vitro and in-vivo studies, it can be assumed that CYP3A, CYP2E and CYP2C are involved in the metabolism of levonorgestrel. Likewise, inducers or inhibitors of these enzymes may either, respectively, decrease the therapeutic effects or resultin side effects). Products include:

Ethosuximide (Inducers of CYP3A4 may reduce plasma concentrations of estrogens, possibly resulting in a decrease in therapeutic effects and/or changes in the uterine bleeding profile). No products indexed under this heading.

Ethynodiol Diacetate (Based on in-vitro and in-vivo studies, it can be assumed that CYP3A, CYP2E and CYP2C are involved in the metabolism of levonorgestrel. Likewise, inducers or inhibitors of these enzymes may either, respectively, decrease the therapeutic effects or resultin side effects). No products indexed under this heading.

Felbamate (Inducers of CYP3A4 may reduce plasma concentrations of estrogens, possibly resulting in a decrease in therapeutic effects and/or changes in the uterine bleeding profile). No products indexed under this heading.

Fenofibrate (Based on in-vitro and in-vivo studies, it can be assumed that CYP3A, CYP2E and CYP2C are involved in the metabolism of levonorgestrel. Likewise, inducers or inhibitors of these enzymes may either, respectively, decrease the therapeutic effects or resultin side effects). Products include:

Fluconazole (Inhibitors of CYP3A4 such as erythromycin, clarithromycin, ketoconazole, itraconazole, ritonavir and grapefruit juice may increase plasma concentrations of estrogens and may result in side effects). No products indexed under this heading.

Fludrocortisone Acetate (Inducers of CYP3A4 may reduce plasma concentrations of estrogens, possibly resulting in a decrease in therapeutic effects and/or changes in the uterine bleeding profile). No products indexed under this heading.

Fluorouracil (Based on in-vitro and in-vivo studies, it can be assumed that CYP3A, CYP2E and CYP2C are involved in the metabolism of levonorgestrel. Likewise, inducers or inhibitors of these enzymes may either, respectively, decrease the therapeutic effects or resultin side effects). Products include:

Fluoxetine (Inhibitors of CYP3A4 such as erythromycin, clarithromycin, ketoconazole, itraconazole, ritonavir and grapefruit juice may increase plasma concentrations of estrogens and may result in side effects). No products indexed under this heading.

IMPORTANT NOTE: Always consult each drug listing in the patient's regimen for possible interactions.

Climara Pro Interactions Index 360

Fluoxetine Hydrochloride (Inhibitors of CYP3A4 such as erythromycin, clarithromycin, ketoconazole, itraconazole, ritonavir and grapefruit juice may increase plasma concentrations of estrogens and may result in side effects). Products include:
Prozac Weekly ... 1941
Prozac Pulvules ... 1941
Symbyax ... 1965

Flurbiprofen (Based on in-vitro and in-vivo studies, it can be assumed that CYP3A, CYP2E and CYP2C are involved in the metabolism of levonorgestrel. Likewise, inducers or inhibitors of these enzymes may either, respectively, decrease the therapeutic effects or resultin side effects).
No products indexed under this heading.

Flurbiprofen Sodium (Based on in-vitro and in-vivo studies, it can be assumed that CYP3A, CYP2E and CYP2C are involved in the metabolism of levonorgestrel. Likewise, inducers or inhibitors of these enzymes may either, respectively, decrease the therapeutic effects or resultin side effects).
No products indexed under this heading.

Fluvastatin Sodium (Based on in-vitro and in-vivo studies, it can be assumed that CYP3A, CYP2E and CYP2C are involved in the metabolism of levonorgestrel. Likewise, inducers or inhibitors of these enzymes may either, respectively, decrease the therapeutic effects or resultin side effects).
No products indexed under this heading.

Fluvoxamine (Based on in-vitro and in-vivo studies, it can be assumed that CYP3A, CYP2E and CYP2C are involved in the metabolism of levonorgestrel. Likewise, inducers or inhibitors of these enzymes may either, respectively, decrease the therapeutic effects or resultin side effects).
No products indexed under this heading.

Fluvoxamine Maleate (Inhibitors of CYP3A4 such as erythromycin, clarithromycin, ketoconazole, itraconazole, ritonavir and grapefruit juice may increase plasma concentrations of estrogens and may result in side effects).
No products indexed under this heading.

Fosamprenavir Calcium (Inhibitors of CYP3A4 such as erythromycin, clarithromycin, ketoconazole, itraconazole, ritonavir and grapefruit juice may increase plasma concentrations of estrogens and may result in side effects). Products include:
Lexiva Oral Suspension ... 1558
Lexiva ... 1558

Fosphenytoin Sodium (Inducers of CYP3A4 may reduce plasma concentrations of estrogens, possibly resulting in a decrease in therapeutic effects and/or changes in the uterine bleeding profile).
No products indexed under this heading.

Garlic Extract (Inducers of CYP3A4 may reduce plasma concentrations of estrogens, possibly resulting in a decrease in therapeutic effects and/or changes in the uterine bleeding profile).
No products indexed under this heading.

Garlic Oil (Inducers of CYP3A4 may reduce plasma concentrations of estrogens, possibly resulting in a decrease in therapeutic effects and/or changes in the uterine bleeding profile).
No products indexed under this heading.

Gemfibrozil (Based on in-vitro and in-vivo studies, it can be assumed that CYP3A, CYP2E and CYP2C are involved in the metabolism of levonorgestrel. Likewise, inducers or inhibitors of these enzymes may either, respectively, decrease the therapeutic effects or resultin side effects).
No products indexed under this heading.

Glipizide (Based on in-vitro and in-vivo studies, it can be assumed that CYP3A, CYP2E and CYP2C are involved in the metabolism of levonorgestrel. Likewise, inducers or inhibitors of these enzymes may either, respectively, decrease the therapeutic effects or resultin side effects).
No products indexed under this heading.

Glyburide (Based on in-vitro and in-vivo studies, it can be assumed that CYP3A, CYP2E and CYP2C are involved in the metabolism of levonorgestrel. Likewise, inducers or inhibitors of these enzymes may either, respectively, decrease the therapeutic effects or resultin side effects).
No products indexed under this heading.

Hydrochlorothiazide (Based on in-vitro and in-vivo studies, it can be assumed that CYP3A, CYP2E and CYP2C are involved in the metabolism of levonorgestrel. Likewise, inducers or inhibitors of these enzymes may either, respectively, decrease the therapeutic effects or resultin side effects).
Products include:
Atacand HCT ... 700
Avalide ... 2956
Benicar HCT ... 1017
Diovan HCT ... 2419
Dyazide ... 1429
Exforge HCT ... 2449
Hyzaar ... 2162
Hyzaar 100-12.5 ... 2162
Micardis HCT ... 889
Prinzide ... 2246
Tekturna HCT ... 2541
Teveten HCT ... 541

Hydrochlorothiazide Hydrochloride (Based on in-vitro and in-vivo studies, it can be assumed that CYP3A, CYP2E and CYP2C are involved in the metabolism of levonorgestrel. Likewise, inducers or inhibitors of these enzymes may either, respectively, decrease the therapeutic effects or resultin side effects).
No products indexed under this heading.

Hydrocortisone (Inducers of CYP3A4 may reduce plasma concentrations of estrogens, possibly resulting in a decrease in therapeutic effects and/or changes in the uterine bleeding profile).
No products indexed under this heading.

Hydrocortisone (Alcohol) (Inducers of CYP3A4 may reduce plasma concentrations of estrogens, possibly resulting in a decrease in therapeutic effects and/or changes in the uterine bleeding profile).
No products indexed under this heading.

Hydrocortisone Acetate (Inducers of CYP3A4 may reduce plasma concentrations of estrogens, possibly resulting in a decrease in therapeutic effects and/or changes in the uterine bleeding profile).
No products indexed under this heading.

Hydrocortisone Butyrate (Inducers of CYP3A4 may reduce plasma concentrations of estrogens, possibly resulting in a decrease in therapeutic effects and/or changes in the uterine bleeding profile).
No products indexed under this heading.

Hydrocortisone Cypionate (Inducers of CYP3A4 may reduce plasma concentrations of estrogens, possibly resulting in a decrease in therapeutic effects and/or changes in the uterine bleeding profile).
No products indexed under this heading.

Hydrocortisone Hemisuccinate (Inducers of CYP3A4 may reduce plasma concentrations of estrogens, possibly resulting in a decrease in therapeutic effects and/or changes in the uterine bleeding profile).
No products indexed under this heading.

Hydrocortisone Probutate (Inducers of CYP3A4 may reduce plasma concentrations of estrogens, possibly resulting in a decrease in therapeutic effects and/or changes in the uterine bleeding profile).
No products indexed under this heading.

Hydrocortisone Sodium Phosphate (Inducers of CYP3A4 may reduce plasma concentrations of estrogens, possibly resulting in a decrease in therapeutic effects and/or changes in the uterine bleeding profile).
No products indexed under this heading.

Hydrocortisone Sodium Succinate (Inducers of CYP3A4 may reduce plasma concentrations of estrogens, possibly resulting in a decrease in therapeutic effects and/or changes in the uterine bleeding profile).
No products indexed under this heading.

Hydrocortisone Valerate (Inducers of CYP3A4 may reduce plasma concentrations of estrogens, possibly resulting in a decrease in therapeutic effects and/or changes in the uterine bleeding profile).
No products indexed under this heading.

Hydroflumethiazide (Based on in-vitro and in-vivo studies, it can be assumed that CYP3A, CYP2E and CYP2C are involved in the metabolism of levonorgestrel. Likewise, inducers or inhibitors of these enzymes may either, respectively, decrease the therapeutic effects or resultin side effects).
No products indexed under this heading.

Hypericum (Inducers of CYP3A4 may reduce plasma concentrations of estrogens, possibly resulting in a decrease in therapeutic effects and/or changes in the uterine bleeding profile).
No products indexed under this heading.

Hypericum Perforatum (Inducers of CYP3A4 may reduce plasma concentrations of estrogens, possibly resulting in a decrease in therapeutic effects and/or changes in the uterine bleeding profile). Products include:
Traumeel ... 1800

Imatinib Mesylate (Inhibitors of CYP3A4 such as erythromycin, clarithromycin, ketoconazole, itraconazole, ritonavir and grapefruit juice may increase plasma concentrations of estrogens and may result in side effects). Products include:
Gleevec ... 2477

Indinavir Sulfate (Inhibitors of CYP3A4 such as erythromycin, clarithromycin, ketoconazole, itraconazole, ritonavir and grapefruit juice may increase plasma concentrations of estrogens and may result in side effects). Products include:
Crixivan ... 2113

Indomethacin (Based on in-vitro and in-vivo studies, it can be assumed that CYP3A, CYP2E and CYP2C are involved in the metabolism of levonorgestrel. Likewise, inducers or inhibitors of these enzymes may either, respectively, decrease the therapeutic effects or resultin side effects). Products include:
Indocin ... 2167

Indomethacin Sodium Trihydrate (Based on in-vitro and in-vivo studies, it can be assumed that CYP3A, CYP2E and CYP2C are involved in the metabolism of levonorgestrel. Likewise, inducers or inhibitors of these enzymes may either, respectively, decrease the therapeutic effects or resultin side effects).
Products include:
Indocin I.V. ... 2007

Isoniazid (Inhibitors of CYP3A4 such as erythromycin, clarithromycin, ketoconazole, itraconazole, ritonavir and grapefruit juice may increase plasma concentrations of estrogens and may result in side effects).
No products indexed under this heading.

Itraconazole (Inhibitors of CYP3A4 such as erythromycin, clarithromycin, ketoconazole, itraconazole, ritonavir and grapefruit juice may increase plasma concentrations of estrogens and may result in side effects).
No products indexed under this heading.

Ketoconazole (Inhibitors of CYP3A4 such as erythromycin, clarithromycin, ketoconazole, itraconazole, ritonavir and grapefruit juice may increase plasma concentrations of estrogens and may result in side effects). Products include:
Extina ... 3319
Xolegel ... 3337

Ketoprofen (Based on in-vitro and in-vivo studies, it can be assumed that CYP3A, CYP2E and CYP2C are involved in the metabolism of levonorgestrel. Likewise, inducers or inhibitors of these enzymes may either, respectively, decrease the therapeutic effects or resultin side effects).
No products indexed under this heading.

Lansoprazole (Based on in-vitro and in-vivo studies, it can be assumed that CYP3A, CYP2E and CYP2C are involved in the metabolism of levonorgestrel. Likewise, inducers or inhibitors of these enzymes may either, respectively, decrease the therapeutic effects or resultin side effects).
No products indexed under this heading.

Lapatinib (Inhibitors of CYP3A4 such as erythromycin, clarithromycin, ketoconazole, itraconazole, ritonavir and grapefruit juice may increase plasma concentrations of estrogens and may result in side effects). Products include:
Tykerb ... 1698

Leflunomide (Based on in-vitro and in-vivo studies, it can be assumed that CYP3A, CYP2E and CYP2C are involved in the metabolism of levonorgestrel. Likewise, inducers or inhibitors of these enzymes may either, respectively, decrease the therapeutic effects or resultin side effects).
No products indexed under this heading.

Letrozole (Based on in-vitro and in-vivo studies, it can be assumed that CYP3A, CYP2E and CYP2C are involved in the metabolism of levonorgestrel. Likewise, inducers or inhibitors of these enzymes may either, respectively, decrease the therapeutic effects or resultin side effects). Products include:
Femara ... 2466

Lopinavir (Inhibitors of CYP3A4 such as erythromycin, clarithromycin, ketoconazole, itraconazole, ritonavir and grapefruit juice may increase plasma concentrations of estrogens and may result in side effects). Products include:
Kaletra ... 458

Loratadine (Inhibitors of CYP3A4 such as erythromycin, clarithromycin, ketoconazole, itraconazole, ritonavir and grapefruit juice may increase plasma concentrations of estrogens and may result in side effects).
No products indexed under this heading.

Lovastatin (Based on in-vitro and in-vivo studies, it can be assumed that CYP3A, CYP2E and CYP2C are involved in the metabolism of levonorgestrel. Likewise, inducers or inhibitors of these enzymes may either, respectively, decrease the therapeutic effects or resultin side effects). Products include:
Advicor ... 402
Mevacor ... 2212

Mephenytoin (Inducers of CYP3A4 may reduce plasma concentrations of estrogens, possibly resulting in a decrease in therapeutic effects and/or changes in the uterine bleeding profile).
No products indexed under this heading.

Mestranol (Based on in-vitro and in-vivo studies, it can be assumed that CYP3A, CYP2E and CYP2C are involved in the metabolism of levonorgestrel. Likewise, inducers or inhibitors of these enzymes may either, respectively, decrease the therapeutic effects or resultin side effects).
No products indexed under this heading.

Methsuximide (Inducers of CYP3A4 may reduce plasma concentrations of estrogens, possibly resulting in a decrease in therapeutic effects and/or changes in the uterine bleeding profile).
No products indexed under this heading.

Methyclothiazide (Based on in-vitro and in-vivo studies, it can be assumed that CYP3A, CYP2E and CYP2C are involved in the metabolism of levonorgestrel. Likewise, inducers or inhibitors of these enzymes may either, respectively, decrease the therapeutic effects or resultin side effects).
No products indexed under this heading.

Methylprednisolone (Inducers of CYP3A4 may reduce plasma concentrations of estrogens, possibly resulting in a decrease in therapeutic effects and/or changes in the uterine bleeding profile).
No products indexed under this heading.

Methylprednisolone Acetate (Inducers of CYP3A4 may reduce plasma concentrations of estrogens, possibly resulting in a decrease in therapeutic effects and/or changes in the uterine bleeding profile).
No products indexed under this heading.

Methylprednisolone Sodium Succinate (Inducers of CYP3A4 may reduce plasma concentrations of estrogens, possibly resulting in a decrease in therapeutic effects and/or changes in the uterine bleeding profile).
No products indexed under this heading.

Metronidazole (Inhibitors of CYP3A4 such as erythromycin, clarithromycin, ketoconazole, itraconazole, ritonavir and grapefruit juice may increase plasma concentrations of estrogens and may result in side effects). Products include:
Pylera 793

Metronidazole Benzoate (Inhibitors of CYP3A4 such as erythromycin, clarithromycin, ketoconazole, itraconazole, ritonavir and grapefruit juice may increase plasma concentrations of estrogens and may result in side effects).
No products indexed under this heading.

Metronidazole Hydrochloride (Inhibitors of CYP3A4 such as erythromycin, clarithromycin, ketoconazole, itraconazole, ritonavir and grapefruit juice may increase plasma concentrations of estrogens and may result in side effects).
No products indexed under this heading.

Metronidazole Sodium (Inhibitors of CYP3A4 such as erythromycin, clarithromycin, ketoconazole, itraconazole, ritonavir and grapefruit juice may increase plasma concentrations of estrogens and may result in side effects).
No products indexed under this heading.

Miconazole (Inhibitors of CYP3A4 such as erythromycin, clarithromycin, ketoconazole, itraconazole, ritonavir and grapefruit juice may increase plasma concentrations of estrogens and may result in side effects).
No products indexed under this heading.

Miconazole Nitrate (Inhibitors of CYP3A4 such as erythromycin, clarithromycin, ketoconazole, itraconazole, ritonavir and grapefruit juice may increase plasma concentrations of estrogens and may result in side effects). Products include:
Vusion Ointment 3335

Mifepristone (Inhibitors of CYP3A4 such as erythromycin, clarithromycin, ketoconazole, itraconazole, ritonavir and grapefruit juice may increase plasma concentrations of estrogens and may result in side effects).
No products indexed under this heading.

Modafinil (Inducers of CYP3A4 may reduce plasma concentrations of estrogens, possibly resulting in a decrease in therapeutic effects and/or changes in the uterine bleeding profile). Products include:
Provigil 983

Nafcillin Sodium (Inducers of CYP3A4 may reduce plasma concentrations of estrogens, possibly resulting in a decrease in therapeutic effects and/or changes in the uterine bleeding profile).
No products indexed under this heading.

Nefazodone Hydrochloride (Inhibitors of CYP3A4 such as erythromycin, clarithromycin, ketoconazole, itraconazole, ritonavir and grapefruit juice may increase plasma concentrations of estrogens and may result in side effects).
No products indexed under this heading.

Nelfinavir Mesylate (Inhibitors of CYP3A4 such as erythromycin, clarithromycin, ketoconazole, itraconazole, ritonavir and grapefruit juice may increase plasma concentrations of estrogens and may result in side effects).
No products indexed under this heading.

Nevirapine (Inducers of CYP3A4 may reduce plasma concentrations of estrogens, possibly resulting in a decrease in therapeutic effects and/or changes in the uterine bleeding profile). Products include:
Viramune Oral Suspension 897
Viramune Tablets 897

Niacin (Inhibitors of CYP3A4 such as erythromycin, clarithromycin, ketoconazole, itraconazole, ritonavir and grapefruit juice may increase plasma concentrations of estrogens and may result in side effects). Products include:
Advicor 402
Cardio Basics 3455
Niaspan 497
Simcor 524

Niacinamide (Inhibitors of CYP3A4 such as erythromycin, clarithromycin, ketoconazole, itraconazole, ritonavir and grapefruit juice may increase plasma concentrations of estrogens and may result in side effects). Products include:
CitraNatal 90 DHA Capsules 2332
CitraNatal Assure 2332
CitraNatal Rx 2332
Heplive 607

Niacinamide Hydroiodide (Inhibitors of CYP3A4 such as erythromycin, clarithromycin, ketoconazole, itraconazole, ritonavir and grapefruit juice may increase plasma concentrations of estrogens and may result in side effects).
No products indexed under this heading.

Nicardipine (Based on in-vitro and in-vivo studies, it can be assumed that CYP3A, CYP2E and CYP2C are involved in the metabolism of levonorgestrel. Likewise, inducers or inhibitors of these enzymes may either, respectively, decrease the therapeutic effects or resultin side effects).
No products indexed under this heading.

Nicardipine Hydrochloride (Based on in-vitro and in-vivo studies, it can be assumed that CYP3A, CYP2E and CYP2C are involved in the metabolism of levonorgestrel. Likewise, inducers or inhibitors of these enzymes may either, respectively, decrease the therapeutic effects or resultin side effects).
No products indexed under this heading.

Nicotinamide (Inhibitors of CYP3A4 such as erythromycin, clarithromycin, ketoconazole, itraconazole, ritonavir and grapefruit juice may increase plasma concentrations of estrogens and may result in side effects).
No products indexed under this heading.

Nifedipine (Inhibitors of CYP3A4 such as erythromycin, clarithromycin, ketoconazole, itraconazole, ritonavir and grapefruit juice may increase plasma concentrations of estrogens and may result in side effects).
No products indexed under this heading.

Norethindrone (Based on in-vitro and in-vivo studies, it can be assumed that CYP3A, CYP2E and CYP2C are involved in the metabolism of levonorgestrel. Likewise, inducers or inhibitors of these enzymes may either, respectively, decrease the therapeutic effects or resultin side effects). Products include:
Ortho Micronor 2660

Norethindrone Acetate (Based on in-vitro and in-vivo studies, it can be assumed that CYP3A, CYP2E and CYP2C are involved in the metabolism of levonorgestrel. Likewise, inducers or inhibitors of these enzymes may either, respectively, decrease the therapeutic effects or resultin side effects). Products include:
Activella 2561

Norethynodrel (Based on in-vitro and in-vivo studies, it can be assumed that CYP3A, CYP2E and CYP2C are involved in the metabolism of levonorgestrel. Likewise, inducers or inhibitors of these enzymes may either, respectively, decrease the therapeutic effects or resultin side effects).
No products indexed under this heading.

Norfloxacin (Inhibitors of CYP3A4 such as erythromycin, clarithromycin, ketoconazole, itraconazole, ritonavir and grapefruit juice may increase plasma concentrations of estrogens and may result in side effects). Products include:
Noroxin 2220

Norgestimate (Based on in-vitro and in-vivo studies, it can be assumed that CYP3A, CYP2E and CYP2C are involved in the metabolism of levonorgestrel. Likewise, inducers or inhibitors of these enzymes may either, respectively, decrease the therapeutic effects or resultin side effects). Products include:
Ortho-Cyclen/Ortho Tri-Cyclen 2663
Ortho Tri-Cyclen Lo Tablets 2673

Norgestrel (Based on in-vitro and in-vivo studies, it can be assumed that CYP3A, CYP2E and CYP2C are involved in the metabolism of levonorgestrel. Likewise, inducers or inhibitors of these enzymes may either, respectively, decrease the therapeutic effects or resultin side effects).
No products indexed under this heading.

Omeprazole (Inhibitors of CYP3A4 such as erythromycin, clarithromycin, ketoconazole, itraconazole, ritonavir and grapefruit juice may increase plasma concentrations of estrogens and may result in side effects).
No products indexed under this heading.

Oxcarbazepine (Inducers of CYP3A4 may reduce plasma concentrations of estrogens, possibly resulting in a decrease in therapeutic effects and/or changes in the uterine bleeding profile).
No products indexed under this heading.

Oxiconazole Nitrate (Based on in-vitro and in-vivo studies, it can be assumed that CYP3A, CYP2E and CYP2C are involved in the metabolism of levonorgestrel. Likewise, inducers or inhibitors of these enzymes may either, respectively, decrease the therapeutic effects or resultin side effects).
No products indexed under this heading.

Paroxetine Hydrochloride (Inhibitors of CYP3A4 such as erythromycin, clarithromycin, ketoconazole, itraconazole, ritonavir and grapefruit juice may increase plasma concentrations of estrogens and may result in side effects). Products include:
Paroxetine CR 2361
Paroxetine ER 2371
Paxil 1586
Paxil CR 1596

Phenobarbital (Inducers of CYP3A4 may reduce plasma concentrations of estrogens, possibly resulting in a decrease in therapeutic effects and/or changes in the uterine bleeding profile). Products include:
Donnatal 2711

Phenobarbital Sodium (Inducers of CYP3A4 may reduce plasma concentrations of estrogens, possibly resulting in a decrease in therapeutic effects and/or changes in the uterine bleeding profile).
No products indexed under this heading.

Phenylbutazone (Based on in-vitro and in-vivo studies, it can be assumed that CYP3A, CYP2E and CYP2C are involved in the metabolism of levonorgestrel. Likewise, inducers or inhibitors of these enzymes may either, respectively, decrease the therapeutic effects or resultin side effects).
No products indexed under this heading.

Phenytoin (Inducers of CYP3A4 may reduce plasma concentrations of estrogens, possibly resulting in a decrease in therapeutic effects and/or changes in the uterine bleeding profile).
No products indexed under this heading.

Phenytoin Sodium (Inducers of CYP3A4 may reduce plasma concentrations of estrogens, possibly resulting in a decrease in therapeutic effects and/or changes in the uterine bleeding profile). Products include:
Phenytek Capsules 2380

Polythiazide (Based on in-vitro and in-vivo studies, it can be assumed that CYP3A, CYP2E and CYP2C are involved in the metabolism of levonorgestrel. Likewise, inducers or inhibitors of these enzymes may either, respectively, decrease the therapeutic effects or resultin side effects).
No products indexed under this heading.

Posaconazole (Inhibitors of CYP3A4 such as erythromycin, clarithromycin, ketoconazole, itraconazole, ritonavir and grapefruit juice may increase plasma concentrations of estrogens and may result in side effects). Products include:
Noxafil 3172

Prednisolone (Inducers of CYP3A4 may reduce plasma concentrations of estrogens, possibly resulting in a decrease in therapeutic effects and/or changes in the uterine bleeding profile).
No products indexed under this heading.

Prednisolone Acetate (Inducers of CYP3A4 may reduce plasma concentrations of estrogens, possibly resulting in a decrease in therapeutic effects and/or changes in the uterine bleeding profile). Products include:
Blephamide .... ⊙212, ⊙214
Pred Forte .... ⊙225
Pred Mild .... ⊙230
Pred-G .... ⊙226, ⊙227

IMPORTANT NOTE: Always consult each drug listing in the patient's regimen for possible interactions.

Prednisolone Sodium Phosphate (Inducers of CYP3A4 may reduce plasma concentrations of estrogens, possibly resulting in a decrease in therapeutic effects and/or changes in the uterine bleeding profile).
     No products indexed under this heading.

Prednisolone Tebutate (Inducers of CYP3A4 may reduce plasma concentrations of estrogens, possibly resulting in a decrease in therapeutic effects and/or changes in the uterine bleeding profile).
     No products indexed under this heading.

Prednisone (Inducers of CYP3A4 may reduce plasma concentrations of estrogens, possibly resulting in a decrease in therapeutic effects and/or changes in the uterine bleeding profile).
     No products indexed under this heading.

Prednisone sodium phosphate (Inducers of CYP3A4 may reduce plasma concentrations of estrogens, possibly resulting in a decrease in therapeutic effects and/or changes in the uterine bleeding profile).
     No products indexed under this heading.

Primidone (Inducers of CYP3A4 may reduce plasma concentrations of estrogens, possibly resulting in a decrease in therapeutic effects and/or changes in the uterine bleeding profile).
     No products indexed under this heading.

Propoxyphene Hydrochloride (Inhibitors of CYP3A4 such as erythromycin, clarithromycin, ketoconazole, itraconazole, ritonavir and grapefruit juice may increase plasma concentrations of estrogens and may result in side effects).
     No products indexed under this heading.

Propoxyphene Napsylate (Inhibitors of CYP3A4 such as erythromycin, clarithromycin, ketoconazole, itraconazole, ritonavir and grapefruit juice may increase plasma concentrations of estrogens and may result in side effects).
     No products indexed under this heading.

Quercetin (Based on in-vitro and in-vivo studies, it can be assumed that CYP3A, CYP2E and CYP2C are involved in the metabolism of levonorgestrel. Likewise, inducers or inhibitors of these enzymes may either, respectively, decrease the therapeutic effects or resultin side effects).
     No products indexed under this heading.

Quinidine (Inhibitors of CYP3A4 such as erythromycin, clarithromycin, ketoconazole, itraconazole, ritonavir and grapefruit juice may increase plasma concentrations of estrogens and may result in side effects).
     No products indexed under this heading.

Quinidine Gluconate (Based on in-vitro and in-vivo studies, it can be assumed that CYP3A, CYP2E and CYP2C are involved in the metabolism of levonorgestrel. Likewise, inducers or inhibitors of these enzymes may either, respectively, decrease the therapeutic effects or resultin side effects).
     No products indexed under this heading.

Quinidine Hydrochloride (Inhibitors of CYP3A4 such as erythromycin, clarithromycin, ketoconazole, itraconazole, ritonavir and grapefruit juice may increase plasma concentrations of estrogens and may result in side effects).
     No products indexed under this heading.

Quinidine Polygalacturonate (Inhibitors of CYP3A4 such as erythromycin, clarithromycin, ketoconazole, itraconazole, ritonavir and grapefruit juice may increase plasma concentrations of estrogens and may result in side effects).
     No products indexed under this heading.

Quinidine Sulfate (Inhibitors of CYP3A4 such as erythromycin, clarithromycin, ketoconazole, itraconazole, ritonavir and grapefruit juice may increase plasma concentrations of estrogens and may result in side effects).
     No products indexed under this heading.

Quinine (Inhibitors of CYP3A4 such as erythromycin, clarithromycin, ketoconazole, itraconazole, ritonavir and grapefruit juice may increase plasma concentrations of estrogens and may result in side effects). Products include:
     Hyland's Leg Cramps PM with Quinine 3315

Quinine Sulfate (Inhibitors of CYP3A4 such as erythromycin, clarithromycin, ketoconazole, itraconazole, ritonavir and grapefruit juice may increase plasma concentrations of estrogens and may result in side effects).
     No products indexed under this heading.

Quinupristin (Inhibitors of CYP3A4 such as erythromycin, clarithromycin, ketoconazole, itraconazole, ritonavir and grapefruit juice may increase plasma concentrations of estrogens and may result in side effects).
     No products indexed under this heading.

Ranitidine Bismuth Citrate (Inhibitors of CYP3A4 such as erythromycin, clarithromycin, ketoconazole, itraconazole, ritonavir and grapefruit juice may increase plasma concentrations of estrogens and may result in side effects).
     No products indexed under this heading.

Ranitidine Hydrochloride (Inhibitors of CYP3A4 such as erythromycin, clarithromycin, ketoconazole, itraconazole, ritonavir and grapefruit juice may increase plasma concentrations of estrogens and may result in side effects). Products include:
     Zantac 1737
     Zantac Injection 1732
     Zantac Pharmacy 1735

Rifabutin (Inducers of CYP3A4 may reduce plasma concentrations of estrogens, possibly resulting in a decrease in therapeutic effects and/or changes in the uterine bleeding profile).
     No products indexed under this heading.

Rifampicin (Inducers of CYP3A4 may reduce plasma concentrations of estrogens, possibly resulting in a decrease in therapeutic effects and/or changes in the uterine bleeding profile).
     No products indexed under this heading.

Rifampin (Inducers of CYP3A4 may reduce plasma concentrations of estrogens, possibly resulting in a decrease in therapeutic effects and/or changes in the uterine bleeding profile).
     No products indexed under this heading.

Rifapentine (Inducers of CYP3A4 may reduce plasma concentrations of estrogens, possibly resulting in a decrease in therapeutic effects and/or changes in the uterine bleeding profile).
     No products indexed under this heading.

Ritonavir (Inhibitors of CYP3A4 such as erythromycin, clarithromycin, ketoconazole, itraconazole, ritonavir and grapefruit juice may increase plasma concentrations of estrogens and may result in side effects). Products include:
     Kaletra 458
     Norvir 509

Saquinavir (Inhibitors of CYP3A4 such as erythromycin, clarithromycin, ketoconazole, itraconazole, ritonavir and grapefruit juice may increase plasma concentrations of estrogens and may result in side effects).
     No products indexed under this heading.

Saquinavir Mesylate (Inhibitors of CYP3A4 such as erythromycin, clarithromycin, ketoconazole, itraconazole, ritonavir and grapefruit juice may increase plasma concentrations of estrogens and may result in side effects).
     No products indexed under this heading.

Secobarbital Sodium (Based on in-vitro and in-vivo studies, it can be assumed that CYP3A, CYP2E and CYP2C are involved in the metabolism of levonorgestrel. Likewise, inducers or inhibitors of these enzymes may either, respectively, decrease the therapeutic effects or resultin side effects).
     No products indexed under this heading.

Sertraline Hydrochloride (Inhibitors of CYP3A4 such as erythromycin, clarithromycin, ketoconazole, itraconazole, ritonavir and grapefruit juice may increase plasma concentrations of estrogens and may result in side effects).
     No products indexed under this heading.

Sildenafil Citrate (Inhibitors of CYP3A4 such as erythromycin, clarithromycin, ketoconazole, itraconazole, ritonavir and grapefruit juice may increase plasma concentrations of estrogens and may result in side effects).
     No products indexed under this heading.

Sulfacytine (Based on in-vitro and in-vivo studies, it can be assumed that CYP3A, CYP2E and CYP2C are involved in the metabolism of levonorgestrel. Likewise, inducers or inhibitors of these enzymes may either, respectively, decrease the therapeutic effects or resultin side effects).
     No products indexed under this heading.

Sulfamethizole (Based on in-vitro and in-vivo studies, it can be assumed that CYP3A, CYP2E and CYP2C are involved in the metabolism of levonorgestrel. Likewise, inducers or inhibitors of these enzymes may either, respectively, decrease the therapeutic effects or resultin side effects).
     No products indexed under this heading.

Sulfamethoxazole (Based on in-vitro and in-vivo studies, it can be assumed that CYP3A, CYP2E and CYP2C are involved in the metabolism of levonorgestrel. Likewise, inducers or inhibitors of these enzymes may either, respectively, decrease the therapeutic effects or resultin side effects).
     No products indexed under this heading.

Sulfaphenazole (Based on in-vitro and in-vivo studies, it can be assumed that CYP3A, CYP2E and CYP2C are involved in the metabolism of levonorgestrel. Likewise, inducers or inhibitors of these enzymes may either, respectively, decrease the therapeutic effects or resultin side effects).
     No products indexed under this heading.

Sulfasalazine (Based on in-vitro and in-vivo studies, it can be assumed that CYP3A, CYP2E and CYP2C are involved in the metabolism of levonorgestrel. Likewise, inducers or inhibitors of these enzymes may either, respectively, decrease the therapeutic effects or resultin side effects).
     No products indexed under this heading.

Sulfinpyrazone (Inducers of CYP3A4 may reduce plasma concentrations of estrogens, possibly resulting in a decrease in therapeutic effects and/or changes in the uterine bleeding profile).
     No products indexed under this heading.

Sulfisoxazole Acetyl (Based on in-vitro and in-vivo studies, it can be assumed that CYP3A, CYP2E and CYP2C are involved in the metabolism of levonorgestrel. Likewise, inducers or inhibitors of these enzymes may either, respectively, decrease the therapeutic effects or resultin side effects).
     No products indexed under this heading.

Sulfisoxazole Diolamine (Based on in-vitro and in-vivo studies, it can be assumed that CYP3A, CYP2E and CYP2C are involved in the metabolism of levonorgestrel. Likewise, inducers or inhibitors of these enzymes may either, respectively, decrease the therapeutic effects or resultin side effects).
     No products indexed under this heading.

Telithromycin (Inhibitors of CYP3A4 such as erythromycin, clarithromycin, ketoconazole, itraconazole, ritonavir and grapefruit juice may increase plasma concentrations of estrogens and may result in side effects). Products include:
     Ketek 2991

Telmisartan (Based on in-vitro and in-vivo studies, it can be assumed that CYP3A, CYP2E and CYP2C are involved in the metabolism of levonorgestrel. Likewise, inducers or inhibitors of these enzymes may either, respectively, decrease the therapeutic effects or resultin side effects). Products include:
     Micardis 887
     Micardis HCT 889

Terconazole (Based on in-vitro and in-vivo studies, it can be assumed that CYP3A, CYP2E and CYP2C are involved in the metabolism of levonorgestrel. Likewise, inducers or inhibitors of these enzymes may either, respectively, decrease the therapeutic effects or resultin side effects).
     No products indexed under this heading.

Theophyllinate (Inducers of CYP3A4 may reduce plasma concentrations of estrogens, possibly resulting in a decrease in therapeutic effects and/or changes in the uterine bleeding profile).
     No products indexed under this heading.

Theophylline (Inducers of CYP3A4 may reduce plasma concentrations of estrogens, possibly resulting in a decrease in therapeutic effects and/or changes in the uterine bleeding profile).
     No products indexed under this heading.

Theophylline Anhydrous (Inducers of CYP3A4 may reduce plasma concentrations of estrogens, possibly resulting in a decrease in therapeutic effects and/or changes in the uterine bleeding profile). Products include:
     Uniphyl 2817

Theophylline Calcium Salicylate (Inducers of CYP3A4 may reduce plasma concentrations of estrogens, possibly resulting in a decrease in therapeutic effects and/or changes in the uterine bleeding profile).
     No products indexed under this heading.

Theophylline Dihydroxypropyl (Glyceryl) (Inducers of CYP3A4 may reduce plasma concentrations of estrogens, possibly resulting in a decrease in therapeutic effects and/or changes in the uterine bleeding profile).
     No products indexed under this heading.

Theophylline Ethylenediamine (Inducers of CYP3A4 may reduce plasma concentrations of estrogens, possibly resulting in a decrease in therapeutic effects and/or changes in the uterine bleeding profile).
     No products indexed under this heading.

(⊙ Described in PDR® for Ophthalmic Medicines)

363 Interactions Index Clinoril

Theophylline Sodium Glycinate (Inducers of CYP3A4 may reduce plasma concentrations of estrogens, possibly resulting in a decrease in therapeutic effects and/or changes in the uterine bleeding profile).
No products indexed under this heading.

Ticlopidine Hydrochloride (Based on in-vitro and in-vivo studies, it can be assumed that CYP3A, CYP2E and CYP2C are involved in the metabolism of levonorgestrel. Likewise, inducers or inhibitors of these enzymes may either, respectively, decrease the therapeutic effects or resultin side effects).
No products indexed under this heading.

Tolazamide (Based on in-vitro and in-vivo studies, it can be assumed that CYP3A, CYP2E and CYP2C are involved in the metabolism of levonorgestrel. Likewise, inducers or inhibitors of these enzymes may either, respectively, decrease the therapeutic effects or resultin side effects).
No products indexed under this heading.

Tolbutamide (Based on in-vitro and in-vivo studies, it can be assumed that CYP3A, CYP2E and CYP2C are involved in the metabolism of levonorgestrel. Likewise, inducers or inhibitors of these enzymes may either, respectively, decrease the therapeutic effects or resultin side effects).
No products indexed under this heading.

Tolbutamide Sodium (Based on in-vitro and in-vivo studies, it can be assumed that CYP3A, CYP2E and CYP2C are involved in the metabolism of levonorgestrel. Likewise, inducers or inhibitors of these enzymes may either, respectively, decrease the therapeutic effects or resultin side effects).
No products indexed under this heading.

Topiramate (Based on in-vitro and in-vivo studies, it can be assumed that CYP3A, CYP2E and CYP2C are involved in the metabolism of levonorgestrel. Likewise, inducers or inhibitors of these enzymes may either, respectively, decrease the therapeutic effects or resultin side effects).
No products indexed under this heading.

Tranylcypromine Sulfate (Based on in-vitro and in-vivo studies, it can be assumed that CYP3A, CYP2E and CYP2C are involved in the metabolism of levonorgestrel. Likewise, inducers or inhibitors of these enzymes may either, respectively, decrease the therapeutic effects or resultin side effects). Products include:
Parnate 1584

Triamcinolone (Inducers of CYP3A4 may reduce plasma concentrations of estrogens, possibly resulting in a decrease in therapeutic effects and/or changes in the uterine bleeding profile).
No products indexed under this heading.

Triamcinolone Acetonide (Inducers of CYP3A4 may reduce plasma concentrations of estrogens, possibly resulting in a decrease in therapeutic effects and/or changes in the uterine bleeding profile). Products include:
Azmacort 408
Nasacort AQ 3019

Triamcinolone Diacetate (Inducers of CYP3A4 may reduce plasma concentrations of estrogens, possibly resulting in a decrease in therapeutic effects and/or changes in the uterine bleeding profile).
No products indexed under this heading.

Triamcinolone Hexacetonide (Inducers of CYP3A4 may reduce plasma concentrations of estrogens, possibly resulting in a decrease in therapeutic effects and/or changes in the uterine bleeding profile).
No products indexed under this heading.

Trimethoprim (Based on in-vitro and in-vivo studies, it can be assumed that CYP3A, CYP2E and CYP2C are involved in the metabolism of levonorgestrel. Likewise, inducers or inhibitors of these enzymes may either, respectively, decrease the therapeutic effects or resultin side effects).
No products indexed under this heading.

Trimethoprim Hydrochloride (Based on in-vitro and in-vivo studies, it can be assumed that CYP3A, CYP2E and CYP2C are involved in the metabolism of levonorgestrel. Likewise, inducers or inhibitors of these enzymes may either, respectively, decrease the therapeutic effects or resultin side effects).
No products indexed under this heading.

Trimethoprim Sulfate (Based on in-vitro and in-vivo studies, it can be assumed that CYP3A, CYP2E and CYP2C are involved in the metabolism of levonorgestrel. Likewise, inducers or inhibitors of these enzymes may either, respectively, decrease the therapeutic effects or resultin side effects).
No products indexed under this heading.

Troglitazone (Inducers of CYP3A4 may reduce plasma concentrations of estrogens, possibly resulting in a decrease in therapeutic effects and/or changes in the uterine bleeding profile).
No products indexed under this heading.

Troleandomycin (Inhibitors of CYP3A4 such as erythromycin, clarithromycin, ketoconazole, itraconazole, ritonavir and grapefruit juice may increase plasma concentrations of estrogens and may result in side effects).
No products indexed under this heading.

Valproate Sodium (Inhibitors of CYP3A4 such as erythromycin, clarithromycin, ketoconazole, itraconazole, ritonavir and grapefruit juice may increase plasma concentrations of estrogens and may result in side effects).
No products indexed under this heading.

Vardenafil Hydrochloride (Inhibitors of CYP3A4 such as erythromycin, clarithromycin, ketoconazole, itraconazole, ritonavir and grapefruit juice may increase plasma concentrations of estrogens and may result in side effects). Products include:
Levitra 3157

Verapamil Hydrochloride (Inhibitors of CYP3A4 such as erythromycin, clarithromycin, ketoconazole, itraconazole, ritonavir and grapefruit juice may increase plasma concentrations of estrogens and may result in side effects). Products include:
Tarka 534

Voriconazole (Inhibitors of CYP3A4 such as erythromycin, clarithromycin, ketoconazole, itraconazole, ritonavir and grapefruit juice may increase plasma concentrations of estrogens and may result in side effects).
No products indexed under this heading.

Zafirlukast (Inhibitors of CYP3A4 such as erythromycin, clarithromycin, ketoconazole, itraconazole, ritonavir and grapefruit juice may increase plasma concentrations of estrogens and may result in side effects). Products include:
Accolate 3612

Zileuton (Inhibitors of CYP3A4 such as erythromycin, clarithromycin, ketoconazole, itraconazole, ritonavir and grapefruit juice may increase plasma concentrations of estrogens and may result in side effects).
No products indexed under this heading.

Food Interactions

Grapefruit (Inhibitors of CYP3A4 such as erythromycin, clarithromycin, ketoconazole, itraconazole, ritonavir and grapefruit juice may increase plasma concentrations of estrogens and may result in side effects).

Grapefruit Juice (Inhibitors of CYP3A4 such as erythromycin, clarithromycin, ketoconazole, itraconazole, ritonavir and grapefruit juice may increase plasma concentrations of estrogens and may result in side effects).

CLINORIL TABLETS

(Sulindac) 2098
May interact with ACE inhibitors, alcohols, angiotensin-II receptor antagonists, anticoagulants, aspirin-acetylsalicylic acid, corticosteroids, diuretics, lithium preparations, non-steroidal anti-inflammatory agents, oral anticoagulants, oral hypoglycemic agents, thiazides, and certain other agents. Compounds in these categories include:

Acarbose (Studies in which sulindac was given at a dose of 400 mg daily have shown no clinically significant interaction with oral hypoglycemic agents. However, patients should be monitored carefully until it is certain that no change in their hypoglycemic dosage is required. Special attention should be paid to patients taking higher doses than those recommended and to patients with renal impairment or other metabolic defects that might increase sulindac blood levels).
No products indexed under this heading.

Alclometasone Dipropionate (Concomitant use of oral corticosteroids may increase the risk of GI bleeding).
No products indexed under this heading.

Amiloride Hydrochloride (Clinical studies, as well as post-marketing observations, have shown that sulindac can reduce the natriuretic effect of furosemide and thiazides in some patients. This response has been attributed to inhibition of renal prostaglandin synthesis. During concomitant therapy with NSAIDs, the patient should be observed closely for signs of renal failure, as well as to assure diuretic efficacy).
No products indexed under this heading.

Anisindione (Studies in which sulindac was given at a dose of 400 mg daily have shown no clinically significant interaction with oral anticoagulants. However, patients should be monitored carefully until it is certain that no change in their anticoagulant dosage is required. Special attention should be paid to patients taking higher doses than those recommended and to patients with renal impairment or other metabolic defects that might increase sulindac blood levels. In addition, concomitant use of anticoagulants may increase the incidence of GI bleeding).
No products indexed under this heading.

Ardeparin Sodium (Concomitant use of anticoagulants may increase the risk of GI bleeding).
No products indexed under this heading.

Aspirin (The concomitant administration of aspirin with sulindac significantly depressed the plasma levels of the active sulfide metabolite. A double-blind study compared the safety and efficacy of sulindac 300 or 400 mg daily given alone with or alone with aspirin 2.4 g/day for the treatment of osteoarthritis. The addition of aspirin did not alter the types of clinical or laboratory adverse experiences for sulindac; however, the combination showed an increase in the incidence of gastrointestinal adverse experiences. Since the addition of aspirin did not have a favorable effect on the therapeutic response to sulindac, the combination is not recommended). Products include:
Aggrenox 880
Bayer Aspirin 829
Percodan 1124
St. Joseph Aspirin 2045

Aspirin, Enteric Coated (The concomitant administration of aspirin with sulindac significantly depressed the plasma levels of the active sulfide metabolite. A double-blind study compared the safety and efficacy of sulindac 300 or 400 mg daily given alone with or alone with aspirin 2.4 g/day for the treatment of osteoarthritis. The addition of aspirin did not alter the types of clinical or laboratory adverse experiences for sulindac; however, the combination showed an increase in the incidence of gastrointestinal adverse experiences. Since the addition of aspirin did not have a favorable effect on the therapeutic response to sulindac, the combination is not recommended).
No products indexed under this heading.

Aspirin Buffered (The concomitant administration of aspirin with sulindac significantly depressed the plasma levels of the active sulfide metabolite. A double-blind study compared the safety and efficacy of sulindac 300 or 400 mg daily given alone with or alone with aspirin 2.4 g/day for the treatment of osteoarthritis. The addition of aspirin did not alter the types of clinical or laboratory adverse experiences for sulindac; however, the combination showed an increase in the incidence of gastrointestinal adverse experiences. Since the addition of aspirin did not have a favorable effect on the therapeutic response to sulindac, the combination is not recommended).
No products indexed under this heading.

Beclomethasone Dipropionate (Concomitant use of oral corticosteroids may increase the risk of GI bleeding). Products include:
Qvar 3398

Beclomethasone Dipropionate Monohydrate (Concomitant use of oral corticosteroids may increase the risk of GI bleeding). Products include:
Beconase AQ 1386

Benazepril Hydrochloride (Reports suggest that NSAIDs may diminish the antihypertensive effect of ACE-inhibitors. This interaction should be given consideration in patients taking NSAIDS concomitantly with ACE-inhibitors. In some patients with compromised renal function, the co-administration of an NSAID and an ACE-inhibitor may result in further deterioration of renal function, including possible acute renal failure, which is usually reversible).
No products indexed under this heading.

Bendroflumethiazide (Clinical studies, as well as post-marketing observations, have shown that sulindac can reduce the natriuretic effect of thiazides in some patients. This response has been attributed to inhibition of renal prostaglandin synthesis. During concomitant therapy with NSAIDs, the patient should be observed closely for signs of renal failure, as well as to assure diuretic efficacy).
No products indexed under this heading.

Betamethasone (Concomitant use of oral corticosteroids may increase the risk of GI bleeding).
No products indexed under this heading.

Betamethasone Acetate (Concomitant use of oral corticosteroids may increase the risk of GI bleeding).
No products indexed under this heading.

Betamethasone Benzoate (Concomitant use of oral corticosteroids may increase the risk of GI bleeding).
No products indexed under this heading.

Betamethasone Dipropionate (Concomitant use of oral corticosteroids may increase the risk of GI bleeding). Products include:

IMPORTANT NOTE: Always consult each drug listing in the patient's regimen for possible interactions.

Betamethasone Sodium Phosphate (Concomitant use of oral corticosteroids may increase the risk of GI bleeding).
No products indexed under this heading.

Betamethasone Valerate (Concomitant use of oral corticosteroids may increase the risk of GI bleeding). Products include:

Budesonide (Concomitant use of oral corticosteroids may increase the risk of GI bleeding). Products include:

Bumetanide (Clinical studies, as well as post-marketing observations, have shown that sulindac can reduce the natriuretic effect of furosemide and thiazides in some patients. This response has been attributed to inhibition of renal prostaglandin synthesis. During concomitant therapy with NSAIDs, the patient should be observed closely for signs of renal failure, as well as to assure diuretic efficacy).
No products indexed under this heading.

Candesartan Cilexetil (Reports suggest that NSAIDs may diminish the antihypertensive effect of angiotensin II antagonists. This interaction should be given consideration in patients taking NSAIDs concomitantly with angiotensin II antagonists. In some patients with compromised renal function, the co-administration of an NSAID and an angiotensin II antagonist may result in further deterioration of renal function, including possible acute renal failure, which is usually reversible). Products include:

Captopril (Reports suggest that NSAIDs may diminish the antihypertensive effect of ACE-inhibitors. This interaction should be given consideration in patients taking NSAIDS concomitantly with ACE-inhibitors. In some patients with compromised renal function, the co-administration of an NSAID and an ACE-inhibitor may result in further deterioration of renal function, including possible acute renal failure, which is usually reversible). Products include:

Celecoxib (The concomitant use of sulindac with other NSAIDs is not recommended due to the increased possibility of gastrointestinal toxicity, with little or no increase in efficacy). Products include:

Chlorothiazide (Clinical studies, as well as post-marketing observations, have shown that sulindac can reduce the natriuretic effect of thiazides in some patients. This response has been attributed to inhibition of renal prostaglandin synthesis. During concomitant therapy with NSAIDs, the patient should be observed closely for signs of renal failure, as well as to assure diuretic efficacy).
No products indexed under this heading.

Chlorothiazide Sodium (Clinical studies, as well as post-marketing observations, have shown that sulindac can reduce the natriuretic effect of thiazides in some patients. This response has been attributed to inhibition of renal prostaglandin synthesis. During concomitant therapy with NSAIDs, the patient should be observed closely for signs of renal failure, as well as to assure diuretic efficacy). Products include:

Chlorpropamide (Studies in which sulindac was given at a dose of 400 mg daily have shown no clinically significant interaction with oral hypoglycemic agents. However, patients should be monitored carefully until it is certain that no change in their hypoglycemic dosage is required. Special attention should be paid to patients taking higher doses than those recommended and to patients with renal impairment or other metabolic defects that might increase sulindac blood levels).
No products indexed under this heading.

Chlorthalidone (Clinical studies, as well as post-marketing observations, have shown that sulindac can reduce the natriuretic effect of furosemide and thiazides in some patients. This response has been attributed to inhibition of renal prostaglandin synthesis. During concomitant therapy with NSAIDs, the patient should be observed closely for signs of renal failure, as well as to assure diuretic efficacy). Products include:

Ciclesonide (Concomitant use of oral corticosteroids may increase the risk of GI bleeding).
No products indexed under this heading.

Cortisone Acetate (Concomitant use of oral corticosteroids may increase the risk of GI bleeding).
No products indexed under this heading.

Cyclosporine (Administration of non-steroidal anti-inflammatory drugs concomitantly with cyclosporine has been associated with an increase in cyclosporine-induced toxicity, possibly due to decreased synthesis of renal prostacyclin. NSAIDs should be used with caution in patients taking cyclosporine and renal funciton should be carefully monitored). Products include:

Dalteparin Sodium (Concomitant use of anticoagulants may increase the risk of GI bleeding). Products include:

Danaparoid Sodium (Concomitant use of anticoagulants may increase the risk of GI bleeding).
No products indexed under this heading.

Desoximetasone (Concomitant use of oral corticosteroids may increase the risk of GI bleeding).
No products indexed under this heading.

Dexamethasone (Concomitant use of oral corticosteroids may increase the risk of GI bleeding). Products include:

Dexamethasone Acetate (Concomitant use of oral corticosteroids may increase the risk of GI bleeding).
No products indexed under this heading.

Dexamethasone Phosphate (Concomitant use of oral corticosteroids may increase the risk of GI bleeding).
No products indexed under this heading.

Dexamethasone Sodium (Concomitant use of oral corticosteroids may increase the risk of GI bleeding).
No products indexed under this heading.

Dexamethasone Sodium Phosphate (Concomitant use of oral corticosteroids may increase the risk of GI bleeding).
No products indexed under this heading.

Dexamethasone Sodium Phosphate Injection (Concomitant use of oral corticosteroids may increase the risk of GI bleeding).
No products indexed under this heading.

Diclofenac Epolamine (The concomitant use of sulindac with other NSAIDs is not recommended due to the increased possibility of gastrointestinal toxicity, with little or no increase in efficacy). Products include:

Diclofenac Potassium (The concomitant use of sulindac with other NSAIDs is not recommended due to the increased possibility of gastrointestinal toxicity, with little or no increase in efficacy).
No products indexed under this heading.

Diclofenac Sodium (The concomitant use of sulindac with other NSAIDs is not recommended due to the increased possibility of gastrointestinal toxicity, with little or no increase in efficacy).
No products indexed under this heading.

Dicumarol (Studies in which sulindac was given at a dose of 400 mg daily have shown no clinically significant interaction with oral anticoagulants. However, patients should be monitored carefully until it is certain that no change in their anticoagulant dosage is required. Special attention should be paid to patients taking higher doses than those recommended and to patients with renal impairment or other metabolic defects that might increase sulindac blood levels. In addition, concomitant use of anticoagulants may increase the incidence of GI bleeding).
No products indexed under this heading.

Diflorasone Diacetate (Concomitant use of oral corticosteroids may increase the risk of GI bleeding).
No products indexed under this heading.

Diflunisal (The concomitant administration of sulindac and diflunisal in normal volunteers resulted in lowering of the plasma levels of the active sulindac sulfide metabolite by approximately one-third).
No products indexed under this heading.

DMSO (DMSO should not be used with sulindac. Concomitant administration has been reported to reduce the plasma levels of the active sulfide and potentially reduce efficacy. In addition, this combination has been reported to cause peripheral neuropathy).
No products indexed under this heading.

Enalapril Maleate (Reports suggest that NSAIDs may diminish the antihypertensive effect of ACE-inhibitors. This interaction should be given consideration in patients taking NSAIDS concomitantly with ACE-inhibitors. In some patients with compromised renal function, the co-administration of an NSAID and an ACE-inhibitor may result in further deterioration of renal function, including possible acute renal failure, which is usually reversible).
No products indexed under this heading.

Enalaprilat (Reports suggest that NSAIDs may diminish the antihypertensive effect of ACE-inhibitors. This interaction should be given consideration in patients taking NSAIDS concomitantly with ACE-inhibitors. In some patients with compromised renal function, the co-administration of an NSAID and an ACE-inhibitor may result in further deterioration of renal function, including possible acute renal failure, which is usually reversible).
No products indexed under this heading.

Enoxaparin Sodium (Concomitant use of anticoagulants may increase the risk of GI bleeding). Products include:

Eprosartan Mesylate (Reports suggest that NSAIDs may diminish the antihypertensive effect of angiotensin II antagonists. This interaction should be given consideration in patients taking NSAIDS concomitantly with angiotensin

II antagonists. In some patients with compromised renal function, the co-administration of an NSAID and an angiotensin II antagonist may result in further deterioration of renal function, including possible acute renal failure, which is usually reversible). Products include:

Ethacrynic Acid (Clinical studies, as well as post-marketing observations, have shown that sulindac can reduce the natriuretic effect of furosemide and thiazides in some patients. This response has been attributed to inhibition of renal prostaglandin synthesis. During concomitant therapy with NSAIDs, the patient should be observed closely for signs of renal failure, as well as to assure diuretic efficacy).
No products indexed under this heading.

Ethanol (Concomitant use of alcohol may increase the risk of GI bleeding).
No products indexed under this heading.

Ethyl Alcohol (Concomitant use of alcohol may increase the risk of GI bleeding).
No products indexed under this heading.

Etodolac (The concomitant use of sulindac with other NSAIDs is not recommended due to the increased possibility of gastrointestinal toxicity, with little or no increase in efficacy).
No products indexed under this heading.

Fenoprofen Calcium (The concomitant use of sulindac with other NSAIDs is not recommended due to the increased possibility of gastrointestinal toxicity, with little or no increase in efficacy).
No products indexed under this heading.

Fludrocortisone Acetate (Concomitant use of oral corticosteroids may increase the risk of GI bleeding).
No products indexed under this heading.

Flumethasone Pivalate (Concomitant use of oral corticosteroids may increase the risk of GI bleeding).
No products indexed under this heading.

Flunisolide Hemihydrate (Concomitant use of oral corticosteroids may increase the risk of GI bleeding).
No products indexed under this heading.

Flurbiprofen (The concomitant use of sulindac with other NSAIDs is not recommended due to the increased possibility of gastrointestinal toxicity, with little or no increase in efficacy).
No products indexed under this heading.

Fluticasone Furoate (Concomitant use of oral corticosteroids may increase the risk of GI bleeding). Products include:

Fluticasone Propionate (Concomitant use of oral corticosteroids may increase the risk of GI bleeding). Products include:

Fondaparinux Sodium (Concomitant use of anticoagulants may increase the risk of GI bleeding). Products include:

Fosinopril Sodium (Reports suggest that NSAIDs may diminish the antihypertensive effect of ACE-inhibitors. This interaction should be given consideration in patients taking NSAIDS concomitantly with ACE-inhibitors. In some patients with compromised renal function, the co-administration of an NSAID

and an ACE-inhibitor may result in further deterioration of renal function, including possible acute renal failure, which is usually reversible).

No products indexed under this heading.

Furosemide (Clinical studies, as well as post-marketing observations, have shown that sulindac can reduce the natriuretic effect of furosemide in some patients. This response has been attributed to inhibition of renal prostaglandin synthesis. During concomitant therapy with NSAIDs, the patient should be observed closely for signs of renal failure, as well as to assure diuretic efficacy). Products include:

Glibenclamide (Studies in which sulindac was given at a dose of 400 mg daily have shown no clinically significant interaction with oral hypoglycemic agents. However, patients should be monitored carefully until it is certain that no change in their hypoglycemic dosage is required. Special attention should be paid to patients taking higher doses than those recommended and to patients with renal impairment or other metabolic defects that might increase sulindac blood levels).

No products indexed under this heading.

Glimepiride (Studies in which sulindac was given at a dose of 400 mg daily have shown no clinically significant interaction with oral hypoglycemic agents. However, patients should be monitored carefully until it is certain that no change in their hypoglycemic dosage is required. Special attention should be paid to patients taking higher doses than those recommended and to patients with renal impairment or other metabolic defects that might increase sulindac blood levels). Products include:

Glipizide (Studies in which sulindac was given at a dose of 400 mg daily have shown no clinically significant interaction with oral hypoglycemic agents. However, patients should be monitored carefully until it is certain that no change in their hypoglycemic dosage is required. Special attention should be paid to patients taking higher doses than those recommended and to patients with renal impairment or other metabolic defects that might increase sulindac blood levels).

No products indexed under this heading.

Glyburide (Studies in which sulindac was given at a dose of 400 mg daily have shown no clinically significant interaction with oral hypoglycemic agents. However, patients should be monitored carefully until it is certain that no change in their hypoglycemic dosage is required. Special attention should be paid to patients taking higher doses than those recommended and to patients with renal impairment or other metabolic defects that might increase sulindac blood levels).

No products indexed under this heading.

Heparin Calcium (Concomitant use of anticoagulants may increase the risk of GI bleeding).

No products indexed under this heading.

Heparin Sodium (Concomitant use of anticoagulants may increase the risk of GI bleeding).

No products indexed under this heading.

Hydrochlorothiazide (Clinical studies, as well as post-marketing observations, have shown that sulindac can reduce the natriuretic effect of thiazides in some patients. This response has been attributed to inhibition of renal prostaglandin synthesis. During concomitant therapy with NSAIDs, the patient should be observed closely for

signs of renal failure, as well as to assure diuretic efficacy). Products include:

Hydrocortisone (Concomitant use of oral corticosteroids may increase the risk of GI bleeding).

No products indexed under this heading.

Hydrocortisone (Alcohol) (Concomitant use of oral corticosteroids may increase the risk of GI bleeding).

No products indexed under this heading.

Hydrocortisone Acetate (Concomitant use of oral corticosteroids may increase the risk of GI bleeding).

No products indexed under this heading.

Hydrocortisone Butyrate (Concomitant use of oral corticosteroids may increase the risk of GI bleeding).

No products indexed under this heading.

Hydrocortisone Cypionate (Concomitant use of oral corticosteroids may increase the risk of GI bleeding).

No products indexed under this heading.

Hydrocortisone Hemisuccinate (Concomitant use of oral corticosteroids may increase the risk of GI bleeding).

No products indexed under this heading.

Hydrocortisone Probutate (Concomitant use of oral corticosteroids may increase the risk of GI bleeding).

No products indexed under this heading.

Hydrocortisone Sodium Phosphate (Concomitant use of oral corticosteroids may increase the risk of GI bleeding).

No products indexed under this heading.

Hydrocortisone Sodium Succinate (Concomitant use of oral corticosteroids may increase the risk of GI bleeding).

No products indexed under this heading.

Hydrocortisone Valerate (Concomitant use of oral corticosteroids may increase the risk of GI bleeding).

No products indexed under this heading.

Hydroflumethiazide (Clinical studies, as well as post-marketing observations, have shown that sulindac can reduce the natriuretic effect of thiazides in some patients. This response has been attributed to inhibition of renal prostaglandin synthesis. During concomitant therapy with NSAIDs, the patient should be observed closely for signs of renal failure, as well as to assure diuretic efficacy).

No products indexed under this heading.

Ibuprofen (The concomitant use of sulindac with other NSAIDs is not recommended due to the increased possibility of gastrointestinal toxicity, with little or no increase in efficacy). Products include:

Indapamide (Clinical studies, as well as post-marketing observations, have shown that sulindac can reduce the natriuretic effect of furosemide and thiazides in some patients. This response has been attributed to inhibition of renal

prostaglandin synthesis. During concomitant therapy with NSAIDs, the patient should be observed closely for signs of renal failure, as well as to assure diuretic efficacy). Products include:

Indomethacin (The concomitant use of sulindac with other NSAIDs is not recommended due to the increased possibility of gastrointestinal toxicity, with little or no increase in efficacy). Products include:

Indomethacin Sodium Trihydrate (The concomitant use of sulindac with other NSAIDs is not recommended due to the increased possibility of gastrointestinal toxicity, with little or no increase in efficacy). Products include:

Irbesartan (Reports suggest that NSAIDs may diminish the antihypertensive effect of angiotensin II antagonists. This interaction should be given consideration in patients taking NSAIDS concomitantly with angiotensin II antagonists. In some patients with compromised renal function, the co-administration of an NSAID and an angiotensin II antagonist may result in further deterioration of renal function, including possible acute renal failure, which is usually reversible). Products include:

Ketoprofen (The concomitant use of sulindac with other NSAIDs is not recommended due to the increased possibility of gastrointestinal toxicity, with little or no increase in efficacy).

No products indexed under this heading.

Ketorolac Tromethamine (The concomitant use of sulindac with other NSAIDs is not recommended due to the increased possibility of gastrointestinal toxicity, with little or no increase in efficacy). Products include:

Lisinopril (Reports suggest that NSAIDs may diminish the antihypertensive effect of ACE-inhibitors. This interaction should be given consideration in patients taking NSAIDS concomitantly with ACE-inhibitors. In some patients with compromised renal function, the co-administration of an NSAID and an ACE-inhibitor may result in further deterioration of renal function, including possible acute renal failure, which is usually reversible). Products include:

Lithium (NSAIDs have produced an elevation of plasma lithium levels and a reduction in renal lithium clearance. The mean minimum lithium concentration increased 15% and the renal clearance was decreased by approximately 20%. These effects have been attributed to inhibition of renal prostaglandin synthesis by the NSAID. Thus, when NSAIDs and lithium are administered concurrently, subjects should be observed carefully for signs of lithium toxicity).

No products indexed under this heading.

Lithium Carbonate (NSAIDs have produced an elevation of plasma lithium levels and a reduction in renal lithium clearance. The mean minimum lithium concentration increased 15% and the renal clearance was decreased by approximately 20%. These effects have been attributed to inhibition of renal prostaglandin synthesis by the NSAID. Thus, when NSAIDs and lithium are administered concurrently, subjects should be observed carefully for signs of lithium toxicity).

No products indexed under this heading.

Lithium Citrate (NSAIDs have produced an elevation of plasma lithium levels and a reduction in renal lithium clearance. The mean minimum lithium concentration increased 15% and the renal clearance was decreased by approximately 20%. These effects have been attributed to inhibition of renal prostaglandin synthesis by the NSAID. Thus, when NSAIDs and lithium are administered concurrently, subjects should be observed carefully for signs of lithium toxicity).

No products indexed under this heading.

Losartan Potassium (Reports suggest that NSAIDs may diminish the antihypertensive effect of angiotensin II antagonists. This interaction should be given consideration in patients taking NSAIDs concomitantly with angiotensin II antagonists. In some patients with compromised renal function, the co-administration of an NSAID and an angiotensin II antagonist may result in further deterioration of renal function, including possible acute renal failure, which is usually reversible). Products include:

Low Molecular Weight Heparins (Concomitant use of anticoagulants may increase the risk of GI bleeding).

No products indexed under this heading.

Meclofenamate Sodium (The concomitant use of sulindac with other NSAIDs is not recommended due to the increased possibility of gastrointestinal toxicity, with little or no increase in efficacy).

No products indexed under this heading.

Mefenamic Acid (The concomitant use of sulindac with other NSAIDs is not recommended due to the increased possibility of gastrointestinal toxicity, with little or no increase in efficacy).

No products indexed under this heading.

Meloxicam (The concomitant use of sulindac with other NSAIDs is not recommended due to the increased possibility of gastrointestinal toxicity, with little or no increase in efficacy).

No products indexed under this heading.

Metformin Hydrochloride (Studies in which sulindac was given at a dose of 400 mg daily have shown no clinically significant interaction with oral hypoglycemic agents. However, patients should be monitored carefully until it is certain that no change in their hypoglycemic dosage is required. Special attention should be paid to patients taking higher doses than those recommended and to patients with renal impairment or other metabolic defects that might increase sulindac blood levels). Products include:

Methotrexate (Concomitant use could enhance the toxicity of methotrexate. Caution should be used when NSAIDs are administered concomitantly with methotrexate).

No products indexed under this heading.

Methotrexate Sodium (Concomitant use could enhance the toxicity of methotrexate. Caution should be used when NSAIDs are administered concomitantly with methotrexate).

No products indexed under this heading.

Methyclothiazide (Clinical studies, as well as post-marketing observations, have shown that sulindac can reduce the natriuretic effect of thiazides in some patients. This response has been attributed to inhibition of renal prostaglandin synthesis. During concomitant therapy with NSAIDs, the patient should

be observed closely for signs of renal failure, as well as to assure diuretic efficacy).
No products indexed under this heading.

Methylprednisolone (Concomitant use of oral corticosteroids may increase the risk of GI bleeding).
No products indexed under this heading.

Methylprednisolone Acetate (Concomitant use of oral corticosteroids may increase the risk of GI bleeding).
No products indexed under this heading.

Methylprednisolone Sodium Succinate (Concomitant use of oral corticosteroids may increase the risk of GI bleeding).
No products indexed under this heading.

Metolazone (Clinical studies, as well as post-marketing observations, have shown that sulindac can reduce the natriuretic effect of furosemide and thiazides in some patients. This response has been attributed to inhibition of renal prostaglandin synthesis. During concomitant therapy with NSAIDs, the patient should be observed closely for signs of renal failure, as well as to assure diuretic efficacy).
No products indexed under this heading.

Miglitol (Studies in which sulindac was given at a dose of 400 mg daily have shown no clinically significant interaction with oral hypoglycemic agents. However, patients should be monitored carefully until it is certain that no change in their hypoglycemic dosage is required. Special attention should be paid to patients taking higher doses than those recommended and to patients with renal impairment or other metabolic defects that might increase sulindac blood levels).
No products indexed under this heading.

Moexipril Hydrochloride (Reports suggest that NSAIDs may diminish the antihypertensive effect of ACE-inhibitors. This interaction should be given consideration in patients taking NSAIDS concomitantly with ACE-inhibitors. In some patients with compromised renal function, the co-administration of an NSAID and an ACE-inhibitor may result in further deterioration of renal function, including possible acute renal failure, which is usually reversible).
No products indexed under this heading.

Mometasone Furoate (Concomitant use of oral corticosteroids may increase the risk of GI bleeding).
Products include:

Asmanex 3058
Elocon Cream 3111
Elocon Lotion 3112
Elocon Ointment 3114

Mometasone Furoate Monohydrate (Concomitant use of oral corticosteroids may increase the risk of GI bleeding). Products include:

Nasonex 3166

Nabumetone (The concomitant use of sulindac with other NSAIDs is not recommended due to the increased possibility of gastrointestinal toxicity, with little or no increase in efficacy).
No products indexed under this heading.

Naproxen (The concomitant use of sulindac with other NSAIDs is not recommended due to the increased possibility of gastrointestinal toxicity, with little or no increase in efficacy).
Products include:

EC-Naprosyn 2850
Naprosyn 2850
Anaprox/Naprosyn 2850

Naproxen Sodium (The concomitant use of sulindac with other NSAIDs is not recommended due to the increased possibility of gastrointestinal toxicity, with little or no increase in efficacy).
Products include:

Anaprox 2850
Anaprox DS 2850
Treximet 1681

Nateglinide (Studies in which sulindac was given at a dose of 400 mg daily have shown no clinically significant interaction with oral hypoglycemic agents. However, patients should be monitored carefully until it is certain that no change in their hypoglycemic dosage is required. Special attention should be paid to patients taking higher doses than those recommended and to patients with renal impairment or other metabolic defects that might increase sulindac blood levels).
No products indexed under this heading.

Oxaprozin (The concomitant use of sulindac with other NSAIDs is not recommended due to the increased possibility of gastrointestinal toxicity, with little or no increase in efficacy).
No products indexed under this heading.

Perindopril Erbumine (Reports suggest that NSAIDs may diminish the antihypertensive effect of ACE-inhibitors. This interaction should be given consideration in patients taking NSAIDS concomitantly with ACE-inhibitors. In some patients with compromised renal function, the co-administration of an NSAID and an ACE-inhibitor may result in further deterioration of renal function, including possible acute renal failure, which is usually reversible).
No products indexed under this heading.

Phenylbutazone (The concomitant use of sulindac with other NSAIDs is not recommended due to the increased possibility of gastrointestinal toxicity, with little or no increase in efficacy).
No products indexed under this heading.

Pioglitazone Hydrochloride (Studies in which sulindac was given at a dose of 400 mg daily have shown no clinically significant interaction with oral hypoglycemic agents. However, patients should be monitored carefully until it is certain that no change in their hypoglycemic dosage is required. Special attention should be paid to patients taking higher doses than those recommended and to patients with renal impairment or other metabolic defects that might increase sulindac blood levels). Products include:

ActoPlus 3338
Actos 3345
Duetact 3354

Piroxicam (The concomitant use of sulindac with other NSAIDs is not recommended due to the increased possibility of gastrointestinal toxicity, with little or no increase in efficacy).
No products indexed under this heading.

Polythiazide (Clinical studies, as well as post-marketing observations, have shown that sulindac can reduce the natriuretic effect of thiazides in some patients. This response has been attributed to inhibition of renal prostaglandin synthesis. During concomitant therapy with NSAIDs, the patient should be observed closely for signs of renal failure, as well as to assure diuretic efficacy).
No products indexed under this heading.

Prednisolone (Concomitant use of oral corticosteroids may increase the risk of GI bleeding).
No products indexed under this heading.

Prednisolone Acetate (Concomitant use of oral corticosteroids may increase the risk of GI bleeding).
Products include:

Blephamide .... ⊙212, ⊙214
Pred Forte .... ⊙225
Pred Mild .... ⊙230
Pred-G .... ⊙226, ⊙227

Prednisolone Sodium Phosphate (Concomitant use of oral corticosteroids may increase the risk of GI bleeding).
No products indexed under this heading.

Prednisolone Tebutate (Concomitant use of oral corticosteroids may increase the risk of GI bleeding).
No products indexed under this heading.

Prednisone (Concomitant use of oral corticosteroids may increase the risk of GI bleeding).
No products indexed under this heading.

Prednisone sodium phosphate (Concomitant use of oral corticosteroids may increase the risk of GI bleeding).
No products indexed under this heading.

Probenecid (Probenecid given concomitantly with sulindac had only a slight effect on plasma sulfide levels, while plasma levels of sulindac and sulfone were increased. Sulindac was shown to produce a modest reduction in the uricosuric action of probenecid, which probably is not significant under most circumstances).
No products indexed under this heading.

Quinapril Hydrochloride (Reports suggest that NSAIDs may diminish the antihypertensive effect of ACE-inhibitors. This interaction should be given consideration in patients taking NSAIDS concomitantly with ACE-inhibitors. In some patients with compromised renal function, the co-administration of an NSAID and an ACE-inhibitor may result in further deterioration of renal function, including possible acute renal failure, which is usually reversible).
No products indexed under this heading.

Ramipril (Reports suggest that NSAIDs may diminish the antihypertensive effect of ACE-inhibitors. This interaction should be given consideration in patients taking NSAIDS concomitantly with ACE-inhibitors. In some patients with compromised renal function, the co-administration of an NSAID and an ACE-inhibitor may result in further deterioration of renal function, including possible acute renal failure, which is usually reversible).
No products indexed under this heading.

Repaglinide (Studies in which sulindac was given at a dose of 400 mg daily have shown no clinically significant interaction with oral hypoglycemic agents. However, patients should be monitored carefully until it is certain that no change in their hypoglycemic dosage is required. Special attention should be paid to patients taking higher doses than those recommended and to patients with renal impairment or other metabolic defects that might increase sulindac blood levels).
No products indexed under this heading.

Rofecoxib (The concomitant use of sulindac with other NSAIDs is not recommended due to the increased possibility of gastrointestinal toxicity, with little or no increase in efficacy).
No products indexed under this heading.

Rosiglitazone Maleate (Studies in which sulindac was given at a dose of 400 mg daily have shown no clinically significant interaction with oral hypoglycemic agents. However, patients should be monitored carefully until it is certain that no change in their hypoglycemic dosage is required. Special attention should be paid to patients taking higher doses than those recommended and to patients with renal impairment or other metabolic defects that might increase sulindac blood levels). Products include:

Avandamet 1345
Avandaryl 1356
Avandia 1366

Sitagliptin Phosphate (Studies in which sulindac was given at a dose of 400 mg daily have shown no clinically significant interaction with oral hypoglycemic agents. However, patients should be monitored carefully until it is certain that no change in their hypoglycemic dosage is required. Special attention should be paid to patients taking higher doses than those recommended and to patients with renal impairment or other metabolic defects that might increase sulindac blood levels). Products include:

Janumet 2188
Januvia 2196

Spirapril Hydrochloride (Reports suggest that NSAIDs may diminish the antihypertensive effect of ACE-inhibitors. This interaction should be given consideration in patients taking NSAIDS concomitantly with ACE-inhibitors. In some patients with compromised renal function, the co-administration of an NSAID and an ACE-inhibitor may result in further deterioration of renal function, including possible acute renal failure, which is usually reversible).
No products indexed under this heading.

Spironolactone (Clinical studies, as well as post-marketing observations, have shown that sulindac can reduce the natriuretic effect of furosemide and thiazides in some patients. This response has been attributed to inhibition of renal prostaglandin synthesis. During concomitant therapy with NSAIDs, the patient should be observed closely for signs of renal failure, as well as to assure diuretic efficacy).
No products indexed under this heading.

Telmisartan (Reports suggest that NSAIDs may diminish the antihypertensive effect of angiotensin II antagonists. This interaction should be given consideration in patients taking NSAIDS concomitantly with angiotensin II antagonists. In some patients with compromised renal function, the co-administration of an NSAID and an angiotensin II antagonist may result in further deterioration of renal function, including possible acute renal failure, which is usually reversible). Products include:

Micardis 887
Micardis HCT 889

Tinzaparin Sodium (Concomitant use of anticoagulants may increase the risk of GI bleeding).
No products indexed under this heading.

Tolazamide (Studies in which sulindac was given at a dose of 400 mg daily have shown no clinically significant interaction with oral hypoglycemic agents. However, patients should be monitored carefully until it is certain that no change in their hypoglycemic dosage is required. Special attention should be paid to patients taking higher doses than those recommended and to patients with renal impairment or other metabolic defects that might increase sulindac blood levels).
No products indexed under this heading.

Tolbutamide (Studies in which sulindac was given at a dose of 400 mg daily have shown no clinically significant interaction with oral hypoglycemic agents. However, patients should be monitored carefully until it is certain that no change in their hypoglycemic dosage is required. Special attention should be paid to patients taking higher doses than those recommended and to patients with renal impairment or other metabolic defects that might increase sulindac blood levels).
No products indexed under this heading.

(⊙ Described in PDR® for Ophthalmic Medicines)

Tolmetin Sodium (The concomitant use of sulindac with other NSAIDs is not recommended due to the increased possibility of gastrointestinal toxicity, with little or no increase in efficacy). No products indexed under this heading.

Torsemide (Clinical studies, as well as post-marketing observations, have shown that sulindac can reduce the natriuretic effect of furosemide and thiazides in some patients. This response has been attributed to inhibition of renal prostaglandin synthesis. During concomitant therapy with NSAIDs, the patient should be observed closely for signs of renal failure, as well as to assure diuretic efficacy). No products indexed under this heading.

Trandolapril (Reports suggest that NSAIDs may diminish the antihypertensive effect of ACE-inhibitors. This interaction should be given consideration in patients taking NSAIDS concomitantly with ACE-inhibitors. In some patients with compromised renal function, the co-administration of an NSAID and an ACE-inhibitor may result in further deterioration of renal function, including possible acute renal failure, which is usually reversible). Products include:

Triamcinolone (Concomitant use of oral corticosteroids may increase the risk of GI bleeding). No products indexed under this heading.

Triamcinolone Acetonide (Concomitant use of oral corticosteroids may increase the risk of GI bleeding). Products include:

Triamcinolone Diacetate (Concomitant use of oral corticosteroids may increase the risk of GI bleeding). No products indexed under this heading.

Triamcinolone Hexacetonide (Concomitant use of oral corticosteroids may increase the risk of GI bleeding). No products indexed under this heading.

Triamterene (Clinical studies, as well as post-marketing observations, have shown that sulindac can reduce the natriuretic effect of furosemide and thiazides in some patients. This response has been attributed to inhibition of renal prostaglandin synthesis. During concomitant therapy with NSAIDs, the patient should be observed closely for signs of renal failure, as well as to assure diuretic efficacy). Products include:

Troglitazone (Studies in which sulindac was given at a dose of 400 mg daily have shown no clinically significant interaction with oral hypoglycemic agents. However, patients should be monitored carefully until it is certain that no change in their hypoglycemic dosage is required. Special attention should be paid to patients taking higher doses than those recommended and to patients with renal impairment or other metabolic defects that might increase sulindac blood levels). No products indexed under this heading.

Valdecoxib (The concomitant use of sulindac with other NSAIDs is not recommended due to the increased possibility of gastrointestinal toxicity, with little or no increase in efficacy). No products indexed under this heading.

Valsartan (Reports suggest that NSAIDs may diminish the antihypertensive effect of angiotensin II antagonists. This interaction should be given consideration in patients taking NSAIDS concomitantly with angiotensin II antagonists. In some patients with compromised renal function, the co-

administration of an NSAID and an angiotensin II antagonist may result in further deterioration of renal function, including possible acute renal failure, which is usually reversible). Products include:

Warfarin Sodium (Studies in which sulindac was given at a dose of 400 mg daily have shown no clinically significant interaction with oral anticoagulants. However, patients should be monitored carefully until it is certain that no change in their anticoagulant dosage is required. Special attention should be paid to patients taking higher doses than those recommended and to patients with renal impairment or other metabolic defects that might increase sulindac blood levels. The effects of warfarin and NSAIDs on GI bleeding are synergistic, such that users of both drugs together have a risk of serious GI bleeding higher than users of either drug alone). No products indexed under this heading.

Food Interactions

Alcohol (Concomitant use of alcohol may increase the risk of GI bleeding).

Beer, reduced-alcohol (Concomitant use of alcohol may increase the risk of GI bleeding).

Beer, unspecified (Concomitant use of alcohol may increase the risk of GI bleeding).

Wine, Chianti (Concomitant use of alcohol may increase the risk of GI bleeding).

Wine, Red (Concomitant use of alcohol may increase the risk of GI bleeding).

Wine, unspecified (Concomitant use of alcohol may increase the risk of GI bleeding).

Wine products (Concomitant use of alcohol may increase the risk of GI bleeding).

CLOLAR FOR INTRAVENOUS INFUSION

(Clofarabine) 1234
May interact with antibiotics, antihypertensives, hepatotoxic drugs, nephrotoxic agents, and certain other agents. Compounds in these categories include:

Abacavir Sulfate (Nephrotoxic medications may contribute to renal toxicity in patients taking clofarabine. Patients should avoid medications including over the counter and herbal medications, which may be nephrotoxic, during the 5 days of clofarabine administration). Products include:

Acebutolol Hydrochloride (Patients taking medications known to affect blood pressure should be monitored during administration of clofarabine). No products indexed under this heading.

Acyclovir (Nephrotoxic medications may contribute to renal toxicity in patients taking clofarabine. Patients should avoid medications including over the counter and herbal medications, which may be nephrotoxic, during the 5 days of clofarabine administration). Products include:

Acyclovir Sodium (Nephrotoxic medications may contribute to renal toxicity in patients taking clofarabine. Patients should avoid medications including over the counter and herbal medications, which may be nephrotoxic, during the 5 days of clofarabine administration). No products indexed under this heading.

Alatrofloxacin Mesylate (Nephrotoxic medications may contribute to renal toxicity in patients taking clofarabine. Patients should avoid medications including over the counter and herbal medications, which may be nephrotoxic, during the 5 days of clofarabine administration). No products indexed under this heading.

Aldesleukin (Nephrotoxic medications may contribute to renal toxicity in patients taking clofarabine. Patients should avoid medications including over the counter and herbal medications, which may be nephrotoxic, during the 5 days of clofarabine administration). Products include:

Aliskiren (Patients taking medications known to affect blood pressure should be monitored during administration of clofarabine). Products include:

Allopurinol (Occurrences of Stevens-Johnson Syndrome (SJS) and toxic epidermal necrolysis (TEN) have been reported in patients who were receiving or had recently been treated with clofarabine and other medications (eg, allopurinol) known to cause these syndromes). No products indexed under this heading.

Allopurinol Sodium (Occurrences of Stevens-Johnson Syndrome (SJS) and toxic epidermal necrolysis (TEN) have been reported in patients who were receiving or had recently been treated with clofarabine and other medications (eg, allopurinol) known to cause these syndromes). No products indexed under this heading.

Amikacin Sulfate (Nephrotoxic medications may contribute to renal toxicity in patients taking clofarabine. Patients should avoid medications including over the counter and herbal medications, which may be nephrotoxic, during the 5 days of clofarabine administration). No products indexed under this heading.

Amiodarone Hydrochloride (Patients should avoid medications, including over the counter and herbal medications, which may be hepatotoxic, during the 5 days of clofarabine administration). No products indexed under this heading.

Amitriptyline Hydrochloride (Patients should avoid medications, including over the counter and herbal medications, which may be hepatotoxic, during the 5 days of clofarabine administration). No products indexed under this heading.

Amlodipine Besylate (Patients taking medications known to affect blood pressure should be monitored during administration of clofarabine). Products include:

Amoxapine (Patients should avoid medications, including over the counter and herbal medications, which may be hepatotoxic, during the 5 days of clofarabine administration). No products indexed under this heading.

Amoxicillin (Nephrotoxic medications may contribute to renal toxicity in patients taking clofarabine. Patients should avoid medications including over

the counter and herbal medications, which may be nephrotoxic, during the 5 days of clofarabine administration). Products include:

Amoxicillin Trihydrate (Nephrotoxic medications may contribute to renal toxicity in patients taking clofarabine. Patients should avoid medications including over the counter and herbal medications, which may be nephrotoxic, during the 5 days of clofarabine administration). No products indexed under this heading.

Amphotericin B (Nephrotoxic medications may contribute to renal toxicity in patients taking clofarabine. Patients should avoid medications including over the counter and herbal medications, which may be nephrotoxic, during the 5 days of clofarabine administration). No products indexed under this heading.

Amphotericin B, liposomal (Nephrotoxic medications may contribute to renal toxicity in patients taking clofarabine. Patients should avoid medications including over the counter and herbal medications, which may be nephrotoxic, during the 5 days of clofarabine administration). Products include:

Amphotericin B Cholesteryl Sulfate (Nephrotoxic medications may contribute to renal toxicity in patients taking clofarabine. Patients should avoid medications including over the counter and herbal medications, which may be nephrotoxic, during the 5 days of clofarabine administration). No products indexed under this heading.

Amphotericin B Lipid Complex (Nephrotoxic medications may contribute to renal toxicity in patients taking clofarabine. Patients should avoid medications including over the counter and herbal medications, which may be nephrotoxic, during the 5 days of clofarabine administration). No products indexed under this heading.

Ampicillin (Nephrotoxic medications may contribute to renal toxicity in patients taking clofarabine. Patients should avoid medications including over the counter and herbal medications, which may be nephrotoxic, during the 5 days of clofarabine administration). No products indexed under this heading.

Ampicillin Sodium (Nephrotoxic medications may contribute to renal toxicity in patients taking clofarabine. Patients should avoid medications including over the counter and herbal medications, which may be nephrotoxic, during the 5 days of clofarabine administration). No products indexed under this heading.

Ampicillin Trihydrate (Nephrotoxic medications may contribute to renal toxicity in patients taking clofarabine. Patients should avoid medications including over the counter and herbal medications, which may be nephrotoxic, during the 5 days of clofarabine administration). No products indexed under this heading.

Amprenavir (Nephrotoxic medications may contribute to renal toxicity in patients taking clofarabine. Patients should avoid medications including over the counter and herbal medications, which may be nephrotoxic, during the 5 days of clofarabine administration). No products indexed under this heading.

Antibiotics, non-penicillin, unspecified (Occurrences of Stevens-Johnson Syndrome (SJS) and toxic epidermal necrolysis (TEN) have been reported in patients who were receiving or had recently been treated with clofarabine and other medications (eg, antibiotics) known to cause these syndromes).
No products indexed under this heading.

Aspirin (Nephrotoxic medications may contribute to renal toxicity in patients taking clofarabine. Patients should avoid medications including over the counter and herbal medications, which may be nephrotoxic, during the 5 days of clofarabine administration). Products include:
Aggrenox 880
Bayer Aspirin 829
Percodan 1124
St. Joseph Aspirin 2045

Atazanavir (Nephrotoxic medications may contribute to renal toxicity in patients taking clofarabine. Patients should avoid medications including over the counter and herbal medications, which may be nephrotoxic, during the 5 days of clofarabine administration).
No products indexed under this heading.

Atazanavir Sulfate (Patients should avoid medications, including over the counter and herbal medications, which may be hepatotoxic, during the 5 days of clofarabine administration).
No products indexed under this heading.

Atenolol (Patients taking medications known to affect blood pressure should be monitored during administration of clofarabine).
No products indexed under this heading.

Atorvastatin Calcium (Nephrotoxic medications may contribute to renal toxicity in patients taking clofarabine. Patients should avoid medications including over the counter and herbal medications, which may be nephrotoxic, during the 5 days of clofarabine administration). Products include:
Lipitor 2703

Azathioprine (Patients should avoid medications, including over the counter and herbal medications, which may be hepatotoxic, during the 5 days of clofarabine administration).
No products indexed under this heading.

Azathioprine Sodium (Patients should avoid medications, including over the counter and herbal medications, which may be hepatotoxic, during the 5 days of clofarabine administration).
No products indexed under this heading.

Azithromycin Dihydrate (Nephrotoxic medications may contribute to renal toxicity in patients taking clofarabine. Patients should avoid medications including over the counter and herbal medications, which may be nephrotoxic, during the 5 days of clofarabine administration).
No products indexed under this heading.

Azlocillin Sodium (Nephrotoxic medications may contribute to renal toxicity in patients taking clofarabine. Patients should avoid medications including over the counter and herbal medications, which may be nephrotoxic, during the 5 days of clofarabine administration).
No products indexed under this heading.

Aztreonam (Nephrotoxic medications may contribute to renal toxicity in patients taking clofarabine. Patients should avoid medications including over the counter and herbal medications, which may be nephrotoxic, during the 5 days of clofarabine administration).
No products indexed under this heading.

Bacampicillin Hydrochloride (Nephrotoxic medications may contribute to renal toxicity in patients taking clofarabine. Patients should avoid medications including over the counter and herbal medications, which may be nephrotoxic, during the 5 days of clofarabine administration).
No products indexed under this heading.

Bacitracin (Nephrotoxic medications may contribute to renal toxicity in patients taking clofarabine. Patients should avoid medications including over the counter and herbal medications, which may be nephrotoxic, during the 5 days of clofarabine administration).
No products indexed under this heading.

Bacitracin Zinc (Nephrotoxic medications may contribute to renal toxicity in patients taking clofarabine. Patients should avoid medications including over the counter and herbal medications, which may be nephrotoxic, during the 5 days of clofarabine administration).
No products indexed under this heading.

Balsalazide Disodium (Nephrotoxic medications may contribute to renal toxicity in patients taking clofarabine. Patients should avoid medications including over the counter and herbal medications, which may be nephrotoxic, during the 5 days of clofarabine administration).
No products indexed under this heading.

Benazepril Hydrochloride (Nephrotoxic medications may contribute to renal toxicity in patients taking clofarabine. Patients should avoid medications including over the counter and herbal medications, which may be nephrotoxic, during the 5 days of clofarabine administration).
No products indexed under this heading.

Bendroflumethiazide (Nephrotoxic medications may contribute to renal toxicity in patients taking clofarabine. Patients should avoid medications including over the counter and herbal medications, which may be nephrotoxic, during the 5 days of clofarabine administration).
No products indexed under this heading.

Betaxolol Hydrochloride (Patients taking medications known to affect blood pressure should be monitored during administration of clofarabine).
No products indexed under this heading.

Bisoprolol Fumarate (Patients taking medications known to affect blood pressure should be monitored during administration of clofarabine).
No products indexed under this heading.

Bupropion (Patients should avoid medications, including over the counter and herbal medications, which may be hepatotoxic, during the 5 days of clofarabine administration).
No products indexed under this heading.

Bupropion Hydrochloride (Patients should avoid medications, including over the counter and herbal medications, which may be hepatotoxic, during the 5 days of clofarabine administration). Products include:
Aplenzin 2948
Wellbutrin 1719
Wellbutrin SR 1725
Zyban 1762

Busulfan (Serious hepatotoxic adverse reactions of veno-occlusive disease have been reported in adult patients following hematopoietic stem cell transplant. These patients received conditioning regimens that included busulfan, melphalan, and/or the combination of cyclophosphamide and total body irradiation). Products include:
Myleran 1581

Caffeine (Nephrotoxic medications may contribute to renal toxicity in patients taking clofarabine. Patients should avoid medications including over the counter and herbal medications, which may be nephrotoxic, during the 5 days of clofarabine administration).
No products indexed under this heading.

Candesartan Cilexetil (Patients taking medications known to affect blood pressure should be monitored during administration of clofarabine). Products include:
Atacand 697
Atacand HCT 700

Captopril (Nephrotoxic medications may contribute to renal toxicity in patients taking clofarabine. Patients should avoid medications including over the counter and herbal medications, which may be nephrotoxic, during the 5 days of clofarabine administration). Products include:
Captopril 2341

Carbamazepine (Patients should avoid medications, including over the counter and herbal medications, which may be hepatotoxic, during the 5 days of clofarabine administration). Products include:
Carbatrol 3280
Equetro 3477

Carbenicillin Disodium (Nephrotoxic medications may contribute to renal toxicity in patients taking clofarabine. Patients should avoid medications including over the counter and herbal medications, which may be nephrotoxic, during the 5 days of clofarabine administration).
No products indexed under this heading.

Carbenicillin Indanyl Sodium (Nephrotoxic medications may contribute to renal toxicity in patients taking clofarabine. Patients should avoid medications including over the counter and herbal medications, which may be nephrotoxic, during the 5 days of clofarabine administration).
No products indexed under this heading.

Carboplatin (Nephrotoxic medications may contribute to renal toxicity in patients taking clofarabine. Patients should avoid medications including over the counter and herbal medications, which may be nephrotoxic, during the 5 days of clofarabine administration).
No products indexed under this heading.

Carmustine (BCNU) (Nephrotoxic medications may contribute to renal toxicity in patients taking clofarabine. Patients should avoid medications including over the counter and herbal medications, which may be nephrotoxic, during the 5 days of clofarabine administration).
No products indexed under this heading.

Carteolol Hydrochloride (Patients taking medications known to affect blood pressure should be monitored during administration of clofarabine).
No products indexed under this heading.

Carvedilol (Patients taking medications known to affect blood pressure should be monitored during administration of clofarabine). Products include:
Coreg 1409

Carvedilol Phosphate (Patients taking medications known to affect blood pressure should be monitored during administration of clofarabine). Products include:
Coreg CR 1416

Cefaclor (Nephrotoxic medications may contribute to renal toxicity in patients taking clofarabine. Patients should avoid medications including over the counter and herbal medications, which may be nephrotoxic, during the 5 days of clofarabine administration).
No products indexed under this heading.

Cefadroxil (Nephrotoxic medications may contribute to renal toxicity in patients taking clofarabine. Patients should avoid medications including over the counter and herbal medications, which may be nephrotoxic, during the 5 days of clofarabine administration).
No products indexed under this heading.

Cefamandole Nafate (Nephrotoxic medications may contribute to renal toxicity in patients taking clofarabine. Patients should avoid medications including over the counter and herbal medications, which may be nephrotoxic, during the 5 days of clofarabine administration).
No products indexed under this heading.

Cefazolin Sodium (Nephrotoxic medications may contribute to renal toxicity in patients taking clofarabine. Patients should avoid medications including over the counter and herbal medications, which may be nephrotoxic, during the 5 days of clofarabine administration).
No products indexed under this heading.

Cefdinir (Nephrotoxic medications may contribute to renal toxicity in patients taking clofarabine. Patients should avoid medications including over the counter and herbal medications, which may be nephrotoxic, during the 5 days of clofarabine administration). Products include:
Omnicef Capsules 518
Omnicef Oral Suspension 518

Cefepime Hydrochloride (Nephrotoxic medications may contribute to renal toxicity in patients taking clofarabine. Patients should avoid medications including over the counter and herbal medications, which may be nephrotoxic, during the 5 days of clofarabine administration).
No products indexed under this heading.

Cefixime (Nephrotoxic medications may contribute to renal toxicity in patients taking clofarabine. Patients should avoid medications including over the counter and herbal medications, which may be nephrotoxic, during the 5 days of clofarabine administration). Products include:
Suprax for Oral Suspension 2038
Suprax Tablets 2038

Cefmetazole Sodium (Nephrotoxic medications may contribute to renal toxicity in patients taking clofarabine. Patients should avoid medications including over the counter and herbal medications, which may be nephrotoxic, during the 5 days of clofarabine administration).
No products indexed under this heading.

Cefonicid Sodium (Nephrotoxic medications may contribute to renal toxicity in patients taking clofarabine. Patients should avoid medications including over the counter and herbal medications, which may be nephrotoxic, during the 5 days of clofarabine administration).
No products indexed under this heading.

Cefoperazone Sodium (Nephrotoxic medications may contribute to renal toxicity in patients taking clofarabine. Patients should avoid medications including over the counter and herbal medications, which may be nephrotoxic, during the 5 days of clofarabine administration).
No products indexed under this heading.

Ceforanide (Nephrotoxic medications may contribute to renal toxicity in patients taking clofarabine. Patients should avoid medications including over the counter and herbal medications, which may be nephrotoxic, during the 5 days of clofarabine administration).
No products indexed under this heading.

369 Interactions Index Clolar

Cefotaxime Sodium (Nephrotoxic medications may contribute to renal toxicity in patients taking clofarabine. Patients should avoid medications including over the counter and herbal medications, which may be nephrotoxic, during the 5 days of clofarabine administration).
No products indexed under this heading.

Cefotetan (Nephrotoxic medications may contribute to renal toxicity in patients taking clofarabine. Patients should avoid medications including over the counter and herbal medications, which may be nephrotoxic, during the 5 days of clofarabine administration).
No products indexed under this heading.

Cefoxitin Sodium (Nephrotoxic medications may contribute to renal toxicity in patients taking clofarabine. Patients should avoid medications including over the counter and herbal medications, which may be nephrotoxic, during the 5 days of clofarabine administration).
No products indexed under this heading.

Cefpodoxime Proxetil (Nephrotoxic medications may contribute to renal toxicity in patients taking clofarabine. Patients should avoid medications including over the counter and herbal medications, which may be nephrotoxic, during the 5 days of clofarabine administration).
No products indexed under this heading.

Cefprozil (Nephrotoxic medications may contribute to renal toxicity in patients taking clofarabine. Patients should avoid medications including over the counter and herbal medications, which may be nephrotoxic, during the 5 days of clofarabine administration).
No products indexed under this heading.

Ceftazidime (Nephrotoxic medications may contribute to renal toxicity in patients taking clofarabine. Patients should avoid medications including over the counter and herbal medications, which may be nephrotoxic, during the 5 days of clofarabine administration). Products include:
Fortaz 1481

Ceftizoxime Sodium (Nephrotoxic medications may contribute to renal toxicity in patients taking clofarabine. Patients should avoid medications including over the counter and herbal medications, which may be nephrotoxic, during the 5 days of clofarabine administration).
No products indexed under this heading.

Ceftriaxone Sodium (Nephrotoxic medications may contribute to renal toxicity in patients taking clofarabine. Patients should avoid medications including over the counter and herbal medications, which may be nephrotoxic, during the 5 days of clofarabine administration). Products include:
Rocephin 2859

Cefuroxime Axetil (Nephrotoxic medications may contribute to renal toxicity in patients taking clofarabine. Patients should avoid medications including over the counter and herbal medications, which may be nephrotoxic, during the 5 days of clofarabine administration). Products include:
Ceftin 1399

Cefuroxime Sodium (Nephrotoxic medications may contribute to renal toxicity in patients taking clofarabine. Patients should avoid medications including over the counter and herbal medications, which may be nephrotoxic, during the 5 days of clofarabine administration).
No products indexed under this heading.

Celecoxib (Nephrotoxic medications may contribute to renal toxicity in patients taking clofarabine. Patients should avoid medications including over the counter and herbal medications, which may be nephrotoxic, during the 5 days of clofarabine administration). Products include:
Celebrex 3272

Cephalexin (Nephrotoxic medications may contribute to renal toxicity in patients taking clofarabine. Patients should avoid medications including over the counter and herbal medications, which may be nephrotoxic, during the 5 days of clofarabine administration).
No products indexed under this heading.

Cephalothin Sodium (Nephrotoxic medications may contribute to renal toxicity in patients taking clofarabine. Patients should avoid medications including over the counter and herbal medications, which may be nephrotoxic, during the 5 days of clofarabine administration).
No products indexed under this heading.

Cephapirin Sodium (Nephrotoxic medications may contribute to renal toxicity in patients taking clofarabine. Patients should avoid medications including over the counter and herbal medications, which may be nephrotoxic, during the 5 days of clofarabine administration).
No products indexed under this heading.

Cephradine (Nephrotoxic medications may contribute to renal toxicity in patients taking clofarabine. Patients should avoid medications including over the counter and herbal medications, which may be nephrotoxic, during the 5 days of clofarabine administration).
No products indexed under this heading.

Cerivastatin Sodium (Nephrotoxic medications may contribute to renal toxicity in patients taking clofarabine. Patients should avoid medications including over the counter and herbal medications, which may be nephrotoxic, during the 5 days of clofarabine administration).
No products indexed under this heading.

Chloramphenicol (Occurrences of Stevens-Johnson Syndrome (SJS) and toxic epidermal necrolysis (TEN) have been reported in patients who were receiving or had recently been treated with clofarabine and other medications (eg, antibiotics) known to cause these syndromes).
No products indexed under this heading.

Chloramphenicol Palmitate (Occurrences of Stevens-Johnson Syndrome (SJS) and toxic epidermal necrolysis (TEN) have been reported in patients who were receiving or had recently been treated with clofarabine and other medications (eg, antibiotics) known to cause these syndromes).
No products indexed under this heading.

Chloramphenicol Sodium Succinate (Occurrences of Stevens-Johnson Syndrome (SJS) and toxic epidermal necrolysis (TEN) have been reported in patients who were receiving or had recently been treated with clofarabine and other medications (eg, antibiotics) known to cause these syndromes).
No products indexed under this heading.

Chlorothiazide (Nephrotoxic medications may contribute to renal toxicity in patients taking clofarabine. Patients should avoid medications including over the counter and herbal medications, which may be nephrotoxic, during the 5 days of clofarabine administration).
No products indexed under this heading.

Chlorothiazide Sodium (Nephrotoxic medications may contribute to renal toxicity in patients taking clofarabine. Patients should avoid medications including over the counter and herbal medications, which may be nephrotoxic, during the 5 days of clofarabine administration). Products include:
Diuril Intravenous 2009

Chlorpromazine (Patients should avoid medications, including over the counter and herbal medications, which may be hepatotoxic, during the 5 days of clofarabine administration).
No products indexed under this heading.

Chlorpromazine Hydrochloride (Patients should avoid medications, including over the counter and herbal medications, which may be hepatotoxic, during the 5 days of clofarabine administration).
No products indexed under this heading.

Chlorpropamide (Nephrotoxic medications may contribute to renal toxicity in patients taking clofarabine. Patients should avoid medications including over the counter and herbal medications, which may be nephrotoxic, during the 5 days of clofarabine administration).
No products indexed under this heading.

Chlorthalidone (Patients taking medications known to affect blood pressure should be monitored during administration of clofarabine). Products include:
Clorpres 2344

Cidofovir (Nephrotoxic medications may contribute to renal toxicity in patients taking clofarabine. Patients should avoid medications including over the counter and herbal medications, which may be nephrotoxic, during the 5 days of clofarabine administration).
No products indexed under this heading.

Cilastatin Sodium (Nephrotoxic medications may contribute to renal toxicity in patients taking clofarabine. Patients should avoid medications including over the counter and herbal medications, which may be nephrotoxic, during the 5 days of clofarabine administration).
Products include:
Primaxin I.M. 2232
Primaxin I.V. 2235

Cimetidine (Nephrotoxic medications may contribute to renal toxicity in patients taking clofarabine. Patients should avoid medications including over the counter and herbal medications, which may be nephrotoxic, during the 5 days of clofarabine administration).
No products indexed under this heading.

Cimetidine Hydrochloride (Nephrotoxic medications may contribute to renal toxicity in patients taking clofarabine. Patients should avoid medications including over the counter and herbal medications, which may be nephrotoxic, during the 5 days of clofarabine administration).
No products indexed under this heading.

Ciprofloxacin (Occurrences of Stevens-Johnson Syndrome (SJS) and toxic epidermal necrolysis (TEN) have been reported in patients who were receiving or had recently been treated with clofarabine and other medications (eg, antibiotics) known to cause these syndromes). Products include:
Cipro I.V. 3082
Cipro 3073
Cipro XR 3091
Ciprodex 583

Ciprofloxacin Hydrochloride (Occurrences of Stevens-Johnson Syndrome (SJS) and toxic epidermal necrolysis (TEN) have been reported in patients who were receiving or had recently been treated with clofarabine and other medications (eg, antibiotics) known to cause these syndromes).
Products include:
Cipro 3073

Cisplatin (Nephrotoxic medications may contribute to renal toxicity in patients taking clofarabine. Patients should avoid medications including over the counter and herbal medications, which may be nephrotoxic, during the 5 days of clofarabine administration).
No products indexed under this heading.

Cladribine (Nephrotoxic medications may contribute to renal toxicity in patients taking clofarabine. Patients should avoid medications including over the counter and herbal medications, which may be nephrotoxic, during the 5 days of clofarabine administration).
Products include:
Leustatin 946

Clarithromycin (Occurrences of Stevens-Johnson Syndrome (SJS) and toxic epidermal necrolysis (TEN) have been reported in patients who were receiving or had recently been treated with clofarabine and other medications (eg, antibiotics) known to cause these syndromes). Products include:
Biaxin/Biaxin XL 412

Clomipramine Hydrochloride (Patients should avoid medications, including over the counter and herbal medications, which may be hepatotoxic, during the 5 days of clofarabine administration).
No products indexed under this heading.

Clonidine (Patients taking medications known to affect blood pressure should be monitored during administration of clofarabine). Products include:
Catapres-TTS 884

Clonidine Hydrochloride (Patients taking medications known to affect blood pressure should be monitored during administration of clofarabine).
Products include:
Clorpres 2344

Clotrimazole (Occurrences of Stevens-Johnson Syndrome (SJS) and toxic epidermal necrolysis (TEN) have been reported in patients who were receiving or had recently been treated with clofarabine and other medications (eg, antibiotics) known to cause these syndromes). Products include:
Lotrisone 3163

Cloxacillin (Patients should avoid medications, including over the counter and herbal medications, which may be hepatotoxic, during the 5 days of clofarabine administration).
No products indexed under this heading.

Cloxacillin Sodium (Patients should avoid medications, including over the counter and herbal medications, which may be hepatotoxic, during the 5 days of clofarabine administration).
No products indexed under this heading.

Cloxacillin Sodium Monohydrate (Patients should avoid medications, including over the counter and herbal medications, which may be hepatotoxic, during the 5 days of clofarabine administration).
No products indexed under this heading.

Clozapine (Nephrotoxic medications may contribute to renal toxicity in patients taking clofarabine. Patients should avoid medications including over the counter and herbal medications, which may be nephrotoxic, during the 5 days of clofarabine administration).
No products indexed under this heading.

Colistimethate Sodium (Nephrotoxic medications may contribute to renal toxicity in patients taking clofarabine. Patients should avoid medications including over the counter and herbal medications, which may be nephrotoxic, during the 5 days of clofarabine administration).
No products indexed under this heading.

Colistin Sulfate (Nephrotoxic medications may contribute to renal toxicity in patients taking clofarabine. Patients should avoid medications including over the counter and herbal medications, which may be nephrotoxic, during the 5 days of clofarabine administration).
No products indexed under this heading.

Cyclophosphamide (Patients who have previously received a hematopo-

Clolar Interactions Index 370

etic stem cell transplant may be at higher risk for hepatotoxicity suggestive of veno-occlusive disease following treatment with clofarabine (40 mg/m^2) when used in combination with etoposide (100 mg/m^2) and cyclophosphamide (440 mg/m^2). In addition, serious hepatotoxic adverse reactions of veno-occlusive disease have been reported in adult patients following hematopoietic stem cell transplant; these patients received conditioning regimens that included busulfan, melphalan, and/or the combination of cyclophosphamide and total body irradiation).
No products indexed under this heading.

Cyclosporine (Nephrotoxic medications may contribute to renal toxicity in patients taking clofarabine. Patients should avoid medications including over the counter and herbal medications, which may be nephrotoxic, during the 5 days of clofarabine administration).
Products include:
Gengraf 440
Neoral Oral Solution 2496
Neoral Capsules 2496
Restasis 605

Cytarabine (Nephrotoxic medications may contribute to renal toxicity in patients taking clofarabine. Patients should avoid medications including over the counter and herbal medications, which may be nephrotoxic, during the 5 days of clofarabine administration).
No products indexed under this heading.

Cytarabine Liposome (Nephrotoxic medications may contribute to renal toxicity in patients taking clofarabine. Patients should avoid medications including over the counter and herbal medications, which may be nephrotoxic, during the 5 days of clofarabine administration).
No products indexed under this heading.

Darunavir (Patients should avoid medications, including over the counter and herbal medications, which may be hepatotoxic, during the 5 days of clofarabine administration).
No products indexed under this heading.

Daunorubicin Hydrochloride (Occurrences of Stevens-Johnson Syndrome (SJS) and toxic epidermal necrolysis (TEN) have been reported in patients who were receiving or had recently been treated with clofarabine and other medications (eg, antibiotics) known to cause these syndromes).
No products indexed under this heading.

Delavirdine Mesylate (Nephrotoxic medications may contribute to renal toxicity in patients taking clofarabine. Patients should avoid medications including over the counter and herbal medications, which may be nephrotoxic, during the 5 days of clofarabine administration).
No products indexed under this heading.

Demeclocycline Hydrochloride (Patients should avoid medications, including over the counter and herbal medications, which may be hepatotoxic, during the 5 days of clofarabine administration).
No products indexed under this heading.

Deserpidine (Patients taking medications known to affect blood pressure should be monitored during administration of clofarabine).
No products indexed under this heading.

Desipramine Hydrochloride (Patients should avoid medications, including over the counter and herbal medications, which may be hepatotoxic, during the 5 days of clofarabine administration).
No products indexed under this heading.

Diatrizoate Meglumine (Nephrotoxic medications may contribute to renal toxicity in patients taking clofarabine. Patients should avoid medications including over the counter and herbal medications, which may be nephrotoxic, during the 5 days of clofarabine administration).
No products indexed under this heading.

Diatrizoate Sodium (Nephrotoxic medications may contribute to renal toxicity in patients taking clofarabine. Patients should avoid medications including over the counter and herbal medications, which may be nephrotoxic, during the 5 days of clofarabine administration).
No products indexed under this heading.

Diazoxide (Patients taking medications known to affect blood pressure should be monitored during administration of clofarabine). Products include:
Proglycem 1179
Proglycem Suspension 1179

Diclofenac Epolamine (Patients should avoid medications, including over the counter and herbal medications, which may be hepatotoxic, during the 5 days of clofarabine administration). Products include:
Flector 1839

Diclofenac Potassium (Nephrotoxic medications may contribute to renal toxicity in patients taking clofarabine. Patients should avoid medications including over the counter and herbal medications, which may be nephrotoxic, during the 5 days of clofarabine administration).
No products indexed under this heading.

Diclofenac Sodium (Nephrotoxic medications may contribute to renal toxicity in patients taking clofarabine. Patients should avoid medications including over the counter and herbal medications, which may be nephrotoxic, during the 5 days of clofarabine administration).
No products indexed under this heading.

Dicloxacillin (Patients should avoid medications, including over the counter and herbal medications, which may be hepatotoxic, during the 5 days of clofarabine administration).
No products indexed under this heading.

Dicloxacillin Sodium (Nephrotoxic medications may contribute to renal toxicity in patients taking clofarabine. Patients should avoid medications including over the counter and herbal medications, which may be nephrotoxic, during the 5 days of clofarabine administration).
No products indexed under this heading.

Didanosine (Nephrotoxic medications may contribute to renal toxicity in patients taking clofarabine. Patients should avoid medications including over the counter and herbal medications, which may be nephrotoxic, during the 5 days of clofarabine administration).
No products indexed under this heading.

Diltiazem Hydrochloride (Patients taking medications known to affect blood pressure should be monitored during administration of clofarabine).
Products include:
Cardizem LA 423

Diltiazem Maleate (Patients taking medications known to affect blood pressure should be monitored during administration of clofarabine).
No products indexed under this heading.

Dirithromycin (Occurrences of Stevens-Johnson Syndrome (SJS) and toxic epidermal necrolysis (TEN) have been reported in patients who were receiving or had recently been treated with clofarabine and other medications (eg, antibiotics) known to cause these syndromes).
No products indexed under this heading.

Disodium Carbenicillin (Patients should avoid medications, including over the counter and herbal medications, which may be hepatotoxic, during the 5 days of clofarabine administration).
No products indexed under this heading.

Divalproex Sodium (Patients should avoid medications, including over the counter and herbal medications, which may be hepatotoxic, during the 5 days of clofarabine administration). Products include:
Depakote ER 426

Doxazosin Mesylate (Patients taking medications known to affect blood pressure should be monitored during administration of clofarabine).
No products indexed under this heading.

Doxepin Hydrochloride (Patients should avoid medications, including over the counter and herbal medications, which may be hepatotoxic, during the 5 days of clofarabine administration).
No products indexed under this heading.

Doxycycline (Patients should avoid medications, including over the counter and herbal medications, which may be hepatotoxic, during the 5 days of clofarabine administration).
No products indexed under this heading.

Doxycycline Calcium (Patients should avoid medications, including over the counter and herbal medications, which may be hepatotoxic, during the 5 days of clofarabine administration).
No products indexed under this heading.

Doxycycline Hyclate (Patients should avoid medications, including over the counter and herbal medications, which may be hepatotoxic, during the 5 days of clofarabine administration).
No products indexed under this heading.

Doxycycline Monohydrate (Patients should avoid medications, including over the counter and herbal medications, which may be hepatotoxic, during the 5 days of clofarabine administration).
No products indexed under this heading.

Duloxetine Hydrochloride (Patients should avoid medications, including over the counter and herbal medications, which may be hepatotoxic, during the 5 days of clofarabine administration). Products include:
Cymbalta 1871

Efavirenz (Nephrotoxic medications may contribute to renal toxicity in patients taking clofarabine. Patients should avoid medications including over the counter and herbal medications, which may be nephrotoxic, during the 5 days of clofarabine administration).
Products include:
Atripla 906

Emtricitabine (Nephrotoxic medications may contribute to renal toxicity in patients taking clofarabine. Patients should avoid medications including over the counter and herbal medications, which may be nephrotoxic, during the 5 days of clofarabine administration).
Products include:
Atripla 906
Emtriva 1238
Emtriva Oral Solution 1238
Truvada 1258

Enalapril Maleate (Nephrotoxic medications may contribute to renal toxicity in patients taking clofarabine. Patients should avoid medications including over the counter and herbal medications, which may be nephrotoxic, during the 5 days of clofarabine administration).
No products indexed under this heading.

Enalaprilat (Nephrotoxic medications may contribute to renal toxicity in patients taking clofarabine. Patients should avoid medications including over the counter and herbal medications, which may be nephrotoxic, during the 5 days of clofarabine administration).
No products indexed under this heading.

Enfuvirtide (Nephrotoxic medications may contribute to renal toxicity in patients taking clofarabine. Patients should avoid medications including over the counter and herbal medications, which may be nephrotoxic, during the 5 days of clofarabine administration).
No products indexed under this heading.

Enoxacin (Occurrences of Stevens-Johnson Syndrome (SJS) and toxic epidermal necrolysis (TEN) have been reported in patients who were receiving or had recently been treated with clofarabine and other medications (eg, antibiotics) known to cause these syndromes).
No products indexed under this heading.

Epirubicin Hydrochloride (Occurrences of Stevens-Johnson Syndrome (SJS) and toxic epidermal necrolysis (TEN) have been reported in patients who were receiving or had recently been treated with clofarabine and other medications (eg, antibiotics) known to cause these syndromes).
No products indexed under this heading.

Eprosartan Mesylate (Patients taking medications known to affect blood pressure should be monitored during administration of clofarabine). Products include:
Teveten 538
Teveten HCT 541

Erythromycin (Patients should avoid medications, including over the counter and herbal medications, which may be hepatotoxic, during the 5 days of clofarabine administration).
No products indexed under this heading.

Erythromycin, Topical (Patients should avoid medications, including over the counter and herbal medications, which may be hepatotoxic, during the 5 days of clofarabine administration).
No products indexed under this heading.

Erythromycin Estolate (Patients should avoid medications, including over the counter and herbal medications, which may be hepatotoxic, during the 5 days of clofarabine administration).
No products indexed under this heading.

Erythromycin Ethylsuccinate (Patients should avoid medications, including over the counter and herbal medications, which may be hepatotoxic, during the 5 days of clofarabine administration). Products include:
E.E.S. 437
EryPed 435

Erythromycin Gluceptate (Patients should avoid medications, including over the counter and herbal medications, which may be hepatotoxic, during the 5 days of clofarabine administration).
No products indexed under this heading.

Erythromycin Lactobionate (Patients should avoid medications, including over the counter and herbal medications, which may be hepatotoxic, during the 5 days of clofarabine administration).
No products indexed under this heading.

(⊙ Described in PDR® for Ophthalmic Medicines)

Erythromycin Stearate (Patients should avoid medications, including over the counter and herbal medications, which may be hepatotoxic, during the 5 days of clofarabine administration).
No products indexed under this heading.

Esmolol Hydrochloride (Patients taking medications known to affect blood pressure should be monitored during administration of clofarabine).
No products indexed under this heading.

Ethiodized Oil (Nephrotoxic medications may contribute to renal toxicity in patients taking clofarabine. Patients should avoid medications including over the counter and herbal medications, which may be nephrotoxic, during the 5 days of clofarabine administration).
No products indexed under this heading.

Etodolac (Nephrotoxic medications may contribute to renal toxicity in patients taking clofarabine. Patients should avoid medications including over the counter and herbal medications, which may be nephrotoxic, during the 5 days of clofarabine administration).
No products indexed under this heading.

Etoposide (Patients who have previously received a hematopoietic stem cell transplant may be at higher risk for hepatotoxicity suggestive of veno-occlusive disease following treatment with clofarabine (40 mg/m^2) when used in combination with etoposide (100 mg/m^2) and cyclophosphamide (440 mg/m^2)).
No products indexed under this heading.

Etoposide Phosphate (Patients who have previously received a hematopoietic stem cell transplant may be at higher risk for hepatotoxicity suggestive of veno-occlusive disease following treatment with clofarabine (40 mg/m^2) when used in combination with etoposide (100 mg/m^2) and cyclophosphamide (440 mg/m^2)).
No products indexed under this heading.

Felbamate (Patients should avoid medications, including over the counter and herbal medications, which may be hepatotoxic, during the 5 days of clofarabine administration).
No products indexed under this heading.

Felodipine (Patients taking medications known to affect blood pressure should be monitored during administration of clofarabine).
No products indexed under this heading.

Fenofibrate (Patients should avoid medications, including over the counter and herbal medications, which may be hepatotoxic, during the 5 days of clofarabine administration). Products include:
Fenoglide 3263
Tricor 544
Trilipix 548

Fenoprofen Calcium (Nephrotoxic medications may contribute to renal toxicity in patients taking clofarabine. Patients should avoid medications including over the counter and herbal medications, which may be nephrotoxic, during the 5 days of clofarabine administration).
No products indexed under this heading.

Filgrastim (Nephrotoxic medications may contribute to renal toxicity in patients taking clofarabine. Patients should avoid medications including over the counter and herbal medications, which may be nephrotoxic, during the 5 days of clofarabine administration). Products include:
Neupogen 631

Fluconazole (Patients should avoid medications, including over the counter and herbal medications, which may be hepatotoxic, during the 5 days of clofarabine administration).
No products indexed under this heading.

Fluorouracil (Nephrotoxic medications may contribute to renal toxicity in patients taking clofarabine. Patients should avoid medications including over the counter and herbal medications, which may be nephrotoxic, during the 5 days of clofarabine administration). Products include:
Carac 2966

Flurbiprofen (Nephrotoxic medications may contribute to renal toxicity in patients taking clofarabine. Patients should avoid medications including over the counter and herbal medications, which may be nephrotoxic, during the 5 days of clofarabine administration).
No products indexed under this heading.

Flurbiprofen Sodium (Patients should avoid medications, including over the counter and herbal medications, which may be hepatotoxic, during the 5 days of clofarabine administration).
No products indexed under this heading.

Fluvastatin Sodium (Nephrotoxic medications may contribute to renal toxicity in patients taking clofarabine. Patients should avoid medications including over the counter and herbal medications, which may be nephrotoxic, during the 5 days of clofarabine administration).
No products indexed under this heading.

Fosamprenavir Calcium (Patients should avoid medications, including over the counter and herbal medications, which may be hepatotoxic, during the 5 days of clofarabine administration). Products include:
Lexiva Oral Suspension 1558
Lexiva 1558

Foscarnet Sodium (Nephrotoxic medications may contribute to renal toxicity in patients taking clofarabine. Patients should avoid medications including over the counter and herbal medications, which may be nephrotoxic, during the 5 days of clofarabine administration).
No products indexed under this heading.

Fosinopril Sodium (Nephrotoxic medications may contribute to renal toxicity in patients taking clofarabine. Patients should avoid medications including over the counter and herbal medications, which may be nephrotoxic, during the 5 days of clofarabine administration).
No products indexed under this heading.

Fosphenytoin (Patients should avoid medications, including over the counter and herbal medications, which may be hepatotoxic, during the 5 days of clofarabine administration).
No products indexed under this heading.

Fosphenytoin Sodium (Patients should avoid medications, including over the counter and herbal medications, which may be hepatotoxic, during the 5 days of clofarabine administration).
No products indexed under this heading.

Furosemide (Nephrotoxic medications may contribute to renal toxicity in patients taking clofarabine. Patients should avoid medications including over the counter and herbal medications, which may be nephrotoxic, during the 5 days of clofarabine administration). Products include:
Furosemide 2354

Gadopentetate Dimeglumine (Nephrotoxic medications may contribute to renal toxicity in patients taking clofarabine. Patients should avoid medications including over the counter and herbal medications, which may be nephrotoxic, during the 5 days of clofarabine administration).
No products indexed under this heading.

Gatifloxacin (Occurrences of Stevens-Johnson Syndrome (SJS) and toxic epidermal necrolysis (TEN) have been reported in patients who were receiving or had recently been treated with clofarabine and other medications (eg, antibiotics) known to cause these syndromes).
No products indexed under this heading.

Gemfibrozil (Patients should avoid medications, including over the counter and herbal medications, which may be hepatotoxic, during the 5 days of clofarabine administration).
No products indexed under this heading.

Gemifloxacin Mesylate (Occurrences of Stevens-Johnson Syndrome (SJS) and toxic epidermal necrolysis (TEN) have been reported in patients who were receiving or had recently been treated with clofarabine and other medications (eg, antibiotics) known to cause these syndromes).
No products indexed under this heading.

Gentamicin (Nephrotoxic medications may contribute to renal toxicity in patients taking clofarabine. Patients should avoid medications including over the counter and herbal medications, which may be nephrotoxic, during the 5 days of clofarabine administration).
No products indexed under this heading.

Gentamicin Sulfate (Nephrotoxic medications may contribute to renal toxicity in patients taking clofarabine. Patients should avoid medications including over the counter and herbal medications, which may be nephrotoxic, during the 5 days of clofarabine administration). Products include:
Pred-G .... ⊙226, ⊙227

Glimepiride (Patients should avoid medications, including over the counter and herbal medications, which may be hepatotoxic, during the 5 days of clofarabine administration). Products include:
Avandaryl 1356
Duetact 3354

Glipizide (Nephrotoxic medications may contribute to renal toxicity in patients taking clofarabine. Patients should avoid medications including over the counter and herbal medications, which may be nephrotoxic, during the 5 days of clofarabine administration).
No products indexed under this heading.

Globulin, Immune (Human) (Nephrotoxic medications may contribute to renal toxicity in patients taking clofarabine. Patients should avoid medications including over the counter and herbal medications, which may be nephrotoxic, during the 5 days of clofarabine administration). Products include:

Glyburide (Nephrotoxic medications may contribute to renal toxicity in patients taking clofarabine. Patients should avoid medications including over the counter and herbal medications, which may be nephrotoxic, during the 5 days of clofarabine administration).
No products indexed under this heading.

Gold Therapy (Nephrotoxic medications may contribute to renal toxicity in patients taking clofarabine. Patients should avoid medications including over the counter and herbal medications, which may be nephrotoxic, during the 5 days of clofarabine administration).
No products indexed under this heading.

Grepafloxacin Hydrochloride (Occurrences of Stevens-Johnson Syndrome (SJS) and toxic epidermal necrolysis (TEN) have been reported in patients who were receiving or had recently been treated with clofarabine and other medications (eg, antibiotics) known to cause these syndromes).
No products indexed under this heading.

Griseofulvin (Patients should avoid medications, including over the counter and herbal medications, which may be hepatotoxic, during the 5 days of clofarabine administration).
No products indexed under this heading.

Guanabenz Acetate (Patients taking medications known to affect blood pressure should be monitored during administration of clofarabine).
No products indexed under this heading.

Guanethidine (Patients taking medications known to affect blood pressure should be monitored during administration of clofarabine).
No products indexed under this heading.

Guanethidine Monosulfate (Patients taking medications known to affect blood pressure should be monitored during administration of clofarabine).
No products indexed under this heading.

Guanethidine Sulfate (Patients taking medications known to affect blood pressure should be monitored during administration of clofarabine).
No products indexed under this heading.

Halothane (Patients should avoid medications, including over the counter and herbal medications, which may be hepatotoxic, during the 5 days of clofarabine administration).
No products indexed under this heading.

Heparin (Patients should avoid medications, including over the counter and herbal medications, which may be hepatotoxic, during the 5 days of clofarabine administration).
No products indexed under this heading.

Heparin Calcium (Patients should avoid medications, including over the counter and herbal medications, which may be hepatotoxic, during the 5 days of clofarabine administration).
No products indexed under this heading.

Heparin Sodium (Patients should avoid medications, including over the counter and herbal medications, which may be hepatotoxic, during the 5 days of clofarabine administration).
No products indexed under this heading.

HMG-CoA Reductase Inhibitors (Nephrotoxic medications may contribute to renal toxicity in patients taking clofarabine. Patients should avoid medications including over the counter and herbal medications, which may be nephrotoxic, during the 5 days of clofarabine administration).
No products indexed under this heading.

Hydralazine (Patients should avoid medications, including over the counter and herbal medications, which may be hepatotoxic, during the 5 days of clofarabine administration).
No products indexed under this heading.

Hydralazine Hydrochloride (Patients should avoid medications, including over the counter and herbal medications, which may be hepatotoxic, during the 5 days of clofarabine administration).
No products indexed under this heading.

Hydrochlorothiazide (Nephrotoxic medications may contribute to renal toxicity in patients taking clofarabine. Patients should avoid medications including over the counter and herbal medications, which may be nephrotoxic, during the 5 days of clofarabine administration). Products include:

IMPORTANT NOTE: Always consult each drug listing in the patient's regimen for possible interactions.

Hydrochlorothiazide Hydrochloride (Patients should avoid medications, including over the counter and herbal medications, which may be hepatotoxic, during the 5 days of clofarabine administration).
   No products indexed under this heading.

Hydroflumethiazide (Nephrotoxic medications may contribute to renal toxicity in patients taking clofarabine. Patients should avoid medications including over the counter and herbal medications, which may be nephrotoxic, during the 5 days of clofarabine administration).
   No products indexed under this heading.

Ibuprofen (Nephrotoxic medications may contribute to renal toxicity in patients taking clofarabine. Patients should avoid medications including over the counter and herbal medications, which may be nephrotoxic, during the 5 days of clofarabine administration). Products include:

Idarubicin Hydrochloride (Nephrotoxic medications may contribute to renal toxicity in patients taking clofarabine. Patients should avoid medications including over the counter and herbal medications, which may be nephrotoxic, during the 5 days of clofarabine administration).
   No products indexed under this heading.

Ifosfamide (Nephrotoxic medications may contribute to renal toxicity in patients taking clofarabine. Patients should avoid medications including over the counter and herbal medications, which may be nephrotoxic, during the 5 days of clofarabine administration).
   No products indexed under this heading.

Imatinib Mesylate (Patients should avoid medications, including over the counter and herbal medications, which may be hepatotoxic, during the 5 days of clofarabine administration). Products include:

Imipenem (Nephrotoxic medications may contribute to renal toxicity in patients taking clofarabine. Patients should avoid medications including over the counter and herbal medications, which may be nephrotoxic, during the 5 days of clofarabine administration). Products include:

Imipramine Hydrochloride (Patients should avoid medications, including over the counter and herbal medications, which may be hepatotoxic, during the 5 days of clofarabine administration).
   No products indexed under this heading.

Imipramine Pamoate (Patients should avoid medications, including over the counter and herbal medications, which may be hepatotoxic, during the 5 days of clofarabine administration).
   No products indexed under this heading.

Immune Globulin Intravenous (Human) (Nephrotoxic medications may contribute to renal toxicity in patients taking clofarabine. Patients should avoid medications including over the counter and herbal medications, which may be nephrotoxic, during the 5 days of clofarabine administration). Products include:

Indapamide (Patients taking medications known to affect blood pressure should be monitored during administration of clofarabine). Products include:

Indinavir Sulfate (Nephrotoxic medications may contribute to renal toxicity in patients taking clofarabine. Patients should avoid medications including over the counter and herbal medications, which may be nephrotoxic, during the 5 days of clofarabine administration). Products include:

Indomethacin (Nephrotoxic medications may contribute to renal toxicity in patients taking clofarabine. Patients should avoid medications including over the counter and herbal medications, which may be nephrotoxic, during the 5 days of clofarabine administration). Products include:

Indomethacin Sodium Trihydrate (Nephrotoxic medications may contribute to renal toxicity in patients taking clofarabine. Patients should avoid medications including over the counter and herbal medications, which may be nephrotoxic, during the 5 days of clofarabine administration). Products include:

Interferon Beta-1a (Patients should avoid medications, including over the counter and herbal medications, which may be hepatotoxic, during the 5 days of clofarabine administration). Products include:

Interferon Beta-1b (Nephrotoxic medications may contribute to renal toxicity in patients taking clofarabine. Patients should avoid medications including over the counter and herbal medications, which may be nephrotoxic, during the 5 days of clofarabine administration). Products include:

Interleukin-2 (Nephrotoxic medications may contribute to renal toxicity in patients taking clofarabine. Patients should avoid medications including over the counter and herbal medications, which may be nephrotoxic, during the 5 days of clofarabine administration).
   No products indexed under this heading.

Iodamide Meglumine (Nephrotoxic medications may contribute to renal toxicity in patients taking clofarabine. Patients should avoid medications including over the counter and herbal medications, which may be nephrotoxic, during the 5 days of clofarabine administration).
   No products indexed under this heading.

Iohexol (Nephrotoxic medications may contribute to renal toxicity in patients taking clofarabine. Patients should avoid medications including over the counter and herbal medications, which may be nephrotoxic, during the 5 days of clofarabine administration).
   No products indexed under this heading.

Iopamidol (Nephrotoxic medications may contribute to renal toxicity in patients taking clofarabine. Patients should avoid medications including over the counter and herbal medications, which may be nephrotoxic, during the 5 days of clofarabine administration).
   No products indexed under this heading.

Iopanoic Acid (Nephrotoxic medications may contribute to renal toxicity in patients taking clofarabine. Patients should avoid medications including over the counter and herbal medications, which may be nephrotoxic, during the 5 days of clofarabine administration).
   No products indexed under this heading.

Iothalamate Meglumine (Nephrotoxic medications may contribute to renal toxicity in patients taking clofarabine. Patients should avoid medications including over the counter and herbal medications, which may be nephrotoxic, during the 5 days of clofarabine administration).
   No products indexed under this heading.

Ioxaglate Meglumine (Nephrotoxic medications may contribute to renal toxicity in patients taking clofarabine. Patients should avoid medications including over the counter and herbal medications, which may be nephrotoxic, during the 5 days of clofarabine administration).
   No products indexed under this heading.

Ioxaglate Sodium (Nephrotoxic medications may contribute to renal toxicity in patients taking clofarabine. Patients should avoid medications including over the counter and herbal medications, which may be nephrotoxic, during the 5 days of clofarabine administration).
   No products indexed under this heading.

Irbesartan (Patients taking medications known to affect blood pressure should be monitored during administration of clofarabine). Products include:

Isoniazid (Patients should avoid medications, including over the counter and herbal medications, which may be hepatotoxic, during the 5 days of clofarabine administration).
   No products indexed under this heading.

Isotretinoin (Patients should avoid medications, including over the counter and herbal medications, which may be hepatotoxic, during the 5 days of clofarabine administration). Products include:

Isradipine (Patients taking medications known to affect blood pressure should be monitored during administration of clofarabine). Products include:

Itraconazole (Patients should avoid medications, including over the counter and herbal medications, which may be hepatotoxic, during the 5 days of clofarabine administration).
   No products indexed under this heading.

Kanamycin Sulfate (Nephrotoxic medications may contribute to renal toxicity in patients taking clofarabine. Patients should avoid medications including over the counter and herbal medications, which may be nephrotoxic, during the 5 days of clofarabine administration).
   No products indexed under this heading.

Ketoconazole (Patients should avoid medications, including over the counter and herbal medications, which may be hepatotoxic, during the 5 days of clofarabine administration). Products include:

Ketoprofen (Nephrotoxic medications may contribute to renal toxicity in patients taking clofarabine. Patients should avoid medications including over the counter and herbal medications, which may be nephrotoxic, during the 5 days of clofarabine administration).
   No products indexed under this heading.

Ketorolac Tromethamine (Nephrotoxic medications may contribute to renal toxicity in patients taking clofarabine. Patients should avoid medications including over the counter and herbal medications, which may be nephrotoxic, during the 5 days of clofarabine administration). Products include:

Labetalol Hydrochloride (Patients should avoid medications, including over the counter and herbal medications, which may be hepatotoxic, during the 5 days of clofarabine administration).
   No products indexed under this heading.

Lamium album (Nephrotoxic medications may contribute to renal toxicity in patients taking clofarabine. Patients should avoid medications including over the counter and herbal medications, which may be nephrotoxic, during the 5 days of clofarabine administration).
   No products indexed under this heading.

Leflunomide (Patients should avoid medications, including over the counter and herbal medications, which may be hepatotoxic, during the 5 days of clofarabine administration).
   No products indexed under this heading.

Levofloxacin (Occurrences of Stevens-Johnson Syndrome (SJS) and toxic epidermal necrolysis (TEN) have been reported in patients who were receiving or had recently been treated with clofarabine and other medications (eg, antibiotics) known to cause these syndromes). Products include:

Lisinopril (Nephrotoxic medications may contribute to renal toxicity in patients taking clofarabine. Patients should avoid medications including over the counter and herbal medications, which may be nephrotoxic, during the 5 days of clofarabine administration). Products include:

Lithium (Nephrotoxic medications may contribute to renal toxicity in patients taking clofarabine. Patients should avoid medications including over the counter and herbal medications, which may be nephrotoxic, during the 5 days of clofarabine administration).
   No products indexed under this heading.

Lithium Carbonate (Nephrotoxic medications may contribute to renal toxicity in patients taking clofarabine. Patients should avoid medications including over the counter and herbal medications, which may be nephrotoxic, during the 5 days of clofarabine administration).
   No products indexed under this heading.

Lithium Citrate (Nephrotoxic medications may contribute to renal toxicity in patients taking clofarabine. Patients should avoid medications including over the counter and herbal medications, which may be nephrotoxic, during the 5 days of clofarabine administration).
   No products indexed under this heading.

373 Interactions Index Clolar

Lomefloxacin Hydrochloride (Occurrences of Stevens-Johnson Syndrome (SJS) and toxic epidermal necrolysis (TEN) have been reported in patients who were receiving or had recently been treated with clofarabine and other medications (eg, antibiotics) known to cause these syndromes).
No products indexed under this heading.

Lopinavir (Nephrotoxic medications may contribute to renal toxicity in patients taking clofarabine. Patients should avoid medications including over the counter and herbal medications, which may be nephrotoxic, during the 5 days of clofarabine administration). Products include:
Kaletra 458

Loracarbef (Nephrotoxic medications may contribute to renal toxicity in patients taking clofarabine. Patients should avoid medications including over the counter and herbal medications, which may be nephrotoxic, during the 5 days of clofarabine administration).
No products indexed under this heading.

Losartan Potassium (Patients taking medications known to affect blood pressure should be monitored during administration of clofarabine). Products include:
Cozaar 2106
Hyzaar 2162
Hyzaar 100-12.5 2162

Lovastatin (Nephrotoxic medications may contribute to renal toxicity in patients taking clofarabine. Patients should avoid medications including over the counter and herbal medications, which may be nephrotoxic, during the 5 days of clofarabine administration). Products include:
Advicor 402
Mevacor 2212

Maprotiline Hydrochloride (Patients should avoid medications, including over the counter and herbal medications, which may be hepatotoxic, during the 5 days of clofarabine administration).
No products indexed under this heading.

Maraviroc (Patients should avoid medications, including over the counter and herbal medications, which may be hepatotoxic, during the 5 days of clofarabine administration). Products include:
Selzentry 2740

Mecamylamine Hydrochloride (Patients taking medications known to affect blood pressure should be monitored during administration of clofarabine).
No products indexed under this heading.

Meclofenamate Sodium (Nephrotoxic medications may contribute to renal toxicity in patients taking clofarabine. Patients should avoid medications including over the counter and herbal medications, which may be nephrotoxic, during the 5 days of clofarabine administration).
No products indexed under this heading.

Mefenamic Acid (Nephrotoxic medications may contribute to renal toxicity in patients taking clofarabine. Patients should avoid medications including over the counter and herbal medications, which may be nephrotoxic, during the 5 days of clofarabine administration).
No products indexed under this heading.

Meloxicam (Nephrotoxic medications may contribute to renal toxicity in patients taking clofarabine. Patients should avoid medications including over the counter and herbal medications, which may be nephrotoxic, during the 5 days of clofarabine administration).
No products indexed under this heading.

Melphalan (Serious hepatotoxic adverse reactions of veno-occlusive disease have been reported in adult patients following hematopoietic stem cell transplant. These patients received conditioning regimens that included busulfan, melphalan, and/or the combination of cyclophosphamide and total body irradiation). Products include:
Alkeran 1302

Melphalan Hydrochloride (Serious hepatotoxic adverse reactions of veno-occlusive disease have been reported in adult patients following hematopoietic stem cell transplant. These patients received conditioning regimens that included busulfan, melphalan, and/or the combination of cyclophosphamide and total body irradiation). Products include:
Alkeran for Injection 1300

Mephenytoin (Patients should avoid medications, including over the counter and herbal medications, which may be hepatotoxic, during the 5 days of clofarabine administration).
No products indexed under this heading.

Mesalamine (Nephrotoxic medications may contribute to renal toxicity in patients taking clofarabine. Patients should avoid medications including over the counter and herbal medications, which may be nephrotoxic, during the 5 days of clofarabine administration). Products include:
Apriso 2899
Asacol 2786
Asacol HD 2787
Canasa 782
Lialda 3295
Pentasa 3297

Methacycline Hydrochloride (Patients should avoid medications, including over the counter and herbal medications, which may be hepatotoxic, during the 5 days of clofarabine administration).
No products indexed under this heading.

Methicillin Sodium (Patients should avoid medications, including over the counter and herbal medications, which may be hepatotoxic, during the 5 days of clofarabine administration).
No products indexed under this heading.

Methimazole (Nephrotoxic medications may contribute to renal toxicity in patients taking clofarabine. Patients should avoid medications including over the counter and herbal medications, which may be nephrotoxic, during the 5 days of clofarabine administration).
No products indexed under this heading.

Methotrexate (Nephrotoxic medications may contribute to renal toxicity in patients taking clofarabine. Patients should avoid medications including over the counter and herbal medications, which may be nephrotoxic, during the 5 days of clofarabine administration).
No products indexed under this heading.

Methotrexate Sodium (Nephrotoxic medications may contribute to renal toxicity in patients taking clofarabine. Patients should avoid medications including over the counter and herbal medications, which may be nephrotoxic, during the 5 days of clofarabine administration).
No products indexed under this heading.

Methyclothiazide (Nephrotoxic medications may contribute to renal toxicity in patients taking clofarabine. Patients should avoid medications including over the counter and herbal medications, which may be nephrotoxic, during the 5 days of clofarabine administration).
No products indexed under this heading.

Methyldopa (Patients taking medications known to affect blood pressure should be monitored during administration of clofarabine).
No products indexed under this heading.

Methyldopate Hydrochloride (Patients taking medications known to affect blood pressure should be monitored during administration of clofarabine).
No products indexed under this heading.

Metolazone (Patients taking medications known to affect blood pressure should be monitored during administration of clofarabine).
No products indexed under this heading.

Metoprolol Succinate (Patients taking medications known to affect blood pressure should be monitored during administration of clofarabine). Products include:
Toprol XL 732

Metoprolol Tartrate (Patients taking medications known to affect blood pressure should be monitored during administration of clofarabine).
No products indexed under this heading.

Metyrosine (Patients taking medications known to affect blood pressure should be monitored during administration of clofarabine).
No products indexed under this heading.

Mezlocillin Sodium (Nephrotoxic medications may contribute to renal toxicity in patients taking clofarabine. Patients should avoid medications including over the counter and herbal medications, which may be nephrotoxic, during the 5 days of clofarabine administration).
No products indexed under this heading.

Mibefradil Dihydrochloride (Patients taking medications known to affect blood pressure should be monitored during administration of clofarabine).
No products indexed under this heading.

Minocycline Hydrochloride (Nephrotoxic medications may contribute to renal toxicity in patients taking clofarabine. Patients should avoid medications including over the counter and herbal medications, which may be nephrotoxic, during the 5 days of clofarabine administration). Products include:
Solodyn 2073

Minoxidil (Patients taking medications known to affect blood pressure should be monitored during administration of clofarabine).
No products indexed under this heading.

Mitomycin (Mitomycin-C) (Nephrotoxic medications may contribute to renal toxicity in patients taking clofarabine. Patients should avoid medications including over the counter and herbal medications, which may be nephrotoxic, during the 5 days of clofarabine administration).
No products indexed under this heading.

Moexipril Hydrochloride (Nephrotoxic medications may contribute to renal toxicity in patients taking clofarabine. Patients should avoid medications including over the counter and herbal medications, which may be nephrotoxic, during the 5 days of clofarabine administration).
No products indexed under this heading.

Moxifloxacin Hydrochloride (Occurrences of Stevens-Johnson Syndrome (SJS) and toxic epidermal necrolysis (TEN) have been reported in patients who were receiving or had recently been treated with clofarabine and other medications (eg, antibiotics) known to cause these syndromes). Products include:
Avelox 3064
Vigamox 589

Muromonab-CD3 (Nephrotoxic medications may contribute to renal toxicity in patients taking clofarabine. Patients should avoid medications including over the counter and herbal medications, which may be nephrotoxic, during the 5 days of clofarabine administration). Products include:
Orthoclone OKT3 949

Nabumetone (Nephrotoxic medications may contribute to renal toxicity in patients taking clofarabine. Patients should avoid medications including over the counter and herbal medications, which may be nephrotoxic, during the 5 days of clofarabine administration).
No products indexed under this heading.

Nadolol (Patients taking medications known to affect blood pressure should be monitored during administration of clofarabine). Products include:
Nadolol 2359

Nafcillin Sodium (Nephrotoxic medications may contribute to renal toxicity in patients taking clofarabine. Patients should avoid medications including over the counter and herbal medications, which may be nephrotoxic, during the 5 days of clofarabine administration).
No products indexed under this heading.

Naproxen (Nephrotoxic medications may contribute to renal toxicity in patients taking clofarabine. Patients should avoid medications including over the counter and herbal medications, which may be nephrotoxic, during the 5 days of clofarabine administration). Products include:
EC-Naprosyn 2850
Naprosyn 2850
Anaprox/Naprosyn 2850

Naproxen Sodium (Nephrotoxic medications may contribute to renal toxicity in patients taking clofarabine. Patients should avoid medications including over the counter and herbal medications, which may be nephrotoxic, during the 5 days of clofarabine administration). Products include:
Anaprox 2850
Anaprox DS 2850
Treximet 1681

Nebivolol (Patients taking medications known to affect blood pressure should be monitored during administration of clofarabine). Products include:
Bystolic 1147

Nefazodone Hydrochloride (Patients should avoid medications, including over the counter and herbal medications, which may be hepatotoxic, during the 5 days of clofarabine administration).
No products indexed under this heading.

Nelfinavir Mesylate (Nephrotoxic medications may contribute to renal toxicity in patients taking clofarabine. Patients should avoid medications including over the counter and herbal medications, which may be nephrotoxic, during the 5 days of clofarabine administration).
No products indexed under this heading.

Neomycin (Nephrotoxic medications may contribute to renal toxicity in patients taking clofarabine. Patients should avoid medications including over the counter and herbal medications, which may be nephrotoxic, during the 5 days of clofarabine administration).
No products indexed under this heading.

Neomycin, oral (Nephrotoxic medications may contribute to renal toxicity in patients taking clofarabine. Patients should avoid medications including over the counter and herbal medications, which may be nephrotoxic, during the 5 days of clofarabine administration).
No products indexed under this heading.

IMPORTANT NOTE: Always consult each drug listing in the patient's regimen for possible interactions.

Neomycin Sulfate (Nephrotoxic medications may contribute to renal toxicity in patients taking clofarabine. Patients should avoid medications including over the counter and herbal medications, which may be nephrotoxic, during the 5 days of clofarabine administration).
No products indexed under this heading.

Nevirapine (Nephrotoxic medications may contribute to renal toxicity in patients taking clofarabine. Patients should avoid medications including over the counter and herbal medications, which may be nephrotoxic, during the 5 days of clofarabine administration). Products include:

Niacin (Patients should avoid medications, including over the counter and herbal medications, which may be hepatotoxic, during the 5 days of clofarabine administration). Products include:

Niacinamide (Patients should avoid medications, including over the counter and herbal medications, which may be hepatotoxic, during the 5 days of clofarabine administration). Products include:

Niacinamide Hydroiodide (Patients should avoid medications, including over the counter and herbal medications, which may be hepatotoxic, during the 5 days of clofarabine administration).
No products indexed under this heading.

Nicardipine Hydrochloride (Patients taking medications known to affect blood pressure should be monitored during administration of clofarabine).
No products indexed under this heading.

Nicotinic Acid (Patients should avoid medications, including over the counter and herbal medications, which may be hepatotoxic, during the 5 days of clofarabine administration).
No products indexed under this heading.

Nifedipine (Patients taking medications known to affect blood pressure should be monitored during administration of clofarabine).
No products indexed under this heading.

Nisoldipine (Patients taking medications known to affect blood pressure should be monitored during administration of clofarabine).
No products indexed under this heading.

Nitrofurantoin (Patients should avoid medications, including over the counter and herbal medications, which may be hepatotoxic, during the 5 days of clofarabine administration).
No products indexed under this heading.

Nitrofurantoin Macrocrystals (Patients should avoid medications, including over the counter and herbal medications, which may be hepatotoxic, during the 5 days of clofarabine administration).
No products indexed under this heading.

Nitrofurantoin Monohydrate (Patients should avoid medications, including over the counter and herbal medications, which may be hepatotoxic, during the 5 days of clofarabine administration).
No products indexed under this heading.

Nitrofurantoin Sodium (Patients should avoid medications, including over the counter and herbal medications, which may be hepatotoxic, during the 5 days of clofarabine administration).
No products indexed under this heading.

Nitroglycerin (Patients taking medications known to affect blood pressure should be monitored during administration of clofarabine). Products include:

Norfloxacin (Nephrotoxic medications may contribute to renal toxicity in patients taking clofarabine. Patients should avoid medications including over the counter and herbal medications, which may be nephrotoxic, during the 5 days of clofarabine administration). Products include:

Nortriptyline Hydrochloride (Patients should avoid medications, including over the counter and herbal medications, which may be hepatotoxic, during the 5 days of clofarabine administration).
No products indexed under this heading.

Ofloxacin (Occurrences of Stevens-Johnson Syndrome (SJS) and toxic epidermal necrolysis (TEN) have been reported in patients who were receiving or had recently been treated with clofarabine and other medications (eg, antibiotics) known to cause these syndromes).
No products indexed under this heading.

Olsalazine Sodium (Nephrotoxic medications may contribute to renal toxicity in patients taking clofarabine. Patients should avoid medications including over the counter and herbal medications, which may be nephrotoxic, during the 5 days of clofarabine administration).
No products indexed under this heading.

Omeprazole (Nephrotoxic medications may contribute to renal toxicity in patients taking clofarabine. Patients should avoid medications including over the counter and herbal medications, which may be nephrotoxic, during the 5 days of clofarabine administration).
No products indexed under this heading.

Oxacillin (Patients should avoid medications, including over the counter and herbal medications, which may be hepatotoxic, during the 5 days of clofarabine administration).
No products indexed under this heading.

Oxacillin Sodium (Patients should avoid medications, including over the counter and herbal medications, which may be hepatotoxic, during the 5 days of clofarabine administration).
No products indexed under this heading.

Oxaprozin (Nephrotoxic medications may contribute to renal toxicity in patients taking clofarabine. Patients should avoid medications including over the counter and herbal medications, which may be nephrotoxic, during the 5 days of clofarabine administration).
No products indexed under this heading.

Oxymetholone (Patients should avoid medications, including over the counter and herbal medications, which may be hepatotoxic, during the 5 days of clofarabine administration).
No products indexed under this heading.

Oxytetracycline (Patients should avoid medications, including over the counter and herbal medications, which may be hepatotoxic, during the 5 days of clofarabine administration).
No products indexed under this heading.

Oxytetracycline Hydrochloride (Patients should avoid medications, including over the counter and herbal medications, which may be hepatotoxic, during the 5 days of clofarabine administration).
No products indexed under this heading.

Pamidronate Disodium (Nephrotoxic medications may contribute to renal toxicity in patients taking clofarabine. Patients should avoid medications including over the counter and herbal medications, which may be nephrotoxic, during the 5 days of clofarabine administration).
No products indexed under this heading.

Paroxetine Hydrochloride (Nephrotoxic medications may contribute to renal toxicity in patients taking clofarabine. Patients should avoid medications including over the counter and herbal medications, which may be nephrotoxic, during the 5 days of clofarabine administration). Products include:

Penbutolol Sulfate (Patients taking medications known to affect blood pressure should be monitored during administration of clofarabine).
No products indexed under this heading.

Penicillamine (Nephrotoxic medications may contribute to renal toxicity in patients taking clofarabine. Patients should avoid medications including over the counter and herbal medications, which may be nephrotoxic, during the 5 days of clofarabine administration).
No products indexed under this heading.

Penicillin, Potassium Phenoxymethyl (Patients should avoid medications, including over the counter and herbal medications, which may be hepatotoxic, during the 5 days of clofarabine administration).
No products indexed under this heading.

Penicillin G Benzathine (Nephrotoxic medications may contribute to renal toxicity in patients taking clofarabine. Patients should avoid medications including over the counter and herbal medications, which may be nephrotoxic, during the 5 days of clofarabine administration). Products include:

Penicillin G Dibenzylethyenedi-amine (Patients should avoid medications, including over the counter and herbal medications, which may be hepatotoxic, during the 5 days of clofarabine administration).
No products indexed under this heading.

Penicillin G Potassium (Nephrotoxic medications may contribute to renal toxicity in patients taking clofarabine. Patients should avoid medications including over the counter and herbal medications, which may be nephrotoxic, during the 5 days of clofarabine administration).
No products indexed under this heading.

Penicillin G Procaine (Nephrotoxic medications may contribute to renal toxicity in patients taking clofarabine. Patients should avoid medications including over the counter and herbal medications, which may be nephrotoxic, during the 5 days of clofarabine administration). Products include:

Penicillin G Sodium (Nephrotoxic medications may contribute to renal toxicity in patients taking clofarabine. Patients should avoid medications including over the counter and herbal medications, which may be nephrotoxic, during the 5 days of clofarabine administration).
No products indexed under this heading.

Penicillin V (Patients should avoid medications, including over the counter and herbal medications, which may be hepatotoxic, during the 5 days of clofarabine administration).
No products indexed under this heading.

Penicillin V Potassium (Nephrotoxic medications may contribute to renal toxicity in patients taking clofarabine. Patients should avoid medications including over the counter and herbal medications, which may be nephrotoxic, during the 5 days of clofarabine administration).
No products indexed under this heading.

Penicillins (Patients should avoid medications, including over the counter and herbal medications, which may be hepatotoxic, during the 5 days of clofarabine administration).
No products indexed under this heading.

Pentamidine Isethionate (Nephrotoxic medications may contribute to renal toxicity in patients taking clofarabine. Patients should avoid medications including over the counter and herbal medications, which may be nephrotoxic, during the 5 days of clofarabine administration).
No products indexed under this heading.

Perindopril Erbumine (Nephrotoxic medications may contribute to renal toxicity in patients taking clofarabine. Patients should avoid medications including over the counter and herbal medications, which may be nephrotoxic, during the 5 days of clofarabine administration).
No products indexed under this heading.

Phenoxybenzamine Hydrochloride (Patients taking medications known to affect blood pressure should be monitored during administration of clofarabine). Products include:

Phentolamine Mesylate (Patients taking medications known to affect blood pressure should be monitored during administration of clofarabine).
No products indexed under this heading.

Phenylbutazone (Nephrotoxic medications may contribute to renal toxicity in patients taking clofarabine. Patients should avoid medications including over the counter and herbal medications, which may be nephrotoxic, during the 5 days of clofarabine administration).
No products indexed under this heading.

Phenytoin (Patients should avoid medications, including over the counter and herbal medications, which may be hepatotoxic, during the 5 days of clofarabine administration).
No products indexed under this heading.

Phenytoin Sodium (Patients should avoid medications, including over the counter and herbal medications, which may be hepatotoxic, during the 5 days of clofarabine administration). Products include:

Pindolol (Patients taking medications known to affect blood pressure should be monitored during administration of clofarabine).
No products indexed under this heading.

Pioglitazone Hydrochloride (Patients should avoid medications, including over the counter and herbal medications, which may be hepatotoxic, during the 5 days of clofarabine administration). Products include:

ActoPlus 3338
Actos 3345
Duetact 3354

Piperacillin Sodium (Patients should avoid medications, including over the counter and herbal medications, which may be hepatotoxic, during the 5 days of clofarabine administration). Products include:
Zosyn 3607

Piroxicam (Nephrotoxic medications may contribute to renal toxicity in patients taking clofarabine. Patients should avoid medications including over the counter and herbal medications, which may be nephrotoxic, during the 5 days of clofarabine administration).
No products indexed under this heading.

Plicamycin (Nephrotoxic medications may contribute to renal toxicity in patients taking clofarabine. Patients should avoid medications including over the counter and herbal medications, which may be nephrotoxic, during the 5 days of clofarabine administration).
No products indexed under this heading.

Polymyxin (Nephrotoxic medications may contribute to renal toxicity in patients taking clofarabine. Patients should avoid medications including over the counter and herbal medications, which may be nephrotoxic, during the 5 days of clofarabine administration).
No products indexed under this heading.

Polymyxin B Sulfate (Nephrotoxic medications may contribute to renal toxicity in patients taking clofarabine. Patients should avoid medications including over the counter and herbal medications, which may be nephrotoxic, during the 5 days of clofarabine administration).
No products indexed under this heading.

Polythiazide (Nephrotoxic medications may contribute to renal toxicity in patients taking clofarabine. Patients should avoid medications including over the counter and herbal medications, which may be nephrotoxic, during the 5 days of clofarabine administration).
No products indexed under this heading.

Pravastatin Sodium (Nephrotoxic medications may contribute to renal toxicity in patients taking clofarabine. Patients should avoid medications including over the counter and herbal medications, which may be nephrotoxic, during the 5 days of clofarabine administration).
No products indexed under this heading.

Prazosin Hydrochloride (Patients taking medications known to affect blood pressure should be monitored during administration of clofarabine).
No products indexed under this heading.

Procainamide (Patients should avoid medications, including over the counter and herbal medications, which may be hepatotoxic, during the 5 days of clofarabine administration).
No products indexed under this heading.

Procainamide Hydrochloride (Patients should avoid medications, including over the counter and herbal medications, which may be hepatotoxic, during the 5 days of clofarabine administration).
No products indexed under this heading.

Propranolol Hydrochloride (Patients taking medications known to affect blood pressure should be monitored during administration of clofarabine). Products include:
InnoPran XL 1517

Propylthiouracil (Patients should avoid medications, including over the counter and herbal medications, which may be hepatotoxic, during the 5 days of clofarabine administration).
No products indexed under this heading.

Protriptyline Hydrochloride (Patients should avoid medications, including over the counter and herbal medications, which may be hepatotoxic, during the 5 days of clofarabine administration).
No products indexed under this heading.

Quinapril Hydrochloride (Nephrotoxic medications may contribute to renal toxicity in patients taking clofarabine. Patients should avoid medications including over the counter and herbal medications, which may be nephrotoxic, during the 5 days of clofarabine administration).
No products indexed under this heading.

Rabeprazole Sodium (Nephrotoxic medications may contribute to renal toxicity in patients taking clofarabine. Patients should avoid medications including over the counter and herbal medications, which may be nephrotoxic, during the 5 days of clofarabine administration). Products include:
Aciphex 1035

Radiation (Serious hepatotoxic adverse reactions of veno-occlusive disease have been reported in adult patients following hematopoietic stem cell transplant. These patients received conditioning regimens that included busulfan, melphalan, and/or the combination of cyclophosphamide and total body irradiation).
No products indexed under this heading.

Ramipril (Nephrotoxic medications may contribute to renal toxicity in patients taking clofarabine. Patients should avoid medications including over the counter and herbal medications, which may be nephrotoxic, during the 5 days of clofarabine administration).
No products indexed under this heading.

Rauwolfia Serpentina (Patients taking medications known to affect blood pressure should be monitored during administration of clofarabine).
No products indexed under this heading.

Rescinnamine (Patients taking medications known to affect blood pressure should be monitored during administration of clofarabine).
No products indexed under this heading.

Reserpine (Patients taking medications known to affect blood pressure should be monitored during administration of clofarabine).
No products indexed under this heading.

Rifampin (Nephrotoxic medications may contribute to renal toxicity in patients taking clofarabine. Patients should avoid medications including over the counter and herbal medications, which may be nephrotoxic, during the 5 days of clofarabine administration).
No products indexed under this heading.

Riluzole (Nephrotoxic medications may contribute to renal toxicity in patients taking clofarabine. Patients should avoid medications including over the counter and herbal medications, which may be nephrotoxic, during the 5 days of clofarabine administration). Products include:
Rilutek 3032

Ritonavir (Nephrotoxic medications may contribute to renal toxicity in patients taking clofarabine. Patients should avoid medications including over the counter and herbal medications, which may be nephrotoxic, during the 5 days of clofarabine administration). Products include:
Kaletra 458
Norvir 509

Rofecoxib (Nephrotoxic medications may contribute to renal toxicity in patients taking clofarabine. Patients should avoid medications including over the counter and herbal medications, which may be nephrotoxic, during the 5 days of clofarabine administration).
No products indexed under this heading.

Rosuvastatin Calcium (Patients should avoid medications, including over the counter and herbal medications, which may be hepatotoxic, during the 5 days of clofarabine administration). Products include:
Crestor 736

Saquinavir (Nephrotoxic medications may contribute to renal toxicity in patients taking clofarabine. Patients should avoid medications including over the counter and herbal medications, which may be nephrotoxic, during the 5 days of clofarabine administration).
No products indexed under this heading.

Saquinavir Mesylate (Patients should avoid medications, including over the counter and herbal medications, which may be hepatotoxic, during the 5 days of clofarabine administration).
No products indexed under this heading.

Sibutramine Hydrochloride Monohydrate (Nephrotoxic medications may contribute to renal toxicity in patients taking clofarabine. Patients should avoid medications including over the counter and herbal medications, which may be nephrotoxic, during the 5 days of clofarabine administration). Products include:
Meridia 492

Simvastatin (Nephrotoxic medications may contribute to renal toxicity in patients taking clofarabine. Patients should avoid medications including over the counter and herbal medications, which may be nephrotoxic, during the 5 days of clofarabine administration). Products include:
Simcor 524
Vytorin 10/10 .... 2303, 3240
Vytorin 10/20 .... 2303, 3240
Vytorin 10/40 .... 2303, 3240
Vytorin 10/80 .... 2303, 3240
Zocor 2289

Sodium Cloxacillin Monohydrate (Patients should avoid medications, including over the counter and herbal medications, which may be hepatotoxic, during the 5 days of clofarabine administration).
No products indexed under this heading.

Sodium Nitroprusside (Patients taking medications known to affect blood pressure should be monitored during administration of clofarabine).
No products indexed under this heading.

Sotalol Hydrochloride (Patients taking medications known to affect blood pressure should be monitored during administration of clofarabine).
No products indexed under this heading.

Sparfloxacin (Occurrences of Stevens-Johnson Syndrome (SJS) and toxic epidermal necrolysis (TEN) have been reported in patients who were receiving or had recently been treated with clofarabine and other medications (eg, antibiotics) known to cause these syndromes).
No products indexed under this heading.

Spirapril Hydrochloride (Nephrotoxic medications may contribute to renal toxicity in patients taking clofarabine. Patients should avoid medications including over the counter and herbal medications, which may be nephrotoxic, during the 5 days of clofarabine administration).
No products indexed under this heading.

Statins (Patients should avoid medications, including over the counter and herbal medications, which may be hepatotoxic, during the 5 days of clofarabine administration).
No products indexed under this heading.

Stavudine (Nephrotoxic medications may contribute to renal toxicity in patients taking clofarabine. Patients should avoid medications including over the counter and herbal medications, which may be nephrotoxic, during the 5 days of clofarabine administration).
No products indexed under this heading.

Streptomycin Sulfate (Nephrotoxic medications may contribute to renal toxicity in patients taking clofarabine. Patients should avoid medications including over the counter and herbal medications, which may be nephrotoxic, during the 5 days of clofarabine administration).
No products indexed under this heading.

Streptozocin (Nephrotoxic medications may contribute to renal toxicity in patients taking clofarabine. Patients should avoid medications including over the counter and herbal medications, which may be nephrotoxic, during the 5 days of clofarabine administration).
No products indexed under this heading.

Sulfacytine (Nephrotoxic medications may contribute to renal toxicity in patients taking clofarabine. Patients should avoid medications including over the counter and herbal medications, which may be nephrotoxic, during the 5 days of clofarabine administration).
No products indexed under this heading.

Sulfamethizole (Nephrotoxic medications may contribute to renal toxicity in patients taking clofarabine. Patients should avoid medications including over the counter and herbal medications, which may be nephrotoxic, during the 5 days of clofarabine administration).
No products indexed under this heading.

Sulfamethoxazole (Nephrotoxic medications may contribute to renal toxicity in patients taking clofarabine. Patients should avoid medications including over the counter and herbal medications, which may be nephrotoxic, during the 5 days of clofarabine administration).
No products indexed under this heading.

Sulfasalazine (Nephrotoxic medications may contribute to renal toxicity in patients taking clofarabine. Patients should avoid medications including over the counter and herbal medications, which may be nephrotoxic, during the 5 days of clofarabine administration).
No products indexed under this heading.

Sulfinpyrazone (Nephrotoxic medications may contribute to renal toxicity in patients taking clofarabine. Patients should avoid medications including over the counter and herbal medications, which may be nephrotoxic, during the 5 days of clofarabine administration).
No products indexed under this heading.

Sulfisoxazole Acetyl (Nephrotoxic medications may contribute to renal toxicity in patients taking clofarabine. Patients should avoid medications including over the counter and herbal medications, which may be nephrotoxic, during the 5 days of clofarabine administration).
No products indexed under this heading.

Sulfisoxazole Diolamine (Nephrotoxic medications may contribute to renal toxicity in patients taking clofarabine. Patients should avoid medications including over the counter and herbal medications, which may be nephrotoxic, during the 5 days of clofarabine administration).
No products indexed under this heading.

IMPORTANT NOTE: Always consult each drug listing in the patient's regimen for possible interactions.

Clolar Interactions Index 376

Sulindac (Nephrotoxic medications may contribute to renal toxicity in patients taking clofarabine. Patients should avoid medications including over the counter and herbal medications, which may be nephrotoxic, during the 5 days of clofarabine administration). Products include:
Clinoril 2098

Tacrine Hydrochloride (Patients should avoid medications, including over the counter and herbal medications, which may be hepatotoxic, during the 5 days of clofarabine administration).
No products indexed under this heading.

Tacrolimus (Nephrotoxic medications may contribute to renal toxicity in patients taking clofarabine. Patients should avoid medications including over the counter and herbal medications, which may be nephrotoxic, during the 5 days of clofarabine administration). Products include:
Prograf Capsules 677
Prograf Injection 677
Protopic 685

Tamoxifen Citrate (Patients should avoid medications, including over the counter and herbal medications, which may be hepatotoxic, during the 5 days of clofarabine administration).
No products indexed under this heading.

Telithromycin (Patients should avoid medications, including over the counter and herbal medications, which may be hepatotoxic, during the 5 days of clofarabine administration). Products include:
Ketek 2991

Telmisartan (Patients taking medications known to affect blood pressure should be monitored during administration of clofarabine). Products include:
Micardis 887
Micardis HCT 889

Tenofovir Disoproxil Fumarate (Nephrotoxic medications may contribute to renal toxicity in patients taking clofarabine. Patients should avoid medications including over the counter and herbal medications, which may be nephrotoxic, during the 5 days of clofarabine administration). Products include:
Atripla 906
Truvada 1258
Viread 1266

Terazosin Hydrochloride (Patients taking medications known to affect blood pressure should be monitored during administration of clofarabine).
No products indexed under this heading.

Tetracycline Hydrochloride (Patients should avoid medications, including over the counter and herbal medications, which may be hepatotoxic, during the 5 days of clofarabine administration). Products include:
Pylera 793

Tetracycline Phosphate Complex (Patients should avoid medications, including over the counter and herbal medications, which may be hepatotoxic, during the 5 days of clofarabine administration).
No products indexed under this heading.

Thiazide Diuretics (Patients should avoid medications, including over the counter and herbal medications, which may be hepatotoxic, during the 5 days of clofarabine administration).
No products indexed under this heading.

Thiazides (Patients should avoid medications, including over the counter and herbal medications, which may be hepatotoxic, during the 5 days of clofarabine administration).
No products indexed under this heading.

Thioguanine (Nephrotoxic medications may contribute to renal toxicity in patients taking clofarabine. Patients should avoid medications including over the counter and herbal medications, which may be nephrotoxic, during the 5 days of clofarabine administration). Products include:
Tabloid 1664

Ticarcillin Disodium (Nephrotoxic medications may contribute to renal toxicity in patients taking clofarabine. Patients should avoid medications including over the counter and herbal medications, which may be nephrotoxic, during the 5 days of clofarabine administration). Products include:
Timentin ADD-Vantage 1670
Timentin Galaxy 1674
Timentin 1666
Timentin Pharmacy 1678

Timolol Maleate (Patients taking medications known to affect blood pressure should be monitored during administration of clofarabine). Products include:
Combigan 601
Dorzolamide Hydrochloride/Timolol Maleate Ophthalmic Solution .... ⊙243
Timoptic in Ocudose .... ⊙231

Tipranavir (Patients should avoid medications, including over the counter and herbal medications, which may be hepatotoxic, during the 5 days of clofarabine administration).
No products indexed under this heading.

Tobramycin (Nephrotoxic medications may contribute to renal toxicity in patients taking clofarabine. Patients should avoid medications including over the counter and herbal medications, which may be nephrotoxic, during the 5 days of clofarabine administration). Products include:
Tobi Nebulizer 2546
Tobramycin and Dexamethasone Ophthalmic Suspension .... ⊙251
Zylet .... ⊙252

Tobramycin Sulfate (Nephrotoxic medications may contribute to renal toxicity in patients taking clofarabine. Patients should avoid medications including over the counter and herbal medications, which may be nephrotoxic, during the 5 days of clofarabine administration).
No products indexed under this heading.

Tolazamide (Nephrotoxic medications may contribute to renal toxicity in patients taking clofarabine. Patients should avoid medications including over the counter and herbal medications, which may be nephrotoxic, during the 5 days of clofarabine administration).
No products indexed under this heading.

Tolbutamide (Nephrotoxic medications may contribute to renal toxicity in patients taking clofarabine. Patients should avoid medications including over the counter and herbal medications, which may be nephrotoxic, during the 5 days of clofarabine administration).
No products indexed under this heading.

Tolbutamide Sodium (Patients should avoid medications, including over the counter and herbal medications, which may be hepatotoxic, during the 5 days of clofarabine administration).
No products indexed under this heading.

Tolmetin Sodium (Nephrotoxic medications may contribute to renal toxicity in patients taking clofarabine. Patients should avoid medications including over the counter and herbal medications, which may be nephrotoxic, during the 5 days of clofarabine administration).
No products indexed under this heading.

Torsemide (Patients taking medications known to affect blood pressure should be monitored during administration of clofarabine).
No products indexed under this heading.

Trandolapril (Nephrotoxic medications may contribute to renal toxicity in patients taking clofarabine. Patients should avoid medications including over the counter and herbal medications, which may be nephrotoxic, during the 5 days of clofarabine administration). Products include:
Mavik 489
Tarka 534

Triamterene (Nephrotoxic medications may contribute to renal toxicity in patients taking clofarabine. Patients should avoid medications including over the counter and herbal medications, which may be nephrotoxic, during the 5 days of clofarabine administration). Products include:
Dyazide 1429
Dyrenium 3495

Trimethadione (Nephrotoxic medications may contribute to renal toxicity in patients taking clofarabine. Patients should avoid medications including over the counter and herbal medications, which may be nephrotoxic, during the 5 days of clofarabine administration).
No products indexed under this heading.

Trimethaphan Camsylate (Patients taking medications known to affect blood pressure should be monitored during administration of clofarabine).
No products indexed under this heading.

Trimethoprim (Patients should avoid medications, including over the counter and herbal medications, which may be hepatotoxic, during the 5 days of clofarabine administration).
No products indexed under this heading.

Trimethoprim Hydrochloride (Patients should avoid medications, including over the counter and herbal medications, which may be hepatotoxic, during the 5 days of clofarabine administration).
No products indexed under this heading.

Trimethoprim Sulfate (Patients should avoid medications, including over the counter and herbal medications, which may be hepatotoxic, during the 5 days of clofarabine administration).
No products indexed under this heading.

Trimipramine Maleate (Patients should avoid medications, including over the counter and herbal medications, which may be hepatotoxic, during the 5 days of clofarabine administration).
No products indexed under this heading.

Troleandomycin (Occurrences of Stevens-Johnson Syndrome (SJS) and toxic epidermal necrolysis (TEN) have been reported in patients who were receiving or had recently been treated with clofarabine and other medications (eg, antibiotics) known to cause these syndromes).
No products indexed under this heading.

Trovafloxacin Mesylate (Nephrotoxic medications may contribute to renal toxicity in patients taking clofarabine. Patients should avoid medications including over the counter and herbal medications, which may be nephrotoxic, during the 5 days of clofarabine administration).
No products indexed under this heading.

Tyropanoate Sodium (Nephrotoxic medications may contribute to renal toxicity in patients taking clofarabine. Patients should avoid medications including over the counter and herbal medications, which may be nephrotoxic, during the 5 days of clofarabine administration).
No products indexed under this heading.

Valacyclovir Hydrochloride (Nephrotoxic medications may contribute to renal toxicity in patients taking clofarabine. Patients should avoid medications including over the counter and herbal medications, which may be nephrotoxic, during the 5 days of clofarabine administration). Products include:
Valtrex 1702

Valdecoxib (Nephrotoxic medications may contribute to renal toxicity in patients taking clofarabine. Patients should avoid medications including over the counter and herbal medications, which may be nephrotoxic, during the 5 days of clofarabine administration).
No products indexed under this heading.

Valproate Sodium (Patients should avoid medications, including over the counter and herbal medications, which may be hepatotoxic, during the 5 days of clofarabine administration).
No products indexed under this heading.

Valproic Acid (Patients should avoid medications, including over the counter and herbal medications, which may be hepatotoxic, during the 5 days of clofarabine administration).
No products indexed under this heading.

Valsartan (Patients taking medications known to affect blood pressure should be monitored during administration of clofarabine). Products include:
Diovan 2413
Diovan HCT 2419
Exforge 2443
Exforge HCT 2449
Valturna 3637

Vancomycin Hydrochloride (Nephrotoxic medications may contribute to renal toxicity in patients taking clofarabine. Patients should avoid medications including over the counter and herbal medications, which may be nephrotoxic, during the 5 days of clofarabine administration).
No products indexed under this heading.

Verapamil Hydrochloride (Patients taking medications known to affect blood pressure should be monitored during administration of clofarabine). Products include:
Tarka 534

Voriconazole (Nephrotoxic medications may contribute to renal toxicity in patients taking clofarabine. Patients should avoid medications including over the counter and herbal medications, which may be nephrotoxic, during the 5 days of clofarabine administration).
No products indexed under this heading.

Zalcitabine (Nephrotoxic medications may contribute to renal toxicity in patients taking clofarabine. Patients should avoid medications including over the counter and herbal medications, which may be nephrotoxic, during the 5 days of clofarabine administration).
No products indexed under this heading.

Zidovudine (Nephrotoxic medications may contribute to renal toxicity in patients taking clofarabine. Patients should avoid medications including over the counter and herbal medications, which may be nephrotoxic, during the 5 days of clofarabine administration). Products include:
Combivir 1404
Retrovir 1634
Retrovir IV 1640
Trizivir 1688

Zoledronic Acid (Nephrotoxic medications may contribute to renal toxicity in patients taking clofarabine. Patients should avoid medications including over the counter and herbal medications, which may be nephrotoxic, during the 5 days of clofarabine administration). Products include:
Reclast 2509
Zometa 2554

CLORPACTIN WCS-90

(Sodium Oxychlorosene) 1799
None cited in PDR database.

(⊙ Described in PDR® for Ophthalmic Medicines)

CLORPRES TABLETS

(Chlorthalidone, Clonidine
Hydrochloride)...................................... 2344
May interact with alcohols, antihypertensives, barbiturates, beta-blockers, cardiac glycosides, hypnotics and sedatives, insulin, lithium preparations, narcotic analgesics, oral hypoglycemic agents, tricyclic antidepressants, and certain other agents. Compounds in these categories include:

Acarbose (Higher dosage of oral hypoglycemic agents may be required when co-administered with chlorthalidone).
No products indexed under this heading.

Acebutolol Hydrochloride (Chlorthalidone may add to or potentiate the action of other antihypertensives).
No products indexed under this heading.

Alfentanil Hydrochloride (Orthostatic hypotension may be aggravated by narcotics).
No products indexed under this heading.

Aliskiren (Chlorthalidone may add to or potentiate the action of other antihypertensives). Products include:
Tekturna 2538
Tekturna HCT 2541
Valturna 3637

Amitriptyline Hydrochloride (Amitriptyline in combination with clonidine enhances the manifestation of corneal lesions. Co-administration of clonidine with tricyclic antidepressants may result in reduced effect of clonidine, necessitating an increase in dosage).
No products indexed under this heading.

Amlodipine Besylate (Chlorthalidone may add to or potentiate the action of other antihypertensives). Products include:
Azor 1010
Exforge 2443
Exforge HCT 2449

Amobarbital (Clonidine may enhance the CNS-depressive effects of barbiturates; orthostatic hypotension may be aggravated by barbiturates).
No products indexed under this heading.

Amobarbital Sodium (Clonidine may enhance the CNS-depressive effects of barbiturates; orthostatic hypotension may be aggravated by barbiturates).
No products indexed under this heading.

Amoxapine (Co-administration of clonidine with tricyclic antidepressants may result in reduced effect of clonidine, necessitating an increase in dosage).
No products indexed under this heading.

Apomorphine (Orthostatic hypotension may be aggravated by narcotics).
No products indexed under this heading.

Apomorphine Hydrochloride (Orthostatic hypotension may be aggravated by narcotics).
No products indexed under this heading.

Aprobarbital (Clonidine may enhance the CNS-depressive effects of barbiturates; orthostatic hypotension may be aggravated by barbiturates).
No products indexed under this heading.

Atenolol (Chlorthalidone may add to or potentiate the action of other antihypertensives).
No products indexed under this heading.

Benazepril Hydrochloride (Chlorthalidone may add to or potentiate the action of other antihypertensives).
No products indexed under this heading.

Bendroflumethiazide (Chlorthalidone may add to or potentiate the action of other antihypertensives).
No products indexed under this heading.

Betaxolol Hydrochloride (Chlorthalidone may add to or potentiate the action of other antihypertensives).
No products indexed under this heading.

Bisoprolol Fumarate (Chlorthalidone may add to or potentiate the action of other antihypertensives).
No products indexed under this heading.

Buprenorphine Hydrochloride (Orthostatic hypotension may be aggravated by narcotics).
No products indexed under this heading.

Butabarbital (Clonidine may enhance the CNS-depressive effects of barbiturates; orthostatic hypotension may be aggravated by barbiturates).
No products indexed under this heading.

Butabarbital Sodium (Clonidine may enhance the CNS-depressive effects of barbiturates; orthostatic hypotension may be aggravated by barbiturates).
No products indexed under this heading.

Butalbital (Clonidine may enhance the CNS-depressive effects of barbiturates; orthostatic hypotension may be aggravated by barbiturates).
No products indexed under this heading.

Candesartan Cilexetil (Chlorthalidone may add to or potentiate the action of other antihypertensives). Products include:
Atacand 697
Atacand HCT 700

Captopril (Chlorthalidone may add to or potentiate the action of other antihypertensives). Products include:
Captopril 2341

Carteolol Hydrochloride (Chlorthalidone may add to or potentiate the action of other antihypertensives).
No products indexed under this heading.

Carvedilol (Chlorthalidone may add to or potentiate the action of other antihypertensives). Products include:
Coreg 1409

Carvedilol Phosphate (Chlorthalidone may add to or potentiate the action of other antihypertensives). Products include:
Coreg CR 1416

Chloral Hydrate (Clonidine may enhance the CNS-depressive effects of other sedatives).
No products indexed under this heading.

Chlorothiazide (Chlorthalidone may add to or potentiate the action of other antihypertensives).
No products indexed under this heading.

Chlorothiazide Sodium (Chlorthalidone may add to or potentiate the action of other antihypertensives). Products include:
Diuril Intravenous 2009

Chlorpropamide (Higher dosage of oral hypoglycemic agents may be required when co-administered with chlorthalidone).
No products indexed under this heading.

Clomipramine Hydrochloride (Co-administration of clonidine with tricyclic antidepressants may result in reduced effect of clonidine, necessitating an increase in dosage).
No products indexed under this heading.

Clonidine (Chlorthalidone may add to or potentiate the action of other antihypertensives). Products include:
Catapres-TTS 884

Codeine Phosphate (Orthostatic hypotension may be aggravated by narcotics). Products include:
Tylenol with Codeine 2691

Codeine Sulfate (Orthostatic hypotension may be aggravated by narcotics).
No products indexed under this heading.

Deserpidine (Chlorthalidone may add to or potentiate the action of other antihypertensives).
No products indexed under this heading.

Desipramine Hydrochloride (Co-administration of clonidine with tricyclic antidepressants may result in reduced effect of clonidine, necessitating an increase in dosage).
No products indexed under this heading.

Deslanoside (Hypokalemia and other electrolyte abnormalities are common in patients receiving chlorthalidone. Digitalis therapy may exaggerate the metabolic effects of hypokalemia especially with reference to myocardial activity).
No products indexed under this heading.

Dezocine (Orthostatic hypotension may be aggravated by narcotics).
No products indexed under this heading.

Diazoxide (Chlorthalidone may add to or potentiate the action of other antihypertensives). Products include:
Proglycem 1179
Proglycem Suspension 1179

Digitalis Glycoside Preparations (Hypokalemia and other electrolyte abnormalities are common in patients receiving chlorthalidone. Digitalis therapy may exaggerate the metabolic effects of hypokalemia especially with reference to myocardial activity).
No products indexed under this heading.

Digitalis Lanata (Hypokalemia and other electrolyte abnormalities are common in patients receiving chlorthalidone. Digitalis therapy may exaggerate the metabolic effects of hypokalemia especially with reference to myocardial activity).
No products indexed under this heading.

Digitalis Purpurea (Hypokalemia and other electrolyte abnormalities are common in patients receiving chlorthalidone. Digitalis therapy may exaggerate the metabolic effects of hypokalemia especially with reference to myocardial activity).
No products indexed under this heading.

Digitoxin (Hypokalemia and other electrolyte abnormalities are common in patients receiving chlorthalidone. Digitalis therapy may exaggerate the metabolic effects of hypokalemia especially with reference to myocardial activity).
No products indexed under this heading.

Digoxin (Hypokalemia and other electrolyte abnormalities are common in patients receiving chlorthalidone. Digitalis therapy may exaggerate the metabolic effects of hypokalemia especially with reference to myocardial activity). Products include:
Lanoxin Injection 1546
Lanoxin Injection Pediatric 1549
Lanoxin Tablets 1553

Dihydrocodeine Bitartrate (Orthostatic hypotension may be aggravated by narcotics).
No products indexed under this heading.

Dihydrocodeinone Bitartrate (Orthostatic hypotension may be aggravated by narcotics).
No products indexed under this heading.

Diltiazem Hydrochloride (Chlorthalidone may add to or potentiate the action of other antihypertensives). Products include:
Cardizem LA 423

Diltiazem Maleate (Chlorthalidone may add to or potentiate the action of other antihypertensives).
No products indexed under this heading.

Doxazosin Mesylate (Chlorthalidone may add to or potentiate the action of other antihypertensives).
No products indexed under this heading.

Doxepin Hydrochloride (Co-administration of clonidine with tricyclic antidepressants may result in reduced effect of clonidine, necessitating an increase in dosage).
No products indexed under this heading.

Enalapril Maleate (Chlorthalidone may add to or potentiate the action of other antihypertensives).
No products indexed under this heading.

Enalaprilat (Chlorthalidone may add to or potentiate the action of other antihypertensives).
No products indexed under this heading.

Eprosartan Mesylate (Chlorthalidone may add to or potentiate the action of other antihypertensives). Products include:
Teveten 538
Teveten HCT 541

Esmolol Hydrochloride (Chlorthalidone may add to or potentiate the action of other antihypertensives).
No products indexed under this heading.

Estazolam (Clonidine may enhance the CNS-depressive effects of other sedatives).
No products indexed under this heading.

Ethanol (Clonidine may enhance the CNS-depressive effects of alcohol; orthostatic hypotension may be aggravated by alcohol).
No products indexed under this heading.

Ethchlorvynol (Clonidine may enhance the CNS-depressive effects of other sedatives).
No products indexed under this heading.

Ethinamate (Clonidine may enhance the CNS-depressive effects of other sedatives).
No products indexed under this heading.

Ethyl Alcohol (Clonidine may enhance the CNS-depressive effects of alcohol; orthostatic hypotension may be aggravated by alcohol).
No products indexed under this heading.

Felodipine (Chlorthalidone may add to or potentiate the action of other antihypertensives).
No products indexed under this heading.

Fentanyl (Orthostatic hypotension may be aggravated by narcotics). Products include:
Duragesic 2604
Fentanyl Transdermal System 2346
Onsolis 2054

Fentanyl Citrate (Orthostatic hypotension may be aggravated by narcotics). Products include:
Fentora 966

Flurazepam Hydrochloride (Clonidine may enhance the CNS-depressive effects of other sedatives).
No products indexed under this heading.

Fosinopril Sodium (Chlorthalidone may add to or potentiate the action of other antihypertensives).
No products indexed under this heading.

Furosemide (Chlorthalidone may add to or potentiate the action of other antihypertensives). Products include:
Furosemide 2354

Glibenclamide (Higher dosage of oral hypoglycemic agents may be required when co-administered with chlorthalidone).
No products indexed under this heading.

Glimepiride (Higher dosage of oral hypoglycemic agents may be required when co-administered with chlorthalidone). Products include:
Avandaryl 1356
Duetact 3354

Glipizide (Higher dosage of oral hypoglycemic agents may be required when co-administered with chlorthalidone).
No products indexed under this heading.

Glutethimide (Clonidine may enhance the CNS-depressive effects of other sedatives).
No products indexed under this heading.

IMPORTANT NOTE: Always consult each drug listing in the patient's regimen for possible interactions.

Food Interactions

Alcohol (Clonidine may enhance the CNS-depressive effects of alcohol; orthostatic hypotension may be aggravated by alcohol).

Beer, reduced-alcohol (Clonidine may enhance the CNS-depressive effects of alcohol; orthostatic hypotension may be aggravated by alcohol).

Beer, unspecified (Clonidine may enhance the CNS-depressive effects of alcohol; orthostatic hypotension may be aggravated by alcohol).

Wine, Chianti (Clonidine may enhance the CNS-depressive effects of alcohol; orthostatic hypotension may be aggravated by alcohol).

Wine, Red (Clonidine may enhance the CNS-depressive effects of alcohol; orthostatic hypotension may be aggravated by alcohol).

IMPORTANT NOTE: Always consult each drug listing in the patient's regimen for possible interactions.

Wine, unspecified (Clonidine may enhance the CNS-depressive effects of alcohol; orthostatic hypotension may be aggravated by alcohol).

Wine products (Clonidine may enhance the CNS-depressive effects of alcohol; orthostatic hypotension may be aggravated by alcohol).

CM PLEX CREAM
(Fatty Acids, Olive Oil) 3455
None cited in PDR database.

CM PLEX SOFTGELS
(Fatty Acids, Salmon Oil, Soy oil) 3455
None cited in PDR database.

COARTEM TABLETS
(Artemether, Lumefantrine) 2403
May interact with antibiotics, antidepressant drugs, antifungals, antihistamines, antimalarials, antipsychotic agents, antiretroviral agents, azole antifungals, class 1A antiarrhythmics, class III antiarrhythmics, cytochrome p450 2b6 substrates (selected), cytochrome p450 3a4 inducers (selected), cytochrome p450 3a4 inhibitors (selected), cytochrome p450 3a4 inhibitors, potent (selected), cytochrome p450 3a4 substrates (selected), drugs that prolong the QT interval, fluoroquinolone antibiotics, imidazoles, macrolide antibiotics, Non-nucleoside reverse transcriptase inhibtors, oral contraceptives, protease inhibitors, quinidine, and certain other agents. Compounds in these categories include:

Abacavir Sulfate (Drugs that have a mixed effect on CYP3A4, especially anti-retroviral drugs, and those that have an effect on the QT interval should be used with caution in patients taking Coartem Tablets). Products include:
Epzicom	1448
Trizivir	1688
Ziagen	1740

Acetazolamide (When Coartem Tablets are co-administered with an inhibitor of CYP3A4, including grapefruit juice, it may result in increased concentrations of artemether and/or lumefantrine and potentiate QT prolongation).
No products indexed under this heading.

Acetazolamide Sodium (When Coartem Tablets are co-administered with an inhibitor of CYP3A4, including grapefruit juice, it may result in increased concentrations of artemether and/or lumefantrine and potentiate QT prolongation).
No products indexed under this heading.

Acrivastine (Coartem Tablets should be avoided in patients receiving other medications that prolong the QT interval, such as certain non-sedating antihistaminics (terfenadine, astemizole)).
No products indexed under this heading.

Alatrofloxacin Mesylate (Coartem Tablets should be avoided in patients receiving other medications that prolong the QT interval, such as certain antibiotics (macrolide antibiotics, fluoroquinolone antibiotics, imidazole, and triazole antifungal agents)).
No products indexed under this heading.

Alfentanil Hydrochloride (When Coartem Tablets are co-administered with substrates of CYP3A4 it may result in decreased concentrations of the substrate and potential loss of substrate efficacy).
No products indexed under this heading.

Allium sativum (When Coartem Tablets are co-administered with inducers of CYP3A4 it may result in decreased concentrations of artemether and/or lumefantrine and loss of anti-malarial efficacy).
No products indexed under this heading.

Alprazolam (Drugs that prolong the QT interval, including antimalarials such as quinine and quinidine, should be used cautiously following Coartem Tablets, due to the long elimination half-life of lumefantrine (3-6 days) and the potential for additive effects on the QT interval).
No products indexed under this heading.

Amikacin Sulfate (Coartem Tablets should be avoided in patients receiving other medications that prolong the QT interval, such as certain antibiotics (macrolide antibiotics, fluoroquinolone antibiotics, imidazole, and triazole antifungal agents)).
No products indexed under this heading.

Aminoglutethimide (When Coartem Tablets are co-administered with inducers of CYP3A4 it may result in decreased concentrations of artemether and/or lumefantrine and loss of anti-malarial efficacy).
No products indexed under this heading.

Amiodarone Hydrochloride (Coartem Tablets should be avoided in patients receiving other medications that prolong the QT interval, such as class III (amiodarone, sotalol) antiarrhythmic agents).
No products indexed under this heading.

Amitriptyline Hydrochloride (Coartem Tablets should be avoided in patients receiving other medications that prolong the QT interval, such as antidepressants).
No products indexed under this heading.

Amlodipine Besylate (When Coartem Tablets are co-administered with substrates of CYP3A4 it may result in decreased concentrations of the substrate and potential loss of substrate efficacy). Products include:
Azor	1010
Exforge	2443
Exforge HCT	2449

Amoxapine (Coartem Tablets should be avoided in patients receiving other medications that prolong the QT interval, such as antidepressants).
No products indexed under this heading.

Amoxicillin (Coartem Tablets should be avoided in patients receiving other medications that prolong the QT interval, such as certain antibiotics (macrolide antibiotics, fluoroquinolone antibiotics, imidazole, and triazole antifungal agents)). Products include:
Amoxil Capsules	1311
Amoxil Chewable Tablets	1311
Amoxil	1311
Amoxil Powder	1311
Augmentin	1331
Augmentin Tablets	1335
Augmentin ES-600	1338
Augmentin XR	1342
Moxatag	2321

Amoxicillin Trihydrate (Coartem Tablets should be avoided in patients receiving other medications that prolong the QT interval, such as certain antibiotics (macrolide antibiotics, fluoroquinolone antibiotics, imidazole, and triazole antifungal agents)).
No products indexed under this heading.

Amphotericin B (Coartem Tablets should be avoided in patients receiving other medications that prolong the QT interval, such as certain antibiotics (macrolide antibiotics, fluoroquinolone antibiotics, imidazole, and triazole antifungal agents)).
No products indexed under this heading.

Amphotericin B, liposomal (Coartem Tablets should be avoided in patients receiving other medications that prolong the QT interval, such as certain antibiotics (macrolide antibiotics, fluoroquinolone antibiotics, imidazole, and triazole antifungal agents)).
Products include:

AmBisome 659

Amphotericin B Cholesteryl Sulfate (Coartem Tablets should be avoided in patients receiving other medications that prolong the QT interval, such as certain antibiotics (macrolide antibiotics, fluoroquinolone antibiotics, imidazole, and triazole antifungal agents)).
No products indexed under this heading.

Amphotericin B Lipid Complex (Coartem Tablets should be avoided in patients receiving other medications that prolong the QT interval, such as certain antibiotics (macrolide antibiotics, fluoroquinolone antibiotics, imidazole, and triazole antifungal agents)).
No products indexed under this heading.

Ampicillin (Coartem Tablets should be avoided in patients receiving other medications that prolong the QT interval, such as certain antibiotics (macrolide antibiotics, fluoroquinolone antibiotics, imidazole, and triazole antifungal agents)).
No products indexed under this heading.

Ampicillin Sodium (Coartem Tablets should be avoided in patients receiving other medications that prolong the QT interval, such as certain antibiotics (macrolide antibiotics, fluoroquinolone antibiotics, imidazole, and triazole antifungal agents)).
No products indexed under this heading.

Ampicillin Trihydrate (Coartem Tablets should be avoided in patients receiving other medications that prolong the QT interval, such as certain antibiotics (macrolide antibiotics, fluoroquinolone antibiotics, imidazole, and triazole antifungal agents)).
No products indexed under this heading.

Amprenavir (When Coartem Tablets are co-administered with an inhibitor of CYP3A4, including grapefruit juice, it may result in increased concentrations of artemether and/or lumefantrine and potentiate QT prolongation).
No products indexed under this heading.

Anastrozole (When Coartem Tablets are co-administered with an inhibitor of CYP3A4, including grapefruit juice, it may result in increased concentrations of artemether and/or lumefantrine and potentiate QT prolongation).
No products indexed under this heading.

Anidulafungin (Coartem Tablets should be avoided in patients receiving other medications that prolong the QT interval, such as certain antibiotics (macrolide antibiotics, fluoroquinolone antibiotics, imidazole, and triazole antifungal agents)).
No products indexed under this heading.

Antibiotics, non-penicillin, unspecified (Coartem Tablets should be avoided in patients receiving other medications that prolong the QT interval, such as certain antibiotics (macrolide antibiotics, fluoroquinolone antibiotics, imidazole, and triazole antifungal agents)).
No products indexed under this heading.

Aprepitant (When Coartem Tablets are co-administered with substrates of CYP3A4 it may result in decreased concentrations of the substrate and potential loss of substrate efficacy). Products include:
Emend	2124

Aripiprazole (Coartem Tablets should be avoided in patients receiving other medications that prolong the QT interval, such as antipsychotics (pimozide, ziprasidone)).
No products indexed under this heading.

Astemizole (Coartem Tablets should be avoided in patients receiving other medications that prolong the QT interval, such as certain non-sedating antihistaminics (terfenadine, astemizole)).
No products indexed under this heading.

Atazanavir (When Coartem Tablets are co-administered with an inhibitor of CYP3A4, including grapefruit juice, it may result in increased concentrations of artemether and/or lumefantrine and potentiate QT prolongation).
No products indexed under this heading.

Atazanavir Sulfate (When Coartem Tablets are co-administered with an inhibitor of CYP3A4, including grapefruit juice, it may result in increased concentrations of artemether and/or lumefantrine and potentiate QT prolongation).
No products indexed under this heading.

Atorvastatin Calcium (When Coartem Tablets are co-administered with substrates of CYP3A4 it may result in decreased concentrations of the substrate and potential loss of substrate efficacy). Products include:
Lipitor	2703

Azatadine Maleate (Coartem Tablets should be avoided in patients receiving other medications that prolong the QT interval, such as certain non-sedating antihistaminics (terfenadine, astemizole)).
No products indexed under this heading.

Azithromycin Dihydrate (Coartem Tablets should be avoided in patients receiving other medications that prolong the QT interval, such as certain antibiotics (macrolide antibiotics, fluoroquinolone antibiotics, imidazole, and triazole antifungal agents)).
No products indexed under this heading.

Azlocillin Sodium (Coartem Tablets should be avoided in patients receiving other medications that prolong the QT interval, such as certain antibiotics (macrolide antibiotics, fluoroquinolone antibiotics, imidazole, and triazole antifungal agents)).
No products indexed under this heading.

Aztreonam (Coartem Tablets should be avoided in patients receiving other medications that prolong the QT interval, such as certain antibiotics (macrolide antibiotics, fluoroquinolone antibiotics, imidazole, and triazole antifungal agents)).
No products indexed under this heading.

Bacampicillin Hydrochloride (Coartem Tablets should be avoided in patients receiving other medications that prolong the QT interval, such as certain antibiotics (macrolide antibiotics, fluoroquinolone antibiotics, imidazole, and triazole antifungal agents)).
No products indexed under this heading.

Belladonna Ergotamine (When Coartem Tablets are co-administered with substrates of CYP3A4 it may result in decreased concentrations of the substrate and potential loss of substrate efficacy).
No products indexed under this heading.

Betamethasone (When Coartem Tablets are co-administered with inducers of CYP3A4 it may result in decreased concentrations of artemether and/or lumefantrine and loss of anti-malarial efficacy).
No products indexed under this heading.

Betamethasone Acetate (When Coartem Tablets are co-administered with inducers of CYP3A4 it may result in decreased concentrations of artemether and/or lumefantrine and loss of anti-malarial efficacy).
No products indexed under this heading.

381 Interactions Index Coartem

Betamethasone Benzoate (When Coartem Tablets are co-administered with inducers of CYP3A4 it may result in decreased concentrations of artemether and/or lumefantrine and loss of anti-malarial efficacy).
No products indexed under this heading.

Betamethasone Dipropionate (When Coartem Tablets are co-administered with inducers of CYP3A4 it may result in decreased concentrations of artemether and/or lumefantrine and loss of anti-malarial efficacy). Products include:
Diprolene Lotion 0.05% ... 3108
Diprolene Ointment 0.05% ... 3109
Diprolene AF Cream 0.05% ... 3107
Lotrisone ... 3163

Betamethasone Sodium Phosphate (When Coartem Tablets are co-administered with inducers of CYP3A4 it may result in decreased concentrations of artemether and/or lumefantrine and loss of anti-malarial efficacy).
No products indexed under this heading.

Betamethasone Valerate (When Coartem Tablets are co-administered with inducers of CYP3A4 it may result in decreased concentrations of artemether and/or lumefantrine and loss of anti-malarial efficacy). Products include:
Luxíq ... 3321

Bosentan (When Coartem Tablets are co-administered with inducers of CYP3A4 it may result in decreased concentrations of artemether and/or lumefantrine and loss of anti-malarial efficacy). Products include:
Tracleer ... 573

Bretylium Tosylate (Coartem Tablets should be avoided in patients receiving other medications that prolong the QT interval, such as class III (amiodarone, sotalol) antiarrhythmic agents).
No products indexed under this heading.

Bromodiphenhydramine Hydrochloride (Coartem Tablets should be avoided in patients receiving other medications that prolong the QT interval, such as certain non-sedating antihistaminics (terfenadine, astemizole)).
No products indexed under this heading.

Brompheniramine Maleate (Coartem Tablets should be avoided in patients receiving other medications that prolong the QT interval, such as certain non-sedating antihistaminics (terfenadine, astemizole)).
No products indexed under this heading.

Bupropion (Administration of Coartem Tablets with drugs that are metabolized by CYP2D6 maysignificantly increase plasma concentrations of the co-administered drug and increase the risk of adverse effects. Many of the drugs metabolized by CYP2D6 can prolong the QT interval and should not be administered with Coartem Tablets due to the potential additive effect on the QT interval (eg, flecainide, imipramine, amitriptyline, clomipramine)).
No products indexed under this heading.

Bupropion Hydrochloride (Coartem Tablets should be avoided in patients receiving other medications that prolong the QT interval, such as antidepressants). Products include:
Aplenzin ... 2948
Wellbutrin ... 1719
Wellbutrin SR ... 1725
Zyban ... 1762

Buspirone Hydrochloride (Drugs that prolong the QT interval, including antimalarials such as quinine and quinidine, should be used cautiously following Coartem Tablets, due to the long elimination half-life of lumefantrine (3-6 days) and the potential for additive effects on the QT interval).
No products indexed under this heading.

Busulfan (When Coartem Tablets are co-administered with substrates of CYP3A4 it may result in decreased concentrations of the substrate and potential loss of substrate efficacy). Products include:
Myleran ... 1581

Butoconazole Nitrate (Coartem Tablets should be avoided in patients receiving other medications that prolong the QT interval, such as certain antibiotics (macrolide antibiotics, fluoroquinolone antibiotics, imidazole, and triazole antifungal agents)).
No products indexed under this heading.

Carbamazepine (When Coartem Tablets are co-administered with substrates of CYP3A4 it may result in decreased concentrations of the substrate and potential loss of substrate efficacy). Products include:
Carbatrol ... 3280
Equetro ... 3477

Carbenicillin Disodium (Coartem Tablets should be avoided in patients receiving other medications that prolong the QT interval, such as certain antibiotics (macrolide antibiotics, fluoroquinolone antibiotics, imidazole, and triazole antifungal agents)).
No products indexed under this heading.

Carbenicillin Indanyl Sodium (Coartem Tablets should be avoided in patients receiving other medications that prolong the QT interval, such as certain antibiotics (macrolide antibiotics, fluoroquinolone antibiotics, imidazole, and triazole antifungal agents)).
No products indexed under this heading.

Caspofungin acetate (Coartem Tablets should be avoided in patients receiving other medications that prolong the QT interval, such as certain antibiotics (macrolide antibiotics, fluoroquinolone antibiotics, imidazole, and triazole antifungal agents)). Products include:
Cancidas ... 2088

Cefaclor (Coartem Tablets should be avoided in patients receiving other medications that prolong the QT interval, such as certain antibiotics (macrolide antibiotics, fluoroquinolone antibiotics, imidazole, and triazole antifungal agents)).
No products indexed under this heading.

Cefadroxil (Coartem Tablets should be avoided in patients receiving other medications that prolong the QT interval, such as certain antibiotics (macrolide antibiotics, fluoroquinolone antibiotics, imidazole, and triazole antifungal agents)).
No products indexed under this heading.

Cefamandole Nafate (Coartem Tablets should be avoided in patients receiving other medications that prolong the QT interval, such as certain antibiotics (macrolide antibiotics, fluoroquinolone antibiotics, imidazole, and triazole antifungal agents)).
No products indexed under this heading.

Cefazolin Sodium (Coartem Tablets should be avoided in patients receiving other medications that prolong the QT interval, such as certain antibiotics (macrolide antibiotics, fluoroquinolone antibiotics, imidazole, and triazole antifungal agents)).
No products indexed under this heading.

Cefixime (Coartem Tablets should be avoided in patients receiving other medications that prolong the QT interval, such as certain antibiotics (macrolide antibiotics, fluoroquinolone antibiotics, imidazole, and triazole antifungal agents)). Products include:
Suprax for Oral Suspension ... 2038
Suprax Tablets ... 2038

Cefmetazole Sodium (Coartem Tablets should be avoided in patients receiving other medications that prolong the QT interval, such as certain antibiotics (macrolide antibiotics, fluoroquinolone antibiotics, imidazole, and triazole antifungal agents)).
No products indexed under this heading.

Cefonicid Sodium (Coartem Tablets should be avoided in patients receiving other medications that prolong the QT interval, such as certain antibiotics (macrolide antibiotics, fluoroquinolone antibiotics, imidazole, and triazole antifungal agents)).
No products indexed under this heading.

Cefoperazone Sodium (Coartem Tablets should be avoided in patients receiving other medications that prolong the QT interval, such as certain antibiotics (macrolide antibiotics, fluoroquinolone antibiotics, imidazole, and triazole antifungal agents)).
No products indexed under this heading.

Ceforanide (Coartem Tablets should be avoided in patients receiving other medications that prolong the QT interval, such as certain antibiotics (macrolide antibiotics, fluoroquinolone antibiotics, imidazole, and triazole antifungal agents)).
No products indexed under this heading.

Cefotaxime Sodium (Coartem Tablets should be avoided in patients receiving other medications that prolong the QT interval, such as certain antibiotics (macrolide antibiotics, fluoroquinolone antibiotics, imidazole, and triazole antifungal agents)).
No products indexed under this heading.

Cefotetan (Coartem Tablets should be avoided in patients receiving other medications that prolong the QT interval, such as certain antibiotics (macrolide antibiotics, fluoroquinolone antibiotics, imidazole, and triazole antifungal agents)).
No products indexed under this heading.

Cefoxitin Sodium (Coartem Tablets should be avoided in patients receiving other medications that prolong the QT interval, such as certain antibiotics (macrolide antibiotics, fluoroquinolone antibiotics, imidazole, and triazole antifungal agents)).
No products indexed under this heading.

Cefpodoxime Proxetil (Coartem Tablets should be avoided in patients receiving other medications that prolong the QT interval, such as certain antibiotics (macrolide antibiotics, fluoroquinolone antibiotics, imidazole, and triazole antifungal agents)).
No products indexed under this heading.

Cefprozil (Coartem Tablets should be avoided in patients receiving other medications that prolong the QT interval, such as certain antibiotics (macrolide antibiotics, fluoroquinolone antibiotics, imidazole, and triazole antifungal agents)).
No products indexed under this heading.

Ceftazidime (Coartem Tablets should be avoided in patients receiving other medications that prolong the QT interval, such as certain antibiotics (macrolide antibiotics, fluoroquinolone antibiotics, imidazole, and triazole antifungal agents)). Products include:
Fortaz ... 1481

Ceftizoxime Sodium (Coartem Tablets should be avoided in patients receiving other medications that prolong the QT interval, such as certain antibiotics (macrolide antibiotics, fluoroquinolone antibiotics, imidazole, and triazole antifungal agents)).
No products indexed under this heading.

Ceftriaxone Sodium (Coartem Tablets should be avoided in patients receiving other medications that prolong the QT interval, such as certain antibiotics (macrolide antibiotics, fluoroquinolone antibiotics, imidazole, and triazole antifungal agents)). Products include:
Rocephin ... 2859

Cefuroxime Axetil (Coartem Tablets should be avoided in patients receiving other medications that prolong the QT interval, such as certain antibiotics (macrolide antibiotics, fluoroquinolone antibiotics, imidazole, and triazole antifungal agents)). Products include:
Ceftin ... 1399

Cefuroxime Sodium (Coartem Tablets should be avoided in patients receiving other medications that prolong the QT interval, such as certain antibiotics (macrolide antibiotics, fluoroquinolone antibiotics, imidazole, and triazole antifungal agents)).
No products indexed under this heading.

Cephalexin (Coartem Tablets should be avoided in patients receiving other medications that prolong the QT interval, such as certain antibiotics (macrolide antibiotics, fluoroquinolone antibiotics, imidazole, and triazole antifungal agents)).
No products indexed under this heading.

Cephalothin Sodium (Coartem Tablets should be avoided in patients receiving other medications that prolong the QT interval, such as certain antibiotics (macrolide antibiotics, fluoroquinolone antibiotics, imidazole, and triazole antifungal agents)).
No products indexed under this heading.

Cephapirin Sodium (Coartem Tablets should be avoided in patients receiving other medications that prolong the QT interval, such as certain antibiotics (macrolide antibiotics, fluoroquinolone antibiotics, imidazole, and triazole antifungal agents)).
No products indexed under this heading.

Cephradine (Coartem Tablets should be avoided in patients receiving other medications that prolong the QT interval, such as certain antibiotics (macrolide antibiotics, fluoroquinolone antibiotics, imidazole, and triazole antifungal agents)).
No products indexed under this heading.

Cerivastatin Sodium (When Coartem Tablets are co-administered with substrates of CYP3A4 it may result in decreased concentrations of the substrate and potential loss of substrate efficacy).
No products indexed under this heading.

Cetirizine Hydrochloride (Coartem Tablets should be avoided in patients receiving other medications that prolong the QT interval, such as certain non-sedating antihistaminics (terfenadine, astemizole)). Products include:
Zyrtec Allergy ... 2052
Children's Zyrtec Allergy Syrup ... 2053
Children's Zyrtec Allergy ... 2053
Children's Zyrtec Hives Relief ... 2053
Zyrtec-D Allergy & Congestion ... 2054

Chloramphenicol (Coartem Tablets should be avoided in patients receiving other medications that prolong the QT interval, such as certain antibiotics (macrolide antibiotics, fluoroquinolone antibiotics, imidazole, and triazole antifungal agents)).
No products indexed under this heading.

Chloramphenicol Palmitate (Coartem Tablets should be avoided in patients receiving other medications that prolong the QT interval, such as certain antibiotics (macrolide antibiotics, fluoroquinolone antibiotics, imidazole, and triazole antifungal agents)).
No products indexed under this heading.

IMPORTANT NOTE: Always consult each drug listing in the patient's regimen for possible interactions.

(⊙ Described in PDR® for Ophthalmic Medicines)

Desipramine Hydrochloride (Coartem Tablets should be avoided in patients receiving other medications that prolong the QT interval, such as antidepressants).
No products indexed under this heading.

Desloratadine (When Coartem Tablets are co-administered with an inhibitor of CYP3A4, including grapefruit juice, it may result in increased concentrations of artemether and/or lumefantrine and potentiate QT prolongation). Products include:
Clarinex Syrup 3098
Clarinex 3098
Clarinex Reditabs 3098
Clarinex-D 12-Hour 3101
Clarinex-D 3104

Desogestrel (When Coartem Tablets are co-administered with substrates of CYP3A4 it may result in decreased concentrations of the substrate and potential loss of substrate efficacy).
No products indexed under this heading.

Dexamethasone (When Coartem Tablets are co-administered with inducers of CYP3A4 it may result in decreased concentrations of artemether and/or lumefantrine and loss of anti-malarial efficacy). Products include:
Ciprodex 583
Ozurdex .... ⊙ 223
Tobramycin and Dexamethasone Ophthalmic Suspension .... ⊙ 251

Dexamethasone Acetate (When Coartem Tablets are co-administered with inducers of CYP3A4 it may result in decreased concentrations of artemether and/or lumefantrine and loss of anti-malarial efficacy).
No products indexed under this heading.

Dexamethasone Phosphate (When Coartem Tablets are co-administered with inducers of CYP3A4 it may result in decreased concentrations of artemether and/or lumefantrine and loss of anti-malarial efficacy).
No products indexed under this heading.

Dexamethasone Sodium (When Coartem Tablets are co-administered with inducers of CYP3A4 it may result in decreased concentrations of artemether and/or lumefantrine and loss of anti-malarial efficacy).
No products indexed under this heading.

Dexamethasone Sodium Phosphate (When Coartem Tablets are co-administered with inducers of CYP3A4 it may result in decreased concentrations of artemether and/or lumefantrine and loss of anti-malarial efficacy).
No products indexed under this heading.

Dexamethasone Sodium Phosphate Injection (When Coartem Tablets are co-administered with inducers of CYP3A4 it may result in decreased concentrations of artemether and/or lumefantrine and loss of anti-malarial efficacy).
No products indexed under this heading.

Dexchlorpheniramine Maleate (Coartem Tablets should be avoided in patients receiving other medications that prolong the QT interval, such as certain non-sedating antihistaminics (terfenadine, astemizole)).
No products indexed under this heading.

Diazepam (Drugs that prolong the QT interval, including antimalarials such as quinine and quinidine, should be used cautiously following Coartem Tablets, due to the long elimination half-life of lumefantrine (3-6 days) and the potential for additive effects on the QT interval). Products include:
Valium Tablets 2880

Diclofenac Epolamine (Administration of Coartem Tablets with drugs that are metabolized by CYP2D6 maysignificantly increase plasma concentrations of the co-administered drug and increase the risk of adverse effects. Many of the drugs metabolized by CYP2D6 can prolong the QT interval and should not be administered with Coartem Tablets due to the potential additive effect on the QT interval (eg, flecainide, imipramine, amitriptyline, clomipramine)). Products include:
Flector 1839

Diclofenac Potassium (Administration of Coartem Tablets with drugs that are metabolized by CYP2D6 maysignificantly increase plasma concentrations of the co-administered drug and increase the risk of adverse effects. Many of the drugs metabolized by CYP2D6 can prolong the QT interval and should not be administered with Coartem Tablets due to the potential additive effect on the QT interval (eg, flecainide, imipramine, amitriptyline, clomipramine)).
No products indexed under this heading.

Diclofenac Sodium (Administration of Coartem Tablets with drugs that are metabolized by CYP2D6 maysignificantly increase plasma concentrations of the co-administered drug and increase the risk of adverse effects. Many of the drugs metabolized by CYP2D6 can prolong the QT interval and should not be administered with Coartem Tablets due to the potential additive effect on the QT interval (eg, flecainide, imipramine, amitriptyline, clomipramine)).
No products indexed under this heading.

Dicloxacillin (Coartem Tablets should be avoided in patients receiving other medications that prolong the QT interval, such as certain antibiotics (macrolide antibiotics, fluoroquinolone antibiotics, imidazole, and triazole antifungal agents)).
No products indexed under this heading.

Dicloxacillin Sodium (Coartem Tablets should be avoided in patients receiving other medications that prolong the QT interval, such as certain antibiotics (macrolide antibiotics, fluoroquinolone antibiotics, imidazole, and triazole antifungal agents)).
No products indexed under this heading.

Didanosine (Drugs that have a mixed effect on CYP3A4, especially antiretroviral drugs, and those that have an effect on the QT interval should be used with caution in patients taking Coartem Tablets).
No products indexed under this heading.

Dihydroergotamine Mesylate (When Coartem Tablets are co-administered with substrates of CYP3A4 it may result in decreased concentrations of the substrate and potential loss of substrate efficacy).
No products indexed under this heading.

Diltiazem Hydrochloride (When Coartem Tablets are co-administered with substrates of CYP3A4 it may result in decreased concentrations of the substrate and potential loss of substrate efficacy). Products include:
Cardizem LA 423

Diltiazem Maleate (When Coartem Tablets are co-administered with substrates of CYP3A4 it may result in decreased concentrations of the substrate and potential loss of substrate efficacy).
No products indexed under this heading.

Diphenhydramine Hydrochloride (Coartem Tablets should be avoided in patients receiving other medications that prolong the QT interval, such as certain non-sedating antihistaminics (terfenadine, astemizole)). Products include:
Benadryl Allergy Ultratab 2042
Children's Benadryl Allergy Liquid 2042

Diphenylpyraline Hydrochloride (Coartem Tablets should be avoided in patients receiving other medications that prolong the QT interval, such as certain non-sedating antihistaminics (terfenadine, astemizole)).
No products indexed under this heading.

Dirithromycin (Coartem Tablets should be avoided in patients receiving other medications that prolong the QT interval, such as certain antibiotics (macrolide antibiotics, fluoroquinolone antibiotics, imidazole, and triazole antifungal agents)).
No products indexed under this heading.

Disodium Carbenicillin (Coartem Tablets should be avoided in patients receiving other medications that prolong the QT interval, such as certain antibiotics (macrolide antibiotics, fluoroquinolone antibiotics, imidazole, and triazole antifungal agents)).
No products indexed under this heading.

Disopyramide (Coartem Tablets should be avoided in patients receiving other medications that prolong the QT interval, such as class IA (quinidine, procainamide, disopyramide) antiarrhythmic agents).
No products indexed under this heading.

Disopyramide Phosphate (Coartem Tablets should be avoided in patients receiving other medications that prolong the QT interval, such as class IA (quinidine, procainamide, disopyramide) antiarrhythmic agents).
No products indexed under this heading.

Disulfiram (When Coartem Tablets are co-administered with substrates of CYP3A4 it may result in decreased concentrations of the substrate and potential loss of substrate efficacy).
No products indexed under this heading.

Divalproex Sodium (Administration of Coartem Tablets with drugs that are metabolized by CYP2D6 maysignificantly increase plasma concentrations of the co-administered drug and increase the risk of adverse effects. Many of the drugs metabolized by CYP2D6 can prolong the QT interval and should not be administered with Coartem Tablets due to the potential additive effect on the QT interval (eg, flecainide, imipramine, amitriptyline, clomipramine)). Products include:
Depakote ER 426

Dofetilide (Drugs that prolong the QT interval, including antimalarials such as quinine and quinidine, should be used cautiously following Coartem Tablets, due to the long elimination half-life of lumefantrine (3-6 days) and the potential for additive effects on the QT interval).
No products indexed under this heading.

Doxepin Hydrochloride (Coartem Tablets should be avoided in patients receiving other medications that prolong the QT interval, such as antidepressants).
No products indexed under this heading.

Doxorubicin Hydrochloride (When Coartem Tablets are co-administered with substrates of CYP3A4 it may result in decreased concentrations of the substrate and potential loss of substrate efficacy).
No products indexed under this heading.

Doxycycline Calcium (Coartem Tablets should be avoided in patients receiving other medications that prolong the QT interval, such as certain antibiotics (macrolide antibiotics, fluoroquinolone antibiotics, imidazole, and triazole antifungal agents)).
No products indexed under this heading.

Doxycycline Hyclate (Coartem Tablets should be avoided in patients receiving other medications that prolong the QT interval, such as certain antibiotics (macrolide antibiotics, fluoroquinolone antibiotics, imidazole, and triazole antifungal agents)).
No products indexed under this heading.

Doxycycline Monohydrate (Coartem Tablets should be avoided in patients receiving other medications that prolong the QT interval, such as certain antibiotics (macrolide antibiotics, fluoroquinolone antibiotics, imidazole, and triazole antifungal agents)).
No products indexed under this heading.

Dronabinol (When Coartem Tablets are co-administered with substrates of CYP3A4 it may result in decreased concentrations of the substrate and potential loss of substrate efficacy).
No products indexed under this heading.

Droperidol (Drugs that prolong the QT interval, including antimalarials such as quinine and quinidine, should be used cautiously following Coartem Tablets, due to the long elimination half-life of lumefantrine (3-6 days) and the potential for additive effects on the QT interval).
No products indexed under this heading.

Econazole Nitrate (Coartem Tablets should be avoided in patients receiving other medications that prolong the QT interval, such as certain antibiotics (macrolide antibiotics, fluoroquinolone antibiotics, imidazole, and triazole antifungal agents)).
No products indexed under this heading.

Efavirenz (When Coartem Tablets are co-administered with an inhibitor of CYP3A4, including grapefruit juice, it may result in increased concentrations of artemether and/or lumefantrine and potentiate QT prolongation). Products include:
Atripla 906

Emtricitabine (Drugs that have a mixed effect on CYP3A4, especially anti-retroviral drugs, and those that have an effect on the QT interval should be used with caution in patients taking Coartem Tablets). Products include:
Atripla 906
Emtriva 1238
Emtriva Oral Solution 1238
Truvada 1258

Enfuvirtide (Drugs that have a mixed effect on CYP3A4, especially antiretroviral drugs, and those that have an effect on the QT interval should be used with caution in patients taking Coartem Tablets).
No products indexed under this heading.

Enoxacin (Coartem Tablets should be avoided in patients receiving other medications that prolong the QT interval, such as certain antibiotics (macrolide antibiotics, fluoroquinolone antibiotics, imidazole, and triazole antifungal agents)).
No products indexed under this heading.

Epirubicin Hydrochloride (Coartem Tablets should be avoided in patients receiving other medications that prolong the QT interval, such as certain antibiotics (macrolide antibiotics, fluoroquinolone antibiotics, imidazole, and triazole antifungal agents)).
No products indexed under this heading.

Ergotamine Tartrate (When Coartem Tablets are co-administered with substrates of CYP3A4 it may result in decreased concentrations of the substrate and potential loss of substrate efficacy).
No products indexed under this heading.

IMPORTANT NOTE: Always consult each drug listing in the patient's regimen for possible interactions.

Fluoxetine (When Coartem Tablets are co-administered with an inhibitor of CYP3A4, including grapefruit juice, it may result in increased concentrations of artemether and/or lumefantrine and potentiate QT prolongation).
No products indexed under this heading.

Fluoxetine Hydrochloride (Coartem Tablets should be avoided in patients receiving other medications that prolong the QT interval, such as antidepressants). Products include:
Prozac Weekly 1941
Prozac Pulvules 1941
Symbyax 1965

Fluphenazine Decanoate (Coartem Tablets should be avoided in patients receiving other medications that prolong the QT interval, such as antipsychotics (pimozide, ziprasidone)).
No products indexed under this heading.

Fluphenazine Enanthate (Coartem Tablets should be avoided in patients receiving other medications that prolong the QT interval, such as antipsychotics (pimozide, ziprasidone)).
No products indexed under this heading.

Fluphenazine Hydrochloride (Coartem Tablets should be avoided in patients receiving other medications that prolong the QT interval, such as antipsychotics (pimozide, ziprasidone)).
No products indexed under this heading.

Fluvoxamine (Coartem Tablets should be avoided in patients receiving other medications that prolong the QT interval, such as antidepressants).
No products indexed under this heading.

Fluvoxamine Maleate (Coartem Tablets should be avoided in patients receiving other medications that prolong the QT interval, such as antidepressants).
No products indexed under this heading.

Fosamprenavir Calcium (When Coartem Tablets are co-administered with an inhibitor of CYP3A4, including grapefruit juice, it may result in increased concentrations of artemether and/or lumefantrine and potentiate QT prolongation). Products include:
Lexiva Oral Suspension 1558
Lexiva 1558

Fosphenytoin Sodium (When Coartem Tablets are co-administered with inducers of CYP3A4 it may result in decreased concentrations of artemether and/or lumefantrine and loss of anti-malarial efficacy).
No products indexed under this heading.

Garlic Extract (When Coartem Tablets are co-administered with inducers of CYP3A4 it may result in decreased concentrations of artemether and/or lumefantrine and loss of anti-malarial efficacy).
No products indexed under this heading.

Garlic Oil (When Coartem Tablets are co-administered with inducers of CYP3A4 it may result in decreased concentrations of artemether and/or lumefantrine and loss of anti-malarial efficacy).
No products indexed under this heading.

Gatifloxacin (Coartem Tablets should be avoided in patients receiving other medications that prolong the QT interval, such as certain antibiotics (macrolide antibiotics, fluoroquinolone antibiotics, imidazole, and triazole antifungal agents)).
No products indexed under this heading.

Gemifloxacin Mesylate (Coartem Tablets should be avoided in patients receiving other medications that prolong the QT interval, such as certain antibiotics (macrolide antibiotics, fluoroquinolone antibiotics, imidazole, and triazole antifungal agents)).
No products indexed under this heading.

Gentamicin Sulfate (Coartem Tablets should be avoided in patients receiving other medications that prolong the QT interval, such as certain antibiotics (macrolide antibiotics, fluoroquinolone antibiotics, imidazole, and triazole antifungal agents)). Products include:
Pred-G .... ⊙226, ⊙227

Grepafloxacin Hydrochloride (Coartem Tablets should be avoided in patients receiving other medications that prolong the QT interval, such as certain antibiotics (macrolide antibiotics, fluoroquinolone antibiotics, imidazole, and triazole antifungal agents)).
No products indexed under this heading.

Griseofulvin (Coartem Tablets should be avoided in patients receiving other medications that prolong the QT interval, such as certain antibiotics (macrolide antibiotics, fluoroquinolone antibiotics, imidazole, and triazole antifungal agents)).
No products indexed under this heading.

Halofantrine (Halofantrine and Coartem Tablets should not be administered within one month of each other due to the long elimination half-life of lumefantrine (3-6 days) and potential additive effects on the QT interval).
No products indexed under this heading.

Halofantrine Hydrochloride (Halofantrine and Coartem Tablets should not be administered within one month of each other due to the long elimination half-life of lumefantrine (3-6 days) and potential additive effects on the QT interval).
No products indexed under this heading.

Haloperidol (Coartem Tablets should be avoided in patients receiving other medications that prolong the QT interval, such as antipsychotics (pimozide, ziprasidone)).
No products indexed under this heading.

Haloperidol Decanoate (Coartem Tablets should be avoided in patients receiving other medications that prolong the QT interval, such as antipsychotics (pimozide, ziprasidone)).
No products indexed under this heading.

Haloperidol Lactate (Coartem Tablets should be avoided in patients receiving other medications that prolong the QT interval, such as antipsychotics (pimozide, ziprasidone)).
No products indexed under this heading.

Halothane (Administration of Coartem Tablets with drugs that are metabolized by CYP2D6 maysignificantly increase plasma concentrations of the co-administered drug and increase the risk of adverse effects. Many of the drugs metabolized by CYP2D6 can prolong the QT interval and should not be administered with Coartem Tablets due to the potential additive effect on the QT interval (eg, flecainide, imipramine, amitriptyline, clomipramine)).
No products indexed under this heading.

Hydrocortisone (When Coartem Tablets are co-administered with inducers of CYP3A4 it may result in decreased concentrations of artemether and/or lumefantrine and loss of anti-malarial efficacy).
No products indexed under this heading.

Hydrocortisone (Alcohol) (When Coartem Tablets are co-administered with inducers of CYP3A4 it may result in decreased concentrations of artemether and/or lumefantrine and loss of anti-malarial efficacy).
No products indexed under this heading.

Hydrocortisone Acetate (When Coartem Tablets are co-administered with inducers of CYP3A4 it may result in decreased concentrations of artemether and/or lumefantrine and loss of anti-malarial efficacy).
No products indexed under this heading.

Hydrocortisone Butyrate (When Coartem Tablets are co-administered with inducers of CYP3A4 it may result in decreased concentrations of artemether and/or lumefantrine and loss of anti-malarial efficacy).
No products indexed under this heading.

Hydrocortisone Cypionate (When Coartem Tablets are co-administered with inducers of CYP3A4 it may result in decreased concentrations of artemether and/or lumefantrine and loss of anti-malarial efficacy).
No products indexed under this heading.

Hydrocortisone Hemisuccinate (When Coartem Tablets are co-administered with inducers of CYP3A4 it may result in decreased concentrations of artemether and/or lumefantrine and loss of anti-malarial efficacy).
No products indexed under this heading.

Hydrocortisone Probutate (When Coartem Tablets are co-administered with inducers of CYP3A4 it may result in decreased concentrations of artemether and/or lumefantrine and loss of anti-malarial efficacy).
No products indexed under this heading.

Hydrocortisone Sodium Phosphate (When Coartem Tablets are co-administered with inducers of CYP3A4 it may result in decreased concentrations of artemether and/or lumefantrine and loss of anti-malarial efficacy).
No products indexed under this heading.

Hydrocortisone Sodium Succinate (When Coartem Tablets are co-administered with inducers of CYP3A4 it may result in decreased concentrations of artemether and/or lumefantrine and loss of anti-malarial efficacy).
No products indexed under this heading.

Hydrocortisone Valerate (When Coartem Tablets are co-administered with inducers of CYP3A4 it may result in decreased concentrations of artemether and/or lumefantrine and loss of anti-malarial efficacy).
No products indexed under this heading.

Hydroxyzine Hydrochloride (Drugs that prolong the QT interval, including antimalarials such as quinine and quinidine, should be used cautiously following Coartem Tablets, due to the long elimination half-life of lumefantrine (3-6 days) and the potential for additive effects on the QT interval).
No products indexed under this heading.

Hypericum (When Coartem Tablets are co-administered with inducers of CYP3A4 it may result in decreased concentrations of artemether and/or lumefantrine and loss of anti-malarial efficacy).
No products indexed under this heading.

Hypericum Perforatum (When Coartem Tablets are co-administered with inducers of CYP3A4 it may result in decreased concentrations of artemether and/or lumefantrine and loss of anti-malarial efficacy). Products include:
Traumeel 1800

Idarubicin Hydrochloride (Coartem Tablets should be avoided in patients receiving other medications that prolong the QT interval, such as certain antibiotics (macrolide antibiotics, fluoroquinolone antibiotics, imidazole, and triazole antifungal agents)).
No products indexed under this heading.

Ifosfamide (Administration of Coartem Tablets with drugs that are metabolized by CYP2D6 maysignificantly increase plasma concentrations of the co-administered drug and increase the risk of adverse effects. Many of the drugs metabolized by CYP2D6 can prolong the QT interval and should not be administered with Coartem Tablets due to the

potential additive effect on the QT interval (eg, flecainide, imipramine, amitriptyline, clomipramine)).
No products indexed under this heading.

Imatinib Mesylate (When Coartem Tablets are co-administered with an inhibitor of CYP3A4, including grapefruit juice, it may result in increased concentrations of artemether and/or lumefantrine and potentiate QT prolongation). Products include:
Gleevec 2477

Imipenem (Coartem Tablets should be avoided in patients receiving other medications that prolong the QT interval, such as certain antibiotics (macrolide antibiotics, fluoroquinolone antibiotics, imidazole, and triazole antifungal agents)). Products include:
Primaxin I.M. 2232
Primaxin I.V. 2235

Imipramine Hydrochloride (Coartem Tablets should be avoided in patients receiving other medications that prolong the QT interval, such as antidepressants).
No products indexed under this heading.

Imipramine Pamoate (Coartem Tablets should be avoided in patients receiving other medications that prolong the QT interval, such as antidepressants).
No products indexed under this heading.

Indinavir Sulfate (When Coartem Tablets are co-administered with substrates of CYP3A4 it may result in decreased concentrations of the substrate and potential loss of substrate efficacy). Products include:
Crixivan 2113

Irinotecan Hydrochloride (Administration of Coartem Tablets with drugs that are metabolized by CYP2D6 maysignificantly increase plasma concentrations of the co-administered drug and increase the risk of adverse effects. Many of the drugs metabolized by CYP2D6 can prolong the QT interval and should not be administered with Coartem Tablets due to the potential additive effect on the QT interval (eg, flecainide, imipramine, amitriptyline, clomipramine)).
No products indexed under this heading.

Isocarboxazid (Coartem Tablets should be avoided in patients receiving other medications that prolong the QT interval, such as antidepressants). Products include:
Marplan 3481

Isoniazid (When Coartem Tablets are co-administered with an inhibitor of CYP3A4, including grapefruit juice, it may result in increased concentrations of artemether and/or lumefantrine and potentiate QT prolongation).
No products indexed under this heading.

Isotretinoin (Administration of Coartem Tablets with drugs that are metabolized by CYP2D6 maysignificantly increase plasma concentrations of the co-administered drug and increase the risk of adverse effects. Many of the drugs metabolized by CYP2D6 can prolong the QT interval and should not be administered with Coartem Tablets due to the potential additive effect on the QT interval (eg, flecainide, imipramine, amitriptyline, clomipramine)). Products include:
Accutane 2832

Isradipine (When Coartem Tablets are co-administered with substrates of CYP3A4 it may result in decreased concentrations of the substrate and potential loss of substrate efficacy). Products include:
DynaCirc CR 1432

IMPORTANT NOTE: Always consult each drug listing in the patient's regimen for possible interactions.

Coartem Interactions Index 386

Itraconazole (Coartem Tablets should be avoided in patients receiving other medications that prolong the QT interval, such as certain antibiotics (macrolide antibiotics, fluoroquinolone antibiotics, imidazole, and triazole antifungal agents)).
No products indexed under this heading.

Ixabepilone (When Coartem Tablets are co-administered with substrates of CYP3A4 it may result in decreased concentrations of the substrate and potential loss of substrate efficacy).
No products indexed under this heading.

Kanamycin Sulfate (Coartem Tablets should be avoided in patients receiving other medications that prolong the QT interval, such as certain antibiotics (macrolide antibiotics, fluoroquinolone antibiotics, imidazole, and triazole antifungal agents)).
No products indexed under this heading.

Ketamine (Administration of Coartem Tablets with drugs that are metabolized by CYP2D6 maysignificantly increase plasma concentrations of the co-administered drug and increase the risk of adverse effects. Many of the drugs metabolized by CYP2D6 can prolong the QT interval and should not be administered with Coartem Tablets due to the potential additive effect on the QT interval (eg, flecainide, imipramine, amitriptyline, clomipramine)).
No products indexed under this heading.

Ketamine Hydrochloride (Administration of Coartem Tablets with drugs that are metabolized by CYP2D6 maysignificantly increase plasma concentrations of the co-administered drug and increase the risk of adverse effects. Many of the drugs metabolized by CYP2D6 can prolong the QT interval and should not be administered with Coartem Tablets due to the potential additive effect on the QT interval (eg, flecainide, imipramine, amitriptyline, clomipramine)).
No products indexed under this heading.

Ketoconazole (Concurrent oral administration of ketoconazole, a potent CYP3A4 inhibitor, with a single dose of Coartem Tablets resulted in a moderate increase in exposure to artemether, dihydroartemisinin (DHA, metabolite of artemether), and lumefantrine in a study of 15 healthy subjects. No dose adjustment of Coartem Tablets is necessary when administered with ketoconazole or other potent CYP3A4 inhibitors. However, due to the potential for increased concentrations of lumefantrine which could lead to QT prolongation, Coartem Tablets should be used cautiously with drugs that inhibit CYP3A4). Products include:
Extina 3319
Xolegel 3337

Lamium album (Drugs that have a mixed effect on CYP3A4, especially anti-retroviral drugs, and those that have an effect on the QT interval should be used with caution in patients taking Coartem Tablets).
No products indexed under this heading.

Lapatinib (When Coartem Tablets are co-administered with an inhibitor of CYP3A4, including grapefruit juice, it may result in increased concentrations of artemether and/or lumefantrine and potentiate QT prolongation). Products include:
Tykerb 1698

Levofloxacin (Coartem Tablets should be avoided in patients receiving other medications that prolong the QT interval, such as certain antibiotics (macrolide antibiotics, fluoroquinolone antibiotics, imidazole, and triazole antifungal agents)). Products include:
Iquix 3492
Levaquin 2629
Levaquin in 5% Dextrose 2629
Quixin 3493

Levonorgestrel (When Coartem Tablets are co-administered with substrates of CYP3A4 it may result in decreased concentrations of the substrate and potential loss of substrate efficacy). Products include:
Climara Pro 847
LoSeasonique 3407
Lybrel 3514
Mirena 854
Plan B 3416
Seasonique 3418

Lidocaine (Drugs that prolong the QT interval, including antimalarials such as quinine and quinidine, should be used cautiously following Coartem Tablets, due to the long elimination half-life of lumefantrine (3-6 days) and the potential for additive effects on the QT interval). Products include:
Lidoderm 1107

Lidocaine Base (Administration of Coartem Tablets with drugs that are metabolized by CYP2D6 maysignificantly increase plasma concentrations of the co-administered drug and increase the risk of adverse effects. Many of the drugs metabolized by CYP2D6 can prolong the QT interval and should not be administered with Coartem Tablets due to the potential additive effect on the QT interval (eg, flecainide, imipramine, amitriptyline, clomipramine)).
No products indexed under this heading.

Lidocaine Hydrochloride (Drugs that prolong the QT interval, including antimalarials such as quinine and quinidine, should be used cautiously following Coartem Tablets, due to the long elimination half-life of lumefantrine (3-6 days) and the potential for additive effects on the QT interval).
No products indexed under this heading.

Lithium (Coartem Tablets should be avoided in patients receiving other medications that prolong the QT interval, such as antipsychotics (pimozide, ziprasidone)).
No products indexed under this heading.

Lithium Carbonate (Coartem Tablets should be avoided in patients receiving other medications that prolong the QT interval, such as antipsychotics (pimozide, ziprasidone)).
No products indexed under this heading.

Lithium Citrate (Coartem Tablets should be avoided in patients receiving other medications that prolong the QT interval, such as antipsychotics (pimozide, ziprasidone)).
No products indexed under this heading.

Lomefloxacin Hydrochloride (Coartem Tablets should be avoided in patients receiving other medications that prolong the QT interval, such as certain antibiotics (macrolide antibiotics, fluoroquinolone antibiotics, imidazole, and triazole antifungal agents)).
No products indexed under this heading.

Lopinavir (When Coartem Tablets are co-administered with an inhibitor of CYP3A4, including grapefruit juice, it may result in increased concentrations of artemether and/or lumefantrine and potentiate QT prolongation). Products include:
Kaletra 458

Loracarbef (Coartem Tablets should be avoided in patients receiving other medications that prolong the QT interval, such as certain antibiotics (macrolide antibiotics, fluoroquinolone antibiotics, imidazole, and triazole antifungal agents)).
No products indexed under this heading.

Loratadine (Coartem Tablets should be avoided in patients receiving other medications that prolong the QT interval, such as certain non-sedating antihistaminics (terfenadine, astemizole)).
No products indexed under this heading.

Lorazepam (Drugs that prolong the QT interval, including antimalarials such as quinine and quinidine, should be used cautiously following Coartem Tablets, due to the long elimination half-life of lumefantrine (3-6 days) and the potential for additive effects on the QT interval).
No products indexed under this heading.

Lovastatin (When Coartem Tablets are co-administered with substrates of CYP3A4 it may result in decreased concentrations of the substrate and potential loss of substrate efficacy). Products include:
Advicor 402
Mevacor 2212

Loxapine Hydrochloride (Coartem Tablets should be avoided in patients receiving other medications that prolong the QT interval, such as antipsychotics (pimozide, ziprasidone)).
No products indexed under this heading.

Loxapine Succinate (Coartem Tablets should be avoided in patients receiving other medications that prolong the QT interval, such as antipsychotics (pimozide, ziprasidone)).
No products indexed under this heading.

Maprotiline Hydrochloride (Coartem Tablets should be avoided in patients receiving other medications that prolong the QT interval, such as antidepressants).
No products indexed under this heading.

Mefloquine Hydrochloride (If mefloquine is administered immediately prior to Coartem Tablets there may be a decreased exposure to lumefantrine, possibly due to a mefloquine-induced decrease in bile production. Therefore, patients should be monitored for decreased efficacy and food consumption should be encouraged while taking Coartem Tablets).
No products indexed under this heading.

Meperidine Hydrochloride (Administration of Coartem Tablets with drugs that are metabolized by CYP2D6 maysignificantly increase plasma concentrations of the co-administered drug and increase the risk of adverse effects. Many of the drugs metabolized by CYP2D6 can prolong the QT interval and should not be administered with Coartem Tablets due to the potential additive effect on the QT interval (eg, flecainide, imipramine, amitriptyline, clomipramine)).
No products indexed under this heading.

Mephenytoin (When Coartem Tablets are co-administered with inducers of CYP3A4 it may result in decreased concentrations of artemether and/or lumefantrine and loss of anti-malarial efficacy).
No products indexed under this heading.

Mephobarbital (Administration of Coartem Tablets with drugs that are metabolized by CYP2D6 maysignificantly increase plasma concentrations of the co-administered drug and increase the risk of adverse effects. Many of the drugs metabolized by CYP2D6 can prolong the QT interval and should not be administered with Coartem Tablets due to the potential additive effect on the QT interval (eg, flecainide, imipramine, amitriptyline, clomipramine)).
No products indexed under this heading.

Meprobamate (Drugs that prolong the QT interval, including antimalarials such as quinine and quinidine, should be used cautiously following Coartem Tablets, due to the long elimination half-life of lumefantrine (3-6 days) and the potential for additive effects on the QT interval).
No products indexed under this heading.

Mesoridazine Besylate (Coartem Tablets should be avoided in patients receiving other medications that prolong the QT interval, such as antipsychotics (pimozide, ziprasidone)).
No products indexed under this heading.

Mestranol (When Coartem Tablets are co-administered with substrates of CYP3A4 it may result in decreased concentrations of the substrate and potential loss of substrate efficacy).
No products indexed under this heading.

Methacycline Hydrochloride (Coartem Tablets should be avoided in patients receiving other medications that prolong the QT interval, such as certain antibiotics (macrolide antibiotics, fluoroquinolone antibiotics, imidazole, and triazole antifungal agents)).
No products indexed under this heading.

Methadone Hydrochloride (When Coartem Tablets are co-administered with substrates of CYP3A4 it may result in decreased concentrations of the substrate and potential loss of substrate efficacy).
No products indexed under this heading.

Methdilazine Hydrochloride (Coartem Tablets should be avoided in patients receiving other medications that prolong the QT interval, such as certain non-sedating antihistaminics (terfenadine, astemizole)).
No products indexed under this heading.

Methicillin Sodium (Coartem Tablets should be avoided in patients receiving other medications that prolong the QT interval, such as certain antibiotics (macrolide antibiotics, fluoroquinolone antibiotics, imidazole, and triazole antifungal agents)).
No products indexed under this heading.

Methotrimeprazine (Coartem Tablets should be avoided in patients receiving other medications that prolong the QT interval, such as antipsychotics (pimozide, ziprasidone)).
No products indexed under this heading.

Methsuximide (When Coartem Tablets are co-administered with inducers of CYP3A4 it may result in decreased concentrations of artemether and/or lumefantrine and loss of anti-malarial efficacy).
No products indexed under this heading.

Methylprednisolone (When Coartem Tablets are co-administered with inducers of CYP3A4 it may result in decreased concentrations of artemether and/or lumefantrine and loss of anti-malarial efficacy).
No products indexed under this heading.

Methylprednisolone Acetate (When Coartem Tablets are co-administered with inducers of CYP3A4 it may result in decreased concentrations of artemether and/or lumefantrine and loss of anti-malarial efficacy).
No products indexed under this heading.

Methylprednisolone Sodium Succinate (When Coartem Tablets are co-administered with inducers of CYP3A4 it may result in decreased concentrations of artemether and/or lumefantrine and loss of anti-malarial efficacy).
No products indexed under this heading.

Methyltestosterone (Administration of Coartem Tablets with drugs that are metabolized by CYP2D6 maysignificantly increase plasma concentrations of the co-administered drug and

387 Interactions Index Coartem

increase the risk of adverse effects. Many of the drugs metabolized by CYP2D6 can prolong the QT interval and should not be administered with Coartem Tablets due to the potential additive effect on the QT interval (eg, flecainide, imipramine, amitriptyline, clomipramine)).
No products indexed under this heading.

Metronidazole (When Coartem Tablets are co-administered with an inhibitor of CYP3A4, including grapefruit juice, it may result in increased concentrations of artemether and/or lumefantrine and potentiate QT prolongation). Products include:
Pylera ... 793

Metronidazole Benzoate (When Coartem Tablets are co-administered with an inhibitor of CYP3A4, including grapefruit juice, it may result in increased concentrations of artemether and/or lumefantrine and potentiate QT prolongation).
No products indexed under this heading.

Metronidazole Hydrochloride (When Coartem Tablets are co-administered with an inhibitor of CYP3A4, including grapefruit juice, it may result in increased concentrations of artemether and/or lumefantrine and potentiate QT prolongation).
No products indexed under this heading.

Metronidazole Sodium (When Coartem Tablets are co-administered with an inhibitor of CYP3A4, including grapefruit juice, it may result in increased concentrations of artemether and/or lumefantrine and potentiate QT prolongation).
No products indexed under this heading.

Mexiletine Hydrochloride (Drugs that prolong the QT interval, including antimalarials such as quinine and quinidine, should be used cautiously following Coartem Tablets, due to the long elimination half-life of lumefantrine (3-6 days) and the potential for additive effects on the QT interval).
No products indexed under this heading.

Mezlocillin Sodium (Coartem Tablets should be avoided in patients receiving other medications that prolong the QT interval, such as certain antibiotics (macrolide antibiotics, fluoroquinolone antibiotics, imidazole, and triazole antifungal agents)).
No products indexed under this heading.

Micafungin Sodium (Coartem Tablets should be avoided in patients receiving other medications that prolong the QT interval, such as certain antibiotics (macrolide antibiotics, fluoroquinolone antibiotics, imidazole, and triazole antifungal agents)). Products include:
Mycamine ... 670

Miconazole (Coartem Tablets should be avoided in patients receiving other medications that prolong the QT interval, such as certain antibiotics (macrolide antibiotics, fluoroquinolone antibiotics, imidazole, and triazole antifungal agents)).
No products indexed under this heading.

Miconazole Nitrate (Coartem Tablets should be avoided in patients receiving other medications that prolong the QT interval, such as certain antibiotics (macrolide antibiotics, fluoroquinolone antibiotics, imidazole, and triazole antifungal agents)). Products include:
Vusion Ointment ... 3335

Midazolam Hydrochloride (Drugs that prolong the QT interval, including antimalarials such as quinine and quinidine, should be used cautiously following Coartem Tablets, due to the long elimination half-life of lumefantrine (3-6 days) and the potential for additive effects on the QT interval).
No products indexed under this heading.

Mifepristone (When Coartem Tablets are co-administered with an inhibitor of CYP3A4, including grapefruit juice, it may result in increased concentrations of artemether and/or lumefantrine and potentiate QT prolongation).
No products indexed under this heading.

Minocycline Hydrochloride (Coartem Tablets should be avoided in patients receiving other medications that prolong the QT interval, such as certain antibiotics (macrolide antibiotics, fluoroquinolone antibiotics, imidazole, and triazole antifungal agents)). Products include:
Solodyn ... 2073

Mirtazapine (Coartem Tablets should be avoided in patients receiving other medications that prolong the QT interval, such as antidepressants). Products include:
Remeron Tablets ... 3214
RemeronSolTab Tablets ... 3219

Modafinil (When Coartem Tablets are co-administered with inducers of CYP3A4 it may result in decreased concentrations of artemether and/or lumefantrine and loss of anti-malarial efficacy). Products include:
Provigil ... 983

Molindone Hydrochloride (Coartem Tablets should be avoided in patients receiving other medications that prolong the QT interval, such as antipsychotics (pimozide, ziprasidone)). Products include:
Moban ... 1108

Moricizine Hydrochloride (Coartem Tablets should be avoided in patients receiving other medications that prolong the QT interval, such as class IA (quinidine, procainamide, disopyramide) antiarrhythmic agents).
No products indexed under this heading.

Moxifloxacin Hydrochloride (Coartem Tablets should be avoided in patients receiving other medications that prolong the QT interval, such as certain antibiotics (macrolide antibiotics, fluoroquinolone antibiotics, imidazole, and triazole antifungal agents)). Products include:
Avelox ... 3064
Vigamox ... 589

Nafcillin Sodium (Coartem Tablets should be avoided in patients receiving other medications that prolong the QT interval, such as certain antibiotics (macrolide antibiotics, fluoroquinolone antibiotics, imidazole, and triazole antifungal agents)).
No products indexed under this heading.

Nefazodone Hydrochloride (Coartem Tablets should be avoided in patients receiving other medications that prolong the QT interval, such as antidepressants).
No products indexed under this heading.

Nelfinavir Mesylate (When Coartem Tablets are co-administered with substrates of CYP3A4 it may result in decreased concentrations of the substrate and potential loss of substrate efficacy).
No products indexed under this heading.

Nevirapine (When Coartem Tablets are co-administered with an inhibitor of CYP3A4, including grapefruit juice, it may result in increased concentrations of artemether and/or lumefantrine and potentiate QT prolongation). Products include:
Viramune Oral Suspension ... 897
Viramune Tablets ... 897

Niacin (When Coartem Tablets are co-administered with an inhibitor of CYP3A4, including grapefruit juice, it may result in increased concentrations of artemether and/or lumefantrine and potentiate QT prolongation). Products include:
Advicor ... 402
Cardio Basics ... 3455
Niaspan ... 497
Simcor ... 524

Niacinamide (When Coartem Tablets are co-administered with an inhibitor of CYP3A4, including grapefruit juice, it may result in increased concentrations of artemether and/or lumefantrine and potentiate QT prolongation). Products include:
CitraNatal 90 DHA Capsules ... 2332
CitraNatal Assure ... 2332
CitraNatal Rx ... 2332
Heplive ... 607

Niacinamide Hydroiodide (When Coartem Tablets are co-administered with an inhibitor of CYP3A4, including grapefruit juice, it may result in increased concentrations of artemether and/or lumefantrine and potentiate QT prolongation).
No products indexed under this heading.

Nicardipine (When Coartem Tablets are co-administered with substrates of CYP3A4 it may result in decreased concentrations of the substrate and potential loss of substrate efficacy).
No products indexed under this heading.

Nicardipine Hydrochloride (When Coartem Tablets are co-administered with substrates of CYP3A4 it may result in decreased concentrations of the substrate and potential loss of substrate efficacy).
No products indexed under this heading.

Nicotinamide (When Coartem Tablets are co-administered with an inhibitor of CYP3A4, including grapefruit juice, it may result in increased concentrations of artemether and/or lumefantrine and potentiate QT prolongation).
No products indexed under this heading.

Nicotine (Administration of Coartem Tablets with drugs that are metabolized by CYP2D6 maysignificantly increase plasma concentrations of the co-administered drug and increase the risk of adverse effects. Many of the drugs metabolized by CYP2D6 can prolong the QT interval and should not be administered with Coartem Tablets due to the potential additive effect on the QT interval (eg, flecainide, imipramine, amitriptyline, clomipramine)).
No products indexed under this heading.

Nicotine Polacrilex (Administration of Coartem Tablets with drugs that are metabolized by CYP2D6 maysignificantly increase plasma concentrations of the co-administered drug and increase the risk of adverse effects. Many of the drugs metabolized by CYP2D6 can prolong the QT interval and should not be administered with Coartem Tablets due to the potential additive effect on the QT interval (eg, flecainide, imipramine, amitriptyline, clomipramine)).
No products indexed under this heading.

Nicotine Salicylate (Administration of Coartem Tablets with drugs that are metabolized by CYP2D6 maysignificantly increase plasma concentrations of the co-administered drug and increase the risk of adverse effects. Many of the drugs metabolized by CYP2D6 can prolong the QT interval and should not be administered with Coartem Tablets due to the potential additive effect on the QT interval (eg, flecainide, imipramine, amitriptyline, clomipramine)).
No products indexed under this heading.

Nicotine Sulfate (Administration of Coartem Tablets with drugs that are metabolized by CYP2D6 maysignificantly increase plasma concentrations of the co-administered drug and increase the risk of adverse effects. Many of the drugs metabolized by CYP2D6 can prolong the QT interval and should not be administered with Coartem Tablets due to the potential additive effect on the QT interval (eg, flecainide, imipramine, amitriptyline, clomipramine)).
No products indexed under this heading.

Nifedipine (When Coartem Tablets are co-administered with substrates of CYP3A4 it may result in decreased concentrations of the substrate and potential loss of substrate efficacy).
No products indexed under this heading.

Nimodipine (When Coartem Tablets are co-administered with substrates of CYP3A4 it may result in decreased concentrations of the substrate and potential loss of substrate efficacy).
No products indexed under this heading.

Nisoldipine (When Coartem Tablets are co-administered with substrates of CYP3A4 it may result in decreased concentrations of the substrate and potential loss of substrate efficacy).
No products indexed under this heading.

Nitrendipine (When Coartem Tablets are co-administered with substrates of CYP3A4 it may result in decreased concentrations of the substrate and potential loss of substrate efficacy).
No products indexed under this heading.

Norethindrone (When Coartem Tablets are co-administered with substrates of CYP3A4 it may result in decreased concentrations of the substrate and potential loss of substrate efficacy). Products include:
Ortho Micronor ... 2660

Norethindrone Acetate (When Coartem Tablets are co-administered with substrates of CYP3A4 it may result in decreased concentrations of the substrate and potential loss of substrate efficacy). Products include:
Activella ... 2561

Norethynodrel (Coartem Tablets may reduce the effectiveness of hormonal contraceptives. Therefore, patients using oral, transdermal patch, or other systemic hormonal contraceptives should be advised to use an additional non-hormonal method of birth control).
No products indexed under this heading.

Norfloxacin (Coartem Tablets should be avoided in patients receiving other medications that prolong the QT interval, such as certain antibiotics (macrolide antibiotics, fluoroquinolone antibiotics, imidazole, and triazole antifungal agents)). Products include:
Noroxin ... 2220

Norgestimate (Coartem Tablets may reduce the effectiveness of hormonal contraceptives. Therefore, patients using oral, transdermal patch, or other systemic hormonal contraceptives should be advised to use an additional non-hormonal method of birth control). Products include:
Ortho-Cyclen/Ortho Tri-Cyclen ... 2663
Ortho Tri-Cyclen Lo Tablets ... 2673

Norgestrel (When Coartem Tablets are co-administered with substrates of CYP3A4 it may result in decreased concentrations of the substrate and potential loss of substrate efficacy).
No products indexed under this heading.

Nortriptyline Hydrochloride (Coartem Tablets should be avoided in patients receiving other medications that prolong the QT interval, such as antidepressants).
No products indexed under this heading.

Ofloxacin (Coartem Tablets should be avoided in patients receiving other medications that prolong the QT interval, such as certain antibiotics (macrolide antibiotics, fluoroquinolone antibiotics, imidazole, and triazole antifungal agents)).
No products indexed under this heading.

IMPORTANT NOTE: Always consult each drug listing in the patient's regimen for possible interactions.

Olanzapine (Coartem Tablets should be avoided in patients receiving other medications that prolong the QT interval, such as antipsychotics (pimozide, ziprasidone)). Products include:

Omeprazole (When Coartem Tablets are co-administered with an inhibitor of CYP3A4, including grapefruit juice, it may result in increased concentrations of artemether and/or lumefantrine and potentiate QT prolongation).
No products indexed under this heading.

Ondansetron (When Coartem Tablets are co-administered with substrates of CYP3A4 it may result in decreased concentrations of the substrate and potential loss of substrate efficacy).
No products indexed under this heading.

Ondansetron Hydrochloride (When Coartem Tablets are co-administered with substrates of CYP3A4 it may result in decreased concentrations of the substrate and potential loss of substrate efficacy). Products include:

Orphenadrine Citrate (Administration of Coartem Tablets with drugs that are metabolized by CYP2D6 maysignificantly increase plasma concentrations of the co-administered drug and increase the risk of adverse effects. Many of the drugs metabolized by CYP2D6 can prolong the QT interval and should not be administered with Coartem Tablets due to the potential additive effect on the QT interval (eg, flecainide, imipramine, amitriptyline, clomipramine)).
No products indexed under this heading.

Orphenadrine Hydrochloride (Administration of Coartem Tablets with drugs that are metabolized by CYP2D6 maysignificantly increase plasma concentrations of the co-administered drug and increase the risk of adverse effects. Many of the drugs metabolized by CYP2D6 can prolong the QT interval and should not be administered with Coartem Tablets due to the potential additive effect on the QT interval (eg, flecainide, imipramine, amitriptyline, clomipramine)).
No products indexed under this heading.

Oxacillin (Coartem Tablets should be avoided in patients receiving other medications that prolong the QT interval, such as certain antibiotics (macrolide antibiotics, fluoroquinolone antibiotics, imidazole, and triazole antifungal agents)).
No products indexed under this heading.

Oxacillin Sodium (Coartem Tablets should be avoided in patients receiving other medications that prolong the QT interval, such as certain antibiotics (macrolide antibiotics, fluoroquinolone antibiotics, imidazole, and triazole antifungal agents)).
No products indexed under this heading.

Oxazepam (Drugs that prolong the QT interval, including antimalarials such as quinine and quinidine, should be used cautiously following Coartem Tablets, due to the long elimination half-life of lumefantrine (3-6 days) and the potential for additive effects on the QT interval).
No products indexed under this heading.

Oxcarbazepine (When Coartem Tablets are co-administered with inducers of CYP3A4 it may result in decreased concentrations of artemether and/or lumefantrine and loss of anti-malarial efficacy).
No products indexed under this heading.

Oxiconazole Nitrate (Coartem Tablets should be avoided in patients receiving other medications that prolong the QT interval, such as certain antibiotics (macrolide antibiotics, fluoroquinolone antibiotics, imidazole, and triazole antifungal agents)).
No products indexed under this heading.

Oxytetracycline Hydrochloride (Coartem Tablets should be avoided in patients receiving other medications that prolong the QT interval, such as certain antibiotics (macrolide antibiotics, fluoroquinolone antibiotics, imidazole, and triazole antifungal agents)).
No products indexed under this heading.

Paclitaxel (When Coartem Tablets are co-administered with substrates of CYP3A4 it may result in decreased concentrations of the substrate and potential loss of substrate efficacy).
No products indexed under this heading.

Paliperidone (Coartem Tablets should be avoided in patients receiving other medications that prolong the QT interval, such as antipsychotics (pimozide, ziprasidone)). Products include:

Paroxetine (Coartem Tablets should be avoided in patients receiving other medications that prolong the QT interval, such as antidepressants).
No products indexed under this heading.

Paroxetine Hydrochloride (Coartem Tablets should be avoided in patients receiving other medications that prolong the QT interval, such as antidepressants). Products include:

Paroxetine Mesylate (Coartem Tablets should be avoided in patients receiving other medications that prolong the QT interval, such as antidepressants).
No products indexed under this heading.

Penicillin, Potassium Phenoxymethyl (Coartem Tablets should be avoided in patients receiving other medications that prolong the QT interval, such as certain antibiotics (macrolide antibiotics, fluoroquinolone antibiotics, imidazole, and triazole antifungal agents)).
No products indexed under this heading.

Penicillin G Benzathine (Coartem Tablets should be avoided in patients receiving other medications that prolong the QT interval, such as certain antibiotics (macrolide antibiotics, fluoroquinolone antibiotics, imidazole, and triazole antifungal agents)). Products include:

Penicillin G Dibenzylethyenediamine (Coartem Tablets should be avoided in patients receiving other medications that prolong the QT interval, such as certain antibiotics (macrolide antibiotics, fluoroquinolone antibiotics, imidazole, and triazole antifungal agents)).
No products indexed under this heading.

Penicillin G Potassium (Coartem Tablets should be avoided in patients receiving other medications that prolong the QT interval, such as certain antibiotics (macrolide antibiotics, fluoroquinolone antibiotics, imidazole, and triazole antifungal agents)).
No products indexed under this heading.

Penicillin G Procaine (Coartem Tablets should be avoided in patients receiving other medications that prolong the QT interval, such as certain antibiotics (macrolide antibiotics, fluoro-

quinolone antibiotics, imidazole, and triazole antifungal agents)). Products include:

Penicillin G Sodium (Coartem Tablets should be avoided in patients receiving other medications that prolong the QT interval, such as certain antibiotics (macrolide antibiotics, fluoroquinolone antibiotics, imidazole, and triazole antifungal agents)).
No products indexed under this heading.

Penicillin V (Coartem Tablets should be avoided in patients receiving other medications that prolong the QT interval, such as certain antibiotics (macrolide antibiotics, fluoroquinolone antibiotics, imidazole, and triazole antifungal agents)).
No products indexed under this heading.

Penicillin V Potassium (Coartem Tablets should be avoided in patients receiving other medications that prolong the QT interval, such as certain antibiotics (macrolide antibiotics, fluoroquinolone antibiotics, imidazole, and triazole antifungal agents)).
No products indexed under this heading.

Penicillins (Coartem Tablets should be avoided in patients receiving other medications that prolong the QT interval, such as certain antibiotics (macrolide antibiotics, fluoroquinolone antibiotics, imidazole, and triazole antifungal agents)).
No products indexed under this heading.

Perphenazine (Coartem Tablets should be avoided in patients receiving other medications that prolong the QT interval, such as antipsychotics (pimozide, ziprasidone)).
No products indexed under this heading.

Phenelzine Sulfate (Coartem Tablets should be avoided in patients receiving other medications that prolong the QT interval, such as antidepressants).
No products indexed under this heading.

Phenobarbital (When Coartem Tablets are co-administered with inducers of CYP3A4 it may result in decreased concentrations of artemether and/or lumefantrine and loss of anti-malarial efficacy). Products include:

Phenobarbital Sodium (When Coartem Tablets are co-administered with inducers of CYP3A4 it may result in decreased concentrations of artemether and/or lumefantrine and loss of anti-malarial efficacy).
No products indexed under this heading.

Phenytoin (When Coartem Tablets are co-administered with inducers of CYP3A4 it may result in decreased concentrations of artemether and/or lumefantrine and loss of anti-malarial efficacy).
No products indexed under this heading.

Phenytoin Sodium (When Coartem Tablets are co-administered with inducers of CYP3A4 it may result in decreased concentrations of artemether and/or lumefantrine and loss of anti-malarial efficacy). Products include:

Pimozide (Coartem Tablets should be avoided in patients receiving other medications that prolong the QT interval, such as antipsychotics (pimozide, ziprasidone)).
No products indexed under this heading.

Piperacillin Sodium (Coartem Tablets should be avoided in patients receiving other medications that prolong the QT interval, such as certain antibiotics (macrolide antibiotics, fluoroquinolone antibiotics, imidazole, and triazole antifungal agents)). Products include:

Polyestradiol Phosphate (When Coartem Tablets are co-administered with substrates of CYP3A4 it may result in decreased concentrations of the substrate and potential loss of substrate efficacy).
No products indexed under this heading.

Posaconazole (Coartem Tablets should be avoided in patients receiving other medications that prolong the QT interval, such as certain antibiotics (macrolide antibiotics, fluoroquinolone antibiotics, imidazole, and triazole antifungal agents)). Products include:

Prazepam (Drugs that prolong the QT interval, including antimalarials such as quinine and quinidine, should be used cautiously following Coartem Tablets, due to the long elimination half-life of lumefantrine (3-6 days) and the potential for additive effects on the QT interval).
No products indexed under this heading.

Prednisolone (When Coartem Tablets are co-administered with inducers of CYP3A4 it may result in decreased concentrations of artemether and/or lumefantrine and loss of anti-malarial efficacy).
No products indexed under this heading.

Prednisolone Acetate (When Coartem Tablets are co-administered with inducers of CYP3A4 it may result in decreased concentrations of artemether and/or lumefantrine and loss of anti-malarial efficacy). Products include:

Prednisolone Sodium Phosphate (When Coartem Tablets are co-administered with inducers of CYP3A4 it may result in decreased concentrations of artemether and/or lumefantrine and loss of anti-malarial efficacy).
No products indexed under this heading.

Prednisolone Tebutate (When Coartem Tablets are co-administered with inducers of CYP3A4 it may result in decreased concentrations of artemether and/or lumefantrine and loss of anti-malarial efficacy).
No products indexed under this heading.

Prednisone (When Coartem Tablets are co-administered with inducers of CYP3A4 it may result in decreased concentrations of artemether and/or lumefantrine and loss of anti-malarial efficacy).
No products indexed under this heading.

Prednisone sodium phosphate (When Coartem Tablets are co-administered with inducers of CYP3A4 it may result in decreased concentrations of artemether and/or lumefantrine and loss of anti-malarial efficacy).
No products indexed under this heading.

Primidone (When Coartem Tablets are co-administered with inducers of CYP3A4 it may result in decreased concentrations of artemether and/or lumefantrine and loss of anti-malarial efficacy).
No products indexed under this heading.

Procainamide (Coartem Tablets should be avoided in patients receiving other medications that prolong the QT interval, such as class IA (quinidine, procainamide, disopyramide) antiarrhythmic agents).
No products indexed under this heading.

389 Interactions Index Coartem

Procainamide Hydrochloride (Drugs that prolong the QT interval, including antimalarials such as quinine and quinidine, should be used cautiously following Coartem Tablets, due to the long elimination half-life of lumefantrine (3-6 days) and the potential for additive effects on the QT interval).
No products indexed under this heading.

Prochlorperazine (Coartem Tablets should be avoided in patients receiving other medications that prolong the QT interval, such as antipsychotics (pimozide, ziprasidone)).
No products indexed under this heading.

Promethazine (Administration of Coartem Tablets with drugs that are metabolized by CYP2D6 maysignificantly increase plasma concentrations of the co-administered drug and increase the risk of adverse effects. Many of the drugs metabolized by CYP2D6 can prolong the QT interval and should not be administered with Coartem Tablets due to the potential additive effect on the QT interval (eg, flecainide, imipramine, amitriptyline, clomipramine)).
No products indexed under this heading.

Promethazine Hydrochloride (Coartem Tablets should be avoided in patients receiving other medications that prolong the QT interval, such as certain non-sedating antihistaminics (terfenadine, astemizole)).
No products indexed under this heading.

Propafenone Hydrochloride (Drugs that prolong the QT interval, including antimalarials such as quinine and quinidine, should be used cautiously following Coartem Tablets, due to the long elimination half-life of lumefantrine (3-6 days) and the potential for additive effects on the QT interval). Products include:
Rythmol 1648
Rythmol SR 1652

Propofol (Administration of Coartem Tablets with drugs that are metabolized by CYP2D6 maysignificantly increase plasma concentrations of the co-administered drug and increase the risk of adverse effects. Many of the drugs metabolized by CYP2D6 can prolong the QT interval and should not be administered with Coartem Tablets due to the potential additive effect on the QT interval (eg, flecainide, imipramine, amitriptyline, clomipramine)).
No products indexed under this heading.

Propoxyphene Hydrochloride (When Coartem Tablets are co-administered with an inhibitor of CYP3A4, including grapefruit juice, it may result in increased concentrations of artemether and/or lumefantrine and potentiate QT prolongation).
No products indexed under this heading.

Propoxyphene Napsylate (When Coartem Tablets are co-administered with an inhibitor of CYP3A4, including grapefruit juice, it may result in increased concentrations of artemether and/or lumefantrine and potentiate QT prolongation).
No products indexed under this heading.

Protriptyline Hydrochloride (Coartem Tablets should be avoided in patients receiving other medications that prolong the QT interval, such as antidepressants).
No products indexed under this heading.

Pyrilamine Maleate (Coartem Tablets should be avoided in patients receiving other medications that prolong the QT interval, such as certain non-sedating antihistaminics (terfenadine, astemizole)).
No products indexed under this heading.

Pyrilamine Tannate (Coartem Tablets should be avoided in patients receiving other medications that prolong the QT interval, such as certain non-sedating antihistaminics (terfenadine, astemizole)).
No products indexed under this heading.

Pyrimethamine (Drugs that prolong the QT interval, including antimalarials such as quinine and quinidine, should be used cautiously following Coartem Tablets, due to the long elimination half-life of lumefantrine (3-6 days) and the potential for additive effects on the QT interval). Products include:
Daraprim 1423

Quetiapine Fumarate (Coartem Tablets should be avoided in patients receiving other medications that prolong the QT interval, such as antipsychotics (pimozide, ziprasidone)). Products include:
Seroquel 750
Seroquel XR 759

Quinidine (Coartem Tablets should be avoided in patients receiving other medications that prolong the QT interval, such as class IA (quinidine, procainamide, disopyramide) antiarrhythmic agents).
No products indexed under this heading.

Quinidine Gluconate (Coartem Tablets should be avoided in patients receiving other medications that prolong the QT interval, such as class IA (quinidine, procainamide, disopyramide) antiarrhythmic agents).
No products indexed under this heading.

Quinidine Hydrochloride (Coartem Tablets should be avoided in patients receiving other medications that prolong the QT interval, such as class IA (quinidine, procainamide, disopyramide) antiarrhythmic agents).
No products indexed under this heading.

Quinidine Polygalacturonate (Coartem Tablets should be avoided in patients receiving other medications that prolong the QT interval, such as class IA (quinidine, procainamide, disopyramide) antiarrhythmic agents).
No products indexed under this heading.

Quinidine Sulfate (Coartem Tablets should be avoided in patients receiving other medications that prolong the QT interval, such as class IA (quinidine, procainamide, disopyramide) antiarrhythmic agents).
No products indexed under this heading.

Quinine (A single dose of intravenous quinine (10 mg/kg bodyweight) concurrent with the final dose of a 6-dose regimen of Coartem Tablets demonstrated no effect of intravenous quinine on the systemic exposure of DHA or lumefantrine. Quinine exposure was also not altered. Exposure to artemether was decreased. This decrease in artemether exposure is not thought to be clinically significant. However, quinine and other drugs that prolong the QT interval should be used cautiously following treatment with Coartem Tablets due to the long elimination half life of lumefantrine and the potential for additive QT effects). Products include:
Hyland's Leg Cramps PM with Quinine 3315

Quinine Sulfate (A single dose of intravenous quinine (10 mg/kg bodyweight) concurrent with the final dose of a 6-dose regimen of Coartem Tablets demonstrated no effect of intravenous quinine on the systemic exposure of DHA or lumefantrine. Quinine exposure was also not altered. Exposure to artemether was decreased. This decrease in artemether exposure is not thought to be clinically significant. However, quinine and other drugs that prolong the QT interval should be used cautiously following treatment with Coartem Tablets due to the long elimination half life of lumefantrine and the potential for additive QT effects).
No products indexed under this heading.

Quinupristin (When Coartem Tablets are co-administered with an inhibitor of CYP3A4, including grapefruit juice, it may result in increased concentrations of artemether and/or lumefantrine and potentiate QT prolongation).
No products indexed under this heading.

Ranitidine Bismuth Citrate (When Coartem Tablets are co-administered with an inhibitor of CYP3A4, including grapefruit juice, it may result in increased concentrations of artemether and/or lumefantrine and potentiate QT prolongation).
No products indexed under this heading.

Ranitidine Hydrochloride (When Coartem Tablets are co-administered with an inhibitor of CYP3A4, including grapefruit juice, it may result in increased concentrations of artemether and/or lumefantrine and potentiate QT prolongation). Products include:
Zantac 1737
Zantac Injection 1732
Zantac Pharmacy 1735

Rifabutin (When Coartem Tablets are co-administered with substrates of CYP3A4 it may result in decreased concentrations of the substrate and potential loss of substrate efficacy).
No products indexed under this heading.

Rifampicin (When Coartem Tablets are co-administered with inducers of CYP3A4 it may result in decreased concentrations of artemether and/or lumefantrine and loss of anti-malarial efficacy).
No products indexed under this heading.

Rifampin (When Coartem Tablets are co-administered with inducers of CYP3A4 it may result in decreased concentrations of artemether and/or lumefantrine and loss of anti-malarial efficacy).
No products indexed under this heading.

Rifapentine (When Coartem Tablets are co-administered with inducers of CYP3A4 it may result in decreased concentrations of artemether and/or lumefantrine and loss of anti-malarial efficacy).
No products indexed under this heading.

Risperidone (Coartem Tablets should be avoided in patients receiving other medications that prolong the QT interval, such as antipsychotics (pimozide, ziprasidone)). Products include:
Risperdal Consta 2682

Ritonavir (When Coartem Tablets are co-administered with substrates of CYP3A4 it may result in decreased concentrations of the substrate and potential loss of substrate efficacy). Products include:
Kaletra 458
Norvir 509

Ropivacaine Hydrochloride (Administration of Coartem Tablets with drugs that are metabolized by CYP2D6 maysignificantly increase plasma concentrations of the co-administered drug and increase the risk of adverse effects. Many of the drugs metabolized by CYP2D6 can prolong the QT interval and should not be administered with Coartem Tablets due to the potential additive effect on the QT interval (eg, flecainide, imipramine, amitriptyline, clomipramine)).
No products indexed under this heading.

Saquinavir (When Coartem Tablets are co-administered with substrates of CYP3A4 it may result in decreased concentrations of the substrate and potential loss of substrate efficacy).
No products indexed under this heading.

Saquinavir Mesylate (When Coartem Tablets are co-administered with substrates of CYP3A4 it may result in decreased concentrations of the substrate and potential loss of substrate efficacy).
No products indexed under this heading.

Selegiline (Coartem Tablets should be avoided in patients receiving other medications that prolong the QT interval, such as antidepressants). Products include:
Emsam 3623

Selegiline Hydrochloride (Coartem Tablets should be avoided in patients receiving other medications that prolong the QT interval, such as antidepressants). Products include:
Eldepryl 3312

Sertaconazole Nitrate (Coartem Tablets should be avoided in patients receiving other medications that prolong the QT interval, such as certain antibiotics (macrolide antibiotics, fluoroquinolone antibiotics, imidazole, and triazole antifungal agents)).
No products indexed under this heading.

Sertraline Hydrochloride (Coartem Tablets should be avoided in patients receiving other medications that prolong the QT interval, such as antidepressants).
No products indexed under this heading.

Sevoflurane (Administration of Coartem Tablets with drugs that are metabolized by CYP2D6 maysignificantly increase plasma concentrations of the co-administered drug and increase the risk of adverse effects. Many of the drugs metabolized by CYP2D6 can prolong the QT interval and should not be administered with Coartem Tablets due to the potential additive effect on the QT interval (eg, flecainide, imipramine, amitriptyline, clomipramine)). Products include:
Ultane 554

Sildenafil Citrate (When Coartem Tablets are co-administered with substrates of CYP3A4 it may result in decreased concentrations of the substrate and potential loss of substrate efficacy).
No products indexed under this heading.

Simvastatin (When Coartem Tablets are co-administered with substrates of CYP3A4 it may result in decreased concentrations of the substrate and potential loss of substrate efficacy). Products include:
Simcor 524
Vytorin 10/10 .... 2303, 3240
Vytorin 10/20 .... 2303, 3240
Vytorin 10/40 .... 2303, 3240
Vytorin 10/80 .... 2303, 3240
Zocor 2289

Sirolimus (When Coartem Tablets are co-administered with substrates of CYP3A4 it may result in decreased concentrations of the substrate and potential loss of substrate efficacy). Products include:
Rapamune 3579

Sodium Cloxacillin Monohydrate (Coartem Tablets should be avoided in patients receiving other medications that prolong the QT interval, such as certain antibiotics (macrolide antibiotics, fluoroquinolone antibiotics, imidazole, and triazole antifungal agents)).
No products indexed under this heading.

Sotalol Hydrochloride (Coartem Tablets should be avoided in patients receiving other medications that prolong the QT interval, such as class III (amiodarone, sotalol) antiarrhythmic agents).
No products indexed under this heading.

IMPORTANT NOTE: Always consult each drug listing in the patient's regimen for possible interactions.

Coartem Interactions Index 390

Sparfloxacin (Coartem Tablets should be avoided in patients receiving other medications that prolong the QT interval, such as certain antibiotics (macrolide antibiotics, fluoroquinolone antibiotics, imidazole, and triazole antifungal agents)).
No products indexed under this heading.

Stavudine (Drugs that have a mixed effect on CYP3A4, especially anti-retroviral drugs, and those that have an effect on the QT interval should be used with caution in patients taking Coartem Tablets).
No products indexed under this heading.

Streptomycin Sulfate (Coartem Tablets should be avoided in patients receiving other medications that prolong the QT interval, such as certain antibiotics (macrolide antibiotics, fluoroquinolone antibiotics, imidazole, and triazole antifungal agents)).
No products indexed under this heading.

Sulfamethizole (Coartem Tablets should be avoided in patients receiving other medications that prolong the QT interval, such as certain antibiotics (macrolide antibiotics, fluoroquinolone antibiotics, imidazole, and triazole antifungal agents)).
No products indexed under this heading.

Sulfamethoxazole (Coartem Tablets should be avoided in patients receiving other medications that prolong the QT interval, such as certain antibiotics (macrolide antibiotics, fluoroquinolone antibiotics, imidazole, and triazole antifungal agents)).
No products indexed under this heading.

Sulfinpyrazone (When Coartem Tablets are co-administered with inducers of CYP3A4 it may result in decreased concentrations of artemether and/or lumefantrine and loss of anti-malarial efficacy).
No products indexed under this heading.

Sulfisoxazole Acetyl (Coartem Tablets should be avoided in patients receiving other medications that prolong the QT interval, such as certain antibiotics (macrolide antibiotics, fluoroquinolone antibiotics, imidazole, and triazole antifungal agents)).
No products indexed under this heading.

Sulfisoxazole Diolamine (Coartem Tablets should be avoided in patients receiving other medications that prolong the QT interval, such as certain antibiotics (macrolide antibiotics, fluoroquinolone antibiotics, imidazole, and triazole antifungal agents)).
No products indexed under this heading.

Tacrolimus (When Coartem Tablets are co-administered with substrates of CYP3A4 it may result in decreased concentrations of the substrate and potential loss of substrate efficacy). Products include:
Prograf Capsules 677
Prograf Injection 677
Protopic 685

Tadalafil (When Coartem Tablets are co-administered with substrates of CYP3A4 it may result in decreased concentrations of the substrate and potential loss of substrate efficacy). Products include:
Adcirca 3461
Cialis 1861

Tamoxifen Citrate (When Coartem Tablets are co-administered with substrates of CYP3A4 it may result in decreased concentrations of the substrate and potential loss of substrate efficacy).
No products indexed under this heading.

Telithromycin (When Coartem Tablets are co-administered with an inhibitor of CYP3A4, including grapefruit juice, it may result in increased concentrations of artemether and/or lumefantrine and potentiate QT prolongation). Products include:
Ketek 2991

Temazepam (Administration of Coartem Tablets with drugs that are metabolized by CYP2D6 maysignificantly increase plasma concentrations of the co-administered drug and increase the risk of adverse effects. Many of the drugs metabolized by CYP2D6 can prolong the QT interval and should not be administered with Coartem Tablets due to the potential additive effect on the QT interval (eg, flecainide, imipramine, amitriptyline, clomipramine)).
No products indexed under this heading.

Tenofovir Disoproxil Fumarate (Drugs that have a mixed effect on CYP3A4, especially anti-retroviral drugs, and those that have an effect on the QT interval should be used with caution in patients taking Coartem Tablets). Products include:
Atripla 906
Truvada 1258
Viread 1266

Terbinafine Hydrochloride (Coartem Tablets should be avoided in patients receiving other medications that prolong the QT interval, such as certain antibiotics (macrolide antibiotics, fluoroquinolone antibiotics, imidazole, and triazole antifungal agents)).
No products indexed under this heading.

Terconazole (Coartem Tablets should be avoided in patients receiving other medications that prolong the QT interval, such as certain antibiotics (macrolide antibiotics, fluoroquinolone antibiotics, imidazole, and triazole antifungal agents)).
No products indexed under this heading.

Terfenadine (Coartem Tablets should be avoided in patients receiving other medications that prolong the QT interval, such as certain non-sedating antihistaminics (terfenadine, astemizole)).
No products indexed under this heading.

Testosterone (Administration of Coartem Tablets with drugs that are metabolized by CYP2D6 maysignificantly increase plasma concentrations of the co-administered drug and increase the risk of adverse effects. Many of the drugs metabolized by CYP2D6 can prolong the QT interval and should not be administered with Coartem Tablets due to the potential additive effect on the QT interval (eg, flecainide, imipramine, amitriptyline, clomipramine)). Products include:
AndroGel 3456

Testosterone Cypionate (Administration of Coartem Tablets with drugs that are metabolized by CYP2D6 maysignificantly increase plasma concentrations of the co-administered drug and increase the risk of adverse effects. Many of the drugs metabolized by CYP2D6 can prolong the QT interval and should not be administered with Coartem Tablets due to the potential additive effect on the QT interval (eg, flecainide, imipramine, amitriptyline, clomipramine)).
No products indexed under this heading.

Testosterone Enanthate (Administration of Coartem Tablets with drugs that are metabolized by CYP2D6 maysignificantly increase plasma concentrations of the co-administered drug and increase the risk of adverse effects. Many of the drugs metabolized by CYP2D6 can prolong the QT interval and should not be administered with Coartem Tablets due to the potential additive effect on the QT interval (eg, flecainide, imipramine, amitriptyline, clomipramine)). Products include:
Delatestryl 1102

Testosterone Propionate (Administration of Coartem Tablets with drugs that are metabolized by CYP2D6 may significantly increase plasma concentrations of the co-administered drug and increase the risk of adverse effects. Many of the drugs metabolized by CYP2D6 can prolong the QT interval and should not be administered with Coartem Tablets due to the potential additive effect on the QT interval (eg, flecainide, imipramine, amitriptyline, clomipramine)).
No products indexed under this heading.

Tetracycline Hydrochloride (Coartem Tablets should be avoided in patients receiving other medications that prolong the QT interval, such as certain antibiotics (macrolide antibiotics, fluoroquinolone antibiotics, imidazole, and triazole antifungal agents)). Products include:
Pylera 793

Theophyllinate (When Coartem Tablets are co-administered with inducers of CYP3A4 it may result in decreased concentrations of artemether and/or lumefantrine and loss of anti-malarial efficacy).
No products indexed under this heading.

Theophylline (When Coartem Tablets are co-administered with substrates of CYP3A4 it may result in decreased concentrations of the substrate and potential loss of substrate efficacy).
No products indexed under this heading.

Theophylline Anhydrous (When Coartem Tablets are co-administered with substrates of CYP3A4 it may result in decreased concentrations of the substrate and potential loss of substrate efficacy). Products include:
Uniphyl 2817

Theophylline Calcium Salicylate (When Coartem Tablets are co-administered with substrates of CYP3A4 it may result in decreased concentrations of the substrate and potential loss of substrate efficacy).
No products indexed under this heading.

Theophylline Dihydroxypropyl (Glyceryl) (When Coartem Tablets are co-administered with substrates of CYP3A4 it may result in decreased concentrations of the substrate and potential loss of substrate efficacy).
No products indexed under this heading.

Theophylline Ethylenediamine (When Coartem Tablets are co-administered with substrates of CYP3A4 it may result in decreased concentrations of the substrate and potential loss of substrate efficacy).
No products indexed under this heading.

Theophylline Sodium Glycinate (When Coartem Tablets are co-administered with substrates of CYP3A4 it may result in decreased concentrations of the substrate and potential loss of substrate efficacy).
No products indexed under this heading.

Thioridazine Hydrochloride (Coartem Tablets should be avoided in patients receiving other medications that prolong the QT interval, such as antipsychotics (pimozide, ziprasidone)). Products include:
Thioridazine Hydrochloride 2384

Thiothixene (Coartem Tablets should be avoided in patients receiving other medications that prolong the QT interval, such as antipsychotics (pimozide, ziprasidone)). Products include:
Thiothixene 2386

Tiagabine Hydrochloride (When Coartem Tablets are co-administered with substrates of CYP3A4 it may result in decreased concentrations of the substrate and potential loss of substrate efficacy). Products include:
Gabitril 972

Ticarcillin Disodium (Coartem Tablets should be avoided in patients receiving other medications that prolong the QT interval, such as certain antibiotics (macrolide antibiotics, fluoroquinolone antibiotics, imidazole, and triazole antifungal agents)). Products include:
Timentin ADD-Vantage 1670
Timentin Galaxy 1674
Timentin 1666
Timentin Pharmacy 1678

Tipranavir (Drugs that have a mixed effect on CYP3A4, especially anti-retroviral drugs, and those that have an effect on the QT interval should be used with caution in patients taking Coartem Tablets).
No products indexed under this heading.

Tobramycin (Coartem Tablets should be avoided in patients receiving other medications that prolong the QT interval, such as certain antibiotics (macrolide antibiotics, fluoroquinolone antibiotics, imidazole, and triazole antifungal agents)). Products include:
Tobi Nebulizer 2546
Tobramycin and Dexamethasone Ophthalmic Suspension .... ⊙251
Zylet .... ⊙252

Tobramycin Sulfate (Coartem Tablets should be avoided in patients receiving other medications that prolong the QT interval, such as certain antibiotics (macrolide antibiotics, fluoroquinolone antibiotics, imidazole, and triazole antifungal agents)).
No products indexed under this heading.

Tocainide Hydrochloride (Drugs that prolong the QT interval, including antimalarials such as quinine and quinidine, should be used cautiously following Coartem Tablets, due to the long elimination half-life of lumefantrine (3-6 days) and the potential for additive effects on the QT interval).
No products indexed under this heading.

Tolterodine Tartrate (When Coartem Tablets are co-administered with substrates of CYP3A4 it may result in decreased concentrations of the substrate and potential loss of substrate efficacy).
No products indexed under this heading.

Tranylcypromine Sulfate (Coartem Tablets should be avoided in patients receiving other medications that prolong the QT interval, such as antidepressants). Products include:
Parnate 1584

Trazodone Hydrochloride (Coartem Tablets should be avoided in patients receiving other medications that prolong the QT interval, such as antidepressants).
No products indexed under this heading.

Tretinoin (Administration of Coartem Tablets with drugs that are metabolized by CYP2D6 maysignificantly increase plasma concentrations of the co-administered drug and increase the risk of adverse effects. Many of the drugs metabolized by CYP2D6 can prolong the QT interval and should not be administered with Coartem Tablets due to the potential additive effect on the QT interval (eg, flecainide, imipramine, amitriptyline, clomipramine)).
No products indexed under this heading.

Triamcinolone (When Coartem Tablets are co-administered with inducers of CYP3A4 it may result in decreased concentrations of artemether and/or lumefantrine and loss of anti-malarial efficacy).
No products indexed under this heading.

Triamcinolone Acetonide (When Coartem Tablets are co-administered with inducers of CYP3A4 it may result in decreased concentrations of artemether and/or lumefantrine and loss of anti-malarial efficacy). Products include:

Azmacort 408
Nasacort AQ 3019

Triamcinolone Diacetate (When Coartem Tablets are co-administered with inducers of CYP3A4 it may result in decreased concentrations of artemether and/or lumefantrine and loss of anti-malarial efficacy).
No products indexed under this heading.

Triamcinolone Hexacetonide (When Coartem Tablets are co-administered with inducers of CYP3A4 it may result in decreased concentrations of artemether and/or lumefantrine and loss of anti-malarial efficacy).
No products indexed under this heading.

Triazolam (When Coartem Tablets are co-administered with substrates of CYP3A4 it may result in decreased concentrations of the substrate and potential loss of substrate efficacy).
No products indexed under this heading.

Trifluoperazine Hydrochloride (Coartem Tablets should be avoided in patients receiving other medications that prolong the QT interval, such as antipsychotics (pimozide, ziprasidone)).
No products indexed under this heading.

Trimeprazine Tartrate (Coartem Tablets should be avoided in patients receiving other medications that prolong the QT interval, such as certain non-sedating antihistaminics (terfenadine, astemizole)).
No products indexed under this heading.

Trimipramine Maleate (Coartem Tablets should be avoided in patients receiving other medications that prolong the QT interval, such as antidepressants).
No products indexed under this heading.

Tripelennamine Hydrochloride (Coartem Tablets should be avoided in patients receiving other medications that prolong the QT interval, such as certain non-sedating antihistaminics (terfenadine, astemizole)).
No products indexed under this heading.

Triprolidine Hydrochloride (Coartem Tablets should be avoided in patients receiving other medications that prolong the QT interval, such as certain non-sedating antihistaminics (terfenadine, astemizole)).
No products indexed under this heading.

Troglitazone (When Coartem Tablets are co-administered with an inhibitor of CYP3A4, including grapefruit juice, it may result in increased concentrations of artemether and/or lumefantrine and potentiate QT prolongation).
No products indexed under this heading.

Troleandomycin (Coartem Tablets should be avoided in patients receiving other medications that prolong the QT interval, such as certain antibiotics (macrolide antibiotics, fluoroquinolone antibiotics, imidazole, and triazole antifungal agents)).
No products indexed under this heading.

Trovafloxacin Mesylate (Coartem Tablets should be avoided in patients receiving other medications that prolong the QT interval, such as certain antibiotics (macrolide antibiotics, fluoroquinolone antibiotics, imidazole, and triazole antifungal agents)).
No products indexed under this heading.

Valproate Sodium (When Coartem Tablets are co-administered with an inhibitor of CYP3A4, including grapefruit juice, it may result in increased concentrations of artemether and/or lumefantrine and potentiate QT prolongation).
No products indexed under this heading.

Valproic Acid (Administration of Coartem Tablets with drugs that are metabolized by CYP2D6 maysignificantly increase plasma concentrations of the co-administered drug and increase the risk of adverse effects. Many of the drugs metabolized by CYP2D6 can prolong the QT interval and should not be administered with Coartem Tablets due to the potential additive effect on the QT interval (eg, flecainide, imipramine, amitriptyline, clomipramine)).
No products indexed under this heading.

Vardenafil Hydrochloride (When Coartem Tablets are co-administered with substrates of CYP3A4 it may result in decreased concentrations of the substrate and potential loss of substrate efficacy). Products include:
Levitra 3157

Venlafaxine Hydrochloride (Coartem Tablets should be avoided in patients receiving other medications that prolong the QT interval, such as antidepressants). Products include:
Effexor XR 3504
Venlafaxine Hydrochloride Tablets ... 2388

Verapamil Hydrochloride (When Coartem Tablets are co-administered with substrates of CYP3A4 it may result in decreased concentrations of the substrate and potential loss of substrate efficacy). Products include:
Tarka 534

Vinblastine Sulfate (When Coartem Tablets are co-administered with substrates of CYP3A4 it may result in decreased concentrations of the substrate and potential loss of substrate efficacy).
No products indexed under this heading.

Vincristine Sulfate (When Coartem Tablets are co-administered with substrates of CYP3A4 it may result in decreased concentrations of the substrate and potential loss of substrate efficacy).
No products indexed under this heading.

Voriconazole (Coartem Tablets should be avoided in patients receiving other medications that prolong the QT interval, such as certain antibiotics (macrolide antibiotics, fluoroquinolone antibiotics, imidazole, and triazole antifungal agents)).
No products indexed under this heading.

Warfarin Sodium (When Coartem Tablets are co-administered with substrates of CYP3A4 it may result in decreased concentrations of the substrate and potential loss of substrate efficacy).
No products indexed under this heading.

Zafirlukast (When Coartem Tablets are co-administered with an inhibitor of CYP3A4, including grapefruit juice, it may result in increased concentrations of artemether and/or lumefantrine and potentiate QT prolongation). Products include:
Accolate 3612

Zalcitabine (Drugs that have a mixed effect on CYP3A4, especially antiretroviral drugs, and those that have an effect on the QT interval should be used with caution in patients taking Coartem Tablets).
No products indexed under this heading.

Zidovudine (Drugs that have a mixed effect on CYP3A4, especially antiretroviral drugs, and those that have an effect on the QT interval should be used with caution in patients taking Coartem Tablets). Products include:
Combivir 1404
Retrovir 1634
Retrovir IV 1640
Trizivir 1688

Zileuton (When Coartem Tablets are co-administered with an inhibitor of CYP3A4, including grapefruit juice, it may result in increased concentrations of artemether and/or lumefantrine and potentiate QT prolongation).
No products indexed under this heading.

Ziprasidone Hydrochloride (Coartem Tablets should be avoided in patients receiving other medications that prolong the QT interval, such as antipsychotics (pimozide, ziprasidone)). Products include:
Geodon 2723

Food Interactions

Food, unspecified (Food enhances absorption of artemether and lumefantrine following administration of Coartem Tablets. Patients who remain averse to food during treatment should be closely monitored, as the risk of recrudescence may be greater).

Grapefruit (When Coartem Tablets are co-administered with an inhibitor of CYP3A4, including grapefruit juice, it may result in increased concentrations of artemether and/or lumefantrine and potentiate QT prolongation).

Grapefruit Juice (When Coartem Tablets are co-administered with an inhibitor of CYP3A4, including grapefruit juice, it may result in increased concentrations of artemether and/or lumefantrine and potentiate QT prolongation).

COMBIGAN OPHTHALMIC SOLUTION

(Brimonidine Tartrate, Timolol Maleate) 601
May interact with alcohols, anesthetics, antihypertensives, barbiturates, beta-blockers, calcium channel blockers, cardiac glycosides, catecholamine-depleting drugs, central nervous system depressants, cytochrome p450 2d6 inhibitors (selected), hypnotics and sedatives, insulin, monoamine oxidase inhibitors, narcotic analgesics, oral hypoglycemic agents, tricyclic antidepressants. Compounds in these categories include:

Acarbose (Beta-adrenergic blocking agents should be administered with caution in patients subject to spontaneous hypoglycemia or to diabetic patients (especially those with labile diabetes) who are receiving insulin or oral hypoglycemic agents. Beta-adrenergic receptor blocking agents may mask the signs and symptoms of acute hypoglycemia).
No products indexed under this heading.

Acebutolol Hydrochloride (Patients who are receiving a beta-adrenergic blocking agent orally and Combigan should be observed for potential additive effects of beta-blockade, both systemic and on intraocular pressure. The concomitant use of two topical beta-adrenergic blocking agents is not recommended).
No products indexed under this heading.

Alfentanil Hydrochloride (Although specific drug interaction studies have not been conducted with Combigan, the possibility of an additive or potentiating effect with CNS depressants (alcohol, barbiturates, opiates, sedatives or anesthetics) should be considered).
No products indexed under this heading.

Aliskiren (Because Combigan may reduce blood pressure, caution in using drugs such as antihypertensives with Combigan is advised). Products include:
Tekturna 2538
Tekturna HCT 2541
Valturna 3637

Alprazolam (Although specific drug interaction studies have not been conducted with Combigan, the possibility of an additive or potentiating effect with CNS depressants (alcohol, barbiturates, opiates, sedatives or anesthetics) should be considered).
No products indexed under this heading.

Amiodarone Hydrochloride (Potentiated systemic beta-blockade (eg, decreased heart rate, depression) has been reported during combined treatment with CYP2D6 inhibitors (eg, quinidine, SSRIs) and timolol).
No products indexed under this heading.

Amitriptyline Hydrochloride (Tricyclic antidepressants have been reported to blunt the hypotensive effect of systemic clonidine. It is not known whether the concurrent use of these agents with Combigan in humans can lead to resulting interference with the IOP lowering effect. Caution, however, is advised in patients taking tricyclic antidepressants which can affect the metabolism and uptake of circulating amines).
No products indexed under this heading.

Amlodipine Besylate (Caution should be used in the co-administration of beta-adrenergic blocking agents, such as Combigan, and oral or intravenous calcium antagonists because of possible atrioventricular conduction disturbances, left ventricular failure and hypotension. In patients with impaired cardiac function, co-administration should be avoided. The concomitant use of beta-adrenergic blocking agents with calcium antagonists may have additive effects in proloning atrioventricular conduction time). Products include:
Azor 1010
Exforge 2443
Exforge HCT 2449

Amobarbital (Although specific drug interaction studies have not been conducted with Combigan, the possibility of an additive or potentiating effect with CNS depressants (alcohol, barbiturates, opiates, sedatives or anesthetics) should be considered).
No products indexed under this heading.

Amobarbital Sodium (Although specific drug interaction studies have not been conducted with Combigan, the possibility of an additive or potentiating effect with CNS depressants (alcohol, barbiturates, opiates, sedatives or anesthetics) should be considered).
No products indexed under this heading.

Amoxapine (Tricyclic antidepressants have been reported to blunt the hypotensive effect of systemic clonidine. It is not known whether the concurrent use of these agents with Combigan in humans can lead to resulting interference with the IOP lowering effect. Caution, however, is advised in patients taking tricyclic antidepressants which can affect the metabolism and uptake of circulating amines).
No products indexed under this heading.

Apomorphine (Although specific drug interaction studies have not been conducted with Combigan, the possibility of an additive or potentiating effect with CNS depressants (alcohol, barbiturates, opiates, sedatives or anesthetics) should be considered).
No products indexed under this heading.

Apomorphine Hydrochloride (Although specific drug interaction studies have not been conducted with Combigan, the possibility of an additive or potentiating effect with CNS depressants (alcohol, barbiturates, opiates, sedatives or anesthetics) should be considered).
No products indexed under this heading.

Aprobarbital (Although specific drug interaction studies have not been conducted with Combigan, the possibility of an additive or potentiating effect with CNS depressants (alcohol, barbiturates, opiates, sedatives or anesthetics) should be considered).
No products indexed under this heading.

IMPORTANT NOTE: Always consult each drug listing in the patient's regimen for possible interactions.

Articaine Hydrochloride (Although specific drug interaction studies have not been conducted with Combigan, the possibility of an additive or potentiating effect with CNS depressants (alcohol, barbiturates, opiates, sedatives or anesthetics) should be considered).
No products indexed under this heading.

Atenolol (Patients who are receiving a beta-adrenergic blocking agent orally and Combigan should be observed for potential additive effects of beta-blockade, both systemic and on intraocular pressure. The concomitant use of two topical beta-adrenergic blocking agents is not recommended.
No products indexed under this heading.

Benazepril Hydrochloride (Because Combigan may reduce blood pressure, caution in using drugs such as antihypertensives with Combigan is advised).
No products indexed under this heading.

Bendroflumethiazide (Because Combigan may reduce blood pressure, caution in using drugs such as antihypertensives with Combigan is advised).
No products indexed under this heading.

Benzocaine (Although specific drug interaction studies have not been conducted with Combigan, the possibility of an additive or potentiating effect with CNS depressants (alcohol, barbiturates, opiates, sedatives or anesthetics) should be considered).
No products indexed under this heading.

Bepridil Hydrochloride (Caution should be used in the co-administration of beta-adrenergic blocking agents, such as Combigan, and oral or intravenous calcium antagonists because of possible atrioventricular conduction disturbances, left ventricular failure and hypotension. In patients with impaired cardiac function, co-administration should be avoided. The concomitant use of beta-adrenergic blocking agents with calcium antagonists may have additive effects in prolonging atrioventricular conduction time).
No products indexed under this heading.

Betaxolol Hydrochloride (Patients who are receiving a beta-adrenergic blocking agent orally and Combigan should be observed for potential additive effects of beta-blockade, both systemic and on intraocular pressure. The concomitant use of two topical beta-adrenergic blocking agents is not recommended.
No products indexed under this heading.

Bisoprolol Fumarate (Patients who are receiving a beta-adrenergic blocking agent orally and Combigan should be observed for potential additive effects of beta-blockade, both systemic and on intraocular pressure. The concomitant use of two topical beta-adrenergic blocking agents is not recommended).
No products indexed under this heading.

Bupivacaine Hydrochloride (Although specific drug interaction studies have not been conducted with Combigan, the possibility of an additive or potentiating effect with CNS depressants (alcohol, barbiturates, opiates, sedatives or anesthetics) should be considered).
No products indexed under this heading.

Buprenorphine Hydrochloride (Although specific drug interaction studies have not been conducted with Combigan, the possibility of an additive or potentiating effect with CNS depressants (alcohol, barbiturates, opiates, sedatives or anesthetics) should be considered).
No products indexed under this heading.

Bupropion Hydrochloride (Potentiated systemic beta-blockade (eg, decreased heart rate, depression) has been reported during combined treat-

ment with CYP2D6 inhibitors (eg, quinidine, SSRIs) and timolol). Products include:
Aplenzin 2948
Wellbutrin 1719
Wellbutrin SR 1725
Zyban 1762

Buspirone Hydrochloride (Although specific drug interaction studies have not been conducted with Combigan, the possibility of an additive or potentiating effect with CNS depressants (alcohol, barbiturates, opiates, sedatives or anesthetics) should be considered).
No products indexed under this heading.

Butabarbital (Although specific drug interaction studies have not been conducted with Combigan, the possibility of an additive or potentiating effect with CNS depressants (alcohol, barbiturates, opiates, sedatives or anesthetics) should be considered).
No products indexed under this heading.

Butabarbital Sodium (Although specific drug interaction studies have not been conducted with Combigan, the possibility of an additive or potentiating effect with CNS depressants (alcohol, barbiturates, opiates, sedatives or anesthetics) should be considered).
No products indexed under this heading.

Butalbital (Although specific drug interaction studies have not been conducted with Combigan, the possibility of an additive or potentiating effect with CNS depressants (alcohol, barbiturates, opiates, sedatives or anesthetics) should be considered).
No products indexed under this heading.

Candesartan Cilexetil (Because Combigan may reduce blood pressure, caution in using drugs such as antihypertensives with Combigan is advised).
Products include:
Atacand 697
Atacand HCT 700

Captopril (Because Combigan may reduce blood pressure, caution in using drugs such as antihypertensives with Combigan is advised). Products include:
Captopril 2341

Carteolol Hydrochloride (Patients who are receiving a beta-adrenergic blocking agent orally and Combigan should be observed for potential additive effects of beta-blockade, both systemic and on intraocular pressure. The concomitant use of two topical beta-adrenergic blocking agents is not recommended).
No products indexed under this heading.

Carvedilol (Patients who are receiving a beta-adrenergic blocking agent orally and Combigan should be observed for potential additive effects of beta-blockade, both systemic and on intraocular pressure. The concomitant use of two topical beta-adrenergic blocking agents is not recommended). Products include:
Coreg 1409

Carvedilol Phosphate (Patients who are receiving a beta-adrenergic blocking agent orally and Combigan should be observed for potential additive effects of beta-blockade, both systemic and on intraocular pressure. The concomitant use of two topical beta-adrenergic blocking agents is not recommended).
Products include:
Coreg CR 1416

Celecoxib (Potentiated systemic beta-blockade (eg, decreased heart rate, depression) has been reported during combined treatment with CYP2D6 inhibitors (eg, quinidine, SSRIs) and timolol). Products include:
Celebrex 3272

Chloral Hydrate (Although specific drug interaction studies have not been conducted with Combigan, the possibility of an additive or potentiating effect with CNS depressants (alcohol, barbiturates, opiates, sedatives or anesthetics) should be considered).
No products indexed under this heading.

Chlordiazepoxide (Although specific drug interaction studies have not been conducted with Combigan, the possibility of an additive or potentiating effect with CNS depressants (alcohol, barbiturates, opiates, sedatives or anesthetics) should be considered).
No products indexed under this heading.

Chlordiazepoxide Hydrochloride (Although specific drug interaction studies have not been conducted with Combigan, the possibility of an additive or potentiating effect with CNS depressants (alcohol, barbiturates, opiates, sedatives or anesthetics) should be considered).
No products indexed under this heading.

Chloroprocaine Hydrochloride (Although specific drug interaction studies have not been conducted with Combigan, the possibility of an additive or potentiating effect with CNS depressants (alcohol, barbiturates, opiates, sedatives or anesthetics) should be considered).
No products indexed under this heading.

Chloroquine (Potentiated systemic beta-blockade (eg, decreased heart rate, depression) has been reported during combined treatment with CYP2D6 inhibitors (eg, quinidine, SSRIs) and timolol).
No products indexed under this heading.

Chloroquine Hydrochloride (Potentiated systemic beta-blockade (eg, decreased heart rate, depression) has been reported during combined treatment with CYP2D6 inhibitors (eg, quinidine, SSRIs) and timolol).
No products indexed under this heading.

Chloroquine Phosphate (Potentiated systemic beta-blockade (eg, decreased heart rate, depression) has been reported during combined treatment with CYP2D6 inhibitors (eg, quinidine, SSRIs) and timolol).
No products indexed under this heading.

Chlorothiazide (Because Combigan may reduce blood pressure, caution in using drugs such as antihypertensives with Combigan is advised).
No products indexed under this heading.

Chlorothiazide Sodium (Because Combigan may reduce blood pressure, caution in using drugs such as antihypertensives with Combigan is advised).
Products include:
Diuril Intravenous 2009

Chlorpheniramine (Potentiated systemic beta-blockade (eg, decreased heart rate, depression) has been reported during combined treatment with CYP2D6 inhibitors (eg, quinidine, SSRIs) and timolol).
No products indexed under this heading.

Chlorpheniramine Maleate (Potentiated systemic beta-blockade (eg, decreased heart rate, depression) has been reported during combined treatment with CYP2D6 inhibitors (eg, quinidine, SSRIs) and timolol).
No products indexed under this heading.

Chlorpheniramine Polistirex (Potentiated systemic beta-blockade (eg, decreased heart rate, depression) has been reported during combined treatment with CYP2D6 inhibitors (eg, quinidine, SSRIs) and timolol). Products include:
Tussionex 3443

Chlorpheniramine Tannate (Potentiated systemic beta-blockade (eg, decreased heart rate, depression) has been reported during combined treatment with CYP2D6 inhibitors (eg, quinidine, SSRIs) and timolol).
No products indexed under this heading.

Chlorpromazine (Although specific drug interaction studies have not been conducted with Combigan, the possibility of an additive or potentiating effect with CNS depressants (alcohol, barbiturates, opiates, sedatives or anesthetics) should be considered).
No products indexed under this heading.

Chlorpromazine Hydrochloride (Although specific drug interaction studies have not been conducted with Combigan, the possibility of an additive or potentiating effect with CNS depressants (alcohol, barbiturates, opiates, sedatives or anesthetics) should be considered).
No products indexed under this heading.

Chlorpropamide (Beta-adrenergic blocking agents should be administered with caution in patients subject to spontaneous hypoglycemia or to diabetic patients (especially those with labile diabetes) who are receiving insulin or oral hypoglycemic agents. Beta-adrenergic receptor blocking agents may mask the signs and symptoms of acute hypoglycemia).
No products indexed under this heading.

Chlorprothixene (Although specific drug interaction studies have not been conducted with Combigan, the possibility of an additive or potentiating effect with CNS depressants (alcohol, barbiturates, opiates, sedatives or anesthetics) should be considered).
No products indexed under this heading.

Chlorprothixene Hydrochloride (Although specific drug interaction studies have not been conducted with Combigan, the possibility of an additive or potentiating effect with CNS depressants (alcohol, barbiturates, opiates, sedatives or anesthetics) should be considered).
No products indexed under this heading.

Chlorprothixene Lactate (Although specific drug interaction studies have not been conducted with Combigan, the possibility of an additive or potentiating effect with CNS depressants (alcohol, barbiturates, opiates, sedatives or anesthetics) should be considered).
No products indexed under this heading.

Chlorthalidone (Because Combigan may reduce blood pressure, caution in using drugs such as antihypertensives with Combigan is advised). Products include:
Clorpres 2344

Cimetidine (Potentiated systemic beta-blockade (eg, decreased heart rate, depression) has been reported during combined treatment with CYP2D6 inhibitors (eg, quinidine, SSRIs) and timolol).
No products indexed under this heading.

Cimetidine Hydrochloride (Potentiated systemic beta-blockade (eg, decreased heart rate, depression) has been reported during combined treatment with CYP2D6 inhibitors (eg, quinidine, SSRIs) and timolol).
No products indexed under this heading.

Citalopram Hydrobromide (Potentiated systemic beta-blockade (eg, decreased heart rate, depression) has been reported during combined treatment with CYP2D6 inhibitors (eg, quinidine, SSRIs) and timolol). Products include:
Celexa 1153

Clomipramine Hydrochloride (Tricyclic antidepressants have been reported to blunt the hypotensive effect

of systemic clonidine. It is not known whether the concurrent use of these agents with Combigan in humans can lead to resulting interference with the IOP lowering effect. Caution, however, is advised in patients taking tricyclic antidepressants which can affect the metabolism and uptake of circulating amines).
No products indexed under this heading.

Clonazepam (Although specific drug interaction studies have not been conducted with Combigan, the possibility of an additive or potentiating effect with CNS depressants (alcohol, barbiturates, opiates, sedatives or anesthetics) should be considered). Products include:
Klonopin **2855**

Clonidine (Because Combigan may reduce blood pressure, caution in using drugs such as antihypertensives with Combigan is advised). Products include:
Catapres-TTS **884**

Clonidine Hydrochloride (Because Combigan may reduce blood pressure, caution in using drugs such as antihypertensives with Combigan is advised). Products include:
Clorpres **2344**

Clorazepate Dipotassium (Although specific drug interaction studies have not been conducted with Combigan, the possibility of an additive or potentiating effect with CNS depressants (alcohol, barbiturates, opiates, sedatives or anesthetics) should be considered).
No products indexed under this heading.

Clozapine (Although specific drug interaction studies have not been conducted with Combigan, the possibility of an additive or potentiating effect with CNS depressants (alcohol, barbiturates, opiates, sedatives or anesthetics) should be considered).
No products indexed under this heading.

Cocaine Hydrochloride (Although specific drug interaction studies have not been conducted with Combigan, the possibility of an additive or potentiating effect with CNS depressants (alcohol, barbiturates, opiates, sedatives or anesthetics) should be considered).
No products indexed under this heading.

Codeine Phosphate (Although specific drug interaction studies have not been conducted with Combigan, the possibility of an additive or potentiating effect with CNS depressants (alcohol, barbiturates, opiates, sedatives or anesthetics) should be considered). Products include:
Tylenol with Codeine **2691**

Codeine Sulfate (Although specific drug interaction studies have not been conducted with Combigan, the possibility of an additive or potentiating effect with CNS depressants (alcohol, barbiturates, opiates, sedatives or anesthetics) should be considered).
No products indexed under this heading.

Deserpidine (Because Combigan may reduce blood pressure, caution in using drugs such as antihypertensives with Combigan is advised).
No products indexed under this heading.

Desflurane (Although specific drug interaction studies have not been conducted with Combigan, the possibility of an additive or potentiating effect with CNS depressants (alcohol, barbiturates, opiates, sedatives or anesthetics) should be considered).
No products indexed under this heading.

Desipramine Hydrochloride (Tricyclic antidepressants have been reported to blunt the hypotensive effect of systemic clonidine. It is not known whether the concurrent use of these agents with Combigan in humans can lead to resulting interference with the IOP lowering effect. Caution, however, is advised in patients taking tricyclic antidepressants which can affect the metabolism and uptake of circulating amines).
No products indexed under this heading.

Deslanoside (Because Combigan may reduce blood pressure, caution in using drugs such as cardiac glycosides with Combigan is advised. The concomitant use of beta-adrenergic blocking agents with digitalis may have additive effects in prolonging atrioventricular conduction time).
No products indexed under this heading.

Dezocine (Although specific drug interaction studies have not been conducted with Combigan, the possibility of an additive or potentiating effect with CNS depressants (alcohol, barbiturates, opiates, sedatives or anesthetics) should be considered).
No products indexed under this heading.

Diazepam (Although specific drug interaction studies have not been conducted with Combigan, the possibility of an additive or potentiating effect with CNS depressants (alcohol, barbiturates, opiates, sedatives or anesthetics) should be considered). Products include:
Valium Tablets **2880**

Diazoxide (Because Combigan may reduce blood pressure, caution in using drugs such as antihypertensives with Combigan is advised). Products include:
Proglycem **1179**
Proglycem Suspension **1179**

Dibucaine (Although specific drug interaction studies have not been conducted with Combigan, the possibility of an additive or potentiating effect with CNS depressants (alcohol, barbiturates, opiates, sedatives or anesthetics) should be considered).
No products indexed under this heading.

Dibucaine Hydrochloride (Although specific drug interaction studies have not been conducted with Combigan, the possibility of an additive or potentiating effect with CNS depressants (alcohol, barbiturates, opiates, sedatives or anesthetics) should be considered).
No products indexed under this heading.

Digitalis Glycoside Preparations (Because Combigan may reduce blood pressure, caution in using drugs such as cardiac glycosides with Combigan is advised. The concomitant use of beta-adrenergic blocking agents with digitalis may have additive effects in prolonging atrioventricular conduction time).
No products indexed under this heading.

Digitalis Lanata (Because Combigan may reduce blood pressure, caution in using drugs such as cardiac glycosides with Combigan is advised. The concomitant use of beta-adrenergic blocking agents with digitalis may have additive effects in prolonging atrioventricular conduction time).
No products indexed under this heading.

Digitalis Purpurea (Because Combigan may reduce blood pressure, caution in using drugs such as cardiac glycosides with Combigan is advised. The concomitant use of beta-adrenergic blocking agents with digitalis may have additive effects in prolonging atrioventricular conduction time).
No products indexed under this heading.

Digitoxin (Because Combigan may reduce blood pressure, caution in using drugs such as cardiac glycosides with Combigan is advised. The concomitant use of beta-adrenergic blocking agents with digitalis may have additive effects in prolonging atrioventricular conduction time).
No products indexed under this heading.

Digoxin (Because Combigan may reduce blood pressure, caution in using drugs such as cardiac glycosides with Combigan is advised. The concomitant use of beta-adrenergic blocking agents with digitalis may have additive effects in prolonging atrioventricular conduction time). Products include:
Lanoxin Injection **1546**
Lanoxin Injection Pediatric **1549**
Lanoxin Tablets **1553**

Dihydrocodeine Bitartrate (Although specific drug interaction studies have not been conducted with Combigan, the possibility of an additive or potentiating effect with CNS depressants (alcohol, barbiturates, opiates, sedatives or anesthetics) should be considered).
No products indexed under this heading.

Dihydrocodeinone Bitartrate (Although specific drug interaction studies have not been conducted with Combigan, the possibility of an additive or potentiating effect with CNS depressants (alcohol, barbiturates, opiates, sedatives or anesthetics) should be considered).
No products indexed under this heading.

Diltiazem Hydrochloride (Caution should be used in the co-administration of beta-adrenergic blocking agents, such as Combigan, and oral or intravenous calcium antagonists because of possible atrioventricular conduction disturbances, left ventricular failure and hypotension. In patients with impaired cardiac function, co-administration should be avoided. The concomitant use of beta-adrenergic blocking agents with calcium antagonists may have additive effects in proloning atrioventricular conduction time). Products include:
Cardizem LA **423**

Diltiazem Maleate (Because Combigan may reduce blood pressure, caution in using drugs such as antihypertensives with Combigan is advised).
No products indexed under this heading.

Diphenhydramine (Potentiated systemic beta-blockade (eg, decreased heart rate, depression) has been reported during combined treatment with CYP2D6 inhibitors (eg, quinidine, SSRIs) and timolol).
No products indexed under this heading.

Diphenhydramine Hydrochloride (Potentiated systemic beta-blockade (eg, decreased heart rate, depression) has been reported during combined treatment with CYP2D6 inhibitors (eg, quinidine, SSRIs) and timolol). Products include:
Benadryl Allergy Ultratab **2042**
Children's Benadryl Allergy Liquid **2042**

Doxazosin Mesylate (Because Combigan may reduce blood pressure, caution in using drugs such as antihypertensives with Combigan is advised).
No products indexed under this heading.

Doxepin Hydrochloride (Tricyclic antidepressants have been reported to blunt the hypotensive effect of systemic clonidine. It is not known whether the concurrent use of these agents with Combigan in humans can lead to resulting interference with the IOP lowering effect. Caution, however, is advised in patients taking tricyclic antidepressants which can affect the metabolism and uptake of circulating amines).
No products indexed under this heading.

Droperidol (Although specific drug interaction studies have not been conducted with Combigan, the possibility of an additive or potentiating effect with CNS depressants (alcohol, barbiturates, opiates, sedatives or anesthetics) should be considered).
No products indexed under this heading.

Enalapril Maleate (Because Combigan may reduce blood pressure, caution in using drugs such as antihypertensives with Combigan is advised).
No products indexed under this heading.

Enalaprilat (Because Combigan may reduce blood pressure, caution in using drugs such as antihypertensives with Combigan is advised).
No products indexed under this heading.

Enflurane (Although specific drug interaction studies have not been conducted with Combigan, the possibility of an additive or potentiating effect with CNS depressants (alcohol, barbiturates, opiates, sedatives or anesthetics) should be considered).
No products indexed under this heading.

Eprosartan Mesylate (Because Combigan may reduce blood pressure, caution in using drugs such as antihypertensives with Combigan is advised). Products include:
Teveten **538**
Teveten HCT **541**

Escitalopram Oxalate (Potentiated systemic beta-blockade (eg, decreased heart rate, depression) has been reported during combined treatment with CYP2D6 inhibitors (eg, quinidine, SSRIs) and timolol). Products include:
Lexapro Oral Suspension **1160**
Lexapro Tablets **1160**

Esmolol Hydrochloride (Patients who are receiving a beta-adrenergic blocking agent orally and Combigan should be observed for potential additive effects of beta-blockade, both systemic and on intraocular pressure. The concomitant use of two topical beta-adrenergic blocking agents is not recommended).
No products indexed under this heading.

Estazolam (Although specific drug interaction studies have not been conducted with Combigan, the possibility of an additive or potentiating effect with CNS depressants (alcohol, barbiturates, opiates, sedatives or anesthetics) should be considered).
No products indexed under this heading.

Ethanol (Although specific drug interaction studies have not been conducted with Combigan, the possibility of an additive or potentiating effect with CNS depressants (alcohol, barbiturates, opiates, sedatives or anesthetics) should be considered).
No products indexed under this heading.

Ethchlorvynol (Although specific drug interaction studies have not been conducted with Combigan, the possibility of an additive or potentiating effect with CNS depressants (alcohol, barbiturates, opiates, sedatives or anesthetics) should be considered).
No products indexed under this heading.

Ethinamate (Although specific drug interaction studies have not been conducted with Combigan, the possibility of an additive or potentiating effect with CNS depressants (alcohol, barbiturates, opiates, sedatives or anesthetics) should be considered).
No products indexed under this heading.

Ethyl Alcohol (Although specific drug interaction studies have not been conducted with Combigan, the possibility of an additive or potentiating effect with CNS depressants (alcohol, barbiturates, opiates, sedatives or anesthetics) should be considered).
No products indexed under this heading.

Etidocaine Hydrochloride (Although specific drug interaction studies have not been conducted with Combigan, the possibility of an additive or potentiating effect with CNS depressants (alcohol, barbiturates, opiates, sedatives or anesthetics) should be considered).
No products indexed under this heading.

IMPORTANT NOTE: Always consult each drug listing in the patient's regimen for possible interactions.

Felodipine (Caution should be used in the co-administration of beta-adrenergic blocking agents, such as Combigan, and oral or intravenous calcium antagonists because of possible atrioventricular conduction disturbances, left ventricular failure and hypotension. In patients with impaired cardiac function, co-administration should be avoided. The concomitant use of beta-adrenergic blocking agents with calcium antagonists may have additive effects in proloning atrioventricular conduction time).
No products indexed under this heading.

Fentanyl (Although specific drug interaction studies have not been conducted with Combigan, the possibility of an additive or potentiating effect with CNS depressants (alcohol, barbiturates, opiates, sedatives or anesthetics) should be considered). Products include:

Fentanyl Citrate (Although specific drug interaction studies have not been conducted with Combigan, the possibility of an additive or potentiating effect with CNS depressants (alcohol, barbiturates, opiates, sedatives or anesthetics) should be considered). Products include:

Fluoxetine (Potentiated systemic beta-blockade (eg, decreased heart rate, depression) has been reported during combined treatment with CYP2D6 inhibitors (eg, quinidine, SSRIs) and timolol).
No products indexed under this heading.

Fluoxetine Hydrochloride (Potentiated systemic beta-blockade (eg, decreased heart rate, depression) has been reported during combined treatment with CYP2D6 inhibitors (eg, quinidine, SSRIs) and timolol). Products include:

Fluphenazine Decanoate (Although specific drug interaction studies have not been conducted with Combigan, the possibility of an additive or potentiating effect with CNS depressants (alcohol, barbiturates, opiates, sedatives or anesthetics) should be considered).
No products indexed under this heading.

Fluphenazine Enanthate (Although specific drug interaction studies have not been conducted with Combigan, the possibility of an additive or potentiating effect with CNS depressants (alcohol, barbiturates, opiates, sedatives or anesthetics) should be considered).
No products indexed under this heading.

Fluphenazine Hydrochloride (Although specific drug interaction studies have not been conducted with Combigan, the possibility of an additive or potentiating effect with CNS depressants (alcohol, barbiturates, sedatives or anesthetics) should be considered).
No products indexed under this heading.

Flurazepam Hydrochloride (Although specific drug interaction studies have not been conducted with Combigan, the possibility of an additive or potentiating effect with CNS depressants (alcohol, barbiturates, opiates, sedatives or anesthetics) should be considered).
No products indexed under this heading.

Fluvoxamine Maleate (Potentiated systemic beta-blockade (eg, decreased heart rate, depression) has been reported during combined treatment with CYP2D6 inhibitors (eg, quinidine, SSRIs) and timolol).
No products indexed under this heading.

Fosinopril Sodium (Because Combigan may reduce blood pressure, caution in using drugs such as antihypertensives with Combigan is advised).
No products indexed under this heading.

Furosemide (Because Combigan may reduce blood pressure, caution in using drugs such as antihypertensives with Combigan is advised). Products include:

Glibenclamide (Beta-adrenergic blocking agents should be administered with caution in patients subject to spontaneous hypoglycemia or to diabetic patients (especially those with labile diabetes) who are receiving insulin or oral hypoglycemic agents. Beta-adrenergic receptor blocking agents may mask the signs and symptoms of acute hypoglycemia).
No products indexed under this heading.

Glimepiride (Beta-adrenergic blocking agents should be administered with caution in patients subject to spontaneous hypoglycemia or to diabetic patients (especially those with labile diabetes) who are receiving insulin or oral hypoglycemic agents. Beta-adrenergic receptor blocking agents may mask the signs and symptoms of acute hypoglycemia). Products include:

Glipizide (Beta-adrenergic blocking agents should be administered with caution in patients subject to spontaneous hypoglycemia or to diabetic patients (especially those with labile diabetes) who are receiving insulin or oral hypoglycemic agents. Beta-adrenergic receptor blocking agents may mask the signs and symptoms of acute hypoglycemia).
No products indexed under this heading.

Glutethimide (Although specific drug interaction studies have not been conducted with Combigan, the possibility of an additive or potentiating effect with CNS depressants (alcohol, barbiturates, opiates, sedatives or anesthetics) should be considered).
No products indexed under this heading.

Glyburide (Beta-adrenergic blocking agents should be administered with caution in patients subject to spontaneous hypoglycemia or to diabetic patients (especially those with labile diabetes) who are receiving insulin or oral hypoglycemic agents. Beta-adrenergic receptor blocking agents may mask the signs and symptoms of acute hypoglycemia).
No products indexed under this heading.

Guanabenz Acetate (Because Combigan may reduce blood pressure, caution in using drugs such as antihypertensives with Combigan is advised).
No products indexed under this heading.

Guanethidine (Because Combigan may reduce blood pressure, caution in using drugs such as antihypertensives with Combigan is advised).
No products indexed under this heading.

Guanethidine Monosulfate (Because Combigan may reduce blood pressure, caution in using drugs such as antihypertensives with Combigan is advised).
No products indexed under this heading.

Guanethidine Sulfate (Because Combigan may reduce blood pressure, caution in using drugs such as antihypertensives with Combigan is advised).
No products indexed under this heading.

Halazepam (Although specific drug interaction studies have not been conducted with Combigan, the possibility of an additive or potentiating effect with CNS depressants (alcohol, barbiturates, opiates, sedatives or anesthetics) should be considered).
No products indexed under this heading.

Halofantrine Hydrochloride (Potentiated systemic beta-blockade (eg, decreased heart rate, depression) has been reported during combined treatment with CYP2D6 inhibitors (eg, quinidine, SSRIs) and timolol).
No products indexed under this heading.

Haloperidol (Although specific drug interaction studies have not been conducted with Combigan, the possibility of an additive or potentiating effect with CNS depressants (alcohol, barbiturates, opiates, sedatives or anesthetics) should be considered).
No products indexed under this heading.

Haloperidol Decanoate (Although specific drug interaction studies have not been conducted with Combigan, the possibility of an additive or potentiating effect with CNS depressants (alcohol, barbiturates, opiates, sedatives or anesthetics) should be considered).
No products indexed under this heading.

Haloperidol Lactate (Although specific drug interaction studies have not been conducted with Combigan, the possibility of an additive or potentiating effect with CNS depressants (alcohol, barbiturates, opiates, sedatives or anesthetics) should be considered).
No products indexed under this heading.

Halothane (Although specific drug interaction studies have not been conducted with Combigan, the possibility of an additive or potentiating effect with CNS depressants (alcohol, barbiturates, opiates, sedatives or anesthetics) should be considered).
No products indexed under this heading.

Hexobarbital (Although specific drug interaction studies have not been conducted with Combigan, the possibility of an additive or potentiating effect with CNS depressants (alcohol, barbiturates, opiates, sedatives or anesthetics) should be considered).
No products indexed under this heading.

Hydralazine Hydrochloride (Because Combigan may reduce blood pressure, caution in using drugs such as antihypertensives with Combigan is advised).
No products indexed under this heading.

Hydrochlorothiazide (Because Combigan may reduce blood pressure, caution in using drugs such as antihypertensives with Combigan is advised). Products include:

Hydrocodone Bitartrate (Although specific drug interaction studies have not been conducted with Combigan, the possibility of an additive or potentiating effect with CNS depressants (alcohol, barbiturates, opiates, sedatives or anesthetics) should be considered). Products include:

Hydrocodone Polistirex (Although specific drug interaction studies have not been conducted with Combigan, the possibility of an additive or potentiating effect with CNS depressants (alcohol, barbiturates, opiates, sedatives or anesthetics) should be considered). Products include:

Hydroflumethiazide (Because Combigan may reduce blood pressure, caution in using drugs such as antihypertensives with Combigan is advised).
No products indexed under this heading.

Hydromorphone (Although specific drug interaction studies have not been conducted with Combigan, the possibility of an additive or potentiating effect with CNS depressants (alcohol, barbiturates, opiates, sedatives or anesthetics) should be considered).
No products indexed under this heading.

Hydromorphone Hydrochloride (Although specific drug interaction studies have not been conducted with Combigan, the possibility of an additive or potentiating effect with CNS depressants (alcohol, barbiturates, opiates, sedatives or anesthetics) should be considered). Products include:

Hydroxychloroquine Sulfate (Potentiated systemic beta-blockade (eg, decreased heart rate, depression) has been reported during combined treatment with CYP2D6 inhibitors (eg, quinidine, SSRIs) and timolol).
No products indexed under this heading.

Hydroxyzine Hydrochloride (Although specific drug interaction studies have not been conducted with Combigan, the possibility of an additive or potentiating effect with CNS depressants (alcohol, barbiturates, opiates, sedatives or anesthetics) should be considered).
No products indexed under this heading.

Imatinib Mesylate (Potentiated systemic beta-blockade (eg, decreased heart rate, depression) has been reported during combined treatment with CYP2D6 inhibitors (eg, quinidine, SSRIs) and timolol). Products include:

Imipramine Hydrochloride (Tricyclic antidepressants have been reported to blunt the hypotensive effect of systemic clonidine. It is not known whether the concurrent use of these agents with Combigan in humans can lead to resulting interference with the IOP lowering effect. Caution, however, is advised in patients taking tricyclic antidepressants which can affect the metabolism and uptake of circulating amines).
No products indexed under this heading.

Imipramine Pamoate (Tricyclic antidepressants have been reported to blunt the hypotensive effect of systemic clonidine. It is not known whether the concurrent use of these agents with Combigan in humans can lead to resulting interference with the IOP lowering effect. Caution, however, is advised in patients taking tricyclic antidepressants which can affect the metabolism and uptake of circulating amines).
No products indexed under this heading.

Indapamide (Because Combigan may reduce blood pressure, caution in using drugs such as antihypertensives with Combigan is advised). Products include:

395 Interactions Index Combigan

Insulin (Beta-adrenergic blocking agents should be administered with caution in patients subject to spontaneous hypoglycemia or to diabetic patients (especially those with labile diabetes) who are receiving insulin or oral hypoglycemic agents. Beta-adrenergic receptor blocking agents may mask the signs and symptoms of acute hypoglycemia).
No products indexed under this heading.

Insulin, Human, Zinc Suspension (Beta-adrenergic blocking agents should be administered with caution in patients subject to spontaneous hypoglycemia or to diabetic patients (especially those with labile diabetes) who are receiving insulin or oral hypoglycemic agents. Beta-adrenergic receptor blocking agents may mask the signs and symptoms of acute hypoglycemia).
No products indexed under this heading.

Insulin, Human (rDNA origin) (Beta-adrenergic blocking agents should be administered with caution in patients subject to spontaneous hypoglycemia or to diabetic patients (especially those with labile diabetes) who are receiving insulin or oral hypoglycemic agents. Beta-adrenergic receptor blocking agents may mask the signs and symptoms of acute hypoglycemia). Products include:
Exubera 2717

Insulin, Human NPH (Beta-adrenergic blocking agents should be administered with caution in patients subject to spontaneous hypoglycemia or to diabetic patients (especially those with labile diabetes) who are receiving insulin or oral hypoglycemic agents. Beta-adrenergic receptor blocking agents may mask the signs and symptoms of acute hypoglycemia). Products include:
Humulin N Vial 1934

Insulin, Human Regular (Beta-adrenergic blocking agents should be administered with caution in patients subject to spontaneous hypoglycemia or to diabetic patients (especially those with labile diabetes) who are receiving insulin or oral hypoglycemic agents. Beta-adrenergic receptor blocking agents may mask the signs and symptoms of acute hypoglycemia). Products include:
Humulin R 1937
Humulin R (U-500) 1939

Insulin, Human Regular and Human NPH Mixture (Beta-adrenergic blocking agents should be administered with caution in patients subject to spontaneous hypoglycemia or to diabetic patients (especially those with labile diabetes) who are receiving insulin or oral hypoglycemic agents. Beta-adrenergic receptor blocking agents may mask the signs and symptoms of acute hypoglycemia). Products include:
Humulin 50/50 1930
Humulin 70/30 Vial 1931

Insulin, NPH (Beta-adrenergic blocking agents should be administered with caution in patients subject to spontaneous hypoglycemia or to diabetic patients (especially those with labile diabetes) who are receiving insulin or oral hypoglycemic agents. Beta-adrenergic receptor blocking agents may mask the signs and symptoms of acute hypoglycemia).
No products indexed under this heading.

Insulin, Regular (Beta-adrenergic blocking agents should be administered with caution in patients subject to spontaneous hypoglycemia or to diabetic patients (especially those with labile diabetes) who are receiving insulin or oral hypoglycemic agents. Beta-adrenergic receptor blocking agents may mask the signs and symptoms of acute hypoglycemia).
No products indexed under this heading.

Insulin, Regular and NPH mixture (Beta-adrenergic blocking agents should be administered with caution in patients subject to spontaneous hypoglycemia or to diabetic patients (especially those with labile diabetes) who are receiving insulin or oral hypoglycemic agents. Beta-adrenergic receptor blocking agents may mask the signs and symptoms of acute hypoglycemia).
No products indexed under this heading.

Insulin, Zinc Crystals (Beta-adrenergic blocking agents should be administered with caution in patients subject to spontaneous hypoglycemia or to diabetic patients (especially those with labile diabetes) who are receiving insulin or oral hypoglycemic agents. Beta-adrenergic receptor blocking agents may mask the signs and symptoms of acute hypoglycemia).
No products indexed under this heading.

Insulin, Zinc Suspension (Beta-adrenergic blocking agents should be administered with caution in patients subject to spontaneous hypoglycemia or to diabetic patients (especially those with labile diabetes) who are receiving insulin or oral hypoglycemic agents. Beta-adrenergic receptor blocking agents may mask the signs and symptoms of acute hypoglycemia).
No products indexed under this heading.

Insulin Aspart (Beta-adrenergic blocking agents should be administered with caution in patients subject to spontaneous hypoglycemia or to diabetic patients (especially those with labile diabetes) who are receiving insulin or oral hypoglycemic agents. Beta-adrenergic receptor blocking agents may mask the signs and symptoms of acute hypoglycemia).
No products indexed under this heading.

Insulin Aspart, Human (Beta-adrenergic blocking agents should be administered with caution in patients subject to spontaneous hypoglycemia or to diabetic patients (especially those with labile diabetes) who are receiving insulin or oral hypoglycemic agents. Beta-adrenergic receptor blocking agents may mask the signs and symptoms of acute hypoglycemia). Products include:
NovoLog Mix 70/30 2581

Insulin Aspart, Human Regular (Beta-adrenergic blocking agents should be administered with caution in patients subject to spontaneous hypoglycemia or to diabetic patients (especially those with labile diabetes) who are receiving insulin or oral hypoglycemic agents. Beta-adrenergic receptor blocking agents may mask the signs and symptoms of acute hypoglycemia). Products include:
NovoLog 2575

Insulin Aspart Protamine, Human (Beta-adrenergic blocking agents should be administered with caution in patients subject to spontaneous hypoglycemia or to diabetic patients (especially those with labile diabetes) who are receiving insulin or oral hypoglycemic agents. Beta-adrenergic receptor blocking agents may mask the signs and symptoms of acute hypoglycemia). Products include:
NovoLog Mix 70/30 2581

Insulin Detemir (rDNA Origin) (Beta-adrenergic blocking agents should be administered with caution in patients subject to spontaneous hypoglycemia or to diabetic patients (especially those with labile diabetes) who are receiving insulin or oral hypoglycemic agents. Beta-adrenergic receptor blocking agents may mask the signs and symptoms of acute hypoglycemia). Products include:
Levemir 2566

Insulin Glargine (Beta-adrenergic blocking agents should be administered with caution in patients subject to spontaneous hypoglycemia or to diabetic patients (especially those with labile diabetes) who are receiving insulin or oral hypoglycemic agents. Beta-adrenergic receptor blocking agents may mask the signs and symptoms of acute hypoglycemia). Products include:
Lantus 2996

Insulin Glulisine (Beta-adrenergic blocking agents should be administered with caution in patients subject to spontaneous hypoglycemia or to diabetic patients (especially those with labile diabetes) who are receiving insulin or oral hypoglycemic agents. Beta-adrenergic receptor blocking agents may mask the signs and symptoms of acute hypoglycemia). Products include:
Apidra 2937
Apidra SoloStar 2937

Insulin Lispro, Human (Beta-adrenergic blocking agents should be administered with caution in patients subject to spontaneous hypoglycemia or to diabetic patients (especially those with labile diabetes) who are receiving insulin or oral hypoglycemic agents. Beta-adrenergic receptor blocking agents may mask the signs and symptoms of acute hypoglycemia). Products include:
Humalog 1910
Humalog Mix 1914
Humalog Mix75/25 1917

Insulin Lispro Protamine, Human (Beta-adrenergic blocking agents should be administered with caution in patients subject to spontaneous hypoglycemia or to diabetic patients (especially those with labile diabetes) who are receiving insulin or oral hypoglycemic agents. Beta-adrenergic receptor blocking agents may mask the signs and symptoms of acute hypoglycemia). Products include:
Humalog Mix 1914
Humalog Mix75/25 1917

Irbesartan (Because Combigan may reduce blood pressure, caution in using drugs such as antihypertensives with Combigan is advised). Products include:
Avalide 2956
Avapro 2962

Isocarboxazid (Monoamine oxidase (MAO) inhibitors may theoretically interfere with the metabolism of brimonidine and potentially result in an increased systemic side-effect such as hypotension. Caution is advised in patients taking MAO inhibitors which can affect the metabolism and uptake of circulating amines). Products include:
Marplan 3481

Isoflurane (Although specific drug interaction studies have not been conducted with Combigan, the possibility of an additive or potentiating effect with CNS depressants (alcohol, barbiturates, opiates, sedatives or anesthetics) should be considered).
No products indexed under this heading.

Isradipine (Caution should be used in the co-administration of beta-adrenergic blocking agents, such as Combigan, and oral or intravenous calcium antagonists because of possible atrioventricular conduction disturbances, left ventricular failure and hypotension. In patients with impaired cardiac function, co-administration should be avoided. The concomitant use of beta-adrenergic blocking agents with calcium antagonists may have additive effects in prolonging atrioventricular conduction time). Products include:
DynaCirc CR 1432

Ketamine Hydrochloride (Although specific drug interaction studies have not been conducted with Combigan, the possibility of an additive or potentiating effect with CNS depressants (alcohol, barbiturates, opiates, sedatives or anesthetics) should be considered).
No products indexed under this heading.

Labetalol Hydrochloride (Patients who are receiving a beta-adrenergic blocking agent orally and Combigan should be observed for potential additive effects of beta-blockade, both systemic and on intraocular pressure. The concomitant use of two topical beta-adrenergic blocking agents is not recommended).
No products indexed under this heading.

Levobunolol Hydrochloride (Patients who are receiving a beta-adrenergic blocking agent orally and Combigan should be observed for potential additive effects of beta-blockade, both systemic and on intraocular pressure. The concomitant use of two topical beta-adrenergic blocking agents is not recommended).
No products indexed under this heading.

Levobupivacaine Hydrochloride (Although specific drug interaction studies have not been conducted with Combigan, the possibility of an additive or potentiating effect with CNS depressants (alcohol, barbiturates, opiates, sedatives or anesthetics) should be considered).
No products indexed under this heading.

Levomethadyl Acetate Hydrochloride (Although specific drug interaction studies have not been conducted with Combigan, the possibility of an additive or potentiating effect with CNS depressants (alcohol, barbiturates, opiates, sedatives or anesthetics) should be considered).
No products indexed under this heading.

Levorphanol Tartrate (Although specific drug interaction studies have not been conducted with Combigan, the possibility of an additive or potentiating effect with CNS depressants (alcohol, barbiturates, opiates, sedatives or anesthetics) should be considered).
No products indexed under this heading.

Lidocaine (Although specific drug interaction studies have not been conducted with Combigan, the possibility of an additive or potentiating effect with CNS depressants (alcohol, barbiturates, opiates, sedatives or anesthetics) should be considered). Products include:
Lidoderm 1107

Lidocaine Base (Although specific drug interaction studies have not been conducted with Combigan, the possibility of an additive or potentiating effect with CNS depressants (alcohol, barbiturates, opiates, sedatives or anesthetics) should be considered).
No products indexed under this heading.

Lidocaine Hydrochloride (Although specific drug interaction studies have not been conducted with Combigan, the possibility of an additive or potentiating effect with CNS depressants (alcohol, barbiturates, opiates, sedatives or anesthetics) should be considered).
No products indexed under this heading.

Lisinopril (Because Combigan may reduce blood pressure, caution in using drugs such as antihypertensives with Combigan is advised). Products include:
Prinivil 2241
Prinzide 2246

IMPORTANT NOTE: Always consult each drug listing in the patient's regimen for possible interactions.

Combigan Interactions Index 396

Lorazepam (Although specific drug interaction studies have not been conducted with Combigan, the possibility of an additive or potentiating effect with CNS depressants (alcohol, barbiturates, opiates, sedatives or anesthetics) should be considered).
No products indexed under this heading.

Losartan Potassium (Because Combigan may reduce blood pressure, caution in using drugs such as antihypertensives with Combigan is advised). Products include:
Cozaar ... 2106
Hyzaar ... 2162
Hyzaar 100-12.5 ... 2162

Loxapine Hydrochloride (Although specific drug interaction studies have not been conducted with Combigan, the possibility of an additive or potentiating effect with CNS depressants (alcohol, barbiturates, opiates, sedatives or anesthetics) should be considered).
No products indexed under this heading.

Loxapine Succinate (Although specific drug interaction studies have not been conducted with Combigan, the possibility of an additive or potentiating effect with CNS depressants (alcohol, barbiturates, opiates, sedatives or anesthetics) should be considered).
No products indexed under this heading.

Maprotiline Hydrochloride (Tricyclic antidepressants have been reported to blunt the hypotensive effect of systemic clonidine. It is not known whether the concurrent use of these agents with Combigan in humans can lead to resulting interference with the IOP lowering effect. Caution, however, is advised in patients taking tricyclic antidepressants which can affect the metabolism and uptake of circulating amines).
No products indexed under this heading.

Mecamylamine Hydrochloride (Because Combigan may reduce blood pressure, caution in using drugs such as antihypertensives with Combigan is advised).
No products indexed under this heading.

Meperidine Hydrochloride (Although specific drug interaction studies have not been conducted with Combigan, the possibility of an additive or potentiating effect with CNS depressants (alcohol, barbiturates, opiates, sedatives or anesthetics) should be considered).
No products indexed under this heading.

Mephobarbital (Although specific drug interaction studies have not been conducted with Combigan, the possibility of an additive or potentiating effect with CNS depressants (alcohol, barbiturates, opiates, sedatives or anesthetics) should be considered).
No products indexed under this heading.

Mepivacaine Hydrochloride (Although specific drug interaction studies have not been conducted with Combigan, the possibility of an additive or potentiating effect with CNS depressants (alcohol, barbiturates, opiates, sedatives or anesthetics) should be considered).
No products indexed under this heading.

Meprobamate (Although specific drug interaction studies have not been conducted with Combigan, the possibility of an additive or potentiating effect with CNS depressants (alcohol, barbiturates, opiates, sedatives or anesthetics) should be considered).
No products indexed under this heading.

Mesoridazine Besylate (Although specific drug interaction studies have not been conducted with Combigan, the possibility of an additive or potentiating effect with CNS depressants (alcohol, barbiturates, opiates, sedatives or anesthetics) should be considered).
No products indexed under this heading.

Metformin Hydrochloride (Beta-adrenergic blocking agents should be administered with caution in patients subject to spontaneous hypoglycemia or to diabetic patients (especially those with labile diabetes) who are receiving insulin or oral hypoglycemic agents. Beta-adrenergic receptor blocking agents may mask the signs and symptoms of acute hypoglycemia). Products include:
ActoPlus ... 3338
Avandamet ... 1345
Janumet ... 2188

Methadone Hydrochloride (Although specific drug interaction studies have not been conducted with Combigan, the possibility of an additive or potentiating effect with CNS depressants (alcohol, barbiturates, opiates, sedatives or anesthetics) should be considered).
No products indexed under this heading.

Methohexital Sodium (Although specific drug interaction studies have not been conducted with Combigan, the possibility of an additive or potentiating effect with CNS depressants (alcohol, barbiturates, opiates, sedatives or anesthetics) should be considered).
No products indexed under this heading.

Methotrimeprazine (Although specific drug interaction studies have not been conducted with Combigan, the possibility of an additive or potentiating effect with CNS depressants (alcohol, barbiturates, opiates, sedatives or anesthetics) should be considered).
No products indexed under this heading.

Methoxyflurane (Although specific drug interaction studies have not been conducted with Combigan, the possibility of an additive or potentiating effect with CNS depressants (alcohol, barbiturates, opiates, sedatives or anesthetics) should be considered).
No products indexed under this heading.

Methyclothiazide (Because Combigan may reduce blood pressure, caution in using drugs such as antihypertensives with Combigan is advised).
No products indexed under this heading.

Methyldopa (Because Combigan may reduce blood pressure, caution in using drugs such as antihypertensives with Combigan is advised).
No products indexed under this heading.

Methyldopate Hydrochloride (Because Combigan may reduce blood pressure, caution in using drugs such as antihypertensives with Combigan is advised).
No products indexed under this heading.

Metipranolol Hydrochloride (Patients who are receiving a beta-adrenergic blocking agent orally and Combigan should be observed for potential additive effects of beta-blockade, both systemic and on intraocular pressure. The concomitant use of two topical beta-adrenergic blocking agents is not recommended).
No products indexed under this heading.

Metolazone (Because Combigan may reduce blood pressure, caution in using drugs such as antihypertensives with Combigan is advised).
No products indexed under this heading.

Metoprolol Succinate (Patients who are receiving a beta-adrenergic blocking agent orally and Combigan should be observed for potential additive effects of beta-blockade, both systemic and on intraocular pressure. The concomitant use of two topical beta-adrenergic blocking agents is not recommended). Products include:
Toprol XL ... 732

Metoprolol Tartrate (Patients who are receiving a beta-adrenergic blocking agent orally and Combigan should be observed for potential additive effects of beta-blockade, both systemic and on intraocular pressure. The concomitant use of two topical beta-adrenergic blocking agents is not recommended).
No products indexed under this heading.

Metyrosine (Because Combigan may reduce blood pressure, caution in using drugs such as antihypertensives with Combigan is advised).
No products indexed under this heading.

Mibefradil Dihydrochloride (Caution should be used in the co-administration of beta-adrenergic blocking agents, such as Combigan, and oral or intravenous calcium antagonists because of possible atrioventricular conduction disturbances, left ventricular failure and hypotension. In patients with impaired cardiac function, co-administration should be avoided. The concomitant use of beta-adrenergic blocking agents with calcium antagonists may have additive effects in proloning atrioventricular conduction time).
No products indexed under this heading.

Midazolam Hydrochloride (Although specific drug interaction studies have not been conducted with Combigan, the possibility of an additive or potentiating effect with CNS depressants (alcohol, barbiturates, opiates, sedatives or anesthetics) should be considered).
No products indexed under this heading.

Miglitol (Beta-adrenergic blocking agents should be administered with caution in patients subject to spontaneous hypoglycemia or to diabetic patients (especially those with labile diabetes) who are receiving insulin or oral hypoglycemic agents. Beta-adrenergic receptor blocking agents may mask the signs and symptoms of acute hypoglycemia).
No products indexed under this heading.

Minoxidil (Because Combigan may reduce blood pressure, caution in using drugs such as antihypertensives with Combigan is advised).
No products indexed under this heading.

Moclobemide (Monoamine oxidase (MAO) inhibitors may theoretically interfere with the metabolism of brimonidine and potentially result in an increased systemic side-effect such as hypotension. Caution is advised in patients taking MAO inhibitors which can affect the metabolism and uptake of circulating amines).
No products indexed under this heading.

Moexipril Hydrochloride (Because Combigan may reduce blood pressure, caution in using drugs such as antihypertensives with Combigan is advised).
No products indexed under this heading.

Molindone Hydrochloride (Although specific drug interaction studies have not been conducted with Combigan, the possibility of an additive or potentiating effect with CNS depressants (alcohol, barbiturates, opiates, sedatives or anesthetics) should be considered). Products include:
Moban ... 1108

Morphine Sulfate (Although specific drug interaction studies have not been conducted with Combigan, the possibility of an additive or potentiating effect with CNS depressants (alcohol, barbiturates, opiates, sedatives or anesthetics) should be considered). Products include:
Avinza ... 1822
Embeda ... 1831
MS Contin ... 2803

Morphine Sulfate, Liposomal (Although specific drug interaction studies have not been conducted with Combigan, the possibility of an additive or potentiating effect with CNS depressants (alcohol, barbiturates, opiates, sedatives or anesthetics) should be considered).
No products indexed under this heading.

Nadolol (Patients who are receiving a beta-adrenergic blocking agent orally and Combigan should be observed for potential additive effects of beta-blockade, both systemic and on intraocular pressure. The concomitant use of two topical beta-adrenergic blocking agents is not recommended). Products include:
Nadolol ... 2359

Nateglinide (Beta-adrenergic blocking agents should be administered with caution in patients subject to spontaneous hypoglycemia or to diabetic patients (especially those with labile diabetes) who are receiving insulin or oral hypoglycemic agents. Beta-adrenergic receptor blocking agents may mask the signs and symptoms of acute hypoglycemia).
No products indexed under this heading.

Nebivolol (Patients who are receiving a beta-adrenergic blocking agent orally and Combigan should be observed for potential additive effects of beta-blockade, both systemic and on intraocular pressure. The concomitant use of two topical beta-adrenergic blocking agents is not recommended). Products include:
Bystolic ... 1147

Nicardipine (Caution should be used in the co-administration of beta-adrenergic blocking agents, such as Combigan, and oral or intravenous calcium antagonists because of possible atrioventricular conduction disturbances, left ventricular failure and hypotension. In patients with impaired cardiac function, co-administration should be avoided. The concomitant use of beta-adrenergic blocking agents with calcium antagonists may have additive effects in proloning atrioventricular conduction time).
No products indexed under this heading.

Nicardipine Hydrochloride (Caution should be used in the co-administration of beta-adrenergic blocking agents, such as Combigan, and oral or intravenous calcium antagonists because of possible atrioventricular conduction disturbances, left ventricular failure and hypotension. In patients with impaired cardiac function, co-administration should be avoided. The concomitant use of beta-adrenergic blocking agents with calcium antagonists may have additive effects in proloning atrioventricular conduction time).
No products indexed under this heading.

Nifedipine (Caution should be used in the co-administration of beta-adrenergic blocking agents, such as Combigan, and oral or intravenous calcium antagonists because of possible atrioventricular conduction disturbances, left ventricular failure and hypotension. In patients with impaired cardiac function, co-administration should be avoided. The concomitant use of beta-adrenergic blocking agents with calcium antagonists may have additive effects in proloning atrioventricular conduction time).
No products indexed under this heading.

Nimodipine (Caution should be used in the co-administration of beta-adrenergic blocking agents, such as Combigan, and oral or intravenous calcium antagonists because of possible atrioventricular conduction disturbances, left ventricular failure and hypotension. In patients with impaired cardiac function, co-administration should be avoided. The concomitant use of beta-adrenergic

blocking agents with calcium antagonists may have additive effects in proloning atrioventricular conduction time). No products indexed under this heading.

Nisoldipine (Caution should be used in the co-administration of beta-adrenergic blocking agents, such as Combigan, and oral or intravenous calcium antagonists because of possible atrioventricular conduction disturbances, left ventricular failure and hypotension. In patients with impaired cardiac function, co-administration should be avoided. The concomitant use of beta-adrenergic blocking agents with calcium antagonists may have additive effects in proloning atrioventricular conduction time). No products indexed under this heading.

Nitroglycerin (Because Combigan may reduce blood pressure, caution in using drugs such as antihypertensives with Combigan is advised). Products include:

Nitro-Dur	3170
Nitrolingual	3266

Nortriptyline Hydrochloride (Tricyclic antidepressants have been reported to blunt the hypotensive effect of systemic clonidine. It is not known whether the concurrent use of these agents with Combigan in humans can lead to resulting interference with the IOP lowering effect. Caution, however, is advised in patients taking tricyclic antidepressants which can affect the metabolism and uptake of circulating amines). No products indexed under this heading.

Olanzapine (Although specific drug interaction studies have not been conducted with Combigan, the possibility of an additive or potentiating effect with CNS depressants (alcohol, barbiturates, opiates, sedatives or anesthetics) should be considered). Products include:

Symbyax	1965
Zyprexa	1984
Zyprexa IntraMuscular	1984
Zyprexa ZYDIS	1984

Oxazepam (Although specific drug interaction studies have not been conducted with Combigan, the possibility of an additive or potentiating effect with CNS depressants (alcohol, barbiturates, opiates, sedatives or anesthetics) should be considered). No products indexed under this heading.

Oxycodone Hydrochloride (Although specific drug interaction studies have not been conducted with Combigan, the possibility of an additive or potentiating effect with CNS depressants (alcohol, barbiturates, opiates, sedatives or anesthetics) should be considered). Products include:

OxyContin	2807
Percocet	1121
Percodan	1124

Oxycodone Terephthalate (Although specific drug interaction studies have not been conducted with Combigan, the possibility of an additive or potentiating effect with CNS depressants (alcohol, barbiturates, opiates, sedatives or anesthetics) should be considered). No products indexed under this heading.

Oxymorphone Hydrochloride (Although specific drug interaction studies have not been conducted with Combigan, the possibility of an additive or potentiating effect with CNS depressants (alcohol, barbiturates, opiates, sedatives or anesthetics) should be considered). Products include:

Opana	1110
Opana ER	1114

Pargyline Hydrochloride (Monoamine oxidase (MAO) inhibitors may theoretically interfere with the metabolism of brimonidine and potentially result in an increased systemic side-effect such as hypotension. Caution is advised in patients taking MAO inhibitors which can affect the metabolism and uptake of circulating amines). No products indexed under this heading.

Paroxetine Hydrochloride (Potentiated systemic beta-blockade (eg, decreased heart rate, depression) has been reported during combined treatment with CYP2D6 inhibitors (eg, quinidine, SSRIs) and timolol). Products include:

Paroxetine CR	2361
Paroxetine ER	2371
Paxil	1586
Paxil CR	1596

Penbutolol Sulfate (Patients who are receiving a beta-adrenergic blocking agent orally and Combigan should be observed for potential additive effects of beta-blockade, both systemic and on intraocular pressure. The concomitant use of two topical beta-adrenergic blocking agents is not recommended). No products indexed under this heading.

Pentobarbital (Although specific drug interaction studies have not been conducted with Combigan, the possibility of an additive or potentiating effect with CNS depressants (alcohol, barbiturates, opiates, sedatives or anesthetics) should be considered). No products indexed under this heading.

Pentobarbital Sodium (Although specific drug interaction studies have not been conducted with Combigan, the possibility of an additive or potentiating effect with CNS depressants (alcohol, barbiturates, opiates, sedatives or anesthetics) should be considered). Products include:

Nembutal	2012

Perindopril Erbumine (Because Combigan may reduce blood pressure, caution in using drugs such as antihypertensives with Combigan is advised). No products indexed under this heading.

Perphenazine (Although specific drug interaction studies have not been conducted with Combigan, the possibility of an additive or potentiating effect with CNS depressants (alcohol, barbiturates, opiates, sedatives or anesthetics) should be considered). No products indexed under this heading.

Phenelzine Sulfate (Monoamine oxidase (MAO) inhibitors may theoretically interfere with the metabolism of brimonidine and potentially result in an increased systemic side-effect such as hypotension. Caution is advised in patients taking MAO inhibitors which can affect the metabolism and uptake of circulating amines). No products indexed under this heading.

Phenobarbital (Although specific drug interaction studies have not been conducted with Combigan, the possibility of an additive or potentiating effect with CNS depressants (alcohol, barbiturates, opiates, sedatives or anesthetics) should be considered). Products include:

Donnatal	2711

Phenobarbital Sodium (Although specific drug interaction studies have not been conducted with Combigan, the possibility of an additive or potentiating effect with CNS depressants (alcohol, barbiturates, opiates, sedatives or anesthetics) should be considered). No products indexed under this heading.

Phenoxybenzamine Hydrochloride (Because Combigan may reduce blood pressure, caution in using drugs such as antihypertensives with Combigan is advised). Products include:

Dibenzyline	3495

Phentolamine Mesylate (Because Combigan may reduce blood pressure, caution in using drugs such as antihypertensives with Combigan is advised). No products indexed under this heading.

Pindolol (Patients who are receiving a beta-adrenergic blocking agent orally and Combigan should be observed for potential additive effects of beta-blockade, both systemic and on intraocular pressure. The concomitant use of two topical beta-adrenergic blocking agents is not recommended). No products indexed under this heading.

Pioglitazone Hydrochloride (Beta-adrenergic blocking agents should be administered with caution in patients subject to spontaneous hypoglycemia or to diabetic patients (especially those with labile diabetes) who are receiving insulin or oral hypoglycemic agents. Beta-adrenergic receptor blocking agents may mask the signs and symptoms of acute hypoglycemia). Products include:

ActoPlus	3338
Actos	3345
Duetact	3354

Polythiazide (Because Combigan may reduce blood pressure, caution in using drugs such as antihypertensives with Combigan is advised). No products indexed under this heading.

Prazepam (Although specific drug interaction studies have not been conducted with Combigan, the possibility of an additive or potentiating effect with CNS depressants (alcohol, barbiturates, opiates, sedatives or anesthetics) should be considered). No products indexed under this heading.

Prazosin Hydrochloride (Because Combigan may reduce blood pressure, caution in using drugs such as antihypertensives with Combigan is advised). No products indexed under this heading.

Prilocaine (Although specific drug interaction studies have not been conducted with Combigan, the possibility of an additive or potentiating effect with CNS depressants (alcohol, barbiturates, opiates, sedatives or anesthetics) should be considered). No products indexed under this heading.

Prilocaine Hydrochloride (Although specific drug interaction studies have not been conducted with Combigan, the possibility of an additive or potentiating effect with CNS depressants (alcohol, barbiturates, opiates, sedatives or anesthetics) should be considered). No products indexed under this heading.

Procaine (Although specific drug interaction studies have not been conducted with Combigan, the possibility of an additive or potentiating effect with CNS depressants (alcohol, barbiturates, opiates, sedatives or anesthetics) should be considered). No products indexed under this heading.

Procaine Hydrochloride (Although specific drug interaction studies have not been conducted with Combigan, the possibility of an additive or potentiating effect with CNS depressants (alcohol, barbiturates, opiates, sedatives or anesthetics) should be considered). No products indexed under this heading.

Procarbazine Hydrochloride (Monoamine oxidase (MAO) inhibitors may theoretically interfere with the metabolism of brimonidine and potentially result in an increased systemic side-effect such as hypotension. Caution is advised in patients taking MAO inhibitors which can affect the metabolism and uptake of circulating amines). No products indexed under this heading.

Prochlorperazine (Although specific drug interaction studies have not been conducted with Combigan, the possibility of an additive or potentiating effect with CNS depressants (alcohol, barbiturates, opiates, sedatives or anesthetics) should be considered). No products indexed under this heading.

Prochlorperazine Edisylate (Although specific drug interaction studies have not been conducted with Combigan, the possibility of an additive or potentiating effect with CNS depressants (alcohol, barbiturates, opiates, sedatives or anesthetics) should be considered). No products indexed under this heading.

Prochlorperazine Maleate (Although specific drug interaction studies have not been conducted with Combigan, the possibility of an additive or potentiating effect with CNS depressants (alcohol, barbiturates, opiates, sedatives or anesthetics) should be considered). No products indexed under this heading.

Promethazine (Although specific drug interaction studies have not been conducted with Combigan, the possibility of an additive or potentiating effect with CNS depressants (alcohol, barbiturates, opiates, sedatives or anesthetics) should be considered). No products indexed under this heading.

Promethazine Hydrochloride (Although specific drug interaction studies have not been conducted with Combigan, the possibility of an additive or potentiating effect with CNS depressants (alcohol, barbiturates, opiates, sedatives or anesthetics) should be considered). No products indexed under this heading.

Propafenone Hydrochloride (Potentiated systemic beta-blockade (eg, decreased heart rate, depression) has been reported during combined treatment with CYP2D6 inhibitors (eg, quinidine, SSRIs) and timolol). Products include:

Rythmol	1648
Rythmol SR	1652

Proparacaine Hydrochloride (Although specific drug interaction studies have not been conducted with Combigan, the possibility of an additive or potentiating effect with CNS depressants (alcohol, barbiturates, opiates, sedatives or anesthetics) should be considered). No products indexed under this heading.

Propofol (Although specific drug interaction studies have not been conducted with Combigan, the possibility of an additive or potentiating effect with CNS depressants (alcohol, barbiturates, opiates, sedatives or anesthetics) should be considered). No products indexed under this heading.

Propoxyphene Hydrochloride (Although specific drug interaction studies have not been conducted with Combigan, the possibility of an additive or potentiating effect with CNS depressants (alcohol, barbiturates, opiates, sedatives or anesthetics) should be considered). No products indexed under this heading.

Propoxyphene Napsylate (Although specific drug interaction studies have not been conducted with Combigan, the possibility of an additive or potentiating effect with CNS depressants (alcohol, barbiturates, opiates, sedatives or anesthetics) should be considered). No products indexed under this heading.

Propranolol Hydrochloride (Patients who are receiving a beta-adrenergic blocking agent orally and Combigan should be observed for potential additive effects of beta-blockade, both

IMPORTANT NOTE: Always consult each drug listing in the patient's regimen for possible interactions.

(☉ Described in PDR® for Ophthalmic Medicines)

Tetracaine (Although specific drug interaction studies have not been conducted with Combigan, the possibility of an additive or potentiating effect with CNS depressants (alcohol, barbiturates, opiates, sedatives or anesthetics) should be considered).
No products indexed under this heading.

Tetracaine Hydrochloride (Although specific drug interaction studies have not been conducted with Combigan, the possibility of an additive or potentiating effect with CNS depressants (alcohol, barbiturates, opiates, sedatives or anesthetics) should be considered).
No products indexed under this heading.

Thiamylal Sodium (Although specific drug interaction studies have not been conducted with Combigan, the possibility of an additive or potentiating effect with CNS depressants (alcohol, barbiturates, opiates, sedatives or anesthetics) should be considered).
No products indexed under this heading.

Thioridazine (Although specific drug interaction studies have not been conducted with Combigan, the possibility of an additive or potentiating effect with CNS depressants (alcohol, barbiturates, opiates, sedatives or anesthetics) should be considered).
No products indexed under this heading.

Thioridazine Hydrochloride (Although specific drug interaction studies have not been conducted with Combigan, the possibility of an additive or potentiating effect with CNS depressants (alcohol, barbiturates, opiates, sedatives or anesthetics) should be considered). Products include:
Thioridazine Hydrochloride 2384

Thiothixene (Although specific drug interaction studies have not been conducted with Combigan, the possibility of an additive or potentiating effect with CNS depressants (alcohol, barbiturates, opiates, sedatives or anesthetics) should be considered). Products include:
Thiothixene 2386

Thiothixene Hydrochloride (Although specific drug interaction studies have not been conducted with Combigan, the possibility of an additive or potentiating effect with CNS depressants (alcohol, barbiturates, opiates, sedatives or anesthetics) should be considered).
No products indexed under this heading.

Timolol Hemihydrate (Patients who are receiving a beta-adrenergic blocking agent orally and Combigan should be observed for potential additive effects of beta-blockade, both systemic and on intraocular pressure. The concomitant use of two topical beta-adrenergic blocking agents is not recommended). Products include:
Betimol 3490

Tolazamide (Beta-adrenergic blocking agents should be administered with caution in patients subject to spontaneous hypoglycemia or to diabetic patients (especially those with labile diabetes) who are receiving insulin or oral hypoglycemic agents. Beta-adrenergic receptor blocking agents may mask the signs and symptoms of acute hypoglycemia).
No products indexed under this heading.

Tolbutamide (Beta-adrenergic blocking agents should be administered with caution in patients subject to spontaneous hypoglycemia or to diabetic patients (especially those with labile diabetes) who are receiving insulin or oral hypoglycemic agents. Beta-adrenergic receptor blocking agents may mask the signs and symptoms of acute hypoglycemia).
No products indexed under this heading.

Torsemide (Because Combigan may reduce blood pressure, caution in using drugs such as antihypertensives with Combigan is advised).
No products indexed under this heading.

Trandolapril (Because Combigan may reduce blood pressure, caution in using drugs such as antihypertensives with Combigan is advised). Products include:
Mavik 489
Tarka 534

Tranylcypromine Sulfate (Monoamine oxidase (MAO) inhibitors may theoretically interfere with the metabolism of brimonidine and potentially result in an increased systemic side-effect such as hypotension. Caution is advised in patients taking MAO inhibitors which can affect the metabolism and uptake of circulating amines). Products include:
Parnate 1584

Triazolam (Although specific drug interaction studies have not been conducted with Combigan, the possibility of an additive or potentiating effect with CNS depressants (alcohol, barbiturates, opiates, sedatives or anesthetics) should be considered).
No products indexed under this heading.

Trifluoperazine Hydrochloride (Although specific drug interaction studies have not been conducted with Combigan, the possibility of an additive or potentiating effect with CNS depressants (alcohol, barbiturates, opiates, sedatives or anesthetics) should be considered).
No products indexed under this heading.

Trimethaphan Camsylate (Because Combigan may reduce blood pressure, caution in using drugs such as antihypertensives with Combigan is advised).
No products indexed under this heading.

Trimipramine Maleate (Tricyclic antidepressants have been reported to blunt the hypotensive effect of systemic clonidine. It is not known whether the concurrent use of these agents with Combigan in humans can lead to resulting interference with the IOP lowering effect. Caution, however, is advised in patients taking tricyclic antidepressants which can affect the metabolism and uptake of circulating amines).
No products indexed under this heading.

Troglitazone (Beta-adrenergic blocking agents should be administered with caution in patients subject to spontaneous hypoglycemia or to diabetic patients (especially those with labile diabetes) who are receiving insulin or oral hypoglycemic agents. Beta-adrenergic receptor blocking agents may mask the signs and symptoms of acute hypoglycemia).
No products indexed under this heading.

Valsartan (Because Combigan may reduce blood pressure, caution in using drugs such as antihypertensives with Combigan is advised). Products include:
Diovan 2413
Diovan HCT 2419
Exforge 2443
Exforge HCT 2449
Valturna 3637

Vardenafil Hydrochloride (Potentiated systemic beta-blockade (eg, decreased heart rate, depression) has been reported during combined treatment with CYP2D6 inhibitors (eg, quinidine, SSRIs) and timolol). Products include:
Levitra 3157

Verapamil Hydrochloride (Caution should be used in the co-administration of beta-adrenergic blocking agents, such as Combigan, and oral or intravenous calcium antagonists because of possible atrioventricular conduction disturbances, left ventricular failure and hypotension. In patients with impaired cardiac function, co-administration should be avoided. The concomitant use of beta-adrenergic blocking agents with calcium antagonists may have additive effects in proloning atrioventricular conduction time). Products include:
Tarka 534

Zaleplon (Although specific drug interaction studies have not been conducted with Combigan, the possibility of an additive or potentiating effect with CNS depressants (alcohol, barbiturates, opiates, sedatives or anesthetics) should be considered).
No products indexed under this heading.

Ziprasidone Hydrochloride (Although specific drug interaction studies have not been conducted with Combigan, the possibility of an additive or potentiating effect with CNS depressants (alcohol, barbiturates, opiates, sedatives or anesthetics) should be considered). Products include:
Geodon 2723

Zolpidem Tartrate (Although specific drug interaction studies have not been conducted with Combigan, the possibility of an additive or potentiating effect with CNS depressants (alcohol, barbiturates, opiates, sedatives or anesthetics) should be considered). Products include:
Ambien 2920
Ambien CR 2925

Food Interactions

Alcohol (Although specific drug interaction studies have not been conducted with Combigan, the possibility of an additive or potentiating effect with CNS depressants (alcohol, barbiturates, opiates, sedatives or anesthetics) should be considered).

Beer, reduced-alcohol (Although specific drug interaction studies have not been conducted with Combigan, the possibility of an additive or potentiating effect with CNS depressants (alcohol, barbiturates, opiates, sedatives or anesthetics) should be considered).

Beer, unspecified (Although specific drug interaction studies have not been conducted with Combigan, the possibility of an additive or potentiating effect with CNS depressants (alcohol, barbiturates, opiates, sedatives or anesthetics) should be considered).

Wine, Chianti (Although specific drug interaction studies have not been conducted with Combigan, the possibility of an additive or potentiating effect with CNS depressants (alcohol, barbiturates, opiates, sedatives or anesthetics) should be considered).

Wine, Red (Although specific drug interaction studies have not been conducted with Combigan, the possibility of an additive or potentiating effect with CNS depressants (alcohol, barbiturates, opiates, sedatives or anesthetics) should be considered).

Wine, unspecified (Although specific drug interaction studies have not been conducted with Combigan, the possibility of an additive or potentiating effect with CNS depressants (alcohol, barbiturates, opiates, sedatives or anesthetics) should be considered).

Wine products (Although specific drug interaction studies have not been conducted with Combigan, the possibility of an additive or potentiating effect with CNS depressants (alcohol, barbiturates, opiates, sedatives or anesthetics) should be considered).

COMBIVIR TABLETS

(Lamivudine, Zidovudine) 1404

May interact with agents associated with myelosuppression, cytotoxic drugs, interferon alpha, nucleoside analogues, nucleoside/nucleotide analogue reverse transcriptase inhibitors, valproate, and certain other agents. Compounds in these categories include:

Abacavir Sulfate (Some nucleoside analogues affecting DNA replication antagonize the *in vitro* antiviral activity of zidovudine against HIV-1; concomitant use of such drugs should be avoided). Products include:
Epzicom 1448
Trizivir 1688
Ziagen 1740

Acyclovir (Some nucleoside analogues affecting DNA replication antagonize the *in vitro* antiviral activity of zidovudine against HIV-1; concomitant use of such drugs should be avoided). Products include:
Zovirax 1760

Acyclovir Sodium (Some nucleoside analogues affecting DNA replication antagonize the *in vitro* antiviral activity of zidovudine against HIV-1; concomitant use of such drugs should be avoided).
No products indexed under this heading.

Adefovir dipivoxil (Some nucleoside analogues affecting DNA replication antagonize the *in vitro* antiviral activity of zidovudine against HIV-1; concomitant use of such drugs should be avoided). Products include:
Hepsera 1244

Altretamine (Co-administration of Combivir (zidovudine) with other bone marrow suppressive agents may increase the hematologic toxicity of zidovudine). Products include:
Hexalen 1066

Atovaquone (Co-administration results in an increased AUC of zidovudine by 31%. Routine dose modification of zidovudine is not warranted). Products include:
Malarone Pediatric Tablets 1572
Malarone 1572
Mepron Suspension 1576

Bleomycin Sulfate (Co-administration of Combivir (zidovudine) with cytotoxic agents may increase the hematologic toxicity of zidovudine).
No products indexed under this heading.

Bone Marrow Suppressants, unspecified (Co-administration of Combivir (zidovudine) with other bone marrow suppressive agents may increase the hematologic toxicity of zidovudine).
No products indexed under this heading.

Busulfan (Co-administration of Combivir (zidovudine) with other bone marrow suppressive agents may increase the hematologic toxicity of zidovudine). Products include:
Myleran 1581

Chlorambucil (Co-administration of Combivir (zidovudine) with other bone marrow suppressive agents may increase the hematologic toxicity of zidovudine). Products include:
Leukeran 1557

Chloramphenicol (Co-administration of Combivir (zidovudine) with other bone marrow suppressive agents may increase the hematologic toxicity of zidovudine).
No products indexed under this heading.

Chloramphenicol Palmitate (Co-administration of Combivir (zidovudine) with other bone marrow suppressive agents may increase the hematologic toxicity of zidovudine).
No products indexed under this heading.

IMPORTANT NOTE: Always consult each drug listing in the patient's regimen for possible interactions.

(⊙ Described in PDR® for Ophthalmic Medicines)

epinephrine-containing products, erythromycin, nonselective MAO inhibitors, and certain other agents. Compounds in these categories include:

Alatrofloxacin Mesylate (As most entacapone excretion is via the bile, caution should be exercised when drugs known to interfere with biliary excretion, glucuronidation, and intestinal β-glucuronidase are given concurrently with entacapone. This includes some antibiotics (eg, erythromycin, rifampicin, ampicillin and chloramphenicol).
No products indexed under this heading.

Alfentanil Hydrochloride (Due to the possible additive sedative effects, caution should be used when concomitantly taking other CNS depressants in combination with entacapone).
No products indexed under this heading.

Alprazolam (Due to the possible additive sedative effects, caution should be used when concomitantly taking other CNS depressants in combination with entacapone).
No products indexed under this heading.

Amikacin Sulfate (As most entacapone excretion is via the bile, caution should be exercised when drugs known to interfere with biliary excretion, glucuronidation, and intestinal β-glucuronidase are given concurrently with entacapone. This includes some antibiotics (eg, erythromycin, rifampicin, ampicillin and chloramphenicol)).
No products indexed under this heading.

Amobarbital (Due to the possible additive sedative effects, caution should be used when concomitantly taking other CNS depressants in combination with entacapone).
No products indexed under this heading.

Amobarbital Sodium (Due to the possible additive sedative effects, caution should be used when concomitantly taking other CNS depressants in combination with entacapone).
No products indexed under this heading.

Amoxicillin (As most entacapone excretion is via the bile, caution should be exercised when drugs known to interfere with biliary excretion, glucuronidation, and intestinal β-glucuronidase are given concurrently with entacapone. This includes some antibiotics (eg, erythromycin, rifampicin, ampicillin and chloramphenicol)).
Products include:

Amoxicillin Trihydrate (As most entacapone excretion is via the bile, caution should be exercised when drugs known to interfere with biliary excretion, glucuronidation, and intestinal β-glucuronidase are given concurrently with entacapone. This includes some antibiotics (eg, erythromycin, rifampicin, ampicillin and chloramphenicol)).
No products indexed under this heading.

Ampicillin (As most entacapone excretion is via the bile, caution should be exercised when drugs known to interfere with biliary excretion, glucuronidation, and intestinal β-glucuronidase are given concurrently with entacapone. This includes some antibiotics (eg, ampicillin)).
No products indexed under this heading.

Ampicillin Sodium (As most entacapone excretion is via the bile, caution should be exercised when drugs known to interfere with biliary excretion, glucuronidation, and intestinal β-glucuronidase are given concurrently with entacapone. This includes some antibiotics (eg, ampicillin)).
No products indexed under this heading.

Ampicillin Trihydrate (As most entacapone excretion is via the bile, caution should be exercised when drugs known to interfere with biliary excretion, glucuronidation, and intestinal β-glucuronidase are given concurrently with entacapone. This includes some antibiotics (eg, ampicillin)).
No products indexed under this heading.

Antibiotics, non-penicillin, unspecified (As most entacapone excretion is via the bile, caution should be exercised when drugs known to interfere with biliary excretion, glucuronidation, and intestinal β-glucuronidase are given concurrently with entacapone. This includes some antibiotics (eg, erythromycin, rifampicin, ampicillin and chloramphenicol)).
No products indexed under this heading.

Apomorphine (Co-administration of drugs that are metabolized by catechol-O-methyltransferase (COMT), such as apomorphine, should be administered with caution in patients receiving entacapone regardless of the route of administration. Concomitant administration may result in increased heart rates, possibly arrhythmias, and excessive changes in blood pressure).
No products indexed under this heading.

Apomorphine Hydrochloride (Co-administration of drugs that are metabolized by catechol-O-methyltransferase (COMT), such as apomorphine, should be administered with caution in patients receiving entacapone regardless of the route of administration. Concomitant administration may result in increased heart rates, possibly arrhythmias, and excessive changes in blood pressure).
No products indexed under this heading.

Aprobarbital (Due to the possible additive sedative effects, caution should be used when concomitantly taking other CNS depressants in combination with entacapone).
No products indexed under this heading.

Azithromycin Dihydrate (As most entacapone excretion is via the bile, caution should be exercised when drugs known to interfere with biliary excretion, glucuronidation, and intestinal β-glucuronidase are given concurrently with entacapone. This includes some antibiotics (eg, erythromycin, rifampicin, ampicillin and chloramphenicol)).
No products indexed under this heading.

Azlocillin Sodium (As most entacapone excretion is via the bile, caution should be exercised when drugs known to interfere with biliary excretion, glucuronidation, and intestinal β-glucuronidase are given concurrently with entacapone. This includes some antibiotics (eg, erythromycin, rifampicin, ampicillin and chloramphenicol)).
No products indexed under this heading.

Aztreonam (As most entacapone excretion is via the bile, caution should be exercised when drugs known to interfere with biliary excretion, glucuronidation, and intestinal β-glucuronidase are given concurrently with entacapone. This includes some antibiotics (eg, erythromycin, rifampicin, ampicillin and chloramphenicol)).
No products indexed under this heading.

Bacampicillin Hydrochloride (As most entacapone excretion is via the bile, caution should be exercised when drugs known to interfere with biliary excretion, glucuronidation, and intestinal β-glucuronidase are given concurrently with entacapone. This includes some antibiotics (eg, ampicillin)).
No products indexed under this heading.

Bitolterol Mesylate (Co-administration of drugs that are metabolized by catechol-O-methyltransferase (COMT), such as bitolterol, should be administered with caution in patients receiving entacapone regardless of the route of administration. Concomitant administration may result in increased heart rates, possibly arrhythmias, and excessive changes in blood pressure).
No products indexed under this heading.

Buprenorphine Hydrochloride (Due to the possible additive sedative effects, caution should be used when concomitantly taking other CNS depressants in combination with entacapone).
No products indexed under this heading.

Buspirone Hydrochloride (Due to the possible additive sedative effects, caution should be used when concomitantly taking other CNS depressants in combination with entacapone).
No products indexed under this heading.

Butabarbital (Due to the possible additive sedative effects, caution should be used when concomitantly taking other CNS depressants in combination with entacapone).
No products indexed under this heading.

Butabarbital Sodium (Due to the possible additive sedative effects, caution should be used when concomitantly taking other CNS depressants in combination with entacapone).
No products indexed under this heading.

Butalbital (Due to the possible additive sedative effects, caution should be used when concomitantly taking other CNS depressants in combination with entacapone).
No products indexed under this heading.

Carbenicillin Disodium (As most entacapone excretion is via the bile, caution should be exercised when drugs known to interfere with biliary excretion, glucuronidation, and intestinal β-glucuronidase are given concurrently with entacapone. This includes some antibiotics (eg, erythromycin, rifampicin, ampicillin and chloramphenicol)).
No products indexed under this heading.

Carbenicillin Indanyl Sodium (As most entacapone excretion is via the bile, caution should be exercised when drugs known to interfere with biliary excretion, glucuronidation, and intestinal β-glucuronidase are given concurrently with entacapone. This includes some antibiotics (eg, erythromycin, rifampicin, ampicillin and chloramphenicol)).
No products indexed under this heading.

Cefaclor (As most entacapone excretion is via the bile, caution should be exercised when drugs known to interfere with biliary excretion, glucuronidation, and intestinal β-glucuronidase are given concurrently with entacapone. This includes some antibiotics (eg, erythromycin, rifampicin, ampicillin and chloramphenicol)).
No products indexed under this heading.

Cefadroxil (As most entacapone excretion is via the bile, caution should be exercised when drugs known to interfere with biliary excretion, glucuronidation, and intestinal β-glucuronidase are given concurrently with entacapone. This includes some antibiotics (eg, erythromycin, rifampicin, ampicillin and chloramphenicol)).
No products indexed under this heading.

Cefamandole Nafate (As most entacapone excretion is via the bile, caution should be exercised when drugs known to interfere with biliary excretion, glucuronidation, and intestinal β-glucuronidase are given concurrently with entacapone. This includes some antibiotics (eg, erythromycin, rifampicin, ampicillin and chloramphenicol)).
No products indexed under this heading.

Cefazolin Sodium (As most entacapone excretion is via the bile, caution should be exercised when drugs known to interfere with biliary excretion, glucuronidation, and intestinal β-glucuronidase are given concurrently with entacapone. This includes some antibiotics (eg, erythromycin, rifampicin, ampicillin and chloramphenicol)).
No products indexed under this heading.

Cefixime (As most entacapone excretion is via the bile, caution should be exercised when drugs known to interfere with biliary excretion, glucuronidation, and intestinal β-glucuronidase are given concurrently with entacapone. This includes some antibiotics (eg, erythromycin, rifampicin, ampicillin and chloramphenicol)). Products include:

Cefmetazole Sodium (As most entacapone excretion is via the bile, caution should be exercised when drugs known to interfere with biliary excretion, glucuronidation, and intestinal β-glucuronidase are given concurrently with entacapone. This includes some antibiotics (eg, erythromycin, rifampicin, ampicillin and chloramphenicol)).
No products indexed under this heading.

Cefonicid Sodium (As most entacapone excretion is via the bile, caution should be exercised when drugs known to interfere with biliary excretion, glucuronidation, and intestinal β-glucuronidase are given concurrently with entacapone. This includes some antibiotics (eg, erythromycin, rifampicin, ampicillin and chloramphenicol)).
No products indexed under this heading.

Cefoperazone Sodium (As most entacapone excretion is via the bile, caution should be exercised when drugs known to interfere with biliary excretion, glucuronidation, and intestinal β-glucuronidase are given concurrently with entacapone. This includes some antibiotics (eg, erythromycin, rifampicin, ampicillin and chloramphenicol)).
No products indexed under this heading.

Ceforanide (As most entacapone excretion is via the bile, caution should be exercised when drugs known to interfere with biliary excretion, glucuronidation, and intestinal β-glucuronidase are given concurrently with entacapone. This includes some antibiotics (eg, erythromycin, rifampicin, ampicillin and chloramphenicol)).
No products indexed under this heading.

Cefotaxime Sodium (As most entacapone excretion is via the bile, caution should be exercised when drugs known to interfere with biliary excretion, glucuronidation, and intestinal β-glucuronidase are given concurrently with entacapone. This includes some antibiotics (eg, erythromycin, rifampicin, ampicillin and chloramphenicol)).
No products indexed under this heading.

IMPORTANT NOTE: Always consult each drug listing in the patient's regimen for possible interactions.

Cefotetan (As most entacapone excretion is via the bile, caution should be exercised when drugs known to interfere with biliary excretion, glucuronidation, and intestinal β-glucuronidase are given concurrently with entacapone. This includes some antibiotics (eg, erythromycin, rifampicin, ampicillin and chloramphenicol)).
No products indexed under this heading.

Cefoxitin Sodium (As most entacapone excretion is via the bile, caution should be exercised when drugs known to interfere with biliary excretion, glucuronidation, and intestinal β-glucuronidase are given concurrently with entacapone. This includes some antibiotics (eg, erythromycin, rifampicin, ampicillin and chloramphenicol)).
No products indexed under this heading.

Cefpodoxime Proxetil (As most entacapone excretion is via the bile, caution should be exercised when drugs known to interfere with biliary excretion, glucuronidation, and intestinal β-glucuronidase are given concurrently with entacapone. This includes some antibiotics (eg, erythromycin, rifampicin, ampicillin and chloramphenicol)).
No products indexed under this heading.

Cefprozil (As most entacapone excretion is via the bile, caution should be exercised when drugs known to interfere with biliary excretion, glucuronidation, and intestinal β-glucuronidase are given concurrently with entacapone. This includes some antibiotics (eg, erythromycin, rifampicin, ampicillin and chloramphenicol)).
No products indexed under this heading.

Ceftazidime (As most entacapone excretion is via the bile, caution should be exercised when drugs known to interfere with biliary excretion, glucuronidation, and intestinal β-glucuronidase are given concurrently with entacapone. This includes some antibiotics (eg, erythromycin, rifampicin, ampicillin and chloramphenicol)).
Products include:
Fortaz 1481

Ceftizoxime Sodium (As most entacapone excretion is via the bile, caution should be exercised when drugs known to interfere with biliary excretion, glucuronidation, and intestinal β-glucuronidase are given concurrently with entacapone. This includes some antibiotics (eg, erythromycin, rifampicin, ampicillin and chloramphenicol)).
No products indexed under this heading.

Ceftriaxone Sodium (As most entacapone excretion is via the bile, caution should be exercised when drugs known to interfere with biliary excretion, glucuronidation, and intestinal β-glucuronidase are given concurrently with entacapone. This includes some antibiotics (eg, erythromycin, rifampicin, ampicillin and chloramphenicol)).
Products include:
Rocephin 2859

Cefuroxime Axetil (As most entacapone excretion is via the bile, caution should be exercised when drugs known to interfere with biliary excretion, glucuronidation, and intestinal β-glucuronidase are given concurrently with entacapone. This includes some antibiotics (eg, erythromycin, rifampicin, ampicillin and chloramphenicol)).
Products include:
Ceftin 1399

Cefuroxime Sodium (As most entacapone excretion is via the bile, caution should be exercised when drugs known to interfere with biliary excretion, glucuronidation, and intestinal β-glucuronidase are given concurrently with entacapone. This includes some antibiotics (eg, erythromycin, rifampicin, ampicillin and chloramphenicol)).
No products indexed under this heading.

Cephalexin (As most entacapone excretion is via the bile, caution should be exercised when drugs known to interfere with biliary excretion, glucuronidation, and intestinal β-glucuronidase are given concurrently with entacapone. This includes some antibiotics (eg, erythromycin, rifampicin, ampicillin and chloramphenicol)).
No products indexed under this heading.

Cephalothin Sodium (As most entacapone excretion is via the bile, caution should be exercised when drugs known to interfere with biliary excretion, glucuronidation, and intestinal β-glucuronidase are given concurrently with entacapone. This includes some antibiotics (eg, erythromycin, rifampicin, ampicillin and chloramphenicol)).
No products indexed under this heading.

Cephapirin Sodium (As most entacapone excretion is via the bile, caution should be exercised when drugs known to interfere with biliary excretion, glucuronidation, and intestinal β-glucuronidase are given concurrently with entacapone. This includes some antibiotics (eg, erythromycin, rifampicin, ampicillin and chloramphenicol)).
No products indexed under this heading.

Cephradine (As most entacapone excretion is via the bile, caution should be exercised when drugs known to interfere with biliary excretion, glucuronidation, and intestinal β-glucuronidase are given concurrently with entacapone. This includes some antibiotics (eg, erythromycin, rifampicin, ampicillin and chloramphenicol)).
No products indexed under this heading.

Chloramphenicol (As most entacapone excretion is via the bile, caution should be exercised when drugs known to interfere with biliary excretion, glucuronidation, and intestinal β-glucuronidase are given concurrently with entacapone. This includes some antibiotics (eg, chloramphenicol)).
No products indexed under this heading.

Chloramphenicol Palmitate (As most entacapone excretion is via the bile, caution should be exercised when drugs known to interfere with biliary excretion, glucuronidation, and intestinal β-glucuronidase are given concurrently with entacapone. This includes some antibiotics (eg, chloramphenicol)).
No products indexed under this heading.

Chloramphenicol Sodium Succinate (As most entacapone excretion is via the bile, caution should be exercised when drugs known to interfere with biliary excretion, glucuronidation, and intestinal β-glucuronidase are given concurrently with entacapone. This includes some antibiotics (eg, chloramphenicol)).
No products indexed under this heading.

Chlordiazepoxide (Due to the possible additive sedative effects, caution should be used when concomitantly taking other CNS depressants in combination with entacapone).
No products indexed under this heading.

Chlordiazepoxide Hydrochloride (Due to the possible additive sedative effects, caution should be used when concomitantly taking other CNS depressants in combination with entacapone).
No products indexed under this heading.

Chlorpromazine (Due to the possible additive sedative effects, caution should be used when concomitantly taking other CNS depressants in combination with entacapone).
No products indexed under this heading.

Chlorpromazine Hydrochloride (Due to the possible additive sedative effects, caution should be used when concomitantly taking other CNS depressants in combination with entacapone).
No products indexed under this heading.

Chlorprothixene (Due to the possible additive sedative effects, caution should be used when concomitantly taking other CNS depressants in combination with entacapone).
No products indexed under this heading.

Chlorprothixene Hydrochloride (Due to the possible additive sedative effects, caution should be used when concomitantly taking other CNS depressants in combination with entacapone).
No products indexed under this heading.

Chlorprothixene Lactate (Due to the possible additive sedative effects, caution should be used when concomitantly taking other CNS depressants in combination with entacapone).
No products indexed under this heading.

Cholestyramine (As most entacapone excretion is via the bile, caution should be exercised when drugs known to interfere with biliary excretion, glucuronidation, and intestinal β-glucuronidase are given concurrently with entacapone. This includes cholestyramine).
No products indexed under this heading.

Cilastatin Sodium (As most entacapone excretion is via the bile, caution should be exercised when drugs known to interfere with biliary excretion, glucuronidation, and intestinal β-glucuronidase are given concurrently with entacapone. This includes some antibiotics (eg, erythromycin, rifampicin, ampicillin and chloramphenicol)).
Products include:
Primaxin I.M. 2232
Primaxin I.V. 2235

Ciprofloxacin (As most entacapone excretion is via the bile, caution should be exercised when drugs known to interfere with biliary excretion, glucuronidation, and intestinal β-glucuronidase are given concurrently with entacapone. This includes some antibiotics (eg, erythromycin, rifampicin, ampicillin and chloramphenicol)).
Products include:
Cipro I.V. 3082
Cipro 3073
Cipro XR 3091
Ciprodex 583

Ciprofloxacin Hydrochloride (As most entacapone excretion is via the bile, caution should be exercised when drugs known to interfere with biliary excretion, glucuronidation, and intestinal β-glucuronidase are given concurrently with entacapone. This includes some antibiotics (eg, erythromycin, rifampicin, ampicillin and chloramphenicol)). Products include:
Cipro 3073

Clarithromycin (As most entacapone excretion is via the bile, caution should be exercised when drugs known to interfere with biliary excretion, glucuronidation, and intestinal β-glucuronidase are given concurrently with entacapone. This includes some antibiotics (eg, erythromycin, rifampicin, ampicillin and chloramphenicol)).
Products include:
Biaxin/Biaxin XL 412

Clonazepam (Due to the possible additive sedative effects, caution should

be used when concomitantly taking other CNS depressants in combination with entacapone). Products include:
Klonopin 2855

Clorazepate Dipotassium (Due to the possible additive sedative effects, caution should be used when concomitantly taking other CNS depressants in combination with entacapone).
No products indexed under this heading.

Clotrimazole (As most entacapone excretion is via the bile, caution should be exercised when drugs known to interfere with biliary excretion, glucuronidation, and intestinal β-glucuronidase are given concurrently with entacapone. This includes some antibiotics (eg, erythromycin, rifampicin, ampicillin and chloramphenicol)).
Products include:
Lotrisone 3163

Cloxacillin (As most entacapone excretion is via the bile, caution should be exercised when drugs known to interfere with biliary excretion, glucuronidation, and intestinal β-glucuronidase are given concurrently with entacapone. This includes some antibiotics (eg, erythromycin, rifampicin, ampicillin and chloramphenicol)).
No products indexed under this heading.

Cloxacillin Sodium (As most entacapone excretion is via the bile, caution should be exercised when drugs known to interfere with biliary excretion, glucuronidation, and intestinal β-glucuronidase are given concurrently with entacapone. This includes some antibiotics (eg, erythromycin, rifampicin, ampicillin and chloramphenicol)).
No products indexed under this heading.

Cloxacillin Sodium Monohydrate (As most entacapone excretion is via the bile, caution should be exercised when drugs known to interfere with biliary excretion, glucuronidation, and intestinal β-glucuronidase are given concurrently with entacapone. This includes some antibiotics (eg, erythromycin, rifampicin, ampicillin and chloramphenicol)).
No products indexed under this heading.

Clozapine (Due to the possible additive sedative effects, caution should be used when concomitantly taking other CNS depressants in combination with entacapone).
No products indexed under this heading.

Codeine Phosphate (Due to the possible additive sedative effects, caution should be used when concomitantly taking other CNS depressants in combination with entacapone). Products include:
Tylenol with Codeine 2691

Codeine Sulfate (Due to the possible additive sedative effects, caution should be used when concomitantly taking other CNS depressants in combination with entacapone).
No products indexed under this heading.

Daunorubicin Hydrochloride (As most entacapone excretion is via the bile, caution should be exercised when drugs known to interfere with biliary excretion, glucuronidation, and intestinal β-glucuronidase are given concurrently with entacapone. This includes some antibiotics (eg, erythromycin, rifampicin, ampicillin and chloramphenicol)).
No products indexed under this heading.

Demeclocycline Hydrochloride (As most entacapone excretion is via the bile, caution should be exercised when drugs known to interfere with biliary excretion, glucuronidation, and intestinal β-glucuronidase are given concurrently with entacapone. This includes some antibiotics (eg, erythromycin, rifampicin, ampicillin and chloramphenicol)).
No products indexed under this heading.

Desflurane (Due to the possible additive sedative effects, caution should be used when concomitantly taking other CNS depressants in combination with entacapone).
No products indexed under this heading.

Dezocine (Due to the possible additive sedative effects, caution should be used when concomitantly taking other CNS depressants in combination with entacapone).
No products indexed under this heading.

Diazepam (Due to the possible additive sedative effects, caution should be used when concomitantly taking other CNS depressants in combination with entacapone). Products include:
Valium Tablets 2880

Dicloxacillin (As most entacapone excretion is via the bile, caution should be exercised when drugs known to interfere with biliary excretion, glucuronidation, and intestinal β-glucuronidase are given concurrently with entacapone. This includes some antibiotics (eg, erythromycin, rifampicin, ampicillin and chloramphenicol)).
No products indexed under this heading.

Dicloxacillin Sodium (As most entacapone excretion is via the bile, caution should be exercised when drugs known to interfere with biliary excretion, glucuronidation, and intestinal β-glucuronidase are given concurrently with entacapone. This includes some antibiotics (eg, erythromycin, rifampicin, ampicillin and chloramphenicol)).
No products indexed under this heading.

Dirithromycin (As most entacapone excretion is via the bile, caution should be exercised when drugs known to interfere with biliary excretion, glucuronidation, and intestinal β-glucuronidase are given concurrently with entacapone. This includes some antibiotics (eg, erythromycin, rifampicin, ampicillin and chloramphenicol)).
No products indexed under this heading.

Disodium Carbenicillin (As most entacapone excretion is via the bile, caution should be exercised when drugs known to interfere with biliary excretion, glucuronidation, and intestinal β-glucuronidase are given concurrently with entacapone. This includes some antibiotics (eg, erythromycin, rifampicin, ampicillin and chloramphenicol)).
No products indexed under this heading.

Dobutamine (Co-administration of drugs that are metabolized by catechol-O-methyltransferase (COMT), such as dobutamine, should be administered with caution in patients receiving entacapone regardless of the route of administration. Concomitant administration may result in increased heart rates, possibly arrhythmias, and excessive changes in blood pressure).
No products indexed under this heading.

Dobutamine Hydrochloride (Co-administration of drugs that are metabolized by catechol-O-methyltransferase (COMT), such as dobutamine, should be administered with caution in patients receiving entacapone regardless of the route of administration. Concomitant administration may result in increased heart rates, possibly arrhythmias, and excessive changes in blood pressure).
No products indexed under this heading.

Dopamine Hydrochloride (Co-administration of drugs that are metabolized by catechol-O-methyltransferase (COMT), such as dopamine, should be administered with caution in patients receiving entacapone regardless of the route of administration. Concomitant administration may result in increased heart rates, possibly arrhythmias, and excessive changes in blood pressure).
No products indexed under this heading.

Doxycycline Calcium (As most entacapone excretion is via the bile, caution should be exercised when drugs known to interfere with biliary excretion, glucuronidation, and intestinal β-glucuronidase are given concurrently with entacapone. This includes some antibiotics (eg, erythromycin, rifampicin, ampicillin and chloramphenicol)).
No products indexed under this heading.

Doxycycline Hyclate (As most entacapone excretion is via the bile, caution should be exercised when drugs known to interfere with biliary excretion, glucuronidation, and intestinal β-glucuronidase are given concurrently with entacapone. This includes some antibiotics (eg, erythromycin, rifampicin, ampicillin and chloramphenicol)).
No products indexed under this heading.

Doxycycline Monohydrate (As most entacapone excretion is via the bile, caution should be exercised when drugs known to interfere with biliary excretion, glucuronidation, and intestinal β-glucuronidase are given concurrently with entacapone. This includes some antibiotics (eg, erythromycin, rifampicin, ampicillin and chloramphenicol)).
No products indexed under this heading.

Droperidol (Due to the possible additive sedative effects, caution should be used when concomitantly taking other CNS depressants in combination with entacapone).
No products indexed under this heading.

Enflurane (Due to the possible additive sedative effects, caution should be used when concomitantly taking other CNS depressants in combination with entacapone).
No products indexed under this heading.

Enoxacin (As most entacapone excretion is via the bile, caution should be exercised when drugs known to interfere with biliary excretion, glucuronidation, and intestinal β-glucuronidase are given concurrently with entacapone. This includes some antibiotics (eg, erythromycin, rifampicin, ampicillin and chloramphenicol)).
No products indexed under this heading.

Epinephrine (Co-administration of drugs that are metabolized by catechol-O-methyltransferase (COMT), such as epinephrine, should be administered with caution in patients receiving entacapone regardless of the route of administration. Concomitant administration may result in increased heart rates, possibly arrhythmias, and excessive changes in blood pressure. Ventricular tachycardia was noted in one 32-year-old healthy male volunteer in an interaction study after epinephrine infusion and oral entacapone administration. Treatment with propranolol was required. A causal relationship to entacapone administration appears probable but cannot be attributed with certainty). Products include:
EpiPen 3631
Twinject 3268

Epinephrine, Racemic (Co-administration of drugs that are metabolized by catechol-O-methyltransferase (COMT), such as epinephrine, should be administered with caution in patients receiving entacapone regardless of the route of administration. Concomitant

administration may result in increased heart rates, possibly arrhythmias, and excessive changes in blood pressure. Ventricular tachycardia was noted in one 32-year-old healthy male volunteer in an interaction study after epinephrine infusion and oral entacapone administration. Treatment with propranolol was required. A causal relationship to entacapone administration appears probable but cannot be attributed with certainty).
No products indexed under this heading.

Epinephrine Bitartrate (Co-administration of drugs that are metabolized by catechol-O-methyltransferase (COMT), such as epinephrine, should be administered with caution in patients receiving entacapone regardless of the route of administration. Concomitant administration may result in increased heart rates, possibly arrhythmias, and excessive changes in blood pressure. Ventricular tachycardia was noted in one 32-year-old healthy male volunteer in an interaction study after epinephrine infusion and oral entacapone administration. Treatment with propranolol was required. A causal relationship to entacapone administration appears probable but cannot be attributed with certainty).
No products indexed under this heading.

Epinephrine Hydrochloride (Co-administration of drugs that are metabolized by catechol-O-methyltransferase (COMT), such as epinephrine, should be administered with caution in patients receiving entacapone regardless of the route of administration. Concomitant administration may result in increased heart rates, possibly arrhythmias, and excessive changes in blood pressure. Ventricular tachycardia was noted in one 32-year-old healthy male volunteer in an interaction study after epinephrine infusion and oral entacapone administration. Treatment with propranolol was required. A causal relationship to entacapone administration appears probable but cannot be attributed with certainty).
No products indexed under this heading.

Epirubicin Hydrochloride (As most entacapone excretion is via the bile, caution should be exercised when drugs known to interfere with biliary excretion, glucuronidation, and intestinal β-glucuronidase are given concurrently with entacapone. This includes some antibiotics (eg, erythromycin, rifampicin, ampicillin and chloramphenicol)).
No products indexed under this heading.

Erythromycin (As most entacapone excretion is via the bile, caution should be exercised when drugs known to interfere with biliary excretion, glucuronidation, and intestinal β-glucuronidase are given concurrently with entacapone. This includes some antibiotics (eg, erythromycin)).
No products indexed under this heading.

Erythromycin, Topical (As most entacapone excretion is via the bile, caution should be exercised when drugs known to interfere with biliary excretion, glucuronidation, and intestinal β-glucuronidase are given concurrently with entacapone. This includes some antibiotics (eg, erythromycin)).
No products indexed under this heading.

Erythromycin Estolate (As most entacapone excretion is via the bile, caution should be exercised when drugs known to interfere with biliary excretion, glucuronidation, and intestinal β-glucuronidase are given concurrently with entacapone. This includes some antibiotics (eg, erythromycin)).
No products indexed under this heading.

Erythromycin Ethylsuccinate (As most entacapone excretion is via the

bile, caution should be exercised when drugs known to interfere with biliary excretion, glucuronidation, and intestinal β-glucuronidase are given concurrently with entacapone. This includes some antibiotics (eg, erythromycin)). Products include:
E.E.S. 437
EryPed 435

Erythromycin Gluceptate (As most entacapone excretion is via the bile, caution should be exercised when drugs known to interfere with biliary excretion, glucuronidation, and intestinal β-glucuronidase are given concurrently with entacapone. This includes some antibiotics (eg, erythromycin)).
No products indexed under this heading.

Erythromycin Lactobionate (As most entacapone excretion is via the bile, caution should be exercised when drugs known to interfere with biliary excretion, glucuronidation, and intestinal β-glucuronidase are given concurrently with entacapone. This includes some antibiotics (eg, erythromycin)).
No products indexed under this heading.

Erythromycin Stearate (As most entacapone excretion is via the bile, caution should be exercised when drugs known to interfere with biliary excretion, glucuronidation, and intestinal β-glucuronidase are given concurrently with entacapone. This includes some antibiotics (eg, erythromycin)).
No products indexed under this heading.

Estazolam (Due to the possible additive sedative effects, caution should be used when concomitantly taking other CNS depressants in combination with entacapone).
No products indexed under this heading.

Ethanol (Due to the possible additive sedative effects, caution should be used when concomitantly taking other CNS depressants in combination with entacapone).
No products indexed under this heading.

Ethchlorvynol (Due to the possible additive sedative effects, caution should be used when concomitantly taking other CNS depressants in combination with entacapone).
No products indexed under this heading.

Ethinamate (Due to the possible additive sedative effects, caution should be used when concomitantly taking other CNS depressants in combination with entacapone).
No products indexed under this heading.

Ethyl Alcohol (Due to the possible additive sedative effects, caution should be used when concomitantly taking other CNS depressants in combination with entacapone).
No products indexed under this heading.

Fentanyl (Due to the possible additive sedative effects, caution should be used when concomitantly taking other CNS depressants in combination with entacapone). Products include:
Duragesic 2604
Fentanyl Transdermal System 2346
Onsolis 2054

Fentanyl Citrate (Due to the possible additive sedative effects, caution should be used when concomitantly taking other CNS depressants in combination with entacapone). Products include:
Fentora 966

Fluphenazine Decanoate (Due to the possible additive sedative effects, caution should be used when concomitantly taking other CNS depressants in combination with entacapone).
No products indexed under this heading.

IMPORTANT NOTE: Always consult each drug listing in the patient's regimen for possible interactions.

Fluphenazine Enanthate (Due to the possible additive sedative effects, caution should be used when concomitantly taking other CNS depressants in combination with entacapone).
No products indexed under this heading.

Fluphenazine Hydrochloride (Due to the possible additive sedative effects, caution should be used when concomitantly taking other CNS depressants in combination with entacapone).
No products indexed under this heading.

Flurazepam Hydrochloride (Due to the possible additive sedative effects, caution should be used when concomitantly taking other CNS depressants in combination with entacapone).
No products indexed under this heading.

Gatifloxacin (As most entacapone excretion is via the bile, caution should be exercised when drugs known to interfere with biliary excretion, glucuronidation, and intestinal β-glucuronidase are given concurrently with entacapone. This includes some antibiotics (eg, erythromycin, rifampicin, ampicillin and chloramphenicol)).
No products indexed under this heading.

Gemifloxacin Mesylate (As most entacapone excretion is via the bile, caution should be exercised when drugs known to interfere with biliary excretion, glucuronidation, and intestinal β-glucuronidase are given concurrently with entacapone. This includes some antibiotics (eg, erythromycin, rifampicin, ampicillin and chloramphenicol)).
No products indexed under this heading.

Gentamicin Sulfate (As most entacapone excretion is via the bile, caution should be exercised when drugs known to interfere with biliary excretion, glucuronidation, and intestinal β-glucuronidase are given concurrently with entacapone. This includes some antibiotics (eg, erythromycin, rifampicin, ampicillin and chloramphenicol)).
Products include:
Pred-G .... ⊙226, ⊙227

Glutethimide (Due to the possible additive sedative effects, caution should be used when concomitantly taking other CNS depressants in combination with entacapone).
No products indexed under this heading.

Grepafloxacin Hydrochloride (As most entacapone excretion is via the bile, caution should be exercised when drugs known to interfere with biliary excretion, glucuronidation, and intestinal β-glucuronidase are given concurrently with entacapone. This includes some antibiotics (eg, erythromycin, rifampicin, ampicillin and chloramphenicol)).
No products indexed under this heading.

Griseofulvin (As most entacapone excretion is via the bile, caution should be exercised when drugs known to interfere with biliary excretion, glucuronidation, and intestinal β-glucuronidase are given concurrently with entacapone. This includes some antibiotics (eg, erythromycin, rifampicin, ampicillin and chloramphenicol)).
No products indexed under this heading.

Halazepam (Due to the possible additive sedative effects, caution should be used when concomitantly taking other CNS depressants in combination with entacapone).
No products indexed under this heading.

Haloperidol (Due to the possible additive sedative effects, caution should be used when concomitantly taking other CNS depressants in combination with entacapone).
No products indexed under this heading.

Haloperidol Decanoate (Due to the possible additive sedative effects, caution should be used when concomitantly taking other CNS depressants in combination with entacapone).
No products indexed under this heading.

Haloperidol Lactate (Due to the possible additive sedative effects, caution should be used when concomitantly taking other CNS depressants in combination with entacapone).
No products indexed under this heading.

Hexobarbital (Due to the possible additive sedative effects, caution should be used when concomitantly taking other CNS depressants in combination with entacapone).
No products indexed under this heading.

Hydrocodone Bitartrate (Due to the possible additive sedative effects, caution should be used when concomitantly taking other CNS depressants in combination with entacapone). Products include:
Vicodin 560
Vicodin ES 561
Vicodin HP 563
Vicoprofen 564
Zydone 1138

Hydrocodone Polistirex (Due to the possible additive sedative effects, caution should be used when concomitantly taking other CNS depressants in combination with entacapone). Products include:
Tussionex 3443

Hydromorphone (Due to the possible additive sedative effects, caution should be used when concomitantly taking other CNS depressants in combination with entacapone).
No products indexed under this heading.

Hydromorphone Hydrochloride (Due to the possible additive sedative effects, caution should be used when concomitantly taking other CNS depressants in combination with entacapone). Products include:
Dilaudid Injection 2800
Dilaudid Oral 2797
Dilaudid Tablets 2797
Dilaudid-HP 2800

Hydroxyzine Hydrochloride (Due to the possible additive sedative effects, caution should be used when concomitantly taking other CNS depressants in combination with entacapone).
No products indexed under this heading.

Idarubicin Hydrochloride (As most entacapone excretion is via the bile, caution should be exercised when drugs known to interfere with biliary excretion, glucuronidation, and intestinal β-glucuronidase are given concurrently with entacapone. This includes some antibiotics (eg, erythromycin, rifampicin, ampicillin and chloramphenicol)).
No products indexed under this heading.

Imipenem (As most entacapone excretion is via the bile, caution should be exercised when drugs known to interfere with biliary excretion, glucuronidation, and intestinal β-glucuronidase are given concurrently with entacapone. This includes some antibiotics (eg, erythromycin, rifampicin, ampicillin and chloramphenicol)). Products include:
Primaxin I.M. 2232
Primaxin I.V. 2235

Isocarboxazid (Monoamine oxidase (MAO) and COMT are the two major enzyme systems involved in the metabolism of catecholamines. It is theoretically possible, therefore, that the combination of entacapone and a non-selective MAO inhibitor (eg, phenelzine, tranylcypromine) would result in inhibition of the majority of the pathways responsible for normal catechol-

amine metabolism. For this reason, patients should ordinarily not be treated concomitantly with entacapone and a non-selective MAO inhibitor). Products include:
Marplan 3481

Isoetharine (Co-administration of drugs that are metabolized by catechol-O-methyltransferase (COMT), such as isoetharine, should be administered with caution in patients receiving entacapone regardless of the route of administration. Concomitant administration may result in increased heart rates, possibly arrhythmias, and excessive changes in blood pressure).
No products indexed under this heading.

Isoflurane (Due to the possible additive sedative effects, caution should be used when concomitantly taking other CNS depressants in combination with entacapone).
No products indexed under this heading.

Isoproterenol Hydrochloride (Co-administration of drugs that are metabolized by catechol-O-methyltransferase (COMT), such as isoproterenol, should be administered with caution in patients receiving entacapone regardless of the route of administration. Concomitant administration may result in increased heart rates, possibly arrhythmias, and excessive changes in blood pressure).
No products indexed under this heading.

Isoproterenol Sulfate (Co-administration of drugs that are metabolized by catechol-O-methyltransferase (COMT), such as isoproterenol, should be administered with caution in patients receiving entacapone regardless of the route of administration. Concomitant administration may result in increased heart rates, possibly arrhythmias, and excessive changes in blood pressure).
No products indexed under this heading.

Kanamycin Sulfate (As most entacapone excretion is via the bile, caution should be exercised when drugs known to interfere with biliary excretion, glucuronidation, and intestinal β-glucuronidase are given concurrently with entacapone. This includes some antibiotics (eg, erythromycin, rifampicin, ampicillin and chloramphenicol)).
No products indexed under this heading.

Ketamine Hydrochloride (Due to the possible additive sedative effects, caution should be used when concomitantly taking other CNS depressants in combination with entacapone).
No products indexed under this heading.

Levodopa (Entacapone enhances levodopa bioavailability and, therefore, might be expected to increase the occurence of orthostatic hypotension). Products include:
Stalevo 2526

Levofloxacin (As most entacapone excretion is via the bile, caution should be exercised when drugs known to interfere with biliary excretion, glucuronidation, and intestinal β-glucuronidase are given concurrently with entacapone. This includes some antibiotics (eg, erythromycin, rifampicin, ampicillin and chloramphenicol)). Products include:
Iquix 3492
Levaquin 2629
Levaquin in 5% Dextrose 2629
Quixin 3493

Levomethadyl Acetate Hydrochloride (Due to the possible additive sedative effects, caution should be used when concomitantly taking other CNS depressants in combination with entacapone).
No products indexed under this heading.

Levorphanol Tartrate (Due to the possible additive sedative effects, caution should be used when concomitantly taking other CNS depressants in combination with entacapone).
No products indexed under this heading.

Lomefloxacin Hydrochloride (As most entacapone excretion is via the bile, caution should be exercised when drugs known to interfere with biliary excretion, glucuronidation, and intestinal β-glucuronidase are given concurrently with entacapone. This includes some antibiotics (eg, erythromycin, rifampicin, ampicillin and chloramphenicol)).
No products indexed under this heading.

Loracarbef (As most entacapone excretion is via the bile, caution should be exercised when drugs known to interfere with biliary excretion, glucuronidation, and intestinal β-glucuronidase are given concurrently with entacapone. This includes some antibiotics (eg, erythromycin, rifampicin, ampicillin and chloramphenicol)).
No products indexed under this heading.

Lorazepam (Due to the possible additive sedative effects, caution should be used when concomitantly taking other CNS depressants in combination with entacapone).
No products indexed under this heading.

Loxapine Hydrochloride (Due to the possible additive sedative effects, caution should be used when concomitantly taking other CNS depressants in combination with entacapone).
No products indexed under this heading.

Loxapine Succinate (Due to the possible additive sedative effects, caution should be used when concomitantly taking other CNS depressants in combination with entacapone).
No products indexed under this heading.

Meperidine Hydrochloride (Due to the possible additive sedative effects, caution should be used when concomitantly taking other CNS depressants in combination with entacapone).
No products indexed under this heading.

Mephobarbital (Due to the possible additive sedative effects, caution should be used when concomitantly taking other CNS depressants in combination with entacapone).
No products indexed under this heading.

Meprobamate (Due to the possible additive sedative effects, caution should be used when concomitantly taking other CNS depressants in combination with entacapone).
No products indexed under this heading.

Mesoridazine Besylate (Due to the possible additive sedative effects, caution should be used when concomitantly taking other CNS depressants in combination with entacapone).
No products indexed under this heading.

Methacycline Hydrochloride (As most entacapone excretion is via the bile, caution should be exercised when drugs known to interfere with biliary excretion, glucuronidation, and intestinal β-glucuronidase are given concurrently with entacapone. This includes some antibiotics (eg, erythromycin, rifampicin, ampicillin and chloramphenicol)).
No products indexed under this heading.

Methadone Hydrochloride (Due to the possible additive sedative effects, caution should be used when concomitantly taking other CNS depressants in combination with entacapone).
No products indexed under this heading.

Methicillin Sodium (As most entacapone excretion is via the bile, caution should be exercised when drugs known to interfere with biliary excretion, glucuronidation, and intestinal β-glucuronidase are given concurrently with entacapone. This includes some antibiotics (eg, erythromycin, rifampicin, ampicillin and chloramphenicol)).
No products indexed under this heading.

Methohexital Sodium (Due to the possible additive sedative effects, caution should be used when concomitantly taking other CNS depressants in combination with entacapone).
No products indexed under this heading.

Methotrimeprazine (Due to the possible additive sedative effects, caution should be used when concomitantly taking other CNS depressants in combination with entacapone).
No products indexed under this heading.

Methoxyflurane (Due to the possible additive sedative effects, caution should be used when concomitantly taking other CNS depressants in combination with entacapone).
No products indexed under this heading.

Methyldopa (Co-administration of drugs that are metabolized by catechol-O-methyltransferase (COMT), such as α-methyldopa, should be administered with caution in patients receiving entacapone regardless of the route of administration. Concomitant administration may result in increased heart rates, possibly arrhythmias, and excessive changes in blood pressure).
No products indexed under this heading.

Mezlocillin Sodium (As most entacapone excretion is via the bile, caution should be exercised when drugs known to interfere with biliary excretion, glucuronidation, and intestinal β-glucuronidase are given concurrently with entacapone. This includes some antibiotics (eg, erythromycin, rifampicin, ampicillin and chloramphenicol)).
No products indexed under this heading.

Midazolam Hydrochloride (Due to the possible additive sedative effects, caution should be used when concomitantly taking other CNS depressants in combination with entacapone).
No products indexed under this heading.

Minocycline Hydrochloride (As most entacapone excretion is via the bile, caution should be exercised when drugs known to interfere with biliary excretion, glucuronidation, and intestinal β-glucuronidase are given concurrently with entacapone. This includes some antibiotics (eg, erythromycin, rifampicin, ampicillin and chloramphenicol)). Products include:
Solodyn 2073

Molindone Hydrochloride (Due to the possible additive sedative effects, caution should be used when concomitantly taking other CNS depressants in combination with entacapone). Products include:
Moban 1108

Morphine Sulfate (Due to the possible additive sedative effects, caution should be used when concomitantly taking other CNS depressants in combination with entacapone). Products include:
Avinza 1822
Embeda 1831
MS Contin 2803

Morphine Sulfate, Liposomal (Due to the possible additive sedative effects, caution should be used when concomitantly taking other CNS depressants in combination with entacapone).
No products indexed under this heading.

Moxifloxacin Hydrochloride (As most entacapone excretion is via the bile, caution should be exercised when

drugs known to interfere with biliary excretion, glucuronidation, and intestinal β-glucuronidase are given concurrently with entacapone. This includes some antibiotics (eg, erythromycin, rifampicin, ampicillin and chloramphenicol)). Products include:
Avelox 3064
Vigamox 589

Nafcillin Sodium (As most entacapone excretion is via the bile, caution should be exercised when drugs known to interfere with biliary excretion, glucuronidation, and intestinal β-glucuronidase are given concurrently with entacapone. This includes some antibiotics (eg, erythromycin, rifampicin, ampicillin and chloramphenicol)).
No products indexed under this heading.

Norepinephrine Bitartrate (Co-administration of drugs that are metabolized by catechol-O-methyltransferase (COMT), such as norepinephrine, should be administered with caution in patients receiving entacapone regardless of the route of administration. Concomitant administration may result in increased heart rates, possibly arrhythmias, and excessive changes in blood pressure).
No products indexed under this heading.

Norepinephrine Hydrochloride (Co-administration of drugs that are metabolized by catechol-O-methyltransferase (COMT), such as norepinephrine, should be administered with caution in patients receiving entacapone regardless of the route of administration. Concomitant administration may result in increased heart rates, possibly arrhythmias, and excessive changes in blood pressure).
No products indexed under this heading.

Norfloxacin (As most entacapone excretion is via the bile, caution should be exercised when drugs known to interfere with biliary excretion, glucuronidation, and intestinal β-glucuronidase are given concurrently with entacapone. This includes some antibiotics (eg, erythromycin, rifampicin, ampicillin and chloramphenicol)). Products include:
Noroxin 2220

Ofloxacin (As most entacapone excretion is via the bile, caution should be exercised when drugs known to interfere with biliary excretion, glucuronidation, and intestinal β-glucuronidase are given concurrently with entacapone. This includes some antibiotics (eg, erythromycin, rifampicin, ampicillin and chloramphenicol)).
No products indexed under this heading.

Olanzapine (Due to the possible additive sedative effects, caution should be used when concomitantly taking other CNS depressants in combination with entacapone). Products include:
Symbyax 1965
Zyprexa 1984
Zyprexa IntraMuscular 1984
Zyprexa ZYDIS 1984

Oxacillin (As most entacapone excretion is via the bile, caution should be exercised when drugs known to interfere with biliary excretion, glucuronidation, and intestinal β-glucuronidase are given concurrently with entacapone. This includes some antibiotics (eg, erythromycin, rifampicin, ampicillin and chloramphenicol)).
No products indexed under this heading.

Oxacillin Sodium (As most entacapone excretion is via the bile, caution should be exercised when drugs known to interfere with biliary excretion, glucuronidation, and intestinal β-glucuronidase are given concurrently with entacapone. This includes some antibiotics (eg, erythromycin, rifampicin, ampicillin and chloramphenicol)).
No products indexed under this heading.

Oxazepam (Due to the possible additive sedative effects, caution should be used when concomitantly taking other CNS depressants in combination with entacapone).
No products indexed under this heading.

Oxycodone Hydrochloride (Due to the possible additive sedative effects, caution should be used when concomitantly taking other CNS depressants in combination with entacapone). Products include:
OxyContin 2807
Percocet 1121
Percodan 1124

Oxycodone Terephthalate (Due to the possible additive sedative effects, caution should be used when concomitantly taking other CNS depressants in combination with entacapone).
No products indexed under this heading.

Oxymorphone Hydrochloride (Due to the possible additive sedative effects, caution should be used when concomitantly taking other CNS depressants in combination with entacapone). Products include:
Opana 1110
Opana ER 1114

Oxytetracycline Hydrochloride (As most entacapone excretion is via the bile, caution should be exercised when drugs known to interfere with biliary excretion, glucuronidation, and intestinal β-glucuronidase are given concurrently with entacapone. This includes some antibiotics (eg, erythromycin, rifampicin, ampicillin and chloramphenicol)).
No products indexed under this heading.

Pargyline Hydrochloride (Monoamine oxidase (MAO) and COMT are the two major enzyme systems involved in the metabolism of catecholamines. It is theoretically possible, therefore, that the combination of entacapone and a non-selective MAO inhibitor (eg, phenelzine, tranylcypromine) would result in inhibition of the majority of the pathways responsible for normal catecholamine metabolism. For this reason, patients should ordinarily not be treated concomitantly with entacapone and a non-selective MAO inhibitor).
No products indexed under this heading.

Penicillin, Potassium Phenoxymethyl (As most entacapone excretion is via the bile, caution should be exercised when drugs known to interfere with biliary excretion, glucuronidation, and intestinal β-glucuronidase are given concurrently with entacapone. This includes some antibiotics (eg, erythromycin, rifampicin, ampicillin and chloramphenicol)).
No products indexed under this heading.

Penicillin G Benzathine (As most entacapone excretion is via the bile, caution should be exercised when drugs known to interfere with biliary excretion, glucuronidation, and intestinal β-glucuronidase are given concurrently with entacapone. This includes some antibiotics (eg, erythromycin, rifampicin, ampicillin and chloramphenicol)). Products include:
Bicillin C-R Injectable Suspension 1826
Bicillin L-A 1828

Penicillin G Dibenzylethyenediamine (As most entacapone excretion is via the bile, caution should be exercised when drugs known to interfere with biliary excretion, glucuronidation, and intestinal β-glucuronidase are given concurrently with entacapone. This includes some antibiotics (eg, erythromycin, rifampicin, ampicillin and chloramphenicol)).
No products indexed under this heading.

Penicillin G Potassium (As most entacapone excretion is via the bile, caution should be exercised when drugs known to interfere with biliary excretion, glucuronidation, and intestinal β-glucuronidase are given concurrently with entacapone. This includes some antibiotics (eg, erythromycin, rifampicin, ampicillin and chloramphenicol)).
No products indexed under this heading.

Penicillin G Procaine (As most entacapone excretion is via the bile, caution should be exercised when drugs known to interfere with biliary excretion, glucuronidation, and intestinal β-glucuronidase are given concurrently with entacapone. This includes some antibiotics (eg, erythromycin, rifampicin, ampicillin and chloramphenicol)). Products include:
Bicillin C-R Injectable Suspension 1826
Bicillin L-A 1828

Penicillin G Sodium (As most entacapone excretion is via the bile, caution should be exercised when drugs known to interfere with biliary excretion, glucuronidation, and intestinal β-glucuronidase are given concurrently with entacapone. This includes some antibiotics (eg, erythromycin, rifampicin, ampicillin and chloramphenicol)).
No products indexed under this heading.

Penicillin V (As most entacapone excretion is via the bile, caution should be exercised when drugs known to interfere with biliary excretion, glucuronidation, and intestinal β-glucuronidase are given concurrently with entacapone. This includes some antibiotics (eg, erythromycin, rifampicin, ampicillin and chloramphenicol)).
No products indexed under this heading.

Penicillin V Potassium (As most entacapone excretion is via the bile, caution should be exercised when drugs known to interfere with biliary excretion, glucuronidation, and intestinal β-glucuronidase are given concurrently with entacapone. This includes some antibiotics (eg, erythromycin, rifampicin, ampicillin and chloramphenicol)).
No products indexed under this heading.

Penicillins (As most entacapone excretion is via the bile, caution should be exercised when drugs known to interfere with biliary excretion, glucuronidation, and intestinal β-glucuronidase are given concurrently with entacapone. This includes some antibiotics (eg, erythromycin, rifampicin, ampicillin and chloramphenicol)).
No products indexed under this heading.

Pentobarbital (Due to the possible additive sedative effects, caution should be used when concomitantly taking other CNS depressants in combination with entacapone).
No products indexed under this heading.

Pentobarbital Sodium (Due to the possible additive sedative effects, caution should be used when concomitantly taking other CNS depressants in combination with entacapone). Products include:
Nembutal 2012

Perphenazine (Due to the possible additive sedative effects, caution should be used when concomitantly taking other CNS depressants in combination with entacapone).
No products indexed under this heading.

Phenelzine Sulfate (Monoamine oxidase (MAO) and catechol-O-methyltransferase (COMT) are the two major enzyme systems involved in the metabolism of catecholamines. It is theoretically possible, therefore, that the combination of entacapone and a non-selective MAO inhibitor (eg, phenelzine) would result in inhibition of the

IMPORTANT NOTE: Always consult each drug listing in the patient's regimen for possible interactions.

majority of the pathways responsible for normal catecholamine metabolism. For this reason, patients should ordinarily not be treated concomitantly with entacapone and a non-selective MAO inhibitor).

No products indexed under this heading.

Phenobarbital (Due to the possible additive sedative effects, caution should be used when concomitantly taking other CNS depressants in combination with entacapone). Products include:

Donnatal 2711

Phenobarbital Sodium (Due to the possible additive sedative effects, caution should be used when concomitantly taking other CNS depressants in combination with entacapone).

No products indexed under this heading.

Piperacillin Sodium (As most entacapone excretion is via the bile, caution should be exercised when drugs known to interfere with biliary excretion, glucuronidation, and intestinal β-glucuronidase are given concurrently with entacapone. This includes some antibiotics (eg, erythromycin, rifampicin, ampicillin and chloramphenicol)). Products include:

Zosyn 3607

Prazepam (Due to the possible additive sedative effects, caution should be used when concomitantly taking other CNS depressants in combination with entacapone).

No products indexed under this heading.

Probenecid (As most entacapone excretion is via the bile, caution should be exercised when drugs known to interfere with biliary excretion, glucuronidation, and intestinal β-glucuronidase are given concurrently with entacapone. This includes probenecid).

No products indexed under this heading.

Procarbazine Hydrochloride (Monoamine oxidase (MAO) and COMT are the two major enzyme systems involved in the metabolism of catecholamines. It is theoretically possible, therefore, that the combination of entacapone and a non-selective MAO inhibitor (eg, phenelzine, tranylcypromine) would result in inhibition of the majority of the pathways responsible for normal catecholamine metabolism. For this reason, patients should ordinarily not be treated concomitantly with entacapone and a non-selective MAO inhibitor).

No products indexed under this heading.

Prochlorperazine (Due to the possible additive sedative effects, caution should be used when concomitantly taking other CNS depressants in combination with entacapone).

No products indexed under this heading.

Prochlorperazine Edisylate (Due to the possible additive sedative effects, caution should be used when concomitantly taking other CNS depressants in combination with entacapone).

No products indexed under this heading.

Prochlorperazine Maleate (Due to the possible additive sedative effects, caution should be used when concomitantly taking other CNS depressants in combination with entacapone).

No products indexed under this heading.

Promethazine (Due to the possible additive sedative effects, caution should be used when concomitantly taking other CNS depressants in combination with entacapone).

No products indexed under this heading.

Promethazine Hydrochloride (Due to the possible additive sedative effects, caution should be used when concomitantly taking other CNS depressants in combination with entacapone).

No products indexed under this heading.

Propofol (Due to the possible additive sedative effects, caution should be used when concomitantly taking other CNS depressants in combination with entacapone).

No products indexed under this heading.

Propoxyphene Hydrochloride (Due to the possible additive sedative effects, caution should be used when concomitantly taking other CNS depressants in combination with entacapone).

No products indexed under this heading.

Propoxyphene Napsylate (Due to the possible additive sedative effects, caution should be used when concomitantly taking other CNS depressants in combination with entacapone).

No products indexed under this heading.

Quazepam (Due to the possible additive sedative effects, caution should be used when concomitantly taking other CNS depressants in combination with entacapone).

No products indexed under this heading.

Quetiapine Fumarate (Due to the possible additive sedative effects, caution should be used when concomitantly taking other CNS depressants in combination with entacapone). Products include:

Seroquel 750
Seroquel XR 759

Remifentanil Hydrochloride (Due to the possible additive sedative effects, caution should be used when concomitantly taking other CNS depressants in combination with entacapone).

No products indexed under this heading.

Rifampicin (As most entacapone excretion is via the bile, caution should be exercised when drugs known to interfere with biliary excretion, glucuronidation, and intestinal β-glucuronidase are given concurrently with entacapone. This includes some antibiotics (eg, rifampicin)).

No products indexed under this heading.

Risperidone (Due to the possible additive sedative effects, caution should be used when concomitantly taking other CNS depressants in combination with entacapone). Products include:

Risperdal Consta 2682

Secobarbital Sodium (Due to the possible additive sedative effects, caution should be used when concomitantly taking other CNS depressants in combination with entacapone).

No products indexed under this heading.

Sevoflurane (Due to the possible additive sedative effects, caution should be used when concomitantly taking other CNS depressants in combination with entacapone). Products include:

Ultane 554

Sodium Butabarbital (Due to the possible additive sedative effects, caution should be used when concomitantly taking other CNS depressants in combination with entacapone).

No products indexed under this heading.

Sodium Cloxacillin Monohydrate (As most entacapone excretion is via the bile, caution should be exercised when drugs known to interfere with biliary excretion, glucuronidation, and intestinal β-glucuronidase are given concurrently with entacapone. This includes some antibiotics (eg, erythromycin, rifampicin, ampicillin and chloramphenicol)).

No products indexed under this heading.

Sodium Oxybate (Due to the possible additive sedative effects, caution should be used when concomitantly taking other CNS depressants in combination with entacapone).

No products indexed under this heading.

Sodium Pentobarbital (Due to the possible additive sedative effects, caution should be used when concomitantly taking other CNS depressants in combination with entacapone).

No products indexed under this heading.

Sparfloxacin (As most entacapone excretion is via the bile, caution should be exercised when drugs known to interfere with biliary excretion, glucuronidation, and intestinal β-glucuronidase are given concurrently with entacapone. This includes some antibiotics (eg, erythromycin, rifampicin, ampicillin and chloramphenicol)).

No products indexed under this heading.

Streptomycin Sulfate (As most entacapone excretion is via the bile, caution should be exercised when drugs known to interfere with biliary excretion, glucuronidation, and intestinal β-glucuronidase are given concurrently with entacapone. This includes some antibiotics (eg, erythromycin, rifampicin, ampicillin and chloramphenicol)).

No products indexed under this heading.

Sufentanil Citrate (Due to the possible additive sedative effects, caution should be used when concomitantly taking other CNS depressants in combination with entacapone).

No products indexed under this heading.

Sulfamethizole (As most entacapone excretion is via the bile, caution should be exercised when drugs known to interfere with biliary excretion, glucuronidation, and intestinal β-glucuronidase are given concurrently with entacapone. This includes some antibiotics (eg, erythromycin, rifampicin, ampicillin and chloramphenicol)).

No products indexed under this heading.

Sulfamethoxazole (As most entacapone excretion is via the bile, caution should be exercised when drugs known to interfere with biliary excretion, glucuronidation, and intestinal β-glucuronidase are given concurrently with entacapone. This includes some antibiotics (eg, erythromycin, rifampicin, ampicillin and chloramphenicol)).

No products indexed under this heading.

Sulfisoxazole Acetyl (As most entacapone excretion is via the bile, caution should be exercised when drugs known to interfere with biliary excretion, glucuronidation, and intestinal β-glucuronidase are given concurrently with entacapone. This includes some antibiotics (eg, erythromycin, rifampicin, ampicillin and chloramphenicol)).

No products indexed under this heading.

Sulfisoxazole Diolamine (As most entacapone excretion is via the bile, caution should be exercised when drugs known to interfere with biliary excretion, glucuronidation, and intestinal β-glucuronidase are given concurrently with entacapone. This includes some antibiotics (eg, erythromycin, rifampicin, ampicillin and chloramphenicol)).

No products indexed under this heading.

Talbutal (Due to the possible additive sedative effects, caution should be used when concomitantly taking other CNS depressants in combination with entacapone).

No products indexed under this heading.

Temazepam (Due to the possible additive sedative effects, caution should be used when concomitantly taking other CNS depressants in combination with entacapone).

No products indexed under this heading.

Tetracycline Hydrochloride (As most entacapone excretion is via the bile, caution should be exercised when drugs known to interfere with biliary excretion, glucuronidation, and intestinal β-glucuronidase are given concur-

rently with entacapone. This includes some antibiotics (eg, erythromycin, rifampicin, ampicillin and chloramphenicol)). Products include:

Pylera 793

Thiamylal Sodium (Due to the possible additive sedative effects, caution should be used when concomitantly taking other CNS depressants in combination with entacapone).

No products indexed under this heading.

Thioridazine (Due to the possible additive sedative effects, caution should be used when concomitantly taking other CNS depressants in combination with entacapone).

No products indexed under this heading.

Thioridazine Hydrochloride (Due to the possible additive sedative effects, caution should be used when concomitantly taking other CNS depressants in combination with entacapone). Products include:

Thioridazine Hydrochloride 2384

Thiothixene (Due to the possible additive sedative effects, caution should be used when concomitantly taking other CNS depressants in combination with entacapone). Products include:

Thiothixene 2386

Thiothixene Hydrochloride (Due to the possible additive sedative effects, caution should be used when concomitantly taking other CNS depressants in combination with entacapone).

No products indexed under this heading.

Ticarcillin Disodium (As most entacapone excretion is via the bile, caution should be exercised when drugs known to interfere with biliary excretion, glucuronidation, and intestinal β-glucuronidase are given concurrently with entacapone. This includes some antibiotics (eg, erythromycin, rifampicin, ampicillin and chloramphenicol)). Products include:

Timentin ADD-Vantage 1670
Timentin Galaxy 1674
Timentin 1666
Timentin Pharmacy 1678

Tobramycin (As most entacapone excretion is via the bile, caution should be exercised when drugs known to interfere with biliary excretion, glucuronidation, and intestinal β-glucuronidase are given concurrently with entacapone. This includes some antibiotics (eg, erythromycin, rifampicin, ampicillin and chloramphenicol)). Products include:

Tobi Nebulizer 2546
Tobramycin and Dexamethasone Ophthalmic Suspension .... ⊙251
Zylet ....⊙252

Tobramycin Sulfate (As most entacapone excretion is via the bile, caution should be exercised when drugs known to interfere with biliary excretion, glucuronidation, and intestinal β-glucuronidase are given concurrently with entacapone. This includes some antibiotics (eg, erythromycin, rifampicin, ampicillin and chloramphenicol)).

No products indexed under this heading.

Tranylcypromine Sulfate (Monoamine oxidase (MAO) and COMT are the two major enzyme systems involved in the metabolism of catecholamines. It is theoretically possible, therefore, that the combination of entacapone and a non-selective MAO inhibitor (eg, tranylcypromine) would result in inhibition of the majority of the pathways responsible for normal catecholamine metabolism. For this reason, patients should ordinarily not be treated concomitantly with entacapone and a non-selective MAO inhibitor). Products include:

Parnate 1584

IMPORTANT NOTE: Always consult each drug listing in the patient's regimen for possible interactions.

Concerta Interactions Index 408

Maprotiline Hydrochloride (Studies have shown that methylphenidate may inhibit the metabolism of some antidepressants (eg, tricyclics). It may be necessary to downward dose adjust the dosage and monitor plasma drug concentrations when initiating or discontinuing concomitant methylphenidate).
No products indexed under this heading.

Mephentermine Sulfate (Methylphenidate causes a rise in blood pressure; co-administration with other pressor agents should be undertaken with caution).
No products indexed under this heading.

Metaraminol Bitartrate (Methylphenidate causes a rise in blood pressure; co-administration with other pressor agents should be undertaken with caution).
No products indexed under this heading.

Methoxamine Hydrochloride (Methylphenidate causes a rise in blood pressure; co-administration with other pressor agents should be undertaken with caution).
No products indexed under this heading.

Moclobemide (Co-administration with MOA inhibitors may result in hypertensive crises; concurrent and/or sequential use is contraindicated. Methylphenidate HCl is contraindicated during treatment with monoamine oxidase (MAO) inhibitors, and also with a minimum of 14 days following discontinuation of an MAO inhibitor. Co-administration is not recommended).
No products indexed under this heading.

Norepinephrine Bitartrate (Methylphenidate causes a rise in blood pressure; co-administration with other pressor agents should be undertaken with caution).
No products indexed under this heading.

Nortriptyline Hydrochloride (Studies have shown that methylphenidate may inhibit the metabolism of some antidepressants (eg, tricyclics). It may be necessary to downward dose adjust the dosage and monitor plasma drug concentrations when initiating or discontinuing concomitant methylphenidate).
No products indexed under this heading.

Pargyline Hydrochloride (Co-administration with MOA inhibitors may result in hypertensive crises; concurrent and/or sequential use is contraindicated. Methylphenidate HCl is contraindicated during treatment with monoamine oxidase (MAO) inhibitors, and also with a minimum of 14 days following discontinuation of an MAO inhibitor. Co-administration is not recommended).
No products indexed under this heading.

Paroxetine (Studies have shown that methylphenidate may inhibit the metabolism of antidepressants (eg, selective serotoinin reuptate inhibitors). It may be necessary to downward dose adjust the dosage and monitor plasma drug concentrations when initiating or discontinuing concomitant methylphenidate).
No products indexed under this heading.

Paroxetine Hydrochloride (Studies have shown that methylphenidate may inhibit the metabolism of antidepressants (eg, selective serotoinin reuptate inhibitors). It may be necessary to downward dose adjust the dosage and monitor plasma drug concentrations when initiating or discontinuing concomitant methylphenidate). Products include:
Paroxetine CR 2361
Paroxetine ER 2371
Paxil 1586
Paxil CR 1596

Paroxetine Mesylate (Studies have shown that methylphenidate may inhibit the metabolism of antidepressants (eg, selective serotoinin reuptate inhibitors). It may be necessary to downward dose adjust the dosage and monitor plasma drug concentrations when initiating or discontinuing concomitant methylphenidate).
No products indexed under this heading.

Phenelzine Sulfate (Co-administration with MOA inhibitors may result in hypertensive crises; concurrent and/or sequential use is contraindicated. Methylphenidate HCl is contraindicated during treatment with monoamine oxidase (MAO) inhibitors, and also with a minimum of 14 days following discontinuation of an MAO inhibitor. Co-administration is not recommended).
No products indexed under this heading.

Phenobarbital (Studies have shown that methylphenidate may inhibit the metabolism of anticonvulsants (eg, phenobarbital). It may be necessary to downward dose adjust the dosage and monitor plasma drug concentrations when initiating or discontinuing concomitant methylphenidate). Products include:
Donnatal 2711

Phenylephrine Hydrochloride (Methylphenidate causes a rise in blood pressure; co-administration with other pressor agents should be undertaken with caution). Products include:
Sudafed PE Nasal Decongestant 2048
Children's Sudafed PE Nasal Decongestant 2047

Phenytoin (Studies have shown that methylphenidate may inhibit the metabolism of anticonvulsants (eg, phenytoin). It may be necessary to downward dose adjust the dosage and monitor plasma drug concentrations when initiating or discontinuing concomitant methylphenidate).
No products indexed under this heading.

Phenytoin Sodium (Studies have shown that methylphenidate may inhibit the metabolism of anticonvulsants (eg, phenytoin). It may be necessary to downward dose adjust the dosage and monitor plasma drug concentrations when initiating or discontinuing concomitant methylphenidate). Products include:
Phenytek Capsules 2380

Primidone (Studies have shown that methylphenidate may inhibit the metabolism of anticonvulsants (eg, primidone). It may be necessary to downward dose adjust the dosage and monitor plasma drug concentrations when initiating or discontinuing concomitant methylphenidate).
No products indexed under this heading.

Procarbazine Hydrochloride (Co-administration with MOA inhibitors may result in hypertensive crises; concurrent and/or sequential use is contraindicated. Methylphenidate HCl is contraindicated during treatment with monoamine oxidase (MAO) inhibitors, and also with a minimum of 14 days following discontinuation of an MAO inhibitor. Co-administration is not recommended).
No products indexed under this heading.

Protriptyline Hydrochloride (Studies have shown that methylphenidate may inhibit the metabolism of some antidepressants (eg, tricyclics). It may be necessary to downward dose adjust the dosage and monitor plasma drug concentrations when initiating or discontinuing concomitant methylphenidate).
No products indexed under this heading.

Rasagiline Mesylate (Co-administration with MOA inhibitors may result in hypertensive crises; concurrent and/or sequential use is contraindicated. Methylphenidate HCl is contraindicated during treatment with monoamine oxidase (MAO) inhibitors, and also with a minimum of 14 days following discontinuation of an MAO inhibitor. Co-administration is not recommended). Products include:
Azilect 3383

Selegiline (Co-administration with MOA inhibitors may result in hypertensive crises; concurrent and/or sequential use is contraindicated. Methylphenidate HCl is contraindicated during treatment with monoamine oxidase (MAO) inhibitors, and also with a minimum of 14 days following discontinuation of an MAO inhibitor. Co-administration is not recommended). Products include:
Emsam 3623

Selegiline Hydrochloride (Co-administration with MOA inhibitors may result in hypertensive crises; concurrent and/or sequential use is contraindicated. Methylphenidate HCl is contraindicated during treatment with monoamine oxidase (MAO) inhibitors, and also with a minimum of 14 days following discontinuation of an MAO inhibitor. Co-administration is not recommended). Products include:
Eldepryl 3312

Sertraline Hydrochloride (Studies have shown that methylphenidate may inhibit the metabolism of antidepressants (eg, selective serotoinin reuptate inhibitors). It may be necessary to downward dose adjust the dosage and monitor plasma drug concentrations when initiating or discontinuing concomitant methylphenidate).
No products indexed under this heading.

Tranylcypromine Sulfate (Co-administration with MOA inhibitors may result in hypertensive crises; concurrent and/or sequential use is contraindicated. Methylphenidate HCl is contraindicated during treatment with monoamine oxidase (MAO) inhibitors, and also with a minimum of 14 days following discontinuation of an MAO inhibitor. Co-administration is not recommended). Products include:
Parnate 1584

Trimipramine Maleate (Studies have shown that methylphenidate may inhibit the metabolism of some antidepressants (eg, tricyclics). It may be necessary to downward dose adjust the dosage and monitor plasma drug concentrations when initiating or discontinuing concomitant methylphenidate).
No products indexed under this heading.

Warfarin Sodium (Methylphenidate may inhibit the metabolism of coumarin anticoagulants; downward dosage adjustment of anticoagulants may be required. Dosage adjustment and plasma drug concentrations monitoring may be necessary when initiating or discontinuing concomitant methylphenidate).
No products indexed under this heading.

COPAXONE FOR INJECTION

(Glatiramer Acetate) 3388
None cited in PDR database. ().

COQUINONE 30 CAPSULES

(Coenzyme Q-10, Lipoic Acid) 3476
None cited in PDR database.

CORDYMAX CS-4 CAPSULES

(Herbals, Multiple) 2778
May interact with monoamine oxidase inhibitors, oral anticoagulants. Compounds in these categories include:

Anisindione (Concurrent use with anticoagulants requires consultation with a physician).
No products indexed under this heading.

Dicumarol (Concurrent use with anticoagulants requires consultation with a physician).
No products indexed under this heading.

Isocarboxazid (Concurrent use with MAO inhibitors requires consultation with a physician). Products include:
Marplan 3481

Moclobemide (Concurrent use with MAO inhibitors requires consultation with a physician).
No products indexed under this heading.

Pargyline Hydrochloride (Concurrent use with MAO inhibitors requires consultation with a physician).
No products indexed under this heading.

Phenelzine Sulfate (Concurrent use with MAO inhibitors requires consultation with a physician).
No products indexed under this heading.

Procarbazine Hydrochloride (Concurrent use with MAO inhibitors requires consultation with a physician).
No products indexed under this heading.

Rasagiline Mesylate (Concurrent use with MAO inhibitors requires consultation with a physician). Products include:
Azilect 3383

Selegiline (Concurrent use with MAO inhibitors requires consultation with a physician). Products include:
Emsam 3623

Selegiline Hydrochloride (Concurrent use with MAO inhibitors requires consultation with a physician). Products include:
Eldepryl 3312

Tranylcypromine Sulfate (Concurrent use with MAO inhibitors requires consultation with a physician). Products include:
Parnate 1584

Warfarin Sodium (Concurrent use with anticoagulants requires consultation with a physician).
No products indexed under this heading.

COREG TABLETS

(Carvedilol) 1409
May interact with ACE inhibitors, anesthetics, calcium channel blockers that are metabolized by CYP3A4, cardiac glycosides, catecholamine-depleting drugs, cytochrome p450 2c9 inhibitors (selected), cytochrome p450 2d6 inhibitors (selected), diuretics, epinephrine-containing products, insulin, monoamine oxidase inhibitors, oral hypoglycemic agents, quinidine, and certain other agents. Compounds in these categories include:

Acarbose (Agents with β-blocking properties may enhance the blood sugar reducing effect of oral hypoglycemics. Therefore, in patients taking oral hypoglycemics, regular monitoring of blood glucose is recommended).
No products indexed under this heading.

Alfentanil Hydrochloride (If treatment with carvedilol is to be continued perioperatively, particular care should be taken when anesthetic agents which depress myocardial function, such as ether, cyclopropane, and trichloroethylene, are used).
No products indexed under this heading.

Amiloride Hydrochloride (Concomitant administration with a diuretic can be expected to produce additive effects and exaggerate the orthostatic component of carvedilol action).
No products indexed under this heading.

Amiodarone Hydrochloride (Amiodarone, and its metabolite desethyl amiodarone, inhibitors of CYP2C9 and P-glycoprotein, increased concentrations of the S(-)-enantiomer of carvedilol by at least 2-fold. The concomitant administration of amiodarone or other CYP2C9 inhibitors such as fluconazole with carvedilol may enhance the

β-blocking properties of carvedilol resulting in further slowing of the heart rate or cardiac conduction. Patients should be observed for signs of bradycardia or heart block, particularly when one agent is added to pre-existing treatment with the other).

No products indexed under this heading.

Amitriptyline Hydrochloride (Concomitant use with CYP2D6 enzyme inhibitors may increase carvedilol levels).

No products indexed under this heading.

Amlodipine Besylate (As with other agents with β-blocking properties, if carvedilol is to be administered orally with calcium channel blockers of the verapamil or diltiazem type, it is recommended that ECG and blood pressure be monitored). Products include:

Azor 1010
Exforge 2443
Exforge HCT 2449

Amoxapine (Concomitant use with CYP2D6 enzyme inhibitors may increase carvedilol levels).

No products indexed under this heading.

Anastrozole (Amiodarone, and its metabolite desethyl amiodarone, inhibitors of CYP2C9 and P-glycoprotein, increased concentrations of the (S)-enantiomer of carvedilol by at least 2-fold. The concomitant administration of amiodarone or other CYP2C9 inhibitors, such as fluconazole, with carvedilol may enhance the β-blocking properties of carvedilol resulting in further slowing of the heart rate or cardiac conduction. Patients should be observed for signs of bradycardia or heart block, particularly when one agent is added to pre-existing treatment with the other).

No products indexed under this heading.

Articaine Hydrochloride (If treatment with carvedilol is to be continued perioperatively, particular care should be taken when anesthetic agents which depress myocardial function, such as ether, cyclopropane, and trichloroethylene, are used).

No products indexed under this heading.

Benazepril Hydrochloride (Vasodilatory symptoms often do not require treatment, but it may be useful to separate the time of dosing of carvedilol from that of the ACE inhibitor or to reduce temporarily the dose of the ACE inhibitor. The dose of carvedilol should not be increased until symptoms of worsening heart failure or vasodilation have been stabilized).

No products indexed under this heading.

Bendroflumethiazide (Concomitant administration with a diuretic can be expected to produce additive effects and exaggerate the orthostatic component of carvedilol action).

No products indexed under this heading.

Benzocaine (If treatment with carvedilol is to be continued perioperatively, particular care should be taken when anesthetic agents which depress myocardial function, such as ether, cyclopropane, and trichloroethylene, are used).

No products indexed under this heading.

Bumetanide (Concomitant administration with a diuretic can be expected to produce additive effects and exaggerate the orthostatic component of carvedilol action).

No products indexed under this heading.

Bupivacaine Hydrochloride (If treatment with carvedilol is to be continued perioperatively, particular care should be taken when anesthetic agents which depress myocardial function, such as ether, cyclopropane, and trichloroethylene, are used).

No products indexed under this heading.

Bupropion Hydrochloride (Concomitant use with CYP2D6 enzyme inhibitors may increase carvedilol levels).
Products include:

Aplenzin 2948
Wellbutrin 1719
Wellbutrin SR 1725
Zyban 1762

Captopril (Vasodilatory symptoms often do not require treatment, but it may be useful to separate the time of dosing of carvedilol from that of the ACE inhibitor or to reduce temporarily the dose of the ACE inhibitor. The dose of carvedilol should not be increased until symptoms of worsening heart failure or vasodilation have been stabilized). Products include:

Captopril 2341

Celecoxib (Concomitant use with CYP2D6 enzyme inhibitors may increase carvedilol levels). Products include:

Celebrex 3272

Chloramphenicol (Amiodarone, and its metabolite desethyl amiodarone, inhibitors of CYP2C9 and P-glycoprotein, increased concentrations of the (S)-enantiomer of carvedilol by at least 2-fold. The concomitant administration of amiodarone or other CYP2C9 inhibitors, such as fluconazole, with carvedilol may enhance the β-blocking properties of carvedilol resulting in further slowing of the heart rate or cardiac conduction. Patients should be observed for signs of bradycardia or heart block, particularly when one agent is added to pre-existing treatment with the other).

No products indexed under this heading.

Chloramphenicol Palmitate (Amiodarone, and its metabolite desethyl amiodarone, inhibitors of CYP2C9 and P-glycoprotein, increased concentrations of the (S)-enantiomer of carvedilol by at least 2-fold. The concomitant administration of amiodarone or other CYP2C9 inhibitors, such as fluconazole, with carvedilol may enhance the β-blocking properties of carvedilol resulting in further slowing of the heart rate or cardiac conduction. Patients should be observed for signs of bradycardia or heart block, particularly when one agent is added to pre-existing treatment with the other).

No products indexed under this heading.

Chloramphenicol Sodium Succinate (Amiodarone, and its metabolite desethyl amiodarone, inhibitors of CYP2C9 and P-glycoprotein, increased concentrations of the (S)-enantiomer of carvedilol by at least 2-fold. The concomitant administration of amiodarone or other CYP2C9 inhibitors, such as fluconazole, with carvedilol may enhance the β-blocking properties of carvedilol resulting in further slowing of the heart rate or cardiac conduction. Patients should be observed for signs of bradycardia or heart block, particularly when one agent is added to pre-existing treatment with the other).

No products indexed under this heading.

Chloroprocaine Hydrochloride (If treatment with carvedilol is to be continued perioperatively, particular care should be taken when anesthetic agents which depress myocardial function, such as ether, cyclopropane, and trichloroethylene, are used).

No products indexed under this heading.

Chloroquine (Concomitant use with CYP2D6 enzyme inhibitors may increase carvedilol levels).

No products indexed under this heading.

Chloroquine Hydrochloride (Concomitant use with CYP2D6 enzyme inhibitors may increase carvedilol levels).

No products indexed under this heading.

Chloroquine Phosphate (Concomitant use with CYP2D6 enzyme inhibitors may increase carvedilol levels).

No products indexed under this heading.

Chlorothiazide (Concomitant administration with a diuretic can be expected to produce additive effects and exaggerate the orthostatic component of carvedilol action).

No products indexed under this heading.

Chlorothiazide Sodium (Concomitant administration with a diuretic can be expected to produce additive effects and exaggerate the orthostatic component of carvedilol action). Products include:

Diuril Intravenous 2009

Chlorpheniramine (Concomitant use with CYP2D6 enzyme inhibitors may increase carvedilol levels).

No products indexed under this heading.

Chlorpheniramine Maleate (Concomitant use with CYP2D6 enzyme inhibitors may increase carvedilol levels).

No products indexed under this heading.

Chlorpheniramine Polistirex (Concomitant use with CYP2D6 enzyme inhibitors may increase carvedilol levels). Products include:

Tussionex 3443

Chlorpheniramine Tannate (Concomitant use with CYP2D6 enzyme inhibitors may increase carvedilol levels).

No products indexed under this heading.

Chlorpropamide (Agents with β-blocking properties may enhance the blood sugar reducing effect of oral hypoglycemics. Therefore, in patients taking oral hypoglycemics, regular monitoring of blood glucose is recommended).

No products indexed under this heading.

Chlorthalidone (Concomitant administration with a diuretic can be expected to produce additive effects and exaggerate the orthostatic component of carvedilol action). Products include:

Clorpres 2344

Cimetidine (In a pharmacokinetic study conducted in 10 healthy male subjects, cimetidine (1000 mg/day) increased the steady state AUC of carvedilol by 30% with no change in C_{max}).

No products indexed under this heading.

Cimetidine Hydrochloride (In a pharmacokinetic study conducted in 10 healthy male subjects, cimetidine (1000 mg/day) increased the steady state AUC of carvedilol by 30% with no change in C_{max}).

No products indexed under this heading.

Citalopram Hydrobromide (Concomitant use with CYP2D6 enzyme inhibitors may increase carvedilol levels). Products include:

Celexa 1153

Clomipramine Hydrochloride (Concomitant use with CYP2D6 enzyme inhibitors may increase carvedilol levels).

No products indexed under this heading.

Clonidine (Concomitant administration of clonidine with agents with β-blocking properties may potentiate blood pressure- and heart rate-lowering effects. When concomitant treatment with agents with β-blocking properties and clonidine is terminated, the β-blocking agent should be discontinued first. Clonidine therapy can then be discontinued several days later by gradually decreasing the dosage). Products include:

Catapres-TTS 884

Clonidine Hydrochloride (Concomitant administration of clonidine with agents with β-blocking properties may potentiate blood pressure- and heart rate-lowering effects. When concomitant treatment with agents with β-blocking properties and clonidine is terminated, the β-blocking agent should be discontinued first. Clonidine therapy can then be discontinued several days later by gradually decreasing the dosage). Products include:

Clorpres 2344

Clopidogrel Bisulfate (Amiodarone, and its metabolite desethyl amiodarone, inhibitors of CYP2C9 and P-glycoprotein, increased concentrations of the (S)-enantiomer of carvedilol by at least 2-fold. The concomitant administration of amiodarone or other CYP2C9 inhibitors, such as fluconazole, with carvedilol may enhance the β-blocking properties of carvedilol resulting in further slowing of the heart rate or cardiac conduction. Patients should be observed for signs of bradycardia or heart block, particularly when one agent is added to pre-existing treatment with the other). Products include:

Plavix 3027

Clopidogrel Hydrogen Sulfate (Amiodarone, and its metabolite desethyl amiodarone, inhibitors of CYP2C9 and P-glycoprotein, increased concentrations of the (S)-enantiomer of carvedilol by at least 2-fold. The concomitant administration of amiodarone or other CYP2C9 inhibitors, such as fluconazole, with carvedilol may enhance the β-blocking properties of carvedilol resulting in further slowing of the heart rate or cardiac conduction. Patients should be observed for signs of bradycardia or heart block, particularly when one agent is added to pre-existing treatment with the other).

No products indexed under this heading.

Clotrimazole (Amiodarone, and its metabolite desethyl amiodarone, inhibitors of CYP2C9 and P-glycoprotein, increased concentrations of the (S)-enantiomer of carvedilol by at least 2-fold. The concomitant administration of amiodarone or other CYP2C9 inhibitors, such as fluconazole, with carvedilol may enhance the β-blocking properties of carvedilol resulting in further slowing of the heart rate or cardiac conduction. Patients should be observed for signs of bradycardia or heart block, particularly when one agent is added to pre-existing treatment with the other). Products include:

Lotrisone 3163

Cocaine Hydrochloride (If treatment with carvedilol is to be continued perioperatively, particular care should be taken when anesthetic agents which depress myocardial function, such as ether, cyclopropane, and trichloroethylene, are used).

No products indexed under this heading.

Cyclopropane (If treatment with carvedilol is to be continued perioperatively, particular care should be taken when anesthetic agents which depress myocardial function, such as cyclopropane, are used).

No products indexed under this heading.

Cyclosporine (Modest increases in mean trough cyclosporine concentrations were observed following initiation of carvedilol treatment in 21 renal transplant patients. In about 30% of patients, the dose of cyclosporine had to be reduced in order to maintain cyclosporine concentrations within the therapeutic range. On the average for the group, the dose of cyclosporine was reduced about 20%. Due to wide interindividual variability in the dose adjustment required, it is recommended that cyclosporine concentrations be monitored closely after initiation of carvedilol

therapy and that the dose of cyclosporine be adjusted as appropriate). Products include:

Gengraf 440
Neoral Oral Solution 2496
Neoral Capsules 2496
Restasis 605

Deserpidine (Patients taking both agents with β-blocking properties and a drug that can deplete catecholamines should be observed closely for signs of hypotension and/or severe bradycardia).
No products indexed under this heading.

Desipramine Hydrochloride (Concomitant use with CYP2D6 enzyme inhibitors may increase carvedilol levels).
No products indexed under this heading.

Deslanoside (Both digitalis glycosides and β-blockers slow atrioventricular conduction and decrease heart rate. Concomitant use can increase the risk of bradycardia).
No products indexed under this heading.

Dibucaine (If treatment with carvedilol is to be continued perioperatively, particular care should be taken when anesthetic agents which depress myocardial function, such as ether, cyclopropane, and trichloroethylene, are used).
No products indexed under this heading.

Dibucaine Hydrochloride (If treatment with carvedilol is to be continued perioperatively, particular care should be taken when anesthetic agents which depress myocardial function, such as ether, cyclopropane, and trichloroethylene, are used).
No products indexed under this heading.

Diclofenac Epolamine (Amiodarone, and its metabolite desethyl amiodarone, inhibitors of CYP2C9 and P-glycoprotein, increased concentrations of the (S)-enantiomer of carvedilol by at least 2-fold. The concomitant administration of amiodarone or other CYP2C9 inhibitors, such as fluconazole, with carvedilol may enhance the β-blocking properties of carvedilol resulting in further slowing of the heart rate or cardiac conduction. Patients should be observed for signs of bradycardia or heart block, particularly when one agent is added to pre-existing treatment with the other). Products include:

Flector 1839

Diclofenac Potassium (Amiodarone, and its metabolite desethyl amiodarone, inhibitors of CYP2C9 and P-glycoprotein, increased concentrations of the (S)-enantiomer of carvedilol by at least 2-fold. The concomitant administration of amiodarone or other CYP2C9 inhibitors, such as fluconazole, with carvedilol may enhance the β-blocking properties of carvedilol resulting in further slowing of the heart rate or cardiac conduction. Patients should be observed for signs of bradycardia or heart block, particularly when one agent is added to pre-existing treatment with the other).
No products indexed under this heading.

Diclofenac Sodium (Amiodarone, and its metabolite desethyl amiodarone, inhibitors of CYP2C9 and P-glycoprotein, increased concentrations of the (S)-enantiomer of carvedilol by at least 2-fold. The concomitant administration of amiodarone or other CYP2C9 inhibitors, such as fluconazole, with carvedilol may enhance the β-blocking properties of carvedilol resulting in further slowing of the heart rate or cardiac conduction. Patients should be observed for signs of bradycardia or heart block, particularly when one agent is added to pre-existing treatment with the other).
No products indexed under this heading.

Digitalis Glycoside Preparations (Both digitalis glycosides and β-blockers slow atrioventricular conduction and decrease heart rate. Concomitant use can increase the risk of bradycardia. Digoxin concentrations are increased by about 15% when digoxin and carvedilol are administered concomitantly. Therefore, increased monitoring of digoxin is recommended when initiating, adjusting or discontinuing carvedilol).
No products indexed under this heading.

Digitalis Lanata (Both digitalis glycosides and β-blockers slow atrioventricular conduction and decrease heart rate. Concomitant use can increase the risk of bradycardia).
No products indexed under this heading.

Digitalis Purpurea (Both digitalis glycosides and β-blockers slow atrioventricular conduction and decrease heart rate. Concomitant use can increase the risk of bradycardia).
No products indexed under this heading.

Digitoxin (Both digitalis glycosides and β-blockers slow atrioventricular conduction and decrease heart rate. Concomitant use can increase the risk of bradycardia).
No products indexed under this heading.

Digoxin (Both digitalis glycosides and β-blockers slow atrioventricular conduction and decrease heart rate. Concomitant use can increase the risk of bradycardia. Digoxin concentrations are increased by about 15% when digoxin and carvedilol are administered concomitantly. Therefore, increased monitoring of digoxin is recommended when initiating, adjusting or discontinuing carvedilol). Products include:

Lanoxin Injection 1546
Lanoxin Injection Pediatric 1549
Lanoxin Tablets 1553

Diltiazem Hydrochloride (Conduction disturbance (rarely with hemodynamic compromise) has been observed when carvedilol is co-administered with diltiazem. As with other agents with β-blocking properties, if carvedilol is to be administered with calcium channel blockers of the verapamil or diltiazem type, it is recommended that ECG and blood pressure be monitored). Products include:

Cardizem LA 423

Diphenhydramine (Concomitant use with CYP2D6 enzyme inhibitors may increase carvedilol levels).
No products indexed under this heading.

Diphenhydramine Hydrochloride (Concomitant use with CYP2D6 enzyme inhibitors may increase carvedilol levels). Products include:

Benadryl Allergy Ultratab 2042
Children's Benadryl Allergy Liquid 2042

Disulfiram (Amiodarone, and its metabolite desethyl amiodarone, inhibitors of CYP2C9 and P-glycoprotein, increased concentrations of the (S)-enantiomer of carvedilol by at least 2-fold. The concomitant administration of amiodarone or other CYP2C9 inhibitors, such as fluconazole, with carvedilol may enhance the β-blocking properties of carvedilol resulting in further slowing of the heart rate or cardiac conduction. Patients should be observed for signs of bradycardia or heart block, particularly when one agent is added to pre-existing treatment with the other).
No products indexed under this heading.

Doxepin Hydrochloride (Concomitant use with CYP2D6 enzyme inhibitors may increase carvedilol levels).
No products indexed under this heading.

Efavirenz (Amiodarone, and its metabolite desethyl amiodarone, inhibitors of CYP2C9 and P-glycoprotein, increased concentrations of the (S)-enantiomer of carvedilol by at least 2-fold. The concomitant administration of amiodarone or other CYP2C9 inhibitors, such as fluconazole, with carvedilol may enhance the β-blocking properties of carvedilol resulting in further slowing of the heart rate or cardiac conduction. Patients should be observed for signs of bradycardia or heart block, particularly when one agent is added to pre-existing treatment with the other). Products include:

Atripla 906

Enalapril Maleate (Vasodilatory symptoms often do not require treatment, but it may be useful to separate the time of dosing of carvedilol from that of the ACE inhibitor or to reduce temporarily the dose of the ACE inhibitor. The dose of carvedilol should not be increased until symptoms of worsening heart failure or vasodilation have been stabilized).
No products indexed under this heading.

Enalaprilat (Vasodilatory symptoms often do not require treatment, but it may be useful to separate the time of dosing of carvedilol from that of the ACE inhibitor or to reduce temporarily the dose of the ACE inhibitor. The dose of carvedilol should not be increased until symptoms of worsening heart failure or vasodilation have been stabilized).
No products indexed under this heading.

Enflurane (If treatment with carvedilol is to be continued perioperatively, particular care should be taken when anesthetic agents which depress myocardial function, such as ether, cyclopropane, and trichloroethylene, are used).
No products indexed under this heading.

Epinephrine (Patients on β-blocker therapy and with a history of severe anaphylactic reactions to a variety of allergens may be unresponsive to the usual doses of epinephrine used to treat allergic reactions). Products include:

EpiPen 3631
Twinject 3268

Epinephrine, Racemic (Patients on β-blocker therapy and with a history of severe anaphylactic reactions to a variety of allergens may be unresponsive to the usual doses of epinephrine used to treat allergic reactions).
No products indexed under this heading.

Epinephrine Bitartrate (Patients on β-blocker therapy and with a history of severe anaphylactic reactions to a variety of allergens may be unresponsive to the usual doses of epinephrine used to treat allergic reactions).
No products indexed under this heading.

Epinephrine Hydrochloride (Patients on β-blocker therapy and with a history of severe anaphylactic reactions to a variety of allergens may be unresponsive to the usual doses of epinephrine used to treat allergic reactions).
No products indexed under this heading.

Escitalopram Oxalate (Concomitant use with CYP2D6 enzyme inhibitors may increase carvedilol levels). Products include:

Lexapro Oral Suspension 1160
Lexapro Tablets 1160

Ethacrynic Acid (Concomitant administration with a diuretic can be expected to produce additive effects and exaggerate the orthostatic component of carvedilol action).
No products indexed under this heading.

Ether (If treatment with carvedilol is to be continued perioperatively, particular care should be taken when anesthetic agents which depress myocardial function, such as ether, are used).
No products indexed under this heading.

Etidocaine Hydrochloride (If treatment with carvedilol is to be continued perioperatively, particular care should be taken when anesthetic agents which depress myocardial function, such as ether, cyclopropane, and trichloroethylene, are used).
No products indexed under this heading.

Felodipine (As with other agents with β-blocking properties, if carvedilol is to be administered orally with calcium channel blockers of the verapamil or diltiazem type, it is recommended that ECG and blood pressure be monitored).
No products indexed under this heading.

Fenofibrate (Amiodarone, and its metabolite desethyl amiodarone, inhibitors of CYP2C9 and P-glycoprotein, increased concentrations of the (S)-enantiomer of carvedilol by at least 2-fold. The concomitant administration of amiodarone or other CYP2C9 inhibitors, such as fluconazole, with carvedilol may enhance the β-blocking properties of carvedilol resulting in further slowing of the heart rate or cardiac conduction. Patients should be observed for signs of bradycardia or heart block, particularly when one agent is added to pre-existing treatment with the other). Products include:

Fenoglide 3263
Tricor 544
Trilipix 548

Fentanyl Citrate (If treatment with carvedilol is to be continued perioperatively, particular care should be taken when anesthetic agents which depress myocardial function, such as ether, cyclopropane, and trichloroethylene, are used). Products include:

Fentora 966

Fluconazole (The concomitant administration of amiodarone or other CYP2C9 inhibitors such as fluconazole with carvedilol may enhance the β-blocking properties of carvedilol resulting in further slowing of the heart rate or cardiac conduction. Patients should be observed for signs of bradycardia or heart block, particularly when one agent is added to pre-existing treatment with the other).
No products indexed under this heading.

Fluorouracil (Amiodarone, and its metabolite desethyl amiodarone, inhibitors of CYP2C9 and P-glycoprotein, increased concentrations of the (S)-enantiomer of carvedilol by at least 2-fold. The concomitant administration of amiodarone or other CYP2C9 inhibitors, such as fluconazole, with carvedilol may enhance the β-blocking properties of carvedilol resulting in further slowing of the heart rate or cardiac conduction. Patients should be observed for signs of bradycardia or heart block, particularly when one agent is added to pre-existing treatment with the other). Products include:

Carac 2966

Fluoxetine (Concomitant use with CYP2D6 enzyme inhibitors, such as fluoxetine, may increase carvedilol levels).
No products indexed under this heading.

Fluoxetine Hydrochloride (Concomitant use with CYP2D6 enzyme inhibitors, such as fluoxetine, may increase carvedilol levels). Products include:

Prozac Weekly 1941
Prozac Pulvules 1941
Symbyax 1965

Fluphenazine Decanoate (Concomitant use with CYP2D6 enzyme inhibitors may increase carvedilol levels).
No products indexed under this heading.

Fluphenazine Enanthate (Concomitant use with CYP2D6 enzyme inhibitors may increase carvedilol levels).
No products indexed under this heading.

Fluphenazine Hydrochloride (Concomitant use with CYP2D6 enzyme inhibitors may increase carvedilol levels).

No products indexed under this heading.

Flurbiprofen (Amiodarone, and its metabolite desethyl amiodarone, inhibitors of CYP2C9 and P-glycoprotein, increased concentrations of the (S)-enantiomer of carvedilol by at least 2-fold. The concomitant administration of amiodarone or other CYP2C9 inhibitors, such as fluconazole, with carvedilol may enhance the β-blocking properties of carvedilol resulting in further slowing of the heart rate or cardiac conduction. Patients should be observed for signs of bradycardia or heart block, particularly when one agent is added to pre-existing treatment with the other).

No products indexed under this heading.

Flurbiprofen Sodium (Amiodarone, and its metabolite desethyl amiodarone, inhibitors of CYP2C9 and P-glycoprotein, increased concentrations of the (S)-enantiomer of carvedilol by at least 2-fold. The concomitant administration of amiodarone or other CYP2C9 inhibitors, such as fluconazole, with carvedilol may enhance the β-blocking properties of carvedilol resulting in further slowing of the heart rate or cardiac conduction. Patients should be observed for signs of bradycardia or heart block, particularly when one agent is added to pre-existing treatment with the other).

No products indexed under this heading.

Fluvastatin Sodium (Amiodarone, and its metabolite desethyl amiodarone, inhibitors of CYP2C9 and P-glycoprotein, increased concentrations of the (S)-enantiomer of carvedilol by at least 2-fold. The concomitant administration of amiodarone or other CYP2C9 inhibitors, such as fluconazole, with carvedilol may enhance the β-blocking properties of carvedilol resulting in further slowing of the heart rate or cardiac conduction. Patients should be observed for signs of bradycardia or heart block, particularly when one agent is added to pre-existing treatment with the other).

No products indexed under this heading.

Fluvoxamine Maleate (Amiodarone, and its metabolite desethyl amiodarone, inhibitors of CYP2C9 and P-glycoprotein, increased concentrations of the (S)-enantiomer of carvedilol by at least 2-fold. The concomitant administration of amiodarone or other CYP2C9 inhibitors, such as fluconazole, with carvedilol may enhance the β-blocking properties of carvedilol resulting in further slowing of the heart rate or cardiac conduction. Patients should be observed for signs of bradycardia or heart block, particularly when one agent is added to pre-existing treatment with the other).

No products indexed under this heading.

Fosinopril Sodium (Vasodilatory symptoms often do not require treatment, but it may be useful to separate the time of dosing of carvedilol from that of the ACE inhibitor or to reduce temporarily the dose of the ACE inhibitor. The dose of carvedilol should not be increased until symptoms of worsening heart failure or vasodilation have been stabilized).

No products indexed under this heading.

Furosemide (Concomitant administration with a diuretic can be expected to produce additive effects and exaggerate the orthostatic component of carvedilol action). Products include:
Furosemide 2354

Gemfibrozil (Amiodarone, and its metabolite desethyl amiodarone, inhibi-

tors of CYP2C9 and P-glycoprotein, increased concentrations of the (S)-enantiomer of carvedilol by at least 2-fold. The concomitant administration of amiodarone or other CYP2C9 inhibitors, such as fluconazole, with carvedilol may enhance the β-blocking properties of carvedilol resulting in further slowing of the heart rate or cardiac conduction. Patients should be observed for signs of bradycardia or heart block, particularly when one agent is added to pre-existing treatment with the other).

No products indexed under this heading.

Glibenclamide (Agents with β-blocking properties may enhance the blood sugar reducing effect of oral hypoglycemics. Therefore, in patients taking oral hypoglycemics, regular monitoring of blood glucose is recommended).

No products indexed under this heading.

Glimepiride (Agents with β-blocking properties may enhance the blood sugar reducing effect of oral hypoglycemics. Therefore, in patients taking oral hypoglycemics, regular monitoring of blood glucose is recommended). Products include:
Avandaryl 1356
Duetact 3354

Glipizide (Agents with β-blocking properties may enhance the blood sugar reducing effect of oral hypoglycemics. Therefore, in patients taking oral hypoglycemics, regular monitoring of blood glucose is recommended).

No products indexed under this heading.

Glyburide (Agents with β-blocking properties may enhance the blood sugar reducing effect of oral hypoglycemics. Therefore, in patients taking oral hypoglycemics, regular monitoring of blood glucose is recommended).

No products indexed under this heading.

Guanethidine (Patients taking both agents with β-blocking properties and a drug that can deplete catecholamines should be observed closely for signs of hypotension and/or severe bradycardia).

No products indexed under this heading.

Guanethidine Monosulfate (Patients taking both agents with β-blocking properties and a drug that can deplete catecholamines should be observed closely for signs of hypotension and/or severe bradycardia).

No products indexed under this heading.

Guanethidine Sulfate (Patients taking both agents with β-blocking properties and a drug that can deplete catecholamines should be observed closely for signs of hypotension and/or severe bradycardia).

No products indexed under this heading.

Halofantrine Hydrochloride (Concomitant use with CYP2D6 enzyme inhibitors may increase carvedilol levels).

No products indexed under this heading.

Haloperidol (Concomitant use with CYP2D6 enzyme inhibitors may increase carvedilol levels).

No products indexed under this heading.

Haloperidol Decanoate (Concomitant use with CYP2D6 enzyme inhibitors may increase carvedilol levels).

No products indexed under this heading.

Haloperidol Lactate (Concomitant use with CYP2D6 enzyme inhibitors may increase carvedilol levels).

No products indexed under this heading.

Halothane (If treatment with carvedilol is to be continued perioperatively, particular care should be taken when anesthetic agents which depress myocardial function, such as ether, cyclopropane, and trichloroethylene, are used).

No products indexed under this heading.

Hydrochlorothiazide (Concomitant administration with a diuretic can be expected to produce additive effects and exaggerate the orthostatic component of carvedilol action). Products include:

Atacand HCT	700
Avalide	2956
Benicar HCT	1017
Diovan HCT	2419
Dyazide	1429
Exforge HCT	2449
Hyzaar	2162
Hyzaar 100-12.5	2162
Micardis HCT	889
Prinzide	2246
Tekturna HCT	2541
Teveten HCT	541

Hydrochlorothiazide Hydrochloride (Amiodarone, and its metabolite desethyl amiodarone, inhibitors of CYP2C9 and P-glycoprotein, increased concentrations of the (S)-enantiomer of carvedilol by at least 2-fold. The concomitant administration of amiodarone or other CYP2C9 inhibitors, such as fluconazole, with carvedilol may enhance the β-blocking properties of carvedilol resulting in further slowing of the heart rate or cardiac conduction. Patients should be observed for signs of bradycardia or heart block, particularly when one agent is added to pre-existing treatment with the other).

No products indexed under this heading.

Hydroflumethiazide (Concomitant administration with a diuretic can be expected to produce additive effects and exaggerate the orthostatic component of carvedilol action).

No products indexed under this heading.

Hydroxychloroquine Sulfate (Concomitant use with CYP2D6 enzyme inhibitors may increase carvedilol levels).

No products indexed under this heading.

Imatinib Mesylate (Amiodarone, and its metabolite desethyl amiodarone, inhibitors of CYP2C9 and P-glycoprotein, increased concentrations of the (S)-enantiomer of carvedilol by at least 2-fold. The concomitant administration of amiodarone or other CYP2C9 inhibitors, such as fluconazole, with carvedilol may enhance the β-blocking properties of carvedilol resulting in further slowing of the heart rate or cardiac conduction. Patients should be observed for signs of bradycardia or heart block, particularly when one agent is added to pre-existing treatment with the other). Products include:
Gleevec 2477

Imipramine Hydrochloride (Concomitant use with CYP2D6 enzyme inhibitors may increase carvedilol levels).

No products indexed under this heading.

Imipramine Pamoate (Concomitant use with CYP2D6 enzyme inhibitors may increase carvedilol levels).

No products indexed under this heading.

Indapamide (Concomitant administration with a diuretic can be expected to produce additive effects and exaggerate the orthostatic component of carvedilol action). Products include:
Indapamide 2356

Insulin (Agents with β-blocking properties may enhance the blood sugar reducing effect of insulin. Therefore, in patients taking insulin, regular monitoring of blood glucose is recommended).

No products indexed under this heading.

Insulin, Human, Zinc Suspension (Agents with β-blocking properties may enhance the blood sugar reducing effect of insulin. Therefore, in patients taking insulin, regular monitoring of blood glucose is recommended).

No products indexed under this heading.

Insulin, Human (rDNA origin) (Agents with β-blocking properties may enhance the blood sugar reducing effect of insulin. Therefore, in patients taking insulin, regular monitoring of blood glucose is recommended). Products include:
Exubera 2717

Insulin, Human NPH (Agents with β-blocking properties may enhance the blood sugar reducing effect of insulin. Therefore, in patients taking insulin, regular monitoring of blood glucose is recommended). Products include:
Humulin N Vial 1934

Insulin, Human Regular (Agents with β-blocking properties may enhance the blood sugar reducing effect of insulin. Therefore, in patients taking insulin, regular monitoring of blood glucose is recommended). Products include:
Humulin R 1937
Humulin R (U-500) 1939

Insulin, Human Regular and Human NPH Mixture (Agents with β-blocking properties may enhance the blood sugar reducing effect of insulin. Therefore, in patients taking insulin, regular monitoring of blood glucose is recommended). Products include:
Humulin 50/50 1930
Humulin 70/30 Vial 1931

Insulin, NPH (Agents with β-blocking properties may enhance the blood sugar reducing effect of insulin. Therefore, in patients taking insulin, regular monitoring of blood glucose is recommended).

No products indexed under this heading.

Insulin, Regular (Agents with β-blocking properties may enhance the blood sugar reducing effect of insulin. Therefore, in patients taking insulin, regular monitoring of blood glucose is recommended).

No products indexed under this heading.

Insulin, Regular and NPH mixture (Agents with β-blocking properties may enhance the blood sugar reducing effect of insulin. Therefore, in patients taking insulin, regular monitoring of blood glucose is recommended).

No products indexed under this heading.

Insulin, Zinc Crystals (Agents with β-blocking properties may enhance the blood sugar reducing effect of insulin. Therefore, in patients taking insulin, regular monitoring of blood glucose is recommended).

No products indexed under this heading.

Insulin, Zinc Suspension (Agents with β-blocking properties may enhance the blood sugar reducing effect of insulin. Therefore, in patients taking insulin, regular monitoring of blood glucose is recommended).

No products indexed under this heading.

Insulin Aspart (Agents with β-blocking properties may enhance the blood sugar reducing effect of insulin. Therefore, in patients taking insulin, regular monitoring of blood glucose is recommended).

No products indexed under this heading.

Insulin Aspart, Human (Agents with β-blocking properties may enhance the blood sugar reducing effect of insulin. Therefore, in patients taking insulin, regular monitoring of blood glucose is recommended). Products include:
NovoLog Mix 70/30 2581

Insulin Aspart, Human Regular (Agents with β-blocking properties may enhance the blood sugar reducing effect of insulin. Therefore, in patients taking insulin, regular monitoring of blood glucose is recommended). Products include:
NovoLog 2575

Insulin Aspart Protamine, Human (Agents with β-blocking properties may

enhance the blood sugar reducing effect of insulin. Therefore, in patients taking insulin, regular monitoring of blood glucose is recommended). Products include:

Insulin Detemir (rDNA Origin)
(Agents with β-blocking properties may enhance the blood sugar reducing effect of insulin. Therefore, in patients taking insulin, regular monitoring of blood glucose is recommended). Products include:

Insulin Glargine (Agents with β-blocking properties may enhance the blood sugar reducing effect of insulin. Therefore, in patients taking insulin, regular monitoring of blood glucose is recommended). Products include:

Insulin Glulisine (Agents with β-blocking properties may enhance the blood sugar reducing effect of insulin. Therefore, in patients taking insulin, regular monitoring of blood glucose is recommended). Products include:

Insulin Lispro, Human (Agents with β-blocking properties may enhance the blood sugar reducing effect of insulin. Therefore, in patients taking insulin, regular monitoring of blood glucose is recommended). Products include:

Insulin Lispro Protamine, Human
(Agents with β-blocking properties may enhance the blood sugar reducing effect of insulin. Therefore, in patients taking insulin, regular monitoring of blood glucose is recommended). Products include:

Isocarboxazid (Patients taking both agents with β-blocking properties and a drug that may deplete catecholamines, such as MAO Inhibitors, should be observed closely for signs of hypotension and/or severe bradycardia). Products include:

Isoflurane (If treatment with carvedilol is to be continued perioperatively, particular care should be taken when anesthetic agents which depress myocardial function, such as ether, cyclopropane, and trichloroethylene, are used).
No products indexed under this heading.

Isoniazid (Amiodarone, and its metabolite desethyl amiodarone, inhibitors of CYP2C9 and P-glycoprotein, increased concentrations of the (S)-enantiomer of carvedilol by at least 2-fold. The concomitant administration of amiodarone or other CYP2C9 inhibitors, such as fluconazole, with carvedilol may enhance the β-blocking properties of carvedilol resulting in further slowing of the heart rate or cardiac conduction. Patients should be observed for signs of bradycardia or heart block, particularly when one agent is added to pre-existing treatment with the other).
No products indexed under this heading.

Itraconazole (Amiodarone, and its metabolite desethyl amiodarone, inhibitors of CYP2C9 and P-glycoprotein, increased concentrations of the (S)-enantiomer of carvedilol by at least 2-fold. The concomitant administration of amiodarone or other CYP2C9 inhibitors, such as fluconazole, with carvedilol may enhance the β-blocking properties of carvedilol resulting in further slowing of the heart rate or cardiac conduction. Patients should be observed for signs of bradycardia or

heart block, particularly when one agent is added to pre-existing treatment with the other).
No products indexed under this heading.

Ketamine Hydrochloride (If treatment with carvedilol is to be continued perioperatively, particular care should be taken when anesthetic agents which depress myocardial function, such as ether, cyclopropane, and trichloroethylene, are used).
No products indexed under this heading.

Ketoconazole (Amiodarone, and its metabolite desethyl amiodarone, inhibitors of CYP2C9 and P-glycoprotein, increased concentrations of the (S)-enantiomer of carvedilol by at least 2-fold. The concomitant administration of amiodarone or other CYP2C9 inhibitors, such as fluconazole, with carvedilol may enhance the β-blocking properties of carvedilol resulting in further slowing of the heart rate or cardiac conduction. Patients should be observed for signs of bradycardia or heart block, particularly when one agent is added to pre-existing treatment with the other). Products include:

Ketoprofen (Amiodarone, and its metabolite desethyl amiodarone, inhibitors of CYP2C9 and P-glycoprotein, increased concentrations of the (S)-enantiomer of carvedilol by at least 2-fold. The concomitant administration of amiodarone or other CYP2C9 inhibitors, such as fluconazole, with carvedilol may enhance the β-blocking properties of carvedilol resulting in further slowing of the heart rate or cardiac conduction. Patients should be observed for signs of bradycardia or heart block, particularly when one agent is added to pre-existing treatment with the other).
No products indexed under this heading.

Leflunomide (Amiodarone, and its metabolite desethyl amiodarone, inhibitors of CYP2C9 and P-glycoprotein, increased concentrations of the (S)-enantiomer of carvedilol by at least 2-fold. The concomitant administration of amiodarone or other CYP2C9 inhibitors, such as fluconazole, with carvedilol may enhance the β-blocking properties of carvedilol resulting in further slowing of the heart rate or cardiac conduction. Patients should be observed for signs of bradycardia or heart block, particularly when one agent is added to pre-existing treatment with the other).
No products indexed under this heading.

Levobupivacaine Hydrochloride (If treatment with carvedilol is to be continued perioperatively, particular care should be taken when anesthetic agents which depress myocardial function, such as ether, cyclopropane, and trichloroethylene, are used).
No products indexed under this heading.

Lidocaine (If treatment with carvedilol is to be continued perioperatively, particular care should be taken when anesthetic agents which depress myocardial function, such as ether, cyclopropane, and trichloroethylene, are used). Products include:

Lidocaine Base (If treatment with carvedilol is to be continued perioperatively, particular care should be taken when anesthetic agents which depress myocardial function, such as ether, cyclopropane, and trichloroethylene, are used).
No products indexed under this heading.

Lidocaine Hydrochloride (If treatment with carvedilol is to be continued perioperatively, particular care should be taken when anesthetic agents which depress myocardial function, such as ether, cyclopropane, and trichloroethylene, are used).
No products indexed under this heading.

Lisinopril (Vasodilatory symptoms often do not require treatment, but it may be useful to separate the time of dosing of carvedilol from that of the ACE inhibitor or to reduce temporarily the dose of the ACE inhibitor. The dose of carvedilol should not be increased until symptoms of worsening heart failure or vasodilation have been stabilized). Products include:

Lovastatin (Amiodarone, and its metabolite desethyl amiodarone, inhibitors of CYP2C9 and P-glycoprotein, increased concentrations of the (S)-enantiomer of carvedilol by at least 2-fold. The concomitant administration of amiodarone or other CYP2C9 inhibitors, such as fluconazole, with carvedilol may enhance the β-blocking properties of carvedilol resulting in further slowing of the heart rate or cardiac conduction. Patients should be observed for signs of bradycardia or heart block, particularly when one agent is added to pre-existing treatment with the other). Products include:

Maprotiline Hydrochloride (Concomitant use with CYP2D6 enzyme inhibitors may increase carvedilol levels).
No products indexed under this heading.

Mepivacaine Hydrochloride (If treatment with carvedilol is to be continued perioperatively, particular care should be taken when anesthetic agents which depress myocardial function, such as ether, cyclopropane, and trichloroethylene, are used).
No products indexed under this heading.

Metformin Hydrochloride (Agents with β-blocking properties may enhance the blood sugar reducing effect of oral hypoglycemics. Therefore, in patients taking oral hypoglycemics, regular monitoring of blood glucose is recommended). Products include:

Methadone Hydrochloride (Concomitant use with CYP2D6 enzyme inhibitors may increase carvedilol levels).
No products indexed under this heading.

Methohexital Sodium (If treatment with carvedilol is to be continued perioperatively, particular care should be taken when anesthetic agents which depress myocardial function, such as ether, cyclopropane, and trichloroethylene, are used).
No products indexed under this heading.

Methyclothiazide (Concomitant administration with a diuretic can be expected to produce additive effects and exaggerate the orthostatic component of carvedilol action).
No products indexed under this heading.

Metolazone (Concomitant administration with a diuretic can be expected to produce additive effects and exaggerate the orthostatic component of carvedilol action).
No products indexed under this heading.

Metronidazole (Amiodarone, and its metabolite desethyl amiodarone, inhibitors of CYP2C9 and P-glycoprotein, increased concentrations of the (S)-enantiomer of carvedilol by at least

2-fold. The concomitant administration of amiodarone or other CYP2C9 inhibitors, such as fluconazole, with carvedilol may enhance the β-blocking properties of carvedilol resulting in further slowing of the heart rate or cardiac conduction. Patients should be observed for signs of bradycardia or heart block, particularly when one agent is added to pre-existing treatment with the other). Products include:

Metronidazole Benzoate (Amiodarone, and its metabolite desethyl amiodarone, inhibitors of CYP2C9 and P-glycoprotein, increased concentrations of the (S)-enantiomer of carvedilol by at least 2-fold. The concomitant administration of amiodarone or other CYP2C9 inhibitors, such as fluconazole, with carvedilol may enhance the β-blocking properties of carvedilol resulting in further slowing of the heart rate or cardiac conduction. Patients should be observed for signs of bradycardia or heart block, particularly when one agent is added to pre-existing treatment with the other).
No products indexed under this heading.

Metronidazole Hydrochloride (Amiodarone, and its metabolite desethyl amiodarone, inhibitors of CYP2C9 and P-glycoprotein, increased concentrations of the (S)-enantiomer of carvedilol by at least 2-fold. The concomitant administration of amiodarone or other CYP2C9 inhibitors, such as fluconazole, with carvedilol may enhance the β-blocking properties of carvedilol resulting in further slowing of the heart rate or cardiac conduction. Patients should be observed for signs of bradycardia or heart block, particularly when one agent is added to pre-existing treatment with the other).
No products indexed under this heading.

Metronidazole Sodium (Amiodarone, and its metabolite desethyl amiodarone, inhibitors of CYP2C9 and P-glycoprotein, increased concentrations of the (S)-enantiomer of carvedilol by at least 2-fold. The concomitant administration of amiodarone or other CYP2C9 inhibitors, such as fluconazole, with carvedilol may enhance the β-blocking properties of carvedilol resulting in further slowing of the heart rate or cardiac conduction. Patients should be observed for signs of bradycardia or heart block, particularly when one agent is added to pre-existing treatment with the other).
No products indexed under this heading.

Mibefradil Dihydrochloride (Concomitant use with CYP2D6 enzyme inhibitors may increase carvedilol levels).
No products indexed under this heading.

Miconazole (Amiodarone, and its metabolite desethyl amiodarone, inhibitors of CYP2C9 and P-glycoprotein, increased concentrations of the (S)-enantiomer of carvedilol by at least 2-fold. The concomitant administration of amiodarone or other CYP2C9 inhibitors, such as fluconazole, with carvedilol may enhance the β-blocking properties of carvedilol resulting in further slowing of the heart rate or cardiac conduction. Patients should be observed for signs of bradycardia or heart block, particularly when one agent is added to pre-existing treatment with the other).
No products indexed under this heading.

Miconazole Nitrate (Amiodarone, and its metabolite desethyl amiodarone, inhibitors of CYP2C9 and P-glycoprotein, increased concentrations of the (S)-enantiomer of carvedilol by at least 2-fold. The concomitant administration of amiodarone or other CYP2C9 inhibitors, such as fluconazole,

413 Interactions Index Coreg

with carvedilol may enhance the β-blocking properties of carvedilol resulting in further slowing of the heart rate or cardiac conduction. Patients should be observed for signs of bradycardia or heart block, particularly when one agent is added to pre-existing treatment with the other). Products include:
Vusion Ointment 3335

Midazolam Hydrochloride (If treatment with carvedilol is to be continued perioperatively, particular care should be taken when anesthetic agents which depress myocardial function, such as ether, cyclopropane, and trichloroethylene, are used).
No products indexed under this heading.

Miglitol (Agents with β-blocking properties may enhance the blood sugar reducing effect of oral hypoglycemics. Therefore, in patients taking oral hypoglycemics, regular monitoring of blood glucose is recommended).
No products indexed under this heading.

Moclobemide (Patients taking both agents with β-blocking properties and a drug that may deplete catecholamines, such as MAO Inhibitors, should be observed closely for signs of hypotension and/or severe bradycardia).
No products indexed under this heading.

Modafinil (Amiodarone, and its metabolite desethyl amiodarone, inhibitors of CYP2C9 and P-glycoprotein, increased concentrations of the (S)-enantiomer of carvedilol by at least 2-fold. The concomitant administration of amiodarone or other CYP2C9 inhibitors, such as fluconazole, with carvedilol may enhance the β-blocking properties of carvedilol resulting in further slowing of the heart rate or cardiac conduction. Patients should be observed for signs of bradycardia or heart block, particularly when one agent is added to pre-existing treatment with the other). Products include:
Provigil 983

Moexipril Hydrochloride (Vasodilatory symptoms often do not require treatment, but it may be useful to separate the time of dosing of carvedilol from that of the ACE inhibitor or to reduce temporarily the dose of the ACE inhibitor. The dose of carvedilol should not be increased until symptoms of worsening heart failure or vasodilation have been stabilized).
No products indexed under this heading.

Nateglinide (Agents with β-blocking properties may enhance the blood sugar reducing effect of oral hypoglycemics. Therefore, in patients taking oral hypoglycemics, regular monitoring of blood glucose is recommended).
No products indexed under this heading.

Nifedipine (Amiodarone, and its metabolite desethyl amiodarone, inhibitors of CYP2C9 and P-glycoprotein, increased concentrations of the (S)-enantiomer of carvedilol by at least 2-fold. The concomitant administration of amiodarone or other CYP2C9 inhibitors, such as fluconazole, with carvedilol may enhance the β-blocking properties of carvedilol resulting in further slowing of the heart rate or cardiac conduction. Patients should be observed for signs of bradycardia or heart block, particularly when one agent is added to pre-existing treatment with the other).
No products indexed under this heading.

Nisoldipine (As with other agents with β-blocking properties, if carvedilol is to be administered orally with calcium channel blockers of the verapamil or diltiazem type, it is recommended that ECG and blood pressure be monitored).
No products indexed under this heading.

Norepinephrine Bitartrate (Patients on β-blocker therapy and with a history of severe anaphylactic reactions to a variety of allergens may be unresponsive to the usual doses of epinephrine used to treat allergic reactions).
No products indexed under this heading.

Norepinephrine Hydrochloride (Patients on β-blocker therapy and with a history of severe anaphylactic reactions to a variety of allergens may be unresponsive to the usual doses of epinephrine used to treat allergic reactions).
No products indexed under this heading.

Nortriptyline Hydrochloride (Concomitant use with CYP2D6 enzyme inhibitors may increase carvedilol levels).
No products indexed under this heading.

Omeprazole (Amiodarone, and its metabolite desethyl amiodarone, inhibitors of CYP2C9 and P-glycoprotein, increased concentrations of the (S)-enantiomer of carvedilol by at least 2-fold. The concomitant administration of amiodarone or other CYP2C9 inhibitors, such as fluconazole, with carvedilol may enhance the β-blocking properties of carvedilol resulting in further slowing of the heart rate or cardiac conduction. Patients should be observed for signs of bradycardia or heart block, particularly when one agent is added to pre-existing treatment with the other).
No products indexed under this heading.

Oxiconazole Nitrate (Amiodarone, and its metabolite desethyl amiodarone, inhibitors of CYP2C9 and P-glycoprotein, increased concentrations of the (S)-enantiomer of carvedilol by at least 2-fold. The concomitant administration of amiodarone or other CYP2C9 inhibitors, such as fluconazole, with carvedilol may enhance the β-blocking properties of carvedilol resulting in further slowing of the heart rate or cardiac conduction. Patients should be observed for signs of bradycardia or heart block, particularly when one agent is added to pre-existing treatment with the other).
No products indexed under this heading.

Pargyline Hydrochloride (Patients taking both agents with β-blocking properties and a drug that may deplete catecholamines, such as MAO Inhibitors, should be observed closely for signs of hypotension and/or severe bradycardia).
No products indexed under this heading.

Paroxetine (Concomitant use with CYP2D6 enzyme inhibitors, such as paroxetine, may increase carvedilol levels).
No products indexed under this heading.

Paroxetine Hydrochloride (Concomitant use with CYP2D6 enzyme inhibitors, such as paroxetine, may increase carvedilol levels). Products include:
Paroxetine CR 2361
Paroxetine ER 2371
Paxil 1586
Paxil CR 1596

Paroxetine Mesylate (Concomitant use with CYP2D6 enzyme inhibitors, such as paroxetine, may increase carvedilol levels).
No products indexed under this heading.

Perindopril Erbumine (Vasodilatory symptoms often do not require treatment, but it may be useful to separate the time of dosing of carvedilol from that of the ACE inhibitor or to reduce temporarily the dose of the ACE inhibitor. The dose of carvedilol should not be increased until symptoms of worsening heart failure or vasodilation have been stabilized).
No products indexed under this heading.

Perphenazine (Concomitant use with CYP2D6 enzyme inhibitors may increase carvedilol levels).
No products indexed under this heading.

Phenelzine Sulfate (Patients taking both agents with β-blocking properties and a drug that may deplete catecholamines, such as MAO Inhibitors, should be observed closely for signs of hypotension and/or severe bradycardia).
No products indexed under this heading.

Phenylbutazone (Amiodarone, and its metabolite desethyl amiodarone, inhibitors of CYP2C9 and P-glycoprotein, increased concentrations of the (S)-enantiomer of carvedilol by at least 2-fold. The concomitant administration of amiodarone or other CYP2C9 inhibitors, such as fluconazole, with carvedilol may enhance the β-blocking properties of carvedilol resulting in further slowing of the heart rate or cardiac conduction. Patients should be observed for signs of bradycardia or heart block, particularly when one agent is added to pre-existing treatment with the other).
No products indexed under this heading.

Pioglitazone Hydrochloride (Agents with β-blocking properties may enhance the blood sugar reducing effect of oral hypoglycemics. Therefore, in patients taking oral hypoglycemics, regular monitoring of blood glucose is recommended). Products include:
ActoPlus 3338
Actos 3345
Duetact 3354

Polythiazide (Concomitant administration with a diuretic can be expected to produce additive effects and exaggerate the orthostatic component of carvedilol action).
No products indexed under this heading.

Prilocaine (If treatment with carvedilol is to be continued perioperatively, particular care should be taken when anesthetic agents which depress myocardial function, such as ether, cyclopropane, and trichloroethylene, are used).
No products indexed under this heading.

Prilocaine Hydrochloride (If treatment with carvedilol is to be continued perioperatively, particular care should be taken when anesthetic agents which depress myocardial function, such as ether, cyclopropane, and trichloroethylene, are used).
No products indexed under this heading.

Procaine (If treatment with carvedilol is to be continued perioperatively, particular care should be taken when anesthetic agents which depress myocardial function, such as ether, cyclopropane, and trichloroethylene, are used).
No products indexed under this heading.

Procaine Hydrochloride (If treatment with carvedilol is to be continued perioperatively, particular care should be taken when anesthetic agents which depress myocardial function, such as ether, cyclopropane, and trichloroethylene, are used).
No products indexed under this heading.

Procarbazine Hydrochloride (Patients taking both agents with β-blocking properties and a drug that may deplete catecholamines, such as MAO Inhibitors, should be observed closely for signs of hypotension and/or severe bradycardia).
No products indexed under this heading.

Propafenone Hydrochloride (Concomitant use with CYP2D6 enzyme inhibitors, such as propafenone, may increase carvedilol levels). Products include:
Rythmol 1648
Rythmol SR 1652

Proparacaine Hydrochloride (If treatment with carvedilol is to be continued perioperatively, particular care should be taken when anesthetic agents which depress myocardial function, such as ether, cyclopropane, and trichloroethylene, are used).
No products indexed under this heading.

Propofol (If treatment with carvedilol is to be continued perioperatively, particular care should be taken when anesthetic agents which depress myocardial function, such as ether, cyclopropane, and trichloroethylene, are used).
No products indexed under this heading.

Propoxyphene Hydrochloride (Concomitant use with CYP2D6 enzyme inhibitors may increase carvedilol levels).
No products indexed under this heading.

Propoxyphene Napsylate (Concomitant use with CYP2D6 enzyme inhibitors may increase carvedilol levels).
No products indexed under this heading.

Protriptyline Hydrochloride (Concomitant use with CYP2D6 enzyme inhibitors may increase carvedilol levels).
No products indexed under this heading.

Quinacrine Hydrochloride (Concomitant use with CYP2D6 enzyme inhibitors may increase carvedilol levels).
No products indexed under this heading.

Quinapril Hydrochloride (Vasodilatory symptoms often do not require treatment, but it may be useful to separate the time of dosing of carvedilol from that of the ACE inhibitor or to reduce temporarily the dose of the ACE inhibitor. The dose of carvedilol should not be increased until symptoms of worsening heart failure or vasodilation have been stabilized).
No products indexed under this heading.

Quinidine (Concomitant use with CYP2D6 enzyme inhibitors, such as quinidine, may increase carvedilol levels).
No products indexed under this heading.

Quinidine Gluconate (Concomitant use with CYP2D6 enzyme inhibitors, such as quinidine, may increase carvedilol levels).
No products indexed under this heading.

Quinidine Hydrochloride (Concomitant use with CYP2D6 enzyme inhibitors, such as quinidine, may increase carvedilol levels).
No products indexed under this heading.

Quinidine Polygalacturonate (Concomitant use with CYP2D6 enzyme inhibitors, such as quinidine, may increase carvedilol levels).
No products indexed under this heading.

Quinidine Sulfate (Concomitant use with CYP2D6 enzyme inhibitors, such as quinidine, may increase carvedilol levels).
No products indexed under this heading.

Ramipril (Vasodilatory symptoms often do not require treatment, but it may be useful to separate the time of dosing of carvedilol from that of the ACE inhibitor or to reduce temporarily the dose of the ACE inhibitor. The dose of carvedilol should not be increased until symptoms of worsening heart failure or vasodilation have been stabilized).
No products indexed under this heading.

Ranitidine Bismuth Citrate (Concomitant use with CYP2D6 enzyme inhibitors may increase carvedilol levels).
No products indexed under this heading.

Ranitidine Hydrochloride (Concomitant use with CYP2D6 enzyme inhibitors may increase carvedilol levels). Products include:

IMPORTANT NOTE: Always consult each drug listing in the patient's regimen for possible interactions.

Coreg **Interactions Index** 414

Zantac 1737
Zantac Injection 1732
Zantac Pharmacy 1735

Rasagiline Mesylate (Patients taking both agents with β-blocking properties and a drug that may deplete catecholamines, such as MAO Inhibitors, should be observed closely for signs of hypotension and/or severe bradycardia). Products include:
Azilect 3383

Rauwolfia Serpentina (Patients taking both agents with β-blocking properties and a drug that can deplete catecholamines should be observed closely for signs of hypotension and/or severe bradycardia).
No products indexed under this heading.

Remifentanil Hydrochloride (If treatment with carvedilol is to be continued perioperatively, particular care should be taken when anesthetic agents which depress myocardial function, such as ether, cyclopropane, and trichloroethylene, are used).
No products indexed under this heading.

Repaglinide (Agents with β-blocking properties may enhance the blood sugar reducing effect of oral hypoglycemics. Therefore, in patients taking oral hypoglycemics, regular monitoring of blood glucose is recommended).
No products indexed under this heading.

Rescinnamine (Patients taking both agents with β-blocking properties and a drug that can deplete catecholamines should be observed closely for signs of hypotension and/or severe bradycardia).
No products indexed under this heading.

Reserpine (Patients taking both agents with β-blocking properties and a drug that can deplete catecholamines, such as reserpine, should be observed closely for signs of hypotension and/or severe bradycardia).
No products indexed under this heading.

Rifampin (In a pharmacokinetic study conducted in 8 healthy males, rifampin (600 mg for 12 days) decreased the AUC and C_{max} of carvedilol by about 70%).
No products indexed under this heading.

Ritonavir (Amiodarone, and its metabolite desethyl amiodarone, inhibitors of CYP2C9 and P-glycoprotein, increased concentrations of the (S)-enantiomer of carvedilol by at least 2-fold. The concomitant administration of amiodarone or other CYP2C9 inhibitors, such as fluconazole, with carvedilol may enhance the β-blocking properties of carvedilol resulting in further slowing of the heart rate or cardiac conduction. Patients should be observed for signs of bradycardia or heart block, particularly when one agent is added to pre-existing treatment with the other). Products include:
Kaletra 458
Norvir 509

Ropivacaine Hydrochloride (If treatment with carvedilol is to be continued perioperatively, particular care should be taken when anesthetic agents which depress myocardial function, such as ether, cyclopropane, and trichloroethylene, are used).
No products indexed under this heading.

Rosiglitazone Maleate (Agents with β-blocking properties may enhance the blood sugar reducing effect of oral hypoglycemics. Therefore, in patients taking oral hypoglycemics, regular monitoring of blood glucose is recommended). Products include:
Avandamet 1345
Avandaryl 1356
Avandia 1366

Selegiline (Patients taking both agents with β-blocking properties and a drug that may deplete catecholamines, such as MAO Inhibitors, should be observed closely for signs of hypotension and/or severe bradycardia). Products include:
Emsam 3623

Selegiline Hydrochloride (Patients taking both agents with β-blocking properties and a drug that may deplete catecholamines, such as MAO Inhibitors, should be observed closely for signs of hypotension and/or severe bradycardia). Products include:
Eldepryl 3312

Sertraline Hydrochloride (Amiodarone, and its metabolite desethyl amiodarone, inhibitors of CYP2C9 and P-glycoprotein, increased concentrations of the (S)-enantiomer of carvedilol by at least 2-fold. The concomitant administration of amiodarone or other CYP2C9 inhibitors, such as fluconazole, with carvedilol may enhance the β-blocking properties of carvedilol resulting in further slowing of the heart rate or cardiac conduction. Patients should be observed for signs of bradycardia or heart block, particularly when one agent is added to pre-existing treatment with the other).
No products indexed under this heading.

Sildenafil Citrate (Amiodarone, and its metabolite desethyl amiodarone, inhibitors of CYP2C9 and P-glycoprotein, increased concentrations of the (S)-enantiomer of carvedilol by at least 2-fold. The concomitant administration of amiodarone or other CYP2C9 inhibitors, such as fluconazole, with carvedilol may enhance the β-blocking properties of carvedilol resulting in further slowing of the heart rate or cardiac conduction. Patients should be observed for signs of bradycardia or heart block, particularly when one agent is added to pre-existing treatment with the other).
No products indexed under this heading.

Sitagliptin Phosphate (Agents with β-blocking properties may enhance the blood sugar reducing effect of oral hypoglycemics. Therefore, in patients taking oral hypoglycemics, regular monitoring of blood glucose is recommended). Products include:
Janumet 2188
Januvia 2196

Spirapril Hydrochloride (Vasodilatory symptoms often do not require treatment, but it may be useful to separate the time of dosing of carvedilol from that of the ACE inhibitor or to reduce temporarily the dose of the ACE inhibitor. The dose of carvedilol should not be increased until symptoms of worsening heart failure or vasodilation have been stabilized).
No products indexed under this heading.

Spironolactone (Concomitant administration with a diuretic can be expected to produce additive effects and exaggerate the orthostatic component of carvedilol action).
No products indexed under this heading.

Sufentanil Citrate (If treatment with carvedilol is to be continued perioperatively, particular care should be taken when anesthetic agents which depress myocardial function, such as ether, cyclopropane, and trichloroethylene, are used).
No products indexed under this heading.

Sulfacytine (Amiodarone, and its metabolite desethyl amiodarone, inhibitors of CYP2C9 and P-glycoprotein, increased concentrations of the (S)-enantiomer of carvedilol by at least 2-fold. The concomitant administration of amiodarone or other CYP2C9 inhibitors, such as fluconazole, with carvedilol may enhance the β-blocking properties of carvedilol resulting in further slowing of the heart rate or cardiac conduction. Patients should be observed for signs of bradycardia or heart block, particularly when one agent is added to pre-existing treatment with the other).
No products indexed under this heading.

Sulfamethizole (Amiodarone, and its metabolite desethyl amiodarone, inhibitors of CYP2C9 and P-glycoprotein, increased concentrations of the (S)-enantiomer of carvedilol by at least 2-fold. The concomitant administration of amiodarone or other CYP2C9 inhibitors, such as fluconazole, with carvedilol may enhance the β-blocking properties of carvedilol resulting in further slowing of the heart rate or cardiac conduction. Patients should be observed for signs of bradycardia or heart block, particularly when one agent is added to pre-existing treatment with the other).
No products indexed under this heading.

Sulfamethoxazole (Amiodarone, and its metabolite desethyl amiodarone, inhibitors of CYP2C9 and P-glycoprotein, increased concentrations of the (S)-enantiomer of carvedilol by at least 2-fold. The concomitant administration of amiodarone or other CYP2C9 inhibitors, such as fluconazole, with carvedilol may enhance the β-blocking properties of carvedilol resulting in further slowing of the heart rate or cardiac conduction. Patients should be observed for signs of bradycardia or heart block, particularly when one agent is added to pre-existing treatment with the other).
No products indexed under this heading.

Sulfasalazine (Amiodarone, and its metabolite desethyl amiodarone, inhibitors of CYP2C9 and P-glycoprotein, increased concentrations of the (S)-enantiomer of carvedilol by at least 2-fold. The concomitant administration of amiodarone or other CYP2C9 inhibitors, such as fluconazole, with carvedilol may enhance the β-blocking properties of carvedilol resulting in further slowing of the heart rate or cardiac conduction. Patients should be observed for signs of bradycardia or heart block, particularly when one agent is added to pre-existing treatment with the other).
No products indexed under this heading.

Sulfinpyrazone (Amiodarone, and its metabolite desethyl amiodarone, inhibitors of CYP2C9 and P-glycoprotein, increased concentrations of the (S)-enantiomer of carvedilol by at least 2-fold. The concomitant administration of amiodarone or other CYP2C9 inhibitors, such as fluconazole, with carvedilol may enhance the β-blocking properties of carvedilol resulting in further slowing of the heart rate or cardiac conduction. Patients should be observed for signs of bradycardia or heart block, particularly when one agent is added to pre-existing treatment with the other).
No products indexed under this heading.

Sulfisoxazole Acetyl (Amiodarone, and its metabolite desethyl amiodarone, inhibitors of CYP2C9 and P-glycoprotein, increased concentrations of the (S)-enantiomer of carvedilol by at least 2-fold. The concomitant administration of amiodarone or other CYP2C9 inhibitors, such as fluconazole, with carvedilol may enhance the β-blocking properties of carvedilol resulting in further slowing of the heart rate or cardiac conduction. Patients should be observed for signs of bradycardia or heart block, particularly when one agent is added to pre-existing treatment with the other).
No products indexed under this heading.

Sulfisoxazole Diolamine (Amiodarone, and its metabolite desethyl amiodarone, inhibitors of CYP2C9 and P-glycoprotein, increased concentrations of the (S)-enantiomer of carvedilol by at least 2-fold. The concomitant administration of amiodarone or other CYP2C9 inhibitors, such as fluconazole, with carvedilol may enhance the β-blocking properties of carvedilol resulting in further slowing of the heart rate or cardiac conduction. Patients should be observed for signs of bradycardia or heart block, particularly when one agent is added to pre-existing treatment with the other).
No products indexed under this heading.

Terbinafine Hydrochloride (Concomitant use with CYP2D6 enzyme inhibitors may increase carvedilol levels).
No products indexed under this heading.

Terconazole (Amiodarone, and its metabolite desethyl amiodarone, inhibitors of CYP2C9 and P-glycoprotein, increased concentrations of the (S)-enantiomer of carvedilol by at least 2-fold. The concomitant administration of amiodarone or other CYP2C9 inhibitors, such as fluconazole, with carvedilol may enhance the β-blocking properties of carvedilol resulting in further slowing of the heart rate or cardiac conduction. Patients should be observed for signs of bradycardia or heart block, particularly when one agent is added to pre-existing treatment with the other).
No products indexed under this heading.

Tetracaine (If treatment with carvedilol is to be continued perioperatively, particular care should be taken when anesthetic agents which depress myocardial function, such as ether, cyclopropane, and trichloroethylene, are used).
No products indexed under this heading.

Tetracaine Hydrochloride (If treatment with carvedilol is to be continued perioperatively, particular care should be taken when anesthetic agents which depress myocardial function, such as ether, cyclopropane, and trichloroethylene, are used).
No products indexed under this heading.

Thiamylal Sodium (If treatment with carvedilol is to be continued perioperatively, particular care should be taken when anesthetic agents which depress myocardial function, such as ether, cyclopropane, and trichloroethylene, are used).
No products indexed under this heading.

Thioridazine Hydrochloride (Concomitant use with CYP2D6 enzyme inhibitors may increase carvedilol levels). Products include:
Thioridazine Hydrochloride 2384

Ticlopidine Hydrochloride (Amiodarone, and its metabolite desethyl amiodarone, inhibitors of CYP2C9 and P-glycoprotein, increased concentrations of the (S)-enantiomer of carvedilol by at least 2-fold. The concomitant administration of amiodarone or other CYP2C9 inhibitors, such as fluconazole, with carvedilol may enhance the β-blocking properties of carvedilol resulting in further slowing of the heart rate or cardiac conduction. Patients should be observed for signs of bradycardia or heart block, particularly when one agent is added to pre-existing treatment with the other).
No products indexed under this heading.

Tolazamide (Agents with β-blocking properties may enhance the blood sugar reducing effect of oral hypoglycemics. Therefore, in patients taking oral hypoglycemics, regular monitoring of blood glucose is recommended).
No products indexed under this heading.

Tolbutamide (Agents with β-blocking properties may enhance the blood sugar reducing effect of oral hypoglycemics. Therefore, in patients taking oral hypoglycemics, regular monitoring of blood glucose is recommended).
No products indexed under this heading.

Tolbutamide Sodium (Amiodarone, and its metabolite desethyl amiodarone, inhibitors of CYP2C9 and P-glycoprotein, increased concentrations of the (S)-enantiomer of carvedilol by at least 2-fold. The concomitant administration of amiodarone or other CYP2C9 inhibitors, such as fluconazole, with carvedilol may enhance the β-blocking properties of carvedilol resulting in further slowing of the heart rate or cardiac conduction. Patients should be observed for signs of bradycardia or heart block, particularly when one agent is added to pre-existing treatment with the other).
No products indexed under this heading.

Torsemide (Concomitant administration with a diuretic can be expected to produce additive effects and exaggerate the orthostatic component of carvedilol action).
No products indexed under this heading.

Trandolapril (Vasodilatory symptoms often do not require treatment, but it may be useful to separate the time of dosing of carvedilol from that of the ACE inhibitor or to reduce temporarily the dose of the ACE inhibitor. The dose of carvedilol should not be increased until symptoms of worsening heart failure or vasodilation have been stabilized). Products include:
Mavik 489
Tarka 534

Tranylcypromine Sulfate (Patients taking both agents with β-blocking properties and a drug that may deplete catecholamines, such as MAO Inhibitors, should be observed closely for signs of hypotension and/or severe bradycardia). Products include:
Parnate 1584

Triamterene (Concomitant administration with a diuretic can be expected to produce additive effects and exaggerate the orthostatic component of carvedilol action). Products include:
Dyazide 1429
Dyrenium 3495

Trichloroethylene (If treatment with carvedilol is to be continued perioperatively, particular care should be taken when anesthetic agents which depress myocardial function, such as trichloroethylene, are used).
No products indexed under this heading.

Trimipramine Maleate (Concomitant use with CYP2D6 enzyme inhibitors may increase carvedilol levels).
No products indexed under this heading.

Troglitazone (Agents with β-blocking properties may enhance the blood sugar reducing effect of oral hypoglycemics. Therefore, in patients taking oral hypoglycemics, regular monitoring of blood glucose is recommended).
No products indexed under this heading.

Vardenafil Hydrochloride (Amiodarone, and its metabolite desethyl amiodarone, inhibitors of CYP2C9 and P-glycoprotein, increased concentrations of the (S)-enantiomer of carvedilol by at least 2-fold. The concomitant administration of amiodarone or other CYP2C9 inhibitors, such as fluconazole, with carvedilol may enhance the β-blocking properties of carvedilol resulting in further slowing of the heart rate or cardiac conduction. Patients should be observed for signs of bradycardia or heart block, particularly when one agent is added to pre-existing treatment with the other). Products include:
Levitra 3157

Verapamil Hydrochloride (Conduction disturbance (rarely with hemodynamic compromise) has been observed when carvedilol is co-administered with diltiazem. As with other agents with β-blocking properties, if carvedilol is to be administered with calcium channel blockers of the verapamil or diltiazem type, it is recommended that ECG and blood pressure be monitored). Products include:
Tarka 534

Voriconazole (Amiodarone, and its metabolite desethyl amiodarone, inhibitors of CYP2C9 and P-glycoprotein, increased concentrations of the (S)-enantiomer of carvedilol by at least 2-fold. The concomitant administration of amiodarone or other CYP2C9 inhibitors, such as fluconazole, with carvedilol may enhance the β-blocking properties of carvedilol resulting in further slowing of the heart rate or cardiac conduction. Patients should be observed for signs of bradycardia or heart block, particularly when one agent is added to pre-existing treatment with the other).
No products indexed under this heading.

Zafirlukast (Amiodarone, and its metabolite desethyl amiodarone, inhibitors of CYP2C9 and P-glycoprotein, increased concentrations of the (S)-enantiomer of carvedilol by at least 2-fold. The concomitant administration of amiodarone or other CYP2C9 inhibitors, such as fluconazole, with carvedilol may enhance the β-blocking properties of carvedilol resulting in further slowing of the heart rate or cardiac conduction. Patients should be observed for signs of bradycardia or heart block, particularly when one agent is added to pre-existing treatment with the other). Products include:
Accolate 3612

COREG CR EXTENDED-RELEASE CAPSULES

(Carvedilol Phosphate) 1416

May interact with ACE inhibitors, anesthetics, cardiac glycosides, catecholamine-depleting drugs, cytochrome p450 2c9 inhibitors (selected), cytochrome p450 2d6 inhibitors (selected), diuretics, epinephrine-containing products, insulin, monoamine oxidase inhibitors, oral hypoglycemic agents, quinidine, and certain other agents. Compounds in these categories include:

Acarbose (Agents with β-blocking properties may enhance the blood sugar reducing effect of oral hypoglycemics. Therefore, in patients taking oral hypoglycemics, regular monitoring of blood glucose is recommended).
No products indexed under this heading.

Alfentanil Hydrochloride (If treatment with carvedilol is to be continued perioperatively, particular care should be taken when anesthetic agents which depress myocardial function, such as ether, cyclopropane, and trichloroethylene, are used).
No products indexed under this heading.

Amiloride Hydrochloride (Concomitant administration with a diuretic can be expected to produce additive effects and exaggerate the orthostatic component of carvedilol action).
No products indexed under this heading.

Amiodarone Hydrochloride (Amiodarone, and its metabolite desethyl amiodarone, inhibitors of CYP2C9 and P-glycoprotein, increased concentrations of the (S)-enantiomer of carvedilol by at least 2-fold. The concomitant administration of amiodarone or other CYP2C9 inhibitors, such as fluconazole, with carvedilol may enhance the β-blocking properties of carvedilol resulting in further slowing of the heart rate or cardiac conduction. Patients should be observed for signs of bradycardia or heart block, particularly when one agent is added to pre-existing treatment with the other).
No products indexed under this heading.

Amitriptyline Hydrochloride (Concomitant use with CYP2D6 enzyme inhibitors may increase carvedilol levels).
No products indexed under this heading.

Amoxapine (Concomitant use with CYP2D6 enzyme inhibitors may increase carvedilol levels).
No products indexed under this heading.

Anastrozole (Amiodarone, and its metabolite desethyl amiodarone, inhibitors of CYP2C9 and P-glycoprotein, increased concentrations of the (S)-enantiomer of carvedilol by at least 2-fold. The concomitant administration of amiodarone or other CYP2C9 inhibitors, such as fluconazole, with carvedilol may enhance the β-blocking properties of carvedilol resulting in further slowing of the heart rate or cardiac conduction. Patients should be observed for signs of bradycardia or heart block, particularly when one agent is added to pre-existing treatment with the other).
No products indexed under this heading.

Articaine Hydrochloride (If treatment with carvedilol is to be continued perioperatively, particular care should be taken when anesthetic agents which depress myocardial function, such as ether, cyclopropane, and trichloroethylene, are used).
No products indexed under this heading.

Benazepril Hydrochloride (Vasodilatory symptoms often do not require treatment, but it may be useful to separate the time of dosing of carvedilol from that of the ACE inhibitor or to reduce temporarily the dose of the ACE inhibitor. The dose of carvedilol should not be increased until symptoms of worsening heart failure or vasodilation have been stabilized).
No products indexed under this heading.

Bendroflumethiazide (Concomitant administration with a diuretic can be expected to produce additive effects and exaggerate the orthostatic component of carvedilol action).
No products indexed under this heading.

Benzocaine (If treatment with carvedilol is to be continued perioperatively, particular care should be taken when anesthetic agents which depress myocardial function, such as ether, cyclopropane, and trichloroethylene, are used).
No products indexed under this heading.

Bumetanide (Concomitant administration with a diuretic can be expected to produce additive effects and exaggerate the orthostatic component of carvedilol action).
No products indexed under this heading.

Bupivacaine Hydrochloride (If treatment with carvedilol is to be continued perioperatively, particular care should be taken when anesthetic agents which depress myocardial function, such as ether, cyclopropane, and trichloroethylene, are used).
No products indexed under this heading.

Bupropion Hydrochloride (Concomitant use with CYP2D6 enzyme inhibitors may increase carvedilol levels). Products include:
Aplenzin 2948
Wellbutrin 1719
Wellbutrin SR 1725
Zyban 1762

Captopril (Vasodilatory symptoms often do not require treatment, but it may be useful to separate the time of dosing of carvedilol from that of the ACE inhibitor or to reduce temporarily the dose of the ACE inhibitor. The dose of carvedilol should not be increased until symptoms of worsening heart failure or vasodilation have been stabilized). Products include:
Captopril 2341

Celecoxib (Concomitant use with CYP2D6 enzyme inhibitors may increase carvedilol levels). Products include:
Celebrex 3272

Chloramphenicol (Amiodarone, and its metabolite desethyl amiodarone, inhibitors of CYP2C9 and P-glycoprotein, increased concentrations of the (S)-enantiomer of carvedilol by at least 2-fold. The concomitant administration of amiodarone or other CYP2C9 inhibitors, such as fluconazole, with carvedilol may enhance the β-blocking properties of carvedilol resulting in further slowing of the heart rate or cardiac conduction. Patients should be observed for signs of bradycardia or heart block, particularly when one agent is added to pre-existing treatment with the other).
No products indexed under this heading.

Chloramphenicol Palmitate (Amiodarone, and its metabolite desethyl amiodarone, inhibitors of CYP2C9 and P-glycoprotein, increased concentrations of the (S)-enantiomer of carvedilol by at least 2-fold. The concomitant administration of amiodarone or other CYP2C9 inhibitors, such as fluconazole, with carvedilol may enhance the β-blocking properties of carvedilol resulting in further slowing of the heart rate or cardiac conduction. Patients should be observed for signs of bradycardia or heart block, particularly when one agent is added to pre-existing treatment with the other).
No products indexed under this heading.

Chloramphenicol Sodium Succinate (Amiodarone, and its metabolite desethyl amiodarone, inhibitors of CYP2C9 and P-glycoprotein, increased concentrations of the (S)-enantiomer of carvedilol by at least 2-fold. The concomitant administration of amiodarone or other CYP2C9 inhibitors, such as fluconazole, with carvedilol may enhance the β-blocking properties of carvedilol resulting in further slowing of the heart rate or cardiac conduction. Patients should be observed for signs of bradycardia or heart block, particularly when one agent is added to pre-existing treatment with the other).
No products indexed under this heading.

Chloroprocaine Hydrochloride (If treatment with carvedilol is to be continued perioperatively, particular care should be taken when anesthetic agents which depress myocardial function, such as ether, cyclopropane, and trichloroethylene, are used).
No products indexed under this heading.

Chloroquine (Concomitant use with CYP2D6 enzyme inhibitors may increase carvedilol levels).
No products indexed under this heading.

Chloroquine Hydrochloride (Concomitant use with CYP2D6 enzyme inhibitors may increase carvedilol levels).
No products indexed under this heading.

Chloroquine Phosphate (Concomitant use with CYP2D6 enzyme inhibitors may increase carvedilol levels).
No products indexed under this heading.

Chlorothiazide (Concomitant administration with a diuretic can be expected to produce additive effects and exaggerate the orthostatic component of carvedilol action).
No products indexed under this heading.

IMPORTANT NOTE: Always consult each drug listing in the patient's regimen for possible interactions.

Chlorothiazide Sodium (Concomitant administration with a diuretic can be expected to produce additive effects and exaggerate the orthostatic component of carvedilol action). Products include:

Diuril Intravenous **2009**

Chlorpheniramine (Concomitant use with CYP2D6 enzyme inhibitors may increase carvedilol levels).

No products indexed under this heading.

Chlorpheniramine Maleate (Concomitant use with CYP2D6 enzyme inhibitors may increase carvedilol levels).

No products indexed under this heading.

Chlorpheniramine Polistirex (Concomitant use with CYP2D6 enzyme inhibitors may increase carvedilol levels). Products include:

Tussionex **3443**

Chlorpheniramine Tannate (Concomitant use with CYP2D6 enzyme inhibitors may increase carvedilol levels).

No products indexed under this heading.

Chlorpropamide (Agents with β-blocking properties may enhance the blood sugar reducing effect of oral hypoglycemics. Therefore, in patients taking oral hypoglycemics, regular monitoring of blood glucose is recommended).

No products indexed under this heading.

Chlorthalidone (Concomitant administration with a diuretic can be expected to produce additive effects and exaggerate the orthostatic component of carvedilol action). Products include:

Clorpres **2344**

Cimetidine (In a pharmacokinetic study conducted in 10 healthy male subjects, cimetidine (1000 mg/day) increased the steady state AUC of carvedilol by 30% with no change in C_{max}).

No products indexed under this heading.

Cimetidine Hydrochloride (In a pharmacokinetic study conducted in 10 healthy male subjects, cimetidine (1000 mg/day) increased the steady state AUC of carvedilol by 30% with no change in C_{max}).

No products indexed under this heading.

Citalopram Hydrobromide (Concomitant use with CYP2D6 enzyme inhibitors may increase carvedilol levels). Products include:

Celexa **1153**

Clomipramine Hydrochloride (Concomitant use with CYP2D6 enzyme inhibitors may increase carvedilol levels).

No products indexed under this heading.

Clonidine (Concomitant administration of clonidine with agents with β-blocking properties may potentiate blood-pressure- and heart-rate-lowering effects. When concomitant treatment with agents with β-blocking properties and clonidine terminated, the β-blocking agent should be discontinued first. Clonidine therapy can then be discontinued several days later by gradually decreasing the dosage). Products include:

Catapres-TTS **884**

Clonidine Hydrochloride (Concomitant administration of clonidine with agents with β-blocking properties may potentiate blood-pressure- and heart-rate-lowering effects. When concomitant treatment with agents with β-blocking properties and clonidine terminated, the β-blocking agent should be discontinued first. Clonidine therapy can then be discontinued several days later by gradually decreasing the dosage). Products include:

Clorpres **2344**

Clopidogrel Bisulfate (Amiodarone, and its metabolite desethyl amiodarone, inhibitors of CYP2C9 and P-glycoprotein, increased concentrations of the (S)-enantiomer of carvedilol by at least 2-fold. The concomitant administration of amiodarone or other CYP2C9 inhibitors, such as fluconazole, with carvedilol may enhance the β-blocking properties of carvedilol resulting in further slowing of the heart rate or cardiac conduction. Patients should be observed for signs of bradycardia or heart block, particularly when one agent is added to pre-existing treatment with the other). Products include:

Plavix **3027**

Clopidogrel Hydrogen Sulfate (Amiodarone, and its metabolite desethyl amiodarone, inhibitors of CYP2C9 and P-glycoprotein, increased concentrations of the (S)-enantiomer of carvedilol by at least 2-fold. The concomitant administration of amiodarone or other CYP2C9 inhibitors, such as fluconazole, with carvedilol may enhance the β-blocking properties of carvedilol resulting in further slowing of the heart rate or cardiac conduction. Patients should be observed for signs of bradycardia or heart block, particularly when one agent is added to pre-existing treatment with the other).

No products indexed under this heading.

Clotrimazole (Amiodarone, and its metabolite desethyl amiodarone, inhibitors of CYP2C9 and P-glycoprotein, increased concentrations of the (S)-enantiomer of carvedilol by at least 2-fold. The concomitant administration of amiodarone or other CYP2C9 inhibitors, such as fluconazole, with carvedilol may enhance the β-blocking properties of carvedilol resulting in further slowing of the heart rate or cardiac conduction. Patients should be observed for signs of bradycardia or heart block, particularly when one agent is added to pre-existing treatment with the other). Products include:

Lotrisone **3163**

Cocaine Hydrochloride (If treatment with carvedilol is to be continued perioperatively, particular care should be taken when anesthetic agents which depress myocardial function, such as ether, cyclopropane, and trichloroethylene, are used).

No products indexed under this heading.

Cyclopropane (If treatment with carvedilol is to be continued perioperatively, particular care should be taken when anesthetic agents which depress myocardial funciton, such as cyclopropane, are used).

No products indexed under this heading.

Cyclosporine (Modest increases in mean trough cyclosporine concentrations were observed following initiation of carvedilol treatment in 21 renal transplant patients. In about 30% of patients, the dose of cyclosporine had to be reduced in order to maintain cyclosporine concentrations within the therapeutic range. On the average for the group, the dose of cyclosporine was reduced about 20%. Due to wide interindividual variability in the dose adjustment required, it is recommended that cyclosporine concentrations be monitored closely after initiation of carvedilol therapy and that the dose of cyclosporine be adjusted as appropriate). Products include:

Gengraf **440**
Neoral Oral Solution **2496**
Neoral Capsules **2496**
Restasis **605**

Deserpidine (Patients taking both agents with β-blocking properties and a drug that can deplete catecholamines should be observed closely for signs of hypotension and/or severe bradycardia).

No products indexed under this heading.

Desipramine Hydrochloride (Concomitant use with CYP2D6 enzyme inhibitors may increase carvedilol levels).

No products indexed under this heading.

Deslanoside (Both digitalis glycosides and β-blockers slow atrioventricular conduction and decrease heart rate. Concomitant use can increase the risk of bradycardia).

No products indexed under this heading.

Dibucaine (If treatment with carvedilol is to be continued perioperatively, particular care should be taken when anesthetic agents which depress myocardial function, such as ether, cyclopropane, and trichloroethylene, are used).

No products indexed under this heading.

Dibucaine Hydrochloride (If treatment with carvedilol is to be continued perioperatively, particular care should be taken when anesthetic agents which depress myocardial function, such as ether, cyclopropane, and trichloroethylene, are used).

No products indexed under this heading.

Diclofenac Epolamine (Amiodarone, and its metabolite desethyl amiodarone, inhibitors of CYP2C9 and P-glycoprotein, increased concentrations of the (S)-enantiomer of carvedilol by at least 2-fold. The concomitant administration of amiodarone or other CYP2C9 inhibitors, such as fluconazole, with carvedilol may enhance the β-blocking properties of carvedilol resulting in further slowing of the heart rate or cardiac conduction. Patients should be observed for signs of bradycardia or heart block, particularly when one agent is added to pre-existing treatment with the other). Products include:

Flector **1839**

Diclofenac Potassium (Amiodarone, and its metabolite desethyl amiodarone, inhibitors of CYP2C9 and P-glycoprotein, increased concentrations of the (S)-enantiomer of carvedilol by at least 2-fold. The concomitant administration of amiodarone or other CYP2C9 inhibitors, such as fluconazole, with carvedilol may enhance the β-blocking properties of carvedilol resulting in further slowing of the heart rate or cardiac conduction. Patients should be observed for signs of bradycardia or heart block, particularly when one agent is added to pre-existing treatment with the other).

No products indexed under this heading.

Diclofenac Sodium (Amiodarone, and its metabolite desethyl amiodarone, inhibitors of CYP2C9 and P-glycoprotein, increased concentrations of the (S)-enantiomer of carvedilol by at least 2-fold. The concomitant administration of amiodarone or other CYP2C9 inhibitors, such as fluconazole, with carvedilol may enhance the β-blocking properties of carvedilol resulting in further slowing of the heart rate or cardiac conduction. Patients should be observed for signs of bradycardia or heart block, particularly when one agent is added to pre-existing treatment with the other).

No products indexed under this heading.

Digitalis Glycoside Preparations (Both digitalis glycosides and β-blockers slow atrioventricular conduction and decrease heart rate. Concomitant use can increase the risk of bradycardia. Digoxin concentrations are increased by about 15% when digoxin and carvedilol are administered con-

comitantly. Therefore, increased monitoring of digoxin is recommended when initiating, adjusting or discontinuing carvedilol).

No products indexed under this heading.

Digitalis Lanata (Both digitalis glycosides and β-blockers slow atrioventricular conduction and decrease heart rate. Concomitant use can increase the risk of bradycardia).

No products indexed under this heading.

Digitalis Purpurea (Both digitalis glycosides and β-blockers slow atrioventricular conduction and decrease heart rate. Concomitant use can increase the risk of bradycardia).

No products indexed under this heading.

Digitoxin (Both digitalis glycosides and β-blockers slow atrioventricular conduction and decrease heart rate. Concomitant use can increase the risk of bradycardia).

No products indexed under this heading.

Digoxin (Both digitalis glycosides and β-blockers slow atrioventricular conduction and decrease heart rate. Concomitant use can increase the risk of bradycardia. Digoxin concentrations are increased by about 15% when digoxin and carvedilol are administered concomitantly. Therefore, increased monitoring of digoxin is recommended when initiating, adjusting or discontinuing carvedilol). Products include:

Lanoxin Injection **1546**
Lanoxin Injection Pediatric **1549**
Lanoxin Tablets **1553**

Diltiazem Hydrochloride (Conduction disturbance (rarely with hemodynamic compromise) has been observed when carvedilol is co-administered with diltiazem. As with other agents with β-blocking properties, if carvedilol is to be administered with calcium channel blockers of the verapamil or diltiazem type, it is recommended that ECG and blood pressure be monitored). Products include:

Cardizem LA **423**

Diphenhydramine (Concomitant use with CYP2D6 enzyme inhibitors may increase carvedilol levels).

No products indexed under this heading.

Diphenhydramine Hydrochloride (Concomitant use with CYP2D6 enzyme inhibitors may increase carvedilol levels). Products include:

Benadryl Allergy Ultratab **2042**
Children's Benadryl Allergy Liquid **2042**

Disulfiram (Amiodarone, and its metabolite desethyl amiodarone, inhibitors of CYP2C9 and P-glycoprotein, increased concentrations of the (S)-enantiomer of carvedilol by at least 2-fold. The concomitant administration of amiodarone or other CYP2C9 inhibitors, such as fluconazole, with carvedilol may enhance the β-blocking properties of carvedilol resulting in further slowing of the heart rate or cardiac conduction. Patients should be observed for signs of bradycardia or heart block, particularly when one agent is added to pre-existing treatment with the other).

No products indexed under this heading.

Doxepin Hydrochloride (Concomitant use with CYP2D6 enzyme inhibitors may increase carvedilol levels).

No products indexed under this heading.

Efavirenz (Amiodarone, and its metabolite desethyl amiodarone, inhibitors of CYP2C9 and P-glycoprotein, increased concentrations of the (S)-enantiomer of carvedilol by at least 2-fold. The concomitant administration of amiodarone or other CYP2C9 inhibitors, such as fluconazole, with carvedilol may enhance the β-blocking properties of carvedilol resulting in further slowing of the heart rate or cardiac conduction. Patients should be observed for signs

of bradycardia or heart block, particularly when one agent is added to pre-existing treatment with the other). Products include:

Enalapril Maleate (Vasodilatory symptoms often do not require treatment, but it may be useful to separate the time of dosing of carvedilol from that of the ACE inhibitor or to reduce temporarily the dose of the ACE inhibitor. The dose of carvedilol should not be increased until symptoms of worsening heart failure or vasodilation have been stabilized).

No products indexed under this heading.

Enalaprilat (Vasodilatory symptoms often do not require treatment, but it may be useful to separate the time of dosing of carvedilol from that of the ACE inhibitor or to reduce temporarily the dose of the ACE inhibitor. The dose of carvedilol should not be increased until symptoms of worsening heart failure or vasodilation have been stabilized).

No products indexed under this heading.

Enflurane (If treatment with carvedilol is to be continued perioperatively, particular care should be taken when anesthetic agents which depress myocardial function, such as ether, cyclopropane, and trichloroethylene, are used).

No products indexed under this heading.

Epinephrine (Patients on β-blocker therapy and with a history of severe anaphylactic reactions to a variety of allergens may be unresponsive to the usual doses of epinephrine used to treat allergic reactions). Products include:

Epinephrine, Racemic (Patients on β-blocker therapy and with a history of severe anaphylactic reactions to a variety of allergens may be unresponsive to the usual doses of epinephrine used to treat allergic reactions).

No products indexed under this heading.

Epinephrine Bitartrate (Patients on β-blocker therapy and with a history of severe anaphylactic reactions to a variety of allergens may be unresponsive to the usual doses of epinephrine used to treat allergic reactions).

No products indexed under this heading.

Epinephrine Hydrochloride (Patients on β-blocker therapy and with a history of severe anaphylactic reactions to a variety of allergens may be unresponsive to the usual doses of epinephrine used to treat allergic reactions).

No products indexed under this heading.

Escitalopram Oxalate (Concomitant use with CYP2D6 enzyme inhibitors may increase carvedilol levels). Products include:

Ethacrynic Acid (Concomitant administration with a diuretic can be expected to produce additive effects and exaggerate the orthostatic component of carvedilol action).

No products indexed under this heading.

Ether (If treatment with carvedilol is to be continued perioperatively, particular care should be taken when anesthetic agents which depress myocardial function, such as ether, are used).

No products indexed under this heading.

Etidocaine Hydrochloride (If treatment with carvedilol is to be continued perioperatively, particular care should be taken when anesthetic agents which depress myocardial function, such as ether, cyclopropane, and trichloroethylene, are used).

No products indexed under this heading.

Fat (Administration of carvedilol with a high-fat meal resulted in increases (~20%) in AUC and C_{max} compared to carvedilol administered with a standard meal. Decreases in AUC (27%) and C_{max} (43%) were observed when carvedilol was administered in the fasted state compared to administration after a standard meal. Carvedilol should be taken with food).

No products indexed under this heading.

Fenofibrate (Amiodarone, and its metabolite desethyl amiodarone, inhibitors of CYP2C9 and P-glycoprotein, increased concentrations of the (S)-enantiomer of carvedilol by at least 2-fold. The concomitant administration of amiodarone or other CYP2C9 inhibitors, such as fluconazole, with carvedilol may enhance the β-blocking properties of carvedilol resulting in further slowing of the heart rate or cardiac conduction. Patients should be observed for signs of bradycardia or heart block, particularly when one agent is added to pre-existing treatment with the other). Products include:

Fentanyl Citrate (If treatment with carvedilol is to be continued perioperatively, particular care should be taken when anesthetic agents which depress myocardial function, such as ether, cyclopropane, and trichloroethylene, are used). Products include:

Fluconazole (The concomitant administration of amiodarone or other CYP2C9 inhibitors, such as fluconazole, with carvedilol may enhance the β-blocking properties of carvedilol resulting in further slowing of the heart rate or cardiac conduction. Patients should be observed for signs of bradycardia or heart block, particularly when one agent is added to pre-existing treatment with the other).

No products indexed under this heading.

Fluorouracil (Amiodarone, and its metabolite desethyl amiodarone, inhibitors of CYP2C9 and P-glycoprotein, increased concentrations of the (S)-enantiomer of carvedilol by at least 2-fold. The concomitant administration of amiodarone or other CYP2C9 inhibitors, such as fluconazole, with carvedilol may enhance the β-blocking properties of carvedilol resulting in further slowing of the heart rate or cardiac conduction. Patients should be observed for signs of bradycardia or heart block, particularly when one agent is added to pre-existing treatment with the other). Products include:

Fluoxetine (Concomitant use with CYP2D6 enzyme inhibitors, such as fluoxetine, may increase carvedilol levels).

No products indexed under this heading.

Fluoxetine Hydrochloride (Concomitant use with CYP2D6 enzyme inhibitors, such as fluoxetine, may increase carvedilol levels). Products include:

Fluphenazine Decanoate (Concomitant use with CYP2D6 enzyme inhibitors may increase carvedilol levels).

No products indexed under this heading.

Fluphenazine Enanthate (Concomitant use with CYP2D6 enzyme inhibitors may increase carvedilol levels).

No products indexed under this heading.

Fluphenazine Hydrochloride (Concomitant use with CYP2D6 enzyme inhibitors may increase carvedilol levels).

No products indexed under this heading.

Flurbiprofen (Amiodarone, and its metabolite desethyl amiodarone, inhibitors of CYP2C9 and P-glycoprotein, increased concentrations of the (S)-enantiomer of carvedilol by at least 2-fold. The concomitant administration of amiodarone or other CYP2C9 inhibitors, such as fluconazole, with carvedilol may enhance the β-blocking properties of carvedilol resulting in further slowing of the heart rate or cardiac conduction. Patients should be observed for signs of bradycardia or heart block, particularly when one agent is added to pre-existing treatment with the other).

No products indexed under this heading.

Flurbiprofen Sodium (Amiodarone, and its metabolite desethyl amiodarone, inhibitors of CYP2C9 and P-glycoprotein, increased concentrations of the (S)-enantiomer of carvedilol by at least 2-fold. The concomitant administration of amiodarone or other CYP2C9 inhibitors, such as fluconazole, with carvedilol may enhance the β-blocking properties of carvedilol resulting in further slowing of the heart rate or cardiac conduction. Patients should be observed for signs of bradycardia or heart block, particularly when one agent is added to pre-existing treatment with the other).

No products indexed under this heading.

Fluvastatin Sodium (Amiodarone, and its metabolite desethyl amiodarone, inhibitors of CYP2C9 and P-glycoprotein, increased concentrations of the (S)-enantiomer of carvedilol by at least 2-fold. The concomitant administration of amiodarone or other CYP2C9 inhibitors, such as fluconazole, with carvedilol may enhance the β-blocking properties of carvedilol resulting in further slowing of the heart rate or cardiac conduction. Patients should be observed for signs of bradycardia or heart block, particularly when one agent is added to pre-existing treatment with the other).

No products indexed under this heading.

Fluvoxamine Maleate (Amiodarone, and its metabolite desethyl amiodarone, inhibitors of CYP2C9 and P-glycoprotein, increased concentrations of the (S)-enantiomer of carvedilol by at least 2-fold. The concomitant administration of amiodarone or other CYP2C9 inhibitors, such as fluconazole, with carvedilol may enhance the β-blocking properties of carvedilol resulting in further slowing of the heart rate or cardiac conduction. Patients should be observed for signs of bradycardia or heart block, particularly when one agent is added to pre-existing treatment with the other).

No products indexed under this heading.

Fosinopril Sodium (Vasodilatory symptoms often do not require treatment, but it may be useful to separate the time of dosing of carvedilol from that of the ACE inhibitor or to reduce temporarily the dose of the ACE inhibitor. The dose of carvedilol should not be increased until symptoms of worsening heart failure or vasodilation have been stabilized).

No products indexed under this heading.

Furosemide (Concomitant administration with a diuretic can be expected to produce additive effects and exaggerate the orthostatic component of carvedilol action). Products include:

Gemfibrozil (Amiodarone, and its metabolite desethyl amiodarone, inhibitors of CYP2C9 and P-glycoprotein, increased concentrations of the (S)-enantiomer of carvedilol by at least 2-fold. The concomitant administration of amiodarone or other CYP2C9 inhibitors, such as fluconazole, with

carvedilol may enhance the β-blocking properties of carvedilol resulting in further slowing of the heart rate or cardiac conduction. Patients should be observed for signs of bradycardia or heart block, particularly when one agent is added to pre-existing treatment with the other).

No products indexed under this heading.

Glibenclamide (Agents with β-blocking properties may enhance the blood sugar reducing effect of oral hypoglycemics. Therefore, in patients taking oral hypoglycemics, regular monitoring of blood glucose is recommended).

No products indexed under this heading.

Glimepiride (Agents with β-blocking properties may enhance the blood sugar reducing effect of oral hypoglycemics. Therefore, in patients taking oral hypoglycemics, regular monitoring of blood glucose is recommended). Products include:

Glipizide (Agents with β-blocking properties may enhance the blood sugar reducing effect of oral hypoglycemics. Therefore, in patients taking oral hypoglycemics, regular monitoring of blood glucose is recommended).

No products indexed under this heading.

Glyburide (Agents with β-blocking properties may enhance the blood sugar reducing effect of oral hypoglycemics. Therefore, in patients taking oral hypoglycemics, regular monitoring of blood glucose is recommended).

No products indexed under this heading.

Guanethidine (Patients taking both agents with β-blocking properties and a drug that can deplete catecholamines should be observed closely for signs of hypotension and/or severe bradycardia).

No products indexed under this heading.

Guanethidine Monosulfate (Patients taking both agents with β-blocking properties and a drug that can deplete catecholamines should be observed closely for signs of hypotension and/or severe bradycardia).

No products indexed under this heading.

Guanethidine Sulfate (Patients taking both agents with β-blocking properties and a drug that can deplete catecholamines should be observed closely for signs of hypotension and/or severe bradycardia).

No products indexed under this heading.

Halofantrine Hydrochloride (Concomitant use with CYP2D6 enzyme inhibitors may increase carvedilol levels).

No products indexed under this heading.

Haloperidol (Concomitant use with CYP2D6 enzyme inhibitors may increase carvedilol levels).

No products indexed under this heading.

Haloperidol Decanoate (Concomitant use with CYP2D6 enzyme inhibitors may increase carvedilol levels).

No products indexed under this heading.

Haloperidol Lactate (Concomitant use with CYP2D6 enzyme inhibitors may increase carvedilol levels).

No products indexed under this heading.

Halothane (If treatment with carvedilol is to be continued perioperatively, particular care should be taken when anesthetic agents which depress myocardial function, such as ether, cyclopropane, and trichloroethylene, are used).

No products indexed under this heading.

Hydrochlorothiazide (Concomitant administration with a diuretic can be expected to produce additive effects and exaggerate the orthostatic component of carvedilol action). Products include:

IMPORTANT NOTE: Always consult each drug listing in the patient's regimen for possible interactions.

Coreg CR Interactions Index 418

Atacand HCT 700
Avalide 2956
Benicar HCT 1017
Diovan HCT 2419
Dyazide 1429
Exforge HCT 2449
Hyzaar 2162
Hyzaar 100-12.5 2162
Micardis HCT 889
Prinzide 2246
Tekturna HCT 2541
Teveten HCT 541

Hydrochlorothiazide Hydrochloride (Amiodarone, and its metabolite desethyl amiodarone, inhibitors of CYP2C9 and P-glycoprotein, increased concentrations of the (S)-enantiomer of carvedilol by at least 2-fold. The concomitant administration of amiodarone or other CYP2C9 inhibitors, such as fluconazole, with carvedilol may enhance the β-blocking properties of carvedilol resulting in further slowing of the heart rate or cardiac conduction. Patients should be observed for signs of bradycardia or heart block, particularly when one agent is added to pre-existing treatment with the other).
No products indexed under this heading.

Hydroflumethiazide (Concomitant administration with a diuretic can be expected to produce additive effects and exaggerate the orthostatic component of carvedilol action).
No products indexed under this heading.

Hydroxychloroquine Sulfate (Concomitant use with CYP2D6 enzyme inhibitors may increase carvedilol levels).
No products indexed under this heading.

Imatinib Mesylate (Amiodarone, and its metabolite desethyl amiodarone, inhibitors of CYP2C9 and P-glycoprotein, increased concentrations of the (S)-enantiomer of carvedilol by at least 2-fold. The concomitant administration of amiodarone or other CYP2C9 inhibitors, such as fluconazole, with carvedilol may enhance the β-blocking properties of carvedilol resulting in further slowing of the heart rate or cardiac conduction. Patients should be observed for signs of bradycardia or heart block, particularly when one agent is added to pre-existing treatment with the other). Products include:
Gleevec 2477

Imipramine Hydrochloride (Concomitant use with CYP2D6 enzyme inhibitors may increase carvedilol levels).
No products indexed under this heading.

Imipramine Pamoate (Concomitant use with CYP2D6 enzyme inhibitors may increase carvedilol levels).
No products indexed under this heading.

Indapamide (Concomitant administration with a diuretic can be expected to produce additive effects and exaggerate the orthostatic component of carvedilol action). Products include:
Indapamide 2356

Insulin (Agents with β-blocking properties may enhance the blood sugar reducing effect of insulin. Therefore, in patients taking insulin, regular monitoring of blood glucose is recommended).
No products indexed under this heading.

Insulin, Human, Zinc Suspension (Agents with β-blocking properties may enhance the blood sugar reducing effect of insulin. Therefore, in patients taking insulin, regular monitoring of blood glucose is recommended).
No products indexed under this heading.

Insulin, Human (rDNA origin) (Agents with β-blocking properties may enhance the blood sugar reducing effect of insulin. Therefore, in patients taking insulin, regular monitoring of blood glucose is recommended). Products include:
Exubera 2717

Insulin, Human NPH (Agents with β-blocking properties may enhance the blood sugar reducing effect of insulin. Therefore, in patients taking insulin, regular monitoring of blood glucose is recommended). Products include:
Humulin N Vial 1934

Insulin, Human Regular (Agents with β-blocking properties may enhance the blood sugar reducing effect of insulin. Therefore, in patients taking insulin, regular monitoring of blood glucose is recommended). Products include:
Humulin R 1937
Humulin R (U-500) 1939

Insulin, Human Regular and Human NPH Mixture (Agents with β-blocking properties may enhance the blood sugar reducing effect of insulin. Therefore, in patients taking insulin, regular monitoring of blood glucose is recommended). Products include:
Humulin 50/50 1930
Humulin 70/30 Vial 1931

Insulin, NPH (Agents with β-blocking properties may enhance the blood sugar reducing effect of insulin. Therefore, in patients taking insulin, regular monitoring of blood glucose is recommended).
No products indexed under this heading.

Insulin, Regular (Agents with β-blocking properties may enhance the blood sugar reducing effect of insulin. Therefore, in patients taking insulin, regular monitoring of blood glucose is recommended).
No products indexed under this heading.

Insulin, Regular and NPH mixture (Agents with β-blocking properties may enhance the blood sugar reducing effect of insulin. Therefore, in patients taking insulin, regular monitoring of blood glucose is recommended).
No products indexed under this heading.

Insulin, Zinc Crystals (Agents with β-blocking properties may enhance the blood sugar reducing effect of insulin. Therefore, in patients taking insulin, regular monitoring of blood glucose is recommended).
No products indexed under this heading.

Insulin, Zinc Suspension (Agents with β-blocking properties may enhance the blood sugar reducing effect of insulin. Therefore, in patients taking insulin, regular monitoring of blood glucose is recommended).
No products indexed under this heading.

Insulin Aspart (Agents with β-blocking properties may enhance the blood sugar reducing effect of insulin. Therefore, in patients taking insulin, regular monitoring of blood glucose is recommended).
No products indexed under this heading.

Insulin Aspart, Human (Agents with β-blocking properties may enhance the blood sugar reducing effect of insulin. Therefore, in patients taking insulin, regular monitoring of blood glucose is recommended). Products include:
NovoLog Mix 70/30 2581

Insulin Aspart, Human Regular (Agents with β-blocking properties may enhance the blood sugar reducing effect of insulin. Therefore, in patients taking insulin, regular monitoring of blood glucose is recommended). Products include:
NovoLog 2575

Insulin Aspart Protamine, Human (Agents with β-blocking properties may enhance the blood sugar reducing effect of insulin. Therefore, in patients taking insulin, regular monitoring of blood glucose is recommended). Products include:
NovoLog Mix 70/30 2581

Insulin Detemir (rDNA Origin) (Agents with β-blocking properties may enhance the blood sugar reducing effect of insulin. Therefore, in patients taking insulin, regular monitoring of blood glucose is recommended). Products include:
Levemir 2566

Insulin Glargine (Agents with β-blocking properties may enhance the blood sugar reducing effect of insulin. Therefore, in patients taking insulin, regular monitoring of blood glucose is recommended). Products include:
Lantus 2996

Insulin Glulisine (Agents with β-blocking properties may enhance the blood sugar reducing effect of insulin. Therefore, in patients taking insulin, regular monitoring of blood glucose is recommended). Products include:
Apidra 2937
Apidra SoloStar 2937

Insulin Lispro, Human (Agents with β-blocking properties may enhance the blood sugar reducing effect of insulin. Therefore, in patients taking insulin, regular monitoring of blood glucose is recommended). Products include:
Humalog 1910
Humalog Mix 1914
Humalog Mix75/25 1917

Insulin Lispro Protamine, Human (Agents with β-blocking properties may enhance the blood sugar reducing effect of insulin. Therefore, in patients taking insulin, regular monitoring of blood glucose is recommended). Products include:
Humalog Mix 1914
Humalog Mix75/25 1917

Isocarboxazid (Patients taking both agents with β-blocking properties and a drug that may deplete catecholamines, such as MAO Inhibitors, should be observed closely for signs of hypotension and/or severe bradycardia). Products include:
Marplan 3481

Isoflurane (If treatment with carvedilol is to be continued perioperatively, particular care should be taken when anesthetic agents which depress myocardial function, such as ether, cyclopropane, and trichloroethylene, are used).
No products indexed under this heading.

Isoniazid (Amiodarone, and its metabolite desethyl amiodarone, inhibitors of CYP2C9 and P-glycoprotein, increased concentrations of the (S)-enantiomer of carvedilol by at least 2-fold. The concomitant administration of amiodarone or other CYP2C9 inhibitors, such as fluconazole, with carvedilol may enhance the β-blocking properties of carvedilol resulting in further slowing of the heart rate or cardiac conduction. Patients should be observed for signs of bradycardia or heart block, particularly when one agent is added to pre-existing treatment with the other).
No products indexed under this heading.

Itraconazole (Amiodarone, and its metabolite desethyl amiodarone, inhibitors of CYP2C9 and P-glycoprotein, increased concentrations of the (S)-enantiomer of carvedilol by at least 2-fold. The concomitant administration of amiodarone or other CYP2C9 inhibitors, such as fluconazole, with carvedilol may enhance the β-blocking properties of carvedilol resulting in further slowing of the heart rate or cardiac conduction. Patients should be observed for signs of bradycardia or heart block, particularly when one agent is added to pre-existing treatment with the other).
No products indexed under this heading.

Ketamine Hydrochloride (If treatment with carvedilol is to be continued perioperatively, particular care should be taken when anesthetic agents which depress myocardial function, such as ether, cyclopropane, and trichloroethylene, are used).
No products indexed under this heading.

Ketoconazole (Amiodarone, and its metabolite desethyl amiodarone, inhibitors of CYP2C9 and P-glycoprotein, increased concentrations of the (S)-enantiomer of carvedilol by at least 2-fold. The concomitant administration of amiodarone or other CYP2C9 inhibitors, such as fluconazole, with carvedilol may enhance the β-blocking properties of carvedilol resulting in further slowing of the heart rate or cardiac conduction. Patients should be observed for signs of bradycardia or heart block, particularly when one agent is added to pre-existing treatment with the other). Products include:
Extina 3319
Xolegel 3337

Ketoprofen (Amiodarone, and its metabolite desethyl amiodarone, inhibitors of CYP2C9 and P-glycoprotein, increased concentrations of the (S)-enantiomer of carvedilol by at least 2-fold. The concomitant administration of amiodarone or other CYP2C9 inhibitors, such as fluconazole, with carvedilol may enhance the β-blocking properties of carvedilol resulting in further slowing of the heart rate or cardiac conduction. Patients should be observed for signs of bradycardia or heart block, particularly when one agent is added to pre-existing treatment with the other).
No products indexed under this heading.

Leflunomide (Amiodarone, and its metabolite desethyl amiodarone, inhibitors of CYP2C9 and P-glycoprotein, increased concentrations of the (S)-enantiomer of carvedilol by at least 2-fold. The concomitant administration of amiodarone or other CYP2C9 inhibitors, such as fluconazole, with carvedilol may enhance the β-blocking properties of carvedilol resulting in further slowing of the heart rate or cardiac conduction. Patients should be observed for signs of bradycardia or heart block, particularly when one agent is added to pre-existing treatment with the other).
No products indexed under this heading.

Levobupivacaine Hydrochloride (If treatment with carvedilol is to be continued perioperatively, particular care should be taken when anesthetic agents which depress myocardial function, such as ether, cyclopropane, and trichloroethylene, are used).
No products indexed under this heading.

Lidocaine (If treatment with carvedilol is to be continued perioperatively, particular care should be taken when anesthetic agents which depress myocardial function, such as ether, cyclopropane, and trichloroethylene, are used). Products include:
Lidoderm 1107

Lidocaine Base (If treatment with carvedilol is to be continued perioperatively, particular care should be taken when anesthetic agents which depress myocardial function, such as ether, cyclopropane, and trichloroethylene, are used).
No products indexed under this heading.

Lidocaine Hydrochloride (If treatment with carvedilol is to be continued perioperatively, particular care should be taken when anesthetic agents which depress myocardial function, such as ether, cyclopropane, and trichloroethylene, are used).
No products indexed under this heading.

Lisinopril (Vasodilatory symptoms often do not require treatment, but it may be useful to separate the time of dosing of carvedilol from that of the ACE inhibitor or to reduce temporarily the dose of the ACE inhibitor. The dose of carvedilol should not be increased until symptoms of worsening heart failure or vasodilation have been stabilized). Products include:
Prinivil 2241
Prinzide 2246

Lovastatin (Amiodarone, and its metabolite desethyl amiodarone, inhibitors of CYP2C9 and P-glycoprotein, increased concentrations of the (S)-enantiomer of carvedilol by at least 2-fold. The concomitant administration of amiodarone or other CYP2C9 inhibitors, such as fluconazole, with carvedilol may enhance the β-blocking properties of carvedilol resulting in further slowing of the heart rate or cardiac conduction. Patients should be observed for signs of bradycardia or heart block, particularly when one agent is added to pre-existing treatment with the other). Products include:
Advicor 402
Mevacor 2212

Maprotiline Hydrochloride (Concomitant use with CYP2D6 enzyme inhibitors may increase carvedilol levels).
No products indexed under this heading.

Mepivacaine Hydrochloride (If treatment with carvedilol is to be continued perioperatively, particular care should be taken when anesthetic agents which depress myocardial function, such as ether, cyclopropane, and trichloroethylene, are used).
No products indexed under this heading.

Metformin Hydrochloride (Agents with β-blocking properties may enhance the blood sugar reducing effect of oral hypoglycemics. Therefore, in patients taking oral hypoglycemics, regular monitoring of blood glucose is recommended). Products include:
ActoPlus 3338
Avandamet 1345
Janumet 2188

Methadone Hydrochloride (Concomitant use with CYP2D6 enzyme inhibitors may increase carvedilol levels).
No products indexed under this heading.

Methohexital Sodium (If treatment with carvedilol is to be continued perioperatively, particular care should be taken when anesthetic agents which depress myocardial function, such as ether, cyclopropane, and trichloroethylene, are used).
No products indexed under this heading.

Methyclothiazide (Concomitant administration with a diuretic can be expected to produce additive effects and exaggerate the orthostatic component of carvedilol action).
No products indexed under this heading.

Metolazone (Concomitant administration with a diuretic can be expected to produce additive effects and exaggerate the orthostatic component of carvedilol action).
No products indexed under this heading.

Metronidazole (Amiodarone, and its metabolite desethyl amiodarone, inhibitors of CYP2C9 and P-glycoprotein, increased concentrations of the (S)-enantiomer of carvedilol by at least 2-fold. The concomitant administration of amiodarone or other CYP2C9 inhibitors, such as fluconazole, with carvedilol may enhance the β-blocking properties of carvedilol resulting in further slowing of the heart rate or cardiac conduction. Patients should be observed for signs of bradycardia or heart block, particularly when one agent is added to pre-existing treatment with the other). Products include:
Pylera 793

Metronidazole Benzoate (Amiodarone, and its metabolite desethyl amiodarone, inhibitors of CYP2C9 and P-glycoprotein, increased concentrations of the (S)-enantiomer of carvedilol by at least 2-fold. The concomitant administration of amiodarone or other CYP2C9 inhibitors, such as fluconazole, with carvedilol may enhance the β-blocking properties of carvedilol resulting in further slowing of the heart rate or cardiac conduction. Patients should be observed for signs of bradycardia or heart block, particularly when one agent is added to pre-existing treatment with the other).
No products indexed under this heading.

Metronidazole Hydrochloride (Amiodarone, and its metabolite desethyl amiodarone, inhibitors of CYP2C9 and P-glycoprotein, increased concentrations of the (S)-enantiomer of carvedilol by at least 2-fold. The concomitant administration of amiodarone or other CYP2C9 inhibitors, such as fluconazole, with carvedilol may enhance the β-blocking properties of carvedilol resulting in further slowing of the heart rate or cardiac conduction. Patients should be observed for signs of bradycardia or heart block, particularly when one agent is added to pre-existing treatment with the other).
No products indexed under this heading.

Metronidazole Sodium (Amiodarone, and its metabolite desethyl amiodarone, inhibitors of CYP2C9 and P-glycoprotein, increased concentrations of the (S)-enantiomer of carvedilol by at least 2-fold. The concomitant administration of amiodarone or other CYP2C9 inhibitors, such as fluconazole, with carvedilol may enhance the β-blocking properties of carvedilol resulting in further slowing of the heart rate or cardiac conduction. Patients should be observed for signs of bradycardia or heart block, particularly when one agent is added to pre-existing treatment with the other).
No products indexed under this heading.

Mibefradil Dihydrochloride (Concomitant use with CYP2D6 enzyme inhibitors may increase carvedilol levels).
No products indexed under this heading.

Miconazole (Amiodarone, and its metabolite desethyl amiodarone, inhibitors of CYP2C9 and P-glycoprotein, increased concentrations of the (S)-enantiomer of carvedilol by at least 2-fold. The concomitant administration of amiodarone or other CYP2C9 inhibitors, such as fluconazole, with carvedilol may enhance the β-blocking properties of carvedilol resulting in further slowing of the heart rate or cardiac conduction. Patients should be observed for signs of bradycardia or heart block, particularly when one agent is added to pre-existing treatment with the other).
No products indexed under this heading.

Miconazole Nitrate (Amiodarone, and its metabolite desethyl amiodarone, inhibitors of CYP2C9 and P-glycoprotein, increased concentrations of the (S)-enantiomer of carvedilol by at least 2-fold. The concomitant administration of amiodarone or other CYP2C9 inhibitors, such as fluconazole, with carvedilol may enhance the β-blocking properties of carvedilol resulting in further slowing of the heart rate or cardiac conduction. Patients should be observed for signs of bradycardia or heart block, particularly when one agent is added to pre-existing treatment with the other). Products include:
Vusion Ointment 3335

Midazolam Hydrochloride (If treatment with carvedilol is to be continued perioperatively, particular care should be taken when anesthetic agents which depress myocardial function, such as ether, cyclopropane, and trichloroethylene, are used).
No products indexed under this heading.

Miglitol (Agents with β-blocking properties may enhance the blood sugar reducing effect of oral hypoglycemics. Therefore, in patients taking oral hypoglycemics, regular monitoring of blood glucose is recommended).
No products indexed under this heading.

Moclobemide (Patients taking both agents with β-blocking properties and a drug that may deplete catecholamines, such as MAO Inhibitors, should be observed closely for signs of hypotension and/or severe bradycardia).
No products indexed under this heading.

Modafinil (Amiodarone, and its metabolite desethyl amiodarone, inhibitors of CYP2C9 and P-glycoprotein, increased concentrations of the (S)-enantiomer of carvedilol by at least 2-fold. The concomitant administration of amiodarone or other CYP2C9 inhibitors, such as fluconazole, with carvedilol may enhance the β-blocking properties of carvedilol resulting in further slowing of the heart rate or cardiac conduction. Patients should be observed for signs of bradycardia or heart block, particularly when one agent is added to pre-existing treatment with the other). Products include:
Provigil 983

Moexipril Hydrochloride (Vasodilatory symptoms often do not require treatment, but it may be useful to separate the time of dosing of carvedilol from that of the ACE inhibitor or to reduce temporarily the dose of the ACE inhibitor. The dose of carvedilol should not be increased until symptoms of worsening heart failure or vasodilation have been stabilized).
No products indexed under this heading.

Nateglinide (Agents with β-blocking properties may enhance the blood sugar reducing effect of oral hypoglycemics. Therefore, in patients taking oral hypoglycemics, regular monitoring of blood glucose is recommended).
No products indexed under this heading.

Nifedipine (Amiodarone, and its metabolite desethyl amiodarone, inhibitors of CYP2C9 and P-glycoprotein, increased concentrations of the (S)-enantiomer of carvedilol by at least 2-fold. The concomitant administration of amiodarone or other CYP2C9 inhibitors, such as fluconazole, with carvedilol may enhance the β-blocking properties of carvedilol resulting in further slowing of the heart rate or cardiac conduction. Patients should be observed for signs of bradycardia or heart block, particularly when one agent is added to pre-existing treatment with the other).
No products indexed under this heading.

Norepinephrine Bitartrate (Patients on β-blocker therapy and with a history of severe anaphylactic reactions to a variety of allergens may be unresponsive to the usual doses of epinephrine used to treat allergic reactions).
No products indexed under this heading.

Norepinephrine Hydrochloride (Patients on β-blocker therapy and with a history of severe anaphylactic reactions to a variety of allergens may be unresponsive to the usual doses of epinephrine used to treat allergic reactions).
No products indexed under this heading.

Nortriptyline Hydrochloride (Concomitant use with CYP2D6 enzyme inhibitors may increase carvedilol levels).
No products indexed under this heading.

Omeprazole (Amiodarone, and its metabolite desethyl amiodarone, inhibitors of CYP2C9 and P-glycoprotein, increased concentrations of the (S)-enantiomer of carvedilol by at least 2-fold. The concomitant administration of amiodarone or other CYP2C9 inhibitors, such as fluconazole, with carvedilol may enhance the β-blocking properties of carvedilol resulting in further slowing of the heart rate or cardiac conduction. Patients should be observed for signs of bradycardia or heart block, particularly when one agent is added to pre-existing treatment with the other).
No products indexed under this heading.

Oxiconazole Nitrate (Amiodarone, and its metabolite desethyl amiodarone, inhibitors of CYP2C9 and P-glycoprotein, increased concentrations of the (S)-enantiomer of carvedilol by at least 2-fold. The concomitant administration of amiodarone or other CYP2C9 inhibitors, such as fluconazole, with carvedilol may enhance the β-blocking properties of carvedilol resulting in further slowing of the heart rate or cardiac conduction. Patients should be observed for signs of bradycardia or heart block, particularly when one agent is added to pre-existing treatment with the other).
No products indexed under this heading.

Pargyline Hydrochloride (Patients taking both agents with β-blocking properties and a drug that may deplete catecholamines, such as MAO Inhibitors, should be observed closely for signs of hypotension and/or severe bradycardia).
No products indexed under this heading.

Paroxetine (Concomitant use with CYP2D6 enzyme inhibitors, such as paroxetine, may increase carvedilol levels).
No products indexed under this heading.

Paroxetine Hydrochloride (Concomitant use with CYP2D6 enzyme inhibitors, such as paroxetine, may increase carvedilol levels). Products include:
Paroxetine CR 2361
Paroxetine ER 2371
Paxil 1586
Paxil CR 1596

Paroxetine Mesylate (Concomitant use with CYP2D6 enzyme inhibitors, such as paroxetine, may increase carvedilol levels).
No products indexed under this heading.

Perindopril Erbumine (Vasodilatory symptoms often do not require treatment, but it may be useful to separate the time of dosing of carvedilol from that of the ACE inhibitor or to reduce temporarily the dose of the ACE inhibitor. The dose of carvedilol should not be increased until symptoms of worsening heart failure or vasodilation have been stabilized).
No products indexed under this heading.

Perphenazine (Concomitant use with CYP2D6 enzyme inhibitors may increase carvedilol levels).
No products indexed under this heading.

Phenelzine Sulfate (Patients taking both agents with β-blocking properties and a drug that may deplete catecholamines, such as MAO Inhibitors, should be observed closely for signs of hypotension and/or severe bradycardia).
No products indexed under this heading.

Phenylbutazone (Amiodarone, and its metabolite desethyl amiodarone, inhibitors of CYP2C9 and P-glycoprotein, increased concentrations of the

IMPORTANT NOTE: Always consult each drug listing in the patient's regimen for possible interactions.

Coreg CR Interactions Index 420

(S)-enantiomer of carvedilol by at least 2-fold. The concomitant administration of amiodarone or other CYP2C9 inhibitors, such as fluconazole, with carvedilol may enhance the β-blocking properties of carvedilol resulting in further slowing of the heart rate or cardiac conduction. Patients should be observed for signs of bradycardia or heart block, particularly when one agent is added to pre-existing treatment with the other).
No products indexed under this heading.

Pioglitazone Hydrochloride (Agents with β-blocking properties may enhance the blood sugar reducing effect of oral hypoglycemics. Therefore, in patients taking oral hypoglycemics, regular monitoring of blood glucose is recommended). Products include:
ActoPlus 3338
Actos 3345
Duetact 3354

Polythiazide (Concomitant administration with a diuretic can be expected to produce additive effects and exaggerate the orthostatic component of carvedilol action).
No products indexed under this heading.

Prilocaine (If treatment with carvedilol is to be continued perioperatively, particular care should be taken when anesthetic agents which depress myocardial function, such as ether, cyclopropane, and trichloroethylene, are used).
No products indexed under this heading.

Prilocaine Hydrochloride (If treatment with carvedilol is to be continued perioperatively, particular care should be taken when anesthetic agents which depress myocardial function, such as ether, cyclopropane, and trichloroethylene, are used).
No products indexed under this heading.

Procaine (If treatment with carvedilol is to be continued perioperatively, particular care should be taken when anesthetic agents which depress myocardial function, such as ether, cyclopropane, and trichloroethylene, are used).
No products indexed under this heading.

Procaine Hydrochloride (If treatment with carvedilol is to be continued perioperatively, particular care should be taken when anesthetic agents which depress myocardial function, such as ether, cyclopropane, and trichloroethylene, are used).
No products indexed under this heading.

Procarbazine Hydrochloride (Patients taking both agents with β-blocking properties and a drug that may deplete catecholamines, such as MAO Inhibitors, should be observed closely for signs of hypotension and/or severe bradycardia).
No products indexed under this heading.

Propafenone Hydrochloride (Concomitant use with CYP2D6 enzyme inhibitors, such as propafenone, may increase carvedilol levels). Products include:
Rythmol 1648
Rythmol SR 1652

Proparacaine Hydrochloride (If treatment with carvedilol is to be continued perioperatively, particular care should be taken when anesthetic agents which depress myocardial function, such as ether, cyclopropane, and trichloroethylene, are used).
No products indexed under this heading.

Propofol (If treatment with carvedilol is to be continued perioperatively, particular care should be taken when anesthetic agents which depress myocardial function, such as ether, cyclopropane, and trichloroethylene, are used).
No products indexed under this heading.

Propoxyphene Hydrochloride (Concomitant use with CYP2D6 enzyme inhibitors may increase carvedilol levels).
No products indexed under this heading.

Propoxyphene Napsylate (Concomitant use with CYP2D6 enzyme inhibitors may increase carvedilol levels).
No products indexed under this heading.

Protriptyline Hydrochloride (Concomitant use with CYP2D6 enzyme inhibitors may increase carvedilol levels).
No products indexed under this heading.

Quinacrine Hydrochloride (Concomitant use with CYP2D6 enzyme inhibitors may increase carvedilol levels).
No products indexed under this heading.

Quinapril Hydrochloride (Vasodilatory symptoms often do not require treatment, but it may be useful to separate the time of dosing of carvedilol from that of the ACE inhibitor or to reduce temporarily the dose of the ACE inhibitor. The dose of carvedilol should not be increased until symptoms of worsening heart failure or vasodilation have been stabilized).
No products indexed under this heading.

Quinidine (Concomitant use with CYP2D6 enzyme inhibitors such as quinidine may increase carvedilol levels).
No products indexed under this heading.

Quinidine Gluconate (Concomitant use with CYP2D6 enzyme inhibitors such as quinidine may increase carvedilol levels).
No products indexed under this heading.

Quinidine Hydrochloride (Concomitant use with CYP2D6 enzyme inhibitors such as quinidine may increase carvedilol levels).
No products indexed under this heading.

Quinidine Polygalacturonate (Concomitant use with CYP2D6 enzyme inhibitors such as quinidine may increase carvedilol levels).
No products indexed under this heading.

Quinidine Sulfate (Concomitant use with CYP2D6 enzyme inhibitors such as quinidine may increase carvedilol levels).
No products indexed under this heading.

Ramipril (Vasodilatory symptoms often do not require treatment, but it may be useful to separate the time of dosing of carvedilol from that of the ACE inhibitor or to reduce temporarily the dose of the ACE inhibitor. The dose of carvedilol should not be increased until symptoms of worsening heart failure or vasodilation have been stabilized).
No products indexed under this heading.

Ranitidine Bismuth Citrate (Concomitant use with CYP2D6 enzyme inhibitors may increase carvedilol levels).
No products indexed under this heading.

Ranitidine Hydrochloride (Concomitant use with CYP2D6 enzyme inhibitors may increase carvedilol levels). Products include:
Zantac 1737
Zantac Injection 1732
Zantac Pharmacy 1735

Rasagiline Mesylate (Patients taking both agents with β-blocking properties and a drug that may deplete catecholamines, such as MAO Inhibitors, should be observed closely for signs of hypotension and/or severe bradycardia). Products include:
Azilect 3383

Rauwolfia Serpentina (Patients taking both agents with β-blocking properties and a drug that can deplete catecholamines should be observed closely for signs of hypotension and/or severe bradycardia).
No products indexed under this heading.

Remifentanil Hydrochloride (If treatment with carvedilol is to be continued perioperatively, particular care should be taken when anesthetic agents which depress myocardial function, such as ether, cyclopropane, and trichloroethylene, are used).
No products indexed under this heading.

Repaglinide (Agents with β-blocking properties may enhance the blood sugar reducing effect of oral hypoglycemics. Therefore, in patients taking oral hypoglycemics, regular monitoring of blood glucose is recommended).
No products indexed under this heading.

Rescinnamine (Patients taking both agents with β-blocking properties and a drug that can deplete catecholamines should be observed closely for signs of hypotension and/or severe bradycardia).
No products indexed under this heading.

Reserpine (Patients taking both agents with β-blocking properties and a drug that can deplete catecholamines, such as reserpine, should be observed closely for signs of hypotension and/or severe bradycardia).
No products indexed under this heading.

Rifampin (In a pharmacokinetic study conducted in 8 healthy males, rifampin (600 mg for 12 days) decreased the AUC and C_{max} of carvedilol by about 70%).
No products indexed under this heading.

Ritonavir (Amiodarone, and its metabolite desethyl amiodarone, inhibitors of CYP2C9 and P-glycoprotein, increased concentrations of the (S)-enantiomer of carvedilol by at least 2-fold. The concomitant administration of amiodarone or other CYP2C9 inhibitors, such as fluconazole, with carvedilol may enhance the β-blocking properties of carvedilol resulting in further slowing of the heart rate or cardiac conduction. Patients should be observed for signs of bradycardia or heart block, particularly when one agent is added to preexisting treatment with the other). Products include:
Kaletra 458
Norvir 509

Ropivacaine Hydrochloride (If treatment with carvedilol is to be continued perioperatively, particular care should be taken when anesthetic agents which depress myocardial function, such as ether, cyclopropane, and trichloroethylene, are used).
No products indexed under this heading.

Rosiglitazone Maleate (Agents with β-blocking properties may enhance the blood sugar reducing effect of oral hypoglycemics. Therefore, in patients taking oral hypoglycemics, regular monitoring of blood glucose is recommended). Products include:
Avandamet 1345
Avandaryl 1356
Avandia 1366

Selegiline (Patients taking both agents with β-blocking properties and a drug that may deplete catecholamines, such as MAO Inhibitors, should be observed closely for signs of hypotension and/or severe bradycardia). Products include:
Emsam 3623

Selegiline Hydrochloride (Patients taking both agents with β-blocking properties and a drug that can deplete catecholamines, such as MAO Inhibitors, should be observed closely for signs of hypotension and/or severe bradycardia). Products include:
Eldepryl 3312

Sertraline Hydrochloride (Amiodarone, and its metabolite desethyl amiodarone, inhibitors of CYP2C9 and P-glycoprotein, increased concentrations of the (S)-enantiomer of carvedilol by at least 2-fold. The concomitant administration of amiodarone or other CYP2C9 inhibitors, such as fluconazole, with carvedilol may enhance the β-blocking properties of carvedilol resulting in further slowing of the heart rate or cardiac conduction. Patients should be observed for signs of bradycardia or heart block, particularly when one agent is added to pre-existing treatment with the other).
No products indexed under this heading.

Sildenafil Citrate (Amiodarone, and its metabolite desethyl amiodarone, inhibitors of CYP2C9 and P-glycoprotein, increased concentrations of the (S)-enantiomer of carvedilol by at least 2-fold. The concomitant administration of amiodarone or other CYP2C9 inhibitors, such as fluconazole, with carvedilol may enhance the β-blocking properties of carvedilol resulting in further slowing of the heart rate or cardiac conduction. Patients should be observed for signs of bradycardia or heart block, particularly when one agent is added to pre-existing treatment with the other).
No products indexed under this heading.

Sitagliptin Phosphate (Agents with β-blocking properties may enhance the blood sugar reducing effect of oral hypoglycemics. Therefore, in patients taking oral hypoglycemics, regular monitoring of blood glucose is recommended). Products include:
Janumet 2188
Januvia 2196

Spirapril Hydrochloride (Vasodilatory symptoms often do not require treatment, but it may be useful to separate the time of dosing of carvedilol from that of the ACE inhibitor or to reduce temporarily the dose of the ACE inhibitor. The dose of carvedilol should not be increased until symptoms of worsening heart failure or vasodilation have been stabilized).
No products indexed under this heading.

Spironolactone (Concomitant administration with a diuretic can be expected to produce additive effects and exaggerate the orthostatic component of carvedilol action).
No products indexed under this heading.

Sufentanil Citrate (If treatment with carvedilol is to be continued perioperatively, particular care should be taken when anesthetic agents which depress myocardial function, such as ether, cyclopropane, and trichloroethylene, are used).
No products indexed under this heading.

Sulfacytine (Amiodarone, and its metabolite desethyl amiodarone, inhibitors of CYP2C9 and P-glycoprotein, increased concentrations of the (S)-enantiomer of carvedilol by at least 2-fold. The concomitant administration of amiodarone or other CYP2C9 inhibitors, such as fluconazole, with carvedilol may enhance the β-blocking properties of carvedilol resulting in further slowing of the heart rate or cardiac conduction. Patients should be observed for signs of bradycardia or heart block, particularly when one agent is added to pre-existing treatment with the other).
No products indexed under this heading.

Sulfamethizole (Amiodarone, and its metabolite desethyl amiodarone, inhibitors of CYP2C9 and P-glycoprotein,

421 Interactions Index Correctol

increased concentrations of the (S)-enantiomer of carvedilol by at least 2-fold. The concomitant administration of amiodarone or other CYP2C9 inhibitors, such as fluconazole, with carvedilol may enhance the β-blocking properties of carvedilol resulting in further slowing of the heart rate or cardiac conduction. Patients should be observed for signs of bradycardia or heart block, particularly when one agent is added to pre-existing treatment with the other).
No products indexed under this heading.

Sulfamethoxazole (Amiodarone, and its metabolite desethyl amiodarone, inhibitors of CYP2C9 and P-glycoprotein, increased concentrations of the (S)-enantiomer of carvedilol by at least 2-fold. The concomitant administration of amiodarone or other CYP2C9 inhibitors, such as fluconazole, with carvedilol may enhance the β-blocking properties of carvedilol resulting in further slowing of the heart rate or cardiac conduction. Patients should be observed for signs of bradycardia or heart block, particularly when one agent is added to pre-existing treatment with the other).
No products indexed under this heading.

Sulfasalazine (Amiodarone, and its metabolite desethyl amiodarone, inhibitors of CYP2C9 and P-glycoprotein, increased concentrations of the (S)-enantiomer of carvedilol by at least 2-fold. The concomitant administration of amiodarone or other CYP2C9 inhibitors, such as fluconazole, with carvedilol may enhance the β-blocking properties of carvedilol resulting in further slowing of the heart rate or cardiac conduction. Patients should be observed for signs of bradycardia or heart block, particularly when one agent is added to pre-existing treatment with the other).
No products indexed under this heading.

Sulfinpyrazone (Amiodarone, and its metabolite desethyl amiodarone, inhibitors of CYP2C9 and P-glycoprotein, increased concentrations of the (S)-enantiomer of carvedilol by at least 2-fold. The concomitant administration of amiodarone or other CYP2C9 inhibitors, such as fluconazole, with carvedilol may enhance the β-blocking properties of carvedilol resulting in further slowing of the heart rate or cardiac conduction. Patients should be observed for signs of bradycardia or heart block, particularly when one agent is added to pre-existing treatment with the other).
No products indexed under this heading.

Sulfisoxazole Acetyl (Amiodarone, and its metabolite desethyl amiodarone, inhibitors of CYP2C9 and P-glycoprotein, increased concentrations of the (S)-enantiomer of carvedilol by at least 2-fold. The concomitant administration of amiodarone or other CYP2C9 inhibitors, such as fluconazole, with carvedilol may enhance the β-blocking properties of carvedilol resulting in further slowing of the heart rate or cardiac conduction. Patients should be observed for signs of bradycardia or heart block, particularly when one agent is added to pre-existing treatment with the other).
No products indexed under this heading.

Sulfisoxazole Diolamine (Amiodarone, and its metabolite desethyl amiodarone, inhibitors of CYP2C9 and P-glycoprotein, increased concentrations of the (S)-enantiomer of carvedilol by at least 2-fold. The concomitant administration of amiodarone or other CYP2C9 inhibitors, such as fluconazole, with carvedilol may enhance the β-blocking properties of carvedilol resulting in further slowing of the heart rate or cardiac conduction. Patients should be observed for signs of bradycardia or heart block, particularly when one agent is added to pre-existing treatment with the other).
No products indexed under this heading.

Terbinafine Hydrochloride (Concomitant use with CYP2D6 enzyme inhibitors may increase carvedilol levels).
No products indexed under this heading.

Terconazole (Amiodarone, and its metabolite desethyl amiodarone, inhibitors of CYP2C9 and P-glycoprotein, increased concentrations of the (S)-enantiomer of carvedilol by at least 2-fold. The concomitant administration of amiodarone or other CYP2C9 inhibitors, such as fluconazole, with carvedilol may enhance the β-blocking properties of carvedilol resulting in further slowing of the heart rate or cardiac conduction. Patients should be observed for signs of bradycardia or heart block, particularly when one agent is added to pre-existing treatment with the other).
No products indexed under this heading.

Tetracaine (If treatment with carvedilol is to be continued perioperatively, particular care should be taken when anesthetic agents which depress myocardial function, such as ether, cyclopropane, and trichloroethylene, are used).
No products indexed under this heading.

Tetracaine Hydrochloride (If treatment with carvedilol is to be continued perioperatively, particular care should be taken when anesthetic agents which depress myocardial function, such as ether, cyclopropane, and trichloroethylene, are used).
No products indexed under this heading.

Thiamylal Sodium (If treatment with carvedilol is to be continued perioperatively, particular care should be taken when anesthetic agents which depress myocardial function, such as ether, cyclopropane, and trichloroethylene, are used).
No products indexed under this heading.

Thioridazine Hydrochloride (Concomitant use with CYP2D6 enzyme inhibitors may increase carvedilol levels). Products include:
Thioridazine Hydrochloride 2384

Ticlopidine Hydrochloride (Amiodarone, and its metabolite desethyl amiodarone, inhibitors of CYP2C9 and P-glycoprotein, increased concentrations of the (S)-enantiomer of carvedilol by at least 2-fold. The concomitant administration of amiodarone or other CYP2C9 inhibitors, such as fluconazole, with carvedilol may enhance the β-blocking properties of carvedilol resulting in further slowing of the heart rate or cardiac conduction. Patients should be observed for signs of bradycardia or heart block, particularly when one agent is added to pre-existing treatment with the other).
No products indexed under this heading.

Tolazamide (Agents with β-blocking properties may enhance the blood sugar reducing effect of oral hypoglycemics. Therefore, in patients taking oral hypoglycemics, regular monitoring of blood glucose is recommended).
No products indexed under this heading.

Tolbutamide (Agents with β-blocking properties may enhance the blood sugar reducing effect of oral hypoglycemics. Therefore, in patients taking oral hypoglycemics, regular monitoring of blood glucose is recommended).
No products indexed under this heading.

Tolbutamide Sodium (Amiodarone, and its metabolite desethyl amiodarone, inhibitors of CYP2C9 and P-glycoprotein, increased concentrations of the (S)-enantiomer of carvedilol by at least 2-fold. The concomitant administration of amiodarone or other CYP2C9 inhibitors, such as fluconazole, with carvedilol may enhance the β-blocking properties of carvedilol resulting in further slowing of the heart rate or cardiac conduction. Patients should be observed for signs of bradycardia or heart block, particularly when one agent is added to pre-existing treatment with the other).
No products indexed under this heading.

Torsemide (Concomitant administration with a diuretic can be expected to produce additive effects and exaggerate the orthostatic component of carvedilol action).
No products indexed under this heading.

Trandolapril (Vasodilatory symptoms often do not require treatment, but it may be useful to separate the time of dosing of carvedilol from that of the ACE inhibitor or to reduce temporarily the dose of the ACE inhibitor. The dose of carvedilol should not be increased until symptoms of worsening heart failure or vasodilation have been stabilized). Products include:
Mavik 489
Tarka 534

Tranylcypromine Sulfate (Patients taking both agents with β-blocking properties and a drug that may deplete catecholamines, such as MAO Inhibitors, should be observed closely for signs of hypotension and/or severe bradycardia). Products include:
Parnate 1584

Triamterene (Concomitant administration with a diuretic can be expected to produce additive effects and exaggerate the orthostatic component of carvedilol action). Products include:
Dyazide 1429
Dyrenium 3495

Trichloroethylene (If treatment with carvedilol is to be continued perioperatively, particular care should be taken when anesthetic agents which depress myocardial function, such as trichloroethylene, are used).
No products indexed under this heading.

Trimipramine Maleate (Concomitant use with CYP2D6 enzyme inhibitors may increase carvedilol levels).
No products indexed under this heading.

Troglitazone (Agents with β-blocking properties may enhance the blood sugar reducing effect of oral hypoglycemics. Therefore, in patients taking oral hypoglycemics, regular monitoring of blood glucose is recommended).
No products indexed under this heading.

Vardenafil Hydrochloride (Amiodarone, and its metabolite desethyl amiodarone, inhibitors of CYP2C9 and P-glycoprotein, increased concentrations of the (S)-enantiomer of carvedilol by at least 2-fold. The concomitant administration of amiodarone or other CYP2C9 inhibitors, such as fluconazole, with carvedilol may enhance the β-blocking properties of carvedilol resulting in further slowing of the heart rate or cardiac conduction. Patients should be observed for signs of bradycardia or heart block, particularly when one agent is added to pre-existing treatment with the other). Products include:
Levitra 3157

Verapamil Hydrochloride (Conduction disturbance (rarely with hemodynamic compromise) has been observed when carvedilol is co-administered with diltiazem. As with other agents with β-blocking properties, if carvedilol is to be administered with calcium channel blockers of the verapamil or diltiazem type, it is recommended that ECG and blood pressure be monitored). Products include:
Tarka 534

Voriconazole (Amiodarone, and its metabolite desethyl amiodarone, inhibitors of CYP2C9 and P-glycoprotein, increased concentrations of the (S)-enantiomer of carvedilol by at least 2-fold. The concomitant administration of amiodarone or other CYP2C9 inhibitors, such as fluconazole, with carvedilol may enhance the β-blocking properties of carvedilol resulting in further slowing of the heart rate or cardiac conduction. Patients should be observed for signs of bradycardia or heart block, particularly when one agent is added to pre-existing treatment with the other).
No products indexed under this heading.

Zafirlukast (Amiodarone, and its metabolite desethyl amiodarone, inhibitors of CYP2C9 and P-glycoprotein, increased concentrations of the (S)-enantiomer of carvedilol by at least 2-fold. The concomitant administration of amiodarone or other CYP2C9 inhibitors, such as fluconazole, with carvedilol may enhance the β-blocking properties of carvedilol resulting in further slowing of the heart rate or cardiac conduction. Patients should be observed for signs of bradycardia or heart block, particularly when one agent is added to pre-existing treatment with the other). Products include:
Accolate 3612

Food Interactions

Food, unspecified (Administration of carvedilol with a high-fat meal resulted in increases (~20%) in AUC and C_{max} compared to carvedilol administered with a standard meal. Decreases in AUC (27%) and C_{max} (43%) were observed when carvedilol was administered in the fasted state compared to administration after a standard meal. Carvedilol should be taken with food).

Meal, unspecified (Administration of carvedilol with a high-fat meal resulted in increases (~20%) in AUC and C_{max} compared to carvedilol administered with a standard meal. Decreases in AUC (27%) and C_{max} (43%) were observed when carvedilol was administered in the fasted state compared to administration after a standard meal. Carvedilol should be taken with food).

CORRECTOL DELAYED-RELEASE TABLETS, USP

(Bisacodyl) 3263
May interact with antacids, and certain other agents. Compounds in these categories include:

Aluminum Carbonate (Patients should not take bisacodyl within 1 hour after taking an antacid or milk).
No products indexed under this heading.

Aluminum Hydroxide (Patients should not take bisacodyl within 1 hour after taking an antacid or milk).
No products indexed under this heading.

Calcium Carbonate (Patients should not take bisacodyl within 1 hour after taking an antacid or milk). Products include:
Chelated Mineral 3476
Pepcid Complete 1822
Extra Strength Rolaids Softchews Vanilla Creme 2045

Magaldrate (Patients should not take bisacodyl within 1 hour after taking an antacid or milk).
No products indexed under this heading.

Magnesium Carbonate (Patients should not take bisacodyl within 1 hour after taking an antacid or milk).
No products indexed under this heading.

IMPORTANT NOTE: Always consult each drug listing in the patient's regimen for possible interactions.

Magnesium Hydroxide (Patients should not take bisacodyl within 1 hour after taking an antacid or milk). Products include:
Fleet Pedia-Lax Chewable Tablets 1144
Pepcid Complete 1822

Magnesium Oxide (Patients should not take bisacodyl within 1 hour after taking an antacid or milk). Products include:
Beelith 873

Magnesium Trisilicate (Patients should not take bisacodyl within 1 hour after taking an antacid or milk).
No products indexed under this heading.

Sodium Bicarbonate (Patients should not take bisacodyl within 1 hour after taking an antacid or milk).
No products indexed under this heading.

Food Interactions

Dairy products (Patients should not take bisacodyl within 1 hour after taking an antacid or milk).

COSMEGEN FOR INJECTION

(Dactinomycin) 2003
May interact with vaccines, live, and certain other agents. Compounds in these categories include:

BCG Vaccine (Live virus vaccines should not be administered during drug therapy with dactinomycin).
No products indexed under this heading.

Influenza Vaccine, Live Attenuated (Live virus vaccines should not be administered during drug therapy with dactinomycin).
No products indexed under this heading.

Influenza Virus Vaccine Live, Intranasal (Live virus vaccines should not be administered during drug therapy with dactinomycin). Products include:
FluMist 2078

Measles, Mumps, Rubella and Varicella Virus Vaccine Live (Live virus vaccines should not be administered during drug therapy with dactinomycin). Products include:
ProQuad 2254

Measles, Mumps & Rubella Virus Vaccine, Live (Live virus vaccines should not be administered during drug therapy with dactinomycin). Products include:
M-M-R II 2203
ProQuad 2254

Measles & Rubella Virus Vaccine Live (Live virus vaccines should not be administered during drug therapy with dactinomycin).
No products indexed under this heading.

Measles Virus Vaccine Live (Live virus vaccines should not be administered during drug therapy with dactinomycin). Products include:
Attenuvax 2086

Mumps Virus Vaccine, Live (Live virus vaccines should not be administered during drug therapy with dactinomycin). Products include:
Mumpsvax 2218

Poliovirus Vaccine, Live, Oral, Trivalent, Types 1,2,3 (Sabin) (Live virus vaccines should not be administered during drug therapy with dactinomycin).
No products indexed under this heading.

Radiation (An increased incidence of gastrointestinal toxicity and marrow suppression has been reported with combined therapy incorporating dactinomycin and radiation. Moreover, the normal skin, as well as the buccal and pharyngeal mucosa, may show early erythema. A smaller than usual radiation dose administered in combination with dactinomycin causes erythema and vesiculation, which progress more rapidly through the stages of tanning and desquamation. Particular caution is necessary when administering dactinomycin within two months of irradiation for the treatment of right-sided Wilms' tumor, since hepatomegaly and elevated AST levels have been noted. In general, dactinomycin should not be concomitantly administered with radiotherapy in the treatment of Wilms' tumor unless the benefit outweighs the risk).
No products indexed under this heading.

Rotavirus Vaccine, Live, Oral, Tetravalent (Live virus vaccines should not be administered during drug therapy with dactinomycin).
No products indexed under this heading.

Rubella & Mumps Virus Vaccine Live (Live virus vaccines should not be administered during drug therapy with dactinomycin).
No products indexed under this heading.

Rubella Virus Vaccine Live (Live virus vaccines should not be administered during drug therapy with dactinomycin). Products include:
Meruvax II 2210

Smallpox Vaccine (Live virus vaccines should not be administered during drug therapy with dactinomycin).
No products indexed under this heading.

Typhoid Vaccine (Live virus vaccines should not be administered during drug therapy with dactinomycin).
No products indexed under this heading.

Varicella Virus Vaccine, Live (Live virus vaccines should not be administered during drug therapy with dactinomycin). Products include:
Varivax 2285

Yellow Fever Vaccine (Live virus vaccines should not be administered during drug therapy with dactinomycin).
No products indexed under this heading.

Zoster Vaccine Live (Live virus vaccines should not be administered during drug therapy with dactinomycin). Products include:
Zostavax 2299

COZAAR TABLETS

(Losartan Potassium) 2106
May interact with lithium preparations, non-steroidal anti-inflammatory agents, potassium preparations, potassium sparing diuretics, and certain other agents. Compounds in these categories include:

Amiloride Hydrochloride (Concomitant use with potassium-sparing diuretics may lead to hyperkalemia).
No products indexed under this heading.

Celecoxib (In some patients with compromised renal function who are being treated with non-steroidal anti-inflammatory drugs (NSAIDs), including those that selectively inhibit cyclooxygenase-2 inhibitors (COX-2 inhibitors), the co-administration of angiotensin II receptor antagonists including losartan may result in a further deterioration of renal function. These effects are usually reversible. Reports suggest that NSAIDs, including selective COX-2 inhibitors, may diminish the antihypertensive effect of angiotensin II receptor antagonists, including losartan. This interaction should be given consideration in patients taking NSAIDs, including selective COX-2 inhibitors, concomitantly with angiotensin II receptor antagonists). Products include:
Celebrex 3272

Cimetidine (Co-administration leads to an increase of about 18% in AUC of losartan with no effect on pharmacokinetics of its active metabolites).
No products indexed under this heading.

Cimetidine Hydrochloride (Co-administration leads to an increase of about 18% in AUC of losartan with no effect on pharmacokinetics of its active metabolites).
No products indexed under this heading.

Diclofenac Epolamine (In some patients with compromised renal function who are being treated with non-steroidal anti-inflammatory drugs (NSAIDs), including those that selectively inhibit cyclooxygenase-2 inhibitors (COX-2 inhibitors), the co-administration of angiotensin II receptor antagonists including losartan may result in a further deterioration of renal function. These effects are usually reversible. Reports suggest that NSAIDs, including selective COX-2 inhibitors, may diminish the antihypertensive effect of angiotensin II receptor antagonists, including losartan. This interaction should be given consideration in patients taking NSAIDs, including selective COX-2 inhibitors, concomitantly with angiotensin II receptor antagonists). Products include:
Flector 1839

Diclofenac Potassium (In some patients with compromised renal function who are being treated with non-steroidal anti-inflammatory drugs (NSAIDs), including those that selectively inhibit cyclooxygenase-2 inhibitors (COX-2 inhibitors), the co-administration of angiotensin II receptor antagonists including losartan may result in a further deterioration of renal function. These effects are usually reversible. Reports suggest that NSAIDs, including selective COX-2 inhibitors, may diminish the antihypertensive effect of angiotensin II receptor antagonists, including losartan. This interaction should be given consideration in patients taking NSAIDs, including selective COX-2 inhibitors, concomitantly with angiotensin II receptor antagonists).
No products indexed under this heading.

Diclofenac Sodium (In some patients with compromised renal function who are being treated with non-steroidal anti-inflammatory drugs (NSAIDs), including those that selectively inhibit cyclooxygenase-2 inhibitors (COX-2 inhibitors), the co-administration of angiotensin II receptor antagonists including losartan may result in a further deterioration of renal function. These effects are usually reversible. Reports suggest that NSAIDs, including selective COX-2 inhibitors, may diminish the antihypertensive effect of angiotensin II receptor antagonists, including losartan. This interaction should be given consideration in patients taking NSAIDs, including selective COX-2 inhibitors, concomitantly with angiotensin II receptor antagonists).
No products indexed under this heading.

Etodolac (In some patients with compromised renal function who are being treated with non-steroidal anti-inflammatory drugs (NSAIDs), including those that selectively inhibit cyclooxygenase-2 inhibitors (COX-2 inhibitors), the co-administration of angiotensin II receptor antagonists including losartan may result in a further deterioration of renal function. These effects are usually reversible. Reports suggest that NSAIDs, including selective COX-2 inhibitors, may diminish the antihypertensive effect of angiotensin II receptor antagonists, including losartan. This interaction should be given consideration in patients taking NSAIDs, including selective COX-2 inhibitors, concomitantly with angiotensin II receptor antagonists).
No products indexed under this heading.

Fenoprofen Calcium (In some patients with compromised renal function who are being treated with non-steroidal anti-inflammatory drugs (NSAIDs), including those that selectively inhibit cyclooxygenase-2 inhibitors (COX-2 inhibitors), the co-administration of angiotensin II receptor antagonists including losartan may result in a further deterioration of renal function. These effects are usually reversible. Reports suggest that NSAIDs, including selective COX-2 inhibitors, may diminish the antihypertensive effect of angiotensin II receptor antagonists, including losartan. This interaction should be given consideration in patients taking NSAIDs, including selective COX-2 inhibitors, concomitantly with angiotensin II receptor antagonists).
No products indexed under this heading.

Fluconazole (Fluconazole, an inhibitor of cytochrome P450 2C9, decreased the AUC of the active metabolite by approximately 40%, but increased the AUC of losartan by approximately 70% following multiple doses).
No products indexed under this heading.

Flurbiprofen (In some patients with compromised renal function who are being treated with non-steroidal anti-inflammatory drugs (NSAIDs), including those that selectively inhibit cyclooxygenase-2 inhibitors (COX-2 inhibitors), the co-administration of angiotensin II receptor antagonists including losartan may result in a further deterioration of renal function. These effects are usually reversible. Reports suggest that NSAIDs, including selective COX-2 inhibitors, may diminish the antihypertensive effect of angiotensin II receptor antagonists, including losartan. This interaction should be given consideration in patients taking NSAIDs, including selective COX-2 inhibitors, concomitantly with angiotensin II receptor antagonists).
No products indexed under this heading.

Ibuprofen (In some patients with compromised renal function who are being treated with non-steroidal anti-inflammatory drugs (NSAIDs), including those that selectively inhibit cyclooxygenase-2 inhibitors (COX-2 inhibitors), the co-administration of angiotensin II receptor antagonists including losartan may result in a further deterioration of renal function. These effects are usually reversible. Reports suggest that NSAIDs, including selective COX-2 inhibitors, may diminish the antihypertensive effect of angiotensin II receptor antagonists, including losartan. This interaction should be given consideration in patients taking NSAIDs, including selective COX-2 inhibitors, concomitantly with angiotensin II receptor antagonists). Products include:
Motrin IB 2043
Children's Motrin 2044
Children's Motrin Non-Staining Dye-Free 2044
Infants' Motrin 2044
Infants' Motrin Dye-Free 2044
Junior Strength Motrin 2044
Vicoprofen 564

Indomethacin (In some patients with compromised renal function who are being treated with non-steroidal anti-inflammatory drugs (NSAIDs), including those that selectively inhibit cyclooxygenase-2 inhibitors (COX-2 inhibitors), the co-administration of angiotensin II receptor antagonists including losartan may result in a further deterioration of renal function. These effects are usually reversible. Reports suggest that NSAIDs, including selective COX-2 inhibitors, may diminish the antihypertensive effect of angiotensin II receptor antagonists, including losartan. This interaction should be given consideration in patients taking NSAIDs,

including selective COX-2 inhibitors, concomitantly with angiotensin II receptor antagonists). Products include:
Indocin 2167

Indomethacin Sodium Trihydrate (In some patients with compromised renal function who are being treated with non-steroidal anti-inflammatory drugs (NSAIDs), including those that selectively inhibit cyclooxygenase-2 inhibitors (COX-2 inhibitors), the co-administration of angiotensin II receptor antagonists including losartan may result in a further deterioration of renal function. These effects are usually reversible. Reports suggest that NSAIDs, including selective COX-2 inhibitors, may diminish the antihypertensive effect of angiotensin II receptor antagonists, including losartan. This interaction should be given consideration in patients taking NSAIDs, including selective COX-2 inhibitors, concomitantly with angiotensin II receptor antagonists). Products include:
Indocin I.V. 2007

Ketoprofen (In some patients with compromised renal function who are being treated with non-steroidal anti-inflammatory drugs (NSAIDs), including those that selectively inhibit cyclooxygenase-2 inhibitors (COX-2 inhibitors), the co-administration of angiotensin II receptor antagonists including losartan may result in a further deterioration of renal function. These effects are usually reversible. Reports suggest that NSAIDs, including selective COX-2 inhibitors, may diminish the antihypertensive effect of angiotensin II receptor antagonists, including losartan. This interaction should be given consideration in patients taking NSAIDs, including selective COX-2 inhibitors, concomitantly with angiotensin II receptor antagonists).
No products indexed under this heading.

Ketorolac Tromethamine (In some patients with compromised renal function who are being treated with non-steroidal anti-inflammatory drugs (NSAIDs), including those that selectively inhibit cyclooxygenase-2 inhibitors (COX-2 inhibitors), the co-administration of angiotensin II receptor antagonists including losartan may result in a further deterioration of renal function. These effects are usually reversible. Reports suggest that NSAIDs, including selective COX-2 inhibitors, may diminish the antihypertensive effect of angiotensin II receptor antagonists, including losartan. This interaction should be given consideration in patients taking NSAIDs, including selective COX-2 inhibitors, concomitantly with angiotensin II receptor antagonists). Products include:
Acuvail .... ⊙209

Lithium (As with other drugs which affect the excretion of sodium, lithium excretion may be reduced. Therefore, serum lithium levels should be monitored carefully if lithium salts are to be co-administered with angiotensin II receptor antagonists).
No products indexed under this heading.

Lithium Carbonate (As with other drugs which affect the excretion of sodium, lithium excretion may be reduced. Therefore, serum lithium levels should be monitored carefully if lithium salts are to be co-administered with angiotensin II receptor antagonists).
No products indexed under this heading.

Lithium Citrate (As with other drugs which affect the excretion of sodium, lithium excretion may be reduced. Therefore, serum lithium levels should be monitored carefully if lithium salts are to be co-administered with angiotensin II receptor antagonists).
No products indexed under this heading.

Meclofenamate Sodium (In some patients with compromised renal function who are being treated with non-steroidal anti-inflammatory drugs (NSAIDs), including those that selectively inhibit cyclooxygenase-2 inhibitors (COX-2 inhibitors), the co-administration of angiotensin II receptor antagonists including losartan may result in a further deterioration of renal function. These effects are usually reversible. Reports suggest that NSAIDs, including selective COX-2 inhibitors, may diminish the antihypertensive effect of angiotensin II receptor antagonists, including losartan. This interaction should be given consideration in patients taking NSAIDs, including selective COX-2 inhibitors, concomitantly with angiotensin II receptor antagonists).
No products indexed under this heading.

Mefenamic Acid (In some patients with compromised renal function who are being treated with non-steroidal anti-inflammatory drugs (NSAIDs), including those that selectively inhibit cyclooxygenase-2 inhibitors (COX-2 inhibitors), the co-administration of angiotensin II receptor antagonists including losartan may result in a further deterioration of renal function. These effects are usually reversible. Reports suggest that NSAIDs, including selective COX-2 inhibitors, may diminish the antihypertensive effect of angiotensin II receptor antagonists, including losartan. This interaction should be given consideration in patients taking NSAIDs, including selective COX-2 inhibitors, concomitantly with angiotensin II receptor antagonists).
No products indexed under this heading.

Meloxicam (In some patients with compromised renal function who are being treated with non-steroidal anti-inflammatory drugs (NSAIDs), including those that selectively inhibit cyclooxygenase-2 inhibitors (COX-2 inhibitors), the co-administration of angiotensin II receptor antagonists including losartan may result in a further deterioration of renal function. These effects are usually reversible. Reports suggest that NSAIDs, including selective COX-2 inhibitors, may diminish the antihypertensive effect of angiotensin II receptor antagonists, including losartan. This interaction should be given consideration in patients taking NSAIDs, including selective COX-2 inhibitors, concomitantly with angiotensin II receptor antagonists).
No products indexed under this heading.

Nabumetone (In some patients with compromised renal function who are being treated with non-steroidal anti-inflammatory drugs (NSAIDs), including those that selectively inhibit cyclooxygenase-2 inhibitors (COX-2 inhibitors), the co-administration of angiotensin II receptor antagonists including losartan may result in a further deterioration of renal function. These effects are usually reversible. Reports suggest that NSAIDs, including selective COX-2 inhibitors, may diminish the antihypertensive effect of angiotensin II receptor antagonists, including losartan. This interaction should be given consideration in patients taking NSAIDs, including selective COX-2 inhibitors, concomitantly with angiotensin II receptor antagonists).
No products indexed under this heading.

Naproxen (In some patients with compromised renal function who are being treated with non-steroidal anti-inflammatory drugs (NSAIDs), including those that selectively inhibit cyclooxygenase-2 inhibitors (COX-2 inhibitors), the co-administration of angiotensin II receptor antagonists including losartan may result in a further deterioration of renal function. These effects are usually reversible. Reports suggest that NSAIDs, including selective COX-2 inhibitors, may diminish the antihypertensive effect of angiotensin II receptor antagonists, including losartan. This interaction should be given consideration in patients taking NSAIDs, including selective COX-2 inhibitors, concomitantly with angiotensin II receptor antagonists). Products include:
EC-Naprosyn 2850
Naprosyn 2850
Anaprox/Naprosyn 2850

Naproxen Sodium (In some patients with compromised renal function who are being treated with non-steroidal anti-inflammatory drugs (NSAIDs), including those that selectively inhibit cyclooxygenase-2 inhibitors (COX-2 inhibitors), the co-administration of angiotensin II receptor antagonists including losartan may result in a further deterioration of renal function. These effects are usually reversible. Reports suggest that NSAIDs, including selective COX-2 inhibitors, may diminish the antihypertensive effect of angiotensin II receptor antagonists, including losartan. This interaction should be given consideration in patients taking NSAIDs, including selective COX-2 inhibitors, concomitantly with angiotensin II receptor antagonists). Products include:
Anaprox 2850
Anaprox DS 2850
Treximet 1681

Oxaprozin (In some patients with compromised renal function who are being treated with non-steroidal anti-inflammatory drugs (NSAIDs), including those that selectively inhibit cyclooxygenase-2 inhibitors (COX-2 inhibitors), the co-administration of angiotensin II receptor antagonists including losartan may result in a further deterioration of renal function. These effects are usually reversible. Reports suggest that NSAIDs, including selective COX-2 inhibitors, may diminish the antihypertensive effect of angiotensin II receptor antagonists, including losartan. This interaction should be given consideration in patients taking NSAIDs, including selective COX-2 inhibitors, concomitantly with angiotensin II receptor antagonists).
No products indexed under this heading.

Phenobarbital (Co-administration leads to a reduction of about 20% in AUC of losartan and that of its active metabolites). Products include:
Donnatal 2711

Phenylbutazone (In some patients with compromised renal function who are being treated with non-steroidal anti-inflammatory drugs (NSAIDs), including those that selectively inhibit cyclooxygenase-2 inhibitors (COX-2 inhibitors), the co-administration of angiotensin II receptor antagonists including losartan may result in a further deterioration of renal function. These effects are usually reversible. Reports suggest that NSAIDs, including selective COX-2 inhibitors, may diminish the antihypertensive effect of angiotensin II receptor antagonists, including losartan. This interaction should be given consideration in patients taking NSAIDs, including selective COX-2 inhibitors, concomitantly with angiotensin II receptor antagonists).
No products indexed under this heading.

Piroxicam (In some patients with compromised renal function who are being treated with non-steroidal anti-inflammatory drugs (NSAIDs), including those that selectively inhibit cyclooxygenase-2 inhibitors (COX-2 inhibitors), the co-administration of angiotensin II receptor antagonists including losartan may result in a further deterioration of renal function. These effects are usually reversible. Reports suggest that NSAIDs, including selective COX-2 inhibitors, may diminish the antihypertensive effect of angiotensin II receptor antagonists, including losartan. This interaction should be given consideration in patients taking NSAIDs, including selective COX-2 inhibitors, concomitantly with angiotensin II receptor antagonists).
No products indexed under this heading.

Potassium Acid Phosphate (Concomitant use with potassium supplements or salt substitute containing potassium may lead to hyperkalemia; patients should be advised to avoid these potassium-containing preparations). Products include:
K-Phos Original 874

Potassium Bicarbonate (Concomitant use with potassium supplements or salt substitute containing potassium may lead to hyperkalemia; patients should be advised to avoid these potassium-containing preparations).
No products indexed under this heading.

Potassium Chloride (Concomitant use with potassium supplements or salt substitute containing potassium may lead to hyperkalemia; patients should be advised to avoid these potassium-containing preparations). Products include:
MoviPrep Oral Solution 2905

Potassium Citrate (Concomitant use with potassium supplements or salt substitute containing potassium may lead to hyperkalemia; patients should be advised to avoid these potassium-containing preparations). Products include:
Urocit-K 2333

Potassium Gluconate (Concomitant use with potassium supplements or salt substitute containing potassium may lead to hyperkalemia; patients should be advised to avoid these potassium-containing preparations).
No products indexed under this heading.

Potassium Phosphate (Concomitant use with potassium supplements or salt substitute containing potassium may lead to hyperkalemia; patients should be advised to avoid these potassium-containing preparations). Products include:
K-Phos Neutral 873

Rifampin (Approximately 40% reduction in the AUC of losartan has been reported with rifampin).
No products indexed under this heading.

Rofecoxib (In some patients with compromised renal function who are being treated with non-steroidal anti-inflammatory drugs (NSAIDs), including those that selectively inhibit cyclooxygenase-2 inhibitors (COX-2 inhibitors), the co-administration of angiotensin II receptor antagonists including losartan may result in a further deterioration of renal function. These effects are usually reversible. Reports suggest that NSAIDs, including selective COX-2 inhibitors, may diminish the antihypertensive effect of angiotensin II receptor antagonists, including losartan. This interaction should be given consideration in patients taking NSAIDs, including selective COX-2 inhibitors, concomitantly with angiotensin II receptor antagonists).
No products indexed under this heading.

Spironolactone (Concomitant use with potassium-sparing diuretics may lead to hyperkalemia).
No products indexed under this heading.

Sulindac (In some patients with compromised renal function who are being treated with non-steroidal anti-inflammatory drugs (NSAIDs), including those that selectively inhibit cyclooxygenase-2

inhibitors (COX-2 inhibitors), the co-administration of angiotensin II receptor antagonists including losartan may result in a further deterioration of renal function. These effects are usually reversible. Reports suggest that NSAIDs, including selective COX-2 inhibitors, may diminish the antihypertensive effect of angiotensin II receptor antagonists, including losartan. This interaction should be given consideration in patients taking NSAIDs, including selective COX-2 inhibitors, concomitantly with angiotensin II receptor antagonists). Products include:

Tolmetin Sodium (In some patients with compromised renal function who are being treated with non-steroidal anti-inflammatory drugs (NSAIDs), including those that selectively inhibit cyclooxygenase-2 inhibitors (COX-2 inhibitors), the co-administration of angiotensin II receptor antagonists including losartan may result in a further deterioration of renal function. These effects are usually reversible. Reports suggest that NSAIDs, including selective COX-2 inhibitors, may diminish the antihypertensive effect of angiotensin II receptor antagonists, including losartan. This interaction should be given consideration in patients taking NSAIDs, including selective COX-2 inhibitors, concomitantly with angiotensin II receptor antagonists).

No products indexed under this heading.

Triamterene (Concomitant use with potassium-sparing diuretics may lead to hyperkalemia). Products include:

Valdecoxib (In some patients with compromised renal function who are being treated with non-steroidal anti-inflammatory drugs (NSAIDs), including those that selectively inhibit cyclooxygenase-2 inhibitors (COX-2 inhibitors), the co-administration of angiotensin II receptor antagonists including losartan may result in a further deterioration of renal function. These effects are usually reversible. Reports suggest that NSAIDs, including selective COX-2 inhibitors, may diminish the antihypertensive effect of angiotensin II receptor antagonists, including losartan. This interaction should be given consideration in patients taking NSAIDs, including selective COX-2 inhibitors, concomitantly with angiotensin II receptor antagonists).

No products indexed under this heading.

Food Interactions

Salt Substitutes, Potassium-Containing (Concomitant use with salt substitutes containing potassium may lead to hyperkalemia).

CREON DELAYED-RELEASE CAPSULES

May interact with macrolide antibiotics, and certain other agents. Compounds in these categories include:

Azithromycin Dihydrate (Transient neutropenia without clinical sequelae was observed as an abnormal laboratory finding in one patient receiving pancrelipase and a macrolide antibiotic).

No products indexed under this heading.

Clarithromycin (Transient neutropenia without clinical sequelae was observed as an abnormal laboratory finding in one patient receiving pancrelipase and a macrolide antibiotic). Products include:

Dirithromycin (Transient neutropenia without clinical sequelae was observed as an abnormal laboratory finding in one patient receiving pancrelipase and a macrolide antibiotic).

No products indexed under this heading.

Erythromycin (Transient neutropenia without clinical sequelae was observed as an abnormal laboratory finding in one patient receiving pancrelipase and a macrolide antibiotic).

No products indexed under this heading.

Erythromycin Estolate (Transient neutropenia without clinical sequelae was observed as an abnormal laboratory finding in one patient receiving pancrelipase and a macrolide antibiotic).

No products indexed under this heading.

Erythromycin Ethylsuccinate (Transient neutropenia without clinical sequelae was observed as an abnormal laboratory finding in one patient receiving pancrelipase and a macrolide antibiotic). Products include:

Erythromycin Gluceptate (Transient neutropenia without clinical sequelae was observed as an abnormal laboratory finding in one patient receiving pancrelipase and a macrolide antibiotic).

No products indexed under this heading.

Erythromycin Stearate (Transient neutropenia without clinical sequelae was observed as an abnormal laboratory finding in one patient receiving pancrelipase and a macrolide antibiotic).

No products indexed under this heading.

Troleandomycin (Transient neutropenia without clinical sequelae was observed as an abnormal laboratory finding in one patient receiving pancrelipase and a macrolide antibiotic).

No products indexed under this heading.

Food Interactions

Food having a pH greater than 5.5 (Pancrelipase should not be crushed or chewed or mixed in foods having a pH greater than 4. These actions can disrupt the protective enteric coating, resulting in early release of enzymes, irritation of oral mucosa, and/or loss or enzyme activity.)

CRESTOR TABLETS

May interact with alcohols, antacids containing aluminum, calcium and magnesium, erythromycin, fibrates, lipid-lowering drugs, oral anticoagulants, oral contraceptives, and certain other agents. Compounds in these categories include:

Aluminum Carbonate (Co-administration with an aluminum and magnesium hydroxide combination antacid may lead to decreased rosuvastatin calcium levels. Studies showed that the aluminium hydroxide/magnesium hydroxide antacid reduced AUC and C_{max} of rosuvastatin by 50%. Separate administration by at least two hours is recommended).

No products indexed under this heading.

Aluminum Hydroxide (Co-administration with an aluminum and magnesium hydroxide combination antacid may lead to decreased rosuvastatin calcium levels. Studies showed that the aluminium hydroxide/magnesium hydroxide antacid reduced AUC and C_{max} of rosuvastatin by 50%. Separate administration by at least two hours is recommended).

No products indexed under this heading.

Anisindione (Rosuvastatin calcium significantly increased INR in patients receiving coumarin anticoagulants. Therefore caution should be exercised when coumarin anticoagulants are given

in conjunction with rosuvastatin calcium. In patients taking coumarin anticoagulants and rosuvastatin calcium concomitantly, INR should be determined before starting rosuvastatin calcium and frequently enough during early therapy to ensure that no significant alteration of INR occurs).

No products indexed under this heading.

Atorvastatin Calcium (The risk of myopathy during treatment with rosuvastatin calcium may be increased with concurrent administration of some other lipid-lowering therapies (fibrates or niacin)). Products include:

Calcium Carbonate (Co-administration with an aluminum and magnesium hydroxide combination antacid may lead to decreased rosuvastatin calcium levels. Studies showed that the aluminium hydroxide/magnesium hydroxide antacid reduced AUC and C_{max} of rosuvastatin by 50%. Separate administration by at least two hours is recommended). Products include:

Cerivastatin Sodium (The risk of myopathy during treatment with rosuvastatin calcium may be increased with concurrent administration of some other lipid-lowering therapies (fibrates or niacin)).

No products indexed under this heading.

Cholestyramine (The risk of myopathy during treatment with rosuvastatin calcium may be increased with concurrent administration of some other lipid-lowering therapies (fibrates or niacin)).

No products indexed under this heading.

Cimetidine (Although clinical studies have shown that rosuvastatin calcium alone does not reduce basal plasma cortisol concentration or impair adrenal reserve, caution should be exercised if rosuvastatin calcium is administered concomitantly with drugs that may decrease the levels or activity of endogenous steroid hormones such as ketoconazole, spironolactone, and cimetidine).

No products indexed under this heading.

Cimetidine Hydrochloride (Although clinical studies have shown that rosuvastatin calcium alone does not reduce basal plasma cortisol concentration or impair adrenal reserve, caution should be exercised if rosuvastatin calcium is administered concomitantly with drugs that may decrease the levels or activity of endogenous steroid hormones such as ketoconazole, spironolactone, and cimetidine).

No products indexed under this heading.

Clofibrate (When rosuvastatin calcium was co-administered with fenofibrate, no clinically significant increase in the AUC of rosuvastatin or fenofibrate was observed. However, the risk of skeletal muscle effects may be enhanced when rosuvastatin calcium is used in combination with fenofibrate. The benefit of further alterations in lipid levels by the combined use of rosuvastatin calcium with fibrates should be carefully weighed against the potential risks of this combination; a reduction in rosuvastatin calcium dosage should be considered in this setting).

No products indexed under this heading.

Colestipol Hydrochloride (The risk of myopathy during treatment with rosuvastatin calcium may be increased with concurrent administration of some other lipid-lowering therapies (fibrates or niacin)).

No products indexed under this heading.

Cyclosporine (Cyclosporine significantly increased rosuvastatin exposure.

Concurrent administration of rosuvastatin and cyclosporine also increases the risk of myopathy. Therefore, in patients taking cyclosporine, therapy should be limited to rosuvastatin calcium 5 mg once daily). Products include:

Desogestrel (Co-administration may lead to increased ethinyl estradiol and norgestrel levels).

No products indexed under this heading.

Dicumarol (Rosuvastatin calcium significantly increased INR in patients receiving coumarin anticoagulants. Therefore caution should be exercised when coumarin anticoagulants are given in conjunction with rosuvastatin calcium. In patients taking coumarin anticoagulants and rosuvastatin calcium concomitantly, INR should be determined before starting rosuvastatin calcium and frequently enough during early therapy to ensure that no significant alteration of INR occurs).

No products indexed under this heading.

Digoxin (Co-administration with digoxin and rosuvastatin calcium may lead to increased digoxin levels). Products include:

Erythromycin (Co-administration with erythromycin may lead to decreased rosuvastatin calcium levels).

No products indexed under this heading.

Erythromycin, Topical (Co-administration with erythromycin may lead to decreased rosuvastatin calcium levels).

No products indexed under this heading.

Erythromycin Estolate (Co-administration with erythromycin may lead to decreased rosuvastatin calcium levels).

No products indexed under this heading.

Erythromycin Ethylsuccinate (Co-administration with erythromycin may lead to decreased rosuvastatin calcium levels). Products include:

Erythromycin Gluceptate (Co-administration with erythromycin may lead to decreased rosuvastatin calcium levels).

No products indexed under this heading.

Erythromycin Lactobionate (Co-administration with erythromycin may lead to decreased rosuvastatin calcium levels).

No products indexed under this heading.

Erythromycin Stearate (Co-administration with erythromycin may lead to decreased rosuvastatin calcium levels).

No products indexed under this heading.

Ethanol (Rosuvastatin calcium should be used with caution in patients who consume substantial quantities of alcohol).

No products indexed under this heading.

Ethinyl Estradiol (Co-administration may lead to increased ethinyl estradiol and norgestrel levels). Products include:

Ethyl Alcohol (Rosuvastatin calcium should be used with caution in patients who consume substantial quantities of alcohol).

No products indexed under this heading.

Ethynodiol Diacetate (Co-administration may lead to increased ethinyl estradiol and norgestrel levels).

No products indexed under this heading.

Fenofibrate (When rosuvastatin calcium was co-administered with fenofibrate, no clinically significant increase in the AUC of rosuvastatin or fenofibrate was observed. However, the risk of skeletal muscle effects may be enhanced when rosuvastatin calcium is used in combination with fenofibrate. The benefit of further alterations in lipid levels by the combined use of rosuvastatin calcium with fibrates should be carefully weighed against the potential risks of this combination; a reduction in rosuvastatin calcium dosage should be considered in this setting). Products include:

Fluconazole (Co-administration of fluconazole may lead to increased rosuvastatin calcium levels).

No products indexed under this heading.

Fluvastatin Sodium (The risk of myopathy during treatment with rosuvastatin calcium may be increased with concurrent administration of some other lipid-lowering therapies (fibrates or niacin)).

No products indexed under this heading.

Gemfibrozil (Gemfibrozil significantly increased rosuvastatin exposure. Therefore, combination therapy with rosuvastatin calcium and gemfibrozil should be avoided. If used, do not exceed rosuvastatin calcium 10 mg once daily).

No products indexed under this heading.

Itraconazole (Co-administration of itraconazole may lead to increased rosuvastatin calcium levels).

No products indexed under this heading.

Ketoconazole (Interaction studies with rosuvastatin and ketoconazole have shown minor or no increases in rosuvastatin exposure. However, caution should be exercised if rosuvastatin is administered concomitantly with drugs that may decrease the levels or activity of endogenous steroid hormones such as ketoconazole, spironolactone, and cimetidine since rosuvastatin may decrease basal plasma cortisol concentration and impair adrenal reserve). Products include:

Levonorgestrel (Co-administration may lead to increased ethinyl estradiol and norgestrel levels). Products include:

Lopinavir (The combination of lopinavir and ritonavir significantly increased rosuvastatin exposure and increases the risk of myopathy. Therefore, in patients taking a combination of lopinavir and ritonavir, the dose of rosuvastatin calcium should be limited to 10 mg once daily. The effect of other protease inhibitors on rosuvastatin pharmacokinetics has not been examined). Products include:

Lovastatin (The risk of myopathy during treatment with rosuvastatin calcium may be increased with concurrent

administration of some other lipid-lowering therapies (fibrates or niacin)). Products include:

Magaldrate (Co-administration with an aluminum and magnesium hydroxide combination antacid may lead to decreased rosuvastatin calcium levels. Studies showed that the aluminium hydroxide/magnesium hydroxide antacid reduced AUC and C_{max} of rosuvastatin by 50%. Separate administration by at least two hours is recommended).

No products indexed under this heading.

Magnesium Carbonate (Co-administration with an aluminum and magnesium hydroxide combination antacid may lead to decreased rosuvastatin calcium levels. Studies showed that the aluminium hydroxide/magnesium hydroxide antacid reduced AUC and C_{max} of rosuvastatin by 50%. Separate administration by at least two hours is recommended).

No products indexed under this heading.

Magnesium Hydroxide (Co-administration with an aluminum and magnesium hydroxide combination antacid may lead to decreased rosuvastatin calcium levels. Studies showed that the aluminium hydroxide/magnesium hydroxide antacid reduced AUC and C_{max} of rosuvastatin by 50%. Separate administration by at least two hours is recommended). Products include:

Magnesium Oxide (Co-administration with an aluminum and magnesium hydroxide combination antacid may lead to decreased rosuvastatin calcium levels. Studies showed that the aluminium hydroxide/magnesium hydroxide antacid reduced AUC and C_{max} of rosuvastatin by 50%. Separate administration by at least two hours is recommended). Products include:

Magnesium Trisilicate (Co-administration with an aluminum and magnesium hydroxide combination antacid may lead to decreased rosuvastatin calcium levels. Studies showed that the aluminium hydroxide/magnesium hydroxide antacid reduced AUC and C_{max} of rosuvastatin by 50%. Separate administration by at least two hours is recommended).

No products indexed under this heading.

Mestranol (Co-administration may lead to increased ethinyl estradiol and norgestrel levels).

No products indexed under this heading.

Niacin (The risk of skeletal muscle effects may be enhanced when rosuvastatin calcium is used in combination with niacin; a reduction in rosuvastatin calcium dosage should be considered in this setting). Products include:

Niacinamide (The risk of skeletal muscle effects may be enhanced when rosuvastatin calcium is used in combination with niacin; a reduction in rosuvastatin calcium dosage should be considered in this setting). Products include:

Norethindrone (Co-administration may lead to increased ethinyl estradiol and norgestrel levels). Products include:

Norethynodrel (Co-administration may lead to increased ethinyl estradiol and norgestrel levels).

No products indexed under this heading.

Norgestimate (Co-administration may lead to increased ethinyl estradiol and norgestrel levels). Products include:

Norgestrel (Co-administration may lead to increased ethinyl estradiol and norgestrel levels).

No products indexed under this heading.

Pravastatin Sodium (The risk of myopathy during treatment with rosuvastatin calcium may be increased with concurrent administration of some other lipid-lowering therapies (fibrates or niacin)).

No products indexed under this heading.

Probucol (The risk of myopathy during treatment with rosuvastatin calcium may be increased with concurrent administration of some other lipid-lowering therapies (fibrates or niacin)).

No products indexed under this heading.

Ritonavir (The combination of lopinavir and ritonavir significantly increased rosuvastatin exposure and increases the risk of myopathy. Therefore, in patients taking a combination of lopinavir and ritonavir, the dose of rosuvastatin calcium should be limited to 10 mg once daily. The effect of other protease inhibitors on rosuvastatin pharmacokinetics has not been examined). Products include:

Simvastatin (The risk of myopathy during treatment with rosuvastatin calcium may be increased with concurrent administration of some other lipid-lowering therapies (fibrates or niacin)). Products include:

Spironolactone (Although clinical studies have shown that rosuvastatin calcium alone does not reduce basal plasma cortisol concentration or impair adrenal reserve, caution should be exercised if rosuvastatin calcium is administered concomitantly with drugs that may decrease the levels or activity of endogenous steroid hormones such as ketoconazole, spironolactone, and cimetidine).

No products indexed under this heading.

Warfarin Sodium (Rosuvastatin calcium significantly increased INR in patients receiving coumarin anticoagulants. Therefore caution should be exercised when coumarin anticoagulants are given in conjunction with rosuvastatin calcium. In patients taking coumarin anticoagulants and rosuvastatin calcium concomitantly, INR should be determined before starting rosuvastatin calcium and frequently enough during early therapy to ensure that no significant alteration of INR occurs).

No products indexed under this heading.

Food Interactions

Alcohol (Rosuvastatin calcium should be used with caution in patients who consume substantial quantities of alcohol).

Beer, reduced-alcohol (Rosuvastatin calcium should be used with caution in patients who consume substantial quantities of alcohol).

Beer, unspecified (Rosuvastatin calcium should be used with caution in patients who consume substantial quantities of alcohol).

Wine, Chianti (Rosuvastatin calcium should be used with caution in patients who consume substantial quantities of alcohol).

Wine, Red (Rosuvastatin calcium should be used with caution in patients who consume substantial quantities of alcohol).

Wine, unspecified (Rosuvastatin calcium should be used with caution in patients who consume substantial quantities of alcohol).

Wine products (Rosuvastatin calcium should be used with caution in patients who consume substantial quantities of alcohol).

CRINONE 4% GEL

None cited in PDR database.

CRINONE 8% GEL

None cited in PDR database.

CRIXIVAN CAPSULES

May interact with cytochrome p450 3a4 inducers (selected), cytochrome p450 3a4 inhibitors (selected), cytochrome p450 3a4 substrates (selected), dihydropyridine calcium channel blockers, phenytoin, quinidine, and certain other agents. Compounds in these categories include:

Acetazolamide (Indinavir is metabolized by CYP3A4. Co-administration of indinavir and other drugs that inhibit CYP3A4 may decrease the clearance of indinavir and may result in increased plasma concentrations of indinavir).

No products indexed under this heading.

Acetazolamide Sodium (Indinavir is metabolized by CYP3A4. Co-administration of indinavir and other drugs that inhibit CYP3A4 may decrease the clearance of indinavir and may result in increased plasma concentrations of indinavir).

No products indexed under this heading.

Alfentanil Hydrochloride (Indinavir is an inhibitor of CYP3A4. Co-administration of indinavir and drugs primarily metabolized by CYP3A4 may result in increased plasma concentrations of the other drug, which could increase or prolong its therapeutic and adverse effects).

No products indexed under this heading.

Allium sativum (Indinavir is metabolized by CYP3A4. Drugs that induce CYP3A4 activity would be expected to increase the clearance of indinavir, resulting in lowered plasma concentrations of indinavir).

No products indexed under this heading.

Alprazolam (Co-administration of indinavir with alprazolam is contraindicated. Inhibition by CYP3A4 by indinavir can result in elevated plasma concentrations of alprazolam. Co-administration is contraindicated due to potential for serious and/or life-threatening reactions such as prolonged or increased sedation or respiratory depression).

No products indexed under this heading.

Aminoglutethimide (Indinavir is metabolized by CYP3A4. Drugs that induce CYP3A4 activity would be expected to increase the clearance of indinavir, resulting in lowered plasma concentrations of indinavir).

No products indexed under this heading.

IMPORTANT NOTE: Always consult each drug listing in the patient's regimen for possible interactions.

Amiodarone Hydrochloride (Co-administration of amiodarone with indinavir is contraindicated. Inhibition of CYP3A4 by indinavir can result in elevated plasma concentrations of amiodarone. Co-administration has the potential for serious and/or life threatening reactions such as cardiac arrhythmias).
No products indexed under this heading.

Amitriptyline Hydrochloride (Indinavir is an inhibitor of CYP3A4. Co-administration of indinavir and drugs primarily metabolized by CYP3A4 may result in increased plasma concentrations of the other drug, which could increase or prolong its therapeutic and adverse effects).
No products indexed under this heading.

Amlodipine Besylate (Co-administration with dihydropyridine calcium channel blockers may increase the concentration of the dihydropyridine calcium channel blocker. Caution is warranted and clinical monitoring of patients is recommended). Products include:
Azor ... 1010
Exforge ... 2443
Exforge HCT ... 2449

Amprenavir (Indinavir is metabolized by CYP3A4. Co-administration of indinavir and other drugs that inhibit CYP3A4 may decrease the clearance of indinavir and may result in increased plasma concentrations of indinavir).
No products indexed under this heading.

Anastrozole (Indinavir is metabolized by CYP3A4. Co-administration of indinavir and other drugs that inhibit CYP3A4 may decrease the clearance of indinavir and may result in increased plasma concentrations of indinavir).
No products indexed under this heading.

Aprepitant (Indinavir is metabolized by CYP3A4. Drugs that induce CYP3A4 activity would be expected to increase the clearance of indinavir, resulting in lowered plasma concentrations of indinavir). Products include:
Emend ... 2124

Astemizole (Indinavir is an inhibitor of CYP3A4. Co-administration of indinavir and drugs primarily metabolized by CYP3A4 may result in increased plasma concentrations of the other drug, which could increase or prolong its therapeutic and adverse effects).
No products indexed under this heading.

Atazanavir (Both indinavir sulfate and atazanavir are associated with indirect (unconjugated) hyperbilirubinemia. Combinations of these drugs have not been studied and co-administration of indinavir and atazanavir is not recommended).
No products indexed under this heading.

Atazanavir Sulfate (Both indinavir sulfate and atazanavir are associated with indirect (unconjugated) hyperbilirubinemia. Combinations of these drugs have not been studied and co-administration of indinavir and atazanavir is not recommended).
No products indexed under this heading.

Atorvastatin Calcium (Caution should be exercised if HIV protease inhibitors, including indinavir are used concurrently with atorvastatin. The risk of myopathy, including rhabdomyolysis, may be increased when HIV protease inhibitors, including indinavir are used in combination with atorvastatin. Use the lowest possible dose of atorvastatin with careful monitoring). Products include:
Lipitor ... 2703

Belladonna Ergotamine (Indinavir is an inhibitor of CYP3A4. Co-administration of indinavir and drugs primarily metabolized by CYP3A4 may result in increased plasma concentrations of the other drug, which could increase or prolong its therapeutic and adverse effects).
No products indexed under this heading.

Bepridil Hydrochloride (Co-administration may lead to increased bepridil concentrations. Caution is warranted and therapeutic concentration monitoring is recommended for bepridil when co-administered with indinavir).
No products indexed under this heading.

Betamethasone (Indinavir is metabolized by CYP3A4. Drugs that induce CYP3A4 activity would be expected to increase the clearance of indinavir, resulting in lowered plasma concentrations of indinavir).
No products indexed under this heading.

Betamethasone Acetate (Indinavir is metabolized by CYP3A4. Drugs that induce CYP3A4 activity would be expected to increase the clearance of indinavir, resulting in lowered plasma concentrations of indinavir).
No products indexed under this heading.

Betamethasone Benzoate (Indinavir is metabolized by CYP3A4. Drugs that induce CYP3A4 activity would be expected to increase the clearance of indinavir, resulting in lowered plasma concentrations of indinavir).
No products indexed under this heading.

Betamethasone Dipropionate (Indinavir is metabolized by CYP3A4. Drugs that induce CYP3A4 activity would be expected to increase the clearance of indinavir, resulting in lowered plasma concentrations of indinavir). Products include:
Diprolene Lotion 0.05% ... 3108
Diprolene Ointment 0.05% ... 3109
Diprolene AF Cream 0.05% ... 3107
Lotrisone ... 3163

Betamethasone Sodium Phosphate (Indinavir is metabolized by CYP3A4. Drugs that induce CYP3A4 activity would be expected to increase the clearance of indinavir, resulting in lowered plasma concentrations of indinavir).
No products indexed under this heading.

Betamethasone Valerate (Indinavir is metabolized by CYP3A4. Drugs that induce CYP3A4 activity would be expected to increase the clearance of indinavir, resulting in lowered plasma concentrations of indinavir). Products include:
Luxíq ... 3321

Bosentan (Indinavir is metabolized by CYP3A4. Drugs that induce CYP3A4 activity would be expected to increase the clearance of indinavir, resulting in lowered plasma concentrations of indinavir). Products include:
Tracleer ... 573

Buspirone Hydrochloride (Indinavir is an inhibitor of CYP3A4. Co-administration of indinavir and drugs primarily metabolized by CYP3A4 may result in increased plasma concentrations of the other drug, which could increase or prolong its therapeutic and adverse effects).
No products indexed under this heading.

Busulfan (Indinavir is an inhibitor of CYP3A4. Co-administration of indinavir and drugs primarily metabolized by CYP3A4 may result in increased plasma concentrations of the other drug, which could increase or prolong its therapeutic and adverse effects). Products include:
Myleran ... 1581

Carbamazepine (Co-administration with carbamazepine may reduce indinavir concentrations. Concomitant use should be used with caution. Indinavir may not be effective due to decreased indinavir in patients taking these agents concomitantly). Products include:
Carbatrol ... 3280
Equetro ... 3477

Cerivastatin Sodium (The risk of myopathy including rhabdomyolysis may be increased when protease inhibitors, including indinavir, are used in combination with HMG-CoA inhibitors that are metabolized by the CYP3A4 pathway).
No products indexed under this heading.

Chlorpheniramine (Indinavir is an inhibitor of CYP3A4. Co-administration of indinavir and drugs primarily metabolized by CYP3A4 may result in increased plasma concentrations of the other drug, which could increase or prolong its therapeutic and adverse effects).
No products indexed under this heading.

Chlorpheniramine Maleate (Indinavir is an inhibitor of CYP3A4. Co-administration of indinavir and drugs primarily metabolized by CYP3A4 may result in increased plasma concentrations of the other drug, which could increase or prolong its therapeutic and adverse effects).
No products indexed under this heading.

Chlorpheniramine Polistirex (Indinavir is an inhibitor of CYP3A4. Co-administration of indinavir and drugs primarily metabolized by CYP3A4 may result in increased plasma concentrations of the other drug, which could increase or prolong its therapeutic and adverse effects). Products include:
Tussionex ... 3443

Chlorpheniramine Tannate (Indinavir is an inhibitor of CYP3A4. Co-administration of indinavir and drugs primarily metabolized by CYP3A4 may result in increased plasma concentrations of the other drug, which could increase or prolong its therapeutic and adverse effects).
No products indexed under this heading.

Cimetidine (Indinavir is metabolized by CYP3A4. Co-administration of indinavir and other drugs that inhibit CYP3A4 may decrease the clearance of indinavir and may result in increased plasma concentrations of indinavir).
No products indexed under this heading.

Cimetidine Hydrochloride (Indinavir is metabolized by CYP3A4. Co-administration of indinavir and other drugs that inhibit CYP3A4 may decrease the clearance of indinavir and may result in increased plasma concentrations of indinavir).
No products indexed under this heading.

Ciprofloxacin (Indinavir is metabolized by CYP3A4. Drugs that induce CYP3A4 activity would be expected to increase the clearance of indinavir, resulting in lowered plasma concentrations of indinavir). Products include:
Cipro I.V. ... 3082
Cipro ... 3073
Cipro XR ... 3091
Ciprodex ... 583

Ciprofloxacin Hydrochloride (Indinavir is metabolized by CYP3A4. Drugs that induce CYP3A4 activity would be expected to increase the clearance of indinavir, resulting in lowered plasma concentrations of indinavir). Products include:
Cipro ... 3073

Cisapride (Co-administration of indinavir with cisapride is contraindicated. Inhibition of CYP3A4 by indinavir can result in elevated plasma concentrations of cisapride. Indinavir is contraindicated with cisapride due to the potential for serious and/or life-threatening reactions such as cardiac arrhythmias).
No products indexed under this heading.

Cisplatin (Indinavir is metabolized by CYP3A4. Drugs that induce CYP3A4 activity would be expected to increase the clearance of indinavir, resulting in lowered plasma concentrations of indinavir).
No products indexed under this heading.

Clarithromycin (Co-administration of indinavir and clarithromycin may lead to increased clarithromycin and indinavir concentrations. The appropriate doses for this combination, with respect to safety and efficacy, have not been established). Products include:
Biaxin/Biaxin XL ... 412

Clotrimazole (Indinavir is metabolized by CYP3A4. Co-administration of indinavir and other drugs that inhibit CYP3A4 may decrease the clearance of indinavir and may result in increased plasma concentrations of indinavir). Products include:
Lotrisone ... 3163

Conivaptan Hydrochloride (Indinavir is metabolized by CYP3A4. Co-administration of indinavir and other drugs that inhibit CYP3A4 may decrease the clearance of indinavir and may result in increased plasma concentrations of indinavir). Products include:
Vaprisol ... 689

Cortisone Acetate (Indinavir is metabolized by CYP3A4. Drugs that induce CYP3A4 activity would be expected to increase the clearance of indinavir, resulting in lowered plasma concentrations of indinavir).
No products indexed under this heading.

Cyclosporine (Co-administration of indinavir and cyclosporine may lead to increased cyclosporine concentrations). Products include:
Gengraf ... 440
Neoral Oral Solution ... 2496
Neoral Capsules ... 2496
Restasis ... 605

Dalfopristin (Indinavir is metabolized by CYP3A4. Co-administration of indinavir and other drugs that inhibit CYP3A4 may decrease the clearance of indinavir and may result in increased plasma concentrations of indinavir).
No products indexed under this heading.

Danazol (Indinavir is metabolized by CYP3A4. Co-administration of indinavir and other drugs that inhibit CYP3A4 may decrease the clearance of indinavir and may result in increased plasma concentrations of indinavir).
No products indexed under this heading.

Darunavir (Indinavir is metabolized by CYP3A4. Co-administration of indinavir and other drugs that inhibit CYP3A4 may decrease the clearance of indinavir and may result in increased plasma concentrations of indinavir).
No products indexed under this heading.

Dasatinib (Indinavir is metabolized by CYP3A4. Co-administration of indinavir and other drugs that inhibit CYP3A4 may decrease the clearance of indinavir and may result in increased plasma concentrations of indinavir).
No products indexed under this heading.

Delavirdine Mesylate (Co-administration results in inhibition of indinavir metabolism producing an increase in indinavir concentrations. A dose reduction of indinavir to 600 mg every 8 hours should be considered when taking delavirdine 400 mg three times a day).
No products indexed under this heading.

(⊙ Described in PDR® for Ophthalmic Medicines)

Delavirine (Indinavir is metabolized by CYP3A4. Co-administration of indinavir and other drugs that inhibit CYP3A4 may decrease the clearance of indinavir and may result in increased plasma concentrations of indinavir).
No products indexed under this heading.

Desloratadine (Indinavir is metabolized by CYP3A4. Co-administration of indinavir and other drugs that inhibit CYP3A4 may decrease the clearance of indinavir and may result in increased plasma concentrations of indinavir). Products include:

Desogestrel (Indinavir is an inhibitor of CYP3A4. Co-administration of indinavir and drugs primarily metabolized by CYP3A4 may result in increased plasma concentrations of the other drug, which could increase or prolong its therapeutic and adverse effects).
No products indexed under this heading.

Dexamethasone (Indinavir is metabolized by CYP3A4. Drugs that induce CYP3A4 activity would be expected to increase the clearance of indinavir, resulting in lowered plasma concentrations of indinavir). Products include:

Dexamethasone Acetate (Indinavir is metabolized by CYP3A4. Drugs that induce CYP3A4 activity would be expected to increase the clearance of indinavir, resulting in lowered plasma concentrations of indinavir).
No products indexed under this heading.

Dexamethasone Phosphate (Indinavir is metabolized by CYP3A4. Drugs that induce CYP3A4 activity would be expected to increase the clearance of indinavir, resulting in lowered plasma concentrations of indinavir).
No products indexed under this heading.

Dexamethasone Sodium (Indinavir is metabolized by CYP3A4. Drugs that induce CYP3A4 activity would be expected to increase the clearance of indinavir, resulting in lowered plasma concentrations of indinavir).
No products indexed under this heading.

Dexamethasone Sodium Phosphate (Indinavir is metabolized by CYP3A4. Drugs that induce CYP3A4 activity would be expected to increase the clearance of indinavir, resulting in lowered plasma concentrations of indinavir).
No products indexed under this heading.

Dexamethasone Sodium Phosphate Injection (Indinavir is metabolized by CYP3A4. Drugs that induce CYP3A4 activity would be expected to increase the clearance of indinavir, resulting in lowered plasma concentrations of indinavir).
No products indexed under this heading.

Diazepam (Indinavir is an inhibitor of CYP3A4. Co-administration of indinavir and drugs primarily metabolized by CYP3A4 may result in increased plasma concentrations of the other drug, which could increase or prolong its therapeutic and adverse effects). Products include:

Didanosine (Indinavir and didanosine formulations containing buffer should be administered at least one hour apart on an empty stomach).
No products indexed under this heading.

Dihydroergotamine Mesylate (Concomitant use with dihydroergotamine is contraindicated. Inhibition of CYP3A4 by indinavir can result in elevated plasma concentrations of dihydroergotamine. Concomitant use has the potential for serious and/or life threatening reactions such as acute ergot toxicity characterized by peripheral vasospasm and ischemia of the extremities and other tissues).
No products indexed under this heading.

Diltiazem Hydrochloride (Indinavir is metabolized by CYP3A4. Co-administration of indinavir and other drugs that inhibit CYP3A4 may decrease the clearance of indinavir and may result in increased plasma concentrations of indinavir). Products include:

Diltiazem Maleate (Indinavir is metabolized by CYP3A4. Co-administration of indinavir and other drugs that inhibit CYP3A4 may decrease the clearance of indinavir and may result in increased plasma concentrations of indinavir).
No products indexed under this heading.

Disopyramide (Indinavir is an inhibitor of CYP3A4. Co-administration of indinavir and drugs primarily metabolized by CYP3A4 may result in increased plasma concentrations of the other drug, which could increase or prolong its therapeutic and adverse effects).
No products indexed under this heading.

Disopyramide Phosphate (Indinavir is an inhibitor of CYP3A4. Co-administration of indinavir and drugs primarily metabolized by CYP3A4 may result in increased plasma concentrations of the other drug, which could increase or prolong its therapeutic and adverse effects).
No products indexed under this heading.

Disulfiram (Indinavir is an inhibitor of CYP3A4. Co-administration of indinavir and drugs primarily metabolized by CYP3A4 may result in increased plasma concentrations of the other drug, which could increase or prolong its therapeutic and adverse effects).
No products indexed under this heading.

Doxorubicin Hydrochloride (Indinavir is metabolized by CYP3A4. Drugs that induce CYP3A4 activity would be expected to increase the clearance of indinavir, resulting in lowered plasma concentrations of indinavir).
No products indexed under this heading.

Dronabinol (Indinavir is an inhibitor of CYP3A4. Co-administration of indinavir and drugs primarily metabolized by CYP3A4 may result in increased plasma concentrations of the other drug, which could increase or prolong its therapeutic and adverse effects).
No products indexed under this heading.

Efavirenz (Co-administration results in decreased concentrations of indinavir. The optimal dose of indinavir, when given in combination with efavirenz, is not known. Increasing the indinavir dose to 1000 mg every 8 hours does not compensate for the increased indinavir metabolism due to efavirenz). Products include:

Ergonovine Maleate (Co-administration with ergonovine is contraindicated. Inhibition of CYP3A4 by indinavir can result in elevated plasma concentrations of ergonovine. Co-administration has the potential for serious and/or life threatening reactions such as acute ergot toxicity characterized by peripheral vasospasm and ischemia of the extremities and other tissues).
No products indexed under this heading.

Ergotamine Tartrate (Co-administration with ergotamine is contraindicated. Inhibition of CYP3A4 by indinavir can result in elevated plasma concentrations of ergotamine. Co-administration has the potential for serious and/or life threatening reactions such as acute ergot toxicity characterized by peripheral vasospasm and ischemia of the extremities and other tissues).
No products indexed under this heading.

Erythromycin (Indinavir is metabolized by CYP3A4. Co-administration of indinavir and other drugs that inhibit CYP3A4 may decrease the clearance of indinavir and may result in increased plasma concentrations of indinavir).
No products indexed under this heading.

Erythromycin Estolate (Indinavir is metabolized by CYP3A4. Co-administration of indinavir and other drugs that inhibit CYP3A4 may decrease the clearance of indinavir and may result in increased plasma concentrations of indinavir).
No products indexed under this heading.

Erythromycin Ethylsuccinate (Indinavir is metabolized by CYP3A4. Co-administration of indinavir and other drugs that inhibit CYP3A4 may decrease the clearance of indinavir and may result in increased plasma concentrations of indinavir). Products include:

Erythromycin Glucceptate (Indinavir is metabolized by CYP3A4. Co-administration of indinavir and other drugs that inhibit CYP3A4 may decrease the clearance of indinavir and may result in increased plasma concentrations of indinavir).
No products indexed under this heading.

Erythromycin Lactobionate (Indinavir is metabolized by CYP3A4. Co-administration of indinavir and other drugs that inhibit CYP3A4 may decrease the clearance of indinavir and may result in increased plasma concentrations of indinavir).
No products indexed under this heading.

Erythromycin Stearate (Indinavir is metabolized by CYP3A4. Co-administration of indinavir and other drugs that inhibit CYP3A4 may decrease the clearance of indinavir and may result in increased plasma concentrations of indinavir).
No products indexed under this heading.

Esomeprazole Magnesium (Indinavir is metabolized by CYP3A4. Co-administration of indinavir and other drugs that inhibit CYP3A4 may decrease the clearance of indinavir and may result in increased plasma concentrations of indinavir). Products include:

Esomeprazole Sodium (Indinavir is metabolized by CYP3A4. Co-administration of indinavir and other drugs that inhibit CYP3A4 may decrease the clearance of indinavir and may result in increased plasma concentrations of indinavir). Products include:

Estradiol (Indinavir is an inhibitor of CYP3A4. Co-administration of indinavir and drugs primarily metabolized by CYP3A4 may result in increased plasma concentrations of the other drug, which could increase or prolong its therapeutic and adverse effects). Products include:

Estradiol Benzoate (Indinavir is an inhibitor of CYP3A4. Co-administration of indinavir and drugs primarily metabolized by CYP3A4 may result in increased plasma concentrations of the other drug, which could increase or prolong its therapeutic and adverse effects).
No products indexed under this heading.

Estradiol Cypionate (Indinavir is an inhibitor of CYP3A4. Co-administration of indinavir and drugs primarily metabolized by CYP3A4 may result in increased plasma concentrations of the other drug, which could increase or prolong its therapeutic and adverse effects).
No products indexed under this heading.

Estradiol Valerate (Indinavir is an inhibitor of CYP3A4. Co-administration of indinavir and drugs primarily metabolized by CYP3A4 may result in increased plasma concentrations of the other drug, which could increase or prolong its therapeutic and adverse effects).
No products indexed under this heading.

Ethinyl Estradiol (Indinavir is an inhibitor of CYP3A4. Co-administration of indinavir and drugs primarily metabolized by CYP3A4 may result in increased plasma concentrations of the other drug, which could increase or prolong its therapeutic and adverse effects). Products include:

Ethosuximide (Indinavir is metabolized by CYP3A4. Drugs that induce CYP3A4 activity would be expected to increase the clearance of indinavir, resulting in lowered plasma concentrations of indinavir).
No products indexed under this heading.

Ethynodiol Diacetate (Indinavir is an inhibitor of CYP3A4. Co-administration of indinavir and drugs primarily metabolized by CYP3A4 may result in increased plasma concentrations of the other drug, which could increase or prolong its therapeutic and adverse effects).
No products indexed under this heading.

Etoposide (Indinavir is an inhibitor of CYP3A4. Co-administration of indinavir and drugs primarily metabolized by CYP3A4 may result in increased plasma concentrations of the other drug, which could increase or prolong its therapeutic and adverse effects).
No products indexed under this heading.

Etoposide Phosphate (Indinavir is an inhibitor of CYP3A4. Co-administration of indinavir and drugs primarily metabolized by CYP3A4 may result in increased plasma concentrations of the other drug, which could increase or prolong its therapeutic and adverse effects).
No products indexed under this heading.

Felbamate (Indinavir is metabolized by CYP3A4. Drugs that induce CYP3A4 activity would be expected to increase the clearance of indinavir, resulting in lowered plasma concentrations of indinavir).
No products indexed under this heading.

Felodipine (Co-administration with dihydropyridine calcium channel blockers may increase the concentration of the dihydropyridine calcium channel blocker. Caution is warranted and clinical monitoring of patients is recommended).
No products indexed under this heading.

IMPORTANT NOTE: Always consult each drug listing in the patient's regimen for possible interactions.

Fentanyl (Indinavir is an inhibitor of CYP3A4. Co-administration of indinavir and drugs primarily metabolized by CYP3A4 may result in increased plasma concentrations of the other drug, which could increase or prolong its therapeutic and adverse effects). Products include:

Fentanyl Citrate (Indinavir is an inhibitor of CYP3A4. Co-administration of indinavir and drugs primarily metabolized by CYP3A4 may result in increased plasma concentrations of the other drug, which could increase or prolong its therapeutic and adverse effects). Products include:

Fluconazole (Indinavir is metabolized by CYP3A4. Co-administration of indinavir and other drugs that inhibit CYP3A4 may decrease the clearance of indinavir and may result in increased plasma concentrations of indinavir).

No products indexed under this heading.

Fludrocortisone Acetate (Indinavir is metabolized by CYP3A4. Drugs that induce CYP3A4 activity would be expected to increase the clearance of indinavir, resulting in lowered plasma concentrations of indinavir).

No products indexed under this heading.

Fluoxetine (Indinavir is metabolized by CYP3A4. Co-administration of indinavir and other drugs that inhibit CYP3A4 may decrease the clearance of indinavir and may result in increased plasma concentrations of indinavir).

No products indexed under this heading.

Fluoxetine Hydrochloride (Indinavir is metabolized by CYP3A4. Co-administration of indinavir and other drugs that inhibit CYP3A4 may decrease the clearance of indinavir and may result in increased plasma concentrations of indinavir). Products include:

Fluticasone Furoate (Concomitant use may increase fluticasone concentrations. Fluticasone is not recommended in situations where indinavir is co-administered with a potent CYP3A4 inhibitor, such as ritonavir, unless the potential benefit outweighs the risk of systemic corticosteroid side effects). Products include:

Fluticasone Propionate (Concomitant use of fluticasone propionate and indinavir may increase fluticasone concentrations of fluticasone propionate; co-administer with caution. Consider alternatives to fluticasone propionate, particularly for long-term use. Fluticasone is not recommended in situations where indinavir is co-administered with a potent CYP3A4 inhibitor such as ritonavir unless the potential benefit outweighs the risk of systemic corticosteroid side effects). Products include:

Fluvastatin Sodium (Co-administration of indinavir with fluvastatin has not been studied. If no alternative treatment is available, use with careful monitoring).

No products indexed under this heading.

Fluvoxamine Maleate (Indinavir is metabolized by CYP3A4. Co-administration of indinavir and other drugs that inhibit CYP3A4 may decrease the clearance of indinavir and may result in increased plasma concentrations of indinavir).

No products indexed under this heading.

Fosamprenavir Calcium (Indinavir is metabolized by CYP3A4. Co-administration of indinavir and other drugs that inhibit CYP3A4 may decrease the clearance of indinavir and may result in increased plasma concentrations of indinavir). Products include:

Fosphenytoin (Co-administration with phenytoin may decrease indinavir concentrations. Concurrent use should be used with caution. Indinavir may not be effective due to decreased indinavir concentrations in patients taking these agents concomitantly).

No products indexed under this heading.

Fosphenytoin Sodium (Co-administration with phenytoin may decrease indinavir concentrations. Concurrent use should be used with caution. Indinavir may not be effective due to decreased indinavir concentrations in patients taking these agents concomitantly).

No products indexed under this heading.

Garlic Extract (Indinavir is metabolized by CYP3A4. Drugs that induce CYP3A4 activity would be expected to increase the clearance of indinavir, resulting in lowered plasma concentrations of indinavir).

No products indexed under this heading.

Garlic Oil (Indinavir is metabolized by CYP3A4. Drugs that induce CYP3A4 activity would be expected to increase the clearance of indinavir, resulting in lowered plasma concentrations of indinavir).

No products indexed under this heading.

Haloperidol (Indinavir is an inhibitor of CYP3A4. Co-administration of indinavir and drugs primarily metabolized by CYP3A4 may result in increased plasma concentrations of the other drug, which could increase or prolong its therapeutic and adverse effects).

No products indexed under this heading.

Haloperidol Decanoate (Indinavir is an inhibitor of CYP3A4. Co-administration of indinavir and drugs primarily metabolized by CYP3A4 may result in increased plasma concentrations of the other drug, which could increase or prolong its therapeutic and adverse effects).

No products indexed under this heading.

Haloperidol Lactate (Indinavir is an inhibitor of CYP3A4. Co-administration of indinavir and drugs primarily metabolized by CYP3A4 may result in increased plasma concentrations of the other drug, which could increase or prolong its therapeutic and adverse effects).

No products indexed under this heading.

Hydrocortisone (Indinavir is metabolized by CYP3A4. Drugs that induce CYP3A4 activity would be expected to increase the clearance of indinavir, resulting in lowered plasma concentrations of indinavir).

No products indexed under this heading.

Hydrocortisone (Alcohol) (Indinavir is metabolized by CYP3A4. Drugs that induce CYP3A4 activity would be expected to increase the clearance of indinavir, resulting in lowered plasma concentrations of indinavir).

No products indexed under this heading.

Hydrocortisone Acetate (Indinavir is metabolized by CYP3A4. Drugs that induce CYP3A4 activity would be expected to increase the clearance of indinavir, resulting in lowered plasma concentrations of indinavir).

No products indexed under this heading.

Hydrocortisone Butyrate (Indinavir is metabolized by CYP3A4. Drugs that induce CYP3A4 activity would be expected to increase the clearance of indinavir, resulting in lowered plasma concentrations of indinavir).

No products indexed under this heading.

Hydrocortisone Cypionate (Indinavir is metabolized by CYP3A4. Drugs that induce CYP3A4 activity would be expected to increase the clearance of indinavir, resulting in lowered plasma concentrations of indinavir).

No products indexed under this heading.

Hydrocortisone Hemisuccinate (Indinavir is metabolized by CYP3A4. Drugs that induce CYP3A4 activity would be expected to increase the clearance of indinavir, resulting in lowered plasma concentrations of indinavir).

No products indexed under this heading.

Hydrocortisone Probutate (Indinavir is metabolized by CYP3A4. Drugs that induce CYP3A4 activity would be expected to increase the clearance of indinavir, resulting in lowered plasma concentrations of indinavir).

No products indexed under this heading.

Hydrocortisone Sodium Phosphate (Indinavir is metabolized by CYP3A4. Drugs that induce CYP3A4 activity would be expected to increase the clearance of indinavir, resulting in lowered plasma concentrations of indinavir).

No products indexed under this heading.

Hydrocortisone Sodium Succinate (Indinavir is metabolized by CYP3A4. Drugs that induce CYP3A4 activity would be expected to increase the clearance of indinavir, resulting in lowered plasma concentrations of indinavir).

No products indexed under this heading.

Hydrocortisone Valerate (Indinavir is metabolized by CYP3A4. Drugs that induce CYP3A4 activity would be expected to increase the clearance of indinavir, resulting in lowered plasma concentrations of indinavir).

No products indexed under this heading.

Hypericum (Co-administration of indinavir and St. John's Wort (hypericum perforatum) or products containing St. John's Wort has been shown to substantially decrease indinavir concentrations and may lead to loss of virologic response and possible resistance to indinavir or to the class of protease inhibitors; co-administration is not recommended).

No products indexed under this heading.

Hypericum Perforatum (Concomitant use of indinavir and St. John's wort (Hypericum perforatum) or products containing St. John's wort is not recommended. Co-administration of indinavir and St. John's wort has been shown to substantially decrease indinavir concentrations and may lead to loss of virologic response and possible resistance to indinavir or to the class of protease inhibitors). Products include:

Imatinib Mesylate (Indinavir is metabolized by CYP3A4. Co-administration of indinavir and other drugs that inhibit CYP3A4 may decrease the clearance of indinavir and may result in increased plasma concentrations of indinavir). Products include:

Isoniazid (Indinavir is metabolized by CYP3A4. Co-administration of indinavir and other drugs that inhibit CYP3A4 may decrease the clearance of indinavir and may result in increased plasma concentrations of indinavir).

No products indexed under this heading.

Isradipine (Co-administration with dihydropyridine calcium channel blockers may increase the concentration of the dihydropyridine calcium channel blocker. Caution is warranted and clinical monitoring of patients is recommended). Products include:

Itraconazole (Co-administration of indinavir and itraconazole may lead to increased indinavir concentrations. Dose reduction of indinavir to 600 mg every 8 hours is recommended when administering itraconazole concurrently).

No products indexed under this heading.

Ixabepilone (Indinavir is an inhibitor of CYP3A4. Co-administration of indinavir and drugs primarily metabolized by CYP3A4 may result in increased plasma concentrations of the other drug, which could increase or prolong its therapeutic and adverse effects).

No products indexed under this heading.

Ketoconazole (Co-administration of indinavir and ketoconazole may lead to increased indinavir concentrations. Dose reduction of indinavir to 600 mg every 8 hours should be considered when administering ketoconazole concomitantly). Products include:

Lapatinib (Indinavir is metabolized by CYP3A4. Co-administration of indinavir and other drugs that inhibit CYP3A4 may decrease the clearance of indinavir and may result in increased plasma concentrations of indinavir). Products include:

Levonorgestrel (Indinavir is an inhibitor of CYP3A4. Co-administration of indinavir and drugs primarily metabolized by CYP3A4 may result in increased plasma concentrations of the other drug, which could increase or prolong its therapeutic and adverse effects). Products include:

Lidocaine (Co-administration with systemic lidocaine may lead to increased lidocaine concentrations. Caution is warranted and therapeutic concentration monitoring is recommended for systemic lidocaine when co-administered with indinavir). Products include:

Lidocaine Hydrochloride (Co-administration with systemic lidocaine may lead to increased lidocaine concentrations. Caution is warranted and therapeutic concentration monitoring is recommended for systemic lidocaine when co-administered with indinavir).

No products indexed under this heading.

Lopinavir (Indinavir is metabolized by CYP3A4. Co-administration of indinavir and other drugs that inhibit CYP3A4 may decrease the clearance of indinavir and may result in increased plasma concentrations of indinavir). Products include:

429 Interactions Index Crixivan

Loratadine (Indinavir is metabolized by CYP3A4. Co-administration of indinavir and other drugs that inhibit CYP3A4 may decrease the clearance of indinavir and may result in increased plasma concentrations of indinavir).
No products indexed under this heading.

Lovastatin (Concomitant use of indinavir with lovastatin is not recommended. The risk of myopathy including rhabdomyolysis may be increased when HIV protease inhibitors, including indinavir, is used with lovastatin). Products include:
Advicor 402
Mevacor 2212

Mephenytoin (Indinavir is metabolized by CYP3A4. Drugs that induce CYP3A4 activity would be expected to increase the clearance of indinavir, resulting in lowered plasma concentrations of indinavir).
No products indexed under this heading.

Mestranol (Indinavir is an inhibitor of CYP3A4. Co-administration of indinavir and drugs primarily metabolized by CYP3A4 may result in increased plasma concentrations of the other drug, which could increase or prolong its therapeutic and adverse effects).
No products indexed under this heading.

Methadone Hydrochloride (Indinavir is an inhibitor of CYP3A4. Co-administration of indinavir and drugs primarily metabolized by CYP3A4 may result in increased plasma concentrations of the other drug, which could increase or prolong its therapeutic and adverse effects).
No products indexed under this heading.

Methsuximide (Indinavir is metabolized by CYP3A4. Drugs that induce CYP3A4 activity would be expected to increase the clearance of indinavir, resulting in lowered plasma concentrations of indinavir).
No products indexed under this heading.

Methylergonovine Maleate (Co-administration with methylergonovine is contraindicated. Inhibition of CYP3A4 by indinavir can result in elevated plasma concentrations of methylergonovineine. Co-administration has the potential for serious and/or life threatening reactions, such as acute ergot toxicity characterized by peripheral vasospasm and ischemia of the extremities and other tissues).
No products indexed under this heading.

Methylprednisolone (Indinavir is metabolized by CYP3A4. Drugs that induce CYP3A4 activity would be expected to increase the clearance of indinavir, resulting in lowered plasma concentrations of indinavir).
No products indexed under this heading.

Methylprednisolone Acetate (Indinavir is metabolized by CYP3A4. Drugs that induce CYP3A4 activity would be expected to increase the clearance of indinavir, resulting in lowered plasma concentrations of indinavir).
No products indexed under this heading.

Methylprednisolone Sodium Succinate (Indinavir is metabolized by CYP3A4. Drugs that induce CYP3A4 activity would be expected to increase the clearance of indinavir, resulting in lowered plasma concentrations of indinavir).
No products indexed under this heading.

Metronidazole (Indinavir is metabolized by CYP3A4. Co-administration of indinavir and other drugs that inhibit CYP3A4 may decrease the clearance of indinavir and may result in increased plasma concentrations of indinavir). Products include:
Pylera 793

Metronidazole Benzoate (Indinavir is metabolized by CYP3A4. Co-administration of indinavir and other drugs that inhibit CYP3A4 may decrease the clearance of indinavir and may result in increased plasma concentrations of indinavir).
No products indexed under this heading.

Metronidazole Hydrochloride (Indinavir is metabolized by CYP3A4. Co-administration of indinavir and other drugs that inhibit CYP3A4 may decrease the clearance of indinavir and may result in increased plasma concentrations of indinavir).
No products indexed under this heading.

Metronidazole Sodium (Indinavir is metabolized by CYP3A4. Co-administration of indinavir and other drugs that inhibit CYP3A4 may decrease the clearance of indinavir and may result in increased plasma concentrations of indinavir).
No products indexed under this heading.

Miconazole (Indinavir is metabolized by CYP3A4. Co-administration of indinavir and other drugs that inhibit CYP3A4 may decrease the clearance of indinavir and may result in increased plasma concentrations of indinavir).
No products indexed under this heading.

Miconazole Nitrate (Indinavir is metabolized by CYP3A4. Co-administration of indinavir and other drugs that inhibit CYP3A4 may decrease the clearance of indinavir and may result in increased plasma concentrations of indinavir). Products include:
Vusion Ointment 3335

Midazolam Hydrochloride (Co-administration with oral midazolam is contraindicated. Midazolam is extensively metabolized by CYP3A4. Co-administration with indinavir with or without ritonavir may cause a large increase in the concentration. Based on data from other CYP3A4 inhibitors, plasma concentrations of midazolam are expected to be significantly higher when midazolam is given orally. Therefore, indinavir should not be co-administered with orally administered midazolam, whereas caution should be used with co-administration of indinavir and parenteral midazolam. Data from concomitant use of parenteral midazolam with other protease inhibitors suggest a possible 3-4 fold increase in midazolam plasma levels. If indinavir with or without ritonavir is co-administered with parenteral midazolam, it should be done in a setting which ensures close clinical monitoring and appropriate medical management in case of respiratory depression and/or prolonged sedation. Dosage reduction for midazolam should be considered, especially if more than a single dose of midazolam is administered).
No products indexed under this heading.

Mifepristone (Indinavir is metabolized by CYP3A4. Co-administration of indinavir and other drugs that inhibit CYP3A4 may decrease the clearance of indinavir and may result in increased plasma concentrations of indinavir).
No products indexed under this heading.

Modafinil (Indinavir is metabolized by CYP3A4. Drugs that induce CYP3A4 activity would be expected to increase the clearance of indinavir, resulting in lowered plasma concentrations of indinavir). Products include:
Provigil 983

Nafcillin Sodium (Indinavir is metabolized by CYP3A4. Drugs that induce CYP3A4 activity would be expected to increase the clearance of indinavir, resulting in lowered plasma concentrations of indinavir).
No products indexed under this heading.

Nefazodone Hydrochloride (Indinavir is metabolized by CYP3A4. Co-administration of indinavir and other drugs that inhibit CYP3A4 may decrease the clearance of indinavir and may result in increased plasma concentrations of indinavir).
No products indexed under this heading.

Nelfinavir Mesylate (Co-administration of indinavir and nelfinavir increases indinavir concentrations. The appropriate doses for this combination, with respect to safety and efficacy, have not been established).
No products indexed under this heading.

Nevirapine (Co-administration of indinavir and nevirapine may lead to decreased indinavir concentrations. The appropriate doses for this combination, with respect to safety and efficacy, have not been established). Products include:
Viramune Oral Suspension 897
Viramune Tablets 897

Niacin (Indinavir is metabolized by CYP3A4. Co-administration of indinavir and other drugs that inhibit CYP3A4 may decrease the clearance of indinavir and may result in increased plasma concentrations of indinavir). Products include:
Advicor 402
Cardio Basics 3455
Niaspan 497
Simcor 524

Niacinamide (Indinavir is metabolized by CYP3A4. Co-administration of indinavir and other drugs that inhibit CYP3A4 may decrease the clearance of indinavir and may result in increased plasma concentrations of indinavir). Products include:
CitraNatal 90 DHA Capsules 2332
CitraNatal Assure 2332
CitraNatal Rx 2332
Heplive 607

Niacinamide Hydroiodide (Indinavir is metabolized by CYP3A4. Co-administration of indinavir and other drugs that inhibit CYP3A4 may decrease the clearance of indinavir and may result in increased plasma concentrations of indinavir).
No products indexed under this heading.

Nicardipine (Indinavir is an inhibitor of CYP3A4. Co-administration of indinavir and drugs primarily metabolized by CYP3A4 may result in increased plasma concentrations of the other drug, which could increase or prolong its therapeutic and adverse effects).
No products indexed under this heading.

Nicardipine Hydrochloride (Co-administration with dihydropyridine calcium channel blockers may increase the concentration of the dihydropyridine calcium channel blocker. Caution is warranted and clinical monitoring of patients is recommended).
No products indexed under this heading.

Nicotinamide (Indinavir is metabolized by CYP3A4. Co-administration of indinavir and other drugs that inhibit CYP3A4 may decrease the clearance of indinavir and may result in increased plasma concentrations of indinavir).
No products indexed under this heading.

Nifedipine (Co-administration with dihydropyridine calcium channel blockers may increase the concentration of the dihydropyridine calcium channel blocker. Caution is warranted and clinical monitoring of patients is recommended).
No products indexed under this heading.

Nimodipine (Co-administration with dihydropyridine calcium channel blockers may increase the concentration of the dihydropyridine calcium channel blocker. Caution is warranted and clinical monitoring of patients is recommended).
No products indexed under this heading.

Nisoldipine (Indinavir is an inhibitor of CYP3A4. Co-administration of indinavir and drugs primarily metabolized by CYP3A4 may result in increased plasma concentrations of the other drug, which could increase or prolong its therapeutic and adverse effects).
No products indexed under this heading.

Nitrendipine (Indinavir is an inhibitor of CYP3A4. Co-administration of indinavir and drugs primarily metabolized by CYP3A4 may result in increased plasma concentrations of the other drug, which could increase or prolong its therapeutic and adverse effects).
No products indexed under this heading.

Norethindrone (Indinavir is an inhibitor of CYP3A4. Co-administration of indinavir and drugs primarily metabolized by CYP3A4 may result in increased plasma concentrations of the other drug, which could increase or prolong its therapeutic and adverse effects). Products include:
Ortho Micronor 2660

Norethindrone Acetate (Indinavir is an inhibitor of CYP3A4. Co-administration of indinavir and drugs primarily metabolized by CYP3A4 may result in increased plasma concentrations of the other drug, which could increase or prolong its therapeutic and adverse effects). Products include:
Activella 2561

Norfloxacin (Indinavir is metabolized by CYP3A4. Co-administration of indinavir and other drugs that inhibit CYP3A4 may decrease the clearance of indinavir and may result in increased plasma concentrations of indinavir). Products include:
Noroxin 2220

Norgestrel (Indinavir is an inhibitor of CYP3A4. Co-administration of indinavir and drugs primarily metabolized by CYP3A4 may result in increased plasma concentrations of the other drug, which could increase or prolong its therapeutic and adverse effects).
No products indexed under this heading.

Omeprazole (Indinavir is metabolized by CYP3A4. Co-administration of indinavir and other drugs that inhibit CYP3A4 may decrease the clearance of indinavir and may result in increased plasma concentrations of indinavir).
No products indexed under this heading.

Ondansetron (Indinavir is an inhibitor of CYP3A4. Co-administration of indinavir and drugs primarily metabolized by CYP3A4 may result in increased plasma concentrations of the other drug, which could increase or prolong its therapeutic and adverse effects).
No products indexed under this heading.

Ondansetron Hydrochloride (Indinavir is an inhibitor of CYP3A4. Co-administration of indinavir and drugs primarily metabolized by CYP3A4 may result in increased plasma concentrations of the other drug, which could increase or prolong its therapeutic and adverse effects). Products include:
Zofran Injection 1750
Zofran 1756
Zofran ODT 1756

Oxcarbazepine (Indinavir is metabolized by CYP3A4. Drugs that induce CYP3A4 activity would be expected to increase the clearance of indinavir, resulting in lowered plasma concentrations of indinavir).
No products indexed under this heading.

IMPORTANT NOTE: Always consult each drug listing in the patient's regimen for possible interactions.

Paclitaxel (Indinavir is an inhibitor of CYP3A4. Co-administration of indinavir and drugs primarily metabolized by CYP3A4 may result in increased plasma concentrations of the other drug, which could increase or prolong its therapeutic and adverse effects).
No products indexed under this heading.

Paroxetine Hydrochloride (Indinavir is metabolized by CYP3A4. Co-administration of indinavir and other drugs that inhibit CYP3A4 may decrease the clearance of indinavir and may result in increased plasma concentrations of indinavir). Products include:
Paroxetine CR 2361
Paroxetine ER 2371
Paxil 1586
Paxil CR 1596

Phenobarbital (Co-administration may decrease concentrations of indinavir. Concurrent use should be used with caution. Indinavir may not be effective due to decreased indinavir concentrations in patients taking these agents concomitantly). Products include:
Donnatal 2711

Phenobarbital Sodium (Co-administration may decrease concentrations of indinavir. Concurrent use should be used with caution. Indinavir may not be effective due to decreased indinavir concentrations in patients taking these agents concomitantly).
No products indexed under this heading.

Phenytoin (Co-administration with phenytoin may decrease indinavir concentrations. Concurrent use should be used with caution. Indinavir may not be effective due to decreased indinavir concentrations in patients taking these agents concomitantly).
No products indexed under this heading.

Phenytoin Sodium (Co-administration with phenytoin may decrease indinavir concentrations. Concurrent use should be used with caution. Indinavir may not be effective due to decreased indinavir concentrations in patients taking these agents concomitantly). Products include:
Phenytek Capsules 2380

Pimozide (Co-administration of indinavir with pimozide is contraindicated. Inhibition of CYP3A4 by indinavir can result in elevated plasma concentrations of pimozide. Co-administration is contraindicated due to potential for serious and/or life-threatening reactions, such as cardiac arrhythmias).
No products indexed under this heading.

Polyestradiol Phosphate (Indinavir is an inhibitor of CYP3A4. Co-administration of indinavir and drugs primarily metabolized by CYP3A4 may result in increased plasma concentrations of the other drug, which could increase or prolong its therapeutic and adverse effects).
No products indexed under this heading.

Posaconazole (Indinavir is metabolized by CYP3A4. Co-administration of indinavir and other drugs that inhibit CYP3A4 may decrease the clearance of indinavir and may result in increased plasma concentrations of indinavir). Products include:
Noxafil 3172

Pravastatin Sodium (Co-administration of indinavir with pravastatin has not been studied. If no alternative treatment is available, use with careful monitoring).
No products indexed under this heading.

Prednisolone (Indinavir is metabolized by CYP3A4. Drugs that induce CYP3A4 activity would be expected to increase the clearance of indinavir, resulting in lowered plasma concentrations of indinavir).
No products indexed under this heading.

Prednisolone Acetate (Indinavir is metabolized by CYP3A4. Drugs that induce CYP3A4 activity would be expected to increase the clearance of indinavir, resulting in lowered plasma concentrations of indinavir). Products include:
Blephamide .... ⊙212, ⊙214
Pred Forte .... ⊙225
Pred Mild .... ⊙230
Pred-G .... ⊙226, ⊙227

Prednisolone Sodium Phosphate (Indinavir is metabolized by CYP3A4. Drugs that induce CYP3A4 activity would be expected to increase the clearance of indinavir, resulting in lowered plasma concentrations of indinavir).
No products indexed under this heading.

Prednisolone Tebutate (Indinavir is metabolized by CYP3A4. Drugs that induce CYP3A4 activity would be expected to increase the clearance of indinavir, resulting in lowered plasma concentrations of indinavir).
No products indexed under this heading.

Prednisone (Indinavir is metabolized by CYP3A4. Drugs that induce CYP3A4 activity would be expected to increase the clearance of indinavir, resulting in lowered plasma concentrations of indinavir).
No products indexed under this heading.

Prednisone sodium phosphate (Indinavir is metabolized by CYP3A4. Drugs that induce CYP3A4 activity would be expected to increase the clearance of indinavir, resulting in lowered plasma concentrations of indinavir).
No products indexed under this heading.

Primidone (Indinavir is metabolized by CYP3A4. Drugs that induce CYP3A4 activity would be expected to increase the clearance of indinavir, resulting in lowered plasma concentrations of indinavir).
No products indexed under this heading.

Propoxyphene Hydrochloride (Indinavir is metabolized by CYP3A4. Co-administration of indinavir and other drugs that inhibit CYP3A4 may decrease the clearance of indinavir and may result in increased plasma concentrations of indinavir).
No products indexed under this heading.

Propoxyphene Napsylate (Indinavir is metabolized by CYP3A4. Co-administration of indinavir and other drugs that inhibit CYP3A4 may decrease the clearance of indinavir and may result in increased plasma concentrations of indinavir).
No products indexed under this heading.

Quinidine (Co-administration with quinidine may increase quinidine concentrations. Caution is warranted and therapeutic concentration monitoring is recommended for quinidine when co-administered with indinavir).
No products indexed under this heading.

Quinidine Gluconate (Co-administration with quinidine may increase quinidine concentrations. Caution is warranted and therapeutic concentration monitoring is recommended for quinidine when co-administered with indinavir).
No products indexed under this heading.

Quinidine Hydrochloride (Co-administration with quinidine may increase quinidine concentrations. Caution is warranted and therapeutic concentration monitoring is recommended for quinidine when co-administered with indinavir).
No products indexed under this heading.

Quinidine Polygalacturonate (Co-administration with quinidine may increase quinidine concentrations. Caution is warranted and therapeutic concentration monitoring is recommended for quinidine when co-administered with indinavir).
No products indexed under this heading.

Quinidine Sulfate (Co-administration with quinidine may increase quinidine concentrations. Caution is warranted and therapeutic concentration monitoring is recommended for quinidine when co-administered with indinavir).
No products indexed under this heading.

Quinine (Indinavir is metabolized by CYP3A4. Co-administration of indinavir and other drugs that inhibit CYP3A4 may decrease the clearance of indinavir and may result in increased plasma concentrations of indinavir). Products include:
Hyland's Leg Cramps PM with
Quinine 3315

Quinine Sulfate (Indinavir is metabolized by CYP3A4. Co-administration of indinavir and other drugs that inhibit CYP3A4 may decrease the clearance of indinavir and may result in increased plasma concentrations of indinavir).
No products indexed under this heading.

Quinupristin (Indinavir is metabolized by CYP3A4. Co-administration of indinavir and other drugs that inhibit CYP3A4 may decrease the clearance of indinavir and may result in increased plasma concentrations of indinavir).
No products indexed under this heading.

Ranitidine Bismuth Citrate (Indinavir is metabolized by CYP3A4. Co-administration of indinavir and other drugs that inhibit CYP3A4 may decrease the clearance of indinavir and may result in increased plasma concentrations of indinavir).
No products indexed under this heading.

Ranitidine Hydrochloride (Indinavir is metabolized by CYP3A4. Co-administration of indinavir and other drugs that inhibit CYP3A4 may decrease the clearance of indinavir and may result in increased plasma concentrations of indinavir). Products include:
Zantac 1737
Zantac Injection 1732
Zantac Pharmacy 1735

Rifabutin (Co-administration of indinavir and rifabutin may lead to decreased indinavir and increased rifabutin concentrations. Dose reduction of rifabutin to half the standard dose and a dose increase of indinavir to 1000 mg (three 333-mg capsules) every 8 hours are recommended when rifabutin and indinavir are co-administered).
No products indexed under this heading.

Rifampicin (Indinavir is metabolized by CYP3A4. Drugs that induce CYP3A4 activity would be expected to increase the clearance of indinavir, resulting in lowered plasma concentrations of indinavir).
No products indexed under this heading.

Rifampin (Co-administration of indinavir with rifampin may lead to loss of virologic response and possible resistance to indinavir or to the class of protease inhibitors or other co-administered antiretroviral agents).
No products indexed under this heading.

Rifapentine (Indinavir is metabolized by CYP3A4. Drugs that induce CYP3A4 activity would be expected to increase the clearance of indinavir, resulting in lowered plasma concentrations of indinavir).
No products indexed under this heading.

Ritonavir (Co-administration of indinavir and ritonavir may lead to increased indinavir and ritonavir concen-

trations. The appropriate doses for this combination, with respect to safety and efficacy, have not been established. Preliminary clinical data suggest that the incidence of nephrolithiasis is higher in patients receiving indinavir in combination with ritonavir than those receiving indinavir 800 mg q8h). Products include:
Kaletra 458
Norvir 509

Rosuvastatin Calcium (Concomitant use of indinavir with rosuvastatin is not recommended. The risk of myopathy including rhabdomyolysis may be increased when HIV protease inhibitors, including indinavir, is used in combination with rosuvastatin). Products include:
Crestor 736

Saquinavir (Co-administration of indinavir and saquinavir may lead to increased saquinavir concentrations. The appropriate doses for this combination, with respect to efficacy and safety, have not been established).
No products indexed under this heading.

Saquinavir Mesylate (Co-administration of indinavir and saquinavir may lead to increased saquinavir concentrations. The appropriate doses for this combination, with respect to efficacy and safety, have not been established).
No products indexed under this heading.

Sertraline Hydrochloride (Indinavir is metabolized by CYP3A4. Co-administration of indinavir and other drugs that inhibit CYP3A4 may decrease the clearance of indinavir and may result in increased plasma concentrations of indinavir).
No products indexed under this heading.

Sildenafil Citrate (Co-administration of sildenafil with indinavir may substantially increase plasma concentrations of sildenafil. This may result in an increase in adverse events including hypotension, visual changes, and priapism. The sildenafil dose should not exceed a maximum of 25 mg in a 48-hour period in patients receiving concomitant indinavir therapy).
No products indexed under this heading.

Simvastatin (Concomitant use of indinavir with simvastatin is not recommended. The risk of myopathy including rhabdomyolysis may be increased when HIV protease inhibitors, including indinavir, is used in combination with simvastatin). Products include:
Simcor 524
Vytorin 10/10 .... 2303, 3240
Vytorin 10/20 .... 2303, 3240
Vytorin 10/40 .... 2303, 3240
Vytorin 10/80 .... 2303, 3240
Zocor 2289

Sirolimus (Co-administration of indinavir and sirolimus may lead to increased sirolimus concentrations). Products include:
Rapamune 3579

Sulfinpyrazone (Indinavir is metabolized by CYP3A4. Drugs that induce CYP3A4 activity would be expected to increase the clearance of indinavir, resulting in lowered plasma concentrations of indinavir).
No products indexed under this heading.

Tacrolimus (Co-administration of indinavir and tacrolimus may lead to increased tacrolimus concentrations). Products include:
Prograf Capsules 677
Prograf Injection 677
Protopic 685

Tadalafil (Co-administration of indinavir and tadalafil is expected to substantially increase plasma concentrations of tadalafil and may result in an increase in adverse events, including hypotension,

visual changes, and priapism. Tadalafil dose should not exceed a maximum of 10 mg in a 72-hour period in patients receiving concomitant indinavir therapy). Products include:
Adcirca 3461
Cialis 1861

Tamoxifen Citrate (Indinavir is an inhibitor of CYP3A4. Co-administration of indinavir and drugs primarily metabolized by CYP3A4 may result in increased plasma concentrations of the other drug, which could increase or prolong its therapeutic and adverse effects).
No products indexed under this heading.

Telithromycin (Indinavir is metabolized by CYP3A4. Co-administration of indinavir and other drugs that inhibit CYP3A4 may decrease the clearance of indinavir and may result in increased plasma concentrations of indinavir). Products include:
Ketek 2991

Terfenadine (Indinavir is an inhibitor of CYP3A4. Co-administration of indinavir and drugs primarily metabolized by CYP3A4 may result in increased plasma concentrations of the other drug, which could increase or prolong its therapeutic and adverse effects).
No products indexed under this heading.

Theophyllinate (Indinavir is metabolized by CYP3A4. Drugs that induce CYP3A4 activity would be expected to increase the clearance of indinavir, resulting in lowered plasma concentrations of indinavir).
No products indexed under this heading.

Theophylline (Indinavir is metabolized by CYP3A4. Drugs that induce CYP3A4 activity would be expected to increase the clearance of indinavir, resulting in lowered plasma concentrations of indinavir).
No products indexed under this heading.

Theophylline Anhydrous (Indinavir is metabolized by CYP3A4. Drugs that induce CYP3A4 activity would be expected to increase the clearance of indinavir, resulting in lowered plasma concentrations of indinavir). Products include:
Uniphyl 2817

Theophylline Calcium Salicylate (Indinavir is metabolized by CYP3A4. Drugs that induce CYP3A4 activity would be expected to increase the clearance of indinavir, resulting in lowered plasma concentrations of indinavir).
No products indexed under this heading.

Theophylline Dihydroxypropyl (Glyceryl) (Indinavir is metabolized by CYP3A4. Drugs that induce CYP3A4 activity would be expected to increase the clearance of indinavir, resulting in lowered plasma concentrations of indinavir).
No products indexed under this heading.

Theophylline Ethylenediamine (Indinavir is metabolized by CYP3A4. Drugs that induce CYP3A4 activity would be expected to increase the clearance of indinavir, resulting in lowered plasma concentrations of indinavir).
No products indexed under this heading.

Theophylline Sodium Glycinate (Indinavir is metabolized by CYP3A4. Drugs that induce CYP3A4 activity would be expected to increase the clearance of indinavir, resulting in lowered plasma concentrations of indinavir).
No products indexed under this heading.

Tiagabine Hydrochloride (Indinavir is an inhibitor of CYP3A4. Co-administration of indinavir and drugs primarily metabolized by CYP3A4 may result in increased plasma concentrations of the other drug, which could increase or prolong its therapeutic and adverse effects). Products include:
Gabitril 972

Tolterodine Tartrate (Indinavir is an inhibitor of CYP3A4. Co-administration of indinavir and drugs primarily metabolized by CYP3A4 may result in increased plasma concentrations of the other drug, which could increase or prolong its therapeutic and adverse effects).
No products indexed under this heading.

Trazodone Hydrochloride (Concomitant use of trazodone and indinavir may increase plasma concentrations of trazodone. If trazodone is used with a CYP3A4 inhibitor, such as indinavir, the combination should be used with caution and a lower dose of trazodone should be considered).
No products indexed under this heading.

Triamcinolone (Indinavir is metabolized by CYP3A4. Drugs that induce CYP3A4 activity would be expected to increase the clearance of indinavir, resulting in lowered plasma concentrations of indinavir).
No products indexed under this heading.

Triamcinolone Acetonide (Indinavir is metabolized by CYP3A4. Drugs that induce CYP3A4 activity would be expected to increase the clearance of indinavir, resulting in lowered plasma concentrations of indinavir). Products include:
Azmacort 408
Nasacort AQ 3019

Triamcinolone Diacetate (Indinavir is metabolized by CYP3A4. Drugs that induce CYP3A4 activity would be expected to increase the clearance of indinavir, resulting in lowered plasma concentrations of indinavir).
No products indexed under this heading.

Triamcinolone Hexacetonide (Indinavir is metabolized by CYP3A4. Drugs that induce CYP3A4 activity would be expected to increase the clearance of indinavir, resulting in lowered plasma concentrations of indinavir).
No products indexed under this heading.

Triazolam (Co-administration of indinavir with triazolam is contraindicated. Inhibition by CYP3A4 by indinavir can result in elevated plasma concentrations of triazolam. Co-administration is contraindicated due to potential for serious and/or life-threatening reactions, such as prolonged or increased sedation or respiratory depression).
No products indexed under this heading.

Troglitazone (Indinavir is metabolized by CYP3A4. Drugs that induce CYP3A4 activity would be expected to increase the clearance of indinavir, resulting in lowered plasma concentrations of indinavir).
No products indexed under this heading.

Troleandomycin (Indinavir is metabolized by CYP3A4. Co-administration of indinavir and other drugs that inhibit CYP3A4 may decrease the clearance of indinavir and may result in increased plasma concentrations of indinavir).
No products indexed under this heading.

Valproate Sodium (Indinavir is metabolized by CYP3A4. Co-administration of indinavir and other drugs that inhibit CYP3A4 may decrease the clearance of indinavir and may result in increased plasma concentrations of indinavir).
No products indexed under this heading.

Vardenafil Hydrochloride (Co-administration of indinavir and vardenafil is expected to substantially increase plasma concentrations of vardenafil and may result in an increase in adverse events, including hypotension, visual changes, and priapism. Vardenafil dose should not exceed a maximum of 2.5 mg in a 24-hour period in patient receiving concomitant indinavir therapy). Products include:
Levitra 3157

Venlafaxine Hydrochloride (Concomitant use with venlafaxine may reduce the concentration of indinavir. In a study, venlafaxine administered under steady-state conditions at 150 mg/day resulted in a 28% decrease in the AUC of a single 800 mg oral dose of indinavir and a 36% decrease in indinavir C_{max}. Indinavir did not affect the pharmacokinetics of venlafaxine). Products include:
Effexor XR 3504
Venlafaxine Hydrochloride Tablets ... 2388

Verapamil Hydrochloride (Indinavir is metabolized by CYP3A4. Co-administration of indinavir and other drugs that inhibit CYP3A4 may decrease the clearance of indinavir and may result in increased plasma concentrations of indinavir). Products include:
Tarka 534

Vinblastine Sulfate (Indinavir is an inhibitor of CYP3A4. Co-administration of indinavir and drugs primarily metabolized by CYP3A4 may result in increased plasma concentrations of the other drug, which could increase or prolong its therapeutic and adverse effects).
No products indexed under this heading.

Vincristine Sulfate (Indinavir is an inhibitor of CYP3A4. Co-administration of indinavir and drugs primarily metabolized by CYP3A4 may result in increased plasma concentrations of the other drug, which could increase or prolong its therapeutic and adverse effects).
No products indexed under this heading.

Voriconazole (Indinavir is metabolized by CYP3A4. Co-administration of indinavir and other drugs that inhibit CYP3A4 may decrease the clearance of indinavir and may result in increased plasma concentrations of indinavir).
No products indexed under this heading.

Warfarin Sodium (Indinavir is an inhibitor of CYP3A4. Co-administration of indinavir and drugs primarily metabolized by CYP3A4 may result in increased plasma concentrations of the other drug, which could increase or prolong its therapeutic and adverse effects).
No products indexed under this heading.

Zafirlukast (Indinavir is metabolized by CYP3A4. Co-administration of indinavir and other drugs that inhibit CYP3A4 may decrease the clearance of indinavir and may result in increased plasma concentrations of indinavir). Products include:
Accolate 3612

Zileuton (Indinavir is metabolized by CYP3A4. Co-administration of indinavir and other drugs that inhibit CYP3A4 may decrease the clearance of indinavir and may result in increased plasma concentrations of indinavir).
No products indexed under this heading.

Food Interactions

Food, unspecified (Co-administration of indinavir with a meal high in calories, fat, and protein, may reduce the absorption of indinavir; administer without food but with water one hour before or 2 hours after a meal).

Grapefruit (Indinavir is metabolized by CYP3A4. Co-administration of indinavir and other drugs that inhibit CYP3A4 may decrease the clearance of indinavir and may result in increased plasma concentrations of indinavir).

Grapefruit Juice (Indinavir is metabolized by CYP3A4. Co-administration of indinavir and other drugs that inhibit CYP3A4 may decrease the clearance of indinavir and may result in increased plasma concentrations of indinavir).

CUBICIN FOR INJECTION

(Daptomycin) 999
May interact with aminoglycosides, beta-lactams antibiotics, HMG-CoA reductase inhibitors, and certain other agents. Compounds in these categories include:

Amikacin Sulfate (*In vitro* synergistic interactions of daptomycin with aminoglycosides, β-lactam antibiotics, and rifampin have been shown against some isolates of staphylococci (including some methicillin-resistant isolates) and enterococci (including some vancomycin-resistant isolates)).
No products indexed under this heading.

Amoxicillin (*In vitro* synergistic interactions of daptomycin with aminoglycosides, β-lactam antibiotics, and rifampin have been shown against some isolates of staphylococci (including some methicillin-resistant isolates) and enterococci (including some vancomycin-resistant isolates). Products include:
Amoxil Capsules 1311
Amoxil Chewable Tablets 1311
Amoxil 1311
Amoxil Powder 1311
Augmentin 1331
Augmentin Tablets 1335
Augmentin ES-600 1338
Augmentin XR 1342
Moxatag 2321

Amoxicillin Trihydrate (*In vitro* synergistic interactions of daptomycin with aminoglycosides, β-lactam antibiotics, and rifampin have been shown against some isolates of staphylococci (including some methicillin-resistant isolates) and enterococci (including some vancomycin-resistant isolates).
No products indexed under this heading.

Ampicillin (*In vitro* synergistic interactions of daptomycin with aminoglycosides, β-lactam antibiotics, and rifampin have been shown against some isolates of staphylococci (including some methicillin-resistant isolates) and enterococci (including some vancomycin-resistant isolates).
No products indexed under this heading.

Ampicillin Sodium (*In vitro* synergistic interactions of daptomycin with aminoglycosides, β-lactam antibiotics, and rifampin have been shown against some isolates of staphylococci (including some methicillin-resistant isolates) and enterococci (including some vancomycin-resistant isolates).
No products indexed under this heading.

Ampicillin Trihydrate (*In vitro* synergistic interactions of daptomycin with aminoglycosides, β-lactam antibiotics, and rifampin have been shown against some isolates of staphylococci (including some methicillin-resistant isolates) and enterococci (including some vancomycin-resistant isolates).
No products indexed under this heading.

Atorvastatin Calcium (In a clinical trial, 5/22 daptomycin-treated patients who received prior or concomitant therapy with an HMG-CoA reductase inhibitor developed CPK elevations>500 U/L. Experience with co-administration of HMG-CoA reductase inhibitors and daptomycin is limited; therefore, consideration should be given to temporarily suspending use of HMG-CoA reductase inhibitors in patients receiving daptomycin). Products include:
Lipitor 2703

IMPORTANT NOTE: Always consult each drug listing in the patient's regimen for possible interactions.

Cubicin **Interactions Index** **432**

Azlocillin Sodium (*In vitro* synergistic interactions of daptomycin with aminoglycosides, β-lactam antibiotics, and rifampin have been shown against some isolates of staphylococci (including some methicillin-resistant isolates) and enterococci (including some vancomycin-resistant isolates).
No products indexed under this heading.

Aztreonam (*In vitro* synergistic interactions of daptomycin with aminoglycosides, β-lactam antibiotics, and rifampin have been shown against some isolates of staphylococci (including some methicillin-resistant isolates) and enterococci (including some vancomycin-resistant isolates).
No products indexed under this heading.

Bacampicillin Hydrochloride (*In vitro* synergistic interactions of daptomycin with aminoglycosides, β-lactam antibiotics, and rifampin have been shown against some isolates of staphylococci (including some methicillin-resistant isolates) and enterococci (including some vancomycin-resistant isolates).
No products indexed under this heading.

Carbenicillin Disodium (*In vitro* synergistic interactions of daptomycin with aminoglycosides, β-lactam antibiotics, and rifampin have been shown against some isolates of staphylococci (including some methicillin-resistant isolates) and enterococci (including some vancomycin-resistant isolates).
No products indexed under this heading.

Carbenicillin Indanyl Sodium (*In vitro* synergistic interactions of daptomycin with aminoglycosides, β-lactam antibiotics, and rifampin have been shown against some isolates of staphylococci (including some methicillin-resistant isolates) and enterococci (including some vancomycin-resistant isolates).
No products indexed under this heading.

Cefaclor (*In vitro* synergistic interactions of daptomycin with aminoglycosides, β-lactam antibiotics, and rifampin have been shown against some isolates of staphylococci (including some methicillin-resistant isolates) and enterococci (including some vancomycin-resistant isolates).
No products indexed under this heading.

Cefadroxil (*In vitro* synergistic interactions of daptomycin with aminoglycosides, β-lactam antibiotics, and rifampin have been shown against some isolates of staphylococci (including some methicillin-resistant isolates) and enterococci (including some vancomycin-resistant isolates).
No products indexed under this heading.

Cefamandole Nafate (*In vitro* synergistic interactions of daptomycin with aminoglycosides, β-lactam antibiotics, and rifampin have been shown against some isolates of staphylococci (including some methicillin-resistant isolates) and enterococci (including some vancomycin-resistant isolates).
No products indexed under this heading.

Cefazolin Sodium (*In vitro* synergistic interactions of daptomycin with aminoglycosides, β-lactam antibiotics, and rifampin have been shown against some isolates of staphylococci (including some methicillin-resistant isolates) and enterococci (including some vancomycin-resistant isolates).
No products indexed under this heading.

Cefixime (*In vitro* synergistic interactions of daptomycin with aminoglycosides, β-lactam antibiotics, and rifampin have been shown against some isolates of staphylococci (including some methicillin-resistant isolates) and enterococci (including some vancomycin-resistant isolates). Products include:
Suprax for Oral Suspension **2038**
Suprax Tablets **2038**

Cefmetazole Sodium (*In vitro* synergistic interactions of daptomycin with aminoglycosides, β-lactam antibiotics, and rifampin have been shown against some isolates of staphylococci (including some methicillin-resistant isolates) and enterococci (including some vancomycin-resistant isolates).
No products indexed under this heading.

Cefonicid Sodium (*In vitro* synergistic interactions of daptomycin with aminoglycosides, β-lactam antibiotics, and rifampin have been shown against some isolates of staphylococci (including some methicillin-resistant isolates) and enterococci (including some vancomycin-resistant isolates).
No products indexed under this heading.

Cefoperazone Sodium (*In vitro* synergistic interactions of daptomycin with aminoglycosides, β-lactam antibiotics, and rifampin have been shown against some isolates of staphylococci (including some methicillin-resistant isolates) and enterococci (including some vancomycin-resistant isolates).
No products indexed under this heading.

Ceforanide (*In vitro* synergistic interactions of daptomycin with aminoglycosides, β-lactam antibiotics, and rifampin have been shown against some isolates of staphylococci (including some methicillin-resistant isolates) and enterococci (including some vancomycin-resistant isolates).
No products indexed under this heading.

Cefotaxime Sodium (*In vitro* synergistic interactions of daptomycin with aminoglycosides, β-lactam antibiotics, and rifampin have been shown against some isolates of staphylococci (including some methicillin-resistant isolates) and enterococci (including some vancomycin-resistant isolates).
No products indexed under this heading.

Cefotetan (*In vitro* synergistic interactions of daptomycin with aminoglycosides, β-lactam antibiotics, and rifampin have been shown against some isolates of staphylococci (including some methicillin-resistant isolates) and enterococci (including some vancomycin-resistant isolates).
No products indexed under this heading.

Cefoxitin Sodium (*In vitro* synergistic interactions of daptomycin with aminoglycosides, β-lactam antibiotics, and rifampin have been shown against some isolates of staphylococci (including some methicillin-resistant isolates) and enterococci (including some vancomycin-resistant isolates).
No products indexed under this heading.

Cefpodoxime Proxetil (*In vitro* synergistic interactions of daptomycin with aminoglycosides, β-lactam antibiotics, and rifampin have been shown against some isolates of staphylococci (including some methicillin-resistant isolates) and enterococci (including some vancomycin-resistant isolates).
No products indexed under this heading.

Cefprozil (*In vitro* synergistic interactions of daptomycin with aminoglycosides, β-lactam antibiotics, and rifampin have been shown against some isolates of staphylococci (including some methicillin-resistant isolates) and enterococci (including some vancomycin-resistant isolates).
No products indexed under this heading.

Ceftazidime (*In vitro* synergistic interactions of daptomycin with aminoglycosides, β-lactam antibiotics, and rifampin have been shown against some isolates of staphylococci (including some methicillin-resistant isolates) and enterococci (including some vancomycin-resistant isolates). Products include:
Fortaz **1481**

Ceftizoxime Sodium (*In vitro* synergistic interactions of daptomycin with aminoglycosides, β-lactam antibiotics, and rifampin have been shown against some isolates of staphylococci (including some methicillin-resistant isolates) and enterococci (including some vancomycin-resistant isolates).
No products indexed under this heading.

Ceftriaxone Sodium (*In vitro* synergistic interactions of daptomycin with aminoglycosides, β-lactam antibiotics, and rifampin have been shown against some isolates of staphylococci (including some methicillin-resistant isolates) and enterococci (including some vancomycin-resistant isolates).
Products include:
Rocephin **2859**

Cefuroxime Axetil (*In vitro* synergistic interactions of daptomycin with aminoglycosides, β-lactam antibiotics, and rifampin have been shown against some isolates of staphylococci (including some methicillin-resistant isolates) and enterococci (including some vancomycin-resistant isolates).
Products include:
Ceftin **1399**

Cefuroxime Sodium (*In vitro* synergistic interactions of daptomycin with aminoglycosides, β-lactam antibiotics, and rifampin have been shown against some isolates of staphylococci (including some methicillin-resistant isolates) and enterococci (including some vancomycin-resistant isolates).
No products indexed under this heading.

Cephalexin (*In vitro* synergistic interactions of daptomycin with aminoglycosides, β-lactam antibiotics, and rifampin have been shown against some isolates of staphylococci (including some methicillin-resistant isolates) and enterococci (including some vancomycin-resistant isolates).
No products indexed under this heading.

Cephalothin Sodium (*In vitro* synergistic interactions of daptomycin with aminoglycosides, β-lactam antibiotics, and rifampin have been shown against some isolates of staphylococci (including some methicillin-resistant isolates) and enterococci (including some vancomycin-resistant isolates).
No products indexed under this heading.

Cephapirin Sodium (*In vitro* synergistic interactions of daptomycin with aminoglycosides, β-lactam antibiotics, and rifampin have been shown against some isolates of staphylococci (including some methicillin-resistant isolates) and enterococci (including some vancomycin-resistant isolates).
No products indexed under this heading.

Cephradine (*In vitro* synergistic interactions of daptomycin with aminoglycosides, β-lactam antibiotics, and rifampin have been shown against some isolates of staphylococci (including some methicillin-resistant isolates) and enterococci (including some vancomycin-resistant isolates).
No products indexed under this heading.

Cerivastatin Sodium (In a clinical trial, 5/22 daptomycin-treated patients who received prior or concomitant therapy with an HMG-CoA reductase inhibitor developed CPK elevations>500 U/L. Experience with co-administration of HMG-CoA reductase inhibitors and daptomycin is limited; therefore, consideration should be given to temporarily suspending use of HMG-CoA reductase inhibitors in patients receiving daptomycin).
No products indexed under this heading.

Cilastatin Sodium (*In vitro* synergistic interactions of daptomycin with aminoglycosides, β-lactam antibiotics, and rifampin have been shown against some isolates of staphylococci (including some methicillin-resistant isolates) and enterococci (including some vancomycin-resistant isolates).
Products include:
Primaxin I.M. **2232**
Primaxin I.V. **2235**

Cloxacillin (*In vitro* synergistic interactions of daptomycin with aminoglycosides, β-lactam antibiotics, and rifampin have been shown against some isolates of staphylococci (including some methicillin-resistant isolates) and enterococci (including some vancomycin-resistant isolates).
No products indexed under this heading.

Cloxacillin Sodium (*In vitro* synergistic interactions of daptomycin with aminoglycosides, β-lactam antibiotics, and rifampin have been shown against some isolates of staphylococci (including some methicillin-resistant isolates) and enterococci (including some vancomycin-resistant isolates).
No products indexed under this heading.

Cloxacillin Sodium Monohydrate (*In vitro* synergistic interactions of daptomycin with aminoglycosides, β-lactam antibiotics, and rifampin have been shown against some isolates of staphylococci (including some methicillin-resistant isolates) and enterococci (including some vancomycin-resistant isolates).
No products indexed under this heading.

Dicloxacillin (*In vitro* synergistic interactions of daptomycin with aminoglycosides, β-lactam antibiotics, and rifampin have been shown against some isolates of staphylococci (including some methicillin-resistant isolates) and enterococci (including some vancomycin-resistant isolates).
No products indexed under this heading.

Dicloxacillin Sodium (*In vitro* synergistic interactions of daptomycin with aminoglycosides, β-lactam antibiotics, and rifampin have been shown against some isolates of staphylococci (including some methicillin-resistant isolates) and enterococci (including some vancomycin-resistant isolates).
No products indexed under this heading.

Dihydrostreptomycin (*In vitro* synergistic interactions of daptomycin with aminoglycosides, β-lactam antibiotics, and rifampin have been shown against some isolates of staphylococci (including some methicillin-resistant isolates) and enterococci (including some vancomycin-resistant isolates)).
No products indexed under this heading.

Disodium Carbenicillin (*In vitro* synergistic interactions of daptomycin with aminoglycosides, β-lactam antibiotics, and rifampin have been shown against some isolates of staphylococci (including some methicillin-resistant isolates) and enterococci (including some vancomycin-resistant isolates).
No products indexed under this heading.

Fluvastatin Sodium (In a clinical trial, 5/22 daptomycin-treated patients who received prior or concomitant therapy with an HMG-CoA reductase inhibitor developed CPK elevations>500 U/L. Experience with co-administration of HMG-CoA reductase inhibitors and daptomycin is limited; therefore, consideration should be given to temporarily suspending use of HMG-CoA reductase inhibitors in patients receiving daptomycin).
No products indexed under this heading.

Gentamicin (*In vitro* synergistic interactions of daptomycin with aminoglycosides, β-lactam antibiotics, and rifampin have been shown against some isolates of staphylococci (including some methicillin-resistant isolates) and enterococci (including some vancomycin-resistant isolates).
    No products indexed under this heading.

Gentamicin Sulfate (*In vitro* synergistic interactions of daptomycin with aminoglycosides, β-lactam antibiotics, and rifampin have been shown against some isolates of staphylococci (including some methicillin-resistant isolates) and enterococci (including some vancomycin-resistant isolates)).
Products include:
    Pred-G .... ⊙226, ⊙227

Imipenem (*In vitro* synergistic interactions of daptomycin with aminoglycosides, β-lactam antibiotics, and rifampin have been shown against some isolates of staphylococci (including some methicillin-resistant isolates) and enterococci (including some vancomycin-resistant isolates). Products include:
    Primaxin I.M. 2232
    Primaxin I.V. 2235

Kanamycin Sulfate (*In vitro* synergistic interactions of daptomycin with aminoglycosides, β-lactam antibiotics, and rifampin have been shown against some isolates of staphylococci (including some methicillin-resistant isolates) and enterococci (including some vancomycin-resistant isolates)).
    No products indexed under this heading.

Loracarbef (*In vitro* synergistic interactions of daptomycin with aminoglycosides, β-lactam antibiotics, and rifampin have been shown against some isolates of staphylococci (including some methicillin-resistant isolates) and enterococci (including some vancomycin-resistant isolates).
    No products indexed under this heading.

Lovastatin (In a clinical trial, 5/22 daptomycin-treated patients who received prior or concomitant therapy with an HMG-CoA reductase inhibitor developed CPK elevations>500 U/L. Experience with co-administration of HMG-CoA reductase inhibitors and daptomycin is limited; therefore, consideration should be given to temporarily suspending use of HMG-CoA reductase inhibitors in patients receiving daptomycin). Products include:
    Advicor 402
    Mevacor 2212

Methicillin Sodium (*In vitro* synergistic interactions of daptomycin with aminoglycosides, β-lactam antibiotics, and rifampin have been shown against some isolates of staphylococci (including some methicillin-resistant isolates) and enterococci (including some vancomycin-resistant isolates).
    No products indexed under this heading.

Mezlocillin Sodium (*In vitro* synergistic interactions of daptomycin with aminoglycosides, β-lactam antibiotics, and rifampin have been shown against some isolates of staphylococci (including some methicillin-resistant isolates) and enterococci (including some vancomycin-resistant isolates).
    No products indexed under this heading.

Nafcillin Sodium (*In vitro* synergistic interactions of daptomycin with aminoglycosides, β-lactam antibiotics, and rifampin have been shown against some isolates of staphylococci (including some methicillin-resistant isolates) and enterococci (including some vancomycin-resistant isolates).
    No products indexed under this heading.

Neomycin (*In vitro* synergistic interactions of daptomycin with aminoglycosides, β-lactam antibiotics, and rifampin have been shown against some isolates of staphylococci (including some methicillin-resistant isolates) and enterococci (including some vancomycin-resistant isolates).
    No products indexed under this heading.

Neomycin, oral (*In vitro* synergistic interactions of daptomycin with aminoglycosides, β-lactam antibiotics, and rifampin have been shown against some isolates of staphylococci (including some methicillin-resistant isolates) and enterococci (including some vancomycin-resistant isolates).
    No products indexed under this heading.

Neomycin Sulfate (*In vitro* synergistic interactions of daptomycin with aminoglycosides, β-lactam antibiotics, and rifampin have been shown against some isolates of staphylococci (including some methicillin-resistant isolates) and enterococci (including some vancomycin-resistant isolates)).
    No products indexed under this heading.

Oxacillin (*In vitro* synergistic interactions of daptomycin with aminoglycosides, β-lactam antibiotics, and rifampin have been shown against some isolates of staphylococci (including some methicillin-resistant isolates) and enterococci (including some vancomycin-resistant isolates).
    No products indexed under this heading.

Oxacillin Sodium (*In vitro* synergistic interactions of daptomycin with aminoglycosides, β-lactam antibiotics, and rifampin have been shown against some isolates of staphylococci (including some methicillin-resistant isolates) and enterococci (including some vancomycin-resistant isolates).
    No products indexed under this heading.

Penicillin, Potassium Phenoxymethyl (*In vitro* synergistic interactions of daptomycin with aminoglycosides, β-lactam antibiotics, and rifampin have been shown against some isolates of staphylococci (including some methicillin-resistant isolates) and enterococci (including some vancomycin-resistant isolates).
    No products indexed under this heading.

Penicillin G Benzathine (*In vitro* synergistic interactions of daptomycin with aminoglycosides, β-lactam antibiotics, and rifampin have been shown against some isolates of staphylococci (including some methicillin-resistant isolates) and enterococci (including some vancomycin-resistant isolates). Products include:
    Bicillin C-R Injectable Suspension 1826
    Bicillin L-A 1828

Penicillin G Dibenzylethyenedi-amine (*In vitro* synergistic interactions of daptomycin with aminoglycosides, β-lactam antibiotics, and rifampin have been shown against some isolates of staphylococci (including some methicillin-resistant isolates) and enterococci (including some vancomycin-resistant isolates).
    No products indexed under this heading.

Penicillin G Potassium (*In vitro* synergistic interactions of daptomycin with aminoglycosides, β-lactam antibiotics, and rifampin have been shown against some isolates of staphylococci (including some methicillin-resistant isolates) and enterococci (including some vancomycin-resistant isolates).
    No products indexed under this heading.

Penicillin G Procaine (*In vitro* synergistic interactions of daptomycin with aminoglycosides, β-lactam antibiotics, and rifampin have been shown against some isolates of staphylococci (including some methicillin-resistant isolates)

and enterococci (including some vancomycin-resistant isolates).
Products include:
    Bicillin C-R Injectable Suspension 1826
    Bicillin L-A 1828

Penicillin G Sodium (*In vitro* synergistic interactions of daptomycin with aminoglycosides, β-lactam antibiotics, and rifampin have been shown against some isolates of staphylococci (including some methicillin-resistant isolates) and enterococci (including some vancomycin-resistant isolates).
    No products indexed under this heading.

Penicillin V (*In vitro* synergistic interactions of daptomycin with aminoglycosides, β-lactam antibiotics, and rifampin have been shown against some isolates of staphylococci (including some methicillin-resistant isolates) and enterococci (including some vancomycin-resistant isolates).
    No products indexed under this heading.

Penicillin V Potassium (*In vitro* synergistic interactions of daptomycin with aminoglycosides, β-lactam antibiotics, and rifampin have been shown against some isolates of staphylococci (including some methicillin-resistant isolates) and enterococci (including some vancomycin-resistant isolates).
    No products indexed under this heading.

Penicillins (*In vitro* synergistic interactions of daptomycin with aminoglycosides, β-lactam antibiotics, and rifampin have been shown against some isolates of staphylococci (including some methicillin-resistant isolates) and enterococci (including some vancomycin-resistant isolates).
    No products indexed under this heading.

Piperacillin Sodium (*In vitro* synergistic interactions of daptomycin with aminoglycosides, β-lactam antibiotics, and rifampin have been shown against some isolates of staphylococci (including some methicillin-resistant isolates) and enterococci (including some vancomycin-resistant isolates).
Products include:
    Zosyn 3607

Pravastatin Sodium (In a clinical trial, 5/22 daptomycin-treated patients who received prior or concomitant therapy with an HMG-CoA reductase inhibitor developed CPK elevations>500 U/L. Experience with co-administration of HMG-CoA reductase inhibitors and daptomycin is limited; therefore, consideration should be given to temporarily suspending use of HMG-CoA reductase inhibitors in patients receiving daptomycin).
    No products indexed under this heading.

Rifampin (*In vitro* synergistic interactions of daptomycin with aminoglycosides, β-lactam antibiotics, and rifampin have been shown against some isolates of staphylococci (including some methicillin-resistant isolates) and enterococci (including some vancomycin-resistant isolates)).
    No products indexed under this heading.

Rosuvastatin Calcium (In a clinical trial, 5/22 daptomycin-treated patients who received prior or concomitant therapy with an HMG-CoA reductase inhibitor developed CPK elevations>500 U/L. Experience with co-administration of HMG-CoA reductase inhibitors and daptomycin is limited; therefore, consideration should be given to temporarily suspending use of HMG-CoA reductase inhibitors in patients receiving daptomycin). Products include:
    Crestor 736

Simvastatin (In a clinical trial, 5/22 daptomycin-treated patients who received prior or concomitant therapy with an HMG-CoA reductase inhibitor developed CPK elevations>500 U/L. Experience with co-administration of

HMG-CoA reductase inhibitors and daptomycin is limited; therefore, consideration should be given to temporarily suspending use of HMG-CoA reductase inhibitors in patients receiving daptomycin). Products include:
    Simcor 524
    Vytorin 10/10 .... 2303, 3240
    Vytorin 10/20 .... 2303, 3240
    Vytorin 10/40 .... 2303, 3240
    Vytorin 10/80 .... 2303, 3240
    Zocor 2289

Sodium Cloxacillin Monohydrate (*In vitro* synergistic interactions of daptomycin with aminoglycosides, β-lactam antibiotics, and rifampin have been shown against some isolates of staphylococci (including some methicillin-resistant isolates) and enterococci (including some vancomycin-resistant isolates).
    No products indexed under this heading.

Streptomycin Sulfate (*In vitro* synergistic interactions of daptomycin with aminoglycosides, β-lactam antibiotics, and rifampin have been shown against some isolates of staphylococci (including some methicillin-resistant isolates) and enterococci (including some vancomycin-resistant isolates)).
    No products indexed under this heading.

Ticarcillin Disodium (*In vitro* synergistic interactions of daptomycin with aminoglycosides, β-lactam antibiotics, and rifampin have been shown against some isolates of staphylococci (including some methicillin-resistant isolates) and enterococci (including some vancomycin-resistant isolates).
Products include:
    Timentin ADD-Vantage 1670
    Timentin Galaxy 1674
    Timentin 1666
    Timentin Pharmacy 1678

Tobramycin (In a study in which 6 healthy adult males received a single dose of daptomycin 2 mg/kg IV, tobramycin 1 mg/kg IV, and both in combination, the mean C_{max} and AUC(0-infinity) of daptomycin increased 12.7% and 8.7%, respectively, when administered with tobramycin. The mean C_{max} and AUC(0-infinity) of tobramycin decreased 10.7% and 6.6%, respectively, when administered with daptomycin. These differences were not statistically significant. The interaction between daptomycin and tobramycin with a clinical dose of daptomycin is unknown. Caution is warranted when daptomycin is co-administered with tobramycin). Products include:
    Tobi Nebulizer 2546
    Tobramycin and Dexamethasone Ophthalmic Suspension............... ⊙251
    Zylet .... ⊙252

Tobramycin Sulfate (In a study in which 6 healthy adult males received a single dose of daptomycin 2 mg/kg IV, tobramycin 1 mg/kg IV, and both in combination, the mean C_{max} and AUC(0-infinity) of daptomycin increased 12.7% and 8.7%, respectively, when administered with tobramycin. The mean C_{max} and AUC(0-infinity) of tobramycin decreased 10.7% and 6.6%, respectively, when administered with daptomycin. These differences were not statistically significant. The interaction between daptomycin and tobramycin with a clinical dose of daptomycin is unknown. Caution is warranted when daptomycin is co-administered with tobramycin).
    No products indexed under this heading.

Warfarin Sodium (As experience with the concomitant administration of daptomycin and warfarin is limited, anticoagulant activity in patients receiving daptomycin and warfarin should be monitored for the first several days after initiating therapy with daptomycin).
    No products indexed under this heading.

IMPORTANT NOTE: Always consult each drug listing in the patient's regimen for possible interactions.

CYMBALTA DELAYED-RELEASE CAPSULES

(Duloxetine Hydrochloride) 1871
May interact with alcohols, anticoagulants, antipsychotic agents, aspirin-acetylsalicylic acid, central nervous system depressants, central nervous system stimulants, class IC antiarrhythmics, cytochrome p450 1a2 inhibitors (selected), cytochrome p450 2d6 inhibitors (selected), cytochrome p450 2d6 substrates (selected), diuretics, dopamine antagonists, drugs that reduce gastric acidity, highly protein bound drugs (selected), lithium preparations, monoamine oxidase inhibitors, non-steroidal anti-inflammatory agents, phenothiazines, selective serotonin reuptake inhibitors, serotonin and norepinephrine reuptake inhibitors, serotoninergic agents, theophyllines, tricyclic antidepressants, triptans, and certain other agents. Compounds in these categories include:

Alatrofloxacin Mesylate (Both CYP1A2 and CYP2D6 are responsible for duloxetine metabolism. When duloxetine 60 mg was co-administered with fluvoxamine 100 mg, a potent CYP1A2 inhibitor to male subjects, duloxetine AUC was increased approximately 6-fold, the C_{max} was increased approximately 2.5-fold and duloxetine $t_{1/2}$ was increased approximately 3-fold. Co-administration of duloxetine with potent CYP1A2 inhibitors should be avoided).
No products indexed under this heading.

Alfentanil Hydrochloride (Given the primary CNS effects of duloxetine, it should be used with caution when it is taken in combination with or substituted for other centrally acting drugs, including those with a similar mechanism of action).
No products indexed under this heading.

Almotriptan Malate (There have been rare post-marketing reports of serotonin syndrome with the use of an SSRI and a triptan. If concomitant treatment is clinically warranted, careful observation of the patient is advised, particularly during treatment initiation and dose increases). Products include:
Axert 2593

Alprazolam (Given the primary CNS effects of duloxetine, it should be used with caution when it is taken in combination with or substituted for other centrally acting drugs, including those with a similar mechanism of action).
No products indexed under this heading.

Aluminum Carbonate (Duloxetine has an enteric coating that resists dissolution until reaching a segment of the gastrointestinal tract where the pH exceeds 5.5. Drugs that raise the gastrointestinal pH may lead to an earlier release of duloxetine).
No products indexed under this heading.

Aluminum Hydroxide (Duloxetine has an enteric coating that resists dissolution until reaching a segment of the gastrointestinal tract where the pH exceeds 5.5. Drugs that raise the gastrointestinal pH may lead to an earlier release of duloxetine).
No products indexed under this heading.

Amiloride Hydrochloride (Hyponatremia may occur as a result of treatment with duloxetine. Patients taking diuretics may be at greater risk. Discontinuation of duloxetine should be considered in patients with symptomatic hyponatremia and appropriate medical intervention should be instituted).
No products indexed under this heading.

Amiodarone Hydrochloride (Both CYP1A2 and CYP2D6 are responsible for duloxetine metabolism. When duloxetine 60 mg was co-administered with fluvoxamine 100 mg, a potent CYP1A2 inhibitor to male subjects, duloxetine

AUC was increased approximately 6-fold, the C_{max} was increased approximately 2.5-fold and duloxetine $t_{1/2}$ was increased approximately 3-fold. Co-administration of duloxetine with potent CYP1A2 inhibitors should be avoided).
No products indexed under this heading.

Amitriptyline Hydrochloride (Duloxetine is a moderate inhibitor of CYP2D6. Co-administration of duloxetine with other drugs that are extensively metabolized by CYP2D6 and have a narrow therapeutic window, including tricyclic antidepressants, should be approached with caution. Plasma tricyclic antidepressant concentrations may need to be monitored, and the dose of the TCA may need to be reduced, if a TCA is co-administered with duloxetine).
No products indexed under this heading.

Amobarbital (Given the primary CNS effects of duloxetine, it should be used with caution when it is taken in combination with or substituted for other centrally acting drugs, including those with a similar mechanism of action).
No products indexed under this heading.

Amobarbital Sodium (Given the primary CNS effects of duloxetine, it should be used with caution when it is taken in combination with or substituted for other centrally acting drugs, including those with a similar mechanism of action).
No products indexed under this heading.

Amoxapine (Duloxetine is a moderate inhibitor of CYP2D6. Co-administration of duloxetine with other drugs that are extensively metabolized by CYP2D6 and have a narrow therapeutic window, including tricyclic antidepressants, should be approached with caution. Plasma tricyclic antidepressant concentrations may need to be monitored, and the dose of the TCA may need to be reduced, if a TCA is co-administered with duloxetine).
No products indexed under this heading.

Amphetamine Aspartate (Given the primary CNS effects of duloxetine, it should be used with caution when it is taken in combination with or substituted for other centrally acting drugs, including those with a similar mechanism of action).
No products indexed under this heading.

Amphetamine Aspartate Monohydrate (Given the primary CNS effects of duloxetine, it should be used with caution when it is taken in combination with or substituted for other centrally acting drugs, including those with a similar mechanism of action).
No products indexed under this heading.

Amphetamine Resins (Given the primary CNS effects of duloxetine, it should be used with caution when it is taken in combination with or substituted for other centrally acting drugs, including those with a similar mechanism of action).
No products indexed under this heading.

Amphetamine Sulfate (Given the primary CNS effects of duloxetine, it should be used with caution when it is taken in combination with or substituted for other centrally acting drugs, including those with a similar mechanism of action).
No products indexed under this heading.

Anastrozole (Both CYP1A2 and CYP2D6 are responsible for duloxetine metabolism. When duloxetine 60 mg was co-administered with fluvoxamine 100 mg, a potent CYP1A2 inhibitor to male subjects, duloxetine AUC was increased approximately 6-fold, the C_{max} was increased approximately 2.5-fold and duloxetine $t_{1/2}$ was

increased approximately 3-fold. Co-administration of duloxetine with potent CYP1A2 inhibitors should be avoided).
No products indexed under this heading.

Anisindione (Duloxetine may increase the risk of bleeding events. Concomitant use of anticoagulants may add to this risk. Case reports and epidemiological studies have demonstrated an association between use of drugs that interfere with serotonin reuptake and the occurrence of gastrointestinal bleeding. Patients should be cautioned about the risk of bleeding associated with concomitant use of duloxetine and anticoagulants).
No products indexed under this heading.

Aprobarbital (Given the primary CNS effects of duloxetine, it should be used with caution when it is taken in combination with or substituted for other centrally acting drugs, including those with a similar mechanism of action).
No products indexed under this heading.

Ardeparin Sodium (Duloxetine may increase the risk of bleeding events. Concomitant use of anticoagulants may add to this risk. Case reports and epidemiological studies have demonstrated an association between use of drugs that interfere with serotonin reuptake and the occurrence of gastrointestinal bleeding. Patients should be cautioned about the risk of bleeding associated with concomitant use of duloxetine and anticoagulants).
No products indexed under this heading.

Aripiprazole (Development of a potentially life-threatening serotonin syndrome or Neuroleptic Malignant Syndrome-like reactions have been reported with duloxetine, and with concomitant use of antipsychotics. Serotonin syndrome symptoms may include mental status changes, autonomic instability, neuromuscular aberrations, and/or gastrointestinal symptoms. Serotonin syndrome in its most severe form can resemble neuroleptic malignant syndrome. Patients should be monitored for the emergence of serotonin syndrome or NMS-like signs and symptoms. Treatment with duloxetine and any antipsychotic agent should be discontinued immediately if the above events occur and supportive symptomatic treatment should be initiated).
No products indexed under this heading.

Aspirin (Duloxetine may increase the risk of bleeding events. Concomitant use of aspirin may add to this risk. Case reports and epidemiological studies have demonstrated an association between use of drugs that interfere with serotonin reuptake and the occurrence of gastrointestinal bleeding. Patients should be cautioned about the risk of bleeding associated with concomitant use of duloxetine and aspirin). Products include:
Aggrenox 880
Bayer Aspirin 829
Percodan 1124
St. Joseph Aspirin 2045

Aspirin, Enteric Coated (Duloxetine may increase the risk of bleeding events. Concomitant use of aspirin may add to this risk. Case reports and epidemiological studies have demonstrated an association between use of drugs that interfere with serotonin reuptake and the occurrence of gastrointestinal bleeding. Patients should be cautioned about the risk of bleeding associated with concomitant use of duloxetine and aspirin).
No products indexed under this heading.

Aspirin Buffered (Duloxetine may increase the risk of bleeding events. Concomitant use of aspirin may add to this risk. Case reports and epidemiological studies have demonstrated an asso-

ciation between use of drugs that interfere with serotonin reuptake and the occurrence of gastrointestinal bleeding. Patients should be cautioned about the risk of bleeding associated with concomitant use of duloxetine and aspirin).
No products indexed under this heading.

Atomoxetine Hydrochloride (Duloxetine is a moderate inhibitor of CYP2D6. Co-administration of duloxetine with other drugs that are extensively metabolized by CYP2D6 isoenzyme, and which have a narrow therapeutic window, should be approached with caution). Products include:
Strattera 1957

Atovaquone (Because duloxetine is highly bound to plasma protein, administration of duloxetine to a patient taking another drug that is highly protein bound may cause increased free concentration of the other drug, potentially resulting in serious adverse reactions). Products include:
Malarone Pediatric Tablets 1572
Malarone 1572
Mepron Suspension 1576

Bendroflumethiazide (Hyponatremia may occur as a result of treatment with duloxetine. Patients taking diuretics may be at greater risk. Discontinuation of duloxetine should be considered in patients with symptomatic hyponatremia and appropriate medical intervention should be instituted).
No products indexed under this heading.

Bisoprolol Fumarate (Duloxetine is a moderate inhibitor of CYP2D6. Co-administration of duloxetine with other drugs that are extensively metabolized by CYP2D6 isoenzyme, and which have a narrow therapeutic window, should be approached with caution).
No products indexed under this heading.

Bumetanide (Hyponatremia may occur as a result of treatment with duloxetine. Patients taking diuretics may be at greater risk. Discontinuation of duloxetine should be considered in patients with symptomatic hyponatremia and appropriate medical intervention should be instituted).
No products indexed under this heading.

Buprenorphine Hydrochloride (Given the primary CNS effects of duloxetine, it should be used with caution when it is taken in combination with or substituted for other centrally acting drugs, including those with a similar mechanism of action).
No products indexed under this heading.

Bupropion Hydrochloride (Because CYP2D6 is involved in duloxetine metabolism, concomitant use of duloxetine with potent inhibitors of CYP2D6 would be expected to, and does, result in higher concentrations (on average of 60%) of duloxetine). Products include:
Aplenzin 2948
Wellbutrin 1719
Wellbutrin SR 1725
Zyban 1762

Buspirone Hydrochloride (Given the primary CNS effects of duloxetine, it should be used with caution when it is taken in combination with or substituted for other centrally acting drugs, including those with a similar mechanism of action).
No products indexed under this heading.

Butabarbital (Given the primary CNS effects of duloxetine, it should be used with caution when it is taken in combination with or substituted for other centrally acting drugs, including those with a similar mechanism of action).
No products indexed under this heading.

(⊙ Described in PDR® for Ophthalmic Medicines)

Butabarbital Sodium (Given the primary CNS effects of duloxetine, it should be used with caution when it is taken in combination with or substituted for other centrally acting drugs, including those with a similar mechanism of action).
No products indexed under this heading.

Butalbital (Given the primary CNS effects of duloxetine, it should be used with caution when it is taken in combination with or substituted for other centrally acting drugs, including those with a similar mechanism of action).
No products indexed under this heading.

Captopril (Duloxetine is a moderate inhibitor of CYP2D6. Co-administration of duloxetine with other drugs that are extensively metabolized by CYP2D6 isoenzyme, and which have a narrow therapeutic window, should be approached with caution). Products include:
Captopril 2341

Carvedilol (Duloxetine is a moderate inhibitor of CYP2D6. Co-administration of duloxetine with other drugs that are extensively metabolized by CYP2D6 isoenzyme, and which have a narrow therapeutic window, should be approached with caution). Products include:
Coreg 1409

Cefonicid Sodium (Because duloxetine is highly bound to plasma protein, administration of duloxetine to a patient taking another drug that is highly protein bound may cause increased free concentration of the other drug, potentially resulting in serious adverse reactions).
No products indexed under this heading.

Celecoxib (Duloxetine may increase the risk of bleeding events. Concomitant use of non-steroidal anti-inflammatory drugs may add to this risk. Case reports and epidemiological studies have demonstrated an association between use of drugs that interfere with serotonin reuptake and the occurrence of gastrointestinal bleeding. Patients should be cautioned about the risk of bleeding associated with concomitant use of duloxetine and NSAIDs). Products include:
Celebrex 3272

Cevimeline Hydrochloride (Duloxetine is a moderate inhibitor of CYP2D6. Co-administration of duloxetine with other drugs that are extensively metabolized by CYP2D6 isoenzyme, and which have a narrow therapeutic window, should be approached with caution). Products include:
Evoxac 1027

Chlordiazepoxide (Given the primary CNS effects of duloxetine, it should be used with caution when it is taken in combination with or substituted for other centrally acting drugs, including those with a similar mechanism of action).
No products indexed under this heading.

Chlordiazepoxide Hydrochloride (Given the primary CNS effects of duloxetine, it should be used with caution when it is taken in combination with or substituted for other centrally acting drugs, including those with a similar mechanism of action).
No products indexed under this heading.

Chloroquine (Because CYP2D6 is involved in duloxetine metabolism, concomitant use of duloxetine with potent inhibitors of CYP2D6 would be expected to, and does, result in higher concentrations (on average of 60%) of duloxetine).
No products indexed under this heading.

Chloroquine Hydrochloride (Because CYP2D6 is involved in duloxetine metabolism, concomitant use of duloxetine with potent inhibitors of CYP2D6 would be expected to, and does, result in higher concentrations (on average of 60%) of duloxetine).
No products indexed under this heading.

Chloroquine Phosphate (Because CYP2D6 is involved in duloxetine metabolism, concomitant use of duloxetine with potent inhibitors of CYP2D6 would be expected to, and does, result in higher concentrations (on average of 60%) of duloxetine).
No products indexed under this heading.

Chlorothiazide (Hyponatremia may occur as a result of treatment with duloxetine. Patients taking diuretics may be at greater risk. Discontinuation of duloxetine should be considered in patients with symptomatic hyponatremia and appropriate medical intervention should be instituted).
No products indexed under this heading.

Chlorothiazide Sodium (Hyponatremia may occur as a result of treatment with duloxetine. Patients taking diuretics may be at greater risk. Discontinuation of duloxetine should be considered in patients with symptomatic hyponatremia and appropriate medical intervention should be instituted). Products include:
Diuril Intravenous 2009

Chlorpheniramine (Because CYP2D6 is involved in duloxetine metabolism, concomitant use of duloxetine with potent inhibitors of CYP2D6 would be expected to, and does, result in higher concentrations (on average of 60%) of duloxetine).
No products indexed under this heading.

Chlorpheniramine Maleate (Because CYP2D6 is involved in duloxetine metabolism, concomitant use of duloxetine with potent inhibitors of CYP2D6 would be expected to, and does, result in higher concentrations (on average of 60%) of duloxetine).
No products indexed under this heading.

Chlorpheniramine Polistirex (Because CYP2D6 is involved in duloxetine metabolism, concomitant use of duloxetine with potent inhibitors of CYP2D6 would be expected to, and does, result in higher concentrations (on average of 60%) of duloxetine). Products include:
Tussionex 3443

Chlorpheniramine Tannate (Because CYP2D6 is involved in duloxetine metabolism, concomitant use of duloxetine with potent inhibitors of CYP2D6 would be expected to, and does, result in higher concentrations (on average of 60%) of duloxetine).
No products indexed under this heading.

Chlorpromazine (Development of a potentially life-threatening serotonin syndrome or Neuroleptic Malignant Syndrome-like reactions have been reported with duloxetine, and with concomitant use of dopamine antagonists. Serotonin syndrome symptoms may include mental status changes, autonomic instability, neuromuscular aberrations, and/or gastrointestinal symptoms. Serotonin syndrome in its most severe form can resemble neuroleptic malignant syndrome. Patients should be monitored for the emergence of serotonin syndrome or NMS-like signs and symptoms. Treatment with duloxetine and any antidopaminergic agents should be discontinued immediately if the above events occur and supportive symptomatic treatment should be initiated).
No products indexed under this heading.

Chlorpromazine Hydrochloride (Development of a potentially life-threatening serotonin syndrome or Neuroleptic Malignant Syndrome-like reactions have been reported with duloxetine, and with concomitant use of dopamine antagonists. Serotonin syndrome symptoms may include mental status changes, autonomic instability, neuromuscular aberrations, and/or gastrointestinal symptoms. Serotonin syndrome in its most severe form can resemble neuroleptic malignant syndrome. Patients should be monitored for the emergence of serotonin syndrome or NMS-like signs and symptoms. Treatment with duloxetine and any antidopaminergic agents should be discontinued immediately if the above events occur and supportive symptomatic treatment should be initiated).
No products indexed under this heading.

Chlorpropamide (Duloxetine is a moderate inhibitor of CYP2D6. Co-administration of duloxetine with other drugs that are extensively metabolized by CYP2D6 isoenzyme, and which have a narrow therapeutic window, should be approached with caution).
No products indexed under this heading.

Chlorprothixene (Development of a potentially life-threatening serotonin syndrome or Neuroleptic Malignant Syndrome-like reactions have been reported with duloxetine, and with concomitant use of antipsychotics. Serotonin syndrome symptoms may include mental status changes, autonomic instability, neuromuscular aberrations, and/or gastrointestinal symptoms. Serotonin syndrome in its most severe form can resemble neuroleptic malignant syndrome. Patients should be monitored for the emergence of serotonin syndrome or NMS-like signs and symptoms. Treatment with duloxetine and any antipsychotic agent should be discontinued immediately if the above events occur and supportive symptomatic treatment should be initiated).
No products indexed under this heading.

Chlorprothixene Hydrochloride (Development of a potentially life-threatening serotonin syndrome or Neuroleptic Malignant Syndrome-like reactions have been reported with duloxetine, and with concomitant use of antipsychotics. Serotonin syndrome symptoms may include mental status changes, autonomic instability, neuromuscular aberrations, and/or gastrointestinal symptoms. Serotonin syndrome in its most severe form can resemble neuroleptic malignant syndrome. Patients should be monitored for the emergence of serotonin syndrome or NMS-like signs and symptoms. Treatment with duloxetine and any antipsychotic agent should be discontinued immediately if the above events occur and supportive symptomatic treatment should be initiated).
No products indexed under this heading.

Chlorprothixene Lactate (Development of a potentially life-threatening serotonin syndrome or Neuroleptic Malignant Syndrome-like reactions have been reported with duloxetine, and with concomitant use of antipsychotics. Serotonin syndrome symptoms may include mental status changes, autonomic instability, neuromuscular aberrations, and/or gastrointestinal symptoms. Serotonin syndrome in its most severe form can resemble neuroleptic malignant syndrome. Patients should be monitored for the emergence of serotonin syndrome or NMS-like signs and symptoms. Treatment with duloxetine and any antipsychotic agent should be discontinued immediately if the above events occur and supportive symptomatic treatment should be initiated).
No products indexed under this heading.

Chlorthalidone (Hyponatremia may occur as a result of treatment with duloxetine. Patients taking diuretics may be at greater risk. Discontinuation of duloxetine should be considered in patients with symptomatic hyponatremia and appropriate medical intervention should be instituted). Products include:
Clorpres 2344

Cimetidine (Both CYP1A2 and CYP2D6 are responsible for duloxetine metabolism. When duloxetine 60 mg was co-administered with fluvoxamine 100 mg, a potent CYP1A2 inhibitor to male subjects, duloxetine AUC was increased approximately 6-fold, the C_{max} was increased approximately 2.5-fold and duloxetine $t_{1/2}$ was increased approximately 3-fold. Co-administration of duloxetine with potent CYP1A2 inhibitors should be avoided).
No products indexed under this heading.

Cimetidine Hydrochloride (Both CYP1A2 and CYP2D6 are responsible for duloxetine metabolism. When duloxetine 60 mg was co-administered with fluvoxamine 100 mg, a potent CYP1A2 inhibitor to male subjects, duloxetine AUC was increased approximately 6-fold, the C_{max} was increased approximately 2.5-fold and duloxetine $t_{1/2}$ was increased approximately 3-fold. Co-administration of duloxetine with potent CYP1A2 inhibitors should be avoided).
No products indexed under this heading.

Ciprofloxacin (Both CYP1A2 and CYP2D6 are responsible for duloxetine metabolism. When duloxetine 60 mg was co-administered with fluvoxamine 100 mg, a potent CYP1A2 inhibitor to male subjects, duloxetine AUC was increased approximately 6-fold, the C_{max} was increased approximately 2.5-fold and duloxetine $t_{1/2}$ was increased approximately 3-fold. Co-administration of duloxetine with potent CYP1A2 inhibitors should be avoided). Products include:
Cipro I.V. 3082
Cipro 3073
Cipro XR 3091
Ciprodex 583

Ciprofloxacin Hydrochloride (Both CYP1A2 and CYP2D6 are responsible for duloxetine metabolism. When duloxetine 60 mg was co-administered with fluvoxamine 100 mg, a potent CYP1A2 inhibitor to male subjects, duloxetine AUC was increased approximately 6-fold, the C_{max} was increased approximately 2.5-fold and duloxetine $t_{1/2}$ was increased approximately 3-fold. Co-administration of duloxetine with potent CYP1A2 inhibitors should be avoided). Products include:
Cipro 3073

Citalopram Hydrobromide (The development of a potentially life-threatening serotonin syndrome or Neuroleptic Malignant Syndrome-like reactions have been reported with duloxetine, but particularly with concomitant use of serotonergic drugs. Serotonin syndrome symptoms may include mental status changes, autonomic instability, and/or gastrointestinal symptoms. Serotonin syndrome, in its most severe form can resemble neuroleptic malignant syndrome. The concomitant use of duloxetine with SSRIs is not recommended). Products include:
Celexa 1153

Clarithromycin (Both CYP1A2 and CYP2D6 are responsible for duloxetine metabolism. When duloxetine 60 mg was co-administered with fluvoxamine 100 mg, a potent CYP1A2 inhibitor to male subjects, duloxetine AUC was increased approximately 6-fold, the C_{max} was increased approximately 2.5-fold and duloxetine $t_{1/2}$ was increased approximately 3-fold. Co-

---

IMPORTANT NOTE: Always consult each drug listing in the patient's regimen for possible interactions.

administration of duloxetine with potent CYP1A2 inhibitors should be avoided). Products include:
Biaxin/Biaxin XL 412

Clomipramine Hydrochloride
(Duloxetine is a moderate inhibitor of CYP2D6. Co-administration of duloxetine with other drugs that are extensively metabolized by CYP2D6 and have a narrow therapeutic window, including tricyclic antidepressants, should be approached with caution. Plasma tricyclic antidepressant concentrations may need to be monitored, and the dose of the TCA may need to be reduced, if a TCA is co-administered with duloxetine). No products indexed under this heading.

Clonazepam (Given the primary CNS effects of duloxetine, it should be used with caution when it is taken in combination with or substituted for other centrally acting drugs, including those with a similar mechanism of action). Products include:
Klonopin 2855

Clorazepate Dipotassium (Given the primary CNS effects of duloxetine, it should be used with caution when it is taken in combination with or substituted for other centrally acting drugs, including those with a similar mechanism of action). No products indexed under this heading.

Clozapine (Development of a potentially life-threatening serotonin syndrome or Neuroleptic Malignant Syndrome-like reactions have been reported with duloxetine, and with concomitant use of dopamine antagonists. Serotonin syndrome symptoms may include mental status changes, autonomic instability, neuromuscular aberrations, and/or gastrointestinal symptoms. Serotonin syndrome in its most severe form can resemble neuroleptic malignant syndrome. Patients should be monitored for the emergence of serotonin syndrome or NMS-like signs and symptoms. Treatment with duloxetine and any antidopaminergic agents should be discontinued immediately if the above events occur and supportive symptomatic treatment should be initiated). No products indexed under this heading.

Cocaine Hydrochloride (Because CYP2D6 is involved in duloxetine metabolism, concomitant use of duloxetine with potent inhibitors of CYP2D6 would be expected to, and does, result in higher concentrations (on average of 60%) of duloxetine). No products indexed under this heading.

Codeine Phosphate (Given the primary CNS effects of duloxetine, it should be used with caution when it is taken in combination with or substituted for other centrally acting drugs, including those with a similar mechanism of action). Products include:
Tylenol with Codeine 2691

Codeine Sulfate (Given the primary CNS effects of duloxetine, it should be used with caution when it is taken in combination with or substituted for other centrally acting drugs, including those with a similar mechanism of action). No products indexed under this heading.

Cyclobenzaprine Hydrochloride (Duloxetine is a moderate inhibitor of CYP2D6. Co-administration of duloxetine with other drugs that are extensively metabolized by CYP2D6 isoenzyme, and which have a narrow therapeutic window, should be approached with caution). Products include:
Amrix 964

Cyclosporine (Because duloxetine is highly bound to plasma protein, administration of duloxetine to a patient taking another drug that is highly protein

bound may cause increased free concentration of the other drug, potentially resulting in serious adverse reactions). Products include:
Gengraf 440
Neoral Oral Solution 2496
Neoral Capsules 2496
Restasis 605

Dalteparin Sodium (Duloxetine may increase the risk of bleeding events. Concomitant use of anticoagulants may add to this risk. Case reports and epidemiological studies have demonstrated an association between use of drugs that interfere with serotonin reuptake and the occurrence of gastrointestinal bleeding. Patients should be cautioned about the risk of bleeding associated with concomitant use of duloxetine and anticoagulants). Products include:
Fragmin 1058

Danaparoid Sodium (Duloxetine may increase the risk of bleeding events. Concomitant use of anticoagulants may add to this risk. Case reports and epidemiological studies have demonstrated an association between use of drugs that interfere with serotonin reuptake and the occurrence of gastrointestinal bleeding. Patients should be cautioned about the risk of bleeding associated with concomitant use of duloxetine and anticoagulants). No products indexed under this heading.

Debrisoquine (Duloxetine is a moderate inhibitor of CYP2D6. Co-administration of duloxetine with other drugs that are extensively metabolized by CYP2D6 isoenzyme, and which have a narrow therapeutic window, should be approached with caution). No products indexed under this heading.

Desflurane (Given the primary CNS effects of duloxetine, it should be used with caution when it is taken in combination with or substituted for other centrally acting drugs, including those with a similar mechanism of action). No products indexed under this heading.

Desipramine Hydrochloride (Duloxetine is a moderate inhibitor of CYP2D6. Co-administration of duloxetine with other drugs that are extensively metabolized by CYP2D6 and have a narrow therapeutic window, including tricyclic antidepressants, should be approached with caution. Plasma tricyclic antidepressant concentrations may need to be monitored, and the dose of the TCA may need to be reduced, if a TCA is co-administered with duloxetine). No products indexed under this heading.

Desogestrel (Both CYP1A2 and CYP2D6 are responsible for duloxetine metabolism. When duloxetine 60 mg was co-administered with fluvoxamine 100 mg, a potent CYP1A2 inhibitor to male subjects, duloxetine AUC was increased approximately 6-fold, the C_{max} was increased approximately 2.5-fold and duloxetine $t_{1/2}$ was increased approximately 3-fold. Co-administration of duloxetine with potent CYP1A2 inhibitors should be avoided). No products indexed under this heading.

Desvenlafaxine Succinate (The development of a potentially life-threatening serotonin syndrome or Neuroleptic Malignant Syndrome-like reactions have been reported with duloxetine, but particularly with concomitant use of serotonergic drugs. Serotonin syndrome symptoms may include mental status changes, autonomic instability, and/or gastrointestinal symptoms. Serotonin syndrome, in its most severe form can resemble neuroleptic malignant syndrome. The concomitant use of duloxetine with SNRIs is not recommended). Products include:
Pristiq 3564

Dexfenfluramine Hydrochloride (Duloxetine is a moderate inhibitor of CYP2D6. Co-administration of duloxetine with other drugs that are extensively metabolized by CYP2D6 isoenzyme, and which have a narrow therapeutic window, should be approached with caution). No products indexed under this heading.

Dexmethylphenidate Hydrochloride (Given the primary CNS effects of duloxetine, it should be used with caution when it is taken in combination with or substituted for other centrally acting drugs, including those with a similar mechanism of action). Products include:
Focalin XR 2472

Dextroamphetamine (Given the primary CNS effects of duloxetine, it should be used with caution when it is taken in combination with or substituted for other centrally acting drugs, including those with a similar mechanism of action). No products indexed under this heading.

Dextroamphetamine Saccharate (Given the primary CNS effects of duloxetine, it should be used with caution when it is taken in combination with or substituted for other centrally acting drugs, including those with a similar mechanism of action). No products indexed under this heading.

Dextroamphetamine Sulfate (Given the primary CNS effects of duloxetine, it should be used with caution when it is taken in combination with or substituted for other centrally acting drugs, including those with a similar mechanism of action). Products include:
Dexedrine 1425

Dextromethorphan Hydrobromide (Duloxetine is a moderate inhibitor of CYP2D6. Co-administration of duloxetine with other drugs that are extensively metabolized by CYP2D6 isoenzyme, and which have a narrow therapeutic window, should be approached with caution). No products indexed under this heading.

Dextromethorphan Polistirex (Duloxetine is a moderate inhibitor of CYP2D6. Co-administration of duloxetine with other drugs that are extensively metabolized by CYP2D6 isoenzyme, and which have a narrow therapeutic window, should be approached with caution). No products indexed under this heading.

Dezocine (Given the primary CNS effects of duloxetine, it should be used with caution when it is taken in combination with or substituted for other centrally acting drugs, including those with a similar mechanism of action). No products indexed under this heading.

Diazepam (Given the primary CNS effects of duloxetine, it should be used with caution when it is taken in combination with or substituted for other centrally acting drugs, including those with a similar mechanism of action). Products include:
Valium Tablets 2880

Diclofenac Epolamine (Duloxetine may increase the risk of bleeding events. Concomitant use of non-steroidal anti-inflammatory drugs may add to this risk. Case reports and epidemiological studies have demonstrated an association between use of drugs that interfere with serotonin reuptake and the occurrence of gastrointestinal bleeding. Patients should be cautioned about the risk of bleeding associated with concomitant use of duloxetine and NSAIDs). Products include:
Flector 1839

Diclofenac Potassium (Duloxetine may increase the risk of bleeding events. Concomitant use of non-steroidal anti-inflammatory drugs may

add to this risk. Case reports and epidemiological studies have demonstrated an association between use of drugs that interfere with serotonin reuptake and the occurrence of gastrointestinal bleeding. Patients should be cautioned about the risk of bleeding associated with concomitant use of duloxetine and NSAIDs). No products indexed under this heading.

Diclofenac Sodium (Duloxetine may increase the risk of bleeding events. Concomitant use of non-steroidal anti-inflammatory drugs may add to this risk. Case reports and epidemiological studies have demonstrated an association between use of drugs that interfere with serotonin reuptake and the occurrence of gastrointestinal bleeding. Patients should be cautioned about the risk of bleeding associated with concomitant use of duloxetine and NSAIDs). No products indexed under this heading.

Dicumarol (Duloxetine may increase the risk of bleeding events. Concomitant use of anticoagulants may add to this risk. Case reports and epidemiological studies have demonstrated an association between use of drugs that interfere with serotonin reuptake and the occurrence of gastrointestinal bleeding. Patients should be cautioned about the risk of bleeding associated with concomitant use of duloxetine and anticoagulants). No products indexed under this heading.

Digitalis Glycoside Preparations (Because duloxetine is highly bound to plasma protein, administration of duloxetine to a patient taking another drug that is highly protein bound may cause increased free concentration of the other drug, potentially resulting in serious adverse reactions). No products indexed under this heading.

Digitalis Lanata (Because duloxetine is highly bound to plasma protein, administration of duloxetine to a patient taking another drug that is highly protein bound may cause increased free concentration of the other drug, potentially resulting in serious adverse reactions). No products indexed under this heading.

Digitalis Purpurea (Because duloxetine is highly bound to plasma protein, administration of duloxetine to a patient taking another drug that is highly protein bound may cause increased free concentration of the other drug, potentially resulting in serious adverse reactions). No products indexed under this heading.

Diphenhydramine (Because CYP2D6 is involved in duloxetine metabolism, concomitant use of duloxetine with potent inhibitors of CYP2D6 would be expected to, and does, result in higher concentrations (on average of 60%) of duloxetine). No products indexed under this heading.

Diphenhydramine Hydrochloride (Because CYP2D6 is involved in duloxetine metabolism, concomitant use of duloxetine with potent inhibitors of CYP2D6 would be expected to, and does, result in higher concentrations (on average of 60%) of duloxetine). Products include:
Benadryl Allergy Ultratab 2042
Children's Benadryl Allergy Liquid 2042

Dipyridamole (Because duloxetine is highly bound to plasma protein, administration of duloxetine to a patient taking another drug that is highly protein bound may cause increased free concentration of the other drug, potentially resulting in serious adverse reactions). Products include:
Aggrenox 880

Dolasetron Mesylate (Duloxetine is a moderate inhibitor of CYP2D6. Co-administration of duloxetine with other drugs that are extensively metabolized

by CYP2D6 isoenzyme, and which have a narrow therapeutic window, should be approached with caution). Products include:

Anzemet Injection **2931**
Anzemet Tablets **2934**

Donepezil Hydrochloride (Duloxetine is a moderate inhibitor of CYP2D6. Co-administration of duloxetine with other drugs that are extensively metabolized by CYP2D6 isoenzyme, and which have a narrow therapeutic window, should be approached with caution). Products include:

Aricept **1045**
Aricept ODT **1045**

Doxepin Hydrochloride (Duloxetine is a moderate inhibitor of CYP2D6. Co-administration of duloxetine with other drugs that are extensively metabolized by CYP2D6 and have a narrow therapeutic window, including tricyclic antidepressants, should be approached with caution. Plasma tricyclic antidepressant concentrations may need to be monitored, and the dose of the TCA may need to be reduced, if a TCA is co-administered with duloxetine).

No products indexed under this heading.

Droperidol (Given the primary CNS effects of duloxetine, it should be used with caution when it is taken in combination with or substituted for other centrally acting drugs, including those with a similar mechanism of action).

No products indexed under this heading.

Eletriptan Hydrobromide (There have been rare post-marketing reports of serotonin syndrome with the use of an SSRI and a triptan. If concomitant treatment is clinically warranted, careful observation of the patient is advised, particularly during treatment initiation and dose increases).

No products indexed under this heading.

Encainide Hydrochloride (Duloxetine is a moderate inhibitor of CYP2D6. Co-administration of duloxetine with drugs that are extensively metabolized by CYP2D6 and that have a narrow therapeutic index, including Type 1C antiarrhythmics, should be approached with caution).

No products indexed under this heading.

Enflurane (Given the primary CNS effects of duloxetine, it should be used with caution when it is taken in combination with or substituted for other centrally acting drugs, including those with a similar mechanism of action).

No products indexed under this heading.

Enoxacin (Both CYP1A2 and CYP2D6 are responsible for duloxetine metabolism. When duloxetine 60 mg was co-administered with fluvoxamine 100 mg, a potent CYP1A2 inhibitor to male subjects, duloxetine AUC was increased approximately 6-fold, the C_{max} was increased approximately 2.5-fold and duloxetine $t_{1/2}$ was increased approximately 3-fold. Co-administration of duloxetine with potent CYP1A2 inhibitors should be avoided).

No products indexed under this heading.

Enoxaparin Sodium (Duloxetine may increase the risk of bleeding events. Concomitant use of anticoagulants may add to this risk. Case reports and epidemiological studies have demonstrated an association between use of drugs that interfere with serotonin reuptake and the occurrence of gastrointestinal bleeding. Patients should be cautioned about the risk of bleeding associated with concomitant use of duloxetine and anticoagulants). Products include:

Lovenox **3005**

Escitalopram Oxalate (The development of a potentially life-threatening serotonin syndrome or Neuroleptic Malignant Syndrome-like reactions have been reported with duloxetine, but particularly with concomitant use of serotonergic drugs. Serotonin syndrome symptoms may include mental status changes, autonomic instability, and/or gastrointestinal symptoms. Serotonin syndrome, in its most severe form can resemble neuroleptic malignant syndrome. The concomitant use of duloxetine with SSRIs is not recommended). Products include:

Lexapro Oral Suspension **1160**
Lexapro Tablets **1160**

Esomeprazole Magnesium (Both CYP1A2 and CYP2D6 are responsible for duloxetine metabolism. When duloxetine 60 mg was co-administered with fluvoxamine 100 mg, a potent CYP1A2 inhibitor to male subjects, duloxetine AUC was increased approximately 6-fold, the C_{max} was increased approximately 2.5-fold and duloxetine $t_{1/2}$ was increased approximately 3-fold. Co-administration of duloxetine with potent CYP1A2 inhibitors should be avoided). Products include:

Nexium Capsules **704**
Nexium Oral Suspension **704**

Esomeprazole Sodium (Both CYP1A2 and CYP2D6 are responsible for duloxetine metabolism. When duloxetine 60 mg was co-administered with fluvoxamine 100 mg, a potent CYP1A2 inhibitor to male subjects, duloxetine AUC was increased approximately 6-fold, the C_{max} was increased approximately 2.5-fold and duloxetine $t_{1/2}$ was increased approximately 3-fold. Co-administration of duloxetine with potent CYP1A2 inhibitors should be avoided). Products include:

Nexium I.V. **712**

Estazolam (Given the primary CNS effects of duloxetine, it should be used with caution when it is taken in combination with or substituted for other centrally acting drugs, including those with a similar mechanism of action).

No products indexed under this heading.

Ethacrynic Acid (Hyponatremia may occur as a result of treatment with duloxetine. Patients taking diuretics may be at greater risk. Discontinuation of duloxetine should be considered in patients with symptomatic hyponatremia and appropriate medical intervention should be instituted).

No products indexed under this heading.

Ethanol (Use of duloxetine concomitantly with heavy alcohol intake may be associated with severe liver injury. For this reason, duloxetine should ordinarily not be prescribed for patients with substantial alcohol use).

No products indexed under this heading.

Ethchlorvynol (Given the primary CNS effects of duloxetine, it should be used with caution when it is taken in combination with or substituted for other centrally acting drugs, including those with a similar mechanism of action).

No products indexed under this heading.

Ethinamate (Given the primary CNS effects of duloxetine, it should be used with caution when it is taken in combination with or substituted for other centrally acting drugs, including those with a similar mechanism of action).

No products indexed under this heading.

Ethinyl Estradiol (Both CYP1A2 and CYP2D6 are responsible for duloxetine metabolism. When duloxetine 60 mg was co-administered with fluvoxamine 100 mg, a potent CYP1A2 inhibitor to male subjects, duloxetine AUC was increased approximately 6-fold, the C_{max} was increased approximately 2.5-fold and duloxetine $t_{1/2}$ was increased approximately 3-fold. Co-administration of duloxetine with potent CYP1A2 inhibitors should be avoided). Products include:

LoSeasonique **3407**
Lybrel **3514**
NuvaRing **3181**
Ortho Evra **2648**
Ortho-Cyclen/Ortho Tri-Cyclen **2663**
Ortho Tri-Cyclen Lo Tablets **2673**
Seasonique **3418**
Yaz **864**

Ethyl Alcohol (Use of duloxetine concomitantly with heavy alcohol intake may be associated with severe liver injury. For this reason, duloxetine should ordinarily not be prescribed for patients with substantial alcohol use).

No products indexed under this heading.

Etodolac (Duloxetine may increase the risk of bleeding events. Concomitant use of non-steroidal anti-inflammatory drugs may add to this risk. Case reports and epidemiological studies have demonstrated an association between use of drugs that interfere with serotonin reuptake and the occurrence of gastrointestinal bleeding. Patients should be cautioned about the risk of bleeding associated with concomitant use of duloxetine and NSAIDs).

No products indexed under this heading.

Famotidine (Duloxetine has an enteric coating that resists dissolution until reaching a segment of the gastrointestinal tract where the pH exceeds 5.5. Drugs that raise the gastrointestinal pH may lead to an earlier release of duloxetine). Products include:

Pepcid **2227**
Original Strength Pepcid AC
Gelcaps **1821**
Original Strength Pepcid AC **1821**
Maximum Strength Pepcid AC **1821**
Pepcid Complete **1822**

Fenoprofen Calcium (Duloxetine may increase the risk of bleeding events. Concomitant use of non-steroidal anti-inflammatory drugs may add to this risk. Case reports and epidemiological studies have demonstrated an association between use of drugs that interfere with serotonin reuptake and the occurrence of gastrointestinal bleeding. Patients should be cautioned about the risk of bleeding associated with concomitant use of duloxetine and NSAIDs).

No products indexed under this heading.

Fentanyl (Given the primary CNS effects of duloxetine, it should be used with caution when it is taken in combination with or substituted for other centrally acting drugs, including those with a similar mechanism of action). Products include:

Duragesic **2604**
Fentanyl Transdermal System **2346**
Onsolis **2054**

Fentanyl Citrate (Given the primary CNS effects of duloxetine, it should be used with caution when it is taken in combination with or substituted for other centrally acting drugs, including those with a similar mechanism of action). Products include:

Fentora **966**

Flecainide Acetate (Duloxetine is a moderate inhibitor of CYP2D6. Co-administration of duloxetine with drugs that are extensively metabolized by CYP2D6 and that have a narrow therapeutic index, including Type 1C antiarrhythmics, should be approached with caution).

No products indexed under this heading.

Fluoxetine (The development of a potentially life-threatening serotonin syndrome or Neuroleptic Malignant Syndrome-like reactions have been reported with duloxetine, but particularly with concomitant use of serotonergic drugs. Serotonin syndrome symptoms may include mental status changes, autonomic instability, and/or gastrointestinal symptoms. Serotonin syndrome, in its most severe form can resemble neuroleptic malignant syndrome. The concomitant use of duloxetine with SSRIs is not recommended).

No products indexed under this heading.

Fluoxetine Hydrochloride (The development of a potentially life-threatening serotonin syndrome or Neuroleptic Malignant Syndrome-like reactions have been reported with duloxetine, but particularly with concomitant use of serotonergic drugs. Serotonin syndrome symptoms may include mental status changes, autonomic instability, and/or gastrointestinal symptoms. Serotonin syndrome, in its most severe form can resemble neuroleptic malignant syndrome. The concomitant use of duloxetine with SSRIs is not recommended). Products include:

Prozac Weekly **1941**
Prozac Pulvules **1941**
Symbyax **1965**

Fluphenazine Decanoate (Development of a potentially life-threatening serotonin syndrome or Neuroleptic Malignant Syndrome-like reactions have been reported with duloxetine, and with concomitant use of dopamine antagonists. Serotonin syndrome symptoms may include mental status changes, autonomic instability, neuromuscular aberrations, and/or gastrointestinal symptoms. Serotonin syndrome in its most severe form can resemble neuroleptic malignant syndrome. Patients should be monitored for the emergence of serotonin syndrome or NMS-like signs and symptoms. Treatment with duloxetine and any antidopaminergic agents should be discontinued immediately if the above events occur and supportive symptomatic treatment should be initiated).

No products indexed under this heading.

Fluphenazine Enanthate (Development of a potentially life-threatening serotonin syndrome or Neuroleptic Malignant Syndrome-like reactions have been reported with duloxetine, and with concomitant use of dopamine antagonists. Serotonin syndrome symptoms may include mental status changes, autonomic instability, neuromuscular aberrations, and/or gastrointestinal symptoms. Serotonin syndrome in its most severe form can resemble neuroleptic malignant syndrome. Patients should be monitored for the emergence of serotonin syndrome or NMS-like signs and symptoms. Treatment with duloxetine and any antidopaminergic agents should be discontinued immediately if the above events occur and supportive symptomatic treatment should be initiated).

No products indexed under this heading.

Fluphenazine Hydrochloride (Development of a potentially life-threatening serotonin syndrome or Neuroleptic Malignant Syndrome-like reactions have been reported with duloxetine, and with concomitant use of dopamine antagonists. Serotonin syndrome symptoms may include mental status changes, autonomic instability, neuromuscular aberrations, and/or gastrointestinal symptoms. Serotonin syndrome in its most severe form can resemble neuroleptic malignant syndrome. Patients should be monitored for the emergence of serotonin syndrome or NMS-like signs and symptoms. Treatment with duloxetine and any antidopaminergic agents should be discontinued immediately if the above events occur and supportive symptomatic treatment should be initiated).

No products indexed under this heading.

Cymbalta Interactions Index 438

Flurazepam Hydrochloride (Given the primary CNS effects of duloxetine, it should be used with caution when it is taken in combination with or substituted for other centrally acting drugs, including those with a similar mechanism of action).
No products indexed under this heading.

Flurbiprofen (Duloxetine may increase the risk of bleeding events. Concomitant use of non-steroidal anti-inflammatory drugs may add to this risk. Case reports and epidemiological studies have demonstrated an association between use of drugs that interfere with serotonin reuptake and the occurrence of gastrointestinal bleeding. Patients should be cautioned about the risk of bleeding associated with concomitant use of duloxetine and NSAIDs).
No products indexed under this heading.

Fluvoxamine (When duloxetine 60 mg was co-administered with fluvoxamine 100 mg, a potent inhibitor of CYP1A2, to male subjects, duloxetine AUC was increased approximately 6-fold, the C_{max} was increased about 2.5-fold, and duloxetine $t_{1/2}$ was increased approximately 3-fold. Co-administration of duloxetine with potent CYP1A2 inhibitors should be avoided).
No products indexed under this heading.

Fluvoxamine Maleate (When duloxetine 60 mg was co-administered with fluvoxamine 100 mg, a potent inhibitor of CYP1A2, to male subjects, duloxetine AUC was increased approximately 6-fold, the C_{max} was increased about 2.5-fold, and duloxetine t1/2 was increased approximately 3-fold. Co-administration of duloxetine with potent CYP1A2 inhibitors should be avoided).
No products indexed under this heading.

Fondaparinux Sodium (Duloxetine may increase the risk of bleeding events. Concomitant use of anticoagulants may add to this risk. Case reports and epidemiological studies have demonstrated an association between use of drugs that interfere with serotonin reuptake and the occurrence of gastrointestinal bleeding. Patients should be cautioned about the risk of bleeding associated with concomitant use of duloxetine and anticoagulants). Products include:
Arixtra 1320

Formoterol Fumarate (Duloxetine is a moderate inhibitor of CYP2D6. Co-administration of duloxetine with other drugs that are extensively metabolized by CYP2D6 isoenzyme, and which have a narrow therapeutic window, should be approached with caution). Products include:
Foradil 3121
Perforomist 3634

Frovatriptan Succinate (There have been rare post-marketing reports of serotonin syndrome with the use of an SSRI and a triptan. If concomitant treatment is clinically warranted, careful observation of the patient is advised, particularly during treatment initiation and dose increases). Products include:
Frova 1103

Furosemide (Hyponatremia may occur as a result of treatment with duloxetine. Patients taking diuretics may be at greater risk. Discontinuation of duloxetine should be considered in patients with symptomatic hyponatremia and appropriate medical intervention should be instituted). Products include:
Furosemide 2354

Galantamine Hydrobromide (Duloxetine is a moderate inhibitor of CYP2D6. Co-administration of duloxetine with other drugs that are extensively metabolized by CYP2D6 isoenzyme, and which have a narrow therapeutic window, should be approached with caution).
No products indexed under this heading.

Gatifloxacin (Both CYP1A2 and CYP2D6 are responsible for duloxetine metabolism. When duloxetine 60 mg was co-administered with fluvoxamine 100 mg, a potent CYP1A2 inhibitor to male subjects, duloxetine AUC was increased approximately 6-fold, the C_{max} was increased approximately 2.5-fold and duloxetine $t_{1/2}$ was increased approximately 3-fold. Co-administration of duloxetine with potent CYP1A2 inhibitors should be avoided).
No products indexed under this heading.

Gemifloxacin Mesylate (Both CYP1A2 and CYP2D6 are responsible for duloxetine metabolism. When duloxetine 60 mg was co-administered with fluvoxamine 100 mg, a potent CYP1A2 inhibitor to male subjects, duloxetine AUC was increased approximately 6-fold, the C_{max} was increased approximately 2.5-fold and duloxetine $t_{1/2}$ was increased approximately 3-fold. Co-administration of duloxetine with potent CYP1A2 inhibitors should be avoided).
No products indexed under this heading.

Glipizide (Because duloxetine is highly bound to plasma protein, administration of duloxetine to a patient taking another drug that is highly protein bound may cause increased free concentration of the other drug, potentially resulting in serious adverse reactions).
No products indexed under this heading.

Glutethimide (Given the primary CNS effects of duloxetine, it should be used with caution when it is taken in combination with or substituted for other centrally acting drugs, including those with a similar mechanism of action).
No products indexed under this heading.

Grepafloxacin Hydrochloride (Both CYP1A2 and CYP2D6 are responsible for duloxetine metabolism. When duloxetine 60 mg was co-administered with fluvoxamine 100 mg, a potent CYP1A2 inhibitor to male subjects, duloxetine AUC was increased approximately 6-fold, the C_{max} was increased approximately 2.5-fold and duloxetine $t_{1/2}$ was increased approximately 3-fold. Co-administration of duloxetine with potent CYP1A2 inhibitors should be avoided).
No products indexed under this heading.

Halazepam (Given the primary CNS effects of duloxetine, it should be used with caution when it is taken in combination with or substituted for other centrally acting drugs, including those with a similar mechanism of action).
No products indexed under this heading.

Halofantrine Hydrochloride (Because CYP2D6 is involved in duloxetine metabolism, concomitant use of duloxetine with potent inhibitors of CYP2D6 would be expected to, and does, result in higher concentrations (on average of 60%) of duloxetine).
No products indexed under this heading.

Haloperidol (Development of a potentially life-threatening serotonin syndrome or Neuroleptic Malignant Syndrome-like reactions have been reported with duloxetine, and with concomitant use of dopamine antagonists. Serotonin syndrome symptoms may include mental status changes, autonomic instability, neuromuscular aberrations, and/or gastrointestinal symptoms. Serotonin syndrome in its most severe form can resemble neuroleptic malignant syndrome. Patients should be monitored for the emergence of serotonin syndrome or NMS-like signs and symptoms. Treatment with duloxetine and any antidopaminergic agents should be discontinued immediately if the above events occur and supportive symptomatic treatment should be initiated).
No products indexed under this heading.

Haloperidol Decanoate (Development of a potentially life-threatening serotonin syndrome or Neuroleptic Malignant Syndrome-like reactions have been reported with duloxetine, and with concomitant use of dopamine antagonists. Serotonin syndrome symptoms may include mental status changes, autonomic instability, neuromuscular aberrations, and/or gastrointestinal symptoms. Serotonin syndrome in its most severe form can resemble neuroleptic malignant syndrome. Patients should be monitored for the emergence of serotonin syndrome or NMS-like signs and symptoms. Treatment with duloxetine and any antidopaminergic agents should be discontinued immediately if the above events occur and supportive symptomatic treatment should be initiated).
No products indexed under this heading.

Haloperidol Lactate (Development of a potentially life-threatening serotonin syndrome or Neuroleptic Malignant Syndrome-like reactions have been reported with duloxetine, and with concomitant use of antipsychotics. Serotonin syndrome symptoms may include mental status changes, autonomic instability, neuromuscular aberrations, and/or gastrointestinal symptoms. Serotonin syndrome in its most severe form can resemble neuroleptic malignant syndrome. Patients should be monitored for the emergence of serotonin syndrome or NMS-like signs and symptoms. Treatment with duloxetine and any antipsychotic agent should be discontinued immediately if the above events occur and supportive symptomatic treatment should be initiated).
No products indexed under this heading.

Heparin Calcium (Duloxetine may increase the risk of bleeding events. Concomitant use of anticoagulants may add to this risk. Case reports and epidemiological studies have demonstrated an association between use of drugs that interfere with serotonin reuptake and the occurrence of gastrointestinal bleeding. Patients should be cautioned about the risk of bleeding associated with concomitant use of duloxetine and anticoagulants).
No products indexed under this heading.

Heparin Sodium (Duloxetine may increase the risk of bleeding events. Concomitant use of anticoagulants may add to this risk. Case reports and epidemiological studies have demonstrated an association between use of drugs that interfere with serotonin reuptake and the occurrence of gastrointestinal bleeding. Patients should be cautioned about the risk of bleeding associated with concomitant use of duloxetine and anticoagulants).
No products indexed under this heading.

Hexobarbital (Given the primary CNS effects of duloxetine, it should be used with caution when it is taken in combination with or substituted for other centrally acting drugs, including those with a similar mechanism of action).
No products indexed under this heading.

Hydrochlorothiazide (Hyponatremia may occur as a result of treatment with duloxetine. Patients taking diuretics may be at greater risk. Discontinuation of duloxetine should be considered in patients with symptomatic hyponatremia and appropriate medical intervention should be instituted). Products include:
Atacand HCT 700
Avalide 2956
Benicar HCT 1017
Diovan HCT 2419
Dyazide 1429
Exforge HCT 2449
Hyzaar 2162
Hyzaar 100-12.5 2162
Micardis HCT 889
Prinzide 2246
Tekturna HCT 2541
Teveten HCT 541

Hydrocodone Bitartrate (Given the primary CNS effects of duloxetine, it should be used with caution when it is taken in combination with or substituted for other centrally acting drugs, including those with a similar mechanism of action). Products include:
Vicodin 560
Vicodin ES 561
Vicodin HP 563
Vicoprofen 564
Zydone 1138

Hydrocodone Polistirex (Given the primary CNS effects of duloxetine, it should be used with caution when it is taken in combination with or substituted for other centrally acting drugs, including those with a similar mechanism of action). Products include:
Tussionex 3443

Hydroflumethiazide (Hyponatremia may occur as a result of treatment with duloxetine. Patients taking diuretics may be at greater risk. Discontinuation of duloxetine should be considered in patients with symptomatic hyponatremia and appropriate medical intervention should be instituted).
No products indexed under this heading.

Hydromorphone (Given the primary CNS effects of duloxetine, it should be used with caution when it is taken in combination with or substituted for other centrally acting drugs, including those with a similar mechanism of action).
No products indexed under this heading.

Hydromorphone Hydrochloride (Given the primary CNS effects of duloxetine, it should be used with caution when it is taken in combination with or substituted for other centrally acting drugs, including those with a similar mechanism of action). Products include:
Dilaudid Injection 2800
Dilaudid Oral 2797
Dilaudid Tablets 2797
Dilaudid-HP 2800

Hydroxyamphetamine Hydrobromide (Given the primary CNS effects of duloxetine, it should be used with caution when it is taken in combination with or substituted for other centrally acting drugs, including those with a similar mechanism of action).
No products indexed under this heading.

Hydroxychloroquine Sulfate (Because CYP2D6 is involved in duloxetine metabolism, concomitant use of duloxetine with potent inhibitors of CYP2D6 would be expected to, and does, result in higher concentrations (on average of 60%) of duloxetine).
No products indexed under this heading.

Hydroxyzine Hydrochloride (Given the primary CNS effects of duloxetine, it should be used with caution when it is taken in combination with or substituted for other centrally acting drugs, including those with a similar mechanism of action).
No products indexed under this heading.

Hypericum (Based on the mechanism of action of duloxetine and the potential for serotonin syndrome, caution is advised when duloxetine is co-administered with drugs that may affect the serotonergic neurotransmitter systems, such as St. John's Wort).
No products indexed under this heading.

(⊙ Described in PDR® for Ophthalmic Medicines)

439 Interactions Index Cymbalta

Ibuprofen (Duloxetine may increase the risk of bleeding events. Concomitant use of non-steroidal anti-inflammatory drugs may add to this risk. Case reports and epidemiological studies have demonstrated an association between use of drugs that interfere with serotonin reuptake and the occurrence of gastrointestinal bleeding. Patients should be cautioned about the risk of bleeding associated with concomitant use of duloxetine and NSAIDs). Products include:

Motrin IB 2043
Children's Motrin 2044
Children's Motrin Non-Staining Dye-Free........ 2044
Infants' Motrin 2044
Infants' Motrin Dye-Free 2044
Junior Strength Motrin 2044
Vicoprofen 564

Imatinib Mesylate (Because CYP2D6 is involved in duloxetine metabolism, concomitant use of duloxetine with potent inhibitors of CYP2D6 would be expected to, and does, result in higher concentrations (on average of 60%) of duloxetine). Products include:

Gleevec 2477

Imipramine Hydrochloride (Duloxetine is a moderate inhibitor of CYP2D6. Co-administration of duloxetine with other drugs that are extensively metabolized by CYP2D6 and have a narrow therapeutic window, including tricyclic antidepressants, should be approached with caution. Plasma tricyclic antidepressant concentrations may need to be monitored, and the dose of the TCA may need to be reduced, if a TCA is co-administered with duloxetine).

No products indexed under this heading.

Imipramine Pamoate (Duloxetine is a moderate inhibitor of CYP2D6. Co-administration of duloxetine with other drugs that are extensively metabolized by CYP2D6 and have a narrow therapeutic window, including tricyclic antidepressants, should be approached with caution. Plasma tricyclic antidepressant concentrations may need to be monitored, and the dose of the TCA may need to be reduced, if a TCA is co-administered with duloxetine).

No products indexed under this heading.

Indapamide (Hyponatremia may occur as a result of treatment with duloxetine. Patients taking diuretics may be at greater risk. Discontinuation of duloxetine should be considered in patients with symptomatic hyponatremia and appropriate medical intervention should be instituted). Products include:

Indapamide 2356

Indomethacin (Duloxetine may increase the risk of bleeding events. Concomitant use of non-steroidal anti-inflammatory drugs may add to this risk. Case reports and epidemiological studies have demonstrated an association between use of drugs that interfere with serotonin reuptake and the occurrence of gastrointestinal bleeding. Patients should be cautioned about the risk of bleeding associated with concomitant use of duloxetine and NSAIDs). Products include:

Indocin 2167

Indomethacin Sodium Trihydrate (Duloxetine may increase the risk of bleeding events. Concomitant use of non-steroidal anti-inflammatory drugs may add to this risk. Case reports and epidemiological studies have demonstrated an association between use of drugs that interfere with serotonin reuptake and the occurrence of gastrointestinal bleeding. Patients should be cautioned about the risk of bleeding associated with concomitant use of duloxetine and NSAIDs). Products include:

Indocin I.V. 2007

Indoramin Hydrochloride (Duloxetine is a moderate inhibitor of CYP2D6. Co-administration of duloxetine with other drugs that are extensively metabolized by CYP2D6 isoenzyme, and which have a narrow therapeutic window, should be approached with caution).

No products indexed under this heading.

Isocarboxazid (Concomitant use in patients taking MAO inhibitors is contraindicated due to the risk of serious, sometimes fatal, drug interactions with serotonergic drugs. These interactions may include hyperthermia, rigidity, myoclonus, autonomic instability, and mental status changes that include extreme agitation progressing to delirium and coma. These reactions have also been reported in patients who have recently discontinued serotonin reuptake inhibitors and are started on an MAOI. At least 14 days should elapse between discontinuation of an MAO inhibitor and initiation of therapy with duloxetine. In addition, at least 5 days should be allowed after stopping duloxetine before starting an MAO inhibitor). Products include:

Marplan 3481

Isoflurane (Given the primary CNS effects of duloxetine, it should be used with caution when it is taken in combination with or substituted for other centrally acting drugs, including those with a similar mechanism of action).

No products indexed under this heading.

Isoniazid (Both CYP1A2 and CYP2D6 are responsible for duloxetine metabolism. When duloxetine 60 mg was co-administered with fluvoxamine 100 mg, a potent CYP1A2 inhibitor to male subjects, duloxetine AUC was increased approximately 6-fold, the C_{max} was increased approximately 2.5-fold and duloxetine $t_{1/2}$ was increased approximately 3-fold. Co-administration of duloxetine with potent CYP1A2 inhibitors should be avoided).

No products indexed under this heading.

Ketamine Hydrochloride (Given the primary CNS effects of duloxetine, it should be used with caution when it is taken in combination with or substituted for other centrally acting drugs, including those with a similar mechanism of action).

No products indexed under this heading.

Ketoconazole (Both CYP1A2 and CYP2D6 are responsible for duloxetine metabolism. When duloxetine 60 mg was co-administered with fluvoxamine 100 mg, a potent CYP1A2 inhibitor to male subjects, duloxetine AUC was increased approximately 6-fold, the C_{max} was increased approximately 2.5-fold and duloxetine $t_{1/2}$ was increased approximately 3-fold. Co-administration of duloxetine with potent CYP1A2 inhibitors should be avoided). Products include:

Extina 3319
Xolegel 3337

Ketoprofen (Duloxetine may increase the risk of bleeding events. Concomitant use of non-steroidal anti-inflammatory drugs may add to this risk. Case reports and epidemiological studies have demonstrated an association between use of drugs that interfere with serotonin reuptake and the occurrence of gastrointestinal bleeding. Patients should be cautioned about the risk of bleeding associated with concomitant use of duloxetine and NSAIDs).

No products indexed under this heading.

Ketorolac Tromethamine (Duloxetine may increase the risk of bleeding events. Concomitant use of non-steroidal anti-inflammatory drugs may add to this risk. Case reports and epidemiological studies have demonstrated an association between use of drugs that interfere with serotonin reuptake and the occurrence of gastrointestinal bleeding. Patients should be cautioned about the risk of bleeding associated with concomitant use of duloxetine and NSAIDs). Products include:

Acuvail .... ⊙ 209

Labetalol Hydrochloride (Duloxetine is a moderate inhibitor of CYP2D6. Co-administration of duloxetine with other drugs that are extensively metabolized by CYP2D6 isoenzyme, and which have a narrow therapeutic window, should be approached with caution).

No products indexed under this heading.

Lansoprazole (Duloxetine has an enteric coating that resists dissolution until reaching a segment of the gastrointestinal tract where the pH exceeds 5.5. Drugs that raise the gastrointestinal pH may lead to an earlier release of duloxetine).

No products indexed under this heading.

Levofloxacin (Both CYP1A2 and CYP2D6 are responsible for duloxetine metabolism. When duloxetine 60 mg was co-administered with fluvoxamine 100 mg, a potent CYP1A2 inhibitor to male subjects, duloxetine AUC was increased approximately 6-fold, the C_{max} was increased approximately 2.5-fold and duloxetine $t_{1/2}$ was increased approximately 3-fold. Co-administration of duloxetine with potent CYP1A2 inhibitors should be avoided). Products include:

Iquix 3492
Levaquin 2629
Levaquin in 5% Dextrose 2629
Quixin 3493

Levomethadyl Acetate Hydrochloride (Given the primary CNS effects of duloxetine, it should be used with caution when it is taken in combination with or substituted for other centrally acting drugs, including those with a similar mechanism of action).

No products indexed under this heading.

Levonorgestrel (Both CYP1A2 and CYP2D6 are responsible for duloxetine metabolism. When duloxetine 60 mg was co-administered with fluvoxamine 100 mg, a potent CYP1A2 inhibitor to male subjects, duloxetine AUC was increased approximately 6-fold, the C_{max} was increased approximately 2.5-fold and duloxetine $t_{1/2}$ was increased approximately 3-fold. Co-administration of duloxetine with potent CYP1A2 inhibitors should be avoided). Products include:

Climara Pro 847
LoSeasonique 3407
Lybrel 3514
Mirena 854
Plan B 3416
Seasonique 3418

Levorphanol Tartrate (Given the primary CNS effects of duloxetine, it should be used with caution when it is taken in combination with or substituted for other centrally acting drugs, including those with a similar mechanism of action).

No products indexed under this heading.

Lidocaine (Duloxetine is a moderate inhibitor of CYP2D6. Co-administration of duloxetine with other drugs that are extensively metabolized by CYP2D6 isoenzyme, and which have a narrow therapeutic window, should be approached with caution). Products include:

Lidoderm 1107

Lidocaine Hydrochloride (Duloxetine is a moderate inhibitor of CYP2D6. Co-administration of duloxetine with other drugs that are extensively metabolized by CYP2D6 isoenzyme, and which have a narrow therapeutic window, should be approached with caution).

No products indexed under this heading.

Linezolid (Based on the mechanism of action of duloxetine and the potential for serotonin syndrome, caution is advised when duloxetine is co-administered with other drugs that may affect the serotonergic neurotransmitter systems, such as linezolid). Products include:

Zyvox 2769

Lisdexamfetamine Dimesylate (Given the primary CNS effects of duloxetine, it should be used with caution when it is taken in combination with or substituted for other centrally acting drugs, including those with a similar mechanism of action). Products include:

Vyvanse 3298

Lithium (Based on the mechanism of action of duloxetine and the potential for serotonin syndrome, caution is advised when duloxetine is co-administered with other drugs that may affect the serotonergic neurotransmitter systems, such as lithium).

No products indexed under this heading.

Lithium Carbonate (Based on the mechanism of action of duloxetine and the potential for serotonin syndrome, caution is advised when duloxetine is co-administered with other drugs that may affect the serotonergic neurotransmitter systems, such as lithium).

No products indexed under this heading.

Lithium Citrate (Based on the mechanism of action of duloxetine and the potential for serotonin syndrome, caution is advised when duloxetine is co-administered with other drugs that may affect the serotonergic neurotransmitter systems, such as lithium).

No products indexed under this heading.

Lomefloxacin Hydrochloride (Both CYP1A2 and CYP2D6 are responsible for duloxetine metabolism. When duloxetine 60 mg was co-administered with fluvoxamine 100 mg, a potent CYP1A2 inhibitor to male subjects, duloxetine AUC was increased approximately 6-fold, the C_{max} was increased approximately 2.5-fold and duloxetine $t_{1/2}$ was increased approximately 3-fold. Co-administration of duloxetine with potent CYP1A2 inhibitors should be avoided).

No products indexed under this heading.

Lorazepam (Given the primary CNS effects of duloxetine, it should be used with caution when it is taken in combination with or substituted for other centrally acting drugs, including those with a similar mechanism of action).

No products indexed under this heading.

Low Molecular Weight Heparins (Duloxetine may increase the risk of bleeding events. Concomitant use of anticoagulants may add to this risk. Case reports and epidemiological studies have demonstrated an association between use of drugs that interfere with serotonin reuptake and the occurrence of gastrointestinal bleeding. Patients should be cautioned about the risk of bleeding associated with concomitant use of duloxetine and anticoagulants).

No products indexed under this heading.

Loxapine Hydrochloride (Development of a potentially life-threatening serotonin syndrome or Neuroleptic Malignant Syndrome-like reactions have been reported with duloxetine, and with concomitant use of antipsychotics. Serotonin syndrome symptoms may include mental status changes, autonomic instability, neuromuscular aberra-

IMPORTANT NOTE: Always consult each drug listing in the patient's regimen for possible interactions.

tions, and/or gastrointestinal symptoms. Serotonin syndrome in its most severe form can resemble neuroleptic malignant syndrome. Patients should be monitored for the emergence of serotonin syndrome or NMS-like signs and symptoms. Treatment with duloxetine and any antipsychotic agent should be discontinued immediately if the above events occur and supportive symptomatic treatment should be initiated).

No products indexed under this heading.

Loxapine Succinate (Development of a potentially life-threatening serotonin syndrome or Neuroleptic Malignant Syndrome-like reactions have been reported with duloxetine, and with concomitant use of antipsychotics. Serotonin syndrome symptoms may include mental status changes, autonomic instability, neuromuscular aberrations, and/or gastrointestinal symptoms. Serotonin syndrome in its most severe form can resemble neuroleptic malignant syndrome. Patients should be monitored for the emergence of serotonin syndrome or NMS-like signs and symptoms. Treatment with duloxetine and any antipsychotic agent should be discontinued immediately if the above events occur and supportive symptomatic treatment should be initiated).

No products indexed under this heading.

Magnesium Hydroxide (Duloxetine has an enteric coating that resists dissolution until reaching a segment of the gastrointestinal tract where the pH exceeds 5.5. Drugs that raise the gastrointestinal pH may lead to an earlier release of duloxetine). Products include:

Fleet Pedia-Lax Chewable Tablets 1144
Pepcid Complete 1822

Maprotiline Hydrochloride (Duloxetine is a moderate inhibitor of CYP2D6. Co-administration of duloxetine with other drugs that are extensively metabolized by CYP2D6 and have a narrow therapeutic window, including tricyclic antidepressants, should be approached with caution. Plasma tricyclic antidepressant concentrations may need to be monitored, and the dose of the TCA may need to be reduced, if a TCA is co-administered with duloxetine).

No products indexed under this heading.

Meclofenamate Sodium (Duloxetine may increase the risk of bleeding events. Concomitant use of non-steroidal anti-inflammatory drugs may add to this risk. Case reports and epidemiological studies have demonstrated an association between use of drugs that interfere with serotonin reuptake and the occurrence of gastrointestinal bleeding. Patients should be cautioned about the risk of bleeding associated with concomitant use of duloxetine and NSAIDs).

No products indexed under this heading.

Mefenamic Acid (Duloxetine may increase the risk of bleeding events. Concomitant use of non-steroidal anti-inflammatory drugs may add to this risk. Case reports and epidemiological studies have demonstrated an association between use of drugs that interfere with serotonin reuptake and the occurrence of gastrointestinal bleeding. Patients should be cautioned about the risk of bleeding associated with concomitant use of duloxetine and NSAIDs).

No products indexed under this heading.

Meloxicam (Duloxetine may increase the risk of bleeding events. Concomitant use of non-steroidal anti-inflammatory drugs may add to this risk. Case reports and epidemiological studies have demonstrated an association between use of drugs that interfere with serotonin reuptake and the occurrence of gastrointestinal bleeding. Patients

should be cautioned about the risk of bleeding associated with concomitant use of duloxetine and NSAIDs).

No products indexed under this heading.

Meperidine Hydrochloride (Given the primary CNS effects of duloxetine, it should be used with caution when it is taken in combination with or substituted for other centrally acting drugs, including those with a similar mechanism of action).

No products indexed under this heading.

Mephobarbital (Given the primary CNS effects of duloxetine, it should be used with caution when it is taken in combination with or substituted for other centrally acting drugs, including those with a similar mechanism of action).

No products indexed under this heading.

Meprobamate (Given the primary CNS effects of duloxetine, it should be used with caution when it is taken in combination with or substituted for other centrally acting drugs, including those with a similar mechanism of action).

No products indexed under this heading.

Mesoridazine Besylate (Development of a potentially life-threatening serotonin syndrome or Neuroleptic Malignant Syndrome-like reactions have been reported with duloxetine, and with concomitant use of dopamine antagonists. Serotonin syndrome symptoms may include mental status changes, autonomic instability, neuromuscular aberrations, and/or gastrointestinal symptoms. Serotonin syndrome in its most severe form can resemble neuroleptic malignant syndrome. Patients should be monitored for the emergence of serotonin syndrome or NMS-like signs and symptoms. Treatment with duloxetine and any antidopaminergic agents should be discontinued immediately if the above events occur and supportive symptomatic treatment should be initiated).

No products indexed under this heading.

Mestranol (Both CYP1A2 and CYP2D6 are responsible for duloxetine metabolism. When duloxetine 60 mg was co-administered with fluvoxamine 100 mg, a potent CYP1A2 inhibitor to male subjects, duloxetine AUC was increased approximately 6-fold, the C_{max} was increased approximately 2.5-fold and duloxetine $t_{1/2}$ was increased approximately 3-fold. Co-administration of duloxetine with potent CYP1A2 inhibitors should be avoided).

No products indexed under this heading.

Methadone Hydrochloride (Given the primary CNS effects of duloxetine, it should be used with caution when it is taken in combination with or substituted for other centrally acting drugs, including those with a similar mechanism of action).

No products indexed under this heading.

Methamphetamine Hydrochloride (Given the primary CNS effects of duloxetine, it should be used with caution when it is taken in combination with or substituted for other centrally acting drugs, including those with a similar mechanism of action).

No products indexed under this heading.

Methohexital Sodium (Given the primary CNS effects of duloxetine, it should be used with caution when it is taken in combination with or substituted for other centrally acting drugs, including those with a similar mechanism of action).

No products indexed under this heading.

Methotrimeprazine (Development of a potentially life-threatening serotonin syndrome or Neuroleptic Malignant Syndrome-like reactions have been

reported with duloxetine, and with concomitant use of dopamine antagonists. Serotonin syndrome symptoms may include mental status changes, autonomic instability, neuromuscular aberrations, and/or gastrointestinal symptoms. Serotonin syndrome in its most severe form can resemble neuroleptic malignant syndrome. Patients should be monitored for the emergence of serotonin syndrome or NMS-like signs and symptoms. Treatment with duloxetine and any antidopaminergic agents should be discontinued immediately if the above events occur and supportive symptomatic treatment should be initiated).

No products indexed under this heading.

Methoxsalen (Both CYP1A2 and CYP2D6 are responsible for duloxetine metabolism. When duloxetine 60 mg was co-administered with fluvoxamine 100 mg, a potent CYP1A2 inhibitor to male subjects, duloxetine AUC was increased approximately 6-fold, the C_{max} was increased approximately 2.5-fold and duloxetine $t_{1/2}$ was increased approximately 3-fold. Co-administration of duloxetine with potent CYP1A2 inhibitors should be avoided).

No products indexed under this heading.

Methoxyflurane (Given the primary CNS effects of duloxetine, it should be used with caution when it is taken in combination with or substituted for other centrally acting drugs, including those with a similar mechanism of action).

No products indexed under this heading.

Methoxyphenamine (Duloxetine is a moderate inhibitor of CYP2D6. Co-administration of duloxetine with other drugs that are extensively metabolized by CYP2D6 isoenzyme, and which have a narrow therapeutic window, should be approached with caution).

No products indexed under this heading.

Methyclothiazide (Hyponatremia may occur as a result of treatment with duloxetine. Patients taking diuretics may be at greater risk. Discontinuation of duloxetine should be considered in patients with symptomatic hyponatremia and appropriate medical intervention should be instituted).

No products indexed under this heading.

Methylphenidate (Given the primary CNS effects of duloxetine, it should be used with caution when it is taken in combination with or substituted for other centrally acting drugs, including those with a similar mechanism of action). Products include:

Daytrana 3283

Methylphenidate Hydrochloride (Given the primary CNS effects of duloxetine, it should be used with caution when it is taken in combination with or substituted for other centrally acting drugs, including those with a similar mechanism of action). Products include:

Concerta 2598
Metadate CD 3439

Metoclopramide Hydrochloride (Development of a potentially life-threatening serotonin syndrome or Neuroleptic Malignant Syndrome-like reactions have been reported with duloxetine, and with concomitant use of dopamine antagonists. Serotonin syndrome symptoms may include mental status changes, autonomic instability, neuromuscular aberrations, and/or gastrointestinal symptoms. Serotonin syndrome in its most severe form can resemble neuroleptic malignant syndrome. Patients should be monitored for the emergence of serotonin syndrome or NMS-like signs and symptoms. Treatment with duloxetine and any antidopaminergic agents should be discontinued immediately if the above

events occur and supportive symptomatic treatment should be initiated). Products include:

Metozolv ODT 2901

Metolazone (Hyponatremia may occur as a result of treatment with duloxetine. Patients taking diuretics may be at greater risk. Discontinuation of duloxetine should be considered in patients with symptomatic hyponatremia and appropriate medical intervention should be instituted).

No products indexed under this heading.

Metoprolol Succinate (Duloxetine is a moderate inhibitor of CYP2D6. Co-administration of duloxetine with other drugs that are extensively metabolized by CYP2D6 isoenzyme, and which have a narrow therapeutic window, should be approached with caution). Products include:

Toprol XL **732**

Metoprolol Tartrate (Duloxetine is a moderate inhibitor of CYP2D6. Co-administration of duloxetine with other drugs that are extensively metabolized by CYP2D6 isoenzyme, and which have a narrow therapeutic window, should be approached with caution).

No products indexed under this heading.

Mexiletine Hydrochloride (Both CYP1A2 and CYP2D6 are responsible for duloxetine metabolism. When duloxetine 60 mg was co-administered with fluvoxamine 100 mg, a potent CYP1A2 inhibitor to male subjects, duloxetine AUC was increased approximately 6-fold, the C_{max} was increased approximately 2.5-fold and duloxetine $t_{1/2}$ was increased approximately 3-fold. Co-administration of duloxetine with potent CYP1A2 inhibitors should be avoided).

No products indexed under this heading.

Mibefradil Dihydrochloride (Both CYP1A2 and CYP2D6 are responsible for duloxetine metabolism. When duloxetine 60 mg was co-administered with fluvoxamine 100 mg, a potent CYP1A2 inhibitor to male subjects, duloxetine AUC was increased approximately 6-fold, the C_{max} was increased approximately 2.5-fold and duloxetine $t_{1/2}$ was increased approximately 3-fold. Co-administration of duloxetine with potent CYP1A2 inhibitors should be avoided).

No products indexed under this heading.

Midazolam Hydrochloride (Given the primary CNS effects of duloxetine, it should be used with caution when it is taken in combination with or substituted for other centrally acting drugs, including those with a similar mechanism of action).

No products indexed under this heading.

Mirtazapine (Duloxetine is a moderate inhibitor of CYP2D6. Co-administration of duloxetine with other drugs that are extensively metabolized by CYP2D6 isoenzyme, and which have a narrow therapeutic window, should be approached with caution). Products include:

Remeron Tablets **3214**
RemeronSolTab Tablets **3219**

Moclobemide (Concomitant use in patients taking MAO inhibitors is contraindicated due to the risk of serious, sometimes fatal, drug interactions with serotonergic drugs. These interactions may include hyperthermia, rigidity, myoclonus, autonomic instability, and mental status changes that include extreme agitation progressing to delirium and coma. These reactions have also been reported in patients who have recently discontinued serotonin reuptake inhibitors and are started on an MAOI. At least 14 days should elapse between discontinuation of an MAO inhibitor and initiation of therapy with duloxetine. In addition, at least 5

441 **Interactions Index** **Cymbalta**

days should be allowed after stopping duloxetine before starting an MAO inhibitor).
No products indexed under this heading.

Molindone Hydrochloride (Development of a potentially life-threatening serotonin syndrome or Neuroleptic Malignant Syndrome-like reactions have been reported with duloxetine, and with concomitant use of antipsychotics. Serotonin syndrome symptoms may include mental status changes, autonomic instability, neuromuscular aberrations, and/or gastrointestinal symptoms. Serotonin syndrome in its most severe form can resemble neuroleptic malignant syndrome. Patients should be monitored for the emergence of serotonin syndrome or NMS-like signs and symptoms. Treatment with duloxetine and any antipsychotic agent should be discontinued immediately if the above events occur and supportive symptomatic treatment should be initiated). Products include:
Moban 1108

Morphine Sulfate (Given the primary CNS effects of duloxetine, it should be used with caution when it is taken in combination with or substituted for other centrally acting drugs, including those with a similar mechanism of action). Products include:
Avinza 1822
Embeda 1831
MS Contin 2803

Morphine Sulfate, Liposomal (Given the primary CNS effects of duloxetine, it should be used with caution when it is taken in combination with or substituted for other centrally acting drugs, including those with a similar mechanism of action).
No products indexed under this heading.

Moxifloxacin Hydrochloride (Both CYP1A2 and CYP2D6 are responsible for duloxetine metabolism. When duloxetine 60 mg was co-administered with fluvoxamine 100 mg, a potent CYP1A2 inhibitor to male subjects, duloxetine AUC was increased approximately 6-fold, the C_{max} was increased approximately 2.5-fold and duloxetine $t_{1/2}$ was increased approximately 3-fold. Co-administration of duloxetine with potent CYP1A2 inhibitors should be avoided). Products include:
Avelox 3064
Vigamox 589

Nabumetone (Duloxetine may increase the risk of bleeding events. Concomitant use of non-steroidal anti-inflammatory drugs may add to this risk. Case reports and epidemiological studies have demonstrated an association between use of drugs that interfere with serotonin reuptake and the occurrence of gastrointestinal bleeding. Patients should be cautioned about the risk of bleeding associated with concomitant use of duloxetine and NSAIDs).
No products indexed under this heading.

Nalidixic Acid (Both CYP1A2 and CYP2D6 are responsible for duloxetine metabolism. When duloxetine 60 mg was co-administered with fluvoxamine 100 mg, a potent CYP1A2 inhibitor to male subjects, duloxetine AUC was increased approximately 6-fold, the C_{max} was increased approximately 2.5-fold and duloxetine $t_{1/2}$ was increased approximately 3-fold. Co-administration of duloxetine with potent CYP1A2 inhibitors should be avoided).
No products indexed under this heading.

Naproxen (Duloxetine may increase the risk of bleeding events. Concomitant use of non-steroidal anti-inflammatory drugs may add to this risk. Case reports and epidemiological studies have demonstrated an association between use of drugs that interfere with serotonin reuptake and the occurrence of gastrointestinal bleeding. Patients should be cautioned about the risk of bleeding associated with concomitant use of duloxetine and NSAIDs). Products include:
EC-Naprosyn 2850
Naprosyn 2850
Anaprox/Naprosyn 2850

Naproxen Sodium (Duloxetine may increase the risk of bleeding events. Concomitant use of non-steroidal anti-inflammatory drugs may add to this risk. Case reports and epidemiological studies have demonstrated an association between use of drugs that interfere with serotonin reuptake and the occurrence of gastrointestinal bleeding. Patients should be cautioned about the risk of bleeding associated with concomitant use of duloxetine and NSAIDs). Products include:
Anaprox 2850
Anaprox DS 2850
Treximet 1681

Naratriptan Hydrochloride (There have been rare post-marketing reports of serotonin syndrome with the use of an SSRI and a triptan. If concomitant treatment is clinically warranted, careful observation of the patient is advised, particularly during treatment initiation and dose increases). Products include:
Amerge 1306

Nefazodone Hydrochloride (The development of a potentially life-threatening serotonin syndrome or Neuroleptic Malignant Syndrome-like reactions have been reported with duloxetine, but particularly with concomitant use of serotonergic drugs. Serotonin syndrome symptoms may include mental status changes, autonomic instability, and/or gastrointestinal symptoms. Serotonin syndrome, in its most severe form can resemble neuroleptic malignant syndrome. The concomitant use of duloxetine with SNRIs is not recommended).
No products indexed under this heading.

Nelfinavir Mesylate (Duloxetine is a moderate inhibitor of CYP2D6. Co-administration of duloxetine with other drugs that are extensively metabolized by CYP2D6 isoenzyme, and which have a narrow therapeutic window, should be approached with caution).
No products indexed under this heading.

Nizatidine (Duloxetine has an enteric coating that resists dissolution until reaching a segment of the gastrointestinal tract where the pH exceeds 5.5. Drugs that raise the gastrointestinal pH may lead to an earlier release of duloxetine). Products include:
Axid 1381

Norethindrone (Both CYP1A2 and CYP2D6 are responsible for duloxetine metabolism. When duloxetine 60 mg was co-administered with fluvoxamine 100 mg, a potent CYP1A2 inhibitor to male subjects, duloxetine AUC was increased approximately 6-fold, the C_{max} was increased approximately 2.5-fold and duloxetine $t_{1/2}$ was increased approximately 3-fold. Co-administration of duloxetine with potent CYP1A2 inhibitors should be avoided). Products include:
Ortho Micronor 2660

Norethindrone Acetate (Both CYP1A2 and CYP2D6 are responsible for duloxetine metabolism. When duloxetine 60 mg was co-administered with fluvoxamine 100 mg, a potent CYP1A2 inhibitor to male subjects, duloxetine AUC was increased approximately 6-fold, the C_{max} was increased approximately 2.5-fold and duloxetine $t_{1/2}$ was increased approximately 3-fold. Co-administration of duloxetine with potent CYP1A2 inhibitors should be avoided). Products include:
Activella 2561

Norfloxacin (Both CYP1A2 and CYP2D6 are responsible for duloxetine metabolism. When duloxetine 60 mg was co-administered with fluvoxamine 100 mg, a potent CYP1A2 inhibitor to male subjects, duloxetine AUC was increased approximately 6-fold, the C_{max} was increased approximately 2.5-fold and duloxetine $t_{1/2}$ was increased approximately 3-fold. Co-administration of duloxetine with potent CYP1A2 inhibitors should be avoided). Products include:
Noroxin 2220

Norgestrel (Both CYP1A2 and CYP2D6 are responsible for duloxetine metabolism. When duloxetine 60 mg was co-administered with fluvoxamine 100 mg, a potent CYP1A2 inhibitor to male subjects, duloxetine AUC was increased approximately 6-fold, the C_{max} was increased approximately 2.5-fold and duloxetine $t_{1/2}$ was increased approximately 3-fold. Co-administration of duloxetine with potent CYP1A2 inhibitors should be avoided).
No products indexed under this heading.

Nortriptyline Hydrochloride (Duloxetine is a moderate inhibitor of CYP2D6. Co-administration of duloxetine with other drugs that are extensively metabolized by CYP2D6 and have a narrow therapeutic window, including tricyclic antidepressants, should be approached with caution. Plasma tricyclic antidepressant concentrations may need to be monitored, and the dose of the TCA may need to be reduced, if a TCA is co-administered with duloxetine).
No products indexed under this heading.

Ofloxacin (Both CYP1A2 and CYP2D6 are responsible for duloxetine metabolism. When duloxetine 60 mg was co-administered with fluvoxamine 100 mg, a potent CYP1A2 inhibitor to male subjects, duloxetine AUC was increased approximately 6-fold, the C_{max} was increased approximately 2.5-fold and duloxetine $t_{1/2}$ was increased approximately 3-fold. Co-administration of duloxetine with potent CYP1A2 inhibitors should be avoided).
No products indexed under this heading.

Olanzapine (Development of a potentially life-threatening serotonin syndrome or Neuroleptic Malignant Syndrome-like reactions have been reported with duloxetine, and with concomitant use of dopamine antagonists. Serotonin syndrome symptoms may include mental status changes, autonomic instability, neuromuscular aberrations, and/or gastrointestinal symptoms. Serotonin syndrome in its most severe form can resemble neuroleptic malignant syndrome. Patients should be monitored for the emergence of serotonin syndrome or NMS-like signs and symptoms. Treatment with duloxetine and any antidopaminergic agents should be discontinued immediately if the above events occur and supportive symptomatic treatment should be initiated). Products include:
Symbyax 1965
Zyprexa 1984
Zyprexa IntraMuscular 1984
Zyprexa ZYDIS 1984

Omeprazole (Both CYP1A2 and CYP2D6 are responsible for duloxetine metabolism. When duloxetine 60 mg was co-administered with fluvoxamine 100 mg, a potent CYP1A2 inhibitor to male subjects, duloxetine AUC was increased approximately 6-fold, the C_{max} was increased approximately 2.5-fold and duloxetine $t_{1/2}$ was increased approximately 3-fold. Co-administration of duloxetine with potent CYP1A2 inhibitors should be avoided).
No products indexed under this heading.

Omeprazole Magnesium (Both CYP1A2 and CYP2D6 are responsible for duloxetine metabolism. When duloxetine 60 mg was co-administered with fluvoxamine 100 mg, a potent CYP1A2 inhibitor to male subjects, duloxetine AUC was increased approximately 6-fold, the C_{max} was increased approximately 2.5-fold and duloxetine $t_{1/2}$ was increased approximately 3-fold. Co-administration of duloxetine with potent CYP1A2 inhibitors should be avoided).
No products indexed under this heading.

Ondansetron (Duloxetine is a moderate inhibitor of CYP2D6. Co-administration of duloxetine with other drugs that are extensively metabolized by CYP2D6 isoenzyme, and which have a narrow therapeutic window, should be approached with caution).
No products indexed under this heading.

Ondansetron Hydrochloride (Duloxetine is a moderate inhibitor of CYP2D6. Co-administration of duloxetine with other drugs that are extensively metabolized by CYP2D6 isoenzyme, and which have a narrow therapeutic window, should be approached with caution). Products include:
Zofran Injection 1750
Zofran 1756
Zofran ODT 1756

Oxaprozin (Duloxetine may increase the risk of bleeding events. Concomitant use of non-steroidal anti-inflammatory drugs may add to this risk. Case reports and epidemiological studies have demonstrated an association between use of drugs that interfere with serotonin reuptake and the occurrence of gastrointestinal bleeding. Patients should be cautioned about the risk of bleeding associated with concomitant use of duloxetine and NSAIDs).
No products indexed under this heading.

Oxazepam (Given the primary CNS effects of duloxetine, it should be used with caution when it is taken in combination with or substituted for other centrally acting drugs, including those with a similar mechanism of action).
No products indexed under this heading.

Oxycodone Hydrochloride (Given the primary CNS effects of duloxetine, it should be used with caution when it is taken in combination with or substituted for other centrally acting drugs, including those with a similar mechanism of action). Products include:
OxyContin 2807
Percocet 1121
Percodan 1124

Oxycodone Terephthalate (Given the primary CNS effects of duloxetine, it should be used with caution when it is taken in combination with or substituted for other centrally acting drugs, including those with a similar mechanism of action).
No products indexed under this heading.

Oxymorphone Hydrochloride (Given the primary CNS effects of duloxetine, it should be used with caution when it is taken in combination with or substituted for other centrally acting drugs, including those with a similar mechanism of action). Products include:
Opana 1110
Opana ER 1114

Paclitaxel (Duloxetine is a moderate inhibitor of CYP2D6. Co-administration of duloxetine with other drugs that are extensively metabolized by CYP2D6 isoenzyme, and which have a narrow therapeutic window, should be approached with caution).
No products indexed under this heading.

Paliperidone (Development of a potentially life-threatening serotonin syndrome or Neuroleptic Malignant Syndrome-like reactions have been reported with duloxetine, and with con-

IMPORTANT NOTE: Always consult each drug listing in the patient's regimen for possible interactions.

Cymbalta Interactions Index 442

comitant use of antipsychotics. Serotonin syndrome symptoms may include mental status changes, autonomic instability, neuromuscular aberrations, and/or gastrointestinal symptoms. Serotonin syndrome in its most severe form can resemble neuroleptic malignant syndrome. Patients should be monitored for the emergence of serotonin syndrome or NMS-like signs and symptoms. Treatment with duloxetine and any antipsychotic agent should be discontinued immediately if the above events occur and supportive symptomatic treatment should be initiated). Products include:
Invega 2613
Invega Sustenna 2621

Pargyline Hydrochloride (Concomitant use in patients taking MAO inhibitors is contradindicated due to the risk of serious, sometimes fatal, drug interactions with serotonergic drugs. These interactions may include hyperthermia, rigidity, myoclonus, autonomic instability, and mental status changes that include extreme agitation progressing to delirium and coma. These reactions have also been reported in patients who have recently discontinued serotonin reuptake inhibitors and are started on an MAOI. At least 14 days should elapse between discontinuation of an MAO inhibitor and initiation of therapy with duloxetine. In addition, at least 5 days should be allowed after stopping duloxetine before starting an MAO inhibitor).
No products indexed under this heading.

Paroxetine (The development of a potentially life-threatening serotonin syndrome or Neuroleptic Malignant Syndrome-like reactions have been reported with duloxetine, but particularly with concomitant use of serotonergic drugs. Serotonin syndrome symptoms may include mental status changes, autonomic instability, and/or gastrointestinal symptoms. Serotonin syndrome, in its most severe form can resemble neuroleptic malignant syndrome. The concomitant use of duloxetine with SSRIs is not recommended).
No products indexed under this heading.

Paroxetine Hydrochloride (The development of a potentially life-threatening serotonin syndrome or Neuroleptic Malignant Syndrome-like reactions have been reported with duloxetine, but particularly with concomitant use of serotonergic drugs. Serotonin syndrome symptoms may include mental status changes, autonomic instability, and/or gastrointestinal symptoms. Serotonin syndrome, in its most severe form can resemble neuroleptic malignant syndrome. The concomitant use of duloxetine with SSRIs is not recommended). Products include:
Paroxetine CR 2361
Paroxetine ER 2371
Paxil 1586
Paxil CR 1596

Paroxetine Mesylate (The development of a potentially life-threatening serotonin syndrome or Neuroleptic Malignant Syndrome-like reactions have been reported with duloxetine, but particularly with concomitant use of serotonergic drugs. Serotonin syndrome symptoms may include mental status changes, autonomic instability, and/or gastrointestinal symptoms. Serotonin syndrome, in its most severe form can resemble neuroleptic malignant syndrome. The concomitant use of duloxetine with SSRIs is not recommended).
No products indexed under this heading.

Pemoline (Given the primary CNS effects of duloxetine, it should be used with caution when it is taken in combination with or substituted for other centrally acting drugs, including those with a similar mechanism of action).
No products indexed under this heading.

Pentobarbital (Given the primary CNS effects of duloxetine, it should be used with caution when it is taken in combination with or substituted for other centrally acting drugs, including those with a similar mechanism of action).
No products indexed under this heading.

Pentobarbital Sodium (Given the primary CNS effects of duloxetine, it should be used with caution when it is taken in combination with or substituted for other centrally acting drugs, including those with a similar mechanism of action). Products include:
Nembutal 2012

Perphenazine (Development of a potentially life-threatening serotonin syndrome or Neuroleptic Malignant Syndrome-like reactions have been reported with duloxetine, and with concomitant use of dopamine antagonists. Serotonin syndrome symptoms may include mental status changes, autonomic instability, neuromuscular aberrations, and/or gastrointestinal symptoms. Serotonin syndrome in its most severe form can resemble neuroleptic malignant syndrome. Patients should be monitored for the emergence of serotonin syndrome or NMS-like signs and symptoms. Treatment with duloxetine and any antidopaminergic agents should be discontinued immediately if the above events occur and supportive symptomatic treatment should be initiated).
No products indexed under this heading.

Phenelzine Sulfate (Concomitant use in patients taking MAO inhibitors is contradindicated due to the risk of serious, sometimes fatal, drug interactions with serotonergic drugs. These interactions may include hyperthermia, rigidity, myoclonus, autonomic instability, and mental status changes that include extreme agitation progressing to delirium and coma. These reactions have also been reported in patients who have recently discontinued serotonin reuptake inhibitors and are started on an MAOI. At least 14 days should elapse between discontinuation of an MAO inhibitor and initiation of therapy with duloxetine. In addition, at least 5 days should be allowed after stopping duloxetine before starting an MAO inhibitor).
No products indexed under this heading.

Phenobarbital (Given the primary CNS effects of duloxetine, it should be used with caution when it is taken in combination with or substituted for other centrally acting drugs, including those with a similar mechanism of action). Products include:
Donnatal 2711

Phenobarbital Sodium (Given the primary CNS effects of duloxetine, it should be used with caution when it is taken in combination with or substituted for other centrally acting drugs, including those with a similar mechanism of action).
No products indexed under this heading.

Phenothiazine Derivatives (Duloxetine is a moderate inhibitor of CYP2D6. Co-administration of duloxetine with other drugs that are extensively metabolized by this isoenzyme, and which have a narrow therapeutic window including phenthiazines, should be approached with caution).
No products indexed under this heading.

Phenothiazines (Duloxetine is a moderate inhibitor of CYP2D6. Co-administration of duloxetine with other drugs that are extensively metabolized by this isoenzyme, and which have a narrow therapeutic window including phenthiazines, should be approached with caution).
No products indexed under this heading.

Phenylbutazone (Duloxetine may increase the risk of bleeding events. Concomitant use of non-steroidal anti-inflammatory drugs may add to this risk. Case reports and epidemiological studies have demonstrated an association between use of drugs that interfere with serotonin reuptake and the occurrence of gastrointestinal bleeding. Patients should be cautioned about the risk of bleeding associated with concomitant use of duloxetine and NSAIDs).
No products indexed under this heading.

Pimozide (Development of a potentially life-threatening serotonin syndrome or Neuroleptic Malignant Syndrome-like reactions have been reported with duloxetine, and with concomitant use of dopamine antagonists. Serotonin syndrome symptoms may include mental status changes, autonomic instability, neuromuscular aberrations, and/or gastrointestinal symptoms. Serotonin syndrome in its most severe form can resemble neuroleptic malignant syndrome. Patients should be monitored for the emergence of serotonin syndrome or NMS-like signs and symptoms. Treatment with duloxetine and any antidopaminergic agents should be discontinued immediately if the above events occur and supportive symptomatic treatment should be initiated).
No products indexed under this heading.

Pindolol (Duloxetine is a moderate inhibitor of CYP2D6. Co-administration of duloxetine with other drugs that are extensively metabolized by CYP2D6 isoenzyme, and which have a narrow therapeutic window, should be approached with caution).
No products indexed under this heading.

Piroxicam (Duloxetine may increase the risk of bleeding events. Concomitant use of non-steroidal anti-inflammatory drugs may add to this risk. Case reports and epidemiological studies have demonstrated an association between use of drugs that interfere with serotonin reuptake and the occurrence of gastrointestinal bleeding. Patients should be cautioned about the risk of bleeding associated with concomitant use of duloxetine and NSAIDs).
No products indexed under this heading.

Polythiazide (Hyponatremia may occur as a result of treatment with duloxetine. Patients taking diuretics may be at greater risk. Discontinuation of duloxetine should be considered in patients with symptomatic hyponatremia and appropriate medical intervention should be instituted).
No products indexed under this heading.

Prazepam (Given the primary CNS effects of duloxetine, it should be used with caution when it is taken in combination with or substituted for other centrally acting drugs, including those with a similar mechanism of action).
No products indexed under this heading.

Procarbazine Hydrochloride (Concomitant use in patients taking MAO inhibitors is contradindicated due to the risk of serious, sometimes fatal, drug interactions with serotonergic drugs. These interactions may include hyperthermia, rigidity, myoclonus, autonomic instability, and mental status changes that include extreme agitation progressing to delirium and coma. These reactions have also been reported in patients who have recently discontinued serotonin reuptake inhibitors and are started on an MAOI. At least 14 days should elapse between discontinuation of an MAO inhibitor and initiation of therapy with duloxetine. In addition, at least 5 days should be allowed after stopping duloxetine before starting an MAO inhibitor).
No products indexed under this heading.

Prochlorperazine (Development of a potentially life-threatening serotonin syndrome or Neuroleptic Malignant Syndrome-like reactions have been reported with duloxetine, and with concomitant use of dopamine antagonists. Serotonin syndrome symptoms may include mental status changes, autonomic instability, neuromuscular aberrations, and/or gastrointestinal symptoms. Serotonin syndrome in its most severe form can resemble neuroleptic malignant syndrome. Patients should be monitored for the emergence of serotonin syndrome or NMS-like signs and symptoms. Treatment with duloxetine and any antidopaminergic agents should be discontinued immediately if the above events occur and supportive symptomatic treatment should be initiated).
No products indexed under this heading.

Prochlorperazine Edisylate (Duloxetine is a moderate inhibitor of CYP2D6. Co-administration of duloxetine with other drugs that are extensively metabolized by this isoenzyme, and which have a narrow therapeutic window including phenthiazines, should be approached with caution).
No products indexed under this heading.

Prochlorperazine Maleate (Duloxetine is a moderate inhibitor of CYP2D6. Co-administration of duloxetine with other drugs that are extensively metabolized by this isoenzyme, and which have a narrow therapeutic window including phenthiazines, should be approached with caution).
No products indexed under this heading.

Promethazine (Development of a potentially life-threatening serotonin syndrome or Neuroleptic Malignant Syndrome-like reactions have been reported with duloxetine, and with concomitant use of dopamine antagonists. Serotonin syndrome symptoms may include mental status changes, autonomic instability, neuromuscular aberrations, and/or gastrointestinal symptoms. Serotonin syndrome in its most severe form can resemble neuroleptic malignant syndrome. Patients should be monitored for the emergence of serotonin syndrome or NMS-like signs and symptoms. Treatment with duloxetine and any antidopaminergic agents should be discontinued immediately if the above events occur and supportive symptomatic treatment should be initiated).
No products indexed under this heading.

Promethazine Hydrochloride (Development of a potentially life-threatening serotonin syndrome or Neuroleptic Malignant Syndrome-like reactions have been reported with duloxetine, and with concomitant use of dopamine antagonists. Serotonin syndrome symptoms may include mental status changes, autonomic instability, neuromuscular aberrations, and/or gastrointestinal symptoms. Serotonin syndrome in its most severe form can resemble neuroleptic malignant syndrome. Patients should be monitored for the emergence of serotonin syndrome or NMS-like signs and symptoms. Treatment with duloxetine and any antidopaminergic agents should be discontinued immediately if the above events occur and supportive symptomatic treatment should be initiated).
No products indexed under this heading.

IMPORTANT NOTE: Always consult each drug listing in the patient's regimen for possible interactions.

Sodium Pentobarbital (Given the primary CNS effects of duloxetine, it should be used with caution when it is taken in combination with or substituted for other centrally acting drugs, including those with a similar mechanism of action).
No products indexed under this heading.

Sparfloxacin (Both CYP1A2 and CYP2D6 are responsible for duloxetine metabolism. When duloxetine 60 mg was co-administered with fluvoxamine 100 mg, a potent CYP1A2 inhibitor to male subjects, duloxetine AUC was increased approximately 6-fold, the C_{max} was increased approximately 2.5-fold and duloxetine $t_{1/2}$ was increased approximately 3-fold. Co-administration of duloxetine with potent CYP1A2 inhibitors should be avoided).
No products indexed under this heading.

Spironolactone (Hyponatremia may occur as a result of treatment with duloxetine. Patients taking diuretics may be at greater risk. Discontinuation of duloxetine should be considered in patients with symptomatic hyponatremia and appropriate medical intervention should be instituted).
No products indexed under this heading.

Sufentanil Citrate (Given the primary CNS effects of duloxetine, it should be used with caution when it is taken in combination with or substituted for other centrally acting drugs, including those with a similar mechanism of action).
No products indexed under this heading.

Sulindac (Duloxetine may increase the risk of bleeding events. Concomitant use of non-steroidal anti-inflammatory drugs may add to this risk. Case reports and epidemiological studies have demonstrated an association between use of drugs that interfere with serotonin reuptake and the occurrence of gastrointestinal bleeding. Patients should be cautioned about the risk of bleeding associated with concomitant use of duloxetine and NSAIDs). Products include:
Clinoril 2098

Sumatriptan (There have been rare post-marketing reports of serotonin syndrome with the use of an SSRI and a triptan. If concomitant treatment is clinically warranted, careful observation of the patient is advised, particularly during treatment initiation and dose increases). Products include:
Imitrex Nasal 1503

Sumatriptan Succinate (There have been rare post-marketing reports of serotonin syndrome with the use of an SSRI and a triptan. If concomitant treatment is clinically warranted, careful observation of the patient is advised, particularly during treatment initiation and dose increases). Products include:
Imitrex 1497
Imitrex Tablets 1508
Treximet 1681

Tacrine Hydrochloride (Both CYP1A2 and CYP2D6 are responsible for duloxetine metabolism. When duloxetine 60 mg was co-administered with fluvoxamine 100 mg, a potent CYP1A2 inhibitor to male subjects, duloxetine AUC was increased approximately 6-fold, the C_{max} was increased approximately 2.5-fold and duloxetine $t_{1/2}$ was increased approximately 3-fold. Co-administration of duloxetine with potent CYP1A2 inhibitors should be avoided).
No products indexed under this heading.

Talbutal (Given the primary CNS effects of duloxetine, it should be used with caution when it is taken in combination with or substituted for other centrally acting drugs, including those with a similar mechanism of action).
No products indexed under this heading.

Tamoxifen Citrate (Duloxetine is a moderate inhibitor of CYP2D6. Co-administration of duloxetine with other drugs that are extensively metabolized by CYP2D6 isoenzyme, and which have a narrow therapeutic window, should be approached with caution).
No products indexed under this heading.

Temazepam (Given the primary CNS effects of duloxetine, it should be used with caution when it is taken in combination with or substituted for other centrally acting drugs, including those with a similar mechanism of action).
No products indexed under this heading.

Teniposide (Duloxetine is a moderate inhibitor of CYP2D6. Co-administration of duloxetine with other drugs that are extensively metabolized by CYP2D6 isoenzyme, and which have a narrow therapeutic window, should be approached with caution).
No products indexed under this heading.

Terbinafine Hydrochloride (Because CYP2D6 is involved in duloxetine metabolism, concomitant use of duloxetine with potent inhibitors of CYP2D6 would be expected to, and does, result in higher concentrations (on average of 60%) of duloxetine).
No products indexed under this heading.

Testosterone (Duloxetine is a moderate inhibitor of CYP2D6. Co-administration of duloxetine with other drugs that are extensively metabolized by CYP2D6 isoenzyme, and which have a narrow therapeutic window, should be approached with caution). Products include:
AndroGel 3456

Testosterone Cypionate (Duloxetine is a moderate inhibitor of CYP2D6. Co-administration of duloxetine with other drugs that are extensively metabolized by CYP2D6 isoenzyme, and which have a narrow therapeutic window, should be approached with caution).
No products indexed under this heading.

Testosterone Enanthate (Duloxetine is a moderate inhibitor of CYP2D6. Co-administration of duloxetine with other drugs that are extensively metabolized by CYP2D6 isoenzyme, and which have a narrow therapeutic window, should be approached with caution). Products include:
Delatestryl 1102

Testosterone Propionate (Duloxetine is a moderate inhibitor of CYP2D6. Co-administration of duloxetine with other drugs that are extensively metabolized by CYP2D6 isoenzyme, and which have a narrow therapeutic window, should be approached with caution).
No products indexed under this heading.

Theophylline (*In vitro* drug interaction studies demonstrate that duloxetine does not induce CYP1A2 activity. Therefore, an increase in the metabolism of CYP1A2 substrates (eg, theophylline) resulting from induction is not anticipated, although clinical studies of induction have not been performed. Duloxetine is an inhibitor of the CYP1A2 isoform in *in vitro* studies, and in two clinical studies the average increase in theophylline AUC was 7% (1%-15%) and 20% (13%-27%) when co-administered with duloxetine (60 mg twice daily)).
No products indexed under this heading.

Theophylline Anhydrous (*In vitro* drug interaction studies demonstrate that duloxetine does not induce CYP1A2 activity. Therefore, an increase in the metabolism of CYP1A2 substrates (eg, theophylline) resulting from induction is not anticipated, although clinical studies of induction have not been performed. Duloxetine is an inhibitor of the CYP1A2 isoform in *in vitro* studies, and in two clinical studies the average increase in theophylline AUC was 7% (1%-15%) and 20% (13%-27%) when co-administered with duloxetine (60 mg twice daily)). Products include:
Uniphyl 2817

Theophylline Calcium Salicylate (*In vitro* drug interaction studies demonstrate that duloxetine does not induce CYP1A2 activity. Therefore, an increase in the metabolism of CYP1A2 substrates (eg, theophylline) resulting from induction is not anticipated, although clinical studies of induction have not been performed. Duloxetine is an inhibitor of the CYP1A2 isoform in *in vitro* studies, and in two clinical studies the average increase in theophylline AUC was 7% (1%-15%) and 20% (13%-27%) when co-administered with duloxetine (60 mg twice daily)).
No products indexed under this heading.

Theophylline Dihydroxypropyl (Glyceryl) (*In vitro* drug interaction studies demonstrate that duloxetine does not induce CYP1A2 activity. Therefore, an increase in the metabolism of CYP1A2 substrates (eg, theophylline) resulting from induction is not anticipated, although clinical studies of induction have not been performed. Duloxetine is an inhibitor of the CYP1A2 isoform in *in vitro* studies, and in two clinical studies the average increase in theophylline AUC was 7% (1%-15%) and 20% (13%-27%) when co-administered with duloxetine (60 mg twice daily)).
No products indexed under this heading.

Theophylline Ethylenediamine (*In vitro* drug interaction studies demonstrate that duloxetine does not induce CYP1A2 activity. Therefore, an increase in the metabolism of CYP1A2 substrates (eg, theophylline) resulting from induction is not anticipated, although clinical studies of induction have not been performed. Duloxetine is an inhibitor of the CYP1A2 isoform in *in vitro* studies, and in two clinical studies the average increase in theophylline AUC was 7% (1%-15%) and 20% (13%-27%) when co-administered with duloxetine (60 mg twice daily)).
No products indexed under this heading.

Theophylline Sodium Glycinate (*In vitro* drug interaction studies demonstrate that duloxetine does not induce CYP1A2 activity. Therefore, an increase in the metabolism of CYP1A2 substrates (eg, theophylline) resulting from induction is not anticipated, although clinical studies of induction have not been performed. Duloxetine is an inhibitor of the CYP1A2 isoform in *in vitro* studies, and in two clinical studies the average increase in theophylline AUC was 7% (1%-15%) and 20% (13%-27%) when co-administered with duloxetine (60 mg twice daily)).
No products indexed under this heading.

Thiamylal Sodium (Given the primary CNS effects of duloxetine, it should be used with caution when it is taken in combination with or substituted for other centrally acting drugs, including those with a similar mechanism of action).
No products indexed under this heading.

Thioridazine (Duloxetine is a moderate inhibitor of CYP2D6. Because of the risk of serious ventricular arrhythmias and sudden death potentially associated with elevated plasma levels of thioridazine, duloxetine and thioridazine should not be co-administered).
No products indexed under this heading.

Thioridazine Hydrochloride (Duloxetine is a moderate inhibitor of CYP2D6. Because of the risk of serious ventricular arrhythmias and sudden death potentially associated with elevated plasma levels of thioridazine, duloxetine and thioridazine should not be co-administered). Products include:
Thioridazine Hydrochloride 2384

Thiothixene (Development of a potentially life-threatening serotonin syndrome or Neuroleptic Malignant Syndrome-like reactions have been reported with duloxetine, and with concomitant use of antipsychotics. Serotonin syndrome symptoms may include mental status changes, autonomic instability, neuromuscular aberrations, and/or gastrointestinal symptoms. Serotonin syndrome in its most severe form can resemble neuroleptic malignant syndrome. Patients should be monitored for the emergence of serotonin syndrome or NMS-like signs and symptoms. Treatment with duloxetine and any antipsychotic agent should be discontinued immediately if the above events occur and supportive symptomatic treatment should be initiated). Products include:
Thiothixene 2386

Thiothixene Hydrochloride (Given the primary CNS effects of duloxetine, it should be used with caution when it is taken in combination with or substituted for other centrally acting drugs, including those with a similar mechanism of action).
No products indexed under this heading.

Ticlopidine Hydrochloride (Both CYP1A2 and CYP2D6 are responsible for duloxetine metabolism. When duloxetine 60 mg was co-administered with fluvoxamine 100 mg, a potent CYP1A2 inhibitor to male subjects, duloxetine AUC was increased approximately 6-fold, the C_{max} was increased approximately 2.5-fold and duloxetine $t_{1/2}$ was increased approximately 3-fold. Co-administration of duloxetine with potent CYP1A2 inhibitors should be avoided).
No products indexed under this heading.

Timolol Maleate (Duloxetine is a moderate inhibitor of CYP2D6. Co-administration of duloxetine with other drugs that are extensively metabolized by CYP2D6 isoenzyme, and which have a narrow therapeutic window, should be approached with caution). Products include:
Combigan 601
Dorzolamide Hydrochloride/Timolol Maleate Ophthalmic Solution .... ⊙243
Timoptic in Ocudose .... ⊙231

Tinzaparin Sodium (Duloxetine may increase the risk of bleeding events. Concomitant use of anticoagulants may add to this risk. Case reports and epidemiological studies have demonstrated an association between use of drugs that interfere with serotonin reuptake and the occurrence of gastrointestinal bleeding. Patients should be cautioned about the risk of bleeding associated with concomitant use of duloxetine and anticoagulants).
No products indexed under this heading.

Tolbutamide (Because duloxetine is highly bound to plasma protein, administration of duloxetine to a patient taking another drug that is highly protein bound may cause increased free concentration of the other drug, potentially resulting in serious adverse reactions).
No products indexed under this heading.

Tolmetin Sodium (Duloxetine may increase the risk of bleeding events. Concomitant use of non-steroidal anti-inflammatory drugs may add to this risk. Case reports and epidemiological studies have demonstrated an association between use of drugs that interfere with serotonin reuptake and the occurrence of gastrointestinal bleeding. Patients should be cautioned about the risk of bleeding associated with concomitant use of duloxetine and NSAIDs).
No products indexed under this heading.

Tolterodine Tartrate (Duloxetine is a moderate inhibitor of CYP2D6. Co-administration of duloxetine with other drugs that are extensively metabolized by CYP2D6 isoenzyme, and which have a narrow therapeutic window, should be approached with caution).
No products indexed under this heading.

Torsemide (Hyponatremia may occur as a result of treatment with duloxetine. Patients taking diuretics may be at greater risk. Discontinuation of duloxetine should be considered in patients with symptomatic hyponatremia and appropriate medical intervention should be instituted).
No products indexed under this heading.

Tramadol Hydrochloride (Based on the mechanism of action of duloxetine and the potential for serotonin syndrome, caution is advised when duloxetine is co-administered with drugs that may affect the serotonergic neurotransmitter systems, such as tramadol). Products include:
Ryzolt 2813
Ultram ER 2693

Tranylcypromine Sulfate (Concomitant use in patients taking MAO inhibitors is contradindicated due to the risk of serious, sometimes fatal, drug interactions with serotonergic drugs. These interactions may include hyperthermia, rigidity, myoclonus, autonomic instability, and mental status changes that include extreme agitation progressing to delirium and coma. These reactions have also been reported in patients who have recently discontinued serotonin reuptake inhibitors and are started on an MAOI. At least 14 days should elapse between discontinuation of an MAO inhibitor and initiation of therapy with duloxetine. In addition, at least 5 days should be allowed after stopping duloxetine before starting an MAO inhibitor). Products include:
Parnate 1584

Trazodone Hydrochloride (Duloxetine is a moderate inhibitor of CYP2D6. Co-administration of duloxetine with other drugs that are extensively metabolized by CYP2D6 isoenzyme, and which have a narrow therapeutic window, should be approached with caution).
No products indexed under this heading.

Triamterene (Hyponatremia may occur as a result of treatment with duloxetine. Patients taking diuretics may be at greater risk. Discontinuation of duloxetine should be considered in patients with symptomatic hyponatremia and appropriate medical intervention should be instituted). Products include:
Dyazide 1429
Dyrenium 3495

Triazolam (Given the primary CNS effects of duloxetine, it should be used with caution when it is taken in combination with or substituted for other centrally acting drugs, including those with a similar mechanism of action).
No products indexed under this heading.

Trifluoperazine Hydrochloride (Development of a potentially life-threatening serotonin syndrome or Neuroleptic Malignant Syndrome-like reactions have been reported with duloxetine, and with concomitant use of dopamine antagonists. Serotonin syndrome symptoms may include mental status changes, autonomic instability, neuromuscular aberrations, and/or gastrointestinal symptoms. Serotonin syndrome in its most severe form can resemble neuroleptic malignant syndrome. Patients should be monitored for the emergence of serotonin syndrome or NMS-like signs and symptoms. Treatment with duloxetine and any antidopaminergic agents should be discontinued immediately if the above events occur and supportive symptomatic treatment should be initiated).
No products indexed under this heading.

Trimipramine Maleate (Duloxetine is a moderate inhibitor of CYP2D6. Co-administration of duloxetine with other drugs that are extensively metabolized by CYP2D6 and have a narrow therapeutic window, including tricyclic antidepressants, should be approached with caution. Plasma tricyclic antidepressant concentrations may need to be monitored, and the dose of the TCA may need to be reduced, if a TCA is co-administered with duloxetine).
No products indexed under this heading.

Troleandomycin (Both CYP1A2 and CYP2D6 are responsible for duloxetine metabolism. When duloxetine 60 mg was co-administered with fluvoxamine 100 mg, a potent CYP1A2 inhibitor to male subjects, duloxetine AUC was increased approximately 6-fold, the C_{max} was increased approximately 2.5-fold and duloxetine $t_{1/2}$ was increased approximately 3-fold. Co-administration of duloxetine with potent CYP1A2 inhibitors should be avoided).
No products indexed under this heading.

Trovafloxacin Mesylate (Both CYP1A2 and CYP2D6 are responsible for duloxetine metabolism. When duloxetine 60 mg was co-administered with fluvoxamine 100 mg, a potent CYP1A2 inhibitor to male subjects, duloxetine AUC was increased approximately 6-fold, the C_{max} was increased approximately 2.5-fold and duloxetine $t_{1/2}$ was increased approximately 3-fold. Co-administration of duloxetine with potent CYP1A2 inhibitors should be avoided).
No products indexed under this heading.

Tryptophan (The concomitant use of duloxetine with serotonin precursors (eg, tryptophan) is not recommended).
No products indexed under this heading.

Valdecoxib (Duloxetine may increase the risk of bleeding events. Concomitant use of non-steroidal anti-inflammatory drugs may add to this risk. Case reports and epidemiological studies have demonstrated an association between use of drugs that interfere with serotonin reuptake and the occurrence of gastrointestinal bleeding. Patients should be cautioned about the risk of bleeding associated with concomitant use of duloxetine and NSAIDs).
No products indexed under this heading.

Vardenafil Hydrochloride (Both CYP1A2 and CYP2D6 are responsible for duloxetine metabolism. When duloxetine 60 mg was co-administered with fluvoxamine 100 mg, a potent CYP1A2 inhibitor to male subjects, duloxetine AUC was increased approximately 6-fold, the C_{max} was increased approximately 2.5-fold and duloxetine $t_{1/2}$ was increased approximately 3-fold. Co-administration of duloxetine with potent CYP1A2 inhibitors should be avoided). Products include:
Levitra 3157

Venlafaxine Hydrochloride (The development of a potentially life-threatening serotonin syndrome or Neuroleptic Malignant Syndrome-like reactions have been reported with duloxetine, but particularly with concomitant use of serotonergic drugs. Serotonin syndrome symptoms may include mental status changes, autonomic instability, and/or gastrointestinal symptoms. Serotonin syndrome, in its most severe form can resemble neuroleptic malignant syndrome. The concomitant use of duloxetine with SNRIs is not recommended). Products include:
Effexor XR 3504
Venlafaxine Hydrochloride Tablets ... 2388

Vinblastine Sulfate (Duloxetine is a moderate inhibitor of CYP2D6. Co-administration of duloxetine with other drugs that are extensively metabolized by CYP2D6 isoenzyme, and which have a narrow therapeutic window, should be approached with caution).
No products indexed under this heading.

Warfarin Sodium (Altered anticoagulant effects, including increased bleeding have been reported when SSRIs or SNRIs are co-administered with warfarin. Patients receiving warfarin therapy should be carefully monitored when duloxetine is initiated or discontinued).
No products indexed under this heading.

Zaleplon (Given the primary CNS effects of duloxetine, it should be used with caution when it is taken in combination with or substituted for other centrally acting drugs, including those with a similar mechanism of action).
No products indexed under this heading.

Zileuton (Both CYP1A2 and CYP2D6 are responsible for duloxetine metabolism. When duloxetine 60 mg was co-administered with fluvoxamine 100 mg, a potent CYP1A2 inhibitor to male subjects, duloxetine AUC was increased approximately 6-fold, the C_{max} was increased approximately 2.5-fold and duloxetine $t_{1/2}$ was increased approximately 3-fold. Co-administration of duloxetine with potent CYP1A2 inhibitors should be avoided).
No products indexed under this heading.

Ziprasidone Hydrochloride (Development of a potentially life-threatening serotonin syndrome or Neuroleptic Malignant Syndrome-like reactions have been reported with duloxetine, and with concomitant use of antipsychotics. Serotonin syndrome symptoms may include mental status changes, autonomic instability, neuromuscular aberrations, and/or gastrointestinal symptoms. Serotonin syndrome in its most severe form can resemble neuroleptic malignant syndrome. Patients should be monitored for the emergence of serotonin syndrome or NMS-like signs and symptoms. Treatment with duloxetine and any antipsychotic agent should be discontinued immediately if the above events occur and supportive symptomatic treatment should be initiated). Products include:
Geodon 2723

Zolmitriptan (There have been rare post-marketing reports of serotonin syndrome with the use of an SSRI and a triptan. If concomitant treatment is clinically warranted, careful observation of the patient is advised, particularly during treatment initiation and dose increases). Products include:
Zomig Tablets 773
Zomig Nasal Spray 768
Zomig-ZMT Tablets 773

Zolpidem Tartrate (Given the primary CNS effects of duloxetine, it should be used with caution when it is taken in combination with or substituted for other centrally acting drugs, including those with a similar mechanism of action). Products include:
Ambien 2920
Ambien CR 2925

Zonisamide (Duloxetine is a moderate inhibitor of CYP2D6. Co-administration of duloxetine with other drugs that are extensively metabolized by CYP2D6 isoenzyme, and which have a narrow therapeutic window, should be approached with caution). Products include:
Zonegran 1081

Food Interactions

Alcohol (Use of duloxetine concomitantly with heavy alcohol intake may be associated with severe liver injury. For this reason, duloxetine should ordinarily not be prescribed for patients with substantial alcohol use).

Beer, reduced-alcohol (Use of duloxetine concomitantly with heavy alcohol intake may be associated with severe liver injury. For this reason, duloxetine should ordinarily not be prescribed for patients with substantial alcohol use).

Beer, unspecified (Use of duloxetine concomitantly with heavy alcohol intake may be associated with severe liver injury. For this reason, duloxetine should ordinarily not be prescribed for patients with substantial alcohol use).

Grapefruit (Both CYP1A2 and CYP2D6 are responsible for duloxetine metabolism. When duloxetine 60 mg was co-administered with fluvoxamine 100 mg, a potent CYP1A2 inhibitor to male subjects, duloxetine AUC was increased approximately 6-fold, the C_{max} was increased approximately 2.5-fold and duloxetine $t_{1/2}$ was increased approximately 3-fold. Co-administration of duloxetine with potent CYP1A2 inhibitors should be avoided).

Grapefruit Juice (Both CYP1A2 and CYP2D6 are responsible for duloxetine metabolism. When duloxetine 60 mg was co-administered with fluvoxamine 100 mg, a potent CYP1A2 inhibitor to male subjects, duloxetine AUC was increased approximately 6-fold, the C_{max} was increased approximately 2.5-fold and duloxetine $t_{1/2}$ was increased approximately 3-fold. Co-administration of duloxetine with potent CYP1A2 inhibitors should be avoided).

Wine, Chianti (Use of duloxetine concomitantly with heavy alcohol intake may be associated with severe liver injury. For this reason, duloxetine should ordinarily not be prescribed for patients with substantial alcohol use).

Wine, Red (Use of duloxetine concomitantly with heavy alcohol intake may be associated with severe liver injury. For this reason, duloxetine should ordinarily not be prescribed for patients with substantial alcohol use).

Wine, unspecified (Use of duloxetine concomitantly with heavy alcohol intake may be associated with severe liver injury. For this reason, duloxetine should ordinarily not be prescribed for patients with substantial alcohol use).

Wine products (Use of duloxetine concomitantly with heavy alcohol intake may be associated with severe liver injury. For this reason, duloxetine should ordinarily not be prescribed for patients with substantial alcohol use).

CYTOMEL TABLETS

(Liothyronine Sodium) 1830
May interact with cardiac glycosides, estrogens, insulin, oral anticoagulants, oral hypoglycemic agents, tricyclic antidepressants, and certain other agents. Compounds in these categories include:

Acarbose (Initiating thyroid replacement therapy may cause increases in oral hypoglycemic requirements).
No products indexed under this heading.

Amitriptyline Hydrochloride (Use of thyroid hormones may increase receptor sensitivity and enhance antidepressant activity; transient cardiac arrhythmias; thyroid hormone activity may also be enhanced).
No products indexed under this heading.

Amoxapine (Use of thyroid hormones may increase receptor sensitivity and enhance antidepressant activity; transient cardiac arrhythmias; thyroid hormone activity may also be enhanced).
No products indexed under this heading.

IMPORTANT NOTE: Always consult each drug listing in the patient's regimen for possible interactions.

(⊙ Described in PDR® for Ophthalmic Medicines)

Miglitol (Initiating thyroid replacement therapy may cause increases in oral hypoglycemic requirements).
No products indexed under this heading.

Nateglinide (Initiating thyroid replacement therapy may cause increases in oral hypoglycemic requirements).
No products indexed under this heading.

Norepinephrine Hydrochloride (Thyroxine increases the adrenergic effect of catecholamines, such as norepinephrine).
No products indexed under this heading.

Nortriptyline Hydrochloride (Use of thyroid hormones may increase receptor sensitivity and enhance antidepressant activity; transient cardiac arrhythmias; thyroid hormone activity may also be enhanced).
No products indexed under this heading.

Pioglitazone Hydrochloride (Initiating thyroid replacement therapy may cause increases in oral hypoglycemic requirements). Products include:

Polyestradiol Phosphate (Estrogens tend to increase serum thyroxine-binding globulin in a patient with a nonfunctioning thyroid gland who is receiving thyroid replacement therapy; patients without functioning thyroid gland who are on thyroid replacement therapy may need to increase their thyroid dose if estrogens or estrogen-containing oral contraceptives are given).
No products indexed under this heading.

Protriptyline Hydrochloride (Use of thyroid hormones may increase receptor sensitivity and enhance antidepressant activity; transient cardiac arrhythmias; thyroid hormone activity may also be enhanced).
No products indexed under this heading.

Quinestrol (Estrogens tend to increase serum thyroxine-binding globulin in a patient with a nonfunctioning thyroid gland who is receiving thyroid replacement therapy; patients without functioning thyroid gland who are on thyroid replacement therapy may need to increase their thyroid dose if estrogens or estrogen-containing oral contraceptives are given).
No products indexed under this heading.

Repaglinide (Initiating thyroid replacement therapy may cause increases in oral hypoglycemic requirements).
No products indexed under this heading.

Rosiglitazone Maleate (Initiating thyroid replacement therapy may cause increases in oral hypoglycemic requirements). Products include:

Sitagliptin Phosphate (Initiating thyroid replacement therapy may cause increases in oral hypoglycemic requirements). Products include:

Tolazamide (Initiating thyroid replacement therapy may cause increases in oral hypoglycemic requirements).
No products indexed under this heading.

Tolbutamide (Initiating thyroid replacement therapy may cause increases in oral hypoglycemic requirements).
No products indexed under this heading.

Trimipramine Maleate (Use of thyroid hormones may increase receptor sensitivity and enhance antidepressant activity; transient cardiac arrhythmias; thyroid hormone activity may also be enhanced).
No products indexed under this heading.

Troglitazone (Initiating thyroid replacement therapy may cause increases in oral hypoglycemic requirements).
No products indexed under this heading.

Warfarin Sodium (Thyroid hormones appear to increase catabolism of vitamin K-dependent clotting factor; if oral anticoagulants are also given compensatory increases in clotting factor synthesis are impaired).
No products indexed under this heading.

DACOGEN INJECTION

(Decitabine) 1054
None cited in PDR database.

DAPSONE TABLETS USP

(Dapsone) 1819
May interact with Folic acid antagonists, and certain other agents. Compounds in these categories include:

Carbamazepine (Folic acid antagonists may increase the likelihood of hematologic reactions). Products include:

Fosphenytoin (Folic acid antagonists may increase the likelihood of hematologic reactions).
No products indexed under this heading.

Fosphenytoin Sodium (Folic acid antagonists may increase the likelihood of hematologic reactions).
No products indexed under this heading.

Mephenytoin (Folic acid antagonists may increase the likelihood of hematologic reactions).
No products indexed under this heading.

Methotrexate (Folic acid antagonists may increase the likelihood of hematologic reactions).
No products indexed under this heading.

Methotrexate Sodium (Folic acid antagonists may increase the likelihood of hematologic reactions).
No products indexed under this heading.

Phenobarbital (Folic acid antagonists may increase the likelihood of hematologic reactions). Products include:

Phenobarbital Sodium (Folic acid antagonists may increase the likelihood of hematologic reactions).
No products indexed under this heading.

Phenytoin (Folic acid antagonists may increase the likelihood of hematologic reactions).
No products indexed under this heading.

Phenytoin Sodium (Folic acid antagonists may increase the likelihood of hematologic reactions). Products include:

Primidone (Folic acid antagonists may increase the likelihood of hematologic reactions).
No products indexed under this heading.

Pyrimethamine (Agranulocytosis reported; may increase likelihood of hematologic reactions). Products include:

Rifampin (Rifampin lowers dapsone levels 7 to 10-fold by accelerating plasma clearance).
No products indexed under this heading.

Triamterene (Folic acid antagonists may increase the likelihood of hematologic reactions). Products include:

Trimethoprim (Mutual interaction between dapsone and trimethoprim exists in which each raises the level of the other about 1.5 times).
No products indexed under this heading.

Trimethoprim Hydrochloride (Mutual interaction between dapsone and trimethoprim exists in which each raises the level of the other about 1.5 times).
No products indexed under this heading.

Trimethoprim Sulfate (Mutual interaction between dapsone and trimethoprim exists in which each raises the level of the other about 1.5 times).
No products indexed under this heading.

DARAPRIM TABLETS

(Pyrimethamine) 1423
May interact with agents associated with myelosuppression, cytotoxic drugs, dihydrofolate reductase inhibitors, phenytoin, sulfonamides, and certain other agents. Compounds in these categories include:

Altretamine (The concomitant use of other antifolic drugs or agents associated with myelosuppression including cytostatic agents while the patient is receiving pyrimethamine, may increase the risk of bone marrow suppression). Products include:

Bendroflumethiazide (Co-administration of other antifolic drugs, such as sulfonamides, may increase the risk of bone marrow suppression; potential for hypersensitivity reactions such as Stevens-Johnson syndrome, toxic epidermal necrolysis, erythema multiforme, and anaphylaxis).
No products indexed under this heading.

Bleomycin Sulfate (The concomitant use of other antifolic drugs or agents associated with myelosuppression including cytostatic agents while the patient is receiving pyrimethamine, may increase the risk of bone marrow suppression).
No products indexed under this heading.

Busulfan (The concomitant use of other antifolic drugs or agents associated with myelosuppression including cytostatic agents while the patient is receiving pyrimethamine, may increase the risk of bone marrow suppression). Products include:

Chlorambucil (The concomitant use of other antifolic drugs or agents associated with myelosuppression including cytostatic agents while the patient is receiving pyrimethamine, may increase the risk of bone marrow suppression). Products include:

Chloramphenicol (The concomitant use of other antifolic drugs or agents associated with myelosuppression including cytostatic agents while the patient is receiving pyrimethamine, may increase the risk of bone marrow suppression).
No products indexed under this heading.

Chloramphenicol Palmitate (The concomitant use of other antifolic drugs or agents associated with myelosuppression including cytostatic agents while the patient is receiving pyrimethamine, may increase the risk of bone marrow suppression).
No products indexed under this heading.

Chloramphenicol Sodium Succinate (The concomitant use of other antifolic drugs or agents associated with myelosuppression including cytostatic agents while the patient is receiving pyrimethamine, may increase the risk of bone marrow suppression).
No products indexed under this heading.

Chlorothiazide (Co-administration of other antifolic drugs, such as sulfonamides, may increase the risk of bone marrow suppression; potential for hypersensitivity reactions such as Stevens-Johnson syndrome, toxic epidermal necrolysis, erythema multiforme, and anaphylaxis).
No products indexed under this heading.

Chlorothiazide Sodium (Co-administration of other antifolic drugs, such as sulfonamides, may increase the risk of bone marrow suppression; potential for hypersensitivity reactions such as Stevens-Johnson syndrome, toxic epidermal necrolysis, erythema multiforme, and anaphylaxis). Products include:

Chlorpropamide (Co-administration of other antifolic drugs, such as sulfonamides, may increase the risk of bone marrow suppression; potential for hypersensitivity reactions such as Stevens-Johnson syndrome, toxic epidermal necrolysis, erythema multiforme, and anaphylaxis).
No products indexed under this heading.

Cladribine (The concomitant use of other antifolic drugs or agents associated with myelosuppression including cytostatic agents while the patient is receiving pyrimethamine, may increase the risk of bone marrow suppression). Products include:

Cyclophosphamide (The concomitant use of other antifolic drugs or agents associated with myelosuppression including cytostatic agents while the patient is receiving pyrimethamine, may increase the risk of bone marrow suppression).
No products indexed under this heading.

Daunorubicin Citrate Liposome (The concomitant use of other antifolic drugs or agents associated with myelosuppression including cytostatic agents while the patient is receiving pyrimethamine, may increase the risk of bone marrow suppression).
No products indexed under this heading.

Daunorubicin Hydrochloride (The concomitant use of other antifolic drugs or agents associated with myelosuppression including cytostatic agents while the patient is receiving pyrimethamine, may increase the risk of bone marrow suppression).
No products indexed under this heading.

Dexrazoxane (The concomitant use of other antifolic drugs or agents associated with myelosuppression including cytostatic agents while the patient is receiving pyrimethamine, may increase the risk of bone marrow suppression).
No products indexed under this heading.

Doxorubicin Hydrochloride (The concomitant use of other antifolic drugs or agents associated with myelosuppression including cytostatic agents while the patient is receiving pyrimethamine, may increase the risk of bone marrow suppression).
No products indexed under this heading.

Doxorubicin Hydrochloride Liposome (The concomitant use of other antifolic drugs or agents associated with myelosuppression including cytostatic agents while the patient is receiving pyrimethamine, may increase the risk of bone marrow suppression). Products include:

Epirubicin Hydrochloride (The concomitant use of other antifolic drugs or agents associated with myelosuppression including cytostatic agents while the patient is receiving pyrimethamine, may increase the risk of bone marrow suppression).
No products indexed under this heading.

(⊙ Described in PDR® for Ophthalmic Medicines)

Felodipine (Methylphenidate may decrease the effectiveness of drugs used to treat hypertension).
No products indexed under this heading.

Fluoxetine (Human pharmacologic studies have shown that methylphenidate may inhibit the metabolism of selective serotonin reuptake inhibitors. Downward dose adjustments of these drugs may be required when given concomitantly with methylphenidate. It may be necessary to adjust the dosage and monitor plasma drug concentrations when initiating or discontinuing methylphenidate).
No products indexed under this heading.

Fluoxetine Hydrochloride (Human pharmacologic studies have shown that methylphenidate may inhibit the metabolism of selective serotonin reuptake inhibitors. Downward dose adjustments of these drugs may be required when given concomitantly with methylphenidate. It may be necessary to adjust the dosage and monitor plasma drug concentrations when initiating or discontinuing methylphenidate). Products include:
Prozac Weekly 1941
Prozac Pulvules 1941
Symbyax 1965

Fluvoxamine (Human pharmacologic studies have shown that methylphenidate may inhibit the metabolism of selective serotonin reuptake inhibitors. Downward dose adjustments of these drugs may be required when given concomitantly with methylphenidate. It may be necessary to adjust the dosage and monitor plasma drug concentrations when initiating or discontinuing methylphenidate).
No products indexed under this heading.

Fluvoxamine Maleate (Human pharmacologic studies have shown that methylphenidate may inhibit the metabolism of selective serotonin reuptake inhibitors. Downward dose adjustments of these drugs may be required when given concomitantly with methylphenidate. It may be necessary to adjust the dosage and monitor plasma drug concentrations when initiating or discontinuing methylphenidate).
No products indexed under this heading.

Fosinopril Sodium (Methylphenidate may decrease the effectiveness of drugs used to treat hypertension).
No products indexed under this heading.

Fosphenytoin (Human pharmacologic studies have shown that methylphenidate may inhibit the metabolism of anticonvulsants (eg, phenobarbital, phenytoin, primidone). Downward dose adjustments of these drugs may be required when given concomitantly with methylphenidate. It may be necessary to adjust the dosage and monitor plasma drug concentrations when initiating or discontinuing methylphenidate).
No products indexed under this heading.

Fosphenytoin Sodium (Human pharmacologic studies have shown that methylphenidate may inhibit the metabolism of anticonvulsants (eg, phenobarbital, phenytoin, primidone). Downward dose adjustments of these drugs may be required when given concomitantly with methylphenidate. It may be necessary to adjust the dosage and monitor plasma drug concentrations when initiating or discontinuing methylphenidate).
No products indexed under this heading.

Furosemide (Methylphenidate may decrease the effectiveness of drugs used to treat hypertension). Products include:
Furosemide 2354

Gabapentin (Human pharmacologic studies have shown that methylphenidate may inhibit the metabolism of anticonvulsants (eg, phenobarbital, phenytoin, primidone). Downward dose

adjustments of these drugs may be required when given concomitantly with methylphenidate. It may be necessary to adjust the dosage and monitor plasma drug concentrations when initiating or discontinuing methylphenidate).
No products indexed under this heading.

Guanabenz Acetate (Methylphenidate may decrease the effectiveness of drugs used to treat hypertension).
No products indexed under this heading.

Guanethidine (Methylphenidate may decrease the effectiveness of drugs used to treat hypertension).
No products indexed under this heading.

Guanethidine Monosulfate (Methylphenidate may decrease the effectiveness of drugs used to treat hypertension).
No products indexed under this heading.

Guanethidine Sulfate (Methylphenidate may decrease the effectiveness of drugs used to treat hypertension).
No products indexed under this heading.

Hydralazine Hydrochloride (Methylphenidate may decrease the effectiveness of drugs used to treat hypertension).
No products indexed under this heading.

Hydrochlorothiazide (Methylphenidate may decrease the effectiveness of drugs used to treat hypertension). Products include:
Atacand HCT 700
Avalide 2956
Benicar HCT 1017
Diovan HCT 2419
Dyazide 1429
Exforge HCT 2449
Hyzaar 2162
Hyzaar 100-12.5 2162
Micardis HCT 889
Prinzide 2246
Tekturna HCT 2541
Teveten HCT 541

Hydroflumethiazide (Methylphenidate may decrease the effectiveness of drugs used to treat hypertension).
No products indexed under this heading.

Imipramine Hydrochloride (Human pharmacologic studies have shown that methylphenidate may inhibit the metabolism of some tricyclic drugs (eg, imipramine, clomipramine, desipramine). Downward dose adjustments of these drugs may be required when given concomitantly with methylphenidate. It may be necessary to adjust the dosage and monitor plasma drug concentrations when initiating or discontinuing methylphenidate).
No products indexed under this heading.

Imipramine Pamoate (Human pharmacologic studies have shown that methylphenidate may inhibit the metabolism of some tricyclic drugs (eg, imipramine, clomipramine, desipramine). Downward dose adjustments of these drugs may be required when given concomitantly with methylphenidate. It may be necessary to adjust the dosage and monitor plasma drug concentrations when initiating or discontinuing methylphenidate).
No products indexed under this heading.

Indapamide (Methylphenidate may decrease the effectiveness of drugs used to treat hypertension). Products include:
Indapamide 2356

Irbesartan (Methylphenidate may decrease the effectiveness of drugs used to treat hypertension). Products include:
Avalide 2956
Avapro 2962

Isocarboxazid (Methylphenidate transdermal system is contraindicated during treatment with monoamine oxidase inhibitors and also within a mini-

mum of 14 days following discontinuation of treatment with a MAO inhibitor (hypertensive crises may occur)). Products include:
Marplan 3481

Isoproterenol Hydrochloride (Because of a possible effect on blood pressure, methylphenidate transdermal system should be used cautiously with pressor agents).
No products indexed under this heading.

Isoproterenol Sulfate (Because of a possible effect on blood pressure, methylphenidate transdermal system should be used cautiously with pressor agents).
No products indexed under this heading.

Isradipine (Methylphenidate may decrease the effectiveness of drugs used to treat hypertension). Products include:
DynaCirc CR 1432

Labetalol Hydrochloride (Methylphenidate may decrease the effectiveness of drugs used to treat hypertension).
No products indexed under this heading.

Lamotrigine (Human pharmacologic studies have shown that methylphenidate may inhibit the metabolism of anticonvulsants (eg, phenobarbital, phenytoin, primidone). Downward dose adjustments of these drugs may be required when given concomitantly with methylphenidate. It may be necessary to adjust the dosage and monitor plasma drug concentrations when initiating or discontinuing methylphenidate). Products include:
Lamictal 1522
Lamictal ODT 1522
Lamictal XR 1536

Levetiracetam (Human pharmacologic studies have shown that methylphenidate may inhibit the metabolism of anticonvulsants (eg, phenobarbital, phenytoin, primidone). Downward dose adjustments of these drugs may be required when given concomitantly with methylphenidate. It may be necessary to adjust the dosage and monitor plasma drug concentrations when initiating or discontinuing methylphenidate). Products include:
Keppra XR 3434

Lisinopril (Methylphenidate may decrease the effectiveness of drugs used to treat hypertension). Products include:
Prinivil 2241
Prinzide 2246

Losartan Potassium (Methylphenidate may decrease the effectiveness of drugs used to treat hypertension). Products include:
Cozaar 2106
Hyzaar 2162
Hyzaar 100-12.5 2162

Maprotiline Hydrochloride (Human pharmacologic studies have shown that methylphenidate may inhibit the metabolism of some tricyclic drugs (eg, imipramine, clomipramine, desipramine). Downward dose adjustments of these drugs may be required when given concomitantly with methylphenidate. It may be necessary to adjust the dosage and monitor plasma drug concentrations when initiating or discontinuing methylphenidate).
No products indexed under this heading.

Mecamylamine Hydrochloride (Methylphenidate may decrease the effectiveness of drugs used to treat hypertension).
No products indexed under this heading.

Mephentermine Sulfate (Because of a possible effect on blood pressure, methylphenidate transdermal system should be used cautiously with pressor agents).
No products indexed under this heading.

Mephenytoin (Human pharmacologic studies have shown that methylphenidate may inhibit the metabolism of anticonvulsants (eg, phenobarbital, phenytoin, primidone). Downward dose adjustments of these drugs may be required when given concomitantly with methylphenidate. It may be necessary to adjust the dosage and monitor plasma drug concentrations when initiating or discontinuing methylphenidate).
No products indexed under this heading.

Metaraminol Bitartrate (Because of a possible effect on blood pressure, methylphenidate transdermal system should be used cautiously with pressor agents).
No products indexed under this heading.

Methoxamine Hydrochloride (Because of a possible effect on blood pressure, methylphenidate transdermal system should be used cautiously with pressor agents).
No products indexed under this heading.

Methsuximide (Human pharmacologic studies have shown that methylphenidate may inhibit the metabolism of anticonvulsants (eg, phenobarbital, phenytoin, primidone). Downward dose adjustments of these drugs may be required when given concomitantly with methylphenidate. It may be necessary to adjust the dosage and monitor plasma drug concentrations when initiating or discontinuing methylphenidate).
No products indexed under this heading.

Methyclothiazide (Methylphenidate may decrease the effectiveness of drugs used to treat hypertension).
No products indexed under this heading.

Methyldopa (Methylphenidate may decrease the effectiveness of drugs used to treat hypertension).
No products indexed under this heading.

Methyldopate Hydrochloride (Methylphenidate may decrease the effectiveness of drugs used to treat hypertension).
No products indexed under this heading.

Metolazone (Methylphenidate may decrease the effectiveness of drugs used to treat hypertension).
No products indexed under this heading.

Metoprolol Succinate (Methylphenidate may decrease the effectiveness of drugs used to treat hypertension). Products include:
Toprol XL 732

Metoprolol Tartrate (Methylphenidate may decrease the effectiveness of drugs used to treat hypertension).
No products indexed under this heading.

Metyrosine (Methylphenidate may decrease the effectiveness of drugs used to treat hypertension).
No products indexed under this heading.

Mibefradil Dihydrochloride (Methylphenidate may decrease the effectiveness of drugs used to treat hypertension).
No products indexed under this heading.

Minoxidil (Methylphenidate may decrease the effectiveness of drugs used to treat hypertension).
No products indexed under this heading.

Moclobemide (Methylphenidate transdermal system is contraindicated during treatment with monoamine oxidase inhibitors and also within a minimum of 14 days following discontinuation of treatment with a MAO inhibitor (hypertensive crises may occur)).
No products indexed under this heading.

Moexipril Hydrochloride (Methylphenidate may decrease the effectiveness of drugs used to treat hypertension).
No products indexed under this heading.

IMPORTANT NOTE: Always consult each drug listing in the patient's regimen for possible interactions.

(⊙ Described in PDR® for Ophthalmic Medicines)

DENAVIR CREAM

(Penciclovir) 2395
None cited in PDR database.

DEPAKOTE ER EXTENDED RELEASE TABLETS

(Divalproex Sodium) 426
May interact with alcohols, anticonvulsants, aspirin-acetylsalicylic acid, barbiturates, carbapenems, central nervous system depressants, phenytoin, and certain other agents. Compounds in these categories include:

Alfentanil Hydrochloride (Since valproate products may produce CNS depression, especially when combined with another CNS depressant (eg, alcohol), patients should be advised not to engage in hazardous activities, such as driving an automobile or operating dangerous machinery, until it is known that they do not become drowsy from the drug).
No products indexed under this heading.

Depakote Interactions Index 454

Alprazolam (Since valproate products may produce CNS depression, especially when combined with another CNS depressant (eg, alcohol), patients should be advised not to engage in hazardous activities, such as driving an automobile or operating dangerous machinery, until it is known that they do not become drowsy from the drug).
No products indexed under this heading.

Amitriptyline Hydrochloride (Rare postmarketing reports of concurrent use of valproate and amitriptyline resulting in an increased amitriptyline level have been received. Concurrent use of valproate and amitriptyline has rarely been associated with toxicity. Monitoring of amitriptyline levels should be considered for patients taking valproate concomitantly with amitriptyline. Consideration should be given to lowering the dose of amitriptyline/nortriptyline in the presence of valproate).
No products indexed under this heading.

Amobarbital (Since valproate products may produce CNS depression, especially when combined with another CNS depressant (eg, alcohol), patients should be advised not to engage in hazardous activities, such as driving an automobile or operating dangerous machinery, until it is known that they do not become drowsy from the drug).
No products indexed under this heading.

Amobarbital Sodium (Since valproate products may produce CNS depression, especially when combined with another CNS depressant (eg, alcohol), patients should be advised not to engage in hazardous activities, such as driving an automobile or operating dangerous machinery, until it is known that they do not become drowsy from the drug).
No products indexed under this heading.

Aprobarbital (Since valproate products may produce CNS depression, especially when combined with another CNS depressant (eg, alcohol), patients should be advised not to engage in hazardous activities, such as driving an automobile or operating dangerous machinery, until it is known that they do not become drowsy from the drug).
No products indexed under this heading.

Aspirin (A study involving the co-administration of aspirin at antipyretic doses (11 to 16 mg/kg) with valproate to pediatric patients (n=6) revealed a decrease in protein binding and an inhibition of metabolism of valproate. Valproate free fraction was increased 4-fold in the presence of aspirin compared to valproate alone. Whether or not the interaction observed in this study applies to adults is unknown, but caution should be observed if valproate and aspirin are to be co-administered). Products include:
Aggrenox 880
Bayer Aspirin 829
Percodan 1124
St. Joseph Aspirin 2045

Aspirin, Enteric Coated (A study involving the co-administration of aspirin at antipyretic doses (11 to 16 mg/kg) with valproate to pediatric patients (n=6) revealed a decrease in protein binding and an inhibition of metabolism of valproate. Valproate free fraction was increased 4-fold in the presence of aspirin compared to valproate alone. Whether or not the interaction observed in this study applies to adults is unknown, but caution should be observed if valproate and aspirin are to be co-administered).
No products indexed under this heading.

Aspirin Buffered (A study involving the co-administration of aspirin at antipyretic doses (11 to 16 mg/kg) with valproate to pediatric patients (n=6) revealed a decrease in protein binding and an inhibition of metabolism of valproate. Valproate free fraction was increased 4-fold in the presence of aspirin compared to valproate alone. Whether or not the interaction observed in this study applies to adults is unknown, but caution should be observed if valproate and aspirin are to be co-administered).
No products indexed under this heading.

Buprenorphine Hydrochloride (Since valproate products may produce CNS depression, especially when combined with another CNS depressant (eg, alcohol), patients should be advised not to engage in hazardous activities, such as driving an automobile or operating dangerous machinery, until it is known that they do not become drowsy from the drug).
No products indexed under this heading.

Buspirone Hydrochloride (Since valproate products may produce CNS depression, especially when combined with another CNS depressant (eg, alcohol), patients should be advised not to engage in hazardous activities, such as driving an automobile or operating dangerous machinery, until it is known that they do not become drowsy from the drug).
No products indexed under this heading.

Butabarbital (Since valproate products may produce CNS depression, especially when combined with another CNS depressant (eg, alcohol), patients should be advised not to engage in hazardous activities, such as driving an automobile or operating dangerous machinery, until it is known that they do not become drowsy from the drug).
No products indexed under this heading.

Butabarbital Sodium (Since valproate products may produce CNS depression, especially when combined with another CNS depressant (eg, alcohol), patients should be advised not to engage in hazardous activities, such as driving an automobile or operating dangerous machinery, until it is known that they do not become drowsy from the drug).
No products indexed under this heading.

Butalbital (Since valproate products may produce CNS depression, especially when combined with another CNS depressant (eg, alcohol), patients should be advised not to engage in hazardous activities, such as driving an automobile or operating dangerous machinery, until it is known that they do not become drowsy from the drug).
No products indexed under this heading.

Carbamazepine (Co-administration has resulted in decreased serum levels of carbamazepine and increased serum levels of carbamazepine 10,11-epoxide; drugs that affect the levels of expression of hepatic enzymes, particularly those that elevate levels of glucuronosyltransferases, such as carbamazepine, may increase the clearance of valproate). Products include:
Carbatrol 3280
Equetro 3477

Chlordiazepoxide (Since valproate products may produce CNS depression, especially when combined with another CNS depressant (eg, alcohol), patients should be advised not to engage in hazardous activities, such as driving an automobile or operating dangerous machinery, until it is known that they do not become drowsy from the drug).
No products indexed under this heading.

Chlordiazepoxide Hydrochloride (Since valproate products may produce CNS depression, especially when combined with another CNS depressant (eg, alcohol), patients should be advised not to engage in hazardous activities, such as driving an automobile or operating dangerous machinery, until it is known that they do not become drowsy from the drug).
No products indexed under this heading.

Chlorpromazine (A study involving the administration of 100 to 300 mg/day of chlorpromazine to schizophrenic patients already receiving valproate (200 mg BID) revealed a 15% increase in trough plasma levels of valproate).
No products indexed under this heading.

Chlorpromazine Hydrochloride (A study involving the administration of 100 to 300 mg/day of chlorpromazine to schizophrenic patients already receiving valproate (200 mg BID) revealed a 15% increase in trough plasma levels of valproate).
No products indexed under this heading.

Chlorprothixene (Since valproate products may produce CNS depression, especially when combined with another CNS depressant (eg, alcohol), patients should be advised not to engage in hazardous activities, such as driving an automobile or operating dangerous machinery, until it is known that they do not become drowsy from the drug).
No products indexed under this heading.

Chlorprothixene Hydrochloride (Since valproate products may produce CNS depression, especially when combined with another CNS depressant (eg, alcohol), patients should be advised not to engage in hazardous activities, such as driving an automobile or operating dangerous machinery, until it is known that they do not become drowsy from the drug).
No products indexed under this heading.

Chlorprothixene Lactate (Since valproate products may produce CNS depression, especially when combined with another CNS depressant (eg, alcohol), patients should be advised not to engage in hazardous activities, such as driving an automobile or operating dangerous machinery, until it is known that they do not become drowsy from the drug).
No products indexed under this heading.

Clonazepam (Concomitant use of valproic acid and clonazepam may induce absence status in patients with a history of absence type seizures). Products include:
Klonopin 2855

Clorazepate Dipotassium (Since valproate products may produce CNS depression, especially when combined with another CNS depressant (eg, alcohol), patients should be advised not to engage in hazardous activities, such as driving an automobile or operating dangerous machinery, until it is known that they do not become drowsy from the drug).
No products indexed under this heading.

Clozapine (Since valproate products may produce CNS depression, especially when combined with another CNS depressant (eg, alcohol), patients should be advised not to engage in hazardous activities, such as driving an automobile or operating dangerous machinery, until it is known that they do not become drowsy from the drug).
No products indexed under this heading.

Codeine Phosphate (Since valproate products may produce CNS depression, especially when combined with another CNS depressant (eg, alcohol), patients should be advised not to engage in hazardous activities, such as driving an automobile or operating dangerous machinery, until it is known that they do not become drowsy from the drug). Products include:
Tylenol with Codeine 2691

Codeine Sulfate (Since valproate products may produce CNS depression, especially when combined with another CNS depressant (eg, alcohol), patients should be advised not to engage in hazardous activities, such as driving an automobile or operating dangerous machinery, until it is known that they do not become drowsy from the drug).
No products indexed under this heading.

Desflurane (Since valproate products may produce CNS depression, especially when combined with another CNS depressant (eg, alcohol), patients should be advised not to engage in hazardous activities, such as driving an automobile or operating dangerous machinery, until it is known that they do not become drowsy from the drug).
No products indexed under this heading.

Dezocine (Since valproate products may produce CNS depression, especially when combined with another CNS depressant (eg, alcohol), patients should be advised not to engage in hazardous activities, such as driving an automobile or operating dangerous machinery, until it is known that they do not become drowsy from the drug).
No products indexed under this heading.

Diazepam (Valproate displaces diazepam from its plasma albumin binding sites and inhibits its metabolism. Co-administration of valproate (1500 mg daily) increased the free fraction of diazepam (10 mg) by 90% in healthy volunteers (n=6). Plasma clearance and volume of distribution for free diazepam were reduced by 25% and 20%, respectively, in the presence of valproate. The elimination half-life of diazepam remained unchanged upon addition of valproate). Products include:
Valium Tablets 2880

Doripenem (Co-administration of valproic acid with carbapenem antibiotics (ertapenem, imipenem, meropenem) has lead to a clinically significant reduction in serum valproic acid concentration and may result in loss of seizure control. The mechanism of this interaction is not well understood. Serum valproic acid concentrations should be monitored frequently after initiating carbapenem therapy. Alternative antibacterial or anticonvulsant therapy should be considered if serum valproic acid concentrations drop significantly or seizure control deteriorates).
No products indexed under this heading.

Droperidol (Since valproate products may produce CNS depression, especially when combined with another CNS depressant (eg, alcohol), patients should be advised not to engage in hazardous activities, such as driving an automobile or operating dangerous machinery, until it is known that they do not become drowsy from the drug).
No products indexed under this heading.

Enflurane (Since valproate products may produce CNS depression, especially when combined with another CNS depressant (eg, alcohol), patients should be advised not to engage in hazardous activities, such as driving an automobile or operating dangerous machinery, until it is known that they do not become drowsy from the drug).
No products indexed under this heading.

Ertapenem (Co-administration of valproic acid with carbapenem antibiotics (ertapenem, imipenem, meropenem) has lead to a clinically significant reduction in serum valproic acid concentration and may result in loss of seizure control. The mechanism of this interaction is not well understood. Serum valp-

(⊙ Described in PDR® for Ophthalmic Medicines)

455 **Interactions Index** **Depakote**

roic acid concentrations should be monitored frequently after initiating carbapenem therapy. Alternative antibacterial or anticonvulsant therapy should be considered if serum valproic acid concentrations drop significantly or seizure control deteriorates). Products include:
Invanz 2172

Estazolam (Since valproate products may produce CNS depression, especially when combined with another CNS depressant (eg, alcohol), patients should be advised not to engage in hazardous activities, such as driving an automobile or operating dangerous machinery, until it is known that they do not become drowsy from the drug).
No products indexed under this heading.

Ethanol (Since valproate products may produce CNS depression, especially when combined with another CNS depressant (eg, alcohol), patients should be advised not to engage in hazardous activities, such as driving an automobile or operating dangerous machinery, until it is known that they do not become drowsy from the drug).
No products indexed under this heading.

Ethchlorvynol (Since valproate products may produce CNS depression, especially when combined with another CNS depressant (eg, alcohol), patients should be advised not to engage in hazardous activities, such as driving an automobile or operating dangerous machinery, until it is known that they do not become drowsy from the drug).
No products indexed under this heading.

Ethinamate (Since valproate products may produce CNS depression, especially when combined with another CNS depressant (eg, alcohol), patients should be advised not to engage in hazardous activities, such as driving an automobile or operating dangerous machinery, until it is known that they do not become drowsy from the drug).
No products indexed under this heading.

Ethosuximide (Valproate inhibits the metabolism of ethosuximide. Administration of a single ethosuximide dose of 500 mg with valproate (800 to 1600 mg/day) to healthy volunteers (n=6) was accompanied by a 25% increase in elimination half-life of ethosuximide and a 15% decrease in its total clearance as compared to ethosuximide alone. Patients receiving valproate and ethosuximide, especially along with other anticonvulsants, should be monitored for alterations in serum concentrations of both drugs).
No products indexed under this heading.

Ethotoin (Hepatic failure resulting in fatalities has occurred in patients receiving valproic acid and its derivatives. Children under the age of two years are at a considerably increased risk of developing fatal hepatotoxicity, especially those on multiple anticonvulsants, those with congenital metabolic disorders, those with severe seizure disorders accompanied by mental retardation, and those with organic brain disease).
No products indexed under this heading.

Ethyl Alcohol (Since valproate products may produce CNS depression, especially when combined with another CNS depressant (eg, alcohol), patients should be advised not to engage in hazardous activities, such as driving an automobile or operating dangerous machinery, until it is known that they do not become drowsy from the drug).
No products indexed under this heading.

Felbamate (A study involving the coadministration of 1200 mg/day of felbamate with valproate to patients with epilepsy (n=10) revealed an increase in mean valproate peak concentration by 35% (from 86 to 115 mcg/mL) compared to valproate alone. Increasing the felbamate dose to 2400 mg/day increased the mean valproate peak concentration to 133 mcg/mL (another 16% increase). A decrease in valproate dosage may be necessary when felbamate therapy is initiated).
No products indexed under this heading.

Fentanyl (Since valproate products may produce CNS depression, especially when combined with another CNS depressant (eg, alcohol), patients should be advised not to engage in hazardous activities, such as driving an automobile or operating dangerous machinery, until it is known that they do not become drowsy from the drug). Products include:
Duragesic 2604
Fentanyl Transdermal System 2346
Onsolis 2054

Fentanyl Citrate (Since valproate products may produce CNS depression, especially when combined with another CNS depressant (eg, alcohol), patients should be advised not to engage in hazardous activities, such as driving an automobile or operating dangerous machinery, until it is known that they do not become drowsy from the drug). Products include:
Fentora 966

Fluphenazine Decanoate (Since valproate products may produce CNS depression, especially when combined with another CNS depressant (eg, alcohol), patients should be advised not to engage in hazardous activities, such as driving an automobile or operating dangerous machinery, until it is known that they do not become drowsy from the drug).
No products indexed under this heading.

Fluphenazine Enanthate (Since valproate products may produce CNS depression, especially when combined with another CNS depressant (eg, alcohol), patients should be advised not to engage in hazardous activities, such as driving an automobile or operating dangerous machinery, until it is known that they do not become drowsy from the drug).
No products indexed under this heading.

Fluphenazine Hydrochloride (Since valproate products may produce CNS depression, especially when combined with another CNS depressant (eg, alcohol), patients should be advised not to engage in hazardous activities, such as driving an automobile or operating dangerous machinery, until it is known that they do not become drowsy from the drug).
No products indexed under this heading.

Flurazepam Hydrochloride (Since valproate products may produce CNS depression, especially when combined with another CNS depressant (eg, alcohol), patients should be advised not to engage in hazardous activities, such as driving an automobile or operating dangerous machinery, until it is known that they do not become drowsy from the drug).
No products indexed under this heading.

Fosphenytoin (Co-administration with drugs that affect the levels of expression of hepatic enzymes, particularly those that elevate levels of glucuronosyltransferases, such as phenytoin, may increase the clearance of valproate. Valproate displaces phenytoin from its plasma binding sites and inhibits its hepatic metabolism. Concurrent use has resulted in breakthrough seizures. The dosage of phenytoin should be adjusted as required by the clinical situation).
No products indexed under this heading.

Fosphenytoin Sodium (Co-administration with drugs that affect the levels of expression of hepatic enzymes, particularly those that elevate levels of glucuronosyltransferases, such as phenytoin, may increase the clearance of valproate. Valproate displaces phenytoin from its plasma binding sites and inhibits its hepatic metabolism. Concurrent use has resulted in breakthrough seizures. The dosage of phenytoin should be adjusted as required by the clinical situation).
No products indexed under this heading.

Gabapentin (Hepatic failure resulting in fatalities has occurred in patients receiving valproic acid and its derivatives. Children under the age of two years are at a considerably increased risk of developing fatal hepatotoxicity, especially those on multiple anticonvulsants, those with congenital metabolic disorders, those with severe seizure disorders accompanied by mental retardation, and those with organic brain disease).
No products indexed under this heading.

Glutethimide (Since valproate products may produce CNS depression, especially when combined with another CNS depressant (eg, alcohol), patients should be advised not to engage in hazardous activities, such as driving an automobile or operating dangerous machinery, until it is known that they do not become drowsy from the drug).
No products indexed under this heading.

Halazepam (Since valproate products may produce CNS depression, especially when combined with another CNS depressant (eg, alcohol), patients should be advised not to engage in hazardous activities, such as driving an automobile or operating dangerous machinery, until it is known that they do not become drowsy from the drug).
No products indexed under this heading.

Haloperidol (Since valproate products may produce CNS depression, especially when combined with another CNS depressant (eg, alcohol), patients should be advised not to engage in hazardous activities, such as driving an automobile or operating dangerous machinery, until it is known that they do not become drowsy from the drug).
No products indexed under this heading.

Haloperidol Decanoate (Since valproate products may produce CNS depression, especially when combined with another CNS depressant (eg, alcohol), patients should be advised not to engage in hazardous activities, such as driving an automobile or operating dangerous machinery, until it is known that they do not become drowsy from the drug).
No products indexed under this heading.

Haloperidol Lactate (Since valproate products may produce CNS depression, especially when combined with another CNS depressant (eg, alcohol), patients should be advised not to engage in hazardous activities, such as driving an automobile or operating dangerous machinery, until it is known that they do not become drowsy from the drug).
No products indexed under this heading.

Hexobarbital (Since valproate products may produce CNS depression, especially when combined with another CNS depressant (eg, alcohol), patients should be advised not to engage in hazardous activities, such as driving an automobile or operating dangerous machinery, until it is known that they do not become drowsy from the drug).
No products indexed under this heading.

Hydrocodone Bitartrate (Since valproate products may produce CNS depression, especially when combined with another CNS depressant (eg, alcohol), patients should be advised not to engage in hazardous activities, such as driving an automobile or operating dangerous machinery, until it is known that they do not become drowsy from the drug). Products include:
Vicodin 560
Vicodin ES 561
Vicodin HP 563
Vicoprofen 564
Zydone 1138

Hydrocodone Polistirex (Since valproate products may produce CNS depression, especially when combined with another CNS depressant (eg, alcohol), patients should be advised not to engage in hazardous activities, such as driving an automobile or operating dangerous machinery, until it is known that they do not become drowsy from the drug). Products include:
Tussionex 3443

Hydromorphone (Since valproate products may produce CNS depression, especially when combined with another CNS depressant (eg, alcohol), patients should be advised not to engage in hazardous activities, such as driving an automobile or operating dangerous machinery, until it is known that they do not become drowsy from the drug).
No products indexed under this heading.

Hydromorphone Hydrochloride (Since valproate products may produce CNS depression, especially when combined with another CNS depressant (eg, alcohol), patients should be advised not to engage in hazardous activities, such as driving an automobile or operating dangerous machinery, until it is known that they do not become drowsy from the drug). Products include:
Dilaudid Injection 2800
Dilaudid Oral 2797
Dilaudid Tablets 2797
Dilaudid-HP 2800

Hydroxyzine Hydrochloride (Since valproate products may produce CNS depression, especially when combined with another CNS depressant (eg, alcohol), patients should be advised not to engage in hazardous activities, such as driving an automobile or operating dangerous machinery, until it is known that they do not become drowsy from the drug).
No products indexed under this heading.

Imipenem (Co-administration of valproic acid with carbapenem antibiotics (ertapenem, imipenem, meropenem) has lead to a clinically significant reduction in serum valproic acid concentration and may result in loss of seizure control. The mechanism of this interaction is not well understood. Serum valproic acid concentrations should be monitored frequently after initiating carbapenem therapy. Alternative antibacterial or anticonvulsant therapy should be considered if serum valproic acid concentrations drop significantly or seizure control deteriorates). Products include:
Primaxin I.M. 2232
Primaxin I.V. 2235

Isoflurane (Since valproate products may produce CNS depression, especially when combined with another CNS depressant (eg, alcohol), patients should be advised not to engage in hazardous activities, such as driving an automobile or operating dangerous machinery, until it is known that they do not become drowsy from the drug).
No products indexed under this heading.

IMPORTANT NOTE: Always consult each drug listing in the patient's regimen for possible interactions.

Ketamine Hydrochloride (Since valproate products may produce CNS depression, especially when combined with another CNS depressant (eg, alcohol), patients should be advised not to engage in hazardous activities, such as driving an automobile or operating dangerous machinery, until it is known that they do not become drowsy from the drug).
No products indexed under this heading.

Lamotrigine (In a steady-state study involving 10 healthy volunteers, the elimination half-life of lamotrigine increased from 26 to 70 hours with valproate co-administration (a 165% increase). The dose of lamotrigine should be reduced when co-administered with valproate. Serious skin reactions (such as Stevens - Johnson syndrome and toxic epidermal necrolysis) have been reported with concomitant lamotrigine and valproate administration). Products include:
Lamictal **1522**
Lamictal ODT **1522**
Lamictal XR **1536**

Levetiracetam (Hepatic failure resulting in fatalities has occurred in patients receiving valproic acid and its derivatives. Children under the age of two years are at a considerably increased risk of developing fatal hepatotoxicity, especially those on multiple anticonvulsants, those with congenital metabolic disorders, those with severe seizure disorders accompanied by mental retardation, and those with organic brain disease). Products include:
Keppra XR **3434**

Levomethadyl Acetate Hydrochloride (Since valproate products may produce CNS depression, especially when combined with another CNS depressant (eg, alcohol), patients should be advised not to engage in hazardous activities, such as driving an automobile or operating dangerous machinery, until it is known that they do not become drowsy from the drug).
No products indexed under this heading.

Levorphanol Tartrate (Since valproate products may produce CNS depression, especially when combined with another CNS depressant (eg, alcohol), patients should be advised not to engage in hazardous activities, such as driving an automobile or operating dangerous machinery, until it is known that they do not become drowsy from the drug).
No products indexed under this heading.

Lorazepam (Co-administration was accompanied by a 17% decrease in the plasma clearance of lorazepam).
No products indexed under this heading.

Loxapine Hydrochloride (Since valproate products may produce CNS depression, especially when combined with another CNS depressant (eg, alcohol), patients should be advised not to engage in hazardous activities, such as driving an automobile or operating dangerous machinery, until it is known that they do not become drowsy from the drug).
No products indexed under this heading.

Loxapine Succinate (Since valproate products may produce CNS depression, especially when combined with another CNS depressant (eg, alcohol), patients should be advised not to engage in hazardous activities, such as driving an automobile or operating dangerous machinery, until it is known that they do not become drowsy from the drug).
No products indexed under this heading.

Meperidine Hydrochloride (Since valproate products may produce CNS depression, especially when combined with another CNS depressant (eg, alcohol), patients should be advised not to engage in hazardous activities, such as driving an automobile or operating dangerous machinery, until it is known that they do not become drowsy from the drug).
No products indexed under this heading.

Mephenytoin (Hepatic failure resulting in fatalities has occurred in patients receiving valproic acid and its derivatives. Children under the age of two years are at a considerably increased risk of developing fatal hepatotoxicity, especially those on multiple anticonvulsants, those with congenital metabolic disorders, those with severe seizure disorders accompanied by mental retardation, and those with organic brain disease).
No products indexed under this heading.

Mephobarbital (Since valproate products may produce CNS depression, especially when combined with another CNS depressant (eg, alcohol), patients should be advised not to engage in hazardous activities, such as driving an automobile or operating dangerous machinery, until it is known that they do not become drowsy from the drug).
No products indexed under this heading.

Meprobamate (Since valproate products may produce CNS depression, especially when combined with another CNS depressant (eg, alcohol), patients should be advised not to engage in hazardous activities, such as driving an automobile or operating dangerous machinery, until it is known that they do not become drowsy from the drug).
No products indexed under this heading.

Meropenem (Co-administration of valproic acid with carbapenem antibiotics (ertapenem, imipenem, meropenem) has lead to a clinically significant reduction in serum valproic acid concentration and may result in loss of seizure control. The mechanism of this interaction is not well understood. Serum valproic acid concentrations should be monitored frequently after initiating carbapenem therapy. Alternative antibacterial or anticonvulsant therapy should be considered if serum valproic acid concentrations drop significantly or seizure control deteriorates). Products include:
Merrem I.V. **745**

Mesoridazine Besylate (Since valproate products may produce CNS depression, especially when combined with another CNS depressant (eg, alcohol), patients should be advised not to engage in hazardous activities, such as driving an automobile or operating dangerous machinery, until it is known that they do not become drowsy from the drug).
No products indexed under this heading.

Methadone Hydrochloride (Since valproate products may produce CNS depression, especially when combined with another CNS depressant (eg, alcohol), patients should be advised not to engage in hazardous activities, such as driving an automobile or operating dangerous machinery, until it is known that they do not become drowsy from the drug).
No products indexed under this heading.

Methohexital Sodium (Since valproate products may produce CNS depression, especially when combined with another CNS depressant (eg, alcohol), patients should be advised not to engage in hazardous activities, such as driving an automobile or operating dangerous machinery, until it is known that they do not become drowsy from the drug).
No products indexed under this heading.

Methotrimeprazine (Since valproate products may produce CNS depression, especially when combined with another CNS depressant (eg, alcohol), patients should be advised not to engage in hazardous activities, such as driving an automobile or operating dangerous machinery, until it is known that they do not become drowsy from the drug).
No products indexed under this heading.

Methoxyflurane (Since valproate products may produce CNS depression, especially when combined with another CNS depressant (eg, alcohol), patients should be advised not to engage in hazardous activities, such as driving an automobile or operating dangerous machinery, until it is known that they do not become drowsy from the drug).
No products indexed under this heading.

Methsuximide (Hepatic failure resulting in fatalities has occurred in patients receiving valproic acid and its derivatives. Children under the age of two years are at a considerably increased risk of developing fatal hepatotoxicity, especially those on multiple anticonvulsants, those with congenital metabolic disorders, those with severe seizure disorders accompanied by mental retardation, and those with organic brain disease).
No products indexed under this heading.

Midazolam Hydrochloride (Since valproate products may produce CNS depression, especially when combined with another CNS depressant (eg, alcohol), patients should be advised not to engage in hazardous activities, such as driving an automobile or operating dangerous machinery, until it is known that they do not become drowsy from the drug).
No products indexed under this heading.

Molindone Hydrochloride (Since valproate products may produce CNS depression, especially when combined with another CNS depressant (eg, alcohol), patients should be advised not to engage in hazardous activities, such as driving an automobile or operating dangerous machinery, until it is known that they do not become drowsy from the drug). Products include:
Moban **1108**

Morphine Sulfate (Since valproate products may produce CNS depression, especially when combined with another CNS depressant (eg, alcohol), patients should be advised not to engage in hazardous activities, such as driving an automobile or operating dangerous machinery, until it is known that they do not become drowsy from the drug). Products include:
Avinza **1822**
Embeda **1831**
MS Contin **2803**

Morphine Sulfate, Liposomal (Since valproate products may produce CNS depression, especially when combined with another CNS depressant (eg, alcohol), patients should be advised not to engage in hazardous activities, such as driving an automobile or operating dangerous machinery, until it is known that they do not become drowsy from the drug).
No products indexed under this heading.

Nortriptyline Hydrochloride (Administration of a single oral 50 mg dose of amitriptyline to 15 normal volunteers (10 males and 5 females) who received valproate (500 mg BID) resulted in a 21% decrease in plasma clearance of amitriptyline and a 34% decrease in the net clearance of nortriptyline).
No products indexed under this heading.

Olanzapine (Since valproate products may produce CNS depression, especially when combined with another CNS depressant (eg, alcohol), patients should be advised not to engage in hazardous activities, such as driving an automobile or operating dangerous machinery, until it is known that they do not become drowsy from the drug). Products include:
Symbyax **1965**
Zyprexa **1984**
Zyprexa IntraMuscular **1984**
Zyprexa ZYDIS **1984**

Oxazepam (Since valproate products may produce CNS depression, especially when combined with another CNS depressant (eg, alcohol), patients should be advised not to engage in hazardous activities, such as driving an automobile or operating dangerous machinery, until it is known that they do not become drowsy from the drug).
No products indexed under this heading.

Oxcarbazepine (Hepatic failure resulting in fatalities has occurred in patients receiving valproic acid and its derivatives. Children under the age of two years are at a considerably increased risk of developing fatal hepatotoxicity, especially those on multiple anticonvulsants, those with congenital metabolic disorders, those with severe seizure disorders accompanied by mental retardation, and those with organic brain disease).
No products indexed under this heading.

Oxycodone Hydrochloride (Since valproate products may produce CNS depression, especially when combined with another CNS depressant (eg, alcohol), patients should be advised not to engage in hazardous activities, such as driving an automobile or operating dangerous machinery, until it is known that they do not become drowsy from the drug). Products include:
OxyContin **2807**
Percocet **1121**
Percodan **1124**

Oxycodone Terephthalate (Since valproate products may produce CNS depression, especially when combined with another CNS depressant (eg, alcohol), patients should be advised not to engage in hazardous activities, such as driving an automobile or operating dangerous machinery, until it is known that they do not become drowsy from the drug).
No products indexed under this heading.

Oxymorphone Hydrochloride (Since valproate products may produce CNS depression, especially when combined with another CNS depressant (eg, alcohol), patients should be advised not to engage in hazardous activities, such as driving an automobile or operating dangerous machinery, until it is known that they do not become drowsy from the drug). Products include:
Opana **1110**
Opana ER **1114**

Paramethadione (Hepatic failure resulting in fatalities has occurred in patients receiving valproic acid and its derivatives. Children under the age of two years are at a considerably increased risk of developing fatal hepatotoxicity, especially those on multiple anticonvulsants, those with congenital metabolic disorders, those with severe

457 **Interactions Index** **Depakote**

seizure disorders accompanied by mental retardation, and those with organic brain disease).
No products indexed under this heading.

Pentobarbital (Since valproate products may produce CNS depression, especially when combined with another CNS depressant (eg, alcohol), patients should be advised not to engage in hazardous activities, such as driving an automobile or operating dangerous machinery, until it is known that they do not become drowsy from the drug).
No products indexed under this heading.

Pentobarbital Sodium (Since valproate products may produce CNS depression, especially when combined with another CNS depressant (eg, alcohol), patients should be advised not to engage in hazardous activities, such as driving an automobile or operating dangerous machinery, until it is known that they do not become drowsy from the drug). Products include:
Nembutal 2012

Perphenazine (Since valproate products may produce CNS depression, especially when combined with another CNS depressant (eg, alcohol), patients should be advised not to engage in hazardous activities, such as driving an automobile or operating dangerous machinery, until it is known that they do not become drowsy from the drug).
No products indexed under this heading.

Phenacemide (Hepatic failure resulting in fatalities has occurred in patients receiving valproic acid and its derivatives. Children under the age of two years are at a considerably increased risk of developing fatal hepatotoxicity, especially those on multiple anticonvulsants, those with congenital metabolic disorders, those with severe seizure disorders accompanied by mental retardation, and those with organic brain disease).
No products indexed under this heading.

Phenobarbital (Co-administration with drugs that affect the levels of expression of hepatic enzymes, particularly those that elevate levels of glucuronosyltransferases, such as phenobarbital, may increase the clearance of valproate. Valproate inhibits the metabolism of phenobarbital. Co-administration has resulted in an increase in half-life and a decrease in plasma clearance of phenobarbital; all patients should be monitored for neurological toxicity because of severe CNS depression). Products include:
Donnatal 2711

Phenobarbital Sodium (Co-administration with drugs that affect the levels of expression of hepatic enzymes, particularly those that elevate levels of glucuronosyltransferases, such as phenobarbital, may increase the clearance of valproate. Valproate inhibits the metabolism of phenobarbital. Co-administration has resulted in an increase in half-life and a decrease in plasma clearance of phenobarbital. All patients should be monitored for neurological toxicity because of severe CNS depression).
No products indexed under this heading.

Phensuximide (Hepatic failure resulting in fatalities has occurred in patients receiving valproic acid and its derivatives. Children under the age of two years are at a considerably increased risk of developing fatal hepatotoxicity, especially those on multiple anticonvulsants, those with congenital metabolic disorders, those with severe seizure disorders accompanied by mental retardation, and those with organic brain disease).
No products indexed under this heading.

Phenytoin (Co-administration with drugs that affect the levels of expression of hepatic enzymes, particularly those that elevate levels of glucuronosyltransferases, such as phenytoin, may increase the clearance of valproate. Valproate displaces phenytoin from its plasma binding sites and inhibits its hepatic metabolism. Concurrent use has resulted in breakthrough seizures. The dosage of phenytoin should be adjusted as required by the clinical situation).
No products indexed under this heading.

Phenytoin Sodium (Co-administration with drugs that affect the levels of expression of hepatic enzymes, particularly those that elevate levels of glucuronosyltransferases, such as phenytoin, may increase the clearance of valproate. Valproate displaces phenytoin from its plasma binding sites and inhibits its hepatic metabolism. Concurrent use has resulted in breakthrough seizures. The dosage of phenytoin should be adjusted as required by the clinical situation). Products include:
Phenytek Capsules 2380

Prazepam (Since valproate products may produce CNS depression, especially when combined with another CNS depressant (eg, alcohol), patients should be advised not to engage in hazardous activities, such as driving an automobile or operating dangerous machinery, until it is known that they do not become drowsy from the drug).
No products indexed under this heading.

Primidone (Drugs that affect the level of expression of hepatic enzymes, particularly those that elevate levels of glucuronosyltransferases, such as phenobarbital (or primidone) may increase the clearance of valproate. Phenobarbital (or primidone) can double the clearance of valproate. Thus, patients on monotherapy will generally have longer half-lives and higher concentrations than patients receiving polytherapy with antiepilepsy drugs. Primidone, which is metabolized to a barbiturate, may be involved in a similar interaction with valproate).
No products indexed under this heading.

Prochlorperazine (Since valproate products may produce CNS depression, especially when combined with another CNS depressant (eg, alcohol), patients should be advised not to engage in hazardous activities, such as driving an automobile or operating dangerous machinery, until it is known that they do not become drowsy from the drug).
No products indexed under this heading.

Prochlorperazine Edisylate (Since valproate products may produce CNS depression, especially when combined with another CNS depressant (eg, alcohol), patients should be advised not to engage in hazardous activities, such as driving an automobile or operating dangerous machinery, until it is known that they do not become drowsy from the drug).
No products indexed under this heading.

Prochlorperazine Maleate (Since valproate products may produce CNS depression, especially when combined with another CNS depressant (eg, alcohol), patients should be advised not to engage in hazardous activities, such as driving an automobile or operating dangerous machinery, until it is known that they do not become drowsy from the drug).
No products indexed under this heading.

Promethazine (Since valproate products may produce CNS depression, especially when combined with another CNS depressant (eg, alcohol), patients should be advised not to engage in hazardous activities, such as driving an automobile or operating dangerous machinery, until it is known that they do not become drowsy from the drug).
No products indexed under this heading.

Promethazine Hydrochloride (Since valproate products may produce CNS depression, especially when combined with another CNS depressant (eg, alcohol), patients should be advised not to engage in hazardous activities, such as driving an automobile or operating dangerous machinery, until it is known that they do not become drowsy from the drug).
No products indexed under this heading.

Propofol (Since valproate products may produce CNS depression, especially when combined with another CNS depressant (eg, alcohol), patients should be advised not to engage in hazardous activities, such as driving an automobile or operating dangerous machinery, until it is known that they do not become drowsy from the drug).
No products indexed under this heading.

Propoxyphene Hydrochloride (Since valproate products may produce CNS depression, especially when combined with another CNS depressant (eg, alcohol), patients should be advised not to engage in hazardous activities, such as driving an automobile or operating dangerous machinery, until it is known that they do not become drowsy from the drug).
No products indexed under this heading.

Propoxyphene Napsylate (Since valproate products may produce CNS depression, especially when combined with another CNS depressant (eg, alcohol), patients should be advised not to engage in hazardous activities, such as driving an automobile or operating dangerous machinery, until it is known that they do not become drowsy from the drug).
No products indexed under this heading.

Quazepam (Since valproate products may produce CNS depression, especially when combined with another CNS depressant (eg, alcohol), patients should be advised not to engage in hazardous activities, such as driving an automobile or operating dangerous machinery, until it is known that they do not become drowsy from the drug).
No products indexed under this heading.

Quetiapine Fumarate (Since valproate products may produce CNS depression, especially when combined with another CNS depressant (eg, alcohol), patients should be advised not to engage in hazardous activities, such as driving an automobile or operating dangerous machinery, until it is known that they do not become drowsy from the drug). Products include:
Seroquel 750
Seroquel XR 759

Remifentanil Hydrochloride (Since valproate products may produce CNS depression, especially when combined with another CNS depressant (eg, alcohol), patients should be advised not to engage in hazardous activities, such as driving an automobile or operating dangerous machinery, until it is known that they do not become drowsy from the drug).
No products indexed under this heading.

Rifampin (A study involving the administration of a single dose of valproate (7 mg/kg) 36 hours after 5 nights of daily dosing with rifampin (600 mg) revealed a 40% increase in the oral clearance of valproate. Valproate dosage adjustment may be necessary when it is co-administered with rifampin).
No products indexed under this heading.

Risperidone (Since valproate products may produce CNS depression, especially when combined with another CNS depressant (eg, alcohol), patients should be advised not to engage in hazardous activities, such as driving an automobile or operating dangerous machinery, until it is known that they do not become drowsy from the drug). Products include:
Risperdal Consta 2682

Rufinamide (Hepatic failure resulting in fatalities has occurred in patients receiving valproic acid and its derivatives. Children under the age of two years are at a considerably increased risk of developing fatal hepatotoxicity, especially those on multiple anticonvulsants, those with congenital metabolic disorders, those with severe seizure disorders accompanied by mental retardation, and those with organic brain disease). Products include:
Banzel 1050

Secobarbital Sodium (Since valproate products may produce CNS depression, especially when combined with another CNS depressant (eg, alcohol), patients should be advised not to engage in hazardous activities, such as driving an automobile or operating dangerous machinery, until it is known that they do not become drowsy from the drug).
No products indexed under this heading.

Sevoflurane (Since valproate products may produce CNS depression, especially when combined with another CNS depressant (eg, alcohol), patients should be advised not to engage in hazardous activities, such as driving an automobile or operating dangerous machinery, until it is known that they do not become drowsy from the drug). Products include:
Ultane 554

Sodium Butabarbital (Since valproate products may produce CNS depression, especially when combined with another CNS depressant (eg, alcohol), patients should be advised not to engage in hazardous activities, such as driving an automobile or operating dangerous machinery, until it is known that they do not become drowsy from the drug).
No products indexed under this heading.

Sodium Oxybate (Since valproate products may produce CNS depression, especially when combined with another CNS depressant (eg, alcohol), patients should be advised not to engage in hazardous activities, such as driving an automobile or operating dangerous machinery, until it is known that they do not become drowsy from the drug).
No products indexed under this heading.

Sodium Pentobarbital (Since valproate products may produce CNS depression, especially when combined with another CNS depressant (eg, alcohol), patients should be advised not to engage in hazardous activities, such as driving an automobile or operating dangerous machinery, until it is known that they do not become drowsy from the drug).
No products indexed under this heading.

IMPORTANT NOTE: Always consult each drug listing in the patient's regimen for possible interactions.

Sufentanil Citrate (Since valproate products may produce CNS depression, especially when combined with another CNS depressant (eg, alcohol), patients should be advised not to engage in hazardous activities, such as driving an automobile or operating dangerous machinery, until it is known that they do not become drowsy from the drug).
No products indexed under this heading.

Talbutal (Since valproate products may produce CNS depression, especially when combined with another CNS depressant (eg, alcohol), patients should be advised not to engage in hazardous activities, such as driving an automobile or operating dangerous machinery, until it is known that they do not become drowsy from the drug).
No products indexed under this heading.

Temazepam (Since valproate products may produce CNS depression, especially when combined with another CNS depressant (eg, alcohol), patients should be advised not to engage in hazardous activities, such as driving an automobile or operating dangerous machinery, until it is known that they do not become drowsy from the drug).
No products indexed under this heading.

Thiamylal Sodium (Since valproate products may produce CNS depression, especially when combined with another CNS depressant (eg, alcohol), patients should be advised not to engage in hazardous activities, such as driving an automobile or operating dangerous machinery, until it is known that they do not become drowsy from the drug).
No products indexed under this heading.

Thioridazine (Since valproate products may produce CNS depression, especially when combined with another CNS depressant (eg, alcohol), patients should be advised not to engage in hazardous activities, such as driving an automobile or operating dangerous machinery, until it is known that they do not become drowsy from the drug).
No products indexed under this heading.

Thioridazine Hydrochloride (Since valproate products may produce CNS depression, especially when combined with another CNS depressant (eg, alcohol), patients should be advised not to engage in hazardous activities, such as driving an automobile or operating dangerous machinery, until it is known that they do not become drowsy from the drug). Products include:
Thioridazine Hydrochloride 2384

Thiothixene (Since valproate products may produce CNS depression, especially when combined with another CNS depressant (eg, alcohol), patients should be advised not to engage in hazardous activities, such as driving an automobile or operating dangerous machinery, until it is known that they do not become drowsy from the drug). Products include:
Thiothixene 2386

Thiothixene Hydrochloride (Since valproate products may produce CNS depression, especially when combined with another CNS depressant (eg, alcohol), patients should be advised not to engage in hazardous activities, such as driving an automobile or operating dangerous machinery, until it is known that they do not become drowsy from the drug).
No products indexed under this heading.

Tiagabine Hydrochloride (Hepatic failure resulting in fatalities has occurred in patients receiving valproic acid and its derivatives. Children under the age of two years are at a considerably increased risk of developing fatal hepatotoxicity, especially those on multiple anticonvulsants, those with congenital metabolic disorders, those with

severe seizure disorders accompanied by mental retardation, and those with organic brain disease). Products include:
Gabitril 972

Tolbutamide (Co-administration in *in vitro* experiments has resulted in increased unbound fraction of tolbutamide).
No products indexed under this heading.

Topiramate (Concomitant administration of topiramate and valproic acid has been associated with hyperammonemia and hypothermia with or without encephalopathy in patients who have tolerated either drug alone. It may be prudent to examine blood ammonia levels in patients in whom the onset of hypothermia has been reported).
No products indexed under this heading.

Triazolam (Since valproate products may produce CNS depression, especially when combined with another CNS depressant (eg, alcohol), patients should be advised not to engage in hazardous activities, such as driving an automobile or operating dangerous machinery, until it is known that they do not become drowsy from the drug).
No products indexed under this heading.

Trifluoperazine Hydrochloride (Since valproate products may produce CNS depression, especially when combined with another CNS depressant (eg, alcohol), patients should be advised not to engage in hazardous activities, such as driving an automobile or operating dangerous machinery, until it is known that they do not become drowsy from the drug).
No products indexed under this heading.

Trimethadione (Hepatic failure resulting in fatalities has occurred in patients receiving valproic acid and its derivatives. Children under the age of two years are at a considerably increased risk of developing fatal hepatotoxicity, especially those on multiple anticonvulsants, those with congenital metabolic disorders, those with severe seizure disorders accompanied by mental retardation, and those with organic brain disease).
No products indexed under this heading.

Valproate Sodium (Hepatic failure resulting in fatalities has occurred in patients receiving valproic acid and its derivatives. Children under the age of two years are at a considerably increased risk of developing fatal hepatotoxicity, especially those on multiple anticonvulsants, those with congenital metabolic disorders, those with severe seizure disorders accompanied by mental retardation, and those with organic brain disease).
No products indexed under this heading.

Valproic Acid (Hepatic failure resulting in fatalities has occurred in patients receiving valproic acid and its derivatives. Children under the age of two years are at a considerably increased risk of developing fatal hepatotoxicity, especially those on multiple anticonvulsants, those with congenital metabolic disorders, those with severe seizure disorders accompanied by mental retardation, and those with organic brain disease).
No products indexed under this heading.

Warfarin Sodium (In an *in vitro* study, valproate increased the unbound fraction of warfarin by up to 32.6%. The therapeutic relevance of this is unknown; however, coagulation tests should be monitored if valproic acid therapy is instituted in patients taking anticoagulants).
No products indexed under this heading.

Zaleplon (Since valproate products may produce CNS depression, especially when combined with another CNS depressant (eg, alcohol), patients should be advised not to engage in hazardous activities, such as driving an automobile or operating dangerous machinery, until it is known that they do not become drowsy from the drug).
No products indexed under this heading.

Zidovudine (In six patients who were seropositive for HIV, the clearance of zidovudine (100 mg q8h) was decreased by 38% after administration of valproate (250 or 500 mg q8h); the half-life of zidovudine was unaffected). Products include:
Combivir 1404
Retrovir 1634
Retrovir IV 1640
Trizivir 1688

Ziprasidone Hydrochloride (Since valproate products may produce CNS depression, especially when combined with another CNS depressant (eg, alcohol), patients should be advised not to engage in hazardous activities, such as driving an automobile or operating dangerous machinery, until it is known that they do not become drowsy from the drug). Products include:
Geodon 2723

Zolpidem Tartrate (Since valproate products may produce CNS depression, especially when combined with another CNS depressant (eg, alcohol), patients should be advised not to engage in hazardous activities, such as driving an automobile or operating dangerous machinery, until it is known that they do not become drowsy from the drug). Products include:
Ambien 2920
Ambien CR 2925

Zonisamide (Hepatic failure resulting in fatalities has occurred in patients receiving valproic acid and its derivatives. Children under the age of two years are at a considerably increased risk of developing fatal hepatotoxicity, especially those on multiple anticonvulsants, those with congenital metabolic disorders, those with severe seizure disorders accompanied by mental retardation, and those with organic brain disease). Products include:
Zonegran 1081

Food Interactions

Alcohol (Since valproate products may produce CNS depression, especially when combined with another CNS depressant (eg, alcohol), patients should be advised not to engage in hazardous activities, such as driving an automobile or operating dangerous machinery, until it is known that they do not become drowsy from the drug).

Beer, reduced-alcohol (Since valproate products may produce CNS depression, especially when combined with another CNS depressant (eg, alcohol), patients should be advised not to engage in hazardous activities, such as driving an automobile or operating dangerous machinery, until it is known that they do not become drowsy from the drug).

Beer, unspecified (Since valproate products may produce CNS depression, especially when combined with another CNS depressant (eg, alcohol), patients should be advised not to engage in hazardous activities, such as driving an automobile or operating dangerous machinery, until it is known that they do not become drowsy from the drug).

Wine, Chianti (Since valproate products may produce CNS depression, especially when combined with another CNS depressant (eg, alcohol), patients

should be advised not to engage in hazardous activities, such as driving an automobile or operating dangerous machinery, until it is known that they do not become drowsy from the drug).

Wine, Red (Since valproate products may produce CNS depression, especially when combined with another CNS depressant (eg, alcohol), patients should be advised not to engage in hazardous activities, such as driving an automobile or operating dangerous machinery, until it is known that they do not become drowsy from the drug).

Wine, unspecified (Since valproate products may produce CNS depression, especially when combined with another CNS depressant (eg, alcohol), patients should be advised not to engage in hazardous activities, such as driving an automobile or operating dangerous machinery, until it is known that they do not become drowsy from the drug).

Wine products (Since valproate products may produce CNS depression, especially when combined with another CNS depressant (eg, alcohol), patients should be advised not to engage in hazardous activities, such as driving an automobile or operating dangerous machinery, until it is known that they do not become drowsy from the drug).

DEXEDRINE SPANSULE SUSTAINED-RELEASE CAPSULES

(Dextroamphetamine Sulfate) 1425
May interact with alpha adrenergic blockers, antihistamines, antihypertensives, beta-blockers, monoamine oxidase inhibitors, peripheral adrenergic blockers, phenytoin, sympathomimetics, thiazides, tricyclic antidepressants, urinary alkalinizing agents, veratrum alkaloids, and certain other agents. Compounds in these categories include:

Acebutolol Hydrochloride (Adrenergic blockers are inhibited by amphetamines; amphetamines may antagonize the hypotensive effects of antihypertensives).
No products indexed under this heading.

Acetazolamide (Urinary alkalinizing agents (eg, acetazolamide) increase the concentration of the non-ionized species of the amphetamine molecule, thereby decreasing urinary excretion. Urinary alkalinizing agents increase blood levels and, therefore, potentiate the actions of amphetamines).
No products indexed under this heading.

Acetazolamide Sodium (Urinary alkalinizing agents (eg, acetazolamide) increase the concentration of the non-ionized species of the amphetamine molecule, thereby decreasing urinary excretion. Urinary alkalinizing agents increase blood levels and, therefore, potentiate the actions of amphetamines).
No products indexed under this heading.

Acrivastine (Amphetamines may counteract the sedative effects of antihistamines).
No products indexed under this heading.

Albuterol (Amphetamines may enhance the activity of sympathomimetic agents).
No products indexed under this heading.

Albuterol Sulfate (Amphetamines may enhance the activity of sympathomimetic agents). Products include:
ProAir HFA 3393
Proventil HFA 3204
Ventolin HFA 1708

Alfuzosin Hydrochloride (Adrenergic blockers are inhibited by amphetamines). Products include:
Uroxatral 3050

(☉ Described in PDR® for Ophthalmic Medicines)

IMPORTANT NOTE: Always consult each drug listing in the patient's regimen for possible interactions.

Dexedrine Interactions Index 460

Fosphenytoin Sodium (Amphetamines may delay intestinal absorption of phenytoin; co-administration of phenytoin may produce a synergistic anticonvulsant).
No products indexed under this heading.

Furazolidone (A metabolite of furazolidone slows amphetamine metabolism. This slowing potentiates amphetamines, increasing their effect on the release of norepinephrine and other monoamines from adrenergic nerve endings; this can cause headaches and other signs of hypertensive crisis).
No products indexed under this heading.

Furosemide (Amphetamines may antagonize the hypotensive effects of antihypertensives). Products include:
Furosemide 2354

Glutamic Acid Hydrochloride (Gastrointestinal acidifying agents (eg, glutamic acid hydrochloride) lower the absorption of amphetamines. Gastrointestinal acidifying agents lower blood levels and efficacy of amphetamines).
No products indexed under this heading.

Guanabenz Acetate (Amphetamines may antagonize the hypotensive effects of antihypertensives).
No products indexed under this heading.

Guanethidine (Gastrointestinal acidifying agents (eg, guanethidine) lower the absorption of amphetamines. Gastrointestinal acidifying agents lower blood levels and efficacy of amphetamines).
No products indexed under this heading.

Guanethidine Monosulfate (Gastrointestinal acidifying agents (eg, guanethidine) lower the absorption of amphetamines. Gastrointestinal acidifying agents lower blood levels and efficacy of amphetamines).
No products indexed under this heading.

Guanethidine Sulfate (Gastrointestinal acidifying agents (eg, guanethidine) lower the absorption of amphetamines. Gastrointestinal acidifying agents lower blood levels and efficacy of amphetamines).
No products indexed under this heading.

Haloperidol (Haloperidol blocks dopamine and norepinephrine reuptake, thus inhibiting the central effects of amphetamines).
No products indexed under this heading.

Haloperidol Decanoate (Haloperidol blocks dopamine and norepinephrine reuptake, thus inhibiting the central effects of amphetamines).
No products indexed under this heading.

Haloperidol Lactate (Haloperidol blocks dopamine and norepinephrine reuptake, thus inhibiting the central effects of amphetamines).
No products indexed under this heading.

Hydralazine Hydrochloride (Amphetamines may antagonize the hypotensive effects of antihypertensives).
No products indexed under this heading.

Hydrochlorothiazide (Urinary alkalinizing agents (eg, some thiazides) increase the concentration of the non-ionized species of the amphetamine molecule, thereby decreasing urinary excretion. Urinary alkalinizing agents increase blood levels and, therefore, potentiate the actions of amphetamines). Products include:
Atacand HCT 700
Avalide 2956
Benicar HCT 1017
Diovan HCT 2419
Dyazide 1429
Exforge HCT 2449
Hyzaar 2162
Hyzaar 100-12.5 2162
Micardis HCT 889
Prinzide 2246
Tekturna HCT 2541
Teveten HCT 541

Hydroflumethiazide (Urinary alkalinizing agents (eg, some thiazides) increase the concentration of the non-ionized species of the amphetamine molecule, thereby decreasing urinary excretion. Urinary alkalinizing agents increase blood levels and, therefore, potentiate the actions of amphetamines).
No products indexed under this heading.

Imipramine Hydrochloride (Amphetamines may enhance the activity of tricyclic agents; d-amphetamine with desipramine or protriptyline and possibly other tricyclics cause striking and sustained increases in the concentration of d-amphetamine in the brain; cardiovascular effects can be potentiated).
No products indexed under this heading.

Imipramine Pamoate (Amphetamines may enhance the activity of tricyclic agents; d-amphetamine with desipramine or protriptyline and possibly other tricyclics cause striking and sustained increases in the concentration of d-amphetamine in the brain; cardiovascular effects can be potentiated).
No products indexed under this heading.

Indapamide (Amphetamines may antagonize the hypotensive effects of antihypertensives). Products include:
Indapamide 2356

Irbesartan (Amphetamines may antagonize the hypotensive effects of antihypertensives). Products include:
Avalide 2956
Avapro 2962

Isocarboxazid (Dextroamphetamine sulfate is contraindicated during or within 14 days following the administration of monoamine oxidase inhibitor (MAOI). MAOI antidepressants slow amphetamine metabolism. This slowing potentiates amphetamines, increasing their effect on the release of norepinephrine and other monoamines from adrenergic nerve endings; this can cause headaches and other signs of hypertensive crisis. A variety of neurological toxic effects and malignant hyperpyrexia can occur, sometimes with fatal results). Products include:
Marplan 3481

Isoproterenol Hydrochloride (Amphetamines may enhance the activity of sympathomimetic agents).
No products indexed under this heading.

Isoproterenol Sulfate (Amphetamines may enhance the activity of sympathomimetic agents).
No products indexed under this heading.

Isradipine (Amphetamines may antagonize the hypotensive effects of antihypertensives). Products include:
DynaCirc CR 1432

Labetalol Hydrochloride (Adrenergic blockers are inhibited by amphetamines; amphetamines may antagonize the hypotensive effects of antihypertensives).
No products indexed under this heading.

Levalbuterol Hydrochloride (Amphetamines may enhance the activity of sympathomimetic agents).
No products indexed under this heading.

Levobetaxolol Hydrochloride (Adrenergic blockers are inhibited by amphetamines).
No products indexed under this heading.

Levobunolol Hydrochloride (Adrenergic blockers are inhibited by amphetamines; amphetamines may antagonize the hypotensive effects of antihypertensives).
No products indexed under this heading.

Lisinopril (Amphetamines may antagonize the hypotensive effects of antihypertensives). Products include:
Prinivil 2241
Prinzide 2246

Lithium Carbonate (The stimulatory effects of amphetamines may be inhibited by lithium carbonate).
No products indexed under this heading.

Loratadine (Amphetamines may counteract the sedative effects of antihistamines).
No products indexed under this heading.

Losartan Potassium (Amphetamines may antagonize the hypotensive effects of antihypertensives). Products include:
Cozaar 2106
Hyzaar 2162
Hyzaar 100-12.5 2162

Maprotiline Hydrochloride (Amphetamines may enhance the activity of tricyclic agents; d-amphetamine with desipramine or protriptyline and possibly other tricyclics cause striking and sustained increases in the concentration of d-amphetamine in the brain; cardiovascular effects can be potentiated).
No products indexed under this heading.

Mecamylamine Hydrochloride (Amphetamines may antagonize the hypotensive effects of antihypertensives).
No products indexed under this heading.

Meperidine Hydrochloride (Amphetamines potentiate the analgesic effect of meperidine).
No products indexed under this heading.

Metaproterenol Sulfate (Amphetamines may enhance the activity of sympathomimetic agents).
No products indexed under this heading.

Metaraminol Bitartrate (Amphetamines may enhance the activity of sympathomimetic agents).
No products indexed under this heading.

Methdilazine Hydrochloride (Amphetamines may counteract the sedative effects of antihistamines).
No products indexed under this heading.

Methenamine (Urinary excretion of amphetamines is increased and efficacy is reduced by acidifying agents used in methenamine therapy).
No products indexed under this heading.

Methenamine Hippurate (Urinary excretion of amphetamines is increased and efficacy is reduced by acidifying agents used in methenamine therapy).
No products indexed under this heading.

Methenamine Mandelate (Urinary excretion of amphetamines is increased and efficacy is reduced by acidifying agents used in methenamine therapy). Products include:
Uroqid-Acid 874

Methoxamine Hydrochloride (Amphetamines may enhance the activity of sympathomimetic agents).
No products indexed under this heading.

Methyclothiazide (Urinary alkalinizing agents (eg, some thiazides) increase the concentration of the non-ionized species of the amphetamine molecule, thereby decreasing urinary excretion. Urinary alkalinizing agents increase blood levels and, therefore, potentiate the actions of amphetamines).
No products indexed under this heading.

Methyldopa (Amphetamines may antagonize the hypotensive effects of antihypertensives).
No products indexed under this heading.

Methyldopate Hydrochloride (Amphetamines may antagonize the hypotensive effects of antihypertensives).
No products indexed under this heading.

Metipranolol (Adrenergic blockers are inhibited by amphetamines). Products include:
Optipranolol .... ⊙249

Metipranolol Hydrochloride (Adrenergic blockers are inhibited by amphetamines; amphetamines may antagonize the hypotensive effects of antihypertensives).
No products indexed under this heading.

Metolazone (Amphetamines may antagonize the hypotensive effects of antihypertensives).
No products indexed under this heading.

Metoprolol Succinate (Adrenergic blockers are inhibited by amphetamines; amphetamines may antagonize the hypotensive effects of antihypertensives). Products include:
Toprol XL 732

Metoprolol Tartrate (Adrenergic blockers are inhibited by amphetamines; amphetamines may antagonize the hypotensive effects of antihypertensives).
No products indexed under this heading.

Metyrosine (Amphetamines may antagonize the hypotensive effects of antihypertensives).
No products indexed under this heading.

Mibefradil Dihydrochloride (Amphetamines may antagonize the hypotensive effects of antihypertensives).
No products indexed under this heading.

Minoxidil (Amphetamines may antagonize the hypotensive effects of antihypertensives).
No products indexed under this heading.

Moclobemide (Dextroamphetamine sulfate is contraindicated during or within 14 days following the administration of monoamine oxidase inhibitor (MAOI). MAOI antidepressants slow amphetamine metabolism. This slowing potentiates amphetamines, increasing their effect on the release of norepinephrine and other monoamines from adrenergic nerve endings; this can cause headaches and other signs of hypertensive crisis. A variety of neurological toxic effects and malignant hyperpyrexia can occur, sometimes with fatal results).
No products indexed under this heading.

Moexipril Hydrochloride (Amphetamines may antagonize the hypotensive effects of antihypertensives).
No products indexed under this heading.

Nadolol (Adrenergic blockers are inhibited by amphetamines; amphetamines may antagonize the hypotensive effects of antihypertensives). Products include:
Nadolol 2359

Nebivolol (Adrenergic blockers are inhibited by amphetamines; amphetamines may antagonize the hypotensive effects of antihypertensives). Products include:
Bystolic 1147

Nicardipine Hydrochloride (Amphetamines may antagonize the hypotensive effects of antihypertensives).
No products indexed under this heading.

Nifedipine (Amphetamines may antagonize the hypotensive effects of antihypertensives).
No products indexed under this heading.

Nisoldipine (Amphetamines may antagonize the hypotensive effects of antihypertensives).
No products indexed under this heading.

Nitroglycerin (Amphetamines may antagonize the hypotensive effects of antihypertensives). Products include:
Nitro-Dur 3170
Nitrolingual 3266

Norepinephrine Bitartrate (Amphetamines enhance the adrenergic effects of norepinephrine).
No products indexed under this heading.

(⊙ Described in PDR® for Ophthalmic Medicines)

IMPORTANT NOTE: Always consult each drug listing in the patient's regimen for possible interactions.

mines; amphetamines may antagonize the hypotensive effects of antihypertensives). Products include:

Timolol Maleate (Adrenergic blockers are inhibited by amphetamines; amphetamines may antagonize the hypotensive effects of antihypertensives). Products include:

Torsemide (Amphetamines may antagonize the hypotensive effects of antihypertensives).

No products indexed under this heading.

Trandolapril (Amphetamines may antagonize the hypotensive effects of antihypertensives). Products include:

Tranylcypromine Sulfate (Dextroamphetamine sulfate is contraindicated during or within 14 days following the administration of monoamine oxidase inhibitor (MAOI). MAOI antidepressants slow amphetamine metabolism. This slowing potentiates amphetamines, increasing their effect on the release of norepinephrine and other monoamines from adrenergic nerve endings; this can cause headaches and other signs of hypertensive crisis. A variety of neurological toxic effects and malignant hyperpyrexia can occur, sometimes with fatal results). Products include:

Trimeprazine Tartrate (Amphetamines may counteract the sedative effects of antihistamines).

No products indexed under this heading.

Trimethaphan Camsylate (Amphetamines may antagonize the hypotensive effects of antihypertensives).

No products indexed under this heading.

Trimipramine Maleate (Amphetamines may enhance the activity of tricyclic agents; d-amphetamine with desipramine or protriptyline and possibly other tricyclics cause striking and sustained increases in the concentration of d-amphetamine in the brain; cardiovascular effects can be potentiated).

No products indexed under this heading.

Tripelennamine Hydrochloride (Amphetamines may counteract the sedative effects of antihistamines).

No products indexed under this heading.

Triprolidine Hydrochloride (Amphetamines may counteract the sedative effects of antihistamines).

No products indexed under this heading.

Valsartan (Amphetamines may antagonize the hypotensive effects of antihypertensives). Products include:

Verapamil Hydrochloride (Amphetamines may antagonize the hypotensive effects of antihypertensives). Products include:

Vitamin C (Gastrointestinal acidifying agents (eg, ascorbic acid) lower the absorption of amphetamines. Gastrointestinal acidifying agents lower blood levels and efficacy of amphetamines). Products include:

Food Interactions

Fruit juices, unspecified (Gastrointestinal acidifying agents (eg, fruit juices) lower the absorption of amphetamines. Gastrointestinal acidifying agents lower blood levels and efficacy of amphetamines).

DIBENZYLINE CAPSULES

(Phenoxybenzamine Hydrochloride) 3495
May interact with epinephrine-containing products, and certain other agents. Compounds in these categories include:

Alpha and Beta Adrenergic Stimulators (Phenoxybenzamine hydrochloride may interact with compounds that stimulate both alpha- and beta-adrenergic receptors to produce an exaggerated hypotensive response and tachycardia).

No products indexed under this heading.

Epinephrine (Phenoxybenzamine hydrochloride may interact with compounds that stimulate both alpha- and beta-adrenergic receptors (eg, epinephrine) to produce an exaggerated hypotensive response and tachycardia). Products include:

Epinephrine, Racemic (Phenoxybenzamine hydrochloride may interact with compounds that stimulate both alpha- and beta-adrenergic receptors (eg, epinephrine) to produce an exaggerated hypotensive response and tachycardia).

No products indexed under this heading.

Epinephrine Bitartrate (Phenoxybenzamine hydrochloride may interact with compounds that stimulate both alpha- and beta-adrenergic receptors (eg, epinephrine) to produce an exaggerated hypotensive response and tachycardia).

No products indexed under this heading.

Epinephrine Hydrochloride (Phenoxybenzamine hydrochloride may interact with compounds that stimulate both alpha- and beta-adrenergic receptors (eg, epinephrine) to produce an exaggerated hypotensive response and tachycardia).

No products indexed under this heading.

Levarterenol (Phenoxybenzamine hydrochloride blocks hyperthermia production by levarterenol).

No products indexed under this heading.

Norepinephrine Bitartrate (Phenoxybenzamine hydrochloride may interact with compounds that stimulate both alpha- and beta-adrenergic receptors (eg, epinephrine) to produce an exaggerated hypotensive response and tachycardia).

No products indexed under this heading.

Norepinephrine Hydrochloride (Phenoxybenzamine hydrochloride may interact with compounds that stimulate both alpha- and beta-adrenergic receptors (eg, epinephrine) to produce an exaggerated hypotensive response and tachycardia).

No products indexed under this heading.

Reserpine (Phenoxybenzamine hydrochloride blocks hypothermia production by reserpine).

No products indexed under this heading.

DIDRONEL TABLETS

(Etidronate Disodium) 2790

Warfarin Sodium (Co-administration has resulted in isolated reports of increase in prothrombin time without clinically significant sequelae).

No products indexed under this heading.

DIGIBIND FOR INJECTION

(Digoxin Immune Fab (Ovine)) 1427
None cited in PDR database.

DILAUDID INJECTION

(Hydromorphone Hydrochloride) 2800
See Dilaudid-HP Injection

DILAUDID ORAL LIQUID

(Hydromorphone Hydrochloride) 2797
May interact with alcohols, central nervous system depressants, general anesthetics, hypnotics and sedatives, mixed agonist/antagonist opioid analgesics, narcotic analgesics, neuromuscular blocking agents, phenothiazines, tranquilizers, and certain other agents. Compounds in these categories include:

Alfentanil Hydrochloride (Concomitant use of other central nervous system depressants, including sedatives or hypnotics, general anesthetics, phenothiazines, tranquilizers and alcohol with hydromorphone, may produce an additive depressant effect. Respiratory depression, hypotension and profound sedation or coma may occur. When such combined therapy is contemplated, the dose of one or both agents should be reduced. Hydromorphone should not be taken with alcohol).

No products indexed under this heading.

Alprazolam (Concomitant use of tranquilizers with hydromorphone, may produce an additive depressant effect. Respiratory depression, hypotension and profound sedation or coma may occur. When such combined therapy is contemplated, the dose of one or both agents should be reduced).

No products indexed under this heading.

Amobarbital (Concomitant use of other central nervous system depressants, including sedatives or hypnotics, general anesthetics, phenothiazines, tranquilizers and alcohol with hydromorphone, may produce an additive depressant effect. Respiratory depression, hypotension and profound sedation or coma may occur. When such combined therapy is contemplated, the dose of one or both agents should be reduced. Hydromorphone should not be taken with alcohol).

No products indexed under this heading.

Amobarbital Sodium (Concomitant use of other central nervous system depressants, including sedatives or hypnotics, general anesthetics, phenothiazines, tranquilizers and alcohol with hydromorphone, may produce an additive depressant effect. Respiratory depression, hypotension and profound sedation or coma may occur. When such combined therapy is contemplated, the dose of one or both agents should be reduced. Hydromorphone should not be taken with alcohol).

No products indexed under this heading.

Apomorphine (Hydromorphone may be expected to have additive effects when used in conjunction with other alcohol. Other opioids potentiate the respiratory depressant effects of hydromorphone, increasing the risk of respiratory depression that might result in death).

No products indexed under this heading.

Apomorphine Hydrochloride (Hydromorphone may be expected to have additive effects when used in conjunction with other alcohol. Other opioids potentiate the respiratory depressant effects of hydromorphone, increasing the risk of respiratory depression that might result in death).

No products indexed under this heading.

Aprobarbital (Concomitant use of other central nervous system depressants, including sedatives or hypnotics, general anesthetics, phenothiazines, tranquilizers and alcohol with hydromorphone, may produce an additive depressant effect. Respiratory depression, hypotension and profound sedation or coma may occur. When such combined therapy is contemplated, the dose of one or both agents should be reduced. Hydromorphone should not be taken with alcohol).

No products indexed under this heading.

Atracurium Besylate (Opioid analgesics, including hydromorphone, may enhance the action of neuromuscular blocking agents and produce an excessive degree of respiratory depression).

No products indexed under this heading.

Buprenorphine Hydrochloride (Concomitant use of other central nervous system depressants, including sedatives or hypnotics, general anesthetics, phenothiazines, tranquilizers and alcohol with hydromorphone, may produce an additive depressant effect. Respiratory depression, hypotension and profound sedation or coma may occur. When such combined therapy is contemplated, the dose of one or both agents should be reduced. Hydromorphone should not be taken with alcohol).

No products indexed under this heading.

Buspirone Hydrochloride (Concomitant use of tranquilizers with hydromorphone, may produce an additive depressant effect. Respiratory depression, hypotension and profound sedation or coma may occur. When such combined therapy is contemplated, the dose of one or both agents should be reduced).

No products indexed under this heading.

Butabarbital (Concomitant use of other central nervous system depressants, including sedatives or hypnotics with hydromorphone, may produce an additive depressant effect. Respiratory depression, hypotension and profound sedation or coma may occur. When such combined therapy is contemplated, the dose of one or both agents should be reduced).

No products indexed under this heading.

Butabarbital Sodium (Concomitant use of other central nervous system depressants, including sedatives or hypnotics with hydromorphone, may produce an additive depressant effect. Respiratory depression, hypotension and profound sedation or coma may occur. When such combined therapy is contemplated, the dose of one or both agents should be reduced).

No products indexed under this heading.

Butalbital (Concomitant use of other central nervous system depressants, including sedatives or hypnotics with hydromorphone, may produce an additive depressant effect. Respiratory depression, hypotension and profound sedation or coma may occur. When such combined therapy is contemplated, the dose of one or both agents should be reduced).

No products indexed under this heading.

Butorphanol Tartrate (Agonist/antagonist analgesics (eg, pentazocine, nalbuphine, butorphanol, buprenorphine) should be administered with caution to a patient who has received or is receiving a course of therapy with a pure opioid agonist analgesic such as

hydromorphone. In this situation, mixed agonist/antagonist analgesics may reduce the analgesic effect of hydromorphone and/or may precipitate withdrawal symptoms in these patients).

No products indexed under this heading.

Chloral Hydrate (Concomitant use of other central nervous system depressants, including sedatives or hypnotics with hydromorphone, may produce an additive depressant effect. Respiratory depression, hypotension and profound sedation or coma may occur. When such combined therapy is contemplated, the dose of one or both agents should be reduced).

No products indexed under this heading.

Chlordiazepoxide (Concomitant use of tranquilizers with hydromorphone, may produce an additive depressant effect. Respiratory depression, hypotension and profound sedation or coma may occur. When such combined therapy is contemplated, the dose of one or both agents should be reduced).

No products indexed under this heading.

Chlordiazepoxide Hydrochloride (Concomitant use of tranquilizers with hydromorphone, may produce an additive depressant effect. Respiratory depression, hypotension and profound sedation or coma may occur. When such combined therapy is contemplated, the dose of one or both agents should be reduced).

No products indexed under this heading.

Chlorpromazine (Concomitant use of phenothiazines with hydromorphone, may produce an additive depressant effect. Respiratory depression, hypotension and profound sedation or coma may occur. When such combined therapy is contemplated, the dose of one or both agents should be reduced. Administer with caution to patients in circulatory shock, since vasodilation produced by the drug may further reduce cardiac output and blood pressure).

No products indexed under this heading.

Chlorpromazine Hydrochloride (Concomitant use of phenothiazines with hydromorphone, may produce an additive depressant effect. Respiratory depression, hypotension and profound sedation or coma may occur. When such combined therapy is contemplated, the dose of one or both agents should be reduced. Administer with caution to patients in circulatory shock, since vasodilation produced by the drug may further reduce cardiac output and blood pressure).

No products indexed under this heading.

Chlorprothixene (Concomitant use of tranquilizers with hydromorphone, may produce an additive depressant effect. Respiratory depression, hypotension and profound sedation or coma may occur. When such combined therapy is contemplated, the dose of one or both agents should be reduced).

No products indexed under this heading.

Chlorprothixene Hydrochloride (Concomitant use of tranquilizers with hydromorphone, may produce an additive depressant effect. Respiratory depression, hypotension and profound sedation or coma may occur. When such combined therapy is contemplated, the dose of one or both agents should be reduced).

No products indexed under this heading.

Chlorprothixene Lactate (Concomitant use of tranquilizers with hydromorphone, may produce an additive depressant effect. Respiratory depression, hypotension and profound sedation or coma may occur. When such combined therapy is contemplated, the dose of one or both agents should be reduced).

No products indexed under this heading.

Cisatracurium Besylate (Opioid analgesics, including hydromorphone, may enhance the action of neuromuscular blocking agents and produce an excessive degree of respiratory depression). Products include:

Nimbex 503

Clonazepam (Concomitant use of other central nervous system depressants, including sedatives or hypnotics, general anesthetics, phenothiazines, tranquilizers and alcohol with hydromorphone, may produce an additive depressant effect. Respiratory depression, hypotension and profound sedation or coma may occur. When such combined therapy is contemplated, the dose of one or both agents should be reduced. Hydromorphone should not be taken with alcohol). Products include:

Klonopin 2855

Clorazepate Dipotassium (Concomitant use of tranquilizers with hydromorphone, may produce an additive depressant effect. Respiratory depression, hypotension and profound sedation or coma may occur. When such combined therapy is contemplated, the dose of one or both agents should be reduced).

No products indexed under this heading.

Clozapine (Concomitant use of other central nervous system depressants, including sedatives or hypnotics, general anesthetics, phenothiazines, tranquilizers and alcohol with hydromorphone, may produce an additive depressant effect. Respiratory depression, hypotension and profound sedation or coma may occur. When such combined therapy is contemplated, the dose of one or both agents should be reduced. Hydromorphone should not be taken with alcohol).

No products indexed under this heading.

Codeine Phosphate (Concomitant use of other central nervous system depressants, including sedatives or hypnotics, general anesthetics, phenothiazines, tranquilizers and alcohol with hydromorphone, may produce an additive depressant effect. Respiratory depression, hypotension and profound sedation or coma may occur. When such combined therapy is contemplated, the dose of one or both agents should be reduced. Hydromorphone should not be taken with alcohol). Products include:

Tylenol with Codeine 2691

Codeine Sulfate (Concomitant use of other central nervous system depressants, including sedatives or hypnotics, general anesthetics, phenothiazines, tranquilizers and alcohol with hydromorphone, may produce an additive depressant effect. Respiratory depression, hypotension and profound sedation or coma may occur. When such combined therapy is contemplated, the dose of one or both agents should be reduced. Hydromorphone should not be taken with alcohol).

No products indexed under this heading.

Decamethonium (Opioid analgesics, including hydromorphone, may enhance the action of neuromuscular blocking agents and produce an excessive degree of respiratory depression).

No products indexed under this heading.

Desflurane (Concomitant use of general anesthetics with hydromorphone, may produce an additive depressant effect. Respiratory depression, hypotension and profound sedation or coma may occur. When such combined therapy is contemplated, the dose of one or both agents should be reduced. Administer with caution to patients in circulatory shock, since vasodilation produced by the drug may further reduce cardiac output and blood pressure).

No products indexed under this heading.

Dezocine (Concomitant use of other central nervous system depressants, including sedatives or hypnotics, general anesthetics, phenothiazines, tranquilizers and alcohol with hydromorphone, may produce an additive depressant effect. Respiratory depression, hypotension and profound sedation or coma may occur. When such combined therapy is contemplated, the dose of one or both agents should be reduced. Hydromorphone should not be taken with alcohol).

No products indexed under this heading.

Diazepam (Concomitant use of tranquilizers with hydromorphone, may produce an additive depressant effect. Respiratory depression, hypotension and profound sedation or coma may occur. When such combined therapy is contemplated, the dose of one or both agents should be reduced). Products include:

Valium Tablets 2880

Dihydrocodeine Bitartrate (Hydromorphone may be expected to have additive effects when used in conjunction with other alcohol. Other opioids potentiate the respiratory depressant effects of hydromorphone, increasing the risk of respiratory depression that might result in death).

No products indexed under this heading.

Dihydrocodeinone Bitartrate (Hydromorphone may be expected to have additive effects when used in conjunction with other alcohol. Other opioids potentiate the respiratory depressant effects of hydromorphone, increasing the risk of respiratory depression that might result in death).

No products indexed under this heading.

Doxacurium Chloride (Opioid analgesics, including hydromorphone, may enhance the action of neuromuscular blocking agents and produce an excessive degree of respiratory depression).

No products indexed under this heading.

Droperidol (Concomitant use of tranquilizers with hydromorphone, may produce an additive depressant effect. Respiratory depression, hypotension and profound sedation or coma may occur. When such combined therapy is contemplated, the dose of one or both agents should be reduced).

No products indexed under this heading.

d-Tubocurarine (Opioid analgesics, including hydromorphone, may enhance the action of neuromuscular blocking agents and produce an excessive degree of respiratory depression).

No products indexed under this heading.

Enflurane (Concomitant use of general anesthetics with hydromorphone, may produce an additive depressant effect. Respiratory depression, hypotension and profound sedation or coma may occur. When such combined therapy is contemplated, the dose of one or both agents should be reduced. Administer with caution to patients in circulatory shock, since vasodilation produced by the drug may further reduce cardiac output and blood pressure).

No products indexed under this heading.

Estazolam (Concomitant use of other central nervous system depressants, including sedatives or hypnotics with hydromorphone, may produce an additive depressant effect. Respiratory depression, hypotension and profound sedation or coma may occur. When such combined therapy is contemplated, the dose of one or both agents should be reduced).

No products indexed under this heading.

Ethanol (Hydromorphone may be expected to have additive effects when used in conjunction with alcohol. Alcohol potentiates the respiratory depressant effects of hydromorphone, increasing the risk of respiratory depression that might result in death).

No products indexed under this heading.

Ethchlorvynol (Concomitant use of other central nervous system depressants, including sedatives or hypnotics with hydromorphone, may produce an additive depressant effect. Respiratory depression, hypotension and profound sedation or coma may occur. When such combined therapy is contemplated, the dose of one or both agents should be reduced).

No products indexed under this heading.

Ethinamate (Concomitant use of other central nervous system depressants, including sedatives or hypnotics with hydromorphone, may produce an additive depressant effect. Respiratory depression, hypotension and profound sedation or coma may occur. When such combined therapy is contemplated, the dose of one or both agents should be reduced).

No products indexed under this heading.

Ethyl Alcohol (Hydromorphone may be expected to have additive effects when used in conjunction with alcohol. Alcohol potentiates the respiratory depressant effects of hydromorphone, increasing the risk of respiratory depression that might result in death).

No products indexed under this heading.

Fentanyl (Concomitant use of other central nervous system depressants, including sedatives or hypnotics, general anesthetics, phenothiazines, tranquilizers and alcohol with hydromorphone, may produce an additive depressant effect. Respiratory depression, hypotension and profound sedation or coma may occur. When such combined therapy is contemplated, the dose of one or both agents should be reduced. Hydromorphone should not be taken with alcohol). Products include:

Duragesic 2604
Fentanyl Transdermal System 2346
Onsolis 2054

Fentanyl Citrate (Concomitant use of other central nervous system depressants, including sedatives or hypnotics, general anesthetics, phenothiazines, tranquilizers and alcohol with hydromorphone, may produce an additive depressant effect. Respiratory depression, hypotension and profound sedation or coma may occur. When such combined therapy is contemplated, the dose of one or both agents should be reduced. Hydromorphone should not be taken with alcohol). Products include:

Fentora 966

Fluphenazine Decanoate (Concomitant use of phenothiazines with hydromorphone, may produce an additive depressant effect. Respiratory depression, hypotension and profound sedation or coma may occur. When such combined therapy is contemplated, the dose of one or both agents should be reduced. Administer with caution to patients in circulatory shock, since vasodilation produced by the drug may further reduce cardiac output and blood pressure).

No products indexed under this heading.

Fluphenazine Enanthate (Concomitant use of phenothiazines with hydromorphone, may produce an additive depressant effect. Respiratory depression, hypotension and profound sedation or coma may occur. When such combined therapy is contemplated, the dose of one or both agents should be reduced. Administer with caution to patients in circulatory shock, since

---

IMPORTANT NOTE: Always consult each drug listing in the patient's regimen for possible interactions.

Dilaudid Interactions Index 464

vasodilation produced by the drug may further reduce cardiac output and blood pressure).
No products indexed under this heading.

Fluphenazine Hydrochloride (Concomitant use of phenothiazines with hydromorphone, may produce an additive depressant effect. Respiratory depression, hypotension and profound sedation or coma may occur. When such combined therapy is contemplated, the dose of one or both agents should be reduced. Administer with caution to patients in circulatory shock, since vasodilation produced by the drug may further reduce cardiac output and blood pressure).
No products indexed under this heading.

Flurazepam Hydrochloride (Concomitant use of other central nervous system depressants, including sedatives or hypnotics with hydromorphone, may produce an additive depressant effect. Respiratory depression, hypotension and profound sedation or coma may occur. When such combined therapy is contemplated, the dose of one or both agents should be reduced).
No products indexed under this heading.

Gallamine (Opioid analgesics, including hydromorphone, may enhance the action of neuromuscular blocking agents and produce an excessive degree of respiratory depression).
No products indexed under this heading.

Gallamine Triethiodide (Opioid analgesics, including hydromorphone, may enhance the action of neuromuscular blocking agents and produce an excessive degree of respiratory depression).
No products indexed under this heading.

Glutethimide (Concomitant use of other central nervous system depressants, including sedatives or hypnotics with hydromorphone, may produce an additive depressant effect. Respiratory depression, hypotension and profound sedation or coma may occur. When such combined therapy is contemplated, the dose of one or both agents should be reduced).
No products indexed under this heading.

Halazepam (Concomitant use of other central nervous system depressants, including sedatives or hypnotics, general anesthetics, phenothiazines, tranquilizers and alcohol with hydromorphone, may produce an additive depressant effect. Respiratory depression, hypotension and profound sedation or coma may occur. When such combined therapy is contemplated, the dose of one or both agents should be reduced. Hydromorphone should not be taken with alcohol).
No products indexed under this heading.

Haloperidol (Concomitant use of tranquilizers with hydromorphone, may produce an additive depressant effect. Respiratory depression, hypotension and profound sedation or coma may occur. When such combined therapy is contemplated, the dose of one or both agents should be reduced).
No products indexed under this heading.

Haloperidol Decanoate (Concomitant use of tranquilizers with hydromorphone, may produce an additive depressant effect. Respiratory depression, hypotension and profound sedation or coma may occur. When such combined therapy is contemplated, the dose of one or both agents should be reduced).
No products indexed under this heading.

Haloperidol Lactate (Concomitant use of other central nervous system depressants, including sedatives or hypnotics, general anesthetics, phenothiazines, tranquilizers and alcohol with hydromorphone, may produce an additive depressant effect. Respiratory depression, hypotension and profound sedation or coma may occur. When such combined therapy is contemplated, the dose of one or both agents should be reduced. Hydromorphone should not be taken with alcohol).
No products indexed under this heading.

Halothane (Concomitant use of general anesthetics with hydromorphone, may produce an additive depressant effect. Respiratory depression, hypotension and profound sedation or coma may occur. When such combined therapy is contemplated, the dose of one or both agents should be reduced. Administer with caution to patients in circulatory shock, since vasodilation produced by the drug may further reduce cardiac output and blood pressure).
No products indexed under this heading.

Hexobarbital (Concomitant use of other central nervous system depressants, including sedatives or hypnotics, general anesthetics, phenothiazines, tranquilizers and alcohol with hydromorphone, may produce an additive depressant effect. Respiratory depression, hypotension and profound sedation or coma may occur. When such combined therapy is contemplated, the dose of one or both agents should be reduced. Hydromorphone should not be taken with alcohol).
No products indexed under this heading.

Hydrocodone Bitartrate (Concomitant use of other central nervous system depressants, including sedatives or hypnotics, general anesthetics, phenothiazines, tranquilizers and alcohol with hydromorphone, may produce an additive depressant effect. Respiratory depression, hypotension and profound sedation or coma may occur. When such combined therapy is contemplated, the dose of one or both agents should be reduced. Hydromorphone should not be taken with alcohol).
Products include:
Vicodin 560
Vicodin ES 561
Vicodin HP 563
Vicoprofen 564
Zydone 1138

Hydrocodone Polistirex (Concomitant use of other central nervous system depressants, including sedatives or hypnotics, general anesthetics, phenothiazines, tranquilizers and alcohol with hydromorphone, may produce an additive depressant effect. Respiratory depression, hypotension and profound sedation or coma may occur. When such combined therapy is contemplated, the dose of one or both agents should be reduced. Hydromorphone should not be taken with alcohol).
Products include:
Tussionex 3443

Hydromorphone (Concomitant use of other central nervous system depressants, including sedatives or hypnotics, general anesthetics, phenothiazines, tranquilizers and alcohol with hydromorphone, may produce an additive depressant effect. Respiratory depression, hypotension and profound sedation or coma may occur. When such combined therapy is contemplated, the dose of one or both agents should be reduced. Hydromorphone should not be taken with alcohol).
No products indexed under this heading.

Hydroxyzine Hydrochloride (Concomitant use of tranquilizers with hydromorphone, may produce an additive depressant effect. Respiratory depression, hypotension and profound sedation or coma may occur. When such combined therapy is contemplated, the dose of one or both agents should be reduced).
No products indexed under this heading.

Isoflurane (Concomitant use of general anesthetics with hydromorphone, may produce an additive depressant effect. Respiratory depression, hypotension and profound sedation or coma may occur. When such combined therapy is contemplated, the dose of one or both agents should be reduced. Administer with caution to patients in circulatory shock, since vasodilation produced by the drug may further reduce cardiac output and blood pressure).
No products indexed under this heading.

Ketamine Hydrochloride (Concomitant use of general anesthetics with hydromorphone, may produce an additive depressant effect. Respiratory depression, hypotension and profound sedation or coma may occur. When such combined therapy is contemplated, the dose of one or both agents should be reduced. Administer with caution to patients in circulatory shock, since vasodilation produced by the drug may further reduce cardiac output and blood pressure).
No products indexed under this heading.

Levomethadyl Acetate Hydrochloride (Concomitant use of other central nervous system depressants, including sedatives or hypnotics, general anesthetics, phenothiazines, tranquilizers and alcohol with hydromorphone, may produce an additive depressant effect. Respiratory depression, hypotension and profound sedation or coma may occur. When such combined therapy is contemplated, the dose of one or both agents should be reduced. Hydromorphone should not be taken with alcohol).
No products indexed under this heading.

Levorphanol Tartrate (Concomitant use of other central nervous system depressants, including sedatives or hypnotics, general anesthetics, phenothiazines, tranquilizers and alcohol with hydromorphone, may produce an additive depressant effect. Respiratory depression, hypotension and profound sedation or coma may occur. When such combined therapy is contemplated, the dose of one or both agents should be reduced. Hydromorphone should not be taken with alcohol).
No products indexed under this heading.

Lorazepam (Concomitant use of other central nervous system depressants, including sedatives or hypnotics with hydromorphone, may produce an additive depressant effect. Respiratory depression, hypotension and profound sedation or coma may occur. When such combined therapy is contemplated, the dose of one or both agents should be reduced).
No products indexed under this heading.

Loxapine Hydrochloride (Concomitant use of tranquilizers with hydromorphone, may produce an additive depressant effect. Respiratory depression, hypotension and profound sedation or coma may occur. When such combined therapy is contemplated, the dose of one or both agents should be reduced).
No products indexed under this heading.

Loxapine Succinate (Concomitant use of tranquilizers with hydromorphone, may produce an additive depressant effect. Respiratory depression, hypotension and profound sedation or coma may occur. When such combined therapy is contemplated, the dose of one or both agents should be reduced).
No products indexed under this heading.

Meperidine Hydrochloride (Concomitant use of other central nervous system depressants, including sedatives or hypnotics, general anesthetics, phenothiazines, tranquilizers and alcohol with hydromorphone, may produce an additive depressant effect. Respiratory depression, hypotension and profound sedation or coma may occur. When such combined therapy is contemplated, the dose of one or both agents should be reduced. Hydromorphone should not be taken with alcohol).
No products indexed under this heading.

Mephobarbital (Concomitant use of other central nervous system depressants, including sedatives or hypnotics, general anesthetics, phenothiazines, tranquilizers and alcohol with hydromorphone, may produce an additive depressant effect. Respiratory depression, hypotension and profound sedation or coma may occur. When such combined therapy is contemplated, the dose of one or both agents should be reduced. Hydromorphone should not be taken with alcohol).
No products indexed under this heading.

Meprobamate (Concomitant use of tranquilizers with hydromorphone, may produce an additive depressant effect. Respiratory depression, hypotension and profound sedation or coma may occur. When such combined therapy is contemplated, the dose of one or both agents should be reduced).
No products indexed under this heading.

Mesoridazine Besylate (Concomitant use of phenothiazines with hydromorphone, may produce an additive depressant effect. Respiratory depression, hypotension and profound sedation or coma may occur. When such combined therapy is contemplated, the dose of one or both agents should be reduced. Administer with caution to patients in circulatory shock, since vasodilation produced by the drug may further reduce cardiac output and blood pressure).
No products indexed under this heading.

Methadone Hydrochloride (Concomitant use of other central nervous system depressants, including sedatives or hypnotics, general anesthetics, phenothiazines, tranquilizers and alcohol with hydromorphone, may produce an additive depressant effect. Respiratory depression, hypotension and profound sedation or coma may occur. When such combined therapy is contemplated, the dose of one or both agents should be reduced. Hydromorphone should not be taken with alcohol).
No products indexed under this heading.

Methohexital Sodium (Concomitant use of general anesthetics with hydromorphone, may produce an additive depressant effect. Respiratory depression, hypotension and profound sedation or coma may occur. When such combined therapy is contemplated, the dose of one or both agents should be reduced. Administer with caution to patients in circulatory shock, since vasodilation produced by the drug may further reduce cardiac output and blood pressure).
No products indexed under this heading.

Methotrimeprazine (Concomitant use of phenothiazines with hydromorphone, may produce an additive depressant effect. Respiratory depression, hypotension and profound sedation or coma may occur. When such combined therapy is contemplated, the dose of one or both agents should be reduced. Administer with caution to patients in circulatory shock, since vasodilation produced by the drug may further reduce cardiac output and blood pressure).
No products indexed under this heading.

Methoxyflurane (Concomitant use of general anesthetics with hydromorphone, may produce an additive depressant effect. Respiratory depression, hypotension and profound sedation or coma may occur. When such combined therapy is contemplated, the dose of

one or both agents should be reduced. Administer with caution to patients in circulatory shock, since vasodilation produced by the drug may further reduce cardiac output and blood pressure).

No products indexed under this heading.

Metocurine Iodide (Opioid analgesics, including hydromorphone, may enhance the action of neuromuscular blocking agents and produce an excessive degree of respiratory depression).

No products indexed under this heading.

Midazolam Hydrochloride (Concomitant use of other central nervous system depressants, including sedatives or hypnotics with hydromorphone, may produce an additive depressant effect. Respiratory depression, hypotension and profound sedation or coma may occur. When such combined therapy is contemplated, the dose of one or both agents should be reduced).

No products indexed under this heading.

Mivacurium Chloride (Opioid analgesics, including hydromorphone, may enhance the action of neuromuscular blocking agents and produce an excessive degree of respiratory depression).

No products indexed under this heading.

Molindone Hydrochloride (Concomitant use of tranquilizers with hydromorphone, may produce an additive depressant effect. Respiratory depression, hypotension and profound sedation or coma may occur. When such combined therapy is contemplated, the dose of one or both agents should be reduced). Products include:

Moban 1108

Morphine Sulfate (Concomitant use of other central nervous system depressants, including sedatives or hypnotics, general anesthetics, phenothiazines, tranquilizers and alcohol with hydromorphone, may produce an additive depressant effect. Respiratory depression, hypotension and profound sedation or coma may occur. When such combined therapy is contemplated, the dose of one or both agents should be reduced. Hydromorphone should not be taken with alcohol). Products include:

Avinza 1822
Embeda 1831
MS Contin 2803

Morphine Sulfate, Liposomal (Concomitant use of other central nervous system depressants, including sedatives or hypnotics, general anesthetics, phenothiazines, tranquilizers and alcohol with hydromorphone, may produce an additive depressant effect. Respiratory depression, hypotension and profound sedation or coma may occur. When such combined therapy is contemplated, the dose of one or both agents should be reduced. Hydromorphone should not be taken with alcohol).

No products indexed under this heading.

Nalbuphine Hydrochloride (Agonist/antagonist analgesics (eg, pentazocine, nalbuphine, butorphanol, buprenorphine) should be administered with caution to a patient who has received or is receiving a course of therapy with a pure opioid agonist analgesic such as hydromorphone. In this situation, mixed agonist/antagonist analgesics may reduce the analgesic effect of hydromorphone and/or may precipitate withdrawal symptoms in these patients).

No products indexed under this heading.

Nitrous Oxide (Concomitant use of general anesthetics with hydromorphone, may produce an additive depressant effect. Respiratory depression, hypotension and profound sedation or coma may occur. When such combined therapy is contemplated, the dose of one or both agents should be reduced.

Administer with caution to patients in circulatory shock, since vasodilation produced by the drug may further reduce cardiac output and blood pressure).

No products indexed under this heading.

Olanzapine (Concomitant use of other central nervous system depressants, including sedatives or hypnotics, general anesthetics, phenothiazines, tranquilizers and alcohol with hydromorphone, may produce an additive depressant effect. Respiratory depression, hypotension and profound sedation or coma may occur. When such combined therapy is contemplated, the dose of one or both agents should be reduced. Hydromorphone should not be taken with alcohol). Products include:

Symbyax 1965
Zyprexa 1984
Zyprexa IntraMuscular 1984
Zyprexa ZYDIS 1984

Oxazepam (Concomitant use of tranquilizers with hydromorphone, may produce an additive depressant effect. Respiratory depression, hypotension and profound sedation or coma may occur. When such combined therapy is contemplated, the dose of one or both agents should be reduced).

No products indexed under this heading.

Oxycodone Hydrochloride (Concomitant use of other central nervous system depressants, including sedatives or hypnotics, general anesthetics, phenothiazines, tranquilizers and alcohol with hydromorphone, may produce an additive depressant effect. Respiratory depression, hypotension and profound sedation or coma may occur. When such combined therapy is contemplated, the dose of one or both agents should be reduced. Hydromorphone should not be taken with alcohol). Products include:

OxyContin 2807
Percocet 1121
Percodan 1124

Oxycodone Terephthalate (Concomitant use of other central nervous system depressants, including sedatives or hypnotics, general anesthetics, phenothiazines, tranquilizers and alcohol with hydromorphone, may produce an additive depressant effect. Respiratory depression, hypotension and profound sedation or coma may occur. When such combined therapy is contemplated, the dose of one or both agents should be reduced. Hydromorphone should not be taken with alcohol).

No products indexed under this heading.

Oxymorphone Hydrochloride (Concomitant use of other central nervous system depressants, including sedatives or hypnotics, general anesthetics, phenothiazines, tranquilizers and alcohol with hydromorphone, may produce an additive depressant effect. Respiratory depression, hypotension and profound sedation or coma may occur. When such combined therapy is contemplated, the dose of one or both agents should be reduced. Hydromorphone should not be taken with alcohol). Products include:

Opana 1110
Opana ER 1114

Pancuronium Bromide (Opioid analgesics, including hydromorphone, may enhance the action of neuromuscular blocking agents and produce an excessive degree of respiratory depression).

No products indexed under this heading.

Pentazocine Hydrochloride (Agonist/antagonist analgesics (eg, pentazocine, nalbuphine, butorphanol, buprenorphine) should be administered with caution to a patient who has received or is receiving a course of therapy with a pure opioid agonist analgesic such as hydromorphone. In this

situation, mixed agonist/antagonist analgesics may reduce the analgesic effect of hydromorphone and/or may precipitate withdrawal symptoms in these patients).

No products indexed under this heading.

Pentazocine Lactate (Agonist/antagonist analgesics (eg, pentazocine, nalbuphine, butorphanol, buprenorphine) should be administered with caution to a patient who has received or is receiving a course of therapy with a pure opioid agonist analgesic such as hydromorphone. In this situation, mixed agonist/antagonist analgesics may reduce the analgesic effect of hydromorphone and/or may precipitate withdrawal symptoms in these patients).

No products indexed under this heading.

Pentobarbital (Concomitant use of other central nervous system depressants, including sedatives or hypnotics, general anesthetics, phenothiazines, tranquilizers and alcohol with hydromorphone, may produce an additive depressant effect. Respiratory depression, hypotension and profound sedation or coma may occur. When such combined therapy is contemplated, the dose of one or both agents should be reduced. Hydromorphone should not be taken with alcohol).

No products indexed under this heading.

Pentobarbital Sodium (Concomitant use of other central nervous system depressants, including sedatives or hypnotics, general anesthetics, phenothiazines, tranquilizers and alcohol with hydromorphone, may produce an additive depressant effect. Respiratory depression, hypotension and profound sedation or coma may occur. When such combined therapy is contemplated, the dose of one or both agents should be reduced. Hydromorphone should not be taken with alcohol). Products include:

Nembutal 2012

Perphenazine (Concomitant use of phenothiazines with hydromorphone, may produce an additive depressant effect. Respiratory depression, hypotension and profound sedation or coma may occur. When such combined therapy is contemplated, the dose of one or both agents should be reduced. Administer with caution to patients in circulatory shock, since vasodilation produced by the drug may further reduce cardiac output and blood pressure).

No products indexed under this heading.

Phenobarbital (Concomitant use of other central nervous system depressants, including sedatives or hypnotics, general anesthetics, phenothiazines, tranquilizers and alcohol with hydromorphone, may produce an additive depressant effect. Respiratory depression, hypotension and profound sedation or coma may occur. When such combined therapy is contemplated, the dose of one or both agents should be reduced. Hydromorphone should not be taken with alcohol). Products include:

Donnatal 2711

Phenobarbital Sodium (Concomitant use of other central nervous system depressants, including sedatives or hypnotics, general anesthetics, phenothiazines, tranquilizers and alcohol with hydromorphone, may produce an additive depressant effect. Respiratory depression, hypotension and profound sedation or coma may occur. When such combined therapy is contemplated, the dose of one or both agents should be reduced. Hydromorphone should not be taken with alcohol).

No products indexed under this heading.

Phenothiazine Derivatives (Concomitant use of phenothiazines with hydromorphone, may produce an addi-

tive depressant effect. Respiratory depression, hypotension and profound sedation or coma may occur. When such combined therapy is contemplated, the dose of one or both agents should be reduced. Administer with caution to patients in circulatory shock, since vasodilation produced by the drug may further reduce cardiac output and blood pressure).

No products indexed under this heading.

Phenothiazines (Concomitant use of phenothiazines with hydromorphone, may produce an additive depressant effect. Respiratory depression, hypotension and profound sedation or coma may occur. When such combined therapy is contemplated, the dose of one or both agents should be reduced. Administer with caution to patients in circulatory shock, since vasodilation produced by the drug may further reduce cardiac output and blood pressure).

No products indexed under this heading.

Prazepam (Concomitant use of tranquilizers with hydromorphone, may produce an additive depressant effect. Respiratory depression, hypotension and profound sedation or coma may occur. When such combined therapy is contemplated, the dose of one or both agents should be reduced).

No products indexed under this heading.

Prochlorperazine (Concomitant use of phenothiazines with hydromorphone, may produce an additive depressant effect. Respiratory depression, hypotension and profound sedation or coma may occur. When such combined therapy is contemplated, the dose of one or both agents should be reduced. Administer with caution to patients in circulatory shock, since vasodilation produced by the drug may further reduce cardiac output and blood pressure).

No products indexed under this heading.

Prochlorperazine Edisylate (Concomitant use of phenothiazines with hydromorphone, may produce an additive depressant effect. Respiratory depression, hypotension and profound sedation or coma may occur. When such combined therapy is contemplated, the dose of one or both agents should be reduced. Administer with caution to patients in circulatory shock, since vasodilation produced by the drug may further reduce cardiac output and blood pressure).

No products indexed under this heading.

Prochlorperazine Maleate (Concomitant use of phenothiazines with hydromorphone, may produce an additive depressant effect. Respiratory depression, hypotension and profound sedation or coma may occur. When such combined therapy is contemplated, the dose of one or both agents should be reduced. Administer with caution to patients in circulatory shock, since vasodilation produced by the drug may further reduce cardiac output and blood pressure).

No products indexed under this heading.

Promethazine (Concomitant use of phenothiazines with hydromorphone, may produce an additive depressant effect. Respiratory depression, hypotension and profound sedation or coma may occur. When such combined therapy is contemplated, the dose of one or both agents should be reduced. Administer with caution to patients in circulatory shock, since vasodilation produced by the drug may further reduce cardiac output and blood pressure).

No products indexed under this heading.

Promethazine Hydrochloride (Concomitant use of phenothiazines with hydromorphone, may produce an additive depressant effect. Respiratory depression, hypotension and profound

sedation or coma may occur. When such combined therapy is contemplated, the dose of one or both agents should be reduced. Administer with caution to patients in circulatory shock, since vasodilation produced by the drug may further reduce cardiac output and blood pressure).

No products indexed under this heading.

Propofol (Concomitant use of other central nervous system depressants, including sedatives or hypnotics with hydromorphone, may produce an additive depressant effect. Respiratory depression, hypotension and profound sedation or coma may occur. When such combined therapy is contemplated, the dose of one or both agents should be reduced.)

No products indexed under this heading.

Propoxyphene Hydrochloride (Concomitant use of other central nervous system depressants, including sedatives or hypnotics, general anesthetics, phenothiazines, tranquilizers and alcohol with hydromorphone, may produce an additive depressant effect. Respiratory depression, hypotension and profound sedation or coma may occur. When such combined therapy is contemplated, the dose of one or both agents should be reduced. Hydromorphone should not be taken with alcohol).

No products indexed under this heading.

Propoxyphene Napsylate (Concomitant use of other central nervous system depressants, including sedatives or hypnotics, general anesthetics, phenothiazines, tranquilizers and alcohol with hydromorphone, may produce an additive depressant effect. Respiratory depression, hypotension and profound sedation or coma may occur. When such combined therapy is contemplated, the dose of one or both agents should be reduced. Hydromorphone should not be taken with alcohol).

No products indexed under this heading.

Quazepam (Concomitant use of other central nervous system depressants, including sedatives or hypnotics with hydromorphone, may produce an additive depressant effect. Respiratory depression, hypotension and profound sedation or coma may occur. When such combined therapy is contemplated, the dose of one or both agents should be reduced.)

No products indexed under this heading.

Quetiapine Fumarate (Concomitant use of other central nervous system depressants, including sedatives or hypnotics, general anesthetics, phenothiazines, tranquilizers and alcohol with hydromorphone, may produce an additive depressant effect. Respiratory depression, hypotension and profound sedation or coma may occur. When such combined therapy is contemplated, the dose of one or both agents should be reduced. Hydromorphone should not be taken with alcohol). Products include:

Seroquel 750
Seroquel XR 759

Ramelteon (Concomitant use of other central nervous system depressants, including sedatives or hypnotics with hydromorphone, may produce an additive depressant effect. Respiratory depression, hypotension and profound sedation or coma may occur. When such combined therapy is contemplated, the dose of one or both agents should be reduced). Products include:

Rozerem 3366

Rapacuronium Bromide (Opioid analgesics, including hydromorphone, may enhance the action of neuromuscular blocking agents and produce an excessive degree of respiratory depression).

No products indexed under this heading.

Remifentanil Hydrochloride (Concomitant use of other central nervous system depressants, including sedatives or hypnotics, general anesthetics, phenothiazines, tranquilizers and alcohol with hydromorphone, may produce an additive depressant effect. Respiratory depression, hypotension and profound sedation or coma may occur. When such combined therapy is contemplated, the dose of one or both agents should be reduced. Hydromorphone should not be taken with alcohol).

No products indexed under this heading.

Risperidone (Concomitant use of other central nervous system depressants, including sedatives or hypnotics, general anesthetics, phenothiazines, tranquilizers and alcohol with hydromorphone, may produce an additive depressant effect. Respiratory depression, hypotension and profound sedation or coma may occur. When such combined therapy is contemplated, the dose of one or both agents should be reduced. Hydromorphone should not be taken with alcohol). Products include:

Risperdal Consta 2682

Rocuronium Bromide (Opioid analgesics, including hydromorphone, may enhance the action of neuromuscular blocking agents and produce an excessive degree of respiratory depression). Products include:

Zemuron 3249

Secobarbital Sodium (Concomitant use of other central nervous system depressants, including sedatives or hypnotics with hydromorphone, may produce an additive depressant effect. Respiratory depression, hypotension and profound sedation or coma may occur. When such combined therapy is contemplated, the dose of one or both agents should be reduced.)

No products indexed under this heading.

Sevoflurane (Concomitant use of general anesthetics with hydromorphone, may produce an additive depressant effect. Respiratory depression, hypotension and profound sedation or coma may occur. When such combined therapy is contemplated, the dose of one or both agents should be reduced. Administer with caution to patients in circulatory shock, since vasodilation produced by the drug may further reduce cardiac output and blood pressure). Products include:

Ultane 554

Sodium Butabarbital (Concomitant use of other central nervous system depressants, including sedatives or hypnotics with hydromorphone, may produce an additive depressant effect. Respiratory depression, hypotension and profound sedation or coma may occur. When such combined therapy is contemplated, the dose of one or both agents should be reduced.)

No products indexed under this heading.

Sodium Oxybate (Concomitant use of other central nervous system depressants, including sedatives or hypnotics, general anesthetics, phenothiazines, tranquilizers and alcohol with hydromorphone, may produce an additive depressant effect. Respiratory depression, hypotension and profound sedation or coma may occur. When such combined therapy is contemplated, the dose of one or both agents should be reduced. Hydromorphone should not be taken with alcohol).

No products indexed under this heading.

Sodium Pentobarbital (Concomitant use of other central nervous system depressants, including sedatives or hypnotics, general anesthetics, phenothiazines, tranquilizers and alcohol with hydromorphone, may produce an additive depressant effect. Respiratory depression, hypotension and profound sedation or coma may occur. When such combined therapy is contemplated, the dose of one or both agents should be reduced. Hydromorphone should not be taken with alcohol).

No products indexed under this heading.

Succinylcholine Chloride (Opioid analgesics, including hydromorphone, may enhance the action of neuromuscular blocking agents and produce an excessive degree of respiratory depression).

No products indexed under this heading.

Sufentanil Citrate (Concomitant use of other central nervous system depressants, including sedatives or hypnotics, general anesthetics, phenothiazines, tranquilizers and alcohol with hydromorphone, may produce an additive depressant effect. Respiratory depression, hypotension and profound sedation or coma may occur. When such combined therapy is contemplated, the dose of one or both agents should be reduced. Hydromorphone should not be taken with alcohol).

No products indexed under this heading.

Talbutal (Concomitant use of other central nervous system depressants, including sedatives or hypnotics, general anesthetics, phenothiazines, tranquilizers and alcohol with hydromorphone, may produce an additive depressant effect. Respiratory depression, hypotension and profound sedation or coma may occur. When such combined therapy is contemplated, the dose of one or both agents should be reduced. Hydromorphone should not be taken with alcohol).

No products indexed under this heading.

Temazepam (Concomitant use of other central nervous system depressants, including sedatives or hypnotics with hydromorphone, may produce an additive depressant effect. Respiratory depression, hypotension and profound sedation or coma may occur. When such combined therapy is contemplated, the dose of one or both agents should be reduced.)

No products indexed under this heading.

Thiamylal Sodium (Concomitant use of other central nervous system depressants, including sedatives or hypnotics, general anesthetics, phenothiazines, tranquilizers and alcohol with hydromorphone, may produce an additive depressant effect. Respiratory depression, hypotension and profound sedation or coma may occur. When such combined therapy is contemplated, the dose of one or both agents should be reduced. Hydromorphone should not be taken with alcohol).

No products indexed under this heading.

Thioridazine (Concomitant use of phenothiazines with hydromorphone, may produce an additive depressant effect. Respiratory depression, hypotension and profound sedation or coma may occur. When such combined therapy is contemplated, the dose of one or both agents should be reduced. Administer with caution to patients in circulatory shock, since vasodilation produced by the drug may further reduce cardiac output and blood pressure).

No products indexed under this heading.

Thioridazine Hydrochloride (Concomitant use of phenothiazines with hydromorphone, may produce an additive depressant effect. Respiratory depression, hypotension and profound

sedation or coma may occur. When such combined therapy is contemplated, the dose of one or both agents should be reduced. Administer with caution to patients in circulatory shock, since vasodilation produced by the drug may further reduce cardiac output and blood pressure). Products include:

Thioridazine Hydrochloride 2384

Thiothixene (Concomitant use of tranquilizers with hydromorphone, may produce an additive depressant effect. Respiratory depression, hypotension and profound sedation or coma may occur. When such combined therapy is contemplated, the dose of one or both agents should be reduced). Products include:

Thiothixene 2386

Thiothixene Hydrochloride (Concomitant use of other central nervous system depressants, including sedatives or hypnotics, general anesthetics, phenothiazines, tranquilizers and alcohol with hydromorphone, may produce an additive depressant effect. Respiratory depression, hypotension and profound sedation or coma may occur. When such combined therapy is contemplated, the dose of one or both agents should be reduced. Hydromorphone should not be taken with alcohol).

No products indexed under this heading.

Triazolam (Concomitant use of other central nervous system depressants, including sedatives or hypnotics with hydromorphone, may produce an additive depressant effect. Respiratory depression, hypotension and profound sedation or coma may occur. When such combined therapy is contemplated, the dose of one or both agents should be reduced.)

No products indexed under this heading.

Trifluoperazine Hydrochloride (Concomitant use of phenothiazines with hydromorphone, may produce an additive depressant effect. Respiratory depression, hypotension and profound sedation or coma may occur. When such combined therapy is contemplated, the dose of one or both agents should be reduced. Administer with caution to patients in circulatory shock, since vasodilation produced by the drug may further reduce cardiac output and blood pressure).

No products indexed under this heading.

Tubocurarine Chloride (Opioid analgesics, including hydromorphone, may enhance the action of neuromuscular blocking agents and produce an excessive degree of respiratory depression).

No products indexed under this heading.

Vecuronium Bromide (Opioid analgesics, including hydromorphone, may enhance the action of neuromuscular blocking agents and produce an excessive degree of respiratory depression).

No products indexed under this heading.

Zaleplon (Concomitant use of other central nervous system depressants, including sedatives or hypnotics with hydromorphone, may produce an additive depressant effect. Respiratory depression, hypotension and profound sedation or coma may occur. When such combined therapy is contemplated, the dose of one or both agents should be reduced.)

No products indexed under this heading.

Ziprasidone Hydrochloride (Concomitant use of other central nervous system depressants, including sedatives or hypnotics, general anesthetics, phenothiazines, tranquilizers and alcohol with hydromorphone, may produce an additive depressant effect. Respiratory depression, hypotension and profound sedation or coma may occur. When such combined therapy is contemplated, the dose of one or both

467 Interactions Index Dilaudid-HP

agents should be reduced. Hydromorphone should not be taken with alcohol). Products include:
Geodon 2723

Zolpidem Tartrate (Concomitant use of other central nervous system depressants, including sedatives or hypnotics with hydromorphone, may produce an additive depressant effect. Respiratory depression, hypotension and profound sedation or coma may occur. When such combined therapy is contemplated, the dose of one or both agents should be reduced). Products include:
Ambien 2920
Ambien CR 2925

Food Interactions

Alcohol (Hydromorphone may be expected to have additive effects when used in conjunction with alcohol. Alcohol potentiates the respiratory depressant effects of hydromorphone, increasing the risk of respiratory depression that might result in death).

Beer, reduced-alcohol (Hydromorphone may be expected to have additive effects when used in conjunction with alcohol. Alcohol potentiates the respiratory depressant effects of hydromorphone, increasing the risk of respiratory depression that might result in death).

Beer, unspecified (Hydromorphone may be expected to have additive effects when used in conjunction with alcohol. Alcohol potentiates the respiratory depressant effects of hydromorphone, increasing the risk of respiratory depression that might result in death).

Food, unspecified (In a study conducted with a single 8 mg dose of hydromorphone (2 mg tablets), food lowered C_{max} by 25%, prolonged T_{max} by 0.8 hour, and increased AUC by 35%. The effects may not be clinically relevant).

Meal, unspecified (In a study conducted with a single 8 mg dose of hydromorphone (2 mg tablets), food lowered C_{max} by 25%, prolonged T_{max} by 0.8 hour, and increased AUC by 35%. The effects may not be clinically relevant).

Wine, Chianti (Hydromorphone may be expected to have additive effects when used in conjunction with alcohol. Alcohol potentiates the respiratory depressant effects of hydromorphone, increasing the risk of respiratory depression that might result in death).

Wine, Red (Hydromorphone may be expected to have additive effects when used in conjunction with alcohol. Alcohol potentiates the respiratory depressant effects of hydromorphone, increasing the risk of respiratory depression that might result in death).

Wine, unspecified (Hydromorphone may be expected to have additive effects when used in conjunction with alcohol. Alcohol potentiates the respiratory depressant effects of hydromorphone, increasing the risk of respiratory depression that might result in death).

Wine products (Hydromorphone may be expected to have additive effects when used in conjunction with alcohol. Alcohol potentiates the respiratory depressant effects of hydromorphone, increasing the risk of respiratory depression that might result in death).

DILAUDID TABLETS
(Hydromorphone Hydrochloride) 2797
See Dilaudid Oral Liquid

DILAUDID-HP INJECTION
(Hydromorphone Hydrochloride) 2800
May interact with alcohols, central nervous system depressants, general anesthetics, hypnotics and sedatives, mixed agonist/antagonist opioid analgesics, narcotic analgesics, neuromuscular blocking agents, phenothiazines, skeletal muscle relaxants, tranquilizers, and certain other agents. Compounds in these categories include:

Alfentanil Hydrochloride (Concomitant use of other central nervous system depressants, including sedatives or hypnotics, general anesthetics, phenothiazines, tranquilizers and alcohol with hydromorphone, may produce an additive depressant effect. Respiratory depression, hypotension and profound sedation or coma may occur. When such combined therapy is contemplated, the dose of one or both agents should be reduced. Hydromorphone should not be taken with alcohol).
No products indexed under this heading.

Alprazolam (Concomitant use of tranquilizers with hydromorphone, may produce an additive depressant effect. Respiratory depression, hypotension and profound sedation or coma may occur. When such combined therapy is contemplated, the dose of one or both agents should be reduced).
No products indexed under this heading.

Amobarbital (Concomitant use of other central nervous system depressants, including sedatives or hypnotics, general anesthetics, phenothiazines, tranquilizers and alcohol with hydromorphone, may produce an additive depressant effect. Respiratory depression, hypotension and profound sedation or coma may occur. When such combined therapy is contemplated, the dose of one or both agents should be reduced. Hydromorphone should not be taken with alcohol).
No products indexed under this heading.

Amobarbital Sodium (Concomitant use of other central nervous system depressants, including sedatives or hypnotics, general anesthetics, phenothiazines, tranquilizers and alcohol with hydromorphone, may produce an additive depressant effect. Respiratory depression, hypotension and profound sedation or coma may occur. When such combined therapy is contemplated, the dose of one or both agents should be reduced. Hydromorphone should not be taken with alcohol).
No products indexed under this heading.

Apomorphine (Hydromorphone may be expected to have additive effects when used in conjunction with other opioids or illicit drugs that cause central nervous depression. Additional opioids potentiate the respiratory depressant effects of hydromorphone, increasing the risk of respiratory depression that might result in death).
No products indexed under this heading.

Apomorphine Hydrochloride (Hydromorphone may be expected to have additive effects when used in conjunction with other opioids or illicit drugs that cause central nervous depression. Additional opioids potentiate the respiratory depressant effects of hydromorphone, increasing the risk of respiratory depression that might result in death).
No products indexed under this heading.

Aprobarbital (Concomitant use of other central nervous system depressants, including sedatives or hypnotics, general anesthetics, phenothiazines, tranquilizers and alcohol with hydromorphone, may produce an additive depressant effect. Respiratory depression, hypotension and profound sedation or coma may occur. When such combined therapy is contemplated, the dose of one or both agents should be reduced. Hydromorphone should not be taken with alcohol).
No products indexed under this heading.

Atracurium Besylate (Opioid analgesics, including hydromorphone, may enhance the action of neuromuscular blocking agents and produce an excessive degree of respiratory depression).
No products indexed under this heading.

Baclofen (Other central nervous system depressants (eg, skeletal muscle relaxants) can potentiate the respiratory-depressant effects of hydromorphone and increase the risk of adverse outcomes, including death).
No products indexed under this heading.

Buprenorphine Hydrochloride (Concomitant use of other central nervous system depressants, including sedatives or hypnotics, general anesthetics, phenothiazines, tranquilizers and alcohol with hydromorphone, may produce an additive depressant effect. Respiratory depression, hypotension and profound sedation or coma may occur. When such combined therapy is contemplated, the dose of one or both agents should be reduced. Hydromorphone should not be taken with alcohol).
No products indexed under this heading.

Buspirone Hydrochloride (Concomitant use of tranquilizers with hydromorphone, may produce an additive depressant effect. Respiratory depression, hypotension and profound sedation or coma may occur. When such combined therapy is contemplated, the dose of one or both agents should be reduced).
No products indexed under this heading.

Butabarbital (Concomitant use of other central nervous system depressants, including sedatives or hypnotics with hydromorphone, may produce an additive depressant effect. Respiratory depression, hypotension and profound sedation or coma may occur. When such combined therapy is contemplated, the dose of one or both agents should be reduced).
No products indexed under this heading.

Butabarbital Sodium (Concomitant use of other central nervous system depressants, including sedatives or hypnotics with hydromorphone, may produce an additive depressant effect. Respiratory depression, hypotension and profound sedation or coma may occur. When such combined therapy is contemplated, the dose of one or both agents should be reduced).
No products indexed under this heading.

Butalbital (Concomitant use of other central nervous system depressants, including sedatives or hypnotics with hydromorphone, may produce an additive depressant effect. Respiratory depression, hypotension and profound sedation or coma may occur. When such combined therapy is contemplated, the dose of one or both agents should be reduced).
No products indexed under this heading.

Butorphanol Tartrate (Agonist/antagonist analgesics (eg, pentazocine, nalbuphine, butorphanol, buprenorphine) should be administered with caution to a patient who has received or is receiving a course of therapy with a pure opioid agonist analgesic such as hydromorphone. In this situation, mixed agonist/antagonist analgesics may reduce the analgesic effect of hydromorphone and/or may precipitate withdrawal symptoms in these patients).
No products indexed under this heading.

Carisoprodol (Other central nervous system depressants (eg, skeletal muscle relaxants) can potentiate the respiratory-depressant effects of hydromorphone and increase the risk of adverse outcomes, including death).
No products indexed under this heading.

Chloral Hydrate (Concomitant use of other central nervous system depressants, including sedatives or hypnotics with hydromorphone, may produce an additive depressant effect. Respiratory depression, hypotension and profound sedation or coma may occur. When such combined therapy is contemplated, the dose of one or both agents should be reduced).
No products indexed under this heading.

Chlordiazepoxide (Concomitant use of tranquilizers with hydromorphone, may produce an additive depressant effect. Respiratory depression, hypotension and profound sedation or coma may occur. When such combined therapy is contemplated, the dose of one or both agents should be reduced).
No products indexed under this heading.

Chlordiazepoxide Hydrochloride (Concomitant use of tranquilizers with hydromorphone, may produce an additive depressant effect. Respiratory depression, hypotension and profound sedation or coma may occur. When such combined therapy is contemplated, the dose of one or both agents should be reduced).
No products indexed under this heading.

Chlorpromazine (Concomitant use of phenothiazines with hydromorphone, may produce an additive depressant effect. Respiratory depression, hypotension and profound sedation or coma may occur. When such combined therapy is contemplated, the dose of one or both agents should be reduced. Administer with caution to patients in circulatory shock, since vasodilation produced by the drug may further reduce cardiac output and blood pressure).
No products indexed under this heading.

Chlorpromazine Hydrochloride (Concomitant use of phenothiazines with hydromorphone, may produce an additive depressant effect. Respiratory depression, hypotension and profound sedation or coma may occur. When such combined therapy is contemplated, the dose of one or both agents should be reduced. Administer with caution to patients in circulatory shock, since vasodilation produced by the drug may further reduce cardiac output and blood pressure).
No products indexed under this heading.

Chlorprothixene (Concomitant use of tranquilizers with hydromorphone, may produce an additive depressant effect. Respiratory depression, hypotension and profound sedation or coma may occur. When such combined therapy is contemplated, the dose of one or both agents should be reduced).
No products indexed under this heading.

Chlorprothixene Hydrochloride (Concomitant use of tranquilizers with hydromorphone, may produce an additive depressant effect. Respiratory depression, hypotension and profound sedation or coma may occur. When such combined therapy is contemplated, the dose of one or both agents should be reduced).
No products indexed under this heading.

Chlorprothixene Lactate (Concomitant use of tranquilizers with hydromorphone, may produce an additive depressant effect. Respiratory depression, hypotension and profound sedation or coma may occur. When such combined therapy is contemplated, the dose of one or both agents should be reduced).
No products indexed under this heading.

Chlorzoxazone (Other central nervous system depressants (eg, skeletal muscle relaxants) can potentiate the respiratory-depressant effects of hydromorphone and increase the risk of adverse outcomes, including death).
No products indexed under this heading.

IMPORTANT NOTE: Always consult each drug listing in the patient's regimen for possible interactions.

Cisatracurium Besylate (Opioid analgesics, including hydromorphone, may enhance the action of neuromuscular blocking agents and produce an excessive degree of respiratory depression). Products include:
Nimbex 503

Clonazepam (Concomitant use of other central nervous system depressants, including sedatives or hypnotics, general anesthetics, phenothiazines, tranquilizers and alcohol with hydromorphone, may produce an additive depressant effect. Respiratory depression, hypotension and profound sedation or coma may occur. When such combined therapy is contemplated, the dose of one or both agents should be reduced. Hydromorphone should not be taken with alcohol). Products include:
Klonopin 2855

Clorazepate Dipotassium (Concomitant use of tranquilizers with hydromorphone, may produce an additive depressant effect. Respiratory depression, hypotension and profound sedation or coma may occur. When such combined therapy is contemplated, the dose of one or both agents should be reduced).
No products indexed under this heading.

Clozapine (Concomitant use of other central nervous system depressants, including sedatives or hypnotics, general anesthetics, phenothiazines, tranquilizers and alcohol with hydromorphone, may produce an additive depressant effect. Respiratory depression, hypotension and profound sedation or coma may occur. When such combined therapy is contemplated, the dose of one or both agents should be reduced. Hydromorphone should not be taken with alcohol).
No products indexed under this heading.

Codeine Phosphate (Concomitant use of other central nervous system depressants, including sedatives or hypnotics, general anesthetics, phenothiazines, tranquilizers and alcohol with hydromorphone, may produce an additive depressant effect. Respiratory depression, hypotension and profound sedation or coma may occur. When such combined therapy is contemplated, the dose of one or both agents should be reduced. Hydromorphone should not be taken with alcohol). Products include:
Tylenol with Codeine 2691

Codeine Sulfate (Concomitant use of other central nervous system depressants, including sedatives or hypnotics, general anesthetics, phenothiazines, tranquilizers and alcohol with hydromorphone, may produce an additive depressant effect. Respiratory depression, hypotension and profound sedation or coma may occur. When such combined therapy is contemplated, the dose of one or both agents should be reduced. Hydromorphone should not be taken with alcohol).
No products indexed under this heading.

Cyclobenzaprine Hydrochloride (Other central nervous system depressants (eg, skeletal muscle relaxants) can potentiate the respiratory-depressant effects of hydromorphone and increase the risk of adverse outcomes, including death). Products include:
Amrix 964

Dantrolene Sodium (Other central nervous system depressants (eg, skeletal muscle relaxants) can potentiate the respiratory-depressant effects of hydromorphone and increase the risk of adverse outcomes, including death).
No products indexed under this heading.

Decamethonium (Opioid analgesics, including hydromorphone, may enhance the action of neuromuscular blocking agents and produce an excessive degree of respiratory depression).
No products indexed under this heading.

Desflurane (Concomitant use of general anesthetics with hydromorphone, may produce an additive depressant effect. Respiratory depression, hypotension and profound sedation or coma may occur. When such combined therapy is contemplated, the dose of one or both agents should be reduced. Administer with caution to patients in circulatory shock, since vasodilation produced by the drug may further reduce cardiac output and blood pressure).
No products indexed under this heading.

Dezocine (Concomitant use of other central nervous system depressants, including sedatives or hypnotics, general anesthetics, phenothiazines, tranquilizers and alcohol with hydromorphone, may produce an additive depressant effect. Respiratory depression, hypotension and profound sedation or coma may occur. When such combined therapy is contemplated, the dose of one or both agents should be reduced. Hydromorphone should not be taken with alcohol).
No products indexed under this heading.

Diazepam (Concomitant use of tranquilizers with hydromorphone, may produce an additive depressant effect. Respiratory depression, hypotension and profound sedation or coma may occur. When such combined therapy is contemplated, the dose of one or both agents should be reduced). Products include:
Valium Tablets 2880

Dihydrocodeine Bitartrate (Hydromorphone may be expected to have additive effects when used in conjunction with other opioids or illicit drugs that cause central nervous depression. Additional opioids potentiate the respiratory depressant effects of hydromorphone, increasing the risk of respiratory depression that might result in death).
No products indexed under this heading.

Dihydrocodeinone Bitartrate (Hydromorphone may be expected to have additive effects when used in conjunction with other opioids or illicit drugs that cause central nervous depression. Additional opioids potentiate the respiratory depressant effects of hydromorphone, increasing the risk of respiratory depression that might result in death).
No products indexed under this heading.

Doxacurium Chloride (Opioid analgesics, including hydromorphone, may enhance the action of neuromuscular blocking agents and produce an excessive degree of respiratory depression).
No products indexed under this heading.

Droperidol (Concomitant use of tranquilizers with hydromorphone, may produce an additive depressant effect. Respiratory depression, hypotension and profound sedation or coma may occur. When such combined therapy is contemplated, the dose of one or both agents should be reduced).
No products indexed under this heading.

d-Tubocurarine (Opioid analgesics, including hydromorphone, may enhance the action of neuromuscular blocking agents and produce an excessive degree of respiratory depression).
No products indexed under this heading.

Enflurane (Concomitant use of general anesthetics with hydromorphone, may produce an additive depressant effect. Respiratory depression, hypotension and profound sedation or coma may occur. When such combined thera-

py is contemplated, the dose of one or both agents should be reduced. Administer with caution to patients in circulatory shock, since vasodilation produced by the drug may further reduce cardiac output and blood pressure).
No products indexed under this heading.

Estazolam (Concomitant use of other central nervous system depressants, including sedatives or hypnotics with hydromorphone, may produce an additive depressant effect. Respiratory depression, hypotension and profound sedation or coma may occur. When such combined therapy is contemplated, the dose of one or both agents should be reduced).
No products indexed under this heading.

Ethanol (Ethanol, other opioids, and other central nervous system depressants (eg, sedative-hypnotics, skeletal muscle relaxants) can potentiate the respiratory-depressant effects of hydromorphone and increase the risk of adverse outcomes, including death).
No products indexed under this heading.

Ethchlorvynol (Concomitant use of other central nervous system depressants, including sedatives or hypnotics with hydromorphone, may produce an additive depressant effect. Respiratory depression, hypotension and profound sedation or coma may occur. When such combined therapy is contemplated, the dose of one or both agents should be reduced).
No products indexed under this heading.

Ethinamate (Concomitant use of other central nervous system depressants, including sedatives or hypnotics with hydromorphone, may produce an additive depressant effect. Respiratory depression, hypotension and profound sedation or coma may occur. When such combined therapy is contemplated, the dose of one or both agents should be reduced).
No products indexed under this heading.

Ethyl Alcohol (Hydromorphone may be expected to have additive effects when used in conjunction with alcohol. Alcohol potentiates the respiratory depressant effects of hydromorphone, increasing the risk of respiratory depression that might result in death).
No products indexed under this heading.

Fentanyl (Concomitant use of other central nervous system depressants, including sedatives or hypnotics, general anesthetics, phenothiazines, tranquilizers and alcohol with hydromorphone, may produce an additive depressant effect. Respiratory depression, hypotension and profound sedation or coma may occur. When such combined therapy is contemplated, the dose of one or both agents should be reduced. Hydromorphone should not be taken with alcohol). Products include:
Duragesic 2604
Fentanyl Transdermal System 2346
Onsolis 2054

Fentanyl Citrate (Concomitant use of other central nervous system depressants, including sedatives or hypnotics, general anesthetics, phenothiazines, tranquilizers and alcohol with hydromorphone, may produce an additive depressant effect. Respiratory depression, hypotension and profound sedation or coma may occur. When such combined therapy is contemplated, the dose of one or both agents should be reduced. Hydromorphone should not be taken with alcohol). Products include:
Fentora 966

Fluphenazine Decanoate (Concomitant use of phenothiazines with hydromorphone, may produce an additive depressant effect. Respiratory depression, hypotension and profound sedation or coma may occur. When such

combined therapy is contemplated, the dose of one or both agents should be reduced. Administer with caution to patients in circulatory shock, since vasodilation produced by the drug may further reduce cardiac output and blood pressure).
No products indexed under this heading.

Fluphenazine Enanthate (Concomitant use of phenothiazines with hydromorphone, may produce an additive depressant effect. Respiratory depression, hypotension and profound sedation or coma may occur. When such combined therapy is contemplated, the dose of one or both agents should be reduced. Administer with caution to patients in circulatory shock, since vasodilation produced by the drug may further reduce cardiac output and blood pressure).
No products indexed under this heading.

Fluphenazine Hydrochloride (Concomitant use of phenothiazines with hydromorphone, may produce an additive depressant effect. Respiratory depression, hypotension and profound sedation or coma may occur. When such combined therapy is contemplated, the dose of one or both agents should be reduced. Administer with caution to patients in circulatory shock, since vasodilation produced by the drug may further reduce cardiac output and blood pressure).
No products indexed under this heading.

Flurazepam Hydrochloride (Concomitant use of other central nervous system depressants, including sedatives or hypnotics with hydromorphone, may produce an additive depressant effect. Respiratory depression, hypotension and profound sedation or coma may occur. When such combined therapy is contemplated, the dose of one or both agents should be reduced).
No products indexed under this heading.

Gallamine (Opioid analgesics, including hydromorphone, may enhance the action of neuromuscular blocking agents and produce an excessive degree of respiratory depression).
No products indexed under this heading.

Gallamine Triethiodide (Opioid analgesics, including hydromorphone, may enhance the action of neuromuscular blocking agents and produce an excessive degree of respiratory depression).
No products indexed under this heading.

Glutethimide (Concomitant use of other central nervous system depressants, including sedatives or hypnotics with hydromorphone, may produce an additive depressant effect. Respiratory depression, hypotension and profound sedation or coma may occur. When such combined therapy is contemplated, the dose of one or both agents should be reduced).
No products indexed under this heading.

Halazepam (Concomitant use of other central nervous system depressants, including sedatives or hypnotics, general anesthetics, phenothiazines, tranquilizers and alcohol with hydromorphone, may produce an additive depressant effect. Respiratory depression, hypotension and profound sedation or coma may occur. When such combined therapy is contemplated, the dose of one or both agents should be reduced. Hydromorphone should not be taken with alcohol).
No products indexed under this heading.

Haloperidol (Concomitant use of tranquilizers with hydromorphone, may produce an additive depressant effect. Respiratory depression, hypotension and profound sedation or coma may occur. When such combined therapy is contemplated, the dose of one or both agents should be reduced).
No products indexed under this heading.

Haloperidol Decanoate (Concomitant use of tranquilizers with hydromorphone, may produce an additive depressant effect. Respiratory depression, hypotension and profound sedation or coma may occur. When such combined therapy is contemplated, the dose of one or both agents should be reduced).
No products indexed under this heading.

Haloperidol Lactate (Concomitant use of other central nervous system depressants, including sedatives or hypnotics, general anesthetics, phenothiazines, tranquilizers and alcohol with hydromorphone, may produce an additive depressant effect. Respiratory depression, hypotension and profound sedation or coma may occur. When such combined therapy is contemplated, the dose of one or both agents should be reduced. Hydromorphone should not be taken with alcohol).
No products indexed under this heading.

Halothane (Concomitant use of general anesthetics with hydromorphone, may produce an additive depressant effect. Respiratory depression, hypotension and profound sedation or coma may occur. When such combined therapy is contemplated, the dose of one or both agents should be reduced. Administer with caution to patients in circulatory shock, since vasodilation produced by the drug may further reduce cardiac output and blood pressure).
No products indexed under this heading.

Hexobarbital (Concomitant use of other central nervous system depressants, including sedatives or hypnotics, general anesthetics, phenothiazines, tranquilizers and alcohol with hydromorphone, may produce an additive depressant effect. Respiratory depression, hypotension and profound sedation or coma may occur. When such combined therapy is contemplated, the dose of one or both agents should be reduced. Hydromorphone should not be taken with alcohol).
No products indexed under this heading.

Hydrocodone Bitartrate (Concomitant use of other central nervous system depressants, including sedatives or hypnotics, general anesthetics, phenothiazines, tranquilizers and alcohol with hydromorphone, may produce an additive depressant effect. Respiratory depression, hypotension and profound sedation or coma may occur. When such combined therapy is contemplated, the dose of one or both agents should be reduced. Hydromorphone should not be taken with alcohol).
Products include:
Vicodin **560**
Vicodin ES **561**
Vicodin HP **563**
Vicoprofen **564**
Zydone **1138**

Hydrocodone Polistirex (Concomitant use of other central nervous system depressants, including sedatives or hypnotics, general anesthetics, phenothiazines, tranquilizers and alcohol with hydromorphone, may produce an additive depressant effect. Respiratory depression, hypotension and profound sedation or coma may occur. When such combined therapy is contemplated, the dose of one or both agents should be reduced. Hydromorphone should not be taken with alcohol).
Products include:
Tussionex **3443**

Hydromorphone (Concomitant use of other central nervous system depressants, including sedatives or hypnotics, general anesthetics, phenothiazines, tranquilizers and alcohol with hydromorphone, may produce an additive depressant effect. Respiratory depression, hypotension and profound sedation or coma may occur. When such combined therapy is contemplated, the dose of one or both agents should be reduced. Hydromorphone should not be taken with alcohol).
No products indexed under this heading.

Hydroxyzine Hydrochloride (Concomitant use of tranquilizers with hydromorphone, may produce an additive depressant effect. Respiratory depression, hypotension and profound sedation or coma may occur. When such combined therapy is contemplated, the dose of one or both agents should be reduced).
No products indexed under this heading.

Isoflurane (Concomitant use of general anesthetics with hydromorphone, may produce an additive depressant effect. Respiratory depression, hypotension and profound sedation or coma may occur. When such combined therapy is contemplated, the dose of one or both agents should be reduced. Administer with caution to patients in circulatory shock, since vasodilation produced by the drug may further reduce cardiac output and blood pressure).
No products indexed under this heading.

Ketamine Hydrochloride (Concomitant use of general anesthetics with hydromorphone, may produce an additive depressant effect. Respiratory depression, hypotension and profound sedation or coma may occur. When such combined therapy is contemplated, the dose of one or both agents should be reduced. Administer with caution to patients in circulatory shock, since vasodilation produced by the drug may further reduce cardiac output and blood pressure).
No products indexed under this heading.

Levomethadyl Acetate Hydrochloride (Concomitant use of other central nervous system depressants, including sedatives or hypnotics, general anesthetics, phenothiazines, tranquilizers and alcohol with hydromorphone, may produce an additive depressant effect. Respiratory depression, hypotension and profound sedation or coma may occur. When such combined therapy is contemplated, the dose of one or both agents should be reduced. Hydromorphone should not be taken with alcohol).
No products indexed under this heading.

Levorphanol Tartrate (Concomitant use of other central nervous system depressants, including sedatives or hypnotics, general anesthetics, phenothiazines, tranquilizers and alcohol with hydromorphone, may produce an additive depressant effect. Respiratory depression, hypotension and profound sedation or coma may occur. When such combined therapy is contemplated, the dose of one or both agents should be reduced. Hydromorphone should not be taken with alcohol).
No products indexed under this heading.

Lorazepam (Concomitant use of other central nervous system depressants, including sedatives or hypnotics with hydromorphone, may produce an additive depressant effect. Respiratory depression, hypotension and profound sedation or coma may occur. When such combined therapy is contemplated, the dose of one or both agents should be reduced).
No products indexed under this heading.

Loxapine Hydrochloride (Concomitant use of tranquilizers with hydromorphone, may produce an additive depressant effect. Respiratory depression, hypotension and profound sedation or coma may occur. When such combined therapy is contemplated, the dose of one or both agents should be reduced).
No products indexed under this heading.

Loxapine Succinate (Concomitant use of tranquilizers with hydromorphone, may produce an additive depressant effect. Respiratory depression, hypotension and profound sedation or coma may occur. When such combined therapy is contemplated, the dose of one or both agents should be reduced).
No products indexed under this heading.

Meperidine Hydrochloride (Concomitant use of other central nervous system depressants, including sedatives or hypnotics, general anesthetics, phenothiazines, tranquilizers and alcohol with hydromorphone, may produce an additive depressant effect. Respiratory depression, hypotension and profound sedation or coma may occur. When such combined therapy is contemplated, the dose of one or both agents should be reduced. Hydromorphone should not be taken with alcohol).
No products indexed under this heading.

Mephobarbital (Concomitant use of other central nervous system depressants, including sedatives or hypnotics, general anesthetics, phenothiazines, tranquilizers and alcohol with hydromorphone, may produce an additive depressant effect. Respiratory depression, hypotension and profound sedation or coma may occur. When such combined therapy is contemplated, the dose of one or both agents should be reduced. Hydromorphone should not be taken with alcohol).
No products indexed under this heading.

Meprobamate (Concomitant use of tranquilizers with hydromorphone, may produce an additive depressant effect. Respiratory depression, hypotension and profound sedation or coma may occur. When such combined therapy is contemplated, the dose of one or both agents should be reduced).
No products indexed under this heading.

Mesoridazine Besylate (Concomitant use of phenothiazines with hydromorphone, may produce an additive depressant effect. Respiratory depression, hypotension and profound sedation or coma may occur. When such combined therapy is contemplated, the dose of one or both agents should be reduced. Administer with caution to patients in circulatory shock, since vasodilation produced by the drug may further reduce cardiac output and blood pressure).
No products indexed under this heading.

Metaxalone (Other central nervous system depressants (eg, skeletal muscle relaxants) can potentiate the respiratory-depressant effects of hydromorphone and increase the risk of adverse outcomes, including death).
Products include:
Skelaxin **1848**

Methadone Hydrochloride (Concomitant use of other central nervous system depressants, including sedatives or hypnotics, general anesthetics, phenothiazines, tranquilizers and alcohol with hydromorphone, may produce an additive depressant effect. Respiratory depression, hypotension and profound sedation or coma may occur. When such combined therapy is contemplated, the dose of one or both agents should be reduced. Hydromorphone should not be taken with alcohol).
No products indexed under this heading.

Methocarbamol (Other central nervous system depressants (eg, skeletal muscle relaxants) can potentiate the respiratory-depressant effects of hydromorphone and increase the risk of adverse outcomes, including death).
No products indexed under this heading.

Methohexital Sodium (Concomitant use of general anesthetics with hydromorphone, may produce an additive depressant effect. Respiratory depression, hypotension and profound sedation or coma may occur. When such combined therapy is contemplated, the dose of one or both agents should be reduced. Administer with caution to patients in circulatory shock, since vasodilation produced by the drug may further reduce cardiac output and blood pressure).
No products indexed under this heading.

Methotrimeprazine (Concomitant use of phenothiazines with hydromorphone, may produce an additive depressant effect. Respiratory depression, hypotension and profound sedation or coma may occur. When such combined therapy is contemplated, the dose of one or both agents should be reduced. Administer with caution to patients in circulatory shock, since vasodilation produced by the drug may further reduce cardiac output and blood pressure).
No products indexed under this heading.

Methoxyflurane (Concomitant use of general anesthetics with hydromorphone, may produce an additive depressant effect. Respiratory depression, hypotension and profound sedation or coma may occur. When such combined therapy is contemplated, the dose of one or both agents should be reduced. Administer with caution to patients in circulatory shock, since vasodilation produced by the drug may further reduce cardiac output and blood pressure).
No products indexed under this heading.

Metocurine Iodide (Opioid analgesics, including hydromorphone, may enhance the action of neuromuscular blocking agents and produce an excessive degree of respiratory depression).
No products indexed under this heading.

Midazolam Hydrochloride (Concomitant use of other central nervous system depressants, including sedatives or hypnotics with hydromorphone, may produce an additive depressant effect. Respiratory depression, hypotension and profound sedation or coma may occur. When such combined therapy is contemplated, the dose of one or both agents should be reduced).
No products indexed under this heading.

Mivacurium Chloride (Opioid analgesics, including hydromorphone, may enhance the action of neuromuscular blocking agents and produce an excessive degree of respiratory depression).
No products indexed under this heading.

Molindone Hydrochloride (Concomitant use of tranquilizers with hydromorphone, may produce an additive depressant effect. Respiratory depression, hypotension and profound sedation or coma may occur. When such combined therapy is contemplated, the dose of one or both agents should be reduced).
Products include:
Moban **1108**

Morphine Sulfate (Concomitant use of other central nervous system depressants, including sedatives or hypnotics, general anesthetics, phenothiazines, tranquilizers and alcohol with hydromorphone, may produce an additive depressant effect. Respiratory depression, hypotension and profound sedation or coma may occur. When such combined therapy is contemplated, the dose of

IMPORTANT NOTE: Always consult each drug listing in the patient's regimen for possible interactions.

one or both agents should be reduced. Hydromorphone should not be taken with alcohol). Products include:

Morphine Sulfate, Liposomal (Concomitant use of other central nervous system depressants, including sedatives or hypnotics, general anesthetics, phenothiazines, tranquilizers and alcohol with hydromorphone, may produce an additive depressant effect. Respiratory depression, hypotension and profound sedation or coma may occur. When such combined therapy is contemplated, the dose of one or both agents should be reduced. Hydromorphone should not be taken with alcohol).
No products indexed under this heading.

Nalbuphine Hydrochloride (Agonist/antagonist analgesics (eg, pentazocine, nalbuphine, butorphanol, buprenorphine) should be administered with caution to a patient who has received or is receiving a course of therapy with a pure opioid agonist analgesic such as hydromorphone. In this situation, mixed agonist/antagonist analgesics may reduce the analgesic effect of hydromorphone and/or may precipitate withdrawal symptoms in these patients).
No products indexed under this heading.

Nitrous Oxide (Concomitant use of general anesthetics with hydromorphone, may produce an additive depressant effect. Respiratory depression, hypotension and profound sedation or coma may occur. When such combined therapy is contemplated, the dose of one or both agents should be reduced. Administer with caution to patients in circulatory shock, since vasodilation produced by the drug may further reduce cardiac output and blood pressure).
No products indexed under this heading.

Olanzapine (Concomitant use of other central nervous system depressants, including sedatives or hypnotics, general anesthetics, phenothiazines, tranquilizers and alcohol with hydromorphone, may produce an additive depressant effect. Respiratory depression, hypotension and profound sedation or coma may occur. When such combined therapy is contemplated, the dose of one or both agents should be reduced. Hydromorphone should not be taken with alcohol). Products include:

Orphenadrine Citrate (Other central nervous system depressants (eg, skeletal muscle relaxants) can potentiate the respiratory-depressant effects of hydromorphone and increase the risk of adverse outcomes, including death).
No products indexed under this heading.

Oxazepam (Concomitant use of tranquilizers with hydromorphone, may produce an additive depressant effect. Respiratory depression, hypotension and profound sedation or coma may occur. When such combined therapy is contemplated, the dose of one or both agents should be reduced).
No products indexed under this heading.

Oxycodone Hydrochloride (Concomitant use of other central nervous system depressants, including sedatives or hypnotics, general anesthetics, phenothiazines, tranquilizers and alcohol with hydromorphone, may produce an additive depressant effect. Respiratory depression, hypotension and profound sedation or coma may occur. When such combined therapy is contemplated, the dose of one or both

agents should be reduced. Hydromorphone should not be taken with alcohol). Products include:

Oxycodone Terephthalate (Concomitant use of other central nervous system depressants, including sedatives or hypnotics, general anesthetics, phenothiazines, tranquilizers and alcohol with hydromorphone, may produce an additive depressant effect. Respiratory depression, hypotension and profound sedation or coma may occur. When such combined therapy is contemplated, the dose of one or both agents should be reduced. Hydromorphone should not be taken with alcohol).
No products indexed under this heading.

Oxymorphone Hydrochloride (Concomitant use of other central nervous system depressants, including sedatives or hypnotics, general anesthetics, phenothiazines, tranquilizers and alcohol with hydromorphone, may produce an additive depressant effect. Respiratory depression, hypotension and profound sedation or coma may occur. When such combined therapy is contemplated, the dose of one or both agents should be reduced. Hydromorphone should not be taken with alcohol). Products include:

Pancuronium Bromide (Opioid analgesics, including hydromorphone, may enhance the action of neuromuscular blocking agents and produce an excessive degree of respiratory depression).
No products indexed under this heading.

Pentazocine Hydrochloride (Agonist/antagonist analgesics (eg, pentazocine, nalbuphine, butorphanol, buprenorphine) should be administered with caution to a patient who has received or is receiving a course of therapy with a pure opioid agonist analgesic such as hydromorphone. In this situation, mixed agonist/antagonist analgesics may reduce the analgesic effect of hydromorphone and/or may precipitate withdrawal symptoms in these patients).
No products indexed under this heading.

Pentazocine Lactate (Agonist/antagonist analgesics (eg, pentazocine, nalbuphine, butorphanol, buprenorphine) should be administered with caution to a patient who has received or is receiving a course of therapy with a pure opioid agonist analgesic such as hydromorphone. In this situation, mixed agonist/antagonist analgesics may reduce the analgesic effect of hydromorphone and/or may precipitate withdrawal symptoms in these patients).
No products indexed under this heading.

Pentobarbital (Concomitant use of other central nervous system depressants, including sedatives or hypnotics, general anesthetics, phenothiazines, tranquilizers and alcohol with hydromorphone, may produce an additive depressant effect. Respiratory depression, hypotension and profound sedation or coma may occur. When such combined therapy is contemplated, the dose of one or both agents should be reduced. Hydromorphone should not be taken with alcohol).
No products indexed under this heading.

Pentobarbital Sodium (Concomitant use of other central nervous system depressants, including sedatives or hypnotics, general anesthetics, phenothiazines, tranquilizers and alcohol with hydromorphone, may produce an additive depressant effect. Respiratory depression, hypotension and profound sedation or coma may occur. When

such combined therapy is contemplated, the dose of one or both agents should be reduced. Hydromorphone should not be taken with alcohol). Products include:

Perphenazine (Concomitant use of phenothiazines with hydromorphone, may produce an additive depressant effect. Respiratory depression, hypotension and profound sedation or coma may occur. When such combined therapy is contemplated, the dose of one or both agents should be reduced. Administer with caution to patients in circulatory shock, since vasodilation produced by the drug may further reduce cardiac output and blood pressure).
No products indexed under this heading.

Phenobarbital (Concomitant use of other central nervous system depressants, including sedatives or hypnotics, general anesthetics, phenothiazines, tranquilizers and alcohol with hydromorphone, may produce an additive depressant effect. Respiratory depression, hypotension and profound sedation or coma may occur. When such combined therapy is contemplated, the dose of one or both agents should be reduced. Hydromorphone should not be taken with alcohol). Products include:

Phenobarbital Sodium (Concomitant use of other central nervous system depressants, including sedatives or hypnotics, general anesthetics, phenothiazines, tranquilizers and alcohol with hydromorphone, may produce an additive depressant effect. Respiratory depression, hypotension and profound sedation or coma may occur. When such combined therapy is contemplated, the dose of one or both agents should be reduced. Hydromorphone should not be taken with alcohol).
No products indexed under this heading.

Phenothiazine Derivatives (Concomitant use of phenothiazines with hydromorphone, may produce an additive depressant effect. Respiratory depression, hypotension and profound sedation or coma may occur. When such combined therapy is contemplated, the dose of one or both agents should be reduced. Administer with caution to patients in circulatory shock, since vasodilation produced by the drug may further reduce cardiac output and blood pressure).
No products indexed under this heading.

Phenothiazines (Concomitant use of phenothiazines with hydromorphone, may produce an additive depressant effect. Respiratory depression, hypotension and profound sedation or coma may occur. When such combined therapy is contemplated, the dose of one or both agents should be reduced. Administer with caution to patients in circulatory shock, since vasodilation produced by the drug may further reduce cardiac output and blood pressure).
No products indexed under this heading.

Pipecuronium Bromide (Other central nervous system depressants (eg, skeletal muscle relaxants) can potentiate the respiratory-depressant effects of hydromorphone and increase the risk of adverse outcomes, including death).
No products indexed under this heading.

Prazepam (Concomitant use of tranquilizers with hydromorphone, may produce an additive depressant effect. Respiratory depression, hypotension and profound sedation or coma may occur. When such combined therapy is contemplated, the dose of one or both agents should be reduced).
No products indexed under this heading.

Prochlorperazine (Concomitant use of phenothiazines with hydromorphone,

may produce an additive depressant effect. Respiratory depression, hypotension and profound sedation or coma may occur. When such combined therapy is contemplated, the dose of one or both agents should be reduced. Administer with caution to patients in circulatory shock, since vasodilation produced by the drug may further reduce cardiac output and blood pressure).
No products indexed under this heading.

Prochlorperazine Edisylate (Concomitant use of phenothiazines with hydromorphone, may produce an additive depressant effect. Respiratory depression, hypotension and profound sedation or coma may occur. When such combined therapy is contemplated, the dose of one or both agents should be reduced. Administer with caution to patients in circulatory shock, since vasodilation produced by the drug may further reduce cardiac output and blood pressure).
No products indexed under this heading.

Prochlorperazine Maleate (Concomitant use of phenothiazines with hydromorphone, may produce an additive depressant effect. Respiratory depression, hypotension and profound sedation or coma may occur. When such combined therapy is contemplated, the dose of one or both agents should be reduced. Administer with caution to patients in circulatory shock, since vasodilation produced by the drug may further reduce cardiac output and blood pressure).
No products indexed under this heading.

Promethazine (Concomitant use of phenothiazines with hydromorphone, may produce an additive depressant effect. Respiratory depression, hypotension and profound sedation or coma may occur. When such combined therapy is contemplated, the dose of one or both agents should be reduced. Administer with caution to patients in circulatory shock, since vasodilation produced by the drug may further reduce cardiac output and blood pressure).
No products indexed under this heading.

Promethazine Hydrochloride (Concomitant use of phenothiazines with hydromorphone, may produce an additive depressant effect. Respiratory depression, hypotension and profound sedation or coma may occur. When such combined therapy is contemplated, the dose of one or both agents should be reduced. Administer with caution to patients in circulatory shock, since vasodilation produced by the drug may further reduce cardiac output and blood pressure).
No products indexed under this heading.

Propofol (Concomitant use of other central nervous system depressants, including sedatives or hypnotics with hydromorphone, may produce an additive depressant effect. Respiratory depression, hypotension and profound sedation or coma may occur. When such combined therapy is contemplated, the dose of one or both agents should be reduced).
No products indexed under this heading.

Propoxyphene Hydrochloride (Concomitant use of other central nervous system depressants, including sedatives or hypnotics, general anesthetics, phenothiazines, tranquilizers and alcohol with hydromorphone, may produce an additive depressant effect. Respiratory depression, hypotension and profound sedation or coma may occur. When such combined therapy is contemplated, the dose of one or both agents should be reduced. Hydromorphone should not be taken with alcohol).
No products indexed under this heading.

Propoxyphene Napsylate (Concomitant use of other central nervous sys-

tem depressants, including sedatives or hypnotics, general anesthetics, phenothiazines, tranquilizers and alcohol with hydromorphone, may produce an additive depressant effect. Respiratory depression, hypotension and profound sedation or coma may occur. When such combined therapy is contemplated, the dose of one or both agents should be reduced. Hydromorphone should not be taken with alcohol).
No products indexed under this heading.

Quazepam (Concomitant use of other central nervous system depressants, including sedatives or hypnotics with hydromorphone, may produce an additive depressant effect. Respiratory depression, hypotension and profound sedation or coma may occur. When such combined therapy is contemplated, the dose of one or both agents should be reduced).
No products indexed under this heading.

Quetiapine Fumarate (Concomitant use of other central nervous system depressants, including sedatives or hypnotics, general anesthetics, phenothiazines, tranquilizers and alcohol with hydromorphone, may produce an additive depressant effect. Respiratory depression, hypotension and profound sedation or coma may occur. When such combined therapy is contemplated, the dose of one or both agents should be reduced. Hydromorphone should not be taken with alcohol).
Products include:

Ramelteon (Concomitant use of other central nervous system depressants, including sedatives or hypnotics with hydromorphone, may produce an additive depressant effect. Respiratory depression, hypotension and profound sedation or coma may occur. When such combined therapy is contemplated, the dose of one or both agents should be reduced). Products include:

Rapacuronium Bromide (Opioid analgesics, including hydromorphone, may enhance the action of neuromuscular blocking agents and produce an excessive degree of respiratory depression).
No products indexed under this heading.

Remifentanil Hydrochloride (Concomitant use of other central nervous system depressants, including sedatives or hypnotics, general anesthetics, phenothiazines, tranquilizers and alcohol with hydromorphone, may produce an additive depressant effect. Respiratory depression, hypotension and profound sedation or coma may occur. When such combined therapy is contemplated, the dose of one or both agents should be reduced. Hydromorphone should not be taken with alcohol).
No products indexed under this heading.

Risperidone (Concomitant use of other central nervous system depressants, including sedatives or hypnotics, general anesthetics, phenothiazines, tranquilizers and alcohol with hydromorphone, may produce an additive depressant effect. Respiratory depression, hypotension and profound sedation or coma may occur. When such combined therapy is contemplated, the dose of one or both agents should be reduced. Hydromorphone should not be taken with alcohol). Products include:

Rocuronium Bromide (Opioid analgesics, including hydromorphone, may enhance the action of neuromuscular blocking agents and produce an excessive degree of respiratory depression). Products include:

Secobarbital Sodium (Concomitant use of other central nervous system depressants, including sedatives or hypnotics with hydromorphone, may produce an additive depressant effect. Respiratory depression, hypotension and profound sedation or coma may occur. When such combined therapy is contemplated, the dose of one or both agents should be reduced).
No products indexed under this heading.

Sevoflurane (Concomitant use of general anesthetics with hydromorphone, may produce an additive depressant effect. Respiratory depression, hypotension and profound sedation or coma may occur. When such combined therapy is contemplated, the dose of one or both agents should be reduced. Administer with caution to patients in circulatory shock, since vasodilation produced by the drug may further reduce cardiac output and blood pressure). Products include:

Sodium Butabarbital (Concomitant use of other central nervous system depressants, including sedatives or hypnotics with hydromorphone, may produce an additive depressant effect. Respiratory depression, hypotension and profound sedation or coma may occur. When such combined therapy is contemplated, the dose of one or both agents should be reduced).
No products indexed under this heading.

Sodium Oxybate (Concomitant use of other central nervous system depressants, including sedatives or hypnotics, general anesthetics, phenothiazines, tranquilizers and alcohol with hydromorphone, may produce an additive depressant effect. Respiratory depression, hypotension and profound sedation or coma may occur. When such combined therapy is contemplated, the dose of one or both agents should be reduced. Hydromorphone should not be taken with alcohol).
No products indexed under this heading.

Sodium Pentobarbital (Concomitant use of other central nervous system depressants, including sedatives or hypnotics, general anesthetics, phenothiazines, tranquilizers and alcohol with hydromorphone, may produce an additive depressant effect. Respiratory depression, hypotension and profound sedation or coma may occur. When such combined therapy is contemplated, the dose of one or both agents should be reduced. Hydromorphone should not be taken with alcohol).
No products indexed under this heading.

Succinylcholine Chloride (Opioid analgesics, including hydromorphone, may enhance the action of neuromuscular blocking agents and produce an excessive degree of respiratory depression).
No products indexed under this heading.

Sufentanil Citrate (Concomitant use of other central nervous system depressants, including sedatives or hypnotics, general anesthetics, phenothiazines, tranquilizers and alcohol with hydromorphone, may produce an additive depressant effect. Respiratory depression, hypotension and profound sedation or coma may occur. When such combined therapy is contemplated, the dose of one or both agents should be reduced. Hydromorphone should not be taken with alcohol).
No products indexed under this heading.

Talbutal (Concomitant use of other central nervous system depressants, including sedatives or hypnotics, general anesthetics, phenothiazines, tranquilizers and alcohol with hydromorphone, may produce an additive depressant effect. Respiratory depression, hypoten-

sion and profound sedation or coma may occur. When such combined therapy is contemplated, the dose of one or both agents should be reduced. Hydromorphone should not be taken with alcohol).
No products indexed under this heading.

Temazepam (Concomitant use of other central nervous system depressants, including sedatives or hypnotics with hydromorphone, may produce an additive depressant effect. Respiratory depression, hypotension and profound sedation or coma may occur. When such combined therapy is contemplated, the dose of one or both agents should be reduced).
No products indexed under this heading.

Thiamylal Sodium (Concomitant use of other central nervous system depressants, including sedatives or hypnotics, general anesthetics, phenothiazines, tranquilizers and alcohol with hydromorphone, may produce an additive depressant effect. Respiratory depression, hypotension and profound sedation or coma may occur. When such combined therapy is contemplated, the dose of one or both agents should be reduced. Hydromorphone should not be taken with alcohol).
No products indexed under this heading.

Thioridazine (Concomitant use of phenothiazines with hydromorphone, may produce an additive depressant effect. Respiratory depression, hypotension and profound sedation or coma may occur. When such combined therapy is contemplated, the dose of one or both agents should be reduced. Administer with caution to patients in circulatory shock, since vasodilation produced by the drug may further reduce cardiac output and blood pressure).
No products indexed under this heading.

Thioridazine Hydrochloride (Concomitant use of phenothiazines with hydromorphone, may produce an additive depressant effect. Respiratory depression, hypotension and profound sedation or coma may occur. When such combined therapy is contemplated, the dose of one or both agents should be reduced. Administer with caution to patients in circulatory shock, since vasodilation produced by the drug may further reduce cardiac output and blood pressure). Products include:

Thiothixene (Concomitant use of tranquilizers with hydromorphone, may produce an additive depressant effect. Respiratory depression, hypotension and profound sedation or coma may occur. When such combined therapy is contemplated, the dose of one or both agents should be reduced). Products include:

Thiothixene Hydrochloride (Concomitant use of other central nervous system depressants, including sedatives or hypnotics, general anesthetics, phenothiazines, tranquilizers and alcohol with hydromorphone, may produce an additive depressant effect. Respiratory depression, hypotension and profound sedation or coma may occur. When such combined therapy is contemplated, the dose of one or both agents should be reduced. Hydromorphone should not be taken with alcohol).
No products indexed under this heading.

Tizanidine (Other central nervous system depressants (eg, skeletal muscle relaxants) can potentiate the respiratory-depressant effects of hydromorphone and increase the risk of adverse outcomes, including death).
No products indexed under this heading.

Tizanidine Hydrochloride (Other central nervous system depressants (eg, skeletal muscle relaxants) can potentiate the respiratory-depressant effects of hydromorphone and increase the risk of adverse outcomes, including death).
No products indexed under this heading.

Triazolam (Concomitant use of other central nervous system depressants, including sedatives or hypnotics with hydromorphone, may produce an additive depressant effect. Respiratory depression, hypotension and profound sedation or coma may occur. When such combined therapy is contemplated, the dose of one or both agents should be reduced).
No products indexed under this heading.

Trifluoperazine Hydrochloride (Concomitant use of phenothiazines with hydromorphone, may produce an additive depressant effect. Respiratory depression, hypotension and profound sedation or coma may occur. When such combined therapy is contemplated, the dose of one or both agents should be reduced. Administer with caution to patients in circulatory shock, since vasodilation produced by the drug may further reduce cardiac output and blood pressure).
No products indexed under this heading.

Tubocurarine Chloride (Opioid analgesics, including hydromorphone, may enhance the action of neuromuscular blocking agents and produce an excessive degree of respiratory depression).
No products indexed under this heading.

Vecuronium Bromide (Opioid analgesics, including hydromorphone, may enhance the action of neuromuscular blocking agents and produce an excessive degree of respiratory depression).
No products indexed under this heading.

Zaleplon (Concomitant use of other central nervous system depressants, including sedatives or hypnotics with hydromorphone, may produce an additive depressant effect. Respiratory depression, hypotension and profound sedation or coma may occur. When such combined therapy is contemplated, the dose of one or both agents should be reduced).
No products indexed under this heading.

Ziprasidone Hydrochloride (Concomitant use of other central nervous system depressants, including sedatives or hypnotics, general anesthetics, phenothiazines, tranquilizers and alcohol with hydromorphone, may produce an additive depressant effect. Respiratory depression, hypotension and profound sedation or coma may occur. When such combined therapy is contemplated, the dose of one or both agents should be reduced. Hydromorphone should not be taken with alcohol). Products include:

Zolpidem Tartrate (Concomitant use of other central nervous system depressants, including sedatives or hypnotics with hydromorphone, may produce an additive depressant effect. Respiratory depression, hypotension and profound sedation or coma may occur. When such combined therapy is contemplated, the dose of one or both agents should be reduced). Products include:

Food Interactions

Alcohol (Hydromorphone may be expected to have additive effects when used in conjunction with alcohol. Alcohol potentiates the respiratory depressant effects of hydromorphone, increasing the risk of respiratory depression that might result in death).

IMPORTANT NOTE: Always consult each drug listing in the patient's regimen for possible interactions.

Beer, reduced-alcohol (Hydromorphone may be expected to have additive effects when used in conjunction with alcohol. Alcohol potentiates the respiratory depressant effects of hydromorphone, increasing the risk of respiratory depression that might result in death).

Beer, unspecified (Hydromorphone may be expected to have additive effects when used in conjunction with alcohol. Alcohol potentiates the respiratory depressant effects of hydromorphone, increasing the risk of respiratory depression that might result in death).

Wine, Chianti (Hydromorphone may be expected to have additive effects when used in conjunction with alcohol. Alcohol potentiates the respiratory depressant effects of hydromorphone, increasing the risk of respiratory depression that might result in death).

Wine, Red (Hydromorphone may be expected to have additive effects when used in conjunction with alcohol. Alcohol potentiates the respiratory depressant effects of hydromorphone, increasing the risk of respiratory depression that might result in death).

Wine, unspecified (Hydromorphone may be expected to have additive effects when used in conjunction with alcohol. Alcohol potentiates the respiratory depressant effects of hydromorphone, increasing the risk of respiratory depression that might result in death).

Wine products (Hydromorphone may be expected to have additive effects when used in conjunction with alcohol. Alcohol potentiates the respiratory depressant effects of hydromorphone, increasing the risk of respiratory depression that might result in death).

DILAUDID-HP LYOPHILIZED POWDER 250 MG

(Hydromorphone Hydrochloride) 2800
See Dilaudid-HP Injection

DIOVAN TABLETS

(Valsartan) 2413
May interact with diuretics, potassium preparations, potassium sparing diuretics, and certain other agents. Compounds in these categories include:

Amiloride Hydrochloride (Concomitant use of potassium sparing diuretics (eg, amiloride) may lead to increases in serum potassium and in heart failure patients to increases in serum creatinine).
No products indexed under this heading.

Atenolol (Combination therapy is more antihypertensive than either component, but does not lower the heart rate more than atenolol alone).
No products indexed under this heading.

Bendroflumethiazide (In patients with an activated renin-angiotensin system, such as volume- and/or salt-depleted patients receiving high doses of diuretics, symptomatic hypotension may occur).
No products indexed under this heading.

Bumetanide (In patients with an activated renin-angiotensin system, such as volume- and/or salt-depleted patients receiving high doses of diuretics, symptomatic hypotension may occur).
No products indexed under this heading.

Chlorothiazide (In patients with an activated renin-angiotensin system, such as volume- and/or salt-depleted patients receiving high doses of diuretics, symptomatic hypotension may occur).
No products indexed under this heading.

Chlorothiazide Sodium (In patients with an activated renin-angiotensin sys-

tem, such as volume- and/or salt-depleted patients receiving high doses of diuretics, symptomatic hypotension may occur). Products include:
Diuril Intravenous 2009

Chlorthalidone (In patients with an activated renin-angiotensin system, such as volume- and/or salt-depleted patients receiving high doses of diuretics, symptomatic hypotension may occur). Products include:
Clorpres 2344

Cyclosporine (The results from an *in vitro* study with human liver tissue indicate that valsartan is a substrate of the hepatic uptake transporter OATP1B1 and the hepatic efflux transporter MRP2. Co-administration of inhibitors of the uptake transporter (eg, rifampin, cyclosporine) or efflux transporter (eg, ritonavir) may increase the systemic exposure to valsartan). Products include:
Gengraf 440
Neoral Oral Solution 2496
Neoral Capsules 2496
Restasis 605

Ethacrynic Acid (In patients with an activated renin-angiotensin system, such as volume- and/or salt-depleted patients receiving high doses of diuretics, symptomatic hypotension may occur).
No products indexed under this heading.

Furosemide (In patients with an activated renin-angiotensin system, such as volume- and/or salt-depleted patients receiving high doses of diuretics, symptomatic hypotension may occur). Products include:
Furosemide 2354

Hydrochlorothiazide (In patients with an activated renin-angiotensin system, such as volume- and/or salt-depleted patients receiving high doses of diuretics, symptomatic hypotension may occur). Products include:
Atacand HCT 700
Avalide 2956
Benicar HCT 1017
Diovan HCT 2419
Dyazide 1429
Exforge HCT 2449
Hyzaar 2162
Hyzaar 100-12.5 2162
Micardis HCT 889
Prinzide 2246
Tekturna HCT 2541
Teveten HCT 541

Hydroflumethiazide (In patients with an activated renin-angiotensin system, such as volume- and/or salt-depleted patients receiving high doses of diuretics, symptomatic hypotension may occur).
No products indexed under this heading.

Indapamide (In patients with an activated renin-angiotensin system, such as volume- and/or salt-depleted patients receiving high doses of diuretics, symptomatic hypotension may occur). Products include:
Indapamide 2356

Methyclothiazide (In patients with an activated renin-angiotensin system, such as volume- and/or salt-depleted patients receiving high doses of diuretics, symptomatic hypotension may occur).
No products indexed under this heading.

Metolazone (In patients with an activated renin-angiotensin system, such as volume- and/or salt-depleted patients receiving high doses of diuretics, symptomatic hypotension may occur).
No products indexed under this heading.

Polythiazide (In patients with an activated renin-angiotensin system, such as volume- and/or salt-depleted patients receiving high doses of diuretics, symptomatic hypotension may occur).
No products indexed under this heading.

Potassium Acid Phosphate (Concomitant use of potassium supplements may lead to increases in serum potassium and in heart failure patients to increases in serum creatinine). Products include:
K-Phos Original 874

Potassium Bicarbonate (Concomitant use of potassium supplements may lead to increases in serum potassium and in heart failure patients to increases in serum creatinine).
No products indexed under this heading.

Potassium Chloride (Concomitant use of potassium supplements may lead to increases in serum potassium and in heart failure patients to increases in serum creatinine). Products include:
MoviPrep Oral Solution 2905

Potassium Citrate (Concomitant use of potassium supplements may lead to increases in serum potassium and in heart failure patients to increases in serum creatinine). Products include:
Urocit-K 2333

Potassium Gluconate (Concomitant use of potassium supplements may lead to increases in serum potassium and in heart failure patients to increases in serum creatinine).
No products indexed under this heading.

Potassium Phosphate (Concomitant use of potassium supplements may lead to increases in serum potassium and in heart failure patients to increases in serum creatinine). Products include:
K-Phos Neutral 873

Rifampin (The results from an *in vitro* study with human liver tissue indicate that valsartan is a substrate of the hepatic uptake transporter OATP1B1 and the hepatic efflux transporter MRP2. Co-administration of inhibitors of the uptake transporter (eg, rifampin, cyclosporine) or efflux transporter (eg, ritonavir) may increase the systemic exposure to valsartan).
No products indexed under this heading.

Ritonavir (The results from an *in vitro* study with human liver tissue indicate that valsartan is a substrate of the hepatic uptake transporter OATP1B1 and the hepatic efflux transporter MRP2. Co-administration of inhibitors of the uptake transporter (eg, rifampin, cyclosporine) or efflux transporter (eg, ritonavir) may increase the systemic exposure to valsartan). Products include:
Kaletra 458
Norvir 509

Salt Substitutes (Concomitant use of salt substitutes containing potassium may lead to increases in serum potassium and in heart failure patients to increases in serum creatinine).
No products indexed under this heading.

Spironolactone (Concomitant use of potassium sparing diuretics (eg, spironolactone) may lead to increases in serum potassium and in heart failure patients to increases in serum creatinine).
No products indexed under this heading.

Torsemide (In patients with an activated renin-angiotensin system, such as volume- and/or salt-depleted patients receiving high doses of diuretics, symptomatic hypotension may occur).
No products indexed under this heading.

Triamterene (Concomitant use of potassium sparing diuretics (eg, triamterene) may lead to increases in serum potassium and in heart failure patients to increases in serum creatinine). Products include:
Dyazide 1429
Dyrenium 3495

Food Interactions

Food, unspecified (Food decreases the exposure (as measured by AUC) to valsartan about 40% and peak plasma concentration (C_{max}) by about 50%; valsartan may be administered with or without food).

Meal, unspecified (Food decreases the exposure (as measured by AUC) to valsartan about 40% and peak plasma concentration (C_{max}) by about 50%; valsartan may be administered with or without food).

DIOVAN HCT TABLETS

(Hydrochlorothiazide, Valsartan) 2419
May interact with alcohols, antihypertensives, barbiturates, cardiac glycosides, corticosteroids, insulin, lithium preparations, narcotic analgesics, nonsteroidal anti-inflammatory agents, nondepolarizing neuromuscular blocking agents, oral hypoglycemic agents, potassium preparations, and certain other agents. Compounds in these categories include:

Acarbose (Concurrent use of thiazide diuretics with antidiabetic drugs (eg, oral agents, insulin) may require a dosage adjustment of the antidiabetic drug).
No products indexed under this heading.

Acebutolol Hydrochloride (Concurrent use of thiazide diuretics with other antihypertensive drugs may result in an additive effect or potentiation).
No products indexed under this heading.

ACTH (Concurrent administration of thiazide diuretics with ACTH may intensify electrolyte depletion, particularly hypokalemia).
No products indexed under this heading.

Alclometasone Dipropionate (Concurrent administration of thiazide diuretics with corticosteroids may intensify electrolyte depletion, particularly hypokalemia).
No products indexed under this heading.

Alfentanil Hydrochloride (Concurrent use of thiazide diuretics with narcotics may result in potentiation of orthostatic hypotension).
No products indexed under this heading.

Aliskiren (Concurrent use of thiazide diuretics with other antihypertensive drugs may result in an additive effect or potentiation). Products include:
Tekturna 2538
Tekturna HCT 2541
Valturna 3637

Amlodipine Besylate (Concurrent use of thiazide diuretics with other antihypertensive drugs may result in an additive effect or potentiation). Products include:
Azor 1010
Exforge 2443
Exforge HCT 2449

Amobarbital (Concurrent use of thiazide diuretics with barbiturates may result in potentiation of orthostatic hypotension).
No products indexed under this heading.

Amobarbital Sodium (Concurrent use of thiazide diuretics with barbiturates may result in potentiation of orthostatic hypotension).
No products indexed under this heading.

Antidiabetic Drugs, unspecified (Concurrent use of thiazide diuretics with antidiabetic drugs (eg, oral agents, insulin) may require a dosage adjustment of the antidiabetic drug).
No products indexed under this heading.

Apomorphine (Concurrent use of thiazide diuretics with narcotics may result in potentiation of orthostatic hypotension).
No products indexed under this heading.

IMPORTANT NOTE: Always consult each drug listing in the patient's regimen for possible interactions.

Diovan **Interactions Index** 474

observed closely to determine if the desired effect of the diuretic is obtained).
No products indexed under this heading.

Diflorasone Diacetate (Concurrent administration of thiazide diuretics with corticosteroids may intensify electrolyte depletion, particularly hypokalemia).
No products indexed under this heading.

Digitalis Glycoside Preparations (Hypokalemia induced by thiazides may cause cardiac arrhythmia and may sensitize or exaggerate the response of the heart to the toxic effects of digitalis, such as increased ventricular irritability).
No products indexed under this heading.

Digitalis Lanata (Hypokalemia induced by thiazides may cause cardiac arrhythmia and may sensitize or exaggerate the response of the heart to the toxic effects of digitalis, such as increased ventricular irritability).
No products indexed under this heading.

Digitalis Purpurea (Hypokalemia induced by thiazides may cause cardiac arrhythmia and may sensitize or exaggerate the response of the heart to the toxic effects of digitalis, such as increased ventricular irritability).
No products indexed under this heading.

Digitoxin (Hypokalemia induced by thiazides may cause cardiac arrhythmia and may sensitize or exaggerate the response of the heart to the toxic effects of digitalis, such as increased ventricular irritability).
No products indexed under this heading.

Digoxin (Hypokalemia induced by thiazides may cause cardiac arrhythmia and may sensitize or exaggerate the response of the heart to the toxic effects of digitalis, such as increased ventricular irritability). Products include:
Lanoxin Injection **1546**
Lanoxin Injection Pediatric **1549**
Lanoxin Tablets **1553**

Dihydrocodeine Bitartrate (Concurrent use of thiazide diuretics with narcotics may result in potentiation of orthostatic hypotension).
No products indexed under this heading.

Dihydrocodeinone Bitartrate (Concurrent use of thiazide diuretics with narcotics may result in potentiation of orthostatic hypotension).
No products indexed under this heading.

Diltiazem Hydrochloride (Concurrent use of thiazide diuretics with other antihypertensive drugs may result in an additive effect or potentiation).
Products include:
Cardizem LA **423**

Diltiazem Maleate (Concurrent use of thiazide diuretics with other antihypertensive drugs may result in an additive effect or potentiation).
No products indexed under this heading.

Doxacurium Chloride (Concurrent administration of thiazide diuretics with nondepolarizing skeletal muscle relaxants may possibly increase responsiveness to the muscle relaxant).
No products indexed under this heading.

Doxazosin Mesylate (Concurrent use of thiazide diuretics with other antihypertensive drugs may result in an additive effect or potentiation).
No products indexed under this heading.

d-Tubocurarine (Concurrent administration of thiazide diuretics with nondepolarizing skeletal muscle relaxants may possibly increase responsiveness to the muscle relaxant).
No products indexed under this heading.

Enalapril Maleate (Concurrent use of thiazide diuretics with other antihypertensive drugs may result in an additive effect or potentiation).
No products indexed under this heading.

Enalaprilat (Concurrent use of thiazide diuretics with other antihypertensive drugs may result in an additive effect or potentiation).
No products indexed under this heading.

Eprosartan Mesylate (Concurrent use of thiazide diuretics with other antihypertensive drugs may result in an additive effect or potentiation).
Products include:
Teveten **538**
Teveten HCT **541**

Esmolol Hydrochloride (Concurrent use of thiazide diuretics with other antihypertensive drugs may result in an additive effect or potentiation).
No products indexed under this heading.

Ethanol (Concurrent use of thiazide diuretics with alcohol may result in potentiation of orthostatic hypotension).
No products indexed under this heading.

Ethyl Alcohol (Concurrent use of thiazide diuretics with alcohol may result in potentiation of orthostatic hypotension).
No products indexed under this heading.

Etodolac (In some patients, the administration of a nonsteroidal anti-inflammatory agent can reduce the diuretic, natriuretic, and antihypertensive effects of loop, potassium-sparing and thiazide diuretics. Therefore, when Diovan HCT and nonsteroidal anti-inflammatory agents are used concomitantly, the patient should be observed closely to determine if the desired effect of the diuretic is obtained).
No products indexed under this heading.

Felodipine (Concurrent use of thiazide diuretics with other antihypertensive drugs may result in an additive effect or potentiation).
No products indexed under this heading.

Fenoprofen Calcium (In some patients, the administration of a nonsteroidal anti-inflammatory agent can reduce the diuretic, natriuretic, and antihypertensive effects of loop, potassium-sparing and thiazide diuretics. Therefore, when Diovan HCT and nonsteroidal anti-inflammatory agents are used concomitantly, the patient should be observed closely to determine if the desired effect of the diuretic is obtained).
No products indexed under this heading.

Fentanyl (Concurrent use of thiazide diuretics with narcotics may result in potentiation of orthostatic hypotension).
Products include:
Duragesic **2604**
Fentanyl Transdermal System **2346**
Onsolis **2054**

Fentanyl Citrate (Concurrent use of thiazide diuretics with narcotics may result in potentiation of orthostatic hypotension). Products include:
Fentora **966**

Fludrocortisone Acetate (Concurrent administration of thiazide diuretics with corticosteroids may intensify electrolyte depletion, particularly hypokalemia).
No products indexed under this heading.

Flumethasone Pivalate (Concurrent administration of thiazide diuretics with corticosteroids may intensify electrolyte depletion, particularly hypokalemia).
No products indexed under this heading.

Flunisolide Hemihydrate (Concurrent administration of thiazide diuretics with corticosteroids may intensify electrolyte depletion, particularly hypokalemia).
No products indexed under this heading.

Flurbiprofen (In some patients, the administration of a nonsteroidal anti-inflammatory agent can reduce the diuretic, natriuretic, and antihypertensive effects of loop, potassium-sparing and thiazide diuretics. Therefore, when Diovan HCT and nonsteroidal anti-inflammatory agents are used concomitantly, the patient should be observed closely to determine if the desired effect of the diuretic is obtained).
No products indexed under this heading.

Fluticasone Furoate (Concurrent administration of thiazide diuretics with corticosteroids may intensify electrolyte depletion, particularly hypokalemia).
Products include:
Veramyst **1713**

Fluticasone Propionate (Concurrent administration of thiazide diuretics with corticosteroids may intensify electrolyte depletion, particularly hypokalemia).
Products include:
Advair 100/50 .... **1275**
Advair 250/50 .... **1275**
Advair 500/50 .... **1275**
Advair HFA 45/21 .... **1288**
Advair HFA 115/21 .... **1288**
Advair HFA 230/21 .... **1288**
Flonase **1459**
Flovent Diskus **1463**
Flovent HFA **1470**

Fosinopril Sodium (Concurrent use of thiazide diuretics with other antihypertensive drugs may result in an additive effect or potentiation).
No products indexed under this heading.

Furosemide (Concurrent use of thiazide diuretics with other antihypertensive drugs may result in an additive effect or potentiation). Products include:
Furosemide **2354**

Gallamine (Concurrent administration of thiazide diuretics with nondepolarizing skeletal muscle relaxants may possibly increase responsiveness to the muscle relaxant).
No products indexed under this heading.

Gallamine Triethiodide (Concurrent administration of thiazide diuretics with nondepolarizing skeletal muscle relaxants may possibly increase responsiveness to the muscle relaxant).
No products indexed under this heading.

Glibenclamide (Concurrent use of thiazide diuretics with antidiabetic drugs (eg, oral agents, insulin) may require a dosage adjustment of the antidiabetic drug).
No products indexed under this heading.

Glimepiride (Concurrent use of thiazide diuretics with antidiabetic drugs (eg, oral agents, insulin) may require a dosage adjustment of the antidiabetic drug). Products include:
Avandaryl **1356**
Duetact **3354**

Glipizide (Concurrent use of thiazide diuretics with antidiabetic drugs (eg, oral agents, insulin) may require a dosage adjustment of the antidiabetic drug).
No products indexed under this heading.

Glyburide (Concurrent use of thiazide diuretics with antidiabetic drugs (eg, oral agents, insulin) may require a dosage adjustment of the antidiabetic drug).
No products indexed under this heading.

Guanabenz Acetate (Concurrent use of thiazide diuretics with other antihypertensive drugs may result in an additive effect or potentiation).
No products indexed under this heading.

Guanethidine (Concurrent use of thiazide diuretics with other antihypertensive drugs may result in an additive effect or potentiation).
No products indexed under this heading.

Guanethidine Monosulfate (Concurrent use of thiazide diuretics with other antihypertensive drugs may result in an additive effect or potentiation).
No products indexed under this heading.

Guanethidine Sulfate (Concurrent use of thiazide diuretics with other antihypertensive drugs may result in an additive effect or potentiation).
No products indexed under this heading.

Hexobarbital (Concurrent use of thiazide diuretics with barbiturates may result in potentiation of orthostatic hypotension).
No products indexed under this heading.

Hydralazine Hydrochloride (Concurrent use of thiazide diuretics with other antihypertensive drugs may result in an additive effect or potentiation).
No products indexed under this heading.

Hydrocodone Bitartrate (Concurrent use of thiazide diuretics with narcotics may result in potentiation of orthostatic hypotension). Products include:
Vicodin **560**
Vicodin ES **561**
Vicodin HP **563**
Vicoprofen **564**
Zydone **1138**

Hydrocodone Polistirex (Concurrent use of thiazide diuretics with narcotics may result in potentiation of orthostatic hypotension). Products include:
Tussionex **3443**

Hydrocortisone (Concurrent administration of thiazide diuretics with corticosteroids may intensify electrolyte depletion, particularly hypokalemia).
No products indexed under this heading.

Hydrocortisone (Alcohol) (Concurrent administration of thiazide diuretics with corticosteroids may intensify electrolyte depletion, particularly hypokalemia).
No products indexed under this heading.

Hydrocortisone Acetate (Concurrent administration of thiazide diuretics with corticosteroids may intensify electrolyte depletion, particularly hypokalemia).
No products indexed under this heading.

Hydrocortisone Butyrate (Concurrent administration of thiazide diuretics with corticosteroids may intensify electrolyte depletion, particularly hypokalemia).
No products indexed under this heading.

Hydrocortisone Cypionate (Concurrent administration of thiazide diuretics with corticosteroids may intensify electrolyte depletion, particularly hypokalemia).
No products indexed under this heading.

Hydrocortisone Hemisuccinate (Concurrent administration of thiazide diuretics with corticosteroids may intensify electrolyte depletion, particularly hypokalemia).
No products indexed under this heading.

Hydrocortisone Probutate (Concurrent administration of thiazide diuretics with corticosteroids may intensify electrolyte depletion, particularly hypokalemia).
No products indexed under this heading.

Hydrocortisone Sodium Phosphate (Concurrent administration of thiazide diuretics with corticosteroids may intensify electrolyte depletion, particularly hypokalemia).
No products indexed under this heading.

Hydrocortisone Sodium Succinate (Concurrent administration of thiazide diuretics with corticosteroids may intensify electrolyte depletion, particularly hypokalemia).
No products indexed under this heading.

Hydrocortisone Valerate (Concurrent administration of thiazide diuretics with corticosteroids may intensify electrolyte depletion, particularly hypokalemia).
No products indexed under this heading.

(⊙ Described in PDR® for Ophthalmic Medicines)

Hydroflumethiazide (Concurrent use of thiazide diuretics with other antihypertensive drugs may result in an additive effect or potentiation).
No products indexed under this heading.

Hydromorphone (Concurrent use of thiazide diuretics with narcotics may result in potentiation of orthostatic hypotension).
No products indexed under this heading.

Hydromorphone Hydrochloride (Concurrent use of thiazide diuretics with narcotics may result in potentiation of orthostatic hypotension). Products include:

Ibuprofen (In some patients, the administration of a nonsteroidal anti-inflammatory agent can reduce the diuretic, natriuretic, and antihypertensive effects of loop, potassium-sparing and thiazide diuretics. Therefore, when Diovan HCT and nonsteroidal anti-inflammatory agents are used concomitantly, the patient should be observed closely to determine if the desired effect of the diuretic is obtained). Products include:

Indapamide (Concurrent use of thiazide diuretics with other antihypertensive drugs may result in an additive effect or potentiation). Products include:

Indomethacin (In some patients, the administration of a nonsteroidal anti-inflammatory agent can reduce the diuretic, natriuretic, and antihypertensive effects of loop, potassium-sparing and thiazide diuretics. Therefore, when Diovan HCT and nonsteroidal anti-inflammatory agents are used concomitantly, the patient should be observed closely to determine if the desired effect of the diuretic is obtained). Products include:

Indomethacin Sodium Trihydrate (In some patients, the administration of a nonsteroidal anti-inflammatory agent can reduce the diuretic, natriuretic, and antihypertensive effects of loop, potassium-sparing and thiazide diuretics. Therefore, when Diovan HCT and nonsteroidal anti-inflammatory agents are used concomitantly, the patient should be observed closely to determine if the desired effect of the diuretic is obtained). Products include:

Insulin (Concurrent use of thiazide diuretics with antidiabetic drugs (eg, oral agents, insulin) may require a dosage adjustment of the antidiabetic drug).
No products indexed under this heading.

Insulin, Human, Zinc Suspension (Concurrent use of thiazide diuretics with antidiabetic drugs (eg, oral agents, insulin) may require a dosage adjustment of the antidiabetic drug).
No products indexed under this heading.

Insulin, Human (rDNA origin) (Concurrent use of thiazide diuretics with antidiabetic drugs (eg, oral agents, insulin) may require a dosage adjustment of the antidiabetic drug). Products include:

Insulin, Human NPH (Concurrent use of thiazide diuretics with antidiabetic drugs (eg, oral agents, insulin) may require a dosage adjustment of the antidiabetic drug). Products include:

Insulin, Human Regular (Concurrent use of thiazide diuretics with antidiabetic drugs (eg, oral agents, insulin) may require a dosage adjustment of the antidiabetic drug). Products include:

Insulin, Human Regular and Human NPH Mixture (Concurrent use of thiazide diuretics with antidiabetic drugs (eg, oral agents, insulin) may require a dosage adjustment of the antidiabetic drug). Products include:

Insulin, NPH (Concurrent use of thiazide diuretics with antidiabetic drugs (eg, oral agents, insulin) may require a dosage adjustment of the antidiabetic drug).
No products indexed under this heading.

Insulin, Regular (Concurrent use of thiazide diuretics with antidiabetic drugs (eg, oral agents, insulin) may require a dosage adjustment of the antidiabetic drug).
No products indexed under this heading.

Insulin, Regular and NPH mixture (Concurrent use of thiazide diuretics with antidiabetic drugs (eg, oral agents, insulin) may require a dosage adjustment of the antidiabetic drug).
No products indexed under this heading.

Insulin, Zinc Crystals (Concurrent use of thiazide diuretics with antidiabetic drugs (eg, oral agents, insulin) may require a dosage adjustment of the antidiabetic drug).
No products indexed under this heading.

Insulin, Zinc Suspension (Concurrent use of thiazide diuretics with antidiabetic drugs (eg, oral agents, insulin) may require a dosage adjustment of the antidiabetic drug).
No products indexed under this heading.

Insulin Aspart (Concurrent use of thiazide diuretics with antidiabetic drugs (eg, oral agents, insulin) may require a dosage adjustment of the antidiabetic drug).
No products indexed under this heading.

Insulin Aspart, Human (Concurrent use of thiazide diuretics with antidiabetic drugs (eg, oral agents, insulin) may require a dosage adjustment of the antidiabetic drug). Products include:

Insulin Aspart, Human Regular (Concurrent use of thiazide diuretics with antidiabetic drugs (eg, oral agents, insulin) may require a dosage adjustment of the antidiabetic drug). Products include:

Insulin Aspart Protamine, Human (Concurrent use of thiazide diuretics with antidiabetic drugs (eg, oral agents, insulin) may require a dosage adjustment of the antidiabetic drug). Products include:

Insulin Detemir (rDNA Origin) (Concurrent use of thiazide diuretics with antidiabetic drugs (eg, oral agents, insulin) may require a dosage adjustment of the antidiabetic drug). Products include:

Insulin Glargine (Concurrent use of thiazide diuretics with antidiabetic drugs (eg, oral agents, insulin) may require a dosage adjustment of the antidiabetic drug). Products include:

Insulin Glulisine (Concurrent use of thiazide diuretics with antidiabetic drugs (eg, oral agents, insulin) may require a dosage adjustment of the antidiabetic drug). Products include:

Insulin Lispro, Human (Concurrent use of thiazide diuretics with antidiabetic drugs (eg, oral agents, insulin) may require a dosage adjustment of the antidiabetic drug). Products include:

Insulin Lispro Protamine, Human (Concurrent use of thiazide diuretics with antidiabetic drugs (eg, oral agents, insulin) may require a dosage adjustment of the antidiabetic drug). Products include:

Irbesartan (Concurrent use of thiazide diuretics with other antihypertensive drugs may result in an additive effect or potentiation). Products include:

Isradipine (Concurrent use of thiazide diuretics with other antihypertensive drugs may result in an additive effect or potentiation). Products include:

Ketoprofen (In some patients, the administration of a nonsteroidal anti-inflammatory agent can reduce the diuretic, natriuretic, and antihypertensive effects of loop, potassium-sparing and thiazide diuretics. Therefore, when Diovan HCT and nonsteroidal anti-inflammatory agents are used concomitantly, the patient should be observed closely to determine if the desired effect of the diuretic is obtained).
No products indexed under this heading.

Ketorolac Tromethamine (In some patients, the administration of a nonsteroidal anti-inflammatory agent can reduce the diuretic, natriuretic, and antihypertensive effects of loop, potassium-sparing and thiazide diuretics. Therefore, when Diovan HCT and nonsteroidal anti-inflammatory agents are used concomitantly, the patient should be observed closely to determine if the desired effect of the diuretic is obtained). Products include:

Labetalol Hydrochloride (Concurrent use of thiazide diuretics with other antihypertensive drugs may result in an additive effect or potentiation).
No products indexed under this heading.

Levorphanol Tartrate (Concurrent use of thiazide diuretics with narcotics may result in potentiation of orthostatic hypotension).
No products indexed under this heading.

Lisinopril (Concurrent use of thiazide diuretics with other antihypertensive drugs may result in an additive effect or potentiation). Products include:

Lithium (Lithium generally should not be given with diuretics. Diuretic agents reduce the renal clearance of lithium and add a high risk of lithium toxicity).
No products indexed under this heading.

Lithium Carbonate (Lithium generally should not be given with diuretics. Diuretic agents reduce the renal clearance of lithium and add a high risk of lithium toxicity).
No products indexed under this heading.

Lithium Citrate (Lithium generally should not be given with diuretics. Diuretic agents reduce the renal clearance of lithium and add a high risk of lithium toxicity).
No products indexed under this heading.

Losartan Potassium (Concurrent use of thiazide diuretics with other antihypertensive drugs may result in an additive effect or potentiation). Products include:

Mecamylamine Hydrochloride (Concurrent use of thiazide diuretics with other antihypertensive drugs may result in an additive effect or potentiation).
No products indexed under this heading.

Meclofenamate Sodium (In some patients, the administration of a nonsteroidal anti-inflammatory agent can reduce the diuretic, natriuretic, and antihypertensive effects of loop, potassium-sparing and thiazide diuretics. Therefore, when Diovan HCT and nonsteroidal anti-inflammatory agents are used concomitantly, the patient should be observed closely to determine if the desired effect of the diuretic is obtained).
No products indexed under this heading.

Mefenamic Acid (In some patients, the administration of a nonsteroidal anti-inflammatory agent can reduce the diuretic, natriuretic, and antihypertensive effects of loop, potassium-sparing and thiazide diuretics. Therefore, when Diovan HCT and nonsteroidal anti-inflammatory agents are used concomitantly, the patient should be observed closely to determine if the desired effect of the diuretic is obtained).
No products indexed under this heading.

Meloxicam (In some patients, the administration of a nonsteroidal anti-inflammatory agent can reduce the diuretic, natriuretic, and antihypertensive effects of loop, potassium-sparing and thiazide diuretics. Therefore, when Diovan HCT and nonsteroidal anti-inflammatory agents are used concomitantly, the patient should be observed closely to determine if the desired effect of the diuretic is obtained).
No products indexed under this heading.

Meperidine Hydrochloride (Concurrent use of thiazide diuretics with narcotics may result in potentiation of orthostatic hypotension).
No products indexed under this heading.

Mephobarbital (Concurrent use of thiazide diuretics with barbiturates may result in potentiation of orthostatic hypotension).
No products indexed under this heading.

Metformin Hydrochloride (Concurrent use of thiazide diuretics with antidiabetic drugs (eg, oral agents, insulin) may require a dosage adjustment of the antidiabetic drug). Products include:

Methadone Hydrochloride (Concurrent use of thiazide diuretics with narcotics may result in potentiation of orthostatic hypotension).
No products indexed under this heading.

Methyclothiazide (Concurrent use of thiazide diuretics with other antihypertensive drugs may result in an additive effect or potentiation).
No products indexed under this heading.

Methyldopa (Concurrent use of thiazide diuretics with other antihypertensive drugs may result in an additive effect or potentiation).
No products indexed under this heading.

Methyldopate Hydrochloride (Concurrent use of thiazide diuretics with other antihypertensive drugs may result in an additive effect or potentiation).
No products indexed under this heading.

Methylprednisolone (Concurrent administration of thiazide diuretics with corticosteroids may intensify electrolyte depletion, particularly hypokalemia).
No products indexed under this heading.

IMPORTANT NOTE: Always consult each drug listing in the patient's regimen for possible interactions.

Prednisolone Acetate (Concurrent administration of thiazide diuretics with corticosteroids may intensify electrolyte depletion, particularly hypokalemia). Products include:

Prednisolone Sodium Phosphate (Concurrent administration of thiazide diuretics with corticosteroids may intensify electrolyte depletion, particularly hypokalemia).
No products indexed under this heading.

Prednisolone Tebutate (Concurrent administration of thiazide diuretics with corticosteroids may intensify electrolyte depletion, particularly hypokalemia).
No products indexed under this heading.

Prednisone (Concurrent administration of thiazide diuretics with corticosteroids may intensify electrolyte depletion, particularly hypokalemia).
No products indexed under this heading.

Prednisone sodium phosphate (Concurrent administration of thiazide diuretics with corticosteroids may intensify electrolyte depletion, particularly hypokalemia).
No products indexed under this heading.

Propoxyphene Hydrochloride (Concurrent use of thiazide diuretics with narcotics may result in potentiation of orthostatic hypotension).
No products indexed under this heading.

Propoxyphene Napsylate (Concurrent use of thiazide diuretics with narcotics may result in potentiation of orthostatic hypotension).
No products indexed under this heading.

Propranolol Hydrochloride (Concurrent use of thiazide diuretics with other antihypertensive drugs may result in an additive effect or potentiation). Products include:

Quinapril Hydrochloride (Concurrent use of thiazide diuretics with other antihypertensive drugs may result in an additive effect or potentiation).
No products indexed under this heading.

Ramipril (Concurrent use of thiazide diuretics with other antihypertensive drugs may result in an additive effect or potentiation).
No products indexed under this heading.

Rapacuronium Bromide (Concurrent administration of thiazide diuretics with nondepolarizing skeletal muscle relaxants may possibly increase responsiveness to the muscle relaxant).
No products indexed under this heading.

Rauwolfia Serpentina (Concurrent use of thiazide diuretics with other antihypertensive drugs may result in an additive effect or potentiation).
No products indexed under this heading.

Remifentanil Hydrochloride (Concurrent use of thiazide diuretics with narcotics may result in potentiation of orthostatic hypotension).
No products indexed under this heading.

Repaglinide (Concurrent use of thiazide diuretics with antidiabetic drugs (eg, oral agents, insulin) may require a dosage adjustment of the antidiabetic drug).
No products indexed under this heading.

Rescinnamine (Concurrent use of thiazide diuretics with other antihypertensive drugs may result in an additive effect or potentiation).
No products indexed under this heading.

Reserpine (Concurrent use of thiazide diuretics with other antihypertensive drugs may result in an additive effect or potentiation).
No products indexed under this heading.

Rocuronium Bromide (Concurrent administration of thiazide diuretics with nondepolarizing skeletal muscle relaxants may possibly increase responsiveness to the muscle relaxant). Products include:

Rofecoxib (In some patients, the administration of a nonsteroidal anti-inflammatory agent can reduce the diuretic, natriuretic, and antihypertensive effects of loop, potassium-sparing and thiazide diuretics. Therefore, when Diovan HCT and nonsteroidal anti-inflammatory agents are used concomitantly, the patient should be observed closely to determine if the desired effect of the diuretic is obtained).
No products indexed under this heading.

Rosiglitazone Maleate (Concurrent use of thiazide diuretics with antidiabetic drugs (eg, oral agents, insulin) may require a dosage adjustment of the antidiabetic drug). Products include:

Secobarbital Sodium (Concurrent use of thiazide diuretics with barbiturates may result in potentiation of orthostatic hypotension).
No products indexed under this heading.

Sitagliptin Phosphate (Concurrent use of thiazide diuretics with antidiabetic drugs (eg, oral agents, insulin) may require a dosage adjustment of the antidiabetic drug). Products include:

Sodium Butabarbital (Concurrent use of thiazide diuretics with barbiturates may result in potentiation of orthostatic hypotension).
No products indexed under this heading.

Sodium Nitroprusside (Concurrent use of thiazide diuretics with other antihypertensive drugs may result in an additive effect or potentiation).
No products indexed under this heading.

Sodium Pentobarbital (Concurrent use of thiazide diuretics with barbiturates may result in potentiation of orthostatic hypotension).
No products indexed under this heading.

Sotalol Hydrochloride (Concurrent use of thiazide diuretics with other antihypertensive drugs may result in an additive effect or potentiation).
No products indexed under this heading.

Spirapril Hydrochloride (Concurrent use of thiazide diuretics with other antihypertensive drugs may result in an additive effect or potentiation).
No products indexed under this heading.

Sufentanil Citrate (Concurrent use of thiazide diuretics with narcotics may result in potentiation of orthostatic hypotension).
No products indexed under this heading.

Sulindac (In some patients, the administration of a nonsteroidal anti-inflammatory agent can reduce the diuretic, natriuretic, and antihypertensive effects of loop, potassium-sparing and thiazide diuretics. Therefore, when Diovan HCT and nonsteroidal anti-inflammatory agents are used concomitantly, the patient should be observed closely to determine if the desired effect of the diuretic is obtained). Products include:

Telmisartan (Concurrent use of thiazide diuretics with other antihypertensive drugs may result in an additive effect or potentiation). Products include:

Terazosin Hydrochloride (Concurrent use of thiazide diuretics with other antihypertensive drugs may result in an additive effect or potentiation).
No products indexed under this heading.

Thiamylal Sodium (Concurrent use of thiazide diuretics with barbiturates may result in potentiation of orthostatic hypotension).
No products indexed under this heading.

Timolol Maleate (Concurrent use of thiazide diuretics with other antihypertensive drugs may result in an additive effect or potentiation). Products include:

Tolazamide (Concurrent use of thiazide diuretics with antidiabetic drugs (eg, oral agents, insulin) may require a dosage adjustment of the antidiabetic drug).
No products indexed under this heading.

Tolbutamide (Concurrent use of thiazide diuretics with antidiabetic drugs (eg, oral agents, insulin) may require a dosage adjustment of the antidiabetic drug).
No products indexed under this heading.

Tolmetin Sodium (In some patients, the administration of a nonsteroidal anti-inflammatory agent can reduce the diuretic, natriuretic, and antihypertensive effects of loop, potassium-sparing and thiazide diuretics. Therefore, when Diovan HCT and nonsteroidal anti-inflammatory agents are used concomitantly, the patient should be observed closely to determine if the desired effect of the diuretic is obtained).
No products indexed under this heading.

Torsemide (Concurrent use of thiazide diuretics with other antihypertensive drugs may result in an additive effect or potentiation).
No products indexed under this heading.

Trandolapril (Concurrent use of thiazide diuretics with other antihypertensive drugs may result in an additive effect or potentiation). Products include:

Triamcinolone (Concurrent administration of thiazide diuretics with corticosteroids may intensify electrolyte depletion, particularly hypokalemia).
No products indexed under this heading.

Triamcinolone Acetonide (Concurrent administration of thiazide diuretics with corticosteroids may intensify electrolyte depletion, particularly hypokalemia). Products include:

Triamcinolone Diacetate (Concurrent administration of thiazide diuretics with corticosteroids may intensify electrolyte depletion, particularly hypokalemia).
No products indexed under this heading.

Triamcinolone Hexacetonide (Concurrent administration of thiazide diuretics with corticosteroids may intensify electrolyte depletion, particularly hypokalemia).
No products indexed under this heading.

Trimethaphan Camsylate (Concurrent use of thiazide diuretics with other antihypertensive drugs may result in an additive effect or potentiation).
No products indexed under this heading.

Troglitazone (Concurrent use of thiazide diuretics with antidiabetic drugs (eg, oral agents, insulin) may require a dosage adjustment of the antidiabetic drug).
No products indexed under this heading.

Tubocurarine Chloride (Concurrent administration of thiazide diuretics with nondepolarizing skeletal muscle relaxants (eg, tubocurarine) may possibly increase responsiveness to the muscle relaxant).
No products indexed under this heading.

Valdecoxib (In some patients, the administration of a nonsteroidal anti-inflammatory agent can reduce the diuretic, natriuretic, and antihypertensive effects of loop, potassium-sparing and thiazide diuretics. Therefore, when Diovan HCT and nonsteroidal anti-inflammatory agents are used concomitantly, the patient should be observed closely to determine if the desired effect of the diuretic is obtained).
No products indexed under this heading.

Vecuronium Bromide (Concurrent administration of thiazide diuretics with nondepolarizing skeletal muscle relaxants may possibly increase responsiveness to the muscle relaxant).
No products indexed under this heading.

Verapamil Hydrochloride (Concurrent use of thiazide diuretics with other antihypertensive drugs may result in an additive effect or potentiation). Products include:

Food Interactions

Alcohol (Concurrent use of thiazide diuretics with alcohol may result in potentiation of orthostatic hypotension).

Beer, reduced-alcohol (Concurrent use of thiazide diuretics with alcohol may result in potentiation of orthostatic hypotension).

Beer, unspecified (Concurrent use of thiazide diuretics with alcohol may result in potentiation of orthostatic hypotension).

Wine, Chianti (Concurrent use of thiazide diuretics with alcohol may result in potentiation of orthostatic hypotension).

Wine, Red (Concurrent use of thiazide diuretics with alcohol may result in potentiation of orthostatic hypotension).

Wine, unspecified (Concurrent use of thiazide diuretics with alcohol may result in potentiation of orthostatic hypotension).

Wine products (Concurrent use of thiazide diuretics with alcohol may result in potentiation of orthostatic hypotension).

DIPROLENE LOTION 0.05%
None cited in PDR database.

DIPROLENE OINTMENT 0.05%
None cited in PDR database.

DIPROLENE AF CREAM 0.05%
None cited in PDR database.

DIVIGEL
May interact with cytochrome p450 3a4 inducers (selected), cytochrome p450 3a4 inhibitors (selected), and certain other agents. Compounds in these categories include:

Acetazolamide (Inhibitors of CYP3A4, such as erythromycin, clarithromycin, ketoconazole, itraconazole, ritonavir, and grapefruit juice, may increase plasma concentrations of estrogens and result in side effects).
No products indexed under this heading.

479 Interactions Index Divigel

Diltiazem Maleate (Inhibitors of CYP3A4, such as erythromycin, clarithromycin, ketoconazole, itraconazole, ritonavir, and grapefruit juice, may increase plasma concentrations of estrogens and result in side effects).
No products indexed under this heading.

Doxorubicin Hydrochloride (Inducers of CYP3A4, such as St. John's Wort preparations (Hypericum perforatum), phenobarbital and rifampin, may reduce plasma concentrations of estrogens, possibly resulting in a decrease in therapeutic effects and/or changes in the uterine bleeding profile).
No products indexed under this heading.

Efavirenz (Inhibitors of CYP3A4, such as erythromycin, clarithromycin, ketoconazole, itraconazole, ritonavir, and grapefruit juice, may increase plasma concentrations of estrogens and result in side effects). Products include:
Atripla 906

Erythromycin (Inhibitors of CYP3A4, such as erythromycin, clarithromycin, ketoconazole, itraconazole, ritonavir, and grapefruit juice, may increase plasma concentrations of estrogens and result in side effects).
No products indexed under this heading.

Erythromycin Estolate (Inhibitors of CYP3A4, such as erythromycin, clarithromycin, ketoconazole, itraconazole, ritonavir, and grapefruit juice, may increase plasma concentrations of estrogens and result in side effects).
No products indexed under this heading.

Erythromycin Ethylsuccinate (Inhibitors of CYP3A4, such as erythromycin, clarithromycin, ketoconazole, itraconazole, ritonavir, and grapefruit juice, may increase plasma concentrations of estrogens and result in side effects). Products include:
E.E.S. 437
EryPed 435

Erythromycin Gluceptate (Inhibitors of CYP3A4, such as erythromycin, clarithromycin, ketoconazole, itraconazole, ritonavir, and grapefruit juice, may increase plasma concentrations of estrogens and result in side effects).
No products indexed under this heading.

Erythromycin Lactobionate (Inhibitors of CYP3A4, such as erythromycin, clarithromycin, ketoconazole, itraconazole, ritonavir, and grapefruit juice, may increase plasma concentrations of estrogens and result in side effects).
No products indexed under this heading.

Erythromycin Stearate (Inhibitors of CYP3A4, such as erythromycin, clarithromycin, ketoconazole, itraconazole, ritonavir, and grapefruit juice, may increase plasma concentrations of estrogens and result in side effects).
No products indexed under this heading.

Esomeprazole Magnesium (Inhibitors of CYP3A4, such as erythromycin, clarithromycin, ketoconazole, itraconazole, ritonavir, and grapefruit juice, may increase plasma concentrations of estrogens and result in side effects). Products include:
Nexium Capsules 704
Nexium Oral Suspension 704

Esomeprazole Sodium (Inhibitors of CYP3A4, such as erythromycin, clarithromycin, ketoconazole, itraconazole, ritonavir, and grapefruit juice, may increase plasma concentrations of estrogens and result in side effects). Products include:
Nexium I.V. 712

Ethosuximide (Inducers of CYP3A4, such as St. John's Wort preparations (Hypericum perforatum), phenobarbital and rifampin, may reduce plasma concentrations of estrogens, possibly resulting in a decrease in therapeutic effects and/or changes in the uterine bleeding profile).
No products indexed under this heading.

Felbamate (Inducers of CYP3A4, such as St. John's Wort preparations (Hypericum perforatum), phenobarbital and rifampin, may reduce plasma concentrations of estrogens, possibly resulting in a decrease in therapeutic effects and/or changes in the uterine bleeding profile).
No products indexed under this heading.

Fluconazole (Inhibitors of CYP3A4, such as erythromycin, clarithromycin, ketoconazole, itraconazole, ritonavir, and grapefruit juice, may increase plasma concentrations of estrogens and result in side effects).
No products indexed under this heading.

Fludrocortisone Acetate (Inducers of CYP3A4, such as St. John's Wort preparations (Hypericum perforatum), phenobarbital and rifampin, may reduce plasma concentrations of estrogens, possibly resulting in a decrease in therapeutic effects and/or changes in the uterine bleeding profile).
No products indexed under this heading.

Fluoxetine (Inhibitors of CYP3A4, such as erythromycin, clarithromycin, ketoconazole, itraconazole, ritonavir, and grapefruit juice, may increase plasma concentrations of estrogens and result in side effects).
No products indexed under this heading.

Fluoxetine Hydrochloride (Inhibitors of CYP3A4, such as erythromycin, clarithromycin, ketoconazole, itraconazole, ritonavir, and grapefruit juice, may increase plasma concentrations of estrogens and result in side effects). Products include:
Prozac Weekly 1941
Prozac Pulvules 1941
Symbyax 1965

Fluvoxamine Maleate (Inhibitors of CYP3A4, such as erythromycin, clarithromycin, ketoconazole, itraconazole, ritonavir, and grapefruit juice, may increase plasma concentrations of estrogens and result in side effects).
No products indexed under this heading.

Fosamprenavir Calcium (Inhibitors of CYP3A4, such as erythromycin, clarithromycin, ketoconazole, itraconazole, ritonavir, and grapefruit juice, may increase plasma concentrations of estrogens and result in side effects). Products include:
Lexiva Oral Suspension 1558
Lexiva 1558

Fosphenytoin Sodium (Inducers of CYP3A4, such as St. John's Wort preparations (Hypericum perforatum), phenobarbital and rifampin, may reduce plasma concentrations of estrogens, possibly resulting in a decrease in therapeutic effects and/or changes in the uterine bleeding profile).
No products indexed under this heading.

Garlic Extract (Inducers of CYP3A4, such as St. John's Wort preparations (Hypericum perforatum), phenobarbital and rifampin, may reduce plasma concentrations of estrogens, possibly resulting in a decrease in therapeutic effects and/or changes in the uterine bleeding profile).
No products indexed under this heading.

Garlic Oil (Inducers of CYP3A4, such as St. John's Wort preparations (Hypericum perforatum), phenobarbital and rifampin, may reduce plasma concentrations of estrogens, possibly resulting in a decrease in therapeutic effects and/or changes in the uterine bleeding profile).
No products indexed under this heading.

Hydrocortisone (Inducers of CYP3A4, such as St. John's Wort preparations (Hypericum perforatum), phenobarbital and rifampin, may reduce plasma concentrations of estrogens, possibly resulting in a decrease in therapeutic effects and/or changes in the uterine bleeding profile).
No products indexed under this heading.

Hydrocortisone (Alcohol) (Inducers of CYP3A4, such as St. John's Wort preparations (Hypericum perforatum), phenobarbital and rifampin, may reduce plasma concentrations of estrogens, possibly resulting in a decrease in therapeutic effects and/or changes in the uterine bleeding profile).
No products indexed under this heading.

Hydrocortisone Acetate (Inducers of CYP3A4, such as St. John's Wort preparations (Hypericum perforatum), phenobarbital and rifampin, may reduce plasma concentrations of estrogens, possibly resulting in a decrease in therapeutic effects and/or changes in the uterine bleeding profile).
No products indexed under this heading.

Hydrocortisone Butyrate (Inducers of CYP3A4, such as St. John's Wort preparations (Hypericum perforatum), phenobarbital and rifampin, may reduce plasma concentrations of estrogens, possibly resulting in a decrease in therapeutic effects and/or changes in the uterine bleeding profile).
No products indexed under this heading.

Hydrocortisone Cypionate (Inducers of CYP3A4, such as St. John's Wort preparations (Hypericum perforatum), phenobarbital and rifampin, may reduce plasma concentrations of estrogens, possibly resulting in a decrease in therapeutic effects and/or changes in the uterine bleeding profile).
No products indexed under this heading.

Hydrocortisone Hemisuccinate (Inducers of CYP3A4, such as St. John's Wort preparations (Hypericum perforatum), phenobarbital and rifampin, may reduce plasma concentrations of estrogens, possibly resulting in a decrease in therapeutic effects and/or changes in the uterine bleeding profile).
No products indexed under this heading.

Hydrocortisone Probutate (Inducers of CYP3A4, such as St. John's Wort preparations (Hypericum perforatum), phenobarbital and rifampin, may reduce plasma concentrations of estrogens, possibly resulting in a decrease in therapeutic effects and/or changes in the uterine bleeding profile).
No products indexed under this heading.

Hydrocortisone Sodium Phosphate (Inducers of CYP3A4, such as St. John's Wort preparations (Hypericum perforatum), phenobarbital and rifampin, may reduce plasma concentrations of estrogens, possibly resulting in a decrease in therapeutic effects and/or changes in the uterine bleeding profile).
No products indexed under this heading.

Hydrocortisone Sodium Succinate (Inducers of CYP3A4, such as St. John's Wort preparations (Hypericum perforatum), phenobarbital and rifampin, may reduce plasma concentrations of estrogens, possibly resulting in a decrease in therapeutic effects and/or changes in the uterine bleeding profile).
No products indexed under this heading.

Hydrocortisone Valerate (Inducers of CYP3A4, such as St. John's Wort preparations (Hypericum perforatum), phenobarbital and rifampin, may reduce plasma concentrations of estrogens, possibly resulting in a decrease in therapeutic effects and/or changes in the uterine bleeding profile).
No products indexed under this heading.

Hypericum (Inducers of CYP3A4, such as St. John's Wort preparations (Hypericum perforatum), phenobarbital and rifampin, may reduce plasma concentrations of estrogens, possibly resulting in a decrease in therapeutic effects and/or changes in the uterine bleeding profile).
No products indexed under this heading.

Hypericum Perforatum (Inducers of CYP3A4, such as St. John's Wort preparations (Hypericum perforatum), phenobarbital and rifampin, may reduce plasma concentrations of estrogens, possibly resulting in a decrease in therapeutic effects and/or changes in the uterine bleeding profile). Products include:
Traumeel 1800

Imatinib Mesylate (Inhibitors of CYP3A4, such as erythromycin, clarithromycin, ketoconazole, itraconazole, ritonavir, and grapefruit juice, may increase plasma concentrations of estrogens and result in side effects). Products include:
Gleevec 2477

Indinavir Sulfate (Inhibitors of CYP3A4, such as erythromycin, clarithromycin, ketoconazole, itraconazole, ritonavir, and grapefruit juice, may increase plasma concentrations of estrogens and result in side effects). Products include:
Crixivan 2113

Isoniazid (Inhibitors of CYP3A4, such as erythromycin, clarithromycin, ketoconazole, itraconazole, ritonavir, and grapefruit juice, may increase plasma concentrations of estrogens and result in side effects).
No products indexed under this heading.

Itraconazole (Inhibitors of CYP3A4, such as erythromycin, clarithromycin, ketoconazole, itraconazole, ritonavir, and grapefruit juice, may increase plasma concentrations of estrogens and result in side effects).
No products indexed under this heading.

Ketoconazole (Inhibitors of CYP3A4, such as erythromycin, clarithromycin, ketoconazole, itraconazole, ritonavir, and grapefruit juice, may increase plasma concentrations of estrogens and result in side effects). Products include:
Extina 3319
Xolegel 3337

Lapatinib (Inhibitors of CYP3A4, such as erythromycin, clarithromycin, ketoconazole, itraconazole, ritonavir, and grapefruit juice, may increase plasma concentrations of estrogens and result in side effects). Products include:
Tykerb 1698

Lopinavir (Inhibitors of CYP3A4, such as erythromycin, clarithromycin, ketoconazole, itraconazole, ritonavir, and grapefruit juice, may increase plasma concentrations of estrogens and result in side effects). Products include:
Kaletra 458

Loratadine (Inhibitors of CYP3A4, such as erythromycin, clarithromycin, ketoconazole, itraconazole, ritonavir, and grapefruit juice, may increase plasma concentrations of estrogens and result in side effects).
No products indexed under this heading.

IMPORTANT NOTE: Always consult each drug listing in the patient's regimen for possible interactions.

Mephenytoin (Inducers of CYP3A4, such as St. John's Wort preparations (Hypericum perforatum), phenobarbital and rifampin, may reduce plasma concentrations of estrogens, possibly resulting in a decrease in therapeutic effects and/or changes in the uterine bleeding profile).
No products indexed under this heading.

Methsuximide (Inducers of CYP3A4, such as St. John's Wort preparations (Hypericum perforatum), phenobarbital and rifampin, may reduce plasma concentrations of estrogens, possibly resulting in a decrease in therapeutic effects and/or changes in the uterine bleeding profile).
No products indexed under this heading.

Methylprednisolone (Inducers of CYP3A4, such as St. John's Wort preparations (Hypericum perforatum), phenobarbital and rifampin, may reduce plasma concentrations of estrogens, possibly resulting in a decrease in therapeutic effects and/or changes in the uterine bleeding profile).
No products indexed under this heading.

Methylprednisolone Acetate (Inducers of CYP3A4, such as St. John's Wort preparations (Hypericum perforatum), phenobarbital and rifampin, may reduce plasma concentrations of estrogens, possibly resulting in a decrease in therapeutic effects and/or changes in the uterine bleeding profile).
No products indexed under this heading.

Methylprednisolone Sodium Succinate (Inducers of CYP3A4, such as St. John's Wort preparations (Hypericum perforatum), phenobarbital and rifampin, may reduce plasma concentrations of estrogens, possibly resulting in a decrease in therapeutic effects and/or changes in the uterine bleeding profile).
No products indexed under this heading.

Metronidazole (Inhibitors of CYP3A4, such as erythromycin, clarithromycin, ketoconazole, itraconazole, ritonavir, and grapefruit juice, may increase plasma concentrations of estrogens and result in side effects). Products include:
Pylera 793

Metronidazole Benzoate (Inhibitors of CYP3A4, such as erythromycin, clarithromycin, ketoconazole, itraconazole, ritonavir, and grapefruit juice, may increase plasma concentrations of estrogens and result in side effects).
No products indexed under this heading.

Metronidazole Hydrochloride (Inhibitors of CYP3A4, such as erythromycin, clarithromycin, ketoconazole, itraconazole, ritonavir, and grapefruit juice, may increase plasma concentrations of estrogens and result in side effects).
No products indexed under this heading.

Metronidazole Sodium (Inhibitors of CYP3A4, such as erythromycin, clarithromycin, ketoconazole, itraconazole, ritonavir, and grapefruit juice, may increase plasma concentrations of estrogens and result in side effects).
No products indexed under this heading.

Miconazole (Inhibitors of CYP3A4, such as erythromycin, clarithromycin, ketoconazole, itraconazole, ritonavir, and grapefruit juice, may increase plasma concentrations of estrogens and result in side effects).
No products indexed under this heading.

Miconazole Nitrate (Inhibitors of CYP3A4, such as erythromycin, clarithromycin, ketoconazole, itraconazole, ritonavir, and grapefruit juice, may increase plasma concentrations of estrogens and result in side effects). Products include:
Vusion Ointment 3335

Mifepristone (Inhibitors of CYP3A4, such as erythromycin, clarithromycin, ketoconazole, itraconazole, ritonavir, and grapefruit juice, may increase plasma concentrations of estrogens and result in side effects).
No products indexed under this heading.

Modafinil (Inducers of CYP3A4, such as St. John's Wort preparations (Hypericum perforatum), phenobarbital and rifampin, may reduce plasma concentrations of estrogens, possibly resulting in a decrease in therapeutic effects and/or changes in the uterine bleeding profile). Products include:
Provigil 983

Nafcillin Sodium (Inducers of CYP3A4, such as St. John's Wort preparations (Hypericum perforatum), phenobarbital and rifampin, may reduce plasma concentrations of estrogens, possibly resulting in a decrease in therapeutic effects and/or changes in the uterine bleeding profile).
No products indexed under this heading.

Nefazodone Hydrochloride (Inhibitors of CYP3A4, such as erythromycin, clarithromycin, ketoconazole, itraconazole, ritonavir, and grapefruit juice, may increase plasma concentrations of estrogens and result in side effects).
No products indexed under this heading.

Nelfinavir Mesylate (Inhibitors of CYP3A4, such as erythromycin, clarithromycin, ketoconazole, itraconazole, ritonavir, and grapefruit juice, may increase plasma concentrations of estrogens and result in side effects).
No products indexed under this heading.

Nevirapine (Inhibitors of CYP3A4, such as erythromycin, clarithromycin, ketoconazole, itraconazole, ritonavir, and grapefruit juice, may increase plasma concentrations of estrogens and result in side effects). Products include:
Viramune Oral Suspension 897
Viramune Tablets 897

Niacin (Inhibitors of CYP3A4, such as erythromycin, clarithromycin, ketoconazole, itraconazole, ritonavir, and grapefruit juice, may increase plasma concentrations of estrogens and result in side effects). Products include:
Advicor 402
Cardio Basics 3455
Niaspan 497
Simcor 524

Niacinamide (Inhibitors of CYP3A4, such as erythromycin, clarithromycin, ketoconazole, itraconazole, ritonavir, and grapefruit juice, may increase plasma concentrations of estrogens and result in side effects). Products include:
CitraNatal 90 DHA Capsules 2332
CitraNatal Assure 2332
CitraNatal Rx 2332
Heplive 607

Niacinamide Hydroiodide (Inhibitors of CYP3A4, such as erythromycin, clarithromycin, ketoconazole, itraconazole, ritonavir, and grapefruit juice, may increase plasma concentrations of estrogens and result in side effects).
No products indexed under this heading.

Nicotinamide (Inhibitors of CYP3A4, such as erythromycin, clarithromycin, ketoconazole, itraconazole, ritonavir, and grapefruit juice, may increase plasma concentrations of estrogens and result in side effects).
No products indexed under this heading.

Nifedipine (Inhibitors of CYP3A4, such as erythromycin, clarithromycin, ketoconazole, itraconazole, ritonavir, and grapefruit juice, may increase plasma concentrations of estrogens and result in side effects).
No products indexed under this heading.

Norfloxacin (Inhibitors of CYP3A4, such as erythromycin, clarithromycin, ketoconazole, itraconazole, ritonavir,
and grapefruit juice, may increase plasma concentrations of estrogens and result in side effects). Products include:
Noroxin 2220

Omeprazole (Inhibitors of CYP3A4, such as erythromycin, clarithromycin, ketoconazole, itraconazole, ritonavir, and grapefruit juice, may increase plasma concentrations of estrogens and result in side effects).
No products indexed under this heading.

Oxcarbazepine (Inducers of CYP3A4, such as St. John's Wort preparations (Hypericum perforatum), phenobarbital and rifampin, may reduce plasma concentrations of estrogens, possibly resulting in a decrease in therapeutic effects and/or changes in the uterine bleeding profile).
No products indexed under this heading.

Paroxetine Hydrochloride (Inhibitors of CYP3A4, such as erythromycin, clarithromycin, ketoconazole, itraconazole, ritonavir, and grapefruit juice, may increase plasma concentrations of estrogens and result in side effects). Products include:
Paroxetine CR 2361
Paroxetine ER 2371
Paxil 1586
Paxil CR 1596

Phenobarbital (Inducers of CYP3A4, such as St. John's Wort preparations (Hypericum perforatum), phenobarbital and rifampin, may reduce plasma concentrations of estrogens, possibly resulting in a decrease in therapeutic effects and/or changes in the uterine bleeding profile). Products include:
Donnatal 2711

Phenobarbital Sodium (Inducers of CYP3A4, such as St. John's Wort preparations (Hypericum perforatum), phenobarbital and rifampin, may reduce plasma concentrations of estrogens, possibly resulting in a decrease in therapeutic effects and/or changes in the uterine bleeding profile).
No products indexed under this heading.

Phenytoin (Inducers of CYP3A4, such as St. John's Wort preparations (Hypericum perforatum), phenobarbital and rifampin, may reduce plasma concentrations of estrogens, possibly resulting in a decrease in therapeutic effects and/or changes in the uterine bleeding profile).
No products indexed under this heading.

Phenytoin Sodium (Inducers of CYP3A4, such as St. John's Wort preparations (Hypericum perforatum), phenobarbital and rifampin, may reduce plasma concentrations of estrogens, possibly resulting in a decrease in therapeutic effects and/or changes in the uterine bleeding profile). Products include:
Phenytek Capsules 2380

Posaconazole (Inhibitors of CYP3A4, such as erythromycin, clarithromycin, ketoconazole, itraconazole, ritonavir, and grapefruit juice, may increase plasma concentrations of estrogens and result in side effects). Products include:
Noxafil 3172

Prednisolone (Inducers of CYP3A4, such as St. John's Wort preparations (Hypericum perforatum), phenobarbital and rifampin, may reduce plasma concentrations of estrogens, possibly resulting in a decrease in therapeutic effects and/or changes in the uterine bleeding profile).
No products indexed under this heading.

Prednisolone Acetate (Inducers of CYP3A4, such as St. John's Wort preparations (Hypericum perforatum), phenobarbital and rifampin, may reduce plasma concentrations of estrogens, possibly resulting in a decrease in thera-
peutic effects and/or changes in the uterine bleeding profile). Products include:
Blephamide .... ⊙212, ⊙214
Pred Forte .... ⊙225
Pred Mild .... ⊙230
Pred-G .... ⊙226, ⊙227

Prednisolone Sodium Phosphate (Inducers of CYP3A4, such as St. John's Wort preparations (Hypericum perforatum), phenobarbital and rifampin, may reduce plasma concentrations of estrogens, possibly resulting in a decrease in therapeutic effects and/or changes in the uterine bleeding profile).
No products indexed under this heading.

Prednisolone Tebutate (Inducers of CYP3A4, such as St. John's Wort preparations (Hypericum perforatum), phenobarbital and rifampin, may reduce plasma concentrations of estrogens, possibly resulting in a decrease in therapeutic effects and/or changes in the uterine bleeding profile).
No products indexed under this heading.

Prednisone (Inducers of CYP3A4, such as St. John's Wort preparations (Hypericum perforatum), phenobarbital and rifampin, may reduce plasma concentrations of estrogens, possibly resulting in a decrease in therapeutic effects and/or changes in the uterine bleeding profile).
No products indexed under this heading.

Prednisone sodium phosphate (Inducers of CYP3A4, such as St. John's Wort preparations (Hypericum perforatum), phenobarbital and rifampin, may reduce plasma concentrations of estrogens, possibly resulting in a decrease in therapeutic effects and/or changes in the uterine bleeding profile).
No products indexed under this heading.

Primidone (Inducers of CYP3A4, such as St. John's Wort preparations (Hypericum perforatum), phenobarbital and rifampin, may reduce plasma concentrations of estrogens, possibly resulting in a decrease in therapeutic effects and/or changes in the uterine bleeding profile).
No products indexed under this heading.

Propoxyphene Hydrochloride (Inhibitors of CYP3A4, such as erythromycin, clarithromycin, ketoconazole, itraconazole, ritonavir, and grapefruit juice, may increase plasma concentrations of estrogens and result in side effects).
No products indexed under this heading.

Propoxyphene Napsylate (Inhibitors of CYP3A4, such as erythromycin, clarithromycin, ketoconazole, itraconazole, ritonavir, and grapefruit juice, may increase plasma concentrations of estrogens and result in side effects).
No products indexed under this heading.

Quinidine (Inhibitors of CYP3A4, such as erythromycin, clarithromycin, ketoconazole, itraconazole, ritonavir, and grapefruit juice, may increase plasma concentrations of estrogens and result in side effects).
No products indexed under this heading.

Quinidine Hydrochloride (Inhibitors of CYP3A4, such as erythromycin, clarithromycin, ketoconazole, itraconazole, ritonavir, and grapefruit juice, may increase plasma concentrations of estrogens and result in side effects).
No products indexed under this heading.

Quinidine Polygalacturonate (Inhibitors of CYP3A4, such as erythromycin, clarithromycin, ketoconazole, itraconazole, ritonavir, and grapefruit juice, may increase plasma concentrations of estrogens and result in side effects).
No products indexed under this heading.

Food Interactions

DIVISTA SOFTGEL CAPSULES

May interact with antacids, antibiotics, anticoagulants, anticonvulsants, aspirin-acetylsalicylic acid, iron containing oral preparations, iron salts, phenytoin, valproate, and certain other agents. Compounds in these categories include:

Danaparoid Sodium (Ingestion of more than 3 grams of omega-3 fatty acids from fish oils per day may have potential antithrombotic effects, including an increased in bleeding time and INR (international normalized ratio). DHA should be avoided in patients with taking anticoagulants).
No products indexed under this heading.

Daunorubicin Hydrochloride (Long-term treatment with sulfa drugs or other antibiotics may decrease bacterial synthesis of biotin, potentially increasing the requirement for dietary biotin).
No products indexed under this heading.

Demeclocycline Hydrochloride (Long-term treatment with sulfa drugs or other antibiotics may decrease bacterial synthesis of biotin, potentially increasing the requirement for dietary biotin).
No products indexed under this heading.

Dicloxacillin (Long-term treatment with sulfa drugs or other antibiotics may decrease bacterial synthesis of biotin, potentially increasing the requirement for dietary biotin).
No products indexed under this heading.

Dicloxacillin Sodium (Long-term treatment with sulfa drugs or other antibiotics may decrease bacterial synthesis of biotin, potentially increasing the requirement for dietary biotin).
No products indexed under this heading.

Dicumarol (Ingestion of more than 3 grams of omega-3 fatty acids from fish oils per day may have potential antithrombotic effects, including an increased in bleeding time and INR (international normalized ratio). DHA should be avoided in patients with taking anticoagulants).
No products indexed under this heading.

Dirithromycin (Long-term treatment with sulfa drugs or other antibiotics may decrease bacterial synthesis of biotin, potentially increasing the requirement for dietary biotin).
No products indexed under this heading.

Disodium Carbenicillin (Long-term treatment with sulfa drugs or other antibiotics may decrease bacterial synthesis of biotin, potentially increasing the requirement for dietary biotin).
No products indexed under this heading.

Divalproex Sodium (Use of the anticonvulsant valproic acid has been associated with decreased biotinidase activity in children). Products include:
Depakote ER 426

Doxycycline Calcium (Long-term treatment with sulfa drugs or other antibiotics may decrease bacterial synthesis of biotin, potentially increasing the requirement for dietary biotin).
No products indexed under this heading.

Doxycycline Hyclate (Long-term treatment with sulfa drugs or other antibiotics may decrease bacterial synthesis of biotin, potentially increasing the requirement for dietary biotin).
No products indexed under this heading.

Doxycycline Monohydrate (Long-term treatment with sulfa drugs or other antibiotics may decrease bacterial synthesis of biotin, potentially increasing the requirement for dietary biotin).
No products indexed under this heading.

Enoxacin (Long-term treatment with sulfa drugs or other antibiotics may decrease bacterial synthesis of biotin, potentially increasing the requirement for dietary biotin).
No products indexed under this heading.

Enoxaparin Sodium (Ingestion of more than 3 grams of omega-3 fatty acids from fish oils per day may have potential antithrombotic effects, including an increased in bleeding time and

INR (international normalized ratio). DHA should be avoided in patients with taking anticoagulants). Products include:
Lovenox 3005

Epirubicin Hydrochloride (Long-term treatment with sulfa drugs or other antibiotics may decrease bacterial synthesis of biotin, potentially increasing the requirement for dietary biotin).
No products indexed under this heading.

Erythromycin (Long-term treatment with sulfa drugs or other antibiotics may decrease bacterial synthesis of biotin, potentially increasing the requirement for dietary biotin).
No products indexed under this heading.

Erythromycin, Topical (Long-term treatment with sulfa drugs or other antibiotics may decrease bacterial synthesis of biotin, potentially increasing the requirement for dietary biotin).
No products indexed under this heading.

Erythromycin Estolate (Long-term treatment with sulfa drugs or other antibiotics may decrease bacterial synthesis of biotin, potentially increasing the requirement for dietary biotin).
No products indexed under this heading.

Erythromycin Ethylsuccinate (Long-term treatment with sulfa drugs or other antibiotics may decrease bacterial synthesis of biotin, potentially increasing the requirement for dietary biotin). Products include:
E.E.S. 437
EryPed 435

Erythromycin Gluceptate (Long-term treatment with sulfa drugs or other antibiotics may decrease bacterial synthesis of biotin, potentially increasing the requirement for dietary biotin).
No products indexed under this heading.

Erythromycin Lactobionate (Long-term treatment with sulfa drugs or other antibiotics may decrease bacterial synthesis of biotin, potentially increasing the requirement for dietary biotin).
No products indexed under this heading.

Erythromycin Stearate (Long-term treatment with sulfa drugs or other antibiotics may decrease bacterial synthesis of biotin, potentially increasing the requirement for dietary biotin).
No products indexed under this heading.

Ethosuximide (Individuals on long-term anticonvulsant therapy may have reduced levels of biotin in their blood and urinary excretion of organic acids consistent with decreased carboxylase activity).
No products indexed under this heading.

Ethotoin (Individuals on long-term anticonvulsant therapy may have reduced levels of biotin in their blood and urinary excretion of organic acids consistent with decreased carboxylase activity).
No products indexed under this heading.

Felbamate (Individuals on long-term anticonvulsant therapy may have reduced levels of biotin in their blood and urinary excretion of organic acids consistent with decreased carboxylase activity).
No products indexed under this heading.

Ferrous Fumarate (Chromium may compete for one of the binding sites on the iron transport protein, transferrin. Serum iron concentrations and serum ferritin concentrations were unchanged by either resistive training or chromium picolinate supplementation. The high-dose chromium picolinate supplementation for 12 week did not influence hematologic indexes or indexes of iron metabolism). Products include:
PreNexa 3473

Ferrous Gluconate (Chromium may compete for one of the binding sites on the iron transport protein, transferrin. Serum iron concentrations and serum

ferritin concentrations were unchanged by either resistive training or chromium picolinate supplementation. The high-dose chromium picolinate supplementation for 12 week did not influence hematologic indexes or indexes of iron metabolism). Products include:
CitraNatal Assure 2332
CitraNatal Rx 2332

Ferrous Sulfate (Chromium may compete for one of the binding sites on the iron transport protein, transferrin. Serum iron concentrations and serum ferritin concentrations were unchanged by either resistive training or chromium picolinate supplementation. The high-dose chromium picolinate supplementation for 12 week did not influence hematologic indexes or indexes of iron metabolism).
No products indexed under this heading.

Fondaparinux Sodium (Ingestion of more than 3 grams of omega-3 fatty acids from fish oils per day may have potential antithrombotic effects, including an increased in bleeding time and INR (international normalized ratio). DHA should be avoided in patients with taking anticoagulants). Products include:
Arixtra 1320

Fosphenytoin (Concomitant use with phenytoin may increase urinary excretion of biotin).
No products indexed under this heading.

Fosphenytoin Sodium (Concomitant use with phenytoin may increase urinary excretion of biotin).
No products indexed under this heading.

Gabapentin (Individuals on long-term anticonvulsant therapy may have reduced levels of biotin in their blood and urinary excretion of organic acids consistent with decreased carboxylase activity).
No products indexed under this heading.

Gatifloxacin (Long-term treatment with sulfa drugs or other antibiotics may decrease bacterial synthesis of biotin, potentially increasing the requirement for dietary biotin).
No products indexed under this heading.

Gemifloxacin Mesylate (Long-term treatment with sulfa drugs or other antibiotics may decrease bacterial synthesis of biotin, potentially increasing the requirement for dietary biotin).
No products indexed under this heading.

Gentamicin Sulfate (Long-term treatment with sulfa drugs or other antibiotics may decrease bacterial synthesis of biotin, potentially increasing the requirement for dietary biotin). Products include:
Pred-G .... ⊙226, ⊙227

Grepafloxacin Hydrochloride (Long-term treatment with sulfa drugs or other antibiotics may decrease bacterial synthesis of biotin, potentially increasing the requirement for dietary biotin).
No products indexed under this heading.

Griseofulvin (Long-term treatment with sulfa drugs or other antibiotics may decrease bacterial synthesis of biotin, potentially increasing the requirement for dietary biotin).
No products indexed under this heading.

Heparin Calcium (Ingestion of more than 3 grams of omega-3 fatty acids from fish oils per day may have potential antithrombotic effects, including an increased in bleeding time and INR (international normalized ratio). DHA should be avoided in patients with taking anticoagulants).
No products indexed under this heading.

Heparin Sodium (Ingestion of more than 3 grams of omega-3 fatty acids from fish oils per day may have potential antithrombotic effects, including an increased in bleeding time and INR (international normalized ratio). DHA should be avoided in patients with taking anticoagulants).
No products indexed under this heading.

Idarubicin Hydrochloride (Long-term treatment with sulfa drugs or other antibiotics may decrease bacterial synthesis of biotin, potentially increasing the requirement for dietary biotin).
No products indexed under this heading.

Imipenem (Long-term treatment with sulfa drugs or other antibiotics may decrease bacterial synthesis of biotin, potentially increasing the requirement for dietary biotin). Products include:
Primaxin I.M. 2232
Primaxin I.V. 2235

Iron (Chromium may compete for one of the binding sites on the iron transport protein, transferrin. Serum iron concentrations and serum ferritin concentrations were unchanged by either resistive training or chromium picolinate supplementation. The high-dose chromium picolinate supplementation for 12 week did not influence hematologic indexes or indexes of iron metabolism).
No products indexed under this heading.

Iron, Peptonized (Chromium may compete for one of the binding sites on the iron transport protein, transferrin. Serum iron concentrations and serum ferritin concentrations were unchanged by either resistive training or chromium picolinate supplementation. The high-dose chromium picolinate supplementation for 12 week did not influence hematologic indexes or indexes of iron metabolism).
No products indexed under this heading.

Iron Cacodylate (Chromium may compete for one of the binding sites on the iron transport protein, transferrin. Serum iron concentrations and serum ferritin concentrations were unchanged by either resistive training or chromium picolinate supplementation. The high-dose chromium picolinate supplementation for 12 week did not influence hematologic indexes or indexes of iron metabolism).
No products indexed under this heading.

Iron Carbonyl (Chromium may compete for one of the binding sites on the iron transport protein, transferrin. Serum iron concentrations and serum ferritin concentrations were unchanged by either resistive training or chromium picolinate supplementation. The high-dose chromium picolinate supplementation for 12 week did not influence hematologic indexes or indexes of iron metabolism). Products include:
CitraNatal 90 DHA Capsules 2332
CitraNatal Assure 2332
CitraNatal Harmony 2332
CitraNatal Rx 2332
Ferralet 2333

Iron Dextran (Chromium may compete for one of the binding sites on the iron transport protein, transferrin. Serum iron concentrations and serum ferritin concentrations were unchanged by either resistive training or chromium picolinate supplementation. The high-dose chromium picolinate supplementation for 12 week did not influence hematologic indexes or indexes of iron metabolism).
No products indexed under this heading.

Iron Polysaccharide Complex (Chromium may compete for one of the binding sites on the iron transport protein, transferrin. Serum iron concentrations and serum ferritin concentrations were unchanged by either resistive training or chromium picolinate supple-

IMPORTANT NOTE: Always consult each drug listing in the patient's regimen for possible interactions.

mentation. The high-dose chromium picolinate supplementation for 12 week did not influence hematologic indexes or indexes of iron metabolism).
No products indexed under this heading.

Iron Sucrose (Chromium may compete for one of the binding sites on the iron transport protein, transferrin. Serum iron concentrations and serum ferritin concentrations were unchanged by either resistive training or chromium picolinate supplementation. The high-dose chromium picolinate supplementation for 12 week did not influence hematologic indexes or indexes of iron metabolism).
No products indexed under this heading.

Iron Supplements (Chromium may compete for one of the binding sites on the iron transport protein, transferrin. Serum iron concentrations and serum ferritin concentrations were unchanged by either resistive training or chromium picolinate supplementation. The high-dose chromium picolinate supplementation for 12 week did not influence hematologic indexes or indexes of iron metabolism).
No products indexed under this heading.

Kanamycin Sulfate (Long-term treatment with sulfa drugs or other antibiotics may decrease bacterial synthesis of biotin, potentially increasing the requirement for dietary biotin).
No products indexed under this heading.

Lamotrigine (Individuals on long-term anticonvulsant therapy may have reduced levels of biotin in their blood and urinary excretion of organic acids consistent with decreased carboxylase activity). Products include:
Lamictal ... **1522**
Lamictal ODT ... **1522**
Lamictal XR ... **1536**

Levetiracetam (Individuals on long-term anticonvulsant therapy may have reduced levels of biotin in their blood and urinary excretion of organic acids consistent with decreased carboxylase activity). Products include:
Keppra XR ... **3434**

Levofloxacin (Long-term treatment with sulfa drugs or other antibiotics may decrease bacterial synthesis of biotin, potentially increasing the requirement for dietary biotin). Products include:
Iquix ... **3492**
Levaquin ... **2629**
Levaquin in 5% Dextrose ... **2629**
Quixin ... **3493**

Lomefloxacin Hydrochloride (Long-term treatment with sulfa drugs or other antibiotics may decrease bacterial synthesis of biotin, potentially increasing the requirement for dietary biotin).
No products indexed under this heading.

Loracarbef (Long-term treatment with sulfa drugs or other antibiotics may decrease bacterial synthesis of biotin, potentially increasing the requirement for dietary biotin).
No products indexed under this heading.

Low Molecular Weight Heparins (Ingestion of more than 3 grams of omega-3 fatty acids from fish oils per day may have potential antithrombotic effects, including an increased in bleeding time and INR (international normalized ratio). DHA should be avoided in patients with taking anticoagulants).
No products indexed under this heading.

Magaldrate (Concomitant use with antacids interferes with the absorption of chromium. However, the overall interference is not of clinically relevant concern).
No products indexed under this heading.

Magnesium Carbonate (Concomitant use with antacids interferes with the absorption of chromium. However, the overall interference is not of clinically relevant concern).
No products indexed under this heading.

Magnesium Hydroxide (Concomitant use with antacids interferes with the absorption of chromium. However, the overall interference is not of clinically relevant concern). Products include:
Fleet Pedia-Lax Chewable Tablets ... **1144**
Pepcid Complete ... **1822**

Magnesium Oxide (Concomitant use with antacids interferes with the absorption of chromium. However, the overall interference is not of clinically relevant concern). Products include:
Beelith ... **873**

Magnesium Trisilicate (Concomitant use with antacids interferes with the absorption of chromium. However, the overall interference is not of clinically relevant concern).
No products indexed under this heading.

Mephenytoin (Individuals on long-term anticonvulsant therapy may have reduced levels of biotin in their blood and urinary excretion of organic acids consistent with decreased carboxylase activity).
No products indexed under this heading.

Methacycline Hydrochloride (Long-term treatment with sulfa drugs or other antibiotics may decrease bacterial synthesis of biotin, potentially increasing the requirement for dietary biotin).
No products indexed under this heading.

Methicillin Sodium (Long-term treatment with sulfa drugs or other antibiotics may decrease bacterial synthesis of biotin, potentially increasing the requirement for dietary biotin).
No products indexed under this heading.

Methsuximide (Individuals on long-term anticonvulsant therapy may have reduced levels of biotin in their blood and urinary excretion of organic acids consistent with decreased carboxylase activity).
No products indexed under this heading.

Mezlocillin Sodium (Long-term treatment with sulfa drugs or other antibiotics may decrease bacterial synthesis of biotin, potentially increasing the requirement for dietary biotin).
No products indexed under this heading.

Minocycline Hydrochloride (Long-term treatment with sulfa drugs or other antibiotics may decrease bacterial synthesis of biotin, potentially increasing the requirement for dietary biotin). Products include:
Solodyn ... **2073**

Moxifloxacin Hydrochloride (Long-term treatment with sulfa drugs or other antibiotics may decrease bacterial synthesis of biotin, potentially increasing the requirement for dietary biotin). Products include:
Avelox ... **3064**
Vigamox ... **589**

Nafcillin Sodium (Long-term treatment with sulfa drugs or other antibiotics may decrease bacterial synthesis of biotin, potentially increasing the requirement for dietary biotin).
No products indexed under this heading.

Norfloxacin (Long-term treatment with sulfa drugs or other antibiotics may decrease bacterial synthesis of biotin, potentially increasing the requirement for dietary biotin). Products include:
Noroxin ... **2220**

Ofloxacin (Long-term treatment with sulfa drugs or other antibiotics may decrease bacterial synthesis of biotin, potentially increasing the requirement for dietary biotin).
No products indexed under this heading.

Oxacillin (Long-term treatment with sulfa drugs or other antibiotics may decrease bacterial synthesis of biotin, potentially increasing the requirement for dietary biotin).
No products indexed under this heading.

Oxacillin Sodium (Long-term treatment with sulfa drugs or other antibiotics may decrease bacterial synthesis of biotin, potentially increasing the requirement for dietary biotin).
No products indexed under this heading.

Oxcarbazepine (Individuals on long-term anticonvulsant therapy may have reduced levels of biotin in their blood and urinary excretion of organic acids consistent with decreased carboxylase activity).
No products indexed under this heading.

Oxytetracycline Hydrochloride (Long-term treatment with sulfa drugs or other antibiotics may decrease bacterial synthesis of biotin, potentially increasing the requirement for dietary biotin).
No products indexed under this heading.

Pantothenic Acid (Large doses of the nutrient pantothenic acid have the potential to compete with biotin for intestinal and cellular uptake due to their similar structures). Products include:
Heplive ... **607**

Paramethadione (Individuals on long-term anticonvulsant therapy may have reduced levels of biotin in their blood and urinary excretion of organic acids consistent with decreased carboxylase activity).
No products indexed under this heading.

Penicillin, Potassium Phenoxymethyl (Long-term treatment with sulfa drugs or other antibiotics may decrease bacterial synthesis of biotin, potentially increasing the requirement for dietary biotin).
No products indexed under this heading.

Penicillin G Benzathine (Long-term treatment with sulfa drugs or other antibiotics may decrease bacterial synthesis of biotin, potentially increasing the requirement for dietary biotin). Products include:
Bicillin C-R Injectable Suspension ... **1826**
Bicillin L-A ... **1828**

Penicillin G Dibenzylethyenediamine (Long-term treatment with sulfa drugs or other antibiotics may decrease bacterial synthesis of biotin, potentially increasing the requirement for dietary biotin).
No products indexed under this heading.

Penicillin G Potassium (Long-term treatment with sulfa drugs or other antibiotics may decrease bacterial synthesis of biotin, potentially increasing the requirement for dietary biotin).
No products indexed under this heading.

Penicillin G Procaine (Long-term treatment with sulfa drugs or other antibiotics may decrease bacterial synthesis of biotin, potentially increasing the requirement for dietary biotin). Products include:
Bicillin C-R Injectable Suspension ... **1826**
Bicillin L-A ... **1828**

Penicillin G Sodium (Long-term treatment with sulfa drugs or other antibiotics may decrease bacterial synthesis of biotin, potentially increasing the requirement for dietary biotin).
No products indexed under this heading.

Penicillin V (Long-term treatment with sulfa drugs or other antibiotics may decrease bacterial synthesis of biotin, potentially increasing the requirement for dietary biotin).
No products indexed under this heading.

Penicillin V Potassium (Long-term treatment with sulfa drugs or other antibiotics may decrease bacterial synthesis of biotin, potentially increasing the requirement for dietary biotin).
No products indexed under this heading.

Penicillins (Long-term treatment with sulfa drugs or other antibiotics may decrease bacterial synthesis of biotin, potentially increasing the requirement for dietary biotin).
No products indexed under this heading.

Phenacemide (Individuals on long-term anticonvulsant therapy may have reduced levels of biotin in their blood and urinary excretion of organic acids consistent with decreased carboxylase activity).
No products indexed under this heading.

Phenobarbital (Concomitant use with phenobarbital may increase urinary excretion of biotin). Products include:
Donnatal ... **2711**

Phenobarbital Sodium (Concomitant use with phenobarbital may increase urinary excretion of biotin).
No products indexed under this heading.

Phensuximide (Individuals on long-term anticonvulsant therapy may have reduced levels of biotin in their blood and urinary excretion of organic acids consistent with decreased carboxylase activity).
No products indexed under this heading.

Phenytoin (Concomitant use with phenytoin may increase urinary excretion of biotin).
No products indexed under this heading.

Phenytoin Sodium (Concomitant use with phenytoin may increase urinary excretion of biotin). Products include:
Phenytek Capsules ... **2380**

Piperacillin Sodium (Long-term treatment with sulfa drugs or other antibiotics may decrease bacterial synthesis of biotin, potentially increasing the requirement for dietary biotin). Products include:
Zosyn ... **3607**

Polysaccharide Iron Complex (Chromium may compete for one of the binding sites on the iron transport protein, transferrin. Serum iron concentrations and serum ferritin concentrations were unchanged by either resistive training or chromium picolinate supplementation. The high-dose chromium picolinate supplementation for 12 week did not influence hematologic indexes or indexes of iron metabolism). Products include:
Nu-Iron 150 ... **2321**

Primidone (Individuals on long-term anticonvulsant therapy may have reduced levels of biotin in their blood and urinary excretion of organic acids consistent with decreased carboxylase activity).
No products indexed under this heading.

Rufinamide (Individuals on long-term anticonvulsant therapy may have reduced levels of biotin in their blood and urinary excretion of organic acids consistent with decreased carboxylase activity). Products include:
Banzel ... **1050**

Sodium Bicarbonate (Concomitant use with antacids interferes with the absorption of chromium. However, the overall interference is not of clinically relevant concern).
No products indexed under this heading.

Sodium Cloxacillin Monohydrate (Long-term treatment with sulfa drugs or other antibiotics may decrease bacterial synthesis of biotin, potentially increasing the requirement for dietary biotin).
No products indexed under this heading.

Sparfloxacin (Long-term treatment with sulfa drugs or other antibiotics may decrease bacterial synthesis of biotin, potentially increasing the requirement for dietary biotin).

No products indexed under this heading.

Streptomycin Sulfate (Long-term treatment with sulfa drugs or other antibiotics may decrease bacterial synthesis of biotin, potentially increasing the requirement for dietary biotin).

No products indexed under this heading.

Sucrose (Diets high in simple sugars (eg sucrose), compared to diets high in complex carbohydrates (eg, whole grains) increase urinary chromium excretion in adults. This effect may be related to increase insulin secretion response to the consumption of simple sugars compared to complex carbohydrates).

No products indexed under this heading.

Sulfamethizole (Long-term treatment with sulfa drugs or other antibiotics may decrease bacterial synthesis of biotin, potentially increasing the requirement for dietary biotin).

No products indexed under this heading.

Sulfamethoxazole (Long-term treatment with sulfa drugs or other antibiotics may decrease bacterial synthesis of biotin, potentially increasing the requirement for dietary biotin).

No products indexed under this heading.

Sulfisoxazole Acetyl (Long-term treatment with sulfa drugs or other antibiotics may decrease bacterial synthesis of biotin, potentially increasing the requirement for dietary biotin).

No products indexed under this heading.

Sulfisoxazole Diolamine (Long-term treatment with sulfa drugs or other antibiotics may decrease bacterial synthesis of biotin, potentially increasing the requirement for dietary biotin).

No products indexed under this heading.

Tetracycline Hydrochloride (Long-term treatment with sulfa drugs or other antibiotics may decrease bacterial synthesis of biotin, potentially increasing the requirement for dietary biotin).
Products include:

Tiagabine Hydrochloride (Individuals on long-term anticonvulsant therapy may have reduced levels of biotin in their blood and urinary excretion of organic acids consistent with decreased carboxylase activity).
Products include:

Ticarcillin Disodium (Long-term treatment with sulfa drugs or other antibiotics may decrease bacterial synthesis of biotin, potentially increasing the requirement for dietary biotin). Products include:

Tinzaparin Sodium (Ingestion of more than 3 grams of omega-3 fatty acids from fish oils per day may have potential antithrombotic effects, including an increased in bleeding time and INR (international normalized ratio). DHA should be avoided in patients with taking anticoagulants).

No products indexed under this heading.

Tobramycin (Long-term treatment with sulfa drugs or other antibiotics may decrease bacterial synthesis of biotin, potentially increasing the requirement for dietary biotin). Products include:

Tobramycin Sulfate (Long-term treatment with sulfa drugs or other antibiotics may decrease bacterial synthesis of biotin, potentially increasing the requirement for dietary biotin).

No products indexed under this heading.

Topiramate (Individuals on long-term anticonvulsant therapy may have reduced levels of biotin in their blood and urinary excretion of organic acids consistent with decreased carboxylase activity).

No products indexed under this heading.

Trimethadione (Individuals on long-term anticonvulsant therapy may have reduced levels of biotin in their blood and urinary excretion of organic acids consistent with decreased carboxylase activity).

No products indexed under this heading.

Troleandomycin (Long-term treatment with sulfa drugs or other antibiotics may decrease bacterial synthesis of biotin, potentially increasing the requirement for dietary biotin).

No products indexed under this heading.

Trovafloxacin Mesylate (Long-term treatment with sulfa drugs or other antibiotics may decrease bacterial synthesis of biotin, potentially increasing the requirement for dietary biotin).

No products indexed under this heading.

Valproate Sodium (Use of the anticonvulsant valproic acid has been associated with decreased biotinidase activity in children).

No products indexed under this heading.

Valproic Acid (Use of the anticonvulsant valproic acid has been associated with decreased biotinidase activity in children).

No products indexed under this heading.

Vitamin C (Co-administration with vitamin C potentiates the absorption of chromium. However, the overall potentiation is minimal and not of clinically relevant concern. Administration of 100 mg vitamin C with 1 mg of chromium resulted in higher plasma levels of chromium than with 1 mg of chromium alone).
Products include:

Warfarin Sodium (Ingestion of more than 3 grams of omega-3 fatty acids from fish oils per day may have potential antithrombotic effects, including an increased in bleeding time and INR (international normalized ratio). DHA should be avoided in patients with taking anticoagulants).

No products indexed under this heading.

Zonisamide (Individuals on long-term anticonvulsant therapy may have reduced levels of biotin in their blood and urinary excretion of organic acids consistent with decreased carboxylase activity). Products include:

Food Interactions

Eggs (Egg whites contain avidin substance that binds to biotin and block absorption resulting to altered levels of biotin).

Food, unspecified (Diets high in simple sugars (eg, sucrose), compared to diets high in complex carbohydrates (eg, whole grains) increase urinary chromium

excretion in adults. This effect may be related to increase insulin secretion response to the consumption of simple sugars compared to complex carbohydrates).

Meal, unspecified (Diets high in simple sugars (eg, sucrose), compared to diets high in complex carbohydrates (eg, whole grains) increase urinary chromium excretion in adults. This effect may be related to increase insulin secretion response to the consumption of simple sugars compared to complex carbohydrates).

DONNATAL EXTENTABS
May interact with anticoagulants. Compounds in these categories include:

Anisindione (Phenobarbital may decrease the effect of anticoagulants and necessitate larger doses of the anticoagulant for optimal effect. When phenobarbital is discontinued, the dose of the anticoagulant may have to be decreased).

No products indexed under this heading.

Ardeparin Sodium (Phenobarbital may decrease the effect of anticoagulants and necessitate larger doses of the anticoagulant for optimal effect. When phenobarbital is discontinued, the dose of the anticoagulant may have to be decreased).

No products indexed under this heading.

Dalteparin Sodium (Phenobarbital may decrease the effect of anticoagulants and necessitate larger doses of the anticoagulant for optimal effect. When phenobarbital is discontinued, the dose of the anticoagulant may have to be decreased). Products include:

Danaparoid Sodium (Phenobarbital may decrease the effect of anticoagulants and necessitate larger doses of the anticoagulant for optimal effect. When phenobarbital is discontinued, the dose of the anticoagulant may have to be decreased).

No products indexed under this heading.

Dicumarol (Phenobarbital may decrease the effect of anticoagulants and necessitate larger doses of the anticoagulant for optimal effect. When phenobarbital is discontinued, the dose of the anticoagulant may have to be decreased).

No products indexed under this heading.

Enoxaparin Sodium (Phenobarbital may decrease the effect of anticoagulants and necessitate larger doses of the anticoagulant for optimal effect. When phenobarbital is discontinued, the dose of the anticoagulant may have to be decreased). Products include:

Fondaparinux Sodium (Phenobarbital may decrease the effect of anticoagulants and necessitate larger doses of the anticoagulant for optimal effect. When phenobarbital is discontinued, the dose of the anticoagulant may have to be decreased). Products include:

Heparin Calcium (Phenobarbital may decrease the effect of anticoagulants and necessitate larger doses of the anticoagulant for optimal effect. When phenobarbital is discontinued, the dose of the anticoagulant may have to be decreased).

No products indexed under this heading.

Heparin Sodium (Phenobarbital may decrease the effect of anticoagulants and necessitate larger doses of the anticoagulant for optimal effect. When phenobarbital is discontinued, the dose of the anticoagulant may have to be decreased).

No products indexed under this heading.

Low Molecular Weight Heparins (Phenobarbital may decrease the effect of anticoagulants and necessitate larger doses of the anticoagulant for optimal effect. When phenobarbital is discontinued, the dose of the anticoagulant may have to be decreased).

No products indexed under this heading.

Tinzaparin Sodium (Phenobarbital may decrease the effect of anticoagulants and necessitate larger doses of the anticoagulant for optimal effect. When phenobarbital is discontinued, the dose of the anticoagulant may have to be decreased).

No products indexed under this heading.

Warfarin Sodium (Phenobarbital may decrease the effect of anticoagulants and necessitate larger doses of the anticoagulant for optimal effect. When phenobarbital is discontinued, the dose of the anticoagulant may have to be decreased).

No products indexed under this heading.

DORZOLAMIDE HYDROCHLORIDE OPHTHALMIC SOLUTION, 2%
May interact with carbonic anhydrase inhibitors, salicylates, and certain other agents. Compounds in these categories include:

Acetazolamide (There is a potential for an additive effect on the known systemic effects of carbonic anhydrase inhibition in patients receiving an oral carbonic anhydrase inhibitor and dorzolamide hydrochloride ophthalmic solution. The concomitant administration of dorzolamide hydrochloride ophthalmic solution and oral carbonic anhydrase inhibitors is not recommended).

No products indexed under this heading.

Aspirin (Although acid-base and electrolyte disturbances were not reported in the clinical trials with dorzolamide hydrochloride ophthalmic solution, these disturbances have been reported with oral carbonic anhydrase inhibitors and have, in some instances, resulted in drug interactions (eg, toxicity associated with high-dose salicylate therapy). Therefore, the potential for such drug interactions should be considered in patients receiving dorzolamide hydrochloride ophthalmic solution). Products include:

Aspirin, Enteric Coated (Although acid-base and electrolyte disturbances were not reported in the clinical trials with dorzolamide hydrochloride ophthalmic solution, these disturbances have been reported with oral carbonic anhydrase inhibitors and have, in some instances, resulted in drug interactions (eg, toxicity associated with high-dose salicylate therapy). Therefore, the potential for such drug interactions should be considered in patients receiving dorzolamide hydrochloride ophthalmic solution).

No products indexed under this heading.

Aspirin Buffered (Although acid-base and electrolyte disturbances were not reported in the clinical trials with dorzolamide hydrochloride ophthalmic solution, these disturbances have been

reported with oral carbonic anhydrase inhibitors and have, in some instances, resulted in drug interactions (eg, toxicity associated with high-dose salicylate therapy). Therefore, the potential for such drug interactions should be considered in patients receiving dorzolamide hydrochloride ophthalmic solution).

No products indexed under this heading.

Choline Magnesium Trisalicylate (Although acid-base and electrolyte disturbances were not reported in the clinical trials with dorzolamide hydrochloride ophthalmic solution, these disturbances have been reported with oral carbonic anhydrase inhibitors and have, in some instances, resulted in drug interactions (eg, toxicity associated with high-dose salicylate therapy). Therefore, the potential for such drug interactions should be considered in patients receiving dorzolamide hydrochloride ophthalmic solution).

No products indexed under this heading.

Dichlorphenamide (There is a potential for an additive effect on the known systemic effects of carbonic anhydrase inhibition in patients receiving an oral carbonic anhydrase inhibitor and dorzolamide hydrochloride ophthalmic solution. The concomitant administration of dorzolamide hydrochloride ophthalmic solution and oral carbonic anhydrase inhibitors is not recommended).

No products indexed under this heading.

Diflunisal (Although acid-base and electrolyte disturbances were not reported in the clinical trials with dorzolamide hydrochloride ophthalmic solution, these disturbances have been reported with oral carbonic anhydrase inhibitors and have, in some instances, resulted in drug interactions (eg, toxicity associated with high-dose salicylate therapy). Therefore, the potential for such drug interactions should be considered in patients receiving dorzolamide hydrochloride ophthalmic solution).

No products indexed under this heading.

Drugs, unspecified (Although acid-base and electrolyte disturbances were not reported in the clinical trials with dorzolamide hydrochloride ophthalmic solution, these disturbances have been reported with oral carbonic anhydrase inhibitors and have, in some instances, resulted in drug interactions (eg, toxicity associated with high-dose salicylate therapy). Therefore, the potential for such drug interactions should be considered in patients receiving dorzolamide hydrochloride ophthalmic solution).

No products indexed under this heading.

Magnesium Salicylate (Although acid-base and electrolyte disturbances were not reported in the clinical trials with dorzolamide hydrochloride ophthalmic solution, these disturbances have been reported with oral carbonic anhydrase inhibitors and have, in some instances, resulted in drug interactions (eg, toxicity associated with high-dose salicylate therapy). Therefore, the potential for such drug interactions should be considered in patients receiving dorzolamide hydrochloride ophthalmic solution).

No products indexed under this heading.

Methazolamide (There is a potential for an additive effect on the known systemic effects of carbonic anhydrase inhibition in patients receiving an oral carbonic anhydrase inhibitor and dorzolamide hydrochloride ophthalmic solution. The concomitant administration of dorzolamide hydrochloride ophthalmic solution and oral carbonic anhydrase inhibitors is not recommended).

No products indexed under this heading.

Salsalate (Although acid-base and electrolyte disturbances were not reported in the clinical trials with dorzolamide hydrochloride ophthalmic solution, these disturbances have been reported with oral carbonic anhydrase inhibitors and have, in some instances, resulted in drug interactions (eg, toxicity associated with high-dose salicylate therapy). Therefore, the potential for such drug interactions should be considered in patients receiving dorzolamide hydrochloride ophthalmic solution).

No products indexed under this heading.

Topical Medications (If more than one topical ophthalmic drug is being used, the drugs should be administered at least ten minutes apart).

No products indexed under this heading.

Torsemide (There is a potential for an additive effect on the known systemic effects of carbonic anhydrase inhibition in patients receiving an oral carbonic anhydrase inhibitor and dorzolamide hydrochloride ophthalmic solution. The concomitant administration of dorzolamide hydrochloride ophthalmic solution and oral carbonic anhydrase inhibitors is not recommended).

No products indexed under this heading.

DORZOLAMIDE HYDROCHLORIDE/ TIMOLOL MALEATE OPHTHALMIC SOLUTION

(Dorzolamide Hydrochloride, Timolol Maleate) ....⊙243
May interact with beta-blockers, calcium channel blockers, carbonic anhydrase inhibitors, cardiac glycosides, catecholamine-depleting drugs, cytochrome p450 2d6 inhibitors (selected), epinephrine-containing products, general anesthetics, insulin, oral hypoglycemic agents, quinidine, salicylates, selective serotonin reuptake inhibitors, and certain other agents. Compounds in these categories include:

Acarbose (β-adrenergic blocking agents should be administered with caution in patients subject to spontaneous hypoglycemia or to diabetic patients (especially those with labile diabetes) who are receiving insulin or oral hypoglycemic agents. β-adrenergic receptor blocking agents may mask the signs and symptoms of acute hypoglycemia).

No products indexed under this heading.

Acebutolol Hydrochloride (Patients who are receiving a β-adrenergic blocking agent orally and dorzolamide hydrochloride/timolol maleate ophthalmic solution should be observed for potential additive effects of β-blockade, both systemic and on intraocular pressure. The concomitant use of two topical β-adrenergic blocking agents is not recommended).

No products indexed under this heading.

Acetazolamide (There is a potential for an additive effect on the known systemic effects of carbonic anhydrase inhibition in patients receiving an oral carbonic anhydrase inhibitor and dorzolamide hydrochloride/timolol maleate ophthalmic solution. The concomitant administration of dorzolamide hydrochloride/timolol maleate ophthalmic solution and oral carbonic anhydrase inhibitors is not recommended).

No products indexed under this heading.

Amiodarone Hydrochloride (Potentiated systemic β-blockade (eg, decreased heart rate, depression) has been reported during combined treatment with CYP2D6 inhibitors (eg, quinidine, SSRIs) and timolol).

No products indexed under this heading.

Amitriptyline Hydrochloride (Potentiated systemic β-blockade (eg, decreased heart rate, depression) has been reported during combined treatment with CYP2D6 inhibitors (eg, quinidine, SSRIs) and timolol).

No products indexed under this heading.

Amlodipine Besylate (The concomitant use of β-adrenergic blocking agents with digitalisand calcium antagonists may have additive effects in prolonging atrioventricular conduction time. Caution should be used in the co-administration of β-adrenergic blocking agents, such as dorzolamide hydrochloride/timolol maleate ophthalmic solution, and oral or intravenous calcium antagonists because of possible atrioventricular conduction disturbances, left ventricular failure, and hypotension. In patients with impaired cardiac function, co-administration should be avoided). Products include:

    Azor 1010
    Exforge 2443
    Exforge HCT 2449

Amoxapine (Potentiated systemic β-blockade (eg, decreased heart rate, depression) has been reported during combined treatment with CYP2D6 inhibitors (eg, quinidine, SSRIs) and timolol).

No products indexed under this heading.

Aspirin (Although acid-base and electrolyte disturbances were not reported in the clinical trials with dorzolamide hydrochloride ophthalmic solution, these disturbances have been reported with oral carbonic anhydrase inhibitors and have, in some instances, resulted in drug interactions (eg, toxicity associated with high-dose salicylate therapy). Therefore, the potential for such drug interactions should be considered in patients receiving dorzolamide hydrochloride/timolol maleate ophthalmic solution). Products include:

    Aggrenox 880
    Bayer Aspirin 829
    Percodan 1124
    St. Joseph Aspirin 2045

Aspirin, Enteric Coated (Although acid-base and electrolyte disturbances were not reported in the clinical trials with dorzolamide hydrochloride ophthalmic solution, these disturbances have been reported with oral carbonic anhydrase inhibitors and have, in some instances, resulted in drug interactions (eg, toxicity associated with high-dose salicylate therapy). Therefore, the potential for such drug interactions should be considered in patients receiving dorzolamide hydrochloride/timolol maleate ophthalmic solution).

No products indexed under this heading.

Aspirin Buffered (Although acid-base and electrolyte disturbances were not reported in the clinical trials with dorzolamide hydrochloride ophthalmic solution, these disturbances have been reported with oral carbonic anhydrase inhibitors and have, in some instances, resulted in drug interactions (eg, toxicity associated with high-dose salicylate therapy). Therefore, the potential for such drug interactions should be considered in patients receiving dorzolamide hydrochloride/timolol maleate ophthalmic solution).

No products indexed under this heading.

Atenolol (Patients who are receiving a β-adrenergic blocking agent orally and dorzolamide hydrochloride/timolol maleate ophthalmic solution should be observed for potential additive effects of β-blockade, both systemic and on intraocular pressure. The concomitant use of two topical β-adrenergic blocking agents is not recommended).

No products indexed under this heading.

Bepridil Hydrochloride (The concomitant use of β-adrenergic blocking agents with digitalisand calcium antago-

nists may have additive effects in prolonging atrioventricular conduction time. Caution should be used in the co-administration of β-adrenergic blocking agents, such as dorzolamide hydrochloride/timolol maleate ophthalmic solution, and oral or intravenous calcium antagonists because of possible atrioventricular conduction disturbances, left ventricular failure, and hypotension. In patients with impaired cardiac function, co-administration should be avoided).

No products indexed under this heading.

Betaxolol Hydrochloride (Patients who are receiving a β-adrenergic blocking agent orally and dorzolamide hydrochloride/timolol maleate ophthalmic solution should be observed for potential additive effects of β-blockade, both systemic and on intraocular pressure. The concomitant use of two topical β-adrenergic blocking agents is not recommended).

No products indexed under this heading.

Bisoprolol Fumarate (Patients who are receiving a β-adrenergic blocking agent orally and dorzolamide hydrochloride/timolol maleate ophthalmic solution should be observed for potential additive effects of β-blockade, both systemic and on intraocular pressure. The concomitant use of two topical β-adrenergic blocking agents is not recommended).

No products indexed under this heading.

Bupropion Hydrochloride (Potentiated systemic β-blockade (eg, decreased heart rate, depression) has been reported during combined treatment with CYP2D6 inhibitors (eg, quinidine, SSRIs) and timolol). Products include:

    Aplenzin 2948
    Wellbutrin 1719
    Wellbutrin SR 1725
    Zyban 1762

Carteolol Hydrochloride (Patients who are receiving a β-adrenergic blocking agent orally and dorzolamide hydrochloride/timolol maleate ophthalmic solution should be observed for potential additive effects of β-blockade, both systemic and on intraocular pressure. The concomitant use of two topical β-adrenergic blocking agents is not recommended).

No products indexed under this heading.

Carvedilol (Patients who are receiving a β-adrenergic blocking agent orally and dorzolamide hydrochloride/timolol maleate ophthalmic solution should be observed for potential additive effects of β-blockade, both systemic and on intraocular pressure. The concomitant use of two topical β-adrenergic blocking agents is not recommended). Products include:
    Coreg 1409

Carvedilol Phosphate (Patients who are receiving a β-adrenergic blocking agent orally and dorzolamide hydrochloride/timolol maleate ophthalmic solution should be observed for potential additive effects of β-blockade, both systemic and on intraocular pressure. The concomitant use of two topical β-adrenergic blocking agents is not recommended). Products include:
    Coreg CR 1416

Celecoxib (Potentiated systemic β-blockade (eg, decreased heart rate, depression) has been reported during combined treatment with CYP2D6 inhibitors (eg, quinidine, SSRIs) and timolol). Products include:
    Celebrex 3272

Chloroquine (Potentiated systemic β-blockade (eg, decreased heart rate, depression) has been reported during combined treatment with CYP2D6 inhibitors (eg, quinidine, SSRIs) and timolol).

No products indexed under this heading.

Chloroquine Hydrochloride (Potentiated systemic β-blockade (eg, decreased heart rate, depression) has been reported during combined treatment with CYP2D6 inhibitors (eg, quinidine, SSRIs) and timolol).
No products indexed under this heading.

Chloroquine Phosphate (Potentiated systemic β-blockade (eg, decreased heart rate, depression) has been reported during combined treatment with CYP2D6 inhibitors (eg, quinidine, SSRIs) and timolol).
No products indexed under this heading.

Chlorpheniramine (Potentiated systemic β-blockade (eg, decreased heart rate, depression) has been reported during combined treatment with CYP2D6 inhibitors (eg, quinidine, SSRIs) and timolol).
No products indexed under this heading.

Chlorpheniramine Maleate (Potentiated systemic β-blockade (eg, decreased heart rate, depression) has been reported during combined treatment with CYP2D6 inhibitors (eg, quinidine, SSRIs) and timolol).
No products indexed under this heading.

Chlorpheniramine Polistirex (Potentiated systemic β-blockade (eg, decreased heart rate, depression) has been reported during combined treatment with CYP2D6 inhibitors (eg, quinidine, SSRIs) and timolol). Products include:
Tussionex **3443**

Chlorpheniramine Tannate (Potentiated systemic β-blockade (eg, decreased heart rate, depression) has been reported during combined treatment with CYP2D6 inhibitors (eg, quinidine, SSRIs) and timolol).
No products indexed under this heading.

Chlorpropamide (β-adrenergic blocking agents should be administered with caution in patients subject to spontaneous hypoglycemia or to diabetic patients (especially those with labile diabetes) who are receiving insulin or oral hypoglycemic agents. β-adrenergic receptor blocking agents may mask the signs and symptoms of acute hypoglycemia).
No products indexed under this heading.

Choline Magnesium Trisalicylate (Although acid-base and electrolyte disturbances were not reported in the clinical trials with dorzolamide hydrochloride ophthalmic solution, these disturbances have been reported with oral carbonic anhydrase inhibitors and have, in some instances, resulted in drug interactions (eg, toxicity associated with high-dose salicylate therapy). Therefore, the potential for such drug interactions should be considered in patients receiving dorzolamide hydrochloride/timolol maleate ophthalmic solution).
No products indexed under this heading.

Cimetidine (Potentiated systemic β-blockade (eg, decreased heart rate, depression) has been reported during combined treatment with CYP2D6 inhibitors (eg, quinidine, SSRIs) and timolol).
No products indexed under this heading.

Cimetidine Hydrochloride (Potentiated systemic β-blockade (eg, decreased heart rate, depression) has been reported during combined treatment with CYP2D6 inhibitors (eg, quinidine, SSRIs) and timolol).
No products indexed under this heading.

Citalopram Hydrobromide (Potentiated systemic β-blockade (eg, decreased heart rate, depression) has been reported during combined treatment with CYP2D6 inhibitors (eg, quinidine, SSRIs) and timolol). Products include:
Celexa **1153**

Clomipramine Hydrochloride (Potentiated systemic β-blockade (eg, decreased heart rate, depression) has been reported during combined treatment with CYP2D6 inhibitors (eg, quinidine, SSRIs) and timolol).
No products indexed under this heading.

Clonidine (Oral β-adrenergic blocking agents may exacerbate the rebound hypertension which can follow the withdrawal of clonidine. There have been no reports of exacerbation of rebound hypertension with ophthalmic timolol maleate). Products include:
Catapres-TTS **884**

Clonidine Hydrochloride (Oral β-adrenergic blocking agents may exacerbate the rebound hypertension which can follow the withdrawal of clonidine. There have been no reports of exacerbation of rebound hypertension with ophthalmic timolol maleate). Products include:
Clorpres **2344**

Cocaine Hydrochloride (Potentiated systemic β-blockade (eg, decreased heart rate, depression) has been reported during combined treatment with CYP2D6 inhibitors (eg, quinidine, SSRIs) and timolol).
No products indexed under this heading.

Deserpidine (Close observation of the patient is recommended when a β-blocker is administered to patients receiving catecholamine depleting drugs, such as reserpine, because of possible additive effects and the production of hypotension and/ or marked bradycardia, which may result in vertigo, syncope, or postural hypotension).
No products indexed under this heading.

Desflurane (β-adrenergic receptor blockade impairs the ability of the heart to respond to β-adrenergically mediated reflex stimuli. This may augment the risk of general anesthesia in surgical procedures. Some patients receiving β-adrenergic receptor blocking agents have experienced protracted severe hypotension during anesthesia. Difficulty in restarting and maintaining the heartbeat has also been reported. For these reasons, in patients undergoing elective surgery, some authorities recommend gradual withdrawal of β-adrenergic receptor blocking agents).
No products indexed under this heading.

Desipramine Hydrochloride (Potentiated systemic β-blockade (eg, decreased heart rate, depression) has been reported during combined treatment with CYP2D6 inhibitors (eg, quinidine, SSRIs) and timolol).
No products indexed under this heading.

Deslanoside (The concomitant use of β-adrenergic blocking agents with digitalisand calcium antagonists may have additive effects in prolonging atrioventricular conduction time).
No products indexed under this heading.

Dichlorphenamide (There is a potential for an additive effect on the known systemic effects of carbonic anhydrase inhibition in patients receiving an oral carbonic anhydrase inhibitor and dorzolamide hydrochloride/timolol maleate ophthalmic solution. The concomitant administration of dorzolamide hydrochloride/timolol maleate ophthalmic solution and oral carbonic anhydrase inhibitors is not recommended).
No products indexed under this heading.

Diflunisal (Although acid-base and electrolyte disturbances were not reported in the clinical trials with dorzolamide hydrochloride ophthalmic solution, these disturbances have been reported with oral carbonic anhydrase inhibitors and have, in some instances, resulted in drug interactions (eg, toxicity associated with high-dose salicylate therapy). Therefore, the potential for such drug interactions should be considered in patients receiving dorzolamide hydrochloride/timolol maleate ophthalmic solution).
No products indexed under this heading.

Digitalis Glycoside Preparations (The concomitant use of β-adrenergic blocking agents with digitalisand calcium antagonists may have additive effects in prolonging atrioventricular conduction time).
No products indexed under this heading.

Digitalis Lanata (The concomitant use of β-adrenergic blocking agents with digitalisand calcium antagonists may have additive effects in prolonging atrioventricular conduction time).
No products indexed under this heading.

Digitalis Purpurea (The concomitant use of β-adrenergic blocking agents with digitalisand calcium antagonists may have additive effects in prolonging atrioventricular conduction time).
No products indexed under this heading.

Digitoxin (The concomitant use of β-adrenergic blocking agents with digitalisand calcium antagonists may have additive effects in prolonging atrioventricular conduction time).
No products indexed under this heading.

Digoxin (The concomitant use of β-adrenergic blocking agents with digitalisand calcium antagonists may have additive effects in prolonging atrioventricular conduction time). Products include:
Lanoxin Injection **1546**
Lanoxin Injection Pediatric **1549**
Lanoxin Tablets **1553**

Diltiazem Hydrochloride (The concomitant use of β-adrenergic blocking agents with digitalisand calcium antagonists may have additive effects in prolonging atrioventricular conduction time. Caution should be used in the co-administration of β-adrenergic blocking agents, such as dorzolamide hydrochloride/timolol maleate ophthalmic solution, and oral or intravenous calcium antagonists because of possible atrioventricular conduction disturbances, left ventricular failure, and hypotension. In patients with impaired cardiac function, co-administration should be avoided). Products include:
Cardizem LA **423**

Diphenhydramine (Potentiated systemic β-blockade (eg, decreased heart rate, depression) has been reported during combined treatment with CYP2D6 inhibitors (eg, quinidine, SSRIs) and timolol).
No products indexed under this heading.

Diphenhydramine Hydrochloride (Potentiated systemic β-blockade (eg, decreased heart rate, depression) has been reported during combined treatment with CYP2D6 inhibitors (eg, quinidine, SSRIs) and timolol). Products include:
Benadryl Allergy Ultratab **2042**
Children's Benadryl Allergy Liquid **2042**

Doxepin Hydrochloride (Potentiated systemic β-blockade (eg, decreased heart rate, depression) has been reported during combined treatment with CYP2D6 inhibitors (eg, quinidine, SSRIs) and timolol).
No products indexed under this heading.

Drugs, unspecified (Although acid-base and electrolyte disturbances were not reported in the clinicaltrials with dorzolamide hydrochloride ophthalmic solution, these disturbances have been reported with oral carbonic anhydrase inhibitors and have, in someinstances, resulted in drug interactions (eg, toxicity associated with high-dose salicylate therapy). Therefore, the potential for such drug interactions shouldbe considered in patients receiving dorzolamide hydrochloride/timolol maleate ophthalmic solution).
No products indexed under this heading.

Enflurane (β-adrenergic receptor blockade impairs the ability of the heart to respond to β-adrenergically mediated reflex stimuli. This may augment the risk of general anesthesia in surgical procedures. Some patients receiving β-adrenergic receptor blocking agents have experienced protracted severe hypotension during anesthesia. Difficulty in restarting and maintaining the heartbeat has also been reported. For these reasons, in patients undergoing elective surgery, some authorities recommend gradual withdrawal of β-adrenergic receptor blocking agents).
No products indexed under this heading.

Epinephrine (While taking β-blockers, patients with a history of atopy or a history of severe anaphylactic reactions to a variety of allergens may be more reactive to repeated accidental, diagnostic, or therapeutic challenge with such allergens. Such patients may be unresponsive to the usual doses of epinephrine used to treat anaphylactic reactions). Products include:
EpiPen **3631**
Twinject **3268**

Epinephrine, Racemic (While taking β-blockers, patients with a history of atopy or a history of severe anaphylactic reactions to a variety of allergens may be more reactive to repeated accidental, diagnostic, or therapeutic challenge with such allergens. Such patients may be unresponsive to the usual doses of epinephrine used to treat anaphylactic reactions).
No products indexed under this heading.

Epinephrine Bitartrate (While taking β-blockers, patients with a history of atopy or a history of severe anaphylactic reactions to a variety of allergens may be more reactive to repeated accidental, diagnostic, or therapeutic challenge with such allergens. Such patients may be unresponsive to the usual doses of epinephrine used to treat anaphylactic reactions).
No products indexed under this heading.

Epinephrine Hydrochloride (While taking β-blockers, patients with a history of atopy or a history of severe anaphylactic reactions to a variety of allergens may be more reactive to repeated accidental, diagnostic, or therapeutic challenge with such allergens. Such patients may be unresponsive to the usual doses of epinephrine used to treat anaphylactic reactions).
No products indexed under this heading.

Escitalopram Oxalate (Potentiated systemic β-blockade (eg, decreased heart rate, depression) has been reported during combined treatment with CYP2D6 inhibitors (eg, quinidine, SSRIs) and timolol). Products include:
Lexapro Oral Suspension **1160**
Lexapro Tablets **1160**

Esmolol Hydrochloride (Patients who are receiving a β-adrenergic blocking agent orally and dorzolamide hydrochloride/timolol maleate ophthalmic solution should be observed for potential additive effects of β-blockade, both systemic and on intraocular pressure. The concomitant use of two topical β-adrenergic blocking agents is not recommended).
No products indexed under this heading.

Felodipine (The concomitant use of β-adrenergic blocking agents with digitalisand calcium antagonists may have additive effects in prolonging atrioventricular conduction time. Caution should be used in the co-administration of β-adrenergic blocking agents, such as dorzolamide hydrochloride/timolol mal-

Dorzolamide/Timolol Interactions Index 488

eate ophthalmic solution, and oral or intravenous calcium antagonists because of possible atrioventricular conduction disturbances, left ventricular failure, and hypotension. In patients with impaired cardiac function, co-administration should be avoided).
No products indexed under this heading.

Fluoxetine (Potentiated systemic β-blockade (eg, decreased heart rate, depression) has been reported during combined treatment with CYP2D6 inhibitors (eg, quinidine, SSRIs) and timolol).
No products indexed under this heading.

Fluoxetine Hydrochloride (Potentiated systemic β-blockade (eg, decreased heart rate, depression) has been reported during combined treatment with CYP2D6 inhibitors (eg, quinidine, SSRIs) and timolol). Products include:
Prozac Weekly 1941
Prozac Pulvules 1941
Symbyax 1965

Fluphenazine Decanoate (Potentiated systemic β-blockade (eg, decreased heart rate, depression) has been reported during combined treatment with CYP2D6 inhibitors (eg, quinidine, SSRIs) and timolol).
No products indexed under this heading.

Fluphenazine Enanthate (Potentiated systemic β-blockade (eg, decreased heart rate, depression) has been reported during combined treatment with CYP2D6 inhibitors (eg, quinidine, SSRIs) and timolol).
No products indexed under this heading.

Fluphenazine Hydrochloride (Potentiated systemic β-blockade (eg, decreased heart rate, depression) has been reported during combined treatment with CYP2D6 inhibitors (eg, quinidine, SSRIs) and timolol).
No products indexed under this heading.

Fluvoxamine (Potentiated systemic β-blockade (eg, decreased heart rate, depression) has been reported during combined treatment with CYP2D6 inhibitors (eg, quinidine, SSRIs) and timolol).
No products indexed under this heading.

Fluvoxamine Maleate (Potentiated systemic β-blockade (eg, decreased heart rate, depression) has been reported during combined treatment with CYP2D6 inhibitors (eg, quinidine, SSRIs) and timolol).
No products indexed under this heading.

Glibenclamide (β-adrenergic blocking agents should be administered with caution in patients subject to spontaneous hypoglycemia or to diabetic patients (especially those with labile diabetes) who are receiving insulin or oral hypoglycemic agents. β-adrenergic receptor blocking agents may mask the signs and symptoms of acute hypoglycemia).
No products indexed under this heading.

Glimepiride (β-adrenergic blocking agents should be administered with caution in patients subject to spontaneous hypoglycemia or to diabetic patients (especially those with labile diabetes) who are receiving insulin or oral hypoglycemic agents. β-adrenergic receptor blocking agents may mask the signs and symptoms of acute hypoglycemia). Products include:
Avandaryl 1356
Duetact 3354

Glipizide (β-adrenergic blocking agents should be administered with caution in patients subject to spontaneous hypoglycemia or to diabetic patients (especially those with labile diabetes) who are receiving insulin or oral hypoglycemic agents. β-adrenergic receptor blocking agents may mask the signs and symptoms of acute hypoglycemia).
No products indexed under this heading.

Glyburide (β-adrenergic blocking agents should be administered with caution in patients subject to spontaneous hypoglycemia or to diabetic patients (especially those with labile diabetes) who are receiving insulin or oral hypoglycemic agents. β-adrenergic receptor blocking agents may mask the signs and symptoms of acute hypoglycemia).
No products indexed under this heading.

Guanethidine (Close observation of the patient is recommended when a β-blocker is administered to patients receiving catecholamine depleting drugs, such as reserpine, because of possible additive effects and the production of hypotension and/ or marked bradycardia, which may result in vertigo, syncope, or postural hypotension).
No products indexed under this heading.

Guanethidine Monosulfate (Close observation of the patient is recommended when a β-blocker is administered to patients receiving catecholamine depleting drugs, such as reserpine, because of possible additive effects and the production of hypotension and/ or marked bradycardia, which may result in vertigo, syncope, or postural hypotension).
No products indexed under this heading.

Guanethidine Sulfate (Close observation of the patient is recommended when a β-blocker is administered to patients receiving catecholamine depleting drugs, such as reserpine, because of possible additive effects and the production of hypotension and/ or marked bradycardia, which may result in vertigo, syncope, or postural hypotension).
No products indexed under this heading.

Halofantrine Hydrochloride (Potentiated systemic β-blockade (eg, decreased heart rate, depression) has been reported during combined treatment with CYP2D6 inhibitors (eg, quinidine, SSRIs) and timolol).
No products indexed under this heading.

Haloperidol (Potentiated systemic β-blockade (eg, decreased heart rate, depression) has been reported during combined treatment with CYP2D6 inhibitors (eg, quinidine, SSRIs) and timolol).
No products indexed under this heading.

Haloperidol Decanoate (Potentiated systemic β-blockade (eg, decreased heart rate, depression) has been reported during combined treatment with CYP2D6 inhibitors (eg, quinidine, SSRIs) and timolol).
No products indexed under this heading.

Haloperidol Lactate (Potentiated systemic β-blockade (eg, decreased heart rate, depression) has been reported during combined treatment with CYP2D6 inhibitors (eg, quinidine, SSRIs) and timolol).
No products indexed under this heading.

Halothane (β-adrenergic receptor blockade impairs the ability of the heart to respond to β-adrenergically mediated reflex stimuli. This may augment the risk of general anesthesia in surgical procedures. Some patients receiving β-adrenergic receptor blocking agents have experienced protracted severe hypotension during anesthesia. Difficulty in restarting and maintaining the heartbeat has also been reported. For these reasons, in patients undergoing elective surgery, some authorities recommend gradual withdrawal of β-adrenergic receptor blocking agents).
No products indexed under this heading.

Hydroxychloroquine Sulfate (Potentiated systemic β-blockade (eg, decreased heart rate, depression) has been reported during combined treatment with CYP2D6 inhibitors (eg, quinidine, SSRIs) and timolol).
No products indexed under this heading.

Imatinib Mesylate (Potentiated systemic β-blockade (eg, decreased heart rate, depression) has been reported during combined treatment with CYP2D6 inhibitors (eg, quinidine, SSRIs) and timolol). Products include:
Gleevec 2477

Imipramine Hydrochloride (Potentiated systemic β-blockade (eg, decreased heart rate, depression) has been reported during combined treatment with CYP2D6 inhibitors (eg, quinidine, SSRIs) and timolol).
No products indexed under this heading.

Imipramine Pamoate (Potentiated systemic β-blockade (eg, decreased heart rate, depression) has been reported during combined treatment with CYP2D6 inhibitors (eg, quinidine, SSRIs) and timolol).
No products indexed under this heading.

Insulin (β-adrenergic blocking agents should be administered with caution in patients subject to spontaneous hypoglycemia or to diabetic patients (especially those with labile diabetes) who are receiving insulin or oral hypoglycemic agents. β-adrenergic receptor blocking agents may mask the signs and symptoms of acute hypoglycemia).
No products indexed under this heading.

Insulin, Human, Zinc Suspension (β-adrenergic blocking agents should be administered with caution in patients subject to spontaneous hypoglycemia or to diabetic patients (especially those with labile diabetes) who are receiving insulin or oral hypoglycemic agents. β-adrenergic receptor blocking agents may mask the signs and symptoms of acute hypoglycemia).
No products indexed under this heading.

Insulin, Human (rDNA origin) (β-adrenergic blocking agents should be administered with caution in patients subject to spontaneous hypoglycemia or to diabetic patients (especially those with labile diabetes) who are receiving insulin or oral hypoglycemic agents. β-adrenergic receptor blocking agents may mask the signs and symptoms of acute hypoglycemia). Products include:
Exubera 2717

Insulin, Human NPH (β-adrenergic blocking agents should be administered with caution in patients subject to spontaneous hypoglycemia or to diabetic patients (especially those with labile diabetes) who are receiving insulin or oral hypoglycemic agents. β-adrenergic receptor blocking agents may mask the signs and symptoms of acute hypoglycemia). Products include:
Humulin N Vial 1934

Insulin, Human Regular (β-adrenergic blocking agents should be administered with caution in patients subject to spontaneous hypoglycemia or to diabetic patients (especially those with labile diabetes) who are receiving insulin or oral hypoglycemic agents. β-adrenergic receptor blocking agents may mask the signs and symptoms of acute hypoglycemia). Products include:
Humulin R 1937
Humulin R (U-500) 1939

Insulin, Human Regular and Human NPH Mixture (β-adrenergic blocking agents should be administered with caution in patients subject to spontaneous hypoglycemia or to diabetic patients (especially those with labile diabetes) who are receiving insulin or oral hypoglycemic agents. β-adrenergic receptor blocking agents may mask the signs and symptoms of acute hypoglycemia). Products include:
Humulin 50/50 1930
Humulin 70/30 Vial 1931

Insulin, NPH (β-adrenergic blocking agents should be administered with caution in patients subject to spontaneous hypoglycemia or to diabetic patients (especially those with labile diabetes) who are receiving insulin or oral hypoglycemic agents. β-adrenergic receptor blocking agents may mask the signs and symptoms of acute hypoglycemia).
No products indexed under this heading.

Insulin, Regular (β-adrenergic blocking agents should be administered with caution in patients subject to spontaneous hypoglycemia or to diabetic patients (especially those with labile diabetes) who are receiving insulin or oral hypoglycemic agents. β-adrenergic receptor blocking agents may mask the signs and symptoms of acute hypoglycemia).
No products indexed under this heading.

Insulin, Regular and NPH mixture (β-adrenergic blocking agents should be administered with caution in patients subject to spontaneous hypoglycemia or to diabetic patients (especially those with labile diabetes) who are receiving insulin or oral hypoglycemic agents. β-adrenergic receptor blocking agents may mask the signs and symptoms of acute hypoglycemia).
No products indexed under this heading.

Insulin, Zinc Crystals (β-adrenergic blocking agents should be administered with caution in patients subject to spontaneous hypoglycemia or to diabetic patients (especially those with labile diabetes) who are receiving insulin or oral hypoglycemic agents. β-adrenergic receptor blocking agents may mask the signs and symptoms of acute hypoglycemia).
No products indexed under this heading.

Insulin, Zinc Suspension (β-adrenergic blocking agents should be administered with caution in patients subject to spontaneous hypoglycemia or to diabetic patients (especially those with labile diabetes) who are receiving insulin or oral hypoglycemic agents. β-adrenergic receptor blocking agents may mask the signs and symptoms of acute hypoglycemia).
No products indexed under this heading.

Insulin Aspart (β-adrenergic blocking agents should be administered with caution in patients subject to spontaneous hypoglycemia or to diabetic patients (especially those with labile diabetes) who are receiving insulin or oral hypoglycemic agents. β-adrenergic receptor blocking agents may mask the signs and symptoms of acute hypoglycemia).
No products indexed under this heading.

Insulin Aspart, Human (β-adrenergic blocking agents should be administered with caution in patients subject to spontaneous hypoglycemia or to diabetic patients (especially those with labile diabetes) who are receiving insulin or oral hypoglycemic agents. β-adrenergic receptor blocking agents may mask the signs and symptoms of acute hypoglycemia). Products include:
NovoLog Mix 70/30 2581

Insulin Aspart, Human Regular (β-adrenergic blocking agents should be administered with caution in patients subject to spontaneous hypoglycemia or to diabetic patients (especially those with labile diabetes) who are receiving insulin or oral hypoglycemic agents. β-adrenergic receptor blocking agents may mask the signs and symptoms of acute hypoglycemia). Products include:
NovoLog 2575

Insulin Aspart Protamine, Human (β-adrenergic blocking agents should be administered with caution in patients subject to spontaneous hypoglycemia or to diabetic patients (especially those with labile diabetes) who are receiving

insulin or oral hypoglycemic agents. β-adrenergic receptor blocking agents may mask the signs and symptoms of acute hypoglycemia). Products include:
NovoLog Mix 70/30 2581

Insulin Detemir (rDNA Origin) (β-adrenergic blocking agents should be administered with caution in patients subject to spontaneous hypoglycemia or to diabetic patients (especially those with labile diabetes) who are receiving insulin or oral hypoglycemic agents. β-adrenergic receptor blocking agents may mask the signs and symptoms of acute hypoglycemia). Products include:
Levemir 2566

Insulin Glargine (β-adrenergic blocking agents should be administered with caution in patients subject to spontaneous hypoglycemia or to diabetic patients (especially those with labile diabetes) who are receiving insulin or oral hypoglycemic agents. β-adrenergic receptor blocking agents may mask the signs and symptoms of acute hypoglycemia). Products include:
Lantus 2996

Insulin Glulisine (β-adrenergic blocking agents should be administered with caution in patients subject to spontaneous hypoglycemia or to diabetic patients (especially those with labile diabetes) who are receiving insulin or oral hypoglycemic agents. β-adrenergic receptor blocking agents may mask the signs and symptoms of acute hypoglycemia). Products include:
Apidra 2937
Apidra SoloStar 2937

Insulin Lispro, Human (β-adrenergic blocking agents should be administered with caution in patients subject to spontaneous hypoglycemia or to diabetic patients (especially those with labile diabetes) who are receiving insulin or oral hypoglycemic agents. β-adrenergic receptor blocking agents may mask the signs and symptoms of acute hypoglycemia). Products include:
Humalog 1910
Humalog Mix 1914
Humalog Mix75/25 1917

Insulin Lispro Protamine, Human (β-adrenergic blocking agents should be administered with caution in patients subject to spontaneous hypoglycemia or to diabetic patients (especially those with labile diabetes) who are receiving insulin or oral hypoglycemic agents. β-adrenergic receptor blocking agents may mask the signs and symptoms of acute hypoglycemia). Products include:
Humalog Mix 1914
Humalog Mix75/25 1917

Isoflurane (β-adrenergic receptor blockade impairs the ability of the heart to respond to β-adrenergically mediated reflex stimuli. This may augment the risk of general anesthesia in surgical procedures. Some patients receiving β-adrenergic receptor blocking agents have experienced protracted severe hypotension during anesthesia. Difficulty in restarting and maintaining the heartbeat has also been reported. For these reasons, in patients undergoing elective surgery, some authorities recommend gradual withdrawal of β-adrenergic receptor blocking agents).
No products indexed under this heading.

Isradipine (The concomitant use of β-adrenergic blocking agents with digitalisand calcium antagonists may have additive effects in prolonging atrioventricular conduction time. Caution should be used in the co-administration of β-adrenergic blocking agents, such as dorzolamide hydrochloride/timolol maleate ophthalmic solution, and oral or intravenous calcium antagonists because of possible atrioventricular conduction disturbances, left ventricular failure, and hypotension. In patients with impaired cardiac function, co-administration should be avoided). Products include:
DynaCirc CR 1432

Ketamine Hydrochloride (β-adrenergic receptor blockade impairs the ability of the heart to respond to β-adrenergically mediated reflex stimuli. This may augment the risk of general anesthesia in surgical procedures. Some patients receiving β-adrenergic receptor blocking agents have experienced protracted severe hypotension during anesthesia. Difficulty in restarting and maintaining the heartbeat has also been reported. For these reasons, in patients undergoing elective surgery, some authorities recommend gradual withdrawal of β-adrenergic receptor blocking agents).
No products indexed under this heading.

Labetalol Hydrochloride (Patients who are receiving a β-adrenergic blocking agent orally and dorzolamide hydrochloride/timolol maleate ophthalmic solution should be observed for potential additive effects of β-blockade, both systemic and on intraocular pressure. The concomitant use of two topical β-adrenergic blocking agents is not recommended).
No products indexed under this heading.

Levobunolol Hydrochloride (Patients who are receiving a β-adrenergic blocking agent orally and dorzolamide hydrochloride/timolol maleate ophthalmic solution should be observed for potential additive effects of β-blockade, both systemic and on intraocular pressure. The concomitant use of two topical β-adrenergic blocking agents is not recommended).
No products indexed under this heading.

Magnesium Salicylate (Although acid-base and electrolyte disturbances were not reported in the clinical trials with dorzolamide hydrochloride ophthalmic solution, these disturbances have been reported with oral carbonic anhydrase inhibitors and have, in some instances, resulted in drug interactions (eg, toxicity associated with high-dose salicylate therapy). Therefore, the potential for such drug interactions should be considered in patients receiving dorzolamide hydrochloride/timolol maleate ophthalmic solution).
No products indexed under this heading.

Maprotiline Hydrochloride (Potentiated systemic β-blockade (eg, decreased heart rate, depression) has been reported during combined treatment with CYP2D6 inhibitors (eg, quinidine, SSRIs) and timolol).
No products indexed under this heading.

Metformin Hydrochloride (β-adrenergic blocking agents should be administered with caution in patients subject to spontaneous hypoglycemia or to diabetic patients (especially those with labile diabetes) who are receiving insulin or oral hypoglycemic agents. β-adrenergic receptor blocking agents may mask the signs and symptoms of acute hypoglycemia). Products include:
ActoPlus 3338
Avandamet 1345
Janumet 2188

Methadone Hydrochloride (Potentiated systemic β-blockade (eg, decreased heart rate, depression) has been reported during combined treatment with CYP2D6 inhibitors (eg, quinidine, SSRIs) and timolol).
No products indexed under this heading.

Methazolamide (There is a potential for an additive effect on the known systemic effects of carbonic anhydrase inhibition in patients receiving an oral carbonic anhydrase inhibitor and dorzolamide hydrochloride/timolol maleate ophthalmic solution. The concomitant administration of dorzolamide hydrochloride/timolol maleate ophthalmic solution and oral carbonic anhydrase inhibitors is not recommended).
No products indexed under this heading.

Methohexital Sodium (β-adrenergic receptor blockade impairs the ability of the heart to respond to β-adrenergically mediated reflex stimuli. This may augment the risk of general anesthesia in surgical procedures. Some patients receiving β-adrenergic receptor blocking agents have experienced protracted severe hypotension during anesthesia. Difficulty in restarting and maintaining the heartbeat has also been reported. For these reasons, in patients undergoing elective surgery, some authorities recommend gradual withdrawal of β-adrenergic receptor blocking agents).
No products indexed under this heading.

Methoxyflurane (β-adrenergic receptor blockade impairs the ability of the heart to respond to β-adrenergically mediated reflex stimuli. This may augment the risk of general anesthesia in surgical procedures. Some patients receiving β-adrenergic receptor blocking agents have experienced protracted severe hypotension during anesthesia. Difficulty in restarting and maintaining the heartbeat has also been reported. For these reasons, in patients undergoing elective surgery, some authorities recommend gradual withdrawal of β-adrenergic receptor blocking agents).
No products indexed under this heading.

Metipranolol Hydrochloride (Patients who are receiving a β-adrenergic blocking agent orally and dorzolamide hydrochloride/timolol maleate ophthalmic solution should be observed for potential additive effects of β-blockade, both systemic and on intraocular pressure. The concomitant use of two topical β-adrenergic blocking agents is not recommended).
No products indexed under this heading.

Metoprolol Succinate (Patients who are receiving a β-adrenergic blocking agent orally and dorzolamide hydrochloride/timolol maleate ophthalmic solution should be observed for potential additive effects of β-blockade, both systemic and on intraocular pressure. The concomitant use of two topical β-adrenergic blocking agents is not recommended). Products include:
Toprol XL 732

Metoprolol Tartrate (Patients who are receiving a β-adrenergic blocking agent orally and dorzolamide hydrochloride/timolol maleate ophthalmic solution should be observed for potential additive effects of β-blockade, both systemic and on intraocular pressure. The concomitant use of two topical β-adrenergic blocking agents is not recommended).
No products indexed under this heading.

Mibefradil Dihydrochloride (The concomitant use of β-adrenergic blocking agents with digitalisand calcium antagonists may have additive effects in prolonging atrioventricular conduction time. Caution should be used in the co-administration of β-adrenergic blocking agents, such as dorzolamide hydrochloride/timolol maleate ophthalmic solution, and oral or intravenous calcium antagonists because of possible atrioventricular conduction disturbances, left ventricular failure, and hypotension. In patients with impaired cardiac function, co-administration should be avoided).
No products indexed under this heading.

Miglitol (β-adrenergic blocking agents should be administered with caution in patients subject to spontaneous hypoglycemia or to diabetic patients (especially those with labile diabetes) who are receiving insulin or oral hypoglycemic agents. β-adrenergic receptor blocking agents may mask the signs and symptoms of acute hypoglycemia).
No products indexed under this heading.

Moclobemide (Potentiated systemic β-blockade (eg, decreased heart rate, depression) has been reported during combined treatment with CYP2D6 inhibitors (eg, quinidine, SSRIs) and timolol).
No products indexed under this heading.

Nadolol (Patients who are receiving a β-adrenergic blocking agent orally and dorzolamide hydrochloride/timolol maleate ophthalmic solution should be observed for potential additive effects of β-blockade, both systemic and on intraocular pressure. The concomitant use of two topical β-adrenergic blocking agents is not recommended). Products include:
Nadolol 2359

Nateglinide (β-adrenergic blocking agents should be administered with caution in patients subject to spontaneous hypoglycemia or to diabetic patients (especially those with labile diabetes) who are receiving insulin or oral hypoglycemic agents. β-adrenergic receptor blocking agents may mask the signs and symptoms of acute hypoglycemia).
No products indexed under this heading.

Nebivolol (Patients who are receiving a β-adrenergic blocking agent orally and dorzolamide hydrochloride/timolol maleate ophthalmic solution should be observed for potential additive effects of β-blockade, both systemic and on intraocular pressure. The concomitant use of two topical β-adrenergic blocking agents is not recommended). Products include:
Bystolic 1147

Nicardipine (The concomitant use of β-adrenergic blocking agents with digitalisand calcium antagonists may have additive effects in prolonging atrioventricular conduction time. Caution should be used in the co-administration of β-adrenergic blocking agents, such as dorzolamide hydrochloride/timolol maleate ophthalmic solution, and oral or intravenous calcium antagonists because of possible atrioventricular conduction disturbances, left ventricular failure, and hypotension. In patients with impaired cardiac function, co-administration should be avoided).
No products indexed under this heading.

Nicardipine Hydrochloride (The concomitant use of β-adrenergic blocking agents with digitalisand calcium antagonists may have additive effects in prolonging atrioventricular conduction time. Caution should be used in the co-administration of β-adrenergic blocking agents, such as dorzolamide hydrochloride/timolol maleate ophthalmic solution, and oral or intravenous calcium antagonists because of possible atrioventricular conduction disturbances, left ventricular failure, and hypotension. In patients with impaired cardiac function, co-administration should be avoided).
No products indexed under this heading.

Nifedipine (The concomitant use of β-adrenergic blocking agents with digitalisand calcium antagonists may have additive effects in prolonging atrioventricular conduction time. Caution should be used in the co-administration of β-adrenergic blocking agents, such as dorzolamide hydrochloride/timolol maleate ophthalmic solution, and oral or intravenous calcium antagonists because of possible atrioventricular conduction disturbances, left ventricular

Dorzolamide/Timolol Interactions Index 490

failure, and hypotension. In patients with impaired cardiac function, co-administration should be avoided).
No products indexed under this heading.

Nimodipine (The concomitant use of β-adrenergic blocking agents with digitalisand calcium antagonists may have additive effects in prolonging atrioventricular conduction time. Caution should be used in the co-administration of β-adrenergic blocking agents, such as dorzolamide hydrochloride/timolol maleate ophthalmic solution, and oral or intravenous calcium antagonists because of possible atrioventricular conduction disturbances, left ventricular failure, and hypotension. In patients with impaired cardiac function, co-administration should be avoided).
No products indexed under this heading.

Nisoldipine (The concomitant use of β-adrenergic blocking agents with digitalisand calcium antagonists may have additive effects in prolonging atrioventricular conduction time. Caution should be used in the co-administration of β-adrenergic blocking agents, such as dorzolamide hydrochloride/timolol maleate ophthalmic solution, and oral or intravenous calcium antagonists because of possible atrioventricular conduction disturbances, left ventricular failure, and hypotension. In patients with impaired cardiac function, co-administration should be avoided).
No products indexed under this heading.

Nitrous Oxide (β-adrenergic receptor blockade impairs the ability of the heart to respond to β-adrenergically mediated reflex stimuli. This may augment the risk of general anesthesia in surgical procedures. Some patients receiving β-adrenergic receptor blocking agents have experienced protracted severe hypotension during anesthesia. Difficulty in restarting and maintaining the heartbeat has also been reported. For these reasons, in patients undergoing elective surgery, some authorities recommend gradual withdrawal of β-adrenergic receptor blocking agents).
No products indexed under this heading.

Norepinephrine Bitartrate (While taking β-blockers, patients with a history of atopy or a history of severe anaphylactic reactions to a variety of allergens may be more reactive to repeated accidental, diagnostic, or therapeutic challenge with such allergens. Such patients may be unresponsive to the usual doses of epinephrine used to treat anaphylactic reactions).
No products indexed under this heading.

Norepinephrine Hydrochloride (While taking β-blockers, patients with a history of atopy or a history of severe anaphylactic reactions to a variety of allergens may be more reactive to repeated accidental, diagnostic, or therapeutic challenge with such allergens. Such patients may be unresponsive to the usual doses of epinephrine used to treat anaphylactic reactions).
No products indexed under this heading.

Nortriptyline Hydrochloride (Potentiated systemic β-blockade (eg, decreased heart rate, depression) has been reported during combined treatment with CYP2D6 inhibitors (eg, quinidine, SSRIs) and timolol).
No products indexed under this heading.

Paroxetine (Potentiated systemic β-blockade (eg, decreased heart rate, depression) has been reported during combined treatment with CYP2D6 inhibitors (eg, quinidine, SSRIs) and timolol).
No products indexed under this heading.

Paroxetine Hydrochloride (Potentiated systemic β-blockade (eg, decreased heart rate, depression) has been reported during combined treatment with CYP2D6 inhibitors (eg, quinidine, SSRIs) and timolol). Products include:
Paroxetine CR **2361**
Paroxetine ER **2371**
Paxil **1586**
Paxil CR **1596**

Paroxetine Mesylate (Potentiated systemic β-blockade (eg, decreased heart rate, depression) has been reported during combined treatment with CYP2D6 inhibitors (eg, quinidine, SSRIs) and timolol).
No products indexed under this heading.

Penbutolol Sulfate (Patients who are receiving a β-adrenergic blocking agent orally and dorzolamide hydrochloride/timolol maleate ophthalmic solution should be observed for potential additive effects of β-blockade, both systemic and on intraocular pressure. The concomitant use of two topical β-adrenergic blocking agents is not recommended).
No products indexed under this heading.

Perphenazine (Potentiated systemic β-blockade (eg, decreased heart rate, depression) has been reported during combined treatment with CYP2D6 inhibitors (eg, quinidine, SSRIs) and timolol).
No products indexed under this heading.

Pindolol (Patients who are receiving a β-adrenergic blocking agent orally and dorzolamide hydrochloride/timolol maleate ophthalmic solution should be observed for potential additive effects of β-blockade, both systemic and on intraocular pressure. The concomitant use of two topical β-adrenergic blocking agents is not recommended).
No products indexed under this heading.

Pioglitazone Hydrochloride (β-adrenergic blocking agents should be administered with caution in patients subject to spontaneous hypoglycemia or to diabetic patients (especially those with labile diabetes) who are receiving insulin or oral hypoglycemic agents. β-adrenergic receptor blocking agents may mask the signs and symptoms of acute hypoglycemia). Products include:
ActoPlus **3338**
Actos **3345**
Duetact **3354**

Propafenone Hydrochloride (Potentiated systemic β-blockade (eg, decreased heart rate, depression) has been reported during combined treatment with CYP2D6 inhibitors (eg, quinidine, SSRIs) and timolol). Products include:
Rythmol **1648**
Rythmol SR **1652**

Propofol (β-adrenergic receptor blockade impairs the ability of the heart to respond to β-adrenergically mediated reflex stimuli. This may augment the risk of general anesthesia in surgical procedures. Some patients receiving β-adrenergic receptor blocking agents have experienced protracted severe hypotension during anesthesia. Difficulty in restarting and maintaining the heartbeat has also been reported. For these reasons, in patients undergoing elective surgery, some authorities recommend gradual withdrawal of β-adrenergic receptor blocking agents).
No products indexed under this heading.

Propoxyphene Hydrochloride (Potentiated systemic β-blockade (eg, decreased heart rate, depression) has been reported during combined treatment with CYP2D6 inhibitors (eg, quinidine, SSRIs) and timolol).
No products indexed under this heading.

Propoxyphene Napsylate (Potentiated systemic β-blockade (eg, decreased heart rate, depression) has been reported during combined treatment with CYP2D6 inhibitors (eg, quinidine, SSRIs) and timolol).
No products indexed under this heading.

Propranolol Hydrochloride (Patients who are receiving a β-adrenergic blocking agent orally and dorzolamide hydrochloride/timolol maleate ophthalmic solution should be observed for potential additive effects of β-blockade, both systemic and on intraocular pressure. The concomitant use of two topical β-adrenergic blocking agents is not recommended). Products include:
InnoPran XL **1517**

Protriptyline Hydrochloride (Potentiated systemic β-blockade (eg, decreased heart rate, depression) has been reported during combined treatment with CYP2D6 inhibitors (eg, quinidine, SSRIs) and timolol).
No products indexed under this heading.

Quinacrine Hydrochloride (Potentiated systemic β-blockade (eg, decreased heart rate, depression) has been reported during combined treatment with CYP2D6 inhibitors (eg, quinidine, SSRIs) and timolol).
No products indexed under this heading.

Quinidine (Potentiated systemic β-blockade (eg, decreased heart rate, depression) has been reported during combined treatment with CYP2D6 inhibitors (eg, quinidine, SSRIs) and timolol).
No products indexed under this heading.

Quinidine Gluconate (Potentiated systemic β-blockade (eg, decreased heart rate, depression) has been reported during combined treatment with CYP2D6 inhibitors (eg, quinidine, SSRIs) and timolol).
No products indexed under this heading.

Quinidine Hydrochloride (Potentiated systemic β-blockade (eg, decreased heart rate, depression) has been reported during combined treatment with CYP2D6 inhibitors (eg, quinidine, SSRIs) and timolol).
No products indexed under this heading.

Quinidine Polygalacturonate (Potentiated systemic β-blockade (eg, decreased heart rate, depression) has been reported during combined treatment with CYP2D6 inhibitors (eg, quinidine, SSRIs) and timolol).
No products indexed under this heading.

Quinidine Sulfate (Potentiated systemic β-blockade (eg, decreased heart rate, depression) has been reported during combined treatment with CYP2D6 inhibitors (eg, quinidine, SSRIs) and timolol).
No products indexed under this heading.

Ranitidine Bismuth Citrate (Potentiated systemic β-blockade (eg, decreased heart rate, depression) has been reported during combined treatment with CYP2D6 inhibitors (eg, quinidine, SSRIs) and timolol).
No products indexed under this heading.

Ranitidine Hydrochloride (Potentiated systemic β-blockade (eg, decreased heart rate, depression) has been reported during combined treatment with CYP2D6 inhibitors (eg, quinidine, SSRIs) and timolol). Products include:
Zantac **1737**
Zantac Injection **1732**
Zantac Pharmacy **1735**

Rauwolfia Serpentina (Close observation of the patient is recommended when a β-blocker is administered to patients receiving catecholamine depleting drugs, such as reserpine, because of possible additive effects and the production of hypotension and/ or marked bradycardia, which may result in vertigo, syncope, or postural hypotension).
No products indexed under this heading.

Repaglinide (β-adrenergic blocking agents should be administered with caution in patients subject to spontaneous hypoglycemia or to diabetic patients (especially those with labile diabetes) who are receiving insulin or oral hypoglycemic agents. β-adrenergic receptor blocking agents may mask the signs and symptoms of acute hypoglycemia).
No products indexed under this heading.

Rescinnamine (Close observation of the patient is recommended when a β-blocker is administered to patients receiving catecholamine depleting drugs, such as reserpine, because of possible additive effects and the production of hypotension and/ or marked bradycardia, which may result in vertigo, syncope, or postural hypotension).
No products indexed under this heading.

Reserpine (Close observation of the patient is recommended when a β-blocker is administered to patients receiving catecholamine depleting drugs, such as reserpine, because of possible additive effects and the production of hypotension and/or marked bradycardia, which may result in vertigo, syncope, or postural hypotension).
No products indexed under this heading.

Ritonavir (Potentiated systemic β-blockade (eg, decreased heart rate, depression) has been reported during combined treatment with CYP2D6 inhibitors (eg, quinidine, SSRIs) and timolol). Products include:
Kaletra **458**
Norvir **509**

Rosiglitazone Maleate (β-adrenergic blocking agents should be administered with caution in patients subject to spontaneous hypoglycemia or to diabetic patients (especially those with labile diabetes) who are receiving insulin or oral hypoglycemic agents. β-adrenergic receptor blocking agents may mask the signs and symptoms of acute hypoglycemia). Products include:
Avandamet **1345**
Avandaryl **1356**
Avandia **1366**

Salsalate (Although acid-base and electrolyte disturbances were not reported in the clinical trials with dorzolamide hydrochloride ophthalmic solution, these disturbances have been reported with oral carbonic anhydrase inhibitors and have, in some instances, resulted in drug interactions (eg, toxicity associated with high-dose salicylate therapy). Therefore, the potential for such drug interactions should be considered in patients receiving dorzolamide hydrochloride/timolol maleate ophthalmic solution).
No products indexed under this heading.

Sertraline Hydrochloride (Potentiated systemic β-blockade (eg, decreased heart rate, depression) has been reported during combined treatment with CYP2D6 inhibitors (eg, quinidine, SSRIs) and timolol).
No products indexed under this heading.

Sevoflurane (β-adrenergic receptor blockade impairs the ability of the heart to respond to β-adrenergically mediated reflex stimuli. This may augment the risk of general anesthesia in surgical procedures. Some patients receiving β-adrenergic receptor blocking agents have experienced protracted severe hypotension during anesthesia. Difficul-

(⊙ Described in PDR® for Ophthalmic Medicines)

491 Interactions Index Doxil

ty in restarting and maintaining the heartbeat has also been reported. For these reasons, in patients undergoing elective surgery, some authorities recommend gradual withdrawal of β-adrenergic receptor blocking agents). Products include:
Ultane 554

Sildenafil Citrate (Potentiated systemic β-blockade (eg, decreased heart rate, depression) has been reported during combined treatment with CYP2D6 inhibitors (eg, quinidine, SSRIs) and timolol).
No products indexed under this heading.

Sitagliptin Phosphate (β-adrenergic blocking agents should be administered with caution in patients subject to spontaneous hypoglycemia or to diabetic patients (especially those with labile diabetes) who are receiving insulin or oral hypoglycemic agents. β-adrenergic receptor blocking agents may mask the signs and symptoms of acute hypoglycemia). Products include:
Janumet 2188
Januvia 2196

Sotalol Hydrochloride (Patients who are receiving a β-adrenergic blocking agent orally and dorzolamide hydrochloride/timolol maleate ophthalmic solution should be observed for potential additive effects of β-blockade, both systemic and on intraocular pressure. The concomitant use of two topical β-adrenergic blocking agents is not recommended).
No products indexed under this heading.

Terbinafine Hydrochloride (Potentiated systemic β-blockade (eg, decreased heart rate, depression) has been reported during combined treatment with CYP2D6 inhibitors (eg, quinidine, SSRIs) and timolol).
No products indexed under this heading.

Thioridazine Hydrochloride (Potentiated systemic β-blockade (eg, decreased heart rate, depression) has been reported during combined treatment with CYP2D6 inhibitors (eg, quinidine, SSRIs) and timolol). Products include:
Thioridazine Hydrochloride 2384

Timolol Hemihydrate (Patients who are receiving a β-adrenergic blocking agent orally and dorzolamide hydrochloride/timolol maleate ophthalmic solution should be observed for potential additive effects of β-blockade, both systemic and on intraocular pressure. The concomitant use of two topical β-adrenergic blocking agents is not recommended). Products include:
Betimol 3490

Tolazamide (β-adrenergic blocking agents should be administered with caution in patients subject to spontaneous hypoglycemia or to diabetic patients (especially those with labile diabetes) who are receiving insulin or oral hypoglycemic agents. β-adrenergic receptor blocking agents may mask the signs and symptoms of acute hypoglycemia).
No products indexed under this heading.

Tolbutamide (β-adrenergic blocking agents should be administered with caution in patients subject to spontaneous hypoglycemia or to diabetic patients (especially those with labile diabetes) who are receiving insulin or oral hypoglycemic agents. β-adrenergic receptor blocking agents may mask the signs and symptoms of acute hypoglycemia).
No products indexed under this heading.

Topical Medications (If more than one topical ophthalmic drug is being used, the drugs should be administered at least ten minutes apart).
No products indexed under this heading.

Torsemide (There is a potential for an additive effect on the known systemic effects of carbonic anhydrase inhibition in patients receiving an oral carbonic anhydrase inhibitor and dorzolamide hydrochloride/timolol maleate ophthalmic solution. The concomitant administration of dorzolamide hydrochloride/timolol maleate ophthalmic solution and oral carbonic anhydrase inhibitors is not recommended).
No products indexed under this heading.

Trimipramine Maleate (Potentiated systemic β-blockade (eg, decreased heart rate, depression) has been reported during combined treatment with CYP2D6 inhibitors (eg, quinidine, SSRIs) and timolol).
No products indexed under this heading.

Troglitazone (β-adrenergic blocking agents should be administered with caution in patients subject to spontaneous hypoglycemia or to diabetic patients (especially those with labile diabetes) who are receiving insulin or oral hypoglycemic agents. β-adrenergic receptor blocking agents may mask the signs and symptoms of acute hypoglycemia).
No products indexed under this heading.

Vardenafil Hydrochloride (Potentiated systemic β-blockade (eg, decreased heart rate, depression) has been reported during combined treatment with CYP2D6 inhibitors (eg, quinidine, SSRIs) and timolol). Products include:
Levitra 3157

Verapamil Hydrochloride (The concomitant use of β-adrenergic blocking agents with digitalisand calcium antagonists may have additive effects in prolonging atrioventricular conduction time. Caution should be used in the coadministration of β-adrenergic blocking agents, such as dorzolamide hydrochloride/timolol maleate ophthalmic solution, and oral or intravenous calcium antagonists because of possible atrioventricular conduction disturbances, left ventricular failure, and hypotension. In patients with impaired cardiac function, co-administration should be avoided). Products include:
Tarka 534

DOXIL INJECTION

(Doxorubicin Hydrochloride Liposome) 939
May interact with antineoplastics, and certain other agents. Compounds in these categories include:

Altretamine (Co-administration with the conventional formulation of doxorubicin results in potentiation of the toxicity of other anti-cancer therapies; this interaction may occur with Doxil). Products include:
Hexalen 1066

Anastrozole (Co-administration with the conventional formulation of doxorubicin results in potentiation of the toxicity of other anti-cancer therapies; this interaction may occur with Doxil).
No products indexed under this heading.

Asparaginase (Co-administration with the conventional formulation of doxorubicin results in potentiation of the toxicity of other anti-cancer therapies; this interaction may occur with Doxil). Products include:
Elspar 2005, 2122

Bicalutamide (Co-administration with the conventional formulation of doxorubicin results in potentiation of the toxicity of other anti-cancer therapies; this interaction may occur with Doxil).
No products indexed under this heading.

Bleomycin Sulfate (Co-administration with the conventional formulation of doxorubicin results in potentiation of the toxicity of other anti-cancer therapies; this interaction may occur with Doxil).
No products indexed under this heading.

Busulfan (Co-administration with the conventional formulation of doxorubicin results in potentiation of the toxicity of other anti-cancer therapies; this interaction may occur with Doxil). Products include:
Myleran 1581

Carboplatin (Co-administration with the conventional formulation of doxorubicin results in potentiation of the toxicity of other anti-cancer therapies; this interaction may occur with Doxil).
No products indexed under this heading.

Carmustine (BCNU) (Co-administration with the conventional formulation of doxorubicin results in potentiation of the toxicity of other anti-cancer therapies; this interaction may occur with Doxil).
No products indexed under this heading.

Chlorambucil (Co-administration with the conventional formulation of doxorubicin results in potentiation of the toxicity of other anti-cancer therapies; this interaction may occur with Doxil). Products include:
Leukeran 1557

Cisplatin (Co-administration with the conventional formulation of doxorubicin results in potentiation of the toxicity of other anti-cancer therapies; this interaction may occur with Doxil).
No products indexed under this heading.

Cyclophosphamide (Co-administration of conventional formulation of doxorubicin with cyclophosphamide has resulted in exacerbation of cyclophosphamide-induced hemorrhagic cystitis; cardiac toxicity may occur at lower cumulative doses in patients who are receiving cyclophosphamide).
No products indexed under this heading.

Cyclosporine (Co-administration of conventional formulation of doxorubicin may result in increases in AUC for both doxorubicin and doxorubicinol possibly due to a decrease in clearance of parent drug and a decrease in metabolism of doxorubicin; potential for more profound and prolonged hematologic toxicity is associated with combined use; coma and seizures have also been reported). Products include:
Gengraf 440
Neoral Oral Solution 2496
Neoral Capsules 2496
Restasis 605

Dacarbazine (Co-administration with the conventional formulation of doxorubicin results in potentiation of the toxicity of other anti-cancer therapies; this interaction may occur with Doxil).
No products indexed under this heading.

Daunorubicin Citrate (Co-administration with the conventional formulation of doxorubicin results in potentiation of the toxicity of other anti-cancer therapies; this interaction may occur with Doxil).
No products indexed under this heading.

Daunorubicin Hydrochloride (Co-administration with the conventional formulation of doxorubicin results in potentiation of the toxicity of other anti-cancer therapies; this interaction may occur with Doxil).
No products indexed under this heading.

Denileukin Diftitox (Co-administration with the conventional formulation of doxorubicin results in potentiation of the toxicity of other anti-cancer therapies; this interaction may occur with Doxil). Products include:
Ontak 1068

Docetaxel (Co-administration with the conventional formulation of doxorubicin results in potentiation of the toxicity of other anti-cancer therapies; this interaction may occur with Doxil). Products include:
Taxotere 3035

Doxorubicin Hydrochloride (Co-administration with the conventional formulation of doxorubicin results in potentiation of the toxicity of other anti-cancer therapies; this interaction may occur with Doxil).
No products indexed under this heading.

Epirubicin Hydrochloride (Co-administration with the conventional formulation of doxorubicin results in potentiation of the toxicity of other anti-cancer therapies; this interaction may occur with Doxil).
No products indexed under this heading.

Estramustine Phosphate Sodium (Co-administration with the conventional formulation of doxorubicin results in potentiation of the toxicity of other anti-cancer therapies; this interaction may occur with Doxil).
No products indexed under this heading.

Etoposide (Co-administration with the conventional formulation of doxorubicin results in potentiation of the toxicity of other anti-cancer therapies; this interaction may occur with Doxil).
No products indexed under this heading.

Exemestane (Co-administration with the conventional formulation of doxorubicin results in potentiation of the toxicity of other anti-cancer therapies; this interaction may occur with Doxil). Products include:
Aromasin 2758

Floxuridine (Co-administration with the conventional formulation of doxorubicin results in potentiation of the toxicity of other anti-cancer therapies; this interaction may occur with Doxil).
No products indexed under this heading.

Fluorouracil (Co-administration with the conventional formulation of doxorubicin results in potentiation of the toxicity of other anti-cancer therapies; this interaction may occur with Doxil). Products include:
Carac 2966

Flutamide (Co-administration with the conventional formulation of doxorubicin results in potentiation of the toxicity of other anti-cancer therapies; this interaction may occur with Doxil).
No products indexed under this heading.

Gemcitabine Hydrochloride (Co-administration with the conventional formulation of doxorubicin results in potentiation of the toxicity of other anti-cancer therapies; this interaction may occur with Doxil). Products include:
Gemzar 1900

Hydroxyurea (Co-administration with the conventional formulation of doxorubicin results in potentiation of the toxicity of other anti-cancer therapies; this interaction may occur with Doxil).
No products indexed under this heading.

Idarubicin Hydrochloride (Co-administration with the conventional formulation of doxorubicin results in potentiation of the toxicity of other anti-cancer therapies; this interaction may occur with Doxil).
No products indexed under this heading.

Ifosfamide (Co-administration with the conventional formulation of doxorubicin results in potentiation of the toxicity of other anti-cancer therapies; this interaction may occur with Doxil).
No products indexed under this heading.

Interferon alfa-2a, Recombinant (Co-administration with the conventional formulation of doxorubicin results in potentiation of the toxicity of other anti-cancer therapies; this interaction may occur with Doxil).
No products indexed under this heading.

Interferon alfa-2b, Recombinant (Co-administration with the conventional formulation of doxorubicin results in

IMPORTANT NOTE: Always consult each drug listing in the patient's regimen for possible interactions.

Doxil **Interactions Index** **492**

potentiation of the toxicity of other anti-cancer therapies; this interaction may occur with Doxil). Products include:
Intron A 3140

Irinotecan Hydrochloride (Co-administration with the conventional formulation of doxorubicin results in potentiation of the toxicity of other anti-cancer therapies; this interaction may occur with Doxil).
No products indexed under this heading.

Levamisole Hydrochloride (Co-administration with the conventional formulation of doxorubicin results in potentiation of the toxicity of other anti-cancer therapies; this interaction may occur with Doxil).
No products indexed under this heading.

Lomustine (CCNU) (Co-administration with the conventional formulation of doxorubicin results in potentiation of the toxicity of other anti-cancer therapies; this interaction may occur with Doxil).
No products indexed under this heading.

Mechlorethamine Hydrochloride (Co-administration with the conventional formulation of doxorubicin results in potentiation of the toxicity of other anti-cancer therapies; this interaction may occur with Doxil). Products include:
Mustargen 2010

Medroxyprogesterone Acetate (Co-administration of intravenous progesterone to patients with advanced malignancies at high doses with conventional formulation of fixed doxorubicin dose via bolus enhances doxorubicin-induced neutropenia and thrombocytopenia; this interaction may occur with Doxil). Products include:
Premphase 3549
Prempro 3549

Megestrol Acetate (Co-administration with the conventional formulation of doxorubicin results in potentiation of the toxicity of other anti-cancer therapies; this interaction may occur with Doxil). Products include:
Megace ES 2698

Melphalan (Co-administration with the conventional formulation of doxorubicin results in potentiation of the toxicity of other anti-cancer therapies; this interaction may occur with Doxil). Products include:
Alkeran 1302

Mercaptopurine (Co-administration of conventional formulation of doxorubicin with 6-mercaptopurine has resulted in enhancement of hepatotoxicity of 6-mercaptopurine).
No products indexed under this heading.

Methotrexate (Co-administration with the conventional formulation of doxorubicin results in potentiation of the toxicity of other anti-cancer therapies; this interaction may occur with Doxil).
No products indexed under this heading.

Methotrexate Sodium (Co-administration with the conventional formulation of doxorubicin results in potentiation of the toxicity of other anti-cancer therapies; this interaction may occur with Doxil).
No products indexed under this heading.

Mitomycin (Mitomycin-C) (Co-administration with the conventional formulation of doxorubicin results in potentiation of the toxicity of other anti-cancer therapies; this interaction may occur with Doxil).
No products indexed under this heading.

Mitotane (Co-administration with the conventional formulation of doxorubicin results in potentiation of the toxicity of other anti-cancer therapies; this interaction may occur with Doxil).
No products indexed under this heading.

Mitoxantrone Hydrochloride (Co-administration with the conventional formulation of doxorubicin results in potentiation of the toxicity of other anti-cancer therapies; this interaction may occur with Doxil). Products include:
Novantrone 1088

Oxaliplatin (Co-administration with the conventional formulation of doxorubicin results in potentiation of the toxicity of other anti-cancer therapies; this interaction may occur with Doxil). Products include:
Eloxatin 2975

Paclitaxel (Administration of paclitaxel infused over 24 hours followed by conventional formulation of doxorubicin administered over 48 hours resulted in a significant decrease in doxorubicin clearance with more profound neutropenic and stomatitis episodes than the reverse sequence of administration; this interaction may occur with Doxil).
No products indexed under this heading.

Phenobarbital (Co-administration with the conventional formulation of doxorubicin results in increased elimination of doxorubicin; this interaction may occur with Doxil). Products include:
Donnatal 2711

Phenytoin (Co-administration with the conventional formulation of doxorubicin results in decreased phenytoin levels; this interaction may occur with Doxil).
No products indexed under this heading.

Phenytoin Sodium (Co-administration with the conventional formulation of doxorubicin results in decreased phenytoin levels; this interaction may occur with Doxil). Products include:
Phenytek Capsules 2380

Procarbazine Hydrochloride (Co-administration with the conventional formulation of doxorubicin results in potentiation of the toxicity of other anti-cancer therapies; this interaction may occur with Doxil).
No products indexed under this heading.

Progesterone (Co-administration of intravenous progesterone to patients with advanced malignancies at high doses with conventional formulation of fixed doxorubicin dose via bolus enhances doxorubicin-induced neutropenia and thrombocytopenia; this interaction may occur with Doxil). Products include:
Crinone 4% 996
Crinone 8% 996
Prometrium 3307

Streptozocin (Co-administration with the conventional formulation of doxorubicin results in inhibition of hepatic metabolism; this interaction may occur with Doxil).
No products indexed under this heading.

Tamoxifen Citrate (Co-administration with the conventional formulation of doxorubicin results in potentiation of the toxicity of other anti-cancer therapies; this interaction may occur with Doxil).
No products indexed under this heading.

Teniposide (Co-administration with the conventional formulation of doxorubicin results in potentiation of the toxicity of other anti-cancer therapies; this interaction may occur with Doxil).
No products indexed under this heading.

Thioguanine (Co-administration with the conventional formulation of doxorubicin results in potentiation of the toxicity of other anti-cancer therapies; this interaction may occur with Doxil). Products include:
Tabloid 1664

Thiotepa (Co-administration with the conventional formulation of doxorubicin results in potentiation of the toxicity of other anti-cancer therapies; this interaction may occur with Doxil).
No products indexed under this heading.

Topotecan Hydrochloride (Co-administration with the conventional formulation of doxorubicin results in potentiation of the toxicity of other anti-cancer therapies; this interaction may occur with Doxil). Products include:
Hycamtin 1491
Hycamtin Capsules 1488

Toremifene Citrate (Co-administration with the conventional formulation of doxorubicin results in potentiation of the toxicity of other anti-cancer therapies; this interaction may occur with Doxil).
No products indexed under this heading.

Valrubicin (Co-administration with the conventional formulation of doxorubicin results in potentiation of the toxicity of other anti-cancer therapies; this interaction may occur with Doxil). Products include:
Valstar 1131

Verapamil Hydrochloride (Co-administration of conventional formulation of doxorubicin in animal studies has resulted in higher initial peak concentrations of doxorubicin in the heart with a higher incidence and severity of degenerative changes in cardiac tissue resulting in a shorter survival; this interaction may occur with Doxil). Products include:
Tarka 534

Vincristine Sulfate (Co-administration with the conventional formulation of doxorubicin results in potentiation of the toxicity of other anti-cancer therapies; this interaction may occur with Doxil).
No products indexed under this heading.

Vinorelbine Tartrate (Co-administration with the conventional formulation of doxorubicin results in potentiation of the toxicity of other anti-cancer therapies; this interaction may occur with Doxil).
No products indexed under this heading.

DUAC TOPICAL GEL

(Benzoyl Peroxide, Clindamycin) 3317
May interact with erythromycin, and certain other agents. Compounds in these categories include:

Concomitant Topical Acne Therapy (Concomitant topical acne therapy should be used with caution because a possible cumulative irritancy effect may occur, especially with the use of peeling, desquamating, or abrasive agents).
No products indexed under this heading.

Erythromycin (Clindamycin- and erythromycin-containing products should not be used in combination. In vitro studies have shown antagonism between these two antimicrobials. The clinical significance of this *in vitro* antagonism is not known).
No products indexed under this heading.

Erythromycin, Topical (Clindamycin- and erythromycin-containing products should not be used in combination. In vitro studies have shown antagonism between these two antimicrobials. The clinical significance of this *in vitro* antagonism is not known).
No products indexed under this heading.

Erythromycin Estolate (Clindamycin- and erythromycin-containing products should not be used in combination. In vitro studies have shown antagonism between these two antimicrobials. The clinical significance of this *in vitro* antagonism is not known).
No products indexed under this heading.

Erythromycin Ethylsuccinate (Clindamycin- and erythromycin-containing products should not be used in combination. In vitro studies have shown antagonism between these two antimicrobials. The clinical significance of this *in vitro* antagonism is not known). Products include:
E.E.S. 437
EryPed 435

Erythromycin Gluceptate (Clindamycin- and erythromycin-containing products should not be used in combination. In vitro studies have shown antagonism between these two antimicrobials. The clinical significance of this *in vitro* antagonism is not known).
No products indexed under this heading.

Erythromycin Lactobionate (Clindamycin- and erythromycin-containing products should not be used in combination. In vitro studies have shown antagonism between these two antimicrobials. The clinical significance of this *in vitro* antagonism is not known).
No products indexed under this heading.

Erythromycin Stearate (Clindamycin- and erythromycin-containing products should not be used in combination. In vitro studies have shown antagonism between these two antimicrobials. The clinical significance of this *in vitro* antagonism is not known).
No products indexed under this heading.

DUETACT TABLETS

(Glimepiride, Pioglitazone Hydrochloride) 3354
May interact with alcohols, aspirin-acetylsalicylic acid, beta-blockers, chloramphenicol, corticosteroids, cytochrome p450 2c8 inducers (selected), cytochrome p450 2c8 inhibitors (selected), cytochrome p450 2c9 inducers (selected), cytochrome p450 2c9 inhibitors (selected), cytochrome p450 3a4 substrates (selected), diuretics, estrogens, highly protein bound drugs (selected), insulin, monoamine oxidase inhibitors, non-steroidal anti-inflammatory agents, oral anticoagulants, oral contraceptives, oral hypoglycemic agents, phenothiazines, phenytoin, salicylates, sulfonamides, sympathomimetics, thiazides, thyroid preparations, and certain other agents. Compounds in these categories include:

Acarbose (Patients receiving pioglitazone in combination with oral hypoglycemic agents may be at risk for hypoglycemia, and a reduction in the dose of the concomitant agent may be necessary).
No products indexed under this heading.

Acebutolol Hydrochloride (The hypoglycemic action of sulfonylureas may be potentiated by certain drugs, including other drugs that are highly protein bound, such as β adrenergic blocking agents. Due to the potential drug interaction between these drugs and glimepiride, the patient should be observed closely for hypoglycemia when these drugs are co-administered. Conversely, when these drugs are withdrawn, the patient should be observed closely for loss of glycemic control).
No products indexed under this heading.

Albuterol (Certain drugs tend to produce hyperglycemia and may lead to loss of control. These drugs include sympathomimetics. Due to the potential drug interaction between sympathomimetics and glimepiride, the patient should be observed closely for loss of glycemic control when these drugs are co-administered. Conversely, when sympathomimetics are withdrawn, the patient should be observed closely for hypoglycemia).
No products indexed under this heading.

Albuterol Sulfate (Certain drugs tend to produce hyperglycemia and may lead to loss of control. These drugs include sympathomimetics. Due to the potential drug interaction between sympathomimetics and glimepiride, the patient should be observed closely for loss of glycemic control when these drugs are co-administered. Conversely, when sym-

493 Interactions Index Duetact

pathomimetics are withdrawn, the patient should be observed closely for hypoglycemia). Products include:
ProAir HFA 3393
Proventil HFA 3204
Ventolin HFA 1708

Alclometasone Dipropionate (Certain drugs tend to produce hyperglycemia and may lead to loss of control. These drugs include corticosteroids. Due to the potential drug interaction between corticosteroids and glimepiride, the patient should be observed closely for loss of glycemic control when these drugs are co-administered. Conversely, when corticosteroids are withdrawn, the patient should be observed closely for hypoglycemia).
No products indexed under this heading.

Alfentanil Hydrochloride (*In vivo* drug-drug interaction studies have suggested that pioglitazone may be a weak inducer of CYP 450 isoform 3A4 substrate).
No products indexed under this heading.

Alprazolam (*In vivo* drug-drug interaction studies have suggested that pioglitazone may be a weak inducer of CYP 450 isoform 3A4 substrate).
No products indexed under this heading.

Amiloride Hydrochloride (Certain drugs tend to produce hyperglycemia and may lead to loss of control. These drugs include diuretics. Due to the potential drug interaction between diuretics and glimepiride, the patient should be observed closely for loss of glycemic control when these drugs are co-administered. Conversely, when diuretics are withdrawn, the patient should be observed closely for hypoglycemia).
No products indexed under this heading.

Amiodarone Hydrochloride (The hypoglycemic action of sulfonylureas may be potentiated by certain drugs, including drugs that are highly protein bound. Due to the potential drug interaction between these drugs and glimepiride, the patient should be observed closely for hypoglycemia when these drugs are co-administered. Conversely, when these drugs are withdrawn, the patient should be observed closely for loss of glycemic control).
No products indexed under this heading.

Amitriptyline Hydrochloride (The hypoglycemic action of sulfonylureas may be potentiated by certain drugs, including drugs that are highly protein bound. Due to the potential drug interaction between these drugs and glimepiride, the patient should be observed closely for hypoglycemia when these drugs are co-administered. Conversely, when these drugs are withdrawn, the patient should be observed closely for loss of glycemic control).
No products indexed under this heading.

Amlodipine Besylate (*In vivo* drug-drug interaction studies have suggested that pioglitazone may be a weak inducer of CYP 450 isoform 3A4 substrate). Products include:
Azor 1010
Exforge 2443
Exforge HCT 2449

Anastrozole (An enzyme inhibitor of CYP2C8 (such as gemfibrozil) may significantly increase the AUC of pioglitazone. Therefore, if an inhibitor of CYP2C8 is started or stopped during treatment with pioglitazone, changes in diabetes treatment may be needed based on clinical response).
No products indexed under this heading.

Anisindione (The hypoglycemic action of sulfonylureas may be potentiated by certain drugs, including other drugs that are highly protein bound, such as coumarins. Due to the potential drug interaction between these drugs and glimepiride, the patient should be observed closely for hypoglycemia when these drugs are co-administered. Conversely, when these drugs are withdrawn, the patient should be observed closely for loss of glycemic control).
No products indexed under this heading.

Aprepitant (There is a potential interaction of glimepiride with inducers (eg, rifampicin) of cytochrome P450 2C9). Products include:
Emend 2124

Aspirin (Co-administration of aspirin (1 g three times daily) and glimepiride led to a 34% decrease in the mean glimepiride AUC and, therefore, a 34% increase in the mean CL/f. The mean C_{max} had a decrease of 4%. In addition, the hypoglycemic action of sulfonylureas may be potentiated by certain drugs, including drugs that are highly protein bound, such as salicylates. Due to the potential drug interaction between these drugs and glimepiride, the patient should be observed closely for hypoglycemia when these drugs are co-administered. Conversely, when these drugs are withdrawn, the patient should be observed closely for loss of glycemic control). Products include:
Aggrenox 880
Bayer Aspirin 829
Percodan 1124
St. Joseph Aspirin 2045

Aspirin, Enteric Coated (Co-administration of aspirin (1 g three times daily) and glimepiride led to a 34% decrease in the mean glimepiride AUC and, therefore, a 34% increase in the mean CL/f. The mean C_{max} had a decrease of 4%. In addition, the hypoglycemic action of sulfonylureas may be potentiated by certain drugs, including drugs that are highly protein bound, such as salicylates. Due to the potential drug interaction between these drugs and glimepiride, the patient should be observed closely for hypoglycemia when these drugs are co-administered. Conversely, when these drugs are withdrawn, the patient should be observed closely for loss of glycemic control).
No products indexed under this heading.

Aspirin Buffered (Co-administration of aspirin (1 g three times daily) and glimepiride led to a 34% decrease in the mean glimepiride AUC and, therefore, a 34% increase in the mean CL/f. The mean C_{max} had a decrease of 4%. In addition, the hypoglycemic action of sulfonylureas may be potentiated by certain drugs, including drugs that are highly protein bound, such as salicylates. Due to the potential drug interaction between these drugs and glimepiride, the patient should be observed closely for hypoglycemia when these drugs are co-administered. Conversely, when these drugs are withdrawn, the patient should be observed closely for loss of glycemic control).
No products indexed under this heading.

Astemizole (*In vivo* drug-drug interaction studies have suggested that pioglitazone may be a weak inducer of CYP 450 isoform 3A4 substrate).
No products indexed under this heading.

Atenolol (The hypoglycemic action of sulfonylureas may be potentiated by certain drugs, including other drugs that are highly protein bound, such as β adrenergic blocking agents. Due to the potential drug interaction between these drugs and glimepiride, the patient should be observed closely for hypoglycemia when these drugs are co-administered. Conversely, when these drugs are withdrawn, the patient should be observed closely for loss of glycemic control).
No products indexed under this heading.

Atorvastatin Calcium (Co-administration of pioglitazone for 7 days with atorvastatin calcium 80 mg once daily resulted in a ratio of least square mean (90% CI) values for unchanged pioglitazone of 0.69 (0.57-0.85) for C_{max}, 0.76 (0.65-0.88) for AUC, and 0.96 (0.87-1.05) for C_{min}. For unchanged atorvastatin, the ratio of least square mean (90% CI) values were 0.77 (0.66-0.90) for C_{max}, 0.86 (0.78-0.94) for AUC, and 0.92 (0.82-1.02) for C_{min}). Products include:
Lipitor 2703

Atovaquone (The hypoglycemic action of sulfonylureas may be potentiated by certain drugs, including drugs that are highly protein bound. Due to the potential drug interaction between these drugs and glimepiride, the patient should be observed closely for hypoglycemia when these drugs are co-administered. Conversely, when these drugs are withdrawn, the patient should be observed closely for loss of glycemic control). Products include:
Malarone Pediatric Tablets 1572
Malarone 1572
Mepron Suspension 1576

Beclomethasone Dipropionate (Certain drugs tend to produce hyperglycemia and may lead to loss of control. These drugs include corticosteroids. Due to the potential drug interaction between corticosteroids and glimepiride, the patient should be observed closely for loss of glycemic control when these drugs are co-administered. Conversely, when corticosteroids are withdrawn, the patient should be observed closely for hypoglycemia). Products include:
Qvar 3398

Beclomethasone Dipropionate Monohydrate (Certain drugs tend to produce hyperglycemia and may lead to loss of control. These drugs include corticosteroids. Due to the potential drug interaction between corticosteroids and glimepiride, the patient should be observed closely for loss of glycemic control when these drugs are co-administered. Conversely, when corticosteroids are withdrawn, the patient should be observed closely for hypoglycemia). Products include:
Beconase AQ 1386

Belladonna Ergotamine (*In vivo* drug-drug interaction studies have suggested that pioglitazone may be a weak inducer of CYP 450 isoform 3A4 substrate).
No products indexed under this heading.

Bendroflumethiazide (Certain drugs tend to produce hyperglycemia and may lead to loss of control. These drugs include thiazides. Due to the potential drug interaction between thiazides and glimepiride, the patient should be observed closely for loss of glycemic control when these drugs are co-administered. Conversely, when thiazides are withdrawn, the patient should be observed closely for hypoglycemia).
No products indexed under this heading.

Betamethasone (Certain drugs tend to produce hyperglycemia and may lead to loss of control. These drugs include corticosteroids. Due to the potential drug interaction between corticosteroids and glimepiride, the patient should be observed closely for loss of glycemic control when these drugs are co-administered. Conversely, when corticosteroids are withdrawn, the patient should be observed closely for hypoglycemia).
No products indexed under this heading.

Betamethasone Acetate (Certain drugs tend to produce hyperglycemia and may lead to loss of control. These drugs include corticosteroids. Due to the potential drug interaction between corticosteroids and glimepiride, the patient should be observed closely for loss of glycemic control when these drugs are co-administered. Conversely, when corticosteroids are withdrawn, the patient should be observed closely for hypoglycemia).
No products indexed under this heading.

Betamethasone Benzoate (Certain drugs tend to produce hyperglycemia and may lead to loss of control. These drugs include corticosteroids. Due to the potential drug interaction between corticosteroids and glimepiride, the patient should be observed closely for loss of glycemic control when these drugs are co-administered. Conversely, when corticosteroids are withdrawn, the patient should be observed closely for hypoglycemia).
No products indexed under this heading.

Betamethasone Dipropionate (Certain drugs tend to produce hyperglycemia and may lead to loss of control. These drugs include corticosteroids. Due to the potential drug interaction between corticosteroids and glimepiride, the patient should be observed closely for loss of glycemic control when these drugs are co-administered. Conversely, when corticosteroids are withdrawn, the patient should be observed closely for hypoglycemia). Products include:
Diprolene Lotion 0.05% 3108
Diprolene Ointment 0.05% 3109
Diprolene AF Cream 0.05% 3107
Lotrisone 3163

Betamethasone Sodium Phosphate (Certain drugs tend to produce hyperglycemia and may lead to loss of control. These drugs include corticosteroids. Due to the potential drug interaction between corticosteroids and glimepiride, the patient should be observed closely for loss of glycemic control when these drugs are co-administered. Conversely, when corticosteroids are withdrawn, the patient should be observed closely for hypoglycemia).
No products indexed under this heading.

Betamethasone Valerate (Certain drugs tend to produce hyperglycemia and may lead to loss of control. These drugs include corticosteroids. Due to the potential drug interaction between corticosteroids and glimepiride, the patient should be observed closely for loss of glycemic control when these drugs are co-administered. Conversely, when corticosteroids are withdrawn, the patient should be observed closely for hypoglycemia). Products include:
Luxiq 3321

Betaxolol Hydrochloride (The hypoglycemic action of sulfonylureas may be potentiated by certain drugs, including other drugs that are highly protein bound, such as β adrenergic blocking agents. Due to the potential drug interaction between these drugs and glimepiride, the patient should be observed closely for hypoglycemia when these drugs are co-administered. Conversely, when these drugs are withdrawn, the patient should be observed closely for loss of glycemic control).
No products indexed under this heading.

Bisoprolol Fumarate (The hypoglycemic action of sulfonylureas may be potentiated by certain drugs, including other drugs that are highly protein bound, such as β adrenergic blocking agents. Due to the potential drug interaction between these drugs and glimepiride, the patient should be observed closely for hypoglycemia when these drugs are co-administered. Conversely, when these drugs are withdrawn, the patient should be observed closely for loss of glycemic control).
No products indexed under this heading.

Budesonide (Certain drugs tend to produce hyperglycemia and may lead to

loss of control. These drugs include corticosteroids. Due to the potential drug interaction between corticosteroids and glimepiride, the patient should be observed closely for loss of glycemic control when these drugs are co-administered. Conversely, when corticosteroids are withdrawn, the patient should be observed closely for hypoglycemia). Products include:

Pulmicort Flexhaler 714
Symbicort 80/4.5 720
Symbicort 160/4.5 720

Bumetanide (Certain drugs tend to produce hyperglycemia and may lead to loss of control. These drugs include diuretics. Due to the potential drug interaction between diuretics and glimepiride, the patient should be observed closely for loss of glycemic control when these drugs are co-administered. Conversely, when diuretics are withdrawn, the patient should be observed closely for hypoglycemia).

No products indexed under this heading.

Buspirone Hydrochloride (*In vivo* drug-drug interaction studies have suggested that pioglitazone may be a weak inducer of CYP 450 isoform 3A4 substrate).

No products indexed under this heading.

Busulfan (*In vivo* drug-drug interaction studies have suggested that pioglitazone may be a weak inducer of CYP 450 isoform 3A4 substrate). Products include:

Myleran 1581

Carbamazepine (An enzyme inducer of CYP2C8 (such as rifampin) may significantly decrease the AUC of pioglitazone. Therefore, if an inducer of CYP2C8 is started or stopped during treatment with pioglitazone, changes in diabetes treatment may be needed based on clinical response). Products include:

Carbatrol 3280
Equetro 3477

Carteolol Hydrochloride (The hypoglycemic action of sulfonylureas may be potentiated by certain drugs, including other drugs that are highly protein bound, such as β adrenergic blocking agents. Due to the potential drug interaction between these drugs and glimepiride, the patient should be observed closely for hypoglycemia when these drugs are co-administered. Conversely, when these drugs are withdrawn, the patient should be observed closely for loss of glycemic control).

No products indexed under this heading.

Carvedilol (The hypoglycemic action of sulfonylureas may be potentiated by certain drugs, including other drugs that are highly protein bound, such as β adrenergic blocking agents. Due to the potential drug interaction between these drugs and glimepiride, the patient should be observed closely for hypoglycemia when these drugs are co-administered. Conversely, when these drugs are withdrawn, the patient should be observed closely for loss of glycemic control). Products include:

Coreg 1409

Carvedilol Phosphate (The hypoglycemic action of sulfonylureas may be potentiated by certain drugs, including other drugs that are highly protein bound, such as β adrenergic blocking agents. Due to the potential drug interaction between these drugs and glimepiride, the patient should be observed closely for hypoglycemia when these drugs are co-administered. Conversely, when these drugs are withdrawn, the patient should be observed closely for loss of glycemic control). Products include:

Coreg CR 1416

Cefonicid Sodium (The hypoglycemic action of sulfonylureas may be potentiated by certain drugs, including drugs that are highly protein bound. Due to the potential drug interaction between these drugs and glimepiride, the patient should be observed closely for hypoglycemia when these drugs are co-administered. Conversely, when these drugs are withdrawn, the patient should be observed closely for loss of glycemic control).

No products indexed under this heading.

Celecoxib (The hypoglycemic action of sulfonylureas may be potentiated by certain drugs, including nonsteroidal anti-inflammatory drugs. Due to the potential drug interaction between these drugs and glimepiride, the patient should be observed closely for hypoglycemia when these drugs are co-administered. Conversely, when these drugs are withdrawn, the patient should be observed closely for loss of glycemic control). Products include:

Celebrex 3272

Cerivastatin Sodium (*In vivo* drug-drug interaction studies have suggested that pioglitazone may be a weak inducer of CYP 450 isoform 3A4 substrate).

No products indexed under this heading.

Chloramphenicol (The hypoglycemic action of sulfonylureas may be potentiated by certain drugs, including other drugs that are highly protein bound, such as chloramphenicol. Due to the potential drug interaction between these drugs and glimepiride, the patient should be observed closely for hypoglycemia when these drugs are co-administered. Conversely, when these drugs are withdrawn, the patient should be observed closely for loss of glycemic control).

No products indexed under this heading.

Chloramphenicol Palmitate (The hypoglycemic action of sulfonylureas may be potentiated by certain drugs, including other drugs that are highly protein bound, such as chloramphenicol. Due to the potential drug interaction between these drugs and glimepiride, the patient should be observed closely for hypoglycemia when these drugs are co-administered. Conversely, when these drugs are withdrawn, the patient should be observed closely for loss of glycemic control).

No products indexed under this heading.

Chloramphenicol Sodium Succinate (The hypoglycemic action of sulfonylureas may be potentiated by certain drugs, including other drugs that are highly protein bound, such as chloramphenicol. Due to the potential drug interaction between these drugs and glimepiride, the patient should be observed closely for hypoglycemia when these drugs are co-administered. Conversely, when these drugs are withdrawn, the patient should be observed closely for loss of glycemic control).

No products indexed under this heading.

Chlordiazepoxide (The hypoglycemic action of sulfonylureas may be potentiated by certain drugs, including drugs that are highly protein bound. Due to the potential drug interaction between these drugs and glimepiride, the patient should be observed closely for hypoglycemia when these drugs are co-administered. Conversely, when these drugs are withdrawn, the patient should be observed closely for loss of glycemic control).

No products indexed under this heading.

Chlordiazepoxide Hydrochloride (The hypoglycemic action of sulfonylureas may be potentiated by certain drugs, including drugs that are highly protein bound. Due to the potential drug interaction between these drugs and glimepiride, the patient should be observed closely for hypoglycemia when these drugs are co-administered. Conversely, when these drugs are withdrawn, the patient should be observed closely for loss of glycemic control).

No products indexed under this heading.

Chlorothiazide (Certain drugs tend to produce hyperglycemia and may lead to loss of control. These drugs include thiazides. Due to the potential drug interaction between thiazides and glimepiride, the patient should be observed closely for loss of glycemic control when these drugs are co-administered. Conversely, when thiazides are withdrawn, the patient should be observed closely for hypoglycemia).

No products indexed under this heading.

Chlorothiazide Sodium (Certain drugs tend to produce hyperglycemia and may lead to loss of control. These drugs include thiazides. Due to the potential drug interaction between thiazides and glimepiride, the patient should be observed closely for loss of glycemic control when these drugs are co-administered. Conversely, when thiazides are withdrawn, the patient should be observed closely for hypoglycemia). Products include:

Diuril Intravenous 2009

Chlorotrianisene (Certain drugs tend to produce hyperglycemia and may lead to loss of control. These drugs include estrogens. Due to the potential drug interaction between estrogens and glimepiride, the patient should be observed closely for loss of glycemic control when these drugs are co-administered. Conversely, when estrogens are withdrawn, the patient should be observed closely for hypoglycemia).

No products indexed under this heading.

Chlorpheniramine (*In vivo* drug-drug interaction studies have suggested that pioglitazone may be a weak inducer of CYP 450 isoform 3A4 substrate).

No products indexed under this heading.

Chlorpheniramine Maleate (*In vivo* drug-drug interaction studies have suggested that pioglitazone may be a weak inducer of CYP 450 isoform 3A4 substrate).

No products indexed under this heading.

Chlorpheniramine Polistirex (*In vivo* drug-drug interaction studies have suggested that pioglitazone may be a weak inducer of CYP 450 isoform 3A4 substrate). Products include:

Tussionex 3443

Chlorpheniramine Tannate (*In vivo* drug-drug interaction studies have suggested that pioglitazone may be a weak inducer of CYP 450 isoform 3A4 substrate).

No products indexed under this heading.

Chlorpromazine (Certain drugs tend to produce hyperglycemia and may lead to loss of control. These drugs include phenothiazines. Due to the potential drug interaction between phenothiazines and glimepiride, the patient should be observed closely for loss of glycemic control when these drugs are co-administered. Conversely, when phenothiazines are withdrawn, the patient should be observed closely for hypoglycemia).

No products indexed under this heading.

Chlorpromazine Hydrochloride (Certain drugs tend to produce hyperglycemia and may lead to loss of control. These drugs include phenothiazines. Due to the potential drug interaction between phenothiazines and glimepiride, the patient should be observed closely for loss of glycemic control when these drugs are co-administered. Conversely, when phenothiazines are withdrawn, the patient should be observed closely for hypoglycemia).

No products indexed under this heading.

Chlorpropamide (Patients receiving pioglitazone in combination with oral hypoglycemic agents may be at risk for hypoglycemia, and a reduction in the dose of the concomitant agent may be necessary).

No products indexed under this heading.

Chlorthalidone (Certain drugs tend to produce hyperglycemia and may lead to loss of control. These drugs include diuretics. Due to the potential drug interaction between diuretics and glimepiride, the patient should be observed closely for loss of glycemic control when these drugs are co-administered. Conversely, when diuretics are withdrawn, the patient should be observed closely for hypoglycemia). Products include:

Clorpres 2344

Choline Magnesium Trisalicylate (The hypoglycemic action of sulfonylureas may be potentiated by certain drugs, including drugs that are highly protein bound, such as salicylates. Due to the potential drug interaction between these drugs and glimepiride, the patient should be observed closely for hypoglycemia when these drugs are co-administered. Conversely, when these drugs are withdrawn, the patient should be observed closely for loss of glycemic control).

No products indexed under this heading.

Ciclesonide (Certain drugs tend to produce hyperglycemia and may lead to loss of control. These drugs include corticosteroids. Due to the potential drug interaction between corticosteroids and glimepiride, the patient should be observed closely for loss of glycemic control when these drugs are co-administered. Conversely, when corticosteroids are withdrawn, the patient should be observed closely for hypoglycemia).

No products indexed under this heading.

Cimetidine (An enzyme inhibitor of CYP2C8 (such as gemfibrozil) may significantly increase the AUC of pioglitazone. Therefore, if an inhibitor of CYP2C8 is started or stopped during treatment with pioglitazone, changes in diabetes treatment may be needed based on clinical response).

No products indexed under this heading.

Cimetidine Hydrochloride (An enzyme inhibitor of CYP2C8 (such as gemfibrozil) may significantly increase the AUC of pioglitazone. Therefore, if an inhibitor of CYP2C8 is started or stopped during treatment with pioglitazone, changes in diabetes treatment may be needed based on clinical response).

No products indexed under this heading.

Cisapride (*In vivo* drug-drug interaction studies have suggested that pioglitazone may be a weak inducer of CYP 450 isoform 3A4 substrate).

No products indexed under this heading.

Clarithromycin (*In vivo* drug-drug interaction studies have suggested that pioglitazone may be a weak inducer of CYP 450 isoform 3A4 substrate). Products include:

Biaxin/Biaxin XL 412

Clomipramine Hydrochloride (The hypoglycemic action of sulfonylureas may be potentiated by certain drugs, including drugs that are highly protein bound. Due to the potential drug interaction between these drugs and glimepiride, the patient should be observed closely for hypoglycemia when these drugs are co-administered. Conversely,

when these drugs are withdrawn, the patient should be observed closely for loss of glycemic control).

No products indexed under this heading.

Clopidogrel Bisulfate (There is a potential interaction of glimepiride with inhibitors (eg, fluconazole) of cytochrome P450 2C9). Products include:

Plavix 3027

Clopidogrel Hydrogen Sulfate (There is a potential interaction of glimepiride with inhibitors (eg, fluconazole) of cytochrome P450 2C9).

No products indexed under this heading.

Clotrimazole (There is a potential interaction of glimepiride with inhibitors (eg, fluconazole) of cytochrome P450 2C9). Products include:

Lotrisone 3163

Clozapine (The hypoglycemic action of sulfonylureas may be potentiated by certain drugs, including drugs that are highly protein bound. Due to the potential drug interaction between these drugs and glimepiride, the patient should be observed closely for hypoglycemia when these drugs are co-administered. Conversely, when these drugs are withdrawn, the patient should be observed closely for loss of glycemic control).

No products indexed under this heading.

Cortisone Acetate (Certain drugs tend to produce hyperglycemia and may lead to loss of control. These drugs include corticosteroids. Due to the potential drug interaction between corticosteroids and glimepiride, the patient should be observed closely for loss of glycemic control when these drugs are co-administered. Conversely, when corticosteroids are withdrawn, the patient should be observed closely for hypoglycemia).

No products indexed under this heading.

Cyclosporine (The hypoglycemic action of sulfonylureas may be potentiated by certain drugs, including drugs that are highly protein bound. Due to the potential drug interaction between these drugs and glimepiride, the patient should be observed closely for hypoglycemia when these drugs are co-administered. Conversely, when these drugs are withdrawn, the patient should be observed closely for loss of glycemic control). Products include:

Gengraf 440
Neoral Oral Solution 2496
Neoral Capsules 2496
Restasis 605

Desogestrel (Co-administration of pioglitazone (45 mg qd) and an oral contraceptive (1 mg norethindrone plus 0.035 mg ethinyl estradiol qd) for 21 days, resulted in 11% and 11-14% decrease in ethinyl estradiol AUC (0-24h) and C_{max} respectively. In view of the high variability of ethinyl estradiol pharmacokinetics, the clinical significance of this finding is unknown. In addition, certain drugs tend to produce hyperglycemia and may lead to loss of control. These drugs include oral contraceptives. Due to the potential drug interaction between oral contraceptives and glimepiride, the patient should be observed closely for loss of glycemic control when these drugs are co-administered. Conversely, when oral contraceptives are withdrawn, the patient should be observed closely for hypoglycemia).

No products indexed under this heading.

Desoximetasone (Certain drugs tend to produce hyperglycemia and may lead to loss of control. These drugs include corticosteroids. Due to the potential drug interaction between corticosteroids and glimepiride, the patient should be observed closely for loss of glycemic control when these drugs are co-

administered. Conversely, when corticosteroids are withdrawn, the patient should be observed closely for hypoglycemia).

No products indexed under this heading.

Dexamethasone (Certain drugs tend to produce hyperglycemia and may lead to loss of control. These drugs include corticosteroids. Due to the potential drug interaction between corticosteroids and glimepiride, the patient should be observed closely for loss of glycemic control when these drugs are co-administered. Conversely, when corticosteroids are withdrawn, the patient should be observed closely for hypoglycemia). Products include:

Ciprodex 583
Ozurdex .... ⊙223
Tobramycin and Dexamethasone Ophthalmic Suspension .... ⊙251

Dexamethasone Acetate (Certain drugs tend to produce hyperglycemia and may lead to loss of control. These drugs include corticosteroids. Due to the potential drug interaction between corticosteroids and glimepiride, the patient should be observed closely for loss of glycemic control when these drugs are co-administered. Conversely, when corticosteroids are withdrawn, the patient should be observed closely for hypoglycemia).

No products indexed under this heading.

Dexamethasone Phosphate (Certain drugs tend to produce hyperglycemia and may lead to loss of control. These drugs include corticosteroids. Due to the potential drug interaction between corticosteroids and glimepiride, the patient should be observed closely for loss of glycemic control when these drugs are co-administered. Conversely, when corticosteroids are withdrawn, the patient should be observed closely for hypoglycemia).

No products indexed under this heading.

Dexamethasone Sodium (Certain drugs tend to produce hyperglycemia and may lead to loss of control. These drugs include corticosteroids. Due to the potential drug interaction between corticosteroids and glimepiride, the patient should be observed closely for loss of glycemic control when these drugs are co-administered. Conversely, when corticosteroids are withdrawn, the patient should be observed closely for hypoglycemia).

No products indexed under this heading.

Dexamethasone Sodium Phosphate (Certain drugs tend to produce hyperglycemia and may lead to loss of control. These drugs include corticosteroids. Due to the potential drug interaction between corticosteroids and glimepiride, the patient should be observed closely for loss of glycemic control when these drugs are co-administered. Conversely, when corticosteroids are withdrawn, the patient should be observed closely for hypoglycemia).

No products indexed under this heading.

Dexamethasone Sodium Phosphate Injection (Certain drugs tend to produce hyperglycemia and may lead to loss of control. These drugs include corticosteroids. Due to the potential drug interaction between corticosteroids and glimepiride, the patient should be observed closely for loss of glycemic control when these drugs are co-administered. Conversely, when corticosteroids are withdrawn, the patient should be observed closely for hypoglycemia).

No products indexed under this heading.

Diazepam (The hypoglycemic action of sulfonylureas may be potentiated by certain drugs, including drugs that are highly protein bound. Due to the poten-

tial drug interaction between these drugs and glimepiride, the patient should be observed closely for hypoglycemia when these drugs are co-administered. Conversely, when these drugs are withdrawn, the patient should be observed closely for loss of glycemic control). Products include:

Valium Tablets 2880

Diclofenac Epolamine (The hypoglycemic action of sulfonylureas may be potentiated by certain drugs, including nonsteroidal anti-inflammatory drugs. Due to the potential drug interaction between these drugs and glimepiride, the patient should be observed closely for hypoglycemia when these drugs are co-administered. Conversely, when these drugs are withdrawn, the patient should be observed closely for loss of glycemic control). Products include:

Flector 1839

Diclofenac Potassium (The hypoglycemic action of sulfonylureas may be potentiated by certain drugs, including nonsteroidal anti-inflammatory drugs. Due to the potential drug interaction between these drugs and glimepiride, the patient should be observed closely for hypoglycemia when these drugs are co-administered. Conversely, when these drugs are withdrawn, the patient should be observed closely for loss of glycemic control).

No products indexed under this heading.

Diclofenac Sodium (The hypoglycemic action of sulfonylureas may be potentiated by certain drugs, including nonsteroidal anti-inflammatory drugs. Due to the potential drug interaction between these drugs and glimepiride, the patient should be observed closely for hypoglycemia when these drugs are co-administered. Conversely, when these drugs are withdrawn, the patient should be observed closely for loss of glycemic control).

No products indexed under this heading.

Dicumarol (The hypoglycemic action of sulfonylureas may be potentiated by certain drugs, including other drugs that are highly protein bound, such as coumarins. Due to the potential drug interaction between these drugs and glimepiride, the patient should be observed closely for hypoglycemia when these drugs are co-administered. Conversely, when these drugs are withdrawn, the patient should be observed closely for loss of glycemic control).

No products indexed under this heading.

Dienestrol (Certain drugs tend to produce hyperglycemia and may lead to loss of control. These drugs include estrogens. Due to the potential drug interaction between estrogens and glimepiride, the patient should be observed closely for loss of glycemic control when these drugs are co-administered. Conversely, when estrogens are withdrawn, the patient should be observed closely for hypoglycemia).

No products indexed under this heading.

Diethylstilbestrol (Certain drugs tend to produce hyperglycemia and may lead to loss of control. These drugs include estrogens. Due to the potential drug interaction between estrogens and glimepiride, the patient should be observed closely for loss of glycemic control when these drugs are co-administered. Conversely, when estrogens are withdrawn, the patient should be observed closely for hypoglycemia).

No products indexed under this heading.

Diflorasone Diacetate (Certain drugs tend to produce hyperglycemia and may lead to loss of control. These drugs include corticosteroids. Due to the potential drug interaction between corticosteroids and glimepiride, the patient should be observed closely for

loss of glycemic control when these drugs are co-administered. Conversely, when corticosteroids are withdrawn, the patient should be observed closely for hypoglycemia).

No products indexed under this heading.

Diflunisal (The hypoglycemic action of sulfonylureas may be potentiated by certain drugs, including drugs that are highly protein bound, such as salicylates. Due to the potential drug interaction between these drugs and glimepiride, the patient should be observed closely for hypoglycemia when these drugs are co-administered. Conversely, when these drugs are withdrawn, the patient should be observed closely for loss of glycemic control).

No products indexed under this heading.

Digitalis Glycoside Preparations (The hypoglycemic action of sulfonylureas may be potentiated by certain drugs, including drugs that are highly protein bound. Due to the potential drug interaction between these drugs and glimepiride, the patient should be observed closely for hypoglycemia when these drugs are co-administered. Conversely, when these drugs are withdrawn, the patient should be observed closely for loss of glycemic control).

No products indexed under this heading.

Digitalis Lanata (The hypoglycemic action of sulfonylureas may be potentiated by certain drugs, including drugs that are highly protein bound. Due to the potential drug interaction between these drugs and glimepiride, the patient should be observed closely for hypoglycemia when these drugs are co-administered. Conversely, when these drugs are withdrawn, the patient should be observed closely for loss of glycemic control).

No products indexed under this heading.

Digitalis Purpurea (The hypoglycemic action of sulfonylureas may be potentiated by certain drugs, including drugs that are highly protein bound. Due to the potential drug interaction between these drugs and glimepiride, the patient should be observed closely for hypoglycemia when these drugs are co-administered. Conversely, when these drugs are withdrawn, the patient should be observed closely for loss of glycemic control).

No products indexed under this heading.

Dihydroergotamine Mesylate (In vivo drug-drug interaction studies have suggested that pioglitazone may be a weak inducer of CYP 450 isoform 3A4 substrate).

No products indexed under this heading.

Diltiazem Hydrochloride (In vivo drug-drug interaction studies have suggested that pioglitazone may be a weak inducer of CYP 450 isoform 3A4 substrate). Products include:

Cardizem LA 423

Diltiazem Maleate (In vivo drug-drug interaction studies have suggested that pioglitazone may be a weak inducer of CYP 450 isoform 3A4 substrate).

No products indexed under this heading.

Dipyridamole (The hypoglycemic action of sulfonylureas may be potentiated by certain drugs, including drugs that are highly protein bound. Due to the potential drug interaction between these drugs and glimepiride, the patient should be observed closely for hypoglycemia when these drugs are co-administered. Conversely, when these drugs are withdrawn, the patient should be observed closely for loss of glycemic control). Products include:

Aggrenox 880

IMPORTANT NOTE: Always consult each drug listing in the patient's regimen for possible interactions.

Duetact | Interactions Index | 496

Disopyramide (*In vivo* drug-drug interaction studies have suggested that pioglitazone may be a weak inducer of CYP 450 isoform 3A4 substrate).
No products indexed under this heading.

Disopyramide Phosphate (*In vivo* drug-drug interaction studies have suggested that pioglitazone may be a weak inducer of CYP 450 isoform 3A4 substrate).
No products indexed under this heading.

Disulfiram (There is a potential interaction of glimepiride with inhibitors (eg, fluconazole) of cytochrome P450 2C9).
No products indexed under this heading.

Dobutamine Hydrochloride (Certain drugs tend to produce hyperglycemia and may lead to loss of control. These drugs include sympathomimetics. Due to the potential drug interaction between sympathomimetics and glimepiride, the patient should be observed closely for loss of glycemic control when these drugs are co-administered. Conversely, when sympathomimetics are withdrawn, the patient should be observed closely for hypoglycemia).
No products indexed under this heading.

Dopamine Hydrochloride (Certain drugs tend to produce hyperglycemia and may lead to loss of control. These drugs include sympathomimetics. Due to the potential drug interaction between sympathomimetics and glimepiride, the patient should be observed closely for loss of glycemic control when these drugs are co-administered. Conversely, when sympathomimetics are withdrawn, the patient should be observed closely for hypoglycemia).
No products indexed under this heading.

Doxorubicin Hydrochloride (*In vivo* drug-drug interaction studies have suggested that pioglitazone may be a weak inducer of CYP 450 isoform 3A4 substrate).
No products indexed under this heading.

Dronabinol (*In vivo* drug-drug interaction studies have suggested that pioglitazone may be a weak inducer of CYP 450 isoform 3A4 substrate).
No products indexed under this heading.

Efavirenz (There is a potential interaction of glimepiride with inhibitors (eg, fluconazole) of cytochrome P450 2C9). Products include:
Atripla 906

Ephedrine Hydrochloride (Certain drugs tend to produce hyperglycemia and may lead to loss of control. These drugs include sympathomimetics. Due to the potential drug interaction between sympathomimetics and glimepiride, the patient should be observed closely for loss of glycemic control when these drugs are co-administered. Conversely, when sympathomimetics are withdrawn, the patient should be observed closely for hypoglycemia).
No products indexed under this heading.

Ephedrine Sulfate (Certain drugs tend to produce hyperglycemia and may lead to loss of control. These drugs include sympathomimetics. Due to the potential drug interaction between sympathomimetics and glimepiride, the patient should be observed closely for loss of glycemic control when these drugs are co-administered. Conversely, when sympathomimetics are withdrawn, the patient should be observed closely for hypoglycemia).
No products indexed under this heading.

Ephedrine Tannate (Certain drugs tend to produce hyperglycemia and may lead to loss of control. These drugs include sympathomimetics. Due to the potential drug interaction between sympathomimetics and glimepiride, the patient should be observed closely for loss of glycemic control when these drugs are co-administered. Conversely, when sympathomimetics are withdrawn, the patient should be observed closely for hypoglycemia).
No products indexed under this heading.

Epinephrine (Certain drugs tend to produce hyperglycemia and may lead to loss of control. These drugs include sympathomimetics. Due to the potential drug interaction between sympathomimetics and glimepiride, the patient should be observed closely for loss of glycemic control when these drugs are co-administered. Conversely, when sympathomimetics are withdrawn, the patient should be observed closely for hypoglycemia). Products include:
EpiPen 3631
Twinject 3268

Epinephrine Bitartrate (Certain drugs tend to produce hyperglycemia and may lead to loss of control. These drugs include sympathomimetics. Due to the potential drug interaction between sympathomimetics and glimepiride, the patient should be observed closely for loss of glycemic control when these drugs are co-administered. Conversely, when sympathomimetics are withdrawn, the patient should be observed closely for hypoglycemia).
No products indexed under this heading.

Epinephrine Hydrochloride (Certain drugs tend to produce hyperglycemia and may lead to loss of control. These drugs include sympathomimetics. Due to the potential drug interaction between sympathomimetics and glimepiride, the patient should be observed closely for loss of glycemic control when these drugs are co-administered. Conversely, when sympathomimetics are withdrawn, the patient should be observed closely for hypoglycemia).
No products indexed under this heading.

Ergotamine Tartrate (*In vivo* drug-drug interaction studies have suggested that pioglitazone may be a weak inducer of CYP 450 isoform 3A4 substrate).
No products indexed under this heading.

Erythromycin (*In vivo* drug-drug interaction studies have suggested that pioglitazone may be a weak inducer of CYP 450 isoform 3A4 substrate).
No products indexed under this heading.

Erythromycin Estolate (*In vivo* drug-drug interaction studies have suggested that pioglitazone may be a weak inducer of CYP 450 isoform 3A4 substrate).
No products indexed under this heading.

Erythromycin Ethylsuccinate (*In vivo* drug-drug interaction studies have suggested that pioglitazone may be a weak inducer of CYP 450 isoform 3A4 substrate). Products include:
E.E.S. 437
EryPed 435

Erythromycin Gluceptate (*In vivo* drug-drug interaction studies have suggested that pioglitazone may be a weak inducer of CYP 450 isoform 3A4 substrate).
No products indexed under this heading.

Erythromycin Lactobionate (*In vivo* drug-drug interaction studies have suggested that pioglitazone may be a weak inducer of CYP 450 isoform 3A4 substrate).
No products indexed under this heading.

Erythromycin Stearate (*In vivo* drug-drug interaction studies have suggested that pioglitazone may be a weak inducer of CYP 450 isoform 3A4 substrate).
No products indexed under this heading.

Esmolol Hydrochloride (The hypoglycemic action of sulfonylureas may be potentiated by certain drugs, including other drugs that are highly protein bound, such as β adrenergic blocking agents. Due to the potential drug interaction between these drugs and glimepiride, the patient should be observed closely for hypoglycemia when these drugs are co-administered. Conversely, when these drugs are withdrawn, the patient should be observed closely for loss of glycemic control).
No products indexed under this heading.

Estradiol (Certain drugs tend to produce hyperglycemia and may lead to loss of control. These drugs include estrogens. Due to the potential drug interaction between estrogens and glimepiride, the patient should be observed closely for loss of glycemic control when these drugs are co-administered. Conversely, when estrogens are withdrawn, the patient should be observed closely for hypoglycemia). Products include:
Activella 2561
Angeliq 831
Climara 841
Climara Pro 847
Divigel 3467
Estrasorb 1777
Vagifem 2589

Estradiol Benzoate (*In vivo* drug-drug interaction studies have suggested that pioglitazone may be a weak inducer of CYP 450 isoform 3A4 substrate).
No products indexed under this heading.

Estradiol Cypionate (*In vivo* drug-drug interaction studies have suggested that pioglitazone may be a weak inducer of CYP 450 isoform 3A4 substrate).
No products indexed under this heading.

Estradiol Valerate (*In vivo* drug-drug interaction studies have suggested that pioglitazone may be a weak inducer of CYP 450 isoform 3A4 substrate).
No products indexed under this heading.

Estrogens, Conjugated (Certain drugs tend to produce hyperglycemia and may lead to loss of control. These drugs include estrogens. Due to the potential drug interaction between estrogens and glimepiride, the patient should be observed closely for loss of glycemic control when these drugs are co-administered. Conversely, when estrogens are withdrawn, the patient should be observed closely for hypoglycemia). Products include:
Premarin Intravenous 3528
Premarin Tablets 3533
Premarin Vaginal Cream 3540
Premphase 3549
Prempro 3549

Estrogens, Esterified (Certain drugs tend to produce hyperglycemia and may lead to loss of control. These drugs include estrogens. Due to the potential drug interaction between estrogens and glimepiride, the patient should be observed closely for loss of glycemic control when these drugs are co-administered. Conversely, when estrogens are withdrawn, the patient should be observed closely for hypoglycemia).
No products indexed under this heading.

Estropipate (Certain drugs tend to produce hyperglycemia and may lead to loss of control. These drugs include estrogens. Due to the potential drug interaction between estrogens and glimepiride, the patient should be observed closely for loss of glycemic control when these drugs are co-administered. Conversely, when estrogens are withdrawn, the patient should be observed closely for hypoglycemia).
No products indexed under this heading.

Ethacrynic Acid (Certain drugs tend to produce hyperglycemia and may lead to loss of control. These drugs include diuretics. Due to the potential drug interaction between diuretics and glimepiride, the patient should be observed closely for loss of glycemic control when these drugs are co-administered. Conversely, when diuretics are withdrawn, the patient should be observed closely for hypoglycemia).
No products indexed under this heading.

Ethanol (All sulfonylurea drugs are capable of producing hypoglycemia; hypoglycemia is more likely to occur when alcohol is ingested).
No products indexed under this heading.

Ethinyl Estradiol (Co-administration of pioglitazone (45 mg qd) and an oral contraceptive (1 mg norethindrone plus 0.035 mg ethinyl estradiol qd) for 21 days, resulted in 11% and 11-14% decrease in ethinyl estradiol AUC (0-24h) and C_{max}, respectively. In view of the high variability of ethinyl estradiol pharmacokinetics, the clinical significance of this finding is unknown. In addition, certain drugs tend to produce hyperglycemia and may lead to loss of control. These drugs include estrogens. Due to the potential drug interaction between these drugs and glimepiride, the patient should be observed closely for loss of glycemic control when these drugs are co-administered. Conversely, when these drugs are withdrawn, the patient should be observed closely for hypoglycemia). Products include:
LoSeasonique 3407
Lybrel 3514
NuvaRing 3181
Ortho Evra 2648
Ortho-Cyclen/Ortho Tri-Cyclen 2663
Ortho Tri-Cyclen Lo Tablets 2673
Seasonique 3418
Yaz 864

Ethosuximide (*In vivo* drug-drug interaction studies have suggested that pioglitazone may be a weak inducer of CYP 450 isoform 3A4 substrate).
No products indexed under this heading.

Ethyl Alcohol (All sulfonylurea drugs are capable of producing hypoglycemia; hypoglycemia is more likely to occur when alcohol is ingested).
No products indexed under this heading.

Ethynodiol Diacetate (Co-administration of pioglitazone (45 mg qd) and an oral contraceptive (1 mg norethindrone plus 0.035 mg ethinyl estradiol qd) for 21 days, resulted in 11% and 11-14% decrease in ethinyl estradiol AUC (0-24h) and C_{max} respectively. In view of the high variability of ethinyl estradiol pharmacokinetics, the clinical significance of this finding is unknown. In addition, certain drugs tend to produce hyperglycemia and may lead to loss of control. These drugs include oral contraceptives. Due to the potential drug interaction between oral contraceptives and glimepiride, the patient should be observed closely for loss of glycemic control when these drugs are co-administered. Conversely, when oral contraceptives are withdrawn, the patient should be observed closely for hypoglycemia).
No products indexed under this heading.

Etodolac (The hypoglycemic action of sulfonylureas may be potentiated by certain drugs, including nonsteroidal anti-inflammatory drugs. Due to the potential drug interaction between these drugs and glimepiride, the patient should be observed closely for hypoglycemia when these drugs are co-administered. Conversely, when these drugs are withdrawn, the patient should be observed closely for loss of glycemic control).
No products indexed under this heading.

Etoposide (*In vivo* drug-drug interaction studies have suggested that pioglitazone may be a weak inducer of CYP 450 isoform 3A4 substrate).
No products indexed under this heading.

patient should be observed closely for loss of glycemic control when these drugs are co-administered. Conversely, when corticosteroids are withdrawn, the patient should be observed closely for hypoglycemia).

No products indexed under this heading.

Hydrocortisone Butyrate (Certain drugs tend to produce hyperglycemia and may lead to loss of control. These drugs include corticosteroids. Due to the potential drug interaction between corticosteroids and glimepiride, the patient should be observed closely for loss of glycemic control when these drugs are co-administered. Conversely, when corticosteroids are withdrawn, the patient should be observed closely for hypoglycemia).

No products indexed under this heading.

Hydrocortisone Cypionate (Certain drugs tend to produce hyperglycemia and may lead to loss of control. These drugs include corticosteroids. Due to the potential drug interaction between corticosteroids and glimepiride, the patient should be observed closely for loss of glycemic control when these drugs are co-administered. Conversely, when corticosteroids are withdrawn, the patient should be observed closely for hypoglycemia).

No products indexed under this heading.

Hydrocortisone Hemisuccinate (Certain drugs tend to produce hyperglycemia and may lead to loss of control. These drugs include corticosteroids. Due to the potential drug interaction between corticosteroids and glimepiride, the patient should be observed closely for loss of glycemic control when these drugs are co-administered. Conversely, when corticosteroids are withdrawn, the patient should be observed closely for hypoglycemia).

No products indexed under this heading.

Hydrocortisone Probutate (Certain drugs tend to produce hyperglycemia and may lead to loss of control. These drugs include corticosteroids. Due to the potential drug interaction between corticosteroids and glimepiride, the patient should be observed closely for loss of glycemic control when these drugs are co-administered. Conversely, when corticosteroids are withdrawn, the patient should be observed closely for hypoglycemia).

No products indexed under this heading.

Hydrocortisone Sodium Phosphate (Certain drugs tend to produce hyperglycemia and may lead to loss of control. These drugs include corticosteroids. Due to the potential drug interaction between corticosteroids and glimepiride, the patient should be observed closely for loss of glycemic control when these drugs are co-administered. Conversely, when corticosteroids are withdrawn, the patient should be observed closely for hypoglycemia).

No products indexed under this heading.

Hydrocortisone Sodium Succinate (Certain drugs tend to produce hyperglycemia and may lead to loss of control. These drugs include corticosteroids. Due to the potential drug interaction between corticosteroids and glimepiride, the patient should be observed closely for loss of glycemic control when these drugs are co-administered. Conversely, when corticosteroids are withdrawn, the patient should be observed closely for hypoglycemia).

No products indexed under this heading.

Hydrocortisone Valerate (Certain drugs tend to produce hyperglycemia and may lead to loss of control. These drugs include corticosteroids. Due to

the potential drug interaction between corticosteroids and glimepiride, the patient should be observed closely for loss of glycemic control when these drugs are co-administered. Conversely, when corticosteroids are withdrawn, the patient should be observed closely for hypoglycemia).

No products indexed under this heading.

Hydroflumethiazide (Certain drugs tend to produce hyperglycemia and may lead to loss of control. These drugs include thiazides. Due to the potential drug interaction between thiazides and glimepiride, the patient should be observed closely for loss of glycemic control when these drugs are co-administered. Conversely, when thiazides are withdrawn, the patient should be observed closely for hypoglycemia).

No products indexed under this heading.

Ibuprofen (The hypoglycemic action of sulfonylureas may be potentiated by certain drugs, including nonsteroidal anti-inflammatory drugs. Due to the potential drug interaction between these drugs and glimepiride, the patient should be observed closely for hypoglycemia when these drugs are co-administered. Conversely, when these drugs are withdrawn, the patient should be observed closely for loss of glycemic control). Products include:

Imatinib Mesylate (There is a potential interaction of glimepiride with inhibitors (eg, fluconazole) of cytochrome P450 2C9). Products include:

Imipramine Hydrochloride (The hypoglycemic action of sulfonylureas may be potentiated by certain drugs, including drugs that are highly protein bound. Due to the potential drug interaction between these drugs and glimepiride, the patient should be observed closely for hypoglycemia when these drugs are co-administered. Conversely, when these drugs are withdrawn, the patient should be observed closely for loss of glycemic control).

No products indexed under this heading.

Imipramine Pamoate (The hypoglycemic action of sulfonylureas may be potentiated by certain drugs, including drugs that are highly protein bound. Due to the potential drug interaction between these drugs and glimepiride, the patient should be observed closely for hypoglycemia when these drugs are co-administered. Conversely, when these drugs are withdrawn, the patient should be observed closely for loss of glycemic control).

No products indexed under this heading.

Indapamide (Certain drugs tend to produce hyperglycemia and may lead to loss of control. These drugs include diuretics. Due to the potential drug interaction between diuretics and glimepiride, the patient should be observed closely for loss of glycemic control when these drugs are co-administered. Conversely, when diuretics are withdrawn, the patient should be observed closely for hypoglycemia). Products include:

Indinavir Sulfate (In vivo drug-drug interaction studies have suggested that pioglitazone may be a weak inducer of CYP 450 isoform 3A4 substrate). Products include:

Indomethacin (The hypoglycemic action of sulfonylureas may be potentiated by certain drugs, including nonsteroidal anti-inflammatory drugs. Due to the potential drug interaction between these drugs and glimepiride, the patient should be observed closely for hypoglycemia when these drugs are co-administered. Conversely, when these drugs are withdrawn, the patient should be observed closely for loss of glycemic control). Products include:

Indomethacin Sodium Trihydrate (The hypoglycemic action of sulfonylureas may be potentiated by certain drugs, including nonsteroidal anti-inflammatory drugs. Due to the potential drug interaction between these drugs and glimepiride, the patient should be observed closely for hypoglycemia when these drugs are co-administered. Conversely, when these drugs are withdrawn, the patient should be observed closely for loss of glycemic control). Products include:

Insulin (Patients receiving pioglitazone in combination with insulin may be at risk for hypoglycemia, and a reduction in the dose of the concomitant agent may be necessary).

No products indexed under this heading.

Insulin, Human, Zinc Suspension (Patients receiving pioglitazone in combination with insulin may be at risk for hypoglycemia, and a reduction in the dose of the concomitant agent may be necessary).

No products indexed under this heading.

Insulin, Human (rDNA origin) (Patients receiving pioglitazone in combination with insulin may be at risk for hypoglycemia, and a reduction in the dose of the concomitant agent may be necessary). Products include:

Insulin, Human NPH (Patients receiving pioglitazone in combination with insulin may be at risk for hypoglycemia, and a reduction in the dose of the concomitant agent may be necessary). Products include:

Insulin, Human Regular (Patients receiving pioglitazone in combination with insulin may be at risk for hypoglycemia, and a reduction in the dose of the concomitant agent may be necessary). Products include:

Insulin, Human Regular and Human NPH Mixture (Patients receiving pioglitazone in combination with insulin may be at risk for hypoglycemia, and a reduction in the dose of the concomitant agent may be necessary). Products include:

Insulin, NPH (Patients receiving pioglitazone in combination with insulin may be at risk for hypoglycemia, and a reduction in the dose of the concomitant agent may be necessary).

No products indexed under this heading.

Insulin, Regular (Patients receiving pioglitazone in combination with insulin may be at risk for hypoglycemia, and a reduction in the dose of the concomitant agent may be necessary).

No products indexed under this heading.

Insulin, Regular and NPH mixture (Patients receiving pioglitazone in combination with insulin may be at risk for hypoglycemia, and a reduction in the dose of the concomitant agent may be necessary).

No products indexed under this heading.

Insulin, Zinc Crystals (Patients receiving pioglitazone in combination with insulin may be at risk for hypoglycemia, and a reduction in the dose of the concomitant agent may be necessary).

No products indexed under this heading.

Insulin, Zinc Suspension (Patients receiving pioglitazone in combination with insulin may be at risk for hypoglycemia, and a reduction in the dose of the concomitant agent may be necessary).

No products indexed under this heading.

Insulin Aspart (Patients receiving pioglitazone in combination with insulin may be at risk for hypoglycemia, and a reduction in the dose of the concomitant agent may be necessary).

No products indexed under this heading.

Insulin Aspart, Human (Patients receiving pioglitazone in combination with insulin may be at risk for hypoglycemia, and a reduction in the dose of the concomitant agent may be necessary). Products include:

Insulin Aspart, Human Regular (Patients receiving pioglitazone in combination with insulin may be at risk for hypoglycemia, and a reduction in the dose of the concomitant agent may be necessary). Products include:

Insulin Aspart Protamine, Human (Patients receiving pioglitazone in combination with insulin may be at risk for hypoglycemia, and a reduction in the dose of the concomitant agent may be necessary). Products include:

Insulin Detemir (rDNA Origin) (Patients receiving pioglitazone in combination with insulin may be at risk for hypoglycemia, and a reduction in the dose of the concomitant agent may be necessary). Products include:

Insulin Glargine (Patients receiving pioglitazone in combination with insulin may be at risk for hypoglycemia, and a reduction in the dose of the concomitant agent may be necessary). Products include:

Insulin Glulisine (Patients receiving pioglitazone in combination with insulin may be at risk for hypoglycemia, and a reduction in the dose of the concomitant agent may be necessary). Products include:

Insulin Lispro, Human (Patients receiving pioglitazone in combination with insulin may be at risk for hypoglycemia, and a reduction in the dose of the concomitant agent may be necessary). Products include:

Insulin Lispro Protamine, Human (Patients receiving pioglitazone in combination with insulin may be at risk for hypoglycemia, and a reduction in the dose of the concomitant agent may be necessary). Products include:

Isocarboxazid (The hypoglycemic action of sulfonylureas may be potentiated by certain drugs, including other drugs that are highly protein bound, such as monoamine oxidase inhibitors. Due to the potential drug interaction between these drugs and glimepiride, the patient should be observed closely for hypoglycemia when these drugs are co-administered. Conversely, when

these drugs are withdrawn, the patient should be observed closely for loss of glycemic control). Products include:
Marplan 3481

Isoniazid (Certain drugs tend to produce hyperglycemia and may lead to loss of control. These drugs include isoniazid. Due to the potential drug interaction between isoniazid and glimepiride, the patient should be observed closely for loss of glycemic control when these drugs are co-administered. Conversely, when isoniazid is withdrawn, the patient should be observed closely for hypoglycemia).
No products indexed under this heading.

Isoproterenol Hydrochloride (Certain drugs tend to produce hyperglycemia and may lead to loss of control. These drugs include sympathomimetics. Due to the potential drug interaction between sympathomimetics and glimepiride, the patient should be observed closely for loss of glycemic control when these drugs are co-administered. Conversely, when sympathomimetics are withdrawn, the patient should be observed closely for hypoglycemia).
No products indexed under this heading.

Isoproterenol Sulfate (Certain drugs tend to produce hyperglycemia and may lead to loss of control. These drugs include sympathomimetics. Due to the potential drug interaction between sympathomimetics and glimepiride, the patient should be observed closely for loss of glycemic control when these drugs are co-administered. Conversely, when sympathomimetics are withdrawn, the patient should be observed closely for hypoglycemia).
No products indexed under this heading.

Isradipine (*In vivo* drug-drug interaction studies have suggested that pioglitazone may be a weak inducer of CYP 450 isoform 3A4 substrate). Products include:
DynaCirc CR 1432

Itraconazole (There is a potential interaction of glimepiride with inhibitors (eg, fluconazole) of cytochrome P450 2C9).
No products indexed under this heading.

Ixabepilone (*In vivo* drug-drug interaction studies have suggested that pioglitazone may be a weak inducer of CYP 450 isoform 3A4 substrate).
No products indexed under this heading.

Ketoconazole (Co-administration of pioglitazone for 7 days with ketoconazole 200 mg administered twice daily resulted in a ratio of least square mean (90% CI) values for unchanged pioglitazone of 1.14 (1.06-1.23) for C_{max}, 1.34 (1.26-1.41) for AUC, and 1.87 (1.71-2.04) for C_{min}). Products include:
Extina 3319
Xolegel 3337

Ketoprofen (The hypoglycemic action of sulfonylureas may be potentiated by certain drugs, including nonsteroidal anti-inflammatory drugs. Due to the potential drug interaction between these drugs and glimepiride, the patient should be observed closely for hypoglycemia when these drugs are co-administered. Conversely, when these drugs are withdrawn, the patient should be observed closely for loss of glycemic control).
No products indexed under this heading.

Ketorolac Tromethamine (The hypoglycemic action of sulfonylureas may be potentiated by certain drugs, including nonsteroidal anti-inflammatory drugs. Due to the potential drug interaction between these drugs and glimepiride, the patient should be observed closely for hypoglycemia when these drugs are co-administered. Conversely, when these drugs are withdrawn, the patient should be observed closely for loss of glycemic control). Products include:
Acuvail .... ⊙ 209

Labetalol Hydrochloride (The hypoglycemic action of sulfonylureas may be potentiated by certain drugs, including other drugs that are highly protein bound, such as β adrenergic blocking agents. Due to the potential drug interaction between these drugs and glimepiride, the patient should be observed closely for hypoglycemia when these drugs are co-administered. Conversely, when these drugs are withdrawn, the patient should be observed closely for loss of glycemic control).
No products indexed under this heading.

Leflunomide (There is a potential interaction of glimepiride with inhibitors (eg, fluconazole) of cytochrome P450 2C9).
No products indexed under this heading.

Levalbuterol Hydrochloride (Certain drugs tend to produce hyperglycemia and may lead to loss of control. These drugs include sympathomimetics. Due to the potential drug interaction between sympathomimetics and glimepiride, the patient should be observed closely for loss of glycemic control when these drugs are co-administered. Conversely, when sympathomimetics are withdrawn, the patient should be observed closely for hypoglycemia).
No products indexed under this heading.

Levobunolol Hydrochloride (The hypoglycemic action of sulfonylureas may be potentiated by certain drugs, including other drugs that are highly protein bound, such as β adrenergic blocking agents. Due to the potential drug interaction between these drugs and glimepiride, the patient should be observed closely for hypoglycemia when these drugs are co-administered. Conversely, when these drugs are withdrawn, the patient should be observed closely for loss of glycemic control).
No products indexed under this heading.

Levonorgestrel (Co-administration of pioglitazone (45 mg qd) and an oral contraceptive (1 mg norethindrone plus 0.035 mg ethinyl estradiol qd) for 21 days, resulted in 11% and 11-14% decrease in ethinyl estradiol AUC (0-24h) and C_{max} respectively. In view of the high variability of ethinyl estradiol pharmacokinetics, the clinical significance of this finding is unknown. In addition, certain drugs tend to produce hyperglycemia and may lead to loss of control. These drugs include oral contraceptives. Due to the potential drug interaction between oral contraceptives and glimepiride, the patient should be observed closely for loss of glycemic control when these drugs are co-administered. Conversely, when oral contraceptives are withdrawn, the patient should be observed closely for hypoglycemia). Products include:
Climara Pro 847
LoSeasonique 3407
Lybrel 3514
Mirena 854
Plan B 3416
Seasonique 3418

Levothyroxine Sodium (Certain drugs tend to produce hyperglycemia and may lead to loss of control. These drugs include thyroid products. Due to the potential drug interaction between thyroid products and glimepiride, the patient should be observed closely for loss of glycemic control when these drugs are co-administered. Conversely, when thyroid products are withdrawn, the patient should be observed closely for hypoglycemia). Products include:
Levoxyl Tablets 1843
Synthroid 529

Lidocaine (*In vivo* drug-drug interaction studies have suggested that pioglitazone may be a weak inducer of CYP 450 isoform 3A4 substrate). Products include:
Lidoderm 1107

Lidocaine Hydrochloride (*In vivo* drug-drug interaction studies have suggested that pioglitazone may be a weak inducer of CYP 450 isoform 3A4 substrate).
No products indexed under this heading.

Liothyronine Sodium (Certain drugs tend to produce hyperglycemia and may lead to loss of control. These drugs include thyroid products. Due to the potential drug interaction between thyroid products and glimepiride, the patient should be observed closely for loss of glycemic control when these drugs are co-administered. Conversely, when thyroid products are withdrawn, the patient should be observed closely for hypoglycemia). Products include:
Cytomel 1830

Liotrix (Certain drugs tend to produce hyperglycemia and may lead to loss of control. These drugs include thyroid products. Due to the potential drug interaction between thyroid products and glimepiride, the patient should be observed closely for loss of glycemic control when these drugs are co-administered. Conversely, when thyroid products are withdrawn, the patient should be observed closely for hypoglycemia).
No products indexed under this heading.

Lovastatin (There is a potential interaction of glimepiride with inhibitors (eg, fluconazole) of cytochrome P450 2C9). Products include:
Advicor 402
Mevacor 2212

Magnesium Salicylate (The hypoglycemic action of sulfonylureas may be potentiated by certain drugs, including drugs that are highly protein bound, such as salicylates. Due to the potential drug interaction between these drugs and glimepiride, the patient should be observed closely for hypoglycemia when these drugs are co-administered. Conversely, when these drugs are withdrawn, the patient should be observed closely for loss of glycemic control).
No products indexed under this heading.

Meclofenamate Sodium (The hypoglycemic action of sulfonylureas may be potentiated by certain drugs, including nonsteroidal anti-inflammatory drugs. Due to the potential drug interaction between these drugs and glimepiride, the patient should be observed closely for hypoglycemia when these drugs are co-administered. Conversely, when these drugs are withdrawn, the patient should be observed closely for loss of glycemic control).
No products indexed under this heading.

Mefenamic Acid (The hypoglycemic action of sulfonylureas may be potentiated by certain drugs, including nonsteroidal anti-inflammatory drugs. Due to the potential drug interaction between these drugs and glimepiride, the patient should be observed closely for hypoglycemia when these drugs are co-administered. Conversely, when these drugs are withdrawn, the patient should be observed closely for loss of glycemic control).
No products indexed under this heading.

Meloxicam (The hypoglycemic action of sulfonylureas may be potentiated by certain drugs, including nonsteroidal anti-inflammatory drugs. Due to the potential drug interaction between these drugs and glimepiride, the patient should be observed closely for hypoglycemia when these drugs are co-administered. Conversely, when these drugs are withdrawn, the patient should be observed closely for loss of glycemic control).
No products indexed under this heading.

Mesoridazine Besylate (Certain drugs tend to produce hyperglycemia and may lead to loss of control. These drugs include phenothiazines. Due to the potential drug interaction between phenothiazines and glimepiride, the patient should be observed closely for loss of glycemic control when these drugs are co-administered. Conversely, when phenothiazines are withdrawn, the patient should be observed closely for hypoglycemia).
No products indexed under this heading.

Mestranol (Co-administration of pioglitazone (45 mg qd) and an oral contraceptive (1 mg norethindrone plus 0.035 mg ethinyl estradiol qd) for 21 days, resulted in 11% and 11-14% decrease in ethinyl estradiol AUC (0-24h) and C_{max} respectively. In view of the high variability of ethinyl estradiol pharmacokinetics, the clinical significance of this finding is unknown. In addition, certain drugs tend to produce hyperglycemia and may lead to loss of control. These drugs include oral contraceptives. Due to the potential drug interaction between oral contraceptives and glimepiride, the patient should be observed closely for loss of glycemic control when these drugs are co-administered. Conversely, when oral contraceptives are withdrawn, the patient should be observed closely for hypoglycemia).
No products indexed under this heading.

Metaproterenol Sulfate (Certain drugs tend to produce hyperglycemia and may lead to loss of control. These drugs include sympathomimetics. Due to the potential drug interaction between sympathomimetics and glimepiride, the patient should be observed closely for loss of glycemic control when these drugs are co-administered. Conversely, when sympathomimetics are withdrawn, the patient should be observed closely for hypoglycemia).
No products indexed under this heading.

Metaraminol Bitartrate (Certain drugs tend to produce hyperglycemia and may lead to loss of control. These drugs include sympathomimetics. Due to the potential drug interaction between sympathomimetics and glimepiride, the patient should be observed closely for loss of glycemic control when these drugs are co-administered. Conversely, when sympathomimetics are withdrawn, the patient should be observed closely for hypoglycemia).
No products indexed under this heading.

Metformin (Combined use of glimepiride with metformin may increase the potential for hypoglycemia).
No products indexed under this heading.

Metformin Hydrochloride (Combined use of glimepiride with metformin may increase the potential for hypoglycemia). Products include:
ActoPlus 3338
Avandamet 1345
Janumet 2188

Methadone Hydrochloride (*In vivo* drug-drug interaction studies have suggested that pioglitazone may be a weak inducer of CYP 450 isoform 3A4 substrate).
No products indexed under this heading.

Methotrimeprazine (Certain drugs tend to produce hyperglycemia and may lead to loss of control. These drugs include phenothiazines. Due to the potential drug interaction between phenothiazines and glimepiride, the patient should be observed closely for loss of glycemic control when these drugs are

IMPORTANT NOTE: Always consult each drug listing in the patient's regimen for possible interactions.

Duetact Interactions Index 500

co-administered. Conversely, when phenothiazines are withdrawn, the patient should be observed closely for hypoglycemia).
No products indexed under this heading.

Methoxamine Hydrochloride (Certain drugs tend to produce hyperglycemia and may lead to loss of control. These drugs include sympathomimetics. Due to the potential drug interaction between sympathomimetics and glimepiride, the patient should be observed closely for loss of glycemic control when these drugs are co-administered. Conversely, when sympathomimetics are withdrawn, the patient should be observed closely for hypoglycemia).
No products indexed under this heading.

Methyclothiazide (Certain drugs tend to produce hyperglycemia and may lead to loss of control. These drugs include thiazides. Due to the potential drug interaction between thiazides and glimepiride, the patient should be observed closely for loss of glycemic control when these drugs are co-administered. Conversely, when thiazides are withdrawn, the patient should be observed closely for hypoglycemia).
No products indexed under this heading.

Methylprednisolone (Certain drugs tend to produce hyperglycemia and may lead to loss of control. These drugs include corticosteroids. Due to the potential drug interaction between corticosteroids and glimepiride, the patient should be observed closely for loss of glycemic control when these drugs are co-administered. Conversely, when corticosteroids are withdrawn, the patient should be observed closely for hypoglycemia).
No products indexed under this heading.

Methylprednisolone Acetate (Certain drugs tend to produce hyperglycemia and may lead to loss of control. These drugs include corticosteroids. Due to the potential drug interaction between corticosteroids and glimepiride, the patient should be observed closely for loss of glycemic control when these drugs are co-administered. Conversely, when corticosteroids are withdrawn, the patient should be observed closely for hypoglycemia).
No products indexed under this heading.

Methylprednisolone Sodium Succinate (Certain drugs tend to produce hyperglycemia and may lead to loss of control. These drugs include corticosteroids. Due to the potential drug interaction between corticosteroids and glimepiride, the patient should be observed closely for loss of glycemic control when these drugs are co-administered. Conversely, when corticosteroids are withdrawn, the patient should be observed closely for hypoglycemia).
No products indexed under this heading.

Metipranolol Hydrochloride (The hypoglycemic action of sulfonylureas may be potentiated by certain drugs, including other drugs that are highly protein bound, such as β adrenergic blocking agents. Due to the potential drug interaction between these drugs and glimepiride, the patient should be observed closely for hypoglycemia when these drugs are co-administered. Conversely, when these drugs are withdrawn, the patient should be observed closely for loss of glycemic control).
No products indexed under this heading.

Metolazone (Certain drugs tend to produce hyperglycemia and may lead to loss of control. These drugs include diuretics. Due to the potential drug interaction between diuretics and glimepiride, the patient should be observed closely for loss of glycemic control when these drugs are co-administered. Conversely, when diuretics are withdrawn, the patient should be observed closely for hypoglycemia).
No products indexed under this heading.

Metoprolol Succinate (The hypoglycemic action of sulfonylureas may be potentiated by certain drugs, including other drugs that are highly protein bound, such as β adrenergic blocking agents. Due to the potential drug interaction between these drugs and glimepiride, the patient should be observed closely for hypoglycemia when these drugs are co-administered. Conversely, when these drugs are withdrawn, the patient should be observed closely for loss of glycemic control). Products include:
Toprol XL 732

Metoprolol Tartrate (The hypoglycemic action of sulfonylureas may be potentiated by certain drugs, including other drugs that are highly protein bound, such as β adrenergic blocking agents. Due to the potential drug interaction between these drugs and glimepiride, the patient should be observed closely for hypoglycemia when these drugs are co-administered. Conversely, when these drugs are withdrawn, the patient should be observed closely for loss of glycemic control).
No products indexed under this heading.

Metronidazole (There is a potential interaction of glimepiride with inhibitors (eg, fluconazole) of cytochrome P450 2C9). Products include:
Pylera 793

Metronidazole Benzoate (There is a potential interaction of glimepiride with inhibitors (eg, fluconazole) of cytochrome P450 2C9).
No products indexed under this heading.

Metronidazole Hydrochloride (There is a potential interaction of glimepiride with inhibitors (eg, fluconazole) of cytochrome P450 2C9).
No products indexed under this heading.

Metronidazole Sodium (There is a potential interaction of glimepiride with inhibitors (eg, fluconazole) of cytochrome P450 2C9).
No products indexed under this heading.

Miconazole (A potential interaction between oral miconazole and oral hypoglycemic agents leading to severe hypoglycemia has been reported. Whether this interaction also occurs with the intravenous, topical, or vaginal preparations of miconazole is not known).
No products indexed under this heading.

Miconazole Nitrate (A potential interaction between oral miconazole and oral hypoglycemic agents leading to severe hypoglycemia has been reported. Whether this interaction also occurs with intravenous, topical, or vaginal preparations of miconazole is not known). Products include:
Vusion Ointment 3335

Midazolam Hydrochloride (Administration of pioglitazone for 15 days followed by a single 7.5 mg dose of midazolam syrup resulted in a 26% reduction in midazolam C_{max} and AUC).
No products indexed under this heading.

Miglitol (Patients receiving pioglitazone in combination with oral hypoglycemic agents may be at risk for hypoglycemia, and a reduction in the dose of the concomitant agent may be necessary).
No products indexed under this heading.

Moclobemide (The hypoglycemic action of sulfonylureas may be potentiated by certain drugs, including other drugs that are highly protein bound, such as monoamine oxidase inhibitors. Due to the potential drug interaction between these drugs and glimepiride, the patient should be observed closely for hypoglycemia when these drugs are co-administered. Conversely, when these drugs are withdrawn, the patient should be observed closely for loss of glycemic control).
No products indexed under this heading.

Modafinil (There is a potential interaction of glimepiride with inhibitors (eg, fluconazole) of cytochrome P450 2C9). Products include:
Provigil 983

Mometasone Furoate (Certain drugs tend to produce hyperglycemia and may lead to loss of control. These drugs include corticosteroids. Due to the potential drug interaction between corticosteroids and glimepiride, the patient should be observed closely for loss of glycemic control when these drugs are co-administered. Conversely, when corticosteroids are withdrawn, the patient should be observed closely for hypoglycemia). Products include:
Asmanex 3058
Elocon Cream 3111
Elocon Lotion 3112
Elocon Ointment 3114

Mometasone Furoate Monohydrate (Certain drugs tend to produce hyperglycemia and may lead to loss of control. These drugs include corticosteroids. Due to the potential drug interaction between corticosteroids and glimepiride, the patient should be observed closely for loss of glycemic control when these drugs are co-administered. Conversely, when corticosteroids are withdrawn, the patient should be observed closely for hypoglycemia). Products include:
Nasonex 3166

Nabumetone (The hypoglycemic action of sulfonylureas may be potentiated by certain drugs, including nonsteroidal anti-inflammatory drugs. Due to the potential drug interaction between these drugs and glimepiride, the patient should be observed closely for hypoglycemia when these drugs are co-administered. Conversely, when these drugs are withdrawn, the patient should be observed closely for loss of glycemic control).
No products indexed under this heading.

Nadolol (The hypoglycemic action of sulfonylureas may be potentiated by certain drugs, including other drugs that are highly protein bound, such as β adrenergic blocking agents. Due to the potential drug interaction between these drugs and glimepiride, the patient should be observed closely for hypoglycemia when these drugs are co-administered. Conversely, when these drugs are withdrawn, the patient should be observed closely for loss of glycemic control). Products include:
Nadolol 2359

Naproxen (The hypoglycemic action of sulfonylureas may be potentiated by certain drugs, including nonsteroidal anti-inflammatory drugs. Due to the potential drug interaction between these drugs and glimepiride, the patient should be observed closely for hypoglycemia when these drugs are co-administered. Conversely, when these drugs are withdrawn, the patient should be observed closely for loss of glycemic control). Products include:
EC-Naprosyn 2850
Naprosyn 2850
Anaprox/Naprosyn 2850

Naproxen Sodium (The hypoglycemic action of sulfonylureas may be potentiated by certain drugs, including nonsteroidal anti-inflammatory drugs. Due to the potential drug interaction between these drugs and glimepiride, the patient should be observed closely for hypoglycemia when these drugs are co-administered. Conversely, when these drugs are withdrawn, the patient should be observed closely for loss of glycemic control). Products include:
Anaprox 2850
Anaprox DS 2850
Treximet 1681

Nateglinide (Patients receiving pioglitazone in combination with oral hypoglycemic agents may be at risk for hypoglycemia, and a reduction in the dose of the concomitant agent may be necessary).
No products indexed under this heading.

Nebivolol (The hypoglycemic action of sulfonylureas may be potentiated by certain drugs, including other drugs that are highly protein bound, such as β adrenergic blocking agents. Due to the potential drug interaction between these drugs and glimepiride, the patient should be observed closely for hypoglycemia when these drugs are co-administered. Conversely, when these drugs are withdrawn, the patient should be observed closely for loss of glycemic control). Products include:
Bystolic 1147

Nefazodone Hydrochloride (*In vivo* drug-drug interaction studies have suggested that pioglitazone may be a weak inducer of CYP 450 isoform 3A4 substrate).
No products indexed under this heading.

Nelfinavir Mesylate (*In vivo* drug-drug interaction studies have suggested that pioglitazone may be a weak inducer of CYP 450 isoform 3A4 substrate).
No products indexed under this heading.

Nicardipine (An enzyme inhibitor of CYP2C8 (such as gemfibrozil) may significantly increase the AUC of pioglitazone. Therefore, if an inhibitor of CYP2C8 is started or stopped during treatment with pioglitazone, changes in diabetes treatment may be needed based on clinical response).
No products indexed under this heading.

Nicardipine Hydrochloride (An enzyme inhibitor of CYP2C8 (such as gemfibrozil) may significantly increase the AUC of pioglitazone. Therefore, if an inhibitor of CYP2C8 is started or stopped during treatment with pioglitazone, changes in diabetes treatment may be needed based on clinical response).
No products indexed under this heading.

Nicotinic Acid (Certain drugs tend to produce hyperglycemia and may lead to loss of control. These drugs include nicotinic acid. Due to the potential drug interaction between nicotinic acid and glimepiride, the patient should be observed closely for loss of glycemic control when these drugs are co-administered. Conversely, when nicotinic acid is withdrawn, the patient should be observed closely for hypoglycemia).
No products indexed under this heading.

Nifedipine (Co-administration of pioglitazone for 7 days with 30 mg nifedipine ER administered orally once daily for 4 days to male and female volunteers resulted in a ratio of least square mean (90% CI) values for unchanged nifedipine of 0.83 (0.73-0.95) for C_{max} and 0.88 (0.80 - 0.96) for AUC. In view of the high variability of nifedipine pharmacokinetics, the clinical significance of this finding is unknown).
No products indexed under this heading.

Nimodipine (*In vivo* drug-drug interaction studies have suggested that pioglitazone may be a weak inducer of CYP 450 isoform 3A4 substrate).
No products indexed under this heading.

(⊙ Described in PDR® for Ophthalmic Medicines)

501 Interactions Index Duetact

Nisoldipine (*In vivo* drug-drug interaction studies have suggested that pioglitazone may be a weak inducer of CYP 450 isoform 3A4 substrate).
No products indexed under this heading.

Nitrendipine (*In vivo* drug-drug interaction studies have suggested that pioglitazone may be a weak inducer of CYP 450 isoform 3A4 substrate).
No products indexed under this heading.

Norepinephrine Bitartrate (Certain drugs tend to produce hyperglycemia and may lead to loss of control. These drugs include sympathomimetics. Due to the potential drug interaction between sympathomimetics and glimepiride, the patient should be observed closely for loss of glycemic control when these drugs are co-administered. Conversely, when sympathomimetics are withdrawn, the patient should be observed closely for hypoglycemia).
No products indexed under this heading.

Norethindrone (Co-administration of pioglitazone (45 mg qd) and an oral contraceptive (1 mg norethindrone plus 0.035 mg ethinyl estradiol qd) for 21 days, resulted in 11% and 11-14% decrease in ethinyl estradiol AUC (0-24h) and C_{max} respectively. In view of the high variability of ethinyl estradiol pharmacokinetics, the clinical significance of this finding is unknown. In addition, certain drugs tend to produce hyperglycemia and may lead to loss of control. These drugs include oral contraceptives. Due to the potential drug interaction between oral contraceptives and glimepiride, the patient should be observed closely for loss of glycemic control when these drugs are co-administered. Conversely, when oral contraceptives are withdrawn, the patient should be observed closely for hypoglycemia). Products include:
Ortho Micronor 2660

Norethindrone Acetate (*In vivo* drug-drug interaction studies have suggested that pioglitazone may be a weak inducer of CYP 450 isoform 3A4 substrate). Products include:
Activella 2561

Norethynodrel (Co-administration of pioglitazone (45 mg qd) and an oral contraceptive (1 mg norethindrone plus 0.035 mg ethinyl estradiol qd) for 21 days, resulted in 11% and 11-14% decrease in ethinyl estradiol AUC (0-24h) and C_{max} respectively. In view of the high variability of ethinyl estradiol pharmacokinetics, the clinical significance of this finding is unknown. In addition, certain drugs tend to produce hyperglycemia and may lead to loss of control. These drugs include oral contraceptives. Due to the potential drug interaction between oral contraceptives and glimepiride, the patient should be observed closely for loss of glycemic control when these drugs are co-administered. Conversely, when oral contraceptives are withdrawn, the patient should be observed closely for hypoglycemia).
No products indexed under this heading.

Norgestimate (Co-administration of pioglitazone (45 mg qd) and an oral contraceptive (1 mg norethindrone plus 0.035 mg ethinyl estradiol qd) for 21 days, resulted in 11% and 11-14% decrease in ethinyl estradiol AUC (0-24h) and C_{max} respectively. In view of the high variability of ethinyl estradiol pharmacokinetics, the clinical significance of this finding is unknown. In addition, certain drugs tend to produce hyperglycemia and may lead to loss of control. These drugs include oral contraceptives. Due to the potential drug interaction between oral contraceptives and glimepiride, the patient should be observed closely for loss of glycemic control when these drugs are co-administered. Conversely, when oral contraceptives are withdrawn, the patient should be observed closely for hypoglycemia). Products include:
Ortho-Cyclen/Ortho Tri-Cyclen 2663
Ortho Tri-Cyclen Lo Tablets 2673

Norgestrel (Co-administration of pioglitazone (45 mg qd) and an oral contraceptive (1 mg norethindrone plus 0.035 mg ethinyl estradiol qd) for 21 days, resulted in 11% and 11-14% decrease in ethinyl estradiol AUC (0-24h) and C_{max} respectively. In view of the high variability of ethinyl estradiol pharmacokinetics, the clinical significance of this finding is unknown. In addition, certain drugs tend to produce hyperglycemia and may lead to loss of control. These drugs include oral contraceptives. Due to the potential drug interaction between oral contraceptives and glimepiride, the patient should be observed closely for loss of glycemic control when these drugs are co-administered. Conversely, when oral contraceptives are withdrawn, the patient should be observed closely for hypoglycemia).
No products indexed under this heading.

Nortriptyline Hydrochloride (The hypoglycemic action of sulfonylureas may be potentiated by certain drugs, including drugs that are highly protein bound. Due to the potential drug interaction between these drugs and glimepiride, the patient should be observed closely for hypoglycemia when these drugs are co-administered. Conversely, when these drugs are withdrawn, the patient should be observed closely for loss of glycemic control).
No products indexed under this heading.

Omeprazole (An enzyme inhibitor of CYP2C8 (such as gemfibrozil) may significantly increase the AUC of pioglitazone. Therefore, if an inhibitor of CYP2C8 is started or stopped during treatment with pioglitazone, changes in diabetes treatment may be needed based on clinical response).
No products indexed under this heading.

Ondansetron (*In vivo* drug-drug interaction studies have suggested that pioglitazone may be a weak inducer of CYP 450 isoform 3A4 substrate).
No products indexed under this heading.

Ondansetron Hydrochloride (*In vivo* drug-drug interaction studies have suggested that pioglitazone may be a weak inducer of CYP 450 isoform 3A4 substrate). Products include:
Zofran Injection 1750
Zofran 1756
Zofran ODT 1756

Oxaprozin (The hypoglycemic action of sulfonylureas may be potentiated by certain drugs, including nonsteroidal anti-inflammatory drugs. Due to the potential drug interaction between these drugs and glimepiride, the patient should be observed closely for hypoglycemia when these drugs are co-administered. Conversely, when these drugs are withdrawn, the patient should be observed closely for loss of glycemic control).
No products indexed under this heading.

Oxazepam (The hypoglycemic action of sulfonylureas may be potentiated by certain drugs, including drugs that are highly protein bound. Due to the potential drug interaction between these drugs and glimepiride, the patient should be observed closely for hypoglycemia when these drugs are co-administered. Conversely, when these drugs are withdrawn, the patient should be observed closely for loss of glycemic control).
No products indexed under this heading.

Oxiconazole Nitrate (There is a potential interaction of glimepiride with inhibitors (eg, fluconazole) of cytochrome P450 2C9).
No products indexed under this heading.

Paclitaxel (*In vivo* drug-drug interaction studies have suggested that pioglitazone may be a weak inducer of CYP 450 isoform 3A4 substrate).
No products indexed under this heading.

Pargyline Hydrochloride (The hypoglycemic action of sulfonylureas may be potentiated by certain drugs, including other drugs that are highly protein bound, such as monoamine oxidase inhibitors. Due to the potential drug interaction between these drugs and glimepiride, the patient should be observed closely for hypoglycemia when these drugs are co-administered. Conversely, when these drugs are withdrawn, the patient should be observed closely for loss of glycemic control).
No products indexed under this heading.

Paroxetine Hydrochloride (There is a potential interaction of glimepiride with inhibitors (eg, fluconazole) of cytochrome P450 2C9). Products include:
Paroxetine CR 2361
Paroxetine ER 2371
Paxil 1586
Paxil CR 1596

Penbutolol Sulfate (The hypoglycemic action of sulfonylureas may be potentiated by certain drugs, including other drugs that are highly protein bound, such as β adrenergic blocking agents. Due to the potential drug interaction between these drugs and glimepiride, the patient should be observed closely for hypoglycemia when these drugs are co-administered. Conversely, when these drugs are withdrawn, the patient should be observed closely for loss of glycemic control).
No products indexed under this heading.

Perphenazine (Certain drugs tend to produce hyperglycemia and may lead to loss of control. These drugs include phenothiazines. Due to the potential drug interaction between phenothiazines and glimepiride, the patient should be observed closely for loss of glycemic control when these drugs are co-administered. Conversely, when phenothiazines are withdrawn, the patient should be observed closely for hypoglycemia).
No products indexed under this heading.

Phenelzine Sulfate (The hypoglycemic action of sulfonylureas may be potentiated by certain drugs, including other drugs that are highly protein bound, such as monoamine oxidase inhibitors. Due to the potential drug interaction between these drugs and glimepiride, the patient should be observed closely for hypoglycemia when these drugs are co-administered. Conversely, when these drugs are withdrawn, the patient should be observed closely for loss of glycemic control).
No products indexed under this heading.

Phenobarbital (An enzyme inducer of CYP2C8 (such as rifampin) may significantly decrease the AUC of pioglitazone. Therefore, if an inducer of CYP2C8 is started or stopped during treatment with pioglitazone, changes in diabetes treatment may be needed based on clinical response). Products include:
Donnatal 2711

Phenobarbital Sodium (An enzyme inducer of CYP2C8 (such as rifampin) may significantly decrease the AUC of pioglitazone. Therefore, if an inducer of CYP2C8 is started or stopped during treatment with pioglitazone, changes in diabetes treatment may be needed based on clinical response).
No products indexed under this heading.

Phenothiazine Derivatives (Certain drugs tend to produce hyperglycemia and may lead to loss of control. These drugs include phenothiazines. Due to the potential drug interaction between phenothiazines and glimepiride, the patient should be observed closely for loss of glycemic control when these drugs are co-administered. Conversely, when phenothiazines are withdrawn, the patient should be observed closely for hypoglycemia).
No products indexed under this heading.

Phenothiazines (Certain drugs tend to produce hyperglycemia and may lead to loss of control. These drugs include phenothiazines. Due to the potential drug interaction between phenothiazines and glimepiride, the patient should be observed closely for loss of glycemic control when these drugs are co-administered. Conversely, when phenothiazines are withdrawn, the patient should be observed closely for hypoglycemia).
No products indexed under this heading.

Phenylbutazone (The hypoglycemic action of sulfonylureas may be potentiated by certain drugs, including nonsteroidal anti-inflammatory drugs. Due to the potential drug interaction between these drugs and glimepiride, the patient should be observed closely for hypoglycemia when these drugs are co-administered. Conversely, when these drugs are withdrawn, the patient should be observed closely for loss of glycemic control).
No products indexed under this heading.

Phenylephrine Bitartrate (Certain drugs tend to produce hyperglycemia and may lead to loss of control. These drugs include sympathomimetics. Due to the potential drug interaction between sympathomimetics and glimepiride, the patient should be observed closely for loss of glycemic control when these drugs are co-administered. Conversely, when sympathomimetics are withdrawn, the patient should be observed closely for hypoglycemia).
No products indexed under this heading.

Phenylephrine Hydrochloride (Certain drugs tend to produce hyperglycemia and may lead to loss of control. These drugs include sympathomimetics. Due to the potential drug interaction between sympathomimetics and glimepiride, the patient should be observed closely for loss of glycemic control when these drugs are co-administered. Conversely, when sympathomimetics are withdrawn, the patient should be observed closely for hypoglycemia). Products include:
Sudafed PE Nasal Decongestant 2048
Children's Sudafed PE Nasal Decongestant 2047

Phenylephrine Tannate (Certain drugs tend to produce hyperglycemia and may lead to loss of control. These drugs include sympathomimetics. Due to the potential drug interaction between sympathomimetics and glimepiride, the patient should be observed closely for loss of glycemic control when these drugs are co-administered. Conversely, when sympathomimetics are withdrawn, the patient should be observed closely for hypoglycemia).
No products indexed under this heading.

Phenylpropanolamine Hydrochloride (Certain drugs tend to produce hyperglycemia and may lead to loss of control. These drugs include sympathomimetics. Due to the potential drug interaction between sympathomimetics and glimepiride, the patient should be observed closely for loss of glycemic control when these drugs are co-administered. Conversely, when sym-

IMPORTANT NOTE: Always consult each drug listing in the patient's regimen for possible interactions.

pathomimetics are withdrawn, the patient should be observed closely for hypoglycemia).
No products indexed under this heading.

Phenytoin (Certain drugs tend to produce hyperglycemia and may lead to loss of control. These drugs include phenytoin. Due to the potential drug interaction between phenytoin and glimepiride, the patient should be observed closely for loss of glycemic control when these drugs are co-administered. Conversely, when phenytoin is withdrawn, the patient should be observed closely for hypoglycemia).
No products indexed under this heading.

Phenytoin Sodium (Certain drugs tend to produce hyperglycemia and may lead to loss of control. These drugs include phenytoin. Due to the potential drug interaction between phenytoin and glimepiride, the patient should be observed closely for loss of glycemic control when these drugs are co-administered. Conversely, when phenytoin is withdrawn, the patient should be observed closely for hypoglycemia). Products include:
Phenytek Capsules **2380**

Pimozide (*In vivo* drug-drug interaction studies have suggested that pioglitazone may be a weak inducer of CYP 450 isoform 3A4 substrate).
No products indexed under this heading.

Pindolol (The hypoglycemic action of sulfonylureas may be potentiated by certain drugs, including other drugs that are highly protein bound, such as β adrenergic blocking agents. Due to the potential drug interaction between these drugs and glimepiride, the patient should be observed closely for hypoglycemia when these drugs are co-administered. Conversely, when these drugs are withdrawn, the patient should be observed closely for loss of glycemic control).
No products indexed under this heading.

Pirbuterol Acetate (Certain drugs tend to produce hyperglycemia and may lead to loss of control. These drugs include sympathomimetics. Due to the potential drug interaction between sympathomimetics and glimepiride, the patient should be observed closely for loss of glycemic control when these drugs are co-administered. Conversely, when sympathomimetics are withdrawn, the patient should be observed closely for hypoglycemia). Products include:
Maxair Autohaler **1782**

Piroxicam (The hypoglycemic action of sulfonylureas may be potentiated by certain drugs, including nonsteroidal anti-inflammatory drugs. Due to the potential drug interaction between these drugs and glimepiride, the patient should be observed closely for hypoglycemia when these drugs are co-administered. Conversely, when these drugs are withdrawn, the patient should be observed closely for loss of glycemic control).
No products indexed under this heading.

Polyestradiol Phosphate (Certain drugs tend to produce hyperglycemia and may lead to loss of control. These drugs include estrogens. Due to the potential drug interaction between estrogens and glimepiride, the patient should be observed closely for loss of glycemic control when these drugs are co-administered. Conversely, when estrogens are withdrawn, the patient should be observed closely for hypoglycemia).
No products indexed under this heading.

Polythiazide (Certain drugs tend to produce hyperglycemia and may lead to loss of control. These drugs include thiazides. Due to the potential drug interaction between thiazides and glimepiride, the patient should be observed closely for loss of glycemic control when these drugs are co-administered. Conversely, when thiazides are withdrawn, the patient should be observed closely for hypoglycemia).
No products indexed under this heading.

Prednisolone (Certain drugs tend to produce hyperglycemia and may lead to loss of control. These drugs include corticosteroids. Due to the potential drug interaction between corticosteroids and glimepiride, the patient should be observed closely for loss of glycemic control when these drugs are co-administered. Conversely, when corticosteroids are withdrawn, the patient should be observed closely for hypoglycemia).
No products indexed under this heading.

Prednisolone Acetate (Certain drugs tend to produce hyperglycemia and may lead to loss of control. These drugs include corticosteroids. Due to the potential drug interaction between corticosteroids and glimepiride, the patient should be observed closely for loss of glycemic control when these drugs are co-administered. Conversely, when corticosteroids are withdrawn, the patient should be observed closely for hypoglycemia). Products include:
Blephamide .... ⊙**212**, ⊙**214**
Pred Forte .... ⊙**225**
Pred Mild .... ⊙**230**
Pred-G .... ⊙**226**, ⊙**227**

Prednisolone Sodium Phosphate (Certain drugs tend to produce hyperglycemia and may lead to loss of control. These drugs include corticosteroids. Due to the potential drug interaction between corticosteroids and glimepiride, the patient should be observed closely for loss of glycemic control when these drugs are co-administered. Conversely, when corticosteroids are withdrawn, the patient should be observed closely for hypoglycemia).
No products indexed under this heading.

Prednisolone Tebutate (Certain drugs tend to produce hyperglycemia and may lead to loss of control. These drugs include corticosteroids. Due to the potential drug interaction between corticosteroids and glimepiride, the patient should be observed closely for loss of glycemic control when these drugs are co-administered. Conversely, when corticosteroids are withdrawn, the patient should be observed closely for hypoglycemia).
No products indexed under this heading.

Prednisone (Certain drugs tend to produce hyperglycemia and may lead to loss of control. These drugs include corticosteroids. Due to the potential drug interaction between corticosteroids and glimepiride, the patient should be observed closely for loss of glycemic control when these drugs are co-administered. Conversely, when corticosteroids are withdrawn, the patient should be observed closely for hypoglycemia).
No products indexed under this heading.

Prednisone sodium phosphate (Certain drugs tend to produce hyperglycemia and may lead to loss of control. These drugs include corticosteroids. Due to the potential drug interaction between corticosteroids and glimepiride, the patient should be observed closely for loss of glycemic control when these drugs are co-administered. Conversely, when corticosteroids are withdrawn, the patient should be observed closely for hypoglycemia).
No products indexed under this heading.

Primidone (An enzyme inducer of CYP2C8 (such as rifampin) may significantly decrease the AUC of pioglitazone. Therefore, if an inducer of CYP2C8 is started or stopped during treatment with pioglitazone, changes in diabetes treatment may be needed based on clinical response).
No products indexed under this heading.

Probenecid (The hypoglycemic action of sulfonylureas may be potentiated by certain drugs, including other drugs that are highly protein bound, such as probenecid. Due to the potential drug interaction between these drugs and glimepiride, the patient should be observed closely for hypoglycemia when these drugs are co-administered. Conversely, when these drugs are withdrawn, the patient should be observed closely for loss of glycemic control).
No products indexed under this heading.

Procarbazine Hydrochloride (The hypoglycemic action of sulfonylureas may be potentiated by certain drugs, including other drugs that are highly protein bound, such as monoamine oxidase inhibitors. Due to the potential drug interaction between these drugs and glimepiride, the patient should be observed closely for hypoglycemia when these drugs are co-administered. Conversely, when these drugs are withdrawn, the patient should be observed closely for loss of glycemic control).
No products indexed under this heading.

Prochlorperazine (Certain drugs tend to produce hyperglycemia and may lead to loss of control. These drugs include phenothiazines. Due to the potential drug interaction between phenothiazines and glimepiride, the patient should be observed closely for loss of glycemic control when these drugs are co-administered. Conversely, when phenothiazines are withdrawn, the patient should be observed closely for hypoglycemia).
No products indexed under this heading.

Prochlorperazine Edisylate (Certain drugs tend to produce hyperglycemia and may lead to loss of control. These drugs include phenothiazines. Due to the potential drug interaction between phenothiazines and glimepiride, the patient should be observed closely for loss of glycemic control when these drugs are co-administered. Conversely, when phenothiazines are withdrawn, the patient should be observed closely for hypoglycemia).
No products indexed under this heading.

Prochlorperazine Maleate (Certain drugs tend to produce hyperglycemia and may lead to loss of control. These drugs include phenothiazines. Due to the potential drug interaction between phenothiazines and glimepiride, the patient should be observed closely for loss of glycemic control when these drugs are co-administered. Conversely, when phenothiazines are withdrawn, the patient should be observed closely for hypoglycemia).
No products indexed under this heading.

Promethazine (Certain drugs tend to produce hyperglycemia and may lead to loss of control. These drugs include phenothiazines. Due to the potential drug interaction between phenothiazines and glimepiride, the patient should be observed closely for loss of glycemic control when these drugs are co-administered. Conversely, when phenothiazines are withdrawn, the patient should be observed closely for hypoglycemia).
No products indexed under this heading.

Promethazine Hydrochloride (Certain drugs tend to produce hyperglycemia and may lead to loss of control. These drugs include phenothiazines. Due to the potential drug interaction between phenothiazines and glimepiride, the patient should be observed closely for loss of glycemic control when these drugs are co-administered. Conversely, when phenothiazines are withdrawn, the patient should be observed closely for hypoglycemia).
No products indexed under this heading.

Propranolol (Concomitant administration of propranolol (40 mg three times daily) and glimepiride significantly increased C_{max}, AUC, and $T_{1/2}$ of glimepiride by 23%, 22%, and 15%, respectively, and it decreased CL/f by 18%. The recovery of M1 and M2 from urine, however, did not change. The pharmacodynamic responses to glimepiride were nearly identical in normal subjects receiving propranolol and placebo. Pooled data from clinical trials in patients with type 2 diabetes showed no evidence of clinically significant adverse interactions with uncontrolled concurrent administration of β-blockers. However, if beta-blockers are used, caution should be exercised and patients should be warned about the potential for hypoglycemia).
No products indexed under this heading.

Propranolol Hydrochloride (Concomitant administration of propranolol (40 mg three times daily) and glimepiride significantly increased C_{max}, AUC, and $T_{1/2}$ of glimepiride by 23%, 22%, and 15%, respectively, and it decreased CL/f by 18%. The recovery of M1 and M2 from urine, however, did not change. The pharmacodynamic responses to glimepiride were nearly identical in normal subjects receiving propranolol and placebo. Pooled data from clinical trials in patients with type 2 diabetes showed no evidence of clinically significant adverse interactions with uncontrolled concurrent administration of β-blockers. However, if beta-blockers are used, caution should be exercised and patients should be warned about the potential for hypoglycemia). Products include:
InnoPran XL **1517**

Pseudoephedrine Hydrochloride (Certain drugs tend to produce hyperglycemia and may lead to loss of control. These drugs include sympathomimetics. Due to the potential drug interaction between sympathomimetics and glimepiride, the patient should be observed closely for loss of glycemic control when these drugs are co-administered. Conversely, when sympathomimetics are withdrawn, the patient should be observed closely for hypoglycemia). Products include:
Allegra-D **2915**
Allegra-D 24 .... **2918**
Sudafed 12 Hour Nasal Decongestant Non-Drowsy **2048**
Sudafed 24 Hour **2048**
Sudafed Nasal Decongestant **2047**
Children's Sudafed Nasal Decongestant Liquid **2047**
Zyrtec-D Allergy & Congestion **2054**

Pseudoephedrine Sulfate (Certain drugs tend to produce hyperglycemia and may lead to loss of control. These drugs include sympathomimetics. Due to the potential drug interaction between sympathomimetics and glimepiride, the patient should be observed closely for loss of glycemic control when these drugs are co-administered. Conversely, when sympathomimetics are withdrawn, the patient should be observed closely for hypoglycemia). Products include:
Clarinex-D 12-Hour **3101**
Clarinex-D **3104**

(⊙ Described in PDR® for Ophthalmic Medicines)

503 Interactions Index Duetact

Quercetin (An enzyme inhibitor of CYP2C8 (such as gemfibrozil) may significantly increase the AUC of pioglitazone. Therefore, if an inhibitor of CYP2C8 is started or stopped during treatment with pioglitazone, changes in diabetes treatment may be needed based on clinical response).
No products indexed under this heading.

Quinestrol (Certain drugs tend to produce hyperglycemia and may lead to loss of control. These drugs include estrogens. Due to the potential drug interaction between estrogens and glimepiride, the patient should be observed closely for loss of glycemic control when these drugs are co-administered. Conversely, when estrogens are withdrawn, the patient should be observed closely for hypoglycemia).
No products indexed under this heading.

Quinidine Gluconate (*In vivo* drug-drug interaction studies have suggested that pioglitazone may be a weak inducer of CYP 450 isoform 3A4 substrate).
No products indexed under this heading.

Quinidine Polygalacturonate (*In vivo* drug-drug interaction studies have suggested that pioglitazone may be a weak inducer of CYP 450 isoform 3A4 substrate).
No products indexed under this heading.

Quinidine Sulfate (*In vivo* drug-drug interaction studies have suggested that pioglitazone may be a weak inducer of CYP 450 isoform 3A4 substrate).
No products indexed under this heading.

Rasagiline Mesylate (The hypoglycemic action of sulfonylureas may be potentiated by certain drugs, including other drugs that are highly protein bound, such as monoamine oxidase inhibitors. Due to the potential drug interaction between these drugs and glimepiride, the patient should be observed closely for hypoglycemia when these drugs are co-administered. Conversely, when these drugs are withdrawn, the patient should be observed closely for loss of glycemic control). Products include:
Azilect 3383

Repaglinide (Patients receiving pioglitazone in combination with oral hypoglycemic agents may be at risk for hypoglycemia, and a reduction in the dose of the concomitant agent may be necessary).
No products indexed under this heading.

Rifabutin (An enzyme inducer of CYP2C8 (such as rifampin) may significantly decrease the AUC of pioglitazone. Therefore, if an inducer of CYP2C8 is started or stopped during treatment with pioglitazone, changes in diabetes treatment may be needed based on clinical response).
No products indexed under this heading.

Rifampicin (There is a potential interaction of glimepiride with inducers (eg, rifampicin) of cytochrome P450 2C9).
No products indexed under this heading.

Rifampin (Concomitant administration of rifampin (oral 600 mg once daily), an inducer of CYP2C8, with pioglitazone (oral 30 mg) in 10 healthy volunteers pre-treated for 5 days prior with rifampin (oral 600 mg once daily) resulted in a decrease in the AUC of pioglitazone by 54%. An enzyme inducer of CYP2C8 (such as rifampin) may significantly decrease the AUC of pioglitazone. Therefore, if an inducer of CYP2C8 is started or stopped during treatment with pioglitazone, changes in diabetes treatment may be needed based on clinical response).
No products indexed under this heading.

Rifapentine (There is a potential interaction of glimepiride with inducers (eg, rifampicin) of cytochrome P450 2C9).
No products indexed under this heading.

Ritonavir (There is a potential interaction of glimepiride with inhibitors (eg, fluconazole) of cytochrome P450 2C9). Products include:
Kaletra 458
Norvir 509

Rofecoxib (The hypoglycemic action of sulfonylureas may be potentiated by certain drugs, including nonsteroidal anti-inflammatory drugs. Due to the potential drug interaction between these drugs and glimepiride, the patient should be observed closely for hypoglycemia when these drugs are co-administered. Conversely, when these drugs are withdrawn, the patient should be observed closely for loss of glycemic control).
No products indexed under this heading.

Rosiglitazone Maleate (Patients receiving pioglitazone in combination with oral hypoglycemic agents may be at risk for hypoglycemia, and a reduction in the dose of the concomitant agent may be necessary). Products include:
Avandamet 1345
Avandaryl 1356
Avandia 1366

Salmeterol Xinafoate (Certain drugs tend to produce hyperglycemia and may lead to loss of control. These drugs include sympathomimetics. Due to the potential drug interaction between sympathomimetics and glimepiride, the patient should be observed closely for loss of glycemic control when these drugs are co-administered. Conversely, when sympathomimetics are withdrawn, the patient should be observed closely for hypoglycemia). Products include:
Advair 100/50 1275
Advair 250/50 1275
Advair 500/50 1275
Advair HFA 45/21 1288
Advair HFA 115/21 1288
Advair HFA 230/21 1288
Serevent Diskus 1656

Salsalate (The hypoglycemic action of sulfonylureas may be potentiated by certain drugs, including drugs that are highly protein bound, such as salicylates. Due to the potential drug interaction between these drugs and glimepiride, the patient should be observed closely for hypoglycemia when these drugs are co-administered. Conversely, when these drugs are withdrawn, the patient should be observed closely for loss of glycemic control).
No products indexed under this heading.

Saquinavir (*In vivo* drug-drug interaction studies have suggested that pioglitazone may be a weak inducer of CYP 450 isoform 3A4 substrate).
No products indexed under this heading.

Saquinavir Mesylate (*In vivo* drug-drug interaction studies have suggested that pioglitazone may be a weak inducer of CYP 450 isoform 3A4 substrate).
No products indexed under this heading.

Secobarbital Sodium (There is a potential interaction of glimepiride with inducers (eg, rifampicin) of cytochrome P450 2C9).
No products indexed under this heading.

Selegiline (The hypoglycemic action of sulfonylureas may be potentiated by certain drugs, including other drugs that are highly protein bound, such as monoamine oxidase inhibitors. Due to the potential drug interaction between these drugs and glimepiride, the patient should be observed closely for hypoglycemia when these drugs are co-administered. Conversely, when these drugs are withdrawn, the patient should be observed closely for loss of glycemic control). Products include:
Emsam 3623

Selegiline Hydrochloride (The hypoglycemic action of sulfonylureas may be potentiated by certain drugs, including other drugs that are highly protein bound, such as monoamine oxidase inhibitors. Due to the potential drug interaction between these drugs and glimepiride, the patient should be observed closely for hypoglycemia when these drugs are co-administered. Conversely, when these drugs are withdrawn, the patient should be observed closely for loss of glycemic control). Products include:
Eldepryl 3312

Sertraline Hydrochloride (There is a potential interaction of glimepiride with inhibitors (eg, fluconazole) of cytochrome P450 2C9).
No products indexed under this heading.

Sildenafil Citrate (There is a potential interaction of glimepiride with inhibitors (eg, fluconazole) of cytochrome P450 2C9).
No products indexed under this heading.

Simvastatin (*In vivo* drug-drug interaction studies have suggested that pioglitazone may be a weak inducer of CYP 450 isoform 3A4 substrate). Products include:
Simcor 524
Vytorin 10/10 .... 2303, 3240
Vytorin 10/20 .... 2303, 3240
Vytorin 10/40 .... 2303, 3240
Vytorin 10/80 .... 2303, 3240
Zocor 2289

Sirolimus (*In vivo* drug-drug interaction studies have suggested that pioglitazone may be a weak inducer of CYP 450 isoform 3A4 substrate). Products include:
Rapamune 3579

Sitagliptin Phosphate (Patients receiving pioglitazone in combination with oral hypoglycemic agents may be at risk for hypoglycemia, and a reduction in the dose of the concomitant agent may be necessary). Products include:
Janumet 2188
Januvia 2196

Sotalol Hydrochloride (The hypoglycemic action of sulfonylureas may be potentiated by certain drugs, including other drugs that are highly protein bound, such as β adrenergic blocking agents. Due to the potential drug interaction between these drugs and glimepiride, the patient should be observed closely for hypoglycemia when these drugs are co-administered. Conversely, when these drugs are withdrawn, the patient should be observed closely for loss of glycemic control).
No products indexed under this heading.

Spironolactone (Certain drugs tend to produce hyperglycemia and may lead to loss of control. These drugs include diuretics. Due to the potential drug interaction between diuretics and glimepiride, the patient should be observed closely for loss of glycemic control when these drugs are co-administered. Conversely, when diuretics are withdrawn, the patient should be observed closely for hypoglycemia).
No products indexed under this heading.

Sulfacytine (The hypoglycemic action of sulfonylureas may be potentiated by certain drugs, including other drugs that are highly protein bound, such as sulfonamides. Due to the potential drug interaction between these drugs and glimepiride, the patient should be observed closely for hypoglycemia when these drugs are co-administered. Conversely, when these drugs are withdrawn, the patient should be observed closely for loss of glycemic control).
No products indexed under this heading.

Sulfamethizole (The hypoglycemic action of sulfonylureas may be potentiated by certain drugs, including other drugs that are highly protein bound, such as sulfonamides. Due to the potential drug interaction between these drugs and glimepiride, the patient should be observed closely for hypoglycemia when these drugs are co-administered. Conversely, when these drugs are withdrawn, the patient should be observed closely for loss of glycemic control).
No products indexed under this heading.

Sulfamethoxazole (The hypoglycemic action of sulfonylureas may be potentiated by certain drugs, including other drugs that are highly protein bound, such as sulfonamides. Due to the potential drug interaction between these drugs and glimepiride, the patient should be observed closely for hypoglycemia when these drugs are co-administered. Conversely, when these drugs are withdrawn, the patient should be observed closely for loss of glycemic control).
No products indexed under this heading.

Sulfaphenazole (An enzyme inhibitor of CYP2C8 (such as gemfibrozil) may significantly increase the AUC of pioglitazone. Therefore, if an inhibitor of CYP2C8 is started or stopped during treatment with pioglitazone, changes in diabetes treatment may be needed based on clinical response).
No products indexed under this heading.

Sulfasalazine (The hypoglycemic action of sulfonylureas may be potentiated by certain drugs, including other drugs that are highly protein bound, such as sulfonamides. Due to the potential drug interaction between these drugs and glimepiride, the patient should be observed closely for hypoglycemia when these drugs are co-administered. Conversely, when these drugs are withdrawn, the patient should be observed closely for loss of glycemic control).
No products indexed under this heading.

Sulfinpyrazone (The hypoglycemic action of sulfonylureas may be potentiated by certain drugs, including other drugs that are highly protein bound, such as sulfonamides. Due to the potential drug interaction between these drugs and glimepiride, the patient should be observed closely for hypoglycemia when these drugs are co-administered. Conversely, when these drugs are withdrawn, the patient should be observed closely for loss of glycemic control).
No products indexed under this heading.

Sulfisoxazole Acetyl (The hypoglycemic action of sulfonylureas may be potentiated by certain drugs, including other drugs that are highly protein bound, such as sulfonamides. Due to the potential drug interaction between these drugs and glimepiride, the patient should be observed closely for hypoglycemia when these drugs are co-administered. Conversely, when these drugs are withdrawn, the patient should be observed closely for loss of glycemic control).
No products indexed under this heading.

Sulfisoxazole Diolamine (The hypoglycemic action of sulfonylureas may be potentiated by certain drugs, including other drugs that are highly protein bound, such as sulfonamides. Due to the potential drug interaction between these drugs and glimepiride, the patient should be observed closely for hypoglycemia when these drugs are co-

IMPORTANT NOTE: Always consult each drug listing in the patient's regimen for possible interactions.

Duetact
Interactions Index
504

administered. Conversely, when these drugs are withdrawn, the patient should be observed closely for loss of glycemic control).
No products indexed under this heading.

Sulindac (The hypoglycemic action of sulfonylureas may be potentiated by certain drugs, including nonsteroidal anti-inflammatory drugs. Due to the potential drug interaction between these drugs and glimepiride, the patient should be observed closely for hypoglycemia when these drugs are co-administered. Conversely, when these drugs are withdrawn, the patient should be observed closely for loss of glycemic control). Products include:
Clinoril 2098

Tacrolimus (*In vivo* drug-drug interaction studies have suggested that pioglitazone may be a weak inducer of CYP 450 isoform 3A4 substrate). Products include:
Prograf Capsules 677
Prograf Injection 677
Protopic 685

Tadalafil (*In vivo* drug-drug interaction studies have suggested that pioglitazone may be a weak inducer of CYP 450 isoform 3A4 substrate). Products include:
Adcirca 3461
Cialis 1861

Tamoxifen Citrate (*In vivo* drug-drug interaction studies have suggested that pioglitazone may be a weak inducer of CYP 450 isoform 3A4 substrate).
No products indexed under this heading.

Temazepam (The hypoglycemic action of sulfonylureas may be potentiated by certain drugs, including drugs that are highly protein bound. Due to the potential drug interaction between these drugs and glimepiride, the patient should be observed closely for hypoglycemia when these drugs are co-administered. Conversely, when these drugs are withdrawn, the patient should be observed closely for loss of glycemic control).
No products indexed under this heading.

Terbutaline Sulfate (Certain drugs tend to produce hyperglycemia and may lead to loss of control. These drugs include sympathomimetics. Due to the potential drug interaction between sympathomimetics and glimepiride, the patient should be observed closely for loss of glycemic control when these drugs are co-administered. Conversely, when sympathomimetics are withdrawn, the patient should be observed closely for hypoglycemia).
No products indexed under this heading.

Terconazole (There is a potential interaction of glimepiride with inhibitors (eg, fluconazole) of cytochrome P450 2C9).
No products indexed under this heading.

Terfenadine (*In vivo* drug-drug interaction studies have suggested that pioglitazone may be a weak inducer of CYP 450 isoform 3A4 substrate).
No products indexed under this heading.

Theophylline (*In vivo* drug-drug interaction studies have suggested that pioglitazone may be a weak inducer of CYP 450 isoform 3A4 substrate).
No products indexed under this heading.

Theophylline Anhydrous (*In vivo* drug-drug interaction studies have suggested that pioglitazone may be a weak inducer of CYP 450 isoform 3A4 substrate). Products include:
Uniphyl 2817

Theophylline Calcium Salicylate (*In vivo* drug-drug interaction studies have suggested that pioglitazone may be a weak inducer of CYP 450 isoform 3A4 substrate).
No products indexed under this heading.

Theophylline Dihydroxypropyl (Glyceryl) (*In vivo* drug-drug interaction studies have suggested that pioglitazone may be a weak inducer of CYP 450 isoform 3A4 substrate).
No products indexed under this heading.

Theophylline Ethylenediamine (*In vivo* drug-drug interaction studies have suggested that pioglitazone may be a weak inducer of CYP 450 isoform 3A4 substrate).
No products indexed under this heading.

Theophylline Sodium Glycinate (*In vivo* drug-drug interaction studies have suggested that pioglitazone may be a weak inducer of CYP 450 isoform 3A4 substrate).
No products indexed under this heading.

Thioridazine (Certain drugs tend to produce hyperglycemia and may lead to loss of control. These drugs include phenothiazines. Due to the potential drug interaction between phenothiazines and glimepiride, the patient should be observed closely for loss of glycemic control when these drugs are co-administered. Conversely, when phenothiazines are withdrawn, the patient should be observed closely for hypoglycemia).
No products indexed under this heading.

Thioridazine Hydrochloride (Certain drugs tend to produce hyperglycemia and may lead to loss of control. These drugs include phenothiazines. Due to the potential drug interaction between phenothiazines and glimepiride, the patient should be observed closely for loss of glycemic control when these drugs are co-administered. Conversely, when phenothiazines are withdrawn, the patient should be observed closely for hypoglycemia). Products include:
Thioridazine Hydrochloride 2384

Thyroglobulin (Certain drugs tend to produce hyperglycemia and may lead to loss of control. These drugs include thyroid products. Due to the potential drug interaction between thyroid products and glimepiride, the patient should be observed closely for loss of glycemic control when these drugs are co-administered. Conversely, when thyroid products are withdrawn, the patient should be observed closely for hypoglycemia).
No products indexed under this heading.

Thyroid (Certain drugs tend to produce hyperglycemia and may lead to loss of control. These drugs include thyroid products. Due to the potential drug interaction between thyroid products and glimepiride, the patient should be observed closely for loss of glycemic control when these drugs are co-administered. Conversely, when thyroid products are withdrawn, the patient should be observed closely for hypoglycemia). Products include:
Naturethroid 2830

Thyroxine (Certain drugs tend to produce hyperglycemia and may lead to loss of control. These drugs include thyroid products. Due to the potential drug interaction between thyroid products and glimepiride, the patient should be observed closely for loss of glycemic control when these drugs are co-administered. Conversely, when thyroid products are withdrawn, the patient should be observed closely for hypoglycemia).
No products indexed under this heading.

Thyroxine Sodium (Certain drugs tend to produce hyperglycemia and may lead to loss of control. These drugs include thyroid products. Due to the potential drug interaction between thyroid products and glimepiride, the patient should be observed closely for loss of glycemic control when these drugs are co-administered. Conversely, when thyroid products are withdrawn, the patient should be observed closely for hypoglycemia).
No products indexed under this heading.

Tiagabine Hydrochloride (*In vivo* drug-drug interaction studies have suggested that pioglitazone may be a weak inducer of CYP 450 isoform 3A4 substrate). Products include:
Gabitril 972

Ticlopidine Hydrochloride (There is a potential interaction of glimepiride with inhibitors (eg, fluconazole) of cytochrome P450 2C9).
No products indexed under this heading.

Timolol Hemihydrate (The hypoglycemic action of sulfonylureas may be potentiated by certain drugs, including other drugs that are highly protein bound, such as β adrenergic blocking agents. Due to the potential drug interaction between these drugs and glimepiride, the patient should be observed closely for hypoglycemia when these drugs are co-administered. Conversely, when these drugs are withdrawn, the patient should be observed closely for loss of glycemic control). Products include:
Betimol 3490

Timolol Maleate (The hypoglycemic action of sulfonylureas may be potentiated by certain drugs, including other drugs that are highly protein bound, such as β adrenergic blocking agents. Due to the potential drug interaction between these drugs and glimepiride, the patient should be observed closely for hypoglycemia when these drugs are co-administered. Conversely, when these drugs are withdrawn, the patient should be observed closely for loss of glycemic control). Products include:
Combigan 601
Dorzolamide Hydrochloride/Timolol Maleate Ophthalmic Solution .... ⊙243
Timoptic in Ocudose .... ⊙231

Tolazamide (Patients receiving pioglitazone in combination with oral hypoglycemic agents may be at risk for hypoglycemia, and a reduction in the dose of the concomitant agent may be necessary).
No products indexed under this heading.

Tolbutamide (Patients receiving pioglitazone in combination with oral hypoglycemic agents may be at risk for hypoglycemia, and a reduction in the dose of the concomitant agent may be necessary).
No products indexed under this heading.

Tolbutamide Sodium (There is a potential interaction of glimepiride with inhibitors (eg, fluconazole) of cytochrome P450 2C9).
No products indexed under this heading.

Tolmetin Sodium (The hypoglycemic action of sulfonylureas may be potentiated by certain drugs, including nonsteroidal anti-inflammatory drugs. Due to the potential drug interaction between these drugs and glimepiride, the patient should be observed closely for hypoglycemia when these drugs are co-administered. Conversely, when these drugs are withdrawn, the patient should be observed closely for loss of glycemic control).
No products indexed under this heading.

Tolterodine Tartrate (*In vivo* drug-drug interaction studies have suggested that pioglitazone may be a weak inducer of CYP 450 isoform 3A4 substrate).
No products indexed under this heading.

Torsemide (Certain drugs tend to produce hyperglycemia and may lead to loss of control. These drugs include diuretics. Due to the potential drug interaction between diuretics and glimepiride, the patient should be observed closely for loss of glycemic control when these drugs are co-administered. Conversely, when diuretics are withdrawn, the patient should be observed closely for hypoglycemia).
No products indexed under this heading.

Tranylcypromine Sulfate (The hypoglycemic action of sulfonylureas may be potentiated by certain drugs, including other drugs that are highly protein bound, such as monoamine oxidase inhibitors. Due to the potential drug interaction between these drugs and glimepiride, the patient should be observed closely for hypoglycemia when these drugs are co-administered. Conversely, when these drugs are withdrawn, the patient should be observed closely for loss of glycemic control). Products include:
Parnate 1584

Trazodone Hydrochloride (*In vivo* drug-drug interaction studies have suggested that pioglitazone may be a weak inducer of CYP 450 isoform 3A4 substrate).
No products indexed under this heading.

Triamcinolone (Certain drugs tend to produce hyperglycemia and may lead to loss of control. These drugs include corticosteroids. Due to the potential drug interaction between corticosteroids and glimepiride, the patient should be observed closely for loss of glycemic control when these drugs are co-administered. Conversely, when corticosteroids are withdrawn, the patient should be observed closely for hypoglycemia).
No products indexed under this heading.

Triamcinolone Acetonide (Certain drugs tend to produce hyperglycemia and may lead to loss of control. These drugs include corticosteroids. Due to the potential drug interaction between corticosteroids and glimepiride, the patient should be observed closely for loss of glycemic control when these drugs are co-administered. Conversely, when corticosteroids are withdrawn, the patient should be observed closely for hypoglycemia). Products include:
Azmacort 408
Nasacort AQ 3019

Triamcinolone Diacetate (Certain drugs tend to produce hyperglycemia and may lead to loss of control. These drugs include corticosteroids. Due to the potential drug interaction between corticosteroids and glimepiride, the patient should be observed closely for loss of glycemic control when these drugs are co-administered. Conversely, when corticosteroids are withdrawn, the patient should be observed closely for hypoglycemia).
No products indexed under this heading.

Triamcinolone Hexacetonide (Certain drugs tend to produce hyperglycemia and may lead to loss of control. These drugs include corticosteroids. Due to the potential drug interaction between corticosteroids and glimepiride, the patient should be observed closely for loss of glycemic control when these drugs are co-administered. Conversely, when corticosteroids are withdrawn, the patient should be observed closely for hypoglycemia).
No products indexed under this heading.

Triamterene (Certain drugs tend to produce hyperglycemia and may lead to loss of control. These drugs include diuretics. Due to the potential drug interaction between diuretics and glimepiride, the patient should be observed closely for loss of glycemic control when these drugs are co-administered. Conversely, when diuretics are with-

505 Interactions Index Duragesic

drawn, the patient should be observed closely for hypoglycemia). Products include:
Dyazide 1429
Dyrenium 3495

Triazolam (*In vivo* drug-drug interaction studies have suggested that pioglitazone may be a weak inducer of CYP 450 isoform 3A4 substrate).
No products indexed under this heading.

Trifluoperazine Hydrochloride (Certain drugs tend to produce hyperglycemia and may lead to loss of control. These drugs include phenothiazines. Due to the potential drug interaction between phenothiazines and glimepiride, the patient should be observed closely for loss of glycemic control when these drugs are co-administered. Conversely, when phenothiazines are withdrawn, the patient should be observed closely for hypoglycemia).
No products indexed under this heading.

Trimethoprim (An enzyme inhibitor of CYP2C8 (such as gemfibrozil) may significantly increase the AUC of pioglitazone. Therefore, if an inhibitor of CYP2C8 is started or stopped during treatment with pioglitazone, changes in diabetes treatment may be needed based on clinical response).
No products indexed under this heading.

Trimethoprim Hydrochloride (An enzyme inhibitor of CYP2C8 (such as gemfibrozil) may significantly increase the AUC of pioglitazone. Therefore, if an inhibitor of CYP2C8 is started or stopped during treatment with pioglitazone, changes in diabetes treatment may be needed based on clinical response).
No products indexed under this heading.

Trimethoprim Sulfate (An enzyme inhibitor of CYP2C8 (such as gemfibrozil) may significantly increase the AUC of pioglitazone. Therefore, if an inhibitor of CYP2C8 is started or stopped during treatment with pioglitazone, changes in diabetes treatment may be needed based on clinical response).
No products indexed under this heading.

Trimipramine Maleate (The hypoglycemic action of sulfonylureas may be potentiated by certain drugs, including drugs that are highly protein bound. Due to the potential drug interaction between these drugs and glimepiride, the patient should be observed closely for hypoglycemia when these drugs are co-administered. Conversely, when these drugs are withdrawn, the patient should be observed closely for loss of glycemic control).
No products indexed under this heading.

Troglitazone (Patients receiving pioglitazone in combination with oral hypoglycemic agents may be at risk for hypoglycemia, and a reduction in the dose of the concomitant agent may be necessary).
No products indexed under this heading.

Valdecoxib (The hypoglycemic action of sulfonylureas may be potentiated by certain drugs, including nonsteroidal anti-inflammatory drugs. Due to the potential drug interaction between these drugs and glimepiride, the patient should be observed closely for hypoglycemia when these drugs are co-administered. Conversely, when these drugs are withdrawn, the patient should be observed closely for loss of glycemic control).
No products indexed under this heading.

Vardenafil Hydrochloride (There is a potential interaction of glimepiride with inhibitors (eg, fluconazole) of cytochrome P450 2C9). Products include:
Levitra 3157

Verapamil Hydrochloride (*In vivo* drug-drug interaction studies have suggested that pioglitazone may be a weak inducer of CYP 450 isoform 3A4 substrate). Products include:
Tarka 534

Vinblastine Sulfate (*In vivo* drug-drug interaction studies have suggested that pioglitazone may be a weak inducer of CYP 450 isoform 3A4 substrate).
No products indexed under this heading.

Vincristine Sulfate (*In vivo* drug-drug interaction studies have suggested that pioglitazone may be a weak inducer of CYP 450 isoform 3A4 substrate).
No products indexed under this heading.

Voriconazole (There is a potential interaction of glimepiride with inhibitors (eg, fluconazole) of cytochrome P450 2C9).
No products indexed under this heading.

Warfarin Sodium (Concomitant administration of glimepiride with warfarin result in a slight, but statistically significant, decrease in the pharmacodynamic response to warfarin. The reductions in mean area under the prothrombin time (PT) curve and maximum PT values during glimepiride treatment were very small (3.3% and 9.9%, respectively) and are unlikely to be clinically important).
No products indexed under this heading.

Zafirlukast (There is a potential interaction of glimepiride with inhibitors (eg, fluconazole) of cytochrome P450 2C9). Products include:
Accolate 3612

Food Interactions

Alcohol (All sulfonylurea drugs are capable of producing hypoglycemia; hypoglycemia is more likely to occur when alcohol is ingested).

Beer, reduced-alcohol (All sulfonylurea drugs are capable of producing hypoglycemia; hypoglycemia is more likely to occur when alcohol is ingested).

Beer, unspecified (All sulfonylurea drugs are capable of producing hypoglycemia; hypoglycemia is more likely to occur when alcohol is ingested).

Food, unspecified (Food did not change the systemic exposures of glimepiride or pioglitazone. However, for glimepiride, there was a 22% increase in C_{max} when Duetact was administered with food).

Meal, unspecified (Food did not change the systemic exposures of glimepiride or pioglitazone. However, for glimepiride, there was a 22% increase in C_{max} when Duetact was administered with food).

Wine, Chianti (All sulfonylurea drugs are capable of producing hypoglycemia; hypoglycemia is more likely to occur when alcohol is ingested).

Wine, Red (All sulfonylurea drugs are capable of producing hypoglycemia; hypoglycemia is more likely to occur when alcohol is ingested).

Wine, unspecified (All sulfonylurea drugs are capable of producing hypoglycemia; hypoglycemia is more likely to occur when alcohol is ingested).

Wine products (All sulfonylurea drugs are capable of producing hypoglycemia; hypoglycemia is more likely to occur when alcohol is ingested).

DURAGESIC TRANSDERMAL SYSTEM

(Fentanyl) 2604
May interact with alcohols, benzodiazepines, central nervous system depressants, centrally-acting drugs, cytochrome p450 3a4 inducers (selected), cytochrome p450 3a4 inhibitors (selected), erythromycin, general anesthetics, hypnotics and sedatives, monoamine oxidase inhibitors, narcotic analgesics, phenothiazines, skeletal muscle relaxants, tranquilizers, and certain other agents. Compounds in these categories include:

Acetazolamide (The concomitant use of fentanyl with all CYP3A4 inhibitors may result in an increase in fentanyl plasma concentrations, which could increase or prolong adverse drug effects and may cause potentially fatal respiratory depression. Patients receiving fentanyl and any CYP3A4 inhibitor should be monitored for an extended period of time and dosage adjustments should be made if warranted).
No products indexed under this heading.

Acetazolamide Sodium (The concomitant use of fentanyl with all CYP3A4 inhibitors may result in an increase in fentanyl plasma concentrations, which could increase or prolong adverse drug effects and may cause potentially fatal respiratory depression. Patients receiving fentanyl and any CYP3A4 inhibitor should be monitored for an extended period of time and dosage adjustments should be made if warranted).
No products indexed under this heading.

Alfentanil Hydrochloride (The concomitant use of fentanyl with other CNS depressants, including other opioids, may cause repiratory depression, hypotension, and profound sedation or potentially result in coma. When such combined therapy is contemplated, the dose of one or both agents should be significantly reduced. The use of concomitant CNS active drugs requires special patient care and observation).
No products indexed under this heading.

Allium sativum (Co-administration with agents that induce CYP 3A4 activity may reduce the efficacy of fentanyl).
No products indexed under this heading.

Alprazolam (The concomitant use of fentanyl with other central nervous system depressants, including tranquilizers (eg, benzodiazepines) may cause respiratory depression, hypotension, and profound sedation, or potentially result in coma or death. When such combined therapy is contemplated, the dose of one or both agents should be significantly reduced. The use of concomitant CNS active drugs requires special patient care and observation).
No products indexed under this heading.

Aminoglutethimide (Co-administration with agents that induce CYP 3A4 activity may reduce the efficacy of fentanyl).
No products indexed under this heading.

Amiodarone Hydrochloride (The concomitant use of fentanyl with all CYP3A4 inhibitors (eg, amiodarone) may result in an increase in fentanyl plasma concentrations, which could increase or prolong adverse drug effects and may cause potentially fatal respiratory depression. Patients receiving fentanyl and any CYP3A4 inhibitor should be monitored for an extended period of time and dosage adjustments should be made if warranted).
No products indexed under this heading.

Amobarbital (The comcomitant use of fentanyl with other CNS depressants may cause respiratory depression, hypotension, and profound sedation or potentially result in coma. When such combined therapy is contemplated, the dose of one or both agents should be significantly reduced. The use of concomitant CNS active drugs requires special patient care and observation).
No products indexed under this heading.

Amobarbital Sodium (The comcomitant use of fentanyl with other CNS depressants may cause respiratory depression, hypotension, and profound sedation or potentially result in coma. When such combined therapy is contemplated, the dose of one or both agents should be significantly reduced. The use of concomitant CNS active drugs requires special patient care and observation).
No products indexed under this heading.

Amphetamine Aspartate (The use of concomitant CNS active drugs requires special patient care and observation).
No products indexed under this heading.

Amphetamine Aspartate Monohydrate (The use of concomitant CNS active drugs requires special patient care and observation).
No products indexed under this heading.

Amphetamine Resins (The use of concomitant CNS active drugs requires special patient care and observation).
No products indexed under this heading.

Amphetamine Sulfate (The use of concomitant CNS active drugs requires special patient care and observation).
No products indexed under this heading.

Amprenavir (The concomitant use of fentanyl with all CYP3A4 inhibitors (eg, amprenavir) may result in an increase in fentanyl plasma concentrations, which could increase or prolong adverse drug effects and may cause potentially fatal respiratory depression. Patients receiving fentanyl and any CYP3A4 inhibitor should be monitored for an extended period of time and dosage adjustments should be made if warranted).
No products indexed under this heading.

Anastrozole (The concomitant use of fentanyl with all CYP3A4 inhibitors may result in an increase in fentanyl plasma concentrations, which could increase or prolong adverse drug effects and may cause potentially fatal respiratory depression. Patients receiving fentanyl and any CYP3A4 inhibitor should be monitored for an extended period of time and dosage adjustments should be made if warranted).
No products indexed under this heading.

Apomorphine (The concomitant use of fentanyl with other CNS depressants, including other opioids, may cause repiratory depression, hypotension, and profound sedation or potentially result in coma. When such combined therapy is contemplated, the dose of one or both agents should be significantly reduced. The use of concomitant CNS active drugs requires special patient care and observation).
No products indexed under this heading.

Apomorphine Hydrochloride (The concomitant use of fentanyl with other CNS depressants, including other opioids, may cause repiratory depression, hypotension, and profound sedation or potentially result in coma. When such combined therapy is contemplated, the dose of one or both agents should be significantly reduced. The use of concomitant CNS active drugs requires special patient care and observation).
No products indexed under this heading.

Aprepitant (The concomitant use of fentanyl with all CYP3A4 inhibitors (eg, aprepitant) may result in an increase in fentanyl plasma concentrations, which could increase or prolong adverse drug effects and may cause potentially fatal respiratory depression. Patients receiving fentanyl and any CYP3A4 inhibitor should be monitored for an extended period of time and dosage adjustments should be made if warranted). Products include:
Emend 2124

IMPORTANT NOTE: Always consult each drug listing in the patient's regimen for possible interactions.

Aprobarbital (The comcomitant use of fentanyl with other CNS depressants may cause respiratory depression, hypotension, and profound sedation or potentially result in coma. When such combined therapy is contemplated, the dose of one or both agents should be significantly reduced. The use of concomitant CNS active drugs requires special patient care and observation).
No products indexed under this heading.

Atazanavir (The concomitant use of fentanyl with all CYP3A4 inhibitors may result in an increase in fentanyl plasma concentrations, which could increase or prolong adverse drug effects and may cause potentially fatal respiratory depression. Patients receiving fentanyl and any CYP3A4 inhibitor should be monitored for an extended period of time and dosage adjustments should be made if warranted).
No products indexed under this heading.

Atazanavir Sulfate (The concomitant use of fentanyl with all CYP3A4 inhibitors may result in an increase in fentanyl plasma concentrations, which could increase or prolong adverse drug effects and may cause potentially fatal respiratory depression. Patients receiving fentanyl and any CYP3A4 inhibitor should be monitored for an extended period of time and dosage adjustments should be made if warranted).
No products indexed under this heading.

Atracurium Besylate (The concomitant use of fentanyl with other CNS depressants, including skeletal muscle relaxants, may cause respiratory depression, hypotension, and profound sedation or potentially result in coma. When such combined therapy is contemplated, the dose of one or both agents should be significantly reduced. The use of concomitant CNS active drugs requires special patient care and observation).
No products indexed under this heading.

Baclofen (The concomitant use of fentanyl with other CNS depressants, including skeletal muscle relaxants, may cause respiratory depression, hypotension, and profound sedation or potentially result in coma. When such combined therapy is contemplated, the dose of one or both agents should be significantly reduced. The use of concomitant CNS active drugs requires special patient care and observation).
No products indexed under this heading.

Betamethasone (Co-administration with agents that induce CYP 3A4 activity may reduce the efficacy of fentanyl).
No products indexed under this heading.

Betamethasone Acetate (Co-administration with agents that induce CYP 3A4 activity may reduce the efficacy of fentanyl).
No products indexed under this heading.

Betamethasone Benzoate (Co-administration with agents that induce CYP 3A4 activity may reduce the efficacy of fentanyl).
No products indexed under this heading.

Betamethasone Dipropionate (Co-administration with agents that induce CYP 3A4 activity may reduce the efficacy of fentanyl). Products include:
Diprolene Lotion 0.05% 3108
Diprolene Ointment 0.05% 3109
Diprolene AF Cream 0.05% 3107
Lotrisone 3163

Betamethasone Sodium Phosphate (Co-administration with agents that induce CYP 3A4 activity may reduce the efficacy of fentanyl).
No products indexed under this heading.

Betamethasone Valerate (Co-administration with agents that induce CYP 3A4 activity may reduce the efficacy of fentanyl). Products include:
Luxiq 3321

Bosentan (Co-administration with agents that induce CYP 3A4 activity may reduce the efficacy of fentanyl). Products include:
Tracleer 573

Buprenorphine Hydrochloride (The concomitant use of fentanyl with other CNS depressants, including other opioids, may cause repiratory depression, hypotension, and profound sedation or potentially result in coma. When such combined therapy is contemplated, the dose of one or both agents should be significantly reduced. The use of concomitant CNS active drugs requires special patient care and observation).
No products indexed under this heading.

Buspirone Hydrochloride (The concomitant use of fentanyl with other CNS depressants, including tranquilizers, may cause respiratory depression, hypotension, and profound sedation or potentially result in coma. When such combined therapy is contemplated, the dose of one or both agents should be significantly reduced. The use of concomitant CNS active drugs requires special patient care and observation).
No products indexed under this heading.

Butabarbital (The concomitant use of fentanyl with other CNS depressants, including sedatives and hypnotics, may cause respiratory depression, hypotension, and profound sedation or potentially result in coma. When such combined therapy is contemplated, the dose of one or both agents should be significantly reduced. The use of concomitant CNS active drugs requires special patient care and observation).
No products indexed under this heading.

Butabarbital Sodium (The concomitant use of fentanyl with other CNS depressants, including sedatives and hypnotics, may cause respiratory depression, hypotension, and profound sedation or potentially result in coma. When such combined therapy is contemplated, the dose of one or both agents should be significantly reduced. The use of concomitant CNS active drugs requires special patient care and observation).
No products indexed under this heading.

Butalbital (The concomitant use of fentanyl with other CNS depressants, including sedatives and hypnotics, may cause respiratory depression, hypotension, and profound sedation or potentially result in coma. When such combined therapy is contemplated, the dose of one or both agents should be significantly reduced. The use of concomitant CNS active drugs requires special patient care and observation).
No products indexed under this heading.

Carbamazepine (Co-administration with agents that induce CYP 3A4 activity may reduce the efficacy of fentanyl). Products include:
Carbatrol 3280
Equetro 3477

Carisoprodol (The concomitant use of fentanyl with other CNS depressants, including skeletal muscle relaxants, may cause respiratory depression, hypotension, and profound sedation or potentially result in coma. When such combined therapy is contemplated, the dose of one or both agents should be significantly reduced. The use of concomitant CNS active drugs requires special patient care and observation).
No products indexed under this heading.

Chloral Hydrate (The concomitant use of fentanyl with other CNS depressants, including sedatives and hypnotics, may cause respiratory depression, hypotension, and profound sedation or potentially result in coma. When such combined therapy is contemplated, the dose of one or both agents should be significantly reduced. The use of concomitant CNS active drugs requires special patient care and observation).
No products indexed under this heading.

Chlordiazepoxide (The concomitant use of fentanyl with other central nervous system depressants, including tranquilizers (eg, benzodiazepines) may cause respiratory depression, hypotension, and profound sedation, or potentially result in coma or death. When such combined therapy is contemplated, the dose of one or both agents should be significantly reduced. The use of concomitant CNS active drugs requires special patient care and observation).
No products indexed under this heading.

Chlordiazepoxide Hydrochloride (The concomitant use of fentanyl with other central nervous system depressants, including tranquilizers (eg, benzodiazepines) may cause respiratory depression, hypotension, and profound sedation, or potentially result in coma or death. When such combined therapy is contemplated, the dose of one or both agents should be significantly reduced. The use of concomitant CNS active drugs requires special patient care and observation).
No products indexed under this heading.

Chlorpromazine (The concomitant use of fentanyl with other CNS depressants, including tranquilizers, may cause respiratory depression, hypotension, and profound sedation or potentially result in coma. When such combined therapy is contemplated, the dose of one or both agents should be significantly reduced. The use of concomitant CNS active drugs requires special patient care and observation).
No products indexed under this heading.

Chlorpromazine Hydrochloride (The concomitant use of fentanyl with other CNS depressants, including tranquilizers, may cause respiratory depression, hypotension, and profound sedation or potentially result in coma. When such combined therapy is contemplated, the dose of one or both agents should be significantly reduced. The use of concomitant CNS active drugs requires special patient care and observation).
No products indexed under this heading.

Chlorprothixene (The concomitant use of fentanyl with other CNS depressants, including tranquilizers, may cause respiratory depression, hypotension, and profound sedation or potentially result in coma. When such combined therapy is contemplated, the dose of one or both agents should be significantly reduced. The use of concomitant CNS active drugs requires special patient care and observation).
No products indexed under this heading.

Chlorprothixene Hydrochloride (The concomitant use of fentanyl with other CNS depressants, including tranquilizers, may cause respiratory depression, hypotension, and profound sedation or potentially result in coma. When such combined therapy is contemplated, the dose of one or both agents should be significantly reduced. The use of concomitant CNS active drugs requires special patient care and observation).
No products indexed under this heading.

Chlorprothixene Lactate (The concomitant use of fentanyl with other CNS depressants, including tranquilizers, may cause respiratory depression, hypotension, and profound sedation or potentially result in coma. When such combined therapy is contemplated, the dose of one or both agents should be significantly reduced. The use of concomitant CNS active drugs requires special patient care and observation).
No products indexed under this heading.

Chlorzoxazone (The concomitant use of fentanyl with other CNS depressants, including skeletal muscle relaxants, may cause respiratory depression, hypotension, and profound sedation or potentially result in coma. When such combined therapy is contemplated, the dose of one or both agents should be significantly reduced. The use of concomitant CNS active drugs requires special patient care and observation).
No products indexed under this heading.

Cimetidine (The concomitant use of fentanyl with all CYP3A4 inhibitors may result in an increase in fentanyl plasma concentrations, which could increase or prolong adverse drug effects and may cause potentially fatal respiratory depression. Patients receiving fentanyl and any CYP3A4 inhibitor should be monitored for an extended period of time and dosage adjustments should be made if warranted).
No products indexed under this heading.

Cimetidine Hydrochloride (The concomitant use of fentanyl with all CYP3A4 inhibitors may result in an increase in fentanyl plasma concentrations, which could increase or prolong adverse drug effects and may cause potentially fatal respiratory depression. Patients receiving fentanyl and any CYP3A4 inhibitor should be monitored for an extended period of time and dosage adjustments should be made if warranted).
No products indexed under this heading.

Ciprofloxacin (The concomitant use of fentanyl with all CYP3A4 inhibitors may result in an increase in fentanyl plasma concentrations, which could increase or prolong adverse drug effects and may cause potentially fatal respiratory depression. Patients receiving fentanyl and any CYP3A4 inhibitor should be monitored for an extended period of time and dosage adjustments should be made if warranted). Products include:
Cipro I.V. 3082
Cipro 3073
Cipro XR 3091
Ciprodex 583

Ciprofloxacin Hydrochloride (Co-administration with agents that induce CYP 3A4 activity may reduce the efficacy of fentanyl). Products include:
Cipro 3073

Cisatracurium Besylate (The concomitant use of fentanyl with other CNS depressants, including skeletal muscle relaxants, may cause respiratory depression, hypotension, and profound sedation or potentially result in coma. When such combined therapy is contemplated, the dose of one or both agents should be significantly reduced. The use of concomitant CNS active drugs requires special patient care and observation). Products include:
Nimbex 503

Cisplatin (Co-administration with agents that induce CYP 3A4 activity may reduce the efficacy of fentanyl).
No products indexed under this heading.

Clarithromycin (The concomitant use of fentanyl with all CYP3A4 inhibitors (eg, clarithromycin) may result in an increase in fentanyl plasma concentrations, which could increase or prolong adverse drug effects and may cause potentially fatal respiratory depression. Patients receiving fentanyl and any CYP3A4 inhibitor should be monitored for an extended period of time and dosage adjustments should be made if warranted). Products include:
Biaxin/Biaxin XL 412

507 Interactions Index Duragesic

Clonazepam (The comcomitant use of fentanyl with other CNS depressants may cause respiratory depression, hypotension, and profound sedation or potentially result in coma. When such combined therapy is contemplated, the dose of one or both agents should be significantly reduced. The use of concomitant CNS active drugs requires special patient care and observation). Products include:
Klonopin 2855

Clorazepate Dipotassium (The concomitant use of fentanyl with other central nervous system depressants, including tranquilizers (eg, benzodiazepines) may cause repiratory depression, hypotension, and profound sedation, or potentially result in coma or death. When such combined therapy is contemplated, the dose of one or both agents should be significantly reduced. The use of concomitant CNS active drugs requires special patient care and observation).
No products indexed under this heading.

Clotrimazole (The concomitant use of fentanyl with all CYP3A4 inhibitors may result in an increase in fentanyl plasma concentrations, which could increase or prolong adverse drug effects and may cause potentially fatal respiratory depression. Patients receiving fentanyl and any CYP3A4 inhibitor should be monitored for an extended period of time and dosage adjustments should be made if warranted). Products include:
Lotrisone 3163

Clozapine (The comcomitant use of fentanyl with other CNS depressants may cause respiratory depression, hypotension, and profound sedation or potentially result in coma. When such combined therapy is contemplated, the dose of one or both agents should be significantly reduced. The use of concomitant CNS active drugs requires special patient care and observation).
No products indexed under this heading.

Codeine Phosphate (The concomitant use of fentanyl with other CNS depressants, including other opioids, may cause repiratory depression, hypotension, and profound sedation or potentially result in coma. When such combined therapy is contemplated, the dose of one or both agents should be significantly reduced. The use of concomitant CNS active drugs requires special patient care and observation). Products include:
Tylenol with Codeine 2691

Codeine Sulfate (The concomitant use of fentanyl with other CNS depressants, including other opioids, may cause repiratory depression, hypotension, and profound sedation or potentially result in coma. When such combined therapy is contemplated, the dose of one or both agents should be significantly reduced. The use of concomitant CNS active drugs requires special patient care and observation).
No products indexed under this heading.

Conivaptan Hydrochloride (The concomitant use of fentanyl with all CYP3A4 inhibitors may result in an increase in fentanyl plasma concentrations, which could increase or prolong adverse drug effects and may cause potentially fatal respiratory depression. Patients receiving fentanyl and any CYP3A4 inhibitor should be monitored for an extended period of time and dosage adjustments should be made if warranted). Products include:
Vaprisol 689

Cortisone Acetate (Co-administration with agents that induce CYP 3A4 activity may reduce the efficacy of fentanyl).
No products indexed under this heading.

Cyclobenzaprine Hydrochloride (The concomitant use of fentanyl with other CNS depressants, including skeletal muscle relaxants, may cause respiratory depression, hypotension, and profound sedation or potentially result in coma. When such combined therapy is contemplated, the dose of one or both agents should be significantly reduced. The use of concomitant CNS active drugs requires special patient care and observation). Products include:
Amrix 964

Cyclosporine (The concomitant use of fentanyl with all CYP3A4 inhibitors may result in an increase in fentanyl plasma concentrations, which could increase or prolong adverse drug effects and may cause potentially fatal respiratory depression. Patients receiving fentanyl and any CYP3A4 inhibitor should be monitored for an extended period of time and dosage adjustments should be made if warranted). Products include:
Gengraf 440
Neoral Oral Solution 2496
Neoral Capsules 2496
Restasis 605

Dalfopristin (The concomitant use of fentanyl with all CYP3A4 inhibitors may result in an increase in fentanyl plasma concentrations, which could increase or prolong adverse drug effects and may cause potentially fatal respiratory depression. Patients receiving fentanyl and any CYP3A4 inhibitor should be monitored for an extended period of time and dosage adjustments should be made if warranted).
No products indexed under this heading.

Danazol (The concomitant use of fentanyl with all CYP3A4 inhibitors may result in an increase in fentanyl plasma concentrations, which could increase or prolong adverse drug effects and may cause potentially fatal respiratory depression. Patients receiving fentanyl and any CYP3A4 inhibitor should be monitored for an extended period of time and dosage adjustments should be made if warranted).
No products indexed under this heading.

Dantrolene Sodium (The concomitant use of fentanyl with other CNS depressants, including skeletal muscle relaxants, may cause respiratory depression, hypotension, and profound sedation or potentially result in coma. When such combined therapy is contemplated, the dose of one or both agents should be significantly reduced. The use of concomitant CNS active drugs requires special patient care and observation).
No products indexed under this heading.

Darunavir (The concomitant use of fentanyl with all CYP3A4 inhibitors may result in an increase in fentanyl plasma concentrations, which could increase or prolong adverse drug effects and may cause potentially fatal respiratory depression. Patients receiving fentanyl and any CYP3A4 inhibitor should be monitored for an extended period of time and dosage adjustments should be made if warranted).
No products indexed under this heading.

Dasatinib (The concomitant use of fentanyl with all CYP3A4 inhibitors may result in an increase in fentanyl plasma concentrations, which could increase or prolong adverse drug effects and may cause potentially fatal respiratory depression. Patients receiving fentanyl and any CYP3A4 inhibitor should be monitored for an extended period of time and dosage adjustments should be made if warranted).
No products indexed under this heading.

Delavirdine Mesylate (The concomitant use of fentanyl with all CYP3A4 inhibitors may result in an increase in fentanyl plasma concentrations, which could increase or prolong adverse drug effects and may cause potentially fatal respiratory depression. Patients receiving fentanyl and any CYP3A4 inhibitor should be monitored for an extended period of time and dosage adjustments should be made if warranted).
No products indexed under this heading.

Delavirine (The concomitant use of fentanyl with all CYP3A4 inhibitors may result in an increase in fentanyl plasma concentrations, which could increase or prolong adverse drug effects and may cause potentially fatal respiratory depression. Patients receiving fentanyl and any CYP3A4 inhibitor should be monitored for an extended period of time and dosage adjustments should be made if warranted).
No products indexed under this heading.

Desflurane (The concomitant use of fentanyl with other CNS depressants, including general anesthetics, may cause respiratory depression, hypotension, and profound sedation or potentially result in coma. When such combined therapy is contemplated, the dose of one or both agents should be significantly reduced. The use of concomitant CNS active drugs requires special patient care and observation).
No products indexed under this heading.

Desloratadine (The concomitant use of fentanyl with all CYP3A4 inhibitors may result in an increase in fentanyl plasma concentrations, which could increase or prolong adverse drug effects and may cause potentially fatal respiratory depression. Patients receiving fentanyl and any CYP3A4 inhibitor should be monitored for an extended period of time and dosage adjustments should be made if warranted). Products include:
Clarinex Syrup 3098
Clarinex 3098
Clarinex Reditabs 3098
Clarinex-D 12-Hour 3101
Clarinex-D 3104

Dexamethasone (Co-administration with agents that induce CYP 3A4 activity may reduce the efficacy of fentanyl). Products include:
Ciprodex 583
Ozurdex .... ⊙ 223
Tobramycin and Dexamethasone Ophthalmic Suspension .... ⊙ 251

Dexamethasone Acetate (Co-administration with agents that induce CYP 3A4 activity may reduce the efficacy of fentanyl).
No products indexed under this heading.

Dexamethasone Phosphate (Co-administration with agents that induce CYP 3A4 activity may reduce the efficacy of fentanyl).
No products indexed under this heading.

Dexamethasone Sodium (Co-administration with agents that induce CYP 3A4 activity may reduce the efficacy of fentanyl).
No products indexed under this heading.

Dexamethasone Sodium Phosphate (Co-administration with agents that induce CYP 3A4 activity may reduce the efficacy of fentanyl).
No products indexed under this heading.

Dexamethasone Sodium Phosphate Injection (Co-administration with agents that induce CYP 3A4 activity may reduce the efficacy of fentanyl).
No products indexed under this heading.

Dexmethylphenidate Hydrochloride (The use of concomitant CNS active drugs requires special patient care and observation). Products include:
Focalin XR 2472

Dextroamphetamine (The use of concomitant CNS active drugs requires special patient care and observation).
No products indexed under this heading.

Dextroamphetamine Saccharate (The use of concomitant CNS active drugs requires special patient care and observation).
No products indexed under this heading.

Dextroamphetamine Sulfate (The use of concomitant CNS active drugs requires special patient care and observation). Products include:
Dexedrine 1425

Dezocine (The concomitant use of fentanyl with other CNS depressants, including other opioids, may cause repiratory depression, hypotension, and profound sedation or potentially result in coma. When such combined therapy is contemplated, the dose of one or both agents should be significantly reduced. The use of concomitant CNS active drugs requires special patient care and observation).
No products indexed under this heading.

Diazepam (The concomitant use of fentanyl with other central nervous system depressants, including tranquilizers (eg, benzodiazepines) may cause respiratory depression, hypotension, and profound sedation, or potentially result in coma or death. When such combined therapy is contemplated, the dose of one or both agents should be significantly reduced. The use of concomitant CNS active drugs requires special patient care and observation). Products include:
Valium Tablets 2880

Dihydrocodeine Bitartrate (The concomitant use of fentanyl with other CNS depressants, including other opioids, may cause repiratory depression, hypotension, and profound sedation or potentially result in coma. When such combined therapy is contemplated, the dose of one or both agents should be significantly reduced. The use of concomitant CNS active drugs requires special patient care and observation).
No products indexed under this heading.

Dihydrocodeinone Bitartrate (The concomitant use of fentanyl with other CNS depressants, including other opioids, may cause repiratory depression, hypotension, and profound sedation or potentially result in coma. When such combined therapy is contemplated, the dose of one or both agents should be significantly reduced. The use of concomitant CNS active drugs requires special patient care and observation).
No products indexed under this heading.

Diltiazem Hydrochloride (The concomitant use of fentanyl with all CYP3A4 inhibitors (eg, diltiazem) may result in an increase in fentanyl plasma concentrations, which could increase or prolong adverse drug effects and may cause potentially fatal respiratory depression. Patients receiving fentanyl and any CYP3A4 inhibitor should be monitored for an extended period of time and dosage adjustments should be made if warranted). Products include:
Cardizem LA 423

Diltiazem Maleate (The concomitant use of fentanyl with all CYP3A4 inhibitors (eg, diltiazem) may result in an increase in fentanyl plasma concentrations, which could increase or prolong adverse drug effects and may cause potentially fatal respiratory depression. Patients receiving fentanyl and any CYP3A4 inhibitor should be monitored for an extended period of time and dosage adjustments should be made if warranted).
No products indexed under this heading.

Doxacurium Chloride (The concomitant use of fentanyl with other CNS

IMPORTANT NOTE: Always consult each drug listing in the patient's regimen for possible interactions.

depressants, including skeletal muscle relaxants, may cause respiratory depression, hypotension, and profound sedation or potentially result in coma. When such combined therapy is contemplated, the dose of one or both agents should be significantly reduced. The use of concomitant CNS active drugs requires special patient care and observation).
No products indexed under this heading.

Doxorubicin Hydrochloride (Co-administration with agents that induce CYP 3A4 activity may reduce the efficacy of fentanyl).
No products indexed under this heading.

Droperidol (The concomitant use of fentanyl with other CNS depressants, including tranquilizers, may cause respiratory depression, hypotension, and profound sedation or potentially result in coma. When such combined therapy is contemplated, the dose of one or both agents should be significantly reduced. The use of concomitant CNS active drugs requires special patient care and observation).
No products indexed under this heading.

d-Tubocurarine (The concomitant use of fentanyl with other CNS depressants, including skeletal muscle relaxants, may cause respiratory depression, hypotension, and profound sedation or potentially result in coma. When such combined therapy is contemplated, the dose of one or both agents should be significantly reduced. The use of concomitant CNS active drugs requires special patient care and observation).
No products indexed under this heading.

Efavirenz (The concomitant use of fentanyl with all CYP3A4 inhibitors may result in an increase in fentanyl plasma concentrations, which could increase or prolong adverse drug effects and may cause potentially fatal respiratory depression. Patients receiving fentanyl and any CYP3A4 inhibitor should be monitored for an extended period of time and dosage adjustments should be made if warranted). Products include:
Atripla 906

Enflurane (The concomitant use of fentanyl with other CNS depressants, including general anesthetics, may cause respiratory depression, hypotension, and profound sedation or potentially result in coma. When such combined therapy is contemplated, the dose of one or both agents should be significantly reduced. The use of concomitant CNS active drugs requires special patient care and observation).
No products indexed under this heading.

Erythromycin (The concomitant use of fentanyl with all CYP3A4 inhibitors (eg, erythromycin) may result in an increase in fentanyl plasma concentrations, which could increase or prolong adverse drug effects and may cause potentially fatal respiratory depression. Patients receiving fentanyl and any CYP3A4 inhibitor should be monitored for an extended period of time and dosage adjustments should be made if warranted).
No products indexed under this heading.

Erythromycin, Topical (The concomitant use of fentanyl with all CYP3A4 inhibitors (eg, erythromycin) may result in an increase in fentanyl plasma concentrations, which could increase or prolong adverse drug effects and may cause potentially fatal respiratory depression. Patients receiving fentanyl and any CYP3A4 inhibitor should be monitored for an extended period of time and dosage adjustments should be made if warranted).
No products indexed under this heading.

Erythromycin Estolate (The concomitant use of fentanyl with all CYP3A4 inhibitors (eg, erythromycin) may result in an increase in fentanyl plasma concentrations, which could increase or prolong adverse drug effects and may cause potentially fatal respiratory depression. Patients receiving fentanyl and any CYP3A4 inhibitor should be monitored for an extended period of time and dosage adjustments should be made if warranted).
No products indexed under this heading.

Erythromycin Ethylsuccinate (The concomitant use of fentanyl with all CYP3A4 inhibitors (eg, erythromycin) may result in an increase in fentanyl plasma concentrations, which could increase or prolong adverse drug effects and may cause potentially fatal respiratory depression. Patients receiving fentanyl and any CYP3A4 inhibitor should be monitored for an extended period of time and dosage adjustments should be made if warranted). Products include:
E.E.S. 437
EryPed 435

Erythromycin Gluceptate (The concomitant use of fentanyl with all CYP3A4 inhibitors (eg, erythromycin) may result in an increase in fentanyl plasma concentrations, which could increase or prolong adverse drug effects and may cause potentially fatal respiratory depression. Patients receiving fentanyl and any CYP3A4 inhibitor should be monitored for an extended period of time and dosage adjustments should be made if warranted).
No products indexed under this heading.

Erythromycin Lactobionate (The concomitant use of fentanyl with all CYP3A4 inhibitors (eg, erythromycin) may result in an increase in fentanyl plasma concentrations, which could increase or prolong adverse drug effects and may cause potentially fatal respiratory depression. Patients receiving fentanyl and any CYP3A4 inhibitor should be monitored for an extended period of time and dosage adjustments should be made if warranted).
No products indexed under this heading.

Erythromycin Stearate (The concomitant use of fentanyl with all CYP3A4 inhibitors (eg, erythromycin) may result in an increase in fentanyl plasma concentrations, which could increase or prolong adverse drug effects and may cause potentially fatal respiratory depression. Patients receiving fentanyl and any CYP3A4 inhibitor should be monitored for an extended period of time and dosage adjustments should be made if warranted).
No products indexed under this heading.

Esomeprazole Magnesium (The concomitant use of fentanyl with all CYP3A4 inhibitors may result in an increase in fentanyl plasma concentrations, which could increase or prolong adverse drug effects and may cause potentially fatal respiratory depression. Patients receiving fentanyl and any CYP3A4 inhibitor should be monitored for an extended period of time and dosage adjustments should be made if warranted). Products include:
Nexium Capsules 704
Nexium Oral Suspension 704

Esomeprazole Sodium (The concomitant use of fentanyl with all CYP3A4 inhibitors may result in an increase in fentanyl plasma concentrations, which could increase or prolong adverse drug effects and may cause potentially fatal respiratory depression. Patients receiving fentanyl and any CYP3A4 inhibitor should be monitored for an extended period of time and dosage adjustments should be made if warranted). Products include:

Nexium I.V. 712

Estazolam (The concomitant use of fentanyl with other central nervous system depressants, including tranquilizers (eg, benzodiazepines) may cause respiratory depression, hypotension, and profound sedation, or potentially result in coma or death. When such combined therapy is contemplated, the dose of one or both agents should be significantly reduced. The use of concomitant CNS active drugs requires special patient care and observation).
No products indexed under this heading.

Ethanol (The comcomitant use of fentanyl with other CNS depressants may cause respiratory depression, hypotension, and profound sedation or potentially result in coma. When such combined therapy is contemplated, the dose of one or both agents should be significantly reduced. The use of concomitant CNS active drugs requires special patient care and observation).
No products indexed under this heading.

Ethchlorvynol (The concomitant use of fentanyl with other CNS depressants, including sedatives and hypnotics, may cause respiratory depression, hypotension, and profound sedation or potentially result in coma. When such combined therapy is contemplated, the dose of one or both agents should be significantly reduced. The use of concomitant CNS active drugs requires special patient care and observation).
No products indexed under this heading.

Ethinamate (The concomitant use of fentanyl with other CNS depressants, including sedatives and hypnotics, may cause respiratory depression, hypotension, and profound sedation or potentially result in coma. When such combined therapy is contemplated, the dose of one or both agents should be significantly reduced. The use of concomitant CNS active drugs requires special patient care and observation).
No products indexed under this heading.

Ethosuximide (Co-administration with agents that induce CYP 3A4 activity may reduce the efficacy of fentanyl).
No products indexed under this heading.

Ethyl Alcohol (The comcomitant use of fentanyl with other CNS depressants may cause respiratory depression, hypotension, and profound sedation or potentially result in coma. When such combined therapy is contemplated, the dose of one or both agents should be significantly reduced. The use of concomitant CNS active drugs requires special patient care and observation).
No products indexed under this heading.

Felbamate (Co-administration with agents that induce CYP 3A4 activity may reduce the efficacy of fentanyl).
No products indexed under this heading.

Fentanyl Citrate (The concomitant use of fentanyl with other CNS depressants, including other opioids, may cause repiratory depression, hypotension, and profound sedation or potentially result in coma. When such combined therapy is contemplated, the dose of one or both agents should be significantly reduced. The use of concomitant CNS active drugs requires special patient care and observation). Products include:
Fentora 966

Fluconazole (The concomitant use of fentanyl with all CYP3A4 inhibitors (eg, fluconazole) may result in an increase in fentanyl plasma concentrations, which could increase or prolong adverse drug effects and may cause potentially fatal respiratory depression. Patients receiving fentanyl and any CYP3A4 inhibitor

should be monitored for an extended period of time and dosage adjustments should be made if warranted.
No products indexed under this heading.

Fludrocortisone Acetate (Co-administration with agents that induce CYP 3A4 activity may reduce the efficacy of fentanyl).
No products indexed under this heading.

Fluoxetine (The concomitant use of fentanyl with all CYP3A4 inhibitors may result in an increase in fentanyl plasma concentrations, which could increase or prolong adverse drug effects and may cause potentially fatal respiratory depression. Patients receiving fentanyl and any CYP3A4 inhibitor should be monitored for an extended period of time and dosage adjustments should be made if warranted).
No products indexed under this heading.

Fluoxetine Hydrochloride (The concomitant use of fentanyl with all CYP3A4 inhibitors may result in an increase in fentanyl plasma concentrations, which could increase or prolong adverse drug effects and may cause potentially fatal respiratory depression. Patients receiving fentanyl and any CYP3A4 inhibitor should be monitored for an extended period of time and dosage adjustments should be made if warranted). Products include:
Prozac Weekly 1941
Prozac Pulvules 1941
Symbyax 1965

Fluphenazine Decanoate (The concomitant use of fentanyl with other CNS depressants, including tranquilizers, may cause respiratory depression, hypotension, and profound sedation or potentially result in coma. When such combined therapy is contemplated, the dose of one or both agents should be significantly reduced. The use of concomitant CNS active drugs requires special patient care and observation).
No products indexed under this heading.

Fluphenazine Enanthate (The concomitant use of fentanyl with other CNS depressants, including tranquilizers, may cause respiratory depression, hypotension, and profound sedation or potentially result in coma. When such combined therapy is contemplated, the dose of one or both agents should be significantly reduced. The use of concomitant CNS active drugs requires special patient care and observation).
No products indexed under this heading.

Fluphenazine Hydrochloride (The concomitant use of fentanyl with other CNS depressants, including tranquilizers, may cause respiratory depression, hypotension, and profound sedation or potentially result in coma. When such combined therapy is contemplated, the dose of one or both agents should be significantly reduced. The use of concomitant CNS active drugs requires special patient care and observation).
No products indexed under this heading.

Flurazepam Hydrochloride (The concomitant use of fentanyl with other central nervous system depressants, including tranquilizers (eg, benzodiazepines) may cause respiratory depression, hypotension, and profound sedation, or potentially result in coma or death. When such combined therapy is contemplated, the dose of one or both agents should be significantly reduced. The use of concomitant CNS active drugs requires special patient care and observation).
No products indexed under this heading.

Fluvoxamine Maleate (The concomitant use of fentanyl with all CYP3A4 inhibitors may result in an increase in fentanyl plasma concentrations, which could increase or prolong adverse drug effects and may cause potentially fatal

respiratory depression. Patients receiving fentanyl and any CYP3A4 inhibitor should be monitored for an extended period of time and dosage adjustments should be made if warranted).
No products indexed under this heading.

Fosamprenavir Calcium (The concomitant use of fentanyl with all CYP3A4 inhibitors (eg, fosamprenavir) may result in an increase in fentanyl plasma concentrations, which could increase or prolong adverse drug effects and may cause potentially fatal respiratory depression. Patients receiving fentanyl and any CYP3A4 inhibitor should be monitored for an extended period of time and dosage adjustments should be made if warranted). Products include:
Lexiva Oral Suspension 1558
Lexiva 1558

Fosphenytoin Sodium (Co-administration with agents that induce CYP 3A4 activity may reduce the efficacy of fentanyl).
No products indexed under this heading.

Gallamine (The concomitant use of fentanyl with other CNS depressants, including skeletal muscle relaxants, may cause respiratory depression, hypotension, and profound sedation or potentially result in coma. When such combined therapy is contemplated, the dose of one or both agents should be significantly reduced. The use of concomitant CNS active drugs requires special patient care and observation).
No products indexed under this heading.

Gallamine Triethiodide (The concomitant use of fentanyl with other CNS depressants, including skeletal muscle relaxants, may cause respiratory depression, hypotension, and profound sedation or potentially result in coma. When such combined therapy is contemplated, the dose of one or both agents should be significantly reduced. The use of concomitant CNS active drugs requires special patient care and observation).
No products indexed under this heading.

Garlic Extract (Co-administration with agents that induce CYP 3A4 activity may reduce the efficacy of fentanyl).
No products indexed under this heading.

Garlic Oil (Co-administration with agents that induce CYP 3A4 activity may reduce the efficacy of fentanyl).
No products indexed under this heading.

Glutethimide (The concomitant use of fentanyl with other CNS depressants, including sedatives and hypnotics, may cause respiratory depression, hypotension, and profound sedation or potentially result in coma. When such combined therapy is contemplated, the dose of one or both agents should be significantly reduced. The use of concomitant CNS active drugs requires special patient care and observation).
No products indexed under this heading.

Halazepam (The concomitant use of fentanyl with other central nervous system depressants, including tranquilizers (eg, benzodiazepines) may cause respiratory depression, hypotension, and profound sedation, or potentially result in coma or death. When such combined therapy is contemplated, the dose of one or both agents should be significantly reduced. The use of concomitant CNS active drugs requires special patient care and observation).
No products indexed under this heading.

Haloperidol (The concomitant use of fentanyl with other CNS depressants, including tranquilizers, may cause respiratory depression, hypotension, and profound sedation or potentially result in coma. When such combined therapy is contemplated, the dose of one or both agents should be significantly reduced. The use of concomitant CNS active drugs requires special patient care and observation).
No products indexed under this heading.

Haloperidol Decanoate (The concomitant use of fentanyl with other CNS depressants, including tranquilizers, may cause respiratory depression, hypotension, and profound sedation or potentially result in coma. When such combined therapy is contemplated, the dose of one or both agents should be significantly reduced. The use of concomitant CNS active drugs requires special patient care and observation).
No products indexed under this heading.

Haloperidol Lactate (The comcomitant use of fentanyl with other CNS depressants may cause respiratory depression, hypotension, and profound sedation or potentially result in coma. When such combined therapy is contemplated, the dose of one or both agents should be significantly reduced. The use of concomitant CNS active drugs requires special patient care and observation).
No products indexed under this heading.

Halothane (The concomitant use of fentanyl with other CNS depressants, including general anesthetics, may cause respiratory depression, hypotension, and profound sedation or potentially result in coma. When such combined therapy is contemplated, the dose of one or both agents should be significantly reduced. The use of concomitant CNS active drugs requires special patient care and observation).
No products indexed under this heading.

Hexobarbital (The comcomitant use of fentanyl with other CNS depressants may cause respiratory depression, hypotension, and profound sedation or potentially result in coma. When such combined therapy is contemplated, the dose of one or both agents should be significantly reduced. The use of concomitant CNS active drugs requires special patient care and observation).
No products indexed under this heading.

Hydrocodone Bitartrate (The concomitant use of fentanyl with other CNS depressants, including other opioids, may cause repiratory depression, hypotension, and profound sedation or potentially result in coma. When such combined therapy is contemplated, the dose of one or both agents should be significantly reduced. The use of concomitant CNS active drugs requires special patient care and observation). Products include:
Vicodin 560
Vicodin ES 561
Vicodin HP 563
Vicoprofen 564
Zydone 1138

Hydrocodone Polistirex (The concomitant use of fentanyl with other CNS depressants, including other opioids, may cause repiratory depression, hypotension, and profound sedation or potentially result in coma. When such combined therapy is contemplated, the dose of one or both agents should be significantly reduced. The use of concomitant CNS active drugs requires special patient care and observation). Products include:
Tussionex 3443

Hydrocortisone (Co-administration with agents that induce CYP 3A4 activity may reduce the efficacy of fentanyl).
No products indexed under this heading.

Hydrocortisone (Alcohol) (Co-administration with agents that induce CYP 3A4 activity may reduce the efficacy of fentanyl).
No products indexed under this heading.

Hydrocortisone Acetate (Co-administration with agents that induce CYP 3A4 activity may reduce the efficacy of fentanyl).
No products indexed under this heading.

Hydrocortisone Butyrate (Co-administration with agents that induce CYP 3A4 activity may reduce the efficacy of fentanyl).
No products indexed under this heading.

Hydrocortisone Cypionate (Co-administration with agents that induce CYP 3A4 activity may reduce the efficacy of fentanyl).
No products indexed under this heading.

Hydrocortisone Hemisuccinate (Co-administration with agents that induce CYP 3A4 activity may reduce the efficacy of fentanyl).
No products indexed under this heading.

Hydrocortisone Probutate (Co-administration with agents that induce CYP 3A4 activity may reduce the efficacy of fentanyl).
No products indexed under this heading.

Hydrocortisone Sodium Phosphate (Co-administration with agents that induce CYP 3A4 activity may reduce the efficacy of fentanyl).
No products indexed under this heading.

Hydrocortisone Sodium Succinate (Co-administration with agents that induce CYP 3A4 activity may reduce the efficacy of fentanyl).
No products indexed under this heading.

Hydrocortisone Valerate (Co-administration with agents that induce CYP 3A4 activity may reduce the efficacy of fentanyl).
No products indexed under this heading.

Hydromorphone (The concomitant use of fentanyl with other CNS depressants, including other opioids, may cause repiratory depression, hypotension, and profound sedation or potentially result in coma. When such combined therapy is contemplated, the dose of one or both agents should be significantly reduced. The use of concomitant CNS active drugs requires special patient care and observation).
No products indexed under this heading.

Hydromorphone Hydrochloride (The concomitant use of fentanyl with other CNS depressants, including other opioids, may cause repiratory depression, hypotension, and profound sedation or potentially result in coma. When such combined therapy is contemplated, the dose of one or both agents should be significantly reduced. The use of concomitant CNS active drugs requires special patient care and observation). Products include:
Dilaudid Injection 2800
Dilaudid Oral 2797
Dilaudid Tablets 2797
Dilaudid-HP 2800

Hydroxyamphetamine Hydrobromide (The use of concomitant CNS active drugs requires special patient care and observation).
No products indexed under this heading.

Hydroxyzine Hydrochloride (The concomitant use of fentanyl with other CNS depressants, including tranquilizers, may cause respiratory depression, hypotension, and profound sedation or potentially result in coma. When such combined therapy is contemplated, the dose of one or both agents should be significantly reduced. The use of concomitant CNS active drugs requires special patient care and observation).
No products indexed under this heading.

Hypericum (Co-administration with agents that induce CYP 3A4 activity may reduce the efficacy of fentanyl).
No products indexed under this heading.

Hypericum Perforatum (Co-administration with agents that induce CYP 3A4 activity may reduce the efficacy of fentanyl). Products include:
Traumeel 1800

Imatinib Mesylate (The concomitant use of fentanyl with all CYP3A4 inhibitors may result in an increase in fentanyl plasma concentrations, which could increase or prolong adverse drug effects and may cause potentially fatal respiratory depression. Patients receiving fentanyl and any CYP3A4 inhibitor should be monitored for an extended period of time and dosage adjustments should be made if warranted). Products include:
Gleevec 2477

Indinavir Sulfate (The concomitant use of fentanyl with all CYP3A4 inhibitors may result in an increase in fentanyl plasma concentrations, which could increase or prolong adverse drug effects and may cause potentially fatal respiratory depression. Patients receiving fentanyl and any CYP3A4 inhibitor should be monitored for an extended period of time and dosage adjustments should be made if warranted). Products include:
Crixivan 2113

Isocarboxazid (Fentanyl is not recommended for use in patients who have received monoamine oxidase (MAO) inhibitors within 14 days because severe and unpredictable potentiation by MAO inhibitors has been reported with opioid analgesics). Products include:
Marplan 3481

Isoflurane (The concomitant use of fentanyl with other CNS depressants, including general anesthetics, may cause respiratory depression, hypotension, and profound sedation or potentially result in coma. When such combined therapy is contemplated, the dose of one or both agents should be significantly reduced. The use of concomitant CNS active drugs requires special patient care and observation).
No products indexed under this heading.

Isoniazid (The concomitant use of fentanyl with all CYP3A4 inhibitors may result in an increase in fentanyl plasma concentrations, which could increase or prolong adverse drug effects and may cause potentially fatal respiratory depression. Patients receiving fentanyl and any CYP3A4 inhibitor should be monitored for an extended period of time and dosage adjustments should be made if warranted).
No products indexed under this heading.

Itraconazole (The concomitant use of fentanyl with all CYP3A4 inhibitors (eg, itraconazole) may result in an increase in fentanyl plasma concentrations, which could increase or prolong adverse drug effects and may cause potentially fatal respiratory depression. Patients receiving fentanyl and any CYP3A4 inhibitor should be monitored for an extended period of time and dosage adjustments should be made if warranted).
No products indexed under this heading.

Ketamine Hydrochloride (The concomitant use of fentanyl with other CNS depressants, including general anesthetics, may cause respiratory depression, hypotension, and profound sedation or potentially result in coma. When such combined therapy is contemplated, the dose of one or both agents should be significantly reduced. The use of concomitant CNS active drugs requires special patient care and observation).
No products indexed under this heading.

Ketoconazole (The concomitant use of fentanyl with all CYP3A4 inhibitors

(eg, ketoconazole) may result in an increase in fentanyl plasma concentrations, which could increase or prolong adverse drug effects and may cause potentially fatal respiratory depression. Patients receiving fentanyl and any CYP3A4 inhibitor should be monitored for an extended period of time and dosage adjustments should be made if warranted). Products include:

Extina 3319
Xolegel 3337

Lapatinib (The concomitant use of fentanyl with all CYP3A4 inhibitors may result in an increase in fentanyl plasma concentrations, which could increase or prolong adverse drug effects and may cause potentially fatal respiratory depression. Patients receiving fentanyl and any CYP3A4 inhibitor should be monitored for an extended period of time and dosage adjustments should be made if warranted). Products include:

Tykerb 1698

Levomethadyl Acetate Hydrochloride (The comcomitant use of fentanyl with other CNS depressants may cause respiratory depression, hypotension, and profound sedation or potentially result in coma. When such combined therapy is contemplated, the dose of one or both agents should be significantly reduced. The use of concomitant CNS active drugs requires special patient care and observation).
No products indexed under this heading.

Levorphanol Tartrate (The concomitant use of fentanyl with other CNS depressants, including other opioids, may cause repiratory depression, hypotension, and profound sedation or potentially result in coma. When such combined therapy is contemplated, the dose of one or both agents should be significantly reduced. The use of concomitant CNS active drugs requires special patient care and observation).
No products indexed under this heading.

Lisdexamfetamine Dimesylate (The use of concomitant CNS active drugs requires special patient care and observation). Products include:

Vyvanse 3298

Lopinavir (The concomitant use of fentanyl with all CYP3A4 inhibitors may result in an increase in fentanyl plasma concentrations, which could increase or prolong adverse drug effects and may cause potentially fatal respiratory depression. Patients receiving fentanyl and any CYP3A4 inhibitor should be monitored for an extended period of time and dosage adjustments should be made if warranted). Products include:

Kaletra 458

Loratadine (The concomitant use of fentanyl with all CYP3A4 inhibitors may result in an increase in fentanyl plasma concentrations, which could increase or prolong adverse drug effects and may cause potentially fatal respiratory depression. Patients receiving fentanyl and any CYP3A4 inhibitor should be monitored for an extended period of time and dosage adjustments should be made if warranted).
No products indexed under this heading.

Lorazepam (The concomitant use of fentanyl with other central nervous system depressants, including tranquilizers (eg, benzodiazepines) may cause respiratory depression, hypotension, and profound sedation, or potentially result in coma or death. When such combined therapy is contemplated, the dose of one or both agents should be significantly reduced. The use of concomitant CNS active drugs requires special patient care and observation).
No products indexed under this heading.

Loxapine Hydrochloride (The concomitant use of fentanyl with other CNS depressants, including tranquilizers, may cause respiratory depression, hypotension, and profound sedation or potentially result in coma. When such combined therapy is contemplated, the dose of one or both agents should be significantly reduced. The use of concomitant CNS active drugs requires special patient care and observation).
No products indexed under this heading.

Loxapine Succinate (The concomitant use of fentanyl with other CNS depressants, including tranquilizers, may cause respiratory depression, hypotension, and profound sedation or potentially result in coma. When such combined therapy is contemplated, the dose of one or both agents should be significantly reduced. The use of concomitant CNS active drugs requires special patient care and observation).
No products indexed under this heading.

Meperidine Hydrochloride (The concomitant use of fentanyl with other CNS depressants, including other opioids, may cause repiratory depression, hypotension, and profound sedation or potentially result in coma. When such combined therapy is contemplated, the dose of one or both agents should be significantly reduced. The use of concomitant CNS active drugs requires special patient care and observation).
No products indexed under this heading.

Mephenytoin (Co-administration with agents that induce CYP 3A4 activity may reduce the efficacy of fentanyl).
No products indexed under this heading.

Mephobarbital (The comcomitant use of fentanyl with other CNS depressants may cause respiratory depression, hypotension, and profound sedation or potentially result in coma. When such combined therapy is contemplated, the dose of one or both agents should be significantly reduced. The use of concomitant CNS active drugs requires special patient care and observation).
No products indexed under this heading.

Meprobamate (The concomitant use of fentanyl with other CNS depressants, including tranquilizers, may cause respiratory depression, hypotension, and profound sedation or potentially result in coma. When such combined therapy is contemplated, the dose of one or both agents should be significantly reduced. The use of concomitant CNS active drugs requires special patient care and observation).
No products indexed under this heading.

Mesoridazine Besylate (The concomitant use of fentanyl with other CNS depressants, including tranquilizers, may cause respiratory depression, hypotension, and profound sedation or potentially result in coma. When such combined therapy is contemplated, the dose of one or both agents should be significantly reduced. The use of concomitant CNS active drugs requires special patient care and observation).
No products indexed under this heading.

Metaxalone (The concomitant use of fentanyl with other CNS depressants, including skeletal muscle relaxants, may cause respiratory depression, hypotension, and profound sedation or potentially result in coma. When such combined therapy is contemplated, the dose of one or both agents should be significantly reduced. The use of concomitant CNS active drugs requires special patient care and observation). Products include:

Skelaxin 1848

Methadone Hydrochloride (The concomitant use of fentanyl with other CNS depressants, including other opioids, may cause repiratory depression, hypotension, and profound sedation or potentially result in coma. When such combined therapy is contemplated, the dose of one or both agents should be significantly reduced. The use of concomitant CNS active drugs requires special patient care and observation).
No products indexed under this heading.

Methamphetamine Hydrochloride (The use of concomitant CNS active drugs requires special patient care and observation).
No products indexed under this heading.

Methocarbamol (The concomitant use of fentanyl with other CNS depressants, including skeletal muscle relaxants, may cause respiratory depression, hypotension, and profound sedation or potentially result in coma. When such combined therapy is contemplated, the dose of one or both agents should be significantly reduced. The use of concomitant CNS active drugs requires special patient care and observation).
No products indexed under this heading.

Methohexital Sodium (The concomitant use of fentanyl with other CNS depressants, including general anesthetics, may cause respiratory depression, hypotension, and profound sedation or potentially result in coma. When such combined therapy is contemplated, the dose of one or both agents should be significantly reduced. The use of concomitant CNS active drugs requires special patient care and observation).
No products indexed under this heading.

Methotrimeprazine (The concomitant use of fentanyl with other CNS depressants, including phenothiazines, may cause respiratory depression, hypotension, and profound sedation or potentially result in coma. When such combined therapy is contemplated, the dose of one or both agents should be significantly reduced. The use of concomitant CNS active drugs requires special patient care and observation).
No products indexed under this heading.

Methoxyflurane (The concomitant use of fentanyl with other CNS depressants, including general anesthetics, may cause respiratory depression, hypotension, and profound sedation or potentially result in coma. When such combined therapy is contemplated, the dose of one or both agents should be significantly reduced. The use of concomitant CNS active drugs requires special patient care and observation).
No products indexed under this heading.

Methsuximide (Co-administration with agents that induce CYP 3A4 activity may reduce the efficacy of fentanyl).
No products indexed under this heading.

Methylphenidate (The use of concomitant CNS active drugs requires special patient care and observation). Products include:

Daytrana 3283

Methylphenidate Hydrochloride (The use of concomitant CNS active drugs requires special patient care and observation). Products include:

Concerta 2598
Metadate CD 3439

Methylprednisolone (Co-administration with agents that induce CYP 3A4 activity may reduce the efficacy of fentanyl).
No products indexed under this heading.

Methylprednisolone Acetate (Co-administration with agents that induce CYP 3A4 activity may reduce the efficacy of fentanyl).
No products indexed under this heading.

Methylprednisolone Sodium Succinate (Co-administration with agents that induce CYP 3A4 activity may reduce the efficacy of fentanyl).
No products indexed under this heading.

Metocurine Iodide (The concomitant use of fentanyl with other CNS depressants, including skeletal muscle relaxants, may cause respiratory depression, hypotension, and profound sedation or potentially result in coma. When such combined therapy is contemplated, the dose of one or both agents should be significantly reduced. The use of concomitant CNS active drugs requires special patient care and observation).
No products indexed under this heading.

Metronidazole (The concomitant use of fentanyl with all CYP3A4 inhibitors may result in an increase in fentanyl plasma concentrations, which could increase or prolong adverse drug effects and may cause potentially fatal respiratory depression. Patients receiving fentanyl and any CYP3A4 inhibitor should be monitored for an extended period of time and dosage adjustments should be made if warranted). Products include:

Pylera 793

Metronidazole Benzoate (The concomitant use of fentanyl with all CYP3A4 inhibitors may result in an increase in fentanyl plasma concentrations, which could increase or prolong adverse drug effects and may cause potentially fatal respiratory depression. Patients receiving fentanyl and any CYP3A4 inhibitor should be monitored for an extended period of time and dosage adjustments should be made if warranted).
No products indexed under this heading.

Metronidazole Hydrochloride (The concomitant use of fentanyl with all CYP3A4 inhibitors may result in an increase in fentanyl plasma concentrations, which could increase or prolong adverse drug effects and may cause potentially fatal respiratory depression. Patients receiving fentanyl and any CYP3A4 inhibitor should be monitored for an extended period of time and dosage adjustments should be made if warranted).
No products indexed under this heading.

Metronidazole Sodium (The concomitant use of fentanyl with all CYP3A4 inhibitors may result in an increase in fentanyl plasma concentrations, which could increase or prolong adverse drug effects and may cause potentially fatal respiratory depression. Patients receiving fentanyl and any CYP3A4 inhibitor should be monitored for an extended period of time and dosage adjustments should be made if warranted).
No products indexed under this heading.

Miconazole (The concomitant use of fentanyl with all CYP3A4 inhibitors may result in an increase in fentanyl plasma concentrations, which could increase or prolong adverse drug effects and may cause potentially fatal respiratory depression. Patients receiving fentanyl and any CYP3A4 inhibitor should be monitored for an extended period of time and dosage adjustments should be made if warranted).
No products indexed under this heading.

Miconazole Nitrate (The concomitant use of fentanyl with all CYP3A4 inhibitors may result in an increase in fentanyl plasma concentrations, which could increase or prolong adverse drug effects and may cause potentially fatal respiratory depression. Patients receiving fentanyl and any CYP3A4 inhibitor should be monitored for an extended period of time and dosage adjustments should be made if warranted). Products include:

Vusion Ointment 3335

Midazolam Hydrochloride (The concomitant use of fentanyl with other cen-

511 **Interactions Index** **Duragesic**

tral nervous system depressants, including tranquilizers (eg, benzodiazepines) may cause respiratory depression, hypotension, and profound sedation, or potentially result in coma or death. When such combined therapy is contemplated, the dose of one or both agents should be significantly reduced. The use of concomitant CNS active drugs requires special patient care and observation).
No products indexed under this heading.

Mifepristone (The concomitant use of fentanyl with all CYP3A4 inhibitors may result in an increase in fentanyl plasma concentrations, which could increase or prolong adverse drug effects and may cause potentially fatal respiratory depression. Patients receiving fentanyl and any CYP3A4 inhibitor should be monitored for an extended period of time and dosage adjustments should be made if warranted).
No products indexed under this heading.

Mivacurium Chloride (The concomitant use of fentanyl with other CNS depressants, including skeletal muscle relaxants, may cause respiratory depression, hypotension, and profound sedation or potentially result in coma. When such combined therapy is contemplated, the dose of one or both agents should be significantly reduced. The use of concomitant CNS active drugs requires special patient care and observation).
No products indexed under this heading.

Moclobemide (Fentanyl is not recommended for use in patients who have received monoamine oxidase (MAO) inhibitors within 14 days because severe and unpredictable potentiation by MAO inhibitors has been reported with opioid analgesics).
No products indexed under this heading.

Modafinil (Co-administration with agents that induce CYP 3A4 activity may reduce the efficacy of fentanyl). Products include:
Provigil 983

Molindone Hydrochloride (The concomitant use of fentanyl with other CNS depressants, including tranquilizers, may cause respiratory depression, hypotension, and profound sedation or potentially result in coma. When such combined therapy is contemplated, the dose of one or both agents should be significantly reduced. The use of concomitant CNS active drugs requires special patient care and observation). Products include:
Moban 1108

Morphine Sulfate (The concomitant use of fentanyl with other CNS depressants, including other opioids, may cause repiratory depression, hypotension, and profound sedation or potentially result in coma. When such combined therapy is contemplated, the dose of one or both agents should be significantly reduced. The use of concomitant CNS active drugs requires special patient care and observation). Products include:
Avinza 1822
Embeda 1831
MS Contin 2803

Morphine Sulfate, Liposomal (The concomitant use of fentanyl with other CNS depressants, including other opioids, may cause repiratory depression, hypotension, and profound sedation or potentially result in coma. When such combined therapy is contemplated, the dose of one or both agents should be significantly reduced. The use of concomitant CNS active drugs requires special patient care and observation).
No products indexed under this heading.

Nafcillin Sodium (Co-administration with agents that induce CYP 3A4 activity may reduce the efficacy of fentanyl).
No products indexed under this heading.

Nefazodone Hydrochloride (The concomitant use of fentanyl with all CYP3A4 inhibitors (eg, nefazodone) may result in an increase in fentanyl plasma concentrations, which could increase or prolong adverse drug effects and may cause potentially fatal respiratory depression. Patients receiving fentanyl and any CYP3A4 inhibitor should be monitored for an extended period of time and dosage adjustments should be made if warranted).
No products indexed under this heading.

Nelfinavir Mesylate (The concomitant use of fentanyl with all CYP3A4 inhibitors (eg, nelfinavir) may result in an increase in fentanyl plasma concentrations, which could increase or prolong adverse drug effects and may cause potentially fatal respiratory depression. Patients receiving fentanyl and any CYP3A4 inhibitor should be monitored for an extended period of time and dosage adjustments should be made if warranted).
No products indexed under this heading.

Nevirapine (The concomitant use of fentanyl with all CYP3A4 inhibitors may result in an increase in fentanyl plasma concentrations, which could increase or prolong adverse drug effects and may cause potentially fatal respiratory depression. Patients receiving fentanyl and any CYP3A4 inhibitor should be monitored for an extended period of time and dosage adjustments should be made if warranted). Products include:
Viramune Oral Suspension 897
Viramune Tablets 897

Niacin (The concomitant use of fentanyl with all CYP3A4 inhibitors may result in an increase in fentanyl plasma concentrations, which could increase or prolong adverse drug effects and may cause potentially fatal respiratory depression. Patients receiving fentanyl and any CYP3A4 inhibitor should be monitored for an extended period of time and dosage adjustments should be made if warranted). Products include:
Advicor 402
Cardio Basics 3455
Niaspan 497
Simcor 524

Niacinamide (The concomitant use of fentanyl with all CYP3A4 inhibitors may result in an increase in fentanyl plasma concentrations, which could increase or prolong adverse drug effects and may cause potentially fatal respiratory depression. Patients receiving fentanyl and any CYP3A4 inhibitor should be monitored for an extended period of time and dosage adjustments should be made if warranted). Products include:
CitraNatal 90 DHA Capsules 2332
CitraNatal Assure 2332
CitraNatal Rx 2332
Heplive 607

Niacinamide Hydroiodide (The concomitant use of fentanyl with all CYP3A4 inhibitors may result in an increase in fentanyl plasma concentrations, which could increase or prolong adverse drug effects and may cause potentially fatal respiratory depression. Patients receiving fentanyl and any CYP3A4 inhibitor should be monitored for an extended period of time and dosage adjustments should be made if warranted).
No products indexed under this heading.

Nicotinamide (The concomitant use of fentanyl with all CYP3A4 inhibitors may result in an increase in fentanyl plasma concentrations, which could increase or prolong adverse drug effects and may cause potentially fatal respiratory depression. Patients receiving fentanyl and any CYP3A4 inhibitor should be monitored for an extended period of time and dosage adjustments should be made if warranted).
No products indexed under this heading.

Nifedipine (The concomitant use of fentanyl with all CYP3A4 inhibitors may result in an increase in fentanyl plasma concentrations, which could increase or prolong adverse drug effects and may cause potentially fatal respiratory depression. Patients receiving fentanyl and any CYP3A4 inhibitor should be monitored for an extended period of time and dosage adjustments should be made if warranted).
No products indexed under this heading.

Nitrous Oxide (The concomitant use of fentanyl with other CNS depressants, including general anesthetics, may cause respiratory depression, hypotension, and profound sedation or potentially result in coma. When such combined therapy is contemplated, the dose of one or both agents should be significantly reduced. The use of concomitant CNS active drugs requires special patient care and observation).
No products indexed under this heading.

Norfloxacin (The concomitant use of fentanyl with all CYP3A4 inhibitors may result in an increase in fentanyl plasma concentrations, which could increase or prolong adverse drug effects and may cause potentially fatal respiratory depression. Patients receiving fentanyl and any CYP3A4 inhibitor should be monitored for an extended period of time and dosage adjustments should be made if warranted). Products include:
Noroxin 2220

Olanzapine (The comcomitant use of fentanyl with other CNS depressants may cause respiratory depression, hypotension, and profound sedation or potentially result in coma. When such combined therapy is contemplated, the dose of one or both agents should be significantly reduced. The use of concomitant CNS active drugs requires special patient care and observation). Products include:
Symbyax 1965
Zyprexa 1984
Zyprexa IntraMuscular 1984
Zyprexa ZYDIS 1984

Omeprazole (The concomitant use of fentanyl with all CYP3A4 inhibitors may result in an increase in fentanyl plasma concentrations, which could increase or prolong adverse drug effects and may cause potentially fatal respiratory depression. Patients receiving fentanyl and any CYP3A4 inhibitor should be monitored for an extended period of time and dosage adjustments should be made if warranted).
No products indexed under this heading.

Orphenadrine Citrate (The concomitant use of fentanyl with other CNS depressants, including skeletal muscle relaxants, may cause respiratory depression, hypotension, and profound sedation or potentially result in coma. When such combined therapy is contemplated, the dose of one or both agents should be significantly reduced. The use of concomitant CNS active drugs requires special patient care and observation).
No products indexed under this heading.

Oxazepam (The concomitant use of fentanyl with other central nervous system depressants, including tranquilizers (eg, benzodiazepines) may cause respiratory depression, hypotension, and profound sedation, or potentially result in coma or death. When such combined therapy is contemplated, the dose of one or both agents should be significantly reduced. The use of concomitant CNS active drugs requires special patient care and observation).
No products indexed under this heading.

Oxcarbazepine (Co-administration with agents that induce CYP 3A4 activity may reduce the efficacy of fentanyl).
No products indexed under this heading.

Oxycodone Hydrochloride (The concomitant use of fentanyl with other CNS depressants, including other opioids, may cause repiratory depression, hypotension, and profound sedation or potentially result in coma. When such combined therapy is contemplated, the dose of one or both agents should be significantly reduced. The use of concomitant CNS active drugs requires special patient care and observation). Products include:
OxyContin 2807
Percocet 1121
Percodan 1124

Oxycodone Terephthalate (The concomitant use of fentanyl with other CNS depressants, including other opioids, may cause repiratory depression, hypotension, and profound sedation or potentially result in coma. When such combined therapy is contemplated, the dose of one or both agents should be significantly reduced. The use of concomitant CNS active drugs requires special patient care and observation).
No products indexed under this heading.

Oxymorphone Hydrochloride (The concomitant use of fentanyl with other CNS depressants, including other opioids, may cause repiratory depression, hypotension, and profound sedation or potentially result in coma. When such combined therapy is contemplated, the dose of one or both agents should be significantly reduced. The use of concomitant CNS active drugs requires special patient care and observation). Products include:
Opana 1110
Opana ER 1114

Pancuronium Bromide (The concomitant use of fentanyl with other CNS depressants, including skeletal muscle relaxants, may cause respiratory depression, hypotension, and profound sedation or potentially result in coma. When such combined therapy is contemplated, the dose of one or both agents should be significantly reduced. The use of concomitant CNS active drugs requires special patient care and observation).
No products indexed under this heading.

Pargyline Hydrochloride (Fentanyl is not recommended for use in patients who have received monoamine oxidase (MAO) inhibitors within 14 days because severe and unpredictable potentiation by MAO inhibitors has been reported with opioid analgesics).
No products indexed under this heading.

Paroxetine Hydrochloride (The concomitant use of fentanyl with all CYP3A4 inhibitors may result in an increase in fentanyl plasma concentrations, which could increase or prolong adverse drug effects and may cause potentially fatal respiratory depression. Patients receiving fentanyl and any CYP3A4 inhibitor should be monitored for an extended period of time and dosage adjustments should be made if warranted). Products include:
Paroxetine CR 2361
Paroxetine ER 2371
Paxil 1586
Paxil CR 1596

Pemoline (The use of concomitant CNS active drugs requires special patient care and observation).
No products indexed under this heading.

IMPORTANT NOTE: Always consult each drug listing in the patient's regimen for possible interactions.

(⊙ Described in PDR® for Ophthalmic Medicines)

IMPORTANT NOTE: Always consult each drug listing in the patient's regimen for possible interactions.

Theophylline Calcium Salicylate (Co-administration with agents that induce CYP 3A4 activity may reduce the efficacy of fentanyl).
No products indexed under this heading.

Theophylline Dihydroxypropyl (Glyceryl) (Co-administration with agents that induce CYP 3A4 activity may reduce the efficacy of fentanyl).
No products indexed under this heading.

Theophylline Ethylenediamine (Co-administration with agents that induce CYP 3A4 activity may reduce the efficacy of fentanyl).
No products indexed under this heading.

Theophylline Sodium Glycinate (Co-administration with agents that induce CYP 3A4 activity may reduce the efficacy of fentanyl).
No products indexed under this heading.

Thiamylal Sodium (The comcomitant use of fentanyl with other CNS depressants may cause respiratory depression, hypotension, and profound sedation or potentially result in coma. When such combined therapy is contemplated, the dose of one or both agents should be significantly reduced. The use of concomitant CNS active drugs requires special patient care and observation).
No products indexed under this heading.

Thioridazine (The concomitant use of fentanyl with other CNS depressants, including phenothiazines, may cause repiratory depression, hypotension, and profound sedation or potentially result in coma. When such combined therapy is contemplated, the dose of one or both agents should be significantly reduced. The use of concomitant CNS active drugs requires special patient care and observation).
No products indexed under this heading.

Thioridazine Hydrochloride (The concomitant use of fentanyl with other CNS depressants, including tranquilizers, may cause respiratory depression, hypotension, and profound sedation or potentially result in coma. When such combined therapy is contemplated, the dose of one or both agents should be significantly reduced. The use of concomitant CNS active drugs requires special patient care and observation). Products include:
Thioridazine Hydrochloride 2384

Thiothixene (The concomitant use of fentanyl with other CNS depressants, including tranquilizers, may cause respiratory depression, hypotension, and profound sedation or potentially result in coma. When such combined therapy is contemplated, the dose of one or both agents should be significantly reduced. The use of concomitant CNS active drugs requires special patient care and observation). Products include:
Thiothixene 2386

Thiothixene Hydrochloride (The comcomitant use of fentanyl with other CNS depressants may cause respiratory depression, hypotension, and profound sedation or potentially result in coma. When such combined therapy is contemplated, the dose of one or both agents should be significantly reduced. The use of concomitant CNS active drugs requires special patient care and observation).
No products indexed under this heading.

Tizanidine (The concomitant use of fentanyl with other CNS depressants, including skeletal muscle relaxants, may cause respiratory depression, hypotension, and profound sedation or potentially result in coma. When such combined therapy is contemplated, the dose of one or both agents should be significantly reduced. The use of concomitant CNS active drugs requires special patient care and observation).
No products indexed under this heading.

Tizanidine Hydrochloride (The concomitant use of fentanyl with other CNS depressants, including skeletal muscle relaxants, may cause respiratory depression, hypotension, and profound sedation or potentially result in coma. When such combined therapy is contemplated, the dose of one or both agents should be significantly reduced. The use of concomitant CNS active drugs requires special patient care and observation).
No products indexed under this heading.

Tranylcypromine Sulfate (Fentanyl is not recommended for use in patients who have received monoamine oxidase (MAO) inhibitors within 14 days because severe and unpredictable potentiation by MAO inhibitors has been reported with opioid analgesics). Products include:
Parnate 1584

Triamcinolone (Co-administration with agents that induce CYP 3A4 activity may reduce the efficacy of fentanyl).
No products indexed under this heading.

Triamcinolone Acetonide (Co-administration with agents that induce CYP 3A4 activity may reduce the efficacy of fentanyl). Products include:
Azmacort 408
Nasacort AQ 3019

Triamcinolone Diacetate (Co-administration with agents that induce CYP 3A4 activity may reduce the efficacy of fentanyl).
No products indexed under this heading.

Triamcinolone Hexacetonide (Co-administration with agents that induce CYP 3A4 activity may reduce the efficacy of fentanyl).
No products indexed under this heading.

Triazolam (The concomitant use of fentanyl with other central nervous system depressants, including tranquilizers (eg, benzodiazepines) may cause respiratory depression, hypotension, and profound sedation, or potentially result in coma or death. When such combined therapy is contemplated, the dose of one or both agents should be significantly reduced. The use of concomitant CNS active drugs requires special patient care and observation).
No products indexed under this heading.

Trifluoperazine Hydrochloride (The concomitant use of fentanyl with other CNS depressants, including tranquilizers, may cause respiratory depression, hypotension, and profound sedation or potentially result in coma. When such combined therapy is contemplated, the dose of one or both agents should be significantly reduced. The use of concomitant CNS active drugs requires special patient care and observation).
No products indexed under this heading.

Troglitazone (The concomitant use of fentanyl with all CYP3A4 inhibitors may result in an increase in fentanyl plasma concentrations, which could increase or prolong adverse drug effects and may cause potentially fatal respiratory depression. Patients receiving fentanyl and any CYP3A4 inhibitor should be monitored for an extended period of time and dosage adjustments should be made if warranted).
No products indexed under this heading.

Troleandomycin (The concomitant use of fentanyl with all CYP3A4 inhibitors (eg, troleandomycin) may result in an increase in fentanyl plasma concentrations, which could increase or prolong adverse drug effects and may cause potentially fatal respiratory depression. Patients receiving fentanyl and any CYP3A4 inhibitor should be monitored for an extended period of time and dosage adjustments should be made if warranted).
No products indexed under this heading.

Tubocurarine Chloride (The concomitant use of fentanyl with other CNS depressants, including skeletal muscle relaxants, may cause respiratory depression, hypotension, and profound sedation or potentially result in coma. When such combined therapy is contemplated, the dose of one or both agents should be significantly reduced. The use of concomitant CNS active drugs requires special patient care and observation).
No products indexed under this heading.

Valproate Sodium (The concomitant use of fentanyl with all CYP3A4 inhibitors may result in an increase in fentanyl plasma concentrations, which could increase or prolong adverse drug effects and may cause potentially fatal respiratory depression. Patients receiving fentanyl and any CYP3A4 inhibitor should be monitored for an extended period of time and dosage adjustments should be made if warranted).
No products indexed under this heading.

Vardenafil Hydrochloride (The concomitant use of fentanyl with all CYP3A4 inhibitors may result in an increase in fentanyl plasma concentrations, which could increase or prolong adverse drug effects and may cause potentially fatal respiratory depression. Patients receiving fentanyl and any CYP3A4 inhibitor should be monitored for an extended period of time and dosage adjustments should be made if warranted). Products include:
Levitra 3157

Vecuronium Bromide (The concomitant use of fentanyl with other CNS depressants, including skeletal muscle relaxants, may cause respiratory depression, hypotension, and profound sedation or potentially result in coma. When such combined therapy is contemplated, the dose of one or both agents should be significantly reduced. The use of concomitant CNS active drugs requires special patient care and observation).
No products indexed under this heading.

Verapamil Hydrochloride (The concomitant use of fentanyl with all CYP3A4 inhibitors (eg, verapamil) may result in an increase in fentanyl plasma concentrations, which could increase or prolong adverse drug effects and may cause potentially fatal respiratory depression. Patients receiving fentanyl and any CYP3A4 inhibitor should be monitored for an extended period of time and dosage adjustments should be made if warranted). Products include:
Tarka 534

Voriconazole (The concomitant use of fentanyl with all CYP3A4 inhibitors may result in an increase in fentanyl plasma concentrations, which could increase or prolong adverse drug effects and may cause potentially fatal respiratory depression. Patients receiving fentanyl and any CYP3A4 inhibitor should be monitored for an extended period of time and dosage adjustments should be made if warranted).
No products indexed under this heading.

Zafirlukast (The concomitant use of fentanyl with all CYP3A4 inhibitors may result in an increase in fentanyl plasma concentrations, which could increase or prolong adverse drug effects and may cause potentially fatal respiratory depression. Patients receiving fentanyl and any CYP3A4 inhibitor should be monitored for an extended period of time and dosage adjustments should be made if warranted). Products include:
Accolate 3612

Zaleplon (The concomitant use of fentanyl with other CNS depressants, including sedatives and hypnotics, may cause respiratory depression, hypotension, and profound sedation or potentially result in coma. When such combined therapy is contemplated, the dose of one or both agents should be significantly reduced. The use of concomitant CNS active drugs requires special patient care and observation).
No products indexed under this heading.

Zileuton (The concomitant use of fentanyl with all CYP3A4 inhibitors may result in an increase in fentanyl plasma concentrations, which could increase or prolong adverse drug effects and may cause potentially fatal respiratory depression. Patients receiving fentanyl and any CYP3A4 inhibitor should be monitored for an extended period of time and dosage adjustments should be made if warranted).
No products indexed under this heading.

Ziprasidone Hydrochloride (The comcomitant use of fentanyl with other CNS depressants may cause respiratory depression, hypotension, and profound sedation or potentially result in coma. When such combined therapy is contemplated, the dose of one or both agents should be significantly reduced. The use of concomitant CNS active drugs requires special patient care and observation). Products include:
Geodon 2723

Zolpidem Tartrate (The concomitant use of fentanyl with other CNS depressants, including sedatives and hypnotics, may cause respiratory depression, hypotension, and profound sedation or potentially result in coma. When such combined therapy is contemplated, the dose of one or both agents should be significantly reduced. The use of concomitant CNS active drugs requires special patient care and observation). Products include:
Ambien 2920
Ambien CR 2925

Food Interactions

Alcohol (The comcomitant use of fentanyl with other CNS depressants may cause respiratory depression, hypotension, and profound sedation or potentially result in coma. When such combined therapy is contemplated, the dose of one or both agents should be significantly reduced. The use of concomitant CNS active drugs requires special patient care and observation).

Beer, reduced-alcohol (Fentanyl may be expected to have additive CNS depressant effects when used in conjunction with alcohol. The concomitant use of fentanyl with alcohol may cause respiratory depression, hypotension, and profound sedation or potentially result in coma).

Beer, unspecified (Fentanyl may be expected to have additive CNS depressant effects when used in conjunction with alcohol. The concomitant use of fentanyl with alcohol may cause respiratory depression, hypotension, and profound sedation or potentially result in coma).

Grapefruit (The concomitant use of fentanyl with all CYP3A4 inhibitors may result in an increase in fentanyl plasma concentrations, which could increase or prolong adverse drug effects and may cause potentially fatal respiratory depression. Patients receiving fentanyl and any CYP3A4 inhibitor should be monitored for an extended period of time and dosage adjustments should be made if warranted).

Grapefruit Juice (The concomitant use of fentanyl with all CYP3A4 inhibitors (eg, grapefruit juice) may result in an increase in fentanyl plasma concentrations, which could increase or prolong adverse drug effects and may cause potentially fatal respiratory depression. Patients receiving fentanyl and any CYP3A4 inhibitor should be monitored for an extended period of time and dosage adjustments should be made if warranted).

Wine, Chianti (Fentanyl may be expected to have additive CNS depressant effects when used in conjunction with alcohol. The concomitant use of fentanyl with alcohol may cause respiratory depression, hypotension, and profound sedation or potentially result in coma).

Wine, Red (Fentanyl may be expected to have additive CNS depressant effects when used in conjunction with alcohol. The concomitant use of fentanyl with alcohol may cause respiratory depression, hypotension, and profound sedation or potentially result in coma).

Wine, unspecified (Fentanyl may be expected to have additive CNS depressant effects when used in conjunction with alcohol. The concomitant use of fentanyl with alcohol may cause respiratory depression, hypotension, and profound sedation or potentially result in coma).

Wine products (Fentanyl may be expected to have additive CNS depressant effects when used in conjunction with alcohol. The concomitant use of fentanyl with alcohol may cause respiratory depression, hypotension, and profound sedation or potentially result in coma).

DUREZOL OPHTHALMIC EMULSION

(Difluprednate) .... ⊙275
May interact with corticosteroids. Compounds in these categories include:

Alclometasone Dipropionate (Corticosteroid use may result in glaucoma with damage to the optic nerve, defects in visual acuity and fields of vision, and in posterior subcapsular cataract formation. Steroids should be used with caution in the presence of glaucoma and thus increase the hazard of secondary ocular infections. Employment of a corticosteroid medication in the treatment of patients with a history of herpes simplex requires great caution. The use of steroids after cataract surgery may delay healing and increase the incidence of bleb formation).
No products indexed under this heading.

Beclomethasone Dipropionate (Corticosteroid use may result in glaucoma with damage to the optic nerve, defects in visual acuity and fields of vision, and in posterior subcapsular cataract formation. Steroids should be used with caution in the presence of glaucoma and thus increase the hazard of secondary ocular infections. Employment of a corticosteroid medication in the treatment of patients with a history of herpes simplex requires great caution. The use of steroids after cataract surgery may delay healing and increase the incidence of bleb formation).
Products include:
Qvar 3398

Beclomethasone Dipropionate Monohydrate (Corticosteroid use may result in glaucoma with damage to the optic nerve, defects in visual acuity and fields of vision, and in posterior subcapsular cataract formation. Steroids should be used with caution in the

presence of glaucoma and thus increase the hazard of secondary ocular infections. Employment of a corticosteroid medication in the treatment of patients with a history of herpes simplex requires great caution. The use of steroids after cataract surgery may delay healing and increase the incidence of bleb formation). Products include:
Beconase AQ 1386

Betamethasone (Corticosteroid use may result in glaucoma with damage to the optic nerve, defects in visual acuity and fields of vision, and in posterior subcapsular cataract formation. Steroids should be used with caution in the presence of glaucoma and thus increase the hazard of secondary ocular infections. Employment of a corticosteroid medication in the treatment of patients with a history of herpes simplex requires great caution. The use of steroids after cataract surgery may delay healing and increase the incidence of bleb formation).
No products indexed under this heading.

Betamethasone Acetate (Corticosteroid use may result in glaucoma with damage to the optic nerve, defects in visual acuity and fields of vision, and in posterior subcapsular cataract formation. Steroids should be used with caution in the presence of glaucoma and thus increase the hazard of secondary ocular infections. Employment of a corticosteroid medication in the treatment of patients with a history of herpes simplex requires great caution. The use of steroids after cataract surgery may delay healing and increase the incidence of bleb formation).
No products indexed under this heading.

Betamethasone Benzoate (Corticosteroid use may result in glaucoma with damage to the optic nerve, defects in visual acuity and fields of vision, and in posterior subcapsular cataract formation. Steroids should be used with caution in the presence of glaucoma and thus increase the hazard of secondary ocular infections. Employment of a corticosteroid medication in the treatment of patients with a history of herpes simplex requires great caution. The use of steroids after cataract surgery may delay healing and increase the incidence of bleb formation).
No products indexed under this heading.

Betamethasone Dipropionate (Corticosteroid use may result in glaucoma with damage to the optic nerve, defects in visual acuity and fields of vision, and in posterior subcapsular cataract formation. Steroids should be used with caution in the presence of glaucoma and thus increase the hazard of secondary ocular infections. Employment of a corticosteroid medication in the treatment of patients with a history of herpes simplex requires great caution. The use of steroids after cataract surgery may delay healing and increase the incidence of bleb formation). Products include:
Diprolene Lotion 0.05% 3108
Diprolene Ointment 0.05% 3109
Diprolene AF Cream 0.05% 3107
Lotrisone 3163

Betamethasone Sodium Phosphate (Corticosteroid use may result in glaucoma with damage to the optic nerve, defects in visual acuity and fields of vision, and in posterior subcapsular cataract formation. Steroids should be used with caution in the presence of glaucoma and thus increase the hazard of secondary ocular infections. Employment of a corticosteroid medication in the treatment of patients with a history of herpes simplex requires great cau-

tion. The use of steroids after cataract surgery may delay healing and increase the incidence of bleb formation).
No products indexed under this heading.

Betamethasone Valerate (Corticosteroid use may result in glaucoma with damage to the optic nerve, defects in visual acuity and fields of vision, and in posterior subcapsular cataract formation. Steroids should be used with caution in the presence of glaucoma and thus increase the hazard of secondary ocular infections. Employment of a corticosteroid medication in the treatment of patients with a history of herpes simplex requires great caution. The use of steroids after cataract surgery may delay healing and increase the incidence of bleb formation). Products include:
Luxiq 3321

Budesonide (Corticosteroid use may result in glaucoma with damage to the optic nerve, defects in visual acuity and fields of vision, and in posterior subcapsular cataract formation. Steroids should be used with caution in the presence of glaucoma and thus increase the hazard of secondary ocular infections. Employment of a corticosteroid medication in the treatment of patients with a history of herpes simplex requires great caution. The use of steroids after cataract surgery may delay healing and increase the incidence of bleb formation). Products include:
Pulmicort Flexhaler 714
Symbicort 80/4.5 720
Symbicort 160/4.5 720

Ciclesonide (Corticosteroid use may result in glaucoma with damage to the optic nerve, defects in visual acuity and fields of vision, and in posterior subcapsular cataract formation. Steroids should be used with caution in the presence of glaucoma and thus increase the hazard of secondary ocular infections. Employment of a corticosteroid medication in the treatment of patients with a history of herpes simplex requires great caution. The use of steroids after cataract surgery may delay healing and increase the incidence of bleb formation).
No products indexed under this heading.

Cortisone Acetate (Corticosteroid use may result in glaucoma with damage to the optic nerve, defects in visual acuity and fields of vision, and in posterior subcapsular cataract formation. Steroids should be used with caution in the presence of glaucoma and thus increase the hazard of secondary ocular infections. Employment of a corticosteroid medication in the treatment of patients with a history of herpes simplex requires great caution. The use of steroids after cataract surgery may delay healing and increase the incidence of bleb formation).
No products indexed under this heading.

Desoximetasone (Corticosteroid use may result in glaucoma with damage to the optic nerve, defects in visual acuity and fields of vision, and in posterior subcapsular cataract formation. Steroids should be used with caution in the presence of glaucoma and thus increase the hazard of secondary ocular infections. Employment of a corticosteroid medication in the treatment of patients with a history of herpes simplex requires great caution. The use of steroids after cataract surgery may delay healing and increase the incidence of bleb formation).
No products indexed under this heading.

Dexamethasone (Corticosteroid use may result in glaucoma with damage to the optic nerve, defects in visual acuity and fields of vision, and in posterior subcapsular cataract formation. Steroids should be used with caution in the

presence of glaucoma and thus increase the hazard of secondary ocular infections. Employment of a corticosteroid medication in the treatment of patients with a history of herpes simplex requires great caution. The use of steroids after cataract surgery may delay healing and increase the incidence of bleb formation). Products include:
Ciprodex 583
Ozurdex .... ⊙223
Tobramycin and Dexamethasone Ophthalmic Suspension.............. ⊙251

Dexamethasone Acetate (Corticosteroid use may result in glaucoma with damage to the optic nerve, defects in visual acuity and fields of vision, and in posterior subcapsular cataract formation. Steroids should be used with caution in the presence of glaucoma and thus increase the hazard of secondary ocular infections. Employment of a corticosteroid medication in the treatment of patients with a history of herpes simplex requires great caution. The use of steroids after cataract surgery may delay healing and increase the incidence of bleb formation).
No products indexed under this heading.

Dexamethasone Phosphate (Corticosteroid use may result in glaucoma with damage to the optic nerve, defects in visual acuity and fields of vision, and in posterior subcapsular cataract formation. Steroids should be used with caution in the presence of glaucoma and thus increase the hazard of secondary ocular infections. Employment of a corticosteroid medication in the treatment of patients with a history of herpes simplex requires great caution. The use of steroids after cataract surgery may delay healing and increase the incidence of bleb formation).
No products indexed under this heading.

Dexamethasone Sodium (Corticosteroid use may result in glaucoma with damage to the optic nerve, defects in visual acuity and fields of vision, and in posterior subcapsular cataract formation. Steroids should be used with caution in the presence of glaucoma and thus increase the hazard of secondary ocular infections. Employment of a corticosteroid medication in the treatment of patients with a history of herpes simplex requires great caution. The use of steroids after cataract surgery may delay healing and increase the incidence of bleb formation).
No products indexed under this heading.

Dexamethasone Sodium Phosphate (Corticosteroid use may result in glaucoma with damage to the optic nerve, defects in visual acuity and fields of vision, and in posterior subcapsular cataract formation. Steroids should be used with caution in the presence of glaucoma and thus increase the hazard of secondary ocular infections. Employment of a corticosteroid medication in the treatment of patients with a history of herpes simplex requires great caution. The use of steroids after cataract surgery may delay healing and increase the incidence of bleb formation).
No products indexed under this heading.

Dexamethasone Sodium Phosphate Injection (Corticosteroid use may result in glaucoma with damage to the optic nerve, defects in visual acuity and fields of vision, and in posterior subcapsular cataract formation. Steroids should be used with caution in the presence of glaucoma and thus increase the hazard of secondary ocular infections. Employment of a corticosteroid medication in the treatment of patients with a history of herpes simplex requires great caution. The use of

---

IMPORTANT NOTE: Always consult each drug listing in the patient's regimen for possible interactions.

steroids after cataract surgery may delay healing and increase the incidence of bleb formation).
No products indexed under this heading.

Diflorasone Diacetate (Corticosteroid use may result in glaucoma with damage to the optic nerve, defects in visual acuity and fields of vision, and in posterior subcapsular cataract formation. Steroids should be used with caution in the presence of glaucoma and thus increase the hazard of secondary ocular infections. Employment of a corticosteroid medication in the treatment of patients with a history of herpes simplex requires great caution. The use of steroids after cataract surgery may delay healing and increase the incidence of bleb formation).
No products indexed under this heading.

Fludrocortisone Acetate (Corticosteroid use may result in glaucoma with damage to the optic nerve, defects in visual acuity and fields of vision, and in posterior subcapsular cataract formation. Steroids should be used with caution in the presence of glaucoma and thus increase the hazard of secondary ocular infections. Employment of a corticosteroid medication in the treatment of patients with a history of herpes simplex requires great caution. The use of steroids after cataract surgery may delay healing and increase the incidence of bleb formation).
No products indexed under this heading.

Flumethasone Pivalate (Corticosteroid use may result in glaucoma with damage to the optic nerve, defects in visual acuity and fields of vision, and in posterior subcapsular cataract formation. Steroids should be used with caution in the presence of glaucoma and thus increase the hazard of secondary ocular infections. Employment of a corticosteroid medication in the treatment of patients with a history of herpes simplex requires great caution. The use of steroids after cataract surgery may delay healing and increase the incidence of bleb formation).
No products indexed under this heading.

Flunisolide Hemihydrate (Corticosteroid use may result in glaucoma with damage to the optic nerve, defects in visual acuity and fields of vision, and in posterior subcapsular cataract formation. Steroids should be used with caution in the presence of glaucoma and thus increase the hazard of secondary ocular infections. Employment of a corticosteroid medication in the treatment of patients with a history of herpes simplex requires great caution. The use of steroids after cataract surgery may delay healing and increase the incidence of bleb formation).
No products indexed under this heading.

Fluticasone Furoate (Corticosteroid use may result in glaucoma with damage to the optic nerve, defects in visual acuity and fields of vision, and in posterior subcapsular cataract formation. Steroids should be used with caution in the presence of glaucoma and thus increase the hazard of secondary ocular infections. Employment of a corticosteroid medication in the treatment of patients with a history of herpes simplex requires great caution. The use of steroids after cataract surgery may delay healing and increase the incidence of bleb formation). Products include:
Veramyst 1713

Fluticasone Propionate (Corticosteroid use may result in glaucoma with damage to the optic nerve, defects in visual acuity and fields of vision, and in posterior subcapsular cataract formation. Steroids should be used with caution in the presence of glaucoma and thus increase the hazard of secondary ocular infections. Employment of a corticosteroid medication in the treatment of patients with a history of herpes simplex requires great caution. The use of steroids after cataract surgery may delay healing and increase the incidence of bleb formation). Products include:
Advair 100/50 1275
Advair 250/50 1275
Advair 500/50 1275
Advair HFA 45/21 1288
Advair HFA 115/21 1288
Advair HFA 230/21 1288
Flonase 1459
Flovent Diskus 1463
Flovent HFA 1470

Hydrocortisone (Corticosteroid use may result in glaucoma with damage to the optic nerve, defects in visual acuity and fields of vision, and in posterior subcapsular cataract formation. Steroids should be used with caution in the presence of glaucoma and thus increase the hazard of secondary ocular infections. Employment of a corticosteroid medication in the treatment of patients with a history of herpes simplex requires great caution. The use of steroids after cataract surgery may delay healing and increase the incidence of bleb formation).
No products indexed under this heading.

Hydrocortisone (Alcohol) (Corticosteroid use may result in glaucoma with damage to the optic nerve, defects in visual acuity and fields of vision, and in posterior subcapsular cataract formation. Steroids should be used with caution in the presence of glaucoma and thus increase the hazard of secondary ocular infections. Employment of a corticosteroid medication in the treatment of patients with a history of herpes simplex requires great caution. The use of steroids after cataract surgery may delay healing and increase the incidence of bleb formation).
No products indexed under this heading.

Hydrocortisone Acetate (Corticosteroid use may result in glaucoma with damage to the optic nerve, defects in visual acuity and fields of vision, and in posterior subcapsular cataract formation. Steroids should be used with caution in the presence of glaucoma and thus increase the hazard of secondary ocular infections. Employment of a corticosteroid medication in the treatment of patients with a history of herpes simplex requires great caution. The use of steroids after cataract surgery may delay healing and increase the incidence of bleb formation).
No products indexed under this heading.

Hydrocortisone Butyrate (Corticosteroid use may result in glaucoma with damage to the optic nerve, defects in visual acuity and fields of vision, and in posterior subcapsular cataract formation. Steroids should be used with caution in the presence of glaucoma and thus increase the hazard of secondary ocular infections. Employment of a corticosteroid medication in the treatment of patients with a history of herpes simplex requires great caution. The use of steroids after cataract surgery may delay healing and increase the incidence of bleb formation).
No products indexed under this heading.

Hydrocortisone Cypionate (Corticosteroid use may result in glaucoma with damage to the optic nerve, defects in visual acuity and fields of vision, and in posterior subcapsular cataract formation. Steroids should be used with caution in the presence of glaucoma and thus increase the hazard of secondary ocular infections. Employment of a corticosteroid medication in the treatment of patients with a history of herpes simplex requires great caution. The use of steroids after cataract surgery may delay healing and increase the incidence of bleb formation).
No products indexed under this heading.

Hydrocortisone Hemisuccinate (Corticosteroid use may result in glaucoma with damage to the optic nerve, defects in visual acuity and fields of vision, and in posterior subcapsular cataract formation. Steroids should be used with caution in the presence of glaucoma and thus increase the hazard of secondary ocular infections. Employment of a corticosteroid medication in the treatment of patients with a history of herpes simplex requires great caution. The use of steroids after cataract surgery may delay healing and increase the incidence of bleb formation).
No products indexed under this heading.

Hydrocortisone Probutate (Corticosteroid use may result in glaucoma with damage to the optic nerve, defects in visual acuity and fields of vision, and in posterior subcapsular cataract formation. Steroids should be used with caution in the presence of glaucoma and thus increase the hazard of secondary ocular infections. Employment of a corticosteroid medication in the treatment of patients with a history of herpes simplex requires great caution. The use of steroids after cataract surgery may delay healing and increase the incidence of bleb formation).
No products indexed under this heading.

Hydrocortisone Sodium Phosphate (Corticosteroid use may result in glaucoma with damage to the optic nerve, defects in visual acuity and fields of vision, and in posterior subcapsular cataract formation. Steroids should be used with caution in the presence of glaucoma and thus increase the hazard of secondary ocular infections. Employment of a corticosteroid medication in the treatment of patients with a history of herpes simplex requires great caution. The use of steroids after cataract surgery may delay healing and increase the incidence of bleb formation).
No products indexed under this heading.

Hydrocortisone Sodium Succinate (Corticosteroid use may result in glaucoma with damage to the optic nerve, defects in visual acuity and fields of vision, and in posterior subcapsular cataract formation. Steroids should be used with caution in the presence of glaucoma and thus increase the hazard of secondary ocular infections. Employment of a corticosteroid medication in the treatment of patients with a history of herpes simplex requires great caution. The use of steroids after cataract surgery may delay healing and increase the incidence of bleb formation).
No products indexed under this heading.

Hydrocortisone Valerate (Corticosteroid use may result in glaucoma with damage to the optic nerve, defects in visual acuity and fields of vision, and in posterior subcapsular cataract formation. Steroids should be used with caution in the presence of glaucoma and thus increase the hazard of secondary ocular infections. Employment of a corticosteroid medication in the treatment of patients with a history of herpes simplex requires great caution. The use of steroids after cataract surgery may delay healing and increase the incidence of bleb formation).
No products indexed under this heading.

Methylprednisolone (Corticosteroid use may result in glaucoma with damage to the optic nerve, defects in visual acuity and fields of vision, and in posterior subcapsular cataract formation. Steroids should be used with caution in the presence of glaucoma and thus increase the hazard of secondary ocular infections. Employment of a corticosteroid medication in the treatment of patients with a history of herpes simplex requires great caution. The use of steroids after cataract surgery may delay healing and increase the incidence of bleb formation).
No products indexed under this heading.

Methylprednisolone Acetate (Corticosteroid use may result in glaucoma with damage to the optic nerve, defects in visual acuity and fields of vision, and in posterior subcapsular cataract formation. Steroids should be used with caution in the presence of glaucoma and thus increase the hazard of secondary ocular infections. Employment of a corticosteroid medication in the treatment of patients with a history of herpes simplex requires great caution. The use of steroids after cataract surgery may delay healing and increase the incidence of bleb formation).
No products indexed under this heading.

Methylprednisolone Sodium Succinate (Corticosteroid use may result in glaucoma with damage to the optic nerve, defects in visual acuity and fields of vision, and in posterior subcapsular cataract formation. Steroids should be used with caution in the presence of glaucoma and thus increase the hazard of secondary ocular infections. Employment of a corticosteroid medication in the treatment of patients with a history of herpes simplex requires great caution. The use of steroids after cataract surgery may delay healing and increase the incidence of bleb formation).
No products indexed under this heading.

Mometasone Furoate (Corticosteroid use may result in glaucoma with damage to the optic nerve, defects in visual acuity and fields of vision, and in posterior subcapsular cataract formation. Steroids should be used with caution in the presence of glaucoma and thus increase the hazard of secondary ocular infections. Employment of a corticosteroid medication in the treatment of patients with a history of herpes simplex requires great caution. The use of steroids after cataract surgery may delay healing and increase the incidence of bleb formation). Products include:
Asmanex 3058
Elocon Cream 3111
Elocon Lotion 3112
Elocon Ointment 3114

Mometasone Furoate Monohydrate (Corticosteroid use may result in glaucoma with damage to the optic nerve, defects in visual acuity and fields of vision, and in posterior subcapsular cataract formation. Steroids should be used with caution in the presence of glaucoma and thus increase the hazard of secondary ocular infections. Employment of a corticosteroid medication in the treatment of patients with a history of herpes simplex requires great caution. The use of steroids after cataract surgery may delay healing and increase the incidence of bleb formation). Products include:
Nasonex 3166

Prednisolone (Corticosteroid use may result in glaucoma with damage to the optic nerve, defects in visual acuity and fields of vision, and in posterior subcapsular cataract formation. Steroids should be used with caution in the presence of glaucoma and thus increase the hazard of secondary ocular infections. Employment of a corticosteroid medication in the treatment of patients with a history of herpes simplex requires great caution. The use of steroids after cataract surgery may delay healing and increase the incidence of bleb formation).
No products indexed under this heading.

Prednisolone Acetate (Corticosteroid use may result in glaucoma with damage to the optic nerve, defects in visual acuity and fields of vision, and in posterior subcapsular cataract formation. Steroids should be used with caution in the presence of glaucoma and thus increase the hazard of secondary ocular infections. Employment of a corticosteroid medication in the treatment of patients with a history of herpes simplex requires great caution. The use of steroids after cataract surgery may delay healing and increase the incidence of bleb formation). Products include:

Prednisolone Sodium Phosphate (Corticosteroid use may result in glaucoma with damage to the optic nerve, defects in visual acuity and fields of vision, and in posterior subcapsular cataract formation. Steroids should be used with caution in the presence of glaucoma and thus increase the hazard of secondary ocular infections. Employment of a corticosteroid medication in the treatment of patients with a history of herpes simplex requires great caution. The use of steroids after cataract surgery may delay healing and increase the incidence of bleb formation).

No products indexed under this heading.

Prednisolone Tebutate (Corticosteroid use may result in glaucoma with damage to the optic nerve, defects in visual acuity and fields of vision, and in posterior subcapsular cataract formation. Steroids should be used with caution in the presence of glaucoma and thus increase the hazard of secondary ocular infections. Employment of a corticosteroid medication in the treatment of patients with a history of herpes simplex requires great caution. The use of steroids after cataract surgery may delay healing and increase the incidence of bleb formation).

No products indexed under this heading.

Prednisone (Corticosteroid use may result in glaucoma with damage to the optic nerve, defects in visual acuity and fields of vision, and in posterior subcapsular cataract formation. Steroids should be used with caution in the presence of glaucoma and thus increase the hazard of secondary ocular infections. Employment of a corticosteroid medication in the treatment of patients with a history of herpes simplex requires great caution. The use of steroids after cataract surgery may delay healing and increase the incidence of bleb formation).

No products indexed under this heading.

Prednisone sodium phosphate (Corticosteroid use may result in glaucoma with damage to the optic nerve, defects in visual acuity and fields of vision, and in posterior subcapsular cataract formation. Steroids should be used with caution in the presence of glaucoma and thus increase the hazard of secondary ocular infections. Employment of a corticosteroid medication in the treatment of patients with a history of herpes simplex requires great caution. The use of steroids after cataract surgery may delay healing and increase the incidence of bleb formation).

No products indexed under this heading.

Triamcinolone (Corticosteroid use may result in glaucoma with damage to the optic nerve, defects in visual acuity and fields of vision, and in posterior subcapsular cataract formation. Steroids should be used with caution in the presence of glaucoma and thus increase the hazard of secondary ocular infections. Employment of a cortico-

steroid medication in the treatment of patients with a history of herpes simplex requires great caution. The use of steroids after cataract surgery may delay healing and increase the incidence of bleb formation).

No products indexed under this heading.

Triamcinolone Acetonide (Corticosteroid use may result in glaucoma with damage to the optic nerve, defects in visual acuity and fields of vision, and in posterior subcapsular cataract formation. Steroids should be used with caution in the presence of glaucoma and thus increase the hazard of secondary ocular infections. Employment of a corticosteroid medication in the treatment of patients with a history of herpes simplex requires great caution. The use of steroids after cataract surgery may delay healing and increase the incidence of bleb formation). Products include:

Triamcinolone Diacetate (Corticosteroid use may result in glaucoma with damage to the optic nerve, defects in visual acuity and fields of vision, and in posterior subcapsular cataract formation. Steroids should be used with caution in the presence of glaucoma and thus increase the hazard of secondary ocular infections. Employment of a corticosteroid medication in the treatment of patients with a history of herpes simplex requires great caution. The use of steroids after cataract surgery may delay healing and increase the incidence of bleb formation).

No products indexed under this heading.

Triamcinolone Hexacetonide (Corticosteroid use may result in glaucoma with damage to the optic nerve, defects in visual acuity and fields of vision, and in posterior subcapsular cataract formation. Steroids should be used with caution in the presence of glaucoma and thus increase the hazard of secondary ocular infections. Employment of a corticosteroid medication in the treatment of patients with a history of herpes simplex requires great caution. The use of steroids after cataract surgery may delay healing and increase the incidence of bleb formation).

No products indexed under this heading.

DYAZIDE CAPSULES

(Hydrochlorothiazide, Triamterene) .... 1429 May interact with ACE inhibitors, antigout agents, antihypertensives, corticosteroids, insulin, lithium preparations, non-steroidal anti-inflammatory agents, nondepolarizing neuromuscular blocking agents, oral anticoagulants, oral hypoglycemic agents, potassium preparations, potassium sparing diuretics, and certain other agents. Compounds in these categories include:

Acarbose (Increased risk of severe hyponatremia).

No products indexed under this heading.

Acebutolol Hydrochloride (May add to potentiate the action of other hypertensives).

No products indexed under this heading.

ACTH (May intensify electrolyte imbalance, particularly hypokalemia).

No products indexed under this heading.

Alclometasone Dipropionate (May intensify electrolyte imbalance, particularly hypokalemia).

No products indexed under this heading.

Aliskiren (May add to potentiate the action of other hypertensives). Products include:

Allopurinol (Dyazide may raise the level of blood uric acid; may require dosage adjustment of antigout agent).

No products indexed under this heading.

Amiloride Hydrochloride (Concurrent use is contraindicated).

No products indexed under this heading.

Amlodipine Besylate (May add to potentiate the action of other hypertensives). Products include:

Amphotericin B (May intensify electrolyte imbalance, particularly hypokalemia).

No products indexed under this heading.

Anisindione (Effects of oral anticoagulants may be decreased).

No products indexed under this heading.

Atenolol (May add to potentiate the action of other hypertensives).

No products indexed under this heading.

Atracurium Besylate (Increased paralyzing effect).

No products indexed under this heading.

Beclomethasone Dipropionate (May intensify electrolyte imbalance, particularly hypokalemia). Products include:

Beclomethasone Dipropionate Monohydrate (May intensify electrolyte imbalance, particularly hypokalemia). Products include:

Benazepril Hydrochloride (May add to potentiate the action of other hypertensives).

No products indexed under this heading.

Benazepril Hydrochloride (May add to potentiate the action of other hypertensives; increased risk of hyperkalemia).

No products indexed under this heading.

Bendroflumethiazide (May add to potentiate the action of other hypertensives).

No products indexed under this heading.

Betamethasone (May intensify electrolyte imbalance, particularly hypokalemia).

No products indexed under this heading.

Betamethasone Acetate (May intensify electrolyte imbalance, particularly hypokalemia).

No products indexed under this heading.

Betamethasone Benzoate (May intensify electrolyte imbalance, particularly hypokalemia).

No products indexed under this heading.

Betamethasone Dipropionate (May intensify electrolyte imbalance, particularly hypokalemia). Products include:

Betamethasone Sodium Phosphate (May intensify electrolyte imbalance, particularly hypokalemia).

No products indexed under this heading.

Betamethasone Valerate (May intensify electrolyte imbalance, particularly hypokalemia). Products include:

Betaxolol Hydrochloride (May add to potentiate the action of other hypertensives).

No products indexed under this heading.

Bisoprolol Fumarate (May add to potentiate the action of other hypertensives).

No products indexed under this heading.

Blood, whole (Concurrent use of whole blood from blood bank with triamterene may result in hyperkalemia, especially in patients with renal insufficiency).

No products indexed under this heading.

Budesonide (May intensify electrolyte imbalance, particularly hypokalemia). Products include:

Candesartan Cilexetil (May add to potentiate the action of other hypertensives). Products include:

Captopril (May add to potentiate the action of other hypertensives). Products include:

Captopril (May add to potentiate the action of other hypertensives; increased risk of hyperkalemia). Products include:

Carteolol Hydrochloride (May add to potentiate the action of other hypertensives).

No products indexed under this heading.

Carvedilol (May add to potentiate the action of other hypertensives). Products include:

Carvedilol Phosphate (May add to potentiate the action of other hypertensives). Products include:

Celecoxib (Potential for acute renal failure). Products include:

Chlorothiazide (May add to potentiate the action of other hypertensives).

No products indexed under this heading.

Chlorothiazide Sodium (May add to potentiate the action of other hypertensives). Products include:

Chlorpropamide (Increased risk of severe hyponatremia).

No products indexed under this heading.

Chlorthalidone (May add to potentiate the action of other hypertensives). Products include:

Ciclesonide (May intensify electrolyte imbalance, particularly hypokalemia).

No products indexed under this heading.

Cisatracurium Besylate (Increased paralyzing effect). Products include:

Clonidine (May add to potentiate the action of other hypertensives). Products include:

Clonidine Hydrochloride (May add to potentiate the action of other hypertensives). Products include:

Colchicine (Dyazide may raise the level of blood uric acid; may require dosage adjustment of antigout agent).

No products indexed under this heading.

Cortisone Acetate (May intensify electrolyte imbalance, particularly hypokalemia).

No products indexed under this heading.

Deserpidine (May add to potentiate the action of other hypertensives).

No products indexed under this heading.

Desoximetasone (May intensify electrolyte imbalance, particularly hypokalemia).

No products indexed under this heading.

Dexamethasone (May intensify electrolyte imbalance, particularly hypokalemia). Products include:

IMPORTANT NOTE: Always consult each drug listing in the patient's regimen for possible interactions.

Dexamethasone Acetate (May intensify electrolyte imbalance, particularly hypokalemia).
  No products indexed under this heading.

Dexamethasone Phosphate (May intensify electrolyte imbalance, particularly hypokalemia).
  No products indexed under this heading.

Dexamethasone Sodium (May intensify electrolyte imbalance, particularly hypokalemia).
  No products indexed under this heading.

Dexamethasone Sodium Phosphate (May intensify electrolyte imbalance, particularly hypokalemia).
  No products indexed under this heading.

Dexamethasone Sodium Phosphate Injection (May intensify electrolyte imbalance, particularly hypokalemia).
  No products indexed under this heading.

Diazoxide (May add to potentiate the action of other hypertensives). Products include:

Diclofenac Epolamine (Potential for acute renal failure). Products include:

Diclofenac Potassium (Potential for acute renal failure).
  No products indexed under this heading.

Diclofenac Sodium (Potential for acute renal failure).
  No products indexed under this heading.

Dicumarol (Effects of oral anticoagulants may be decreased).
  No products indexed under this heading.

Diflorasone Diacetate (May intensify electrolyte imbalance, particularly hypokalemia).
  No products indexed under this heading.

Diltiazem Hydrochloride (May add to potentiate the action of other hypertensives). Products include:

Diltiazem Maleate (May add to potentiate the action of other hypertensives).
  No products indexed under this heading.

Doxacurium Chloride (Increased paralyzing effect).
  No products indexed under this heading.

Doxazosin Mesylate (May add to potentiate the action of other hypertensives).
  No products indexed under this heading.

d-Tubocurarine (Increased paralyzing effect).
  No products indexed under this heading.

Enalapril Maleate (May add to potentiate the action of other hypertensives).
  No products indexed under this heading.

Enalapril Maleate (May add to potentiate the action of other hypertensives; increased risk of hyperkalemia).
  No products indexed under this heading.

Enalaprilat (May add to potentiate the action of other hypertensives).
  No products indexed under this heading.

Enalaprilat (May add to potentiate the action of other hypertensives; increased risk of hyperkalemia).
  No products indexed under this heading.

Eprosartan Mesylate (May add to potentiate the action of other hypertensives). Products include:

Esmolol Hydrochloride (May add to potentiate the action of other hypertensives).
  No products indexed under this heading.

Etodolac (Potential for acute renal failure).
  No products indexed under this heading.

Febuxostat (Dyazide may raise the level of blood uric acid; may require dosage adjustment of antigout agent). Products include:

Felodipine (May add to potentiate the action of other hypertensives).
  No products indexed under this heading.

Fenoprofen Calcium (Potential for acute renal failure).
  No products indexed under this heading.

Fludrocortisone Acetate (May intensify electrolyte imbalance, particularly hypokalemia).
  No products indexed under this heading.

Flumethasone Pivalate (May intensify electrolyte imbalance, particularly hypokalemia).
  No products indexed under this heading.

Flunisolide Hemihydrate (May intensify electrolyte imbalance, particularly hypokalemia).
  No products indexed under this heading.

Flurbiprofen (Potential for acute renal failure).
  No products indexed under this heading.

Fluticasone Furoate (May intensify electrolyte imbalance, particularly hypokalemia). Products include:

Fluticasone Propionate (May intensify electrolyte imbalance, particularly hypokalemia). Products include:

Fosinopril Sodium (May add to potentiate the action of other hypertensives).
  No products indexed under this heading.

Fosinopril Sodium (May add to potentiate the action of other hypertensives; increased risk of hyperkalemia).
  No products indexed under this heading.

Furosemide (May add to potentiate the action of other hypertensives). Products include:

Gallamine (Increased paralyzing effect).
  No products indexed under this heading.

Gallamine Triethiodide (Increased paralyzing effect).
  No products indexed under this heading.

Glibenclamide (Thiazides may cause hyperglycemia and glycosuria; dosage alteration of oral antidiabetic agents may be required).
  No products indexed under this heading.

Glimepiride (Thiazides may cause hyperglycemia and glycosuria; dosage alteration of oral antidiabetic agents may be required). Products include:

Glipizide (Thiazides may cause hyperglycemia and glycosuria; dosage alteration of oral antidiabetic agents may be required).
  No products indexed under this heading.

Glyburide (Thiazides may cause hyperglycemia and glycosuria; dosage alteration of oral antidiabetic agents may be required).
  No products indexed under this heading.

Guanabenz Acetate (May add to potentiate the action of other hypertensives).
  No products indexed under this heading.

Guanethidine (May add to potentiate the action of other hypertensives).
  No products indexed under this heading.

Guanethidine Monosulfate (May add to potentiate the action of other hypertensives).
  No products indexed under this heading.

Guanethidine Sulfate (May add to potentiate the action of other hypertensives).
  No products indexed under this heading.

Hydralazine Hydrochloride (May add to potentiate the action of other hypertensives).
  No products indexed under this heading.

Hydrocortisone (May intensify electrolyte imbalance, particularly hypokalemia).
  No products indexed under this heading.

Hydrocortisone (Alcohol) (May intensify electrolyte imbalance, particularly hypokalemia).
  No products indexed under this heading.

Hydrocortisone Acetate (May intensify electrolyte imbalance, particularly hypokalemia).
  No products indexed under this heading.

Hydrocortisone Butyrate (May intensify electrolyte imbalance, particularly hypokalemia).
  No products indexed under this heading.

Hydrocortisone Cypionate (May intensify electrolyte imbalance, particularly hypokalemia).
  No products indexed under this heading.

Hydrocortisone Hemisuccinate (May intensify electrolyte imbalance, particularly hypokalemia).
  No products indexed under this heading.

Hydrocortisone Probutate (May intensify electrolyte imbalance, particularly hypokalemia).
  No products indexed under this heading.

Hydrocortisone Sodium Phosphate (May intensify electrolyte imbalance, particularly hypokalemia).
  No products indexed under this heading.

Hydrocortisone Sodium Succinate (May intensify electrolyte imbalance, particularly hypokalemia).
  No products indexed under this heading.

Hydrocortisone Valerate (May intensify electrolyte imbalance, particularly hypokalemia).
  No products indexed under this heading.

Hydroflumethiazide (May add to potentiate the action of other hypertensives).
  No products indexed under this heading.

Ibuprofen (Potential for acute renal failure). Products include:

Indapamide (May add to potentiate the action of other hypertensives). Products include:

Indomethacin (Potential for acute renal failure). Products include:

Indomethacin Sodium Trihydrate (Potential for acute renal failure). Products include:

Insulin (Thiazides may cause hyperglycemia, glycosuria and alter insulin requirements in diabetes; diabetes mellitus may become manifest during thiazide administration).
  No products indexed under this heading.

Insulin, Human, Zinc Suspension (Thiazides may cause hyperglycemia, glycosuria and alter insulin requirements in diabetes; diabetes mellitus may become manifest during thiazide administration).
  No products indexed under this heading.

Insulin, Human (rDNA origin) (Thiazides may cause hyperglycemia, glycosuria and alter insulin requirements in diabetes; diabetes mellitus may become manifest during thiazide administration). Products include:

Insulin, Human NPH (Thiazides may cause hyperglycemia, glycosuria and alter insulin requirements in diabetes; diabetes mellitus may become manifest during thiazide administration). Products include:

Insulin, Human Regular (Thiazides may cause hyperglycemia, glycosuria and alter insulin requirements in diabetes; diabetes mellitus may become manifest during thiazide administration). Products include:

Insulin, Human Regular and Human NPH Mixture (Thiazides may cause hyperglycemia, glycosuria and alter insulin requirements in diabetes; diabetes mellitus may become manifest during thiazide administration). Products include:

Insulin, NPH (Thiazides may cause hyperglycemia, glycosuria and alter insulin requirements in diabetes; diabetes mellitus may become manifest during thiazide administration).
  No products indexed under this heading.

Insulin, Regular (Thiazides may cause hyperglycemia, glycosuria and alter insulin requirements in diabetes; diabetes mellitus may become manifest during thiazide administration).
  No products indexed under this heading.

Insulin, Regular and NPH mixture (Thiazides may cause hyperglycemia, glycosuria and alter insulin requirements in diabetes; diabetes mellitus may become manifest during thiazide administration).
  No products indexed under this heading.

Insulin, Zinc Crystals (Thiazides may cause hyperglycemia, glycosuria and alter insulin requirements in diabetes; diabetes mellitus may become manifest during thiazide administration).
  No products indexed under this heading.

Insulin, Zinc Suspension (Thiazides may cause hyperglycemia, glycosuria and alter insulin requirements in diabetes; diabetes mellitus may become manifest during thiazide administration).
  No products indexed under this heading.

Insulin Aspart (Thiazides may cause hyperglycemia, glycosuria and alter insulin requirements in diabetes; diabetes mellitus may become manifest during thiazide administration).
  No products indexed under this heading.

Insulin Aspart, Human (Thiazides may cause hyperglycemia, glycosuria and alter insulin requirements in diabetes; diabetes mellitus may become manifest during thiazide administration). Products include:

Insulin Aspart, Human Regular (Thiazides may cause hyperglycemia, glycosuria and alter insulin requirements in diabetes; diabetes mellitus may become manifest during thiazide administration). Products include:

Insulin Aspart Protamine, Human (Thiazides may cause hyperglycemia,

IMPORTANT NOTE: Always consult each drug listing in the patient's regimen for possible interactions.

Prednisolone Sodium Phosphate (May intensify electrolyte imbalance, particularly hypokalemia).
No products indexed under this heading.

Prednisolone Tebutate (May intensify electrolyte imbalance, particularly hypokalemia).
No products indexed under this heading.

Prednisone (May intensify electrolyte imbalance, particularly hypokalemia).
No products indexed under this heading.

Prednisone sodium phosphate (May intensify electrolyte imbalance, particularly hypokalemia).
No products indexed under this heading.

Probenecid (Dyazide may raise the level of blood uric acid; may require dosage adjustment of antigout agent).
No products indexed under this heading.

Propranolol Hydrochloride (May add to potentiate the action of other hypertensives). Products include:
InnoPran XL 1517

Quinapril Hydrochloride (May add to potentiate the action of other hypertensives; increased risk of hyperkalemia).
No products indexed under this heading.

Quinapril Hydrochloride (May add to potentiate the action of other hypertensives).
No products indexed under this heading.

Ramipril (May add to potentiate the action of other hypertensives).
No products indexed under this heading.

Ramipril (May add to potentiate the action of other hypertensives; increased risk of hyperkalemia).
No products indexed under this heading.

Rapacuronium Bromide (Increased paralyzing effect).
No products indexed under this heading.

Rauwolfia Serpentina (May add to potentiate the action of other hypertensives).
No products indexed under this heading.

Repaglinide (Thiazides may cause hyperglycemia and glycosuria; dosage alteration of oral antidiabetic agents may be required).
No products indexed under this heading.

Rescinnamine (May add to potentiate the action of other hypertensives).
No products indexed under this heading.

Reserpine (May add to potentiate the action of other hypertensives).
No products indexed under this heading.

Rocuronium Bromide (Increased paralyzing effect). Products include:
Zemuron 3249

Rofecoxib (Potential for acute renal failure).
No products indexed under this heading.

Rosiglitazone Maleate (Thiazides may cause hyperglycemia and glycosuria; dosage alteration of oral antidiabetic agents may be required). Products include:
Avandamet 1345
Avandaryl 1356
Avandia 1366

Salt Substitutes (Concurrent use of salt substitues with triamterene may result in hyperkalemia, especially in patients with renal insufficiency).
No products indexed under this heading.

Sitagliptin Phosphate (Thiazides may cause hyperglycemia and glycosuria; dosage alteration of oral antidiabetic agents may be required). Products include:
Janumet 2188
Januvia 2196

Sodium Nitroprusside (May add to potentiate the action of other hypertensives).
No products indexed under this heading.

Sodium Polystyrene Sulfonate (May result in fluid retention).
No products indexed under this heading.

Sotalol Hydrochloride (May add to potentiate the action of other hypertensives).
No products indexed under this heading.

Spirapril Hydrochloride (May add to potentiate the action of other hypertensives).
No products indexed under this heading.

Spirapril Hydrochloride (May add to potentiate the action of other hypertensives; increased risk of hyperkalemia).
No products indexed under this heading.

Spironolactone (Concurrent use is contraindicated).
No products indexed under this heading.

Sulfinpyrazone (Dyazide may raise the level of blood uric acid; may require dosage adjustment of antigout agent).
No products indexed under this heading.

Sulindac (Potential for acute renal failure). Products include:
Clinoril 2098

Telmisartan (May add to potentiate the action of other hypertensives). Products include:
Micardis 887
Micardis HCT 889

Terazosin Hydrochloride (May add to potentiate the action of other hypertensives).
No products indexed under this heading.

Timolol Maleate (May add to potentiate the action of other hypertensives). Products include:
Combigan 601
Dorzolamide Hydrochloride/Timolol Maleate Ophthalmic Solution .... ⊙243
Timoptic in Ocudose .... ⊙231

Tolazamide (Thiazides may cause hyperglycemia and glycosuria; dosage alteration of oral antidiabetic agents may be required).
No products indexed under this heading.

Tolbutamide (Thiazides may cause hyperglycemia and glycosuria; dosage alteration of oral antidiabetic agents may be required).
No products indexed under this heading.

Tolmetin Sodium (Potential for acute renal failure).
No products indexed under this heading.

Torsemide (May add to potentiate the action of other hypertensives).
No products indexed under this heading.

Trandolapril (May add to potentiate the action of other hypertensives). Products include:
Mavik 489
Tarka 534

Trandolapril (May add to potentiate the action of other hypertensives; increased risk of hyperkalemia). Products include:
Mavik 489
Tarka 534

Triamcinolone (May intensify electrolyte imbalance, particularly hypokalemia).
No products indexed under this heading.

Triamcinolone Acetonide (May intensify electrolyte imbalance, particularly hypokalemia). Products include:
Azmacort 408
Nasacort AQ 3019

Triamcinolone Diacetate (May intensify electrolyte imbalance, particularly hypokalemia).
No products indexed under this heading.

Triamcinolone Hexacetonide (May intensify electrolyte imbalance, particularly hypokalemia).
No products indexed under this heading.

Trimethaphan Camsylate (May add to potentiate the action of other hypertensives).
No products indexed under this heading.

Troglitazone (Thiazides may cause hyperglycemia and glycosuria; dosage alteration of oral antidiabetic agents may be required).
No products indexed under this heading.

Tubocurarine Chloride (Increased paralyzing effect).
No products indexed under this heading.

Valdecoxib (Potential for acute renal failure).
No products indexed under this heading.

Valsartan (May add to potentiate the action of other hypertensives). Products include:
Diovan 2413
Diovan HCT 2419
Exforge 2443
Exforge HCT 2449
Valturna 3637

Vecuronium Bromide (Increased paralyzing effect).
No products indexed under this heading.

Verapamil Hydrochloride (May add to potentiate the action of other hypertensives). Products include:
Tarka 534

Warfarin Sodium (Effects of oral anticoagulants may be decreased).
No products indexed under this heading.

Food Interactions

Milk, low salt (Concurrent use of low-salt milk with triamterene may result in hyperkalemia, especially in patients with renal insufficiency).

DYNACIRC CR CONTROLLED RELEASE TABLETS

(Isradipine) 1432
May interact with beta-blockers, and certain other agents. Compounds in these categories include:

Acebutolol Hydrochloride (Caution should be exercised when using isradipine in congestive heart failure patients, particularly in combination with a β-blocker. Severe hypotension has been reported during fentanyl anesthesia with concomitant use of a β-blocker and a calcium channel blocker. An increased volume of circulating fluids might be required if such an interaction were to occur).
No products indexed under this heading.

Atenolol (Caution should be exercised when using isradipine in congestive heart failure patients, particularly in combination with a β-blocker. Severe hypotension has been reported during fentanyl anesthesia with concomitant use of a β-blocker and a calcium channel blocker. An increased volume of circulating fluids might be required if such an interaction were to occur).
No products indexed under this heading.

Betaxolol Hydrochloride (Caution should be exercised when using isradipine in congestive heart failure patients, particularly in combination with a β-blocker. Severe hypotension has been reported during fentanyl anesthesia with concomitant use of a β-blocker and a calcium channel blocker. An increased volume of circulating fluids might be required if such an interaction were to occur).
No products indexed under this heading.

Bisoprolol Fumarate (Caution should be exercised when using isradipine in congestive heart failure patients, particularly in combination with a β-blocker. Severe hypotension has been reported during fentanyl anesthesia with concomitant use of a β-blocker and a calcium channel blocker. An increased volume of circulating fluids might be required if such an interaction were to occur).
No products indexed under this heading.

Carteolol Hydrochloride (Caution should be exercised when using isradipine in congestive heart failure patients, particularly in combination with a β-blocker. Severe hypotension has been reported during fentanyl anesthesia with concomitant use of a β-blocker and a calcium channel blocker. An increased volume of circulating fluids might be required if such an interaction were to occur).
No products indexed under this heading.

Carvedilol (Caution should be exercised when using isradipine in congestive heart failure patients, particularly in combination with a β-blocker. Severe hypotension has been reported during fentanyl anesthesia with concomitant use of a β-blocker and a calcium channel blocker. An increased volume of circulating fluids might be required if such an interaction were to occur). Products include:
Coreg 1409

Carvedilol Phosphate (Caution should be exercised when using isradipine in congestive heart failure patients, particularly in combination with a β-blocker. Severe hypotension has been reported during fentanyl anesthesia with concomitant use of a β-blocker and a calcium channel blocker. An increased volume of circulating fluids might be required if such an interaction were to occur). Products include:
Coreg CR 1416

Esmolol Hydrochloride (Caution should be exercised when using isradipine in congestive heart failure patients, particularly in combination with a β-blocker. Severe hypotension has been reported during fentanyl anesthesia with concomitant use of a β-blocker and a calcium channel blocker. An increased volume of circulating fluids might be required if such an interaction were to occur).
No products indexed under this heading.

Fentanyl (Severe hypotension has been reported during fentanyl anesthesia with concomitant use of β-blocker and a calcium channel blocker. An increased volume of circulating fluids might be required if such an interaction were to occur). Products include:
Duragesic 2604
Fentanyl Transdermal System 2346
Onsolis 2054

Fentanyl Citrate (Severe hypotension has been reported during fentanyl anesthesia with concomitant use of β-blocker and a calcium channel blocker. An increased volume of circulating fluids might be required if such an interaction were to occur). Products include:
Fentora 966

Hydrochlorothiazide (In a study in hypertensive patients, addition of isradipine to existing hydrochlorothiazide therapy did not result in any unexpected adverse effects, and isradipine had an additional antihypertensive effect). Products include:
Atacand HCT 700
Avalide 2956
Benicar HCT 1017
Diovan HCT 2419
Dyazide 1429
Exforge HCT 2449
Hyzaar 2162
Hyzaar 100-12.5 2162
Micardis HCT 889
Prinzide 2246
Tekturna HCT 2541
Teveten HCT 541

Labetalol Hydrochloride (Caution should be exercised when using isradipine in congestive heart failure

patients, particularly in combination with a β-blocker. Severe hypotension has been reported during fentanyl anesthesia with concomitant use of a β-blocker and a calcium channel blocker. An increased volume of circulating fluids might be required if such an interaction were to occur).

No products indexed under this heading.

Levobunolol Hydrochloride (Caution should be exercised when using isradipine in congestive heart failure patients, particularly in combination with a β-blocker. Severe hypotension has been reported during fentanyl anesthesia with concomitant use of a β-blocker and a calcium channel blocker. An increased volume of circulating fluids might be required if such an interaction were to occur).

No products indexed under this heading.

Metipranolol Hydrochloride (Caution should be exercised when using isradipine in congestive heart failure patients, particularly in combination with a β-blocker. Severe hypotension has been reported during fentanyl anesthesia with concomitant use of a β-blocker and a calcium channel blocker. An increased volume of circulating fluids might be required if such an interaction were to occur).

No products indexed under this heading.

Metoprolol Succinate (Caution should be exercised when using isradipine in congestive heart failure patients, particularly in combination with a β-blocker. Severe hypotension has been reported during fentanyl anesthesia with concomitant use of a β-blocker and a calcium channel blocker. An increased volume of circulating fluids might be required if such an interaction were to occur). Products include:
Toprol XL 732

Metoprolol Tartrate (Caution should be exercised when using isradipine in congestive heart failure patients, particularly in combination with a β-blocker. Severe hypotension has been reported during fentanyl anesthesia with concomitant use of a β-blocker and a calcium channel blocker. An increased volume of circulating fluids might be required if such an interaction were to occur).

No products indexed under this heading.

Nadolol (Caution should be exercised when using isradipine in congestive heart failure patients, particularly in combination with a β-blocker. Severe hypotension has been reported during fentanyl anesthesia with concomitant use of a β-blocker and a calcium channel blocker. An increased volume of circulating fluids might be required if such an interaction were to occur). Products include:
Nadolol 2359

Nebivolol (Caution should be exercised when using isradipine in congestive heart failure patients, particularly in combination with a β-blocker. Severe hypotension has been reported during fentanyl anesthesia with concomitant use of a β-blocker and a calcium channel blocker. An increased volume of circulating fluids might be required if such an interaction were to occur). Products include:
Bystolic 1147

Penbutolol Sulfate (Caution should be exercised when using isradipine in congestive heart failure patients, particularly in combination with a β-blocker. Severe hypotension has been reported during fentanyl anesthesia with concomitant use of a β-blocker and a calcium channel blocker. An increased volume of circulating fluids might be required if such an interaction were to occur).

No products indexed under this heading.

Pindolol (Caution should be exercised when using isradipine in congestive heart failure patients, particularly in combination with a β-blocker. Severe hypotension has been reported during fentanyl anesthesia with concomitant use of a β-blocker and a calcium channel blocker. An increased volume of circulating fluids might be required if such an interaction were to occur).

No products indexed under this heading.

Propranolol (Co-administration of propranolol had a small effect on the rate but no effect on the extent of isradipine bioavailability. Significant increases in AUC (27%) and C_{max} (58%) and decreases in T_{max} (23%) of propranolol were noted).

No products indexed under this heading.

Propranolol Hydrochloride (Co-administration of propranolol had a small effect on the rate but no effect on the extent of isradipine bioavailability. Significant increases in AUC (27%) and C_{max} (58%) and decreases in T_{max} (23%) of propranolol were noted). Products include:
InnoPran XL 1517

Sotalol Hydrochloride (Caution should be exercised when using isradipine in congestive heart failure patients, particularly in combination with a β-blocker. Severe hypotension has been reported during fentanyl anesthesia with concomitant use of a β-blocker and a calcium channel blocker. An increased volume of circulating fluids might be required if such an interaction were to occur).

No products indexed under this heading.

Timolol Hemihydrate (Caution should be exercised when using isradipine in congestive heart failure patients, particularly in combination with a β-blocker. Severe hypotension has been reported during fentanyl anesthesia with concomitant use of a β-blocker and a calcium channel blocker. An increased volume of circulating fluids might be required if such an interaction were to occur). Products include:
Betimol 3490

Timolol Maleate (Caution should be exercised when using isradipine in congestive heart failure patients, particularly in combination with a β-blocker. Severe hypotension has been reported during fentanyl anesthesia with concomitant use of a β-blocker and a calcium channel blocker. An increased volume of circulating fluids might be required if such an interaction were to occur). Products include:
Combigan 601
Dorzolamide
Hydrochloride/Timolol Maleate
Ophthalmic Solution .... ⊙243
Timoptic in Ocudose .... ⊙231

Food Interactions

Food, unspecified (Food has been shown to decrease the extent of bioavailability of isradipine by up to 25%).

Meal, unspecified (Food has been shown to decrease the extent of bioavailability of isradipine by up to 25%).

DYRENIUM CAPSULES

(Triamterene) 3495

May interact with ACE inhibitors, anesthetics, antihypertensives, diuretics, insulin, lithium preparations, non-steroidal anti-inflammatory agents, nondepolarizing neuromuscular blocking agents, oral hypoglycemic agents, potassium preparations, potassium sparing diuretics, preanesthetic medications, and certain other agents. Compounds in these categories include:

Acarbose (Triamterene may raise blood glucose levels; for adult-onset diabetes, dosage adjustments of hypoglycemic agents may be necessary during and/or after therapy).

No products indexed under this heading.

Acebutolol Hydrochloride (The effects of anti-hypertensive medication may be potentiated when given together with triamterene).

No products indexed under this heading.

Alfentanil Hydrochloride (The effects of anesthetic agents may be potentiated when given together with triamterene).

No products indexed under this heading.

Aliskiren (The effects of anti-hypertensive medication may be potentiated when given together with triamterene). Products include:
Tekturna 2538
Tekturna HCT 2541
Valturna 3637

Amiloride Hydrochloride (Concomitant use with other potassium sparing agents such as amiloride hydrochloride is contraindicated. Two deaths have been reported in patients receiving concomitant spironolactone and triamterene or triamterene with hydrochlorothiazide).

No products indexed under this heading.

Amlodipine Besylate (The effects of anti-hypertensive medication may be potentiated when given together with triamterene). Products include:
Azor 1010
Exforge 2443
Exforge HCT 2449

Articaine Hydrochloride (The effects of anesthetic agents may be potentiated when given together with triamterene).

No products indexed under this heading.

Atenolol (The effects of anti-hypertensive medication may be potentiated when given together with triamterene).

No products indexed under this heading.

Atracurium Besylate (The effects of skeletal muscle relaxants (nondepolarizing) may be potentiated when given together with triamterene).

No products indexed under this heading.

Benazepril Hydrochloride (Potassium-sparing agents should be used with caution in conjunction with angiotensin-converting enzyme (ACE) inhibitors due to an increased risk of hyperkalemia).

No products indexed under this heading.

Bendroflumethiazide (The effects of other diuretics may be potentiated when given together with triamterene).

No products indexed under this heading.

Benzocaine (The effects of anesthetic agents may be potentiated when given together with triamterene).

No products indexed under this heading.

Betaxolol Hydrochloride (The effects of anti-hypertensive medication may be potentiated when given together with triamterene).

No products indexed under this heading.

Bisoprolol Fumarate (The effects of anti-hypertensive medication may be potentiated when given together with triamterene).

No products indexed under this heading.

Blood, whole (Co-administration of triamterene with blood from blood bank (may contain up to 30 mEq of potassium per liter of plasma or up to 65 mEq per liter of whole blood when stored for more than 10 days) may promote serum potassium accumulation and possibly result in hyperkalemia, especially in patients with renal insufficiency).

No products indexed under this heading.

Bumetanide (The effects of other diuretics may be potentiated when given together with triamterene).

No products indexed under this heading.

Bupivacaine Hydrochloride (The effects of anesthetic agents may be potentiated when given together with triamterene).

No products indexed under this heading.

Candesartan Cilexetil (The effects of anti-hypertensive medication may be potentiated when given together with triamterene). Products include:
Atacand 697
Atacand HCT 700

Captopril (Potassium-sparing agents should be used with caution in conjunction with angiotensin-converting enzyme (ACE) inhibitors due to an increased risk of hyperkalemia). Products include:
Captopril 2341

Carteolol Hydrochloride (The effects of anti-hypertensive medication may be potentiated when given together with triamterene).

No products indexed under this heading.

Carvedilol (The effects of anti-hypertensive medication may be potentiated when given together with triamterene). Products include:
Coreg 1409

Carvedilol Phosphate (The effects of anti-hypertensive medication may be potentiated when given together with triamterene). Products include:
Coreg CR 1416

Celecoxib (A possible interaction resulting in acute renal failure has been reported in a few subjects when indomethacin, a nonsteroidal anti-inflammatory agent, was given with triamterene. Caution is advised in administering non-steroidal anti-inflammatory agents with triamterene). Products include:
Celebrex 3272

Chloroprocaine Hydrochloride (The effects of anesthetic agents may be potentiated when given together with triamterene).

No products indexed under this heading.

Chlorothiazide (The effects of other diuretics may be potentiated when given together with triamterene).

No products indexed under this heading.

Chlorothiazide Sodium (The effects of other diuretics may be potentiated when given together with triamterene). Products include:
Diuril Intravenous 2009

Chlorpropamide (Concurrent use of triamterene with chlorpropamide may increase the risk of severe hyponatremia).

No products indexed under this heading.

Chlorthalidone (The effects of other diuretics may be potentiated when given together with triamterene). Products include:
Clorpres 2344

Cisatracurium Besylate (The effects of skeletal muscle relaxants (nondepolarizing) may be potentiated when given together with triamterene). Products include:
Nimbex 503

Clonidine (The effects of anti-hypertensive medication may be potentiated when given together with triamterene). Products include:
Catapres-TTS 884

Clonidine Hydrochloride (The effects of anti-hypertensive medication may be potentiated when given together with triamterene). Products include:
Clorpres 2344

Cocaine Hydrochloride (The effects of anesthetic agents may be potentiated when given together with triamterene).

No products indexed under this heading.

IMPORTANT NOTE: Always consult each drug listing in the patient's regimen for possible interactions.

523 Interactions Index Dyrenium

Insulin, Regular and NPH mixture (Triamterene may raise blood glucose levels; for adult-onset diabetes, dosage adjustments of hypoglycemic agents may be necessary during and/or after therapy).
No products indexed under this heading.

Insulin, Zinc Crystals (Triamterene may raise blood glucose levels; for adult-onset diabetes, dosage adjustments of hypoglycemic agents may be necessary during and/or after therapy).
No products indexed under this heading.

Insulin, Zinc Suspension (Triamterene may raise blood glucose levels; for adult-onset diabetes, dosage adjustments of hypoglycemic agents may be necessary during and/or after therapy).
No products indexed under this heading.

Insulin Aspart (Triamterene may raise blood glucose levels; for adult-onset diabetes, dosage adjustments of hypoglycemic agents may be necessary during and/or after therapy).
No products indexed under this heading.

Insulin Aspart, Human (Triamterene may raise blood glucose levels; for adult-onset diabetes, dosage adjustments of hypoglycemic agents may be necessary during and/or after therapy). Products include:
NovoLog Mix 70/30 2581

Insulin Aspart, Human Regular (Triamterene may raise blood glucose levels; for adult-onset diabetes, dosage adjustments of hypoglycemic agents may be necessary during and/or after therapy). Products include:
NovoLog 2575

Insulin Aspart Protamine, Human (Triamterene may raise blood glucose levels; for adult-onset diabetes, dosage adjustments of hypoglycemic agents may be necessary during and/or after therapy). Products include:
NovoLog Mix 70/30 2581

Insulin Detemir (rDNA Origin) (Triamterene may raise blood glucose levels; for adult-onset diabetes, dosage adjustments of hypoglycemic agents may be necessary during and/or after therapy). Products include:
Levemir 2566

Insulin Glargine (Triamterene may raise blood glucose levels; for adult-onset diabetes, dosage adjustments of hypoglycemic agents may be necessary during and/or after therapy). Products include:
Lantus 2996

Insulin Glulisine (Triamterene may raise blood glucose levels; for adult-onset diabetes, dosage adjustments of hypoglycemic agents may be necessary during and/or after therapy). Products include:
Apidra 2937
Apidra SoloStar 2937

Insulin Lispro, Human (Triamterene may raise blood glucose levels; for adult-onset diabetes, dosage adjustments of hypoglycemic agents may be necessary during and/or after therapy). Products include:
Humalog 1910
Humalog Mix 1914
Humalog Mix75/25 1917

Insulin Lispro Protamine, Human (Triamterene may raise blood glucose levels; for adult-onset diabetes, dosage adjustments of hypoglycemic agents may be necessary during and/or after therapy). Products include:
Humalog Mix 1914
Humalog Mix75/25 1917

Irbesartan (The effects of anti-hypertensive medication may be potentiated when given together with triamterene). Products include:
Avalide 2956
Avapro 2962

Isoflurane (The effects of anesthetic agents may be potentiated when given together with triamterene).
No products indexed under this heading.

Isradipine (The effects of anti-hypertensive medication may be potentiated when given together with triamterene). Products include:
DynaCirc CR 1432

Ketamine Hydrochloride (The effects of anesthetic agents may be potentiated when given together with triamterene).
No products indexed under this heading.

Ketoprofen (A possible interaction resulting in acute renal failure has been reported in a few subjects when indomethacin, a nonsteroidal anti-inflammatory agent, was given with triamterene. Caution is advised in administering nonsteroidal anti-inflammatory agents with triamterene).
No products indexed under this heading.

Ketorolac Tromethamine (A possible interaction resulting in acute renal failure has been reported in a few subjects when indomethacin, a nonsteroidal anti-inflammatory agent, was given with triamterene. Caution is advised in administering nonsteroidal anti-inflammatory agents with triamterene). Products include:
Acuvail .... ⊙ 209

Labetalol Hydrochloride (The effects of anti-hypertensive medication may be potentiated when given together with triamterene).
No products indexed under this heading.

Levobupivacaine Hydrochloride (The effects of anesthetic agents may be potentiated when given together with triamterene).
No products indexed under this heading.

Lidocaine (The effects of anesthetic agents may be potentiated when given together with triamterene). Products include:
Lidoderm 1107

Lidocaine Base (The effects of anesthetic agents may be potentiated when given together with triamterene).
No products indexed under this heading.

Lidocaine Hydrochloride (The effects of anesthetic agents may be potentiated when given together with triamterene).
No products indexed under this heading.

Lisinopril (Potassium-sparing agents should be used with caution in conjunction with angiotensin-converting enzyme (ACE) inhibitors due to an increased risk of hyperkalemia). Products include:
Prinivil 2241
Prinzide 2246

Lithium (Caution should be used when lithium and diuretics are used concomitantly because diuretic-induced sodium loss may reduce the renal clearance of lithium and increase serum lithium levels with risk of lithium toxicity. Patients receiving such combined therapy should have serum lithium levels monitored closely and the lithium dosage adjusted if necessary).
No products indexed under this heading.

Lithium Carbonate (Caution should be used when lithium and diuretics are used concomitantly because diuretic-induced sodium loss may reduce the renal clearance of lithium and increase serum lithium levels with risk of lithium toxicity. Patients receiving such combined therapy should have serum lithium levels monitored closely and the lithium dosage adjusted if necessary).
No products indexed under this heading.

Lithium Citrate (Caution should be used when lithium and diuretics are used concomitantly because diuretic-induced sodium loss may reduce the renal clearance of lithium and increase serum lithium levels with risk of lithium toxicity. Patients receiving such combined therapy should have serum lithium levels monitored closely and the lithium dosage adjusted if necessary).
No products indexed under this heading.

Lorazepam (The effects of preanesthetic drugs may be potentiated when given together with triamterene).
No products indexed under this heading.

Losartan Potassium (The effects of anti-hypertensive medication may be potentiated when given together with triamterene). Products include:
Cozaar 2106
Hyzaar 2162
Hyzaar 100-12.5 2162

Mecamylamine Hydrochloride (The effects of anti-hypertensive medication may be potentiated when given together with triamterene).
No products indexed under this heading.

Meclofenamate Sodium (A possible interaction resulting in acute renal failure has been reported in a few subjects when indomethacin, a nonsteroidal anti-inflammatory agent, was given with triamterene. Caution is advised in administering nonsteroidal anti-inflammatory agents with triamterene).
No products indexed under this heading.

Mefenamic Acid (A possible interaction resulting in acute renal failure has been reported in a few subjects when indomethacin, a nonsteroidal anti-inflammatory agent, was given with triamterene. Caution is advised in administering nonsteroidal anti-inflammatory agents with triamterene).
No products indexed under this heading.

Meloxicam (A possible interaction resulting in acute renal failure has been reported in a few subjects when indomethacin, a nonsteroidal anti-inflammatory agent, was given with triamterene. Caution is advised in administering nonsteroidal anti-inflammatory agents with triamterene).
No products indexed under this heading.

Meperidine Hydrochloride (The effects of preanesthetic drugs may be potentiated when given together with triamterene).
No products indexed under this heading.

Mepivacaine Hydrochloride (The effects of anesthetic agents may be potentiated when given together with triamterene).
No products indexed under this heading.

Metformin Hydrochloride (Triamterene may raise blood glucose levels; for adult-onset diabetes, dosage adjustments of hypoglycemic agents may be necessary during and/or after therapy). Products include:
ActoPlus 3338
Avandamet 1345
Janumet 2188

Methohexital Sodium (The effects of anesthetic agents may be potentiated when given together with triamterene).
No products indexed under this heading.

Methyclothiazide (The effects of other diuretics may be potentiated when given together with triamterene).
No products indexed under this heading.

Methyldopa (The effects of anti-hypertensive medication may be potentiated when given together with triamterene).
No products indexed under this heading.

Methyldopate Hydrochloride (The effects of anti-hypertensive medication may be potentiated when given together with triamterene).
No products indexed under this heading.

Metocurine Iodide (The effects of skeletal muscle relaxants (non-depolarizing) may be potentiated when given together with triamterene).
No products indexed under this heading.

Metolazone (The effects of other diuretics may be potentiated when given together with triamterene).
No products indexed under this heading.

Metoprolol Succinate (The effects of anti-hypertensive medication may be potentiated when given together with triamterene). Products include:
Toprol XL 732

Metoprolol Tartrate (The effects of anti-hypertensive medication may be potentiated when given together with triamterene).
No products indexed under this heading.

Metyrosine (The effects of anti-hypertensive medication may be potentiated when given together with triamterene).
No products indexed under this heading.

Mibefradil Dihydrochloride (The effects of anti-hypertensive medication may be potentiated when given together with triamterene).
No products indexed under this heading.

Midazolam Hydrochloride (The effects of anesthetic agents may be potentiated when given together with triamterene).
No products indexed under this heading.

Miglitol (Triamterene may raise blood glucose levels; for adult-onset diabetes, dosage adjustments of hypoglycemic agents may be necessary during and/or after therapy).
No products indexed under this heading.

Minoxidil (The effects of anti-hypertensive medication may be potentiated when given together with triamterene).
No products indexed under this heading.

Mivacurium Chloride (The effects of skeletal muscle relaxants (non-depolarizing) may be potentiated when given together with triamterene).
No products indexed under this heading.

Moexipril Hydrochloride (Potassium-sparing agents should be used with caution in conjunction with angiotensin-converting enzyme (ACE) inhibitors due to an increased risk of hyperkalemia).
No products indexed under this heading.

Morphine Sulfate (The effects of preanesthetic drugs may be potentiated when given together with triamterene). Products include:
Avinza 1822
Embeda 1831
MS Contin 2803

Nabumetone (A possible interaction resulting in acute renal failure has been reported in a few subjects when indomethacin, a nonsteroidal anti-inflammatory agent, was given with triamterene. Caution is advised in administering nonsteroidal anti-inflammatory agents with triamterene).
No products indexed under this heading.

Nadolol (The effects of anti-hypertensive medication may be potentiated when given together with triamterene). Products include:
Nadolol 2359

Naproxen (A possible interaction resulting in acute renal failure has been reported in a few subjects when indomethacin, a nonsteroidal anti-inflammatory agent, was given with triamterene.

IMPORTANT NOTE: Always consult each drug listing in the patient's regimen for possible interactions.

Caution is advised in administering non-steroidal anti-inflammatory agents with triamterene). Products include:

Naproxen Sodium (A possible interaction resulting in acute renal failure has been reported in a few subjects when indomethacin, a nonsteroidal anti-inflammatory agent, was given with triamterene. Caution is advised in administering nonsteroidal anti-inflammatory agents with triamterene). Products include:

Nateglinide (Triamterene may raise blood glucose levels; for adult-onset diabetes, dosage adjustments of hypoglycemic agents may be necessary during and/or after therapy).
No products indexed under this heading.

Nebivolol (The effects of anti-hypertensive medication may be potentiated when given together with triamterene). Products include:

Nicardipine Hydrochloride (The effects of anti-hypertensive medication may be potentiated when given together with triamterene).
No products indexed under this heading.

Nifedipine (The effects of anti-hypertensive medication may be potentiated when given together with triamterene).
No products indexed under this heading.

Nisoldipine (The effects of anti-hypertensive medication may be potentiated when given together with triamterene).
No products indexed under this heading.

Nitroglycerin (The effects of anti-hypertensive medication may be potentiated when given together with triamterene). Products include:

Oxaprozin (A possible interaction resulting in acute renal failure has been reported in a few subjects when indomethacin, a nonsteroidal anti-inflammatory agent, was given with triamterene. Caution is advised in administering nonsteroidal anti-inflammatory agents with triamterene).
No products indexed under this heading.

Pancuronium Bromide (The effects of skeletal muscle relaxants (non-depolarizing) may be potentiated when given together with triamterene).
No products indexed under this heading.

Penbutolol Sulfate (The effects of anti-hypertensive medication may be potentiated when given together with triamterene).
No products indexed under this heading.

Penicillin G Potassium (Co-administration of triamterene with potassium-containing medications (such as parenteral penicillin G potassium) may promote serum potassium accumulation and possibly result in hyperkalemia because of the potassium-sparing nature of triamterene, especially in patients with renal insufficiency).
No products indexed under this heading.

Pentobarbital Sodium (The effects of preanesthetic drugs may be potentiated when given together with triamterene). Products include:

Perindopril Erbumine (Potassium-sparing agents should be used with caution in conjunction with angiotensin-converting enzyme (ACE) inhibitors due to an increased risk of hyperkalemia).
No products indexed under this heading.

Phenoxybenzamine Hydrochloride (The effects of anti-hypertensive medication may be potentiated when given together with triamterene). Products include:

Phentolamine Mesylate (The effects of anti-hypertensive medication may be potentiated when given together with triamterene).
No products indexed under this heading.

Phenylbutazone (A possible interaction resulting in acute renal failure has been reported in a few subjects when indomethacin, a nonsteroidal anti-inflammatory agent, was given with triamterene. Caution is advised in administering nonsteroidal anti-inflammatory agents with triamterene).
No products indexed under this heading.

Pindolol (The effects of anti-hypertensive medication may be potentiated when given together with triamterene).
No products indexed under this heading.

Pioglitazone Hydrochloride (Triamterene may raise blood glucose levels; for adult-onset diabetes, dosage adjustments of hypoglycemic agents may be necessary during and/or after therapy). Products include:

Pipecuronium Bromide (The effects of skeletal muscle relaxants (non-depolarizing) may be potentiated when given together with triamterene).
No products indexed under this heading.

Piroxicam (A possible interaction resulting in acute renal failure has been reported in a few subjects when indomethacin, a nonsteroidal anti-inflammatory agent, was given with triamterene. Caution is advised in administering nonsteroidal anti-inflammatory agents with triamterene).
No products indexed under this heading.

Polythiazide (The effects of other diuretics may be potentiated when given together with triamterene).
No products indexed under this heading.

Potassium Acid Phosphate (Co-administration of triamterene with dietary potassium supplements, potassium salts, or potassium containing salt substitutes is contraindicated. Concomitant use may promote serum potassium accumulation and possibly result in hyperkalemia because of the potassium-sparing nature of triamterene, especially in patients with renal insufficiency). Products include:

Potassium Bicarbonate (Co-administration of triamterene with dietary potassium supplements, potassium salts, or potassium containing salt substitutes is contraindicated. Concomitant use may promote serum potassium accumulation and possibly result in hyperkalemia because of the potassium-sparing nature of triamterene, especially in patients with renal insufficiency).
No products indexed under this heading.

Potassium Chloride (Co-administration of triamterene with dietary potassium supplements, potassium salts, or potassium containing salt substitutes is contraindicated. Concomitant use may promote serum potassium accumulation and possibly result in hyperkalemia because of the potassium-sparing nature of triamterene, especially in patients with renal insufficiency). Products include:

Potassium Citrate (Co-administration of triamterene with dietary potassium supplements, potassium salts, or potassium containing salt substitutes is contraindicated. Concomitant use may promote serum potassium accumulation and possibly result in hyperkalemia because of the potassium-sparing nature of triamterene, especially in patients with renal insufficiency). Products include:

Potassium Gluconate (Co-administration of triamterene with dietary potassium supplements, potassium salts, or potassium containing salt substitutes is contraindicated. Concomitant use may promote serum potassium accumulation and possibly result in hyperkalemia because of the potassium-sparing nature of triamterene, especially in patients with renal insufficiency).
No products indexed under this heading.

Potassium Phosphate (Co-administration of triamterene with dietary potassium supplements, potassium salts, or potassium containing salt substitutes is contraindicated. Concomitant use may promote serum potassium accumulation and possibly result in hyperkalemia because of the potassium-sparing nature of triamterene, especially in patients with renal insufficiency). Products include:

Prazosin Hydrochloride (The effects of anti-hypertensive medication may be potentiated when given together with triamterene).
No products indexed under this heading.

Prilocaine (The effects of anesthetic agents may be potentiated when given together with triamterene).
No products indexed under this heading.

Prilocaine Hydrochloride (The effects of anesthetic agents may be potentiated when given together with triamterene).
No products indexed under this heading.

Procaine (The effects of anesthetic agents may be potentiated when given together with triamterene).
No products indexed under this heading.

Procaine Hydrochloride (The effects of anesthetic agents may be potentiated when given together with triamterene).
No products indexed under this heading.

Promethazine Hydrochloride (The effects of preanesthetic drugs may be potentiated when given together with triamterene).
No products indexed under this heading.

Proparacaine Hydrochloride (The effects of anesthetic agents may be potentiated when given together with triamterene).
No products indexed under this heading.

Propofol (The effects of anesthetic agents may be potentiated when given together with triamterene).
No products indexed under this heading.

Propranolol Hydrochloride (The effects of anti-hypertensive medication may be potentiated when given together with triamterene). Products include:

Quinapril Hydrochloride (Potassium-sparing agents should be used with caution in conjunction with angiotensin-converting enzyme (ACE) inhibitors due to an increased risk of hyperkalemia).
No products indexed under this heading.

Ramipril (Potassium-sparing agents should be used with caution in conjunction with angiotensin-converting enzyme (ACE) inhibitors due to an increased risk of hyperkalemia).
No products indexed under this heading.

Rapacuronium Bromide (The effects of skeletal muscle relaxants (non-depolarizing) may be potentiated when given together with triamterene).
No products indexed under this heading.

Rauwolfia Serpentina (The effects of anti-hypertensive medication may be potentiated when given together with triamterene).
No products indexed under this heading.

Remifentanil Hydrochloride (The effects of anesthetic agents may be potentiated when given together with triamterene).
No products indexed under this heading.

Repaglinide (Triamterene may raise blood glucose levels; for adult-onset diabetes, dosage adjustments of hypoglycemic agents may be necessary during and/or after therapy).
No products indexed under this heading.

Rescinnamine (The effects of anti-hypertensive medication may be potentiated when given together with triamterene).
No products indexed under this heading.

Reserpine (The effects of anti-hypertensive medication may be potentiated when given together with triamterene).
No products indexed under this heading.

Rocuronium Bromide (The effects of skeletal muscle relaxants (non-depolarizing) may be potentiated when given together with triamterene). Products include:

Rofecoxib (A possible interaction resulting in acute renal failure has been reported in a few subjects when indomethacin, a nonsteroidal anti-inflammatory agent, was given with triamterene. Caution is advised in administering nonsteroidal anti-inflammatory agents with triamterene).
No products indexed under this heading.

Ropivacaine Hydrochloride (The effects of anesthetic agents may be potentiated when given together with triamterene).
No products indexed under this heading.

Rosiglitazone Maleate (Triamterene may raise blood glucose levels; for adult-onset diabetes, dosage adjustments of hypoglycemic agents may be necessary during and/or after therapy). Products include:

Salt Substitutes (Co-administration of triamterene with dietary potassium supplements, potassium salts, or potassium containing salt substitutes is contraindicated. Concomitant use may promote serum potassium accumulation and possibly result in hyperkalemia because of the potassium-sparing nature of triamterene, especially in patients with renal insufficiency).
No products indexed under this heading.

Secobarbital Sodium (The effects of preanesthetic drugs may be potentiated when given together with triamterene).
No products indexed under this heading.

Sitagliptin Phosphate (Triamterene may raise blood glucose levels; for adult-onset diabetes, dosage adjustments of hypoglycemic agents may be necessary during and/or after therapy). Products include:

Sodium Nitroprusside (The effects of anti-hypertensive medication may be potentiated when given together with triamterene).
No products indexed under this heading.

(⊙ Described in PDR® for Ophthalmic Medicines)

Sotalol Hydrochloride (The effects of anti-hypertensive medication may be potentiated when given together with triamterene).
No products indexed under this heading.

Spirapril Hydrochloride (Potassium-sparing agents should be used with caution in conjunction with angiotensin-converting enzyme (ACE) inhibitors due to an increased risk of hyperkalemia).
No products indexed under this heading.

Spironolactone (Concomitant use with other potassium sparing agents such as spironolactone is contraindicated. Two deaths have been reported in patients receiving concomitant spironolactone and triamterene or triamterene with hydrochlorothiazide).
No products indexed under this heading.

Sufentanil Citrate (The effects of anesthetic agents may be potentiated when given together with triamterene).
No products indexed under this heading.

Sulindac (A possible interaction resulting in acute renal failure has been reported in a few subjects when indomethacin, a nonsteroidal anti-inflammatory agent, was given with triamterene. Caution is advised in administering nonsteroidal anti-inflammatory agents with triamterene). Products include:
Clinoril 2098

Telmisartan (The effects of anti-hypertensive medication may be potentiated when given together with triamterene). Products include:
Micardis 887
Micardis HCT 889

Terazosin Hydrochloride (The effects of anti-hypertensive medication may be potentiated when given together with triamterene).
No products indexed under this heading.

Tetracaine (The effects of anesthetic agents may be potentiated when given together with triamterene).
No products indexed under this heading.

Tetracaine Hydrochloride (The effects of anesthetic agents may be potentiated when given together with triamterene).
No products indexed under this heading.

Thiamylal Sodium (The effects of anesthetic agents may be potentiated when given together with triamterene).
No products indexed under this heading.

Timolol Maleate (The effects of anti-hypertensive medication may be potentiated when given together with triamterene). Products include:
Combigan 601
Dorzolamide
Hydrochloride/Timolol Maleate
Ophthalmic Solution .... ⊙243
Timoptic in Ocudose .... ⊙231

Tolazamide (Triamterene may raise blood glucose levels; for adult-onset diabetes, dosage adjustments of hypoglycemic agents may be necessary during and/or after therapy).
No products indexed under this heading.

Tolbutamide (Triamterene may raise blood glucose levels; for adult-onset diabetes, dosage adjustments of hypoglycemic agents may be necessary during and/or after therapy).
No products indexed under this heading.

Tolmetin Sodium (A possible interaction resulting in acute renal failure has been reported in a few subjects when indomethacin, a nonsteroidal anti-inflammatory agent, was given with triamterene. Caution is advised in administering nonsteroidal anti-inflammatory agents with triamterene).
No products indexed under this heading.

Torsemide (The effects of other diuretics may be potentiated when given together with triamterene).
No products indexed under this heading.

Trandolapril (Potassium-sparing agents should be used with caution in conjunction with angiotensin-converting enzyme (ACE) inhibitors due to an increased risk of hyperkalemia). Products include:
Mavik 489
Tarka 534

Trimethaphan Camsylate (The effects of anti-hypertensive medication may be potentiated when given together with triamterene).
No products indexed under this heading.

Troglitazone (Triamterene may raise blood glucose levels; for adult-onset diabetes, dosage adjustments of hypoglycemic agents may be necessary during and/or after therapy).
No products indexed under this heading.

Tubocurarine Chloride (The effects of skeletal muscle relaxants (nondepolarizing) may be potentiated when given together with triamterene).
No products indexed under this heading.

Valdecoxib (A possible interaction resulting in acute renal failure has been reported in a few subjects when indomethacin, a nonsteroidal anti-inflammatory agent, was given with triamterene. Caution is advised in administering nonsteroidal anti-inflammatory agents with triamterene).
No products indexed under this heading.

Valsartan (The effects of anti-hypertensive medication may be potentiated when given together with triamterene). Products include:
Diovan 2413
Diovan HCT 2419
Exforge 2443
Exforge HCT 2449
Valturna 3637

Vecuronium Bromide (The effects of skeletal muscle relaxants (nondepolarizing) may be potentiated when given together with triamterene).
No products indexed under this heading.

Verapamil Hydrochloride (The effects of anti-hypertensive medication may be potentiated when given together with triamterene). Products include:
Tarka 534

Food Interactions

Milk, low salt (Co-administration of triamterene with low-salt milk (may contain up to 60 mEq of potassium per liter) may promote serum potassium accumulation and possibly result in hyperkalemia because of the potassium-sparing nature of triamterene, especially in patients with renal insufficiency).

Salt Substitutes, Potassium-Containing (Co-administration of triamterene with dietary potassium supplements, potassium salts, or potassium containing salt substitutes is contraindicated. Concomitant use may promote serum potassium accumulation and possibly result in hyperkalemia because of the potassium-sparing nature of triamterene, especially in patients with renal insufficiency).

DYSPORT FOR INJECTION

(Botulinum Toxin Type A) 2067
May interact with aminoglycosides, anticholinergics, curariform skeletal muscle relaxants, neuromuscular blocking agents, skeletal muscle relaxants, spasmolytic muscle relaxants, and certain other agents. Compounds in these categories include:

Amikacin Sulfate (Patients treated concomitantly with botulinum toxins and aminoglycosides should be observed closely because the effect of the botulinum toxin may be potentiated).
No products indexed under this heading.

Atracurium Besylate (Patients treated concomitantly with botulinum toxins and other agents interfering with neuromuscular transmission (eg, curare-like agents) should be observed closely because the effect of the botulinum toxin may be potentiated. Excessive weakness may be exaggerated by administration of a muscle relaxant before or after administration of botulinum toxin type a).
No products indexed under this heading.

Atropine Sulfate (Use of anticholinergic drugs after administration of botulinum toxin type a may potentiate systemic anticholinergic effects such as blurred vision). Products include:
Donnatal 2711

Baclofen (Excessive weakness may be exaggerated by administration of a muscle relaxant before or after administration of botulinum toxins).
No products indexed under this heading.

Belladonna Alkaloids (Use of anticholinergic drugs after administration of botulinum toxin type a may potentiate systemic anticholinergic effects such as blurred vision). Products include:
Hyland's Teething Tablets 3316

Benztropine Mesylate (Use of anticholinergic drugs after administration of botulinum toxin type a may potentiate systemic anticholinergic effects such as blurred vision).
No products indexed under this heading.

Biperiden Hydrochloride (Use of anticholinergic drugs after administration of botulinum toxin type a may potentiate systemic anticholinergic effects such as blurred vision).
No products indexed under this heading.

Botulinum Toxin Type B (The effect of administering different botulinum neurotoxin products at the same time or within several months of each other is unknown. Excessive weakness may be exacerbated by another administration of botulinum toxin prior to the resolution of the effects of a previously administered botulinum toxin).
No products indexed under this heading.

Carisoprodol (Excessive weakness may be exaggerated by administration of a muscle relaxant before or after administration of botulinum toxins).
No products indexed under this heading.

Chlorzoxazone (Excessive weakness may be exaggerated by administration of a muscle relaxant before or after administration of botulinum toxins).
No products indexed under this heading.

Cisatracurium Besylate (Patients treated concomitantly with botulinum toxins and other agents interfering with neuromuscular transmission (eg, curare-like agents) should be observed closely because the effect of the botulinum toxin may be potentiated. Excessive weakness may be exaggerated by administration of a muscle relaxant before or after administration of botulinum toxin type a). Products include:
Nimbex 503

Clidinium Bromide (Use of anticholinergic drugs after administration of botulinum toxin type a may potentiate systemic anticholinergic effects such as blurred vision).
No products indexed under this heading.

Cyclobenzaprine Hydrochloride (Excessive weakness may be exaggerated by administration of a muscle relaxant before or after administration of botulinum toxins). Products include:
Amrix 964

Dantrolene Sodium (Excessive weakness may be exaggerated by administration of a muscle relaxant before or after administration of botulinum toxins).
No products indexed under this heading.

Decamethonium (Patients treated concomitantly with botulinum toxins and other agents interfering with neuromuscular transmission (eg, curare-like agents) should be observed closely because the effect of the botulinum toxin may be potentiated).
No products indexed under this heading.

Dicyclomine Hydrochloride (Use of anticholinergic drugs after administration of botulinum toxin type a may potentiate systemic anticholinergic effects such as blurred vision). Products include:
Bentyl Capsules 780
Bentyl Injection 780
Bentyl Syrup 780
Bentyl Tablets 780

Dihydrostreptomycin (Patients treated concomitantly with botulinum toxins and aminoglycosides should be observed closely because the effect of the botulinum toxin may be potentiated).
No products indexed under this heading.

Doxacurium Chloride (Patients treated concomitantly with botulinum toxins and other agents interfering with neuromuscular transmission (eg, curare-like agents) should be observed closely because the effect of the botulinum toxin may be potentiated. Excessive weakness may be exaggerated by administration of a muscle relaxant before or after administration of botulinum toxin type a).
No products indexed under this heading.

d-Tubocurarine (Patients treated concomitantly with botulinum toxins and other agents interfering with neuromuscular transmission (eg, curare-like agents) should be observed closely because the effect of the botulinum toxin may be potentiated. Excessive weakness may be exaggerated by administration of a muscle relaxant before or after administration of botulinum toxin type a).
No products indexed under this heading.

Gallamine (Patients treated concomitantly with botulinum toxins and other agents interfering with neuromuscular transmission (eg, curare-like agents) should be observed closely because the effect of the botulinum toxin may be potentiated. Excessive weakness may be exaggerated by administration of a muscle relaxant before or after administration of botulinum toxin type a).
No products indexed under this heading.

Gallamine Triethiodide (Patients treated concomitantly with botulinum toxins and other agents interfering with neuromuscular transmission (eg, curare-like agents) should be observed closely because the effect of the botulinum toxin may be potentiated. Excessive weakness may be exaggerated by administration of a muscle relaxant before or after administration of botulinum toxin type a).
No products indexed under this heading.

Gentamicin (Patients treated concomitantly with botulinum toxins and aminoglycosides should be observed closely because the effect of the botulinum toxin may be potentiated).
No products indexed under this heading.

Gentamicin Sulfate (Patients treated concomitantly with botulinum toxins and aminoglycosides should be observed closely because the effect of the botulinum toxin may be potentiated). Products include:
Pred-G .... ⊙226, ⊙227

Glycopyrrolate (Use of anticholinergic drugs after administration of botulinum toxin type a may potentiate systemic anticholinergic effects such as blurred vision).
No products indexed under this heading.

IMPORTANT NOTE: Always consult each drug listing in the patient's regimen for possible interactions.

Hyoscyamine (Use of anticholinergic drugs after administration of botulinum toxin type a may potentiate systemic anticholinergic effects such as blurred vision).
No products indexed under this heading.

Hyoscyamine Sulfate (Use of anticholinergic drugs after administration of botulinum toxin type a may potentiate systemic anticholinergic effects such as blurred vision). Products include:
Donnatal 2711

Ipratropium Bromide (Use of anticholinergic drugs after administration of botulinum toxin type a may potentiate systemic anticholinergic effects such as blurred vision).
No products indexed under this heading.

Kanamycin Sulfate (Patients treated concomitantly with botulinum toxins and aminoglycosides should be observed closely because the effect of the botulinum toxin may be potentiated).
No products indexed under this heading.

Mepenzolate Bromide (Use of anticholinergic drugs after administration of botulinum toxin type a may potentiate systemic anticholinergic effects such as blurred vision).
No products indexed under this heading.

Metaxalone (Excessive weakness may be exaggerated by administration of a muscle relaxant before or after administration of botulinum toxins). Products include:
Skelaxin 1848

Methocarbamol (Excessive weakness may be exaggerated by administration of a muscle relaxant before or after administration of botulinum toxins).
No products indexed under this heading.

Metocurine Iodide (Patients treated concomitantly with botulinum toxins and other agents interfering with neuromuscular transmission (eg, curare-like agents) should be observed closely because the effect of the botulinum toxin may be potentiated. Excessive weakness may be exaggerated by administration of a muscle relaxant before or after administration of botulinum toxin type a).
No products indexed under this heading.

Mivacurium Chloride (Patients treated concomitantly with botulinum toxins and other agents interfering with neuromuscular transmission (eg, curare-like agents) should be observed closely because the effect of the botulinum toxin may be potentiated. Excessive weakness may be exaggerated by administration of a muscle relaxant before or after administration of botulinum toxin type a).
No products indexed under this heading.

Neomycin (Patients treated concomitantly with botulinum toxins and aminoglycosides should be observed closely because the effect of the botulinum toxin may be potentiated).
No products indexed under this heading.

Neomycin, oral (Patients treated concomitantly with botulinum toxins and aminoglycosides should be observed closely because the effect of the botulinum toxin may be potentiated).
No products indexed under this heading.

Neomycin Sulfate (Patients treated concomitantly with botulinum toxins and aminoglycosides should be observed closely because the effect of the botulinum toxin may be potentiated).
No products indexed under this heading.

Orphenadrine Citrate (Excessive weakness may be exaggerated by administration of a muscle relaxant before or after administration of botulinum toxins).
No products indexed under this heading.

Oxybutynin Chloride (Use of anticholinergic drugs after administration of botulinum toxin type a may potentiate systemic anticholinergic effects such as blurred vision).
No products indexed under this heading.

Pancuronium Bromide (Patients treated concomitantly with botulinum toxins and other agents interfering with neuromuscular transmission (eg, curare-like agents) should be observed closely because the effect of the botulinum toxin may be potentiated. Excessive weakness may be exaggerated by administration of a muscle relaxant before or after administration of botulinum toxin type a).
No products indexed under this heading.

Pipecuronium Bromide (Patients treated concomitantly with botulinum toxins and other agents interfering with neuromuscular transmission (eg, curare-like agents) should be observed closely because the effect of the botulinum toxin may be potentiated. Excessive weakness may be exaggerated by administration of a muscle relaxant before or after administration of botulinum toxin type a).
No products indexed under this heading.

Procyclidine Hydrochloride (Use of anticholinergic drugs after administration of botulinum toxin type a may potentiate systemic anticholinergic effects such as blurred vision).
No products indexed under this heading.

Propantheline Bromide (Use of anticholinergic drugs after administration of botulinum toxin type a may potentiate systemic anticholinergic effects such as blurred vision).
No products indexed under this heading.

Rapacuronium Bromide (Patients treated concomitantly with botulinum toxins and other agents interfering with neuromuscular transmission (eg, curare-like agents) should be observed closely because the effect of the botulinum toxin may be potentiated. Excessive weakness may be exaggerated by administration of a muscle relaxant before or after administration of botulinum toxin type a).
No products indexed under this heading.

Rocuronium Bromide (Patients treated concomitantly with botulinum toxins and other agents interfering with neuromuscular transmission (eg, curare-like agents) should be observed closely because the effect of the botulinum toxin may be potentiated. Excessive weakness may be exaggerated by administration of a muscle relaxant before or after administration of botulinum toxin type a). Products include:
Zemuron 3249

Scopolamine (Use of anticholinergic drugs after administration of botulinum toxin type a may potentiate systemic anticholinergic effects such as blurred vision). Products include:
Transderm Scōp 2397

Scopolamine Hydrobromide (Use of anticholinergic drugs after administration of botulinum toxin type a may potentiate systemic anticholinergic effects such as blurred vision). Products include:
Donnatal 2711

Streptomycin Sulfate (Patients treated concomitantly with botulinum toxins and aminoglycosides should be observed closely because the effect of the botulinum toxin may be potentiated).
No products indexed under this heading.

Succinylcholine Chloride (Patients treated concomitantly with botulinum toxins and other agents interfering with neuromuscular transmission (eg, curare-like agents) should be observed closely because the effect of the botulinum toxin may be potentiated).
No products indexed under this heading.

Tizanidine (Excessive weakness may be exaggerated by administration of a muscle relaxant before or after administration of botulinum toxins).
No products indexed under this heading.

Tizanidine Hydrochloride (Excessive weakness may be exaggerated by administration of a muscle relaxant before or after administration of botulinum toxins).
No products indexed under this heading.

Tobramycin (Patients treated concomitantly with botulinum toxins and aminoglycosides should be observed closely because the effect of the botulinum toxin may be potentiated). Products include:
Tobi Nebulizer 2546
Tobramycin and Dexamethasone Ophthalmic Suspension .... ⊙ 251
Zylet .... ⊙ 252

Tobramycin Sulfate (Patients treated concomitantly with botulinum toxins and aminoglycosides should be observed closely because the effect of the botulinum toxin may be potentiated).
No products indexed under this heading.

Tolterodine Tartrate (Use of anticholinergic drugs after administration of botulinum toxin type a may potentiate systemic anticholinergic effects such as blurred vision).
No products indexed under this heading.

Tridihexethyl Chloride (Use of anticholinergic drugs after administration of botulinum toxin type a may potentiate systemic anticholinergic effects such as blurred vision).
No products indexed under this heading.

Trihexyphenidyl Hydrochloride (Use of anticholinergic drugs after administration of botulinum toxin type a may potentiate systemic anticholinergic effects such as blurred vision).
No products indexed under this heading.

Tubocurarine Chloride (Patients treated concomitantly with botulinum toxins and other agents interfering with neuromuscular transmission (eg, curare-like agents) should be observed closely because the effect of the botulinum toxin may be potentiated. Excessive weakness may be exaggerated by administration of a muscle relaxant before or after administration of botulinum toxin type a).
No products indexed under this heading.

Vecuronium Bromide (Patients treated concomitantly with botulinum toxins and other agents interfering with neuromuscular transmission (eg, curare-like agents) should be observed closely because the effect of the botulinum toxin may be potentiated. Excessive weakness may be exaggerated by administration of a muscle relaxant before or after administration of botulinum toxin type a).
No products indexed under this heading.

DYSPORT FOR INJECTION

(Abobotulinumtoxina) 1813
May interact with aminoglycosides, anticholinergics, curariform skeletal muscle relaxants, neuromuscular blocking agents, skeletal muscle relaxants, spasmolytic muscle relaxants, and certain other agents. Compounds in these categories include:

Amikacin Sulfate (Patients treated concomitantly with botulinum toxins and aminoglycosides should be observed closely because the effect of the botulinum toxin may be potentiated).
No products indexed under this heading.

Atracurium Besylate (Patients treated concomitantly with botulinum toxins and other agents interfering with neuromuscular transmission (eg, curare-like agents) should be observed closely because the effect of the botulinum toxin may be potentiated).
No products indexed under this heading.

Atropine Sulfate (Use of anticholinergic drugs after administration of abobotulinumtoxinA may potentiate systemic anticholinergic effects such as blurred vision). Products include:
Donnatal 2711

Baclofen (Excessive weakness may also be exaggerated by administration of a muscle relaxant before or after administration of abobotulinumtoxinA).
No products indexed under this heading.

Belladonna Alkaloids (Use of anticholinergic drugs after administration of abobotulinumtoxinA may potentiate systemic anticholinergic effects such as blurred vision). Products include:
Hyland's Teething Tablets 3316

Benztropine Mesylate (Use of anticholinergic drugs after administration of abobotulinumtoxinA may potentiate systemic anticholinergic effects such as blurred vision).
No products indexed under this heading.

Biperiden Hydrochloride (Use of anticholinergic drugs after administration of abobotulinumtoxinA may potentiate systemic anticholinergic effects such as blurred vision).
No products indexed under this heading.

Botulinum Toxin Type B (The effect of administering different botulinum neurotoxin products at the same time or within several months of each other is unknown. Excessive weakness may be exacerbated by another administration of botulinum toxin prior to the resolution of the effects of a previously administered botulinum toxin).
No products indexed under this heading.

Carisoprodol (Excessive weakness may also be exaggerated by administration of a muscle relaxant before or after administration of abobotulinumtoxinA).
No products indexed under this heading.

Chlorzoxazone (Excessive weakness may also be exaggerated by administration of a muscle relaxant before or after administration of abobotulinumtoxinA).
No products indexed under this heading.

Cisatracurium Besylate (Patients treated concomitantly with botulinum toxins and other agents interfering with neuromuscular transmission (eg, curare-like agents) should be observed closely because the effect of the botulinum toxin may be potentiated). Products include:
Nimbex 503

Clidinium Bromide (Use of anticholinergic drugs after administration of abobotulinumtoxinA may potentiate systemic anticholinergic effects such as blurred vision).
No products indexed under this heading.

Cyclobenzaprine Hydrochloride (Excessive weakness may also be exaggerated by administration of a muscle relaxant before or after administration of abobotulinumtoxinA). Products include:
Amrix 964

Dantrolene Sodium (Excessive weakness may also be exaggerated by administration of a muscle relaxant before or after administration of abobotulinumtoxinA).
No products indexed under this heading.

Decamethonium (Patients treated concomitantly with botulinum toxins and other agents interfering with neuromuscular transmission (eg, curare-like agents) should be observed closely because the effect of the botulinum toxin may be potentiated).
No products indexed under this heading.

Dicyclomine Hydrochloride (Use of anticholinergic drugs after administration of abobotulinumtoxinA may potentiate systemic anticholinergic effects such as blurred vision). Products include:
Bentyl Capsules 780
Bentyl Injection 780
Bentyl Syrup 780
Bentyl Tablets 780

Dihydrostreptomycin (Patients treated concomitantly with botulinum toxins and aminoglycosides should be observed closely because the effect of the botulinum toxin may be potentiated).
No products indexed under this heading.

Doxacurium Chloride (Patients treated concomitantly with botulinum toxins and other agents interfering with neuromuscular transmission (eg, curare-like agents) should be observed closely because the effect of the botulinum toxin may be potentiated).
No products indexed under this heading.

d-Tubocurarine (Patients treated concomitantly with botulinum toxins and other agents interfering with neuromuscular transmission (eg, curare-like agents) should be observed closely because the effect of the botulinum toxin may be potentiated).
No products indexed under this heading.

Gallamine (Patients treated concomitantly with botulinum toxins and other agents interfering with neuromuscular transmission (eg, curare-like agents) should be observed closely because the effect of the botulinum toxin may be potentiated).
No products indexed under this heading.

Gallamine Triethiodide (Patients treated concomitantly with botulinum toxins and other agents interfering with neuromuscular transmission (eg, curare-like agents) should be observed closely because the effect of the botulinum toxin may be potentiated).
No products indexed under this heading.

Gentamicin (Patients treated concomitantly with botulinum toxins and aminoglycosides should be observed closely because the effect of the botulinum toxin may be potentiated).
No products indexed under this heading.

Gentamicin Sulfate (Patients treated concomitantly with botulinum toxins and aminoglycosides should be observed closely because the effect of the botulinum toxin may be potentiated).
Products include:
Pred-G .... ⊙ 226, ⊙ 227

Glycopyrrolate (Use of anticholinergic drugs after administration of abobotulinumtoxinA may potentiate systemic anticholinergic effects such as blurred vision).
No products indexed under this heading.

Hyoscyamine (Use of anticholinergic drugs after administration of abobotulinumtoxinA may potentiate systemic anticholinergic effects such as blurred vision).
No products indexed under this heading.

Hyoscyamine Sulfate (Use of anticholinergic drugs after administration of abobotulinumtoxinA may potentiate systemic anticholinergic effects such as blurred vision). Products include:
Donnatal 2711

Ipratropium Bromide (Use of anticholinergic drugs after administration of abobotulinumtoxinA may potentiate systemic anticholinergic effects such as blurred vision).
No products indexed under this heading.

Kanamycin Sulfate (Patients treated concomitantly with botulinum toxins and aminoglycosides should be observed closely because the effect of the botulinum toxin may be potentiated).
No products indexed under this heading.

Mepenzolate Bromide (Use of anticholinergic drugs after administration of abobotulinumtoxinA may potentiate systemic anticholinergic effects such as blurred vision).
No products indexed under this heading.

Metaxalone (Excessive weakness may also be exaggerated by administration of a muscle relaxant before or after administration of abobotulinumtoxinA). Products include:
Skelaxin 1848

Methocarbamol (Excessive weakness may also be exaggerated by administration of a muscle relaxant before or after administration of abobotulinumtoxinA).
No products indexed under this heading.

Metocurine Iodide (Patients treated concomitantly with botulinum toxins and other agents interfering with neuromuscular transmission (eg, curare-like agents) should be observed closely because the effect of the botulinum toxin may be potentiated).
No products indexed under this heading.

Mivacurium Chloride (Patients treated concomitantly with botulinum toxins and other agents interfering with neuromuscular transmission (eg, curare-like agents) should be observed closely because the effect of the botulinum toxin may be potentiated).
No products indexed under this heading.

Neomycin (Patients treated concomitantly with botulinum toxins and aminoglycosides should be observed closely because the effect of the botulinum toxin may be potentiated).
No products indexed under this heading.

Neomycin, oral (Patients treated concomitantly with botulinum toxins and aminoglycosides should be observed closely because the effect of the botulinum toxin may be potentiated).
No products indexed under this heading.

Neomycin Sulfate (Patients treated concomitantly with botulinum toxins and aminoglycosides should be observed closely because the effect of the botulinum toxin may be potentiated).
No products indexed under this heading.

Orphenadrine Citrate (Excessive weakness may also be exaggerated by administration of a muscle relaxant before or after administration of abobotulinumtoxinA).
No products indexed under this heading.

Oxybutynin Chloride (Use of anticholinergic drugs after administration of abobotulinumtoxinA may potentiate systemic anticholinergic effects such as blurred vision).
No products indexed under this heading.

Pancuronium Bromide (Patients treated concomitantly with botulinum toxins and other agents interfering with neuromuscular transmission (eg, curare-like agents) should be observed closely because the effect of the botulinum toxin may be potentiated).
No products indexed under this heading.

Pipecuronium Bromide (Patients treated concomitantly with botulinum toxins and other agents interfering with neuromuscular transmission (eg, curare-like agents) should be observed closely because the effect of the botulinum toxin may be potentiated).
No products indexed under this heading.

Procyclidine Hydrochloride (Use of anticholinergic drugs after administration of abobotulinumtoxinA may potentiate systemic anticholinergic effects such as blurred vision).
No products indexed under this heading.

Propantheline Bromide (Use of anticholinergic drugs after administration of abobotulinumtoxinA may potentiate systemic anticholinergic effects such as blurred vision).
No products indexed under this heading.

Rapacuronium Bromide (Patients treated concomitantly with botulinum toxins and other agents interfering with neuromuscular transmission (eg, curare-like agents) should be observed closely because the effect of the botulinum toxin may be potentiated).
No products indexed under this heading.

Rocuronium Bromide (Patients treated concomitantly with botulinum toxins and other agents interfering with neuromuscular transmission (eg, curare-like agents) should be observed closely because the effect of the botulinum toxin may be potentiated). Products include:
Zemuron 3249

Scopolamine (Use of anticholinergic drugs after administration of abobotulinumtoxinA may potentiate systemic anticholinergic effects such as blurred vision). Products include:
Transderm Scōp 2397

Scopolamine Hydrobromide (Use of anticholinergic drugs after administration of abobotulinumtoxinA may potentiate systemic anticholinergic effects such as blurred vision).
Products include:
Donnatal 2711

Streptomycin Sulfate (Patients treated concomitantly with botulinum toxins and aminoglycosides should be observed closely because the effect of the botulinum toxin may be potentiated).
No products indexed under this heading.

Succinylcholine Chloride (Patients treated concomitantly with botulinum toxins and other agents interfering with neuromuscular transmission (eg, curare-like agents) should be observed closely because the effect of the botulinum toxin may be potentiated).
No products indexed under this heading.

Tizanidine (Excessive weakness may also be exaggerated by administration of a muscle relaxant before or after administration of abobotulinumtoxinA).
No products indexed under this heading.

Tizanidine Hydrochloride (Excessive weakness may also be exaggerated by administration of a muscle relaxant before or after administration of abobotulinumtoxinA).
No products indexed under this heading.

Tobramycin (Patients treated concomitantly with botulinum toxins and aminoglycosides should be observed closely because the effect of the botulinum toxin may be potentiated). Products include:
Tobi Nebulizer 2546
Tobramycin and Dexamethasone Ophthalmic Suspension .... ⊙ 251
Zylet .... ⊙ 252

Tobramycin Sulfate (Patients treated concomitantly with botulinum toxins and aminoglycosides should be observed closely because the effect of the botulinum toxin may be potentiated).
No products indexed under this heading.

Tolterodine Tartrate (Use of anticholinergic drugs after administration of abobotulinumtoxinA may potentiate systemic anticholinergic effects such as blurred vision).
No products indexed under this heading.

Tridihexethyl Chloride (Use of anticholinergic drugs after administration of abobotulinumtoxinA may potentiate systemic anticholinergic effects such as blurred vision).
No products indexed under this heading.

Trihexyphenidyl Hydrochloride (Use of anticholinergic drugs after administration of abobotulinumtoxinA may potentiate systemic anticholinergic effects such as blurred vision).
No products indexed under this heading.

Tubocurarine Chloride (Patients treated concomitantly with botulinum toxins and other agents interfering with neuromuscular transmission (eg, curare-like agents) should be observed closely because the effect of the botulinum toxin may be potentiated).
No products indexed under this heading.

Vecuronium Bromide (Patients treated concomitantly with botulinum toxins and other agents interfering with neuromuscular transmission (eg, curare-like agents) should be observed closely because the effect of the botulinum toxin may be potentiated).
No products indexed under this heading.

EC-NAPROSYN DELAYED-RELEASE TABLETS

(Naproxen) 2850
May interact with ACE inhibitors, antacids containing aluminum, calcium and magnesium, beta-blockers, histamine H2-receptor antagonists, hydantoin anticonvulsants, lithium preparations, oral anticoagulants, selective serotonin reuptake inhibitors, sulfonylureas, thiazides, and certain other agents. Compounds in these categories include:

Acebutolol Hydrochloride (Reduced antihypertensive effect of beta blockers).
No products indexed under this heading.

Aluminum Carbonate (Due to the gastric pH elevating effects of intensive antacids therapy, concomitant administration of EC-Naprosyn is not recommended).
No products indexed under this heading.

Aluminum Hydroxide (Due to the gastric pH elevating effects of intensive antacids therapy, concomitant administration of EC-Naprosyn is not recommended).
No products indexed under this heading.

Anisindione (Short-term studies have failed to show any significant effect of concurrent use on prothrombin time; caution is advised since interactions have been seen with other NSAIDs).
No products indexed under this heading.

Aspirin (Naproxen is displaced from its binding sites during the concomitant administration of aspirin resulting in lower plasma concentrations and peak plasma levels; concurrent use is not recommended). Products include:
Aggrenox 880
Bayer Aspirin 829
Percodan 1124
St. Joseph Aspirin 2045

Atenolol (Reduced antihypertensive effect of beta blockers).
No products indexed under this heading.

Benazepril Hydrochloride (Reports suggest that NSAIDs may diminish the antihypertensive effect of ACE-inhibitors. The use of NSAIDs in patients who are receiving ACE-inhibitors may potentiate renal dise states).
No products indexed under this heading.

Paroxetine (There is an increased risk of GI bleeding when selective serotonin reuptake inhibitors (SSRIs) are combined with NSAIDs. Caution should be used when NSAIDs are administered concomitantly with SSRIs).
No products indexed under this heading.

Paroxetine Hydrochloride (There is an increased risk of GI bleeding when selective serotonin reuptake inhibitors (SSRIs) are combined with NSAIDs. Caution should be used when NSAIDs are administered concomitantly with SSRIs). Products include:

Paroxetine Mesylate (There is an increased risk of GI bleeding when selective serotonin reuptake inhibitors (SSRIs) are combined with NSAIDs. Caution should be used when NSAIDs are administered concomitantly with SSRIs).
No products indexed under this heading.

Penbutolol Sulfate (Reduced antihypertensive effect of beta blockers).
No products indexed under this heading.

Perindopril Erbumine (Reports suggest that NSAIDs may diminish the antihypertensive effect of ACE-inhibitors. The use of NSAIDs in patients who are receiving ACE-inhibitors may potentiate renal dise states).
No products indexed under this heading.

Phenytoin (Potential for hydantoin toxicity).
No products indexed under this heading.

Phenytoin Sodium (Potential for hydantoin toxicity). Products include:

Pindolol (Reduced antihypertensive effect of beta blockers).
No products indexed under this heading.

Polythiazide (Clinical studies, as well as postmarketing observations, have shown that Naproxen can reduce the natriuretic effect of furosemide and thiazides in some patients. Response has been attributed to inhibition of renal prostaglandin synthesis. Patients should be observed closely for signs of renal failure, as well as to assure diuretic efficacy).
No products indexed under this heading.

Probenecid (Probenecid given concurrently increases naproxen anion plasma levels and extends its plasma half-life significantly).
No products indexed under this heading.

Propranolol Hydrochloride (Reduced antihypertensive effect of beta blockers). Products include:

Quinapril Hydrochloride (Reports suggest that NSAIDs may diminish the antihypertensive effect of ACE-inhibitors. The use of NSAIDs in patients who are receiving ACE-inhibitors may potentiate renal dise states).
No products indexed under this heading.

Ramipril (Reports suggest that NSAIDs may diminish the antihypertensive effect of ACE-inhibitors. The use of NSAIDs in patients who are receiving ACE-inhibitors may potentiate renal dise states).
No products indexed under this heading.

Ranitidine Bismuth Citrate (Due to the gastric pH elevating effects of H2-blockers concomitant administration of EC-Naprosyn is not recommended).
No products indexed under this heading.

Ranitidine Hydrochloride (Due to the gastric pH elevating effects of H2-blockers concomitant administration of EC-Naprosyn is not recommended). Products include:

Sertraline Hydrochloride (There is an increased risk of GI bleeding when selective serotonin reuptake inhibitors (SSRIs) are combined with NSAIDs. Caution should be used when NSAIDs are administered concomitantly with SSRIs).
No products indexed under this heading.

Sotalol Hydrochloride (Reduced antihypertensive effect of beta blockers).
No products indexed under this heading.

Spirapril Hydrochloride (Reports suggest that NSAIDs may diminish the antihypertensive effect of ACE-inhibitors. The use of NSAIDs in patients who are receiving ACE-inhibitors may potentiate renal dise states).
No products indexed under this heading.

Sucralfate (Due to the gastric pH elevating effects of sucralfate, concomitant administration of EC-Naprosyn is not recommended). Products include:

Sulfamethoxazole (Potential for sulfonamide toxicity).
No products indexed under this heading.

Sulfisoxazole Acetyl (Potential for sulfonamide toxicity).
No products indexed under this heading.

Timolol Hemihydrate (Reduced antihypertensive effect of beta blockers). Products include:

Timolol Maleate (Reduced antihypertensive effect of beta blockers). Products include:

Tolazamide (Potential for sulfonylurea toxicity).
No products indexed under this heading.

Tolbutamide (Potential for sulfonylurea toxicity).
No products indexed under this heading.

Trandolapril (Co-administration of NSAIDs and ACE inhibitors may potentiate renal disease states). Products include:

Warfarin Sodium (Short-term studies have failed to show any significant effect of concurrent use on prothrombin time; caution is advised since interactions have been seen with other NSAIDs).
No products indexed under this heading.

Food Interactions

Food, unspecified (The presence of food prolonged the time the EC-Naprosyn remained in the stomach, time to first detectable serum naproxen levels, and time to maximal naproxen levels (T_{max}), but did not affect peak naproxen levels (C_{max})).

E.E.S. 200 LIQUID
(Erythromycin Ethylsuccinate) 437
See E.E.S. 400 Filmtab Tablets

E.E.S. 400 LIQUID
(Erythromycin Ethylsuccinate) 437
See E.E.S. 400 Filmtab Tablets

E.E.S. 400 FILMTAB TABLETS
(Erythromycin Ethylsuccinate) 437
May interact with cytochrome p450 3a substrates (selected), HMG-CoA reductase inhibitors, methylprednisolone, oral anticoagulants, phenytoin, quinidine, theophyllines, triazolobenzodiazepines, valproate, and certain other agents. Compounds in these categories include:

Alfentanil Hydrochloride (There have been spontaneous or published reports of CYP3A based interactions of erythromycin with alfentanil).
No products indexed under this heading.

Alprazolam (Erythromycin has been reported to decrease the clearance of triazolam and midazolam, and thus, may increase the pharmacologic effect of these benzodiazepines).
No products indexed under this heading.

Aminophylline (Co-administration of erythromycin and a drug primarily metabolized by CYP3A may be associated with elevations in drug concentrations that could increase or prolong both the therapeutic and adverse effects of the concomitant drug. Dosage adjustments may be considered, and when possible, serum concentrations of drugs primarily metabolized by CYP3A should be monitored closely in patients concurrently receiving erythromycin).
No products indexed under this heading.

Amitriptyline Hydrochloride (Co-administration of erythromycin and a drug primarily metabolized by CYP3A may be associated with elevations in drug concentrations that could increase or prolong both the therapeutic and adverse effects of the concomitant drug. Dosage adjustments may be considered, and when possible, serum concentrations of drugs primarily metabolized by CYP3A should be monitored closely in patients concurrently receiving erythromycin).
No products indexed under this heading.

Amlodipine Besylate (Co-administration of erythromycin and a drug primarily metabolized by CYP3A may be associated with elevations in drug concentrations that could increase or prolong both the therapeutic and adverse effects of the concomitant drug. Dosage adjustments may be considered, and when possible, serum concentrations of drugs primarily metabolized by CYP3A should be monitored closely in patients concurrently receiving erythromycin). Products include:

Anisindione (There have been reports of increased anticoagulant effects when erythromycin and oral anticoagulants were used concomitantly. Increased anticoagulation effects due to interactions of erythromycin with various oral anticoagulants may be more pronounced in the elderly).
No products indexed under this heading.

Aprepitant (Co-administration of erythromycin and a drug primarily metabolized by CYP3A may be associated with elevations in drug concentrations that could increase or prolong both the therapeutic and adverse effects of the concomitant drug. Dosage adjustments may be considered, and when possible, serum concentrations of drugs primarily metabolized by CYP3A should be monitored closely in patients concurrently receiving erythromycin). Products include:

Astemizole (Co-administration of erythromycin with astemizole is contraindicated. Erythromycin has been reported to significantly alter the metabolism of the non-sedating antihistamines terfenadine and astemizole when taken concomitantly. Rare cases of serious cardiovascular adverse events, including electrocardiographic QT/QT_c interval prolongation, cardiac arrest, torsades de pointes, and other ventricular arrhythmias have been observed).
No products indexed under this heading.

Atorvastatin Calcium (Erythromycin has been reported to increase concentrations of HMG-CoA reductase inhibitors (eg, lovastatin and simvastatin). Rare reports of rhabdomyolysis have been reported in patients taking these drugs concomitantly). Products include:

Bromocriptine Mesylate (There have been spontaneous or published reports of CYP3A based interactions of erythromycin with bromocriptine).
No products indexed under this heading.

Buspirone Hydrochloride (Co-administration of erythromycin and a drug primarily metabolized by CYP3A may be associated with elevations in drug concentrations that could increase or prolong both the therapeutic and adverse effects of the concomitant drug. Dosage adjustments may be considered, and when possible, serum concentrations of drugs primarily metabolized by CYP3A should be monitored closely in patients concurrently receiving erythromycin).
No products indexed under this heading.

Busulfan (Co-administration of erythromycin and a drug primarily metabolized by CYP3A may be associated with elevations in drug concentrations that could increase or prolong both the therapeutic and adverse effects of the concomitant drug. Dosage adjustments may be considered, and when possible, serum concentrations of drugs primarily metabolized by CYP3A should be monitored closely in patients concurrently receiving erythromycin). Products include:

Carbamazepine (There have been spontaneous or published reports of CYP3A based interactions of erythromycin with carbamazepine). Products include:

Cerivastatin Sodium (Erythromycin has been reported to increase concentrations of HMG-CoA reductase inhibitors (eg, lovastatin and simvastatin). Rare reports of rhabdomyolysis have been reported in patients taking these drugs concomitantly).
No products indexed under this heading.

Chlorpheniramine (Co-administration of erythromycin and a drug primarily metabolized by CYP3A may be associated with elevations in drug concentrations that could increase or prolong both the therapeutic and adverse effects of the concomitant drug. Dosage adjustments may be considered, and when possible, serum concentrations of drugs primarily metabolized by CYP3A should be monitored closely in patients concurrently receiving erythromycin).
No products indexed under this heading.

Chlorpheniramine Maleate (Co-administration of erythromycin and a drug primarily metabolized by CYP3A may be associated with elevations in drug concentrations that could increase or prolong both the therapeutic and adverse effects of the concomitant drug. Dosage adjustments may be considered, and when possible, serum concentrations of drugs primarily metabolized by CYP3A should be monitored closely in patients concurrently receiving erythromycin).
No products indexed under this heading.

Chlorpheniramine Polistirex (Co-administration of erythromycin and a drug primarily metabolized by CYP3A may be associated with elevations in drug concentrations that could increase or prolong both the therapeutic and adverse effects of the concomitant drug. Dosage adjustments may be con-

sidered, and when possible, serum concentrations of drugs primarily metabolized by CYP3A should be monitored closely in patients concurrently receiving erythromycin). Products include:
Tussionex 3443

Chlorpheniramine Tannate (Co-administration of erythromycin and a drug primarily metabolized by CYP3A may be associated with elevations in drug concentrations that could increase or prolong both the therapeutic and adverse effects of the concomitant drug. Dosage adjustments may be considered, and when possible, serum concentrations of drugs primarily metabolized by CYP3A should be monitored closely in patients concurrently receiving erythromycin).
No products indexed under this heading.

Cilostazol (There have been spontaneous or published reports of CYP3A based interactions of erythromycin with cilostazol).
No products indexed under this heading.

Cisapride (Co-administration of erythromycin with cisapride is contraindicated. There have been post-marketing reports of drug interactions when erythromycin is co-administered with cisapride, resulting in QT prolongation, cardiac arrhythmias, ventricular tachycardia, ventricular fibrillation, and torsades de pointes, most likely due to inhibition of hepatic metabolism of cisapride by erythromycin. Fatalities have been reported).
No products indexed under this heading.

Clarithromycin (Co-administration of erythromycin and a drug primarily metabolized by CYP3A may be associated with elevations in drug concentrations that could increase or prolong both the therapeutic and adverse effects of the concomitant drug. Dosage adjustments may be considered, and when possible, serum concentrations of drugs primarily metabolized by CYP3A should be monitored closely in patients concurrently receiving erythromycin). Products include:
Biaxin/Biaxin XL 412

Cyclosporine (There have been spontaneous or published reports of CYP3A based interactions of erythromycin with cyclosporine). Products include:
Gengraf 440
Neoral Oral Solution 2496
Neoral Capsules 2496
Restasis 605

Desogestrel (Co-administration of erythromycin and a drug primarily metabolized by CYP3A may be associated with elevations in drug concentrations that could increase or prolong both the therapeutic and adverse effects of the concomitant drug. Dosage adjustments may be considered, and when possible, serum concentrations of drugs primarily metabolized by CYP3A should be monitored closely in patients concurrently receiving erythromycin).
No products indexed under this heading.

Dexamethasone (Co-administration of erythromycin and a drug primarily metabolized by CYP3A may be associated with elevations in drug concentrations that could increase or prolong both the therapeutic and adverse effects of the concomitant drug. Dosage adjustments may be considered, and when possible, serum concentrations of drugs primarily metabolized by CYP3A should be monitored closely in patients concurrently receiving erythromycin). Products include:
Ciprodex 583
Ozurdex .... ⊙ 223
Tobramycin and Dexamethasone Ophthalmic Suspension .... ⊙ 251

Dexamethasone Acetate (Co-administration of erythromycin and a drug primarily metabolized by CYP3A may be associated with elevations in drug concentrations that could increase or prolong both the therapeutic and adverse effects of the concomitant drug. Dosage adjustments may be considered, and when possible, serum concentrations of drugs primarily metabolized by CYP3A should be monitored closely in patients concurrently receiving erythromycin).
No products indexed under this heading.

Dexamethasone Phosphate (Co-administration of erythromycin and a drug primarily metabolized by CYP3A may be associated with elevations in drug concentrations that could increase or prolong both the therapeutic and adverse effects of the concomitant drug. Dosage adjustments may be considered, and when possible, serum concentrations of drugs primarily metabolized by CYP3A should be monitored closely in patients concurrently receiving erythromycin).
No products indexed under this heading.

Dexamethasone Sodium (Co-administration of erythromycin and a drug primarily metabolized by CYP3A may be associated with elevations in drug concentrations that could increase or prolong both the therapeutic and adverse effects of the concomitant drug. Dosage adjustments may be considered, and when possible, serum concentrations of drugs primarily metabolized by CYP3A should be monitored closely in patients concurrently receiving erythromycin).
No products indexed under this heading.

Dexamethasone Sodium Phosphate (Co-administration of erythromycin and a drug primarily metabolized by CYP3A may be associated with elevations in drug concentrations that could increase or prolong both the therapeutic and adverse effects of the concomitant drug. Dosage adjustments may be considered, and when possible, serum concentrations of drugs primarily metabolized by CYP3A should be monitored closely in patients concurrently receiving erythromycin).
No products indexed under this heading.

Diazepam (Co-administration of erythromycin and a drug primarily metabolized by CYP3A may be associated with elevations in drug concentrations that could increase or prolong both the therapeutic and adverse effects of the concomitant drug. Dosage adjustments may be considered, and when possible, serum concentrations of drugs primarily metabolized by CYP3A should be monitored closely in patients concurrently receiving erythromycin). Products include:
Valium Tablets 2880

Dicumarol (There have been reports of increased anticoagulant effects when erythromycin and oral anticoagulants were used concomitantly. Increased anticoagulation effects due to interactions of erythromycin with various oral anticoagulants may be more pronounced in the elderly).
No products indexed under this heading.

Digoxin (Concomitant administration of erythromycin and digoxin has been reported to result in elevated digoxin serum levels). Products include:
Lanoxin Injection 1546
Lanoxin Injection Pediatric 1549
Lanoxin Tablets 1553

Dihydroergotamine Mesylate (Concurrent use of erythromycin and ergotamine or dihydroergotamine has been associated in some patients with acute ergot toxicity characterized by severe peripheral vasospasm and dysesthesia).
No products indexed under this heading.

Diltiazem Hydrochloride (Co-administration of erythromycin and a drug primarily metabolized by CYP3A may be associated with elevations in drug concentrations that could increase or prolong both the therapeutic and adverse effects of the concomitant drug. Dosage adjustments may be considered, and when possible, serum concentrations of drugs primarily metabolized by CYP3A should be monitored closely in patients concurrently receiving erythromycin). Products include:
Cardizem LA 423

Diltiazem Maleate (Co-administration of erythromycin and a drug primarily metabolized by CYP3A may be associated with elevations in drug concentrations that could increase or prolong both the therapeutic and adverse effects of the concomitant drug. Dosage adjustments may be considered, and when possible, serum concentrations of drugs primarily metabolized by CYP3A should be monitored closely in patients concurrently receiving erythromycin).
No products indexed under this heading.

Disopyramide (There have been spontaneous or published reports of CYP3A based interactions of erythromycin with disopyramide).
No products indexed under this heading.

Disopyramide Phosphate (There have been spontaneous or published reports of CYP3A based interactions of erythromycin with disopyramide).
No products indexed under this heading.

Divalproex Sodium (There have been reports of interactions of erythromycin with drugs not thought to be metabolized by CYP3A, including valproate). Products include:
Depakote ER 426

Doxorubicin Hydrochloride (Co-administration of erythromycin and a drug primarily metabolized by CYP3A may be associated with elevations in drug concentrations that could increase or prolong both the therapeutic and adverse effects of the concomitant drug. Dosage adjustments may be considered, and when possible, serum concentrations of drugs primarily metabolized by CYP3A should be monitored closely in patients concurrently receiving erythromycin).
No products indexed under this heading.

Dronabinol (Co-administration of erythromycin and a drug primarily metabolized by CYP3A may be associated with elevations in drug concentrations that could increase or prolong both the therapeutic and adverse effects of the concomitant drug. Dosage adjustments may be considered, and when possible, serum concentrations of drugs primarily metabolized by CYP3A should be monitored closely in patients concurrently receiving erythromycin).
No products indexed under this heading.

Dyphylline (Co-administration of erythromycin and a drug primarily metabolized by CYP3A may be associated with elevations in drug concentrations that could increase or prolong both the therapeutic and adverse effects of the concomitant drug. Dosage adjustments may be considered, and when possible, serum concentrations of drugs primarily metabolized by CYP3A should be monitored closely in patients concurrently receiving erythromycin).
No products indexed under this heading.

Ergotamine Tartrate (Concurrent use of erythromycin and ergotamine or dihydroergotamine has been associated in some patients with acute ergot toxicity characterized by severe peripheral vasospasm and dysesthesia).
No products indexed under this heading.

Erythromycin (Co-administration of erythromycin and a drug primarily metabolized by CYP3A may be associated with elevations in drug concentrations that could increase or prolong both the therapeutic and adverse effects of the concomitant drug. Dosage adjustments may be considered, and when possible, serum concentrations of drugs primarily metabolized by CYP3A should be monitored closely in patients concurrently receiving erythromycin).
No products indexed under this heading.

Erythromycin Estolate (Co-administration of erythromycin and a drug primarily metabolized by CYP3A may be associated with elevations in drug concentrations that could increase or prolong both the therapeutic and adverse effects of the concomitant drug. Dosage adjustments may be considered, and when possible, serum concentrations of drugs primarily metabolized by CYP3A should be monitored closely in patients concurrently receiving erythromycin).
No products indexed under this heading.

Erythromycin Gluceptate (Co-administration of erythromycin and a drug primarily metabolized by CYP3A may be associated with elevations in drug concentrations that could increase or prolong both the therapeutic and adverse effects of the concomitant drug. Dosage adjustments may be considered, and when possible, serum concentrations of drugs primarily metabolized by CYP3A should be monitored closely in patients concurrently receiving erythromycin).
No products indexed under this heading.

Erythromycin Lactobionate (Co-administration of erythromycin and a drug primarily metabolized by CYP3A may be associated with elevations in drug concentrations that could increase or prolong both the therapeutic and adverse effects of the concomitant drug. Dosage adjustments may be considered, and when possible, serum concentrations of drugs primarily metabolized by CYP3A should be monitored closely in patients concurrently receiving erythromycin).
No products indexed under this heading.

Erythromycin Stearate (Co-administration of erythromycin and a drug primarily metabolized by CYP3A may be associated with elevations in drug concentrations that could increase or prolong both the therapeutic and adverse effects of the concomitant drug. Dosage adjustments may be considered, and when possible, serum concentrations of drugs primarily metabolized by CYP3A should be monitored closely in patients concurrently receiving erythromycin).
No products indexed under this heading.

Estrogen (Co-administration of erythromycin and a drug primarily metabolized by CYP3A may be associated with elevations in drug concentrations that could increase or prolong both the therapeutic and adverse effects of the concomitant drug. Dosage adjustments may be considered, and when possible, serum concentrations of drugs primarily

metabolized by CYP3A should be monitored closely in patients concurrently receiving erythromycin).
No products indexed under this heading.

Estrogens, Conjugated (Co-administration of erythromycin and a drug primarily metabolized by CYP3A may be associated with elevations in drug concentrations that could increase or prolong both the therapeutic and adverse effects of the concomitant drug. Dosage adjustments may be considered, and when possible, serum concentrations of drugs primarily metabolized by CYP3A should be monitored closely in patients concurrently receiving erythromycin). Products include:
Premarin Intravenous 3528
Premarin Tablets 3533
Premarin Vaginal Cream 3540
Premphase 3549
Prempro 3549

Estrogens, Conjugated, Synthetic A (Co-administration of erythromycin and a drug primarily metabolized by CYP3A may be associated with elevations in drug concentrations that could increase or prolong both the therapeutic and adverse effects of the concomitant drug. Dosage adjustments may be considered, and when possible, serum concentrations of drugs primarily metabolized by CYP3A should be monitored closely in patients concurrently receiving erythromycin).
No products indexed under this heading.

Estrogens, Esterified (Co-administration of erythromycin and a drug primarily metabolized by CYP3A may be associated with elevations in drug concentrations that could increase or prolong both the therapeutic and adverse effects of the concomitant drug. Dosage adjustments may be considered, and when possible, serum concentrations of drugs primarily metabolized by CYP3A should be monitored closely in patients concurrently receiving erythromycin).
No products indexed under this heading.

Ethinyl Estradiol (Co-administration of erythromycin and a drug primarily metabolized by CYP3A may be associated with elevations in drug concentrations that could increase or prolong both the therapeutic and adverse effects of the concomitant drug. Dosage adjustments may be considered, and when possible, serum concentrations of drugs primarily metabolized by CYP3A should be monitored closely in patients concurrently receiving erythromycin). Products include:
LoSeasonique 3407
Lybrel 3514
NuvaRing 3181
Ortho Evra 2648
Ortho-Cyclen/Ortho Tri-Cyclen 2663
Ortho Tri-Cyclen Lo Tablets 2673
Seasonique 3418
Yaz 864

Ethosuximide (Co-administration of erythromycin and a drug primarily metabolized by CYP3A may be associated with elevations in drug concentrations that could increase or prolong both the therapeutic and adverse effects of the concomitant drug. Dosage adjustments may be considered, and when possible, serum concentrations of drugs primarily metabolized by CYP3A should be monitored closely in patients concurrently receiving erythromycin).
No products indexed under this heading.

Ethynodiol Diacetate (Co-administration of erythromycin and a drug primarily metabolized by CYP3A may be associated with elevations in drug concentrations that could increase or prolong both the therapeutic and adverse effects of the concomitant drug. Dosage adjustments may be considered, and when possible, serum concentrations of drugs primarily metabolized by CYP3A should be monitored closely in patients concurrently receiving erythromycin).
No products indexed under this heading.

Etoposide (Co-administration of erythromycin and a drug primarily metabolized by CYP3A may be associated with elevations in drug concentrations that could increase or prolong both the therapeutic and adverse effects of the concomitant drug. Dosage adjustments may be considered, and when possible, serum concentrations of drugs primarily metabolized by CYP3A should be monitored closely in patients concurrently receiving erythromycin).
No products indexed under this heading.

Etoposide Phosphate (Co-administration of erythromycin and a drug primarily metabolized by CYP3A may be associated with elevations in drug concentrations that could increase or prolong both the therapeutic and adverse effects of the concomitant drug. Dosage adjustments may be considered, and when possible, serum concentrations of drugs primarily metabolized by CYP3A should be monitored closely in patients concurrently receiving erythromycin).
No products indexed under this heading.

Felodipine (Co-administration of erythromycin and a drug primarily metabolized by CYP3A may be associated with elevations in drug concentrations that could increase or prolong both the therapeutic and adverse effects of the concomitant drug. Dosage adjustments may be considered, and when possible, serum concentrations of drugs primarily metabolized by CYP3A should be monitored closely in patients concurrently receiving erythromycin).
No products indexed under this heading.

Fentanyl (Co-administration of erythromycin and a drug primarily metabolized by CYP3A may be associated with elevations in drug concentrations that could increase or prolong both the therapeutic and adverse effects of the concomitant drug. Dosage adjustments may be considered, and when possible, serum concentrations of drugs primarily metabolized by CYP3A should be monitored closely in patients concurrently receiving erythromycin). Products include:
Duragesic 2604
Fentanyl Transdermal System 2346
Onsolis 2054

Fentanyl Citrate (Co-administration of erythromycin and a drug primarily metabolized by CYP3A may be associated with elevations in drug concentrations that could increase or prolong both the therapeutic and adverse effects of the concomitant drug. Dosage adjustments may be considered, and when possible, serum concentrations of drugs primarily metabolized by CYP3A should be monitored closely in patients concurrently receiving erythromycin). Products include:
Fentora 966

Fluvastatin Sodium (Erythromycin has been reported to increase concentrations of HMG-CoA reductase inhibitors (eg, lovastatin and simvastatin). Rare reports of rhabdomyolysis have been reported in patients taking these drugs concomitantly).
No products indexed under this heading.

Fosphenytoin (There have been reports of interactions of erythromycin with drugs not thought to be metabolized by CYP3A, including phenytoin).
No products indexed under this heading.

Fosphenytoin Sodium (There have been reports of interactions of erythromycin with drugs not thought to be metabolized by CYP3A, including phenytoin).
No products indexed under this heading.

Glyburide (Co-administration of erythromycin and a drug primarily metabolized by CYP3A may be associated with elevations in drug concentrations that could increase or prolong both the therapeutic and adverse effects of the concomitant drug. Dosage adjustments may be considered, and when possible, serum concentrations of drugs primarily metabolized by CYP3A should be monitored closely in patients concurrently receiving erythromycin).
No products indexed under this heading.

Haloperidol (Co-administration of erythromycin and a drug primarily metabolized by CYP3A may be associated with elevations in drug concentrations that could increase or prolong both the therapeutic and adverse effects of the concomitant drug. Dosage adjustments may be considered, and when possible, serum concentrations of drugs primarily metabolized by CYP3A should be monitored closely in patients concurrently receiving erythromycin).
No products indexed under this heading.

Haloperidol Decanoate (Co-administration of erythromycin and a drug primarily metabolized by CYP3A may be associated with elevations in drug concentrations that could increase or prolong both the therapeutic and adverse effects of the concomitant drug. Dosage adjustments may be considered, and when possible, serum concentrations of drugs primarily metabolized by CYP3A should be monitored closely in patients concurrently receiving erythromycin).
No products indexed under this heading.

Hexobarbital (There have been reports of interactions of erythromycin with drugs not thought to be metabolized by CYP3A, including hexobarbital).
No products indexed under this heading.

Imipramine Hydrochloride (Co-administration of erythromycin and a drug primarily metabolized by CYP3A may be associated with elevations in drug concentrations that could increase or prolong both the therapeutic and adverse effects of the concomitant drug. Dosage adjustments may be considered, and when possible, serum concentrations of drugs primarily metabolized by CYP3A should be monitored closely in patients concurrently receiving erythromycin).
No products indexed under this heading.

Imipramine Pamoate (Co-administration of erythromycin and a drug primarily metabolized by CYP3A may be associated with elevations in drug concentrations that could increase or prolong both the therapeutic and adverse effects of the concomitant drug. Dosage adjustments may be considered, and when possible, serum concentrations of drugs primarily metabolized by CYP3A should be monitored closely in patients concurrently receiving erythromycin).
No products indexed under this heading.

Indinavir Sulfate (Co-administration of erythromycin and a drug primarily metabolized by CYP3A may be associated with elevations in drug concentrations that could increase or prolong both the therapeutic and adverse effects of the concomitant drug. Dosage adjustments may be considered, and when possible, serum concentrations of drugs primarily metabolized by CYP3A should be monitored closely in patients concurrently receiving erythromycin). Products include:
Crixivan 2113

Isradipine (Co-administration of erythromycin and a drug primarily metabolized by CYP3A may be associated with elevations in drug concentrations that could increase or prolong both the therapeutic and adverse effects of the concomitant drug. Dosage adjustments may be considered, and when possible, serum concentrations of drugs primarily metabolized by CYP3A should be monitored closely in patients concurrently receiving erythromycin). Products include:
DynaCirc CR 1432

Itraconazole (Co-administration of erythromycin and a drug primarily metabolized by CYP3A may be associated with elevations in drug concentrations that could increase or prolong both the therapeutic and adverse effects of the concomitant drug. Dosage adjustments may be considered, and when possible, serum concentrations of drugs primarily metabolized by CYP3A should be monitored closely in patients concurrently receiving erythromycin).
No products indexed under this heading.

Ketoconazole (Co-administration of erythromycin and a drug primarily metabolized by CYP3A may be associated with elevations in drug concentrations that could increase or prolong both the therapeutic and adverse effects of the concomitant drug. Dosage adjustments may be considered, and when possible, serum concentrations of drugs primarily metabolized by CYP3A should be monitored closely in patients concurrently receiving erythromycin). Products include:
Extina 3319
Xolegel 3337

Levonorgestrel (Co-administration of erythromycin and a drug primarily metabolized by CYP3A may be associated with elevations in drug concentrations that could increase or prolong both the therapeutic and adverse effects of the concomitant drug. Dosage adjustments may be considered, and when possible, serum concentrations of drugs primarily metabolized by CYP3A should be monitored closely in patients concurrently receiving erythromycin). Products include:
Climara Pro 847
LoSeasonique 3407
Lybrel 3514
Mirena 854
Plan B 3416
Seasonique 3418

Lidocaine (Co-administration of erythromycin and a drug primarily metabolized by CYP3A may be associated with elevations in drug concentrations that could increase or prolong both the therapeutic and adverse effects of the concomitant drug. Dosage adjustments may be considered, and when possible, serum concentrations of drugs primarily metabolized by CYP3A should be monitored closely in patients concurrently receiving erythromycin). Products include:
Lidoderm 1107

Lidocaine Hydrochloride (Co-administration of erythromycin and a drug primarily metabolized by CYP3A may be associated with elevations in drug concentrations that could increase or prolong both the therapeutic and adverse effects of the concomitant drug. Dosage adjustments may be considered, and when possible, serum concentrations of drugs primarily metabolized by CYP3A should be monitored closely in patients concurrently receiving erythromycin).
No products indexed under this heading.

Lovastatin (Rhabdomyolysis with or without renal impairment has been

E.E.S. Interactions Index 532

reported in seriously ill patients receiving erythromycin concomitantly with lovastatin. Therefore, patients receiving concomitant lovastatin and erythromycin should be carefully monitored for creatine kinase (CK) and serum transaminase levels). Products include:

Advicor 402
Mevacor 2212

Mestranol (Co-administration of erythromycin and a drug primarily metabolized by CYP3A may be associated with elevations in drug concentrations that could increase or prolong both the therapeutic and adverse effects of the concomitant drug. Dosage adjustments may be considered, and when possible, serum concentrations of drugs primarily metabolized by CYP3A should be monitored closely in patients concurrently receiving erythromycin).
No products indexed under this heading.

Methadone Hydrochloride (Co-administration of erythromycin and a drug primarily metabolized by CYP3A may be associated with elevations in drug concentrations that could increase or prolong both the therapeutic and adverse effects of the concomitant drug. Dosage adjustments may be considered, and when possible, serum concentrations of drugs primarily metabolized by CYP3A should be monitored closely in patients concurrently receiving erythromycin).
No products indexed under this heading.

Methylprednisolone (There have been spontaneous or published reports of CYP3A based interactions of erythromycin with methylprednisolone).
No products indexed under this heading.

Methylprednisolone Acetate (There have been spontaneous or published reports of CYP3A based interactions of erythromycin with methylprednisolone).
No products indexed under this heading.

Methylprednisolone Sodium Succinate (There have been spontaneous or published reports of CYP3A based interactions of erythromycin with methylprednisolone).
No products indexed under this heading.

Midazolam Hydrochloride (Erythromycin has been reported to decrease the clearance of triazolam and midazolam, and thus, may increase the pharmacologic effect of these benzodiazepines).
No products indexed under this heading.

Nefazodone Hydrochloride (Co-administration of erythromycin and a drug primarily metabolized by CYP3A may be associated with elevations in drug concentrations that could increase or prolong both the therapeutic and adverse effects of the concomitant drug. Dosage adjustments may be considered, and when possible, serum concentrations of drugs primarily metabolized by CYP3A should be monitored closely in patients concurrently receiving erythromycin).
No products indexed under this heading.

Nelfinavir Mesylate (Co-administration of erythromycin and a drug primarily metabolized by CYP3A may be associated with elevations in drug concentrations that could increase or prolong both the therapeutic and adverse effects of the concomitant drug. Dosage adjustments may be considered, and when possible, serum concentrations of drugs primarily metabolized by CYP3A should be monitored closely in patients concurrently receiving erythromycin).
No products indexed under this heading.

Nicardipine (Co-administration of erythromycin and a drug primarily metabolized by CYP3A may be associated with elevations in drug concentrations that could increase or prolong both the therapeutic and adverse effects of the concomitant drug. Dosage adjustments may be considered, and when possible, serum concentrations of drugs primarily metabolized by CYP3A should be monitored closely in patients concurrently receiving erythromycin).
No products indexed under this heading.

Nicardipine Hydrochloride (Co-administration of erythromycin and a drug primarily metabolized by CYP3A may be associated with elevations in drug concentrations that could increase or prolong both the therapeutic and adverse effects of the concomitant drug. Dosage adjustments may be considered, and when possible, serum concentrations of drugs primarily metabolized by CYP3A should be monitored closely in patients concurrently receiving erythromycin).
No products indexed under this heading.

Nifedipine (Co-administration of erythromycin and a drug primarily metabolized by CYP3A may be associated with elevations in drug concentrations that could increase or prolong both the therapeutic and adverse effects of the concomitant drug. Dosage adjustments may be considered, and when possible, serum concentrations of drugs primarily metabolized by CYP3A should be monitored closely in patients concurrently receiving erythromycin).
No products indexed under this heading.

Nimodipine (Co-administration of erythromycin and a drug primarily metabolized by CYP3A may be associated with elevations in drug concentrations that could increase or prolong both the therapeutic and adverse effects of the concomitant drug. Dosage adjustments may be considered, and when possible, serum concentrations of drugs primarily metabolized by CYP3A should be monitored closely in patients concurrently receiving erythromycin).
No products indexed under this heading.

Nisoldipine (Co-administration of erythromycin and a drug primarily metabolized by CYP3A may be associated with elevations in drug concentrations that could increase or prolong both the therapeutic and adverse effects of the concomitant drug. Dosage adjustments may be considered, and when possible, serum concentrations of drugs primarily metabolized by CYP3A should be monitored closely in patients concurrently receiving erythromycin).
No products indexed under this heading.

Norethindrone (Co-administration of erythromycin and a drug primarily metabolized by CYP3A may be associated with elevations in drug concentrations that could increase or prolong both the therapeutic and adverse effects of the concomitant drug. Dosage adjustments may be considered, and when possible, serum concentrations of drugs primarily metabolized by CYP3A should be monitored closely in patients concurrently receiving erythromycin). Products include:

Ortho Micronor 2660

Norgestrel (Co-administration of erythromycin and a drug primarily metabolized by CYP3A may be associated with elevations in drug concentrations that could increase or prolong both the therapeutic and adverse effects of the concomitant drug. Dosage adjustments may be considered, and when possible, serum concentrations of drugs primarily metabolized by CYP3A should be monitored closely in patients concurrently receiving erythromycin).
No products indexed under this heading.

Ondansetron Hydrochloride (Co-administration of erythromycin and a drug primarily metabolized by CYP3A may be associated with elevations in drug concentrations that could increase or prolong both the therapeutic and adverse effects of the concomitant drug. Dosage adjustments may be considered, and when possible, serum concentrations of drugs primarily metabolized by CYP3A should be monitored closely in patients concurrently receiving erythromycin). Products include:

Zofran Injection 1750
Zofran 1756
Zofran ODT 1756

Paclitaxel (Co-administration of erythromycin and a drug primarily metabolized by CYP3A may be associated with elevations in drug concentrations that could increase or prolong both the therapeutic and adverse effects of the concomitant drug. Dosage adjustments may be considered, and when possible, serum concentrations of drugs primarily metabolized by CYP3A should be monitored closely in patients concurrently receiving erythromycin).
No products indexed under this heading.

Phenytoin (There have been reports of interactions of erythromycin with drugs not thought to be metabolized by CYP3A, including phenytoin).
No products indexed under this heading.

Phenytoin Sodium (There have been reports of interactions of erythromycin with drugs not thought to be metabolized by CYP3A, including phenytoin). Products include:

Phenytek Capsules 2380

Pimozide (Co-administration of erythromycin with pimozide is contraindicated).
No products indexed under this heading.

Pravastatin Sodium (Erythromycin has been reported to increase concentrations of HMG-CoA reductase inhibitors (eg, lovastatin and simvastatin). Rare reports of rhabdomyolysis have been reported in patients taking these drugs concomitantly).
No products indexed under this heading.

Quinidine (There have been spontaneous or published reports of CYP3A based interactions of erythromycin with quinidine).
No products indexed under this heading.

Quinidine Gluconate (There have been spontaneous or published reports of CYP3A based interactions of erythromycin with quinidine).
No products indexed under this heading.

Quinidine Hydrochloride (There have been spontaneous or published reports of CYP3A based interactions of erythromycin with quinidine).
No products indexed under this heading.

Quinidine Polygalacturonate (There have been spontaneous or published reports of CYP3A based interactions of erythromycin with quinidine).
No products indexed under this heading.

Quinidine Sulfate (There have been spontaneous or published reports of CYP3A based interactions of erythromycin with quinidine).
No products indexed under this heading.

Quinine (Co-administration of erythromycin and a drug primarily metabolized by CYP3A may be associated with elevations in drug concentrations that could increase or prolong both the therapeutic and adverse effects of the concomitant drug. Dosage adjustments may be considered, and when possible, serum concentrations of drugs primarily metabolized by CYP3A should be monitored closely in patients concurrently receiving erythromycin). Products include:

Hyland's Leg Cramps PM with Quinine 3315

Quinine Sulfate (Co-administration of erythromycin and a drug primarily metabolized by CYP3A may be associated with elevations in drug concentrations that could increase or prolong both the therapeutic and adverse effects of the concomitant drug. Dosage adjustments may be considered, and when possible, serum concentrations of drugs primarily metabolized by CYP3A should be monitored closely in patients concurrently receiving erythromycin).
No products indexed under this heading.

Rifabutin (There have been spontaneous or published reports of CYP3A based interactions of erythromycin with rifabutin).
No products indexed under this heading.

Ritonavir (Co-administration of erythromycin and a drug primarily metabolized by CYP3A may be associated with elevations in drug concentrations that could increase or prolong both the therapeutic and adverse effects of the concomitant drug. Dosage adjustments may be considered, and when possible, serum concentrations of drugs primarily metabolized by CYP3A should be monitored closely in patients concurrently receiving erythromycin). Products include:

Kaletra 458
Norvir 509

Rosuvastatin Calcium (Erythromycin has been reported to increase concentrations of HMG-CoA reductase inhibitors (eg, lovastatin and simvastatin). Rare reports of rhabdomyolysis have been reported in patients taking these drugs concomitantly). Products include:

Crestor 736

Saquinavir (Co-administration of erythromycin and a drug primarily metabolized by CYP3A may be associated with elevations in drug concentrations that could increase or prolong both the therapeutic and adverse effects of the concomitant drug. Dosage adjustments may be considered, and when possible, serum concentrations of drugs primarily metabolized by CYP3A should be monitored closely in patients concurrently receiving erythromycin).
No products indexed under this heading.

Saquinavir Mesylate (Co-administration of erythromycin and a drug primarily metabolized by CYP3A may be associated with elevations in drug concentrations that could increase or prolong both the therapeutic and adverse effects of the concomitant drug. Dosage adjustments may be considered, and when possible, serum concentrations of drugs primarily metabolized by CYP3A should be monitored closely in patients concurrently receiving erythromycin).
No products indexed under this heading.

Sertraline Hydrochloride (Co-administration of erythromycin and a drug primarily metabolized by CYP3A may be associated with elevations in drug concentrations that could increase or prolong both the therapeutic and adverse effects of the concomitant drug. Dosage adjustments may be considered, and when possible, serum concentrations of drugs primarily metabolized by CYP3A should be monitored closely in patients concurrently receiving erythromycin).
No products indexed under this heading.

Sildenafil Citrate (Erythromycin has been reported to increase the systemic exposure (AUC) of sildenafil. Reduction of sildenafil dosage should be considered).
No products indexed under this heading.

IMPORTANT NOTE: Always consult each drug listing in the patient's regimen for possible interactions.

Effexor Interactions Index 534

Alfentanil Hydrochloride (The risk of using venlafaxine in combination with other CNS active drugs has not been systematically evaluated. Consequently, caution is advised if the concomitant administration of venlafaxine and such drugs is required).
No products indexed under this heading.

Almotriptan Malate (There have been rare post-marketing reports of serotonin syndrome with use of an SSRI and a triptan. If concomitant treatment of venlafaxine with a triptan is clinically warranted, careful observation of the patient is advised, particularly during treatment initiation and dose increases. Patients should be cautioned about the risk of serotonin syndrome with the concomitant use of venlafaxine and triptans, tramadol, tryptophan supplements or other serotonergic agents). Products include:
Axert 2593

Alprazolam (The risk of using venlafaxine in combination with other CNS active drugs has not been systematically evaluated. Consequently, caution is advised if the concomitant administration of venlafaxine and such drugs is required).
No products indexed under this heading.

Amiloride Hydrochloride (Elderly patients may be at greater risk of developing hyponatremia with SSRIs and SNRIs. Also patients taking diuretics or who are otherwise volume depleted may be at greater risk. Discontinuation of venlafaxine should be considered in patients with symptomatic hyponatremia and appropriate medical intervention should be instituted).
No products indexed under this heading.

Amiodarone Hydrochloride (Studies indicate that venlafaxine is metabolized to its active metabolite, ODV, by CYP2D6. Thus the potential exists for a drug interaction between drugs that inhibit CYP2D6-mediated metabolism and venlafaxine. However, although imipramine partially inhibited the CYP2D6-mediated metabolism of venlafaxine, resulting in higher plasma concentrations of venlafaxine and lower plasma concentrations of ODV, the total concentration of active compounds (venlafaxine plus ODV) was not affected. Also, in a clinical study involving CYP2D6 poor and extensive metabolizers, the total concentration of active compounds (venlafaxine plus ODV), was similar in both groups. No dosage adjustment is required when venlafaxine is co-administered with a CYP2D6 inhibitor. Caution is advised should a patient's therapy include venlafaxine and CYP2D6 inhibitor).
No products indexed under this heading.

Amitriptyline Hydrochloride (Studies indicate that venlafaxine is metabolized to its active metabolite, ODV, by CYP2D6. Thus the potential exists for a drug interaction between drugs that inhibit CYP2D6-mediated metabolism and venlafaxine. However, although imipramine partially inhibited the CYP2D6-mediated metabolism of venlafaxine, resulting in higher plasma concentrations of venlafaxine and lower plasma concentrations of ODV, the total concentration of active compounds (venlafaxine plus ODV) was not affected. Also, in a clinical study involving CYP2D6 poor and extensive metabolizers, the total concentration of active compounds (venlafaxine plus ODV), was similar in both groups. No dosage adjustment is required when venlafaxine is co-administered with a CYP2D6 inhibitor. Caution is advised should a patient's therapy include venlafaxine and CYP2D6 inhibitor).
No products indexed under this heading.

Amoxapine (Studies indicate that venlafaxine is metabolized to its active metabolite, ODV, by CYP2D6. Thus the potential exists for a drug interaction between drugs that inhibit CYP2D6-mediated metabolism and venlafaxine. However, although imipramine partially inhibited the CYP2D6-mediated metabolism of venlafaxine, resulting in higher plasma concentrations of venlafaxine and lower plasma concentrations of ODV, the total concentration of active compounds (venlafaxine plus ODV) was not affected. Also, in a clinical study involving CYP2D6 poor and extensive metabolizers, the total concentration of active compounds (venlafaxine plus ODV), was similar in both groups. No dosage adjustment is required when venlafaxine is co-administered with a CYP2D6 inhibitor. Caution is advised should a patient's therapy include venlafaxine and CYP2D6 inhibitor).
No products indexed under this heading.

Amphetamine Aspartate (The risk of using venlafaxine in combination with other CNS active drugs has not been systematically evaluated. Consequently, caution is advised if the concomitant administration of venlafaxine and such drugs is required).
No products indexed under this heading.

Amphetamine Aspartate Monohydrate (The risk of using venlafaxine in combination with other CNS active drugs has not been systematically evaluated. Consequently, caution is advised if the concomitant administration of venlafaxine and such drugs is required).
No products indexed under this heading.

Amphetamine Resins (The risk of using venlafaxine in combination with other CNS active drugs has not been systematically evaluated. Consequently, caution is advised if the concomitant administration of venlafaxine and such drugs is required).
No products indexed under this heading.

Amphetamine Sulfate (The risk of using venlafaxine in combination with other CNS active drugs has not been systematically evaluated. Consequently, caution is advised if the concomitant administration of venlafaxine and such drugs is required).
No products indexed under this heading.

Amprenavir (Concomitant use of CYP3A4 inhibitors and venlafaxine may increase levels of venlafaxine and ODV. Therefore, caution is advised if a patient's therapy includes a CYP3A4 inhibitor and venlafaxine concomitantly. The concomitant use of venlafaxine with a drug treatment(s) that potently inhibits both CYP2D6 and CYP3A4, the primary metabolizing enzymes for venlafaxine, has not been studied. Therefore, caution is advised should a patient's therapy include venlafaxine and any agent(s) that produce potent simultaneous inhibition of these two enzyme systems).
No products indexed under this heading.

Anastrozole (Concomitant use of CYP3A4 inhibitors and venlafaxine may increase levels of venlafaxine and ODV. Therefore, caution is advised if a patient's therapy includes a CYP3A4 inhibitor and venlafaxine concomitantly. The concomitant use of venlafaxine with a drug treatment(s) that potently inhibits both CYP2D6 and CYP3A4, the primary metabolizing enzymes for venlafaxine, has not been studied. Therefore, caution is advised should a patient's therapy include venlafaxine and any agent(s) that produce potent simultaneous inhibition of these two enzyme systems).
No products indexed under this heading.

Anisindione (Patients should be cautioned about the concomitant use of venlafaxine and anti-coagulants since combined use of psychotropic drugs that interfere with serotonin reuptake and this agent has been associated with an increased risk of bleeding. SSRIs and SNRIs, including venlafaxine, may increase the risk of bleeding events. Concomitant use of anti-coagulants may add to this risk. Case reports and epidemiological studies (case-control and cohort design) have demonstrated an association between use of drugs that interfere with serotonin reuptake and the occurrence of gastrointestinal bleeding).
No products indexed under this heading.

Aprepitant (Concomitant use of CYP3A4 inhibitors and venlafaxine may increase levels of venlafaxine and ODV. Therefore, caution is advised if a patient's therapy includes a CYP3A4 inhibitor and venlafaxine concomitantly. The concomitant use of venlafaxine with a drug treatment(s) that potently inhibits both CYP2D6 and CYP3A4, the primary metabolizing enzymes for venlafaxine, has not been studied. Therefore, caution is advised should a patient's therapy include venlafaxine and any agent(s) that produce potent simultaneous inhibition of these two enzyme systems). Products include:
Emend 2124

Aprobarbital (The risk of using venlafaxine in combination with other CNS active drugs has not been systematically evaluated. Consequently, caution is advised if the concomitant administration of venlafaxine and such drugs is required).
No products indexed under this heading.

Ardeparin Sodium (Patients should be cautioned about the concomitant use of venlafaxine and anti-coagulants since combined use of psychotropic drugs that interfere with serotonin reuptake and this agent has been associated with an increased risk of bleeding. SSRIs and SNRIs, including venlafaxine, may increase the risk of bleeding events. Concomitant use of anti-coagulants may add to this risk. Case reports and epidemiological studies (case-control and cohort design) have demonstrated an association between use of drugs that interfere with serotonin reuptake and the occurrence of gastrointestinal bleeding).
No products indexed under this heading.

Aripiprazole (The development of a potentially life-threatening serotonin syndrome or Neuroleptic Malignant Syndrome (NMS)-like reactions have been reported with SNRIs and SSRIs alone, including venlafaxine, but particularly with concomitant use of antipsychotics).
No products indexed under this heading.

Aspirin (Patients should be cautioned about the concomitant use of venlafaxine and aspirin since combined use of psychotropic drugs that interfere with serotonin reuptake and this agent has been associated with an increased risk of bleeding. SSRIs and SNRIs, including venlafaxine, may increase the risk of bleeding events. Concomitant use of aspirin may add to this risk. Case reports and epidemiological studies (case-control and cohort design) have demonstrated an association between use of drugs that interfere with serotonin reuptake and the occurrence of gastrointestinal bleeding). Products include:
Aggrenox 880
Bayer Aspirin 829
Percodan 1124
St. Joseph Aspirin 2045

Aspirin, Enteric Coated (Patients should be cautioned about the concomitant use of venlafaxine and aspirin since combined use of psychotropic drugs that interfere with serotonin reuptake and this agent has been associated with an increased risk of bleeding. SSRIs and SNRIs, including venlafaxine, may increase the risk of bleeding events. Concomitant use of aspirin may add to this risk. Case reports and epidemiological studies (case-control and cohort design) have demonstrated an association between use of drugs that interfere with serotonin reuptake and the occurrence of gastrointestinal bleeding).
No products indexed under this heading.

Aspirin Buffered (Patients should be cautioned about the concomitant use of venlafaxine and aspirin since combined use of psychotropic drugs that interfere with serotonin reuptake and this agent has been associated with an increased risk of bleeding. SSRIs and SNRIs, including venlafaxine, may increase the risk of bleeding events. Concomitant use of aspirin may add to this risk. Case reports and epidemiological studies (case-control and cohort design) have demonstrated an association between use of drugs that interfere with serotonin reuptake and the occurrence of gastrointestinal bleeding).
No products indexed under this heading.

Atazanavir (Concomitant use of CYP3A4 inhibitors and venlafaxine may increase levels of venlafaxine and ODV. Therefore, caution is advised if a patient's therapy includes a CYP3A4 inhibitor and venlafaxine concomitantly. The concomitant use of venlafaxine with a drug treatment(s) that potently inhibits both CYP2D6 and CYP3A4, the primary metabolizing enzymes for venlafaxine, has not been studied. Therefore, caution is advised should a patient's therapy include venlafaxine and any agent(s) that produce potent simultaneous inhibition of these two enzyme systems).
No products indexed under this heading.

Atazanavir Sulfate (Concomitant use of CYP3A4 inhibitors and venlafaxine may increase levels of venlafaxine and ODV. Therefore, caution is advised if a patient's therapy includes a CYP3A4 inhibitor and venlafaxine concomitantly. The concomitant use of venlafaxine with a drug treatment(s) that potently inhibits both CYP2D6 and CYP3A4, the primary metabolizing enzymes for venlafaxine, has not been studied. Therefore, caution is advised should a patient's therapy include venlafaxine and any agent(s) that produce potent simultaneous inhibition of these two enzyme systems).
No products indexed under this heading.

Atomoxetine Hydrochloride (*In vitro* studies indicate that venlafaxine is a relatively weak inhibitor of CYP2D6. These findings have been confirmed in a clinical drug interaction study comparing the effect of venlafaxine to that of fluoxetine on the CYP2D6-mediated metabolism of dextromethorphan to dextrophan). Products include:
Strattera 1957

Bendroflumethiazide (Elderly patients may be at greater risk of developing hyponatremia with SSRIs and SNRIs. Also patients taking diuretics or who are otherwise volume depleted may be at greater risk. Discontinuation of venlafaxine should be considered in patients with symptomatic hyponatremia and appropriate medical intervention should be instituted).
No products indexed under this heading.

Benzphetamine Hydrochloride (The safety and efficacy of venlafaxine therapy in combination with weight loss agents, including phentermine, have not been established. Co-administration of venlafaxine and weight loss agents is not recommended. Venlafaxine is not indicated for weight loss alone or in combination with other products).
No products indexed under this heading.

Bisoprolol Fumarate (*In vitro* studies indicate that venlafaxine is a relatively weak inhibitor of CYP2D6. These findings have been confirmed in a clinical drug interaction study comparing the effect of venlafaxine to that of fluoxetine on the CYP2D6-mediated metabolism of dextrometrophan to dextrophan).
No products indexed under this heading.

Bumetanide (Elderly patients may be at greater risk of developing hyponatremia with SSRIs and SNRIs. Also patients taking diuretics or who are otherwise volume depleted may be at greater risk. Discontinuation of venlafaxine should be considered in patients with symptomatic hyponatremia and appropriate medical intervention should be instituted).
No products indexed under this heading.

Buprenorphine Hydrochloride (The risk of using venlafaxine in combination with other CNS active drugs has not been systematically evaluated. Consequently, caution is advised if the concomitant administration of venlafaxine and such drugs is required).
No products indexed under this heading.

Bupropion Hydrochloride (Studies indicate that venlafaxine is metabolized to its active metabolite, ODV, by CYP2D6. Thus the potential exists for a drug interaction between drugs that inhibit CYP2D6-mediated metabolism and venlafaxine. However, although imipramine partially inhibited the CYP2D6-mediated metabolism of venlafaxine, resulting in higher plasma concentrations of venlafaxine and lower plasma concentrations of ODV, the total concentration of active compounds (venlafaxine plus ODV) was not affected. Also, in a clinical study involving CYP2D6 poor and extensive metabolizers, the total concentration of active compounds (venlafaxine plus ODV), was similar in both groups. No dosage adjustment is required when venlafaxine is co-administered with a CYP2D6 inhibitor. Caution is advised should a patient's therapy include venlafaxine and CYP2D6 inhibitor). Products include:
Aplenzin 2948
Wellbutrin 1719
Wellbutrin SR 1725
Zyban 1762

Buspirone Hydrochloride (The risk of using venlafaxine in combination with other CNS active drugs has not been systematically evaluated. Consequently, caution is advised if the concomitant administration of venlafaxine and such drugs is required).
No products indexed under this heading.

Butabarbital (The risk of using venlafaxine in combination with other CNS active drugs has not been systematically evaluated. Consequently, caution is advised if the concomitant administration of venlafaxine and such drugs is required).
No products indexed under this heading.

Butalbital (The risk of using venlafaxine in combination with other CNS active drugs has not been systematically evaluated. Consequently, caution is advised if the concomitant administration of venlafaxine and such drugs is required).
No products indexed under this heading.

Captopril (*In vitro* studies indicate that venlafaxine is a relatively weak inhibitor of CYP2D6. These findings have been confirmed in a clinical drug interaction study comparing the effect of venlafaxine to that of fluoxetine on the CYP2D6-mediated metabolism of dextrometrophan to dextrophan). Products include:
Captopril 2341

Carvedilol (*In vitro* studies indicate that venlafaxine is a relatively weak inhibitor of CYP2D6. These findings have been confirmed in a clinical drug interaction study comparing the effect of venlafaxine to that of fluoxetine on the CYP2D6-mediated metabolism of dextrometrophan to dextrophan). Products include:
Coreg 1409

Celecoxib (Patients should be cautioned about the concomitant use of venlafaxine and NSAIDs since combined use of psychotropic drugs that interfere with serotonin reuptake and this agent has been associated with an increased risk of bleeding. SSRIs and SNRIs, including venlafaxine, may increase the risk of bleeding events. Concomitant use of nonsteroidal anti-inflammatory drugs may add to this risk. Case reports and epidemiological studies (case-control and cohort design) have demonstrated an association between use of drugs that interfere with serotonin reuptake and the occurrence of gastrointestinal bleeding). Products include:
Celebrex 3272

Cevimeline Hydrochloride (*In vitro* studies indicate that venlafaxine is a relatively weak inhibitor of CYP2D6. These findings have been confirmed in a clinical drug interaction study comparing the effect of venlafaxine to that of fluoxetine on the CYP2D6-mediated metabolism of dextrometrophan to dextrophan). Products include:
Evoxac 1027

Chlordiazepoxide (The risk of using venlafaxine in combination with other CNS active drugs has not been systematically evaluated. Consequently, caution is advised if the concomitant administration of venlafaxine and such drugs is required).
No products indexed under this heading.

Chlordiazepoxide Hydrochloride (The risk of using venlafaxine in combination with other CNS active drugs has not been systematically evaluated. Consequently, caution is advised if the concomitant administration of venlafaxine and such drugs is required).
No products indexed under this heading.

Chloroquine (Studies indicate that venlafaxine is metabolized to its active metabolite, ODV, by CYP2D6. Thus the potential exists for a drug interaction between drugs that inhibit CYP2D6-mediated metabolism and venlafaxine. However, although imipramine partially inhibited the CYP2D6-mediated metabolism of venlafaxine, resulting in higher plasma concentrations of venlafaxine and lower plasma concentrations of ODV, the total concentration of active compounds (venlafaxine plus ODV) was not affected. Also, in a clinical study involving CYP2D6 poor and extensive metabolizers, the total concentration of active compounds (venlafaxine plus ODV), was similar in both groups. No dosage adjustment is required when venlafaxine is co-administered with a CYP2D6 inhibitor. Caution is advised should a patient's therapy include venlafaxine and CYP2D6 inhibitor).
No products indexed under this heading.

Chloroquine Hydrochloride (Studies indicate that venlafaxine is metabolized to its active metabolite, ODV, by CYP2D6. Thus the potential exists for a drug interaction between drugs that inhibit CYP2D6-mediated metabolism and venlafaxine. However, although imipramine partially inhibited the CYP2D6-mediated metabolism of venlafaxine, resulting in higher plasma concentrations of venlafaxine and lower plasma concentrations of ODV, the total concentration of active compounds (venlafaxine plus ODV) was not affected. Also, in a clinical study involving CYP2D6 poor and extensive metabolizers, the total concentration of active compounds (venlafaxine plus ODV), was similar in both groups. No dosage adjustment is required when venlafaxine is co-administered with a CYP2D6 inhibitor. Caution is advised should a patient's therapy include venlafaxine and CYP2D6 inhibitor).
No products indexed under this heading.

Chloroquine Phosphate (Studies indicate that venlafaxine is metabolized to its active metabolite, ODV, by CYP2D6. Thus the potential exists for a drug interaction between drugs that inhibit CYP2D6-mediated metabolism and venlafaxine. However, although imipramine partially inhibited the CYP2D6-mediated metabolism of venlafaxine, resulting in higher plasma concentrations of venlafaxine and lower plasma concentrations of ODV, the total concentration of active compounds (venlafaxine plus ODV) was not affected. Also, in a clinical study involving CYP2D6 poor and extensive metabolizers, the total concentration of active compounds (venlafaxine plus ODV), was similar in both groups. No dosage adjustment is required when venlafaxine is co-administered with a CYP2D6 inhibitor. Caution is advised should a patient's therapy include venlafaxine and CYP2D6 inhibitor).
No products indexed under this heading.

Chlorothiazide (Elderly patients may be at greater risk of developing hyponatremia with SSRIs and SNRIs. Also patients taking diuretics or who are otherwise volume depleted may be at greater risk. Discontinuation of venlafaxine should be considered in patients with symptomatic hyponatremia and appropriate medical intervention should be instituted).
No products indexed under this heading.

Chlorothiazide Sodium (Elderly patients may be at greater risk of developing hyponatremia with SSRIs and SNRIs. Also patients taking diuretics or who are otherwise volume depleted may be at greater risk. Discontinuation of venlafaxine should be considered in patients with symptomatic hyponatremia and appropriate medical intervention should be instituted). Products include:
Diuril Intravenous 2009

Chlorpheniramine (Studies indicate that venlafaxine is metabolized to its active metabolite, ODV, by CYP2D6. Thus the potential exists for a drug interaction between drugs that inhibit CYP2D6-mediated metabolism and venlafaxine. However, although imipramine partially inhibited the CYP2D6-mediated metabolism of venlafaxine, resulting in higher plasma concentrations of venlafaxine and lower plasma concentrations of ODV, the total concentration of active compounds (venlafaxine plus ODV) was not affected. Also, in a clinical study involving CYP2D6 poor and extensive metabolizers, the total concentration of active compounds (venlafaxine plus ODV), was similar in both groups. No dosage adjustment is required when venlafaxine is co-administered with a CYP2D6 inhibitor. Caution is advised should a patient's therapy include venlafaxine and CYP2D6 inhibitor).
No products indexed under this heading.

Chlorpheniramine Maleate (Studies indicate that venlafaxine is metabolized to its active metabolite, ODV, by CYP2D6. Thus the potential exists for a drug interaction between drugs that inhibit CYP2D6-mediated metabolism and venlafaxine. However, although imipramine partially inhibited the CYP2D6-mediated metabolism of venlafaxine, resulting in higher plasma concentrations of venlafaxine and lower plasma concentrations of ODV, the total concentration of active compounds (venlafaxine plus ODV) was not affected. Also, in a clinical study involving CYP2D6 poor and extensive metabolizers, the total concentration of active compounds (venlafaxine plus ODV), was similar in both groups. No dosage adjustment is required when venlafaxine is co-administered with a CYP2D6 inhibitor. Caution is advised should a patient's therapy include venlafaxine and CYP2D6 inhibitor).
No products indexed under this heading.

Chlorpheniramine Polistirex (Studies indicate that venlafaxine is metabolized to its active metabolite, ODV, by CYP2D6. Thus the potential exists for a drug interaction between drugs that inhibit CYP2D6-mediated metabolism and venlafaxine. However, although imipramine partially inhibited the CYP2D6-mediated metabolism of venlafaxine, resulting in higher plasma concentrations of venlafaxine and lower plasma concentrations of ODV, the total concentration of active compounds (venlafaxine plus ODV) was not affected. Also, in a clinical study involving CYP2D6 poor and extensive metabolizers, the total concentration of active compounds (venlafaxine plus ODV), was similar in both groups. No dosage adjustment is required when venlafaxine is co-administered with a CYP2D6 inhibitor. Caution is advised should a patient's therapy include venlafaxine and CYP2D6 inhibitor). Products include:
Tussionex 3443

Chlorpheniramine Tannate (Studies indicate that venlafaxine is metabolized to its active metabolite, ODV, by CYP2D6. Thus the potential exists for a drug interaction between drugs that inhibit CYP2D6-mediated metabolism and venlafaxine. However, although imipramine partially inhibited the CYP2D6-mediated metabolism of venlafaxine, resulting in higher plasma concentrations of venlafaxine and lower plasma concentrations of ODV, the total concentration of active compounds (venlafaxine plus ODV) was not affected. Also, in a clinical study involving CYP2D6 poor and extensive metabolizers, the total concentration of active compounds (venlafaxine plus ODV), was similar in both groups. No dosage adjustment is required when venlafaxine is co-administered with a CYP2D6 inhibitor. Caution is advised should a patient's therapy include venlafaxine and CYP2D6 inhibitor).
No products indexed under this heading.

Chlorpromazine (The risk of using venlafaxine in combination with other CNS active drugs has not been systematically evaluated. Consequently, caution is advised if the concomitant administration of venlafaxine and such drugs is required).
No products indexed under this heading.

Chlorpromazine Hydrochloride (The risk of using venlafaxine in combination with other CNS active drugs has not been systematically evaluated. Consequently, caution is advised if the concomitant administration of venlafaxine and such drugs is required).
No products indexed under this heading.

Chlorpropamide (*In vitro* studies indicate that venlafaxine is a relatively weak inhibitor of CYP2D6. These findings have been confirmed in a clinical drug interaction study comparing the effect of venlafaxine to that of fluoxetine on the CYP2D6-mediated metabolism of dextrometrophan to dextrophan).
No products indexed under this heading.

IMPORTANT NOTE: Always consult each drug listing in the patient's regimen for possible interactions.

Chlorprothixene (The risk of using venlafaxine in combination with other CNS active drugs has not been systematically evaluated. Consequently, caution is advised if the concomitant administration of venlafaxine and such drugs is required).

No products indexed under this heading.

Chlorprothixene Hydrochloride (The risk of using venlafaxine in combination with other CNS active drugs has not been systematically evaluated. Consequently, caution is advised if the concomitant administration of venlafaxine and such drugs is required).

No products indexed under this heading.

Chlorprothixene Lactate (The risk of using venlafaxine in combination with other CNS active drugs has not been systematically evaluated. Consequently, caution is advised if the concomitant administration of venlafaxine and such drugs is required).

No products indexed under this heading.

Chlorthalidone (Elderly patients may be at greater risk of developing hyponatremia with SSRIs and SNRIs. Also patients taking diuretics or who are otherwise volume depleted may be at greater risk. Discontinuation of venlafaxine should be considered in patients with symptomatic hyponatremia and appropriate medical intervention should be instituted). Products include:

Clorpres 2344

Cimetidine (Concomitant administration of cimetidine and venlafaxine resulted in inhibition of first-pass metabolism of venlafaxine. The oral clearance of venlafaxine was reduced by about 43%, and the exposure (AUC) and maximum concentration (C_{max}) of the drug were increased by about 60%. However, co-administration of cimetidine had no apparent effect on the pharmacokinetics of O-desmethylvenlafaxine (ODV). The overall pharmacological activity of venlafaxine plus ODV is expected to increase only slightly, and no dosage adjustment should be necessary for most normal adults. However, in elderly patients, patients with pre-existing hypertension or hepatic dysfunction, the interaction of venlafaxine and cimetidine is not known and potentially could be more pronounced).

No products indexed under this heading.

Cimetidine Hydrochloride (Concomitant administration of cimetidine and venlafaxine resulted in inhibition of first-pass metabolism of venlafaxine. The oral clearance of venlafaxine was reduced by about 43%, and the exposure (AUC) and maximum concentration (C_{max}) of the drug were increased by about 60%. However, co-administration of cimetidine had no apparent effect on the pharmacokinetics of O-desmethylvenlafaxine (ODV). The overall pharmacological activity of venlafaxine plus ODV is expected to increase only slightly, and no dosage adjustment should be necessary for most normal adults. However, in elderly patients, patients with pre-existing hypertension or hepatic dysfunction, the interaction of venlafaxine and cimetidine is not known and potentially could be more pronounced).

No products indexed under this heading.

Ciprofloxacin (Concomitant use of CYP3A4 inhibitors and venlafaxine may increase levels of venlafaxine and ODV. Therefore, caution is advised if a patient's therapy includes a CYP3A4 inhibitor and venlafaxine concomitantly. The concomitant use of venlafaxine with a drug treatment(s) that potently inhibits both CYP2D6 and CYP3A4, the primary metabolizing enzymes for venlafaxine, has not been studied. Therefore, caution is advised should a patient's therapy include venlafaxine and any agent(s)

that produce potent simultaneous inhibition of these two enzyme systems). Products include:

Cipro I.V. 3082
Cipro 3073
Cipro XR 3091
Ciprodex 583

Citalopram Hydrobromide (Based on the mechanism of action of venlafaxine and the potential for serotonin syndrome, caution is advised when venlafaxine is co-administered with other drugs that may affect the serotonergic neurotransmitter systems, such as SSRIs. If concomitant treatment of venlafaxine with an SSRI is clinically warranted, careful observation of the patient is advised, particularly during treatment initiation and dose increases). Products include:

Celexa 1153

Clarithromycin (Concomitant use of CYP3A4 inhibitors and venlafaxine may increase levels of venlafaxine and ODV. Therefore, caution is advised if a patient's therapy includes a CYP3A4 inhibitor and venlafaxine concomitantly. The concomitant use of venlafaxine with a drug treatment(s) that potently inhibits both CYP2D6 and CYP3A4, the primary metabolizing enzymes for venlafaxine, has not been studied. Therefore, caution is advised should a patient's therapy include venlafaxine and any agent(s) that produce potent simultaneous inhibition of these two enzyme systems). Products include:

Biaxin/Biaxin XL 412

Clomipramine Hydrochloride (Studies indicate that venlafaxine is metabolized to its active metabolite, ODV, by CYP2D6. Thus the potential exists for a drug interaction between drugs that inhibit CYP2D6-mediated metabolism and venlafaxine. However, although imipramine partially inhibited the CYP2D6-mediated metabolism of venlafaxine, resulting in higher plasma concentrations of venlafaxine and lower plasma concentrations of ODV, the total concentration of active compounds (venlafaxine plus ODV) was not affected. Also, in a clinical study involving CYP2D6 poor and extensive metabolizers, the total concentration of active compounds (venlafaxine plus ODV), was similar in both groups. No dosage adjustment is required when venlafaxine is co-administered with a CYP2D6 inhibitor. Caution is advised should a patient's therapy include venlafaxine and CYP2D6 inhibitor).

No products indexed under this heading.

Clorazepate Dipotassium (The risk of using venlafaxine in combination with other CNS active drugs has not been systematically evaluated. Consequently, caution is advised if the concomitant administration of venlafaxine and such drugs is required).

No products indexed under this heading.

Clotrimazole (Concomitant use of CYP3A4 inhibitors and venlafaxine may increase levels of venlafaxine and ODV. Therefore, caution is advised if a patient's therapy includes a CYP3A4 inhibitor and venlafaxine concomitantly. The concomitant use of venlafaxine with a drug treatment(s) that potently inhibits both CYP2D6 and CYP3A4, the primary metabolizing enzymes for venlafaxine, has not been studied. Therefore, caution is advised should a patient's therapy include venlafaxine and any agent(s) that produce potent simultaneous inhibition of these two enzyme systems). Products include:

Lotrisone 3163

Clozapine (There have been reports of elevated clozapine levels that were temporally associated with adverse events, including seizures, following the addition of venlafaxine).

No products indexed under this heading.

Cocaine Hydrochloride (Studies indicate that venlafaxine is metabolized to its active metabolite, ODV, by CYP2D6. Thus the potential exists for a drug interaction between drugs that inhibit CYP2D6-mediated metabolism and venlafaxine. However, although imipramine partially inhibited the CYP2D6-mediated metabolism of venlafaxine, resulting in higher plasma concentrations of venlafaxine and lower plasma concentrations of ODV, the total concentration of active compounds (venlafaxine plus ODV) was not affected. Also, in a clinical study involving CYP2D6 poor and extensive metabolizers, the total concentration of active compounds (venlafaxine plus ODV), was similar in both groups. No dosage adjustment is required when venlafaxine is co-administered with a CYP2D6 inhibitor. Caution is advised should a patient's therapy include venlafaxine and CYP2D6 inhibitor).

No products indexed under this heading.

Codeine Phosphate (The risk of using venlafaxine in combination with other CNS active drugs has not been systematically evaluated. Consequently, caution is advised if the concomitant administration of venlafaxine and such drugs is required). Products include:

Tylenol with Codeine 2691

Codeine Sulfate (The risk of using venlafaxine in combination with other CNS active drugs has not been systematically evaluated. Consequently, caution is advised if the concomitant administration of venlafaxine and such drugs is required).

No products indexed under this heading.

Conivaptan Hydrochloride (Concomitant use of CYP3A4 inhibitors and venlafaxine may increase levels of venlafaxine and ODV. Therefore, caution is advised if a patient's therapy includes a CYP3A4 inhibitor and venlafaxine concomitantly. The concomitant use of venlafaxine with a drug treatment(s) that potently inhibits both CYP2D6 and CYP3A4, the primary metabolizing enzymes for venlafaxine, has not been studied. Therefore, caution is advised should a patient's therapy include venlafaxine and any agent(s) that produce potent simultaneous inhibition of these two enzyme systems). Products include:

Vaprisol 689

Cyclobenzaprine Hydrochloride (In vitro studies indicate that venlafaxine is a relatively weak inhibitor of CYP2D6. These findings have been confirmed in a clinical drug interaction study comparing the effect of venlafaxine to that of fluoxetine on the CYP2D6-mediated metabolism of dextrometrophan to dextrophan). Products include:

Amrix 964

Cyclosporine (Concomitant use of CYP3A4 inhibitors and venlafaxine may increase levels of venlafaxine and ODV. Therefore, caution is advised if a patient's therapy includes a CYP3A4 inhibitor and venlafaxine concomitantly. The concomitant use of venlafaxine with a drug treatment(s) that potently inhibits both CYP2D6 and CYP3A4, the primary metabolizing enzymes for venlafaxine, has not been studied. Therefore, caution is advised should a patient's therapy include venlafaxine and any agent(s) that produce potent simultaneous inhibition of these two enzyme systems). Products include:

Gengraf 440

Neoral Oral Solution 2496
Neoral Capsules 2496
Restasis 605

Dalfopristin (Concomitant use of CYP3A4 inhibitors and venlafaxine may increase levels of venlafaxine and ODV. Therefore, caution is advised if a patient's therapy includes a CYP3A4 inhibitor and venlafaxine concomitantly. The concomitant use of venlafaxine with a drug treatment(s) that potently inhibits both CYP2D6 and CYP3A4, the primary metabolizing enzymes for venlafaxine, has not been studied. Therefore, caution is advised should a patient's therapy include venlafaxine and any agent(s) that produce potent simultaneous inhibition of these two enzyme systems).

No products indexed under this heading.

Dalteparin Sodium (Patients should be cautioned about the concomitant use of venlafaxine and anti-coagulants since combined use of psychotropic drugs that interfere with serotonin reuptake and this agent has been associated with an increased risk of bleeding. SSRIs and SNRIs, including venlafaxine, may increase the risk of bleeding events. Concomitant use of anti-coagulants may add to this risk. Case reports and epidemiological studies (case-control and cohort design) have demonstrated an association between use of drugs that interfere with serotonin reuptake and the occurrence of gastrointestinal bleeding). Products include:

Fragmin 1058

Danaparoid Sodium (Patients should be cautioned about the concomitant use of venlafaxine and anti-coagulants since combined use of psychotropic drugs that interfere with serotonin reuptake and this agent has been associated with an increased risk of bleeding. SSRIs and SNRIs, including venlafaxine, may increase the risk of bleeding events. Concomitant use of anti-coagulants may add to this risk. Case reports and epidemiological studies (case-control and cohort design) have demonstrated an association between use of drugs that interfere with serotonin reuptake and the occurrence of gastrointestinal bleeding).

No products indexed under this heading.

Danazol (Concomitant use of CYP3A4 inhibitors and venlafaxine may increase levels of venlafaxine and ODV. Therefore, caution is advised if a patient's therapy includes a CYP3A4 inhibitor and venlafaxine concomitantly. The concomitant use of venlafaxine with a drug treatment(s) that potently inhibits both CYP2D6 and CYP3A4, the primary metabolizing enzymes for venlafaxine, has not been studied. Therefore, caution is advised should a patient's therapy include venlafaxine and any agent(s) that produce potent simultaneous inhibition of these two enzyme systems).

No products indexed under this heading.

Darunavir (Concomitant use of CYP3A4 inhibitors and venlafaxine may increase levels of venlafaxine and ODV. Therefore, caution is advised if a patient's therapy includes a CYP3A4 inhibitor and venlafaxine concomitantly. The concomitant use of venlafaxine with a drug treatment(s) that potently inhibits both CYP2D6 and CYP3A4, the primary metabolizing enzymes for venlafaxine, has not been studied. Therefore, caution is advised should a patient's therapy include venlafaxine and any agent(s) that produce potent simultaneous inhibition of these two enzyme systems).

No products indexed under this heading.

Dasatinib (Concomitant use of CYP3A4 inhibitors and venlafaxine may increase levels of venlafaxine and ODV. Therefore, caution is advised if a patient's therapy includes a CYP3A4

inhibitor and venlafaxine concomitantly. The concomitant use of venlafaxine with a drug treatment(s) that potently inhibits both CYP2D6 and CYP3A4, the primary metabolizing enzymes for venlafaxine, has not been studied. Therefore, caution is advised should a patient's therapy include venlafaxine and any agent(s) that produce potent simultaneous inhibition of these two enzyme systems).
No products indexed under this heading.

Debrisoquine (*In vitro* studies indicate that venlafaxine is a relatively weak inhibitor of CYP2D6. These findings have been confirmed in a clinical drug interaction study comparing the effect of venlafaxine to that of fluoxetine on the CYP2D6-mediated metabolism of dextrometrophan to dextrophan).
No products indexed under this heading.

Delavirdine Mesylate (Concomitant use of CYP3A4 inhibitors and venlafaxine may increase levels of venlafaxine and ODV. Therefore, caution is advised if a patient's therapy includes a CYP3A4 inhibitor and venlafaxine concomitantly. The concomitant use of venlafaxine with a drug treatment(s) that potently inhibits both CYP2D6 and CYP3A4, the primary metabolizing enzymes for venlafaxine, has not been studied. Therefore, caution is advised should a patient's therapy include venlafaxine and any agent(s) that produce potent simultaneous inhibition of these two enzyme systems).
No products indexed under this heading.

Delavirine (Concomitant use of CYP3A4 inhibitors and venlafaxine may increase levels of venlafaxine and ODV. Therefore, caution is advised if a patient's therapy includes a CYP3A4 inhibitor and venlafaxine concomitantly. The concomitant use of venlafaxine with a drug treatment(s) that potently inhibits both CYP2D6 and CYP3A4, the primary metabolizing enzymes for venlafaxine, has not been studied. Therefore, caution is advised should a patient's therapy include venlafaxine and any agent(s) that produce potent simultaneous inhibition of these two enzyme systems).
No products indexed under this heading.

Desflurane (The risk of using venlafaxine in combination with other CNS active drugs has not been systematically evaluated. Consequently, caution is advised if the concomitant administration of venlafaxine and such drugs is required).
No products indexed under this heading.

Desipramine Hydrochloride (Desipramine AUC, C_{max}, and C_{min} increased by about 35% in the presence of venlafaxine. The 2-OH-desipramine AUCs increased by at least 2.5 fold (with venlafaxine 37.5 mg q12h) and by 4.5 fold (with venlafaxine 75 mg q12h)).
No products indexed under this heading.

Desloratadine (Concomitant use of CYP3A4 inhibitors and venlafaxine may increase levels of venlafaxine and ODV. Therefore, caution is advised if a patient's therapy includes a CYP3A4 inhibitor and venlafaxine concomitantly. The concomitant use of venlafaxine with a drug treatment(s) that potently inhibits both CYP2D6 and CYP3A4, the primary metabolizing enzymes for venlafaxine, has not been studied. Therefore, caution is advised should a patient's therapy include venlafaxine and any agent(s) that produce potent simultaneous inhibition of these two enzyme systems). Products include:
Clarinex Syrup 3098
Clarinex 3098
Clarinex Reditabs 3098
Clarinex-D 12-Hour 3101
Clarinex-D 3104

Desvenlafaxine Succinate (Based on the mechanism of action of venlafaxine and the potential for serotonin syndrome, caution is advised when venlafaxine is co-administered with other drugs that may affect the serotonergic neurotransmitter systems, such as other SNRIs. If concomitant treatment of venlafaxine with another SNRI is clinically warranted, careful observation of the patient is advised, particularly during treatment initiation and dose increases). Products include:
Pristiq 3564

Dexfenfluramine Hydrochloride (*In vitro* studies indicate that venlafaxine is a relatively weak inhibitor of CYP2D6. These findings have been confirmed in a clinical drug interaction study comparing the effect of venlafaxine to that of fluoxetine on the CYP2D6-mediated metabolism of dextrometrophan to dextrophan).
No products indexed under this heading.

Dexmethylphenidate Hydrochloride (The risk of using venlafaxine in combination with other CNS active drugs has not been systematically evaluated. Consequently, caution is advised if the concomitant administration of venlafaxine and such drugs is required). Products include:
Focalin XR 2472

Dextroamphetamine (The risk of using venlafaxine in combination with other CNS active drugs has not been systematically evaluated. Consequently, caution is advised if the concomitant administration of venlafaxine and such drugs is required).
No products indexed under this heading.

Dextroamphetamine Saccharate (The risk of using venlafaxine in combination with other CNS active drugs has not been systematically evaluated. Consequently, caution is advised if the concomitant administration of venlafaxine and such drugs is required).
No products indexed under this heading.

Dextroamphetamine Sulfate (The risk of using venlafaxine in combination with other CNS active drugs has not been systematically evaluated. Consequently, caution is advised if the concomitant administration of venlafaxine and such drugs is required). Products include:
Dexedrine 1425

Dextromethorphan Hydrobromide (*In vitro* studies indicate that venlafaxine is a relatively weak inhibitor of CYP2D6. These findings have been confirmed in a clinical drug interaction study comparing the effect of venlafaxine to that of fluoxetine on the CYP2D6-mediated metabolism of dextrometrophan to dextrophan).
No products indexed under this heading.

Dextromethorphan Polistirex (*In vitro* studies indicate that venlafaxine is a relatively weak inhibitor of CYP2D6. These findings have been confirmed in a clinical drug interaction study comparing the effect of venlafaxine to that of fluoxetine on the CYP2D6-mediated metabolism of dextrometrophan to dextrophan).
No products indexed under this heading.

Dezocine (The risk of using venlafaxine in combination with other CNS active drugs has not been systematically evaluated. Consequently, caution is advised if the concomitant administration of venlafaxine and such drugs is required).
No products indexed under this heading.

Diazepam (The risk of using venlafaxine in combination with other CNS active drugs has not been systematically evaluated. Consequently, caution is advised if the concomitant administration of venlafaxine and such drugs is required). Products include:
Valium Tablets 2880

Diclofenac Epolamine (Patients should be cautioned about the concomitant use of venlafaxine and NSAIDs since combined use of psychotropic drugs that interfere with serotonin reuptake and this agent has been associated with an increased risk of bleeding. SSRIs and SNRIs, including venlafaxine, may increase the risk of bleeding events. Concomitant use of nonsteroidal anti-inflammatory drugs may add to this risk. Case reports and epidemiological studies (case-control and cohort design) have demonstrated an association between use of drugs that interfere with serotonin reuptake and the occurrence of gastrointestinal bleeding). Products include:
Flector 1839

Diclofenac Potassium (Patients should be cautioned about the concomitant use of venlafaxine and NSAIDs since combined use of psychotropic drugs that interfere with serotonin reuptake and this agent has been associated with an increased risk of bleeding. SSRIs and SNRIs, including venlafaxine, may increase the risk of bleeding events. Concomitant use of nonsteroidal anti-inflammatory drugs may add to this risk. Case reports and epidemiological studies (case-control and cohort design) have demonstrated an association between use of drugs that interfere with serotonin reuptake and the occurrence of gastrointestinal bleeding).
No products indexed under this heading.

Diclofenac Sodium (Patients should be cautioned about the concomitant use of venlafaxine and NSAIDs since combined use of psychotropic drugs that interfere with serotonin reuptake and this agent has been associated with an increased risk of bleeding. SSRIs and SNRIs, including venlafaxine, may increase the risk of bleeding events. Concomitant use of nonsteroidal anti-inflammatory drugs may add to this risk. Case reports and epidemiological studies (case-control and cohort design) have demonstrated an association between use of drugs that interfere with serotonin reuptake and the occurrence of gastrointestinal bleeding).
No products indexed under this heading.

Dicumarol (Patients should be cautioned about the concomitant use of venlafaxine and anti-coagulants since combined use of psychotropic drugs that interfere with serotonin reuptake and this agent has been associated with an increased risk of bleeding. SSRIs and SNRIs, including venlafaxine, may increase the risk of bleeding events. Concomitant use of anti-coagulants may add to this risk. Case reports and epidemiological studies (case-control and cohort design) have demonstrated an association between use of drugs that interfere with serotonin reuptake and the occurrence of gastrointestinal bleeding).
No products indexed under this heading.

Diethylpropion Hydrochloride (The safety and efficacy of venlafaxine therapy in combination with weight loss agents, including phentermine, have not been established. Co-administration of venlafaxine and weight loss agents is not recommended. Venlafaxine is not indicated for weight loss alone or in combination with other products).
No products indexed under this heading.

Diltiazem Hydrochloride (Concomitant use of CYP3A4 inhibitors and venlafaxine may increase levels of venlafaxine and ODV. Therefore, caution is advised if a patient's therapy includes a CYP3A4 inhibitor and venlafaxine concomitantly. The concomitant use of venlafaxine with a drug treatment(s) that potently inhibits both CYP2D6 and CYP3A4, the primary metabolizing enzymes for venlafaxine, has not been studied. Therefore, caution is advised should a patient's therapy include venlafaxine and any agent(s) that produce potent simultaneous inhibition of these two enzyme systems). Products include:
Cardizem LA 423

Diltiazem Maleate (Concomitant use of CYP3A4 inhibitors and venlafaxine may increase levels of venlafaxine and ODV. Therefore, caution is advised if a patient's therapy includes a CYP3A4 inhibitor and venlafaxine concomitantly. The concomitant use of venlafaxine with a drug treatment(s) that potently inhibits both CYP2D6 and CYP3A4, the primary metabolizing enzymes for venlafaxine, has not been studied. Therefore, caution is advised should a patient's therapy include venlafaxine and any agent(s) that produce potent simultaneous inhibition of these two enzyme systems).
No products indexed under this heading.

Diphenhydramine (Studies indicate that venlafaxine is metabolized to its active metabolite, ODV, by CYP2D6. Thus the potential exists for a drug interaction between drugs that inhibit CYP2D6-mediated metabolism and venlafaxine. However, although imipramine partially inhibited the CYP2D6-mediated metabolism of venlafaxine, resulting in higher plasma concentrations of venlafaxine and lower plasma concentrations of ODV, the total concentration of active compounds (venlafaxine plus ODV) was not affected. Also, in a clinical study involving CYP2D6 poor and extensive metabolizers, the total concentration of active compounds (venlafaxine plus ODV), was similar in both groups. No dosage adjustment is required when venlafaxine is co-administered with a CYP2D6 inhibitor. Caution is advised should a patient's therapy include venlafaxine and CYP2D6 inhibitor).
No products indexed under this heading.

Diphenhydramine Hydrochloride (Studies indicate that venlafaxine is metabolized to its active metabolite, ODV, by CYP2D6. Thus the potential exists for a drug interaction between drugs that inhibit CYP2D6-mediated metabolism and venlafaxine. However, although imipramine partially inhibited the CYP2D6-mediated metabolism of venlafaxine, resulting in higher plasma concentrations of venlafaxine and lower plasma concentrations of ODV, the total concentration of active compounds (venlafaxine plus ODV) was not affected. Also, in a clinical study involving CYP2D6 poor and extensive metabolizers, the total concentration of active compounds (venlafaxine plus ODV), was similar in both groups. No dosage adjustment is required when venlafaxine is co-administered with a CYP2D6 inhibitor. Caution is advised should a patient's therapy include venlafaxine and CYP2D6 inhibitor). Products include:
Benadryl Allergy Ultratab 2042
Children's Benadryl Allergy Liquid 2042

Dolasetron Mesylate (*In vitro* studies indicate that venlafaxine is a relatively weak inhibitor of CYP2D6. These findings have been confirmed in a clinical drug interaction study comparing the effect of venlafaxine to that of fluoxetine on the CYP2D6-mediated metabolism of dextrometrophan to dextrophan). Products include:
Anzemet Injection 2931
Anzemet Tablets 2934

Donepezil Hydrochloride (*In vitro* studies indicate that venlafaxine is a relatively weak inhibitor of CYP2D6. These findings have been confirmed in a clinical drug interaction study comparing the effect of venlafaxine to that of

Effexor Interactions Index 538

fluoxetine on the CYP2D6-mediated metabolism of dextrometrophan to dextrophan). Products include:
Aricept 1045
Aricept ODT 1045

Doxepin Hydrochloride (Studies indicate that venlafaxine is metabolized to its active metabolite, ODV, by CYP2D6. Thus the potential exists for a drug interaction between drugs that inhibit CYP2D6-mediated metabolism and venlafaxine. However, although imipramine partially inhibited the CYP2D6-mediated metabolism of venlafaxine, resulting in higher plasma concentrations of venlafaxine and lower plasma concentrations of ODV, the total concentration of active compounds (venlafaxine plus ODV) was not affected. Also, in a clinical study involving CYP2D6 poor and extensive metabolizers, the total concentration of active compounds (venlafaxine plus ODV), was similar in both groups. No dosage adjustment is required when venlafaxine is co-administered with a CYP2D6 inhibitor. Caution is advised should a patient's therapy include venlafaxine and CYP2D6 inhibitor).
No products indexed under this heading.

Droperidol (The risk of using venlafaxine in combination with other CNS active drugs has not been systematically evaluated. Consequently, caution is advised if the concomitant administration of venlafaxine and such drugs is required).
No products indexed under this heading.

Duloxetine Hydrochloride (Based on the mechanism of action of venlafaxine and the potential for serotonin syndrome, caution is advised when venlafaxine is co-administered with other drugs that may affect the serotonergic neurotransmitter systems, such as other SNRIs. If concomitant treatment of venlafaxine with another SNRI is clinically warranted, careful observation of the patient is advised, particularly during treatment initiation and dose increases). Products include:
Cymbalta 1871

Efavirenz (Concomitant use of CYP3A4 inhibitors and venlafaxine may increase levels of venlafaxine and ODV. Therefore, caution is advised if a patient's therapy includes a CYP3A4 inhibitor and venlafaxine concomitantly. The concomitant use of venlafaxine with a drug treatment(s) that potently inhibits both CYP2D6 and CYP3A4, the primary metabolizing enzymes for venlafaxine, has not been studied. Therefore, caution is advised should a patient's therapy include venlafaxine and any agent(s) that produce potent simultaneous inhibition of these two enzyme systems). Products include:
Atripla 906

Eletriptan Hydrobromide (There have been rare post-marketing reports of serotonin syndrome with use of an SSRI and a triptan. If concomitant treatment of venlafaxine with a triptan is clinically warranted, careful observation of the patient is advised, particularly during treatment initiation and dose increases. Patients should be cautioned about the risk of serotonin syndrome with the concomitant use of venlafaxine and triptans, tramadol, tryptophan supplements or other serotonergic agents).
No products indexed under this heading.

Encainide Hydrochloride (*In vitro* studies indicate that venlafaxine is a relatively weak inhibitor of CYP2D6. These findings have been confirmed in a clinical drug interaction study comparing the effect of venlafaxine to that of fluoxetine on the CYP2D6-mediated metabolism of dextrometrophan to dextrophan).
No products indexed under this heading.

Enflurane (The risk of using venlafaxine in combination with other CNS active drugs has not been systematically evaluated. Consequently, caution is advised if the concomitant administration of venlafaxine and such drugs is required).
No products indexed under this heading.

Enoxaparin Sodium (Patients should be cautioned about the concomitant use of venlafaxine and anti-coagulants since combined use of psychotropic drugs that interfere with serotonin reuptake and this agent has been associated with an increased risk of bleeding. SSRIs and SNRIs, including venlafaxine, may increase the risk of bleeding events. Concomitant use of anti-coagulants may add to this risk. Case reports and epidemiological studies (case-control and cohort design) have demonstrated an association between use of drugs that interfere with serotonin reuptake and the occurrence of gastrointestinal bleeding). Products include:
Lovenox 3005

Erythromycin (Concomitant use of CYP3A4 inhibitors and venlafaxine may increase levels of venlafaxine and ODV. Therefore, caution is advised if a patient's therapy includes a CYP3A4 inhibitor and venlafaxine concomitantly. The concomitant use of venlafaxine with a drug treatment(s) that potently inhibits both CYP2D6 and CYP3A4, the primary metabolizing enzymes for venlafaxine, has not been studied. Therefore, caution is advised should a patient's therapy include venlafaxine and any agent(s) that produce potent simultaneous inhibition of these two enzyme systems).
No products indexed under this heading.

Erythromycin Estolate (Concomitant use of CYP3A4 inhibitors and venlafaxine may increase levels of venlafaxine and ODV. Therefore, caution is advised if a patient's therapy includes a CYP3A4 inhibitor and venlafaxine concomitantly. The concomitant use of venlafaxine with a drug treatment(s) that potently inhibits both CYP2D6 and CYP3A4, the primary metabolizing enzymes for venlafaxine, has not been studied. Therefore, caution is advised should a patient's therapy include venlafaxine and any agent(s) that produce potent simultaneous inhibition of these two enzyme systems).
No products indexed under this heading.

Erythromycin Ethylsuccinate (Concomitant use of CYP3A4 inhibitors and venlafaxine may increase levels of venlafaxine and ODV. Therefore, caution is advised if a patient's therapy includes a CYP3A4 inhibitor and venlafaxine concomitantly. The concomitant use of venlafaxine with a drug treatment(s) that potently inhibits both CYP2D6 and CYP3A4, the primary metabolizing enzymes for venlafaxine, has not been studied. Therefore, caution is advised should a patient's therapy include venlafaxine and any agent(s) that produce potent simultaneous inhibition of these two enzyme systems). Products include:
E.E.S. 437
EryPed 435

Erythromycin Gluceptate (Concomitant use of CYP3A4 inhibitors and venlafaxine may increase levels of venlafaxine and ODV. Therefore, caution is advised if a patient's therapy includes a CYP3A4 inhibitor and venlafaxine concomitantly. The concomitant use of venlafaxine with a drug treatment(s) that potently inhibits both CYP2D6 and CYP3A4, the primary metabolizing enzymes for venlafaxine, has not been studied. Therefore, caution is advised should a patient's therapy include venlafaxine and any agent(s) that produce potent simultaneous inhibition of these two enzyme systems).
No products indexed under this heading.

Erythromycin Lactobionate (Concomitant use of CYP3A4 inhibitors and venlafaxine may increase levels of venlafaxine and ODV. Therefore, caution is advised if a patient's therapy includes a CYP3A4 inhibitor and venlafaxine concomitantly. The concomitant use of venlafaxine with a drug treatment(s) that potently inhibits both CYP2D6 and CYP3A4, the primary metabolizing enzymes for venlafaxine, has not been studied. Therefore, caution is advised should a patient's therapy include venlafaxine and any agent(s) that produce potent simultaneous inhibition of these two enzyme systems).
No products indexed under this heading.

Erythromycin Stearate (Concomitant use of CYP3A4 inhibitors and venlafaxine may increase levels of venlafaxine and ODV. Therefore, caution is advised if a patient's therapy includes a CYP3A4 inhibitor and venlafaxine concomitantly. The concomitant use of venlafaxine with a drug treatment(s) that potently inhibits both CYP2D6 and CYP3A4, the primary metabolizing enzymes for venlafaxine, has not been studied. Therefore, caution is advised should a patient's therapy include venlafaxine and any agent(s) that produce potent simultaneous inhibition of these two enzyme systems).
No products indexed under this heading.

Escitalopram Oxalate (Based on the mechanism of action of venlafaxine and the potential for serotonin syndrome, caution is advised when venlafaxine is co-administered with other drugs that may affect the serotonergic neurotransmitter systems, such as SSRIs. If concomitant treatment of venlafaxine with an SSRI is clinically warranted, careful observation of the patient is advised, particularly during treatment initiation and dose increases). Products include:
Lexapro Oral Suspension 1160
Lexapro Tablets 1160

Esomeprazole Magnesium (Concomitant use of CYP3A4 inhibitors and venlafaxine may increase levels of venlafaxine and ODV. Therefore, caution is advised if a patient's therapy includes a CYP3A4 inhibitor and venlafaxine concomitantly. The concomitant use of venlafaxine with a drug treatment(s) that potently inhibits both CYP2D6 and CYP3A4, the primary metabolizing enzymes for venlafaxine, has not been studied. Therefore, caution is advised should a patient's therapy include venlafaxine and any agent(s) that produce potent simultaneous inhibition of these two enzyme systems). Products include:
Nexium Capsules 704
Nexium Oral Suspension 704

Esomeprazole Sodium (Concomitant use of CYP3A4 inhibitors and venlafaxine may increase levels of venlafaxine and ODV. Therefore, caution is advised if a patient's therapy includes a CYP3A4 inhibitor and venlafaxine concomitantly. The concomitant use of venlafaxine with a drug treatment(s) that potently inhibits both CYP2D6 and CYP3A4, the primary metabolizing enzymes for venlafaxine, has not been studied. Therefore, caution is advised should a patient's therapy include venlafaxine and any agent(s) that produce potent simultaneous inhibition of these two enzyme systems). Products include:
Nexium I.V. 712

Estazolam (The risk of using venlafaxine in combination with other CNS active drugs has not been systematically evaluated. Consequently, caution is advised if the concomitant administration of venlafaxine and such drugs is required).
No products indexed under this heading.

Ethacrynic Acid (Elderly patients may be at greater risk of developing hyponatremia with SSRIs and SNRIs. Also patients taking diuretics or who are otherwise volume depleted may be at greater risk. Discontinuation of venlafaxine should be considered in patients with symptomatic hyponatremia and appropriate medical intervention should be instituted).
No products indexed under this heading.

Ethanol (Although venlafaxine has not been shown to increase the impairment of mental and motor skills caused by alcohol, patients should be advised to avoid alcohol while taking venlafaxine).
No products indexed under this heading.

Ethchlorvynol (The risk of using venlafaxine in combination with other CNS active drugs has not been systematically evaluated. Consequently, caution is advised if the concomitant administration of venlafaxine and such drugs is required).
No products indexed under this heading.

Ethinamate (The risk of using venlafaxine in combination with other CNS active drugs has not been systematically evaluated. Consequently, caution is advised if the concomitant administration of venlafaxine and such drugs is required).
No products indexed under this heading.

Ethyl Alcohol (Although venlafaxine has not been shown to increase the impairment of mental and motor skills caused by alcohol, patients should be advised to avoid alcohol while taking venlafaxine).
No products indexed under this heading.

Etodolac (Patients should be cautioned about the concomitant use of venlafaxine and NSAIDs since combined use of psychotropic drugs that interfere with serotonin reuptake and this agent has been associated with an increased risk of bleeding. SSRIs and SNRIs, including venlafaxine, may increase the risk of bleeding events. Concomitant use of nonsteroidal anti-inflammatory drugs may add to this risk. Case reports and epidemiological studies (case-control and cohort design) have demonstrated an association between use of drugs that interfere with serotonin reuptake and the occurrence of gastrointestinal bleeding).
No products indexed under this heading.

Fenfluramine Hydrochloride (The safety and efficacy of venlafaxine therapy in combination with weight loss agents, including phentermine, have not been established. Co-administration of venlafaxine and weight loss agents is not recommended. Venlafaxine is not indicated for weight loss alone or in combination with other products).
No products indexed under this heading.

Fenoprofen Calcium (Patients should be cautioned about the concomitant use of venlafaxine and NSAIDs since combined use of psychotropic drugs that interfere with serotonin reuptake and this agent has been associated with an increased risk of bleeding. SSRIs and SNRIs, including venlafaxine, may increase the risk of bleeding events. Concomitant use of nonsteroidal anti-inflammatory drugs

may add to this risk. Case reports and epidemiological studies (case-control and cohort design) have demonstrated an association between use of drugs that interfere with serotonin reuptake and the occurrence of gastrointestinal bleeding).
No products indexed under this heading.

Fentanyl (The risk of using venlafaxine in combination with other CNS active drugs has not been systematically evaluated. Consequently, caution is advised if the concomitant administration of venlafaxine and such drugs is required). Products include:
Duragesic 2604
Fentanyl Transdermal System 2346
Onsolis 2054

Fentanyl Citrate (The risk of using venlafaxine in combination with other CNS active drugs has not been systematically evaluated. Consequently, caution is advised if the concomitant administration of venlafaxine and such drugs is required). Products include:
Fentora 966

Flecainide Acetate (*In vitro* studies indicate that venlafaxine is a relatively weak inhibitor of CYP2D6. These findings have been confirmed in a clinical drug interaction study comparing the effect of venlafaxine to that of fluoxetine on the CYP2D6-mediated metabolism of dextrometrophan to dextrophan).
No products indexed under this heading.

Fluconazole (Concomitant use of CYP3A4 inhibitors and venlafaxine may increase levels of venlafaxine and ODV. Therefore, caution is advised if a patient's therapy includes a CYP3A4 inhibitor and venlafaxine concomitantly. The concomitant use of venlafaxine with a drug treatment(s) that potently inhibits both CYP2D6 and CYP3A4, the primary metabolizing enzymes for venlafaxine, has not been studied. Therefore, caution is advised should a patient's therapy include venlafaxine and any agent(s) that produce potent simultaneous inhibition of these two enzyme systems).
No products indexed under this heading.

Fluoxetine (Based on the mechanism of action of venlafaxine and the potential for serotonin syndrome, caution is advised when venlafaxine is co-administered with other drugs that may affect the serotonergic neurotransmitter systems, such as SSRIs. If concomitant treatment of venlafaxine with an SSRI is clinically warranted, careful observation of the patient is advised, particularly during treatment initiation and dose increases).
No products indexed under this heading.

Fluoxetine Hydrochloride (Based on the mechanism of action of venlafaxine and the potential for serotonin syndrome, caution is advised when venlafaxine is co-administered with other drugs that may affect the serotonergic neurotransmitter systems, such as SSRIs. If concomitant treatment of venlafaxine with an SSRI is clinically warranted, careful observation of the patient is advised, particularly during treatment initiation and dose increases). Products include:
Prozac Weekly 1941
Prozac Pulvules 1941
Symbyax 1965

Fluphenazine Decanoate (The risk of using venlafaxine in combination with other CNS active drugs has not been systematically evaluated. Consequently, caution is advised if the concomitant administration of venlafaxine and such drugs is required).
No products indexed under this heading.

Fluphenazine Enanthate (The risk of using venlafaxine in combination with other CNS active drugs has not been systematically evaluated. Consequently, caution is advised if the concomitant administration of venlafaxine and such drugs is required).
No products indexed under this heading.

Fluphenazine Hydrochloride (The risk of using venlafaxine in combination with other CNS active drugs has not been systematically evaluated. Consequently, caution is advised if the concomitant administration of venlafaxine and such drugs is required).
No products indexed under this heading.

Flurazepam Hydrochloride (The risk of using venlafaxine in combination with other CNS active drugs has not been systematically evaluated. Consequently, caution is advised if the concomitant administration of venlafaxine and such drugs is required).
No products indexed under this heading.

Flurbiprofen (Patients should be cautioned about the concomitant use of venlafaxine and NSAIDs since combined use of psychotropic drugs that interfere with serotonin reuptake and this agent has been associated with an increased risk of bleeding. SSRIs and SNRIs, including venlafaxine, may increase the risk of bleeding events. Concomitant use of nonsteroidal anti-inflammatory drugs may add to this risk. Case reports and epidemiological studies (case-control and cohort design) have demonstrated an association between use of drugs that interfere with serotonin reuptake and the occurrence of gastrointestinal bleeding).
No products indexed under this heading.

Fluvoxamine (Based on the mechanism of action of venlafaxine and the potential for serotonin syndrome, caution is advised when venlafaxine is co-administered with other drugs that may affect the serotonergic neurotransmitter systems, such as SSRIs. If concomitant treatment of venlafaxine with an SSRI is clinically warranted, careful observation of the patient is advised, particularly during treatment initiation and dose increases).
No products indexed under this heading.

Fluvoxamine Maleate (Based on the mechanism of action of venlafaxine and the potential for serotonin syndrome, caution is advised when venlafaxine is co-administered with other drugs that may affect the serotonergic neurotransmitter systems, such as SSRIs. If concomitant treatment of venlafaxine with an SSRI is clinically warranted, careful observation of the patient is advised, particularly during treatment initiation and dose increases).
No products indexed under this heading.

Fondaparinux Sodium (Patients should be cautioned about the concomitant use of venlafaxine and anti-coagulants since combined use of psychotropic drugs that interfere with serotonin reuptake and this agent has been associated with an increased risk of bleeding. SSRIs and SNRIs, including venlafaxine, may increase the risk of bleeding events. Concomitant use of anti-coagulants may add to this risk. Case reports and epidemiological studies (case-control and cohort design) have demonstrated an association between use of drugs that interfere with serotonin reuptake and the occurrence of gastrointestinal bleeding). Products include:
Arixtra 1320

Formoterol Fumarate (*In vitro* studies indicate that venlafaxine is a relatively weak inhibitor of CYP2D6. These findings have been confirmed in a clinical drug interaction study comparing the effect of venlafaxine to that of fluoxetine on the CYP2D6-mediated metabolism of dextrometrophan to dextrophan). Products include:
Foradil 3121
Perforomist 3634

Fosamprenavir Calcium (Concomitant use of CYP3A4 inhibitors and venlafaxine may increase levels of venlafaxine and ODV. Therefore, caution is advised if a patient's therapy includes a CYP3A4 inhibitor and venlafaxine concomitantly. The concomitant use of venlafaxine with a drug treatment(s) that potently inhibits both CYP2D6 and CYP3A4, the primary metabolizing enzymes for venlafaxine, has not been studied. Therefore, caution is advised should a patient's therapy include venlafaxine and any agent(s) that produce potent simultaneous inhibition of these two enzyme systems). Products include:
Lexiva Oral Suspension 1558
Lexiva 1558

Frovatriptan Succinate (There have been rare post-marketing reports of serotonin syndrome with use of an SSRI and a triptan. If concomitant treatment of venlafaxine with a triptan is clinically warranted, careful observation of the patient is advised, particularly during treatment initiation and dose increases. Patients should be cautioned about the risk of serotonin syndrome with the concomitant use of venlafaxine and triptans, tramadol, tryptophan supplements or other serotonergic agents). Products include:
Frova 1103

Furosemide (Elderly patients may be at greater risk of developing hyponatremia with SSRIs and SNRIs. Also patients taking diuretics or who are otherwise volume depleted may be at greater risk. Discontinuation of venlafaxine should be considered in patients with symptomatic hyponatremia and appropriate medical intervention should be instituted). Products include:
Furosemide 2354

Galantamine Hydrobromide (*In vitro* studies indicate that venlafaxine is a relatively weak inhibitor of CYP2D6. These findings have been confirmed in a clinical drug interaction study comparing the effect of venlafaxine to that of fluoxetine on the CYP2D6-mediated metabolism of dextrometrophan to dextrophan).
No products indexed under this heading.

Glutethimide (The risk of using venlafaxine in combination with other CNS active drugs has not been systematically evaluated. Consequently, caution is advised if the concomitant administration of venlafaxine and such drugs is required).
No products indexed under this heading.

Halofantrine Hydrochloride (Studies indicate that venlafaxine is metabolized to its active metabolite, ODV, by CYP2D6. Thus the potential exists for a drug interaction between drugs that inhibit CYP2D6-mediated metabolism and venlafaxine. However, although imipramine partially inhibited the CYP2D6-mediated metabolism of venlafaxine, resulting in higher plasma concentrations of venlafaxine and lower plasma concentrations of ODV, the total concentration of active compounds (venlafaxine plus ODV) was not affected. Also, in a clinical study involving CYP2D6 poor and extensive metabolizers, the total concentration of active compounds (venlafaxine plus ODV), was similar in both groups. No dosage adjustment is required when venlafaxine is co-administered with a CYP2D6 inhibitor. Caution is advised should a patient's therapy include venlafaxine and CYP2D6 inhibitor).
No products indexed under this heading.

Haloperidol (The risk of using venlafaxine in combination with other CNS active drugs has not been systematically evaluated. Consequently, caution is advised if the concomitant administration of venlafaxine and such drugs is required).
No products indexed under this heading.

Haloperidol Decanoate (The risk of using venlafaxine in combination with other CNS active drugs has not been systematically evaluated. Consequently, caution is advised if the concomitant administration of venlafaxine and such drugs is required).
No products indexed under this heading.

Haloperidol Lactate (Venlafaxine administered under steady-state conditions at 150 mg/day in 24 healthy subjects decreased total oral-dose clearance (Cl/F) of a single 2 mg dose of haloperidol by 42%, which resulted in a 70% increase in haloperidol AUC. In addition, the haloperidol C_{max} increased 88% when co-administered with venlafaxine, but the haloperidol elimination half-life ($t_{1/2}$) was unchanged. The mechanism explaining this finding is unknown).
No products indexed under this heading.

Heparin Calcium (Patients should be cautioned about the concomitant use of venlafaxine and anti-coagulants since combined use of psychotropic drugs that interfere with serotonin reuptake and this agent has been associated with an increased risk of bleeding. SSRIs and SNRIs, including venlafaxine, may increase the risk of bleeding events. Concomitant use of anti-coagulants may add to this risk. Case reports and epidemiological studies (case-control and cohort design) have demonstrated an association between use of drugs that interfere with serotonin reuptake and the occurrence of gastrointestinal bleeding).
No products indexed under this heading.

Heparin Sodium (Patients should be cautioned about the concomitant use of venlafaxine and anti-coagulants since combined use of psychotropic drugs that interfere with serotonin reuptake and this agent has been associated with an increased risk of bleeding. SSRIs and SNRIs, including venlafaxine, may increase the risk of bleeding events. Concomitant use of anti-coagulants may add to this risk. Case reports and epidemiological studies (case-control and cohort design) have demonstrated an association between use of drugs that interfere with serotonin reuptake and the occurrence of gastrointestinal bleeding).
No products indexed under this heading.

Herbal Medicines, unspecified (Patients should be advised to inform their physicians if they are taking, or plan to take, any prescription or over-the-counter drugs, including herbal preparations since there is a potential for interactions).
No products indexed under this heading.

Hydrochlorothiazide (Elderly patients may be at greater risk of developing hyponatremia with SSRIs and SNRIs. Also patients taking diuretics or who are otherwise volume depleted may be at greater risk. Discontinuation of venlafaxine should be considered in patients with symptomatic hyponatremia and appropriate medical intervention should be instituted). Products include:
Atacand HCT 700
Avalide 2956
Benicar HCT 1017

IMPORTANT NOTE: Always consult each drug listing in the patient's regimen for possible interactions.

Hydrocodone Bitartrate (The risk of using venlafaxine in combination with other CNS active drugs has not been systematically evaluated. Consequently, caution is advised if the concomitant administration of venlafaxine and such drugs is required). Products include:

Hydrocodone Polistirex (The risk of using venlafaxine in combination with other CNS active drugs has not been systematically evaluated. Consequently, caution is advised if the concomitant administration of venlafaxine and such drugs is required). Products include:

Hydroflumethiazide (Elderly patients may be at greater risk of developing hyponatremia with SSRIs and SNRIs. Also patients taking diuretics or who are otherwise volume depleted may be at greater risk. Discontinuation of venlafaxine should be considered in patients with symptomatic hyponatremia and appropriate medical intervention should be instituted).
No products indexed under this heading.

Hydromorphone Hydrochloride (The risk of using venlafaxine in combination with other CNS active drugs has not been systematically evaluated. Consequently, caution is advised if the concomitant administration of venlafaxine and such drugs is required). Products include:

Hydroxyamphetamine Hydrobromide (The risk of using venlafaxine in combination with other CNS active drugs has not been systematically evaluated. Consequently, caution is advised if the concomitant administration of venlafaxine and such drugs is required).
No products indexed under this heading.

Hydroxychloroquine Sulfate (Studies indicate that venlafaxine is metabolized to its active metabolite, ODV, by CYP2D6. Thus the potential exists for a drug interaction between drugs that inhibit CYP2D6-mediated metabolism and venlafaxine. However, although imipramine partially inhibited the CYP2D6-mediated metabolism of venlafaxine, resulting in higher plasma concentrations of venlafaxine and lower plasma concentrations of ODV, the total concentration of active compounds (venlafaxine plus ODV) was not affected. Also, in a clinical study involving CYP2D6 poor and extensive metabolizers, the total concentration of active compounds (venlafaxine plus ODV), was similar in both groups. No dosage adjustment is required when venlafaxine is co-administered with a CYP2D6 inhibitor. Caution is advised should a patient's therapy include venlafaxine and CYP2D6 inhibitor).
No products indexed under this heading.

Hydroxyzine Hydrochloride (The risk of using venlafaxine in combination with other CNS active drugs has not been systematically evaluated. Consequently, caution is advised if the concomitant administration of venlafaxine and such drugs is required).
No products indexed under this heading.

Hypericum (Based on the mechanism of action of venlafaxine and the potential for serotonin syndrome, caution is advised when venlafaxine is co-administered with other drugs that may affect the serotonergic neurotransmitter systems, such as St. John's Wort. If concomitant treatment of venlafaxine with St. John's Wort is clinically warranted, careful observation of the patient is advised, particularly during treatment initiation and dose increases).
No products indexed under this heading.

Hypericum Perforatum (Based on the mechanism of action of venlafaxine and the potential for serotonin syndrome, caution is advised when venlafaxine is co-administered with other drugs that may affect the serotonergic neurotransmitter systems, such as St. John's Wort. If concomitant treatment of venlafaxine with St. John's Wort is clinically warranted, careful observation of the patient is advised, particularly during treatment initiation and dose increases). Products include:

Ibuprofen (Patients should be cautioned about the concomitant use of venlafaxine and NSAIDs since combined use of psychotropic drugs that interfere with serotonin reuptake and this agent has been associated with an increased risk of bleeding. SSRIs and SNRIs, including venlafaxine, may increase the risk of bleeding events. Concomitant use of nonsteroidal anti-inflammatory drugs may add to this risk. Case reports and epidemiological studies (case-control and cohort design) have demonstrated an association between use of drugs that interfere with serotonin reuptake and the occurrence of gastrointestinal bleeding). Products include:

Imatinib Mesylate (Studies indicate that venlafaxine is metabolized to its active metabolite, ODV, by CYP2D6. Thus the potential exists for a drug interaction between drugs that inhibit CYP2D6-mediated metabolism and venlafaxine. However, although imipramine partially inhibited the CYP2D6-mediated metabolism of venlafaxine, resulting in higher plasma concentrations of venlafaxine and lower plasma concentrations of ODV, the total concentration of active compounds (venlafaxine plus ODV) was not affected. Also, in a clinical study involving CYP2D6 poor and extensive metabolizers, the total concentration of active compounds (venlafaxine plus ODV), was similar in both groups. No dosage adjustment is required when venlafaxine is co-administered with a CYP2D6 inhibitor. Caution is advised should a patient's therapy include venlafaxine and CYP2D6 inhibitor). Products include:

Imipramine Hydrochloride (Venlafaxine did not affect the pharmacokinetics of imipramine and 2-OH-imipramine. However desipramine AUC, C_{max}, and C_{min} increased by about 35% in the presence of venlafaxine. The 2-OH-desipramine AUCs increased by at least 2.5-fold (with venlafaxine 37.5 mg q 12h) and 4.5-fold (with venlafaxine 75 mg q 12h). Imipramine did not affect the pharmacokinetics of venlafaxine and ODV. The clinical significance of elevated 2-OH-desipramine levels is unknown).
No products indexed under this heading.

Imipramine Pamoate (Venlafaxine did not affect the pharmacokinetics of imipramine and 2-OH-imipramine. However desipramine AUC, C_{max}, and C_{min} increased by about 35% in the presence of venlafaxine. The 2-OH-desipramine AUCs increased by at least 2.5-fold (with venlafaxine 37.5 mg q 12h) and 4.5-fold (with venlafaxine 75 mg q 12h). Imipramine did not affect the pharmacokinetics of venlafaxine and ODV. The clinical significance of elevated 2-OH-desipramine levels is unknown).
No products indexed under this heading.

Indapamide (Elderly patients may be at greater risk of developing hyponatremia with SSRIs and SNRIs. Also patients taking diuretics or who are otherwise volume depleted may be at greater risk. Discontinuation of venlafaxine should be considered in patients with symptomatic hyponatremia and appropriate medical intervention should be instituted). Products include:

Indinavir Sulfate (In a study of nine healthy volunteers, venlafaxine administered under steady-state conditions at 150 mg/day resulted in a 28% decrease in the AUC of a single 800 mg dose of indinavir and a 36% decrease in indinavir C_{max}. Indinavir did not affect the pharmacokinetics of venlafaxine and ODV. The clinical significance of this finding is unknown). Products include:

Indomethacin (Patients should be cautioned about the concomitant use of venlafaxine and NSAIDs since combined use of psychotropic drugs that interfere with serotonin reuptake and this agent has been associated with an increased risk of bleeding. SSRIs and SNRIs, including venlafaxine, may increase the risk of bleeding events. Concomitant use of nonsteroidal anti-inflammatory drugs may add to this risk. Case reports and epidemiological studies (case-control and cohort design) have demonstrated an association between use of drugs that interfere with serotonin reuptake and the occurrence of gastrointestinal bleeding). Products include:

Indomethacin Sodium Trihydrate (Patients should be cautioned about the concomitant use of venlafaxine and NSAIDs since combined use of psychotropic drugs that interfere with serotonin reuptake and this agent has been associated with an increased risk of bleeding. SSRIs and SNRIs, including venlafaxine, may increase the risk of bleeding events. Concomitant use of nonsteroidal anti-inflammatory drugs may add to this risk. Case reports and epidemiological studies (case-control and cohort design) have demonstrated an association between use of drugs that interfere with serotonin reuptake and the occurrence of gastrointestinal bleeding). Products include:

Indoramin Hydrochloride (*In vitro* studies indicate that venlafaxine is a relatively weak inhibitor of CYP2D6. These findings have been confirmed in a clinical drug interaction study comparing the effect of venlafaxine to that of fluoxetine on the CYP2D6-mediated metabolism of dextrometrophan to dextrophan).
No products indexed under this heading.

Isocarboxazid (Concomitant use in patients taking monoamine oxidase inhibitors (MAOIs) is contraindicated. Adverse reactions, some of which were serious, have been reported in patients who have recently been discontinued from a monoamine oxidase inhibitor (MAOI) and started on venlafaxine hydrochloride, or who have recently had venlafaxine hydrochloride therapy discontinued prior to initiation of a MAOI. It is recommended that venlafaxine hydrochloride not be used in combination with a MAOI, or within at least 14 days of discontinuing treatment with a MAOI. Based on the half-life of venlafaxine hydrochloride, at least 7 days should be allowed after stopping venlafaxine hydrochloride before starting an MAOI). Products include:

Isoflurane (The risk of using venlafaxine in combination with other CNS active drugs has not been systematically evaluated. Consequently, caution is advised if the concomitant administration of venlafaxine and such drugs is required).
No products indexed under this heading.

Isoniazid (Concomitant use of CYP3A4 inhibitors and venlafaxine may increase levels of venlafaxine and ODV. Therefore, caution is advised if a patient's therapy includes a CYP3A4 inhibitor and venlafaxine concomitantly. The concomitant use of venlafaxine with a drug treatment(s) that potently inhibits both CYP2D6 and CYP3A4, the primary metabolizing enzymes for venlafaxine, has not been studied. Therefore, caution is advised should a patient's therapy include venlafaxine and any agent(s) that produce potent simultaneous inhibition of these two enzyme systems).
No products indexed under this heading.

Itraconazole (Concomitant use of CYP3A4 inhibitors and venlafaxine may increase levels of venlafaxine and ODV. Therefore, caution is advised if a patient's therapy includes a CYP3A4 inhibitor and venlafaxine concomitantly. The concomitant use of venlafaxine with a drug treatment(s) that potently inhibits both CYP2D6 and CYP3A4, the primary metabolizing enzymes for venlafaxine, has not been studied. Therefore, caution is advised should a patient's therapy include venlafaxine and any agent(s) that produce potent simultaneous inhibition of these two enzyme systems).
No products indexed under this heading.

Ketamine Hydrochloride (The risk of using venlafaxine in combination with other CNS active drugs has not been systematically evaluated. Consequently, caution is advised if the concomitant administration of venlafaxine and such drugs is required).
No products indexed under this heading.

Ketoconazole (A study of ketoconazole 100 mg b.i.d. with a single dose of venlafaxine 50 mg in extensive metabolizers and 25 mg in poor metabolizers of CYP2D6 resulted in higher plasma concentrations of both venlafaxine and O-desvenlafaxine (ODV) in most subjects following administration of ketoconazole. Venlafaxine C_{max} increased by 26% in EM subjects and 48% in PM subjects. C_{max} values for ODV increased by 14% and 29% in EM and PM subjects, respectively. Venlafaxine AUC increased by 21% in EM subjects and 70% in PM subjects, and AUC values for ODV increased by 23% and 33% in EM and PM subjects, respectively. Combined AUCs of venlafaxine and ODV increased on an average of approximately 23% in EMs and 53% in PMs). Products include:

Ketoprofen (Patients should be cautioned about the concomitant use of venlafaxine and NSAIDs since combined use of psychotropic drugs that interfere with serotonin reuptake and this agent has been associated with an increased risk of bleeding. SSRIs and SNRIs, including venlafaxine, may increase the risk of bleeding events. Concomitant use of nonsteroidal anti-inflammatory drugs may add to this risk. Case reports and epidemiological studies (case-control and cohort design) have demonstrated an association between

use of drugs that interfere with serotonin reuptake and the occurrence of gastrointestinal bleeding).
No products indexed under this heading.

Ketorolac Tromethamine (Patients should be cautioned about the concomitant use of venlafaxine and NSAIDs since combined use of psychotropic drugs that interfere with serotonin reuptake and this agent has been associated with an increased risk of bleeding. SSRIs and SNRIs, including venlafaxine, may increase the risk of bleeding events. Concomitant use of nonsteroidal anti-inflammatory drugs may add to this risk. Case reports and epidemiological studies (case-control and cohort design) have demonstrated an association between use of drugs that interfere with serotonin reuptake and the occurrence of gastrointestinal bleeding). Products include:
Acuvail .... ⊙209

Labetalol Hydrochloride (*In vitro* studies indicate that venlafaxine is a relatively weak inhibitor of CYP2D6. These findings have been confirmed in a clinical drug interaction study comparing the effect of venlafaxine to that of fluoxetine on the CYP2D6-mediated metabolism of dextrometrophan to dextrophan).
No products indexed under this heading.

Lapatinib (Concomitant use of CYP3A4 inhibitors and venlafaxine may increase levels of venlafaxine and ODV. Therefore, caution is advised if a patient's therapy includes a CYP3A4 inhibitor and venlafaxine concomitantly. The concomitant use of venlafaxine with a drug treatment(s) that potently inhibits both CYP2D6 and CYP3A4, the primary metabolizing enzymes for venlafaxine, has not been studied. Therefore, caution is advised should a patient's therapy include venlafaxine and any agent(s) that produce potent simultaneous inhibition of these two enzyme systems). Products include:
Tykerb 1698

Levomethadyl Acetate Hydrochloride (The risk of using venlafaxine in combination with other CNS active drugs has not been systematically evaluated. Consequently, caution is advised if the concomitant administration of venlafaxine and such drugs is required).
No products indexed under this heading.

Levorphanol Tartrate (The risk of using venlafaxine in combination with other CNS active drugs has not been systematically evaluated. Consequently, caution is advised if the concomitant administration of venlafaxine and such drugs is required).
No products indexed under this heading.

Lidocaine (*In vitro* studies indicate that venlafaxine is a relatively weak inhibitor of CYP2D6. These findings have been confirmed in a clinical drug interaction study comparing the effect of venlafaxine to that of fluoxetine on the CYP2D6-mediated metabolism of dextrometrophan to dextrophan). Products include:
Lidoderm 1107

Lidocaine Hydrochloride (*In vitro* studies indicate that venlafaxine is a relatively weak inhibitor of CYP2D6. These findings have been confirmed in a clinical drug interaction study comparing the effect of venlafaxine to that of fluoxetine on the CYP2D6-mediated metabolism of dextrometrophan to dextrophan).
No products indexed under this heading.

Linezolid (Based on the mechanism of action of venlafaxine and the potential for serotonin syndrome, caution is advised when venlafaxine is co-administered with other drugs that may affect the serotonergic neurotransmitter systems, such as linezolid (an antibiotic which is a reversible non-selective MAOI). If concomitant treatment of venlafaxine with linezolid is clinically warranted, careful observation of the patient is advised, particularly during treatment initiation and dose increases). Products include:
Zyvox 2769

Lisdexamfetamine Dimesylate (The risk of using venlafaxine in combination with other CNS active drugs has not been systematically evaluated. Consequently, caution is advised if the concomitant administration of venlafaxine and such drugs is required). Products include:
Vyvanse 3298

Lithium (Based on the mechanism of action of venlafaxine and the potential for serotonin syndrome, caution is advised when venlafaxine is co-administered with other drugs that may affect the serotonergic neurotransmitter systems, such as lithium. If concomitant treatment of venlafaxine with lithium is clinically warranted, careful observation of the patient is advised, particularly during treatment initiation and dose increases).
No products indexed under this heading.

Lithium Carbonate (Based on the mechanism of action of venlafaxine and the potential for serotonin syndrome, caution is advised when venlafaxine is co-administered with other drugs that may affect the serotonergic neurotransmitter systems, such as lithium. If concomitant treatment of venlafaxine with lithium is clinically warranted, careful observation of the patient is advised, particularly during treatment initiation and dose increases).
No products indexed under this heading.

Lithium Citrate (Based on the mechanism of action of venlafaxine and the potential for serotonin syndrome, caution is advised when venlafaxine is co-administered with other drugs that may affect the serotonergic neurotransmitter systems, such as lithium. If concomitant treatment of venlafaxine with lithium is clinically warranted, careful observation of the patient is advised, particularly during treatment initiation and dose increases).
No products indexed under this heading.

Lopinavir (Concomitant use of CYP3A4 inhibitors and venlafaxine may increase levels of venlafaxine and ODV. Therefore, caution is advised if a patient's therapy includes a CYP3A4 inhibitor and venlafaxine concomitantly. The concomitant use of venlafaxine with a drug treatment(s) that potently inhibits both CYP2D6 and CYP3A4, the primary metabolizing enzymes for venlafaxine, has not been studied. Therefore, caution is advised should a patient's therapy include venlafaxine and any agent(s) that produce potent simultaneous inhibition of these two enzyme systems). Products include:
Kaletra 458

Loratadine (Concomitant use of CYP3A4 inhibitors and venlafaxine may increase levels of venlafaxine and ODV. Therefore, caution is advised if a patient's therapy includes a CYP3A4 inhibitor and venlafaxine concomitantly. The concomitant use of venlafaxine with a drug treatment(s) that potently inhibits both CYP2D6 and CYP3A4, the primary metabolizing enzymes for venlafaxine, has not been studied. Therefore, caution is advised should a patient's therapy include venlafaxine and any agent(s) that produce potent simultaneous inhibition of these two enzyme systems).
No products indexed under this heading.

Lorazepam (The risk of using venlafaxine in combination with other CNS active drugs has not been systematically evaluated. Consequently, caution is advised if the concomitant administration of venlafaxine and such drugs is required).
No products indexed under this heading.

Low Molecular Weight Heparins (Patients should be cautioned about the concomitant use of venlafaxine and anti-coagulants since combined use of psychotropic drugs that interfere with serotonin reuptake and this agent has been associated with an increased risk of bleeding. SSRIs and SNRIs, including venlafaxine, may increase the risk of bleeding events. Concomitant use of anti-coagulants may add to this risk. Case reports and epidemiological studies (case-control and cohort design) have demonstrated an association between use of drugs that interfere with serotonin reuptake and the occurrence of gastrointestinal bleeding).
No products indexed under this heading.

Loxapine Hydrochloride (The risk of using venlafaxine in combination with other CNS active drugs has not been systematically evaluated. Consequently, caution is advised if the concomitant administration of venlafaxine and such drugs is required).
No products indexed under this heading.

Loxapine Succinate (The risk of using venlafaxine in combination with other CNS active drugs has not been systematically evaluated. Consequently, caution is advised if the concomitant administration of venlafaxine and such drugs is required).
No products indexed under this heading.

Maprotiline Hydrochloride (Studies indicate that venlafaxine is metabolized to its active metabolite, ODV, by CYP2D6. Thus the potential exists for a drug interaction between drugs that inhibit CYP2D6-mediated metabolism and venlafaxine. However, although imipramine partially inhibited the CYP2D6-mediated metabolism of venlafaxine, resulting in higher plasma concentrations of venlafaxine and lower plasma concentrations of ODV, the total concentration of active compounds (venlafaxine plus ODV) was not affected. Also, in a clinical study involving CYP2D6 poor and extensive metabolizers, the total concentration of active compounds (venlafaxine plus ODV), was similar in both groups. No dosage adjustment is required when venlafaxine is co-administered with a CYP2D6 inhibitor. Caution is advised should a patient's therapy include venlafaxine and CYP2D6 inhibitor).
No products indexed under this heading.

Mazindol (The safety and efficacy of venlafaxine therapy in combination with weight loss agents, including phentermine, have not been established. Co-administration of venlafaxine and weight loss agents is not recommended. Venlafaxine is not indicated for weight loss alone or in combination with other products).
No products indexed under this heading.

Meclofenamate Sodium (Patients should be cautioned about the concomitant use of venlafaxine and NSAIDs since combined use of psychotropic drugs that interfere with serotonin reuptake and this agent has been associated with an increased risk of bleeding. SSRIs and SNRIs, including venlafaxine, may increase the risk of bleeding events. Concomitant use of nonsteroidal anti-inflammatory drugs may add to this risk. Case reports and epidemiological studies (case-control and cohort design) have demonstrated an association between use of drugs that interfere with serotonin reuptake and the occurrence of gastrointestinal bleeding).
No products indexed under this heading.

Mefenamic Acid (Patients should be cautioned about the concomitant use of venlafaxine and NSAIDs since combined use of psychotropic drugs that interfere with serotonin reuptake and this agent has been associated with an increased risk of bleeding. SSRIs and SNRIs, including venlafaxine, may increase the risk of bleeding events. Concomitant use of nonsteroidal anti-inflammatory drugs may add to this risk. Case reports and epidemiological studies (case-control and cohort design) have demonstrated an association between use of drugs that interfere with serotonin reuptake and the occurrence of gastrointestinal bleeding).
No products indexed under this heading.

Meloxicam (Patients should be cautioned about the concomitant use of venlafaxine and NSAIDs since combined use of psychotropic drugs that interfere with serotonin reuptake and this agent has been associated with an increased risk of bleeding. SSRIs and SNRIs, including venlafaxine, may increase the risk of bleeding events. Concomitant use of nonsteroidal anti-inflammatory drugs may add to this risk. Case reports and epidemiological studies (case-control and cohort design) have demonstrated an association between use of drugs that interfere with serotonin reuptake and the occurrence of gastrointestinal bleeding).
No products indexed under this heading.

Meperidine Hydrochloride (The risk of using venlafaxine in combination with other CNS active drugs has not been systematically evaluated. Consequently, caution is advised if the concomitant administration of venlafaxine and such drugs is required).
No products indexed under this heading.

Mephobarbital (The risk of using venlafaxine in combination with other CNS active drugs has not been systematically evaluated. Consequently, caution is advised if the concomitant administration of venlafaxine and such drugs is required).
No products indexed under this heading.

Meprobamate (The risk of using venlafaxine in combination with other CNS active drugs has not been systematically evaluated. Consequently, caution is advised if the concomitant administration of venlafaxine and such drugs is required).
No products indexed under this heading.

Mesoridazine Besylate (The risk of using venlafaxine in combination with other CNS active drugs has not been systematically evaluated. Consequently, caution is advised if the concomitant administration of venlafaxine and such drugs is required).
No products indexed under this heading.

Methadone Hydrochloride (The risk of using venlafaxine in combination with other CNS active drugs has not been systematically evaluated. Consequently, caution is advised if the concomitant administration of venlafaxine and such drugs is required).
No products indexed under this heading.

Methamphetamine Hydrochloride (The risk of using venlafaxine in combination with other CNS active drugs has not been systematically evaluated. Consequently, caution is advised if the concomitant administration of venlafaxine and such drugs is required).
No products indexed under this heading.

IMPORTANT NOTE: Always consult each drug listing in the patient's regimen for possible interactions.

Methohexital Sodium (The risk of using venlafaxine in combination with other CNS active drugs has not been systematically evaluated. Consequently, caution is advised if the concomitant administration of venlafaxine and such drugs is required).
No products indexed under this heading.

Methotrimeprazine (The risk of using venlafaxine in combination with other CNS active drugs has not been systematically evaluated. Consequently, caution is advised if the concomitant administration of venlafaxine and such drugs is required).
No products indexed under this heading.

Methoxyflurane (The risk of using venlafaxine in combination with other CNS active drugs has not been systematically evaluated. Consequently, caution is advised if the concomitant administration of venlafaxine and such drugs is required).
No products indexed under this heading.

Methoxyphenamine (In vitro studies indicate that venlafaxine is a relatively weak inhibitor of CYP2D6. These findings have been confirmed in a clinical drug interaction study comparing the effect of venlafaxine to that of fluoxetine on the CYP2D6-mediated metabolism of dextrometrophan to dextrophan).
No products indexed under this heading.

Methyclothiazide (Elderly patients may be at greater risk of developing hyponatremia with SSRIs and SNRIs. Also patients taking diuretics or who are otherwise volume depleted may be at greater risk. Discontinuation of venlafaxine should be considered in patients with symptomatic hyponatremia and appropriate medical intervention should be instituted).
No products indexed under this heading.

Methylphenidate (The risk of using venlafaxine in combination with other CNS active drugs has not been systematically evaluated. Consequently, caution is advised if the concomitant administration of venlafaxine and such drugs is required). Products include:
Daytrana 3283

Methylphenidate Hydrochloride (The risk of using venlafaxine in combination with other CNS active drugs has not been systematically evaluated. Consequently, caution is advised if the concomitant administration of venlafaxine and such drugs is required). Products include:
Concerta 2598
Metadate CD 3439

Metoclopramide Hydrochloride (The development of a potentially life-threatening serotonin syndrome or Neuroleptic Malignant Syndrome (NMS)-like reactions have been reported with SNRIs and SSRIs alone, including venlafaxine, but particularly with concomitant use other dopamine antagonists. Products include:
Metozolv ODT 2901

Metolazone (Elderly patients may be at greater risk of developing hyponatremia with SSRIs and SNRIs. Also patients taking diuretics or who are otherwise volume depleted may be at greater risk. Discontinuation of venlafaxine should be considered in patients with symptomatic hyponatremia and appropriate medical intervention should be instituted).
No products indexed under this heading.

Metoprolol Succinate (Concomitant administration of venlafaxine (50 mg every 8 hours for 5 days) and metoprolol (100 mg every 24 hours for 5 days) to 18 healthy male subjects in a pharmacokinetic interaction study for both drugs resulted in an increase of plasma concentrations of metoprolol by approximately 30% to 40% without altering the plasma concentrations of

its active metabolite, alpha-hydroxymetoprolol. Metoprolol did not alter the pharmacokinetic profile of venlafaxine or its active metabolite, O-desmethylvenlafaxine. Venlafaxine appeared to reduce the blood pressure-lowering effect of metoprolol in this study. The clinical relevance of this finding for hypertensive patients is unknown. Caution should be exercised with co-administration of venlafaxine and metoprolol. It is recommended that patients receiving venlafaxine hydrochloride have regular monitoring of blood pressure). Products include:
Toprol XL 732

Metoprolol Tartrate (Concomitant administration of venlafaxine (50 mg every 8 hours for 5 days) and metoprolol (100 mg every 24 hours for 5 days) to 18 healthy male subjects in a pharmacokinetic interaction study for both drugs resulted in an increase of plasma concentrations of metoprolol by approximately 30% to 40% without altering the plasma concentrations of its active metabolite, alpha-hydroxymetoprolol. Metoprolol did not alter the pharmacokinetic profile of venlafaxine or its active metabolite, O-desmethylvenlafaxine. Venlafaxine appeared to reduce the blood pressure-lowering effect of metoprolol in this study. The clinical relevance of this finding for hypertensive patients is unknown. Caution should be exercised with co-administration of venlafaxine and metoprolol. It is recommended that patients receiving venlafaxine hydrochloride have regular monitoring of blood pressure).
No products indexed under this heading.

Metronidazole (Concomitant use of CYP3A4 inhibitors and venlafaxine may increase levels of venlafaxine and ODV. Therefore, caution is advised if a patient's therapy includes a CYP3A4 inhibitor and venlafaxine concomitantly. The concomitant use of venlafaxine with a drug treatment(s) that potently inhibits both CYP2D6 and CYP3A4, the primary metabolizing enzymes for venlafaxine, has not been studied. Therefore, caution is advised should a patient's therapy include venlafaxine and any agent(s) that produce potent simultaneous inhibition of these two enzyme systems). Products include:
Pylera 793

Metronidazole Benzoate (Concomitant use of CYP3A4 inhibitors and venlafaxine may increase levels of venlafaxine and ODV. Therefore, caution is advised if a patient's therapy includes a CYP3A4 inhibitor and venlafaxine concomitantly. The concomitant use of venlafaxine with a drug treatment(s) that potently inhibits both CYP2D6 and CYP3A4, the primary metabolizing enzymes for venlafaxine, has not been studied. Therefore, caution is advised should a patient's therapy include venlafaxine and any agent(s) that produce potent simultaneous inhibition of these two enzyme systems).
No products indexed under this heading.

Metronidazole Hydrochloride (Concomitant use of CYP3A4 inhibitors and venlafaxine may increase levels of venlafaxine and ODV. Therefore, caution is advised if a patient's therapy includes a CYP3A4 inhibitor and venlafaxine concomitantly. The concomitant use of venlafaxine with a drug treatment(s) that potently inhibits both CYP2D6 and CYP3A4, the primary metabolizing enzymes for venlafaxine, has not been studied. Therefore, caution is advised should a patient's therapy include venlafaxine and any agent(s) that produce potent simultaneous inhibition of these two enzyme systems).
No products indexed under this heading.

Metronidazole Sodium (Concomitant use of CYP3A4 inhibitors and venlafaxine may increase levels of venlafaxine and ODV. Therefore, caution is advised if a patient's therapy includes a CYP3A4 inhibitor and venlafaxine concomitantly. The concomitant use of venlafaxine with a drug treatment(s) that potently inhibits both CYP2D6 and CYP3A4, the primary metabolizing enzymes for venlafaxine, has not been studied. Therefore, caution is advised should a patient's therapy include venlafaxine and any agent(s) that produce potent simultaneous inhibition of these two enzyme systems).
No products indexed under this heading.

Mexiletine Hydrochloride (In vitro studies indicate that venlafaxine is a relatively weak inhibitor of CYP2D6. These findings have been confirmed in a clinical drug interaction study comparing the effect of venlafaxine to that of fluoxetine on the CYP2D6-mediated metabolism of dextrometrophan to dextrophan).
No products indexed under this heading.

Mibefradil Dihydrochloride (Studies indicate that venlafaxine is metabolized to its active metabolite, ODV, by CYP2D6. Thus the potential exists for a drug interaction between drugs that inhibit CYP2D6-mediated metabolism and venlafaxine. However, although imipramine partially inhibited the CYP2D6-mediated metabolism of venlafaxine, resulting in higher plasma concentrations of venlafaxine and lower plasma concentrations of ODV, the total concentration of active compounds (venlafaxine plus ODV) was not affected. Also, in a clinical study involving CYP2D6 poor and extensive metabolizers, the total concentration of active compounds (venlafaxine plus ODV), was similar in both groups. No dosage adjustment is required when venlafaxine is co-administered with a CYP2D6 inhibitor. Caution is advised should a patient's therapy include venlafaxine and CYP2D6 inhibitor).
No products indexed under this heading.

Miconazole (Concomitant use of CYP3A4 inhibitors and venlafaxine may increase levels of venlafaxine and ODV. Therefore, caution is advised if a patient's therapy includes a CYP3A4 inhibitor and venlafaxine concomitantly. The concomitant use of venlafaxine with a drug treatment(s) that potently inhibits both CYP2D6 and CYP3A4, the primary metabolizing enzymes for venlafaxine, has not been studied. Therefore, caution is advised should a patient's therapy include venlafaxine and any agent(s) that produce potent simultaneous inhibition of these two enzyme systems).
No products indexed under this heading.

Miconazole Nitrate (Concomitant use of CYP3A4 inhibitors and venlafaxine may increase levels of venlafaxine and ODV. Therefore, caution is advised if a patient's therapy includes a CYP3A4 inhibitor and venlafaxine concomitantly. The concomitant use of venlafaxine with a drug treatment(s) that potently inhibits both CYP2D6 and CYP3A4, the primary metabolizing enzymes for venlafaxine, has not been studied. Therefore, caution is advised should a patient's therapy include venlafaxine and any agent(s) that produce potent simultaneous inhibition of these two enzyme systems). Products include:
Vusion Ointment 3335

Midazolam Hydrochloride (The risk of using venlafaxine in combination with other CNS active drugs has not been systematically evaluated. Consequently, caution is advised if the concomitant administration of venlafaxine and such drugs is required).
No products indexed under this heading.

Mifepristone (Concomitant use of CYP3A4 inhibitors and venlafaxine may increase levels of venlafaxine and ODV. Therefore, caution is advised if a patient's therapy includes a CYP3A4 inhibitor and venlafaxine concomitantly. The concomitant use of venlafaxine with a drug treatment(s) that potently inhibits both CYP2D6 and CYP3A4, the primary metabolizing enzymes for venlafaxine, has not been studied. Therefore, caution is advised should a patient's therapy include venlafaxine and any agent(s) that produce potent simultaneous inhibition of these two enzyme systems).
No products indexed under this heading.

Mirtazapine (In vitro studies indicate that venlafaxine is a relatively weak inhibitor of CYP2D6. These findings have been confirmed in a clinical drug interaction study comparing the effect of venlafaxine to that of fluoxetine on the CYP2D6-mediated metabolism of dextrometrophan to dextrophan). Products include:
Remeron Tablets 3214
RemeronSolTab Tablets 3219

Moclobemide (Concomitant use in patients taking monoamine oxidase inhibitors (MAOIs) is contraindicated. Adverse reactions, some of which were serious, have been reported in patients who have recently been discontinued from a monoamine oxidase inhibitor (MAOI) and started on venlafaxine hydrochloride, or who have recently had venlafaxine hydrochloride therapy discontinued prior to initiation of a MAOI. It is recommended that venlafaxine hydrochloride not be used in combination with a MAOI, or within at least 14 days of discontinuing treatment with a MAOI. Based on the half-life of venlafaxine hydrochloride, at least 7 days should be allowed after stopping venlafaxine hydrochloride before starting an MAOI).
No products indexed under this heading.

Molindone Hydrochloride (The risk of using venlafaxine in combination with other CNS active drugs has not been systematically evaluated. Consequently, caution is advised if the concomitant administration of venlafaxine and such drugs is required). Products include:
Moban 1108

Morphine Sulfate (The risk of using venlafaxine in combination with other CNS active drugs has not been systematically evaluated. Consequently, caution is advised if the concomitant administration of venlafaxine and such drugs is required). Products include:
Avinza 1822
Embeda 1831
MS Contin 2803

Nabumetone (Patients should be cautioned about the concomitant use of venlafaxine and NSAIDs since combined use of psychotropic drugs that interfere with serotonin reuptake and this agent has been associated with an increased risk of bleeding. SSRIs and SNRIs, including venlafaxine, may increase the risk of bleeding events. Concomitant use of nonsteroidal anti-inflammatory drugs may add to this risk. Case reports and epidemiological studies (case-control and cohort design) have demonstrated an association between use of drugs that interfere with serotonin reuptake and the occurrence of gastrointestinal bleeding).
No products indexed under this heading.

Naproxen (Patients should be cautioned about the concomitant use of venlafaxine and NSAIDs since combined use of psychotropic drugs that interfere with serotonin reuptake and this agent has been associated with an increased risk of bleeding. SSRIs and SNRIs, including venlafaxine, may increase the risk of bleeding events. Concomitant use of nonsteroidal anti-inflammatory

drugs may add to this risk. Case reports and epidemiological studies (case-control and cohort design) have demonstrated an association between use of drugs that interfere with serotonin reuptake and the occurrence of gastrointestinal bleeding). Products include:

- EC-Naprosyn 2850
- Naprosyn 2850
- Anaprox/Naprosyn 2850

Naproxen Sodium (Patients should be cautioned about the concomitant use of venlafaxine and NSAIDs since combined use of psychotropic drugs that interfere with serotonin reuptake and this agent has been associated with an increased risk of bleeding. SSRIs and SNRIs, including venlafaxine, may increase the risk of bleeding events. Concomitant use of nonsteroidal anti-inflammatory drugs may add to this risk. Case reports and epidemiological studies (case-control and cohort design) have demonstrated an association between use of drugs that interfere with serotonin reuptake and the occurrence of gastrointestinal bleeding). Products include:

- Anaprox 2850
- Anaprox DS 2850
- Treximet 1681

Naratriptan Hydrochloride (There have been rare post-marketing reports of serotonin syndrome with use of an SSRI and a triptan. If concomitant treatment of venlafaxine with a triptan is clinically warranted, careful observation of the patient is advised, particularly during treatment initiation and dose increases. Patients should be cautioned about the risk of serotonin syndrome with the concomitant use of venlafaxine and triptans, tramadol, tryptophan supplements or other serotonergic agents). Products include:

- Amerge 1306

Nefazodone Hydrochloride (Based on the mechanism of action of venlafaxine and the potential for serotonin syndrome, caution is advised when venlafaxine is co-administered with other drugs that may affect the serotonergic neurotransmitter systems, such as other SNRIs. If concomitant treatment of venlafaxine with another SNRI is clinically warranted, careful observation of the patient is advised, particularly during treatment initiation and dose increases).
No products indexed under this heading.

Nelfinavir Mesylate (Concomitant use of CYP3A4 inhibitors and venlafaxine may increase levels of venlafaxine and ODV. Therefore, caution is advised if a patient's therapy includes a CYP3A4 inhibitor and venlafaxine concomitantly. The concomitant use of venlafaxine with a drug treatment(s) that potently inhibits both CYP2D6 and CYP3A4, the primary metabolizing enzymes for venlafaxine, has not been studied. Therefore, caution is advised should a patient's therapy include venlafaxine and any agent(s) that produce potent simultaneous inhibition of these two enzyme systems).
No products indexed under this heading.

Nevirapine (Concomitant use of CYP3A4 inhibitors and venlafaxine may increase levels of venlafaxine and ODV. Therefore, caution is advised if a patient's therapy includes a CYP3A4 inhibitor and venlafaxine concomitantly. The concomitant use of venlafaxine with a drug treatment(s) that potently inhibits both CYP2D6 and CYP3A4, the primary metabolizing enzymes for venlafaxine, has not been studied. Therefore, caution is advised should a patient's therapy include venlafaxine and any agent(s) that produce potent simultaneous inhibition of these two enzyme systems). Products include:

- Viramune Oral Suspension 897
- Viramune Tablets 897

Niacin (Concomitant use of CYP3A4 inhibitors and venlafaxine may increase levels of venlafaxine and ODV. Therefore, caution is advised if a patient's therapy includes a CYP3A4 inhibitor and venlafaxine concomitantly. The concomitant use of venlafaxine with a drug treatment(s) that potently inhibits both CYP2D6 and CYP3A4, the primary metabolizing enzymes for venlafaxine, has not been studied. Therefore, caution is advised should a patient's therapy include venlafaxine and any agent(s) that produce potent simultaneous inhibition of these two enzyme systems). Products include:

- Advicor 402
- Cardio Basics 3455
- Niaspan 497
- Simcor 524

Niacinamide (Concomitant use of CYP3A4 inhibitors and venlafaxine may increase levels of venlafaxine and ODV. Therefore, caution is advised if a patient's therapy includes a CYP3A4 inhibitor and venlafaxine concomitantly. The concomitant use of venlafaxine with a drug treatment(s) that potently inhibits both CYP2D6 and CYP3A4, the primary metabolizing enzymes for venlafaxine, has not been studied. Therefore, caution is advised should a patient's therapy include venlafaxine and any agent(s) that produce potent simultaneous inhibition of these two enzyme systems). Products include:

- CitraNatal 90 DHA Capsules 2332
- CitraNatal Assure 2332
- CitraNatal Rx 2332
- Heplive 607

Niacinamide Hydroiodide (Concomitant use of CYP3A4 inhibitors and venlafaxine may increase levels of venlafaxine and ODV. Therefore, caution is advised if a patient's therapy includes a CYP3A4 inhibitor and venlafaxine concomitantly. The concomitant use of venlafaxine with a drug treatment(s) that potently inhibits both CYP2D6 and CYP3A4, the primary metabolizing enzymes for venlafaxine, has not been studied. Therefore, caution is advised should a patient's therapy include venlafaxine and any agent(s) that produce potent simultaneous inhibition of these two enzyme systems).
No products indexed under this heading.

Nicotinamide (Concomitant use of CYP3A4 inhibitors and venlafaxine may increase levels of venlafaxine and ODV. Therefore, caution is advised if a patient's therapy includes a CYP3A4 inhibitor and venlafaxine concomitantly. The concomitant use of venlafaxine with a drug treatment(s) that potently inhibits both CYP2D6 and CYP3A4, the primary metabolizing enzymes for venlafaxine, has not been studied. Therefore, caution is advised should a patient's therapy include venlafaxine and any agent(s) that produce potent simultaneous inhibition of these two enzyme systems).
No products indexed under this heading.

Nifedipine (Concomitant use of CYP3A4 inhibitors and venlafaxine may increase levels of venlafaxine and ODV. Therefore, caution is advised if a patient's therapy includes a CYP3A4 inhibitor and venlafaxine concomitantly. The concomitant use of venlafaxine with a drug treatment(s) that potently inhibits both CYP2D6 and CYP3A4, the primary metabolizing enzymes for venlafaxine, has not been studied. Therefore, caution is advised should a patient's therapy include venlafaxine and any agent(s) that produce potent simultaneous inhibition of these two enzyme systems).
No products indexed under this heading.

Norfloxacin (Concomitant use of CYP3A4 inhibitors and venlafaxine may increase levels of venlafaxine and ODV. Therefore, caution is advised if a patient's therapy includes a CYP3A4 inhibitor and venlafaxine concomitantly. The concomitant use of venlafaxine with a drug treatment(s) that potently inhibits both CYP2D6 and CYP3A4, the primary metabolizing enzymes for venlafaxine, has not been studied. Therefore, caution is advised should a patient's therapy include venlafaxine and any agent(s) that produce potent simultaneous inhibition of these two enzyme systems). Products include:

- Noroxin 2220

Nortriptyline Hydrochloride (Studies indicate that venlafaxine is metabolized to its active metabolite, ODV, by CYP2D6. Thus the potential exists for a drug interaction between drugs that inhibit CYP2D6-mediated metabolism and venlafaxine. However, although imipramine partially inhibited the CYP2D6-mediated metabolism of venlafaxine, resulting in higher plasma concentrations of venlafaxine and lower plasma concentrations of ODV, the total concentration of active compounds (venlafaxine plus ODV) was not affected. Also, in a clinical study involving CYP2D6 poor and extensive metabolizers, the total concentration of active compounds (venlafaxine plus ODV), was similar in both groups. No dosage adjustment is required when venlafaxine is co-administered with a CYP2D6 inhibitor. Caution is advised should a patient's therapy include venlafaxine and CYP2D6 inhibitor).
No products indexed under this heading.

Nutritional Supplement (Patients should be advised to inform their physicians if they are taking, or plan to take, any prescription or over-the-counter drugs, including nutritional supplements, since there is a potential for interactions).
No products indexed under this heading.

Olanzapine (The risk of using venlafaxine in combination with other CNS active drugs has not been systematically evaluated. Consequently, caution is advised if the concomitant administration of venlafaxine and such drugs is required). Products include:

- Symbyax 1965
- Zyprexa 1984
- Zyprexa IntraMuscular 1984
- Zyprexa ZYDIS 1984

Omeprazole (Concomitant use of CYP3A4 inhibitors and venlafaxine may increase levels of venlafaxine and ODV. Therefore, caution is advised if a patient's therapy includes a CYP3A4 inhibitor and venlafaxine concomitantly. The concomitant use of venlafaxine with a drug treatment(s) that potently inhibits both CYP2D6 and CYP3A4, the primary metabolizing enzymes for venlafaxine, has not been studied. Therefore, caution is advised should a patient's therapy include venlafaxine and any agent(s) that produce potent simultaneous inhibition of these two enzyme systems).
No products indexed under this heading.

Ondansetron (*In vitro* studies indicate that venlafaxine is a relatively weak inhibitor of CYP2D6. These findings have been confirmed in a clinical drug interaction study comparing the effect of venlafaxine to that of fluoxetine on the CYP2D6-mediated metabolism of dextrometrophan to dextrophan).
No products indexed under this heading.

Ondansetron Hydrochloride (*In vitro* studies indicate that venlafaxine is a relatively weak inhibitor of CYP2D6. These findings have been confirmed in a clinical drug interaction study comparing the effect of venlafaxine to that of fluoxetine on the CYP2D6-mediated metabolism of dextrometrophan to dextrophan). Products include:

- Zofran Injection 1750
- Zofran 1756
- Zofran ODT 1756

Oxaprozin (Patients should be cautioned about the concomitant use of venlafaxine and NSAIDs since combined use of psychotropic drugs that interfere with serotonin reuptake and this agent has been associated with an increased risk of bleeding. SSRIs and SNRIs, including venlafaxine, may increase the risk of bleeding events. Concomitant use of nonsteroidal anti-inflammatory drugs may add to this risk. Case reports and epidemiological studies (case-control and cohort design) have demonstrated an association between use of drugs that interfere with serotonin reuptake and the occurrence of gastrointestinal bleeding).
No products indexed under this heading.

Oxazepam (The risk of using venlafaxine in combination with other CNS active drugs has not been systematically evaluated. Consequently, caution is advised if the concomitant administration of venlafaxine and such drugs is required).
No products indexed under this heading.

Oxycodone Hydrochloride (The risk of using venlafaxine in combination with other CNS active drugs has not been systematically evaluated. Consequently, caution is advised if the concomitant administration of venlafaxine and such drugs is required). Products include:

- OxyContin 2807
- Percocet 1121
- Percodan 1124

Paclitaxel (*In vitro* studies indicate that venlafaxine is a relatively weak inhibitor of CYP2D6. These findings have been confirmed in a clinical drug interaction study comparing the effect of venlafaxine to that of fluoxetine on the CYP2D6-mediated metabolism of dextrometrophan to dextrophan).
No products indexed under this heading.

Paliperidone (The development of a potentially life-threatening serotonin syndrome or Neuroleptic Malignant Syndrome (NMS)-like reactions have been reported with SNRIs and SSRIs alone, including venlafaxine, but particularly with concomitant use of antipsychotics). Products include:

- Invega 2613
- Invega Sustenna 2621

Pargyline Hydrochloride (Concomitant use in patients taking monoamine oxidase inhibitors (MAOIs) is contraindicated. Adverse reactions, some of which were serious, have been reported in patients who have recently been discontinued from a monoamine oxidase inhibitor (MAOI) and started on venlafaxine hydrochloride, or who have recently had venlafaxine hydrochloride therapy discontinued prior to initiation of a MAOI. It is recommended that venlafaxine hydrochloride not be used in combination with a MAOI, or within at least 14 days of discontinuing treatment with a MAOI. Based on the half-life of venlafaxine hydrochloride, at least 7 days should be allowed after stopping venlafaxine hydrochloride before starting an MAOI).
No products indexed under this heading.

Paroxetine (Based on the mechanism of action of venlafaxine and the potential for serotonin syndrome, caution is advised when venlafaxine is co-administered with other drugs that may affect the serotonergic neurotransmitter systems, such as SSRIs. If concomitant treatment of venlafaxine with an SSRI is clinically warranted, careful observation of the patient is advised, particularly during treatment initiation and dose increases).
No products indexed under this heading.

IMPORTANT NOTE: Always consult each drug listing in the patient's regimen for possible interactions.

Paroxetine Hydrochloride (Based on the mechanism of action of venlafaxine and the potential for serotonin syndrome, caution is advised when venlafaxine is co-administered with other drugs that may affect the serotonergic neurotransmitter systems, such as SSRIs. If concomitant treatment of venlafaxine with an SSRI is clinically warranted, careful observation of the patient is advised, particularly during treatment initiation and dose increases). Products include:

Paroxetine CR **2361**
Paroxetine ER **2371**
Paxil **1586**
Paxil CR **1596**

Paroxetine Mesylate (Based on the mechanism of action of venlafaxine and the potential for serotonin syndrome, caution is advised when venlafaxine is co-administered with other drugs that may affect the serotonergic neurotransmitter systems, such as SSRIs. If concomitant treatment of venlafaxine with an SSRI is clinically warranted, careful observation of the patient is advised, particularly during treatment initiation and dose increases).
No products indexed under this heading.

Pemoline (The risk of using venlafaxine in combination with other CNS active drugs has not been systematically evaluated. Consequently, caution is advised if the concomitant administration of venlafaxine and such drugs is required).
No products indexed under this heading.

Pentobarbital Sodium (The risk of using venlafaxine in combination with other CNS active drugs has not been systematically evaluated. Consequently, caution is advised if the concomitant administration of venlafaxine and such drugs is required). Products include:

Nembutal **2012**

Perphenazine (The risk of using venlafaxine in combination with other CNS active drugs has not been systematically evaluated. Consequently, caution is advised if the concomitant administration of venlafaxine and such drugs is required).
No products indexed under this heading.

Phendimetrazine Tartrate (The safety and efficacy of venlafaxine therapy in combination with weight loss agents, including phentermine, have not been established. Co-administration of venlafaxine and weight loss agents is not recommended. Venlafaxine is not indicated for weight loss alone or in combination with other products).
No products indexed under this heading.

Phenelzine Sulfate (Concomitant use in patients taking monoamine oxidase inhibitors (MAOIs) is contraindicated. Adverse reactions, some of which were serious, have been reported in patients who have recently been discontinued from a monoamine oxidase inhibitor (MAOI) and started on venlafaxine hydrochloride, or who have recently had venlafaxine hydrochloride therapy discontinued prior to initiation of a MAOI. It is recommended that venlafaxine hydrochloride not be used in combination with a MAOI, or within at least 14 days of discontinuing treatment with a MAOI. Based on the half-life of venlafaxine hydrochloride, at least 7 days should be allowed after stopping venlafaxine hydrochloride before starting an MAOI).
No products indexed under this heading.

Phenmetrazine Hydrochloride (The safety and efficacy of venlafaxine therapy in combination with weight loss agents, including phentermine, have not been established. Co-administration of venlafaxine and weight loss agents is not recommended. Venlafaxine is not indicated for weight loss alone or in combination with other products).
No products indexed under this heading.

Phenobarbital (The risk of using venlafaxine in combination with other CNS active drugs has not been systematically evaluated. Consequently, caution is advised if the concomitant administration of venlafaxine and such drugs is required). Products include:

Donnatal **2711**

Phenobarbital Sodium (The risk of using venlafaxine in combination with other CNS active drugs has not been systematically evaluated. Consequently, caution is advised if the concomitant administration of venlafaxine and such drugs is required).
No products indexed under this heading.

Phentermine Hydrochloride (The safety and efficacy of venlafaxine therapy in combination with weight loss agents, including phentermine, have not been established. Co-administration of venlafaxine and weight loss agents is not recommended). Products include:

Adipex-P **1178**

Phenylbutazone (Patients should be cautioned about the concomitant use of venlafaxine and NSAIDs since combined use of psychotropic drugs that interfere with serotonin reuptake and this agent has been associated with an increased risk of bleeding. SSRIs and SNRIs, including venlafaxine, may increase the risk of bleeding events. Concomitant use of nonsteroidal anti-inflammatory drugs may add to this risk. Case reports and epidemiological studies (case-control and cohort design) have demonstrated an association between use of drugs that interfere with serotonin reuptake and the occurrence of gastrointestinal bleeding).
No products indexed under this heading.

Pimozide (The development of a potentially life-threatening serotonin syndrome or Neuroleptic Malignant Syndrome (NMS)-like reactions have been reported with SNRIs and SSRIs alone, including venlafaxine, but particularly with concomitant use of antipsychotics).
No products indexed under this heading.

Pindolol (*In vitro* studies indicate that venlafaxine is a relatively weak inhibitor of CYP2D6. These findings have been confirmed in a clinical drug interaction study comparing the effect of venlafaxine to that of fluoxetine on the CYP2D6-mediated metabolism of dextrometrophan to dextrophan).
No products indexed under this heading.

Piroxicam (Patients should be cautioned about the concomitant use of venlafaxine and NSAIDs since combined use of psychotropic drugs that interfere with serotonin reuptake and this agent has been associated with an increased risk of bleeding. SSRIs and SNRIs, including venlafaxine, may increase the risk of bleeding events. Concomitant use of nonsteroidal anti-inflammatory drugs may add to this risk. Case reports and epidemiological studies (case-control and cohort design) have demonstrated an association between use of drugs that interfere with serotonin reuptake and the occurrence of gastrointestinal bleeding).
No products indexed under this heading.

Polythiazide (Elderly patients may be at greater risk of developing hyponatremia with SSRIs and SNRIs. Also patients taking diuretics or who are otherwise volume depleted may be at greater risk. Discontinuation of venlafaxine should be considered in patients with symptomatic hyponatremia and appropriate medical intervention should be instituted).
No products indexed under this heading.

Posaconazole (Concomitant use of CYP3A4 inhibitors and venlafaxine may increase levels of venlafaxine and ODV. Therefore, caution is advised if a patient's therapy includes a CYP3A4 inhibitor and venlafaxine concomitantly. The concomitant use of venlafaxine with a drug treatment(s) that potently inhibits both CYP2D6 and CYP3A4, the primary metabolizing enzymes for venlafaxine, has not been studied. Therefore, caution is advised should a patient's therapy include venlafaxine and any agent(s) that produce potent simultaneous inhibition of these two enzyme systems). Products include:

Noxafil **3172**

Prazepam (The risk of using venlafaxine in combination with other CNS active drugs has not been systematically evaluated. Consequently, caution is advised if the concomitant administration of venlafaxine and such drugs is required).
No products indexed under this heading.

Procarbazine Hydrochloride (Concomitant use in patients taking monoamine oxidase inhibitors (MAOIs) is contraindicated. Adverse reactions, some of which were serious, have been reported in patients who have recently been discontinued from a monoamine oxidase inhibitor (MAOI) and started on venlafaxine hydrochloride, or who have recently had venlafaxine hydrochloride therapy discontinued prior to initiation of a MAOI. It is recommended that venlafaxine hydrochloride not be used in combination with a MAOI, or within at least 14 days of discontinuing treatment with a MAOI. Based on the half-life of venlafaxine hydrochloride, at least 7 days should be allowed after stopping venlafaxine hydrochloride before starting an MAOI).
No products indexed under this heading.

Prochlorperazine (The risk of using venlafaxine in combination with other CNS active drugs has not been systematically evaluated. Consequently, caution is advised if the concomitant administration of venlafaxine and such drugs is required).
No products indexed under this heading.

Promethazine (The development of a potentially life-threatening serotonin syndrome or Neuroleptic Malignant Syndrome (NMS)-like reactions have been reported with SNRIs and SSRIs alone, including venlafaxine, but particularly with concomitant use other dopamine antagonists).
No products indexed under this heading.

Promethazine Hydrochloride (The risk of using venlafaxine in combination with other CNS active drugs has not been systematically evaluated. Consequently, caution is advised if the concomitant administration of venlafaxine and such drugs is required).
No products indexed under this heading.

Propafenone Hydrochloride (Studies indicate that venlafaxine is metabolized to its active metabolite, ODV, by CYP2D6. Thus the potential exists for a drug interaction between drugs that inhibit CYP2D6-mediated metabolism and venlafaxine. However, although imipramine partially inhibited the CYP2D6-mediated metabolism of venlafaxine, resulting in higher plasma concentrations of venlafaxine and lower plasma concentrations of ODV, the total concentration of active compounds (venlafaxine plus ODV) was not affected. Also, in a clinical study involving CYP2D6 poor and extensive metabolizers, the total concentration of active compounds (venlafaxine plus ODV), was similar in both groups. No dosage adjustment is required when venlafaxine is co-administered with a CYP2D6 inhibitor. Caution is advised should a patient's therapy include venlafaxine and CYP2D6 inhibitor). Products include:

Rythmol **1648**
Rythmol SR **1652**

Propofol (The risk of using venlafaxine in combination with other CNS active drugs has not been systematically evaluated. Consequently, caution is advised if the concomitant administration of venlafaxine and such drugs is required).
No products indexed under this heading.

Propoxyphene Hydrochloride (The risk of using venlafaxine in combination with other CNS active drugs has not been systematically evaluated. Consequently, caution is advised if the concomitant administration of venlafaxine and such drugs is required).
No products indexed under this heading.

Propoxyphene Napsylate (The risk of using venlafaxine in combination with other CNS active drugs has not been systematically evaluated. Consequently, caution is advised if the concomitant administration of venlafaxine and such drugs is required).
No products indexed under this heading.

Propranolol Hydrochloride (*In vitro* studies indicate that venlafaxine is a relatively weak inhibitor of CYP2D6. These findings have been confirmed in a clinical drug interaction study comparing the effect of venlafaxine to that of fluoxetine on the CYP2D6-mediated metabolism of dextromethorphan to dextrophan). Products include:

InnoPran XL **1517**

Protriptyline Hydrochloride (Studies indicate that venlafaxine is metabolized to its active metabolite, ODV, by CYP2D6. Thus the potential exists for a drug interaction between drugs that inhibit CYP2D6-mediated metabolism and venlafaxine. However, although imipramine partially inhibited the CYP2D6-mediated metabolism of venlafaxine, resulting in higher plasma concentrations of venlafaxine and lower plasma concentrations of ODV, the total concentration of active compounds (venlafaxine plus ODV) was not affected. Also, in a clinical study involving CYP2D6 poor and extensive metabolizers, the total concentration of active compounds (venlafaxine plus ODV), was similar in both groups. No dosage adjustment is required when venlafaxine is co-administered with a CYP2D6 inhibitor. Caution is advised should a patient's therapy include venlafaxine and CYP2D6 inhibitor).
No products indexed under this heading.

Quazepam (The risk of using venlafaxine in combination with other CNS active drugs has not been systematically evaluated. Consequently, caution is advised if the concomitant administration of venlafaxine and such drugs is required).
No products indexed under this heading.

Quetiapine Fumarate (The risk of using venlafaxine in combination with other CNS active drugs has not been systematically evaluated. Consequently, caution is advised if the concomitant administration of venlafaxine and such drugs is required). Products include:

Seroquel **750**
Seroquel XR **759**

(⊙ Described in PDR® for Ophthalmic Medicines)

Quinacrine Hydrochloride (Studies indicate that venlafaxine is metabolized to its active metabolite, ODV, by CYP2D6. Thus the potential exists for a drug interaction between drugs that inhibit CYP2D6-mediated metabolism and venlafaxine. However, although imipramine partially inhibited the CYP2D6-mediated metabolism of venlafaxine, resulting in higher plasma concentrations of venlafaxine and lower plasma concentrations of ODV, the total concentration of active compounds (venlafaxine plus ODV) was not affected. Also, in a clinical study involving CYP2D6 poor and extensive metabolizers, the total concentration of active compounds (venlafaxine plus ODV), was similar in both groups. No dosage adjustment is required when venlafaxine is co-administered with a CYP2D6 inhibitor. Caution is advised should a patient's therapy include venlafaxine and CYP2D6 inhibitor).

No products indexed under this heading.

Quinidine (Studies indicate that venlafaxine is metabolized to its active metabolite, ODV, by CYP2D6. Thus the potential exists for a drug interaction between drugs that inhibit CYP2D6-mediated metabolism and venlafaxine. However, although imipramine partially inhibited the CYP2D6-mediated metabolism of venlafaxine, resulting in higher plasma concentrations of venlafaxine and lower plasma concentrations of ODV, the total concentration of active compounds (venlafaxine plus ODV) was not affected. Also, in a clinical study involving CYP2D6 poor and extensive metabolizers, the total concentration of active compounds (venlafaxine plus ODV), was similar in both groups. No dosage adjustment is required when venlafaxine is co-administered with a CYP2D6 inhibitor. Caution is advised should a patient's therapy include venlafaxine and CYP2D6 inhibitor).

No products indexed under this heading.

Quinidine Gluconate (Studies indicate that venlafaxine is metabolized to its active metabolite, ODV, by CYP2D6. Thus the potential exists for a drug interaction between drugs that inhibit CYP2D6-mediated metabolism and venlafaxine. However, although imipramine partially inhibited the CYP2D6-mediated metabolism of venlafaxine, resulting in higher plasma concentrations of venlafaxine and lower plasma concentrations of ODV, the total concentration of active compounds (venlafaxine plus ODV) was not affected. Also, in a clinical study involving CYP2D6 poor and extensive metabolizers, the total concentration of active compounds (venlafaxine plus ODV), was similar in both groups. No dosage adjustment is required when venlafaxine is co-administered with a CYP2D6 inhibitor. Caution is advised should a patient's therapy include venlafaxine and CYP2D6 inhibitor).

No products indexed under this heading.

Quinidine Hydrochloride (Studies indicate that venlafaxine is metabolized to its active metabolite, ODV, by CYP2D6. Thus the potential exists for a drug interaction between drugs that inhibit CYP2D6-mediated metabolism and venlafaxine. However, although imipramine partially inhibited the CYP2D6-mediated metabolism of venlafaxine, resulting in higher plasma concentrations of venlafaxine and lower plasma concentrations of ODV, the total concentration of active compounds (venlafaxine plus ODV) was not affected. Also, in a clinical study involving CYP2D6 poor and extensive metabolizers, the total concentration of active compounds (venlafaxine plus ODV), was similar in both groups. No dosage adjustment is required when venlafaxine is co-administered with a CYP2D6 inhibi-

tor. Caution is advised should a patient's therapy include venlafaxine and CYP2D6 inhibitor).

No products indexed under this heading.

Quinidine Polygalacturonate (Studies indicate that venlafaxine is metabolized to its active metabolite, ODV, by CYP2D6. Thus the potential exists for a drug interaction between drugs that inhibit CYP2D6-mediated metabolism and venlafaxine. However, although imipramine partially inhibited the CYP2D6-mediated metabolism of venlafaxine, resulting in higher plasma concentrations of venlafaxine and lower plasma concentrations of ODV, the total concentration of active compounds (venlafaxine plus ODV) was not affected. Also, in a clinical study involving CYP2D6 poor and extensive metabolizers, the total concentration of active compounds (venlafaxine plus ODV), was similar in both groups. No dosage adjustment is required when venlafaxine is co-administered with a CYP2D6 inhibitor. Caution is advised should a patient's therapy include venlafaxine and CYP2D6 inhibitor).

No products indexed under this heading.

Quinidine Sulfate (Studies indicate that venlafaxine is metabolized to its active metabolite, ODV, by CYP2D6. Thus the potential exists for a drug interaction between drugs that inhibit CYP2D6-mediated metabolism and venlafaxine. However, although imipramine partially inhibited the CYP2D6-mediated metabolism of venlafaxine, resulting in higher plasma concentrations of venlafaxine and lower plasma concentrations of ODV, the total concentration of active compounds (venlafaxine plus ODV) was not affected. Also, in a clinical study involving CYP2D6 poor and extensive metabolizers, the total concentration of active compounds (venlafaxine plus ODV), was similar in both groups. No dosage adjustment is required when venlafaxine is co-administered with a CYP2D6 inhibitor. Caution is advised should a patient's therapy include venlafaxine and CYP2D6 inhibitor).

No products indexed under this heading.

Quinine (Concomitant use of CYP3A4 inhibitors and venlafaxine may increase levels of venlafaxine and ODV. Therefore, caution is advised if a patient's therapy includes a CYP3A4 inhibitor and venlafaxine concomitantly. The concomitant use of venlafaxine with a drug treatment(s) that potently inhibits both CYP2D6 and CYP3A4, the primary metabolizing enzymes for venlafaxine, has not been studied. Therefore, caution is advised should a patient's therapy include venlafaxine and any agent(s) that produce potent simultaneous inhibition of these two enzyme systems). Products include:

Hyland's Leg Cramps PM with
    Quinine 3315

Quinine Sulfate (Concomitant use of CYP3A4 inhibitors and venlafaxine may increase levels of venlafaxine and ODV. Therefore, caution is advised if a patient's therapy includes a CYP3A4 inhibitor and venlafaxine concomitantly. The concomitant use of venlafaxine with a drug treatment(s) that potently inhibits both CYP2D6 and CYP3A4, the primary metabolizing enzymes for venlafaxine, has not been studied. Therefore, caution is advised should a patient's therapy include venlafaxine and any agent(s) that produce potent simultaneous inhibition of these two enzyme systems).

No products indexed under this heading.

Quinupristin (Concomitant use of CYP3A4 inhibitors and venlafaxine may increase levels of venlafaxine and ODV. Therefore, caution is advised if a patient's therapy includes a CYP3A4 inhibitor and venlafaxine concomitantly.

The concomitant use of venlafaxine with a drug treatment(s) that potently inhibits both CYP2D6 and CYP3A4, the primary metabolizing enzymes for venlafaxine, has not been studied. Therefore, caution is advised should a patient's therapy include venlafaxine and any agent(s) that produce potent simultaneous inhibition of these two enzyme systems).

No products indexed under this heading.

Ranitidine Bismuth Citrate (Studies indicate that venlafaxine is metabolized to its active metabolite, ODV, by CYP2D6. Thus the potential exists for a drug interaction between drugs that inhibit CYP2D6-mediated metabolism and venlafaxine. However, although imipramine partially inhibited the CYP2D6-mediated metabolism of venlafaxine, resulting in higher plasma concentrations of venlafaxine and lower plasma concentrations of ODV, the total concentration of active compounds (venlafaxine plus ODV) was not affected. Also, in a clinical study involving CYP2D6 poor and extensive metabolizers, the total concentration of active compounds (venlafaxine plus ODV), was similar in both groups. No dosage adjustment is required when venlafaxine is co-administered with a CYP2D6 inhibitor. Caution is advised should a patient's therapy include venlafaxine and CYP2D6 inhibitor).

No products indexed under this heading.

Ranitidine Hydrochloride (Studies indicate that venlafaxine is metabolized to its active metabolite, ODV, by CYP2D6. Thus the potential exists for a drug interaction between drugs that inhibit CYP2D6-mediated metabolism and venlafaxine. However, although imipramine partially inhibited the CYP2D6-mediated metabolism of venlafaxine, resulting in higher plasma concentrations of venlafaxine and lower plasma concentrations of ODV, the total concentration of active compounds (venlafaxine plus ODV) was not affected. Also, in a clinical study involving CYP2D6 poor and extensive metabolizers, the total concentration of active compounds (venlafaxine plus ODV), was similar in both groups. No dosage adjustment is required when venlafaxine is co-administered with a CYP2D6 inhibitor. Caution is advised should a patient's therapy include venlafaxine and CYP2D6 inhibitor). Products include:

Zantac 1737
Zantac Injection 1732
Zantac Pharmacy 1735

Rasagiline Mesylate (Concomitant use in patients taking monoamine oxidase inhibitors (MAOIs) is contraindicated. Adverse reactions, some of which were serious, have been reported in patients who have recently been discontinued from a monoamine oxidase inhibitor (MAOI) and started on venlafaxine hydrochloride, or who have recently had venlafaxine hydrochloride therapy discontinued prior to initiation of a MAOI. It is recommended that venlafaxine hydrochloride not be used in combination with a MAOI, or within at least 14 days of discontinuing treatment with a MAOI. Based on the half-life of venlafaxine hydrochloride, at least 7 days should be allowed after stopping venlafaxine hydrochloride before starting an MAOI). Products include:

Azilect 3383

Remifentanil Hydrochloride (The risk of using venlafaxine in combination with other CNS active drugs has not been systematically evaluated. Consequently, caution is advised if the concomitant administration of venlafaxine and such drugs is required).

No products indexed under this heading.

Risperidone (Venlafaxine administered under steady-state conditions at 150 mg/day slightly inhibited the CYP2D6-mediated metabolism of risperidone (administered as a single 1 mg oral dose) to its active metabolite, 9-hydroxyrisperidone, resulting in an approximately 32% increase in risperidone AUC. However venlafaxine co-administration did not significantly alter the pharmacokinetic profile of the total active moiety (risperidone plus 9-hydroxyrisperidone)). Products include:

Risperdal Consta 2682

Ritonavir (Studies indicate that venlafaxine is metabolized to its active metabolite, ODV, by CYP2D6. Thus the potential exists for a drug interaction between drugs that inhibit CYP2D6-mediated metabolism and venlafaxine. However, although imipramine partially inhibited the CYP2D6-mediated metabolism of venlafaxine, resulting in higher plasma concentrations of venlafaxine and lower plasma concentrations of ODV, the total concentration of active compounds (venlafaxine plus ODV) was not affected. Also, in a clinical study involving CYP2D6 poor and extensive metabolizers, the total concentration of active compounds (venlafaxine plus ODV), was similar in both groups. No dosage adjustment is required when venlafaxine is co-administered with a CYP2D6 inhibitor. Caution is advised should a patient's therapy include venlafaxine and CYP2D6 inhibitor). Products include:

Kaletra 458
Norvir 509

Rizatriptan Benzoate (There have been rare post-marketing reports of serotonin syndrome with use of an SSRI and a triptan. If concomitant treatment of venlafaxine with a triptan is clinically warranted, careful observation of the patient is advised, particularly during treatment initiation and dose increases. Patients should be cautioned about the risk of serotonin syndrome with the concomitant use of venlafaxine and triptans, tramadol, tryptophan supplements or other serotonergic agents). Products include:

Maxalt 2206
Maxalt-MLT 2206

Rofecoxib (Patients should be cautioned about the concomitant use of venlafaxine and NSAIDs since combined use of psychotropic drugs that interfere with serotonin reuptake and this agent has been associated with an increased risk of bleeding. SSRIs and SNRIs, including venlafaxine, may increase the risk of bleeding events. Concomitant use of nonsteroidal anti-inflammatory drugs may add to this risk. Case reports and epidemiological studies (case-control and cohort design) have demonstrated an association between use of drugs that interfere with serotonin reuptake and the occurrence of gastrointestinal bleeding).

No products indexed under this heading.

Saquinavir (Concomitant use of CYP3A4 inhibitors and venlafaxine may increase levels of venlafaxine and ODV. Therefore, caution is advised if a patient's therapy includes a CYP3A4 inhibitor and venlafaxine concomitantly. The concomitant use of venlafaxine with a drug treatment(s) that potently inhibits both CYP2D6 and CYP3A4, the primary metabolizing enzymes for venlafaxine, has not been studied. Therefore, caution is advised should a patient's therapy include venlafaxine and any agent(s) that produce potent simultaneous inhibition of these two enzyme systems).

No products indexed under this heading.

Saquinavir Mesylate (Concomitant use of CYP3A4 inhibitors and venlafax-

---

IMPORTANT NOTE: Always consult each drug listing in the patient's regimen for possible interactions.

ine may increase levels of venlafaxine and ODV. Therefore, caution is advised if a patient's therapy includes a CYP3A4 inhibitor and venlafaxine concomitantly. The concomitant use of venlafaxine with a drug treatment(s) that potently inhibits both CYP2D6 and CYP3A4, the primary metabolizing enzymes for venlafaxine, has not been studied. Therefore, caution is advised should a patient's therapy include venlafaxine and any agent(s) that produce potent simultaneous inhibition of these two enzyme systems).

No products indexed under this heading.

Secobarbital Sodium (The risk of using venlafaxine in combination with other CNS active drugs has not been systematically evaluated. Consequently, caution is advised if the concomitant administration of venlafaxine and such drugs is required).

No products indexed under this heading.

Selegiline (Concomitant use in patients taking monoamine oxidase inhibitors (MAOIs) is contraindicated. Adverse reactions, some of which were serious, have been reported in patients who have recently been discontinued from a monoamine oxidase inhibitor (MAOI) and started on venlafaxine hydrochloride, or who have recently had venlafaxine hydrochloride therapy discontinued prior to initiation of a MAOI. It is recommended that venlafaxine hydrochloride not be used in combination with a MAOI, or within at least 14 days of discontinuing treatment with a MAOI. Based on the half-life of venlafaxine hydrochloride, at least 7 days should be allowed after stopping venlafaxine hydrochloride before starting an MAOI). Products include:
Emsam 3623

Selegiline Hydrochloride (Concomitant use in patients taking monoamine oxidase inhibitors (MAOIs) is contraindicated. Adverse reactions, some of which were serious, have been reported in patients who have recently been discontinued from a monoamine oxidase inhibitor (MAOI) and started on venlafaxine hydrochloride, or who have recently had venlafaxine hydrochloride therapy discontinued prior to initiation of a MAOI. It is recommended that venlafaxine hydrochloride not be used in combination with a MAOI, or within at least 14 days of discontinuing treatment with a MAOI. Based on the half-life of venlafaxine hydrochloride, at least 7 days should be allowed after stopping venlafaxine hydrochloride before starting an MAOI). Products include:
Eldepryl 3312

Sertraline Hydrochloride (Based on the mechanism of action of venlafaxine and the potential for serotonin syndrome, caution is advised when venlafaxine is co-administered with other drugs that may affect the serotonergic neurotransmitter systems, such as SSRIs. If concomitant treatment of venlafaxine with an SSRI is clinically warranted, careful observation of the patient is advised, particularly during treatment initiation and dose increases).

No products indexed under this heading.

Sevoflurane (The risk of using venlafaxine in combination with other CNS active drugs has not been systematically evaluated. Consequently, caution is advised if the concomitant administration of venlafaxine and such drugs is required). Products include:
Ultane 554

Sibutramine Hydrochloride Monohydrate (The safety and efficacy of venlafaxine therapy in combination with weight loss agents, including phentermine, have not been established. Co-administration of venlafaxine and weight loss agents is not recommended. Ven-

lafaxine is not indicated for weight loss alone or in combination with other products). Products include:
Meridia 492

Sildenafil Citrate (Studies indicate that venlafaxine is metabolized to its active metabolite, ODV, by CYP2D6. Thus the potential exists for a drug interaction between drugs that inhibit CYP2D6-mediated metabolism and venlafaxine. However, although imipramine partially inhibited the CYP2D6-mediated metabolism of venlafaxine, resulting in higher plasma concentrations of venlafaxine and lower plasma concentrations of ODV, the total concentration of active compounds (venlafaxine plus ODV) was not affected. Also, in a clinical study involving CYP2D6 poor and extensive metabolizers, the total concentration of active compounds (venlafaxine plus ODV), was similar in both groups. No dosage adjustment is required when venlafaxine is co-administered with a CYP2D6 inhibitor. Caution is advised should a patient's therapy include venlafaxine and CYP2D6 inhibitor).

No products indexed under this heading.

Sodium Oxybate (The risk of using venlafaxine in combination with other CNS active drugs has not been systematically evaluated. Consequently, caution is advised if the concomitant administration of venlafaxine and such drugs is required).

No products indexed under this heading.

Spironolactone (Elderly patients may be at greater risk of developing hyponatremia with SSRIs and SNRIs. Also patients taking diuretics or who are otherwise volume depleted may be at greater risk. Discontinuation of venlafaxine should be considered in patients with symptomatic hyponatremia and appropriate medical intervention should be instituted).

No products indexed under this heading.

Sufentanil Citrate (The risk of using venlafaxine in combination with other CNS active drugs has not been systematically evaluated. Consequently, caution is advised if the concomitant administration of venlafaxine and such drugs is required).

No products indexed under this heading.

Sulindac (Patients should be cautioned about the concomitant use of venlafaxine and NSAIDs since combined use of psychotropic drugs that interfere with serotonin reuptake and this agent has been associated with an increased risk of bleeding. SSRIs and SNRIs, including venlafaxine, may increase the risk of bleeding events. Concomitant use of nonsteroidal anti-inflammatory drugs may add to this risk. Case reports and epidemiological studies (case-control and cohort design) have demonstrated an association between use of drugs that interfere with serotonin reuptake and the occurrence of gastrointestinal bleeding). Products include:
Clinoril 2098

Sumatriptan (There have been rare post-marketing reports of serotonin syndrome with use of an SSRI and a triptan. If concomitant treatment of venlafaxine with a triptan is clinically warranted, careful observation of the patient is advised, particularly during treatment initiation and dose increases. Patients should be cautioned about the risk of serotonin syndrome with the concomitant use of venlafaxine and triptans, tramadol, tryptophan supplements or other serotonergic agents). Products include:
Imitrex Nasal 1503

Sumatriptan Succinate (There have been rare post-marketing reports of serotonin syndrome with use of an SSRI and a triptan. If concomitant treatment of venlafaxine with a triptan is clinically

warranted, careful observation of the patient is advised, particularly during treatment initiation and dose increases. Patients should be cautioned about the risk of serotonin syndrome with the concomitant use of venlafaxine and triptans, tramadol, tryptophan supplements or other serotonergic agents). Products include:
Imitrex 1497
Imitrex Tablets 1508
Treximet 1681

Tamoxifen Citrate (In vitro studies indicate that venlafaxine is a relatively weak inhibitor of CYP2D6. These findings have been confirmed in a clinical drug interaction study comparing the effect of venlafaxine to that of fluoxetine on the CYP2D6-mediated metabolism of dextrometrophan to dextrophan).

No products indexed under this heading.

Telithromycin (Concomitant use of CYP3A4 inhibitors and venlafaxine may increase levels of venlafaxine and ODV. Therefore, caution is advised if a patient's therapy includes a CYP3A4 inhibitor and venlafaxine concomitantly. The concomitant use of venlafaxine with a drug treatment(s) that potently inhibits both CYP2D6 and CYP3A4, the primary metabolizing enzymes for venlafaxine, has not been studied. Therefore, caution is advised should a patient's therapy include venlafaxine and any agent(s) that produce potent simultaneous inhibition of these two enzyme systems). Products include:
Ketek 2991

Temazepam (The risk of using venlafaxine in combination with other CNS active drugs has not been systematically evaluated. Consequently, caution is advised if the concomitant administration of venlafaxine and such drugs is required).

No products indexed under this heading.

Teniposide (In vitro studies indicate that venlafaxine is a relatively weak inhibitor of CYP2D6. These findings have been confirmed in a clinical drug interaction study comparing the effect of venlafaxine to that of fluoxetine on the CYP2D6-mediated metabolism of dextrometrophan to dextrophan).

No products indexed under this heading.

Terbinafine Hydrochloride (Studies indicate that venlafaxine is metabolized to its active metabolite, ODV, by CYP2D6. Thus the potential exists for a drug interaction between drugs that inhibit CYP2D6-mediated metabolism and venlafaxine. However, although imipramine partially inhibited the CYP2D6-mediated metabolism of venlafaxine, resulting in higher plasma concentrations of venlafaxine and lower plasma concentrations of ODV, the total concentration of active compounds (venlafaxine plus ODV) was not affected. Also, in a clinical study involving CYP2D6 poor and extensive metabolizers, the total concentration of active compounds (venlafaxine plus ODV), was similar in both groups. No dosage adjustment is required when venlafaxine is co-administered with a CYP2D6 inhibitor. Caution is advised should a patient's therapy include venlafaxine and CYP2D6 inhibitor).

No products indexed under this heading.

Testosterone (In vitro studies indicate that venlafaxine is a relatively weak inhibitor of CYP2D6. These findings have been confirmed in a clinical drug interaction study comparing the effect of venlafaxine to that of fluoxetine on the CYP2D6-mediated metabolism of dextrometrophan to dextrophan).
Products include:
AndroGel 3456

Testosterone Cypionate (In vitro studies indicate that venlafaxine is a relatively weak inhibitor of CYP2D6. These findings have been confirmed in a clinical drug interaction study comparing the effect of venlafaxine to that of fluoxetine on the CYP2D6-mediated metabolism of dextrometrophan to dextrophan).

No products indexed under this heading.

Testosterone Enanthate (In vitro studies indicate that venlafaxine is a relatively weak inhibitor of CYP2D6. These findings have been confirmed in a clinical drug interaction study comparing the effect of venlafaxine to that of fluoxetine on the CYP2D6-mediated metabolism of dextrometrophan to dextrophan). Products include:
Delatestryl 1102

Testosterone Propionate (In vitro studies indicate that venlafaxine is a relatively weak inhibitor of CYP2D6. These findings have been confirmed in a clinical drug interaction study comparing the effect of venlafaxine to that of fluoxetine on the CYP2D6-mediated metabolism of dextrometrophan to dextrophan).

No products indexed under this heading.

Thiamylal Sodium (The risk of using venlafaxine in combination with other CNS active drugs has not been systematically evaluated. Consequently, caution is advised if the concomitant administration of venlafaxine and such drugs is required).

No products indexed under this heading.

Thioridazine (In vitro studies indicate that venlafaxine is a relatively weak inhibitor of CYP2D6. These findings have been confirmed in a clinical drug interaction study comparing the effect of venlafaxine to that of fluoxetine on the CYP2D6-mediated metabolism of dextrometrophan to dextrophan).

No products indexed under this heading.

Thioridazine Hydrochloride (The risk of using venlafaxine in combination with other CNS active drugs has not been systematically evaluated. Consequently, caution is advised if the concomitant administration of venlafaxine and such drugs is required). Products include:
Thioridazine Hydrochloride 2384

Thiothixene (The risk of using venlafaxine in combination with other CNS active drugs has not been systematically evaluated. Consequently, caution is advised if the concomitant administration of venlafaxine and such drugs is required). Products include:
Thiothixene 2386

Timolol Maleate (In vitro studies indicate that venlafaxine is a relatively weak inhibitor of CYP2D6. These findings have been confirmed in a clinical drug interaction study comparing the effect of venlafaxine to that of fluoxetine on the CYP2D6-mediated metabolism of dextrometrophan to dextrophan). Products include:
Combigan 601
Dorzolamide
  Hydrochloride/Timolol Maleate
  Ophthalmic Solution .... ☉243
Timoptic in Ocudose .... ☉231

Tinzaparin Sodium (Patients should be cautioned about the concomitant use of venlafaxine and anti-coagulants since combined use of psychotropic drugs that interfere with serotonin reuptake and this agent has been associated with an increased risk of bleeding. SSRIs and SNRIs, including venlafaxine, may increase the risk of bleeding events. Concomitant use of anti-coagulants may add to this risk. Case reports and epidemiological studies (case-control and cohort design) have demonstrated an association

547 Interactions Index Effexor

between use of drugs that interfere with serotonin reuptake and the occurrence of gastrointestinal bleeding).
No products indexed under this heading.

Tolmetin Sodium (Patients should be cautioned about the concomitant use of venlafaxine and NSAIDs since combined use of psychotropic drugs that interfere with serotonin reuptake and this agent has been associated with an increased risk of bleeding. SSRIs and SNRIs, including venlafaxine, may increase the risk of bleeding events. Concomitant use of nonsteroidal anti-inflammatory drugs may add to this risk. Case reports and epidemiological studies (case-control and cohort design) have demonstrated an association between use of drugs that interfere with serotonin reuptake and the occurrence of gastrointestinal bleeding).
No products indexed under this heading.

Tolterodine Tartrate (*In vitro* studies indicate that venlafaxine is a relatively weak inhibitor of CYP2D6. These findings have been confirmed in a clinical drug interaction study comparing the effect of venlafaxine to that of fluoxetine on the CYP2D6-mediated metabolism of dextrometrophan to dextrophan).
No products indexed under this heading.

Torsemide (Elderly patients may be at greater risk of developing hyponatremia with SSRIs and SNRIs. Also patients taking diuretics or who are otherwise volume depleted may be at greater risk. Discontinuation of venlafaxine should be considered in patients with symptomatic hyponatremia and appropriate medical intervention should be instituted).
No products indexed under this heading.

Tramadol Hydrochloride (Based on the mechanism of action of venlafaxine and the potential for serotonin syndrome, caution is advised when venlafaxine is co-administered with other drugs that may affect the serotonergic neurotransmitter systems, such as tramadol. If concomitant treatment of venlafaxine with tramadol is clinically warranted, careful observation of the patient is advised, particularly during treatment initiation and dose increases). Products include:
Ryzolt 2813
Ultram ER 2693

Tranylcypromine Sulfate (Concomitant use in patients taking monoamine oxidase inhibitors (MAOIs) is contraindicated. Adverse reactions, some of which were serious, have been reported in patients who have recently been discontinued from a monoamine oxidase inhibitor (MAOI) and started on venlafaxine hydrochloride, or who have recently had venlafaxine hydrochloride therapy discontinued prior to initiation of a MAOI. It is recommended that venlafaxine hydrochloride not be used in combination with a MAOI, or within at least 14 days of discontinuing treatment with a MAOI. Based on the half-life of venlafaxine hydrochloride, at least 7 days should be allowed after stopping venlafaxine hydrochloride before starting an MAOI). Products include:
Parnate 1584

Trazodone Hydrochloride (*In vitro* studies indicate that venlafaxine is a relatively weak inhibitor of CYP2D6. These findings have been confirmed in a clinical drug interaction study comparing the effect of venlafaxine to that of fluoxetine on the CYP2D6-mediated metabolism of dextrometrophan to dextrophan).
No products indexed under this heading.

Triamterene (Elderly patients may be at greater risk of developing hyponatremia with SSRIs and SNRIs. Also patients taking diuretics or who are otherwise volume depleted may be at greater risk. Discontinuation of venlafaxine should be considered in patients with symptomatic hyponatremia and appropriate medical intervention should be instituted). Products include:
Dyazide 1429
Dyrenium 3495

Triazolam (The risk of using venlafaxine in combination with other CNS active drugs has not been systematically evaluated. Consequently, caution is advised if the concomitant administration of venlafaxine and such drugs is required).
No products indexed under this heading.

Trifluoperazine Hydrochloride (The risk of using venlafaxine in combination with other CNS active drugs has not been systematically evaluated. Consequently, caution is advised if the concomitant administration of venlafaxine and such drugs is required).
No products indexed under this heading.

Trimipramine Maleate (Studies indicate that venlafaxine is metabolized to its active metabolite, ODV, by CYP2D6. Thus the potential exists for a drug interaction between drugs that inhibit CYP2D6-mediated metabolism and venlafaxine. However, although imipramine partially inhibited the CYP2D6-mediated metabolism of venlafaxine, resulting in higher plasma concentrations of venlafaxine and lower plasma concentrations of ODV, the total concentration of active compounds (venlafaxine plus ODV) was not affected. Also, in a clinical study involving CYP2D6 poor and extensive metabolizers, the total concentration of active compounds (venlafaxine plus ODV), was similar in both groups. No dosage adjustment is required when venlafaxine is co-administered with a CYP2D6 inhibitor. Caution is advised should a patient's therapy include venlafaxine and CYP2D6 inhibitor).
No products indexed under this heading.

Troglitazone (Concomitant use of CYP3A4 inhibitors and venlafaxine may increase levels of venlafaxine and ODV. Therefore, caution is advised if a patient's therapy includes a CYP3A4 inhibitor and venlafaxine concomitantly. The concomitant use of venlafaxine with a drug treatment(s) that potently inhibits both CYP2D6 and CYP3A4, the primary metabolizing enzymes for venlafaxine, has not been studied. Therefore, caution is advised should a patient's therapy include venlafaxine and any agent(s) that produce potent simultaneous inhibition of these two enzyme systems).
No products indexed under this heading.

Troleandomycin (Concomitant use of CYP3A4 inhibitors and venlafaxine may increase levels of venlafaxine and ODV. Therefore, caution is advised if a patient's therapy includes a CYP3A4 inhibitor and venlafaxine concomitantly. The concomitant use of venlafaxine with a drug treatment(s) that potently inhibits both CYP2D6 and CYP3A4, the primary metabolizing enzymes for venlafaxine, has not been studied. Therefore, caution is advised should a patient's therapy include venlafaxine and any agent(s) that produce potent simultaneous inhibition of these two enzyme systems).
No products indexed under this heading.

Tryptophan (Patients should be cautioned about the risk of serotonin syndrome with the concomitant use of venlafaxine and tryptophan supplements. The concomitant use of venlafaxine with serotonin precursors (such as tryptophan) is not recommended).
No products indexed under this heading.

L-Tryptophan (Patients should be cautioned about the risk of serotonin syndrome with the concomitant use of venlafaxine and tryptophan supplements. The concomitant use of venlafaxine with serotonin precursors (such as tryptophan) is not recommended).
No products indexed under this heading.

Valdecoxib (Patients should be cautioned about the concomitant use of venlafaxine and NSAIDs since combined use of psychotropic drugs that interfere with serotonin reuptake and this agent has been associated with an increased risk of bleeding. SSRIs and SNRIs, including venlafaxine, may increase the risk of bleeding events. Concomitant use of nonsteroidal anti-inflammatory drugs may add to this risk. Case reports and epidemiological studies (case-control and cohort design) have demonstrated an association between use of drugs that interfere with serotonin reuptake and the occurrence of gastrointestinal bleeding).
No products indexed under this heading.

Valproate Sodium (Concomitant use of CYP3A4 inhibitors and venlafaxine may increase levels of venlafaxine and ODV. Therefore, caution is advised if a patient's therapy includes a CYP3A4 inhibitor and venlafaxine concomitantly. The concomitant use of venlafaxine with a drug treatment(s) that potently inhibits both CYP2D6 and CYP3A4, the primary metabolizing enzymes for venlafaxine, has not been studied. Therefore, caution is advised should a patient's therapy include venlafaxine and any agent(s) that produce potent simultaneous inhibition of these two enzyme systems).
No products indexed under this heading.

Vardenafil Hydrochloride (Studies indicate that venlafaxine is metabolized to its active metabolite, ODV, by CYP2D6. Thus the potential exists for a drug interaction between drugs that inhibit CYP2D6-mediated metabolism and venlafaxine. However, although imipramine partially inhibited the CYP2D6-mediated metabolism of venlafaxine, resulting in higher plasma concentrations of venlafaxine and lower plasma concentrations of ODV, the total concentration of active compounds (venlafaxine plus ODV) was not affected. Also, in a clinical study involving CYP2D6 poor and extensive metabolizers, the total concentration of active compounds (venlafaxine plus ODV), was similar in both groups. No dosage adjustment is required when venlafaxine is co-administered with a CYP2D6 inhibitor. Caution is advised should a patient's therapy include venlafaxine and CYP2D6 inhibitor). Products include:
Levitra 3157

Verapamil Hydrochloride (Concomitant use of CYP3A4 inhibitors and venlafaxine may increase levels of venlafaxine and ODV. Therefore, caution is advised if a patient's therapy includes a CYP3A4 inhibitor and venlafaxine concomitantly. The concomitant use of venlafaxine with a drug treatment(s) that potently inhibits both CYP2D6 and CYP3A4, the primary metabolizing enzymes for venlafaxine, has not been studied. Therefore, caution is advised should a patient's therapy include venlafaxine and any agent(s) that produce potent simultaneous inhibition of these two enzyme systems). Products include:
Tarka 534

Vinblastine Sulfate (*In vitro* studies indicate that venlafaxine is a relatively weak inhibitor of CYP2D6. These findings have been confirmed in a clinical drug interaction study comparing the effect of venlafaxine to that of fluoxetine on the CYP2D6-mediated metabolism of dextrometrophan to dextrophan).
No products indexed under this heading.

Voriconazole (Concomitant use of CYP3A4 inhibitors and venlafaxine may increase levels of venlafaxine and ODV. Therefore, caution is advised if a patient's therapy includes a CYP3A4 inhibitor and venlafaxine concomitantly. The concomitant use of venlafaxine with a drug treatment(s) that potently inhibits both CYP2D6 and CYP3A4, the primary metabolizing enzymes for venlafaxine, has not been studied. Therefore, caution is advised should a patient's therapy include venlafaxine and any agent(s) that produce potent simultaneous inhibition of these two enzyme systems).
No products indexed under this heading.

Warfarin Sodium (Patients should be cautioned about the concomitant use of venlafaxine and warfarin since combined use of psychotropic drugs that interfere with serotonin reuptake and this agent has been associated with an increased risk of bleeding. SSRIs and SNRIs, including venlafaxine, may increase the risk of bleeding events. Concomitant use of warfarin may add to this risk. Case reports and epidemiological studies (case-control and cohort design) have demonstrated an association between use of drugs that interfere with serotonin reuptake and the occurrence of gastrointestinal bleeding. Altered anticoagulant effects, including increased bleeding, have been reported when SSRIs and SNRIs are co-administered with warfarin. Patients receiving warfarin therapy should be carefully monitored when venlafaxine is initiated or discontinued).
No products indexed under this heading.

Zafirlukast (Concomitant use of CYP3A4 inhibitors and venlafaxine may increase levels of venlafaxine and ODV. Therefore, caution is advised if a patient's therapy includes a CYP3A4 inhibitor and venlafaxine concomitantly. The concomitant use of venlafaxine with a drug treatment(s) that potently inhibits both CYP2D6 and CYP3A4, the primary metabolizing enzymes for venlafaxine, has not been studied. Therefore, caution is advised should a patient's therapy include venlafaxine and any agent(s) that produce potent simultaneous inhibition of these two enzyme systems). Products include:
Accolate 3612

Zaleplon (The risk of using venlafaxine in combination with other CNS active drugs has not been systematically evaluated. Consequently, caution is advised if the concomitant administration of venlafaxine and such drugs is required).
No products indexed under this heading.

Zileuton (Concomitant use of CYP3A4 inhibitors and venlafaxine may increase levels of venlafaxine and ODV. Therefore, caution is advised if a patient's therapy includes a CYP3A4 inhibitor and venlafaxine concomitantly. The concomitant use of venlafaxine with a drug treatment(s) that potently inhibits both CYP2D6 and CYP3A4, the primary metabolizing enzymes for venlafaxine, has not been studied. Therefore, caution is advised should a patient's therapy include venlafaxine and any agent(s) that produce potent simultaneous inhibition of these two enzyme systems).
No products indexed under this heading.

Ziprasidone Hydrochloride (The risk of using venlafaxine in combination with other CNS active drugs has not been systematically evaluated. Conse-

IMPORTANT NOTE: Always consult each drug listing in the patient's regimen for possible interactions.

quently, caution is advised if the concomitant administration of venlafaxine and such drugs is required). Products include:

Zolmitriptan (There have been rare post-marketing reports of serotonin syndrome with the use of an SSRI and a triptan. If concomitant treatment of venlafaxine with a triptan is clinically warranted, careful observation of the patient is advised, particularly during treatment initiation and dose increases. Patients should be cautioned about the risk of serotonin syndrome with the concomitant use of venlafaxine and triptans, tramadol, tryptophan supplements or other serotonergic agents). Products include:

Zolpidem Tartrate (The risk of using venlafaxine in combination with other CNS active drugs has not been systematically evaluated. Consequently, caution is advised if the concomitant administration of venlafaxine and such drugs is required). Products include:

Zonisamide (*In vitro* studies indicate that venlafaxine is a relatively weak inhibitor of CYP2D6. These findings have been confirmed in a clinical drug interaction study comparing the effect of venlafaxine to that of fluoxetine on the CYP2D6-mediated metabolism of dextrometrophan to dextrophan). Products include:

Food Interactions

Alcohol (Although venlafaxine has not been shown to increase the impairment of mental and motor skills caused by alcohol, patients should be advised to avoid alcohol while taking venlafaxine).

Beer, reduced-alcohol (Although venlafaxine has not been shown to increase the impairment of mental and motor skills caused by alcohol, patients should be advised to avoid alcohol while taking venlafaxine).

Beer, unspecified (Although venlafaxine has not been shown to increase the impairment of mental and motor skills caused by alcohol, patients should be advised to avoid alcohol while taking venlafaxine).

Grapefruit (Concomitant use of CYP3A4 inhibitors and venlafaxine may increase levels of venlafaxine and ODV. Therefore, caution is advised if a patient's therapy includes a CYP3A4 inhibitor and venlafaxine concomitantly. The concomitant use of venlafaxine with a drug treatment(s) that potently inhibits both CYP2D6 and CYP3A4, the primary metabolizing enzymes for venlafaxine, has not been studied. Therefore, caution is advised should a patient's therapy include venlafaxine and any agent(s) that produce potent simultaneous inhibition of these two enzyme systems).

Grapefruit Juice (Concomitant use of CYP3A4 inhibitors and venlafaxine may increase levels of venlafaxine and ODV. Therefore, caution is advised if a patient's therapy includes a CYP3A4 inhibitor and venlafaxine concomitantly. The concomitant use of venlafaxine with a drug treatment(s) that potently inhibits both CYP2D6 and CYP3A4, the primary metabolizing enzymes for venlafaxine, has not been studied. Therefore, caution is advised should a patient's therapy include venlafaxine and any agent(s) that produce potent simultaneous inhibition of these two enzyme systems).

Wine, Chianti (Although venlafaxine has not been shown to increase the impairment of mental and motor skills caused by alcohol, patients should be advised to avoid alcohol while taking venlafaxine).

Wine, Red (Although venlafaxine has not been shown to increase the impairment of mental and motor skills caused by alcohol, patients should be advised to avoid alcohol while taking venlafaxine).

Wine, unspecified (Although venlafaxine has not been shown to increase the impairment of mental and motor skills caused by alcohol, patients should be advised to avoid alcohol while taking venlafaxine).

Wine products (Although venlafaxine has not been shown to increase the impairment of mental and motor skills caused by alcohol, patients should be advised to avoid alcohol while taking venlafaxine).

EFFIENT TABLETS

May interact with aspirin-acetylsalicylic acid, fibrinolytic agents, non-steroidal anti-inflammatory agents, oral anticoagulants, and certain other agents. Compounds in these categories include:

Alteplase (Co-administration of prasugrel hydrochloride and fibrinolytic agents may increase the risk of bleeding). Products include:

Anisindione (Co-administration of prasugrel hydrochloride and oral anticoagulants may increase the risk of bleeding).
No products indexed under this heading.

Anistreplase (Co-administration of prasugrel hydrochloride and fibrinolytic agents may increase the risk of bleeding).
No products indexed under this heading.

Aspirin (Aspirin 150 mg daily did not alter prasugrel-mediated inhibition of plateletaggregation; however, bleeding time was increased compared with either drug alone). Products include:

Aspirin, Enteric Coated (Aspirin 150 mg daily did not alter prasugrel-mediated inhibition of plateletaggregation; however, bleeding time was increased compared with either drug alone).
No products indexed under this heading.

Aspirin Buffered (Aspirin 150 mg daily did not alter prasugrel-mediated inhibition of plateletaggregation; however, bleeding time was increased compared with either drug alone).
No products indexed under this heading.

Celecoxib (Co-administration of prasugrel hydrochloride and NSAIDs (used chronically) may increase the risk of bleeding). Products include:

Diclofenac Epolamine (Co-administration of prasugrel hydrochloride and NSAIDs (used chronically) may increase the risk of bleeding). Products include:

Diclofenac Potassium (Co-administration of prasugrel hydrochloride and NSAIDs (used chronically) may increase the risk of bleeding).
No products indexed under this heading.

Diclofenac Sodium (Co-administration of prasugrel hydrochloride and NSAIDs (used chronically) may increase the risk of bleeding).
No products indexed under this heading.

Dicumarol (Co-administration of prasugrel hydrochloride and oral anticoagulants may increase the risk of bleeding).
No products indexed under this heading.

Etodolac (Co-administration of prasugrel hydrochloride and NSAIDs (used chronically) may increase the risk of bleeding).
No products indexed under this heading.

Fat (In a study of healthy subjects given a single 15 mg dose, the AUC of the active metabolite was unaffected by a high fat, high calorie meal, but C_{max} was decreased by 49% and T_{max} was increased from 0.5 to 1.5 hours. Prasugrel hydrochloride can be administered without regard to food. The active metabolite is bound about 98% to human serum albumin).
No products indexed under this heading.

Fenoprofen Calcium (Co-administration of prasugrel hydrochloride and NSAIDs (used chronically) may increase the risk of bleeding).
No products indexed under this heading.

Flurbiprofen (Co-administration of prasugrel hydrochloride and NSAIDs (used chronically) may increase the risk of bleeding).
No products indexed under this heading.

Heparin (A single intravenous dose of unfractionated heparin (100 U/kg) did not significantly alter coagulation or the prasugrel-mediated inhibition of platelet aggregation; however, bleeding time was increased compared with either drug alone).
No products indexed under this heading.

Heparin Calcium (A single intravenous dose of unfractionated heparin (100 U/kg) did not significantly alter coagulation or the prasugrel-mediated inhibition of platelet aggregation; however, bleeding time was increased compared with either drug alone).
No products indexed under this heading.

Heparin Sodium (A single intravenous dose of unfractionated heparin (100 U/kg) did not significantly alter coagulation or the prasugrel-mediated inhibition of platelet aggregation; however, bleeding time was increased compared with either drug alone).
No products indexed under this heading.

Ibuprofen (Co-administration of prasugrel hydrochloride and NSAIDs (used chronically) may increase the risk of bleeding). Products include:

Indomethacin (Co-administration of prasugrel hydrochloride and NSAIDs (used chronically) may increase the risk of bleeding). Products include:

Indomethacin Sodium Trihydrate (Co-administration of prasugrel hydrochloride and NSAIDs (used chronically) may increase the risk of bleeding). Products include:

Ketoconazole (Ketoconazole (400 mg daily), a selective and potent inhibitor of CYP3A4 and CYP3A5, did not affect prasugrel-mediated inhibition of platelet aggregation or the active metabolite's AUC and T_{max}, but decreased the C_{max} by 34% to 46%). Products include:

Ketoprofen (Co-administration of prasugrel hydrochloride and NSAIDs (used chronically) may increase the risk of bleeding).
No products indexed under this heading.

Ketorolac Tromethamine (Co-administration of prasugrel hydrochloride and NSAIDs (used chronically) may increase the risk of bleeding). Products include:

Lansoprazole (Daily co-administration of ranitidine (an H_2 blocker) or lansoprazole (a proton pump inhibitor) decreased the C_{max} of the prasugrel active metabolite by 14% and 29%, respectively, but did not change the active metabolite's AUC and T_{max}).
No products indexed under this heading.

Meclofenamate Sodium (Co-administration of prasugrel hydrochloride and NSAIDs (used chronically) may increase the risk of bleeding).
No products indexed under this heading.

Mefenamic Acid (Co-administration of prasugrel hydrochloride and NSAIDs (used chronically) may increase the risk of bleeding).
No products indexed under this heading.

Meloxicam (Co-administration of prasugrel hydrochloride and NSAIDs (used chronically) may increase the risk of bleeding).
No products indexed under this heading.

Nabumetone (Co-administration of prasugrel hydrochloride and NSAIDs (used chronically) may increase the risk of bleeding).
No products indexed under this heading.

Naproxen (Co-administration of prasugrel hydrochloride and NSAIDs (used chronically) may increase the risk of bleeding). Products include:

Naproxen Sodium (Co-administration of prasugrel hydrochloride and NSAIDs (used chronically) may increase the risk of bleeding). Products include:

Oxaprozin (Co-administration of prasugrel hydrochloride and NSAIDs (used chronically) may increase the risk of bleeding).
No products indexed under this heading.

Phenylbutazone (Co-administration of prasugrel hydrochloride and NSAIDs (used chronically) may increase the risk of bleeding).
No products indexed under this heading.

Piroxicam (Co-administration of prasugrel hydrochloride and NSAIDs (used chronically) may increase the risk of bleeding).
No products indexed under this heading.

Ranitidine Bismuth Citrate (Daily co-administration of ranitidine (an H_2 blocker) or lansoprazole (a proton pump inhibitor) decreased the C_{max} of the prasugrel active metabolite by 14% and 29%, respectively, but did not change the active metabolite's AUC and T_{max}).
No products indexed under this heading.

Ranitidine Hydrochloride (Daily co-administration of ranitidine (an H_2 blocker) or lansoprazole (a proton pump inhibitor) decreased the C_{max} of the prasugrel active metabolite by 14% and 29%, respectively, but did not change the active metabolite's AUC and T_{max}). Products include:

(⊙ Described in PDR® for Ophthalmic Medicines)

Rofecoxib (Co-administration of prasugrel hydrochloride and NSAIDs (used chronically) may increase the risk of bleeding).
No products indexed under this heading.

Streptokinase (Co-administration of prasugrel hydrochloride and fibrinolytic agents may increase the risk of bleeding).
No products indexed under this heading.

Sulindac (Co-administration of prasugrel hydrochloride and NSAIDs (used chronically) may increase the risk of bleeding). Products include:
Clinoril 2098

Tolmetin Sodium (Co-administration of prasugrel hydrochloride and NSAIDs (used chronically) may increase the risk of bleeding).
No products indexed under this heading.

Urokinase (Co-administration of prasugrel hydrochloride and fibrinolytic agents may increase the risk of bleeding).
No products indexed under this heading.

Valdecoxib (Co-administration of prasugrel hydrochloride and NSAIDs (used chronically) may increase the risk of bleeding).
No products indexed under this heading.

Warfarin Sodium (Co-administration of prasugrel hydrochloride and warfarin may increase the risk of bleeding. A significant prolongation of the bleeding time was observed when prasugrel was co-administered with 15 mg of warfarin).
No products indexed under this heading.

Food Interactions

Food, unspecified (In a study of healthy subjects given a single 15 mg dose, the AUC of the active metabolite was unaffected by a high fat, high calorie meal, but C_{max} was decreased by 49% and T_{max} was increased from 0.5 to 1.5 hours. Prasugrel hydrochloride can be administered without regard to food. The active metabolite is bound about 98% to human serum albumin).

Meal, unspecified (In a study of healthy subjects given a single 15 mg dose, the AUC of the active metabolite was unaffected by a high fat, high calorie meal, but C_{max} was decreased by 49% and T_{max} was increased from 0.5 to 1.5 hours. Prasugrel hydrochloride can be administered without regard to food. The active metabolite is bound about 98% to human serum albumin).

EFFIENT TABLETS

(Prasugrel Hydrochloride) 1881
May interact with aspirin-acetylsalicylic acid, fibrinolytic agents, non-steroidal anti-inflammatory agents, oral anticoagulants, and certain other agents. Compounds in these categories include:

Alteplase (Co-administration of prasugrel hydrochloride and fibrinolytic agents may increase the risk of bleeding). Products include:
Activase 1183
Cathflo 1192

Anisindione (Co-administration of prasugrel hydrochloride and oral anticoagulants may increase the risk of bleeding).
No products indexed under this heading.

Anistreplase (Co-administration of prasugrel hydrochloride and fibrinolytic agents may increase the risk of bleeding).
No products indexed under this heading.

Aspirin (Aspirin 150 mg daily did not alter prasugrel-mediated inhibition of plateletaggregation; however, bleeding time was increased compared with either drug alone). Products include:

Aggrenox 880
Bayer Aspirin 829
Percodan 1124
St. Joseph Aspirin 2045

Aspirin, Enteric Coated (Aspirin 150 mg daily did not alter prasugrel-mediated inhibition of plateletaggregation; however, bleeding time was increased compared with either drug alone).
No products indexed under this heading.

Aspirin Buffered (Aspirin 150 mg daily did not alter prasugrel-mediated inhibition of plateletaggregation; however, bleeding time was increased compared with either drug alone).
No products indexed under this heading.

Celecoxib (Co-administration of prasugrel hydrochloride and NSAIDs (used chronically) may increase the risk of bleeding). Products include:
Celebrex 3272

Diclofenac Epolamine (Co-administration of prasugrel hydrochloride and NSAIDs (used chronically) may increase the risk of bleeding). Products include:
Flector 1839

Diclofenac Potassium (Co-administration of prasugrel hydrochloride and NSAIDs (used chronically) may increase the risk of bleeding).
No products indexed under this heading.

Diclofenac Sodium (Co-administration of prasugrel hydrochloride and NSAIDs (used chronically) may increase the risk of bleeding).
No products indexed under this heading.

Dicumarol (Co-administration of prasugrel hydrochloride and oral anticoagulants may increase the risk of bleeding).
No products indexed under this heading.

Etodolac (Co-administration of prasugrel hydrochloride and NSAIDs (used chronically) may increase the risk of bleeding).
No products indexed under this heading.

Fat (In a study of healthy subjects given a single 15 mg dose, the AUC of the active metabolite was unaffected by a high fat, high calorie meal, but C_{max} was decreased by 49% and T_{max} was increased from 0.5 to 1.5 hours. Prasugrel hydrochloride can be administered without regard to food. The active metabolite is bound about 98% to human serum albumin).
No products indexed under this heading.

Fenoprofen Calcium (Co-administration of prasugrel hydrochloride and NSAIDs (used chronically) may increase the risk of bleeding).
No products indexed under this heading.

Flurbiprofen (Co-administration of prasugrel hydrochloride and NSAIDs (used chronically) may increase the risk of bleeding).
No products indexed under this heading.

Heparin (A single intravenous dose of unfractionated heparin (100 U/kg) did not significantly alter coagulation or the prasugrel-mediated inhibition of platelet aggregation; however, bleeding time was increased compared with either drug alone).
No products indexed under this heading.

Heparin Calcium (A single intravenous dose of unfractionated heparin (100 U/kg) did not significantly alter coagulation or the prasugrel-mediated inhibition of platelet aggregation; however, bleeding time was increased compared with either drug alone).
No products indexed under this heading.

Heparin Sodium (A single intravenous dose of unfractionated heparin (100 U/kg) did not significantly alter coagulation or the prasugrel-mediated inhibition of platelet aggregation; however, bleeding time was increased compared with either drug alone).
No products indexed under this heading.

Ibuprofen (Co-administration of prasugrel hydrochloride and NSAIDs (used chronically) may increase the risk of bleeding). Products include:
Motrin IB 2043
Children's Motrin 2044
Children's Motrin Non-Staining
   Dye-Free 2044
Infants' Motrin 2044
Infants' Motrin Dye-Free 2044
Junior Strength Motrin 2044
Vicoprofen 564

Indomethacin (Co-administration of prasugrel hydrochloride and NSAIDs (used chronically) may increase the risk of bleeding). Products include:
Indocin 2167

Indomethacin Sodium Trihydrate (Co-administration of prasugrel hydrochloride and NSAIDs (used chronically) may increase the risk of bleeding). Products include:
Indocin I.V. 2007

Ketoconazole (Ketoconazole (400 mg daily), a selective and potent inhibitor of CYP3A4 and CYP3A5, did not affect prasugrel-mediated inhibition of platelet aggregation or the active metabolite's AUC and T_{max}, but decreased the C_{max} by 34% to 46%). Products include:
Extina 3319
Xolegel 3337

Ketoprofen (Co-administration of prasugrel hydrochloride and NSAIDs (used chronically) may increase the risk of bleeding).
No products indexed under this heading.

Ketorolac Tromethamine (Co-administration of prasugrel hydrochloride and NSAIDs (used chronically) may increase the risk of bleeding). Products include:
Acuvail .... ⊙ 209

Lansoprazole (Daily co-administration of ranitidine (an H_2 blocker) or lansoprazole (a proton pump inhibitor) decreased the C_{max} of the prasugrel active metabolite by 14% and 29%, respectively, but did not change the active metabolite's AUC and T_{max}).
No products indexed under this heading.

Meclofenamate Sodium (Co-administration of prasugrel hydrochloride and NSAIDs (used chronically) may increase the risk of bleeding).
No products indexed under this heading.

Mefenamic Acid (Co-administration of prasugrel hydrochloride and NSAIDs (used chronically) may increase the risk of bleeding).
No products indexed under this heading.

Meloxicam (Co-administration of prasugrel hydrochloride and NSAIDs (used chronically) may increase the risk of bleeding).
No products indexed under this heading.

Nabumetone (Co-administration of prasugrel hydrochloride and NSAIDs (used chronically) may increase the risk of bleeding).
No products indexed under this heading.

Naproxen (Co-administration of prasugrel hydrochloride and NSAIDs (used chronically) may increase the risk of bleeding). Products include:
EC-Naprosyn 2850
Naprosyn 2850
Anaprox/Naprosyn 2850

Naproxen Sodium (Co-administration of prasugrel hydrochloride and NSAIDs (used chronically) may increase the risk of bleeding). Products include:

Anaprox 2850
Anaprox DS 2850
Treximet 1681

Oxaprozin (Co-administration of prasugrel hydrochloride and NSAIDs (used chronically) may increase the risk of bleeding).
No products indexed under this heading.

Phenylbutazone (Co-administration of prasugrel hydrochloride and NSAIDs (used chronically) may increase the risk of bleeding).
No products indexed under this heading.

Piroxicam (Co-administration of prasugrel hydrochloride and NSAIDs (used chronically) may increase the risk of bleeding).
No products indexed under this heading.

Ranitidine Bismuth Citrate (Daily co-administration of ranitidine (an H_2 blocker) or lansoprazole (a proton pump inhibitor) decreased the C_{max} of the prasugrel active metabolite by 14% and 29%, respectively, but did not change the active metabolite's AUC and T_{max}).
No products indexed under this heading.

Ranitidine Hydrochloride (Daily co-administration of ranitidine (an H_2 blocker) or lansoprazole (a proton pump inhibitor) decreased the C_{max} of the prasugrel active metabolite by 14% and 29%, respectively, but did not change the active metabolite's AUC and T_{max}). Products include:
Zantac 1737
Zantac Injection 1732
Zantac Pharmacy 1735

Rofecoxib (Co-administration of prasugrel hydrochloride and NSAIDs (used chronically) may increase the risk of bleeding).
No products indexed under this heading.

Streptokinase (Co-administration of prasugrel hydrochloride and fibrinolytic agents may increase the risk of bleeding).
No products indexed under this heading.

Sulindac (Co-administration of prasugrel hydrochloride and NSAIDs (used chronically) may increase the risk of bleeding). Products include:
Clinoril 2098

Tolmetin Sodium (Co-administration of prasugrel hydrochloride and NSAIDs (used chronically) may increase the risk of bleeding).
No products indexed under this heading.

Urokinase (Co-administration of prasugrel hydrochloride and fibrinolytic agents may increase the risk of bleeding).
No products indexed under this heading.

Valdecoxib (Co-administration of prasugrel hydrochloride and NSAIDs (used chronically) may increase the risk of bleeding).
No products indexed under this heading.

Warfarin Sodium (Co-administration of prasugrel hydrochloride and warfarin may increase the risk of bleeding. A significant prolongation of the bleeding time was observed when prasugrel was co-administered with 15 mg of warfarin).
No products indexed under this heading.

Food Interactions

Food, unspecified (In a study of healthy subjects given a single 15 mg dose, the AUC of the active metabolite was unaffected by a high fat, high calorie meal, but C_{max} was decreased by 49% and T_{max} was increased from 0.5 to 1.5 hours. Prasugrel hydrochloride can be administered without regard to food. The active metabolite is bound about 98% to human serum albumin).

IMPORTANT NOTE: Always consult each drug listing in the patient's regimen for possible interactions.

Meal, unspecified (In a study of healthy subjects given a single 15 mg dose, the AUC of the active metabolite was unaffected by a high fat, high calorie meal, but C_{max} was decreased by 49% and T_{max} was increased from 0.5 to 1.5 hours. Prasugrel hydrochloride can be administered without regard to food. The active metabolite is bound about 98% to human serum albumin).

ELDEPRYL CAPSULES

(Selegiline Hydrochloride) 3312
May interact with ephedrine, narcotic analgesics, selective serotonin re-uptake inhibitors, sympathomimetics, tricyclic antidepressants, and certain other agents. Compounds in these categories include:

Albuterol (One case of hypertensive crisis has been reported in a patient taking the recommended doses of selegiline and ephedrine, a sympathomimetic medication).
No products indexed under this heading.

Albuterol Sulfate (One case of hypertensive crisis has been reported in a patient taking the recommended doses of selegiline and ephedrine, a sympathomimetic medication). Products include:
ProAir HFA 3393
Proventil HFA 3204
Ventolin HFA 1708

Alfentanil Hydrochloride (Selegiline hydrochloride is contraindicated for use with meperidine. This contraindication is often extended to other opioids).
No products indexed under this heading.

Amitriptyline Hydrochloride (Severe CNS toxicity associated with hyperpyrexia and death have been reported with the combination of tricyclic antidepressants and non-selective MAOIs. A similar reaction has been reported for a patient on amitriptyline and selegiline hydrochloride. Related adverse events including hypertension, syncope, asystole, diaphoresis, seizures, changes in behavioral and mental status, and muscular rigidity have also been reported in some patients receiving selegiline hydrochloride and various tricyclic antidepressants. At least 14 days should elapse between discontinuation of selegiline and initiation of treatment with tricyclic antidepressants).
No products indexed under this heading.

Amoxapine (Severe toxicity has been reported with the combination of tricyclic antidepressants and selegiline hydrochloride. Adverse events including hypertension, syncope, asystole, diaphoresis, seizures, changes in behavioral and mental status, and muscular rigidity have been reported in some patients receiving selegiline hydrochloride and various tricyclic antidepressants. The combination of selegiline hydrochloride and tricyclic antidepressants should, in general, be avoided. At least 14 days should elapse between discontinuation of selegiline and initiation of treatment with tricyclic antidepressants).
No products indexed under this heading.

Apomorphine (Selegiline hydrochloride is contraindicated for use with meperidine. This contraindication is often extended to other opioids).
No products indexed under this heading.

Apomorphine Hydrochloride (Selegiline hydrochloride is contraindicated for use with meperidine. This contraindication is often extended to other opioids).
No products indexed under this heading.

Buprenorphine Hydrochloride (Selegiline hydrochloride is contraindicated for use with meperidine. This contraindication is often extended to other opioids).
No products indexed under this heading.

Citalopram Hydrobromide (Severe toxicity has been reported with the combination of selective serotonin reuptake inhibitors and selegiline hydrochloride. The combination of selegiline hydrochloride and SSRIs should, in general, be avoided. At least 14 days should elapse between discontinuation of selegiline and initiation of treatment with selective serotonin re-uptake inhibitors). Products include:
Celexa 1153

Clomipramine Hydrochloride (Severe toxicity has been reported with the combination of tricyclic antidepressants and selegiline hydrochloride. Adverse events including hypertension, syncope, asystole, diaphoresis, seizures, changes in behavioral and mental status, and muscular rigidity have been reported in some patients receiving selegiline hydrochloride and various tricyclic antidepressants. The combination of selegiline hydrochloride and tricyclic antidepressants should, in general, be avoided. At least 14 days should elapse between discontinuation of selegiline and initiation of treatment with tricyclic antidepressants).
No products indexed under this heading.

Codeine Phosphate (Selegiline hydrochloride is contraindicated for use with meperidine. This contraindication is often extended to other opioids). Products include:
Tylenol with Codeine 2691

Codeine Sulfate (Selegiline hydrochloride is contraindicated for use with meperidine. This contraindication is often extended to other opioids).
No products indexed under this heading.

Desipramine Hydrochloride (Severe toxicity has been reported with the combination of tricyclic antidepressants and selegiline hydrochloride. Adverse events including hypertension, syncope, asystole, diaphoresis, seizures, changes in behavioral and mental status, and muscular rigidity have been reported in some patients receiving selegiline hydrochloride and various tricyclic antidepressants. The combination of selegiline hydrochloride and tricyclic antidepressants should, in general, be avoided. At least 14 days should elapse between discontinuation of selegiline and initiation of treatment with tricyclic antidepressants).
No products indexed under this heading.

Dezocine (Selegiline hydrochloride is contraindicated for use with meperidine. This contraindication is often extended to other opioids).
No products indexed under this heading.

Dihydrocodeine Bitartrate (Selegiline hydrochloride is contraindicated for use with meperidine. This contraindication is often extended to other opioids).
No products indexed under this heading.

Dihydrocodeinone Bitartrate (Selegiline hydrochloride is contraindicated for use with meperidine. This contraindication is often extended to other opioids).
No products indexed under this heading.

Dobutamine Hydrochloride (One case of hypertensive crisis has been reported in a patient taking the recommended doses of selegiline and ephedrine, a sympathomimetic medication).
No products indexed under this heading.

Dopamine Hydrochloride (One case of hypertensive crisis has been reported in a patient taking the recommended doses of selegiline and ephedrine, a sympathomimetic medication).
No products indexed under this heading.

Doxepin Hydrochloride (Severe toxicity has been reported with the combination of tricyclic antidepressants and selegiline hydrochloride. Adverse events including hypertension, syncope, asystole, diaphoresis, seizures, changes in behavioral and mental status, and muscular rigidity have been reported in some patients receiving selegiline hydrochloride and various tricyclic antidepressants. The combination of selegiline hydrochloride and tricyclic antidepressants should, in general, be avoided. At least 14 days should elapse between discontinuation of selegiline and initiation of treatment with tricyclic antidepressants).
No products indexed under this heading.

Ephedrine Hydrochloride (One case of hypertensive crisis has been reported in a patient taking the recommended doses of selegiline and ephedrine, a sympathomimetic medication).
No products indexed under this heading.

Ephedrine Sulfate (One case of hypertensive crisis has been reported in a patient taking the recommended doses of selegiline and ephedrine, a sympathomimetic medication).
No products indexed under this heading.

Ephedrine Tannate (One case of hypertensive crisis has been reported in a patient taking the recommended doses of selegiline and ephedrine, a sympathomimetic medication).
No products indexed under this heading.

Epinephrine (One case of hypertensive crisis has been reported in a patient taking the recommended doses of selegiline and ephedrine, a sympathomimetic medication). Products include:
EpiPen 3631
Twinject 3268

Epinephrine Bitartrate (One case of hypertensive crisis has been reported in a patient taking the recommended doses of selegiline and ephedrine, a sympathomimetic medication).
No products indexed under this heading.

Epinephrine Hydrochloride (One case of hypertensive crisis has been reported in a patient taking the recommended doses of selegiline and ephedrine, a sympathomimetic medication).
No products indexed under this heading.

Escitalopram Oxalate (Severe toxicity has been reported with the combination of selective serotonin reuptake inhibitors and selegiline hydrochloride. The combination of selegiline hydrochloride and SSRIs should, in general, be avoided. At least 14 days should elapse between discontinuation of selegiline and initiation of treatment with selective serotonin re-uptake inhibitors). Products include:
Lexapro Oral Suspension 1160
Lexapro Tablets 1160

Fentanyl (Selegiline hydrochloride is contraindicated for use with meperidine. This contraindication is often extended to other opioids). Products include:
Duragesic 2604
Fentanyl Transdermal System 2346
Onsolis 2054

Fentanyl Citrate (Selegiline hydrochloride is contraindicated for use with meperidine. This contraindication is often extended to other opioids). Products include:
Fentora 966

Fluoxetine (Serious, sometimes fatal, reactions with signs and symptoms that may include hyperthermia, rigidity, autonomic instability with rapid fluctuations of the vital signs, and mental status changes that include extreme agitation progressing to delirium and coma have been reported with patients receiving a combination of fluoxetine hydrochloride and non-selective MAOIs. Similar signs have been reported in some patients on the combination of selegiline hydrochloride (10 mg/day) and fluoxetine. Because of the long half-lives of fluoxetine and its active metabolite, at least five weeks should elapse between discontinuation of fluoxetine and initiation of treatment with selegiline hydrochloride).
No products indexed under this heading.

Fluoxetine Hydrochloride (Serious, sometimes fatal, reactions with signs and symptoms that may include hyperthermia, rigidity, autonomic instability with rapid fluctuations of the vital signs, and mental status changes that include extreme agitation progressing to delirium and coma have been reported with patients receiving a combination of fluoxetine hydrochloride and non-selective MAOIs. Similar signs have been reported in some patients on the combination of selegiline hydrochloride (10 mg/day) and fluoxetine. Because of the long half-lives of fluoxetine and its active metabolite, at least five weeks should elapse between discontinuation of fluoxetine and initiation of treatment with selegiline hydrochloride). Products include:
Prozac Weekly 1941
Prozac Pulvules 1941
Symbyax 1965

Fluvoxamine (Severe toxicity has been reported with the combination of selective serotonin reuptake inhibitors and selegiline hydrochloride. The combination of selegiline hydrochloride and SSRIs should, in general, be avoided. At least 14 days should elapse between discontinuation of selegiline and initiation of treatment with selective serotonin re-uptake inhibitors).
No products indexed under this heading.

Fluvoxamine Maleate (Severe toxicity has been reported with the combination of selective serotonin reuptake inhibitors and selegiline hydrochloride. The combination of selegiline hydrochloride and SSRIs should, in general, be avoided. At least 14 days should elapse between discontinuation of selegiline and initiation of treatment with selective serotonin re-uptake inhibitors).
No products indexed under this heading.

Hydrocodone Bitartrate (Selegiline hydrochloride is contraindicated for use with meperidine. This contraindication is often extended to other opioids). Products include:
Vicodin 560
Vicodin ES 561
Vicodin HP 563
Vicoprofen 564
Zydone 1138

Hydrocodone Polistirex (Selegiline hydrochloride is contraindicated for use with meperidine. This contraindication is often extended to other opioids). Products include:
Tussionex 3443

Hydromorphone (Selegiline hydrochloride is contraindicated for use with meperidine. This contraindication is often extended to other opioids).
No products indexed under this heading.

Hydromorphone Hydrochloride (Selegiline hydrochloride is contraindicated for use with meperidine. This contraindication is often extended to other opioids). Products include:
Dilaudid Injection 2800
Dilaudid Oral 2797
Dilaudid Tablets 2797
Dilaudid-HP 2800

(⊙ Described in PDR® for Ophthalmic Medicines)

551 Interactions Index Eldepryl

Imipramine Hydrochloride (Severe toxicity has been reported with the combination of tricyclic antidepressants and selegiline hydrochloride. Adverse events including hypertension, syncope, asystole, diaphoresis, seizures, changes in behavioral and mental status, and muscular rigidity have been reported in some patients receiving selegiline hydrochloride and various tricyclic antidepressants. The combination of selegiline hydrochloride and tricyclic antidepressants should, in general, be avoided. At least 14 days should elapse between discontinuation of selegiline and initiation of treatment with tricyclic antidepressants).
No products indexed under this heading.

Imipramine Pamoate (Severe toxicity has been reported with the combination of tricyclic antidepressants and selegiline hydrochloride. Adverse events including hypertension, syncope, asystole, diaphoresis, seizures, changes in behavioral and mental status, and muscular rigidity have been reported in some patients receiving selegiline hydrochloride and various tricyclic antidepressants. The combination of selegiline hydrochloride and tricyclic antidepressants should, in general, be avoided. At least 14 days should elapse between discontinuation of selegiline and initiation of treatment with tricyclic antidepressants).
No products indexed under this heading.

Isoproterenol Hydrochloride (One case of hypertensive crisis has been reported in a patient taking the recommended doses of selegiline and ephedrine, a sympathomimetic medication).
No products indexed under this heading.

Isoproterenol Sulfate (One case of hypertensive crisis has been reported in a patient taking the recommended doses of selegiline and ephedrine, a sympathomimetic medication).
No products indexed under this heading.

Levalbuterol Hydrochloride (One case of hypertensive crisis has been reported in a patient taking the recommended doses of selegiline and ephedrine, a sympathomimetic medication).
No products indexed under this heading.

Levodopa (Co-administration in some patients may exacerbate levodopa-associated side effects. After two to three days of treatment with selegiline, an attempt may be made to reduce the dose of levodopa/carbidopa). Products include:
Stalevo 2526

Levorphanol Tartrate (Selegiline hydrochloride is contraindicated for use with meperidine. This contraindication is often extended to other opioids).
No products indexed under this heading.

Maprotiline Hydrochloride (Severe toxicity has been reported with the combination of tricyclic antidepressants and selegiline hydrochloride. Adverse events including hypertension, syncope, asystole, diaphoresis, seizures, changes in behavioral and mental status, and muscular rigidity have been reported in some patients receiving selegiline hydrochloride and various tricyclic antidepressants. The combination of selegiline hydrochloride and tricyclic antidepressants should, in general, be avoided. At least 14 days should elapse between discontinuation of selegiline and initiation of treatment with tricyclic antidepressants).
No products indexed under this heading.

Meperidine Hydrochloride (Co-administration of meperidine and selegiline hydrochloride is contraindicated. The occurence of stupor, muscular rigidity, severe agitation, and elevated temperature has been reported in some patients receiving the combination of selegiline and meperidine. Symptoms usually resolve over days when the combination is discontinued. This is typical of the interaction of meperidine and MAOIs. Other serious reactions (including severe agitation, hallucinations and death) have been reported in patients receiving this combination).
No products indexed under this heading.

Metaproterenol Sulfate (One case of hypertensive crisis has been reported in a patient taking the recommended doses of selegiline and ephedrine, a sympathomimetic medication).
No products indexed under this heading.

Metaraminol Bitartrate (One case of hypertensive crisis has been reported in a patient taking the recommended doses of selegiline and ephedrine, a sympathomimetic medication).
No products indexed under this heading.

Methadone Hydrochloride (Selegiline hydrochloride is contraindicated for use with meperidine. This contraindication is often extended to other opioids).
No products indexed under this heading.

Methoxamine Hydrochloride (One case of hypertensive crisis has been reported in a patient taking the recommended doses of selegiline and ephedrine, a sympathomimetic medication).
No products indexed under this heading.

Morphine Sulfate (Selegiline hydrochloride is contraindicated for use with meperidine. This contraindication is often extended to other opioids). Products include:
Avinza 1822
Embeda 1831
MS Contin 2803

Morphine Sulfate, Liposomal (Selegiline hydrochloride is contraindicated for use with meperidine. This contraindication is often extended to other opioids).
No products indexed under this heading.

Norepinephrine Bitartrate (One case of hypertensive crisis has been reported in a patient taking the recommended doses of selegiline and ephedrine, a sympathomimetic medication).
No products indexed under this heading.

Nortriptyline Hydrochioride (Severe toxicity has been reported with the combination of tricyclic antidepressants and selegiline hydrochloride. Adverse events including hypertension, syncope, asystole, diaphoresis, seizures, changes in behavioral and mental status, and muscular rigidity have been reported in some patients receiving selegiline hydrochloride and various tricyclic antidepressants. The combination of selegiline hydrochloride and tricyclic antidepressants should, in general, be avoided. At least 14 days should elapse between discontinuation of selegiline and initiation of treatment with tricyclic antidepressants).
No products indexed under this heading.

Oxycodone Hydrochloride (Selegiline hydrochloride is contraindicated for use with meperidine. This contraindication is often extended to other opioids). Products include:
OxyContin 2807
Percocet 1121
Percodan 1124

Oxycodone Terephthalate (Selegiline hydrochloride is contraindicated for use with meperidine. This contraindication is often extended to other opioids).
No products indexed under this heading.

Oxymorphone Hydrochloride (Selegiline hydrochloride is contraindicated for use with meperidine. This contraindication is often extended to other opioids). Products include:
Opana 1110
Opana ER 1114

Paroxetine (Serious, sometimes fatal, reactions with signs and symptoms that may include hyperthermia, rigidity, autonomic instability with rapid fluctuations of the vital signs, and mental status changes that include extreme agitation progressing to delirium and coma have been reported with patients receiving a combination of fluoxetine hydrochloride and non-selective MAOIs. Similar signs have been reported in some patients on the combination of selegiline hydrochloride (10 mg/day) and paroxetine. At least 14 days should elapse between discontinuation of selegiline and initiation of treatment with SSRIs).
No products indexed under this heading.

Paroxetine Hydrochloride (Serious, sometimes fatal, reactions with signs and symptoms that may include hyperthermia, rigidity, autonomic instability with rapid fluctuations of the vital signs, and mental status changes that include extreme agitation progressing to delirium and coma have been reported with patients receiving a combination of fluoxetine hydrochloride and non-selective MAOIs. Similar signs have been reported in some patients on the combination of selegiline hydrochloride (10 mg/day) and paroxetine. At least 14 days should elapse between discontinuation of selegiline and initiation of treatment with SSRIs). Products include:
Paroxetine CR 2361
Paroxetine ER 2371
Paxil 1586
Paxil CR 1596

Paroxetine Mesylate (Serious, sometimes fatal, reactions with signs and symptoms that may include hyperthermia, rigidity, autonomic instability with rapid fluctuations of the vital signs, and mental status changes that include extreme agitation progressing to delirium and coma have been reported with patients receiving a combination of fluoxetine hydrochloride and non-selective MAOIs. Similar signs have been reported in some patients on the combination of selegiline hydrochloride (10 mg/day) and paroxetine. At least 14 days should elapse between discontinuation of selegiline and initiation of treatment with SSRIs).
No products indexed under this heading.

Phenylephrine Bitartrate (One case of hypertensive crisis has been reported in a patient taking the recommended doses of selegiline and ephedrine, a sympathomimetic medication).
No products indexed under this heading.

Phenylephrine Hydrochloride (One case of hypertensive crisis has been reported in a patient taking the recommended doses of selegiline and ephedrine, a sympathomimetic medication). Products include:
Sudafed PE Nasal Decongestant 2048
Children's Sudafed PE Nasal Decongestant 2047

Phenylephrine Tannate (One case of hypertensive crisis has been reported in a patient taking the recommended doses of selegiline and ephedrine, a sympathomimetic medication).
No products indexed under this heading.

Phenylpropanolamine Hydrochloride (One case of hypertensive crisis has been reported in a patient taking the recommended doses of selegiline and ephedrine, a sympathomimetic medication).
No products indexed under this heading.

Pirbuterol Acetate (One case of hypertensive crisis has been reported in a patient taking the recommended doses of selegiline and ephedrine, a sympathomimetic medication). Products include:
Maxair Autohaler 1782

Propoxyphene Hydrochloride (Selegiline hydrochloride is contraindicated for use with meperidine. This contraindication is often extended to other opioids).
No products indexed under this heading.

Propoxyphene Napsylate (Selegiline hydrochloride is contraindicated for use with meperidine. This contraindication is often extended to other opioids).
No products indexed under this heading.

Protriptyline Hydrochloride (A patient receiving protriptyline and selegiline hydrochloride developed tremors, agitation, and restlessness followed by unresponsiveness and death two weeks after selegiline hydrochloride was added. Related adverse events including hypertension, syncope, asystole, diaphoresis, seizures, changes in behavioral and mental status, and muscular rigidity have also been reported in some patients receiving selegiline hydrochloride and various tricyclic antidepressants. At least 14 days should elapse between discontinuation of selegiline and initiation of treatment with tricyclic antidepressants).
No products indexed under this heading.

Pseudoephedrine Hydrochloride (One case of hypertensive crisis has been reported in a patient taking the recommended doses of selegiline and ephedrine, a sympathomimetic medication). Products include:
Allegra-D 2915
Allegra-D 24 2918
Sudafed 12 Hour Nasal Decongestant Non-Drowsy 2048
Sudafed 24 Hour 2048
Sudafed Nasal Decongestant 2047
Children's Sudafed Nasal Decongestant Liquid 2047
Zyrtec-D Allergy & Congestion 2054

Pseudoephedrine Sulfate (One case of hypertensive crisis has been reported in a patient taking the recommended doses of selegiline and ephedrine, a sympathomimetic medication). Products include:
Clarinex-D 12-Hour 3101
Clarinex-D 3104

Remifentanil Hydrochloride (Selegiline hydrochloride is contraindicated for use with meperidine. This contraindication is often extended to other opioids).
No products indexed under this heading.

Salmeterol Xinafoate (One case of hypertensive crisis has been reported in a patient taking the recommended doses of selegiline and ephedrine, a sympathomimetic medication). Products include:
Advair 100/50 1275
Advair 250/50 1275
Advair 500/50 1275
Advair HFA 45/21 1288
Advair HFA 115/21 1288
Advair HFA 230/21 1288
Serevent Diskus 1656

Sertraline Hydrochloride (Serious, sometimes fatal, reactions with signs and symptoms that may include hyperthermia, rigidity, autonomic instability with rapid fluctuations of the vital signs, and mental status changes that include extreme agitation progressing to delirium and coma have been reported with patients receiving a combination of fluoxetine hydrochloride (PROZAC) and non-selective MAOIs. Similar signs have been reported in some patients on the combination of selegiline hydrochloride (10 mg a day) and selective serotonin re-uptake inhibitors including fluoxetine, sertraline and paroxetine. At least 14 days should elapse between discontinu-

IMPORTANT NOTE: Always consult each drug listing in the patient's regimen for possible interactions.

Eldepryl Interactions Index 552

ation of selegiline and initiation of treatment with selective serotonin re-uptake inhibitors).
No products indexed under this heading.

Sufentanil Citrate (Selegiline hydrochloride is contraindicated for use with meperidine. This contraindication is often extended to other opioids).
No products indexed under this heading.

Terbutaline Sulfate (One case of hypertensive crisis has been reported in a patient taking the recommended doses of selegiline and ephedrine, a sympathomimetic medication).
No products indexed under this heading.

Trimipramine Maleate (Severe toxicity has been reported with the combination of tricyclic antidepressants and selegiline hydrochloride. Adverse events including hypertension, syncope, asystole, diaphoresis, seizures, changes in behavioral and mental status, and muscular rigidity have been reported in some patients receiving selegiline hydrochloride and various tricyclic antidepressants. The combination of selegiline hydrochloride and tricyclic antidepressants should, in general, be avoided. At least 14 days should elapse between discontinuation of selegiline and initiation of treatment with tricyclic antidepressants).
No products indexed under this heading.

Tyramine (Rare cases of hypertensive reactions associated with ingestion of tyramine-containing foods have been reported in patients taking the recommended daily dose of selegiline hydrochloride).
No products indexed under this heading.

Food Interactions

Beverages with high tyramine (Rare cases of hypertensive reactions associated with ingestion of tyramine-containing foods have been reported in patients taking the recommended daily dose of selegiline hydrochloride).

Food, unspecified (The bioavailability of selegiline is increased 3 to 4 fold when it is taken with food).

Food high in tyramine (Rare cases of hypertensive reactions associated with ingestion of tyramine-containing foods have been reported in patients taking the recommended daily dose of selegiline).

Food with high concentration of tyramine (Rare cases of hypertensive reactions associated with ingestion of tyramine-containing foods have been reported in patients taking the recommended daily dose of selegiline hydrochloride).

Meal, unspecified (The bioavailability of selegiline is increased 3 to 4 fold when it is taken with food).

ELESTAT OPHTHALMIC SOLUTION
(Epinastine Hydrochloride) 1808
None cited in PDR database.

ELIDEL CREAM 1%
(Pimecrolimus) 2424
May interact with alcohols, calcium channel blockers, cytochrome p450 3a inhibitors (selected), erythromycin, and certain other agents. Compounds in these categories include:

Amiodarone Hydrochloride (The concomitant administration of known CYP3A family of inhibitors in patients with widespread and/or erythrodermic disease should be done with caution. Some examples of such drugs are erythromycin, itraconazole, ketoconazole, fluconazole, calcium channel blockers and cimetidine).
No products indexed under this heading.

Amlodipine Besylate (The concomitant administration of known CYP3A family of inhibitors in patients with widespread and/or erythrodermic disease should be done with caution. Some examples of such drugs are erythromycin, itraconazole, ketoconazole, fluconazole, calcium channel blockers and cimetidine). Products include:
Azor 1010
Exforge 2443
Exforge HCT 2449

Amprenavir (The concomitant administration of known CYP3A family of inhibitors in patients with widespread and/or erythrodermic disease should be done with caution. Some examples of such drugs are erythromycin, itraconazole, ketoconazole, fluconazole, calcium channel blockers and cimetidine).
No products indexed under this heading.

Aprepitant (The concomitant administration of known CYP3A family of inhibitors in patients with widespread and/or erythrodermic disease should be done with caution. Some examples of such drugs are erythromycin, itraconazole, ketoconazole, fluconazole, calcium channel blockers and cimetidine). Products include:
Emend 2124

Bepridil Hydrochloride (The concomitant administration of known CYP3A family of inhibitors in patients with widespread and/or erythrodermic disease should be done with caution. Some examples of such drugs are erythromycin, itraconazole, ketoconazole, fluconazole, calcium channel blockers and cimetidine).
No products indexed under this heading.

Cimetidine (The concomitant administration of known CYP3A family of inhibitors in patients with widespread and/or erythrodermic disease should be done with caution. Some examples of such drugs are erythromycin, itraconazole, ketoconazole, fluconazole, calcium channel blockers and cimetidine).
No products indexed under this heading.

Cimetidine Hydrochloride (The concomitant administration of known CYP3A family of inhibitors in patients with widespread and/or erythrodermic disease should be done with caution. Some examples of such drugs are erythromycin, itraconazole, ketoconazole, fluconazole, calcium channel blockers and cimetidine).
No products indexed under this heading.

Ciprofloxacin (The concomitant administration of known CYP3A family of inhibitors in patients with widespread and/or erythrodermic disease should be done with caution. Some examples of such drugs are erythromycin, itraconazole, ketoconazole, fluconazole, calcium channel blockers and cimetidine). Products include:
Cipro I.V. 3082
Cipro 3073
Cipro XR 3091
Ciprodex 583

Ciprofloxacin Hydrochloride (The concomitant administration of known CYP3A family of inhibitors in patients with widespread and/or erythrodermic disease should be done with caution. Some examples of such drugs are erythromycin, itraconazole, ketoconazole, fluconazole, calcium channel blockers and cimetidine). Products include:
Cipro 3073

Clarithromycin (The concomitant administration of known CYP3A family of inhibitors in patients with widespread and/or erythrodermic disease should be done with caution. Some examples of such drugs are erythromycin, itraconazole, ketoconazole, fluconazole, calcium channel blockers and cimetidine). Products include:
Biaxin/Biaxin XL 412

Cyclosporine (The concomitant administration of known CYP3A family of inhibitors in patients with widespread and/or erythrodermic disease should be done with caution. Some examples of such drugs are erythromycin, itraconazole, ketoconazole, fluconazole, calcium channel blockers and cimetidine). Products include:
Gengraf 440
Neoral Oral Solution 2496
Neoral Capsules 2496
Restasis 605

Delavirdine Mesylate (The concomitant administration of known CYP3A family of inhibitors in patients with widespread and/or erythrodermic disease should be done with caution. Some examples of such drugs are erythromycin, itraconazole, ketoconazole, fluconazole, calcium channel blockers and cimetidine).
No products indexed under this heading.

Diltiazem Hydrochloride (The concomitant administration of known CYP3A family of inhibitors in patients with widespread and/or erythrodermic disease should be done with caution. Some examples of such drugs are erythromycin, itraconazole, ketoconazole, fluconazole, calcium channel blockers and cimetidine). Products include:
Cardizem LA 423

Diltiazem Maleate (The concomitant administration of known CYP3A family of inhibitors in patients with widespread and/or erythrodermic disease should be done with caution. Some examples of such drugs are erythromycin, itraconazole, ketoconazole, fluconazole, calcium channel blockers and cimetidine).
No products indexed under this heading.

Efavirenz (The concomitant administration of known CYP3A family of inhibitors in patients with widespread and/or erythrodermic disease should be done with caution. Some examples of such drugs are erythromycin, itraconazole, ketoconazole, fluconazole, calcium channel blockers and cimetidine). Products include:
Atripla 906

Erythromycin (The concomitant administration of known CYP3A family of inhibitors in patients with widespread and/or erythrodermic disease should be done with caution. Some examples of such drugs are erythromycin, itraconazole, ketoconazole, fluconazole, calcium channel blockers and cimetidine).
No products indexed under this heading.

Erythromycin, Topical (The concomitant administration of known CYP3A family of inhibitors in patients with widespread and/or erythrodermic disease should be done with caution. Some examples of such drugs are erythromycin, itraconazole, ketoconazole, fluconazole, calcium channel blockers and cimetidine).
No products indexed under this heading.

Erythromycin Estolate (The concomitant administration of known CYP3A family of inhibitors in patients with widespread and/or erythrodermic disease should be done with caution. Some examples of such drugs are erythromycin, itraconazole, ketoconazole, fluconazole, calcium channel blockers and cimetidine).
No products indexed under this heading.

Erythromycin Ethylsuccinate (The concomitant administration of known CYP3A family of inhibitors in patients with widespread and/or erythrodermic disease should be done with caution. Some examples of such drugs are erythromycin, itraconazole, ketoconazole, fluconazole, calcium channel blockers and cimetidine). Products include:
E.E.S. 437
EryPed 435

Erythromycin Gluceptate (The concomitant administration of known CYP3A family of inhibitors in patients with widespread and/or erythrodermic disease should be done with caution. Some examples of such drugs are erythromycin, itraconazole, ketoconazole, fluconazole, calcium channel blockers and cimetidine).
No products indexed under this heading.

Erythromycin Lactobionate (The concomitant administration of known CYP3A family of inhibitors in patients with widespread and/or erythrodermic disease should be done with caution. Some examples of such drugs are erythromycin, itraconazole, ketoconazole, fluconazole, calcium channel blockers and cimetidine).
No products indexed under this heading.

Erythromycin Stearate (The concomitant administration of known CYP3A family of inhibitors in patients with widespread and/or erythrodermic disease should be done with caution. Some examples of such drugs are erythromycin, itraconazole, ketoconazole, fluconazole, calcium channel blockers and cimetidine).
No products indexed under this heading.

Ethanol (Skin flushing due to pimecrolimus is associated with alcohol use).
No products indexed under this heading.

Ethyl Alcohol (Skin flushing due to pimecrolimus is associated with alcohol use).
No products indexed under this heading.

Felodipine (The concomitant administration of known CYP3A family of inhibitors in patients with widespread and/or erythrodermic disease should be done with caution. Some examples of such drugs are erythromycin, itraconazole, ketoconazole, fluconazole, calcium channel blockers and cimetidine).
No products indexed under this heading.

Fluconazole (The concomitant administration of known CYP3A family of inhibitors in patients with widespread and/or erythrodermic disease should be done with caution. Some examples of such drugs are erythromycin, itraconazole, ketoconazole, fluconazole, calcium channel blockers and cimetidine).
No products indexed under this heading.

Fluoxetine (The concomitant administration of known CYP3A family of inhibitors in patients with widespread and/or erythrodermic disease should be done with caution. Some examples of such drugs are erythromycin, itraconazole, ketoconazole, fluconazole, calcium channel blockers and cimetidine).
No products indexed under this heading.

Fluoxetine Hydrochloride (The concomitant administration of known CYP3A family of inhibitors in patients with widespread and/or erythrodermic disease should be done with caution. Some examples of such drugs are erythromycin, itraconazole, ketoconazole, fluconazole, calcium channel blockers and cimetidine). Products include:
Prozac Weekly 1941
Prozac Pulvules 1941
Symbyax 1965

(⊙ Described in PDR® for Ophthalmic Medicines)

Fluvoxamine Maleate (The concomitant administration of known CYP3A family of inhibitors in patients with widespread and/or erythrodermic disease should be done with caution. Some examples of such drugs are erythromycin, itraconazole, ketoconazole, fluconazole, calcium channel blockers and cimetidine).
No products indexed under this heading.

Indinavir Sulfate (The concomitant administration of known CYP3A family of inhibitors in patients with widespread and/or erythrodermic disease should be done with caution. Some examples of such drugs are erythromycin, itraconazole, ketoconazole, fluconazole, calcium channel blockers and cimetidine). Products include:
Crixivan 2113

Isoniazid (The concomitant administration of known CYP3A family of inhibitors in patients with widespread and/or erythrodermic disease should be done with caution. Some examples of such drugs are erythromycin, itraconazole, ketoconazole, fluconazole, calcium channel blockers and cimetidine).
No products indexed under this heading.

Isradipine (The concomitant administration of known CYP3A family of inhibitors in patients with widespread and/or erythrodermic disease should be done with caution. Some examples of such drugs are erythromycin, itraconazole, ketoconazole, fluconazole, calcium channel blockers and cimetidine).
Products include:
DynaCirc CR 1432

Itraconazole (The concomitant administration of known CYP3A family of inhibitors in patients with widespread and/or erythrodermic disease should be done with caution. Some examples of such drugs are erythromycin, itraconazole, ketoconazole, fluconazole, calcium channel blockers and cimetidine).
No products indexed under this heading.

Ketoconazole (The concomitant administration of known CYP3A family of inhibitors in patients with widespread and/or erythrodermic disease should be done with caution. Some examples of such drugs are erythromycin, itraconazole, ketoconazole, fluconazole, calcium channel blockers and cimetidine). Products include:
Extina 3319
Xolegel 3337

Lopinavir (The concomitant administration of known CYP3A family of inhibitors in patients with widespread and/or erythrodermic disease should be done with caution. Some examples of such drugs are erythromycin, itraconazole, ketoconazole, fluconazole, calcium channel blockers and cimetidine).
Products include:
Kaletra 458

Metronidazole (The concomitant administration of known CYP3A family of inhibitors in patients with widespread and/or erythrodermic disease should be done with caution. Some examples of such drugs are erythromycin, itraconazole, ketoconazole, fluconazole, calcium channel blockers and cimetidine). Products include:
Pylera 793

Metronidazole Benzoate (The concomitant administration of known CYP3A family of inhibitors in patients with widespread and/or erythrodermic disease should be done with caution. Some examples of such drugs are erythromycin, itraconazole, ketoconazole, fluconazole, calcium channel blockers and cimetidine).
No products indexed under this heading.

Metronidazole Hydrochloride (The concomitant administration of known CYP3A family of inhibitors in patients with widespread and/or erythrodermic disease should be done with caution. Some examples of such drugs are erythromycin, itraconazole, ketoconazole, fluconazole, calcium channel blockers and cimetidine).
No products indexed under this heading.

Mibefradil Dihydrochloride (The concomitant administration of known CYP3A family of inhibitors in patients with widespread and/or erythrodermic disease should be done with caution. Some examples of such drugs are erythromycin, itraconazole, ketoconazole, fluconazole, calcium channel blockers and cimetidine).
No products indexed under this heading.

Miconazole (The concomitant administration of known CYP3A family of inhibitors in patients with widespread and/or erythrodermic disease should be done with caution. Some examples of such drugs are erythromycin, itraconazole, ketoconazole, fluconazole, calcium channel blockers and cimetidine).
No products indexed under this heading.

Nefazodone Hydrochloride (The concomitant administration of known CYP3A family of inhibitors in patients with widespread and/or erythrodermic disease should be done with caution. Some examples of such drugs are erythromycin, itraconazole, ketoconazole, fluconazole, calcium channel blockers and cimetidine).
No products indexed under this heading.

Nelfinavir Mesylate (The concomitant administration of known CYP3A family of inhibitors in patients with widespread and/or erythrodermic disease should be done with caution. Some examples of such drugs are erythromycin, itraconazole, ketoconazole, fluconazole, calcium channel blockers and cimetidine).
No products indexed under this heading.

Nicardipine (The concomitant administration of known CYP3A family of inhibitors in patients with widespread and/or erythrodermic disease should be done with caution. Some examples of such drugs are erythromycin, itraconazole, ketoconazole, fluconazole, calcium channel blockers and cimetidine).
No products indexed under this heading.

Nicardipine Hydrochloride (The concomitant administration of known CYP3A family of inhibitors in patients with widespread and/or erythrodermic disease should be done with caution. Some examples of such drugs are erythromycin, itraconazole, ketoconazole, fluconazole, calcium channel blockers and cimetidine).
No products indexed under this heading.

Nifedipine (The concomitant administration of known CYP3A family of inhibitors in patients with widespread and/or erythrodermic disease should be done with caution. Some examples of such drugs are erythromycin, itraconazole, ketoconazole, fluconazole, calcium channel blockers and cimetidine).
No products indexed under this heading.

Nimodipine (The concomitant administration of known CYP3A family of inhibitors in patients with widespread and/or erythrodermic disease should be done with caution. Some examples of such drugs are erythromycin, itraconazole, ketoconazole, fluconazole, calcium channel blockers and cimetidine).
No products indexed under this heading.

Nisoldipine (The concomitant administration of known CYP3A family of inhibitors in patients with widespread and/or erythrodermic disease should be done with caution. Some examples of such drugs are erythromycin, itraconazole, ketoconazole, fluconazole, calcium channel blockers and cimetidine).
No products indexed under this heading.

Norfloxacin (The concomitant administration of known CYP3A family of inhibitors in patients with widespread and/or erythrodermic disease should be done with caution. Some examples of such drugs are erythromycin, itraconazole, ketoconazole, fluconazole, calcium channel blockers and cimetidine). Products include:
Noroxin 2220

Paroxetine Hydrochloride (The concomitant administration of known CYP3A family of inhibitors in patients with widespread and/or erythrodermic disease should be done with caution. Some examples of such drugs are erythromycin, itraconazole, ketoconazole, fluconazole, calcium channel blockers and cimetidine). Products include:
Paroxetine CR 2361
Paroxetine ER 2371
Paxil 1586
Paxil CR 1596

Quinine (The concomitant administration of known CYP3A family of inhibitors in patients with widespread and/or erythrodermic disease should be done with caution. Some examples of such drugs are erythromycin, itraconazole, ketoconazole, fluconazole, calcium channel blockers and cimetidine).
Products include:
Hyland's Leg Cramps PM with
Quinine 3315

Quinine Sulfate (The concomitant administration of known CYP3A family of inhibitors in patients with widespread and/or erythrodermic disease should be done with caution. Some examples of such drugs are erythromycin, itraconazole, ketoconazole, fluconazole, calcium channel blockers and cimetidine).
No products indexed under this heading.

Ritonavir (The concomitant administration of known CYP3A family of inhibitors in patients with widespread and/or erythrodermic disease should be done with caution. Some examples of such drugs are erythromycin, itraconazole, ketoconazole, fluconazole, calcium channel blockers and cimetidine).
Products include:
Kaletra 458
Norvir 509

Saquinavir (The concomitant administration of known CYP3A family of inhibitors in patients with widespread and/or erythrodermic disease should be done with caution. Some examples of such drugs are erythromycin, itraconazole, ketoconazole, fluconazole, calcium channel blockers and cimetidine).
No products indexed under this heading.

Saquinavir Mesylate (The concomitant administration of known CYP3A family of inhibitors in patients with widespread and/or erythrodermic disease should be done with caution. Some examples of such drugs are erythromycin, itraconazole, ketoconazole, fluconazole, calcium channel blockers and cimetidine).
No products indexed under this heading.

Sertraline Hydrochloride (The concomitant administration of known CYP3A family of inhibitors in patients with widespread and/or erythrodermic disease should be done with caution. Some examples of such drugs are erythromycin, itraconazole, ketoconazole, fluconazole, calcium channel blockers and cimetidine).
No products indexed under this heading.

Troleandomycin (The concomitant administration of known CYP3A family of inhibitors in patients with widespread and/or erythrodermic disease should be done with caution. Some examples of such drugs are erythromycin, itraconazole, ketoconazole, fluconazole, calcium channel blockers and cimetidine).
No products indexed under this heading.

Venlafaxine Hydrochloride (The concomitant administration of known CYP3A family of inhibitors in patients with widespread and/or erythrodermic disease should be done with caution. Some examples of such drugs are erythromycin, itraconazole, ketoconazole, fluconazole, calcium channel blockers and cimetidine). Products include:
Effexor XR 3504
Venlafaxine Hydrochloride Tablets ... 2388

Verapamil Hydrochloride (The concomitant administration of known CYP3A family of inhibitors in patients with widespread and/or erythrodermic disease should be done with caution. Some examples of such drugs are erythromycin, itraconazole, ketoconazole, fluconazole, calcium channel blockers and cimetidine). Products include:
Tarka 534

Voriconazole (The concomitant administration of known CYP3A family of inhibitors in patients with widespread and/or erythrodermic disease should be done with caution. Some examples of such drugs are erythromycin, itraconazole, ketoconazole, fluconazole, calcium channel blockers and cimetidine).
No products indexed under this heading.

Zafirlukast (The concomitant administration of known CYP3A family of inhibitors in patients with widespread and/or erythrodermic disease should be done with caution. Some examples of such drugs are erythromycin, itraconazole, ketoconazole, fluconazole, calcium channel blockers and cimetidine).
Products include:
Accolate 3612

Zileuton (The concomitant administration of known CYP3A family of inhibitors in patients with widespread and/or erythrodermic disease should be done with caution. Some examples of such drugs are erythromycin, itraconazole, ketoconazole, fluconazole, calcium channel blockers and cimetidine).
No products indexed under this heading.

Food Interactions

Alcohol (Skin flushing due to pimecrolimus is associated with alcohol use).

Beer, reduced-alcohol (Skin flushing due to pimecrolimus is associated with alcohol use).

Beer, unspecified (Skin flushing due to pimecrolimus is associated with alcohol use).

Grapefruit (The concomitant administration of known CYP3A family of inhibitors in patients with widespread and/or erythrodermic disease should be done with caution. Some examples of such drugs are erythromycin, itraconazole, ketoconazole, fluconazole, calcium channel blockers and cimetidine).

IMPORTANT NOTE: Always consult each drug listing in the patient's regimen for possible interactions.

Grapefruit Juice (The concomitant administration of known CYP3A family of inhibitors in patients with widespread and/or erythrodermic disease should be done with caution. Some examples of such drugs are erythromycin, itraconazole, ketoconazole, fluconazole, calcium channel blockers and cimetidine).

Wine, Chianti (Skin flushing due to pimecrolimus is associated with alcohol use).

Wine, Red (Skin flushing due to pimecrolimus is associated with alcohol use).

Wine, unspecified (Skin flushing due to pimecrolimus is associated with alcohol use).

Wine products (Skin flushing due to pimecrolimus is associated with alcohol use).

ELIGARD 7.5 MG
(Leuprolide Acetate) 2968
None cited in PDR database.

ELIGARD 22.5 MG
(Leuprolide Acetate) 2968
None cited in PDR database.

ELIGARD 30 MG
(Leuprolide Acetate) 2968
None cited in PDR database.

ELIGARD 45 MG
(Leuprolide Acetate) 2968
None cited in PDR database.

ELITEK
(Rasburicase) 2973
None cited in PDR database.

ELMIRON CAPSULES
(Pentosan Polysulfate Sodium) 2611
May interact with anticoagulants, aspirin-acetylsalicylic acid, non-steroidal anti-inflammatory agents, oral anticoagulants, and certain other agents. Compounds in these categories include:

Alteplase (Pentosan polysulfate sodium is a weak anticoagulant. Bleeding complications of ecchymosis, epistaxis, and gum hemorrhage have been reported. Patients undergoing invasive procedures or having signs/symptoms of underlying coagulopathy or other increased risk of bleeding (due to other therapies such as coumarin anticoagulants, heparin, t-PA, streptokinase, high dose aspirin, or nonsteroidal anti-inflammatory drugs) should be evaluated for hemorrhage). Products include:
Activase 1183
Cathflo 1192

Anisindione (Pentosan polysulfate sodium is a weak anticoagulant. Bleeding complications of ecchymosis, epistaxis, and gum hemorrhage have been reported. Patients undergoing invasive procedures or having signs/symptoms of underlying coagulopathy or other increased risk of bleeding (due to other therapies such as coumarin anticoagulants or heparin) should be evaluated for hemorrhage).
No products indexed under this heading.

Ardeparin Sodium (Pentosan polysulfate sodium is a weak anticoagulant. Bleeding complications of ecchymosis, epistaxis, and gum hemorrhage have been reported. Patients undergoing invasive procedures or having signs/symptoms of underlying coagulopathy or other increased risk of bleeding (due to other therapies such as coumarin anticoagulants or heparin) should be evaluated for hemorrhage).
No products indexed under this heading.

Aspirin (Pentosan polysulfate sodium is a weak anticoagulant. Bleeding com-

plications of ecchymosis, epistaxis, and gum hemorrhage have been reported. Patients undergoing invasive procedures or having signs/symptoms of underlying coagulopathy or other increased risk of bleeding (due to other therapies such as high dose aspirin) should be evaluated for hemorrhage). Products include:
Aggrenox 880
Bayer Aspirin 829
Percodan 1124
St. Joseph Aspirin 2045

Aspirin, Enteric Coated (Pentosan polysulfate sodium is a weak anticoagulant. Bleeding complications of ecchymosis, epistaxis, and gum hemorrhage have been reported. Patients undergoing invasive procedures or having signs/symptoms of underlying coagulopathy or other increased risk of bleeding (due to other therapies such as high dose aspirin) should be evaluated for hemorrhage).
No products indexed under this heading.

Aspirin Buffered (Pentosan polysulfate sodium is a weak anticoagulant. Bleeding complications of ecchymosis, epistaxis, and gum hemorrhage have been reported. Patients undergoing invasive procedures or having signs/symptoms of underlying coagulopathy or other increased risk of bleeding (due to other therapies such as high dose aspirin) should be evaluated for hemorrhage).
No products indexed under this heading.

Celecoxib (Pentosan polysulfate sodium is a weak anticoagulant. Bleeding complications of ecchymosis, epistaxis, and gum hemorrhage have been reported. Patients undergoing invasive procedures or having signs/symptoms of underlying coagulopathy or other increased risk of bleeding (due to other therapies such as nonsteroidal anti-inflammatory drugs) should be evaluated for hemorrhage). Products include:
Celebrex 3272

Dalteparin Sodium (Pentosan polysulfate sodium is a weak anticoagulant. Bleeding complications of ecchymosis, epistaxis, and gum hemorrhage have been reported. Patients undergoing invasive procedures or having signs/symptoms of underlying coagulopathy or other increased risk of bleeding (due to other therapies such as coumarin anticoagulants or heparin) should be evaluated for hemorrhage). Products include:
Fragmin 1058

Danaparoid Sodium (Pentosan polysulfate sodium is a weak anticoagulant. Bleeding complications of ecchymosis, epistaxis, and gum hemorrhage have been reported. Patients undergoing invasive procedures or having signs/symptoms of underlying coagulopathy or other increased risk of bleeding (due to other therapies such as coumarin anticoagulants or heparin) should be evaluated for hemorrhage).
No products indexed under this heading.

Diclofenac Epolamine (Pentosan polysulfate sodium is a weak anticoagulant. Bleeding complications of ecchymosis, epistaxis, and gum hemorrhage have been reported. Patients undergoing invasive procedures or having signs/symptoms of underlying coagulopathy or other increased risk of bleeding (due to other therapies such as nonsteroidal anti-inflammatory drugs) should be evaluated for hemorrhage). Products include:
Flector 1839

Diclofenac Potassium (Pentosan polysulfate sodium is a weak anticoagulant. Bleeding complications of ecchymosis, epistaxis, and gum hemorrhage have been reported. Patients undergoing invasive procedures or having

signs/symptoms of underlying coagulopathy or other increased risk of bleeding (due to other therapies such as nonsteroidal anti-inflammatory drugs) should be evaluated for hemorrhage).
No products indexed under this heading.

Diclofenac Sodium (Pentosan polysulfate sodium is a weak anticoagulant. Bleeding complications of ecchymosis, epistaxis, and gum hemorrhage have been reported. Patients undergoing invasive procedures or having signs/symptoms of underlying coagulopathy or other increased risk of bleeding (due to other therapies such as nonsteroidal anti-inflammatory drugs) should be evaluated for hemorrhage).
No products indexed under this heading.

Dicumarol (Pentosan polysulfate sodium is a weak anticoagulant. Bleeding complications of ecchymosis, epistaxis, and gum hemorrhage have been reported. Patients undergoing invasive procedures or having signs/symptoms of underlying coagulopathy or other increased risk of bleeding (due to other therapies such as coumarin anticoagulants or heparin) should be evaluated for hemorrhage).
No products indexed under this heading.

Enoxaparin Sodium (Pentosan polysulfate sodium is a weak anticoagulant. Bleeding complications of ecchymosis, epistaxis, and gum hemorrhage have been reported. Patients undergoing invasive procedures or having signs/symptoms of underlying coagulopathy or other increased risk of bleeding (due to other therapies such as coumarin anticoagulants or heparin) should be evaluated for hemorrhage). Products include:
Lovenox 3005

Etodolac (Pentosan polysulfate sodium is a weak anticoagulant. Bleeding complications of ecchymosis, epistaxis, and gum hemorrhage have been reported. Patients undergoing invasive procedures or having signs/symptoms of underlying coagulopathy or other increased risk of bleeding (due to other therapies such as nonsteroidal anti-inflammatory drugs) should be evaluated for hemorrhage).
No products indexed under this heading.

Fenoprofen Calcium (Pentosan polysulfate sodium is a weak anticoagulant. Bleeding complications of ecchymosis, epistaxis, and gum hemorrhage have been reported. Patients undergoing invasive procedures or having signs/symptoms of underlying coagulopathy or other increased risk of bleeding (due to other therapies such as nonsteroidal anti-inflammatory drugs) should be evaluated for hemorrhage).
No products indexed under this heading.

Flurbiprofen (Pentosan polysulfate sodium is a weak anticoagulant. Bleeding complications of ecchymosis, epistaxis, and gum hemorrhage have been reported. Patients undergoing invasive procedures or having signs/symptoms of underlying coagulopathy or other increased risk of bleeding (due to other therapies such as nonsteroidal anti-inflammatory drugs) should be evaluated for hemorrhage).
No products indexed under this heading.

Fondaparinux Sodium (Pentosan polysulfate sodium is a weak anticoagulant. Bleeding complications of ecchymosis, epistaxis, and gum hemorrhage have been reported. Patients undergoing invasive procedures or having signs/symptoms of underlying coagulopathy or other increased risk of bleeding (due to other therapies such as coumarin anticoagulants or heparin) should be evaluated for hemorrhage). Products include:
Arixtra 1320

Heparin Calcium (Pentosan polysulfate sodium is a weak anticoagulant. Bleeding complications of ecchymosis, epistaxis, and gum hemorrhage have been reported. Patients undergoing invasive procedures or having signs/symptoms of underlying coagulopathy or other increased risk of bleeding (due to other therapies such as coumarin anticoagulants or heparin) should be evaluated for hemorrhage).
No products indexed under this heading.

Heparin Sodium (Pentosan polysulfate sodium is a weak anticoagulant. Bleeding complications of ecchymosis, epistaxis, and gum hemorrhage have been reported. Patients undergoing invasive procedures or having signs/symptoms of underlying coagulopathy or other increased risk of bleeding (due to other therapies such as coumarin anticoagulants or heparin) should be evaluated for hemorrhage).
No products indexed under this heading.

Ibuprofen (Pentosan polysulfate sodium is a weak anticoagulant. Bleeding complications of ecchymosis, epistaxis, and gum hemorrhage have been reported. Patients undergoing invasive procedures or having signs/symptoms of underlying coagulopathy or other increased risk of bleeding (due to other therapies such as nonsteroidal anti-inflammatory drugs) should be evaluated for hemorrhage). Products include:
Motrin IB 2043
Children's Motrin 2044
Children's Motrin Non-Staining
Dye-Free 2044
Infants' Motrin 2044
Infants' Motrin Dye-Free 2044
Junior Strength Motrin 2044
Vicoprofen 564

Indomethacin (Pentosan polysulfate sodium is a weak anticoagulant. Bleeding complications of ecchymosis, epistaxis, and gum hemorrhage have been reported. Patients undergoing invasive procedures or having signs/symptoms of underlying coagulopathy or other increased risk of bleeding (due to other therapies such as nonsteroidal anti-inflammatory drugs) should be evaluated for hemorrhage). Products include:
Indocin 2167

Indomethacin Sodium Trihydrate (Pentosan polysulfate sodium is a weak anticoagulant. Bleeding complications of ecchymosis, epistaxis, and gum hemorrhage have been reported. Patients undergoing invasive procedures or having signs/symptoms of underlying coagulopathy or other increased risk of bleeding (due to other therapies such as nonsteroidal anti-inflammatory drugs) should be evaluated for hemorrhage). Products include:
Indocin I.V. 2007

Ketoprofen (Pentosan polysulfate sodium is a weak anticoagulant. Bleeding complications of ecchymosis, epistaxis, and gum hemorrhage have been reported. Patients undergoing invasive procedures or having signs/symptoms of underlying coagulopathy or other increased risk of bleeding (due to other therapies such as nonsteroidal anti-inflammatory drugs) should be evaluated for hemorrhage).
No products indexed under this heading.

Ketorolac Tromethamine (Pentosan polysulfate sodium is a weak anticoagulant. Bleeding complications of ecchymosis, epistaxis, and gum hemorrhage have been reported. Patients undergoing invasive procedures or having signs/symptoms of underlying coagulopathy or other increased risk of bleeding (due to other therapies such as nonsteroidal anti-inflammatory drugs) should be evaluated for hemorrhage). Products include:
Acuvail ....⊙209

Low Molecular Weight Heparins (Pentosan polysulfate sodium is a weak anticoagulant. Bleeding complications of ecchymosis, epistaxis, and gum hemorrhage have been reported. Patients undergoing invasive procedures or having signs/symptoms of underlying coagulopathy or other increased risk of bleeding (due to other therapies such as coumarin anticoagulants or heparin) should be evaluated for hemorrhage).

No products indexed under this heading.

Meclofenamate Sodium (Pentosan polysulfate sodium is a weak anticoagulant. Bleeding complications of ecchymosis, epistaxis, and gum hemorrhage have been reported. Patients undergoing invasive procedures or having signs/symptoms of underlying coagulopathy or other increased risk of bleeding (due to other therapies such as nonsteroidal anti-inflammatory drugs) should be evaluated for hemorrhage).

No products indexed under this heading.

Mefenamic Acid (Pentosan polysulfate sodium is a weak anticoagulant. Bleeding complications of ecchymosis, epistaxis, and gum hemorrhage have been reported. Patients undergoing invasive procedures or having signs/symptoms of underlying coagulopathy or other increased risk of bleeding (due to other therapies such as nonsteroidal anti-inflammatory drugs) should be evaluated for hemorrhage).

No products indexed under this heading.

Meloxicam (Pentosan polysulfate sodium is a weak anticoagulant. Bleeding complications of ecchymosis, epistaxis, and gum hemorrhage have been reported. Patients undergoing invasive procedures or having signs/symptoms of underlying coagulopathy or other increased risk of bleeding (due to other therapies such as nonsteroidal anti-inflammatory drugs) should be evaluated for hemorrhage).

No products indexed under this heading.

Nabumetone (Pentosan polysulfate sodium is a weak anticoagulant. Bleeding complications of ecchymosis, epistaxis, and gum hemorrhage have been reported. Patients undergoing invasive procedures or having signs/symptoms of underlying coagulopathy or other increased risk of bleeding (due to other therapies such as nonsteroidal anti-inflammatory drugs) should be evaluated for hemorrhage).

No products indexed under this heading.

Naproxen (Pentosan polysulfate sodium is a weak anticoagulant. Bleeding complications of ecchymosis, epistaxis, and gum hemorrhage have been reported. Patients undergoing invasive procedures or having signs/symptoms of underlying coagulopathy or other increased risk of bleeding (due to other therapies such as nonsteroidal anti-inflammatory drugs) should be evaluated for hemorrhage). Products include:

Naproxen Sodium (Pentosan polysulfate sodium is a weak anticoagulant. Bleeding complications of ecchymosis, epistaxis, and gum hemorrhage have been reported. Patients undergoing invasive procedures or having signs/symptoms of underlying coagulopathy or other increased risk of bleeding (due to other therapies such as nonsteroidal anti-inflammatory drugs) should be evaluated for hemorrhage). Products include:

Oxaprozin (Pentosan polysulfate sodium is a weak anticoagulant. Bleeding complications of ecchymosis, epistaxis, and gum hemorrhage have been reported. Patients undergoing invasive procedures or having signs/symptoms of underlying coagulopathy or other increased risk of bleeding (due to other therapies such as nonsteroidal anti-inflammatory drugs) should be evaluated for hemorrhage).

No products indexed under this heading.

Phenylbutazone (Pentosan polysulfate sodium is a weak anticoagulant. Bleeding complications of ecchymosis, epistaxis, and gum hemorrhage have been reported. Patients undergoing invasive procedures or having signs/symptoms of underlying coagulopathy or other increased risk of bleeding (due to other therapies such as nonsteroidal anti-inflammatory drugs) should be evaluated for hemorrhage).

No products indexed under this heading.

Piroxicam (Pentosan polysulfate sodium is a weak anticoagulant. Bleeding complications of ecchymosis, epistaxis, and gum hemorrhage have been reported. Patients undergoing invasive procedures or having signs/symptoms of underlying coagulopathy or other increased risk of bleeding (due to other therapies such as nonsteroidal anti-inflammatory drugs) should be evaluated for hemorrhage).

No products indexed under this heading.

Rofecoxib (Pentosan polysulfate sodium is a weak anticoagulant. Bleeding complications of ecchymosis, epistaxis, and gum hemorrhage have been reported. Patients undergoing invasive procedures or having signs/symptoms of underlying coagulopathy or other increased risk of bleeding (due to other therapies such as nonsteroidal anti-inflammatory drugs) should be evaluated for hemorrhage).

No products indexed under this heading.

Streptokinase (Pentosan polysulfate sodium is a weak anticoagulant. Bleeding complications of ecchymosis, epistaxis, and gum hemorrhage have been reported. Patients undergoing invasive procedures or having signs/symptoms of underlying coagulopathy or other increased risk of bleeding (due to other therapies such as streptokinase) should be evaluated for hemorrhage).

No products indexed under this heading.

Sulindac (Pentosan polysulfate sodium is a weak anticoagulant. Bleeding complications of ecchymosis, epistaxis, and gum hemorrhage have been reported. Patients undergoing invasive procedures or having signs/symptoms of underlying coagulopathy or other increased risk of bleeding (due to other therapies such as nonsteroidal anti-inflammatory drugs) should be evaluated for hemorrhage). Products include:

Tinzaparin Sodium (Pentosan polysulfate sodium is a weak anticoagulant. Bleeding complications of ecchymosis, epistaxis, and gum hemorrhage have been reported. Patients undergoing invasive procedures or having signs/symptoms of underlying coagulopathy or other increased risk of bleeding (due to other therapies such as coumarin anticoagulants or heparin) should be evaluated for hemorrhage).

No products indexed under this heading.

Tissue Plasminogen Activator (Pentosan polysulfate sodium is a weak anticoagulant. Bleeding complications of ecchymosis, epistaxis, and gum hemorrhage have been reported. Patients undergoing invasive procedures or having signs/symptoms of underlying coagulopathy or other increased risk of bleeding (due to other therapies such as t-PA) should be evaluated for hemorrhage).

No products indexed under this heading.

Tolmetin Sodium (Pentosan polysulfate sodium is a weak anticoagulant. Bleeding complications of ecchymosis, epistaxis, and gum hemorrhage have been reported. Patients undergoing invasive procedures or having signs/symptoms of underlying coagulopathy or other increased risk of bleeding (due to other therapies such as nonsteroidal anti-inflammatory drugs) should be evaluated for hemorrhage).

No products indexed under this heading.

Valdecoxib (Pentosan polysulfate sodium is a weak anticoagulant. Bleeding complications of ecchymosis, epistaxis, and gum hemorrhage have been reported. Patients undergoing invasive procedures or having signs/symptoms of underlying coagulopathy or other increased risk of bleeding (due to other therapies such as nonsteroidal anti-inflammatory drugs) should be evaluated for hemorrhage).

No products indexed under this heading.

Warfarin Sodium (Pentosan polysulfate sodium is a weak anticoagulant (1/15 the activity of heparin). At a daily dose of 300 mg (n-128), rectal hemorrhage was reported as an adverse event in 6.3% of patients. Bleeding complications of ecchymosis, epistaxis, and gum hemorrhage have been reported. Patients undergoing invasive procedures or having signs/symptoms of underlying coagulopathy or other increased risk of bleeding (due to other therapies such as coumarin anticoagulants, heparin, t-PA, streptokinase, high dose aspirin, or nonsteroidal anti-inflammatory drugs) should be evaluated for hemorrhage. In a study in which healthy subjects received pentosan polysulfate sodium 100 mg capsule or placebo every 8 hours for 7 days, and were titrated with warfarin to an INR of 1.4 to 1.8, the pharmacokinetic parameters of R-warfarin and S-warfarin were similar in the absence and presence of pentosan polysulfate sodium. INR for warfarin + placebo and warfarin + pentosan polysulfate were comparable).

No products indexed under this heading.

ELOCON CREAM 0.1%
(Mometasone Furoate) 3111
None cited in PDR database.

ELOCON LOTION 0.1%
(Mometasone Furoate) 3112
None cited in PDR database.

ELOCON OINTMENT 0.1%
(Mometasone Furoate) 3114
None cited in PDR database.

ELOXATIN FOR INJECTION
(Oxaliplatin) 2975
May interact with anticoagulants, nephrotoxic agents, and certain other agents. Compounds in these categories include:

Abacavir Sulfate (Because platinum-containing species are eliminated primarily through the kidney, clearance of these products may be decreased by co-administration of potentially nephrotoxic compounds, although this has not been specifically studied). Products include:

Acyclovir (Because platinum-containing species are eliminated primarily through the kidney, clearance of these products may be decreased by co-administration of potentially nephrotoxic compounds, although this has not been specifically studied). Products include:

Acyclovir Sodium (Because platinum-containing species are eliminated primarily through the kidney, clearance of these products may be decreased by co-administration of potentially nephrotoxic compounds, although this has not been specifically studied).

No products indexed under this heading.

Alatrofloxacin Mesylate (Because platinum-containing species are eliminated primarily through the kidney, clearance of these products may be decreased by co-administration of potentially nephrotoxic compounds, although this has not been specifically studied).

No products indexed under this heading.

Aldesleukin (Because platinum-containing species are eliminated primarily through the kidney, clearance of these products may be decreased by co-administration of potentially nephrotoxic compounds, although this has not been specifically studied). Products include:

Amikacin Sulfate (Because platinum-containing species are eliminated primarily through the kidney, clearance of these products may be decreased by co-administration of potentially nephrotoxic compounds, although this has not been specifically studied).

No products indexed under this heading.

Amoxicillin (Because platinum-containing species are eliminated primarily through the kidney, clearance of these products may be decreased by co-administration of potentially nephrotoxic compounds, although this has not been specifically studied). Products include:

Amoxicillin Trihydrate (Because platinum-containing species are eliminated primarily through the kidney, clearance of these products may be decreased by co-administration of potentially nephrotoxic compounds, although this has not been specifically studied).

No products indexed under this heading.

Amphotericin B (Because platinum-containing species are eliminated primarily through the kidney, clearance of these products may be decreased by co-administration of potentially nephrotoxic compounds, although this has not been specifically studied).

No products indexed under this heading.

Amphotericin B, liposomal (Because platinum-containing species are eliminated primarily through the kidney, clearance of these products may be decreased by co-administration of potentially nephrotoxic compounds, although this has not been specifically studied). Products include:

IMPORTANT NOTE: Always consult each drug listing in the patient's regimen for possible interactions.

Amphotericin B Cholesteryl Sulfate (Because platinum-containing species are eliminated primarily through the kidney, clearance of these products may be decreased by co-administration of potentially nephrotoxic compounds, although this has not been specifically studied).
No products indexed under this heading.

Amphotericin B Lipid Complex (Because platinum-containing species are eliminated primarily through the kidney, clearance of these products may be decreased by co-administration of potentially nephrotoxic compounds, although this has not been specifically studied).
No products indexed under this heading.

Ampicillin (Because platinum-containing species are eliminated primarily through the kidney, clearance of these products may be decreased by co-administration of potentially nephrotoxic compounds, although this has not been specifically studied).
No products indexed under this heading.

Ampicillin Sodium (Because platinum-containing species are eliminated primarily through the kidney, clearance of these products may be decreased by co-administration of potentially nephrotoxic compounds, although this has not been specifically studied).
No products indexed under this heading.

Ampicillin Trihydrate (Because platinum-containing species are eliminated primarily through the kidney, clearance of these products may be decreased by co-administration of potentially nephrotoxic compounds, although this has not been specifically studied).
No products indexed under this heading.

Amprenavir (Because platinum-containing species are eliminated primarily through the kidney, clearance of these products may be decreased by co-administration of potentially nephrotoxic compounds, although this has not been specifically studied).
No products indexed under this heading.

Anisindione (There have been reports while on study and from post-marketing surveillance of prolonged prothrombin time and INR occasionally associated with hemorrhage in patients who received oxaliplatin plus 5-FU/LV while on anticoagulants. Patients receiving oxaliplatin plus 5-FU/LV and requiring oral anticoagulants may require closer monitoring).
No products indexed under this heading.

Ardeparin Sodium (There have been reports while on study and from post-marketing surveillance of prolonged prothrombin time and INR occasionally associated with hemorrhage in patients who received oxaliplatin plus 5-FU/LV while on anticoagulants. Patients receiving oxaliplatin plus 5-FU/LV and requiring oral anticoagulants may require closer monitoring).
No products indexed under this heading.

Aspirin (Because platinum-containing species are eliminated primarily through the kidney, clearance of these products may be decreased by co-administration of potentially nephrotoxic compounds, although this has not been specifically studied). Products include:

Atazanavir (Because platinum-containing species are eliminated primarily through the kidney, clearance of these products may be decreased by co-administration of potentially nephrotoxic compounds, although this has not been specifically studied).
No products indexed under this heading.

Atorvastatin Calcium (Because platinum-containing species are eliminated primarily through the kidney, clearance of these products may be decreased by co-administration of potentially nephrotoxic compounds, although this has not been specifically studied). Products include:

Azithromycin Dihydrate (Because platinum-containing species are eliminated primarily through the kidney, clearance of these products may be decreased by co-administration of potentially nephrotoxic compounds, although this has not been specifically studied).
No products indexed under this heading.

Azlocillin Sodium (Because platinum-containing species are eliminated primarily through the kidney, clearance of these products may be decreased by co-administration of potentially nephrotoxic compounds, although this has not been specifically studied).
No products indexed under this heading.

Aztreonam (Because platinum-containing species are eliminated primarily through the kidney, clearance of these products may be decreased by co-administration of potentially nephrotoxic compounds, although this has not been specifically studied).
No products indexed under this heading.

Bacampicillin Hydrochloride (Because platinum-containing species are eliminated primarily through the kidney, clearance of these products may be decreased by co-administration of potentially nephrotoxic compounds, although this has not been specifically studied).
No products indexed under this heading.

Bacitracin (Because platinum-containing species are eliminated primarily through the kidney, clearance of these products may be decreased by co-administration of potentially nephrotoxic compounds, although this has not been specifically studied).
No products indexed under this heading.

Bacitracin Zinc (Because platinum-containing species are eliminated primarily through the kidney, clearance of these products may be decreased by co-administration of potentially nephrotoxic compounds, although this has not been specifically studied).
No products indexed under this heading.

Balsalazide Disodium (Because platinum-containing species are eliminated primarily through the kidney, clearance of these products may be decreased by co-administration of potentially nephrotoxic compounds, although this has not been specifically studied).
No products indexed under this heading.

Benazepril Hydrochloride (Because platinum-containing species are eliminated primarily through the kidney, clearance of these products may be decreased by co-administration of potentially nephrotoxic compounds, although this has not been specifically studied).
No products indexed under this heading.

Bendroflumethiazide (Because platinum-containing species are eliminated primarily through the kidney, clearance of these products may be decreased by co-administration of potentially nephrotoxic compounds, although this has not been specifically studied).
No products indexed under this heading.

Caffeine (Because platinum-containing species are eliminated primarily through the kidney, clearance of these products may be decreased by co-administration of potentially nephrotoxic compounds, although this has not been specifically studied).
No products indexed under this heading.

Captopril (Because platinum-containing species are eliminated primarily through the kidney, clearance of these products may be decreased by co-administration of potentially nephrotoxic compounds, although this has not been specifically studied). Products include:

Carbenicillin Disodium (Because platinum-containing species are eliminated primarily through the kidney, clearance of these products may be decreased by co-administration of potentially nephrotoxic compounds, although this has not been specifically studied).
No products indexed under this heading.

Carbenicillin Indanyl Sodium (Because platinum-containing species are eliminated primarily through the kidney, clearance of these products may be decreased by co-administration of potentially nephrotoxic compounds, although this has not been specifically studied).
No products indexed under this heading.

Carboplatin (Because platinum-containing species are eliminated primarily through the kidney, clearance of these products may be decreased by co-administration of potentially nephrotoxic compounds, although this has not been specifically studied).
No products indexed under this heading.

Carmustine (BCNU) (Because platinum-containing species are eliminated primarily through the kidney, clearance of these products may be decreased by co-administration of potentially nephrotoxic compounds, although this has not been specifically studied).
No products indexed under this heading.

Cefaclor (Because platinum-containing species are eliminated primarily through the kidney, clearance of these products may be decreased by co-administration of potentially nephrotoxic compounds, although this has not been specifically studied).
No products indexed under this heading.

Cefadroxil (Because platinum-containing species are eliminated primarily through the kidney, clearance of these products may be decreased by co-administration of potentially nephrotoxic compounds, although this has not been specifically studied).
No products indexed under this heading.

Cefamandole Nafate (Because platinum-containing species are eliminated primarily through the kidney, clearance of these products may be decreased by co-administration of potentially nephrotoxic compounds, although this has not been specifically studied).
No products indexed under this heading.

Cefazolin Sodium (Because platinum-containing species are eliminated primarily through the kidney, clearance of these products may be decreased by co-administration of potentially nephrotoxic compounds, although this has not been specifically studied).
No products indexed under this heading.

Cefdinir (Because platinum-containing species are eliminated primarily through the kidney, clearance of these products may be decreased by co-administration of potentially nephrotoxic compounds, although this has not been specifically studied). Products include:

Cefepime Hydrochloride (Because platinum-containing species are eliminated primarily through the kidney, clearance of these products may be decreased by co-administration of potentially nephrotoxic compounds, although this has not been specifically studied).
No products indexed under this heading.

Cefixime (Because platinum-containing species are eliminated primarily through the kidney, clearance of these products may be decreased by co-administration of potentially nephrotoxic compounds, although this has not been specifically studied). Products include:

Cefmetazole Sodium (Because platinum-containing species are eliminated primarily through the kidney, clearance of these products may be decreased by co-administration of potentially nephrotoxic compounds, although this has not been specifically studied).
No products indexed under this heading.

Cefonicid Sodium (Because platinum-containing species are eliminated primarily through the kidney, clearance of these products may be decreased by co-administration of potentially nephrotoxic compounds, although this has not been specifically studied).
No products indexed under this heading.

Cefoperazone Sodium (Because platinum-containing species are eliminated primarily through the kidney, clearance of these products may be decreased by co-administration of potentially nephrotoxic compounds, although this has not been specifically studied).
No products indexed under this heading.

Ceforanide (Because platinum-containing species are eliminated primarily through the kidney, clearance of these products may be decreased by co-administration of potentially nephrotoxic compounds, although this has not been specifically studied).
No products indexed under this heading.

Cefotaxime Sodium (Because platinum-containing species are eliminated primarily through the kidney, clearance of these products may be decreased by co-administration of potentially nephrotoxic compounds, although this has not been specifically studied).
No products indexed under this heading.

Cefotetan (Because platinum-containing species are eliminated primarily through the kidney, clearance of these products may be decreased by co-administration of potentially nephrotoxic compounds, although this has not been specifically studied).
No products indexed under this heading.

Cefoxitin Sodium (Because platinum-containing species are eliminated primarily through the kidney, clearance of these products may be decreased by co-administration of potentially nephrotoxic compounds, although this has not been specifically studied).
    No products indexed under this heading.

Cefpodoxime Proxetil (Because platinum-containing species are eliminated primarily through the kidney, clearance of these products may be decreased by co-administration of potentially nephrotoxic compounds, although this has not been specifically studied).
    No products indexed under this heading.

Cefprozil (Because platinum-containing species are eliminated primarily through the kidney, clearance of these products may be decreased by co-administration of potentially nephrotoxic compounds, although this has not been specifically studied).
    No products indexed under this heading.

Ceftazidime (Because platinum-containing species are eliminated primarily through the kidney, clearance of these products may be decreased by co-administration of potentially nephrotoxic compounds, although this has not been specifically studied). Products include:

Ceftizoxime Sodium (Because platinum-containing species are eliminated primarily through the kidney, clearance of these products may be decreased by co-administration of potentially nephrotoxic compounds, although this has not been specifically studied).
    No products indexed under this heading.

Ceftriaxone Sodium (Because platinum-containing species are eliminated primarily through the kidney, clearance of these products may be decreased by co-administration of potentially nephrotoxic compounds, although this has not been specifically studied). Products include:

Cefuroxime Axetil (Because platinum-containing species are eliminated primarily through the kidney, clearance of these products may be decreased by co-administration of potentially nephrotoxic compounds, although this has not been specifically studied). Products include:

Cefuroxime Sodium (Because platinum-containing species are eliminated primarily through the kidney, clearance of these products may be decreased by co-administration of potentially nephrotoxic compounds, although this has not been specifically studied).
    No products indexed under this heading.

Celecoxib (Because platinum-containing species are eliminated primarily through the kidney, clearance of these products may be decreased by co-administration of potentially nephrotoxic compounds, although this has not been specifically studied). Products include:

Cephalexin (Because platinum-containing species are eliminated primarily through the kidney, clearance of these products may be decreased by co-administration of potentially nephrotoxic compounds, although this has not been specifically studied).
    No products indexed under this heading.

Cephalothin Sodium (Because platinum-containing species are eliminated primarily through the kidney, clearance of these products may be decreased by co-administration of potentially nephrotoxic compounds, although this has not been specifically studied).
    No products indexed under this heading.

Cephapirin Sodium (Because platinum-containing species are eliminated primarily through the kidney, clearance of these products may be decreased by co-administration of potentially nephrotoxic compounds, although this has not been specifically studied).
    No products indexed under this heading.

Cephradine (Because platinum-containing species are eliminated primarily through the kidney, clearance of these products may be decreased by co-administration of potentially nephrotoxic compounds, although this has not been specifically studied).
    No products indexed under this heading.

Cerivastatin Sodium (Because platinum-containing species are eliminated primarily through the kidney, clearance of these products may be decreased by co-administration of potentially nephrotoxic compounds, although this has not been specifically studied).
    No products indexed under this heading.

Chlorothiazide (Because platinum-containing species are eliminated primarily through the kidney, clearance of these products may be decreased by co-administration of potentially nephrotoxic compounds, although this has not been specifically studied).
    No products indexed under this heading.

Chlorothiazide Sodium (Because platinum-containing species are eliminated primarily through the kidney, clearance of these products may be decreased by co-administration of potentially nephrotoxic compounds, although this has not been specifically studied). Products include:

Chlorpropamide (Because platinum-containing species are eliminated primarily through the kidney, clearance of these products may be decreased by co-administration of potentially nephrotoxic compounds, although this has not been specifically studied).
    No products indexed under this heading.

Cidofovir (Because platinum-containing species are eliminated primarily through the kidney, clearance of these products may be decreased by co-administration of potentially nephrotoxic compounds, although this has not been specifically studied).
    No products indexed under this heading.

Cilastatin Sodium (Because platinum-containing species are eliminated primarily through the kidney, clearance of these products may be decreased by co-administration of potentially nephrotoxic compounds, although this has not been specifically studied). Products include:

Cimetidine (Because platinum-containing species are eliminated primarily through the kidney, clearance of these products may be decreased by co-administration of potentially nephrotoxic compounds, although this has not been specifically studied).
    No products indexed under this heading.

Cimetidine Hydrochloride (Because platinum-containing species are eliminated primarily through the kidney, clearance of these products may be decreased by co-administration of potentially nephrotoxic compounds, although this has not been specifically studied).
    No products indexed under this heading.

Cisplatin (Because platinum-containing species are eliminated primarily through the kidney, clearance of these products may be decreased by co-administration of potentially nephrotoxic compounds, although this has not been specifically studied).
    No products indexed under this heading.

Cladribine (Because platinum-containing species are eliminated primarily through the kidney, clearance of these products may be decreased by co-administration of potentially nephrotoxic compounds, although this has not been specifically studied). Products include:

Clozapine (Because platinum-containing species are eliminated primarily through the kidney, clearance of these products may be decreased by co-administration of potentially nephrotoxic compounds, although this has not been specifically studied).
    No products indexed under this heading.

Colistimethate Sodium (Because platinum-containing species are eliminated primarily through the kidney, clearance of these products may be decreased by co-administration of potentially nephrotoxic compounds, although this has not been specifically studied).
    No products indexed under this heading.

Colistin Sulfate (Because platinum-containing species are eliminated primarily through the kidney, clearance of these products may be decreased by co-administration of potentially nephrotoxic compounds, although this has not been specifically studied).
    No products indexed under this heading.

Cyclophosphamide (Because platinum-containing species are eliminated primarily through the kidney, clearance of these products may be decreased by co-administration of potentially nephrotoxic compounds, although this has not been specifically studied).
    No products indexed under this heading.

Cyclosporine (Because platinum-containing species are eliminated primarily through the kidney, clearance of these products may be decreased by co-administration of potentially nephrotoxic compounds, although this has not been specifically studied). Products include:

Cytarabine (Because platinum-containing species are eliminated primarily through the kidney, clearance of these products may be decreased by co-administration of potentially nephrotoxic compounds, although this has not been specifically studied).
    No products indexed under this heading.

Cytarabine Liposome (Because platinum-containing species are eliminated primarily through the kidney, clearance of these products may be decreased by co-administration of potentially nephrotoxic compounds, although this has not been specifically studied).
    No products indexed under this heading.

Dalteparin Sodium (There have been reports while on study and from post-marketing surveillance of prolonged prothrombin time and INR occasionally associated with hemorrhage in patients who received oxaliplatin plus 5-FU/LV while on anticoagulants. Patients receiving oxaliplatin plus 5-FU/LV and requiring oral anticoagulants may require closer monitoring). Products include:

Danaparoid Sodium (There have been reports while on study and from post-marketing surveillance of prolonged prothrombin time and INR occasionally associated with hemorrhage in patients who received oxaliplatin plus 5-FU/LV while on anticoagulants. Patients receiving oxaliplatin plus 5-FU/LV and requiring oral anticoagulants may require closer monitoring).
    No products indexed under this heading.

Delavirdine Mesylate (Because platinum-containing species are eliminated primarily through the kidney, clearance of these products may be decreased by co-administration of potentially nephrotoxic compounds, although this has not been specifically studied).
    No products indexed under this heading.

Diatrizoate Meglumine (Because platinum-containing species are eliminated primarily through the kidney, clearance of these products may be decreased by co-administration of potentially nephrotoxic compounds, although this has not been specifically studied).
    No products indexed under this heading.

Diatrizoate Sodium (Because platinum-containing species are eliminated primarily through the kidney, clearance of these products may be decreased by co-administration of potentially nephrotoxic compounds, although this has not been specifically studied).
    No products indexed under this heading.

Diclofenac Potassium (Because platinum-containing species are eliminated primarily through the kidney, clearance of these products may be decreased by co-administration of potentially nephrotoxic compounds, although this has not been specifically studied).
    No products indexed under this heading.

Diclofenac Sodium (Because platinum-containing species are eliminated primarily through the kidney, clearance of these products may be decreased by co-administration of potentially nephrotoxic compounds, although this has not been specifically studied).
    No products indexed under this heading.

Dicloxacillin Sodium (Because platinum-containing species are eliminated primarily through the kidney, clearance of these products may be decreased by co-administration of potentially nephrotoxic compounds, although this has not been specifically studied).
    No products indexed under this heading.

Dicumarol (There have been reports while on study and from post-marketing surveillance of prolonged prothrombin time and INR occasionally associated with hemorrhage in patients who received oxaliplatin plus 5-FU/LV while on anticoagulants. Patients receiving oxaliplatin plus 5-FU/LV and requiring oral anticoagulants may require closer monitoring).
    No products indexed under this heading.

IMPORTANT NOTE: Always consult each drug listing in the patient's regimen for possible interactions.

IMPORTANT NOTE: Always consult each drug listing in the patient's regimen for possible interactions.

Sulfamethizole (Because platinum-containing species are eliminated primarily through the kidney, clearance of these products may be decreased by co-administration of potentially nephrotoxic compounds, although this has not been specifically studied).
No products indexed under this heading.

Sulfamethoxazole (Because platinum-containing species are eliminated primarily through the kidney, clearance of these products may be decreased by co-administration of potentially nephrotoxic compounds, although this has not been specifically studied).
No products indexed under this heading.

Sulfasalazine (Because platinum-containing species are eliminated primarily through the kidney, clearance of these products may be decreased by co-administration of potentially nephrotoxic compounds, although this has not been specifically studied).
No products indexed under this heading.

Sulfinpyrazone (Because platinum-containing species are eliminated primarily through the kidney, clearance of these products may be decreased by co-administration of potentially nephrotoxic compounds, although this has not been specifically studied).
No products indexed under this heading.

Sulfisoxazole Acetyl (Because platinum-containing species are eliminated primarily through the kidney, clearance of these products may be decreased by co-administration of potentially nephrotoxic compounds, although this has not been specifically studied).
No products indexed under this heading.

Sulfisoxazole Diolamine (Because platinum-containing species are eliminated primarily through the kidney, clearance of these products may be decreased by co-administration of potentially nephrotoxic compounds, although this has not been specifically studied).
No products indexed under this heading.

Sulindac (Because platinum-containing species are eliminated primarily through the kidney, clearance of these products may be decreased by co-administration of potentially nephrotoxic compounds, although this has not been specifically studied). Products include:

Tacrolimus (Because platinum-containing species are eliminated primarily through the kidney, clearance of these products may be decreased by co-administration of potentially nephrotoxic compounds, although this has not been specifically studied). Products include:

Tenofovir Disoproxil Fumarate (Because platinum-containing species are eliminated primarily through the kidney, clearance of these products may be decreased by co-administration of potentially nephrotoxic compounds, although this has not been specifically studied). Products include:

Thioguanine (Because platinum-containing species are eliminated primarily through the kidney, clearance of these products may be decreased by co-administration of potentially nephrotoxic compounds, although this has not been specifically studied). Products include:

Ticarcillin Disodium (Because platinum-containing species are eliminated primarily through the kidney, clearance of these products may be decreased by co-administration of potentially nephrotoxic compounds, although this has not been specifically studied). Products include:

Tinzaparin Sodium (There have been reports while on study and from post-marketing surveillance of prolonged prothrombin time and INR occasionally associated with hemorrhage in patients who received oxaliplatin plus 5-FU/LV while on anticoagulants. Patients receiving oxaliplatin plus 5-FU/LV and requiring oral anticoagulants may require closer monitoring).
No products indexed under this heading.

Tobramycin (Because platinum-containing species are eliminated primarily through the kidney, clearance of these products may be decreased by co-administration of potentially nephrotoxic compounds, although this has not been specifically studied). Products include:

Tobramycin Sulfate (Because platinum-containing species are eliminated primarily through the kidney, clearance of these products may be decreased by co-administration of potentially nephrotoxic compounds, although this has not been specifically studied).
No products indexed under this heading.

Tolazamide (Because platinum-containing species are eliminated primarily through the kidney, clearance of these products may be decreased by co-administration of potentially nephrotoxic compounds, although this has not been specifically studied).
No products indexed under this heading.

Tolbutamide (Because platinum-containing species are eliminated primarily through the kidney, clearance of these products may be decreased by co-administration of potentially nephrotoxic compounds, although this has not been specifically studied).
No products indexed under this heading.

Tolmetin Sodium (Because platinum-containing species are eliminated primarily through the kidney, clearance of these products may be decreased by co-administration of potentially nephrotoxic compounds, although this has not been specifically studied).
No products indexed under this heading.

Trandolapril (Because platinum-containing species are eliminated primarily through the kidney, clearance of these products may be decreased by co-administration of potentially nephrotoxic compounds, although this has not been specifically studied). Products include:

Triamterene (Because platinum-containing species are eliminated primarily through the kidney, clearance of these products may be decreased by co-administration of potentially nephrotoxic compounds, although this has not been specifically studied). Products include:

Trimethadione (Because platinum-containing species are eliminated primarily through the kidney, clearance of these products may be decreased by co-administration of potentially nephrotoxic compounds, although this has not been specifically studied).
No products indexed under this heading.

Trovafloxacin Mesylate (Because platinum-containing species are eliminated primarily through the kidney, clearance of these products may be decreased by co-administration of potentially nephrotoxic compounds, although this has not been specifically studied).
No products indexed under this heading.

Tyropanoate Sodium (Because platinum-containing species are eliminated primarily through the kidney, clearance of these products may be decreased by co-administration of potentially nephrotoxic compounds, although this has not been specifically studied).
No products indexed under this heading.

Valacyclovir Hydrochloride (Because platinum-containing species are eliminated primarily through the kidney, clearance of these products may be decreased by co-administration of potentially nephrotoxic compounds, although this has not been specifically studied). Products include:

Valdecoxib (Because platinum-containing species are eliminated primarily through the kidney, clearance of these products may be decreased by co-administration of potentially nephrotoxic compounds, although this has not been specifically studied).
No products indexed under this heading.

Vancomycin Hydrochloride (Because platinum-containing species are eliminated primarily through the kidney, clearance of these products may be decreased by co-administration of potentially nephrotoxic compounds, although this has not been specifically studied).
No products indexed under this heading.

Voriconazole (Because platinum-containing species are eliminated primarily through the kidney, clearance of these products may be decreased by co-administration of potentially nephrotoxic compounds, although this has not been specifically studied).
No products indexed under this heading.

Warfarin Sodium (There have been reports while on study and from post-marketing surveillance of prolonged prothrombin time and INR occasionally associated with hemorrhage in patients who received oxaliplatin plus 5-FU/LV while on anticoagulants. Patients receiving oxaliplatin plus 5-FU/LV and requiring oral anticoagulants may require closer monitoring).
No products indexed under this heading.

Zalcitabine (Because platinum-containing species are eliminated primarily through the kidney, clearance of these products may be decreased by co-administration of potentially nephrotoxic compounds, although this has not been specifically studied).
No products indexed under this heading.

Zidovudine (Because platinum-containing species are eliminated primarily through the kidney, clearance of these products may be decreased by co-administration of potentially nephrotoxic compounds, although this has not been specifically studied). Products include:

Zoledronic Acid (Because platinum-containing species are eliminated primarily through the kidney, clearance of these products may be decreased by co-administration of potentially nephrotoxic compounds, although this has not been specifically studied). Products include:

ELSPAR FOR INJECTION

Methotrexate Sodium (Tissue culture and animal studies indicate that asparaginase can diminish or abolish the effect of methotrexate on malignant cells).
No products indexed under this heading.

Prednisone (The administration of asparaginase intravenously and concurrently with or immediately before a course of prednisone may be associated with increased toxicity).
No products indexed under this heading.

Vincristine Sulfate (The administration of asparaginase intravenouosly and concurrently with or immediately before a course of prednisone may be associated with increased toxicity).
No products indexed under this heading.

ELSPAR FOR INJECTION
None cited in PDR database.

EMBEDA EXTENDED RELEASE CAPSULES
May interact with alcohols, anticholinergics, antiemetics, central nervous system depressants, diuretics, general anesthetics, hypnotics and sedatives, mixed agonist/antagonist opioid analgesics, monoamine oxidase inhibitors, P-glycoprotein inhibitors, phenothiazines, quinidine, skeletal muscle relaxants, tranquilizers, and certain other agents. Compounds in these categories include:

Alfentanil Hydrochloride (Embeda should be used with great caution and in reduced dosage in patients who are concurrently receiving other central nervous system (CNS) depressants including sedatives, hypnotics, general anesthetics, antiemetics, phenothiazines, other tranquilizers, and alcohol because of the risk of respiratory depression, hypotension, and profound sedation or coma. When such combined therapy is contemplated, the initial dose of one or both agents should be reduced by at least 50%).
No products indexed under this heading.

Alprazolam (Embeda should be used with great caution and in reduced dosage in patients who are concurrently receiving other central nervous system (CNS) depressants including other tranquilizers because of the risk of respiratory depression, hypotension, and profound sedation or coma. When such combined therapy is contemplated, the initial dose of one or both agents should be reduced by at least 50%).
No products indexed under this heading.

Amiloride Hydrochloride (Morphine can reduce the efficacy of diuretics by inducing the release of antidiuretic hormone. Morphine may also lead to acute retention of urine by causing spasm of the sphincter of the bladder, particularly in men with prostatism).
No products indexed under this heading.

563 Interactions Index Embeda

sedation or coma. When such combined therapy is contemplated, the initial dose of one or both agents should be reduced by at least 50%).
No products indexed under this heading.

Chlorprothixene Lactate (Embeda should be used with great caution and in reduced dosage in patients who are concurrently receiving other central nervous system (CNS) depressants including other tranquilizers because of the risk of respiratory depression, hypotension, and profound sedation or coma. When such combined therapy is contemplated, the initial dose of one or both agents should be reduced by at least 50%).
No products indexed under this heading.

Chlorthalidone (Morphine can reduce the efficacy of diuretics by inducing the release of antidiuretic hormone. Morphine may also lead to acute retention of urine by causing spasm of the sphincter of the bladder, particularly in men with prostatism). Products include:
Clorpres **2344**

Chlorzoxazone (Embeda may enhance the neuromuscular blocking action of skeletal relaxants and produce an increased degree of respiratory depression).
No products indexed under this heading.

Cimetidine (There is an isolated report of confusion and severe respiratory depression when a hemodialysis patient was concurrently administered morphine and cimetidine).
No products indexed under this heading.

Cimetidine Hydrochloride (There is an isolated report of confusion and severe respiratory depression when a hemodialysis patient was concurrently administered morphine and cimetidine).
No products indexed under this heading.

Cisatracurium Besylate (Embeda may enhance the neuromuscular blocking action of skeletal relaxants and produce an increased degree of respiratory depression). Products include:
Nimbex **503**

Clarithromycin (Based on published reports, PGP inhibitors may increase the absorption/exposure of morphine sulfate by about two fold. Therefore, caution should be exercised when morphine sulfate is co-administered with PGP inhibitors). Products include:
Biaxin/Biaxin XL **412**

Clidinium Bromide (Anticholinergics or other medications with anticholinergic activity when used concurrently with opioid analgesics may result in increased risk of urinary retention and/or severe constipation, which may lead to paralytic ileus).
No products indexed under this heading.

Clonazepam (Embeda should be used with great caution and in reduced dosage in patients who are concurrently receiving other central nervous system (CNS) depressants including sedatives, hypnotics, general anesthetics, antiemetics, phenothiazines, other tranquilizers, and alcohol because of the risk of respiratory depression, hypotension, and profound sedation or coma. When such combined therapy is contemplated, the initial dose of one or both agents should be reduced by at least 50%). Products include:
Klonopin **2855**

Clorazepate Dipotassium (Embeda should be used with great caution and in reduced dosage in patients who are concurrently receiving other central nervous system (CNS) depressants including other tranquilizers because of the risk of respiratory depression, hypotension, and profound sedation or coma. When such combined therapy is contemplated, the initial dose of one or both agents should be reduced by at least 50%).
No products indexed under this heading.

Clozapine (Embeda should be used with great caution and in reduced dosage in patients who are concurrently receiving other central nervous system (CNS) depressants including sedatives, hypnotics, general anesthetics, antiemetics, phenothiazines, other tranquilizers, and alcohol because of the risk of respiratory depression, hypotension, and profound sedation or coma. When such combined therapy is contemplated, the initial dose of one or both agents should be reduced by at least 50%).
No products indexed under this heading.

Codeine Phosphate (Embeda should be used with great caution and in reduced dosage in patients who are concurrently receiving other central nervous system (CNS) depressants including sedatives, hypnotics, general anesthetics, antiemetics, phenothiazines, other tranquilizers, and alcohol because of the risk of respiratory depression, hypotension, and profound sedation or coma. When such combined therapy is contemplated, the initial dose of one or both agents should be reduced by at least 50%). Products include:
Tylenol with Codeine **2691**

Codeine Sulfate (Embeda should be used with great caution and in reduced dosage in patients who are concurrently receiving other central nervous system (CNS) depressants including sedatives, hypnotics, general anesthetics, antiemetics, phenothiazines, other tranquilizers, and alcohol because of the risk of respiratory depression, hypotension, and profound sedation or coma. When such combined therapy is contemplated, the initial dose of one or both agents should be reduced by at least 50%).
No products indexed under this heading.

Cyclobenzaprine Hydrochloride (Embeda may enhance the neuromuscular blocking action of skeletal relaxants and produce an increased degree of respiratory depression). Products include:
Amrix **964**

Cyclosporine (Based on published reports, PGP inhibitors may increase the absorption/exposure of morphine sulfate by about two fold. Therefore, caution should be exercised when morphine sulfate is co-administered with PGP inhibitors). Products include:
Gengraf **440**
Neoral Oral Solution **2496**
Neoral Capsules **2496**
Restasis **605**

Dantrolene Sodium (Embeda may enhance the neuromuscular blocking action of skeletal relaxants and produce an increased degree of respiratory depression).
No products indexed under this heading.

Desflurane (Embeda should be used with great caution and in reduced dosage in patients who are concurrently receiving other central nervous system (CNS) depressants including general anesthetics because of the risk of respiratory depression, hypotension, and profound sedation or coma. When such combined therapy is contemplated, the initial dose of one or both agents should be reduced by at least 50%).
No products indexed under this heading.

Dezocine (Embeda should be used with great caution and in reduced dosage in patients who are concurrently receiving other central nervous system (CNS) depressants including sedatives, hypnotics, general anesthetics, antiemetics, phenothiazines, other tranquilizers, and alcohol because of the risk of respiratory depression, hypotension, and profound sedation or coma. When such combined therapy is contemplated, the initial dose of one or both agents should be reduced by at least 50%).
No products indexed under this heading.

Diazepam (Embeda should be used with great caution and in reduced dosage in patients who are concurrently receiving other central nervous system (CNS) depressants including other tranquilizers because of the risk of respiratory depression, hypotension, and profound sedation or coma. When such combined therapy is contemplated, the initial dose of one or both agents should be reduced by at least 50%). Products include:
Valium Tablets **2880**

Dicyclomine Hydrochloride (Anticholinergics or other medications with anticholinergic activity when used concurrently with opioid analgesics may result in increased risk of urinary retention and/or severe constipation, which may lead to paralytic ileus). Products include:
Bentyl Capsules **780**
Bentyl Injection **780**
Bentyl Syrup **780**
Bentyl Tablets **780**

Digoxin (Based on published reports, PGP inhibitors may increase the absorption/exposure of morphine sulfate by about two fold. Therefore, caution should be exercised when morphine sulfate is co-administered with PGP inhibitors). Products include:
Lanoxin Injection **1546**
Lanoxin Injection Pediatric **1549**
Lanoxin Tablets **1553**

Diltiazem Hydrochloride (Based on published reports, PGP inhibitors may increase the absorption/exposure of morphine sulfate by about two fold. Therefore, caution should be exercised when morphine sulfate is co-administered with PGP inhibitors). Products include:
Cardizem LA **423**

Diltiazem Maleate (Based on published reports, PGP inhibitors may increase the absorption/exposure of morphine sulfate by about two fold. Therefore, caution should be exercised when morphine sulfate is co-administered with PGP inhibitors).
No products indexed under this heading.

Dimenhydrinate (Embeda should be used with great caution and in reduced dosage in patients who are concurrently receiving other central nervous system (CNS) depressants including antiemetic because of the risk of respiratory depression, hypotension, and profound sedation or coma. When such combined therapy is contemplated, the initial dose of one or both agents should be reduced by at least 50%).
No products indexed under this heading.

Diphenhydramine (Embeda should be used with great caution and in reduced dosage in patients who are concurrently receiving other central nervous system (CNS) depressants including antiemetic because of the risk of respiratory depression, hypotension, and profound sedation or coma. When such combined therapy is contemplated, the initial dose of one or both agents should be reduced by at least 50%).
No products indexed under this heading.

Diphenhydramine Hydrochloride (Embeda should be used with great caution and in reduced dosage in patients who are concurrently receiving other central nervous system (CNS) depressants including antiemetic because of the risk of respiratory depression, hypotension, and profound sedation or coma. When such combined therapy is contemplated, the initial dose of one or both agents should be reduced by at least 50%). Products include:
Benadryl Allergy Ultratab **2042**
Children's Benadryl Allergy Liquid **2042**

Dirithromycin (Based on published reports, PGP inhibitors may increase the absorption/exposure of morphine sulfate by about two fold. Therefore, caution should be exercised when morphine sulfate is co-administered with PGP inhibitors).
No products indexed under this heading.

Dolasetron Mesylate (Embeda should be used with great caution and in reduced dosage in patients who are concurrently receiving other central nervous system (CNS) depressants including antiemetic because of the risk of respiratory depression, hypotension, and profound sedation or coma. When such combined therapy is contemplated, the initial dose of one or both agents should be reduced by at least 50%). Products include:
Anzemet Injection **2931**
Anzemet Tablets **2934**

Doxacurium Chloride (Embeda may enhance the neuromuscular blocking action of skeletal relaxants and produce an increased degree of respiratory depression).
No products indexed under this heading.

Dronabinol (Embeda should be used with great caution and in reduced dosage in patients who are concurrently receiving other central nervous system (CNS) depressants including antiemetic because of the risk of respiratory depression, hypotension, and profound sedation or coma. When such combined therapy is contemplated, the initial dose of one or both agents should be reduced by at least 50%).
No products indexed under this heading.

Droperidol (Embeda should be used with great caution and in reduced dosage in patients who are concurrently receiving other central nervous system (CNS) depressants including antiemetic because of the risk of respiratory depression, hypotension, and profound sedation or coma. When such combined therapy is contemplated, the initial dose of one or both agents should be reduced by at least 50%).
No products indexed under this heading.

d-Tubocurarine (Embeda may enhance the neuromuscular blocking action of skeletal relaxants and produce an increased degree of respiratory depression).
No products indexed under this heading.

Elacridar (Based on published reports, PGP inhibitors may increase the absorption/exposure of morphine sulfate by about two fold. Therefore, caution should be exercised when morphine sulfate is co-administered with PGP inhibitors).
No products indexed under this heading.

Enflurane (Embeda should be used with great caution and in reduced dosage in patients who are concurrently receiving other central nervous system (CNS) depressants including general anesthetics because of the risk of respiratory depression, hypotension, and profound sedation or coma. When such combined therapy is contemplated, the initial dose of one or both agents should be reduced by at least 50%).
No products indexed under this heading.

Embeda Interactions Index 564

Erythromycin (Based on published reports, PGP inhibitors may increase the absorption/exposure of morphine sulfate by about two fold. Therefore, caution should be exercised when morphine sulfate is co-administered with PGP inhibitors).
No products indexed under this heading.

Erythromycin, Topical (Based on published reports, PGP inhibitors may increase the absorption/exposure of morphine sulfate by about two fold. Therefore, caution should be exercised when morphine sulfate is co-administered with PGP inhibitors).
No products indexed under this heading.

Erythromycin Estolate (Based on published reports, PGP inhibitors may increase the absorption/exposure of morphine sulfate by about two fold. Therefore, caution should be exercised when morphine sulfate is co-administered with PGP inhibitors).
No products indexed under this heading.

Erythromycin Ethylsuccinate (Based on published reports, PGP inhibitors may increase the absorption/exposure of morphine sulfate by about two fold. Therefore, caution should be exercised when morphine sulfate is co-administered with PGP inhibitors). Products include:
E.E.S. **437**
EryPed **435**

Erythromycin Gluceptate (Based on published reports, PGP inhibitors may increase the absorption/exposure of morphine sulfate by about two fold. Therefore, caution should be exercised when morphine sulfate is co-administered with PGP inhibitors).
No products indexed under this heading.

Erythromycin Lactobionate (Based on published reports, PGP inhibitors may increase the absorption/exposure of morphine sulfate by about two fold. Therefore, caution should be exercised when morphine sulfate is co-administered with PGP inhibitors).
No products indexed under this heading.

Erythromycin Stearate (Based on published reports, PGP inhibitors may increase the absorption/exposure of morphine sulfate by about two fold. Therefore, caution should be exercised when morphine sulfate is co-administered with PGP inhibitors).
No products indexed under this heading.

Estazolam (Embeda should be used with great caution and in reduced dosage in patients who are concurrently receiving other central nervous system (CNS) depressants including sedatives and hypnotics because of the risk of respiratory depression, hypotension, and profound sedation or coma. When such combined therapy is contemplated, the initial dose of one or both agents should be reduced by at least 50%).
No products indexed under this heading.

Ethacrynic Acid (Morphine can reduce the efficacy of diuretics by inducing the release of antidiuretic hormone. Morphine may also lead to acute retention of urine by causing spasm of the sphincter of the bladder, particularly in men with prostatism).
No products indexed under this heading.

Ethanol (Embeda should be used with great caution and in reduced dosage in patients who are concurrently receiving other central nervous system (CNS) depressants including alcohol because of the risk of respiratory depression, hypotension, and profound sedation or coma. When such combined therapy is contemplated, the initial dose of one or both agents should be reduced by at least 50%).
No products indexed under this heading.

Ethchlorvynol (Embeda should be used with great caution and in reduced dosage in patients who are concurrently receiving other central nervous system (CNS) depressants including sedatives and hypnotics because of the risk of respiratory depression, hypotension, and profound sedation or coma. When such combined therapy is contemplated, the initial dose of one or both agents should be reduced by at least 50%).
No products indexed under this heading.

Ethinamate (Embeda should be used with great caution and in reduced dosage in patients who are concurrently receiving other central nervous system (CNS) depressants including sedatives and hypnotics because of the risk of respiratory depression, hypotension, and profound sedation or coma. When such combined therapy is contemplated, the initial dose of one or both agents should be reduced by at least 50%).
No products indexed under this heading.

Ethyl Alcohol (Embeda should be used with great caution and in reduced dosage in patients who are concurrently receiving other central nervous system (CNS) depressants including alcohol because of the risk of respiratory depression, hypotension, and profound sedation or coma. When such combined therapy is contemplated, the initial dose of one or both agents should be reduced by at least 50%).
No products indexed under this heading.

Fentanyl (Embeda should be used with great caution and in reduced dosage in patients who are concurrently receiving other central nervous system (CNS) depressants including sedatives, hypnotics, general anesthetics, antiemetics, phenothiazines, other tranquilizers, and alcohol because of the risk of respiratory depression, hypotension, and profound sedation or coma. When such combined therapy is contemplated, the initial dose of one or both agents should be reduced by at least 50%). Products include:
Duragesic **2604**
Fentanyl Transdermal System **2346**
Onsolis **2054**

Fentanyl Citrate (Embeda should be used with great caution and in reduced dosage in patients who are concurrently receiving other central nervous system (CNS) depressants including sedatives, hypnotics, general anesthetics, antiemetics, phenothiazines, other tranquilizers, and alcohol because of the risk of respiratory depression, hypotension, and profound sedation or coma. When such combined therapy is contemplated, the initial dose of one or both agents should be reduced by at least 50%). Products include:
Fentora **966**

Fluphenazine Decanoate (Embeda should be used with great caution and in reduced dosage in patients who are concurrently receiving other central nervous system (CNS) depressants including phenothiazines because of the risk of respiratory depression, hypotension, and profound sedation or coma. When such combined therapy is contemplated, the initial dose of one or both agents should be reduced by at least 50%).
No products indexed under this heading.

Fluphenazine Enanthate (Embeda should be used with great caution and in reduced dosage in patients who are concurrently receiving other central nervous system (CNS) depressants including phenothiazines because of the risk of respiratory depression, hypotension, and profound sedation or coma. When such combined therapy is contemplated, the initial dose of one or both agents should be reduced by at least 50%).
No products indexed under this heading.

Fluphenazine Hydrochloride (Embeda should be used with great caution and in reduced dosage in patients who are concurrently receiving other central nervous system (CNS) depressants including phenothiazines because of the risk of respiratory depression, hypotension, and profound sedation or coma. When such combined therapy is contemplated, the initial dose of one or both agents should be reduced by at least 50%).
No products indexed under this heading.

Flurazepam Hydrochloride (Embeda should be used with great caution and in reduced dosage in patients who are concurrently receiving other central nervous system (CNS) depressants including sedatives and hypnotics because of the risk of respiratory depression, hypotension, and profound sedation or coma. When such combined therapy is contemplated, the initial dose of one or both agents should be reduced by at least 50%).
No products indexed under this heading.

Furosemide (Morphine can reduce the efficacy of diuretics by inducing the release of antidiuretic hormone. Morphine may also lead to acute retention of urine by causing spasm of the sphincter of the bladder, particularly in men with prostatism). Products include:
Furosemide **2354**

Gallamine (Embeda may enhance the neuromuscular blocking action of skeletal relaxants and produce an increased degree of respiratory depression).
No products indexed under this heading.

Gallamine Triethiodide (Embeda may enhance the neuromuscular blocking action of skeletal relaxants and produce an increased degree of respiratory depression).
No products indexed under this heading.

Glutethimide (Embeda should be used with great caution and in reduced dosage in patients who are concurrently receiving other central nervous system (CNS) depressants including sedatives and hypnotics because of the risk of respiratory depression, hypotension, and profound sedation or coma. When such combined therapy is contemplated, the initial dose of one or both agents should be reduced by at least 50%).
No products indexed under this heading.

Glycopyrrolate (Anticholinergics or other medications with anticholinergic activity when used concurrently with opioid analgesics may result in increased risk of urinary retention and/or severe constipation, which may lead to paralytic ileus).
No products indexed under this heading.

Granisetron Hydrochloride (Embeda should be used with great caution and in reduced dosage in patients who are concurrently receiving other central nervous system (CNS) depressants including antiemetic because of the risk of respiratory depression, hypotension, and profound sedation or coma. When such combined therapy is contemplated, the initial dose of one or both agents should be reduced by at least 50%).
No products indexed under this heading.

Halazepam (Embeda should be used with great caution and in reduced dosage in patients who are concurrently receiving other central nervous system (CNS) depressants including sedatives, hypnotics, general anesthetics, antiemetics, phenothiazines, other tranquilizers, and alcohol because of the risk of respiratory depression, hypotension, and profound sedation or coma. When such combined therapy is contemplated, the initial dose of one or both agents should be reduced by at least 50%).
No products indexed under this heading.

Haloperidol (Embeda should be used with great caution and in reduced dosage in patients who are concurrently receiving other central nervous system (CNS) depressants including other tranquilizers because of the risk of respiratory depression, hypotension, and profound sedation or coma. When such combined therapy is contemplated, the initial dose of one or both agents should be reduced by at least 50%).
No products indexed under this heading.

Haloperidol Decanoate (Embeda should be used with great caution and in reduced dosage in patients who are concurrently receiving other central nervous system (CNS) depressants including other tranquilizers because of the risk of respiratory depression, hypotension, and profound sedation or coma. When such combined therapy is contemplated, the initial dose of one or both agents should be reduced by at least 50%).
No products indexed under this heading.

Haloperidol Lactate (Embeda should be used with great caution and in reduced dosage in patients who are concurrently receiving other central nervous system (CNS) depressants including sedatives, hypnotics, general anesthetics, antiemetics, phenothiazines, other tranquilizers, and alcohol because of the risk of respiratory depression, hypotension, and profound sedation or coma. When such combined therapy is contemplated, the initial dose of one or both agents should be reduced by at least 50%).
No products indexed under this heading.

Halothane (Embeda should be used with great caution and in reduced dosage in patients who are concurrently receiving other central nervous system (CNS) depressants including general anesthetics because of the risk of respiratory depression, hypotension, and profound sedation or coma. When such combined therapy is contemplated, the initial dose of one or both agents should be reduced by at least 50%).
No products indexed under this heading.

Hexobarbital (Embeda should be used with great caution and in reduced dosage in patients who are concurrently receiving other central nervous system (CNS) depressants including sedatives, hypnotics, general anesthetics, antiemetics, phenothiazines, other tranquilizers, and alcohol because of the risk of respiratory depression, hypotension, and profound sedation or coma. When such combined therapy is contemplated, the initial dose of one or both agents should be reduced by at least 50%).
No products indexed under this heading.

Hydrochlorothiazide (Morphine can reduce the efficacy of diuretics by inducing the release of antidiuretic hormone. Morphine may also lead to acute retention of urine by causing spasm of the sphincter of the bladder, particularly in men with prostatism). Products include:
Atacand HCT **700**
Avalide **2956**
Benicar HCT **1017**
Diovan HCT **2419**
Dyazide **1429**
Exforge HCT **2449**
Hyzaar **2162**
Hyzaar 100-12.5 .... **2162**
Micardis HCT **889**
Prinzide **2246**

565 **Interactions Index** **Embeda**

Tekturna HCT 2541
Teveten HCT 541

Hydrocodone Bitartrate (Embeda should be used with great caution and in reduced dosage in patients who are concurrently receiving other central nervous system (CNS) depressants including sedatives, hypnotics, general anesthetics, antiemetics, phenothiazines, other tranquilizers, and alcohol because of the risk of respiratory depression, hypotension, and profound sedation or coma. When such combined therapy is contemplated, the initial dose of one or both agents should be reduced by at least 50%). Products include:
Vicodin 560
Vicodin ES 561
Vicodin HP 563
Vicoprofen 564
Zydone 1138

Hydrocodone Polistirex (Embeda should be used with great caution and in reduced dosage in patients who are concurrently receiving other central nervous system (CNS) depressants including sedatives, hypnotics, general anesthetics, antiemetics, phenothiazines, other tranquilizers, and alcohol because of the risk of respiratory depression, hypotension, and profound sedation or coma. When such combined therapy is contemplated, the initial dose of one or both agents should be reduced by at least 50%). Products include:
Tussionex 3443

Hydroflumethiazide (Morphine can reduce the efficacy of diuretics by inducing the release of antidiuretic hormone. Morphine may also lead to acute retention of urine by causing spasm of the sphincter of the bladder, particularly in men with prostatism).
No products indexed under this heading.

Hydromorphone (Embeda should be used with great caution and in reduced dosage in patients who are concurrently receiving other central nervous system (CNS) depressants including sedatives, hypnotics, general anesthetics, antiemetics, phenothiazines, other tranquilizers, and alcohol because of the risk of respiratory depression, hypotension, and profound sedation or coma. When such combined therapy is contemplated, the initial dose of one or both agents should be reduced by at least 50%).
No products indexed under this heading.

Hydromorphone Hydrochloride (Embeda should be used with great caution and in reduced dosage in patients who are concurrently receiving other central nervous system (CNS) depressants including sedatives, hypnotics, general anesthetics, antiemetics, phenothiazines, other tranquilizers, and alcohol because of the risk of respiratory depression, hypotension, and profound sedation or coma. When such combined therapy is contemplated, the initial dose of one or both agents should be reduced by at least 50%). Products include:
Dilaudid Injection 2800
Dilaudid Oral 2797
Dilaudid Tablets 2797
Dilaudid-HP 2800

Hydroxyzine Hydrochloride (Embeda should be used with great caution and in reduced dosage in patients who are concurrently receiving other central nervous system (CNS) depressants including antiemetic because of the risk of respiratory depression, hypotension, and profound sedation or coma. When such combined therapy is contemplated, the initial dose of one or both agents should be reduced by at least 50%).
No products indexed under this heading.

Hyoscyamine (Anticholinergics or other medications with anticholinergic activity when used concurrently with opioid analgesics may result in increased risk of urinary retention and/or severe constipation, which may lead to paralytic ileus).
No products indexed under this heading.

Hyoscyamine Sulfate (Anticholinergics or other medications with anticholinergic activity when used concurrently with opioid analgesics may result in increased risk of urinary retention and/or severe constipation, which may lead to paralytic ileus). Products include:
Donnatal 2711

Indapamide (Morphine can reduce the efficacy of diuretics by inducing the release of antidiuretic hormone. Morphine may also lead to acute retention of urine by causing spasm of the sphincter of the bladder, particularly in men with prostatism). Products include:
Indapamide 2356

Ipratropium Bromide (Anticholinergics or other medications with anticholinergic activity when used concurrently with opioid analgesics may result in increased risk of urinary retention and/or severe constipation, which may lead to paralytic ileus).
No products indexed under this heading.

Isocarboxazid (MAOIs have been reported to potentiate the effects of morphine anxiety, confusion, and significant depression of respiration or coma. Embeda should not be used in patients taking MAOIs or within 14 days of stopping such treatment). Products include:
Marplan 3481

Isoflurane (Embeda should be used with great caution and in reduced dosage in patients who are concurrently receiving other central nervous system (CNS) depressants including general anesthetics because of the risk of respiratory depression, hypotension, and profound sedation or coma. When such combined therapy is contemplated, the initial dose of one or both agents should be reduced by at least 50%).
No products indexed under this heading.

Itraconazole (Based on published reports, PGP inhibitors may increase the absorption/exposure of morphine sulfate by about two fold. Therefore, caution should be exercised when morphine sulfate is co-administered with PGP inhibitors).
No products indexed under this heading.

Ketamine Hydrochloride (Embeda should be used with great caution and in reduced dosage in patients who are concurrently receiving other central nervous system (CNS) depressants including general anesthetics because of the risk of respiratory depression, hypotension, and profound sedation or coma. When such combined therapy is contemplated, the initial dose of one or both agents should be reduced by at least 50%).
No products indexed under this heading.

Ketoconazole (Based on published reports, PGP inhibitors may increase the absorption/exposure of morphine sulfate by about two fold. Therefore, caution should be exercised when morphine sulfate is co-administered with PGP inhibitors). Products include:
Extina 3319
Xolegel 3337

Levomethadyl Acetate Hydrochloride (Embeda should be used with great caution and in reduced dosage in patients who are concurrently receiving other central nervous system (CNS) depressants including sedatives, hypnotics, general anesthetics, antiemetics, phenothiazines, other tranquilizers, and alcohol because of the risk of respiratory depression, hypotension, and profound sedation or coma. When such combined therapy is contemplated, the initial dose of one or both agents should be reduced by at least 50%).
No products indexed under this heading.

Levorphanol Tartrate (Embeda should be used with great caution and in reduced dosage in patients who are concurrently receiving other central nervous system (CNS) depressants including sedatives, hypnotics, general anesthetics, antiemetics, phenothiazines, other tranquilizers, and alcohol because of the risk of respiratory depression, hypotension, and profound sedation or coma. When such combined therapy is contemplated, the initial dose of one or both agents should be reduced by at least 50%).
No products indexed under this heading.

Lorazepam (Embeda should be used with great caution and in reduced dosage in patients who are concurrently receiving other central nervous system (CNS) depressants including sedatives and hypnotics because of the risk of respiratory depression, hypotension, and profound sedation or coma. When such combined therapy is contemplated, the initial dose of one or both agents should be reduced by at least 50%).
No products indexed under this heading.

Loxapine Hydrochloride (Embeda should be used with great caution and in reduced dosage in patients who are concurrently receiving other central nervous system (CNS) depressants including other tranquilizers because of the risk of respiratory depression, hypotension, and profound sedation or coma. When such combined therapy is contemplated, the initial dose of one or both agents should be reduced by at least 50%).
No products indexed under this heading.

Loxapine Succinate (Embeda should be used with great caution and in reduced dosage in patients who are concurrently receiving other central nervous system (CNS) depressants including other tranquilizers because of the risk of respiratory depression, hypotension, and profound sedation or coma. When such combined therapy is contemplated, the initial dose of one or both agents should be reduced by at least 50%).
No products indexed under this heading.

Meclizine Hydrochloride (Embeda should be used with great caution and in reduced dosage in patients who are concurrently receiving other central nervous system (CNS) depressants including antiemetic because of the risk of respiratory depression, hypotension, and profound sedation or coma. When such combined therapy is contemplated, the initial dose of one or both agents should be reduced by at least 50%).
No products indexed under this heading.

Mepenzolate Bromide (Anticholinergics or other medications with anticholinergic activity when used concurrently with opioid analgesics may result in increased risk of urinary retention and/or severe constipation, which may lead to paralytic ileus).
No products indexed under this heading.

Meperidine Hydrochloride (Embeda should be used with great caution and in reduced dosage in patients who are concurrently receiving other central nervous system (CNS) depressants including sedatives, hypnotics, general anesthetics, antiemetics, phenothiazines, other tranquilizers, and alcohol because of the risk of respiratory depression, hypotension, and profound sedation or coma. When such combined therapy is contemplated, the initial dose of one or both agents should be reduced by at least 50%).
No products indexed under this heading.

Mephobarbital (Embeda should be used with great caution and in reduced dosage in patients who are concurrently receiving other central nervous system (CNS) depressants including sedatives, hypnotics, general anesthetics, antiemetics, phenothiazines, other tranquilizers, and alcohol because of the risk of respiratory depression, hypotension, and profound sedation or coma. When such combined therapy is contemplated, the initial dose of one or both agents should be reduced by at least 50%).
No products indexed under this heading.

Meprobamate (Embeda should be used with great caution and in reduced dosage in patients who are concurrently receiving other central nervous system (CNS) depressants including other tranquilizers because of the risk of respiratory depression, hypotension, and profound sedation or coma. When such combined therapy is contemplated, the initial dose of one or both agents should be reduced by at least 50%).
No products indexed under this heading.

Mesoridazine Besylate (Embeda should be used with great caution and in reduced dosage in patients who are concurrently receiving other central nervous system (CNS) depressants including phenothiazines because of the risk of respiratory depression, hypotension, and profound sedation or coma. When such combined therapy is contemplated, the initial dose of one or both agents should be reduced by at least 50%).
No products indexed under this heading.

Metaxalone (Embeda may enhance the neuromuscular blocking action of skeletal relaxants and produce an increased degree of respiratory depression). Products include:
Skelaxin 1848

Methadone Hydrochloride (Embeda should be used with great caution and in reduced dosage in patients who are concurrently receiving other central nervous system (CNS) depressants including sedatives, hypnotics, general anesthetics, antiemetics, phenothiazines, other tranquilizers, and alcohol because of the risk of respiratory depression, hypotension, and profound sedation or coma. When such combined therapy is contemplated, the initial dose of one or both agents should be reduced by at least 50%).
No products indexed under this heading.

Methocarbamol (Embeda may enhance the neuromuscular blocking action of skeletal relaxants and produce an increased degree of respiratory depression).
No products indexed under this heading.

Methohexital Sodium (Embeda should be used with great caution and in reduced dosage in patients who are concurrently receiving other central nervous system (CNS) depressants including general anesthetics because of the risk of respiratory depression, hypotension, and profound sedation or coma. When such combined therapy is contemplated, the initial dose of one or both agents should be reduced by at least 50%).
No products indexed under this heading.

Methotrimeprazine (Embeda should be used with great caution and in reduced dosage in patients who are concurrently receiving other central nervous system (CNS) depressants including phenothiazines because of the risk of respiratory depression, hypotension, and profound sedation or coma.

IMPORTANT NOTE: Always consult each drug listing in the patient's regimen for possible interactions.

Embeda Interactions Index 566

When such combined therapy is contemplated, the initial dose of one or both agents should be reduced by at least 50%).
No products indexed under this heading.

Methoxyflurane (Embeda should be used with great caution and in reduced dosage in patients who are concurrently receiving other central nervous system (CNS) depressants including general anesthetics because of the risk of respiratory depression, hypotension, and profound sedation or coma. When such combined therapy is contemplated, the initial dose of one or both agents should be reduced by at least 50%).
No products indexed under this heading.

Methyclothiazide (Morphine can reduce the efficacy of diuretics by inducing the release of antidiuretic hormone. Morphine may also lead to acute retention of urine by causing spasm of the sphincter of the bladder, particularly in men with prostatism).
No products indexed under this heading.

Metoclopramide Hydrochloride (Embeda should be used with great caution and in reduced dosage in patients who are concurrently receiving other central nervous system (CNS) depressants including antiemetic because of the risk of respiratory depression, hypotension, and profound sedation or coma. When such combined therapy is contemplated, the initial dose of one or both agents should be reduced by at least 50%). Products include:
Metozolv ODT 2901

Metocurine Iodide (Embeda may enhance the neuromuscular blocking action of skeletal relaxants and produce an increased degree of respiratory depression).
No products indexed under this heading.

Metolazone (Morphine can reduce the efficacy of diuretics by inducing the release of antidiuretic hormone. Morphine may also lead to acute retention of urine by causing spasm of the sphincter of the bladder, particularly in men with prostatism).
No products indexed under this heading.

Mibefradil Dihydrochloride (Based on published reports, PGP inhibitors may increase the absorption/exposure of morphine sulfate by about two fold. Therefore, caution should be exercised when morphine sulfate is co-administered with PGP inhibitors).
No products indexed under this heading.

Midazolam Hydrochloride (Embeda should be used with great caution and in reduced dosage in patients who are concurrently receiving other central nervous system (CNS) depressants including sedatives and hypnotics because of the risk of respiratory depression, hypotension, and profound sedation or coma. When such combined therapy is contemplated, the initial dose of one or both agents should be reduced by at least 50%).
No products indexed under this heading.

Mivacurium Chloride (Embeda may enhance the neuromuscular blocking action of skeletal relaxants and produce an increased degree of respiratory depression).
No products indexed under this heading.

Moclobemide (MAOIs have been reported to potentiate the effects of morphine anxiety, confusion, and significant depression of respiration or coma. Embeda should not be used in patients taking MAOIs or within 14 days of stopping such treatment).
No products indexed under this heading.

Molindone Hydrochloride (Embeda should be used with great caution and in reduced dosage in patients who are concurrently receiving other central nervous system (CNS) depressants including other tranquilizers because of the risk of respiratory depression, hypotension, and profound sedation or coma. When such combined therapy is contemplated, the initial dose of one or both agents should be reduced by at least 50%). Products include:
Moban 1108

Morphine Sulfate, Liposomal (Embeda should be used with great caution and in reduced dosage in patients who are concurrently receiving other central nervous system (CNS) depressants including sedatives, hypnotics, general anesthetics, antiemetics, phenothiazines, other tranquilizers, and alcohol because of the risk of respiratory depression, hypotension, and profound sedation or coma. When such combined therapy is contemplated, the initial dose of one or both agents should be reduced by at least 50%).
No products indexed under this heading.

Nabilone (Embeda should be used with great caution and in reduced dosage in patients who are concurrently receiving other central nervous system (CNS) depressants including antiemetic because of the risk of respiratory depression, hypotension, and profound sedation or coma. When such combined therapy is contemplated, the initial dose of one or both agents should be reduced by at least 50%).
No products indexed under this heading.

Nalbuphine Hydrochloride (Agonist/antagonist analgesics (ie, pentazocine, nalbuphine, butorphanol) should be administered with caution to a patient who has received or is receiving a course of therapy with Embeda. In this situation, mixed agonist/antagonist analgesics may reduce the analgesic effect of Embeda and/or may precipitate withdrawal symptoms in these patients).
No products indexed under this heading.

Nitrous Oxide (Embeda should be used with great caution and in reduced dosage in patients who are concurrently receiving other central nervous system (CNS) depressants including general anesthetics because of the risk of respiratory depression, hypotension, and profound sedation or coma. When such combined therapy is contemplated, the initial dose of one or both agents should be reduced by at least 50%).
No products indexed under this heading.

Olanzapine (Embeda should be used with great caution and in reduced dosage in patients who are concurrently receiving other central nervous system (CNS) depressants including sedatives, hypnotics, general anesthetics, antiemetics, phenothiazines, other tranquilizers, and alcohol because of the risk of respiratory depression, hypotension, and profound sedation or coma. When such combined therapy is contemplated, the initial dose of one or both agents should be reduced by at least 50%). Products include:
Symbyax 1965
Zyprexa 1984
Zyprexa IntraMuscular 1984
Zyprexa ZYDIS 1984

Ondansetron (Embeda should be used with great caution and in reduced dosage in patients who are concurrently receiving other central nervous system (CNS) depressants including antiemetic because of the risk of respiratory depression, hypotension, and profound sedation or coma. When such combined therapy is contemplated, the initial dose of one or both agents should be reduced by at least 50%).
No products indexed under this heading.

Ondansetron Hydrochloride (Embeda should be used with great caution and in reduced dosage in patients who are concurrently receiving other central nervous system (CNS) depressants including antiemetic because of the risk of respiratory depression, hypotension, and profound sedation or coma. When such combined therapy is contemplated, the initial dose of one or both agents should be reduced by at least 50%). Products include:
Zofran Injection 1750
Zofran 1756
Zofran ODT 1756

Orphenadrine Citrate (Embeda may enhance the neuromuscular blocking action of skeletal relaxants and produce an increased degree of respiratory depression).
No products indexed under this heading.

Oxazepam (Embeda should be used with great caution and in reduced dosage in patients who are concurrently receiving other central nervous system (CNS) depressants including other tranquilizers because of the risk of respiratory depression, hypotension, and profound sedation or coma. When such combined therapy is contemplated, the initial dose of one or both agents should be reduced by at least 50%).
No products indexed under this heading.

Oxybutynin Chloride (Anticholinergics or other medications with anticholinergic activity when used concurrently with opioid analgesics may result in increased risk of urinary retention and/or severe constipation, which may lead to paralytic ileus).
No products indexed under this heading.

Oxycodone Hydrochloride (Embeda should be used with great caution and in reduced dosage in patients who are concurrently receiving other central nervous system (CNS) depressants including sedatives, hypnotics, general anesthetics, antiemetics, phenothiazines, other tranquilizers, and alcohol because of the risk of respiratory depression, hypotension, and profound sedation or coma. When such combined therapy is contemplated, the initial dose of one or both agents should be reduced by at least 50%). Products include:
OxyContin 2807
Percocet 1121
Percodan 1124

Oxycodone Terephthalate (Embeda should be used with great caution and in reduced dosage in patients who are concurrently receiving other central nervous system (CNS) depressants including sedatives, hypnotics, general anesthetics, antiemetics, phenothiazines, other tranquilizers, and alcohol because of the risk of respiratory depression, hypotension, and profound sedation or coma. When such combined therapy is contemplated, the initial dose of one or both agents should be reduced by at least 50%).
No products indexed under this heading.

Oxymorphone Hydrochloride (Embeda should be used with great caution and in reduced dosage in patients who are concurrently receiving other central nervous system (CNS) depressants including sedatives, hypnotics, general anesthetics, antiemetics, phenothiazines, other tranquilizers, and alcohol because of the risk of respiratory depression, hypotension, and profound sedation or coma. When such combined therapy is contemplated, the initial dose of one or both agents should be reduced by at least 50%). Products include:
Opana 1110
Opana ER 1114

Palonosetron Hydrochloride (Embeda should be used with great caution and in reduced dosage in patients who are concurrently receiving other central nervous system (CNS) depressants including antiemetic because of the risk of respiratory depression, hypotension, and profound sedation or coma. When such combined therapy is contemplated, the initial dose of one or both agents should be reduced by at least 50%). Products include:
Aloxi 1042

Pancuronium Bromide (Embeda may enhance the neuromuscular blocking action of skeletal relaxants and produce an increased degree of respiratory depression).
No products indexed under this heading.

Pargyline Hydrochloride (MAOIs have been reported to potentiate the effects of morphine anxiety, confusion, and significant depression of respiration or coma. Embeda should not be used in patients taking MAOIs or within 14 days of stopping such treatment).
No products indexed under this heading.

Pentazocine Hydrochloride (Agonist/antagonist analgesics (ie, pentazocine, nalbuphine, butorphanol) should be administered with caution to a patient who has received or is receiving a course of therapy with Embeda. In this situation, mixed agonist/antagonist analgesics may reduce the analgesic effect of Embeda and/or may precipitate withdrawal symptoms in these patients).
No products indexed under this heading.

Pentazocine Lactate (Agonist/antagonist analgesics (ie, pentazocine, nalbuphine, butorphanol) should be administered with caution to a patient who has received or is receiving a course of therapy with Embeda. In this situation, mixed agonist/antagonist analgesics may reduce the analgesic effect of Embeda and/or may precipitate withdrawal symptoms in these patients).
No products indexed under this heading.

Pentobarbital (Embeda should be used with great caution and in reduced dosage in patients who are concurrently receiving other central nervous system (CNS) depressants including sedatives, hypnotics, general anesthetics, antiemetics, phenothiazines, other tranquilizers, and alcohol because of the risk of respiratory depression, hypotension, and profound sedation or coma. When such combined therapy is contemplated, the initial dose of one or both agents should be reduced by at least 50%).
No products indexed under this heading.

Pentobarbital Sodium (Embeda should be used with great caution and in reduced dosage in patients who are concurrently receiving other central nervous system (CNS) depressants including sedatives, hypnotics, general anesthetics, antiemetics, phenothiazines, other tranquilizers, and alcohol because of the risk of respiratory depression, hypotension, and profound sedation or coma. When such combined therapy is contemplated, the initial dose of one or both agents should be reduced by at least 50%). Products include:
Nembutal 2012

Perphenazine (Embeda should be used with great caution and in reduced dosage in patients who are concurrently receiving other central nervous system (CNS) depressants including antiemetic because of the risk of respiratory depression, hypotension, and profound sedation or coma. When such combined therapy is contemplated, the initial dose of one or both agents should be reduced by at least 50%).
No products indexed under this heading.

(⊙ Described in PDR® for Ophthalmic Medicines)

567 Interactions Index Embeda

Phenelzine Sulfate (MAOIs have been reported to potentiate the effects of morphine anxiety, confusion, and significant depression of respiration or coma. Embeda should not be used in patients taking MAOIs or within 14 days of stopping such treatment).
No products indexed under this heading.

Phenobarbital (Embeda should be used with great caution and in reduced dosage in patients who are concurrently receiving other central nervous system (CNS) depressants including sedatives, hypnotics, general anesthetics, antiemetics, phenothiazines, other tranquilizers, and alcohol because of the risk of respiratory depression, hypotension, and profound sedation or coma. When such combined therapy is contemplated, the initial dose of one or both agents should be reduced by at least 50%). Products include:
Donnatal 2711

Phenobarbital Sodium (Embeda should be used with great caution and in reduced dosage in patients who are concurrently receiving other central nervous system (CNS) depressants including sedatives, hypnotics, general anesthetics, antiemetics, phenothiazines, other tranquilizers, and alcohol because of the risk of respiratory depression, hypotension, and profound sedation or coma. When such combined therapy is contemplated, the initial dose of one or both agents should be reduced by at least 50%).
No products indexed under this heading.

Phenothiazine Derivatives (Embeda should be used with great caution and in reduced dosage in patients who are concurrently receiving other central nervous system (CNS) depressants including phenothiazines because of the risk of respiratory depression, hypotension, and profound sedation or coma. When such combined therapy is contemplated, the initial dose of one or both agents should be reduced by at least 50%).
No products indexed under this heading.

Phenothiazines (Embeda should be used with great caution and in reduced dosage in patients who are concurrently receiving other central nervous system (CNS) depressants including phenothiazines because of the risk of respiratory depression, hypotension, and profound sedation or coma. When such combined therapy is contemplated, the initial dose of one or both agents should be reduced by at least 50%).
No products indexed under this heading.

Pipecuronium Bromide (Embeda may enhance the neuromuscular blocking action of skeletal relaxants and produce an increased degree of respiratory depression).
No products indexed under this heading.

Polythiazide (Morphine can reduce the efficacy of diuretics by inducing the release of antidiuretic hormone. Morphine may also lead to acute retention of urine by causing spasm of the sphincter of the bladder, particularly in men with prostatism).
No products indexed under this heading.

Prazepam (Embeda should be used with great caution and in reduced dosage in patients who are concurrently receiving other central nervous system (CNS) depressants including other tranquilizers because of the risk of respiratory depression, hypotension, and profound sedation or coma. When such combined therapy is contemplated, the initial dose of one or both agents should be reduced by at least 50%).
No products indexed under this heading.

Procarbazine Hydrochloride (MAOIs have been reported to potentiate the effects of morphine anxiety, confusion, and significant depression of respiration or coma. Embeda should not be used in patients taking MAOIs or within 14 days of stopping such treatment).
No products indexed under this heading.

Prochlorperazine (Embeda should be used with great caution and in reduced dosage in patients who are concurrently receiving other central nervous system (CNS) depressants including antiemetic because of the risk of respiratory depression, hypotension, and profound sedation or coma. When such combined therapy is contemplated, the initial dose of one or both agents should be reduced by at least 50%).
No products indexed under this heading.

Prochlorperazine Edisylate (Embeda should be used with great caution and in reduced dosage in patients who are concurrently receiving other central nervous system (CNS) depressants including antiemetic because of the risk of respiratory depression, hypotension, and profound sedation or coma. When such combined therapy is contemplated, the initial dose of one or both agents should be reduced by at least 50%).
No products indexed under this heading.

Prochlorperazine Maleate (Embeda should be used with great caution and in reduced dosage in patients who are concurrently receiving other central nervous system (CNS) depressants including antiemetic because of the risk of respiratory depression, hypotension, and profound sedation or coma. When such combined therapy is contemplated, the initial dose of one or both agents should be reduced by at least 50%).
No products indexed under this heading.

Procyclidine Hydrochloride (Anticholinergics or other medications with anticholinergic activity when used concurrently with opioid analgesics may result in increased risk of urinary retention and/or severe constipation, which may lead to paralytic ileus).
No products indexed under this heading.

Promethazine (Embeda should be used with great caution and in reduced dosage in patients who are concurrently receiving other central nervous system (CNS) depressants including antiemetic because of the risk of respiratory depression, hypotension, and profound sedation or coma. When such combined therapy is contemplated, the initial dose of one or both agents should be reduced by at least 50%).
No products indexed under this heading.

Promethazine Hydrochloride (Embeda should be used with great caution and in reduced dosage in patients who are concurrently receiving other central nervous system (CNS) depressants including antiemetic because of the risk of respiratory depression, hypotension, and profound sedation or coma. When such combined therapy is contemplated, the initial dose of one or both agents should be reduced by at least 50%).
No products indexed under this heading.

Propantheline Bromide (Anticholinergics or other medications with anticholinergic activity when used concurrently with opioid analgesics may result in increased risk of urinary retention and/or severe constipation, which may lead to paralytic ileus).
No products indexed under this heading.

Propofol (Embeda should be used with great caution and in reduced dosage in patients who are concurrently receiving other central nervous system (CNS) depressants including sedatives and hypnotics because of the risk of respiratory depression, hypotension, and profound sedation or coma. When such combined therapy is contemplated, the initial dose of one or both agents should be reduced by at least 50%).
No products indexed under this heading.

Propoxyphene Hydrochloride (Embeda should be used with great caution and in reduced dosage in patients who are concurrently receiving other central nervous system (CNS) depressants including sedatives, hypnotics, general anesthetics, antiemetics, phenothiazines, other tranquilizers, and alcohol because of the risk of respiratory depression, hypotension, and profound sedation or coma. When such combined therapy is contemplated, the initial dose of one or both agents should be reduced by at least 50%).
No products indexed under this heading.

Propoxyphene Napsylate (Embeda should be used with great caution and in reduced dosage in patients who are concurrently receiving other central nervous system (CNS) depressants including sedatives, hypnotics, general anesthetics, antiemetics, phenothiazines, other tranquilizers, and alcohol because of the risk of respiratory depression, hypotension, and profound sedation or coma. When such combined therapy is contemplated, the initial dose of one or both agents should be reduced by at least 50%).
No products indexed under this heading.

Quazepam (Embeda should be used with great caution and in reduced dosage in patients who are concurrently receiving other central nervous system (CNS) depressants including sedatives and hypnotics because of the risk of respiratory depression, hypotension, and profound sedation or coma. When such combined therapy is contemplated, the initial dose of one or both agents should be reduced by at least 50%).
No products indexed under this heading.

Quetiapine Fumarate (Embeda should be used with great caution and in reduced dosage in patients who are concurrently receiving other central nervous system (CNS) depressants including sedatives, hypnotics, general anesthetics, antiemetics, phenothiazines, other tranquilizers, and alcohol because of the risk of respiratory depression, hypotension, and profound sedation or coma. When such combined therapy is contemplated, the initial dose of one or both agents should be reduced by at least 50%). Products include:
Seroquel 750
Seroquel XR 759

Quinidine (Based on published reports, PGP inhibitors (eg, quinidine) may increase the absorption/exposure of morphine sulfate by about two fold. Therefore, caution should be exercised when morphine sulfate is co-administered with PGP inhibitors).
No products indexed under this heading.

Quinidine Gluconate (Based on published reports, PGP inhibitors (eg, quinidine) may increase the absorption/exposure of morphine sulfate by about two fold. Therefore, caution should be exercised when morphine sulfate is co-administered with PGP inhibitors).
No products indexed under this heading.

Quinidine Hydrochloride (Based on published reports, PGP inhibitors (eg, quinidine) may increase the absorption/exposure of morphine sulfate by about two fold. Therefore, caution should be exercised when morphine sulfate is co-administered with PGP inhibitors).
No products indexed under this heading.

Quinidine Polygalacturonate (Based on published reports, PGP inhibitors (eg, quinidine) may increase the absorption/exposure of morphine sulfate by about two fold. Therefore, caution should be exercised when morphine sulfate is co-administered with PGP inhibitors).
No products indexed under this heading.

Quinidine Sulfate (Based on published reports, PGP inhibitors (eg, quinidine) may increase the absorption/exposure of morphine sulfate by about two fold. Therefore, caution should be exercised when morphine sulfate is co-administered with PGP inhibitors).
No products indexed under this heading.

Ramelteon (Embeda should be used with great caution and in reduced dosage in patients who are concurrently receiving other central nervous system (CNS) depressants including sedatives and hypnotics because of the risk of respiratory depression, hypotension, and profound sedation or coma. When such combined therapy is contemplated, the initial dose of one or both agents should be reduced by at least 50%). Products include:
Rozerem 3366

Rapacuronium Bromide (Embeda may enhance the neuromuscular blocking action of skeletal relaxants and produce an increased degree of respiratory depression).
No products indexed under this heading.

Rasagiline Mesylate (MAOIs have been reported to potentiate the effects of morphine anxiety, confusion, and significant depression of respiration or coma. Embeda should not be used in patients taking MAOIs or within 14 days of stopping such treatment). Products include:
Azilect 3383

Remifentanil Hydrochloride (Embeda should be used with great caution and in reduced dosage in patients who are concurrently receiving other central nervous system (CNS) depressants including sedatives, hypnotics, general anesthetics, antiemetics, phenothiazines, other tranquilizers, and alcohol because of the risk of respiratory depression, hypotension, and profound sedation or coma. When such combined therapy is contemplated, the initial dose of one or both agents should be reduced by at least 50%).
No products indexed under this heading.

Risperidone (Embeda should be used with great caution and in reduced dosage in patients who are concurrently receiving other central nervous system (CNS) depressants including sedatives, hypnotics, general anesthetics, antiemetics, phenothiazines, other tranquilizers, and alcohol because of the risk of respiratory depression, hypotension, and profound sedation or coma. When such combined therapy is contemplated, the initial dose of one or both agents should be reduced by at least 50%). Products include:
Risperdal Consta 2682

Ritonavir (Based on published reports, PGP inhibitors may increase the absorption/exposure of morphine sulfate by about two fold. Therefore, caution should be exercised when morphine sulfate is co-administered with PGP inhibitors). Products include:
Kaletra 458
Norvir 509

Rocuronium Bromide (Embeda may enhance the neuromuscular blocking action of skeletal relaxants and produce an increased degree of respiratory depression). Products include:
Zemuron 3249

Scopolamine (Embeda should be used with great caution and in reduced

IMPORTANT NOTE: Always consult each drug listing in the patient's regimen for possible interactions.

dosage in patients who are concurrently receiving other central nervous system (CNS) depressants including antiemetic because of the risk of respiratory depression, hypotension, and profound sedation or coma. When such combined therapy is contemplated, the initial dose of one or both agents should be reduced by at least 50%). Products include:

Transderm Scōp 2397

Scopolamine Hydrobromide (Embeda should be used with great caution and in reduced dosage in patients who are concurrently receiving other central nervous system (CNS) depressants including antiemetic because of the risk of respiratory depression, hypotension, and profound sedation or coma. When such combined therapy is contemplated, the initial dose of one or both agents should be reduced by at least 50%). Products include:

Donnatal 2711

Secobarbital Sodium (Embeda should be used with great caution and in reduced dosage in patients who are concurrently receiving other central nervous system (CNS) depressants including sedatives and hypnotics because of the risk of respiratory depression, hypotension, and profound sedation or coma. When such combined therapy is contemplated, the initial dose of one or both agents should be reduced by at least 50%).

No products indexed under this heading.

Selegiline (MAOIs have been reported to potentiate the effects of morphine anxiety, confusion, and significant depression of respiration or coma. Embeda should not be used in patients taking MAOIs or within 14 days of stopping such treatment). Products include:

Emsam 3623

Selegiline Hydrochloride (MAOIs have been reported to potentiate the effects of morphine anxiety, confusion, and significant depression of respiration or coma. Embeda should not be used in patients taking MAOIs or within 14 days of stopping such treatment). Products include:

Eldepryl 3312

Sevoflurane (Embeda should be used with great caution and in reduced dosage in patients who are concurrently receiving other central nervous system (CNS) depressants including general anesthetics because of the risk of respiratory depression, hypotension, and profound sedation or coma. When such combined therapy is contemplated, the initial dose of one or both agents should be reduced by at least 50%). Products include:

Ultane 554

Sodium Butabarbital (Embeda should be used with great caution and in reduced dosage in patients who are concurrently receiving other central nervous system (CNS) depressants including sedatives and hypnotics because of the risk of respiratory depression, hypotension, and profound sedation or coma. When such combined therapy is contemplated, the initial dose of one or both agents should be reduced by at least 50%).

No products indexed under this heading.

Sodium Oxybate (Embeda should be used with great caution and in reduced dosage in patients who are concurrently receiving other central nervous system (CNS) depressants including sedatives, hypnotics, general anesthetics, antiemetics, phenothiazines, other tranquilizers, and alcohol because of the risk of respiratory depression, hypotension, and profound sedation or coma. When such combined therapy is contemplated, the initial dose of one or both agents should be reduced by at least 50%).

No products indexed under this heading.

Sodium Pentobarbital (Embeda should be used with great caution and in reduced dosage in patients who are concurrently receiving other central nervous system (CNS) depressants including sedatives, hypnotics, general anesthetics, antiemetics, phenothiazines, other tranquilizers, and alcohol because of the risk of respiratory depression, hypotension, and profound sedation or coma. When such combined therapy is contemplated, the initial dose of one or both agents should be reduced by at least 50%).

No products indexed under this heading.

Spironolactone (Morphine can reduce the efficacy of diuretics by inducing the release of antidiuretic hormone. Morphine may also lead to acute retention of urine by causing spasm of the sphincter of the bladder, particularly in men with prostatism).

No products indexed under this heading.

Succinylcholine Chloride (Embeda may enhance the neuromuscular blocking action of skeletal relaxants and produce an increased degree of respiratory depression).

No products indexed under this heading.

Sufentanil Citrate (Embeda should be used with great caution and in reduced dosage in patients who are concurrently receiving other central nervous system (CNS) depressants including sedatives, hypnotics, general anesthetics, antiemetics, phenothiazines, other tranquilizers, and alcohol because of the risk of respiratory depression, hypotension, and profound sedation or coma. When such combined therapy is contemplated, the initial dose of one or both agents should be reduced by at least 50%).

No products indexed under this heading.

Talbutal (Embeda should be used with great caution and in reduced dosage in patients who are concurrently receiving other central nervous system (CNS) depressants including sedatives, hypnotics, general anesthetics, antiemetics, phenothiazines, other tranquilizers, and alcohol because of the risk of respiratory depression, hypotension, and profound sedation or coma. When such combined therapy is contemplated, the initial dose of one or both agents should be reduced by at least 50%).

No products indexed under this heading.

Tamoxifen Citrate (Based on published reports, PGP inhibitors may increase the absorption/exposure of morphine sulfate by about two fold. Therefore, caution should be exercised when morphine sulfate is co-administered with PGP inhibitors).

No products indexed under this heading.

Temazepam (Embeda should be used with great caution and in reduced dosage in patients who are concurrently receiving other central nervous system (CNS) depressants including sedatives and hypnotics because of the risk of respiratory depression, hypotension, and profound sedation or coma. When such combined therapy is contemplated, the initial dose of one or both agents should be reduced by at least 50%).

No products indexed under this heading.

Thiamylal Sodium (Embeda should be used with great caution and in reduced dosage in patients who are concurrently receiving other central nervous system (CNS) depressants including sedatives, hypnotics, general anesthetics, antiemetics, phenothiazines, other tranquilizers, and alcohol because of the risk of respiratory depression, hypotension, and profound sedation or coma. When such combined therapy is contemplated, the initial dose of one or both agents should be reduced by at least 50%).

No products indexed under this heading.

Thioridazine (Embeda should be used with great caution and in reduced dosage in patients who are concurrently receiving other central nervous system (CNS) depressants including phenothiazines because of the risk of respiratory depression, hypotension, and profound sedation or coma. When such combined therapy is contemplated, the initial dose of one or both agents should be reduced by at least 50%).

No products indexed under this heading.

Thioridazine Hydrochloride (Embeda should be used with great caution and in reduced dosage in patients who are concurrently receiving other central nervous system (CNS) depressants including phenothiazines because of the risk of respiratory depression, hypotension, and profound sedation or coma. When such combined therapy is contemplated, the initial dose of one or both agents should be reduced by at least 50%). Products include:

Thioridazine Hydrochloride 2384

Thiothixene (Embeda should be used with great caution and in reduced dosage in patients who are concurrently receiving other central nervous system (CNS) depressants including other tranquilizers because of the risk of respiratory depression, hypotension, and profound sedation or coma. When such combined therapy is contemplated, the initial dose of one or both agents should be reduced by at least 50%). Products include:

Thiothixene 2386

Thiothixene Hydrochloride (Embeda should be used with great caution and in reduced dosage in patients who are concurrently receiving other central nervous system (CNS) depressants including sedatives, hypnotics, general anesthetics, antiemetics, phenothiazines, other tranquilizers, and alcohol because of the risk of respiratory depression, hypotension, and profound sedation or coma. When such combined therapy is contemplated, the initial dose of one or both agents should be reduced by at least 50%).

No products indexed under this heading.

Tizanidine (Embeda may enhance the neuromuscular blocking action of skeletal relaxants and produce an increased degree of respiratory depression).

No products indexed under this heading.

Tizanidine Hydrochloride (Embeda may enhance the neuromuscular blocking action of skeletal relaxants and produce an increased degree of respiratory depression).

No products indexed under this heading.

Tolterodine Tartrate (Anticholinergics or other medications with anticholinergic activity when used concurrently with opioid analgesics may result in increased risk of urinary retention and/or severe constipation, which may lead to paralytic ileus).

No products indexed under this heading.

Torsemide (Morphine can reduce the efficacy of diuretics by inducing the release of antidiuretic hormone. Morphine may also lead to acute retention of urine by causing spasm of the sphincter of the bladder, particularly in men with prostatism).

No products indexed under this heading.

Tranylcypromine Sulfate (MAOIs have been reported to potentiate the effects of morphine anxiety, confusion, and significant depression of respiration or coma. Embeda should not be used in patients taking MAOIs or within 14 days of stopping such treatment). Products include:

Parnate 1584

Triamterene (Morphine can reduce the efficacy of diuretics by inducing the release of antidiuretic hormone. Morphine may also lead to acute retention of urine by causing spasm of the sphincter of the bladder, particularly in men with prostatism). Products include:

Dyazide 1429
Dyrenium 3495

Triazolam (Embeda should be used with great caution and in reduced dosage in patients who are concurrently receiving other central nervous system (CNS) depressants including sedatives and hypnotics because of the risk of respiratory depression, hypotension, and profound sedation or coma. When such combined therapy is contemplated, the initial dose of one or both agents should be reduced by at least 50%).

No products indexed under this heading.

Tridihexethyl Chloride (Anticholinergics or other medications with anticholinergic activity when used concurrently with opioid analgesics may result in increased risk of urinary retention and/or severe constipation, which may lead to paralytic ileus).

No products indexed under this heading.

Trifluoperazine Hydrochloride (Embeda should be used with great caution and in reduced dosage in patients who are concurrently receiving other central nervous system (CNS) depressants including phenothiazines because of the risk of respiratory depression, hypotension, and profound sedation or coma. When such combined therapy is contemplated, the initial dose of one or both agents should be reduced by at least 50%).

No products indexed under this heading.

Trihexyphenidyl Hydrochloride (Anticholinergics or other medications with anticholinergic activity when used concurrently with opioid analgesics may result in increased risk of urinary retention and/or severe constipation, which may lead to paralytic ileus).

No products indexed under this heading.

Trimethobenzamide Hydrochloride (Embeda should be used with great caution and in reduced dosage in patients who are concurrently receiving other central nervous system (CNS) depressants including antiemetic because of the risk of respiratory depression, hypotension, and profound sedation or coma. When such combined therapy is contemplated, the initial dose of one or both agents should be reduced by at least 50%).

No products indexed under this heading.

Troleandomycin (Based on published reports, PGP inhibitors may increase the absorption/exposure of morphine sulfate by about two fold. Therefore, caution should be exercised when morphine sulfate is co-administered with PGP inhibitors).

No products indexed under this heading.

Tubocurarine Chloride (Embeda may enhance the neuromuscular blocking action of skeletal relaxants and produce an increased degree of respiratory depression).

No products indexed under this heading.

Vecuronium Bromide (Embeda may enhance the neuromuscular blocking action of skeletal relaxants and produce an increased degree of respiratory depression).

No products indexed under this heading.

Verapamil Hydrochloride (Based on published reports, PGP inhibitors may increase the absorption/exposure of

569 **Interactions Index** **Emend**

morphine sulfate by about two fold. Therefore, caution should be exercised when morphine sulfate is co-administered with PGP inhibitors).
Products include:
Tarka 534

Zaleplon (Embeda should be used with great caution and in reduced dosage in patients who are concurrently receiving other central nervous system (CNS) depressants including sedatives and hypnotics because of the risk of respiratory depression, hypotension, and profound sedation or coma. When such combined therapy is contemplated, the initial dose of one or both agents should be reduced by at least 50%).
No products indexed under this heading.

Ziprasidone Hydrochloride (Embeda should be used with great caution and in reduced dosage in patients who are concurrently receiving other central nervous system (CNS) depressants including sedatives, hypnotics, general anesthetics, antiemetics, phenothiazines, other tranquilizers, and alcohol because of the risk of respiratory depression, hypotension, and profound sedation or coma. When such combined therapy is contemplated, the initial dose of one or both agents should be reduced by at least 50%). Products include:
Geodon 2723

Zolpidem Tartrate (Embeda should be used with great caution and in reduced dosage in patients who are concurrently receiving other central nervous system (CNS) depressants including sedatives and hypnotics because of the risk of respiratory depression, hypotension, and profound sedation or coma. When such combined therapy is contemplated, the initial dose of one or both agents should be reduced by at least 50%). Products include:
Ambien 2920
Ambien CR 2925

Food Interactions

Alcohol (Embeda should be used with great caution and in reduced dosage in patients who are concurrently receiving other central nervous system (CNS) depressants including alcohol because of the risk of respiratory depression, hypotension, and profound sedation or coma. When such combined therapy is contemplated, the initial dose of one or both agents should be reduced by at least 50%).

Beer, reduced-alcohol (Embeda should be used with great caution and in reduced dosage in patients who are concurrently receiving other central nervous system (CNS) depressants including alcohol because of the risk of respiratory depression, hypotension, and profound sedation or coma. When such combined therapy is contemplated, the initial dose of one or both agents should be reduced by at least 50%).

Beer, unspecified (Embeda should be used with great caution and in reduced dosage in patients who are concurrently receiving other central nervous system (CNS) depressants including alcohol because of the risk of respiratory depression, hypotension, and profound sedation or coma. When such combined therapy is contemplated, the initial dose of one or both agents should be reduced by at least 50%).

Wine, Chianti (Embeda should be used with great caution and in reduced dosage in patients who are concurrently receiving other central nervous system (CNS) depressants including alcohol because of the risk of respiratory depression, hypotension, and profound sedation or coma. When such combined therapy is contemplated, the initial dose of one or both agents should be reduced by at least 50%).

Wine, Red (Embeda should be used with great caution and in reduced dosage in patients who are concurrently receiving other central nervous system (CNS) depressants including alcohol because of the risk of respiratory depression, hypotension, and profound sedation or coma. When such combined therapy is contemplated, the initial dose of one or both agents should be reduced by at least 50%).

Wine, unspecified (Embeda should be used with great caution and in reduced dosage in patients who are concurrently receiving other central nervous system (CNS) depressants including alcohol because of the risk of respiratory depression, hypotension, and profound sedation or coma. When such combined therapy is contemplated, the initial dose of one or both agents should be reduced by at least 50%).

Wine products (Embeda should be used with great caution and in reduced dosage in patients who are concurrently receiving other central nervous system (CNS) depressants including alcohol because of the risk of respiratory depression, hypotension, and profound sedation or coma. When such combined therapy is contemplated, the initial dose of one or both agents should be reduced by at least 50%).

EMEND CAPSULES

(Aprepitant) 2124
May interact with benzodiazepine that are metabolized by CYP3A4, cytochrome p450 2c9 substrates (selected), cytochrome p450 3a4 inducers (selected), cytochrome p450 3a4 inhibitors (selected), cytochrome p450 3a4 inhibitors, potent (selected), cytochrome p450 3a4 substrates (selected), dexamethasones, methylprednisolone, oral contraceptives, phenytoin, and certain other agents. Compounds in these categories include:

Acarbose (Co-administration of fosaprepitant or oral aprepitant with drugs that are known to be metabolized by CYP2C9 may result in lower plasma concentrations of these drugs).
No products indexed under this heading.

Acetazolamide (Aprepitant is a substrate for CYP3A4; therefore, co-administration of fosaprepitant or aprepitant with drugs that inhibit CYP3A4 activity may result in increased plasma concentrations of aprepitant. Consequently, concomitant administration of fosaprepitant or aprepitant with strong CYP3A4 inhibitors (eg, ketoconazole, itraconazole, nefazodone, troleandomycin, clarithromycin, ritonavir, nelfinavir) should be approached with caution. Because moderate CYP3A4 inhibitors (eg, diltiazem) result in a 2-fold increase in plasma concentrations of aprepitant, concomitant administration should also be approached with caution).
No products indexed under this heading.

Acetazolamide Sodium (Aprepitant is a substrate for CYP3A4; therefore, co-administration of fosaprepitant or aprepitant with drugs that inhibit CYP3A4 activity may result in increased plasma concentrations of aprepitant. Consequently, concomitant administration of fosaprepitant or aprepitant with strong CYP3A4 inhibitors (eg, ketoconazole, itraconazole, nefazodone, troleandomycin, clarithromycin, ritonavir, nelfinavir) should be approached with caution. Because moderate CYP3A4 inhibitors (eg, diltiazem) result in a 2-fold increase in plasma concentrations of aprepitant, concomitant administration should also be approached with caution).
No products indexed under this heading.

Alfentanil Hydrochloride (As a moderate inhibitor of CYP3A4, aprepitant can increase plasma concentrations of orally co-administered medicinal products that are metabolized through CYP3A4).
No products indexed under this heading.

Allium sativum (Aprepitant is substrate for CYP3A4; therefore, co-administration of fosaprepitant or aprepitant with drugs that strongly induce CYP3A4 activity (eg, rifampin, carbamazepine, phenytoin) may result in reduced plasma concentrations and decreased efficacy).
No products indexed under this heading.

Alprazolam (Fosaprepitant and oral aprepitant may increase the AUC of midazolam. The potential effects of increased plasma concentrations of midazolam or other benzodiazepines metabolized via CYP3A4 (alprazolam, triazolam) should be considered when co-administeringthese agents with a 3-day regimen of fosaprepitant followed by aprepitant).
No products indexed under this heading.

Aminoglutethimide (Aprepitant is substrate for CYP3A4; therefore, co-administration of fosaprepitant or aprepitant with drugs that strongly induce CYP3A4 activity (eg, rifampin, carbamazepine, phenytoin) may result in reduced plasma concentrations and decreased efficacy).
No products indexed under this heading.

Amiodarone Hydrochloride (Aprepitant is a substrate for CYP3A4; therefore, co-administration of fosaprepitant or aprepitant with drugs that inhibit CYP3A4 activity may result in increased plasma concentrations of aprepitant. Consequently, concomitant administration of fosaprepitant or aprepitant with strong CYP3A4 inhibitors (eg, ketoconazole, itraconazole, nefazodone, troleandomycin, clarithromycin, ritonavir, nelfinavir) should be approached with caution. Because moderate CYP3A4 inhibitors (eg, diltiazem) result in a 2-fold increase in plasma concentrations of aprepitant, concomitant administration should also be approached with caution).
No products indexed under this heading.

Amitriptyline Hydrochloride (Co-administration of fosaprepitant or oral aprepitant with drugs that are known to be metabolized by CYP2C9 may result in lower plasma concentrations of these drugs).
No products indexed under this heading.

Amlodipine Besylate (As a moderate inhibitor of CYP3A4, aprepitant can increase plasma concentrations of orally co-administered medicinal products that are metabolized through CYP3A4).
Products include:
Azor 1010
Exforge 2443
Exforge HCT 2449

Amprenavir (Aprepitant is a substrate for CYP3A4; therefore, co-administration of fosaprepitant or aprepitant with drugs that inhibit CYP3A4 activity may result in increased plasma concentrations of aprepitant. Consequently, concomitant administration of fosaprepitant or apreitant with strong CYP3A4 inhibitors (eg, ketoconazole, itraconzole, nefazodone, troleandomycin, clarithromycin, ritonavir, nelfinavir) should be approached with caution).
No products indexed under this heading.

Anastrozole (Aprepitant is a substrate for CYP3A4; therefore, co-administration of fosaprepitant or aprepitant with drugs that inhibit CYP3A4 activity may result in increased plasma concentrations of aprepitant. Consequently, concomitant administration of fosaprepitant or aprepitant with strong CYP3A4 inhibitors (eg, ketoconazole, itraconazole, nefazodone, troleandomycin, clarithromycin, ritonavir, nelfinavir) should be approached with caution. Because moderate CYP3A4 inhibitors (eg, diltiazem) result in a 2-fold increase in plasma concentrations of aprepitant, concomitant administration should also be approached with caution).
No products indexed under this heading.

Astemizole (EMEND is a moderate CYP3A4 inhibitor; concurrent use with EMEND could result in elevated plasma concentrations of astemizole, potentially causing serious or life-threatening reactions, and is contraindicated).
No products indexed under this heading.

Atazanavir (Aprepitant is a substrate for CYP3A4; therefore, co-administration of fosaprepitant or aprepitant with drugs that inhibit CYP3A4 activity may result in increased plasma concentrations of aprepitant. Consequently, concomitant administration of fosaprepitant or apreitant with strong CYP3A4 inhibitors (eg, ketoconazole, itraconzole, nefazodone, troleandomycin, clarithromycin, ritonavir, nelfinavir) should be approached with caution).
No products indexed under this heading.

Atazanavir Sulfate (Aprepitant is a substrate for CYP3A4; therefore, co-administration of fosaprepitant or aprepitant with drugs that inhibit CYP3A4 activity may result in increased plasma concentrations of aprepitant. Consequently, concomitant administration of fosaprepitant or apreitant with strong CYP3A4 inhibitors (eg, ketoconazole, itraconzole, nefazodone, troleandomycin, clarithromycin, ritonavir, nelfinavir) should be approached with caution).
No products indexed under this heading.

Atorvastatin Calcium (As a moderate inhibitor of CYP3A4, aprepitant can increase plasma concentrations of orally co-administered medicinal products that are metabolized through CYP3A4).
Products include:
Lipitor 2703

Belladonna Ergotamine (As a moderate inhibitor of CYP3A4, aprepitant can increase plasma concentrations of orally co-administered medicinal products that are metabolized through CYP3A4).
No products indexed under this heading.

Betamethasone (Aprepitant is substrate for CYP3A4; therefore, co-administration of fosaprepitant or aprepitant with drugs that strongly induce CYP3A4 activity (eg, rifampin, carbamazepine, phenytoin) may result in reduced plasma concentrations and decreased efficacy).
No products indexed under this heading.

Betamethasone Acetate (Aprepitant is substrate for CYP3A4; therefore, co-administration of fosaprepitant or aprepitant with drugs that strongly induce CYP3A4 activity (eg, rifampin, carbamazepine, phenytoin) may result in reduced plasma concentrations and decreased efficacy).
No products indexed under this heading.

IMPORTANT NOTE: Always consult each drug listing in the patient's regimen for possible interactions.

571 Interactions Index Emend

fosaprepitant or aprepitant with drugs that inhibit CYP3A4 activity may result in increased plasma concentrations of aprepitant. Consequently, concomitant administration of fosaprepitant or aprepitant with strong CYP3A4 inhibitors (eg, ketoconazole, itraconazole, nefazodone, troleandomycin, clarithromycin, ritonavir, nelfinavir) should be approached with caution. Because moderate CYP3A4 inhibitors (eg, diltiazem) result in a 2-fold increase in plasma concentrations of aprepitant, concomitant administration should also be approached with caution).
No products indexed under this heading.

Delavirdine Mesylate (Aprepitant is a substrate for CYP3A4; therefore, co-administration of fosaprepitant or aprepitant with drugs that inhibit CYP3A4 activity may result in increased plasma concentrations of aprepitant. Consequently, concomitant administration of fosaprepitant or apreitant with strong CYP3A4 inhibitors (eg, ketoconazole, itraconzole, nefazodone, troleandomycin, clarithromycin, ritonavir, nelfinavir) should be approached with caution).
No products indexed under this heading.

Delavirine (Aprepitant is a substrate for CYP3A4; therefore, co-administration of fosaprepitant or aprepitant with drugs that inhibit CYP3A4 activity may result in increased plasma concentrations of aprepitant. Consequently, concomitant administration of fosaprepitant or apreitant with strong CYP3A4 inhibitors (eg, ketoconazole, itraconzole, nefazodone, troleandomycin, clarithromycin, ritonavir, nelfinavir) should be approached with caution).
No products indexed under this heading.

Desloratadine (Aprepitant is a substrate for CYP3A4; therefore, co-administration of fosaprepitant or aprepitant with drugs that inhibit CYP3A4 activity may result in increased plasma concentrations of aprepitant. Consequently, concomitant administration of fosaprepitant or aprepitant with strong CYP3A4 inhibitors (eg, ketoconazole, itraconazole, nefazodone, troleandomycin, clarithromycin, ritonavir, nelfinavir) should be approached with caution. Because moderate CYP3A4 inhibitors (eg, diltiazem) result in a 2-fold increase in plasma concentrations of aprepitant, concomitant administration should also be approached with caution). Products include:
Clarinex Syrup **3098**
Clarinex **3098**
Clarinex Reditabs **3098**
Clarinex-D 12-Hour **3101**
Clarinex-D **3104**

Desogestrel (The co-administration of fosaprepitant or aprepitant may reduce the efficacy of hormonal contraceptives during and for 28 days after administration of the last dose of either. Alternative or back-up methods of contraception should be used during treatment with fosaprepitant or aprepitant and for one month following the last dose of aprepitant).
No products indexed under this heading.

Dexamethasone (Oral aprepitant may increase the AUC of dexamethasone, a CYP3A4 substrate. The oral dexamethasone should be reduced by approximately 50% when co-administered with regimen of fosaprepitant followed by aprepitant, to achieve exposures of dexamethasone similar to those obtained when dexamethasone is given without aprepitant). Products include:
Ciprodex **583**
Ozurdex .... ⊙**223**
Tobramycin and Dexamethasone Ophthalmic Suspension .... ⊙**251**

Dexamethasone Acetate (Oral aprepitant may increase the AUC of dexamethasone, a CYP3A4 substrate. The oral dexamethasone should be reduced by approximately 50% when co-administered with regimen of fosaprepitant followed by aprepitant, to achieve exposures of dexamethasone similar to those obtained when dexamethasone is given without aprepitant).
No products indexed under this heading.

Dexamethasone Phosphate (Oral aprepitant may increase the AUC of dexamethasone, a CYP3A4 substrate. The oral dexamethasone should be reduced by approximately 50% when co-administered with regimen of fosaprepitant followed by aprepitant, to achieve exposures of dexamethasone similar to those obtained when dexamethasone is given without aprepitant).
No products indexed under this heading.

Dexamethasone Sodium (Oral aprepitant may increase the AUC of dexamethasone, a CYP3A4 substrate. The oral dexamethasone should be reduced by approximately 50% when co-administered with regimen of fosaprepitant followed by aprepitant, to achieve exposures of dexamethasone similar to those obtained when dexamethasone is given without aprepitant).
No products indexed under this heading.

Dexamethasone Sodium Phosphate (Oral aprepitant may increase the AUC of dexamethasone, a CYP3A4 substrate. The oral dexamethasone should be reduced by approximately 50% when co-administered with regimen of fosaprepitant followed by aprepitant, to achieve exposures of dexamethasone similar to those obtained when dexamethasone is given without aprepitant).
No products indexed under this heading.

Dexamethasone Sodium Phosphate Injection (Oral aprepitant may increase the AUC of dexamethasone, a CYP3A4 substrate. The oral dexamethasone should be reduced by approximately 50% when co-administered with regimen of fosaprepitant followed by aprepitant, to achieve exposures of dexamethasone similar to those obtained when dexamethasone is given without aprepitant).
No products indexed under this heading.

Dextromethorphan (Co-administration of fosaprepitant or oral aprepitant with drugs that are known to be metabolized by CYP2C9 may result in lower plasma concentrations of these drugs).
No products indexed under this heading.

Diazepam (Fosaprepitant and oral aprepitant may increase the AUC of midazolam. The potential effects of increased plasma concentrations of midazolam or other benzodiazepines metabolized via CYP3A4 (alprazolam, triazolam) should be considered when co-administeringthese agents with a 3-day regimen of fosaprepitant followed by aprepitant). Products include:
Valium Tablets **2880**

Diclofenac Potassium (Co-administration of fosaprepitant or oral aprepitant with drugs that are known to be metabolized by CYP2C9 may result in lower plasma concentrations of these drugs).
No products indexed under this heading.

Diclofenac Sodium (Co-administration of fosaprepitant or oral aprepitant with drugs that are known to be metabolized by CYP2C9 may result in lower plasma concentrations of these drugs).
No products indexed under this heading.

Dihydroergotamine Mesylate (As a moderate inhibitor of CYP3A4, aprepitant can increase plasma concentrations of orally co-administered medicinal products that are metabolized through CYP3A4).
No products indexed under this heading.

Diltiazem Hydrochloride (Aprepitant is a substrate for CYP3A4; therefore, co-administration of fosaprepitant or aprepitant with drugs that inhibit CYP3A4 activity may result in increased plasma concentrations of aprepitant. Consequently, concomitant administration of fosaprepitant or aprepitant with strong CYP3A4 inhibitors (eg, ketoconazole, itraconazole, nefazodone, troleandomycin, clarithromycin, ritonavir, nelfinavir) should be approached with caution. Because moderate CYP3A4 inhibitors (eg, diltiazem) result in a 2-fold increase in plasma concentrations of aprepitant, concomitant administration should also be approached with caution). Products include:
Cardizem LA **423**

Diltiazem Maleate (Aprepitant is a substrate for CYP3A4; therefore, co-administration of fosaprepitant or aprepitant with drugs that inhibit CYP3A4 activity may result in increased plasma concentrations of aprepitant. Consequently, concomitant administration of fosaprepitant or aprepitant with strong CYP3A4 inhibitors (eg, ketoconazole, itraconazole, nefazodone, troleandomycin, clarithromycin, ritonavir, nelfinavir) should be approached with caution. Because moderate CYP3A4 inhibitors (eg, diltiazem) result in a 2-fold increase in plasma concentrations of aprepitant, concomitant administration should also be approached with caution).
No products indexed under this heading.

Disopyramide (As a moderate inhibitor of CYP3A4, aprepitant can increase plasma concentrations of orally co-administered medicinal products that are metabolized through CYP3A4).
No products indexed under this heading.

Disopyramide Phosphate (As a moderate inhibitor of CYP3A4, aprepitant can increase plasma concentrations of orally co-administered medicinal products that are metabolized through CYP3A4).
No products indexed under this heading.

Disulfiram (As a moderate inhibitor of CYP3A4, aprepitant can increase plasma concentrations of orally co-administered medicinal products that are metabolized through CYP3A4).
No products indexed under this heading.

Docetaxel (Particular caution and careful monitoring are advised in patients receiving chemotherapy agents metabolized primarily by CYP3A4, like docetaxel). Products include:
Taxotere **3035**

Doxorubicin Hydrochloride (Aprepitant is substrate for CYP3A4; therefore, co-administration of fosaprepitant or aprepitant with drugs that strongly induce CYP3A4 activity (eg, rifampin, carbamazepine, phenytoin) may result in reduced plasma concentrations and decreased efficacy).
No products indexed under this heading.

Dronabinol (Co-administration of fosaprepitant or oral aprepitant with drugs that are known to be metabolized by CYP2C9 may result in lower plasma concentrations of these drugs).
No products indexed under this heading.

Efavirenz (Aprepitant is a substrate for CYP3A4; therefore, co-administration of fosaprepitant or aprepitant with drugs that inhibit CYP3A4 activity may result in increased plasma concentrations of aprepitant. Consequently, concomitant administration of fosaprepitant or aprepitant with strong CYP3A4 inhibitors (eg, ketoconazole, itraconazole, nefazodone, troleandomycin, clarithromycin, ritonavir, nelfinavir) should be approached with caution. Because moderate CYP3A4 inhibitors (eg, diltiazem) result in a 2-fold increase in plasma concentrations of aprepitant, concomitant administration should also be approached with caution). Products include:
Atripla **906**

Eprosartan Mesylate (Co-administration of fosaprepitant or oral aprepitant with drugs that are known to be metabolized by CYP2C9 may result in lower plasma concentrations of these drugs). Products include:
Teveten **538**
Teveten HCT **541**

Ergotamine Tartrate (As a moderate inhibitor of CYP3A4, aprepitant can increase plasma concentrations of orally co-administered medicinal products that are metabolized through CYP3A4).
No products indexed under this heading.

Erythromycin (Aprepitant is a substrate for CYP3A4; therefore, co-administration of fosaprepitant or aprepitant with drugs that inhibit CYP3A4 activity may result in increased plasma concentrations of aprepitant. Consequently, concomitant administration of fosaprepitant or aprepitant with strong CYP3A4 inhibitors (eg, ketoconazole, itraconazole, nefazodone, troleandomycin, clarithromycin, ritonavir, nelfinavir) should be approached with caution. Because moderate CYP3A4 inhibitors (eg, diltiazem) result in a 2-fold increase in plasma concentrations of aprepitant, concomitant administration should also be approached with caution).
No products indexed under this heading.

Erythromycin Estolate (Aprepitant is a substrate for CYP3A4; therefore, co-administration of fosaprepitant or aprepitant with drugs that inhibit CYP3A4 activity may result in increased plasma concentrations of aprepitant. Consequently, concomitant administration of fosaprepitant or aprepitant with strong CYP3A4 inhibitors (eg, ketoconazole, itraconazole, nefazodone, troleandomycin, clarithromycin, ritonavir, nelfinavir) should be approached with caution. Because moderate CYP3A4 inhibitors (eg, diltiazem) result in a 2-fold increase in plasma concentrations of aprepitant, concomitant administration should also be approached with caution).
No products indexed under this heading.

Erythromycin Ethylsuccinate (Aprepitant is a substrate for CYP3A4; therefore, co-administration of fosaprepitant or aprepitant with drugs that inhibit CYP3A4 activity may result in increased plasma concentrations of aprepitant. Consequently, concomitant administration of fosaprepitant or aprepitant with strong CYP3A4 inhibitors (eg, ketoconazole, itraconazole, nefazodone, troleandomycin, clarithromycin, ritonavir, nelfinavir) should be approached with caution. Because moderate CYP3A4 inhibitors (eg, diltiazem) result in a 2-fold increase in plasma concentrations of aprepitant, concomitant administration should also be approached with caution). Products include:
E.E.S. **437**
EryPed **435**

Erythromycin Gluceptate (Aprepitant is a substrate for CYP3A4; therefore, co-administration of fosaprepitant or aprepitant with drugs that inhibit CYP3A4 activity may result in increased plasma concentrations of aprepitant. Consequently, concomitant administration of fosaprepitant or aprepitant with

strong CYP3A4 inhibitors (eg, ketocona-zole, itraconazole, nefazodone, trolean-domycin, clarithromycin, ritonavir, nelfi-navir) should be approached with caution. Because moderate CYP3A4 inhibitors (eg, diltiazem) result in a 2-fold increase in plasma concentra-tions of aprepitant, concomitant admin-istration should also be approached with caution).

No products indexed under this heading.

Erythromycin Lactobionate (Aprepi-tant is a substrate for CYP3A4; there-fore, co-administration of fosaprepitant or aprepitant with drugs that inhibit CYP3A4 activity may result in increased plasma concentrations of aprepitant. Consequently, concomitant administra-tion of fosaprepitant or aprepitant with strong CYP3A4 inhibitors (eg, ketocona-zole, itraconazole, nefazodone, trolean-domycin, clarithromycin, ritonavir, nelfi-navir) should be approached with caution. Because moderate CYP3A4 inhibitors (eg, diltiazem) result in a 2-fold increase in plasma concentra-tions of aprepitant, concomitant admin-istration should also be approached with caution).

No products indexed under this heading.

Erythromycin Stearate (Aprepitant is a substrate for CYP3A4; therefore, co-administration of fosaprepitant or aprepitant with drugs that inhibit CYP3A4 activity may result in increased plasma concentrations of aprepitant. Consequently, concomitant administra-tion of fosaprepitant or aprepitant with strong CYP3A4 inhibitors (eg, ketocona-zole, itraconazole, nefazodone, trolean-domycin, clarithromycin, ritonavir, nelfi-navir) should be approached with caution. Because moderate CYP3A4 inhibitors (eg, diltiazem) result in a 2-fold increase in plasma concentra-tions of aprepitant, concomitant admin-istration should also be approached with caution).

No products indexed under this heading.

Esomeprazole Magnesium (Aprepi-tant is a substrate for CYP3A4; there-fore, co-administration of fosaprepitant or aprepitant with drugs that inhibit CYP3A4 activity may result in increased plasma concentrations of aprepitant. Consequently, concomitant administra-tion of fosaprepitant or aprepitant with strong CYP3A4 inhibitors (eg, ketocona-zole, itraconazole, nefazodone, trolean-domycin, clarithromycin, ritonavir, nelfi-navir) should be approached with caution. Because moderate CYP3A4 inhibitors (eg, diltiazem) result in a 2-fold increase in plasma concentra-tions of aprepitant, concomitant admin-istration should also be approached with caution). Products include:

Esomeprazole Sodium (Aprepitant is a substrate for CYP3A4; therefore, co-administration of fosaprepitant or aprepitant with drugs that inhibit CYP3A4 activity may result in increased plasma concentrations of aprepitant. Consequently, concomitant administra-tion of fosaprepitant or aprepitant with strong CYP3A4 inhibitors (eg, ketocona-zole, itraconazole, nefazodone, trolean-domycin, clarithromycin, ritonavir, nelfi-navir) should be approached with caution. Because moderate CYP3A4 inhibitors (eg, diltiazem) result in a 2-fold increase in plasma concentra-tions of aprepitant, concomitant admin-istration should also be approached with caution). Products include:

Estradiol (As a moderate inhibitor of CYP3A4, aprepitant can increase plas-ma concentrations of orally co-

administered medicinal products that are metabolized through CYP3A4). Products include:

Estradiol Benzoate (As a moderate inhibitor of CYP3A4, aprepitant can increase plasma concentrations of oral-ly co-administered medicinal products that are metabolized through CYP3A4).

No products indexed under this heading.

Estradiol Cypionate (As a moderate inhibitor of CYP3A4, aprepitant can increase plasma concentrations of oral-ly co-administered medicinal products that are metabolized through CYP3A4).

No products indexed under this heading.

Estradiol Valerate (As a moderate inhibitor of CYP3A4, aprepitant can increase plasma concentrations of oral-ly co-administered medicinal products that are metabolized through CYP3A4).

No products indexed under this heading.

Ethinyl Estradiol (The co-administration of fosaprepitant or aprepitant may reduce the efficacy of hormonal contraceptives during and for 28 days after administration of the last dose of either. Alternative or back-up methods of contraception should be used during treatment with fosaprepi-tant or aprepitant and for one month following the last dose of aprepitant). Products include:

Ethosuximide (Aprepitant is substrate for CYP3A4; therefore, co-administration of fosaprepitant or aprepitant with drugs that strongly induce CYP3A4 activity (eg, rifampin, carbamazepine, phenytoin) may result in reduced plasma concentrations and decreased efficacy).

No products indexed under this heading.

Ethynodiol Diacetate (The co-administration of fosaprepitant or aprepitant may reduce the efficacy of hormonal contraceptives during and for 28 days after administration of the last dose of either. Alternative or back-up methods of contraception should be used during treatment with fosaprepi-tant or aprepitant and for one month following the last dose of aprepitant).

No products indexed under this heading.

Etodolac (Co-administration of fos-aprepitant or oral aprepitant with drugs that are known to be metabolized by CYP2C9 may result in lower plasma concentrations of these drugs).

No products indexed under this heading.

Etoposide (Particular caution and careful monitoring are advised in patients receiving chemotherapy agents metabolized primarily by CYP3A4, like etoposide).

No products indexed under this heading.

Etoposide Phosphate (As a moder-ate inhibitor of CYP3A4, aprepitant can increase plasma concentrations of oral-ly co-administered medicinal products that are metabolized through CYP3A4).

No products indexed under this heading.

Felbamate (Aprepitant is substrate for CYP3A4; therefore, co-administration of fosaprepitant or aprepitant with drugs that strongly induce CYP3A4 activity (eg, rifampin, carbamazepine, phenyto-in) may result in reduced plasma con-centrations and decreased efficacy).

No products indexed under this heading.

Felodipine (As a moderate inhibitor of CYP3A4, aprepitant can increase plas-ma concentrations of orally co-administered medicinal products that are metabolized through CYP3A4).

No products indexed under this heading.

Fenoprofen Calcium (Co-administration of fosaprepitant or oral aprepitant with drugs that are known to be metabolized by CYP2C9 may result in lower plasma concentrations of these drugs).

No products indexed under this heading.

Fentanyl (As a moderate inhibitor of CYP3A4, aprepitant can increase plas-ma concentrations of orally co-administered medicinal products that are metabolized through CYP3A4). Products include:

Fentanyl Citrate (As a moderate inhibitor of CYP3A4, aprepitant can increase plasma concentrations of oral-ly co-administered medicinal products that are metabolized through CYP3A4). Products include:

Fluconazole (Aprepitant is a substrate for CYP3A4; therefore, co-administration of fosaprepitant or aprepitant with drugs that inhibit CYP3A4 activity may result in increased plasma concentrations of aprepitant. Consequently, concomitant administra-tion of fosaprepitant or aprepitant with strong CYP3A4 inhibitors (eg, ketocona-zole, itraconazole, nefazodone, trolean-domycin, clarithromycin, ritonavir, nelfi-navir) should be approached with caution. Because moderate CYP3A4 inhibitors (eg, diltiazem) result in a 2-fold increase in plasma concentra-tions of aprepitant, concomitant admin-istration should also be approached with caution).

No products indexed under this heading.

Fludrocortisone Acetate (Aprepitant is substrate for CYP3A4; therefore, co-administration of fosaprepitant or aprepitant with drugs that strongly induce CYP3A4 activity (eg, rifampin, carbamazepine, phenytoin) may result in reduced plasma concentrations and decreased efficacy).

No products indexed under this heading.

Fluoxetine (Aprepitant is a substrate for CYP3A4; therefore, co-administration of fosaprepitant or aprepitant with drugs that inhibit CYP3A4 activity may result in increased plasma concentrations of aprepitant. Consequently, concomitant administra-tion of fosaprepitant or aprepitant with strong CYP3A4 inhibitors (eg, ketocona-zole, itraconazole, nefazodone, trolean-domycin, clarithromycin, ritonavir, nelfi-navir) should be approached with caution. Because moderate CYP3A4 inhibitors (eg, diltiazem) result in a 2-fold increase in plasma concentra-tions of aprepitant, concomitant admin-istration should also be approached with caution).

No products indexed under this heading.

Fluoxetine Hydrochloride (Aprepi-tant is a substrate for CYP3A4; there-fore, co-administration of fosaprepitant or aprepitant with drugs that inhibit CYP3A4 activity may result in increased plasma concentrations of aprepitant. Consequently, concomitant administra-tion of fosaprepitant or aprepitant with

strong CYP3A4 inhibitors (eg, ketocona-zole, itraconazole, nefazodone, trolean-domycin, clarithromycin, ritonavir, nelfi-navir) should be approached with caution. Because moderate CYP3A4 inhibitors (eg, diltiazem) result in a 2-fold increase in plasma concentra-tions of aprepitant, concomitant admin-istration should also be approached with caution). Products include:

Flurbiprofen (Co-administration of fosaprepitant or oral aprepitant with drugs that are known to be metabolized by CYP2C9 may result in lower plasma concentrations of these drugs).

No products indexed under this heading.

Flurbiprofen Sodium (Co-administration of fosaprepitant or oral aprepitant with drugs that are known to be metabolized by CYP2C9 may result in lower plasma concentrations of these drugs).

No products indexed under this heading.

Fluvastatin Sodium (Co-administration of fosaprepitant or oral aprepitant with drugs that are known to be metabolized by CYP2C9 may result in lower plasma concentrations of these drugs).

No products indexed under this heading.

Fluvoxamine Maleate (Aprepitant is a substrate for CYP3A4; therefore, co-administration of fosaprepitant or aprepitant with drugs that inhibit CYP3A4 activity may result in increased plasma concentrations of aprepitant. Consequently, concomitant administra-tion of fosaprepitant or aprepitant with strong CYP3A4 inhibitors (eg, ketocona-zole, itraconazole, nefazodone, trolean-domycin, clarithromycin, ritonavir, nelfi-navir) should be approached with caution. Because moderate CYP3A4 inhibitors (eg, diltiazem) result in a 2-fold increase in plasma concentra-tions of aprepitant, concomitant admin-istration should also be approached with caution).

No products indexed under this heading.

Fosamprenavir Calcium (Aprepitant is a substrate for CYP3A4; therefore, co-administration of fosaprepitant or aprepitant with drugs that inhibit CYP3A4 activity may result in increased plasma concentrations of aprepitant. Consequently, concomitant administra-tion of fosaprepitant or apreitant with strong CYP3A4 inhibitors (eg, ketocona-zole, itraconzole, nefazodone, trolean-domycin, clarithromycin, ritonavir, nelfi-navir) should be approached with caution). Products include:

Fosphenytoin (Aprepitant has been shown to induce the metabolism of S(-) warfarin and tolbutamide, which are metabolized through CYP2C9. Co-administration of aprepitant with these drugs or other drugs that are known to be metabolized by CYP2C9, such as phenytoin, may result in lower plasma concentrations of these drugs).

No products indexed under this heading.

Fosphenytoin Sodium (Aprepitant has been shown to induce the metabo-lism of S(-) warfarin and tolbutamide, which are metabolized through CYP2C9. Co-administration of aprepi-tant with these drugs or other drugs that are known to be metabolized by CYP2C9, such as phenytoin, may result in lower plasma concentrations of these drugs).

No products indexed under this heading.

Garlic Extract (Aprepitant is substrate for CYP3A4; therefore, co-administration of fosaprepitant or aprepitant with drugs that strongly induce CYP3A4 activity (eg, rifampin, carbamazepine, phenytoin) may result in reduced plasma concentrations and decreased efficacy).
No products indexed under this heading.

Garlic Oil (Aprepitant is substrate for CYP3A4; therefore, co-administration of fosaprepitant or aprepitant with drugs that strongly induce CYP3A4 activity (eg, rifampin, carbamazepine, phenytoin) may result in reduced plasma concentrations and decreased efficacy).
No products indexed under this heading.

Glimepiride (Co-administration of fosaprepitant or oral aprepitant with drugs that are known to be metabolized by CYP2C9 may result in lower plasma concentrations of these drugs). Products include:
Avandaryl 1356
Duetact 3354

Glipizide (Co-administration of fosaprepitant or oral aprepitant with drugs that are known to be metabolized by CYP2C9 may result in lower plasma concentrations of these drugs).
No products indexed under this heading.

Haloperidol (As a moderate inhibitor of CYP3A4, aprepitant can increase plasma concentrations of orally co-administered medicinal products that are metabolized through CYP3A4).
No products indexed under this heading.

Haloperidol Decanoate (As a moderate inhibitor of CYP3A4, aprepitant can increase plasma concentrations of orally co-administered medicinal products that are metabolized through CYP3A4).
No products indexed under this heading.

Haloperidol Lactate (As a moderate inhibitor of CYP3A4, aprepitant can increase plasma concentrations of orally co-administered medicinal products that are metabolized through CYP3A4).
No products indexed under this heading.

Hydrocortisone (Aprepitant is substrate for CYP3A4; therefore, co-administration of fosaprepitant or aprepitant with drugs that strongly induce CYP3A4 activity (eg, rifampin, carbamazepine, phenytoin) may result in reduced plasma concentrations and decreased efficacy).
No products indexed under this heading.

Hydrocortisone (Alcohol) (Aprepitant is substrate for CYP3A4; therefore, co-administration of fosaprepitant or aprepitant with drugs that strongly induce CYP3A4 activity (eg, rifampin, carbamazepine, phenytoin) may result in reduced plasma concentrations and decreased efficacy).
No products indexed under this heading.

Hydrocortisone Acetate (Aprepitant is substrate for CYP3A4; therefore, co-administration of fosaprepitant or aprepitant with drugs that strongly induce CYP3A4 activity (eg, rifampin, carbamazepine, phenytoin) may result in reduced plasma concentrations and decreased efficacy).
No products indexed under this heading.

Hydrocortisone Butyrate (Aprepitant is substrate for CYP3A4; therefore, co-administration of fosaprepitant or aprepitant with drugs that strongly induce CYP3A4 activity (eg, rifampin, carbamazepine, phenytoin) may result in reduced plasma concentrations and decreased efficacy).
No products indexed under this heading.

Hydrocortisone Cypionate (Aprepitant is substrate for CYP3A4; therefore, co-administration of fosaprepitant or aprepitant with drugs that strongly induce CYP3A4 activity (eg, rifampin, carbamazepine, phenytoin) may result in reduced plasma concentrations and decreased efficacy).
No products indexed under this heading.

Hydrocortisone Hemisuccinate (Aprepitant is substrate for CYP3A4; therefore, co-administration of fosaprepitant or aprepitant with drugs that strongly induce CYP3A4 activity (eg, rifampin, carbamazepine, phenytoin) may result in reduced plasma concentrations and decreased efficacy).
No products indexed under this heading.

Hydrocortisone Probutate (Aprepitant is substrate for CYP3A4; therefore, co-administration of fosaprepitant or aprepitant with drugs that strongly induce CYP3A4 activity (eg, rifampin, carbamazepine, phenytoin) may result in reduced plasma concentrations and decreased efficacy).
No products indexed under this heading.

Hydrocortisone Sodium Phosphate (Aprepitant is substrate for CYP3A4; therefore, co-administration of fosaprepitant or aprepitant with drugs that strongly induce CYP3A4 activity (eg, rifampin, carbamazepine, phenytoin) may result in reduced plasma concentrations and decreased efficacy).
No products indexed under this heading.

Hydrocortisone Sodium Succinate (Aprepitant is substrate for CYP3A4; therefore, co-administration of fosaprepitant or aprepitant with drugs that strongly induce CYP3A4 activity (eg, rifampin, carbamazepine, phenytoin) may result in reduced plasma concentrations and decreased efficacy).
No products indexed under this heading.

Hydrocortisone Valerate (Aprepitant is substrate for CYP3A4; therefore, co-administration of fosaprepitant or aprepitant with drugs that strongly induce CYP3A4 activity (eg, rifampin, carbamazepine, phenytoin) may result in reduced plasma concentrations and decreased efficacy).
No products indexed under this heading.

Hypericum (Aprepitant is substrate for CYP3A4; therefore, co-administration of fosaprepitant or aprepitant with drugs that strongly induce CYP3A4 activity (eg, rifampin, carbamazepine, phenytoin) may result in reduced plasma concentrations and decreased efficacy).
No products indexed under this heading.

Hypericum Perforatum (Aprepitant is substrate for CYP3A4; therefore, co-administration of fosaprepitant or aprepitant with drugs that strongly induce CYP3A4 activity (eg, rifampin, carbamazepine, phenytoin) may result in reduced plasma concentrations and decreased efficacy). Products include:
Traumeel 1800

Ibuprofen (Co-administration of fosaprepitant or oral aprepitant with drugs that are known to be metabolized by CYP2C9 may result in lower plasma concentrations of these drugs). Products include:
Motrin IB 2043
Children's Motrin 2044
Children's Motrin Non-Staining Dye-Free 2044
Infants' Motrin 2044
Infants' Motrin Dye-Free 2044
Junior Strength Motrin 2044
Vicoprofen 564

Ifosfamide (Particular caution and careful monitoring are advised in patients receiving chemotherapy agents metabolized primarily by CYP3A4, like ifosfamide).
No products indexed under this heading.

Imatinib Mesylate (Particular caution and careful monitoring are advised in patients receiving chemotherapy agents metabolized primarily by CYP3A4, like imatinib). Products include:
Gleevec 2477

Imipramine Hydrochloride (Co-administration of fosaprepitant or oral aprepitant with drugs that are known to be metabolized by CYP2C9 may result in lower plasma concentrations of these drugs).
No products indexed under this heading.

Indinavir Sulfate (Aprepitant is a substrate for CYP3A4; therefore, co-administration of fosaprepitant or aprepitant with drugs that inhibit CYP3A4 activity may result in increased plasma concentrations of aprepitant. Consequently, concomitant administration of fosaprepitant or apreitant with strong CYP3A4 inhibitors (eg, ketoconazole, itraconzole, nefazodone, troleandomycin, clarithromycin, ritonavir, nelfinavir) should be approached with caution). Products include:
Crixivan 2113

Indomethacin (Co-administration of fosaprepitant or oral aprepitant with drugs that are known to be metabolized by CYP2C9 may result in lower plasma concentrations of these drugs). Products include:
Indocin 2167

Indomethacin Sodium Trihydrate (Co-administration of fosaprepitant or oral aprepitant with drugs that are known to be metabolized by CYP2C9 may result in lower plasma concentrations of these drugs). Products include:
Indocin I.V. 2007

Irbesartan (Co-administration of fosaprepitant or oral aprepitant with drugs that are known to be metabolized by CYP2C9 may result in lower plasma concentrations of these drugs). Products include:
Avalide 2956
Avapro 2962

Irinotecan Hydrochloride (Particular caution and careful monitoring are advised in patients receiving chemotherapy agents metabolized primarily by CYP3A4, like irinotecan).
No products indexed under this heading.

Isoniazid (Aprepitant is a substrate for CYP3A4; therefore, co-administration of fosaprepitant or aprepitant with drugs that inhibit CYP3A4 activity may result in increased plasma concentrations of aprepitant. Consequently, concomitant administration of fosaprepitant or aprepitant with strong CYP3A4 inhibitors (eg, ketoconazole, itraconazole, nefazodone, troleandomycin, clarithromycin, ritonavir, nelfinavir) should be approached with caution. Because moderate CYP3A4 inhibitors (eg, diltiazem) result in a 2-fold increase in plasma concentrations of aprepitant, concomitant administration should also be approached with caution).
No products indexed under this heading.

Isradipine (As a moderate inhibitor of CYP3A4, aprepitant can increase plasma concentrations of orally co-administered medicinal products that are metabolized through CYP3A4). Products include:
DynaCirc CR 1432

Itraconazole (Aprepitant is a substrate for CYP3A4; therefore, co-administration of fosaprepitant or aprepitant with drugs that inhibit CYP3A4 activity may result in increased plasma concentrations of aprepitant. Consequently, concomitant administration of fosaprepitant or apreitant with strong CYP3A4 inhibitors (eg, ketoconazole, itraconzole, nefazodone, troleandomycin, clarithromycin, ritonavir, nelfinavir) should be approached with caution).
No products indexed under this heading.

Ixabepilone (As a moderate inhibitor of CYP3A4, aprepitant can increase plasma concentrations of orally co-administered medicinal products that are metabolized through CYP3A4).
No products indexed under this heading.

Ketoconazole (Aprepitant is a substrate for CYP3A4; therefore, co-administration of fosaprepitant or aprepitant with drugs that inhibit CYP3A4 activity may result in increased plasma concentrations of aprepitant. Consequently, concomitant administration of fosaprepitant or apreitant with strong CYP3A4 inhibitors (eg, ketoconazole, itraconzole, nefazodone, troleandomycin, clarithromycin, ritonavir, nelfinavir) should be approached with caution). Products include:
Extina 3319
Xolegel 3337

Ketoprofen (Co-administration of fosaprepitant or oral aprepitant with drugs that are known to be metabolized by CYP2C9 may result in lower plasma concentrations of these drugs).
No products indexed under this heading.

Ketorolac Tromethamine (Co-administration of fosaprepitant or oral aprepitant with drugs that are known to be metabolized by CYP2C9 may result in lower plasma concentrations of these drugs). Products include:
Acuvail .... ⊙ 209

Lansoprazole (Co-administration of fosaprepitant or oral aprepitant with drugs that are known to be metabolized by CYP2C9 may result in lower plasma concentrations of these drugs).
No products indexed under this heading.

Lapatinib (Aprepitant is a substrate for CYP3A4; therefore, co-administration of fosaprepitant or aprepitant with drugs that inhibit CYP3A4 activity may result in increased plasma concentrations of aprepitant. Consequently, concomitant administration of fosaprepitant or aprepitant with strong CYP3A4 inhibitors (eg, ketoconazole, itraconazole, nefazodone, troleandomycin, clarithromycin, ritonavir, nelfinavir) should be approached with caution. Because moderate CYP3A4 inhibitors (eg, diltiazem) result in a 2-fold increase in plasma concentrations of aprepitant, concomitant administration should also be approached with caution). Products include:
Tykerb 1698

Levonorgestrel (The co-administration of fosaprepitant or aprepitant may reduce the efficacy of hormonal contraceptives during and for 28 days after administration of the last dose of either. Alternative or back-up methods of contraception should be used during treatment with fosaprepitant or aprepitant and for one month following the last dose of aprepitant). Products include:
Climara Pro 847
LoSeasonique 3407
Lybrel 3514
Mirena 854
Plan B 3416
Seasonique 3418

Lidocaine (As a moderate inhibitor of CYP3A4, aprepitant can increase plasma concentrations of orally co-administered medicinal products that are metabolized through CYP3A4). Products include:
Lidoderm 1107

IMPORTANT NOTE: Always consult each drug listing in the patient's regimen for possible interactions.

Lidocaine Hydrochloride (As a moderate inhibitor of CYP3A4, aprepitant can increase plasma concentrations of orally co-administered medicinal products that are metabolized through CYP3A4).
No products indexed under this heading.

Lopinavir (Aprepitant is a substrate for CYP3A4; therefore, co-administration of fosaprepitant or aprepitant with drugs that inhibit CYP3A4 activity may result in increased plasma concentrations of aprepitant. Consequently, concomitant administration of fosaprepitant or apreitant with strong CYP3A4 inhibitors (eg, ketoconazole, itraconzole, nefazodone, troleandomycin, clarithromycin, ritonavir, nelfinavir) should be approached with caution). Products include:
Kaletra 458

Loratadine (Aprepitant is a substrate for CYP3A4; therefore, co-administration of fosaprepitant or aprepitant with drugs that inhibit CYP3A4 activity may result in increased plasma concentrations of aprepitant. Consequently, concomitant administration of fosaprepitant or aprepitant with strong CYP3A4 inhibitors (eg, ketoconazole, itraconazole, nefazodone, troleandomycin, clarithromycin, ritonavir, nelfinavir) should be approached with caution. Because moderate CYP3A4 inhibitors (eg, diltiazem) result in a 2-fold increase in plasma concentrations of aprepitant, concomitant administration should also be approached with caution).
No products indexed under this heading.

Losartan Potassium (Co-administration of fosaprepitant or oral aprepitant with drugs that are known to be metabolized by CYP2C9 may result in lower plasma concentrations of these drugs). Products include:
Cozaar 2106
Hyzaar 2162
Hyzaar 100-12.5 2162

Lovastatin (As a moderate inhibitor of CYP3A4, aprepitant can increase plasma concentrations of orally co-administered medicinal products that are metabolized through CYP3A4). Products include:
Advicor 402
Mevacor 2212

Meclofenamate Sodium (Co-administration of fosaprepitant or oral aprepitant with drugs that are known to be metabolized by CYP2C9 may result in lower plasma concentrations of these drugs).
No products indexed under this heading.

Mefenamic Acid (Co-administration of fosaprepitant or oral aprepitant with drugs that are known to be metabolized by CYP2C9 may result in lower plasma concentrations of these drugs).
No products indexed under this heading.

Meloxicam (Co-administration of fosaprepitant or oral aprepitant with drugs that are known to be metabolized by CYP2C9 may result in lower plasma concentrations of these drugs).
No products indexed under this heading.

Mephenytoin (Aprepitant is substrate for CYP3A4; therefore, co-administration of fosaprepitant or aprepitant with drugs that strongly induce CYP3A4 activity (eg, rifampin, carbamazepine, phenytoin) may result in reduced plasma concentrations and decreased efficacy).
No products indexed under this heading.

Mestranol (The co-administration of fosaprepitant or aprepitant may reduce the efficacy of hormonal contraceptives during and for 28 days after administration of the last dose of either. Alternative or back-up methods of contraception should be used during treatment with fosaprepitant or aprepitant and for one month following the last dose of aprepitant).
No products indexed under this heading.

Metformin Hydrochloride (Co-administration of fosaprepitant or oral aprepitant with drugs that are known to be metabolized by CYP2C9 may result in lower plasma concentrations of these drugs). Products include:
ActoPlus 3338
Avandamet 1345
Janumet 2188

Methadone Hydrochloride (As a moderate inhibitor of CYP3A4, aprepitant can increase plasma concentrations of orally co-administered medicinal products that are metabolized through CYP3A4).
No products indexed under this heading.

Methsuximide (Aprepitant is substrate for CYP3A4; therefore, co-administration of fosaprepitant or aprepitant with drugs that strongly induce CYP3A4 activity (eg, rifampin, carbamazepine, phenytoin) may result in reduced plasma concentrations and decreased efficacy).
No products indexed under this heading.

Methylprednisolone (Oral aprepitant may increase the AUC of methylprednisolone, a CYP3A4 substrate. The IV methylprednisolone doses should be reduced by approximately 25% and the oral methylprednisolone dose should be reduced by approximately 50% when co-administered with a regimen of fosaprepitant followed by aprepitant to achieve exposures of methylprednisolone similar to those obtained when it is given without aprepitant).
No products indexed under this heading.

Methylprednisolone Acetate (Oral aprepitant may increase the AUC of methylprednisolone, a CYP3A4 substrate. The IV methylprednisolone doses should be reduced by approximately 25% and the oral methylprednisolone dose should be reduced by approximately 50% when co-administered with a regimen of fosaprepitant followed by aprepitant to achieve exposures of methylprednisolone similar to those obtained when it is given without aprepitant).
No products indexed under this heading.

Methylprednisolone Sodium Succinate (Oral aprepitant may increase the AUC of methylprednisolone, a CYP3A4 substrate. The IV methylprednisolone doses should be reduced by approximately 25% and the oral methylprednisolone dose should be reduced by approximately 50% when co-administered with a regimen of fosaprepitant followed by aprepitant to achieve exposures of methylprednisolone similar to those obtained when it is given without aprepitant).
No products indexed under this heading.

Metronidazole (Aprepitant is a substrate for CYP3A4; therefore, co-administration of fosaprepitant or aprepitant with drugs that inhibit CYP3A4 activity may result in increased plasma concentrations of aprepitant. Consequently, concomitant administration of fosaprepitant or aprepitant with strong CYP3A4 inhibitors (eg, ketoconazole, itraconazole, nefazodone, troleandomycin, clarithromycin, ritonavir, nelfinavir) should be approached with caution. Because moderate CYP3A4 inhibitors (eg, diltiazem) result in a 2-fold increase in plasma concentrations of aprepitant, concomitant administration should also be approached with caution). Products include:
Pylera 793

Metronidazole Benzoate (Aprepitant is a substrate for CYP3A4; therefore, co-administration of fosaprepitant or aprepitant with drugs that inhibit CYP3A4 activity may result in increased plasma concentrations of aprepitant. Consequently, concomitant administration of fosaprepitant or aprepitant with strong CYP3A4 inhibitors (eg, ketoconazole, itraconazole, nefazodone, troleandomycin, clarithromycin, ritonavir, nelfinavir) should be approached with caution. Because moderate CYP3A4 inhibitors (eg, diltiazem) result in a 2-fold increase in plasma concentrations of aprepitant, concomitant administration should also be approached with caution).
No products indexed under this heading.

Metronidazole Hydrochloride (Aprepitant is a substrate for CYP3A4; therefore, co-administration of fosaprepitant or aprepitant with drugs that inhibit CYP3A4 activity may result in increased plasma concentrations of aprepitant. Consequently, concomitant administration of fosaprepitant or aprepitant with strong CYP3A4 inhibitors (eg, ketoconazole, itraconazole, nefazodone, troleandomycin, clarithromycin, ritonavir, nelfinavir) should be approached with caution. Because moderate CYP3A4 inhibitors (eg, diltiazem) result in a 2-fold increase in plasma concentrations of aprepitant, concomitant administration should also be approached with caution).
No products indexed under this heading.

Metronidazole Sodium (Aprepitant is a substrate for CYP3A4; therefore, co-administration of fosaprepitant or aprepitant with drugs that inhibit CYP3A4 activity may result in increased plasma concentrations of aprepitant. Consequently, concomitant administration of fosaprepitant or aprepitant with strong CYP3A4 inhibitors (eg, ketoconazole, itraconazole, nefazodone, troleandomycin, clarithromycin, ritonavir, nelfinavir) should be approached with caution. Because moderate CYP3A4 inhibitors (eg, diltiazem) result in a 2-fold increase in plasma concentrations of aprepitant, concomitant administration should also be approached with caution).
No products indexed under this heading.

Miconazole (Aprepitant is a substrate for CYP3A4; therefore, co-administration of fosaprepitant or aprepitant with drugs that inhibit CYP3A4 activity may result in increased plasma concentrations of aprepitant. Consequently, concomitant administration of fosaprepitant or aprepitant with strong CYP3A4 inhibitors (eg, ketoconazole, itraconazole, nefazodone, troleandomycin, clarithromycin, ritonavir, nelfinavir) should be approached with caution. Because moderate CYP3A4 inhibitors (eg, diltiazem) result in a 2-fold increase in plasma concentrations of aprepitant, concomitant administration should also be approached with caution).
No products indexed under this heading.

Miconazole Nitrate (Aprepitant is a substrate for CYP3A4; therefore, co-administration of fosaprepitant or aprepitant with drugs that inhibit CYP3A4 activity may result in increased plasma concentrations of aprepitant. Consequently, concomitant administration of fosaprepitant or aprepitant with strong CYP3A4 inhibitors (eg, ketoconazole, itraconazole, nefazodone, troleandomycin, clarithromycin, ritonavir, nelfinavir) should be approached with caution. Because moderate CYP3A4 inhibitors (eg, diltiazem) result in a 2-fold increase in plasma concentrations of aprepitant, concomitant administration should also be approached with caution). Products include:
Vusion Ointment 3335

Midazolam Hydrochloride (Fosaprepitant and oral aprepitant may increase the AUC of midazolam. The potential effects of increased plasma concentrations of midazolam or other benzodiazepines metabolized via CYP3A4 (alprazolam, triazolam) should be considered when co-administeringthese agents with a 3-day regimen of fosaprepitant followed by aprepitant).
No products indexed under this heading.

Mifepristone (Aprepitant is a substrate for CYP3A4; therefore, co-administration of fosaprepitant or aprepitant with drugs that inhibit CYP3A4 activity may result in increased plasma concentrations of aprepitant. Consequently, concomitant administration of fosaprepitant or aprepitant with strong CYP3A4 inhibitors (eg, ketoconazole, itraconazole, nefazodone, troleandomycin, clarithromycin, ritonavir, nelfinavir) should be approached with caution. Because moderate CYP3A4 inhibitors (eg, diltiazem) result in a 2-fold increase in plasma concentrations of aprepitant, concomitant administration should also be approached with caution).
No products indexed under this heading.

Miglitol (Co-administration of fosaprepitant or oral aprepitant with drugs that are known to be metabolized by CYP2C9 may result in lower plasma concentrations of these drugs).
No products indexed under this heading.

Mirtazapine (Co-administration of fosaprepitant or oral aprepitant with drugs that are known to be metabolized by CYP2C9 may result in lower plasma concentrations of these drugs). Products include:
Remeron Tablets 3214
RemeronSolTab Tablets 3219

Modafinil (Aprepitant is substrate for CYP3A4; therefore, co-administration of fosaprepitant or aprepitant with drugs that strongly induce CYP3A4 activity (eg, rifampin, carbamazepine, phenytoin) may result in reduced plasma concentrations and decreased efficacy). Products include:
Provigil 983

Montelukast Sodium (Co-administration of fosaprepitant or oral aprepitant with drugs that are known to be metabolized by CYP2C9 may result in lower plasma concentrations of these drugs). Products include:
Singulair 2270

Nabumetone (Co-administration of fosaprepitant or oral aprepitant with drugs that are known to be metabolized by CYP2C9 may result in lower plasma concentrations of these drugs).
No products indexed under this heading.

Nafcillin Sodium (Aprepitant is substrate for CYP3A4; therefore, co-administration of fosaprepitant or aprepitant with drugs that strongly induce CYP3A4 activity (eg, rifampin, carbamazepine, phenytoin) may result in reduced plasma concentrations and decreased efficacy).
No products indexed under this heading.

Naproxen (Co-administration of fosaprepitant or oral aprepitant with drugs that are known to be metabolized by CYP2C9 may result in lower plasma concentrations of these drugs). Products include:
EC-Naprosyn 2850
Naprosyn 2850
Anaprox/Naprosyn 2850

Naproxen Sodium (Co-administration of fosapreppitant or oral aprepitant with drugs that are known to be metabolized by CYP2C9 may result in lower plasma concentrations of these drugs). Products include:
- Anaprox ... 2850
- Anaprox DS ... 2850
- Treximet ... 1681

Nateglinide (Co-administration of fosaprepitant or oral aprepitant with drugs that are known to be metabolized by CYP2C9 may result in lower plasma concentrations of these drugs).
No products indexed under this heading.

Nefazodone Hydrochloride (Aprepitant is a substrate for CYP3A4; therefore, co-administration of fosaprepitant or aprepitant with drugs that inhibit CYP3A4 activity may result in increased plasma concentrations of aprepitant. Consequently, concomitant administration of fosaprepitant or apreitant with strong CYP3A4 inhibitors (eg, ketoconazole, itraconzole, nefazodone, troleandomycin, clarithromycin, ritonavir, nelfinavir) should be approached with caution).
No products indexed under this heading.

Nelfinavir Mesylate (Aprepitant is a substrate for CYP3A4; therefore, co-administration of fosaprepitant or aprepitant with drugs that inhibit CYP3A4 activity may result in increased plasma concentrations of aprepitant. Consequently, concomitant administration of fosaprepitant or apreitant with strong CYP3A4 inhibitors (eg, ketoconazole, itraconzole, nefazodone, troleandomycin, clarithromycin, ritonavir, nelfinavir) should be approached with caution).
No products indexed under this heading.

Nevirapine (Aprepitant is a substrate for CYP3A4; therefore, co-administration of fosaprepitant or aprepitant with drugs that inhibit CYP3A4 activity may result in increased plasma concentrations of aprepitant. Consequently, concomitant administration of fosaprepitant or aprepitant with strong CYP3A4 inhibitors (eg, ketoconazole, itraconazole, nefazodone, troleandomycin, clarithromycin, ritonavir, nelfinavir) should be approached with caution. Because moderate CYP3A4 inhibitors (eg, diltiazem) result in a 2-fold increase in plasma concentrations of aprepitant, concomitant administration should also be approached with caution). Products include:
- Viramune Oral Suspension ... 897
- Viramune Tablets ... 897

Niacin (Aprepitant is a substrate for CYP3A4; therefore, co-administration of fosaprepitant or aprepitant with drugs that inhibit CYP3A4 activity may result in increased plasma concentrations of aprepitant. Consequently, concomitant administration of fosaprepitant or aprepitant with strong CYP3A4 inhibitors (eg, ketoconazole, itraconazole, nefazodone, troleandomycin, clarithromycin, ritonavir, nelfinavir) should be approached with caution. Because moderate CYP3A4 inhibitors (eg, diltiazem) result in a 2-fold increase in plasma concentrations of aprepitant, concomitant administration should also be approached with caution). Products include:
- Advicor ... 402
- Cardio Basics ... 3455
- Niaspan ... 497
- Simcor ... 524

Niacinamide (Aprepitant is a substrate for CYP3A4; therefore, co-administration of fosaprepitant or aprepitant with drugs that inhibit CYP3A4 activity may result in increased plasma concentrations of aprepitant. Consequently, concomitant administration of fosaprepitant or aprepitant with strong CYP3A4 inhibitors (eg, ketoconazole, itraconazole, nefazodone, troleandomycin, clarithromycin, ritonavir, nelfinavir) should be approached with caution. Because moderate CYP3A4 inhibitors (eg, diltiazem) result in a 2-fold increase in plasma concentrations of aprepitant, concomitant administration should also be approached with caution). Products include:
- CitraNatal 90 DHA Capsules ... 2332
- CitraNatal Assure ... 2332
- CitraNatal Rx ... 2332
- Heplive ... 607

Niacinamide Hydroiodide (Aprepitant is a substrate for CYP3A4; therefore, co-administration of fosaprepitant or aprepitant with drugs that inhibit CYP3A4 activity may result in increased plasma concentrations of aprepitant. Consequently, concomitant administration of fosaprepitant or aprepitant with strong CYP3A4 inhibitors (eg, ketoconazole, itraconazole, nefazodone, troleandomycin, clarithromycin, ritonavir, nelfinavir) should be approached with caution. Because moderate CYP3A4 inhibitors (eg, diltiazem) result in a 2-fold increase in plasma concentrations of aprepitant, concomitant administration should also be approached with caution).
No products indexed under this heading.

Nicardipine (As a moderate inhibitor of CYP3A4, aprepitant can increase plasma concentrations of orally co-administered medicinal products that are metabolized through CYP3A4).
No products indexed under this heading.

Nicardipine Hydrochloride (As a moderate inhibitor of CYP3A4, aprepitant can increase plasma concentrations of orally co-administered medicinal products that are metabolized through CYP3A4).
No products indexed under this heading.

Nicotinamide (Aprepitant is a substrate for CYP3A4; therefore, co-administration of fosaprepitant or aprepitant with drugs that inhibit CYP3A4 activity may result in increased plasma concentrations of aprepitant. Consequently, concomitant administration of fosaprepitant or aprepitant with strong CYP3A4 inhibitors (eg, ketoconazole, itraconazole, nefazodone, troleandomycin, clarithromycin, ritonavir, nelfinavir) should be approached with caution. Because moderate CYP3A4 inhibitors (eg, diltiazem) result in a 2-fold increase in plasma concentrations of aprepitant, concomitant administration should also be approached with caution).
No products indexed under this heading.

Nifedipine (Aprepitant is a substrate for CYP3A4; therefore, co-administration of fosaprepitant or aprepitant with drugs that inhibit CYP3A4 activity may result in increased plasma concentrations of aprepitant. Consequently, concomitant administration of fosaprepitant or aprepitant with strong CYP3A4 inhibitors (eg, ketoconazole, itraconazole, nefazodone, troleandomycin, clarithromycin, ritonavir, nelfinavir) should be approached with caution. Because moderate CYP3A4 inhibitors (eg, diltiazem) result in a 2-fold increase in plasma concentrations of aprepitant, concomitant administration should also be approached with caution).
No products indexed under this heading.

Nimodipine (As a moderate inhibitor of CYP3A4, aprepitant can increase plasma concentrations of orally co-administered medicinal products that are metabolized through CYP3A4).
No products indexed under this heading.

Nisoldipine (As a moderate inhibitor of CYP3A4, aprepitant can increase plasma concentrations of orally co-administered medicinal products that are metabolized through CYP3A4).
No products indexed under this heading.

Nitrendipine (As a moderate inhibitor of CYP3A4, aprepitant can increase plasma concentrations of orally co-administered medicinal products that are metabolized through CYP3A4).
No products indexed under this heading.

Norethindrone (The co-administration of fosaprepitant or aprepitant may reduce the efficacy of hormonal contraceptives during and for 28 days after administration of the last dose of either. Alternative or back-up methods of contraception should be used during treatment with fosaprepitant or aprepitant and for one month following the last dose of aprepitant). Products include:
- Ortho Micronor ... 2660

Norethindrone Acetate (As a moderate inhibitor of CYP3A4, aprepitant can increase plasma concentrations of orally co-administered medicinal products that are metabolized through CYP3A4). Products include:
- Activella ... 2561

Norethynodrel (The co-administration of fosaprepitant or aprepitant may reduce the efficacy of hormonal contraceptives during and for 28 days after administration of the last dose of either. Alternative or back-up methods of contraception should be used during treatment with fosaprepitant or aprepitant and for one month following the last dose of aprepitant).
No products indexed under this heading.

Norfloxacin (Aprepitant is a substrate for CYP3A4; therefore, co-administration of fosaprepitant or aprepitant with drugs that inhibit CYP3A4 activity may result in increased plasma concentrations of aprepitant. Consequently, concomitant administration of fosaprepitant or aprepitant with strong CYP3A4 inhibitors (eg, ketoconazole, itraconazole, nefazodone, troleandomycin, clarithromycin, ritonavir, nelfinavir) should be approached with caution. Because moderate CYP3A4 inhibitors (eg, diltiazem) result in a 2-fold increase in plasma concentrations of aprepitant, concomitant administration should also be approached with caution). Products include:
- Noroxin ... 2220

Norgestimate (The co-administration of fosaprepitant or aprepitant may reduce the efficacy of hormonal contraceptives during and for 28 days after administration of the last dose of either. Alternative or back-up methods of contraception should be used during treatment with fosaprepitant or aprepitant and for one month following the last dose of aprepitant). Products include:
- Ortho-Cyclen/Ortho Tri-Cyclen ... 2663
- Ortho Tri-Cyclen Lo Tablets ... 2673

Norgestrel (The co-administration of fosaprepitant or aprepitant may reduce the efficacy of hormonal contraceptives during and for 28 days after administration of the last dose of either. Alternative or back-up methods of contraception should be used during treatment with fosaprepitant or aprepitant and for one month following the last dose of aprepitant).
No products indexed under this heading.

Omeprazole (Aprepitant is a substrate for CYP3A4; therefore, co-administration of fosaprepitant or aprepitant with drugs that inhibit CYP3A4 activity may result in increased plasma concentrations of aprepitant. Consequently, concomitant administration of fosaprepitant or aprepitant with strong CYP3A4 inhibitors (eg, ketoconazole, itraconazole, nefazodone, troleandomycin, clarithromycin, ritonavir, nelfinavir) should be approached with caution. Because moderate CYP3A4 inhibitors (eg, diltiazem) result in a 2-fold increase in plasma concentrations of aprepitant, concomitant administration should also be approached with caution).
No products indexed under this heading.

Ondansetron (As a moderate inhibitor of CYP3A4, aprepitant can increase plasma concentrations of orally co-administered medicinal products that are metabolized through CYP3A4).
No products indexed under this heading.

Ondansetron Hydrochloride (As a moderate inhibitor of CYP3A4, aprepitant can increase plasma concentrations of orally co-administered medicinal products that are metabolized through CYP3A4). Products include:
- Zofran Injection ... 1750
- Zofran ... 1756
- Zofran ODT ... 1756

Oxaprozin (Co-administration of fosaprepitant or oral aprepitant with drugs that are known to be metabolized by CYP2C9 may result in lower plasma concentrations of these drugs).
No products indexed under this heading.

Oxcarbazepine (Aprepitant is substrate for CYP3A4; therefore, co-administration of fosaprepitant or aprepitant with drugs that strongly induce CYP3A4 activity (eg, rifampin, carbamazepine, phenytoin) may result in reduced plasma concentrations and decreased efficacy).
No products indexed under this heading.

Paclitaxel (Particular caution and careful monitoring are advised in patients receiving chemotherapy agents metabolized primarily by CYP3A4, like paclitaxel).
No products indexed under this heading.

Paroxetine Hydrochloride (Co-administration resulted in a decrease in AUC by approximately 25% and C_{max} by approximately 20% of both aprepitant and paroxetine). Products include:
- Paroxetine CR ... 2361
- Paroxetine ER ... 2371
- Paxil ... 1586
- Paxil CR ... 1596

Phenobarbital (Aprepitant is substrate for CYP3A4; therefore, co-administration of fosaprepitant or aprepitant with drugs that strongly induce CYP3A4 activity (eg, rifampin, carbamazepine, phenytoin) may result in reduced plasma concentrations and decreased efficacy). Products include:
- Donnatal ... 2711

Phenobarbital Sodium (Aprepitant is substrate for CYP3A4; therefore, co-administration of fosaprepitant or aprepitant with drugs that strongly induce CYP3A4 activity (eg, rifampin, carbamazepine, phenytoin) may result in reduced plasma concentrations and decreased efficacy).
No products indexed under this heading.

Phenylbutazone (Co-administration of fosaprepitant or oral aprepitant with drugs that are known to be metabolized by CYP2C9 may result in lower plasma concentrations of these drugs).
No products indexed under this heading.

Phenytoin (Aprepitant has been shown to induce the metabolism of S(-) warfarin and tolbutamide, which are metabolized through CYP2C9. Co-administration of aprepitant with these drugs or other drugs that are known to be metabolized by CYP2C9, such as phenytoin, may result in lower plasma concentrations of these drugs).
No products indexed under this heading.

Phenytoin Sodium (Aprepitant has been shown to induce the metabolism

IMPORTANT NOTE: Always consult each drug listing in the patient's regimen for possible interactions.

of S(-) warfarin and tolbutamide, which are metabolized through CYP2C9. Co-administration of aprepitant with these drugs or other drugs that are known to be metabolized by CYP2C9, such as phenytoin, may result in lower plasma concentrations of these drugs).
Products include:
Phenytek Capsules 2380

Pimozide (EMEND is a moderate CYP3A4 inhibitor; concurrent use with EMEND could result in elevated plasma concentrations of pimozide, potentially causing serious or life-threatening reactions, and is contraindicated).
No products indexed under this heading.

Pioglitazone Hydrochloride (Co-administration of fosaprepitant or oral aprepitant with drugs that are known to be metabolized by CYP2C9 may result in lower plasma concentrations of these drugs). Products include:
ActoPlus 3338
Actos 3345
Duetact 3354

Piroxicam (Co-administration of fosaprepitant or oral aprepitant with drugs that are known to be metabolized by CYP2C9 may result in lower plasma concentrations of these drugs).
No products indexed under this heading.

Polyestradiol Phosphate (As a moderate inhibitor of CYP3A4, aprepitant can increase plasma concentrations of orally co-administered medicinal products that are metabolized through CYP3A4).
No products indexed under this heading.

Posaconazole (Aprepitant is a substrate for CYP3A4; therefore, co-administration of fosaprepitant or aprepitant with drugs that inhibit CYP3A4 activity may result in increased plasma concentrations of aprepitant. Consequently, concomitant administration of fosaprepitant or aprepitant with strong CYP3A4 inhibitors (eg, ketoconazole, itraconazole, nefazodone, troleandomycin, clarithromycin, ritonavir, nelfinavir) should be approached with caution. Because moderate CYP3A4 inhibitors (eg, diltiazem) result in a 2-fold increase in plasma concentrations of aprepitant, concomitant administration should also be approached with caution). Products include:
Noxafil 3172

Prednisolone (Aprepitant is substrate for CYP3A4; therefore, co-administration of fosaprepitant or aprepitant with drugs that strongly induce CYP3A4 activity (eg, rifampin, carbamazepine, phenytoin) may result in reduced plasma concentrations and decreased efficacy).
No products indexed under this heading.

Prednisolone Acetate (Aprepitant is substrate for CYP3A4; therefore, co-administration of fosaprepitant or aprepitant with drugs that strongly induce CYP3A4 activity (eg, rifampin, carbamazepine, phenytoin) may result in reduced plasma concentrations and decreased efficacy). Products include:
Blephamide .... ⊙ 212, ⊙ 214
Pred Forte .... ⊙ 225
Pred Mild .... ⊙ 230
Pred-G .... ⊙ 226, ⊙ 227

Prednisolone Sodium Phosphate (Aprepitant is substrate for CYP3A4; therefore, co-administration of fosaprepitant or aprepitant with drugs that strongly induce CYP3A4 activity (eg, rifampin, carbamazepine, phenytoin) may result in reduced plasma concentrations and decreased efficacy).
No products indexed under this heading.

Prednisolone Tebutate (Aprepitant is substrate for CYP3A4; therefore, co-administration of fosaprepitant or aprepitant with drugs that strongly induce CYP3A4 activity (eg, rifampin, carbamazepine, phenytoin) may result in reduced plasma concentrations and decreased efficacy).
No products indexed under this heading.

Prednisone (Aprepitant is substrate for CYP3A4; therefore, co-administration of fosaprepitant or aprepitant with drugs that strongly induce CYP3A4 activity (eg, rifampin, carbamazepine, phenytoin) may result in reduced plasma concentrations and decreased efficacy).
No products indexed under this heading.

Prednisone sodium phosphate (Aprepitant is substrate for CYP3A4; therefore, co-administration of fosaprepitant or aprepitant with drugs that strongly induce CYP3A4 activity (eg, rifampin, carbamazepine, phenytoin) may result in reduced plasma concentrations and decreased efficacy).
No products indexed under this heading.

Primidone (Aprepitant is substrate for CYP3A4; therefore, co-administration of fosaprepitant or aprepitant with drugs that strongly induce CYP3A4 activity (eg, rifampin, carbamazepine, phenytoin) may result in reduced plasma concentrations and decreased efficacy).
No products indexed under this heading.

Propoxyphene Hydrochloride (Aprepitant is a substrate for CYP3A4; therefore, co-administration of fosaprepitant or aprepitant with drugs that inhibit CYP3A4 activity may result in increased plasma concentrations of aprepitant. Consequently, concomitant administration of fosaprepitant or aprepitant with strong CYP3A4 inhibitors (eg, ketoconazole, itraconazole, nefazodone, troleandomycin, clarithromycin, ritonavir, nelfinavir) should be approached with caution. Because moderate CYP3A4 inhibitors (eg, diltiazem) result in a 2-fold increase in plasma concentrations of aprepitant, concomitant administration should also be approached with caution).
No products indexed under this heading.

Propoxyphene Napsylate (Aprepitant is a substrate for CYP3A4; therefore, co-administration of fosaprepitant or aprepitant with drugs that inhibit CYP3A4 activity may result in increased plasma concentrations of aprepitant. Consequently, concomitant administration of fosaprepitant or aprepitant with strong CYP3A4 inhibitors (eg, ketoconazole, itraconazole, nefazodone, troleandomycin, clarithromycin, ritonavir, nelfinavir) should be approached with caution. Because moderate CYP3A4 inhibitors (eg, diltiazem) result in a 2-fold increase in plasma concentrations of aprepitant, concomitant administration should also be approached with caution).
No products indexed under this heading.

Quinidine (Aprepitant is a substrate for CYP3A4; therefore, co-administration of fosaprepitant or aprepitant with drugs that inhibit CYP3A4 activity may result in increased plasma concentrations of aprepitant. Consequently, concomitant administration of fosaprepitant or aprepitant with strong CYP3A4 inhibitors (eg, ketoconazole, itraconazole, nefazodone, troleandomycin, clarithromycin, ritonavir, nelfinavir) should be approached with caution. Because moderate CYP3A4 inhibitors (eg, diltiazem) result in a 2-fold increase in plasma concentrations of aprepitant, concomitant administration should also be approached with caution).
No products indexed under this heading.

Quinidine Gluconate (As a moderate inhibitor of CYP3A4, aprepitant can increase plasma concentrations of orally co-administered medicinal products that are metabolized through CYP3A4).
No products indexed under this heading.

Quinidine Hydrochloride (Aprepitant is a substrate for CYP3A4; therefore, co-administration of fosaprepitant or aprepitant with drugs that inhibit CYP3A4 activity may result in increased plasma concentrations of aprepitant. Consequently, concomitant administration of fosaprepitant or aprepitant with strong CYP3A4 inhibitors (eg, ketoconazole, itraconazole, nefazodone, troleandomycin, clarithromycin, ritonavir, nelfinavir) should be approached with caution. Because moderate CYP3A4 inhibitors (eg, diltiazem) result in a 2-fold increase in plasma concentrations of aprepitant, concomitant administration should also be approached with caution).
No products indexed under this heading.

Quinidine Polygalacturonate (Aprepitant is a substrate for CYP3A4; therefore, co-administration of fosaprepitant or aprepitant with drugs that inhibit CYP3A4 activity may result in increased plasma concentrations of aprepitant. Consequently, concomitant administration of fosaprepitant or aprepitant with strong CYP3A4 inhibitors (eg, ketoconazole, itraconazole, nefazodone, troleandomycin, clarithromycin, ritonavir, nelfinavir) should be approached with caution. Because moderate CYP3A4 inhibitors (eg, diltiazem) result in a 2-fold increase in plasma concentrations of aprepitant, concomitant administration should also be approached with caution).
No products indexed under this heading.

Quinidine Sulfate (Aprepitant is a substrate for CYP3A4; therefore, co-administration of fosaprepitant or aprepitant with drugs that inhibit CYP3A4 activity may result in increased plasma concentrations of aprepitant. Consequently, concomitant administration of fosaprepitant or aprepitant with strong CYP3A4 inhibitors (eg, ketoconazole, itraconazole, nefazodone, troleandomycin, clarithromycin, ritonavir, nelfinavir) should be approached with caution. Because moderate CYP3A4 inhibitors (eg, diltiazem) result in a 2-fold increase in plasma concentrations of aprepitant, concomitant administration should also be approached with caution).
No products indexed under this heading.

Quinine (Aprepitant is a substrate for CYP3A4; therefore, co-administration of fosaprepitant or aprepitant with drugs that inhibit CYP3A4 activity may result in increased plasma concentrations of aprepitant. Consequently, concomitant administration of fosaprepitant or aprepitant with strong CYP3A4 inhibitors (eg, ketoconazole, itraconazole, nefazodone, troleandomycin, clarithromycin, ritonavir, nelfinavir) should be approached with caution. Because moderate CYP3A4 inhibitors (eg, diltiazem) result in a 2-fold increase in plasma concentrations of aprepitant, concomitant administration should also be approached with caution). Products include:
Hyland's Leg Cramps PM with Quinine 3315

Quinine Sulfate (Aprepitant is a substrate for CYP3A4; therefore, co-administration of fosaprepitant or aprepitant with drugs that inhibit CYP3A4 activity may result in increased plasma concentrations of aprepitant. Consequently, concomitant administration of fosaprepitant or aprepitant with strong CYP3A4 inhibitors (eg, ketoconazole, itraconazole, nefazodone, troleandomycin, clarithromycin, ritonavir, nelfinavir) should be approached with caution. Because moderate CYP3A4 inhibitors (eg, diltiazem) result in a 2-fold increase in plasma concentrations of aprepitant, concomitant administration should also be approached with caution).
No products indexed under this heading.

Quinupristin (Aprepitant is a substrate for CYP3A4; therefore, co-administration of fosaprepitant or aprepitant with drugs that inhibit CYP3A4 activity may result in increased plasma concentrations of aprepitant. Consequently, concomitant administration of fosaprepitant or aprepitant with strong CYP3A4 inhibitors (eg, ketoconazole, itraconazole, nefazodone, troleandomycin, clarithromycin, ritonavir, nelfinavir) should be approached with caution. Because moderate CYP3A4 inhibitors (eg, diltiazem) result in a 2-fold increase in plasma concentrations of aprepitant, concomitant administration should also be approached with caution).
No products indexed under this heading.

Ranitidine Bismuth Citrate (Aprepitant is a substrate for CYP3A4; therefore, co-administration of fosaprepitant or aprepitant with drugs that inhibit CYP3A4 activity may result in increased plasma concentrations of aprepitant. Consequently, concomitant administration of fosaprepitant or aprepitant with strong CYP3A4 inhibitors (eg, ketoconazole, itraconazole, nefazodone, troleandomycin, clarithromycin, ritonavir, nelfinavir) should be approached with caution. Because moderate CYP3A4 inhibitors (eg, diltiazem) result in a 2-fold increase in plasma concentrations of aprepitant, concomitant administration should also be approached with caution).
No products indexed under this heading.

Ranitidine Hydrochloride (Aprepitant is a substrate for CYP3A4; therefore, co-administration of fosaprepitant or aprepitant with drugs that inhibit CYP3A4 activity may result in increased plasma concentrations of aprepitant. Consequently, concomitant administration of fosaprepitant or aprepitant with strong CYP3A4 inhibitors (eg, ketoconazole, itraconazole, nefazodone, troleandomycin, clarithromycin, ritonavir, nelfinavir) should be approached with caution. Because moderate CYP3A4 inhibitors (eg, diltiazem) result in a 2-fold increase in plasma concentrations of aprepitant, concomitant administration should also be approached with caution). Products include:
Zantac 1737
Zantac Injection 1732
Zantac Pharmacy 1735

Repaglinide (Co-administration of fosaprepitant or oral aprepitant with drugs that are known to be metabolized by CYP2C9 may result in lower plasma concentrations of these drugs).
No products indexed under this heading.

Rifabutin (Aprepitant is substrate for CYP3A4; therefore, co-administration of fosaprepitant or aprepitant with drugs that strongly induce CYP3A4 activity (eg, rifampin, carbamazepine, phenytoin) may result in reduced plasma concentrations and decreased efficacy).
No products indexed under this heading.

Rifampicin (Aprepitant is substrate for CYP3A4; therefore, co-administration of fosaprepitant or aprepitant with drugs that strongly induce CYP3A4 activity (eg, rifampin, carbamazepine, phenytoin) may result in reduced plasma concentrations and decreased efficacy).
No products indexed under this heading.

IMPORTANT NOTE: Always consult each drug listing in the patient's regimen for possible interactions.

Triamcinolone Hexacetonide (Aprepitant is substrate for CYP3A4; therefore, co-administration of fosaprepitant or aprepitant with drugs that strongly induce CYP3A4 activity (eg, rifampin, carbamazepine, phenytoin) may result in reduced plasma concentrations and decreased efficacy).
No products indexed under this heading.

Triazolam (Fosaprepitant and oral aprepitant may increase the AUC of midazolam. The potential effects of increased plasma concentrations of midazolam or other benzodiazepines metabolized via CYP3A4 (alprazolam, triazolam) should be considered when co-administeringthese agents with a 3-day regimen of fosaprepitant followed by aprepitant).
No products indexed under this heading.

Troglitazone (Aprepitant is a substrate for CYP3A4; therefore, co-administration of fosaprepitant or aprepitant with drugs that inhibit CYP3A4 activity may result in increased plasma concentrations of aprepitant. Consequently, concomitant administration of fosaprepitant or aprepitant with strong CYP3A4 inhibitors (eg, ketoconazole, itraconazole, nefazodone, troleandomycin, clarithromycin, ritonavir, nelfinavir) should be approached with caution. Because moderate CYP3A4 inhibitors (eg, diltiazem) result in a 2-fold increase in plasma concentrations of aprepitant, concomitant administration should also be approached with caution).
No products indexed under this heading.

Troleandomycin (Aprepitant is a substrate for CYP3A4; therefore, co-administration of fosaprepitant or aprepitant with drugs that inhibit CYP3A4 activity may result in increased plasma concentrations of aprepitant. Consequently, concomitant administration of fosaprepitant or apreitant with strong CYP3A4 inhibitors (eg, ketoconazole, itraconzole, nefazodone, troleandomycin, clarithromycin, ritonavir, nelfinavir) should be approached with caution).
No products indexed under this heading.

Valdecoxib (Co-administration of fosaprepitant or oral aprepitant with drugs that are known to be metabolized by CYP2C9 may result in lower plasma concentrations of these drugs).
No products indexed under this heading.

Valproate Sodium (Aprepitant is a substrate for CYP3A4; therefore, co-administration of fosaprepitant or aprepitant with drugs that inhibit CYP3A4 activity may result in increased plasma concentrations of aprepitant. Consequently, concomitant administration of fosaprepitant or aprepitant with strong CYP3A4 inhibitors (eg, ketoconazole, itraconazole, nefazodone, troleandomycin, clarithromycin, ritonavir, nelfinavir) should be approached with caution. Because moderate CYP3A4 inhibitors (eg, diltiazem) result in a 2-fold increase in plasma concentrations of aprepitant, concomitant administration should also be approached with caution).
No products indexed under this heading.

Valsartan (Co-administration of fosaprepitant or oral aprepitant with drugs that are known to be metabolized by CYP2C9 may result in lower plasma concentrations of these drugs).
Products include:
Diovan 2413
Diovan HCT 2419
Exforge 2443
Exforge HCT 2449
Valturna 3637

Vardenafil Hydrochloride (Aprepitant is a substrate for CYP3A4; therefore, co-administration of fosaprepitant or aprepitant with drugs that inhibit CYP3A4 activity may result in increased plasma concentrations of aprepitant. Consequently, concomitant administration of fosaprepitant or aprepitant with strong CYP3A4 inhibitors (eg, ketoconazole, itraconazole, nefazodone, troleandomycin, clarithromycin, ritonavir, nelfinavir) should be approached with caution. Because moderate CYP3A4 inhibitors (eg, diltiazem) result in a 2-fold increase in plasma concentrations of aprepitant, concomitant administration should also be approached with caution). Products include:
Levitra 3157

Verapamil Hydrochloride (Aprepitant is a substrate for CYP3A4; therefore, co-administration of fosaprepitant or aprepitant with drugs that inhibit CYP3A4 activity may result in increased plasma concentrations of aprepitant. Consequently, concomitant administration of fosaprepitant or aprepitant with strong CYP3A4 inhibitors (eg, ketoconazole, itraconazole, nefazodone, troleandomycin, clarithromycin, ritonavir, nelfinavir) should be approached with caution. Because moderate CYP3A4 inhibitors (eg, diltiazem) result in a 2-fold increase in plasma concentrations of aprepitant, concomitant administration should also be approached with caution). Products include:
Tarka 534

Vinblastine Sulfate (Particular caution and careful monitoring are advised in patients receiving chemotherapy agents metabolized primarily by CYP3A4, like vinblastine).
No products indexed under this heading.

Vincristine Sulfate (Particular caution and careful monitoring are advised in patients receiving chemotherapy agents metabolized primarily by CYP3A4, like vincristine).
No products indexed under this heading.

Voriconazole (Aprepitant is a substrate for CYP3A4; therefore, co-administration of fosaprepitant or aprepitant with drugs that inhibit CYP3A4 activity may result in increased plasma concentrations of aprepitant. Consequently, concomitant administration of fosaprepitant or apreitant with strong CYP3A4 inhibitors (eg, ketoconazole, itraconazole, nefazodone, troleandomycin, clarithromycin, ritonavir, nelfinavir) should be approached with caution).
No products indexed under this heading.

Warfarin Sodium (Aprepitant is an inducer of CYP2C9; co-administration has been shown to induce the metabolism of S(-) warfarin which is metabolized through CYP2C9; may result in a clinically significant decrease in INR of prothrombin time. In patients on chronic warfarin therapy, prothrombin time (INR) should be closely monitored in the 2-week period, particularly at 7-10 days, following initiation of the 3-day regimen of fosaprepitant followed by aprepitant with each chemotherapy cycle).
No products indexed under this heading.

Zafirlukast (Aprepitant is a substrate for CYP3A4; therefore, co-administration of fosaprepitant or aprepitant with drugs that inhibit CYP3A4 activity may result in increased plasma concentrations of aprepitant. Consequently, concomitant administration of fosaprepitant or aprepitant with strong CYP3A4 inhibitors (eg, ketoconazole, itraconazole, nefazodone, troleandomycin, clarithromycin, ritonavir, nelfinavir) should be approached with caution. Because moderate CYP3A4 inhibitors (eg, diltiazem) result in a 2-fold increase in plasma concentrations of aprepitant, concomitant administration should also be approached with caution). Products include:
Accolate 3612

Zileuton (Aprepitant is a substrate for CYP3A4; therefore, co-administration of fosaprepitant or aprepitant with drugs that inhibit CYP3A4 activity may result in increased plasma concentrations of aprepitant. Consequently, concomitant administration of fosaprepitant or aprepitant with strong CYP3A4 inhibitors (eg, ketoconazole, itraconazole, nefazodone, troleandomycin, clarithromycin, ritonavir, nelfinavir) should be approached with caution. Because moderate CYP3A4 inhibitors (eg, diltiazem) result in a 2-fold increase in plasma concentrations of aprepitant, concomitant administration should also be approached with caution).
No products indexed under this heading.

Food Interactions

Grapefruit (Aprepitant is a substrate for CYP3A4; therefore, co-administration of fosaprepitant or aprepitant with drugs that inhibit CYP3A4 activity may result in increased plasma concentrations of aprepitant. Consequently, concomitant administration of fosaprepitant or aprepitant with strong CYP3A4 inhibitors (eg, ketoconazole, itraconazole, nefazodone, troleandomycin, clarithromycin, ritonavir, nelfinavir) should be approached with caution. Because moderate CYP3A4 inhibitors (eg, diltiazem) result in a 2-fold increase in plasma concentrations of aprepitant, concomitant administration should also be approached with caution).

Grapefruit Juice (Aprepitant is a substrate for CYP3A4; therefore, co-administration of fosaprepitant or aprepitant with drugs that inhibit CYP3A4 activity may result in increased plasma concentrations of aprepitant. Consequently, concomitant administration of fosaprepitant or aprepitant with strong CYP3A4 inhibitors (eg, ketoconazole, itraconazole, nefazodone, troleandomycin, clarithromycin, ritonavir, nelfinavir) should be approached with caution. Because moderate CYP3A4 inhibitors (eg, diltiazem) result in a 2-fold increase in plasma concentrations of aprepitant, concomitant administration should also be approached with caution).

EMEND FOR INJECTION

(Fosaprepitant Dimeglumine) 2132
See Emend Capsules

EMSAM TRANSDERMAL SYSTEM

(Selegiline) 3623
May interact with alcohols, amphetamines, ephedrine, general anesthetics, local anesthetics, monoamine oxidase inhibitors, narcotic analgesics, phenylpropanolamine containing anorectics, phenylpropanolamines, selective serotonin reuptake inhibitors, serotonin and norepinephrine reuptake inhibitors, sympathomimetics, tricyclic antidepressants, vasopressors, and certain other agents. Compounds in these categories include:

Albuterol (Concomitant use of sympathomimetic agents with selegiline transdermal system is contraindicated).
No products indexed under this heading.

Albuterol Sulfate (Concomitant use of sympathomimetic agents with selegiline transdermal system is contraindicated). Products include:
ProAir HFA 3393
Proventil HFA 3204
Ventolin HFA 1708

Alfentanil Hydrochloride (Selegiline transdermal system is contraindicated with analgesic agents such as tramadol, methadone, and propoxyphene).
No products indexed under this heading.

Amitriptyline Hydrochloride (Selegiline transdermal system is contraindicated with tricyclic antidepressants. Serious, sometimes fatal, central nervous system (CNS) toxicity referred to as the "serotonin syndrome" has been reported with the combination of non-selective MAOIs with certain other drugs, including selective serotonin reuptake inhibitor antidepressants).
No products indexed under this heading.

Amoxapine (Selegiline transdermal system is contraindicated with tricyclic antidepressants. Serious, sometimes fatal, central nervous system (CNS) toxicity referred to as the "serotonin syndrome" has been reported with the combination of non-selective MAOIs with certain other drugs, including selective serotonin reuptake inhibitor antidepressants).
No products indexed under this heading.

Amphetamine Aspartate (Selegiline transdermal system is contraindicated for use with sympathomimetic amines, including amphetamines. Serious, sometimes fatal, central nervous system (CNS) toxicity referred to as the "serotonin syndrome" has been reported with the combination of non-selective MAOIs with certain other drugs, including amphetamines).
No products indexed under this heading.

Amphetamine Aspartate Monohydrate (Selegiline transdermal system is contraindicated for use with sympathomimetic amines, including amphetamines. Serious, sometimes fatal, central nervous system (CNS) toxicity referred to as the "serotonin syndrome" has been reported with the combination of non-selective MAOIs with certain other drugs, including amphetamines).
No products indexed under this heading.

Amphetamine Resins (Selegiline transdermal system is contraindicated for use with sympathomimetic amines, including amphetamines. Serious, sometimes fatal, central nervous system (CNS) toxicity referred to as the "serotonin syndrome" has been reported with the combination of non-selective MAOIs with certain other drugs, including amphetamines).
No products indexed under this heading.

Amphetamine Sulfate (Selegiline transdermal system is contraindicated for use with sympathomimetic amines, including amphetamines. Serious, sometimes fatal, central nervous system (CNS) toxicity referred to as the "serotonin syndrome" has been reported with the combination of non-selective MAOIs with certain other drugs, including amphetamines).
No products indexed under this heading.

Apomorphine (Selegiline transdermal system is contraindicated with analgesic agents such as tramadol, methadone, and propoxyphene).
No products indexed under this heading.

Apomorphine Hydrochloride (Selegiline transdermal system is contraindicated with analgesic agents such as tramadol, methadone, and propoxyphene).
No products indexed under this heading.

Articaine Hydrochloride (Patients taking selegiline transdermal system should not be given local anesthesia containing sympathomimetic vasoconstrictors).
No products indexed under this heading.

579 Interactions Index Emsam

Bupivacaine Hydrochloride (Patients taking selegiline transdermal system should not be given local anesthesia containing sympathomimetic vasoconstrictors).
No products indexed under this heading.

Buprenorphine Hydrochloride (Selegiline transdermal system is contraindicated with analgesic agents such as tramadol, methadone, and propoxyphene).
No products indexed under this heading.

Bupropion (Selegiline transdermal system is contraindicated with bupropion hydrochloride. Concomitant use of selegiline with buspirone hydrochloride is not advised since several cases of elevated blood pressure have been reported in patients taking MAOIs who were then given buspirone hydrochloride).
No products indexed under this heading.

Bupropion Hydrochloride (Selegiline transdermal system is contraindicated with bupropion hydrochloride. Concomitant use of selegiline with buspirone hydrochloride is not advised since several cases of elevated blood pressure have been reported in patients taking MAOIs who were then given buspirone hydrochloride). Products include:
Aplenzin 2948
Wellbutrin 1719
Wellbutrin SR 1725
Zyban 1762

Carbamazepine (Carbamazepine is contraindicated in patients taking selegiline. Carbamazepine is an enzyme inducer and typically causes decreases in drug exposure; however, slightly increased levels of selegiline and its metabolites were seen after single application of selegiline 6 mg/24 hours in subjects who had received carbamazepine (400 mg/day) for 14 days. Changes in plasma selegiline concentrations were nearly two-fold, and variable across the subject population. The clinical relevance of these observations is unknown). Products include:
Carbatrol 3280
Equetro 3477

Chloroprocaine Hydrochloride (Patients taking selegiline transdermal system should not be given local anesthesia containing sympathomimetic vasoconstrictors).
No products indexed under this heading.

Citalopram Hydrobromide (Selegiline transdermal system is contraindicated with selective serotonin reuptake inhibitors. Serious, sometimes fatal, central nervous system (CNS) toxicity referred to as the "serotonin syndrome" has been reported with the combination of non-selective MAOIs with certain other drugs, including selective serotonin reuptake inhibitor antidepressants). Products include:
Celexa 1153

Clomipramine Hydrochloride (Selegiline transdermal system is contraindicated with tricyclic antidepressants. Serious, sometimes fatal, central nervous system (CNS) toxicity referred to as the "serotonin syndrome" has been reported with the combination of non-selective MAOIs with certain other drugs, including selective serotonin reuptake inhibitor antidepressants).
No products indexed under this heading.

Cocaine Hydrochloride (Patients taking selegiline transdermal system should not be given cocaine).
No products indexed under this heading.

Codeine Phosphate (Selegiline transdermal system is contraindicated with analgesic agents such as tramadol, methadone, and propoxyphene).
Products include:
Tylenol with Codeine 2691

Codeine Sulfate (Selegiline transdermal system is contraindicated with analgesic agents such as tramadol, methadone, and propoxyphene).
No products indexed under this heading.

Cold remedy (As with other MAOIs, selegiline is contraindicated for use with sympathomimetic amines, including amphetamines as well as cold products).
No products indexed under this heading.

Cyclobenzaprine (Selegiline transdermal system is contraindicated with cyclobenzaprine).
No products indexed under this heading.

Cyclobenzaprine Hydrochloride (Selegiline transdermal system is contraindicated with cyclobenzaprine). Products include:
Amrix 964

Desflurane (Patients taking selegiline transdermal system should not undergo elective surgery requiring general anesthesia).
No products indexed under this heading.

Desipramine Hydrochloride (Selegiline transdermal system is contraindicated with tricyclic antidepressants. Serious, sometimes fatal, central nervous system (CNS) toxicity referred to as the "serotonin syndrome" has been reported with the combination of non-selective MAOIs with certain other drugs, including selective serotonin reuptake inhibitor antidepressants).
No products indexed under this heading.

Desvenlafaxine Succinate (Selegiline transdermal system is contraindicated with dual serotonin and norepinephrine reuptake inhibitors). Products include:
Pristiq 3564

Dextroamphetamine Sulfate (Selegiline transdermal system is contraindicated for use with sympathomimetic amines, including amphetamines). Products include:
Dexedrine 1425

Dextromethorphan (Selegiline transdermal system is contraindicated with the antitussive agent dextromethorphan).
No products indexed under this heading.

Dextromethorphan Hydrobromide (Selegiline transdermal system is contraindicated with the antitussive agent dextromethorphan).
No products indexed under this heading.

Dextromethorphan Polistirex (Selegiline transdermal system is contraindicated with the antitussive agent dextromethorphan).
No products indexed under this heading.

Dextromethorphan Tannate (Selegiline transdermal system is contraindicated with the antitussive agent dextromethorphan).
No products indexed under this heading.

Dezocine (Selegiline transdermal system is contraindicated with analgesic agents such as tramadol, methadone, and propoxyphene).
No products indexed under this heading.

Dihydrocodeine Bitartrate (Selegiline transdermal system is contraindicated with analgesic agents such as tramadol, methadone, and propoxyphene).
No products indexed under this heading.

Dihydrocodeinone Bitartrate (Selegiline transdermal system is contraindicated with analgesic agents such as tramadol, methadone, and propoxyphene).
No products indexed under this heading.

Dobutamine (Selegiline transdermal system is contraindicated with the use of drugs or products containing vasoconstrictors).
No products indexed under this heading.

Dobutamine Hydrochloride (Concomitant use of sympathomimetic agents with selegiline transdermal system is contraindicated).
No products indexed under this heading.

Dopamine Hydrochloride (Concomitant use of sympathomimetic agents with selegiline transdermal system is contraindicated).
No products indexed under this heading.

Doxepin Hydrochloride (Selegiline transdermal system is contraindicated with tricyclic antidepressants. Serious, sometimes fatal, central nervous system (CNS) toxicity referred to as the "serotonin syndrome" has been reported with the combination of non-selective MAOIs with certain other drugs, including selective serotonin reuptake inhibitor antidepressants).
No products indexed under this heading.

Duloxetine Hydrochloride (Selegiline transdermal system is contraindicated with dual serotonin and norepinephrine reuptake inhibitors). Products include:
Cymbalta 1871

Enflurane (Patients taking selegiline transdermal system should not undergo elective surgery requiring general anesthesia).
No products indexed under this heading.

Ephedrine Hydrochloride (Selegiline transdermal system is contraindicated for use with ephedrine).
No products indexed under this heading.

Ephedrine Sulfate (Selegiline transdermal system is contraindicated for use with ephedrine).
No products indexed under this heading.

Ephedrine Tannate (Selegiline transdermal system is contraindicated for use with ephedrine).
No products indexed under this heading.

Epinephrine (Concomitant use of sympathomimetic agents with selegiline transdermal system is contraindicated). Products include:
EpiPen 3631
Twinject 3268

Epinephrine Bitartrate (Concomitant use of sympathomimetic agents with selegiline transdermal system is contraindicated).
No products indexed under this heading.

Epinephrine Hydrochloride (Concomitant use of sympathomimetic agents with selegiline transdermal system is contraindicated).
No products indexed under this heading.

Escitalopram Oxalate (Selegiline transdermal system is contraindicated with selective serotonin reuptake inhibitors. Serious, sometimes fatal, central nervous system (CNS) toxicity referred to as the "serotonin syndrome" has been reported with the combination of non-selective MAOIs with certain other drugs, including selective serotonin reuptake inhibitor antidepressants). Products include:
Lexapro Oral Suspension 1160
Lexapro Tablets 1160

Ethanol (The use of alcohol is not recommended while using selegiline transdermal system).
No products indexed under this heading.

Ethyl Alcohol (The use of alcohol is not recommended while using selegiline transdermal system).
No products indexed under this heading.

Etidocaine Hydrochloride (Patients taking selegiline transdermal system should not be given local anesthesia containing sympathomimetic vasoconstrictors).
No products indexed under this heading.

Fentanyl (Selegiline transdermal system is contraindicated with analgesic agents such as tramadol, methadone, and propoxyphene). Products include:
Duragesic 2604
Fentanyl Transdermal System 2346
Onsolis 2054

Fentanyl Citrate (Selegiline transdermal system is contraindicated with analgesic agents such as tramadol, methadone, and propoxyphene). Products include:
Fentora 966

Fluoxetine (Selegiline transdermal system is contraindicated with selective serotonin reuptake inhibitors. Serious, sometimes fatal, central nervous system (CNS) toxicity referred to as the "serotonin syndrome" has been reported with the combination of non-selective MAOIs with certain other drugs, including selective serotonin reuptake inhibitor antidepressants).
No products indexed under this heading.

Fluoxetine Hydrochloride (Selegiline transdermal system is contraindicated with selective serotonin reuptake inhibitors. Serious, sometimes fatal, central nervous system (CNS) toxicity referred to as the "serotonin syndrome" has been reported with the combination of non-selective MAOIs with certain other drugs, including selective serotonin reuptake inhibitor antidepressants). Products include:
Prozac Weekly 1941
Prozac Pulvules 1941
Symbyax 1965

Fluvoxamine (Selegiline transdermal system is contraindicated with selective serotonin reuptake inhibitors. Serious, sometimes fatal, central nervous system (CNS) toxicity referred to as the "serotonin syndrome" has been reported with the combination of non-selective MAOIs with certain other drugs, including selective serotonin reuptake inhibitor antidepressants).
No products indexed under this heading.

Fluvoxamine Maleate (Selegiline transdermal system is contraindicated with selective serotonin reuptake inhibitors. Serious, sometimes fatal, central nervous system (CNS) toxicity referred to as the "serotonin syndrome" has been reported with the combination of non-selective MAOIs with certain other drugs, including selective serotonin reuptake inhibitor antidepressants).
No products indexed under this heading.

Halothane (Patients taking selegiline transdermal system should not undergo elective surgery requiring general anesthesia).
No products indexed under this heading.

Herbal Medicines, unspecified (Patients should be advised to notify their physician if they are taking, or plan to take, any prescription or over-the-counter drugs, including herbals, because of the potential for drug interactions with selegiline).
No products indexed under this heading.

Hydrocodone Bitartrate (Selegiline transdermal system is contraindicated with analgesic agents such as tramadol, methadone, and propoxyphene).
Products include:
Vicodin 560
Vicodin ES 561
Vicodin HP 563
Vicoprofen 564
Zydone 1138

Hydrocodone Polistirex (Selegiline transdermal system is contraindicated with analgesic agents such as tramadol, methadone, and propoxyphene).
Products include:
Tussionex 3443

Hydromorphone (Selegiline transdermal system is contraindicated with analgesic agents such as tramadol, methadone, and propoxyphene).
No products indexed under this heading.

Hydromorphone Hydrochloride (Selegiline transdermal system is contraindicated with analgesic agents such as tramadol, methadone, and propoxyphene). Products include:

Hypericum (Selegiline transdermal system is contraindicated with St. John's wort).
No products indexed under this heading.

Hypericum Perforatum (Selegiline transdermal system is contraindicated with St. John's wort). Products include:

Imipramine Hydrochloride (Selegiline transdermal system is contraindicated with tricyclic antidepressants. Serious, sometimes fatal, central nervous system (CNS) toxicity referred to as the "serotonin syndrome" has been reported with the combination of non-selective MAOIs with certain other drugs, including selective serotonin reuptake inhibitor antidepressants).
No products indexed under this heading.

Imipramine Pamoate (Selegiline transdermal system is contraindicated with tricyclic antidepressants. Serious, sometimes fatal, central nervous system (CNS) toxicity referred to as the "serotonin syndrome" has been reported with the combination of non-selective MAOIs with certain other drugs, including selective serotonin reuptake inhibitor antidepressants).
No products indexed under this heading.

Isocarboxazid (Selegiline transdermal system should not be used with oral selegiline or other MAO inhibitors). Products include:

Isoflurane (Patients taking selegiline transdermal system should not undergo elective surgery requiring general anesthesia).
No products indexed under this heading.

Isoproterenol Hydrochloride (Concomitant use of sympathomimetic agents with selegiline transdermal system is contraindicated).
No products indexed under this heading.

Isoproterenol Sulfate (Concomitant use of sympathomimetic agents with selegiline transdermal system is contraindicated).
No products indexed under this heading.

Ketamine Hydrochloride (Patients taking selegiline transdermal system should not undergo elective surgery requiring general anesthesia).
No products indexed under this heading.

Levalbuterol Hydrochloride (Concomitant use of sympathomimetic agents with selegiline transdermal system is contraindicated).
No products indexed under this heading.

Levobupivacaine Hydrochloride (Patients taking selegiline transdermal system should not be given local anesthesia containing sympathomimetic vasoconstrictors).
No products indexed under this heading.

Levorphanol Tartrate (Selegiline transdermal system is contraindicated with analgesic agents such as tramadol, methadone, and propoxyphene).
No products indexed under this heading.

Lidocaine Hydrochloride (Patients taking selegiline transdermal system should not be given local anesthesia containing sympathomimetic vasoconstrictors).
No products indexed under this heading.

Maprotiline Hydrochloride (Selegiline transdermal system is contraindicated with tricyclic antidepressants. Serious, sometimes fatal, central nervous system (CNS) toxicity referred to as the "serotonin syndrome" has been reported with the combination of non-selective MAOIs with certain other drugs, including selective serotonin reuptake inhibitor antidepressants).
No products indexed under this heading.

Meperidine Hydrochloride (Selegiline transdermal system is contraindicated with meperidine. Serious, sometimes fatal, central nervous system (CNS) toxicity referred to as the "serotonin syndrome" has been reported with the combination of non-selective MAOIs with certain other drugs, including tricyclic or selective serotonin reuptake inhibitor antidepressants, amphetamines, meperidine, or pentazocine).
No products indexed under this heading.

Mephentermine Sulfate (Selegiline transdermal system is contraindicated with the use of drugs or products containing vasoconstrictors).
No products indexed under this heading.

Mepivacaine Hydrochloride (Patients taking selegiline transdermal system should not be given local anesthesia containing sympathomimetic vasoconstrictors).
No products indexed under this heading.

Metaproterenol Sulfate (Concomitant use of sympathomimetic agents with selegiline transdermal system is contraindicated).
No products indexed under this heading.

Metaraminol Bitartrate (Concomitant use of sympathomimetic agents with selegiline transdermal system is contraindicated).
No products indexed under this heading.

Methadone Hydrochloride (Selegiline transdermal system is contraindicated with analgesic agents such as tramadol, methadone, and propoxyphene).
No products indexed under this heading.

Methamphetamine Hydrochloride (Selegiline transdermal system is contraindicated for use with sympathomimetic amines, including amphetamines).
No products indexed under this heading.

Methohexital Sodium (Patients taking selegiline transdermal system should not undergo elective surgery requiring general anesthesia).
No products indexed under this heading.

Methoxamine Hydrochloride (Concomitant use of sympathomimetic agents with selegiline transdermal system is contraindicated).
No products indexed under this heading.

Methoxyflurane (Patients taking selegiline transdermal system should not undergo elective surgery requiring general anesthesia).
No products indexed under this heading.

Mirtazapine (Selegiline transdermal system is contraindicated with mirtazapine). Products include:

Moclobemide (Selegiline transdermal system should not be used with oral selegiline or other MAO inhibitors).
No products indexed under this heading.

Morphine Sulfate (Selegiline transdermal system is contraindicated with analgesic agents such as tramadol, methadone, and propoxyphene). Products include:

Morphine Sulfate, Liposomal (Selegiline transdermal system is contraindicated with analgesic agents such as tramadol, methadone, and propoxyphene).
No products indexed under this heading.

Nasal decongestants, unspecified (It is prudent to avoid the concomitant use of sympathomimetic agents, such as some decongestants with selegiline).
No products indexed under this heading.

Nefazodone Hydrochloride (Selegiline transdermal system is contraindicated with dual serotonin and norepinephrine reuptake inhibitors).
No products indexed under this heading.

Nitrous Oxide (Patients taking selegiline transdermal system should not undergo elective surgery requiring general anesthesia).
No products indexed under this heading.

Norepinephrine Bitartrate (Concomitant use of sympathomimetic agents with selegiline transdermal system is contraindicated).
No products indexed under this heading.

Nortriptyline Hydrochloride (Selegiline transdermal system is contraindicated with tricyclic antidepressants. Serious, sometimes fatal, central nervous system (CNS) toxicity referred to as the "serotonin syndrome" has been reported with the combination of non-selective MAOIs with certain other drugs, including selective serotonin reuptake inhibitor antidepressants).
No products indexed under this heading.

Oxcarbazepine (Oxcarbazepine is contraindicated in patients taking selegiline).
No products indexed under this heading.

Oxycodone Hydrochloride (Selegiline transdermal system is contraindicated with analgesic agents such as tramadol, methadone, and propoxyphene). Products include:

Oxycodone Terephthalate (Selegiline transdermal system is contraindicated with analgesic agents such as tramadol, methadone, and propoxyphene).
No products indexed under this heading.

Oxymorphone Hydrochloride (Selegiline transdermal system is contraindicated with analgesic agents such as tramadol, methadone, and propoxyphene). Products include:

Pargyline Hydrochloride (Selegiline transdermal system should not be used with oral selegiline or other MAO inhibitors).
No products indexed under this heading.

Paroxetine (Selegiline transdermal system is contraindicated with selective serotonin reuptake inhibitors. Serious, sometimes fatal, central nervous system (CNS) toxicity referred to as the "serotonin syndrome" has been reported with the combination of non-selective MAOIs with certain other drugs, including selective serotonin reuptake inhibitor antidepressants).
No products indexed under this heading.

Paroxetine Hydrochloride (Selegiline transdermal system is contraindicated with selective serotonin reuptake inhibitors. Serious, sometimes fatal, central nervous system (CNS) toxicity referred to as the "serotonin syndrome" has been reported with the combination of non-selective MAOIs with

certain other drugs, including selective serotonin reuptake inhibitor antidepressants). Products include:

Paroxetine Mesylate (Selegiline transdermal system is contraindicated with selective serotonin reuptake inhibitors. Serious, sometimes fatal, central nervous system (CNS) toxicity referred to as the "serotonin syndrome" has been reported with the combination of non-selective MAOIs with certain other drugs, including selective serotonin reuptake inhibitor antidepressants).
No products indexed under this heading.

Pentazocine Hydrochloride (Serious, sometimes fatal, central nervous system (CNS) toxicity referred to as the "serotonin syndrome" has been reported with the combination of non-selective MAOIs with certain other drugs, including pentazocine).
No products indexed under this heading.

Pentazocine Lactate (Serious, sometimes fatal, central nervous system (CNS) toxicity referred to as the "serotonin syndrome" has been reported with the combination of non-selective MAOIs with certain other drugs, including pentazocine).
No products indexed under this heading.

Phenelzine Sulfate (Selegiline transdermal system should not be used with oral selegiline or other MAO inhibitors).
No products indexed under this heading.

Phenylephrine (Selegiline transdermal system is contraindicated for use with phenylephrine).
No products indexed under this heading.

Phenylephrine Bitartrate (Selegiline transdermal system is contraindicated for use with phenylephrine).
No products indexed under this heading.

Phenylephrine Hydrobromide (Selegiline transdermal system is contraindicated for use with phenylephrine).
No products indexed under this heading.

Phenylephrine Hydrochloride (Selegiline transdermal system is contraindicated for use with phenylephrine). Products include:

Phenylephrine Tannate (Selegiline transdermal system is contraindicated for use with phenylephrine).
No products indexed under this heading.

Phenylpropanolamine (Selegiline transdermal system is contraindicated for use with phenylpropanolamine).
No products indexed under this heading.

Phenylpropanolamine Bitartrate (Selegiline transdermal system is contraindicated for use with phenylpropanolamine).
No products indexed under this heading.

Phenylpropanolamine Containing Anorectics (Selegiline transdermal system is contraindicated for use with phenylpropanolamine).
No products indexed under this heading.

Phenylpropanolamine Hydrochloride (Selegiline transdermal system is contraindicated for use with phenylpropanolamine).
No products indexed under this heading.

Phenylpropanolamine Polistirex (Selegiline transdermal system is contraindicated for use with phenylpropanolamine).
No products indexed under this heading.

Pirbuterol Acetate (Concomitant use of sympathomimetic agents with selegiline transdermal system is contraindicated). Products include:

IMPORTANT NOTE: Always consult each drug listing in the patient's regimen for possible interactions.

(⊙ Described in PDR® for Ophthalmic Medicines)

Digoxin (Darifenacin (30 mg daily) co-administered with digoxin (0.25 mg) at steady state resulted in a 16% increase in digoxin exposure. Routine therapeutic drug monitoring for digoxin should be continued). Products include:

Dolasetron Mesylate (Caution should be taken when darifenacin is used concomitantly with medications that are predominantly metabolized by CYP2D6 and that have a narrow therapeutic window). Products include:

Donepezil Hydrochloride (Caution should be taken when darifenacin is used concomitantly with medications that are predominantly metabolized by CYP2D6 and that have a narrow therapeutic window). Products include:

Doxepin Hydrochloride (Caution should be taken when darifenacin is used concomitantly with medications that are predominantly metabolized by CYP2D6 and which have a narrow therapeutic window, such as tricyclic antidepressants).
No products indexed under this heading.

Doxorubicin Hydrochloride (Darifenacin metabolism is primarily mediated by the cytochrome P450 enzymes CYP2D6 and CYP3A4. Therefore, inducers of CYP3A4 may alter darifenacin pharmacokinetics).
No products indexed under this heading.

Efavirenz (Darifenacin metabolism is primarily mediated by the cytochrome P450 enzymes CYP2D6 and CYP3A4. Therefore, inducers of CYP3A4 may alter darifenacin pharmacokinetics). Products include:

Encainide Hydrochloride (Caution should be taken when darifenacin is used concomitantly with medications that are predominantly metabolized by CYP2D6 and that have a narrow therapeutic window).
No products indexed under this heading.

Ethosuximide (Darifenacin metabolism is primarily mediated by the cytochrome P450 enzymes CYP2D6 and CYP3A4. Therefore, inducers of CYP3A4 may alter darifenacin pharmacokinetics).
No products indexed under this heading.

Felbamate (Darifenacin metabolism is primarily mediated by the cytochrome P450 enzymes CYP2D6 and CYP3A4. Therefore, inducers of CYP3A4 may alter darifenacin pharmacokinetics).
No products indexed under this heading.

Fentanyl (Caution should be taken when darifenacin is used concomitantly with medications that are predominantly metabolized by CYP2D6 and that have a narrow therapeutic window). Products include:

Fentanyl Citrate (Caution should be taken when darifenacin is used concomitantly with medications that are predominantly metabolized by CYP2D6 and that have a narrow therapeutic window). Products include:

Flecainide Acetate (Caution should be taken when darifenacin is used concomitantly with medications that are predominantly metabolized by CYP2D6 and which have a narrow therapeutic window, such as flecainide).
No products indexed under this heading.

Fludrocortisone Acetate (Darifenacin metabolism is primarily mediated by the cytochrome P450 enzymes CYP2D6 and CYP3A4. Therefore, inducers of CYP3A4 may alter darifenacin pharmacokinetics).
No products indexed under this heading.

Fluoxetine (Caution should be taken when darifenacin is used concomitantly with medications that are predominantly metabolized by CYP2D6 and that have a narrow therapeutic window).
No products indexed under this heading.

Fluoxetine Hydrochloride (Caution should be taken when darifenacin is used concomitantly with medications that are predominantly metabolized by CYP2D6 and that have a narrow therapeutic window). Products include:

Fluphenazine Decanoate (Caution should be taken when darifenacin is used concomitantly with medications that are predominantly metabolized by CYP2D6 and that have a narrow therapeutic window).
No products indexed under this heading.

Fluphenazine Enanthate (Caution should be taken when darifenacin is used concomitantly with medications that are predominantly metabolized by CYP2D6 and that have a narrow therapeutic window).
No products indexed under this heading.

Fluphenazine Hydrochloride (Caution should be taken when darifenacin is used concomitantly with medications that are predominantly metabolized by CYP2D6 and that have a narrow therapeutic window).
No products indexed under this heading.

Fluvoxamine Maleate (Caution should be taken when darifenacin is used concomitantly with medications that are predominantly metabolized by CYP2D6 and that have a narrow therapeutic window).
No products indexed under this heading.

Formoterol Fumarate (Caution should be taken when darifenacin is used concomitantly with medications that are predominantly metabolized by CYP2D6 and that have a narrow therapeutic window). Products include:

Fosamprenavir Calcium (The daily dose of darifenacin should not exceed 7.5 mg when co-administered with potent CYP3A4 inhibitors). Products include:

Fosphenytoin Sodium (Darifenacin metabolism is primarily mediated by the cytochrome P450 enzymes CYP2D6 and CYP3A4. Therefore, inducers of CYP3A4 may alter darifenacin pharmacokinetics).
No products indexed under this heading.

Galantamine Hydrobromide (Caution should be taken when darifenacin is used concomitantly with medications that are predominantly metabolized by CYP2D6 and that have a narrow therapeutic window).
No products indexed under this heading.

Garlic Extract (Darifenacin metabolism is primarily mediated by the cytochrome P450 enzymes CYP2D6 and CYP3A4. Therefore, inducers of CYP3A4 may alter darifenacin pharmacokinetics).
No products indexed under this heading.

Garlic Oil (Darifenacin metabolism is primarily mediated by the cytochrome P450 enzymes CYP2D6 and CYP3A4. Therefore, inducers of CYP3A4 may alter darifenacin pharmacokinetics).
No products indexed under this heading.

Glycopyrrolate (The concomitant use of darifenacin with other anticholinergic agents may increase the frequency and/or severity of dry mouth, constipation, blurred vision and other anticholinergic pharmacological effects. Anticholinergic agents may potentially alter the absorption of some concomitantly administered drugs due to effects on gastrointestinal motility).
No products indexed under this heading.

Haloperidol (Caution should be taken when darifenacin is used concomitantly with medications that are predominantly metabolized by CYP2D6 and that have a narrow therapeutic window).
No products indexed under this heading.

Haloperidol Decanoate (Caution should be taken when darifenacin is used concomitantly with medications that are predominantly metabolized by CYP2D6 and that have a narrow therapeutic window).
No products indexed under this heading.

Hydrocodone Bitartrate (Caution should be taken when darifenacin is used concomitantly with medications that are predominantly metabolized by CYP2D6 and that have a narrow therapeutic window). Products include:

Hydrocortisone (Darifenacin metabolism is primarily mediated by the cytochrome P450 enzymes CYP2D6 and CYP3A4. Therefore, inducers of CYP3A4 may alter darifenacin pharmacokinetics).
No products indexed under this heading.

Hydrocortisone (Alcohol) (Darifenacin metabolism is primarily mediated by the cytochrome P450 enzymes CYP2D6 and CYP3A4. Therefore, inducers of CYP3A4 may alter darifenacin pharmacokinetics).
No products indexed under this heading.

Hydrocortisone Acetate (Darifenacin metabolism is primarily mediated by the cytochrome P450 enzymes CYP2D6 and CYP3A4. Therefore, inducers of CYP3A4 may alter darifenacin pharmacokinetics).
No products indexed under this heading.

Hydrocortisone Butyrate (Darifenacin metabolism is primarily mediated by the cytochrome P450 enzymes CYP2D6 and CYP3A4. Therefore, inducers of CYP3A4 may alter darifenacin pharmacokinetics).
No products indexed under this heading.

Hydrocortisone Cypionate (Darifenacin metabolism is primarily mediated by the cytochrome P450 enzymes CYP2D6 and CYP3A4. Therefore, inducers of CYP3A4 may alter darifenacin pharmacokinetics).
No products indexed under this heading.

Hydrocortisone Hemisuccinate (Darifenacin metabolism is primarily mediated by the cytochrome P450 enzymes CYP2D6 and CYP3A4. Therefore, inducers of CYP3A4 may alter darifenacin pharmacokinetics).
No products indexed under this heading.

Hydrocortisone Probutate (Darifenacin metabolism is primarily mediated by the cytochrome P450 enzymes CYP2D6 and CYP3A4. Therefore, inducers of CYP3A4 may alter darifenacin pharmacokinetics).
No products indexed under this heading.

Hydrocortisone Sodium Phosphate (Darifenacin metabolism is primarily mediated by the cytochrome P450 enzymes CYP2D6 and CYP3A4. Therefore, inducers of CYP3A4 may alter darifenacin pharmacokinetics).
No products indexed under this heading.

Hydrocortisone Sodium Succinate (Darifenacin metabolism is primarily mediated by the cytochrome P450 enzymes CYP2D6 and CYP3A4. Therefore, inducers of CYP3A4 may alter darifenacin pharmacokinetics).
No products indexed under this heading.

Hydrocortisone Valerate (Darifenacin metabolism is primarily mediated by the cytochrome P450 enzymes CYP2D6 and CYP3A4. Therefore, inducers of CYP3A4 may alter darifenacin pharmacokinetics).
No products indexed under this heading.

Hyoscyamine (The concomitant use of darifenacin with other anticholinergic agents may increase the frequency and/or severity of dry mouth, constipation, blurred vision and other anticholinergic pharmacological effects. Anticholinergic agents may potentially alter the absorption of some concomitantly administered drugs due to effects on gastrointestinal motility).
No products indexed under this heading.

Hyoscyamine Sulfate (The concomitant use of darifenacin with other anticholinergic agents may increase the frequency and/or severity of dry mouth, constipation, blurred vision and other anticholinergic pharmacological effects. Anticholinergic agents may potentially alter the absorption of some concomitantly administered drugs due to effects on gastrointestinal motility). Products include:

Hypericum (Darifenacin metabolism is primarily mediated by the cytochrome P450 enzymes CYP2D6 and CYP3A4. Therefore, inducers of CYP3A4 may alter darifenacin pharmacokinetics).
No products indexed under this heading.

Hypericum Perforatum (Darifenacin metabolism is primarily mediated by the cytochrome P450 enzymes CYP2D6 and CYP3A4. Therefore, inducers of CYP3A4 may alter darifenacin pharmacokinetics). Products include:

Imipramine Hydrochloride (Caution should be taken when darifenacin is used concomitantly with medications that are predominantly metabolized by CYP2D6 and which have a narrow therapeutic window, such as tricyclic antidepressants. The mean C_{max} and AUC of imipramine, a CYP2D6 substrate, were increased 57% and 70%, respectively, in the presence of steady-state darifenacin 30 mg once daily. This was accompanied by a 3.6-fold increase in the mean C_{max} and AUC of desipramine, the active metabolite of imipramine).
No products indexed under this heading.

Imipramine Pamoate (Caution should be taken when darifenacin is used concomitantly with medications that are predominantly metabolized by CYP2D6 and which have a narrow therapeutic window, such as tricyclic antidepressants. The mean C_{max} and AUC of imipramine, a CYP2D6 substrate, were increased 57% and 70%, respectively, in the presence of steady-state darifenacin 30 mg once daily. This was accom-

Enablex Interactions Index 584

panied by a 3.6-fold increase in the mean C_{max} and AUC of desipramine, the active metabolite of imipramine).
No products indexed under this heading.

Indinavir Sulfate (The daily dose of darifenacin should not exceed 7.5 mg when co-administered with potent CYP3A4 inhibitors). Products include:
Crixivan 2113

Indoramin Hydrochloride (Caution should be taken when darifenacin is used concomitantly with medications that are predominantly metabolized by CYP2D6 and that have a narrow therapeutic window).
No products indexed under this heading.

Ipratropium Bromide (The concomitant use of darifenacin with other anticholinergic agents may increase the frequency and/or severity of dry mouth, constipation, blurred vision and other anticholinergic pharmacological effects. Anticholinergic agents may potentially alter the absorption of some concomitantly administered drugs due to effects on gastrointestinal motility).
No products indexed under this heading.

Itraconazole (The daily dose of darifenacin should not exceed 7.5 mg when co-administered with potent CYP3A4 inhibitors).
No products indexed under this heading.

Ketoconazole (The daily dose of darifenacin should not exceed 7.5 mg when co-administered with potent CYP3A4 inhibitors. In a drug interaction study, when a 7.5 mg q.d. dose of darifenacin was given to steady state and co-administered with the potent CYP3A4 inhibitor ketoconazole 400 mg, mean darifenacin C_{max} increased to 11.2 ng/mL for extensive metabolizers (EM) (n=10) and 55.4 ng/mL for one poor metabolizer (PM) subject (n=1). Mean AUC increased to 143 and 939 ng.h/mL for EMs and for one PM subject, respectively. When a 15 mg daily dose of darifenacin was given with ketoconazole, mean darifenacin C_{max} increased to 67.6 ng/mL and 58.9 ng.mL for EMs (n=3)). Products include:
Extina 3319
Xolegel 3337

Labetalol Hydrochloride (Caution should be taken when darifenacin is used concomitantly with medications that are predominantly metabolized by CYP2D6 and that have a narrow therapeutic window).
No products indexed under this heading.

Lidocaine (Caution should be taken when darifenacin is used concomitantly with medications that are predominantly metabolized by CYP2D6 and that have a narrow therapeutic window). Products include:
Lidoderm 1107

Lidocaine Hydrochloride (Caution should be taken when darifenacin is used concomitantly with medications that are predominantly metabolized by CYP2D6 and that have a narrow therapeutic window).
No products indexed under this heading.

Lopinavir (The daily dose of darifenacin should not exceed 7.5 mg when co-administered with potent CYP3A4 inhibitors). Products include:
Kaletra 458

Maprotiline Hydrochloride (Caution should be taken when darifenacin is used concomitantly with medications that are predominantly metabolized by CYP2D6 and which have a narrow therapeutic window, such as tricyclic antidepressants).
No products indexed under this heading.

Mepenzolate Bromide (The concomitant use of darifenacin with other anticholinergic agents may increase the frequency and/or severity of dry mouth, constipation, blurred vision and other anticholinergic pharmacological effects. Anticholinergic agents may potentially alter the absorption of some concomitantly administered drugs due to effects on gastrointestinal motility).
No products indexed under this heading.

Meperidine Hydrochloride (Caution should be taken when darifenacin is used concomitantly with medications that are predominantly metabolized by CYP2D6 and that have a narrow therapeutic window).
No products indexed under this heading.

Mephenytoin (Darifenacin metabolism is primarily mediated by the cytochrome P450 enzymes CYP2D6 and CYP3A4. Therefore, inducers of CYP3A4 may alter darifenacin pharmacokinetics).
No products indexed under this heading.

Methadone Hydrochloride (Caution should be taken when darifenacin is used concomitantly with medications that are predominantly metabolized by CYP2D6 and that have a narrow therapeutic window).
No products indexed under this heading.

Methamphetamine Hydrochloride (Caution should be taken when darifenacin is used concomitantly with medications that are predominantly metabolized by CYP2D6 and that have a narrow therapeutic window).
No products indexed under this heading.

Methoxyphenamine (Caution should be taken when darifenacin is used concomitantly with medications that are predominantly metabolized by CYP2D6 and that have a narrow therapeutic window).
No products indexed under this heading.

Methsuximide (Darifenacin metabolism is primarily mediated by the cytochrome P450 enzymes CYP2D6 and CYP3A4. Therefore, inducers of CYP3A4 may alter darifenacin pharmacokinetics).
No products indexed under this heading.

Methylprednisolone (Darifenacin metabolism is primarily mediated by the cytochrome P450 enzymes CYP2D6 and CYP3A4. Therefore, inducers of CYP3A4 may alter darifenacin pharmacokinetics).
No products indexed under this heading.

Methylprednisolone Acetate (Darifenacin metabolism is primarily mediated by the cytochrome P450 enzymes CYP2D6 and CYP3A4. Therefore, inducers of CYP3A4 may alter darifenacin pharmacokinetics).
No products indexed under this heading.

Methylprednisolone Sodium Succinate (Darifenacin metabolism is primarily mediated by the cytochrome P450 enzymes CYP2D6 and CYP3A4. Therefore, inducers of CYP3A4 may alter darifenacin pharmacokinetics).
No products indexed under this heading.

Metoprolol Succinate (Caution should be taken when darifenacin is used concomitantly with medications that are predominantly metabolized by CYP2D6 and that have a narrow therapeutic window). Products include:
Toprol XL 732

Metoprolol Tartrate (Caution should be taken when darifenacin is used concomitantly with medications that are predominantly metabolized by CYP2D6 and that have a narrow therapeutic window).
No products indexed under this heading.

Mexiletine Hydrochloride (Caution should be taken when darifenacin is used concomitantly with medications that are predominantly metabolized by CYP2D6 and that have a narrow therapeutic window).
No products indexed under this heading.

Midazolam Hydrochloride (Darifenacin (30 mg daily) co-administered with a single oral dose of midazolam 7.5 mg resulted in a 17% increase in midazolam exposure).
No products indexed under this heading.

Mirtazapine (Caution should be taken when darifenacin is used concomitantly with medications that are predominantly metabolized by CYP2D6 and that have a narrow therapeutic window). Products include:
Remeron Tablets 3214
RemeronSolTab Tablets 3219

Modafinil (Darifenacin metabolism is primarily mediated by the cytochrome P450 enzymes CYP2D6 and CYP3A4. Therefore, inducers of CYP3A4 may alter darifenacin pharmacokinetics). Products include:
Provigil 983

Morphine Sulfate (Caution should be taken when darifenacin is used concomitantly with medications that are predominantly metabolized by CYP2D6 and that have a narrow therapeutic window). Products include:
Avinza 1822
Embeda 1831
MS Contin 2803

Nafcillin Sodium (Darifenacin metabolism is primarily mediated by the cytochrome P450 enzymes CYP2D6 and CYP3A4. Therefore, inducers of CYP3A4 may alter darifenacin pharmacokinetics).
No products indexed under this heading.

Nefazodone Hydrochloride (The daily dose of darifenacin should not exceed 7.5 mg when co-administered with potent CYP3A4 inhibitors).
No products indexed under this heading.

Nelfinavir Mesylate (The daily dose of darifenacin should not exceed 7.5 mg when co-administered with potent CYP3A4 inhibitors).
No products indexed under this heading.

Nevirapine (Darifenacin metabolism is primarily mediated by the cytochrome P450 enzymes CYP2D6 and CYP3A4. Therefore, inducers of CYP3A4 may alter darifenacin pharmacokinetics). Products include:
Viramune Oral Suspension 897
Viramune Tablets 897

Nortriptyline Hydrochloride (Caution should be taken when darifenacin is used concomitantly with medications that are predominantly metabolized by CYP2D6 and which have a narrow therapeutic window, such as tricyclic antidepressants).
No products indexed under this heading.

Olanzapine (Caution should be taken when darifenacin is used concomitantly with medications that are predominantly metabolized by CYP2D6 and that have a narrow therapeutic window). Products include:
Symbyax 1965
Zyprexa 1984
Zyprexa IntraMuscular 1984
Zyprexa ZYDIS 1984

Omeprazole (Caution should be taken when darifenacin is used concomitantly with medications that are predominantly metabolized by CYP2D6 and that have a narrow therapeutic window).
No products indexed under this heading.

Ondansetron (Caution should be taken when darifenacin is used concomitantly with medications that are predominantly metabolized by CYP2D6 and that have a narrow therapeutic window).
No products indexed under this heading.

Ondansetron Hydrochloride (Caution should be taken when darifenacin is used concomitantly with medications that are predominantly metabolized by CYP2D6 and that have a narrow therapeutic window). Products include:
Zofran Injection 1750
Zofran 1756
Zofran ODT 1756

Oxcarbazepine (Darifenacin metabolism is primarily mediated by the cytochrome P450 enzymes CYP2D6 and CYP3A4. Therefore, inducers of CYP3A4 may alter darifenacin pharmacokinetics).
No products indexed under this heading.

Oxybutynin Chloride (The concomitant use of darifenacin with other anticholinergic agents may increase the frequency and/or severity of dry mouth, constipation, blurred vision and other anticholinergic pharmacological effects. Anticholinergic agents may potentially alter the absorption of some concomitantly administered drugs due to effects on gastrointestinal motility).
No products indexed under this heading.

Oxycodone Hydrochloride (Caution should be taken when darifenacin is used concomitantly with medications that are predominantly metabolized by CYP2D6 and that have a narrow therapeutic window). Products include:
OxyContin 2807
Percocet 1121
Percodan 1124

Paclitaxel (Caution should be taken when darifenacin is used concomitantly with medications that are predominantly metabolized by CYP2D6 and that have a narrow therapeutic window).
No products indexed under this heading.

Paroxetine Hydrochloride (Caution should be taken when darifenacin is used concomitantly with medications that are predominantly metabolized by CYP2D6 and that have a narrow therapeutic window). Products include:
Paroxetine CR 2361
Paroxetine ER 2371
Paxil 1586
Paxil CR 1596

Phenobarbital (Darifenacin metabolism is primarily mediated by the cytochrome P450 enzymes CYP2D6 and CYP3A4. Therefore, inducers of CYP3A4 may alter darifenacin pharmacokinetics). Products include:
Donnatal 2711

Phenobarbital Sodium (Darifenacin metabolism is primarily mediated by the cytochrome P450 enzymes CYP2D6 and CYP3A4. Therefore, inducers of CYP3A4 may alter darifenacin pharmacokinetics).
No products indexed under this heading.

Phenytoin (Darifenacin metabolism is primarily mediated by the cytochrome P450 enzymes CYP2D6 and CYP3A4. Therefore, inducers of CYP3A4 may alter darifenacin pharmacokinetics).
No products indexed under this heading.

Phenytoin Sodium (Darifenacin metabolism is primarily mediated by the cytochrome P450 enzymes CYP2D6 and CYP3A4. Therefore, inducers of CYP3A4 may alter darifenacin pharmacokinetics). Products include:
Phenytek Capsules 2380

Pindolol (Caution should be taken when darifenacin is used concomitantly with medications that are predominantly metabolized by CYP2D6 and that have a narrow therapeutic window).
No products indexed under this heading.

Prednisolone (Darifenacin metabolism is primarily mediated by the cytochrome P450 enzymes CYP2D6 and CYP3A4. Therefore, inducers of CYP3A4 may alter darifenacin pharmacokinetics).
No products indexed under this heading.

Prednisolone Acetate (Darifenacin metabolism is primarily mediated by the cytochrome P450 enzymes CYP2D6 and CYP3A4. Therefore, inducers of CYP3A4 may alter darifenacin pharmacokinetics). Products include:
Blephamide .... ⊙212, ⊙214
Pred Forte .... ⊙225
Pred Mild .... ⊙230
Pred-G .... ⊙226, ⊙227

Prednisolone Sodium Phosphate (Darifenacin metabolism is primarily mediated by the cytochrome P450 enzymes CYP2D6 and CYP3A4. Therefore, inducers of CYP3A4 may alter darifenacin pharmacokinetics).
No products indexed under this heading.

Prednisolone Tebutate (Darifenacin metabolism is primarily mediated by the cytochrome P450 enzymes CYP2D6 and CYP3A4. Therefore, inducers of CYP3A4 may alter darifenacin pharmacokinetics).
No products indexed under this heading.

Prednisone (Darifenacin metabolism is primarily mediated by the cytochrome P450 enzymes CYP2D6 and CYP3A4. Therefore, inducers of CYP3A4 may alter darifenacin pharmacokinetics).
No products indexed under this heading.

Prednisone sodium phosphate (Darifenacin metabolism is primarily mediated by the cytochrome P450 enzymes CYP2D6 and CYP3A4. Therefore, inducers of CYP3A4 may alter darifenacin pharmacokinetics).
No products indexed under this heading.

Primidone (Darifenacin metabolism is primarily mediated by the cytochrome P450 enzymes CYP2D6 and CYP3A4. Therefore, inducers of CYP3A4 may alter darifenacin pharmacokinetics).
No products indexed under this heading.

Procyclidine Hydrochloride (The concomitant use of darifenacin with other anticholinergic agents may increase the frequency and/or severity of dry mouth, constipation, blurred vision and other anticholinergic pharmacological effects. Anticholinergic agents may potentially alter the absorption of some concomitantly administered drugs due to effects on gastrointestinal motility).
No products indexed under this heading.

Propafenone Hydrochloride (Caution should be taken when darifenacin is used concomitantly with medications that are predominantly metabolized by CYP2D6 and that have a narrow therapeutic window). Products include:
Rythmol 1648
Rythmol SR 1652

Propantheline Bromide (The concomitant use of darifenacin with other anticholinergic agents may increase the frequency and/or severity of dry mouth, constipation, blurred vision and other anticholinergic pharmacological effects. Anticholinergic agents may potentially alter the absorption of some concomitantly administered drugs due to effects on gastrointestinal motility).
No products indexed under this heading.

Propoxyphene Hydrochloride (Caution should be taken when darifenacin is used concomitantly with medications that are predominantly metabolized by CYP2D6 and that have a narrow therapeutic window).
No products indexed under this heading.

Propoxyphene Napsylate (Caution should be taken when darifenacin is used concomitantly with medications that are predominantly metabolized by CYP2D6 and that have a narrow therapeutic window).
No products indexed under this heading.

Propranolol Hydrochloride (Caution should be taken when darifenacin is used concomitantly with medications that are predominantly metabolized by CYP2D6 and that have a narrow therapeutic window). Products include:
InnoPran XL 1517

Protriptyline Hydrochloride (Caution should be taken when darifenacin is used concomitantly with medications that are predominantly metabolized by CYP2D6 and which have a narrow therapeutic window, such as tricyclic antidepressants).
No products indexed under this heading.

Quetiapine Fumarate (Caution should be taken when darifenacin is used concomitantly with medications that are predominantly metabolized by CYP2D6 and that have a narrow therapeutic window). Products include:
Seroquel 750
Seroquel XR 759

Quinidine Gluconate (Caution should be taken when darifenacin is used concomitantly with medications that are predominantly metabolized by CYP2D6 and that have a narrow therapeutic window).
No products indexed under this heading.

Quinidine Hydrochloride (Caution should be taken when darifenacin is used concomitantly with medications that are predominantly metabolized by CYP2D6 and that have a narrow therapeutic window).
No products indexed under this heading.

Quinidine Polygalacturonate (Caution should be taken when darifenacin is used concomitantly with medications that are predominantly metabolized by CYP2D6 and that have a narrow therapeutic window).
No products indexed under this heading.

Quinidine Sulfate (Caution should be taken when darifenacin is used concomitantly with medications that are predominantly metabolized by CYP2D6 and that have a narrow therapeutic window).
No products indexed under this heading.

Rifabutin (Darifenacin metabolism is primarily mediated by the cytochrome P450 enzymes CYP2D6 and CYP3A4. Therefore, inducers of CYP3A4 may alter darifenacin pharmacokinetics).
No products indexed under this heading.

Rifampicin (Darifenacin metabolism is primarily mediated by the cytochrome P450 enzymes CYP2D6 and CYP3A4. Therefore, inducers of CYP3A4 may alter darifenacin pharmacokinetics).
No products indexed under this heading.

Rifampin (Darifenacin metabolism is primarily mediated by the cytochrome P450 enzymes CYP2D6 and CYP3A4. Therefore, inducers of CYP3A4 may alter darifenacin pharmacokinetics).
No products indexed under this heading.

Rifapentine (Darifenacin metabolism is primarily mediated by the cytochrome P450 enzymes CYP2D6 and CYP3A4. Therefore, inducers of CYP3A4 may alter darifenacin pharmacokinetics).
No products indexed under this heading.

Risperidone (Caution should be taken when darifenacin is used concomitantly with medications that are predominantly metabolized by CYP2D6 and that have a narrow therapeutic window). Products include:
Risperdal Consta 2682

Ritonavir (The daily dose of darifenacin should not exceed 7.5 mg when co-administered with potent CYP3A4 inhibitors). Products include:
Kaletra 458
Norvir 509

Saquinavir (The daily dose of darifenacin should not exceed 7.5 mg when co-administered with potent CYP3A4 inhibitors).
No products indexed under this heading.

Saquinavir Mesylate (The daily dose of darifenacin should not exceed 7.5 mg when co-administered with potent CYP3A4 inhibitors).
No products indexed under this heading.

Scopolamine (The concomitant use of darifenacin with other anticholinergic agents may increase the frequency and/or severity of dry mouth, constipation, blurred vision and other anticholinergic pharmacological effects. Anticholinergic agents may potentially alter the absorption of some concomitantly administered drugs due to effects on gastrointestinal motility). Products include:
Transderm Scōp 2397

Scopolamine Hydrobromide (The concomitant use of darifenacin with other anticholinergic agents may increase the frequency and/or severity of dry mouth, constipation, blurred vision and other anticholinergic pharmacological effects. Anticholinergic agents may potentially alter the absorption of some concomitantly administered drugs due to effects on gastrointestinal motility). Products include:
Donnatal 2711

Sulfinpyrazone (Darifenacin metabolism is primarily mediated by the cytochrome P450 enzymes CYP2D6 and CYP3A4. Therefore, inducers of CYP3A4 may alter darifenacin pharmacokinetics).
No products indexed under this heading.

Tamoxifen Citrate (Caution should be taken when darifenacin is used concomitantly with medications that are predominantly metabolized by CYP2D6 and that have a narrow therapeutic window).
No products indexed under this heading.

Telithromycin (The daily dose of darifenacin should not exceed 7.5 mg when co-administered with potent CYP3A4 inhibitors). Products include:
Ketek 2991

Teniposide (Caution should be taken when darifenacin is used concomitantly with medications that are predominantly metabolized by CYP2D6 and that have a narrow therapeutic window).
No products indexed under this heading.

Testosterone (Caution should be taken when darifenacin is used concomitantly with medications that are predominantly metabolized by CYP2D6 and that have a narrow therapeutic window). Products include:
AndroGel 3456

Testosterone Cypionate (Caution should be taken when darifenacin is used concomitantly with medications that are predominantly metabolized by CYP2D6 and that have a narrow therapeutic window).
No products indexed under this heading.

Testosterone Enanthate (Caution should be taken when darifenacin is used concomitantly with medications that are predominantly metabolized by CYP2D6 and that have a narrow therapeutic window). Products include:
Delatestryl 1102

Testosterone Propionate (Caution should be taken when darifenacin is used concomitantly with medications that are predominantly metabolized by CYP2D6 and that have a narrow therapeutic window).
No products indexed under this heading.

Theophyllinate (Darifenacin metabolism is primarily mediated by the cytochrome P450 enzymes CYP2D6 and CYP3A4. Therefore, inducers of CYP3A4 may alter darifenacin pharmacokinetics).
No products indexed under this heading.

Theophylline (Darifenacin metabolism is primarily mediated by the cytochrome P450 enzymes CYP2D6 and CYP3A4. Therefore, inducers of CYP3A4 may alter darifenacin pharmacokinetics).
No products indexed under this heading.

Theophylline Anhydrous (Darifenacin metabolism is primarily mediated by the cytochrome P450 enzymes CYP2D6 and CYP3A4. Therefore, inducers of CYP3A4 may alter darifenacin pharmacokinetics). Products include:
Uniphyl 2817

Theophylline Calcium Salicylate (Darifenacin metabolism is primarily mediated by the cytochrome P450 enzymes CYP2D6 and CYP3A4. Therefore, inducers of CYP3A4 may alter darifenacin pharmacokinetics).
No products indexed under this heading.

Theophylline Dihydroxypropyl (Glyceryl) (Darifenacin metabolism is primarily mediated by the cytochrome P450 enzymes CYP2D6 and CYP3A4. Therefore, inducers of CYP3A4 may alter darifenacin pharmacokinetics).
No products indexed under this heading.

Theophylline Ethylenediamine (Darifenacin metabolism is primarily mediated by the cytochrome P450 enzymes CYP2D6 and CYP3A4. Therefore, inducers of CYP3A4 may alter darifenacin pharmacokinetics).
No products indexed under this heading.

Theophylline Sodium Glycinate (Darifenacin metabolism is primarily mediated by the cytochrome P450 enzymes CYP2D6 and CYP3A4. Therefore, inducers of CYP3A4 may alter darifenacin pharmacokinetics).
No products indexed under this heading.

Thioridazine (Caution should be taken when darifenacin is used concomitantly with medications that are predominantly metabolized by CYP2D6 and which have a narrow therapeutic window, such as thioridazine).
No products indexed under this heading.

Thioridazine Hydrochloride (Caution should be taken when darifenacin is used concomitantly with medications that are predominantly metabolized by CYP2D6 and which have a narrow therapeutic window, such as thioridazine). Products include:
Thioridazine Hydrochloride 2384

Timolol Maleate (Caution should be taken when darifenacin is used concomitantly with medications that are predominantly metabolized by CYP2D6 and that have a narrow therapeutic window). Products include:
Combigan 601
Dorzolamide
Hydrochloride/Timolol Maleate
Ophthalmic Solution .... ⊙243
Timoptic in Ocudose .... ⊙231

IMPORTANT NOTE: Always consult each drug listing in the patient's regimen for possible interactions.

Tolterodine Tartrate (The concomitant use of darifenacin with other anticholinergic agents may increase the frequency and/or severity of dry mouth, constipation, blurred vision and other anticholinergic pharmacological effects. Anticholinergic agents may potentially alter the absorption of some concomitantly administered drugs due to effects on gastrointestinal motility).
No products indexed under this heading.

Tramadol Hydrochloride (Caution should be taken when darifenacin is used concomitantly with medications that are predominantly metabolized by CYP2D6 and that have a narrow therapeutic window). Products include:

Trazodone Hydrochloride (Caution should be taken when darifenacin is used concomitantly with medications that are predominantly metabolized by CYP2D6 and that have a narrow therapeutic window).
No products indexed under this heading.

Triamcinolone (Darifenacin metabolism is primarily mediated by the cytochrome P450 enzymes CYP2D6 and CYP3A4. Therefore, inducers of CYP3A4 may alter darifenacin pharmacokinetics).
No products indexed under this heading.

Triamcinolone Acetonide (Darifenacin metabolism is primarily mediated by the cytochrome P450 enzymes CYP2D6 and CYP3A4. Therefore, inducers of CYP3A4 may alter darifenacin pharmacokinetics). Products include:

Triamcinolone Diacetate (Darifenacin metabolism is primarily mediated by the cytochrome P450 enzymes CYP2D6 and CYP3A4. Therefore, inducers of CYP3A4 may alter darifenacin pharmacokinetics).
No products indexed under this heading.

Triamcinolone Hexacetonide (Darifenacin metabolism is primarily mediated by the cytochrome P450 enzymes CYP2D6 and CYP3A4. Therefore, inducers of CYP3A4 may alter darifenacin pharmacokinetics).
No products indexed under this heading.

Triazolam (Caution should be taken when darifenacin is used concomitantly with medications that are predominantly metabolized by CYP2D6 and that have a narrow therapeutic window).
No products indexed under this heading.

Tridihexethyl Chloride (The concomitant use of darifenacin with other anticholinergic agents may increase the frequency and/or severity of dry mouth, constipation, blurred vision and other anticholinergic pharmacological effects. Anticholinergic agents may potentially alter the absorption of some concomitantly administered drugs due to effects on gastrointestinal motility).
No products indexed under this heading.

Trihexyphenidyl Hydrochloride (The concomitant use of darifenacin with other anticholinergic agents may increase the frequency and/or severity of dry mouth, constipation, blurred vision and other anticholinergic pharmacological effects. Anticholinergic agents may potentially alter the absorption of some concomitantly administered drugs due to effects on gastrointestinal motility).
No products indexed under this heading.

Trimipramine Maleate (Caution should be taken when darifenacin is used concomitantly with medications that are predominantly metabolized by CYP2D6 and which have a narrow therapeutic window, such as tricyclic antidepressants).
No products indexed under this heading.

Troglitazone (Darifenacin metabolism is primarily mediated by the cytochrome P450 enzymes CYP2D6 and CYP3A4. Therefore, inducers of CYP3A4 may alter darifenacin pharmacokinetics).
No products indexed under this heading.

Troleandomycin (The daily dose of darifenacin should not exceed 7.5 mg when co-administered with potent CYP3A4 inhibitors).
No products indexed under this heading.

Venlafaxine Hydrochloride (Caution should be taken when darifenacin is used concomitantly with medications that are predominantly metabolized by CYP2D6 and that have a narrow therapeutic window). Products include:

Vinblastine Sulfate (Caution should be taken when darifenacin is used concomitantly with medications that are predominantly metabolized by CYP2D6 and that have a narrow therapeutic window).
No products indexed under this heading.

Voriconazole (The daily dose of darifenacin should not exceed 7.5 mg when co-administered with potent CYP3A4 inhibitors).
No products indexed under this heading.

Zonisamide (Caution should be taken when darifenacin is used concomitantly with medications that are predominantly metabolized by CYP2D6 and that have a narrow therapeutic window). Products include:

ENBREL FOR SUBCUTANEOUS INJECTION

May interact with immunosuppressive agents, vaccines, live, and certain other agents. Compounds in these categories include:

Anakinra (In a study in which patients with active rheumatoid arthritis were treated for up to 24 weeks with concurrent etanercept and anakinra therapy, a 7% rate of serious infections was observed, which was higher than that observed with etanercept alone (0%). Two percent of patients treated concurrently with etanercept and anakinra developed neutropenia (ANC < 1 x 109/L)). Products include:

Azathioprine (The use of etanercept in patients with Wegener's granulomatosis receiving immunosuppressive agents is not recommended).
No products indexed under this heading.

Basiliximab (The use of etanercept in patients with Wegener's granulomatosis receiving immunosuppressive agents is not recommended). Products include:

BCG Vaccine (Most psoriatic arthritis patients receiving etanercept were able to mount effective B-cell immune responses to pneumococcal polysaccharide vaccine, but titers in aggregate were moderately lower and fewer patients had two-fold rises in titers compared to patients not receiving etanercept. The clinical significance of this is unknown. Patients receiving etanercept may receive concurrent vaccinations, except for live vaccines).
No products indexed under this heading.

Cyclophosphamide (In a study of patients with Wegener's granulomatosis, the addition of etanercept to standard therapy (including cyclophosphamide) was associated with a higher incidence of non-cutaneous solid malignancies. The use of etanercept in patients receiving concurrent cyclophosphamide therapy is not recommended).
No products indexed under this heading.

Cyclosporine (The use of etanercept in patients with Wegener's granulomatosis receiving immunosuppressive agents is not recommended). Products include:

Influenza Vaccine, Live Attenuated (Most psoriatic arthritis patients receiving etanercept were able to mount effective B-cell immune responses to pneumococcal polysaccharide vaccine, but titers in aggregate were moderately lower and fewer patients had two-fold rises in titers compared to patients not receiving etanercept. The clinical significance of this is unknown. Patients receiving etanercept may receive concurrent vaccinations, except for live vaccines).
No products indexed under this heading.

Influenza Virus Vaccine Live, Intranasal (Most psoriatic arthritis patients receiving etanercept were able to mount effective B-cell immune responses to pneumococcal polysaccharide vaccine, but titers in aggregate were moderately lower and fewer patients had two-fold rises in titers compared to patients not receiving etanercept. The clinical significance of this is unknown. Patients receiving etanercept may receive concurrent vaccinations, except for live vaccines). Products include:

Measles, Mumps, Rubella and Varicella Virus Vaccine Live (Most psoriatic arthritis patients receiving etanercept were able to mount effective B-cell immune responses to pneumococcal polysaccharide vaccine, but titers in aggregate were moderately lower and fewer patients had two-fold rises in titers compared to patients not receiving etanercept. The clinical significance of this is unknown. Patients receiving etanercept may receive concurrent vaccinations, except for live vaccines). Products include:

Measles, Mumps & Rubella Virus Vaccine, Live (Most psoriatic arthritis patients receiving etanercept were able to mount effective B-cell immune responses to pneumococcal polysaccharide vaccine, but titers in aggregate were moderately lower and fewer patients had two-fold rises in titers compared to patients not receiving etanercept. The clinical significance of this is unknown. Patients receiving etanercept may receive concurrent vaccinations, except for live vaccines). Products include:

Measles & Rubella Virus Vaccine Live (Most psoriatic arthritis patients receiving etanercept were able to mount effective B-cell immune responses to pneumococcal polysaccharide vaccine, but titers in aggregate were moderately lower and fewer patients had two-fold rises in titers compared to patients not receiving etanercept. The clinical significance of this is

unknown. Patients receiving etanercept may receive concurrent vaccinations, except for live vaccines).
No products indexed under this heading.

Measles Virus Vaccine Live (Most psoriatic arthritis patients receiving etanercept were able to mount effective B-cell immune responses to pneumococcal polysaccharide vaccine, but titers in aggregate were moderately lower and fewer patients had two-fold rises in titers compared to patients not receiving etanercept. The clinical significance of this is unknown. Patients receiving etanercept may receive concurrent vaccinations, except for live vaccines). Products include:

Mumps Virus Vaccine, Live (Most psoriatic arthritis patients receiving etanercept were able to mount effective B-cell immune responses to pneumococcal polysaccharide vaccine, but titers in aggregate were moderately lower and fewer patients had two-fold rises in titers compared to patients not receiving etanercept. The clinical significance of this is unknown. Patients receiving etanercept may receive concurrent vaccinations, except for live vaccines). Products include:

Muromonab-CD3 (The use of etanercept in patients with Wegener's granulomatosis receiving immunosuppressive agents is not recommended). Products include:

Mycophenolate Mofetil (The use of etanercept in patients with Wegener's granulomatosis receiving immunosuppressive agents is not recommended).
No products indexed under this heading.

Pneumococcal Vaccine, Polyvalent (Most psoriatic arthritis patients receiving etanercept were able to mount effective B-cell immune responses to pneumococcal polysaccharide vaccine, but titers in aggregate were moderately lower and fewer patients had two-fold rises in titers compared to patients not receiving etanercept. The clinical significance of this is unknown. Patients receiving etanercept may receive concurrent vaccinations, except for live vaccines). Products include:

Poliovirus Vaccine, Live, Oral, Trivalent, Types 1,2,3 (Sabin) (Most psoriatic arthritis patients receiving etanercept were able to mount effective B-cell immune responses to pneumococcal polysaccharide vaccine, but titers in aggregate were moderately lower and fewer patients had two-fold rises in titers compared to patients not receiving etanercept. The clinical significance of this is unknown. Patients receiving etanercept may receive concurrent vaccinations, except for live vaccines).
No products indexed under this heading.

Rapamycin (The use of etanercept in patients with Wegener's granulomatosis receiving immunosuppressive agents is not recommended).
No products indexed under this heading.

Rotavirus Vaccine, Live, Oral, Tetravalent (Most psoriatic arthritis patients receiving etanercept were able to mount effective B-cell immune responses to pneumococcal polysaccharide vaccine, but titers in aggregate were moderately lower and fewer patients had two-fold rises in titers compared to patients not receiving etanercept. The clinical significance of this is unknown. Patients receiving etanercept may receive concurrent vaccinations, except for live vaccines).
No products indexed under this heading.

587 Interactions Index Enjuvia

Rubella & Mumps Virus Vaccine Live (Most psoriatic arthritis patients receiving etanercept were able to mount effective B-cell immune responses to pneumococcal polysaccharide vaccine, but titers in aggregate were moderately lower and fewer patients had two-fold rises in titers compared to patients not receiving etanercept. The clinical significance of this is unknown. Patients receiving etanercept may receive concurrent vaccinations, except for live vaccines).
No products indexed under this heading.

Rubella Virus Vaccine Live (Most psoriatic arthritis patients receiving etanercept were able to mount effective B-cell immune responses to pneumococcal polysaccharide vaccine, but titers in aggregate were moderately lower and fewer patients had two-fold rises in titers compared to patients not receiving etanercept. The clinical significance of this is unknown. Patients receiving etanercept may receive concurrent vaccinations, except for live vaccines). Products include:
Meruvax II 2210

Sirolimus (The use of etanercept in patients with Wegener's granulomatosis receiving immunosuppressive agents is not recommended). Products include:
Rapamune 3579

Smallpox Vaccine (Most psoriatic arthritis patients receiving etanercept were able to mount effective B-cell immune responses to pneumococcal polysaccharide vaccine, but titers in aggregate were moderately lower and fewer patients had two-fold rises in titers compared to patients not receiving etanercept. The clinical significance of this is unknown. Patients receiving etanercept may receive concurrent vaccinations, except for live vaccines).
No products indexed under this heading.

Sulfasalazine (Patients in a clinical study who were on established therapy with sulfasalazine, to which etanercept was added, were noted to develop a mild decrease in mean neutrophil counts in comparison to groups treated with either etanercept or sulfasalazine alone. The clinical significance of this observation is unknown).
No products indexed under this heading.

Tacrolimus (The use of etanercept in patients with Wegener's granulomatosis receiving immunosuppressive agents is not recommended). Products include:
Prograf Capsules 677
Prograf Injection 677
Protopic 685

Typhoid Vaccine (Most psoriatic arthritis patients receiving etanercept were able to mount effective B-cell immune responses to pneumococcal polysaccharide vaccine, but titers in aggregate were moderately lower and fewer patients had two-fold rises in titers compared to patients not receiving etanercept. The clinical significance of this is unknown. Patients receiving etanercept may receive concurrent vaccinations, except for live vaccines).
No products indexed under this heading.

Varicella Virus Vaccine, Live (Most psoriatic arthritis patients receiving etanercept were able to mount effective B-cell immune responses to pneumococcal polysaccharide vaccine, but titers in aggregate were moderately lower and fewer patients had two-fold rises in titers compared to patients not receiving etanercept. The clinical significance of this is unknown. Patients receiving etanercept may receive concurrent vaccinations, except for live vaccines). Products include:
Varivax 2285

Yellow Fever Vaccine (Most psoriatic arthritis patients receiving etanercept were able to mount effective B-cell immune responses to pneumococcal polysaccharide vaccine, but titers in aggregate were moderately lower and fewer patients had two-fold rises in titers compared to patients not receiving etanercept. The clinical significance of this is unknown. Patients receiving etanercept may receive concurrent vaccinations, except for live vaccines).
No products indexed under this heading.

Zoster Vaccine Live (Most psoriatic arthritis patients receiving etanercept were able to mount effective B-cell immune responses to pneumococcal polysaccharide vaccine, but titers in aggregate were moderately lower and fewer patients had two-fold rises in titers compared to patients not receiving etanercept. The clinical significance of this is unknown. Patients receiving etanercept may receive concurrent vaccinations, except for live vaccines). Products include:
Zostavax 2299

ENGERIX-B VACCINE

(Hepatitis B Vaccine, Recombinant) 1434
None cited in PDR database.

ENJUVIA TABLETS

(Estrogens, Conjugated, Synthetic B) ... 3401
May interact with cytochrome p450 3a4 inducers (selected), cytochrome p450 3a4 inhibitors (selected), thyroid preparations. Compounds in these categories include:

Acetazolamide (Inhibitors of CYP3A4 such as erythromycin, clarithromycin, ketoconazole, itraconazole, ritonavir and grapefruit juice may increase plasma concentrations of estrogens and may result in side effects).
No products indexed under this heading.

Acetazolamide Sodium (Inhibitors of CYP3A4 such as erythromycin, clarithromycin, ketoconazole, itraconazole, ritonavir and grapefruit juice may increase plasma concentrations of estrogens and may result in side effects).
No products indexed under this heading.

Allium sativum (Inducers of CYP3A4 such as St. John's Wort preparations (hypericum perforatum), phenobarbital, carbamazepine and rifampin may reduce plasma concentrations of estrogens, possibly resulting in a decrease in therapeutic effects and/or changes in the uterine bleeding profile).
No products indexed under this heading.

Aminoglutethimide (Inducers of CYP3A4 such as St. John's Wort preparations (hypericum perforatum), phenobarbital, carbamazepine and rifampin may reduce plasma concentrations of estrogens, possibly resulting in a decrease in therapeutic effects and/or changes in the uterine bleeding profile).
No products indexed under this heading.

Amiodarone Hydrochloride (Inhibitors of CYP3A4 such as erythromycin, clarithromycin, ketoconazole, itraconazole, ritonavir and grapefruit juice may increase plasma concentrations of estrogens and may result in side effects).
No products indexed under this heading.

Amprenavir (Inhibitors of CYP3A4 such as erythromycin, clarithromycin, ketoconazole, itraconazole, ritonavir and grapefruit juice may increase plasma concentrations of estrogens and may result in side effects).
No products indexed under this heading.

Anastrozole (Inhibitors of CYP3A4 such as erythromycin, clarithromycin, ketoconazole, itraconazole, ritonavir and grapefruit juice may increase plasma concentrations of estrogens and may result in side effects).
No products indexed under this heading.

Aprepitant (Inducers of CYP3A4 such as St. John's Wort preparations (hypericum perforatum), phenobarbital, carbamazepine and rifampin may reduce plasma concentrations of estrogens, possibly resulting in a decrease in therapeutic effects and/or changes in the uterine bleeding profile). Products include:
Emend 2124

Atazanavir (Inhibitors of CYP3A4 such as erythromycin, clarithromycin, ketoconazole, itraconazole, ritonavir and grapefruit juice may increase plasma concentrations of estrogens and may result in side effects).
No products indexed under this heading.

Atazanavir Sulfate (Inhibitors of CYP3A4 such as erythromycin, clarithromycin, ketoconazole, itraconazole, ritonavir and grapefruit juice may increase plasma concentrations of estrogens and may result in side effects).
No products indexed under this heading.

Betamethasone (Inducers of CYP3A4 such as St. John's Wort preparations (hypericum perforatum), phenobarbital, carbamazepine and rifampin may reduce plasma concentrations of estrogens, possibly resulting in a decrease in therapeutic effects and/or changes in the uterine bleeding profile).
No products indexed under this heading.

Betamethasone Acetate (Inducers of CYP3A4 such as St. John's Wort preparations (hypericum perforatum), phenobarbital, carbamazepine and rifampin may reduce plasma concentrations of estrogens, possibly resulting in a decrease in therapeutic effects and/or changes in the uterine bleeding profile).
No products indexed under this heading.

Betamethasone Benzoate (Inducers of CYP3A4 such as St. John's Wort preparations (hypericum perforatum), phenobarbital, carbamazepine and rifampin may reduce plasma concentrations of estrogens, possibly resulting in a decrease in therapeutic effects and/or changes in the uterine bleeding profile).
No products indexed under this heading.

Betamethasone Dipropionate (Inducers of CYP3A4 such as St. John's Wort preparations (hypericum perforatum), phenobarbital, carbamazepine and rifampin may reduce plasma concentrations of estrogens, possibly resulting in a decrease in therapeutic effects and/or changes in the uterine bleeding profile). Products include:
Diprolene Lotion 0.05% 3108
Diprolene Ointment 0.05% 3109
Diprolene AF Cream 0.05% 3107
Lotrisone 3163

Betamethasone Sodium Phosphate (Inducers of CYP3A4 such as St. John's Wort preparations (hypericum perforatum), phenobarbital, carbamazepine and rifampin may reduce plasma concentrations of estrogens, possibly resulting in a decrease in therapeutic effects and/or changes in the uterine bleeding profile).
No products indexed under this heading.

Betamethasone Valerate (Inducers of CYP3A4 such as St. John's Wort preparations (hypericum perforatum), phenobarbital, carbamazepine and rifampin may reduce plasma concentrations of estrogens, possibly resulting in a decrease in therapeutic effects and/or changes in the uterine bleeding profile). Products include:
Luxíq 3321

Bosentan (Inducers of CYP3A4 such as St. John's Wort preparations (hypericum perforatum), phenobarbital, carbamazepine and rifampin may reduce plasma concentrations of estrogens, possibly resulting in a decrease in therapeutic effects and/or changes in the uterine bleeding profile). Products include:
Tracleer 573

Carbamazepine (Inducers of CYP3A4 such as St. John's Wort preparations (hypericum perforatum), phenobarbital, carbamazepine and rifampin may reduce plasma concentrations of estrogens, possibly resulting in a decrease in therapeutic effects and/or changes in the uterine bleeding profile). Products include:
Carbatrol 3280
Equetro 3477

Cimetidine (Inhibitors of CYP3A4 such as erythromycin, clarithromycin, ketoconazole, itraconazole, ritonavir and grapefruit juice may increase plasma concentrations of estrogens and may result in side effects).
No products indexed under this heading.

Cimetidine Hydrochloride (Inhibitors of CYP3A4 such as erythromycin, clarithromycin, ketoconazole, itraconazole, ritonavir and grapefruit juice may increase plasma concentrations of estrogens and may result in side effects).
No products indexed under this heading.

Ciprofloxacin (Inducers of CYP3A4 such as St. John's Wort preparations (hypericum perforatum), phenobarbital, carbamazepine and rifampin may reduce plasma concentrations of estrogens, possibly resulting in a decrease in therapeutic effects and/or changes in the uterine bleeding profile). Products include:
Cipro I.V. 3082
Cipro 3073
Cipro XR 3091
Ciprodex 583

Ciprofloxacin Hydrochloride (Inducers of CYP3A4 such as St. John's Wort preparations (hypericum perforatum), phenobarbital, carbamazepine and rifampin may reduce plasma concentrations of estrogens, possibly resulting in a decrease in therapeutic effects and/or changes in the uterine bleeding profile). Products include:
Cipro 3073

Cisplatin (Inducers of CYP3A4 such as St. John's Wort preparations (hypericum perforatum), phenobarbital, carbamazepine and rifampin may reduce plasma concentrations of estrogens, possibly resulting in a decrease in therapeutic effects and/or changes in the uterine bleeding profile).
No products indexed under this heading.

Clarithromycin (Inhibitors of CYP3A4 such as erythromycin, clarithromycin, ketoconazole, itraconazole, ritonavir and grapefruit juice may increase plasma concentrations of estrogens and may result in side effects). Products include:
Biaxin/Biaxin XL 412

Clotrimazole (Inhibitors of CYP3A4 such as erythromycin, clarithromycin, ketoconazole, itraconazole, ritonavir and grapefruit juice may increase plasma concentrations of estrogens and may result in side effects). Products include:
Lotrisone 3163

Conivaptan Hydrochloride (Inhibitors of CYP3A4 such as erythromycin, clarithromycin, ketoconazole, itraconazole, ritonavir and grapefruit juice may

IMPORTANT NOTE: Always consult each drug listing in the patient's regimen for possible interactions.

Enjuvia Interactions Index 588

increase plasma concentrations of estrogens and may result in side effects). Products include:
Vaprisol 689

Cortisone Acetate (Inducers of CYP3A4 such as St. John's Wort preparations (hypericum perforatum), phenobarbital, carbamazepine and rifampin may reduce plasma concentrations of estrogens, possibly resulting in a decrease in therapeutic effects and/or changes in the uterine bleeding profile).
No products indexed under this heading.

Cyclosporine (Inhibitors of CYP3A4 such as erythromycin, clarithromycin, ketoconazole, itraconazole, ritonavir and grapefruit juice may increase plasma concentrations of estrogens and may result in side effects). Products include:
Gengraf 440
Neoral Oral Solution 2496
Neoral Capsules 2496
Restasis 605

Dalfopristin (Inhibitors of CYP3A4 such as erythromycin, clarithromycin, ketoconazole, itraconazole, ritonavir and grapefruit juice may increase plasma concentrations of estrogens and may result in side effects).
No products indexed under this heading.

Danazol (Inhibitors of CYP3A4 such as erythromycin, clarithromycin, ketoconazole, itraconazole, ritonavir and grapefruit juice may increase plasma concentrations of estrogens and may result in side effects).
No products indexed under this heading.

Darunavir (Inhibitors of CYP3A4 such as erythromycin, clarithromycin, ketoconazole, itraconazole, ritonavir and grapefruit juice may increase plasma concentrations of estrogens and may result in side effects).
No products indexed under this heading.

Dasatinib (Inhibitors of CYP3A4 such as erythromycin, clarithromycin, ketoconazole, itraconazole, ritonavir and grapefruit juice may increase plasma concentrations of estrogens and may result in side effects).
No products indexed under this heading.

Delavirdine Mesylate (Inhibitors of CYP3A4 such as erythromycin, clarithromycin, ketoconazole, itraconazole, ritonavir and grapefruit juice may increase plasma concentrations of estrogens and may result in side effects).
No products indexed under this heading.

Delavirine (Inhibitors of CYP3A4 such as erythromycin, clarithromycin, ketoconazole, itraconazole, ritonavir and grapefruit juice may increase plasma concentrations of estrogens and may result in side effects).
No products indexed under this heading.

Desloratadine (Inhibitors of CYP3A4 such as erythromycin, clarithromycin, ketoconazole, itraconazole, ritonavir and grapefruit juice may increase plasma concentrations of estrogens and may result in side effects). Products include:
Clarinex Syrup 3098
Clarinex 3098
Clarinex Reditabs 3098
Clarinex-D 12-Hour 3101
Clarinex-D 3104

Dexamethasone (Inducers of CYP3A4 such as St. John's Wort preparations (hypericum perforatum), phenobarbital, carbamazepine and rifampin may reduce plasma concentrations of estrogens, possibly resulting in a decrease in therapeutic effects and/or changes in the uterine bleeding profile). Products include:
Ciprodex 583
Ozurdex .... ⊙223
Tobramycin and Dexamethasone Ophthalmic Suspension .... ⊙251

Dexamethasone Acetate (Inducers of CYP3A4 such as St. John's Wort preparations (hypericum perforatum), phenobarbital, carbamazepine and rifampin may reduce plasma concentrations of estrogens, possibly resulting in a decrease in therapeutic effects and/or changes in the uterine bleeding profile).
No products indexed under this heading.

Dexamethasone Phosphate (Inducers of CYP3A4 such as St. John's Wort preparations (hypericum perforatum), phenobarbital, carbamazepine and rifampin may reduce plasma concentrations of estrogens, possibly resulting in a decrease in therapeutic effects and/or changes in the uterine bleeding profile).
No products indexed under this heading.

Dexamethasone Sodium (Inducers of CYP3A4 such as St. John's Wort preparations (hypericum perforatum), phenobarbital, carbamazepine and rifampin may reduce plasma concentrations of estrogens, possibly resulting in a decrease in therapeutic effects and/or changes in the uterine bleeding profile).
No products indexed under this heading.

Dexamethasone Sodium Phosphate (Inducers of CYP3A4 such as St. John's Wort preparations (hypericum perforatum), phenobarbital, carbamazepine and rifampin may reduce plasma concentrations of estrogens, possibly resulting in a decrease in therapeutic effects and/or changes in the uterine bleeding profile).
No products indexed under this heading.

Dexamethasone Sodium Phosphate Injection (Inducers of CYP3A4 such as St. John's Wort preparations (hypericum perforatum), phenobarbital, carbamazepine and rifampin may reduce plasma concentrations of estrogens, possibly resulting in a decrease in therapeutic effects and/or changes in the uterine bleeding profile).
No products indexed under this heading.

Diltiazem Hydrochloride (Inhibitors of CYP3A4 such as erythromycin, clarithromycin, ketoconazole, itraconazole, ritonavir and grapefruit juice may increase plasma concentrations of estrogens and may result in side effects). Products include:
Cardizem LA 423

Diltiazem Maleate (Inhibitors of CYP3A4 such as erythromycin, clarithromycin, ketoconazole, itraconazole, ritonavir and grapefruit juice may increase plasma concentrations of estrogens and may result in side effects).
No products indexed under this heading.

Doxorubicin Hydrochloride (Inducers of CYP3A4 such as St. John's Wort preparations (hypericum perforatum), phenobarbital, carbamazepine and rifampin may reduce plasma concentrations of estrogens, possibly resulting in a decrease in therapeutic effects and/or changes in the uterine bleeding profile).
No products indexed under this heading.

Efavirenz (Inducers of CYP3A4 such as St. John's Wort preparations (hypericum perforatum), phenobarbital, carbamazepine and rifampin may reduce plasma concentrations of estrogens, possibly resulting in a decrease in therapeutic effects and/or changes in the uterine bleeding profile). Products include:
Atripla 906

Erythromycin (Inhibitors of CYP3A4 such as erythromycin, clarithromycin, ketoconazole, itraconazole, ritonavir and grapefruit juice may increase plasma concentrations of estrogens and may result in side effects).
No products indexed under this heading.

Erythromycin Estolate (Inhibitors of CYP3A4 such as erythromycin, clarithromycin, ketoconazole, itraconazole, ritonavir and grapefruit juice may increase plasma concentrations of estrogens and may result in side effects).
No products indexed under this heading.

Erythromycin Ethylsuccinate (Inhibitors of CYP3A4 such as erythromycin, clarithromycin, ketoconazole, itraconazole, ritonavir and grapefruit juice may increase plasma concentrations of estrogens and may result in side effects). Products include:
E.E.S. 437
EryPed 435

Erythromycin Gluceptate (Inhibitors of CYP3A4 such as erythromycin, clarithromycin, ketoconazole, itraconazole, ritonavir and grapefruit juice may increase plasma concentrations of estrogens and may result in side effects).
No products indexed under this heading.

Erythromycin Lactobionate (Inhibitors of CYP3A4 such as erythromycin, clarithromycin, ketoconazole, itraconazole, ritonavir and grapefruit juice may increase plasma concentrations of estrogens and may result in side effects).
No products indexed under this heading.

Erythromycin Stearate (Inhibitors of CYP3A4 such as erythromycin, clarithromycin, ketoconazole, itraconazole, ritonavir and grapefruit juice may increase plasma concentrations of estrogens and may result in side effects).
No products indexed under this heading.

Esomeprazole Magnesium (Inhibitors of CYP3A4 such as erythromycin, clarithromycin, ketoconazole, itraconazole, ritonavir and grapefruit juice may increase plasma concentrations of estrogens and may result in side effects). Products include:
Nexium Capsules 704
Nexium Oral Suspension 704

Esomeprazole Sodium (Inhibitors of CYP3A4 such as erythromycin, clarithromycin, ketoconazole, itraconazole, ritonavir and grapefruit juice may increase plasma concentrations of estrogens and may result in side effects). Products include:
Nexium I.V. 712

Ethosuximide (Inducers of CYP3A4 such as St. John's Wort preparations (hypericum perforatum), phenobarbital, carbamazepine and rifampin may reduce plasma concentrations of estrogens, possibly resulting in a decrease in therapeutic effects and/or changes in the uterine bleeding profile).
No products indexed under this heading.

Felbamate (Inducers of CYP3A4 such as St. John's Wort preparations (hypericum perforatum), phenobarbital, carbamazepine and rifampin may reduce plasma concentrations of estrogens, possibly resulting in a decrease in therapeutic effects and/or changes in the uterine bleeding profile).
No products indexed under this heading.

Fluconazole (Inhibitors of CYP3A4 such as erythromycin, clarithromycin, ketoconazole, itraconazole, ritonavir and grapefruit juice may increase plasma concentrations of estrogens and may result in side effects).
No products indexed under this heading.

Fludrocortisone Acetate (Inducers of CYP3A4 such as St. John's Wort preparations (hypericum perforatum), phenobarbital, carbamazepine and rifampin may reduce plasma concentrations of estrogens, possibly resulting in a decrease in therapeutic effects and/or changes in the uterine bleeding profile).
No products indexed under this heading.

Fluoxetine (Inhibitors of CYP3A4 such as erythromycin, clarithromycin, ketoconazole, itraconazole, ritonavir and grapefruit juice may increase plasma concentrations of estrogens and may result in side effects).
No products indexed under this heading.

Fluoxetine Hydrochloride (Inhibitors of CYP3A4 such as erythromycin, clarithromycin, ketoconazole, itraconazole, ritonavir and grapefruit juice may increase plasma concentrations of estrogens and may result in side effects). Products include:
Prozac Weekly 1941
Prozac Pulvules 1941
Symbyax 1965

Fluvoxamine Maleate (Inhibitors of CYP3A4 such as erythromycin, clarithromycin, ketoconazole, itraconazole, ritonavir and grapefruit juice may increase plasma concentrations of estrogens and may result in side effects).
No products indexed under this heading.

Fosamprenavir Calcium (Inhibitors of CYP3A4 such as erythromycin, clarithromycin, ketoconazole, itraconazole, ritonavir and grapefruit juice may increase plasma concentrations of estrogens and may result in side effects). Products include:
Lexiva Oral Suspension 1558
Lexiva 1558

Fosphenytoin Sodium (Inducers of CYP3A4 such as St. John's Wort preparations (hypericum perforatum), phenobarbital, carbamazepine and rifampin may reduce plasma concentrations of estrogens, possibly resulting in a decrease in therapeutic effects and/or changes in the uterine bleeding profile).
No products indexed under this heading.

Garlic Extract (Inducers of CYP3A4 such as St. John's Wort preparations (hypericum perforatum), phenobarbital, carbamazepine and rifampin may reduce plasma concentrations of estrogens, possibly resulting in a decrease in therapeutic effects and/or changes in the uterine bleeding profile).
No products indexed under this heading.

Garlic Oil (Inducers of CYP3A4 such as St. John's Wort preparations (hypericum perforatum), phenobarbital, carbamazepine and rifampin may reduce plasma concentrations of estrogens, possibly resulting in a decrease in therapeutic effects and/or changes in the uterine bleeding profile).
No products indexed under this heading.

Hydrocortisone (Inducers of CYP3A4 such as St. John's Wort preparations (hypericum perforatum), phenobarbital, carbamazepine and rifampin may reduce plasma concentrations of estrogens, possibly resulting in a decrease in therapeutic effects and/or changes in the uterine bleeding profile).
No products indexed under this heading.

Hydrocortisone (Alcohol) (Inducers of CYP3A4 such as St. John's Wort preparations (hypericum perforatum), phenobarbital, carbamazepine and rifampin may reduce plasma concentrations of estrogens, possibly resulting in a decrease in therapeutic effects and/or changes in the uterine bleeding profile).
No products indexed under this heading.

(⊙ Described in PDR® for Ophthalmic Medicines)

589 **Interactions Index** **Enjuvia**

Hydrocortisone Acetate (Inducers of CYP3A4 such as St. John's Wort preparations (hypericum perforatum), phenobarbital, carbamazepine and rifampin may reduce plasma concentrations of estrogens, possibly resulting in a decrease in therapeutic effects and/or changes in the uterine bleeding profile).
No products indexed under this heading.

Hydrocortisone Butyrate (Inducers of CYP3A4 such as St. John's Wort preparations (hypericum perforatum), phenobarbital, carbamazepine and rifampin may reduce plasma concentrations of estrogens, possibly resulting in a decrease in therapeutic effects and/or changes in the uterine bleeding profile).
No products indexed under this heading.

Hydrocortisone Cypionate (Inducers of CYP3A4 such as St. John's Wort preparations (hypericum perforatum), phenobarbital, carbamazepine and rifampin may reduce plasma concentrations of estrogens, possibly resulting in a decrease in therapeutic effects and/or changes in the uterine bleeding profile).
No products indexed under this heading.

Hydrocortisone Hemisuccinate (Inducers of CYP3A4 such as St. John's Wort preparations (hypericum perforatum), phenobarbital, carbamazepine and rifampin may reduce plasma concentrations of estrogens, possibly resulting in a decrease in therapeutic effects and/or changes in the uterine bleeding profile).
No products indexed under this heading.

Hydrocortisone Probutate (Inducers of CYP3A4 such as St. John's Wort preparations (hypericum perforatum), phenobarbital, carbamazepine and rifampin may reduce plasma concentrations of estrogens, possibly resulting in a decrease in therapeutic effects and/or changes in the uterine bleeding profile).
No products indexed under this heading.

Hydrocortisone Sodium Phosphate (Inducers of CYP3A4 such as St. John's Wort preparations (hypericum perforatum), phenobarbital, carbamazepine and rifampin may reduce plasma concentrations of estrogens, possibly resulting in a decrease in therapeutic effects and/or changes in the uterine bleeding profile).
No products indexed under this heading.

Hydrocortisone Sodium Succinate (Inducers of CYP3A4 such as St. John's Wort preparations (hypericum perforatum), phenobarbital, carbamazepine and rifampin may reduce plasma concentrations of estrogens, possibly resulting in a decrease in therapeutic effects and/or changes in the uterine bleeding profile).
No products indexed under this heading.

Hydrocortisone Valerate (Inducers of CYP3A4 such as St. John's Wort preparations (hypericum perforatum), phenobarbital, carbamazepine and rifampin may reduce plasma concentrations of estrogens, possibly resulting in a decrease in therapeutic effects and/or changes in the uterine bleeding profile).
No products indexed under this heading.

Hypericum (Inducers of CYP3A4 such as St. John's Wort preparations (hypericum perforatum), phenobarbital, carbamazepine and rifampin may reduce plasma concentrations of estrogens, possibly resulting in a decrease in therapeutic effects and/or changes in the uterine bleeding profile).
No products indexed under this heading.

Hypericum Perforatum (Inducers of CYP3A4 such as St. John's Wort preparations (hypericum perforatum), phenobarbital, carbamazepine and rifampin may reduce plasma concentrations of estrogens, possibly resulting in a decrease in therapeutic effects and/or changes in the uterine bleeding profile). Products include:
Traumeel ... 1800

Imatinib Mesylate (Inhibitors of CYP3A4 such as erythromycin, clarithromycin, ketoconazole, itraconazole, ritonavir and grapefruit juice may increase plasma concentrations of estrogens and may result in side effects). Products include:
Gleevec ... 2477

Indinavir Sulfate (Inhibitors of CYP3A4 such as erythromycin, clarithromycin, ketoconazole, itraconazole, ritonavir and grapefruit juice may increase plasma concentrations of estrogens and may result in side effects). Products include:
Crixivan ... 2113

Isoniazid (Inhibitors of CYP3A4 such as erythromycin, clarithromycin, ketoconazole, itraconazole, ritonavir and grapefruit juice may increase plasma concentrations of estrogens and may result in side effects).
No products indexed under this heading.

Itraconazole (Inhibitors of CYP3A4 such as erythromycin, clarithromycin, ketoconazole, itraconazole, ritonavir and grapefruit juice may increase plasma concentrations of estrogens and may result in side effects).
No products indexed under this heading.

Ketoconazole (Inhibitors of CYP3A4 such as erythromycin, clarithromycin, ketoconazole, itraconazole, ritonavir and grapefruit juice may increase plasma concentrations of estrogens and may result in side effects). Products include:
Extina ... 3319
Xolegel ... 3337

Lapatinib (Inhibitors of CYP3A4 such as erythromycin, clarithromycin, ketoconazole, itraconazole, ritonavir and grapefruit juice may increase plasma concentrations of estrogens and may result in side effects). Products include:
Tykerb ... 1698

Levothyroxine Sodium (Patients on thyroid replacement therapy may require higher doses of thryoid hormone). Products include:
Levoxyl Tablets ... 1843
Synthroid ... 529

Liothyronine Sodium (Patients on thyroid replacement therapy may require higher doses of thyroid hormone). Products include:
Cytomel ... 1830

Liotrix (Patients on thyroid replacement therapy may require higher doses of thyroid hormone).
No products indexed under this heading.

Lopinavir (Inhibitors of CYP3A4 such as erythromycin, clarithromycin, ketoconazole, itraconazole, ritonavir and grapefruit juice may increase plasma concentrations of estrogens and may result in side effects). Products include:
Kaletra ... 458

Loratadine (Inhibitors of CYP3A4 such as erythromycin, clarithromycin, ketoconazole, itraconazole, ritonavir and grapefruit juice may increase plasma concentrations of estrogens and may result in side effects).
No products indexed under this heading.

Mephenytoin (Inducers of CYP3A4 such as St. John's Wort preparations (hypericum perforatum), phenobarbital, carbamazepine and rifampin may reduce plasma concentrations of estrogens, possibly resulting in a decrease in therapeutic effects and/or changes in the uterine bleeding profile).
No products indexed under this heading.

Methsuximide (Inducers of CYP3A4 such as St. John's Wort preparations (hypericum perforatum), phenobarbital, carbamazepine and rifampin may reduce plasma concentrations of estrogens, possibly resulting in a decrease in therapeutic effects and/or changes in the uterine bleeding profile).
No products indexed under this heading.

Methylprednisolone (Inducers of CYP3A4 such as St. John's Wort preparations (hypericum perforatum), phenobarbital, carbamazepine and rifampin may reduce plasma concentrations of estrogens, possibly resulting in a decrease in therapeutic effects and/or changes in the uterine bleeding profile).
No products indexed under this heading.

Methylprednisolone Acetate (Inducers of CYP3A4 such as St. John's Wort preparations (hypericum perforatum), phenobarbital, carbamazepine and rifampin may reduce plasma concentrations of estrogens, possibly resulting in a decrease in therapeutic effects and/or changes in the uterine bleeding profile).
No products indexed under this heading.

Methylprednisolone Sodium Succinate (Inducers of CYP3A4 such as St. John's Wort preparations (hypericum perforatum), phenobarbital, carbamazepine and rifampin may reduce plasma concentrations of estrogens, possibly resulting in a decrease in therapeutic effects and/or changes in the uterine bleeding profile).
No products indexed under this heading.

Metronidazole (Inhibitors of CYP3A4 such as erythromycin, clarithromycin, ketoconazole, itraconazole, ritonavir and grapefruit juice may increase plasma concentrations of estrogens and may result in side effects). Products include:
Pylera ... 793

Metronidazole Benzoate (Inhibitors of CYP3A4 such as erythromycin, clarithromycin, ketoconazole, itraconazole, ritonavir and grapefruit juice may increase plasma concentrations of estrogens and may result in side effects).
No products indexed under this heading.

Metronidazole Hydrochloride (Inhibitors of CYP3A4 such as erythromycin, clarithromycin, ketoconazole, itraconazole, ritonavir and grapefruit juice may increase plasma concentrations of estrogens and may result in side effects).
No products indexed under this heading.

Metronidazole Sodium (Inhibitors of CYP3A4 such as erythromycin, clarithromycin, ketoconazole, itraconazole, ritonavir and grapefruit juice may increase plasma concentrations of estrogens and may result in side effects).
No products indexed under this heading.

Miconazole (Inhibitors of CYP3A4 such as erythromycin, clarithromycin, ketoconazole, itraconazole, ritonavir and grapefruit juice may increase plasma concentrations of estrogens and may result in side effects).
No products indexed under this heading.

Miconazole Nitrate (Inhibitors of CYP3A4 such as erythromycin, clarithromycin, ketoconazole, itraconazole, ritonavir and grapefruit juice may increase plasma concentrations of estrogens and may result in side effects). Products include:
Vusion Ointment ... 3335

Mifepristone (Inhibitors of CYP3A4 such as erythromycin, clarithromycin, ketoconazole, itraconazole, ritonavir and grapefruit juice may increase plasma concentrations of estrogens and may result in side effects).
No products indexed under this heading.

Modafinil (Inducers of CYP3A4 such as St. John's Wort preparations (hypericum perforatum), phenobarbital, carbamazepine and rifampin may reduce plasma concentrations of estrogens, possibly resulting in a decrease in therapeutic effects and/or changes in the uterine bleeding profile). Products include:
Provigil ... 983

Nafcillin Sodium (Inducers of CYP3A4 such as St. John's Wort preparations (hypericum perforatum), phenobarbital, carbamazepine and rifampin may reduce plasma concentrations of estrogens, possibly resulting in a decrease in therapeutic effects and/or changes in the uterine bleeding profile).
No products indexed under this heading.

Nefazodone Hydrochloride (Inhibitors of CYP3A4 such as erythromycin, clarithromycin, ketoconazole, itraconazole, ritonavir and grapefruit juice may increase plasma concentrations of estrogens and may result in side effects).
No products indexed under this heading.

Nelfinavir Mesylate (Inhibitors of CYP3A4 such as erythromycin, clarithromycin, ketoconazole, itraconazole, ritonavir and grapefruit juice may increase plasma concentrations of estrogens and may result in side effects).
No products indexed under this heading.

Nevirapine (Inducers of CYP3A4 such as St. John's Wort preparations (hypericum perforatum), phenobarbital, carbamazepine and rifampin may reduce plasma concentrations of estrogens, possibly resulting in a decrease in therapeutic effects and/or changes in the uterine bleeding profile). Products include:
Viramune Oral Suspension ... 897
Viramune Tablets ... 897

Niacin (Inhibitors of CYP3A4 such as erythromycin, clarithromycin, ketoconazole, itraconazole, ritonavir and grapefruit juice may increase plasma concentrations of estrogens and may result in side effects). Products include:
Advicor ... 402
Cardio Basics ... 3455
Niaspan ... 497
Simcor ... 524

Niacinamide (Inhibitors of CYP3A4 such as erythromycin, clarithromycin, ketoconazole, itraconazole, ritonavir and grapefruit juice may increase plasma concentrations of estrogens and may result in side effects). Products include:
CitraNatal 90 DHA Capsules ... 2332
CitraNatal Assure ... 2332
CitraNatal Rx ... 2332
Heplive ... 607

Niacinamide Hydroiodide (Inhibitors of CYP3A4 such as erythromycin, clarithromycin, ketoconazole, itraconazole, ritonavir and grapefruit juice may increase plasma concentrations of estrogens and may result in side effects).
No products indexed under this heading.

Nicotinamide (Inhibitors of CYP3A4 such as erythromycin, clarithromycin, ketoconazole, itraconazole, ritonavir and grapefruit juice may increase plasma concentrations of estrogens and may result in side effects).
No products indexed under this heading.

IMPORTANT NOTE: Always consult each drug listing in the patient's regimen for possible interactions.

591 Interactions Index EpiPen

Uniphyl 2817

Theophylline Calcium Salicylate (Inducers of CYP3A4 such as St. John's Wort preparations (hypericum perforatum), phenobarbital, carbamazepine and rifampin may reduce plasma concentrations of estrogens, possibly resulting in a decrease in therapeutic effects and/or changes in the uterine bleeding profile).
No products indexed under this heading.

Theophylline Dihydroxypropyl (Glyceryl) (Inducers of CYP3A4 such as St. John's Wort preparations (hypericum perforatum), phenobarbital, carbamazepine and rifampin may reduce plasma concentrations of estrogens, possibly resulting in a decrease in therapeutic effects and/or changes in the uterine bleeding profile).
No products indexed under this heading.

Theophylline Ethylenediamine (Inducers of CYP3A4 such as St. John's Wort preparations (hypericum perforatum), phenobarbital, carbamazepine and rifampin may reduce plasma concentrations of estrogens, possibly resulting in a decrease in therapeutic effects and/or changes in the uterine bleeding profile).
No products indexed under this heading.

Theophylline Sodium Glycinate (Inducers of CYP3A4 such as St. John's Wort preparations (hypericum perforatum), phenobarbital, carbamazepine and rifampin may reduce plasma concentrations of estrogens, possibly resulting in a decrease in therapeutic effects and/or changes in the uterine bleeding profile).
No products indexed under this heading.

Thyroglobulin (Patients on thyroid replacement therapy may require higher doses of thryoid hormone).
No products indexed under this heading.

Thyroid (Patients on thyroid replacement therapy may require higher doses of thryoid hormone). Products include:
Naturethroid 2830

Thyroxine (Patients on thyroid replacement therapy may require higher doses of thryoid hormone).
No products indexed under this heading.

Thyroxine Sodium (Patients on thyroid replacement therapy may require higher doses of thryoid hormone).
No products indexed under this heading.

Triamcinolone (Inducers of CYP3A4 such as St. John's Wort preparations (hypericum perforatum), phenobarbital, carbamazepine and rifampin may reduce plasma concentrations of estrogens, possibly resulting in a decrease in therapeutic effects and/or changes in the uterine bleeding profile).
No products indexed under this heading.

Triamcinolone Acetonide (Inducers of CYP3A4 such as St. John's Wort preparations (hypericum perforatum), phenobarbital, carbamazepine and rifampin may reduce plasma concentrations of estrogens, possibly resulting in a decrease in therapeutic effects and/or changes in the uterine bleeding profile). Products include:
Azmacort 408
Nasacort AQ 3019

Triamcinolone Diacetate (Inducers of CYP3A4 such as St. John's Wort preparations (hypericum perforatum), phenobarbital, carbamazepine and rifampin may reduce plasma concentrations of estrogens, possibly resulting in a decrease in therapeutic effects and/or changes in the uterine bleeding profile).
No products indexed under this heading.

Triamcinolone Hexacetonide (Inducers of CYP3A4 such as St. John's Wort preparations (hypericum perforatum), phenobarbital, carbamazepine and rifampin may reduce plasma concentrations of estrogens, possibly resulting in a decrease in therapeutic effects and/or changes in the uterine bleeding profile).
No products indexed under this heading.

Troglitazone (Inducers of CYP3A4 such as St. John's Wort preparations (hypericum perforatum), phenobarbital, carbamazepine and rifampin may reduce plasma concentrations of estrogens, possibly resulting in a decrease in therapeutic effects and/or changes in the uterine bleeding profile).
No products indexed under this heading.

Troleandomycin (Inhibitors of CYP3A4 such as erythromycin, clarithromycin, ketoconazole, itraconazole, ritonavir and grapefruit juice may increase plasma concentrations of estrogens and may result in side effects).
No products indexed under this heading.

Valproate Sodium (Inhibitors of CYP3A4 such as erythromycin, clarithromycin, ketoconazole, itraconazole, ritonavir and grapefruit juice may increase plasma concentrations of estrogens and may result in side effects).
No products indexed under this heading.

Vardenafil Hydrochloride (Inhibitors of CYP3A4 such as erythromycin, clarithromycin, ketoconazole, itraconazole, ritonavir and grapefruit juice may increase plasma concentrations of estrogens and may result in side effects). Products include:
Levitra 3157

Verapamil Hydrochloride (Inhibitors of CYP3A4 such as erythromycin, clarithromycin, ketoconazole, itraconazole, ritonavir and grapefruit juice may increase plasma concentrations of estrogens and may result in side effects). Products include:
Tarka 534

Voriconazole (Inhibitors of CYP3A4 such as erythromycin, clarithromycin, ketoconazole, itraconazole, ritonavir and grapefruit juice may increase plasma concentrations of estrogens and may result in side effects).
No products indexed under this heading.

Zafirlukast (Inhibitors of CYP3A4 such as erythromycin, clarithromycin, ketoconazole, itraconazole, ritonavir and grapefruit juice may increase plasma concentrations of estrogens and may result in side effects). Products include:
Accolate 3612

Zileuton (Inhibitors of CYP3A4 such as erythromycin, clarithromycin, ketoconazole, itraconazole, ritonavir and grapefruit juice may increase plasma concentrations of estrogens and may result in side effects).
No products indexed under this heading.

Food Interactions

Grapefruit (Inhibitors of CYP3A4 such as erythromycin, clarithromycin, ketoconazole, itraconazole, ritonavir and grapefruit juice may increase plasma concentrations of estrogens and may result in side effects).

Grapefruit Juice (Inhibitors of CYP3A4 such as erythromycin, clarithromycin, ketoconazole, itraconazole, ritonavir and grapefruit juice may increase plasma concentrations of estrogens and may result in side effects).

ENTEREG CAPSULES

(Alvimopan) 579
None cited in PDR database.

EPIPEN AUTO-INJECTOR

(Epinephrine) 3631

May interact with alpha adrenergic blockers, antiarrhythmics, antihistamines, beta-blockers, cardiac glycosides, diuretics, ergot-containing drugs, monoamine oxidase inhibitors, quinidine, tricyclic antidepressants, and certain other agents. Compounds in these categories include:

Acebutolol Hydrochloride (Epinephrine should be used with caution in patients who have cardiac arrhythmias, coronary artery or organic heart disease, hypertension, or in patients who are on drugs that may sensitize the heart to arrhythmias, eg, anti-arrhythmics. In such patients, epinephrine may precipitate or aggravate angina pectoris as well as produce ventricular arrhythmias).
No products indexed under this heading.

Acrivastine (The effects of epinephrine may be potentiated by certain antihistamines, notably chlorpheniramine, tripelennamine, and diphenhydramine).
No products indexed under this heading.

Adenosine (Epinephrine should be used with caution in patients who have cardiac arrhythmias, coronary artery or organic heart disease, hypertension, or in patients who are on drugs that may sensitize the heart to arrhythmias, eg, anti-arrhythmics. In such patients, epinephrine may precipitate or aggravate angina pectoris as well as produce ventricular arrhythmias). Products include:
Adenocard 656
Adenoscan 657

Alfuzosin Hydrochloride (The vasoconstricting and hypertensive effects of epinephrine are antagonized by α-adrenergic blocking drugs, such as phentolamine). Products include:
Uroxatral 3050

Amiloride Hydrochloride (Patients who receive epinephrine while concomitantly taking diuretics should be carefully observed for the development of cardiac arrhythmias. Epinephrine should be used with caution in patients who have cardiac arrhythmias, coronary artery or organic heart disease, hypertension, or in patients who are on drugs that may sensitize the heart to arrhythmias, eg, diuretics. In such patients, epinephrine may precipitate or aggravate angina pectoris as well as produce ventricular arrhythmias).
No products indexed under this heading.

Amiodarone Hydrochloride (Epinephrine should be used with caution in patients who have cardiac arrhythmias, coronary artery or organic heart disease, hypertension, or in patients who are on drugs that may sensitize the heart to arrhythmias, eg, anti-arrhythmics. In such patients, epinephrine may precipitate or aggravate angina pectoris as well as produce ventricular arrhythmias).
No products indexed under this heading.

Amitriptyline Hydrochloride (The effects of epinephrine may be potentiated by tricyclic antidepressants).
No products indexed under this heading.

Amoxapine (The effects of epinephrine may be potentiated by tricyclic antidepressants).
No products indexed under this heading.

Apraclonidine Hydrochloride (The vasoconstricting and hypertensive effects of epinephrine are antagonized by α-adrenergic blocking drugs, such as phentolamine).
No products indexed under this heading.

Astemizole (The effects of epinephrine may be potentiated by certain antihistamines, notably chlorpheniramine, tripelennamine, and diphenhydramine).
No products indexed under this heading.

Atenolol (The cardiostimulating and bronchodilating effects of epinephrine are antagonized by β-adrenergic blocking drugs, such as propranolol).
No products indexed under this heading.

Azatadine Maleate (The effects of epinephrine may be potentiated by certain antihistamines, notably chlorpheniramine, tripelennamine, and diphenhydramine).
No products indexed under this heading.

Bendroflumethiazide (Patients who receive epinephrine while concomitantly taking diuretics should be carefully observed for the development of cardiac arrhythmias. Epinephrine should be used with caution in patients who have cardiac arrhythmias, coronary artery or organic heart disease, hypertension, or in patients who are on drugs that may sensitize the heart to arrhythmias, eg, diuretics. In such patients, epinephrine may precipitate or aggravate angina pectoris as well as produce ventricular arrhythmias).
No products indexed under this heading.

Betaxolol Hydrochloride (The cardiostimulating and bronchodilating effects of epinephrine are antagonized by β-adrenergic blocking drugs, such as propranolol).
No products indexed under this heading.

Bisoprolol Fumarate (The cardiostimulating and bronchodilating effects of epinephrine are antagonized by β-adrenergic blocking drugs, such as propranolol).
No products indexed under this heading.

Bretylium Tosylate (Epinephrine should be used with caution in patients who have cardiac arrhythmias, coronary artery or organic heart disease, hypertension, or in patients who are on drugs that may sensitize the heart to arrhythmias, eg, anti-arrhythmics. In such patients, epinephrine may precipitate or aggravate angina pectoris as well as produce ventricular arrhythmias).
No products indexed under this heading.

Bromodiphenhydramine Hydrochloride (The effects of epinephrine may be potentiated by certain antihistamines, notably chlorpheniramine, tripelennamine, and diphenhydramine).
No products indexed under this heading.

Brompheniramine Maleate (The effects of epinephrine may be potentiated by certain antihistamines, notably chlorpheniramine, tripelennamine, and diphenhydramine).
No products indexed under this heading.

Bumetanide (Patients who receive epinephrine while concomitantly taking diuretics should be carefully observed for the development of cardiac arrhythmias. Epinephrine should be used with caution in patients who have cardiac arrhythmias, coronary artery or organic heart disease, hypertension, or in patients who are on drugs that may sensitize the heart to arrhythmias, eg, diuretics. In such patients, epinephrine may precipitate or aggravate angina pectoris as well as produce ventricular arrhythmias).
No products indexed under this heading.

Carteolol Hydrochloride (The cardiostimulating and bronchodilating effects of epinephrine are antagonized by β-adrenergic blocking drugs, such as propranolol).
No products indexed under this heading.

Carvedilol (The cardiostimulating and bronchodilating effects of epinephrine are antagonized by β-adrenergic blocking drugs, such as propranolol). Products include:
Coreg 1409

Carvedilol Phosphate (The cardiostimulating and bronchodilating effects

IMPORTANT NOTE: Always consult each drug listing in the patient's regimen for possible interactions.

(⊙ Described in PDR® for Ophthalmic Medicines)

593 Interactions Index EpiPen

Hydroflumethiazide (Patients who receive epinephrine while concomitantly taking diuretics should be carefully observed for the development of cardiac arrhythmias. Epinephrine should be used with caution in patients who have cardiac arrhythmias, coronary artery or organic heart disease, hypertension, or in patients who are on drugs that may sensitize the heart to arrhythmias, eg, diuretics. In such patients, epinephrine may precipitate or aggravate angina pectoris as well as produce ventricular arrhythmias).
No products indexed under this heading.

Imipramine Hydrochloride (The effects of epinephrine may be potentiated by tricyclic antidepressants).
No products indexed under this heading.

Imipramine Pamoate (The effects of epinephrine may be potentiated by tricyclic antidepressants).
No products indexed under this heading.

Indapamide (Patients who receive epinephrine while concomitantly taking diuretics should be carefully observed for the development of cardiac arrhythmias. Epinephrine should be used with caution in patients who have cardiac arrhythmias, coronary artery or organic heart disease, hypertension, or in patients who are on drugs that may sensitize the heart to arrhythmias, eg, diuretics. In such patients, epinephrine may precipitate or aggravate angina pectoris as well as produce ventricular arrhythmias). Products include:
Indapamide 2356

Isocarboxazid (The effects of epinephrine may be potentiated by monoamine oxidase inhibitors). Products include:
Marplan 3481

Labetalol Hydrochloride (The cardiostimulating and bronchodilating effects of epinephrine are antagonized by β-adrenergic blocking drugs, such as propranolol).
No products indexed under this heading.

Levobunolol Hydrochloride (The cardiostimulating and bronchodilating effects of epinephrine are antagonized by β-adrenergic blocking drugs, such as propranolol).
No products indexed under this heading.

Levothyroxine Sodium (The effects of epinephrine may be potentiated by levothyroxine sodium). Products include:
Levoxyl Tablets 1843
Synthroid 529

Lidocaine Hydrochloride (Epinephrine should be used with caution in patients who have cardiac arrhythmias, coronary artery or organic heart disease, hypertension, or in patients who are on drugs that may sensitize the heart to arrhythmias, eg, antiarrhythmics. In such patients, epinephrine may precipitate or aggravate angina pectoris as well as produce ventricular arrhythmias).
No products indexed under this heading.

Loratadine (The effects of epinephrine may be potentiated by certain antihistamines, notably chlorpheniramine, tripelennamine, and diphenhydramine).
No products indexed under this heading.

Maprotiline Hydrochloride (The effects of epinephrine may be potentiated by tricyclic antidepressants).
No products indexed under this heading.

Methdilazine Hydrochloride (The effects of epinephrine may be potentiated by certain antihistamines, notably chlorpheniramine, tripelennamine, and diphenhydramine).
No products indexed under this heading.

Methyclothiazide (Patients who receive epinephrine while concomitantly taking diuretics should be carefully observed for the development of cardiac arrhythmias. Epinephrine should be used with caution in patients who have cardiac arrhythmias, coronary artery or organic heart disease, hypertension, or in patients who are on drugs that may sensitize the heart to arrhythmias, eg, diuretics. In such patients, epinephrine may precipitate or aggravate angina pectoris as well as produce ventricular arrhythmias).
No products indexed under this heading.

Methylergonovine Maleate (Ergot alkaloids may reverse the pressor effects of epinephrine).
No products indexed under this heading.

Methysergide Maleate (Ergot alkaloids may reverse the pressor effects of epinephrine).
No products indexed under this heading.

Metipranolol Hydrochloride (The cardiostimulating and bronchodilating effects of epinephrine are antagonized by β-adrenergic blocking drugs, such as propranolol).
No products indexed under this heading.

Metolazone (Patients who receive epinephrine while concomitantly taking diuretics should be carefully observed for the development of cardiac arrhythmias. Epinephrine should be used with caution in patients who have cardiac arrhythmias, coronary artery or organic heart disease, hypertension, or in patients who are on drugs that may sensitize the heart to arrhythmias, eg, diuretics. In such patients, epinephrine may precipitate or aggravate angina pectoris as well as produce ventricular arrhythmias).
No products indexed under this heading.

Metoprolol Succinate (The cardiostimulating and bronchodilating effects of epinephrine are antagonized by β-adrenergic blocking drugs, such as propranolol). Products include:
Toprol XL 732

Metoprolol Tartrate (The cardiostimulating and bronchodilating effects of epinephrine are antagonized by β-adrenergic blocking drugs, such as propranolol).
No products indexed under this heading.

Mexiletine Hydrochloride (Epinephrine should be used with caution in patients who have cardiac arrhythmias, coronary artery or organic heart disease, hypertension, or in patients who are on drugs that may sensitize the heart to arrhythmias, eg, antiarrhythmics. In such patients, epinephrine may precipitate or aggravate angina pectoris as well as produce ventricular arrhythmias).
No products indexed under this heading.

Moclobemide (The effects of epinephrine may be potentiated by monoamine oxidase inhibitors).
No products indexed under this heading.

Moricizine Hydrochloride (Epinephrine should be used with caution in patients who have cardiac arrhythmias, coronary artery or organic heart disease, hypertension, or in patients who are on drugs that may sensitize the heart to arrhythmias, eg, antiarrhythmics. In such patients, epinephrine may precipitate or aggravate angina pectoris as well as produce ventricular arrhythmias).
No products indexed under this heading.

Nadolol (The cardiostimulating and bronchodilating effects of epinephrine are antagonized by β-adrenergic blocking drugs, such as propranolol). Products include:
Nadolol 2359

Nebivolol (The cardiostimulating and bronchodilating effects of epinephrine are antagonized by β-adrenergic blocking drugs, such as propranolol). Products include:
Bystolic 1147

Nortriptyline Hydrochloride (The effects of epinephrine may be potentiated by tricyclic antidepressants).
No products indexed under this heading.

Pargyline Hydrochloride (The effects of epinephrine may be potentiated by monoamine oxidase inhibitors).
No products indexed under this heading.

Penbutolol Sulfate (The cardiostimulating and bronchodilating effects of epinephrine are antagonized by β-adrenergic blocking drugs, such as propranolol).
No products indexed under this heading.

Phenelzine Sulfate (The effects of epinephrine may be potentiated by monoamine oxidase inhibitors).
No products indexed under this heading.

Phentolamine Mesylate (The vasoconstricting and hypertensive effects of epinephrine are antagonized by α-adrenergic blocking drugs, such as phentolamine).
No products indexed under this heading.

Pindolol (The cardiostimulating and bronchodilating effects of epinephrine are antagonized by β-adrenergic blocking drugs, such as propranolol).
No products indexed under this heading.

Polythiazide (Patients who receive epinephrine while concomitantly taking diuretics should be carefully observed for the development of cardiac arrhythmias. Epinephrine should be used with caution in patients who have cardiac arrhythmias, coronary artery or organic heart disease, hypertension, or in patients who are on drugs that may sensitize the heart to arrhythmias, eg, diuretics. In such patients, epinephrine may precipitate or aggravate angina pectoris as well as produce ventricular arrhythmias).
No products indexed under this heading.

Prazosin Hydrochloride (The vasoconstricting and hypertensive effects of epinephrine are antagonized by α-adrenergic blocking drugs, such as phentolamine).
No products indexed under this heading.

Procainamide Hydrochloride (Epinephrine should be used with caution in patients who have cardiac arrhythmias, coronary artery or organic heart disease, hypertension, or in patients who are on drugs that may sensitize the heart to arrhythmias, eg, antiarrhythmics. In such patients, epinephrine may precipitate or aggravate angina pectoris as well as produce ventricular arrhythmias).
No products indexed under this heading.

Procarbazine Hydrochloride (The effects of epinephrine may be potentiated by monoamine oxidase inhibitors).
No products indexed under this heading.

Promethazine Hydrochloride (The effects of epinephrine may be potentiated by certain antihistamines, notably chlorpheniramine, tripelennamine, and diphenhydramine).
No products indexed under this heading.

Propafenone Hydrochloride (Epinephrine should be used with caution in patients who have cardiac arrhythmias, coronary artery or organic heart disease, hypertension, or in patients who are on drugs that may sensitize the heart to arrhythmias, eg, antiarrhythmics. In such patients, epinephrine may precipitate or aggravate angina pectoris as well as produce ventricular arrhythmias). Products include:
Rythmol 1648
Rythmol SR 1652

Propranolol (The cardiostimulating and bronchodilating effects of epinephrine are antagonized by β-adrenergic blocking drugs, such as propranolol).
No products indexed under this heading.

Propranolol Hydrochloride (The cardiostimulating and bronchodilating effects of epinephrine are antagonized by β-adrenergic blocking drugs, such as propranolol). Products include:
InnoPran XL 1517

Protriptyline Hydrochloride (The effects of epinephrine may be potentiated by tricyclic antidepressants).
No products indexed under this heading.

Pyrilamine Maleate (The effects of epinephrine may be potentiated by certain antihistamines, notably chlorpheniramine, tripelennamine, and diphenhydramine).
No products indexed under this heading.

Pyrilamine Tannate (The effects of epinephrine may be potentiated by certain antihistamines, notably chlorpheniramine, tripelennamine, and diphenhydramine).
No products indexed under this heading.

Quinidine (Epinephrine should be used with caution in patients who have cardiac arrhythmias, coronary artery or organic heart disease, hypertension, or in patients who are on drugs that may sensitize the heart to arrhythmias, eg, quinidine. In such patients, epinephrine may precipitate or aggravate angina pectoris as well as produce ventricular arrhythmias).
No products indexed under this heading.

Quinidine Gluconate (Epinephrine should be used with caution in patients who have cardiac arrhythmias, coronary artery or organic heart disease, hypertension, or in patients who are on drugs that may sensitize the heart to arrhythmias, eg, quinidine. In such patients, epinephrine may precipitate or aggravate angina pectoris as well as produce ventricular arrhythmias).
No products indexed under this heading.

Quinidine Hydrochloride (Epinephrine should be used with caution in patients who have cardiac arrhythmias, coronary artery or organic heart disease, hypertension, or in patients who are on drugs that may sensitize the heart to arrhythmias, eg, quinidine. In such patients, epinephrine may precipitate or aggravate angina pectoris as well as produce ventricular arrhythmias).
No products indexed under this heading.

Quinidine Polygalacturonate (Epinephrine should be used with caution in patients who have cardiac arrhythmias, coronary artery or organic heart disease, hypertension, or in patients who are on drugs that may sensitize the heart to arrhythmias, eg, quinidine. In such patients, epinephrine may precipitate or aggravate angina pectoris as well as produce ventricular arrhythmias).
No products indexed under this heading.

Quinidine Sulfate (Epinephrine should be used with caution in patients who have cardiac arrhythmias, coronary artery or organic heart disease, hypertension, or in patients who are on drugs that may sensitize the heart to arrhythmias, eg, quinidine. In such patients, epinephrine may precipitate or aggravate angina pectoris as well as produce ventricular arrhythmias).
No products indexed under this heading.

Rasagiline Mesylate (The effects of epinephrine may be potentiated by monoamine oxidase inhibitors). Products include:
Azilect 3383

IMPORTANT NOTE: Always consult each drug listing in the patient's regimen for possible interactions.

EpiPen Interactions Index 594

Selegiline (The effects of epinephrine may be potentiated by monoamine oxidase inhibitors). Products include:
Emsam 3623

Selegiline Hydrochloride (The effects of epinephrine may be potentiated by monoamine oxidase inhibitors). Products include:
Eldepryl 3312

Sotalol Hydrochloride (Epinephrine should be used with caution in patients who have cardiac arrhythmias, coronary artery or organic heart disease, hypertension, or in patients who are on drugs that may sensitize the heart to arrhythmias, eg, anti-arrhythmics. In such patients, epinephrine may precipitate or aggravate angina pectoris as well as produce ventricular arrhythmias).
No products indexed under this heading.

Spironolactone (Patients who receive epinephrine while concomitantly taking diuretics should be carefully observed for the development of cardiac arrhythmias. Epinephrine should be used with caution in patients who have cardiac arrhythmias, coronary artery or organic heart disease, hypertension, or in patients who are on drugs that may sensitize the heart to arrhythmias, eg, diuretics. In such patients, epinephrine may precipitate or aggravate angina pectoris as well as produce ventricular arrhythmias).
No products indexed under this heading.

Tamsulosin Hydrochloride (The vasoconstricting and hypertensive effects of epinephrine are antagonized by α-adrenergic blocking drugs, such as phentolamine).
No products indexed under this heading.

Terazosin Hydrochloride (The vasoconstricting and hypertensive effects of epinephrine are antagonized by α-adrenergic blocking drugs, such as phentolamine).
No products indexed under this heading.

Terfenadine (The effects of epinephrine may be potentiated by certain antihistamines, notably chlorpheniramine, tripelennamine, and diphenhydramine).
No products indexed under this heading.

Timolol Hemihydrate (The cardiostimulating and bronchodilating effects of epinephrine are antagonized by β-adrenergic blocking drugs, such as propranolol). Products include:
Betimol 3490

Timolol Maleate (The cardiostimulating and bronchodilating effects of epinephrine are antagonized by β-adrenergic blocking drugs, such as propranolol). Products include:
Combigan 601
Dorzolamide Hydrochloride/Timolol Maleate Ophthalmic Solution .... ⊙243
Timoptic in Ocudose .... ⊙231

Tocainide Hydrochloride (Epinephrine should be used with caution in patients who have cardiac arrhythmias, coronary artery or organic heart disease, hypertension, or in patients who are on drugs that may sensitize the heart to arrhythmias, eg, anti-arrhythmics. In such patients, epinephrine may precipitate or aggravate angina pectoris as well as produce ventricular arrhythmias).
No products indexed under this heading.

Torsemide (Patients who receive epinephrine while concomitantly taking diuretics should be carefully observed for the development of cardiac arrhythmias. Epinephrine should be used with caution in patients who have cardiac arrhythmias, coronary artery or organic heart disease, hypertension, or in patients who are on drugs that may sensitize the heart to arrhythmias, eg, diuretics. In such patients, epinephrine may precipitate or aggravate angina pectoris as well as produce ventricular arrhythmias).
No products indexed under this heading.

Tranylcypromine Sulfate (The effects of epinephrine may be potentiated by monoamine oxidase inhibitors). Products include:
Parnate 1584

Triamterene (Patients who receive epinephrine while concomitantly taking diuretics should be carefully observed for the development of cardiac arrhythmias. Epinephrine should be used with caution in patients who have cardiac arrhythmias, coronary artery or organic heart disease, hypertension, or in patients who are on drugs that may sensitize the heart to arrhythmias, eg, diuretics. In such patients, epinephrine may precipitate or aggravate angina pectoris as well as produce ventricular arrhythmias). Products include:
Dyazide 1429
Dyrenium 3495

Trimeprazine Tartrate (The effects of epinephrine may be potentiated by certain antihistamines, notably chlorpheniramine, tripelennamine, and diphenhydramine).
No products indexed under this heading.

Trimipramine Maleate (The effects of epinephrine may be potentiated by tricyclic antidepressants).
No products indexed under this heading.

Tripelennamine Hydrochloride (The effects of epinephrine may be potentiated by certain antihistamines, notably tripelennamine).
No products indexed under this heading.

Triprolidine Hydrochloride (The effects of epinephrine may be potentiated by certain antihistamines, notably chlorpheniramine, tripelennamine, and diphenhydramine).
No products indexed under this heading.

Verapamil Hydrochloride (Epinephrine should be used with caution in patients who have cardiac arrhythmias, coronary artery or organic heart disease, hypertension, or in patients who are on drugs that may sensitize the heart to arrhythmias, eg, anti-arrhythmics. In such patients, epinephrine may precipitate or aggravate angina pectoris as well as produce ventricular arrhythmias). Products include:
Tarka 534

EPIPEN JR. AUTO-INJECTOR

(Epinephrine) 3631
See EpiPen Auto-Injector

EPIVIR ORAL SOLUTION

(Lamivudine) 1437
See Epivir Tablets

EPIVIR TABLETS

(Lamivudine) 1437
May interact with cationic drugs that are eliminated by renal tubular, interferon alpha, and certain other agents. Compounds in these categories include:

Abacavir Sulfate (Lamivudine should not be administered concomitantly with other lamivudine-containing products including Epzicom (abacavir sulfate and lamivudine), or Trizvir (abacavir sulfate, lamivudine, and zidovudine)). Products include:
Epzicom 1448
Trizivir 1688
Ziagen 1740

Amiloride Hydrochloride (Lamivudine is predominantly eliminated in the urine by active organic cationic secretion. The possibility of interactions with other drugs administered concurrently should be considered, particularly when their main route of elimination is active renal secretion via the organic cationic transport system).
No products indexed under this heading.

Digoxin (Lamivudine is predominantly eliminated in the urine by active organic cationic secretion. The possibility of interactions with other drugs administered concurrently should be considered, particularly when their main route of elimination is active renal secretion via the organic cationic transport system). Products include:
Lanoxin Injection 1546
Lanoxin Injection Pediatric 1549
Lanoxin Tablets 1553

Efavirenz (Lamivudine should not be administered concomitantly with emtricitabine-containing products, including Atripla (efavirenz, emtricitabine, and tenofovir)). Products include:
Atripla 906

Emtricitabine (Lamivudine should not be administered concomitanty with emtricitabine-containing products, including Atripla (efavirenz, emtricitabine, and tenofovir), Emtriva (emtricitabine), or Truvada (emtricitabine and tenofovir)). Products include:
Atripla 906
Emtriva 1238
Emtriva Oral Solution 1238
Truvada 1258

Interferon alfa-2a, Recombinant (Hepatic decompensation (some fatal) has occurred in HIV-1/HCV co-infected patients receiving interferon and ribavirin-based regimens. Monitor for treatment-associated toxicities. Discontinue lamivudine as medically appropriate and consider dose reduction or discontinuation of interferon alfa, ribavirin, or both).
No products indexed under this heading.

Interferon alfa-2b, Recombinant (Hepatic decompensation (some fatal) has occurred in HIV-1/HCV co-infected patients receiving interferon and ribavirin-based regimens. Monitor for treatment-associated toxicities. Discontinue lamivudine as medically appropriate and consider dose reduction or discontinuation of interferon alfa, ribavirin, or both). Products include:
Intron A 3140

Interferon alfa-N3 (Human Leukocyte Derived) (Hepatic decompensation (some fatal) has occurred in HIV-1/HCV co-infected patients receiving interferon and ribavirin-based regimens. Monitor for treatment-associated toxicities. Discontinue lamivudine as medically appropriate and consider dose reduction or discontinuation of interferon alfa, ribavirin, or both). Products include:
Alferon N 1801

Morphine Sulfate (Lamivudine is predominantly eliminated in the urine by active organic cationic secretion. The possibility of interactions with other drugs administered concurrently should be considered, particularly when their main route of elimination is active renal secretion via the organic cationic transport system). Products include:
Avinza 1822
Embeda 1831
MS Contin 2803

Peginterferon Alfa-2b (Hepatic decompensation (some fatal) has occurred in HIV-1/HCV co-infected patients receiving interferon and ribavirin-based regimens. Monitor for treatment-associated toxicities. Discontinue lamivudine as medically appropriate and consider dose reduction or discontinuation of interferon alfa, ribavirin, or both). Products include:
PegIntron 3188

Procainamide Hydrochloride (Lamivudine is predominantly eliminated in the urine by active organic cationic secretion. The possibility of interactions with other drugs administered concurrently should be considered, particularly when their main route of elimination is active renal secretion via the organic cationic transport system).
No products indexed under this heading.

Quinidine Gluconate (Lamivudine is predominantly eliminated in the urine by active organic cationic secretion. The possibility of interactions with other drugs administered concurrently should be considered, particularly when their main route of elimination is active renal secretion via the organic cationic transport system).
No products indexed under this heading.

Quinidine Polygalacturonate (Lamivudine is predominantly eliminated in the urine by active organic cationic secretion. The possibility of interactions with other drugs administered concurrently should be considered, particularly when their main route of elimination is active renal secretion via the organic cationic transport system).
No products indexed under this heading.

Quinidine Sulfate (Lamivudine is predominantly eliminated in the urine by active organic cationic secretion. The possibility of interactions with other drugs administered concurrently should be considered, particularly when their main route of elimination is active renal secretion via the organic cationic transport system).
No products indexed under this heading.

Quinine Sulfate (Lamivudine is predominantly eliminated in the urine by active organic cationic secretion. The possibility of interactions with other drugs administered concurrently should be considered, particularly when their main route of elimination is active renal secretion via the organic cationic transport system).
No products indexed under this heading.

Ranitidine Hydrochloride (Lamivudine is predominantly eliminated in the urine by active organic cationic secretion. The possibility of interactions with other drugs administered concurrently should be considered, particularly when their main route of elimination is active renal secretion via the organic cationic transport system). Products include:
Zantac 1737
Zantac Injection 1732
Zantac Pharmacy 1735

Ribavirin (*In vitro* data indicate ribavirin reduces phosphorylation of lamivudine. Hepatic decompensation (some fatal) has occurred in HIV-1/HCV co-infected patients receiving interferon and ribavirin-based regimens. Monitor for treatment-associated toxicities. Discontinue lamivudine as medically appropriate and consider dose reduction or discontinuation of interferon alfa, ribavirin, or both). Products include:
Rebetol 3207

Sulfamethoxazole (Co-administration of trimethoprim/sulfamethoxazole with lamivudine resulted in an increase of 43% ± 23% (mean ± SD) in lamivudine $AUC_{infinity}$, a decrease of 29% ± 13% in lamivudine oral clearance, and a decrease of 30% ± 36% in lamivudine renal clearance).
No products indexed under this heading.

Tenofovir Disoproxil Fumarate (Lamivudine should not be administered concomitanty with emtricitabine-containing products, including Atripla

(⊙ Described in PDR® for Ophthalmic Medicines)

(efavirenz, emtricitabine, and tenofovir), or Truvada (emtricitabine and tenofovir)). Products include:
- Atripla 906
- Truvada 1258
- Viread 1266

Triamterene (Lamivudine is predominantly eliminated in the urine by active organic cationic secretion. The possibility of interactions with other drugs administered concurrently should be considered, particularly when their main route of elimination is active renal secretion via the organic cationic transport system). Products include:
- Dyazide 1429
- Dyrenium 3495

Trimethoprim (Lamivudine is predominantly eliminated in the urine by active organic cationic secretion. The possibility of interactions with other drugs administered concurrently should be considered, particularly when their main route of elimination is active renal secretion via the organic cationic transport system (eg, trimethoprim). Co-administration of trimethoprim/sulfamethoxazole with lamivudine resulted in an increase of 43% ± 23% (mean ± SD) in lamivudine $AUC_{infinity}$, a decrease of 29% ± 13% in lamivudine oral clearance, and a decrease of 30% ± 36% in lamivudine renal clearance).
No products indexed under this heading.

Trimethoprim Hydrochloride (Lamivudine is predominantly eliminated in the urine by active organic cationic secretion. The possibility of interactions with other drugs administered concurrently should be considered, particularly when their main route of elimination is active renal secretion via the organic cationic transport system (eg, trimethoprim). Co-administration of trimethoprim/sulfamethoxazole with lamivudine resulted in an increase of 43% ± 23% (mean ± SD) in lamivudine $AUC_{infinity}$, a decrease of 29% ± 13% in lamivudine oral clearance, and a decrease of 30% ± 36% in lamivudine renal clearance).
No products indexed under this heading.

Trimethoprim Sulfate (Lamivudine is predominantly eliminated in the urine by active organic cationic secretion. The possibility of interactions with other drugs administered concurrently should be considered, particularly when their main route of elimination is active renal secretion via the organic cationic transport system (eg, trimethoprim). Co-administration of trimethoprim/sulfamethoxazole with lamivudine resulted in an increase of 43% ± 23% (mean ± SD) in lamivudine $AUC_{infinity}$, a decrease of 29% ± 13% in lamivudine oral clearance, and a decrease of 30% ± 36% in lamivudine renal clearance).
No products indexed under this heading.

Vancomycin Hydrochloride (Lamivudine is predominantly eliminated in the urine by active organic cationic secretion. The possibility of interactions with other drugs administered concurrently should be considered, particularly when their main route of elimination is active renal secretion via the organic cationic transport system).
No products indexed under this heading.

Zalcitabine (Lamivudine and zalcitabine may inhibit the intracellular phosphorylation of one another. Therefore, use of lamivudine in combination with zalcitabine is not recommended).
No products indexed under this heading.

Zidovudine (Lamivudine should not be administered concomitantly with other lamivudine-containing products including Combivir (lamivudine/zidovudine) and Trizivir (abacavir sulfate, lamivudine, and zidovudine)). Products include:
- Combivir 1404
- Retrovir 1634
- Retrovir IV 1640
- Trizivir 1688

Food Interactions

Food, unspecified (Absorption of lamivudine was slower in the fed state (T_{max}: 3.2 ± 1.3 hours) compared with the fasted state (T_{max}: 0.9 ± 0.3 hours); C_{max} in the fed state was 40% ± 23% (mean ± SD) lower than in the fasted state. There was no significant difference in systemic exposure ($AUC_{infinity}$) in the fed and fasted states; therefore, lamivudine may be administered with or without food).

Meal, unspecified (Absorption of lamivudine was slower in the fed state (T_{max}: 3.2 ± 1.3 hours) compared with the fasted state (T_{max}: 0.9 ± 0.3 hours); C_{max} in the fed state was 40% ± 23% (mean ± SD) lower than in the fasted state. There was no significant difference in systemic exposure ($AUC_{infinity}$) in the fed and fasted states; therefore, lamivudine may be administered with or without food).

EPIVIR-HBV ORAL SOLUTION

(Lamivudine) 1443
See Epivir-HBV Tablets

EPIVIR-HBV TABLETS

(Lamivudine) 1443
May interact with cationic drugs that are eliminated by renal tubular, and certain other agents. Compounds in these categories include:

Amiloride Hydrochloride (Lamivudine is predominantly eliminated in the urine by active organic secretion; therefore, the possibility of interactions with other drugs whose main route of elimination is active renal secretion via the organic cationic transport system should be considered).
No products indexed under this heading.

Digoxin (Lamivudine is predominantly eliminated in the urine by active organic secretion; therefore, the possibility of interactions with other drugs whose main route of elimination is active renal secretion via the organic cationic transport system should be considered). Products include:
- Lanoxin Injection 1546
- Lanoxin Injection Pediatric 1549
- Lanoxin Tablets 1553

Morphine Sulfate (Lamivudine is predominantly eliminated in the urine by active organic secretion; therefore, the possibility of interactions with other drugs whose main route of elimination is active renal secretion via the organic cationic transport system should be considered). Products include:
- Avinza 1822
- Embeda 1831
- MS Contin 2803

Procainamide Hydrochloride (Lamivudine is predominantly eliminated in the urine by active organic secretion; therefore, the possibility of interactions with other drugs whose main route of elimination is active renal secretion via the organic cationic transport system should be considered).
No products indexed under this heading.

Quinidine Gluconate (Lamivudine is predominantly eliminated in the urine by active organic secretion; therefore, the possibility of interactions with other drugs whose main route of elimination is active renal secretion via the organic cationic transport system should be considered).
No products indexed under this heading.

Quinidine Polygalacturonate (Lamivudine is predominantly eliminated in the urine by active organic secretion; therefore, the possibility of interactions with other drugs whose main route of elimination is active renal secretion via the organic cationic transport system should be considered).
No products indexed under this heading.

Quinidine Sulfate (Lamivudine is predominantly eliminated in the urine by active organic secretion; therefore, the possibility of interactions with other drugs whose main route of elimination is active renal secretion via the organic cationic transport system should be considered).
No products indexed under this heading.

Quinine Sulfate (Lamivudine is predominantly eliminated in the urine by active organic secretion; therefore, the possibility of interactions with other drugs whose main route of elimination is active renal secretion via the organic cationic transport system should be considered).
No products indexed under this heading.

Ranitidine Hydrochloride (Lamivudine is predominantly eliminated in the urine by active organic secretion; therefore, the possibility of interactions with other drugs whose main route of elimination is active renal secretion via the organic cationic transport system should be considered). Products include:
- Zantac 1737
- Zantac Injection 1732
- Zantac Pharmacy 1735

Sulfamethoxazole (Co-administration of lamivudine with 160 mg of trimethoprim and 800 mg of sulfamethoxazole once daily has been shown to increase lamivudine exposure (AUC); the effect of higher doses of TMP/SMX on lamivudine pharmacokinetics has not been investigated; no change in dose of either drug is recommended).
No products indexed under this heading.

Triamterene (Lamivudine is predominantly eliminated in the urine by active organic secretion; therefore, the possibility of interactions with other drugs whose main route of elimination is active renal secretion via the organic cationic transport system should be considered). Products include:
- Dyazide 1429
- Dyrenium 3495

Trimethoprim (Co-administration of lamivudine with 160 mg of trimethoprim and 800 mg of sulfamethoxazole once daily has been shown to increase lamivudine exposure (AUC); the effect of higher doses of TMP/SMX on lamivudine pharmacokinetics has not been investigated; no change in dose of either drug is recommended).
No products indexed under this heading.

Trimethoprim Sulfate (Lamivudine is predominantly eliminated in the urine by active organic secretion; therefore, the possibility of interactions with other drugs whose main route of elimination is active renal secretion via the organic cationic transport system should be considered).
No products indexed under this heading.

Vancomycin Hydrochloride (Lamivudine is predominantly eliminated in the urine by active organic secretion; therefore, the possibility of interactions with other drugs whose main route of elimination is active renal secretion via the organic cationic transport system should be considered).
No products indexed under this heading.

Zalacitabine (Lamivudine and zalcitabine may inhibit the intracellular phosphorylation of one another; co-administration is not recommended).
No products indexed under this heading.

EPOGEN FOR INJECTION

(Epoetin Alfa) 621
None cited in PDR database.

EPZICOM TABLETS

(Abacavir Sulfate, Lamivudine) 1448
May interact with interferon alpha, and certain other agents. Compounds in these categories include:

Ethanol (Ethanol decreased the elimination of abacavir causing an increase in overall exposure. Co-administration of abacavir with ethanol has been shown to increase the AUC of abacavir by 41%).
No products indexed under this heading.

Interferon alfa-2a, Recombinant (Hepatic decompensation has occurred in HIV/HCV co-infected patients receiving combination antiretroviral therapy for HIV and interferon alpha with or without ribavirin. Patients receiving interferon alpha with or without ribavirin and Epzicom should be closely monitored for treatment-associated toxicities, especially hepatic decompensation. Discontinuation of Epzicom should be considered as medically appropriate. Discontinuation of interferon alpha, ribavirin, or both should also be considered if worsening clinical toxicities are observed, including hepatic decompensation (eg, Childs Pugh> 6)).
No products indexed under this heading.

Interferon alfa-2b, Recombinant (Hepatic decompensation has occurred in HIV/HCV co-infected patients receiving combination antiretroviral therapy for HIV and interferon alpha with or without ribavirin. Patients receiving interferon alpha with or without ribavirin and Epzicom should be closely monitored for treatment-associated toxicities, especially hepatic decompensation. Discontinuation of Epzicom should be considered as medically appropriate. Discontinuation of interferon alpha, ribavirin, or both should also be considered if worsening clinical toxicities are observed, including hepatic decompensation (eg, Childs Pugh> 6)). Products include:
- Intron A 3140

Interferon alfa-N3 (Human Leukocyte Derived) (Hepatic decompensation has occurred in HIV/HCV co-infected patients receiving combination antiretroviral therapy for HIV and interferon alpha with or without ribavirin. Patients receiving interferon alpha with or without ribavirin and Epzicom should be closely monitored for treatment-associated toxicities, especially hepatic decompensation. Discontinuation of Epzicom should be considered as medically appropriate. Discontinuation of interferon alpha, ribavirin, or both should also be considered if worsening clinical toxicities are observed, including hepatic decompensation (eg, Childs Pugh> 6)). Products include:
- Alferon N 1801

Methadone Hydrochloride (The addition of methadone has no clinically significant effect on the pharmacokinetic properties of abacavir. A study of 11 HIV-infected patients receiving methadone-maintenance therapy (40 mg and 90 mg daily), 600 mg of Ziagen twice daily (twice the currently recommended dose), oral methadone clearance increased 22% (90% CI 6% to 42%). This alteration will not result in a methadone dose modification in the majority of patients; however, an increased methadone dose may be required in a small number of patients).
No products indexed under this heading.

IMPORTANT NOTE: Always consult each drug listing in the patient's regimen for possible interactions.

Epzicom
Interactions Index
596

Nelfinavir Mesylate (Co-administration of lamivudine with nelfinavir has been shown to increase the AUC of lamivudine by 10%).
No products indexed under this heading.

Peginterferon Alfa-2b (Hepatic decompensation has occurred in HIV/HCV co-infected patients receiving combination antiretroviral therapy for HIV and interferon alpha with or without ribavirin. Patients receiving interferon alpha with or without ribavirin and Epzicom should be closely monitored for treatment-associated toxicities, especially hepatic decompensation. Discontinuation of Epzicom should be considered as medically appropriate. Discontinuation of interferon alpha, ribavirin, or both should also be considered if worsening clinical toxicities are observed, including hepatic decompensation (eg, Childs Pugh> 6)). Products include:
PegIntron 3188

Sulfamethoxazole (Co-administration of lamivudine with 160 mg of trimethoprim and 800 mg of sulfamethoxazole once daily has been shown to increase AUC of lamivudine by 43%. The effect of higher doses of TMP/SMX on lamivudine pharmacokinetics has not been investigated; no change in dose of either drug is recommended).
No products indexed under this heading.

Trimethoprim (Co-administration of lamivudine with 160 mg of trimethoprim and 800 mg of sulfamethoxazole once daily has been shown to increase AUC of lamivudine by 43%. The effect of higher doses of TMP/SMX on lamivudine pharmacokinetics has not been investigated; no change in dose of either drug is recommended).
No products indexed under this heading.

Zalcitabine (Lamivudine and zalcitabine may inhibit the intracellular phosphorylation of one another; concurrent use is not recommended).
No products indexed under this heading.

EQUETRO EXTENDED-RELEASE CAPSULES

(Carbamazepine) 3477
May interact with alcohols, antimalarials, azole antifungals, centrally-acting drugs, cytochrome p450 1a2 substrates (selected), cytochrome p450 3a4 inducers (selected), cytochrome p450 3a4 inhibitors (selected), cytochrome p450 3a4 substrates (selected), erythromycin, glucocorticoids, haloperidols, lithium preparations, monoamine oxidase inhibitors, Non-nucleoside reverse transcriptase inhibitors, oral contraceptives, phenytoin, protease inhibitors, psychotropics, theophyllines, tricyclic antidepressants, valproate, and certain other agents. Compounds in these categories include:

Acetaminophen (Carbamazepine is known to induce CYP1A2 and CYP3A4. Therefore, the potential exists for interaction between carbamazepine and any agent metabolized by one (or more) of these enzymes. Agents that are metabolized by CYP1A2 and CYP3A4, such as acetaminophen, may have decreased plasma levels when administered concomitantly with carbamazepine).
Products include:
Percocet 1121
Tylenol 2049
Tylenol 8 Hour 2049
Extra Strength Tylenol Caplets, Cool Caplets, and EZ Tabs 2049
Extra Strength Tylenol Adult Rapid Blast Liquid 2049
Extra Strength Tylenol Rapid Release 2049
Tylenol with Codeine 2691
Tylenol Arthritis Pain Extended Release Geltabs/Caplets 2049
Children's Tylenol Suspension Liquid 2048
Children's Tylenol Meltaways 2048
Tylenol, Infants' Drops 2048
Junior Tylenol 2048
Vicodin 560
Vicodin ES 561
Vicodin HP 563
Zydone 1138

Acetazolamide (Carbamazepine is metabolized mainly by CYP3A4 the active carbamazepine 10,11-epoxide, which is further metabolized to the trans-diol by epoxide hydrolase. Therefore, the potential exists for interaction between carbamazepine and any agent that inhibits CYP3A4 and/or epoxide hydrolase. Agents that are CYP3A4 inhibitors may increase the plasma levels of carbamazepine).
No products indexed under this heading.

Acetazolamide Sodium (Carbamazepine is metabolized mainly by CYP3A4 the active carbamazepine 10,11-epoxide, which is further metabolized to the trans-diol by epoxide hydrolase. Therefore, the potential exists for interaction between carbamazepine and any agent that inhibits CYP3A4 and/or epoxide hydrolase. Agents that are CYP3A4 inhibitors may increase the plasma levels of carbamazepine).
No products indexed under this heading.

Alatrofloxacin Mesylate (Carbamazepine is known to induce CYP1A2 and CYP3A4. Therefore, the potential exists for interaction between carbamazepine and any agent metabolized by one (or more) of these enzymes. Agents that are metabolized by CYP1A2 and CYP3A4 may have decreased plasma levels when administered concomitantly with carbamazepine).
No products indexed under this heading.

Alfentanil Hydrochloride (Because of its primary CNS effect, caution should be used when carbamazepine is taken with other centrally acting drugs).
No products indexed under this heading.

Allium sativum (Carbamazepine is metabolized by CYP3A4. Therefore, the potential exists for interaction between carbamazepine and any agent that induces CYP3A4. Agents that are CYP3A4 inducers may decrease plasma levels of carbamazepine).
No products indexed under this heading.

Alprazolam (Because of its primary CNS effect, caution should be used when carbamazepine is taken with other centrally acting drugs).
No products indexed under this heading.

Aminoglutethimide (Carbamazepine is metabolized by CYP3A4. Therefore, the potential exists for interaction between carbamazepine and any agent that induces CYP3A4. Agents that are CYP3A4 inducers may decrease plasma levels of carbamazepine).
No products indexed under this heading.

Aminophylline (Carbamazepine is known to induce CYP1A2 and CYP3A4. Therefore, the potential exists for interaction between carbamazepine and any agent metabolized by one (or more) of these enzymes. Agents that are metabolized by CYP1A2 and CYP3A4 may have decreased plasma levels when administered concomitantly with carbamazepine).
No products indexed under this heading.

Amiodarone Hydrochloride (Carbamazepine is known to induce CYP1A2 and CYP3A4. Therefore, the potential exists for interaction between carbamazepine and any agent metabolized by one (or more) of these enzymes. Agents that are metabolized by CYP1A2 and CYP3A4 may have decreased plasma levels when administered concomitantly with carbamazepine).
No products indexed under this heading.

Amitriptyline Hydrochloride (Carbamazepine is contraindicated in patients with a known sensitivity to any of the tricyclic compounds, such as amitriptyline, desipramine, imipramine, protriptyline, and nortriptyline).
No products indexed under this heading.

Amlodipine Besylate (Carbamazepine is known to induce CYP1A2 and CYP3A4. Therefore, the potential exists for interaction between carbamazepine and any agent metabolized by one (or more) of these enzymes. Agents that are metabolized by CYP1A2 and CYP3A4 may have decreased plasma levels when administered concomitantly with carbamazepine). Products include:
Azor 1010
Exforge 2443
Exforge HCT 2449

Amoxapine (Carbamazepine is contraindicated in patients with a known sensitivity to any of the tricyclic compounds, such as amitriptyline, desipramine, imipramine, protriptyline, and nortriptyline).
No products indexed under this heading.

Amphetamine Aspartate (Because of its primary CNS effect, caution should be used when carbamazepine is taken with other centrally acting drugs).
No products indexed under this heading.

Amphetamine Aspartate Monohydrate (Because of its primary CNS effect, caution should be used when carbamazepine is taken with other centrally acting drugs).
No products indexed under this heading.

Amphetamine Resins (Because of its primary CNS effect, caution should be used when carbamazepine is taken with other centrally acting drugs).
No products indexed under this heading.

Amphetamine Sulfate (Because of its primary CNS effect, caution should be used when carbamazepine is taken with other centrally acting drugs).
No products indexed under this heading.

Amprenavir (Carbamazepine is metabolized mainly by CYP3A4 the active carbamazepine 10,11-epoxide, which is further metabolized to the trans-diol by epoxide hydrolase. Therefore, the potential exists for interaction between carbamazepine and any agent that inhibits CYP3A4 and/or epoxide hydrolase. Agents that are CYP3A4 inhibitors, such as protease inhibitors, may increase the plasma levels of carbamazepine).
No products indexed under this heading.

Anagrelide Hydrochloride (Carbamazepine is known to induce CYP1A2 and CYP3A4. Therefore, the potential exists for interaction between carbamazepine and any agent metabolized by one (or more) of these enzymes. Agents that are metabolized by CYP1A2 and CYP3A4 may have decreased plasma levels when administered concomitantly with carbamazepine).
No products indexed under this heading.

Anastrozole (Carbamazepine is metabolized mainly by CYP3A4 the active carbamazepine 10,11-epoxide, which is further metabolized to the trans-diol by epoxide hydrolase. Therefore, the potential exists for interaction between carbamazepine and any agent that inhibits CYP3A4 and/or epoxide hydrolase. Agents that are CYP3A4 inhibitors may increase the plasma levels of carbamazepine).
No products indexed under this heading.

Aprepitant (Carbamazepine is metabolized by CYP3A4. Therefore, the potential exists for interaction between carbamazepine and any agent that induces CYP3A4. Agents that are CYP3A4 inducers may decrease plasma levels of carbamazepine). Products include:
Emend 2124

Aprobarbital (Because of its primary CNS effect, caution should be used when carbamazepine is taken with other centrally acting drugs).
No products indexed under this heading.

Astemizole (Carbamazepine is known to induce CYP1A2 and CYP3A4. Therefore, the potential exists for interaction between carbamazepine and any agent metabolized by one (or more) of these enzymes. Agents that are metabolized by CYP1A2 and CYP3A4 may have decreased plasma levels when administered concomitantly with carbamazepine).
No products indexed under this heading.

Atazanavir (Carbamazepine is metabolized mainly by CYP3A4 the active carbamazepine 10,11-epoxide, which is further metabolized to the trans-diol by epoxide hydrolase. Therefore, the potential exists for interaction between carbamazepine and any agent that inhibits CYP3A4 and/or epoxide hydrolase. Agents that are CYP3A4 inhibitors, such as protease inhibitors, may increase the plasma levels of carbamazepine).
No products indexed under this heading.

Atazanavir Sulfate (Carbamazepine is metabolized mainly by CYP3A4 the active carbamazepine 10,11-epoxide, which is further metabolized to the trans-diol by epoxide hydrolase. Therefore, the potential exists for interaction between carbamazepine and any agent that inhibits CYP3A4 and/or epoxide hydrolase. Agents that are CYP3A4 inhibitors, such as protease inhibitors, may increase the plasma levels of carbamazepine).
No products indexed under this heading.

Atorvastatin Calcium (Carbamazepine is known to induce CYP1A2 and CYP3A4. Therefore, the potential exists for interaction between carbamazepine and any agent metabolized by one (or more) of these enzymes. Agents that are metabolized by CYP1A2 and CYP3A4 may have decreased plasma levels when administered concomitantly with carbamazepine). Products include:
Lipitor 2703

Belladonna Ergotamine (Carbamazepine is known to induce CYP1A2 and CYP3A4. Therefore, the potential exists for interaction between carbamazepine and any agent metabolized by one (or more) of these enzymes. Agents that are metabolized by CYP1A2 and CYP3A4 may have decreased plasma levels when administered concomitantly with carbamazepine).
No products indexed under this heading.

Betamethasone (Carbamazepine is metabolized by CYP3A4. Therefore, the potential exists for interaction between carbamazepine and any agent that induces CYP3A4. Agents that are CYP3A4 inducers may decrease plasma levels of carbamazepine).
No products indexed under this heading.

Betamethasone Acetate (Carbamazepine is known to induce CYP1A2 and CYP3A4. Therefore, the potential exists for interaction between carbamazepine and any agent metabolized by one (or more) of these enzymes. Agents that are metabolized by CYP1A2 and CYP3A4, such as glucocorticoids, may have decreased plasma levels when administered concomitantly with carbamazepine).
No products indexed under this heading.

Betamethasone Benzoate (Carbamazepine is metabolized by CYP3A4. Therefore, the potential exists for interaction between carbamazepine and any agent that induces CYP3A4. Agents that are CYP3A4 inducers may decrease plasma levels of carbamazepine).
No products indexed under this heading.

Betamethasone Dipropionate (Carbamazepine is metabolized by CYP3A4. Therefore, the potential exists for interaction between carbamazepine and any agent that induces CYP3A4. Agents that are CYP3A4 inducers may decrease plasma levels of carbamazepine).
Products include:

Betamethasone Sodium Phosphate (Carbamazepine is known to induce CYP1A2 and CYP3A4. Therefore, the potential exists for interaction between carbamazepine and any agent metabolized by one (or more) of these enzymes. Agents that are metabolized by CYP1A2 and CYP3A4, such as glucocorticoids, may have decreased plasma levels when administered concomitantly with carbamazepine).
No products indexed under this heading.

Betamethasone Valerate (Carbamazepine is metabolized by CYP3A4. Therefore, the potential exists for interaction between carbamazepine and any agent that induces CYP3A4. Agents that are CYP3A4 inducers may decrease plasma levels of carbamazepine).
Products include:

Bosentan (Carbamazepine is metabolized by CYP3A4. Therefore, the potential exists for interaction between carbamazepine and any agent that induces CYP3A4. Agents that are CYP3A4 inducers may decrease plasma levels of carbamazepine). Products include:

Budesonide (Carbamazepine is known to induce CYP1A2 and CYP3A4. Therefore, the potential exists for interaction between carbamazepine and any agent metabolized by one (or more) of these enzymes. Agents that are metabolized by CYP1A2 and CYP3A4, such as glucocorticoids, may have decreased plasma levels when administered concomitantly with carbamazepine). Products include:

Buprenorphine Hydrochloride (Because of its primary CNS effect, caution should be used when carbamazepine is taken with other centrally acting drugs).
No products indexed under this heading.

Buspirone Hydrochloride (Because of its primary CNS effect, caution should be used when carbamazepine is taken with other centrally acting drugs).
No products indexed under this heading.

Busulfan (Carbamazepine is known to induce CYP1A2 and CYP3A4. Therefore, the potential exists for interaction between carbamazepine and any agent metabolized by one (or more) of these enzymes. Agents that are metabolized by CYP1A2 and CYP3A4 may have decreased plasma levels when administered concomitantly with carbamazepine). Products include:

Butabarbital (Because of its primary CNS effect, caution should be used when carbamazepine is taken with other centrally acting drugs).
No products indexed under this heading.

Butalbital (Because of its primary CNS effect, caution should be used when carbamazepine is taken with other centrally acting drugs).
No products indexed under this heading.

Butoconazole Nitrate (Carbamazepine is metabolized mainly by CYP3A4 the active carbamazepine 10,11-epoxide, which is futher metabolized to the trans-diol by epoxide hydrolase. Therefore, the potential exists for

interaction between carbamazepine and any agent that inhibits CYP3A4 and/or epoxide hydrolase. Agents that are CYP3A4 inhibitors, such as azole antifungals, may increase the plasma levels of carbamazepine).
No products indexed under this heading.

Caffeine (Carbamazepine is known to induce CYP1A2 and CYP3A4. Therefore, the potential exists for interaction between carbamazepine and any agent metabolized by one (or more) of these enzymes. Agents that are metabolized by CYP1A2 and CYP3A4 may have decreased plasma levels when administered concomitantly with carbamazepine).
No products indexed under this heading.

Caffeine Anhydrous (Carbamazepine is known to induce CYP1A2 and CYP3A4. Therefore, the potential exists for interaction between carbamazepine and any agent metabolized by one (or more) of these enzymes. Agents that are metabolized by CYP1A2 and CYP3A4 may have decreased plasma levels when administered concomitantly with carbamazepine).
No products indexed under this heading.

Caffeine Citrate (Carbamazepine is known to induce CYP1A2 and CYP3A4. Therefore, the potential exists for interaction between carbamazepine and any agent metabolized by one (or more) of these enzymes. Agents that are metabolized by CYP1A2 and CYP3A4 may have decreased plasma levels when administered concomitantly with carbamazepine).
No products indexed under this heading.

Caffeine-containing medications (Carbamazepine is known to induce CYP1A2 and CYP3A4. Therefore, the potential exists for interaction between carbamazepine and any agent metabolized by one (or more) of these enzymes. Agents that are metabolized by CYP1A2 and CYP3A4 may have decreased plasma levels when administered concomitantly with carbamazepine).
No products indexed under this heading.

Caffeine Sodium Benzoate (Carbamazepine is known to induce CYP1A2 and CYP3A4. Therefore, the potential exists for interaction between carbamazepine and any agent metabolized by one (or more) of these enzymes. Agents that are metabolized by CYP1A2 and CYP3A4 may have decreased plasma levels when administered concomitantly with carbamazepine).
No products indexed under this heading.

Cerivastatin Sodium (Carbamazepine is known to induce CYP1A2 and CYP3A4. Therefore, the potential exists for interaction between carbamazepine and any agent metabolized by one (or more) of these enzymes. Agents that are metabolized by CYP1A2 and CYP3A4 may have decreased plasma levels when administered concomitantly with carbamazepine).
No products indexed under this heading.

Chlordiazepoxide (Because of its primary CNS effect, caution should be used when carbamazepine is taken with other centrally acting drugs).
No products indexed under this heading.

Chlordiazepoxide Hydrochloride (Because of its primary CNS effect, caution should be used when carbamazepine is taken with other centrally acting drugs).
No products indexed under this heading.

Chloroquine (Anti-malarial drugs, such as chloroquine and mefloquine, may antagonize the activity of carbamazepine).
No products indexed under this heading.

Chloroquine Hydrochloride (Antimalarial drugs, such as chloroquine and mefloquine, may antagonize the activity of carbamazepine).
No products indexed under this heading.

Chloroquine Phosphate (Antimalarial drugs, such as chloroquine and mefloquine, may antagonize the activity of carbamazepine).
No products indexed under this heading.

Chlorpheniramine (Carbamazepine is known to induce CYP1A2 and CYP3A4. Therefore, the potential exists for interaction between carbamazepine and any agent metabolized by one (or more) of these enzymes. Agents that are metabolized by CYP1A2 and CYP3A4 may have decreased plasma levels when administered concomitantly with carbamazepine).
No products indexed under this heading.

Chlorpheniramine Maleate (Carbamazepine is known to induce CYP1A2 and CYP3A4. Therefore, the potential exists for interaction between carbamazepine and any agent metabolized by one (or more) of these enzymes. Agents that are metabolized by CYP1A2 and CYP3A4 may have decreased plasma levels when administered concomitantly with carbamazepine).
No products indexed under this heading.

Chlorpheniramine Polistirex (Carbamazepine is known to induce CYP1A2 and CYP3A4. Therefore, the potential exists for interaction between carbamazepine and any agent metabolized by one (or more) of these enzymes. Agents that are metabolized by CYP1A2 and CYP3A4 may have decreased plasma levels when administered concomitantly with carbamazepine). Products include:

Chlorpheniramine Tannate (Carbamazepine is known to induce CYP1A2 and CYP3A4. Therefore, the potential exists for interaction between carbamazepine and any agent metabolized by one (or more) of these enzymes. Agents that are metabolized by CYP1A2 and CYP3A4 may have decreased plasma levels when administered concomitantly with carbamazepine).
No products indexed under this heading.

Chlorpromazine (Because of its primary CNS effect, caution should be used when carbamazepine is taken with other centrally acting drugs).
No products indexed under this heading.

Chlorpromazine Hydrochloride (Because of its primary CNS effect, caution should be used when carbamazepine is taken with other centrally acting drugs).
No products indexed under this heading.

Chlorprothixene (Because of its primary CNS effect, caution should be used when carbamazepine is taken with other centrally acting drugs).
No products indexed under this heading.

Chlorprothixene Hydrochloride (Because of its primary CNS effect, caution should be used when carbamazepine is taken with other centrally acting drugs).
No products indexed under this heading.

Chlorprothixene Lactate (Because of its primary CNS effect, caution should be used when carbamazepine is taken with other centrally acting drugs).
No products indexed under this heading.

Cimetidine (Carbamazepine is metabolized mainly by CYP3A4 the active carbamazepine 10,11-epoxide, which is further metabolized to the trans-diol by epoxide hydrolase. Therefore, the potential exists for interaction between carbamazepine and any agent that inhibits CYP3A4 and/or epoxide hydrolase. Agents that are CYP3A4 inhibitors may increase the plasma levels of carbamazepine).
No products indexed under this heading.

Cimetidine Hydrochloride (Carbamazepine is known to induce CYP1A2 and CYP3A4. Therefore, the potential exists for interaction between carbamazepine and any agent metabolized by one (or more) of these enzymes. Agents that are metabolized by CYP1A2 and CYP3A4 may have decreased plasma levels when administered concomitantly with carbamazepine).
No products indexed under this heading.

Ciprofloxacin (Carbamazepine is metabolized by CYP3A4. Therefore, the potential exists for interaction between carbamazepine and any agent that induces CYP3A4. Agents that are CYP3A4 inducers may decrease plasma levels of carbamazepine). Products include:

Ciprofloxacin Hydrochloride (Carbamazepine is metabolized by CYP3A4. Therefore, the potential exists for interaction between carbamazepine and any agent that induces CYP3A4. Agents that are CYP3A4 inducers may decrease plasma levels of carbamazepine). Products include:

Cisapride (Carbamazepine is known to induce CYP1A2 and CYP3A4. Therefore, the potential exists for interaction between carbamazepine and any agent metabolized by one (or more) of these enzymes. Agents that are metabolized by CYP1A2 and CYP3A4 may have decreased plasma levels when administered concomitantly with carbamazepine).
No products indexed under this heading.

Cisplatin (Carbamazepine is metabolized by CYP3A4. Therefore, the potential exists for interaction between carbamazepine and any agent that induces CYP3A4. Agents that are CYP3A4 inducers may decrease plasma levels of carbamazepine).
No products indexed under this heading.

Clarithromycin (Carbamazepine is known to induce CYP1A2 and CYP3A4. Therefore, the potential exists for interaction between carbamazepine and any agent metabolized by one (or more) of these enzymes. Agents that are metabolized by CYP1A2 and CYP3A4 may have decreased plasma levels when administered concomitantly with carbamazepine). Products include:

Clomipramine Hydrochloride (Carbamazepine increases the plasma levels of clomipramine hydrochloride).
No products indexed under this heading.

Clopidogrel Bisulfate (Carbamazepine is known to induce CYP1A2 and CYP3A4. Therefore, the potential exists for interaction between carbamazepine and any agent metabolized by one (or more) of these enzymes. Agents that are metabolized by CYP1A2 and CYP3A4 may have decreased plasma levels when administered concomitantly with carbamazepine). Products include:

IMPORTANT NOTE: Always consult each drug listing in the patient's regimen for possible interactions.

(⊙ Described in PDR® for Ophthalmic Medicines)

Disulfiram (Carbamazepine is known to induce CYP1A2 and CYP3A4. Therefore, the potential exists for interaction between carbamazepine and any agent metabolized by one (or more) of these enzymes. Agents that are metabolized by CYP1A2 and CYP3A4 may have decreased plasma levels when administered concomitantly with carbamazepine).

No products indexed under this heading.

Divalproex Sodium (Carbamazepine is metabolized mainly by CYP3A4 the active carbamazepine 10,11-epoxide, which is further metabolized to the trans-diol by epoxide hydrolase. Therefore, the potential exists for interaction between carbamazepine and any agent that inhibits CYP3A4 and/or epoxide hydrolase. Agents that are CYP3A4 inhibitors, such as valproate, may increase the plasma levels of carbamazepine. Also inhibits epoxide hydroxylase, resulting in increased levels of the active metabolite carbamazepine-10,11-epoxide).

Products include:
Depakote ER 426

Doxepin Hydrochloride (Carbamazepine is contraindicated in patients with a known sensitivity to any of the tricyclic compounds, such as amitriptyline, desipramine, imipramine, protriptyline, and nortriptyline).

No products indexed under this heading.

Doxorubicin Hydrochloride (Carbamazepine is metabolized by CYP3A4. Therefore, the potential exists for interaction between carbamazepine and any agent that induces CYP3A4. Agents that are CYP3A4 inducers may decrease plasma levels of carbamazepine).

No products indexed under this heading.

Dronabinol (Carbamazepine is known to induce CYP1A2 and CYP3A4. Therefore, the potential exists for interaction between carbamazepine and any agent metabolized by one (or more) of these enzymes. Agents that are metabolized by CYP1A2 and CYP3A4 may have decreased plasma levels when administered concomitantly with carbamazepine).

No products indexed under this heading.

Droperidol (Because of its primary CNS effect, caution should be used when carbamazepine is taken with other centrally acting drugs).

No products indexed under this heading.

Econazole Nitrate (Carbamazepine is metabolized mainly by CYP3A4 the active carbamazepine 10,11-epoxide, which is futher metabolized to the trans-diol by epoxide hydrolase. Therefore, the potential exists for interaction between carbamazepine and any agent that inhibits CYP3A4 and/or epoxide hydrolase. Agents that are CYP3A4 inhibitors, such as azole antifungals, may increase the plasma levels of carbamazepine).

No products indexed under this heading.

Efavirenz (Co-administration of carbamazepine and delavirdine may lead to loss of virologic response and possible resistance to rescriptor or to the class of non-nucleoside reverse transcriptase inhibitors). Products include:
Atripla 906

Enflurane (Because of its primary CNS effect, caution should be used when carbamazepine is taken with other centrally acting drugs).

No products indexed under this heading.

Enoxacin (Carbamazepine is known to induce CYP1A2 and CYP3A4. Therefore, the potential exists for interaction between carbamazepine and any agent metabolized by one (or more) of these enzymes. Agents that are metabolized by CYP1A2 and CYP3A4 may have decreased plasma levels when administered concomitantly with carbamazepine).

No products indexed under this heading.

Ergotamine Tartrate (Carbamazepine is known to induce CYP1A2 and CYP3A4. Therefore, the potential exists for interaction between carbamazepine and any agent metabolized by one (or more) of these enzymes. Agents that are metabolized by CYP1A2 and CYP3A4 may have decreased plasma levels when administered concomitantly with carbamazepine).

No products indexed under this heading.

Erythromycin (Carbamazepine is metabolized mainly by CYP3A4 the active carbamazepine 10,11-epoxide, which is further metabolized to the trans-diol by epoxide hydrolase. Therefore, the potential exists for interaction between carbamazepine and any agent that inhibits CYP3A4 and/or epoxide hydrolase. Agents that are CYP3A4 inhibitors, such as erythromycin, may increase the plasma levels of carbamazepine. Also inhibits epoxide hydroxylase, resulting in increased levels of the active metabolite carbamazepine-10,11-epoxide).

No products indexed under this heading.

Erythromycin, Topical (Carbamazepine is metabolized mainly by CYP3A4 the active carbamazepine 10,11-epoxide, which is further metabolized to the trans-diol by epoxide hydrolase. Therefore, the potential exists for interaction between carbamazepine and any agent that inhibits CYP3A4 and/or epoxide hydrolase. Agents that are CYP3A4 inhibitors, such as erythromycin, may increase the plasma levels of carbamazepine. Also inhibits epoxide hydroxylase, resulting in increased levels of the active metabolite carbamazepine-10,11-epoxide).

No products indexed under this heading.

Erythromycin Estolate (Carbamazepine is metabolized mainly by CYP3A4 the active carbamazepine 10,11-epoxide, which is further metabolized to the trans-diol by epoxide hydrolase. Therefore, the potential exists for interaction between carbamazepine and any agent that inhibits CYP3A4 and/or epoxide hydrolase. Agents that are CYP3A4 inhibitors, such as erythromycin, may increase the plasma levels of carbamazepine. Also inhibits epoxide hydroxylase, resulting in increased levels of the active metabolite carbamazepine-10,11-epoxide).

No products indexed under this heading.

Erythromycin Ethylsuccinate (Carbamazepine is metabolized mainly by CYP3A4 the active carbamazepine 10,11-epoxide, which is further metabolized to the trans-diol by epoxide hydrolase. Therefore, the potential exists for interaction between carbamazepine and any agent that inhibits CYP3A4 and/or epoxide hydrolase. Agents that are CYP3A4 inhibitors, such as erythromycin, may increase the plasma levels of carbamazepine. Also inhibits epoxide hydroxylase, resulting in increased levels of the active metabolite carbamazepine-10,11-epoxide).

Products include:
E.E.S. 437
EryPed 435

Erythromycin Gluceptate (Carbamazepine is metabolized mainly by CYP3A4 the active carbamazepine 10,11-epoxide, which is further metabolized to the trans-diol by epoxide hydro-

lase. Therefore, the potential exists for interaction between carbamazepine and any agent that inhibits CYP3A4 and/or epoxide hydrolase. Agents that are CYP3A4 inhibitors, such as erythromycin, may increase the plasma levels of carbamazepine. Also inhibits epoxide hydroxylase, resulting in increased levels of the active metabolite carbamazepine-10,11-epoxide).

No products indexed under this heading.

Erythromycin Lactobionate (Carbamazepine is metabolized mainly by CYP3A4 the active carbamazepine 10,11-epoxide, which is further metabolized to the trans-diol by epoxide hydrolase. Therefore, the potential exists for interaction between carbamazepine and any agent that inhibits CYP3A4 and/or epoxide hydrolase. Agents that are CYP3A4 inhibitors, such as erythromycin, may increase the plasma levels of carbamazepine. Also inhibits epoxide hydroxylase, resulting in increased levels of the active metabolite carbamazepine-10,11-epoxide).

No products indexed under this heading.

Erythromycin Stearate (Carbamazepine is metabolized mainly by CYP3A4 the active carbamazepine 10,11-epoxide, which is further metabolized to the trans-diol by epoxide hydrolase. Therefore, the potential exists for interaction between carbamazepine and any agent that inhibits CYP3A4 and/or epoxide hydrolase. Agents that are CYP3A4 inhibitors, such as erythromycin, may increase the plasma levels of carbamazepine. Also inhibits epoxide hydroxylase, resulting in increased levels of the active metabolite carbamazepine-10,11-epoxide).

No products indexed under this heading.

Esomeprazole Magnesium (Carbamazepine is metabolized mainly by CYP3A4 the active carbamazepine 10,11-epoxide, which is further metabolized to the trans-diol by epoxide hydrolase. Therefore, the potential exists for interaction between carbamazepine and any agent that inhibits CYP3A4 and/or epoxide hydrolase. Agents that are CYP3A4 inhibitors may increase the plasma levels of carbamazepine).

Products include:
Nexium Capsules 704
Nexium Oral Suspension 704

Esomeprazole Sodium (Carbamazepine is metabolized mainly by CYP3A4 the active carbamazepine 10,11-epoxide, which is further metabolized to the trans-diol by epoxide hydrolase. Therefore, the potential exists for interaction between carbamazepine and any agent that inhibits CYP3A4 and/or epoxide hydrolase. Agents that are CYP3A4 inhibitors may increase the plasma levels of carbamazepine).

Products include:
Nexium I.V. 712

Estazolam (Because of its primary CNS effect, caution should be used when carbamazepine is taken with other centrally acting drugs).

No products indexed under this heading.

Estradiol (Carbamazepine is known to induce CYP1A2 and CYP3A4. Therefore, the potential exists for interaction between carbamazepine and any agent metabolized by one (or more) of these enzymes. Agents that are metabolized by CYP1A2 and CYP3A4 may have decreased plasma levels when administered concomitantly with carbamazepine). Products include:
Activella 2561
Angeliq 831
Climara 841
Climara Pro 847
Divigel 3467
Estrasorb 1777
Vagifem 2589

Estradiol Benzoate (Carbamazepine is known to induce CYP1A2 and CYP3A4. Therefore, the potential exists for interaction between carbamazepine and any agent metabolized by one (or more) of these enzymes. Agents that are metabolized by CYP1A2 and CYP3A4 may have decreased plasma levels when administered concomitantly with carbamazepine).

No products indexed under this heading.

Estradiol Cypionate (Carbamazepine is known to induce CYP1A2 and CYP3A4. Therefore, the potential exists for interaction between carbamazepine and any agent metabolized by one (or more) of these enzymes. Agents that are metabolized by CYP1A2 and CYP3A4 may have decreased plasma levels when administered concomitantly with carbamazepine).

No products indexed under this heading.

Estradiol Valerate (Carbamazepine is known to induce CYP1A2 and CYP3A4. Therefore, the potential exists for interaction between carbamazepine and any agent metabolized by one (or more) of these enzymes. Agents that are metabolized by CYP1A2 and CYP3A4 may have decreased plasma levels when administered concomitantly with carbamazepine).

No products indexed under this heading.

Ethanol (Because of its primary CNS effect, caution should be used when carbamazepine is taken with alcohol).

No products indexed under this heading.

Ethchlorvynol (Because of its primary CNS effect, caution should be used when carbamazepine is taken with other centrally acting drugs).

No products indexed under this heading.

Ethinamate (Because of its primary CNS effect, caution should be used when carbamazepine is taken with other centrally acting drugs).

No products indexed under this heading.

Ethinyl Estradiol (Carbamazepine is known to induce CYP1A2 and CYP3A4. Therefore, the potential exists for interaction between carbamazepine and any agent metabolized by one (or more) of these enzymes. Agents that are metabolized by CYP1A2 or CYP3A4 may have decreased plasma levels when administered concomitantly with carbamazepine. Breakthrough bleeding has been reported among patients receiving concomitant oral contraceptives and their reliability may be adversely affected). Products include:
LoSeasonique 3407
Lybrel 3514
NuvaRing 3181
Ortho Evra 2648
Ortho-Cyclen/Ortho Tri-Cyclen 2663
Ortho Tri-Cyclen Lo Tablets 2673
Seasonique 3418
Yaz 864

Ethosuximide (Carbamazepine is metabolized by CYP3A4. Therefore, the potential exists for interaction between carbamazepine and any agent that induces CYP3A4. Agents that are CYP3A4 inducers may decrease plasma levels of carbamazepine).

No products indexed under this heading.

Ethyl Alcohol (Because of its primary CNS effect, caution should be used when carbamazepine is taken with alcohol).

No products indexed under this heading.

Ethynodiol Diacetate (Carbamazepine is known to induce CYP1A2 and CYP3A4. Therefore, the potential exists for interaction between carbamazepine and any agent metabolized by one (or more) of these enzymes. Agents that are metabolized by CYP1A2 or CYP3A4 may have decreased plasma levels when administered concomitantly with carbamazepine. Breakthrough bleeding

IMPORTANT NOTE: Always consult each drug listing in the patient's regimen for possible interactions.

has been reported among patients receiving concomitant oral contraceptives and their reliability may be adversely affected).
No products indexed under this heading.

Etoposide (Carbamazepine is known to induce CYP1A2 and CYP3A4. Therefore, the potential exists for interaction between carbamazepine and any agent metabolized by one (or more) of these enzymes. Agents that are metabolized by CYP1A2 and CYP3A4 may have decreased plasma levels when administered concomitantly with carbamazepine).
No products indexed under this heading.

Etoposide Phosphate (Carbamazepine is known to induce CYP1A2 and CYP3A4. Therefore, the potential exists for interaction between carbamazepine and any agent metabolized by one (or more) of these enzymes. Agents that are metabolized by CYP1A2 and CYP3A4 may have decreased plasma levels when administered concomitantly with carbamazepine).
No products indexed under this heading.

Etravirine (Co-administration of carbamazepine and delavirdine may lead to loss of virologic response and possible resistance to rescriptor or to the class of non-nucleoside reverse transcriptase inhibitors).
No products indexed under this heading.

Felbamate (Carbamazepine is metabolized by CYP3A4. Therefore, the potential exists for interaction between carbamazepine and any agent that induces CYP3A4. Agents that are CYP3A4 inducers may decrease plasma levels of carbamazepine).
No products indexed under this heading.

Felodipine (Carbamazepine is known to induce CYP1A2 and CYP3A4. Therefore, the potential exists for interaction between carbamazepine and any agent metabolized by one (or more) of these enzymes. Agents that are metabolized by CYP1A2 and CYP3A4 may have decreased plasma levels when administered concomitantly with carbamazepine).
No products indexed under this heading.

Fentanyl (Because of its primary CNS effect, caution should be used when carbamazepine is taken with other centrally acting drugs). Products include:

Duragesic 2604
Fentanyl Transdermal System 2346
Onsolis 2054

Fentanyl Citrate (Because of its primary CNS effect, caution should be used when carbamazepine is taken with other centrally acting drugs). Products include:

Fentora 966

Fluconazole (Carbamazepine is metabolized mainly by CYP3A4 the active carbamazepine 10,11-epoxide, which is futher metabolized to the trans-diol by epoxide hydrolase. Therefore, the potential exists for interaction between carbamazepine and any agent that inhibits CYP3A4 and/or epoxide hydrolase. Agents that are CYP3A4 inhibitors, such as azole antifungals, may increase the plasma levels of carbamazepine).
No products indexed under this heading.

Fludrocortisone Acetate (Carbamazepine is known to induce CYP1A2 and CYP3A4. Therefore, the potential exists for interaction between carbamazepine and any agent metabolized by one (or more) of these enzymes. Agents that are metabolized by CYP1A2 and CYP3A4, such as glucocorticoids, may have decreased plasma levels when administered concomitantly with carbamazepine).
No products indexed under this heading.

Fluoxetine (Carbamazepine is metabolized mainly by CYP3A4 the active carbamazepine 10,11-epoxide, which is further metabolized to the trans-diol by epoxide hydrolase. Therefore, the potential exists for interaction between carbamazepine and any agent that inhibits CYP3A4 and/or epoxide hydrolase. Agents that are CYP3A4 inhibitors may increase the plasma levels of carbamazepine).
No products indexed under this heading.

Fluoxetine Hydrochloride (Carbamazepine is metabolized mainly by CYP3A4 the active carbamazepine 10,11-epoxide, which is further metabolized to the trans-diol by epoxide hydrolase. Therefore, the potential exists for interaction between carbamazepine and any agent that inhibits CYP3A4 and/or epoxide hydrolase. Agents that are CYP3A4 inhibitors may increase the plasma levels of carbamazepine). Products include:

Prozac Weekly 1941
Prozac Pulvules 1941
Symbyax 1965

Fluphenazine Decanoate (Because of its primary CNS effect, caution should be used when carbamazepine is taken with other centrally acting drugs).
No products indexed under this heading.

Fluphenazine Enanthate (Because of its primary CNS effect, caution should be used when carbamazepine is taken with other centrally acting drugs).
No products indexed under this heading.

Fluphenazine Hydrochloride (Because of its primary CNS effect, caution should be used when carbamazepine is taken with other centrally acting drugs).
No products indexed under this heading.

Flurazepam Hydrochloride (Because of its primary CNS effect, caution should be used when carbamazepine is taken with other centrally acting drugs).
No products indexed under this heading.

Flutamide (Carbamazepine is known to induce CYP1A2 and CYP3A4. Therefore, the potential exists for interaction between carbamazepine and any agent metabolized by one (or more) of these enzymes. Agents that are metabolized by CYP1A2 and CYP3A4 may have decreased plasma levels when administered concomitantly with carbamazepine).
No products indexed under this heading.

Fluticasone Propionate (Carbamazepine is known to induce CYP1A2 and CYP3A4. Therefore, the potential exists for interaction between carbamazepine and any agent metabolized by one (or more) of these enzymes. Agents that are metabolized by CYP1A2 and CYP3A4 may have decreased plasma levels when administered concomitantly with carbamazepine). Products include:

Advair 100/50 1275
Advair 250/50 1275
Advair 500/50 1275
Advair HFA 45/21 1288
Advair HFA 115/21 1288
Advair HFA 230/21 1288
Flonase 1459
Flovent Diskus 1463
Flovent HFA 1470

Fluvoxamine Maleate (Carbamazepine is known to induce CYP1A2 and CYP3A4. Therefore, the potential exists for interaction between carbamazepine and any agent metabolized by one (or more) of these enzymes. Agents that are metabolized by CYP1A2 and CYP3A4 may have decreased plasma levels when administered concomitantly with carbamazepine).
No products indexed under this heading.

Fosamprenavir Calcium (Carbamazepine is metabolized mainly by CYP3A4 the active carbamazepine 10,11-epoxide, which is further metabolized to the trans-diol by epoxide hydrolase. Therefore, the potential exists for interaction between carbamazepine and any agent that inhibits CYP3A4 and/or epoxide hydrolase. Agents that are CYP3A4 inhibitors, such as protease inhibitors, may increase the plasma levels of carbamazepine). Products include:

Lexiva Oral Suspension 1558
Lexiva 1558

Fosphenytoin (Carbamazepine is metabolized by CYP3A4. Therefore, the potential exists for interaction between carbamazepine and any agent that induces CYP3A4. Agents that are CYP3A4 inducers may decrease plasma levels of carbamazepine. Carbamazepine may increase the plasma levels of phenytoin; careful monitoring of phenytoin plasma levels following comedication with carbamazepine is advised).
No products indexed under this heading.

Fosphenytoin Sodium (Carbamazepine is metabolized by CYP3A4. Therefore, the potential exists for interaction between carbamazepine and any agent that induces CYP3A4. Agents that are CYP3A4 inducers may decrease plasma levels of carbamazepine. Carbamazepine may increase the plasma levels of phenytoin; careful monitoring of phenytoin plasma levels following comedication with carbamazepine is advised).
No products indexed under this heading.

Garlic Extract (Carbamazepine is metabolized by CYP3A4. Therefore, the potential exists for interaction between carbamazepine and any agent that induces CYP3A4. Agents that are CYP3A4 inducers may decrease plasma levels of carbamazepine).
No products indexed under this heading.

Garlic Oil (Carbamazepine is metabolized by CYP3A4. Therefore, the potential exists for interaction between carbamazepine and any agent that induces CYP3A4. Agents that are CYP3A4 inducers may decrease plasma levels of carbamazepine).
No products indexed under this heading.

Glutethimide (Because of its primary CNS effect, caution should be used when carbamazepine is taken with other centrally acting drugs).
No products indexed under this heading.

Grepafloxacin Hydrochloride (Carbamazepine is known to induce CYP1A2 and CYP3A4. Therefore, the potential exists for interaction between carbamazepine and any agent metabolized by one (or more) of these enzymes. Agents that are metabolized by CYP1A2 and CYP3A4 may have decreased plasma levels when administered concomitantly with carbamazepine).
No products indexed under this heading.

Haloperidol (Because of its primary CNS effect, caution should be used when carbamazepine is taken with other centrally acting drugs).
No products indexed under this heading.

Haloperidol Decanoate (Because of its primary CNS effect, caution should be used when carbamazepine is taken with other centrally acting drugs).
No products indexed under this heading.

Haloperidol Lactate (Carbamazepine is known to induce CYP1A2 and CYP3A4. Therefore, the potential exists for interaction between carbamazepine and any agent metabolized by one (or more) of these enzymes. Agents that are metabolized by CYP1A2 and CYP3A4, such as haloperidol, may have decreased plasma levels when administered concomitantly with carbamazepine).
No products indexed under this heading.

Hydrocodone Bitartrate (Because of its primary CNS effect, caution should be used when carbamazepine is taken with other centrally acting drugs). Products include:

Vicodin 560
Vicodin ES 561
Vicodin HP 563
Vicoprofen 564
Zydone 1138

Hydrocodone Polistirex (Because of its primary CNS effect, caution should be used when carbamazepine is taken with other centrally acting drugs). Products include:

Tussionex 3443

Hydrocortisone (Carbamazepine is known to induce CYP1A2 and CYP3A4. Therefore, the potential exists for interaction between carbamazepine and any agent metabolized by one (or more) of these enzymes. Agents that are metabolized by CYP1A2 and CYP3A4, such as glucocorticoids, may have decreased plasma levels when administered concomitantly with carbamazepine).
No products indexed under this heading.

Hydrocortisone (Alcohol) (Carbamazepine is metabolized by CYP3A4. Therefore, the potential exists for interaction between carbamazepine and any agent that induces CYP3A4. Agents that are CYP3A4 inducers may decrease plasma levels of carbamazepine).
No products indexed under this heading.

Hydrocortisone Acetate (Carbamazepine is known to induce CYP1A2 and CYP3A4. Therefore, the potential exists for interaction between carbamazepine and any agent metabolized by one (or more) of these enzymes. Agents that are metabolized by CYP1A2 and CYP3A4, such as glucocorticoids, may have decreased plasma levels when administered concomitantly with carbamazepine).
No products indexed under this heading.

Hydrocortisone Butyrate (Carbamazepine is metabolized by CYP3A4. Therefore, the potential exists for interaction between carbamazepine and any agent that induces CYP3A4. Agents that are CYP3A4 inducers may decrease plasma levels of carbamazepine).
No products indexed under this heading.

Hydrocortisone Cypionate (Carbamazepine is metabolized by CYP3A4. Therefore, the potential exists for interaction between carbamazepine and any agent that induces CYP3A4. Agents that are CYP3A4 inducers may decrease plasma levels of carbamazepine).
No products indexed under this heading.

Hydrocortisone Hemisuccinate (Carbamazepine is metabolized by CYP3A4. Therefore, the potential exists for interaction between carbamazepine and any agent that induces CYP3A4. Agents that are CYP3A4 inducers may decrease plasma levels of carbamazepine).
No products indexed under this heading.

Hydrocortisone Probutate (Carbamazepine is metabolized by CYP3A4. Therefore, the potential exists for interaction between carbamazepine and any agent that induces CYP3A4. Agents that are CYP3A4 inducers may decrease plasma levels of carbamazepine).
No products indexed under this heading.

Hydrocortisone Sodium Phosphate (Carbamazepine is known to induce CYP1A2 and CYP3A4. Therefore, the potential exists for interaction between carbamazepine and any agent metabolized by one (or more) of these enzymes. Agents that are metabolized by CYP1A2 and CYP3A4, such as glucocorticoids, may have decreased plasma levels when administered concomitantly with carbamazepine).
No products indexed under this heading.

Hydrocortisone Sodium Succinate (Carbamazepine is known to induce CYP1A2 and CYP3A4. Therefore, the potential exists for interaction between carbamazepine and any agent metabolized by one (or more) of these enzymes. Agents that are metabolized by CYP1A2 and CYP3A4, such as glucocorticoids, may have decreased plasma levels when administered concomitantly with carbamazepine).
No products indexed under this heading.

Hydrocortisone Valerate (Carbamazepine is metabolized by CYP3A4. Therefore, the potential exists for interaction between carbamazepine and any agent that induces CYP3A4. Agents that are CYP3A4 inducers may decrease plasma levels of carbamazepine).
No products indexed under this heading.

Hydromorphone Hydrochloride (Because of its primary CNS effect, caution should be used when carbamazepine is taken with other centrally acting drugs). Products include:
Dilaudid Injection 2800
Dilaudid Oral 2797
Dilaudid Tablets 2797
Dilaudid-HP 2800

Hydroxyamphetamine Hydrobromide (Because of its primary CNS effect, caution should be used when carbamazepine is taken with other centrally acting drugs).
No products indexed under this heading.

Hydroxyzine Hydrochloride (Because of its primary CNS effect, caution should be used when carbamazepine is taken with other centrally acting drugs).
No products indexed under this heading.

Hypericum (Carbamazepine is metabolized by CYP3A4. Therefore, the potential exists for interaction between carbamazepine and any agent that induces CYP3A4. Agents that are CYP3A4 inducers may decrease plasma levels of carbamazepine).
No products indexed under this heading.

Hypericum Perforatum (Carbamazepine is metabolized by CYP3A4. Therefore, the potential exists for interaction between carbamazepine and any agent that induces CYP3A4. Agents that are CYP3A4 inducers may decrease plasma levels of carbamazepine). Products include:
Traumeel 1800

Imatinib Mesylate (Carbamazepine is metabolized mainly by CYP3A4 the active carbamazepine 10,11-epoxide, which is further metabolized to the trans-diol by epoxide hydrolase. Therefore, the potential exists for interaction between carbamazepine and any agent that inhibits CYP3A4 and/or epoxide hydrolase. Agents that are CYP3A4 inhibitors may increase the plasma levels of carbamazepine). Products include:
Gleevec 2477

Imipramine Hydrochloride (Carbamazepine is contraindicated in patients with a known sensitivity to any of the tricyclic compounds, such as amitriptyline, desipramine, imipramine, protriptyline, and nortriptyline).
No products indexed under this heading.

Imipramine Pamoate (Carbamazepine is contraindicated in patients with a known sensitivity to any of the tricyclic compounds, such as amitriptyline, desipramine, imipramine, protriptyline, and nortriptyline).
No products indexed under this heading.

Indinavir Sulfate (Carbamazepine is metabolized mainly by CYP3A4 the active carbamazepine 10,11-epoxide, which is further metabolized to the trans-diol by epoxide hydrolase. Therefore, the potential exists for interaction between carbamazepine and any agent that inhibits CYP3A4 and/or epoxide hydrolase. Agents that are CYP3A4 inhibitors, such as protease inhibitors, may increase the plasma levels of carbamazepine). Products include:
Crixivan 2113

Isocarboxazid (Co-administration of carbamazepine with MAO inhibitors is contraindicated. MAO inhibitors should be discontinued for a minimum of 14 days, or longer if the clinical situation permits). Products include:
Marplan 3481

Isoflurane (Because of its primary CNS effect, caution should be used when carbamazepine is taken with other centrally acting drugs).
No products indexed under this heading.

Isoniazid (Carbamazepine is metabolized mainly by CYP3A4 the active carbamazepine 10,11-epoxide, which is further metabolized to the trans-diol by epoxide hydrolase. Therefore, the potential exists for interaction between carbamazepine and any agent that inhibits CYP3A4 and/or epoxide hydrolase. Agents that are CYP3A4 inhibitors may increase the plasma levels of carbamazepine).
No products indexed under this heading.

Isradipine (Carbamazepine is known to induce CYP1A2 and CYP3A4. Therefore, the potential exists for interaction between carbamazepine and any agent metabolized by one (or more) of these enzymes. Agents that are metabolized by CYP1A2 and CYP3A4 may have decreased plasma levels when administered concomitantly with carbamazepine). Products include:
DynaCirc CR 1432

Itraconazole (Carbamazepine is metabolized mainly by CYP3A4 the active carbamazepine 10,11-epoxide, which is futher metabolized to the trans-diol by epoxide hydrolase. Therefore, the potential exists for interaction between carbamazepine and any agent that inhibits CYP3A4 and/or epoxide hydrolase. Agents that are CYP3A4 inhibitors, such as azole antifungals, may increase the plasma levels of carbamazepine).
No products indexed under this heading.

Ixabepilone (Carbamazepine is known to induce CYP1A2 and CYP3A4. Therefore, the potential exists for interaction between carbamazepine and any agent metabolized by one (or more) of these enzymes. Agents that are metabolized by CYP1A2 and CYP3A4 may have decreased plasma levels when administered concomitantly with carbamazepine).
No products indexed under this heading.

Ketamine Hydrochloride (Because of its primary CNS effect, caution should be used when carbamazepine is taken with other centrally acting drugs).
No products indexed under this heading.

Ketoconazole (Carbamazepine is metabolized mainly by CYP3A4 the active carbamazepine 10,11-epoxide, which is futher metabolized to the trans-diol by epoxide hydrolase. Therefore, the potential exists for interaction between carbamazepine and any agent that inhibits CYP3A4 and/or epoxide

hydrolase. Agents that are CYP3A4 inhibitors, such as azole antifungals, may increase the plasma levels of carbamazepine). Products include:
Extina 3319
Xolegel 3337

Lapatinib (Carbamazepine is metabolized mainly by CYP3A4 the active carbamazepine 10,11-epoxide, which is further metabolized to the trans-diol by epoxide hydrolase. Therefore, the potential exists for interaction between carbamazepine and any agent that inhibits CYP3A4 and/or epoxide hydrolase. Agents that are CYP3A4 inhibitors may increase the plasma levels of carbamazepine). Products include:
Tykerb 1698

Levobupivacaine Hydrochloride (Carbamazepine is known to induce CYP1A2 and CYP3A4. Therefore, the potential exists for interaction between carbamazepine and any agent metabolized by one (or more) of these enzymes. Agents that are metabolized by CYP1A2 and CYP3A4 may have decreased plasma levels when administered concomitantly with carbamazepine).
No products indexed under this heading.

Levomethadyl Acetate Hydrochloride (Because of its primary CNS effect, caution should be used when carbamazepine is taken with other centrally acting drugs).
No products indexed under this heading.

Levonorgestrel (Carbamazepine is known to induce CYP1A2 and CYP3A4. Therefore, the potential exists for interaction between carbamazepine and any agent metabolized by one (or more) of these enzymes. Agents that are metabolized by CYP1A2 or CYP3A4 may have decreased plasma levels when administered concomitantly with carbamazepine. Breakthrough bleeding has been reported among patients receiving concomitant oral contraceptives and their reliability may be adversely affected). Products include:
Climara Pro 847
LoSeasonique 3407
Lybrel 3514
Mirena 854
Plan B 3416
Seasonique 3418

Levorphanol Tartrate (Because of its primary CNS effect, caution should be used when carbamazepine is taken with other centrally acting drugs).
No products indexed under this heading.

Lidocaine (Carbamazepine is known to induce CYP1A2 and CYP3A4. Therefore, the potential exists for interaction between carbamazepine and any agent metabolized by one (or more) of these enzymes. Agents that are metabolized by CYP1A2 and CYP3A4 may have decreased plasma levels when administered concomitantly with carbamazepine). Products include:
Lidoderm 1107

Lidocaine Hydrochloride (Carbamazepine is known to induce CYP1A2 and CYP3A4. Therefore, the potential exists for interaction between carbamazepine and any agent metabolized by one (or more) of these enzymes. Agents that are metabolized by CYP1A2 and CYP3A4 may have decreased plasma levels when administered concomitantly with carbamazepine).
No products indexed under this heading.

Lisdexamfetamine Dimesylate (Because of its primary CNS effect, caution should be used when carbamazepine is taken with other centrally acting drugs). Products include:
Vyvanse 3298

Lithium (Concomitant administration of carbamazepine and lithium may increase the risk of neurotoxic side effects).
No products indexed under this heading.

Lithium Carbonate (Concomitant administration of carbamazepine and lithium may increase the risk of neurotoxic side effects).
No products indexed under this heading.

Lithium Citrate (Concomitant administration of carbamazepine and lithium may increase the risk of neurotoxic side effects).
No products indexed under this heading.

Lomefloxacin Hydrochloride (Carbamazepine is known to induce CYP1A2 and CYP3A4. Therefore, the potential exists for interaction between carbamazepine and any agent metabolized by one (or more) of these enzymes. Agents that are metabolized by CYP1A2 and CYP3A4 may have decreased plasma levels when administered concomitantly with carbamazepine).
No products indexed under this heading.

Lopinavir (Carbamazepine is metabolized mainly by CYP3A4 the active carbamazepine 10,11-epoxide, which is further metabolized to the trans-diol by epoxide hydrolase. Therefore, the potential exists for interaction between carbamazepine and any agent that inhibits CYP3A4 and/or epoxide hydrolase. Agents that are CYP3A4 inhibitors, such as protease inhibitors, may increase the plasma levels of carbamazepine). Products include:
Kaletra 458

Loratadine (Carbamazepine is metabolized mainly by CYP3A4 the active carbamazepine 10,11-epoxide, which is further metabolized to the trans-diol by epoxide hydrolase. Therefore, the potential exists for interaction between carbamazepine and any agent that inhibits CYP3A4 and/or epoxide hydrolase. Agents that are CYP3A4 inhibitors may increase the plasma levels of carbamazepine).
No products indexed under this heading.

Lorazepam (Because of its primary CNS effect, caution should be used when carbamazepine is taken with other centrally acting drugs).
No products indexed under this heading.

Lovastatin (Carbamazepine is known to induce CYP1A2 and CYP3A4. Therefore, the potential exists for interaction between carbamazepine and any agent metabolized by one (or more) of these enzymes. Agents that are metabolized by CYP1A2 and CYP3A4 may have decreased plasma levels when administered concomitantly with carbamazepine). Products include:
Advicor 402
Mevacor 2212

Loxapine Hydrochloride (Because of its primary CNS effect, caution should be used when carbamazepine is taken with other centrally acting drugs).
No products indexed under this heading.

Loxapine Succinate (Because of its primary CNS effect, caution should be used when carbamazepine is taken with other centrally acting drugs).
No products indexed under this heading.

Maprotiline Hydrochloride (Carbamazepine is contraindicated in patients with a known sensitivity to any of the tricyclic compounds, such as amitriptyline, desipramine, imipramine, protriptyline, and nortriptyline).
No products indexed under this heading.

Mefloquine Hydrochloride (Antimalarial drugs, such as chloroquine and mefloquine, may antagonize the activity of carbamazepine).
No products indexed under this heading.

IMPORTANT NOTE: Always consult each drug listing in the patient's regimen for possible interactions.

Equetro Interactions Index 602

Meperidine Hydrochloride (Because of its primary CNS effect, caution should be used when carbamazepine is taken with other centrally acting drugs).
No products indexed under this heading.

Mephenytoin (Carbamazepine is metabolized by CYP3A4. Therefore, the potential exists for interaction between carbamazepine and any agent that induces CYP3A4. Agents that are CYP3A4 inducers may decrease plasma levels of carbamazepine).
No products indexed under this heading.

Mephobarbital (Because of its primary CNS effect, caution should be used when carbamazepine is taken with other centrally acting drugs).
No products indexed under this heading.

Meprobamate (Because of its primary CNS effect, caution should be used when carbamazepine is taken with other centrally acting drugs).
No products indexed under this heading.

Mesoridazine Besylate (Because of its primary CNS effect, caution should be used when carbamazepine is taken with other centrally acting drugs).
No products indexed under this heading.

Mestranol (Carbamazepine is known to induce CYP1A2 and CYP3A4. Therefore, the potential exists for interaction between carbamazepine and any agent metabolized by one (or more) of these enzymes. Agents that are metabolized by CYP1A2 or CYP3A4 may have decreased plasma levels when administered concomitantly with carbamazepine. Breakthrough bleeding has been reported among patients receiving concomitant oral contraceptives and their reliability may be adversely affected).
No products indexed under this heading.

Methadone Hydrochloride (Because of its primary CNS effect, caution should be used when carbamazepine is taken with other centrally acting drugs).
No products indexed under this heading.

Methamphetamine Hydrochloride (Because of its primary CNS effect, caution should be used when carbamazepine is taken with other centrally acting drugs).
No products indexed under this heading.

Methohexital Sodium (Because of its primary CNS effect, caution should be used when carbamazepine is taken with other centrally acting drugs).
No products indexed under this heading.

Methotrimeprazine (Because of its primary CNS effect, caution should be used when carbamazepine is taken with other centrally acting drugs).
No products indexed under this heading.

Methoxyflurane (Because of its primary CNS effect, caution should be used when carbamazepine is taken with other centrally acting drugs).
No products indexed under this heading.

Methsuximide (Carbamazepine is metabolized by CYP3A4. Therefore, the potential exists for interaction between carbamazepine and any agent that induces CYP3A4. Agents that are CYP3A4 inducers may decrease plasma levels of carbamazepine).
No products indexed under this heading.

Methylphenidate (Because of its primary CNS effect, caution should be used when carbamazepine is taken with other centrally acting drugs). Products include:
Daytrana **3283**

Methylphenidate Hydrochloride (Because of its primary CNS effect, caution should be used when carbamazepine is taken with other centrally acting drugs). Products include:
Concerta **2598**
Metadate CD **3439**

Methylprednisolone (Carbamazepine is metabolized by CYP3A4. Therefore, the potential exists for interaction between carbamazepine and any agent that induces CYP3A4. Agents that are CYP3A4 inducers may decrease plasma levels of carbamazepine).
No products indexed under this heading.

Methylprednisolone Acetate (Carbamazepine is known to induce CYP1A2 and CYP3A4. Therefore, the potential exists for interaction between carbamazepine and any agent metabolized by one (or more) of these enzymes. Agents that are metabolized by CYP1A2 and CYP3A4, such as glucocorticoids, may have decreased plasma levels when administered concomitantly with carbamazepine).
No products indexed under this heading.

Methylprednisolone Sodium Succinate (Carbamazepine is known to induce CYP1A2 and CYP3A4. Therefore, the potential exists for interaction between carbamazepine and any agent metabolized by one (or more) of these enzymes. Agents that are metabolized by CYP1A2 and CYP3A4, such as glucocorticoids, may have decreased plasma levels when administered concomitantly with carbamazepine).
No products indexed under this heading.

Metronidazole (Carbamazepine is metabolized mainly by CYP3A4 the active carbamazepine 10,11-epoxide, which is further metabolized to the trans-diol by epoxide hydrolase. Therefore, the potential exists for interaction between carbamazepine and any agent that inhibits CYP3A4 and/or epoxide hydrolase. Agents that are CYP3A4 inhibitors may increase the plasma levels of carbamazepine). Products include:
Pylera **793**

Metronidazole Benzoate (Carbamazepine is metabolized mainly by CYP3A4 the active carbamazepine 10,11-epoxide, which is further metabolized to the trans-diol by epoxide hydrolase. Therefore, the potential exists for interaction between carbamazepine and any agent that inhibits CYP3A4 and/or epoxide hydrolase. Agents that are CYP3A4 inhibitors may increase the plasma levels of carbamazepine).
No products indexed under this heading.

Metronidazole Hydrochloride (Carbamazepine is metabolized mainly by CYP3A4 the active carbamazepine 10,11-epoxide, which is further metabolized to the trans-diol by epoxide hydrolase. Therefore, the potential exists for interaction between carbamazepine and any agent that inhibits CYP3A4 and/or epoxide hydrolase. Agents that are CYP3A4 inhibitors may increase the plasma levels of carbamazepine).
No products indexed under this heading.

Metronidazole Sodium (Carbamazepine is metabolized mainly by CYP3A4 the active carbamazepine 10,11-epoxide, which is further metabolized to the trans-diol by epoxide hydrolase. Therefore, the potential exists for interaction between carbamazepine and any agent that inhibits CYP3A4 and/or epoxide hydrolase. Agents that are CYP3A4 inhibitors may increase the plasma levels of carbamazepine).
No products indexed under this heading.

Mexiletine Hydrochloride (Carbamazepine is known to induce CYP1A2 and CYP3A4. Therefore, the potential exists for interaction between carbamazepine and any agent metabolized by one (or more) of these enzymes. Agents that are metabolized by CYP1A2 and CYP3A4 may have decreased plasma levels when administered concomitantly with carbamazepine).
No products indexed under this heading.

Miconazole (Carbamazepine is metabolized mainly by CYP3A4 the active carbamazepine 10,11-epoxide, which is futher metabolized to the trans-diol by epoxide hydrolase. Therefore, the potential exists for interaction between carbamazepine and any agent that inhibits CYP3A4 and/or epoxide hydrolase. Agents that are CYP3A4 inhibitors, such as azole antifungals, may increase the plasma levels of carbamazepine).
No products indexed under this heading.

Miconazole Nitrate (Carbamazepine is metabolized mainly by CYP3A4 the active carbamazepine 10,11-epoxide, which is further metabolized to the trans-diol by epoxide hydrolase. Therefore, the potential exists for interaction between carbamazepine and any agent that inhibits CYP3A4 and/or epoxide hydrolase. Agents that are CYP3A4 inhibitors may increase the plasma levels of carbamazepine). Products include:
Vusion Ointment **3335**

Midazolam Hydrochloride (Because of its primary CNS effect, caution should be used when carbamazepine is taken with other centrally acting drugs).
No products indexed under this heading.

Mifepristone (Carbamazepine is metabolized mainly by CYP3A4 the active carbamazepine 10,11-epoxide, which is further metabolized to the trans-diol by epoxide hydrolase. Therefore, the potential exists for interaction between carbamazepine and any agent that inhibits CYP3A4 and/or epoxide hydrolase. Agents that are CYP3A4 inhibitors may increase the plasma levels of carbamazepine).
No products indexed under this heading.

Mirtazapine (Carbamazepine is known to induce CYP1A2 and CYP3A4. Therefore, the potential exists for interaction between carbamazepine and any agent metabolized by one (or more) of these enzymes. Agents that are metabolized by CYP1A2 and CYP3A4 may have decreased plasma levels when administered concomitantly with carbamazepine). Products include:
Remeron Tablets **3214**
RemeronSolTab Tablets **3219**

Moclobemide (Co-administration of carbamazepine with MAO inhibitors is contraindicated. MAO inhibitors should be discontinued for a minimum of 14 days, or longer if the clinical situation permits).
No products indexed under this heading.

Modafinil (Carbamazepine is metabolized by CYP3A4. Therefore, the potential exists for interaction between carbamazepine and any agent that induces CYP3A4. Agents that are CYP3A4 inducers may decrease plasma levels of carbamazepine). Products include:
Provigil **983**

Molindone Hydrochloride (Because of its primary CNS effect, caution should be used when carbamazepine is taken with other centrally acting drugs). Products include:
Moban **1108**

Morphine Sulfate (Because of its primary CNS effect, caution should be used when carbamazepine is taken with other centrally acting drugs). Products include:
Avinza **1822**
Embeda **1831**
MS Contin **2803**

Moxifloxacin Hydrochloride (Carbamazepine is known to induce CYP1A2 and CYP3A4. Therefore, the potential exists for interaction between carbamazepine and any agent metabolized by one (or more) of these enzymes. Agents that are metabolized by CYP1A2 and CYP3A4 may have decreased plasma levels when administered concomitantly with carbamazepine). Products include:
Avelox **3064**
Vigamox **589**

Nafcillin Sodium (Carbamazepine is metabolized by CYP3A4. Therefore, the potential exists for interaction between carbamazepine and any agent that induces CYP3A4. Agents that are CYP3A4 inducers may decrease plasma levels of carbamazepine).
No products indexed under this heading.

Naproxen (Carbamazepine is known to induce CYP1A2 and CYP3A4. Therefore, the potential exists for interaction between carbamazepine and any agent metabolized by one (or more) of these enzymes. Agents that are metabolized by CYP1A2 and CYP3A4 may have decreased plasma levels when administered concomitantly with carbamazepine). Products include:
EC-Naprosyn **2850**
Naprosyn **2850**
Anaprox/Naprosyn **2850**

Naproxen Sodium (Carbamazepine is known to induce CYP1A2 and CYP3A4. Therefore, the potential exists for interaction between carbamazepine and any agent metabolized by one (or more) of these enzymes. Agents that are metabolized by CYP1A2 and CYP3A4 may have decreased plasma levels when administered concomitantly with carbamazepine). Products include:
Anaprox **2850**
Anaprox DS **2850**
Treximet **1681**

Nefazodone Hydrochloride (Carbamazepine is known to induce CYP1A2 and CYP3A4. Therefore, the potential exists for interaction between carbamazepine and any agent metabolized by one (or more) of these enzymes. Agents that are metabolized by CYP1A2 and CYP3A4 may have decreased plasma levels when administered concomitantly with carbamazepine).
No products indexed under this heading.

Nelfinavir Mesylate (Carbamazepine is metabolized mainly by CYP3A4 the active carbamazepine 10,11-epoxide, which is further metabolized to the trans-diol by epoxide hydrolase. Therefore, the potential exists for interaction between carbamazepine and any agent that inhibits CYP3A4 and/or epoxide hydrolase. Agents that are CYP3A4 inhibitors, such as protease inhibitors, may increase the plasma levels of carbamazepine).
No products indexed under this heading.

Nevirapine (Co-administration of carbamazepine and delavirdine may lead to loss of virologic response and possible resistance to rescriptor or to the class of non-nucleoside reverse transcriptase inhibitors). Products include:
Viramune Oral Suspension **897**
Viramune Tablets **897**

Niacin (Carbamazepine is metabolized mainly by CYP3A4 the active carbamazepine 10,11-epoxide, which is further metabolized to the trans-diol by epoxide hydrolase. Therefore, the potential exists for interaction between carbamazepine and any agent that inhibits CYP3A4 and/or epoxide hydrolase. Agents that are CYP3A4 inhibitors may increase the plasma levels of carbamazepine). Products include:

Niacinamide (Carbamazepine is metabolized mainly by CYP3A4 the active carbamazepine 10,11-epoxide, which is further metabolized to the trans-diol by epoxide hydrolase. Therefore, the potential exists for interaction between carbamazepine and any agent that inhibits CYP3A4 and/or epoxide hydrolase. Agents that are CYP3A4 inhibitors may increase the plasma levels of carbamazepine). Products include:

Niacinamide Hydroiodide (Carbamazepine is metabolized mainly by CYP3A4 the active carbamazepine 10,11-epoxide, which is further metabolized to the trans-diol by epoxide hydrolase. Therefore, the potential exists for interaction between carbamazepine and any agent that inhibits CYP3A4 and/or epoxide hydrolase. Agents that are CYP3A4 inhibitors may increase the plasma levels of carbamazepine).
No products indexed under this heading.

Nicardipine (Carbamazepine is known to induce CYP1A2 and CYP3A4. Therefore, the potential exists for interaction between carbamazepine and any agent metabolized by one (or more) of these enzymes. Agents that are metabolized by CYP1A2 and CYP3A4 may have decreased plasma levels when administered concomitantly with carbamazepine).
No products indexed under this heading.

Nicardipine Hydrochloride (Carbamazepine is known to induce CYP1A2 and CYP3A4. Therefore, the potential exists for interaction between carbamazepine and any agent metabolized by one (or more) of these enzymes. Agents that are metabolized by CYP1A2 and CYP3A4 may have decreased plasma levels when administered concomitantly with carbamazepine).
No products indexed under this heading.

Nicotinamide (Carbamazepine is metabolized mainly by CYP3A4 the active carbamazepine 10,11-epoxide, which is further metabolized to the trans-diol by epoxide hydrolase. Therefore, the potential exists for interaction between carbamazepine and any agent that inhibits CYP3A4 and/or epoxide hydrolase. Agents that are CYP3A4 inhibitors may increase the plasma levels of carbamazepine).
No products indexed under this heading.

Nicotine Polacrilex (Carbamazepine is known to induce CYP1A2 and CYP3A4. Therefore, the potential exists for interaction between carbamazepine and any agent metabolized by one (or more) of these enzymes. Agents that are metabolized by CYP1A2 and CYP3A4 may have decreased plasma levels when administered concomitantly with carbamazepine).
No products indexed under this heading.

Nicotine Salicylate (Carbamazepine is known to induce CYP1A2 and CYP3A4. Therefore, the potential exists for interaction between carbamazepine and any agent metabolized by one (or more) of these enzymes. Agents that are metabolized by CYP1A2 and CYP3A4 may have decreased plasma levels when administered concomitantly with carbamazepine).
No products indexed under this heading.

Nicotine Sulfate (Carbamazepine is known to induce CYP1A2 and CYP3A4. Therefore, the potential exists for interaction between carbamazepine and any agent metabolized by one (or more) of these enzymes. Agents that are metabolized by CYP1A2 and CYP3A4 may have decreased plasma levels when administered concomitantly with carbamazepine).
No products indexed under this heading.

Nifedipine (Carbamazepine is known to induce CYP1A2 and CYP3A4. Therefore, the potential exists for interaction between carbamazepine and any agent metabolized by one (or more) of these enzymes. Agents that are metabolized by CYP1A2 and CYP3A4 may have decreased plasma levels when administered concomitantly with carbamazepine).
No products indexed under this heading.

Nimodipine (Carbamazepine is known to induce CYP1A2 and CYP3A4. Therefore, the potential exists for interaction between carbamazepine and any agent metabolized by one (or more) of these enzymes. Agents that are metabolized by CYP1A2 and CYP3A4 may have decreased plasma levels when administered concomitantly with carbamazepine).
No products indexed under this heading.

Nisoldipine (Carbamazepine is known to induce CYP1A2 and CYP3A4. Therefore, the potential exists for interaction between carbamazepine and any agent metabolized by one (or more) of these enzymes. Agents that are metabolized by CYP1A2 and CYP3A4 may have decreased plasma levels when administered concomitantly with carbamazepine).
No products indexed under this heading.

Nitrendipine (Carbamazepine is known to induce CYP1A2 and CYP3A4. Therefore, the potential exists for interaction between carbamazepine and any agent metabolized by one (or more) of these enzymes. Agents that are metabolized by CYP1A2 and CYP3A4 may have decreased plasma levels when administered concomitantly with carbamazepine).
No products indexed under this heading.

Norethindrone (Carbamazepine is known to induce CYP1A2 and CYP3A4. Therefore, the potential exists for interaction between carbamazepine and any agent metabolized by one (or more) of these enzymes. Agents that are metabolized by CYP1A2 or CYP3A4 may have decreased plasma levels when administered concomitantly with carbamazepine. Breakthrough bleeding has been reported among patients receiving concomitant oral contraceptives and their reliability may be adversely affected). Products include:

Norethindrone Acetate (Carbamazepine is known to induce CYP1A2 and CYP3A4. Therefore, the potential exists for interaction between carbamazepine and any agent metabolized by one (or more) of these enzymes. Agents that are metabolized by CYP1A2 and CYP3A4 may have decreased plasma levels when administered concomitantly with carbamazepine). Products include:

Norethynodrel (Carbamazepine is known to induce CYP1A2 and CYP3A4. Therefore, the potential exists for interaction between carbamazepine and any agent metabolized by one (or more) of these enzymes. Agents that are metabolized by CYP1A2 or CYP3A4 may have decreased plasma levels when administered concomitantly with carbamazepine. Breakthrough bleeding has been reported among patients receiving concomitant oral contraceptives and their reliability may be adversely affected).
No products indexed under this heading.

Norfloxacin (Carbamazepine is known to induce CYP1A2 and CYP3A4. Therefore, the potential exists for interaction between carbamazepine and any agent metabolized by one (or more) of these enzymes. Agents that are metabolized by CYP1A2 and CYP3A4 may have decreased plasma levels when administered concomitantly with carbamazepine). Products include:

Norgestimate (Carbamazepine is known to induce CYP1A2 and CYP3A4. Therefore, the potential exists for interaction between carbamazepine and any agent metabolized by one (or more) of these enzymes. Agents that are metabolized by CYP1A2 or CYP3A4 may have decreased plasma levels when administered concomitantly with carbamazepine. Breakthrough bleeding has been reported among patients receiving concomitant oral contraceptives and their reliability may be adversely affected). Products include:

Norgestrel (Carbamazepine is known to induce CYP1A2 and CYP3A4. Therefore, the potential exists for interaction between carbamazepine and any agent metabolized by one (or more) of these enzymes. Agents that are metabolized by CYP1A2 or CYP3A4 may have decreased plasma levels when administered concomitantly with carbamazepine. Breakthrough bleeding has been reported among patients receiving concomitant oral contraceptives and their reliability may be adversely affected).
No products indexed under this heading.

Nortriptyline Hydrochloride (Carbamazepine is contraindicated in patients with a known sensitivity to any of the tricyclic compounds, such as amitriptyline, desipramine, imipramine, protriptyline, and nortriptyline).
No products indexed under this heading.

Ofloxacin (Carbamazepine is known to induce CYP1A2 and CYP3A4. Therefore, the potential exists for interaction between carbamazepine and any agent metabolized by one (or more) of these enzymes. Agents that are metabolized by CYP1A2 and CYP3A4 may have decreased plasma levels when administered concomitantly with carbamazepine).
No products indexed under this heading.

Olanzapine (Because of its primary CNS effect, caution should be used when carbamazepine is taken with other centrally acting drugs). Products include:

Omeprazole (Carbamazepine is metabolized mainly by CYP3A4 the active carbamazepine 10,11-epoxide, which is further metabolized to the trans-diol by epoxide hydrolase. Therefore, the potential exists for interaction between carbamazepine and any agent that inhibits CYP3A4 and/or epoxide hydrolase. Agents that are CYP3A4 inhibitors may increase the plasma levels of carbamazepine).
No products indexed under this heading.

Ondansetron (Carbamazepine is known to induce CYP1A2 and CYP3A4. Therefore, the potential exists for interaction between carbamazepine and any agent metabolized by one (or more) of these enzymes. Agents that are metabolized by CYP1A2 and CYP3A4 may have decreased plasma levels when administered concomitantly with carbamazepine).
No products indexed under this heading.

Ondansetron Hydrochloride (Carbamazepine is known to induce CYP1A2 and CYP3A4. Therefore, the potential exists for interaction between carbamazepine and any agent metabolized by one (or more) of these enzymes. Agents that are metabolized by CYP1A2 and CYP3A4 may have decreased plasma levels when administered concomitantly with carbamazepine). Products include:

Oxazepam (Because of its primary CNS effect, caution should be used when carbamazepine is taken with other centrally acting drugs).
No products indexed under this heading.

Oxcarbazepine (Carbamazepine is metabolized by CYP3A4. Therefore, the potential exists for interaction between carbamazepine and any agent that induces CYP3A4. Agents that are CYP3A4 inducers may decrease plasma levels of carbamazepine).
No products indexed under this heading.

Oxiconazole Nitrate (Carbamazepine is metabolized mainly by CYP3A4 the active carbamazepine 10,11-epoxide, which is futher metabolized to the trans-diol by epoxide hydrolase. Therefore, the potential exists for interaction between carbamazepine and any agent that inhibits CYP3A4 and/or epoxide hydrolase. Agents that are CYP3A4 inhibitors, such as azole antifungals, may increase the plasma levels of carbamazepine).
No products indexed under this heading.

Oxycodone Hydrochloride (Because of its primary CNS effect, caution should be used when carbamazepine is taken with other centrally acting drugs). Products include:

Paclitaxel (Carbamazepine is known to induce CYP1A2 and CYP3A4. Therefore, the potential exists for interaction between carbamazepine and any agent metabolized by one (or more) of these enzymes. Agents that are metabolized by CYP1A2 and CYP3A4 may have decreased plasma levels when administered concomitantly with carbamazepine).
No products indexed under this heading.

Paliperidone (Isolated cases of neuroleptic malignant syndrome have been reported with concomitant use of psychotropic drugs). Products include:

Pargyline Hydrochloride (Coadministration of carbamazepine with MAO inhibitors is contraindicated. MAO inhibitors should be discontinued for a minimum of 14 days, or longer if the clinical situation permits).
No products indexed under this heading.

Paroxetine Hydrochloride (Carbamazepine is metabolized mainly by CYP3A4 the active carbamazepine 10,11-epoxide, which is further metabolized to the trans-diol by epoxide hydrolase. Therefore, the potential exists for interaction between carbamazepine and any agent that inhibits CYP3A4 and/or epoxide hydrolase. Agents that are

Equetro **Interactions Index** **604**

CYP3A4 inhibitors may increase the plasma levels of carbamazepine). Products include:

Paroxetine CR 2361
Paroxetine ER 2371
Paxil 1586
Paxil CR 1596

Pemoline (Because of its primary CNS effect, caution should be used when carbamazepine is taken with other centrally acting drugs).
No products indexed under this heading.

Pentobarbital Sodium (Because of its primary CNS effect, caution should be used when carbamazepine is taken with other centrally acting drugs). Products include:

Nembutal 2012

Perphenazine (Because of its primary CNS effect, caution should be used when carbamazepine is taken with other centrally acting drugs).
No products indexed under this heading.

Phenelzine Sulfate (Co-administration of carbamazepine with MAO inhibitors is contraindicated. MAO inhibitors should be discontinued for a minimum of 14 days, or longer if the clinical situation permits).
No products indexed under this heading.

Phenobarbital (Because of its primary CNS effect, caution should be used when carbamazepine is taken with other centrally acting drugs). Products include:

Donnatal 2711

Phenobarbital Sodium (Because of its primary CNS effect, caution should be used when carbamazepine is taken with other centrally acting drugs).
No products indexed under this heading.

Phenytoin (Carbamazepine is metabolized by CYP3A4. Therefore, the potential exists for interaction between carbamazepine and any agent that induces CYP3A4. Agents that are CYP3A4 inducers may decrease plasma levels of carbamazepine. Carbamazepine may increase the plasma levels of phenytoin; careful monitoring of phenytoin plasma levels following co-medication with carbamazepine is advised).
No products indexed under this heading.

Phenytoin Sodium (Carbamazepine is metabolized by CYP3A4. Therefore, the potential exists for interaction between carbamazepine and any agent that induces CYP3A4. Agents that are CYP3A4 inducers may decrease plasma levels of carbamazepine. Carbamazepine may increase the plasma levels of phenytoin; careful monitoring of phenytoin plasma levels following co-medication with carbamazepine is advised). Products include:

Phenytek Capsules 2380

Pimozide (Carbamazepine is known to induce CYP1A2 and CYP3A4. Therefore, the potential exists for interaction between carbamazepine and any agent metabolized by one (or more) of these enzymes. Agents that are metabolized by CYP1A2 and CYP3A4 may have decreased plasma levels when administered concomitantly with carbamazepine).
No products indexed under this heading.

Polyestradiol Phosphate (Carbamazepine is known to induce CYP1A2 and CYP3A4. Therefore, the potential exists for interaction between carbamazepine and any agent metabolized by one (or more) of these enzymes. Agents that are metabolized by CYP1A2 and CYP3A4 may have decreased plasma levels when administered concomitantly with carbamazepine).
No products indexed under this heading.

Posaconazole (Carbamazepine is metabolized mainly by CYP3A4 the active carbamazepine 10,11-epoxide, which is futher metabolized to the trans-diol by epoxide hydrolase. Therefore, the potential exists for interaction between carbamazepine and any agent that inhibits CYP3A4 and/or epoxide hydrolase. Agents that are CYP3A4 inhibitors, such as azole antifungals, may increase the plasma levels of carbamazepine). Products include:

Noxafil 3172

Prazepam (Because of its primary CNS effect, caution should be used when carbamazepine is taken with other centrally acting drugs).
No products indexed under this heading.

Prednisolone (Carbamazepine is metabolized by CYP3A4. Therefore, the potential exists for interaction between carbamazepine and any agent that induces CYP3A4. Agents that are CYP3A4 inducers may decrease plasma levels of carbamazepine).
No products indexed under this heading.

Prednisolone Acetate (Carbamazepine is known to induce CYP1A2 and CYP3A4. Therefore, the potential exists for interaction between carbamazepine and any agent metabolized by one (or more) of these enzymes. Agents that are metabolized by CYP1A2 and CYP3A4, such as glucocorticoids, may have decreased plasma levels when administered concomitantly with carbamazepine). Products include:

Blephamide .... ⊙212, ⊙214
Pred Forte .... ⊙225
Pred Mild .... ⊙230
Pred-G .... ⊙226, ⊙227

Prednisolone Sodium Phosphate (Carbamazepine is known to induce CYP1A2 and CYP3A4. Therefore, the potential exists for interaction between carbamazepine and any agent metabolized by one (or more) of these enzymes. Agents that are metabolized by CYP1A2 and CYP3A4, such as glucocorticoids, may have decreased plasma levels when administered concomitantly with carbamazepine).
No products indexed under this heading.

Prednisolone Tebutate (Carbamazepine is known to induce CYP1A2 and CYP3A4. Therefore, the potential exists for interaction between carbamazepine and any agent metabolized by one (or more) of these enzymes. Agents that are metabolized by CYP1A2 and CYP3A4, such as glucocorticoids, may have decreased plasma levels when administered concomitantly with carbamazepine).
No products indexed under this heading.

Prednisone (Carbamazepine is known to induce CYP1A2 and CYP3A4. Therefore, the potential exists for interaction between carbamazepine and any agent metabolized by one (or more) of these enzymes. Agents that are metabolized by CYP1A2 and CYP3A4, such as glucocorticoids, may have decreased plasma levels when administered concomitantly with carbamazepine).
No products indexed under this heading.

Prednisone sodium phosphate (Carbamazepine is metabolized by CYP3A4. Therefore, the potential exists for interaction between carbamazepine and any agent that induces CYP3A4. Agents that are CYP3A4 inducers may decrease plasma levels of carbamazepine).
No products indexed under this heading.

Primidone (Carbamazepine increases the plasma levels of primidone).
No products indexed under this heading.

Procarbazine Hydrochloride (Co-administration of carbamazepine with MAO inhibitors is contraindicated. MAO inhibitors should be discontinued for a minimum of 14 days, or longer if the clinical situation permits).
No products indexed under this heading.

Prochlorperazine (Because of its primary CNS effect, caution should be used when carbamazepine is taken with other centrally acting drugs).
No products indexed under this heading.

Promethazine Hydrochloride (Because of its primary CNS effect, caution should be used when carbamazepine is taken with other centrally acting drugs).
No products indexed under this heading.

Propafenone Hydrochloride (Carbamazepine is known to induce CYP1A2 and CYP3A4. Therefore, the potential exists for interaction between carbamazepine and any agent metabolized by one (or more) of these enzymes. Agents that are metabolized by CYP1A2 and CYP3A4 may have decreased plasma levels when administered concomitantly with carbamazepine). Products include:

Rythmol 1648
Rythmol SR 1652

Propofol (Because of its primary CNS effect, caution should be used when carbamazepine is taken with other centrally acting drugs).
No products indexed under this heading.

Propoxyphene Hydrochloride (Because of its primary CNS effect, caution should be used when carbamazepine is taken with other centrally acting drugs).
No products indexed under this heading.

Propoxyphene Napsylate (Because of its primary CNS effect, caution should be used when carbamazepine is taken with other centrally acting drugs).
No products indexed under this heading.

Propranolol Hydrochloride (Carbamazepine is known to induce CYP1A2 and CYP3A4. Therefore, the potential exists for interaction between carbamazepine and any agent metabolized by one (or more) of these enzymes. Agents that are metabolized by CYP1A2 and CYP3A4 may have decreased plasma levels when administered concomitantly with carbamazepine). Products include:

InnoPran XL 1517

Protriptyline Hydrochloride (Carbamazepine is contraindicated in patients with a known sensitivity to any of the tricyclic compounds, such as amitriptyline, desipramine, imipramine, protriptyline, and nortriptyline).
No products indexed under this heading.

Pyrimethamine (Anti-malarial drugs, such as chloroquine and mefloquine, may antagonize the activity of carbamazepine). Products include:

Daraprim 1423

Quazepam (Because of its primary CNS effect, caution should be used when carbamazepine is taken with other centrally acting drugs).
No products indexed under this heading.

Quetiapine Fumarate (Because of its primary CNS effect, caution should be used when carbamazepine is taken with other centrally acting drugs). Products include:

Seroquel 750
Seroquel XR 759

Quinidine (Carbamazepine is metabolized mainly by CYP3A4 the active carbamazepine 10,11-epoxide, which is further metabolized to the trans-diol by epoxide hydrolase. Therefore, the potential exists for interaction between carbamazepine and any agent that inhibits CYP3A4 and/or epoxide hydrolase. Agents that are CYP3A4 inhibitors may increase the plasma levels of carbamazepine).
No products indexed under this heading.

Quinidine Gluconate (Carbamazepine is known to induce CYP1A2 and CYP3A4. Therefore, the potential exists for interaction between carbamazepine and any agent metabolized by one (or more) of these enzymes. Agents that are metabolized by CYP1A2 and CYP3A4 may have decreased plasma levels when administered concomitantly with carbamazepine).
No products indexed under this heading.

Quinidine Hydrochloride (Carbamazepine is metabolized mainly by CYP3A4 the active carbamazepine 10,11-epoxide, which is further metabolized to the trans-diol by epoxide hydrolase. Therefore, the potential exists for interaction between carbamazepine and any agent that inhibits CYP3A4 and/or epoxide hydrolase. Agents that are CYP3A4 inhibitors may increase the plasma levels of carbamazepine).
No products indexed under this heading.

Quinidine Polygalacturonate (Carbamazepine is known to induce CYP1A2 and CYP3A4. Therefore, the potential exists for interaction between carbamazepine and any agent metabolized by one (or more) of these enzymes. Agents that are metabolized by CYP1A2 and CYP3A4 may have decreased plasma levels when administered concomitantly with carbamazepine).
No products indexed under this heading.

Quinidine Sulfate (Carbamazepine is known to induce CYP1A2 and CYP3A4. Therefore, the potential exists for interaction between carbamazepine and any agent metabolized by one (or more) of these enzymes. Agents that are metabolized by CYP1A2 and CYP3A4 may have decreased plasma levels when administered concomitantly with carbamazepine).
No products indexed under this heading.

Quinine (Carbamazepine is metabolized mainly by CYP3A4 the active carbamazepine 10,11-epoxide, which is further metabolized to the trans-diol by epoxide hydrolase. Therefore, the potential exists for interaction between carbamazepine and any agent that inhibits CYP3A4 and/or epoxide hydrolase. Agents that are CYP3A4 inhibitors may increase the plasma levels of carbamazepine). Products include:

Hyland's Leg Cramps PM with Quinine 3315

Quinine Sulfate (Carbamazepine is metabolized mainly by CYP3A4 the active carbamazepine 10,11-epoxide, which is further metabolized to the trans-diol by epoxide hydrolase. Therefore, the potential exists for interaction between carbamazepine and any agent that inhibits CYP3A4 and/or epoxide hydrolase. Agents that are CYP3A4 inhibitors may increase the plasma levels of carbamazepine).
No products indexed under this heading.

Quinupristin (Carbamazepine is metabolized mainly by CYP3A4 the active carbamazepine 10,11-epoxide, which is further metabolized to the trans-diol by epoxide hydrolase. Therefore, the potential exists for interaction between carbamazepine and any agent that inhibits CYP3A4 and/or epoxide hydrolase. Agents that are CYP3A4 inhibitors may increase the plasma levels of carbamazepine).
No products indexed under this heading.

Ranitidine Bismuth Citrate (Carbamazepine is metabolized mainly by CYP3A4 the active carbamazepine 10,11-epoxide, which is further metabolized to the trans-diol by epoxide hydrolase. Therefore, the potential exists for interaction between carbamazepine and any agent that inhibits CYP3A4 and/or

epoxide hydrolase. Agents that are CYP3A4 inhibitors may increase the plasma levels of carbamazepine).
No products indexed under this heading.

Ranitidine Hydrochloride (Carbamazepine is metabolized mainly by CYP3A4 the active carbamazepine 10,11-epoxide, which is further metabolized to the trans-diol by epoxide hydrolase. Therefore, the potential exists for interaction between carbamazepine and any agent that inhibits CYP3A4 and/or epoxide hydrolase. Agents that are CYP3A4 inhibitors may increase the plasma levels of carbamazepine). Products include:

Rasagiline Mesylate (Co-administration of carbamazepine with MAO inhibitors is contraindicated. MAO inhibitors should be discontinued for a minimum of 14 days, or longer if the clinical situation permits). Products include:

Remifentanil Hydrochloride (Because of its primary CNS effect, caution should be used when carbamazepine is taken with other centrally acting drugs).
No products indexed under this heading.

Rifabutin (Carbamazepine is metabolized by CYP3A4. Therefore, the potential exists for interaction between carbamazepine and any agent that induces CYP3A4. Agents that are CYP3A4 inducers may decrease plasma levels of carbamazepine).
No products indexed under this heading.

Rifampicin (Carbamazepine is metabolized by CYP3A4. Therefore, the potential exists for interaction between carbamazepine and any agent that induces CYP3A4. Agents that are CYP3A4 inducers may decrease plasma levels of carbamazepine).
No products indexed under this heading.

Rifampin (Carbamazepine is metabolized by CYP3A4. Therefore, the potential exists for interaction between carbamazepine and any agent that induces CYP3A4. Agents that are CYP3A4 inducers may decrease plasma levels of carbamazepine).
No products indexed under this heading.

Rifapentine (Carbamazepine is metabolized by CYP3A4. Therefore, the potential exists for interaction between carbamazepine and any agent that induces CYP3A4. Agents that are CYP3A4 inducers may decrease plasma levels of carbamazepine).
No products indexed under this heading.

Riluzole (Carbamazepine is known to induce CYP1A2 and CYP3A4. Therefore, the potential exists for interaction between carbamazepine and any agent metabolized by one (or more) of these enzymes. Agents that are metabolized by CYP1A2 and CYP3A4 may have decreased plasma levels when administered concomitantly with carbamazepine). Products include:

Risperidone (Because of its primary CNS effect, caution should be used when carbamazepine is taken with other centrally acting drugs). Products include:

Ritonavir (Carbamazepine is metabolized mainly by CYP3A4 the active carbamazepine 10,11-epoxide, which is further metabolized to the trans-diol by epoxide hydrolase. Therefore, the potential exists for interaction between carbamazepine and any agent that inhibits CYP3A4 and/or epoxide hydrolase. Agents that are CYP3A4 inhibitors,

such as protease inhibitors, may increase the plasma levels of carbamazepine). Products include:

Ropinirole Hydrochloride (Carbamazepine is known to induce CYP1A2 and CYP3A4. Therefore, the potential exists for interaction between carbamazepine and any agent metabolized by one (or more) of these enzymes. Agents that are metabolized by CYP1A2 and CYP3A4 may have decreased plasma levels when administered concomitantly with carbamazepine). Products include:

Ropivacaine Hydrochloride (Carbamazepine is known to induce CYP1A2 and CYP3A4. Therefore, the potential exists for interaction between carbamazepine and any agent metabolized by one (or more) of these enzymes. Agents that are metabolized by CYP1A2 and CYP3A4 may have decreased plasma levels when administered concomitantly with carbamazepine).
No products indexed under this heading.

Saquinavir (Carbamazepine is metabolized mainly by CYP3A4 the active carbamazepine 10,11-epoxide, which is further metabolized to the trans-diol by epoxide hydrolase. Therefore, the potential exists for interaction between carbamazepine and any agent that inhibits CYP3A4 and/or epoxide hydrolase. Agents that are CYP3A4 inhibitors, such as protease inhibitors, may increase the plasma levels of carbamazepine).
No products indexed under this heading.

Saquinavir Mesylate (Carbamazepine is metabolized mainly by CYP3A4 the active carbamazepine 10,11-epoxide, which is further metabolized to the trans-diol by epoxide hydrolase. Therefore, the potential exists for interaction between carbamazepine and any agent that inhibits CYP3A4 and/or epoxide hydrolase. Agents that are CYP3A4 inhibitors, such as protease inhibitors, may increase the plasma levels of carbamazepine).
No products indexed under this heading.

Secobarbital Sodium (Because of its primary CNS effect, caution should be used when carbamazepine is taken with other centrally acting drugs).
No products indexed under this heading.

Selegiline (Co-administration of carbamazepine with MAO inhibitors is contraindicated. MAO inhibitors should be discontinued for a minimum of 14 days, or longer if the clinical situation permits). Products include:

Selegiline Hydrochloride (Co-administration of carbamazepine with MAO inhibitors is contraindicated. MAO inhibitors should be discontinued for a minimum of 14 days, or longer if the clinical situation permits). Products include:

Sertaconazole Nitrate (Carbamazepine is metabolized mainly by CYP3A4 the active carbamazepine 10,11-epoxide, which is futher metabolized to the trans-diol by epoxide hydrolase. Therefore, the potential exists for interaction between carbamazepine and any agent that inhibits CYP3A4 and/or epoxide hydrolase. Agents that are CYP3A4 inhibitors, such as azole antifungals, may increase the plasma levels of carbamazepine).
No products indexed under this heading.

Sertraline Hydrochloride (Carbamazepine is known to induce CYP1A2 and CYP3A4. Therefore, the potential exists for interaction between carbamazepine and any agent metabolized by one (or more) of these enzymes. Agents that are metabolized by CYP1A2 and CYP3A4 may have decreased plasma levels when administered concomitantly with carbamazepine).
No products indexed under this heading.

Sevoflurane (Because of its primary CNS effect, caution should be used when carbamazepine is taken with other centrally acting drugs). Products include:

Sildenafil Citrate (Carbamazepine is known to induce CYP1A2 and CYP3A4. Therefore, the potential exists for interaction between carbamazepine and any agent metabolized by one (or more) of these enzymes. Agents that are metabolized by CYP1A2 and CYP3A4 may have decreased plasma levels when administered concomitantly with carbamazepine).
No products indexed under this heading.

Simvastatin (Carbamazepine is known to induce CYP1A2 and CYP3A4. Therefore, the potential exists for interaction between carbamazepine and any agent metabolized by one (or more) of these enzymes. Agents that are metabolized by CYP1A2 and CYP3A4 may have decreased plasma levels when administered concomitantly with carbamazepine). Products include:

Sirolimus (Carbamazepine is known to induce CYP1A2 and CYP3A4. Therefore, the potential exists for interaction between carbamazepine and any agent metabolized by one (or more) of these enzymes. Agents that are metabolized by CYP1A2 and CYP3A4 may have decreased plasma levels when administered concomitantly with carbamazepine). Products include:

Sodium Oxybate (Because of its primary CNS effect, caution should be used when carbamazepine is taken with other centrally acting drugs).
No products indexed under this heading.

Sufentanil Citrate (Because of its primary CNS effect, caution should be used when carbamazepine is taken with other centrally acting drugs).
No products indexed under this heading.

Sulfinpyrazone (Carbamazepine is metabolized by CYP3A4. Therefore, the potential exists for interaction between carbamazepine and any agent that induces CYP3A4. Agents that are CYP3A4 inducers may decrease plasma levels of carbamazepine).
No products indexed under this heading.

Tacrine Hydrochloride (Carbamazepine is known to induce CYP1A2 and CYP3A4. Therefore, the potential exists for interaction between carbamazepine and any agent metabolized by one (or more) of these enzymes. Agents that are metabolized by CYP1A2 and CYP3A4 may have decreased plasma levels when administered concomitantly with carbamazepine).
No products indexed under this heading.

Tacrolimus (Carbamazepine is known to induce CYP1A2 and CYP3A4. Therefore, the potential exists for interaction between carbamazepine and any agent metabolized by one (or more) of these enzymes. Agents that are metabolized by CYP1A2 and CYP3A4 may have

decreased plasma levels when administered concomitantly with carbamazepine). Products include:

Tadalafil (Carbamazepine is known to induce CYP1A2 and CYP3A4. Therefore, the potential exists for interaction between carbamazepine and any agent metabolized by one (or more) of these enzymes. Agents that are metabolized by CYP1A2 and CYP3A4 may have decreased plasma levels when administered concomitantly with carbamazepine). Products include:

Tamoxifen Citrate (Carbamazepine is known to induce CYP1A2 and CYP3A4. Therefore, the potential exists for interaction between carbamazepine and any agent metabolized by one (or more) of these enzymes. Agents that are metabolized by CYP1A2 and CYP3A4 may have decreased plasma levels when administered concomitantly with carbamazepine).
No products indexed under this heading.

Telithromycin (Carbamazepine is metabolized mainly by CYP3A4 the active carbamazepine 10,11-epoxide, which is further metabolized to the trans-diol by epoxide hydrolase. Therefore, the potential exists for interaction between carbamazepine and any agent that inhibits CYP3A4 and/or epoxide hydrolase. Agents that are CYP3A4 inhibitors may increase the plasma levels of carbamazepine). Products include:

Temazepam (Because of its primary CNS effect, caution should be used when carbamazepine is taken with other centrally acting drugs).
No products indexed under this heading.

Terconazole (Carbamazepine is metabolized mainly by CYP3A4 the active carbamazepine 10,11-epoxide, which is futher metabolized to the trans-diol by epoxide hydrolase. Therefore, the potential exists for interaction between carbamazepine and any agent that inhibits CYP3A4 and/or epoxide hydrolase. Agents that are CYP3A4 inhibitors, such as azole antifungals, may increase the plasma levels of carbamazepine).
No products indexed under this heading.

Terfenadine (Carbamazepine is known to induce CYP1A2 and CYP3A4. Therefore, the potential exists for interaction between carbamazepine and any agent metabolized by one (or more) of these enzymes. Agents that are metabolized by CYP1A2 and CYP3A4 may have decreased plasma levels when administered concomitantly with carbamazepine).
No products indexed under this heading.

Theobromine (Carbamazepine is known to induce CYP1A2 and CYP3A4. Therefore, the potential exists for interaction between carbamazepine and any agent metabolized by one (or more) of these enzymes. Agents that are metabolized by CYP1A2 and CYP3A4 may have decreased plasma levels when administered concomitantly with carbamazepine).
No products indexed under this heading.

Theophyllinate (Carbamazepine is metabolized by CYP3A4. Therefore, the potential exists for interaction between carbamazepine and any agent that induces CYP3A4. Agents that are CYP3A4 inducers may decrease plasma levels of carbamazepine).
No products indexed under this heading.

IMPORTANT NOTE: Always consult each drug listing in the patient's regimen for possible interactions.

Theophylline (Carbamazepine is metabolized by CYP3A4. Therefore, the potential exists for interaction between carbamazepine and any agent that induces CYP3A4. Agents that are CYP3A4 inducers, such as theophylline, may decrease plasma levels of carbamazepine).

No products indexed under this heading.

Theophylline Anhydrous (Carbamazepine is metabolized by CYP3A4. Therefore, the potential exists for interaction between carbamazepine and any agent that induces CYP3A4. Agents that are CYP3A4 inducers, such as theophylline, may decrease plasma levels of carbamazepine). Products include:
Uniphyl 2817

Theophylline Calcium Salicylate (Carbamazepine is metabolized by CYP3A4. Therefore, the potential exists for interaction between carbamazepine and any agent that induces CYP3A4. Agents that are CYP3A4 inducers, such as theophylline, may decrease plasma levels of carbamazepine).

No products indexed under this heading.

Theophylline Dihydroxypropyl (Glyceryl) (Carbamazepine is metabolized by CYP3A4. Therefore, the potential exists for interaction between carbamazepine and any agent that induces CYP3A4. Agents that are CYP3A4 inducers, such as theophylline, may decrease plasma levels of carbamazepine).

No products indexed under this heading.

Theophylline Ethylenediamine (Carbamazepine is metabolized by CYP3A4. Therefore, the potential exists for interaction between carbamazepine and any agent that induces CYP3A4. Agents that are CYP3A4 inducers, such as theophylline, may decrease plasma levels of carbamazepine).

No products indexed under this heading.

Theophylline Sodium Glycinate (Carbamazepine is metabolized by CYP3A4. Therefore, the potential exists for interaction between carbamazepine and any agent that induces CYP3A4. Agents that are CYP3A4 inducers, such as theophylline, may decrease plasma levels of carbamazepine).

No products indexed under this heading.

Thiamylal Sodium (Because of its primary CNS effect, caution should be used when carbamazepine is taken with other centrally acting drugs).

No products indexed under this heading.

Thioridazine Hydrochloride (Because of its primary CNS effect, caution should be used when carbamazepine is taken with other centrally acting drugs). Products include:
Thioridazine Hydrochloride 2384

Thiothixene (Because of its primary CNS effect, caution should be used when carbamazepine is taken with other centrally acting drugs). Products include:
Thiothixene 2386

Tiagabine Hydrochloride (Carbamazepine is known to induce CYP1A2 and CYP3A4. Therefore, the potential exists for interaction between carbamazepine and any agent metabolized by one (or more) of these enzymes. Agents that are metabolized by CYP1A2 and CYP3A4 may have decreased plasma levels when administered concomitantly with carbamazepine). Products include:
Gabitril 972

Tipranavir (Carbamazepine is metabolized mainly by CYP3A4 the active carbamazepine 10,11-epoxide, which is further metabolized to the trans-diol by epoxide hydrolase. Therefore, the potential exists for interaction between carbamazepine and any agent that inhibits CYP3A4 and/or epoxide hydrolase. Agents that are CYP3A4 inhibitors,

such as protease inhibitors, may increase the plasma levels of carbamazepine).

No products indexed under this heading.

Tizanidine (Carbamazepine is known to induce CYP1A2 and CYP3A4. Therefore, the potential exists for interaction between carbamazepine and any agent metabolized by one (or more) of these enzymes. Agents that are metabolized by CYP1A2 and CYP3A4 may have decreased plasma levels when administered concomitantly with carbamazepine).

No products indexed under this heading.

Tizanidine Hydrochloride (Carbamazepine is known to induce CYP1A2 and CYP3A4. Therefore, the potential exists for interaction between carbamazepine and any agent metabolized by one (or more) of these enzymes. Agents that are metabolized by CYP1A2 and CYP3A4 may have decreased plasma levels when administered concomitantly with carbamazepine).

No products indexed under this heading.

Tolterodine Tartrate (Carbamazepine is known to induce CYP1A2 and CYP3A4. Therefore, the potential exists for interaction between carbamazepine and any agent metabolized by one (or more) of these enzymes. Agents that are metabolized by CYP1A2 and CYP3A4 may have decreased plasma levels when administered concomitantly with carbamazepine).

No products indexed under this heading.

Tranylcypromine Sulfate (Co-administration of carbamazepine with MAO inhibitors is contraindicated. MAO inhibitors should be discontinued for a minimum of 14 days, or longer if the clinical situation permits). Products include:
Parnate 1584

Trazodone Hydrochloride (Carbamazepine is known to induce CYP1A2 and CYP3A4. Agents that are metabolized by CYP1A2 and CYP3A4 may have decreased plasma levels when administered concomitantly with carbamazepine. Following co-administration of carbamazepine 400 mg/day with trazodone 100 mg to 300 mg daily, carbamazepine reduced the plasma concentration of trazodone by 76% and 60%, respectively, compared to pre-carbamazepine values).

No products indexed under this heading.

Triamcinolone (Carbamazepine is known to induce CYP1A2 and CYP3A4. Therefore, the potential exists for interaction between carbamazepine and any agent metabolized by one (or more) of these enzymes. Agents that are metabolized by CYP1A2 and CYP3A4, such as glucocorticoids, may have decreased plasma levels when administered concomitantly with carbamazepine).

No products indexed under this heading.

Triamcinolone Acetonide (Carbamazepine is known to induce CYP1A2 and CYP3A4. Therefore, the potential exists for interaction between carbamazepine and any agent metabolized by one (or more) of these enzymes. Agents that are metabolized by CYP1A2 and CYP3A4, such as glucocorticoids, may have decreased plasma levels when administered concomitantly with carbamazepine). Products include:
Azmacort 408
Nasacort AQ 3019

Triamcinolone Diacetate (Carbamazepine is known to induce CYP1A2 and CYP3A4. Therefore, the potential exists for interaction between carbamazepine and any agent metabolized by one (or more) of these enzymes. Agents that are metabolized by CYP1A2 and CYP3A4, such as glucocorticoids, may have decreased plasma levels when administered concomitantly with carbamazepine).

No products indexed under this heading.

Triamcinolone Hexacetonide (Carbamazepine is known to induce CYP1A2 and CYP3A4. Therefore, the potential exists for interaction between carbamazepine and any agent metabolized by one (or more) of these enzymes. Agents that are metabolized by CYP1A2 and CYP3A4, such as glucocorticoids, may have decreased plasma levels when administered concomitantly with carbamazepine).

No products indexed under this heading.

Triazolam (Because of its primary CNS effect, caution should be used when carbamazepine is taken with other centrally acting drugs).

No products indexed under this heading.

Trifluoperazine Hydrochloride (Because of its primary CNS effect, caution should be used when carbamazepine is taken with other centrally acting drugs).

No products indexed under this heading.

Trimethaphan Camsylate (Carbamazepine is known to induce CYP1A2 and CYP3A4. Therefore, the potential exists for interaction between carbamazepine and any agent metabolized by one (or more) of these enzymes. Agents that are metabolized by CYP1A2 and CYP3A4 may have decreased plasma levels when administered concomitantly with carbamazepine).

No products indexed under this heading.

Trimipramine Maleate (Carbamazepine is contraindicated in patients with a known sensitivity to any of the tricyclic compounds, such as amitriptyline, desipramine, imipramine, protriptyline, and nortriptyline).

No products indexed under this heading.

Troglitazone (Carbamazepine is metabolized by CYP3A4. Therefore, the potential exists for interaction between carbamazepine and any agent that induces CYP3A4. Agents that are CYP3A4 inducers may decrease plasma levels of carbamazepine).

No products indexed under this heading.

Troleandomycin (Carbamazepine is metabolized mainly by CYP3A4 the active carbamazepine 10,11-epoxide, which is further metabolized to the trans-diol by epoxide hydrolase. Therefore, the potential exists for interaction between carbamazepine and any agent that inhibits CYP3A4 and/or epoxide hydrolase. Agents that are CYP3A4 inhibitors may increase the plasma levels of carbamazepine).

No products indexed under this heading.

Trovafloxacin Mesylate (Carbamazepine is known to induce CYP1A2 and CYP3A4. Therefore, the potential exists for interaction between carbamazepine and any agent metabolized by one (or more) of these enzymes. Agents that are metabolized by CYP1A2 and CYP3A4 may have decreased plasma levels when administered concomitantly with carbamazepine).

No products indexed under this heading.

Valproate Sodium (Carbamazepine is metabolized mainly by CYP3A4 the active carbamazepine 10,11-epoxide, which is further metabolized to the trans-diol by epoxide hydrolase. Therefore, the potential exists for interaction between carbamazepine and any agent

that inhibits CYP3A4 and/or epoxide hydrolase. Agents that are CYP3A4 inhibitors, such as valproate, may increase the plasma levels of carbamazepine. Also inhibits epoxide hydroxylase, resulting in increased levels of the active metabolite carbamazepine-10,11-epoxide).

No products indexed under this heading.

Valproic Acid (Carbamazepine is metabolized mainly by CYP3A4 the active carbamazepine 10,11-epoxide, which is further metabolized to the trans-diol by epoxide hydrolase. Therefore, the potential exists for interaction between carbamazepine and any agent that inhibits CYP3A4 and/or epoxide hydrolase. Agents that are CYP3A4 inhibitors, such as valproate, may increase the plasma levels of carbamazepine. Also inhibits epoxide hydroxylase, resulting in increased levels of the active metabolite carbamazepine-10,11-epoxide).

No products indexed under this heading.

Vardenafil Hydrochloride (Carbamazepine is known to induce CYP1A2 and CYP3A4. Therefore, the potential exists for interaction between carbamazepine and any agent metabolized by one (or more) of these enzymes. Agents that are metabolized by CYP1A2 and CYP3A4 may have decreased plasma levels when administered concomitantly with carbamazepine). Products include:
Levitra 3157

Verapamil Hydrochloride (Carbamazepine is known to induce CYP1A2 and CYP3A4. Therefore, the potential exists for interaction between carbamazepine and any agent metabolized by one (or more) of these enzymes. Agents that are metabolized by CYP1A2 and CYP3A4 may have decreased plasma levels when administered concomitantly with carbamazepine). Products include:
Tarka 534

Vinblastine Sulfate (Carbamazepine is known to induce CYP1A2 and CYP3A4. Therefore, the potential exists for interaction between carbamazepine and any agent metabolized by one (or more) of these enzymes. Agents that are metabolized by CYP1A2 and CYP3A4 may have decreased plasma levels when administered concomitantly with carbamazepine).

No products indexed under this heading.

Vincristine Sulfate (Carbamazepine is known to induce CYP1A2 and CYP3A4. Therefore, the potential exists for interaction between carbamazepine and any agent metabolized by one (or more) of these enzymes. Agents that are metabolized by CYP1A2 and CYP3A4 may have decreased plasma levels when administered concomitantly with carbamazepine).

No products indexed under this heading.

Voriconazole (Carbamazepine is metabolized mainly by CYP3A4 the active carbamazepine 10,11-epoxide, which is futher metabolized to the trans-diol by epoxide hydrolase. Therefore, the potential exists for interaction between carbamazepine and any agent that inhibits CYP3A4 and/or epoxide hydrolase. Agents that are CYP3A4 inhibitors, such as azole antifungals, may increase the plasma levels of carbamazepine).

No products indexed under this heading.

Warfarin Sodium (Carbamazepine is known to induce CYP1A2 and CYP3A4. Therefore, the potential exists for interaction between carbamazepine and any agent metabolized by one (or more) of these enzymes. Agents that are metabolized by CYP1A2 or CYP3A4 may have decreased plasma levels when administered concomitantly with carbamazepine. Thus, if a patient has been titrated

to a stable dosage on one of the agents in these categories, and then begins a course of treatment with carbamazepine, it is reasonable to expect that a dose increase for the concomitant agent may be necessary. Therefore, warfarin's anticoagulant effect may be reduced in the presence of carbamazepine and dosage adjustment may be necessary).

No products indexed under this heading.

Zafirlukast (Carbamazepine is metabolized mainly by CYP3A4 the active carbamazepine 10,11-epoxide, which is further metabolized to the trans-diol by epoxide hydrolase. Therefore, the potential exists for interaction between carbamazepine and any agent that inhibits CYP3A4 and/or epoxide hydrolase. Agents that are CYP3A4 inhibitors may increase the plasma levels of carbamazepine). Products include:
Accolate 3612

Zaleplon (Because of its primary CNS effect, caution should be used when carbamazepine is taken with other centrally acting drugs).

No products indexed under this heading.

Zileuton (Carbamazepine is known to induce CYP1A2 and CYP3A4. Therefore, the potential exists for interaction between carbamazepine and any agent metabolized by one (or more) of these enzymes. Agents that are metabolized by CYP1A2 and CYP3A4 may have decreased plasma levels when administered concomitantly with carbamazepine).

No products indexed under this heading.

Ziprasidone Hydrochloride (Because of its primary CNS effect, caution should be used when carbamazepine is taken with other centrally acting drugs). Products include:
Geodon 2723

Zolmitriptan (Carbamazepine is known to induce CYP1A2 and CYP3A4. Therefore, the potential exists for interaction between carbamazepine and any agent metabolized by one (or more) of these enzymes. Agents that are metabolized by CYP1A2 and CYP3A4 may have decreased plasma levels when administered concomitantly with carbamazepine). Products include:
Zomig Tablets 773
Zomig Nasal Spray 768
Zomig-ZMT Tablets 773

Zolpidem Tartrate (Because of its primary CNS effect, caution should be used when carbamazepine is taken with other centrally acting drugs). Products include:
Ambien 2920
Ambien CR 2925

Food Interactions

Alcohol (Because of its primary CNS effect, caution should be used when carbamazepine is taken with alcohol).

Beer, reduced-alcohol (Because of its primary CNS effect, caution should be used when carbamazepine is taken with alcohol).

Beer, unspecified (Because of its primary CNS effect, caution should be used when carbamazepine is taken with alcohol).

Food, caffeine-containing (Carbamazepine is known to induce CYP1A2 and CYP3A4. Therefore, the potential exists for interaction between carbamazepine and any agent metabolized by one (or more) of these enzymes. Agents that are metabolized by CYP1A2 and CYP3A4 may have decreased plasma levels when administered concomitantly with carbamazepine).

Grapefruit (Carbamazepine is metabolized mainly by CYP3A4 the active carbamazepine 10,11-epoxide, which is further metabolized to the trans-diol by epoxide hydrolase. Therefore, the potential exists for interaction between carbamazepine and any agent that inhibits CYP3A4 and/or epoxide hydrolase. Agents that are CYP3A4 inhibitors may increase the plasma levels of carbamazepine).

Grapefruit Juice (Carbamazepine is metabolized mainly by CYP3A4 the active carbamazepine 10,11-epoxide, which is further metabolized to the trans-diol by epoxide hydrolase. Therefore, the potential exists for interaction between carbamazepine and any agent that inhibits CYP3A4 and/or epoxide hydrolase. Agents that are CYP3A4 inhibitors may increase the plasma levels of carbamazepine).

Wine, Chianti (Because of its primary CNS effect, caution should be used when carbamazepine is taken with alcohol).

Wine, Red (Because of its primary CNS effect, caution should be used when carbamazepine is taken with alcohol).

Wine, unspecified (Because of its primary CNS effect, caution should be used when carbamazepine is taken with alcohol).

Wine products (Because of its primary CNS effect, caution should be used when carbamazepine is taken with alcohol).

ERYPED 200 & ERYPED 400 ORAL SUSPENSION
(Erythromycin Ethylsuccinate) 435
See EryPed Drops

ERYPED DROPS
(Erythromycin Ethylsuccinate) 435
May interact with calcium channel blockers, chloramphenicol, clindamycins, cytochrome p450 3a substrates (selected), HMG-CoA reductase inhibitors, methylprednisolone, oral anticoagulants, phenytoin, quinidine, theophyllines, triazolobenzodiazepines, valproate, and certain other agents. Compounds in these categories include:

Alfentanil Hydrochloride (Co-administration of erythromycin and a drug primarily metabolized by CYP3A may be associated with elevations in drug concentrations that could increase or prolong both the therapeutic and adverse effects of the concomitant drug. Dosage adjustments may be considered, and when possible, serum concentrations of drugs primarily metabolized by CYP3A should be monitored closely in patients concurrently receiving erythromycin. There have been spontaneous or published reports of CYP3A based interactions of erythromycin with alfentanil).

No products indexed under this heading.

Alprazolam (Erythromycin has been reported to decrease the clearance of triazolam and midazolam, and thus, may increase the pharmacologic effect of these benzodiazepines).

No products indexed under this heading.

Aminophylline (Co-administration of erythromycin and a drug primarily metabolized by CYP3A may be associated with elevations in drug concentrations that could increase or prolong both the therapeutic and adverse effects of the concomitant drug. Dosage adjustments may be considered, and when possible, serum concentrations of drugs primarily metabolized by CYP3A should be monitored closely in patients concurrently receiving erythromycin).

No products indexed under this heading.

Amitriptyline Hydrochloride (Co-administration of erythromycin and a drug primarily metabolized by CYP3A may be associated with elevations in drug concentrations that could increase or prolong both the therapeutic and adverse effects of the concomitant drug. Dosage adjustments may be considered, and when possible, serum concentrations of drugs primarily metabolized by CYP3A should be monitored closely in patients concurrently receiving erythromycin).

No products indexed under this heading.

Amlodipine Besylate (Hypotension, bradyarrhythmias, and lactic acidosis have been observed in patients receiving concurrent verapamil, belonging to the calcium channel blockers drug class). Products include:
Azor 1010
Exforge 2443
Exforge HCT 2449

Anisindione (There have been reports of increased anticoagulant effects when erythromycin and oral anticoagulants were used concomitantly. Increased anticoagulation effects due to interactions of erythromycin with various oral anticoagulants may be more pronounced in the elderly).

No products indexed under this heading.

Aprepitant (Co-administration of erythromycin and a drug primarily metabolized by CYP3A may be associated with elevations in drug concentrations that could increase or prolong both the therapeutic and adverse effects of the concomitant drug. Dosage adjustments may be considered, and when possible, serum concentrations of drugs primarily metabolized by CYP3A should be monitored closely in patients concurrently receiving erythromycin). Products include:
Emend 2124

Astemizole (Concomitant administration of erythromycin with astemizole is contraindicated. Erythromycin has been reported to significantly alter the metabolism of the non-sedating antihistamines terfenadine and astemizole when taken concomitantly. Rare cases of serious cardiovascular adverse events, including electrocardiographic QT/QTc interval prolongation, cardiac arrest, torsades de pointes, and other ventricular arrhythmias have been observed).

No products indexed under this heading.

Atorvastatin Calcium (Erythromycin has been reported to increase concentrations of HMG-CoA reductase inhibitors (eg, lovastatin and simvastatin). Rare reports of rhabdomyolysis have been reported in patients taking these drugs concomitantly). Products include:
Lipitor 2703

Bepridil Hydrochloride (Hypotension, bradyarrhythmias, and lactic acidosis have been observed in patients receiving concurrent verapamil, belonging to the calcium channel blockers drug class).

No products indexed under this heading.

Bromocriptine Mesylate (Co-administration of erythromycin and a drug primarily metabolized by CYP3A may be associated with elevations in drug concentrations that could increase or prolong both the therapeutic and adverse effects of the concomitant drug. Dosage adjustments may be considered, and when possible, serum concentrations of drugs primarily metabolized by CYP3A should be monitored closely in patients concurrently receiving erythromycin. There have been spontaneous or published reports of CYP3A based interactions of erythromycin with bromocriptine).

No products indexed under this heading.

Buspirone Hydrochloride (Co-administration of erythromycin and a drug primarily metabolized by CYP3A may be associated with elevations in drug concentrations that could increase or prolong both the therapeutic and adverse effects of the concomitant drug. Dosage adjustments may be considered, and when possible, serum concentrations of drugs primarily metabolized by CYP3A should be monitored closely in patients concurrently receiving erythromycin).

No products indexed under this heading.

Busulfan (Co-administration of erythromycin and a drug primarily metabolized by CYP3A may be associated with elevations in drug concentrations that could increase or prolong both the therapeutic and adverse effects of the concomitant drug. Dosage adjustments may be considered, and when possible, serum concentrations of drugs primarily metabolized by CYP3A should be monitored closely in patients concurrently receiving erythromycin). Products include:
Myleran 1581

Carbamazepine (Co-administration of erythromycin and a drug primarily metabolized by CYP3A may be associated with elevations in drug concentrations that could increase or prolong both the therapeutic and adverse effects of the concomitant drug. Dosage adjustments may be considered, and when possible, serum concentrations of drugs primarily metabolized by CYP3A should be monitored closely in patients concurrently receiving erythromycin. There have been spontaneous or published reports of CYP3A based interactions of erythromycin with carbamazepine). Products include:
Carbatrol 3280
Equetro 3477

Cerivastatin Sodium (Erythromycin has been reported to increase concentrations of HMG-CoA reductase inhibitors (eg, lovastatin and simvastatin). Rare reports of rhabdomyolysis have been reported in patients taking these drugs concomitantly).

No products indexed under this heading.

Chloramphenicol (Antagonism has been demonstrated *in vitro* between erythromycin and chloramphenicol).

No products indexed under this heading.

Chloramphenicol Palmitate (Antagonism has been demonstrated *in vitro* between erythromycin and chloramphenicol).

No products indexed under this heading.

Chloramphenicol Sodium Succinate (Antagonism has been demonstrated *in vitro* between erythromycin and chloramphenicol).

No products indexed under this heading.

Chlorpheniramine (Co-administration of erythromycin and a drug primarily metabolized by CYP3A may be associated with elevations in drug concentrations that could increase or prolong both the therapeutic and adverse effects of the concomitant drug. Dosage adjustments may be considered, and when possible, serum concentrations of drugs primarily metabolized by CYP3A should be monitored closely in patients concurrently receiving erythromycin).

No products indexed under this heading.

Chlorpheniramine Maleate (Co-administration of erythromycin and a drug primarily metabolized by CYP3A may be associated with elevations in drug concentrations that could increase or prolong both the therapeutic and adverse effects of the concomitant drug. Dosage adjustments may be considered, and when possible, serum concentrations of drugs primarily metabo-

EryPed Interactions Index 608

lized by CYP3A should be monitored closely in patients concurrently receiving erythromycin).
No products indexed under this heading.

Chlorpheniramine Polistirex (Co-administration of erythromycin and a drug primarily metabolized by CYP3A may be associated with elevations in drug concentrations that could increase or prolong both the therapeutic and adverse effects of the concomitant drug. Dosage adjustments may be considered, and when possible, serum concentrations of drugs primarily metabolized by CYP3A should be monitored closely in patients concurrently receiving erythromycin). Products include:
Tussionex 3443

Chlorpheniramine Tannate (Co-administration of erythromycin and a drug primarily metabolized by CYP3A may be associated with elevations in drug concentrations that could increase or prolong both the therapeutic and adverse effects of the concomitant drug. Dosage adjustments may be considered, and when possible, serum concentrations of drugs primarily metabolized by CYP3A should be monitored closely in patients concurrently receiving erythromycin).
No products indexed under this heading.

Cilostazol (Co-administration of erythromycin and a drug primarily metabolized by CYP3A may be associated with elevations in drug concentrations that could increase or prolong both the therapeutic and adverse effects of the concomitant drug. Dosage adjustments may be considered, and when possible, serum concentrations of drugs primarily metabolized by CYP3A should be monitored closely in patients concurrently receiving erythromycin. There have been spontaneous or published reports of CYP3A based interactions of erythromycin with cilostazol).
No products indexed under this heading.

Cisapride (Concomitant administration of erythromycin with cisapride is contraindicated. There have been postmarketing reports of drug interactions when erythromycin was co-administered with cisapride, resulting in QT prolongation, cardiac arrhythmias, ventricular tachycardia, ventricular fibrillation, and torsades de pointes most likely due to the inhibition of hepatic metabolism of cisapride by erythromycin. Fatalities have been reported).
No products indexed under this heading.

Clarithromycin (Co-administration of erythromycin and a drug primarily metabolized by CYP3A may be associated with elevations in drug concentrations that could increase or prolong both the therapeutic and adverse effects of the concomitant drug. Dosage adjustments may be considered, and when possible, serum concentrations of drugs primarily metabolized by CYP3A should be monitored closely in patients concurrently receiving erythromycin). Products include:
Biaxin/Biaxin XL 412

Clindamycin (Antagonism has been demonstrated *in vitro* between erythromycin and clindamycin). Products include:
Duac 3317

Clindamycin, Topical (Antagonism has been demonstrated *in vitro* between erythromycin and clindamycin).
No products indexed under this heading.

Clindamycin Hydrochloride (Antagonism has been demonstrated *in vitro* between erythromycin and clindamycin).
No products indexed under this heading.

Clindamycin Palmitate Hydrochloride (Antagonism has been demonstrated *in vitro* between erythromycin and clindamycin).
No products indexed under this heading.

Clindamycin Phosphate (Antagonism has been demonstrated *in vitro* between erythromycin and clindamycin). Products include:
Benzaclin 2965
Evoclin 3318

Cyclosporine (Co-administration of erythromycin and a drug primarily metabolized by CYP3A may be associated with elevations in drug concentrations that could increase or prolong both the therapeutic and adverse effects of the concomitant drug. Dosage adjustments may be considered, and when possible, serum concentrations of drugs primarily metabolized by CYP3A should be monitored closely in patients concurrently receiving erythromycin. There have been spontaneous or published reports of CYP3A based interactions of erythromycin with cyclosporine). Products include:
Gengraf 440
Neoral Oral Solution 2496
Neoral Capsules 2496
Restasis 605

Desogestrel (Co-administration of erythromycin and a drug primarily metabolized by CYP3A may be associated with elevations in drug concentrations that could increase or prolong both the therapeutic and adverse effects of the concomitant drug. Dosage adjustments may be considered, and when possible, serum concentrations of drugs primarily metabolized by CYP3A should be monitored closely in patients concurrently receiving erythromycin).
No products indexed under this heading.

Dexamethasone (Co-administration of erythromycin and a drug primarily metabolized by CYP3A may be associated with elevations in drug concentrations that could increase or prolong both the therapeutic and adverse effects of the concomitant drug. Dosage adjustments may be considered, and when possible, serum concentrations of drugs primarily metabolized by CYP3A should be monitored closely in patients concurrently receiving erythromycin). Products include:
Ciprodex 583
Ozurdex .... ⊙223
Tobramycin and Dexamethasone Ophthalmic Suspension .... ⊙251

Dexamethasone Acetate (Co-administration of erythromycin and a drug primarily metabolized by CYP3A may be associated with elevations in drug concentrations that could increase or prolong both the therapeutic and adverse effects of the concomitant drug. Dosage adjustments may be considered, and when possible, serum concentrations of drugs primarily metabolized by CYP3A should be monitored closely in patients concurrently receiving erythromycin).
No products indexed under this heading.

Dexamethasone Phosphate (Co-administration of erythromycin and a drug primarily metabolized by CYP3A may be associated with elevations in drug concentrations that could increase or prolong both the therapeutic and adverse effects of the concomitant drug. Dosage adjustments may be considered, and when possible, serum concentrations of drugs primarily metabolized by CYP3A should be monitored closely in patients concurrently receiving erythromycin).
No products indexed under this heading.

Dexamethasone Sodium (Co-administration of erythromycin and a drug primarily metabolized by CYP3A may be associated with elevations in drug concentrations that could increase or prolong both the therapeutic and adverse effects of the concomitant drug. Dosage adjustments may be considered, and when possible, serum concentrations of drugs primarily metabolized by CYP3A should be monitored closely in patients concurrently receiving erythromycin).
No products indexed under this heading.

Dexamethasone Sodium Phosphate (Co-administration of erythromycin and a drug primarily metabolized by CYP3A may be associated with elevations in drug concentrations that could increase or prolong both the therapeutic and adverse effects of the concomitant drug. Dosage adjustments may be considered, and when possible, serum concentrations of drugs primarily metabolized by CYP3A should be monitored closely in patients concurrently receiving erythromycin).
No products indexed under this heading.

Diazepam (Co-administration of erythromycin and a drug primarily metabolized by CYP3A may be associated with elevations in drug concentrations that could increase or prolong both the therapeutic and adverse effects of the concomitant drug. Dosage adjustments may be considered, and when possible, serum concentrations of drugs primarily metabolized by CYP3A should be monitored closely in patients concurrently receiving erythromycin). Products include:
Valium Tablets 2880

Dicumarol (There have been reports of increased anticoagulant effects when erythromycin and oral anticoagulants were used concomitantly. Increased anticoagulation effects due to interactions of erythromycin with various oral anticoagulants may be more pronounced in the elderly).
No products indexed under this heading.

Digoxin (Concomitant administration of erythromycin and digoxin has been reported to result in elevated digoxin serum levels). Products include:
Lanoxin Injection 1546
Lanoxin Injection Pediatric 1549
Lanoxin Tablets 1553

Dihydroergotamine Mesylate (Concurrent use of erythromycin and ergotamine or dihydroergotamine has been associated in some patients with acute ergot toxicity characterized by severe peripheral vasospasm and dysesthesia).
No products indexed under this heading.

Diltiazem Hydrochloride (Hypotension, bradyarrhythmias, and lactic acidosis have been observed in patients receiving concurrent verapamil, belonging to the calcium channel blockers drug class). Products include:
Cardizem LA 423

Diltiazem Maleate (Co-administration of erythromycin and a drug primarily metabolized by CYP3A may be associated with elevations in drug concentrations that could increase or prolong both the therapeutic and adverse effects of the concomitant drug. Dosage adjustments may be considered, and when possible, serum concentrations of drugs primarily metabolized by CYP3A should be monitored closely in patients concurrently receiving erythromycin).
No products indexed under this heading.

Disopyramide (Co-administration of erythromycin and a drug primarily metabolized by CYP3A may be associated with elevations in drug concentrations that could increase or prolong both the therapeutic and adverse effects of the concomitant drug. Dosage adjustments may be considered, and when possible, serum concentrations of drugs primarily metabolized by CYP3A should be monitored closely in patients concurrently receiving erythromycin. There have been spontaneous or published reports of CYP3A based interactions of erythromycin with disopyramide).
No products indexed under this heading.

Disopyramide Phosphate (Co-administration of erythromycin and a drug primarily metabolized by CYP3A may be associated with elevations in drug concentrations that could increase or prolong both the therapeutic and adverse effects of the concomitant drug. Dosage adjustments may be considered, and when possible, serum concentrations of drugs primarily metabolized by CYP3A should be monitored closely in patients concurrently receiving erythromycin. There have been spontaneous or published reports of CYP3A based interactions of erythromycin with disopyramide).
No products indexed under this heading.

Divalproex Sodium (There have been reports of interactions of erythromycin with drugs not thought to be metabolized by CYP3A, including valproate). Products include:
Depakote ER 426

Doxorubicin Hydrochloride (Co-administration of erythromycin and a drug primarily metabolized by CYP3A may be associated with elevations in drug concentrations that could increase or prolong both the therapeutic and adverse effects of the concomitant drug. Dosage adjustments may be considered, and when possible, serum concentrations of drugs primarily metabolized by CYP3A should be monitored closely in patients concurrently receiving erythromycin).
No products indexed under this heading.

Dronabinol (Co-administration of erythromycin and a drug primarily metabolized by CYP3A may be associated with elevations in drug concentrations that could increase or prolong both the therapeutic and adverse effects of the concomitant drug. Dosage adjustments may be considered, and when possible, serum concentrations of drugs primarily metabolized by CYP3A should be monitored closely in patients concurrently receiving erythromycin).
No products indexed under this heading.

Dyphylline (Co-administration of erythromycin and a drug primarily metabolized by CYP3A may be associated with elevations in drug concentrations that could increase or prolong both the therapeutic and adverse effects of the concomitant drug. Dosage adjustments may be considered, and when possible, serum concentrations of drugs primarily metabolized by CYP3A should be monitored closely in patients concurrently receiving erythromycin).
No products indexed under this heading.

Ergotamine Tartrate (Concurrent use of erythromycin and ergotamine or dihydroergotamine has been associated in some patients with acute ergot toxicity characterized by severe peripheral vasospasm and dysesthesia).
No products indexed under this heading.

Erythromycin (Co-administration of erythromycin and a drug primarily metabolized by CYP3A may be associated with elevations in drug concentrations that could increase or prolong both the therapeutic and adverse effects of the concomitant drug. Dosage adjustments may be considered, and when possible, serum concentrations of drugs primarily metabolized by

(⊙ Described in PDR® for Ophthalmic Medicines)

CYP3A should be monitored closely in patients concurrently receiving erythromycin).

No products indexed under this heading.

Erythromycin Estolate (Co-administration of erythromycin and a drug primarily metabolized by CYP3A may be associated with elevations in drug concentrations that could increase or prolong both the therapeutic and adverse effects of the concomitant drug. Dosage adjustments may be considered, and when possible, serum concentrations of drugs primarily metabolized by CYP3A should be monitored closely in patients concurrently receiving erythromycin).

No products indexed under this heading.

Erythromycin Gluceptate (Co-administration of erythromycin and a drug primarily metabolized by CYP3A may be associated with elevations in drug concentrations that could increase or prolong both the therapeutic and adverse effects of the concomitant drug. Dosage adjustments may be considered, and when possible, serum concentrations of drugs primarily metabolized by CYP3A should be monitored closely in patients concurrently receiving erythromycin).

No products indexed under this heading.

Erythromycin Lactobionate (Co-administration of erythromycin and a drug primarily metabolized by CYP3A may be associated with elevations in drug concentrations that could increase or prolong both the therapeutic and adverse effects of the concomitant drug. Dosage adjustments may be considered, and when possible, serum concentrations of drugs primarily metabolized by CYP3A should be monitored closely in patients concurrently receiving erythromycin).

No products indexed under this heading.

Erythromycin Stearate (Co-administration of erythromycin and a drug primarily metabolized by CYP3A may be associated with elevations in drug concentrations that could increase or prolong both the therapeutic and adverse effects of the concomitant drug. Dosage adjustments may be considered, and when possible, serum concentrations of drugs primarily metabolized by CYP3A should be monitored closely in patients concurrently receiving erythromycin).

No products indexed under this heading.

Estrogen (Co-administration of erythromycin and a drug primarily metabolized by CYP3A may be associated with elevations in drug concentrations that could increase or prolong both the therapeutic and adverse effects of the concomitant drug. Dosage adjustments may be considered, and when possible, serum concentrations of drugs primarily metabolized by CYP3A should be monitored closely in patients concurrently receiving erythromycin).

No products indexed under this heading.

Estrogens, Conjugated (Co-administration of erythromycin and a drug primarily metabolized by CYP3A may be associated with elevations in drug concentrations that could increase or prolong both the therapeutic and adverse effects of the concomitant drug. Dosage adjustments may be considered, and when possible, serum concentrations of drugs primarily metabolized by CYP3A should be monitored closely in patients concurrently receiving erythromycin). Products include:

Premarin Intravenous	3528
Premarin Tablets	3533
Premarin Vaginal Cream	3540
Premphase	3549
Prempro	3549

Estrogens, Conjugated, Synthetic A (Co-administration of erythromycin and a drug primarily metabolized by CYP3A may be associated with elevations in drug concentrations that could increase or prolong both the therapeutic and adverse effects of the concomitant drug. Dosage adjustments may be considered, and when possible, serum concentrations of drugs primarily metabolized by CYP3A should be monitored closely in patients concurrently receiving erythromycin).

No products indexed under this heading.

Estrogens, Esterified (Co-administration of erythromycin and a drug primarily metabolized by CYP3A may be associated with elevations in drug concentrations that could increase or prolong both the therapeutic and adverse effects of the concomitant drug. Dosage adjustments may be considered, and when possible, serum concentrations of drugs primarily metabolized by CYP3A should be monitored closely in patients concurrently receiving erythromycin).

No products indexed under this heading.

Ethinyl Estradiol (Co-administration of erythromycin and a drug primarily metabolized by CYP3A may be associated with elevations in drug concentrations that could increase or prolong both the therapeutic and adverse effects of the concomitant drug. Dosage adjustments may be considered, and when possible, serum concentrations of drugs primarily metabolized by CYP3A should be monitored closely in patients concurrently receiving erythromycin). Products include:

LoSeasonique	3407
Lybrel	3514
NuvaRing	3181
Ortho Evra	2648
Ortho-Cyclen/Ortho Tri-Cyclen	2663
Ortho Tri-Cyclen Lo Tablets	2673
Seasonique	3418
Yaz	864

Ethosuximide (Co-administration of erythromycin and a drug primarily metabolized by CYP3A may be associated with elevations in drug concentrations that could increase or prolong both the therapeutic and adverse effects of the concomitant drug. Dosage adjustments may be considered, and when possible, serum concentrations of drugs primarily metabolized by CYP3A should be monitored closely in patients concurrently receiving erythromycin).

No products indexed under this heading.

Ethynodiol Diacetate (Co-administration of erythromycin and a drug primarily metabolized by CYP3A may be associated with elevations in drug concentrations that could increase or prolong both the therapeutic and adverse effects of the concomitant drug. Dosage adjustments may be considered, and when possible, serum concentrations of drugs primarily metabolized by CYP3A should be monitored closely in patients concurrently receiving erythromycin).

No products indexed under this heading.

Etoposide (Co-administration of erythromycin and a drug primarily metabolized by CYP3A may be associated with elevations in drug concentrations that could increase or prolong both the therapeutic and adverse effects of the concomitant drug. Dosage adjustments may be considered, and when possible, serum concentrations of drugs primarily metabolized by CYP3A should be monitored closely in patients concurrently receiving erythromycin).

No products indexed under this heading.

Etoposide Phosphate (Co-administration of erythromycin and a drug primarily metabolized by CYP3A

may be associated with elevations in drug concentrations that could increase or prolong both the therapeutic and adverse effects of the concomitant drug. Dosage adjustments may be considered, and when possible, serum concentrations of drugs primarily metabolized by CYP3A should be monitored closely in patients concurrently receiving erythromycin).

No products indexed under this heading.

Felodipine (Hypotension, bradyarrhythmias, and lactic acidosis have been observed in patients receiving concurrent verapamil, belonging to the calcium channel blockers drug class).

No products indexed under this heading.

Fentanyl (Co-administration of erythromycin and a drug primarily metabolized by CYP3A may be associated with elevations in drug concentrations that could increase or prolong both the therapeutic and adverse effects of the concomitant drug. Dosage adjustments may be considered, and when possible, serum concentrations of drugs primarily metabolized by CYP3A should be monitored closely in patients concurrently receiving erythromycin). Products include:

Duragesic	2604
Fentanyl Transdermal System	2346
Onsolis	2054

Fentanyl Citrate (Co-administration of erythromycin and a drug primarily metabolized by CYP3A may be associated with elevations in drug concentrations that could increase or prolong both the therapeutic and adverse effects of the concomitant drug. Dosage adjustments may be considered, and when possible, serum concentrations of drugs primarily metabolized by CYP3A should be monitored closely in patients concurrently receiving erythromycin). Products include:

Fentora	966

Fluvastatin Sodium (Erythromycin has been reported to increase concentrations of HMG-CoA reductase inhibitors (eg, lovastatin and simvastatin). Rare reports of rhabdomyolysis have been reported in patients taking these drugs concomitantly).

No products indexed under this heading.

Fosphenytoin (There have been reports of interactions of erythromycin with drugs not thought to be metabolized by CYP3A, including phenytoin).

No products indexed under this heading.

Fosphenytoin Sodium (There have been reports of interactions of erythromycin with drugs not thought to be metabolized by CYP3A, including phenytoin).

No products indexed under this heading.

Glyburide (Co-administration of erythromycin and a drug primarily metabolized by CYP3A may be associated with elevations in drug concentrations that could increase or prolong both the therapeutic and adverse effects of the concomitant drug. Dosage adjustments may be considered, and when possible, serum concentrations of drugs primarily metabolized by CYP3A should be monitored closely in patients concurrently receiving erythromycin).

No products indexed under this heading.

Haloperidol (Co-administration of erythromycin and a drug primarily metabolized by CYP3A may be associated with elevations in drug concentrations that could increase or prolong both the therapeutic and adverse effects of the concomitant drug. Dosage adjustments may be considered, and when possible, serum concentrations of drugs primarily metabolized by

CYP3A should be monitored closely in patients concurrently receiving erythromycin).

No products indexed under this heading.

Haloperidol Decanoate (Co-administration of erythromycin and a drug primarily metabolized by CYP3A may be associated with elevations in drug concentrations that could increase or prolong both the therapeutic and adverse effects of the concomitant drug. Dosage adjustments may be considered, and when possible, serum concentrations of drugs primarily metabolized by CYP3A should be monitored closely in patients concurrently receiving erythromycin).

No products indexed under this heading.

Hexobarbital (There have been reports of interactions of erythromycin with drugs not thought to be metabolized by CYP3A, including hexobarbital).

No products indexed under this heading.

Imipramine Hydrochloride (Co-administration of erythromycin and a drug primarily metabolized by CYP3A may be associated with elevations in drug concentrations that could increase or prolong both the therapeutic and adverse effects of the concomitant drug. Dosage adjustments may be considered, and when possible, serum concentrations of drugs primarily metabolized by CYP3A should be monitored closely in patients concurrently receiving erythromycin).

No products indexed under this heading.

Imipramine Pamoate (Co-administration of erythromycin and a drug primarily metabolized by CYP3A may be associated with elevations in drug concentrations that could increase or prolong both the therapeutic and adverse effects of the concomitant drug. Dosage adjustments may be considered, and when possible, serum concentrations of drugs primarily metabolized by CYP3A should be monitored closely in patients concurrently receiving erythromycin).

No products indexed under this heading.

Indinavir Sulfate (Co-administration of erythromycin and a drug primarily metabolized by CYP3A may be associated with elevations in drug concentrations that could increase or prolong both the therapeutic and adverse effects of the concomitant drug. Dosage adjustments may be considered, and when possible, serum concentrations of drugs primarily metabolized by CYP3A should be monitored closely in patients concurrently receiving erythromycin). Products include:

Crixivan	2113

Isradipine (Hypotension, bradyarrhythmias, and lactic acidosis have been observed in patients receiving concurrent verapamil, belonging to the calcium channel blockers drug class). Products include:

DynaCirc CR	1432

Itraconazole (Co-administration of erythromycin and a drug primarily metabolized by CYP3A may be associated with elevations in drug concentrations that could increase or prolong both the therapeutic and adverse effects of the concomitant drug. Dosage adjustments may be considered, and when possible, serum concentrations of drugs primarily metabolized by CYP3A should be monitored closely in patients concurrently receiving erythromycin).

No products indexed under this heading.

Ketoconazole (Co-administration of erythromycin and a drug primarily metabolized by CYP3A may be associated with elevations in drug concentrations that could increase or prolong both the therapeutic and adverse

---

IMPORTANT NOTE: Always consult each drug listing in the patient's regimen for possible interactions.

EryPed Interactions Index 610

effects of the concomitant drug. Dosage adjustments may be considered, and when possible, serum concentrations of drugs primarily metabolized by CYP3A should be monitored closely in patients concurrently receiving erythromycin). Products include:
Extina 3319
Xolegel 3337

Levonorgestrel (Co-administration of erythromycin and a drug primarily metabolized by CYP3A may be associated with elevations in drug concentrations that could increase or prolong both the therapeutic and adverse effects of the concomitant drug. Dosage adjustments may be considered, and when possible, serum concentrations of drugs primarily metabolized by CYP3A should be monitored closely in patients concurrently receiving erythromycin). Products include:
Climara Pro 847
LoSeasonique 3407
Lybrel 3514
Mirena 854
Plan B 3416
Seasonique 3418

Lidocaine (Co-administration of erythromycin and a drug primarily metabolized by CYP3A may be associated with elevations in drug concentrations that could increase or prolong both the therapeutic and adverse effects of the concomitant drug. Dosage adjustments may be considered, and when possible, serum concentrations of drugs primarily metabolized by CYP3A should be monitored closely in patients concurrently receiving erythromycin). Products include:
Lidoderm 1107

Lidocaine Hydrochloride (Co-administration of erythromycin and a drug primarily metabolized by CYP3A may be associated with elevations in drug concentrations that could increase or prolong both the therapeutic and adverse effects of the concomitant drug. Dosage adjustments may be considered, and when possible, serum concentrations of drugs primarily metabolized by CYP3A should be monitored closely in patients concurrently receiving erythromycin).
No products indexed under this heading.

Lincomycin Hydrochloride (Antagonism has been demonstrated *in vitro* between erythromycin and lincomycin).
No products indexed under this heading.

Lincomycin Hydrochloride Monohydrate (Antagonism has been demonstrated *in vitro* between erythromycin and lincomycin).
No products indexed under this heading.

Lovastatin (Rhabdomyolysis with or without renal impairment has been reported in seriously ill patients receiving erythromycin concomitantly with lovastatin. Therefore, patients receiving concomitant lovastatin and erythromycin should be carefully monitored for creatine kinase (CK) and serum transaminase levels). Products include:
Advicor 402
Mevacor 2212

Mestranol (Co-administration of erythromycin and a drug primarily metabolized by CYP3A may be associated with elevations in drug concentrations that could increase or prolong both the therapeutic and adverse effects of the concomitant drug. Dosage adjustments may be considered, and when possible, serum concentrations of drugs primarily metabolized by CYP3A should be monitored closely in patients concurrently receiving erythromycin).
No products indexed under this heading.

Methadone Hydrochloride (Co-administration of erythromycin and a drug primarily metabolized by CYP3A may be associated with elevations in drug concentrations that could increase or prolong both the therapeutic and adverse effects of the concomitant drug. Dosage adjustments may be considered, and when possible, serum concentrations of drugs primarily metabolized by CYP3A should be monitored closely in patients concurrently receiving erythromycin).
No products indexed under this heading.

Methylprednisolone (Co-administration of erythromycin and a drug primarily metabolized by CYP3A may be associated with elevations in drug concentrations that could increase or prolong both the therapeutic and adverse effects of the concomitant drug. Dosage adjustments may be considered, and when possible, serum concentrations of drugs primarily metabolized by CYP3A should be monitored closely in patients concurrently receiving erythromycin. There have been spontaneous or published reports of CYP3A based interactions of erythromycin with methylprednisolone).
No products indexed under this heading.

Methylprednisolone Acetate (Co-administration of erythromycin and a drug primarily metabolized by CYP3A may be associated with elevations in drug concentrations that could increase or prolong both the therapeutic and adverse effects of the concomitant drug. Dosage adjustments may be considered, and when possible, serum concentrations of drugs primarily metabolized by CYP3A should be monitored closely in patients concurrently receiving erythromycin. There have been spontaneous or published reports of CYP3A based interactions of erythromycin with methylprednisolone).
No products indexed under this heading.

Methylprednisolone Sodium Succinate (Co-administration of erythromycin and a drug primarily metabolized by CYP3A may be associated with elevations in drug concentrations that could increase or prolong both the therapeutic and adverse effects of the concomitant drug. Dosage adjustments may be considered, and when possible, serum concentrations of drugs primarily metabolized by CYP3A should be monitored closely in patients concurrently receiving erythromycin. There have been spontaneous or published reports of CYP3A based interactions of erythromycin with methylprednisolone).
No products indexed under this heading.

Mibefradil Dihydrochloride (Hypotension, bradyarrhythmias, and lactic acidosis have been observed in patients receiving concurrent verapamil, belonging to the calcium channel blockers drug class).
No products indexed under this heading.

Midazolam Hydrochloride (Erythromycin has been reported to decrease the clearance of triazolam and midazolam, and thus, may increase the pharmacologic effect of these benzodiazepines).
No products indexed under this heading.

Nefazodone Hydrochloride (Co-administration of erythromycin and a drug primarily metabolized by CYP3A may be associated with elevations in drug concentrations that could increase or prolong both the therapeutic and adverse effects of the concomitant drug. Dosage adjustments may be considered, and when possible, serum concentrations of drugs primarily metabolized by CYP3A should be monitored closely in patients concurrently receiving erythromycin).
No products indexed under this heading.

Nelfinavir Mesylate (Co-administration of erythromycin and a drug primarily metabolized by CYP3A may be associated with elevations in drug concentrations that could increase or prolong both the therapeutic and adverse effects of the concomitant drug. Dosage adjustments may be considered, and when possible, serum concentrations of drugs primarily metabolized by CYP3A should be monitored closely in patients concurrently receiving erythromycin).
No products indexed under this heading.

Nicardipine (Hypotension, bradyarrhythmias, and lactic acidosis have been observed in patients receiving concurrent verapamil, belonging to the calcium channel blockers drug class).
No products indexed under this heading.

Nicardipine Hydrochloride (Hypotension, bradyarrhythmias, and lactic acidosis have been observed in patients receiving concurrent verapamil, belonging to the calcium channel blockers drug class).
No products indexed under this heading.

Nifedipine (Hypotension, bradyarrhythmias, and lactic acidosis have been observed in patients receiving concurrent verapamil, belonging to the calcium channel blockers drug class).
No products indexed under this heading.

Nimodipine (Hypotension, bradyarrhythmias, and lactic acidosis have been observed in patients receiving concurrent verapamil, belonging to the calcium channel blockers drug class).
No products indexed under this heading.

Nisoldipine (Hypotension, bradyarrhythmias, and lactic acidosis have been observed in patients receiving concurrent verapamil, belonging to the calcium channel blockers drug class).
No products indexed under this heading.

Norethindrone (Co-administration of erythromycin and a drug primarily metabolized by CYP3A may be associated with elevations in drug concentrations that could increase or prolong both the therapeutic and adverse effects of the concomitant drug. Dosage adjustments may be considered, and when possible, serum concentrations of drugs primarily metabolized by CYP3A should be monitored closely in patients concurrently receiving erythromycin). Products include:
Ortho Micronor 2660

Norgestrel (Co-administration of erythromycin and a drug primarily metabolized by CYP3A may be associated with elevations in drug concentrations that could increase or prolong both the therapeutic and adverse effects of the concomitant drug. Dosage adjustments may be considered, and when possible, serum concentrations of drugs primarily metabolized by CYP3A should be monitored closely in patients concurrently receiving erythromycin).
No products indexed under this heading.

Ondansetron Hydrochloride (Co-administration of erythromycin and a drug primarily metabolized by CYP3A may be associated with elevations in drug concentrations that could increase or prolong both the therapeutic and adverse effects of the concomitant drug. Dosage adjustments may be considered, and when possible, serum concentrations of drugs primarily metabolized by CYP3A should be monitored closely in patients concurrently receiving erythromycin). Products include:
Zofran Injection 1750
Zofran 1756
Zofran ODT 1756

Paclitaxel (Co-administration of erythromycin and a drug primarily metabolized by CYP3A may be associated with elevations in drug concentrations that could increase or prolong both the therapeutic and adverse effects of the concomitant drug. Dosage adjustments may be considered, and when possible, serum concentrations of drugs primarily metabolized by CYP3A should be monitored closely in patients concurrently receiving erythromycin).
No products indexed under this heading.

Phenytoin (There have been reports of interactions of erythromycin with drugs not thought to be metabolized by CYP3A, including phenytoin).
No products indexed under this heading.

Phenytoin Sodium (There have been reports of interactions of erythromycin with drugs not thought to be metabolized by CYP3A, including phenytoin). Products include:
Phenytek Capsules 2380

Pimozide (Concomitant administration of erythromycin with pimozide is contraindicated).
No products indexed under this heading.

Pravastatin Sodium (Erythromycin has been reported to increase concentrations of HMG-CoA reductase inhibitors (eg, lovastatin and simvastatin). Rare reports of rhabdomyolysis have been reported in patients taking these drugs concomitantly).
No products indexed under this heading.

Quinidine (Co-administration of erythromycin and a drug primarily metabolized by CYP3A may be associated with elevations in drug concentrations that could increase or prolong both the therapeutic and adverse effects of the concomitant drug. Dosage adjustments may be considered, and when possible, serum concentrations of drugs primarily metabolized by CYP3A should be monitored closely in patients concurrently receiving erythromycin. There have been spontaneous or published reports of CYP3A based interactions of erythromycin with quinidine).
No products indexed under this heading.

Quinidine Gluconate (Co-administration of erythromycin and a drug primarily metabolized by CYP3A may be associated with elevations in drug concentrations that could increase or prolong both the therapeutic and adverse effects of the concomitant drug. Dosage adjustments may be considered, and when possible, serum concentrations of drugs primarily metabolized by CYP3A should be monitored closely in patients concurrently receiving erythromycin. There have been spontaneous or published reports of CYP3A based interactions of erythromycin with quinidine).
No products indexed under this heading.

Quinidine Hydrochloride (Co-administration of erythromycin and a drug primarily metabolized by CYP3A may be associated with elevations in drug concentrations that could increase or prolong both the therapeutic and adverse effects of the concomitant drug. Dosage adjustments may be considered, and when possible, serum concentrations of drugs primarily metabolized by CYP3A should be monitored closely in patients concurrently receiving erythromycin. There have been spontaneous or published reports of CYP3A based interactions of erythromycin with quinidine).
No products indexed under this heading.

Quinidine Polygalacturonate (Co-administration of erythromycin and a drug primarily metabolized by CYP3A may be associated with elevations in drug concentrations that could increase or prolong both the therapeutic and adverse effects of the concomitant drug. Dosage adjustments may be considered, and when possible, serum concentrations of drugs primarily metabolized by CYP3A should be monitored closely in patients concurrently receiv-

611 Interactions Index EryPed

ing erythromycin. There have been spontaneous or published reports of CYP3A based interactions of erythromycin with quinidine).
No products indexed under this heading.

Quinidine Sulfate (Co-administration of erythromycin and a drug primarily metabolized by CYP3A may be associated with elevations in drug concentrations that could increase or prolong both the therapeutic and adverse effects of the concomitant drug. Dosage adjustments may be considered, and when possible, serum concentrations of drugs primarily metabolized by CYP3A should be monitored closely in patients concurrently receiving erythromycin. There have been spontaneous or published reports of CYP3A based interactions of erythromycin with quinidine).
No products indexed under this heading.

Quinine (Co-administration of erythromycin and a drug primarily metabolized by CYP3A may be associated with elevations in drug concentrations that could increase or prolong both the therapeutic and adverse effects of the concomitant drug. Dosage adjustments may be considered, and when possible, serum concentrations of drugs primarily metabolized by CYP3A should be monitored closely in patients concurrently receiving erythromycin). Products include:
Hyland's Leg Cramps PM with Quinine 3315

Quinine Sulfate (Co-administration of erythromycin and a drug primarily metabolized by CYP3A may be associated with elevations in drug concentrations that could increase or prolong both the therapeutic and adverse effects of the concomitant drug. Dosage adjustments may be considered, and when possible, serum concentrations of drugs primarily metabolized by CYP3A should be monitored closely in patients concurrently receiving erythromycin).
No products indexed under this heading.

Rifabutin (Co-administration of erythromycin and a drug primarily metabolized by CYP3A may be associated with elevations in drug concentrations that could increase or prolong both the therapeutic and adverse effects of the concomitant drug. Dosage adjustments may be considered, and when possible, serum concentrations of drugs primarily metabolized by CYP3A should be monitored closely in patients concurrently receiving erythromycin. There have been spontaneous or published reports of CYP3A based interactions of erythromycin with rifabutin).
No products indexed under this heading.

Ritonavir (Co-administration of erythromycin and a drug primarily metabolized by CYP3A may be associated with elevations in drug concentrations that could increase or prolong both the therapeutic and adverse effects of the concomitant drug. Dosage adjustments may be considered, and when possible, serum concentrations of drugs primarily metabolized by CYP3A should be monitored closely in patients concurrently receiving erythromycin). Products include:
Kaletra 458
Norvir 509

Rosuvastatin Calcium (Erythromycin has been reported to increase concentrations of HMG-CoA reductase inhibitors (eg, lovastatin and simvastatin). Rare reports of rhabdomyolysis have been reported in patients taking these drugs concomitantly). Products include:
Crestor 736

Saquinavir (Co-administration of erythromycin and a drug primarily metabolized by CYP3A may be associated with elevations in drug concentrations that could increase or prolong both the therapeutic and adverse effects of the concomitant drug. Dosage adjustments may be considered, and when possible, serum concentrations of drugs primarily metabolized by CYP3A should be monitored closely in patients concurrently receiving erythromycin).
No products indexed under this heading.

Saquinavir Mesylate (Co-administration of erythromycin and a drug primarily metabolized by CYP3A may be associated with elevations in drug concentrations that could increase or prolong both the therapeutic and adverse effects of the concomitant drug. Dosage adjustments may be considered, and when possible, serum concentrations of drugs primarily metabolized by CYP3A should be monitored closely in patients concurrently receiving erythromycin).
No products indexed under this heading.

Sertraline Hydrochloride (Co-administration of erythromycin and a drug primarily metabolized by CYP3A may be associated with elevations in drug concentrations that could increase or prolong both the therapeutic and adverse effects of the concomitant drug. Dosage adjustments may be considered, and when possible, serum concentrations of drugs primarily metabolized by CYP3A should be monitored closely in patients concurrently receiving erythromycin).
No products indexed under this heading.

Sildenafil Citrate (Erythromycin has been reported to increase the systemic exposure (AUC) of sildenafil. Reduction of sildenafil dosage should be considered).
No products indexed under this heading.

Simvastatin (Erythromycin has been reported to increase concentrations of HMG-CoA reductase inhibitors (eg, lovastatin and simvastatin). Rare reports of rhabdomyolysis have been reported in patients taking these drugs concomitantly). Products include:
Simcor 524
Vytorin 10/10 ..... 2303, 3240
Vytorin 10/20 ..... 2303, 3240
Vytorin 10/40 ..... 2303, 3240
Vytorin 10/80 ..... 2303, 3240
Zocor 2289

Sirolimus (Co-administration of erythromycin and a drug primarily metabolized by CYP3A may be associated with elevations in drug concentrations that could increase or prolong both the therapeutic and adverse effects of the concomitant drug. Dosage adjustments may be considered, and when possible, serum concentrations of drugs primarily metabolized by CYP3A should be monitored closely in patients concurrently receiving erythromycin). Products include:
Rapamune 3579

Tacrolimus (Co-administration of erythromycin and a drug primarily metabolized by CYP3A may be associated with elevations in drug concentrations that could increase or prolong both the therapeutic and adverse effects of the concomitant drug. Dosage adjustments may be considered, and when possible, serum concentrations of drugs primarily metabolized by CYP3A should be monitored closely in patients concurrently receiving erythromycin. There have been spontaneous or published reports of CYP3A based interactions of erythromycin with tacrolimus). Products include:
Prograf Capsules 677
Prograf Injection 677
Protopic 685

Tamoxifen Citrate (Co-administration of erythromycin and a drug primarily metabolized by CYP3A may be associated with elevations in drug concentrations that could increase or prolong both the therapeutic and adverse effects of the concomitant drug. Dosage adjustments may be considered, and when possible, serum concentrations of drugs primarily metabolized by CYP3A should be monitored closely in patients concurrently receiving erythromycin).
No products indexed under this heading.

Terfenadine (Concomitant administration of erythromycin with terfenadine is contraindicated. Erythromycin has been reported to significantly alter the metabolism of the non-sedating antihistamines terfenadine and astemizole when taken concomitantly. Rare cases of serious cardiovascular adverse events, including electrocardiographic QT/QTc interval prolongation, cardiac arrest, torsades de pointes, and other ventricular arrhythmias have been observed. In addition, deaths have been reported rarely with concomitant administration of terfenadine and erythromycin).
No products indexed under this heading.

Testosterone (Co-administration of erythromycin and a drug primarily metabolized by CYP3A may be associated with elevations in drug concentrations that could increase or prolong both the therapeutic and adverse effects of the concomitant drug. Dosage adjustments may be considered, and when possible, serum concentrations of drugs primarily metabolized by CYP3A should be monitored closely in patients concurrently receiving erythromycin). Products include:
AndroGel 3456

Testosterone Cypionate (Co-administration of erythromycin and a drug primarily metabolized by CYP3A may be associated with elevations in drug concentrations that could increase or prolong both the therapeutic and adverse effects of the concomitant drug. Dosage adjustments may be considered, and when possible, serum concentrations of drugs primarily metabolized by CYP3A should be monitored closely in patients concurrently receiving erythromycin).
No products indexed under this heading.

Testosterone Enanthate (Co-administration of erythromycin and a drug primarily metabolized by CYP3A may be associated with elevations in drug concentrations that could increase or prolong both the therapeutic and adverse effects of the concomitant drug. Dosage adjustments may be considered, and when possible, serum concentrations of drugs primarily metabolized by CYP3A should be monitored closely in patients concurrently receiving erythromycin). Products include:
Delatestryl 1102

Testosterone Propionate (Co-administration of erythromycin and a drug primarily metabolized by CYP3A may be associated with elevations in drug concentrations that could increase or prolong both the therapeutic and adverse effects of the concomitant drug. Dosage adjustments may be considered, and when possible, serum concentrations of drugs primarily metabolized by CYP3A should be monitored closely in patients concurrently receiving erythromycin).
No products indexed under this heading.

Theophylline (Co-administration of erythromycin in patients who are receiving high doses of theophylline may be associated with an increase in serum theophylline levels and potential theophylline toxicity. In case of theophylline toxicity and/or elevated serum theophylline levels, the dose of theophylline should be reduced while the patient is receiving concomitant erythromycin therapy).
No products indexed under this heading.

Theophylline Anhydrous (Co-administration of erythromycin in patients who are receiving high doses of theophylline may be associated with an increase in serum theophylline levels and potential theophylline toxicity. In case of theophylline toxicity and/or elevated serum theophylline levels, the dose of theophylline should be reduced while the patient is receiving concomitant erythromycin therapy). Products include:
Uniphyl 2817

Theophylline Calcium Salicylate (Co-administration of erythromycin in patients who are receiving high doses of theophylline may be associated with an increase in serum theophylline levels and potential theophylline toxicity. In case of theophylline toxicity and/or elevated serum theophylline levels, the dose of theophylline should be reduced while the patient is receiving concomitant erythromycin therapy).
No products indexed under this heading.

Theophylline Dihydroxypropyl (Glyceryl) (Co-administration of erythromycin in patients who are receiving high doses of theophylline may be associated with an increase in serum theophylline levels and potential theophylline toxicity. In case of theophylline toxicity and/or elevated serum theophylline levels, the dose of theophylline should be reduced while the patient is receiving concomitant erythromycin therapy).
No products indexed under this heading.

Theophylline Ethylenediamine (Co-administration of erythromycin in patients who are receiving high doses of theophylline may be associated with an increase in serum theophylline levels and potential theophylline toxicity. In case of theophylline toxicity and/or elevated serum theophylline levels, the dose of theophylline should be reduced while the patient is receiving concomitant erythromycin therapy).
No products indexed under this heading.

Theophylline Sodium Glycinate (Co-administration of erythromycin in patients who are receiving high doses of theophylline may be associated with an increase in serum theophylline levels and potential theophylline toxicity. In case of theophylline toxicity and/or elevated serum theophylline levels, the dose of theophylline should be reduced while the patient is receiving concomitant erythromycin therapy).
No products indexed under this heading.

Tiagabine Hydrochloride (Co-administration of erythromycin and a drug primarily metabolized by CYP3A may be associated with elevations in drug concentrations that could increase or prolong both the therapeutic and adverse effects of the concomitant drug. Dosage adjustments may be considered, and when possible, serum concentrations of drugs primarily metabolized by CYP3A should be monitored closely in patients concurrently receiving erythromycin). Products include:
Gabitril 972

Tolterodine Tartrate (Co-administration of erythromycin and a drug primarily metabolized by CYP3A may be associated with elevations in drug concentrations that could increase

IMPORTANT NOTE: Always consult each drug listing in the patient's regimen for possible interactions.

EryPed Interactions Index 612

or prolong both the therapeutic and adverse effects of the concomitant drug. Dosage adjustments may be considered, and when possible, serum concentrations of drugs primarily metabolized by CYP3A should be monitored closely in patients concurrently receiving erythromycin).
No products indexed under this heading.

Trazodone Hydrochloride (Co-administration of erythromycin and a drug primarily metabolized by CYP3A may be associated with elevations in drug concentrations that could increase or prolong both the therapeutic and adverse effects of the concomitant drug. Dosage adjustments may be considered, and when possible, serum concentrations of drugs primarily metabolized by CYP3A should be monitored closely in patients concurrently receiving erythromycin).
No products indexed under this heading.

Triazolam (Erythromycin has been reported to decrease the clearance of triazolam and midazolam, and thus, may increase the pharmacologic effect of these benzodiazepines).
No products indexed under this heading.

Valproate Sodium (There have been reports of interactions of erythromycin with drugs not thought to be metabolized by CYP3A, including valproate).
No products indexed under this heading.

Valproic Acid (There have been reports of interactions of erythromycin with drugs not thought to be metabolized by CYP3A, including valproate).
No products indexed under this heading.

Venlafaxine Hydrochloride (Co-administration of erythromycin and a drug primarily metabolized by CYP3A may be associated with elevations in drug concentrations that could increase or prolong both the therapeutic and adverse effects of the concomitant drug. Dosage adjustments may be considered, and when possible, serum concentrations of drugs primarily metabolized by CYP3A should be monitored closely in patients concurrently receiving erythromycin). Products include:
Effexor XR 3504
Venlafaxine Hydrochloride Tablets ... 2388

Verapamil Hydrochloride (Hypotension, bradyarrhythmias, and lactic acidosis have been observed in patients receiving concurrent verapamil, belonging to the calcium channel blockers drug class). Products include:
Tarka 534

Vinblastine Sulfate (Co-administration of erythromycin and a drug primarily metabolized by CYP3A may be associated with elevations in drug concentrations that could increase or prolong both the therapeutic and adverse effects of the concomitant drug. Dosage adjustments may be considered, and when possible, serum concentrations of drugs primarily metabolized by CYP3A should be monitored closely in patients concurrently receiving erythromycin. There have been spontaneous or published reports of CYP3A based interactions of erythromycin with vinblastine).
No products indexed under this heading.

Vincristine Sulfate (Co-administration of erythromycin and a drug primarily metabolized by CYP3A may be associated with elevations in drug concentrations that could increase or prolong both the therapeutic and adverse effects of the concomitant drug. Dosage adjustments may be considered, and when possible, serum concentrations of drugs primarily metabolized by CYP3A should be monitored closely in patients concurrently receiving erythromycin).
No products indexed under this heading.

Warfarin Sodium (There have been reports of increased anticoagulant effects when erythromycin and oral anticoagulants were used concomitantly. Increased anticoagulation effects due to interactions of erythromycin with various oral anticoagulants may be more pronounced in the elderly).
No products indexed under this heading.

ESTRASORB TOPICAL EMULSION

(Estradiol) 1777
May interact with cytochrome p450 3a4 inducers (selected), cytochrome p450 3a4 inhibitors (selected), erythromycin, thyroid preparations, and certain other agents. Compounds in these categories include:

Acetazolamide (*In vitro* and *in vivo* studies have shown that estrogens are metabolized partially by cytochrome P450 3A4 (CYP3A4). Therefore, inhibitors of CYP3A4 may affect estrogen drug metabolism. Inhibitors of CYP3A4, such as erythromycin, clarithromycin, ketoconazole, itraconazole, ritonavir and grapefruit juice may increase plasma concentrations of estrogens and may result in side effects).
No products indexed under this heading.

Acetazolamide Sodium (*In vitro* and *in vivo* studies have shown that estrogens are metabolized partially by cytochrome P450 3A4 (CYP3A4). Therefore, inhibitors of CYP3A4 may affect estrogen drug metabolism. Inhibitors of CYP3A4, such as erythromycin, clarithromycin, ketoconazole, itraconazole, ritonavir and grapefruit juice may increase plasma concentrations of estrogens and may result in side effects).
No products indexed under this heading.

Allium sativum (*In vitro* and *in vivo* studies have shown that estrogens are metabolized partially by cytochrome P450 3A4 (CYP3A4). Therefore, inducers of CYP3A4 may affect estrogen drug metabolism. Inducers of CYP3A4, such as St. John's Wort preparations (Hypericum perforatum), phenobarbital, carbamazepine and rifampin may reduce plasma concentrations of estrogens, possibly resulting in a decrease in therapeutic effects and/or changes in the uterine bleeding profile).
No products indexed under this heading.

Aminoglutethimide (*In vitro* and *in vivo* studies have shown that estrogens are metabolized partially by cytochrome P450 3A4 (CYP3A4). Therefore, inducers of CYP3A4 may affect estrogen drug metabolism. Inducers of CYP3A4, such as St. John's Wort preparations (Hypericum perforatum), phenobarbital, carbamazepine and rifampin may reduce plasma concentrations of estrogens, possibly resulting in a decrease in therapeutic effects and/or changes in the uterine bleeding profile).
No products indexed under this heading.

Amiodarone Hydrochloride (*In vitro* and *in vivo* studies have shown that estrogens are metabolized partially by cytochrome P450 3A4 (CYP3A4). Therefore, inhibitors of CYP3A4 may affect estrogen drug metabolism. Inhibitors of CYP3A4, such as erythromycin, clarithromycin, ketoconazole, itraconazole, ritonavir and grapefruit juice may increase plasma concentrations of estrogens and may result in side effects).
No products indexed under this heading.

Amprenavir (*In vitro* and *in vivo* studies have shown that estrogens are metabolized partially by cytochrome P450 3A4 (CYP3A4). Therefore, inhibitors of CYP3A4 may affect estrogen drug metabolism. Inhibitors of CYP3A4, such as erythromycin, clarithromycin, ketoconazole, itraconazole, ritonavir and grapefruit juice may increase plasma concentrations of estrogens and may result in side effects).
No products indexed under this heading.

Anastrozole (*In vitro* and *in vivo* studies have shown that estrogens are metabolized partially by cytochrome P450 3A4 (CYP3A4). Therefore, inhibitors of CYP3A4 may affect estrogen drug metabolism. Inhibitors of CYP3A4, such as erythromycin, clarithromycin, ketoconazole, itraconazole, ritonavir and grapefruit juice may increase plasma concentrations of estrogens and may result in side effects).
No products indexed under this heading.

Aprepitant (*In vitro* and *in vivo* studies have shown that estrogens are metabolized partially by cytochrome P450 3A4 (CYP3A4). Therefore, inducers of CYP3A4 may affect estrogen drug metabolism. Inducers of CYP3A4, such as St. John's Wort preparations (Hypericum perforatum), phenobarbital, carbamazepine and rifampin may reduce plasma concentrations of estrogens, possibly resulting in a decrease in therapeutic effects and/or changes in the uterine bleeding profile). Products include:
Emend 2124

Atazanavir (*In vitro* and *in vivo* studies have shown that estrogens are metabolized partially by cytochrome P450 3A4 (CYP3A4). Therefore, inhibitors of CYP3A4 may affect estrogen drug metabolism. Inhibitors of CYP3A4, such as erythromycin, clarithromycin, ketoconazole, itraconazole, ritonavir and grapefruit juice may increase plasma concentrations of estrogens and may result in side effects).
No products indexed under this heading.

Atazanavir Sulfate (*In vitro* and *in vivo* studies have shown that estrogens are metabolized partially by cytochrome P450 3A4 (CYP3A4). Therefore, inhibitors of CYP3A4 may affect estrogen drug metabolism. Inhibitors of CYP3A4, such as erythromycin, clarithromycin, ketoconazole, itraconazole, ritonavir and grapefruit juice may increase plasma concentrations of estrogens and may result in side effects).
No products indexed under this heading.

Betamethasone (*In vitro* and *in vivo* studies have shown that estrogens are metabolized partially by cytochrome P450 3A4 (CYP3A4). Therefore, inducers of CYP3A4 may affect estrogen drug metabolism. Inducers of CYP3A4, such as St. John's Wort preparations (Hypericum perforatum), phenobarbital, carbamazepine and rifampin may reduce plasma concentrations of estrogens, possibly resulting in a decrease in therapeutic effects and/or changes in the uterine bleeding profile).
No products indexed under this heading.

Betamethasone Acetate (*In vitro* and *in vivo* studies have shown that estrogens are metabolized partially by cytochrome P450 3A4 (CYP3A4). Therefore, inducers of CYP3A4 may affect estrogen drug metabolism. Inducers of CYP3A4, such as St. John's Wort preparations (Hypericum perforatum), phenobarbital, carbamazepine and rifampin may reduce plasma concentrations of estrogens, possibly resulting in a decrease in therapeutic effects and/or changes in the uterine bleeding profile).
No products indexed under this heading.

Betamethasone Benzoate (*In vitro* and *in vivo* studies have shown that estrogens are metabolized partially by cytochrome P450 3A4 (CYP3A4). Therefore, inducers of CYP3A4 may affect estrogen drug metabolism. Inducers of CYP3A4, such as St. John's Wort preparations (Hypericum perforatum), phenobarbital, carbamazepine and rifampin may reduce plasma concentrations of estrogens, possibly resulting in a decrease in therapeutic effects and/or changes in the uterine bleeding profile).
No products indexed under this heading.

Betamethasone Dipropionate (*In vitro* and *in vivo* studies have shown that estrogens are metabolized partially by cytochrome P450 3A4 (CYP3A4). Therefore, inducers of CYP3A4 may affect estrogen drug metabolism. Inducers of CYP3A4, such as St. John's Wort preparations (Hypericum perforatum), phenobarbital, carbamazepine and rifampin may reduce plasma concentrations of estrogens, possibly resulting in a decrease in therapeutic effects and/or changes in the uterine bleeding profile). Products include:
Diprolene Lotion 0.05% 3108
Diprolene Ointment 0.05% 3109
Diprolene AF Cream 0.05% 3107
Lotrisone 3163

Betamethasone Sodium Phosphate (*In vitro* and *in vivo* studies have shown that estrogens are metabolized partially by cytochrome P450 3A4 (CYP3A4). Therefore, inducers of CYP3A4 may affect estrogen drug metabolism. Inducers of CYP3A4, such as St. John's Wort preparations (Hypericum perforatum), phenobarbital, carbamazepine and rifampin may reduce plasma concentrations of estrogens, possibly resulting in a decrease in therapeutic effects and/or changes in the uterine bleeding profile).
No products indexed under this heading.

Betamethasone Valerate (*In vitro* and *in vivo* studies have shown that estrogens are metabolized partially by cytochrome P450 3A4 (CYP3A4). Therefore, inducers of CYP3A4 may affect estrogen drug metabolism. Inducers of CYP3A4, such as St. John's Wort preparations (Hypericum perforatum), phenobarbital, carbamazepine and rifampin may reduce plasma concentrations of estrogens, possibly resulting in a decrease in therapeutic effects and/or changes in the uterine bleeding profile). Products include:
Luxíq 3321

Bosentan (*In vitro* and *in vivo* studies have shown that estrogens are metabolized partially by cytochrome P450 3A4 (CYP3A4). Therefore, inducers of CYP3A4 may affect estrogen drug metabolism. Inducers of CYP3A4, such as St. John's Wort preparations (Hypericum perforatum), phenobarbital, carbamazepine and rifampin may reduce plasma concentrations of estrogens, possibly resulting in a decrease in therapeutic effects and/or changes in the uterine bleeding profile). Products include:
Tracleer 573

Carbamazepine (*In vitro* and *in vivo* studies have shown that estrogens are metabolized partially by cytochrome P450 3A4 (CYP3A4). Therefore, inducers of CYP3A4 may affect estrogen drug metabolism. Inducers of CYP3A4, such as carbamazepine, may reduce plasma concentrations of estrogens, possibly resulting in a decrease in therapeutic effects and/or changes in the uterine bleeding profile). Products include:
Carbatrol 3280
Equetro 3477

Cimetidine (*In vitro* and *in vivo* studies have shown that estrogens are metabolized partially by cytochrome P450 3A4 (CYP3A4). Therefore, inhibitors of CYP3A4 may affect estrogen drug metabolism. Inhibitors of CYP3A4, such as erythromycin, clarithromycin, ketoconazole, itraconazole, ritonavir and

613 **Interactions Index** **Estrasorb**

grapefruit juice may increase plasma concentrations of estrogens and may result in side effects).
No products indexed under this heading.

Cimetidine Hydrochloride (*In vitro* and *in vivo* studies have shown that estrogens are metabolized partially by cytochrome P450 3A4 (CYP3A4). Therefore, inhibitors of CYP3A4 may affect estrogen drug metabolism. Inhibitors of CYP3A4, such as erythromycin, clarithromycin, ketoconazole, itraconazole, ritonavir and grapefruit juice may increase plasma concentrations of estrogens and may result in side effects).
No products indexed under this heading.

Ciprofloxacin (*In vitro* and *in vivo* studies have shown that estrogens are metabolized partially by cytochrome P450 3A4 (CYP3A4). Therefore, inducers of CYP3A4 may affect estrogen drug metabolism. Inducers of CYP3A4, such as St. John's Wort preparations (Hypericum perforatum), phenobarbital, carbamazepine and rifampin may reduce plasma concentrations of estrogens, possibly resulting in a decrease in therapeutic effects and/or changes in the uterine bleeding profile). Products include:
Cipro I.V. 3082
Cipro 3073
Cipro XR 3091
Ciprodex 583

Ciprofloxacin Hydrochloride (*In vitro* and *in vivo* studies have shown that estrogens are metabolized partially by cytochrome P450 3A4 (CYP3A4). Therefore, inducers of CYP3A4 may affect estrogen drug metabolism. Inducers of CYP3A4, such as St. John's Wort preparations (Hypericum perforatum), phenobarbital, carbamazepine and rifampin may reduce plasma concentrations of estrogens, possibly resulting in a decrease in therapeutic effects and/or changes in the uterine bleeding profile). Products include:
Cipro 3073

Cisplatin (*In vitro* and *in vivo* studies have shown that estrogens are metabolized partially by cytochrome P450 3A4 (CYP3A4). Therefore, inducers of CYP3A4 may affect estrogen drug metabolism. Inducers of CYP3A4, such as St. John's Wort preparations (Hypericum perforatum), phenobarbital, carbamazepine and rifampin may reduce plasma concentrations of estrogens, possibly resulting in a decrease in therapeutic effects and/or changes in the uterine bleeding profile).
No products indexed under this heading.

Clarithromycin (*In vitro* and *in vivo* studies have shown that estrogens are metabolized partially by cytochrome P450 3A4 (CYP3A4). Therefore, inhibitors of CYP3A4 may affect estrogen drug metabolism. Inhibitors of CYP3A4, such as clarithromycin, may increase plasma concentrations of estrogens and may result in side effects). Products include:
Biaxin/Biaxin XL 412

Clotrimazole (*In vitro* and *in vivo* studies have shown that estrogens are metabolized partially by cytochrome P450 3A4 (CYP3A4). Therefore, inhibitors of CYP3A4 may affect estrogen drug metabolism. Inhibitors of CYP3A4, such as erythromycin, clarithromycin, ketoconazole, itraconazole, ritonavir and grapefruit juice may increase plasma concentrations of estrogens and may result in side effects). Products include:
Lotrisone 3163

Conivaptan Hydrochloride (*In vitro* and *in vivo* studies have shown that estrogens are metabolized partially by cytochrome P450 3A4 (CYP3A4). Therefore, inhibitors of CYP3A4 may affect estrogen drug metabolism. Inhibitors of CYP3A4, such as erythromycin, clarithromycin, ketoconazole, itraconazole, ritonavir and grapefruit juice may increase plasma concentrations of estrogens and may result in side effects). Products include:
Vaprisol 689

Cortisone Acetate (*In vitro* and *in vivo* studies have shown that estrogens are metabolized partially by cytochrome P450 3A4 (CYP3A4). Therefore, inducers of CYP3A4 may affect estrogen drug metabolism. Inducers of CYP3A4, such as St. John's Wort preparations (Hypericum perforatum), phenobarbital, carbamazepine and rifampin may reduce plasma concentrations of estrogens, possibly resulting in a decrease in therapeutic effects and/or changes in the uterine bleeding profile).
No products indexed under this heading.

Cyclosporine (*In vitro* and *in vivo* studies have shown that estrogens are metabolized partially by cytochrome P450 3A4 (CYP3A4). Therefore, inhibitors of CYP3A4 may affect estrogen drug metabolism. Inhibitors of CYP3A4, such as erythromycin, clarithromycin, ketoconazole, itraconazole, ritonavir and grapefruit juice may increase plasma concentrations of estrogens and may result in side effects). Products include:
Gengraf 440
Neoral Oral Solution 2496
Neoral Capsules 2496
Restasis 605

Dalfopristin (*In vitro* and *in vivo* studies have shown that estrogens are metabolized partially by cytochrome P450 3A4 (CYP3A4). Therefore, inhibitors of CYP3A4 may affect estrogen drug metabolism. Inhibitors of CYP3A4, such as erythromycin, clarithromycin, ketoconazole, itraconazole, ritonavir and grapefruit juice may increase plasma concentrations of estrogens and may result in side effects).
No products indexed under this heading.

Danazol (*In vitro* and *in vivo* studies have shown that estrogens are metabolized partially by cytochrome P450 3A4 (CYP3A4). Therefore, inhibitors of CYP3A4 may affect estrogen drug metabolism. Inhibitors of CYP3A4, such as erythromycin, clarithromycin, ketoconazole, itraconazole, ritonavir and grapefruit juice may increase plasma concentrations of estrogens and may result in side effects).
No products indexed under this heading.

Darunavir (*In vitro* and *in vivo* studies have shown that estrogens are metabolized partially by cytochrome P450 3A4 (CYP3A4). Therefore, inhibitors of CYP3A4 may affect estrogen drug metabolism. Inhibitors of CYP3A4, such as erythromycin, clarithromycin, ketoconazole, itraconazole, ritonavir and grapefruit juice may increase plasma concentrations of estrogens and may result in side effects).
No products indexed under this heading.

Dasatinib (*In vitro* and *in vivo* studies have shown that estrogens are metabolized partially by cytochrome P450 3A4 (CYP3A4). Therefore, inhibitors of CYP3A4 may affect estrogen drug metabolism. Inhibitors of CYP3A4, such as erythromycin, clarithromycin, ketoconazole, itraconazole, ritonavir and grapefruit juice may increase plasma concentrations of estrogens and may result in side effects).
No products indexed under this heading.

Delavirdine Mesylate (*In vitro* and *in vivo* studies have shown that estrogens are metabolized partially by cytochrome P450 3A4 (CYP3A4). Therefore, inhibitors of CYP3A4 may affect estrogen drug metabolism. Inhibitors of CYP3A4, such as erythromycin, clarithromycin, ketoconazole, itraconazole, ritonavir and grapefruit juice may increase plasma concentrations of estrogens and may result in side effects).
No products indexed under this heading.

Delavirine (*In vitro* and *in vivo* studies have shown that estrogens are metabolized partially by cytochrome P450 3A4 (CYP3A4). Therefore, inhibitors of CYP3A4 may affect estrogen drug metabolism. Inhibitors of CYP3A4, such as erythromycin, clarithromycin, ketoconazole, itraconazole, ritonavir and grapefruit juice may increase plasma concentrations of estrogens and may result in side effects).
No products indexed under this heading.

Desloratadine (*In vitro* and *in vivo* studies have shown that estrogens are metabolized partially by cytochrome P450 3A4 (CYP3A4). Therefore, inhibitors of CYP3A4 may affect estrogen drug metabolism. Inhibitors of CYP3A4, such as erythromycin, clarithromycin, ketoconazole, itraconazole, ritonavir and grapefruit juice may increase plasma concentrations of estrogens and may result in side effects). Products include:
Clarinex Syrup 3098
Clarinex 3098
Clarinex Reditabs 3098
Clarinex-D 12-Hour 3101
Clarinex-D 3104

Dexamethasone (*In vitro* and *in vivo* studies have shown that estrogens are metabolized partially by cytochrome P450 3A4 (CYP3A4). Therefore, inducers of CYP3A4 may affect estrogen drug metabolism. Inducers of CYP3A4, such as St. John's Wort preparations (Hypericum perforatum), phenobarbital, carbamazepine and rifampin may reduce plasma concentrations of estrogens, possibly resulting in a decrease in therapeutic effects and/or changes in the uterine bleeding profile). Products include:
Ciprodex 583
Ozurdex .... ⊙223
Tobramycin and Dexamethasone Ophthalmic Suspension .... ⊙251

Dexamethasone Acetate (*In vitro* and *in vivo* studies have shown that estrogens are metabolized partially by cytochrome P450 3A4 (CYP3A4). Therefore, inducers of CYP3A4 may affect estrogen drug metabolism. Inducers of CYP3A4, such as St. John's Wort preparations (Hypericum perforatum), phenobarbital, carbamazepine and rifampin may reduce plasma concentrations of estrogens, possibly resulting in a decrease in therapeutic effects and/or changes in the uterine bleeding profile).
No products indexed under this heading.

Dexamethasone Phosphate (*In vitro* and *in vivo* studies have shown that estrogens are metabolized partially by cytochrome P450 3A4 (CYP3A4). Therefore, inducers of CYP3A4 may affect estrogen drug metabolism. Inducers of CYP3A4, such as St. John's Wort preparations (Hypericum perforatum), phenobarbital, carbamazepine and rifampin may reduce plasma concentrations of estrogens, possibly resulting in a decrease in therapeutic effects and/or changes in the uterine bleeding profile).
No products indexed under this heading.

Dexamethasone Sodium (*In vitro* and *in vivo* studies have shown that estrogens are metabolized partially by cytochrome P450 3A4 (CYP3A4). Therefore, inducers of CYP3A4 may affect estrogen drug metabolism. Inducers of CYP3A4, such as St. John's Wort preparations (Hypericum perforatum), phenobarbital, carbamazepine and rifampin may reduce plasma concentrations of estrogens, possibly resulting in a decrease in therapeutic effects and/or changes in the uterine bleeding profile).
No products indexed under this heading.

Dexamethasone Sodium Phosphate (*In vitro* and *in vivo* studies have shown that estrogens are metabolized partially by cytochrome P450 3A4 (CYP3A4). Therefore, inducers of CYP3A4 may affect estrogen drug metabolism. Inducers of CYP3A4, such as St. John's Wort preparations (Hypericum perforatum), phenobarbital, carbamazepine and rifampin may reduce plasma concentrations of estrogens, possibly resulting in a decrease in therapeutic effects and/or changes in the uterine bleeding profile).
No products indexed under this heading.

Dexamethasone Sodium Phosphate Injection (*In vitro* and *in vivo* studies have shown that estrogens are metabolized partially by cytochrome P450 3A4 (CYP3A4). Therefore, inducers of CYP3A4 may affect estrogen drug metabolism. Inducers of CYP3A4, such as St. John's Wort preparations (Hypericum perforatum), phenobarbital, carbamazepine and rifampin may reduce plasma concentrations of estrogens, possibly resulting in a decrease in therapeutic effects and/or changes in the uterine bleeding profile).
No products indexed under this heading.

Diltiazem Hydrochloride (*In vitro* and *in vivo* studies have shown that estrogens are metabolized partially by cytochrome P450 3A4 (CYP3A4). Therefore, inhibitors of CYP3A4 may affect estrogen drug metabolism. Inhibitors of CYP3A4, such as erythromycin, clarithromycin, ketoconazole, itraconazole, ritonavir and grapefruit juice may increase plasma concentrations of estrogens and may result in side effects). Products include:
Cardizem LA 423

Diltiazem Maleate (*In vitro* and *in vivo* studies have shown that estrogens are metabolized partially by cytochrome P450 3A4 (CYP3A4). Therefore, inhibitors of CYP3A4 may affect estrogen drug metabolism. Inhibitors of CYP3A4, such as erythromycin, clarithromycin, ketoconazole, itraconazole, ritonavir and grapefruit juice may increase plasma concentrations of estrogens and may result in side effects).
No products indexed under this heading.

Doxorubicin Hydrochloride (*In vitro* and *in vivo* studies have shown that estrogens are metabolized partially by cytochrome P450 3A4 (CYP3A4). Therefore, inducers of CYP3A4 may affect estrogen drug metabolism. Inducers of CYP3A4, such as St. John's Wort preparations (Hypericum perforatum), phenobarbital, carbamazepine and rifampin may reduce plasma concentrations of estrogens, possibly resulting in a decrease in therapeutic effects and/or changes in the uterine bleeding profile).
No products indexed under this heading.

Efavirenz (*In vitro* and *in vivo* studies have shown that estrogens are metabolized partially by cytochrome P450 3A4 (CYP3A4). Therefore, inducers of CYP3A4 may affect estrogen drug metabolism. Inducers of CYP3A4, such as St. John's Wort preparations (Hypericum perforatum), phenobarbital, carbamazepine and rifampin may reduce plasma concentrations of estrogens, possibly resulting in a decrease in therapeutic effects and/or changes in the uterine bleeding profile). Products include:
Atripla 906

IMPORTANT NOTE: Always consult each drug listing in the patient's regimen for possible interactions.

Erythromycin (In vitro and in vivo studies have shown that estrogens are metabolized partially by cytochrome P450 3A4 (CYP3A4). Therefore, inhibitors of CYP3A4 may affect estrogen drug metabolism. Inhibitors of CYP3A4, such as erythromycin, may increase plasma concentrations of estrogens and may result in side effects).
No products indexed under this heading.

Erythromycin, Topical (In vitro and in vivo studies have shown that estrogens are metabolized partially by cytochrome P450 3A4 (CYP3A4). Therefore, inhibitors of CYP3A4 may affect estrogen drug metabolism. Inhibitors of CYP3A4, such as erythromycin, may increase plasma concentrations of estrogens and may result in side effects).
No products indexed under this heading.

Erythromycin Estolate (In vitro and in vivo studies have shown that estrogens are metabolized partially by cytochrome P450 3A4 (CYP3A4). Therefore, inhibitors of CYP3A4 may affect estrogen drug metabolism. Inhibitors of CYP3A4, such as erythromycin, may increase plasma concentrations of estrogens and may result in side effects).
No products indexed under this heading.

Erythromycin Ethylsuccinate (In vitro and in vivo studies have shown that estrogens are metabolized partially by cytochrome P450 3A4 (CYP3A4). Therefore, inhibitors of CYP3A4 may affect estrogen drug metabolism. Inhibitors of CYP3A4, such as erythromycin, may increase plasma concentrations of estrogens and may result in side effects). Products include:

Erythromycin Gluceptate (In vitro and in vivo studies have shown that estrogens are metabolized partially by cytochrome P450 3A4 (CYP3A4). Therefore, inhibitors of CYP3A4 may affect estrogen drug metabolism. Inhibitors of CYP3A4, such as erythromycin, may increase plasma concentrations of estrogens and may result in side effects).
No products indexed under this heading.

Erythromycin Lactobionate (In vitro and in vivo studies have shown that estrogens are metabolized partially by cytochrome P450 3A4 (CYP3A4). Therefore, inhibitors of CYP3A4 may affect estrogen drug metabolism. Inhibitors of CYP3A4, such as erythromycin, may increase plasma concentrations of estrogens and may result in side effects).
No products indexed under this heading.

Erythromycin Stearate (In vitro and in vivo studies have shown that estrogens are metabolized partially by cytochrome P450 3A4 (CYP3A4). Therefore, inhibitors of CYP3A4 may affect estrogen drug metabolism. Inhibitors of CYP3A4, such as erythromycin, may increase plasma concentrations of estrogens and may result in side effects).
No products indexed under this heading.

Esomeprazole Magnesium (In vitro and in vivo studies have shown that estrogens are metabolized partially by cytochrome P450 3A4 (CYP3A4). Therefore, inhibitors of CYP3A4 may affect estrogen drug metabolism. Inhibitors of CYP3A4, such as erythromycin, clarithromycin, ketoconazole, itraconazole, ritonavir and grapefruit juice may increase plasma concentrations of estrogens and may result in side effects). Products include:

Esomeprazole Sodium (In vitro and in vivo studies have shown that estro-

gens are metabolized partially by cytochrome P450 3A4 (CYP3A4). Therefore, inhibitors of CYP3A4 may affect estrogen drug metabolism. Inhibitors of CYP3A4, such as erythromycin, clarithromycin, ketoconazole, itraconazole, ritonavir and grapefruit juice may increase plasma concentrations of estrogens and may result in side effects). Products include:

Ethosuximide (In vitro and in vivo studies have shown that estrogens are metabolized partially by cytochrome P450 3A4 (CYP3A4). Therefore, inducers of CYP3A4 may affect estrogen drug metabolism. Inducers of CYP3A4, such as St. John's Wort preparations (Hypericum perforatum), phenobarbital, carbamazepine and rifampin may reduce plasma concentrations of estrogens, possibly resulting in a decrease in therapeutic effects and/or changes in the uterine bleeding profile).
No products indexed under this heading.

Felbamate (In vitro and in vivo studies have shown that estrogens are metabolized partially by cytochrome P450 3A4 (CYP3A4). Therefore, inducers of CYP3A4 may affect estrogen drug metabolism. Inducers of CYP3A4, such as St. John's Wort preparations (Hypericum perforatum), phenobarbital, carbamazepine and rifampin may reduce plasma concentrations of estrogens, possibly resulting in a decrease in therapeutic effects and/or changes in the uterine bleeding profile).
No products indexed under this heading.

Fluconazole (In vitro and in vivo studies have shown that estrogens are metabolized partially by cytochrome P450 3A4 (CYP3A4). Therefore, inhibitors of CYP3A4 may affect estrogen drug metabolism. Inhibitors of CYP3A4, such as erythromycin, clarithromycin, ketoconazole, itraconazole, ritonavir and grapefruit juice may increase plasma concentrations of estrogens and may result in side effects).
No products indexed under this heading.

Fludrocortisone Acetate (In vitro and in vivo studies have shown that estrogens are metabolized partially by cytochrome P450 3A4 (CYP3A4). Therefore, inducers of CYP3A4 may affect estrogen drug metabolism. Inducers of CYP3A4, such as St. John's Wort preparations (Hypericum perforatum), phenobarbital, carbamazepine and rifampin may reduce plasma concentrations of estrogens, possibly resulting in a decrease in therapeutic effects and/or changes in the uterine bleeding profile).
No products indexed under this heading.

Fluoxetine (In vitro and in vivo studies have shown that estrogens are metabolized partially by cytochrome P450 3A4 (CYP3A4). Therefore, inhibitors of CYP3A4 may affect estrogen drug metabolism. Inhibitors of CYP3A4, such as erythromycin, clarithromycin, ketoconazole, itraconazole, ritonavir and grapefruit juice may increase plasma concentrations of estrogens and may result in side effects).
No products indexed under this heading.

Fluoxetine Hydrochloride (In vitro and in vivo studies have shown that estrogens are metabolized partially by cytochrome P450 3A4 (CYP3A4). Therefore, inhibitors of CYP3A4 may affect estrogen drug metabolism. Inhibitors of CYP3A4, such as erythromycin, clarithromycin, ketoconazole, itraconazole, ritonavir and grapefruit juice may increase plasma concentrations of estrogens and may result in side effects). Products include:

Symbyax 1965

Fluvoxamine Maleate (In vitro and in vivo studies have shown that estrogens are metabolized partially by cytochrome P450 3A4 (CYP3A4). Therefore, inhibitors of CYP3A4 may affect estrogen drug metabolism. Inhibitors of CYP3A4, such as erythromycin, clarithromycin, ketoconazole, itraconazole, ritonavir and grapefruit juice may increase plasma concentrations of estrogens and may result in side effects).
No products indexed under this heading.

Fosamprenavir Calcium (In vitro and in vivo studies have shown that estrogens are metabolized partially by cytochrome P450 3A4 (CYP3A4). Therefore, inhibitors of CYP3A4 may affect estrogen drug metabolism. Inhibitors of CYP3A4, such as erythromycin, clarithromycin, ketoconazole, itraconazole, ritonavir and grapefruit juice may increase plasma concentrations of estrogens and may result in side effects). Products include:

Fosphenytoin Sodium (In vitro and in vivo studies have shown that estrogens are metabolized partially by cytochrome P450 3A4 (CYP3A4). Therefore, inducers of CYP3A4 may affect estrogen drug metabolism. Inducers of CYP3A4, such as St. John's Wort preparations (Hypericum perforatum), phenobarbital, carbamazepine and rifampin may reduce plasma concentrations of estrogens, possibly resulting in a decrease in therapeutic effects and/or changes in the uterine bleeding profile).
No products indexed under this heading.

Garlic Extract (In vitro and in vivo studies have shown that estrogens are metabolized partially by cytochrome P450 3A4 (CYP3A4). Therefore, inducers of CYP3A4 may affect estrogen drug metabolism. Inducers of CYP3A4, such as St. John's Wort preparations (Hypericum perforatum), phenobarbital, carbamazepine and rifampin may reduce plasma concentrations of estrogens, possibly resulting in a decrease in therapeutic effects and/or changes in the uterine bleeding profile).
No products indexed under this heading.

Garlic Oil (In vitro and in vivo studies have shown that estrogens are metabolized partially by cytochrome P450 3A4 (CYP3A4). Therefore, inducers of CYP3A4 may affect estrogen drug metabolism. Inducers of CYP3A4, such as St. John's Wort preparations (Hypericum perforatum), phenobarbital, carbamazepine and rifampin may reduce plasma concentrations of estrogens, possibly resulting in a decrease in therapeutic effects and/or changes in the uterine bleeding profile).
No products indexed under this heading.

Hydrocortisone (In vitro and in vivo studies have shown that estrogens are metabolized partially by cytochrome P450 3A4 (CYP3A4). Therefore, inducers of CYP3A4 may affect estrogen drug metabolism. Inducers of CYP3A4, such as St. John's Wort preparations (Hypericum perforatum), phenobarbital, carbamazepine and rifampin may reduce plasma concentrations of estrogens, possibly resulting in a decrease in therapeutic effects and/or changes in the uterine bleeding profile).
No products indexed under this heading.

Hydrocortisone (Alcohol) (In vitro and in vivo studies have shown that estrogens are metabolized partially by cytochrome P450 3A4 (CYP3A4). Therefore, inducers of CYP3A4 may affect estrogen drug metabolism. Inducers of CYP3A4, such as St. John's Wort preparations (Hypericum perforatum), phenobarbital, carbamazepine and rifampin may reduce plasma concentra-

tions of estrogens, possibly resulting in a decrease in therapeutic effects and/or changes in the uterine bleeding profile).
No products indexed under this heading.

Hydrocortisone Acetate (In vitro and in vivo studies have shown that estrogens are metabolized partially by cytochrome P450 3A4 (CYP3A4). Therefore, inducers of CYP3A4 may affect estrogen drug metabolism. Inducers of CYP3A4, such as St. John's Wort preparations (Hypericum perforatum), phenobarbital, carbamazepine and rifampin may reduce plasma concentrations of estrogens, possibly resulting in a decrease in therapeutic effects and/or changes in the uterine bleeding profile).
No products indexed under this heading.

Hydrocortisone Butyrate (In vitro and in vivo studies have shown that estrogens are metabolized partially by cytochrome P450 3A4 (CYP3A4). Therefore, inducers of CYP3A4 may affect estrogen drug metabolism. Inducers of CYP3A4, such as St. John's Wort preparations (Hypericum perforatum), phenobarbital, carbamazepine and rifampin may reduce plasma concentrations of estrogens, possibly resulting in a decrease in therapeutic effects and/or changes in the uterine bleeding profile).
No products indexed under this heading.

Hydrocortisone Cypionate (In vitro and in vivo studies have shown that estrogens are metabolized partially by cytochrome P450 3A4 (CYP3A4). Therefore, inducers of CYP3A4 may affect estrogen drug metabolism. Inducers of CYP3A4, such as St. John's Wort preparations (Hypericum perforatum), phenobarbital, carbamazepine and rifampin may reduce plasma concentrations of estrogens, possibly resulting in a decrease in therapeutic effects and/or changes in the uterine bleeding profile).
No products indexed under this heading.

Hydrocortisone Hemisuccinate (In vitro and in vivo studies have shown that estrogens are metabolized partially by cytochrome P450 3A4 (CYP3A4). Therefore, inducers of CYP3A4 may affect estrogen drug metabolism. Inducers of CYP3A4, such as St. John's Wort preparations (Hypericum perforatum), phenobarbital, carbamazepine and rifampin may reduce plasma concentrations of estrogens, possibly resulting in a decrease in therapeutic effects and/or changes in the uterine bleeding profile).
No products indexed under this heading.

Hydrocortisone Probutate (In vitro and in vivo studies have shown that estrogens are metabolized partially by cytochrome P450 3A4 (CYP3A4). Therefore, inducers of CYP3A4 may affect estrogen drug metabolism. Inducers of CYP3A4, such as St. John's Wort preparations (Hypericum perforatum), phenobarbital, carbamazepine and rifampin may reduce plasma concentrations of estrogens, possibly resulting in a decrease in therapeutic effects and/or changes in the uterine bleeding profile).
No products indexed under this heading.

Hydrocortisone Sodium Phosphate (In vitro and in vivo studies have shown that estrogens are metabolized partially by cytochrome P450 3A4 (CYP3A4). Therefore, inducers of CYP3A4 may affect estrogen drug metabolism. Inducers of CYP3A4, such as St. John's Wort preparations (Hypericum perforatum), phenobarbital, carbamazepine and rifampin may reduce plasma concentrations of estrogens,

possibly resulting in a decrease in therapeutic effects and/or changes in the uterine bleeding profile).
No products indexed under this heading.

Hydrocortisone Sodium Succinate (*In vitro* and *in vivo* studies have shown that estrogens are metabolized partially by cytochrome P450 3A4 (CYP3A4). Therefore, inducers of CYP3A4 may affect estrogen drug metabolism. Inducers of CYP3A4, such as St. John's Wort preparations (Hypericum perforatum), phenobarbital, carbamazepine and rifampin may reduce plasma concentrations of estrogens, possibly resulting in a decrease in therapeutic effects and/ or changes in the uterine bleeding profile).
No products indexed under this heading.

Hydrocortisone Valerate (*In vitro* and *in vivo* studies have shown that estrogens are metabolized partially by cytochrome P450 3A4 (CYP3A4). Therefore, inducers of CYP3A4 may affect estrogen drug metabolism. Inducers of CYP3A4, such as St. John's Wort preparations (Hypericum perforatum), phenobarbital, carbamazepine and rifampin may reduce plasma concentrations of estrogens, possibly resulting in a decrease in therapeutic effects and/ or changes in the uterine bleeding profile).
No products indexed under this heading.

Hypericum (*In vitro* and *in vivo* studies have shown that estrogens are metabolized partially by cytochrome P450 3A4 (CYP3A4). Therefore, inducers of CYP3A4 may affect estrogen drug metabolism. Inducers of CYP3A4, such as St. John's Wort preparations (Hypericum perforatum), phenobarbital, carbamazepine and rifampin may reduce plasma concentrations of estrogens, possibly resulting in a decrease in therapeutic effects and/or changes in the uterine bleeding profile).
No products indexed under this heading.

Hypericum Perforatum (*In vitro* and *in vivo* studies have shown that estrogens are metabolized partially by cytochrome P450 3A4 (CYP3A4). Therefore, inducers of CYP3A4 may affect estrogen drug metabolism. Inducers of CYP3A4, such as St. John's Wort preparations (Hypericum perforatum), may reduce plasma concentrations of estrogens, possibly resulting in a decrease in therapeutic effects and/or changes in the uterine bleeding profile). Products include:
Traumeel **1800**

Imatinib Mesylate (*In vitro* and *in vivo* studies have shown that estrogens are metabolized partially by cytochrome P450 3A4 (CYP3A4). Therefore, inhibitors of CYP3A4 may affect estrogen drug metabolism. Inhibitors of CYP3A4, such as erythromycin, clarithromycin, ketoconazole, itraconazole, ritonavir and grapefruit juice may increase plasma concentrations of estrogens and may result in side effects). Products include:
Gleevec **2477**

Indinavir Sulfate (*In vitro* and *in vivo* studies have shown that estrogens are metabolized partially by cytochrome P450 3A4 (CYP3A4). Therefore, inhibitors of CYP3A4 may affect estrogen drug metabolism. Inhibitors of CYP3A4, such as erythromycin, clarithromycin, ketoconazole, itraconazole, ritonavir and grapefruit juice may increase plasma concentrations of estrogens and may result in side effects). Products include:
Crixivan **2113**

Isoniazid (*In vitro* and *in vivo* studies have shown that estrogens are metabolized partially by cytochrome P450 3A4 (CYP3A4). Therefore, inhibitors of CYP3A4 may affect estrogen drug metabolism. Inhibitors of CYP3A4, such as erythromycin, clarithromycin, ketoconazole, itraconazole, ritonavir and grapefruit juice may increase plasma concentrations of estrogens and may result in side effects).
No products indexed under this heading.

Itraconazole (*In vitro* and *in vivo* studies have shown that estrogens are metabolized partially by cytochrome P450 3A4 (CYP3A4). Therefore, inhibitors of CYP3A4 may affect estrogen drug metabolism. Inhibitors of CYP3A4, such as itraconazole, may increase plasma concentrations of estrogens and may result in side effects).
No products indexed under this heading.

Ketoconazole (*In vitro* and *in vivo* studies have shown that estrogens are metabolized partially by cytochrome P450 3A4 (CYP3A4). Therefore, inhibitors of CYP3A4 may affect estrogen drug metabolism. Inhibitors of CYP3A4, such as ketoconazole, may increase plasma concentrations of estrogens and may result in side effects). Products include:
Extina **3319**
Xolegel **3337**

Lapatinib (*In vitro* and *in vivo* studies have shown that estrogens are metabolized partially by cytochrome P450 3A4 (CYP3A4). Therefore, inhibitors of CYP3A4 may affect estrogen drug metabolism. Inhibitors of CYP3A4, such as erythromycin, clarithromycin, ketoconazole, itraconazole, ritonavir and grapefruit juice may increase plasma concentrations of estrogens and may result in side effects). Products include:
Tykerb **1698**

Levothyroxine Sodium (Estrogen administration leads to increased thyroid-binding globulin (TBG) levels. Patients dependent on thyroid hormone replacement therapy who are also receiving estrogens may require increased doses of their thyroid replacement therapy). Products include:
Levoxyl Tablets **1843**
Synthroid **529**

Liothyronine Sodium (Estrogen administration leads to increased thyroid-binding globulin (TBG) levels. Patients dependent on thyroid hormone replacement therapy who are also receiving estrogens may require increased doses of their thyroid replacement therapy). Products include:
Cytomel **1830**

Liotrix (Estrogen administration leads to increased thyroid-binding globulin (TBG) levels. Patients dependent on thyroid hormone replacement therapy who are also receiving estrogens may require increased doses of their thyroid replacement therapy).
No products indexed under this heading.

Lopinavir (*In vitro* and *in vivo* studies have shown that estrogens are metabolized partially by cytochrome P450 3A4 (CYP3A4). Therefore, inhibitors of CYP3A4 may affect estrogen drug metabolism. Inhibitors of CYP3A4, such as erythromycin, clarithromycin, ketoconazole, itraconazole, ritonavir and grapefruit juice may increase plasma concentrations of estrogens and may result in side effects). Products include:
Kaletra **458**

Loratadine (*In vitro* and *in vivo* studies have shown that estrogens are metabolized partially by cytochrome P450 3A4 (CYP3A4). Therefore, inhibitors of CYP3A4 may affect estrogen drug metabolism. Inhibitors of CYP3A4, such as erythromycin, clarithromycin, ketoconazole, itraconazole, ritonavir and grapefruit juice may increase plasma concentrations of estrogens and may result in side effects).
No products indexed under this heading.

Mephenytoin (*In vitro* and *in vivo* studies have shown that estrogens are metabolized partially by cytochrome P450 3A4 (CYP3A4). Therefore, inducers of CYP3A4 may affect estrogen drug metabolism. Inducers of CYP3A4, such as St. John's Wort preparations (Hypericum perforatum), phenobarbital, carbamazepine and rifampin may reduce plasma concentrations of estrogens, possibly resulting in a decrease in therapeutic effects and/or changes in the uterine bleeding profile).
No products indexed under this heading.

Methsuximide (*In vitro* and *in vivo* studies have shown that estrogens are metabolized partially by cytochrome P450 3A4 (CYP3A4). Therefore, inducers of CYP3A4 may affect estrogen drug metabolism. Inducers of CYP3A4, such as St. John's Wort preparations (Hypericum perforatum), phenobarbital, carbamazepine and rifampin may reduce plasma concentrations of estrogens, possibly resulting in a decrease in therapeutic effects and/or changes in the uterine bleeding profile).
No products indexed under this heading.

Methylprednisolone (*In vitro* and *in vivo* studies have shown that estrogens are metabolized partially by cytochrome P450 3A4 (CYP3A4). Therefore, inducers of CYP3A4 may affect estrogen drug metabolism. Inducers of CYP3A4, such as St. John's Wort preparations (Hypericum perforatum), phenobarbital, carbamazepine and rifampin may reduce plasma concentrations of estrogens, possibly resulting in a decrease in therapeutic effects and/or changes in the uterine bleeding profile).
No products indexed under this heading.

Methylprednisolone Acetate (*In vitro* and *in vivo* studies have shown that estrogens are metabolized partially by cytochrome P450 3A4 (CYP3A4). Therefore, inducers of CYP3A4 may affect estrogen drug metabolism. Inducers of CYP3A4, such as St. John's Wort preparations (Hypericum perforatum), phenobarbital, carbamazepine and rifampin may reduce plasma concentrations of estrogens, possibly resulting in a decrease in therapeutic effects and/ or changes in the uterine bleeding profile).
No products indexed under this heading.

Methylprednisolone Sodium Succinate (*In vitro* and *in vivo* studies have shown that estrogens are metabolized partially by cytochrome P450 3A4 (CYP3A4). Therefore, inducers of CYP3A4 may affect estrogen drug metabolism. Inducers of CYP3A4, such as St. John's Wort preparations (Hypericum perforatum), phenobarbital, carbamazepine and rifampin may reduce plasma concentrations of estrogens, possibly resulting in a decrease in therapeutic effects and/or changes in the uterine bleeding profile).
No products indexed under this heading.

Metronidazole (*In vitro* and *in vivo* studies have shown that estrogens are metabolized partially by cytochrome P450 3A4 (CYP3A4). Therefore, inhibitors of CYP3A4 may affect estrogen drug metabolism. Inhibitors of CYP3A4, such as erythromycin, clarithromycin, ketoconazole, itraconazole, ritonavir and grapefruit juice may increase plasma concentrations of estrogens and may result in side effects). Products include:
Pylera **793**

Metronidazole Benzoate (*In vitro* and *in vivo* studies have shown that estrogens are metabolized partially by cytochrome P450 3A4 (CYP3A4). Therefore, inhibitors of CYP3A4 may affect estrogen drug metabolism. Inhibitors of CYP3A4, such as erythromycin, clarithromycin, ketoconazole, itraconazole, ritonavir and grapefruit juice may increase plasma concentrations of estrogens and may result in side effects).
No products indexed under this heading.

Metronidazole Hydrochloride (*In vitro* and *in vivo* studies have shown that estrogens are metabolized partially by cytochrome P450 3A4 (CYP3A4). Therefore, inhibitors of CYP3A4 may affect estrogen drug metabolism. Inhibitors of CYP3A4, such as erythromycin, clarithromycin, ketoconazole, itraconazole, ritonavir and grapefruit juice may increase plasma concentrations of estrogens and may result in side effects).
No products indexed under this heading.

Metronidazole Sodium (*In vitro* and *in vivo* studies have shown that estrogens are metabolized partially by cytochrome P450 3A4 (CYP3A4). Therefore, inhibitors of CYP3A4 may affect estrogen drug metabolism. Inhibitors of CYP3A4, such as erythromycin, clarithromycin, ketoconazole, itraconazole, ritonavir and grapefruit juice may increase plasma concentrations of estrogens and may result in side effects).
No products indexed under this heading.

Miconazole (*In vitro* and *in vivo* studies have shown that estrogens are metabolized partially by cytochrome P450 3A4 (CYP3A4). Therefore, inhibitors of CYP3A4 may affect estrogen drug metabolism. Inhibitors of CYP3A4, such as erythromycin, clarithromycin, ketoconazole, itraconazole, ritonavir and grapefruit juice may increase plasma concentrations of estrogens and may result in side effects).
No products indexed under this heading.

Miconazole Nitrate (*In vitro* and *in vivo* studies have shown that estrogens are metabolized partially by cytochrome P450 3A4 (CYP3A4). Therefore, inhibitors of CYP3A4 may affect estrogen drug metabolism. Inhibitors of CYP3A4, such as erythromycin, clarithromycin, ketoconazole, itraconazole, ritonavir and grapefruit juice may increase plasma concentrations of estrogens and may result in side effects). Products include:
Vusion Ointment **3335**

Mifepristone (*In vitro* and *in vivo* studies have shown that estrogens are metabolized partially by cytochrome P450 3A4 (CYP3A4). Therefore, inhibitors of CYP3A4 may affect estrogen drug metabolism. Inhibitors of CYP3A4, such as erythromycin, clarithromycin, ketoconazole, itraconazole, ritonavir and grapefruit juice may increase plasma concentrations of estrogens and may result in side effects).
No products indexed under this heading.

Modafinil (*In vitro* and *in vivo* studies have shown that estrogens are metabolized partially by cytochrome P450 3A4 (CYP3A4). Therefore, inducers of CYP3A4 may affect estrogen drug metabolism. Inducers of CYP3A4, such as St. John's Wort preparations (Hypericum perforatum), phenobarbital, carbamazepine and rifampin may reduce plasma concentrations of estrogens, possibly resulting in a decrease in therapeutic effects and/or changes in the uterine bleeding profile). Products include:
Provigil **983**

Nafcillin Sodium (*In vitro* and *in vivo* studies have shown that estrogens are metabolized partially by cytochrome P450 3A4 (CYP3A4). Therefore, inducers of CYP3A4 may affect estrogen drug metabolism. Inducers of CYP3A4, such as St. John's Wort preparations (Hypericum perforatum), phenobarbital, carbamazepine and rifampin may

IMPORTANT NOTE: Always consult each drug listing in the patient's regimen for possible interactions.

reduce plasma concentrations of estrogens, possibly resulting in a decrease in therapeutic effects and/or changes in the uterine bleeding profile).
No products indexed under this heading.

Nefazodone Hydrochloride (*In vitro* and *in vivo* studies have shown that estrogens are metabolized partially by cytochrome P450 3A4 (CYP3A4). Therefore, inhibitors of CYP3A4 may affect estrogen drug metabolism. Inhibitors of CYP3A4, such as erythromycin, clarithromycin, ketoconazole, itraconazole, ritonavir and grapefruit juice may increase plasma concentrations of estrogens and may result in side effects).
No products indexed under this heading.

Nelfinavir Mesylate (*In vitro* and *in vivo* studies have shown that estrogens are metabolized partially by cytochrome P450 3A4 (CYP3A4). Therefore, inhibitors of CYP3A4 may affect estrogen drug metabolism. Inhibitors of CYP3A4, such as erythromycin, clarithromycin, ketoconazole, itraconazole, ritonavir and grapefruit juice may increase plasma concentrations of estrogens and may result in side effects).
No products indexed under this heading.

Nevirapine (*In vitro* and *in vivo* studies have shown that estrogens are metabolized partially by cytochrome P450 3A4 (CYP3A4). Therefore, inducers of CYP3A4 may affect estrogen drug metabolism. Inducers of CYP3A4, such as St. John's Wort preparations (Hypericum perforatum), phenobarbital, carbamazepine and rifampin may reduce plasma concentrations of estrogens, possibly resulting in a decrease in therapeutic effects and/or changes in the uterine bleeding profile). Products include:
Viramune Oral Suspension **897**
Viramune Tablets **897**

Niacin (*In vitro* and *in vivo* studies have shown that estrogens are metabolized partially by cytochrome P450 3A4 (CYP3A4). Therefore, inhibitors of CYP3A4 may affect estrogen drug metabolism. Inhibitors of CYP3A4, such as erythromycin, clarithromycin, ketoconazole, itraconazole, ritonavir and grapefruit juice may increase plasma concentrations of estrogens and may result in side effects). Products include:
Advicor **402**
Cardio Basics **3455**
Niaspan **497**
Simcor **524**

Niacinamide (*In vitro* and *in vivo* studies have shown that estrogens are metabolized partially by cytochrome P450 3A4 (CYP3A4). Therefore, inhibitors of CYP3A4 may affect estrogen drug metabolism. Inhibitors of CYP3A4, such as erythromycin, clarithromycin, ketoconazole, itraconazole, ritonavir and grapefruit juice may increase plasma concentrations of estrogens and may result in side effects). Products include:
CitraNatal 90 DHA Capsules **2332**
CitraNatal Assure **2332**
CitraNatal Rx **2332**
Heplive **607**

Niacinamide Hydroiodide (*In vitro* and *in vivo* studies have shown that estrogens are metabolized partially by cytochrome P450 3A4 (CYP3A4). Therefore, inhibitors of CYP3A4 may affect estrogen drug metabolism. Inhibitors of CYP3A4, such as erythromycin, clarithromycin, ketoconazole, itraconazole, ritonavir and grapefruit juice may increase plasma concentrations of estrogens and may result in side effects).
No products indexed under this heading.

Nicotinamide (*In vitro* and *in vivo* studies have shown that estrogens are metabolized partially by cytochrome P450 3A4 (CYP3A4). Therefore, inhibitors of CYP3A4 may affect estrogen drug metabolism. Inhibitors of CYP3A4, such as erythromycin, clarithromycin, ketoconazole, itraconazole, ritonavir and grapefruit juice may increase plasma concentrations of estrogens and may result in side effects).
No products indexed under this heading.

Nifedipine (*In vitro* and *in vivo* studies have shown that estrogens are metabolized partially by cytochrome P450 3A4 (CYP3A4). Therefore, inhibitors of CYP3A4 may affect estrogen drug metabolism. Inhibitors of CYP3A4, such as erythromycin, clarithromycin, ketoconazole, itraconazole, ritonavir and grapefruit juice may increase plasma concentrations of estrogens and may result in side effects).
No products indexed under this heading.

Norfloxacin (*In vitro* and *in vivo* studies have shown that estrogens are metabolized partially by cytochrome P450 3A4 (CYP3A4). Therefore, inhibitors of CYP3A4 may affect estrogen drug metabolism. Inhibitors of CYP3A4, such as erythromycin, clarithromycin, ketoconazole, itraconazole, ritonavir and grapefruit juice may increase plasma concentrations of estrogens and may result in side effects). Products include:
Noroxin **2220**

Omeprazole (*In vitro* and *in vivo* studies have shown that estrogens are metabolized partially by cytochrome P450 3A4 (CYP3A4). Therefore, inhibitors of CYP3A4 may affect estrogen drug metabolism. Inhibitors of CYP3A4, such as erythromycin, clarithromycin, ketoconazole, itraconazole, ritonavir and grapefruit juice may increase plasma concentrations of estrogens and may result in side effects).
No products indexed under this heading.

Oxcarbazepine (*In vitro* and *in vivo* studies have shown that estrogens are metabolized partially by cytochrome P450 3A4 (CYP3A4). Therefore, inducers of CYP3A4 may affect estrogen drug metabolism. Inducers of CYP3A4, such as St. John's Wort preparations (Hypericum perforatum), phenobarbital, carbamazepine and rifampin may reduce plasma concentrations of estrogens, possibly resulting in a decrease in therapeutic effects and/or changes in the uterine bleeding profile).
No products indexed under this heading.

Paroxetine Hydrochloride (*In vitro* and *in vivo* studies have shown that estrogens are metabolized partially by cytochrome P450 3A4 (CYP3A4). Therefore, inhibitors of CYP3A4 may affect estrogen drug metabolism. Inhibitors of CYP3A4, such as erythromycin, clarithromycin, ketoconazole, itraconazole, ritonavir and grapefruit juice may increase plasma concentrations of estrogens and may result in side effects). Products include:
Paroxetine CR **2361**
Paroxetine ER **2371**
Paxil **1586**
Paxil CR **1596**

Phenobarbital (*In vitro* and *in vivo* studies have shown that estrogens are metabolized partially by cytochrome P450 3A4 (CYP3A4). Therefore, inducers of CYP3A4 may affect estrogen drug metabolism. Inducers of CYP3A4, such as phenobarbital, may reduce plasma concentrations of estrogens, possibly resulting in a decrease in therapeutic effects and/or changes in the uterine bleeding profile). Products include:
Donnatal **2711**

Phenobarbital Sodium (*In vitro* and *in vivo* studies have shown that estrogens are metabolized partially by cytochrome P450 3A4 (CYP3A4). Therefore, inducers of CYP3A4 may affect estrogen drug metabolism. Inducers of CYP3A4, such as phenobarbital, may reduce plasma concentrations of estrogens, possibly resulting in a decrease in therapeutic effects and/or changes in the uterine bleeding profile).
No products indexed under this heading.

Phenytoin (*In vitro* and *in vivo* studies have shown that estrogens are metabolized partially by cytochrome P450 3A4 (CYP3A4). Therefore, inducers of CYP3A4 may affect estrogen drug metabolism. Inducers of CYP3A4, such as St. John's Wort preparations (Hypericum perforatum), phenobarbital, carbamazepine and rifampin may reduce plasma concentrations of estrogens, possibly resulting in a decrease in therapeutic effects and/or changes in the uterine bleeding profile).
No products indexed under this heading.

Phenytoin Sodium (*In vitro* and *in vivo* studies have shown that estrogens are metabolized partially by cytochrome P450 3A4 (CYP3A4). Therefore, inducers of CYP3A4 may affect estrogen drug metabolism. Inducers of CYP3A4, such as St. John's Wort preparations (Hypericum perforatum), phenobarbital, carbamazepine and rifampin may reduce plasma concentrations of estrogens, possibly resulting in a decrease in therapeutic effects and/or changes in the uterine bleeding profile). Products include:
Phenytek Capsules **2380**

Posaconazole (*In vitro* and *in vivo* studies have shown that estrogens are metabolized partially by cytochrome P450 3A4 (CYP3A4). Therefore, inhibitors of CYP3A4 may affect estrogen drug metabolism. Inhibitors of CYP3A4, such as erythromycin, clarithromycin, ketoconazole, itraconazole, ritonavir and grapefruit juice may increase plasma concentrations of estrogens and may result in side effects). Products include:
Noxafil **3172**

Prednisolone (*In vitro* and *in vivo* studies have shown that estrogens are metabolized partially by cytochrome P450 3A4 (CYP3A4). Therefore, inducers of CYP3A4 may affect estrogen drug metabolism. Inducers of CYP3A4, such as St. John's Wort preparations (Hypericum perforatum), phenobarbital, carbamazepine and rifampin may reduce plasma concentrations of estrogens, possibly resulting in a decrease in therapeutic effects and/or changes in the uterine bleeding profile).
No products indexed under this heading.

Prednisolone Acetate (*In vitro* and *in vivo* studies have shown that estrogens are metabolized partially by cytochrome P450 3A4 (CYP3A4). Therefore, inducers of CYP3A4 may affect estrogen drug metabolism. Inducers of CYP3A4, such as St. John's Wort preparations (Hypericum perforatum), phenobarbital, carbamazepine and rifampin may reduce plasma concentrations of estrogens, possibly resulting in a decrease in therapeutic effects and/or changes in the uterine bleeding profile). Products include:
Blephamide .... ⊙**212**, ⊙**214**
Pred Forte .... ⊙**225**
Pred Mild .... ⊙**230**
Pred-G .... ⊙**226**, ⊙**227**

Prednisolone Sodium Phosphate (*In vitro* and *in vivo* studies have shown that estrogens are metabolized partially by cytochrome P450 3A4 (CYP3A4). Therefore, inducers of CYP3A4 may affect estrogen drug metabolism. Inducers of CYP3A4, such as St. John's Wort preparations (Hypericum perforatum), phenobarbital, carbamazepine and rifampin may reduce plasma concentrations of estrogens, possibly resulting in a decrease in therapeutic effects and/or changes in the uterine bleeding profile).
No products indexed under this heading.

Prednisolone Tebutate (*In vitro* and *in vivo* studies have shown that estrogens are metabolized partially by cytochrome P450 3A4 (CYP3A4). Therefore, inducers of CYP3A4 may affect estrogen drug metabolism. Inducers of CYP3A4, such as St. John's Wort preparations (Hypericum perforatum), phenobarbital, carbamazepine and rifampin may reduce plasma concentrations of estrogens, possibly resulting in a decrease in therapeutic effects and/or changes in the uterine bleeding profile).
No products indexed under this heading.

Prednisone (*In vitro* and *in vivo* studies have shown that estrogens are metabolized partially by cytochrome P450 3A4 (CYP3A4). Therefore, inducers of CYP3A4 may affect estrogen drug metabolism. Inducers of CYP3A4, such as St. John's Wort preparations (Hypericum perforatum), phenobarbital, carbamazepine and rifampin may reduce plasma concentrations of estrogens, possibly resulting in a decrease in therapeutic effects and/or changes in the uterine bleeding profile).
No products indexed under this heading.

Prednisone sodium phosphate (*In vitro* and *in vivo* studies have shown that estrogens are metabolized partially by cytochrome P450 3A4 (CYP3A4). Therefore, inducers of CYP3A4 may affect estrogen drug metabolism. Inducers of CYP3A4, such as St. John's Wort preparations (Hypericum perforatum), phenobarbital, carbamazepine and rifampin may reduce plasma concentrations of estrogens, possibly resulting in a decrease in therapeutic effects and/or changes in the uterine bleeding profile).
No products indexed under this heading.

Primidone (*In vitro* and *in vivo* studies have shown that estrogens are metabolized partially by cytochrome P450 3A4 (CYP3A4). Therefore, inducers of CYP3A4 may affect estrogen drug metabolism. Inducers of CYP3A4, such as St. John's Wort preparations (Hypericum perforatum), phenobarbital, carbamazepine and rifampin may reduce plasma concentrations of estrogens, possibly resulting in a decrease in therapeutic effects and/or changes in the uterine bleeding profile).
No products indexed under this heading.

Propoxyphene Hydrochloride (*In vitro* and *in vivo* studies have shown that estrogens are metabolized partially by cytochrome P450 3A4 (CYP3A4). Therefore, inhibitors of CYP3A4 may affect estrogen drug metabolism. Inhibitors of CYP3A4, such as erythromycin, clarithromycin, ketoconazole, itraconazole, ritonavir and grapefruit juice may increase plasma concentrations of estrogens and may result in side effects).
No products indexed under this heading.

Propoxyphene Napsylate (*In vitro* and *in vivo* studies have shown that estrogens are metabolized partially by cytochrome P450 3A4 (CYP3A4). Therefore, inhibitors of CYP3A4 may affect estrogen drug metabolism. Inhibitors of CYP3A4, such as erythromycin, clarithromycin, ketoconazole, itraconazole, ritonavir and grapefruit juice may increase plasma concentrations of estrogens and may result in side effects).
No products indexed under this heading.

Quinidine (*In vitro* and *in vivo* studies have shown that estrogens are metabolized partially by cytochrome P450 3A4

(CYP3A4). Therefore, inhibitors of CYP3A4 may affect estrogen drug metabolism. Inhibitors of CYP3A4, such as erythromycin, clarithromycin, ketoconazole, itraconazole, ritonavir and grapefruit juice may increase plasma concentrations of estrogens and may result in side effects).

No products indexed under this heading.

Quinidine Hydrochloride (*In vitro* and *in vivo* studies have shown that estrogens are metabolized partially by cytochrome P450 3A4 (CYP3A4). Therefore, inhibitors of CYP3A4 may affect estrogen drug metabolism. Inhibitors of CYP3A4, such as erythromycin, clarithromycin, ketoconazole, itraconazole, ritonavir and grapefruit juice may increase plasma concentrations of estrogens and may result in side effects).

No products indexed under this heading.

Quinidine Polygalacturonate (*In vitro* and *in vivo* studies have shown that estrogens are metabolized partially by cytochrome P450 3A4 (CYP3A4). Therefore, inhibitors of CYP3A4 may affect estrogen drug metabolism. Inhibitors of CYP3A4, such as erythromycin, clarithromycin, ketoconazole, itraconazole, ritonavir and grapefruit juice may increase plasma concentrations of estrogens and may result in side effects).

No products indexed under this heading.

Quinidine Sulfate (*In vitro* and *in vivo* studies have shown that estrogens are metabolized partially by cytochrome P450 3A4 (CYP3A4). Therefore, inhibitors of CYP3A4 may affect estrogen drug metabolism. Inhibitors of CYP3A4, such as erythromycin, clarithromycin, ketoconazole, itraconazole, ritonavir and grapefruit juice may increase plasma concentrations of estrogens and may result in side effects).

No products indexed under this heading.

Quinine (*In vitro* and *in vivo* studies have shown that estrogens are metabolized partially by cytochrome P450 3A4 (CYP3A4). Therefore, inhibitors of CYP3A4 may affect estrogen drug metabolism. Inhibitors of CYP3A4, such as erythromycin, clarithromycin, ketoconazole, itraconazole, ritonavir and grapefruit juice may increase plasma concentrations of estrogens and may result in side effects). Products include:

Hyland's Leg Cramps PM with Quinine **3315**

Quinine Sulfate (*In vitro* and *in vivo* studies have shown that estrogens are metabolized partially by cytochrome P450 3A4 (CYP3A4). Therefore, inhibitors of CYP3A4 may affect estrogen drug metabolism. Inhibitors of CYP3A4, such as erythromycin, clarithromycin, ketoconazole, itraconazole, ritonavir and grapefruit juice may increase plasma concentrations of estrogens and may result in side effects).

No products indexed under this heading.

Quinupristin (*In vitro* and *in vivo* studies have shown that estrogens are metabolized partially by cytochrome P450 3A4 (CYP3A4). Therefore, inhibitors of CYP3A4 may affect estrogen drug metabolism. Inhibitors of CYP3A4, such as erythromycin, clarithromycin, ketoconazole, itraconazole, ritonavir and grapefruit juice may increase plasma concentrations of estrogens and may result in side effects).

No products indexed under this heading.

Ranitidine Bismuth Citrate (*In vitro* and *in vivo* studies have shown that estrogens are metabolized partially by cytochrome P450 3A4 (CYP3A4). Therefore, inhibitors of CYP3A4 may affect estrogen drug metabolism. Inhibitors of CYP3A4, such as erythromycin, clarithromycin, ketoconazole, itraconazole, ritonavir and grapefruit juice may increase plasma concentrations of estrogens and may result in side effects).

No products indexed under this heading.

Ranitidine Hydrochloride (*In vitro* and *in vivo* studies have shown that estrogens are metabolized partially by cytochrome P450 3A4 (CYP3A4). Therefore, inhibitors of CYP3A4 may affect estrogen drug metabolism. Inhibitors of CYP3A4, such as erythromycin, clarithromycin, ketoconazole, itraconazole, ritonavir and grapefruit juice may increase plasma concentrations of estrogens and may result in side effects). Products include:

Zantac **1737**
Zantac Injection **1732**
Zantac Pharmacy **1735**

Rifabutin (*In vitro* and *in vivo* studies have shown that estrogens are metabolized partially by cytochrome P450 3A4 (CYP3A4). Therefore, inducers of CYP3A4 may affect estrogen drug metabolism. Inducers of CYP3A4, such as St. John's Wort preparations (Hypericum perforatum), phenobarbital, carbamazepine and rifampin may reduce plasma concentrations of estrogens, possibly resulting in a decrease in therapeutic effects and/or changes in the uterine bleeding profile).

No products indexed under this heading.

Rifampicin (*In vitro* and *in vivo* studies have shown that estrogens are metabolized partially by cytochrome P450 3A4 (CYP3A4). Therefore, inducers of CYP3A4 may affect estrogen drug metabolism. Inducers of CYP3A4, such as St. John's Wort preparations (Hypericum perforatum), phenobarbital, carbamazepine and rifampin may reduce plasma concentrations of estrogens, possibly resulting in a decrease in therapeutic effects and/or changes in the uterine bleeding profile).

No products indexed under this heading.

Rifampin (*In vitro* and *in vivo* studies have shown that estrogens are metabolized partially by cytochrome P450 3A4 (CYP3A4). Therefore, inducers of CYP3A4 may affect estrogen drug metabolism. Inducers of CYP3A4, such as rifampin, may reduce plasma concentrations of estrogens, possibly resulting in a decrease in therapeutic effects and/or changes in the uterine bleeding profile).

No products indexed under this heading.

Rifapentine (*In vitro* and *in vivo* studies have shown that estrogens are metabolized partially by cytochrome P450 3A4 (CYP3A4). Therefore, inducers of CYP3A4 may affect estrogen drug metabolism. Inducers of CYP3A4, such as St. John's Wort preparations (Hypericum perforatum), phenobarbital, carbamazepine and rifampin may reduce plasma concentrations of estrogens, possibly resulting in a decrease in therapeutic effects and/or changes in the uterine bleeding profile).

No products indexed under this heading.

Ritonavir (*In vitro* and *in vivo* studies have shown that estrogens are metabolized partially by cytochrome P450 3A4 (CYP3A4). Therefore, inhibitors of CYP3A4 may affect estrogen drug metabolism. Inhibitors of CYP3A4, such as ritonavir, may increase plasma concentrations of estrogens and may result in side effects). Products include:

Kaletra **458**
Norvir **509**

Saquinavir (*In vitro* and *in vivo* studies have shown that estrogens are metabolized partially by cytochrome P450 3A4 (CYP3A4). Therefore, inhibitors of CYP3A4 may affect estrogen drug metabolism. Inhibitors of CYP3A4, such as erythromycin, clarithromycin, ketoconazole, itraconazole, ritonavir and grapefruit juice may increase plasma concentrations of estrogens and may result in side effects).

No products indexed under this heading.

Saquinavir Mesylate (*In vitro* and *in vivo* studies have shown that estrogens are metabolized partially by cytochrome P450 3A4 (CYP3A4). Therefore, inhibitors of CYP3A4 may affect estrogen drug metabolism. Inhibitors of CYP3A4, such as erythromycin, clarithromycin, ketoconazole, itraconazole, ritonavir and grapefruit juice may increase plasma concentrations of estrogens and may result in side effects).

No products indexed under this heading.

Sertraline Hydrochloride (*In vitro* and *in vivo* studies have shown that estrogens are metabolized partially by cytochrome P450 3A4 (CYP3A4). Therefore, inhibitors of CYP3A4 may affect estrogen drug metabolism. Inhibitors of CYP3A4, such as erythromycin, clarithromycin, ketoconazole, itraconazole, ritonavir and grapefruit juice may increase plasma concentrations of estrogens and may result in side effects).

No products indexed under this heading.

Sildenafil Citrate (*In vitro* and *in vivo* studies have shown that estrogens are metabolized partially by cytochrome P450 3A4 (CYP3A4). Therefore, inhibitors of CYP3A4 may affect estrogen drug metabolism. Inhibitors of CYP3A4, such as erythromycin, clarithromycin, ketoconazole, itraconazole, ritonavir and grapefruit juice may increase plasma concentrations of estrogens and may result in side effects).

No products indexed under this heading.

Sulfinpyrazone (*In vitro* and *in vivo* studies have shown that estrogens are metabolized partially by cytochrome P450 3A4 (CYP3A4). Therefore, inducers of CYP3A4 may affect estrogen drug metabolism. Inducers of CYP3A4, such as St. John's Wort preparations (Hypericum perforatum), phenobarbital, carbamazepine and rifampin may reduce plasma concentrations of estrogens, possibly resulting in a decrease in therapeutic effects and/or changes in the uterine bleeding profile).

No products indexed under this heading.

Sunscreen (Estradiol hemihydrate emulsion should not be used in close proximity to sunscreen application because estradiol absorption may be increased).

No products indexed under this heading.

Telithromycin (*In vitro* and *in vivo* studies have shown that estrogens are metabolized partially by cytochrome P450 3A4 (CYP3A4). Therefore, inhibitors of CYP3A4 may affect estrogen drug metabolism. Inhibitors of CYP3A4, such as erythromycin, clarithromycin, ketoconazole, itraconazole, ritonavir and grapefruit juice may increase plasma concentrations of estrogens and may result in side effects). Products include:

Ketek **2991**

Theophyllinate (*In vitro* and *in vivo* studies have shown that estrogens are metabolized partially by cytochrome P450 3A4 (CYP3A4). Therefore, inducers of CYP3A4 may affect estrogen drug metabolism. Inducers of CYP3A4, such as St. John's Wort preparations (Hypericum perforatum), phenobarbital, carbamazepine and rifampin may reduce plasma concentrations of estrogens, possibly resulting in a decrease in therapeutic effects and/or changes in the uterine bleeding profile).

No products indexed under this heading.

Theophylline (*In vitro* and *in vivo* studies have shown that estrogens are metabolized partially by cytochrome P450 3A4 (CYP3A4). Therefore, inducers of CYP3A4 may affect estrogen drug metabolism. Inducers of CYP3A4, such as St. John's Wort preparations (Hypericum perforatum), phenobarbital, carbamazepine and rifampin may reduce plasma concentrations of estrogens, possibly resulting in a decrease in therapeutic effects and/or changes in the uterine bleeding profile).

No products indexed under this heading.

Theophylline Anhydrous (*In vitro* and *in vivo* studies have shown that estrogens are metabolized partially by cytochrome P450 3A4 (CYP3A4). Therefore, inducers of CYP3A4 may affect estrogen drug metabolism. Inducers of CYP3A4, such as St. John's Wort preparations (Hypericum perforatum), phenobarbital, carbamazepine and rifampin may reduce plasma concentrations of estrogens, possibly resulting in a decrease in therapeutic effects and/or changes in the uterine bleeding profile). Products include:

Uniphyl **2817**

Theophylline Calcium Salicylate (*In vitro* and *in vivo* studies have shown that estrogens are metabolized partially by cytochrome P450 3A4 (CYP3A4). Therefore, inducers of CYP3A4 may affect estrogen drug metabolism. Inducers of CYP3A4, such as St. John's Wort preparations (Hypericum perforatum), phenobarbital, carbamazepine and rifampin may reduce plasma concentrations of estrogens, possibly resulting in a decrease in therapeutic effects and/or changes in the uterine bleeding profile).

No products indexed under this heading.

Theophylline Dihydroxypropyl (Glyceryl) (*In vitro* and *in vivo* studies have shown that estrogens are metabolized partially by cytochrome P450 3A4 (CYP3A4). Therefore, inducers of CYP3A4 may affect estrogen drug metabolism. Inducers of CYP3A4, such as St. John's Wort preparations (Hypericum perforatum), phenobarbital, carbamazepine and rifampin may reduce plasma concentrations of estrogens, possibly resulting in a decrease in therapeutic effects and/or changes in the uterine bleeding profile).

No products indexed under this heading.

Theophylline Ethylenediamine (*In vitro* and *in vivo* studies have shown that estrogens are metabolized partially by cytochrome P450 3A4 (CYP3A4). Therefore, inducers of CYP3A4 may affect estrogen drug metabolism. Inducers of CYP3A4, such as St. John's Wort preparations (Hypericum perforatum), phenobarbital, carbamazepine and rifampin may reduce plasma concentrations of estrogens, possibly resulting in a decrease in therapeutic effects and/or changes in the uterine bleeding profile).

No products indexed under this heading.

Theophylline Sodium Glycinate (*In vitro* and *in vivo* studies have shown that estrogens are metabolized partially by cytochrome P450 3A4 (CYP3A4). Therefore, inducers of CYP3A4 may affect estrogen drug metabolism. Inducers of CYP3A4, such as St. John's Wort preparations (Hypericum perforatum), phenobarbital, carbamazepine and rifampin may reduce plasma concentrations of estrogens, possibly resulting in a decrease in therapeutic effects and/or changes in the uterine bleeding profile).

No products indexed under this heading.

IMPORTANT NOTE: Always consult each drug listing in the patient's regimen for possible interactions.

Thyroglobulin (Estrogen administration leads to increased thyroid-binding globulin (TBG) levels. Patients dependent on thyroid hormone replacement therapy who are also receiving estrogens may require increased doses of their thyroid replacement therapy).
No products indexed under this heading.

Thyroid (Estrogen administration leads to increased thyroid-binding globulin (TBG) levels. Patients dependent on thyroid hormone replacement therapy who are also receiving estrogens may require increased doses of their thyroid replacement therapy). Products include:

Thyroxine (Estrogen administration leads to increased thyroid-binding globulin (TBG) levels. Patients dependent on thyroid hormone replacement therapy who are also receiving estrogens may require increased doses of their thyroid replacement therapy).
No products indexed under this heading.

Thyroxine Sodium (Estrogen administration leads to increased thyroid-binding globulin (TBG) levels. Patients dependent on thyroid hormone replacement therapy who are also receiving estrogens may require increased doses of their thyroid replacement therapy).
No products indexed under this heading.

Triamcinolone (In vitro and in vivo studies have shown that estrogens are metabolized partially by cytochrome P450 3A4 (CYP3A4). Therefore, inducers of CYP3A4 may affect estrogen drug metabolism. Inducers of CYP3A4, such as St. John's Wort preparations (Hypericum perforatum), phenobarbital, carbamazepine and rifampin may reduce plasma concentrations of estrogens, possibly resulting in a decrease in therapeutic effects and/or changes in the uterine bleeding profile).
No products indexed under this heading.

Triamcinolone Acetonide (In vitro and in vivo studies have shown that estrogens are metabolized partially by cytochrome P450 3A4 (CYP3A4). Therefore, inducers of CYP3A4 may affect estrogen drug metabolism. Inducers of CYP3A4, such as St. John's Wort preparations (Hypericum perforatum), phenobarbital, carbamazepine and rifampin may reduce plasma concentrations of estrogens, possibly resulting in a decrease in therapeutic effects and/or changes in the uterine bleeding profile). Products include:

Triamcinolone Diacetate (In vitro and in vivo studies have shown that estrogens are metabolized partially by cytochrome P450 3A4 (CYP3A4). Therefore, inducers of CYP3A4 may affect estrogen drug metabolism. Inducers of CYP3A4, such as St. John's Wort preparations (Hypericum perforatum), phenobarbital, carbamazepine and rifampin may reduce plasma concentrations of estrogens, possibly resulting in a decrease in therapeutic effects and/or changes in the uterine bleeding profile).
No products indexed under this heading.

Triamcinolone Hexacetonide (In vitro and in vivo studies have shown that estrogens are metabolized partially by cytochrome P450 3A4 (CYP3A4). Therefore, inducers of CYP3A4 may affect estrogen drug metabolism. Inducers of CYP3A4, such as St. John's Wort preparations (Hypericum perforatum), phenobarbital, carbamazepine and rifampin may reduce plasma concentrations of estrogens, possibly resulting in a decrease in therapeutic effects and/or changes in the uterine bleeding profile).
No products indexed under this heading.

Troglitazone (In vitro and in vivo studies have shown that estrogens are metabolized partially by cytochrome P450 3A4 (CYP3A4). Therefore, inducers of CYP3A4 may affect estrogen drug metabolism. Inducers of CYP3A4, such as St. John's Wort preparations (Hypericum perforatum), phenobarbital, carbamazepine and rifampin may reduce plasma concentrations of estrogens, possibly resulting in a decrease in therapeutic effects and/or changes in the uterine bleeding profile).
No products indexed under this heading.

Troleandomycin (In vitro and in vivo studies have shown that estrogens are metabolized partially by cytochrome P450 3A4 (CYP3A4). Therefore, inhibitors of CYP3A4 may affect estrogen drug metabolism. Inhibitors of CYP3A4, such as erythromycin, clarithromycin, ketoconazole, itraconazole, ritonavir and grapefruit juice may increase plasma concentrations of estrogens and may result in side effects).
No products indexed under this heading.

Valproate Sodium (In vitro and in vivo studies have shown that estrogens are metabolized partially by cytochrome P450 3A4 (CYP3A4). Therefore, inhibitors of CYP3A4 may affect estrogen drug metabolism. Inhibitors of CYP3A4, such as erythromycin, clarithromycin, ketoconazole, itraconazole, ritonavir and grapefruit juice may increase plasma concentrations of estrogens and may result in side effects).
No products indexed under this heading.

Vardenafil Hydrochloride (In vitro and in vivo studies have shown that estrogens are metabolized partially by cytochrome P450 3A4 (CYP3A4). Therefore, inhibitors of CYP3A4 may affect estrogen drug metabolism. Inhibitors of CYP3A4, such as erythromycin, clarithromycin, ketoconazole, itraconazole, ritonavir and grapefruit juice may increase plasma concentrations of estrogens and may result in side effects). Products include:

Verapamil Hydrochloride (In vitro and in vivo studies have shown that estrogens are metabolized partially by cytochrome P450 3A4 (CYP3A4). Therefore, inhibitors of CYP3A4 may affect estrogen drug metabolism. Inhibitors of CYP3A4, such as erythromycin, clarithromycin, ketoconazole, itraconazole, ritonavir and grapefruit juice may increase plasma concentrations of estrogens and may result in side effects). Products include:

Voriconazole (In vitro and in vivo studies have shown that estrogens are metabolized partially by cytochrome P450 3A4 (CYP3A4). Therefore, inhibitors of CYP3A4 may affect estrogen drug metabolism. Inhibitors of CYP3A4, such as erythromycin, clarithromycin, ketoconazole, itraconazole, ritonavir and grapefruit juice may increase plasma concentrations of estrogens and may result in side effects).
No products indexed under this heading.

Zafirlukast (In vitro and in vivo studies have shown that estrogens are metabolized partially by cytochrome P450 3A4 (CYP3A4). Therefore, inhibitors of CYP3A4 may affect estrogen drug metabolism. Inhibitors of CYP3A4, such as erythromycin, clarithromycin, ketoconazole, itraconazole, ritonavir and grapefruit juice may increase plasma concentrations of estrogens and may result in side effects). Products include:

Zileuton (In vitro and in vivo studies have shown that estrogens are metabolized partially by cytochrome P450 3A4 (CYP3A4). Therefore, inhibitors of CYP3A4 may affect estrogen drug metabolism. Inhibitors of CYP3A4, such as erythromycin, clarithromycin, ketoconazole, itraconazole, ritonavir and grapefruit juice may increase plasma concentrations of estrogens and may result in side effects).
No products indexed under this heading.

Food Interactions

Grapefruit (In vitro and in vivo studies have shown that estrogens are metabolized partially by cytochrome P450 3A4 (CYP3A4). Therefore, inhibitors of CYP3A4 may affect estrogen drug metabolism. Inhibitors of CYP3A4, such as erythromycin, clarithromycin, ketoconazole, itraconazole, ritonavir and grapefruit juice may increase plasma concentrations of estrogens and may result in side effects).
No products indexed under this heading.

Grapefruit Juice (In vitro and in vivo studies have shown that estrogens are metabolized partially by cytochrome P450 3A4 (CYP3A4). Therefore, inhibitors of CYP3A4 may affect estrogen drug metabolism. Inhibitors of CYP3A4, such as grapefruit juice, may increase plasma concentrations of estrogens and may result in side effects).

EVISTA TABLETS
May interact with estrogens, and certain other agents. Compounds in these categories include:

Chlorotrianisene (The safety and concomitant use of raloxifene hydrochloride with systemic estrogens has not been established and its use is not recommended).
No products indexed under this heading.

Cholestyramine (Co-administration causes a 60% reduction in the absorption and enterohepatic cycling of raloxifene; concurrent use should be avoided).
No products indexed under this heading.

Diazepam (Raloxifene might affect the protein binding of other highly protein-bound drugs such as diazepam; caution should be exercised). Products include:

Diazoxide (Raloxifene might affect the protein binding of other highly protein-bound drugs such as diazoxide; caution should be exercised). Products include:

Dienestrol (The safety and concomitant use of raloxifene hydrochloride with systemic estrogens has not been established and its use is not recommended).
No products indexed under this heading.

Diethylstilbestrol (The safety and concomitant use of raloxifene hydrochloride with systemic estrogens has not been established and its use is not recommended).
No products indexed under this heading.

Estradiol (The safety and concomitant use of raloxifene hydrochloride with systemic estrogens has not been established and its use is not recommended). Products include:

Estrogens, Conjugated (The safety and concomitant use of raloxifene hydrochloride with systemic estrogens has not been established and its use is not recommended). Products include:

Estrogens, Esterified (The safety and concomitant use of raloxifene hydrochloride with systemic estrogens has not been established and its use is not recommended).
No products indexed under this heading.

Estropipate (The safety and concomitant use of raloxifene hydrochloride with systemic estrogens has not been established and its use is not recommended).
No products indexed under this heading.

Ethinyl Estradiol (The safety and concomitant use of raloxifene hydrochloride with systemic estrogens has not been established and its use is not recommended). Products include:

Lidocaine Hydrochloride (Raloxifene might affect the protein binding of other highly protein-bound drugs such as lidocaine; caution should be exercised).
No products indexed under this heading.

Polyestradiol Phosphate (The safety and concomitant use of raloxifene hydrochloride with systemic estrogens has not been established and its use is not recommended).
No products indexed under this heading.

Quinestrol (The safety and concomitant use of raloxifene hydrochloride with systemic estrogens has not been established and its use is not recommended).
No products indexed under this heading.

Warfarin Sodium (Co-administration has resulted in a 10% decrease in prothrombin time in single-dose studies; if used concurrently, prothrombin time should be monitored).
No products indexed under this heading.

Food Interactions

Food, unspecified (Administration of raloxifene with a standardized, high fat meal increases the absorption of raloxifene, but does not lead to clinically meaningful changes in systemic exposure; Evista can be administered without regard to meals).

EVOCLIN FOAM, 1%
May interact with neuromuscular blocking agents, and certain other agents. Compounds in these categories include:

Atracurium Besylate (Clindamycin has been shown to have neuromuscular blocking properties that may enhance the action of other neuromuscular blocking agents; therefore, it should be used with caution in patients receiving such agents).
No products indexed under this heading.

Cisatracurium Besylate (Clindamycin has been shown to have neuromuscular blocking properties that may enhance the action of other neuromuscular blocking agents; therefore, it should be used with caution in patients receiving such agents). Products include:

Decamethonium (Clindamycin has been shown to have neuromuscular blocking properties that may enhance the action of other neuromuscular blocking agents; therefore, it should be used with caution in patients receiving such agents).
No products indexed under this heading.

(⊙ Described in PDR® for Ophthalmic Medicines)

Doxacurium Chloride (Clindamycin has been shown to have neuromuscular blocking properties that may enhance the action of other neuromuscular blocking agents; therefore, it should be used with caution in patients receiving such agents).
   No products indexed under this heading.

d-Tubocurarine (Clindamycin has been shown to have neuromuscular blocking properties that may enhance the action of other neuromuscular blocking agents; therefore, it should be used with caution in patients receiving such agents).
   No products indexed under this heading.

Gallamine (Clindamycin has been shown to have neuromuscular blocking properties that may enhance the action of other neuromuscular blocking agents; therefore, it should be used with caution in patients receiving such agents).
   No products indexed under this heading.

Gallamine Triethiodide (Clindamycin has been shown to have neuromuscular blocking properties that may enhance the action of other neuromuscular blocking agents; therefore, it should be used with caution in patients receiving such agents).
   No products indexed under this heading.

Metocurine Iodide (Clindamycin has been shown to have neuromuscular blocking properties that may enhance the action of other neuromuscular blocking agents; therefore, it should be used with caution in patients receiving such agents).
   No products indexed under this heading.

Mivacurium Chloride (Clindamycin has been shown to have neuromuscular blocking properties that may enhance the action of other neuromuscular blocking agents; therefore, it should be used with caution in patients receiving such agents).
   No products indexed under this heading.

Pancuronium Bromide (Clindamycin has been shown to have neuromuscular blocking properties that may enhance the action of other neuromuscular blocking agents; therefore, it should be used with caution in patients receiving such agents).
   No products indexed under this heading.

Rapacuronium Bromide (Clindamycin has been shown to have neuromuscular blocking properties that may enhance the action of other neuromuscular blocking agents; therefore, it should be used with caution in patients receiving such agents).
   No products indexed under this heading.

Rocuronium Bromide (Clindamycin has been shown to have neuromuscular blocking properties that may enhance the action of other neuromuscular blocking agents; therefore, it should be used with caution in patients receiving such agents). Products include:
   Zemuron 3249

Succinylcholine Chloride (Clindamycin has been shown to have neuromuscular blocking properties that may enhance the action of other neuromuscular blocking agents; therefore, it should be used with caution in patients receiving such agents).
   No products indexed under this heading.

Tubocurarine Chloride (Clindamycin has been shown to have neuromuscular blocking properties that may enhance the action of other neuromuscular blocking agents; therefore, it should be used with caution in patients receiving such agents).
   No products indexed under this heading.

Vecuronium Bromide (Clindamycin has been shown to have neuromuscular blocking properties that may enhance the action of other neuromuscular blocking agents; therefore, it should be used with caution in patients receiving such agents).
   No products indexed under this heading.

EVOXAC CAPSULES

(Cevimeline Hydrochloride) 1027
May interact with antimuscarinic drugs, beta-blockers, cytochrome p450 2d6 inhibitors (selected), cytochrome p450 3a inhibitors (selected), cytochrome p450 3a4 inhibitors (selected), parasympathomimetics, and certain other agents. Compounds in these categories include:

Acebutolol Hydrochloride (Cevimeline should be administered with caution to patients taking β-adrenergic antagonists because of the possibility of conduction disturbances).
   No products indexed under this heading.

Acer rubrum (When administered with food, there is a decrease in the rate of absorption of cevimeline, with a fasting T_{Max} of 1.53 hours and a T_{Max} of 2.86 hours after a meal; the peak concentration is reduced by 17.3%).
   No products indexed under this heading.

Acetazolamide (Drugs which inhibit CYP3A3/4 also inhibit the metabolism of cevimeline).
   No products indexed under this heading.

Acetazolamide Sodium (Drugs which inhibit CYP3A3/4 also inhibit the metabolism of cevimeline).
   No products indexed under this heading.

Amiodarone Hydrochloride (Drugs which inhibit CYP2D6 also inhibit the metabolism of cevimeline. Cevimeline should be used with caution in individuals known or suspected to be deficient in CYP2D6 activity, as they may be at a higher risk of adverse events).
   No products indexed under this heading.

Amitriptyline Hydrochloride (Drugs which inhibit CYP2D6 also inhibit the metabolism of cevimeline. Cevimeline should be used with caution in individuals known or suspected to be deficient in CYP2D6 activity, as they may be at a higher risk of adverse events).
   No products indexed under this heading.

Amoxapine (Drugs which inhibit CYP2D6 also inhibit the metabolism of cevimeline. Cevimeline should be used with caution in individuals known or suspected to be deficient in CYP2D6 activity, as they may be at a higher risk of adverse events).
   No products indexed under this heading.

Amprenavir (Drugs which inhibit CYP3A3/4 also inhibit the metabolism of cevimeline).
   No products indexed under this heading.

Anastrozole (Drugs which inhibit CYP3A3/4 also inhibit the metabolism of cevimeline).
   No products indexed under this heading.

Aprepitant (Drugs which inhibit CYP3A3/4 also inhibit the metabolism of cevimeline). Products include:
   Emend 2124

Atazanavir (Drugs which inhibit CYP3A3/4 also inhibit the metabolism of cevimeline).
   No products indexed under this heading.

Atazanavir Sulfate (Drugs which inhibit CYP3A3/4 also inhibit the metabolism of cevimeline).
   No products indexed under this heading.

Atenolol (Cevimeline should be administered with caution to patients taking β-adrenergic antagonists because of the possibility of conduction disturbances).
   No products indexed under this heading.

Atropine Sulfate (Cevimeline might interfere with the desirable antimuscarinic effects of drugs used concomitantly). Products include:
   Donnatal 2711

Belladonna Alkaloids (Cevimeline might interfere with the desirable antimuscarinic effects of drugs used concomitantly). Products include:
   Hyland's Teething Tablets 3316

Betaxolol Hydrochloride (Cevimeline should be administered with caution to patients taking β-adrenergic antagonists because of the possibility of conduction disturbances).
   No products indexed under this heading.

Bisoprolol Fumarate (Cevimeline should be administered with caution to patients taking β-adrenergic antagonists because of the possibility of conduction disturbances).
   No products indexed under this heading.

Bupropion Hydrochloride (Drugs which inhibit CYP2D6 also inhibit the metabolism of cevimeline. Cevimeline should be used with caution in individuals known or suspected to be deficient in CYP2D6 activity, as they may be at a higher risk of adverse events). Products include:
   Aplenzin 2948
   Wellbutrin 1719
   Wellbutrin SR 1725
   Zyban 1762

Carteolol Hydrochloride (Cevimeline should be administered with caution to patients taking β-adrenergic antagonists because of the possibility of conduction disturbances).
   No products indexed under this heading.

Carvedilol (Cevimeline should be administered with caution to patients taking β-adrenergic antagonists because of the possibility of conduction disturbances). Products include:
   Coreg 1409

Carvedilol Phosphate (Cevimeline should be administered with caution to patients taking β-adrenergic antagonists because of the possibility of conduction disturbances). Products include:
   Coreg CR 1416

Celecoxib (Drugs which inhibit CYP2D6 also inhibit the metabolism of cevimeline. Cevimeline should be used with caution in individuals known or suspected to be deficient in CYP2D6 activity, as they may be at a higher risk of adverse events). Products include:
   Celebrex 3272

Chloroquine (Drugs which inhibit CYP2D6 also inhibit the metabolism of cevimeline. Cevimeline should be used with caution in individuals known or suspected to be deficient in CYP2D6 activity, as they may be at a higher risk of adverse events).
   No products indexed under this heading.

Chloroquine Hydrochloride (Drugs which inhibit CYP2D6 also inhibit the metabolism of cevimeline. Cevimeline should be used with caution in individuals known or suspected to be deficient in CYP2D6 activity, as they may be at a higher risk of adverse events).
   No products indexed under this heading.

Chloroquine Phosphate (Drugs which inhibit CYP2D6 also inhibit the metabolism of cevimeline. Cevimeline should be used with caution in individuals known or suspected to be deficient in CYP2D6 activity, as they may be at a higher risk of adverse events).
   No products indexed under this heading.

Chlorpheniramine (Drugs which inhibit CYP2D6 also inhibit the metabolism of cevimeline. Cevimeline should be used with caution in individuals known or suspected to be deficient in CYP2D6 activity, as they may be at a higher risk of adverse events).
   No products indexed under this heading.

Chlorpheniramine Maleate (Drugs which inhibit CYP2D6 also inhibit the metabolism of cevimeline. Cevimeline should be used with caution in individuals known or suspected to be deficient in CYP2D6 activity, as they may be at a higher risk of adverse events).
   No products indexed under this heading.

Chlorpheniramine Polistirex (Drugs which inhibit CYP2D6 also inhibit the metabolism of cevimeline. Cevimeline should be used with caution in individuals known or suspected to be deficient in CYP2D6 activity, as they may be at a higher risk of adverse events). Products include:
   Tussionex 3443

Chlorpheniramine Tannate (Drugs which inhibit CYP2D6 also inhibit the metabolism of cevimeline. Cevimeline should be used with caution in individuals known or suspected to be deficient in CYP2D6 activity, as they may be at a higher risk of adverse events).
   No products indexed under this heading.

Cimetidine (Drugs which inhibit CYP2D6 also inhibit the metabolism of cevimeline. Cevimeline should be used with caution in individuals known or suspected to be deficient in CYP2D6 activity, as they may be at a higher risk of adverse events).
   No products indexed under this heading.

Cimetidine Hydrochloride (Drugs which inhibit CYP2D6 also inhibit the metabolism of cevimeline. Cevimeline should be used with caution in individuals known or suspected to be deficient in CYP2D6 activity, as they may be at a higher risk of adverse events).
   No products indexed under this heading.

Ciprofloxacin (Drugs which inhibit CYP3A3/4 also inhibit the metabolism of cevimeline). Products include:
   Cipro I.V. 3082
   Cipro 3073
   Cipro XR 3091
   Ciprodex 583

Ciprofloxacin Hydrochloride (Drugs which inhibit CYP3A3/4 also inhibit the metabolism of cevimeline). Products include:
   Cipro 3073

Citalopram Hydrobromide (Drugs which inhibit CYP2D6 also inhibit the metabolism of cevimeline. Cevimeline should be used with caution in individuals known or suspected to be deficient in CYP2D6 activity, as they may be at a higher risk of adverse events). Products include:
   Celexa 1153

Clarithromycin (Drugs which inhibit CYP3A3/4 also inhibit the metabolism of cevimeline). Products include:
   Biaxin/Biaxin XL 412

Clidinium Bromide (Cevimeline might interfere with the desirable antimuscarinic effects of drugs used concomitantly).
   No products indexed under this heading.

Clomipramine Hydrochloride (Drugs which inhibit CYP2D6 also inhibit the metabolism of cevimeline. Cevimeline should be used with caution in individuals known or suspected to be deficient in CYP2D6 activity, as they may be at a higher risk of adverse events).
   No products indexed under this heading.

Clotrimazole (Drugs which inhibit CYP3A3/4 also inhibit the metabolism of cevimeline). Products include:

621 Interactions Index Evoxac

Maprotiline Hydrochloride (Drugs which inhibit CYP2D6 also inhibit the metabolism of cevimeline. Cevimeline should be used with caution in individuals known or suspected to be deficient in CYP2D6 activity, as they may be at a higher risk of adverse events).
No products indexed under this heading.

Mepenzolate Bromide (Cevimeline might interfere with the desirable antimuscarinic effects of drugs used concomitantly).
No products indexed under this heading.

Methadone Hydrochloride (Drugs which inhibit CYP2D6 also inhibit the metabolism of cevimeline. Cevimeline should be used with caution in individuals known or suspected to be deficient in CYP2D6 activity, as they may be at a higher risk of adverse events).
No products indexed under this heading.

Metipranolol Hydrochloride (Cevimeline should be administered with caution to patients taking β-adrenergic antagonists because of the possibility of conduction disturbances).
No products indexed under this heading.

Metoprolol Succinate (Cevimeline should be administered with caution to patients taking β-adrenergic antagonists because of the possibility of conduction disturbances). Products include:
Toprol XL 732

Metoprolol Tartrate (Cevimeline should be administered with caution to patients taking β-adrenergic antagonists because of the possibility of conduction disturbances).
No products indexed under this heading.

Metronidazole (Drugs which inhibit CYP3A3/4 also inhibit the metabolism of cevimeline). Products include:
Pylera 793

Metronidazole Benzoate (Drugs which inhibit CYP3A3/4 also inhibit the metabolism of cevimeline).
No products indexed under this heading.

Metronidazole Hydrochloride (Drugs which inhibit CYP3A3/4 also inhibit the metabolism of cevimeline).
No products indexed under this heading.

Metronidazole Sodium (Drugs which inhibit CYP3A3/4 also inhibit the metabolism of cevimeline).
No products indexed under this heading.

Mibefradil Dihydrochloride (Drugs which inhibit CYP2D6 also inhibit the metabolism of cevimeline. Cevimeline should be used with caution in individuals known or suspected to be deficient in CYP2D6 activity, as they may be at a higher risk of adverse events).
No products indexed under this heading.

Miconazole (Drugs which inhibit CYP3A3/4 also inhibit the metabolism of cevimeline).
No products indexed under this heading.

Miconazole Nitrate (Drugs which inhibit CYP3A3/4 also inhibit the metabolism of cevimeline). Products include:
Vusion Ointment 3335

Mifepristone (Drugs which inhibit CYP3A3/4 also inhibit the metabolism of cevimeline).
No products indexed under this heading.

Moclobemide (Drugs which inhibit CYP2D6 also inhibit the metabolism of cevimeline. Cevimeline should be used with caution in individuals known or suspected to be deficient in CYP2D6 activity, as they may be at a higher risk of adverse events).
No products indexed under this heading.

Nadolol (Cevimeline should be administered with caution to patients taking β-adrenergic antagonists because of the possibility of conduction disturbances). Products include:
Nadolol 2359

Nebivolol (Cevimeline should be administered with caution to patients taking β-adrenergic antagonists because of the possibility of conduction disturbances). Products include:
Bystolic 1147

Nefazodone Hydrochloride (Drugs which inhibit CYP3A3/4 also inhibit the metabolism of cevimeline).
No products indexed under this heading.

Nelfinavir Mesylate (Drugs which inhibit CYP3A3/4 also inhibit the metabolism of cevimeline).
No products indexed under this heading.

Neostigmine Bromide (Drugs with parasympathomimetic effects administered concurrently with cevimeline can be expected to have additive effects).
No products indexed under this heading.

Neostigmine Methylsulfate (Drugs with parasympathomimetic effects administered concurrently with cevimeline can be expected to have additive effects).
No products indexed under this heading.

Nevirapine (Drugs which inhibit CYP3A3/4 also inhibit the metabolism of cevimeline). Products include:
Viramune Oral Suspension 897
Viramune Tablets 897

Niacin (Drugs which inhibit CYP3A3/4 also inhibit the metabolism of cevimeline). Products include:
Advicor 402
Cardio Basics 3455
Niaspan 497
Simcor 524

Niacinamide (Drugs which inhibit CYP3A3/4 also inhibit the metabolism of cevimeline). Products include:
CitraNatal 90 DHA Capsules 2332
CitraNatal Assure 2332
CitraNatal Rx 2332
Heplive 607

Niacinamide Hydroiodide (Drugs which inhibit CYP3A3/4 also inhibit the metabolism of cevimeline).
No products indexed under this heading.

Nicotinamide (Drugs which inhibit CYP3A3/4 also inhibit the metabolism of cevimeline).
No products indexed under this heading.

Nifedipine (Drugs which inhibit CYP3A3/4 also inhibit the metabolism of cevimeline).
No products indexed under this heading.

Norfloxacin (Drugs which inhibit CYP3A3/4 also inhibit the metabolism of cevimeline). Products include:
Noroxin 2220

Nortriptyline Hydrochloride (Drugs which inhibit CYP2D6 also inhibit the metabolism of cevimeline. Cevimeline should be used with caution in individuals known or suspected to be deficient in CYP2D6 activity, as they may be at a higher risk of adverse events).
No products indexed under this heading.

Omeprazole (Drugs which inhibit CYP3A3/4 also inhibit the metabolism of cevimeline).
No products indexed under this heading.

Oxyphenonium Bromide (Cevimeline might interfere with the desirable antimuscarinic effects of drugs used concomitantly).
No products indexed under this heading.

Paroxetine Hydrochloride (Drugs which inhibit CYP2D6 also inhibit the metabolism of cevimeline. Cevimeline should be used with caution in individuals known or suspected to be deficient in CYP2D6 activity, as they may be at a higher risk of adverse events). Products include:
Paroxetine CR 2361
Paroxetine ER 2371
Paxil 1586
Paxil CR 1596

Penbutolol Sulfate (Cevimeline should be administered with caution to patients taking β-adrenergic antagonists because of the possibility of conduction disturbances).
No products indexed under this heading.

Perphenazine (Drugs which inhibit CYP2D6 also inhibit the metabolism of cevimeline. Cevimeline should be used with caution in individuals known or suspected to be deficient in CYP2D6 activity, as they may be at a higher risk of adverse events).
No products indexed under this heading.

Pindolol (Cevimeline should be administered with caution to patients taking β-adrenergic antagonists because of the possibility of conduction disturbances).
No products indexed under this heading.

Posaconazole (Drugs which inhibit CYP3A3/4 also inhibit the metabolism of cevimeline). Products include:
Noxafil 3172

Propafenone Hydrochloride (Drugs which inhibit CYP2D6 also inhibit the metabolism of cevimeline. Cevimeline should be used with caution in individuals known or suspected to be deficient in CYP2D6 activity, as they may be at a higher risk of adverse events). Products include:
Rythmol 1648
Rythmol SR 1652

Propantheline Bromide (Cevimeline might interfere with the desirable antimuscarinic effects of drugs used concomitantly).
No products indexed under this heading.

Propoxyphene Hydrochloride (Drugs which inhibit CYP2D6 also inhibit the metabolism of cevimeline. Cevimeline should be used with caution in individuals known or suspected to be deficient in CYP2D6 activity, as they may be at a higher risk of adverse events).
No products indexed under this heading.

Propoxyphene Napsylate (Drugs which inhibit CYP2D6 also inhibit the metabolism of cevimeline. Cevimeline should be used with caution in individuals known or suspected to be deficient in CYP2D6 activity, as they may be at a higher risk of adverse events).
No products indexed under this heading.

Propranolol Hydrochloride (Cevimeline should be administered with caution to patients taking β-adrenergic antagonists because of the possibility of conduction disturbances). Products include:
InnoPran XL 1517

Protriptyline Hydrochloride (Drugs which inhibit CYP2D6 also inhibit the metabolism of cevimeline. Cevimeline should be used with caution in individuals known or suspected to be deficient in CYP2D6 activity, as they may be at a higher risk of adverse events).
No products indexed under this heading.

Pyridostigmine Bromide (Drugs with parasympathomimetic effects administered concurrently with cevimeline can be expected to have additive effects).
No products indexed under this heading.

Quinacrine Hydrochloride (Drugs which inhibit CYP2D6 also inhibit the metabolism of cevimeline. Cevimeline should be used with caution in individuals known or suspected to be deficient in CYP2D6 activity, as they may be at a higher risk of adverse events).
No products indexed under this heading.

Quinidine (Drugs which inhibit CYP2D6 also inhibit the metabolism of cevimeline. Cevimeline should be used with caution in individuals known or suspected to be deficient in CYP2D6 activity, as they may be at a higher risk of adverse events).
No products indexed under this heading.

Quinidine Gluconate (Drugs which inhibit CYP2D6 also inhibit the metabolism of cevimeline. Cevimeline should be used with caution in individuals known or suspected to be deficient in CYP2D6 activity, as they may be at a higher risk of adverse events).
No products indexed under this heading.

Quinidine Hydrochloride (Drugs which inhibit CYP2D6 also inhibit the metabolism of cevimeline. Cevimeline should be used with caution in individuals known or suspected to be deficient in CYP2D6 activity, as they may be at a higher risk of adverse events).
No products indexed under this heading.

Quinidine Polygalacturonate (Drugs which inhibit CYP2D6 also inhibit the metabolism of cevimeline. Cevimeline should be used with caution in individuals known or suspected to be deficient in CYP2D6 activity, as they may be at a higher risk of adverse events).
No products indexed under this heading.

Quinidine Sulfate (Drugs which inhibit CYP2D6 also inhibit the metabolism of cevimeline. Cevimeline should be used with caution in individuals known or suspected to be deficient in CYP2D6 activity, as they may be at a higher risk of adverse events).
No products indexed under this heading.

Quinine (Drugs which inhibit CYP3A3/4 also inhibit the metabolism of cevimeline). Products include:
Hyland's Leg Cramps PM with Quinine 3315

Quinine Sulfate (Drugs which inhibit CYP3A3/4 also inhibit the metabolism of cevimeline).
No products indexed under this heading.

Quinupristin (Drugs which inhibit CYP3A3/4 also inhibit the metabolism of cevimeline).
No products indexed under this heading.

Ranitidine Bismuth Citrate (Drugs which inhibit CYP2D6 also inhibit the metabolism of cevimeline. Cevimeline should be used with caution in individuals known or suspected to be deficient in CYP2D6 activity, as they may be at a higher risk of adverse events).
No products indexed under this heading.

Ranitidine Hydrochloride (Drugs which inhibit CYP2D6 also inhibit the metabolism of cevimeline. Cevimeline should be used with caution in individuals known or suspected to be deficient in CYP2D6 activity, as they may be at a higher risk of adverse events). Products include:
Zantac 1737
Zantac Injection 1732
Zantac Pharmacy 1735

Ritonavir (Drugs which inhibit CYP2D6 also inhibit the metabolism of cevimeline. Cevimeline should be used with caution in individuals known or suspected to be deficient in CYP2D6 activity, as they may be at a higher risk of adverse events). Products include:
Kaletra 458
Norvir 509

Saquinavir (Drugs which inhibit CYP3A3/4 also inhibit the metabolism of cevimeline).
No products indexed under this heading.

Saquinavir Mesylate (Drugs which inhibit CYP3A3/4 also inhibit the metabolism of cevimeline).
No products indexed under this heading.

Scopolamine (Cevimeline might interfere with the desirable antimuscarinic effects of drugs used concomitantly). Products include:
Transderm Scōp 2397

Scopolamine Hydrobromide (Cevimeline might interfere with the

desirable antimuscarinic effects of drugs used concomitantly). Products include:
Donnatal 2711

Sertraline Hydrochloride (Drugs which inhibit CYP2D6 also inhibit the metabolism of cevimeline. Cevimeline should be used with caution in individuals known or suspected to be deficient in CYP2D6 activity, as they may be at a higher risk of adverse events).
No products indexed under this heading.

Sildenafil Citrate (Drugs which inhibit CYP2D6 also inhibit the metabolism of cevimeline. Cevimeline should be used with caution in individuals known or suspected to be deficient in CYP2D6 activity, as they may be at a higher risk of adverse events).
No products indexed under this heading.

Sotalol Hydrochloride (Cevimeline should be administered with caution to patients taking β-adrenergic antagonists because of the possibility of conduction disturbances).
No products indexed under this heading.

Telithromycin (Drugs which inhibit CYP3A3/4 also inhibit the metabolism of cevimeline). Products include:
Ketek 2991

Terbinafine Hydrochloride (Drugs which inhibit CYP2D6 also inhibit the metabolism of cevimeline. Cevimeline should be used with caution in individuals known or suspected to be deficient in CYP2D6 activity, as they may be at a higher risk of adverse events).
No products indexed under this heading.

Thioridazine Hydrochloride (Drugs which inhibit CYP2D6 also inhibit the metabolism of cevimeline. Cevimeline should be used with caution in individuals known or suspected to be deficient in CYP2D6 activity, as they may be at a higher risk of adverse events). Products include:
Thioridazine Hydrochloride 2384

Timolol Hemihydrate (Cevimeline should be administered with caution to patients taking β-adrenergic antagonists because of the possibility of conduction disturbances). Products include:
Betimol 3490

Timolol Maleate (Cevimeline should be administered with caution to patients taking β-adrenergic antagonists because of the possibility of conduction disturbances). Products include:
Combigan 601
Dorzolamide Hydrochloride/Timolol Maleate Ophthalmic Solution .... ⊙ 243
Timoptic in Ocudose .... ⊙ 231

Tolterodine Tartrate (Cevimeline might interfere with the desirable antimuscarinic effects of drugs used concomitantly).
No products indexed under this heading.

Tridihexethyl Chloride (Cevimeline might interfere with the desirable antimuscarinic effects of drugs used concomitantly).
No products indexed under this heading.

Trimipramine Maleate (Drugs which inhibit CYP2D6 also inhibit the metabolism of cevimeline. Cevimeline should be used with caution in individuals known or suspected to be deficient in CYP2D6 activity, as they may be at a higher risk of adverse events).
No products indexed under this heading.

Troglitazone (Drugs which inhibit CYP3A3/4 also inhibit the metabolism of cevimeline).
No products indexed under this heading.

Troleandomycin (Drugs which inhibit CYP3A3/4 also inhibit the metabolism of cevimeline).
No products indexed under this heading.

Valproate Sodium (Drugs which inhibit CYP3A3/4 also inhibit the metabolism of cevimeline).
No products indexed under this heading.

Vardenafil Hydrochloride (Drugs which inhibit CYP2D6 also inhibit the metabolism of cevimeline. Cevimeline should be used with caution in individuals known or suspected to be deficient in CYP2D6 activity, as they may be at a higher risk of adverse events). Products include:
Levitra 3157

Venlafaxine Hydrochloride (Drugs which inhibit CYP3A3/4 also inhibit the metabolism of cevimeline). Products include:
Effexor XR 3504
Venlafaxine Hydrochloride Tablets ... 2388

Verapamil Hydrochloride (Drugs which inhibit CYP3A3/4 also inhibit the metabolism of cevimeline). Products include:
Tarka 534

Voriconazole (Drugs which inhibit CYP3A3/4 also inhibit the metabolism of cevimeline).
No products indexed under this heading.

Zafirlukast (Drugs which inhibit CYP3A3/4 also inhibit the metabolism of cevimeline). Products include:
Accolate 3612

Zileuton (Drugs which inhibit CYP3A3/4 also inhibit the metabolism of cevimeline).
No products indexed under this heading.

Food Interactions

Food, unspecified (When administered with food, there is a decrease in the rate of absorption of cevimeline, with a fasting T_{Max} of 1.53 hours and a T_{Max} of 2.86 hours after a meal; the peak concentration is reduced by 17.3%).

Grapefruit (Drugs which inhibit CYP3A3/4 also inhibit the metabolism of cevimeline).

Grapefruit Juice (Drugs which inhibit CYP3A3/4 also inhibit the metabolism of cevimeline).

Meal, unspecified (When administered with food, there is a decrease in the rate of absorption of cevimeline, with a fasting T_{Max} of 1.53 hours and a T_{Max} of 2.86 hours after a meal; the peak concentration is reduced by 17.3%).

EXELON CAPSULES

(Rivastigmine Tartrate) 2432
May interact with anticholinergics, and certain other agents. Compounds in these categories include:

Atropine Sulfate (Rivastigmine, a cholinesterase inhibitor, has the potential to interfere with the activity of anticholinergic medications). Products include:
Donnatal 2711

Belladonna Alkaloids (Rivastigmine, a cholinesterase inhibitor, has the potential to interfere with the activity of anticholinergic medications). Products include:
Hyland's Teething Tablets 3316

Benztropine Mesylate (Rivastigmine, a cholinesterase inhibitor, has the potential to interfere with the activity of anticholinergic medications).
No products indexed under this heading.

Bethanechol Chloride (Co-administration with cholinergic agonist, such as bethanechol, can be expected to result in a synergistic effect).
No products indexed under this heading.

Biperiden Hydrochloride (Rivastigmine, a cholinesterase inhibitor, has the potential to interfere with the activity of anticholinergic medications).
No products indexed under this heading.

Clidinium Bromide (Rivastigmine, a cholinesterase inhibitor, has the potential to interfere with the activity of anticholinergic medications).
No products indexed under this heading.

Dicyclomine Hydrochloride (Rivastigmine, a cholinesterase inhibitor, has the potential to interfere with the activity of anticholinergic medications). Products include:
Bentyl Capsules 780
Bentyl Injection 780
Bentyl Syrup 780
Bentyl Tablets 780

Glycopyrrolate (Rivastigmine, a cholinesterase inhibitor, has the potential to interfere with the activity of anticholinergic medications).
No products indexed under this heading.

Hyoscyamine (Rivastigmine, a cholinesterase inhibitor, has the potential to interfere with the activity of anticholinergic medications).
No products indexed under this heading.

Hyoscyamine Sulfate (Rivastigmine, a cholinesterase inhibitor, has the potential to interfere with the activity of anticholinergic medications). Products include:
Donnatal 2711

Ipratropium Bromide (Rivastigmine, a cholinesterase inhibitor, has the potential to interfere with the activity of anticholinergic medications).
No products indexed under this heading.

Mepenzolate Bromide (Rivastigmine, a cholinesterase inhibitor, has the potential to interfere with the activity of anticholinergic medications).
No products indexed under this heading.

Oxybutynin Chloride (Rivastigmine, a cholinesterase inhibitor, has the potential to interfere with the activity of anticholinergic medications).
No products indexed under this heading.

Procyclidine Hydrochloride (Rivastigmine, a cholinesterase inhibitor, has the potential to interfere with the activity of anticholinergic medications).
No products indexed under this heading.

Propantheline Bromide (Rivastigmine, a cholinesterase inhibitor, has the potential to interfere with the activity of anticholinergic medications).
No products indexed under this heading.

Scopolamine (Rivastigmine, a cholinesterase inhibitor, has the potential to interfere with the activity of anticholinergic medications). Products include:
Transderm Scōp 2397

Scopolamine Hydrobromide (Rivastigmine, a cholinesterase inhibitor, has the potential to interfere with the activity of anticholinergic medications). Products include:
Donnatal 2711

Succinylcholine Chloride (Co-administration with succinylcholine can be expected to result in a synergistic effect).
No products indexed under this heading.

Tolterodine Tartrate (Rivastigmine, a cholinesterase inhibitor, has the potential to interfere with the activity of anticholinergic medications).
No products indexed under this heading.

Tridihexethyl Chloride (Rivastigmine, a cholinesterase inhibitor, has the potential to interfere with the activity of anticholinergic medications).
No products indexed under this heading.

Trihexyphenidyl Hydrochloride (Rivastigmine, a cholinesterase inhibitor, has the potential to interfere with the activity of anticholinergic medications).
No products indexed under this heading.

Food Interactions

Food, unspecified (Co-administration with food delays absorption (T_{max}) by 90 minutes, lowers C_{max} by approximately 30% and increases AUC by approximately 30%).

EXELON ORAL SOLUTION

(Rivastigmine Tartrate) 2432
See Exelon Capsules

EXELON PATCH

(Rivastigmine Tartrate) 2437
None cited in PDR database.

EXFORGE TABLETS

(Amlodipine Besylate, Valsartan) 2443
May interact with potassium preparations, potassium sparing diuretics, and certain other agents. Compounds in these categories include:

Amiloride Hydrochloride (As with other drugs that block angiotensin II or its effects, concomitant use of potassium sparing diuretics (eg, amiloride) may lead to increases in serum potassium and in heart failure patients to increases in serum creatinine).
No products indexed under this heading.

Atenolol (The combination of valsartan and atenolol was more antihypertensive than either component, but it did not lower the heart rate more than atenolol alone).
No products indexed under this heading.

Potassium Acid Phosphate (As with other drugs that block angiotensin II or its effects, concomitant use of potassium supplements or salt substitutes containing potassium may lead to increases in serum potassium, and in heart failure patients to increases in serum creatinine). Products include:
K-Phos Original 874

Potassium Bicarbonate (As with other drugs that block angiotensin II or its effects, concomitant use of potassium supplements or salt substitutes containing potassium may lead to increases in serum potassium, and in heart failure patients to increases in serum creatinine).
No products indexed under this heading.

Potassium Chloride (As with other drugs that block angiotensin II or its effects, concomitant use of potassium supplements or salt substitutes containing potassium may lead to increases in serum potassium, and in heart failure patients to increases in serum creatinine). Products include:
MoviPrep Oral Solution 2905

Potassium Citrate (As with other drugs that block angiotensin II or its effects, concomitant use of potassium supplements or salt substitutes containing potassium may lead to increases in serum potassium, and in heart failure patients to increases in serum creatinine). Products include:
Urocit-K 2333

Potassium Gluconate (As with other drugs that block angiotensin II or its effects, concomitant use of potassium supplements or salt substitutes containing potassium may lead to increases in serum potassium, and in heart failure patients to increases in serum creatinine).
No products indexed under this heading.

Potassium Iodide (As with other drugs that block angiotensin II or its effects, concomitant use of potassium supplements or salt substitutes containing potassium may lead to increases in serum potassium. In heart failure patients may lead to increases in serum creatinine). Products include:
Chelated Mineral 3476
CitraNatal Rx 2332

Potassium Phosphate (As with other drugs that block angiotensin II or its effects, concomitant use of potassium supplements or salt substitutes containing potassium may lead to increases in serum potassium, and in heart failure patients to increases in serum creatinine). Products include:
K-Phos Neutral 873

Sildenafil Citrate (A single 100 mg dose of sildenafil in subjects with essential hypertension had no effect on the pharmacokinetic parameters of amlodipine. When amlodipine and sildenafil were used in combination, each agent independently exerted its own blood pressure lowering effect).
No products indexed under this heading.

Spironolactone (As with other drugs that block angiotensin II or its effects, concomitant use of potassium sparing diuretics (eg, spironolactone) may lead to increases in serum potassium and in heart failure patients to increases in serum creatinine).
No products indexed under this heading.

Triamterene (As with other drugs that block angiotensin II or its effects, concomitant use of potassium sparing diuretics (eg, triamterene) may lead to increases in serum potassium and in heart failure patients to increases in serum creatinine). Products include:
Dyazide 1429
Dyrenium 3495

EXFORGE HCT TABLETS

(Amlodipine Besylate, Hydrochlorothiazide, Valsartan) 2449
May interact with alcohols, antihypertensives, barbiturates, corticosteroids, insulin, lithium preparations, narcotic analgesics, non-steroidal anti-inflammatory agents, nondepolarizing neuromuscular blocking agents, oral hypoglycemic agents, potassium preparations, potassium sparing diuretics, skeletal muscle relaxants, vasopressors, and certain other agents. Compounds in these categories include:

Acarbose (Dosage adjustment of the antidiabetic drug may be required when antidiabetic drugs (oral agents) and thiazide diuretics are administered concurrently).
No products indexed under this heading.

Acebutolol Hydrochloride (Additive effect or potentiation may occur when other hypertensive drugs and thiazide diuretics are administered concurrently).
No products indexed under this heading.

ACTH (Intensified electrolyte depletion, particularly hypokalemia may occur when ACTH and thiazide diuretics are administered concurrently).
No products indexed under this heading.

Alclometasone Dipropionate (Intensified electrolyte depletion, particularly hypokalemia, may occur when corticosteroids and thiazide diuretics are administered concurrently).
No products indexed under this heading.

Alfentanil Hydrochloride (Potentiation of orthostatic hypotension may occur when narcotics and thiazide diuretics are administered concurrently).
No products indexed under this heading.

Aliskiren (Additive effect or potentiation may occur when other hypertensive drugs and thiazide diuretics are administered concurrently). Products include:
Tekturna 2538
Tekturna HCT 2541
Valturna 3637

Amiloride Hydrochloride (As with other drugs that block angiotensin II or its effects, concomitant use of potassium sparing diuretics (eg, spironolactone, triamterene, amiloride), potassium supplements, or salt substitutes containing potassium may lead to increases in serum potassium and in heart failure patients to increases in serum creatinine).
No products indexed under this heading.

Amobarbital (Potentiation of orthostatic hypotension may occur when barbiturates and thiazide diuretics are administered concurrently).
No products indexed under this heading.

Amobarbital Sodium (Potentiation of orthostatic hypotension may occur when barbiturates and thiazide diuretics are administered concurrently).
No products indexed under this heading.

Apomorphine (Potentiation of orthostatic hypotension may occur when narcotics and thiazide diuretics are administered concurrently).
No products indexed under this heading.

Apomorphine Hydrochloride (Potentiation of orthostatic hypotension may occur when narcotics and thiazide diuretics are administered concurrently).
No products indexed under this heading.

Aprobarbital (Potentiation of orthostatic hypotension may occur when barbiturates and thiazide diuretics are administered concurrently).
No products indexed under this heading.

Atenolol (Additive effect or potentiation may occur when other hypertensive drugs and thiazide diuretics are administered concurrently).
No products indexed under this heading.

Atracurium Besylate (Possible increased responsiveness to the muscle relaxant may occur when skeletal muscle relaxants and thiazide diuretics are administered concurrently).
No products indexed under this heading.

Baclofen (Possible increased responsiveness to the muscle relaxant may occur when skeletal muscle relaxants and thiazide diuretics are administered concurrently).
No products indexed under this heading.

Beclomethasone Dipropionate (Intensified electrolyte depletion, particularly hypokalemia, may occur when corticosteroids and thiazide diuretics are administered concurrently). Products include:
Qvar 3398

Beclomethasone Dipropionate Monohydrate (Intensified electrolyte depletion, particularly hypokalemia, may occur when corticosteroids and thiazide diuretics are administered concurrently). Products include:
Beconase AQ 1386

Benazepril Hydrochloride (Additive effect or potentiation may occur when other hypertensive drugs and thiazide diuretics are administered concurrently).
No products indexed under this heading.

Bendroflumethiazide (Additive effect or potentiation may occur when other hypertensive drugs and thiazide diuretics are administered concurrently).
No products indexed under this heading.

Betamethasone (Intensified electrolyte depletion, particularly hypokalemia, may occur when corticosteroids and thiazide diuretics are administered concurrently).
No products indexed under this heading.

Betamethasone Acetate (Intensified electrolyte depletion, particularly hypokalemia, may occur when corticosteroids and thiazide diuretics are administered concurrently).
No products indexed under this heading.

Betamethasone Benzoate (Intensified electrolyte depletion, particularly hypokalemia, may occur when corticosteroids and thiazide diuretics are administered concurrently).
No products indexed under this heading.

Betamethasone Dipropionate (Intensified electrolyte depletion, particularly hypokalemia, may occur when corticosteroids and thiazide diuretics are administered concurrently). Products include:
Diprolene Lotion 0.05% 3108
Diprolene Ointment 0.05% 3109
Diprolene AF Cream 0.05% 3107
Lotrisone 3163

Betamethasone Sodium Phosphate (Intensified electrolyte depletion, particularly hypokalemia, may occur when corticosteroids and thiazide diuretics are administered concurrently).
No products indexed under this heading.

Betamethasone Valerate (Intensified electrolyte depletion, particularly hypokalemia, may occur when corticosteroids and thiazide diuretics are administered concurrently). Products include:
Luxíq 3321

Betaxolol Hydrochloride (Additive effect or potentiation may occur when other hypertensive drugs and thiazide diuretics are administered concurrently).
No products indexed under this heading.

Bisoprolol Fumarate (Additive effect or potentiation may occur when other hypertensive drugs and thiazide diuretics are administered concurrently).
No products indexed under this heading.

Budesonide (Intensified electrolyte depletion, particularly hypokalemia, may occur when corticosteroids and thiazide diuretics are administered concurrently). Products include:
Pulmicort Flexhaler 714
Symbicort 80/4.5 720
Symbicort 160/4.5 720

Buprenorphine Hydrochloride (Potentiation of orthostatic hypotension may occur when narcotics and thiazide diuretics are administered concurrently).
No products indexed under this heading.

Butabarbital (Potentiation of orthostatic hypotension may occur when barbiturates and thiazide diuretics are administered concurrently).
No products indexed under this heading.

Butabarbital Sodium (Potentiation of orthostatic hypotension may occur when barbiturates and thiazide diuretics are administered concurrently).
No products indexed under this heading.

Butalbital (Potentiation of orthostatic hypotension may occur when barbiturates and thiazide diuretics are administered concurrently).
No products indexed under this heading.

Candesartan Cilexetil (Additive effect or potentiation may occur when other hypertensive drugs and thiazide diuretics are administered concurrently). Products include:
Atacand 697
Atacand HCT 700

Captopril (Additive effect or potentiation may occur when other hypertensive drugs and thiazide diuretics are administered concurrently). Products include:
Captopril 2341

Carbamazepine (Concurrent administration of carbamazepine and thiazide diuretics may lead to symptomatic hyponatremia). Products include:
Carbatrol 3280
Equetro 3477

Carisoprodol (Possible increased responsiveness to the muscle relaxant may occur when skeletal muscle relaxants and thiazide diuretics are administered concurrently).
No products indexed under this heading.

Carteolol Hydrochloride (Additive effect or potentiation may occur when other hypertensive drugs and thiazide diuretics are administered concurrently).
No products indexed under this heading.

Carvedilol (Additive effect or potentiation may occur when other hypertensive drugs and thiazide diuretics are administered concurrently). Products include:
Coreg 1409

Carvedilol Phosphate (Additive effect or potentiation may occur when other hypertensive drugs and thiazide diuretics are administered concurrently). Products include:
Coreg CR 1416

Celecoxib (In some patients, the administration of a non-steroidal antiinflammatory agent can reduce the diuretic, natriuretic, and antihypertensive effects of loop, potassium-sparing and thiazide diuretics). Products include:
Celebrex 3272

Chlorothiazide (Additive effect or potentiation may occur when other hypertensive drugs and thiazide diuretics are administered concurrently).
No products indexed under this heading.

Chlorothiazide Sodium (Additive effect or potentiation may occur when other hypertensive drugs and thiazide diuretics are administered concurrently). Products include:
Diuril Intravenous 2009

Chlorpropamide (Dosage adjustment of the antidiabetic drug may be required when antidiabetic drugs (oral agents) and thiazide diuretics are administered concurrently).
No products indexed under this heading.

Chlorthalidone (Additive effect or potentiation may occur when other hypertensive drugs and thiazide diuretics are administered concurrently). Products include:
Clorpres 2344

Chlorzoxazone (Possible increased responsiveness to the muscle relaxant may occur when skeletal muscle relaxants and thiazide diuretics are administered concurrently).
No products indexed under this heading.

Cholestyramine (Absorption of hydrochlorothiazide is impaired in the presence of anionic exchange resins. Single doses of either cholestyramine or colestipol resins bind the hydrochlorothiazide and reduce its absorption from the gastrointestinal tract by up to 85% and 43% respectively).
No products indexed under this heading.

Ciclesonide (Intensified electrolyte depletion, particularly hypokalemia, may occur when corticosteroids and thiazide diuretics are administered concurrently).
No products indexed under this heading.

Cisatracurium Besylate (Possible increased responsiveness to the muscle relaxant may occur when skeletal muscle relaxants and thiazide diuretics are administered concurrently). Products include:
Nimbex 503

Clonidine (Additive effect or potentiation may occur when other hypertensive

IMPORTANT NOTE: Always consult each drug listing in the patient's regimen for possible interactions.

drugs and thiazide diuretics are administered concurrently). Products include:
Catapres-TTS **884**

Clonidine Hydrochloride (Additive effect or potentiation may occur when other hypertensive drugs and thiazide diuretics are administered concurrently). Products include:
Clorpres **2344**

Codeine Phosphate (Potentiation of orthostatic hypotension may occur when narcotics and thiazide diuretics are administered concurrently). Products include:
Tylenol with Codeine **2691**

Codeine Sulfate (Potentiation of orthostatic hypotension may occur when narcotics and thiazide diuretics are administered concurrently).
No products indexed under this heading.

Colestipol (Absorption of hydrochlorothiazide is impaired in the presence of anionic exchange resins. Single doses of either cholestyramine or colestipol resins bind the hydrochlorothiazide and reduce its absorption from the gastrointestinal tract by up to 85% and 43% respectively).
No products indexed under this heading.

Colestipol Hydrochloride (Absorption of hydrochlorothiazide is impaired in the presence of anionic exchange resins. Single doses of either cholestyramine or colestipol resins bind the hydrochlorothiazide and reduce its absorption from the gastrointestinal tract by up to 85% and 43% respectively).
No products indexed under this heading.

Cortisone Acetate (Intensified electrolyte depletion, particularly hypokalemia, may occur when corticosteroids and thiazide diuretics are administered concurrently).
No products indexed under this heading.

Cyclobenzaprine Hydrochloride (Possible increased responsiveness to the muscle relaxant may occur when skeletal muscle relaxants and thiazide diuretics are administered concurrently). Products include:
Amrix **964**

Dantrolene Sodium (Possible increased responsiveness to the muscle relaxant may occur when skeletal muscle relaxants and thiazide diuretics are administered concurrently).
No products indexed under this heading.

Deserpidine (Additive effect or potentiation may occur when other hypertensive drugs and thiazide diuretics are administered concurrently).
No products indexed under this heading.

Desoximetasone (Intensified electrolyte depletion, particularly hypokalemia, may occur when corticosteroids and thiazide diuretics are administered concurrently).
No products indexed under this heading.

Dexamethasone (Intensified electrolyte depletion, particularly hypokalemia, may occur when corticosteroids and thiazide diuretics are administered concurrently). Products include:
Ciprodex **583**
Ozurdex .... ⊙**223**
Tobramycin and Dexamethasone Ophthalmic Suspension .... ⊙**251**

Dexamethasone Acetate (Intensified electrolyte depletion, particularly hypokalemia, may occur when corticosteroids and thiazide diuretics are administered concurrently).
No products indexed under this heading.

Dexamethasone Phosphate (Intensified electrolyte depletion, particularly hypokalemia, may occur when corticosteroids and thiazide diuretics are administered concurrently).
No products indexed under this heading.

Dexamethasone Sodium (Intensified electrolyte depletion, particularly hypokalemia, may occur when corticosteroids and thiazide diuretics are administered concurrently).
No products indexed under this heading.

Dexamethasone Sodium Phosphate (Intensified electrolyte depletion, particularly hypokalemia, may occur when corticosteroids and thiazide diuretics are administered concurrently).
No products indexed under this heading.

Dexamethasone Sodium Phosphate Injection (Intensified electrolyte depletion, particularly hypokalemia, may occur when corticosteroids and thiazide diuretics are administered concurrently).
No products indexed under this heading.

Dezocine (Potentiation of orthostatic hypotension may occur when narcotics and thiazide diuretics are administered concurrently).
No products indexed under this heading.

Diazoxide (Additive effect or potentiation may occur when other hypertensive drugs and thiazide diuretics are administered concurrently). Products include:
Proglycem **1179**
Proglycem Suspension **1179**

Diclofenac Epolamine (In some patients, the administration of a non-steroidal antiinflammatory agent can reduce the diuretic, natriuretic, and antihypertensive effects of loop, potassium-sparing and thiazide diuretics). Products include:
Flector **1839**

Diclofenac Potassium (In some patients, the administration of a non-steroidal antiinflammatory agent can reduce the diuretic, natriuretic, and antihypertensive effects of loop, potassium-sparing and thiazide diuretics).
No products indexed under this heading.

Diclofenac Sodium (In some patients, the administration of a non-steroidal antiinflammatory agent can reduce the diuretic, natriuretic, and antihypertensive effects of loop, potassium-sparing and thiazide diuretics).
No products indexed under this heading.

Diflorasone Diacetate (Intensified electrolyte depletion, particularly hypokalemia, may occur when corticosteroids and thiazide diuretics are administered concurrently).
No products indexed under this heading.

Dihydrocodeine Bitartrate (Potentiation of orthostatic hypotension may occur when narcotics and thiazide diuretics are administered concurrently).
No products indexed under this heading.

Dihydrocodeinone Bitartrate (Potentiation of orthostatic hypotension may occur when narcotics and thiazide diuretics are administered concurrently).
No products indexed under this heading.

Diltiazem Hydrochloride (Additive effect or potentiation may occur when other hypertensive drugs and thiazide diuretics are administered concurrently). Products include:
Cardizem LA **423**

Diltiazem Maleate (Additive effect or potentiation may occur when other hypertensive drugs and thiazide diuretics are administered concurrently).
No products indexed under this heading.

Dobutamine (Possible decreased response to pressor amines, but not sufficient to preclude their use, may occur when pressor amines (eg, norepinephrine) and thiazide diuretics are administered concurrently).
No products indexed under this heading.

Dobutamine Hydrochloride (Possible decreased response to pressor amines, but not sufficient to preclude their use, may occur when pressor amines (eg, norepinephrine) and thiazide diuretics are administered concurrently).
No products indexed under this heading.

Dopamine Hydrochloride (Possible decreased response to pressor amines, but not sufficient to preclude their use, may occur when pressor amines (eg, norepinephrine) and thiazide diuretics are administered concurrently).
No products indexed under this heading.

Doxacurium Chloride (Possible increased responsiveness to the muscle relaxant may occur when skeletal muscle relaxants and thiazide diuretics are administered concurrently).
No products indexed under this heading.

Doxazosin Mesylate (Additive effect or potentiation may occur when other hypertensive drugs and thiazide diuretics are administered concurrently).
No products indexed under this heading.

d-Tubocurarine (Possible increased responsiveness to the muscle relaxant may occur when skeletal muscle relaxants and thiazide diuretics are administered concurrently).
No products indexed under this heading.

Enalapril Maleate (Additive effect or potentiation may occur when other hypertensive drugs and thiazide diuretics are administered concurrently).
No products indexed under this heading.

Enalaprilat (Additive effect or potentiation may occur when other hypertensive drugs and thiazide diuretics are administered concurrently).
No products indexed under this heading.

Ephedrine Sulfate (Possible decreased response to pressor amines, but not sufficient to preclude their use, may occur when pressor amines (eg, norepinephrine) and thiazide diuretics are administered concurrently).
No products indexed under this heading.

Epinephrine Bitartrate (Possible decreased response to pressor amines, but not sufficient to preclude their use, may occur when pressor amines (eg, norepinephrine) and thiazide diuretics are administered concurrently).
No products indexed under this heading.

Epinephrine Hydrochloride (Possible decreased response to pressor amines, but not sufficient to preclude their use, may occur when pressor amines (eg, norepinephrine) and thiazide diuretics are administered concurrently).
No products indexed under this heading.

Eprosartan Mesylate (Additive effect or potentiation may occur when other hypertensive drugs and thiazide diuretics are administered concurrently). Products include:
Teveten **538**
Teveten HCT **541**

Esmolol Hydrochloride (Additive effect or potentiation may occur when other hypertensive drugs and thiazide diuretics are administered concurrently).
No products indexed under this heading.

Ethanol (Potentiation of orthostatic hypotension may occur when alcohol and thiazide diuretics are administered concurrently).
No products indexed under this heading.

Ethyl Alcohol (Potentiation of orthostatic hypotension may occur when alcohol and thiazide diuretics are administered concurrently).
No products indexed under this heading.

Etodolac (In some patients, the administration of a non-steroidal antiinflammatory agent can reduce the diuretic, natriuretic, and antihypertensive effects of loop, potassium-sparing and thiazide diuretics).
No products indexed under this heading.

Felodipine (Additive effect or potentiation may occur when other hypertensive drugs and thiazide diuretics are administered concurrently).
No products indexed under this heading.

Fenoprofen Calcium (In some patients, the administration of a non-steroidal antiinflammatory agent can reduce the diuretic, natriuretic, and antihypertensive effects of loop, potassium-sparing and thiazide diuretics).
No products indexed under this heading.

Fentanyl (Potentiation of orthostatic hypotension may occur when narcotics and thiazide diuretics are administered concurrently). Products include:
Duragesic **2604**
Fentanyl Transdermal System **2346**
Onsolis **2054**

Fentanyl Citrate (Potentiation of orthostatic hypotension may occur when narcotics and thiazide diuretics are administered concurrently). Products include:
Fentora **966**

Fludrocortisone Acetate (Intensified electrolyte depletion, particularly hypokalemia, may occur when corticosteroids and thiazide diuretics are administered concurrently).
No products indexed under this heading.

Flumethasone Pivalate (Intensified electrolyte depletion, particularly hypokalemia, may occur when corticosteroids and thiazide diuretics are administered concurrently).
No products indexed under this heading.

Flunisolide Hemihydrate (Intensified electrolyte depletion, particularly hypokalemia, may occur when corticosteroids and thiazide diuretics are administered concurrently).
No products indexed under this heading.

Flurbiprofen (In some patients, the administration of a non-steroidal antiinflammatory agent can reduce the diuretic, natriuretic, and antihypertensive effects of loop, potassium-sparing and thiazide diuretics).
No products indexed under this heading.

Fluticasone Furoate (Intensified electrolyte depletion, particularly hypokalemia, may occur when corticosteroids and thiazide diuretics are administered concurrently). Products include:
Veramyst **1713**

Fluticasone Propionate (Intensified electrolyte depletion, particularly hypokalemia, may occur when corticosteroids and thiazide diuretics are administered concurrently). Products include:
Advair 100/50 .... **1275**
Advair 250/50 .... **1275**
Advair 500/50 .... **1275**
Advair HFA 45/21 .... **1288**
Advair HFA 115/21 .... **1288**
Advair HFA 230/21 .... **1288**
Flonase **1459**
Flovent Diskus **1463**
Flovent HFA **1470**

Fosinopril Sodium (Additive effect or potentiation may occur when other hypertensive drugs and thiazide diuretics are administered concurrently).
No products indexed under this heading.

Furosemide (Additive effect or potentiation may occur when other hypertensive drugs and thiazide diuretics are administered concurrently). Products include:
Furosemide **2354**

Gallamine (Possible increased responsiveness to the muscle relaxant may occur when skeletal muscle relaxants and thiazide diuretics are administered concurrently).
No products indexed under this heading.

Gallamine Triethiodide (Possible increased responsiveness to the muscle relaxant may occur when skeletal muscle relaxants and thiazide diuretics are administered concurrently).
No products indexed under this heading.

Glibenclamide (Dosage adjustment of the antidiabetic drug may be required when antidiabetic drugs (oral agents) and thiazide diuretics are administered concurrently).
No products indexed under this heading.

Glimepiride (Dosage adjustment of the antidiabetic drug may be required when antidiabetic drugs (oral agents) and thiazide diuretics are administered concurrently). Products include:

Glipizide (Dosage adjustment of the antidiabetic drug may be required when antidiabetic drugs (oral agents) and thiazide diuretics are administered concurrently).
No products indexed under this heading.

Glyburide (Dosage adjustment of the antidiabetic drug may be required when antidiabetic drugs (oral agents) and thiazide diuretics are administered concurrently).
No products indexed under this heading.

Guanabenz Acetate (Additive effect or potentiation may occur when other hypertensive drugs and thiazide diuretics are administered concurrently).
No products indexed under this heading.

Guanethidine (Additive effect or potentiation may occur when other hypertensive drugs and thiazide diuretics are administered concurrently).
No products indexed under this heading.

Guanethidine Monosulfate (Additive effect or potentiation may occur when other hypertensive drugs and thiazide diuretics are administered concurrently).
No products indexed under this heading.

Guanethidine Sulfate (Additive effect or potentiation may occur when other hypertensive drugs and thiazide diuretics are administered concurrently).
No products indexed under this heading.

Hexobarbital (Potentiation of orthostatic hypotension may occur when barbiturates and thiazide diuretics are administered concurrently).
No products indexed under this heading.

Hydralazine Hydrochloride (Additive effect or potentiation may occur when other hypertensive drugs and thiazide diuretics are administered concurrently).
No products indexed under this heading.

Hydrocodone Bitartrate (Potentiation of orthostatic hypotension may occur when narcotics and thiazide diuretics are administered concurrently). Products include:

Hydrocodone Polistirex (Potentiation of orthostatic hypotension may occur when narcotics and thiazide diuretics are administered concurrently). Products include:

Hydrocortisone (Intensified electrolyte depletion, particularly hypokalemia, may occur when corticosteroids and thiazide diuretics are administered concurrently).
No products indexed under this heading.

Hydrocortisone (Alcohol) (Intensified electrolyte depletion, particularly hypokalemia, may occur when corticosteroids and thiazide diuretics are administered concurrently).
No products indexed under this heading.

Hydrocortisone Acetate (Intensified electrolyte depletion, particularly hypokalemia, may occur when corticosteroids and thiazide diuretics are administered concurrently).
No products indexed under this heading.

Hydrocortisone Butyrate (Intensified electrolyte depletion, particularly hypokalemia, may occur when corticosteroids and thiazide diuretics are administered concurrently).
No products indexed under this heading.

Hydrocortisone Cypionate (Intensified electrolyte depletion, particularly hypokalemia, may occur when corticosteroids and thiazide diuretics are administered concurrently).
No products indexed under this heading.

Hydrocortisone Hemisuccinate (Intensified electrolyte depletion, particularly hypokalemia, may occur when corticosteroids and thiazide diuretics are administered concurrently).
No products indexed under this heading.

Hydrocortisone Probutate (Intensified electrolyte depletion, particularly hypokalemia, may occur when corticosteroids and thiazide diuretics are administered concurrently).
No products indexed under this heading.

Hydrocortisone Sodium Phosphate (Intensified electrolyte depletion, particularly hypokalemia, may occur when corticosteroids and thiazide diuretics are administered concurrently).
No products indexed under this heading.

Hydrocortisone Sodium Succinate (Intensified electrolyte depletion, particularly hypokalemia, may occur when corticosteroids and thiazide diuretics are administered concurrently).
No products indexed under this heading.

Hydrocortisone Valerate (Intensified electrolyte depletion, particularly hypokalemia, may occur when corticosteroids and thiazide diuretics are administered concurrently).
No products indexed under this heading.

Hydroflumethiazide (Additive effect or potentiation may occur when other hypertensive drugs and thiazide diuretics are administered concurrently).
No products indexed under this heading.

Hydromorphone (Potentiation of orthostatic hypotension may occur when narcotics and thiazide diuretics are administered concurrently).
No products indexed under this heading.

Hydromorphone Hydrochloride (Potentiation of orthostatic hypotension may occur when narcotics and thiazide diuretics are administered concurrently). Products include:

Ibuprofen (In some patients, the administration of a non-steroidal antiinflammatory agent can reduce the diuretic, natriuretic, and antihypertensive effects of loop, potassium-sparing and thiazide diuretics). Products include:

Indapamide (Additive effect or potentiation may occur when other hypertensive drugs and thiazide diuretics are administered concurrently). Products include:

Indomethacin (In some patients, the administration of a non-steroidal antiinflammatory agent can reduce the diuretic, natriuretic, and antihypertensive effects of loop, potassium-sparing and thiazide diuretics). Products include:

Indomethacin Sodium Trihydrate (In some patients, the administration of a non-steroidal antiinflammatory agent can reduce the diuretic, natriuretic, and antihypertensive effects of loop, potassium-sparing and thiazide diuretics). Products include:

Insulin (Dosage adjustment of the antidiabetic drug may be required when antidiabetic drugs (insulin) and thiazide diuretics are administered concurrently).
No products indexed under this heading.

Insulin, Human, Zinc Suspension (Dosage adjustment of the antidiabetic drug may be required when antidiabetic drugs (insulin) and thiazide diuretics are administered concurrently).
No products indexed under this heading.

Insulin, Human (rDNA origin) (Dosage adjustment of the antidiabetic drug may be required when antidiabetic drugs (insulin) and thiazide diuretics are administered concurrently). Products include:

Insulin, Human NPH (Dosage adjustment of the antidiabetic drug may be required when antidiabetic drugs (insulin) and thiazide diuretics are administered concurrently). Products include:

Insulin, Human Regular (Dosage adjustment of the antidiabetic drug may be required when antidiabetic drugs (insulin) and thiazide diuretics are administered concurrently). Products include:

Insulin, Human Regular and Human NPH Mixture (Dosage adjustment of the antidiabetic drug may be required when antidiabetic drugs (insulin) and thiazide diuretics are administered concurrently). Products include:

Insulin, NPH (Dosage adjustment of the antidiabetic drug may be required when antidiabetic drugs (insulin) and thiazide diuretics are administered concurrently).
No products indexed under this heading.

Insulin, Regular (Dosage adjustment of the antidiabetic drug may be required when antidiabetic drugs (insulin) and thiazide diuretics are administered concurrently).
No products indexed under this heading.

Insulin, Regular and NPH mixture (Dosage adjustment of the antidiabetic drug may be required when antidiabetic drugs (insulin) and thiazide diuretics are administered concurrently).
No products indexed under this heading.

Insulin, Zinc Crystals (Dosage adjustment of the antidiabetic drug may be required when antidiabetic drugs (insulin) and thiazide diuretics are administered concurrently).
No products indexed under this heading.

Insulin, Zinc Suspension (Dosage adjustment of the antidiabetic drug may be required when antidiabetic drugs (insulin) and thiazide diuretics are administered concurrently).
No products indexed under this heading.

Insulin Aspart (Dosage adjustment of the antidiabetic drug may be required when antidiabetic drugs (insulin) and thiazide diuretics are administered concurrently).
No products indexed under this heading.

Insulin Aspart, Human (Dosage adjustment of the antidiabetic drug may be required when antidiabetic drugs (insulin) and thiazide diuretics are administered concurrently). Products include:

Insulin Aspart, Human Regular (Dosage adjustment of the antidiabetic drug may be required when antidiabetic drugs (insulin) and thiazide diuretics are administered concurrently). Products include:

Insulin Aspart Protamine, Human (Dosage adjustment of the antidiabetic drug may be required when antidiabetic drugs (insulin) and thiazide diuretics are administered concurrently). Products include:

Insulin Detemir (rDNA Origin) (Dosage adjustment of the antidiabetic drug may be required when antidiabetic drugs (insulin) and thiazide diuretics are administered concurrently). Products include:

Insulin Glargine (Dosage adjustment of the antidiabetic drug may be required when antidiabetic drugs (insulin) and thiazide diuretics are administered concurrently). Products include:

Insulin Glulisine (Dosage adjustment of the antidiabetic drug may be required when antidiabetic drugs (insulin) and thiazide diuretics are administered concurrently). Products include:

Insulin Lispro, Human (Dosage adjustment of the antidiabetic drug may be required when antidiabetic drugs (insulin) and thiazide diuretics are administered concurrently). Products include:

Insulin Lispro Protamine, Human (Dosage adjustment of the antidiabetic drug may be required when antidiabetic drugs (insulin) and thiazide diuretics are administered concurrently). Products include:

Irbesartan (Additive effect or potentiation may occur when other hypertensive drugs and thiazide diuretics are administered concurrently). Products include:

Isoproterenol Hydrochloride (Possible decreased response to pressor amines, but not sufficient to preclude their use, may occur when pressor amines (eg, norepinephrine) and thiazide diuretics are administered concurrently).
No products indexed under this heading.

IMPORTANT NOTE: Always consult each drug listing in the patient's regimen for possible interactions.

Isoproterenol Sulfate (Possible decreased response to pressor amines, but not sufficient to preclude their use, may occur when pressor amines (eg, norepinephrine) and thiazide diuretics are administered concurrently).
No products indexed under this heading.

Isradipine (Additive effect or potentiation may occur when other hypertensive drugs and thiazide diuretics are administered concurrently). Products include:
DynaCirc CR 1432

Ketoprofen (In some patients, the administration of a non-steroidal antiinflammatory agent can reduce the diuretic, natriuretic, and antihypertensive effects of loop, potassium-sparing and thiazide diuretics).
No products indexed under this heading.

Ketorolac Tromethamine (In some patients, the administration of a non-steroidal antiinflammatory agent can reduce the diuretic, natriuretic, and antihypertensive effects of loop, potassium-sparing and thiazide diuretics). Products include:
Acuvail .... ⊙209

Labetalol Hydrochloride (Additive effect or potentiation may occur when other hypertensive drugs and thiazide diuretics are administered concurrently).
No products indexed under this heading.

Levorphanol Tartrate (Potentiation of orthostatic hypotension may occur when narcotics and thiazide diuretics are administered concurrently).
No products indexed under this heading.

Lisinopril (Additive effect or potentiation may occur when other hypertensive drugs and thiazide diuretics are administered concurrently). Products include:
Prinivil 2241
Prinzide 2246

Lithium (Lithium should not generally be given with diuretics. Diuretic agents reduce the renal clearance of lithium and add a high risk of lithium toxicity).
No products indexed under this heading.

Lithium Carbonate (Lithium should not generally be given with diuretics. Diuretic agents reduce the renal clearance of lithium and add a high risk of lithium toxicity).
No products indexed under this heading.

Lithium Citrate (Lithium should not generally be given with diuretics. Diuretic agents reduce the renal clearance of lithium and add a high risk of lithium toxicity).
No products indexed under this heading.

Losartan Potassium (Additive effect or potentiation may occur when other hypertensive drugs and thiazide diuretics are administered concurrently). Products include:
Cozaar 2106
Hyzaar 2162
Hyzaar 100-12.5 2162

Mecamylamine Hydrochloride (Additive effect or potentiation may occur when other hypertensive drugs and thiazide diuretics are administered concurrently).
No products indexed under this heading.

Meclofenamate Sodium (In some patients, the administration of a non-steroidal antiinflammatory agent can reduce the diuretic, natriuretic, and antihypertensive effects of loop, potassium-sparing and thiazide diuretics).
No products indexed under this heading.

Mefenamic Acid (In some patients, the administration of a non-steroidal antiinflammatory agent can reduce the diuretic, natriuretic, and antihypertensive effects of loop, potassium-sparing and thiazide diuretics).
No products indexed under this heading.

Meloxicam (In some patients, the administration of a non-steroidal antiinflammatory agent can reduce the diuretic, natriuretic, and antihypertensive effects of loop, potassium-sparing and thiazide diuretics).
No products indexed under this heading.

Meperidine Hydrochloride (Potentiation of orthostatic hypotension may occur when narcotics and thiazide diuretics are administered concurrently).
No products indexed under this heading.

Mephentermine Sulfate (Possible decreased response to pressor amines, but not sufficient to preclude their use, may occur when pressor amines (eg, norepinephrine) and thiazide diuretics are administered concurrently).
No products indexed under this heading.

Mephobarbital (Potentiation of orthostatic hypotension may occur when barbiturates and thiazide diuretics are administered concurrently).
No products indexed under this heading.

Metaraminol Bitartrate (Possible decreased response to pressor amines, but not sufficient to preclude their use, may occur when pressor amines (eg, norepinephrine) and thiazide diuretics are administered concurrently).
No products indexed under this heading.

Metaxalone (Possible increased responsiveness to the muscle relaxant may occur when skeletal muscle relaxants and thiazide diuretics are administered concurrently). Products include:
Skelaxin 1848

Metformin Hydrochloride (Dosage adjustment of the antidiabetic drug may be required when antidiabetic drugs (oral agents) and thiazide diuretics are administered concurrently). Products include:
ActoPlus 3338
Avandamet 1345
Janumet 2188

Methadone Hydrochloride (Potentiation of orthostatic hypotension may occur when narcotics and thiazide diuretics are administered concurrently).
No products indexed under this heading.

Methocarbamol (Possible increased responsiveness to the muscle relaxant may occur when skeletal muscle relaxants and thiazide diuretics are administered concurrently).
No products indexed under this heading.

Methoxamine Hydrochloride (Possible decreased response to pressor amines, but not sufficient to preclude their use, may occur when pressor amines (eg, norepinephrine) and thiazide diuretics are administered concurrently).
No products indexed under this heading.

Methyclothiazide (Additive effect or potentiation may occur when other hypertensive drugs and thiazide diuretics are administered concurrently).
No products indexed under this heading.

Methyldopa (Additive effect or potentiation may occur when other hypertensive drugs and thiazide diuretics are administered concurrently).
No products indexed under this heading.

Methyldopate Hydrochloride (Additive effect or potentiation may occur when other hypertensive drugs and thiazide diuretics are administered concurrently).
No products indexed under this heading.

Methylprednisolone (Intensified electrolyte depletion, particularly hypokalemia, may occur when corticosteroids and thiazide diuretics are administered concurrently).
No products indexed under this heading.

Methylprednisolone Acetate (Intensified electrolyte depletion, particularly hypokalemia, may occur when corticosteroids and thiazide diuretics are administered concurrently).
No products indexed under this heading.

Methylprednisolone Sodium Succinate (Intensified electrolyte depletion, particularly hypokalemia, may occur when corticosteroids and thiazide diuretics are administered concurrently).
No products indexed under this heading.

Metocurine Iodide (Possible increased responsiveness to the muscle relaxant may occur when skeletal muscle relaxants and thiazide diuretics are administered concurrently).
No products indexed under this heading.

Metolazone (Additive effect or potentiation may occur when other hypertensive drugs and thiazide diuretics are administered concurrently).
No products indexed under this heading.

Metoprolol Succinate (Additive effect or potentiation may occur when other hypertensive drugs and thiazide diuretics are administered concurrently). Products include:
Toprol XL 732

Metoprolol Tartrate (Additive effect or potentiation may occur when other hypertensive drugs and thiazide diuretics are administered concurrently).
No products indexed under this heading.

Metyrosine (Additive effect or potentiation may occur when other hypertensive drugs and thiazide diuretics are administered concurrently).
No products indexed under this heading.

Mibefradil Dihydrochloride (Additive effect or potentiation may occur when other hypertensive drugs and thiazide diuretics are administered concurrently).
No products indexed under this heading.

Miglitol (Dosage adjustment of the antidiabetic drug may be required when antidiabetic drugs (oral agents) and thiazide diuretics are administered concurrently).
No products indexed under this heading.

Minoxidil (Additive effect or potentiation may occur when other hypertensive drugs and thiazide diuretics are administered concurrently).
No products indexed under this heading.

Mivacurium Chloride (Possible increased responsiveness to the muscle relaxant may occur when skeletal muscle relaxants and thiazide diuretics are administered concurrently).
No products indexed under this heading.

Moexipril Hydrochloride (Additive effect or potentiation may occur when other hypertensive drugs and thiazide diuretics are administered concurrently).
No products indexed under this heading.

Mometasone Furoate (Intensified electrolyte depletion, particularly hypokalemia, may occur when corticosteroids and thiazide diuretics are administered concurrently). Products include:
Asmanex 3058
Elocon Cream 3111
Elocon Lotion 3112
Elocon Ointment 3114

Mometasone Furoate Monohydrate (Intensified electrolyte depletion, particularly hypokalemia, may occur when corticosteroids and thiazide diuretics are administered concurrently). Products include:
Nasonex 3166

Morphine Sulfate (Potentiation of orthostatic hypotension may occur

when narcotics and thiazide diuretics are administered concurrently). Products include:
Avinza 1822
Embeda 1831
MS Contin 2803

Morphine Sulfate, Liposomal (Potentiation of orthostatic hypotension may occur when narcotics and thiazide diuretics are administered concurrently).
No products indexed under this heading.

Nabumetone (In some patients, the administration of a non-steroidal antiinflammatory agent can reduce the diuretic, natriuretic, and antihypertensive effects of loop, potassium-sparing and thiazide diuretics).
No products indexed under this heading.

Nadolol (Additive effect or potentiation may occur when other hypertensive drugs and thiazide diuretics are administered concurrently). Products include:
Nadolol 2359

Naproxen (In some patients, the administration of a non-steroidal antiinflammatory agent can reduce the diuretic, natriuretic, and antihypertensive effects of loop, potassium-sparing and thiazide diuretics). Products include:
EC-Naprosyn 2850
Naprosyn 2850
Anaprox/Naprosyn 2850

Naproxen Sodium (In some patients, the administration of a non-steroidal antiinflammatory agent can reduce the diuretic, natriuretic, and antihypertensive effects of loop, potassium-sparing and thiazide diuretics). Products include:
Anaprox 2850
Anaprox DS 2850
Treximet 1681

Nateglinide (Dosage adjustment of the antidiabetic drug may be required when antidiabetic drugs (oral agents) and thiazide diuretics are administered concurrently).
No products indexed under this heading.

Nebivolol (Additive effect or potentiation may occur when other hypertensive drugs and thiazide diuretics are administered concurrently). Products include:
Bystolic 1147

Nicardipine Hydrochloride (Additive effect or potentiation may occur when other hypertensive drugs and thiazide diuretics are administered concurrently).
No products indexed under this heading.

Nifedipine (Additive effect or potentiation may occur when other hypertensive drugs and thiazide diuretics are administered concurrently).
No products indexed under this heading.

Nisoldipine (Additive effect or potentiation may occur when other hypertensive drugs and thiazide diuretics are administered concurrently).
No products indexed under this heading.

Nitroglycerin (Additive effect or potentiation may occur when other hypertensive drugs and thiazide diuretics are administered concurrently). Products include:
Nitro-Dur 3170
Nitrolingual 3266

Norepinephrine Bitartrate (Possible decreased response to pressor amines, but not sufficient to preclude their use, may occur when pressor amines (eg, norepinephrine) and thiazide diuretics are administered concurrently).
No products indexed under this heading.

Orphenadrine Citrate (Possible increased responsiveness to the muscle relaxant may occur when skeletal muscle relaxants and thiazide diuretics are administered concurrently).
No products indexed under this heading.

Oxaprozin (In some patients, the administration of a non-steroidal antiinflammatory agent can reduce the diuretic, natriuretic, and antihypertensive effects of loop, potassium-sparing and thiazide diuretics).
No products indexed under this heading.

Oxycodone Hydrochloride (Potentiation of orthostatic hypotension may occur when narcotics and thiazide diuretics are administered concurrently). Products include:

Oxycodone Terephthalate (Potentiation of orthostatic hypotension may occur when narcotics and thiazide diuretics are administered concurrently).
No products indexed under this heading.

Oxymorphone Hydrochloride (Potentiation of orthostatic hypotension may occur when narcotics and thiazide diuretics are administered concurrently). Products include:

Pancuronium Bromide (Possible increased responsiveness to the muscle relaxant may occur when skeletal muscle relaxants and thiazide diuretics are administered concurrently).
No products indexed under this heading.

Penbutolol Sulfate (Additive effect or potentiation may occur when other hypertensive drugs and thiazide diuretics are administered concurrently).
No products indexed under this heading.

Pentobarbital (Potentiation of orthostatic hypotension may occur when barbiturates and thiazide diuretics are administered concurrently).
No products indexed under this heading.

Pentobarbital Sodium (Potentiation of orthostatic hypotension may occur when barbiturates and thiazide diuretics are administered concurrently). Products include:

Perindopril Erbumine (Additive effect or potentiation may occur when other hypertensive drugs and thiazide diuretics are administered concurrently).
No products indexed under this heading.

Phenobarbital (Potentiation of orthostatic hypotension may occur when barbiturates and thiazide diuretics are administered concurrently). Products include:

Phenobarbital Sodium (Potentiation of orthostatic hypotension may occur when barbiturates and thiazide diuretics are administered concurrently).
No products indexed under this heading.

Phenoxybenzamine Hydrochloride (Additive effect or potentiation may occur when other hypertensive drugs and thiazide diuretics are administered concurrently). Products include:

Phentolamine Mesylate (Additive effect or potentiation may occur when other hypertensive drugs and thiazide diuretics are administered concurrently).
No products indexed under this heading.

Phenylbutazone (In some patients, the administration of a non-steroidal antiinflammatory agent can reduce the diuretic, natriuretic, and antihypertensive effects of loop, potassium-sparing and thiazide diuretics).
No products indexed under this heading.

Phenylephrine Hydrochloride (Possible decreased response to pressor amines, but not sufficient to preclude their use, may occur when pressor

amines (eg, norepinephrine) and thiazide diuretics are administered concurrently). Products include:

Pindolol (Additive effect or potentiation may occur when other hypertensive drugs and thiazide diuretics are administered concurrently).
No products indexed under this heading.

Pioglitazone Hydrochloride (Dosage adjustment of the antidiabetic drug may be required when antidiabetic drugs (oral agents) and thiazide diuretics are administered concurrently). Products include:

Pipecuronium Bromide (Possible increased responsiveness to the muscle relaxant may occur when skeletal muscle relaxants and thiazide diuretics are administered concurrently).
No products indexed under this heading.

Piroxicam (In some patients, the administration of a non-steroidal antiinflammatory agent can reduce the diuretic, natriuretic, and antihypertensive effects of loop, potassium-sparing and thiazide diuretics).
No products indexed under this heading.

Polythiazide (Additive effect or potentiation may occur when other hypertensive drugs and thiazide diuretics are administered concurrently).
No products indexed under this heading.

Potassium Acid Phosphate (As with other drugs that block angiotensin II or its effects, concomitant use of potassium sparing diuretics (eg, spironolactone, triamterene, amiloride), potassium supplements, or salt substitutes containing potassium may lead to increases in serum potassium and in heart failure patients to increases in serum creatinine). Products include:

Potassium Bicarbonate (As with other drugs that block angiotensin II or its effects, concomitant use of potassium sparing diuretics (eg, spironolactone, triamterene, amiloride), potassium supplements, or salt substitutes containing potassium may lead to increases in serum potassium and in heart failure patients to increases in serum creatinine).
No products indexed under this heading.

Potassium Chloride (As with other drugs that block angiotensin II or its effects, concomitant use of potassium sparing diuretics (eg, spironolactone, triamterene, amiloride), potassium supplements, or salt substitutes containing potassium may lead to increases in serum potassium and in heart failure patients to increases in serum creatinine). Products include:

Potassium Citrate (As with other drugs that block angiotensin II or its effects, concomitant use of potassium sparing diuretics (eg, spironolactone, triamterene, amiloride), potassium supplements, or salt substitutes containing potassium may lead to increases in serum potassium and in heart failure patients to increases in serum creatinine). Products include:

Potassium Gluconate (As with other drugs that block angiotensin II or its effects, concomitant use of potassium sparing diuretics (eg, spironolactone, triamterene, amiloride), potassium supplements, or salt substitutes containing potassium may lead to increases in serum potassium and in heart failure patients to increases in serum creatinine).
No products indexed under this heading.

Potassium Iodide (As with other drugs that block angiotensin II or its effects, concomitant use of potassium sparing diuretics (eg, spironolactone, triamterene, amiloride), potassium supplements, or salt substitutes containing potassium may lead to increases in serum potassium and in heart failure patients to increases in serum creatinine). Products include:

Potassium Phosphate (As with other drugs that block angiotensin II or its effects, concomitant use of potassium sparing diuretics (eg, spironolactone, triamterene, amiloride), potassium supplements, or salt substitutes containing potassium may lead to increases in serum potassium and in heart failure patients to increases in serum creatinine). Products include:

Prazosin Hydrochloride (Additive effect or potentiation may occur when other hypertensive drugs and thiazide diuretics are administered concurrently).
No products indexed under this heading.

Prednisolone (Intensified electrolyte depletion, particularly hypokalemia, may occur when corticosteroids and thiazide diuretics are administered concurrently).
No products indexed under this heading.

Prednisolone Acetate (Intensified electrolyte depletion, particularly hypokalemia, may occur when corticosteroids and thiazide diuretics are administered concurrently). Products include:

Prednisolone Sodium Phosphate (Intensified electrolyte depletion, particularly hypokalemia, may occur when corticosteroids and thiazide diuretics are administered concurrently).
No products indexed under this heading.

Prednisolone Tebutate (Intensified electrolyte depletion, particularly hypokalemia, may occur when corticosteroids and thiazide diuretics are administered concurrently).
No products indexed under this heading.

Prednisone (Intensified electrolyte depletion, particularly hypokalemia, may occur when corticosteroids and thiazide diuretics are administered concurrently).
No products indexed under this heading.

Prednisone sodium phosphate (Intensified electrolyte depletion, particularly hypokalemia, may occur when corticosteroids and thiazide diuretics are administered concurrently).
No products indexed under this heading.

Propoxyphene Hydrochloride (Potentiation of orthostatic hypotension may occur when narcotics and thiazide diuretics are administered concurrently).
No products indexed under this heading.

Propoxyphene Napsylate (Potentiation of orthostatic hypotension may occur when narcotics and thiazide diuretics are administered concurrently).
No products indexed under this heading.

Propranolol Hydrochloride (Additive effect or potentiation may occur when other hypertensive drugs and thiazide diuretics are administered concurrently). Products include:

Quinapril Hydrochloride (Additive effect or potentiation may occur when other hypertensive drugs and thiazide diuretics are administered concurrently).
No products indexed under this heading.

Ramipril (Additive effect or potentiation may occur when other hypertensive drugs and thiazide diuretics are administered concurrently).
No products indexed under this heading.

Rapacuronium Bromide (Possible increased responsiveness to the muscle relaxant may occur when skeletal muscle relaxants and thiazide diuretics are administered concurrently).
No products indexed under this heading.

Rauwolfia Serpentina (Additive effect or potentiation may occur when other hypertensive drugs and thiazide diuretics are administered concurrently).
No products indexed under this heading.

Remifentanil Hydrochloride (Potentiation of orthostatic hypotension may occur when narcotics and thiazide diuretics are administered concurrently).
No products indexed under this heading.

Repaglinide (Dosage adjustment of the antidiabetic drug may be required when antidiabetic drugs (oral agents) and thiazide diuretics are administered concurrently).
No products indexed under this heading.

Rescinnamine (Additive effect or potentiation may occur when other hypertensive drugs and thiazide diuretics are administered concurrently).
No products indexed under this heading.

Reserpine (Additive effect or potentiation may occur when other hypertensive drugs and thiazide diuretics are administered concurrently).
No products indexed under this heading.

Rocuronium Bromide (Possible increased responsiveness to the muscle relaxant may occur when skeletal muscle relaxants and thiazide diuretics are administered concurrently). Products include:

Rofecoxib (In some patients, the administration of a non-steroidal antiinflammatory agent can reduce the diuretic, natriuretic, and antihypertensive effects of loop, potassium-sparing and thiazide diuretics).
No products indexed under this heading.

Rosiglitazone Maleate (Dosage adjustment of the antidiabetic drug may be required when antidiabetic drugs (oral agents) and thiazide diuretics are administered concurrently). Products include:

Secobarbital Sodium (Potentiation of orthostatic hypotension may occur when barbiturates and thiazide diuretics are administered concurrently).
No products indexed under this heading.

Sildenafil Citrate (A single 100 mg dose of sildenafil in subjects with essential hypertension had no effect on the pharmacokinetic parameters of amlodipine. When amlodipine and sildenafil were used in combination, each agent independently exerted its own blood pressure lowering effect).
No products indexed under this heading.

Sitagliptin Phosphate (Dosage adjustment of the antidiabetic drug may

be required when antidiabetic drugs (oral agents) and thiazide diuretics are administered concurrently). Products include:

Sodium Butabarbital (Potentiation of orthostatic hypotension may occur when barbiturates and thiazide diuretics are administered concurrently).
No products indexed under this heading.

Sodium Nitroprusside (Additive effect or potentiation may occur when other hypertensive drugs and thiazide diuretics are administered concurrently).
No products indexed under this heading.

Sodium Pentobarbital (Potentiation of orthostatic hypotension may occur when barbiturates and thiazide diuretics are administered concurrently).
No products indexed under this heading.

Sotalol Hydrochloride (Additive effect or potentiation may occur when other hypertensive drugs and thiazide diuretics are administered concurrently).
No products indexed under this heading.

Spirapril Hydrochloride (Additive effect or potentiation may occur when other hypertensive drugs and thiazide diuretics are administered concurrently).
No products indexed under this heading.

Spironolactone (As with other drugs that block angiotensin II or its effects, concomitant use of potassium sparing diuretics (eg, spironolactone, triamterene, amiloride), potassium supplements, or salt substitutes containing potassium may lead to increases in serum potassium and in heart failure patients to increases in serum creatinine).
No products indexed under this heading.

Succinylcholine Chloride (Possible increased responsiveness to the muscle relaxant may occur when skeletal muscle relaxants and thiazide diuretics are administered concurrently).
No products indexed under this heading.

Sufentanil Citrate (Potentiation of orthostatic hypotension may occur when narcotics and thiazide diuretics are administered concurrently).
No products indexed under this heading.

Sulindac (In some patients, the administration of a non-steroidal antiinflammatory agent can reduce the diuretic, natriuretic, and antihypertensive effects of loop, potassium-sparing and thiazide diuretics). Products include:

Telmisartan (Additive effect or potentiation may occur when other hypertensive drugs and thiazide diuretics are administered concurrently). Products include:

Terazosin Hydrochloride (Additive effect or potentiation may occur when other hypertensive drugs and thiazide diuretics are administered concurrently).
No products indexed under this heading.

Thiamylal Sodium (Potentiation of orthostatic hypotension may occur when barbiturates and thiazide diuretics are administered concurrently).
No products indexed under this heading.

Timolol Maleate (Additive effect or potentiation may occur when other hypertensive drugs and thiazide diuretics are administered concurrently). Products include:

Tizanidine (Possible increased responsiveness to the muscle relaxant may occur when skeletal muscle relaxants and thiazide diuretics are administered concurrently).
No products indexed under this heading.

Tizanidine Hydrochloride (Possible increased responsiveness to the muscle relaxant may occur when skeletal muscle relaxants and thiazide diuretics are administered concurrently).
No products indexed under this heading.

Tolazamide (Dosage adjustment of the antidiabetic drug may be required when antidiabetic drugs (oral agents) and thiazide diuretics are administered concurrently).
No products indexed under this heading.

Tolbutamide (Dosage adjustment of the antidiabetic drug may be required when antidiabetic drugs (oral agents) and thiazide diuretics are administered concurrently).
No products indexed under this heading.

Tolmetin Sodium (In some patients, the administration of a non-steroidal antiinflammatory agent can reduce the diuretic, natriuretic, and antihypertensive effects of loop, potassium-sparing and thiazide diuretics).
No products indexed under this heading.

Torsemide (Additive effect or potentiation may occur when other hypertensive drugs and thiazide diuretics are administered concurrently).
No products indexed under this heading.

Trandolapril (Additive effect or potentiation may occur when other hypertensive drugs and thiazide diuretics are administered concurrently). Products include:

Triamcinolone (Intensified electrolyte depletion, particularly hypokalemia, may occur when corticosteroids and thiazide diuretics are administered concurrently).
No products indexed under this heading.

Triamcinolone Acetonide (Intensified electrolyte depletion, particularly hypokalemia, may occur when corticosteroids and thiazide diuretics are administered concurrently). Products include:

Triamcinolone Diacetate (Intensified electrolyte depletion, particularly hypokalemia, may occur when corticosteroids and thiazide diuretics are administered concurrently).
No products indexed under this heading.

Triamcinolone Hexacetonide (Intensified electrolyte depletion, particularly hypokalemia, may occur when corticosteroids and thiazide diuretics are administered concurrently).
No products indexed under this heading.

Triamterene (As with other drugs that block angiotensin II or its effects, concomitant use of potassium sparing diuretics (eg, spironolactone, triamterene, amiloride), potassium supplements, or salt substitutes containing potassium may lead to increases in serum potassium and in heart failure patients to increases in serum creatinine). Products include:

Trimethaphan Camsylate (Additive effect or potentiation may occur when other hypertensive drugs and thiazide diuretics are administered concurrently).
No products indexed under this heading.

Troglitazone (Dosage adjustment of the antidiabetic drug may be required when antidiabetic drugs (oral agents) and thiazide diuretics are administered concurrently).
No products indexed under this heading.

Tubocurarine Chloride (Possible increased responsiveness to the muscle relaxant may occur when skeletal muscle relaxants and thiazide diuretics are administered concurrently).
No products indexed under this heading.

Valdecoxib (In some patients, the administration of a non-steroidal antiinflammatory agent can reduce the diuretic, natriuretic, and antihypertensive effects of loop, potassium-sparing and thiazide diuretics).
No products indexed under this heading.

Vecuronium Bromide (Possible increased responsiveness to the muscle relaxant may occur when skeletal muscle relaxants and thiazide diuretics are administered concurrently).
No products indexed under this heading.

Verapamil Hydrochloride (Additive effect or potentiation may occur when other hypertensive drugs and thiazide diuretics are administered concurrently). Products include:

Food Interactions

Alcohol (Potentiation of orthostatic hypotension may occur when alcohol and thiazide diuretics are administered concurrently).

Beer, reduced-alcohol (Potentiation of orthostatic hypotension may occur when alcohol and thiazide diuretics are administered concurrently).

Beer, unspecified (Potentiation of orthostatic hypotension may occur when alcohol and thiazide diuretics are administered concurrently).

Wine, Chianti (Potentiation of orthostatic hypotension may occur when alcohol and thiazide diuretics are administered concurrently).

Wine, Red (Potentiation of orthostatic hypotension may occur when alcohol and thiazide diuretics are administered concurrently).

Wine, unspecified (Potentiation of orthostatic hypotension may occur when alcohol and thiazide diuretics are administered concurrently).

Wine products (Potentiation of orthostatic hypotension may occur when alcohol and thiazide diuretics are administered concurrently).

EXJADE TABLETS

May interact with antacids containing aluminum, calcium and magnesium, anticoagulants, bisphosphonates, corticosteroids, cytochrome p450 1a2 substrates (selected), cytochrome p450 2a6 substrates (selected), cytochrome p450 2c19 substrates (selected), cytochrome p450 2c8 substrates (selected), cytochrome p450 2d6 substrates (selected), cytochrome p450 3a4 substrates (selected), non-steroidal anti-inflammatory agents, oral contraceptives, phenytoin, UDP-glucuronosyltransferase (UGT) inducers (selected), and certain other agents. Compounds in these categories include:

Acetaminophen (Deferasirox inhibits human CYP1A2 in vitro). Products include:

Alatrofloxacin Mesylate (Deferasirox inhibits human CYP1A2 in vitro).
No products indexed under this heading.

Alclometasone Dipropionate (Caution should be observed when administering deferasirox in combination with drugs that have ulcerogenic or hemorrhagic potential, such as corticosteroids).
No products indexed under this heading.

Alendronate Sodium (Caution should be observed when administering deferasirox in combination with drugs that have ulcerogenic or hemorrhagic potential, such as oral bisphosphonates). Products include:

Alfentanil Hydrochloride (Concomitant administration of deferasirox and midazolam (a CYP3A4 probe substrate) resulted in a decrease of midazolam peak concentration by 23% and exposure by 17%. In the clinical setting, this effect may be more pronounced. Therefore, due to a possible decrease in CYP3A4 substrate concentration and potential loss of effectiveness, caution should be observed when deferasirox is administered with drugs metabolized by CYP3A4 (eg, cyclosporine, simvastatin, hormonal contraceptives)).
No products indexed under this heading.

Alprazolam (Concomitant administration of deferasirox and midazolam (a CYP3A4 probe substrate) resulted in a decrease of midazolam peak concentration by 23% and exposure by 17%. In the clinical setting, this effect may be more pronounced. Therefore, due to a possible decrease in CYP3A4 substrate concentration and potential loss of effectiveness, caution should be observed when deferasirox is administered with drugs metabolized by CYP3A4 (eg, cyclosporine, simvastatin, hormonal contraceptives)).
No products indexed under this heading.

Aluminum Carbonate (Although deferasirox has a lower affinity for aluminum than for iron, deferasirox should not be administered with aluminum-containing antacid preparations).
No products indexed under this heading.

Aluminum Hydroxide (Although deferasirox has a lower affinity for aluminum than for iron, deferasirox should not be administered with aluminum-containing antacid preparations).
No products indexed under this heading.

Aminophylline (Deferasirox inhibits human CYP1A2 in vitro).
No products indexed under this heading.

Amiodarone Hydrochloride (Concomitant administration of deferasirox and midazolam (a CYP3A4 probe substrate) resulted in a decrease of midazolam peak concentration by 23% and exposure by 17%. In the clinical setting, this effect may be more pronounced. Therefore, due to a possible decrease in CYP3A4 substrate concentration and potential loss of effectiveness, caution should be observed when deferasirox is administered with drugs metabolized by CYP3A4 (eg, cyclosporine, simvastatin, hormonal contraceptives)).
No products indexed under this heading.

Amitriptyline Hydrochloride (Concomitant administration of deferasirox and midazolam (a CYP3A4 probe substrate) resulted in a decrease of midazolam peak concentration by 23% and exposure by 17%. In the clinical setting, this effect may be more pronounced. Therefore, due to a possible decrease in CYP3A4 substrate concentration and potential loss of effectiveness, caution should be observed when deferasirox is administered with drugs metabolized by CYP3A4 (eg, cyclosporine, simvastatin, hormonal contraceptives)).
No products indexed under this heading.

Amlodipine Besylate (Concomitant administration of deferasirox and midazolam (a CYP3A4 probe substrate) resulted in a decrease of midazolam peak concentration by 23% and exposure by 17%. In the clinical setting, this effect may be more pronounced. Therefore, due to a possible decrease in CYP3A4 substrate concentration and potential loss of effectiveness, caution should be observed when deferasirox is administered with drugs metabolized by CYP3A4 (eg, cyclosporine, simvastatin, hormonal contraceptives)). Products include:
Azor 1010
Exforge 2443
Exforge HCT 2449

Amoxapine (Concomitant administration of deferasirox and the CYP2C8 probe substrate repaglinide (single dose of 0.5 mg) resulted in an increase in repaglinide systemic exposure (AUC) to 2.3 fold of control and an increase in C_{max} of 62%. If deferasirox and repaglinide are used concomitantly, decreasing the dose of repaglinide should be considered and careful monitoring of blood glucose levels should be performed. Caution should be exercised when deferasirox and other CYP2C8 substrates like paclitaxel are co-administered).
No products indexed under this heading.

Amphetamine Aspartate (Deferasirox inhibits human CYP2D6 *in vitro*).
No products indexed under this heading.

Amphetamine Aspartate Monohydrate (Deferasirox inhibits human CYP2D6 *in vitro*).
No products indexed under this heading.

Amphetamine Sulfate (Deferasirox inhibits human CYP2D6 *in vitro*).
No products indexed under this heading.

Anagrelide Hydrochloride (Deferasirox inhibits human CYP1A2 *in vitro*).
No products indexed under this heading.

Anisindione (Caution should be observed when administering deferasirox in combination with drugs that have ulcerogenic or hemorrhagic potential, such as anticoagulants).
No products indexed under this heading.

Aprepitant (Concomitant administration of deferasirox and midazolam (a CYP3A4 probe substrate) resulted in a decrease of midazolam peak concentration by 23% and exposure by 17%. In the clinical setting, this effect may be more pronounced. Therefore, due to a possible decrease in CYP3A4 substrate concentration and potential loss of effectiveness, caution should be observed when deferasirox is administered with drugs metabolized by CYP3A4 (eg, cyclosporine, simvastatin, hormonal contraceptives)). Products include:
Emend 2124

Ardeparin Sodium (Caution should be observed when administering deferasirox in combination with drugs that have ulcerogenic or hemorrhagic potential, such as anticoagulants).
No products indexed under this heading.

Astemizole (Concomitant administration of deferasirox and midazolam (a CYP3A4 probe substrate) resulted in a decrease of midazolam peak concentration by 23% and exposure by 17%. In the clinical setting, this effect may be more pronounced. Therefore, due to a possible decrease in CYP3A4 substrate concentration and potential loss of effectiveness, caution should be observed when deferasirox is administered with drugs metabolized by CYP3A4 (eg, cyclosporine, simvastatin, hormonal contraceptives)).
No products indexed under this heading.

Atomoxetine Hydrochloride (Deferasirox inhibits human CYP2D6 *in vitro*). Products include:
Strattera 1957

Atorvastatin Calcium (Concomitant administration of deferasirox and midazolam (a CYP3A4 probe substrate) resulted in a decrease of midazolam peak concentration by 23% and exposure by 17%. In the clinical setting, this effect may be more pronounced. Therefore, due to a possible decrease in CYP3A4 substrate concentration and potential loss of effectiveness, caution should be observed when deferasirox is administered with drugs metabolized by CYP3A4 (eg, cyclosporine, simvastatin, hormonal contraceptives)). Products include:
Lipitor 2703

Beclomethasone Dipropionate (Caution should be observed when administering deferasirox in combination with drugs that have ulcerogenic or hemorrhagic potential, such as corticosteroids). Products include:
Qvar 3398

Beclomethasone Dipropionate Monohydrate (Caution should be observed when administering deferasirox in combination with drugs that have ulcerogenic or hemorrhagic potential, such as corticosteroids). Products include:
Beconase AQ 1386

Belladonna Ergotamine (Concomitant administration of deferasirox and midazolam (a CYP3A4 probe substrate) resulted in a decrease of midazolam peak concentration by 23% and exposure by 17%. In the clinical setting, this effect may be more pronounced. Therefore, due to a possible decrease in CYP3A4 substrate concentration and potential loss of effectiveness, caution should be observed when deferasirox is administered with drugs metabolized by CYP3A4 (eg, cyclosporine, simvastatin, hormonal contraceptives)).
No products indexed under this heading.

Benzphetamine Hydrochloride (Concomitant administration of deferasirox and the CYP2C8 probe substrate repaglinide (single dose of 0.5 mg) resulted in an increase in repaglinide systemic exposure (AUC) to 2.3 fold of control and an increase in C_{max} of 62%. If deferasirox and repaglinide are used concomitantly, decreasing the dose of repaglinide should be considered and careful monitoring of blood glucose levels should be performed. Caution should be exercised when deferasirox and other CYP2C8 substrates like paclitaxel are co-administered).
No products indexed under this heading.

Betamethasone (Caution should be observed when administering deferasirox in combination with drugs that have ulcerogenic or hemorrhagic potential, such as corticosteroids).
No products indexed under this heading.

Betamethasone Acetate (Caution should be observed when administering deferasirox in combination with drugs that have ulcerogenic or hemorrhagic potential, such as corticosteroids).
No products indexed under this heading.

Betamethasone Benzoate (Caution should be observed when administering deferasirox in combination with drugs that have ulcerogenic or hemorrhagic potential, such as corticosteroids).
No products indexed under this heading.

Betamethasone Dipropionate (Caution should be observed when administering deferasirox in combination with drugs that have ulcerogenic or hemorrhagic potential, such as corticosteroids). Products include:
Diprolene Lotion 0.05% 3108
Diprolene Ointment 0.05% 3109
Diprolene AF Cream 0.05% 3107
Lotrisone 3163

Betamethasone Sodium Phosphate (Caution should be observed when administering deferasirox in combination with drugs that have ulcerogenic or hemorrhagic potential, such as corticosteroids).
No products indexed under this heading.

Betamethasone Valerate (Caution should be observed when administering deferasirox in combination with drugs that have ulcerogenic or hemorrhagic potential, such as corticosteroids). Products include:
Luxíq 3321

Bisoprolol Fumarate (Deferasirox inhibits human CYP2D6 *in vitro*).
No products indexed under this heading.

Budesonide (Caution should be observed when administering deferasirox in combination with drugs that have ulcerogenic or hemorrhagic potential, such as corticosteroids). Products include:
Pulmicort Flexhaler 714
Symbicort 80/4.5 720
Symbicort 160/4.5 720

Buspirone Hydrochloride (Concomitant administration of deferasirox and midazolam (a CYP3A4 probe substrate) resulted in a decrease of midazolam peak concentration by 23% and exposure by 17%. In the clinical setting, this effect may be more pronounced. Therefore, due to a possible decrease in CYP3A4 substrate concentration and potential loss of effectiveness, caution should be observed when deferasirox is administered with drugs metabolized by CYP3A4 (eg, cyclosporine, simvastatin, hormonal contraceptives)).
No products indexed under this heading.

Busulfan (Concomitant administration of deferasirox and midazolam (a CYP3A4 probe substrate) resulted in a decrease of midazolam peak concentration by 23% and exposure by 17%. In the clinical setting, this effect may be more pronounced. Therefore, due to a possible decrease in CYP3A4 substrate concentration and potential loss of effectiveness, caution should be observed when deferasirox is administered with drugs metabolized by CYP3A4 (eg, cyclosporine, simvastatin, hormonal contraceptives)). Products include:
Myleran 1581

Caffeine (Deferasirox inhibits human CYP1A2 *in vitro*).
No products indexed under this heading.

Caffeine Anhydrous (Deferasirox inhibits human CYP1A2 *in vitro*).
No products indexed under this heading.

Caffeine Citrate (Deferasirox inhibits human CYP1A2 *in vitro*).
No products indexed under this heading.

Caffeine-containing medications (Deferasirox inhibits human CYP1A2 *in vitro*).
No products indexed under this heading.

Caffeine Sodium Benzoate (Deferasirox inhibits human CYP1A2 *in vitro*).
No products indexed under this heading.

Calcium Carbonate (Although deferasirox has a lower affinity for aluminum than for iron, deferasirox should not be administered with aluminum-containing antacid preparations). Products include:
Chelated Mineral 3476
Pepcid Complete 1822
Extra Strength Rolaids Softchews
Vanilla Creme 2045

Captopril (Deferasirox inhibits human CYP2D6 *in vitro*). Products include:
Captopril 2341

Carbamazepine (Concomitant administration of deferasirox and midazolam (a CYP3A4 probe substrate) resulted in a decrease of midazolam peak concentration by 23% and exposure by 17%. In the clinical setting, this effect may be more pronounced. Therefore, due to a possible decrease in CYP3A4 substrate concentration and potential loss of effectiveness, caution should be observed when deferasirox is administered with drugs metabolized by CYP3A4 (eg, cyclosporine, simvastatin, hormonal contraceptives)). Products include:
Carbatrol 3280
Equetro 3477

Carisoprodol (Deferasirox inhibits human CYP2C19 *in vitro*).
No products indexed under this heading.

Carvedilol (Deferasirox inhibits human CYP2D6 *in vitro*). Products include:
Coreg 1409

Celecoxib (Caution should be observed when administering deferasirox in combination with drugs that have ulcerogenic or hemorrhagic potential, such as non-steroidal anti-inflammatory drugs). Products include:
Celebrex 3272

Cerivastatin Sodium (Concomitant administration of deferasirox and midazolam (a CYP3A4 probe substrate) resulted in a decrease of midazolam peak concentration by 23% and exposure by 17%. In the clinical setting, this effect may be more pronounced. Therefore, due to a possible decrease in CYP3A4 substrate concentration and potential loss of effectiveness, caution should be observed when deferasirox is administered with drugs metabolized by CYP3A4 (eg, cyclosporine, simvastatin, hormonal contraceptives)).
No products indexed under this heading.

Cevimeline Hydrochloride (Deferasirox inhibits human CYP2D6 *in vitro*). Products include:
Evoxac 1027

Chlordiazepoxide (Deferasirox inhibits human CYP1A2 *in vitro*).
No products indexed under this heading.

Chlordiazepoxide Hydrochloride (Deferasirox inhibits human CYP1A2 *in vitro*).
No products indexed under this heading.

Chlorpheniramine (Concomitant administration of deferasirox and midazolam (a CYP3A4 probe substrate) resulted in a decrease of midazolam peak concentration by 23% and exposure by 17%. In the clinical setting, this effect may be more pronounced. Therefore, due to a possible decrease in CYP3A4 substrate concentration and potential loss of effectiveness, caution should be observed when deferasirox is administered with drugs metabolized by CYP3A4 (eg, cyclosporine, simvastatin, hormonal contraceptives)).
No products indexed under this heading.

Chlorpheniramine Maleate (Concomitant administration of deferasirox and midazolam (a CYP3A4 probe substrate) resulted in a decrease of midazolam peak concentration by 23% and exposure by 17%. In the clinical setting, this effect may be more pronounced. Therefore, due to a possible decrease in CYP3A4 substrate concentration and potential loss of effectiveness, caution

IMPORTANT NOTE: Always consult each drug listing in the patient's regimen for possible interactions.

631 **Interactions Index** **Exjade**

peak concentration by 23% and exposure by 17%. In the clinical setting, this effect may be more pronounced. Therefore, due to a possible decrease in CYP3A4 substrate concentration and potential loss of effectiveness, caution should be observed when deferasirox is administered with drugs metabolized by CYP3A4 (eg, cyclosporine, simvastatin, hormonal contraceptives)). Products include:

Cardizem LA 423

Diltiazem Maleate (Concomitant administration of deferasirox and midazolam (a CYP3A4 probe substrate) resulted in a decrease of midazolam peak concentration by 23% and exposure by 17%. In the clinical setting, this effect may be more pronounced. Therefore, due to a possible decrease in CYP3A4 substrate concentration and potential loss of effectiveness, caution should be observed when deferasirox is administered with drugs metabolized by CYP3A4 (eg, cyclosporine, simvastatin, hormonal contraceptives)).
No products indexed under this heading.

Disopyramide (Concomitant administration of deferasirox and midazolam (a CYP3A4 probe substrate) resulted in a decrease of midazolam peak concentration by 23% and exposure by 17%. In the clinical setting, this effect may be more pronounced. Therefore, due to a possible decrease in CYP3A4 substrate concentration and potential loss of effectiveness, caution should be observed when deferasirox is administered with drugs metabolized by CYP3A4 (eg, cyclosporine, simvastatin, hormonal contraceptives)).
No products indexed under this heading.

Disopyramide Phosphate (Concomitant administration of deferasirox and midazolam (a CYP3A4 probe substrate) resulted in a decrease of midazolam peak concentration by 23% and exposure by 17%. In the clinical setting, this effect may be more pronounced. Therefore, due to a possible decrease in CYP3A4 substrate concentration and potential loss of effectiveness, caution should be observed when deferasirox is administered with drugs metabolized by CYP3A4 (eg, cyclosporine, simvastatin, hormonal contraceptives)).
No products indexed under this heading.

Disulfiram (Concomitant administration of deferasirox and midazolam (a CYP3A4 probe substrate) resulted in a decrease of midazolam peak concentration by 23% and exposure by 17%. In the clinical setting, this effect may be more pronounced. Therefore, due to a possible decrease in CYP3A4 substrate concentration and potential loss of effectiveness, caution should be observed when deferasirox is administered with drugs metabolized by CYP3A4 (eg, cyclosporine, simvastatin, hormonal contraceptives)).
No products indexed under this heading.

Divalproex Sodium (Deferasirox inhibits human CYP2C19 *in vitro*). Products include:

Depakote ER 426

Docetaxel (Concomitant administration of deferasirox and the CYP2C8 probe substrate repaglinide (single dose of 0.5 mg) resulted in an increase in repaglinide systemic exposure (AUC) to 2.3 fold of control and an increase in C_{max} of 62%. If deferasirox and repaglinide are used concomitantly, decreasing the dose of repaglinide should be considered and careful monitoring of blood glucose levels should be performed. Caution should be exercised when deferasirox and other CYP2C8 substrates like paclitaxel are co-administered). Products include:

Taxotere 3035

Dolasetron Mesylate (Deferasirox inhibits human CYP2D6 *in vitro*). Products include:

Anzemet Injection 2931
Anzemet Tablets 2934

Donepezil Hydrochloride (Deferasirox inhibits human CYP2D6 *in vitro*). Products include:

Aricept 1045
Aricept ODT 1045

Doxepin Hydrochloride (Concomitant administration of deferasirox and the CYP2C8 probe substrate repaglinide (single dose of 0.5 mg) resulted in an increase in repaglinide systemic exposure (AUC) to 2.3 fold of control and an increase in C_{max} of 62%. If deferasirox and repaglinide are used concomitantly, decreasing the dose of repaglinide should be considered and careful monitoring of blood glucose levels should be performed. Caution should be exercised when deferasirox and other CYP2C8 substrates like paclitaxel are co-administered).
No products indexed under this heading.

Doxorubicin Hydrochloride (Concomitant administration of deferasirox and midazolam (a CYP3A4 probe substrate) resulted in a decrease of midazolam peak concentration by 23% and exposure by 17%. In the clinical setting, this effect may be more pronounced. Therefore, due to a possible decrease in CYP3A4 substrate concentration and potential loss of effectiveness, caution should be observed when deferasirox is administered with drugs metabolized by CYP3A4 (eg, cyclosporine, simvastatin, hormonal contraceptives)).
No products indexed under this heading.

Dronabinol (Concomitant administration of deferasirox and midazolam (a CYP3A4 probe substrate) resulted in a decrease of midazolam peak concentration by 23% and exposure by 17%. In the clinical setting, this effect may be more pronounced. Therefore, due to a possible decrease in CYP3A4 substrate concentration and potential loss of effectiveness, caution should be observed when deferasirox is administered with drugs metabolized by CYP3A4 (eg, cyclosporine, simvastatin, hormonal contraceptives)).
No products indexed under this heading.

Encainide Hydrochloride (Deferasirox inhibits human CYP2D6 *in vitro*).
No products indexed under this heading.

Enoxacin (Deferasirox inhibits human CYP1A2 *in vitro*).
No products indexed under this heading.

Enoxaparin Sodium (Caution should be observed when administering deferasirox in combination with drugs that have ulcerogenic or hemorrhagic potential, such as anticoagulants). Products include:

Lovenox 3005

Ergotamine Tartrate (Concomitant administration of deferasirox and midazolam (a CYP3A4 probe substrate) resulted in a decrease of midazolam peak concentration by 23% and exposure by 17%. In the clinical setting, this effect may be more pronounced. Therefore, due to a possible decrease in CYP3A4 substrate concentration and potential loss of effectiveness, caution should be observed when deferasirox is administered with drugs metabolized by CYP3A4 (eg, cyclosporine, simvastatin, hormonal contraceptives)).
No products indexed under this heading.

Erythromycin (Concomitant administration of deferasirox and midazolam (a CYP3A4 probe substrate) resulted in a decrease of midazolam peak concentration by 23% and exposure by 17%. In the clinical setting, this effect may be more pronounced. Therefore, due to a possible decrease in CYP3A4 substrate concentration and potential loss of effectiveness, caution should be observed when deferasirox is administered with drugs metabolized by CYP3A4 (eg, cyclosporine, simvastatin, hormonal contraceptives)).
No products indexed under this heading.

Erythromycin Estolate (Concomitant administration of deferasirox and midazolam (a CYP3A4 probe substrate) resulted in a decrease of midazolam peak concentration by 23% and exposure by 17%. In the clinical setting, this effect may be more pronounced. Therefore, due to a possible decrease in CYP3A4 substrate concentration and potential loss of effectiveness, caution should be observed when deferasirox is administered with drugs metabolized by CYP3A4 (eg, cyclosporine, simvastatin, hormonal contraceptives)).
No products indexed under this heading.

Erythromycin Ethylsuccinate (Concomitant administration of deferasirox and midazolam (a CYP3A4 probe substrate) resulted in a decrease of midazolam peak concentration by 23% and exposure by 17%. In the clinical setting, this effect may be more pronounced. Therefore, due to a possible decrease in CYP3A4 substrate concentration and potential loss of effectiveness, caution should be observed when deferasirox is administered with drugs metabolized by CYP3A4 (eg, cyclosporine, simvastatin, hormonal contraceptives)). Products include:

E.E.S. 437
EryPed 435

Erythromycin Gluceptate (Concomitant administration of deferasirox and midazolam (a CYP3A4 probe substrate) resulted in a decrease of midazolam peak concentration by 23% and exposure by 17%. In the clinical setting, this effect may be more pronounced. Therefore, due to a possible decrease in CYP3A4 substrate concentration and potential loss of effectiveness, caution should be observed when deferasirox is administered with drugs metabolized by CYP3A4 (eg, cyclosporine, simvastatin, hormonal contraceptives)).
No products indexed under this heading.

Erythromycin Lactobionate (Concomitant administration of deferasirox and midazolam (a CYP3A4 probe substrate) resulted in a decrease of midazolam peak concentration by 23% and exposure by 17%. In the clinical setting, this effect may be more pronounced. Therefore, due to a possible decrease in CYP3A4 substrate concentration and potential loss of effectiveness, caution should be observed when deferasirox is administered with drugs metabolized by CYP3A4 (eg, cyclosporine, simvastatin, hormonal contraceptives)).
No products indexed under this heading.

Erythromycin Stearate (Concomitant administration of deferasirox and midazolam (a CYP3A4 probe substrate) resulted in a decrease of midazolam peak concentration by 23% and exposure by 17%. In the clinical setting, this effect may be more pronounced. Therefore, due to a possible decrease in CYP3A4 substrate concentration and potential loss of effectiveness, caution should be observed when deferasirox is administered with drugs metabolized by CYP3A4 (eg, cyclosporine, simvastatin, hormonal contraceptives)).
No products indexed under this heading.

Esomeprazole Magnesium (Deferasirox inhibits human CYP2C19 *in vitro*). Products include:

Nexium Capsules 704
Nexium Oral Suspension 704

Esomeprazole Sodium (Deferasirox inhibits human CYP2C19 *in vitro*). Products include:

Nexium I.V. 712

Estradiol (Concomitant administration of deferasirox and midazolam (a CYP3A4 probe substrate) resulted in a decrease of midazolam peak concentration by 23% and exposure by 17%. In the clinical setting, this effect may be more pronounced. Therefore, due to a possible decrease in CYP3A4 substrate concentration and potential loss of effectiveness, caution should be observed when deferasirox is administered with drugs metabolized by CYP3A4 (eg, cyclosporine, simvastatin, hormonal contraceptives)). Products include:

Activella 2561
Angeliq 831
Climara 841
Climara Pro 847
Divigel 3467
Estrasorb 1777
Vagifem 2589

Estradiol Benzoate (Concomitant administration of deferasirox and midazolam (a CYP3A4 probe substrate) resulted in a decrease of midazolam peak concentration by 23% and exposure by 17%. In the clinical setting, this effect may be more pronounced. Therefore, due to a possible decrease in CYP3A4 substrate concentration and potential loss of effectiveness, caution should be observed when deferasirox is administered with drugs metabolized by CYP3A4 (eg, cyclosporine, simvastatin, hormonal contraceptives)).
No products indexed under this heading.

Estradiol Cypionate (Concomitant administration of deferasirox and midazolam (a CYP3A4 probe substrate) resulted in a decrease of midazolam peak concentration by 23% and exposure by 17%. In the clinical setting, this effect may be more pronounced. Therefore, due to a possible decrease in CYP3A4 substrate concentration and potential loss of effectiveness, caution should be observed when deferasirox is administered with drugs metabolized by CYP3A4 (eg, cyclosporine, simvastatin, hormonal contraceptives)).
No products indexed under this heading.

Estradiol Valerate (Concomitant administration of deferasirox and midazolam (a CYP3A4 probe substrate) resulted in a decrease of midazolam peak concentration by 23% and exposure by 17%. In the clinical setting, this effect may be more pronounced. Therefore, due to a possible decrease in CYP3A4 substrate concentration and potential loss of effectiveness, caution should be observed when deferasirox is administered with drugs metabolized by CYP3A4 (eg, cyclosporine, simvastatin, hormonal contraceptives)).
No products indexed under this heading.

Ethinyl Estradiol (Concomitant administration of deferasirox and midazolam (a CYP3A4 probe substrate) resulted in a decrease of midazolam peak concentration by 23% and exposure by 17%. In the clinical setting, this effect may be more pronounced. Therefore, due to a possible decrease in CYP3A4 substrate concentration and potential loss of effectiveness, caution should be observed when deferasirox is administered with drugs metabolized by CYP3A4 (eg, cyclosporine, simvastatin, hormonal contraceptives)). Products include:

LoSeasonique 3407
Lybrel 3514
NuvaRing 3181
Ortho Evra 2648
Ortho-Cyclen/Ortho Tri-Cyclen 2663
Ortho Tri-Cyclen Lo Tablets 2673
Seasonique 3418
Yaz 864

Ethosuximide (Concomitant administration of deferasirox and midazolam (a

CYP3A4 probe substrate) resulted in a decrease of midazolam peak concentration by 23% and exposure by 17%. In the clinical setting, this effect may be more pronounced. Therefore, due to a possible decrease in CYP3A4 substrate concentration and potential loss of effectiveness, caution should be observed when deferasirox is administered with drugs metabolized by CYP3A4 (eg, cyclosporine, simvastatin, hormonal contraceptives)).

No products indexed under this heading.

Ethotoin (Deferasirox inhibits human CYP2C19 in vitro).

No products indexed under this heading.

Ethynodiol Diacetate (Concomitant administration of deferasirox and midazolam (a CYP3A4 probe substrate) resulted in a decrease of midazolam peak concentration by 23% and exposure by 17%. In the clinical setting, this effect may be more pronounced. Therefore, due to a possible decrease in CYP3A4 substrate concentration and potential loss of effectiveness, caution should be observed when deferasirox is administered with drugs metabolized by CYP3A4 (eg, cyclosporine, simvastatin, hormonal contraceptives)).

No products indexed under this heading.

Etidronate Disodium (Caution should be observed when administering deferasirox in combination with drugs that have ulcerogenic or hemorrhagic potential, such as oral bisphosphonates).
Products include:
Didronel 2790

Etodolac (Caution should be observed when administering deferasirox in combination with drugs that have ulcerogenic or hemorrhagic potential, such as non-steroidal anti-inflammatory drugs).

No products indexed under this heading.

Etoposide (Concomitant administration of deferasirox and midazolam (a CYP3A4 probe substrate) resulted in a decrease of midazolam peak concentration by 23% and exposure by 17%. In the clinical setting, this effect may be more pronounced. Therefore, due to a possible decrease in CYP3A4 substrate concentration and potential loss of effectiveness, caution should be observed when deferasirox is administered with drugs metabolized by CYP3A4 (eg, cyclosporine, simvastatin, hormonal contraceptives)).

No products indexed under this heading.

Etoposide Phosphate (Concomitant administration of deferasirox and midazolam (a CYP3A4 probe substrate) resulted in a decrease of midazolam peak concentration by 23% and exposure by 17%. In the clinical setting, this effect may be more pronounced. Therefore, due to a possible decrease in CYP3A4 substrate concentration and potential loss of effectiveness, caution should be observed when deferasirox is administered with drugs metabolized by CYP3A4 (eg, cyclosporine, simvastatin, hormonal contraceptives)).

No products indexed under this heading.

Felbamate (Deferasirox inhibits human CYP2C19 in vitro).

No products indexed under this heading.

Felodipine (Concomitant administration of deferasirox and midazolam (a CYP3A4 probe substrate) resulted in a decrease of midazolam peak concentration by 23% and exposure by 17%. In the clinical setting, this effect may be more pronounced. Therefore, due to a possible decrease in CYP3A4 substrate concentration and potential loss of effectiveness, caution should be observed when deferasirox is administered with drugs metabolized by CYP3A4 (eg, cyclosporine, simvastatin, hormonal contraceptives)).

No products indexed under this heading.

Fenoprofen Calcium (Caution should be observed when administering deferasirox in combination with drugs that have ulcerogenic or hemorrhagic potential, such as non-steroidal anti-inflammatory drugs).

No products indexed under this heading.

Fentanyl (Concomitant administration of deferasirox and midazolam (a CYP3A4 probe substrate) resulted in a decrease of midazolam peak concentration by 23% and exposure by 17%. In the clinical setting, this effect may be more pronounced. Therefore, due to a possible decrease in CYP3A4 substrate concentration and potential loss of effectiveness, caution should be observed when deferasirox is administered with drugs metabolized by CYP3A4 (eg, cyclosporine, simvastatin, hormonal contraceptives)). Products include:
Duragesic 2604
Fentanyl Transdermal System 2346
Onsolis 2054

Fentanyl Citrate (Concomitant administration of deferasirox and midazolam (a CYP3A4 probe substrate) resulted in a decrease of midazolam peak concentration by 23% and exposure by 17%. In the clinical setting, this effect may be more pronounced. Therefore, due to a possible decrease in CYP3A4 substrate concentration and potential loss of effectiveness, caution should be observed when deferasirox is administered with drugs metabolized by CYP3A4 (eg, cyclosporine, simvastatin, hormonal contraceptives)). Products include:
Fentora 966

Flecainide Acetate (Deferasirox inhibits human CYP2D6 in vitro).

No products indexed under this heading.

Fludrocortisone Acetate (Caution should be observed when administering deferasirox in combination with drugs that have ulcerogenic or hemorrhagic potential, such as corticosteroids).

No products indexed under this heading.

Flumethasone Pivalate (Caution should be observed when administering deferasirox in combination with drugs that have ulcerogenic or hemorrhagic potential, such as corticosteroids).

No products indexed under this heading.

Flunisolide Hemihydrate (Caution should be observed when administering deferasirox in combination with drugs that have ulcerogenic or hemorrhagic potential, such as corticosteroids).

No products indexed under this heading.

Fluoxetine (Deferasirox inhibits human CYP2D6 in vitro).

No products indexed under this heading.

Fluoxetine Hydrochloride (Deferasirox inhibits human CYP2D6 in vitro). Products include:
Prozac Weekly 1941
Prozac Pulvules 1941
Symbyax 1965

Fluphenazine Decanoate (Deferasirox inhibits human CYP2D6 in vitro).

No products indexed under this heading.

Fluphenazine Enanthate (Deferasirox inhibits human CYP2D6 in vitro).

No products indexed under this heading.

Fluphenazine Hydrochloride (Deferasirox inhibits human CYP2D6 in vitro).

No products indexed under this heading.

Flurbiprofen (Caution should be observed when administering deferasirox in combination with drugs that have ulcerogenic or hemorrhagic potential, such as non-steroidal anti-inflammatory drugs).

No products indexed under this heading.

Flutamide (Deferasirox inhibits human CYP1A2 in vitro).

No products indexed under this heading.

Fluticasone Furoate (Caution should be observed when administering deferasirox in combination with drugs that have ulcerogenic or hemorrhagic potential, such as corticosteroids). Products include:
Veramyst 1713

Fluticasone Propionate (Caution should be observed when administering deferasirox in combination with drugs that have ulcerogenic or hemorrhagic potential, such as corticosteroids). Products include:
Advair 100/50 1275
Advair 250/50 1275
Advair 500/50 1275
Advair HFA 45/21 1288
Advair HFA 115/21 1288
Advair HFA 230/21 1288
Flonase 1459
Flovent Diskus 1463
Flovent HFA 1470

Fluvastatin Sodium (Concomitant administration of deferasirox and the CYP2C8 probe substrate repaglinide (single dose of 0.5 mg) resulted in an increase in repaglinide systemic exposure (AUC) to 2.3 fold of control and an increase in C_{max} of 62%. If deferasirox and repaglinide are used concomitantly, decreasing the dose of repaglinide should be considered and careful monitoring of blood glucose levels should be performed. Caution should be exercised when deferasirox and other CYP2C8 substrates like paclitaxel are co-administered).

No products indexed under this heading.

Fluvoxamine Maleate (Deferasirox inhibits human CYP2D6 in vitro).

No products indexed under this heading.

Fondaparinux Sodium (Caution should be observed when administering deferasirox in combination with drugs that have ulcerogenic or hemorrhagic potential, such as anticoagulants). Products include:
Arixtra 1320

Formoterol Fumarate (Deferasirox inhibits human CYP2D6 in vitro). Products include:
Foradil 3121
Perforomist 3634

Fosphenytoin (In a healthy volunteer study, the concomitant administration of deferasirox (single dose of 30 mg/kg) and the potent UDP-glucuronosyltransferase (UGT) inducer rifampicin (600 mg/day for 9 days) resulted in a decrease of deferasirox systemic exposure (AUC) by 44%. Concomitant use of deferasirox with potent UGT inducers (eg, rifampicin, phenytoin, phenobarbital, ritonavir) may result in a decrease of deferasirox. When used concomitantly, the dose of deferasirox should be increased and serum ferritin levels and clinical responses should be monitored for further dose modifications).

No products indexed under this heading.

Fosphenytoin Sodium (In a healthy volunteer study, the concomitant administration of deferasirox (single dose of 30 mg/kg) and the potent UDP-glucuronosyltransferase (UGT) inducer rifampicin (600 mg/day for 9 days) resulted in a decrease of deferasirox systemic exposure (AUC) by 44%. Concomitant use of deferasirox with potent UGT inducers (eg, rifampicin, phenytoin, phenobarbital, ritonavir) may result in a decrease of deferasirox. When used concomitantly, the dose of deferasirox should be increased and serum ferritin levels and clinical responses should be monitored for further dose modifications).

No products indexed under this heading.

Gabapentin (Deferasirox inhibits human CYP2C19 in vitro).

No products indexed under this heading.

Galantamine Hydrobromide (Deferasirox inhibits human CYP2D6 in vitro).

No products indexed under this heading.

Grepafloxacin Hydrochloride (Deferasirox inhibits human CYP1A2 in vitro).

No products indexed under this heading.

Haloperidol (Concomitant administration of deferasirox and midazolam (a CYP3A4 probe substrate) resulted in a decrease of midazolam peak concentration by 23% and exposure by 17%. In the clinical setting, this effect may be more pronounced. Therefore, due to a possible decrease in CYP3A4 substrate concentration and potential loss of effectiveness, caution should be observed when deferasirox is administered with drugs metabolized by CYP3A4 (eg, cyclosporine, simvastatin, hormonal contraceptives)).

No products indexed under this heading.

Haloperidol Decanoate (Concomitant administration of deferasirox and midazolam (a CYP3A4 probe substrate) resulted in a decrease of midazolam peak concentration by 23% and exposure by 17%. In the clinical setting, this effect may be more pronounced. Therefore, due to a possible decrease in CYP3A4 substrate concentration and potential loss of effectiveness, caution should be observed when deferasirox is administered with drugs metabolized by CYP3A4 (eg, cyclosporine, simvastatin, hormonal contraceptives)).

No products indexed under this heading.

Haloperidol Lactate (Concomitant administration of deferasirox and midazolam (a CYP3A4 probe substrate) resulted in a decrease of midazolam peak concentration by 23% and exposure by 17%. In the clinical setting, this effect may be more pronounced. Therefore, due to a possible decrease in CYP3A4 substrate concentration and potential loss of effectiveness, caution should be observed when deferasirox is administered with drugs metabolized by CYP3A4 (eg, cyclosporine, simvastatin, hormonal contraceptives)).

No products indexed under this heading.

Heparin Calcium (Caution should be observed when administering deferasirox in combination with drugs that have ulcerogenic or hemorrhagic potential, such as anticoagulants).

No products indexed under this heading.

Heparin Sodium (Caution should be observed when administering deferasirox in combination with drugs that have ulcerogenic or hemorrhagic potential, such as anticoagulants).

No products indexed under this heading.

Hydrocodone Bitartrate (Deferasirox inhibits human CYP2D6 in vitro). Products include:
Vicodin 560
Vicodin ES 561
Vicodin HP 563
Vicoprofen 564
Zydone 1138

Hydrocortisone (Caution should be observed when administering deferasirox in combination with drugs that have ulcerogenic or hemorrhagic potential, such as corticosteroids).

No products indexed under this heading.

Hydrocortisone (Alcohol) (Caution should be observed when administering deferasirox in combination with drugs that have ulcerogenic or hemorrhagic potential, such as corticosteroids).

No products indexed under this heading.

Hydrocortisone Acetate (Caution should be observed when administering deferasirox in combination with drugs that have ulcerogenic or hemorrhagic potential, such as corticosteroids).

No products indexed under this heading.

IMPORTANT NOTE: Always consult each drug listing in the patient's regimen for possible interactions.

Meclofenamate Sodium (Caution should be observed when administering deferasirox in combination with drugs that have ulcerogenic or hemorrhagic potential, such as non-steroidal anti-inflammatory drugs).
No products indexed under this heading.

Mefenamic Acid (Caution should be observed when administering deferasirox in combination with drugs that have ulcerogenic or hemorrhagic potential, such as non-steroidal anti-inflammatory drugs).
No products indexed under this heading.

Meloxicam (Caution should be observed when administering deferasirox in combination with drugs that have ulcerogenic or hemorrhagic potential, such as non-steroidal anti-inflammatory drugs).
No products indexed under this heading.

Meperidine Hydrochloride (Deferasirox inhibits human CYP2D6 *in vitro*).
No products indexed under this heading.

Mephenytoin (In a healthy volunteer study, the concomitant administration of deferasirox (single dose of 30 mg/kg) and the potent UDP-glucuronosyltransferase (UGT) inducer rifampicin (600 mg/day for 9 days) resulted in a decrease of deferasirox systemic exposure (AUC) by 44%. Concomitant use of deferasirox with potent UGT inducers (eg, rifampicin, phenytoin, phenobarbital, ritonavir) may result in a decrease of deferasirox. When used concomitantly, the dose of deferasirox should be increased and serum ferritin levels and clinical responses should be monitored for further dose modifications).
No products indexed under this heading.

Mephobarbital (Concomitant administration of deferasirox and the CYP2C8 probe substrate repaglinide (single dose of 0.5 mg) resulted in an increase in repaglinide systemic exposure (AUC) to 2.3 fold of control and an increase in C_{max} of 62%. If deferasirox and repaglinide are used concomitantly, decreasing the dose of repaglinide should be considered and careful monitoring of blood glucose levels should be performed. Caution should be exercised when deferasirox and other CYP2C8 substrates like paclitaxel are co-administered).
No products indexed under this heading.

Meprobamate (Deferasirox inhibits human CYP2C19 *in vitro*).
No products indexed under this heading.

Mestranol (Concomitant administration of deferasirox and midazolam (a CYP3A4 probe substrate) resulted in a decrease of midazolam peak concentration by 23% and exposure by 17%. In the clinical setting, this effect may be more pronounced. Therefore, due to a possible decrease in CYP3A4 substrate concentration and potential loss of effectiveness, caution should be observed when deferasirox is administered with drugs metabolized by CYP3A4 (eg, cyclosporine, simvastatin, hormonal contraceptives)).
No products indexed under this heading.

Methadone Hydrochloride (Concomitant administration of deferasirox and midazolam (a CYP3A4 probe substrate) resulted in a decrease of midazolam peak concentration by 23% and exposure by 17%. In the clinical setting, this effect may be more pronounced. Therefore, due to a possible decrease in CYP3A4 substrate concentration and potential loss of effectiveness, caution should be observed when deferasirox is administered with drugs metabolized by CYP3A4 (eg, cyclosporine, simvastatin, hormonal contraceptives)).
No products indexed under this heading.

Methamphetamine Hydrochloride (Deferasirox inhibits human CYP2D6 *in vitro*).
No products indexed under this heading.

Methoxyphenamine (Deferasirox inhibits human CYP2D6 *in vitro*).
No products indexed under this heading.

Methsuximide (Deferasirox inhibits human CYP2C19 *in vitro*).
No products indexed under this heading.

Methylprednisolone (Caution should be observed when administering deferasirox in combination with drugs that have ulcerogenic or hemorrhagic potential, such as corticosteroids).
No products indexed under this heading.

Methylprednisolone Acetate (Caution should be observed when administering deferasirox in combination with drugs that have ulcerogenic or hemorrhagic potential, such as corticosteroids).
No products indexed under this heading.

Methylprednisolone Sodium Succinate (Caution should be observed when administering deferasirox in combination with drugs that have ulcerogenic or hemorrhagic potential, such as corticosteroids).
No products indexed under this heading.

Metoprolol Succinate (Deferasirox inhibits human CYP2D6 *in vitro*). Products include:
Toprol XL 732

Metoprolol Tartrate (Deferasirox inhibits human CYP2D6 *in vitro*).
No products indexed under this heading.

Mexiletine Hydrochloride (Deferasirox inhibits human CYP2D6 *in vitro*).
No products indexed under this heading.

Midazolam Hydrochloride (Concomitant administration of deferasirox and midazolam (a CYP3A4 probe substrate) resulted in a decrease of midazolam peak concentration by 23% and exposure by 17%. In the clinical setting, this effect may be more pronounced).
No products indexed under this heading.

Mirtazapine (Deferasirox inhibits human CYP2D6 *in vitro*). Products include:
Remeron Tablets 3214
RemeronSolTab Tablets 3219

Mometasone Furoate (Caution should be observed when administering deferasirox in combination with drugs that have ulcerogenic or hemorrhagic potential, such as corticosteroids). Products include:
Asmanex 3058
Elocon Cream 3111
Elocon Lotion 3112
Elocon Ointment 3114

Mometasone Furoate Monohydrate (Caution should be observed when administering deferasirox in combination with drugs that have ulcerogenic or hemorrhagic potential, such as corticosteroids). Products include:
Nasonex 3166

Morphine Sulfate (Deferasirox inhibits human CYP2D6 *in vitro*). Products include:
Avinza 1822
Embeda 1831
MS Contin 2803

Moxifloxacin Hydrochloride (Deferasirox inhibits human CYP1A2 *in vitro*). Products include:
Avelox 3064
Vigamox 589

Nabumetone (Caution should be observed when administering deferasirox in combination with drugs that have ulcerogenic or hemorrhagic potential, such as non-steroidal anti-inflammatory drugs).
No products indexed under this heading.

Nafcillin Sodium (Deferasirox inhibits human CYP1A2 *in vitro*).
No products indexed under this heading.

Naproxen (Caution should be observed when administering deferasirox in combination with drugs that have ulcerogenic or hemorrhagic potential, such as non-steroidal anti-inflammatory drugs). Products include:
EC-Naprosyn 2850
Naprosyn 2850
Anaprox/Naprosyn 2850

Naproxen Sodium (Caution should be observed when administering deferasirox in combination with drugs that have ulcerogenic or hemorrhagic potential, such as non-steroidal anti-inflammatory drugs). Products include:
Anaprox 2850
Anaprox DS 2850
Treximet 1681

Nefazodone Hydrochloride (Concomitant administration of deferasirox and midazolam (a CYP3A4 probe substrate) resulted in a decrease of midazolam peak concentration by 23% and exposure by 17%. In the clinical setting, this effect may be more pronounced. Therefore, due to a possible decrease in CYP3A4 substrate concentration and potential loss of effectiveness, caution should be observed when deferasirox is administered with drugs metabolized by CYP3A4 (eg, cyclosporine, simvastatin, hormonal contraceptives)).
No products indexed under this heading.

Nelfinavir Mesylate (Concomitant administration of deferasirox and midazolam (a CYP3A4 probe substrate) resulted in a decrease of midazolam peak concentration by 23% and exposure by 17%. In the clinical setting, this effect may be more pronounced. Therefore, due to a possible decrease in CYP3A4 substrate concentration and potential loss of effectiveness, caution should be observed when deferasirox is administered with drugs metabolized by CYP3A4 (eg, cyclosporine, simvastatin, hormonal contraceptives)).
No products indexed under this heading.

Nicardipine (Concomitant administration of deferasirox and midazolam (a CYP3A4 probe substrate) resulted in a decrease of midazolam peak concentration by 23% and exposure by 17%. In the clinical setting, this effect may be more pronounced. Therefore, due to a possible decrease in CYP3A4 substrate concentration and potential loss of effectiveness, caution should be observed when deferasirox is administered with drugs metabolized by CYP3A4 (eg, cyclosporine, simvastatin, hormonal contraceptives)).
No products indexed under this heading.

Nicardipine Hydrochloride (Concomitant administration of deferasirox and midazolam (a CYP3A4 probe substrate) resulted in a decrease of midazolam peak concentration by 23% and exposure by 17%. In the clinical setting, this effect may be more pronounced. Therefore, due to a possible decrease in CYP3A4 substrate concentration and potential loss of effectiveness, caution should be observed when deferasirox is administered with drugs metabolized by CYP3A4 (eg, cyclosporine, simvastatin, hormonal contraceptives)).
No products indexed under this heading.

Nicotine (Deferasirox inhibits human CYP2A6 *in vitro*).
No products indexed under this heading.

Nicotine Polacrilex (Deferasirox inhibits human CYP2A6 *in vitro*).
No products indexed under this heading.

Nicotine Salicylate (Deferasirox inhibits human CYP2A6 *in vitro*).
No products indexed under this heading.

Nicotine Sulfate (Deferasirox inhibits human CYP2A6 *in vitro*).
No products indexed under this heading.

Nifedipine (Concomitant administration of deferasirox and midazolam (a CYP3A4 probe substrate) resulted in a decrease of midazolam peak concentration by 23% and exposure by 17%. In the clinical setting, this effect may be more pronounced. Therefore, due to a possible decrease in CYP3A4 substrate concentration and potential loss of effectiveness, caution should be observed when deferasirox is administered with drugs metabolized by CYP3A4 (eg, cyclosporine, simvastatin, hormonal contraceptives)).
No products indexed under this heading.

Nilutamide (Deferasirox inhibits human CYP2C19 *in vitro*).
No products indexed under this heading.

Nimodipine (Concomitant administration of deferasirox and midazolam (a CYP3A4 probe substrate) resulted in a decrease of midazolam peak concentration by 23% and exposure by 17%. In the clinical setting, this effect may be more pronounced. Therefore, due to a possible decrease in CYP3A4 substrate concentration and potential loss of effectiveness, caution should be observed when deferasirox is administered with drugs metabolized by CYP3A4 (eg, cyclosporine, simvastatin, hormonal contraceptives)).
No products indexed under this heading.

Nisoldipine (Concomitant administration of deferasirox and midazolam (a CYP3A4 probe substrate) resulted in a decrease of midazolam peak concentration by 23% and exposure by 17%. In the clinical setting, this effect may be more pronounced. Therefore, due to a possible decrease in CYP3A4 substrate concentration and potential loss of effectiveness, caution should be observed when deferasirox is administered with drugs metabolized by CYP3A4 (eg, cyclosporine, simvastatin, hormonal contraceptives)).
No products indexed under this heading.

Nitrendipine (Concomitant administration of deferasirox and midazolam (a CYP3A4 probe substrate) resulted in a decrease of midazolam peak concentration by 23% and exposure by 17%. In the clinical setting, this effect may be more pronounced. Therefore, due to a possible decrease in CYP3A4 substrate concentration and potential loss of effectiveness, caution should be observed when deferasirox is administered with drugs metabolized by CYP3A4 (eg, cyclosporine, simvastatin, hormonal contraceptives)).
No products indexed under this heading.

Norethindrone (Concomitant administration of deferasirox and midazolam (a CYP3A4 probe substrate) resulted in a decrease of midazolam peak concentration by 23% and exposure by 17%. In the clinical setting, this effect may be more pronounced. Therefore, due to a possible decrease in CYP3A4 substrate concentration and potential loss of effectiveness, caution should be observed when deferasirox is administered with drugs metabolized by CYP3A4 (eg, cyclosporine, simvastatin, hormonal contraceptives)). Products include:
Ortho Micronor 2660

Norethindrone Acetate (Concomitant administration of deferasirox and midazolam (a CYP3A4 probe substrate) resulted in a decrease of midazolam peak concentration by 23% and exposure by 17%. In the clinical setting, this effect may be more pronounced. Therefore, due to a possible decrease in CYP3A4 substrate concentration and potential loss of effectiveness, caution

should be observed when deferasirox is administered with drugs metabolized by CYP3A4 (eg, cyclosporine, simvastatin, hormonal contraceptives)). Products include:

Activella **2561**

Norethynodrel (Concomitant administration of deferasirox and midazolam (a CYP3A4 probe substrate) resulted in a decrease of midazolam peak concentration by 23% and exposure by 17%. In the clinical setting, this effect may be more pronounced. Therefore, due to a possible decrease in CYP3A4 substrate concentration and potential loss of effectiveness, caution should be observed when deferasirox is administered with drugs metabolized by CYP3A4 (eg, cyclosporine, simvastatin, hormonal contraceptives)).

No products indexed under this heading.

Norfloxacin (Deferasirox inhibits human CYP1A2 *in vitro*). Products include:

Noroxin **2220**

Norgestimate (Concomitant administration of deferasirox and midazolam (a CYP3A4 probe substrate) resulted in a decrease of midazolam peak concentration by 23% and exposure by 17%. In the clinical setting, this effect may be more pronounced. Therefore, due to a possible decrease in CYP3A4 substrate concentration and potential loss of effectiveness, caution should be observed when deferasirox is administered with drugs metabolized by CYP3A4 (eg, cyclosporine, simvastatin, hormonal contraceptives)). Products include:

Ortho-Cyclen/Ortho Tri-Cyclen **2663**
Ortho Tri-Cyclen Lo Tablets **2673**

Norgestrel (Concomitant administration of deferasirox and midazolam (a CYP3A4 probe substrate) resulted in a decrease of midazolam peak concentration by 23% and exposure by 17%. In the clinical setting, this effect may be more pronounced. Therefore, due to a possible decrease in CYP3A4 substrate concentration and potential loss of effectiveness, caution should be observed when deferasirox is administered with drugs metabolized by CYP3A4 (eg, cyclosporine, simvastatin, hormonal contraceptives)).

No products indexed under this heading.

Nortriptyline Hydrochloride (Concomitant administration of deferasirox and the CYP2C8 probe substrate repaglinide (single dose of 0.5 mg) resulted in an increase in repaglinide systemic exposure (AUC) to 2.3 fold of control and an increase in C_{max} of 62%. If deferasirox and repaglinide are used concomitantly, decreasing the dose of repaglinide should be considered and careful monitoring of blood glucose levels should be performed. Caution should be exercised when deferasirox and other CYP2C8 substrates like paclitaxel are co-administered).

No products indexed under this heading.

Ofloxacin (Deferasirox inhibits human CYP1A2 *in vitro*).

No products indexed under this heading.

Olanzapine (Deferasirox inhibits human CYP2D6 *in vitro*). Products include:

Symbyax **1965**
Zyprexa **1984**
Zyprexa IntraMuscular **1984**
Zyprexa ZYDIS **1984**

Omeprazole (Concomitant administration of deferasirox and the CYP2C8 probe substrate repaglinide (single dose of 0.5 mg) resulted in an increase in repaglinide systemic exposure (AUC) to 2.3 fold of control and an increase in C_{max} of 62%. If deferasirox and repaglinide are used concomitantly, decreasing the dose of repaglinide should be considered and careful monitoring of blood glucose levels should be performed. Caution should be exercised when deferasirox and other CYP2C8 substrates like paclitaxel are co-administered).

No products indexed under this heading.

Omeprazole Magnesium (Deferasirox inhibits human CYP2C19 *in vitro*).

No products indexed under this heading.

Ondansetron (Concomitant administration of deferasirox and midazolam (a CYP3A4 probe substrate) resulted in a decrease of midazolam peak concentration by 23% and exposure by 17%. In the clinical setting, this effect may be more pronounced. Therefore, due to a possible decrease in CYP3A4 substrate concentration and potential loss of effectiveness, caution should be observed when deferasirox is administered with drugs metabolized by CYP3A4 (eg, cyclosporine, simvastatin, hormonal contraceptives)).

No products indexed under this heading.

Ondansetron Hydrochloride (Concomitant administration of deferasirox and midazolam (a CYP3A4 probe substrate) resulted in a decrease of midazolam peak concentration by 23% and exposure by 17%. In the clinical setting, this effect may be more pronounced. Therefore, due to a possible decrease in CYP3A4 substrate concentration and potential loss of effectiveness, caution should be observed when deferasirox is administered with drugs metabolized by CYP3A4 (eg, cyclosporine, simvastatin, hormonal contraceptives)). Products include:

Zofran Injection **1750**
Zofran **1756**
Zofran ODT **1756**

Oxaprozin (Caution should be observed when administering deferasirox in combination with drugs that have ulcerogenic or hemorrhagic potential, such as non-steroidal anti-inflammatory drugs).

No products indexed under this heading.

Oxcarbazepine (Deferasirox inhibits human CYP2C19 *in vitro*).

No products indexed under this heading.

Oxycodone Hydrochloride (Deferasirox inhibits human CYP2D6 *in vitro*). Products include:

OxyContin **2807**
Percocet **1121**
Percodan **1124**

Paclitaxel (Concomitant administration of deferasirox and the CYP2C8 probe substrate repaglinide (single dose of 0.5 mg) resulted in an increase in repaglinide systemic exposure (AUC) to 2.3 fold of control and an increase in C_{max} of 62%. If deferasirox and repaglinide are used concomitantly, decreasing the dose of repaglinide should be considered and careful monitoring of blood glucose levels should be performed. Caution should be exercised when deferasirox and other CYP2C8 substrates like paclitaxel are co-administered).

No products indexed under this heading.

Paclitaxel, protein-bound (Concomitant administration of deferasirox and the CYP2C8 probe substrate repaglinide (single dose of 0.5 mg) resulted in an increase in repaglinide systemic exposure (AUC) to 2.3 fold of control and an increase in C_{max} of 62%. If deferasirox and repaglinide are used concomitantly, decreasing the dose of repaglinide should be considered and careful monitoring of blood glucose levels should be performed. Caution should be exercised when deferasirox and other CYP2C8 substrates like paclitaxel are co-administered).

No products indexed under this heading.

Pantoprazole Sodium (Deferasirox inhibits human CYP2C19 *in vitro*). Products include:

Protonix Tablets **3571**
Protonix **3575**

Paramethadione (Deferasirox inhibits human CYP2C19 *in vitro*).

No products indexed under this heading.

Paroxetine Hydrochloride (Deferasirox inhibits human CYP2D6 *in vitro*). Products include:

Paroxetine CR **2361**
Paroxetine ER **2371**
Paxil **1586**
Paxil CR **1596**

Pentamidine Isethionate (Deferasirox inhibits human CYP2C19 *in vitro*).

No products indexed under this heading.

Phenacemide (Deferasirox inhibits human CYP2C19 *in vitro*).

No products indexed under this heading.

Phenobarbital (In a healthy volunteer study, the concomitant administration of deferasirox (single dose of 30 mg/kg) and the potent UDP-glucuronosyltransferase (UGT) inducer rifampicin (600 mg/day for 9 days) resulted in a decrease of deferasirox systemic exposure (AUC) by 44%. Concomitant use of deferasirox with potent UGT inducers (eg, rifampicin, phenytoin, phenobarbital, ritonavir) may result in a decrease of deferasirox. When used concomitantly, the dose of deferasirox should be increased and serum ferritin levels and clinical responses should be monitored for further dose modifications). Products include:

Donnatal **2711**

Phenobarbital Sodium (In a healthy volunteer study, the concomitant administration of deferasirox (single dose of 30 mg/kg) and the potent UDP-glucuronosyltransferase (UGT) inducer rifampicin (600 mg/day for 9 days) resulted in a decrease of deferasirox systemic exposure (AUC) by 44%. Concomitant use of deferasirox with potent UGT inducers (eg, rifampicin, phenytoin, phenobarbital, ritonavir) may result in a decrease of deferasirox. When used concomitantly, the dose of deferasirox should be increased and serum ferritin levels and clinical responses should be monitored for further dose modifications).

No products indexed under this heading.

Phensuximide (Deferasirox inhibits human CYP2C19 *in vitro*).

No products indexed under this heading.

Phenylbutazone (Caution should be observed when administering deferasirox in combination with drugs that have ulcerogenic or hemorrhagic potential, such as non-steroidal anti-inflammatory drugs).

No products indexed under this heading.

Phenytoin (Concomitant administration of deferasirox and the CYP2C8 probe substrate repaglinide (single dose of 0.5 mg) resulted in an increase in repaglinide systemic exposure (AUC) to 2.3 fold of control and an increase in C_{max} of 62%. If deferasirox and repaglinide are used concomitantly, decreasing the dose of repaglinide should be considered and careful monitoring of blood glucose levels should be performed. Caution should be exercised when deferasirox and other CYP2C8 substrates like paclitaxel are co-administered).

No products indexed under this heading.

Phenytoin Sodium (Concomitant administration of deferasirox and the CYP2C8 probe substrate repaglinide (single dose of 0.5 mg) resulted in an increase in repaglinide systemic exposure (AUC) to 2.3 fold of control and an increase in C_{max} of 62%. If deferasirox and repaglinide are used concomitantly, decreasing the dose of repaglinide should be considered and careful monitoring of blood glucose levels should be performed. Caution should be exercised when deferasirox and other CYP2C8 substrates like paclitaxel are co-administered). Products include:

Phenytek Capsules **2380**

Pimozide (Concomitant administration of deferasirox and midazolam (a CYP3A4 probe substrate) resulted in a decrease of midazolam peak concentration by 23% and exposure by 17%. In the clinical setting, this effect may be more pronounced. Therefore, due to a possible decrease in CYP3A4 substrate concentration and potential loss of effectiveness, caution should be observed when deferasirox is administered with drugs metabolized by CYP3A4 (eg, cyclosporine, simvastatin, hormonal contraceptives)).

No products indexed under this heading.

Pindolol (Deferasirox inhibits human CYP2D6 *in vitro*).

No products indexed under this heading.

Pioglitazone Hydrochloride (Concomitant administration of deferasirox and the CYP2C8 probe substrate repaglinide (single dose of 0.5 mg) resulted in an increase in repaglinide systemic exposure (AUC) to 2.3 fold of control and an increase in C_{max} of 62%. If deferasirox and repaglinide are used concomitantly, decreasing the dose of repaglinide should be considered and careful monitoring of blood glucose levels should be performed. Caution should be exercised when deferasirox and other CYP2C8 substrates like paclitaxel are co-administered). Products include:

ActoPlus **3338**
Actos **3345**
Duetact **3354**

Piroxicam (Caution should be observed when administering deferasirox in combination with drugs that have ulcerogenic or hemorrhagic potential, such as non-steroidal anti-inflammatory drugs).

No products indexed under this heading.

Polyestradiol Phosphate (Concomitant administration of deferasirox and midazolam (a CYP3A4 probe substrate) resulted in a decrease of midazolam peak concentration by 23% and exposure by 17%. In the clinical setting, this effect may be more pronounced. Therefore, due to a possible decrease in CYP3A4 substrate concentration and potential loss of effectiveness, caution should be observed when deferasirox is administered with drugs metabolized by CYP3A4 (eg, cyclosporine, simvastatin, hormonal contraceptives)).

No products indexed under this heading.

Prednisolone (Caution should be observed when administering deferasirox in combination with drugs that have ulcerogenic or hemorrhagic potential, such as corticosteroids).

No products indexed under this heading.

Prednisolone Acetate (Caution should be observed when administering deferasirox in combination with drugs that have ulcerogenic or hemorrhagic potential, such as corticosteroids). Products include:

Blephamide .... ⊙ **212**, ⊙ **214**
Pred Forte .... ⊙ **225**
Pred Mild .... ⊙ **230**
Pred-G .... ⊙ **226**, ⊙ **227**

Prednisolone Sodium Phosphate (Caution should be observed when administering deferasirox in combination with drugs that have ulcerogenic or hemorrhagic potential, such as corticosteroids).

No products indexed under this heading.

IMPORTANT NOTE: Always consult each drug listing in the patient's regimen for possible interactions.

Prednisolone Tebutate (Caution should be observed when administering deferasirox in combination with drugs that have ulcerogenic or hemorrhagic potential, such as corticosteroids).
No products indexed under this heading.

Prednisone (Caution should be observed when administering deferasirox in combination with drugs that have ulcerogenic or hemorrhagic potential, such as corticosteroids).
No products indexed under this heading.

Prednisone sodium phosphate (Caution should be observed when administering deferasirox in combination with drugs that have ulcerogenic or hemorrhagic potential, such as corticosteroids).
No products indexed under this heading.

Primidone (Deferasirox inhibits human CYP2C19 *in vitro*).
No products indexed under this heading.

Progesterone (Deferasirox inhibits human CYP2C19 *in vitro*). Products include:
Crinone 4% 996
Crinone 8% 996
Prometrium 3307

Proguanil Hydrochloride (Deferasirox inhibits human CYP2C19 *in vitro*). Products include:
Malarone Pediatric Tablets 1572
Malarone 1572

Propafenone Hydrochloride (Deferasirox inhibits human CYP2D6 *in vitro*). Products include:
Rythmol 1648
Rythmol SR 1652

Propoxyphene Hydrochloride (Deferasirox inhibits human CYP2D6 *in vitro*).
No products indexed under this heading.

Propoxyphene Napsylate (Deferasirox inhibits human CYP2D6 *in vitro*).
No products indexed under this heading.

Propranolol Hydrochloride (Deferasirox inhibits human CYP2D6 *in vitro*). Products include:
InnoPran XL 1517

Protriptyline Hydrochloride (Concomitant administration of deferasirox and the CYP2C8 probe substrate repaglinide (single dose of 0.5 mg) resulted in an increase in repaglinide systemic exposure (AUC) to 2.3 fold of control and an increase in C_{max} of 62%. If deferasirox and repaglinide are used concomitantly, decreasing the dose of repaglinide should be considered and careful monitoring of blood glucose levels should be performed. Caution should be exercised when deferasirox and other CYP2C8 substrates like paclitaxel are co-administered).
No products indexed under this heading.

Quetiapine Fumarate (Deferasirox inhibits human CYP2D6 *in vitro*). Products include:
Seroquel 750
Seroquel XR 759

Quinidine Gluconate (Concomitant administration of deferasirox and midazolam (a CYP3A4 probe substrate) resulted in a decrease of midazolam peak concentration by 23% and exposure by 17%. In the clinical setting, this effect may be more pronounced. Therefore, due to a possible decrease in CYP3A4 substrate concentration and potential loss of effectiveness, caution should be observed when deferasirox is administered with drugs metabolized by CYP3A4 (eg, cyclosporine, simvastatin, hormonal contraceptives)).
No products indexed under this heading.

Quinidine Hydrochloride (Deferasirox inhibits human CYP2D6 *in vitro*).
No products indexed under this heading.

Quinidine Polygalacturonate (Concomitant administration of deferasirox and midazolam (a CYP3A4 probe substrate) resulted in a decrease of midazolam peak concentration by 23% and exposure by 17%. In the clinical setting, this effect may be more pronounced. Therefore, due to a possible decrease in CYP3A4 substrate concentration and potential loss of effectiveness, caution should be observed when deferasirox is administered with drugs metabolized by CYP3A4 (eg, cyclosporine, simvastatin, hormonal contraceptives)).
No products indexed under this heading.

Quinidine Sulfate (Concomitant administration of deferasirox and midazolam (a CYP3A4 probe substrate) resulted in a decrease of midazolam peak concentration by 23% and exposure by 17%. In the clinical setting, this effect may be more pronounced. Therefore, due to a possible decrease in CYP3A4 substrate concentration and potential loss of effectiveness, caution should be observed when deferasirox is administered with drugs metabolized by CYP3A4 (eg, cyclosporine, simvastatin, hormonal contraceptives)).
No products indexed under this heading.

Rabeprazole Sodium (Deferasirox inhibits human CYP2C19 *in vitro*). Products include:
Aciphex 1035

Repaglinide (Concomitant administration of deferasirox and the CYP2C8 probe substrate repaglinide (single dose of 0.5 mg) resulted in an increase in repaglinide systemic exposure (AUC) to 2.3 fold of control and an increase in C_{max} of 62%. If deferasirox and repaglinide are used concomitantly, decreasing the dose of repaglinide should be considered and careful monitoring of blood glucose levels should be performed).
No products indexed under this heading.

Rifabutin (Concomitant administration of deferasirox and midazolam (a CYP3A4 probe substrate) resulted in a decrease of midazolam peak concentration by 23% and exposure by 17%. In the clinical setting, this effect may be more pronounced. Therefore, due to a possible decrease in CYP3A4 substrate concentration and potential loss of effectiveness, caution should be observed when deferasirox is administered with drugs metabolized by CYP3A4 (eg, cyclosporine, simvastatin, hormonal contraceptives)).
No products indexed under this heading.

Rifampicin (In a healthy volunteer study, the concomitant administration of deferasirox (single dose of 30 mg/kg) and the potent UDP-glucuronosyltransferase (UGT) inducer rifampicin (600 mg/day for 9 days) resulted in a decrease of deferasirox systemic exposure (AUC) by 44%. Concomitant use of deferasirox with potent UGT inducers (eg, rifampicin, phenytoin, phenobarbital, ritonavir) may result in a decrease of deferasirox. When used concomitantly, the dose of deferasirox should be increased and serum ferritin levels and clinical responses should be monitored for further dose modifications).
No products indexed under this heading.

Riluzole (Deferasirox inhibits human CYP1A2 *in vitro*). Products include:
Rilutek 3032

Risedronate Sodium (Caution should be observed when administering deferasirox in combination with drugs that have ulcerogenic or hemorrhagic potential, such as oral bisphosphonates). Products include:
Actonel 2779

Risperidone (Deferasirox inhibits human CYP2D6 *in vitro*). Products include:
Risperdal Consta 2682

Ritonavir (In a healthy volunteer study, the concomitant administration of deferasirox (single dose of 30 mg/kg) and the potent UDP-glucuronosyltransferase (UGT) inducer rifampicin (600 mg/day for 9 days) resulted in a decrease of deferasirox systemic exposure (AUC) by 44%. Concomitant use of deferasirox with potent UGT inducers (eg, rifampicin, phenytoin, phenobarbital, ritonavir) may result in a decrease of deferasirox. When used concomitantly, the dose of deferasirox should be increased and serum ferritin levels and clinical responses should be monitored for further dose modifications). Products include:
Kaletra 458
Norvir 509

Rofecoxib (Caution should be observed when administering deferasirox in combination with drugs that have ulcerogenic or hemorrhagic potential, such as non-steroidal anti-inflammatory drugs).
No products indexed under this heading.

Ropinirole Hydrochloride (Deferasirox inhibits human CYP1A2 *in vitro*). Products include:
Requip 1620
Requip XL 1628

Ropivacaine Hydrochloride (Deferasirox inhibits human CYP1A2 *in vitro*).
No products indexed under this heading.

Rosiglitazone Maleate (Concomitant administration of deferasirox and the CYP2C8 probe substrate repaglinide (single dose of 0.5 mg) resulted in an increase in repaglinide systemic exposure (AUC) to 2.3 fold of control and an increase in C_{max} of 62%. If deferasirox and repaglinide are used concomitantly, decreasing the dose of repaglinide should be considered and careful monitoring of blood glucose levels should be performed. Caution should be exercised when deferasirox and other CYP2C8 substrates like paclitaxel are co-administered). Products include:
Avandamet 1345
Avandaryl 1356
Avandia 1366

Rosiglitazone/Metformin (Concomitant administration of deferasirox and the CYP2C8 probe substrate repaglinide (single dose of 0.5 mg) resulted in an increase in repaglinide systemic exposure (AUC) to 2.3 fold of control and an increase in C_{max} of 62%. If deferasirox and repaglinide are used concomitantly, decreasing the dose of repaglinide should be considered and careful monitoring of blood glucose levels should be performed. Caution should be exercised when deferasirox and other CYP2C8 substrates like paclitaxel are co-administered).
No products indexed under this heading.

Saquinavir (Concomitant administration of deferasirox and midazolam (a CYP3A4 probe substrate) resulted in a decrease of midazolam peak concentration by 23% and exposure by 17%. In the clinical setting, this effect may be more pronounced. Therefore, due to a possible decrease in CYP3A4 substrate concentration and potential loss of effectiveness, caution should be observed when deferasirox is administered with drugs metabolized by CYP3A4 (eg, cyclosporine, simvastatin, hormonal contraceptives)).
No products indexed under this heading.

Saquinavir Mesylate (Concomitant administration of deferasirox and midazolam (a CYP3A4 probe substrate) resulted in a decrease of midazolam peak concentration by 23% and exposure by 17%. In the clinical setting, this effect may be more pronounced. Therefore, due to a possible decrease in CYP3A4 substrate concentration and potential loss of effectiveness, caution should be observed when deferasirox is administered with drugs metabolized by CYP3A4 (eg, cyclosporine, simvastatin, hormonal contraceptives)).
No products indexed under this heading.

Sertraline Hydrochloride (Concomitant administration of deferasirox and midazolam (a CYP3A4 probe substrate) resulted in a decrease of midazolam peak concentration by 23% and exposure by 17%. In the clinical setting, this effect may be more pronounced. Therefore, due to a possible decrease in CYP3A4 substrate concentration and potential loss of effectiveness, caution should be observed when deferasirox is administered with drugs metabolized by CYP3A4 (eg, cyclosporine, simvastatin, hormonal contraceptives)).
No products indexed under this heading.

Sildenafil Citrate (Concomitant administration of deferasirox and midazolam (a CYP3A4 probe substrate) resulted in a decrease of midazolam peak concentration by 23% and exposure by 17%. In the clinical setting, this effect may be more pronounced. Therefore, due to a possible decrease in CYP3A4 substrate concentration and potential loss of effectiveness, caution should be observed when deferasirox is administered with drugs metabolized by CYP3A4 (eg, cyclosporine, simvastatin, hormonal contraceptives)).
No products indexed under this heading.

Simvastatin (Concomitant administration of deferasirox and midazolam (a CYP3A4 probe substrate) resulted in a decrease of midazolam peak concentration by 23% and exposure by 17%. In the clinical setting, this effect may be more pronounced. Therefore, due to a possible decrease in CYP3A4 substrate concentration and potential loss of effectiveness, caution should be observed when deferasirox is administered with drugs metabolized by CYP3A4 (eg, cyclosporine, simvastatin, hormonal contraceptives)). Products include:
Simcor 524
Vytorin 10/10 .... 2303, 3240
Vytorin 10/20 .... 2303, 3240
Vytorin 10/40 .... 2303, 3240
Vytorin 10/80 .... 2303, 3240
Zocor 2289

Sirolimus (Concomitant administration of deferasirox and midazolam (a CYP3A4 probe substrate) resulted in a decrease of midazolam peak concentration by 23% and exposure by 17%. In the clinical setting, this effect may be more pronounced. Therefore, due to a possible decrease in CYP3A4 substrate concentration and potential loss of effectiveness, caution should be observed when deferasirox is administered with drugs metabolized by CYP3A4 (eg, cyclosporine, simvastatin, hormonal contraceptives)). Products include:
Rapamune 3579

Sulindac (Caution should be observed when administering deferasirox in combination with drugs that have ulcerogenic or hemorrhagic potential, such as non-steroidal anti-inflammatory drugs). Products include:
Clinoril 2098

Tacrine Hydrochloride (Deferasirox inhibits human CYP1A2 *in vitro*).
No products indexed under this heading.

Tacrolimus (Concomitant administration of deferasirox and midazolam (a CYP3A4 probe substrate) resulted in a decrease of midazolam peak concentration by 23% and exposure by 17%. In the clinical setting, this effect may be more pronounced. Therefore, due to a possible decrease in CYP3A4 substrate concentration and potential loss of effectiveness, caution should be observed when deferasirox is adminis-

tered with drugs metabolized by CYP3A4 (eg, cyclosporine, simvastatin, hormonal contraceptives)). Products include:

Prograf Capsules 677
Prograf Injection 677
Protopic 685

Tadalafil (Concomitant administration of deferasirox and midazolam (a CYP3A4 probe substrate) resulted in a decrease of midazolam peak concentration by 23% and exposure by 17%. In the clinical setting, this effect may be more pronounced. Therefore, due to a possible decrease in CYP3A4 substrate concentration and potential loss of effectiveness, caution should be observed when deferasirox is administered with drugs metabolized by CYP3A4 (eg, cyclosporine, simvastatin, hormonal contraceptives)). Products include:

Adcirca 3461
Cialis 1861

Tamoxifen Citrate (Concomitant administration of deferasirox and midazolam (a CYP3A4 probe substrate) resulted in a decrease of midazolam peak concentration by 23% and exposure by 17%. In the clinical setting, this effect may be more pronounced. Therefore, due to a possible decrease in CYP3A4 substrate concentration and potential loss of effectiveness, caution should be observed when deferasirox is administered with drugs metabolized by CYP3A4 (eg, cyclosporine, simvastatin, hormonal contraceptives)).
No products indexed under this heading.

Teniposide (Deferasirox inhibits human CYP2D6 *in vitro*).
No products indexed under this heading.

Terfenadine (Concomitant administration of deferasirox and midazolam (a CYP3A4 probe substrate) resulted in a decrease of midazolam peak concentration by 23% and exposure by 17%. In the clinical setting, this effect may be more pronounced. Therefore, due to a possible decrease in CYP3A4 substrate concentration and potential loss of effectiveness, caution should be observed when deferasirox is administered with drugs metabolized by CYP3A4 (eg, cyclosporine, simvastatin, hormonal contraceptives)).
No products indexed under this heading.

Testosterone (Deferasirox inhibits human CYP2D6 *in vitro*). Products include:

AndroGel 3456

Testosterone Cypionate (Deferasirox inhibits human CYP2D6 *in vitro*).
No products indexed under this heading.

Testosterone Enanthate (Deferasirox inhibits human CYP2D6 *in vitro*). Products include:

Delatestryl 1102

Testosterone Propionate (Deferasirox inhibits human CYP2D6 *in vitro*).
No products indexed under this heading.

Theobromine (Deferasirox inhibits human CYP1A2 *in vitro*).
No products indexed under this heading.

Theophylline (Concomitant administration of deferasirox and midazolam (a CYP3A4 probe substrate) resulted in a decrease of midazolam peak concentration by 23% and exposure by 17%. In the clinical setting, this effect may be more pronounced. Therefore, due to a possible decrease in CYP3A4 substrate concentration and potential loss of effectiveness, caution should be observed when deferasirox is administered with drugs metabolized by CYP3A4 (eg, cyclosporine, simvastatin, hormonal contraceptives)).
No products indexed under this heading.

Theophylline Anhydrous (Concomitant administration of deferasirox and midazolam (a CYP3A4 probe substrate) resulted in a decrease of midazolam peak concentration by 23% and exposure by 17%. In the clinical setting, this effect may be more pronounced. Therefore, due to a possible decrease in CYP3A4 substrate concentration and potential loss of effectiveness, caution should be observed when deferasirox is administered with drugs metabolized by CYP3A4 (eg, cyclosporine, simvastatin, hormonal contraceptives)). Products include:

Uniphyl 2817

Theophylline Calcium Salicylate (Concomitant administration of deferasirox and midazolam (a CYP3A4 probe substrate) resulted in a decrease of midazolam peak concentration by 23% and exposure by 17%. In the clinical setting, this effect may be more pronounced. Therefore, due to a possible decrease in CYP3A4 substrate concentration and potential loss of effectiveness, caution should be observed when deferasirox is administered with drugs metabolized by CYP3A4 (eg, cyclosporine, simvastatin, hormonal contraceptives)).
No products indexed under this heading.

Theophylline Dihydroxypropyl (Glyceryl) (Concomitant administration of deferasirox and midazolam (a CYP3A4 probe substrate) resulted in a decrease of midazolam peak concentration by 23% and exposure by 17%. In the clinical setting, this effect may be more pronounced. Therefore, due to a possible decrease in CYP3A4 substrate concentration and potential loss of effectiveness, caution should be observed when deferasirox is administered with drugs metabolized by CYP3A4 (eg, cyclosporine, simvastatin, hormonal contraceptives)).
No products indexed under this heading.

Theophylline Ethylenediamine (Concomitant administration of deferasirox and midazolam (a CYP3A4 probe substrate) resulted in a decrease of midazolam peak concentration by 23% and exposure by 17%. In the clinical setting, this effect may be more pronounced. Therefore, due to a possible decrease in CYP3A4 substrate concentration and potential loss of effectiveness, caution should be observed when deferasirox is administered with drugs metabolized by CYP3A4 (eg, cyclosporine, simvastatin, hormonal contraceptives)).
No products indexed under this heading.

Theophylline Sodium Glycinate (Concomitant administration of deferasirox and midazolam (a CYP3A4 probe substrate) resulted in a decrease of midazolam peak concentration by 23% and exposure by 17%. In the clinical setting, this effect may be more pronounced. Therefore, due to a possible decrease in CYP3A4 substrate concentration and potential loss of effectiveness, caution should be observed when deferasirox is administered with drugs metabolized by CYP3A4 (eg, cyclosporine, simvastatin, hormonal contraceptives)).
No products indexed under this heading.

Thioridazine (Deferasirox inhibits human CYP2D6 *in vitro*).
No products indexed under this heading.

Thioridazine Hydrochloride (Deferasirox inhibits human CYP2D6 *in vitro*). Products include:

Thioridazine Hydrochloride 2384

Tiagabine Hydrochloride (Concomitant administration of deferasirox and midazolam (a CYP3A4 probe substrate) resulted in a decrease of midazolam peak concentration by 23% and exposure by 17%. In the clinical setting, this effect may be more pronounced. Therefore, due to a possible decrease in CYP3A4 substrate concentration and potential loss of effectiveness, caution should be observed when deferasirox is administered with drugs metabolized by CYP3A4 (eg, cyclosporine, simvastatin, hormonal contraceptives)). Products include:

Gabitril 972

Tiludronate Disodium (Caution should be observed when administering deferasirox in combination with drugs that have ulcerogenic or hemorrhagic potential, such as oral bisphosphonates).
No products indexed under this heading.

Timolol Maleate (Deferasirox inhibits human CYP2D6 *in vitro*). Products include:

Combigan 601
Dorzolamide Hydrochloride/Timolol Maleate Ophthalmic Solution .... ⊙243
Timoptic in Ocudose .... ⊙231

Tinzaparin Sodium (Caution should be observed when administering deferasirox in combination with drugs that have ulcerogenic or hemorrhagic potential, such as anticoagulants).
No products indexed under this heading.

Tizanidine (Deferasirox inhibits human CYP1A2 *in vitro*).
No products indexed under this heading.

Tizanidine Hydrochloride (Deferasirox inhibits human CYP1A2 *in vitro*).
No products indexed under this heading.

Tolbutamide (Concomitant administration of deferasirox and the CYP2C8 probe substrate repaglinide (single dose of 0.5 mg) resulted in an increase in repaglinide systemic exposure (AUC) to 2.3 fold of control and an increase in C_{max} of 62%. If deferasirox and repaglinide are used concomitantly, decreasing the dose of repaglinide should be considered and careful monitoring of blood glucose levels should be performed. Caution should be exercised when deferasirox and other CYP2C8 substrates like paclitaxel are co-administered).
No products indexed under this heading.

Tolbutamide Sodium (Concomitant administration of deferasirox and the CYP2C8 probe substrate repaglinide (single dose of 0.5 mg) resulted in an increase in repaglinide systemic exposure (AUC) to 2.3 fold of control and an increase in C_{max} of 62%. If deferasirox and repaglinide are used concomitantly, decreasing the dose of repaglinide should be considered and careful monitoring of blood glucose levels should be performed. Caution should be exercised when deferasirox and other CYP2C8 substrates like paclitaxel are co-administered).
No products indexed under this heading.

Tolmetin Sodium (Caution should be observed when administering deferasirox in combination with drugs that have ulcerogenic or hemorrhagic potential, such as non-steroidal anti-inflammatory drugs).
No products indexed under this heading.

Tolterodine Tartrate (Concomitant administration of deferasirox and midazolam (a CYP3A4 probe substrate) resulted in a decrease of midazolam peak concentration by 23% and exposure by 17%. In the clinical setting, this effect may be more pronounced. Therefore, due to a possible decrease in CYP3A4 substrate concentration and potential loss of effectiveness, caution should be observed when deferasirox is administered with drugs metabolized by CYP3A4 (eg, cyclosporine, simvastatin, hormonal contraceptives)).
No products indexed under this heading.

Topiramate (Deferasirox inhibits human CYP2C19 *in vitro*).
No products indexed under this heading.

Tramadol Hydrochloride (Deferasirox inhibits human CYP2D6 *in vitro*). Products include:

Ryzolt 2813
Ultram ER 2693

Trazodone Hydrochloride (Concomitant administration of deferasirox and midazolam (a CYP3A4 probe substrate) resulted in a decrease of midazolam peak concentration by 23% and exposure by 17%. In the clinical setting, this effect may be more pronounced. Therefore, due to a possible decrease in CYP3A4 substrate concentration and potential loss of effectiveness, caution should be observed when deferasirox is administered with drugs metabolized by CYP3A4 (eg, cyclosporine, simvastatin, hormonal contraceptives)).
No products indexed under this heading.

Tretinoin (Concomitant administration of deferasirox and the CYP2C8 probe substrate repaglinide (single dose of 0.5 mg) resulted in an increase in repaglinide systemic exposure (AUC) to 2.3 fold of control and an increase in C_{max} of 62%. If deferasirox and repaglinide are used concomitantly, decreasing the dose of repaglinide should be considered and careful monitoring of blood glucose levels should be performed. Caution should be exercised when deferasirox and other CYP2C8 substrates like paclitaxel are co-administered).
No products indexed under this heading.

Triamcinolone (Caution should be observed when administering deferasirox in combination with drugs that have ulcerogenic or hemorrhagic potential, such as corticosteroids).
No products indexed under this heading.

Triamcinolone Acetonide (Caution should be observed when administering deferasirox in combination with drugs that have ulcerogenic or hemorrhagic potential, such as corticosteroids). Products include:

Azmacort 408
Nasacort AQ 3019

Triamcinolone Diacetate (Caution should be observed when administering deferasirox in combination with drugs that have ulcerogenic or hemorrhagic potential, such as corticosteroids).
No products indexed under this heading.

Triamcinolone Hexacetonide (Caution should be observed when administering deferasirox in combination with drugs that have ulcerogenic or hemorrhagic potential, such as corticosteroids).
No products indexed under this heading.

Triazolam (Concomitant administration of deferasirox and midazolam (a CYP3A4 probe substrate) resulted in a decrease of midazolam peak concentration by 23% and exposure by 17%. In the clinical setting, this effect may be more pronounced. Therefore, due to a possible decrease in CYP3A4 substrate concentration and potential loss of effectiveness, caution should be observed when deferasirox is administered with drugs metabolized by CYP3A4 (eg, cyclosporine, simvastatin, hormonal contraceptives)).
No products indexed under this heading.

Trimethadione (Deferasirox inhibits human CYP2C19 *in vitro*).
No products indexed under this heading.

Trimethaphan Camsylate (Deferasirox inhibits human CYP1A2 *in vitro*).
No products indexed under this heading.

Trimipramine Maleate (Concomitant administration of deferasirox and the CYP2C8 probe substrate repaglinide (single dose of 0.5 mg) resulted in an

increase in repaglinide systemic exposure (AUC) to 2.3 fold of control and an increase in C_{max} of 62%. If deferasirox and repaglinide are used concomitantly, decreasing the dose of repaglinide should be considered and careful monitoring of blood glucose levels should be performed. Caution should be exercised when deferasirox and other CYP2C8 substrates like paclitaxel are co-administered).
No products indexed under this heading.

Trovafloxacin Mesylate (Deferasirox inhibits human CYP1A2 in vitro).
No products indexed under this heading.

Valdecoxib (Caution should be observed when administering deferasirox in combination with drugs that have ulcerogenic or hemorrhagic potential, such as non-steroidal anti-inflammatory drugs).
No products indexed under this heading.

Valproate Sodium (Deferasirox inhibits human CYP2C19 in vitro).
No products indexed under this heading.

Valproic Acid (Deferasirox inhibits human CYP2C19 in vitro).
No products indexed under this heading.

Vardenafil Hydrochloride (Concomitant administration of deferasirox and midazolam (a CYP3A4 probe substrate) resulted in a decrease of midazolam peak concentration by 23% and exposure by 17%. In the clinical setting, this effect may be more pronounced. Therefore, due to a possible decrease in CYP3A4 substrate concentration and potential loss of effectiveness, caution should be observed when deferasirox is administered with drugs metabolized by CYP3A4 (eg, cyclosporine, simvastatin, hormonal contraceptives)). Products include:
Levitra 3157

Venlafaxine Hydrochloride (Deferasirox inhibits human CYP2D6 in vitro). Products include:
Effexor XR 3504
Venlafaxine Hydrochloride Tablets ... 2388

Verapamil Hydrochloride (Concomitant administration of deferasirox and midazolam (a CYP3A4 probe substrate) resulted in a decrease of midazolam peak concentration by 23% and exposure by 17%. In the clinical setting, this effect may be more pronounced. Therefore, due to a possible decrease in CYP3A4 substrate concentration and potential loss of effectiveness, caution should be observed when deferasirox is administered with drugs metabolized by CYP3A4 (eg, cyclosporine, simvastatin, hormonal contraceptives)). Products include:
Tarka 534

Vinblastine Sulfate (Concomitant administration of deferasirox and midazolam (a CYP3A4 probe substrate) resulted in a decrease of midazolam peak concentration by 23% and exposure by 17%. In the clinical setting, this effect may be more pronounced. Therefore, due to a possible decrease in CYP3A4 substrate concentration and potential loss of effectiveness, caution should be observed when deferasirox is administered with drugs metabolized by CYP3A4 (eg, cyclosporine, simvastatin, hormonal contraceptives)).
No products indexed under this heading.

Vincristine Sulfate (Concomitant administration of deferasirox and midazolam (a CYP3A4 probe substrate) resulted in a decrease of midazolam peak concentration by 23% and exposure by 17%. In the clinical setting, this effect may be more pronounced. Therefore, due to a possible decrease in CYP3A4 substrate concentration and potential loss of effectiveness, caution should be observed when deferasirox is

administered with drugs metabolized by CYP3A4 (eg, cyclosporine, simvastatin, hormonal contraceptives)).
No products indexed under this heading.

Vitamin A (Concomitant administration of deferasirox and the CYP2C8 probe substrate repaglinide (single dose of 0.5 mg) resulted in an increase in repaglinide systemic exposure (AUC) to 2.3 fold of control and an increase in C_{max} of 62%. If deferasirox and repaglinide are used concomitantly, decreasing the dose of repaglinide should be considered and careful monitoring of blood glucose levels should be performed. Caution should be exercised when deferasirox and other CYP2C8 substrates like paclitaxel are co-administered). Products include:
Cardio Basics 3455
Heplive 607
Norwegian Cod Liver Oil 919

Vitamin A Acetate (Concomitant administration of deferasirox and the CYP2C8 probe substrate repaglinide (single dose of 0.5 mg) resulted in an increase in repaglinide systemic exposure (AUC) to 2.3 fold of control and an increase in C_{max} of 62%. If deferasirox and repaglinide are used concomitantly, decreasing the dose of repaglinide should be considered and careful monitoring of blood glucose levels should be performed. Caution should be exercised when deferasirox and other CYP2C8 substrates like paclitaxel are co-administered).
No products indexed under this heading.

Voriconazole (Deferasirox inhibits human CYP2C19 in vitro).
No products indexed under this heading.

Warfarin Sodium (Caution should be observed when administering deferasirox in combination with drugs that have ulcerogenic or hemorrhagic potential, such as anticoagulants).
No products indexed under this heading.

Zileuton (Deferasirox inhibits human CYP1A2 in vitro).
No products indexed under this heading.

Zolmitriptan (Deferasirox inhibits human CYP1A2 in vitro). Products include:
Zomig Tablets 773
Zomig Nasal Spray 768
Zomig-ZMT Tablets 773

Zonisamide (Deferasirox inhibits human CYP2D6 in vitro). Products include:
Zonegran 1081

Zopiclone (Concomitant administration of deferasirox and the CYP2C8 probe substrate repaglinide (single dose of 0.5 mg) resulted in an increase in repaglinide systemic exposure (AUC) to 2.3 fold of control and an increase in C_{max} of 62%. If deferasirox and repaglinide are used concomitantly, decreasing the dose of repaglinide should be considered and careful monitoring of blood glucose levels should be performed. Caution should be exercised when deferasirox and other CYP2C8 substrates like paclitaxel are co-administered).
No products indexed under this heading.

Food Interactions

Food, caffeine-containing (Deferasirox inhibits human CYP1A2 in vitro).

EXTAVIA KIT
(Interferon Beta-1b) 2459
None cited in PDR database.

EXTINA FOAM, 2%
(Ketoconazole) 3319
None cited in PDR database.

EXUBERA INHALATION POWDER
(Insulin, Human (rDNA origin)) 2717

May interact with ACE inhibitors, alcohols, beta-blockers, corticosteroids, diuretics, estrogens, fibrates, lithium preparations, monoamine oxidase inhibitors, oral contraceptives, oral hypoglycemic agents, phenothiazines, progestins, protease inhibitors, salicylates, sympathomimetic aerosol bronchodilators, sympathomimetic bronchodilators, sympathomimetics, thyroid preparations, and certain other agents. Compounds in these categories include:

Acarbose (Oral antidiabetic products may increase the blood glucose-lowering effect of insulin and susceptibility to hypoglycemia. Co-administration may require insulin dose adjustment and particularly close monitoring).
No products indexed under this heading.

Acebutolol Hydrochloride (Beta-blockers may either increase or reduce the blood glucose-lowering effect of insulin. In addition, under the influence of sympatholytic medicinal products such as beta-blockers, the signs and symptoms of hypoglycemia may be reduced or absent. Co-administration may require insulin dose adjustment and particularly close monitoring).
No products indexed under this heading.

Albuterol (Sympathomimetics may reduce the blood glucose-lowering effect of insulin, which may result in hyperglycemia. Co-administration may require insulin dose adjustment and particularly close monitoring).
No products indexed under this heading.

Albuterol Sulfate (Sympathomimetics may reduce the blood glucose-lowering effect of insulin, which may result in hyperglycemia. Co-administration may require insulin dose adjustment and particularly close monitoring). Products include:
ProAir HFA 3393
Proventil HFA 3204
Ventolin HFA 1708

Alclometasone Dipropionate (Corticosteroids may reduce the blood glucose-lowering effect of insulin, which may result in hyperglycemia. Co-administration may require insulin dose adjustment and particularly close monitoring).
No products indexed under this heading.

Amiloride Hydrochloride (Diuretics may reduce the blood glucose-lowering effect of insulin, which may result in hyperglycemia. Co-administration may require insulin dose adjustment and particularly close monitoring).
No products indexed under this heading.

Amprenavir (Protease inhibitors may reduce the blood glucose-lowering effect of insulin, which may result in hyperglycemia. Co-administration may require insulin dose adjustment and particularly close monitoring).
No products indexed under this heading.

Aspirin (Salicylates may increase the blood glucose-lowering effect of insulin and susceptibility to hypoglycemia. Co-administration may require insulin dose adjustment and particularly close monitoring). Products include:
Aggrenox 880
Bayer Aspirin 829
Percodan 1124
St. Joseph Aspirin 2045

Aspirin, Enteric Coated (Salicylates may increase the blood glucose-lowering effect of insulin and susceptibility to hypoglycemia. Co-administration may require insulin dose adjustment and particularly close monitoring).
No products indexed under this heading.

Aspirin Buffered (Salicylates may increase the blood glucose-lowering effect of insulin and susceptibility to hypoglycemia. Co-administration may require insulin dose adjustment and particularly close monitoring).
No products indexed under this heading.

Atazanavir (Protease inhibitors may reduce the blood glucose-lowering effect of insulin, which may result in hyperglycemia. Co-administration may require insulin dose adjustment and particularly close monitoring).
No products indexed under this heading.

Atazanavir Sulfate (Protease inhibitors may reduce the blood glucose-lowering effect of insulin, which may result in hyperglycemia. Co-administration may require insulin dose adjustment and particularly close monitoring).
No products indexed under this heading.

Atenolol (Beta-blockers may either increase or reduce the blood glucose-lowering effect of insulin. In addition, under the influence of sympatholytic medicinal products such as beta-blockers, the signs and symptoms of hypoglycemia may be reduced or absent. Co-administration may require insulin dose adjustment and particularly close monitoring).
No products indexed under this heading.

Beclomethasone Dipropionate (Corticosteroids may reduce the blood glucose-lowering effect of insulin, which may result in hyperglycemia. Co-administration may require insulin dose adjustment and particularly close monitoring). Products include:
Qvar 3398

Beclomethasone Dipropionate Monohydrate (Corticosteroids may reduce the blood glucose-lowering effect of insulin, which may result in hyperglycemia. Co-administration may require insulin dose adjustment and particularly close monitoring). Products include:
Beconase AQ 1386

Benazepril Hydrochloride (ACE inhibitors may increase the blood glucose-lowering effect of insulin and susceptibility to hypoglycemia. Co-administration may require insulin dose adjustment and particularly close monitoring).
No products indexed under this heading.

Bendroflumethiazide (Diuretics may reduce the blood glucose-lowering effect of insulin, which may result in hyperglycemia. Co-administration may require insulin dose adjustment and particularly close monitoring).
No products indexed under this heading.

Betamethasone (Corticosteroids may reduce the blood glucose-lowering effect of insulin, which may result in hyperglycemia. Co-administration may require insulin dose adjustment and particularly close monitoring).
No products indexed under this heading.

Betamethasone Acetate (Corticosteroids may reduce the blood glucose-lowering effect of insulin, which may result in hyperglycemia. Co-administration may require insulin dose adjustment and particularly close monitoring).
No products indexed under this heading.

Betamethasone Benzoate (Corticosteroids may reduce the blood glucose-lowering effect of insulin, which may result in hyperglycemia. Co-administration may require insulin dose adjustment and particularly close monitoring).
No products indexed under this heading.

Betamethasone Dipropionate (Corticosteroids may reduce the blood glucose-lowering effect of insulin, which

may result in hyperglycemia. Co-administration may require insulin dose adjustment and particularly close monitoring). Products include:

Diprolene Lotion 0.05%	3108
Diprolene Ointment 0.05%	3109
Diprolene AF Cream 0.05%	3107
Lotrisone	3163

Betamethasone Sodium Phosphate (Corticosteroids may reduce the blood glucose-lowering effect of insulin, which may result in hyperglycemia. Co-administration may require insulin dose adjustment and particularly close monitoring).
No products indexed under this heading.

Betamethasone Valerate (Corticosteroids may reduce the blood glucose-lowering effect of insulin, which may result in hyperglycemia. Co-administration may require insulin dose adjustment and particularly close monitoring). Products include:

Luxiq	3321

Betaxolol Hydrochloride (Beta-blockers may either increase or reduce the blood glucose-lowering effect of insulin. In addition, under the influence of sympatholytic medicinal products such as beta-blockers, the signs and symptoms of hypoglycemia may be reduced or absent. Co-administration may require insulin dose adjustment and particularly close monitoring).
No products indexed under this heading.

Bisoprolol Fumarate (Beta-blockers may either increase or reduce the blood glucose-lowering effect of insulin. In addition, under the influence of sympatholytic medicinal products such as beta-blockers, the signs and symptoms of hypoglycemia may be reduced or absent. Co-administration may require insulin dose adjustment and particularly close monitoring).
No products indexed under this heading.

Bitolterol Mesylate (Bronchodilators and other inhaled products may alter the absorption of inhaled human insulin. Consistent timing of dosing of bronchodilators relative to Exubera administration, close monitoring of blood glucose concentrations, and dose titration as appropriate are recommended. Co-administration may require insulin dose adjustment and particularly close monitoring).
No products indexed under this heading.

Budesonide (Corticosteroids may reduce the blood glucose-lowering effect of insulin, which may result in hyperglycemia. Co-administration may require insulin dose adjustment and particularly close monitoring). Products include:

Pulmicort Flexhaler	714
Symbicort 80/4.5	720
Symbicort 160/4.5	720

Bumetanide (Diuretics may reduce the blood glucose-lowering effect of insulin, which may result in hyperglycemia. Co-administration may require insulin dose adjustment and particularly close monitoring).
No products indexed under this heading.

Captopril (ACE inhibitors may increase the blood glucose-lowering effect of insulin and susceptibility to hypoglycemia. Co-administration may require insulin dose adjustment and particularly close monitoring). Products include:

Captopril	2341

Carteolol Hydrochloride (Beta-blockers may either increase or reduce the blood glucose-lowering effect of insulin. In addition, under the influence of sympatholytic medicinal products such as beta-blockers, the signs and symptoms of hypoglycemia may be reduced or absent. Co-administration may require insulin dose adjustment and particularly close monitoring).
No products indexed under this heading.

Carvedilol (Beta-blockers may either increase or reduce the blood glucose-lowering effect of insulin. In addition, under the influence of sympatholytic medicinal products such as beta-blockers, the signs and symptoms of hypoglycemia may be reduced or absent. Co-administration may require insulin dose adjustment and particularly close monitoring). Products include:

Coreg	1409

Carvedilol Phosphate (Beta-blockers may either increase or reduce the blood glucose-lowering effect of insulin. In addition, under the influence of sympatholytic medicinal products such as beta-blockers, the signs and symptoms of hypoglycemia may be reduced or absent. Co-administration may require insulin dose adjustment and particularly close monitoring). Products include:

Coreg CR	1416

Chlorothiazide (Diuretics may reduce the blood glucose-lowering effect of insulin, which may result in hyperglycemia. Co-administration may require insulin dose adjustment and particularly close monitoring).
No products indexed under this heading.

Chlorothiazide Sodium (Diuretics may reduce the blood glucose-lowering effect of insulin, which may result in hyperglycemia. Co-administration may require insulin dose adjustment and particularly close monitoring). Products include:

Diuril Intravenous	2009

Chlorotrianisene (Estrogents may reduce the blood glucose-lowering effect of insulin, which may result in hyperglycemia. Co-administration may require insulin dose adjustment and particularly close monitoring).
No products indexed under this heading.

Chlorpromazine (Phenothiazine derivatives may reduce the blood glucose-lowering effect of insulin, which may result in hyperglycemia. Co-administration may require insulin dose adjustment and particularly close monitoring).
No products indexed under this heading.

Chlorpromazine Hydrochloride (Phenothiazine derivatives may reduce the blood glucose-lowering effect of insulin, which may result in hyperglycemia. Co-administration may require insulin dose adjustment and particularly close monitoring).
No products indexed under this heading.

Chlorpropamide (Oral antidiabetic products may increase the blood glucose-lowering effect of insulin and susceptibility to hypoglycemia. Co-administration may require insulin dose adjustment and particularly close monitoring).
No products indexed under this heading.

Chlorthalidone (Diuretics may reduce the blood glucose-lowering effect of insulin, which may result in hyperglycemia. Co-administration may require insulin dose adjustment and particularly close monitoring). Products include:

Clorpres	2344

Choline Magnesium Trisalicylate (Salicylates may increase the blood glucose-lowering effect of insulin and susceptibility to hypoglycemia. Co-administration may require insulin dose adjustment and particularly close monitoring).
No products indexed under this heading.

Ciclesonide (Corticosteroids may reduce the blood glucose-lowering effect of insulin, which may result in hyperglycemia. Co-administration may require insulin dose adjustment and particularly close monitoring).
No products indexed under this heading.

Clofibrate (Fibrates may increase the blood glucose-lowering effect of insulin and susceptibility to hypoglycemia. Co-administration may require insulin dose adjustment and particularly close monitoring).
No products indexed under this heading.

Clonidine (Clonidine may either increase or reduce the blood glucose-lowering effect of insulin. In addition, under the influence of sympatholytic medicinal products such as clonidine, the signs and symptoms of hypoglycemia may be reduced or absent. In addition, under the influence of clonidine, the signs and symptoms of hypoglycemia may be reduced or absent. Co-administration may require insulin dose adjustment and particularly close monitoring). Products include:

Catapres-TTS	884

Clonidine Hydrochloride (Clonidine may either increase or reduce the blood glucose-lowering effect of insulin. In addition, under the influence of sympatholytic medicinal products such as clonidine, the signs and symptoms of hypoglycemia may be reduced or absent. In addition, under the influence of clonidine, the signs and symptoms of hypoglycemia may be reduced or absent. Co-administration may require insulin dose adjustment and particularly close monitoring). Products include:

Clorpres	2344

Clozapine (Atypical antipsychotics, such as clozapine, may reduce the blood glucose-lowering effect of insulin, which may result in hyperglycemia. Co-administration may require insulin dose adjustment and particularly close monitoring).
No products indexed under this heading.

Cortisone Acetate (Corticosteroids may reduce the blood glucose-lowering effect of insulin, which may result in hyperglycemia. Co-administration may require insulin dose adjustment and particularly close monitoring).
No products indexed under this heading.

Danazol (Danazol may reduce the blood glucose-lowering effect of insulin, which may result in hyperglycemia. Co-administration may require insulin dose adjustment and particularly close monitoring).
No products indexed under this heading.

Darunavir (Protease inhibitors may reduce the blood glucose-lowering effect of insulin, which may result in hyperglycemia. Co-administration may require insulin dose adjustment and particularly close monitoring).
No products indexed under this heading.

Desogestrel (Oral contraceptives may reduce the blood glucose-lowering effect of insulin, which may result in hyperglycemia. Co-administration may require insulin dose adjustment and particularly close monitoring).
No products indexed under this heading.

Desoximetasone (Corticosteroids may reduce the blood glucose-lowering effect of insulin, which may result in hyperglycemia. Co-administration may require insulin dose adjustment and particularly close monitoring).
No products indexed under this heading.

Dexamethasone (Corticosteroids may reduce the blood glucose-lowering effect of insulin, which may result in hyperglycemia. Co-administration may require insulin dose adjustment and particularly close monitoring). Products include:

Ciprodex	583
Ozurdex	☉223
Tobramycin and Dexamethasone Ophthalmic Suspension	☉251

Dexamethasone Acetate (Corticosteroids may reduce the blood glucose-lowering effect of insulin, which may result in hyperglycemia. Co-administration may require insulin dose adjustment and particularly close monitoring).
No products indexed under this heading.

Dexamethasone Phosphate (Corticosteroids may reduce the blood glucose-lowering effect of insulin, which may result in hyperglycemia. Co-administration may require insulin dose adjustment and particularly close monitoring).
No products indexed under this heading.

Dexamethasone Sodium (Corticosteroids may reduce the blood glucose-lowering effect of insulin, which may result in hyperglycemia. Co-administration may require insulin dose adjustment and particularly close monitoring).
No products indexed under this heading.

Dexamethasone Sodium Phosphate (Corticosteroids may reduce the blood glucose-lowering effect of insulin, which may result in hyperglycemia. Co-administration may require insulin dose adjustment and particularly close monitoring).
No products indexed under this heading.

Dexamethasone Sodium Phosphate Injection (Corticosteroids may reduce the blood glucose-lowering effect of insulin, which may result in hyperglycemia. Co-administration may require insulin dose adjustment and particularly close monitoring).
No products indexed under this heading.

Diazoxide (Diazoxide may reduce the blood glucose-lowering effect of insulin, which may result in hyperglycemia. Co-administration may require insulin dose adjustment and particularly close monitoring). Products include:

Proglycem	1179
Proglycem Suspension	1179

Dienestrol (Estrogents may reduce the blood glucose-lowering effect of insulin, which may result in hyperglycemia. Co-administration may require insulin dose adjustment and particularly close monitoring).
No products indexed under this heading.

Diethylstilbestrol (Estrogents may reduce the blood glucose-lowering effect of insulin, which may result in hyperglycemia. Co-administration may require insulin dose adjustment and particularly close monitoring).
No products indexed under this heading.

Diflorasone Diacetate (Corticosteroids may reduce the blood glucose-lowering effect of insulin, which may result in hyperglycemia. Co-administration may require insulin dose adjustment and particularly close monitoring).
No products indexed under this heading.

IMPORTANT NOTE: Always consult each drug listing in the patient's regimen for possible interactions.

Diflunisal (Salicylates may increase the blood glucose-lowering effect of insulin and susceptibility to hypoglycemia. Co-administration may require insulin dose adjustment and particularly close monitoring).
No products indexed under this heading.

Disopyramide (Disopyramide may increase the blood glucose-lowering effect of insulin and susceptibility to hypoglycemia. Co-administration may require insulin dose adjustment and particularly close monitoring).
No products indexed under this heading.

Disopyramide Phosphate (Disopyramide may increase the blood glucose-lowering effect of insulin and susceptibility to hypoglycemia. Co-administration may require insulin dose adjustment and particularly close monitoring).
No products indexed under this heading.

Dobutamine Hydrochloride (Sympathomimetics may reduce the blood glucose-lowering effect of insulin, which may result in hyperglycemia. Co-administration may require insulin dose adjustment and particularly close monitoring).
No products indexed under this heading.

Dopamine Hydrochloride (Sympathomimetics may reduce the blood glucose-lowering effect of insulin, which may result in hyperglycemia. Co-administration may require insulin dose adjustment and particularly close monitoring).
No products indexed under this heading.

Enalapril Maleate (ACE inhibitors may increase the blood glucose-lowering effect of insulin and susceptibility to hypoglycemia. Co-administration may require insulin dose adjustment and particularly close monitoring).
No products indexed under this heading.

Enalaprilat (ACE inhibitors may increase the blood glucose-lowering effect of insulin and susceptibility to hypoglycemia. Co-administration may require insulin dose adjustment and particularly close monitoring).
No products indexed under this heading.

Ephedrine Hydrochloride (Sympathomimetics may reduce the blood glucose-lowering effect of insulin, which may result in hyperglycemia. Co-administration may require insulin dose adjustment and particularly close monitoring).
No products indexed under this heading.

Ephedrine Sulfate (Sympathomimetics may reduce the blood glucose-lowering effect of insulin, which may result in hyperglycemia. Co-administration may require insulin dose adjustment and particularly close monitoring).
No products indexed under this heading.

Ephedrine Tannate (Sympathomimetics may reduce the blood glucose-lowering effect of insulin, which may result in hyperglycemia. Co-administration may require insulin dose adjustment and particularly close monitoring).
No products indexed under this heading.

Epinephrine (Sympathomimetics may reduce the blood glucose-lowering effect of insulin, which may result in hyperglycemia. Co-administration may require insulin dose adjustment and particularly close monitoring). Products include:

Epinephrine Bitartrate (Sympathomimetics may reduce the blood glucose-lowering effect of insulin, which may result in hyperglycemia. Co-administration may require insulin dose adjustment and particularly close monitoring).
No products indexed under this heading.

Epinephrine Hydrochloride (Sympathomimetics may reduce the blood glucose-lowering effect of insulin, which may result in hyperglycemia. Co-administration may require insulin dose adjustment and particularly close monitoring).
No products indexed under this heading.

Esmolol Hydrochloride (Beta-blockers may either increase or reduce the blood glucose-lowering effect of insulin. In addition, under the influence of sympatholytic medicinal products such as beta-blockers, the signs and symptoms of hypoglycemia may be reduced or absent. Co-administration may require insulin dose adjustment and particularly close monitoring).
No products indexed under this heading.

Estradiol (Estrogens may reduce the blood glucose-lowering effect of insulin, which may result in hyperglycemia. Co-administration may require insulin dose adjustment and particularly close monitoring). Products include:

Estrogens, Conjugated (Estrogens may reduce the blood glucose-lowering effect of insulin, which may result in hyperglycemia. Co-administration may require insulin dose adjustment and particularly close monitoring). Products include:

Estrogens, Esterified (Estrogens may reduce the blood glucose-lowering effect of insulin, which may result in hyperglycemia. Co-administration may require insulin dose adjustment and particularly close monitoring).
No products indexed under this heading.

Estropipate (Estrogens may reduce the blood glucose-lowering effect of insulin, which may result in hyperglycemia. Co-administration may require insulin dose adjustment and particularly close monitoring).
No products indexed under this heading.

Ethacrynic Acid (Diuretics may reduce the blood glucose-lowering effect of insulin, which may result in hyperglycemia. Co-administration may require insulin dose adjustment and particularly close monitoring).
No products indexed under this heading.

Ethanol (Alcohol may either increase or reduce the blood glucose-lowering effect of insulin. Co-administration may require insulin dose adjustment and particularly close monitoring).
No products indexed under this heading.

Ethinyl Estradiol (Oral contraceptives may reduce the blood glucose-lowering effect of insulin, which may result in hyperglycemia. Co-administration may require insulin dose adjustment and particularly close monitoring). Products include:

Ethyl Alcohol (Alcohol may either increase or reduce the blood glucose-lowering effect of insulin. Co-administration may require insulin dose adjustment and particularly close monitoring).
No products indexed under this heading.

Ethynodiol Diacetate (Oral contraceptives may reduce the blood glucose-lowering effect of insulin, which may result in hyperglycemia. Co-administration may require insulin dose adjustment and particularly close monitoring).
No products indexed under this heading.

Fenofibrate (Fibrates may increase the blood glucose-lowering effect of insulin and susceptibility to hypoglycemia. Co-administration may require insulin dose adjustment and particularly close monitoring). Products include:

Fludrocortisone Acetate (Corticosteroids may reduce the blood glucose-lowering effect of insulin, which may result in hyperglycemia. Co-administration may require insulin dose adjustment and particularly close monitoring).
No products indexed under this heading.

Flumethasone Pivalate (Corticosteroids may reduce the blood glucose-lowering effect of insulin, which may result in hyperglycemia. Co-administration may require insulin dose adjustment and particularly close monitoring).
No products indexed under this heading.

Flunisolide Hemihydrate (Corticosteroids may reduce the blood glucose-lowering effect of insulin, which may result in hyperglycemia. Co-administration may require insulin dose adjustment and particularly close monitoring).
No products indexed under this heading.

Fluoxetine (Fluoxetine may increase the blood glucose-lowering effect of insulin and susceptibility to hypoglycemia. Co-administration may require insulin dose adjustment and particularly close monitoring).
No products indexed under this heading.

Fluoxetine Hydrochloride (Fluoxetine may increase the blood glucose-lowering effect of insulin and susceptibility to hypoglycemia. Co-administration may require insulin dose adjustment and particularly close monitoring). Products include:

Fluphenazine Decanoate (Phenothiazine derivatives may reduce the blood glucose-lowering effect of insulin, which may result in hyperglycemia. Co-administration may require insulin dose adjustment and particularly close monitoring).
No products indexed under this heading.

Fluphenazine Enanthate (Phenothiazine derivatives may reduce the blood glucose-lowering effect of insulin, which may result in hyperglycemia. Co-administration may require insulin dose adjustment and particularly close monitoring).
No products indexed under this heading.

Fluphenazine Hydrochloride (Phenothiazine derivatives may reduce the blood glucose-lowering effect of insulin, which may result in hyperglycemia. Co-administration may require insulin dose adjustment and particularly close monitoring).
No products indexed under this heading.

Fluticasone Furoate (Corticosteroids may reduce the blood glucose-lowering effect of insulin, which may result in hyperglycemia. Co-administration may require insulin dose adjustment and particularly close monitoring). Products include:

Fluticasone Propionate (Corticosteroids may reduce the blood glucose-lowering effect of insulin, which may result in hyperglycemia. Co-administration may require insulin dose adjustment and particularly close monitoring). Products include:

Fosamprenavir Calcium (Protease inhibitors may reduce the blood glucose-lowering effect of insulin, which may result in hyperglycemia. Co-administration may require insulin dose adjustment and particularly close monitoring). Products include:

Fosinopril Sodium (ACE inhibitors may increase the blood glucose-lowering effect of insulin and susceptibility to hypoglycemia. Co-administration may require insulin dose adjustment and particularly close monitoring).
No products indexed under this heading.

Furosemide (Diuretics may reduce the blood glucose-lowering effect of insulin, which may result in hyperglycemia. Co-administration may require insulin dose adjustment and particularly close monitoring). Products include:

Gemfibrozil (Fibrates may increase the blood glucose-lowering effect of insulin and susceptibility to hypoglycemia. Co-administration may require insulin dose adjustment and particularly close monitoring).
No products indexed under this heading.

Glibenclamide (Oral antidiabetic products may increase the blood glucose-lowering effect of insulin and susceptibility to hypoglycemia. Co-administration may require insulin dose adjustment and particularly close monitoring).
No products indexed under this heading.

Glimepiride (Oral antidiabetic products may increase the blood glucose-lowering effect of insulin and susceptibility to hypoglycemia. Co-administration may require insulin dose adjustment and particularly close monitoring). Products include:

Glipizide (Oral antidiabetic products may increase the blood glucose-lowering effect of insulin and susceptibility to hypoglycemia. Co-administration may require insulin dose adjustment and particularly close monitoring).
No products indexed under this heading.

Glucagon (Glucagon may reduce the blood glucose-lowering effect of insulin, which may result in hyperglycemia. Co-

641 **Interactions Index** **Exubera**

administration may require insulin dose adjustment and particularly close monitoring). Products include:
Glucagon for Injection 1908

Glyburide (Oral antidiabetic products may increase the blood glucose-lowering effect of insulin and susceptibility to hypoglycemia. Co-administration may require insulin dose adjustment and particularly close monitoring).
No products indexed under this heading.

Guanethidine (Under the influence of sympatholytic medicinal products, such as guanethidine, the signs and symptoms of hypoglycemia may be reduced or absent. Co-administration may require insulin dose adjustment and particularly close monitoring).
No products indexed under this heading.

Guanethidine Monosulfate (Under the influence of sympatholytic medicinal products, such as guanethidine, the signs and symptoms of hypoglycemia may be reduced or absent. Co-administration may require insulin dose adjustment and particularly close monitoring).
No products indexed under this heading.

Guanethidine Sulfate (Under the influence of sympatholytic medicinal products, such as guanethidine, the signs and symptoms of hypoglycemia may be reduced or absent. Co-administration may require insulin dose adjustment and particularly close monitoring).
No products indexed under this heading.

Hydrochlorothiazide (Diuretics may reduce the blood glucose-lowering effect of insulin, which may result in hyperglycemia. Co-administration may require insulin dose adjustment and particularly close monitoring). Products include:
Atacand HCT 700
Avalide 2956
Benicar HCT 1017
Diovan HCT 2419
Dyazide 1429
Exforge HCT 2449
Hyzaar 2162
Hyzaar 100-12.5 2162
Micardis HCT 889
Prinzide 2246
Tekturna HCT 2541
Teveten HCT 541

Hydrocortisone (Corticosteroids may reduce the blood glucose-lowering effect of insulin, which may result in hyperglycemia. Co-administration may require insulin dose adjustment and particularly close monitoring).
No products indexed under this heading.

Hydrocortisone (Alcohol) (Corticosteroids may reduce the blood glucose-lowering effect of insulin, which may result in hyperglycemia. Co-administration may require insulin dose adjustment and particularly close monitoring).
No products indexed under this heading.

Hydrocortisone Acetate (Corticosteroids may reduce the blood glucose-lowering effect of insulin, which may result in hyperglycemia. Co-administration may require insulin dose adjustment and particularly close monitoring).
No products indexed under this heading.

Hydrocortisone Butyrate (Corticosteroids may reduce the blood glucose-lowering effect of insulin, which may result in hyperglycemia. Co-administration may require insulin dose adjustment and particularly close monitoring).
No products indexed under this heading.

Hydrocortisone Cypionate (Corticosteroids may reduce the blood glucose-lowering effect of insulin, which may result in hyperglycemia. Co-administration may require insulin dose adjustment and particularly close monitoring).
No products indexed under this heading.

Hydrocortisone Hemisuccinate (Corticosteroids may reduce the blood glucose-lowering effect of insulin, which may result in hyperglycemia. Co-administration may require insulin dose adjustment and particularly close monitoring).
No products indexed under this heading.

Hydrocortisone Probutate (Corticosteroids may reduce the blood glucose-lowering effect of insulin, which may result in hyperglycemia. Co-administration may require insulin dose adjustment and particularly close monitoring).
No products indexed under this heading.

Hydrocortisone Sodium Phosphate (Corticosteroids may reduce the blood glucose-lowering effect of insulin, which may result in hyperglycemia. Co-administration may require insulin dose adjustment and particularly close monitoring).
No products indexed under this heading.

Hydrocortisone Sodium Succinate (Corticosteroids may reduce the blood glucose-lowering effect of insulin, which may result in hyperglycemia. Co-administration may require insulin dose adjustment and particularly close monitoring).
No products indexed under this heading.

Hydrocortisone Valerate (Corticosteroids may reduce the blood glucose-lowering effect of insulin, which may result in hyperglycemia. Co-administration may require insulin dose adjustment and particularly close monitoring).
No products indexed under this heading.

Hydroflumethiazide (Diuretics may reduce the blood glucose-lowering effect of insulin, which may result in hyperglycemia. Co-administration may require insulin dose adjustment and particularly close monitoring).
No products indexed under this heading.

Indapamide (Diuretics may reduce the blood glucose-lowering effect of insulin, which may result in hyperglycemia. Co-administration may require insulin dose adjustment and particularly close monitoring). Products include:
Indapamide 2356

Indinavir Sulfate (Protease inhibitors may reduce the blood glucose-lowering effect of insulin, which may result in hyperglycemia. Co-administration may require insulin dose adjustment and particularly close monitoring). Products include:
Crixivan 2113

Isocarboxazid (MAO inhibitors may increase the blood glucose-lowering effect of insulin and susceptibility to hypoglycemia. Co-administration may require insulin dose adjustment and particularly close monitoring). Products include:
Marplan 3481

Isoetharine (Bronchodilators and other inhaled products may alter the absorption of inhaled human insulin. Consistent timing of dosing of bronchodilators relative to Exubera administration, close monitoring of blood glucose concentrations, and dose titration as appropriate are recommended. Co-administration may require insulin dose adjustment and particularly close monitoring).
No products indexed under this heading.

Isoniazid (Isoniazid may reduce the blood glucose-lowering effect of insulin, which may result in hyperglycemia. Co-administration may require insulin dose adjustment and particularly close monitoring).
No products indexed under this heading.

Isoproterenol Hydrochloride (Sympathomimetics may reduce the blood glucose-lowering effect of insulin, which may result in hyperglycemia. Co-administration may require insulin dose adjustment and particularly close monitoring).
No products indexed under this heading.

Isoproterenol Sulfate (Sympathomimetics may reduce the blood glucose-lowering effect of insulin, which may result in hyperglycemia. Co-administration may require insulin dose adjustment and particularly close monitoring).
No products indexed under this heading.

Labetalol Hydrochloride (Beta-blockers may either increase or reduce the blood glucose-lowering effect of insulin. In addition, under the influence of sympatholytic medicinal products such as beta-blockers, the signs and symptoms of hypoglycemia may be reduced or absent. Co-administration may require insulin dose adjustment and particularly close monitoring).
No products indexed under this heading.

Levalbuterol Hydrochloride (Sympathomimetics may reduce the blood glucose-lowering effect of insulin, which may result in hyperglycemia. Co-administration may require insulin dose adjustment and particularly close monitoring).
No products indexed under this heading.

Levobunolol Hydrochloride (Beta-blockers may either increase or reduce the blood glucose-lowering effect of insulin. In addition, under the influence of sympatholytic medicinal products such as beta-blockers, the signs and symptoms of hypoglycemia may be reduced or absent. Co-administration may require insulin dose adjustment and particularly close monitoring).
No products indexed under this heading.

Levonorgestrel (Oral contraceptives may reduce the blood glucose-lowering effect of insulin, which may result in hyperglycemia. Co-administration may require insulin dose adjustment and particularly close monitoring). Products include:
Climara Pro 847
LoSeasonique 3407
Lybrel 3514
Mirena 854
Plan B 3416
Seasonique 3418

Levothyroxine Sodium (Thyroid hormones may reduce the blood glucose-lowering effect of insulin, which may result in hyperglycemia. Co-administration may require insulin dose adjustment and particularly close monitoring). Products include:
Levoxyl Tablets 1843
Synthroid 529

Liothyronine Sodium (Thyroid hormones may reduce the blood glucose-lowering effect of insulin, which may result in hyperglycemia. Co-administration may require insulin dose adjustment and particularly close monitoring). Products include:
Cytomel 1830

Liotrix (Thyroid hormones may reduce the blood glucose-lowering effect of insulin, which may result in hyperglycemia. Co-administration may require insulin dose adjustment and particularly close monitoring).
No products indexed under this heading.

Lisinopril (ACE inhibitors may increase the blood glucose-lowering effect of insulin and susceptibility to hypoglycemia. Co-administration may require insulin dose adjustment and particularly close monitoring). Products include:
Prinivil 2241
Prinzide 2246

Lithium (Lithium salts may either increase or reduce the blood glucose-lowering effect of insulin. Co-administration may require insulin dose adjustment and particularly close monitoring).
No products indexed under this heading.

Lithium Carbonate (Lithium salts may either increase or reduce the blood glucose-lowering effect of insulin. Co-administration may require insulin dose adjustment and particularly close monitoring).
No products indexed under this heading.

Lithium Citrate (Lithium salts may either increase or reduce the blood glucose-lowering effect of insulin. Co-administration may require insulin dose adjustment and particularly close monitoring).
No products indexed under this heading.

Lopinavir (Protease inhibitors may reduce the blood glucose-lowering effect of insulin, which may result in hyperglycemia. Co-administration may require insulin dose adjustment and particularly close monitoring). Products include:
Kaletra 458

Magnesium Salicylate (Salicylates may increase the blood glucose-lowering effect of insulin and susceptibility to hypoglycemia. Co-administration may require insulin dose adjustment and particularly close monitoring).
No products indexed under this heading.

Medroxyprogesterone Acetate (Progestogens may reduce the blood glucose-lowering effect of insulin, which may result in hyperglycemia. Co-administration may require insulin dose adjustment and particularly close monitoring). Products include:
Premphase 3549
Prempro 3549

Megestrol Acetate (Progestogens may reduce the blood glucose-lowering effect of insulin, which may result in hyperglycemia. Co-administration may require insulin dose adjustment and particularly close monitoring). Products include:
Megace ES 2698

Mesoridazine Besylate (Phenothiazine derivatives may reduce the blood glucose-lowering effect of insulin, which may result in hyperglycemia. Co-administration may require insulin dose adjustment and particularly close monitoring).
No products indexed under this heading.

Mestranol (Oral contraceptives may reduce the blood glucose-lowering effect of insulin, which may result in hyperglycemia. Co-administration may require insulin dose adjustment and particularly close monitoring).
No products indexed under this heading.

Metaproterenol Sulfate (Sympathomimetics may reduce the blood glucose-lowering effect of insulin, which may result in hyperglycemia. Co-administration may require insulin dose adjustment and particularly close monitoring).
No products indexed under this heading.

IMPORTANT NOTE: Always consult each drug listing in the patient's regimen for possible interactions.

Metaraminol Bitartrate (Sympathomimetics may reduce the blood glucose-lowering effect of insulin, which may result in hyperglycemia. Co-administration may require insulin dose adjustment and particularly close monitoring).
No products indexed under this heading.

Metformin Hydrochloride (Oral antidiabetic products may increase the blood glucose-lowering effect of insulin and susceptibility to hypoglycemia. Co-administration may require insulin dose adjustment and particularly close monitoring). Products include:
ActoPlus 3338
Avandamet 1345
Janumet 2188

Methotrimeprazine (Phenothiazine derivatives may reduce the blood glucose-lowering effect of insulin, which may result in hyperglycemia. Co-administration may require insulin dose adjustment and particularly close monitoring).
No products indexed under this heading.

Methoxamine Hydrochloride (Sympathomimetics may reduce the blood glucose-lowering effect of insulin, which may result in hyperglycemia. Co-administration may require insulin dose adjustment and particularly close monitoring).
No products indexed under this heading.

Methyclothiazide (Diuretics may reduce the blood glucose-lowering effect of insulin, which may result in hyperglycemia. Co-administration may require insulin dose adjustment and particularly close monitoring).
No products indexed under this heading.

Methylprednisolone (Corticosteroids may reduce the blood glucose-lowering effect of insulin, which may result in hyperglycemia. Co-administration may require insulin dose adjustment and particularly close monitoring).
No products indexed under this heading.

Methylprednisolone Acetate (Corticosteroids may reduce the blood glucose-lowering effect of insulin, which may result in hyperglycemia. Co-administration may require insulin dose adjustment and particularly close monitoring).
No products indexed under this heading.

Methylprednisolone Sodium Succinate (Corticosteroids may reduce the blood glucose-lowering effect of insulin, which may result in hyperglycemia. Co-administration may require insulin dose adjustment and particularly close monitoring).
No products indexed under this heading.

Metipranolol Hydrochloride (Beta-blockers may either increase or reduce the blood glucose-lowering effect of insulin. In addition, under the influence of sympatholytic medicinal products such as beta-blockers, the signs and symptoms of hypoglycemia may be reduced or absent. Co-administration may require insulin dose adjustment and particularly close monitoring).
No products indexed under this heading.

Metolazone (Diuretics may reduce the blood glucose-lowering effect of insulin, which may result in hyperglycemia. Co-administration may require insulin dose adjustment and particularly close monitoring).
No products indexed under this heading.

Metoprolol Succinate (Beta-blockers may either increase or reduce the blood glucose-lowering effect of insulin. In addition, under the influence of sympatholytic medicinal products such as beta-blockers, the signs and symptoms of hypoglycemia may be reduced or absent. Co-administration may require insulin dose adjustment and particularly close monitoring). Products include:
Toprol XL 732

Metoprolol Tartrate (Beta-blockers may either increase or reduce the blood glucose-lowering effect of insulin. In addition, under the influence of sympatholytic medicinal products such as beta-blockers, the signs and symptoms of hypoglycemia may be reduced or absent. Co-administration may require insulin dose adjustment and particularly close monitoring).
No products indexed under this heading.

Miglitol (Oral antidiabetic products may increase the blood glucose-lowering effect of insulin and susceptibility to hypoglycemia. Co-administration may require insulin dose adjustment and particularly close monitoring).
No products indexed under this heading.

Moclobemide (MAO inhibitors may increase the blood glucose-lowering effect of insulin and susceptibility to hypoglycemia. Co-administration may require insulin dose adjustment and particularly close monitoring).
No products indexed under this heading.

Moexipril Hydrochloride (ACE inhibitors may increase the blood glucose-lowering effect of insulin and susceptibility to hypoglycemia.
Co-administration may require insulin dose adjustment and particularly close monitoring).
No products indexed under this heading.

Mometasone Furoate (Corticosteroids may reduce the blood glucose-lowering effect of insulin, which may result in hyperglycemia. Co-administration may require insulin dose adjustment and particularly close monitoring). Products include:
Asmanex 3058
Elocon Cream 3111
Elocon Lotion 3112
Elocon Ointment 3114

Mometasone Furoate Monohydrate (Corticosteroids may reduce the blood glucose-lowering effect of insulin, which may result in hyperglycemia. Co-administration may require insulin dose adjustment and particularly close monitoring). Products include:
Nasonex 3166

Nadolol (Beta-blockers may either increase or reduce the blood glucose-lowering effect of insulin. In addition, under the influence of sympatholytic medicinal products such as beta-blockers, the signs and symptoms of hypoglycemia may be reduced or absent. Co-administration may require insulin dose adjustment and particularly close monitoring). Products include:
Nadolol 2359

Nateglinide (Oral antidiabetic products may increase the blood glucose-lowering effect of insulin and susceptibility to hypoglycemia.
Co-administration may require insulin dose adjustment and particularly close monitoring).
No products indexed under this heading.

Nebivolol (Beta-blockers may either increase or reduce the blood glucose-lowering effect of insulin. In addition, under the influence of sympatholytic medicinal products such as beta-blockers, the signs and symptoms of hypoglycemia may be reduced or absent. Co-administration may require insulin dose adjustment and particularly close monitoring). Products include:
Bystolic 1147

Nelfinavir Mesylate (Protease inhibitors may reduce the blood glucose-lowering effect of insulin, which may result in hyperglycemia. Co-administration may require insulin dose adjustment and particularly close monitoring).
No products indexed under this heading.

Norepinephrine Bitartrate (Sympathomimetics may reduce the blood glucose-lowering effect of insulin, which may result in hyperglycemia. Co-administration may require insulin dose adjustment and particularly close monitoring).
No products indexed under this heading.

Norethindrone (Oral contraceptives may reduce the blood glucose-lowering effect of insulin, which may result in hyperglycemia. Co-administration may require insulin dose adjustment and particularly close monitoring). Products include:
Ortho Micronor 2660

Norethindrone Acetate (Progestogens may reduce the blood glucose-lowering effect of insulin, which may result in hyperglycemia. Co-administration may require insulin dose adjustment and particularly close monitoring). Products include:
Activella 2561

Norethynodrel (Oral contraceptives may reduce the blood glucose-lowering effect of insulin, which may result in hyperglycemia. Co-administration may require insulin dose adjustment and particularly close monitoring).
No products indexed under this heading.

Norgestimate (Oral contraceptives may reduce the blood glucose-lowering effect of insulin, which may result in hyperglycemia. Co-administration may require insulin dose adjustment and particularly close monitoring). Products include:
Ortho-Cyclen/Ortho Tri-Cyclen 2663
Ortho Tri-Cyclen Lo Tablets 2673

Norgestrel (Oral contraceptives may reduce the blood glucose-lowering effect of insulin, which may result in hyperglycemia. Co-administration may require insulin dose adjustment and particularly close monitoring).
No products indexed under this heading.

Olanzapine (Atypical antipsychotics, such as olanzapine, may reduce the blood glucose-lowering effect of insulin, which may result in hyperglycemia. Co-administration may require insulin dose adjustment and particularly close monitoring). Products include:
Symbyax 1965
Zyprexa 1984
Zyprexa IntraMuscular 1984
Zyprexa ZYDIS 1984

Pargyline Hydrochloride (MAO inhibitors may increase the blood glucose-lowering effect of insulin and susceptibility to hypoglycemia. Co-administration may require insulin dose adjustment and particularly close monitoring).
No products indexed under this heading.

Penbutolol Sulfate (Beta-blockers may either increase or reduce the blood glucose-lowering effect of insulin. In addition, under the influence of sympatholytic medicinal products such as beta-blockers, the signs and symptoms of hypoglycemia may be reduced or absent. Co-administration may require insulin dose adjustment and particularly close monitoring).
No products indexed under this heading.

Pentamidine Isethionate (Pentamidine may cause hypoglycemia, which may sometimes be followed by hyperglycemia. Co-administration may require insulin dose adjustment and particularly close monitoring).
No products indexed under this heading.

Pentoxifylline (Pentoxifylline may increase the blood glucose-lowering effect of insulin and susceptibility to hypoglycemia. Co-administration may require insulin dose adjustment and particularly close monitoring).
No products indexed under this heading.

Perindopril Erbumine (ACE inhibitors may increase the blood glucose-lowering effect of insulin and susceptibility to hypoglycemia. Co-administration may require insulin dose adjustment and particularly close monitoring).
No products indexed under this heading.

Perphenazine (Phenothiazine derivatives may reduce the blood glucose-lowering effect of insulin, which may result in hyperglycemia. Co-administration may require insulin dose adjustment and particularly close monitoring).
No products indexed under this heading.

Phenelzine Sulfate (MAO inhibitors may increase the blood glucose-lowering effect of insulin and susceptibility to hypoglycemia. Co-administration may require insulin dose adjustment and particularly close monitoring).
No products indexed under this heading.

Phenothiazine Derivatives (Phenothiazine derivatives may reduce the blood glucose-lowering effect of insulin, which may result in hyperglycemia. Co-administration may require insulin dose adjustment and particularly close monitoring).
No products indexed under this heading.

Phenothiazines (Phenothiazine derivatives may reduce the blood glucose-lowering effect of insulin, which may result in hyperglycemia. Co-administration may require insulin dose adjustment and particularly close monitoring).
No products indexed under this heading.

Phenylephrine Bitartrate (Sympathomimetics may reduce the blood glucose-lowering effect of insulin, which may result in hyperglycemia. Co-administration may require insulin dose adjustment and particularly close monitoring).
No products indexed under this heading.

Phenylephrine Hydrochloride (Sympathomimetics may reduce the blood glucose-lowering effect of insulin, which may result in hyperglycemia. Co-administration may require insulin dose adjustment and particularly close monitoring). Products include:
Sudafed PE Nasal Decongestant 2048
Children's Sudafed PE Nasal Decongestant 2047

Phenylephrine Tannate (Sympathomimetics may reduce the blood glucose-lowering effect of insulin, which may result in hyperglycemia. Co-administration may require insulin dose adjustment and particularly close monitoring).
No products indexed under this heading.

Phenylpropanolamine Hydrochloride (Sympathomimetics may reduce the blood glucose-lowering effect of insulin, which may result in hyperglycemia. Co-administration may require insulin dose adjustment and particularly close monitoring).
No products indexed under this heading.

Pindolol (Beta-blockers may either increase or reduce the blood glucose-lowering effect of insulin. In addition, under the influence of sympatholytic medicinal products such as beta-blockers, the signs and symptoms of hypoglycemia may be reduced or absent. Co-administration may require insulin dose adjustment and particularly close monitoring).
No products indexed under this heading.

Pioglitazone Hydrochloride (Oral antidiabetic products may increase the blood glucose-lowering effect of insulin and susceptibility to hypoglycemia. Co-administration may require insulin dose adjustment and particularly close monitoring). Products include:

IMPORTANT NOTE: Always consult each drug listing in the patient's regimen for possible interactions.

Spironolactone (Diuretics may reduce the blood glucose-lowering effect of insulin, which may result in hyperglycemia. Co-administration may require insulin dose adjustment and particularly close monitoring).
No products indexed under this heading.

Sulfadiazine (Sulfonamide antibiotics may increase the blood glucose-lowering effect of insulin and susceptibility to hypoglycemia. Co-administration may require insulin dose adjustment and particularly close monitoring).
No products indexed under this heading.

Sulfamethizole (Sulfonamide antibiotics may increase the blood glucose-lowering effect of insulin and susceptibility to hypoglycemia. Co-administration may require insulin dose adjustment and particularly close monitoring).
No products indexed under this heading.

Sulfamethoprim (Sulfonamide antibiotics may increase the blood glucose-lowering effect of insulin and susceptibility to hypoglycemia. Co-administration may require insulin dose adjustment and particularly close monitoring).
No products indexed under this heading.

Sulfamethoxazole (Sulfonamide antibiotics may increase the blood glucose-lowering effect of insulin and susceptibility to hypoglycemia. Co-administration may require insulin dose adjustment and particularly close monitoring).
No products indexed under this heading.

Sulfisoxazole Acetyl (Sulfonamide antibiotics may increase the blood glucose-lowering effect of insulin and susceptibility to hypoglycemia. Co-administration may require insulin dose adjustment and particularly close monitoring).
No products indexed under this heading.

Sulfisoxazole Diolamine (Sulfonamide antibiotics may increase the blood glucose-lowering effect of insulin and susceptibility to hypoglycemia. Co-administration may require insulin dose adjustment and particularly close monitoring).
No products indexed under this heading.

Terbutaline Sulfate (Sympathomimetics may reduce the blood glucose-lowering effect of insulin, which may result in hyperglycemia. Co-administration may require insulin dose adjustment and particularly close monitoring).
No products indexed under this heading.

Thioridazine (Phenothiazine derivatives may reduce the blood glucose-lowering effect of insulin, which may result in hyperglycemia. Co-administration may require insulin dose adjustment and particularly close monitoring).
No products indexed under this heading.

Thioridazine Hydrochloride (Phenothiazine derivatives may reduce the blood glucose-lowering effect of insulin, which may result in hyperglycemia. Co-administration may require insulin dose adjustment and particularly close monitoring). Products include:
Thioridazine Hydrochloride 2384

Thyroglobulin (Thyroid hormones may reduce the blood glucose-lowering effect of insulin, which may result in hyperglycemia. Co-administration may require insulin dose adjustment and particularly close monitoring).
No products indexed under this heading.

Thyroid (Thyroid hormones may reduce the blood glucose-lowering effect of insulin, which may result in hyperglycemia. Co-administration may

require insulin dose adjustment and particularly close monitoring). Products include:
Naturethroid 2830

Thyroxine (Thyroid hormones may reduce the blood glucose-lowering effect of insulin, which may result in hyperglycemia. Co-administration may require insulin dose adjustment and particularly close monitoring).
No products indexed under this heading.

Thyroxine Sodium (Thyroid hormones may reduce the blood glucose-lowering effect of insulin, which may result in hyperglycemia. Co-administration may require insulin dose adjustment and particularly close monitoring).
No products indexed under this heading.

Timolol Hemihydrate (Beta-blockers may either increase or reduce the blood glucose-lowering effect of insulin. In addition, under the influence of sympatholytic medicinal products such as beta-blockers, the signs and symptoms of hypoglycemia may be reduced or absent. Co-administration may require insulin dose adjustment and particularly close monitoring). Products include:
Betimol 3490

Timolol Maleate (Beta-blockers may either increase or reduce the blood glucose-lowering effect of insulin. In addition, under the influence of sympatholytic medicinal products such as beta-blockers, the signs and symptoms of hypoglycemia may be reduced or absent. Co-administration may require insulin dose adjustment and particularly close monitoring). Products include:
Combigan 601
Dorzolamide
Hydrochloride/Timolol Maleate
Ophthalmic Solution .... ⊙243
Timoptic in Ocudose .... ⊙231

Tipranavir (Protease inhibitors may reduce the blood glucose-lowering effect of insulin, which may result in hyperglycemia. Co-administration may require insulin dose adjustment and particularly close monitoring).
No products indexed under this heading.

Tolazamide (Oral antidiabetic products may increase the blood glucose-lowering effect of insulin and susceptibility to hypoglycemia. Co-administration may require insulin dose adjustment and particularly close monitoring).
No products indexed under this heading.

Tolbutamide (Oral antidiabetic products may increase the blood glucose-lowering effect of insulin and susceptibility to hypoglycemia. Co-administration may require insulin dose adjustment and particularly close monitoring).
No products indexed under this heading.

Torsemide (Diuretics may reduce the blood glucose-lowering effect of insulin, which may result in hyperglycemia. Co-administration may require insulin dose adjustment and particularly close monitoring).
No products indexed under this heading.

Trandolapril (ACE inhibitors may increase the blood glucose-lowering effect of insulin and susceptibility to hypoglycemia. Co-administration may require insulin dose adjustment and particularly close monitoring). Products include:
Mavik 489
Tarka 534

Tranylcypromine Sulfate (MAO inhibitors may increase the blood glucose-lowering effect of insulin and susceptibility to hypoglycemia. Co-administration may require insulin dose adjustment and particularly close monitoring). Products include:

Parnate 1584

Triamcinolone (Corticosteroids may reduce the blood glucose-lowering effect of insulin, which may result in hyperglycemia. Co-administration may require insulin dose adjustment and particularly close monitoring).
No products indexed under this heading.

Triamcinolone Acetonide (Corticosteroids may reduce the blood glucose-lowering effect of insulin, which may result in hyperglycemia. Co-administration may require insulin dose adjustment and particularly close monitoring). Products include:
Azmacort 408
Nasacort AQ 3019

Triamcinolone Diacetate (Corticosteroids may reduce the blood glucose-lowering effect of insulin, which may result in hyperglycemia. Co-administration may require insulin dose adjustment and particularly close monitoring).
No products indexed under this heading.

Triamcinolone Hexacetonide (Corticosteroids may reduce the blood glucose-lowering effect of insulin, which may result in hyperglycemia. Co-administration may require insulin dose adjustment and particularly close monitoring).
No products indexed under this heading.

Triamterene (Diuretics may reduce the blood glucose-lowering effect of insulin, which may result in hyperglycemia. Co-administration may require insulin dose adjustment and particularly close monitoring). Products include:
Dyazide 1429
Dyrenium 3495

Trifluoperazine Hydrochloride (Phenothiazine derivatives may reduce the blood glucose-lowering effect of insulin, which may result in hyperglycemia. Co-administration may require insulin dose adjustment and particularly close monitoring).
No products indexed under this heading.

Troglitazone (Oral antidiabetic products may increase the blood glucose-lowering effect of insulin and susceptibility to hypoglycemia. Co-administration may require insulin dose adjustment and particularly close monitoring).
No products indexed under this heading.

Food Interactions

Alcohol (Alcohol may either increase or reduce the blood glucose-lowering effect of insulin. Co-administration may require insulin dose adjustment and particularly close monitoring).

Beer, reduced-alcohol (Alcohol may either increase or reduce the blood glucose-lowering effect of insulin. Co-administration may require insulin dose adjustment and particularly close monitoring).

Beer, unspecified (Alcohol may either increase or reduce the blood glucose-lowering effect of insulin. Co-administration may require insulin dose adjustment and particularly close monitoring).

Wine, Chianti (Alcohol may either increase or reduce the blood glucose-lowering effect of insulin. Co-administration may require insulin dose adjustment and particularly close monitoring).

Wine, Red (Alcohol may either increase or reduce the blood glucose-lowering effect of insulin. Co-administration may require insulin dose adjustment and particularly close monitoring).

Wine, unspecified (Alcohol may either increase or reduce the blood glucose-lowering effect of insulin. Co-administration may require insulin dose adjustment and particularly close monitoring).

Wine products (Alcohol may either increase or reduce the blood glucose-lowering effect of insulin. Co-administration may require insulin dose adjustment and particularly close monitoring).

FANAPT TABLETS
(Iloperidone) 3484
May interact with alcohols, antibiotics, antihypertensives, antipsychotic agents, centrally-acting drugs, class 1A antiarrhythmics, class III antiarrhythmics, cytochrome p450 2d6 inhibitors (selected), cytochrome p450 3a4 inhibitors, potent (selected), drugs that prolong the QT interval, quinidine, and certain other agents. Compounds in these categories include:

Acebutolol Hydrochloride (Due to its α1-adrenergic receptor antagonism, iloperidone has the potential to enhance the effect of certain antihypertensive agents).
No products indexed under this heading.

Alatrofloxacin Mesylate (The use of iloperidone should be avoided in combination with other drugs that are known to prolong QTc including antibiotics (eg, gatifloxacin, moxifloxacin)).
No products indexed under this heading.

Alfentanil Hydrochloride (Given the primary CNS effects of iloperidone, caution should be used when it is taken in combination with other centrally acting drugs).
No products indexed under this heading.

Aliskiren (Due to its α1-adrenergic receptor antagonism, iloperidone has the potential to enhance the effect of certain antihypertensive agents). Products include:
Tekturna 2538
Tekturna HCT 2541
Valturna 3637

Alprazolam (The use of iloperidone should be avoided in combination with other drugs that are known to prolong QTc including class of medications known to prolong the QTc interval (eg, pentamidine, levomethadyl acetate, methadone).
No products indexed under this heading.

Amikacin Sulfate (The use of iloperidone should be avoided in combination with other drugs that are known to prolong QTc including antibiotics (eg, gatifloxacin, moxifloxacin)).
No products indexed under this heading.

Amiodarone Hydrochloride (The use of iloperidone should be avoided in combination with other drugs that are known to prolong QTc including Class III (eg, amiodarone) antiarrhythmic medications).
No products indexed under this heading.

Amitriptyline Hydrochloride (The use of iloperidone should be avoided in combination with other drugs that are known to prolong QTc including class of medications known to prolong the QTc interval (eg, pentamidine, levomethadyl acetate, methadone).
No products indexed under this heading.

Amlodipine Besylate (Due to its α1-adrenergic receptor antagonism, iloperidone has the potential to enhance the effect of certain antihypertensive agents). Products include:
Azor 1010
Exforge 2443
Exforge HCT 2449

(⊙ Described in PDR® for Ophthalmic Medicines)

Amoxapine (The use of iloperidone should be avoided in combination with other drugs that are known to prolong QTc including class of medications known to prolong the QTc interval (eg, pentamidine, levomethadyl acetate, methadone).
No products indexed under this heading.

Amoxicillin (The use of iloperidone should be avoided in combination with other drugs that are known to prolong QTc including antibiotics (eg, gatifloxacin, moxifloxacin)). Products include:
Amoxil Capsules **1311**
Amoxil Chewable Tablets **1311**
Amoxil **1311**
Amoxil Powder **1311**
Augmentin **1331**
Augmentin Tablets **1335**
Augmentin ES-600 ..... **1338**
Augmentin XR **1342**
Moxatag **2321**

Amoxicillin Trihydrate (The use of iloperidone should be avoided in combination with other drugs that are known to prolong QTc including antibiotics (eg, gatifloxacin, moxifloxacin)).
No products indexed under this heading.

Amphetamine Aspartate (Given the primary CNS effects of iloperidone, caution should be used when it is taken in combination with other centrally acting drugs).
No products indexed under this heading.

Amphetamine Aspartate Monohydrate (Given the primary CNS effects of iloperidone, caution should be used when it is taken in combination with other centrally acting drugs).
No products indexed under this heading.

Amphetamine Resins (Given the primary CNS effects of iloperidone, caution should be used when it is taken in combination with other centrally acting drugs).
No products indexed under this heading.

Amphetamine Sulfate (Given the primary CNS effects of iloperidone, caution should be used when it is taken in combination with other centrally acting drugs).
No products indexed under this heading.

Ampicillin (The use of iloperidone should be avoided in combination with other drugs that are known to prolong QTc including antibiotics (eg, gatifloxacin, moxifloxacin)).
No products indexed under this heading.

Ampicillin Sodium (The use of iloperidone should be avoided in combination with other drugs that are known to prolong QTc including antibiotics (eg, gatifloxacin, moxifloxacin)).
No products indexed under this heading.

Ampicillin Trihydrate (The use of iloperidone should be avoided in combination with other drugs that are known to prolong QTc including antibiotics (eg, gatifloxacin, moxifloxacin)).
No products indexed under this heading.

Amprenavir (Both CYP3A4 and CYP2D6 are responsible for iloperidone metabolism. Inhibitors of CYP3A4 (eg, ketoconazole) or CYP2D6 (eg, fluoxetine, paroxetine) can inhibit iloperidone elimination and cause increased blood levels).
No products indexed under this heading.

Antibiotics, non-penicillin, unspecified (The use of iloperidone should be avoided in combination with other drugs that are known to prolong QTc including antibiotics (eg, gatifloxacin, moxifloxacin)).
No products indexed under this heading.

Aprobarbital (Given the primary CNS effects of iloperidone, caution should be used when it is taken in combination with other centrally acting drugs).
No products indexed under this heading.

Aripiprazole (The use of iloperidone should be avoided in combination with other drugs that are known to prolong QTc including antipsychotic medications (eg, chlorpromazine, thiordazine)).
No products indexed under this heading.

Astemizole (The use of iloperidone should be avoided in combination with other drugs that are known to prolong QTc including class of medications known to prolong the QTc interval (eg, pentamidine, levomethadyl acetate, methadone).
No products indexed under this heading.

Atazanavir (Both CYP3A4 and CYP2D6 are responsible for iloperidone metabolism. Inhibitors of CYP3A4 (eg, ketoconazole) or CYP2D6 (eg, fluoxetine, paroxetine) can inhibit iloperidone elimination and cause increased blood levels).
No products indexed under this heading.

Atazanavir Sulfate (Both CYP3A4 and CYP2D6 are responsible for iloperidone metabolism. Inhibitors of CYP3A4 (eg, ketoconazole) or CYP2D6 (eg, fluoxetine, paroxetine) can inhibit iloperidone elimination and cause increased blood levels).
No products indexed under this heading.

Atenolol (Due to its α1-adrenergic receptor antagonism, iloperidone has the potential to enhance the effect of certain antihypertensive agents).
No products indexed under this heading.

Azithromycin Dihydrate (The use of iloperidone should be avoided in combination with other drugs that are known to prolong QTc including antibiotics (eg, gatifloxacin, moxifloxacin)).
No products indexed under this heading.

Azlocillin Sodium (The use of iloperidone should be avoided in combination with other drugs that are known to prolong QTc including antibiotics (eg, gatifloxacin, moxifloxacin)).
No products indexed under this heading.

Aztreonam (The use of iloperidone should be avoided in combination with other drugs that are known to prolong QTc including antibiotics (eg, gatifloxacin, moxifloxacin)).
No products indexed under this heading.

Bacampicillin Hydrochloride (The use of iloperidone should be avoided in combination with other drugs that are known to prolong QTc including antibiotics (eg, gatifloxacin, moxifloxacin)).
No products indexed under this heading.

Benazepril Hydrochloride (Due to its α1-adrenergic receptor antagonism, iloperidone has the potential to enhance the effect of certain antihypertensive agents).
No products indexed under this heading.

Bendroflumethiazide (Due to its α1-adrenergic receptor antagonism, iloperidone has the potential to enhance the effect of certain antihypertensive agents).
No products indexed under this heading.

Betaxolol Hydrochloride (Due to its α1-adrenergic receptor antagonism, iloperidone has the potential to enhance the effect of certain antihypertensive agents).
No products indexed under this heading.

Bisoprolol Fumarate (Due to its α1-adrenergic receptor antagonism, iloperidone has the potential to enhance the effect of certain antihypertensive agents).
No products indexed under this heading.

Bretylium Tosylate (The use of iloperidone should be avoided in combination with other drugs that are known to prolong QTc including Class III (eg, amiodarone, sotalol) antiarrhythmic medications).
No products indexed under this heading.

Buprenorphine Hydrochloride (Given the primary CNS effects of iloperidone, caution should be used when it is taken in combination with other centrally acting drugs).
No products indexed under this heading.

Bupropion Hydrochloride (Both CYP3A4 and CYP2D6 are responsible for iloperidone metabolism. Inhibitors of CYP3A4 (eg, ketoconazole) or CYP2D6 (eg, fluoxetine, paroxetine) can inhibit iloperidone elimination and cause increased blood levels). Products include:
Aplenzin **2948**
Wellbutrin **1719**
Wellbutrin SR **1725**
Zyban **1762**

Buspirone Hydrochloride (The use of iloperidone should be avoided in combination with other drugs that are known to prolong QTc including class of medications known to prolong the QTc interval (eg, pentamidine, levomethadyl acetate, methadone).
No products indexed under this heading.

Butabarbital (Given the primary CNS effects of iloperidone, caution should be used when it is taken in combination with other centrally acting drugs).
No products indexed under this heading.

Butalbital (Given the primary CNS effects of iloperidone, caution should be used when it is taken in combination with other centrally acting drugs).
No products indexed under this heading.

Candesartan Cilexetil (Due to its α1-adrenergic receptor antagonism, iloperidone has the potential to enhance the effect of certain antihypertensive agents). Products include:
Atacand **697**
Atacand HCT **700**

Captopril (Due to its α1-adrenergic receptor antagonism, iloperidone has the potential to enhance the effect of certain antihypertensive agents). Products include:
Captopril **2341**

Carbenicillin Disodium (The use of iloperidone should be avoided in combination with other drugs that are known to prolong QTc including antibiotics (eg, gatifloxacin, moxifloxacin)).
No products indexed under this heading.

Carbenicillin Indanyl Sodium (The use of iloperidone should be avoided in combination with other drugs that are known to prolong QTc including antibiotics (eg, gatifloxacin, moxifloxacin)).
No products indexed under this heading.

Carteolol Hydrochloride (Due to its α1-adrenergic receptor antagonism, iloperidone has the potential to enhance the effect of certain antihypertensive agents).
No products indexed under this heading.

Carvedilol (Due to its α1-adrenergic receptor antagonism, iloperidone has the potential to enhance the effect of certain antihypertensive agents). Products include:
Coreg **1409**

Carvedilol Phosphate (Due to its α1-adrenergic receptor antagonism, iloperidone has the potential to enhance the effect of certain antihypertensive agents). Products include:
Coreg CR **1416**

Cefaclor (The use of iloperidone should be avoided in combination with other drugs that are known to prolong QTc including antibiotics (eg, gatifloxacin, moxifloxacin)).
No products indexed under this heading.

Cefadroxil (The use of iloperidone should be avoided in combination with other drugs that are known to prolong QTc including antibiotics (eg, gatifloxacin, moxifloxacin)).
No products indexed under this heading.

Cefamandole Nafate (The use of iloperidone should be avoided in combination with other drugs that are known to prolong QTc including antibiotics (eg, gatifloxacin, moxifloxacin)).
No products indexed under this heading.

Cefazolin Sodium (The use of iloperidone should be avoided in combination with other drugs that are known to prolong QTc including antibiotics (eg, gatifloxacin, moxifloxacin)).
No products indexed under this heading.

Cefixime (The use of iloperidone should be avoided in combination with other drugs that are known to prolong QTc including antibiotics (eg, gatifloxacin, moxifloxacin)). Products include:
Suprax for Oral Suspension **2038**
Suprax Tablets **2038**

Cefmetazole Sodium (The use of iloperidone should be avoided in combination with other drugs that are known to prolong QTc including antibiotics (eg, gatifloxacin, moxifloxacin)).
No products indexed under this heading.

Cefonicid Sodium (The use of iloperidone should be avoided in combination with other drugs that are known to prolong QTc including antibiotics (eg, gatifloxacin, moxifloxacin)).
No products indexed under this heading.

Cefoperazone Sodium (The use of iloperidone should be avoided in combination with other drugs that are known to prolong QTc including antibiotics (eg, gatifloxacin, moxifloxacin)).
No products indexed under this heading.

Ceforanide (The use of iloperidone should be avoided in combination with other drugs that are known to prolong QTc including antibiotics (eg, gatifloxacin, moxifloxacin)).
No products indexed under this heading.

Cefotaxime Sodium (The use of iloperidone should be avoided in combination with other drugs that are known to prolong QTc including antibiotics (eg, gatifloxacin, moxifloxacin)).
No products indexed under this heading.

Cefotetan (The use of iloperidone should be avoided in combination with other drugs that are known to prolong QTc including antibiotics (eg, gatifloxacin, moxifloxacin)).
No products indexed under this heading.

Cefoxitin Sodium (The use of iloperidone should be avoided in combination with other drugs that are known to prolong QTc including antibiotics (eg, gatifloxacin, moxifloxacin)).
No products indexed under this heading.

Cefpodoxime Proxetil (The use of iloperidone should be avoided in combination with other drugs that are known to prolong QTc including antibiotics (eg, gatifloxacin, moxifloxacin)).
No products indexed under this heading.

Cefprozil (The use of iloperidone should be avoided in combination with other drugs that are known to prolong QTc including antibiotics (eg, gatifloxacin, moxifloxacin)).
No products indexed under this heading.

Ceftazidime (The use of iloperidone should be avoided in combination with other drugs that are known to prolong QTc including antibiotics (eg, gatifloxacin, moxifloxacin)). Products include:
Fortaz **1481**

Ceftizoxime Sodium (The use of iloperidone should be avoided in combination with other drugs that are known to prolong QTc including antibiotics (eg, gatifloxacin, moxifloxacin)).
No products indexed under this heading.

Ceftriaxone Sodium (The use of iloperidone should be avoided in combination with other drugs that are known to

Fanapt Interactions Index 646

prolong QTc including antibiotics (eg, gatifloxacin, moxifloxacin)). Products include:
Rocephin 2859

Cefuroxime Axetil (The use of iloperidone should be avoided in combination with other drugs that are known to prolong QTc including antibiotics (eg, gatifloxacin, moxifloxacin)). Products include:
Ceftin 1399

Cefuroxime Sodium (The use of iloperidone should be avoided in combination with other drugs that are known to prolong QTc including antibiotics (eg, gatifloxacin, moxifloxacin)).
No products indexed under this heading.

Celecoxib (Both CYP3A4 and CYP2D6 are responsible for iloperidone metabolism. Inhibitors of CYP3A4 (eg, ketoconazole) or CYP2D6 (eg, fluoxetine, paroxetine) can inhibit iloperidone elimination and cause increased blood levels). Products include:
Celebrex 3272

Cephalexin (The use of iloperidone should be avoided in combination with other drugs that are known to prolong QTc including antibiotics (eg, gatifloxacin, moxifloxacin)).
No products indexed under this heading.

Cephalothin Sodium (The use of iloperidone should be avoided in combination with other drugs that are known to prolong QTc including antibiotics (eg, gatifloxacin, moxifloxacin)).
No products indexed under this heading.

Cephapirin Sodium (The use of iloperidone should be avoided in combination with other drugs that are known to prolong QTc including antibiotics (eg, gatifloxacin, moxifloxacin)).
No products indexed under this heading.

Cephradine (The use of iloperidone should be avoided in combination with other drugs that are known to prolong QTc including antibiotics (eg, gatifloxacin, moxifloxacin)).
No products indexed under this heading.

Chloramphenicol (The use of iloperidone should be avoided in combination with other drugs that are known to prolong QTc including antibiotics (eg, gatifloxacin, moxifloxacin)).
No products indexed under this heading.

Chloramphenicol Palmitate (The use of iloperidone should be avoided in combination with other drugs that are known to prolong QTc including antibiotics (eg, gatifloxacin, moxifloxacin)).
No products indexed under this heading.

Chloramphenicol Sodium Succinate (The use of iloperidone should be avoided in combination with other drugs that are known to prolong QTc including antibiotics (eg, gatifloxacin, moxifloxacin)).
No products indexed under this heading.

Chlordiazepoxide (The use of iloperidone should be avoided in combination with other drugs that are known to prolong QTc including class of medications known to prolong the QTc interval (eg, pentamidine, levomethadyl acetate, methadone).
No products indexed under this heading.

Chlordiazepoxide Hydrochloride (The use of iloperidone should be avoided in combination with other drugs that are known to prolong QTc including class of medications known to prolong the QTc interval (eg, pentamidine, levomethadyl acetate, methadone).
No products indexed under this heading.

Chloroquine (Both CYP3A4 and CYP2D6 are responsible for iloperidone metabolism. Inhibitors of CYP3A4 (eg, ketoconazole) or CYP2D6 (eg, fluoxetine, paroxetine) can inhibit iloperidone elimination and cause increased blood levels).
No products indexed under this heading.

Chloroquine Hydrochloride (Both CYP3A4 and CYP2D6 are responsible for iloperidone metabolism. Inhibitors of CYP3A4 (eg, ketoconazole) or CYP2D6 (eg, fluoxetine, paroxetine) can inhibit iloperidone elimination and cause increased blood levels).
No products indexed under this heading.

Chloroquine Phosphate (Both CYP3A4 and CYP2D6 are responsible for iloperidone metabolism. Inhibitors of CYP3A4 (eg, ketoconazole) or CYP2D6 (eg, fluoxetine, paroxetine) can inhibit iloperidone elimination and cause increased blood levels).
No products indexed under this heading.

Chlorothiazide (Due to its α1-adrenergic receptor antagonism, iloperidone has the potential to enhance the effect of certain antihypertensive agents).
No products indexed under this heading.

Chlorothiazide Sodium (Due to its α1-adrenergic receptor antagonism, iloperidone has the potential to enhance the effect of certain antihypertensive agents). Products include:
Diuril Intravenous 2009

Chlorpheniramine (Both CYP3A4 and CYP2D6 are responsible for iloperidone metabolism. Inhibitors of CYP3A4 (eg, ketoconazole) or CYP2D6 (eg, fluoxetine, paroxetine) can inhibit iloperidone elimination and cause increased blood levels).
No products indexed under this heading.

Chlorpheniramine Maleate (Both CYP3A4 and CYP2D6 are responsible for iloperidone metabolism. Inhibitors of CYP3A4 (eg, ketoconazole) or CYP2D6 (eg, fluoxetine, paroxetine) can inhibit iloperidone elimination and cause increased blood levels).
No products indexed under this heading.

Chlorpheniramine Polistirex (Both CYP3A4 and CYP2D6 are responsible for iloperidone metabolism. Inhibitors of CYP3A4 (eg, ketoconazole) or CYP2D6 (eg, fluoxetine, paroxetine) can inhibit iloperidone elimination and cause increased blood levels). Products include:
Tussionex 3443

Chlorpheniramine Tannate (Both CYP3A4 and CYP2D6 are responsible for iloperidone metabolism. Inhibitors of CYP3A4 (eg, ketoconazole) or CYP2D6 (eg, fluoxetine, paroxetine) can inhibit iloperidone elimination and cause increased blood levels).
No products indexed under this heading.

Chlorpromazine (The use of iloperidone should be avoided in combination with other drugs that are known to prolong QTc including antipsychotic medications (eg, chlorpromazine)).
No products indexed under this heading.

Chlorpromazine Hydrochloride (The use of iloperidone should be avoided in combination with other drugs that are known to prolong QTc including antipsychotic medications (eg, chlorpromazine)).
No products indexed under this heading.

Chlorprothixene (The use of iloperidone should be avoided in combination with other drugs that are known to prolong QTc including antipsychotic medications (eg, chlorpromazine, thiordazine)).
No products indexed under this heading.

Chlorprothixene Hydrochloride (The use of iloperidone should be avoided in combination with other drugs that are known to prolong QTc including antipsychotic medications (eg, chlorpromazine, thiordazine)).
No products indexed under this heading.

Chlorprothixene Lactate (The use of iloperidone should be avoided in combination with other drugs that are known to prolong QTc including antipsychotic medications (eg, chlorpromazine, thiordazine)).
No products indexed under this heading.

Chlorthalidone (Due to its α1-adrenergic receptor antagonism, iloperidone has the potential to enhance the effect of certain antihypertensive agents). Products include:
Clorpres 2344

Cilastatin Sodium (The use of iloperidone should be avoided in combination with other drugs that are known to prolong QTc including antibiotics (eg, gatifloxacin, moxifloxacin)). Products include:
Primaxin I.M. 2232
Primaxin I.V. 2235

Cimetidine (Both CYP3A4 and CYP2D6 are responsible for iloperidone metabolism. Inhibitors of CYP3A4 (eg, ketoconazole) or CYP2D6 (eg, fluoxetine, paroxetine) can inhibit iloperidone elimination and cause increased blood levels).
No products indexed under this heading.

Cimetidine Hydrochloride (Both CYP3A4 and CYP2D6 are responsible for iloperidone metabolism. Inhibitors of CYP3A4 (eg, ketoconazole) or CYP2D6 (eg, fluoxetine, paroxetine) can inhibit iloperidone elimination and cause increased blood levels).
No products indexed under this heading.

Ciprofloxacin (The use of iloperidone should be avoided in combination with other drugs that are known to prolong QTc including antibiotics (eg, gatifloxacin, moxifloxacin)). Products include:
Cipro I.V. 3082
Cipro 3073
Cipro XR 3091
Ciprodex 583

Ciprofloxacin Hydrochloride (The use of iloperidone should be avoided in combination with other drugs that are known to prolong QTc including antibiotics (eg, gatifloxacin, moxifloxacin)). Products include:
Cipro 3073

Citalopram Hydrobromide (Both CYP3A4 and CYP2D6 are responsible for iloperidone metabolism. Inhibitors of CYP3A4 (eg, ketoconazole) or CYP2D6 (eg, fluoxetine, paroxetine) can inhibit iloperidone elimination and cause increased blood levels). Products include:
Celexa 1153

Clarithromycin (The use of iloperidone should be avoided in combination with other drugs that are known to prolong QTc including antibiotics (eg, gatifloxacin, moxifloxacin)). Products include:
Biaxin/Biaxin XL 412

Clomipramine Hydrochloride (The use of iloperidone should be avoided in combination with other drugs that are known to prolong QTc including class of medications known to prolong the QTc interval (eg, pentamidine, levomethadyl acetate, methadone).
No products indexed under this heading.

Clonidine (Due to its α1-adrenergic receptor antagonism, iloperidone has the potential to enhance the effect of certain antihypertensive agents). Products include:
Catapres-TTS 884

Clonidine Hydrochloride (Due to its α1-adrenergic receptor antagonism, iloperidone has the potential to enhance the effect of certain antihypertensive agents). Products include:
Clorpres 2344

Clorazepate Dipotassium (The use of iloperidone should be avoided in combination with other drugs that are known to prolong QTc including class of medications known to prolong the QTc interval (eg, pentamidine, levomethadyl acetate, methadone).
No products indexed under this heading.

Clotrimazole (The use of iloperidone should be avoided in combination with other drugs that are known to prolong QTc including antibiotics (eg, gatifloxacin, moxifloxacin)). Products include:
Lotrisone 3163

Cloxacillin (The use of iloperidone should be avoided in combination with other drugs that are known to prolong QTc including antibiotics (eg, gatifloxacin, moxifloxacin)).
No products indexed under this heading.

Cloxacillin Sodium (The use of iloperidone should be avoided in combination with other drugs that are known to prolong QTc including antibiotics (eg, gatifloxacin, moxifloxacin)).
No products indexed under this heading.

Cloxacillin Sodium Monohydrate (The use of iloperidone should be avoided in combination with other drugs that are known to prolong QTc including antibiotics (eg, gatifloxacin, moxifloxacin)).
No products indexed under this heading.

Clozapine (The use of iloperidone should be avoided in combination with other drugs that are known to prolong QTc including antipsychotic medications (eg, chlorpromazine, thiordazine)).
No products indexed under this heading.

Cocaine Hydrochloride (Both CYP3A4 and CYP2D6 are responsible for iloperidone metabolism. Inhibitors of CYP3A4 (eg, ketoconazole) or CYP2D6 (eg, fluoxetine, paroxetine) can inhibit iloperidone elimination and cause increased blood levels).
No products indexed under this heading.

Codeine Phosphate (Given the primary CNS effects of iloperidone, caution should be used when it is taken in combination with other centrally acting drugs). Products include:
Tylenol with Codeine 2691

Codeine Sulfate (Given the primary CNS effects of iloperidone, caution should be used when it is taken in combination with other centrally acting drugs).
No products indexed under this heading.

Daunorubicin Hydrochloride (The use of iloperidone should be avoided in combination with other drugs that are known to prolong QTc including antibiotics (eg, gatifloxacin, moxifloxacin)).
No products indexed under this heading.

Delavirdine Mesylate (Both CYP3A4 and CYP2D6 are responsible for iloperidone metabolism. Inhibitors of CYP3A4 (eg, ketoconazole) or CYP2D6 (eg, fluoxetine, paroxetine) can inhibit iloperidone elimination and cause increased blood levels).
No products indexed under this heading.

Delavirine (Both CYP3A4 and CYP2D6 are responsible for iloperidone metabolism. Inhibitors of CYP3A4 (eg, ketoconazole) or CYP2D6 (eg, fluoxetine, paroxetine) can inhibit iloperidone elimination and cause increased blood levels).
No products indexed under this heading.

647 Interactions Index Fanapt

Demeclocycline Hydrochloride (The use of iloperidone should be avoided in combination with other drugs that are known to prolong QTc including antibiotics (eg, gatifloxacin, moxifloxacin)).
No products indexed under this heading.

Deserpidine (Due to its α1-adrenergic receptor antagonism, iloperidone has the potential to enhance the effect of certain antihypertensive agents).
No products indexed under this heading.

Desflurane (Given the primary CNS effects of iloperidone, caution should be used when it is taken in combination with other centrally acting drugs).
No products indexed under this heading.

Desipramine Hydrochloride (The use of iloperidone should be avoided in combination with other drugs that are known to prolong QTc including class of medications known to prolong the QTc interval (eg, pentamidine, levomethadyl acetate, methadone).
No products indexed under this heading.

Dexmethylphenidate Hydrochloride (Given the primary CNS effects of iloperidone, caution should be used when it is taken in combination with other centrally acting drugs). Products include:
Focalin XR 2472

Dextroamphetamine (Given the primary CNS effects of iloperidone, caution should be used when it is taken in combination with other centrally acting drugs).
No products indexed under this heading.

Dextroamphetamine Saccharate (Given the primary CNS effects of iloperidone, caution should be used when it is taken in combination with other centrally acting drugs).
No products indexed under this heading.

Dextroamphetamine Sulfate (Given the primary CNS effects of iloperidone, caution should be used when it is taken in combination with other centrally acting drugs). Products include:
Dexedrine 1425

Dextromethorphan (A study in healthy volunteers showed that changes in the pharmacokinetics of dextromethorphan (80 mg dose) when a 3 mg dose of iloperidone was co-administered resulted in a 17% increase in total exposure and a 26% increase in C_{max} of dextromethorphan).
No products indexed under this heading.

Dextromethorphan Hydrobromide (A study in healthy volunteers showed that changes in the pharmacokinetics of dextromethorphan (80 mg dose) when a 3 mg dose of iloperidone was co-administered resulted in a 17% increase in total exposure and a 26% increase in C_{max} of dextromethorphan).
No products indexed under this heading.

Dextromethorphan Polistirex (A study in healthy volunteers showed that changes in the pharmacokinetics of dextromethorphan (80 mg dose) when a 3 mg dose of iloperidone was co-administered resulted in a 17% increase in total exposure and a 26% increase in C_{max} of dextromethorphan).
No products indexed under this heading.

Dextromethorphan Tannate (A study in healthy volunteers showed that changes in the pharmacokinetics of dextromethorphan (80 mg dose) when a 3 mg dose of iloperidone was co-administered resulted in a 17% increase in total exposure and a 26% increase in C_{max} of dextromethorphan).
No products indexed under this heading.

Dezocine (Given the primary CNS effects of iloperidone, caution should be used when it is taken in combination with other centrally acting drugs).
No products indexed under this heading.

Diazepam (The use of iloperidone should be avoided in combination with other drugs that are known to prolong QTc including class of medications known to prolong the QTc interval (eg, pentamidine, levomethadyl acetate, methadone). Products include:
Valium Tablets 2880

Diazoxide (Due to its α1-adrenergic receptor antagonism, iloperidone has the potential to enhance the effect of certain antihypertensive agents). Products include:
Proglycem 1179
Proglycem Suspension 1179

Dicloxacillin (The use of iloperidone should be avoided in combination with other drugs that are known to prolong QTc including antibiotics (eg, gatifloxacin, moxifloxacin)).
No products indexed under this heading.

Dicloxacillin Sodium (The use of iloperidone should be avoided in combination with other drugs that are known to prolong QTc including antibiotics (eg, gatifloxacin, moxifloxacin)).
No products indexed under this heading.

Diltiazem Hydrochloride (Due to its α1-adrenergic receptor antagonism, iloperidone has the potential to enhance the effect of certain antihypertensive agents). Products include:
Cardizem LA 423

Diltiazem Maleate (Due to its α1-adrenergic receptor antagonism, iloperidone has the potential to enhance the effect of certain antihypertensive agents).
No products indexed under this heading.

Diphenhydramine (Both CYP3A4 and CYP2D6 are responsible for iloperidone metabolism. Inhibitors of CYP3A4 (eg, ketoconazole) or CYP2D6 (eg, fluoxetine, paroxetine) can inhibit iloperidone elimination and cause increased blood levels).
No products indexed under this heading.

Diphenhydramine Hydrochloride (Both CYP3A4 and CYP2D6 are responsible for iloperidone metabolism. Inhibitors of CYP3A4 (eg, ketoconazole) or CYP2D6 (eg, fluoxetine, paroxetine) can inhibit iloperidone elimination and cause increased blood levels). Products include:
Benadryl Allergy Ultratab 2042
Children's Benadryl Allergy Liquid 2042

Dirithromycin (The use of iloperidone should be avoided in combination with other drugs that are known to prolong QTc including antibiotics (eg, gatifloxacin, moxifloxacin)).
No products indexed under this heading.

Disodium Carbenicillin (The use of iloperidone should be avoided in combination with other drugs that are known to prolong QTc including antibiotics (eg, gatifloxacin, moxifloxacin)).
No products indexed under this heading.

Disopyramide (The use of iloperidone should be avoided in combination with other drugs that are known to prolong QTc including Class 1A (eg, quinidine, procainamide)antiarrhythmic medications).
No products indexed under this heading.

Disopyramide Phosphate (The use of iloperidone should be avoided in combination with other drugs that are known to prolong QTc including Class 1A (eg, quinidine, procainamide)antiarrhythmic medications).
No products indexed under this heading.

Dofetilide (The use of iloperidone should be avoided in combination with other drugs that are known to prolong QTc including class of medications known to prolong the QTc interval (eg, pentamidine, levomethadyl acetate, methadone).
No products indexed under this heading.

Doxazosin Mesylate (Due to its α1-adrenergic receptor antagonism, iloperidone has the potential to enhance the effect of certain antihypertensive agents).
No products indexed under this heading.

Doxepin Hydrochloride (The use of iloperidone should be avoided in combination with other drugs that are known to prolong QTc including class of medications known to prolong the QTc interval (eg, pentamidine, levomethadyl acetate, methadone).
No products indexed under this heading.

Doxycycline Calcium (The use of iloperidone should be avoided in combination with other drugs that are known to prolong QTc including antibiotics (eg, gatifloxacin, moxifloxacin)).
No products indexed under this heading.

Doxycycline Hyclate (The use of iloperidone should be avoided in combination with other drugs that are known to prolong QTc including antibiotics (eg, gatifloxacin, moxifloxacin)).
No products indexed under this heading.

Doxycycline Monohydrate (The use of iloperidone should be avoided in combination with other drugs that are known to prolong QTc including antibiotics (eg, gatifloxacin, moxifloxacin)).
No products indexed under this heading.

Droperidol (The use of iloperidone should be avoided in combination with other drugs that are known to prolong QTc including class of medications known to prolong the QTc interval (eg, pentamidine, levomethadyl acetate, methadone).
No products indexed under this heading.

Enalapril Maleate (Due to its α1-adrenergic receptor antagonism, iloperidone has the potential to enhance the effect of certain antihypertensive agents).
No products indexed under this heading.

Enalaprilat (Due to its α1-adrenergic receptor antagonism, iloperidone has the potential to enhance the effect of certain antihypertensive agents).
No products indexed under this heading.

Enflurane (Given the primary CNS effects of iloperidone, caution should be used when it is taken in combination with other centrally acting drugs).
No products indexed under this heading.

Enoxacin (The use of iloperidone should be avoided in combination with other drugs that are known to prolong QTc including antibiotics (eg, gatifloxacin, moxifloxacin)).
No products indexed under this heading.

Epirubicin Hydrochloride (The use of iloperidone should be avoided in combination with other drugs that are known to prolong QTc including antibiotics (eg, gatifloxacin, moxifloxacin)).
No products indexed under this heading.

Eprosartan Mesylate (Due to its α1-adrenergic receptor antagonism, iloperidone has the potential to enhance the effect of certain antihypertensive agents). Products include:
Teveten 538
Teveten HCT 541

Erythromycin (The use of iloperidone should be avoided in combination with other drugs that are known to prolong QTc including antibiotics (eg, gatifloxacin, moxifloxacin)).
No products indexed under this heading.

Erythromycin, Topical (The use of iloperidone should be avoided in combination with other drugs that are known to prolong QTc including antibiotics (eg, gatifloxacin, moxifloxacin)).
No products indexed under this heading.

Erythromycin Estolate (The use of iloperidone should be avoided in combination with other drugs that are known to prolong QTc including antibiotics (eg, gatifloxacin, moxifloxacin)).
No products indexed under this heading.

Erythromycin Ethylsuccinate (The use of iloperidone should be avoided in combination with other drugs that are known to prolong QTc including antibiotics (eg, gatifloxacin, moxifloxacin)). Products include:
E.E.S. 437
EryPed 435

Erythromycin Gluceptate (The use of iloperidone should be avoided in combination with other drugs that are known to prolong QTc including antibiotics (eg, gatifloxacin, moxifloxacin)).
No products indexed under this heading.

Erythromycin Lactobionate (The use of iloperidone should be avoided in combination with other drugs that are known to prolong QTc including antibiotics (eg, gatifloxacin, moxifloxacin)).
No products indexed under this heading.

Erythromycin Stearate (The use of iloperidone should be avoided in combination with other drugs that are known to prolong QTc including antibiotics (eg, gatifloxacin, moxifloxacin)).
No products indexed under this heading.

Escitalopram Oxalate (Both CYP3A4 and CYP2D6 are responsible for iloperidone metabolism. Inhibitors of CYP3A4 (eg, ketoconazole) or CYP2D6 (eg, fluoxetine, paroxetine) can inhibit iloperidone elimination and cause increased blood levels). Products include:
Lexapro Oral Suspension 1160
Lexapro Tablets 1160

Esmolol Hydrochloride (Due to its α1-adrenergic receptor antagonism, iloperidone has the potential to enhance the effect of certain antihypertensive agents).
No products indexed under this heading.

Estazolam (Given the primary CNS effects of iloperidone, caution should be used when it is taken in combination with other centrally acting drugs).
No products indexed under this heading.

Ethanol (Given the primary CNS effects of iloperidone, caution should be used when it is taken in combination with alcohol).
No products indexed under this heading.

Ethchlorvynol (Given the primary CNS effects of iloperidone, caution should be used when it is taken in combination with other centrally acting drugs).
No products indexed under this heading.

Ethinamate (Given the primary CNS effects of iloperidone, caution should be used when it is taken in combination with other centrally acting drugs).
No products indexed under this heading.

Ethyl Alcohol (Given the primary CNS effects of iloperidone, caution should be used when it is taken in combination with alcohol).
No products indexed under this heading.

Felodipine (Due to its α1-adrenergic receptor antagonism, iloperidone has the potential to enhance the effect of certain antihypertensive agents).
No products indexed under this heading.

Fentanyl (Given the primary CNS effects of iloperidone, caution should be used when it is taken in combination with other centrally acting drugs). Products include:
Duragesic 2604
Fentanyl Transdermal System 2346
Onsolis 2054

Fentanyl Citrate (Given the primary CNS effects of iloperidone, caution should be used when it is taken in combination with other centrally acting drugs). Products include:

(⊙ Described in PDR® for Ophthalmic Medicines)

IMPORTANT NOTE: Always consult each drug listing in the patient's regimen for possible interactions.

IMPORTANT NOTE: Always consult each drug listing in the patient's regimen for possible interactions.

(⊙ Described in PDR® for Ophthalmic Medicines)

Amprenavir (The benefits and risks of using fenofibrate with immunosuppressants and other potentially nephrotoxic agents should be carefully considered, and the lowest effective dose employed).
No products indexed under this heading.

Anisindione (Caution should be exercised when anticoagulants are given in conjunction with fenofibrate because of the potentiation of coumarin-type anticoagulants in prolonging the prothrombin time/INR. The dosage of the anticoagulant should be reduced to maintain the prothrombin/INR at the desired level to prevent bleeding complications. Frequent prothrombin time/INR determinations are advisable until it has been definitely determined that the prothrombin time/INR has stabilized).
No products indexed under this heading.

Aspirin (The benefits and risks of using fenofibrate with immunosuppressants and other potentially nephrotoxic agents should be carefully considered, and the lowest effective dose employed). Products include:
Aggrenox 880
Bayer Aspirin 829
Percodan 1124
St. Joseph Aspirin 2045

Atazanavir (The benefits and risks of using fenofibrate with immunosuppressants and other potentially nephrotoxic agents should be carefully considered, and the lowest effective dose employed).
No products indexed under this heading.

Atorvastatin Calcium (The combined use of fenofibric acid derivatives, particularly gemfibrozil, and HMG-CoA reductase inhibitors results in an increased risk of rhabdomyolysis and myoglobinuria leading in a high proportion of cases to acute renal failure. The combined use of fenofibrate and HMG-CoA reductase inhibitors should be avoided unless the benefit of further alterations in lipid levels is likely to outweigh the increased risk of this drug combination). Products include:
Lipitor 2703

Azathioprine (The benefits and risks of using fenofibrate with immunosuppressants and other potentially nephrotoxic agents should be carefully considered, and the lowest effective dose employed).
No products indexed under this heading.

Azithromycin Dihydrate (The benefits and risks of using fenofibrate with immunosuppressants and other potentially nephrotoxic agents should be carefully considered, and the lowest effective dose employed).
No products indexed under this heading.

Azlocillin Sodium (The benefits and risks of using fenofibrate with immunosuppressants and other potentially nephrotoxic agents should be carefully considered, and the lowest effective dose employed).
No products indexed under this heading.

Aztreonam (The benefits and risks of using fenofibrate with immunosuppressants and other potentially nephrotoxic agents should be carefully considered, and the lowest effective dose employed).
No products indexed under this heading.

Bacampicillin Hydrochloride (The benefits and risks of using fenofibrate with immunosuppressants and other potentially nephrotoxic agents should be carefully considered, and the lowest effective dose employed).
No products indexed under this heading.

Bacitracin (The benefits and risks of using fenofibrate with immunosuppressants and other potentially nephrotoxic agents should be carefully considered, and the lowest effective dose employed).
No products indexed under this heading.

Bacitracin Zinc (The benefits and risks of using fenofibrate with immunosuppressants and other potentially nephrotoxic agents should be carefully considered, and the lowest effective dose employed).
No products indexed under this heading.

Balsalazide Disodium (The benefits and risks of using fenofibrate with immunosuppressants and other potentially nephrotoxic agents should be carefully considered, and the lowest effective dose employed).
No products indexed under this heading.

Basiliximab (The benefits and risks of using fenofibrate with immunosuppressants and other potentially nephrotoxic agents should be carefully considered, and the lowest effective dose employed). Products include:
Simulect 2524

Benazepril Hydrochloride (The benefits and risks of using fenofibrate with immunosuppressants and other potentially nephrotoxic agents should be carefully considered, and the lowest effective dose employed).
No products indexed under this heading.

Bendroflumethiazide (The benefits and risks of using fenofibrate with immunosuppressants and other potentially nephrotoxic agents should be carefully considered, and the lowest effective dose employed).
No products indexed under this heading.

Caffeine (The benefits and risks of using fenofibrate with immunosuppressants and other potentially nephrotoxic agents should be carefully considered, and the lowest effective dose employed).
No products indexed under this heading.

Captopril (The benefits and risks of using fenofibrate with immunosuppressants and other potentially nephrotoxic agents should be carefully considered, and the lowest effective dose employed). Products include:
Captopril 2341

Carbenicillin Disodium (The benefits and risks of using fenofibrate with immunosuppressants and other potentially nephrotoxic agents should be carefully considered, and the lowest effective dose employed).
No products indexed under this heading.

Carbenicillin Indanyl Sodium (The benefits and risks of using fenofibrate with immunosuppressants and other potentially nephrotoxic agents should be carefully considered, and the lowest effective dose employed).
No products indexed under this heading.

Carboplatin (The benefits and risks of using fenofibrate with immunosuppressants and other potentially nephrotoxic agents should be carefully considered, and the lowest effective dose employed).
No products indexed under this heading.

Carmustine (BCNU) (The benefits and risks of using fenofibrate with immunosuppressants and other potentially nephrotoxic agents should be carefully considered, and the lowest effective dose employed).
No products indexed under this heading.

Cefaclor (The benefits and risks of using fenofibrate with immunosuppressants and other potentially nephrotoxic agents should be carefully considered, and the lowest effective dose employed).
No products indexed under this heading.

Cefadroxil (The benefits and risks of using fenofibrate with immunosuppressants and other potentially nephrotoxic agents should be carefully considered, and the lowest effective dose employed).
No products indexed under this heading.

Cefamandole Nafate (The benefits and risks of using fenofibrate with immunosuppressants and other potentially nephrotoxic agents should be carefully considered, and the lowest effective dose employed).
No products indexed under this heading.

Cefazolin Sodium (The benefits and risks of using fenofibrate with immunosuppressants and other potentially nephrotoxic agents should be carefully considered, and the lowest effective dose employed).
No products indexed under this heading.

Cefdinir (The benefits and risks of using fenofibrate with immunosuppressants and other potentially nephrotoxic agents should be carefully considered, and the lowest effective dose employed). Products include:
Omnicef Capsules 518
Omnicef Oral Suspension 518

Cefepime Hydrochloride (The benefits and risks of using fenofibrate with immunosuppressants and other potentially nephrotoxic agents should be carefully considered, and the lowest effective dose employed).
No products indexed under this heading.

Cefixime (The benefits and risks of using fenofibrate with immunosuppressants and other potentially nephrotoxic agents should be carefully considered, and the lowest effective dose employed). Products include:
Suprax for Oral Suspension 2038
Suprax Tablets 2038

Cefmetazole Sodium (The benefits and risks of using fenofibrate with immunosuppressants and other potentially nephrotoxic agents should be carefully considered, and the lowest effective dose employed).
No products indexed under this heading.

Cefonicid Sodium (The benefits and risks of using fenofibrate with immunosuppressants and other potentially nephrotoxic agents should be carefully considered, and the lowest effective dose employed).
No products indexed under this heading.

Cefoperazone Sodium (The benefits and risks of using fenofibrate with immunosuppressants and other potentially nephrotoxic agents should be carefully considered, and the lowest effective dose employed).
No products indexed under this heading.

Ceforanide (The benefits and risks of using fenofibrate with immunosuppressants and other potentially nephrotoxic agents should be carefully considered, and the lowest effective dose employed).
No products indexed under this heading.

Cefotaxime Sodium (The benefits and risks of using fenofibrate with immunosuppressants and other potentially nephrotoxic agents should be carefully considered, and the lowest effective dose employed).
No products indexed under this heading.

Cefotetan (The benefits and risks of using fenofibrate with immunosuppressants and other potentially nephrotoxic agents should be carefully considered, and the lowest effective dose employed).
No products indexed under this heading.

Cefoxitin Sodium (The benefits and risks of using fenofibrate with immunosuppressants and other potentially nephrotoxic agents should be carefully considered, and the lowest effective dose employed).
No products indexed under this heading.

Cefpodoxime Proxetil (The benefits and risks of using fenofibrate with immunosuppressants and other potentially nephrotoxic agents should be carefully considered, and the lowest effective dose employed).
No products indexed under this heading.

Cefprozil (The benefits and risks of using fenofibrate with immunosuppressants and other potentially nephrotoxic agents should be carefully considered, and the lowest effective dose employed).
No products indexed under this heading.

Ceftazidime (The benefits and risks of using fenofibrate with immunosuppressants and other potentially nephrotoxic agents should be carefully considered, and the lowest effective dose employed). Products include:
Fortaz 1481

Ceftizoxime Sodium (The benefits and risks of using fenofibrate with immunosuppressants and other potentially nephrotoxic agents should be carefully considered, and the lowest effective dose employed).
No products indexed under this heading.

Ceftriaxone Sodium (The benefits and risks of using fenofibrate with immunosuppressants and other potentially nephrotoxic agents should be carefully considered, and the lowest effective dose employed). Products include:
Rocephin 2859

Cefuroxime Axetil (The benefits and risks of using fenofibrate with immunosuppressants and other potentially nephrotoxic agents should be carefully considered, and the lowest effective dose employed). Products include:
Ceftin 1399

Cefuroxime Sodium (The benefits and risks of using fenofibrate with immunosuppressants and other potentially nephrotoxic agents should be carefully considered, and the lowest effective dose employed).
No products indexed under this heading.

Celecoxib (The benefits and risks of using fenofibrate with immunosuppressants and other potentially nephrotoxic agents should be carefully considered, and the lowest effective dose employed). Products include:
Celebrex 3272

Cephalexin (The benefits and risks of using fenofibrate with immunosuppressants and other potentially nephrotoxic agents should be carefully considered, and the lowest effective dose employed).
No products indexed under this heading.

Cephalothin Sodium (The benefits and risks of using fenofibrate with immunosuppressants and other potentially nephrotoxic agents should be carefully considered, and the lowest effective dose employed).
No products indexed under this heading.

Cephapirin Sodium (The benefits and risks of using fenofibrate with immunosuppressants and other potentially nephrotoxic agents should be carefully considered, and the lowest effective dose employed).
No products indexed under this heading.

IMPORTANT NOTE: Always consult each drug listing in the patient's regimen for possible interactions.

Fenoglide Interactions Index 654

Cephradine (The benefits and risks of using fenofibrate with immunosuppressants and other potentially nephrotoxic agents should be carefully considered, and the lowest effective dose employed).
No products indexed under this heading.

Cerivastatin Sodium (The combined use of fenofibric acid derivatives, particularly gemfibrozil, and HMG-CoA reductase inhibitors results in an increased risk of rhabdomyolysis and myoglobinuria leading in a high proportion of cases to acute renal failure. The combined use of fenofibrate and HMG-CoA reductase inhibitors should be avoided unless the benefit of further alterations in lipid levels is likely to outweigh the increased risk of this drug combination).
No products indexed under this heading.

Chlorothiazide (The benefits and risks of using fenofibrate with immunosuppressants and other potentially nephrotoxic agents should be carefully considered, and the lowest effective dose employed).
No products indexed under this heading.

Chlorothiazide Sodium (The benefits and risks of using fenofibrate with immunosuppressants and other potentially nephrotoxic agents should be carefully considered, and the lowest effective dose employed). Products include:
Diuril Intravenous 2009

Chlorpropamide (The benefits and risks of using fenofibrate with immunosuppressants and other potentially nephrotoxic agents should be carefully considered, and the lowest effective dose employed).
No products indexed under this heading.

Cholestyramine (Since bile acid sequestrants may bind other drugs give concurrently, patients should take fenofibrate at least 1 hour before or 4 to 6 hours after a bile acid binding resin to avoid impeding its absorption).
No products indexed under this heading.

Cidofovir (The benefits and risks of using fenofibrate with immunosuppressants and other potentially nephrotoxic agents should be carefully considered, and the lowest effective dose employed).
No products indexed under this heading.

Cilastatin Sodium (The benefits and risks of using fenofibrate with immunosuppressants and other potentially nephrotoxic agents should be carefully considered, and the lowest effective dose employed). Products include:
Primaxin I.M. 2232
Primaxin I.V. 2235

Cimetidine (The benefits and risks of using fenofibrate with immunosuppressants and other potentially nephrotoxic agents should be carefully considered, and the lowest effective dose employed).
No products indexed under this heading.

Cimetidine Hydrochloride (The benefits and risks of using fenofibrate with immunosuppressants and other potentially nephrotoxic agents should be carefully considered, and the lowest effective dose employed).
No products indexed under this heading.

Cisplatin (The benefits and risks of using fenofibrate with immunosuppressants and other potentially nephrotoxic agents should be carefully considered, and the lowest effective dose employed).
No products indexed under this heading.

Cladribine (The benefits and risks of using fenofibrate with immunosuppressants and other potentially nephrotoxic agents should be carefully considered, and the lowest effective dose employed). Products include:
Leustatin 946

Clozapine (The benefits and risks of using fenofibrate with immunosuppressants and other potentially nephrotoxic agents should be carefully considered, and the lowest effective dose employed).
No products indexed under this heading.

Colesevelam Hydrochloride (Since bile acid sequestrants may bind other drugs give concurrently, patients should take fenofibrate at least 1 hour before or 4 to 6 hours after a bile acid binding resin to avoid impeding its absorption). Products include:
Welchol 1029

Colestipol Hydrochloride (Since bile acid sequestrants may bind other drugs give concurrently, patients should take fenofibrate at least 1 hour before or 4 to 6 hours after a bile acid binding resin to avoid impeding its absorption).
No products indexed under this heading.

Colistimethate Sodium (The benefits and risks of using fenofibrate with immunosuppressants and other potentially nephrotoxic agents should be carefully considered, and the lowest effective dose employed).
No products indexed under this heading.

Colistin Sulfate (The benefits and risks of using fenofibrate with immunosuppressants and other potentially nephrotoxic agents should be carefully considered, and the lowest effective dose employed).
No products indexed under this heading.

Cyclophosphamide (The benefits and risks of using fenofibrate with immunosuppressants and other potentially nephrotoxic agents should be carefully considered, and the lowest effective dose employed).
No products indexed under this heading.

Cyclosporine (Because cyclosporine can product nephrotoxicity with decreases in creatinine clearance and rises in serum creatinine, and because renal excretion is the primary elimination route of fibrate drugs including fenofibrate, there is a risk that an interaction will lead to deterioration of renal function. The benefits and risks of using fenofibrate with immunosuppressants and other potentially nephrotoxic agents should be carefully considered, and the lowest effective dose employed). Products include:
Gengraf 440
Neoral Oral Solution 2496
Neoral Capsules 2496
Restasis 605

Cytarabine (The benefits and risks of using fenofibrate with immunosuppressants and other potentially nephrotoxic agents should be carefully considered, and the lowest effective dose employed).
No products indexed under this heading.

Cytarabine Liposome (The benefits and risks of using fenofibrate with immunosuppressants and other potentially nephrotoxic agents should be carefully considered, and the lowest effective dose employed).
No products indexed under this heading.

Delavirdine Mesylate (The benefits and risks of using fenofibrate with immunosuppressants and other potentially nephrotoxic agents should be carefully considered, and the lowest effective dose employed).
No products indexed under this heading.

Diatrizoate Meglumine (The benefits and risks of using fenofibrate with immunosuppressants and other potentially nephrotoxic agents should be carefully considered, and the lowest effective dose employed).
No products indexed under this heading.

Diatrizoate Sodium (The benefits and risks of using fenofibrate with immunosuppressants and other potentially nephrotoxic agents should be carefully considered, and the lowest effective dose employed).
No products indexed under this heading.

Diclofenac Potassium (The benefits and risks of using fenofibrate with immunosuppressants and other potentially nephrotoxic agents should be carefully considered, and the lowest effective dose employed).
No products indexed under this heading.

Diclofenac Sodium (The benefits and risks of using fenofibrate with immunosuppressants and other potentially nephrotoxic agents should be carefully considered, and the lowest effective dose employed).
No products indexed under this heading.

Dicloxacillin Sodium (The benefits and risks of using fenofibrate with immunosuppressants and other potentially nephrotoxic agents should be carefully considered, and the lowest effective dose employed).
No products indexed under this heading.

Dicumarol (Caution should be exercised when anticoagulants are given in conjunction with fenofibrate because of the potentiation of coumarin-type anticoagulants in prolonging the prothrombin time/INR. The dosage of the anticoagulant should be reduced to maintain the prothrombin/INR at the desired level to prevent bleeding complications. Frequent prothrombin time/INR determinations are advisable until it has been definitely determined that the prothrombin time/INR has stabilized).
No products indexed under this heading.

Didanosine (The benefits and risks of using fenofibrate with immunosuppressants and other potentially nephrotoxic agents should be carefully considered, and the lowest effective dose employed).
No products indexed under this heading.

Efavirenz (The benefits and risks of using fenofibrate with immunosuppressants and other potentially nephrotoxic agents should be carefully considered, and the lowest effective dose employed). Products include:
Atripla 906

Emtricitabine (The benefits and risks of using fenofibrate with immunosuppressants and other potentially nephrotoxic agents should be carefully considered, and the lowest effective dose employed). Products include:
Atripla 906
Emtriva 1238
Emtriva Oral Solution 1238
Truvada 1258

Enalapril Maleate (The benefits and risks of using fenofibrate with immunosuppressants and other potentially nephrotoxic agents should be carefully considered, and the lowest effective dose employed).
No products indexed under this heading.

Enalaprilat (The benefits and risks of using fenofibrate with immunosuppressants and other potentially nephrotoxic agents should be carefully considered, and the lowest effective dose employed).
No products indexed under this heading.

Enfuvirtide (The benefits and risks of using fenofibrate with immunosuppressants and other potentially nephrotoxic agents should be carefully considered, and the lowest effective dose employed).
No products indexed under this heading.

Ethiodized Oil (The benefits and risks of using fenofibrate with immunosuppressants and other potentially nephrotoxic agents should be carefully considered, and the lowest effective dose employed).
No products indexed under this heading.

Etodolac (The benefits and risks of using fenofibrate with immunosuppressants and other potentially nephrotoxic agents should be carefully considered, and the lowest effective dose employed).
No products indexed under this heading.

Fenoprofen Calcium (The benefits and risks of using fenofibrate with immunosuppressants and other potentially nephrotoxic agents should be carefully considered, and the lowest effective dose employed).
No products indexed under this heading.

Filgrastim (The benefits and risks of using fenofibrate with immunosuppressants and other potentially nephrotoxic agents should be carefully considered, and the lowest effective dose employed). Products include:
Neupogen 631

Fluorouracil (The benefits and risks of using fenofibrate with immunosuppressants and other potentially nephrotoxic agents should be carefully considered, and the lowest effective dose employed). Products include:
Carac 2966

Flurbiprofen (The benefits and risks of using fenofibrate with immunosuppressants and other potentially nephrotoxic agents should be carefully considered, and the lowest effective dose employed).
No products indexed under this heading.

Fluvastatin Sodium (The combined use of fenofibric acid derivatives, particularly gemfibrozil, and HMG-CoA reductase inhibitors results in an increased risk of rhabdomyolysis and myoglobinuria leading in a high proportion of cases to acute renal failure. The combined use of fenofibrate and HMG-CoA reductase inhibitors should be avoided unless the benefit of further alterations in lipid levels is likely to outweigh the increased risk of this drug combination).
No products indexed under this heading.

Foscarnet Sodium (The benefits and risks of using fenofibrate with immunosuppressants and other potentially nephrotoxic agents should be carefully considered, and the lowest effective dose employed).
No products indexed under this heading.

Fosinopril Sodium (The benefits and risks of using fenofibrate with immunosuppressants and other potentially nephrotoxic agents should be carefully considered, and the lowest effective dose employed).
No products indexed under this heading.

Furosemide (The benefits and risks of using fenofibrate with immunosuppressants and other potentially nephrotoxic agents should be carefully considered, and the lowest effective dose employed). Products include:
Furosemide 2354

Gadopentetate Dimeglumine (The benefits and risks of using fenofibrate with immunosuppressants and other potentially nephrotoxic agents should be carefully considered, and the lowest effective dose employed).
No products indexed under this heading.

(⊙ Described in PDR® for Ophthalmic Medicines)

IMPORTANT NOTE: Always consult each drug listing in the patient's regimen for possible interactions.

FENTANYL TRANSDERMAL SYSTEM PATCHES

May interact with alcohols, benzodiazepines, central nervous system depressants, centrally-acting drugs, cytochrome p450 3a4 inducers (selected), cytochrome p450 3a4 inhibitors (selected), erythromycin, general anesthetics, hypnotics and sedatives, monoamine oxidase inhibitors, narcotic analgesics, phenothiazines, skeletal muscle relaxants, tranquilizers, and certain other agents. Compounds in these categories include:

Acetazolamide (The concomitant use of fentanyl with all CYP3A4 inhibitors may result in an increase in fentanyl plasma concentrations, which could increase or prolong adverse drug effects and may cause potentially fatal respiratory depression. Patients receiving fentanyl and any CYP3A4 inhibitor should be carefully monitored for an extended period of time and dosage adjustments should be made if warranted).
No products indexed under this heading.

Acetazolamide Sodium (The concomitant use of fentanyl with all CYP3A4 inhibitors may result in an increase in fentanyl plasma concentrations, which could increase or prolong adverse drug effects and may cause potentially fatal respiratory depression. Patients receiving fentanyl and any CYP3A4 inhibitor should be carefully monitored for an extended period of time and dosage adjustments should be made if warranted).
No products indexed under this heading.

Alfentanil Hydrochloride (The concomitant use of fentanyl with other CNS depressants, including other opioids, may cause respiratory depression, hypotension, and profound sedation, or potentially result in coma or death. When such combined therapy is contemplated, the dose of one or both agents should be significantly reduced. The use of concomitant CNS active drugs requires special patient care and observation).
No products indexed under this heading.

Allium sativum (Co-administration with agents that induce CYP 3A4 activity may reduce the efficacy of fentanyl).
No products indexed under this heading.

Alprazolam (The concomitant use of fentanyl with other central nervous system depressants, including tranquilizers

(eg, benzodiazepines) may cause respiratory depression, hypotension, and profound sedation, or potentially result in coma or death. When such combined therapy is contemplated, the dose of one or both agents should be significantly reduced. The use of concomitant CNS active drugs requires special patient care and observation).
No products indexed under this heading.

Aminoglutethimide (Co-administration with agents that induce CYP 3A4 activity may reduce the efficacy of fentanyl).
No products indexed under this heading.

Amiodarone Hydrochloride (The concomitant use of fentanyl with all CYP3A4 inhibitors (eg, amiodarone) may result in an increase in fentanyl plasma concentrations, which could increase or prolong adverse drug effects and may cause potentially fatal respiratory depression. Patients receiving fentanyl and any CYP3A4 inhibitor should be carefully monitored for an extended period of time and dosage adjustments should be made if warranted).
No products indexed under this heading.

Amobarbital (The concomitant use of fentanyl with other CNS depressants may cause respiratory depression, hypotension, and profound sedation, or potentially result in coma or death. When such combined therapy is contemplated, the dose of one or both agents should be significantly reduced. The use of concomitant CNS active drugs requires special patient care and observation).
No products indexed under this heading.

Amobarbital Sodium (The concomitant use of fentanyl with other CNS depressants may cause respiratory depression, hypotension, and profound sedation, or potentially result in coma or death. When such combined therapy is contemplated, the dose of one or both agents should be significantly reduced. The use of concomitant CNS active drugs requires special patient care and observation).
No products indexed under this heading.

Amphetamine Aspartate (The use of concomitant CNS active drugs requires special patient care and observation).
No products indexed under this heading.

Amphetamine Aspartate Monohydrate (The use of concomitant CNS active drugs requires special patient care and observation).
No products indexed under this heading.

Amphetamine Resins (The use of concomitant CNS active drugs requires special patient care and observation).
No products indexed under this heading.

Amphetamine Sulfate (The use of concomitant CNS active drugs requires special patient care and observation).
No products indexed under this heading.

Amprenavir (The concomitant use of fentanyl with all CYP3A4 inhibitors (eg, amprenavir) may result in an increase in fentanyl plasma concentrations, which could increase or prolong adverse drug effects and may cause potentially fatal respiratory depression. Patients receiving fentanyl and any CYP3A4 inhibitor should be carefully monitored for an extended period of time and dosage adjustments should be made if warranted).
No products indexed under this heading.

Anastrozole (The concomitant use of fentanyl with all CYP3A4 inhibitors may result in an increase in fentanyl plasma concentrations, which could increase or prolong adverse drug effects and may cause potentially fatal respiratory depression. Patients receiving fentanyl and any CYP3A4 inhibitor should be carefully monitored for an extended period of time and dosage adjustments should be made if warranted).
No products indexed under this heading.

Apomorphine (The concomitant use of fentanyl with other CNS depressants, including other opioids, may cause repiratory depression, hypotension, and profound sedation, or potentially result in coma or death. When such combined therapy is contemplated, the dose of one or both agents should be significantly reduced. The use of concomitant CNS active drugs requires special patient care and observation).
No products indexed under this heading.

Apomorphine Hydrochloride (The concomitant use of fentanyl with other CNS depressants, including other opioids, may cause repiratory depression, hypotension, and profound sedation, or potentially result in coma or death. When such combined therapy is contemplated, the dose of one or both agents should be significantly reduced. The use of concomitant CNS active drugs requires special patient care and observation).
No products indexed under this heading.

Aprepitant (The concomitant use of fentanyl with all CYP3A4 inhibitors (eg, aprepitant) may result in an increase in fentanyl plasma concentrations, which could increase or prolong adverse drug effects and may cause potentially fatal respiratory depression. Patients receiving fentanyl and any CYP3A4 inhibitor should be carefully monitored for an extended period of time and dosage adjustments should be made if warranted). Products include:
Emend **2124**

Aprobarbital (The concomitant use of fentanyl with other CNS depressants may cause respiratory depression, hypotension, and profound sedation, or potentially result in coma or death. When such combined therapy is contemplated, the dose of one or both agents should be significantly reduced. The use of concomitant CNS active drugs requires special patient care and observation).
No products indexed under this heading.

Atazanavir (The concomitant use of fentanyl with all CYP3A4 inhibitors may result in an increase in fentanyl plasma concentrations, which could increase or prolong adverse drug effects and may cause potentially fatal respiratory depression. Patients receiving fentanyl and any CYP3A4 inhibitor should be carefully monitored for an extended period of time and dosage adjustments should be made if warranted).
No products indexed under this heading.

Atazanavir Sulfate (The concomitant use of fentanyl with all CYP3A4 inhibitors may result in an increase in fentanyl plasma concentrations, which could increase or prolong adverse drug effects and may cause potentially fatal respiratory depression. Patients receiving fentanyl and any CYP3A4 inhibitor should be carefully monitored for an extended period of time and dosage adjustments should be made if warranted).
No products indexed under this heading.

Atracurium Besylate (The concomitant use of fentanyl with other CNS depressants, including skeletal muscle relaxants, may cause respiratory depression, hypotension, and profound sedation, or potentially result in coma or death. When such combined therapy is contemplated, the dose of one or both agents should be significantly reduced. The use of concomitant CNS active drugs requires special patient care and observation).
No products indexed under this heading.

Baclofen (The concomitant use of fentanyl with other CNS depressants, including skeletal muscle relaxants, may cause respiratory depression, hypotension, and profound sedation, or potentially result in coma or death. When such combined therapy is contemplated, the dose of one or both agents should be significantly reduced. The use of concomitant CNS active drugs requires special patient care and observation).
No products indexed under this heading.

Betamethasone (Co-administration with agents that induce CYP 3A4 activity may reduce the efficacy of fentanyl).
No products indexed under this heading.

Betamethasone Acetate (Co-administration with agents that induce CYP 3A4 activity may reduce the efficacy of fentanyl).
No products indexed under this heading.

Betamethasone Benzoate (Co-administration with agents that induce CYP 3A4 activity may reduce the efficacy of fentanyl).
No products indexed under this heading.

Betamethasone Dipropionate (Co-administration with agents that induce CYP 3A4 activity may reduce the efficacy of fentanyl). Products include:
Diprolene Lotion 0.05% **3108**
Diprolene Ointment 0.05% **3109**
Diprolene AF Cream 0.05% **3107**
Lotrisone **3163**

Betamethasone Sodium Phosphate (Co-administration with agents that induce CYP 3A4 activity may reduce the efficacy of fentanyl).
No products indexed under this heading.

Betamethasone Valerate (Co-administration with agents that induce CYP 3A4 activity may reduce the efficacy of fentanyl). Products include:
Luxiq **3321**

Bosentan (Co-administration with agents that induce CYP 3A4 activity may reduce the efficacy of fentanyl). Products include:
Tracleer **573**

Buprenorphine Hydrochloride (The concomitant use of fentanyl with other CNS depressants, including other opioids, may cause repiratory depression, hypotension, and profound sedation, or potentially result in coma or death. When such combined therapy is contemplated, the dose of one or both agents should be significantly reduced. The use of concomitant CNS active drugs requires special patient care and observation).
No products indexed under this heading.

Buspirone Hydrochloride (The concomitant use of fentanyl with other CNS depressants, including tranquilizers, may cause respiratory depression, hypotension, and profound sedation, or potentially result in coma or death. When such combined therapy is contemplated, the dose of one or both agents should be significantly reduced. The use of concomitant CNS active drugs requires special patient care and observation).
No products indexed under this heading.

Butabarbital (The concomitant use of fentanyl with other CNS depressants, including sedatives and hypnotics, may cause respiratory depression, hypotension, and profound sedation, or potentially result in coma or death. When such combined therapy is contemplated, the dose of one or both agents should be significantly reduced. The use of concomitant CNS active drugs requires special patient care and observation).
No products indexed under this heading.

Butabarbital Sodium (The concomitant use of fentanyl with other CNS depressants, including sedatives and hypnotics, may cause respiratory depression, hypotension, and profound sedation, or potentially result in coma or death. When such combined therapy is contemplated, the dose of one or both agents should be significantly reduced. The use of concomitant CNS active drugs requires special patient care and observation).
No products indexed under this heading.

Butalbital (The concomitant use of fentanyl with other CNS depressants, including sedatives and hypnotics, may cause respiratory depression, hypotension, and profound sedation, or potentially result in coma or death. When such combined therapy is contemplated, the dose of one or both agents should be significantly reduced. The use of concomitant CNS active drugs requires special patient care and observation).
No products indexed under this heading.

Carbamazepine (Co-administration with agents that induce CYP 3A4 activity may reduce the efficacy of fentanyl). Products include:
Carbatrol **3280**
Equetro **3477**

Carisoprodol (The concomitant use of fentanyl with other CNS depressants, including skeletal muscle relaxants, may cause respiratory depression, hypotension, and profound sedation, or potentially result in coma or death. When such combined therapy is contemplated, the dose of one or both agents should be significantly reduced. The use of concomitant CNS active drugs requires special patient care and observation).
No products indexed under this heading.

Chloral Hydrate (The concomitant use of fentanyl with other CNS depressants, including sedatives and hypnotics, may cause respiratory depression, hypotension, and profound sedation, or potentially result in coma or death. When such combined therapy is contemplated, the dose of one or both agents should be significantly reduced. The use of concomitant CNS active drugs requires special patient care and observation).
No products indexed under this heading.

Chlordiazepoxide (The concomitant use of fentanyl with other central nervous system depressants, including tranquilizers (eg, benzodiazepines) may cause respiratory depression, hypotension, and profound sedation, or potentially result in coma or death. When such combined therapy is contemplated, the dose of one or both agents should be significantly reduced. The use of concomitant CNS active drugs requires special patient care and observation).
No products indexed under this heading.

Chlordiazepoxide Hydrochloride (The concomitant use of fentanyl with other central nervous system depressants, including tranquilizers (eg, benzodiazepines) may cause respiratory depression, hypotension, and profound sedation, or potentially result in coma or death. When such combined therapy is contemplated, the dose of one or both agents should be significantly reduced. The use of concomitant CNS active drugs requires special patient care and observation).
No products indexed under this heading.

Chlorpromazine (The concomitant use of fentanyl with other CNS depressants, including tranquilizers, may cause respiratory depression, hypotension, and profound sedation, or potentially result in coma or death. When such combined therapy is contemplated, the dose of one or both agents

(⊙ Described in PDR® for Ophthalmic Medicines)

should be significantly reduced. The use of concomitant CNS active drugs requires special patient care and observation).

No products indexed under this heading.

Chlorpromazine Hydrochloride (The concomitant use of fentanyl with other CNS depressants, including tranquilizers, may cause respiratory depression, hypotension, and profound sedation, or potentially result in coma or death. When such combined therapy is contemplated, the dose of one or both agents should be significantly reduced. The use of concomitant CNS active drugs requires special patient care and observation).

No products indexed under this heading.

Chlorprothixene (The concomitant use of fentanyl with other CNS depressants, including tranquilizers, may cause respiratory depression, hypotension, and profound sedation, or potentially result in coma or death. When such combined therapy is contemplated, the dose of one or both agents should be significantly reduced. The use of concomitant CNS active drugs requires special patient care and observation).

No products indexed under this heading.

Chlorprothixene Hydrochloride (The concomitant use of fentanyl with other CNS depressants, including tranquilizers, may cause respiratory depression, hypotension, and profound sedation, or potentially result in coma or death. When such combined therapy is contemplated, the dose of one or both agents should be significantly reduced. The use of concomitant CNS active drugs requires special patient care and observation).

No products indexed under this heading.

Chlorprothixene Lactate (The concomitant use of fentanyl with other CNS depressants, including tranquilizers, may cause respiratory depression, hypotension, and profound sedation, or potentially result in coma or death. When such combined therapy is contemplated, the dose of one or both agents should be significantly reduced. The use of concomitant CNS active drugs requires special patient care and observation).

No products indexed under this heading.

Chlorzoxazone (The concomitant use of fentanyl with other CNS depressants, including skeletal muscle relaxants, may cause respiratory depression, hypotension, and profound sedation, or potentially result in coma or death. When such combined therapy is contemplated, the dose of one or both agents should be significantly reduced. The use of concomitant CNS active drugs requires special patient care and observation).

No products indexed under this heading.

Cimetidine (The concomitant use of fentanyl with all CYP3A4 inhibitors may result in an increase in fentanyl plasma concentrations, which could increase or prolong adverse drug effects and may cause potentially fatal respiratory depression. Patients receiving fentanyl and any CYP3A4 inhibitor should be carefully monitored for an extended period of time and dosage adjustments should be made if warranted).

No products indexed under this heading.

Cimetidine Hydrochloride (The concomitant use of fentanyl with all CYP3A4 inhibitors may result in an increase in fentanyl plasma concentrations, which could increase or prolong adverse drug effects and may cause potentially fatal respiratory depression. Patients receiving fentanyl and any CYP3A4 inhibitor should be carefully

monitored for an extended period of time and dosage adjustments should be made if warranted).

No products indexed under this heading.

Ciprofloxacin (The concomitant use of fentanyl with all CYP3A4 inhibitors may result in an increase in fentanyl plasma concentrations, which could increase or prolong adverse drug effects and may cause potentially fatal respiratory depression. Patients receiving fentanyl and any CYP3A4 inhibitor should be carefully monitored for an extended period of time and dosage adjustments should be made if warranted). Products include:

Cipro I.V. 3082
Cipro 3073
Cipro XR 3091
Ciprodex 583

Ciprofloxacin Hydrochloride (Co-administration with agents that induce CYP 3A4 activity may reduce the efficacy of fentanyl). Products include:

Cipro 3073

Cisatracurium Besylate (The concomitant use of fentanyl with other CNS depressants, including skeletal muscle relaxants, may cause respiratory depression, hypotension, and profound sedation, or potentially result in coma or death. When such combined therapy is contemplated, the dose of one or both agents should be significantly reduced. The use of concomitant CNS active drugs requires special patient care and observation). Products include:

Nimbex 503

Cisplatin (Co-administration with agents that induce CYP 3A4 activity may reduce the efficacy of fentanyl).

No products indexed under this heading.

Clarithromycin (The concomitant use of fentanyl with all CYP3A4 inhibitors (eg, clarithromycin) may result in an increase in fentanyl plasma concentrations, which could increase or prolong adverse drug effects and may cause potentially fatal respiratory depression. Patients receiving fentanyl and any CYP3A4 inhibitor should be carefully monitored for an extended period of time and dosage adjustments should be made if warranted). Products include:

Biaxin/Biaxin XL 412

Clonazepam (The concomitant use of fentanyl with other CNS depressants may cause respiratory depression, hypotension, and profound sedation, or potentially result in coma or death. When such combined therapy is contemplated, the dose of one or both agents should be significantly reduced. The use of concomitant CNS active drugs requires special patient care and observation). Products include:

Klonopin 2855

Clorazepate Dipotassium (The concomitant use of fentanyl with other central nervous system depressants, including tranquilizers (eg, benzodiazepines) may cause respiratory depression, hypotension, and profound sedation, or potentially result in coma or death. When such combined therapy is contemplated, the dose of one or both agents should be significantly reduced. The use of concomitant CNS active drugs requires special patient care and observation).

No products indexed under this heading.

Clotrimazole (The concomitant use of fentanyl with all CYP3A4 inhibitors may result in an increase in fentanyl plasma concentrations, which could increase or prolong adverse drug effects and may cause potentially fatal respiratory depression. Patients receiving fentanyl and any CYP3A4 inhibitor should be carefully monitored for an extended

period of time and dosage adjustments should be made if warranted). Products include:

Lotrisone 3163

Clozapine (The concomitant use of fentanyl with other CNS depressants may cause respiratory depression, hypotension, and profound sedation, or potentially result in coma or death. When such combined therapy is contemplated, the dose of one or both agents should be significantly reduced. The use of concomitant CNS active drugs requires special patient care and observation).

No products indexed under this heading.

Codeine Phosphate (The concomitant use of fentanyl with other CNS depressants, including other opioids, may cause repiratory depression, hypotension, and profound sedation, or potentially result in coma or death. When such combined therapy is contemplated, the dose of one or both agents should be significantly reduced. The use of concomitant CNS active drugs requires special patient care and observation). Products include:

Tylenol with Codeine 2691

Codeine Sulfate (The concomitant use of fentanyl with other CNS depressants, including other opioids, may cause repiratory depression, hypotension, and profound sedation, or potentially result in coma or death. When such combined therapy is contemplated, the dose of one or both agents should be significantly reduced. The use of concomitant CNS active drugs requires special patient care and observation).

No products indexed under this heading.

Conivaptan Hydrochloride (The concomitant use of fentanyl with all CYP3A4 inhibitors may result in an increase in fentanyl plasma concentrations, which could increase or prolong adverse drug effects and may cause potentially fatal respiratory depression. Patients receiving fentanyl and any CYP3A4 inhibitor should be carefully monitored for an extended period of time and dosage adjustments should be made if warranted). Products include:

Vaprisol 689

Cortisone Acetate (Co-administration with agents that induce CYP 3A4 activity may reduce the efficacy of fentanyl).

No products indexed under this heading.

Cyclobenzaprine Hydrochloride (The concomitant use of fentanyl with other CNS depressants, including skeletal muscle relaxants, may cause respiratory depression, hypotension, and profound sedation, or potentially result in coma or death. When such combined therapy is contemplated, the dose of one or both agents should be significantly reduced. The use of concomitant CNS active drugs requires special patient care and observation). Products include:

Amrix 964

Cyclosporine (The concomitant use of fentanyl with all CYP3A4 inhibitors may result in an increase in fentanyl plasma concentrations, which could increase or prolong adverse drug effects and may cause potentially fatal respiratory depression. Patients receiving fentanyl and any CYP3A4 inhibitor should be carefully monitored for an extended period of time and dosage adjustments should be made if warranted). Products include:

Gengraf 440
Neoral Oral Solution 2496
Neoral Capsules 2496
Restasis 605

Dalfopristin (The concomitant use of fentanyl with all CYP3A4 inhibitors may result in an increase in fentanyl plasma

concentrations, which could increase or prolong adverse drug effects and may cause potentially fatal respiratory depression. Patients receiving fentanyl and any CYP3A4 inhibitor should be carefully monitored for an extended period of time and dosage adjustments should be made if warranted).

No products indexed under this heading.

Danazol (The concomitant use of fentanyl with all CYP3A4 inhibitors may result in an increase in fentanyl plasma concentrations, which could increase or prolong adverse drug effects and may cause potentially fatal respiratory depression. Patients receiving fentanyl and any CYP3A4 inhibitor should be carefully monitored for an extended period of time and dosage adjustments should be made if warranted).

No products indexed under this heading.

Dantrolene Sodium (The concomitant use of fentanyl with other CNS depressants, including skeletal muscle relaxants, may cause respiratory depression, hypotension, and profound sedation, or potentially result in coma or death. When such combined therapy is contemplated, the dose of one or both agents should be significantly reduced. The use of concomitant CNS active drugs requires special patient care and observation).

No products indexed under this heading.

Darunavir (The concomitant use of fentanyl with all CYP3A4 inhibitors may result in an increase in fentanyl plasma concentrations, which could increase or prolong adverse drug effects and may cause potentially fatal respiratory depression. Patients receiving fentanyl and any CYP3A4 inhibitor should be carefully monitored for an extended period of time and dosage adjustments should be made if warranted).

No products indexed under this heading.

Dasatinib (The concomitant use of fentanyl with all CYP3A4 inhibitors may result in an increase in fentanyl plasma concentrations, which could increase or prolong adverse drug effects and may cause potentially fatal respiratory depression. Patients receiving fentanyl and any CYP3A4 inhibitor should be carefully monitored for an extended period of time and dosage adjustments should be made if warranted).

No products indexed under this heading.

Delavirdine Mesylate (The concomitant use of fentanyl with all CYP3A4 inhibitors may result in an increase in fentanyl plasma concentrations, which could increase or prolong adverse drug effects and may cause potentially fatal respiratory depression. Patients receiving fentanyl and any CYP3A4 inhibitor should be carefully monitored for an extended period of time and dosage adjustments should be made if warranted).

No products indexed under this heading.

Delavirine (The concomitant use of fentanyl with all CYP3A4 inhibitors may result in an increase in fentanyl plasma concentrations, which could increase or prolong adverse drug effects and may cause potentially fatal respiratory depression. Patients receiving fentanyl and any CYP3A4 inhibitor should be carefully monitored for an extended period of time and dosage adjustments should be made if warranted).

No products indexed under this heading.

Desflurane (The concomitant use of fentanyl with other CNS depressants, including general anesthetics, may cause respiratory depression, hypotension, and profound sedation, or potentially result in coma or death. When such combined therapy is contemplated, the dose of one or both agents should be significantly reduced. The use

IMPORTANT NOTE: Always consult each drug listing in the patient's regimen for possible interactions.

of concomitant CNS active drugs requires special patient care and observation).
No products indexed under this heading.

Desloratadine (The concomitant use of fentanyl with all CYP3A4 inhibitors may result in an increase in fentanyl plasma concentrations, which could increase or prolong adverse drug effects and may cause potentially fatal respiratory depression. Patients receiving fentanyl and any CYP3A4 inhibitor should be carefully monitored for an extended period of time and dosage adjustments should be made if warranted). Products include:
Clarinex Syrup **3098**
Clarinex **3098**
Clarinex Reditabs **3098**
Clarinex-D 12-Hour **3101**
Clarinex-D **3104**

Dexamethasone (Co-administration with agents that induce CYP 3A4 activity may reduce the efficacy of fentanyl). Products include:
Ciprodex **583**
Ozurdex .... ⊙ **223**
Tobramycin and Dexamethasone Ophthalmic Suspension .... ⊙ **251**

Dexamethasone Acetate (Co-administration with agents that induce CYP 3A4 activity may reduce the efficacy of fentanyl).
No products indexed under this heading.

Dexamethasone Phosphate (Co-administration with agents that induce CYP 3A4 activity may reduce the efficacy of fentanyl).
No products indexed under this heading.

Dexamethasone Sodium (Co-administration with agents that induce CYP 3A4 activity may reduce the efficacy of fentanyl).
No products indexed under this heading.

Dexamethasone Sodium Phosphate (Co-administration with agents that induce CYP 3A4 activity may reduce the efficacy of fentanyl).
No products indexed under this heading.

Dexamethasone Sodium Phosphate Injection (Co-administration with agents that induce CYP 3A4 activity may reduce the efficacy of fentanyl).
No products indexed under this heading.

Dexmethylphenidate Hydrochloride (The use of concomitant CNS active drugs requires special patient care and observation). Products include:
Focalin XR **2472**

Dextroamphetamine (The use of concomitant CNS active drugs requires special patient care and observation).
No products indexed under this heading.

Dextroamphetamine Saccharate (The use of concomitant CNS active drugs requires special patient care and observation).
No products indexed under this heading.

Dextroamphetamine Sulfate (The use of concomitant CNS active drugs requires special patient care and observation). Products include:
Dexedrine **1425**

Dezocine (The concomitant use of fentanyl with other CNS depressants, including other opioids, may cause repiratory depression, hypotension, and profound sedation, or potentially result in coma or death. When such combined therapy is contemplated, the dose of one or both agents should be significantly reduced. The use of concomitant CNS active drugs requires special patient care and observation).
No products indexed under this heading.

Diazepam (The concomitant use of fentanyl with other central nervous system depressants, including tranquilizers (eg, benzodiazepines) may cause respiratory depression, hypotension, and profound sedation, or potentially result in coma or death. When such combined therapy is contemplated, the dose of one or both agents should be significantly reduced. The use of concomitant CNS active drugs requires special patient care and observation). Products include:
Valium Tablets **2880**

Dihydrocodeine Bitartrate (The concomitant use of fentanyl with other CNS depressants, including other opioids, may cause repiratory depression, hypotension, and profound sedation, or potentially result in coma or death. When such combined therapy is contemplated, the dose of one or both agents should be significantly reduced. The use of concomitant CNS active drugs requires special patient care and observation).
No products indexed under this heading.

Dihydrocodeinone Bitartrate (The concomitant use of fentanyl with other CNS depressants, including other opioids, may cause repiratory depression, hypotension, and profound sedation, or potentially result in coma or death. When such combined therapy is contemplated, the dose of one or both agents should be significantly reduced. The use of concomitant CNS active drugs requires special patient care and observation).
No products indexed under this heading.

Diltiazem Hydrochloride (The concomitant use of fentanyl with all CYP3A4 inhibitors (eg, diltiazem) may result in an increase in fentanyl plasma concentrations, which could increase or prolong adverse drug effects and may cause potentially fatal respiratory depression. Patients receiving fentanyl and any CYP3A4 inhibitor should be carefully monitored for an extended period of time and dosage adjustments should be made if warranted). Products include:
Cardizem LA **423**

Diltiazem Maleate (The concomitant use of fentanyl with all CYP3A4 inhibitors (eg, diltiazem) may result in an increase in fentanyl plasma concentrations, which could increase or prolong adverse drug effects and may cause potentially fatal respiratory depression. Patients receiving fentanyl and any CYP3A4 inhibitor should be carefully monitored for an extended period of time and dosage adjustments should be made if warranted).
No products indexed under this heading.

Doxacurium Chloride (The concomitant use of fentanyl with other CNS depressants, including skeletal muscle relaxants, may cause respiratory depression, hypotension, and profound sedation, or potentially result in coma or death. When such combined therapy is contemplated, the dose of one or both agents should be significantly reduced. The use of concomitant CNS active drugs requires special patient care and observation).
No products indexed under this heading.

Doxorubicin Hydrochloride (Co-administration with agents that induce CYP 3A4 activity may reduce the efficacy of fentanyl).
No products indexed under this heading.

Droperidol (The concomitant use of fentanyl with other CNS depressants, including tranquilizers, may cause respiratory depression, hypotension, and profound sedation, or potentially result in coma or death. When such combined therapy is contemplated, the dose of one or both agents should be significantly reduced. The use of concomitant CNS active drugs requires special patient care and observation).
No products indexed under this heading.

d-Tubocurarine (The concomitant use of fentanyl with other CNS depressants, including skeletal muscle relaxants, may cause respiratory depression, hypotension, and profound sedation, or potentially result in coma or death. When such combined therapy is contemplated, the dose of one or both agents should be significantly reduced. The use of concomitant CNS active drugs requires special patient care and observation).
No products indexed under this heading.

Efavirenz (The concomitant use of fentanyl with all CYP3A4 inhibitors may result in an increase in fentanyl plasma concentrations, which could increase or prolong adverse drug effects and may cause potentially fatal respiratory depression. Patients receiving fentanyl and any CYP3A4 inhibitor should be carefully monitored for an extended period of time and dosage adjustments should be made if warranted). Products include:
Atripla **906**

Enflurane (The concomitant use of fentanyl with other CNS depressants, including general anesthetics, may cause respiratory depression, hypotension, and profound sedation, or potentially result in coma or death. When such combined therapy is contemplated, the dose of one or both agents should be significantly reduced. The use of concomitant CNS active drugs requires special patient care and observation).
No products indexed under this heading.

Erythromycin (The concomitant use of fentanyl with all CYP3A4 inhibitors (eg, erythromycin) may result in an increase in fentanyl plasma concentrations, which could increase or prolong adverse drug effects and may cause potentially fatal respiratory depression. Patients receiving fentanyl and any CYP3A4 inhibitor should be carefully monitored for an extended period of time and dosage adjustments should be made if warranted).
No products indexed under this heading.

Erythromycin, Topical (The concomitant use of fentanyl with all CYP3A4 inhibitors (eg, erythromycin) may result in an increase in fentanyl plasma concentrations, which could increase or prolong adverse drug effects and may cause potentially fatal respiratory depression. Patients receiving fentanyl and any CYP3A4 inhibitor should be carefully monitored for an extended period of time and dosage adjustments should be made if warranted).
No products indexed under this heading.

Erythromycin Estolate (The concomitant use of fentanyl with all CYP3A4 inhibitors (eg, erythromycin) may result in an increase in fentanyl plasma concentrations, which could increase or prolong adverse drug effects and may cause potentially fatal respiratory depression. Patients receiving fentanyl and any CYP3A4 inhibitor should be carefully monitored for an extended period of time and dosage adjustments should be made if warranted).
No products indexed under this heading.

Erythromycin Ethylsuccinate (The concomitant use of fentanyl with all CYP3A4 inhibitors (eg, erythromycin) may result in an increase in fentanyl plasma concentrations, which could increase or prolong adverse drug effects and may cause potentially fatal respiratory depression. Patients receiving fentanyl and any CYP3A4 inhibitor should be carefully monitored for an extended period of time and dosage adjustments should be made if warranted). Products include:
E.E.S. **437**
EryPed **435**

Erythromycin Gluceptate (The concomitant use of fentanyl with all CYP3A4 inhibitors (eg, erythromycin) may result in an increase in fentanyl plasma concentrations, which could increase or prolong adverse drug effects and may cause potentially fatal respiratory depression. Patients receiving fentanyl and any CYP3A4 inhibitor should be carefully monitored for an extended period of time and dosage adjustments should be made if warranted).
No products indexed under this heading.

Erythromycin Lactobionate (The concomitant use of fentanyl with all CYP3A4 inhibitors (eg, erythromycin) may result in an increase in fentanyl plasma concentrations, which could increase or prolong adverse drug effects and may cause potentially fatal respiratory depression. Patients receiving fentanyl and any CYP3A4 inhibitor should be carefully monitored for an extended period of time and dosage adjustments should be made if warranted).
No products indexed under this heading.

Erythromycin Stearate (The concomitant use of fentanyl with all CYP3A4 inhibitors (eg, erythromycin) may result in an increase in fentanyl plasma concentrations, which could increase or prolong adverse drug effects and may cause potentially fatal respiratory depression. Patients receiving fentanyl and any CYP3A4 inhibitor should be carefully monitored for an extended period of time and dosage adjustments should be made if warranted).
No products indexed under this heading.

Esomeprazole Magnesium (The concomitant use of fentanyl with all CYP3A4 inhibitors may result in an increase in fentanyl plasma concentrations, which could increase or prolong adverse drug effects and may cause potentially fatal respiratory depression. Patients receiving fentanyl and any CYP3A4 inhibitor should be carefully monitored for an extended period of time and dosage adjustments should be made if warranted). Products include:
Nexium Capsules **704**
Nexium Oral Suspension **704**

Esomeprazole Sodium (The concomitant use of fentanyl with all CYP3A4 inhibitors may result in an increase in fentanyl plasma concentrations, which could increase or prolong adverse drug effects and may cause potentially fatal respiratory depression. Patients receiving fentanyl and any CYP3A4 inhibitor should be carefully monitored for an extended period of time and dosage adjustments should be made if warranted). Products include:
Nexium I.V. **712**

Estazolam (The concomitant use of fentanyl with other central nervous system depressants, including tranquilizers (eg, benzodiazepines) may cause respiratory depression, hypotension, and profound sedation, or potentially result in coma or death. When such combined therapy is contemplated, the dose of one or both agents should be significantly reduced. The use of concomitant CNS active drugs requires special patient care and observation).
No products indexed under this heading.

Ethanol (Fentanyl may be expected to have additive CNS depressant effects when used in conjunction with alcohol. The concomitant use of fentanyl with alcohol may cause respiratory depression, hypotension, and profound sedation, or potentially result in coma or death).
No products indexed under this heading.

Ethchlorvynol (The concomitant use of fentanyl with other CNS depressants, including sedatives and hypnotics, may cause respiratory depression, hypotension, and profound sedation, or potentially result in coma or death. When such combined therapy is contemplated, the dose of one or both agents should be significantly reduced. The use of concomitant CNS active drugs requires special patient care and observation).

No products indexed under this heading.

Ethinamate (The concomitant use of fentanyl with other CNS depressants, including sedatives and hypnotics, may cause respiratory depression, hypotension, and profound sedation, or potentially result in coma or death. When such combined therapy is contemplated, the dose of one or both agents should be significantly reduced. The use of concomitant CNS active drugs requires special patient care and observation).

No products indexed under this heading.

Ethosuximide (Co-administration with agents that induce CYP 3A4 activity may reduce the efficacy of fentanyl).

No products indexed under this heading.

Ethyl Alcohol (Fentanyl may be expected to have additive CNS depressant effects when used in conjunction with alcohol. The concomitant use of fentanyl with alcohol may cause respiratory depression, hypotension, and profound sedation, or potentially result in coma or death).

No products indexed under this heading.

Felbamate (Co-administration with agents that induce CYP 3A4 activity may reduce the efficacy of fentanyl).

No products indexed under this heading.

Fentanyl Citrate (The concomitant use of fentanyl with other CNS depressants, including other opioids, may cause repiratory depression, hypotension, and profound sedation, or potentially result in coma or death. When such combined therapy is contemplated, the dose of one or both agents should be significantly reduced. The use of concomitant CNS active drugs requires special patient care and observation). Products include:

Fentora 966

Fluconazole (The concomitant use of fentanyl with all CYP3A4 inhibitors (eg, fluconazole) may result in an increase in fentanyl plasma concentrations, which could increase or prolong adverse drug effects and may cause potentially fatal respiratory depression. Patients receiving fentanyl and any CYP3A4 inhibitor should be carefully monitored for an extended period of time and dosage adjustments should be made if warranted).

No products indexed under this heading.

Fludrocortisone Acetate (Co-administration with agents that induce CYP 3A4 activity may reduce the efficacy of fentanyl).

No products indexed under this heading.

Fluoxetine (The concomitant use of fentanyl with all CYP3A4 inhibitors may result in an increase in fentanyl plasma concentrations, which could increase or prolong adverse drug effects and may cause potentially fatal respiratory depression. Patients receiving fentanyl and any CYP3A4 inhibitor should be carefully monitored for an extended period of time and dosage adjustments should be made if warranted).

No products indexed under this heading.

Fluoxetine Hydrochloride (The concomitant use of fentanyl with all CYP3A4 inhibitors may result in an increase in fentanyl plasma concentrations, which could increase or prolong adverse drug effects and may cause

potentially fatal respiratory depression. Patients receiving fentanyl and any CYP3A4 inhibitor should be carefully monitored for an extended period of time and dosage adjustments should be made if warranted). Products include:

Prozac Weekly 1941
Prozac Pulvules 1941
Symbyax 1965

Fluphenazine Decanoate (The concomitant use of fentanyl with other CNS depressants, including tranquilizers, may cause respiratory depression, hypotension, and profound sedation, or potentially result in coma or death. When such combined therapy is contemplated, the dose of one or both agents should be significantly reduced. The use of concomitant CNS active drugs requires special patient care and observation).

No products indexed under this heading.

Fluphenazine Enanthate (The concomitant use of fentanyl with other CNS depressants, including tranquilizers, may cause respiratory depression, hypotension, and profound sedation, or potentially result in coma or death. When such combined therapy is contemplated, the dose of one or both agents should be significantly reduced. The use of concomitant CNS active drugs requires special patient care and observation).

No products indexed under this heading.

Fluphenazine Hydrochloride (The concomitant use of fentanyl with other CNS depressants, including tranquilizers, may cause respiratory depression, hypotension, and profound sedation, or potentially result in coma or death. When such combined therapy is contemplated, the dose of one or both agents should be significantly reduced. The use of concomitant CNS active drugs requires special patient care and observation).

No products indexed under this heading.

Flurazepam Hydrochloride (The concomitant use of fentanyl with other central nervous system depressants, including tranquilizers (eg, benzodiazepines) may cause respiratory depression, hypotension, and profound sedation, or potentially result in coma or death. When such combined therapy is contemplated, the dose of one or both agents should be significantly reduced. The use of concomitant CNS active drugs requires special patient care and observation).

No products indexed under this heading.

Fluvoxamine Maleate (The concomitant use of fentanyl with all CYP3A4 inhibitors may result in an increase in fentanyl plasma concentrations, which could increase or prolong adverse drug effects and may cause potentially fatal respiratory depression. Patients receiving fentanyl and any CYP3A4 inhibitor should be carefully monitored for an extended period of time and dosage adjustments should be made if warranted).

No products indexed under this heading.

Fosamprenavir Calcium (The concomitant use of fentanyl with all CYP3A4 inhibitors (eg, fosamprenavir) may result in an increase in fentanyl plasma concentrations, which could increase or prolong adverse drug effects and may cause potentially fatal respiratory depression. Patients receiving fentanyl and any CYP3A4 inhibitor should be carefully monitored for an extended period of time and dosage adjustments should be made if warranted). Products include:

Lexiva Oral Suspension 1558
Lexiva 1558

Fosphenytoin Sodium (Co-administration with agents that induce CYP 3A4 activity may reduce the efficacy of fentanyl).

No products indexed under this heading.

Gallamine (The concomitant use of fentanyl with other CNS depressants, including skeletal muscle relaxants, may cause respiratory depression, hypotension, and profound sedation, or potentially result in coma or death. When such combined therapy is contemplated, the dose of one or both agents should be significantly reduced. The use of concomitant CNS active drugs requires special patient care and observation).

No products indexed under this heading.

Gallamine Triethiodide (The concomitant use of fentanyl with other CNS depressants, including skeletal muscle relaxants, may cause respiratory depression, hypotension, and profound sedation, or potentially result in coma or death. When such combined therapy is contemplated, the dose of one or both agents should be significantly reduced. The use of concomitant CNS active drugs requires special patient care and observation).

No products indexed under this heading.

Garlic Extract (Co-administration with agents that induce CYP 3A4 activity may reduce the efficacy of fentanyl).

No products indexed under this heading.

Garlic Oil (Co-administration with agents that induce CYP 3A4 activity may reduce the efficacy of fentanyl).

No products indexed under this heading.

Glutethimide (The concomitant use of fentanyl with other CNS depressants, including sedatives and hypnotics, may cause respiratory depression, hypotension, and profound sedation, or potentially result in coma or death. When such combined therapy is contemplated, the dose of one or both agents should be significantly reduced. The use of concomitant CNS active drugs requires special patient care and observation).

No products indexed under this heading.

Halazepam (The concomitant use of fentanyl with other central nervous system depressants, including tranquilizers (eg, benzodiazepines) may cause respiratory depression, hypotension, and profound sedation, or potentially result in coma or death. When such combined therapy is contemplated, the dose of one or both agents should be significantly reduced. The use of concomitant CNS active drugs requires special patient care and observation).

No products indexed under this heading.

Haloperidol (The concomitant use of fentanyl with other CNS depressants, including tranquilizers, may cause respiratory depression, hypotension, and profound sedation, or potentially result in coma or death. When such combined therapy is contemplated, the dose of one or both agents should be significantly reduced. The use of concomitant CNS active drugs requires special patient care and observation).

No products indexed under this heading.

Haloperidol Decanoate (The concomitant use of fentanyl with other CNS depressants, including tranquilizers, may cause respiratory depression, hypotension, and profound sedation, or potentially result in coma or death. When such combined therapy is contemplated, the dose of one or both agents should be significantly reduced. The use of concomitant CNS active drugs requires special patient care and observation).

No products indexed under this heading.

Haloperidol Lactate (The concomitant use of fentanyl with other CNS depressants may cause respiratory depression, hypotension, and profound sedation, or potentially result in coma or death. When such combined therapy is contemplated, the dose of one or both agents should be significantly reduced. The use of concomitant CNS active drugs requires special patient care and observation).

No products indexed under this heading.

Halothane (The concomitant use of fentanyl with other CNS depressants, including general anesthetics, may cause respiratory depression, hypotension, and profound sedation, or potentially result in coma or death. When such combined therapy is contemplated, the dose of one or both agents should be significantly reduced. The use of concomitant CNS active drugs requires special patient care and observation).

No products indexed under this heading.

Hexobarbital (The concomitant use of fentanyl with other CNS depressants may cause respiratory depression, hypotension, and profound sedation, or potentially result in coma or death. When such combined therapy is contemplated, the dose of one or both agents should be significantly reduced. The use of concomitant CNS active drugs requires special patient care and observation).

No products indexed under this heading.

Hydrocodone Bitartrate (The concomitant use of fentanyl with other CNS depressants, including other opioids, may cause respiratory depression, hypotension, and profound sedation, or potentially result in coma or death. When such combined therapy is contemplated, the dose of one or both agents should be significantly reduced. The use of concomitant CNS active drugs requires special patient care and observation). Products include:

Vicodin 560
Vicodin ES 561
Vicodin HP 563
Vicoprofen 564
Zydone 1138

Hydrocodone Polistirex (The concomitant use of fentanyl with other CNS depressants, including other opioids, may cause repiratory depression, hypotension, and profound sedation, or potentially result in coma or death. When such combined therapy is contemplated, the dose of one or both agents should be significantly reduced. The use of concomitant CNS active drugs requires special patient care and observation). Products include:

Tussionex 3443

Hydrocortisone (Co-administration with agents that induce CYP 3A4 activity may reduce the efficacy of fentanyl).

No products indexed under this heading.

Hydrocortisone (Alcohol) (Co-administration with agents that induce CYP 3A4 activity may reduce the efficacy of fentanyl).

No products indexed under this heading.

Hydrocortisone Acetate (Co-administration with agents that induce CYP 3A4 activity may reduce the efficacy of fentanyl).

No products indexed under this heading.

Hydrocortisone Butyrate (Co-administration with agents that induce CYP 3A4 activity may reduce the efficacy of fentanyl).

No products indexed under this heading.

Hydrocortisone Cypionate (Co-administration with agents that induce CYP 3A4 activity may reduce the efficacy of fentanyl).

No products indexed under this heading.

IMPORTANT NOTE: Always consult each drug listing in the patient's regimen for possible interactions.

Hydrocortisone Hemisuccinate (Co-administration with agents that induce CYP 3A4 activity may reduce the efficacy of fentanyl).
No products indexed under this heading.

Hydrocortisone Probutate (Co-administration with agents that induce CYP 3A4 activity may reduce the efficacy of fentanyl).
No products indexed under this heading.

Hydrocortisone Sodium Phosphate (Co-administration with agents that induce CYP 3A4 activity may reduce the efficacy of fentanyl).
No products indexed under this heading.

Hydrocortisone Sodium Succinate (Co-administration with agents that induce CYP 3A4 activity may reduce the efficacy of fentanyl).
No products indexed under this heading.

Hydrocortisone Valerate (Co-administration with agents that induce CYP 3A4 activity may reduce the efficacy of fentanyl).
No products indexed under this heading.

Hydromorphone (The concomitant use of fentanyl with other CNS depressants, including other opioids, may cause repiratory depression, hypotension, and profound sedation, or potentially result in coma or death. When such combined therapy is contemplated, the dose of one or both agents should be significantly reduced. The use of concomitant CNS active drugs requires special patient care and observation).
No products indexed under this heading.

Hydromorphone Hydrochloride (The concomitant use of fentanyl with other CNS depressants, including other opioids, may cause repiratory depression, hypotension, and profound sedation, or potentially result in coma or death. When such combined therapy is contemplated, the dose of one or both agents should be significantly reduced. The use of concomitant CNS active drugs requires special patient care and observation). Products include:
Dilaudid Injection 2800
Dilaudid Oral 2797
Dilaudid Tablets 2797
Dilaudid-HP 2800

Hydroxyamphetamine Hydrobromide (The use of concomitant CNS active drugs requires special patient care and observation).
No products indexed under this heading.

Hydroxyzine Hydrochloride (The concomitant use of fentanyl with other CNS depressants, including tranquilizers, may cause respiratory depression, hypotension, and profound sedation, or potentially result in coma or death. When such combined therapy is contemplated, the dose of one or both agents should be significantly reduced. The use of concomitant CNS active drugs requires special patient care and observation).
No products indexed under this heading.

Hypericum (Co-administration with agents that induce CYP 3A4 activity may reduce the efficacy of fentanyl).
No products indexed under this heading.

Hypericum Perforatum (Co-administration with agents that induce CYP 3A4 activity may reduce the efficacy of fentanyl). Products include:
Traumeel 1800

Imatinib Mesylate (The concomitant use of fentanyl with all CYP3A4 inhibitors may result in an increase in fentanyl plasma concentrations, which could increase or prolong adverse drug effects and may cause potentially fatal respiratory depression. Patients receiving fentanyl and any CYP3A4 inhibitor should be carefully monitored for an extended period of time and dosage adjustments should be made if warranted). Products include:
Gleevec 2477

Indinavir Sulfate (The concomitant use of fentanyl with all CYP3A4 inhibitors may result in an increase in fentanyl plasma concentrations, which could increase or prolong adverse drug effects and may cause potentially fatal respiratory depression. Patients receiving fentanyl and any CYP3A4 inhibitor should be carefully monitored for an extended period of time and dosage adjustments should be made if warranted). Products include:
Crixivan 2113

Isocarboxazid (Fentanyl is not recommended for use in patients who have received monoamine oxidase (MAO) inhibitors within 14 days because severe and unpredictable potentiation by MAO inhibitors has been reported with opioid analgesics). Products include:
Marplan 3481

Isoflurane (The concomitant use of fentanyl with other CNS depressants, including general anesthetics, may cause respiratory depression, hypotension, and profound sedation, or potentially result in coma or death. When such combined therapy is contemplated, the dose of one or both agents should be significantly reduced. The use of concomitant CNS active drugs requires special patient care and observation).
No products indexed under this heading.

Isoniazid (The concomitant use of fentanyl with all CYP3A4 inhibitors may result in an increase in fentanyl plasma concentrations, which could increase or prolong adverse drug effects and may cause potentially fatal respiratory depression. Patients receiving fentanyl and any CYP3A4 inhibitor should be carefully monitored for an extended period of time and dosage adjustments should be made if warranted).
No products indexed under this heading.

Itraconazole (The concomitant use of fentanyl with all CYP3A4 inhibitors (eg, itraconazole) may result in an increase in fentanyl plasma concentrations, which could increase or prolong adverse drug effects and may cause potentially fatal respiratory depression. Patients receiving fentanyl and any CYP3A4 inhibitor should be carefully monitored for an extended period of time and dosage adjustments should be made if warranted).
No products indexed under this heading.

Ketamine Hydrochloride (The concomitant use of fentanyl with other CNS depressants, including general anesthetics, may cause respiratory depression, hypotension, and profound sedation, or potentially result in coma or death. When such combined therapy is contemplated, the dose of one or both agents should be significantly reduced. The use of concomitant CNS active drugs requires special patient care and observation).
No products indexed under this heading.

Ketoconazole (The concomitant use of fentanyl with all CYP3A4 inhibitors (eg, ketoconazole) may result in an increase in fentanyl plasma concentrations, which could increase or prolong adverse drug effects and may cause potentially fatal respiratory depression. Patients receiving fentanyl and any CYP3A4 inhibitor should be carefully monitored for an extended period of time and dosage adjustments should be made if warranted). Products include:
Extina 3319
Xolegel 3337

Lapatinib (The concomitant use of fentanyl with all CYP3A4 inhibitors may result in an increase in fentanyl plasma concentrations, which could increase or prolong adverse drug effects and may cause potentially fatal respiratory depression. Patients receiving fentanyl and any CYP3A4 inhibitor should be carefully monitored for an extended period of time and dosage adjustments should be made if warranted). Products include:
Tykerb 1698

Levomethadyl Acetate Hydrochloride (The concomitant use of fentanyl with other CNS depressants may cause respiratory depression, hypotension, and profound sedation, or potentially result in coma or death. When such combined therapy is contemplated, the dose of one or both agents should be significantly reduced. The use of concomitant CNS active drugs requires special patient care and observation).
No products indexed under this heading.

Levorphanol Tartrate (The concomitant use of fentanyl with other CNS depressants, including other opioids, may cause repiratory depression, hypotension, and profound sedation, or potentially result in coma or death. When such combined therapy is contemplated, the dose of one or both agents should be significantly reduced. The use of concomitant CNS active drugs requires special patient care and observation).
No products indexed under this heading.

Lisdexamfetamine Dimesylate (The use of concomitant CNS active drugs requires special patient care and observation). Products include:
Vyvanse 3298

Lopinavir (The concomitant use of fentanyl with all CYP3A4 inhibitors may result in an increase in fentanyl plasma concentrations, which could increase or prolong adverse drug effects and may cause potentially fatal respiratory depression. Patients receiving fentanyl and any CYP3A4 inhibitor should be carefully monitored for an extended period of time and dosage adjustments should be made if warranted). Products include:
Kaletra 458

Loratadine (The concomitant use of fentanyl with all CYP3A4 inhibitors may result in an increase in fentanyl plasma concentrations, which could increase or prolong adverse drug effects and may cause potentially fatal respiratory depression. Patients receiving fentanyl and any CYP3A4 inhibitor should be carefully monitored for an extended period of time and dosage adjustments should be made if warranted).
No products indexed under this heading.

Lorazepam (The concomitant use of fentanyl with other central nervous system depressants, including tranquilizers (eg, benzodiazepines) may cause respiratory depression, hypotension, and profound sedation, or potentially result in coma or death. When such combined therapy is contemplated, the dose of one or both agents should be significantly reduced. The use of concomitant CNS active drugs requires special patient care and observation).
No products indexed under this heading.

Loxapine Hydrochloride (The concomitant use of fentanyl with other CNS depressants, including tranquilizers, may cause respiratory depression, hypotension, and profound sedation, or potentially result in coma or death. When such combined therapy is contemplated, the dose of one or both agents should be significantly reduced. The use of concomitant CNS active drugs requires special patient care and observation).
No products indexed under this heading.

Loxapine Succinate (The concomitant use of fentanyl with other CNS depressants, including tranquilizers, may cause respiratory depression, hypotension, and profound sedation, or potentially result in coma or death. When such combined therapy is contemplated, the dose of one or both agents should be significantly reduced. The use of concomitant CNS active drugs requires special patient care and observation).
No products indexed under this heading.

Meperidine Hydrochloride (The concomitant use of fentanyl with other CNS depressants, including other opioids, may cause repiratory depression, hypotension, and profound sedation, or potentially result in coma or death. When such combined therapy is contemplated, the dose of one or both agents should be significantly reduced. The use of concomitant CNS active drugs requires special patient care and observation).
No products indexed under this heading.

Mephenytoin (Co-administration with agents that induce CYP 3A4 activity may reduce the efficacy of fentanyl).
No products indexed under this heading.

Mephobarbital (The concomitant use of fentanyl with other CNS depressants may cause respiratory depression, hypotension, and profound sedation, or potentially result in coma or death. When such combined therapy is contemplated, the dose of one or both agents should be significantly reduced. The use of concomitant CNS active drugs requires special patient care and observation).
No products indexed under this heading.

Meprobamate (The concomitant use of fentanyl with other CNS depressants, including tranquilizers, may cause respiratory depression, hypotension, and profound sedation, or potentially result in coma or death. When such combined therapy is contemplated, the dose of one or both agents should be significantly reduced. The use of concomitant CNS active drugs requires special patient care and observation).
No products indexed under this heading.

Mesoridazine Besylate (The concomitant use of fentanyl with other CNS depressants, including tranquilizers, may cause respiratory depression, hypotension, and profound sedation, or potentially result in coma or death. When such combined therapy is contemplated, the dose of one or both agents should be significantly reduced. The use of concomitant CNS active drugs requires special patient care and observation).
No products indexed under this heading.

Metaxalone (The concomitant use of fentanyl with other CNS depressants, including skeletal muscle relaxants, may cause respiratory depression, hypotension, and profound sedation, or potentially result in coma or death. When such combined therapy is contemplated, the dose of one or both agents should be significantly reduced. The use of concomitant CNS active drugs requires special patient care and observation). Products include:
Skelaxin 1848

Methadone Hydrochloride (The concomitant use of fentanyl with other CNS depressants, including other opioids, may cause respiratory depression, hypotension, and profound sedation, or potentially result in coma or death. When such combined therapy is contemplated, the dose of one or both

agents should be significantly reduced. The use of concomitant CNS active drugs requires special patient care and observation).

No products indexed under this heading.

Methamphetamine Hydrochloride (The use of concomitant CNS active drugs requires special patient care and observation).

No products indexed under this heading.

Methocarbamol (The concomitant use of fentanyl with other CNS depressants, including skeletal muscle relaxants, may cause respiratory depression, hypotension, and profound sedation, or potentially result in coma or death. When such combined therapy is contemplated, the dose of one or both agents should be significantly reduced. The use of concomitant CNS active drugs requires special patient care and observation).

No products indexed under this heading.

Methohexital Sodium (The concomitant use of fentanyl with other CNS depressants, including general anesthetics, may cause respiratory depression, hypotension, and profound sedation, or potentially result in coma or death. When such combined therapy is contemplated, the dose of one or both agents should be significantly reduced. The use of concomitant CNS active drugs requires special patient care and observation).

No products indexed under this heading.

Methotrimeprazine (The concomitant use of fentanyl with other CNS depressants, including phenothiazines, may cause repiratory depression, hypotension, and profound sedation, or potentially result in coma or death. When such combined therapy is contemplated, the dose of one or both agents should be significantly reduced. The use of concomitant CNS active drugs requires special patient care and observation).

No products indexed under this heading.

Methoxyflurane (The concomitant use of fentanyl with other CNS depressants, including general anesthetics, may cause respiratory depression, hypotension, and profound sedation, or potentially result in coma or death. When such combined therapy is contemplated, the dose of one or both agents should be significantly reduced. The use of concomitant CNS active drugs requires special patient care and observation).

No products indexed under this heading.

Methsuximide (Co-administration with agents that induce CYP 3A4 activity may reduce the efficacy of fentanyl).

No products indexed under this heading.

Methylphenidate (The use of concomitant CNS active drugs requires special patient care and observation). Products include:
Daytrana 3283

Methylphenidate Hydrochloride (The use of concomitant CNS active drugs requires special patient care and observation). Products include:
Concerta 2598
Metadate CD 3439

Methylprednisolone (Co-administration with agents that induce CYP 3A4 activity may reduce the efficacy of fentanyl).

No products indexed under this heading.

Methylprednisolone Acetate (Co-administration with agents that induce CYP 3A4 activity may reduce the efficacy of fentanyl).

No products indexed under this heading.

Methylprednisolone Sodium Succinate (Co-administration with agents that induce CYP 3A4 activity may reduce the efficacy of fentanyl).

No products indexed under this heading.

Metocurine Iodide (The concomitant use of fentanyl with other CNS depressants, including skeletal muscle relaxants, may cause respiratory depression, hypotension, and profound sedation, or potentially result in coma or death. When such combined therapy is contemplated, the dose of one or both agents should be significantly reduced. The use of concomitant CNS active drugs requires special patient care and observation).

No products indexed under this heading.

Metronidazole (The concomitant use of fentanyl with all CYP3A4 inhibitors may result in an increase in fentanyl plasma concentrations, which could increase or prolong adverse drug effects and may cause potentially fatal respiratory depression. Patients receiving fentanyl and any CYP3A4 inhibitor should be carefully monitored for an extended period of time and dosage adjustments should be made if warranted). Products include:
Pylera 793

Metronidazole Benzoate (The concomitant use of fentanyl with all CYP3A4 inhibitors may result in an increase in fentanyl plasma concentrations, which could increase or prolong adverse drug effects and may cause potentially fatal respiratory depression. Patients receiving fentanyl and any CYP3A4 inhibitor should be carefully monitored for an extended period of time and dosage adjustments should be made if warranted).

No products indexed under this heading.

Metronidazole Hydrochloride (The concomitant use of fentanyl with all CYP3A4 inhibitors may result in an increase in fentanyl plasma concentrations, which could increase or prolong adverse drug effects and may cause potentially fatal respiratory depression. Patients receiving fentanyl and any CYP3A4 inhibitor should be carefully monitored for an extended period of time and dosage adjustments should be made if warranted).

No products indexed under this heading.

Metronidazole Sodium (The concomitant use of fentanyl with all CYP3A4 inhibitors may result in an increase in fentanyl plasma concentrations, which could increase or prolong adverse drug effects and may cause potentially fatal respiratory depression. Patients receiving fentanyl and any CYP3A4 inhibitor should be carefully monitored for an extended period of time and dosage adjustments should be made if warranted).

No products indexed under this heading.

Miconazole (The concomitant use of fentanyl with all CYP3A4 inhibitors may result in an increase in fentanyl plasma concentrations, which could increase or prolong adverse drug effects and may cause potentially fatal respiratory depression. Patients receiving fentanyl and any CYP3A4 inhibitor should be carefully monitored for an extended period of time and dosage adjustments should be made if warranted).

No products indexed under this heading.

Miconazole Nitrate (The concomitant use of fentanyl with all CYP3A4 inhibitors may result in an increase in fentanyl plasma concentrations, which could increase or prolong adverse drug effects and may cause potentially fatal respiratory depression. Patients receiving fentanyl and any CYP3A4 inhibitor should be carefully monitored for an

extended period of time and dosage adjustments should be made if warranted). Products include:
Vusion Ointment 3335

Midazolam Hydrochloride (The concomitant use of fentanyl with other central nervous system depressants, including tranquilizers (eg, benzodiazepines) may cause respiratory depression, hypotension, and profound sedation, or potentially result in coma or death. When such combined therapy is contemplated, the dose of one or both agents should be significantly reduced. The use of concomitant CNS active drugs requires special patient care and observation).

No products indexed under this heading.

Mifepristone (The concomitant use of fentanyl with all CYP3A4 inhibitors may result in an increase in fentanyl plasma concentrations, which could increase or prolong adverse drug effects and may cause potentially fatal respiratory depression. Patients receiving fentanyl and any CYP3A4 inhibitor should be carefully monitored for an extended period of time and dosage adjustments should be made if warranted).

No products indexed under this heading.

Mivacurium Chloride (The concomitant use of fentanyl with other CNS depressants, including skeletal muscle relaxants, may cause respiratory depression, hypotension, and profound sedation, or potentially result in coma or death. When such combined therapy is contemplated, the dose of one or both agents should be significantly reduced. The use of concomitant CNS active drugs requires special patient care and observation).

No products indexed under this heading.

Moclobemide (Fentanyl is not recommended for use in patients who have received monoamine oxidase (MAO) inhibitors within 14 days because severe and unpredictable potentiation by MAO inhibitors has been reported with opioid analgesics).

No products indexed under this heading.

Modafinil (Co-administration with agents that induce CYP 3A4 activity may reduce the efficacy of fentanyl). Products include:
Provigil 983

Molindone Hydrochloride (The concomitant use of fentanyl with other CNS depressants, including tranquilizers, may cause respiratory depression, hypotension, and profound sedation, or potentially result in coma or death. When such combined therapy is contemplated, the dose of one or both agents should be significantly reduced. The use of concomitant CNS active drugs requires special patient care and observation). Products include:
Moban 1108

Morphine Sulfate (The concomitant use of fentanyl with other CNS depressants, including other opioids, may cause repiratory depression, hypotension, and profound sedation, or potentially result in coma or death. When such combined therapy is contemplated, the dose of one or both agents should be significantly reduced. The use of concomitant CNS active drugs requires special patient care and observation). Products include:
Avinza 1822
Embeda 1831
MS Contin 2803

Morphine Sulfate, Liposomal (The concomitant use of fentanyl with other CNS depressants, including other opioids, may cause repiratory depression, hypotension, and profound sedation, or potentially result in coma or death. When such combined therapy is contemplated, the dose of one or both

agents should be significantly reduced. The use of concomitant CNS active drugs requires special patient care and observation).

No products indexed under this heading.

Nafcillin Sodium (Co-administration with agents that induce CYP 3A4 activity may reduce the efficacy of fentanyl).

No products indexed under this heading.

Nefazodone Hydrochloride (The concomitant use of fentanyl with all CYP3A4 inhibitors (eg, nefazodone) may result in an increase in fentanyl plasma concentrations, which could increase or prolong adverse drug effects and may cause potentially fatal respiratory depression. Patients receiving fentanyl and any CYP3A4 inhibitor should be carefully monitored for an extended period of time and dosage adjustments should be made if warranted).

No products indexed under this heading.

Nelfinavir Mesylate (The concomitant use of fentanyl with all CYP3A4 inhibitors (eg, nelfinavir) may result in an increase in fentanyl plasma concentrations, which could increase or prolong adverse drug effects and may cause potentially fatal respiratory depression. Patients receiving fentanyl and any CYP3A4 inhibitor should be carefully monitored for an extended period of time and dosage adjustments should be made if warranted).

No products indexed under this heading.

Nevirapine (The concomitant use of fentanyl with all CYP3A4 inhibitors may result in an increase in fentanyl plasma concentrations, which could increase or prolong adverse drug effects and may cause potentially fatal respiratory depression. Patients receiving fentanyl and any CYP3A4 inhibitor should be carefully monitored for an extended period of time and dosage adjustments should be made if warranted). Products include:
Viramune Oral Suspension 897
Viramune Tablets 897

Niacin (The concomitant use of fentanyl with all CYP3A4 inhibitors may result in an increase in fentanyl plasma concentrations, which could increase or prolong adverse drug effects and may cause potentially fatal respiratory depression. Patients receiving fentanyl and any CYP3A4 inhibitor should be carefully monitored for an extended period of time and dosage adjustments should be made if warranted). Products include:
Advicor 402
Cardio Basics 3455
Niaspan 497
Simcor 524

Niacinamide (The concomitant use of fentanyl with all CYP3A4 inhibitors may result in an increase in fentanyl plasma concentrations, which could increase or prolong adverse drug effects and may cause potentially fatal respiratory depression. Patients receiving fentanyl and any CYP3A4 inhibitor should be carefully monitored for an extended period of time and dosage adjustments should be made if warranted). Products include:
CitraNatal 90 DHA Capsules 2332
CitraNatal Assure 2332
CitraNatal Rx 2332
Heplive 607

Niacinamide Hydroiodide (The concomitant use of fentanyl with all CYP3A4 inhibitors may result in an increase in fentanyl plasma concentrations, which could increase or prolong adverse drug effects and may cause potentially fatal respiratory depression. Patients receiving fentanyl and any CYP3A4 inhibitor should be carefully

---

IMPORTANT NOTE: Always consult each drug listing in the patient's regimen for possible interactions.

monitored for an extended period of time and dosage adjustments should be made if warranted).
No products indexed under this heading.

Nicotinamide (The concomitant use of fentanyl with all CYP3A4 inhibitors may result in an increase in fentanyl plasma concentrations, which could increase or prolong adverse drug effects and may cause potentially fatal respiratory depression. Patients receiving fentanyl and any CYP3A4 inhibitor should be carefully monitored for an extended period of time and dosage adjustments should be made if warranted).
No products indexed under this heading.

Nifedipine (The concomitant use of fentanyl with all CYP3A4 inhibitors may result in an increase in fentanyl plasma concentrations, which could increase or prolong adverse drug effects and may cause potentially fatal respiratory depression. Patients receiving fentanyl and any CYP3A4 inhibitor should be carefully monitored for an extended period of time and dosage adjustments should be made if warranted).
No products indexed under this heading.

Nitrous Oxide (The concomitant use of fentanyl with other CNS depressants, including general anesthetics, may cause respiratory depression, hypotension, and profound sedation, or potentially result in coma or death. When such combined therapy is contemplated, the dose of one or both agents should be significantly reduced. The use of concomitant CNS active drugs requires special patient care and observation).
No products indexed under this heading.

Norfloxacin (The concomitant use of fentanyl with all CYP3A4 inhibitors may result in an increase in fentanyl plasma concentrations, which could increase or prolong adverse drug effects and may cause potentially fatal respiratory depression. Patients receiving fentanyl and any CYP3A4 inhibitor should be carefully monitored for an extended period of time and dosage adjustments should be made if warranted). Products include:
Noroxin 2220

Olanzapine (The concomitant use of fentanyl with other CNS depressants may cause respiratory depression, hypotension, and profound sedation, or potentially result in coma or death. When such combined therapy is contemplated, the dose of one or both agents should be significantly reduced. The use of concomitant CNS active drugs requires special patient care and observation). Products include:
Symbyax 1965
Zyprexa 1984
Zyprexa IntraMuscular 1984
Zyprexa ZYDIS 1984

Omeprazole (The concomitant use of fentanyl with all CYP3A4 inhibitors may result in an increase in fentanyl plasma concentrations, which could increase or prolong adverse drug effects and may cause potentially fatal respiratory depression. Patients receiving fentanyl and any CYP3A4 inhibitor should be carefully monitored for an extended period of time and dosage adjustments should be made if warranted).
No products indexed under this heading.

Orphenadrine Citrate (The concomitant use of fentanyl with other CNS depressants, including skeletal muscle relaxants, may cause respiratory depression, hypotension, and profound sedation, or potentially result in coma or death. When such combined therapy is contemplated, the dose of one or both agents should be significantly reduced. The use of concomitant CNS active drugs requires special patient care and observation).
No products indexed under this heading.

Oxazepam (The concomitant use of fentanyl with other central nervous system depressants, including tranquilizers (eg, benzodiazepines) may cause respiratory depression, hypotension, and profound sedation, or potentially result in coma or death. When such combined therapy is contemplated, the dose of one or both agents should be significantly reduced. The use of concomitant CNS active drugs requires special patient care and observation).
No products indexed under this heading.

Oxcarbazepine (Co-administration with agents that induce CYP 3A4 activity may reduce the efficacy of fentanyl).
No products indexed under this heading.

Oxycodone Hydrochloride (The concomitant use of fentanyl with other CNS depressants, including other opioids, may cause repiratory depression, hypotension, and profound sedation, or potentially result in coma or death. When such combined therapy is contemplated, the dose of one or both agents should be significantly reduced. The use of concomitant CNS active drugs requires special patient care and observation). Products include:
OxyContin 2807
Percocet 1121
Percodan 1124

Oxycodone Terephthalate (The concomitant use of fentanyl with other CNS depressants, including other opioids, may cause repiratory depression, hypotension, and profound sedation, or potentially result in coma or death. When such combined therapy is contemplated, the dose of one or both agents should be significantly reduced. The use of concomitant CNS active drugs requires special patient care and observation).
No products indexed under this heading.

Oxymorphone Hydrochloride (The concomitant use of fentanyl with other CNS depressants, including other opioids, may cause repiratory depression, hypotension, and profound sedation, or potentially result in coma or death. When such combined therapy is contemplated, the dose of one or both agents should be significantly reduced. The use of concomitant CNS active drugs requires special patient care and observation). Products include:
Opana 1110
Opana ER 1114

Pancuronium Bromide (The concomitant use of fentanyl with other CNS depressants, including skeletal muscle relaxants, may cause respiratory depression, hypotension, and profound sedation, or potentially result in coma or death. When such combined therapy is contemplated, the dose of one or both agents should be significantly reduced. The use of concomitant CNS active drugs requires special patient care and observation).
No products indexed under this heading.

Pargyline Hydrochloride (Fentanyl is not recommended for use in patients who have received monoamine oxidase (MAO) inhibitors within 14 days because severe and unpredictable potentiation by MAO inhibitors has been reported with opioid analgesics).
No products indexed under this heading.

Paroxetine Hydrochloride (The concomitant use of fentanyl with all CYP3A4 inhibitors may result in an increase in fentanyl plasma concentrations, which could increase or prolong adverse drug effects and may cause potentially fatal respiratory depression. Patients receiving fentanyl and any CYP3A4 inhibitor should be carefully monitored for an extended period of time and dosage adjustments should be made if warranted). Products include:
Paroxetine CR 2361
Paroxetine ER 2371
Paxil 1586
Paxil CR 1596

Pemoline (The use of concomitant CNS active drugs requires special patient care and observation).
No products indexed under this heading.

Pentobarbital (The concomitant use of fentanyl with other CNS depressants may cause respiratory depression, hypotension, and profound sedation, or potentially result in coma or death. When such combined therapy is contemplated, the dose of one or both agents should be significantly reduced. The use of concomitant CNS active drugs requires special patient care and observation).
No products indexed under this heading.

Pentobarbital Sodium (The concomitant use of fentanyl with other CNS depressants may cause respiratory depression, hypotension, and profound sedation, or potentially result in coma or death. When such combined therapy is contemplated, the dose of one or both agents should be significantly reduced. The use of concomitant CNS active drugs requires special patient care and observation). Products include:
Nembutal 2012

Perphenazine (The concomitant use of fentanyl with other CNS depressants, including tranquilizers, may cause respiratory depression, hypotension, and profound sedation, or potentially result in coma or death. When such combined therapy is contemplated, the dose of one or both agents should be significantly reduced. The use of concomitant CNS active drugs requires special patient care and observation).
No products indexed under this heading.

Phenelzine Sulfate (Fentanyl is not recommended for use in patients who have received monoamine oxidase (MAO) inhibitors within 14 days because severe and unpredictable potentiation by MAO inhibitors has been reported with opioid analgesics).
No products indexed under this heading.

Phenobarbital (The concomitant use of fentanyl with other CNS depressants may cause respiratory depression, hypotension, and profound sedation, or potentially result in coma or death. When such combined therapy is contemplated, the dose of one or both agents should be significantly reduced. The use of concomitant CNS active drugs requires special patient care and observation). Products include:
Donnatal 2711

Phenobarbital Sodium (The concomitant use of fentanyl with other CNS depressants may cause respiratory depression, hypotension, and profound sedation, or potentially result in coma or death. When such combined therapy is contemplated, the dose of one or both agents should be significantly reduced. The use of concomitant CNS active drugs requires special patient care and observation).
No products indexed under this heading.

Phenothiazine Derivatives (The concomitant use of fentanyl with other CNS depressants, including phenothiazines, may cause repiratory depression, hypotension, and profound sedation, or potentially result in coma or death. When such combined therapy is contemplated, the dose of one or both agents should be significantly reduced. The use of concomitant CNS active drugs requires special patient care and observation).
No products indexed under this heading.

Phenothiazines (The concomitant use of fentanyl with other CNS depressants, including phenothiazines, may cause repiratory depression, hypotension, and profound sedation, or potentially result in coma or death. When such combined therapy is contemplated, the dose of one or both agents should be significantly reduced. The use of concomitant CNS active drugs requires special patient care and observation).
No products indexed under this heading.

Phenytoin (Co-administration with agents that induce CYP 3A4 activity may reduce the efficacy of fentanyl).
No products indexed under this heading.

Phenytoin Sodium (Co-administration with agents that induce CYP 3A4 activity may reduce the efficacy of fentanyl). Products include:
Phenytek Capsules 2380

Pipecuronium Bromide (The concomitant use of fentanyl with other CNS depressants, including skeletal muscle relaxants, may cause respiratory depression, hypotension, and profound sedation, or potentially result in coma or death. When such combined therapy is contemplated, the dose of one or both agents should be significantly reduced. The use of concomitant CNS active drugs requires special patient care and observation).
No products indexed under this heading.

Posaconazole (The concomitant use of fentanyl with all CYP3A4 inhibitors may result in an increase in fentanyl plasma concentrations, which could increase or prolong adverse drug effects and may cause potentially fatal respiratory depression. Patients receiving fentanyl and any CYP3A4 inhibitor should be carefully monitored for an extended period of time and dosage adjustments should be made if warranted). Products include:
Noxafil 3172

Prazepam (The concomitant use of fentanyl with other central nervous system depressants, including tranquilizers (eg, benzodiazepines) may cause respiratory depression, hypotension, and profound sedation, or potentially result in coma or death. When such combined therapy is contemplated, the dose of one or both agents should be significantly reduced. The use of concomitant CNS active drugs requires special patient care and observation).
No products indexed under this heading.

Prednisolone (Co-administration with agents that induce CYP 3A4 activity may reduce the efficacy of fentanyl).
No products indexed under this heading.

Prednisolone Acetate (Co-administration with agents that induce CYP 3A4 activity may reduce the efficacy of fentanyl). Products include:
Blephamide .... ⊙212, ⊙214
Pred Forte .... ⊙225
Pred Mild .... ⊙230
Pred-G .... ⊙226, ⊙227

Prednisolone Sodium Phosphate (Co-administration with agents that induce CYP 3A4 activity may reduce the efficacy of fentanyl).
No products indexed under this heading.

Prednisolone Tebutate (Co-administration with agents that induce CYP 3A4 activity may reduce the efficacy of fentanyl).
No products indexed under this heading.

Prednisone (Co-administration with agents that induce CYP 3A4 activity may reduce the efficacy of fentanyl).
No products indexed under this heading.

665 Interactions Index Fentanyl

Prednisone sodium phosphate (Co-administration with agents that induce CYP 3A4 activity may reduce the efficacy of fentanyl).
No products indexed under this heading.

Primidone (Co-administration with agents that induce CYP 3A4 activity may reduce the efficacy of fentanyl).
No products indexed under this heading.

Procarbazine Hydrochloride (Fentanyl is not recommended for use in patients who have received monoamine oxidase (MAO) inhibitors within 14 days because severe and unpredictable potentiation by MAO inhibitors has been reported with opioid analgesics).
No products indexed under this heading.

Prochlorperazine (The concomitant use of fentanyl with other CNS depressants, including tranquilizers, may cause respiratory depression, hypotension, and profound sedation, or potentially result in coma or death. When such combined therapy is contemplated, the dose of one or both agents should be significantly reduced. The use of concomitant CNS active drugs requires special patient care and observation).
No products indexed under this heading.

Prochlorperazine Edisylate (The concomitant use of fentanyl with other CNS depressants, including phenothiazines, may cause repiratory depression, hypotension, and profound sedation, or potentially result in coma or death. When such combined therapy is contemplated, the dose of one or both agents should be significantly reduced. The use of concomitant CNS active drugs requires special patient care and observation).
No products indexed under this heading.

Prochlorperazine Maleate (The concomitant use of fentanyl with other CNS depressants, including phenothiazines, may cause repiratory depression, hypotension, and profound sedation, or potentially result in coma or death. When such combined therapy is contemplated, the dose of one or both agents should be significantly reduced. The use of concomitant CNS active drugs requires special patient care and observation).
No products indexed under this heading.

Promethazine (The concomitant use of fentanyl with other CNS depressants, including phenothiazines, may cause repiratory depression, hypotension, and profound sedation, or potentially result in coma or death. When such combined therapy is contemplated, the dose of one or both agents should be significantly reduced. The use of concomitant CNS active drugs requires special patient care and observation).
No products indexed under this heading.

Promethazine Hydrochloride (The concomitant use of fentanyl with other CNS depressants, including tranquilizers, may cause respiratory depression, hypotension, and profound sedation, or potentially result in coma or death. When such combined therapy is contemplated, the dose of one or both agents should be significantly reduced. The use of concomitant CNS active drugs requires special patient care and observation).
No products indexed under this heading.

Propofol (The concomitant use of fentanyl with other CNS depressants, including sedatives and hypnotics, may cause respiratory depression, hypotension, and profound sedation, or potentially result in coma or death. When such combined therapy is contemplated, the dose of one or both agents should be significantly reduced. The use of concomitant CNS active drugs requires special patient care and observation).
No products indexed under this heading.

Propoxyphene Hydrochloride (The concomitant use of fentanyl with other CNS depressants, including other opioids, may cause repiratory depression, hypotension, and profound sedation, or potentially result in coma or death. When such combined therapy is contemplated, the dose of one or both agents should be significantly reduced. The use of concomitant CNS active drugs requires special patient care and observation).
No products indexed under this heading.

Propoxyphene Napsylate (The concomitant use of fentanyl with other CNS depressants, including other opioids, may cause repiratory depression, hypotension, and profound sedation, or potentially result in coma or death. When such combined therapy is contemplated, the dose of one or both agents should be significantly reduced. The use of concomitant CNS active drugs requires special patient care and observation).
No products indexed under this heading.

Quazepam (The concomitant use of fentanyl with other central nervous system depressants, including tranquilizers (eg, benzodiazepines) may cause respiratory depression, hypotension, and profound sedation, or potentially result in coma or death. When such combined therapy is contemplated, the dose of one or both agents should be significantly reduced. The use of concomitant CNS active drugs requires special patient care and observation).
No products indexed under this heading.

Quetiapine Fumarate (The concomitant use of fentanyl with other CNS depressants may cause respiratory depression, hypotension, and profound sedation, or potentially result in coma or death. When such combined therapy is contemplated, the dose of one or both agents should be significantly reduced. The use of concomitant CNS active drugs requires special patient care and observation). Products include:
Seroquel 750
Seroquel XR 759

Quinidine (The concomitant use of fentanyl with all CYP3A4 inhibitors may result in an increase in fentanyl plasma concentrations, which could increase or prolong adverse drug effects and may cause potentially fatal respiratory depression. Patients receiving fentanyl and any CYP3A4 inhibitor should be carefully monitored for an extended period of time and dosage adjustments should be made if warranted).
No products indexed under this heading.

Quinidine Hydrochloride (The concomitant use of fentanyl with all CYP3A4 inhibitors may result in an increase in fentanyl plasma concentrations, which could increase or prolong adverse drug effects and may cause potentially fatal respiratory depression. Patients receiving fentanyl and any CYP3A4 inhibitor should be carefully monitored for an extended period of time and dosage adjustments should be made if warranted).
No products indexed under this heading.

Quinidine Polygalacturonate (The concomitant use of fentanyl with all CYP3A4 inhibitors may result in an increase in fentanyl plasma concentrations, which could increase or prolong adverse drug effects and may cause potentially fatal respiratory depression. Patients receiving fentanyl and any CYP3A4 inhibitor should be carefully monitored for an extended period of time and dosage adjustments should be made if warranted).
No products indexed under this heading.

Quinidine Sulfate (The concomitant use of fentanyl with all CYP3A4 inhibitors may result in an increase in fentanyl plasma concentrations, which could increase or prolong adverse drug effects and may cause potentially fatal respiratory depression. Patients receiving fentanyl and any CYP3A4 inhibitor should be carefully monitored for an extended period of time and dosage adjustments should be made if warranted).
No products indexed under this heading.

Quinine (The concomitant use of fentanyl with all CYP3A4 inhibitors may result in an increase in fentanyl plasma concentrations, which could increase or prolong adverse drug effects and may cause potentially fatal respiratory depression. Patients receiving fentanyl and any CYP3A4 inhibitor should be carefully monitored for an extended period of time and dosage adjustments should be made if warranted). Products include:
Hyland's Leg Cramps PM with Quinine 3315

Quinine Sulfate (The concomitant use of fentanyl with all CYP3A4 inhibitors may result in an increase in fentanyl plasma concentrations, which could increase or prolong adverse drug effects and may cause potentially fatal respiratory depression. Patients receiving fentanyl and any CYP3A4 inhibitor should be carefully monitored for an extended period of time and dosage adjustments should be made if warranted).
No products indexed under this heading.

Quinupristin (The concomitant use of fentanyl with all CYP3A4 inhibitors may result in an increase in fentanyl plasma concentrations, which could increase or prolong adverse drug effects and may cause potentially fatal respiratory depression. Patients receiving fentanyl and any CYP3A4 inhibitor should be carefully monitored for an extended period of time and dosage adjustments should be made if warranted).
No products indexed under this heading.

Ramelteon (The concomitant use of fentanyl with other CNS depressants, including sedatives and hypnotics, may cause respiratory depression, hypotension, and profound sedation, or potentially result in coma or death. When such combined therapy is contemplated, the dose of one or both agents should be significantly reduced. The use of concomitant CNS active drugs requires special patient care and observation). Products include:
Rozerem 3366

Ranitidine Bismuth Citrate (The concomitant use of fentanyl with all CYP3A4 inhibitors may result in an increase in fentanyl plasma concentrations, which could increase or prolong adverse drug effects and may cause potentially fatal respiratory depression. Patients receiving fentanyl and any CYP3A4 inhibitor should be carefully monitored for an extended period of time and dosage adjustments should be made if warranted).
No products indexed under this heading.

Ranitidine Hydrochloride (The concomitant use of fentanyl with all CYP3A4 inhibitors may result in an increase in fentanyl plasma concentrations, which could increase or prolong adverse drug effects and may cause potentially fatal respiratory depression. Patients receiving fentanyl and any CYP3A4 inhibitor should be carefully monitored for an extended period of time and dosage adjustments should be made if warranted). Products include:
Zantac 1737
Zantac Injection 1732
Zantac Pharmacy 1735

Rapacuronium Bromide (The concomitant use of fentanyl with other CNS depressants, including skeletal muscle relaxants, may cause respiratory depression, hypotension, and profound sedation, or potentially result in coma or death. When such combined therapy is contemplated, the dose of one or both agents should be significantly reduced. The use of concomitant CNS active drugs requires special patient care and observation).
No products indexed under this heading.

Rasagiline Mesylate (Fentanyl is not recommended for use in patients who have received monoamine oxidase (MAO) inhibitors within 14 days because severe and unpredictable potentiation by MAO inhibitors has been reported with opioid analgesics). Products include:
Azilect 3383

Remifentanil Hydrochloride (The concomitant use of fentanyl with other CNS depressants, including other opioids, may cause repiratory depression, hypotension, and profound sedation, or potentially result in coma or death. When such combined therapy is contemplated, the dose of one or both agents should be significantly reduced. The use of concomitant CNS active drugs requires special patient care and observation).
No products indexed under this heading.

Rifabutin (Co-administration with agents that induce CYP 3A4 activity may reduce the efficacy of fentanyl).
No products indexed under this heading.

Rifampicin (Co-administration with agents that induce CYP 3A4 activity may reduce the efficacy of fentanyl).
No products indexed under this heading.

Rifampin (Co-administration with agents that induce CYP 3A4 activity may reduce the efficacy of fentanyl).
No products indexed under this heading.

Rifapentine (Co-administration with agents that induce CYP 3A4 activity may reduce the efficacy of fentanyl).
No products indexed under this heading.

Risperidone (The concomitant use of fentanyl with other CNS depressants may cause respiratory depression, hypotension, and profound sedation, or potentially result in coma or death. When such combined therapy is contemplated, the dose of one or both agents should be significantly reduced. The use of concomitant CNS active drugs requires special patient care and observation). Products include:
Risperdal Consta 2682

Ritonavir (The concomitant use of fentanyl with all CYP3A4 inhibitors (eg, ritonavir) may result in an increase in fentanyl plasma concentrations, which could increase or prolong adverse drug effects and may cause potentially fatal respiratory depression. Patients receiving fentanyl and any CYP3A4 inhibitor should be carefully monitored for an extended period of time and dosage adjustments should be made if warranted). Products include:
Kaletra 458
Norvir 509

Rocuronium Bromide (The concomitant use of fentanyl with other CNS depressants, including skeletal muscle relaxants, may cause respiratory depression, hypotension, and profound sedation, or potentially result in coma or death. When such combined therapy is contemplated, the dose of one or both agents should be significantly

IMPORTANT NOTE: Always consult each drug listing in the patient's regimen for possible interactions.

Fentanyl Interactions Index 666

reduced. The use of concomitant CNS active drugs requires special patient care and observation). Products include:
Zemuron 3249

Saquinavir (The concomitant use of fentanyl with all CYP3A4 inhibitors may result in an increase in fentanyl plasma concentrations, which could increase or prolong adverse drug effects and may cause potentially fatal respiratory depression. Patients receiving fentanyl and any CYP3A4 inhibitor should be carefully monitored for an extended period of time and dosage adjustments should be made if warranted).
No products indexed under this heading.

Saquinavir Mesylate (The concomitant use of fentanyl with all CYP3A4 inhibitors may result in an increase in fentanyl plasma concentrations, which could increase or prolong adverse drug effects and may cause potentially fatal respiratory depression. Patients receiving fentanyl and any CYP3A4 inhibitor should be carefully monitored for an extended period of time and dosage adjustments should be made if warranted).
No products indexed under this heading.

Secobarbital Sodium (The concomitant use of fentanyl with other CNS depressants, including sedatives and hypnotics, may cause respiratory depression, hypotension, and profound sedation, or potentially result in coma or death. When such combined therapy is contemplated, the dose of one or both agents should be significantly reduced. The use of concomitant CNS active drugs requires special patient care and observation).
No products indexed under this heading.

Selegiline (Fentanyl is not recommended for use in patients who have received monoamine oxidase (MAO) inhibitors within 14 days because severe and unpredictable potentiation by MAO inhibitors has been reported with opioid analgesics). Products include:
Emsam 3623

Selegiline Hydrochloride (Fentanyl is not recommended for use in patients who have received monoamine oxidase (MAO) inhibitors within 14 days because severe and unpredictable potentiation by MAO inhibitors has been reported with opioid analgesics). Products include:
Eldepryl 3312

Sertraline Hydrochloride (The concomitant use of fentanyl with all CYP3A4 inhibitors may result in an increase in fentanyl plasma concentrations, which could increase or prolong adverse drug effects and may cause potentially fatal respiratory depression. Patients receiving fentanyl and any CYP3A4 inhibitor should be carefully monitored for an extended period of time and dosage adjustments should be made if warranted).
No products indexed under this heading.

Sevoflurane (The concomitant use of fentanyl with other CNS depressants, including general anesthetics, may cause respiratory depression, hypotension, and profound sedation, or potentially result in coma or death. When such combined therapy is contemplated, the dose of one or both agents should be significantly reduced. The use of concomitant CNS active drugs requires special patient care and observation). Products include:
Ultane 554

Sildenafil Citrate (The concomitant use of fentanyl with all CYP3A4 inhibitors may result in an increase in fentanyl plasma concentrations, which could increase or prolong adverse drug effects and may cause potentially fatal respiratory depression. Patients receiving fentanyl and any CYP3A4 inhibitor should be carefully monitored for an extended period of time and dosage adjustments should be made if warranted).
No products indexed under this heading.

Sodium Butabarbital (The concomitant use of fentanyl with other CNS depressants, including sedatives and hypnotics, may cause respiratory depression, hypotension, and profound sedation, or potentially result in coma or death. When such combined therapy is contemplated, the dose of one or both agents should be significantly reduced. The use of concomitant CNS active drugs requires special patient care and observation).
No products indexed under this heading.

Sodium Oxybate (The concomitant use of fentanyl with other CNS depressants may cause respiratory depression, hypotension, and profound sedation, or potentially result in coma or death. When such combined therapy is contemplated, the dose of one or both agents should be significantly reduced. The use of concomitant CNS active drugs requires special patient care and observation).
No products indexed under this heading.

Sodium Pentobarbital (The concomitant use of fentanyl with other CNS depressants may cause respiratory depression, hypotension, and profound sedation, or potentially result in coma or death. When such combined therapy is contemplated, the dose of one or both agents should be significantly reduced. The use of concomitant CNS active drugs requires special patient care and observation).
No products indexed under this heading.

Succinylcholine Chloride (The concomitant use of fentanyl with other CNS depressants, including skeletal muscle relaxants, may cause respiratory depression, hypotension, and profound sedation, or potentially result in coma or death. When such combined therapy is contemplated, the dose of one or both agents should be significantly reduced. The use of concomitant CNS active drugs requires special patient care and observation).
No products indexed under this heading.

Sufentanil Citrate (The concomitant use of fentanyl with other CNS depressants, including other opioids, may cause repiratory depression, hypotension, and profound sedation, or potentially result in coma or death. When such combined therapy is contemplated, the dose of one or both agents should be significantly reduced. The use of concomitant CNS active drugs requires special patient care and observation).
No products indexed under this heading.

Sulfinpyrazone (Co-administration with agents that induce CYP 3A4 activity may reduce the efficacy of fentanyl).
No products indexed under this heading.

Talbutal (The concomitant use of fentanyl with other CNS depressants may cause respiratory depression, hypotension, and profound sedation, or potentially result in coma or death. When such combined therapy is contemplated, the dose of one or both agents should be significantly reduced. The use of concomitant CNS active drugs requires special patient care and observation).
No products indexed under this heading.

Telithromycin (The concomitant use of fentanyl with all CYP3A4 inhibitors may result in an increase in fentanyl plasma concentrations, which could increase or prolong adverse drug effects and may cause potentially fatal respiratory depression. Patients receiving fentanyl and any CYP3A4 inhibitor should be carefully monitored for an extended period of time and dosage adjustments should be made if warranted). Products include:
Ketek 2991

Temazepam (The concomitant use of fentanyl with other central nervous system depressants, including tranquilizers (eg, benzodiazepines) may cause respiratory depression, hypotension, and profound sedation, or potentially result in coma or death. When such combined therapy is contemplated, the dose of one or both agents should be significantly reduced. The use of concomitant CNS active drugs requires special patient care and observation).
No products indexed under this heading.

Theophyllinate (Co-administration with agents that induce CYP 3A4 activity may reduce the efficacy of fentanyl).
No products indexed under this heading.

Theophylline (Co-administration with agents that induce CYP 3A4 activity may reduce the efficacy of fentanyl).
No products indexed under this heading.

Theophylline Anhydrous (Co-administration with agents that induce CYP 3A4 activity may reduce the efficacy of fentanyl). Products include:
Uniphyl 2817

Theophylline Calcium Salicylate (Co-administration with agents that induce CYP 3A4 activity may reduce the efficacy of fentanyl).
No products indexed under this heading.

Theophylline Dihydroxypropyl (Glyceryl) (Co-administration with agents that induce CYP 3A4 activity may reduce the efficacy of fentanyl).
No products indexed under this heading.

Theophylline Ethylenediamine (Co-administration with agents that induce CYP 3A4 activity may reduce the efficacy of fentanyl).
No products indexed under this heading.

Theophylline Sodium Glycinate (Co-administration with agents that induce CYP 3A4 activity may reduce the efficacy of fentanyl).
No products indexed under this heading.

Thiamylal Sodium (The concomitant use of fentanyl with other CNS depressants may cause respiratory depression, hypotension, and profound sedation, or potentially result in coma or death. When such combined therapy is contemplated, the dose of one or both agents should be significantly reduced. The use of concomitant CNS active drugs requires special patient care and observation).
No products indexed under this heading.

Thioridazine (The concomitant use of fentanyl with other CNS depressants, including phenothiazines, may cause repiratory depression, hypotension, and profound sedation, or potentially result in coma or death. When such combined therapy is contemplated, the dose of one or both agents should be significantly reduced. The use of concomitant CNS active drugs requires special patient care and observation).
No products indexed under this heading.

Thioridazine Hydrochloride (The concomitant use of fentanyl with other CNS depressants, including tranquilizers, may cause respiratory depression, hypotension, and profound sedation, or potentially result in coma or death. When such combined therapy is contemplated, the dose of one or both agents should be significantly reduced. The use of concomitant CNS active drugs requires special patient care and observation). Products include:
Thioridazine Hydrochloride 2384

Thiothixene (The concomitant use of fentanyl with other CNS depressants, including tranquilizers, may cause respiratory depression, hypotension, and profound sedation, or potentially result in coma or death. When such combined therapy is contemplated, the dose of one or both agents should be significantly reduced. The use of concomitant CNS active drugs requires special patient care and observation). Products include:
Thiothixene 2386

Thiothixene Hydrochloride (The concomitant use of fentanyl with other CNS depressants may cause respiratory depression, hypotension, and profound sedation, or potentially result in coma or death. When such combined therapy is contemplated, the dose of one or both agents should be significantly reduced. The use of concomitant CNS active drugs requires special patient care and observation).
No products indexed under this heading.

Tizanidine (The concomitant use of fentanyl with other CNS depressants, including skeletal muscle relaxants, may cause respiratory depression, hypotension, and profound sedation, or potentially result in coma or death. When such combined therapy is contemplated, the dose of one or both agents should be significantly reduced. The use of concomitant CNS active drugs requires special patient care and observation).
No products indexed under this heading.

Tizanidine Hydrochloride (The concomitant use of fentanyl with other CNS depressants, including skeletal muscle relaxants, may cause respiratory depression, hypotension, and profound sedation, or potentially result in coma or death. When such combined therapy is contemplated, the dose of one or both agents should be significantly reduced. The use of concomitant CNS active drugs requires special patient care and observation).
No products indexed under this heading.

Tranylcypromine Sulfate (Fentanyl is not recommended for use in patients who have received monoamine oxidase (MAO) inhibitors within 14 days because severe and unpredictable potentiation by MAO inhibitors has been reported with opioid analgesics). Products include:
Parnate 1584

Triamcinolone (Co-administration with agents that induce CYP 3A4 activity may reduce the efficacy of fentanyl).
No products indexed under this heading.

Triamcinolone Acetonide (Co-administration with agents that induce CYP 3A4 activity may reduce the efficacy of fentanyl). Products include:
Azmacort 408
Nasacort AQ 3019

Triamcinolone Diacetate (Co-administration with agents that induce CYP 3A4 activity may reduce the efficacy of fentanyl).
No products indexed under this heading.

Triamcinolone Hexacetonide (Co-administration with agents that induce CYP 3A4 activity may reduce the efficacy of fentanyl).
No products indexed under this heading.

Triazolam (The concomitant use of fentanyl with other central nervous system depressants, including tranquilizers (eg, benzodiazepines) may cause respiratory depression, hypotension, and profound sedation, or potentially result in coma or death. When such combined therapy is contemplated, the dose of one or both agents should be signifi-

cantly reduced. The use of concomitant CNS active drugs requires special patient care and observation).

No products indexed under this heading.

Trifluoperazine Hydrochloride (The concomitant use of fentanyl with other CNS depressants, including tranquilizers, may cause respiratory depression, hypotension, and profound sedation, or potentially result in coma or death. When such combined therapy is contemplated, the dose of one or both agents should be significantly reduced. The use of concomitant CNS active drugs requires special patient care and observation).

No products indexed under this heading.

Troglitazone (The concomitant use of fentanyl with all CYP3A4 inhibitors may result in an increase in fentanyl plasma concentrations, which could increase or prolong adverse drug effects and may cause potentially fatal respiratory depression. Patients receiving fentanyl and any CYP3A4 inhibitor should be carefully monitored for an extended period of time and dosage adjustments should be made if warranted).

No products indexed under this heading.

Troleandomycin (The concomitant use of fentanyl with all CYP3A4 inhibitors (eg, troleandomycin) may result in an increase in fentanyl plasma concentrations, which could increase or prolong adverse drug effects and may cause potentially fatal respiratory depression. Patients receiving fentanyl and any CYP3A4 inhibitor should be carefully monitored for an extended period of time and dosage adjustments should be made if warranted).

No products indexed under this heading.

Tubocurarine Chloride (The concomitant use of fentanyl with other CNS depressants, including skeletal muscle relaxants, may cause respiratory depression, hypotension, and profound sedation, or potentially result in coma or death. When such combined therapy is contemplated, the dose of one or both agents should be significantly reduced. The use of concomitant CNS active drugs requires special patient care and observation).

No products indexed under this heading.

Valproate Sodium (The concomitant use of fentanyl with all CYP3A4 inhibitors may result in an increase in fentanyl plasma concentrations, which could increase or prolong adverse drug effects and may cause potentially fatal respiratory depression. Patients receiving fentanyl and any CYP3A4 inhibitor should be carefully monitored for an extended period of time and dosage adjustments should be made if warranted).

No products indexed under this heading.

Vardenafil Hydrochloride (The concomitant use of fentanyl with all CYP3A4 inhibitors may result in an increase in fentanyl plasma concentrations, which could increase or prolong adverse drug effects and may cause potentially fatal respiratory depression. Patients receiving fentanyl and any CYP3A4 inhibitor should be carefully monitored for an extended period of time and dosage adjustments should be made if warranted). Products include:

Levitra 3157

Vecuronium Bromide (The concomitant use of fentanyl with other CNS depressants, including skeletal muscle relaxants, may cause respiratory depression, hypotension, and profound sedation, or potentially result in coma or death. When such combined therapy is contemplated, the dose of one or both agents should be significantly reduced. The use of concomitant CNS active drugs requires special patient care and observation).

No products indexed under this heading.

Verapamil Hydrochloride (The concomitant use of fentanyl with all CYP3A4 inhibitors (eg, verapamil) may result in an increase in fentanyl plasma concentrations, which could increase or prolong adverse drug effects and may cause potentially fatal respiratory depression. Patients receiving fentanyl and any CYP3A4 inhibitor should be carefully monitored for an extended period of time and dosage adjustments should be made if warranted). Products include:

Tarka 534

Voriconazole (The concomitant use of fentanyl with all CYP3A4 inhibitors may result in an increase in fentanyl plasma concentrations, which could increase or prolong adverse drug effects and may cause potentially fatal respiratory depression. Patients receiving fentanyl and any CYP3A4 inhibitor should be carefully monitored for an extended period of time and dosage adjustments should be made if warranted).

No products indexed under this heading.

Zafirlukast (The concomitant use of fentanyl with all CYP3A4 inhibitors may result in an increase in fentanyl plasma concentrations, which could increase or prolong adverse drug effects and may cause potentially fatal respiratory depression. Patients receiving fentanyl and any CYP3A4 inhibitor should be carefully monitored for an extended period of time and dosage adjustments should be made if warranted). Products include:

Accolate 3612

Zaleplon (The concomitant use of fentanyl with other CNS depressants, including sedatives and hypnotics, may cause respiratory depression, hypotension, and profound sedation, or potentially result in coma or death. When such combined therapy is contemplated, the dose of one or both agents should be significantly reduced. The use of concomitant CNS active drugs requires special patient care and observation).

No products indexed under this heading.

Zileuton (The concomitant use of fentanyl with all CYP3A4 inhibitors may result in an increase in fentanyl plasma concentrations, which could increase or prolong adverse drug effects and may cause potentially fatal respiratory depression. Patients receiving fentanyl and any CYP3A4 inhibitor should be carefully monitored for an extended period of time and dosage adjustments should be made if warranted).

No products indexed under this heading.

Ziprasidone Hydrochloride (The concomitant use of fentanyl with other CNS depressants may cause respiratory depression, hypotension, and profound sedation, or potentially result in coma or death. When such combined therapy is contemplated, the dose of one or both agents should be significantly reduced. The use of concomitant CNS active drugs requires special patient care and observation). Products include:

Geodon 2723

Zolpidem Tartrate (The concomitant use of fentanyl with other CNS depressants, including sedatives and hypnotics, may cause respiratory depression, hypotension, and profound sedation, or potentially result in coma or death. When such combined therapy is contemplated, the dose of one or both agents should be significantly reduced. The use of concomitant CNS active drugs requires special patient care and observation). Products include:

Ambien 2920

Ambien CR 2925

Food Interactions

Alcohol (Fentanyl may be expected to have additive CNS depressant effects when used in conjunction with alcohol. The concomitant use of fentanyl with alcohol may cause respiratory depression, hypotension, and profound sedation, or potentially result in coma or death).

Beer, reduced-alcohol (Fentanyl may be expected to have additive CNS depressant effects when used in conjunction with alcohol. The concomitant use of fentanyl with alcohol may cause respiratory depression, hypotension, and profound sedation, or potentially result in coma or death).

Beer, unspecified (Fentanyl may be expected to have additive CNS depressant effects when used in conjunction with alcohol. The concomitant use of fentanyl with alcohol may cause respiratory depression, hypotension, and profound sedation, or potentially result in coma or death).

Grapefruit (The concomitant use of fentanyl with all CYP3A4 inhibitors (eg, grapefruit juice) may result in an increase in fentanyl plasma concentrations, which could increase or prolong adverse drug effects and may cause potentially fatal respiratory depression. Patients receiving fentanyl and any CYP3A4 inhibitor should be carefully monitored for an extended period of time and dosage adjustments should be made if warranted).

Grapefruit Juice (The concomitant use of fentanyl with all CYP3A4 inhibitors (eg, grapefruit juice) may result in an increase in fentanyl plasma concentrations, which could increase or prolong adverse drug effects and may cause potentially fatal respiratory depression. Patients receiving fentanyl and any CYP3A4 inhibitor should be carefully monitored for an extended period of time and dosage adjustments should be made if warranted).

Wine, Chianti (Fentanyl may be expected to have additive CNS depressant effects when used in conjunction with alcohol. The concomitant use of fentanyl with alcohol may cause respiratory depression, hypotension, and profound sedation, or potentially result in coma or death).

Wine, Red (Fentanyl may be expected to have additive CNS depressant effects when used in conjunction with alcohol. The concomitant use of fentanyl with alcohol may cause respiratory depression, hypotension, and profound sedation, or potentially result in coma or death).

Wine, unspecified (Fentanyl may be expected to have additive CNS depressant effects when used in conjunction with alcohol. The concomitant use of fentanyl with alcohol may cause respiratory depression, hypotension, and profound sedation, or potentially result in coma or death).

Wine products (Fentanyl may be expected to have additive CNS depressant effects when used in conjunction with alcohol. The concomitant use of fentanyl with alcohol may cause respiratory depression, hypotension, and profound sedation, or potentially result in coma or death).

FENTORA TABLETS

(Fentanyl Citrate) 966

May interact with alcohols, antihistamines, central nervous system depressants, cytochrome p450 3a4 inducers (selected), cytochrome p450 3a4 inhibitors (selected), cytochrome p450 3a4 inhibitors, potent (selected), general anesthetics, hypnotics and sedatives, monoamine oxidase inhibitors, narcotic analgesics, phenothiazines, spasmolytic muscle relaxants, tranquilizers. Compounds in these categories include:

Acetazolamide (The concomitant use of moderate CYP3A4 inhibitors such as amprenavir, aprepitant, diltiazem, erythromycin, fluconazole, fosamprenavir, grapefruit juice, and verapamil with fentanyl citrate may result in an increase in fentanyl plasma concentrations, which could increase or prolong adverse drug effects and may cause potentially fatal respiratory depression. Patients receiving fentanyl citrate and moderate CYP3A4 inhibitors should be carefully monitored for an extended period of time and dosage increase should be done conservatively).

No products indexed under this heading.

Acetazolamide Sodium (The concomitant use of moderate CYP3A4 inhibitors such as amprenavir, aprepitant, diltiazem, erythromycin, fluconazole, fosamprenavir, grapefruit juice, and verapamil with fentanyl citrate may result in an increase in fentanyl plasma concentrations, which could increase or prolong adverse drug effects and may cause potentially fatal respiratory depression. Patients receiving fentanyl citrate and moderate CYP3A4 inhibitors should be carefully monitored for an extended period of time and dosage increase should be done conservatively).

No products indexed under this heading.

Acrivastine (The concomitant use of other CNS depressants, including sedating antihistamines, may produce increased depressant effects. Hypoventilation, hypotension, and profound sedation may occur).

No products indexed under this heading.

Alfentanil Hydrochloride (The concomitant use of other CNS depressants, including other opioids, sedatives or hypnotics, general anesthetics, phenothiazines, tranquilizers, skeletal muscle relaxants, sedating antihistamines, potent inhibitors of cytochrome P450 3A4 isoform (eg,erythromycin, ketoconazole, and certain protease inhibitors), and alcoholic beverages may produce increased depressant effects. Hypoventilation, hypotension, and profound sedation may occur).

No products indexed under this heading.

Allium sativum (Co-administration with agents that induce CYP3A4 activity may reduce the efficacy of fentanyl citrate).

No products indexed under this heading.

Alprazolam (The concomitant use of other CNS depressants, including other opioids, sedatives or hypnotics, general anesthetics, phenothiazines, tranquilizers, skeletal muscle relaxants, sedating antihistamines, potent inhibitors of cytochrome P450 3A4 isoform (eg,erythromycin, ketoconazole, and certain protease inhibitors), and alcoholic beverages may produce increased depressant effects. Hypoventilation, hypotension, and profound sedation may occur).

No products indexed under this heading.

Aminoglutethimide (Co-administration with agents that induce CYP3A4 activity may reduce the efficacy of fentanyl citrate).

No products indexed under this heading.

Amiodarone Hydrochloride (The concomitant use of moderate CYP3A4 inhibitors such as amprenavir, aprepitant, diltiazem, erythromycin, flucona-

zole, fosamprenavir, grapefruit juice, and verapamil with fentanyl citrate may result in an increase in fentanyl plasma concentrations, which could increase or prolong adverse drug effects and may cause potentially fatal respiratory depression. Patients receiving fentanyl citrate and moderate CYP3A4 inhibitors should be carefully monitored for an extended period of time and dosage increase should be done conservatively).
No products indexed under this heading.

Amobarbital (The concomitant use of other CNS depressants, including other opioids, sedatives or hypnotics, general anesthetics, phenothiazines, tranquilizers, skeletal muscle relaxants, sedating antihistamines, potent inhibitors of cytochrome P450 3A4 isoform (eg,erythromycin, ketoconazole, and certain protease inhibitors), and alcoholic beverages may produce increased depressant effects. Hypoventilation, hypotension, and profound sedation may occur).
No products indexed under this heading.

Amobarbital Sodium (The concomitant use of other CNS depressants, including other opioids, sedatives or hypnotics, general anesthetics, phenothiazines, tranquilizers, skeletal muscle relaxants, sedating antihistamines, potent inhibitors of cytochrome P450 3A4 isoform (eg,erythromycin, ketoconazole, and certain protease inhibitors), and alcoholic beverages may produce increased depressant effects. Hypoventilation, hypotension, and profound sedation may occur).
No products indexed under this heading.

Amprenavir (The concomitant use of fentanyl citrate with ritonavir or other strong CYP3A4 inhibitors such as ketoconazole, itraconazole, troleandomycin, clarithromycin, nelfinavir, and nefazadone may result in a potentially dangerous increase in fentanyl plasma concentrations. Patients receiving fentanyl citrate and potent CYP3A4 inhibitors should be carefully monitored for an extended period of time and dosage increase should be done conservatively).
No products indexed under this heading.

Anastrozole (The concomitant use of moderate CYP3A4 inhibitors such as amprenavir, aprepitant, diltiazem, erythromycin, fluconazole, fosamprenavir, grapefruit juice, and verapamil with fentanyl citrate may result in an increase in fentanyl plasma concentrations, which could increase or prolong adverse drug effects and may cause potentially fatal respiratory depression. Patients receiving fentanyl citrate and moderate CYP3A4 inhibitors should be carefully monitored for an extended period of time and dosage increase should be done conservatively).
No products indexed under this heading.

Apomorphine (The concomitant use of other CNS depressants, including other opioids, may produce increased depressant effects. Hypoventilation, hypotension, and profound sedation may occur).
No products indexed under this heading.

Apomorphine Hydrochloride (The concomitant use of other CNS depressants, including other opioids, may produce increased depressant effects. Hypoventilation, hypotension, and profound sedation may occur).
No products indexed under this heading.

Aprepitant (The concomitant use of moderate CYP3A4 inhibitors such as amprenavir, aprepitant, diltiazem, erythromycin, fluconazole, fosamprenavir, grapefruit juice, and verapamil with fentanyl citrate may result in an increase in fentanyl plasma concentrations, which could increase or prolong adverse drug effects and may cause potentially fatal respiratory depression. Patients receiving fentanyl citrate and moderate CYP3A4 inhibitors should be carefully monitored for an extended period of time and dosage increase should be done conservatively). Products include:
Emend 2124

Aprobarbital (The concomitant use of other CNS depressants, including other opioids, sedatives or hypnotics, general anesthetics, phenothiazines, tranquilizers, skeletal muscle relaxants, sedating antihistamines, potent inhibitors of cytochrome P450 3A4 isoform (eg,erythromycin, ketoconazole, and certain protease inhibitors), and alcoholic beverages may produce increased depressant effects. Hypoventilation, hypotension, and profound sedation may occur).
No products indexed under this heading.

Astemizole (The concomitant use of other CNS depressants, including sedating antihistamines, may produce increased depressant effects. Hypoventilation, hypotension, and profound sedation may occur).
No products indexed under this heading.

Atazanavir (The concomitant use of fentanyl citrate with ritonavir or other strong CYP3A4 inhibitors such as ketoconazole, itraconazole, troleandomycin, clarithromycin, nelfinavir, and nefazadone may result in a potentially dangerous increase in fentanyl plasma concentrations. Patients receiving fentanyl citrate and potent CYP3A4 inhibitors should be carefully monitored for an extended period of time and dosage increase should be done conservatively).
No products indexed under this heading.

Atazanavir Sulfate (The concomitant use of fentanyl citrate with ritonavir or other strong CYP3A4 inhibitors such as ketoconazole, itraconazole, troleandomycin, clarithromycin, nelfinavir, and nefazadone may result in a potentially dangerous increase in fentanyl plasma concentrations. Patients receiving fentanyl citrate and potent CYP3A4 inhibitors should be carefully monitored for an extended period of time and dosage increase should be done conservatively).
No products indexed under this heading.

Azatadine Maleate (The concomitant use of other CNS depressants, including sedating antihistamines, may produce increased depressant effects. Hypoventilation, hypotension, and profound sedation may occur).
No products indexed under this heading.

Baclofen (The concomitant use of other CNS depressants, including skeletal muscle relaxants, may produce increased depressant effects. Hypoventilation, hypotension, and profound sedation may occur).
No products indexed under this heading.

Betamethasone (Co-administration with agents that induce CYP3A4 activity may reduce the efficacy of fentanyl citrate).
No products indexed under this heading.

Betamethasone Acetate (Co-administration with agents that induce CYP3A4 activity may reduce the efficacy of fentanyl citrate).
No products indexed under this heading.

Betamethasone Benzoate (Co-administration with agents that induce CYP3A4 activity may reduce the efficacy of fentanyl citrate).
No products indexed under this heading.

Betamethasone Dipropionate (Co-administration with agents that induce CYP3A4 activity may reduce the efficacy of fentanyl citrate). Products include:
Diprolene Lotion 0.05% 3108
Diprolene Ointment 0.05% 3109
Diprolene AF Cream 0.05% 3107
Lotrisone 3163

Betamethasone Sodium Phosphate (Co-administration with agents that induce CYP3A4 activity may reduce the efficacy of fentanyl citrate).
No products indexed under this heading.

Betamethasone Valerate (Co-administration with agents that induce CYP3A4 activity may reduce the efficacy of fentanyl citrate). Products include:
Luxiq 3321

Bosentan (Co-administration with agents that induce CYP3A4 activity may reduce the efficacy of fentanyl citrate). Products include:
Tracleer 573

Bromodiphenhydramine Hydrochloride (The concomitant use of other CNS depressants, including sedating antihistamines, may produce increased depressant effects. Hypoventilation, hypotension, and profound sedation may occur).
No products indexed under this heading.

Brompheniramine Maleate (The concomitant use of other CNS depressants, including sedating antihistamines, may produce increased depressant effects. Hypoventilation, hypotension, and profound sedation may occur).
No products indexed under this heading.

Buprenorphine Hydrochloride (The concomitant use of other CNS depressants, including other opioids, sedatives or hypnotics, general anesthetics, phenothiazines, tranquilizers, skeletal muscle relaxants, sedating antihistamines, potent inhibitors of cytochrome P450 3A4 isoform (eg,erythromycin, ketoconazole, and certain protease inhibitors), and alcoholic beverages may produce increased depressant effects. Hypoventilation, hypotension, and profound sedation may occur).
No products indexed under this heading.

Buspirone Hydrochloride (The concomitant use of other CNS depressants, including other opioids, sedatives or hypnotics, general anesthetics, phenothiazines, tranquilizers, skeletal muscle relaxants, sedating antihistamines, potent inhibitors of cytochrome P450 3A4 isoform (eg,erythromycin, ketoconazole, and certain protease inhibitors), and alcoholic beverages may produce increased depressant effects. Hypoventilation, hypotension, and profound sedation may occur).
No products indexed under this heading.

Butabarbital (The concomitant use of other CNS depressants, including other opioids, sedatives or hypnotics, general anesthetics, phenothiazines, tranquilizers, skeletal muscle relaxants, sedating antihistamines, potent inhibitors of cytochrome P450 3A4 isoform (eg,erythromycin, ketoconazole, and certain protease inhibitors), and alcoholic beverages may produce increased depressant effects. Hypoventilation, hypotension, and profound sedation may occur).
No products indexed under this heading.

Butabarbital Sodium (The concomitant use of other CNS depressants, including other opioids, sedatives or hypnotics, general anesthetics, phenothiazines, tranquilizers, skeletal muscle relaxants, sedating antihistamines, potent inhibitors of cytochrome P450 3A4 isoform (eg,erythromycin, ketoconazole, and certain protease inhibitors), and alcoholic beverages may produce increased depressant effects. Hypoventilation, hypotension, and profound sedation may occur).
No products indexed under this heading.

Butalbital (The concomitant use of other CNS depressants, including other opioids, sedatives or hypnotics, general anesthetics, phenothiazines, tranquilizers, skeletal muscle relaxants, sedating antihistamines, potent inhibitors of cytochrome P450 3A4 isoform (eg,erythromycin, ketoconazole, and certain protease inhibitors), and alcoholic beverages may produce increased depressant effects. Hypoventilation, hypotension, and profound sedation may occur).
No products indexed under this heading.

Carbamazepine (Co-administration with agents that induce CYP3A4 activity may reduce the efficacy of fentanyl citrate). Products include:
Carbatrol 3280
Equetro 3477

Carisoprodol (The concomitant use of other CNS depressants, including skeletal muscle relaxants, may produce increased depressant effects. Hypoventilation, hypotension, and profound sedation may occur).
No products indexed under this heading.

Cetirizine Hydrochloride (The concomitant use of other CNS depressants, including sedating antihistamines, may produce increased depressant effects. Hypoventilation, hypotension, and profound sedation may occur). Products include:
Zyrtec Allergy 2052
Children's Zyrtec Allergy Syrup 2053
Children's Zyrtec Allergy 2053
Children's Zyrtec Hives Relief 2053
Zyrtec-D Allergy & Congestion 2054

Chloral Hydrate (The concomitant use of other CNS depressants, including sedatives or hypnotics, may produce increased depressant effects. Hypoventilation, hypotension, and profound sedation may occur).
No products indexed under this heading.

Chlordiazepoxide (The concomitant use of other CNS depressants, including other opioids, sedatives or hypnotics, general anesthetics, phenothiazines, tranquilizers, skeletal muscle relaxants, sedating antihistamines, potent inhibitors of cytochrome P450 3A4 isoform (eg,erythromycin, ketoconazole, and certain protease inhibitors), and alcoholic beverages may produce increased depressant effects. Hypoventilation, hypotension, and profound sedation may occur).
No products indexed under this heading.

Chlordiazepoxide Hydrochloride (The concomitant use of other CNS depressants, including other opioids, sedatives or hypnotics, general anesthetics, phenothiazines, tranquilizers, skeletal muscle relaxants, sedating antihistamines, potent inhibitors of cytochrome P450 3A4 isoform (eg,erythromycin, ketoconazole, and certain protease inhibitors), and alcoholic beverages may produce increased depressant effects. Hypoventilation, hypotension, and profound sedation may occur).
No products indexed under this heading.

Chlorpheniramine Maleate (The concomitant use of other CNS depressants, including sedating antihistamines, may produce increased depressant effects. Hypoventilation, hypotension, and profound sedation may occur).
No products indexed under this heading.

Chlorpheniramine Polistirex (The concomitant use of other CNS depressants, including sedating antihistamines, may produce increased depressant effects. Hypoventilation, hypotension, and profound sedation may occur). Products include:
Tussionex 3443

669 Interactions Index Fentora

Chlorpheniramine Tannate (The concomitant use of other CNS depressants, including sedating antihistamines, may produce increased depressant effects. Hypoventilation, hypotension, and profound sedation may occur).
No products indexed under this heading.

Chlorpromazine (The concomitant use of other CNS depressants, including other opioids, sedatives or hypnotics, general anesthetics, phenothiazines, tranquilizers, skeletal muscle relaxants, sedating antihistamines, potent inhibitors of cytochrome P450 3A4 isoform (eg,erythromycin, ketoconazole, and certain protease inhibitors), and alcoholic beverages may produce increased depressant effects. Hypoventilation, hypotension, and profound sedation may occur).
No products indexed under this heading.

Chlorpromazine Hydrochloride (The concomitant use of other CNS depressants, including other opioids, sedatives or hypnotics, general anesthetics, phenothiazines, tranquilizers, skeletal muscle relaxants, sedating antihistamines, potent inhibitors of cytochrome P450 3A4 isoform (eg,erythromycin, ketoconazole, and certain protease inhibitors), and alcoholic beverages may produce increased depressant effects. Hypoventilation, hypotension, and profound sedation may occur).
No products indexed under this heading.

Chlorprothixene (The concomitant use of other CNS depressants, including other opioids, sedatives or hypnotics, general anesthetics, phenothiazines, tranquilizers, skeletal muscle relaxants, sedating antihistamines, potent inhibitors of cytochrome P450 3A4 isoform (eg,erythromycin, ketoconazole, and certain protease inhibitors), and alcoholic beverages may produce increased depressant effects. Hypoventilation, hypotension, and profound sedation may occur).
No products indexed under this heading.

Chlorprothixene Hydrochloride (The concomitant use of other CNS depressants, including other opioids, sedatives or hypnotics, general anesthetics, phenothiazines, tranquilizers, skeletal muscle relaxants, sedating antihistamines, potent inhibitors of cytochrome P450 3A4 isoform (eg,erythromycin, ketoconazole, and certain protease inhibitors), and alcoholic beverages may produce increased depressant effects. Hypoventilation, hypotension, and profound sedation may occur).
No products indexed under this heading.

Chlorprothixene Lactate (The concomitant use of other CNS depressants, including other opioids, sedatives or hypnotics, general anesthetics, phenothiazines, tranquilizers, skeletal muscle relaxants, sedating antihistamines, potent inhibitors of cytochrome P450 3A4 isoform (eg,erythromycin, ketoconazole, and certain protease inhibitors), and alcoholic beverages may produce increased depressant effects. Hypoventilation, hypotension, and profound sedation may occur).
No products indexed under this heading.

Chlorzoxazone (The concomitant use of other CNS depressants, including skeletal muscle relaxants, may produce increased depressant effects. Hypoventilation, hypotension, and profound sedation may occur).
No products indexed under this heading.

Cimetidine (The concomitant use of moderate CYP3A4 inhibitors such as amprenavir, aprepitant, diltiazem, erythromycin, fluconazole, fosamprenavir, grapefruit juice, and verapamil with fentanyl citrate may result in an increase in fentanyl plasma concentrations, which could increase or prolong adverse drug effects and may cause potentially fatal respiratory depression. Patients receiving fentanyl citrate and moderate CYP3A4 inhibitors should be carefully monitored for an extended period of time and dosage increase should be done conservatively).
No products indexed under this heading.

Cimetidine Hydrochloride (The concomitant use of moderate CYP3A4 inhibitors such as amprenavir, aprepitant, diltiazem, erythromycin, fluconazole, fosamprenavir, grapefruit juice, and verapamil with fentanyl citrate may result in an increase in fentanyl plasma concentrations, which could increase or prolong adverse drug effects and may cause potentially fatal respiratory depression. Patients receiving fentanyl citrate and moderate CYP3A4 inhibitors should be carefully monitored for an extended period of time and dosage increase should be done conservatively).
No products indexed under this heading.

Ciprofloxacin (The concomitant use of moderate CYP3A4 inhibitors such as amprenavir, aprepitant, diltiazem, erythromycin, fluconazole, fosamprenavir, grapefruit juice, and verapamil with fentanyl citrate may result in an increase in fentanyl plasma concentrations, which could increase or prolong adverse drug effects and may cause potentially fatal respiratory depression. Patients receiving fentanyl citrate and moderate CYP3A4 inhibitors should be carefully monitored for an extended period of time and dosage increase should be done conservatively). Products include:
Cipro I.V. **3082**
Cipro **3073**
Cipro XR **3091**
Ciprodex **583**

Ciprofloxacin Hydrochloride (Co-administration with agents that induce CYP3A4 activity may reduce the efficacy of fentanyl citrate). Products include:
Cipro **3073**

Cisplatin (Co-administration with agents that induce CYP3A4 activity may reduce the efficacy of fentanyl citrate).
No products indexed under this heading.

Clarithromycin (The concomitant use of fentanyl citrate with ritonavir or other strong CYP3A4 inhibitors such as ketoconazole, itraconazole, troleandomycin, clarithromycin, nelfinavir, and nefazadone may result in a potentially dangerous increase in fentanyl plasma concentrations. Patients receiving fentanyl citrate and potent CYP3A4 inhibitors should be carefully monitored for an extended period of time and dosage increase should be done conservatively). Products include:
Biaxin/Biaxin XL **412**

Clemastine Fumarate (The concomitant use of other CNS depressants, including sedating antihistamines, may produce increased depressant effects. Hypoventilation, hypotension, and profound sedation may occur).
No products indexed under this heading.

Clonazepam (The concomitant use of other CNS depressants, including other opioids, sedatives or hypnotics, general anesthetics, phenothiazines, tranquilizers, skeletal muscle relaxants, sedating antihistamines, potent inhibitors of cytochrome P450 3A4 isoform (eg,erythromycin, ketoconazole, and certain protease inhibitors), and alcoholic beverages may produce increased depressant effects. Hypoventilation, hypotension, and profound sedation may occur). Products include:
Klonopin **2855**

Clorazepate Dipotassium (The concomitant use of other CNS depressants, including other opioids, sedatives or hypnotics, general anesthetics, phenothiazines, tranquilizers, skeletal muscle relaxants, sedating antihistamines, potent inhibitors of cytochrome P450 3A4 isoform (eg,erythromycin, ketoconazole, and certain protease inhibitors), and alcoholic beverages may produce increased depressant effects. Hypoventilation, hypotension, and profound sedation may occur).
No products indexed under this heading.

Clotrimazole (The concomitant use of moderate CYP3A4 inhibitors such as amprenavir, aprepitant, diltiazem, erythromycin, fluconazole, fosamprenavir, grapefruit juice, and verapamil with fentanyl citrate may result in an increase in fentanyl plasma concentrations, which could increase or prolong adverse drug effects and may cause potentially fatal respiratory depression. Patients receiving fentanyl citrate and moderate CYP3A4 inhibitors should be carefully monitored for an extended period of time and dosage increase should be done conservatively). Products include:
Lotrisone **3163**

Clozapine (The concomitant use of other CNS depressants, including other opioids, sedatives or hypnotics, general anesthetics, phenothiazines, tranquilizers, skeletal muscle relaxants, sedating antihistamines, potent inhibitors of cytochrome P450 3A4 isoform (eg,erythromycin, ketoconazole, and certain protease inhibitors), and alcoholic beverages may produce increased depressant effects. Hypoventilation, hypotension, and profound sedation may occur).
No products indexed under this heading.

Codeine Phosphate (The concomitant use of other CNS depressants, including other opioids, sedatives or hypnotics, general anesthetics, phenothiazines, tranquilizers, skeletal muscle relaxants, sedating antihistamines, potent inhibitors of cytochrome P450 3A4 isoform (eg,erythromycin, ketoconazole, and certain protease inhibitors), and alcoholic beverages may produce increased depressant effects. Hypoventilation, hypotension, and profound sedation may occur). Products include:
Tylenol with Codeine **2691**

Codeine Sulfate (The concomitant use of other CNS depressants, including other opioids, sedatives or hypnotics, general anesthetics, phenothiazines, tranquilizers, skeletal muscle relaxants, sedating antihistamines, potent inhibitors of cytochrome P450 3A4 isoform (eg,erythromycin, ketoconazole, and certain protease inhibitors), and alcoholic beverages may produce increased depressant effects. Hypoventilation, hypotension, and profound sedation may occur).
No products indexed under this heading.

Conivaptan Hydrochloride (The concomitant use of moderate CYP3A4 inhibitors such as amprenavir, aprepitant, diltiazem, erythromycin, fluconazole, fosamprenavir, grapefruit juice, and verapamil with fentanyl citrate may result in an increase in fentanyl plasma concentrations, which could increase or prolong adverse drug effects and may cause potentially fatal respiratory depression. Patients receiving fentanyl citrate and moderate CYP3A4 inhibitors should be carefully monitored for an extended period of time and dosage increase should be done conservatively). Products include:
Vaprisol **689**

Cortisone Acetate (Co-administration with agents that induce CYP3A4 activity may reduce the efficacy of fentanyl citrate).
No products indexed under this heading.

Cyclobenzaprine Hydrochloride (The concomitant use of other CNS depressants, including skeletal muscle relaxants, may produce increased depressant effects. Hypoventilation, hypotension, and profound sedation may occur). Products include:
Amrix **964**

Cyclosporine (The concomitant use of moderate CYP3A4 inhibitors such as amprenavir, aprepitant, diltiazem, erythromycin, fluconazole, fosamprenavir, grapefruit juice, and verapamil with fentanyl citrate may result in an increase in fentanyl plasma concentrations, which could increase or prolong adverse drug effects and may cause potentially fatal respiratory depression. Patients receiving fentanyl citrate and moderate CYP3A4 inhibitors should be carefully monitored for an extended period of time and dosage increase should be done conservatively). Products include:
Gengraf **440**
Neoral Oral Solution **2496**
Neoral Capsules **2496**
Restasis **605**

Cyproheptadine Hydrochloride (The concomitant use of other CNS depressants, including sedating antihistamines, may produce increased depressant effects. Hypoventilation, hypotension, and profound sedation may occur).
No products indexed under this heading.

Dalfopristin (The concomitant use of moderate CYP3A4 inhibitors such as amprenavir, aprepitant, diltiazem, erythromycin, fluconazole, fosamprenavir, grapefruit juice, and verapamil with fentanyl citrate may result in an increase in fentanyl plasma concentrations, which could increase or prolong adverse drug effects and may cause potentially fatal respiratory depression. Patients receiving fentanyl citrate and moderate CYP3A4 inhibitors should be carefully monitored for an extended period of time and dosage increase should be done conservatively).
No products indexed under this heading.

Danazol (The concomitant use of moderate CYP3A4 inhibitors such as amprenavir, aprepitant, diltiazem, erythromycin, fluconazole, fosamprenavir, grapefruit juice, and verapamil with fentanyl citrate may result in an increase in fentanyl plasma concentrations, which could increase or prolong adverse drug effects and may cause potentially fatal respiratory depression. Patients receiving fentanyl citrate and moderate CYP3A4 inhibitors should be carefully monitored for an extended period of time and dosage increase should be done conservatively).
No products indexed under this heading.

Dantrolene Sodium (The concomitant use of other CNS depressants, including skeletal muscle relaxants, may produce increased depressant effects. Hypoventilation, hypotension, and profound sedation may occur).
No products indexed under this heading.

Darunavir (The concomitant use of moderate CYP3A4 inhibitors such as amprenavir, aprepitant, diltiazem, erythromycin, fluconazole, fosamprenavir, grapefruit juice, and verapamil with fentanyl citrate may result in an increase in fentanyl plasma concentrations, which could increase or prolong adverse drug effects and may cause potentially fatal respiratory depression. Patients receiving fentanyl citrate and moderate CYP3A4 inhibitors should be carefully

IMPORTANT NOTE: Always consult each drug listing in the patient's regimen for possible interactions.

monitored for an extended period of time and dosage increase should be done conservatively).
No products indexed under this heading.

Dasatinib (The concomitant use of moderate CYP3A4 inhibitors such as amprenavir, aprepitant, diltiazem, erythromycin, fluconazole, fosamprenavir, grapefruit juice, and verapamil with fentanyl citrate may result in an increase in fentanyl plasma concentrations, which could increase or prolong adverse drug effects and may cause potentially fatal respiratory depression. Patients receiving fentanyl citrate and moderate CYP3A4 inhibitors should be carefully monitored for an extended period of time and dosage increase should be done conservatively).
No products indexed under this heading.

Delavirdine Mesylate (The concomitant use of fentanyl citrate with ritonavir or other strong CYP3A4 inhibitors such as ketoconazole, itraconazole, troleandomycin, clarithromycin, nelfinavir, and nefazadone may result in a potentially dangerous increase in fentanyl plasma concentrations. Patients receiving fentanyl citrate and potent CYP3A4 inhibitors should be carefully monitored for an extended period of time and dosage increase should be done conservatively).
No products indexed under this heading.

Delavirine (The concomitant use of fentanyl citrate with ritonavir or other strong CYP3A4 inhibitors such as ketoconazole, itraconazole, troleandomycin, clarithromycin, nelfinavir, and nefazadone may result in a potentially dangerous increase in fentanyl plasma concentrations. Patients receiving fentanyl citrate and potent CYP3A4 inhibitors should be carefully monitored for an extended period of time and dosage increase should be done conservatively).
No products indexed under this heading.

Desflurane (The concomitant use of other CNS depressants, including other opioids, sedatives or hypnotics, general anesthetics, phenothiazines, tranquilizers, skeletal muscle relaxants, sedating antihistamines, potent inhibitors of cytochrome P450 3A4 isoform (eg,erythromycin, ketoconazole, and certain protease inhibitors), and alcoholic beverages may produce increased depressant effects. Hypoventilation, hypotension, and profound sedation may occur).
No products indexed under this heading.

Desloratadine (The concomitant use of moderate CYP3A4 inhibitors such as amprenavir, aprepitant, diltiazem, erythromycin, fluconazole, fosamprenavir, grapefruit juice, and verapamil with fentanyl citrate may result in an increase in fentanyl plasma concentrations, which could increase or prolong adverse drug effects and may cause potentially fatal respiratory depression. Patients receiving fentanyl citrate and moderate CYP3A4 inhibitors should be carefully monitored for an extended period of time and dosage increase should be done conservatively). Products include:
Clarinex Syrup 3098
Clarinex 3098
Clarinex Reditabs 3098
Clarinex-D 12-Hour 3101
Clarinex-D 3104

Dexamethasone (Co-administration with agents that induce CYP3A4 activity may reduce the efficacy of fentanyl citrate). Products include:
Ciprodex 583
Ozurdex ..... ⊙ 223
Tobramycin and Dexamethasone Ophthalmic Suspension ..... ⊙ 251

Dexamethasone Acetate (Co-administration with agents that induce CYP3A4 activity may reduce the efficacy of fentanyl citrate).
No products indexed under this heading.

Dexamethasone Phosphate (Co-administration with agents that induce CYP3A4 activity may reduce the efficacy of fentanyl citrate).
No products indexed under this heading.

Dexamethasone Sodium (Co-administration with agents that induce CYP3A4 activity may reduce the efficacy of fentanyl citrate).
No products indexed under this heading.

Dexamethasone Sodium Phosphate (Co-administration with agents that induce CYP3A4 activity may reduce the efficacy of fentanyl citrate).
No products indexed under this heading.

Dexamethasone Sodium Phosphate Injection (Co-administration with agents that induce CYP3A4 activity may reduce the efficacy of fentanyl citrate).
No products indexed under this heading.

Dexchlorpheniramine Maleate (The concomitant use of other CNS depressants, including sedating antihistamines, may produce increased depressant effects. Hypoventilation, hypotension, and profound sedation may occur).
No products indexed under this heading.

Dezocine (The concomitant use of other CNS depressants, including other opioids, sedatives or hypnotics, general anesthetics, phenothiazines, tranquilizers, skeletal muscle relaxants, sedating antihistamines, potent inhibitors of cytochrome P450 3A4 isoform (eg,erythromycin, ketoconazole, and certain protease inhibitors), and alcoholic beverages may produce increased depressant effects. Hypoventilation, hypotension, and profound sedation may occur).
No products indexed under this heading.

Diazepam (The concomitant use of other CNS depressants, including other opioids, sedatives or hypnotics, general anesthetics, phenothiazines, tranquilizers, skeletal muscle relaxants, sedating antihistamines, potent inhibitors of cytochrome P450 3A4 isoform (eg,erythromycin, ketoconazole, and certain protease inhibitors), and alcoholic beverages may produce increased depressant effects. Hypoventilation, hypotension, and profound sedation may occur). Products include:
Valium Tablets 2880

Dihydrocodeine Bitartrate (The concomitant use of other CNS depressants, including other opioids, may produce increased depressant effects. Hypoventilation, hypotension, and profound sedation may occur).
No products indexed under this heading.

Dihydrocodeinone Bitartrate (The concomitant use of other CNS depressants, including other opioids, may produce increased depressant effects. Hypoventilation, hypotension, and profound sedation may occur).
No products indexed under this heading.

Diltiazem Hydrochloride (The concomitant use of moderate CYP3A4 inhibitors such as amprenavir, aprepitant, diltiazem, erythromycin, fluconazole, fosamprenavir, grapefruit juice, and verapamil with fentanyl citrate may result in an increase in fentanyl plasma concentrations, which could increase or prolong adverse drug effects and may cause potentially fatal respiratory depression. Patients receiving fentanyl citrate and moderate CYP3A4 inhibitors should be carefully monitored for an extended period of time and dosage increase should be done conservatively). Products include:
Cardizem LA 423

Diltiazem Maleate (The concomitant use of moderate CYP3A4 inhibitors such as amprenavir, aprepitant, diltiazem, erythromycin, fluconazole, fosamprenavir, grapefruit juice, and verapamil with fentanyl citrate may result in an increase in fentanyl plasma concentrations, which could increase or prolong adverse drug effects and may cause potentially fatal respiratory depression. Patients receiving fentanyl citrate and moderate CYP3A4 inhibitors should be carefully monitored for an extended period of time and dosage increase should be done conservatively).
No products indexed under this heading.

Diphenhydramine Hydrochloride (The concomitant use of other CNS depressants, including sedating antihistamines, may produce increased depressant effects. Hypoventilation, hypotension, and profound sedation may occur). Products include:
Benadryl Allergy Ultratab 2042
Children's Benadryl Allergy Liquid 2042

Diphenylpyraline Hydrochloride (The concomitant use of other CNS depressants, including sedating antihistamines, may produce increased depressant effects. Hypoventilation, hypotension, and profound sedation may occur).
No products indexed under this heading.

Doxorubicin Hydrochloride (Co-administration with agents that induce CYP3A4 activity may reduce the efficacy of fentanyl citrate).
No products indexed under this heading.

Droperidol (The concomitant use of other CNS depressants, including other opioids, sedatives or hypnotics, general anesthetics, phenothiazines, tranquilizers, skeletal muscle relaxants, sedating antihistamines, potent inhibitors of cytochrome P450 3A4 isoform (eg,erythromycin, ketoconazole, and certain protease inhibitors), and alcoholic beverages may produce increased depressant effects. Hypoventilation, hypotension, and profound sedation may occur).
No products indexed under this heading.

Efavirenz (The concomitant use of moderate CYP3A4 inhibitors such as amprenavir, aprepitant, diltiazem, erythromycin, fluconazole, fosamprenavir, grapefruit juice, and verapamil with fentanyl citrate may result in an increase in fentanyl plasma concentrations, which could increase or prolong adverse drug effects and may cause potentially fatal respiratory depression. Patients receiving fentanyl citrate and moderate CYP3A4 inhibitors should be carefully monitored for an extended period of time and dosage increase should be done conservatively). Products include:
Atripla 906

Enflurane (The concomitant use of other CNS depressants, including other opioids, sedatives or hypnotics, general anesthetics, phenothiazines, tranquilizers, skeletal muscle relaxants, sedating antihistamines, potent inhibitors of cytochrome P450 3A4 isoform (eg,erythromycin, ketoconazole, and certain protease inhibitors), and alcoholic beverages may produce increased depressant effects. Hypoventilation, hypotension, and profound sedation may occur).
No products indexed under this heading.

Erythromycin (The concomitant use of moderate CYP3A4 inhibitors such as amprenavir, aprepitant, diltiazem, erythromycin, fluconazole, fosamprenavir, grapefruit juice, and verapamil with fentanyl citrate may result in an increase in fentanyl plasma concentrations, which could increase or prolong adverse drug effects and may cause potentially fatal respiratory depression. Patients receiving fentanyl citrate and moderate CYP3A4 inhibitors should be carefully monitored for an extended period of time and dosage increase should be done conservatively).
No products indexed under this heading.

Erythromycin Estolate (The concomitant use of moderate CYP3A4 inhibitors such as amprenavir, aprepitant, diltiazem, erythromycin, fluconazole, fosamprenavir, grapefruit juice, and verapamil with fentanyl citrate may result in an increase in fentanyl plasma concentrations, which could increase or prolong adverse drug effects and may cause potentially fatal respiratory depression. Patients receiving fentanyl citrate and moderate CYP3A4 inhibitors should be carefully monitored for an extended period of time and dosage increase should be done conservatively).
No products indexed under this heading.

Erythromycin Ethylsuccinate (The concomitant use of moderate CYP3A4 inhibitors such as amprenavir, aprepitant, diltiazem, erythromycin, fluconazole, fosamprenavir, grapefruit juice, and verapamil with fentanyl citrate may result in an increase in fentanyl plasma concentrations, which could increase or prolong adverse drug effects and may cause potentially fatal respiratory depression. Patients receiving fentanyl citrate and moderate CYP3A4 inhibitors should be carefully monitored for an extended period of time and dosage increase should be done conservatively). Products include:
E.E.S. 437
EryPed 435

Erythromycin Gluceptate (The concomitant use of moderate CYP3A4 inhibitors such as amprenavir, aprepitant, diltiazem, erythromycin, fluconazole, fosamprenavir, grapefruit juice, and verapamil with fentanyl citrate may result in an increase in fentanyl plasma concentrations, which could increase or prolong adverse drug effects and may cause potentially fatal respiratory depression. Patients receiving fentanyl citrate and moderate CYP3A4 inhibitors should be carefully monitored for an extended period of time and dosage increase should be done conservatively).
No products indexed under this heading.

Erythromycin Lactobionate (The concomitant use of moderate CYP3A4 inhibitors such as amprenavir, aprepitant, diltiazem, erythromycin, fluconazole, fosamprenavir, grapefruit juice, and verapamil with fentanyl citrate may result in an increase in fentanyl plasma concentrations, which could increase or prolong adverse drug effects and may cause potentially fatal respiratory depression. Patients receiving fentanyl citrate and moderate CYP3A4 inhibitors should be carefully monitored for an extended period of time and dosage increase should be done conservatively).
No products indexed under this heading.

Erythromycin Stearate (The concomitant use of moderate CYP3A4 inhibitors such as amprenavir, aprepitant, diltiazem, erythromycin, fluconazole, fosamprenavir, grapefruit juice, and verapamil with fentanyl citrate may result in an increase in fentanyl plasma concentrations, which could increase or prolong adverse drug effects and may cause potentially fatal respiratory depression. Patients receiving fentanyl citrate and moderate CYP3A4 inhibitors should be carefully monitored for an extended period of time and dosage increase should be done conservatively).
No products indexed under this heading.

(⊙ Described in PDR® for Ophthalmic Medicines)

Esomeprazole Magnesium (The concomitant use of moderate CYP3A4 inhibitors such as amprenavir, aprepitant, diltiazem, erythromycin, fluconazole, fosamprenavir, grapefruit juice, and verapamil with fentanyl citrate may result in an increase in fentanyl plasma concentrations, which could increase or prolong adverse drug effects and may cause potentially fatal respiratory depression. Patients receiving fentanyl citrate and moderate CYP3A4 inhibitors should be carefully monitored for an extended period of time and dosage increase should be done conservatively). Products include:
Nexium Capsules **704**
Nexium Oral Suspension **704**

Esomeprazole Sodium (The concomitant use of moderate CYP3A4 inhibitors such as amprenavir, aprepitant, diltiazem, erythromycin, fluconazole, fosamprenavir, grapefruit juice, and verapamil with fentanyl citrate may result in an increase in fentanyl plasma concentrations, which could increase or prolong adverse drug effects and may cause potentially fatal respiratory depression. Patients receiving fentanyl citrate and moderate CYP3A4 inhibitors should be carefully monitored for an extended period of time and dosage increase should be done conservatively). Products include:
Nexium I.V. **712**

Estazolam (The concomitant use of other CNS depressants, including other opioids, sedatives or hypnotics, general anesthetics, phenothiazines, tranquilizers, skeletal muscle relaxants, sedating antihistamines, potent inhibitors of cytochrome P450 3A4 isoform (eg,erythromycin, ketoconazole, and certain protease inhibitors), and alcoholic beverages may produce increased depressant effects. Hypoventilation, hypotension, and profound sedation may occur).
No products indexed under this heading.

Ethanol (The concomitant use of other CNS depressants, including other opioids, sedatives or hypnotics, general anesthetics, phenothiazines, tranquilizers, skeletal muscle relaxants, sedating antihistamines, potent inhibitors of cytochrome P450 3A4 isoform (eg,erythromycin, ketoconazole, and certain protease inhibitors), and alcoholic beverages may produce increased depressant effects. Hypoventilation, hypotension, and profound sedation may occur).
No products indexed under this heading.

Ethchlorvynol (The concomitant use of other CNS depressants, including other opioids, sedatives or hypnotics, general anesthetics, phenothiazines, tranquilizers, skeletal muscle relaxants, sedating antihistamines, potent inhibitors of cytochrome P450 3A4 isoform (eg,erythromycin, ketoconazole, and certain protease inhibitors), and alcoholic beverages may produce increased depressant effects. Hypoventilation, hypotension, and profound sedation may occur).
No products indexed under this heading.

Ethinamate (The concomitant use of other CNS depressants, including other opioids, sedatives or hypnotics, general anesthetics, phenothiazines, tranquilizers, skeletal muscle relaxants, sedating antihistamines, potent inhibitors of cytochrome P450 3A4 isoform (eg,erythromycin, ketoconazole, and certain protease inhibitors), and alcoholic beverages may produce increased depressant effects. Hypoventilation, hypotension, and profound sedation may occur).
No products indexed under this heading.

Ethosuximide (Co-administration with agents that induce CYP3A4 activity may reduce the efficacy of fentanyl citrate).
No products indexed under this heading.

Ethyl Alcohol (The concomitant use of other CNS depressants, including other opioids, sedatives or hypnotics, general anesthetics, phenothiazines, tranquilizers, skeletal muscle relaxants, sedating antihistamines, potent inhibitors of cytochrome P450 3A4 isoform (eg,erythromycin, ketoconazole, and certain protease inhibitors), and alcoholic beverages may produce increased depressant effects. Hypoventilation, hypotension, and profound sedation may occur).
No products indexed under this heading.

Felbamate (Co-administration with agents that induce CYP3A4 activity may reduce the efficacy of fentanyl citrate).
No products indexed under this heading.

Fentanyl (The concomitant use of other CNS depressants, including other opioids, sedatives or hypnotics, general anesthetics, phenothiazines, tranquilizers, skeletal muscle relaxants, sedating antihistamines, potent inhibitors of cytochrome P450 3A4 isoform (eg,erythromycin, ketoconazole, and certain protease inhibitors), and alcoholic beverages may produce increased depressant effects. Hypoventilation, hypotension, and profound sedation may occur). Products include:
Duragesic **2604**
Fentanyl Transdermal System **2346**
Onsolis **2054**

Fexofenadine Hydrochloride (The concomitant use of other CNS depressants, including sedating antihistamines, may produce increased depressant effects. Hypoventilation, hypotension, and profound sedation may occur). Products include:
Allegra ODT **2911**
Allegra Oral Solution **2911**
Allegra **2911**
Allegra-D **2915**
Allegra-D 24 .... **2918**

Fluconazole (The concomitant use of moderate CYP3A4 inhibitors such as amprenavir, aprepitant, diltiazem, erythromycin, fluconazole, fosamprenavir, grapefruit juice, and verapamil with fentanyl citrate may result in an increase in fentanyl plasma concentrations, which could increase or prolong adverse drug effects and may cause potentially fatal respiratory depression. Patients receiving fentanyl citrate and moderate CYP3A4 inhibitors should be carefully monitored for an extended period of time and dosage increase should be done conservatively).
No products indexed under this heading.

Fludrocortisone Acetate (Co-administration with agents that induce CYP3A4 activity may reduce the efficacy of fentanyl citrate).
No products indexed under this heading.

Fluoxetine (The concomitant use of moderate CYP3A4 inhibitors such as amprenavir, aprepitant, diltiazem, erythromycin, fluconazole, fosamprenavir, grapefruit juice, and verapamil with fentanyl citrate may result in an increase in fentanyl plasma concentrations, which could increase or prolong adverse drug effects and may cause potentially fatal respiratory depression. Patients receiving fentanyl citrate and moderate CYP3A4 inhibitors should be carefully monitored for an extended period of time and dosage increase should be done conservatively).
No products indexed under this heading.

Fluoxetine Hydrochloride (The concomitant use of moderate CYP3A4 inhibitors such as amprenavir, aprepitant, diltiazem, erythromycin, fluconazole, fosamprenavir, grapefruit juice, and verapamil with fentanyl citrate may result in an increase in fentanyl plasma concentrations, which could increase or prolong adverse drug effects and may cause potentially fatal respiratory depression. Patients receiving fentanyl citrate and moderate CYP3A4 inhibitors should be carefully monitored for an extended period of time and dosage increase should be done conservatively). Products include:
Prozac Weekly **1941**
Prozac Pulvules **1941**
Symbyax **1965**

Fluphenazine Decanoate (The concomitant use of other CNS depressants, including other opioids, sedatives or hypnotics, general anesthetics, phenothiazines, tranquilizers, skeletal muscle relaxants, sedating antihistamines, potent inhibitors of cytochrome P450 3A4 isoform (eg,erythromycin, ketoconazole, and certain protease inhibitors), and alcoholic beverages may produce increased depressant effects. Hypoventilation, hypotension, and profound sedation may occur).
No products indexed under this heading.

Fluphenazine Enanthate (The concomitant use of other CNS depressants, including other opioids, sedatives or hypnotics, general anesthetics, phenothiazines, tranquilizers, skeletal muscle relaxants, sedating antihistamines, potent inhibitors of cytochrome P450 3A4 isoform (eg,erythromycin, ketoconazole, and certain protease inhibitors), and alcoholic beverages may produce increased depressant effects. Hypoventilation, hypotension, and profound sedation may occur).
No products indexed under this heading.

Fluphenazine Hydrochloride (The concomitant use of other CNS depressants, including other opioids, sedatives or hypnotics, general anesthetics, phenothiazines, tranquilizers, skeletal muscle relaxants, sedating antihistamines, potent inhibitors of cytochrome P450 3A4 isoform (eg,erythromycin, ketoconazole, and certain protease inhibitors), and alcoholic beverages may produce increased depressant effects. Hypoventilation, hypotension, and profound sedation may occur).
No products indexed under this heading.

Flurazepam Hydrochloride (The concomitant use of other CNS depressants, including other opioids, sedatives or hypnotics, general anesthetics, phenothiazines, tranquilizers, skeletal muscle relaxants, sedating antihistamines, potent inhibitors of cytochrome P450 3A4 isoform (eg,erythromycin, ketoconazole, and certain protease inhibitors), and alcoholic beverages may produce increased depressant effects. Hypoventilation, hypotension, and profound sedation may occur).
No products indexed under this heading.

Fluvoxamine Maleate (The concomitant use of moderate CYP3A4 inhibitors such as amprenavir, aprepitant, diltiazem, erythromycin, fluconazole, fosamprenavir, grapefruit juice, and verapamil with fentanyl citrate may result in an increase in fentanyl plasma concentrations, which could increase or prolong adverse drug effects and may cause potentially fatal respiratory depression. Patients receiving fentanyl citrate and moderate CYP3A4 inhibitors should be carefully monitored for an extended period of time and dosage increase should be done conservatively).
No products indexed under this heading.

Fosamprenavir Calcium (The concomitant use of fentanyl citrate with ritonavir or other strong CYP3A4 inhibitors such as ketoconazole, itraconazole, troleandomycin, clarithromycin, nelfinavir, and nefazadone may result in a potentially dangerous increase in fentanyl plasma concentrations. Patients receiving fentanyl citrate and potent CYP3A4 inhibitors should be carefully monitored for an extended period of time and dosage increase should be done conservatively). Products include:
Lexiva Oral Suspension **1558**
Lexiva **1558**

Fosphenytoin Sodium (Co-administration with agents that induce CYP3A4 activity may reduce the efficacy of fentanyl citrate).
No products indexed under this heading.

Garlic Extract (Co-administration with agents that induce CYP3A4 activity may reduce the efficacy of fentanyl citrate).
No products indexed under this heading.

Garlic Oil (Co-administration with agents that induce CYP3A4 activity may reduce the efficacy of fentanyl citrate).
No products indexed under this heading.

Glutethimide (The concomitant use of other CNS depressants, including other opioids, sedatives or hypnotics, general anesthetics, phenothiazines, tranquilizers, skeletal muscle relaxants, sedating antihistamines, potent inhibitors of cytochrome P450 3A4 isoform (eg,erythromycin, ketoconazole, and certain protease inhibitors), and alcoholic beverages may produce increased depressant effects. Hypoventilation, hypotension, and profound sedation may occur).
No products indexed under this heading.

Halazepam (The concomitant use of other CNS depressants, including other opioids, sedatives or hypnotics, general anesthetics, phenothiazines, tranquilizers, skeletal muscle relaxants, sedating antihistamines, potent inhibitors of cytochrome P450 3A4 isoform (eg,erythromycin, ketoconazole, and certain protease inhibitors), and alcoholic beverages may produce increased depressant effects. Hypoventilation, hypotension, and profound sedation may occur).
No products indexed under this heading.

Haloperidol (The concomitant use of other CNS depressants, including other opioids, sedatives or hypnotics, general anesthetics, phenothiazines, tranquilizers, skeletal muscle relaxants, sedating antihistamines, potent inhibitors of cytochrome P450 3A4 isoform (eg,erythromycin, ketoconazole, and certain protease inhibitors), and alcoholic beverages may produce increased depressant effects. Hypoventilation, hypotension, and profound sedation may occur).
No products indexed under this heading.

Haloperidol Decanoate (The concomitant use of other CNS depressants, including other opioids, sedatives or hypnotics, general anesthetics, phenothiazines, tranquilizers, skeletal muscle relaxants, sedating antihistamines, potent inhibitors of cytochrome P450 3A4 isoform (eg,erythromycin, ketoconazole, and certain protease inhibitors), and alcoholic beverages may produce increased depressant effects. Hypoventilation, hypotension, and profound sedation may occur).
No products indexed under this heading.

Haloperidol Lactate (The concomitant use of other CNS depressants, including other opioids, sedatives or hypnotics, general anesthetics, phenothiazines, tranquilizers, skeletal muscle relaxants, sedating antihistamines, potent inhibitors of cytochrome P450 3A4 isoform (eg,erythromycin, ketoconazole, and certain protease inhibitors), and alcoholic beverages may produce increased depressant effects. Hypoventilation, hypotension, and profound sedation may occur).
No products indexed under this heading.

Halothane (The concomitant use of other CNS depressants, including general anesthetics, may produce increased depressant effects. Hypoventilation, hypotension, and profound sedation may occur).
No products indexed under this heading.

IMPORTANT NOTE: Always consult each drug listing in the patient's regimen for possible interactions.

Hexobarbital (The concomitant use of other CNS depressants, including other opioids, sedatives or hypnotics, general anesthetics, phenothiazines, tranquilizers, skeletal muscle relaxants, sedating antihistamines, potent inhibitors of cytochrome P450 3A4 isoform (eg,erythromycin, ketoconazole, and certain protease inhibitors), and alcoholic beverages may produce increased depressant effects. Hypoventilation, hypotension, and profound sedation may occur).
No products indexed under this heading.

Hydrocodone Bitartrate (The concomitant use of other CNS depressants, including other opioids, sedatives or hypnotics, general anesthetics, phenothiazines, tranquilizers, skeletal muscle relaxants, sedating antihistamines, potent inhibitors of cytochrome P450 3A4 isoform (eg,erythromycin, ketoconazole, and certain protease inhibitors), and alcoholic beverages may produce increased depressant effects. Hypoventilation, hypotension, and profound sedation may occur). Products include:
Vicodin 560
Vicodin ES 561
Vicodin HP 563
Vicoprofen 564
Zydone 1138

Hydrocodone Polistirex (The concomitant use of other CNS depressants, including other opioids, sedatives or hypnotics, general anesthetics, phenothiazines, tranquilizers, skeletal muscle relaxants, sedating antihistamines, potent inhibitors of cytochrome P450 3A4 isoform (eg,erythromycin, ketoconazole, and certain protease inhibitors), and alcoholic beverages may produce increased depressant effects. Hypoventilation, hypotension, and profound sedation may occur). Products include:
Tussionex 3443

Hydrocortisone (Co-administration with agents that induce CYP3A4 activity may reduce the efficacy of fentanyl citrate).
No products indexed under this heading.

Hydrocortisone (Alcohol) (Co-administration with agents that induce CYP3A4 activity may reduce the efficacy of fentanyl citrate).
No products indexed under this heading.

Hydrocortisone Acetate (Co-administration with agents that induce CYP3A4 activity may reduce the efficacy of fentanyl citrate).
No products indexed under this heading.

Hydrocortisone Butyrate (Co-administration with agents that induce CYP3A4 activity may reduce the efficacy of fentanyl citrate).
No products indexed under this heading.

Hydrocortisone Cypionate (Co-administration with agents that induce CYP3A4 activity may reduce the efficacy of fentanyl citrate).
No products indexed under this heading.

Hydrocortisone Hemisuccinate (Co-administration with agents that induce CYP3A4 activity may reduce the efficacy of fentanyl citrate).
No products indexed under this heading.

Hydrocortisone Probutate (Co-administration with agents that induce CYP3A4 activity may reduce the efficacy of fentanyl citrate).
No products indexed under this heading.

Hydrocortisone Sodium Phosphate (Co-administration with agents that induce CYP3A4 activity may reduce the efficacy of fentanyl citrate).
No products indexed under this heading.

Hydrocortisone Sodium Succinate (Co-administration with agents that induce CYP3A4 activity may reduce the efficacy of fentanyl citrate).
No products indexed under this heading.

Hydrocortisone Valerate (Co-administration with agents that induce CYP3A4 activity may reduce the efficacy of fentanyl citrate).
No products indexed under this heading.

Hydromorphone (The concomitant use of other CNS depressants, including other opioids, sedatives or hypnotics, general anesthetics, phenothiazines, tranquilizers, skeletal muscle relaxants, sedating antihistamines, potent inhibitors of cytochrome P450 3A4 isoform (eg,erythromycin, ketoconazole, and certain protease inhibitors), and alcoholic beverages may produce increased depressant effects. Hypoventilation, hypotension, and profound sedation may occur).
No products indexed under this heading.

Hydromorphone Hydrochloride (The concomitant use of other CNS depressants, including other opioids, sedatives or hypnotics, general anesthetics, phenothiazines, tranquilizers, skeletal muscle relaxants, sedating antihistamines, potent inhibitors of cytochrome P450 3A4 isoform (eg,erythromycin, ketoconazole, and certain protease inhibitors), and alcoholic beverages may produce increased depressant effects. Hypoventilation, hypotension, and profound sedation may occur). Products include:
Dilaudid Injection 2800
Dilaudid Oral 2797
Dilaudid Tablets 2797
Dilaudid-HP 2800

Hydroxyzine Hydrochloride (The concomitant use of other CNS depressants, including other opioids, sedatives or hypnotics, general anesthetics, phenothiazines, tranquilizers, skeletal muscle relaxants, sedating antihistamines, potent inhibitors of cytochrome P450 3A4 isoform (eg,erythromycin, ketoconazole, and certain protease inhibitors), and alcoholic beverages may produce increased depressant effects. Hypoventilation, hypotension, and profound sedation may occur).
No products indexed under this heading.

Hypericum (Co-administration with agents that induce CYP3A4 activity may reduce the efficacy of fentanyl citrate).
No products indexed under this heading.

Hypericum Perforatum (Co-administration with agents that induce CYP3A4 activity may reduce the efficacy of fentanyl citrate). Products include:
Traumeel 1800

Imatinib Mesylate (The concomitant use of moderate CYP3A4 inhibitors such as amprenavir, aprepitant, diltiazem, erythromycin, fluconazole, fosamprenavir, grapefruit juice, and verapamil with fentanyl citrate may result in an increase in fentanyl plasma concentrations, which could increase or prolong adverse drug effects and may cause potentially fatal respiratory depression. Patients receiving fentanyl citrate and moderate CYP3A4 inhibitors should be carefully monitored for an extended period of time and dosage increase should be done conservatively). Products include:
Gleevec 2477

Indinavir Sulfate (The concomitant use of fentanyl citrate with ritonavir or other strong CYP3A4 inhibitors such as ketoconazole, itraconazole, troleandomycin, clarithromycin, nelfinavir, and nefazadone may result in a potentially dangerous increase in fentanyl plasma concentrations. Patients receiving fentanyl citrate and potent CYP3A4 inhibitors should be carefully monitored for an extended period of time and dosage increase should be done conservatively). Products include:
Crixivan 2113

Isocarboxazid (Fentanyl citrate is not recommended for use in patients who are receiving or have received MAO inhibitors within 14 days, because severe and unpredictable potentiation by MAO inhibitors has been reported with opioid analgesics). Products include:
Marplan 3481

Isoflurane (The concomitant use of other CNS depressants, including other opioids, sedatives or hypnotics, general anesthetics, phenothiazines, tranquilizers, skeletal muscle relaxants, sedating antihistamines, potent inhibitors of cytochrome P450 3A4 isoform (eg,erythromycin, ketoconazole, and certain protease inhibitors), and alcoholic beverages may produce increased depressant effects. Hypoventilation, hypotension, and profound sedation may occur).
No products indexed under this heading.

Isoniazid (The concomitant use of moderate CYP3A4 inhibitors such as amprenavir, aprepitant, diltiazem, erythromycin, fluconazole, fosamprenavir, grapefruit juice, and verapamil with fentanyl citrate may result in an increase in fentanyl plasma concentrations, which could increase or prolong adverse drug effects and may cause potentially fatal respiratory depression. Patients receiving fentanyl citrate and moderate CYP3A4 inhibitors should be carefully monitored for an extended period of time and dosage increase should be done conservatively).
No products indexed under this heading.

Itraconazole (The concomitant use of fentanyl citrate with ritonavir or other strong CYP3A4 inhibitors such as ketoconazole, itraconazole, troleandomycin, clarithromycin, nelfinavir, and nefazadone may result in a potentially dangerous increase in fentanyl plasma concentrations. Patients receiving fentanyl citrate and potent CYP3A4 inhibitors should be carefully monitored for an extended period of time and dosage increase should be done conservatively).
No products indexed under this heading.

Ketamine Hydrochloride (The concomitant use of other CNS depressants, including other opioids, sedatives or hypnotics, general anesthetics, phenothiazines, tranquilizers, skeletal muscle relaxants, sedating antihistamines, potent inhibitors of cytochrome P450 3A4 isoform (eg,erythromycin, ketoconazole, and certain protease inhibitors), and alcoholic beverages may produce increased depressant effects. Hypoventilation, hypotension, and profound sedation may occur).
No products indexed under this heading.

Ketoconazole (The concomitant use of fentanyl citrate with ritonavir or other strong CYP3A4 inhibitors such as ketoconazole, itraconazole, troleandomycin, clarithromycin, nelfinavir, and nefazadone may result in a potentially dangerous increase in fentanyl plasma concentrations. Patients receiving fentanyl citrate and potent CYP3A4 inhibitors should be carefully monitored for an extended period of time and dosage increase should be done conservatively). Products include:
Extina 3319
Xolegel 3337

Lapatinib (The concomitant use of moderate CYP3A4 inhibitors such as amprenavir, aprepitant, diltiazem, erythromycin, fluconazole, fosamprenavir, grapefruit juice, and verapamil with fentanyl citrate may result in an increase in fentanyl plasma concentrations, which could increase or prolong adverse drug effects and may cause potentially fatal respiratory depression. Patients receiving fentanyl citrate and moderate CYP3A4 inhibitors should be carefully monitored for an extended period of time and dosage increase should be done conservatively). Products include:
Tykerb 1698

Levomethadyl Acetate Hydrochloride (The concomitant use of other CNS depressants, including other opioids, sedatives or hypnotics, general anesthetics, phenothiazines, tranquilizers, skeletal muscle relaxants, sedating antihistamines, potent inhibitors of cytochrome P450 3A4 isoform (eg,erythromycin, ketoconazole, and certain protease inhibitors), and alcoholic beverages may produce increased depressant effects. Hypoventilation, hypotension, and profound sedation may occur).
No products indexed under this heading.

Levorphanol Tartrate (The concomitant use of other CNS depressants, including other opioids, sedatives or hypnotics, general anesthetics, phenothiazines, tranquilizers, skeletal muscle relaxants, sedating antihistamines, potent inhibitors of cytochrome P450 3A4 isoform (eg,erythromycin, ketoconazole, and certain protease inhibitors), and alcoholic beverages may produce increased depressant effects. Hypoventilation, hypotension, and profound sedation may occur).
No products indexed under this heading.

Lopinavir (The concomitant use of fentanyl citrate with ritonavir or other strong CYP3A4 inhibitors such as ketoconazole, itraconazole, troleandomycin, clarithromycin, nelfinavir, and nefazadone may result in a potentially dangerous increase in fentanyl plasma concentrations. Patients receiving fentanyl citrate and potent CYP3A4 inhibitors should be carefully monitored for an extended period of time and dosage increase should be done conservatively). Products include:
Kaletra 458

Loratadine (The concomitant use of moderate CYP3A4 inhibitors such as amprenavir, aprepitant, diltiazem, erythromycin, fluconazole, fosamprenavir, grapefruit juice, and verapamil with fentanyl citrate may result in an increase in fentanyl plasma concentrations, which could increase or prolong adverse drug effects and may cause potentially fatal respiratory depression. Patients receiving fentanyl citrate and moderate CYP3A4 inhibitors should be carefully monitored for an extended period of time and dosage increase should be done conservatively).
No products indexed under this heading.

Lorazepam (The concomitant use of other CNS depressants, including other opioids, sedatives or hypnotics, general anesthetics, phenothiazines, tranquilizers, skeletal muscle relaxants, sedating antihistamines, potent inhibitors of cytochrome P450 3A4 isoform (eg,erythromycin, ketoconazole, and certain protease inhibitors), and alcoholic beverages may produce increased depressant effects. Hypoventilation, hypotension, and profound sedation may occur).
No products indexed under this heading.

Loxapine Hydrochloride (The concomitant use of other CNS depressants, including other opioids, sedatives or hypnotics, general anesthetics, phenothiazines, tranquilizers, skeletal muscle relaxants, sedating antihistamines, potent inhibitors of cytochrome P450 3A4 isoform (eg,erythromycin, ketoconazole, and certain protease inhibitors), and alcoholic beverages may produce increased depressant effects. Hypoventilation, hypotension, and profound sedation may occur).
No products indexed under this heading.

(⊙ Described in PDR® for Ophthalmic Medicines)

Loxapine Succinate (The concomitant use of other CNS depressants, including other opioids, sedatives or hypnotics, general anesthetics, phenothiazines, tranquilizers, skeletal muscle relaxants, sedating antihistamines, potent inhibitors of cytochrome P450 3A4 isoform (eg,erythromycin, ketoconazole, and certain protease inhibitors), and alcoholic beverages may produce increased depressant effects. Hypoventilation, hypotension, and profound sedation may occur).

No products indexed under this heading.

Meperidine Hydrochloride (The concomitant use of other CNS depressants, including other opioids, sedatives or hypnotics, general anesthetics, phenothiazines, tranquilizers, skeletal muscle relaxants, sedating antihistamines, potent inhibitors of cytochrome P450 3A4 isoform (eg,erythromycin, ketoconazole, and certain protease inhibitors), and alcoholic beverages may produce increased depressant effects. Hypoventilation, hypotension, and profound sedation may occur).

No products indexed under this heading.

Mephenytoin (Co-administration with agents that induce CYP3A4 activity may reduce the efficacy of fentanyl citrate).

No products indexed under this heading.

Mephobarbital (The concomitant use of other CNS depressants, including other opioids, sedatives or hypnotics, general anesthetics, phenothiazines, tranquilizers, skeletal muscle relaxants, sedating antihistamines, potent inhibitors of cytochrome P450 3A4 isoform (eg,erythromycin, ketoconazole, and certain protease inhibitors), and alcoholic beverages may produce increased depressant effects. Hypoventilation, hypotension, and profound sedation may occur).

No products indexed under this heading.

Meprobamate (The concomitant use of other CNS depressants, including other opioids, sedatives or hypnotics, general anesthetics, phenothiazines, tranquilizers, skeletal muscle relaxants, sedating antihistamines, potent inhibitors of cytochrome P450 3A4 isoform (eg,erythromycin, ketoconazole, and certain protease inhibitors), and alcoholic beverages may produce increased depressant effects. Hypoventilation, hypotension, and profound sedation may occur).

No products indexed under this heading.

Mesoridazine Besylate (The concomitant use of other CNS depressants, including other opioids, sedatives or hypnotics, general anesthetics, phenothiazines, tranquilizers, skeletal muscle relaxants, sedating antihistamines, potent inhibitors of cytochrome P450 3A4 isoform (eg,erythromycin, ketoconazole, and certain protease inhibitors), and alcoholic beverages may produce increased depressant effects. Hypoventilation, hypotension, and profound sedation may occur).

No products indexed under this heading.

Metaxalone (The concomitant use of other CNS depressants, including skeletal muscle relaxants, may produce increased depressant effects. Hypoventilation, hypotension, and profound sedation may occur). Products include:
Skelaxin 1848

Methadone Hydrochloride (The concomitant use of other CNS depressants, including other opioids, sedatives or hypnotics, general anesthetics, phenothiazines, tranquilizers, skeletal muscle relaxants, sedating antihistamines, potent inhibitors of cytochrome P450 3A4 isoform (eg,erythromycin, ketoconazole, and certain protease inhibitors), and alcoholic beverages

may produce increased depressant effects. Hypoventilation, hypotension, and profound sedation may occur).

No products indexed under this heading.

Methdilazine Hydrochloride (The concomitant use of other CNS depressants, including sedating antihistamines, may produce increased depressant effects. Hypoventilation, hypotension, and profound sedation may occur).

No products indexed under this heading.

Methocarbamol (The concomitant use of other CNS depressants, including skeletal muscle relaxants, may produce increased depressant effects. Hypoventilation, hypotension, and profound sedation may occur).

No products indexed under this heading.

Methohexital Sodium (The concomitant use of other CNS depressants, including other opioids, sedatives or hypnotics, general anesthetics, phenothiazines, tranquilizers, skeletal muscle relaxants, sedating antihistamines, potent inhibitors of cytochrome P450 3A4 isoform (eg,erythromycin, ketoconazole, and certain protease inhibitors), and alcoholic beverages may produce increased depressant effects. Hypoventilation, hypotension, and profound sedation may occur).

No products indexed under this heading.

Methotrimeprazine (The concomitant use of other CNS depressants, including other opioids, sedatives or hypnotics, general anesthetics, phenothiazines, tranquilizers, skeletal muscle relaxants, sedating antihistamines, potent inhibitors of cytochrome P450 3A4 isoform (eg,erythromycin, ketoconazole, and certain protease inhibitors), and alcoholic beverages may produce increased depressant effects. Hypoventilation, hypotension, and profound sedation may occur).

No products indexed under this heading.

Methoxyflurane (The concomitant use of other CNS depressants, including other opioids, sedatives or hypnotics, general anesthetics, phenothiazines, tranquilizers, skeletal muscle relaxants, sedating antihistamines, potent inhibitors of cytochrome P450 3A4 isoform (eg,erythromycin, ketoconazole, and certain protease inhibitors), and alcoholic beverages may produce increased depressant effects. Hypoventilation, hypotension, and profound sedation may occur).

No products indexed under this heading.

Methsuximide (Co-administration with agents that induce CYP3A4 activity may reduce the efficacy of fentanyl citrate).

No products indexed under this heading.

Methylprednisolone (Co-administration with agents that induce CYP3A4 activity may reduce the efficacy of fentanyl citrate).

No products indexed under this heading.

Methylprednisolone Acetate (Co-administration with agents that induce CYP3A4 activity may reduce the efficacy of fentanyl citrate).

No products indexed under this heading.

Methylprednisolone Sodium Succinate (Co-administration with agents that induce CYP3A4 activity may reduce the efficacy of fentanyl citrate).

No products indexed under this heading.

Metronidazole (The concomitant use of moderate CYP3A4 inhibitors such as amprenavir, aprepitant, diltiazem, erythromycin, fluconazole, fosamprenavir, grapefruit juice, and verapamil with fentanyl citrate may result in an increase in fentanyl plasma concentrations, which could increase or prolong adverse drug effects and may cause potentially fatal respiratory depression. Patients receiving fentanyl citrate and moderate

CYP3A4 inhibitors should be carefully monitored for an extended period of time and dosage increase should be done conservatively). Products include:
Pylera 793

Metronidazole Benzoate (The concomitant use of moderate CYP3A4 inhibitors such as amprenavir, aprepitant, diltiazem, erythromycin, fluconazole, fosamprenavir, grapefruit juice, and verapamil with fentanyl citrate may result in an increase in fentanyl plasma concentrations, which could increase or prolong adverse drug effects and may cause potentially fatal respiratory depression. Patients receiving fentanyl citrate and moderate CYP3A4 inhibitors should be carefully monitored for an extended period of time and dosage increase should be done conservatively).

No products indexed under this heading.

Metronidazole Hydrochloride (The concomitant use of moderate CYP3A4 inhibitors such as amprenavir, aprepitant, diltiazem, erythromycin, fluconazole, fosamprenavir, grapefruit juice, and verapamil with fentanyl citrate may result in an increase in fentanyl plasma concentrations, which could increase or prolong adverse drug effects and may cause potentially fatal respiratory depression. Patients receiving fentanyl citrate and moderate CYP3A4 inhibitors should be carefully monitored for an extended period of time and dosage increase should be done conservatively).

No products indexed under this heading.

Metronidazole Sodium (The concomitant use of moderate CYP3A4 inhibitors such as amprenavir, aprepitant, diltiazem, erythromycin, fluconazole, fosamprenavir, grapefruit juice, and verapamil with fentanyl citrate may result in an increase in fentanyl plasma concentrations, which could increase or prolong adverse drug effects and may cause potentially fatal respiratory depression. Patients receiving fentanyl citrate and moderate CYP3A4 inhibitors should be carefully monitored for an extended period of time and dosage increase should be done conservatively).

No products indexed under this heading.

Miconazole (The concomitant use of moderate CYP3A4 inhibitors such as amprenavir, aprepitant, diltiazem, erythromycin, fluconazole, fosamprenavir, grapefruit juice, and verapamil with fentanyl citrate may result in an increase in fentanyl plasma concentrations, which could increase or prolong adverse drug effects and may cause potentially fatal respiratory depression. Patients receiving fentanyl citrate and moderate CYP3A4 inhibitors should be carefully monitored for an extended period of time and dosage increase should be done conservatively).

No products indexed under this heading.

Miconazole Nitrate (The concomitant use of moderate CYP3A4 inhibitors such as amprenavir, aprepitant, diltiazem, erythromycin, fluconazole, fosamprenavir, grapefruit juice, and verapamil with fentanyl citrate may result in an increase in fentanyl plasma concentrations, which could increase or prolong adverse drug effects and may cause potentially fatal respiratory depression. Patients receiving fentanyl citrate and moderate CYP3A4 inhibitors should be carefully monitored for an extended period of time and dosage increase should be done conservatively). Products include:
Vusion Ointment 3335

Midazolam Hydrochloride (The concomitant use of other CNS depressants, including other opioids, sedatives or hypnotics, general anesthetics,

phenothiazines, tranquilizers, skeletal muscle relaxants, sedating antihistamines, potent inhibitors of cytochrome P450 3A4 isoform (eg,erythromycin, ketoconazole, and certain protease inhibitors), and alcoholic beverages may produce increased depressant effects. Hypoventilation, hypotension, and profound sedation may occur).

No products indexed under this heading.

Mifepristone (The concomitant use of moderate CYP3A4 inhibitors such as amprenavir, aprepitant, diltiazem, erythromycin, fluconazole, fosamprenavir, grapefruit juice, and verapamil with fentanyl citrate may result in an increase in fentanyl plasma concentrations, which could increase or prolong adverse drug effects and may cause potentially fatal respiratory depression. Patients receiving fentanyl citrate and moderate CYP3A4 inhibitors should be carefully monitored for an extended period of time and dosage increase should be done conservatively).

No products indexed under this heading.

Moclobemide (Fentanyl citrate is not recommended for use in patients who are receiving or have received MAO inhibitors within 14 days, because severe and unpredictable potentiation by MAO inhibitors has been reported with opioid analgesics).

No products indexed under this heading.

Modafinil (Co-administration with agents that induce CYP3A4 activity may reduce the efficacy of fentanyl citrate). Products include:
Provigil 983

Molindone Hydrochloride (The concomitant use of other CNS depressants, including other opioids, sedatives or hypnotics, general anesthetics, phenothiazines, tranquilizers, skeletal muscle relaxants, sedating antihistamines, potent inhibitors of cytochrome P450 3A4 isoform (eg,erythromycin, ketoconazole, and certain protease inhibitors), and alcoholic beverages may produce increased depressant effects. Hypoventilation, hypotension, and profound sedation may occur). Products include:
Moban 1108

Morphine Sulfate (The concomitant use of other CNS depressants, including other opioids, sedatives or hypnotics, general anesthetics, phenothiazines, tranquilizers, skeletal muscle relaxants, sedating antihistamines, potent inhibitors of cytochrome P450 3A4 isoform (eg,erythromycin, ketoconazole, and certain protease inhibitors), and alcoholic beverages may produce increased depressant effects. Hypoventilation, hypotension, and profound sedation may occur). Products include:
Avinza 1822
Embeda 1831
MS Contin 2803

Morphine Sulfate, Liposomal (The concomitant use of other CNS depressants, including other opioids, sedatives or hypnotics, general anesthetics, phenothiazines, tranquilizers, skeletal muscle relaxants, sedating antihistamines, potent inhibitors of cytochrome P450 3A4 isoform (eg,erythromycin, ketoconazole, and certain protease inhibitors), and alcoholic beverages may produce increased depressant effects. Hypoventilation, hypotension, and profound sedation may occur).

No products indexed under this heading.

Nafcillin Sodium (Co-administration with agents that induce CYP3A4 activity may reduce the efficacy of fentanyl citrate).

No products indexed under this heading.

Nefazodone Hydrochloride (The concomitant use of fentanyl citrate with

---

IMPORTANT NOTE: Always consult each drug listing in the patient's regimen for possible interactions.

ritonavir or other strong CYP3A4 inhibitors such as ketoconazole, itraconazole, troleandomycin, clarithromycin, nelfinavir, and nefazadone may result in a potentially dangerous increase in fentanyl plasma concentrations. Patients receiving fentanyl citrate and potent CYP3A4 inhibitors should be carefully monitored for an extended period of time and dosage increase should be done conservatively).

No products indexed under this heading.

Nelfinavir Mesylate (The concomitant use of fentanyl citrate with ritonavir or other strong CYP3A4 inhibitors such as ketoconazole, itraconazole, troleandomycin, clarithromycin, nelfinavir, and nefazadone may result in a potentially dangerous increase in fentanyl plasma concentrations. Patients receiving fentanyl citrate and potent CYP3A4 inhibitors should be carefully monitored for an extended period of time and dosage increase should be done conservatively).

No products indexed under this heading.

Nevirapine (The concomitant use of moderate CYP3A4 inhibitors such as amprenavir, aprepitant, diltiazem, erythromycin, fluconazole, fosamprenavir, grapefruit juice, and verapamil with fentanyl citrate may result in an increase in fentanyl plasma concentrations, which could increase or prolong adverse drug effects and may cause potentially fatal respiratory depression. Patients receiving fentanyl citrate and moderate CYP3A4 inhibitors should be carefully monitored for an extended period of time and dosage increase should be done conservatively). Products include:

Viramune Oral Suspension	897
Viramune Tablets	897

Niacin (The concomitant use of moderate CYP3A4 inhibitors such as amprenavir, aprepitant, diltiazem, erythromycin, fluconazole, fosamprenavir, grapefruit juice, and verapamil with fentanyl citrate may result in an increase in fentanyl plasma concentrations, which could increase or prolong adverse drug effects and may cause potentially fatal respiratory depression. Patients receiving fentanyl citrate and moderate CYP3A4 inhibitors should be carefully monitored for an extended period of time and dosage increase should be done conservatively). Products include:

Advicor	402
Cardio Basics	3455
Niaspan	497
Simcor	524

Niacinamide (The concomitant use of moderate CYP3A4 inhibitors such as amprenavir, aprepitant, diltiazem, erythromycin, fluconazole, fosamprenavir, grapefruit juice, and verapamil with fentanyl citrate may result in an increase in fentanyl plasma concentrations, which could increase or prolong adverse drug effects and may cause potentially fatal respiratory depression. Patients receiving fentanyl citrate and moderate CYP3A4 inhibitors should be carefully monitored for an extended period of time and dosage increase should be done conservatively). Products include:

CitraNatal 90 DHA Capsules	2332
CitraNatal Assure	2332
CitraNatal Rx	2332
Heplive	607

Niacinamide Hydroiodide (The concomitant use of moderate CYP3A4 inhibitors such as amprenavir, aprepitant, diltiazem, erythromycin, fluconazole, fosamprenavir, grapefruit juice, and verapamil with fentanyl citrate may result in an increase in fentanyl plasma concentrations, which could increase or prolong adverse drug effects and may cause potentially fatal respiratory depression. Patients receiving fentanyl citrate and moderate CYP3A4 inhibitors

should be carefully monitored for an extended period of time and dosage increase should be done conservatively).

No products indexed under this heading.

Nicotinamide (The concomitant use of moderate CYP3A4 inhibitors such as amprenavir, aprepitant, diltiazem, erythromycin, fluconazole, fosamprenavir, grapefruit juice, and verapamil with fentanyl citrate may result in an increase in fentanyl plasma concentrations, which could increase or prolong adverse drug effects and may cause potentially fatal respiratory depression. Patients receiving fentanyl citrate and moderate CYP3A4 inhibitors should be carefully monitored for an extended period of time and dosage increase should be done conservatively).

No products indexed under this heading.

Nifedipine (The concomitant use of moderate CYP3A4 inhibitors such as amprenavir, aprepitant, diltiazem, erythromycin, fluconazole, fosamprenavir, grapefruit juice, and verapamil with fentanyl citrate may result in an increase in fentanyl plasma concentrations, which could increase or prolong adverse drug effects and may cause potentially fatal respiratory depression. Patients receiving fentanyl citrate and moderate CYP3A4 inhibitors should be carefully monitored for an extended period of time and dosage increase should be done conservatively).

No products indexed under this heading.

Nitrous Oxide (The concomitant use of other CNS depressants, including general anesthetics, may produce increased depressant effects. Hypoventilation, hypotension, and profound sedation may occur).

No products indexed under this heading.

Norfloxacin (The concomitant use of moderate CYP3A4 inhibitors such as amprenavir, aprepitant, diltiazem, erythromycin, fluconazole, fosamprenavir, grapefruit juice, and verapamil with fentanyl citrate may result in an increase in fentanyl plasma concentrations, which could increase or prolong adverse drug effects and may cause potentially fatal respiratory depression. Patients receiving fentanyl citrate and moderate CYP3A4 inhibitors should be carefully monitored for an extended period of time and dosage increase should be done conservatively). Products include:

Noroxin	2220

Olanzapine (The concomitant use of other CNS depressants, including other opioids, sedatives or hypnotics, general anesthetics, phenothiazines, tranquilizers, skeletal muscle relaxants, sedating antihistamines, potent inhibitors of cytochrome P450 3A4 isoform (eg,erythromycin, ketoconazole, and certain protease inhibitors), and alcoholic beverages may produce increased depressant effects. Hypoventilation, hypotension, and profound sedation may occur).

Products include:

Symbyax	1965
Zyprexa	1984
Zyprexa IntraMuscular	1984
Zyprexa ZYDIS	1984

Omeprazole (The concomitant use of moderate CYP3A4 inhibitors such as amprenavir, aprepitant, diltiazem, erythromycin, fluconazole, fosamprenavir, grapefruit juice, and verapamil with fentanyl citrate may result in an increase in fentanyl plasma concentrations, which could increase or prolong adverse drug effects and may cause potentially fatal respiratory depression. Patients receiving fentanyl citrate and moderate CYP3A4 inhibitors should be carefully monitored for an extended period of time and dosage increase should be done conservatively).

No products indexed under this heading.

Orphenadrine Citrate (The concomitant use of other CNS depressants, including skeletal muscle relaxants, may produce increased depressant effects. Hypoventilation, hypotension, and profound sedation may occur).

No products indexed under this heading.

Oxazepam (The concomitant use of other CNS depressants, including other opioids, sedatives or hypnotics, general anesthetics, phenothiazines, tranquilizers, skeletal muscle relaxants, sedating antihistamines, potent inhibitors of cytochrome P450 3A4 isoform (eg,erythromycin, ketoconazole, and certain protease inhibitors), and alcoholic beverages may produce increased depressant effects. Hypoventilation, hypotension, and profound sedation may occur).

No products indexed under this heading.

Oxcarbazepine (Co-administration with agents that induce CYP3A4 activity may reduce the efficacy of fentanyl citrate).

No products indexed under this heading.

Oxycodone Hydrochloride (The concomitant use of other CNS depressants, including other opioids, sedatives or hypnotics, general anesthetics, phenothiazines, tranquilizers, skeletal muscle relaxants, sedating antihistamines, potent inhibitors of cytochrome P450 3A4 isoform (eg,erythromycin, ketoconazole, and certain protease inhibitors), and alcoholic beverages may produce increased depressant effects. Hypoventilation, hypotension, and profound sedation may occur). Products include:

OxyContin	2807
Percocet	1121
Percodan	1124

Oxycodone Terephthalate (The concomitant use of other CNS depressants, including other opioids, sedatives or hypnotics, general anesthetics, phenothiazines, tranquilizers, skeletal muscle relaxants, sedating antihistamines, potent inhibitors of cytochrome P450 3A4 isoform (eg,erythromycin, ketoconazole, and certain protease inhibitors), and alcoholic beverages may produce increased depressant effects. Hypoventilation, hypotension, and profound sedation may occur).

No products indexed under this heading.

Oxymorphone Hydrochloride (The concomitant use of other CNS depressants, including other opioids, sedatives or hypnotics, general anesthetics, phenothiazines, tranquilizers, skeletal muscle relaxants, sedating antihistamines, potent inhibitors of cytochrome P450 3A4 isoform (eg,erythromycin, ketoconazole, and certain protease inhibitors), and alcoholic beverages may produce increased depressant effects. Hypoventilation, hypotension, and profound sedation may occur). Products include:

Opana	1110
Opana ER	1114

Pargyline Hydrochloride (Fentanyl citrate is not recommended for use in patients who are receiving or have received MAO inhibitors within 14 days, because severe and unpredictable potentiation by MAO inhibitors has been reported with opioid analgesics).

No products indexed under this heading.

Paroxetine Hydrochloride (The concomitant use of moderate CYP3A4 inhibitors such as amprenavir, aprepitant, diltiazem, erythromycin, fluconazole, fosamprenavir, grapefruit juice, and verapamil with fentanyl citrate may result in an increase in fentanyl plasma concentrations, which could increase or prolong adverse drug effects and may cause potentially fatal respiratory depression. Patients receiving fentanyl citrate and moderate CYP3A4 inhibitors

should be carefully monitored for an extended period of time and dosage increase should be done conservatively). Products include:

Paroxetine CR	2361
Paroxetine ER	2371
Paxil	1586
Paxil CR	1596

Pentobarbital (The concomitant use of other CNS depressants, including other opioids, sedatives or hypnotics, general anesthetics, phenothiazines, tranquilizers, skeletal muscle relaxants, sedating antihistamines, potent inhibitors of cytochrome P450 3A4 isoform (eg,erythromycin, ketoconazole, and certain protease inhibitors), and alcoholic beverages may produce increased depressant effects. Hypoventilation, hypotension, and profound sedation may occur).

No products indexed under this heading.

Pentobarbital Sodium (The concomitant use of other CNS depressants, including other opioids, sedatives or hypnotics, general anesthetics, phenothiazines, tranquilizers, skeletal muscle relaxants, sedating antihistamines, potent inhibitors of cytochrome P450 3A4 isoform (eg,erythromycin, ketoconazole, and certain protease inhibitors), and alcoholic beverages may produce increased depressant effects. Hypoventilation, hypotension, and profound sedation may occur). Products include:

Nembutal	2012

Perphenazine (The concomitant use of other CNS depressants, including other opioids, sedatives or hypnotics, general anesthetics, phenothiazines, tranquilizers, skeletal muscle relaxants, sedating antihistamines, potent inhibitors of cytochrome P450 3A4 isoform (eg,erythromycin, ketoconazole, and certain protease inhibitors), and alcoholic beverages may produce increased depressant effects. Hypoventilation, hypotension, and profound sedation may occur).

No products indexed under this heading.

Phenelzine Sulfate (Fentanyl citrate is not recommended for use in patients who are receiving or have received MAO inhibitors within 14 days, because severe and unpredictable potentiation by MAO inhibitors has been reported with opioid analgesics).

No products indexed under this heading.

Phenobarbital (Co-administration with agents that induce CYP3A4 activity may reduce the efficacy of fentanyl citrate). Products include:

Donnatal	2711

Phenobarbital Sodium (Co-administration with agents that induce CYP3A4 activity may reduce the efficacy of fentanyl citrate).

No products indexed under this heading.

Phenothiazine Derivatives (The concomitant use of other CNS depressants, including phenothiazines, may produce increased depressant effects. Hypoventilation, hypotension, and profound sedation may occur).

No products indexed under this heading.

Phenothiazines (The concomitant use of other CNS depressants, including phenothiazines, may produce increased depressant effects. Hypoventilation, hypotension, and profound sedation may occur).

No products indexed under this heading.

Phenytoin (Co-administration with agents that induce CYP3A4 activity may reduce the efficacy of fentanyl citrate).

No products indexed under this heading.

Phenytoin Sodium (Co-administration with agents that induce CYP3A4 activity may reduce the efficacy of fentanyl citrate). Products include:

Phenytek Capsules 2380

Posaconazole (The concomitant use of moderate CYP3A4 inhibitors such as amprenavir, aprepitant, diltiazem, erythromycin, fluconazole, fosamprenavir, grapefruit juice, and verapamil with fentanyl citrate may result in an increase in fentanyl plasma concentrations, which could increase or prolong adverse drug effects and may cause potentially fatal respiratory depression. Patients receiving fentanyl citrate and moderate CYP3A4 inhibitors should be carefully monitored for an extended period of time and dosage increase should be done conservatively). Products include:

Noxafil 3172

Prazepam (The concomitant use of other CNS depressants, including other opioids, sedatives or hypnotics, general anesthetics, phenothiazines, tranquilizers, skeletal muscle relaxants, sedating antihistamines, potent inhibitors of cytochrome P450 3A4 isoform (eg,erythromycin, ketoconazole, and certain protease inhibitors), and alcoholic beverages may produce increased depressant effects. Hypoventilation, hypotension, and profound sedation may occur).

No products indexed under this heading.

Prednisolone (Co-administration with agents that induce CYP3A4 activity may reduce the efficacy of fentanyl citrate).

No products indexed under this heading.

Prednisolone Acetate (Co-administration with agents that induce CYP3A4 activity may reduce the efficacy of fentanyl citrate). Products include:

Blephamide .... ⊙212, ⊙214

Pred Forte .... ⊙225

Pred Mild .... ⊙230

Pred-G .... ⊙226, ⊙227

Prednisolone Sodium Phosphate (Co-administration with agents that induce CYP3A4 activity may reduce the efficacy of fentanyl citrate).

No products indexed under this heading.

Prednisolone Tebutate (Co-administration with agents that induce CYP3A4 activity may reduce the efficacy of fentanyl citrate).

No products indexed under this heading.

Prednisone (Co-administration with agents that induce CYP3A4 activity may reduce the efficacy of fentanyl citrate).

No products indexed under this heading.

Prednisone sodium phosphate (Co-administration with agents that induce CYP3A4 activity may reduce the efficacy of fentanyl citrate).

No products indexed under this heading.

Primidone (Co-administration with agents that induce CYP3A4 activity may reduce the efficacy of fentanyl citrate).

No products indexed under this heading.

Procarbazine Hydrochloride (Fentanyl citrate is not recommended for use in patients who are receiving or have received MAO inhibitors within 14 days, because severe and unpredictable potentiation by MAO inhibitors has been reported with opioid analgesics).

No products indexed under this heading.

Prochlorperazine (The concomitant use of other CNS depressants, including other opioids, sedatives or hypnotics, general anesthetics, phenothiazines, tranquilizers, skeletal muscle relaxants, sedating antihistamines, potent inhibitors of cytochrome P450 3A4 isoform (eg,erythromycin, ketoconazole, and certain protease inhibitors), and alcoholic beverages may produce increased depressant effects. Hypoventilation, hypotension, and profound sedation may occur).

No products indexed under this heading.

Prochlorperazine Edisylate (The concomitant use of other CNS depressants, including other opioids, sedatives or hypnotics, general anesthetics, phenothiazines, tranquilizers, skeletal muscle relaxants, sedating antihistamines, potent inhibitors of cytochrome P450 3A4 isoform (eg,erythromycin, ketoconazole, and certain protease inhibitors), and alcoholic beverages may produce increased depressant effects. Hypoventilation, hypotension, and profound sedation may occur).

No products indexed under this heading.

Prochlorperazine Maleate (The concomitant use of other CNS depressants, including other opioids, sedatives or hypnotics, general anesthetics, phenothiazines, tranquilizers, skeletal muscle relaxants, sedating antihistamines, potent inhibitors of cytochrome P450 3A4 isoform (eg,erythromycin, ketoconazole, and certain protease inhibitors), and alcoholic beverages may produce increased depressant effects. Hypoventilation, hypotension, and profound sedation may occur).

No products indexed under this heading.

Promethazine (The concomitant use of other CNS depressants, including other opioids, sedatives or hypnotics, general anesthetics, phenothiazines, tranquilizers, skeletal muscle relaxants, sedating antihistamines, potent inhibitors of cytochrome P450 3A4 isoform (eg,erythromycin, ketoconazole, and certain protease inhibitors), and alcoholic beverages may produce increased depressant effects. Hypoventilation, hypotension, and profound sedation may occur).

No products indexed under this heading.

Promethazine Hydrochloride (The concomitant use of other CNS depressants, including other opioids, sedatives or hypnotics, general anesthetics, phenothiazines, tranquilizers, skeletal muscle relaxants, sedating antihistamines, potent inhibitors of cytochrome P450 3A4 isoform (eg,erythromycin, ketoconazole, and certain protease inhibitors), and alcoholic beverages may produce increased depressant effects. Hypoventilation, hypotension, and profound sedation may occur).

No products indexed under this heading.

Propofol (The concomitant use of other CNS depressants, including other opioids, sedatives or hypnotics, general anesthetics, phenothiazines, tranquilizers, skeletal muscle relaxants, sedating antihistamines, potent inhibitors of cytochrome P450 3A4 isoform (eg,erythromycin, ketoconazole, and certain protease inhibitors), and alcoholic beverages may produce increased depressant effects. Hypoventilation, hypotension, and profound sedation may occur).

No products indexed under this heading.

Propoxyphene Hydrochloride (The concomitant use of moderate CYP3A4 inhibitors such as amprenavir, aprepitant, diltiazem, erythromycin, fluconazole, fosamprenavir, grapefruit juice, and verapamil with fentanyl citrate may result in an increase in fentanyl plasma concentrations, which could increase or prolong adverse drug effects and may cause potentially fatal respiratory depression. Patients receiving fentanyl citrate and moderate CYP3A4 inhibitors should be carefully monitored for an extended period of time and dosage increase should be done conservatively).

No products indexed under this heading.

Propoxyphene Napsylate (The concomitant use of moderate CYP3A4 inhibitors such as amprenavir, aprepitant, diltiazem, erythromycin, fluconazole, fosamprenavir, grapefruit juice, and verapamil with fentanyl citrate may result in an increase in fentanyl plasma concentrations, which could increase or prolong adverse drug effects and may cause potentially fatal respiratory depression. Patients receiving fentanyl citrate and moderate CYP3A4 inhibitors should be carefully monitored for an extended period of time and dosage increase should be done conservatively).

No products indexed under this heading.

Pyrilamine Maleate (The concomitant use of other CNS depressants, including sedating antihistamines, may produce increased depressant effects. Hypoventilation, hypotension, and profound sedation may occur).

No products indexed under this heading.

Pyrilamine Tannate (The concomitant use of other CNS depressants, including sedating antihistamines, may produce increased depressant effects. Hypoventilation, hypotension, and profound sedation may occur).

No products indexed under this heading.

Quazepam (The concomitant use of other CNS depressants, including other opioids, sedatives or hypnotics, general anesthetics, phenothiazines, tranquilizers, skeletal muscle relaxants, sedating antihistamines, potent inhibitors of cytochrome P450 3A4 isoform (eg,erythromycin, ketoconazole, and certain protease inhibitors), and alcoholic beverages may produce increased depressant effects. Hypoventilation, hypotension, and profound sedation may occur).

No products indexed under this heading.

Quetiapine Fumarate (The concomitant use of other CNS depressants, including other opioids, sedatives or hypnotics, general anesthetics, phenothiazines, tranquilizers, skeletal muscle relaxants, sedating antihistamines, potent inhibitors of cytochrome P450 3A4 isoform (eg,erythromycin, ketoconazole, and certain protease inhibitors), and alcoholic beverages may produce increased depressant effects. Hypoventilation, hypotension, and profound sedation may occur). Products include:

Seroquel 750

Seroquel XR 759

Quinidine (The concomitant use of moderate CYP3A4 inhibitors such as amprenavir, aprepitant, diltiazem, erythromycin, fluconazole, fosamprenavir, grapefruit juice, and verapamil with fentanyl citrate may result in an increase in fentanyl plasma concentrations, which could increase or prolong adverse drug effects and may cause potentially fatal respiratory depression. Patients receiving fentanyl citrate and moderate CYP3A4 inhibitors should be carefully monitored for an extended period of time and dosage increase should be done conservatively).

No products indexed under this heading.

Quinidine Hydrochloride (The concomitant use of moderate CYP3A4 inhibitors such as amprenavir, aprepitant, diltiazem, erythromycin, fluconazole, fosamprenavir, grapefruit juice, and verapamil with fentanyl citrate may result in an increase in fentanyl plasma concentrations, which could increase or prolong adverse drug effects and may cause potentially fatal respiratory depression. Patients receiving fentanyl citrate and moderate CYP3A4 inhibitors should be carefully monitored for an extended period of time and dosage increase should be done conservatively).

No products indexed under this heading.

Quinidine Polygalacturonate (The concomitant use of moderate CYP3A4 inhibitors such as amprenavir, aprepitant, diltiazem, erythromycin, fluconazole, fosamprenavir, grapefruit juice, and verapamil with fentanyl citrate may result in an increase in fentanyl plasma concentrations, which could increase or prolong adverse drug effects and may cause potentially fatal respiratory depression. Patients receiving fentanyl citrate and moderate CYP3A4 inhibitors should be carefully monitored for an extended period of time and dosage increase should be done conservatively).

No products indexed under this heading.

Quinidine Sulfate (The concomitant use of moderate CYP3A4 inhibitors such as amprenavir, aprepitant, diltiazem, erythromycin, fluconazole, fosamprenavir, grapefruit juice, and verapamil with fentanyl citrate may result in an increase in fentanyl plasma concentrations, which could increase or prolong adverse drug effects and may cause potentially fatal respiratory depression. Patients receiving fentanyl citrate and moderate CYP3A4 inhibitors should be carefully monitored for an extended period of time and dosage increase should be done conservatively).

No products indexed under this heading.

Quinine (The concomitant use of moderate CYP3A4 inhibitors such as amprenavir, aprepitant, diltiazem, erythromycin, fluconazole, fosamprenavir, grapefruit juice, and verapamil with fentanyl citrate may result in an increase in fentanyl plasma concentrations, which could increase or prolong adverse drug effects and may cause potentially fatal respiratory depression. Patients receiving fentanyl citrate and moderate CYP3A4 inhibitors should be carefully monitored for an extended period of time and dosage increase should be done conservatively). Products include:

Hyland's Leg Cramps PM with Quinine 3315

Quinine Sulfate (The concomitant use of moderate CYP3A4 inhibitors such as amprenavir, aprepitant, diltiazem, erythromycin, fluconazole, fosamprenavir, grapefruit juice, and verapamil with fentanyl citrate may result in an increase in fentanyl plasma concentrations, which could increase or prolong adverse drug effects and may cause potentially fatal respiratory depression. Patients receiving fentanyl citrate and moderate CYP3A4 inhibitors should be carefully monitored for an extended period of time and dosage increase should be done conservatively).

No products indexed under this heading.

Quinupristin (The concomitant use of moderate CYP3A4 inhibitors such as amprenavir, aprepitant, diltiazem, erythromycin, fluconazole, fosamprenavir, grapefruit juice, and verapamil with fentanyl citrate may result in an increase in fentanyl plasma concentrations, which could increase or prolong adverse drug effects and may cause potentially fatal respiratory depression. Patients receiving fentanyl citrate and moderate CYP3A4 inhibitors should be carefully monitored for an extended period of time and dosage increase should be done conservatively).

No products indexed under this heading.

Ramelteon (The concomitant use of other CNS depressants, including sedatives or hypnotics, may produce increased depressant effects. Hypoventilation, hypotension, and profound sedation may occur). Products include:

Rozerem 3366

Ranitidine Bismuth Citrate (The concomitant use of moderate CYP3A4 inhibitors such as amprenavir, aprepitant, diltiazem, erythromycin, fluconazole, fosamprenavir, grapefruit juice, and verapamil with fentanyl citrate may result in an increase in fentanyl plasma concentrations, which could increase or prolong adverse drug effects and may cause potentially fatal respiratory depression. Patients receiving fentanyl citrate and moderate CYP3A4 inhibitors

should be carefully monitored for an extended period of time and dosage increase should be done conservatively).
No products indexed under this heading.

Ranitidine Hydrochloride (The concomitant use of moderate CYP3A4 inhibitors such as amprenavir, aprepitant, diltiazem, erythromycin, fluconazole, fosamprenavir, grapefruit juice, and verapamil with fentanyl citrate may result in an increase in fentanyl plasma concentrations, which could increase or prolong adverse drug effects and may cause potentially fatal respiratory depression. Patients receiving fentanyl citrate and moderate CYP3A4 inhibitors should be carefully monitored for an extended period of time and dosage increase should be done conservatively). Products include:
Zantac 1737
Zantac Injection 1732
Zantac Pharmacy 1735

Rasagiline Mesylate (Fentanyl citrate is not recommended for use in patients who are receiving or have received MAO inhibitors within 14 days, because severe and unpredictable potentiation by MAO inhibitors has been reported with opioid analgesics). Products include:
Azilect 3383

Remifentanil Hydrochloride (The concomitant use of other CNS depressants, including other opioids, sedatives or hypnotics, general anesthetics, phenothiazines, tranquilizers, skeletal muscle relaxants, sedating antihistamines, potent inhibitors of cytochrome P450 3A4 isoform (eg,erythromycin, ketoconazole, and certain protease inhibitors), and alcoholic beverages may produce increased depressant effects. Hypoventilation, hypotension, and profound sedation may occur).
No products indexed under this heading.

Rifabutin (Co-administration with agents that induce CYP3A4 activity may reduce the efficacy of fentanyl citrate).
No products indexed under this heading.

Rifampicin (Co-administration with agents that induce CYP3A4 activity may reduce the efficacy of fentanyl citrate).
No products indexed under this heading.

Rifampin (Co-administration with agents that induce CYP3A4 activity may reduce the efficacy of fentanyl citrate).
No products indexed under this heading.

Rifapentine (Co-administration with agents that induce CYP3A4 activity may reduce the efficacy of fentanyl citrate).
No products indexed under this heading.

Risperidone (The concomitant use of other CNS depressants, including other opioids, sedatives or hypnotics, general anesthetics, phenothiazines, tranquilizers, skeletal muscle relaxants, sedating antihistamines, potent inhibitors of cytochrome P450 3A4 isoform (eg,erythromycin, ketoconazole, and certain protease inhibitors), and alcoholic beverages may produce increased depressant effects. Hypoventilation, hypotension, and profound sedation may occur). Products include:
Risperdal Consta 2682

Ritonavir (The concomitant use of fentanyl citrate with ritonavir or other strong CYP3A4 inhibitors such as ketoconazole, itraconazole, troleandomycin, clarithromycin, nelfinavir, and nefazadone may result in a potentially dangerous increase in fentanyl plasma concentrations. Patients receiving fentanyl citrate and potent CYP3A4 inhibitors should be carefully monitored for an extended period of time and dosage increase should be done conservatively). Products include:
Kaletra 458
Norvir 509

Saquinavir (The concomitant use of fentanyl citrate with ritonavir or other strong CYP3A4 inhibitors such as ketoconazole, itraconazole, troleandomycin, clarithromycin, nelfinavir, and nefazadone may result in a potentially dangerous increase in fentanyl plasma concentrations. Patients receiving fentanyl citrate and potent CYP3A4 inhibitors should be carefully monitored for an extended period of time and dosage increase should be done conservatively).
No products indexed under this heading.

Saquinavir Mesylate (The concomitant use of fentanyl citrate with ritonavir or other strong CYP3A4 inhibitors such as ketoconazole, itraconazole, troleandomycin, clarithromycin, nelfinavir, and nefazadone may result in a potentially dangerous increase in fentanyl plasma concentrations. Patients receiving fentanyl citrate and potent CYP3A4 inhibitors should be carefully monitored for an extended period of time and dosage increase should be done conservatively).
No products indexed under this heading.

Secobarbital Sodium (The concomitant use of other CNS depressants, including other opioids, sedatives or hypnotics, general anesthetics, phenothiazines, tranquilizers, skeletal muscle relaxants, sedating antihistamines, potent inhibitors of cytochrome P450 3A4 isoform (eg,erythromycin, ketoconazole, and certain protease inhibitors), and alcoholic beverages may produce increased depressant effects. Hypoventilation, hypotension, and profound sedation may occur).
No products indexed under this heading.

Selegiline (Fentanyl citrate is not recommended for use in patients who are receiving or have received MAO inhibitors within 14 days, because severe and unpredictable potentiation by MAO inhibitors has been reported with opioid analgesics). Products include:
Emsam 3623

Selegiline Hydrochloride (Fentanyl citrate is not recommended for use in patients who are receiving or have received MAO inhibitors within 14 days, because severe and unpredictable potentiation by MAO inhibitors has been reported with opioid analgesics). Products include:
Eldepryl 3312

Sertraline Hydrochloride (The concomitant use of moderate CYP3A4 inhibitors such as amprenavir, aprepitant, diltiazem, erythromycin, fluconazole, fosamprenavir, grapefruit juice, and verapamil with fentanyl citrate may result in an increase in fentanyl plasma concentrations, which could increase or prolong adverse drug effects and may cause potentially fatal respiratory depression. Patients receiving fentanyl citrate and moderate CYP3A4 inhibitors should be carefully monitored for an extended period of time and dosage increase should be done conservatively).
No products indexed under this heading.

Sevoflurane (The concomitant use of other CNS depressants, including other opioids, sedatives or hypnotics, general anesthetics, phenothiazines, tranquilizers, skeletal muscle relaxants, sedating antihistamines, potent inhibitors of cytochrome P450 3A4 isoform (eg,erythromycin, ketoconazole, and certain protease inhibitors), and alcoholic beverages may produce increased depressant effects. Hypoventilation, hypotension, and profound sedation may occur). Products include:
Ultane 554

Sildenafil Citrate (The concomitant use of moderate CYP3A4 inhibitors such as amprenavir, aprepitant, diltiazem, erythromycin, fluconazole, fosamprenavir, grapefruit juice, and verapamil with fentanyl citrate may result in an increase in fentanyl plasma concentrations, which could increase or prolong adverse drug effects and may cause potentially fatal respiratory depression. Patients receiving fentanyl citrate and moderate CYP3A4 inhibitors should be carefully monitored for an extended period of time and dosage increase should be done conservatively).
No products indexed under this heading.

Sodium Butabarbital (The concomitant use of other CNS depressants, including other opioids, sedatives or hypnotics, general anesthetics, phenothiazines, tranquilizers, skeletal muscle relaxants, sedating antihistamines, potent inhibitors of cytochrome P450 3A4 isoform (eg,erythromycin, ketoconazole, and certain protease inhibitors), and alcoholic beverages may produce increased depressant effects. Hypoventilation, hypotension, and profound sedation may occur).
No products indexed under this heading.

Sodium Oxybate (The concomitant use of other CNS depressants, including other opioids, sedatives or hypnotics, general anesthetics, phenothiazines, tranquilizers, skeletal muscle relaxants, sedating antihistamines, potent inhibitors of cytochrome P450 3A4 isoform (eg,erythromycin, ketoconazole, and certain protease inhibitors), and alcoholic beverages may produce increased depressant effects. Hypoventilation, hypotension, and profound sedation may occur).
No products indexed under this heading.

Sodium Pentobarbital (The concomitant use of other CNS depressants, including other opioids, sedatives or hypnotics, general anesthetics, phenothiazines, tranquilizers, skeletal muscle relaxants, sedating antihistamines, potent inhibitors of cytochrome P450 3A4 isoform (eg,erythromycin, ketoconazole, and certain protease inhibitors), and alcoholic beverages may produce increased depressant effects. Hypoventilation, hypotension, and profound sedation may occur).
No products indexed under this heading.

Sufentanil Citrate (The concomitant use of other CNS depressants, including other opioids, sedatives or hypnotics, general anesthetics, phenothiazines, tranquilizers, skeletal muscle relaxants, sedating antihistamines, potent inhibitors of cytochrome P450 3A4 isoform (eg,erythromycin, ketoconazole, and certain protease inhibitors), and alcoholic beverages may produce increased depressant effects. Hypoventilation, hypotension, and profound sedation may occur).
No products indexed under this heading.

Sulfinpyrazone (Co-administration with agents that induce CYP3A4 activity may reduce the efficacy of fentanyl citrate).
No products indexed under this heading.

Talbutal (The concomitant use of other CNS depressants, including other opioids, sedatives or hypnotics, general anesthetics, phenothiazines, tranquilizers, skeletal muscle relaxants, sedating antihistamines, potent inhibitors of cytochrome P450 3A4 isoform (eg,erythromycin, ketoconazole, and certain protease inhibitors), and alcoholic beverages may produce increased depressant effects. Hypoventilation, hypotension, and profound sedation may occur).
No products indexed under this heading.

Telithromycin (The concomitant use of fentanyl citrate with ritonavir or other strong CYP3A4 inhibitors such as ketoconazole, itraconazole, troleandomycin, clarithromycin, nelfinavir, and nefazadone may result in a potentially dangerous increase in fentanyl plasma concentrations. Patients receiving fentanyl citrate and potent CYP3A4 inhibitors should be carefully monitored for an extended period of time and dosage increase should be done conservatively). Products include:
Ketek 2991

Temazepam (The concomitant use of other CNS depressants, including other opioids, sedatives or hypnotics, general anesthetics, phenothiazines, tranquilizers, skeletal muscle relaxants, sedating antihistamines, potent inhibitors of cytochrome P450 3A4 isoform (eg,erythromycin, ketoconazole, and certain protease inhibitors), and alcoholic beverages may produce increased depressant effects. Hypoventilation, hypotension, and profound sedation may occur).
No products indexed under this heading.

Terfenadine (The concomitant use of other CNS depressants, including sedating antihistamines, may produce increased depressant effects. Hypoventilation, hypotension, and profound sedation may occur).
No products indexed under this heading.

Theophyllinate (Co-administration with agents that induce CYP3A4 activity may reduce the efficacy of fentanyl citrate).
No products indexed under this heading.

Theophylline (Co-administration with agents that induce CYP3A4 activity may reduce the efficacy of fentanyl citrate).
No products indexed under this heading.

Theophylline Anhydrous (Co-administration with agents that induce CYP3A4 activity may reduce the efficacy of fentanyl citrate). Products include:
Uniphyl 2817

Theophylline Calcium Salicylate (Co-administration with agents that induce CYP3A4 activity may reduce the efficacy of fentanyl citrate).
No products indexed under this heading.

Theophylline Dihydroxypropyl (Glyceryl) (Co-administration with agents that induce CYP3A4 activity may reduce the efficacy of fentanyl citrate).
No products indexed under this heading.

Theophylline Ethylenediamine (Co-administration with agents that induce CYP3A4 activity may reduce the efficacy of fentanyl citrate).
No products indexed under this heading.

Theophylline Sodium Glycinate (Co-administration with agents that induce CYP3A4 activity may reduce the efficacy of fentanyl citrate).
No products indexed under this heading.

Thiamylal Sodium (The concomitant use of other CNS depressants, including other opioids, sedatives or hypnotics, general anesthetics, phenothiazines, tranquilizers, skeletal muscle relaxants, sedating antihistamines, potent inhibitors of cytochrome P450 3A4 isoform (eg,erythromycin, ketoconazole, and certain protease inhibitors), and alcoholic beverages may produce increased depressant effects. Hypoventilation, hypotension, and profound sedation may occur).
No products indexed under this heading.

Thioridazine (The concomitant use of other CNS depressants, including other opioids, sedatives or hypnotics, general anesthetics, phenothiazines, tranquilizers, skeletal muscle relaxants, sedating antihistamines, potent inhibitors of cytochrome P450 3A4 isoform (eg,erythromycin, ketoconazole, and certain protease inhibitors), and alcoholic beverages

may produce increased depressant effects. Hypoventilation, hypotension, and profound sedation may occur). No products indexed under this heading.

Thioridazine Hydrochloride (The concomitant use of other CNS depressants, including other opioids, sedatives or hypnotics, general anesthetics, phenothiazines, tranquilizers, skeletal muscle relaxants, sedating antihistamines, potent inhibitors of cytochrome P450 3A4 isoform (eg,erythromycin, ketoconazole, and certain protease inhibitors), and alcoholic beverages may produce increased depressant effects. Hypoventilation, hypotension, and profound sedation may occur). Products include:
Thioridazine Hydrochloride 2384

Thiothixene (The concomitant use of other CNS depressants, including other opioids, sedatives or hypnotics, general anesthetics, phenothiazines, tranquilizers, skeletal muscle relaxants, sedating antihistamines, potent inhibitors of cytochrome P450 3A4 isoform (eg,erythromycin, ketoconazole, and certain protease inhibitors), and alcoholic beverages may produce increased depressant effects. Hypoventilation, hypotension, and profound sedation may occur). Products include:
Thiothixene 2386

Thiothixene Hydrochloride (The concomitant use of other CNS depressants, including other opioids, sedatives or hypnotics, general anesthetics, phenothiazines, tranquilizers, skeletal muscle relaxants, sedating antihistamines, potent inhibitors of cytochrome P450 3A4 isoform (eg,erythromycin, ketoconazole, and certain protease inhibitors), and alcoholic beverages may produce increased depressant effects. Hypoventilation, hypotension, and profound sedation may occur). No products indexed under this heading.

Tizanidine (The concomitant use of other CNS depressants, including skeletal muscle relaxants, may produce increased depressant effects. Hypoventilation, hypotension, and profound sedation may occur). No products indexed under this heading.

Tizanidine Hydrochloride (The concomitant use of other CNS depressants, including skeletal muscle relaxants, may produce increased depressant effects. Hypoventilation, hypotension, and profound sedation may occur). No products indexed under this heading.

Tranylcypromine Sulfate (Fentanyl citrate is not recommended for use in patients who are receiving or have received MAO inhibitors within 14 days, because severe and unpredictable potentiation by MAO inhibitors has been reported with opioid analgesics). Products include:
Parnate 1584

Triamcinolone (Co-administration with agents that induce CYP3A4 activity may reduce the efficacy of fentanyl citrate). No products indexed under this heading.

Triamcinolone Acetonide (Co-administration with agents that induce CYP3A4 activity may reduce the efficacy of fentanyl citrate). Products include:
Azmacort 408
Nasacort AQ 3019

Triamcinolone Diacetate (Co-administration with agents that induce CYP3A4 activity may reduce the efficacy of fentanyl citrate). No products indexed under this heading.

Triamcinolone Hexacetonide (Co-administration with agents that induce CYP3A4 activity may reduce the efficacy of fentanyl citrate). No products indexed under this heading.

Triazolam (The concomitant use of other CNS depressants, including other opioids, sedatives or hypnotics, general anesthetics, phenothiazines, tranquilizers, skeletal muscle relaxants, sedating antihistamines, potent inhibitors of cytochrome P450 3A4 isoform (eg,erythromycin, ketoconazole, and certain protease inhibitors), and alcoholic beverages may produce increased depressant effects. Hypoventilation, hypotension, and profound sedation may occur). No products indexed under this heading.

Trifluoperazine Hydrochloride (The concomitant use of other CNS depressants, including other opioids, sedatives or hypnotics, general anesthetics, phenothiazines, tranquilizers, skeletal muscle relaxants, sedating antihistamines, potent inhibitors of cytochrome P450 3A4 isoform (eg,erythromycin, ketoconazole, and certain protease inhibitors), and alcoholic beverages may produce increased depressant effects. Hypoventilation, hypotension, and profound sedation may occur). No products indexed under this heading.

Trimeprazine Tartrate (The concomitant use of other CNS depressants, including sedating antihistamines, may produce increased depressant effects. Hypoventilation, hypotension, and profound sedation may occur). No products indexed under this heading.

Tripelennamine Hydrochloride (The concomitant use of other CNS depressants, including sedating antihistamines, may produce increased depressant effects. Hypoventilation, hypotension, and profound sedation may occur). No products indexed under this heading.

Triprolidine Hydrochloride (The concomitant use of other CNS depressants, including sedating antihistamines, may produce increased depressant effects. Hypoventilation, hypotension, and profound sedation may occur). No products indexed under this heading.

Troglitazone (The concomitant use of moderate CYP3A4 inhibitors such as amprenavir, aprepitant, diltiazem, erythromycin, fluconazole, fosamprenavir, grapefruit juice, and verapamil with fentanyl citrate may result in an increase in fentanyl plasma concentrations, which could increase or prolong adverse drug effects and may cause potentially fatal respiratory depression. Patients receiving fentanyl citrate and moderate CYP3A4 inhibitors should be carefully monitored for an extended period of time and dosage increase should be done conservatively). No products indexed under this heading.

Troleandomycin (The concomitant use of fentanyl citrate with ritonavir or other strong CYP3A4 inhibitors such as ketoconazole, itraconazole, troleandomycin, clarithromycin, nelfinavir, and nefazadone may result in a potentially dangerous increase in fentanyl plasma concentrations. Patients receiving fentanyl citrate and potent CYP3A4 inhibitors should be carefully monitored for an extended period of time and dosage increase should be done conservatively). No products indexed under this heading.

Valproate Sodium (The concomitant use of moderate CYP3A4 inhibitors such as amprenavir, aprepitant, diltiazem, erythromycin, fluconazole, fosamprenavir, grapefruit juice, and verapamil with fentanyl citrate may result in an increase in fentanyl plasma concentrations, which could increase or prolong adverse drug effects and may cause potentially fatal respiratory depression. Patients receiving fentanyl citrate and moderate CYP3A4 inhibitors

should be carefully monitored for an extended period of time and dosage increase should be done conservatively). No products indexed under this heading.

Vardenafil Hydrochloride (The concomitant use of moderate CYP3A4 inhibitors such as amprenavir, aprepitant, diltiazem, erythromycin, fluconazole, fosamprenavir, grapefruit juice, and verapamil with fentanyl citrate may result in an increase in fentanyl plasma concentrations, which could increase or prolong adverse drug effects and may cause potentially fatal respiratory depression. Patients receiving fentanyl citrate and moderate CYP3A4 inhibitors should be carefully monitored for an extended period of time and dosage increase should be done conservatively). Products include:
Levitra 3157

Verapamil Hydrochloride (The concomitant use of moderate CYP3A4 inhibitors such as amprenavir, aprepitant, diltiazem, erythromycin, fluconazole, fosamprenavir, grapefruit juice, and verapamil with fentanyl citrate may result in an increase in fentanyl plasma concentrations, which could increase or prolong adverse drug effects and may cause potentially fatal respiratory depression. Patients receiving fentanyl citrate and moderate CYP3A4 inhibitors should be carefully monitored for an extended period of time and dosage increase should be done conservatively). Products include:
Tarka 534

Voriconazole (The concomitant use of fentanyl citrate with ritonavir or other strong CYP3A4 inhibitors such as ketoconazole, itraconazole, troleandomycin, clarithromycin, nelfinavir, and nefazadone may result in a potentially dangerous increase in fentanyl plasma concentrations. Patients receiving fentanyl citrate and potent CYP3A4 inhibitors should be carefully monitored for an extended period of time and dosage increase should be done conservatively). No products indexed under this heading.

Zafirlukast (The concomitant use of moderate CYP3A4 inhibitors such as amprenavir, aprepitant, diltiazem, erythromycin, fluconazole, fosamprenavir, grapefruit juice, and verapamil with fentanyl citrate may result in an increase in fentanyl plasma concentrations, which could increase or prolong adverse drug effects and may cause potentially fatal respiratory depression. Patients receiving fentanyl citrate and moderate CYP3A4 inhibitors should be carefully monitored for an extended period of time and dosage increase should be done conservatively). Products include:
Accolate 3612

Zaleplon (The concomitant use of other CNS depressants, including other opioids, sedatives or hypnotics, general anesthetics, phenothiazines, tranquilizers, skeletal muscle relaxants, sedating antihistamines, potent inhibitors of cytochrome P450 3A4 isoform (eg,erythromycin, ketoconazole, and certain protease inhibitors), and alcoholic beverages may produce increased depressant effects. Hypoventilation, hypotension, and profound sedation may occur). No products indexed under this heading.

Zileuton (The concomitant use of moderate CYP3A4 inhibitors such as amprenavir, aprepitant, diltiazem, erythromycin, fluconazole, fosamprenavir, grapefruit juice, and verapamil with fentanyl citrate may result in an increase in fentanyl plasma concentrations, which could increase or prolong adverse drug effects and may cause potentially fatal respiratory depression. Patients receiving fentanyl citrate and moderate

CYP3A4 inhibitors should be carefully monitored for an extended period of time and dosage increase should be done conservatively). No products indexed under this heading.

Ziprasidone Hydrochloride (The concomitant use of other CNS depressants, including other opioids, sedatives or hypnotics, general anesthetics, phenothiazines, tranquilizers, skeletal muscle relaxants, sedating antihistamines, potent inhibitors of cytochrome P450 3A4 isoform (eg,erythromycin, ketoconazole, and certain protease inhibitors), and alcoholic beverages may produce increased depressant effects. Hypoventilation, hypotension, and profound sedation may occur). Products include:
Geodon 2723

Zolpidem Tartrate (The concomitant use of other CNS depressants, including other opioids, sedatives or hypnotics, general anesthetics, phenothiazines, tranquilizers, skeletal muscle relaxants, sedating antihistamines, potent inhibitors of cytochrome P450 3A4 isoform (eg,erythromycin, ketoconazole, and certain protease inhibitors), and alcoholic beverages may produce increased depressant effects. Hypoventilation, hypotension, and profound sedation may occur). Products include:
Ambien 2920
Ambien CR 2925

Food Interactions

Alcohol (The concomitant use of other CNS depressants, including other opioids, sedatives or hypnotics, general anesthetics, phenothiazines, tranquilizers, skeletal muscle relaxants, sedating antihistamines, potent inhibitors of cytochrome P450 3A4 isoform (eg,erythromycin, ketoconazole, and certain protease inhibitors), and alcoholic beverages may produce increased depressant effects. Hypoventilation, hypotension, and profound sedation may occur).

Beer, reduced-alcohol (The concomitant use of other CNS depressants, including alcoholic beverages, may produce increased depressant effects. Hypoventilation, hypotension, and profound sedation may occur).

Beer, unspecified (The concomitant use of other CNS depressants, including alcoholic beverages, may produce increased depressant effects. Hypoventilation, hypotension, and profound sedation may occur).

Grapefruit (The concomitant use of moderate CYP3A4 inhibitors such as amprenavir, aprepitant, diltiazem, erythromycin, fluconazole, fosamprenavir, grapefruit juice, and verapamil with fentanyl citrate may result in an increase in fentanyl plasma concentrations, which could increase or prolong adverse drug effects and may cause potentially fatal respiratory depression. Patients receiving fentanyl citrate and moderate CYP3A4 inhibitors should be carefully monitored for an extended period of time and dosage increase should be done conservatively).

Grapefruit Juice (The concomitant use of moderate CYP3A4 inhibitors such as amprenavir, aprepitant, diltiazem, erythromycin, fluconazole, fosamprenavir, grapefruit juice, and verapamil with fentanyl citrate may result in an increase in fentanyl plasma concentrations, which could increase or prolong adverse drug effects and may cause potentially fatal respiratory depression. Patients receiving fentanyl citrate and moderate CYP3A4 inhibitors should be carefully monitored for an extended period of

IMPORTANT NOTE: Always consult each drug listing in the patient's regimen for possible interactions.

time and dosage increase should be done conservatively).

Wine, Chianti (The concomitant use of other CNS depressants, including alcoholic beverages, may produce increased depressant effects. Hypoventilation, hypotension, and profound sedation may occur).

Wine, Red (The concomitant use of other CNS depressants, including alcoholic beverages, may produce increased depressant effects. Hypoventilation, hypotension, and profound sedation may occur).

Wine, unspecified (The concomitant use of other CNS depressants, including alcoholic beverages, may produce increased depressant effects. Hypoventilation, hypotension, and profound sedation may occur).

Wine products (The concomitant use of other CNS depressants, including alcoholic beverages, may produce increased depressant effects. Hypoventilation, hypotension, and profound sedation may occur).

FERRALET 90 TABLETS
(Docusate Sodium, Folic Acid, Iron Carbonyl, Vitamin B12, Vitamin C) 2333
None cited in PDR database.

FINACEA GEL
(Azelaic Acid) 1808
May interact with alcohols, astringents, peeling/desquamating agents, and certain other agents. Compounds in these categories include:

Acitretin (Avoid concurrent use with alcoholic cleansers, tinctures and astringents, abrasives and peeling agents). Products include:
Soriatane 3326

Adapalene (Avoid concurrent use with alcoholic cleansers, tinctures and astringents, abrasives and peeling agents).
No products indexed under this heading.

Aluminum Acetate (Avoid concurrent use with alcoholic cleansers, tinctures and astringents, abrasives and peeling agents).
No products indexed under this heading.

Aluminum Carbonate (Avoid concurrent use with alcoholic cleansers, tinctures and astringents, abrasives and peeling agents).
No products indexed under this heading.

Aluminum Chlorhydroxide (Avoid concurrent use with alcoholic cleansers, tinctures and astringents, abrasives and peeling agents).
No products indexed under this heading.

Aluminum Chloride (Avoid concurrent use with alcoholic cleansers, tinctures and astringents, abrasives and peeling agents).
No products indexed under this heading.

Aluminum Chlorohydrate (Avoid concurrent use with alcoholic cleansers, tinctures and astringents, abrasives and peeling agents).
No products indexed under this heading.

Aluminum Glycinate (Avoid concurrent use with alcoholic cleansers, tinctures and astringents, abrasives and peeling agents).
No products indexed under this heading.

Aluminum Sulfate (Avoid concurrent use with alcoholic cleansers, tinctures and astringents, abrasives and peeling agents).
No products indexed under this heading.

Ammonium Alum (Avoid concurrent use with alcoholic cleansers, tinctures and astringents, abrasives and peeling agents).
No products indexed under this heading.

Benzoyl Peroxide (Avoid concurrent use with alcoholic cleansers, tinctures and astringents, abrasives and peeling agents). Products include:
Benzaclin 2965
Brevoxyl 3316, 3317
Duac 3317

Burow's Solution (Avoid concurrent use with alcoholic cleansers, tinctures and astringents, abrasives and peeling agents).
No products indexed under this heading.

Calamine (Avoid concurrent use with alcoholic cleansers, tinctures and astringents, abrasives and peeling agents).
No products indexed under this heading.

Calcipotriene (Avoid concurrent use with alcoholic cleansers, tinctures and astringents, abrasives and peeling agents).
No products indexed under this heading.

Cleanser (Avoid concurrent use with alcoholic cleansers, tinctures and astringents, abrasives and peeling agents).
No products indexed under this heading.

Clindamycin, Topical (Avoid concurrent use with alcoholic cleansers, tinctures and astringents, abrasives and peeling agents).
No products indexed under this heading.

Clindamycin Phosphate (Avoid concurrent use with alcoholic cleansers, tinctures and astringents, abrasives and peeling agents). Products include:
Benzaclin 2965
Evoclin 3318

Clotrimazole, Topical (Avoid concurrent use with alcoholic cleansers, tinctures and astringents, abrasives and peeling agents).
No products indexed under this heading.

Coal Tar (Avoid concurrent use with alcoholic cleansers, tinctures and astringents, abrasives and peeling agents).
No products indexed under this heading.

Erythromycin, Topical (Avoid concurrent use with alcoholic cleansers, tinctures and astringents, abrasives and peeling agents).
No products indexed under this heading.

Ethanol (Concomitant use with any foods and beverages that might provoke erythema, flushing, and blushing (including spicy food, alcoholic beverages, and thermally hot drinks, including hot coffee and tea) should be avoided).
No products indexed under this heading.

Ethyl Alcohol (Concomitant use with any foods and beverages that might provoke erythema, flushing, and blushing (including spicy food, alcoholic beverages, and thermally hot drinks, including hot coffee and tea) should be avoided).
No products indexed under this heading.

Fluorouracil, Topical (Avoid concurrent use with alcoholic cleansers, tinctures and astringents, abrasives and peeling agents).
No products indexed under this heading.

Hydroquinone (Avoid concurrent use with alcoholic cleansers, tinctures and astringents, abrasives and peeling agents).
No products indexed under this heading.

Isopropyl Alcohol (Avoid concurrent use with alcoholic cleansers, tinctures and astringents, abrasives and peeling agents).
No products indexed under this heading.

Isotretinoin (Avoid concurrent use with alcoholic cleansers, tinctures and astringents, abrasives and peeling agents). Products include:
Accutane 2832

Mequinol (Avoid concurrent use with alcoholic cleansers, tinctures and astringents, abrasives and peeling agents).
No products indexed under this heading.

Podofilox (Avoid concurrent use with alcoholic cleansers, tinctures and astringents, abrasives and peeling agents).
No products indexed under this heading.

Quaternary Aluminum Salts (Avoid concurrent use with alcoholic cleansers, tinctures and astringents, abrasives and peeling agents).
No products indexed under this heading.

Salicylic Acid (Avoid concurrent use with alcoholic cleansers, tinctures and astringents, abrasives and peeling agents).
No products indexed under this heading.

Silver Nitrate (Avoid concurrent use with alcoholic cleansers, tinctures and astringents, abrasives and peeling agents).
No products indexed under this heading.

Sulfur Preparations (Avoid concurrent use with alcoholic cleansers, tinctures and astringents, abrasives and peeling agents).
No products indexed under this heading.

Tannic Acid (Avoid concurrent use with alcoholic cleansers, tinctures and astringents, abrasives and peeling agents).
No products indexed under this heading.

Tazarotene (Avoid concurrent use with alcoholic cleansers, tinctures and astringents, abrasives and peeling agents).
No products indexed under this heading.

Tincture of Benzoin (Avoid concurrent use with alcoholic cleansers, tinctures and astringents, abrasives and peeling agents).
No products indexed under this heading.

Tretinoin (Avoid concurrent use with alcoholic cleansers, tinctures and astringents, abrasives and peeling agents).
No products indexed under this heading.

Witch Hazel (Avoid concurrent use with alcoholic cleansers, tinctures and astringents, abrasives and peeling agents).
No products indexed under this heading.

Zalcitabine (Avoid concurrent use with alcoholic cleansers, tinctures and astringents, abrasives and peeling agents).
No products indexed under this heading.

Zinc Oxide (Avoid concurrent use with alcoholic cleansers, tinctures and astringents, abrasives and peeling agents). Products include:
Bausch & Lomb Ocuvite Adult 50+ .... ⊙238
CitraNatal Rx 2332
Vusion Ointment 3335

Zinc Sulfate (Avoid concurrent use with alcoholic cleansers, tinctures and astringents, abrasives and peeling agents). Products include:
Heplive 607
Zinc-220 606

Food Interactions

Alcohol (Concomitant use with any foods and beverages that might provoke erythema, flushing, and blushing (including spicy food, alcoholic beverages, and thermally hot drinks, including hot coffee and tea) should be avoided).

Beer, reduced-alcohol (Concomitant use with any foods and beverages that might provoke erythema, flushing, and blushing (including spicy food, alcoholic beverages, and thermally hot drinks, including hot coffee and tea) should be avoided).

Beer, unspecified (Concomitant use with any foods and beverages that might provoke erythema, flushing, and blushing (including spicy food, alcoholic bev-

erages, and thermally hot drinks, including hot coffee and tea) should be avoided).

Beverages, hot (Concomitant use with any foods and beverages that might provoke erythema, flushing, and blushing (including spicy food, alcoholic beverages, and thermally hot drinks, including hot coffee and tea) should be avoided).

Beverages, unspecified (Concomitant use with any foods and beverages that might provoke erythema, flushing, and blushing (including spicy food, alcoholic beverages, and thermally hot drinks, including hot coffee and tea) should be avoided).

Drinks, hot, unspecified (Concomitant use with any foods and beverages that might provoke erythema, flushing, and blushing (including spicy food, alcoholic beverages, and thermally hot drinks, including hot coffee and tea) should be avoided).

Food, unspecified (Concomitant use with any foods and beverages that might provoke erythema, flushing, and blushing (including spicy food, alcoholic beverages, and thermally hot drinks, including hot coffee and tea) should be avoided).

Meal, unspecified (Concomitant use with any foods and beverages that might provoke erythema, flushing, and blushing (including spicy food, alcoholic beverages, and thermally hot drinks, including hot coffee and tea) should be avoided).

Tannins (Avoid concurrent use with alcoholic cleansers, tinctures and astringents, abrasives and peeling agents).

Wine, Chianti (Concomitant use with any foods and beverages that might provoke erythema, flushing, and blushing (including spicy food, alcoholic beverages, and thermally hot drinks, including hot coffee and tea) should be avoided).

Wine, Red (Concomitant use with any foods and beverages that might provoke erythema, flushing, and blushing (including spicy food, alcoholic beverages, and thermally hot drinks, including hot coffee and tea) should be avoided).

Wine, unspecified (Concomitant use with any foods and beverages that might provoke erythema, flushing, and blushing (including spicy food, alcoholic beverages, and thermally hot drinks, including hot coffee and tea) should be avoided).

Wine products (Concomitant use with any foods and beverages that might provoke erythema, flushing, and blushing (including spicy food, alcoholic beverages, and thermally hot drinks, including hot coffee and tea) should be avoided).

FLEBOGAMMA 5% DIF
(Immune Globulin Intravenous (Human)) 1794
May interact with vaccines, live. Compounds in these categories include:

BCG Vaccine (Antibodies in immune globulin intravenous (Human) may interfere with the responses to live viral vaccines, such as measles, mumps, and rubella. Physicians should be informed of recent therapy with immune globulin intravenous (Human) so that administration of live viral vaccines, if indicated, can be appropriately delayed 3 or more months from the time of IGIV administration).
No products indexed under this heading.

Influenza Vaccine, Live Attenuated (Antibodies in immune globulin intravenous (Human) may interfere with the responses to live viral vaccines, such as

(⊙ Described in PDR® for Ophthalmic Medicines)

measles, mumps, and rubella. Physicians should be informed of recent therapy with immune globulin intravenous (Human) so that administration of live viral vaccines, if indicated, can be appropriately delayed 3 or more months from the time of IGIV administration).

No products indexed under this heading.

Influenza Virus Vaccine Live, Intranasal (Antibodies in immune globulin intravenous (Human) may interfere with the responses to live viral vaccines, such as measles, mumps, and rubella. Physicians should be informed of recent therapy with immune globulin intravenous (Human) so that administration of live viral vaccines, if indicated, can be appropriately delayed 3 or more months from the time of IGIV administration). Products include:

FluMist 2078

Measles, Mumps, Rubella and Varicella Virus Vaccine Live (Antibodies in immune globulin intravenous (Human) may interfere with the responses to live viral vaccines, such as measles, mumps, and rubella. Physicians should be informed of recent therapy with immune globulin intravenous (Human) so that administration of live viral vaccines, if indicated, can be appropriately delayed 3 or more months from the time of IGIV administration). Products include:

ProQuad 2254

Measles, Mumps & Rubella Virus Vaccine, Live (Antibodies in immune globulin intravenous (Human) may interfere with the responses to live viral vaccines, such as measles, mumps, and rubella. Physicians should be informed of recent therapy with immune globulin intravenous (Human) so that administration of live viral vaccines, if indicated, can be appropriately delayed 3 or more months from the time of IGIV administration). Products include:

M-M-R II 2203
ProQuad 2254

Measles & Rubella Virus Vaccine Live (Antibodies in immune globulin intravenous (Human) may interfere with the responses to live viral vaccines, such as measles, mumps, and rubella. Physicians should be informed of recent therapy with immune globulin intravenous (Human) so that administration of live viral vaccines, if indicated, can be appropriately delayed 3 or more months from the time of IGIV administration).

No products indexed under this heading.

Measles Virus Vaccine Live (Antibodies in immune globulin intravenous (Human) may interfere with the responses to live viral vaccines, such as measles, mumps, and rubella. Physicians should be informed of recent therapy with immune globulin intravenous (Human) so that administration of live viral vaccines, if indicated, can be appropriately delayed 3 or more months from the time of IGIV administration). Products include:

Attenuvax 2086

Mumps Virus Vaccine, Live (Antibodies in immune globulin intravenous (Human) may interfere with the responses to live viral vaccines, such as measles, mumps, and rubella. Physicians should be informed of recent therapy with immune globulin intravenous (Human) so that administration of live viral vaccines, if indicated, can be appropriately delayed 3 or more months from the time of IGIV administration). Products include:

Mumpsvax 2218

Poliovirus Vaccine, Live, Oral, Trivalent, Types 1,2,3 (Sabin) (Antibodies in immune globulin intravenous (Human) may interfere with the responses to live viral vaccines, such as measles, mumps, and rubella. Physicians should be informed of recent therapy with immune globulin intravenous (Human) so that administration of live viral vaccines, if indicated, can be appropriately delayed 3 or more months from the time of IGIV administration).

No products indexed under this heading.

Rotavirus Vaccine, Live, Oral, Tetravalent (Antibodies in immune globulin intravenous (Human) may interfere with the responses to live viral vaccines, such as measles, mumps, and rubella. Physicians should be informed of recent therapy with immune globulin intravenous (Human) so that administration of live viral vaccines, if indicated, can be appropriately delayed 3 or more months from the time of IGIV administration).

No products indexed under this heading.

Rubella & Mumps Virus Vaccine Live (Antibodies in immune globulin intravenous (Human) may interfere with the responses to live viral vaccines, such as measles, mumps, and rubella. Physicians should be informed of recent therapy with immune globulin intravenous (Human) so that administration of live viral vaccines, if indicated, can be appropriately delayed 3 or more months from the time of IGIV administration).

No products indexed under this heading.

Rubella Virus Vaccine Live (Antibodies in immune globulin intravenous (Human) may interfere with the responses to live viral vaccines, such as measles, mumps, and rubella. Physicians should be informed of recent therapy with immune globulin intravenous (Human) so that administration of live viral vaccines, if indicated, can be appropriately delayed 3 or more months from the time of IGIV administration). Products include:

Meruvax II 2210

Smallpox Vaccine (Antibodies in immune globulin intravenous (Human) may interfere with the responses to live viral vaccines, such as measles, mumps, and rubella. Physicians should be informed of recent therapy with immune globulin intravenous (Human) so that administration of live viral vaccines, if indicated, can be appropriately delayed 3 or more months from the time of IGIV administration).

No products indexed under this heading.

Typhoid Vaccine (Antibodies in immune globulin intravenous (Human) may interfere with the responses to live viral vaccines, such as measles, mumps, and rubella. Physicians should be informed of recent therapy with immune globulin intravenous (Human) so that administration of live viral vaccines, if indicated, can be appropriately delayed 3 or more months from the time of IGIV administration).

No products indexed under this heading.

Varicella Virus Vaccine, Live (Antibodies in immune globulin intravenous (Human) may interfere with the responses to live viral vaccines, such as measles, mumps, and rubella. Physicians should be informed of recent therapy with immune globulin intravenous (Human) so that administration of live viral vaccines, if indicated, can be appropriately delayed 3 or more months from the time of IGIV administration). Products include:

Varivax 2285

Yellow Fever Vaccine (Antibodies in immune globulin intravenous (Human) may interfere with the responses to live viral vaccines, such as measles, mumps, and rubella. Physicians should be informed of recent therapy with immune globulin intravenous (Human) so that administration of live viral vaccines, if indicated, can be appropriately delayed 3 or more months from the time of IGIV administration).

No products indexed under this heading.

Zoster Vaccine Live (Antibodies in immune globulin intravenous (Human) may interfere with the responses to live viral vaccines, such as measles, mumps, and rubella. Physicians should be informed of recent therapy with immune globulin intravenous (Human) so that administration of live viral vaccines, if indicated, can be appropriately delayed 3 or more months from the time of IGIV administration). Products include:

Zostavax 2299

FLECTOR PATCH

(Diclofenac Epolamine) 1839
May interact with ACE inhibitors, aspirin-acetylsalicylic acid, lithium preparations, thiazides, and certain other agents. Compounds in these categories include:

Aspirin (When diclofenac epolamine is administered with aspirin, the binding of diclofenac to protein is reduced, although the clearance of free diclofenac is not altered. The clinical significance of this interaction is not known; however, as with other NSAIDs, concomitant administration of diclofenac and aspirin is not generally recommended because of the potential of increased adverse effects). Products include:

Aggrenox 880
Bayer Aspirin 829
Percodan 1124
St. Joseph Aspirin 2045

Aspirin, Enteric Coated (When diclofenac epolamine is administered with aspirin, the binding of diclofenac to protein is reduced, although the clearance of free diclofenac is not altered. The clinical significance of this interaction is not known; however, as with other NSAIDs, concomitant administration of diclofenac and aspirin is not generally recommended because of the potential of increased adverse effects).

No products indexed under this heading.

Aspirin Buffered (When diclofenac epolamine is administered with aspirin, the binding of diclofenac to protein is reduced, although the clearance of free diclofenac is not altered. The clinical significance of this interaction is not known; however, as with other NSAIDs, concomitant administration of diclofenac and aspirin is not generally recommended because of the potential of increased adverse effects).

No products indexed under this heading.

Benazepril Hydrochloride (Reports suggest that NSAIDs may diminish the antihypertensive effect of ACE-inhibitors. This interaction should be given consideration in patients taking NSAIDs concomitantly with ACE-inhibitors).

No products indexed under this heading.

Bendroflumethiazide (Clinical studies, as well as post-marketing observations, have shown that diclofenac epolamine may reduce the natriuretic effect of furosemide and thiazides in some patients. This response has been attributed to inhibition of renal prostaglandin synthesis. During concomitant therapy with NSAIDs, the patient should be ovserved clsoely for signs of renal failure, as well as to assure diuretic efficacy).

No products indexed under this heading.

Captopril (Reports suggest that NSAIDs may diminish the antihypertensive effect of ACE-inhibitors. This interaction should be given consideration in patients taking NSAIDs concomitantly with ACE-inhibitors). Products include:

Captopril 2341

Chlorothiazide (Clinical studies, as well as post-marketing observations, have shown that diclofenac epolamine may reduce the natriuretic effect of furosemide and thiazides in some patients. This response has been attributed to inhibition of renal prostaglandin synthesis. During concomitant therapy with NSAIDs, the patient should be ovserved clsoely for signs of renal failure, as well as to assure diuretic efficacy).

No products indexed under this heading.

Chlorothiazide Sodium (Clinical studies, as well as post-marketing observations, have shown that diclofenac epolamine may reduce the natriuretic effect of furosemide and thiazides in some patients. This response has been attributed to inhibition of renal prostaglandin synthesis. During concomitant therapy with NSAIDs, the patient should be ovserved clsoely for signs of renal failure, as well as to assure diuretic efficacy). Products include:

Diuril Intravenous 2009

Enalapril Maleate (Reports suggest that NSAIDs may diminish the antihypertensive effect of ACE-inhibitors. This interaction should be given consideration in patients taking NSAIDs concomitantly with ACE-inhibitors).

No products indexed under this heading.

Enalaprilat (Reports suggest that NSAIDs may diminish the antihypertensive effect of ACE-inhibitors. This interaction should be given consideration in patients taking NSAIDs concomitantly with ACE-inhibitors).

No products indexed under this heading.

Fosinopril Sodium (Reports suggest that NSAIDs may diminish the antihypertensive effect of ACE-inhibitors. This interaction should be given consideration in patients taking NSAIDs concomitantly with ACE-inhibitors).

No products indexed under this heading.

Furosemide (Clinical studies, as well as post-marketing observations, have shown that diclofenac epolamine may reduce the natriuretic effect of furosemide and thiazides in some patients. This response has been attributed to inhibition of renal prostaglandin synthesis. During concomitant therapy with NSAIDs, the patient should be observed closely for signs of renal failure, as well as to assure diuretic efficacy). Products include:

Furosemide 2354

Hydrochlorothiazide (Clinical studies, as well as post-marketing observations, have shown that diclofenac epolamine may reduce the natriuretic effect of furosemide and thiazides in some patients. This response has been attributed to inhibition of renal prostaglandin synthesis. During concomitant therapy with NSAIDs, the patient should be ovserved clsoely for signs of renal failure, as well as to assure diuretic efficacy). Products include:

Atacand HCT 700
Avalide 2956
Benicar HCT 1017
Diovan HCT 2419
Dyazide 1429
Exforge HCT 2449
Hyzaar 2162
Hyzaar 100-12.5 2162
Micardis HCT 889
Prinzide 2246
Tekturna HCT 2541
Teveten HCT 541

Hydroflumethiazide (Clinical studies, as well as post-marketing observations, have shown that diclofenac epolamine

may reduce the natriuretic effect of furosemide and thiazides in some patients. This response has been attributed to inhibition of renal prostaglandin synthesis. During concomitant therapy with NSAIDs, the patient should be osverved clsoely for signs of renal failure, as well as to assure diuretic efficacy).

No products indexed under this heading.

Lisinopril (Reports suggest that NSAIDs may diminish the antihypertensive effect of ACE-inhibitors. This interaction should be given consideration in patients taking NSAIDs concomitantly with ACE-inhibitors). Products include:

Lithium (NSAIDs have produced an elevation of plasma lithium levels and a reduction in renal lithium clearance. The mean minimum lithium concentration increased 15% and the renal clearance was decreased by approximately 20%. These effects have been attributed to inhibition of renal prostaglandin synthesis by the NSAID. Thus, when NSAIDs and lithium are administered concurrently, subjects should be observed carefully for signs of lithium toxicity).

No products indexed under this heading.

Lithium Carbonate (NSAIDs have produced an elevation of plasma lithium levels and a reduction in renal lithium clearance. The mean minimum lithium concentration increased 15% and the renal clearance was decreased by approximately 20%. These effects have been attributed to inhibition of renal prostaglandin synthesis by the NSAID. Thus, when NSAIDs and lithium are administered concurrently, subjects should be observed carefully for signs of lithium toxicity).

No products indexed under this heading.

Lithium Citrate (NSAIDs have produced an elevation of plasma lithium levels and a reduction in renal lithium clearance. The mean minimum lithium concentration increased 15% and the renal clearance was decreased by approximately 20%. These effects have been attributed to inhibition of renal prostaglandin synthesis by the NSAID. Thus, when NSAIDs and lithium are administered concurrently, subjects should be observed carefully for signs of lithium toxicity).

No products indexed under this heading.

Methotrexate (NSAIDs have been reported to competitively inhibit methotrexate accumulation in rabbit kidney slices. This may indicate that they could enhance the toxicity of methotrexate. Caution should be used when NSAIDs are administered concomitantly with methotrexate).

No products indexed under this heading.

Methotrexate Sodium (NSAIDs have been reported to competitively inhibit methotrexate accumulation in rabbit kidney slices. This may indicate that they could enhance the toxicity of methotrexate. Caution should be used when NSAIDs are administered concomitantly with methotrexate).

No products indexed under this heading.

Methyclothiazide (Clinical studies, as well as post-marketing observations, have shown that diclofenac epolamine may reduce the natriuretic effect of furosemide and thiazides in some patients. This response has been attributed to inhibition of renal prostaglandin synthesis. During concomitant therapy with NSAIDs, the patient should be osverved clsoely for signs of renal failure, as well as to assure diuretic efficacy).

No products indexed under this heading.

Moexipril Hydrochloride (Reports suggest that NSAIDs may diminish the antihypertensive effect of ACE-inhibitors. This interaction should be given consideration in patients taking NSAIDs concomitantly with ACE-inhibitors).

No products indexed under this heading.

Perindopril Erbumine (Reports suggest that NSAIDs may diminish the antihypertensive effect of ACE-inhibitors. This interaction should be given consideration in patients taking NSAIDs concomitantly with ACE-inhibitors).

No products indexed under this heading.

Polythiazide (Clinical studies, as well as post-marketing observations, have shown that diclofenac epolamine may reduce the natriuretic effect of furosemide and thiazides in some patients. This response has been attributed to inhibition of renal prostaglandin synthesis. During concomitant therapy with NSAIDs, the patient should be osverved clsoely for signs of renal failure, as well as to assure diuretic efficacy).

No products indexed under this heading.

Quinapril Hydrochloride (Reports suggest that NSAIDs may diminish the antihypertensive effect of ACE-inhibitors. This interaction should be given consideration in patients taking NSAIDs concomitantly with ACE-inhibitors).

No products indexed under this heading.

Ramipril (Reports suggest that NSAIDs may diminish the antihypertensive effect of ACE-inhibitors. This interaction should be given consideration in patients taking NSAIDs concomitantly with ACE-inhibitors).

No products indexed under this heading.

Spirapril Hydrochloride (Reports suggest that NSAIDs may diminish the antihypertensive effect of ACE-inhibitors. This interaction should be given consideration in patients taking NSAIDs concomitantly with ACE-inhibitors).

No products indexed under this heading.

Trandolapril (Reports suggest that NSAIDs may diminish the antihypertensive effect of ACE-inhibitors. This interaction should be given consideration in patients taking NSAIDs concomitantly with ACE-inhibitors). Products include:

Warfarin Sodium (The effects of warfarin and NSAIDS of GI bleeding are synergistic, such that users of both drugs together have a risk of serious GI bleeding higher than users of either drug alone).

No products indexed under this heading.

FLEET BABYLAX SUPPOSITORIES

None cited in PDR database.

FLEET BISACODYL LAXATIVES

None cited in PDR database.

FLEET ENEMA

May interact with ACE inhibitors, angiotensin-II receptor antagonists, diuretics, lithium preparations, non-steroidal anti-inflammatory agents, oral phosphate supplements. Compounds in these categories include:

Amiloride Hydrochloride (Electrolyte disturbances are a risk associated with this product; concurrent use in patients taking agents known to disturb electrolytes balance requires caution).

No products indexed under this heading.

Benazepril Hydrochloride (Electrolyte disturbances are a risk associated with this product; concurrent use in patients taking agents known to disturb electrolytes balance requires caution).

No products indexed under this heading.

Bendroflumethiazide (Electrolyte disturbances are a risk associated with this product; concurrent use in patients taking agents known to disturb electrolytes balance requires caution).

No products indexed under this heading.

Bumetanide (Electrolyte disturbances are a risk associated with this product; concurrent use in patients taking agents known to disturb electrolytes balance requires caution).

No products indexed under this heading.

Candesartan Cilexetil (Electrolyte disturbances are a risk associated with this product; concurrent use in patients taking agents known to disturb electrolytes balance requires caution). Products include:

Captopril (Electrolyte disturbances are a risk associated with this product; concurrent use in patients taking agents known to disturb electrolytes balance requires caution). Products include:

Celecoxib (Electrolyte disturbances are a risk associated with this product; concurrent use in patients taking agents known to disturb electrolytes balance requires caution). Products include:

Chlorothiazide (Electrolyte disturbances are a risk associated with this product; concurrent use in patients taking agents known to disturb electrolytes balance requires caution).

No products indexed under this heading.

Chlorothiazide Sodium (Electrolyte disturbances are a risk associated with this product; concurrent use in patients taking agents known to disturb electrolytes balance requires caution). Products include:

Chlorthalidone (Electrolyte disturbances are a risk associated with this product; concurrent use in patients taking agents known to disturb electrolytes balance requires caution). Products include:

Diclofenac Epolamine (Electrolyte disturbances are a risk associated with this product; concurrent use in patients taking agents known to disturb electrolytes balance requires caution). Products include:

Diclofenac Potassium (Electrolyte disturbances are a risk associated with this product; concurrent use in patients taking agents known to disturb electrolytes balance requires caution).

No products indexed under this heading.

Diclofenac Sodium (Electrolyte disturbances are a risk associated with this product; concurrent use in patients taking agents known to disturb electrolytes balance requires caution).

No products indexed under this heading.

Enalapril Maleate (Electrolyte disturbances are a risk associated with this product; concurrent use in patients taking agents known to disturb electrolytes balance requires caution).

No products indexed under this heading.

Enalaprilat (Electrolyte disturbances are a risk associated with this product; concurrent use in patients taking agents known to disturb electrolytes balance requires caution).

No products indexed under this heading.

Eprosartan Mesylate (Electrolyte disturbances are a risk associated with

this product; concurrent use in patients taking agents known to disturb electrolytes balance requires caution). Products include:

Ethacrynic Acid (Electrolyte disturbances are a risk associated with this product; concurrent use in patients taking agents known to disturb electrolytes balance requires caution).

No products indexed under this heading.

Etodolac (Electrolyte disturbances are a risk associated with this product; concurrent use in patients taking agents known to disturb electrolytes balance requires caution).

No products indexed under this heading.

Fenoprofen Calcium (Electrolyte disturbances are a risk associated with this product; concurrent use in patients taking agents known to disturb electrolytes balance requires caution).

No products indexed under this heading.

Flurbiprofen (Electrolyte disturbances are a risk associated with this product; concurrent use in patients taking agents known to disturb electrolytes balance requires caution).

No products indexed under this heading.

Fosinopril Sodium (Electrolyte disturbances are a risk associated with this product; concurrent use in patients taking agents known to disturb electrolytes balance requires caution).

No products indexed under this heading.

Furosemide (Electrolyte disturbances are a risk associated with this product; concurrent use in patients taking agents known to disturb electrolytes balance requires caution). Products include:

Hydrochlorothiazide (Electrolyte disturbances are a risk associated with this product; concurrent use in patients taking agents known to disturb electrolytes balance requires caution). Products include:

Hydroflumethiazide (Electrolyte disturbances are a risk associated with this product; concurrent use in patients taking agents known to disturb electrolytes balance requires caution).

No products indexed under this heading.

Ibuprofen (Electrolyte disturbances are a risk associated with this product; concurrent use in patients taking agents known to disturb electrolytes balance requires caution). Products include:

Indapamide (Electrolyte disturbances are a risk associated with this product; concurrent use in patients taking agents known to disturb electrolytes balance requires caution). Products include:

Indomethacin (Electrolyte disturbances are a risk associated with this product; concurrent use in patients taking agents known to disturb electrolytes balance requires caution). Products include:

681 Interactions Index Fleet Pedia-Lax

Indocin 2167

Indomethacin Sodium Trihydrate (Electrolyte disturbances are a risk associated with this product; concurrent use in patients taking agents known to disturb electrolytes balance requires caution). Products include:
Indocin I.V. 2007

Irbesartan (Electrolyte disturbances are a risk associated with this product; concurrent use in patients taking agents known to disturb electrolytes balance requires caution). Products include:
Avalide 2956
Avapro 2962

Ketoprofen (Electrolyte disturbances are a risk associated with this product; concurrent use in patients taking agents known to disturb electrolytes balance requires caution).
No products indexed under this heading.

Ketorolac Tromethamine (Electrolyte disturbances are a risk associated with this product; concurrent use in patients taking agents known to disturb electrolytes balance requires caution). Products include:
Acuvail .... ⊙ 209

Lisinopril (Electrolyte disturbances are a risk associated with this product; concurrent use in patients taking agents known to disturb electrolytes balance requires caution). Products include:
Prinivil 2241
Prinzide 2246

Lithium (Electrolyte disturbances are a risk associated with this product; concurrent use in patients taking agents known to disturb electrolytes balance requires caution).
No products indexed under this heading.

Lithium Carbonate (Electrolyte disturbances are a risk associated with this product; concurrent use in patients taking agents known to disturb electrolytes balance requires caution).
No products indexed under this heading.

Lithium Citrate (Electrolyte disturbances are a risk associated with this product; concurrent use in patients taking agents known to disturb electrolytes balance requires caution).
No products indexed under this heading.

Losartan Potassium (Electrolyte disturbances are a risk associated with this product; concurrent use in patients taking agents known to disturb electrolytes balance requires caution). Products include:
Cozaar 2106
Hyzaar 2162
Hyzaar 100-12.5 2162

Meclofenamate Sodium (Electrolyte disturbances are a risk associated with this product; concurrent use in patients taking agents known to disturb electrolytes balance requires caution).
No products indexed under this heading.

Mefenamic Acid (Electrolyte disturbances are a risk associated with this product; concurrent use in patients taking agents known to disturb electrolytes balance requires caution).
No products indexed under this heading.

Meloxicam (Electrolyte disturbances are a risk associated with this product; concurrent use in patients taking agents known to disturb electrolytes balance requires caution).
No products indexed under this heading.

Methyclothiazide (Electrolyte disturbances are a risk associated with this product; concurrent use in patients taking agents known to disturb electrolytes balance requires caution).
No products indexed under this heading.

Metolazone (Electrolyte disturbances are a risk associated with this product; concurrent use in patients taking agents known to disturb electrolytes balance requires caution).
No products indexed under this heading.

Moexipril Hydrochloride (Electrolyte disturbances are a risk associated with this product; concurrent use in patients taking agents known to disturb electrolytes balance requires caution).
No products indexed under this heading.

Nabumetone (Electrolyte disturbances are a risk associated with this product; concurrent use in patients taking agents known to disturb electrolytes balance requires caution).
No products indexed under this heading.

Naproxen (Electrolyte disturbances are a risk associated with this product; concurrent use in patients taking agents known to disturb electrolytes balance requires caution). Products include:
EC-Naprosyn 2850
Naprosyn 2850
Anaprox/Naprosyn 2850

Naproxen Sodium (Electrolyte disturbances are a risk associated with this product; concurrent use in patients taking agents known to disturb electrolytes balance requires caution). Products include:
Anaprox 2850
Anaprox DS 2850
Treximet 1681

Oxaprozin (Electrolyte disturbances are a risk associated with this product; concurrent use in patients taking agents known to disturb electrolytes balance requires caution).
No products indexed under this heading.

Perindopril Erbumine (Electrolyte disturbances are a risk associated with this product; concurrent use in patients taking agents known to disturb electrolytes balance requires caution).
No products indexed under this heading.

Phenylbutazone (Electrolyte disturbances are a risk associated with this product; concurrent use in patients taking agents known to disturb electrolytes balance requires caution).
No products indexed under this heading.

Piroxicam (Electrolyte disturbances are a risk associated with this product; concurrent use in patients taking agents known to disturb electrolytes balance requires caution).
No products indexed under this heading.

Polythiazide (Electrolyte disturbances are a risk associated with this product; concurrent use in patients taking agents known to disturb electrolytes balance requires caution).
No products indexed under this heading.

Potassium Phosphate (No oral phosphate supplements or other sodium preparations including sodium phosphates-based enemas or tablets should be given concomitantly). Products include:
K-Phos Neutral 873

Quinapril Hydrochloride (Electrolyte disturbances are a risk associated with this product; concurrent use in patients taking agents known to disturb electrolytes balance requires caution).
No products indexed under this heading.

Ramipril (Electrolyte disturbances are a risk associated with this product; concurrent use in patients taking agents known to disturb electrolytes balance requires caution).
No products indexed under this heading.

Rofecoxib (Electrolyte disturbances are a risk associated with this product; concurrent use in patients taking agents known to disturb electrolytes balance requires caution).
No products indexed under this heading.

Spirapril Hydrochloride (Electrolyte disturbances are a risk associated with this product; concurrent use in patients taking agents known to disturb electrolytes balance requires caution).
No products indexed under this heading.

Spironolactone (Electrolyte disturbances are a risk associated with this product; concurrent use in patients taking agents known to disturb electrolytes balance requires caution).
No products indexed under this heading.

Sulindac (Electrolyte disturbances are a risk associated with this product; concurrent use in patients taking agents known to disturb electrolytes balance requires caution). Products include:
Clinoril 2098

Telmisartan (Electrolyte disturbances are a risk associated with this product; concurrent use in patients taking agents known to disturb electrolytes balance requires caution). Products include:
Micardis 887
Micardis HCT 889

Tolmetin Sodium (Electrolyte disturbances are a risk associated with this product; concurrent use in patients taking agents known to disturb electrolytes balance requires caution).
No products indexed under this heading.

Torsemide (Electrolyte disturbances are a risk associated with this product; concurrent use in patients taking agents known to disturb electrolytes balance requires caution).
No products indexed under this heading.

Trandolapril (Electrolyte disturbances are a risk associated with this product; concurrent use in patients taking agents known to disturb electrolytes balance requires caution). Products include:
Mavik 489
Tarka 534

Triamterene (Electrolyte disturbances are a risk associated with this product; concurrent use in patients taking agents known to disturb electrolytes balance requires caution). Products include:
Dyazide 1429
Dyrenium 3495

Valdecoxib (Electrolyte disturbances are a risk associated with this product; concurrent use in patients taking agents known to disturb electrolytes balance requires caution).
No products indexed under this heading.

Valsartan (Electrolyte disturbances are a risk associated with this product; concurrent use in patients taking agents known to disturb electrolytes balance requires caution). Products include:
Diovan 2413
Diovan HCT 2419
Exforge 2443
Exforge HCT 2449
Valturna 3637

FLEET ENEMA EXTRA
(Sodium Phosphate) 1143
See Fleet Enema

FLEET ENEMA FOR CHILDREN
(Sodium Phosphate) 1143
See Fleet Enema

FLEET GLYCERIN LAXATIVES
(Glycerin) 1142
None cited in PDR database.

FLEET GLYCERIN SUPPOSITORIES
(Glycerin) 1142
None cited in PDR database.

FLEET MINERAL OIL ENEMA
(Mineral Oil) 1144
None cited in PDR database.

FLEET PEDIA-LAX CHEWABLE TABLETS
(Magnesium Hydroxide) 1144
None cited in PDR database.

FLEET PEDIA-LAX ENEMA
(Sodium Phosphate) 1143
May interact with ACE inhibitors, angiotensin-II receptor antagonists, diuretics, lithium preparations, non-steroidal anti-inflammatory agents, oral phosphate supplements. Compounds in these categories include:

Amiloride Hydrochloride (Electrolyte disturbances are a risk associated with this product. Concurrent use of medications that may affect electrolyte levels, such as diuretics, may be associated with acute renal failure and requires caution).
No products indexed under this heading.

Benazepril Hydrochloride (Electrolyte disturbances are a risk associated with this product. Concurrent use of medications that may affect electrolyte levels, such as angiotensen converting enzyme inhibitors (ACE-Is), may be associated with acute renal failure and requires caution).
No products indexed under this heading.

Bendroflumethiazide (Electrolyte disturbances are a risk associated with this product. Concurrent use of medications that may affect electrolyte levels, such as diuretics, may be associated with acute renal failure and requires caution).
No products indexed under this heading.

Bumetanide (Electrolyte disturbances are a risk associated with this product. Concurrent use of medications that may affect electrolyte levels, such as diuretics, may be associated with acute renal failure and requires caution).
No products indexed under this heading.

Candesartan Cilexetil (Electrolyte disturbances are a risk associated with this product. Concurrent use of medications that may affect electrolyte levels, such as angiotensen receptor blockers (ARBs), may be associated with acute renal failure and requires caution). Products include:
Atacand 697
Atacand HCT 700

Captopril (Electrolyte disturbances are a risk associated with this product. Concurrent use of medications that may affect electrolyte levels, such as angiotensen converting enzyme inhibitors (ACE-Is), may be associated with acute renal failure and requires caution). Products include:
Captopril 2341

Celecoxib (Electrolyte disturbances are a risk associated with this product. Concurrent use of medications that may affect electrolyte levels, such as NSAIDs, may be associated with acute renal failure). Products include:
Celebrex 3272

Chlorothiazide (Electrolyte disturbances are a risk associated with this product. Concurrent use of medications that may affect electrolyte levels, such as diuretics, may be associated with acute renal failure and requires caution).
No products indexed under this heading.

Chlorothiazide Sodium (Electrolyte disturbances are a risk associated with this product. Concurrent use of medications that may affect electrolyte levels, such as diuretics, may be associated with acute renal failure and requires caution). Products include:
Diuril Intravenous 2009

Chlorthalidone (Electrolyte disturbances are a risk associated with this product. Concurrent use of medications that may affect electrolyte levels, such

as diuretics, may be associated with acute renal failure and requires caution). Products include:

Diclofenac Epolamine (Electrolyte disturbances are a risk associated with this product. Concurrent use of medications that may affect electrolyte levels, such as NSAIDs, may be associated with acute renal failure). Products include:

Diclofenac Potassium (Electrolyte disturbances are a risk associated with this product. Concurrent use of medications that may affect electrolyte levels, such as NSAIDs, may be associated with acute renal failure).
No products indexed under this heading.

Diclofenac Sodium (Electrolyte disturbances are a risk associated with this product. Concurrent use of medications that may affect electrolyte levels, such as NSAIDs, may be associated with acute renal failure).
No products indexed under this heading.

Enalapril Maleate (Electrolyte disturbances are a risk associated with this product. Concurrent use of medications that may affect electrolyte levels, such as angiotensen converting enzyme inhibitors (ACE-Is), may be associated with acute renal failure and requires caution).
No products indexed under this heading.

Enalaprilat (Electrolyte disturbances are a risk associated with this product. Concurrent use of medications that may affect electrolyte levels, such as angiotensen converting enzyme inhibitors (ACE-Is), may be associated with acute renal failure and requires caution).
No products indexed under this heading.

Eprosartan Mesylate (Electrolyte disturbances are a risk associated with this product. Concurrent use of medications that may affect electrolyte levels, such as angiotensen receptor blockers (ARBs), may be associated with acute renal failure and requires caution). Products include:

Ethacrynic Acid (Electrolyte disturbances are a risk associated with this product. Concurrent use of medications that may affect electrolyte levels, such as diuretics, may be associated with acute renal failure and requires caution).
No products indexed under this heading.

Etodolac (Electrolyte disturbances are a risk associated with this product. Concurrent use of medications that may affect electrolyte levels, such as NSAIDs, may be associated with acute renal failure).
No products indexed under this heading.

Fenoprofen Calcium (Electrolyte disturbances are a risk associated with this product. Concurrent use of medications that may affect electrolyte levels, such as NSAIDs, may be associated with acute renal failure).
No products indexed under this heading.

Flurbiprofen (Electrolyte disturbances are a risk associated with this product. Concurrent use of medications that may affect electrolyte levels, such as NSAIDs, may be associated with acute renal failure).
No products indexed under this heading.

Fosinopril Sodium (Electrolyte disturbances are a risk associated with this product. Concurrent use of medications that may affect electrolyte levels, such as angiotensen converting enzyme inhibitors (ACE-Is), may be associated with acute renal failure and requires caution).
No products indexed under this heading.

Furosemide (Electrolyte disturbances are a risk associated with this product. Concurrent use of medications that may affect electrolyte levels, such as diuretics, may be associated with acute renal failure and requires caution). Products include:

Hydrochlorothiazide (Electrolyte disturbances are a risk associated with this product. Concurrent use of medications that may affect electrolyte levels, such as diuretics, may be associated with acute renal failure and requires caution). Products include:

Hydroflumethiazide (Electrolyte disturbances are a risk associated with this product. Concurrent use of medications that may affect electrolyte levels, such as diuretics, may be associated with acute renal failure and requires caution).
No products indexed under this heading.

Ibuprofen (Electrolyte disturbances are a risk associated with this product. Concurrent use of medications that may affect electrolyte levels, such as NSAIDs, may be associated with acute renal failure). Products include:

Indapamide (Electrolyte disturbances are a risk associated with this product. Concurrent use of medications that may affect electrolyte levels, such as diuretics, may be associated with acute renal failure and requires caution). Products include:

Indomethacin (Electrolyte disturbances are a risk associated with this product. Concurrent use of medications that may affect electrolyte levels, such as NSAIDs, may be associated with acute renal failure). Products include:

Indomethacin Sodium Trihydrate (Electrolyte disturbances are a risk associated with this product. Concurrent use of medications that may affect electrolyte levels, such as NSAIDs, may be associated with acute renal failure). Products include:

Irbesartan (Electrolyte disturbances are a risk associated with this product. Concurrent use of medications that may affect electrolyte levels, such as angiotensen receptor blockers (ARBs), may be associated with acute renal failure and requires caution). Products include:

Ketoprofen (Electrolyte disturbances are a risk associated with this product. Concurrent use of medications that may affect electrolyte levels, such as NSAIDs, may be associated with acute renal failure).
No products indexed under this heading.

Ketorolac Tromethamine (Electrolyte disturbances are a risk associated with this product. Concurrent use of medications that may affect electrolyte

levels, such as NSAIDs, may be associated with acute renal failure). Products include:

Lisinopril (Electrolyte disturbances are a risk associated with this product. Concurrent use of medications that may affect electrolyte levels, such as angiotensen converting enzyme inhibitors (ACE-Is), may be associated with acute renal failure and requires caution). Products include:

Lithium (Electrolyte disturbances are a risk associated with this product. Concurrent use of medications that may affect electrolyte levels, such as lithium, may be associated with acute renal failure).
No products indexed under this heading.

Lithium Carbonate (Electrolyte disturbances are a risk associated with this product. Concurrent use of medications that may affect electrolyte levels, such as lithium, may be associated with acute renal failure).
No products indexed under this heading.

Lithium Citrate (Electrolyte disturbances are a risk associated with this product. Concurrent use of medications that may affect electrolyte levels, such as lithium, may be associated with acute renal failure).
No products indexed under this heading.

Losartan Potassium (Electrolyte disturbances are a risk associated with this product. Concurrent use of medications that may affect electrolyte levels, such as angiotensen receptor blockers (ARBs), may be associated with acute renal failure and requires caution). Products include:

Meclofenamate Sodium (Electrolyte disturbances are a risk associated with this product. Concurrent use of medications that may affect electrolyte levels, such as NSAIDs, may be associated with acute renal failure).
No products indexed under this heading.

Mefenamic Acid (Electrolyte disturbances are a risk associated with this product. Concurrent use of medications that may affect electrolyte levels, such as NSAIDs, may be associated with acute renal failure).
No products indexed under this heading.

Meloxicam (Electrolyte disturbances are a risk associated with this product. Concurrent use of medications that may affect electrolyte levels, such as NSAIDs, may be associated with acute renal failure).
No products indexed under this heading.

Methyclothiazide (Electrolyte disturbances are a risk associated with this product. Concurrent use of medications that may affect electrolyte levels, such as diuretics, may be associated with acute renal failure and requires caution).
No products indexed under this heading.

Metolazone (Electrolyte disturbances are a risk associated with this product. Concurrent use of medications that may affect electrolyte levels, such as diuretics, may be associated with acute renal failure and requires caution).
No products indexed under this heading.

Moexipril Hydrochloride (Electrolyte disturbances are a risk associated with this product. Concurrent use of medications that may affect electrolyte levels, such as angiotensen converting enzyme inhibitors (ACE-Is), may be associated with acute renal failure and requires caution).
No products indexed under this heading.

Nabumetone (Electrolyte disturbances are a risk associated with this product. Concurrent use of medications that may affect electrolyte levels, such as NSAIDs, may be associated with acute renal failure).
No products indexed under this heading.

Naproxen (Electrolyte disturbances are a risk associated with this product. Concurrent use of medications that may affect electrolyte levels, such as NSAIDs, may be associated with acute renal failure). Products include:

Naproxen Sodium (Electrolyte disturbances are a risk associated with this product. Concurrent use of medications that may affect electrolyte levels, such as NSAIDs, may be associated with acute renal failure). Products include:

Oxaprozin (Electrolyte disturbances are a risk associated with this product. Concurrent use of medications that may affect electrolyte levels, such as NSAIDs, may be associated with acute renal failure).
No products indexed under this heading.

Perindopril Erbumine (Electrolyte disturbances are a risk associated with this product. Concurrent use of medications that may affect electrolyte levels, such as angiotensen converting enzyme inhibitors (ACE-Is), may be associated with acute renal failure and requires caution).
No products indexed under this heading.

Phenylbutazone (Electrolyte disturbances are a risk associated with this product. Concurrent use of medications that may affect electrolyte levels, such as NSAIDs, may be associated with acute renal failure).
No products indexed under this heading.

Piroxicam (Electrolyte disturbances are a risk associated with this product. Concurrent use of medications that may affect electrolyte levels, such as NSAIDs, may be associated with acute renal failure).
No products indexed under this heading.

Polythiazide (Electrolyte disturbances are a risk associated with this product. Concurrent use of medications that may affect electrolyte levels, such as diuretics, may be associated with acute renal failure and requires caution).
No products indexed under this heading.

Potassium Phosphate (No oral phosphate supplements or other sodium phosphates preparations including sodium phosphates-based enemas or tablets should be given concomitantly). Products include:

Quinapril Hydrochloride (Electrolyte disturbances are a risk associated with this product. Concurrent use of medications that may affect electrolyte levels, such as angiotensen converting enzyme inhibitors (ACE-Is), may be associated with acute renal failure and requires caution).
No products indexed under this heading.

Ramipril (Electrolyte disturbances are a risk associated with this product. Concurrent use of medications that may affect electrolyte levels, such as angiotensen converting enzyme inhibitors (ACE-Is), may be associated with acute renal failure and requires caution).
No products indexed under this heading.

Rofecoxib (Electrolyte disturbances are a risk associated with this product. Concurrent use of medications that may affect electrolyte levels, such as NSAIDs, may be associated with acute renal failure.
No products indexed under this heading.

Spirapril Hydrochloride (Electrolyte disturbances are a risk associated with this product. Concurrent use of medications that may affect electrolyte levels, such as angiotensen converting enzyme inhibitors (ACE-Is), may be associated with acute renal failure and requires caution).
No products indexed under this heading.

Spironolactone (Electrolyte disturbances are a risk associated with this product. Concurrent use of medications that may affect electrolyte levels, such as diuretics, may be associated with acute renal failure and requires caution).
No products indexed under this heading.

Sulindac (Electrolyte disturbances are a risk associated with this product. Concurrent use of medications that may affect electrolyte levels, such as NSAIDs, may be associated with acute renal failure). Products include:
Clinoril 2098

Telmisartan (Electrolyte disturbances are a risk associated with this product. Concurrent use of medications that may affect electrolyte levels, such as angiotensen receptor blockers (ARBs), may be associated with acute renal failure and requires caution). Products include:

Tolmetin Sodium (Electrolyte disturbances are a risk associated with this product. Concurrent use of medications that may affect electrolyte levels, such as NSAIDs, may be associated with acute renal failure.
No products indexed under this heading.

Torsemide (Electrolyte disturbances are a risk associated with this product. Concurrent use of medications that may affect electrolyte levels, such as diuretics, may be associated with acute renal failure and requires caution).
No products indexed under this heading.

Trandolapril (Electrolyte disturbances are a risk associated with this product. Concurrent use of medications that may affect electrolyte levels, such as angiotensen converting enzyme inhibitors (ACE-Is), may be associated with acute renal failure and requires caution). Products include:

Triamterene (Electrolyte disturbances are a risk associated with this product. Concurrent use of medications that may affect electrolyte levels, such as diuretics, may be associated with acute renal failure and requires caution). Products include:

Valdecoxib (Electrolyte disturbances are a risk associated with this product. Concurrent use of medications that may affect electrolyte levels, such as NSAIDs, may be associated with acute renal failure).
No products indexed under this heading.

Valsartan (Electrolyte disturbances are a risk associated with this product. Concurrent use of medications that may affect electrolyte levels, such as angiotensen receptor blockers (ARBs), may be associated with acute renal failure and requires caution). Products include:

FLEET PEDIA-LAX LIQUID STOOL SOFTENER

Mineral Oil (Do not give this product to a child if child is presently taking mineral oil, unless directed by a doctor). Products include:

FLEET PEDIA-LAX SENNA QUICK DISSOLVE STRIPS
None cited in PDR database.

FLEET PEDIA-LAX SUPPOSITORIES
None cited in PDR database.

FLEET PREP KIT 3
May interact with ACE inhibitors, angiotensin-II receptor antagonists, antacids, antibiotics, anticonvulsants, antihypertensives, diuretics, drugs that prolong the QT interval, lithium preparations, non-steroidal anti-inflammatory agents, oral contraceptives, oral hypoglycemic agents, oral phosphate supplements, and certain other agents. Compounds in these categories include:

Acarbose (The absorption of drugs taken concomitantly with sodium phosphate from the gastrointestinal tract may be delayed or even completely prevented. The efficacy of regularly taken oral drugs (eg, oral contraceptives, antiepileptic drugs, diabetic medications, antibiotics) may be reduced or completely absent).
No products indexed under this heading.

Acebutolol Hydrochloride (A rare, but serious form of kidney failure has been associated with the use of oral sodium phosphate products. Many of the reported cases involve patients with pre-existing kidney problems or patients who are taking drugs that can affect kidney function (such as drugs for hypertension or arthritis) or that can affect hydration (fluid) status (such as diuretics-fluid pills)).
No products indexed under this heading.

Alatrofloxacin Mesylate (The absorption of drugs taken concomitantly with sodium phosphate from the gastrointestinal tract may be delayed or even completely prevented. The efficacy of regularly taken oral drugs (eg, oral contraceptives, antiepileptic drugs, diabetic medications, antibiotics) may be reduced or completely absent).
No products indexed under this heading.

Aliskiren (A rare, but serious form of kidney failure has been associated with the use of oral sodium phosphate products. Many of the reported cases involve patients with pre-existing kidney problems or patients who are taking drugs that can affect kidney function (such as drugs for hypertension or arthritis) or that can affect hydration (fluid) status (such as diuretics-fluid pills)). Products include:

Alprazolam (Electrolyte disturbances are a risk associated with Fleet Prep Kit 3; concurrent use in patients taking agents known to prolong QT interval requires caution).
No products indexed under this heading.

Aluminum Carbonate (Concurrent use of antacids and Fleet Prep Kit 3 within one hour should be avoided).
No products indexed under this heading.

Aluminum Hydroxide (Concurrent use of antacids and Fleet Prep Kit 3 within one hour should be avoided).
No products indexed under this heading.

Amikacin Sulfate (The absorption of drugs taken concomitantly with sodium phosphate from the gastrointestinal tract may be delayed or even completely prevented. The efficacy of regularly taken oral drugs (eg, oral contraceptives, antiepileptic drugs, diabetic medications, antibiotics) may be reduced or completely absent).
No products indexed under this heading.

Amiloride Hydrochloride (Some cases occurred in patients without identifiable risk factors, patients at increased risk of acute phosphate nephropathy may include those with increased age, hypovolemia, increased bowel transit time (such as bowel obstruction), active colitis, or baseline kidney disease, and those using medicines that affect renal perfusion or function (such as diuretics, angiotensin converting enzyme [ACE] inhibitors, angiotensin receptor blocker [ARBs], and possibly nonsteroidal anti-inflammatory drugs [NSAIDs]). Patients at increased risk should be managed appropriately. It is important to use the dose and dosing regimen).
No products indexed under this heading.

Amiodarone Hydrochloride (Electrolyte disturbances are a risk associated with Fleet Prep Kit 3; concurrent use in patients taking agents known to prolong QT interval requires caution).
No products indexed under this heading.

Amitriptyline Hydrochloride (Electrolyte disturbances are a risk associated with Fleet Prep Kit 3; concurrent use in patients taking agents known to prolong QT interval requires caution).
No products indexed under this heading.

Amlodipine Besylate (A rare, but serious form of kidney failure has been associated with the use of oral sodium phosphate products. Many of the reported cases involve patients with pre-existing kidney problems or patients who are taking drugs that can affect kidney function (such as drugs for hypertension or arthritis) or that can affect hydration (fluid) status (such as diuretics-fluid pills)). Products include:

Amoxapine (Electrolyte disturbances are a risk associated with Fleet Prep Kit 3; concurrent use in patients taking agents known to prolong QT interval requires caution).
No products indexed under this heading.

Amoxicillin (The absorption of drugs taken concomitantly with sodium phosphate from the gastrointestinal tract may be delayed or even completely prevented. The efficacy of regularly taken oral drugs (eg, oral contraceptives, antiepileptic drugs, diabetic medications, antibiotics) may be reduced or completely absent). Products include:

Amoxicillin Trihydrate (The absorption of drugs taken concomitantly with sodium phosphate from the gastrointestinal tract may be delayed or even completely prevented. The efficacy of regularly taken oral drugs (eg, oral contraceptives, antiepileptic drugs, diabetic medications, antibiotics) may be reduced or completely absent).
No products indexed under this heading.

Ampicillin (The absorption of drugs taken concomitantly with sodium phosphate from the gastrointestinal tract may be delayed or even completely prevented. The efficacy of regularly taken oral drugs (eg, oral contraceptives, antiepileptic drugs, diabetic medications, antibiotics) may be reduced or completely absent).
No products indexed under this heading.

Ampicillin Sodium (The absorption of drugs taken concomitantly with sodium phosphate from the gastrointestinal tract may be delayed or even completely prevented. The efficacy of regularly taken oral drugs (eg, oral contraceptives, antiepileptic drugs, diabetic medications, antibiotics) may be reduced or completely absent).
No products indexed under this heading.

Ampicillin Trihydrate (The absorption of drugs taken concomitantly with sodium phosphate from the gastrointestinal tract may be delayed or even completely prevented. The efficacy of regularly taken oral drugs (eg, oral contraceptives, antiepileptic drugs, diabetic medications, antibiotics) may be reduced or completely absent).
No products indexed under this heading.

Antibiotics, non-penicillin, unspecified (The absorption of drugs taken concomitantly with sodium phosphate from the gastrointestinal tract may be delayed or even completely prevented. The efficacy of regularly taken oral drugs (eg, oral contraceptives, antiepileptic drugs, diabetic medications, antibiotics) may be reduced or completely absent).
No products indexed under this heading.

Astemizole (Electrolyte disturbances are a risk associated with Fleet Prep Kit 3; concurrent use in patients taking agents known to prolong QT interval requires caution).
No products indexed under this heading.

Atenolol (A rare, but serious form of kidney failure has been associated with the use of oral sodium phosphate products. Many of the reported cases involve patients with pre-existing kidney problems or patients who are taking drugs that can affect kidney function (such as drugs for hypertension or arthritis) or that can affect hydration (fluid) status (such as diuretics-fluid pills)).
No products indexed under this heading.

Azithromycin Dihydrate (The absorption of drugs taken concomitantly with sodium phosphate from the gastrointestinal tract may be delayed or even completely prevented. The efficacy of regularly taken oral drugs (eg, oral contraceptives, antiepileptic drugs, diabetic medications, antibiotics) may be reduced or completely absent).
No products indexed under this heading.

Azlocillin Sodium (The absorption of drugs taken concomitantly with sodium phosphate from the gastrointestinal tract may be delayed or even completely prevented. The efficacy of regularly taken oral drugs (eg, oral contraceptives, antiepileptic drugs, diabetic medications, antibiotics) may be reduced or completely absent).
No products indexed under this heading.

IMPORTANT NOTE: Always consult each drug listing in the patient's regimen for possible interactions.

Fleet Prep Kit Interactions Index 684

Aztreonam (The absorption of drugs taken concomitantly with sodium phosphate from the gastrointestinal tract may be delayed or even completely prevented. The efficacy of regularly taken oral drugs (eg, oral contraceptives, antiepileptic drugs, diabetic medications, antibiotics) may be reduced or completely absent).
No products indexed under this heading.

Bacampicillin Hydrochloride (The absorption of drugs taken concomitantly with sodium phosphate from the gastrointestinal tract may be delayed or even completely prevented. The efficacy of regularly taken oral drugs (eg, oral contraceptives, antiepileptic drugs, diabetic medications, antibiotics) may be reduced or completely absent).
No products indexed under this heading.

Benazepril Hydrochloride (Some cases occurred in patients without identifiable risk factors, patients at increased risk of acute phosphate nephropathy may include those using medicines that affect renal perfusion or function (such as angiotensin converting enzyme [ACE] inhibitors). Patients at increased risk should be managed appropriately. It is important to use the dose and dosing regimen).
No products indexed under this heading.

Bendroflumethiazide (Some cases occurred in patients without identifiable risk factors, patients at increased risk of acute phosphate nephropathy may include those with increased age, hypovolemia, increased bowel transit time (such as bowel obstruction), active colitis, or baseline kidney disease, and those using medicines that affect renal perfusion or function (such as diuretics, angiotensin converting enzyme [ACE] inhibitors, angiotensin receptor blocker [ARBs], and possibly nonsteroidal anti-inflammatory drugs [NSAIDs]). Patients at increased risk should be managed appropriately. It is important to use the dose and dosing regimen).
No products indexed under this heading.

Betaxolol Hydrochloride (A rare, but serious form of kidney failure has been associated with the use of oral sodium phosphate products. Many of the reported cases involve patients with pre-existing kidney problems or patients who are taking drugs that can affect kidney function (such as drugs for hypertension or arthritis) or that can affect hydration (fluid) status (such as diuretics-fluid pills)).
No products indexed under this heading.

Bisoprolol Fumarate (A rare, but serious form of kidney failure has been associated with the use of oral sodium phosphate products. Many of the reported cases involve patients with pre-existing kidney problems or patients who are taking drugs that can affect kidney function (such as drugs for hypertension or arthritis) or that can affect hydration (fluid) status (such as diuretics-fluid pills)).
No products indexed under this heading.

Bretylium Tosylate (Electrolyte disturbances are a risk associated with Fleet Prep Kit 3; concurrent use in patients taking agents known to prolong QT interval requires caution).
No products indexed under this heading.

Bumetanide (Some cases occurred in patients without identifiable risk factors, patients at increased risk of acute phosphate nephropathy may include those with increased age, hypovolemia, increased bowel transit time (such as bowel obstruction), active colitis, or baseline kidney disease, and those using medicines that affect renal perfusion or function (such as diuretics, angiotensin converting enzyme [ACE] inhibitors, angiotensin receptor blocker [ARBs], and possibly nonsteroidal anti-inflammatory drugs [NSAIDs]). Patients at increased risk should be managed appropriately. It is important to use the dose and dosing regimen).
No products indexed under this heading.

Buspirone Hydrochloride (Electrolyte disturbances are a risk associated with Fleet Prep Kit 3; concurrent use in patients taking agents known to prolong QT interval requires caution).
No products indexed under this heading.

Calcium Carbonate (Concurrent use of antacids and Fleet Prep Kit 3 within one hour should be avoided). Products include:
Chelated Mineral **3476**
Pepcid Complete **1822**
Extra Strength Rolaids Softchews Vanilla Creme **2045**

Candesartan Cilexetil (Some cases occurred in patients without identifiable risk factors, patients at increased risk of acute phosphate nephropathy may include those using medicines that affect renal perfusion or function (such as angiotensin receptor blocker [ARBs]). Patients at increased risk should be managed appropriately. It is important to use the dose and dosing regimen). Products include:
Atacand **697**
Atacand HCT **700**

Captopril (Some cases occurred in patients without identifiable risk factors, patients at increased risk of acute phosphate nephropathy may include those using medicines that affect renal perfusion or function (such as angiotensin converting enzyme [ACE] inhibitors). Patients at increased risk should be managed appropriately. It is important to use the dose and dosing regimen). Products include:
Captopril **2341**

Carbamazepine (The absorption of drugs taken concomitantly with sodium phosphate from the gastrointestinal tract may be delayed or even completely prevented. The efficacy of regularly taken oral drugs (eg, oral contraceptives, antiepileptic drugs, diabetic medications, antibiotics) may be reduced or completely absent). Products include:
Carbatrol **3280**
Equetro **3477**

Carbenicillin Disodium (The absorption of drugs taken concomitantly with sodium phosphate from the gastrointestinal tract may be delayed or even completely prevented. The efficacy of regularly taken oral drugs (eg, oral contraceptives, antiepileptic drugs, diabetic medications, antibiotics) may be reduced or completely absent).
No products indexed under this heading.

Carbenicillin Indanyl Sodium (The absorption of drugs taken concomitantly with sodium phosphate from the gastrointestinal tract may be delayed or even completely prevented. The efficacy of regularly taken oral drugs (eg, oral contraceptives, antiepileptic drugs, diabetic medications, antibiotics) may be reduced or completely absent).
No products indexed under this heading.

Carteolol Hydrochloride (A rare, but serious form of kidney failure has been associated with the use of oral sodium phosphate products. Many of the reported cases involve patients with pre-existing kidney problems or patients who are taking drugs that can affect kidney function (such as drugs for hypertension or arthritis) or that can affect hydration (fluid) status (such as diuretics-fluid pills)).
No products indexed under this heading.

Carvedilol (A rare, but serious form of kidney failure has been associated with the use of oral sodium phosphate products. Many of the reported cases involve patients with pre-existing kidney problems or patients who are taking drugs that can affect kidney function (such as drugs for hypertension or arthritis) or that can affect hydration (fluid) status (such as diuretics-fluid pills)). Products include:
Coreg **1409**

Carvedilol Phosphate (A rare, but serious form of kidney failure has been associated with the use of oral sodium phosphate products. Many of the reported cases involve patients with pre-existing kidney problems or patients who are taking drugs that can affect kidney function (such as drugs for hypertension or arthritis) or that can affect hydration (fluid) status (such as diuretics-fluid pills)). Products include:
Coreg CR **1416**

Cefaclor (The absorption of drugs taken concomitantly with sodium phosphate from the gastrointestinal tract may be delayed or even completely prevented. The efficacy of regularly taken oral drugs (eg, oral contraceptives, antiepileptic drugs, diabetic medications, antibiotics) may be reduced or completely absent).
No products indexed under this heading.

Cefadroxil (The absorption of drugs taken concomitantly with sodium phosphate from the gastrointestinal tract may be delayed or even completely prevented. The efficacy of regularly taken oral drugs (eg, oral contraceptives, antiepileptic drugs, diabetic medications, antibiotics) may be reduced or completely absent).
No products indexed under this heading.

Cefamandole Nafate (The absorption of drugs taken concomitantly with sodium phosphate from the gastrointestinal tract may be delayed or even completely prevented. The efficacy of regularly taken oral drugs (eg, oral contraceptives, antiepileptic drugs, diabetic medications, antibiotics) may be reduced or completely absent).
No products indexed under this heading.

Cefazolin Sodium (The absorption of drugs taken concomitantly with sodium phosphate from the gastrointestinal tract may be delayed or even completely prevented. The efficacy of regularly taken oral drugs (eg, oral contraceptives, antiepileptic drugs, diabetic medications, antibiotics) may be reduced or completely absent).
No products indexed under this heading.

Cefixime (The absorption of drugs taken concomitantly with sodium phosphate from the gastrointestinal tract may be delayed or even completely prevented. The efficacy of regularly taken oral drugs (eg, oral contraceptives, antiepileptic drugs, diabetic medications, antibiotics) may be reduced or completely absent). Products include:
Suprax for Oral Suspension **2038**
Suprax Tablets **2038**

Cefmetazole Sodium (The absorption of drugs taken concomitantly with sodium phosphate from the gastrointestinal tract may be delayed or even completely prevented. The efficacy of regularly taken oral drugs (eg, oral contraceptives, antiepileptic drugs, diabetic medications, antibiotics) may be reduced or completely absent).
No products indexed under this heading.

Cefonicid Sodium (The absorption of drugs taken concomitantly with sodium phosphate from the gastrointestinal tract may be delayed or even completely prevented. The efficacy of regularly taken oral drugs (eg, oral contraceptives, antiepileptic drugs, diabetic medications, antibiotics) may be reduced or completely absent).
No products indexed under this heading.

Cefoperazone Sodium (The absorption of drugs taken concomitantly with sodium phosphate from the gastrointestinal tract may be delayed or even completely prevented. The efficacy of regularly taken oral drugs (eg, oral contraceptives, antiepileptic drugs, diabetic medications, antibiotics) may be reduced or completely absent).
No products indexed under this heading.

Ceforanide (The absorption of drugs taken concomitantly with sodium phosphate from the gastrointestinal tract may be delayed or even completely prevented. The efficacy of regularly taken oral drugs (eg, oral contraceptives, antiepileptic drugs, diabetic medications, antibiotics) may be reduced or completely absent).
No products indexed under this heading.

Cefotaxime Sodium (The absorption of drugs taken concomitantly with sodium phosphate from the gastrointestinal tract may be delayed or even completely prevented. The efficacy of regularly taken oral drugs (eg, oral contraceptives, antiepileptic drugs, diabetic medications, antibiotics) may be reduced or completely absent).
No products indexed under this heading.

Cefotetan (The absorption of drugs taken concomitantly with sodium phosphate from the gastrointestinal tract may be delayed or even completely prevented. The efficacy of regularly taken oral drugs (eg, oral contraceptives, antiepileptic drugs, diabetic medications, antibiotics) may be reduced or completely absent).
No products indexed under this heading.

Cefoxitin Sodium (The absorption of drugs taken concomitantly with sodium phosphate from the gastrointestinal tract may be delayed or even completely prevented. The efficacy of regularly taken oral drugs (eg, oral contraceptives, antiepileptic drugs, diabetic medications, antibiotics) may be reduced or completely absent).
No products indexed under this heading.

Cefpodoxime Proxetil (The absorption of drugs taken concomitantly with sodium phosphate from the gastrointestinal tract may be delayed or even completely prevented. The efficacy of regularly taken oral drugs (eg, oral contraceptives, antiepileptic drugs, diabetic medications, antibiotics) may be reduced or completely absent).
No products indexed under this heading.

Cefprozil (The absorption of drugs taken concomitantly with sodium phosphate from the gastrointestinal tract may be delayed or even completely prevented. The efficacy of regularly taken oral drugs (eg, oral contraceptives, antiepileptic drugs, diabetic medications, antibiotics) may be reduced or completely absent).
No products indexed under this heading.

Ceftazidime (The absorption of drugs taken concomitantly with sodium phosphate from the gastrointestinal tract may be delayed or even completely prevented. The efficacy of regularly taken oral drugs (eg, oral contraceptives, antiepileptic drugs, diabetic medications, antibiotics) may be reduced or completely absent). Products include:
Fortaz **1481**

Ceftizoxime Sodium (The absorption of drugs taken concomitantly with sodium phosphate from the gastrointestinal tract may be delayed or even completely prevented. The efficacy of regularly taken oral drugs (eg, oral contraceptives, antiepileptic drugs, diabetic medications, antibiotics) may be reduced or completely absent).
No products indexed under this heading.

Ceftriaxone Sodium (The absorption of drugs taken concomitantly with sodi-

(⊙ Described in PDR® for Ophthalmic Medicines)

IMPORTANT NOTE: Always consult each drug listing in the patient's regimen for possible interactions.

Daunorubicin Hydrochloride (The absorption of drugs taken concomitantly with sodium phosphate from the gastrointestinal tract may be delayed or even completely prevented. The efficacy of regularly taken oral drugs (eg, oral contraceptives, antiepileptic drugs, diabetic medications, antibiotics) may be reduced or completely absent).
No products indexed under this heading.

Demeclocycline Hydrochloride (The absorption of drugs taken concomitantly with sodium phosphate from the gastrointestinal tract may be delayed or even completely prevented. The efficacy of regularly taken oral drugs (eg, oral contraceptives, antiepileptic drugs, diabetic medications, antibiotics) may be reduced or completely absent).
No products indexed under this heading.

Deserpidine (A rare, but serious form of kidney failure has been associated with the use of oral sodium phosphate products. Many of the reported cases involve patients with pre-existing kidney problems or patients who are taking drugs that can affect kidney function (such as drugs for hypertension or arthritis) or that can affect hydration (fluid) status (such as diuretics-fluid pills)).
No products indexed under this heading.

Desipramine Hydrochloride (Electrolyte disturbances are a risk associated with Fleet Prep Kit 3; concurrent use in patients taking agents known to prolong QT interval requires caution).
No products indexed under this heading.

Desogestrel (The absorption of drugs taken concomitantly with sodium phosphate from the gastrointestinal tract may be delayed or even completely prevented. The efficacy of regularly taken oral drugs (eg, oral contraceptives, antiepileptic drugs, diabetic medications, antibiotics) may be reduced or completely absent).
No products indexed under this heading.

Diazepam (Electrolyte disturbances are a risk associated with Fleet Prep Kit 3; concurrent use in patients taking agents known to prolong QT interval requires caution). Products include:
Valium Tablets 2880

Diazoxide (A rare, but serious form of kidney failure has been associated with the use of oral sodium phosphate products. Many of the reported cases involve patients with pre-existing kidney problems or patients who are taking drugs that can affect kidney function (such as drugs for hypertension or arthritis) or that can affect hydration (fluid) status (such as diuretics-fluid pills)). Products include:
Proglycem 1179
Proglycem Suspension 1179

Diclofenac Epolamine (Some cases occurred in patients without identifiable risk factors, patients at increased risk of acute phosphate nephropathy may include those with increased age, hypovolemia, increased bowel transit time (such as bowel obstruction), active colitis, or baseline kidney disease, and those using medicines that affect renal perfusion or function (such as diuretics, angiotensin converting enzyme [ACE] inhibitors, angiotensin receptor blocker [ARBs], and possibly nonsteroidal anti-inflammatory drugs [NSAIDs]). Patients at increased risk should be managed appropriately. It is important to use the dose and dosing regimen). Products include:
Flector 1839

Diclofenac Potassium (Some cases occurred in patients without identifiable risk factors, patients at increased risk of acute phosphate nephropathy may include those with increased age, hypovolemia, increased bowel transit time

(such as bowel obstruction), active colitis, or baseline kidney disease, and those using medicines that affect renal perfusion or function (such as diuretics, angiotensin converting enzyme [ACE] inhibitors, angiotensin receptor blocker [ARBs], and possibly nonsteroidal anti-inflammatory drugs [NSAIDs]). Patients at increased risk should be managed appropriately. It is important to use the dose and dosing regimen).
No products indexed under this heading.

Diclofenac Sodium (Some cases occurred in patients without identifiable risk factors, patients at increased risk of acute phosphate nephropathy may include those with increased age, hypovolemia, increased bowel transit time (such as bowel obstruction), active colitis, or baseline kidney disease, and those using medicines that affect renal perfusion or function (such as diuretics, angiotensin converting enzyme [ACE] inhibitors, angiotensin receptor blocker [ARBs], and possibly nonsteroidal anti-inflammatory drugs [NSAIDs]). Patients at increased risk should be managed appropriately. It is important to use the dose and dosing regimen).
No products indexed under this heading.

Dicloxacillin (The absorption of drugs taken concomitantly with sodium phosphate from the gastrointestinal tract may be delayed or even completely prevented. The efficacy of regularly taken oral drugs (eg, oral contraceptives, antiepileptic drugs, diabetic medications, antibiotics) may be reduced or completely absent).
No products indexed under this heading.

Dicloxacillin Sodium (The absorption of drugs taken concomitantly with sodium phosphate from the gastrointestinal tract may be delayed or even completely prevented. The efficacy of regularly taken oral drugs (eg, oral contraceptives, antiepileptic drugs, diabetic medications, antibiotics) may be reduced or completely absent).
No products indexed under this heading.

Diltiazem Hydrochloride (A rare, but serious form of kidney failure has been associated with the use of oral sodium phosphate products. Many of the reported cases involve patients with pre-existing kidney problems or patients who are taking drugs that can affect kidney function (such as drugs for hypertension or arthritis) or that can affect hydration (fluid) status (such as diuretics-fluid pills)). Products include:
Cardizem LA 423

Diltiazem Maleate (A rare, but serious form of kidney failure has been associated with the use of oral sodium phosphate products. Many of the reported cases involve patients with pre-existing kidney problems or patients who are taking drugs that can affect kidney function (such as drugs for hypertension or arthritis) or that can affect hydration (fluid) status (such as diuretics-fluid pills)).
No products indexed under this heading.

Dirithromycin (The absorption of drugs taken concomitantly with sodium phosphate from the gastrointestinal tract may be delayed or even completely prevented. The efficacy of regularly taken oral drugs (eg, oral contraceptives, antiepileptic drugs, diabetic medications, antibiotics) may be reduced or completely absent).
No products indexed under this heading.

Disodium Carbenicillin (The absorption of drugs taken concomitantly with sodium phosphate from the gastrointestinal tract may be delayed or even completely prevented. The efficacy of regularly taken oral drugs (eg, oral contraceptives, antiepileptic drugs, diabetic medications, antibiotics) may be reduced or completely absent).
No products indexed under this heading.

Disopyramide (Electrolyte disturbances are a risk associated with Fleet Prep Kit 3; concurrent use in patients taking agents known to prolong QT interval requires caution).
No products indexed under this heading.

Disopyramide Phosphate (Electrolyte disturbances are a risk associated with Fleet Prep Kit 3; concurrent use in patients taking agents known to prolong QT interval requires caution).
No products indexed under this heading.

Divalproex Sodium (The absorption of drugs taken concomitantly with sodium phosphate from the gastrointestinal tract may be delayed or even completely prevented. The efficacy of regularly taken oral drugs (eg, oral contraceptives, antiepileptic drugs, diabetic medications, antibiotics) may be reduced or completely absent). Products include:
Depakote ER 426

Dofetilide (Electrolyte disturbances are a risk associated with Fleet Prep Kit 3; concurrent use in patients taking agents known to prolong QT interval requires caution).
No products indexed under this heading.

Doxazosin Mesylate (A rare, but serious form of kidney failure has been associated with the use of oral sodium phosphate products. Many of the reported cases involve patients with pre-existing kidney problems or patients who are taking drugs that can affect kidney function (such as drugs for hypertension or arthritis) or that can affect hydration (fluid) status (such as diuretics-fluid pills)).
No products indexed under this heading.

Doxepin Hydrochloride (Electrolyte disturbances are a risk associated with Fleet Prep Kit 3; concurrent use in patients taking agents known to prolong QT interval requires caution).
No products indexed under this heading.

Doxycycline Calcium (The absorption of drugs taken concomitantly with sodium phosphate from the gastrointestinal tract may be delayed or even completely prevented. The efficacy of regularly taken oral drugs (eg, oral contraceptives, antiepileptic drugs, diabetic medications, antibiotics) may be reduced or completely absent).
No products indexed under this heading.

Doxycycline Hyclate (The absorption of drugs taken concomitantly with sodium phosphate from the gastrointestinal tract may be delayed or even completely prevented. The efficacy of regularly taken oral drugs (eg, oral contraceptives, antiepileptic drugs, diabetic medications, antibiotics) may be reduced or completely absent).
No products indexed under this heading.

Doxycycline Monohydrate (The absorption of drugs taken concomitantly with sodium phosphate from the gastrointestinal tract may be delayed or even completely prevented. The efficacy of regularly taken oral drugs (eg, oral contraceptives, antiepileptic drugs, diabetic medications, antibiotics) may be reduced or completely absent).
No products indexed under this heading.

Droperidol (Electrolyte disturbances are a risk associated with Fleet Prep Kit 3; concurrent use in patients taking agents known to prolong QT interval requires caution).
No products indexed under this heading.

Enalapril Maleate (Some cases occurred in patients without identifiable risk factors, patients at increased risk of acute phosphate nephropathy may include those using medicines that affect renal perfusion or function (such as angiotensin converting enzyme [ACE] inhibitors). Patients at increased risk should be managed appropriately. It is important to use the dose and dosing regimen).
No products indexed under this heading.

Enalaprilat (Some cases occurred in patients without identifiable risk factors, patients at increased risk of acute phosphate nephropathy may include those using medicines that affect renal perfusion or function (such as angiotensin converting enzyme [ACE] inhibitors). Patients at increased risk should be managed appropriately. It is important to use the dose and dosing regimen).
No products indexed under this heading.

Enoxacin (The absorption of drugs taken concomitantly with sodium phosphate from the gastrointestinal tract may be delayed or even completely prevented. The efficacy of regularly taken oral drugs (eg, oral contraceptives, antiepileptic drugs, diabetic medications, antibiotics) may be reduced or completely absent).
No products indexed under this heading.

Epirubicin Hydrochloride (The absorption of drugs taken concomitantly with sodium phosphate from the gastrointestinal tract may be delayed or even completely prevented. The efficacy of regularly taken oral drugs (eg, oral contraceptives, antiepileptic drugs, diabetic medications, antibiotics) may be reduced or completely absent).
No products indexed under this heading.

Eprosartan Mesylate (Some cases occurred in patients without identifiable risk factors, patients at increased risk of acute phosphate nephropathy may include those using medicines that affect renal perfusion or function (such as angiotensin receptor blocker [ARBs]). Patients at increased risk should be managed appropriately. It is important to use the dose and dosing regimen). Products include:
Teveten 538
Teveten HCT 541

Erythromycin (The absorption of drugs taken concomitantly with sodium phosphate from the gastrointestinal tract may be delayed or even completely prevented. The efficacy of regularly taken oral drugs (eg, oral contraceptives, antiepileptic drugs, diabetic medications, antibiotics) may be reduced or completely absent).
No products indexed under this heading.

Erythromycin, Topical (The absorption of drugs taken concomitantly with sodium phosphate from the gastrointestinal tract may be delayed or even completely prevented. The efficacy of regularly taken oral drugs (eg, oral contraceptives, antiepileptic drugs, diabetic medications, antibiotics) may be reduced or completely absent).
No products indexed under this heading.

Erythromycin Estolate (The absorption of drugs taken concomitantly with sodium phosphate from the gastrointestinal tract may be delayed or even completely prevented. The efficacy of regularly taken oral drugs (eg, oral contraceptives, antiepileptic drugs, diabetic medications, antibiotics) may be reduced or completely absent).
No products indexed under this heading.

IMPORTANT NOTE: Always consult each drug listing in the patient's regimen for possible interactions.

Griseofulvin (The absorption of drugs taken concomitantly with sodium phosphate from the gastrointestinal tract may be delayed or even completely prevented. The efficacy of regularly taken oral drugs (eg, oral contraceptives, antiepileptic drugs, diabetic medications, antibiotics) may be reduced or completely absent).
   No products indexed under this heading.

Guanabenz Acetate (A rare, but serious form of kidney failure has been associated with the use of oral sodium phosphate products. Many of the reported cases involve patients with pre-existing kidney problems or patients who are taking drugs that can affect kidney function (such as drugs for hypertension or arthritis) or that can affect hydration (fluid) status (such as diuretics-fluid pills)).
   No products indexed under this heading.

Guanethidine (A rare, but serious form of kidney failure has been associated with the use of oral sodium phosphate products. Many of the reported cases involve patients with pre-existing kidney problems or patients who are taking drugs that can affect kidney function (such as drugs for hypertension or arthritis) or that can affect hydration (fluid) status (such as diuretics-fluid pills)).
   No products indexed under this heading.

Guanethidine Monosulfate (A rare, but serious form of kidney failure has been associated with the use of oral sodium phosphate products. Many of the reported cases involve patients with pre-existing kidney problems or patients who are taking drugs that can affect kidney function (such as drugs for hypertension or arthritis) or that can affect hydration (fluid) status (such as diuretics-fluid pills)).
   No products indexed under this heading.

Guanethidine Sulfate (A rare, but serious form of kidney failure has been associated with the use of oral sodium phosphate products. Many of the reported cases involve patients with pre-existing kidney problems or patients who are taking drugs that can affect kidney function (such as drugs for hypertension or arthritis) or that can affect hydration (fluid) status (such as diuretics-fluid pills)).
   No products indexed under this heading.

Haloperidol (Electrolyte disturbances are a risk associated with Fleet Prep Kit 3; concurrent use in patients taking agents known to prolong QT interval requires caution).
   No products indexed under this heading.

Haloperidol Decanoate (Electrolyte disturbances are a risk associated with Fleet Prep Kit 3; concurrent use in patients taking agents known to prolong QT interval requires caution).
   No products indexed under this heading.

Haloperidol Lactate (Electrolyte disturbances are a risk associated with Fleet Prep Kit 3; concurrent use in patients taking agents known to prolong QT interval requires caution).
   No products indexed under this heading.

Hydralazine Hydrochloride (A rare, but serious form of kidney failure has been associated with the use of oral sodium phosphate products. Many of the reported cases involve patients with pre-existing kidney problems or patients who are taking drugs that can affect kidney function (such as drugs for hypertension or arthritis) or that can affect hydration (fluid) status (such as diuretics-fluid pills)).
   No products indexed under this heading.

Hydrochlorothiazide (Some cases occurred in patients without identifiable risk factors, patients at increased risk

of acute phosphate nephropathy may include those with increased age, hypovolemia, increased bowel transit time (such as bowel obstruction), active colitis, or baseline kidney disease, and those using medicines that affect renal perfusion or function (such as diuretics, angiotensin converting enzyme [ACE] inhibitors, angiotensin receptor blocker [ARBs], and possibly nonsteroidal anti-inflammatory drugs [NSAIDs]). Patients at increased risk should be managed appropriately. It is important to use the dose and dosing regimen). Products include:

Atacand HCT	**700**
Avalide	**2956**
Benicar HCT	**1017**
Diovan HCT	**2419**
Dyazide	**1429**
Exforge HCT	**2449**
Hyzaar	**2162**
Hyzaar 100-12.5	**2162**
Micardis HCT	**889**
Prinzide	**2246**
Tekturna HCT	**2541**
Teveten HCT	**541**

Hydroflumethiazide (Some cases occurred in patients without identifiable risk factors, patients at increased risk of acute phosphate nephropathy may include those with increased age, hypovolemia, increased bowel transit time (such as bowel obstruction), active colitis, or baseline kidney disease, and those using medicines that affect renal perfusion or function (such as diuretics, angiotensin converting enzyme [ACE] inhibitors, angiotensin receptor blocker [ARBs], and possibly nonsteroidal anti-inflammatory drugs [NSAIDs]). Patients at increased risk should be managed appropriately. It is important to use the dose and dosing regimen).
   No products indexed under this heading.

Hydroxyzine Hydrochloride (Electrolyte disturbances are a risk associated with Fleet Prep Kit 3; concurrent use in patients taking agents known to prolong QT interval requires caution).
   No products indexed under this heading.

Ibuprofen (Some cases occurred in patients without identifiable risk factors, patients at increased risk of acute phosphate nephropathy may include those with increased age, hypovolemia, increased bowel transit time (such as bowel obstruction), active colitis, or baseline kidney disease, and those using medicines that affect renal perfusion or function (such as diuretics, angiotensin converting enzyme [ACE] inhibitors, angiotensin receptor blocker [ARBs], and possibly nonsteroidal anti-inflammatory drugs [NSAIDs]). Patients at increased risk should be managed appropriately. It is important to use the dose and dosing regimen). Products include:

Motrin IB	**2043**
Children's Motrin	**2044**
Children's Motrin Non-Staining Dye-Free	**2044**
Infants' Motrin	**2044**
Infants' Motrin Dye-Free	**2044**
Junior Strength Motrin	**2044**
Vicoprofen	**564**

Idarubicin Hydrochloride (The absorption of drugs taken concomitantly with sodium phosphate from the gastrointestinal tract may be delayed or even completely prevented. The efficacy of regularly taken oral drugs (eg, oral contraceptives, antiepileptic drugs, diabetic medications, antibiotics) may be reduced or completely absent).
   No products indexed under this heading.

Imipenem (The absorption of drugs taken concomitantly with sodium phosphate from the gastrointestinal tract may be delayed or even completely prevented. The efficacy of regularly taken oral drugs (eg, oral contraceptives,

antiepileptic drugs, diabetic medications, antibiotics) may be reduced or completely absent). Products include:

Primaxin I.M.	**2232**
Primaxin I.V.	**2235**

Imipramine Hydrochloride (Electrolyte disturbances are a risk associated with Fleet Prep Kit 3; concurrent use in patients taking agents known to prolong QT interval requires caution).
   No products indexed under this heading.

Imipramine Pamoate (Electrolyte disturbances are a risk associated with Fleet Prep Kit 3; concurrent use in patients taking agents known to prolong QT interval requires caution).
   No products indexed under this heading.

Indapamide (Some cases occurred in patients without identifiable risk factors, patients at increased risk of acute phosphate nephropathy may include those with increased age, hypovolemia, increased bowel transit time (such as bowel obstruction), active colitis, or baseline kidney disease, and those using medicines that affect renal perfusion or function (such as diuretics, angiotensin converting enzyme [ACE] inhibitors, angiotensin receptor blocker [ARBs], and possibly nonsteroidal anti-inflammatory drugs [NSAIDs]). Patients at increased risk should be managed appropriately. It is important to use the dose and dosing regimen). Products include:

Indapamide	**2356**

Indomethacin (Some cases occurred in patients without identifiable risk factors, patients at increased risk of acute phosphate nephropathy may include those with increased age, hypovolemia, increased bowel transit time (such as bowel obstruction), active colitis, or baseline kidney disease, and those using medicines that affect renal perfusion or function (such as diuretics, angiotensin converting enzyme [ACE] inhibitors, angiotensin receptor blocker [ARBs], and possibly nonsteroidal anti-inflammatory drugs [NSAIDs]). Patients at increased risk should be managed appropriately. It is important to use the dose and dosing regimen). Products include:

Indocin	**2167**

Indomethacin Sodium Trihydrate (Some cases occurred in patients without identifiable risk factors, patients at increased risk of acute phosphate nephropathy may include those with increased age, hypovolemia, increased bowel transit time (such as bowel obstruction), active colitis, or baseline kidney disease, and those using medicines that affect renal perfusion or function (such as diuretics, angiotensin converting enzyme [ACE] inhibitors, angiotensin receptor blocker [ARBs], and possibly nonsteroidal anti-inflammatory drugs [NSAIDs]). Patients at increased risk should be managed appropriately. It is important to use the dose and dosing regimen). Products include:

Indocin I.V.	**2007**

Irbesartan (Some cases occurred in patients without identifiable risk factors, patients at increased risk of acute phosphate nephropathy may include those using medicines that affect renal perfusion or function (such as angiotensin receptor blocker [ARBs]). Patients at increased risk should be managed appropriately. It is important to use the dose and dosing regimen). Products include:

Avalide	**2956**
Avapro	**2962**

Isocarboxazid (Electrolyte disturbances are a risk associated with Fleet Prep Kit 3; concurrent use in patients

taking agents known to prolong QT interval requires caution). Products include:

Marplan	**3481**

Isradipine (A rare, but serious form of kidney failure has been associated with the use of oral sodium phosphate products. Many of the reported cases involve patients with pre-existing kidney problems or patients who are taking drugs that can affect kidney function (such as drugs for hypertension or arthritis) or that can affect hydration (fluid) status (such as diuretics-fluid pills)). Products include:

DynaCirc CR	**1432**

Kanamycin Sulfate (The absorption of drugs taken concomitantly with sodium phosphate from the gastrointestinal tract may be delayed or even completely prevented. The efficacy of regularly taken oral drugs (eg, oral contraceptives, antiepileptic drugs, diabetic medications, antibiotics) may be reduced or completely absent).
   No products indexed under this heading.

Ketoprofen (Some cases occurred in patients without identifiable risk factors, patients at increased risk of acute phosphate nephropathy may include those with increased age, hypovolemia, increased bowel transit time (such as bowel obstruction), active colitis, or baseline kidney disease, and those using medicines that affect renal perfusion or function (such as diuretics, angiotensin converting enzyme [ACE] inhibitors, angiotensin receptor blocker [ARBs], and possibly nonsteroidal anti-inflammatory drugs [NSAIDs]). Patients at increased risk should be managed appropriately. It is important to use the dose and dosing regimen).
   No products indexed under this heading.

Ketorolac Tromethamine (Some cases occurred in patients without identifiable risk factors, patients at increased risk of acute phosphate nephropathy may include those with increased age, hypovolemia, increased bowel transit time (such as bowel obstruction), active colitis, or baseline kidney disease, and those using medicines that affect renal perfusion or function (such as diuretics, angiotensin converting enzyme [ACE] inhibitors, angiotensin receptor blocker [ARBs], and possibly nonsteroidal anti-inflammatory drugs [NSAIDs]). Patients at increased risk should be managed appropriately. It is important to use the dose and dosing regimen). Products include:

Acuvail	⊙ **209**

Labetalol Hydrochloride (A rare, but serious form of kidney failure has been associated with the use of oral sodium phosphate products. Many of the reported cases involve patients with pre-existing kidney problems or patients who are taking drugs that can affect kidney function (such as drugs for hypertension or arthritis) or that can affect hydration (fluid) status (such as diuretics-fluid pills)).
   No products indexed under this heading.

Lamotrigine (The absorption of drugs taken concomitantly with sodium phosphate from the gastrointestinal tract may be delayed or even completely prevented. The efficacy of regularly taken oral drugs (eg, oral contraceptives, antiepileptic drugs, diabetic medications, antibiotics) may be reduced or completely absent). Products include:

Lamictal	**1522**
Lamictal ODT	**1522**
Lamictal XR	**1536**

Levetiracetam (The absorption of drugs taken concomitantly with sodium phosphate from the gastrointestinal tract may be delayed or even completely prevented. The efficacy of regularly

689 **Interactions Index** **Fleet Prep Kit**

taken oral drugs (eg, oral contraceptives, antiepileptic drugs, diabetic medications, antibiotics) may be reduced or completely absent). Products include:

Keppra XR **3434**

Levofloxacin (The absorption of drugs taken concomitantly with sodium phosphate from the gastrointestinal tract may be delayed or even completely prevented. The efficacy of regularly taken oral drugs (eg, oral contraceptives, antiepileptic drugs, diabetic medications, antibiotics) may be reduced or completely absent). Products include:

Iquix **3492**
Levaquin **2629**
Levaquin in 5% Dextrose **2629**
Quixin **3493**

Levonorgestrel (The absorption of drugs taken concomitantly with sodium phosphate from the gastrointestinal tract may be delayed or even completely prevented. The efficacy of regularly taken oral drugs (eg, oral contraceptives, antiepileptic drugs, diabetic medications, antibiotics) may be reduced or completely absent). Products include:

Climara Pro **847**
LoSeasonique **3407**
Lybrel **3514**
Mirena **854**
Plan B **3416**
Seasonique **3418**

Lidocaine (Electrolyte disturbances are a risk associated with Fleet Prep Kit 3; concurrent use in patients taking agents known to prolong QT interval requires caution). Products include:

Lidoderm **1107**

Lidocaine Hydrochloride (Electrolyte disturbances are a risk associated with Fleet Prep Kit 3; concurrent use in patients taking agents known to prolong QT interval requires caution).
No products indexed under this heading.

Lisinopril (Some cases occurred in patients without identifiable risk factors, patients at increased risk of acute phosphate nephropathy may include those using medicines that affect renal perfusion or function (such as angiotensin converting enzyme [ACE] inhibitors). Patients at increased risk should be managed appropriately. It is important to use the dose and dosing regimen). Products include:

Prinivil **2241**
Prinzide **2246**

Lithium (Dehydration and hypovolemia from purgation may be exacerbated by inadequate oral liquid intake, nausea, vomiting, loss of appetite, or use of lithium or other medications that may affect electrolyte levels and may be associated with acute renal failure. There have been reports of acute renal failure associated with bowel purgatives).
No products indexed under this heading.

Lithium Carbonate (Dehydration and hypovolemia from purgation may be exacerbated by inadequate oral liquid intake, nausea, vomiting, loss of appetite, or use of lithium or other medications that may affect electrolyte levels and may be associated with acute renal failure. There have been reports of acute renal failure associated with bowel purgatives).
No products indexed under this heading.

Lithium Citrate (Dehydration and hypovolemia from purgation may be exacerbated by inadequate oral liquid intake, nausea, vomiting, loss of appetite, or use of lithium or other medications that may affect electrolyte levels and may be associated with acute renal failure. There have been reports of acute renal failure associated with bowel purgatives).
No products indexed under this heading.

Lomefloxacin Hydrochloride (The absorption of drugs taken concomitantly with sodium phosphate from the gastrointestinal tract may be delayed or even completely prevented. The efficacy of regularly taken oral drugs (eg, oral contraceptives, antiepileptic drugs, diabetic medications, antibiotics) may be reduced or completely absent).
No products indexed under this heading.

Loracarbef (The absorption of drugs taken concomitantly with sodium phosphate from the gastrointestinal tract may be delayed or even completely prevented. The efficacy of regularly taken oral drugs (eg, oral contraceptives, antiepileptic drugs, diabetic medications, antibiotics) may be reduced or completely absent).
No products indexed under this heading.

Lorazepam (Electrolyte disturbances are a risk associated with Fleet Prep Kit 3; concurrent use in patients taking agents known to prolong QT interval requires caution).
No products indexed under this heading.

Losartan Potassium (Some cases occurred in patients without identifiable risk factors, patients at increased risk of acute phosphate nephropathy may include those using medicines that affect renal perfusion or function (such as angiotensin receptor blocker [ARBs]). Patients at increased risk should be managed appropriately. It is important to use the dose and dosing regimen). Products include:

Cozaar **2106**
Hyzaar **2162**
Hyzaar 100-12.5 ..... **2162**

Loxapine Hydrochloride (Electrolyte disturbances are a risk associated with Fleet Prep Kit 3; concurrent use in patients taking agents known to prolong QT interval requires caution).
No products indexed under this heading.

Loxapine Succinate (Electrolyte disturbances are a risk associated with Fleet Prep Kit 3; concurrent use in patients taking agents known to prolong QT interval requires caution).
No products indexed under this heading.

Magaldrate (Concurrent use of antacids and Fleet Prep Kit 3 within one hour should be avoided).
No products indexed under this heading.

Magnesium Carbonate (Concurrent use of antacids and Fleet Prep Kit 3 within one hour should be avoided).
No products indexed under this heading.

Magnesium Hydroxide (Concurrent use of antacids and Fleet Prep Kit 3 within one hour should be avoided). Products include:

Fleet Pedia-Lax Chewable Tablets **1144**
Pepcid Complete **1822**

Magnesium Oxide (Concurrent use of antacids and Fleet Prep Kit 3 within one hour should be avoided). Products include:

Beelith **873**

Magnesium Trisilicate (Concurrent use of antacids and Fleet Prep Kit 3 within one hour should be avoided).
No products indexed under this heading.

Maprotiline Hydrochloride (Electrolyte disturbances are a risk associated with Fleet Prep Kit 3; concurrent use in patients taking agents known to prolong QT interval requires caution).
No products indexed under this heading.

Mecamylamine Hydrochloride (A rare, but serious form of kidney failure has been associated with the use of oral sodium phosphate products. Many of the reported cases involve patients with pre-existing kidney problems or patients who are taking drugs that can affect kidney function (such as drugs for hypertension or arthritis) or that can affect hydration (fluid) status (such as diuretics-fluid pills)).
No products indexed under this heading.

Meclofenamate Sodium (Some cases occurred in patients without identifiable risk factors, patients at increased risk of acute phosphate nephropathy may include those with increased age, hypovolemia, increased bowel transit time (such as bowel obstruction), active colitis, or baseline kidney disease, and those using medicines that affect renal perfusion or function (such as diuretics, angiotensin converting enzyme [ACE] inhibitors, angiotensin receptor blocker [ARBs], and possibly nonsteroidal anti-inflammatory drugs [NSAIDs]). Patients at increased risk should be managed appropriately. It is important to use the dose and dosing regimen).
No products indexed under this heading.

Mefenamic Acid (Some cases occurred in patients without identifiable risk factors, patients at increased risk of acute phosphate nephropathy may include those with increased age, hypovolemia, increased bowel transit time (such as bowel obstruction), active colitis, or baseline kidney disease, and those using medicines that affect renal perfusion or function (such as diuretics, angiotensin converting enzyme [ACE] inhibitors, angiotensin receptor blocker [ARBs], and possibly nonsteroidal anti-inflammatory drugs [NSAIDs]). Patients at increased risk should be managed appropriately. It is important to use the dose and dosing regimen).
No products indexed under this heading.

Meloxicam (Some cases occurred in patients without identifiable risk factors, patients at increased risk of acute phosphate nephropathy may include those with increased age, hypovolemia, increased bowel transit time (such as bowel obstruction), active colitis, or baseline kidney disease, and those using medicines that affect renal perfusion or function (such as diuretics, angiotensin converting enzyme [ACE] inhibitors, angiotensin receptor blocker [ARBs], and possibly nonsteroidal anti-inflammatory drugs [NSAIDs]). Patients at increased risk should be managed appropriately. It is important to use the dose and dosing regimen).
No products indexed under this heading.

Mephenytoin (The absorption of drugs taken concomitantly with sodium phosphate from the gastrointestinal tract may be delayed or even completely prevented. The efficacy of regularly taken oral drugs (eg, oral contraceptives, antiepileptic drugs, diabetic medications, antibiotics) may be reduced or completely absent).
No products indexed under this heading.

Meprobamate (Electrolyte disturbances are a risk associated with Fleet Prep Kit 3; concurrent use in patients taking agents known to prolong QT interval requires caution).
No products indexed under this heading.

Mesoridazine Besylate (Electrolyte disturbances are a risk associated with Fleet Prep Kit 3; concurrent use in patients taking agents known to prolong QT interval requires caution).
No products indexed under this heading.

Mestranol (The absorption of drugs taken concomitantly with sodium phosphate from the gastrointestinal tract may be delayed or even completely prevented. The efficacy of regularly taken oral drugs (eg, oral contraceptives, antiepileptic drugs, diabetic medications, antibiotics) may be reduced or completely absent).
No products indexed under this heading.

Metformin Hydrochloride (The absorption of drugs taken concomitantly with sodium phosphate from the gastrointestinal tract may be delayed or even completely prevented. The efficacy of regularly taken oral drugs (eg, oral contraceptives, antiepileptic drugs, diabetic medications, antibiotics) may be reduced or completely absent). Products include:

ActoPlus **3338**
Avandamet **1345**
Janumet **2188**

Methacycline Hydrochloride (The absorption of drugs taken concomitantly with sodium phosphate from the gastrointestinal tract may be delayed or even completely prevented. The efficacy of regularly taken oral drugs (eg, oral contraceptives, antiepileptic drugs, diabetic medications, antibiotics) may be reduced or completely absent).
No products indexed under this heading.

Methicillin Sodium (The absorption of drugs taken concomitantly with sodium phosphate from the gastrointestinal tract may be delayed or even completely prevented. The efficacy of regularly taken oral drugs (eg, oral contraceptives, antiepileptic drugs, diabetic medications, antibiotics) may be reduced or completely absent).
No products indexed under this heading.

Methsuximide (The absorption of drugs taken concomitantly with sodium phosphate from the gastrointestinal tract may be delayed or even completely prevented. The efficacy of regularly taken oral drugs (eg, oral contraceptives, antiepileptic drugs, diabetic medications, antibiotics) may be reduced or completely absent).
No products indexed under this heading.

Methyclothiazide (Some cases occurred in patients without identifiable risk factors, patients at increased risk of acute phosphate nephropathy may include those with increased age, hypovolemia, increased bowel transit time (such as bowel obstruction), active colitis, or baseline kidney disease, and those using medicines that affect renal perfusion or function (such as diuretics, angiotensin converting enzyme [ACE] inhibitors, angiotensin receptor blocker [ARBs], and possibly nonsteroidal anti-inflammatory drugs [NSAIDs]). Patients at increased risk should be managed appropriately. It is important to use the dose and dosing regimen).
No products indexed under this heading.

Methyldopa (A rare, but serious form of kidney failure has been associated with the use of oral sodium phosphate products. Many of the reported cases involve patients with pre-existing kidney problems or patients who are taking drugs that can affect kidney function (such as drugs for hypertension or arthritis) or that can affect hydration (fluid) status (such as diuretics-fluid pills)).
No products indexed under this heading.

Methyldopate Hydrochloride (A rare, but serious form of kidney failure has been associated with the use of oral sodium phosphate products. Many of the reported cases involve patients with pre-existing kidney problems or patients who are taking drugs that can affect kidney function (such as drugs for hypertension or arthritis) or that can affect hydration (fluid) status (such as diuretics-fluid pills)).
No products indexed under this heading.

Metolazone (Some cases occurred in patients without identifiable risk factors, patients at increased risk of acute phosphate nephropathy may include those with increased age, hypovolemia, increased bowel transit time (such as bowel obstruction), active colitis, or

IMPORTANT NOTE: Always consult each drug listing in the patient's regimen for possible interactions.

Fleet Prep Kit Interactions Index 690

baseline kidney disease, and those using medicines that affect renal perfusion or function (such as diuretics, angiotensin converting enzyme [ACE] inhibitors, angiotensin receptor blocker [ARBs], and possibly nonsteroidal anti-inflammatory drugs [NSAIDs]). Patients at increased risk should be managed appropriately. It is important to use the dose and dosing regimen).
No products indexed under this heading.

Metoprolol Succinate (A rare, but serious form of kidney failure has been associated with the use of oral sodium phosphate products. Many of the reported cases involve patients with pre-existing kidney problems or patients who are taking drugs that can affect kidney function (such as drugs for hypertension or arthritis) or that can affect hydration (fluid) status (such as diuretics-fluid pills)). Products include:
Toprol XL 732

Metoprolol Tartrate (A rare, but serious form of kidney failure has been associated with the use of oral sodium phosphate products. Many of the reported cases involve patients with pre-existing kidney problems or patients who are taking drugs that can affect kidney function (such as drugs for hypertension or arthritis) or that can affect hydration (fluid) status (such as diuretics-fluid pills)).
No products indexed under this heading.

Metyrosine (A rare, but serious form of kidney failure has been associated with the use of oral sodium phosphate products. Many of the reported cases involve patients with pre-existing kidney problems or patients who are taking drugs that can affect kidney function (such as drugs for hypertension or arthritis) or that can affect hydration (fluid) status (such as diuretics-fluid pills)).
No products indexed under this heading.

Mexiletine Hydrochloride (Electrolyte disturbances are a risk associated with Fleet Prep Kit 3; concurrent use in patients taking agents known to prolong QT interval requires caution).
No products indexed under this heading.

Mezlocillin Sodium (The absorption of drugs taken concomitantly with sodium phosphate from the gastrointestinal tract may be delayed or even completely prevented. The efficacy of regularly taken oral drugs (eg, oral contraceptives, antiepileptic drugs, diabetic medications, antibiotics) may be reduced or completely absent).
No products indexed under this heading.

Mibefradil Dihydrochloride (A rare, but serious form of kidney failure has been associated with the use of oral sodium phosphate products. Many of the reported cases involve patients with pre-existing kidney problems or patients who are taking drugs that can affect kidney function (such as drugs for hypertension or arthritis) or that can affect hydration (fluid) status (such as diuretics-fluid pills)).
No products indexed under this heading.

Midazolam Hydrochloride (Electrolyte disturbances are a risk associated with Fleet Prep Kit 3; concurrent use in patients taking agents known to prolong QT interval requires caution).
No products indexed under this heading.

Miglitol (The absorption of drugs taken concomitantly with sodium phosphate from the gastrointestinal tract may be delayed or even completely prevented. The efficacy of regularly taken oral drugs (eg, oral contraceptives, antiepileptic drugs, diabetic medications, antibiotics) may be reduced or completely absent).
No products indexed under this heading.

Minocycline Hydrochloride (The absorption of drugs taken concomitantly with sodium phosphate from the gastrointestinal tract may be delayed or even completely prevented. The efficacy of regularly taken oral drugs (eg, oral contraceptives, antiepileptic drugs, diabetic medications, antibiotics) may be reduced or completely absent).
Products include:
Solodyn 2073

Minoxidil (A rare, but serious form of kidney failure has been associated with the use of oral sodium phosphate products. Many of the reported cases involve patients with pre-existing kidney problems or patients who are taking drugs that can affect kidney function (such as drugs for hypertension or arthritis) or that can affect hydration (fluid) status (such as diuretics-fluid pills)).
No products indexed under this heading.

Moexipril Hydrochloride (Some cases occurred in patients without identifiable risk factors, patients at increased risk of acute phosphate nephropathy may include those using medicines that affect renal perfusion or function (such as angiotensin converting enzyme [ACE] inhibitors). Patients at increased risk should be managed appropriately. It is important to use the dose and dosing regimen).
No products indexed under this heading.

Molindone Hydrochloride (Electrolyte disturbances are a risk associated with Fleet Prep Kit 3; concurrent use in patients taking agents known to prolong QT interval requires caution). Products include:
Moban 1108

Moxifloxacin Hydrochloride (The absorption of drugs taken concomitantly with sodium phosphate from the gastrointestinal tract may be delayed or even completely prevented. The efficacy of regularly taken oral drugs (eg, oral contraceptives, antiepileptic drugs, diabetic medications, antibiotics) may be reduced or completely absent).
Products include:
Avelox 3064
Vigamox 589

Nabumetone (Some cases occurred in patients without identifiable risk factors, patients at increased risk of acute phosphate nephropathy may include those with increased age, hypovolemia, increased bowel transit time (such as bowel obstruction), active colitis, or baseline kidney disease, and those using medicines that affect renal perfusion or function (such as diuretics, angiotensin converting enzyme [ACE] inhibitors, angiotensin receptor blocker [ARBs], and possibly nonsteroidal anti-inflammatory drugs [NSAIDs]). Patients at increased risk should be managed appropriately. It is important to use the dose and dosing regimen).
No products indexed under this heading.

Nadolol (A rare, but serious form of kidney failure has been associated with the use of oral sodium phosphate products. Many of the reported cases involve patients with pre-existing kidney problems or patients who are taking drugs that can affect kidney function (such as drugs for hypertension or arthritis) or that can affect hydration (fluid) status (such as diuretics-fluid pills)). Products include:
Nadolol 2359

Nafcillin Sodium (The absorption of drugs taken concomitantly with sodium phosphate from the gastrointestinal tract may be delayed or even completely prevented. The efficacy of regularly taken oral drugs (eg, oral contraceptives, antiepileptic drugs, diabetic medications, antibiotics) may be reduced or completely absent).
No products indexed under this heading.

Naproxen (Some cases occurred in patients without identifiable risk factors, patients at increased risk of acute phosphate nephropathy may include those with increased age, hypovolemia, increased bowel transit time (such as bowel obstruction), active colitis, or baseline kidney disease, and those using medicines that affect renal perfusion or function (such as diuretics, angiotensin converting enzyme [ACE] inhibitors, angiotensin receptor blocker [ARBs], and possibly nonsteroidal anti-inflammatory drugs [NSAIDs]). Patients at increased risk should be managed appropriately. It is important to use the dose and dosing regimen). Products include:
EC-Naprosyn 2850
Naprosyn 2850
Anaprox/Naprosyn 2850

Naproxen Sodium (Some cases occurred in patients without identifiable risk factors, patients at increased risk of acute phosphate nephropathy may include those with increased age, hypovolemia, increased bowel transit time (such as bowel obstruction), active colitis, or baseline kidney disease, and those using medicines that affect renal perfusion or function (such as diuretics, angiotensin converting enzyme [ACE] inhibitors, angiotensin receptor blocker [ARBs], and possibly nonsteroidal anti-inflammatory drugs [NSAIDs]). Patients at increased risk should be managed appropriately. It is important to use the dose and dosing regimen). Products include:
Anaprox 2850
Anaprox DS 2850
Treximet 1681

Nateglinide (The absorption of drugs taken concomitantly with sodium phosphate from the gastrointestinal tract may be delayed or even completely prevented. The efficacy of regularly taken oral drugs (eg, oral contraceptives, antiepileptic drugs, diabetic medications, antibiotics) may be reduced or completely absent).
No products indexed under this heading.

Nebivolol (A rare, but serious form of kidney failure has been associated with the use of oral sodium phosphate products. Many of the reported cases involve patients with pre-existing kidney problems or patients who are taking drugs that can affect kidney function (such as drugs for hypertension or arthritis) or that can affect hydration (fluid) status (such as diuretics-fluid pills)). Products include:
Bystolic 1147

Nicardipine Hydrochloride (A rare, but serious form of kidney failure has been associated with the use of oral sodium phosphate products. Many of the reported cases involve patients with pre-existing kidney problems or patients who are taking drugs that can affect kidney function (such as drugs for hypertension or arthritis) or that can affect hydration (fluid) status (such as diuretics-fluid pills)).
No products indexed under this heading.

Nifedipine (A rare, but serious form of kidney failure has been associated with the use of oral sodium phosphate products. Many of the reported cases involve patients with pre-existing kidney problems or patients who are taking drugs that can affect kidney function (such as drugs for hypertension or arthritis) or that can affect hydration (fluid) status (such as diuretics-fluid pills)).
No products indexed under this heading.

Nisoldipine (A rare, but serious form of kidney failure has been associated with the use of oral sodium phosphate products. Many of the reported cases involve patients with pre-existing kidney problems or patients who are taking drugs that can affect kidney function (such as drugs for hypertension or arthritis) or that can affect hydration (fluid) status (such as diuretics-fluid pills)).
No products indexed under this heading.

Nitroglycerin (A rare, but serious form of kidney failure has been associated with the use of oral sodium phosphate products. Many of the reported cases involve patients with pre-existing kidney problems or patients who are taking drugs that can affect kidney function (such as drugs for hypertension or arthritis) or that can affect hydration (fluid) status (such as diuretics-fluid pills)). Products include:
Nitro-Dur 3170
Nitrolingual 3266

Norethindrone (The absorption of drugs taken concomitantly with sodium phosphate from the gastrointestinal tract may be delayed or even completely prevented. The efficacy of regularly taken oral drugs (eg, oral contraceptives, antiepileptic drugs, diabetic medications, antibiotics) may be reduced or completely absent). Products include:
Ortho Micronor 2660

Norethynodrel (The absorption of drugs taken concomitantly with sodium phosphate from the gastrointestinal tract may be delayed or even completely prevented. The efficacy of regularly taken oral drugs (eg, oral contraceptives, antiepileptic drugs, diabetic medications, antibiotics) may be reduced or completely absent).
No products indexed under this heading.

Norfloxacin (The absorption of drugs taken concomitantly with sodium phosphate from the gastrointestinal tract may be delayed or even completely prevented. The efficacy of regularly taken oral drugs (eg, oral contraceptives, antiepileptic drugs, diabetic medications, antibiotics) may be reduced or completely absent). Products include:
Noroxin 2220

Norgestimate (The absorption of drugs taken concomitantly with sodium phosphate from the gastrointestinal tract may be delayed or even completely prevented. The efficacy of regularly taken oral drugs (eg, oral contraceptives, antiepileptic drugs, diabetic medications, antibiotics) may be reduced or completely absent). Products include:
Ortho-Cyclen/Ortho Tri-Cyclen 2663
Ortho Tri-Cyclen Lo Tablets 2673

Norgestrel (The absorption of drugs taken concomitantly with sodium phosphate from the gastrointestinal tract may be delayed or even completely prevented. The efficacy of regularly taken oral drugs (eg, oral contraceptives, antiepileptic drugs, diabetic medications, antibiotics) may be reduced or completely absent).
No products indexed under this heading.

(⊙ Described in PDR® for Ophthalmic Medicines)

691 Interactions Index Fleet Prep Kit

Nortriptyline Hydrochloride (Electrolyte disturbances are a risk associated with Fleet Prep Kit 3; concurrent use in patients taking agents known to prolong QT interval requires caution).
No products indexed under this heading.

Ofloxacin (The absorption of drugs taken concomitantly with sodium phosphate from the gastrointestinal tract may be delayed or even completely prevented. The efficacy of regularly taken oral drugs (eg, oral contraceptives, antiepileptic drugs, diabetic medications, antibiotics) may be reduced or completely absent).
No products indexed under this heading.

Olanzapine (Electrolyte disturbances are a risk associated with Fleet Prep Kit 3; concurrent use in patients taking agents known to prolong QT interval requires caution). Products include:
Symbyax 1965
Zyprexa 1984
Zyprexa IntraMuscular 1984
Zyprexa ZYDIS 1984

Oral Medications, unspecified (During the intake of sodium phosphate, the absorption of drugs from the gastrointestinal tract may be delayed or even completely prevented).
No products indexed under this heading.

Oxacillin (The absorption of drugs taken concomitantly with sodium phosphate from the gastrointestinal tract may be delayed or even completely prevented. The efficacy of regularly taken oral drugs (eg, oral contraceptives, antiepileptic drugs, diabetic medications, antibiotics) may be reduced or completely absent).
No products indexed under this heading.

Oxacillin Sodium (The absorption of drugs taken concomitantly with sodium phosphate from the gastrointestinal tract may be delayed or even completely prevented. The efficacy of regularly taken oral drugs (eg, oral contraceptives, antiepileptic drugs, diabetic medications, antibiotics) may be reduced or completely absent).
No products indexed under this heading.

Oxaprozin (Some cases occurred in patients without identifiable risk factors, patients at increased risk of acute phosphate nephropathy may include those with increased age, hypovolemia, increased bowel transit time (such as bowel obstruction), active colitis, or baseline kidney disease, and those using medicines that affect renal perfusion or function (such as diuretics, angiotensin converting enzyme [ACE] inhibitors, angiotensin receptor blocker [ARBs], and possibly nonsteroidal anti-inflammatory drugs [NSAIDs]). Patients at increased risk should be managed appropriately. It is important to use the dose and dosing regimen).
No products indexed under this heading.

Oxazepam (Electrolyte disturbances are a risk associated with Fleet Prep Kit 3; concurrent use in patients taking agents known to prolong QT interval requires caution).
No products indexed under this heading.

Oxcarbazepine (The absorption of drugs taken concomitantly with sodium phosphate from the gastrointestinal tract may be delayed or even completely prevented. The efficacy of regularly taken oral drugs (eg, oral contraceptives, antiepileptic drugs, diabetic medications, antibiotics) may be reduced or completely absent).
No products indexed under this heading.

Oxytetracycline Hydrochloride (The absorption of drugs taken concomitantly with sodium phosphate from the gastrointestinal tract may be delayed or even completely prevented. The efficacy of regularly taken oral drugs (eg, oral contraceptives, antiepileptic drugs, diabetic medications, antibiotics) may be reduced or completely absent).
No products indexed under this heading.

Paramethadione (The absorption of drugs taken concomitantly with sodium phosphate from the gastrointestinal tract may be delayed or even completely prevented. The efficacy of regularly taken oral drugs (eg, oral contraceptives, antiepileptic drugs, diabetic medications, antibiotics) may be reduced or completely absent).
No products indexed under this heading.

Penbutolol Sulfate (A rare, but serious form of kidney failure has been associated with the use of oral sodium phosphate products. Many of the reported cases involve patients with pre-existing kidney problems or patients who are taking drugs that can affect kidney function (such as drugs for hypertension or arthritis) or that can affect hydration (fluid) status (such as diuretics-fluid pills)).
No products indexed under this heading.

Penicillin, Potassium Phenoxymethyl (The absorption of drugs taken concomitantly with sodium phosphate from the gastrointestinal tract may be delayed or even completely prevented. The efficacy of regularly taken oral drugs (eg, oral contraceptives, antiepileptic drugs, diabetic medications, antibiotics) may be reduced or completely absent).
No products indexed under this heading.

Penicillin G Benzathine (The absorption of drugs taken concomitantly with sodium phosphate from the gastrointestinal tract may be delayed or even completely prevented. The efficacy of regularly taken oral drugs (eg, oral contraceptives, antiepileptic drugs, diabetic medications, antibiotics) may be reduced or completely absent).
Products include:
Bicillin C-R Injectable Suspension 1826
Bicillin L-A 1828

Penicillin G Dibenzylethyenediamine (The absorption of drugs taken concomitantly with sodium phosphate from the gastrointestinal tract may be delayed or even completely prevented. The efficacy of regularly taken oral drugs (eg, oral contraceptives, antiepileptic drugs, diabetic medications, antibiotics) may be reduced or completely absent).
No products indexed under this heading.

Penicillin G Potassium (The absorption of drugs taken concomitantly with sodium phosphate from the gastrointestinal tract may be delayed or even completely prevented. The efficacy of regularly taken oral drugs (eg, oral contraceptives, antiepileptic drugs, diabetic medications, antibiotics) may be reduced or completely absent).
No products indexed under this heading.

Penicillin G Procaine (The absorption of drugs taken concomitantly with sodium phosphate from the gastrointestinal tract may be delayed or even completely prevented. The efficacy of regularly taken oral drugs (eg, oral contraceptives, antiepileptic drugs, diabetic medications, antibiotics) may be reduced or completely absent).
Products include:
Bicillin C-R Injectable Suspension 1826
Bicillin L-A 1828

Penicillin G Sodium (The absorption of drugs taken concomitantly with sodium phosphate from the gastrointestinal tract may be delayed or even completely prevented. The efficacy of regularly taken oral drugs (eg, oral contraceptives, antiepileptic drugs, diabetic medications, antibiotics) may be reduced or completely absent).
No products indexed under this heading.

Penicillin V (The absorption of drugs taken concomitantly with sodium phosphate from the gastrointestinal tract may be delayed or even completely prevented. The efficacy of regularly taken oral drugs (eg, oral contraceptives, antiepileptic drugs, diabetic medications, antibiotics) may be reduced or completely absent).
No products indexed under this heading.

Penicillin V Potassium (The absorption of drugs taken concomitantly with sodium phosphate from the gastrointestinal tract may be delayed or even completely prevented. The efficacy of regularly taken oral drugs (eg, oral contraceptives, antiepileptic drugs, diabetic medications, antibiotics) may be reduced or completely absent).
No products indexed under this heading.

Penicillins (The absorption of drugs taken concomitantly with sodium phosphate from the gastrointestinal tract may be delayed or even completely prevented. The efficacy of regularly taken oral drugs (eg, oral contraceptives, antiepileptic drugs, diabetic medications, antibiotics) may be reduced or completely absent).
No products indexed under this heading.

Perindopril Erbumine (Some cases occurred in patients without identifiable risk factors, patients at increased risk of acute phosphate nephropathy may include those using medicines that affect renal perfusion or function (such as angiotensin converting enzyme [ACE] inhibitors). Patients at increased risk should be managed appropriately. It is important to use the dose and dosing regimen).
No products indexed under this heading.

Perphenazine (Electrolyte disturbances are a risk associated with Fleet Prep Kit 3; concurrent use in patients taking agents known to prolong QT interval requires caution).
No products indexed under this heading.

Phenacemide (The absorption of drugs taken concomitantly with sodium phosphate from the gastrointestinal tract may be delayed or even completely prevented. The efficacy of regularly taken oral drugs (eg, oral contraceptives, antiepileptic drugs, diabetic medications, antibiotics) may be reduced or completely absent).
No products indexed under this heading.

Phenelzine Sulfate (Electrolyte disturbances are a risk associated with Fleet Prep Kit 3; concurrent use in patients taking agents known to prolong QT interval requires caution).
No products indexed under this heading.

Phenobarbital (The absorption of drugs taken concomitantly with sodium phosphate from the gastrointestinal tract may be delayed or even completely prevented. The efficacy of regularly taken oral drugs (eg, oral contraceptives, antiepileptic drugs, diabetic medications, antibiotics) may be reduced or completely absent). Products include:
Donnatal 2711

Phenobarbital Sodium (The absorption of drugs taken concomitantly with sodium phosphate from the gastrointestinal tract may be delayed or even completely prevented. The efficacy of regularly taken oral drugs (eg, oral contraceptives, antiepileptic drugs, diabetic medications, antibiotics) may be reduced or completely absent).
No products indexed under this heading.

Phenoxybenzamine Hydrochloride (A rare, but serious form of kidney failure has been associated with the use of oral sodium phosphate products. Many of the reported cases involve patients with pre-existing kidney problems or patients who are taking drugs that can affect kidney function (such as drugs for hypertension or arthritis) or that can affect hydration (fluid) status (such as diuretics-fluid pills)). Products include:
Dibenzyline 3495

Phensuximide (The absorption of drugs taken concomitantly with sodium phosphate from the gastrointestinal tract may be delayed or even completely prevented. The efficacy of regularly taken oral drugs (eg, oral contraceptives, antiepileptic drugs, diabetic medications, antibiotics) may be reduced or completely absent).
No products indexed under this heading.

Phentolamine Mesylate (A rare, but serious form of kidney failure has been associated with the use of oral sodium phosphate products. Many of the reported cases involve patients with pre-existing kidney problems or patients who are taking drugs that can affect kidney function (such as drugs for hypertension or arthritis) or that can affect hydration (fluid) status (such as diuretics-fluid pills)).
No products indexed under this heading.

Phenylbutazone (Some cases occurred in patients without identifiable risk factors, patients at increased risk of acute phosphate nephropathy may include those with increased age, hypovolemia, increased bowel transit time (such as bowel obstruction), active colitis, or baseline kidney disease, and those using medicines that affect renal perfusion or function (such as diuretics, angiotensin converting enzyme [ACE] inhibitors, angiotensin receptor blocker [ARBs], and possibly nonsteroidal anti-inflammatory drugs [NSAIDs]). Patients at increased risk should be managed appropriately. It is important to use the dose and dosing regimen).
No products indexed under this heading.

Phenytoin (The absorption of drugs taken concomitantly with sodium phosphate from the gastrointestinal tract may be delayed or even completely prevented. The efficacy of regularly taken oral drugs (eg, oral contraceptives, antiepileptic drugs, diabetic medications, antibiotics) may be reduced or completely absent).
No products indexed under this heading.

Phenytoin Sodium (The absorption of drugs taken concomitantly with sodium phosphate from the gastrointestinal tract may be delayed or even completely prevented. The efficacy of regularly taken oral drugs (eg, oral contraceptives, antiepileptic drugs, diabetic medications, antibiotics) may be reduced or completely absent). Products include:
Phenytek Capsules 2380

IMPORTANT NOTE: Always consult each drug listing in the patient's regimen for possible interactions.

Fleet Prep Kit — Interactions Index — 692

Pindolol (A rare, but serious form of kidney failure has been associated with the use of oral sodium phosphate products. Many of the reported cases involve patients with pre-existing kidney problems or patients who are taking drugs that can affect kidney function (such as drugs for hypertension or arthritis) or that can affect hydration (fluid) status (such as diuretics-fluid pills)).
No products indexed under this heading.

Pioglitazone Hydrochloride (The absorption of drugs taken concomitantly with sodium phosphate from the gastrointestinal tract may be delayed or even completely prevented. The efficacy of regularly taken oral drugs (eg, oral contraceptives, antiepileptic drugs, diabetic medications, antibiotics) may be reduced or completely absent).
Products include:
ActoPlus **3338**
Actos **3345**
Duetact **3354**

Piperacillin Sodium (The absorption of drugs taken concomitantly with sodium phosphate from the gastrointestinal tract may be delayed or even completely prevented. The efficacy of regularly taken oral drugs (eg, oral contraceptives, antiepileptic drugs, diabetic medications, antibiotics) may be reduced or completely absent). Products include:
Zosyn **3607**

Piroxicam (Some cases occurred in patients without identifiable risk factors, patients at increased risk of acute phosphate nephropathy may include those with increased age, hypovolemia, increased bowel transit time (such as bowel obstruction), active colitis, or baseline kidney disease, and those using medicines that affect renal perfusion or function (such as diuretics, angiotensin converting enzyme [ACE] inhibitors, angiotensin receptor blocker [ARBs], and possibly nonsteroidal anti-inflammatory drugs [NSAIDs]). Patients at increased risk should be managed appropriately. It is important to use the dose and dosing regimen).
No products indexed under this heading.

Polythiazide (Some cases occurred in patients without identifiable risk factors, patients at increased risk of acute phosphate nephropathy may include those with increased age, hypovolemia, increased bowel transit time (such as bowel obstruction), active colitis, or baseline kidney disease, and those using medicines that affect renal perfusion or function (such as diuretics, angiotensin converting enzyme [ACE] inhibitors, angiotensin receptor blocker [ARBs], and possibly nonsteroidal anti-inflammatory drugs [NSAIDs]). Patients at increased risk should be managed appropriately. It is important to use the dose and dosing regimen).
No products indexed under this heading.

Potassium Phosphate (No other sodium phosphates preparations including sodium phosphates-based enemas or tablets should be given concomitantly). Products include:
K-Phos Neutral **873**

Prazepam (Electrolyte disturbances are a risk associated with Fleet Prep Kit 3; concurrent use in patients taking agents known to prolong QT interval requires caution).
No products indexed under this heading.

Prazosin Hydrochloride (A rare, but serious form of kidney failure has been associated with the use of oral sodium phosphate products. Many of the reported cases involve patients with pre-existing kidney problems or patients who are taking drugs that can affect kidney function (such as drugs for hypertension or arthritis) or that can affect hydration (fluid) status (such as diuretics-fluid pills)).
No products indexed under this heading.

Primidone (The absorption of drugs taken concomitantly with sodium phosphate from the gastrointestinal tract may be delayed or even completely prevented. The efficacy of regularly taken oral drugs (eg, oral contraceptives, antiepileptic drugs, diabetic medications, antibiotics) may be reduced or completely absent).
No products indexed under this heading.

Procainamide Hydrochloride (Electrolyte disturbances are a risk associated with Fleet Prep Kit 3; concurrent use in patients taking agents known to prolong QT interval requires caution).
No products indexed under this heading.

Prochlorperazine (Electrolyte disturbances are a risk associated with Fleet Prep Kit 3; concurrent use in patients taking agents known to prolong QT interval requires caution).
No products indexed under this heading.

Promethazine Hydrochloride (Electrolyte disturbances are a risk associated with Fleet Prep Kit 3; concurrent use in patients taking agents known to prolong QT interval requires caution).
No products indexed under this heading.

Propafenone Hydrochloride (Electrolyte disturbances are a risk associated with Fleet Prep Kit 3; concurrent use in patients taking agents known to prolong QT interval requires caution).
Products include:
Rythmol **1648**
Rythmol SR **1652**

Propranolol Hydrochloride (A rare, but serious form of kidney failure has been associated with the use of oral sodium phosphate products. Many of the reported cases involve patients with pre-existing kidney problems or patients who are taking drugs that can affect kidney function (such as drugs for hypertension or arthritis) or that can affect hydration (fluid) status (such as diuretics-fluid pills)). Products include:
InnoPran XL **1517**

Protriptyline Hydrochloride (Electrolyte disturbances are a risk associated with Fleet Prep Kit 3; concurrent use in patients taking agents known to prolong QT interval requires caution).
No products indexed under this heading.

Quetiapine Fumarate (Electrolyte disturbances are a risk associated with Fleet Prep Kit 3; concurrent use in patients taking agents known to prolong QT interval requires caution). Products include:
Seroquel **750**
Seroquel XR **759**

Quinapril Hydrochloride (Some cases occurred in patients without identifiable risk factors, patients at increased risk of acute phosphate nephropathy may include those using medicines that affect renal perfusion or function (such as angiotensin converting enzyme [ACE] inhibitors). Patients at increased risk should be managed appropriately. It is important to use the dose and dosing regimen).
No products indexed under this heading.

Quinidine (Electrolyte disturbances are a risk associated with Fleet Prep Kit 3; concurrent use in patients taking agents known to prolong QT interval requires caution).
No products indexed under this heading.

Quinidine Gluconate (Electrolyte disturbances are a risk associated with Fleet Prep Kit 3; concurrent use in patients taking agents known to prolong QT interval requires caution).
No products indexed under this heading.

Quinidine Hydrochloride (Electrolyte disturbances are a risk associated with Fleet Prep Kit 3; concurrent use in patients taking agents known to prolong QT interval requires caution).
No products indexed under this heading.

Quinidine Polygalacturonate (Electrolyte disturbances are a risk associated with Fleet Prep Kit 3; concurrent use in patients taking agents known to prolong QT interval requires caution).
No products indexed under this heading.

Quinidine Sulfate (Electrolyte disturbances are a risk associated with Fleet Prep Kit 3; concurrent use in patients taking agents known to prolong QT interval requires caution).
No products indexed under this heading.

Ramipril (Some cases occurred in patients without identifiable risk factors, patients at increased risk of acute phosphate nephropathy may include those using medicines that affect renal perfusion or function (such as angiotensin converting enzyme [ACE] inhibitors). Patients at increased risk should be managed appropriately. It is important to use the dose and dosing regimen).
No products indexed under this heading.

Rauwolfia Serpentina (A rare, but serious form of kidney failure has been associated with the use of oral sodium phosphate products. Many of the reported cases involve patients with pre-existing kidney problems or patients who are taking drugs that can affect kidney function (such as drugs for hypertension or arthritis) or that can affect hydration (fluid) status (such as diuretics-fluid pills)).
No products indexed under this heading.

Repaglinide (The absorption of drugs taken concomitantly with sodium phosphate from the gastrointestinal tract may be delayed or even completely prevented. The efficacy of regularly taken oral drugs (eg, oral contraceptives, antiepileptic drugs, diabetic medications, antibiotics) may be reduced or completely absent).
No products indexed under this heading.

Rescinnamine (A rare, but serious form of kidney failure has been associated with the use of oral sodium phosphate products. Many of the reported cases involve patients with pre-existing kidney problems or patients who are taking drugs that can affect kidney function (such as drugs for hypertension or arthritis) or that can affect hydration (fluid) status (such as diuretics-fluid pills)).
No products indexed under this heading.

Reserpine (A rare, but serious form of kidney failure has been associated with the use of oral sodium phosphate products. Many of the reported cases involve patients with pre-existing kidney problems or patients who are taking drugs that can affect kidney function (such as drugs for hypertension or arthritis) or that can affect hydration (fluid) status (such as diuretics-fluid pills)).
No products indexed under this heading.

Risperidone (Electrolyte disturbances are a risk associated with Fleet Prep Kit 3; concurrent use in patients taking agents known to prolong QT interval requires caution). Products include:
Risperdal Consta **2682**

Rofecoxib (Some cases occurred in patients without identifiable risk factors, patients at increased risk of acute phosphate nephropathy may include those with increased age, hypovolemia, increased bowel transit time (such as bowel obstruction), active colitis, or baseline kidney disease, and those using medicines that affect renal perfusion or function (such as diuretics, angiotensin converting enzyme [ACE] inhibitors, angiotensin receptor blocker [ARBs], and possibly nonsteroidal anti-inflammatory drugs [NSAIDs]). Patients at increased risk should be managed appropriately. It is important to use the dose and dosing regimen).
No products indexed under this heading.

Rosiglitazone Maleate (The absorption of drugs taken concomitantly with sodium phosphate from the gastrointestinal tract may be delayed or even completely prevented. The efficacy of regularly taken oral drugs (eg, oral contraceptives, antiepileptic drugs, diabetic medications, antibiotics) may be reduced or completely absent).
Products include:
Avandamet **1345**
Avandaryl **1356**
Avandia **1366**

Rufinamide (The absorption of drugs taken concomitantly with sodium phosphate from the gastrointestinal tract may be delayed or even completely prevented. The efficacy of regularly taken oral drugs (eg, oral contraceptives, antiepileptic drugs, diabetic medications, antibiotics) may be reduced or completely absent). Products include:
Banzel **1050**

Sitagliptin Phosphate (The absorption of drugs taken concomitantly with sodium phosphate from the gastrointestinal tract may be delayed or even completely prevented. The efficacy of regularly taken oral drugs (eg, oral contraceptives, antiepileptic drugs, diabetic medications, antibiotics) may be reduced or completely absent).
Products include:
Janumet **2188**
Januvia **2196**

Sodium Bicarbonate (Concurrent use of antacids and Fleet Prep Kit 3 within one hour should be avoided).
No products indexed under this heading.

Sodium Cloxacillin Monohydrate (The absorption of drugs taken concomitantly with sodium phosphate from the gastrointestinal tract may be delayed or even completely prevented. The efficacy of regularly taken oral drugs (eg, oral contraceptives, antiepileptic drugs, diabetic medications, antibiotics) may be reduced or completely absent).
No products indexed under this heading.

Sodium Nitroprusside (A rare, but serious form of kidney failure has been associated with the use of oral sodium phosphate products. Many of the reported cases involve patients with pre-existing kidney problems or patients who are taking drugs that can affect kidney function (such as drugs for hypertension or arthritis) or that can affect hydration (fluid) status (such as diuretics-fluid pills)).
No products indexed under this heading.

Sotalol Hydrochloride (A rare, but serious form of kidney failure has been associated with the use of oral sodium phosphate products. Many of the reported cases involve patients with pre-existing kidney problems or patients who are taking drugs that can affect kidney function (such as drugs for hypertension or arthritis) or that can affect hydration (fluid) status (such as diuretics-fluid pills)).
No products indexed under this heading.

Sparfloxacin (The absorption of drugs taken concomitantly with sodium phosphate from the gastrointestinal tract may be delayed or even completely prevented. The efficacy of regularly taken oral drugs (eg, oral contraceptives, antiepileptic drugs, diabetic medications, antibiotics) may be reduced or completely absent).
No products indexed under this heading.

Spirapril Hydrochloride (Some cases occurred in patients without iden-

(⊙ Described in PDR® for Ophthalmic Medicines)

693 Interactions Index Fleet Prep Kit

tifiable risk factors, patients at increased risk of acute phosphate nephropathy may include those using medicines that affect renal perfusion or function (such as angiotensin converting enzyme [ACE] inhibitors). Patients at increased risk should be managed appropriately. It is important to use the dose and dosing regimen).
No products indexed under this heading.

Spironolactone (Some cases occurred in patients without identifiable risk factors, patients at increased risk of acute phosphate nephropathy may include those with increased age, hypovolemia, increased bowel transit time (such as bowel obstruction), active colitis, or baseline kidney disease, and those using medicines that affect renal perfusion or function (such as diuretics, angiotensin converting enzyme [ACE] inhibitors, angiotensin receptor blocker [ARBs], and possibly nonsteroidal anti-inflammatory drugs [NSAIDs]). Patients at increased risk should be managed appropriately. It is important to use the dose and dosing regimen).
No products indexed under this heading.

Streptomycin Sulfate (The absorption of drugs taken concomitantly with sodium phosphate from the gastrointestinal tract may be delayed or even completely prevented. The efficacy of regularly taken oral drugs (eg, oral contraceptives, antiepileptic drugs, diabetic medications, antibiotics) may be reduced or completely absent).
No products indexed under this heading.

Sulfamethizole (The absorption of drugs taken concomitantly with sodium phosphate from the gastrointestinal tract may be delayed or even completely prevented. The efficacy of regularly taken oral drugs (eg, oral contraceptives, antiepileptic drugs, diabetic medications, antibiotics) may be reduced or completely absent).
No products indexed under this heading.

Sulfamethoxazole (The absorption of drugs taken concomitantly with sodium phosphate from the gastrointestinal tract may be delayed or even completely prevented. The efficacy of regularly taken oral drugs (eg, oral contraceptives, antiepileptic drugs, diabetic medications, antibiotics) may be reduced or completely absent).
No products indexed under this heading.

Sulfisoxazole Acetyl (The absorption of drugs taken concomitantly with sodium phosphate from the gastrointestinal tract may be delayed or even completely prevented. The efficacy of regularly taken oral drugs (eg, oral contraceptives, antiepileptic drugs, diabetic medications, antibiotics) may be reduced or completely absent).
No products indexed under this heading.

Sulfisoxazole Diolamine (The absorption of drugs taken concomitantly with sodium phosphate from the gastrointestinal tract may be delayed or even completely prevented. The efficacy of regularly taken oral drugs (eg, oral contraceptives, antiepileptic drugs, diabetic medications, antibiotics) may be reduced or completely absent).
No products indexed under this heading.

Sulindac (Some cases occurred in patients without identifiable risk factors, patients at increased risk of acute phosphate nephropathy may include those with increased age, hypovolemia, increased bowel transit time (such as bowel obstruction), active colitis, or baseline kidney disease, and those using medicines that affect renal perfusion or function (such as diuretics, angiotensin converting enzyme [ACE] inhibitors, angiotensin receptor blocker [ARBs], and possibly nonsteroidal anti-inflammatory drugs [NSAIDs]). Patients at increased risk should be managed appropriately. It is important to use the dose and dosing regimen). Products include:
Clinoril 2098

Telmisartan (Some cases occurred in patients without identifiable risk factors, patients at increased risk of acute phosphate nephropathy may include those using medicines that affect renal perfusion or function (such as angiotensin receptor blocker [ARBs]). Patients at increased risk should be managed appropriately. It is important to use the dose and dosing regimen). Products include:
Micardis 887
Micardis HCT 889

Terazosin Hydrochloride (A rare, but serious form of kidney failure has been associated with the use of oral sodium phosphate products. Many of the reported cases involve patients with pre-existing kidney problems or patients who are taking drugs that can affect kidney function (such as drugs for hypertension or arthritis) or that can affect hydration (fluid) status (such as diuretics-fluid pills)).
No products indexed under this heading.

Tetracycline Hydrochloride (The absorption of drugs taken concomitantly with sodium phosphate from the gastrointestinal tract may be delayed or even completely prevented. The efficacy of regularly taken oral drugs (eg, oral contraceptives, antiepileptic drugs, diabetic medications, antibiotics) may be reduced or completely absent). Products include:
Pylera 793

Thioridazine Hydrochloride (Electrolyte disturbances are a risk associated with Fleet Prep Kit 3; concurrent use in patients taking agents known to prolong QT interval requires caution). Products include:
Thioridazine Hydrochloride 2384

Thiothixene (Electrolyte disturbances are a risk associated with Fleet Prep Kit 3; concurrent use in patients taking agents known to prolong QT interval requires caution). Products include:
Thiothixene 2386

Tiagabine Hydrochloride (The absorption of drugs taken concomitantly with sodium phosphate from the gastrointestinal tract may be delayed or even completely prevented. The efficacy of regularly taken oral drugs (eg, oral contraceptives, antiepileptic drugs, diabetic medications, antibiotics) may be reduced or completely absent). Products include:
Gabitril 972

Ticarcillin Disodium (The absorption of drugs taken concomitantly with sodium phosphate from the gastrointestinal tract may be delayed or even completely prevented. The efficacy of regularly taken oral drugs (eg, oral contraceptives, antiepileptic drugs, diabetic medications, antibiotics) may be reduced or completely absent). Products include:
Timentin ADD-Vantage 1670
Timentin Galaxy 1674
Timentin 1666
Timentin Pharmacy 1678

Timolol Maleate (A rare, but serious form of kidney failure has been associated with the use of oral sodium phosphate products. Many of the reported cases involve patients with pre-existing kidney problems or patients who are taking drugs that can affect kidney function (such as drugs for hypertension or arthritis) or that can affect hydration (fluid) status (such as diuretics-fluid pills)). Products include:
Combigan 601
Dorzolamide Hydrochloride/Timolol Maleate Ophthalmic Solution .... ⊙243
Timoptic in Ocudose .... ⊙231

Tobramycin (The absorption of drugs taken concomitantly with sodium phosphate from the gastrointestinal tract may be delayed or even completely prevented. The efficacy of regularly taken oral drugs (eg, oral contraceptives, antiepileptic drugs, diabetic medications, antibiotics) may be reduced or completely absent). Products include:
Tobi Nebulizer 2546
Tobramycin and Dexamethasone Ophthalmic Suspension .... ⊙251
Zylet .... ⊙252

Tobramycin Sulfate (The absorption of drugs taken concomitantly with sodium phosphate from the gastrointestinal tract may be delayed or even completely prevented. The efficacy of regularly taken oral drugs (eg, oral contraceptives, antiepileptic drugs, diabetic medications, antibiotics) may be reduced or completely absent).
No products indexed under this heading.

Tocainide Hydrochloride (Electrolyte disturbances are a risk associated with Fleet Prep Kit 3; concurrent use in patients taking agents known to prolong QT interval requires caution).
No products indexed under this heading.

Tolazamide (The absorption of drugs taken concomitantly with sodium phosphate from the gastrointestinal tract may be delayed or even completely prevented. The efficacy of regularly taken oral drugs (eg, oral contraceptives, antiepileptic drugs, diabetic medications, antibiotics) may be reduced or completely absent).
No products indexed under this heading.

Tolbutamide (The absorption of drugs taken concomitantly with sodium phosphate from the gastrointestinal tract may be delayed or even completely prevented. The efficacy of regularly taken oral drugs (eg, oral contraceptives, antiepileptic drugs, diabetic medications, antibiotics) may be reduced or completely absent).
No products indexed under this heading.

Tolmetin Sodium (Some cases occurred in patients without identifiable risk factors, patients at increased risk of acute phosphate nephropathy may include those with increased age, hypovolemia, increased bowel transit time (such as bowel obstruction), active colitis, or baseline kidney disease, and those using medicines that affect renal perfusion or function (such as diuretics, angiotensin converting enzyme [ACE] inhibitors, angiotensin receptor blocker [ARBs], and possibly nonsteroidal anti-inflammatory drugs [NSAIDs]). Patients at increased risk should be managed appropriately. It is important to use the dose and dosing regimen).
No products indexed under this heading.

Topiramate (The absorption of drugs taken concomitantly with sodium phosphate from the gastrointestinal tract may be delayed or even completely prevented. The efficacy of regularly taken oral drugs (eg, oral contraceptives, antiepileptic drugs, diabetic medications, antibiotics) may be reduced or completely absent).
No products indexed under this heading.

Torsemide (Some cases occurred in patients without identifiable risk factors, patients at increased risk of acute phosphate nephropathy may include those with increased age, hypovolemia, increased bowel transit time (such as bowel obstruction), active colitis, or baseline kidney disease, and those using medicines that affect renal perfusion or function (such as diuretics, angiotensin converting enzyme [ACE] inhibitors, angiotensin receptor blocker [ARBs], and possibly nonsteroidal anti-inflammatory drugs [NSAIDs]). Patients at increased risk should be managed appropriately. It is important to use the dose and dosing regimen).
No products indexed under this heading.

Trandolapril (Some cases occurred in patients without identifiable risk factors, patients at increased risk of acute phosphate nephropathy may include those using medicines that affect renal perfusion or function (such as angiotensin converting enzyme [ACE] inhibitors). Patients at increased risk should be managed appropriately. It is important to use the dose and dosing regimen). Products include:
Mavik 489
Tarka 534

Tranylcypromine Sulfate (Electrolyte disturbances are a risk associated with Fleet Prep Kit 3; concurrent use in patients taking agents known to prolong QT interval requires caution). Products include:
Parnate 1584

Triamterene (Some cases occurred in patients without identifiable risk factors, patients at increased risk of acute phosphate nephropathy may include those with increased age, hypovolemia, increased bowel transit time (such as bowel obstruction), active colitis, or baseline kidney disease, and those using medicines that affect renal perfusion or function (such as diuretics, angiotensin converting enzyme [ACE] inhibitors, angiotensin receptor blocker [ARBs], and possibly nonsteroidal anti-inflammatory drugs [NSAIDs]). Patients at increased risk should be managed appropriately. It is important to use the dose and dosing regimen). Products include:
Dyazide 1429
Dyrenium 3495

Trifluoperazine Hydrochloride (Electrolyte disturbances are a risk associated with Fleet Prep Kit 3; concurrent use in patients taking agents known to prolong QT interval requires caution).
No products indexed under this heading.

Trimethadione (The absorption of drugs taken concomitantly with sodium phosphate from the gastrointestinal tract may be delayed or even completely prevented. The efficacy of regularly taken oral drugs (eg, oral contraceptives, antiepileptic drugs, diabetic medications, antibiotics) may be reduced or completely absent).
No products indexed under this heading.

Trimethaphan Camsylate (A rare, but serious form of kidney failure has been associated with the use of oral sodium phosphate products. Many of the reported cases involve patients with pre-existing kidney problems or patients who are taking drugs that can affect kidney function (such as drugs for hypertension or arthritis) or that can affect hydration (fluid) status (such as diuretics-fluid pills)).
No products indexed under this heading.

Trimipramine Maleate (Electrolyte disturbances are a risk associated with Fleet Prep Kit 3; concurrent use in patients taking agents known to prolong QT interval requires caution).
No products indexed under this heading.

Troglitazone (The absorption of drugs taken concomitantly with sodium phosphate from the gastrointestinal tract may be delayed or even completely prevented. The efficacy of regularly taken oral drugs (eg, oral contraceptives, antiepileptic drugs, diabetic medications, antibiotics) may be reduced or completely absent).
No products indexed under this heading.

IMPORTANT NOTE: Always consult each drug listing in the patient's regimen for possible interactions.

(☉ Described in PDR® for Ophthalmic Medicines)

IMPORTANT NOTE: Always consult each drug listing in the patient's regimen for possible interactions.

Tolazoline Hydrochloride (Additional reductions in blood pressure may occur).

No products indexed under this heading.

Tolmetin Sodium (Potential for increased risk of bleeding).

No products indexed under this heading.

Torsemide (Additional reductions in blood pressure may occur).

No products indexed under this heading.

Trandolapril (Additional reductions in blood pressure may occur). Products include:

Triamterene (Additional reductions in blood pressure may occur). Products include:

Trimethaphan Camsylate (Additional reductions in blood pressure may occur).

No products indexed under this heading.

Valsartan (Additional reductions in blood pressure may occur). Products include:

Verapamil Hydrochloride (Additional reductions in blood pressure may occur). Products include:

Warfarin Sodium (Potential for increased risk of bleeding).

No products indexed under this heading.

Food Interactions

Alcohol (Additional reductions in blood pressure may occur).

FLONASE NASAL SPRAY

(Fluticasone Propionate) 1459

May interact with cytochrome p450 3a4 inhibitors (selected), and certain other agents. Compounds in these categories include:

Acetazolamide (Caution should be exercised when potent cytochrome P450 3A4 inhibitors are co-administered with fluticasone propionate).

No products indexed under this heading.

Acetazolamide Sodium (Caution should be exercised when potent cytochrome P450 3A4 inhibitors are co-administered with fluticasone propionate).

No products indexed under this heading.

Amiodarone Hydrochloride (Caution should be exercised when potent cytochrome P450 3A4 inhibitors are co-administered with fluticasone propionate).

No products indexed under this heading.

Amprenavir (Caution should be exercised when potent cytochrome P450 3A4 inhibitors are co-administered with fluticasone propionate).

No products indexed under this heading.

Anastrozole (Caution should be exercised when potent cytochrome P450 3A4 inhibitors are co-administered with fluticasone propionate).

No products indexed under this heading.

Aprepitant (Caution should be exercised when potent cytochrome P450 3A4 inhibitors are co-administered with fluticasone propionate). Products include:

Atazanavir (Caution should be exercised when potent cytochrome P450 3A4 inhibitors are co-administered with fluticasone propionate).

No products indexed under this heading.

Atazanavir Sulfate (Caution should be exercised when potent cytochrome P450 3A4 inhibitors are co-administered with fluticasone propionate).

No products indexed under this heading.

Cimetidine (Caution should be exercised when potent cytochrome P450 3A4 inhibitors are co-administered with fluticasone propionate).

No products indexed under this heading.

Cimetidine Hydrochloride (Caution should be exercised when potent cytochrome P450 3A4 inhibitors are co-administered with fluticasone propionate).

No products indexed under this heading.

Ciprofloxacin (Caution should be exercised when potent cytochrome P450 3A4 inhibitors are co-administered with fluticasone propionate). Products include:

Clarithromycin (Caution should be exercised when potent cytochrome P450 3A4 inhibitors are co-administered with fluticasone propionate). Products include:

Clotrimazole (Caution should be exercised when potent cytochrome P450 3A4 inhibitors are co-administered with fluticasone propionate). Products include:

Conivaptan Hydrochloride (Caution should be exercised when potent cytochrome P450 3A4 inhibitors are co-administered with fluticasone propionate). Products include:

Cyclosporine (Caution should be exercised when potent cytochrome P450 3A4 inhibitors are co-administered with fluticasone propionate). Products include:

Dalfopristin (Caution should be exercised when potent cytochrome P450 3A4 inhibitors are co-administered with fluticasone propionate).

No products indexed under this heading.

Danazol (Caution should be exercised when potent cytochrome P450 3A4 inhibitors are co-administered with fluticasone propionate).

No products indexed under this heading.

Darunavir (Caution should be exercised when potent cytochrome P450 3A4 inhibitors are co-administered with fluticasone propionate).

No products indexed under this heading.

Dasatinib (Caution should be exercised when potent cytochrome P450 3A4 inhibitors are co-administered with fluticasone propionate).

No products indexed under this heading.

Delavirdine Mesylate (Caution should be exercised when potent cytochrome P450 3A4 inhibitors are co-administered with fluticasone propionate).

No products indexed under this heading.

Delavirine (Caution should be exercised when potent cytochrome P450 3A4 inhibitors are co-administered with fluticasone propionate).

No products indexed under this heading.

Desloratadine (Caution should be exercised when potent cytochrome P450 3A4 inhibitors are co-administered with fluticasone propionate). Products include:

Diltiazem Hydrochloride (Caution should be exercised when potent cytochrome P450 3A4 inhibitors are co-administered with fluticasone propionate). Products include:

Diltiazem Maleate (Caution should be exercised when potent cytochrome P450 3A4 inhibitors are co-administered with fluticasone propionate).

No products indexed under this heading.

Efavirenz (Caution should be exercised when potent cytochrome P450 3A4 inhibitors are co-administered with fluticasone propionate). Products include:

Erythromycin (Caution should be exercised when potent cytochrome P450 3A4 inhibitors are co-administered with fluticasone propionate).

No products indexed under this heading.

Erythromycin Estolate (Caution should be exercised when potent cytochrome P450 3A4 inhibitors are co-administered with fluticasone propionate).

No products indexed under this heading.

Erythromycin Ethylsuccinate (Caution should be exercised when potent cytochrome P450 3A4 inhibitors are co-administered with fluticasone propionate). Products include:

Erythromycin Glucceptate (Caution should be exercised when potent cytochrome P450 3A4 inhibitors are co-administered with fluticasone propionate).

No products indexed under this heading.

Erythromycin Lactobionate (Caution should be exercised when potent cytochrome P450 3A4 inhibitors are co-administered with fluticasone propionate).

No products indexed under this heading.

Erythromycin Stearate (Caution should be exercised when potent cytochrome P450 3A4 inhibitors are co-administered with fluticasone propionate).

No products indexed under this heading.

Esomeprazole Magnesium (Caution should be exercised when potent cytochrome P450 3A4 inhibitors are co-administered with fluticasone propionate). Products include:

Esomeprazole Sodium (Caution should be exercised when potent cytochrome P450 3A4 inhibitors are co-administered with fluticasone propionate). Products include:

Fluconazole (Caution should be exercised when potent cytochrome P450 3A4 inhibitors are co-administered with fluticasone propionate).

No products indexed under this heading.

Fluoxetine (Caution should be exercised when potent cytochrome P450 3A4 inhibitors are co-administered with fluticasone propionate).

No products indexed under this heading.

Fluoxetine Hydrochloride (Caution should be exercised when potent cytochrome P450 3A4 inhibitors are co-administered with fluticasone propionate). Products include:

Fluvoxamine Maleate (Caution should be exercised when potent cytochrome P450 3A4 inhibitors are co-administered with fluticasone propionate).

No products indexed under this heading.

Fosamprenavir Calcium (Caution should be exercised when potent cytochrome P450 3A4 inhibitors are co-administered with fluticasone propionate). Products include:

Imatinib Mesylate (Caution should be exercised when potent cytochrome P450 3A4 inhibitors are co-administered with fluticasone propionate). Products include:

Indinavir Sulfate (Caution should be exercised when potent cytochrome P450 3A4 inhibitors are co-administered with fluticasone propionate). Products include:

Isoniazid (Caution should be exercised when potent cytochrome P450 3A4 inhibitors are co-administered with fluticasone propionate).

No products indexed under this heading.

Itraconazole (Caution should be exercised when potent cytochrome P450 3A4 inhibitors are co-administered with fluticasone propionate).

No products indexed under this heading.

Ketoconazole (Fluticasone propionate is a substrate of cytochrome P450 3A4. Co-administration with ketoconazole resulted in increased plasma fluticasone propionate exposure, a reduction in plasma cortisol AUC, and no effect on urinary excretion of cortisol. Caution should be exercised when potent cytochrome P450 3A inhibitors are co-administered with fluticasone propionate). Products include:

Lapatinib (Caution should be exercised when potent cytochrome P450 3A4 inhibitors are co-administered with fluticasone propionate). Products include:

Lopinavir (Caution should be exercised when potent cytochrome P450 3A4 inhibitors are co-administered with fluticasone propionate). Products include:

Loratadine (Caution should be exercised when potent cytochrome P450 3A4 inhibitors are co-administered with fluticasone propionate).

No products indexed under this heading.

Metronidazole (Caution should be exercised when potent cytochrome P450 3A4 inhibitors are co-administered with fluticasone propionate). Products include:

Metronidazole Benzoate (Caution should be exercised when potent cytochrome P450 3A4 inhibitors are co-administered with fluticasone propionate).

No products indexed under this heading.

Metronidazole Hydrochloride (Caution should be exercised when potent cytochrome P450 3A4 inhibitors are co-administered with fluticasone propionate).

No products indexed under this heading.

Metronidazole Sodium (Caution should be exercised when potent cytochrome P450 3A4 inhibitors are co-administered with fluticasone propionate).

No products indexed under this heading.

Miconazole (Caution should be exercised when potent cytochrome P450 3A4 inhibitors are co-administered with fluticasone propionate).
No products indexed under this heading.

Miconazole Nitrate (Caution should be exercised when potent cytochrome P450 3A4 inhibitors are co-administered with fluticasone propionate). Products include:
Vusion Ointment 3335

Mifepristone (Caution should be exercised when potent cytochrome P450 3A4 inhibitors are co-administered with fluticasone propionate).
No products indexed under this heading.

Nefazodone Hydrochloride (Caution should be exercised when potent cytochrome P450 3A4 inhibitors are co-administered with fluticasone propionate).
No products indexed under this heading.

Nelfinavir Mesylate (Caution should be exercised when potent cytochrome P450 3A4 inhibitors are co-administered with fluticasone propionate).
No products indexed under this heading.

Nevirapine (Caution should be exercised when potent cytochrome P450 3A4 inhibitors are co-administered with fluticasone propionate). Products include:
Viramune Oral Suspension 897
Viramune Tablets 897

Niacin (Caution should be exercised when potent cytochrome P450 3A4 inhibitors are co-administered with fluticasone propionate). Products include:
Advicor 402
Cardio Basics 3455
Niaspan 497
Simcor 524

Niacinamide (Caution should be exercised when potent cytochrome P450 3A4 inhibitors are co-administered with fluticasone propionate). Products include:
CitraNatal 90 DHA Capsules 2332
CitraNatal Assure 2332
CitraNatal Rx 2332
Heplive 607

Niacinamide Hydroiodide (Caution should be exercised when potent cytochrome P450 3A4 inhibitors are co-administered with fluticasone propionate).
No products indexed under this heading.

Nicotinamide (Caution should be exercised when potent cytochrome P450 3A4 inhibitors are co-administered with fluticasone propionate).
No products indexed under this heading.

Nifedipine (Caution should be exercised when potent cytochrome P450 3A4 inhibitors are co-administered with fluticasone propionate).
No products indexed under this heading.

Norfloxacin (Caution should be exercised when potent cytochrome P450 3A4 inhibitors are co-administered with fluticasone propionate). Products include:
Noroxin 2220

Omeprazole (Caution should be exercised when potent cytochrome P450 3A4 inhibitors are co-administered with fluticasone propionate).
No products indexed under this heading.

Paroxetine Hydrochloride (Caution should be exercised when potent cytochrome P450 3A4 inhibitors are co-administered with fluticasone propionate). Products include:
Paroxetine CR 2361
Paroxetine ER 2371
Paxil 1586
Paxil CR 1596

Posaconazole (Caution should be exercised when potent cytochrome P450 3A4 inhibitors are co-administered with fluticasone propionate). Products include:
Noxafil 3172

Propoxyphene Hydrochloride (Caution should be exercised when potent cytochrome P450 3A4 inhibitors are co-administered with fluticasone propionate).
No products indexed under this heading.

Propoxyphene Napsylate (Caution should be exercised when potent cytochrome P450 3A4 inhibitors are co-administered with fluticasone propionate).
No products indexed under this heading.

Quinidine (Caution should be exercised when potent cytochrome P450 3A4 inhibitors are co-administered with fluticasone propionate).
No products indexed under this heading.

Quinidine Hydrochloride (Caution should be exercised when potent cytochrome P450 3A4 inhibitors are co-administered with fluticasone propionate).
No products indexed under this heading.

Quinidine Polygalacturonate (Caution should be exercised when potent cytochrome P450 3A4 inhibitors are co-administered with fluticasone propionate).
No products indexed under this heading.

Quinidine Sulfate (Caution should be exercised when potent cytochrome P450 3A4 inhibitors are co-administered with fluticasone propionate).
No products indexed under this heading.

Quinine (Caution should be exercised when potent cytochrome P450 3A4 inhibitors are co-administered with fluticasone propionate). Products include:
Hyland's Leg Cramps PM with
Quinine 3315

Quinine Sulfate (Caution should be exercised when potent cytochrome P450 3A4 inhibitors are co-administered with fluticasone propionate).
No products indexed under this heading.

Quinupristin (Caution should be exercised when potent cytochrome P450 3A4 inhibitors are co-administered with fluticasone propionate).
No products indexed under this heading.

Ranitidine Bismuth Citrate (Caution should be exercised when potent cytochrome P450 3A4 inhibitors are co-administered with fluticasone propionate).
No products indexed under this heading.

Ranitidine Hydrochloride (Caution should be exercised when potent cytochrome P450 3A4 inhibitors are co-administered with fluticasone propionate). Products include:
Zantac 1737
Zantac Injection 1732
Zantac Pharmacy 1735

Ritonavir (Fluticasone propionate is a substrate of cytochrome P450 3A4. A drug interaction study has shown that ritonavir (a highly potent cytochrome P450 3A4 inhibitor) can significantly increase plasma fluticasone propionate exposure, resulting in significantly reduced serum cortisol concentrations. Therefore, co-administration of fluticasone propionate and ritonavir is not recommended unless the potential benefit to the patient outweighs the risk of systemic corticosteroid side effects). Products include:
Kaletra 458
Norvir 509

Saquinavir (Caution should be exercised when potent cytochrome P450 3A4 inhibitors are co-administered with fluticasone propionate).
No products indexed under this heading.

Saquinavir Mesylate (Caution should be exercised when potent cytochrome P450 3A4 inhibitors are co-administered with fluticasone propionate).
No products indexed under this heading.

Sertraline Hydrochloride (Caution should be exercised when potent cytochrome P450 3A4 inhibitors are co-administered with fluticasone propionate).
No products indexed under this heading.

Sildenafil Citrate (Caution should be exercised when potent cytochrome P450 3A4 inhibitors are co-administered with fluticasone propionate).
No products indexed under this heading.

Telithromycin (Caution should be exercised when potent cytochrome P450 3A4 inhibitors are co-administered with fluticasone propionate). Products include:
Ketek 2991

Troglitazone (Caution should be exercised when potent cytochrome P450 3A4 inhibitors are co-administered with fluticasone propionate).
No products indexed under this heading.

Troleandomycin (Caution should be exercised when potent cytochrome P450 3A4 inhibitors are co-administered with fluticasone propionate).
No products indexed under this heading.

Valproate Sodium (Caution should be exercised when potent cytochrome P450 3A4 inhibitors are co-administered with fluticasone propionate).
No products indexed under this heading.

Vardenafil Hydrochloride (Caution should be exercised when potent cytochrome P450 3A4 inhibitors are co-administered with fluticasone propionate). Products include:
Levitra 3157

Verapamil Hydrochloride (Caution should be exercised when potent cytochrome P450 3A4 inhibitors are co-administered with fluticasone propionate). Products include:
Tarka 534

Voriconazole (Caution should be exercised when potent cytochrome P450 3A4 inhibitors are co-administered with fluticasone propionate).
No products indexed under this heading.

Zafirlukast (Caution should be exercised when potent cytochrome P450 3A4 inhibitors are co-administered with fluticasone propionate). Products include:
Accolate 3612

Zileuton (Caution should be exercised when potent cytochrome P450 3A4 inhibitors are co-administered with fluticasone propionate).
No products indexed under this heading.

Food Interactions

Grapefruit (Caution should be exercised when potent cytochrome P450 3A4 inhibitors are co-administered with fluticasone propionate).

Grapefruit Juice (Caution should be exercised when potent cytochrome P450 3A4 inhibitors are co-administered with fluticasone propionate).

FLOVENT DISKUS 50 MCG

(Fluticasone Propionate) 1463
May interact with cytochrome p450 3a4 inhibitors, potent (selected), and certain other agents. Compounds in these categories include:

Amprenavir (Caution should be exercised when potent cytochrome P450 3A4 inhibitors are co-administered with fluticasone. Interactions with ritonavir and ketoconazole, both potent CYP3A4 inhibitors, have resulted in increased fluticasone exposure).
No products indexed under this heading.

Atazanavir (Caution should be exercised when potent cytochrome P450 3A4 inhibitors are co-administered with fluticasone. Interactions with ritonavir and ketoconazole, both potent CYP3A4 inhibitors, have resulted in increased fluticasone exposure).
No products indexed under this heading.

Atazanavir Sulfate (Caution should be exercised when potent cytochrome P450 3A4 inhibitors are co-administered with fluticasone. Interactions with ritonavir and ketoconazole, both potent CYP3A4 inhibitors, have resulted in increased fluticasone exposure).
No products indexed under this heading.

Clarithromycin (Caution should be exercised when potent cytochrome P450 3A4 inhibitors are co-administered with fluticasone. Interactions with ritonavir and ketoconazole, both potent CYP3A4 inhibitors, have resulted in increased fluticasone exposure). Products include:
Biaxin/Biaxin XL 412

Delavirdine Mesylate (Caution should be exercised when potent cytochrome P450 3A4 inhibitors are co-administered with fluticasone. Interactions with ritonavir and ketoconazole, both potent CYP3A4 inhibitors, have resulted in increased fluticasone exposure).
No products indexed under this heading.

Delavirine (Caution should be exercised when potent cytochrome P450 3A4 inhibitors are co-administered with fluticasone. Interactions with ritonavir and ketoconazole, both potent CYP3A4 inhibitors, have resulted in increased fluticasone exposure).
No products indexed under this heading.

Fosamprenavir Calcium (Caution should be exercised when potent cytochrome P450 3A4 inhibitors are co-administered with fluticasone. Interactions with ritonavir and ketoconazole, both potent CYP3A4 inhibitors, have resulted in increased fluticasone exposure). Products include:
Lexiva Oral Suspension 1558
Lexiva 1558

Indinavir Sulfate (Caution should be exercised when potent cytochrome P450 3A4 inhibitors are co-administered with fluticasone. Interactions with ritonavir and ketoconazole, both potent CYP3A4 inhibitors, have resulted in increased fluticasone exposure). Products include:
Crixivan 2113

Itraconazole (Caution should be exercised when potent cytochrome P450 3A4 inhibitors are co-administered with fluticasone. Interactions with ritonavir and ketoconazole, both potent CYP3A4 inhibitors, have resulted in increased fluticasone exposure).
No products indexed under this heading.

Ketoconazole (Co-administration of a single dose of fluticasone (1000 mcg) with multiple doses of ketoconazole (200 mg) to steady state has resulted in increased mean fluticasone concentrations, a reduction in plasma cortisol AUC, and no effect on urinary excretion of cortisol). Products include:
Extina 3319
Xolegel 3337

Lopinavir (Caution should be exercised when potent cytochrome P450 3A4 inhibitors are co-administered with

Flovent

Interactions Index

698

fluticasone. Interactions with ritonavir and ketoconazole, both potent CYP3A4 inhibitors, have resulted in increased fluticasone exposure). Products include:
Kaletra **458**

Nefazodone Hydrochloride (Caution should be exercised when potent cytochrome P450 3A4 inhibitors are co-administered with fluticasone. Interactions with ritonavir and ketoconazole, both potent CYP3A4 inhibitors, have resulted in increased fluticasone exposure).
No products indexed under this heading.

Nelfinavir Mesylate (Caution should be exercised when potent cytochrome P450 3A4 inhibitors are co-administered with fluticasone. Interactions with ritonavir and ketoconazole, both potent CYP3A4 inhibitors, have resulted in increased fluticasone exposure).
No products indexed under this heading.

Ritonavir (Ritonavir can significantly increase plasma fluticasone exposure, resulting in significantly reduced serum cortisol concentrations. Cushing syndrome and adrenal suppression have been reported; therefore, co-administration is not recommended unless the potential benefit outweighs the risks). Products include:
Kaletra **458**
Norvir **509**

Saquinavir (Caution should be exercised when potent cytochrome P450 3A4 inhibitors are co-administered with fluticasone. Interactions with ritonavir and ketoconazole, both potent CYP3A4 inhibitors, have resulted in increased fluticasone exposure).
No products indexed under this heading.

Saquinavir Mesylate (Caution should be exercised when potent cytochrome P450 3A4 inhibitors are co-administered with fluticasone. Interactions with ritonavir and ketoconazole, both potent CYP3A4 inhibitors, have resulted in increased fluticasone exposure).
No products indexed under this heading.

Telithromycin (Caution should be exercised when potent cytochrome P450 3A4 inhibitors are co-administered with fluticasone. Interactions with ritonavir and ketoconazole, both potent CYP3A4 inhibitors, have resulted in increased fluticasone exposure). Products include:
Ketek 2991

Troleandomycin (Caution should be exercised when potent cytochrome P450 3A4 inhibitors are co-administered with fluticasone. Interactions with ritonavir and ketoconazole, both potent CYP3A4 inhibitors, have resulted in increased fluticasone exposure).
No products indexed under this heading.

Voriconazole (Caution should be exercised when potent cytochrome P450 3A4 inhibitors are co-administered with fluticasone. Interactions with ritonavir and ketoconazole, both potent CYP3A4 inhibitors, have resulted in increased fluticasone exposure).
No products indexed under this heading.

FLOVENT DISKUS 100 MCG
(Fluticasone Propionate) 1463
See Flovent Diskus 50 mcg

FLOVENT DISKUS 250 MCG
(Fluticasone Propionate) 1463
See Flovent Diskus 50 mcg

FLOVENT HFA 44 MCG INHALATION AEROSOL
(Fluticasone Propionate) 1470

Ketoconazole (Co-administration of a single dose of fluticasone (1000 mcg) with multiple doses of ketoconazole (200 mg) to steady state has resulted in increased mean plasma fluticasone exposure, a reduction in plasma cortisol AUC, and no effect on urinary excretion of cortisol). Products include:
Extina 3319
Xolegel 3337

Ritonavir (Ritonavir can significantly increase plasma fluticasone exposure, resulting in significantly reduced serum cortisol concentrations. Cushing syndrome and adrenal suppression have been reported; therefore, co-administration is not recommended unless the potential benefit outweighs the risks). Products include:
Kaletra **458**
Norvir **509**

FLOVENT HFA 110 MCG INHALATION AEROSOL
(Fluticasone Propionate) 1470
See Flovent HFA 44 mcg Inhalation Aerosol

FLOVENT HFA 220 MCG INHALATION AEROSOL
(Fluticasone Propionate) 1470
See Flovent HFA 44 mcg Inhalation Aerosol

FLUARIX VACCINE
(Influenza Virus Vaccine) 1476
May interact with alkylating agents, anticoagulants, antimetabolites, corticosteroids, cytotoxic drugs, immunosuppressive agents, phenytoin, theophyllines, and certain other agents. Compounds in these categories include:

Alclometasone Dipropionate
(Immunosuppressive therapies, including corticosteroids (used in greater than physiologic doses), may reduce the immune response to vaccines).
No products indexed under this heading.

Anisindione (Influenza vaccinations should not be given to persons on anticoagulant therapy unless the potential benefit clearly outweighs the risk of administration. If the decision is made to administer an influenza vaccination to such persons, steps should be considered to control the risk of hematoma following the injection).
No products indexed under this heading.

Ardeparin Sodium (Influenza vaccinations should not be given to persons on anticoagulant therapy unless the potential benefit clearly outweighs the risk of administration. If the decision is made to administer an influenza vaccination to such persons, steps should be considered to control the risk of hematoma following the injection).
No products indexed under this heading.

Azathioprine (Immunosuppressive therapies, including irradiation, antimetabolites, alkylating agents, cytotoxic drugs, and corticosteroids (used in greater than physiologic doses), may reduce the immune response to vaccines).
No products indexed under this heading.

Basiliximab (Immunosuppressive therapies, including irradiation, antimetabolites, alkylating agents, cytotoxic drugs, and corticosteroids (used in greater than physiologic doses), may reduce the immune response to vaccines). Products include:
Simulect 2524

Beclomethasone Dipropionate
(Immunosuppressive therapies, including corticosteroids (used in greater than physiologic doses), may reduce the immune response to vaccines). Products include:
Qvar 3398

Beclomethasone Dipropionate Monohydrate (Immunosuppressive

therapies, including corticosteroids (used in greater than physiologic doses), may reduce the immune response to vaccines). Products include:
Beconase AQ 1386

Betamethasone (Immunosuppressive therapies, including corticosteroids (used in greater than physiologic doses), may reduce the immune response to vaccines).
No products indexed under this heading.

Betamethasone Acetate (Immunosuppressive therapies, including corticosteroids (used in greater than physiologic doses), may reduce the immune response to vaccines).
No products indexed under this heading.

Betamethasone Benzoate (Immunosuppressive therapies, including corticosteroids (used in greater than physiologic doses), may reduce the immune response to vaccines).
No products indexed under this heading.

Betamethasone Dipropionate
(Immunosuppressive therapies, including corticosteroids (used in greater than physiologic doses), may reduce the immune response to vaccines). Products include:
Diprolene Lotion 0.05% 3108
Diprolene Ointment 0.05% 3109
Diprolene AF Cream 0.05% 3107
Lotrisone 3163

Betamethasone Sodium Phosphate (Immunosuppressive therapies, including corticosteroids (used in greater than physiologic doses), may reduce the immune response to vaccines).
No products indexed under this heading.

Betamethasone Valerate (Immunosuppressive therapies, including corticosteroids (used in greater than physiologic doses), may reduce the immune response to vaccines). Products include:
Luxíq 3321

Bleomycin Sulfate (Immunosuppressive therapies, including cytotoxic drugs, may reduce the immune response to vaccines).
No products indexed under this heading.

Budesonide (Immunosuppressive therapies, including corticosteroids (used in greater than physiologic doses), may reduce the immune response to vaccines). Products include:
Pulmicort Flexhaler **714**
Symbicort 80/4.5 .... **720**
Symbicort 160/4.5 .... **720**

Busulfan (Immunosuppressive therapies, including alkylating agents, may reduce the immune response to vaccines). Products include:
Myleran 1581

Capecitabine (Immunosuppressive therapies, including antimetabolites, may reduce the immune response to vaccines). Products include:
Xeloda 2882

Carmustine (BCNU) (Immunosuppressive therapies, including alkylating agents, may reduce the immune response to vaccines).
No products indexed under this heading.

Chlorambucil (Immunosuppressive therapies, including alkylating agents, may reduce the immune response to vaccines). Products include:
Leukeran 1557

Ciclesonide (Immunosuppressive therapies, including corticosteroids (used in greater than physiologic doses), may reduce the immune response to vaccines).
No products indexed under this heading.

Cladribine (Immunosuppressive therapies, including antimetabolites, may reduce the immune response to vaccines). Products include:

Leustatin 946

Cortisone Acetate (Immunosuppressive therapies, including corticosteroids (used in greater than physiologic doses), may reduce the immune response to vaccines).
No products indexed under this heading.

Cyclophosphamide (Immunosuppressive therapies, including alkylating agents, may reduce the immune response to vaccines).
No products indexed under this heading.

Cyclosporine (Immunosuppressive therapies, including irradiation, antimetabolites, alkylating agents, cytotoxic drugs, and corticosteroids (used in greater than physiologic doses), may reduce the immune response to vaccines). Products include:
Gengraf **440**
Neoral Oral Solution 2496
Neoral Capsules 2496
Restasis **605**

Cytarabine (Immunosuppressive therapies, including antimetabolites, may reduce the immune response to vaccines).
No products indexed under this heading.

Dacarbazine (Immunosuppressive therapies, including alkylating agents, may reduce the immune response to vaccines).
No products indexed under this heading.

Dalteparin Sodium (Influenza vaccinations should not be given to persons on anticoagulant therapy unless the potential benefit clearly outweighs the risk of administration. If the decision is made to administer an influenza vaccination to such persons, steps should be considered to control the risk of hematoma following the injection). Products include:
Fragmin 1058

Danaparoid Sodium (Influenza vaccinations should not be given to persons on anticoagulant therapy unless the potential benefit clearly outweighs the risk of administration. If the decision is made to administer an influenza vaccination to such persons, steps should be considered to control the risk of hematoma following the injection).
No products indexed under this heading.

Daunorubicin Hydrochloride
(Immunosuppressive therapies, including cytotoxic drugs, may reduce the immune response to vaccines).
No products indexed under this heading.

Desoximetasone (Immunosuppressive therapies, including corticosteroids (used in greater than physiologic doses), may reduce the immune response to vaccines).
No products indexed under this heading.

Dexamethasone (Immunosuppressive therapies, including corticosteroids (used in greater than physiologic doses), may reduce the immune response to vaccines). Products include:
Ciprodex **583**
Ozurdex .... ⊙ **223**
Tobramycin and Dexamethasone
Ophthalmic Suspension .... ⊙ 251

Dexamethasone Acetate (Immunosuppressive therapies, including corticosteroids (used in greater than physiologic doses), may reduce the immune response to vaccines).
No products indexed under this heading.

Dexamethasone Phosphate (Immunosuppressive therapies, including corticosteroids (used in greater than physiologic doses), may reduce the immune response to vaccines).
No products indexed under this heading.

(⊙ Described in PDR® for Ophthalmic Medicines)

Dexamethasone Sodium (Immunosuppressive therapies, including corticosteroids (used in greater than physiologic doses), may reduce the immune response to vaccines).
No products indexed under this heading.

Dexamethasone Sodium Phosphate (Immunosuppressive therapies, including corticosteroids (used in greater than physiologic doses), may reduce the immune response to vaccines).
No products indexed under this heading.

Dexamethasone Sodium Phosphate Injection (Immunosuppressive therapies, including corticosteroids (used in greater than physiologic doses), may reduce the immune response to vaccines).
No products indexed under this heading.

Dicumarol (Influenza vaccinations should not be given to persons on anticoagulant therapy unless the potential benefit clearly outweighs the risk of administration. If the decision is made to administer an influenza vaccination to such persons, steps should be considered to control the risk of hematoma following the injection).
No products indexed under this heading.

Diflorasone Diacetate (Immunosuppressive therapies, including corticosteroids (used in greater than physiologic doses), may reduce the immune response to vaccines).
No products indexed under this heading.

Doxorubicin Hydrochloride (Immunosuppressive therapies, including cytotoxic drugs, may reduce the immune response to vaccines).
No products indexed under this heading.

Enoxaparin Sodium (Influenza vaccinations should not be given to persons on anticoagulant therapy unless the potential benefit clearly outweighs the risk of administration. If the decision is made to administer an influenza vaccination to such persons, steps should be considered to control the risk of hematoma following the injection). Products include:
Lovenox 3005

Epirubicin Hydrochloride (Immunosuppressive therapies, including cytotoxic drugs, may reduce the immune response to vaccines).
No products indexed under this heading.

Floxuridine (Immunosuppressive therapies, including antimetabolites, may reduce the immune response to vaccines).
No products indexed under this heading.

Fludarabine Phosphate (Immunosuppressive therapies, including antimetabolites, may reduce the immune response to vaccines). Products include:
Oforta 3023

Fludrocortisone Acetate (Immunosuppressive therapies, including corticosteroids (used in greater than physiologic doses), may reduce the immune response to vaccines).
No products indexed under this heading.

Flumethasone Pivalate (Immunosuppressive therapies, including corticosteroids (used in greater than physiologic doses), may reduce the immune response to vaccines).
No products indexed under this heading.

Flunisolide Hemihydrate (Immunosuppressive therapies, including corticosteroids (used in greater than physiologic doses), may reduce the immune response to vaccines).
No products indexed under this heading.

Fluorouracil (Immunosuppressive therapies, including antimetabolites, may reduce the immune response to vaccines). Products include:
Carac 2966

Fluticasone Furoate (Immunosuppressive therapies, including corticosteroids (used in greater than physiologic doses), may reduce the immune response to vaccines). Products include:
Veramyst 1713

Fluticasone Propionate (Immunosuppressive therapies, including corticosteroids (used in greater than physiologic doses), may reduce the immune response to vaccines). Products include:
Advair 100/50 1275
Advair 250/50 1275
Advair 500/50 1275
Advair HFA 45/21 1288
Advair HFA 115/21 1288
Advair HFA 230/21 1288
Flonase 1459
Flovent Diskus 1463
Flovent HFA 1470

Fondaparinux Sodium (Influenza vaccinations should not be given to persons on anticoagulant therapy unless the potential benefit clearly outweighs the risk of administration. If the decision is made to administer an influenza vaccination to such persons, steps should be considered to control the risk of hematoma following the injection). Products include:
Arixtra 1320

Fosphenytoin (Although it has been reported that influenza vaccination may inhibit the clearance of phenytoin, controlled studies have yielded inconsistent results regarding pharmacokinetic interactions between influenza vaccine and phenytoin. Nevertheless, clinicians should consider the potential for an interaction when influenza vaccine is administered to persons receiving phenytoin).
No products indexed under this heading.

Fosphenytoin Sodium (Although it has been reported that influenza vaccination may inhibit the clearance of phenytoin, controlled studies have yielded inconsistent results regarding pharmacokinetic interactions between influenza vaccine and phenytoin. Nevertheless, clinicians should consider the potential for an interaction when influenza vaccine is administered to persons receiving phenytoin).
No products indexed under this heading.

Gemcitabine Hydrochloride (Immunosuppressive therapies, including antimetabolites, may reduce the immune response to vaccines). Products include:
Gemzar 1900

Heparin Calcium (Influenza vaccinations should not be given to persons on anticoagulant therapy unless the potential benefit clearly outweighs the risk of administration. If the decision is made to administer an influenza vaccination to such persons, steps should be considered to control the risk of hematoma following the injection).
No products indexed under this heading.

Heparin Sodium (Influenza vaccinations should not be given to persons on anticoagulant therapy unless the potential benefit clearly outweighs the risk of administration. If the decision is made to administer an influenza vaccination to such persons, steps should be considered to control the risk of hematoma following the injection).
No products indexed under this heading.

Hydrocortisone (Immunosuppressive therapies, including corticosteroids (used in greater than physiologic doses), may reduce the immune response to vaccines).
No products indexed under this heading.

Hydrocortisone (Alcohol) (Immunosuppressive therapies, including corticosteroids (used in greater than physiologic doses), may reduce the immune response to vaccines).
No products indexed under this heading.

Hydrocortisone Acetate (Immunosuppressive therapies, including corticosteroids (used in greater than physiologic doses), may reduce the immune response to vaccines).
No products indexed under this heading.

Hydrocortisone Butyrate (Immunosuppressive therapies, including corticosteroids (used in greater than physiologic doses), may reduce the immune response to vaccines).
No products indexed under this heading.

Hydrocortisone Cypionate (Immunosuppressive therapies, including corticosteroids (used in greater than physiologic doses), may reduce the immune response to vaccines).
No products indexed under this heading.

Hydrocortisone Hemisuccinate (Immunosuppressive therapies, including corticosteroids (used in greater than physiologic doses), may reduce the immune response to vaccines).
No products indexed under this heading.

Hydrocortisone Probutate (Immunosuppressive therapies, including corticosteroids (used in greater than physiologic doses), may reduce the immune response to vaccines).
No products indexed under this heading.

Hydrocortisone Sodium Phosphate (Immunosuppressive therapies, including corticosteroids (used in greater than physiologic doses), may reduce the immune response to vaccines).
No products indexed under this heading.

Hydrocortisone Sodium Succinate (Immunosuppressive therapies, including corticosteroids (used in greater than physiologic doses), may reduce the immune response to vaccines).
No products indexed under this heading.

Hydrocortisone Valerate (Immunosuppressive therapies, including corticosteroids (used in greater than physiologic doses), may reduce the immune response to vaccines).
No products indexed under this heading.

Hydroxyurea (Immunosuppressive therapies, including cytotoxic drugs, may reduce the immune response to vaccines).
No products indexed under this heading.

Lomustine (CCNU) (Immunosuppressive therapies, including alkylating agents, may reduce the immune response to vaccines).
No products indexed under this heading.

Low Molecular Weight Heparins (Influenza vaccinations should not be given to persons on anticoagulant therapy unless the potential benefit clearly outweighs the risk of administration. If the decision is made to administer an influenza vaccination to such persons, steps should be considered to control the risk of hematoma following the injection).
No products indexed under this heading.

Mechlorethamine Hydrochloride (Immunosuppressive therapies, including alkylating agents, may reduce the immune response to vaccines). Products include:
Mustargen 2010

Melphalan (Immunosuppressive therapies, including alkylating agents, may reduce the immune response to vaccines). Products include:
Alkeran 1302

Mercaptopurine (Immunosuppressive therapies, including antimetabolites, may reduce the immune response to vaccines).
No products indexed under this heading.

Methotrexate (Immunosuppressive therapies, including antimetabolites, may reduce the immune response to vaccines).
No products indexed under this heading.

Methotrexate Sodium (Immunosuppressive therapies, including antimetabolites, may reduce the immune response to vaccines).
No products indexed under this heading.

Methylprednisolone (Immunosuppressive therapies, including corticosteroids (used in greater than physiologic doses), may reduce the immune response to vaccines).
No products indexed under this heading.

Methylprednisolone Acetate (Immunosuppressive therapies, including corticosteroids (used in greater than physiologic doses), may reduce the immune response to vaccines).
No products indexed under this heading.

Methylprednisolone Sodium Succinate (Immunosuppressive therapies, including corticosteroids (used in greater than physiologic doses), may reduce the immune response to vaccines).
No products indexed under this heading.

Mitotane (Immunosuppressive therapies, including cytotoxic drugs, may reduce the immune response to vaccines).
No products indexed under this heading.

Mitoxantrone Hydrochloride (Immunosuppressive therapies, including cytotoxic drugs, may reduce the immune response to vaccines). Products include:
Novantrone 1088

Mometasone Furoate (Immunosuppressive therapies, including corticosteroids (used in greater than physiologic doses), may reduce the immune response to vaccines). Products include:
Asmanex 3058
Elocon Cream 3111
Elocon Lotion 3112
Elocon Ointment 3114

Mometasone Furoate Monohydrate (Immunosuppressive therapies, including corticosteroids (used in greater than physiologic doses), may reduce the immune response to vaccines). Products include:
Nasonex 3166

Muromonab-CD3 (Immunosuppressive therapies, including irradiation, antimetabolites, alkylating agents, cytotoxic drugs, and corticosteroids (used in greater than physiologic doses), may reduce the immune response to vaccines). Products include:
Orthoclone OKT3 949

Mycophenolate Mofetil (Immunosuppressive therapies, including irradiation, antimetabolites, alkylating agents, cytotoxic drugs, and corticosteroids (used in greater than physiologic doses), may reduce the immune response to vaccines).
No products indexed under this heading.

Pentostatin (Immunosuppressive therapies, including antimetabolites, may reduce the immune response to vaccines).
No products indexed under this heading.

IMPORTANT NOTE: Always consult each drug listing in the patient's regimen for possible interactions.

Phenytoin (Although it has been reported that influenza vaccination may inhibit the clearance of phenytoin, controlled studies have yielded inconsistent results regarding pharmacokinetic interactions between influenza vaccine and phenytoin. Nevertheless, clinicians should consider the potential for an interaction when influenza vaccine is administered to persons receiving phenytoin).
No products indexed under this heading.

Phenytoin Sodium (Although it has been reported that influenza vaccination may inhibit the clearance of phenytoin, controlled studies have yielded inconsistent results regarding pharmacokinetic interactions between influenza vaccine and phenytoin. Nevertheless, clinicians should consider the potential for an interaction when influenza vaccine is administered to persons receiving phenytoin). Products include:
Phenytek Capsules **2380**

Prednisolone (Immunosuppressive therapies, including corticosteroids (used in greater than physiologic doses), may reduce the immune response to vaccines).
No products indexed under this heading.

Prednisolone Acetate (Immunosuppressive therapies, including corticosteroids (used in greater than physiologic doses), may reduce the immune response to vaccines). Products include:
Blephamide .... ⊙ **212**, ⊙ **214**
Pred Forte .... ⊙ **225**
Pred Mild .... ⊙ **230**
Pred-G .... ⊙ **226**, ⊙ **227**

Prednisolone Sodium Phosphate (Immunosuppressive therapies, including corticosteroids (used in greater than physiologic doses), may reduce the immune response to vaccines).
No products indexed under this heading.

Prednisolone Tebutate (Immunosuppressive therapies, including corticosteroids (used in greater than physiologic doses), may reduce the immune response to vaccines).
No products indexed under this heading.

Prednisone (Immunosuppressive therapies, including corticosteroids (used in greater than physiologic doses), may reduce the immune response to vaccines).
No products indexed under this heading.

Prednisone sodium phosphate (Immunosuppressive therapies, including corticosteroids (used in greater than physiologic doses), may reduce the immune response to vaccines).
No products indexed under this heading.

Procarbazine Hydrochloride (Immunosuppressive therapies, including cytotoxic drugs, may reduce the immune response to vaccines).
No products indexed under this heading.

Radiation (Immunosuppressive therapies, including irradiation, may reduce the immune response to vaccines).
No products indexed under this heading.

Rapamycin (Immunosuppressive therapies, including irradiation, antimetabolites, alkylating agents, cytotoxic drugs, and corticosteroids (used in greater than physiologic doses), may reduce the immune response to vaccines).
No products indexed under this heading.

Sirolimus (Immunosuppressive therapies, including irradiation, antimetabolites, alkylating agents, cytotoxic drugs, and corticosteroids (used in greater than physiologic doses), may reduce the immune response to vaccines). Products include:
Rapamune **3579**

Tacrolimus (Immunosuppressive therapies, including irradiation, antimetabolites, alkylating agents, cytotoxic drugs, and corticosteroids (used in greater than physiologic doses), may reduce the immune response to vaccines). Products include:
Prograf Capsules **677**
Prograf Injection **677**
Protopic **685**

Tamoxifen Citrate (Immunosuppressive therapies, including cytotoxic drugs, may reduce the immune response to vaccines).
No products indexed under this heading.

Theophylline (Although it has been reported that influenza vaccination may inhibit the clearance of theophylline, controlled studies have yielded inconsistent results regarding pharmacokinetic interactions between influenza vaccine and theophylline. Nevertheless, clinicians should consider the potential for an interaction when influenza vaccine is administered to persons receiving theophylline).
No products indexed under this heading.

Theophylline Anhydrous (Although it has been reported that influenza vaccination may inhibit the clearance of theophylline, controlled studies have yielded inconsistent results regarding pharmacokinetic interactions between influenza vaccine and theophylline. Nevertheless, clinicians should consider the potential for an interaction when influenza vaccine is administered to persons receiving theophylline). Products include:
Uniphyl **2817**

Theophylline Calcium Salicylate (Although it has been reported that influenza vaccination may inhibit the clearance of theophylline, controlled studies have yielded inconsistent results regarding pharmacokinetic interactions between influenza vaccine and theophylline. Nevertheless, clinicians should consider the potential for an interaction when influenza vaccine is administered to persons receiving theophylline).
No products indexed under this heading.

Theophylline Dihydroxypropyl (Glyceryl) (Although it has been reported that influenza vaccination may inhibit the clearance of theophylline, controlled studies have yielded inconsistent results regarding pharmacokinetic interactions between influenza vaccine and theophylline. Nevertheless, clinicians should consider the potential for an interaction when influenza vaccine is administered to persons receiving theophylline).
No products indexed under this heading.

Theophylline Ethylenediamine (Although it has been reported that influenza vaccination may inhibit the clearance of theophylline, controlled studies have yielded inconsistent results regarding pharmacokinetic interactions between influenza vaccine and theophylline. Nevertheless, clinicians should consider the potential for an interaction when influenza vaccine is administered to persons receiving theophylline).
No products indexed under this heading.

Theophylline Sodium Glycinate (Although it has been reported that influenza vaccination may inhibit the clearance of theophylline, controlled studies have yielded inconsistent results regarding pharmacokinetic interactions between influenza vaccine and theophylline. Nevertheless, clinicians should consider the potential for an interaction when influenza vaccine is administered to persons receiving theophylline).
No products indexed under this heading.

Thioguanine (Immunosuppressive therapies, including antimetabolites, may reduce the immune response to vaccines). Products include:
Tabloid **1664**

Thiotepa (Immunosuppressive therapies, including alkylating agents, may reduce the immune response to vaccines).
No products indexed under this heading.

Tinzaparin Sodium (Influenza vaccinations should not be given to persons on anticoagulant therapy unless the potential benefit clearly outweighs the risk of administration. If the decision is made to administer an influenza vaccination to such persons, steps should be considered to control the risk of hematoma following the injection).
No products indexed under this heading.

Triamcinolone (Immunosuppressive therapies, including corticosteroids (used in greater than physiologic doses), may reduce the immune response to vaccines).
No products indexed under this heading.

Triamcinolone Acetonide (Immunosuppressive therapies, including corticosteroids (used in greater than physiologic doses), may reduce the immune response to vaccines). Products include:
Azmacort **408**
Nasacort AQ **3019**

Triamcinolone Diacetate (Immunosuppressive therapies, including corticosteroids (used in greater than physiologic doses), may reduce the immune response to vaccines).
No products indexed under this heading.

Triamcinolone Hexacetonide (Immunosuppressive therapies, including corticosteroids (used in greater than physiologic doses), may reduce the immune response to vaccines).
No products indexed under this heading.

Vinblastine Sulfate (Immunosuppressive therapies, including cytotoxic drugs, may reduce the immune response to vaccines).
No products indexed under this heading.

Vincristine Sulfate (Immunosuppressive therapies, including cytotoxic drugs, may reduce the immune response to vaccines).
No products indexed under this heading.

Vinorelbine Tartrate (Immunosuppressive therapies, including cytotoxic drugs, may reduce the immune response to vaccines).
No products indexed under this heading.

Warfarin Sodium (Although it has been reported that influenza vaccination may inhibit the clearance of warfarin, controlled studies have yielded inconsistent results regarding pharmacokinetic interactions between influenza vaccine and warfarin. Nevertheless, clinicians should consider the potential for an interaction when influenza vaccine is administered to persons receiving warfarin).
No products indexed under this heading.

FLULAVAL INJECTION VACCINE

(Influenza Virus Vaccine) **1479**
See Fluarix Vaccine

FLUMIST VACCINE

(Influenza Virus Vaccine Live, Intranasal) **2078**
May interact with alkylating agents, antimetabolites, antivirals active against influenza, aspirin-acetylsalicylic acid, corticosteroids, immunosuppressive agents, killed/inactivated vaccines, and certain other agents. Compounds in these categories include:

Alclometasone Dipropionate (Administration of FluMist, a live virus vaccine, to immunocompromised persons should be based on careful consideration of potential benefits and risk).
No products indexed under this heading.

Amantadine Hydrochloride (The concurrent use of FluMist with antiviral agents that are active against influenza A and/or B viruses has not been evaluated. However, base upon the potential for antiviral agents to reduce the effectiveness of FluMist, do not administer FluMist until 48 hours after the cessation of antiviral therapy and antiviral agents should not be administered until two weeks after administration of FluMist unless medically indicated. If antiviral agents and Flumist are administered concomitantly, revaccination should be considered when appropriate).
No products indexed under this heading.

Arginine (FluMist is contraindicated in individuals with history of hypersensitivity, especially anaphylactic reactions, to arginine). Products include:
VasoRect Formula **851**

Aspirin (FluMist is contraindicated in children and adolescents (2-17 years of age) receiving aspirin therapy or aspirin-containing therapy, because of the association of Reye's syndrome with aspirin and wild-type influenza infection). Products include:
Aggrenox **880**
Bayer Aspirin **829**
Percodan **1124**
St. Joseph Aspirin **2045**

Aspirin, Enteric Coated (FluMist is contraindicated in children and adolescents (2-17 years of age) receiving aspirin therapy or aspirin-containing therapy, because of the association of Reye's syndrome with aspirin and wild-type influenza infection).
No products indexed under this heading.

Aspirin Buffered (FluMist is contraindicated in children and adolescents (2-17 years of age) receiving aspirin therapy or aspirin-containing therapy, because of the association of Reye's syndrome with aspirin and wild-type influenza infection).
No products indexed under this heading.

Azathioprine (Administration of FluMist, a live virus vaccine, to immunocompromised persons should be based on careful consideration of potential benefits and risks).
No products indexed under this heading.

Basiliximab (Administration of FluMist, a live virus vaccine, to immunocompromised persons should be based on careful consideration of potential benefits and risks). Products include:
Simulect **2524**

Beclomethasone Dipropionate (Administration of FluMist, a live virus vaccine, to immunocompromised persons should be based on careful consideration of potential benefits and risk). Products include:
Qvar **3398**

Beclomethasone Dipropionate Monohydrate (Administration of FluMist, a live virus vaccine, to immunocompromised persons should be based on careful consideration of potential benefits and risk). Products include:
Beconase AQ **1386**

Betamethasone (Administration of FluMist, a live virus vaccine, to immunocompromised persons should be based on careful consideration of potential benefits and risk).
No products indexed under this heading.

Betamethasone Acetate (Administration of FluMist, a live virus vaccine, to immunocompromised persons should be based on careful consideration of potential benefits and risk).
No products indexed under this heading.

Betamethasone Benzoate (Administration of FluMist, a live virus vaccine, to immunocompromised persons should be based on careful consideration of potential benefits and risk).
No products indexed under this heading.

(⊙ Described in PDR® for Ophthalmic Medicines)

IMPORTANT NOTE: Always consult each drug listing in the patient's regimen for possible interactions.

FluMist Interactions Index 702

have not been determined. Studies of FluMist excluded subjects who received any inactivated or subunit vaccine within two weeks of enrollment. Therefore, healthcare providers should consider the risk and benefits of concurrent administration of Flumist with inactivated vaccines).
No products indexed under this heading.

L-Arginine (FluMist is contraindicated in individuals with history of hypersensitivity, especially anaphylactic reactions, to arginine). Products include:
Cardio Basics 3455

Lomustine (CCNU) (Administration of Flumist, a live virus vaccine, to immunocompromised persons should be based on careful consideration of potential benefits and risks).
No products indexed under this heading.

Mechlorethamine Hydrochloride (Administration of Flumist, a live virus vaccine, to immunocompromised persons should be based on careful consideration of potential benefits and risks). Products include:
Mustargen 2010

Melphalan (Administration of Flumist, a live virus vaccine, to immunocompromised persons should be based on careful consideration of potential benefits and risks). Products include:
Alkeran 1302

Mercaptopurine (Administration of Flumist, a live virus vaccine, to immunocompromised persons should be based on careful consideration of potential benefits and risks).
No products indexed under this heading.

Methotrexate (Administration of Flumist, a live virus vaccine, to immunocompromised persons should be based on careful consideration of potential benefits and risks).
No products indexed under this heading.

Methotrexate Sodium (Administration of Flumist, a live virus vaccine, to immunocompromised persons should be based on careful consideration of potential benefits and risks).
No products indexed under this heading.

Methylprednisolone (Administration of FluMist, a live virus vaccine, to immunocompromised persons should be based on careful consideration of potential benefits and risk).
No products indexed under this heading.

Methylprednisolone Acetate (Administration of FluMist, a live virus vaccine, to immunocompromised persons should be based on careful consideration of potential benefits and risk).
No products indexed under this heading.

Methylprednisolone Sodium Succinate (Administration of FluMist, a live virus vaccine, to immunocompromised persons should be based on careful consideration of potential benefits and risk).
No products indexed under this heading.

Mometasone Furoate (Administration of FluMist, a live virus vaccine, to immunocompromised persons should be based on careful consideration of potential benefits and risk). Products include:
Asmanex 3058
Elocon Cream 3111
Elocon Lotion 3112
Elocon Ointment 3114

Mometasone Furoate Monohydrate (Administration of FluMist, a live virus vaccine, to immunocompromised persons should be based on careful consideration of potential benefits and risk). Products include:
Nasonex 3166

Muromonab-CD3 (Administration of FluMist, a live virus vaccine, to immunocompromised persons should be based on careful consideration of potential benefits and risks). Products include:
Orthoclone OKT3 949

Mycophenolate Mofetil (Administration of FluMist, a live virus vaccine, to immunocompromised persons should be based on careful consideration of potential benefits and risks).
No products indexed under this heading.

Oseltamivir Phosphate (The concurrent use of FluMist with antiviral agents that are active against influenza A and/or B viruses has not been evaluated. However, base upon the potential for antiviral agents to reduce the effectiveness of FluMist, do not administer FluMist until 48 hours after the cessation of antiviral therapy and antiviral agents should not be administered until two weeks after administration of FluMist unless medically indicated. If antiviral agents and Flumist are administered concomitantly, revaccination should be considered when appropriate). Products include:
Tamiflu Capsules 2867
Tamiflu Oral 2867

Pentostatin (Administration of Flumist, a live virus vaccine, to immunocompromised persons should be based on careful consideration of potential benefits and risks).
No products indexed under this heading.

Pneumococcal vaccine, diphtheria conjugate (The safety and immunogenicity of Flumist when administered concurrently with inactivated vaccines have not been determined. Studies of FluMist excluded subjects who received any inactivated or subunit vaccine within two weeks of enrollment. Therefore, healthcare providers should consider the risk and benefits of concurrent administration of Flumist with inactivated vaccines). Products include:
Prevnar 3557

Pneumococcal Vaccine, Polyvalent (The safety and immunogenicity of Flumist when administered concurrently with inactivated vaccines have not been determined. Studies of FluMist excluded subjects who received any inactivated or subunit vaccine within two weeks of enrollment. Therefore, healthcare providers should consider the risk and benefits of concurrent administration of Flumist with inactivated vaccines). Products include:
Pneumovax 23 2230

Poliovirus Vaccine Inactivated (The safety and immunogenicity of Flumist when administered concurrently with inactivated vaccines have not been determined. Studies of FluMist excluded subjects who received any inactivated or subunit vaccine within two weeks of enrollment. Therefore, healthcare providers should consider the risk and benefits of concurrent administration of Flumist with inactivated vaccines). Products include:
Pediarix 1606

Prednisolone (Administration of FluMist, a live virus vaccine, to immunocompromised persons should be based on careful consideration of potential benefits and risk).
No products indexed under this heading.

Prednisolone Acetate (Administration of FluMist, a live virus vaccine, to immunocompromised persons should be based on careful consideration of potential benefits and risk). Products include:
Blephamide .... ⊙212, ⊙214
Pred Forte .... ⊙225
Pred Mild .... ⊙230
Pred-G .... ⊙226, ⊙227

Prednisolone Sodium Phosphate (Administration of FluMist, a live virus vaccine, to immunocompromised persons should be based on careful consideration of potential benefits and risk).
No products indexed under this heading.

Prednisolone Tebutate (Administration of FluMist, a live virus vaccine, to immunocompromised persons should be based on careful consideration of potential benefits and risk).
No products indexed under this heading.

Prednisone (Administration of FluMist, a live virus vaccine, to immunocompromised persons should be based on careful consideration of potential benefits and risk).
No products indexed under this heading.

Prednisone sodium phosphate (Administration of FluMist, a live virus vaccine, to immunocompromised persons should be based on careful consideration of potential benefits and risk).
No products indexed under this heading.

Rapamycin (Administration of FluMist, a live virus vaccine, to immunocompromised persons should be based on careful consideration of potential benefits and risk).
No products indexed under this heading.

Rimantadine Hydrochloride (The concurrent use of FluMist with antiviral agents that are active against influenza A and/or B viruses has not been evaluated. However, base upon the potential for antiviral agents to reduce the effectiveness of FluMist, do not administer FluMist until 48 hours after the cessation of antiviral therapy and antiviral agents should not be administered until two weeks after administration of FluMist unless medically indicated. If antiviral agents and Flumist are administered concomitantly, revaccination should be considered when appropriate).
No products indexed under this heading.

Sirolimus (Administration of FluMist, a live virus vaccine, to immunocompromised persons should be based on careful consideration of potential benefits and risks). Products include:
Rapamune 3579

Tacrolimus (Administration of FluMist, a live virus vaccine, to immunocompromised persons should be based on careful consideration of potential benefits and risks). Products include:
Prograf Capsules 677
Prograf Injection 677
Protopic 685

Thioguanine (Administration of Flumist, a live virus vaccine, to immunocompromised persons should be based on careful consideration of potential benefits and risks). Products include:
Tabloid 1664

Thiotepa (Administration of Flumist, a live virus vaccine, to immunocompromised persons should be based on careful consideration of potential benefits and risks).
No products indexed under this heading.

Triamcinolone (Administration of FluMist, a live virus vaccine, to immunocompromised persons should be based on careful consideration of potential benefits and risk).
No products indexed under this heading.

Triamcinolone Acetonide (Administration of FluMist, a live virus vaccine, to immunocompromised persons should be based on careful consideration of potential benefits and risk). Products include:
Azmacort 408
Nasacort AQ 3019

Triamcinolone Diacetate (Administration of FluMist, a live virus vaccine, to immunocompromised persons should be based on careful consideration of potential benefits and risk).
No products indexed under this heading.

Triamcinolone Hexacetonide (Administration of FluMist, a live virus vaccine, to immunocompromised persons should be based on careful consideration of potential benefits and risk).
No products indexed under this heading.

Zanamivir (The concurrent use of FluMist with antiviral agents that are active against influenza A and/or B viruses has not been evaluated. However, base upon the potential for antiviral agents to reduce the effectiveness of FluMist, do not administer FluMist until 48 hours after the cessation of antiviral therapy and antiviral agents should not be administered until two weeks after administration of FluMist unless medically indicated. If antiviral agents and Flumist are administered concomitantly, revaccination should be considered when appropriate). Products include:
Relenza 1615

Food Interactions

Egg Product (FluMist is contraindicated in individuals with history of hypersensitivity, especially anaphylactic reactions, to eggs and egg proteins).

Eggs (FluMist is contraindicated in individuals with history of hypersensitivity, especially anaphylactic reactions, to eggs and egg proteins).

FML OPHTHALMIC OINTMENT

(Fluorometholone) .... ⊙219
None cited in PDR database.

FML OPHTHALMIC SUSPENSION

(Fluorometholone) .... ⊙220
None cited in PDR database.

FML FORTE OPHTHALMIC SUSPENSION

(Fluorometholone) .... ⊙221
None cited in PDR database.

FOCALIN XR CAPSULES

(Dexmethylphenidate Hydrochloride) 2472
May interact with alcohols, antacids, anticonvulsants, antihypertensives, drugs that reduce gastric acidity, monoamine oxidase inhibitors, oral anticoagulants, phenytoin, tricyclic antidepressants, vasopressors, vitamin K antagonists, and certain other agents. Compounds in these categories include:

Acebutolol Hydrochloride (Methylphenidate may decrease the effectiveness of drugs used to treat hypertension).
No products indexed under this heading.

Aliskiren (Methylphenidate may decrease the effectiveness of drugs used to treat hypertension). Products include:
Tekturna 2538
Tekturna HCT 2541
Valturna 3637

Aluminum Carbonate (Since the modified release characteristics of dexmethylphenidate are pH dependent, the co-administration of antacids or acid suppressants could alter the release of dexmethylphenidate).
No products indexed under this heading.

Aluminum Hydroxide (Since the modified release characteristics of dexmethylphenidate are pH dependent, the co-administration of antacids or acid suppressants could alter the release of dexmethylphenidate).
No products indexed under this heading.

(⊙ Described in PDR® for Ophthalmic Medicines)

Amitriptyline Hydrochloride (Racemic methylphenidate may inhibit the metabolism of tricyclic drugs (eg, imipramine, clomipramine, desipramine). Downward dose adjustments of these drugs may be required when given concomitantly with methylphenidate. It may be necessary to adjust the dosage and monitor plasma drug concentration, when initiating or discontinuing methylphenidate).
No products indexed under this heading.

Amlodipine Besylate (Methylphenidate may decrease the effectiveness of drugs used to treat hypertension). Products include:
Azor 1010
Exforge 2443
Exforge HCT 2449

Amoxapine (Racemic methylphenidate may inhibit the metabolism of tricyclic drugs (eg, imipramine, clomipramine, desipramine). Downward dose adjustments of these drugs may be required when given concomitantly with methylphenidate. It may be necessary to adjust the dosage and monitor plasma drug concentration, when initiating or discontinuing methylphenidate).
No products indexed under this heading.

Anisindione (Human pharmacologic studies have shown that racemic methylphenidate may inhibit the metabolism of coumarin anticoagulants. Downward dose adjustments of these drugs may be required when given concomitantly with methylphenidate. It may be necessary to adjust the dosage and monitor plasma drug concentration (or, in the case of coumarin, coagulation times), when initiating or discontinuing methylphenidate).
No products indexed under this heading.

Atenolol (Methylphenidate may decrease the effectiveness of drugs used to treat hypertension).
No products indexed under this heading.

Benazepril Hydrochloride (Methylphenidate may decrease the effectiveness of drugs used to treat hypertension).
No products indexed under this heading.

Bendroflumethiazide (Methylphenidate may decrease the effectiveness of drugs used to treat hypertension).
No products indexed under this heading.

Betaxolol Hydrochloride (Methylphenidate may decrease the effectiveness of drugs used to treat hypertension).
No products indexed under this heading.

Bisoprolol Fumarate (Methylphenidate may decrease the effectiveness of drugs used to treat hypertension).
No products indexed under this heading.

Calcium Carbonate (Since the modified release characteristics of dexmethylphenidate are pH dependent, the co-administration of antacids or acid suppressants could alter the release of dexmethylphenidate). Products include:
Chelated Mineral 3476
Pepcid Complete 1822
Extra Strength Rolaids Softchews Vanilla Creme 2045

Candesartan Cilexetil (Methylphenidate may decrease the effectiveness of drugs used to treat hypertension). Products include:
Atacand 697
Atacand HCT 700

Captopril (Methylphenidate may decrease the effectiveness of drugs used to treat hypertension). Products include:
Captopril 2341

Carbamazepine (Racemic methylphenidate may inhibit the metabolism of anticonvulsants (eg, phenobarbital, phenytoin, primidone). Downward dose

adjustments of these drugs may be required when given concomitantly with methylphenidate. It may be necessary to adjust the dosage and monitor plasma drug concentration, when initiating or discontinuing methylphenidate).
Products include:
Carbatrol 3280
Equetro 3477

Carteolol Hydrochloride (Methylphenidate may decrease the effectiveness of drugs used to treat hypertension).
No products indexed under this heading.

Carvedilol (Methylphenidate may decrease the effectiveness of drugs used to treat hypertension). Products include:
Coreg 1409

Carvedilol Phosphate (Methylphenidate may decrease the effectiveness of drugs used to treat hypertension).
Products include:
Coreg CR 1416

Chlorothiazide (Methylphenidate may decrease the effectiveness of drugs used to treat hypertension).
No products indexed under this heading.

Chlorothiazide Sodium (Methylphenidate may decrease the effectiveness of drugs used to treat hypertension). Products include:
Diuril Intravenous 2009

Chlorthalidone (Methylphenidate may decrease the effectiveness of drugs used to treat hypertension). Products include:
Clorpres 2344

Cimetidine (Since the modified release characteristics of dexmethylphenidate are pH dependent, the co-administration of antacids or acid suppressants could alter the release of dexmethylphenidate).
No products indexed under this heading.

Cimetidine Hydrochloride (Since the modified release characteristics of dexmethylphenidate are pH dependent, the co-administration of antacids or acid suppressants could alter the release of dexmethylphenidate).
No products indexed under this heading.

Clomipramine Hydrochloride (Racemic methylphenidate may inhibit the metabolism of tricyclic drugs (eg, imipramine, clomipramine, desipramine). Downward dose adjustments of these drugs may be required when given concomitantly with methylphenidate. It may be necessary to adjust the dosage and monitor plasma drug concentration, when initiating or discontinuing methylphenidate).
No products indexed under this heading.

Clonidine (Serious adverse events have been reported in concomitant use with clonidine, although no causality for the combination has been established. The safety of using methylphenidate in combination with clonidine has not been systematically evaluated). Products include:
Catapres-TTS 884

Clonidine Hydrochloride (Serious adverse events have been reported in concomitant use with clonidine, although no causality for the combination has been established. The safety of using methylphenidate in combination with clonidine has not been systematically evaluated). Products include:
Clorpres 2344

Deserpidine (Methylphenidate may decrease the effectiveness of drugs used to treat hypertension).
No products indexed under this heading.

Desipramine Hydrochloride (Racemic methylphenidate may inhibit the metabolism of tricyclic drugs (eg, imipramine, clomipramine, desipramine). Downward dose adjustments of these drugs may be required when given concomitantly with methylphenidate. It may be necessary to adjust the dosage and monitor plasma drug concentration, when initiating or discontinuing methylphenidate).
No products indexed under this heading.

Diazoxide (Methylphenidate may decrease the effectiveness of drugs used to treat hypertension). Products include:
Proglycem 1179
Proglycem Suspension 1179

Dicumarol (Racemic methylphenidate may inhibit the metabolism of coumarin anticoagulants. Downward dose adjustments of these drugs may be required when given concomitantly with methylphenidate. It may be necessary to adjust the dosage and monitor plasma drug concentration (or, in the case of coumarin, coagulation times), when initiating or discontinuing methylphenidate).
No products indexed under this heading.

Diltiazem Hydrochloride (Methylphenidate may decrease the effectiveness of drugs used to treat hypertension). Products include:
Cardizem LA 423

Diltiazem Maleate (Methylphenidate may decrease the effectiveness of drugs used to treat hypertension).
No products indexed under this heading.

Divalproex Sodium (Racemic methylphenidate may inhibit the metabolism of anticonvulsants (eg, phenobarbital, phenytoin, primidone). Downward dose adjustments of these drugs may be required when given concomitantly with methylphenidate. It may be necessary to adjust the dosage and monitor plasma drug concentration, when initiating or discontinuing methylphenidate).
Products include:
Depakote ER 426

Dobutamine (Because of possible effects on blood pressure, dexmethylphenidate should be used cautiously with pressor agents).
No products indexed under this heading.

Dobutamine Hydrochloride (Because of possible effects on blood pressure, dexmethylphenidate should be used cautiously with pressor agents).
No products indexed under this heading.

Dopamine Hydrochloride (Because of possible effects on blood pressure, dexmethylphenidate should be used cautiously with pressor agents).
No products indexed under this heading.

Doxazosin Mesylate (Methylphenidate may decrease the effectiveness of drugs used to treat hypertension).
No products indexed under this heading.

Doxepin Hydrochloride (Racemic methylphenidate may inhibit the metabolism of tricyclic drugs (eg, imipramine, clomipramine, desipramine). Downward dose adjustments of these drugs may be required when given concomitantly with methylphenidate. It may be necessary to adjust the dosage and monitor plasma drug concentration, when initiating or discontinuing methylphenidate).
No products indexed under this heading.

Enalapril Maleate (Methylphenidate may decrease the effectiveness of drugs used to treat hypertension).
No products indexed under this heading.

Enalaprilat (Methylphenidate may decrease the effectiveness of drugs used to treat hypertension).
No products indexed under this heading.

Ephedrine Sulfate (Because of possible effects on blood pressure, dexmethylphenidate should be used cautiously with pressor agents).
No products indexed under this heading.

Epinephrine Bitartrate (Because of possible effects on blood pressure, dexmethylphenidate should be used cautiously with pressor agents).
No products indexed under this heading.

Epinephrine Hydrochloride (Because of possible effects on blood pressure, dexmethylphenidate should be used cautiously with pressor agents).
No products indexed under this heading.

Eprosartan Mesylate (Methylphenidate may decrease the effectiveness of drugs used to treat hypertension). Products include:
Teveten 538
Teveten HCT 541

Esmolol Hydrochloride (Methylphenidate may decrease the effectiveness of drugs used to treat hypertension).
No products indexed under this heading.

Esomeprazole Magnesium (Since the modified release characteristics of dexmethylphenidate are pH dependent, the co-administration of antacids or acid suppressants could alter the release of dexmethylphenidate). Products include:
Nexium Capsules 704
Nexium Oral Suspension 704

Ethanol (Dexmethylphenidate hydrochloride should be given cautiously to patients with a history of drug dependence or alcoholism).
No products indexed under this heading.

Ethosuximide (Racemic methylphenidate may inhibit the metabolism of anticonvulsants (eg, phenobarbital, phenytoin, primidone). Downward dose adjustments of these drugs may be required when given concomitantly with methylphenidate. It may be necessary to adjust the dosage and monitor plasma drug concentration, when initiating or discontinuing methylphenidate).
No products indexed under this heading.

Ethotoin (Racemic methylphenidate may inhibit the metabolism of anticonvulsants (eg, phenobarbital, phenytoin, primidone). Downward dose adjustments of these drugs may be required when given concomitantly with methylphenidate. It may be necessary to adjust the dosage and monitor plasma drug concentration, when initiating or discontinuing methylphenidate).
No products indexed under this heading.

Ethyl Alcohol (Dexmethylphenidate hydrochloride should be given cautiously to patients with a history of drug dependence or alcoholism).
No products indexed under this heading.

Famotidine (Since the modified release characteristics of dexmethylphenidate are pH dependent, the co-administration of antacids or acid suppressants could alter the release of dexmethylphenidate). Products include:
Pepcid 2227
Original Strength Pepcid AC Gelcaps 1821
Original Strength Pepcid AC ... 1821
Maximum Strength Pepcid AC .. 1821
Pepcid Complete 1822

Fat (No food effect study was performed with Focalin XR. However, the effect of food has been studied in adults with racemic methylphenidate in the same type of extended-release formulation. The findings of that study are considered applicable to Focalin XR. After a high fat breakfast, there was a longer lag time until absorption began and variable delays in the time until the first peak concentration, the time until the interpeak minimum, and the time until the second peak. The first peak

concentration and the extent of absorption were unchanged after food relative to the fasting state, although the second peak was approximately 25% lower).

No products indexed under this heading.

Felbamate (Racemic methylphenidate may inhibit the metabolism of anticonvulsants (eg, phenobarbital, phenytoin, primidone). Downward dose adjustments of these drugs may be required when given concomitantly with methylphenidate. It may be necessary to adjust the dosage and monitor plasma drug concentration, when initiating or discontinuing methylphenidate).

No products indexed under this heading.

Felodipine (Methylphenidate may decrease the effectiveness of drugs used to treat hypertension).

No products indexed under this heading.

Fosinopril Sodium (Methylphenidate may decrease the effectiveness of drugs used to treat hypertension).

No products indexed under this heading.

Fosphenytoin (Racemic methylphenidate may inhibit the metabolism of anticonvulsants (eg, phenobarbital, phenytoin, primidone). Downward dose adjustments of these drugs may be required when given concomitantly with methylphenidate. It may be necessary to adjust the dosage and monitor plasma drug concentration, when initiating or discontinuing methylphenidate).

No products indexed under this heading.

Fosphenytoin Sodium (Racemic methylphenidate may inhibit the metabolism of anticonvulsants (eg, phenobarbital, phenytoin, primidone). Downward dose adjustments of these drugs may be required when given concomitantly with methylphenidate. It may be necessary to adjust the dosage and monitor plasma drug concentration, when initiating or discontinuing methylphenidate).

No products indexed under this heading.

Furosemide (Methylphenidate may decrease the effectiveness of drugs used to treat hypertension). Products include:

Furosemide 2354

Gabapentin (Racemic methylphenidate may inhibit the metabolism of anticonvulsants (eg, phenobarbital, phenytoin, primidone). Downward dose adjustments of these drugs may be required when given concomitantly with methylphenidate. It may be necessary to adjust the dosage and monitor plasma drug concentration, when initiating or discontinuing methylphenidate).

No products indexed under this heading.

Guanabenz Acetate (Methylphenidate may decrease the effectiveness of drugs used to treat hypertension).

No products indexed under this heading.

Guanethidine (Methylphenidate may decrease the effectiveness of drugs used to treat hypertension).

No products indexed under this heading.

Guanethidine Monosulfate (Methylphenidate may decrease the effectiveness of drugs used to treat hypertension).

No products indexed under this heading.

Guanethidine Sulfate (Methylphenidate may decrease the effectiveness of drugs used to treat hypertension).

No products indexed under this heading.

Hydralazine Hydrochloride (Methylphenidate may decrease the effectiveness of drugs used to treat hypertension).

No products indexed under this heading.

Hydrochlorothiazide (Methylphenidate may decrease the effectiveness of drugs used to treat hypertension). Products include:

Hydroflumethiazide (Methylphenidate may decrease the effectiveness of drugs used to treat hypertension).

No products indexed under this heading.

Imipramine Hydrochloride (Racemic methylphenidate may inhibit the metabolism of tricyclic drugs (eg, imipramine, clomipramine, desipramine). Downward dose adjustments of these drugs may be required when given concomitantly with methylphenidate. It may be necessary to adjust the dosage and monitor plasma drug concentration, when initiating or discontinuing methylphenidate).

No products indexed under this heading.

Imipramine Pamoate (Racemic methylphenidate may inhibit the metabolism of tricyclic drugs (eg, imipramine, clomipramine, desipramine). Downward dose adjustments of these drugs may be required when given concomitantly with methylphenidate. It may be necessary to adjust the dosage and monitor plasma drug concentration, when initiating or discontinuing methylphenidate).

No products indexed under this heading.

Indapamide (Methylphenidate may decrease the effectiveness of drugs used to treat hypertension). Products include:

Irbesartan (Methylphenidate may decrease the effectiveness of drugs used to treat hypertension). Products include:

Isocarboxazid (Dexmethylphenidate is contraindicated during treatment with monoamine oxidase inhibitors, and also within a minimum of 14 days following discontinuation of treatment with a monoamine oxidase inhibitor (hypertensive crises may result)). Products include:

Isoproterenol Hydrochloride (Because of possible effects on blood pressure, dexmethylphenidate should be used cautiously with pressor agents).

No products indexed under this heading.

Isoproterenol Sulfate (Because of possible effects on blood pressure, dexmethylphenidate should be used cautiously with pressor agents).

No products indexed under this heading.

Isradipine (Methylphenidate may decrease the effectiveness of drugs used to treat hypertension). Products include:

Labetalol Hydrochloride (Methylphenidate may decrease the effectiveness of drugs used to treat hypertension).

No products indexed under this heading.

Lamotrigine (Racemic methylphenidate may inhibit the metabolism of anticonvulsants (eg, phenobarbital, phenytoin, primidone). Downward dose adjustments of these drugs may be required when given concomitantly with methylphenidate. It may be necessary to adjust the dosage and monitor plasma drug concentration, when initiating or discontinuing methylphenidate). Products include:

Lansoprazole (Since the modified release characteristics of dexmethylphenidate are pH dependent, the co-administration of antacids or acid suppressants could alter the release of dexmethylphenidate).

No products indexed under this heading.

Levetiracetam (Racemic methylphenidate may inhibit the metabolism of anticonvulsants (eg, phenobarbital, phenytoin, primidone). Downward dose adjustments of these drugs may be required when given concomitantly with methylphenidate. It may be necessary to adjust the dosage and monitor plasma drug concentration, when initiating or discontinuing methylphenidate). Products include:

Lisinopril (Methylphenidate may decrease the effectiveness of drugs used to treat hypertension). Products include:

Losartan Potassium (Methylphenidate may decrease the effectiveness of drugs used to treat hypertension). Products include:

Magaldrate (Since the modified release characteristics of dexmethylphenidate are pH dependent, the co-administration of antacids or acid suppressants could alter the release of dexmethylphenidate).

No products indexed under this heading.

Magnesium Carbonate (Since the modified release characteristics of dexmethylphenidate are pH dependent, the co-administration of antacids or acid suppressants could alter the release of dexmethylphenidate).

No products indexed under this heading.

Magnesium Hydroxide (Since the modified release characteristics of dexmethylphenidate are pH dependent, the co-administration of antacids or acid suppressants could alter the release of dexmethylphenidate). Products include:

Magnesium Oxide (Since the modified release characteristics of dexmethylphenidate are pH dependent, the co-administration of antacids or acid suppressants could alter the release of dexmethylphenidate). Products include:

Magnesium Trisilicate (Since the modified release characteristics of dexmethylphenidate are pH dependent, the co-administration of antacids or acid suppressants could alter the release of dexmethylphenidate).

No products indexed under this heading.

Maprotiline Hydrochloride (Racemic methylphenidate may inhibit the metabolism of tricyclic drugs (eg, imipramine, clomipramine, desipramine). Downward dose adjustments of these drugs may be required when given concomitantly with methylphenidate. It may be necessary to adjust the dosage and monitor plasma drug concentration, when initiating or discontinuing methylphenidate).

No products indexed under this heading.

Mecamylamine Hydrochloride (Methylphenidate may decrease the effectiveness of drugs used to treat hypertension).

No products indexed under this heading.

Mephentermine Sulfate (Because of possible effects on blood pressure, dexmethylphenidate should be used cautiously with pressor agents).

No products indexed under this heading.

Mephenytoin (Racemic methylphenidate may inhibit the metabolism of anticonvulsants (eg, phenobarbital, phenytoin, primidone). Downward dose adjustments of these drugs may be required when given concomitantly with methylphenidate. It may be necessary to adjust the dosage and monitor plasma drug concentration, when initiating or discontinuing methylphenidate).

No products indexed under this heading.

Metaraminol Bitartrate (Because of possible effects on blood pressure, dexmethylphenidate should be used cautiously with pressor agents).

No products indexed under this heading.

Methoxamine Hydrochloride (Because of possible effects on blood pressure, dexmethylphenidate should be used cautiously with pressor agents).

No products indexed under this heading.

Methsuximide (Racemic methylphenidate may inhibit the metabolism of anticonvulsants (eg, phenobarbital, phenytoin, primidone). Downward dose adjustments of these drugs may be required when given concomitantly with methylphenidate. It may be necessary to adjust the dosage and monitor plasma drug concentration, when initiating or discontinuing methylphenidate).

No products indexed under this heading.

Methyclothiazide (Methylphenidate may decrease the effectiveness of drugs used to treat hypertension).

No products indexed under this heading.

Methyldopa (Methylphenidate may decrease the effectiveness of drugs used to treat hypertension).

No products indexed under this heading.

Methyldopate Hydrochloride (Methylphenidate may decrease the effectiveness of drugs used to treat hypertension).

No products indexed under this heading.

Metolazone (Methylphenidate may decrease the effectiveness of drugs used to treat hypertension).

No products indexed under this heading.

Metoprolol Succinate (Methylphenidate may decrease the effectiveness of drugs used to treat hypertension). Products include:

Metoprolol Tartrate (Methylphenidate may decrease the effectiveness of drugs used to treat hypertension).

No products indexed under this heading.

Metyrosine (Methylphenidate may decrease the effectiveness of drugs used to treat hypertension).

No products indexed under this heading.

Mibefradil Dihydrochloride (Methylphenidate may decrease the effectiveness of drugs used to treat hypertension).

No products indexed under this heading.

Minoxidil (Methylphenidate may decrease the effectiveness of drugs used to treat hypertension).

No products indexed under this heading.

Moclobemide (Dexmethylphenidate is contraindicated during treatment with monoamine oxidase inhibitors, and also within a minimum of 14 days following discontinuation of treatment with a monoamine oxidase inhibitor (hypertensive crises may result)).

No products indexed under this heading.

Moexipril Hydrochloride (Methylphenidate may decrease the effectiveness of drugs used to treat hypertension).

No products indexed under this heading.

705 Interactions Index Focalin

Nadolol (Methylphenidate may decrease the effectiveness of drugs used to treat hypertension). Products include:
Nadolol ... 2359

Nebivolol (Methylphenidate may decrease the effectiveness of drugs used to treat hypertension). Products include:
Bystolic ... 1147

Nicardipine Hydrochloride (Methylphenidate may decrease the effectiveness of drugs used to treat hypertension).
No products indexed under this heading.

Nifedipine (Methylphenidate may decrease the effectiveness of drugs used to treat hypertension).
No products indexed under this heading.

Nisoldipine (Methylphenidate may decrease the effectiveness of drugs used to treat hypertension).
No products indexed under this heading.

Nitroglycerin (Methylphenidate may decrease the effectiveness of drugs used to treat hypertension). Products include:
Nitro-Dur ... 3170
Nitrolingual ... 3266

Nizatidine (Since the modified release characteristics of dexmethylphenidate are pH dependent, the co-administration of antacids or acid suppressants could alter the release of dexmethylphenidate). Products include:
Axid ... 1381

Norepinephrine Bitartrate (Because of possible effects on blood pressure, dexmethylphenidate should be used cautiously with pressor agents).
No products indexed under this heading.

Nortriptyline Hydrochloride (Racemic methylphenidate may inhibit the metabolism of tricyclic drugs (eg, imipramine, clomipramine, desipramine). Downward dose adjustments of these drugs may be required when given concomitantly with methylphenidate. It may be necessary to adjust the dosage and monitor plasma drug concentration, when initiating or discontinuing methylphenidate).
No products indexed under this heading.

Omeprazole (Since the modified release characteristics of dexmethylphenidate are pH dependent, the co-administration of antacids or acid suppressants could alter the release of dexmethylphenidate).
No products indexed under this heading.

Oxcarbazepine (Racemic methylphenidate may inhibit the metabolism of anticonvulsants (eg, phenobarbital, phenytoin, primidone). Downward dose adjustments of these drugs may be required when given concomitantly with methylphenidate. It may be necessary to adjust the dosage and monitor plasma drug concentration, when initiating or discontinuing methylphenidate).
No products indexed under this heading.

Paramethadione (Racemic methylphenidate may inhibit the metabolism of anticonvulsants (eg, phenobarbital, phenytoin, primidone). Downward dose adjustments of these drugs may be required when given concomitantly with methylphenidate. It may be necessary to adjust the dosage and monitor plasma drug concentration, when initiating or discontinuing methylphenidate).
No products indexed under this heading.

Pargyline Hydrochloride (Dexmethylphenidate is contraindicated during treatment with monoamine oxidase inhibitors, and also within a minimum of 14 days following discontinuation of treatment with a monoamine oxidase inhibitor (hypertensive crises may result)).
No products indexed under this heading.

Penbutolol Sulfate (Methylphenidate may decrease the effectiveness of drugs used to treat hypertension).
No products indexed under this heading.

Perindopril Erbumine (Methylphenidate may decrease the effectiveness of drugs used to treat hypertension).
No products indexed under this heading.

Phenacemide (Racemic methylphenidate may inhibit the metabolism of anticonvulsants (eg, phenobarbital, phenytoin, primidone). Downward dose adjustments of these drugs may be required when given concomitantly with methylphenidate. It may be necessary to adjust the dosage and monitor plasma drug concentration, when initiating or discontinuing methylphenidate).
No products indexed under this heading.

Phenelzine Sulfate (Dexmethylphenidate is contraindicated during treatment with monoamine oxidase inhibitors, and also within a minimum of 14 days following discontinuation of treatment with a monoamine oxidase inhibitor (hypertensive crises may result)).
No products indexed under this heading.

Phenobarbital (Racemic methylphenidate may inhibit the metabolism of anticonvulsants (eg, phenobarbital, phenytoin, primidone). Downward dose adjustments of these drugs may be required when given concomitantly with methylphenidate. It may be necessary to adjust the dosage and monitor plasma drug concentration, when initiating or discontinuing methylphenidate). Products include:
Donnatal ... 2711

Phenobarbital Sodium (Racemic methylphenidate may inhibit the metabolism of anticonvulsants (eg, phenobarbital, phenytoin, primidone). Downward dose adjustments of these drugs may be required when given concomitantly with methylphenidate. It may be necessary to adjust the dosage and monitor plasma drug concentration, when initiating or discontinuing methylphenidate).
No products indexed under this heading.

Phenoxybenzamine Hydrochloride (Methylphenidate may decrease the effectiveness of drugs used to treat hypertension). Products include:
Dibenzyline ... 3495

Phensuximide (Racemic methylphenidate may inhibit the metabolism of anticonvulsants (eg, phenobarbital, phenytoin, primidone). Downward dose adjustments of these drugs may be required when given concomitantly with methylphenidate. It may be necessary to adjust the dosage and monitor plasma drug concentration, when initiating or discontinuing methylphenidate).
No products indexed under this heading.

Phentolamine Mesylate (Methylphenidate may decrease the effectiveness of drugs used to treat hypertension).
No products indexed under this heading.

Phenylephrine Hydrochloride (Because of possible effects on blood pressure, dexmethylphenidate should be used cautiously with pressor agents). Products include:
Sudafed PE Nasal Decongestant ... 2048
Children's Sudafed PE Nasal Decongestant ... 2047

Phenytoin (Racemic methylphenidate may inhibit the metabolism of anticonvulsants (eg, phenobarbital, phenytoin, primidone). Downward dose adjustments of these drugs may be required when given concomitantly with methylphenidate. It may be necessary to adjust the dosage and monitor plasma drug concentration, when initiating or discontinuing methylphenidate).
No products indexed under this heading.

Phenytoin Sodium (Racemic methylphenidate may inhibit the metabolism of anticonvulsants (eg, phenobarbital, phenytoin, primidone). Downward dose adjustments of these drugs may be required when given concomitantly with methylphenidate. It may be necessary to adjust the dosage and monitor plasma drug concentration, when initiating or discontinuing methylphenidate). Products include:
Phenytek Capsules ... 2380

Pindolol (Methylphenidate may decrease the effectiveness of drugs used to treat hypertension).
No products indexed under this heading.

Polythiazide (Methylphenidate may decrease the effectiveness of drugs used to treat hypertension).
No products indexed under this heading.

Prazosin Hydrochloride (Methylphenidate may decrease the effectiveness of drugs used to treat hypertension).
No products indexed under this heading.

Primidone (Racemic methylphenidate may inhibit the metabolism of anticonvulsants (eg, phenobarbital, phenytoin, primidone). Downward dose adjustments of these drugs may be required when given concomitantly with methylphenidate. It may be necessary to adjust the dosage and monitor plasma drug concentration, when initiating or discontinuing methylphenidate).
No products indexed under this heading.

Procarbazine Hydrochloride (Dexmethylphenidate is contraindicated during treatment with monoamine oxidase inhibitors, and also within a minimum of 14 days following discontinuation of treatment with a monoamine oxidase inhibitor (hypertensive crises may result)).
No products indexed under this heading.

Propranolol Hydrochloride (Methylphenidate may decrease the effectiveness of drugs used to treat hypertension). Products include:
InnoPran XL ... 1517

Protriptyline Hydrochloride (Racemic methylphenidate may inhibit the metabolism of tricyclic drugs (eg, imipramine, clomipramine, desipramine). Downward dose adjustments of these drugs may be required when given concomitantly with methylphenidate. It may be necessary to adjust the dosage and monitor plasma drug concentration, when initiating or discontinuing methylphenidate).
No products indexed under this heading.

Quinapril Hydrochloride (Methylphenidate may decrease the effectiveness of drugs used to treat hypertension).
No products indexed under this heading.

Rabeprazole Sodium (Since the modified release characteristics of dexmethylphenidate are pH dependent, the co-administration of antacids or acid suppressants could alter the release of dexmethylphenidate). Products include:
Aciphex ... 1035

Ramipril (Methylphenidate may decrease the effectiveness of drugs used to treat hypertension).
No products indexed under this heading.

Ranitidine Hydrochloride (Since the modified release characteristics of dexmethylphenidate are pH dependent, the co-administration of antacids or acid suppressants could alter the release of dexmethylphenidate). Products include:
Zantac ... 1737
Zantac Injection ... 1732
Zantac Pharmacy ... 1735

Rasagiline Mesylate (Dexmethylphenidate is contraindicated during treatment with monoamine oxidase inhibitors, and also within a minimum of 14 days following discontinuation of treatment with a monoamine oxidase inhibitor (hypertensive crises may result)). Products include:
Azilect ... 3383

Rauwolfia Serpentina (Methylphenidate may decrease the effectiveness of drugs used to treat hypertension).
No products indexed under this heading.

Rescinnamine (Methylphenidate may decrease the effectiveness of drugs used to treat hypertension).
No products indexed under this heading.

Reserpine (Methylphenidate may decrease the effectiveness of drugs used to treat hypertension).
No products indexed under this heading.

Rufinamide (Racemic methylphenidate may inhibit the metabolism of anticonvulsants (eg, phenobarbital, phenytoin, primidone). Downward dose adjustments of these drugs may be required when given concomitantly with methylphenidate. It may be necessary to adjust the dosage and monitor plasma drug concentration, when initiating or discontinuing methylphenidate). Products include:
Banzel ... 1050

Selegiline (Dexmethylphenidate is contraindicated during treatment with monoamine oxidase inhibitors, and also within a minimum of 14 days following discontinuation of treatment with a monoamine oxidase inhibitor (hypertensive crises may result)). Products include:
Emsam ... 3623

Selegiline Hydrochloride (Dexmethylphenidate is contraindicated during treatment with monoamine oxidase inhibitors, and also within a minimum of 14 days following discontinuation of treatment with a monoamine oxidase inhibitor (hypertensive crises may result)). Products include:
Eldepryl ... 3312

Sodium Bicarbonate (Since the modified release characteristics of dexmethylphenidate are pH dependent, the co-administration of antacids or acid suppressants could alter the release of dexmethylphenidate).
No products indexed under this heading.

Sodium Nitroprusside (Methylphenidate may decrease the effectiveness of drugs used to treat hypertension).
No products indexed under this heading.

Sotalol Hydrochloride (Methylphenidate may decrease the effectiveness of drugs used to treat hypertension).
No products indexed under this heading.

Spirapril Hydrochloride (Methylphenidate may decrease the effectiveness of drugs used to treat hypertension).
No products indexed under this heading.

Telmisartan (Methylphenidate may decrease the effectiveness of drugs used to treat hypertension). Products include:
Micardis ... 887
Micardis HCT ... 889

Terazosin Hydrochloride (Methylphenidate may decrease the effectiveness of drugs used to treat hypertension).
No products indexed under this heading.

Tiagabine Hydrochloride (Racemic methylphenidate may inhibit the metabolism of anticonvulsants (eg, phenobarbital, phenytoin, primidone). Downward

IMPORTANT NOTE: Always consult each drug listing in the patient's regimen for possible interactions.

dose adjustments of these drugs may be required when given concomitantly with methylphenidate. It may be necessary to adjust the dosage and monitor plasma drug concentration, when initiating or discontinuing methylphenidate). Products include:

Timolol Maleate (Methylphenidate may decrease the effectiveness of drugs used to treat hypertension). Products include:

Topiramate (Racemic methylphenidate may inhibit the metabolism of anticonvulsants (eg, phenobarbital, phenytoin, primidone). Downward dose adjustments of these drugs may be required when given concomitantly with methylphenidate. It may be necessary to adjust the dosage and monitor plasma drug concentration, when initiating or discontinuing methylphenidate).
No products indexed under this heading.

Torsemide (Methylphenidate may decrease the effectiveness of drugs used to treat hypertension).
No products indexed under this heading.

Trandolapril (Methylphenidate may decrease the effectiveness of drugs used to treat hypertension). Products include:

Tranylcypromine Sulfate (Dexmethylphenidate is contraindicated during treatment with monoamine oxidase inhibitors, and also within a minimum of 14 days following discontinuation of treatment with a monoamine oxidase inhibitor (hypertensive crises may result)). Products include:

Trimethadione (Racemic methylphenidate may inhibit the metabolism of anticonvulsants (eg, phenobarbital, phenytoin, primidone). Downward dose adjustments of these drugs may be required when given concomitantly with methylphenidate. It may be necessary to adjust the dosage and monitor plasma drug concentration, when initiating or discontinuing methylphenidate).
No products indexed under this heading.

Trimethaphan Camsylate (Methylphenidate may decrease the effectiveness of drugs used to treat hypertension).
No products indexed under this heading.

Trimipramine Maleate (Racemic methylphenidate may inhibit the metabolism of tricyclic drugs (eg, imipramine, clomipramine, desipramine). Downward dose adjustments of these drugs may be required when given concomitantly with methylphenidate. It may be necessary to adjust the dosage and monitor plasma drug concentration, when initiating or discontinuing methylphenidate).
No products indexed under this heading.

Valproate Sodium (Racemic methylphenidate may inhibit the metabolism of anticonvulsants (eg, phenobarbital, phenytoin, primidone). Downward dose adjustments of these drugs may be required when given concomitantly with methylphenidate. It may be necessary to adjust the dosage and monitor plasma drug concentration, when initiating or discontinuing methylphenidate).
No products indexed under this heading.

Valproic Acid (Racemic methylphenidate may inhibit the metabolism of anticonvulsants (eg, phenobarbital, phenytoin, primidone). Downward dose adjustments of these drugs may be required when given concomitantly with methylphenidate. It may be necessary to adjust the dosage and monitor plasma drug concentration, when initiating or discontinuing methylphenidate).
No products indexed under this heading.

Valsartan (Methylphenidate may decrease the effectiveness of drugs used to treat hypertension). Products include:

Venlafaxine Hydrochloride (In a single report, a ten-year-old boy who had been taking methylphenidate for approximately 18 months experienced an NMS-like event within 45 minutes of ingesting his first dose of venlafaxine. It is uncertain whether this case represented a drug-drug interaction, a response to either drug alone, or some other cause). Products include:

Verapamil Hydrochloride (Methylphenidate may decrease the effectiveness of drugs used to treat hypertension). Products include:

Warfarin Sodium (Racemic methylphenidate may inhibit the metabolism of coumarin anticoagulants. Downward dose adjustments of these drugs may be required when given concomitantly with methylphenidate. It may be necessary to adjust the dosage and monitor plasma drug concentration (or, in the case of coumarin, coagulation times), when initiating or discontinuing methylphenidate).
No products indexed under this heading.

Zonisamide (Racemic methylphenidate may inhibit the metabolism of anticonvulsants (eg, phenobarbital, phenytoin, primidone). Downward dose adjustments of these drugs may be required when given concomitantly with methylphenidate. It may be necessary to adjust the dosage and monitor plasma drug concentration, when initiating or discontinuing methylphenidate). Products include:

Food Interactions

Alcohol (Dexmethylphenidate hydrochloride should be given cautiously to patients with a history of drug dependence or alcoholism).

Beer, reduced-alcohol (Dexmethylphenidate hydrochloride should be given cautiously to patients with a history of drug dependence or alcoholism).

Beer, unspecified (Dexmethylphenidate hydrochloride should be given cautiously to patients with a history of drug dependence or alcoholism).

Food, unspecified (No food effect study was performed with Focalin XR. However, the effect of food has been studied in adults with racemic methylphenidate in the same type of extended-release formulation. The findings of that study are considered applicable to Focalin XR. After a high fat breakfast, there was a longer lag time until absorption began and variable delays in the time until the first peak concentration, the time until the interpeak minimum, and the time until the second peak. The first peak concentration and the extent of absorption were unchanged after food relative to the fasting state, although the second peak was approximately 25% lower).

Meal, unspecified (No food effect study was performed with Focalin XR. However, the effect of food has been studied in adults with racemic methylphenidate in the same type of extended-release formulation. The findings of that study are considered applicable to Focalin XR. After a high fat breakfast, there was a longer lag time until absorption began and variable delays in the time until the first peak concentration, the time until the interpeak minimum, and the time until the second peak. The first peak concentration and the extent of absorption were unchanged after food relative to the fasting state, although the second peak was approximately 25% lower).

Wine, Chianti (Dexmethylphenidate hydrochloride should be given cautiously to patients with a history of drug dependence or alcoholism).

Wine, Red (Dexmethylphenidate hydrochloride should be given cautiously to patients with a history of drug dependence or alcoholism).

Wine, unspecified (Dexmethylphenidate hydrochloride should be given cautiously to patients with a history of drug dependence or alcoholism).

Wine products (Dexmethylphenidate hydrochloride should be given cautiously to patients with a history of drug dependence or alcoholism).

FOLLISTIM AQ CARTRIDGE

None cited in PDR database.

FORADIL AEROLIZER

May interact with beta-blockers, diuretics, drugs that prolong the QT interval, glucocorticoids, monoamine oxidase inhibitors, potassium-depleting diuretics, sympathomimetics, tricyclic antidepressants, xanthines. Compounds in these categories include:

Acebutolol Hydrochloride (Co-administration with beta-blockers may inhibit the effect of each other. Beta-blockers not only block the therapeutic effect of beta-agonists, such as formoterol, but may produce severe bronchospasm in patients with asthma).
No products indexed under this heading.

Albuterol (Co-administration with additional adrenergic drugs may potentiate the sympathetic effects of formoterol).
No products indexed under this heading.

Albuterol Sulfate (Co-administration with additional adrenergic drugs may potentiate the sympathetic effects of formoterol). Products include:

Alprazolam (Co-administration with drugs known to prolong the QTc interval may lead to an increased risk of ventricular arrhythmias; co-administer with extreme caution).
No products indexed under this heading.

Amiloride Hydrochloride (Concomitant treatment with diuretics may potentiate any hypokalemic effect of adrenergic agonists).
No products indexed under this heading.

Aminophylline (Co-administration with xanthine derivatives may potentiate hypokalemic effect of adrenergic agonists).
No products indexed under this heading.

Amiodarone Hydrochloride (Co-administration with drugs known to prolong the QTc interval may lead to an increased risk of ventricular arrhythmias; co-administer with extreme caution).
No products indexed under this heading.

Amitriptyline Hydrochloride (Concurrent and/or sequential administration with tricyclic antidepressants may potentiate the action of adrenergic agonists on the cardiovascular system; co-administer with extreme caution).
No products indexed under this heading.

Amoxapine (Concurrent and/or sequential administration with tricyclic antidepressants may potentiate the action of adrenergic agonists on the cardiovascular system; co-administer with extreme caution).
No products indexed under this heading.

Astemizole (Co-administration with drugs known to prolong the QTc interval may lead to an increased risk of ventricular arrhythmias; co-administer with extreme caution).
No products indexed under this heading.

Atenolol (Co-administration with beta-blockers may inhibit the effect of each other. Beta-blockers not only block the therapeutic effect of beta-agonists, such as formoterol, but may produce severe bronchospasm in patients with asthma).
No products indexed under this heading.

Bendroflumethiazide (The ECG changes and/or hypokalemia that may result from the administration of non-potassium sparing diuretics can be acutely worsened by beta-agonists, especially when the recommended dose of beta-agonist is exceeded).
No products indexed under this heading.

Betamethasone Acetate (Co-administration with glucocorticosteroids may potentiate hypokalemic effect of adrenergic agonists).
No products indexed under this heading.

Betamethasone Sodium Phosphate (Co-administration with glucocorticosteroids may potentiate hypokalemic effect of adrenergic agonists).
No products indexed under this heading.

Betaxolol Hydrochloride (Co-administration with beta-blockers may inhibit the effect of each other. Beta-blockers not only block the therapeutic effect of beta-agonists, such as formoterol, but may produce severe bronchospasm in patients with asthma).
No products indexed under this heading.

Bisoprolol Fumarate (Co-administration with beta-blockers may inhibit the effect of each other. Beta-blockers not only block the therapeutic effect of beta-agonists, such as formoterol, but may produce severe bronchospasm in patients with asthma).
No products indexed under this heading.

Bretylium Tosylate (Co-administration with drugs known to prolong the QTc interval may lead to an increased risk of ventricular arrhythmias; co-administer with extreme caution).
No products indexed under this heading.

Budesonide (Co-administration with glucocorticosteroids may potentiate hypokalemic effect of adrenergic agonists). Products include:

Bumetanide (The ECG changes and/or hypokalemia that may result from the administration of non-potassium sparing diuretics can be acutely worsened by beta-agonists, especially when the recommended dose of beta-agonist is exceeded).
No products indexed under this heading.

IMPORTANT NOTE: Always consult each drug listing in the patient's regimen for possible interactions.

Hydrocortisone (Co-administration with glucocorticosteroids may potentiate hypokalemic effect of adrenergic agonists).
No products indexed under this heading.

Hydrocortisone Acetate (Co-administration with glucocorticosteroids may potentiate hypokalemic effect of adrenergic agonists).
No products indexed under this heading.

Hydrocortisone Sodium Phosphate (Co-administration with glucocorticosteroids may potentiate hypokalemic effect of adrenergic agonists).
No products indexed under this heading.

Hydrocortisone Sodium Succinate (Co-administration with glucocorticosteroids may potentiate hypokalemic effect of adrenergic agonists).
No products indexed under this heading.

Hydroflumethiazide (The ECG changes and/or hypokalemia that may result from the administration of non-potassium sparing diuretics can be acutely worsened by beta-agonists, especially when the recommended dose of beta-agonist is exceeded).
No products indexed under this heading.

Hydroxyzine Hydrochloride (Co-administration with drugs known to prolong the QTc interval may lead to an increased risk of ventricular arrhythmias; co-administer with extreme caution).
No products indexed under this heading.

Imipramine Hydrochloride (Concurrent and/or sequential administration with tricyclic antidepressants may potentiate the action of adrenergic agonists on the cardiovascular system; co-administer with extreme caution).
No products indexed under this heading.

Imipramine Pamoate (Concurrent and/or sequential administration with tricyclic antidepressants may potentiate the action of adrenergic agonists on the cardiovascular system; co-administer with extreme caution).
No products indexed under this heading.

Indapamide (Concomitant treatment with diuretics may potentiate any hypokalemic effect of adrenergic agonists). Products include:

Isocarboxazid (Concurrent and/or sequential administration with MAO inhibitors may potentiate the action of adrenergic agonists on the cardiovascular system; co-administer with extreme caution). Products include:

Isoproterenol Hydrochloride (Co-administration with additional adrenergic drugs may potentiate the sympathetic effects of formoterol).
No products indexed under this heading.

Isoproterenol Sulfate (Co-administration with additional adrenergic drugs may potentiate the sympathetic effects of formoterol).
No products indexed under this heading.

Labetalol Hydrochloride (Co-administration with beta-blockers may inhibit the effect of each other. Beta-blockers not only block the therapeutic effect of beta-agonists, such as formoterol, but may produce severe bronchospasm in patients with asthma).
No products indexed under this heading.

Levalbuterol Hydrochloride (Co-administration with additional adrenergic drugs may potentiate the sympathetic effects of formoterol).
No products indexed under this heading.

Levobunolol Hydrochloride (Co-administration with beta-blockers may inhibit the effect of each other. Beta-blockers not only block the therapeutic effect of beta-agonists, such as formoterol, but may produce severe bronchospasm in patients with asthma).
No products indexed under this heading.

Lidocaine (Co-administration with drugs known to prolong the QTc interval may lead to an increased risk of ventricular arrhythmias; co-administer with extreme caution). Products include:

Lidocaine Hydrochloride (Co-administration with drugs known to prolong the QTc interval may lead to an increased risk of ventricular arrhythmias; co-administer with extreme caution).
No products indexed under this heading.

Lithium Carbonate (Co-administration with drugs known to prolong the QTc interval may lead to an increased risk of ventricular arrhythmias; co-administer with extreme caution).
No products indexed under this heading.

Lithium Citrate (Co-administration with drugs known to prolong the QTc interval may lead to an increased risk of ventricular arrhythmias; co-administer with extreme caution).
No products indexed under this heading.

Lorazepam (Co-administration with drugs known to prolong the QTc interval may lead to an increased risk of ventricular arrhythmias; co-administer with extreme caution).
No products indexed under this heading.

Loxapine Hydrochloride (Co-administration with drugs known to prolong the QTc interval may lead to an increased risk of ventricular arrhythmias; co-administer with extreme caution).
No products indexed under this heading.

Loxapine Succinate (Co-administration with drugs known to prolong the QTc interval may lead to an increased risk of ventricular arrhythmias; co-administer with extreme caution).
No products indexed under this heading.

Maprotiline Hydrochloride (Concurrent and/or sequential administration with tricyclic antidepressants may potentiate the action of adrenergic agonists on the cardiovascular system; co-administer with extreme caution).
No products indexed under this heading.

Meprobamate (Co-administration with drugs known to prolong the QTc interval may lead to an increased risk of ventricular arrhythmias; co-administer with extreme caution).
No products indexed under this heading.

Mesoridazine Besylate (Co-administration with drugs known to prolong the QTc interval may lead to an increased risk of ventricular arrhythmias; co-administer with extreme caution).
No products indexed under this heading.

Metaproterenol Sulfate (Co-administration with additional adrenergic drugs may potentiate the sympathetic effects of formoterol).
No products indexed under this heading.

Metaraminol Bitartrate (Co-administration with additional adrenergic drugs may potentiate the sympathetic effects of formoterol).
No products indexed under this heading.

Methoxamine Hydrochloride (Co-administration with additional adrenergic drugs may potentiate the sympathetic effects of formoterol).
No products indexed under this heading.

Methyclothiazide (The ECG changes and/or hypokalemia that may result from the administration of non-potassium sparing diuretics can be acutely worsened by beta-agonists, especially when the recommended dose of beta-agonist is exceeded).
No products indexed under this heading.

Methylprednisolone Acetate (Co-administration with glucocorticosteroids may potentiate hypokalemic effect of adrenergic agonists).
No products indexed under this heading.

Methylprednisolone Sodium Succinate (Co-administration with glucocorticosteroids may potentiate hypokalemic effect of adrenergic agonists).
No products indexed under this heading.

Metipranolol Hydrochloride (Co-administration with beta-blockers may inhibit the effect of each other. Beta-blockers not only block the therapeutic effect of beta-agonists, such as formoterol, but may produce severe bronchospasm in patients with asthma).
No products indexed under this heading.

Metolazone (Concomitant treatment with diuretics may potentiate any hypokalemic effect of adrenergic agonists).
No products indexed under this heading.

Metoprolol Succinate (Co-administration with beta-blockers may inhibit the effect of each other. Beta-blockers not only block the therapeutic effect of beta-agonists, such as formoterol, but may produce severe bronchospasm in patients with asthma). Products include:

Metoprolol Tartrate (Co-administration with beta-blockers may inhibit the effect of each other. Beta-blockers not only block the therapeutic effect of beta-agonists, such as formoterol, but may produce severe bronchospasm in patients with asthma).
No products indexed under this heading.

Mexiletine Hydrochloride (Co-administration with drugs known to prolong the QTc interval may lead to an increased risk of ventricular arrhythmias; co-administer with extreme caution).
No products indexed under this heading.

Midazolam Hydrochloride (Co-administration with drugs known to prolong the QTc interval may lead to an increased risk of ventricular arrhythmias; co-administer with extreme caution).
No products indexed under this heading.

Moclobemide (Concurrent and/or sequential administration with MAO inhibitors may potentiate the action of adrenergic agonists on the cardiovascular system; co-administer with extreme caution).
No products indexed under this heading.

Molindone Hydrochloride (Co-administration with drugs known to prolong the QTc interval may lead to an increased risk of ventricular arrhythmias; co-administer with extreme caution). Products include:

Nadolol (Co-administration with beta-blockers may inhibit the effect of each other. Beta-blockers not only block the therapeutic effect of beta-agonists, such as formoterol, but may produce severe bronchospasm in patients with asthma). Products include:

Nebivolol (Co-administration with beta-blockers may inhibit the effect of each other. Beta-blockers not only block the therapeutic effect of beta-agonists, such as formoterol, but may produce severe bronchospasm in patients with asthma). Products include:

Norepinephrine Bitartrate (Co-administration with additional adrenergic drugs may potentiate the sympathetic effects of formoterol).
No products indexed under this heading.

Nortriptyline Hydrochloride (Concurrent and/or sequential administration with tricyclic antidepressants may potentiate the action of adrenergic agonists on the cardiovascular system; co-administer with extreme caution).
No products indexed under this heading.

Olanzapine (Co-administration with drugs known to prolong the QTc interval may lead to an increased risk of ventricular arrhythmias; co-administer with extreme caution). Products include:

Oxazepam (Co-administration with drugs known to prolong the QTc interval may lead to an increased risk of ventricular arrhythmias; co-administer with extreme caution).
No products indexed under this heading.

Pargyline Hydrochloride (Concurrent and/or sequential administration with MAO inhibitors may potentiate the action of adrenergic agonists on the cardiovascular system; co-administer with extreme caution).
No products indexed under this heading.

Penbutolol Sulfate (Co-administration with beta-blockers may inhibit the effect of each other. Beta-blockers not only block the therapeutic effect of beta-agonists, such as formoterol, but may produce severe bronchospasm in patients with asthma).
No products indexed under this heading.

Perphenazine (Co-administration with drugs known to prolong the QTc interval may lead to an increased risk of ventricular arrhythmias; co-administer with extreme caution).
No products indexed under this heading.

Phenelzine Sulfate (Concurrent and/or sequential administration with MAO inhibitors may potentiate the action of adrenergic agonists on the cardiovascular system; co-administer with extreme caution).
No products indexed under this heading.

Phenylephrine Bitartrate (Co-administration with additional adrenergic drugs may potentiate the sympathetic effects of formoterol).
No products indexed under this heading.

Phenylephrine Hydrochloride (Co-administration with additional adrenergic drugs may potentiate the sympathetic effects of formoterol). Products include:

Phenylephrine Tannate (Co-administration with additional adrenergic drugs may potentiate the sympathetic effects of formoterol).
No products indexed under this heading.

Phenylpropanolamine Hydrochloride (Co-administration with additional adrenergic drugs may potentiate the sympathetic effects of formoterol).
No products indexed under this heading.

Pindolol (Co-administration with beta-blockers may inhibit the effect of each other. Beta-blockers not only block the therapeutic effect of beta-agonists, such as formoterol, but may produce severe bronchospasm in patients with asthma).
No products indexed under this heading.

Pirbuterol Acetate (Co-administration with additional adrenergic drugs may potentiate the sympathetic effects of formoterol). Products include:
Maxair Autohaler 1782

Polythiazide (The ECG changes and/or hypokalemia that may result from the administration of non-potassium sparing diuretics can be acutely worsened by beta-agonists, especially when the recommended dose of beta-agonist is exceeded).
No products indexed under this heading.

Prazepam (Co-administration with drugs known to prolong the QTc interval may lead to an increased risk of ventricular arrhythmias; co-administer with extreme caution).
No products indexed under this heading.

Prednisolone Acetate (Co-administration with glucocorticosteroids may potentiate hypokalemic effect of adrenergic agonists). Products include:
Blephamide .... ⊙212, ⊙214
Pred Forte .... ⊙225
Pred Mild .... ⊙230
Pred-G .... ⊙226, ⊙227

Prednisolone Sodium Phosphate (Co-administration with glucocorticosteroids may potentiate hypokalemic effect of adrenergic agonists).
No products indexed under this heading.

Prednisolone Tebutate (Co-administration with glucocorticosteroids may potentiate hypokalemic effect of adrenergic agonists).
No products indexed under this heading.

Prednisone (Co-administration with glucocorticosteroids may potentiate hypokalemic effect of adrenergic agonists).
No products indexed under this heading.

Procainamide Hydrochloride (Co-administration with drugs known to prolong the QTc interval may lead to an increased risk of ventricular arrhythmias; co-administer with extreme caution).
No products indexed under this heading.

Procarbazine Hydrochloride (Concurrent and/or sequential administration with MAO inhibitors may potentiate the action of adrenergic agonists on the cardiovascular system; co-administer with extreme caution).
No products indexed under this heading.

Prochlorperazine (Co-administration with drugs known to prolong the QTc interval may lead to an increased risk of ventricular arrhythmias; co-administer with extreme caution).
No products indexed under this heading.

Promethazine Hydrochloride (Co-administration with drugs known to prolong the QTc interval may lead to an increased risk of ventricular arrhythmias; co-administer with extreme caution).
No products indexed under this heading.

Propafenone Hydrochloride (Co-administration with drugs known to prolong the QTc interval may lead to an increased risk of ventricular arrhythmias; co-administer with extreme caution). Products include:
Rythmol 1648
Rythmol SR 1652

Propranolol Hydrochloride (Co-administration with beta-blockers may inhibit the effect of each other. Beta-blockers not only block the therapeutic effect of beta-agonists, such as formoterol, but may produce severe bronchospasm in patients with asthma).
Products include:
InnoPran XL 1517

Protriptyline Hydrochloride (Concurrent and/or sequential administration with tricyclic antidepressants may potentiate the action of adrenergic agonists on the cardiovascular system; co-administer with extreme caution).
No products indexed under this heading.

Pseudoephedrine Hydrochloride (Co-administration with additional adrenergic drugs may potentiate the sympathetic effects of formoterol). Products include:
Allegra-D 2915
Allegra-D 24 2918
Sudafed 12 Hour Nasal
  Decongestant Non-Drowsy 2048
Sudafed 24 Hour 2048
Sudafed Nasal Decongestant 2047
Children's Sudafed Nasal
  Decongestant Liquid 2047
Zyrtec-D Allergy & Congestion 2054

Pseudoephedrine Sulfate (Co-administration with additional adrenergic drugs may potentiate the sympathetic effects of formoterol). Products include:
Clarinex-D 12-Hour 3101
Clarinex-D 3104

Quetiapine Fumarate (Co-administration with drugs known to prolong the QTc interval may lead to an increased risk of ventricular arrhythmias; co-administer with extreme caution). Products include:
Seroquel 750
Seroquel XR 759

Quinidine (Co-administration with drugs known to prolong the QTc interval may lead to an increased risk of ventricular arrhythmias; co-administer with extreme caution).
No products indexed under this heading.

Quinidine Gluconate (Co-administration with drugs known to prolong the QTc interval may lead to an increased risk of ventricular arrhythmias; co-administer with extreme caution).
No products indexed under this heading.

Quinidine Hydrochloride (Co-administration with drugs known to prolong the QTc interval may lead to an increased risk of ventricular arrhythmias; co-administer with extreme caution).
No products indexed under this heading.

Quinidine Polygalacturonate (Co-administration with drugs known to prolong the QTc interval may lead to an increased risk of ventricular arrhythmias; co-administer with extreme caution).
No products indexed under this heading.

Quinidine Sulfate (Co-administration with drugs known to prolong the QTc interval may lead to an increased risk of ventricular arrhythmias; co-administer with extreme caution).
No products indexed under this heading.

Rasagiline Mesylate (Concurrent and/or sequential administration with MAO inhibitors may potentiate the action of adrenergic agonists on the cardiovascular system; co-administer with extreme caution). Products include:
Azilect 3383

Risperidone (Co-administration with drugs known to prolong the QTc interval may lead to an increased risk of ventricular arrhythmias; co-administer with extreme caution). Products include:
Risperdal Consta 2682

Salmeterol Xinafoate (Co-administration with additional adrenergic drugs may potentiate the sympathetic effects of formoterol). Products include:
Advair 100/50 1275
Advair 250/50 1275
Advair 500/50 1275
Advair HFA 45/21 1288
Advair HFA 115/21 1288
Advair HFA 230/21 1288
Serevent Diskus 1656

Selegiline (Concurrent and/or sequential administration with MAO inhibitors may potentiate the action of adrenergic agonists on the cardiovascular system; co-administer with extreme caution). Products include:
Emsam 3623

Selegiline Hydrochloride (Concurrent and/or sequential administration with MAO inhibitors may potentiate the action of adrenergic agonists on the cardiovascular system; co-administer with extreme caution). Products include:
Eldepryl 3312

Sotalol Hydrochloride (Co-administration with beta-blockers may inhibit the effect of each other. Beta-blockers not only block the therapeutic effect of beta-agonists, such as formoterol, but may produce severe bronchospasm in patients with asthma).
No products indexed under this heading.

Spironolactone (Concomitant treatment with diuretics may potentiate any hypokalemic effect of adrenergic agonists).
No products indexed under this heading.

Terbutaline Sulfate (Co-administration with additional adrenergic drugs may potentiate the sympathetic effects of formoterol).
No products indexed under this heading.

Theophylline (Co-administration with xanthine derivatives may potentiate hypokalemic effect of adrenergic agonists).
No products indexed under this heading.

Theophylline Anhydrous (Co-administration with xanthine derivatives may potentiate hypokalemic effect of adrenergic agonists). Products include:
Uniphyl 2817

Theophylline Calcium Salicylate (Co-administration with xanthine derivatives may potentiate hypokalemic effect of adrenergic agonists).
No products indexed under this heading.

Theophylline Dihydroxypropyl (Glyceryl) (Co-administration with xanthine derivatives may potentiate hypokalemic effect of adrenergic agonists).
No products indexed under this heading.

Theophylline Ethylenediamine (Co-administration with xanthine derivatives may potentiate hypokalemic effect of adrenergic agonists).
No products indexed under this heading.

Theophylline Sodium Glycinate (Co-administration with xanthine derivatives may potentiate hypokalemic effect of adrenergic agonists).
No products indexed under this heading.

Thioridazine Hydrochloride (Co-administration with drugs known to prolong the QTc interval may lead to an increased risk of ventricular arrhythmias; co-administer with extreme caution). Products include:
Thioridazine Hydrochloride 2384

Thiothixene (Co-administration with drugs known to prolong the QTc interval may lead to an increased risk of ventricular arrhythmias; co-administer with extreme caution). Products include:
Thiothixene 2386

Timolol Hemihydrate (Co-administration with beta-blockers may inhibit the effect of each other. Beta-

blockers not only block the therapeutic effect of beta-agonists, such as formoterol, but may produce severe bronchospasm in patients with asthma).
Products include:
Betimol 3490

Timolol Maleate (Co-administration with beta-blockers may inhibit the effect of each other. Beta-blockers not only block the therapeutic effect of beta-agonists, such as formoterol, but may produce severe bronchospasm in patients with asthma). Products include:
Combigan 601
Dorzolamide
  Hydrochloride/Timolol Maleate
  Ophthalmic Solution..................... ⊙243
Timoptic in Ocudose .... ⊙231

Tocainide Hydrochloride (Co-administration with drugs known to prolong the QTc interval may lead to an increased risk of ventricular arrhythmias; co-administer with extreme caution).
No products indexed under this heading.

Torsemide (The ECG changes and/or hypokalemia that may result from the administration of non-potassium sparing diuretics can be acutely worsened by beta-agonists, especially when the recommended dose of beta-agonist is exceeded).
No products indexed under this heading.

Tranylcypromine Sulfate (Concurrent and/or sequential administration with MAO inhibitors may potentiate the action of adrenergic agonists on the cardiovascular system; co-administer with extreme caution). Products include:
Parnate 1584

Triamcinolone (Co-administration with glucocorticosteroids may potentiate hypokalemic effect of adrenergic agonists).
No products indexed under this heading.

Triamcinolone Acetonide (Co-administration with glucocorticosteroids may potentiate hypokalemic effect of adrenergic agonists). Products include:
Azmacort 408
Nasacort AQ 3019

Triamcinolone Diacetate (Co-administration with glucocorticosteroids may potentiate hypokalemic effect of adrenergic agonists).
No products indexed under this heading.

Triamcinolone Hexacetonide (Co-administration with glucocorticosteroids may potentiate hypokalemic effect of adrenergic agonists).
No products indexed under this heading.

Triamterene (Concomitant treatment with diuretics may potentiate any hypokalemic effect of adrenergic agonists). Products include:
Dyazide 1429
Dyrenium 3495

Trifluoperazine Hydrochloride (Co-administration with drugs known to prolong the QTc interval may lead to an increased risk of ventricular arrhythmias; co-administer with extreme caution).
No products indexed under this heading.

Trimipramine Maleate (Concurrent and/or sequential administration with tricyclic antidepressants may potentiate the action of adrenergic agonists on the cardiovascular system; co-administer with extreme caution).
No products indexed under this heading.

Ziprasidone Hydrochloride (Co-administration with drugs known to prolong the QTc interval may lead to an increased risk of ventricular arrhythmias; co-administer with extreme caution). Products include:
Geodon 2723

FORMADON SOLUTION
(Formaldehyde) 1770
None cited in PDR database.

IMPORTANT NOTE: Always consult each drug listing in the patient's regimen for possible interactions.

(⊙ Described in PDR® for Ophthalmic Medicines)

taking alendronate before taking any other oral medications). Products include:

Bio-C 3454
Procosa II 3476
Proflavanol 90 3476

Calcium Carbaspirin (Products containing calcium and other multivalent cations are likely to interfere with absorption of alendronate; patients must wait at least one-half hour after taking alendronate before taking any other oral medications).
No products indexed under this heading.

Calcium Carbonate (Concomitant use with calcium supplements may interfere with absorption of alendronate. Therefore, patients must wait at least one-half hour after taking alendronate before taking any other oral medications). Products include:

Chelated Mineral 3476
Pepcid Complete 1822
Extra Strength Rolaids Softchews Vanilla Creme 2045

Calcium Carbonate, Precipitated (Products containing calcium and other multivalent cations are likely to interfere with absorption of alendronate; patients must wait at least one-half hour after taking alendronate before taking any other oral medications).
No products indexed under this heading.

Calcium Caseinate (Products containing calcium and other multivalent cations are likely to interfere with absorption of alendronate; patients must wait at least one-half hour after taking alendronate before taking any other oral medications).
No products indexed under this heading.

Calcium Chloride (Concomitant use with calcium supplements may interfere with absorption of alendronate. Therefore, patients must wait at least one-half hour after taking alendronate before taking any other oral medications).
No products indexed under this heading.

Calcium Citrate (Concomitant use with calcium supplements may interfere with absorption of alendronate. Therefore, patients must wait at least one-half hour after taking alendronate before taking any other oral medications). Products include:

Active Calcium 3476
Chelated Mineral 3476
CitraNatal 90 DHA Capsules 2332
CitraNatal Assure 2332
CitraNatal Harmony 2332
CitraNatal Rx 2332

Calcium Disodium Edetate (Products containing calcium and other multivalent cations are likely to interfere with absorption of alendronate; patients must wait at least one-half hour after taking alendronate before taking any other oral medications).
No products indexed under this heading.

Calcium Glubionate (Concomitant use with calcium supplements may interfere with absorption of alendronate. Therefore, patients must wait at least one-half hour after taking alendronate before taking any other oral medications).
No products indexed under this heading.

Calcium Gluconate (Products containing calcium and other multivalent cations are likely to interfere with absorption of alendronate; patients must wait at least one-half hour after taking alendronate before taking any other oral medications).
No products indexed under this heading.

Calcium Glycerophosphate (Products containing calcium and other multivalent cations are likely to interfere with absorption of alendronate; patients must wait at least one-half hour after taking alendronate before taking any other oral medications).
No products indexed under this heading.

Calcium Iodide (Products containing calcium and other multivalent cations are likely to interfere with absorption of alendronate; patients must wait at least one-half hour after taking alendronate before taking any other oral medications).
No products indexed under this heading.

Calcium Lactate (Products containing calcium and other multivalent cations are likely to interfere with absorption of alendronate; patients must wait at least one-half hour after taking alendronate before taking any other oral medications).
No products indexed under this heading.

Calcium Levulinate (Products containing calcium and other multivalent cations are likely to interfere with absorption of alendronate; patients must wait at least one-half hour after taking alendronate before taking any other oral medications).
No products indexed under this heading.

Calcium Pantothenate (Products containing calcium and other multivalent cations are likely to interfere with absorption of alendronate; patients must wait at least one-half hour after taking alendronate before taking any other oral medications). Products include:

Cardio Basics 3455

Calcium Phosphate (Products containing calcium and other multivalent cations are likely to interfere with absorption of alendronate; patients must wait at least one-half hour after taking alendronate before taking any other oral medications).
No products indexed under this heading.

Calcium Phosphate, Dibasic (Products containing calcium and other multivalent cations are likely to interfere with absorption of alendronate; patients must wait at least one-half hour after taking alendronate before taking any other oral medications).
No products indexed under this heading.

Calcium Phosphate, Tribasic (Products containing calcium and other multivalent cations are likely to interfere with absorption of alendronate; patients must wait at least one-half hour after taking alendronate before taking any other oral medications).
No products indexed under this heading.

Calcium Phosphorus Preparations (Products containing calcium and other multivalent cations are likely to interfere with absorption of alendronate; patients must wait at least one-half hour after taking alendronate before taking any other oral medications).
No products indexed under this heading.

Calcium Polycarbophil (Products containing calcium and other multivalent cations are likely to interfere with absorption of alendronate; patients must wait at least one-half hour after taking alendronate before taking any other oral medications).
No products indexed under this heading.

Calcium Salts (Products containing calcium and other multivalent cations are likely to interfere with absorption of alendronate; patients must wait at least one-half hour after taking alendronate before taking any other oral medications).
No products indexed under this heading.

Calcium Sodium Alginate Fiber (Products containing calcium and other multivalent cations are likely to interfere with absorption of alendronate; patients must wait at least one-half hour after taking alendronate before taking any other oral medications).
No products indexed under this heading.

Calcium Undecylenate (Products containing calcium and other multivalent cations are likely to interfere with absorption of alendronate; patients must wait at least one-half hour after taking alendronate before taking any other oral medications).
No products indexed under this heading.

Celecoxib (Since NSAID use is associated with gastrointestinal irritation, caution should be used during concomitant use with alendronate). Products include:

Celebrex 3272

Chlorotrianisene (Concomitant use of hormone replacement therapy (HRT) (estrogen +/- progestin) and alendronate was assessed in two clinical studies of one or two years duration in postmenopausal osteoporotic women. In these studies, the safety and tolerability profile of the combination was consistent with those of the individual treatments; however, the degree of suppression of bone turnover (as assessed by mineralizing surface) was significantly greater with the combination than with either component alone).
No products indexed under this heading.

Cimetidine (Intravenous ranitidine was shown to double the bioavailability of oral alendronate. The clinical significance of this increased bioavailability and whether similar increases will occur in patients given oral H_2-antagonists is unknown).
No products indexed under this heading.

Cimetidine Hydrochloride (Intravenous ranitidine was shown to double the bioavailability of oral alendronate. The clinical significance of this increased bioavailability and whether similar increases will occur in patients given oral H_2-antagonists is unknown).
No products indexed under this heading.

Desogestrel (Concomitant use of hormone replacement therapy (HRT) (estrogen +/- progestin) and alendronate was assessed in two clinical studies of one or two years duration in postmenopausal osteoporotic women. In these studies, the safety and tolerability profile of the combination was consistent with those of the individual treatments; however, the degree of suppression of bone turnover (as assessed by mineralizing surface) was significantly greater with the combination than with either component alone).
No products indexed under this heading.

Diclofenac Epolamine (Since NSAID use is associated with gastrointestinal irritation, caution should be used during concomitant use with alendronate). Products include:

Flector 1839

Diclofenac Potassium (Since NSAID use is associated with gastrointestinal irritation, caution should be used during concomitant use with alendronate).
No products indexed under this heading.

Diclofenac Sodium (Since NSAID use is associated with gastrointestinal irritation, caution should be used during concomitant use with alendronate).
No products indexed under this heading.

Dienestrol (Concomitant use of hormone replacement therapy (HRT) (estrogen +/- progestin) and alendronate was assessed in two clinical studies of one or two years duration in postmenopausal osteoporotic women. In these studies, the safety and tolerability profile of the combination was consistent with those of the individual treatments; however, the degree of suppression of bone turnover (as assessed by mineralizing surface) was significantly greater with the combination than with either component alone).
No products indexed under this heading.

Diethylstilbestrol (Concomitant use of hormone replacement therapy (HRT) (estrogen +/- progestin) and alendronate was assessed in two clinical studies of one or two years duration in postmenopausal osteoporotic women. In these studies, the safety and tolerability profile of the combination was consistent with those of the individual treatments; however, the degree of suppression of bone turnover (as assessed by mineralizing surface) was significantly greater with the combination than with either component alone).
No products indexed under this heading.

Estradiol (Concomitant use of hormone replacement therapy (HRT) (estrogen +/- progestin) and alendronate was assessed in two clinical studies of one or two years duration in postmenopausal osteoporotic women. In these studies, the safety and tolerability profile of the combination was consistent with those of the individual treatments; however, the degree of suppression of bone turnover (as assessed by mineralizing surface) was significantly greater with the combination than with either component alone). Products include:

Activella 2561
Angeliq 831
Climara 841
Climara Pro 847
Divigel 3467
Estrasorb 1777
Vagifem 2589

Estrogens, Conjugated (Concomitant use of hormone replacement therapy (HRT) (estrogen +/- progestin) and alendronate was assessed in two clinical studies of one or two years duration in postmenopausal osteoporotic women. In these studies, the safety and tolerability profile of the combination was consistent with those of the individual treatments; however, the degree of suppression of bone turnover (as assessed by mineralizing surface) was significantly greater with the combination than with either component alone). Products include:

Premarin Intravenous 3528
Premarin Tablets 3533
Premarin Vaginal Cream 3540
Premphase 3549
Prempro 3549

Estrogens, Esterified (Concomitant use of hormone replacement therapy (HRT) (estrogen +/- progestin) and alendronate was assessed in two clinical studies of one or two years duration in postmenopausal osteoporotic women. In these studies, the safety and tolerability profile of the combination was consistent with those of the individual treatments; however, the degree of suppression of bone turnover (as assessed by mineralizing surface) was significantly greater with the combination than with either component alone).
No products indexed under this heading.

Estropipate (Concomitant use of hormone replacement therapy (HRT) (estrogen +/- progestin) and alendronate was assessed in two clinical studies of one or two years duration in postmenopausal osteoporotic women. In these studies, the safety and tolerability profile of the combination was consistent with those of the individual treatments; however, the degree of suppression of bone turnover (as assessed by mineralizing surface) was significantly greater with the combination than with either component alone).
No products indexed under this heading.

IMPORTANT NOTE: Always consult each drug listing in the patient's regimen for possible interactions.

Ethinyl Estradiol (Concomitant use of hormone replacement therapy (HRT) (estrogen +/- progestin) and alendronate was assessed in two clinical studies of one or two years duration in postmenopausal osteoporotic women. In these studies, the safety and tolerability profile of the combination was consistent with those of the individual treatments; however, the degree of suppression of bone turnover (as assessed by mineralizing surface) was significantly greater with the combination than with either component alone). Products include:

Etodolac (Since NSAID use is associated with gastrointestinal irritation, caution should be used during concomitant use with alendronate).

No products indexed under this heading.

Famotidine (Intravenous ranitidine was shown to double the bioavailability of oral alendronate. The clinical significance of this increased bioavailability and whether similar increases will occur in patients given oral H$_2$-antagonists is unknown). Products include:

Fenoprofen Calcium (Since NSAID use is associated with gastrointestinal irritation, caution should be used during concomitant use with alendronate).

No products indexed under this heading.

Ferrous Fumarate (Products containing calcium and other multivalent cations are likely to interfere with absorption of alendronate; patients must wait at least one-half hour after taking alendronate before taking any other oral medications). Products include:

Ferrous Gluconate (Products containing calcium and other multivalent cations are likely to interfere with absorption of alendronate; patients must wait at least one-half hour after taking alendronate before taking any other oral medications). Products include:

Ferrous Sulfate (Products containing calcium and other multivalent cations are likely to interfere with absorption of alendronate; patients must wait at least one-half hour after taking alendronate before taking any other oral medications).

No products indexed under this heading.

Flurbiprofen (Since NSAID use is associated with gastrointestinal irritation, caution should be used during concomitant use with alendronate).

No products indexed under this heading.

Ibuprofen (Since NSAID use is associated with gastrointestinal irritation, caution should be used during concomitant use with alendronate). Products include:

Indomethacin (Since NSAID use is associated with gastrointestinal irrita-

tion, caution should be used during concomitant use with alendronate). Products include:

Indomethacin Sodium Trihydrate (Since NSAID use is associated with gastrointestinal irritation, caution should be used during concomitant use with alendronate). Products include:

Iron (Products containing calcium and other multivalent cations are likely to interfere with absorption of alendronate; patients must wait at least one-half hour after taking alendronate before taking any other oral medications).

No products indexed under this heading.

Iron, Peptonized (Products containing calcium and other multivalent cations are likely to interfere with absorption of alendronate; patients must wait at least one-half hour after taking alendronate before taking any other oral medications).

No products indexed under this heading.

Iron & Ammonium Citrate (Products containing calcium and other multivalent cations are likely to interfere with absorption of alendronate; patients must wait at least one-half hour after taking alendronate before taking any other oral medications).

No products indexed under this heading.

Iron Cacodylate (Products containing calcium and other multivalent cations are likely to interfere with absorption of alendronate; patients must wait at least one-half hour after taking alendronate before taking any other oral medications).

No products indexed under this heading.

Iron Carbonyl (Products containing calcium and other multivalent cations are likely to interfere with absorption of alendronate; patients must wait at least one-half hour after taking alendronate before taking any other oral medications). Products include:

Iron Supplements (Products containing calcium and other multivalent cations are likely to interfere with absorption of alendronate; patients must wait at least one-half hour after taking alendronate before taking any other oral medications).

No products indexed under this heading.

Ketoprofen (Since NSAID use is associated with gastrointestinal irritation, caution should be used during concomitant use with alendronate).

No products indexed under this heading.

Ketorolac Tromethamine (Since NSAID use is associated with gastrointestinal irritation, caution should be used during concomitant use with alendronate). Products include:

Magaldrate (Concomitant use with antacids may interfere with the absorption of alendronate. Therefore, patients must wait at least one-half hour after taking alendronate before taking any other oral medications).

No products indexed under this heading.

Magnesium (Products containing calcium and other multivalent cations are likely to interfere with absorption of alendronate; patients must wait at least one-half hour after taking alendronate before taking any other oral medications). Products include:

Magnesium Aluminum Silicate (Products containing calcium and other multivalent cations are likely to interfere with absorption of alendronate; patients must wait at least one-half hour after taking alendronate before taking any other oral medications).

No products indexed under this heading.

Magnesium Carbonate (Concomitant use with antacids may interfere with the absorption of alendronate. Therefore, patients must wait at least one-half hour after taking alendronate before taking any other oral medications).

No products indexed under this heading.

Magnesium Chloride (Products containing calcium and other multivalent cations are likely to interfere with absorption of alendronate; patients must wait at least one-half hour after taking alendronate before taking any other oral medications).

No products indexed under this heading.

Magnesium Citrate (Products containing calcium and other multivalent cations are likely to interfere with absorption of alendronate; patients must wait at least one-half hour after taking alendronate before taking any other oral medications). Products include:

Magnesium Gluconate (Products containing calcium and other multivalent cations are likely to interfere with absorption of alendronate; patients must wait at least one-half hour after taking alendronate before taking any other oral medications).

No products indexed under this heading.

Magnesium Hydroxide (Concomitant use with antacids may interfere with the absorption of alendronate. Therefore, patients must wait at least one-half hour after taking alendronate before taking any other oral medications). Products include:

Magnesium Lactate (Products containing calcium and other multivalent cations are likely to interfere with absorption of alendronate; patients must wait at least one-half hour after taking alendronate before taking any other oral medications).

No products indexed under this heading.

Magnesium Oxide (Concomitant use with antacids may interfere with the absorption of alendronate. Therefore, patients must wait at least one-half hour after taking alendronate before taking any other oral medications). Products include:

Magnesium Salicylate (Products containing calcium and other multivalent cations are likely to interfere with absorption of alendronate; patients must wait at least one-half hour after taking alendronate before taking any other oral medications).

No products indexed under this heading.

Magnesium Salicylate Tetrahydrate (Products containing calcium and other multivalent cations are likely to interfere with absorption of alendronate; patients must wait at least one-half hour after taking alendronate before taking any other oral medications).

No products indexed under this heading.

Magnesium Salts (Products containing calcium and other multivalent cations are likely to interfere with absorption of alendronate; patients must wait at least one-half hour after taking alendronate before taking any other oral medications).

No products indexed under this heading.

Magnesium Sulfate (Products containing calcium and other multivalent cations are likely to interfere with absorption of alendronate; patients must wait at least one-half hour after taking alendronate before taking any other oral medications).

No products indexed under this heading.

Magnesium Trisilicate (Concomitant use with antacids may interfere with the absorption of alendronate. Therefore, patients must wait at least one-half hour after taking alendronate before taking any other oral medications).

No products indexed under this heading.

Meclofenamate Sodium (Since NSAID use is associated with gastrointestinal irritation, caution should be used during concomitant use with alendronate).

No products indexed under this heading.

Medroxyprogesterone Acetate (Concomitant use of hormone replacement therapy (HRT) (estrogen +/- progestin) and alendronate was assessed in two clinical studies of one or two years duration in postmenopausal osteoporotic women. In these studies, the safety and tolerability profile of the combination was consistent with those of the individual treatments; however, the degree of suppression of bone turnover (as assessed by mineralizing surface) was significantly greater with the combination than with either component alone). Products include:

Mefenamic Acid (Since NSAID use is associated with gastrointestinal irritation, caution should be used during concomitant use with alendronate).

No products indexed under this heading.

Megestrol Acetate (Concomitant use of hormone replacement therapy (HRT) (estrogen +/- progestin) and alendronate was assessed in two clinical studies of one or two years duration in postmenopausal osteoporotic women. In these studies, the safety and tolerability profile of the combination was consistent with those of the individual treatments; however, the degree of suppression of bone turnover (as assessed by mineralizing surface) was significantly greater with the combination than with either component alone). Products include:

Meloxicam (Since NSAID use is associated with gastrointestinal irritation, caution should be used during concomitant use with alendronate).

No products indexed under this heading.

Nabumetone (Since NSAID use is associated with gastrointestinal irritation, caution should be used during concomitant use with alendronate).

No products indexed under this heading.

Naproxen (Since NSAID use is associated with gastrointestinal irritation, caution should be used during concomitant use with alendronate). Products include:

Naproxen Sodium (Since NSAID use is associated with gastrointestinal irritation, caution should be used during concomitant use with alendronate). Products include:

Nizatidine (Intravenous ranitidine was shown to double the bioavailability of oral alendronate. The clinical significance of this increased bioavailability and whether similar increases will occur in patients given oral H$_2$-antagonists is unknown). Products include:

(⊙ Described in PDR® for Ophthalmic Medicines)

Axid 1381

Norethindrone (Concomitant use of hormone replacement therapy (HRT) (estrogen +/- progestin) and alendronate was assessed in two clinical studies of one or two years duration in postmenopausal osteoporotic women. In these studies, the safety and tolerability profile of the combination was consistent with those of the individual treatments; however, the degree of suppression of bone turnover (as assessed by mineralizing surface) was significantly greater with the combination than with either component alone). Products include:
Ortho Micronor 2660

Norethindrone Acetate (Concomitant use of hormone replacement therapy (HRT) (estrogen +/- progestin) and alendronate was assessed in two clinical studies of one or two years duration in postmenopausal osteoporotic women. In these studies, the safety and tolerability profile of the combination was consistent with those of the individual treatments; however, the degree of suppression of bone turnover (as assessed by mineralizing surface) was significantly greater with the combination than with either component alone). Products include:
Activella 2561

Norgestimate (Concomitant use of hormone replacement therapy (HRT) (estrogen +/- progestin) and alendronate was assessed in two clinical studies of one or two years duration in postmenopausal osteoporotic women. In these studies, the safety and tolerability profile of the combination was consistent with those of the individual treatments; however, the degree of suppression of bone turnover (as assessed by mineralizing surface) was significantly greater with the combination than with either component alone). Products include:
Ortho-Cyclen/Ortho Tri-Cyclen 2663
Ortho Tri-Cyclen Lo Tablets 2673

Oral Medications, unspecified (Concomitant use with some oral medications may interfere with absorption of alendronate. Therefore, patients must wait at least one-half hour after taking alendronate before taking any other oral medications).
No products indexed under this heading.

Oxaprozin (Since NSAID use is associated with gastrointestinal irritation, caution should be used during concomitant use with alendronate).
No products indexed under this heading.

Phenylbutazone (Since NSAID use is associated with gastrointestinal irritation, caution should be used during concomitant use with alendronate).
No products indexed under this heading.

Piroxicam (Since NSAID use is associated with gastrointestinal irritation, caution should be used during concomitant use with alendronate).
No products indexed under this heading.

Polyestradiol Phosphate (Concomitant use of hormone replacement therapy (HRT) (estrogen +/- progestin) and alendronate was assessed in two clinical studies of one or two years duration in postmenopausal osteoporotic women. In these studies, the safety and tolerability profile of the combination was consistent with those of the individual treatments; however, the degree of suppression of bone turnover (as assessed by mineralizing surface) was significantly greater with the combination than with either component alone).
No products indexed under this heading.

Quinestrol (Concomitant use of hormone replacement therapy (HRT) (estrogen +/- progestin) and alendronate was assessed in two clinical studies of one

or two years duration in postmenopausal osteoporotic women. In these studies, the safety and tolerability profile of the combination was consistent with those of the individual treatments; however, the degree of suppression of bone turnover (as assessed by mineralizing surface) was significantly greater with the combination than with either component alone).
No products indexed under this heading.

Ranitidine Bismuth Citrate (Intravenous ranitidine was shown to double the bioavailability of oral alendronate. The clinical significance of this increased bioavailability and whether similar increases will occur in patients given oral H_2-antagonists is unknown).
No products indexed under this heading.

Ranitidine Hydrochloride (Intravenous ranitidine was shown to double the bioavailability of oral alendronate. The clinical significance of this increased bioavailability and whether similar increases will occur in patients given oral H_2-antagonists is unknown). Products include:
Zantac 1737
Zantac Injection 1732
Zantac Pharmacy 1735

Rofecoxib (Since NSAID use is associated with gastrointestinal irritation, caution should be used during concomitant use with alendronate).
No products indexed under this heading.

Selenium (Products containing calcium and other multivalent cations are likely to interfere with absorption of alendronate; patients must wait at least one-half hour after taking alendronate before taking any other oral medications). Products include:
Cardio Basics 3455
Chelated Mineral 3476

Selenium Sulfide (Products containing calcium and other multivalent cations are likely to interfere with absorption of alendronate; patients must wait at least one-half hour after taking alendronate before taking any other oral medications).
No products indexed under this heading.

Sodium Bicarbonate (Concomitant use with antacids may interfere with the absorption of alendronate. Therefore, patients must wait at least one-half hour after taking alendronate before taking any other oral medications).
No products indexed under this heading.

Sulindac (Since NSAID use is associated with gastrointestinal irritation, caution should be used during concomitant use with alendronate). Products include:
Clinoril 2098

Tolmetin Sodium (Since NSAID use is associated with gastrointestinal irritation, caution should be used during concomitant use with alendronate).
No products indexed under this heading.

Valdecoxib (Since NSAID use is associated with gastrointestinal irritation, caution should be used during concomitant use with alendronate).
No products indexed under this heading.

Zinc (Products containing calcium and other multivalent cations are likely to interfere with absorption of alendronate; patients must wait at least one-half hour after taking alendronate before taking any other oral medications). Products include:
BoneMate Plus 3454
Cardio Basics 3455
Chelated Mineral 3476
CitraNatal 90 DHA Capsules 2332
CitraNatal Assure 2332
Heplive 607
Visutein 3456

Zinc Acetate (Products containing calcium and other multivalent cations are likely to interfere with absorption of alendronate; patients must wait at least one-half hour after taking alendronate before taking any other oral medications).
No products indexed under this heading.

Zinc Bisglycinate (Products containing calcium and other multivalent cations are likely to interfere with absorption of alendronate; patients must wait at least one-half hour after taking alendronate before taking any other oral medications).
No products indexed under this heading.

Zinc Chloride (Products containing calcium and other multivalent cations are likely to interfere with absorption of alendronate; patients must wait at least one-half hour after taking alendronate before taking any other oral medications).
No products indexed under this heading.

Zinc Citrate (Products containing calcium and other multivalent cations are likely to interfere with absorption of alendronate; patients must wait at least one-half hour after taking alendronate before taking any other oral medications). Products include:
Chelated Mineral 3476

Zinc-Containing Multivitamins (Products containing calcium and other multivalent cations are likely to interfere with absorption of alendronate; patients must wait at least one-half hour after taking alendronate before taking any other oral medications).
No products indexed under this heading.

Zinc Gluconate (Products containing calcium and other multivalent cations are likely to interfere with absorption of alendronate; patients must wait at least one-half hour after taking alendronate before taking any other oral medications).
No products indexed under this heading.

Zinc Oxide (Products containing calcium and other multivalent cations are likely to interfere with absorption of alendronate; patients must wait at least one-half hour after taking alendronate before taking any other oral medications). Products include:
Bausch & Lomb Ocuvite Adult
50+ .... ⊙238
CitraNatal Rx 2332
Vusion Ointment 3335

Zinc Phenosulfonate (Products containing calcium and other multivalent cations are likely to interfere with absorption of alendronate; patients must wait at least one-half hour after taking alendronate before taking any other oral medications).
No products indexed under this heading.

Zinc Sulfate (Products containing calcium and other multivalent cations are likely to interfere with absorption of alendronate; patients must wait at least one-half hour after taking alendronate before taking any other oral medications). Products include:
Heplive 607
Zinc-220 606

Food Interactions

Beverages, caffeine-containing (Concomitant administration of alendronate with coffee reduces bioavailability by approximately 60%).

Iron Amino Acid Chelate (Products containing calcium and other multivalent cations are likely to interfere with absorption of alendronate; patients must wait at least one-half hour after taking alendronate before taking any other oral medications).

Meal, unspecified (Standardized breakfast decreases bioavailability by approximately 40% when alendronate is administered either one-half or 1 hour before breakfast).

Orange Juice (Concomitant administration of alendronate with orange juice reduces bioavailability by approximately 60%).

FOSAMAX PLUS D TABLETS
(Alendronate Sodium, Cholecalciferol) 2147
May interact with antacids containing aluminum, calcium and magnesium, anticonvulsants, aspirin-acetylsalicylic acid, bile acid sequestering agents, calcium preparations, non-steroidal anti-inflammatory agents, thiazides, and certain other agents. Compounds in these categories include:

Aluminum Carbonate (Antacids may interfere with the absorption of alendronate. Therefore, patients must wait at least one-half hour after taking alendronate sodium/cholecalciferol before taking any other oral medications).
No products indexed under this heading.

Aluminum Hydroxide (Antacids may interfere with the absorption of alendronate. Therefore, patients must wait at least one-half hour after taking alendronate sodium/cholecalciferol before taking any other oral medications).
No products indexed under this heading.

Aspirin (Studies have shown an increased incidence of upper gastrointestinal adverse events in patients receiving concomitant therapy with daily doses of alendronate greater than 10 mg and aspirin-containing products). Products include:
Aggrenox 880
Bayer Aspirin 829
Percodan 1124
St. Joseph Aspirin 2045

Aspirin, Enteric Coated (Studies have shown an increased incidence of upper gastrointestinal adverse events in patients receiving concomitant therapy with daily doses of alendronate greater than 10 mg and aspirin-containing products).
No products indexed under this heading.

Aspirin Buffered (Studies have shown an increased incidence of upper gastrointestinal adverse events in patients receiving concomitant therapy with daily doses of alendronate greater than 10 mg and aspirin-containing products).
No products indexed under this heading.

Bendroflumethiazide (Thiazides may increase the catabolism of vitamin D; consider additional vitamin D supplementation when co-administering).
No products indexed under this heading.

Calcium Carbonate (Antacids may interfere with the absorption of alendronate. Therefore, patients must wait at least one-half hour after taking alendronate sodium/cholecalciferol before taking any other oral medications). Products include:
Chelated Mineral 3476
Pepcid Complete 1822
Extra Strength Rolaids Softchews
Vanilla Creme 2045

Calcium Chloride (Calcium supplements may interfere with the absorption of alendronate. Therefore, patients must wait at least one-half hour after taking alendronate sodium/cholecalciferol before taking any other oral medications).
No products indexed under this heading.

Calcium Citrate (Calcium supplements may interfere with the absorption of alendronate. Therefore, patients must wait at least one-half hour after

IMPORTANT NOTE: Always consult each drug listing in the patient's regimen for possible interactions.

incidence of gastrointestinal irritation was reported in clinical trials). Products include:

Olestra (Olestra may impair the absorption of vitamin D; consider additional vitamin D supplementation when co-administering).
No products indexed under this heading.

Oral Medications, unspecified (Some oral medications will interfere with absorption of alendronate. Therefore, patients must wait at least one-half hour after taking alendronate sodium/cholecalciferol before taking any other oral medications).
No products indexed under this heading.

Orlistat (Orlistat may impair the absorption of vitamin D; consider additional vitamin D supplementation when co-administering). Products include:

Oxaprozin (Since NSAID use is associated with gastrointestinal irritation, caution should be used during concomitant use with alendronate sodium/cholecalciferol. No increase in the incidence of gastrointestinal irritation was reported in clinical trials).
No products indexed under this heading.

Oxcarbazepine (Anticonvulsants may increase the catabolism of vitamin D; consider additional vitamin D supplementation when co-administering).
No products indexed under this heading.

Paramethadione (Anticonvulsants may increase the catabolism of vitamin D; consider additional vitamin D supplementation when co-administering).
No products indexed under this heading.

Phenacemide (Anticonvulsants may increase the catabolism of vitamin D; consider additional vitamin D supplementation when co-administering).
No products indexed under this heading.

Phenobarbital (Anticonvulsants may increase the catabolism of vitamin D; consider additional vitamin D supplementation when co-administering). Products include:

Phenobarbital Sodium (Anticonvulsants may increase the catabolism of vitamin D; consider additional vitamin D supplementation when co-administering).
No products indexed under this heading.

Phensuximide (Anticonvulsants may increase the catabolism of vitamin D; consider additional vitamin D supplementation when co-administering).
No products indexed under this heading.

Phenylbutazone (Since NSAID use is associated with gastrointestinal irritation, caution should be used during concomitant use with alendronate sodium/cholecalciferol. No increase in the incidence of gastrointestinal irritation was reported in clinical trials).
No products indexed under this heading.

Phenytoin (Anticonvulsants may increase the catabolism of vitamin D; consider additional vitamin D supplementation when co-administering).
No products indexed under this heading.

Phenytoin Sodium (Anticonvulsants may increase the catabolism of vitamin D; consider additional vitamin D supplementation when co-administering). Products include:

Piroxicam (Since NSAID use is associated with gastrointestinal irritation, caution should be used during concomitant use with alendronate sodium/cholecalciferol. No increase in the incidence of gastrointestinal irritation was reported in clinical trials).
No products indexed under this heading.

Polythiazide (Thiazides may increase the catabolism of vitamin D; consider additional vitamin D supplementation when co-administering).
No products indexed under this heading.

Primidone (Anticonvulsants may increase the catabolism of vitamin D; consider additional vitamin D supplementation when co-administering).
No products indexed under this heading.

Ranitidine Hydrochloride (Intravenous ranitidine was shown to double the bioavailability of oral alendronate. The clinical significance of this increased bioavailability and whether similar increases will occur in patients given oral H2-antagonists is unknown). Products include:

Rofecoxib (Since NSAID use is associated with gastrointestinal irritation, caution should be used during concomitant use with alendronate sodium/cholecalciferol. No increase in the incidence of gastrointestinal irritation was reported in clinical trials).
No products indexed under this heading.

Rufinamide (Anticonvulsants may increase the catabolism of vitamin D; consider additional vitamin D supplementation when co-administering). Products include:

Sulindac (Since NSAID use is associated with gastrointestinal irritation, caution should be used during concomitant use with alendronate sodium/cholecalciferol. No increase in the incidence of gastrointestinal irritation was reported in clinical trials). Products include:

Tiagabine Hydrochloride (Anticonvulsants may increase the catabolism of vitamin D; consider additional vitamin D supplementation when co-administering). Products include:

Tolmetin Sodium (Since NSAID use is associated with gastrointestinal irritation, caution should be used during concomitant use with alendronate sodium/cholecalciferol. No increase in the incidence of gastrointestinal irritation was reported in clinical trials).
No products indexed under this heading.

Topiramate (Anticonvulsants may increase the catabolism of vitamin D; consider additional vitamin D supplementation when co-administering).
No products indexed under this heading.

Trimethadione (Anticonvulsants may increase the catabolism of vitamin D; consider additional vitamin D supplementation when co-administering).
No products indexed under this heading.

Valdecoxib (Since NSAID use is associated with gastrointestinal irritation, caution should be used during concomitant use with alendronate sodium/cholecalciferol. No increase in the incidence of gastrointestinal irritation was reported in clinical trials).
No products indexed under this heading.

Valproate Sodium (Anticonvulsants may increase the catabolism of vitamin D; consider additional vitamin D supplementation when co-administering).
No products indexed under this heading.

Valproic Acid (Anticonvulsants may increase the catabolism of vitamin D; consider additional vitamin D supplementation when co-administering).
No products indexed under this heading.

Zonisamide (Anticonvulsants may increase the catabolism of vitamin D; consider additional vitamin D supplementation when co-administering). Products include:

Food Interactions

Beverages, caffeine-containing (Concomitant administration of alendronate with coffee reduces bioavailability by approximately 60%).

Food, unspecified (Other beverages (including mineral water) and food are likely to reduce the absorption of alendronate).

Meal, unspecified (Bioavailability was decreased (by approximately 40%) when 10 mg alendronate was administered either 0.5 or 1 hour before a standardized breakfast, when compared to dosing 2 hours before eating).

Orange Juice (Concomitant administration of alendronate with orange juice reduces bioavailability by approximately 60%).

FOSRENOL CHEWABLE TABLETS
(Lanthanum Carbonate) 3289
May interact with antacids. Compounds in these categories include:

Aluminum Carbonate (Avoid administering within 2 hours of antacids).
No products indexed under this heading.

Aluminum Hydroxide (Avoid administering within 2 hours of antacids).
No products indexed under this heading.

Calcium Carbonate (Avoid administering within 2 hours of antacids). Products include:

Magaldrate (Avoid administering within 2 hours of antacids).
No products indexed under this heading.

Magnesium Carbonate (Avoid administering within 2 hours of antacids).
No products indexed under this heading.

Magnesium Hydroxide (Avoid administering within 2 hours of antacids). Products include:

Magnesium Oxide (Avoid administering within 2 hours of antacids). Products include:

Magnesium Trisilicate (Avoid administering within 2 hours of antacids).
No products indexed under this heading.

Sodium Bicarbonate (Avoid administering within 2 hours of antacids).
No products indexed under this heading.

FRAGMIN INJECTION
(Dalteparin Sodium) 1058
May interact with anesthetics, oral anticoagulants, platelet inhibitors, thrombolytics. Compounds in these categories include:

Abciximab (Dalteparin sodium should be used with care in patients receiving oral anticoagulants, platelet inhibitors, and thrombolytic agents because of an increased risk of bleeding). Products include:

Alfentanil Hydrochloride (Patients undergoing regional anesthesia should not receive dalteparin sodium for unstable angina or non-Q-wave myocardial infarction due to an increased risk of bleeding associated with the dosage of dalteparin sodium recommended for unstable angina and non-Q-wave myocardial infarction).
No products indexed under this heading.

Alteplase (Dalteparin sodium should be used with care in patients receiving oral anticoagulants, platelet inhibitors, and thrombolytic agents because of an increased risk of bleeding). Products include:

Anisindione (Dalteparin sodium should be used with care in patients receiving oral anticoagulants, platelet inhibitors, and thrombolytic agents because of an increased risk of bleeding).
No products indexed under this heading.

Anistreplase (Dalteparin sodium should be used with care in patients receiving oral anticoagulants, platelet inhibitors, and thrombolytic agents because of an increased risk of bleeding).
No products indexed under this heading.

Articaine Hydrochloride (Patients undergoing regional anesthesia should not receive dalteparin sodium for unstable angina or non-Q-wave myocardial infarction due to an increased risk of bleeding associated with the dosage of dalteparin sodium recommended for unstable angina and non-Q-wave myocardial infarction).
No products indexed under this heading.

Aspirin (Dalteparin sodium should be used with care in patients receiving oral anticoagulants, platelet inhibitors, and thrombolytic agents because of an increased risk of bleeding). Products include:

Aspirin, Enteric Coated (Dalteparin sodium should be used with care in patients receiving oral anticoagulants, platelet inhibitors, and thrombolytic agents because of an increased risk of bleeding).
No products indexed under this heading.

Aspirin Buffered (Dalteparin sodium should be used with care in patients receiving oral anticoagulants, platelet inhibitors, and thrombolytic agents because of an increased risk of bleeding).
No products indexed under this heading.

Azlocillin Sodium (Dalteparin sodium should be used with care in patients receiving oral anticoagulants, platelet inhibitors, and thrombolytic agents because of an increased risk of bleeding).
No products indexed under this heading.

Benzocaine (Patients undergoing regional anesthesia should not receive dalteparin sodium for unstable angina or non-Q-wave myocardial infarction due to an increased risk of bleeding associated with the dosage of dalteparin sodium recommended for unstable angina and non-Q-wave myocardial infarction).
No products indexed under this heading.

Bivalirudin (Dalteparin sodium should be used with care in patients receiving oral anticoagulants, platelet inhibitors, and thrombolytic agents because of an increased risk of bleeding). Products include:

IMPORTANT NOTE: Always consult each drug listing in the patient's regimen for possible interactions.

Bupivacaine Hydrochloride (Patients undergoing regional anesthesia should not receive dalteparin sodium for unstable angina or non-Q-wave myocardial infarction due to an increased risk of bleeding associated with the dosage of dalteparin sodium recommended for unstable angina and non-Q-wave myocardial infarction).
No products indexed under this heading.

Carbenicillin Indanyl Sodium (Dalteparin sodium should be used with care in patients receiving oral anticoagulants, platelet inhibitors, and thrombolytic agents because of an increased risk of bleeding).
No products indexed under this heading.

Chloroprocaine Hydrochloride (Patients undergoing regional anesthesia should not receive dalteparin sodium for unstable angina or non-Q-wave myocardial infarction due to an increased risk of bleeding associated with the dosage of dalteparin sodium recommended for unstable angina and non-Q-wave myocardial infarction).
No products indexed under this heading.

Choline Magnesium Trisalicylate (Dalteparin sodium should be used with care in patients receiving oral anticoagulants, platelet inhibitors, and thrombolytic agents because of an increased risk of bleeding).
No products indexed under this heading.

Clopidogrel Bisulfate (Dalteparin sodium should be used with care in patients receiving oral anticoagulants, platelet inhibitors, and thrombolytic agents because of an increased risk of bleeding). Products include:
Plavix 3027

Cocaine Hydrochloride (Patients undergoing regional anesthesia should not receive dalteparin sodium for unstable angina or non-Q-wave myocardial infarction due to an increased risk of bleeding associated with the dosage of dalteparin sodium recommended for unstable angina and non-Q-wave myocardial infarction).
No products indexed under this heading.

Dextran (Dalteparin sodium should be used with care in patients receiving oral anticoagulants, platelet inhibitors, and thrombolytic agents because of an increased risk of bleeding).
No products indexed under this heading.

Dextran 40 (Dalteparin sodium should be used with care in patients receiving oral anticoagulants, platelet inhibitors, and thrombolytic agents because of an increased risk of bleeding).
No products indexed under this heading.

Dextran 70 (Dalteparin sodium should be used with care in patients receiving oral anticoagulants, platelet inhibitors, and thrombolytic agents because of an increased risk of bleeding).
No products indexed under this heading.

Dextran I (Dalteparin sodium should be used with care in patients receiving oral anticoagulants, platelet inhibitors, and thrombolytic agents because of an increased risk of bleeding).
No products indexed under this heading.

Dextrans (Low Molecular Weight) (Dalteparin sodium should be used with care in patients receiving oral anticoagulants, platelet inhibitors, and thrombolytic agents because of an increased risk of bleeding).
No products indexed under this heading.

Dibucaine (Patients undergoing regional anesthesia should not receive dalteparin sodium for unstable angina or non-Q-wave myocardial infarction due to an increased risk of bleeding associated with the dosage of dalteparin sodium recommended for unstable angina and non-Q-wave myocardial infarction).
No products indexed under this heading.

Dibucaine Hydrochloride (Patients undergoing regional anesthesia should not receive dalteparin sodium for unstable angina or non-Q-wave myocardial infarction due to an increased risk of bleeding associated with the dosage of dalteparin sodium recommended for unstable angina and non-Q-wave myocardial infarction).
No products indexed under this heading.

Diclofenac Potassium (Dalteparin sodium should be used with care in patients receiving oral anticoagulants, platelet inhibitors, and thrombolytic agents because of an increased risk of bleeding).
No products indexed under this heading.

Diclofenac Sodium (Dalteparin sodium should be used with care in patients receiving oral anticoagulants, platelet inhibitors, and thrombolytic agents because of an increased risk of bleeding).
No products indexed under this heading.

Dicumarol (Dalteparin sodium should be used with care in patients receiving oral anticoagulants, platelet inhibitors, and thrombolytic agents because of an increased risk of bleeding).
No products indexed under this heading.

Diflunisal (Dalteparin sodium should be used with care in patients receiving oral anticoagulants, platelet inhibitors, and thrombolytic agents because of an increased risk of bleeding).
No products indexed under this heading.

Dipyridamole (Dalteparin sodium should be used with care in patients receiving oral anticoagulants, platelet inhibitors, and thrombolytic agents because of an increased risk of bleeding). Products include:
Aggrenox 880

Enflurane (Patients undergoing regional anesthesia should not receive dalteparin sodium for unstable angina or non-Q-wave myocardial infarction due to an increased risk of bleeding associated with the dosage of dalteparin sodium recommended for unstable angina and non-Q-wave myocardial infarction).
No products indexed under this heading.

Eptifibatide (Dalteparin sodium should be used with care in patients receiving oral anticoagulants, platelet inhibitors, and thrombolytic agents because of an increased risk of bleeding). Products include:
Integrilin 3135

Etidocaine Hydrochloride (Patients undergoing regional anesthesia should not receive dalteparin sodium for unstable angina or non-Q-wave myocardial infarction due to an increased risk of bleeding associated with the dosage of dalteparin sodium recommended for unstable angina and non-Q-wave myocardial infarction).
No products indexed under this heading.

Fenoprofen Calcium (Dalteparin sodium should be used with care in patients receiving oral anticoagulants, platelet inhibitors, and thrombolytic agents because of an increased risk of bleeding).
No products indexed under this heading.

Fentanyl Citrate (Patients undergoing regional anesthesia should not receive dalteparin sodium for unstable angina or non-Q-wave myocardial infarction due to an increased risk of bleeding associated with the dosage of dalteparin sodium recommended for unstable angina and non-Q-wave myocardial infarction). Products include:
Fentora 966

Flurbiprofen (Dalteparin sodium should be used with care in patients receiving oral anticoagulants, platelet inhibitors, and thrombolytic agents because of an increased risk of bleeding).
No products indexed under this heading.

Halothane (Patients undergoing regional anesthesia should not receive dalteparin sodium for unstable angina or non-Q-wave myocardial infarction due to an increased risk of bleeding associated with the dosage of dalteparin sodium recommended for unstable angina and non-Q-wave myocardial infarction).
No products indexed under this heading.

Hydroxychloroquine Sulfate (Dalteparin sodium should be used with care in patients receiving oral anticoagulants, platelet inhibitors, and thrombolytic agents because of an increased risk of bleeding).
No products indexed under this heading.

Ibuprofen (Dalteparin sodium should be used with care in patients receiving oral anticoagulants, platelet inhibitors, and thrombolytic agents because of an increased risk of bleeding). Products include:
Motrin IB 2043
Children's Motrin 2044
Children's Motrin Non-Staining
    Dye-Free 2044
Infants' Motrin 2044
Infants' Motrin Dye-Free 2044
Junior Strength Motrin 2044
Vicoprofen 564

Indomethacin (Dalteparin sodium should be used with care in patients receiving oral anticoagulants, platelet inhibitors, and thrombolytic agents because of an increased risk of bleeding). Products include:
Indocin 2167

Indomethacin Sodium Trihydrate (Dalteparin sodium should be used with care in patients receiving oral anticoagulants, platelet inhibitors, and thrombolytic agents because of an increased risk of bleeding). Products include:
Indocin I.V. 2007

Isoflurane (Patients undergoing regional anesthesia should not receive dalteparin sodium for unstable angina or non-Q-wave myocardial infarction due to an increased risk of bleeding associated with the dosage of dalteparin sodium recommended for unstable angina and non-Q-wave myocardial infarction).
No products indexed under this heading.

Ketamine Hydrochloride (Patients undergoing regional anesthesia should not receive dalteparin sodium for unstable angina or non-Q-wave myocardial infarction due to an increased risk of bleeding associated with the dosage of dalteparin sodium recommended for unstable angina and non-Q-wave myocardial infarction).
No products indexed under this heading.

Ketoprofen (Dalteparin sodium should be used with care in patients receiving oral anticoagulants, platelet inhibitors, and thrombolytic agents because of an increased risk of bleeding).
No products indexed under this heading.

Levobupivacaine Hydrochloride (Patients undergoing regional anesthesia should not receive dalteparin sodium for unstable angina or non-Q-wave myocardial infarction due to an increased risk of bleeding associated with the dosage of dalteparin sodium recommended for unstable angina and non-Q-wave myocardial infarction).
No products indexed under this heading.

Lidocaine (Patients undergoing regional anesthesia should not receive dalteparin sodium for unstable angina or non-Q-wave myocardial infarction due to an increased risk of bleeding associat-

ed with the dosage of dalteparin sodium recommended for unstable angina and non-Q-wave myocardial infarction). Products include:
Lidoderm 1107

Lidocaine Base (Patients undergoing regional anesthesia should not receive dalteparin sodium for unstable angina or non-Q-wave myocardial infarction due to an increased risk of bleeding associated with the dosage of dalteparin sodium recommended for unstable angina and non-Q-wave myocardial infarction).
No products indexed under this heading.

Lidocaine Hydrochloride (Patients undergoing regional anesthesia should not receive dalteparin sodium for unstable angina or non-Q-wave myocardial infarction due to an increased risk of bleeding associated with the dosage of dalteparin sodium recommended for unstable angina and non-Q-wave myocardial infarction).
No products indexed under this heading.

Magnesium Salicylate (Dalteparin sodium should be used with care in patients receiving oral anticoagulants, platelet inhibitors, and thrombolytic agents because of an increased risk of bleeding).
No products indexed under this heading.

Meclofenamate Sodium (Dalteparin sodium should be used with care in patients receiving oral anticoagulants, platelet inhibitors, and thrombolytic agents because of an increased risk of bleeding).
No products indexed under this heading.

Mefenamic Acid (Dalteparin sodium should be used with care in patients receiving oral anticoagulants, platelet inhibitors, and thrombolytic agents because of an increased risk of bleeding).
No products indexed under this heading.

Mepivacaine Hydrochloride (Patients undergoing regional anesthesia should not receive dalteparin sodium for unstable angina or non-Q-wave myocardial infarction due to an increased risk of bleeding associated with the dosage of dalteparin sodium recommended for unstable angina and non-Q-wave myocardial infarction).
No products indexed under this heading.

Methohexital Sodium (Patients undergoing regional anesthesia should not receive dalteparin sodium for unstable angina or non-Q-wave myocardial infarction due to an increased risk of bleeding associated with the dosage of dalteparin sodium recommended for unstable angina and non-Q-wave myocardial infarction).
No products indexed under this heading.

Mezlocillin Sodium (Dalteparin sodium should be used with care in patients receiving oral anticoagulants, platelet inhibitors, and thrombolytic agents because of an increased risk of bleeding).
No products indexed under this heading.

Midazolam Hydrochloride (Patients undergoing regional anesthesia should not receive dalteparin sodium for unstable angina or non-Q-wave myocardial infarction due to an increased risk of bleeding associated with the dosage of dalteparin sodium recommended for unstable angina and non-Q-wave myocardial infarction).
No products indexed under this heading.

Nafcillin Sodium (Dalteparin sodium should be used with care in patients receiving oral anticoagulants, platelet inhibitors, and thrombolytic agents because of an increased risk of bleeding).
No products indexed under this heading.

Naproxen (Dalteparin sodium should be used with care in patients receiving

oral anticoagulants, platelet inhibitors, and thrombolytic agents because of an increased risk of bleeding). Products include:

Naproxen Sodium (Dalteparin sodium should be used with care in patients receiving oral anticoagulants, platelet inhibitors, and thrombolytic agents because of an increased risk of bleeding). Products include:

Penicillin G Benzathine (Dalteparin sodium should be used with care in patients receiving oral anticoagulants, platelet inhibitors, and thrombolytic agents because of an increased risk of bleeding). Products include:

Penicillin G Procaine (Dalteparin sodium should be used with care in patients receiving oral anticoagulants, platelet inhibitors, and thrombolytic agents because of an increased risk of bleeding). Products include:

Phenylbutazone (Dalteparin sodium should be used with care in patients receiving oral anticoagulants, platelet inhibitors, and thrombolytic agents because of an increased risk of bleeding).
No products indexed under this heading.

Piroxicam (Dalteparin sodium should be used with care in patients receiving oral anticoagulants, platelet inhibitors, and thrombolytic agents because of an increased risk of bleeding).
No products indexed under this heading.

Prilocaine (Patients undergoing regional anesthesia should not receive dalteparin sodium for unstable angina or non-Q-wave myocardial infarction due to an increased risk of bleeding associated with the dosage of dalteparin sodium recommended for unstable angina and non-Q-wave myocardial infarction).
No products indexed under this heading.

Prilocaine Hydrochloride (Patients undergoing regional anesthesia should not receive dalteparin sodium for unstable angina or non-Q-wave myocardial infarction due to an increased risk of bleeding associated with the dosage of dalteparin sodium recommended for unstable angina and non-Q-wave myocardial infarction).
No products indexed under this heading.

Procaine (Patients undergoing regional anesthesia should not receive dalteparin sodium for unstable angina or non-Q-wave myocardial infarction due to an increased risk of bleeding associated with the dosage of dalteparin sodium recommended for unstable angina and non-Q-wave myocardial infarction).
No products indexed under this heading.

Procaine Hydrochloride (Patients undergoing regional anesthesia should not receive dalteparin sodium for unstable angina or non-Q-wave myocardial infarction due to an increased risk of bleeding associated with the dosage of dalteparin sodium recommended for unstable angina and non-Q-wave myocardial infarction).
No products indexed under this heading.

Proparacaine Hydrochloride (Patients undergoing regional anesthesia should not receive dalteparin sodium for unstable angina or non-Q-wave myocardial infarction due to an increased risk of bleeding associated with the dosage of dalteparin sodium recommended for unstable angina and non-Q-wave myocardial infarction).
No products indexed under this heading.

Propofol (Patients undergoing regional anesthesia should not receive dalteparin sodium for unstable angina or non-Q-wave myocardial infarction due to an increased risk of bleeding associated with the dosage of dalteparin sodium recommended for unstable angina and non-Q-wave myocardial infarction).
No products indexed under this heading.

Remifentanil Hydrochloride (Patients undergoing regional anesthesia should not receive dalteparin sodium for unstable angina or non-Q-wave myocardial infarction due to an increased risk of bleeding associated with the dosage of dalteparin sodium recommended for unstable angina and non-Q-wave myocardial infarction).
No products indexed under this heading.

Reteplase (Dalteparin sodium should be used with care in patients receiving oral anticoagulants, platelet inhibitors, and thrombolytic agents because of an increased risk of bleeding).
No products indexed under this heading.

Ropivacaine Hydrochloride (Patients undergoing regional anesthesia should not receive dalteparin sodium for unstable angina or non-Q-wave myocardial infarction due to an increased risk of bleeding associated with the dosage of dalteparin sodium recommended for unstable angina and non-Q-wave myocardial infarction).
No products indexed under this heading.

Salsalate (Dalteparin sodium should be used with care in patients receiving oral anticoagulants, platelet inhibitors, and thrombolytic agents because of an increased risk of bleeding).
No products indexed under this heading.

Streptokinase (Dalteparin sodium should be used with care in patients receiving oral anticoagulants, platelet inhibitors, and thrombolytic agents because of an increased risk of bleeding).
No products indexed under this heading.

Sufentanil Citrate (Patients undergoing regional anesthesia should not receive dalteparin sodium for unstable angina or non-Q-wave myocardial infarction due to an increased risk of bleeding associated with the dosage of dalteparin sodium recommended for unstable angina and non-Q-wave myocardial infarction).
No products indexed under this heading.

Sulindac (Dalteparin sodium should be used with care in patients receiving oral anticoagulants, platelet inhibitors, and thrombolytic agents because of an increased risk of bleeding). Products include:

Tetracaine (Patients undergoing regional anesthesia should not receive dalteparin sodium for unstable angina or non-Q-wave myocardial infarction due to an increased risk of bleeding associated with the dosage of dalteparin sodium recommended for unstable angina and non-Q-wave myocardial infarction).
No products indexed under this heading.

Tetracaine Hydrochloride (Patients undergoing regional anesthesia should not receive dalteparin sodium for unstable angina or non-Q-wave myocardial infarction due to an increased risk of bleeding associated with the dosage of dalteparin sodium recommended for unstable angina and non-Q-wave myocardial infarction).
No products indexed under this heading.

Thiamylal Sodium (Patients undergoing regional anesthesia should not receive dalteparin sodium for unstable angina or non-Q-wave myocardial infarction due to an increased risk of bleeding associated with the dosage of dalteparin sodium recommended for unstable angina and non-Q-wave myocardial infarction).
No products indexed under this heading.

Ticarcillin Disodium (Dalteparin sodium should be used with care in patients receiving oral anticoagulants, platelet inhibitors, and thrombolytic agents because of an increased risk of bleeding). Products include:

Ticlopidine Hydrochloride (Dalteparin sodium should be used with care in patients receiving oral anticoagulants, platelet inhibitors, and thrombolytic agents because of an increased risk of bleeding).
No products indexed under this heading.

Tirofiban Hydrochloride (Dalteparin sodium should be used with care in patients receiving oral anticoagulants, platelet inhibitors, and thrombolytic agents because of an increased risk of bleeding).
No products indexed under this heading.

Tolmetin Sodium (Dalteparin sodium should be used with care in patients receiving oral anticoagulants, platelet inhibitors, and thrombolytic agents because of an increased risk of bleeding).
No products indexed under this heading.

Urokinase (Dalteparin sodium should be used with care in patients receiving oral anticoagulants, platelet inhibitors, and thrombolytic agents because of an increased risk of bleeding).
No products indexed under this heading.

Warfarin Sodium (Dalteparin sodium should be used with care in patients receiving oral anticoagulants, platelet inhibitors, and thrombolytic agents because of an increased risk of bleeding).
No products indexed under this heading.

FRESHKOTE STERILE OPHTHALMIC SOLUTION
(Polyvinyl Alcohol, Povidone) .... ⊙254
None cited in PDR database.

FROVA TABLETS
(Frovatriptan Succinate) 1103
May interact with 5HT1-receptor agonists, ergot-containing drugs, oral contraceptives, selective serotonin reuptake inhibitors, serotonin and norepinephrine reuptake inhibitors, and certain other agents. Compounds in these categories include:

Almotriptan Malate (Co-administration with other 5-HT1 agonists within 24 hours of each other is contraindicated). Products include:

Citalopram Hydrobromide (The development of a potentially life-threatening serotonin syndrome may occur with triptans, including frovatriptan succinate treatment, particularly during combined use with selective serotonin reuptake inhibitors (SSRIs) or serotonin norepinephrine reuptake inhibitors (SNRIs). If concomitant treatment with FROVA and an SSRI (eg, fluoxetine, paroxetine, sertraline, fluvoxamine, citalopram) or SNRI (eg, venlafaxine, duloxetine) is clinically warranted, careful observation of the patient is advised, particularly during treatment initiation and dose increases). Products include:

Desogestrel (Retrospective analysis of pharmacokinetic data indicates that mean C_{max} and AUC of frovatriptan are 30% higher in females taking oral contraceptives).
No products indexed under this heading.

Desvenlafaxine Succinate (The development of a potentially life-threatening serotonin syndrome may occur with triptans, including frovatriptan succinate treatment, particularly during combined use with selective serotonin reuptake inhibitors (SSRIs) or serotonin norepinephrine reuptake inhibitors (SNRIs). If concomitant treatment with FROVA and an SSRI (eg, fluoxetine, paroxetine, sertraline, fluvoxamine, citalopram, escitalopram) or SNRI (eg, venlafaxine, duloxetine) is clinically warranted, careful observation of the patient is advised, particularly during treatment initiation and dose increases). Products include:

Dihydroergotamine Mesylate (Ergot-containing drugs have been reported to cause prolonged vasospastic reactions; because there is a theoretical basis that these effects may be additive, use of ergot-type agents and frovatriptan within 24 hours is contraindicated).
No products indexed under this heading.

Duloxetine Hydrochloride (The development of a potentially life-threatening serotonin syndrome may occur with triptans, including frovatriptan succinate treatment, particularly during combined use with selective serotonin reuptake inhibitors (SSRIs) or serotonin norepinephrine reuptake inhibitors (SNRIs). If concomitant treatment with FROVA and an SSRI (eg, fluoxetine, paroxetine, sertraline, fluvoxamine, citalopram, escitalopram) or SNRI (eg, venlafaxine, duloxetine) is clinically warranted, careful observation of the patient is advised, particularly during treatment initiation and dose increases). Products include:

Eletriptan Hydrobromide (Co-administration with other 5-HT1 agonists within 24 hours of each other is contraindicated).
No products indexed under this heading.

Ergonovine Maleate (Ergot-containing drugs have been reported to cause prolonged vasospastic reactions; because there is a theoretical basis that these effects may be additive, use of ergot-type agents and frovatriptan within 24 hours is contraindicated).
No products indexed under this heading.

Ergotamine Tartrate (Ergot-containing drugs have been reported to cause prolonged vasospastic reactions; because there is a theoretical basis that these effects may be additive, use of ergot-type agents and frovatriptan within 24 hours is contraindicated).
No products indexed under this heading.

Escitalopram Oxalate (The development of a potentially life-threatening serotonin syndrome may occur with triptans, including frovatriptan succinate treatment, particularly during combined use with selective serotonin reuptake inhibitors (SSRIs) or serotonin norepinephrine reuptake inhibitors (SNRIs). If concomitant treatment with FROVA and

an SSRI (eg, fluoxetine, paroxetine, sertraline, fluvoxamine, citalopram, escitalopram) or SNRI (eg, venlafaxine, duloxetine) is clinically warranted, careful observation of the patient is advised, particularly during treatment initiation and dose increases). Products include:

Ethinyl Estradiol (Retrospective analysis of pharmacokinetic data indicates that mean C_{max} and AUC of frovatriptan are 30% higher in females taking oral contraceptives). Products include:

Ethynodiol Diacetate (Retrospective analysis of pharmacokinetic data indicates that mean C_{max} and AUC of frovatriptan are 30% higher in females taking oral contraceptives).

No products indexed under this heading.

Fluoxetine (The development of a potentially life-threatening serotonin syndrome may occur with triptans, including frovatriptan succinate treatment, particularly during combined use with selective serotonin reuptake inhibitors (SSRIs) or serotonin norepinephrine reuptake inhibitors (SNRIs). If concomitant treatment with FROVA and an SSRI (eg, fluoxetine, paroxetine, sertraline, fluvoxamine, citalopram, escitalopram) or SNRI (eg, venlafaxine, duloxetine) is clinically warranted, careful observation of the patient is advised, particularly during treatment initiation and dose increases).

No products indexed under this heading.

Fluoxetine Hydrochloride (The development of a potentially life-threatening serotonin syndrome may occur with triptans, including frovatriptan succinate treatment, particularly during combined use with selective serotonin reuptake inhibitors (SSRIs) or serotonin norepinephrine reuptake inhibitors (SNRIs). If concomitant treatment with FROVA and an SSRI (eg, fluoxetine, paroxetine, sertraline, fluvoxamine, citalopram, escitalopram) or SNRI (eg, venlafaxine, duloxetine) is clinically warranted, careful observation of the patient is advised, particularly during treatment initiation and dose increases). Products include:

Fluvoxamine (The development of a potentially life-threatening serotonin syndrome may occur with triptans, including frovatriptan succinate treatment, particularly during combined use with selective serotonin reuptake inhibitors (SSRIs) or serotonin norepinephrine reuptake inhibitors (SNRIs). If concomitant treatment with FROVA and an SSRI (eg, fluoxetine, paroxetine, sertraline, fluvoxamine, citalopram, escitalopram) or SNRI (eg, venlafaxine, duloxetine) is clinically warranted, careful observation of the patient is advised, particularly during treatment initiation and dose increases).

No products indexed under this heading.

Fluvoxamine Maleate (The development of a potentially life-threatening serotonin syndrome may occur with triptans, including frovatriptan succinate treatment, particularly during combined use with selective serotonin reuptake inhibitors (SSRIs) or serotonin norepinephrine reuptake inhibitors (SNRIs). If concomitant treatment with FROVA and an SSRI (eg, fluoxetine, paroxetine, sertraline, fluvoxamine, citalopram, escit-

alopram) or SNRI (eg, venlafaxine, duloxetine) is clinically warranted, careful observation of the patient is advised, particularly during treatment initiation and dose increases).

No products indexed under this heading.

Levonorgestrel (Retrospective analysis of pharmacokinetic data indicates that mean C_{max} and AUC of frovatriptan are 30% higher in females taking oral contraceptives). Products include:

Mestranol (Retrospective analysis of pharmacokinetic data indicates that mean C_{max} and AUC of frovatriptan are 30% higher in females taking oral contraceptives).

No products indexed under this heading.

Methylergonovine Maleate (Ergot-containing drugs have been reported to cause prolonged vasospastic reactions; because there is a theoretical basis that these effects may be additive, use of ergot-type agents and frovatriptan within 24 hours is contraindicated).

No products indexed under this heading.

Methysergide Maleate (Ergot-containing drugs have been reported to cause prolonged vasospastic reactions; because there is a theoretical basis that these effects may be additive, use of ergot-type agents and frovatriptan within 24 hours is contraindicated).

No products indexed under this heading.

Naratriptan Hydrochloride (Co-administration with other 5-HT1 agonists within 24 hours of each other is contraindicated). Products include:

Nefazodone Hydrochloride (The development of a potentially life-threatening serotonin syndrome may occur with triptans, including frovatriptan succinate treatment, particularly during combined use with selective serotonin reuptake inhibitors (SSRIs) or serotonin norepinephrine reuptake inhibitors (SNRIs). If concomitant treatment with FROVA and an SSRI (eg, fluoxetine, paroxetine, sertraline, fluvoxamine, citalopram, escitalopram) or SNRI (eg, venlafaxine, duloxetine) is clinically warranted, careful observation of the patient is advised, particularly during treatment initiation and dose increases).

No products indexed under this heading.

Norethindrone (Retrospective analysis of pharmacokinetic data indicates that mean C_{max} and AUC of frovatriptan are 30% higher in females taking oral contraceptives). Products include:

Norethynodrel (Retrospective analysis of pharmacokinetic data indicates that mean C_{max} and AUC of frovatriptan are 30% higher in females taking oral contraceptives).

No products indexed under this heading.

Norgestimate (Retrospective analysis of pharmacokinetic data indicates that mean C_{max} and AUC of frovatriptan are 30% higher in females taking oral contraceptives). Products include:

Norgestrel (Retrospective analysis of pharmacokinetic data indicates that mean C_{max} and AUC of frovatriptan are 30% higher in females taking oral contraceptives).

No products indexed under this heading.

Paroxetine (The development of a potentially life-threatening serotonin syndrome may occur with triptans, including frovatriptan succinate treatment, particularly during combined use

with selective serotonin reuptake inhibitors (SSRIs) or serotonin norepinephrine reuptake inhibitors (SNRIs). If concomitant treatment with FROVA and an SSRI (eg, fluoxetine, paroxetine, sertraline, fluvoxamine, citalopram, escitalopram) or SNRI (eg, venlafaxine, duloxetine) is clinically warranted, careful observation of the patient is advised, particularly during treatment initiation and dose increases).

No products indexed under this heading.

Paroxetine Hydrochloride (The development of a potentially life-threatening serotonin syndrome may occur with triptans, including frovatriptan succinate treatment, particularly during combined use with selective serotonin reuptake inhibitors (SSRIs) or serotonin norepinephrine reuptake inhibitors (SNRIs). If concomitant treatment with FROVA and an SSRI (eg, fluoxetine, paroxetine, sertraline, fluvoxamine, citalopram, escitalopram) or SNRI (eg, venlafaxine, duloxetine) is clinically warranted, careful observation of the patient is advised, particularly during treatment initiation and dose increases). Products include:

Paroxetine Mesylate (The development of a potentially life-threatening serotonin syndrome may occur with triptans, including frovatriptan succinate treatment, particularly during combined use with selective serotonin reuptake inhibitors (SSRIs) or serotonin norepinephrine reuptake inhibitors (SNRIs). If concomitant treatment with FROVA and an SSRI (eg, fluoxetine, paroxetine, sertraline, fluvoxamine, citalopram, escitalopram) or SNRI (eg, venlafaxine, duloxetine) is clinically warranted, careful observation of the patient is advised, particularly during treatment initiation and dose increases).

No products indexed under this heading.

Propranolol Hydrochloride (Increases AUC of frovatriptan in males by 60% and in females by 29%; C_{max} was increased by 23% in males and 16% in females). Products include:

Rizatriptan Benzoate (Co-administration with other 5-HT1 agonists within 24 hours of each other is contraindicated). Products include:

Sertraline Hydrochloride (The development of a potentially life-threatening serotonin syndrome may occur with triptans, including frovatriptan succinate treatment, particularly during combined use with selective serotonin reuptake inhibitors (SSRIs) or serotonin norepinephrine reuptake inhibitors (SNRIs). If concomitant treatment with FROVA and an SSRI (eg, fluoxetine, paroxetine, sertraline, fluvoxamine, citalopram, escitalopram) or SNRI (eg, venlafaxine, duloxetine) is clinically warranted, careful observation of the patient is advised, particularly during treatment initiation and dose increases).

No products indexed under this heading.

Sumatriptan (Co-administration with other 5-HT1 agonists within 24 hours of each other is contraindicated). Products include:

Sumatriptan Succinate (Co-administration with other 5-HT1 agonists within 24 hours of each other is contraindicated). Products include:

Venlafaxine Hydrochloride (The development of a potentially life-threatening serotonin syndrome may occur with triptans, including frovatriptan succinate treatment, particularly during combined use with selective serotonin reuptake inhibitors (SSRIs) or serotonin norepinephrine reuptake inhibitors (SNRIs). If concomitant treatment with FROVA and an SSRI (eg, fluoxetine, paroxetine, sertraline, fluvoxamine, citalopram, escitalopram) or SNRI (eg, venlafaxine, duloxetine) is clinically warranted, careful observation of the patient is advised, particularly during treatment initiation and dose increases). Products include:

Zolmitriptan (Co-administration with other 5-HT1 agonists within 24 hours of each other is contraindicated). Products include:

FUROSEMIDE TABLETS

May interact with alcohols, aminoglycosides, antihypertensives, barbiturates, cardiac glycosides, corticosteroids, lithium preparations, narcotic analgesics, non-steroidal anti-inflammatory agents, salicylates, and certain other agents. Compounds in these categories include:

Acebutolol Hydrochloride (Furosemide may add to or potentiate the therapeutic effect of other antihypertensive drugs).

No products indexed under this heading.

ACTH (Co-administration with ACTH may increase the risk of hypokalemia).

No products indexed under this heading.

Alclometasone Dipropionate (Co-administration with corticosteroids may increase the risk of hypokalemia).

No products indexed under this heading.

Alfentanil Hydrochloride (Aggravates orthostatic hypotension).

No products indexed under this heading.

Aliskiren (Furosemide may add to or potentiate the therapeutic effect of other antihypertensive drugs). Products include:

Amikacin Sulfate (Potential for increased risk of ototoxicity with concomitant therapy, especially in the presence of impaired renal function; avoid concurrent use except in presence of life threatening situations).

No products indexed under this heading.

Amlodipine Besylate (Furosemide may add to or potentiate the therapeutic effect of other antihypertensive drugs). Products include:

Amobarbital (Aggravates orthostatic hypotension).

No products indexed under this heading.

Amobarbital Sodium (Aggravates orthostatic hypotension).

No products indexed under this heading.

Apomorphine (Aggravates orthostatic hypotension).

No products indexed under this heading.

Apomorphine Hydrochloride (Aggravates orthostatic hypotension).

No products indexed under this heading.

Aprobarbital (Aggravates orthostatic hypotension).

No products indexed under this heading.

Aspirin (Combination of furosemide and aspirin temporarily reduced creati-

nine clearance in patients with chronic renal insufficiency; co-administration in patients receiving high doses of salicylates may experience salicylate toxicity). Products include:

Aggrenox	880
Bayer Aspirin	829
Percodan	1124
St. Joseph Aspirin	2045

Aspirin, Enteric Coated (Co-administration in patients receiving high doses of salicylates may experience salicylate toxicity).
No products indexed under this heading.

Aspirin Buffered (Co-administration in patients receiving high doses of salicylates may experience salicylate toxicity).
No products indexed under this heading.

Atenolol (Furosemide may add to or potentiate the therapeutic effect of other antihypertensive drugs).
No products indexed under this heading.

Beclomethasone Dipropionate (Co-administration with corticosteroids may increase the risk of hypokalemia). Products include:
Qvar 3398

Beclomethasone Dipropionate Monohydrate (Co-administration with corticosteroids may increase the risk of hypokalemia). Products include:
Beconase AQ 1386

Benazepril Hydrochloride (Furosemide may add to or potentiate the therapeutic effect of other antihypertensive drugs).
No products indexed under this heading.

Bendroflumethiazide (Furosemide may add to or potentiate the therapeutic effect of other antihypertensive drugs).
No products indexed under this heading.

Betamethasone (Co-administration with corticosteroids may increase the risk of hypokalemia).
No products indexed under this heading.

Betamethasone Acetate (Co-administration with corticosteroids may increase the risk of hypokalemia).
No products indexed under this heading.

Betamethasone Benzoate (Co-administration with corticosteroids may increase the risk of hypokalemia).
No products indexed under this heading.

Betamethasone Dipropionate (Co-administration with corticosteroids may increase the risk of hypokalemia). Products include:

Diprolene Lotion 0.05%	3108
Diprolene Ointment 0.05%	3109
Diprolene AF Cream 0.05%	3107
Lotrisone	3163

Betamethasone Sodium Phosphate (Co-administration with corticosteroids may increase the risk of hypokalemia).
No products indexed under this heading.

Betamethasone Valerate (Co-administration with corticosteroids may increase the risk of hypokalemia). Products include:
Luxiq 3321

Betaxolol Hydrochloride (Furosemide may add to or potentiate the therapeutic effect of other antihypertensive drugs).
No products indexed under this heading.

Bisoprolol Fumarate (Furosemide may add to or potentiate the therapeutic effect of other antihypertensive drugs).
No products indexed under this heading.

Budesonide (Co-administration with corticosteroids may increase the risk of hypokalemia). Products include:

Pulmicort Flexhaler	714
Symbicort 80/4.5	720
Symbicort 160/4.5	720

Buprenorphine Hydrochloride (Aggravates orthostatic hypotension).
No products indexed under this heading.

Butabarbital (Aggravates orthostatic hypotension).
No products indexed under this heading.

Butabarbital Sodium (Aggravates orthostatic hypotension).
No products indexed under this heading.

Butalbital (Aggravates orthostatic hypotension).
No products indexed under this heading.

Candesartan Cilexetil (Furosemide may add to or potentiate the therapeutic effect of other antihypertensive drugs). Products include:

Atacand	697
Atacand HCT	700

Captopril (Furosemide may add to or potentiate the therapeutic effect of other antihypertensive drugs). Products include:
Captopril 2341

Carteolol Hydrochloride (Furosemide may add to or potentiate the therapeutic effect of other antihypertensive drugs).
No products indexed under this heading.

Carvedilol (Furosemide may add to or potentiate the therapeutic effect of other antihypertensive drugs). Products include:
Coreg 1409

Carvedilol Phosphate (Furosemide may add to or potentiate the therapeutic effect of other antihypertensive drugs). Products include:
Coreg CR 1416

Celecoxib (Co-administration with NSAIDs has resulted in increased BUN, serum creatinine and serum potassium levels, and weight gain). Products include:
Celebrex 3272

Chlorothiazide (Furosemide may add to or potentiate the therapeutic effect of other antihypertensive drugs).
No products indexed under this heading.

Chlorothiazide Sodium (Furosemide may add to or potentiate the therapeutic effect of other antihypertensive drugs). Products include:
Diuril Intravenous 2009

Chlorthalidone (Furosemide may add to or potentiate the therapeutic effect of other antihypertensive drugs). Products include:
Clorpres 2344

Choline Magnesium Trisalicylate (Co-administration in patients receiving high doses of salicylates may experience salicylate toxicity).
No products indexed under this heading.

Ciclesonide (Co-administration with corticosteroids may increase the risk of hypokalemia).
No products indexed under this heading.

Clonidine (Furosemide may add to or potentiate the therapeutic effect of other antihypertensive drugs). Products include:
Catapres-TTS 884

Clonidine Hydrochloride (Furosemide may add to or potentiate the therapeutic effect of other antihypertensive drugs). Products include:
Clorpres 2344

Codeine Phosphate (Aggravates orthostatic hypotension). Products include:
Tylenol with Codeine 2691

Codeine Sulfate (Aggravates orthostatic hypotension).
No products indexed under this heading.

Cortisone Acetate (Co-administration with corticosteroids may increase the risk of hypokalemia).
No products indexed under this heading.

Deserpidine (Furosemide may add to or potentiate the therapeutic effect of other antihypertensive drugs).
No products indexed under this heading.

Deslanoside (Concurrent digitalis therapy may exaggerate metabolic effects of hypokalemia, especially myocardial effects).
No products indexed under this heading.

Desoximetasone (Co-administration with corticosteroids may increase the risk of hypokalemia).
No products indexed under this heading.

Dexamethasone (Co-administration with corticosteroids may increase the risk of hypokalemia). Products include:

Ciprodex	583
Ozurdex	⊙223
Tobramycin and Dexamethasone Ophthalmic Suspension	⊙251

Dexamethasone Acetate (Co-administration with corticosteroids may increase the risk of hypokalemia).
No products indexed under this heading.

Dexamethasone Phosphate (Co-administration with corticosteroids may increase the risk of hypokalemia).
No products indexed under this heading.

Dexamethasone Sodium (Co-administration with corticosteroids may increase the risk of hypokalemia).
No products indexed under this heading.

Dexamethasone Sodium Phosphate (Co-administration with corticosteroids may increase the risk of hypokalemia).
No products indexed under this heading.

Dexamethasone Sodium Phosphate Injection (Co-administration with corticosteroids may increase the risk of hypokalemia).
No products indexed under this heading.

Dezocine (Aggravates orthostatic hypotension).
No products indexed under this heading.

Diazoxide (Furosemide may add to or potentiate the therapeutic effect of other antihypertensive drugs). Products include:

Proglycem	1179
Proglycem Suspension	1179

Diclofenac Epolamine (Co-administration with NSAIDs has resulted in increased BUN, serum creatinine and serum potassium levels, and weight gain). Products include:
Flector 1839

Diclofenac Potassium (Co-administration with NSAIDs has resulted in increased BUN, serum creatinine and serum potassium levels, and weight gain).
No products indexed under this heading.

Diclofenac Sodium (Co-administration with NSAIDs has resulted in increased BUN, serum creatinine and serum potassium levels, and weight gain).
No products indexed under this heading.

Diflorasone Diacetate (Co-administration with corticosteroids may increase the risk of hypokalemia).
No products indexed under this heading.

Diflunisal (Co-administration in patients receiving high doses of salicylates may experience salicylate toxicity).
No products indexed under this heading.

Digitalis Glycoside Preparations (Concurrent digitalis therapy may exaggerate metabolic effects of hypokalemia, especially myocardial effects).
No products indexed under this heading.

Digitalis Lanata (Concurrent digitalis therapy may exaggerate metabolic effects of hypokalemia, especially myocardial effects).
No products indexed under this heading.

Digitalis Purpurea (Concurrent digitalis therapy may exaggerate metabolic effects of hypokalemia, especially myocardial effects).
No products indexed under this heading.

Digitoxin (Concurrent digitalis therapy may exaggerate metabolic effects of hypokalemia, especially myocardial effects).
No products indexed under this heading.

Digoxin (Concurrent digitalis therapy may exaggerate metabolic effects of hypokalemia, especially myocardial effects). Products include:

Lanoxin Injection	1546
Lanoxin Injection Pediatric	1549
Lanoxin Tablets	1553

Dihydrocodeine Bitartrate (Aggravates orthostatic hypotension).
No products indexed under this heading.

Dihydrocodeinone Bitartrate (Aggravates orthostatic hypotension).
No products indexed under this heading.

Dihydrostreptomycin (Potential for increased risk of ototoxicity with concomitant therapy, especially in the presence of impaired renal function; avoid concurrent use except in presence of life threatening situations).
No products indexed under this heading.

Diltiazem Hydrochloride (Furosemide may add to or potentiate the therapeutic effect of other antihypertensive drugs). Products include:
Cardizem LA 423

Diltiazem Maleate (Furosemide may add to or potentiate the therapeutic effect of other antihypertensive drugs).
No products indexed under this heading.

Doxazosin Mesylate (Furosemide may add to or potentiate the therapeutic effect of other antihypertensive drugs).
No products indexed under this heading.

Enalapril Maleate (Furosemide may add to or potentiate the therapeutic effect of other antihypertensive drugs).
No products indexed under this heading.

Enalaprilat (Furosemide may add to or potentiate the therapeutic effect of other antihypertensive drugs).
No products indexed under this heading.

Eprosartan Mesylate (Furosemide may add to or potentiate the therapeutic effect of other antihypertensive drugs). Products include:

Teveten	538
Teveten HCT	541

Esmolol Hydrochloride (Furosemide may add to or potentiate the therapeutic effect of other antihypertensive drugs).
No products indexed under this heading.

Ethacrynic Acid (Potential for increased risk of ototoxicity with concomitant therapy; concurrent use should be avoided).
No products indexed under this heading.

Ethanol (Aggravates orthostatic hypotension).
No products indexed under this heading.

Ethyl Alcohol (Aggravates orthostatic hypotension).
No products indexed under this heading.

Etodolac (Co-administration with NSAIDs has resulted in increased BUN, serum creatinine and serum potassium levels, and weight gain).
No products indexed under this heading.

Felodipine (Furosemide may add to or potentiate the therapeutic effect of other antihypertensive drugs).
No products indexed under this heading.

Fenoprofen Calcium (Co-administration with NSAIDs has resulted in increased BUN, serum creatinine and serum potassium levels, and weight gain).
No products indexed under this heading.

IMPORTANT NOTE: Always consult each drug listing in the patient's regimen for possible interactions.

(⊙ Described in PDR® for Ophthalmic Medicines)

Moexipril Hydrochloride (Furosemide may add to or potentiate the therapeutic effect of other antihypertensive drugs).
No products indexed under this heading.

Mometasone Furoate (Co-administration with corticosteroids may increase the risk of hypokalemia). Products include:
Asmanex 3058
Elocon Cream 3111
Elocon Lotion 3112
Elocon Ointment 3114

Mometasone Furoate Monohydrate (Co-administration with corticosteroids may increase the risk of hypokalemia). Products include:
Nasonex 3166

Morphine Sulfate (Aggravates orthostatic hypotension). Products include:
Avinza 1822
Embeda 1831
MS Contin 2803

Morphine Sulfate, Liposomal (Aggravates orthostatic hypotension).
No products indexed under this heading.

Nabumetone (Co-administration with NSAIDs has resulted in increased BUN, serum creatinine and serum potassium levels, and weight gain).
No products indexed under this heading.

Nadolol (Furosemide may add to or potentiate the therapeutic effect of other antihypertensive drugs). Products include:
Nadolol 2359

Naproxen (Co-administration with NSAIDs has resulted in increased BUN, serum creatinine and serum potassium levels, and weight gain). Products include:
EC-Naprosyn 2850
Naprosyn 2850
Anaprox/Naprosyn 2850

Naproxen Sodium (Co-administration with NSAIDs has resulted in increased BUN, serum creatinine and serum potassium levels, and weight gain). Products include:
Anaprox 2850
Anaprox DS 2850
Treximet 1681

Nebivolol (Furosemide may add to or potentiate the therapeutic effect of other antihypertensive drugs). Products include:
Bystolic 1147

Neomycin (Potential for increased risk of ototoxicity with concomitant therapy, especially in the presence of impaired renal function; avoid concurrent use except in presence of life threatening situations).
No products indexed under this heading.

Neomycin, oral (Potential for increased risk of ototoxicity with concomitant therapy, especially in the presence of impaired renal function; avoid concurrent use except in presence of life threatening situations).
No products indexed under this heading.

Neomycin Sulfate (Potential for increased risk of ototoxicity with concomitant therapy, especially in the presence of impaired renal function; avoid concurrent use except in presence of life threatening situations).
No products indexed under this heading.

Nicardipine Hydrochloride (Furosemide may add to or potentiate the therapeutic effect of other antihypertensive drugs).
No products indexed under this heading.

Nifedipine (Furosemide may add to or potentiate the therapeutic effect of other antihypertensive drugs).
No products indexed under this heading.

Nisoldipine (Furosemide may add to or potentiate the therapeutic effect of other antihypertensive drugs).
No products indexed under this heading.

Nitroglycerin (Furosemide may add to or potentiate the therapeutic effect of other antihypertensive drugs). Products include:
Nitro-Dur 3170
Nitrolingual 3266

Norepinephrine Bitartrate (Furosemide may decrease arterial responsiveness to norepinephrine).
No products indexed under this heading.

Oxaprozin (Co-administration with NSAIDs has resulted in increased BUN, serum creatinine and serum potassium levels, and weight gain).
No products indexed under this heading.

Oxycodone Hydrochloride (Aggravates orthostatic hypotension). Products include:
OxyContin 2807
Percocet 1121
Percodan 1124

Oxycodone Terephthalate (Aggravates orthostatic hypotension).
No products indexed under this heading.

Oxymorphone Hydrochloride (Aggravates orthostatic hypotension). Products include:
Opana 1110
Opana ER 1114

Penbutolol Sulfate (Furosemide may add to or potentiate the therapeutic effect of other antihypertensive drugs).
No products indexed under this heading.

Pentobarbital (Aggravates orthostatic hypotension).
No products indexed under this heading.

Pentobarbital Sodium (Aggravates orthostatic hypotension). Products include:
Nembutal 2012

Perindopril Erbumine (Furosemide may add to or potentiate the therapeutic effect of other antihypertensive drugs).
No products indexed under this heading.

Phenobarbital (Aggravates orthostatic hypotension). Products include:
Donnatal 2711

Phenobarbital Sodium (Aggravates orthostatic hypotension).
No products indexed under this heading.

Phenoxybenzamine Hydrochloride (Furosemide may add to or potentiate the therapeutic effect of other antihypertensive drugs). Products include:
Dibenzyline 3495

Phentolamine Mesylate (Furosemide may add to or potentiate the therapeutic effect of other antihypertensive drugs).
No products indexed under this heading.

Phenylbutazone (Co-administration with NSAIDs has resulted in increased BUN, serum creatinine and serum potassium levels, and weight gain).
No products indexed under this heading.

Pindolol (Furosemide may add to or potentiate the therapeutic effect of other antihypertensive drugs).
No products indexed under this heading.

Piroxicam (Co-administration with NSAIDs has resulted in increased BUN, serum creatinine and serum potassium levels, and weight gain).
No products indexed under this heading.

Polythiazide (Furosemide may add to or potentiate the therapeutic effect of other antihypertensive drugs).
No products indexed under this heading.

Prazosin Hydrochloride (Furosemide may add to or potentiate the therapeutic effect of other antihypertensive drugs).
No products indexed under this heading.

Prednisolone (Co-administration with corticosteroids may increase the risk of hypokalemia).
No products indexed under this heading.

Prednisolone Acetate (Co-administration with corticosteroids may increase the risk of hypokalemia). Products include:
Blephamide .... ⊙**212**, ⊙**214**
Pred Forte .... ⊙**225**
Pred Mild .... ⊙**230**
Pred-G .... ⊙**226**, ⊙**227**

Prednisolone Sodium Phosphate (Co-administration with corticosteroids may increase the risk of hypokalemia).
No products indexed under this heading.

Prednisolone Tebutate (Co-administration with corticosteroids may increase the risk of hypokalemia).
No products indexed under this heading.

Prednisone (Co-administration with corticosteroids may increase the risk of hypokalemia).
No products indexed under this heading.

Prednisone sodium phosphate (Co-administration with corticosteroids may increase the risk of hypokalemia).
No products indexed under this heading.

Propoxyphene Hydrochloride (Aggravates orthostatic hypotension).
No products indexed under this heading.

Propoxyphene Napsylate (Aggravates orthostatic hypotension).
No products indexed under this heading.

Propranolol Hydrochloride (Furosemide may add to or potentiate the therapeutic effect of other antihypertensive drugs). Products include:
InnoPran XL 1517

Quinapril Hydrochloride (Furosemide may add to or potentiate the therapeutic effect of other antihypertensive drugs).
No products indexed under this heading.

Ramipril (Furosemide may add to or potentiate the therapeutic effect of other antihypertensive drugs).
No products indexed under this heading.

Rauwolfia Serpentina (Furosemide may add to or potentiate the therapeutic effect of other antihypertensive drugs).
No products indexed under this heading.

Remifentanil Hydrochloride (Aggravates orthostatic hypotension).
No products indexed under this heading.

Rescinnamine (Furosemide may add to or potentiate the therapeutic effect of other antihypertensive drugs).
No products indexed under this heading.

Reserpine (Furosemide may add to or potentiate the therapeutic effect of other antihypertensive drugs).
No products indexed under this heading.

Rofecoxib (Co-administration with NSAIDs has resulted in increased BUN, serum creatinine and serum potassium levels, and weight gain).
No products indexed under this heading.

Salsalate (Co-administration in patients receiving high doses of salicylates may experience salicylate toxicity).
No products indexed under this heading.

Secobarbital Sodium (Aggravates orthostatic hypotension).
No products indexed under this heading.

Sodium Butabarbital (Aggravates orthostatic hypotension).
No products indexed under this heading.

Sodium Nitroprusside (Furosemide may add to or potentiate the therapeutic effect of other antihypertensive drugs).
No products indexed under this heading.

Sodium Pentobarbital (Aggravates orthostatic hypotension).
No products indexed under this heading.

Sotalol Hydrochloride (Furosemide may add to or potentiate the therapeutic effect of other antihypertensive drugs).
No products indexed under this heading.

Spirapril Hydrochloride (Furosemide may add to or potentiate the therapeutic effect of other antihypertensive drugs).
No products indexed under this heading.

Streptomycin Sulfate (Potential for increased risk of ototoxicity with concomitant therapy, especially in the presence of impaired renal function; avoid concurrent use except in presence of life threatening situations).
No products indexed under this heading.

Succinylcholine Chloride (Furosemide has a tendency to potentiate the action of succinylcholine).
No products indexed under this heading.

Sucralfate (Simultaneous administration of sucralfate and furosemide may reduce the natriuretic and antihypertensive effects of furosemide; the intake of these two drugs should be separated by at least two hours). Products include:
Carafate Suspension 784
Carafate Tablets 785

Sufentanil Citrate (Aggravates orthostatic hypotension).
No products indexed under this heading.

Sulindac (Co-administration with NSAIDs has resulted in increased BUN, serum creatinine and serum potassium levels, and weight gain). Products include:
Clinoril 2098

Telmisartan (Furosemide may add to or potentiate the therapeutic effect of other antihypertensive drugs). Products include:
Micardis 887
Micardis HCT 889

Terazosin Hydrochloride (Furosemide may add to or potentiate the therapeutic effect of other antihypertensive drugs).
No products indexed under this heading.

Thiamylal Sodium (Aggravates orthostatic hypotension).
No products indexed under this heading.

Timolol Maleate (Furosemide may add to or potentiate the therapeutic effect of other antihypertensive drugs). Products include:
Combigan 601
Dorzolamide Hydrochloride/Timolol Maleate Ophthalmic Solution .... ⊙243
Timoptic in Ocudose .... ⊙231

Tobramycin (Potential for increased risk of ototoxicity with concomitant therapy, especially in the presence of impaired renal function; avoid concurrent use except in presence of life threatening situations). Products include:
Tobi Nebulizer 2546
Tobramycin and Dexamethasone Ophthalmic Suspension .... ⊙251
Zylet .... ⊙252

Tobramycin Sulfate (Potential for increased risk of ototoxicity with concomitant therapy, especially in the presence of impaired renal function; avoid concurrent use except in presence of life threatening situations).
No products indexed under this heading.

Tolmetin Sodium (Co-administration with NSAIDs has resulted in increased BUN, serum creatinine and serum potassium levels, and weight gain).
No products indexed under this heading.

Torsemide (Furosemide may add to or potentiate the therapeutic effect of other antihypertensive drugs).
No products indexed under this heading.

IMPORTANT NOTE: Always consult each drug listing in the patient's regimen for possible interactions.

Trandolapril (Furosemide may add to or potentiate the therapeutic effect of other antihypertensive drugs). Products include:

Mavik	489
Tarka	534

Triamcinolone (Co-administration with corticosteroids may increase the risk of hypokalemia).
No products indexed under this heading.

Triamcinolone Acetonide (Co-administration with corticosteroids may increase the risk of hypokalemia). Products include:

Azmacort	408
Nasacort AQ	3019

Triamcinolone Diacetate (Co-administration with corticosteroids may increase the risk of hypokalemia).
No products indexed under this heading.

Triamcinolone Hexacetonide (Co-administration with corticosteroids may increase the risk of hypokalemia).
No products indexed under this heading.

Trimethaphan Camsylate (Furosemide may add to or potentiate the therapeutic effect of other antihypertensive drugs).
No products indexed under this heading.

Tubocurarine Chloride (Furosemide has a tendency to antagonize the skeletal muscle relaxing effects of tubocurarine).
No products indexed under this heading.

Valdecoxib (Co-administration with NSAIDs has resulted in increased BUN, serum creatinine and serum potassium levels, and weight gain).
No products indexed under this heading.

Valsartan (Furosemide may add to or potentiate the therapeutic effect of other antihypertensive drugs). Products include:

Diovan	2413
Diovan HCT	2419
Exforge	2443
Exforge HCT	2449
Valturna	3637

Verapamil Hydrochloride (Furosemide may add to or potentiate the therapeutic effect of other antihypertensive drugs). Products include:

Tarka	534

Food Interactions

Alcohol (Aggravates orthostatic hypotension).

Beer, reduced-alcohol (Aggravates orthostatic hypotension).

Beer, unspecified (Aggravates orthostatic hypotension).

Wine, Chianti (Aggravates orthostatic hypotension).

Wine, Red (Aggravates orthostatic hypotension).

Wine, unspecified (Aggravates orthostatic hypotension).

Wine products (Aggravates orthostatic hypotension).

GABITRIL TABLETS

(Tiagabine Hydrochloride)	972

May interact with alcohols, anticonvulsants, antidepressant drugs, antipsychotic agents, central nervous system depressants, central nervous system stimulants, cytochrome p450 inducers (selected), cytochrome p450 inhibitors (selected), highly protein bound drugs (selected), narcotic analgesics, phenytoin, valproate, and certain other agents. Compounds in these categories include:

Acetazolamide (Because of the potential for pharmacokinetic interactions between tiagabine hydrochloride and drugs that inhibit hepatic metabolizing enzymes, it may be useful to obtain plasma levels of tiagabine before and after changes are made in the therapeutic regimen).
No products indexed under this heading.

Acetazolamide Sodium (Because of the potential for pharmacokinetic interactions between tiagabine hydrochloride and drugs that inhibit hepatic metabolizing enzymes, it may be useful to obtain plasma levels of tiagabine before and after changes are made in the therapeutic regimen).
No products indexed under this heading.

Alatrofloxacin Mesylate (Because of the potential for pharmacokinetic interactions between tiagabine hydrochloride and drugs that inhibit hepatic metabolizing enzymes, it may be useful to obtain plasma levels of tiagabine before and after changes are made in the therapeutic regimen).
No products indexed under this heading.

Alfentanil Hydrochloride (Because of the possible additive depressive effects, caution should be used when patients are taking other CNS depressants in combination with tiagabine hydrochloride).
No products indexed under this heading.

Allium cepa (Because of the potential for pharmacokinetic interactions between tiagabine hydrochloride and drugs that induce hepatic metabolizing enzymes, it may be useful to obtain plasma levels of tiagabine before and after changes are made in the therapeutic regimen). Products include:

Hyland's Cold 'N Cough	3314
Mederma	2319
Mederma for Kids	2319

Allium sativum (Because of the potential for pharmacokinetic interactions between tiagabine hydrochloride and drugs that induce hepatic metabolizing enzymes, it may be useful to obtain plasma levels of tiagabine before and after changes are made in the therapeutic regimen).
No products indexed under this heading.

Allium schoenoprasum (Because of the potential for pharmacokinetic interactions between tiagabine hydrochloride and drugs that induce hepatic metabolizing enzymes, it may be useful to obtain plasma levels of tiagabine before and after changes are made in the therapeutic regimen).
No products indexed under this heading.

Allium ursinum (Because of the potential for pharmacokinetic interactions between tiagabine hydrochloride and drugs that induce hepatic metabolizing enzymes, it may be useful to obtain plasma levels of tiagabine before and after changes are made in the therapeutic regimen).
No products indexed under this heading.

Alprazolam (Because of the possible additive depressive effects, caution should be used when patients are taking other CNS depressants in combination with tiagabine hydrochloride).
No products indexed under this heading.

Aminoglutethimide (Because of the potential for pharmacokinetic interactions between tiagabine hydrochloride and drugs that induce hepatic metabolizing enzymes, it may be useful to obtain plasma levels of tiagabine before and after changes are made in the therapeutic regimen).
No products indexed under this heading.

Amiodarone Hydrochloride (Tiagabine is 96% bound to human plasma protein and therefore has the potential to interact with other highly protein bound compounds. Such an interaction can potentially lead to higher free fractions of either tiagabine or the competing drug).
No products indexed under this heading.

Amitriptyline Hydrochloride (Tiagabine is 96% bound to human plasma protein and therefore has the potential to interact with other highly protein bound compounds. Such an interaction can potentially lead to higher free fractions of either tiagabine or the competing drug).
No products indexed under this heading.

Amobarbital (Because of the possible additive depressive effects, caution should be used when patients are taking other CNS depressants in combination with tiagabine hydrochloride).
No products indexed under this heading.

Amobarbital Sodium (Because of the possible additive depressive effects, caution should be used when patients are taking other CNS depressants in combination with tiagabine hydrochloride).
No products indexed under this heading.

Amoxapine (Post-marketing reports have shown that tiagabine hydrochloride use has been associated with new onset seizures and status epilepticus in patients without epilepsy. Dose may be an important predisposing factor in the development of seizures, although seizures have been reported in patients taking daily doses of tiagabine hydrochloride as low as 4 mg/day. In most cases, patients were using concomitant medications (antidepressants, antipsychotics, stimulants, narcotics) that are thought to lower the seizure threshold).
No products indexed under this heading.

Amphetamine Aspartate (Post-marketing reports have shown that tiagabine hydrochloride use has been associated with new onset seizures and status epilepticus in patients without epilepsy. Dose may be an important predisposing factor in the development of seizures, although seizures have been reported in patients taking daily doses of tiagabine hydrochloride as low as 4 mg/day. In most cases, patients were using concomitant medications (antidepressants, antipsychotics, stimulants, narcotics) that are thought to lower the seizure threshold).
No products indexed under this heading.

Amphetamine Aspartate Monohydrate (Post-marketing reports have shown that tiagabine hydrochloride use has been associated with new onset seizures and status epilepticus in patients without epilepsy. Dose may be an important predisposing factor in the development of seizures, although seizures have been reported in patients taking daily doses of tiagabine hydrochloride as low as 4 mg/day. In most cases, patients were using concomitant medications (antidepressants, antipsychotics, stimulants, narcotics) that are thought to lower the seizure threshold).
No products indexed under this heading.

Amphetamine Resins (Post-marketing reports have shown that tiagabine hydrochloride use has been associated with new onset seizures and status epilepticus in patients without epilepsy. Dose may be an important predisposing factor in the development of seizures, although seizures have been reported in patients taking daily doses of tiagabine hydrochloride as low as 4 mg/day. In most cases, patients were using concomitant medications

(antidepressants, antipsychotics, stimulants, narcotics) that are thought to lower the seizure threshold).
No products indexed under this heading.

Amphetamine Sulfate (Post-marketing reports have shown that tiagabine hydrochloride use has been associated with new onset seizures and status epilepticus in patients without epilepsy. Dose may be an important predisposing factor in the development of seizures, although seizures have been reported in patients taking daily doses of tiagabine hydrochloride as low as 4 mg/day. In most cases, patients were using concomitant medications (antidepressants, antipsychotics, stimulants, narcotics) that are thought to lower the seizure threshold).
No products indexed under this heading.

Amprenavir (Because of the potential for pharmacokinetic interactions between tiagabine hydrochloride and drugs that inhibit hepatic metabolizing enzymes, it may be useful to obtain plasma levels of tiagabine before and after changes are made in the therapeutic regimen).
No products indexed under this heading.

Anastrozole (Because of the potential for pharmacokinetic interactions between tiagabine hydrochloride and drugs that inhibit hepatic metabolizing enzymes; it may be useful to obtain plasma levels of tiagabine before and after changes are made in the therapeutic regimen).
No products indexed under this heading.

Apomorphine (Post-marketing reports have shown that tiagabine hydrochloride use has been associated with new onset seizures and status epilepticus in patients without epilepsy. Dose may be an important predisposing factor in the development of seizures, although seizures have been reported in patients taking daily doses of tiagabine hydrochloride as low as 4 mg/day. In most cases, patients were using concomitant medications (antidepressants, antipsychotics, stimulants, narcotics) that are thought to lower the seizure threshold).
No products indexed under this heading.

Apomorphine Hydrochloride (Post-marketing reports have shown that tiagabine hydrochloride use has been associated with new onset seizures and status epilepticus in patients without epilepsy. Dose may be an important predisposing factor in the development of seizures, although seizures have been reported in patients taking daily doses of tiagabine hydrochloride as low as 4 mg/day. In most cases, patients were using concomitant medications (antidepressants, antipsychotics, stimulants, narcotics) that are thought to lower the seizure threshold).
No products indexed under this heading.

Aprepitant (Because of the potential for pharmacokinetic interactions between tiagabine hydrochloride and drugs that induce hepatic metabolizing enzymes, it may be useful to obtain plasma levels of tiagabine before and after changes are made in the therapeutic regimen). Products include:

Emend	2124

Aprobarbital (Because of the possible additive depressive effects, caution should be used when patients are taking other CNS depressants in combination with tiagabine hydrochloride).
No products indexed under this heading.

Aripiprazole (Post-marketing reports have shown that tiagabine hydrochloride use has been associated with new onset seizures and status epilepticus in patients without epilepsy. Dose may be an important predisposing factor in the development of seizures, although seizures have been reported in patients

723 Interactions Index Gabitril

taking daily doses of tiagabine hydrochloride as low as 4 mg/day. In most cases, patients were using concomitant medications (antidepressants, antipsychotics, stimulants, narcotics) that are thought to lower the seizure threshold).
No products indexed under this heading.

Atazanavir (Because of the potential for pharmacokinetic interactions between tiagabine hydrochloride and drugs that inhibit hepatic metabolizing enzymes, it may be useful to obtain plasma levels of tiagabine before and after changes are made in the therapeutic regimen).
No products indexed under this heading.

Atazanavir Sulfate (Because of the potential for pharmacokinetic interactions between tiagabine hydrochloride and drugs that inhibit hepatic metabolizing enzymes, it may be useful to obtain plasma levels of tiagabine before and after changes are made in the therapeutic regimen).
No products indexed under this heading.

Atovaquone (Tiagabine is 96% bound to human plasma protein and therefore has the potential to interact with other highly protein bound compounds. Such an interaction can potentially lead to higher free fractions of either tiagabine or the competing drug). Products include:
Malarone Pediatric Tablets 1572
Malarone 1572
Mepron Suspension 1576

Azosulfisoxazole (Because of the potential for pharmacokinetic interactions between tiagabine hydrochloride and drugs that inhibit hepatic metabolizing enzymes, it may be useful to obtain plasma levels of tiagabine before and after changes are made in the therapeutic regimen).
No products indexed under this heading.

Bendroflumethiazide (Because of the potential for pharmacokinetic interactions between tiagabine hydrochloride and drugs that inhibit hepatic metabolizing enzymes, it may be useful to obtain plasma levels of tiagabine before and after changes are made in the therapeutic regimen).
No products indexed under this heading.

Betamethasone (Because of the potential for pharmacokinetic interactions between tiagabine hydrochloride and drugs that induce hepatic metabolizing enzymes, it may be useful to obtain plasma levels of tiagabine before and after changes are made in the therapeutic regimen).
No products indexed under this heading.

Betamethasone Acetate (Because of the potential for pharmacokinetic interactions between tiagabine hydrochloride and drugs that induce hepatic metabolizing enzymes, it may be useful to obtain plasma levels of tiagabine before and after changes are made in the therapeutic regimen).
No products indexed under this heading.

Betamethasone Benzoate (Because of the potential for pharmacokinetic interactions between tiagabine hydrochloride and drugs that induce hepatic metabolizing enzymes, it may be useful to obtain plasma levels of tiagabine before and after changes are made in the therapeutic regimen).
No products indexed under this heading.

Betamethasone Dipropionate (Because of the potential for pharmacokinetic interactions between tiagabine hydrochloride and drugs that induce hepatic metabolizing enzymes, it may be useful to obtain plasma levels of tiagabine before and after changes are made in the therapeutic regimen). Products include:
Diprolene Lotion 0.05% 3108
Diprolene Ointment 0.05% 3109
Diprolene AF Cream 0.05% 3107
Lotrisone 3163

Betamethasone Sodium Phosphate (Because of the potential for pharmacokinetic interactions between tiagabine hydrochloride and drugs that induce hepatic metabolizing enzymes, it may be useful to obtain plasma levels of tiagabine before and after changes are made in the therapeutic regimen).
No products indexed under this heading.

Betamethasone Valerate (Because of the potential for pharmacokinetic interactions between tiagabine hydrochloride and drugs that induce hepatic metabolizing enzymes, it may be useful to obtain plasma levels of tiagabine before and after changes are made in the therapeutic regimen). Products include:
Luxíq 3321

Bosentan (Because of the potential for pharmacokinetic interactions between tiagabine hydrochloride and drugs that induce hepatic metabolizing enzymes, it may be useful to obtain plasma levels of tiagabine before and after changes are made in the therapeutic regimen). Products include:
Tracleer 573

Buprenorphine Hydrochloride (Because of the possible additive depressive effects, caution should be used when patients are taking other CNS depressants in combination with tiagabine hydrochloride).
No products indexed under this heading.

Bupropion Hydrochloride (Post-marketing reports have shown that tiagabine hydrochloride use has been associated with new onset seizures and status epilepticus in patients without epilepsy. Dose may be an important predisposing factor in the development of seizures, although seizures have been reported in patients taking daily doses of tiagabine hydrochloride as low as 4 mg/day. In most cases, patients were using concomitant medications (antidepressants, antipsychotics, stimulants, narcotics) that are thought to lower the seizure threshold). Products include:
Aplenzin 2948
Wellbutrin 1719
Wellbutrin SR 1725
Zyban 1762

Buspirone Hydrochloride (Because of the possible additive depressive effects, caution should be used when patients are taking other CNS depressants in combination with tiagabine hydrochloride).
No products indexed under this heading.

Butabarbital (Because of the possible additive depressive effects, caution should be used when patients are taking other CNS depressants in combination with tiagabine hydrochloride).
No products indexed under this heading.

Butabarbital Sodium (Because of the possible additive depressive effects, caution should be used when patients are taking other CNS depressants in combination with tiagabine hydrochloride).
No products indexed under this heading.

Butalbital (Because of the possible additive depressive effects, caution should be used when patients are taking other CNS depressants in combination with tiagabine hydrochloride).
No products indexed under this heading.

Carbamazepine (Population pharmacokinetic analyses indicate that tiagabine hydrochloride clearance is 60% greater in patients taking carbamazepine with or without other enzyme-inducing antiepileptic drugs. The clearance of tiagabine is affected by the co-administration of hepatic enzyme-inducing antiepilepsy drugs. Tiagabine is eliminated more rapidly in patients who have been taking hepatic enzyme-inducing drugs, (eg, carbamazepine), than in patients not receiving such treatment). Products include:
Carbatrol 3280
Equetro 3477

Cefonicid Sodium (Tiagabine is 96% bound to human plasma protein and therefore has the potential to interact with other highly protein bound compounds. Such an interaction can potentially lead to higher free fractions of either tiagabine or the competing drug).
No products indexed under this heading.

Celecoxib (Tiagabine is 96% bound to human plasma protein and therefore has the potential to interact with other highly protein bound compounds. Such an interaction can potentially lead to higher free fractions of either tiagabine or the competing drug). Products include:
Celebrex 3272

Chloramphenicol (Because of the potential for pharmacokinetic interactions between tiagabine hydrochloride and drugs that inhibit hepatic metabolizing enzymes, it may be useful to obtain plasma levels of tiagabine before and after changes are made in the therapeutic regimen).
No products indexed under this heading.

Chloramphenicol Palmitate (Because of the potential for pharmacokinetic interactions between tiagabine hydrochloride and drugs that inhibit hepatic metabolizing enzymes, it may be useful to obtain plasma levels of tiagabine before and after changes are made in the therapeutic regimen).
No products indexed under this heading.

Chloramphenicol Sodium Succinate (Because of the potential for pharmacokinetic interactions between tiagabine hydrochloride and drugs that inhibit hepatic metabolizing enzymes, it may be useful to obtain plasma levels of tiagabine before and after changes are made in the therapeutic regimen).
No products indexed under this heading.

Chlordiazepoxide (Because of the possible additive depressive effects, caution should be used when patients are taking other CNS depressants in combination with tiagabine hydrochloride).
No products indexed under this heading.

Chlordiazepoxide Hydrochloride (Because of the possible additive depressive effects, caution should be used when patients are taking other CNS depressants in combination with tiagabine hydrochloride).
No products indexed under this heading.

Chloroquine (Because of the potential for pharmacokinetic interactions between tiagabine hydrochloride and drugs that inhibit hepatic metabolizing enzymes, it may be useful to obtain plasma levels of tiagabine before and after changes are made in the therapeutic regimen).
No products indexed under this heading.

Chloroquine Hydrochloride (Because of the potential for pharmacokinetic interactions between tiagabine hydrochloride and drugs that inhibit hepatic metabolizing enzymes, it may be useful to obtain plasma levels of tiagabine before and after changes are made in the therapeutic regimen).
No products indexed under this heading.

Chloroquine Phosphate (Because of the potential for pharmacokinetic interactions between tiagabine hydrochloride and drugs that inhibit hepatic metabolizing enzymes, it may be useful to obtain plasma levels of tiagabine before and after changes are made in the therapeutic regimen).
No products indexed under this heading.

Chlorothiazide (Because of the potential for pharmacokinetic interactions between tiagabine hydrochloride and drugs that inhibit hepatic metabolizing enzymes, it may be useful to obtain plasma levels of tiagabine before and after changes are made in the therapeutic regimen).
No products indexed under this heading.

Chlorothiazide Sodium (Because of the potential for pharmacokinetic interactions between tiagabine hydrochloride and drugs that inhibit hepatic metabolizing enzymes, it may be useful to obtain plasma levels of tiagabine before and after changes are made in the therapeutic regimen). Products include:
Diuril Intravenous 2009

Chlorpheniramine (Because of the potential for pharmacokinetic interactions between tiagabine hydrochloride and drugs that inhibit hepatic metabolizing enzymes, it may be useful to obtain plasma levels of tiagabine before and after changes are made in the therapeutic regimen).
No products indexed under this heading.

Chlorpheniramine Maleate (Because of the potential for pharmacokinetic interactions between tiagabine hydrochloride and drugs that inhibit hepatic metabolizing enzymes, it may be useful to obtain plasma levels of tiagabine before and after changes are made in the therapeutic regimen).
No products indexed under this heading.

Chlorpheniramine Polistirex (Because of the potential for pharmacokinetic interactions between tiagabine hydrochloride and drugs that inhibit hepatic metabolizing enzymes, it may be useful to obtain plasma levels of tiagabine before and after changes are made in the therapeutic regimen). Products include:
Tussionex 3443

Chlorpheniramine Tannate (Because of the potential for pharmacokinetic interactions between tiagabine hydrochloride and drugs that inhibit hepatic metabolizing enzymes, it may be useful to obtain plasma levels of tiagabine before and after changes are made in the therapeutic regimen).
No products indexed under this heading.

Chlorpromazine (Because of the possible additive depressive effects, caution should be used when patients are taking other CNS depressants in combination with tiagabine hydrochloride).
No products indexed under this heading.

Chlorpromazine Hydrochloride (Because of the possible additive depressive effects, caution should be used when patients are taking other CNS depressants in combination with tiagabine hydrochloride).
No products indexed under this heading.

Chlorpropamide (Because of the potential for pharmacokinetic interactions between tiagabine hydrochloride and drugs that inhibit hepatic metabolizing enzymes, it may be useful to obtain plasma levels of tiagabine before and after changes are made in the therapeutic regimen).
No products indexed under this heading.

IMPORTANT NOTE: Always consult each drug listing in the patient's regimen for possible interactions.

Gabitril **Interactions Index** 724

Chlorprothixene (Because of the possible additive depressive effects, caution should be used when patients are taking other CNS depressants in combination with tiagabine hydrochloride).
No products indexed under this heading.

Chlorprothixene Hydrochloride (Because of the possible additive depressive effects, caution should be used when patients are taking other CNS depressants in combination with tiagabine hydrochloride).
No products indexed under this heading.

Chlorprothixene Lactate (Because of the possible additive depressive effects, caution should be used when patients are taking other CNS depressants in combination with tiagabine hydrochloride).
No products indexed under this heading.

Cimetidine (Because of the potential for pharmacokinetic interactions between tiagabine hydrochloride and drugs that inhibit hepatic metabolizing enzymes, it may be useful to obtain plasma levels of tiagabine before and after changes are made in the therapeutic regimen).
No products indexed under this heading.

Cimetidine Hydrochloride (Because of the potential for pharmacokinetic interactions between tiagabine hydrochloride and drugs that inhibit hepatic metabolizing enzymes, it may be useful to obtain plasma levels of tiagabine before and after changes are made in the therapeutic regimen).
No products indexed under this heading.

Ciprofloxacin (Because of the potential for pharmacokinetic interactions between tiagabine hydrochloride and drugs that induce hepatic metabolizing enzymes, it may be useful to obtain plasma levels of tiagabine before and after changes are made in the therapeutic regimen). Products include:
Cipro I.V. 3082
Cipro 3073
Cipro XR 3091
Ciprodex 583

Ciprofloxacin Hydrochloride (Because of the potential for pharmacokinetic interactions between tiagabine hydrochloride and drugs that induce hepatic metabolizing enzymes, it may be useful to obtain plasma levels of tiagabine before and after changes are made in the therapeutic regimen). Products include:
Cipro 3073

Cisplatin (Because of the potential for pharmacokinetic interactions between tiagabine hydrochloride and drugs that induce hepatic metabolizing enzymes, it may be useful to obtain plasma levels of tiagabine before and after changes are made in the therapeutic regimen).
No products indexed under this heading.

Citalopram Hydrobromide (Post-marketing reports have shown that tiagabine hydrochloride use has been associated with new onset seizures and status epilepticus in patients without epilepsy. Dose may be an important predisposing factor in the development of seizures, although seizures have been reported in patients taking daily doses of tiagabine hydrochloride as low as 4 mg/day. In most cases, patients were using concomitant medications (antidepressants, antipsychotics, stimulants, narcotics) that are thought to lower the seizure threshold). Products include:
Celexa 1153

Clarithromycin (Because of the potential for pharmacokinetic interactions between tiagabine hydrochloride and drugs that inhibit hepatic metabolizing enzymes, it may be useful to obtain plasma levels of tiagabine before and after changes are made in the therapeutic regimen). Products include:
Biaxin/Biaxin XL 412

Clomipramine Hydrochloride (Tiagabine is 96% bound to human plasma protein and therefore has the potential to interact with other highly protein bound compounds. Such an interaction can potentially lead to higher free fractions of either tiagabine or the competing drug).
No products indexed under this heading.

Clonazepam (Because of the possible additive depressive effects, caution should be used when patients are taking other CNS depressants in combination with tiagabine hydrochloride). Products include:
Klonopin 2855

Clopidogrel Bisulfate (Because of the potential for pharmacokinetic interactions between tiagabine hydrochloride and drugs that inhibit hepatic metabolizing enzymes, it may be useful to obtain plasma levels of tiagabine before and after changes are made in the therapeutic regimen). Products include:
Plavix 3027

Clopidogrel Hydrogen Sulfate (Because of the potential for pharmacokinetic interactions between tiagabine hydrochloride and drugs that inhibit hepatic metabolizing enzymes, it may be useful to obtain plasma levels of tiagabine before and after changes are made in the therapeutic regimen).
No products indexed under this heading.

Clorazepate Dipotassium (Because of the possible additive depressive effects, caution should be used when patients are taking other CNS depressants in combination with tiagabine hydrochloride).
No products indexed under this heading.

Clotrimazole (Because of the potential for pharmacokinetic interactions between tiagabine hydrochloride and drugs that inhibit hepatic metabolizing enzymes, it may be useful to obtain plasma levels of tiagabine before and after changes are made in the therapeutic regimen). Products include:
Lotrisone 3163

Clozapine (Because of the possible additive depressive effects, caution should be used when patients are taking other CNS depressants in combination with tiagabine hydrochloride).
No products indexed under this heading.

Cocaine Hydrochloride (Because of the potential for pharmacokinetic interactions between tiagabine hydrochloride and drugs that inhibit hepatic metabolizing enzymes, it may be useful to obtain plasma levels of tiagabine before and after changes are made in the therapeutic regimen).
No products indexed under this heading.

Codeine Phosphate (Because of the possible additive depressive effects, caution should be used when patients are taking other CNS depressants in combination with tiagabine hydrochloride). Products include:
Tylenol with Codeine 2691

Codeine Sulfate (Because of the possible additive depressive effects, caution should be used when patients are taking other CNS depressants in combination with tiagabine hydrochloride).
No products indexed under this heading.

Conivaptan Hydrochloride (Because of the potential for pharmacokinetic interactions between tiagabine hydrochloride and drugs that inhibit hepatic metabolizing enzymes, it may be useful to obtain plasma levels of tiagabine before and after changes are made in the therapeutic regimen). Products include:
Vaprisol 689

Cortisone Acetate (Because of the potential for pharmacokinetic interactions between tiagabine hydrochloride and drugs that induce hepatic metabolizing enzymes, it may be useful to obtain plasma levels of tiagabine before and after changes are made in the therapeutic regimen).
No products indexed under this heading.

Cyclosporine (Tiagabine is 96% bound to human plasma protein and therefore has the potential to interact with other highly protein bound compounds. Such an interaction can potentially lead to higher free fractions of either tiagabine or the competing drug). Products include:
Gengraf 440
Neoral Oral Solution 2496
Neoral Capsules 2496
Restasis 605

Dalfopristin (Because of the potential for pharmacokinetic interactions between tiagabine hydrochloride and drugs that inhibit hepatic metabolizing enzymes, it may be useful to obtain plasma levels of tiagabine before and after changes are made in the therapeutic regimen).
No products indexed under this heading.

Danazol (Because of the potential for pharmacokinetic interactions between tiagabine hydrochloride and drugs that inhibit hepatic metabolizing enzymes, it may be useful to obtain plasma levels of tiagabine before and after changes are made in the therapeutic regimen).
No products indexed under this heading.

Darunavir (Because of the potential for pharmacokinetic interactions between tiagabine hydrochloride and drugs that inhibit hepatic metabolizing enzymes, it may be useful to obtain plasma levels of tiagabine before and after changes are made in the therapeutic regimen).
No products indexed under this heading.

Dasatinib (Because of the potential for pharmacokinetic interactions between tiagabine hydrochloride and drugs that inhibit hepatic metabolizing enzymes, it may be useful to obtain plasma levels of tiagabine before and after changes are made in the therapeutic regimen).
No products indexed under this heading.

Delavirdine Mesylate (Because of the potential for pharmacokinetic interactions between tiagabine hydrochloride and drugs that inhibit hepatic metabolizing enzymes, it may be useful to obtain plasma levels of tiagabine before and after changes are made in the therapeutic regimen).
No products indexed under this heading.

Delavirine (Because of the potential for pharmacokinetic interactions between tiagabine hydrochloride and drugs that inhibit hepatic metabolizing enzymes, it may be useful to obtain plasma levels of tiagabine before and after changes are made in the therapeutic regimen).
No products indexed under this heading.

Desflurane (Because of the possible additive depressive effects, caution should be used when patients are taking other CNS depressants in combination with tiagabine hydrochloride).
No products indexed under this heading.

Desipramine Hydrochloride (Post-marketing reports have shown that tiagabine hydrochloride use has been associated with new onset seizures and status epilepticus in patients without epilepsy. Dose may be an important predisposing factor in the development of seizures, although seizures have been reported in patients taking daily doses of tiagabine hydrochloride as low as 4 mg/day. In most cases, patients were using concomitant medications (antidepressants, antipsychotics, stimulants, narcotics) that are thought to lower the seizure threshold).
No products indexed under this heading.

Desloratadine (Because of the potential for pharmacokinetic interactions between tiagabine hydrochloride and drugs that inhibit hepatic metabolizing enzymes, it may be useful to obtain plasma levels of tiagabine before and after changes are made in the therapeutic regimen). Products include:
Clarinex Syrup 3098
Clarinex 3098
Clarinex Reditabs 3098
Clarinex-D 12-Hour 3101
Clarinex-D 3104

Desogestrel (Because of the potential for pharmacokinetic interactions between tiagabine hydrochloride and drugs that inhibit hepatic metabolizing enzymes, it may be useful to obtain plasma levels of tiagabine before and after changes are made in the therapeutic regimen).
No products indexed under this heading.

Dexamethasone (Because of the potential for pharmacokinetic interactions between tiagabine hydrochloride and drugs that induce hepatic metabolizing enzymes, it may be useful to obtain plasma levels of tiagabine before and after changes are made in the therapeutic regimen). Products include:
Ciprodex 583
Ozurdex .... ⊙ 223
Tobramycin and Dexamethasone Ophthalmic Suspension .... ⊙ 251

Dexamethasone Acetate (Because of the potential for pharmacokinetic interactions between tiagabine hydrochloride and drugs that induce hepatic metabolizing enzymes, it may be useful to obtain plasma levels of tiagabine before and after changes are made in the therapeutic regimen).
No products indexed under this heading.

Dexamethasone Phosphate (Because of the potential for pharmacokinetic interactions between tiagabine hydrochloride and drugs that induce hepatic metabolizing enzymes, it may be useful to obtain plasma levels of tiagabine before and after changes are made in the therapeutic regimen).
No products indexed under this heading.

Dexamethasone Sodium (Because of the potential for pharmacokinetic interactions between tiagabine hydrochloride and drugs that induce hepatic metabolizing enzymes, it may be useful to obtain plasma levels of tiagabine before and after changes are made in the therapeutic regimen).
No products indexed under this heading.

Dexamethasone Sodium Phosphate (Because of the potential for pharmacokinetic interactions between tiagabine hydrochloride and drugs that induce hepatic metabolizing enzymes, it may be useful to obtain plasma levels of tiagabine before and after changes are made in the therapeutic regimen).
No products indexed under this heading.

Dexamethasone Sodium Phosphate Injection (Because of the potential for pharmacokinetic interactions between tiagabine hydrochloride and drugs that induce hepatic metabolizing enzymes, it may be useful to obtain plasma levels of tiagabine before and after changes are made in the therapeutic regimen).
No products indexed under this heading.

Dexmethylphenidate Hydrochloride (Post-marketing reports have shown that tiagabine hydrochloride use has been associated with new onset seizures and status epilepticus in patients without epilepsy. Dose may be an important predisposing factor in the

(⊙ Described in PDR® for Ophthalmic Medicines)

725 Interactions Index Gabitril

development of seizures, although seizures have been reported in patients taking daily doses of tiagabine hydrochloride as low as 4 mg/day. In most cases, patients were using concomitant medications (antidepressants, antipsychotics, stimulants, narcotics) that are thought to lower the seizure threshold). Products include:

Focalin XR 2472

Dextroamphetamine (Post-marketing reports have shown that tiagabine hydrochloride use has been associated with new onset seizures and status epilepticus in patients without epilepsy. Dose may be an important predisposing factor in the development of seizures, although seizures have been reported in patients taking daily doses of tiagabine hydrochloride as low as 4 mg/day. In most cases, patients were using concomitant medications (antidepressants, antipsychotics, stimulants, narcotics) that are thought to lower the seizure threshold).

No products indexed under this heading.

Dextroamphetamine Saccharate (Post-marketing reports have shown that tiagabine hydrochloride use has been associated with new onset seizures and status epilepticus in patients without epilepsy. Dose may be an important predisposing factor in the development of seizures, although seizures have been reported in patients taking daily doses of tiagabine hydrochloride as low as 4 mg/day. In most cases, patients were using concomitant medications (antidepressants, antipsychotics, stimulants, narcotics) that are thought to lower the seizure threshold).

No products indexed under this heading.

Dextroamphetamine Sulfate (Post-marketing reports have shown that tiagabine hydrochloride use has been associated with new onset seizures and status epilepticus in patients without epilepsy. Dose may be an important predisposing factor in the development of seizures, although seizures have been reported in patients taking daily doses of tiagabine hydrochloride as low as 4 mg/day. In most cases, patients were using concomitant medications (antidepressants, antipsychotics, stimulants, narcotics) that are thought to lower the seizure threshold). Products include:

Dexedrine 1425

Dezocine (Because of the possible additive depressive effects, caution should be used when patients are taking other CNS depressants in combination with tiagabine hydrochloride).

No products indexed under this heading.

Diazepam (Because of the possible additive depressive effects, caution should be used when patients are taking other CNS depressants in combination with tiagabine hydrochloride). Products include:

Valium Tablets 2880

Diclofenac Epolamine (Because of the potential for pharmacokinetic interactions between tiagabine hydrochloride and drugs that inhibit hepatic metabolizing enzymes, it may be useful to obtain plasma levels of tiagabine before and after changes are made in the therapeutic regimen). Products include:

Flector 1839

Diclofenac Potassium (Tiagabine is 96% bound to human plasma protein and therefore has the potential to interact with other highly protein bound compounds. Such an interaction can potentially lead to higher free fractions of either tiagabine or the competing drug).

No products indexed under this heading.

Diclofenac Sodium (Tiagabine is 96% bound to human plasma protein and therefore has the potential to interact with other highly protein bound compounds. Such an interaction can potentially lead to higher free fractions of either tiagabine or the competing drug).

No products indexed under this heading.

Digitalis Glycoside Preparations (Tiagabine is 96% bound to human plasma protein and therefore has the potential to interact with other highly protein bound compounds. Such an interaction can potentially lead to higher free fractions of either tiagabine or the competing drug).

No products indexed under this heading.

Digitalis Lanata (Tiagabine is 96% bound to human plasma protein and therefore has the potential to interact with other highly protein bound compounds. Such an interaction can potentially lead to higher free fractions of either tiagabine or the competing drug).

No products indexed under this heading.

Digitalis Purpurea (Tiagabine is 96% bound to human plasma protein and therefore has the potential to interact with other highly protein bound compounds. Such an interaction can potentially lead to higher free fractions of either tiagabine or the competing drug).

No products indexed under this heading.

Dihydrocodeine Bitartrate (Post-marketing reports have shown that tiagabine hydrochloride use has been associated with new onset seizures and status epilepticus in patients without epilepsy. Dose may be an important predisposing factor in the development of seizures, although seizures have been reported in patients taking daily doses of tiagabine hydrochloride as low as 4 mg/day. In most cases, patients were using concomitant medications (antidepressants, antipsychotics, stimulants, narcotics) that are thought to lower the seizure threshold).

No products indexed under this heading.

Dihydrocodeinone Bitartrate (Post-marketing reports have shown that tiagabine hydrochloride use has been associated with new onset seizures and status epilepticus in patients without epilepsy. Dose may be an important predisposing factor in the development of seizures, although seizures have been reported in patients taking daily doses of tiagabine hydrochloride as low as 4 mg/day. In most cases, patients were using concomitant medications (antidepressants, antipsychotics, stimulants, narcotics) that are thought to lower the seizure threshold).

No products indexed under this heading.

Diltiazem Hydrochloride (Because of the potential for pharmacokinetic interactions between tiagabine hydrochloride and drugs that induce hepatic metabolizing enzymes, it may be useful to obtain plasma levels of tiagabine before and after changes are made in the therapeutic regimen). Products include:

Cardizem LA 423

Diltiazem Maleate (Because of the potential for pharmacokinetic interactions between tiagabine hydrochloride and drugs that induce hepatic metabolizing enzymes, it may be useful to obtain plasma levels of tiagabine before and after changes are made in the therapeutic regimen).

No products indexed under this heading.

Diphenhydramine (Because of the potential for pharmacokinetic interactions between tiagabine hydrochloride and drugs that inhibit hepatic metabolizing enzymes, it may be useful to obtain plasma levels of tiagabine before and after changes are made in the therapeutic regimen).

No products indexed under this heading.

Diphenhydramine Hydrochloride (Because of the potential for pharmacokinetic interactions between tiagabine hydrochloride and drugs that inhibit hepatic metabolizing enzymes, it may be useful to obtain plasma levels of tiagabine before and after changes are made in the therapeutic regimen). Products include:

Benadryl Allergy Ultratab 2042

Children's Benadryl Allergy Liquid 2042

Dipyridamole (Tiagabine is 96% bound to human plasma protein and therefore has the potential to interact with other highly protein bound compounds. Such an interaction can potentially lead to higher free fractions of either tiagabine or the competing drug). Products include:

Aggrenox 880

Disulfiram (Because of the potential for pharmacokinetic interactions between tiagabine hydrochloride and drugs that inhibit hepatic metabolizing enzymes, it may be useful to obtain plasma levels of tiagabine before and after changes are made in the therapeutic regimen).

No products indexed under this heading.

Divalproex Sodium (Co-administration of tiagabine in patients taking valproate chronically had no effect on tiagabine pharmacokinetics, but valproate significantly decreased tiagabine binding *in vitro* from 96.3% to 94.8%, which resulted in an increase of approximately 40% in the tiagabine concentrations; the clinical relevance of this *in vitro* finding is unknown. Tiagabine hydrochloride causes a slight decrease (about 10%) in steady-state valproate concentrations). Products include:

Depakote ER 426

Doxepin Hydrochloride (Post-marketing reports have shown that tiagabine hydrochloride use has been associated with new onset seizures and status epilepticus in patients without epilepsy. Dose may be an important predisposing factor in the development of seizures, although seizures have been reported in patients taking daily doses of tiagabine hydrochloride as low as 4 mg/day. In most cases, patients were using concomitant medications (antidepressants, antipsychotics, stimulants, narcotics) that are thought to lower the seizure threshold).

No products indexed under this heading.

Doxorubicin Hydrochloride (Because of the potential for pharmacokinetic interactions between tiagabine hydrochloride and drugs that induce hepatic metabolizing enzymes, it may be useful to obtain plasma levels of tiagabine before and after changes are made in the therapeutic regimen).

No products indexed under this heading.

Droperidol (Because of the possible additive depressive effects, caution should be used when patients are taking other CNS depressants in combination with tiagabine hydrochloride).

No products indexed under this heading.

Efavirenz (Because of the potential for pharmacokinetic interactions between tiagabine hydrochloride and drugs that induce hepatic metabolizing enzymes, it may be useful to obtain plasma levels of tiagabine before and after changes are made in the therapeutic regimen). Products include:

Atripla 906

Enflurane (Because of the possible additive depressive effects, caution should be used when patients are taking other CNS depressants in combination with tiagabine hydrochloride).

No products indexed under this heading.

Enoxacin (Because of the potential for pharmacokinetic interactions between tiagabine hydrochloride and drugs that inhibit hepatic metabolizing enzymes, it may be useful to obtain plasma levels of tiagabine before and after changes are made in the therapeutic regimen).

No products indexed under this heading.

Erythromycin (Because of the potential for pharmacokinetic interactions between tiagabine hydrochloride and drugs that induce hepatic metabolizing enzymes, it may be useful to obtain plasma levels of tiagabine before and after changes are made in the therapeutic regimen).

No products indexed under this heading.

Erythromycin, Topical (Because of the potential for pharmacokinetic interactions between tiagabine hydrochloride and drugs that induce hepatic metabolizing enzymes, it may be useful to obtain plasma levels of tiagabine before and after changes are made in the therapeutic regimen).

No products indexed under this heading.

Erythromycin Estolate (Because of the potential for pharmacokinetic interactions between tiagabine hydrochloride and drugs that induce hepatic metabolizing enzymes, it may be useful to obtain plasma levels of tiagabine before and after changes are made in the therapeutic regimen).

No products indexed under this heading.

Erythromycin Ethylsuccinate (Because of the potential for pharmacokinetic interactions between tiagabine hydrochloride and drugs that induce hepatic metabolizing enzymes, it may be useful to obtain plasma levels of tiagabine before and after changes are made in the therapeutic regimen). Products include:

E.E.S. 437

EryPed 435

Erythromycin Gluceptate (Because of the potential for pharmacokinetic interactions between tiagabine hydrochloride and drugs that induce hepatic metabolizing enzymes, it may be useful to obtain plasma levels of tiagabine before and after changes are made in the therapeutic regimen).

No products indexed under this heading.

Erythromycin Lactobionate (Because of the potential for pharmacokinetic interactions between tiagabine hydrochloride and drugs that induce hepatic metabolizing enzymes, it may be useful to obtain plasma levels of tiagabine before and after changes are made in the therapeutic regimen).

No products indexed under this heading.

Erythromycin Stearate (Because of the potential for pharmacokinetic interactions between tiagabine hydrochloride and drugs that induce hepatic metabolizing enzymes, it may be useful to obtain plasma levels of tiagabine before and after changes are made in the therapeutic regimen).

No products indexed under this heading.

Escitalopram Oxalate (Post-marketing reports have shown that tiagabine hydrochloride use has been associated with new onset seizures and status epilepticus in patients without epilepsy. Dose may be an important predisposing factor in the development of seizures, although seizures have been reported in patients taking daily doses of tiagabine hydrochloride as low as 4 mg/day. In most cases, patients were using concomitant medications (antidepressants, antipsychotics, stimu-

IMPORTANT NOTE: Always consult each drug listing in the patient's regimen for possible interactions.

Gabitril | Interactions Index | 726

lants, narcotics) that are thought to lower the seizure threshold). Products include:
Lexapro Oral Suspension 1160
Lexapro Tablets 1160

Esomeprazole Magnesium (Because of the potential for pharmacokinetic interactions between tiagabine hydrochloride and drugs that induce hepatic metabolizing enzymes, it may be useful to obtain plasma levels of tiagabine before and after changes are made in the therapeutic regimen). Products include:
Nexium Capsules 704
Nexium Oral Suspension 704

Esomeprazole Sodium (Because of the potential for pharmacokinetic interactions between tiagabine hydrochloride and drugs that induce hepatic metabolizing enzymes, it may be useful to obtain plasma levels of tiagabine before and after changes are made in the therapeutic regimen). Products include:
Nexium I.V. 712

Estazolam (Because of the possible additive depressive effects, caution should be used when patients are taking other CNS depressants in combination with tiagabine hydrochloride).
No products indexed under this heading.

Ethanol (Because of the possible additive effects of drugs that may depress the nervous system, ethanol should be used cautiously in combination with tiagabine).
No products indexed under this heading.

Ethchlorvynol (Because of the possible additive depressive effects, caution should be used when patients are taking other CNS depressants in combination with tiagabine hydrochloride).
No products indexed under this heading.

Ethinamate (Because of the possible additive depressive effects, caution should be used when patients are taking other CNS depressants in combination with tiagabine hydrochloride).
No products indexed under this heading.

Ethinyl Estradiol (Because of the potential for pharmacokinetic interactions between tiagabine hydrochloride and drugs that inhibit hepatic metabolizing enzymes, it may be useful to obtain plasma levels of tiagabine before and after changes are made in the therapeutic regimen). Products include:
LoSeasonique 3407
Lybrel 3514
NuvaRing 3181
Ortho Evra 2648
Ortho-Cyclen/Ortho Tri-Cyclen 2663
Ortho Tri-Cyclen Lo Tablets 2673
Seasonique 3418
Yaz 864

Ethosuximide (The clearance of tiagabine is affected by the co-administration of hepatic enzyme-inducing antiepilepsy drugs. Tiagabine is eliminated more rapidly in patients who have been taking hepatic enzyme-inducing drugs, (eg, carbamazepine, phenytoin, primidone and phenobarbital) than in patients not receiving such treatment).
No products indexed under this heading.

Ethotoin (The clearance of tiagabine is affected by the co-administration of hepatic enzyme-inducing antiepilepsy drugs. Tiagabine is eliminated more rapidly in patients who have been taking hepatic enzyme-inducing drugs, (eg, carbamazepine, phenytoin, primidone and phenobarbital) than in patients not receiving such treatment).
No products indexed under this heading.

Ethyl Alcohol (Because of the possible additive effects of drugs that may depress the nervous system, ethanol should be used cautiously in combination with tiagabine).
No products indexed under this heading.

Ethynodiol Diacetate (Because of the potential for pharmacokinetic interactions between tiagabine hydrochloride and drugs that inhibit hepatic metabolizing enzymes, it may be useful to obtain plasma levels of tiagabine before and after changes are made in the therapeutic regimen).
No products indexed under this heading.

Fat (Absorption of tiagabine is rapid, with peak plasma concentrations occurring at approximately 45 minutes following an oral dose in the fasting state. Tiagabine is nearly completely absorbed (>95%), with an absolute oral bioavailability of about 90%. A high fat meal decreases the rate (mean T_{max} was prolonged to 2.5 hours, and mean C_{max} was reduced by about 40%) but not the extent (AUC) of tiagabine absorption).
No products indexed under this heading.

Felbamate (The clearance of tiagabine is affected by the co-administration of hepatic enzyme-inducing antiepilepsy drugs. Tiagabine is eliminated more rapidly in patients who have been taking hepatic enzyme-inducing drugs, (eg, carbamazepine, phenytoin, primidone and phenobarbital) than in patients not receiving such treatment).
No products indexed under this heading.

Fenofibrate (Because of the potential for pharmacokinetic interactions between tiagabine hydrochloride and drugs that inhibit hepatic metabolizing enzymes, it may be useful to obtain plasma levels of tiagabine before and after changes are made in the therapeutic regimen). Products include:
Fenoglide 3263
Tricor 544
Trilipix 548

Fenoprofen Calcium (Tiagabine is 96% bound to human plasma protein and therefore has the potential to interact with other highly protein bound compounds. Such an interaction can potentially lead to higher free fractions of either tiagabine or the competing drug).
No products indexed under this heading.

Fentanyl (Because of the possible additive depressive effects, caution should be used when patients are taking other CNS depressants in combination with tiagabine hydrochloride). Products include:
Duragesic 2604
Fentanyl Transdermal System 2346
Onsolis 2054

Fentanyl Citrate (Because of the possible additive depressive effects, caution should be used when patients are taking other CNS depressants in combination with tiagabine hydrochloride). Products include:
Fentora 966

Fluconazole (Because of the potential for pharmacokinetic interactions between tiagabine hydrochloride and drugs that inhibit hepatic metabolizing enzymes, it may be useful to obtain plasma levels of tiagabine before and after changes are made in the therapeutic regimen).
No products indexed under this heading.

Fludrocortisone Acetate (Because of the potential for pharmacokinetic interactions between tiagabine hydrochloride and drugs that induce hepatic metabolizing enzymes, it may be useful to obtain plasma levels of tiagabine before and after changes are made in the therapeutic regimen).
No products indexed under this heading.

Fluorouracil (Because of the potential for pharmacokinetic interactions between tiagabine hydrochloride and drugs that inhibit hepatic metabolizing enzymes, it may be useful to obtain plasma levels of tiagabine before and after changes are made in the therapeutic regimen). Products include:
Carac 2966

Fluoxetine (Because of the potential for pharmacokinetic interactions between tiagabine hydrochloride and drugs that inhibit hepatic metabolizing enzymes, it may be useful to obtain plasma levels of tiagabine before and after changes are made in the therapeutic regimen).
No products indexed under this heading.

Fluoxetine Hydrochloride (Post-marketing reports have shown that tiagabine hydrochloride use has been associated with new onset seizures and status epilepticus in patients without epilepsy. Dose may be an important predisposing factor in the development of seizures, although seizures have been reported in patients taking daily doses of tiagabine hydrochloride as low as 4 mg/day. In most cases, patients were using concomitant medications (antidepressants, antipsychotics, stimulants, narcotics) that are thought to lower the seizure threshold). Products include:
Prozac Weekly 1941
Prozac Pulvules 1941
Symbyax 1965

Fluphenazine Decanoate (Because of the possible additive depressive effects, caution should be used when patients are taking other CNS depressants in combination with tiagabine hydrochloride).
No products indexed under this heading.

Fluphenazine Enanthate (Because of the possible additive depressive effects, caution should be used when patients are taking other CNS depressants in combination with tiagabine hydrochloride).
No products indexed under this heading.

Fluphenazine Hydrochloride (Because of the possible additive depressive effects, caution should be used when patients are taking other CNS depressants in combination with tiagabine hydrochloride).
No products indexed under this heading.

Flurazepam Hydrochloride (Because of the possible additive depressive effects, caution should be used when patients are taking other CNS depressants in combination with tiagabine hydrochloride).
No products indexed under this heading.

Flurbiprofen (Tiagabine is 96% bound to human plasma protein and therefore has the potential to interact with other highly protein bound compounds. Such an interaction can potentially lead to higher free fractions of either tiagabine or the competing drug).
No products indexed under this heading.

Flurbiprofen Sodium (Because of the potential for pharmacokinetic interactions between tiagabine hydrochloride and drugs that inhibit hepatic metabolizing enzymes, it may be useful to obtain plasma levels of tiagabine before and after changes are made in the therapeutic regimen).
No products indexed under this heading.

Fluvastatin Sodium (Because of the potential for pharmacokinetic interactions between tiagabine hydrochloride and drugs that inhibit hepatic metabolizing enzymes, it may be useful to obtain plasma levels of tiagabine before and after changes are made in the therapeutic regimen).
No products indexed under this heading.

Fluvoxamine (Post-marketing reports have shown that tiagabine hydrochloride use has been associated with new onset seizures and status epilepticus in patients without epilepsy. Dose may be an important predisposing factor in the development of seizures, although seizures have been reported in patients taking daily doses of tiagabine hydrochloride as low as 4 mg/day. In most cases, patients were using concomitant medications (antidepressants, antipsychotics, stimulants, narcotics) that are thought to lower the seizure threshold).
No products indexed under this heading.

Fluvoxamine Maleate (Post-marketing reports have shown that tiagabine hydrochloride use has been associated with new onset seizures and status epilepticus in patients without epilepsy. Dose may be an important predisposing factor in the development of seizures, although seizures have been reported in patients taking daily doses of tiagabine hydrochloride as low as 4 mg/day. In most cases, patients were using concomitant medications (antidepressants, antipsychotics, stimulants, narcotics) that are thought to lower the seizure threshold).
No products indexed under this heading.

Fosamprenavir Calcium (Because of the potential for pharmacokinetic interactions between tiagabine hydrochloride and drugs that inhibit hepatic metabolizing enzymes, it may be useful to obtain plasma levels of tiagabine before and after changes are made in the therapeutic regimen). Products include:
Lexiva Oral Suspension 1558
Lexiva 1558

Fosphenytoin (Population pharmacokinetic analyses indicate that tiagabine clearance is 60% greater in patients taking phenytoin with or without other enzyme-inducing antiepileptic drugs. The clearance of tiagabine is affected by the co-administration of hepatic enzyme-inducing antiepilepsy drugs. Tiagabine is eliminated more rapidly in patients who have been taking hepatic enzyme-inducing drugs, (eg, phenytoin), than in patients not receiving such treatment).
No products indexed under this heading.

Fosphenytoin Sodium (Population pharmacokinetic analyses indicate that tiagabine clearance is 60% greater in patients taking phenytoin with or without other enzyme-inducing antiepileptic drugs. The clearance of tiagabine is affected by the co-administration of hepatic enzyme-inducing antiepilepsy drugs. Tiagabine is eliminated more rapidly in patients who have been taking hepatic enzyme-inducing drugs, (eg, phenytoin), than in patients not receiving such treatment).
No products indexed under this heading.

Gabapentin (The clearance of tiagabine is affected by the co-administration of hepatic enzyme-inducing antiepilepsy drugs. Tiagabine is eliminated more rapidly in patients who have been taking hepatic enzyme-inducing drugs, (eg, carbamazepine, phenytoin, primidone and phenobarbital) than in patients not receiving such treatment).
No products indexed under this heading.

Garlic Extract (Because of the potential for pharmacokinetic interactions between tiagabine hydrochloride and drugs that induce hepatic metabolizing enzymes, it may be useful to obtain plasma levels of tiagabine before and after changes are made in the therapeutic regimen).
No products indexed under this heading.

Garlic Oil (Because of the potential for pharmacokinetic interactions between tiagabine hydrochloride and drugs that induce hepatic metabolizing enzymes, it may be useful to obtain plasma levels of tiagabine before and after changes are made in the therapeutic regimen).
No products indexed under this heading.

727 **Interactions Index** **Gabitril**

Gatifloxacin (Because of the potential for pharmacokinetic interactions between tiagabine hydrochloride and drugs that inhibit hepatic metabolizing enzymes, it may be useful to obtain plasma levels of tiagabine before and after changes are made in the therapeutic regimen).
No products indexed under this heading.

Gemfibrozil (Because of the potential for pharmacokinetic interactions between tiagabine hydrochloride and drugs that inhibit hepatic metabolizing enzymes, it may be useful to obtain plasma levels of tiagabine before and after changes are made in the therapeutic regimen).
No products indexed under this heading.

Gemifloxacin Mesylate (Because of the potential for pharmacokinetic interactions between tiagabine hydrochloride and drugs that inhibit hepatic metabolizing enzymes, it may be useful to obtain plasma levels of tiagabine before and after changes are made in the therapeutic regimen).
No products indexed under this heading.

Glipizide (Tiagabine is 96% bound to human plasma protein and therefore has the potential to interact with other highly protein bound compounds. Such an interaction can potentially lead to higher free fractions of either tiagabine or the competing drug).
No products indexed under this heading.

Glutethimide (Because of the possible additive depressive effects, caution should be used when patients are taking other CNS depressants in combination with tiagabine hydrochloride).
No products indexed under this heading.

Glyburide (Because of the potential for pharmacokinetic interactions between tiagabine hydrochloride and drugs that inhibit hepatic metabolizing enzymes, it may be useful to obtain plasma levels of tiagabine before and after changes are made in the therapeutic regimen).
No products indexed under this heading.

Grepafloxacin Hydrochloride (Because of the potential for pharmacokinetic interactions between tiagabine hydrochloride and drugs that inhibit hepatic metabolizing enzymes, it may be useful to obtain plasma levels of tiagabine before and after changes are made in the therapeutic regimen).
No products indexed under this heading.

Halazepam (Because of the possible additive depressive effects, caution should be used when patients are taking other CNS depressants in combination with tiagabine hydrochloride).
No products indexed under this heading.

Halofantrine Hydrochloride (Because of the potential for pharmacokinetic interactions between tiagabine hydrochloride and drugs that inhibit hepatic metabolizing enzymes, it may be useful to obtain plasma levels of tiagabine before and after changes are made in the therapeutic regimen).
No products indexed under this heading.

Haloperidol (Because of the possible additive depressive effects, caution should be used when patients are taking other CNS depressants in combination with tiagabine hydrochloride).
No products indexed under this heading.

Haloperidol Decanoate (Because of the possible additive depressive effects, caution should be used when patients are taking other CNS depressants in combination with tiagabine hydrochloride).
No products indexed under this heading.

Haloperidol Lactate (Because of the possible additive depressive effects, caution should be used when patients are taking other CNS depressants in combination with tiagabine hydrochloride).
No products indexed under this heading.

Hexobarbital (Because of the possible additive depressive effects, caution should be used when patients are taking other CNS depressants in combination with tiagabine hydrochloride).
No products indexed under this heading.

Hydrochlorothiazide (Because of the potential for pharmacokinetic interactions between tiagabine hydrochloride and drugs that inhibit hepatic metabolizing enzymes, it may be useful to obtain plasma levels of tiagabine before and after changes are made in the therapeutic regimen). Products include:
Atacand HCT **700**
Avalide **2956**
Benicar HCT **1017**
Diovan HCT **2419**
Dyazide **1429**
Exforge HCT **2449**
Hyzaar **2162**
Hyzaar 100-12.5 .... **2162**
Micardis HCT **889**
Prinzide **2246**
Tekturna HCT **2541**
Teveten HCT **541**

Hydrochlorothiazide Hydrochloride (Because of the potential for pharmacokinetic interactions between tiagabine hydrochloride and drugs that inhibit hepatic metabolizing enzymes, it may be useful to obtain plasma levels of tiagabine before and after changes are made in the therapeutic regimen).
No products indexed under this heading.

Hydrocodone Bitartrate (Because of the possible additive depressive effects, caution should be used when patients are taking other CNS depressants in combination with tiagabine hydrochloride). Products include:
Vicodin **560**
Vicodin ES **561**
Vicodin HP **563**
Vicoprofen **564**
Zydone **1138**

Hydrocodone Polistirex (Because of the possible additive depressive effects, caution should be used when patients are taking other CNS depressants in combination with tiagabine hydrochloride). Products include:
Tussionex **3443**

Hydrocortisone (Because of the potential for pharmacokinetic interactions between tiagabine hydrochloride and drugs that induce hepatic metabolizing enzymes, it may be useful to obtain plasma levels of tiagabine before and after changes are made in the therapeutic regimen).
No products indexed under this heading.

Hydrocortisone (Alcohol) (Because of the potential for pharmacokinetic interactions between tiagabine hydrochloride and drugs that induce hepatic metabolizing enzymes, it may be useful to obtain plasma levels of tiagabine before and after changes are made in the therapeutic regimen).
No products indexed under this heading.

Hydrocortisone Acetate (Because of the potential for pharmacokinetic interactions between tiagabine hydrochloride and drugs that induce hepatic metabolizing enzymes, it may be useful to obtain plasma levels of tiagabine before and after changes are made in the therapeutic regimen).
No products indexed under this heading.

Hydrocortisone Butyrate (Because of the potential for pharmacokinetic interactions between tiagabine hydrochloride and drugs that induce hepatic metabolizing enzymes, it may be useful to obtain plasma levels of tiagabine before and after changes are made in the therapeutic regimen).
No products indexed under this heading.

Hydrocortisone Cypionate (Because of the potential for pharmacokinetic interactions between tiagabine hydrochloride and drugs that induce hepatic metabolizing enzymes, it may be useful to obtain plasma levels of tiagabine before and after changes are made in the therapeutic regimen).
No products indexed under this heading.

Hydrocortisone Hemisuccinate (Because of the potential for pharmacokinetic interactions between tiagabine hydrochloride and drugs that induce hepatic metabolizing enzymes, it may be useful to obtain plasma levels of tiagabine before and after changes are made in the therapeutic regimen).
No products indexed under this heading.

Hydrocortisone Probutate (Because of the potential for pharmacokinetic interactions between tiagabine hydrochloride and drugs that induce hepatic metabolizing enzymes, it may be useful to obtain plasma levels of tiagabine before and after changes are made in the therapeutic regimen).
No products indexed under this heading.

Hydrocortisone Sodium Phosphate (Because of the potential for pharmacokinetic interactions between tiagabine hydrochloride and drugs that induce hepatic metabolizing enzymes, it may be useful to obtain plasma levels of tiagabine before and after changes are made in the therapeutic regimen).
No products indexed under this heading.

Hydrocortisone Sodium Succinate (Because of the potential for pharmacokinetic interactions between tiagabine hydrochloride and drugs that induce hepatic metabolizing enzymes, it may be useful to obtain plasma levels of tiagabine before and after changes are made in the therapeutic regimen).
No products indexed under this heading.

Hydrocortisone Valerate (Because of the potential for pharmacokinetic interactions between tiagabine hydrochloride and drugs that induce hepatic metabolizing enzymes, it may be useful to obtain plasma levels of tiagabine before and after changes are made in the therapeutic regimen).
No products indexed under this heading.

Hydroflumethiazide (Because of the potential for pharmacokinetic interactions between tiagabine hydrochloride and drugs that inhibit hepatic metabolizing enzymes, it may be useful to obtain plasma levels of tiagabine before and after changes are made in the therapeutic regimen).
No products indexed under this heading.

Hydromorphone (Because of the possible additive depressive effects, caution should be used when patients are taking other CNS depressants in combination with tiagabine hydrochloride).
No products indexed under this heading.

Hydromorphone Hydrochloride (Because of the possible additive depressive effects, caution should be used when patients are taking other CNS depressants in combination with tiagabine hydrochloride). Products include:
Dilaudid Injection **2800**
Dilaudid Oral **2797**
Dilaudid Tablets **2797**
Dilaudid-HP **2800**

Hydroxyamphetamine Hydrobromide (Post-marketing reports have shown that tiagabine hydrochloride use has been associated with new onset seizures and status epilepticus in patients without epilepsy. Dose may be an important predisposing factor in the development of seizures, although seizures have been reported in patients taking daily doses of tiagabine hydrochloride as low as 4 mg/day. In most cases, patients were using concomitant medications (antidepressants, antipsychotics, stimulants, narcotics) that are thought to lower the seizure threshold).
No products indexed under this heading.

Hydroxychloroquine Sulfate (Because of the potential for pharmacokinetic interactions between tiagabine hydrochloride and drugs that inhibit hepatic metabolizing enzymes, it may be useful to obtain plasma levels of tiagabine before and after changes are made in the therapeutic regimen).
No products indexed under this heading.

Hydroxyzine Hydrochloride (Because of the possible additive depressive effects, caution should be used when patients are taking other CNS depressants in combination with tiagabine hydrochloride).
No products indexed under this heading.

Hypericum (Because of the potential for pharmacokinetic interactions between tiagabine hydrochloride and drugs that induce hepatic metabolizing enzymes, it may be useful to obtain plasma levels of tiagabine before and after changes are made in the therapeutic regimen).
No products indexed under this heading.

Hypericum Perforatum (Because of the potential for pharmacokinetic interactions between tiagabine hydrochloride and drugs that induce hepatic metabolizing enzymes, it may be useful to obtain plasma levels of tiagabine before and after changes are made in the therapeutic regimen). Products include:
Traumeel **1800**

Ibuprofen (Tiagabine is 96% bound to human plasma protein and therefore has the potential to interact with other highly protein bound compounds. Such an interaction can potentially lead to higher free fractions of either tiagabine or the competing drug). Products include:
Motrin IB **2043**
Children's Motrin **2044**
Children's Motrin Non-Staining Dye-Free **2044**
Infants' Motrin **2044**
Infants' Motrin Dye-Free **2044**
Junior Strength Motrin **2044**
Vicoprofen **564**

Imatinib Mesylate (Because of the potential for pharmacokinetic interactions between tiagabine hydrochloride and drugs that inhibit hepatic metabolizing enzymes, it may be useful to obtain plasma levels of tiagabine before and after changes are made in the therapeutic regimen). Products include:
Gleevec **2477**

Imipramine Hydrochloride (Tiagabine is 96% bound to human plasma protein and therefore has the potential to interact with other highly protein bound compounds. Such an interaction can potentially lead to higher free fractions of either tiagabine or the competing drug).
No products indexed under this heading.

Imipramine Pamoate (Tiagabine is 96% bound to human plasma protein and therefore has the potential to interact with other highly protein bound compounds. Such an interaction can potentially lead to higher free fractions of either tiagabine or the competing drug).
No products indexed under this heading.

IMPORTANT NOTE: Always consult each drug listing in the patient's regimen for possible interactions.

(⊙ Described in PDR® for Ophthalmic Medicines)

729 Interactions Index Gabitril

plasma levels of tiagabine before and after changes are made in the therapeutic regimen). Products include:
Iquix ... 3492
Levaquin ... 2629
Levaquin in 5% Dextrose ... 2629
Quixin ... 3493

Levomethadyl Acetate Hydrochloride (Because of the possible additive depressive effects, caution should be used when patients are taking other CNS depressants in combination with tiagabine hydrochloride).
No products indexed under this heading.

Levonorgestrel (Because of the potential for pharmacokinetic interactions between tiagabine hydrochloride and drugs that inhibit hepatic metabolizing enzymes, it may be useful to obtain plasma levels of tiagabine before and after changes are made in the therapeutic regimen). Products include:
Climara Pro ... 847
LoSeasonique ... 3407
Lybrel ... 3514
Mirena ... 854
Plan B ... 3416
Seasonique ... 3418

Levorphanol Tartrate (Because of the possible additive depressive effects, caution should be used when patients are taking other CNS depressants in combination with tiagabine hydrochloride).
No products indexed under this heading.

Lisdexamfetamine Dimesylate (Post-marketing reports have shown that tiagabine hydrochloride use has been associated with new onset seizures and status epilepticus in patients without epilepsy. Dose may be an important predisposing factor in the development of seizures, although seizures have been reported in patients taking daily doses of tiagabine hydrochloride as low as 4 mg/day. In most cases, patients were using concomitant medications (antidepressants, antipsychotics, stimulants, narcotics) that are thought to lower the seizure threshold). Products include:
Vyvanse ... 3298

Lithium (Post-marketing reports have shown that tiagabine hydrochloride use has been associated with new onset seizures and status epilepticus in patients without epilepsy. Dose may be an important predisposing factor in the development of seizures, although seizures have been reported in patients taking daily doses of tiagabine hydrochloride as low as 4 mg/day. In most cases, patients were using concomitant medications (antidepressants, antipsychotics, stimulants, narcotics) that are thought to lower the seizure threshold).
No products indexed under this heading.

Lithium Carbonate (Post-marketing reports have shown that tiagabine hydrochloride use has been associated with new onset seizures and status epilepticus in patients without epilepsy. Dose may be an important predisposing factor in the development of seizures, although seizures have been reported in patients taking daily doses of tiagabine hydrochloride as low as 4 mg/day. In most cases, patients were using concomitant medications (antidepressants, antipsychotics, stimulants, narcotics) that are thought to lower the seizure threshold).
No products indexed under this heading.

Lithium Citrate (Post-marketing reports have shown that tiagabine hydrochloride use has been associated with new onset seizures and status epilepticus in patients without epilepsy. Dose may be an important predisposing factor in the development of seizures, although seizures have been reported in patients taking daily doses of tiagabine hydrochloride as low as 4 mg/day. In most cases, patients were using concomitant medications (antidepressants, antipsychotics, stimulants, narcotics) that are thought to lower the seizure threshold).
No products indexed under this heading.

Lomefloxacin Hydrochloride (Because of the potential for pharmacokinetic interactions between tiagabine hydrochloride and drugs that inhibit hepatic metabolizing enzymes, it may be useful to obtain plasma levels of tiagabine before and after changes are made in the therapeutic regimen).
No products indexed under this heading.

Lopinavir (Because of the potential for pharmacokinetic interactions between tiagabine hydrochloride and drugs that inhibit hepatic metabolizing enzymes, it may be useful to obtain plasma levels of tiagabine before and after changes are made in the therapeutic regimen). Products include:
Kaletra ... 458

Loratadine (Because of the potential for pharmacokinetic interactions between tiagabine hydrochloride and drugs that inhibit hepatic metabolizing enzymes, it may be useful to obtain plasma levels of tiagabine before and after changes are made in the therapeutic regimen).
No products indexed under this heading.

Lorazepam (Because of the possible additive depressive effects, caution should be used when patients are taking other CNS depressants in combination with tiagabine hydrochloride).
No products indexed under this heading.

Lovastatin (Because of the potential for pharmacokinetic interactions between tiagabine hydrochloride and drugs that inhibit hepatic metabolizing enzymes, it may be useful to obtain plasma levels of tiagabine before and after changes are made in the therapeutic regimen). Products include:
Advicor ... 402
Mevacor ... 2212

Loxapine Hydrochloride (Because of the possible additive depressive effects, caution should be used when patients are taking other CNS depressants in combination with tiagabine hydrochloride).
No products indexed under this heading.

Loxapine Succinate (Because of the possible additive depressive effects, caution should be used when patients are taking other CNS depressants in combination with tiagabine hydrochloride).
No products indexed under this heading.

Maprotiline Hydrochloride (Post-marketing reports have shown that tiagabine hydrochloride use has been associated with new onset seizures and status epilepticus in patients without epilepsy. Dose may be an important predisposing factor in the development of seizures, although seizures have been reported in patients taking daily doses of tiagabine hydrochloride as low as 4 mg/day. In most cases, patients were using concomitant medications (antidepressants, antipsychotics, stimulants, narcotics) that are thought to lower the seizure threshold).
No products indexed under this heading.

Meclofenamate Sodium (Tiagabine is 96% bound to human plasma protein and therefore has the potential to interact with other highly protein bound compounds. Such an interaction can potentially lead to higher free fractions of either tiagabine or the competing drug).
No products indexed under this heading.

Mefenamic Acid (Tiagabine is 96% bound to human plasma protein and therefore has the potential to interact with other highly protein bound compounds. Such an interaction can potentially lead to higher free fractions of either tiagabine or the competing drug).
No products indexed under this heading.

Meperidine Hydrochloride (Because of the possible additive depressive effects, caution should be used when patients are taking other CNS depressants in combination with tiagabine hydrochloride).
No products indexed under this heading.

Mephenytoin (The clearance of tiagabine is affected by the co-administration of hepatic enzyme-inducing antiepilepsy drugs. Tiagabine is eliminated more rapidly in patients who have been taking hepatic enzyme-inducing drugs, (eg, carbamazepine, phenytoin, primidone and phenobarbital) than in patients not receiving such treatment).
No products indexed under this heading.

Mephobarbital (Because of the possible additive depressive effects, caution should be used when patients are taking other CNS depressants in combination with tiagabine hydrochloride).
No products indexed under this heading.

Meprobamate (Because of the possible additive depressive effects, caution should be used when patients are taking other CNS depressants in combination with tiagabine hydrochloride).
No products indexed under this heading.

Mesoridazine Besylate (Because of the possible additive depressive effects, caution should be used when patients are taking other CNS depressants in combination with tiagabine hydrochloride).
No products indexed under this heading.

Mestranol (Because of the potential for pharmacokinetic interactions between tiagabine hydrochloride and drugs that inhibit hepatic metabolizing enzymes, it may be useful to obtain plasma levels of tiagabine before and after changes are made in the therapeutic regimen).
No products indexed under this heading.

Methadone Hydrochloride (Because of the possible additive depressive effects, caution should be used when patients are taking other CNS depressants in combination with tiagabine hydrochloride).
No products indexed under this heading.

Methamphetamine Hydrochloride (Post-marketing reports have shown that tiagabine hydrochloride use has been associated with new onset seizures and status epilepticus in patients without epilepsy. Dose may be an important predisposing factor in the development of seizures, although seizures have been reported in patients taking daily doses of tiagabine hydrochloride as low as 4 mg/day. In most cases, patients were using concomitant medications (antidepressants, antipsychotics, stimulants, narcotics) that are thought to lower the seizure threshold).
No products indexed under this heading.

Methohexital Sodium (Because of the possible additive depressive effects, caution should be used when patients are taking other CNS depressants in combination with tiagabine hydrochloride).
No products indexed under this heading.

Methotrimeprazine (Because of the possible additive depressive effects, caution should be used when patients are taking other CNS depressants in combination with tiagabine hydrochloride).
No products indexed under this heading.

Methoxsalen (Because of the potential for pharmacokinetic interactions between tiagabine hydrochloride and drugs that inhibit hepatic metabolizing enzymes, it may be useful to obtain plasma levels of tiagabine before and after changes are made in the therapeutic regimen).
No products indexed under this heading.

Methoxyflurane (Because of the possible additive depressive effects, caution should be used when patients are taking other CNS depressants in combination with tiagabine hydrochloride).
No products indexed under this heading.

Methsuximide (The clearance of tiagabine is affected by the co-administration of hepatic enzyme-inducing antiepilepsy drugs. Tiagabine is eliminated more rapidly in patients who have been taking hepatic enzyme-inducing drugs, (eg, carbamazepine, phenytoin, primidone and phenobarbital) than in patients not receiving such treatment).
No products indexed under this heading.

Methyclothiazide (Because of the potential for pharmacokinetic interactions between tiagabine hydrochloride and drugs that inhibit hepatic metabolizing enzymes, it may be useful to obtain plasma levels of tiagabine before and after changes are made in the therapeutic regimen).
No products indexed under this heading.

Methylphenidate (Post-marketing reports have shown that tiagabine hydrochloride use has been associated with new onset seizures and status epilepticus in patients without epilepsy. Dose may be an important predisposing factor in the development of seizures, although seizures have been reported in patients taking daily doses of tiagabine hydrochloride as low as 4 mg/day. In most cases, patients were using concomitant medications (antidepressants, antipsychotics, stimulants, narcotics) that are thought to lower the seizure threshold). Products include:
Daytrana ... 3283

Methylphenidate Hydrochloride (Post-marketing reports have shown that tiagabine hydrochloride use has been associated with new onset seizures and status epilepticus in patients without epilepsy. Dose may be an important predisposing factor in the development of seizures, although seizures have been reported in patients taking daily doses of tiagabine hydrochloride as low as 4 mg/day. In most cases, patients were using concomitant medications (antidepressants, antipsychotics, stimulants, narcotics) that are thought to lower the seizure threshold). Products include:
Concerta ... 2598
Metadate CD ... 3439

Methylprednisolone (Because of the potential for pharmacokinetic interactions between tiagabine hydrochloride and drugs that induce hepatic metabolizing enzymes, it may be useful to obtain plasma levels of tiagabine before and after changes are made in the therapeutic regimen).
No products indexed under this heading.

Methylprednisolone Acetate (Because of the potential for pharmacokinetic interactions between tiagabine hydrochloride and drugs that induce hepatic metabolizing enzymes, it may be useful to obtain plasma levels of tiagabine before and after changes are made in the therapeutic regimen).
No products indexed under this heading.

IMPORTANT NOTE: Always consult each drug listing in the patient's regimen for possible interactions.

Methylprednisolone Sodium Succinate (Because of the potential for pharmacokinetic interactions between tiagabine hydrochloride and drugs that induce hepatic metabolizing enzymes, it may be useful to obtain plasma levels of tiagabine before and after changes are made in the therapeutic regimen).
No products indexed under this heading.

Metronidazole (Because of the potential for pharmacokinetic interactions between tiagabine hydrochloride and drugs that inhibit hepatic metabolizing enzymes, it may be useful to obtain plasma levels of tiagabine before and after changes are made in the therapeutic regimen). Products include:
Pylera 793

Metronidazole Benzoate (Because of the potential for pharmacokinetic interactions between tiagabine hydrochloride and drugs that inhibit hepatic metabolizing enzymes, it may be useful to obtain plasma levels of tiagabine before and after changes are made in the therapeutic regimen).
No products indexed under this heading.

Metronidazole Hydrochloride (Because of the potential for pharmacokinetic interactions between tiagabine hydrochloride and drugs that inhibit hepatic metabolizing enzymes, it may be useful to obtain plasma levels of tiagabine before and after changes are made in the therapeutic regimen).
No products indexed under this heading.

Metronidazole Sodium (Because of the potential for pharmacokinetic interactions between tiagabine hydrochloride and drugs that inhibit hepatic metabolizing enzymes, it may be useful to obtain plasma levels of tiagabine before and after changes are made in the therapeutic regimen).
No products indexed under this heading.

Mexiletine Hydrochloride (Because of the potential for pharmacokinetic interactions between tiagabine hydrochloride and drugs that inhibit hepatic metabolizing enzymes, it may be useful to obtain plasma levels of tiagabine before and after changes are made in the therapeutic regimen).
No products indexed under this heading.

Mibefradil Dihydrochloride (Because of the potential for pharmacokinetic interactions between tiagabine hydrochloride and drugs that inhibit hepatic metabolizing enzymes, it may be useful to obtain plasma levels of tiagabine before and after changes are made in the therapeutic regimen).
No products indexed under this heading.

Miconazole (Because of the potential for pharmacokinetic interactions between tiagabine hydrochloride and drugs that inhibit hepatic metabolizing enzymes, it may be useful to obtain plasma levels of tiagabine before and after changes are made in the therapeutic regimen).
No products indexed under this heading.

Miconazole Nitrate (Because of the potential for pharmacokinetic interactions between tiagabine hydrochloride and drugs that inhibit hepatic metabolizing enzymes, it may be useful to obtain plasma levels of tiagabine before and after changes are made in the therapeutic regimen). Products include:
Vusion Ointment 3335

Midazolam Hydrochloride (Because of the possible additive depressive effects, caution should be used when patients are taking other CNS depressants in combination with tiagabine hydrochloride).
No products indexed under this heading.

Mifepristone (Because of the potential for pharmacokinetic interactions between tiagabine hydrochloride and drugs that inhibit hepatic metabolizing enzymes, it may be useful to obtain plasma levels of tiagabine before and after changes are made in the therapeutic regimen).
No products indexed under this heading.

Mirtazapine (Post-marketing reports have shown that tiagabine hydrochloride use has been associated with new onset seizures and status epilepticus in patients without epilepsy. Dose may be an important predisposing factor in the development of seizures, although seizures have been reported in patients taking daily doses of tiagabine hydrochloride as low as 4 mg/day. In most cases, patients were using concomitant medications (antidepressants, antipsychotics, stimulants, narcotics) that are thought to lower the seizure threshold). Products include:
Remeron Tablets 3214
RemeronSolTab Tablets 3219

Moclobemide (Because of the potential for pharmacokinetic interactions between tiagabine hydrochloride and drugs that inhibit hepatic metabolizing enzymes, it may be useful to obtain plasma levels of tiagabine before and after changes are made in the therapeutic regimen).
No products indexed under this heading.

Modafinil (Because of the potential for pharmacokinetic interactions between tiagabine hydrochloride and drugs that induce hepatic metabolizing enzymes, it may be useful to obtain plasma levels of tiagabine before and after changes are made in the therapeutic regimen). Products include:
Provigil 983

Molindone Hydrochloride (Because of the possible additive depressive effects, caution should be used when patients are taking other CNS depressants in combination with tiagabine hydrochloride). Products include:
Moban 1108

Morphine Sulfate (Because of the possible additive depressive effects, caution should be used when patients are taking other CNS depressants in combination with tiagabine hydrochloride). Products include:
Avinza 1822
Embeda 1831
MS Contin 2803

Morphine Sulfate, Liposomal (Because of the possible additive depressive effects, caution should be used when patients are taking other CNS depressants in combination with tiagabine hydrochloride).
No products indexed under this heading.

Moxifloxacin Hydrochloride (Because of the potential for pharmacokinetic interactions between tiagabine hydrochloride and drugs that inhibit hepatic metabolizing enzymes, it may be useful to obtain plasma levels of tiagabine before and after changes are made in the therapeutic regimen). Products include:
Avelox 3064
Vigamox 589

Nafcillin Sodium (Because of the potential for pharmacokinetic interactions between tiagabine hydrochloride and drugs that induce hepatic metabolizing enzymes, it may be useful to obtain plasma levels of tiagabine before and after changes are made in the therapeutic regimen).
No products indexed under this heading.

Nalidixic Acid (Because of the potential for pharmacokinetic interactions between tiagabine hydrochloride and drugs that inhibit hepatic metabolizing enzymes, it may be useful to obtain plasma levels of tiagabine before and after changes are made in the therapeutic regimen).
No products indexed under this heading.

Naproxen (Tiagabine is 96% bound to human plasma protein and therefore has the potential to interact with other highly protein bound compounds. Such an interaction can potentially lead to higher free fractions of either tiagabine or the competing drug). Products include:
EC-Naprosyn 2850
Naprosyn 2850
Anaprox/Naprosyn 2850

Naproxen Sodium (Tiagabine is 96% bound to human plasma protein and therefore has the potential to interact with other highly protein bound compounds. Such an interaction can potentially lead to higher free fractions of either tiagabine or the competing drug). Products include:
Anaprox 2850
Anaprox DS 2850
Treximet 1681

Nefazodone Hydrochloride (Post-marketing reports have shown that tiagabine hydrochloride use has been associated with new onset seizures and status epilepticus in patients without epilepsy. Dose may be an important predisposing factor in the development of seizures, although seizures have been reported in patients taking daily doses of tiagabine hydrochloride as low as 4 mg/day. In most cases, patients were using concomitant medications (antidepressants, antipsychotics, stimulants, narcotics) that are thought to lower the seizure threshold).
No products indexed under this heading.

Nelfinavir Mesylate (Because of the potential for pharmacokinetic interactions between tiagabine hydrochloride and drugs that inhibit hepatic metabolizing enzymes, it may be useful to obtain plasma levels of tiagabine before and after changes are made in the therapeutic regimen).
No products indexed under this heading.

Nevirapine (Because of the potential for pharmacokinetic interactions between tiagabine hydrochloride and drugs that induce hepatic metabolizing enzymes, it may be useful to obtain plasma levels of tiagabine before and after changes are made in the therapeutic regimen). Products include:
Viramune Oral Suspension 897
Viramune Tablets 897

Niacinamide (Because of the potential for pharmacokinetic interactions between tiagabine hydrochloride and drugs that inhibit hepatic metabolizing enzymes, it may be useful to obtain plasma levels of tiagabine before and after changes are made in the therapeutic regimen). Products include:
CitraNatal 90 DHA Capsules 2332
CitraNatal Assure 2332
CitraNatal Rx 2332
Heplive 607

Niacinamide Hydroiodide (Because of the potential for pharmacokinetic interactions between tiagabine hydrochloride and drugs that inhibit hepatic metabolizing enzymes, it may be useful to obtain plasma levels of tiagabine before and after changes are made in the therapeutic regimen).
No products indexed under this heading.

Nicardipine (Because of the potential for pharmacokinetic interactions between tiagabine hydrochloride and drugs that inhibit hepatic metabolizing enzymes, it may be useful to obtain plasma levels of tiagabine before and after changes are made in the therapeutic regimen).
No products indexed under this heading.

Nicardipine Hydrochloride (Because of the potential for pharmacokinetic interactions between tiagabine hydrochloride and drugs that inhibit hepatic metabolizing enzymes, it may be useful to obtain plasma levels of tiagabine before and after changes are made in the therapeutic regimen).
No products indexed under this heading.

Nicotinamide (Because of the potential for pharmacokinetic interactions between tiagabine hydrochloride and drugs that inhibit hepatic metabolizing enzymes, it may be useful to obtain plasma levels of tiagabine before and after changes are made in the therapeutic regimen).
No products indexed under this heading.

Nicotine (Because of the potential for pharmacokinetic interactions between tiagabine hydrochloride and drugs that induce hepatic metabolizing enzymes, it may be useful to obtain plasma levels of tiagabine before and after changes are made in the therapeutic regimen).
No products indexed under this heading.

Nicotine Polacrilex (Because of the potential for pharmacokinetic interactions between tiagabine hydrochloride and drugs that induce hepatic metabolizing enzymes, it may be useful to obtain plasma levels of tiagabine before and after changes are made in the therapeutic regimen).
No products indexed under this heading.

Nicotine Salicylate (Because of the potential for pharmacokinetic interactions between tiagabine hydrochloride and drugs that induce hepatic metabolizing enzymes, it may be useful to obtain plasma levels of tiagabine before and after changes are made in the therapeutic regimen).
No products indexed under this heading.

Nicotine Sulfate (Because of the potential for pharmacokinetic interactions between tiagabine hydrochloride and drugs that induce hepatic metabolizing enzymes, it may be useful to obtain plasma levels of tiagabine before and after changes are made in the therapeutic regimen).
No products indexed under this heading.

Nifedipine (Because of the potential for pharmacokinetic interactions between tiagabine hydrochloride and drugs that inhibit hepatic metabolizing enzymes, it may be useful to obtain plasma levels of tiagabine before and after changes are made in the therapeutic regimen).
No products indexed under this heading.

Norethindrone (Because of the potential for pharmacokinetic interactions between tiagabine hydrochloride and drugs that induce hepatic metabolizing enzymes, it may be useful to obtain plasma levels of tiagabine before and after changes are made in the therapeutic regimen). Products include:
Ortho Micronor 2660

Norethindrone Acetate (Because of the potential for pharmacokinetic interactions between tiagabine hydrochloride and drugs that induce hepatic metabolizing enzymes, it may be useful to obtain plasma levels of tiagabine before and after changes are made in the therapeutic regimen). Products include:
Activella 2561

IMPORTANT NOTE: Always consult each drug listing in the patient's regimen for possible interactions.

Gabitril Interactions Index 732

zures have been reported in patients taking daily doses of tiagabine hydrochloride as low as 4 mg/day. In most cases, patients were using concomitant medications (antidepressants, antipsychotics, stimulants, narcotics) that are thought to lower the seizure threshold).
No products indexed under this heading.

Piroxicam (Tiagabine is 96% bound to human plasma protein and therefore has the potential to interact with other highly protein bound compounds. Such an interaction can potentially lead to higher free fractions of either tiagabine or the competing drug).
No products indexed under this heading.

Polythiazide (Because of the potential for pharmacokinetic interactions between tiagabine hydrochloride and drugs that inhibit hepatic metabolizing enzymes, it may be useful to obtain plasma levels of tiagabine before and after changes are made in the therapeutic regimen).
No products indexed under this heading.

Posaconazole (Because of the potential for pharmacokinetic interactions between tiagabine hydrochloride and drugs that inhibit hepatic metabolizing enzymes, it may be useful to obtain plasma levels of tiagabine before and after changes are made in the therapeutic regimen). Products include:
Noxafil **3172**

Prazepam (Because of the possible additive depressive effects, caution should be used when patients are taking other CNS depressants in combination with tiagabine hydrochloride).
No products indexed under this heading.

Prednisolone (Because of the potential for pharmacokinetic interactions between tiagabine hydrochloride and drugs that induce hepatic metabolizing enzymes, it may be useful to obtain plasma levels of tiagabine before and after changes are made in the therapeutic regimen).
No products indexed under this heading.

Prednisolone Acetate (Because of the potential for pharmacokinetic interactions between tiagabine hydrochloride and drugs that induce hepatic metabolizing enzymes, it may be useful to obtain plasma levels of tiagabine before and after changes are made in the therapeutic regimen). Products include:
Blephamide .... ⊙ **212**, ⊙ **214**
Pred Forte .... ⊙ **225**
Pred Mild .... ⊙ **230**
Pred-G .... ⊙ **226**, ⊙ **227**

Prednisolone Sodium Phosphate (Because of the potential for pharmacokinetic interactions between tiagabine hydrochloride and drugs that induce hepatic metabolizing enzymes, it may be useful to obtain plasma levels of tiagabine before and after changes are made in the therapeutic regimen).
No products indexed under this heading.

Prednisolone Tebutate (Because of the potential for pharmacokinetic interactions between tiagabine hydrochloride and drugs that induce hepatic metabolizing enzymes, it may be useful to obtain plasma levels of tiagabine before and after changes are made in the therapeutic regimen).
No products indexed under this heading.

Prednisone (Because of the potential for pharmacokinetic interactions between tiagabine hydrochloride and drugs that induce hepatic metabolizing enzymes, it may be useful to obtain plasma levels of tiagabine before and after changes are made in the therapeutic regimen).
No products indexed under this heading.

Prednisone sodium phosphate (Because of the potential for pharmacokinetic interactions between tiagabine hydrochloride and drugs that induce hepatic metabolizing enzymes, it may be useful to obtain plasma levels of tiagabine before and after changes are made in the therapeutic regimen).
No products indexed under this heading.

Primidone (Population pharmacokinetic analyses indicate that tiagabine clearance is 60% greater in patients taking phenobarbital (primidone), with or without other enzyme-inducing antiepileptic drugs. The clearance of tiagabine is affected by the co-administration of hepatic enzyme-inducing antiepilepsy drugs. Tiagabine is eliminated more rapidly in patients who have been taking hepatic enzyme-inducing drugs, (eg, primidone), than in patients not receiving such treatment).
No products indexed under this heading.

Prochlorperazine (Because of the possible additive depressive effects, caution should be used when patients are taking other CNS depressants in combination with tiagabine hydrochloride).
No products indexed under this heading.

Prochlorperazine Edisylate (Because of the possible additive depressive effects, caution should be used when patients are taking other CNS depressants in combination with tiagabine hydrochloride).
No products indexed under this heading.

Prochlorperazine Maleate (Because of the possible additive depressive effects, caution should be used when patients are taking other CNS depressants in combination with tiagabine hydrochloride).
No products indexed under this heading.

Promethazine (Because of the possible additive depressive effects, caution should be used when patients are taking other CNS depressants in combination with tiagabine hydrochloride).
No products indexed under this heading.

Promethazine Hydrochloride (Because of the possible additive depressive effects, caution should be used when patients are taking other CNS depressants in combination with tiagabine hydrochloride).
No products indexed under this heading.

Propafenone Hydrochloride (Because of the potential for pharmacokinetic interactions between tiagabine hydrochloride and drugs that inhibit hepatic metabolizing enzymes, it may be useful to obtain plasma levels of tiagabine before and after changes are made in the therapeutic regimen). Products include:
Rythmol **1648**
Rythmol SR **1652**

Propofol (Because of the possible additive depressive effects, caution should be used when patients are taking other CNS depressants in combination with tiagabine hydrochloride).
No products indexed under this heading.

Propoxyphene Hydrochloride (Because of the possible additive depressive effects, caution should be used when patients are taking other CNS depressants in combination with tiagabine hydrochloride).
No products indexed under this heading.

Propoxyphene Napsylate (Because of the possible additive depressive effects, caution should be used when patients are taking other CNS depressants in combination with tiagabine hydrochloride).
No products indexed under this heading.

Propranolol Hydrochloride (Tiagabine is 96% bound to human plasma protein and therefore has the potential to interact with other highly protein bound compounds. Such an interaction can potentially lead to higher free fractions of either tiagabine or the competing drug). Products include:
InnoPran XL **1517**

Protriptyline Hydrochloride (Postmarketing reports have shown that tiagabine hydrochloride use has been associated with new onset seizures and status epilepticus in patients without epilepsy. Dose may be an important predisposing factor in the development of seizures, although seizures have been reported in patients taking daily doses of tiagabine hydrochloride as low as 4 mg/day. In most cases, patients were using concomitant medications (antidepressants, antipsychotics, stimulants, narcotics) that are thought to lower the seizure threshold).
No products indexed under this heading.

Quazepam (Because of the possible additive depressive effects, caution should be used when patients are taking other CNS depressants in combination with tiagabine hydrochloride).
No products indexed under this heading.

Quercetin (Because of the potential for pharmacokinetic interactions between tiagabine hydrochloride and drugs that inhibit hepatic metabolizing enzymes, it may be useful to obtain plasma levels of tiagabine before and after changes are made in the therapeutic regimen).
No products indexed under this heading.

Quetiapine Fumarate (Because of the possible additive depressive effects, caution should be used when patients are taking other CNS depressants in combination with tiagabine hydrochloride). Products include:
Seroquel **750**
Seroquel XR **759**

Quinacrine Hydrochloride (Because of the potential for pharmacokinetic interactions between tiagabine hydrochloride and drugs that inhibit hepatic metabolizing enzymes, it may be useful to obtain plasma levels of tiagabine before and after changes are made in the therapeutic regimen).
No products indexed under this heading.

Quinidine (Because of the potential for pharmacokinetic interactions between tiagabine hydrochloride and drugs that inhibit hepatic metabolizing enzymes, it may be useful to obtain plasma levels of tiagabine before and after changes are made in the therapeutic regimen).
No products indexed under this heading.

Quinidine Gluconate (Because of the potential for pharmacokinetic interactions between tiagabine hydrochloride and drugs that inhibit hepatic metabolizing enzymes, it may be useful to obtain plasma levels of tiagabine before and after changes are made in the therapeutic regimen).
No products indexed under this heading.

Quinidine Hydrochloride (Because of the potential for pharmacokinetic interactions between tiagabine hydrochloride and drugs that inhibit hepatic metabolizing enzymes, it may be useful to obtain plasma levels of tiagabine before and after changes are made in the therapeutic regimen).
No products indexed under this heading.

Quinidine Polygalacturonate (Because of the potential for pharmacokinetic interactions between tiagabine hydrochloride and drugs that inhibit hepatic metabolizing enzymes, it may be useful to obtain plasma levels of tiagabine before and after changes are made in the therapeutic regimen).
No products indexed under this heading.

Quinidine Sulfate (Because of the potential for pharmacokinetic interactions between tiagabine hydrochloride and drugs that inhibit hepatic metabolizing enzymes, it may be useful to obtain plasma levels of tiagabine before and after changes are made in the therapeutic regimen).
No products indexed under this heading.

Quinine (Because of the potential for pharmacokinetic interactions between tiagabine hydrochloride and drugs that inhibit hepatic metabolizing enzymes, it may be useful to obtain plasma levels of tiagabine before and after changes are made in the therapeutic regimen). Products include:
Hyland's Leg Cramps PM with Quinine **3315**

Quinine Sulfate (Because of the potential for pharmacokinetic interactions between tiagabine hydrochloride and drugs that inhibit hepatic metabolizing enzymes, it may be useful to obtain plasma levels of tiagabine before and after changes are made in the therapeutic regimen).
No products indexed under this heading.

Quinupristin (Because of the potential for pharmacokinetic interactions between tiagabine hydrochloride and drugs that inhibit hepatic metabolizing enzymes, it may be useful to obtain plasma levels of tiagabine before and after changes are made in the therapeutic regimen).
No products indexed under this heading.

Ranitidine Bismuth Citrate (Because of the potential for pharmacokinetic interactions between tiagabine hydrochloride and drugs that inhibit hepatic metabolizing enzymes, it may be useful to obtain plasma levels of tiagabine before and after changes are made in the therapeutic regimen).
No products indexed under this heading.

Ranitidine Hydrochloride (Because of the potential for pharmacokinetic interactions between tiagabine hydrochloride and drugs that inhibit hepatic metabolizing enzymes, it may be useful to obtain plasma levels of tiagabine before and after changes are made in the therapeutic regimen). Products include:
Zantac **1737**
Zantac Injection **1732**
Zantac Pharmacy **1735**

Remifentanil Hydrochloride (Because of the possible additive depressive effects, caution should be used when patients are taking other CNS depressants in combination with tiagabine hydrochloride).
No products indexed under this heading.

Rifabutin (Because of the potential for pharmacokinetic interactions between tiagabine hydrochloride and drugs that induce hepatic metabolizing enzymes, it may be useful to obtain plasma levels of tiagabine before and after changes are made in the therapeutic regimen).
No products indexed under this heading.

Rifampicin (Because of the potential for pharmacokinetic interactions between tiagabine hydrochloride and drugs that induce hepatic metabolizing enzymes, it may be useful to obtain plasma levels of tiagabine before and after changes are made in the therapeutic regimen).
No products indexed under this heading.

Rifampin (Because of the potential for pharmacokinetic interactions between tiagabine hydrochloride and drugs that induce hepatic metabolizing enzymes, it may be useful to obtain plasma levels of tiagabine before and after changes are made in the therapeutic regimen).
No products indexed under this heading.

Rifapentine (Because of the potential for pharmacokinetic interactions between tiagabine hydrochloride and drugs that induce hepatic metabolizing enzymes, it may be useful to obtain plasma levels of tiagabine before and after changes are made in the therapeutic regimen).

No products indexed under this heading.

Risperidone (Because of the possible additive depressive effects, caution should be used when patients are taking other CNS depressants in combination with tiagabine hydrochloride). Products include:

Risperdal Consta 2682

Ritonavir (Because of the potential for pharmacokinetic interactions between tiagabine hydrochloride and drugs that induce hepatic metabolizing enzymes, it may be useful to obtain plasma levels of tiagabine before and after changes are made in the therapeutic regimen). Products include:

Kaletra 458
Norvir 509

Rufinamide (The clearance of tiagabine is affected by the co-administration of hepatic enzyme-inducing antiepilepsy drugs. Tiagabine is eliminated more rapidly in patients who have been taking hepatic enzyme-inducing drugs, (eg, carbamazepine, phenytoin, primidone and phenobarbital) than in patients not receiving such treatment). Products include:

Banzel 1050

Saquinavir (Because of the potential for pharmacokinetic interactions between tiagabine hydrochloride and drugs that inhibit hepatic metabolizing enzymes, it may be useful to obtain plasma levels of tiagabine before and after changes are made in the therapeutic regimen).

No products indexed under this heading.

Saquinavir Mesylate (Because of the potential for pharmacokinetic interactions between tiagabine hydrochloride and drugs that inhibit hepatic metabolizing enzymes, it may be useful to obtain plasma levels of tiagabine before and after changes are made in the therapeutic regimen).

No products indexed under this heading.

Secobarbital Sodium (Because of the possible additive depressive effects, caution should be used when patients are taking other CNS depressants in combination with tiagabine hydrochloride).

No products indexed under this heading.

Selegiline (Post-marketing reports have shown that tiagabine hydrochloride use has been associated with new onset seizures and status epilepticus in patients without epilepsy. Dose may be an important predisposing factor in the development of seizures, although seizures have been reported in patients taking daily doses of tiagabine hydrochloride as low as 4 mg/day. In most cases, patients were using concomitant medications (antidepressants, antipsychotics, stimulants, narcotics) that are thought to lower the seizure threshold). Products include:

Emsam 3623

Selegiline Hydrochloride (Post-marketing reports have shown that tiagabine hydrochloride use has been associated with new onset seizures and status epilepticus in patients without epilepsy. Dose may be an important predisposing factor in the development of seizures, although seizures have been reported in patients taking daily doses of tiagabine hydrochloride as low as 4 mg/day. In most cases, patients were using concomitant medications (antidepressants, antipsychotics, stimu-

lants, narcotics) that are thought to lower the seizure threshold). Products include:

Eldepryl 3312

Sertraline Hydrochloride (Post-marketing reports have shown that tiagabine hydrochloride use has been associated with new onset seizures and status epilepticus in patients without epilepsy. Dose may be an important predisposing factor in the development of seizures, although seizures have been reported in patients taking daily doses of tiagabine hydrochloride as low as 4 mg/day. In most cases, patients were using concomitant medications (antidepressants, antipsychotics, stimulants, narcotics) that are thought to lower the seizure threshold).

No products indexed under this heading.

Sevoflurane (Because of the possible additive depressive effects, caution should be used when patients are taking other CNS depressants in combination with tiagabine hydrochloride). Products include:

Ultane 554

Sildenafil Citrate (Because of the potential for pharmacokinetic interactions between tiagabine hydrochloride and drugs that inhibit hepatic metabolizing enzymes, it may be useful to obtain plasma levels of tiagabine before and after changes are made in the therapeutic regimen).

No products indexed under this heading.

Sodium Butabarbital (Because of the possible additive depressive effects, caution should be used when patients are taking other CNS depressants in combination with tiagabine hydrochloride).

No products indexed under this heading.

Sodium Oxybate (Because of the possible additive depressive effects, caution should be used when patients are taking other CNS depressants in combination with tiagabine hydrochloride).

No products indexed under this heading.

Sodium Pentobarbital (Because of the possible additive depressive effects, caution should be used when patients are taking other CNS depressants in combination with tiagabine hydrochloride).

No products indexed under this heading.

Sparfloxacin (Because of the potential for pharmacokinetic interactions between tiagabine hydrochloride and drugs that inhibit hepatic metabolizing enzymes, it may be useful to obtain plasma levels of tiagabine before and after changes are made in the therapeutic regimen).

No products indexed under this heading.

Sufentanil Citrate (Because of the possible additive depressive effects, caution should be used when patients are taking other CNS depressants in combination with tiagabine hydrochloride).

No products indexed under this heading.

Sulfacytine (Because of the potential for pharmacokinetic interactions between tiagabine hydrochloride and drugs that inhibit hepatic metabolizing enzymes, it may be useful to obtain plasma levels of tiagabine before and after changes are made in the therapeutic regimen).

No products indexed under this heading.

Sulfamethizole (Because of the potential for pharmacokinetic interactions between tiagabine hydrochloride and drugs that inhibit hepatic metabolizing enzymes, it may be useful to obtain plasma levels of tiagabine before and after changes are made in the therapeutic regimen).

No products indexed under this heading.

Sulfamethoxazole (Because of the potential for pharmacokinetic interactions between tiagabine hydrochloride and drugs that inhibit hepatic metabolizing enzymes, it may be useful to obtain plasma levels of tiagabine before and after changes are made in the therapeutic regimen).

No products indexed under this heading.

Sulfaphenazole (Because of the potential for pharmacokinetic interactions between tiagabine hydrochloride and drugs that inhibit hepatic metabolizing enzymes, it may be useful to obtain plasma levels of tiagabine before and after changes are made in the therapeutic regimen).

No products indexed under this heading.

Sulfasalazine (Because of the potential for pharmacokinetic interactions between tiagabine hydrochloride and drugs that inhibit hepatic metabolizing enzymes, it may be useful to obtain plasma levels of tiagabine before and after changes are made in the therapeutic regimen).

No products indexed under this heading.

Sulfinpyrazone (Because of the potential for pharmacokinetic interactions between tiagabine hydrochloride and drugs that induce hepatic metabolizing enzymes, it may be useful to obtain plasma levels of tiagabine before and after changes are made in the therapeutic regimen).

No products indexed under this heading.

Sulfisoxazole Acetyl (Because of the potential for pharmacokinetic interactions between tiagabine hydrochloride and drugs that inhibit hepatic metabolizing enzymes, it may be useful to obtain plasma levels of tiagabine before and after changes are made in the therapeutic regimen).

No products indexed under this heading.

Sulfisoxazole Diolamine (Because of the potential for pharmacokinetic interactions between tiagabine hydrochloride and drugs that inhibit hepatic metabolizing enzymes, it may be useful to obtain plasma levels of tiagabine before and after changes are made in the therapeutic regimen).

No products indexed under this heading.

Sulindac (Tiagabine is 96% bound to human plasma protein and therefore has the potential to interact with other highly protein bound compounds. Such an interaction can potentially lead to higher free fractions of either tiagabine or the competing drug). Products include:

Clinoril 2098

Tacrine Hydrochloride (Because of the potential for pharmacokinetic interactions between tiagabine hydrochloride and drugs that inhibit hepatic metabolizing enzymes, it may be useful to obtain plasma levels of tiagabine before and after changes are made in the therapeutic regimen).

No products indexed under this heading.

Talbutal (Because of the possible additive depressive effects, caution should be used when patients are taking other CNS depressants in combination with tiagabine hydrochloride).

No products indexed under this heading.

Telithromycin (Because of the potential for pharmacokinetic interactions between tiagabine hydrochloride and drugs that inhibit hepatic metabolizing enzymes, it may be useful to obtain plasma levels of tiagabine before and after changes are made in the therapeutic regimen). Products include:

Ketek 2991

Telmisartan (Because of the potential for pharmacokinetic interactions between tiagabine hydrochloride and drugs that inhibit hepatic metabolizing

enzymes, it may be useful to obtain plasma levels of tiagabine before and after changes are made in the therapeutic regimen). Products include:

Micardis 887
Micardis HCT 889

Temazepam (Because of the possible additive depressive effects, caution should be used when patients are taking other CNS depressants in combination with tiagabine hydrochloride).

No products indexed under this heading.

Terbinafine Hydrochloride (Because of the potential for pharmacokinetic interactions between tiagabine hydrochloride and drugs that inhibit hepatic metabolizing enzymes, it may be useful to obtain plasma levels of tiagabine before and after changes are made in the therapeutic regimen).

No products indexed under this heading.

Terconazole (Because of the potential for pharmacokinetic interactions between tiagabine hydrochloride and drugs that inhibit hepatic metabolizing enzymes, it may be useful to obtain plasma levels of tiagabine before and after changes are made in the therapeutic regimen).

No products indexed under this heading.

Theophyllinate (Because of the potential for pharmacokinetic interactions between tiagabine hydrochloride and drugs that induce hepatic metabolizing enzymes, it may be useful to obtain plasma levels of tiagabine before and after changes are made in the therapeutic regimen).

No products indexed under this heading.

Theophylline (Because of the potential for pharmacokinetic interactions between tiagabine hydrochloride and drugs that induce hepatic metabolizing enzymes, it may be useful to obtain plasma levels of tiagabine before and after changes are made in the therapeutic regimen).

No products indexed under this heading.

Theophylline Anhydrous (Because of the potential for pharmacokinetic interactions between tiagabine hydrochloride and drugs that induce hepatic metabolizing enzymes, it may be useful to obtain plasma levels of tiagabine before and after changes are made in the therapeutic regimen). Products include:

Uniphyl 2817

Theophylline Calcium Salicylate (Because of the potential for pharmacokinetic interactions between tiagabine hydrochloride and drugs that induce hepatic metabolizing enzymes, it may be useful to obtain plasma levels of tiagabine before and after changes are made in the therapeutic regimen).

No products indexed under this heading.

Theophylline Dihydroxypropyl (Glyceryl) (Because of the potential for pharmacokinetic interactions between tiagabine hydrochloride and drugs that induce hepatic metabolizing enzymes, it may be useful to obtain plasma levels of tiagabine before and after changes are made in the therapeutic regimen).

No products indexed under this heading.

Theophylline Ethylenediamine (Because of the potential for pharmacokinetic interactions between tiagabine hydrochloride and drugs that induce hepatic metabolizing enzymes, it may be useful to obtain plasma levels of tiagabine before and after changes are made in the therapeutic regimen).

No products indexed under this heading.

IMPORTANT NOTE: Always consult each drug listing in the patient's regimen for possible interactions.

Theophylline Sodium Glycinate (Because of the potential for pharmacokinetic interactions between tiagabine hydrochloride and drugs that induce hepatic metabolizing enzymes, it may be useful to obtain plasma levels of tiagabine before and after changes are made in the therapeutic regimen).
No products indexed under this heading.

Thiamylal Sodium (Because of the possible additive depressive effects, caution should be used when patients are taking other CNS depressants in combination with tiagabine hydrochloride).
No products indexed under this heading.

Thioridazine (Because of the possible additive depressive effects, caution should be used when patients are taking other CNS depressants in combination with tiagabine hydrochloride).
No products indexed under this heading.

Thioridazine Hydrochloride (Because of the possible additive depressive effects, caution should be used when patients are taking other CNS depressants in combination with tiagabine hydrochloride). Products include:
Thioridazine Hydrochloride **2384**

Thiothixene (Because of the possible additive depressive effects, caution should be used when patients are taking other CNS depressants in combination with tiagabine hydrochloride). Products include:
Thiothixene **2386**

Thiothixene Hydrochloride (Because of the possible additive depressive effects, caution should be used when patients are taking other CNS depressants in combination with tiagabine hydrochloride).
No products indexed under this heading.

Ticlopidine Hydrochloride (Because of the potential for pharmacokinetic interactions between tiagabine hydrochloride and drugs that inhibit hepatic metabolizing enzymes, it may be useful to obtain plasma levels of tiagabine before and after changes are made in the therapeutic regimen).
No products indexed under this heading.

Tobacco (Because of the potential for pharmacokinetic interactions between tiagabine hydrochloride and drugs that induce hepatic metabolizing enzymes, it may be useful to obtain plasma levels of tiagabine before and after changes are made in the therapeutic regimen).
No products indexed under this heading.

Tolazamide (Because of the potential for pharmacokinetic interactions between tiagabine hydrochloride and drugs that inhibit hepatic metabolizing enzymes, it may be useful to obtain plasma levels of tiagabine before and after changes are made in the therapeutic regimen).
No products indexed under this heading.

Tolbutamide (Tiagabine is 96% bound to human plasma protein and therefore has the potential to interact with other highly protein bound compounds. Such an interaction can potentially lead to higher free fractions of either tiagabine or the competing drug).
No products indexed under this heading.

Tolbutamide Sodium (Because of the potential for pharmacokinetic interactions between tiagabine hydrochloride and drugs that inhibit hepatic metabolizing enzymes, it may be useful to obtain plasma levels of tiagabine before and after changes are made in the therapeutic regimen).
No products indexed under this heading.

Tolmetin Sodium (Tiagabine is 96% bound to human plasma protein and therefore has the potential to interact with other highly protein bound compounds. Such an interaction can potentially lead to higher free fractions of either tiagabine or the competing drug).
No products indexed under this heading.

Topiramate (The clearance of tiagabine is affected by the co-administration of hepatic enzyme-inducing antiepilepsy drugs. Tiagabine is eliminated more rapidly in patients who have been taking hepatic enzyme-inducing drugs, (eg, carbamazepine, phenytoin, primidone and phenobarbital) than in patients not receiving such treatment).
No products indexed under this heading.

Tranylcypromine Sulfate (Post-marketing reports have shown that tiagabine hydrochloride use has been associated with new onset seizures and status epilepticus in patients without epilepsy. Dose may be an important predisposing factor in the development of seizures, although seizures have been reported in patients taking daily doses of tiagabine hydrochloride as low as 4 mg/day. In most cases, patients were using concomitant medications (antidepressants, antipsychotics, stimulants, narcotics) that are thought to lower the seizure threshold). Products include:
Parnate **1584**

Trazodone Hydrochloride (Post-marketing reports have shown that tiagabine hydrochloride use has been associated with new onset seizures and status epilepticus in patients without epilepsy. Dose may be an important predisposing factor in the development of seizures, although seizures have been reported in patients taking daily doses of tiagabine hydrochloride as low as 4 mg/day. In most cases, patients were using concomitant medications (antidepressants, antipsychotics, stimulants, narcotics) that are thought to lower the seizure threshold).
No products indexed under this heading.

Triamcinolone (Because of the potential for pharmacokinetic interactions between tiagabine hydrochloride and drugs that induce hepatic metabolizing enzymes, it may be useful to obtain plasma levels of tiagabine before and after changes are made in the therapeutic regimen).
No products indexed under this heading.

Triamcinolone Acetonide (Because of the potential for pharmacokinetic interactions between tiagabine hydrochloride and drugs that induce hepatic metabolizing enzymes, it may be useful to obtain plasma levels of tiagabine before and after changes are made in the therapeutic regimen). Products include:
Azmacort **408**
Nasacort AQ **3019**

Triamcinolone Diacetate (Because of the potential for pharmacokinetic interactions between tiagabine hydrochloride and drugs that induce hepatic metabolizing enzymes, it may be useful to obtain plasma levels of tiagabine before and after changes are made in the therapeutic regimen).
No products indexed under this heading.

Triamcinolone Hexacetonide (Because of the potential for pharmacokinetic interactions between tiagabine hydrochloride and drugs that induce hepatic metabolizing enzymes, it may be useful to obtain plasma levels of tiagabine before and after changes are made in the therapeutic regimen).
No products indexed under this heading.

Triazolam (Because of the possible additive effects of drugs that may depress the nervous system, triazolam should be used cautiously in combination with tiagabine).
No products indexed under this heading.

Trifluoperazine Hydrochloride (Because of the possible additive depressive effects, caution should be used when patients are taking other CNS depressants in combination with tiagabine hydrochloride).
No products indexed under this heading.

Trimethadione (The clearance of tiagabine is affected by the co-administration of hepatic enzyme-inducing antiepilepsy drugs. Tiagabine is eliminated more rapidly in patients who have been taking hepatic enzyme-inducing drugs, (eg, carbamazepine, phenytoin, primidone and phenobarbital) than in patients not receiving such treatment).
No products indexed under this heading.

Trimethoprim (Because of the potential for pharmacokinetic interactions between tiagabine hydrochloride and drugs that inhibit hepatic metabolizing enzymes, it may be useful to obtain plasma levels of tiagabine before and after changes are made in the therapeutic regimen).
No products indexed under this heading.

Trimethoprim Hydrochloride (Because of the potential for pharmacokinetic interactions between tiagabine hydrochloride and drugs that inhibit hepatic metabolizing enzymes, it may be useful to obtain plasma levels of tiagabine before and after changes are made in the therapeutic regimen).
No products indexed under this heading.

Trimethoprim Sulfate (Because of the potential for pharmacokinetic interactions between tiagabine hydrochloride and drugs that inhibit hepatic metabolizing enzymes, it may be useful to obtain plasma levels of tiagabine before and after changes are made in the therapeutic regimen).
No products indexed under this heading.

Trimipramine Maleate (Tiagabine is 96% bound to human plasma protein and therefore has the potential to interact with other highly protein bound compounds. Such an interaction can potentially lead to higher free fractions of either tiagabine or the competing drug).
No products indexed under this heading.

Troglitazone (Because of the potential for pharmacokinetic interactions between tiagabine hydrochloride and drugs that induce hepatic metabolizing enzymes, it may be useful to obtain plasma levels of tiagabine before and after changes are made in the therapeutic regimen).
No products indexed under this heading.

Troleandomycin (Because of the potential for pharmacokinetic interactions between tiagabine hydrochloride and drugs that inhibit hepatic metabolizing enzymes, it may be useful to obtain plasma levels of tiagabine before and after changes are made in the therapeutic regimen).
No products indexed under this heading.

Trovafloxacin Mesylate (Because of the potential for pharmacokinetic interactions between tiagabine hydrochloride and drugs that inhibit hepatic metabolizing enzymes, it may be useful to obtain plasma levels of tiagabine before and after changes are made in the therapeutic regimen).
No products indexed under this heading.

Valproate Sodium (Co-administration of tiagabine in patients taking valproate chronically had no effect on tiagabine pharmacokinetics, but valproate significantly decreased tiagabine binding *in vitro* from 96.3% to 94.8%, which resulted in an increase of approximately 40% in the tiagabine concentrations; the clinical relevance of this *in vitro* finding is unknown. Tiagabine hydrochloride causes a slight decrease (about 10%) in steady-state valproate concentrations).
No products indexed under this heading.

Valproic Acid (Co-administration of tiagabine in patients taking valproate chronically had no effect on tiagabine pharmacokinetics, but valproate significantly decreased tiagabine binding *in vitro* from 96.3% to 94.8%, which resulted in an increase of approximately 40% in the tiagabine concentrations; the clinical relevance of this *in vitro* finding is unknown. Tiagabine hydrochloride causes a slight decrease (about 10%) in steady-state valproate concentrations).
No products indexed under this heading.

Vardenafil Hydrochloride (Because of the potential for pharmacokinetic interactions between tiagabine hydrochloride and drugs that inhibit hepatic metabolizing enzymes, it may be useful to obtain plasma levels of tiagabine before and after changes are made in the therapeutic regimen). Products include:
Levitra **3157**

Venlafaxine Hydrochloride (Post-marketing reports have shown that tiagabine hydrochloride use has been associated with new onset seizures and status epilepticus in patients without epilepsy. Dose may be an important predisposing factor in the development of seizures, although seizures have been reported in patients taking daily doses of tiagabine hydrochloride as low as 4 mg/day. In most cases, patients were using concomitant medications (antidepressants, antipsychotics, stimulants, narcotics) that are thought to lower the seizure threshold). Products include:
Effexor XR **3504**
Venlafaxine Hydrochloride Tablets ... **2388**

Verapamil Hydrochloride (Because of the potential for pharmacokinetic interactions between tiagabine hydrochloride and drugs that inhibit hepatic metabolizing enzymes, it may be useful to obtain plasma levels of tiagabine before and after changes are made in the therapeutic regimen). Products include:
Tarka **534**

Voriconazole (Because of the potential for pharmacokinetic interactions between tiagabine hydrochloride and drugs that inhibit hepatic metabolizing enzymes, it may be useful to obtain plasma levels of tiagabine before and after changes are made in the therapeutic regimen).
No products indexed under this heading.

Warfarin Sodium (Tiagabine is 96% bound to human plasma protein and therefore has the potential to interact with other highly protein bound compounds. Such an interaction can potentially lead to higher free fractions of either tiagabine or the competing drug).
No products indexed under this heading.

Zafirlukast (Because of the potential for pharmacokinetic interactions between tiagabine hydrochloride and drugs that inhibit hepatic metabolizing enzymes, it may be useful to obtain plasma levels of tiagabine before and after changes are made in the therapeutic regimen). Products include:
Accolate **3612**

Zaleplon (Because of the possible additive depressive effects, caution should be used when patients are taking other CNS depressants in combination with tiagabine hydrochloride).
No products indexed under this heading.

Zileuton (Because of the potential for pharmacokinetic interactions between tiagabine hydrochloride and drugs that inhibit hepatic metabolizing enzymes, it may be useful to obtain plasma levels of tiagabine before and after changes are made in the therapeutic regimen).
No products indexed under this heading.

Ziprasidone Hydrochloride (Because of the possible additive depressive effects, caution should be used when patients are taking other CNS depressants in combination with tiagabine hydrochloride). Products include:
Geodon 2723

Zolpidem Tartrate (Because of the possible additive depressive effects, caution should be used when patients are taking other CNS depressants in combination with tiagabine hydrochloride). Products include:
Ambien 2920
Ambien CR 2925

Zonisamide (The clearance of tiagabine is affected by the co-administration of hepatic enzyme-inducing antiepilepsy drugs. Tiagabine is eliminated more rapidly in patients who have been taking hepatic enzyme-inducing drugs, (eg, carbamazepine, phenytoin, primidone and phenobarbital) than in patients not receiving such treatment). Products include:
Zonegran 1081

Food Interactions

Alcohol (Because of the possible additive effects of drugs that may depress the nervous system, ethanol should be used cautiously in combination with tiagabine).

Beer, reduced-alcohol (Because of the possible additive effects of drugs that may depress the nervous system, ethanol should be used cautiously in combination with tiagabine).

Beer, unspecified (Because of the possible additive effects of drugs that may depress the nervous system, ethanol should be used cautiously in combination with tiagabine).

Broccoli (Because of the potential for pharmacokinetic interactions between tiagabine hydrochloride and drugs that induce hepatic metabolizing enzymes, it may be useful to obtain plasma levels of tiagabine before and after changes are made in the therapeutic regimen).

Brussel Sprouts (Because of the potential for pharmacokinetic interactions between tiagabine hydrochloride and drugs that induce hepatic metabolizing enzymes, it may be useful to obtain plasma levels of tiagabine before and after changes are made in the therapeutic regimen).

Charbroiled Food (Because of the potential for pharmacokinetic interactions between tiagabine hydrochloride and drugs that induce hepatic metabolizing enzymes, it may be useful to obtain plasma levels of tiagabine before and after changes are made in the therapeutic regimen).

Food, unspecified (Absorption of tiagabine is rapid, with peak plasma concentrations occurring at approximately 45 minutes following an oral dose in the fasting state. Tiagabine is nearly completely absorbed (>95%), with an absolute oral bioavailability of about 90%. A high fat meal decreases the rate (mean T_{max} was prolonged to 2.5 hours, and mean C_{max} was reduced by about 40%) but not the extent (AUC) of tiagabine absorption).

Grapefruit (Because of the potential for pharmacokinetic interactions between tiagabine hydrochloride and drugs that inhibit hepatic metabolizing enzymes, it may be useful to obtain plasma levels of tiagabine before and after changes are made in the therapeutic regimen).

Grapefruit Juice (Because of the potential for pharmacokinetic interactions between tiagabine hydrochloride and drugs that inhibit hepatic metabolizing enzymes, it may be useful to obtain plasma levels of tiagabine before and after changes are made in the therapeutic regimen).

Meal, unspecified (Absorption of tiagabine is rapid, with peak plasma concentrations occurring at approximately 45 minutes following an oral dose in the fasting state. Tiagabine is nearly completely absorbed (>95%), with an absolute oral bioavailability of about 90%. A high fat meal decreases the rate (mean T_{max} was prolonged to 2.5 hours, and mean C_{max} was reduced by about 40%) but not the extent (AUC) of tiagabine absorption).

Wine, Chianti (Because of the possible additive effects of drugs that may depress the nervous system, ethanol should be used cautiously in combination with tiagabine).

Wine, Red (Because of the possible additive effects of drugs that may depress the nervous system, ethanol should be used cautiously in combination with tiagabine).

Wine, unspecified (Because of the possible additive effects of drugs that may depress the nervous system, ethanol should be used cautiously in combination with tiagabine).

Wine products (Because of the possible additive effects of drugs that may depress the nervous system, ethanol should be used cautiously in combination with tiagabine).

GAMMAGARD LIQUID

(Immune Globulin Intravenous (Human)) 812
May interact with vaccines, live. Compounds in these categories include:

BCG Vaccine (Antibodies in immune globulin intravenous products may interfere with patient responses to live vaccines, such as those for measles, mumps and rubella).
No products indexed under this heading.

Influenza Vaccine, Live Attenuated (Antibodies in immune globulin intravenous products may interfere with patient responses to live vaccines, such as those for measles, mumps and rubella).
No products indexed under this heading.

Influenza Virus Vaccine Live, Intranasal (Antibodies in immune globulin intravenous products may interfere with patient responses to live vaccines, such as those for measles, mumps and rubella). Products include:
FluMist 2078

Measles, Mumps, Rubella and Varicella Virus Vaccine Live (Antibodies in immune globulin intravenous products may interfere with patient responses to live vaccines, such as those for measles, mumps and rubella). Products include:
ProQuad 2254

Measles, Mumps & Rubella Virus Vaccine, Live (Antibodies in immune globulin intravenous products may interfere with patient responses to live vaccines, such as those for measles, mumps and rubella). Products include:
M-M-R II 2203
ProQuad 2254

Measles & Rubella Virus Vaccine Live (Antibodies in immune globulin intravenous products may interfere with patient responses to live vaccines, such as those for measles, mumps and rubella).
No products indexed under this heading.

Measles Virus Vaccine Live (Antibodies in immune globulin intravenous products may interfere with patient responses to live vaccines, such as those for measles, mumps and rubella). Products include:
Attenuvax 2086

Mumps Virus Vaccine, Live (Antibodies in immune globulin intravenous products may interfere with patient responses to live vaccines, such as those for measles, mumps and rubella). Products include:
Mumpsvax 2218

Poliovirus Vaccine, Live, Oral, Trivalent, Types 1,2,3 (Sabin) (Antibodies in immune globulin intravenous products may interfere with patient responses to live vaccines, such as those for measles, mumps and rubella).
No products indexed under this heading.

Rotavirus Vaccine, Live, Oral, Tetravalent (Antibodies in immune globulin intravenous products may interfere with patient responses to live vaccines, such as those for measles, mumps and rubella).
No products indexed under this heading.

Rubella & Mumps Virus Vaccine Live (Antibodies in immune globulin intravenous products may interfere with patient responses to live vaccines, such as those for measles, mumps and rubella).
No products indexed under this heading.

Rubella Virus Vaccine Live (Antibodies in immune globulin intravenous products may interfere with patient responses to live vaccines, such as those for measles, mumps and rubella). Products include:
Meruvax II 2210

Smallpox Vaccine (Antibodies in immune globulin intravenous products may interfere with patient responses to live vaccines, such as those for measles, mumps and rubella).
No products indexed under this heading.

Typhoid Vaccine (Antibodies in immune globulin intravenous products may interfere with patient responses to live vaccines, such as those for measles, mumps and rubella).
No products indexed under this heading.

Varicella Virus Vaccine, Live (Antibodies in immune globulin intravenous products may interfere with patient responses to live vaccines, such as those for measles, mumps and rubella). Products include:
Varivax 2285

Yellow Fever Vaccine (Antibodies in immune globulin intravenous products may interfere with patient responses to live vaccines, such as those for measles, mumps and rubella).
No products indexed under this heading.

Zoster Vaccine Live (Antibodies in immune globulin intravenous products may interfere with patient responses to live vaccines, such as those for measles, mumps and rubella). Products include:
Zostavax 2299

GAMMAGARD S/D

(Immune Globulin Intravenous (Human)) 815
May interact with vaccines, live, and certain other agents. Compounds in these categories include:

BCG Vaccine (Antibodies in immune globulin intravenous products may interfere with patient responses to live vaccines).
No products indexed under this heading.

Influenza Vaccine, Live Attenuated (Antibodies in immune globulin intravenous products may interfere with patient responses to live vaccines).
No products indexed under this heading.

Influenza Virus Vaccine Live, Intranasal (Antibodies in immune globulin intravenous products may interfere with patient responses to live vaccines). Products include:
FluMist 2078

Measles, Mumps, Rubella and Varicella Virus Vaccine Live (Antibodies in immune globulin intravenous products may interfere with patient responses to live vaccines). Products include:
ProQuad 2254

Measles, Mumps & Rubella Virus Vaccine, Live (Antibodies in immune globulin intravenous products may interfere with patient responses to live vaccines). Products include:
M-M-R II 2203
ProQuad 2254

Measles & Rubella Virus Vaccine Live (Antibodies in immune globulin intravenous products may interfere with patient responses to live vaccines).
No products indexed under this heading.

Measles Virus Vaccine Live (Antibodies in immune globulin intravenous products may interfere with patient responses to live vaccines). Products include:
Attenuvax 2086

Mumps Virus Vaccine, Live (Antibodies in immune globulin intravenous products may interfere with patient responses to live vaccines). Products include:
Mumpsvax 2218

Poliovirus Vaccine, Live, Oral, Trivalent, Types 1,2,3 (Sabin) (Antibodies in immune globulin intravenous products may interfere with patient responses to live vaccines).
No products indexed under this heading.

Rotavirus Vaccine, Live, Oral, Tetravalent (Antibodies in immune globulin intravenous products may interfere with patient responses to live vaccines).
No products indexed under this heading.

Rubella & Mumps Virus Vaccine Live (Antibodies in immune globulin intravenous products may interfere with patient responses to live vaccines).
No products indexed under this heading.

Rubella Virus Vaccine Live (Antibodies in immune globulin intravenous products may interfere with patient responses to live vaccines). Products include:
Meruvax II 2210

Smallpox Vaccine (Antibodies in immune globulin intravenous products may interfere with patient responses to live vaccines).
No products indexed under this heading.

Typhoid Vaccine (Antibodies in immune globulin intravenous products may interfere with patient responses to live vaccines).
No products indexed under this heading.

Varicella Virus Vaccine, Live (Antibodies in immune globulin intravenous products may interfere with patient responses to live vaccines). Products include:
Varivax 2285

Yellow Fever Vaccine (Antibodies in immune globulin intravenous products may interfere with patient responses to live vaccines).
No products indexed under this heading.

IMPORTANT NOTE: Always consult each drug listing in the patient's regimen for possible interactions.

(⊙ Described in PDR® for Ophthalmic Medicines)

737 Interactions Index Gamunex

Cefotaxime Sodium (Co-administration of nephrotoxic drugs with immune globulin intravenous (human) products may increase the risk of renal dysfunction, acute renal failure, osmotic nephrosis, and death).
No products indexed under this heading.

Cefotetan (Co-administration of nephrotoxic drugs with immune globulin intravenous (human) products may increase the risk of renal dysfunction, acute renal failure, osmotic nephrosis, and death).
No products indexed under this heading.

Cefoxitin Sodium (Co-administration of nephrotoxic drugs with immune globulin intravenous (human) products may increase the risk of renal dysfunction, acute renal failure, osmotic nephrosis, and death).
No products indexed under this heading.

Cefpodoxime Proxetil (Co-administration of nephrotoxic drugs with immune globulin intravenous (human) products may increase the risk of renal dysfunction, acute renal failure, osmotic nephrosis, and death).
No products indexed under this heading.

Cefprozil (Co-administration of nephrotoxic drugs with immune globulin intravenous (human) products may increase the risk of renal dysfunction, acute renal failure, osmotic nephrosis, and death).
No products indexed under this heading.

Ceftazidime (Co-administration of nephrotoxic drugs with immune globulin intravenous (human) products may increase the risk of renal dysfunction, acute renal failure, osmotic nephrosis, and death). Products include:
Fortaz 1481

Ceftizoxime Sodium (Co-administration of nephrotoxic drugs with immune globulin intravenous (human) products may increase the risk of renal dysfunction, acute renal failure, osmotic nephrosis, and death).
No products indexed under this heading.

Ceftriaxone Sodium (Co-administration of nephrotoxic drugs with immune globulin intravenous (human) products may increase the risk of renal dysfunction, acute renal failure, osmotic nephrosis, and death). Products include:
Rocephin 2859

Cefuroxime Axetil (Co-administration of nephrotoxic drugs with immune globulin intravenous (human) products may increase the risk of renal dysfunction, acute renal failure, osmotic nephrosis, and death). Products include:
Ceftin 1399

Cefuroxime Sodium (Co-administration of nephrotoxic drugs with immune globulin intravenous (human) products may increase the risk of renal dysfunction, acute renal failure, osmotic nephrosis, and death).
No products indexed under this heading.

Celecoxib (Co-administration of nephrotoxic drugs with immune globulin intravenous (human) products may increase the risk of renal dysfunction, acute renal failure, osmotic nephrosis, and death). Products include:
Celebrex 3272

Cephalexin (Co-administration of nephrotoxic drugs with immune globulin intravenous (human) products may increase the risk of renal dysfunction, acute renal failure, osmotic nephrosis, and death).
No products indexed under this heading.

Cephalothin Sodium (Co-administration of nephrotoxic drugs with immune globulin intravenous (human) products may increase the risk of renal dysfunction, acute renal failure, osmotic nephrosis, and death).
No products indexed under this heading.

Cephapirin Sodium (Co-administration of nephrotoxic drugs with immune globulin intravenous (human) products may increase the risk of renal dysfunction, acute renal failure, osmotic nephrosis, and death).
No products indexed under this heading.

Cephradine (Co-administration of nephrotoxic drugs with immune globulin intravenous (human) products may increase the risk of renal dysfunction, acute renal failure, osmotic nephrosis, and death).
No products indexed under this heading.

Cerivastatin Sodium (Co-administration of nephrotoxic drugs with immune globulin intravenous (human) products may increase the risk of renal dysfunction, acute renal failure, osmotic nephrosis, and death).
No products indexed under this heading.

Chlorothiazide (Co-administration of nephrotoxic drugs with immune globulin intravenous (human) products may increase the risk of renal dysfunction, acute renal failure, osmotic nephrosis, and death).
No products indexed under this heading.

Chlorothiazide Sodium (Co-administration of nephrotoxic drugs with immune globulin intravenous (human) products may increase the risk of renal dysfunction, acute renal failure, osmotic nephrosis, and death). Products include:
Diuril Intravenous 2009

Chlorpropamide (Co-administration of nephrotoxic drugs with immune globulin intravenous (human) products may increase the risk of renal dysfunction, acute renal failure, osmotic nephrosis, and death).
No products indexed under this heading.

Cidofovir (Co-administration of nephrotoxic drugs with immune globulin intravenous (human) products may increase the risk of renal dysfunction, acute renal failure, osmotic nephrosis, and death).
No products indexed under this heading.

Cilastatin Sodium (Co-administration of nephrotoxic drugs with immune globulin intravenous (human) products may increase the risk of renal dysfunction, acute renal failure, osmotic nephrosis, and death). Products include:
Primaxin I.M. 2232
Primaxin I.V. 2235

Cimetidine (Co-administration of nephrotoxic drugs with immune globulin intravenous (human) products may increase the risk of renal dysfunction, acute renal failure, osmotic nephrosis, and death).
No products indexed under this heading.

Cimetidine Hydrochloride (Co-administration of nephrotoxic drugs with immune globulin intravenous (human) products may increase the risk of renal dysfunction, acute renal failure, osmotic nephrosis, and death).
No products indexed under this heading.

Cisplatin (Co-administration of nephrotoxic drugs with immune globulin intravenous (human) products may increase the risk of renal dysfunction, acute renal failure, osmotic nephrosis, and death).
No products indexed under this heading.

Cladribine (Co-administration of nephrotoxic drugs with immune globulin intravenous (human) products may increase the risk of renal dysfunction, acute renal failure, osmotic nephrosis, and death). Products include:
Leustatin 946

Clozapine (Co-administration of nephrotoxic drugs with immune globulin intravenous (human) products may increase the risk of renal dysfunction, acute renal failure, osmotic nephrosis, and death).
No products indexed under this heading.

Colistimethate Sodium (Co-administration of nephrotoxic drugs with immune globulin intravenous (human) products may increase the risk of renal dysfunction, acute renal failure, osmotic nephrosis, and death).
No products indexed under this heading.

Colistin Sulfate (Co-administration of nephrotoxic drugs with immune globulin intravenous (human) products may increase the risk of renal dysfunction, acute renal failure, osmotic nephrosis, and death).
No products indexed under this heading.

Cyclophosphamide (Co-administration of nephrotoxic drugs with immune globulin intravenous (human) products may increase the risk of renal dysfunction, acute renal failure, osmotic nephrosis, and death).
No products indexed under this heading.

Cyclosporine (Co-administration of nephrotoxic drugs with immune globulin intravenous (human) products may increase the risk of renal dysfunction, acute renal failure, osmotic nephrosis, and death). Products include:
Gengraf 440
Neoral Oral Solution 2496
Neoral Capsules 2496
Restasis 605

Cytarabine (Co-administration of nephrotoxic drugs with immune globulin intravenous (human) products may increase the risk of renal dysfunction, acute renal failure, osmotic nephrosis, and death).
No products indexed under this heading.

Cytarabine Liposome (Co-administration of nephrotoxic drugs with immune globulin intravenous (human) products may increase the risk of renal dysfunction, acute renal failure, osmotic nephrosis, and death).
No products indexed under this heading.

Delavirdine Mesylate (Co-administration of nephrotoxic drugs with immune globulin intravenous (human) products may increase the risk of renal dysfunction, acute renal failure, osmotic nephrosis, and death).
No products indexed under this heading.

Diatrizoate Meglumine (Co-administration of nephrotoxic drugs with immune globulin intravenous (human) products may increase the risk of renal dysfunction, acute renal failure, osmotic nephrosis, and death).
No products indexed under this heading.

Diatrizoate Sodium (Co-administration of nephrotoxic drugs with immune globulin intravenous (human) products may increase the risk of renal dysfunction, acute renal failure, osmotic nephrosis, and death).
No products indexed under this heading.

Diclofenac Potassium (Co-administration of nephrotoxic drugs with immune globulin intravenous (human) products may increase the risk of renal dysfunction, acute renal failure, osmotic nephrosis, and death).
No products indexed under this heading.

Diclofenac Sodium (Co-administration of nephrotoxic drugs with immune globulin intravenous (human) products may increase the risk of renal dysfunction, acute renal failure, osmotic nephrosis, and death).
No products indexed under this heading.

Dicloxacillin Sodium (Co-administration of nephrotoxic drugs with immune globulin intravenous (human) products may increase the risk of renal dysfunction, acute renal failure, osmotic nephrosis, and death).
No products indexed under this heading.

Didanosine (Co-administration of nephrotoxic drugs with immune globulin intravenous (human) products may increase the risk of renal dysfunction, acute renal failure, osmotic nephrosis, and death).
No products indexed under this heading.

Efavirenz (Co-administration of nephrotoxic drugs with immune globulin intravenous (human) products may increase the risk of renal dysfunction, acute renal failure, osmotic nephrosis, and death). Products include:
Atripla 906

Emtricitabine (Co-administration of nephrotoxic drugs with immune globulin intravenous (human) products may increase the risk of renal dysfunction, acute renal failure, osmotic nephrosis, and death). Products include:
Atripla 906
Emtriva 1238
Emtriva Oral Solution 1238
Truvada 1258

Enalapril Maleate (Co-administration of nephrotoxic drugs with immune globulin intravenous (human) products may increase the risk of renal dysfunction, acute renal failure, osmotic nephrosis, and death).
No products indexed under this heading.

Enalaprilat (Co-administration of nephrotoxic drugs with immune globulin intravenous (human) products may increase the risk of renal dysfunction, acute renal failure, osmotic nephrosis, and death).
No products indexed under this heading.

Enfuvirtide (Co-administration of nephrotoxic drugs with immune globulin intravenous (human) products may increase the risk of renal dysfunction, acute renal failure, osmotic nephrosis, and death).
No products indexed under this heading.

Ethiodized Oil (Co-administration of nephrotoxic drugs with immune globulin intravenous (human) products may increase the risk of renal dysfunction, acute renal failure, osmotic nephrosis, and death).
No products indexed under this heading.

Etodolac (Co-administration of nephrotoxic drugs with immune globulin intravenous (human) products may increase the risk of renal dysfunction, acute renal failure, osmotic nephrosis, and death).
No products indexed under this heading.

Fenoprofen Calcium (Co-administration of nephrotoxic drugs with immune globulin intravenous (human) products may increase the risk of renal dysfunction, acute renal failure, osmotic nephrosis, and death).
No products indexed under this heading.

Filgrastim (Co-administration of nephrotoxic drugs with immune globulin intravenous (human) products may increase the risk of renal dysfunction, acute renal failure, osmotic nephrosis, and death). Products include:
Neupogen 631

Fluorouracil (Co-administration of nephrotoxic drugs with immune globulin intravenous (human) products may increase the risk of renal dysfunction, acute renal failure, osmotic nephrosis, and death). Products include:
Carac 2966

Flurbiprofen (Co-administration of nephrotoxic drugs with immune globulin intravenous (human) products may increase the risk of renal dysfunction, acute renal failure, osmotic nephrosis, and death).
No products indexed under this heading.

IMPORTANT NOTE: Always consult each drug listing in the patient's regimen for possible interactions.

Fluvastatin Sodium (Co-administration of nephrotoxic drugs with immune globulin intravenous (human) products may increase the risk of renal dysfunction, acute renal failure, osmotic nephrosis, and death).
No products indexed under this heading.

Foscarnet Sodium (Co-administration of nephrotoxic drugs with immune globulin intravenous (human) products may increase the risk of renal dysfunction, acute renal failure, osmotic nephrosis, and death).
No products indexed under this heading.

Fosinopril Sodium (Co-administration of nephrotoxic drugs with immune globulin intravenous (human) products may increase the risk of renal dysfunction, acute renal failure, osmotic nephrosis, and death).
No products indexed under this heading.

Furosemide (Co-administration of nephrotoxic drugs with immune globulin intravenous (human) products may increase the risk of renal dysfunction, acute renal failure, osmotic nephrosis, and death). Products include:

Gadopentetate Dimeglumine (Co-administration of nephrotoxic drugs with immune globulin intravenous (human) products may increase the risk of renal dysfunction, acute renal failure, osmotic nephrosis, and death).
No products indexed under this heading.

Gentamicin (Co-administration of nephrotoxic drugs with immune globulin intravenous (human) products may increase the risk of renal dysfunction, acute renal failure, osmotic nephrosis, and death).
No products indexed under this heading.

Gentamicin Sulfate (Co-administration of nephrotoxic drugs with immune globulin intravenous (human) products may increase the risk of renal dysfunction, acute renal failure, osmotic nephrosis, and death). Products include:

Glipizide (Co-administration of nephrotoxic drugs with immune globulin intravenous (human) products may increase the risk of renal dysfunction, acute renal failure, osmotic nephrosis, and death).
No products indexed under this heading.

Globulin, Immune (Human) (Co-administration of nephrotoxic drugs with immune globulin intravenous (human) products may increase the risk of renal dysfunction, acute renal failure, osmotic nephrosis, and death). Products include:

Glyburide (Co-administration of nephrotoxic drugs with immune globulin intravenous (human) products may increase the risk of renal dysfunction, acute renal failure, osmotic nephrosis, and death).
No products indexed under this heading.

Gold Therapy (Co-administration of nephrotoxic drugs with immune globulin intravenous (human) products may increase the risk of renal dysfunction, acute renal failure, osmotic nephrosis, and death).
No products indexed under this heading.

HMG-CoA Reductase Inhibitors (Co-administration of nephrotoxic drugs with immune globulin intravenous (human) products may increase the risk of renal dysfunction, acute renal failure, osmotic nephrosis, and death).
No products indexed under this heading.

Hydrochlorothiazide (Co-administration of nephrotoxic drugs with immune globulin intravenous (human) products may increase the risk of renal dysfunction, acute renal failure, osmotic nephrosis, and death). Products include:

Hydroflumethiazide (Co-administration of nephrotoxic drugs with immune globulin intravenous (human) products may increase the risk of renal dysfunction, acute renal failure, osmotic nephrosis, and death).
No products indexed under this heading.

Ibuprofen (Co-administration of nephrotoxic drugs with immune globulin intravenous (human) products may increase the risk of renal dysfunction, acute renal failure, osmotic nephrosis, and death). Products include:

Idarubicin Hydrochloride (Co-administration of nephrotoxic drugs with immune globulin intravenous (human) products may increase the risk of renal dysfunction, acute renal failure, osmotic nephrosis, and death).
No products indexed under this heading.

Ifosfamide (Co-administration of nephrotoxic drugs with immune globulin intravenous (human) products may increase the risk of renal dysfunction, acute renal failure, osmotic nephrosis, and death).
No products indexed under this heading.

Imipenem (Co-administration of nephrotoxic drugs with immune globulin intravenous (human) products may increase the risk of renal dysfunction, acute renal failure, osmotic nephrosis, and death). Products include:

Indinavir Sulfate (Co-administration of nephrotoxic drugs with immune globulin intravenous (human) products may increase the risk of renal dysfunction, acute renal failure, osmotic nephrosis, and death). Products include:

Indomethacin (Co-administration of nephrotoxic drugs with immune globulin intravenous (human) products may increase the risk of renal dysfunction, acute renal failure, osmotic nephrosis, and death). Products include:

Indomethacin Sodium Trihydrate (Co-administration of nephrotoxic drugs with immune globulin intravenous (human) products may increase the risk of renal dysfunction, acute renal failure, osmotic nephrosis, and death). Products include:

Influenza Vaccine, Live Attenuated (Antibodies in immune globulin intravenous (human) may interfere with the response to live viral vaccines, such as measles, mumps and rubella. Physicians should be informed of recent therapy with IGIVs, so that administration of live viral vaccines, if indicated, can be appropriately delayed 3 or more months from the time of IGIV administration).
No products indexed under this heading.

Influenza Virus Vaccine Live, Intranasal (Antibodies in immune globulin intravenous (human) may interfere with the response to live viral vaccines, such as measles, mumps and rubella. Physicians should be informed of recent therapy with IGIVs, so that administration of live viral vaccines, if indicated, can be appropriately delayed 3 or more months from the time of IGIV administration). Products include:

Interferon Beta-1b (Co-administration of nephrotoxic drugs with immune globulin intravenous (human) products may increase the risk of renal dysfunction, acute renal failure, osmotic nephrosis, and death). Products include:

Interleuken-2 (Co-administration of nephrotoxic drugs with immune globulin intravenous (human) products may increase the risk of renal dysfunction, acute renal failure, osmotic nephrosis, and death).
No products indexed under this heading.

Iodamide Meglumine (Co-administration of nephrotoxic drugs with immune globulin intravenous (human) products may increase the risk of renal dysfunction, acute renal failure, osmotic nephrosis, and death).
No products indexed under this heading.

Iohexol (Co-administration of nephrotoxic drugs with immune globulin intravenous (human) products may increase the risk of renal dysfunction, acute renal failure, osmotic nephrosis, and death).
No products indexed under this heading.

Iopamidol (Co-administration of nephrotoxic drugs with immune globulin intravenous (human) products may increase the risk of renal dysfunction, acute renal failure, osmotic nephrosis, and death).
No products indexed under this heading.

Iopanoic Acid (Co-administration of nephrotoxic drugs with immune globulin intravenous (human) products may increase the risk of renal dysfunction, acute renal failure, osmotic nephrosis, and death).
No products indexed under this heading.

Iothalamate Meglumine (Co-administration of nephrotoxic drugs with immune globulin intravenous (human) products may increase the risk of renal dysfunction, acute renal failure, osmotic nephrosis, and death).
No products indexed under this heading.

Ioxaglate Meglumine (Co-administration of nephrotoxic drugs with immune globulin intravenous (human) products may increase the risk of renal dysfunction, acute renal failure, osmotic nephrosis, and death).
No products indexed under this heading.

Ioxaglate Sodium (Co-administration of nephrotoxic drugs with immune globulin intravenous (human) products may increase the risk of renal dysfunction, acute renal failure, osmotic nephrosis, and death).
No products indexed under this heading.

Kanamycin Sulfate (Co-administration of nephrotoxic drugs with immune globulin intravenous (human) products may increase the risk of renal dysfunction, acute renal failure, osmotic nephrosis, and death).
No products indexed under this heading.

Ketoprofen (Co-administration of nephrotoxic drugs with immune globulin intravenous (human) products may increase the risk of renal dysfunction, acute renal failure, osmotic nephrosis, and death).
No products indexed under this heading.

Ketorolac Tromethamine (Co-administration of nephrotoxic drugs with immune globulin intravenous (human)

products may increase the risk of renal dysfunction, acute renal failure, osmotic nephrosis, and death). Products include:

Lamium album (Co-administration of nephrotoxic drugs with immune globulin intravenous (human) products may increase the risk of renal dysfunction, acute renal failure, osmotic nephrosis, and death).
No products indexed under this heading.

Lisinopril (Co-administration of nephrotoxic drugs with immune globulin intravenous (human) products may increase the risk of renal dysfunction, acute renal failure, osmotic nephrosis, and death). Products include:

Lithium (Co-administration of nephrotoxic drugs with immune globulin intravenous (human) products may increase the risk of renal dysfunction, acute renal failure, osmotic nephrosis, and death).
No products indexed under this heading.

Lithium Carbonate (Co-administration of nephrotoxic drugs with immune globulin intravenous (human) products may increase the risk of renal dysfunction, acute renal failure, osmotic nephrosis, and death).
No products indexed under this heading.

Lithium Citrate (Co-administration of nephrotoxic drugs with immune globulin intravenous (human) products may increase the risk of renal dysfunction, acute renal failure, osmotic nephrosis, and death).
No products indexed under this heading.

Lopinavir (Co-administration of nephrotoxic drugs with immune globulin intravenous (human) products may increase the risk of renal dysfunction, acute renal failure, osmotic nephrosis, and death). Products include:

Loracarbef (Co-administration of nephrotoxic drugs with immune globulin intravenous (human) products may increase the risk of renal dysfunction, acute renal failure, osmotic nephrosis, and death).
No products indexed under this heading.

Lovastatin (Co-administration of nephrotoxic drugs with immune globulin intravenous (human) products may increase the risk of renal dysfunction, acute renal failure, osmotic nephrosis, and death). Products include:

Measles, Mumps, Rubella and Varicella Virus Vaccine Live (Antibodies in immune globulin intravenous (human) may interfere with the response to live viral vaccines, such as measles, mumps and rubella. Physicians should be informed of recent therapy with IGIVs, so that administration of live viral vaccines, if indicated, can be appropriately delayed 3 or more months from the time of IGIV administration). Products include:

Measles, Mumps & Rubella Virus Vaccine, Live (Antibodies in immune globulin intravenous (human) may interfere with the response to live viral vaccines, such as measles, mumps and rubella. Physicians should be informed of recent therapy with IGIVs, so that administration of live viral vaccines, if indicated, can be appropriately delayed 3 or more months from the time of IGIV administration). Products include:

Measles & Rubella Virus Vaccine Live (Antibodies in immune globulin intravenous (human) may interfere with the response to live viral vaccines, such as measles, mumps and rubella. Physicians should be informed of recent therapy with IGIVs, so that administration of live viral vaccines, if indicated, can be appropriately delayed 3 or more months from the time of IGIV administration).
No products indexed under this heading.

Measles Virus Vaccine Live (Antibodies in immune globulin intravenous (human) may interfere with the response to live viral vaccines, such as measles, mumps and rubella. Physicians should be informed of recent therapy with IGIVs, so that administration of live viral vaccines, if indicated, can be appropriately delayed 3 or more months from the time of IGIV administration).
Products include:

Meclofenamate Sodium (Co-administration of nephrotoxic drugs with immune globulin intravenous (human) products may increase the risk of renal dysfunction, acute renal failure, osmotic nephrosis, and death).
No products indexed under this heading.

Mefenamic Acid (Co-administration of nephrotoxic drugs with immune globulin intravenous (human) products may increase the risk of renal dysfunction, acute renal failure, osmotic nephrosis, and death).
No products indexed under this heading.

Meloxicam (Co-administration of nephrotoxic drugs with immune globulin intravenous (human) products may increase the risk of renal dysfunction, acute renal failure, osmotic nephrosis, and death).
No products indexed under this heading.

Melphalan Hydrochloride (Co-administration of nephrotoxic drugs with immune globulin intravenous (human) products may increase the risk of renal dysfunction, acute renal failure, osmotic nephrosis, and death). Products include:

Mesalamine (Co-administration of nephrotoxic drugs with immune globulin intravenous (human) products may increase the risk of renal dysfunction, acute renal failure, osmotic nephrosis, and death). Products include:

Methimazole (Co-administration of nephrotoxic drugs with immune globulin intravenous (human) products may increase the risk of renal dysfunction, acute renal failure, osmotic nephrosis, and death).
No products indexed under this heading.

Methotrexate (Co-administration of nephrotoxic drugs with immune globulin intravenous (human) products may increase the risk of renal dysfunction, acute renal failure, osmotic nephrosis, and death).
No products indexed under this heading.

Methotrexate Sodium (Co-administration of nephrotoxic drugs with immune globulin intravenous (human) products may increase the risk of renal dysfunction, acute renal failure, osmotic nephrosis, and death).
No products indexed under this heading.

Methyclothiazide (Co-administration of nephrotoxic drugs with immune globulin intravenous (human) products may increase the risk of renal dysfunction, acute renal failure, osmotic nephrosis, and death).
No products indexed under this heading.

Mezlocillin Sodium (Co-administration of nephrotoxic drugs with immune globulin intravenous (human) products may increase the risk of renal dysfunction, acute renal failure, osmotic nephrosis, and death).
No products indexed under this heading.

Minocycline Hydrochloride (Co-administration of nephrotoxic drugs with immune globulin intravenous (human) products may increase the risk of renal dysfunction, acute renal failure, osmotic nephrosis, and death). Products include:

Mitomycin (Mitomycin-C) (Co-administration of nephrotoxic drugs with immune globulin intravenous (human) products may increase the risk of renal dysfunction, acute renal failure, osmotic nephrosis, and death).
No products indexed under this heading.

Moexipril Hydrochloride (Co-administration of nephrotoxic drugs with immune globulin intravenous (human) products may increase the risk of renal dysfunction, acute renal failure, osmotic nephrosis, and death).
No products indexed under this heading.

Mumps Virus Vaccine, Live (Antibodies in immune globulin intravenous (human) may interfere with the response to live viral vaccines, such as measles, mumps and rubella. Physicians should be informed of recent therapy with IGIVs, so that administration of live viral vaccines, if indicated, can be appropriately delayed 3 or more months from the time of IGIV administration).
Products include:

Muromonab-CD3 (Co-administration of nephrotoxic drugs with immune globulin intravenous (human) products may increase the risk of renal dysfunction, acute renal failure, osmotic nephrosis, and death). Products include:

Nabumetone (Co-administration of nephrotoxic drugs with immune globulin intravenous (human) products may increase the risk of renal dysfunction, acute renal failure, osmotic nephrosis, and death).
No products indexed under this heading.

Nafcillin Sodium (Co-administration of nephrotoxic drugs with immune globulin intravenous (human) products may increase the risk of renal dysfunction, acute renal failure, osmotic nephrosis, and death).
No products indexed under this heading.

Naproxen (Co-administration of nephrotoxic drugs with immune globulin intravenous (human) products may increase the risk of renal dysfunction, acute renal failure, osmotic nephrosis, and death). Products include:

Naproxen Sodium (Co-administration of nephrotoxic drugs with immune globulin intravenous (human) products may increase the risk of renal dysfunction, acute renal failure, osmotic nephrosis, and death). Products include:

Nelfinavir Mesylate (Co-administration of nephrotoxic drugs with immune globulin intravenous (human) products may increase the risk of renal dysfunction, acute renal failure, osmotic nephrosis, and death).
No products indexed under this heading.

Neomycin (Co-administration of nephrotoxic drugs with immune globulin intravenous (human) products may increase the risk of renal dysfunction, acute renal failure, osmotic nephrosis, and death).
No products indexed under this heading.

Neomycin, oral (Co-administration of nephrotoxic drugs with immune globulin intravenous (human) products may increase the risk of renal dysfunction, acute renal failure, osmotic nephrosis, and death).
No products indexed under this heading.

Neomycin Sulfate (Co-administration of nephrotoxic drugs with immune globulin intravenous (human) products may increase the risk of renal dysfunction, acute renal failure, osmotic nephrosis, and death).
No products indexed under this heading.

Nevirapine (Co-administration of nephrotoxic drugs with immune globulin intravenous (human) products may increase the risk of renal dysfunction, acute renal failure, osmotic nephrosis, and death). Products include:

Norfloxacin (Co-administration of nephrotoxic drugs with immune globulin intravenous (human) products may increase the risk of renal dysfunction, acute renal failure, osmotic nephrosis, and death). Products include:

Olsalazine Sodium (Co-administration of nephrotoxic drugs with immune globulin intravenous (human) products may increase the risk of renal dysfunction, acute renal failure, osmotic nephrosis, and death).
No products indexed under this heading.

Omeprazole (Co-administration of nephrotoxic drugs with immune globulin intravenous (human) products may increase the risk of renal dysfunction, acute renal failure, osmotic nephrosis, and death).
No products indexed under this heading.

Oxaprozin (Co-administration of nephrotoxic drugs with immune globulin intravenous (human) products may increase the risk of renal dysfunction, acute renal failure, osmotic nephrosis, and death).
No products indexed under this heading.

Pamidronate Disodium (Co-administration of nephrotoxic drugs with immune globulin intravenous (human) products may increase the risk of renal dysfunction, acute renal failure, osmotic nephrosis, and death).
No products indexed under this heading.

Paroxetine Hydrochloride (Co-administration of nephrotoxic drugs with immune globulin intravenous (human) products may increase the risk of renal dysfunction, acute renal failure, osmotic nephrosis, and death). Products include:

Penicillamine (Co-administration of nephrotoxic drugs with immune globulin intravenous (human) products may increase the risk of renal dysfunction, acute renal failure, osmotic nephrosis, and death).
No products indexed under this heading.

Penicillin G Benzathine (Co-administration of nephrotoxic drugs with immune globulin intravenous (human) products may increase the risk of renal dysfunction, acute renal failure, osmotic nephrosis, and death). Products include:

Penicillin G Potassium (Co-administration of nephrotoxic drugs with immune globulin intravenous (human) products may increase the risk of renal dysfunction, acute renal failure, osmotic nephrosis, and death).
No products indexed under this heading.

Penicillin G Procaine (Co-administration of nephrotoxic drugs with immune globulin intravenous (human) products may increase the risk of renal dysfunction, acute renal failure, osmotic nephrosis, and death). Products include:

Penicillin G Sodium (Co-administration of nephrotoxic drugs with immune globulin intravenous (human) products may increase the risk of renal dysfunction, acute renal failure, osmotic nephrosis, and death).
No products indexed under this heading.

Penicillin V Potassium (Co-administration of nephrotoxic drugs with immune globulin intravenous (human) products may increase the risk of renal dysfunction, acute renal failure, osmotic nephrosis, and death).
No products indexed under this heading.

Pentamidine Isethionate (Co-administration of nephrotoxic drugs with immune globulin intravenous (human) products may increase the risk of renal dysfunction, acute renal failure, osmotic nephrosis, and death).
No products indexed under this heading.

Perindopril Erbumine (Co-administration of nephrotoxic drugs with immune globulin intravenous (human) products may increase the risk of renal dysfunction, acute renal failure, osmotic nephrosis, and death).
No products indexed under this heading.

Phenylbutazone (Co-administration of nephrotoxic drugs with immune globulin intravenous (human) products may increase the risk of renal dysfunction, acute renal failure, osmotic nephrosis, and death).
No products indexed under this heading.

Piroxicam (Co-administration of nephrotoxic drugs with immune globulin intravenous (human) products may increase the risk of renal dysfunction, acute renal failure, osmotic nephrosis, and death).
No products indexed under this heading.

Plicamycin (Co-administration of nephrotoxic drugs with immune globulin intravenous (human) products may increase the risk of renal dysfunction, acute renal failure, osmotic nephrosis, and death).
No products indexed under this heading.

Poliovirus Vaccine, Live, Oral, Trivalent, Types 1,2,3 (Sabin) (Antibodies in immune globulin intravenous (human) may interfere with the response to live viral vaccines, such as measles, mumps and rubella. Physicians should be informed of recent therapy with IGIVs, so that administration of live viral vaccines, if indicated, can be appropriately delayed 3 or more months from the time of IGIV administration).
No products indexed under this heading.

Polymyxin (Co-administration of nephrotoxic drugs with immune globulin intravenous (human) products may increase the risk of renal dysfunction, acute renal failure, osmotic nephrosis, and death).
No products indexed under this heading.

(⊙ Described in PDR® for Ophthalmic Medicines)

products may increase the risk of renal dysfunction, acute renal failure, osmotic nephrosis, and death). Products include:

Valdecoxib (Co-administration of nephrotoxic drugs with immune globulin intravenous (human) products may increase the risk of renal dysfunction, acute renal failure, osmotic nephrosis, and death).
No products indexed under this heading.

Vancomycin Hydrochloride (Co-administration of nephrotoxic drugs with immune globulin intravenous (human) products may increase the risk of renal dysfunction, acute renal failure, osmotic nephrosis, and death).
No products indexed under this heading.

Varicella Virus Vaccine, Live (Antibodies in immune globulin intravenous (human) may interfere with the response to live viral vaccines, such as measles, mumps and rubella. Physicians should be informed of recent therapy with IGIVs, so that administration of live viral vaccines, if indicated, can be appropriately delayed 3 or more months from the time of IGIV administration). Products include:

Voriconazole (Co-administration of nephrotoxic drugs with immune globulin intravenous (human) products may increase the risk of renal dysfunction, acute renal failure, osmotic nephrosis, and death).
No products indexed under this heading.

Yellow Fever Vaccine (Antibodies in immune globulin intravenous (human) may interfere with the response to live viral vaccines, such as measles, mumps and rubella. Physicians should be informed of recent therapy with IGIVs, so that administration of live viral vaccines, if indicated, can be appropriately delayed 3 or more months from the time of IGIV administration).
No products indexed under this heading.

Zalcitabine (Co-administration of nephrotoxic drugs with immune globulin intravenous (human) products may increase the risk of renal dysfunction, acute renal failure, osmotic nephrosis, and death).
No products indexed under this heading.

Zidovudine (Co-administration of nephrotoxic drugs with immune globulin intravenous (human) products may increase the risk of renal dysfunction, acute renal failure, osmotic nephrosis, and death). Products include:

Zoledronic Acid (Co-administration of nephrotoxic drugs with immune globulin intravenous (human) products may increase the risk of renal dysfunction, acute renal failure, osmotic nephrosis, and death). Products include:

Zoster Vaccine Live (Antibodies in immune globulin intravenous (human) may interfere with the response to live viral vaccines, such as measles, mumps and rubella. Physicians should be informed of recent therapy with IGIVs, so that administration of live viral vaccines, if indicated, can be appropriately delayed 3 or more months from the time of IGIV administration). Products include:

GARDASIL INJECTION

(Quadrivalent Human Papillomavirus (Types 6, 11, 16, 18) Recombinant Vaccine) 2154
May interact with alkylating agents, an-

timetabolites, corticosteroids, cytotoxic drugs, immunosuppressive agents, and certain other agents. Compounds in these categories include:

Alclometasone Dipropionate (Immunosuppressive therapies, including corticosteroids (used in greater than physiologic doses), may reduce the immune responses to vaccines).
No products indexed under this heading.

Azathioprine (Immunosuppressive therapies may reduce the immune responses to vaccines).
No products indexed under this heading.

Basiliximab (Immunosuppressive therapies may reduce the immune responses to vaccines). Products include:

Beclomethasone Dipropionate (Immunosuppressive therapies, including corticosteroids (used in greater than physiologic doses), may reduce the immune responses to vaccines). Products include:

Beclomethasone Dipropionate Monohydrate (Immunosuppressive therapies, including corticosteroids (used in greater than physiologic doses), may reduce the immune responses to vaccines). Products include:

Betamethasone (Immunosuppressive therapies, including corticosteroids (used in greater than physiologic doses), may reduce the immune responses to vaccines).
No products indexed under this heading.

Betamethasone Acetate (Immunosuppressive therapies, including corticosteroids (used in greater than physiologic doses), may reduce the immune responses to vaccines).
No products indexed under this heading.

Betamethasone Benzoate (Immunosuppressive therapies, including corticosteroids (used in greater than physiologic doses), may reduce the immune responses to vaccines).
No products indexed under this heading.

Betamethasone Dipropionate (Immunosuppressive therapies, including corticosteroids (used in greater than physiologic doses), may reduce the immune responses to vaccines). Products include:

Betamethasone Sodium Phosphate (Immunosuppressive therapies, including corticosteroids (used in greater than physiologic doses), may reduce the immune responses to vaccines).
No products indexed under this heading.

Betamethasone Valerate (Immunosuppressive therapies, including corticosteroids (used in greater than physiologic doses), may reduce the immune responses to vaccines). Products include:

Bleomycin Sulfate (Immunosuppressive therapies, including cytotoxic drugs, may reduce the immune responses to vaccines).
No products indexed under this heading.

Budesonide (Immunosuppressive therapies, including corticosteroids (used in greater than physiologic doses), may reduce the immune responses to vaccines). Products include:

Busulfan (Immunosuppressive therapies, including alkylating agents, may reduce the immune responses to vaccines). Products include:

Capecitabine (Immunosuppressive therapies, including antimetabolites, may reduce the immune responses to vaccines). Products include:

Carmustine (BCNU) (Immunosuppressive therapies, including alkylating agents, may reduce the immune responses to vaccines).
No products indexed under this heading.

Chlorambucil (Immunosuppressive therapies, including alkylating agents, may reduce the immune responses to vaccines). Products include:

Ciclesonide (Immunosuppressive therapies, including corticosteroids (used in greater than physiologic doses), may reduce the immune responses to vaccines).
No products indexed under this heading.

Cladribine (Immunosuppressive therapies, including antimetabolites, may reduce the immune responses to vaccines). Products include:

Cortisone Acetate (Immunosuppressive therapies, including corticosteroids (used in greater than physiologic doses), may reduce the immune responses to vaccines).
No products indexed under this heading.

Cyclophosphamide (Immunosuppressive therapies, including alkylating agents, may reduce the immune responses to vaccines).
No products indexed under this heading.

Cyclosporine (Immunosuppressive therapies may reduce the immune responses to vaccines). Products include:

Cytarabine (Immunosuppressive therapies, including antimetabolites, may reduce the immune responses to vaccines).
No products indexed under this heading.

Dacarbazine (Immunosuppressive therapies, including alkylating agents, may reduce the immune responses to vaccines).
No products indexed under this heading.

Daunorubicin Hydrochloride (Immunosuppressive therapies, including cytotoxic drugs, may reduce the immune responses to vaccines).
No products indexed under this heading.

Desoximetasone (Immunosuppressive therapies, including corticosteroids (used in greater than physiologic doses), may reduce the immune responses to vaccines).
No products indexed under this heading.

Dexamethasone (Immunosuppressive therapies, including corticosteroids (used in greater than physiologic doses), may reduce the immune responses to vaccines). Products include:

Dexamethasone Acetate (Immunosuppressive therapies, including corticosteroids (used in greater than physiologic doses), may reduce the immune responses to vaccines).
No products indexed under this heading.

Dexamethasone Phosphate (Immunosuppressive therapies, including corticosteroids (used in greater than physiologic doses), may reduce the immune responses to vaccines).
No products indexed under this heading.

Dexamethasone Sodium (Immunosuppressive therapies, including corticosteroids (used in greater than physiologic doses), may reduce the immune responses to vaccines).
No products indexed under this heading.

Dexamethasone Sodium Phosphate (Immunosuppressive therapies, including corticosteroids (used in greater than physiologic doses), may reduce the immune responses to vaccines).
No products indexed under this heading.

Dexamethasone Sodium Phosphate Injection (Immunosuppressive therapies, including corticosteroids (used in greater than physiologic doses), may reduce the immune responses to vaccines).
No products indexed under this heading.

Diflorasone Diacetate (Immunosuppressive therapies, including corticosteroids (used in greater than physiologic doses), may reduce the immune responses to vaccines).
No products indexed under this heading.

Doxorubicin Hydrochloride (Immunosuppressive therapies, including cytotoxic drugs, may reduce the immune responses to vaccines).
No products indexed under this heading.

Epirubicin Hydrochloride (Immunosuppressive therapies, including cytotoxic drugs, may reduce the immune responses to vaccines).
No products indexed under this heading.

Floxuridine (Immunosuppressive therapies, including antimetabolites, may reduce the immune responses to vaccines).
No products indexed under this heading.

Fludarabine Phosphate (Immunosuppressive therapies, including antimetabolites, may reduce the immune responses to vaccines). Products include:

Fludrocortisone Acetate (Immunosuppressive therapies, including corticosteroids (used in greater than physiologic doses), may reduce the immune responses to vaccines).
No products indexed under this heading.

Flumethasone Pivalate (Immunosuppressive therapies, including corticosteroids (used in greater than physiologic doses), may reduce the immune responses to vaccines).
No products indexed under this heading.

Flunisolide Hemihydrate (Immunosuppressive therapies, including corticosteroids (used in greater than physiologic doses), may reduce the immune responses to vaccines).
No products indexed under this heading.

Fluorouracil (Immunosuppressive therapies, including antimetabolites, may reduce the immune responses to vaccines). Products include:

Fluticasone Furoate (Immunosuppressive therapies, including corticosteroids (used in greater than physiologic doses), may reduce the immune responses to vaccines). Products include:

Fluticasone Propionate (Immunosuppressive therapies, including corticosteroids (used in greater than physiologic doses), may reduce the immune responses to vaccines). Products include:

Gemcitabine Hydrochloride (Immunosuppressive therapies, including antimetabolites, may reduce the immune responses to vaccines). Products include:

Hydrocortisone (Immunosuppressive therapies, including corticosteroids (used in greater than physiologic doses), may reduce the immune responses to vaccines).
No products indexed under this heading.

Hydrocortisone (Alcohol) (Immunosuppressive therapies, including corticosteroids (used in greater than physiologic doses), may reduce the immune responses to vaccines).
No products indexed under this heading.

Hydrocortisone Acetate (Immunosuppressive therapies, including corticosteroids (used in greater than physiologic doses), may reduce the immune responses to vaccines).
No products indexed under this heading.

Hydrocortisone Butyrate (Immunosuppressive therapies, including corticosteroids (used in greater than physiologic doses), may reduce the immune responses to vaccines).
No products indexed under this heading.

Hydrocortisone Cypionate (Immunosuppressive therapies, including corticosteroids (used in greater than physiologic doses), may reduce the immune responses to vaccines).
No products indexed under this heading.

Hydrocortisone Hemisuccinate (Immunosuppressive therapies, including corticosteroids (used in greater than physiologic doses), may reduce the immune responses to vaccines).
No products indexed under this heading.

Hydrocortisone Probutate (Immunosuppressive therapies, including corticosteroids (used in greater than physiologic doses), may reduce the immune responses to vaccines).
No products indexed under this heading.

Hydrocortisone Sodium Phosphate (Immunosuppressive therapies, including corticosteroids (used in greater than physiologic doses), may reduce the immune responses to vaccines).
No products indexed under this heading.

Hydrocortisone Sodium Succinate (Immunosuppressive therapies, including corticosteroids (used in greater than physiologic doses), may reduce the immune responses to vaccines).
No products indexed under this heading.

Hydrocortisone Valerate (Immunosuppressive therapies, including corticosteroids (used in greater than physiologic doses), may reduce the immune responses to vaccines).
No products indexed under this heading.

Hydroxyurea (Immunosuppressive therapies, including cytotoxic drugs, may reduce the immune responses to vaccines).
No products indexed under this heading.

Lomustine (CCNU) (Immunosuppressive therapies, including alkylating agents, may reduce the immune responses to vaccines).
No products indexed under this heading.

Mechlorethamine Hydrochloride (Immunosuppressive therapies, including alkylating agents, may reduce the immune responses to vaccines). Products include:

Melphalan (Immunosuppressive therapies, including alkylating agents, may reduce the immune responses to vaccines). Products include:

Mercaptopurine (Immunosuppressive therapies, including antimetabolites, may reduce the immune responses to vaccines).
No products indexed under this heading.

Methotrexate (Immunosuppressive therapies, including antimetabolites, may reduce the immune responses to vaccines).
No products indexed under this heading.

Methotrexate Sodium (Immunosuppressive therapies, including antimetabolites, may reduce the immune responses to vaccines).
No products indexed under this heading.

Methylprednisolone (Immunosuppressive therapies, including corticosteroids (used in greater than physiologic doses), may reduce the immune responses to vaccines).
No products indexed under this heading.

Methylprednisolone Acetate (Immunosuppressive therapies, including corticosteroids (used in greater than physiologic doses), may reduce the immune responses to vaccines).
No products indexed under this heading.

Methylprednisolone Sodium Succinate (Immunosuppressive therapies, including corticosteroids (used in greater than physiologic doses), may reduce the immune responses to vaccines).
No products indexed under this heading.

Mitotane (Immunosuppressive therapies, including cytotoxic drugs, may reduce the immune responses to vaccines).
No products indexed under this heading.

Mitoxantrone Hydrochloride (Immunosuppressive therapies, including cytotoxic drugs, may reduce the immune responses to vaccines). Products include:

Mometasone Furoate (Immunosuppressive therapies, including corticosteroids (used in greater than physiologic doses), may reduce the immune responses to vaccines). Products include:

Mometasone Furoate Monohydrate (Immunosuppressive therapies, including corticosteroids (used in greater than physiologic doses), may reduce the immune responses to vaccines). Products include:

Muromonab-CD3 (Immunosuppressive therapies may reduce the immune responses to vaccines). Products include:

Mycophenolate Mofetil (Immunosuppressive therapies may reduce the immune responses to vaccines).
No products indexed under this heading.

Pentostatin (Immunosuppressive therapies, including antimetabolites, may reduce the immune responses to vaccines).
No products indexed under this heading.

Prednisolone (Immunosuppressive therapies, including corticosteroids (used in greater than physiologic doses), may reduce the immune responses to vaccines).
No products indexed under this heading.

Prednisolone Acetate (Immunosuppressive therapies, including corticosteroids (used in greater than physiologic

doses), may reduce the immune responses to vaccines). Products include:

Prednisolone Sodium Phosphate (Immunosuppressive therapies, including corticosteroids (used in greater than physiologic doses), may reduce the immune responses to vaccines).
No products indexed under this heading.

Prednisolone Tebutate (Immunosuppressive therapies, including corticosteroids (used in greater than physiologic doses), may reduce the immune responses to vaccines).
No products indexed under this heading.

Prednisone (Immunosuppressive therapies, including corticosteroids (used in greater than physiologic doses), may reduce the immune responses to vaccines).
No products indexed under this heading.

Prednisone sodium phosphate (Immunosuppressive therapies, including corticosteroids (used in greater than physiologic doses), may reduce the immune responses to vaccines).
No products indexed under this heading.

Procarbazine Hydrochloride (Immunosuppressive therapies, including cytotoxic drugs, may reduce the immune responses to vaccines).
No products indexed under this heading.

Radiation (Immunosuppressive therapies, including irradiation, may reduce the immune responses to vaccines).
No products indexed under this heading.

Rapamycin (Immunosuppressive therapies may reduce the immune responses to vaccines).
No products indexed under this heading.

Sirolimus (Immunosuppressive therapies may reduce the immune responses to vaccines). Products include:

Tacrolimus (Immunosuppressive therapies may reduce the immune responses to vaccines). Products include:

Tamoxifen Citrate (Immunosuppressive therapies, including cytotoxic drugs, may reduce the immune responses to vaccines).
No products indexed under this heading.

Thioguanine (Immunosuppressive therapies, including antimetabolites, may reduce the immune responses to vaccines). Products include:

Thiotepa (Immunosuppressive therapies, including alkylating agents, may reduce the immune responses to vaccines).
No products indexed under this heading.

Triamcinolone (Immunosuppressive therapies, including corticosteroids (used in greater than physiologic doses), may reduce the immune responses to vaccines).
No products indexed under this heading.

Triamcinolone Acetonide (Immunosuppressive therapies, including corticosteroids (used in greater than physiologic doses), may reduce the immune responses to vaccines). Products include:

Triamcinolone Diacetate (Immunosuppressive therapies, including corticosteroids (used in greater than physiologic doses), may reduce the immune responses to vaccines).
No products indexed under this heading.

Triamcinolone Hexacetonide (Immunosuppressive therapies, including corticosteroids (used in greater than physiologic doses), may reduce the immune responses to vaccines).
No products indexed under this heading.

Vinblastine Sulfate (Immunosuppressive therapies, including cytotoxic drugs, may reduce the immune responses to vaccines).
No products indexed under this heading.

Vincristine Sulfate (Immunosuppressive therapies, including cytotoxic drugs, may reduce the immune responses to vaccines).
No products indexed under this heading.

Vinorelbine Tartrate (Immunosuppressive therapies, including cytotoxic drugs, may reduce the immune responses to vaccines).
No products indexed under this heading.

GEMZAR FOR INJECTION

(Gemcitabine Hydrochloride) **1900**
None cited in PDR database.

GENGRAF CAPSULES

(Cyclosporine) **440**
May interact with ACE inhibitors, angiotensin-II receptor antagonists, calcium channel blockers, cytochrome p450 3a inducers (selected), cytochrome p450 3a inhibitors (selected), erythromycin, HMG-CoA reductase inhibitors, immunosuppressive agents, killed/inactivated vaccines, methylprednisolone, nephrotoxic agents, non-steroidal anti-inflammatory agents, oral contraceptives, phenytoin, potassium preparations, potassium sparing diuretics, prednisolone, protease inhibitors, vaccines, live, and certain other agents. Compounds in these categories include:

Abacavir Sulfate (Care should be taken in using cyclosporine with nephrotoxic drugs). Products include:

Acyclovir (Care should be taken in using cyclosporine with nephrotoxic drugs). Products include:

Acyclovir Sodium (Care should be taken in using cyclosporine with nephrotoxic drugs).
No products indexed under this heading.

Alatrofloxacin Mesylate (Care should be taken in using cyclosporine with nephrotoxic drugs).
No products indexed under this heading.

Aldesleukin (Care should be taken in using cyclosporine with nephrotoxic drugs). Products include:

Allium sativum (Cyclosporine is extensively metabolized by CYP3A. Substances that are inducers of CYP3A could increase metabolism and decrease cyclosporine concentrations).
No products indexed under this heading.

Allopurinol (Cyclosporine is extensively metabolized by CYP450 3A. Substances that inhibit this enzyme could decrease the metabolism and increase cyclosporine concentrations).
No products indexed under this heading.

Amikacin Sulfate (Care should be taken in using cyclosporine with nephrotoxic drugs).
No products indexed under this heading.

Amiloride Hydrochloride (Cyclosporine causes hyperkalemia; concurrent use with potassium-sparing diuretics can result in increased risk of hyperkalemia; co-administration should be avoided).
No products indexed under this heading.

IMPORTANT NOTE: Always consult each drug listing in the patient's regimen for possible interactions.

Gengraf Interactions Index 744

Cerivastatin Sodium (Cyclosporine may reduce the clearance of HMG-CoA reductase inhibitors. Myotoxicity, including muscle pain and weakness, myositis, and rhabdomyolysis, have been reported with concomitant administration of cyclosporine with lovastatin, simvastatin, atorvastatin, pravastatin, and, rarely, fluvastatin. Dosage of these statins should be reduced).
No products indexed under this heading.

Chlorothiazide (Care should be taken in using cyclosporine with nephrotoxic drugs).
No products indexed under this heading.

Chlorothiazide Sodium (Care should be taken in using cyclosporine with nephrotoxic drugs). Products include:
Diuril Intravenous 2009

Chlorpropamide (Care should be taken in using cyclosporine with nephrotoxic drugs).
No products indexed under this heading.

Cidofovir (Care should be taken in using cyclosporine with nephrotoxic drugs).
No products indexed under this heading.

Cilastatin Sodium (Care should be taken in using cyclosporine with nephrotoxic drugs). Products include:
Primaxin I.M. 2232
Primaxin I.V. 2235

Cimetidine (May potentiate renal dysfunction).
No products indexed under this heading.

Cimetidine Hydrochloride (May potentiate renal dysfunction).
No products indexed under this heading.

Ciprofloxacin (May potentiate renal dysfunction). Products include:
Cipro I.V. 3082
Cipro 3073
Cipro XR 3091
Ciprodex 583

Ciprofloxacin Hydrochloride (May potentiate renal dysfunction). Products include:
Cipro 3073

Cisplatin (Care should be taken in using cyclosporine with nephrotoxic drugs).
No products indexed under this heading.

Cladribine (Care should be taken in using cyclosporine with nephrotoxic drugs). Products include:
Leustatin 946

Clarithromycin (Cyclosporine is extensively metabolized by CYP450 3A. Substances that inhibit this enzyme could decrease the metabolism and increase cyclosporine concentrations). Products include:
Biaxin/Biaxin XL 412

Clozapine (Care should be taken in using cyclosporine with nephrotoxic drugs).
No products indexed under this heading.

Coal Tar (Psoriasis patients who are treated with cyclosporine capsules should not receive concomitant coal tar).
No products indexed under this heading.

Colchicine (Cyclosporine may reduce the clearance of colchicine and enhance its toxic effects, such as myopathy and neuropathy, especially in patients with renal dysfunction. Close clinical observation is required during concomitant administration).
No products indexed under this heading.

Colistimethate Sodium (Care should be taken in using cyclosporine with nephrotoxic drugs).
No products indexed under this heading.

Colistin Sulfate (Care should be taken in using cyclosporine with nephrotoxic drugs).
No products indexed under this heading.

Cyclophosphamide (Care should be taken in using cyclosporine with nephrotoxic drugs).
No products indexed under this heading.

Cytarabine (Care should be taken in using cyclosporine with nephrotoxic drugs).
No products indexed under this heading.

Cytarabine Liposome (Care should be taken in using cyclosporine with nephrotoxic drugs).
No products indexed under this heading.

Dalfopristin (Cyclosporine is extensively metabolized by CYP450 3A. Substances that inhibit this enzyme could decrease the metabolism and increase cyclosporine concentrations).
No products indexed under this heading.

Danazol (Cyclosporine is extensively metabolized by CYP450 3A. Substances that inhibit this enzyme could decrease the metabolism and increase cyclosporine concentrations).
No products indexed under this heading.

Darunavir (the HIV protease inhibitors are known to inhibit CYP3A and thus could potentially increase the concentrations of cyclosporine; care should be exercised when these drugs are administered concomitantly).
No products indexed under this heading.

Delavirdine Mesylate (Care should be taken in using cyclosporine with nephrotoxic drugs).
No products indexed under this heading.

Desogestrel (Cyclosporine is extensively metabolized by CYP3A. Substances that inhibit this enzyme could decrease the metabolism and increase cyclosporine concentrations).
No products indexed under this heading.

Dexamethasone (Cyclosporine is extensively metabolized by CYP3A. Substances that are inducers of CYP3A could increase metabolism and decrease cyclosporine concentrations). Products include:
Ciprodex 583
Ozurdex .... ⊙ 223
Tobramycin and Dexamethasone Ophthalmic Suspension .... ⊙ 251

Diatrizoate Meglumine (Care should be taken in using cyclosporine with nephrotoxic drugs).
No products indexed under this heading.

Diatrizoate Sodium (Care should be taken in using cyclosporine with nephrotoxic drugs).
No products indexed under this heading.

Diclofenac Epolamine (Cyclosporine can cause nephrotoxicity; clinical status and serum creatinine should be closely monitored when cyclosporine is used with NSAIDs in rheumatoid arthritis patients). Products include:
Flector 1839

Diclofenac Potassium (May potentiate renal dysfunction; potential for doubling of diclofenac blood levels and occasional reports of reversible decreases in renal function have been reported with concurrent use).
No products indexed under this heading.

Diclofenac Sodium (May potentiate renal dysfunction; potential for doubling of diclofenac blood levels and occasional reports of reversible decreases in renal function have been reported with concurrent use).
No products indexed under this heading.

Dicloxacillin Sodium (Care should be taken in using cyclosporine with nephrotoxic drugs).
No products indexed under this heading.

Didanosine (Care should be taken in using cyclosporine with nephrotoxic drugs).
No products indexed under this heading.

Digoxin (Cyclosporine may reduce the clearance of digoxin. Severe digitalis toxicity has been seen within days of starting cyclosporine. Close clinical observation is required during concomitant administration). Products include:
Lanoxin Injection 1546
Lanoxin Injection Pediatric 1549
Lanoxin Tablets 1553

Diltiazem Hydrochloride (Cyclosporine is extensively metabolized by CYP450 3A. Substances that inhibit this enzyme could decrease the metabolism and increase cyclosporine concentrations). Products include:
Cardizem LA 423

Diltiazem Maleate (Cyclosporine is extensively metabolized by CYP450 3A. Substances that inhibit this enzyme could decrease the metabolism and increase cyclosporine concentrations).
No products indexed under this heading.

Diphtheria & Tetanus Toxoids and Acellular Pertussis Vaccine Adsorbed, Hepatitis B (recombinant) and Inactivated Poliovirus Vaccine Combined (During treatment with cyclosporine, vaccination may be less effective).
No products indexed under this heading.

Efavirenz (Care should be taken in using cyclosporine with nephrotoxic drugs). Products include:
Atripla 906

Emtricitabine (Care should be taken in using cyclosporine with nephrotoxic drugs). Products include:
Atripla 906
Emtriva 1238
Emtriva Oral Solution 1238
Truvada 1258

Enalapril Maleate (Caution is required when co-administering cyclosporine with potassium sparing drugs, such as ACE inhibitors).
No products indexed under this heading.

Enalaprilat (Caution is required when co-administering cyclosporine with potassium sparing drugs, such as ACE inhibitors).
No products indexed under this heading.

Enfuvirtide (Care should be taken in using cyclosporine with nephrotoxic drugs).
No products indexed under this heading.

Eprosartan Mesylate (Caution is required when co-administering cyclosporine with potassium sparing drugs, such as angiotensin II receptor antagonists). Products include:
Teveten 538
Teveten HCT 541

Erythromycin (Cyclosporine is extensively metabolized by CYP450 3A. Substances that inhibit this enzyme could decrease the metabolism and increase cyclosporine concentrations).
No products indexed under this heading.

Erythromycin, Topical (Cyclosporine is extensively metabolized by CYP450 3A. Substances that inhibit this enzyme could decrease the metabolism and increase cyclosporine concentrations).
No products indexed under this heading.

Erythromycin Estolate (Cyclosporine is extensively metabolized by CYP450 3A. Substances that inhibit this enzyme could decrease the metabolism and increase cyclosporine concentrations).
No products indexed under this heading.

Erythromycin Ethylsuccinate (Cyclosporine is extensively metabolized by CYP450 3A. Substances that inhibit this enzyme could decrease the metabolism and increase cyclosporine concentrations). Products include:
E.E.S. 437
EryPed 435

Erythromycin Gluceptate (Cyclosporine is extensively metabolized by CYP450 3A. Substances that inhibit this enzyme could decrease the metabolism and increase cyclosporine concentrations).
No products indexed under this heading.

Erythromycin Lactobionate (Cyclosporine is extensively metabolized by CYP450 3A. Substances that inhibit this enzyme could decrease the metabolism and increase cyclosporine concentrations).
No products indexed under this heading.

Erythromycin Stearate (Cyclosporine is extensively metabolized by CYP450 3A. Substances that inhibit this enzyme could decrease the metabolism and increase cyclosporine concentrations).
No products indexed under this heading.

Ethinyl Estradiol (Cyclosporine is extensively metabolized by CYP3A. Substances that inhibit this enzyme could decrease the metabolism and increase cyclosporine concentrations). Products include:
LoSeasonique 3407
Lybrel 3514
NuvaRing 3181
Ortho Evra 2648
Ortho-Cyclen/Ortho Tri-Cyclen 2663
Ortho Tri-Cyclen Lo Tablets 2673
Seasonique 3418
Yaz 864

Ethiodized Oil (Care should be taken in using cyclosporine with nephrotoxic drugs).
No products indexed under this heading.

Ethosuximide (Cyclosporine is extensively metabolized by CYP3A. Substances that are inducers of CYP3A could increase metabolism and decrease cyclosporine concentrations).
No products indexed under this heading.

Ethynodiol Diacetate (Cyclosporine is extensively metabolized by CYP3A. Substances that inhibit this enzyme could decrease the metabolism and increase cyclosporine concentrations).
No products indexed under this heading.

Etodolac (Cyclosporine can cause nephrotoxicity; clinical status and serum creatinine should be closely monitored when cyclosporine is used with NSAIDs in rheumatoid arthritis patients).
No products indexed under this heading.

Felodipine (While calcium antagonists can be effective agents in treating cyclosporine-associated hypertension, they can interfere with cyclosporine metabolism).
No products indexed under this heading.

Fenoprofen Calcium (Cyclosporine can cause nephrotoxicity; clinical status and serum creatinine should be closely monitored when cyclosporine is used with NSAIDs in rheumatoid arthritis patients).
No products indexed under this heading.

Fibrates (May potentiate renal dysfunction).
No products indexed under this heading.

Filgrastim (Care should be taken in using cyclosporine with nephrotoxic drugs). Products include:
Neupogen 631

Fluconazole (Co-administration with drugs that inhibit CYP450 3A, such as fluconazole, could decrease metabolism of cyclosporine and increase its concentrations).
No products indexed under this heading.

Fluorouracil (Care should be taken in using cyclosporine with nephrotoxic drugs). Products include:
Carac 2966

(⊙ Described in PDR® for Ophthalmic Medicines)

Fluoxetine (Cyclosporine is extensively metabolized by CYP3A. Substances that inhibit this enzyme could decrease the metabolism and increase cyclosporine concentrations).
No products indexed under this heading.

Fluoxetine Hydrochloride (Cyclosporine is extensively metabolized by CYP3A. Substances that inhibit this enzyme could decrease the metabolism and increase cyclosporine concentrations). Products include:
Prozac Weekly 1941
Prozac Pulvules 1941
Symbyax 1965

Flurbiprofen (Cyclosporine can cause nephrotoxicity; clinical status and serum creatinine should be closely monitored when cyclosporine is used with NSAIDs in rheumatoid arthritis patients).
No products indexed under this heading.

Fluvastatin Sodium (Cyclosporine may reduce the clearance of HMG-CoA reductase inhibitors. Myotoxicity, including muscle pain and weakness, myositis, and rhabdomyolysis, have been reported with concomitant administration of cyclosporine with lovastatin, simvastatin, atorvastatin, pravastatin, and, rarely, fluvastatin. Dosage of these statins should be reduced).
No products indexed under this heading.

Fluvoxamine Maleate (Cyclosporine is extensively metabolized by CYP3A. Substances that inhibit this enzyme could decrease the metabolism and increase cyclosporine concentrations).
No products indexed under this heading.

Fosamprenavir Calcium (the HIV protease inhibitors are known to inhibit CYP3A and thus could potentially increase the concentrations of cyclosporine; care should be exercised when these drugs are administered concomitantly). Products include:
Lexiva Oral Suspension 1558
Lexiva 1558

Foscarnet Sodium (Care should be taken in using cyclosporine with nephrotoxic drugs).
No products indexed under this heading.

Fosinopril Sodium (Caution is required when co-administering cyclosporine with potassium sparing drugs, such as ACE inhibitors).
No products indexed under this heading.

Fosphenytoin (Co-administration with drugs that are inducers of CYP450 3A, such as phenytoin, could increase metabolism of cyclosporine and decrease its concentrations).
No products indexed under this heading.

Fosphenytoin Sodium (Co-administration with drugs that are inducers of CYP450 3A, such as phenytoin, could increase metabolism of cyclosporine and decrease its concentrations).
No products indexed under this heading.

Furosemide (Care should be taken in using cyclosporine with nephrotoxic drugs). Products include:
Furosemide 2354

Gadopentetate Dimeglumine (Care should be taken in using cyclosporine with nephrotoxic drugs).
No products indexed under this heading.

Gentamicin (Care should be taken in using cyclosporine with nephrotoxic drugs).
No products indexed under this heading.

Gentamicin Sulfate (May potentiate renal dysfunction). Products include:
Pred-G .... ⊙226, ⊙227

Glipizide (Care should be taken in using cyclosporine with nephrotoxic drugs).
No products indexed under this heading.

Globulin, Immune (Human) (Care should be taken in using cyclosporine with nephrotoxic drugs). Products include:

Glyburide (Care should be taken in using cyclosporine with nephrotoxic drugs).
No products indexed under this heading.

Gold Therapy (Care should be taken in using cyclosporine with nephrotoxic drugs).
No products indexed under this heading.

Hepatitis A Vaccine, Inactivated (During treatment with cyclosporine, vaccination may be less effective). Products include:
Havrix 1485
Twinrix 1694
Vaqta 2281

HMG-CoA Reductase Inhibitors (Care should be taken in using cyclosporine with nephrotoxic drugs).
No products indexed under this heading.

Hydrochlorothiazide (Care should be taken in using cyclosporine with nephrotoxic drugs). Products include:
Atacand HCT 700
Avalide 2956
Benicar HCT 1017
Diovan HCT 2419
Dyazide 1429
Exforge HCT 2449
Hyzaar 2162
Hyzaar 100-12.5 2162
Micardis HCT 889
Prinzide 2246
Tekturna HCT 2541
Teveten HCT 541

Hydroflumethiazide (Care should be taken in using cyclosporine with nephrotoxic drugs).
No products indexed under this heading.

Hypericum (Co-administration with drugs that are inducers of CYP450 3A could increase metabolism of cyclosporine and decrease its concentrations. This interaction has been reported to produce a marked reduction in the blood concentrations of cyclosporine, resulting in subtherapeutic levels, rejection of transplant organs, and graft loss).
No products indexed under this heading.

Ibuprofen (Cyclosporine can cause nephrotoxicity; clinical status and serum creatinine should be closely monitored when cyclosporine is used with NSAIDs in rheumatoid arthritis patients). Products include:
Motrin IB 2043
Children's Motrin 2044
Children's Motrin Non-Staining
Dye-Free 2044
Infants' Motrin 2044
Infants' Motrin Dye-Free 2044
Junior Strength Motrin 2044
Vicoprofen 564

Idarubicin Hydrochloride (Care should be taken in using cyclosporine with nephrotoxic drugs).
No products indexed under this heading.

Ifosfamide (Care should be taken in using cyclosporine with nephrotoxic drugs).
No products indexed under this heading.

Imatinib Mesylate (Cyclosporine is extensively metabolized by CYP3A. Substances that inhibit this enzyme could decrease the metabolism and increase cyclosporine concentrations). Products include:
Gleevec 2477

Imipenem (Care should be taken in using cyclosporine with nephrotoxic drugs). Products include:
Primaxin I.M. 2232
Primaxin I.V. 2235

Immune Globulin Intravenous (Human) (Care should be taken in using cyclosporine with nephrotoxic drugs). Products include:
Flebogamma 5% DIF 1794
Gammagard 812, 815
Gamunex 3374

Indinavir Sulfate (the HIV protease inhibitors are known to inhibit CYP3A and thus could potentially increase the concentrations of cyclosporine; care should be exercised when these drugs are administered concomitantly). Products include:
Crixivan 2113

Indomethacin (Cyclosporine can cause nephrotoxicity; clinical status and serum creatinine should be closely monitored when cyclosporine is used with NSAIDs in rheumatoid arthritis patients). Products include:
Indocin 2167

Indomethacin Sodium Trihydrate (Cyclosporine can cause nephrotoxicity; clinical status and serum creatinine should be closely monitored when cyclosporine is used with NSAIDs in rheumatoid arthritis patients). Products include:
Indocin I.V. 2007

Influenza Vaccine, Live Attenuated (During treatment with cyclosporine, vaccination may be less effective; and the use of live attenuated vaccines avoided).
No products indexed under this heading.

Influenza Virus Vaccine (During treatment with cyclosporine, vaccination may be less effective). Products include:
Fluarix 1476
Flulaval 1479

Influenza Virus Vaccine Live, Intranasal (During treatment with cyclosporine, vaccination may be less effective; and the use of live attenuated vaccines avoided). Products include:
FluMist 2078

Interferon Beta-1b (Care should be taken in using cyclosporine with nephrotoxic drugs). Products include:
Betaseron 836
Extavia 2459

Interleuken-2 (Care should be taken in using cyclosporine with nephrotoxic drugs).
No products indexed under this heading.

Iodamide Meglumine (Care should be taken in using cyclosporine with nephrotoxic drugs).
No products indexed under this heading.

Iohexol (Care should be taken in using cyclosporine with nephrotoxic drugs).
No products indexed under this heading.

Iopamidol (Care should be taken in using cyclosporine with nephrotoxic drugs).
No products indexed under this heading.

Iopanoic Acid (Care should be taken in using cyclosporine with nephrotoxic drugs).
No products indexed under this heading.

Iothalamate Meglumine (Care should be taken in using cyclosporine with nephrotoxic drugs).
No products indexed under this heading.

Ioxaglate Meglumine (Care should be taken in using cyclosporine with nephrotoxic drugs).
No products indexed under this heading.

Ioxaglate Sodium (Care should be taken in using cyclosporine with nephrotoxic drugs).
No products indexed under this heading.

Irbesartan (Caution is required when co-administering cyclosporine with potassium sparing drugs, such as angiotensin II receptor antagonists). Products include:

Avalide 2956
Avapro 2962

Isoniazid (Cyclosporine is extensively metabolized by CYP3A. Substances that inhibit this enzyme could decrease the metabolism and increase cyclosporine concentrations).
No products indexed under this heading.

Isradipine (While calcium antagonists can be effective agents in treating cyclosporine-associated hypertension, they can interfere with cyclosporine metabolism). Products include:
DynaCirc CR 1432

Itraconazole (Co-administration with drugs that inhibit CYP450 3A, such as itraconazole, could decrease metabolism of cyclosporine and increase its concentrations).
No products indexed under this heading.

Japanese Encephalitis Vaccine Inactivated (During treatment with cyclosporine, vaccination may be less effective).
No products indexed under this heading.

Kanamycin Sulfate (Care should be taken in using cyclosporine with nephrotoxic drugs).
No products indexed under this heading.

Ketoconazole (May potentiate renal dysfunction; co-administration with drugs that inhibit CYP4503A, such as ketoconazole, could decrease metabolism of cyclosporine and increase its concentrations). Products include:
Extina 3319
Xolegel 3337

Ketoprofen (Cyclosporine can cause nephrotoxicity; clinical status and serum creatinine should be closely monitored when cyclosporine is used with NSAIDs in rheumatoid arthritis patients).
No products indexed under this heading.

Ketorolac Tromethamine (Cyclosporine can cause nephrotoxicity; clinical status and serum creatinine should be closely monitored when cyclosporine is used with NSAIDs in rheumatoid arthritis patients). Products include:
Acuvail .... ⊙209

Lamium album (Care should be taken in using cyclosporine with nephrotoxic drugs).
No products indexed under this heading.

Levonorgestrel (Cyclosporine is extensively metabolized by CYP3A. Substances that inhibit this enzyme could decrease the metabolism and increase cyclosporine concentrations). Products include:
Climara Pro 847
LoSeasonique 3407
Lybrel 3514
Mirena 854
Plan B 3416
Seasonique 3418

Lisinopril (Caution is required when co-administering cyclosporine with potassium sparing drugs, such as ACE inhibitors). Products include:
Prinivil 2241
Prinzide 2246

Lithium (Care should be taken in using cyclosporine with nephrotoxic drugs).
No products indexed under this heading.

Lithium Carbonate (Care should be taken in using cyclosporine with nephrotoxic drugs).
No products indexed under this heading.

Lithium Citrate (Care should be taken in using cyclosporine with nephrotoxic drugs).
No products indexed under this heading.

Lopinavir (the HIV protease inhibitors are known to inhibit CYP3A and thus could potentially increase the concentrations of cyclosporine; care should be exercised when these drugs are administered concomitantly). Products include:

Gengraf Interactions Index 746

Kaletra 458

Loracarbef (Care should be taken in using cyclosporine with nephrotoxic drugs).
No products indexed under this heading.

Losartan Potassium (Caution is required when co-administering cyclosporine with potassium sparing drugs, such as angiotensin II receptor antagonists). Products include:
Cozaar 2106
Hyzaar 2162
Hyzaar 100-12.5 2162

Lovastatin (Co-administration results in reduced clearance of lovastatin; myositis has been reported with concurrent use). Products include:
Advicor 402
Mevacor 2212

Measles, Mumps, Rubella and Varicella Virus Vaccine Live (During treatment with cyclosporine, vaccination may be less effective; and the use of live attenuated vaccines avoided). Products include:
ProQuad 2254

Measles, Mumps & Rubella Virus Vaccine, Live (During treatment with cyclosporine, vaccination may be less effective; and the use of live attenuated vaccines avoided). Products include:
M-M-R II 2203
ProQuad 2254

Measles & Rubella Virus Vaccine Live (During treatment with cyclosporine, vaccination may be less effective; and the use of live attenuated vaccines avoided).
No products indexed under this heading.

Measles Virus Vaccine Live (During treatment with cyclosporine, vaccination may be less effective; and the use of live attenuated vaccines avoided). Products include:
Attenuvax 2086

Meclofenamate Sodium (Cyclosporine can cause nephrotoxicity; clinical status and serum creatinine should be closely monitored when cyclosporine is used with NSAIDs in rheumatoid arthritis patients).
No products indexed under this heading.

Mefenamic Acid (Cyclosporine can cause nephrotoxicity; clinical status and serum creatinine should be closely monitored when cyclosporine is used with NSAIDs in rheumatoid arthritis patients).
No products indexed under this heading.

Meloxicam (Cyclosporine can cause nephrotoxicity; clinical status and serum creatinine should be closely monitored when cyclosporine is used with NSAIDs in rheumatoid arthritis patients).
No products indexed under this heading.

Melphalan (May potentiate renal dysfunction). Products include:
Alkeran 1302

Melphalan Hydrochloride (Care should be taken in using cyclosporine with nephrotoxic drugs). Products include:
Alkeran for Injection 1300

Mesalamine (Care should be taken in using cyclosporine with nephrotoxic drugs). Products include:
Apriso 2899
Asacol 2786
Asacol HD 2787
Canasa 782
Lialda 3295
Pentasa 3297

Mestranol (Cyclosporine is extensively metabolized by CYP3A. Substances that inhibit this enzyme could decrease the metabolism and increase cyclosporine concentrations).
No products indexed under this heading.

Methimazole (Care should be taken in using cyclosporine with nephrotoxic drugs).
No products indexed under this heading.

Methotrexate (Care should be taken in using cyclosporine with nephrotoxic drugs).
No products indexed under this heading.

Methotrexate Sodium (Psoriasis patients who are treated with cyclosporine capsules should not receive concomitant methotrexate. Co-administration in rheumatoid arthritis patients has resulted in increased concentrations (AUC) of methotrexate by approximately 30% and the concentrations of its metabolite, 7-hydromethotrexate, were decreased by approximately 80%; the clinical significance of this outcome is not known).
No products indexed under this heading.

Methyclothiazide (Care should be taken in using cyclosporine with nephrotoxic drugs).
No products indexed under this heading.

Methylprednisolone (Co-administration with drugs that inhibit CYP450 3A such as methylprednisolone, could decrease metabolism of cyclosporine and increase its concentrations; convulsions have been reported with concurrent high dose methylprednisolone).
No products indexed under this heading.

Methylprednisolone Acetate (Co-administration with drugs that inhibit CYP450 3A such as methylprednisolone, could decrease metabolism of cyclosporine and increase its concentrations; convulsions have been reported with concurrent high dose methylprednisolone).
No products indexed under this heading.

Methylprednisolone Sodium Succinate (Co-administration with drugs that inhibit CYP450 3A such as methylprednisolone, could decrease metabolism of cyclosporine and increase its concentrations; convulsions have been reported with concurrent high dose methylprednisolone).
No products indexed under this heading.

Metoclopramide Hydrochloride (Cyclosporine is extensively metabolized by CYP450 3A. Substances that inhibit this enzyme could decrease the metabolism and increase cyclosporine concentrations). Products include:
Metozolv ODT 2901

Metronidazole (Cyclosporine is extensively metabolized by CYP3A. Substances that inhibit this enzyme could decrease the metabolism and increase cyclosporine concentrations). Products include:
Pylera 793

Metronidazole Benzoate (Cyclosporine is extensively metabolized by CYP3A. Substances that inhibit this enzyme could decrease the metabolism and increase cyclosporine concentrations).
No products indexed under this heading.

Metronidazole Hydrochloride (Cyclosporine is extensively metabolized by CYP3A. Substances that inhibit this enzyme could decrease the metabolism and increase cyclosporine concentrations).
No products indexed under this heading.

Mezlocillin Sodium (Care should be taken in using cyclosporine with nephrotoxic drugs).
No products indexed under this heading.

Mibefradil Dihydrochloride (While calcium antagonists can be effective agents in treating cyclosporine-associated hypertension, they can interfere with cyclosporine metabolism).
No products indexed under this heading.

Miconazole (Cyclosporine is extensively metabolized by CYP3A. Substances that inhibit this enzyme could decrease the metabolism and increase cyclosporine concentrations).
No products indexed under this heading.

Minocycline Hydrochloride (Care should be taken in using cyclosporine with nephrotoxic drugs). Products include:
Solodyn 2073

Mitomycin (Mitomycin-C) (Care should be taken in using cyclosporine with nephrotoxic drugs).
No products indexed under this heading.

Modafinil (Cyclosporine is extensively metabolized by CYP3A. Substances that are inducers of CYP3A could increase metabolism and decrease cyclosporine concentrations). Products include:
Provigil 983

Moexipril Hydrochloride (Caution is required when co-administering cyclosporine with potassium sparing drugs, such as ACE inhibitors).
No products indexed under this heading.

Mumps Virus Vaccine, Live (During treatment with cyclosporine, vaccination may be less effective; and the use of live attenuated vaccines avoided). Products include:
Mumpsvax 2218

Muromonab-CD3 (Psoriasis patients who are treated with cyclosporine capsules should not receive concomitant immunosuppressive agents. Co-administration with other immunosuppressive agents increases the possibility of excessive immunosuppression). Products include:
Orthoclone OKT3 949

Mycophenolate Mofetil (Psoriasis patients who are treated with cyclosporine capsules should not receive concomitant immunosuppressive agents. Co-administration with other immunosuppressive agents increases the possibility of excessive immunosuppression).
No products indexed under this heading.

Nabumetone (Cyclosporine can cause nephrotoxicity; clinical status and serum creatinine should be closely monitored when cyclosporine is used with NSAIDs in rheumatoid arthritis patients).
No products indexed under this heading.

Nafcillin Sodium (Co-administration with drugs that are inducers of CYP450 3A, such as nafcillin, could increase metabolism of cyclosporine and decrease its concentrations).
No products indexed under this heading.

Naproxen (May potentiate renal dysfunction; co-administration is associated with additive decreases in renal function). Products include:
EC-Naprosyn 2850
Naprosyn 2850
Anaprox/Naprosyn 2850

Naproxen Sodium (May potentiate renal dysfunction; co-administration is associated with additive decreases in renal function). Products include:
Anaprox 2850
Anaprox DS 2850
Treximet 1681

Nefazodone Hydrochloride (Cyclosporine is extensively metabolized by CYP3A. Substances that inhibit this enzyme could decrease the metabolism and increase cyclosporine concentrations).
No products indexed under this heading.

Nelfinavir Mesylate (the HIV protease inhibitors are known to inhibit CYP3A and thus could potentially increase the concentrations of cyclosporine; care should be exercised when these drugs are administered concomitantly).
No products indexed under this heading.

Neomycin (Care should be taken in using cyclosporine with nephrotoxic drugs).
No products indexed under this heading.

Neomycin, oral (Care should be taken in using cyclosporine with nephrotoxic drugs).
No products indexed under this heading.

Neomycin Sulfate (Care should be taken in using cyclosporine with nephrotoxic drugs).
No products indexed under this heading.

Nevirapine (Care should be taken in using cyclosporine with nephrotoxic drugs). Products include:
Viramune Oral Suspension 897
Viramune Tablets 897

Nicardipine (While calcium antagonists can be effective agents in treating cyclosporine-associated hypertension, they can interfere with cyclosporine metabolism).
No products indexed under this heading.

Nicardipine Hydrochloride (Cyclosporine is extensively metabolized by CYP450 3A. Substances that inhibit this enzyme could decrease the metabolism and increase cyclosporine concentrations).
No products indexed under this heading.

Nifedipine (Co-administration results in frequent episodes of gingival hyperplasia).
No products indexed under this heading.

Nimodipine (While calcium antagonists can be effective agents in treating cyclosporine-associated hypertension, they can interfere with cyclosporine metabolism).
No products indexed under this heading.

Nisoldipine (While calcium antagonists can be effective agents in treating cyclosporine-associated hypertension, they can interfere with cyclosporine metabolism).
No products indexed under this heading.

Norethindrone (Cyclosporine is extensively metabolized by CYP3A. Substances that inhibit this enzyme could decrease the metabolism and increase cyclosporine concentrations). Products include:
Ortho Micronor 2660

Norethynodrel (Cyclosporine is extensively metabolized by CYP3A. Substances that inhibit this enzyme could decrease the metabolism and increase cyclosporine concentrations).
No products indexed under this heading.

Norfloxacin (Care should be taken in using cyclosporine with nephrotoxic drugs). Products include:
Noroxin 2220

Norgestimate (Cyclosporine is extensively metabolized by CYP3A. Substances that inhibit this enzyme could decrease the metabolism and increase cyclosporine concentrations). Products include:
Ortho-Cyclen/Ortho Tri-Cyclen 2663
Ortho Tri-Cyclen Lo Tablets 2673

Norgestrel (Cyclosporine is extensively metabolized by CYP3A. Substances that inhibit this enzyme could decrease the metabolism and increase cyclosporine concentrations).
No products indexed under this heading.

Octreotide Acetate (Co-administration with drugs that are inducers of CYP450 3A, such as octreotide, could increase metabolism of cyclosporine and decrease its concentrations). Products include:
Sandostatin 2517
Sandostatin LAR 2519

Olsalazine Sodium (Care should be taken in using cyclosporine with nephrotoxic drugs).
No products indexed under this heading.

Omeprazole (Care should be taken in using cyclosporine with nephrotoxic drugs).
No products indexed under this heading.

Orlistat (Compounds that decrease cyclosporine absorption such as orlistat should be avoided). Products include:
Xenical 2893

Oxaprozin (Cyclosporine can cause nephrotoxicity; clinical status and serum creatinine should be closely monitored when cyclosporine is used with NSAIDs in rheumatoid arthritis patients).
No products indexed under this heading.

Pamidronate Disodium (Care should be taken in using cyclosporine with nephrotoxic drugs).
No products indexed under this heading.

Paroxetine Hydrochloride (Care should be taken in using cyclosporine with nephrotoxic drugs). Products include:
Paroxetine CR 2361
Paroxetine ER 2371
Paxil 1586
Paxil CR 1596

Penicillamine (Care should be taken in using cyclosporine with nephrotoxic drugs).
No products indexed under this heading.

Penicillin G Benzathine (Care should be taken in using cyclosporine with nephrotoxic drugs). Products include:
Bicillin C-R Injectable Suspension 1826
Bicillin L-A 1828

Penicillin G Potassium (Care should be taken in using cyclosporine with nephrotoxic drugs).
No products indexed under this heading.

Penicillin G Procaine (Care should be taken in using cyclosporine with nephrotoxic drugs). Products include:
Bicillin C-R Injectable Suspension 1826
Bicillin L-A 1828

Penicillin G Sodium (Care should be taken in using cyclosporine with nephrotoxic drugs).
No products indexed under this heading.

Penicillin V Potassium (Care should be taken in using cyclosporine with nephrotoxic drugs).
No products indexed under this heading.

Pentamidine Isethionate (Care should be taken in using cyclosporine with nephrotoxic drugs).
No products indexed under this heading.

Perindopril Erbumine (Caution is required when co-administering cyclosporine with potassium sparing drugs, such as ACE inhibitors).
No products indexed under this heading.

Phenobarbital (Co-administration with drugs that are inducers of CYP450 3A, such as phenobarbital, could increase metabolism of cyclosporine and decrease its concentrations). Products include:
Donnatal 2711

Phenobarbital Sodium (Cyclosporine is extensively metabolized by CYP3A. Substances that are inducers of CYP3A could increase metabolism and decrease cyclosporine concentrations).
No products indexed under this heading.

Phenylbutazone (Cyclosporine can cause nephrotoxicity; clinical status and serum creatinine should be closely monitored when cyclosporine is used with NSAIDs in rheumatoid arthritis patients).
No products indexed under this heading.

Phenytoin (Co-administration with drugs that are inducers of CYP450 3A, such as phenytoin, could increase metabolism of cyclosporine and decrease its concentrations).
No products indexed under this heading.

Phenytoin Sodium (Co-administration with drugs that are inducers of CYP450 3A, such as phenytoin, could increase

metabolism of cyclosporine and decrease its concentrations). Products include:
Phenytek Capsules 2380

Piroxicam (Cyclosporine can cause nephrotoxicity; clinical status and serum creatinine should be closely monitored when cyclosporine is used with NSAIDs in rheumatoid arthritis patients).
No products indexed under this heading.

Plicamycin (Care should be taken in using cyclosporine with nephrotoxic drugs).
No products indexed under this heading.

Pneumococcal vaccine, diphtheria conjugate (During treatment with cyclosporine, vaccination may be less effective). Products include:
Prevnar 3557

Pneumococcal Vaccine, Polyvalent (During treatment with cyclosporine, vaccination may be less effective). Products include:
Pneumovax 23 2230

Poliovirus Vaccine, Live, Oral, Trivalent, Types 1,2,3 (Sabin) (During treatment with cyclosporine, vaccination may be less effective; and the use of live attenuated vaccines avoided).
No products indexed under this heading.

Poliovirus Vaccine Inactivated (During treatment with cyclosporine, vaccination may be less effective). Products include:
Pediarix 1606

Polymyxin (Care should be taken in using cyclosporine with nephrotoxic drugs).
No products indexed under this heading.

Polymyxin B Sulfate (Care should be taken in using cyclosporine with nephrotoxic drugs).
No products indexed under this heading.

Polythiazide (Care should be taken in using cyclosporine with nephrotoxic drugs).
No products indexed under this heading.

Potassium Acid Phosphate (Caution is required when co-administering cyclosporine with potassium containing drugs, such as angiotensin II receptor antagonists). Products include:
K-Phos Original 874

Potassium Bicarbonate (Caution is required when co-administering cyclosporine with potassium containing drugs, such as angiotensin II receptor antagonists).
No products indexed under this heading.

Potassium Chloride (Caution is required when co-administering cyclosporine with potassium containing drugs, such as angiotensin II receptor antagonists). Products include:
MoviPrep Oral Solution 2905

Potassium Citrate (Caution is required when co-administering cyclosporine with potassium containing drugs, such as angiotensin II receptor antagonists). Products include:
Urocit-K 2333

Potassium Gluconate (Caution is required when co-administering cyclosporine with potassium containing drugs, such as angiotensin II receptor antagonists).
No products indexed under this heading.

Potassium Phosphate (Caution is required when co-administering cyclosporine with potassium containing drugs, such as angiotensin II receptor antagonists). Products include:
K-Phos Neutral 873

Pravastatin Sodium (Cyclosporine may reduce the clearance of HMG-CoA reductase inhibitors. Myotoxicity, including muscle pain and weakness, myositis, and rhabdomyolysis, have been reported with concomitant administration of cyclosporine with lovastatin, simvastatin, atorvastatin, pravastatin, and, rarely, fluvastatin. Dosage of these statins should be reduced).
No products indexed under this heading.

Prednisolone (Co-administration results in reduced clearance of prednisolone).
No products indexed under this heading.

Prednisolone Acetate (Co-administration results in reduced clearance of prednisolone). Products include:
Blephamide .... ⊙**212**, ⊙**214**
Pred Forte .... ⊙**225**
Pred Mild .... ⊙**230**
Pred-G .... ⊙**226**, ⊙**227**

Prednisolone Sodium Phosphate (Co-administration results in reduced clearance of prednisolone).
No products indexed under this heading.

Prednisolone Tebutate (Co-administration results in reduced clearance of prednisolone).
No products indexed under this heading.

Quinapril Hydrochloride (Caution is required when co-administering cyclosporine with potassium sparing drugs, such as ACE inhibitors).
No products indexed under this heading.

Quinine (Cyclosporine is extensively metabolized by CYP3A. Substances that inhibit this enzyme could decrease the metabolism and increase cyclosporine concentrations). Products include:
Hyland's Leg Cramps PM with
Quinine 3315

Quinine Sulfate (Cyclosporine is extensively metabolized by CYP3A. Substances that inhibit this enzyme could decrease the metabolism and increase cyclosporine concentrations).
No products indexed under this heading.

Quinupristin (Cyclosporine is extensively metabolized by CYP450 3A. Substances that inhibit this enzyme could decrease the metabolism and increase cyclosporine concentrations).
No products indexed under this heading.

Rabeprazole Sodium (Care should be taken in using cyclosporine with nephrotoxic drugs). Products include:
Aciphex 1035

Ramipril (Caution is required when co-administering cyclosporine with potassium sparing drugs, such as ACE inhibitors).
No products indexed under this heading.

Ranitidine Hydrochloride (May potentiate renal dysfunction). Products include:
Zantac 1737
Zantac Injection 1732
Zantac Pharmacy 1735

Rapamycin (Psoriasis patients who are treated with cyclosporine capsules should not receive concomitant immunosuppressive agents. Co-administration with other immunosuppressive agents increases the possibility of excessive immunosuppression).
No products indexed under this heading.

Rifabutin (Rifabutin is known to increase the metabolism of other drugs metabolized by CYP450 system; cyclosporine is extensively metabolized by CYP450 3A system, therefore, caution should be exercised).
No products indexed under this heading.

Rifampicin (Cyclosporine is extensively metabolized by CYP3A. Substances that are inducers of CYP3A could increase metabolism and decrease cyclosporine concentrations).
No products indexed under this heading.

Rifampin (Co-administration with drugs that are inducers of CYP450 3A, such as rifampin, could increase metabolism of cyclosporine and decrease its concentrations).
No products indexed under this heading.

Rifapentine (Cyclosporine is extensively metabolized by CYP3A. Substances that are inducers of CYP3A could increase metabolism and decrease cyclosporine concentrations).
No products indexed under this heading.

Riluzole (Care should be taken in using cyclosporine with nephrotoxic drugs). Products include:
Rilutek 3032

Ritonavir (the HIV protease inhibitors are known to inhibit CYP3A and thus could potentially increase the concentrations of cyclosporine; care should be exercised when these drugs are administered concomitantly). Products include:
Kaletra **458**
Norvir **509**

Rofecoxib (Cyclosporine can cause nephrotoxicity; clinical status and serum creatinine should be closely monitored when cyclosporine is used with NSAIDs in rheumatoid arthritis patients).
No products indexed under this heading.

Rosuvastatin Calcium (Cyclosporine may reduce the clearance of HMG-CoA reductase inhibitors. Myotoxicity, including muscle pain and weakness, myositis, and rhabdomyolysis, have been reported with concomitant administration of cyclosporine with lovastatin, simvastatin, atorvastatin, pravastatin, and, rarely, fluvastatin. Dosage of these statins should be reduced). Products include:
Crestor **736**

Rotavirus Vaccine, Live, Oral, Tetravalent (During treatment with cyclosporine, vaccination may be less effective; and the use of live attenuated vaccines avoided).
No products indexed under this heading.

Rubella & Mumps Virus Vaccine Live (During treatment with cyclosporine, vaccination may be less effective; and the use of live attenuated vaccines avoided).
No products indexed under this heading.

Rubella Virus Vaccine Live (During treatment with cyclosporine, vaccination may be less effective; and the use of live attenuated vaccines avoided). Products include:
Meruvax II 2210

Saquinavir (the HIV protease inhibitors are known to inhibit CYP3A and thus could potentially increase the concentrations of cyclosporine; care should be exercised when these drugs are administered concomitantly).
No products indexed under this heading.

Saquinavir Mesylate (the HIV protease inhibitors are known to inhibit CYP3A and thus could potentially increase the concentrations of cyclosporine; care should be exercised when these drugs are administered concomitantly).
No products indexed under this heading.

Sertraline Hydrochloride (Cyclosporine is extensively metabolized by CYP3A. Substances that inhibit this enzyme could decrease the metabolism and increase cyclosporine concentrations).
No products indexed under this heading.

Food Interactions

GENOTROPIN LYOPHILIZED POWDER

(☉ Described in PDR® for Ophthalmic Medicines)

ing is advisable when somatropin is administered in combination with other drugs known to be metabolized by CYP450 liver enzymes). Products include:
- Percocet ... **1121**
- Tylenol ... **2049**
- Tylenol 8 Hour ... **2049**
- Extra Strength Tylenol Caplets, Cool Caplets, and EZ Tabs ... **2049**
- Extra Strength Tylenol Adult Rapid Blast Liquid ... **2049**
- Extra Strength Tylenol Rapid Release ... **2049**
- Tylenol with Codeine ... **2691**
- Tylenol Arthritis Pain Extended Release Geltabs/Caplets ... **2049**
- Children's Tylenol Suspension Liquid ... **2048**
- Children's Tylenol Meltaways ... **2048**
- Tylenol, Infants' Drops ... **2048**
- Junior Tylenol ... **2048**
- Vicodin ... **560**
- Vicodin ES ... **561**
- Vicodin HP ... **563**
- Zydone ... **1138**

Alatrofloxacin Mesylate (Limited published data indicates that somatropin treatment increases cytochrome P450 (CYP450)-mediated antipyrine clearance in man. These data suggest that somatropin administration may alter the clearance of compounds metabolized by CYP450 liver enzymes. Careful monitoring is advisable when somatropin is administered in combination with other drugs known to be metabolized by CYP450 liver enzymes).
No products indexed under this heading.

Alclometasone Dipropionate (Somatropin inhibits 11β-hydroxysteroid dehydrogenase type 1 (11βHSD-1) in adipose/hepatic tissue and may significantly impact the metabolism of cortisol and cortisone. Patients treated with glucocorticoid replacement therapy for previously diagnosed hypoadrenalism may require an increase in their maintenance or stress doses; this may be especially true for patients treated with cortisone acetate and prednisone. In addition, excessive glucocorticoid therapy may attenuate the growth promoting effects of somatropin in children. Therefore, glucocorticoid replacement therapy should be carefully adjusted in children with concomitant GH and glucocorticoid deficiency to avoid both hypoadrenalism and an inhibitory effect on growth. Also, somatropin administration may alter the clearance of compounds known to be metabolized by CYP450 liver enzymes (eg, corticosteroids). Careful monitoring is advisable when somatropin is administered in combination with other drugs known to be metabolized by CYP450 liver enzymes).
No products indexed under this heading.

Alfentanil Hydrochloride (Limited published data indicates that somatropin treatment increases cytochrome P450 (CYP450)-mediated antipyrine clearance in man. These data suggest that somatropin administration may alter the clearance of compounds metabolized by CYP450 liver enzymes. Careful monitoring is advisable when somatropin is administered in combination with other drugs known to be metabolized by CYP450 liver enzymes).
No products indexed under this heading.

Alprazolam (Limited published data indicates that somatropin treatment increases cytochrome P450 (CYP450)-mediated antipyrine clearance in man. These data suggest that somatropin administration may alter the clearance of compounds metabolized by CYP450 liver enzymes. Careful monitoring is advisable when somatropin is administered in combination with other drugs known to be metabolized by CYP450 liver enzymes).
No products indexed under this heading.

Aminophylline (Limited published data indicates that somatropin treatment increases cytochrome P450 (CYP450)-mediated antipyrine clearance in man. These data suggest that somatropin administration may alter the clearance of compounds metabolized by CYP450 liver enzymes. Careful monitoring is advisable when somatropin is administered in combination with other drugs known to be metabolized by CYP450 liver enzymes).
No products indexed under this heading.

Amiodarone Hydrochloride (Limited published data indicates that somatropin treatment increases cytochrome P450 (CYP450)-mediated antipyrine clearance in man. These data suggest that somatropin administration may alter the clearance of compounds metabolized by CYP450 liver enzymes. Careful monitoring is advisable when somatropin is administered in combination with other drugs known to be metabolized by CYP450 liver enzymes).
No products indexed under this heading.

Amitriptyline Hydrochloride (Limited published data indicates that somatropin treatment increases cytochrome P450 (CYP450)-mediated antipyrine clearance in man. These data suggest that somatropin administration may alter the clearance of compounds metabolized by CYP450 liver enzymes. Careful monitoring is advisable when somatropin is administered in combination with other drugs known to be metabolized by CYP450 liver enzymes).
No products indexed under this heading.

Amlodipine Besylate (Limited published data indicates that somatropin treatment increases cytochrome P450 (CYP450)-mediated antipyrine clearance in man. These data suggest that somatropin administration may alter the clearance of compounds metabolized by CYP450 liver enzymes. Careful monitoring is advisable when somatropin is administered in combination with other drugs known to be metabolized by CYP450 liver enzymes). Products include:
- Azor ... **1010**
- Exforge ... **2443**
- Exforge HCT ... **2449**

Amoxapine (Limited published data indicates that somatropin treatment increases cytochrome P450 (CYP450)-mediated antipyrine clearance in man. These data suggest that somatropin administration may alter the clearance of compounds metabolized by CYP450 liver enzymes. Careful monitoring is advisable when somatropin is administered in combination with other drugs known to be metabolized by CYP450 liver enzymes).
No products indexed under this heading.

Amphetamine Aspartate (Limited published data indicates that somatropin treatment increases cytochrome P450 (CYP450)-mediated antipyrine clearance in man. These data suggest that somatropin administration may alter the clearance of compounds metabolized by CYP450 liver enzymes. Careful monitoring is advisable when somatropin is administered in combination with other drugs known to be metabolized by CYP450 liver enzymes).
No products indexed under this heading.

Amphetamine Aspartate Monohydrate (Limited published data indicates that somatropin treatment increases cytochrome P450 (CYP450)-mediated antipyrine clearance in man. These data suggest that somatropin administration may alter the clearance of compounds metabolized by CYP450 liver enzymes. Careful monitoring is advisable when somatropin is administered in combination with other drugs known to be metabolized by CYP450 liver enzymes).
No products indexed under this heading.

Amphetamine Sulfate (Limited published data indicates that somatropin treatment increases cytochrome P450 (CYP450)-mediated antipyrine clearance in man. These data suggest that somatropin administration may alter the clearance of compounds metabolized by CYP450 liver enzymes. Careful monitoring is advisable when somatropin is administered in combination with other drugs known to be metabolized by CYP450 liver enzymes).
No products indexed under this heading.

Anagrelide Hydrochloride (Limited published data indicates that somatropin treatment increases cytochrome P450 (CYP450)-mediated antipyrine clearance in man. These data suggest that somatropin administration may alter the clearance of compounds metabolized by CYP450 liver enzymes. Careful monitoring is advisable when somatropin is administered in combination with other drugs known to be metabolized by CYP450 liver enzymes).
No products indexed under this heading.

Antipyrine (Limited published data indicates that somatropin treatment increases cytochrome P450 (CYP450)-mediated antipyrine clearance in man. These data suggest that somatropin administration may alter the clearance of compounds metabolized by CYP450 liver enzymes. Careful monitoring is advisable when somatropin is administered in combination with other drugs known to be metabolized by CYP450 liver enzymes).
No products indexed under this heading.

Aprepitant (Limited published data indicates that somatropin treatment increases cytochrome P450 (CYP450)-mediated antipyrine clearance in man. These data suggest that somatropin administration may alter the clearance of compounds metabolized by CYP450 liver enzymes. Careful monitoring is advisable when somatropin is administered in combination with other drugs known to be metabolized by CYP450 liver enzymes). Products include:
- Emend ... **2124**

Astemizole (Limited published data indicates that somatropin treatment increases cytochrome P450 (CYP450)-mediated antipyrine clearance in man. These data suggest that somatropin administration may alter the clearance of compounds metabolized by CYP450 liver enzymes. Careful monitoring is advisable when somatropin is administered in combination with other drugs known to be metabolized by CYP450 liver enzymes).
No products indexed under this heading.

Atomoxetine Hydrochloride (Limited published data indicates that somatropin treatment increases cytochrome P450 (CYP450)-mediated antipyrine clearance in man. These data suggest that somatropin administration may alter the clearance of compounds metabolized by CYP450 liver enzymes. Careful monitoring is advisable when somatropin is administered in combination with other drugs known to be metabolized by CYP450 liver enzymes). Products include:
- Strattera ... **1957**

Atorvastatin Calcium (Limited published data indicates that somatropin treatment increases cytochrome P450 (CYP450)-mediated antipyrine clearance in man. These data suggest that somatropin administration may alter the clearance of compounds metabolized by CYP450 liver enzymes. Careful monitoring is advisable when somatropin is administered in combination with other drugs known to be metabolized by CYP450 liver enzymes). Products include:
- Lipitor ... **2703**

Beclomethasone Dipropionate (Somatropin inhibits 11β-hydroxysteroid dehydrogenase type 1 (11βHSD-1) in adipose/hepatic tissue and may significantly impact the metabolism of cortisol and cortisone. Patients treated with glucocorticoid replacement therapy for previously diagnosed hypoadrenalism may require an increase in their maintenance or stress doses; this may be especially true for patients treated with cortisone acetate and prednisone. In addition, excessive glucocorticoid therapy may attenuate the growth promoting effects of somatropin in children. Therefore, glucocorticoid replacement therapy should be carefully adjusted in children with concomitant GH and glucocorticoid deficiency to avoid both hypoadrenalism and an inhibitory effect on growth. Also, somatropin administration may alter the clearance of compounds known to be metabolized by CYP450 liver enzymes (eg, corticosteroids). Careful monitoring is advisable when somatropin is administered in combination with other drugs known to be metabolized by CYP450 liver enzymes). Products include:
- Qvar ... **3398**

Beclomethasone Dipropionate Monohydrate (Somatropin inhibits 11β-hydroxysteroid dehydrogenase type 1 (11βHSD-1) in adipose/hepatic tissue and may significantly impact the metabolism of cortisol and cortisone. Patients treated with glucocorticoid replacement therapy for previously diagnosed hypoadrenalism may require an increase in their maintenance or stress doses; this may be especially true for patients treated with cortisone acetate and prednisone. In addition, excessive glucocorticoid therapy may attenuate the growth promoting effects of somatropin in children. Therefore, glucocorticoid replacement therapy should be carefully adjusted in children with concomitant GH and glucocorticoid deficiency to avoid both hypoadrenalism and an inhibitory effect on growth. Also, somatropin administration may alter the clearance of compounds known to be metabolized by CYP450 liver enzymes (eg, corticosteroids). Careful monitoring is advisable when somatropin is administered in combination with other drugs known to be metabolized by CYP450 liver enzymes). Products include:
- Beconase AQ ... **1386**

Belladonna Ergotamine (Limited published data indicates that somatropin treatment increases cytochrome P450 (CYP450)-mediated antipyrine clearance in man. These data suggest that somatropin administration may alter the clearance of compounds metabolized by CYP450 liver enzymes. Careful monitoring is advisable when somatropin is administered in combination with other drugs known to be metabolized by CYP450 liver enzymes).
No products indexed under this heading.

Benzphetamine Hydrochloride (Limited published data indicates that somatropin treatment increases cytochrome P450 (CYP450)-mediated antipyrine clearance in man. These data suggest that somatropin administration may alter the clearance of compounds metabolized by CYP450 liver enzymes. Careful monitoring is advisable when somatropin is administered in combination with other drugs known to be metabolized by CYP450 liver enzymes).
No products indexed under this heading.

Betamethasone (Somatropin inhibits 11β-hydroxysteroid dehydrogenase

type 1 (11βHSD-1) in adipose/hepatic tissue and may significantly impact the metabolism of cortisol and cortisone. Patients treated with glucocorticoid replacement therapy for previously diagnosed hypoadrenalism may require an increase in their maintenance or stress doses; this may be especially true for patients treated with cortisone acetate and prednisone. In addition, excessive glucocorticoid therapy may attenuate the growth promoting effects of somatropin in children. Therefore, glucocorticoid replacement therapy should be carefully adjusted in children with concomitant GH and glucocorticoid deficiency to avoid both hypoadrenalism and an inhibitory effect on growth. Also, somatropin administration may alter the clearance of compounds known to be metabolized by CYP450 liver enzymes (eg, corticosteroids). Careful monitoring is advisable when somatropin is administered in combination with other drugs known to be metabolized by CYP450 liver enzymes).

No products indexed under this heading.

Betamethasone Acetate (Somatropin inhibits 11β-hydroxysteroid dehydrogenase type 1 (11βHSD-1) in adipose/hepatic tissue and may significantly impact the metabolism of cortisol and cortisone. Patients treated with glucocorticoid replacement therapy for previously diagnosed hypoadrenalism may require an increase in their maintenance or stress doses; this may be especially true for patients treated with cortisone acetate and prednisone. In addition, excessive glucocorticoid therapy may attenuate the growth promoting effects of somatropin in children. Therefore, glucocorticoid replacement therapy should be carefully adjusted in children with concomitant GH and glucocorticoid deficiency to avoid both hypoadrenalism and an inhibitory effect on growth. Also, somatropin administration may alter the clearance of compounds known to be metabolized by CYP450 liver enzymes (eg, corticosteroids). Careful monitoring is advisable when somatropin is administered in combination with other drugs known to be metabolized by CYP450 liver enzymes).

No products indexed under this heading.

Betamethasone Benzoate (Somatropin inhibits 11β-hydroxysteroid dehydrogenase type 1 (11βHSD-1) in adipose/hepatic tissue and may significantly impact the metabolism of cortisol and cortisone. Patients treated with glucocorticoid replacement therapy for previously diagnosed hypoadrenalism may require an increase in their maintenance or stress doses; this may be especially true for patients treated with cortisone acetate and prednisone. In addition, excessive glucocorticoid therapy may attenuate the growth promoting effects of somatropin in children. Therefore, glucocorticoid replacement therapy should be carefully adjusted in children with concomitant GH and glucocorticoid deficiency to avoid both hypoadrenalism and an inhibitory effect on growth. Also, somatropin administration may alter the clearance of compounds known to be metabolized by CYP450 liver enzymes (eg, corticosteroids). Careful monitoring is advisable when somatropin is administered in combination with other drugs known to be metabolized by CYP450 liver enzymes).

No products indexed under this heading.

Betamethasone Dipropionate (Somatropin inhibits 11β-hydroxysteroid dehydrogenase type 1 (11βHSD-1) in adipose/hepatic tissue and may significantly impact the metabolism of cortisol and cortisone. Patients treated with glucocorticoid replacement therapy for previously diagnosed hypoadrenalism may require an increase in their maintenance or stress doses; this may be especially true for patients treated with cortisone acetate and prednisone. In addition, excessive glucocorticoid therapy may attenuate the growth promoting effects of somatropin in children. Therefore, glucocorticoid replacement therapy should be carefully adjusted in children with concomitant GH and glucocorticoid deficiency to avoid both hypoadrenalism and an inhibitory effect on growth. Also, somatropin administration may alter the clearance of compounds known to be metabolized by CYP450 liver enzymes (eg, corticosteroids). Careful monitoring is advisable when somatropin is administered in combination with other drugs known to be metabolized by CYP450 liver enzymes). Products include:

Diprolene Lotion 0.05% **3108**
Diprolene Ointment 0.05% **3109**
Diprolene AF Cream 0.05% **3107**
Lotrisone **3163**

Betamethasone Sodium Phosphate (Somatropin inhibits 11β-hydroxysteroid dehydrogenase type 1 (11βHSD-1) in adipose/hepatic tissue and may significantly impact the metabolism of cortisol and cortisone. Patients treated with glucocorticoid replacement therapy for previously diagnosed hypoadrenalism may require an increase in their maintenance or stress doses; this may be especially true for patients treated with cortisone acetate and prednisone. In addition, excessive glucocorticoid therapy may attenuate the growth promoting effects of somatropin in children. Therefore, glucocorticoid replacement therapy should be carefully adjusted in children with concomitant GH and glucocorticoid deficiency to avoid both hypoadrenalism and an inhibitory effect on growth. Also, somatropin administration may alter the clearance of compounds known to be metabolized by CYP450 liver enzymes (eg, corticosteroids). Careful monitoring is advisable when somatropin is administered in combination with other drugs known to be metabolized by CYP450 liver enzymes).

No products indexed under this heading.

Betamethasone Valerate (Somatropin inhibits 11β-hydroxysteroid dehydrogenase type 1 (11βHSD-1) in adipose/hepatic tissue and may significantly impact the metabolism of cortisol and cortisone. Patients treated with glucocorticoid replacement therapy for previously diagnosed hypoadrenalism may require an increase in their maintenance or stress doses; this may be especially true for patients treated with cortisone acetate and prednisone. In addition, excessive glucocorticoid therapy may attenuate the growth promoting effects of somatropin in children. Therefore, glucocorticoid replacement therapy should be carefully adjusted in children with concomitant GH and glucocorticoid deficiency to avoid both hypoadrenalism and an inhibitory effect on growth. Also, somatropin administration may alter the clearance of compounds known to be metabolized by CYP450 liver enzymes (eg, corticosteroids). Careful monitoring is advisable when somatropin is administered in combination with other drugs known to be metabolized by CYP450 liver enzymes). Products include:

Luxiq **3321**

Bisoprolol Fumarate (Limited published data indicates that somatropin treatment increases cytochrome P450 (CYP450)-mediated antipyrine clearance in man. These data suggest that somatropin administration may alter the clearance of compounds metabolized by CYP450 liver enzymes. Careful monitoring is advisable when somatropin is administered in combination with other drugs known to be metabolized by CYP450 liver enzymes).

No products indexed under this heading.

Bromocriptine Mesylate (Limited published data indicates that somatropin treatment increases cytochrome P450 (CYP450)-mediated antipyrine clearance in man. These data suggest that somatropin administration may alter the clearance of compounds metabolized by CYP450 liver enzymes. Careful monitoring is advisable when somatropin is administered in combination with other drugs known to be metabolized by CYP450 liver enzymes).

No products indexed under this heading.

Budesonide (Somatropin inhibits 11β-hydroxysteroid dehydrogenase type 1 (11βHSD-1) in adipose/hepatic tissue and may significantly impact the metabolism of cortisol and cortisone. Patients treated with glucocorticoid replacement therapy for previously diagnosed hypoadrenalism may require an increase in their maintenance or stress doses; this may be especially true for patients treated with cortisone acetate and prednisone. In addition, excessive glucocorticoid therapy may attenuate the growth promoting effects of somatropin in children. Therefore, glucocorticoid replacement therapy should be carefully adjusted in children with concomitant GH and glucocorticoid deficiency to avoid both hypoadrenalism and an inhibitory effect on growth. Also, somatropin administration may alter the clearance of compounds known to be metabolized by CYP450 liver enzymes (eg, corticosteroids). Careful monitoring is advisable when somatropin is administered in combination with other drugs known to be metabolized by CYP450 liver enzymes). Products include:

Pulmicort Flexhaler **714**
Symbicort 80/4.5 .... **720**
Symbicort 160/4.5 .... **720**

Buspirone Hydrochloride (Limited published data indicates that somatropin treatment increases cytochrome P450 (CYP450)-mediated antipyrine clearance in man. These data suggest that somatropin administration may alter the clearance of compounds metabolized by CYP450 liver enzymes. Careful monitoring is advisable when somatropin is administered in combination with other drugs known to be metabolized by CYP450 liver enzymes).

No products indexed under this heading.

Busulfan (Limited published data indicates that somatropin treatment increases cytochrome P450 (CYP450)-mediated antipyrine clearance in man. These data suggest that somatropin administration may alter the clearance of compounds metabolized by CYP450 liver enzymes. Careful monitoring is advisable when somatropin is administered in combination with other drugs known to be metabolized by CYP450 liver enzymes). Products include:

Myleran **1581**

Caffeine (Limited published data indicates that somatropin treatment increases cytochrome P450 (CYP450)-mediated antipyrine clearance in man. These data suggest that somatropin administration may alter the clearance of compounds metabolized by CYP450 liver enzymes. Careful monitoring is advisable when somatropin is administered in combination with other drugs known to be metabolized by CYP450 liver enzymes).

No products indexed under this heading.

Caffeine Anhydrous (Limited published data indicates that somatropin treatment increases cytochrome P450 (CYP450)-mediated antipyrine clearance in man. These data suggest that somatropin administration may alter the clearance of compounds metabolized by CYP450 liver enzymes. Careful monitoring is advisable when somatropin is administered in combination with other drugs known to be metabolized by CYP450 liver enzymes).

No products indexed under this heading.

Caffeine Citrate (Limited published data indicates that somatropin treatment increases cytochrome P450 (CYP450)-mediated antipyrine clearance in man. These data suggest that somatropin administration may alter the clearance of compounds metabolized by CYP450 liver enzymes. Careful monitoring is advisable when somatropin is administered in combination with other drugs known to be metabolized by CYP450 liver enzymes).

No products indexed under this heading.

Caffeine-containing medications (Limited published data indicates that somatropin treatment increases cytochrome P450 (CYP450)-mediated antipyrine clearance in man. These data suggest that somatropin administration may alter the clearance of compounds metabolized by CYP450 liver enzymes. Careful monitoring is advisable when somatropin is administered in combination with other drugs known to be metabolized by CYP450 liver enzymes).

No products indexed under this heading.

Caffeine Sodium Benzoate (Limited published data indicates that somatropin treatment increases cytochrome P450 (CYP450)-mediated antipyrine clearance in man. These data suggest that somatropin administration may alter the clearance of compounds metabolized by CYP450 liver enzymes. Careful monitoring is advisable when somatropin is administered in combination with other drugs known to be metabolized by CYP450 liver enzymes).

No products indexed under this heading.

Candesartan Cilexetil (Limited published data indicates that somatropin treatment increases cytochrome P450 (CYP450)-mediated antipyrine clearance in man. These data suggest that somatropin administration may alter the clearance of compounds metabolized by CYP450 liver enzymes. Careful monitoring is advisable when somatropin is administered in combination with other drugs known to be metabolized by CYP450 liver enzymes). Products include:

Atacand **697**
Atacand HCT **700**

Captopril (Limited published data indicates that somatropin treatment increases cytochrome P450 (CYP450)-mediated antipyrine clearance in man. These data suggest that somatropin administration may alter the clearance of compounds metabolized by CYP450 liver enzymes. Careful monitoring is advisable when somatropin is administered in combination with other drugs known to be metabolized by CYP450 liver enzymes). Products include:

Captopril **2341**

Carbamazepine (Limited published data indicates that somatropin treatment increases cytochrome P450 (CYP450)-mediated antipyrine clearance in man. These data suggest that somatropin administration may alter the clearance of compounds metabolized by CYP450 liver enzymes (eg, anticonvulsants). Careful monitoring is advisable when somatropin is administered in combination with other drugs known to be metabolized by CYP450 liver enzymes). Products include:

Carbatrol **3280**
Equetro **3477**

Carisoprodol (Limited published data indicates that somatropin treatment increases cytochrome P450 (CYP450)-mediated antipyrine clearance in man. These data suggest that somatropin administration may alter the clearance of compounds metabolized by CYP450 liver enzymes. Careful monitoring is advisable when somatropin is administered in combination with other drugs known to be metabolized by CYP450 liver enzymes).
No products indexed under this heading.

Carvedilol (Limited published data indicates that somatropin treatment increases cytochrome P450 (CYP450)-mediated antipyrine clearance in man. These data suggest that somatropin administration may alter the clearance of compounds metabolized by CYP450 liver enzymes. Careful monitoring is advisable when somatropin is administered in combination with other drugs known to be metabolized by CYP450 liver enzymes). Products include:
Coreg 1409

Celecoxib (Limited published data indicates that somatropin treatment increases cytochrome P450 (CYP450)-mediated antipyrine clearance in man. These data suggest that somatropin administration may alter the clearance of compounds metabolized by CYP450 liver enzymes. Careful monitoring is advisable when somatropin is administered in combination with other drugs known to be metabolized by CYP450 liver enzymes). Products include:
Celebrex 3272

Cerivastatin Sodium (Limited published data indicates that somatropin treatment increases cytochrome P450 (CYP450)-mediated antipyrine clearance in man. These data suggest that somatropin administration may alter the clearance of compounds metabolized by CYP450 liver enzymes. Careful monitoring is advisable when somatropin is administered in combination with other drugs known to be metabolized by CYP450 liver enzymes).
No products indexed under this heading.

Cevimeline Hydrochloride (Limited published data indicates that somatropin treatment increases cytochrome P450 (CYP450)-mediated antipyrine clearance in man. These data suggest that somatropin administration may alter the clearance of compounds metabolized by CYP450 liver enzymes. Careful monitoring is advisable when somatropin is administered in combination with other drugs known to be metabolized by CYP450 liver enzymes). Products include:
Evoxac 1027

Chlordiazepoxide (Limited published data indicates that somatropin treatment increases cytochrome P450 (CYP450)-mediated antipyrine clearance in man. These data suggest that somatropin administration may alter the clearance of compounds metabolized by CYP450 liver enzymes. Careful monitoring is advisable when somatropin is administered in combination with other drugs known to be metabolized by CYP450 liver enzymes).
No products indexed under this heading.

Chlordiazepoxide Hydrochloride (Limited published data indicates that somatropin treatment increases cytochrome P450 (CYP450)-mediated antipyrine clearance in man. These data suggest that somatropin administration may alter the clearance of compounds metabolized by CYP450 liver enzymes. Careful monitoring is advisable when somatropin is administered in combina-

tion with other drugs known to be metabolized by CYP450 liver enzymes).
No products indexed under this heading.

Chlorotrianisene (In patients on oral estrogen replacement, a larger dose of somatropin may be required to achieve the defined treatment goal).
No products indexed under this heading.

Chlorpheniramine (Limited published data indicates that somatropin treatment increases cytochrome P450 (CYP450)-mediated antipyrine clearance in man. These data suggest that somatropin administration may alter the clearance of compounds metabolized by CYP450 liver enzymes. Careful monitoring is advisable when somatropin is administered in combination with other drugs known to be metabolized by CYP450 liver enzymes).
No products indexed under this heading.

Chlorpheniramine Maleate (Limited published data indicates that somatropin treatment increases cytochrome P450 (CYP450)-mediated antipyrine clearance in man. These data suggest that somatropin administration may alter the clearance of compounds metabolized by CYP450 liver enzymes. Careful monitoring is advisable when somatropin is administered in combination with other drugs known to be metabolized by CYP450 liver enzymes).
No products indexed under this heading.

Chlorpheniramine Polistirex (Limited published data indicates that somatropin treatment increases cytochrome P450 (CYP450)-mediated antipyrine clearance in man. These data suggest that somatropin administration may alter the clearance of compounds metabolized by CYP450 liver enzymes. Careful monitoring is advisable when somatropin is administered in combination with other drugs known to be metabolized by CYP450 liver enzymes). Products include:
Tussionex 3443

Chlorpheniramine Tannate (Limited published data indicates that somatropin treatment increases cytochrome P450 (CYP450)-mediated antipyrine clearance in man. These data suggest that somatropin administration may alter the clearance of compounds metabolized by CYP450 liver enzymes. Careful monitoring is advisable when somatropin is administered in combination with other drugs known to be metabolized by CYP450 liver enzymes).
No products indexed under this heading.

Chlorpromazine (Limited published data indicates that somatropin treatment increases cytochrome P450 (CYP450)-mediated antipyrine clearance in man. These data suggest that somatropin administration may alter the clearance of compounds metabolized by CYP450 liver enzymes. Careful monitoring is advisable when somatropin is administered in combination with other drugs known to be metabolized by CYP450 liver enzymes).
No products indexed under this heading.

Chlorpromazine Hydrochloride (Limited published data indicates that somatropin treatment increases cytochrome P450 (CYP450)-mediated antipyrine clearance in man. These data suggest that somatropin administration may alter the clearance of compounds metabolized by CYP450 liver enzymes. Careful monitoring is advisable when somatropin is administered in combination with other drugs known to be metabolized by CYP450 liver enzymes).
No products indexed under this heading.

Chlorpropamide (In patients with diabetes mellitus requiring drug therapy, the dose of insulin and/or oral agent may require adjustment when somatropin therapy is initiated).
No products indexed under this heading.

Ciclesonide (Somatropin inhibits 11β-hydroxysteroid dehydrogenase type 1 (11βHSD-1) in adipose/hepatic tissue and may significantly impact the metabolism of cortisol and cortisone. Patients treated with glucocorticoid replacement therapy for previously diagnosed hypoadrenalism may require an increase in their maintenance or stress doses; this may be especially true for patients treated with cortisone acetate and prednisone. In addition, excessive glucocorticoid therapy may attenuate the growth promoting effects of somatropin in children. Therefore, glucocorticoid replacement therapy should be carefully adjusted in children with concomitant GH and glucocorticoid deficiency to avoid both hypoadrenalism and an inhibitory effect on growth. Also, somatropin administration may alter the clearance of compounds known to be metabolized by CYP450 liver enzymes (eg, corticosteroids). Careful monitoring is advisable when somatropin is administered in combination with other drugs known to be metabolized by CYP450 liver enzymes).
No products indexed under this heading.

Cilostazol (Limited published data indicates that somatropin treatment increases cytochrome P450 (CYP450)-mediated antipyrine clearance in man. These data suggest that somatropin administration may alter the clearance of compounds metabolized by CYP450 liver enzymes. Careful monitoring is advisable when somatropin is administered in combination with other drugs known to be metabolized by CYP450 liver enzymes).
No products indexed under this heading.

Cimetidine Hydrochloride (Limited published data indicates that somatropin treatment increases cytochrome P450 (CYP450)-mediated antipyrine clearance in man. These data suggest that somatropin administration may alter the clearance of compounds metabolized by CYP450 liver enzymes. Careful monitoring is advisable when somatropin is administered in combination with other drugs known to be metabolized by CYP450 liver enzymes).
No products indexed under this heading.

Ciprofloxacin (Limited published data indicates that somatropin treatment increases cytochrome P450 (CYP450)-mediated antipyrine clearance in man. These data suggest that somatropin administration may alter the clearance of compounds metabolized by CYP450 liver enzymes. Careful monitoring is advisable when somatropin is administered in combination with other drugs known to be metabolized by CYP450 liver enzymes). Products include:
Cipro I.V. 3082
Cipro 3073
Cipro XR 3091
Ciprodex 583

Ciprofloxacin Hydrochloride (Limited published data indicates that somatropin treatment increases cytochrome P450 (CYP450)-mediated antipyrine clearance in man. These data suggest that somatropin administration may alter the clearance of compounds metabolized by CYP450 liver enzymes. Careful monitoring is advisable when somatropin is administered in combination with other drugs known to be metabolized by CYP450 liver enzymes). Products include:
Cipro 3073

Cisapride (Limited published data indicates that somatropin treatment increases cytochrome P450 (CYP450)-mediated antipyrine clearance in man. These data suggest that somatropin administration may alter the clearance of compounds metabolized by CYP450 liver enzymes. Careful monitoring is advisable when somatropin is administered in combination with other drugs known to be metabolized by CYP450 liver enzymes).
No products indexed under this heading.

Citalopram Hydrobromide (Limited published data indicates that somatropin treatment increases cytochrome P450 (CYP450)-mediated antipyrine clearance in man. These data suggest that somatropin administration may alter the clearance of compounds metabolized by CYP450 liver enzymes. Careful monitoring is advisable when somatropin is administered in combination with other drugs known to be metabolized by CYP450 liver enzymes). Products include:
Celexa 1153

Clarithromycin (Limited published data indicates that somatropin treatment increases cytochrome P450 (CYP450)-mediated antipyrine clearance in man. These data suggest that somatropin administration may alter the clearance of compounds metabolized by CYP450 liver enzymes. Careful monitoring is advisable when somatropin is administered in combination with other drugs known to be metabolized by CYP450 liver enzymes). Products include:
Biaxin/Biaxin XL 412

Clomipramine Hydrochloride (Limited published data indicates that somatropin treatment increases cytochrome P450 (CYP450)-mediated antipyrine clearance in man. These data suggest that somatropin administration may alter the clearance of compounds metabolized by CYP450 liver enzymes. Careful monitoring is advisable when somatropin is administered in combination with other drugs known to be metabolized by CYP450 liver enzymes).
No products indexed under this heading.

Clopidogrel Bisulfate (Limited published data indicates that somatropin treatment increases cytochrome P450 (CYP450)-mediated antipyrine clearance in man. These data suggest that somatropin administration may alter the clearance of compounds metabolized by CYP450 liver enzymes. Careful monitoring is advisable when somatropin is administered in combination with other drugs known to be metabolized by CYP450 liver enzymes). Products include:
Plavix 3027

Clopidogrel Hydrogen Sulfate (Limited published data indicates that somatropin treatment increases cytochrome P450 (CYP450)-mediated antipyrine clearance in man. These data suggest that somatropin administration may alter the clearance of compounds metabolized by CYP450 liver enzymes. Careful monitoring is advisable when somatropin is administered in combination with other drugs known to be metabolized by CYP450 liver enzymes).
No products indexed under this heading.

Clozapine (Limited published data indicates that somatropin treatment increases cytochrome P450 (CYP450)-mediated antipyrine clearance in man. These data suggest that somatropin administration may alter the clearance of compounds metabolized by CYP450 liver enzymes. Careful monitoring is advisable when somatropin is

IMPORTANT NOTE: Always consult each drug listing in the patient's regimen for possible interactions.

administered in combination with other drugs known to be metabolized by CYP450 liver enzymes).

No products indexed under this heading.

Codeine Phosphate (Limited published data indicates that somatropin treatment increases cytochrome P450 (CYP450)-mediated antipyrine clearance in man. These data suggest that somatropin administration may alter the clearance of compounds metabolized by CYP450 liver enzymes. Careful monitoring is advisable when somatropin is administered in combination with other drugs known to be metabolized by CYP450 liver enzymes). Products include:

Tylenol with Codeine **2691**

Codeine Sulfate (Limited published data indicates that somatropin treatment increases cytochrome P450 (CYP450)-mediated antipyrine clearance in man. These data suggest that somatropin administration may alter the clearance of compounds metabolized by CYP450 liver enzymes. Careful monitoring is advisable when somatropin is administered in combination with other drugs known to be metabolized by CYP450 liver enzymes).

No products indexed under this heading.

Cortisol (Somatropin inhibits 11β-hydroxysteroid dehydrogenase type 1 (11βHSD-1) in adipose/hepatic tissue and may significantly impact the metabolism of cortisol and cortisone. Patients treated with glucocorticoid replacement therapy for previously diagnosed hypoadrenalism may require an increase in their maintenance or stress doses; this may be especially true for patients treated with cortisone acetate and prednisone. In addition, excessive glucocorticoid therapy may attenuate the growth promoting effects of somatropin in children. Therefore, glucocorticoid replacement therapy should be carefully adjusted in children with concomitant GH and glucocorticoid deficiency to avoid both hypoadrenalism and an inhibitory effect on growth. Also, somatropin administration may alter the clearance of compounds known to be metabolized by CYP450 liver enzymes (eg, corticosteroids). Careful monitoring is advisable when somatropin is administered in combination with other drugs known to be metabolized by CYP450 liver enzymes).

No products indexed under this heading.

Cortisone Acetate (Somatropin inhibits 11β-hydroxysteroid dehydrogenase type 1 (11βHSD-1) in adipose/hepatic tissue and may significantly impact the metabolism of cortisol and cortisone. Patients treated with glucocorticoid replacement therapy for previously diagnosed hypoadrenalism may require an increase in their maintenance or stress doses; this may be especially true for patients treated with cortisone acetate and prednisone. In addition, excessive glucocorticoid therapy may attenuate the growth promoting effects of somatropin in children. Therefore, glucocorticoid replacement therapy should be carefully adjusted in children with concomitant GH and glucocorticoid deficiency to avoid both hypoadrenalism and an inhibitory effect on growth. Also, somatropin administration may alter the clearance of compounds known to be metabolized by CYP450 liver enzymes (eg, corticosteroids). Careful monitoring is advisable when somatropin is administered in combination with other drugs known to be metabolized by CYP450 liver enzymes).

No products indexed under this heading.

Cyclobenzaprine (Limited published data indicates that somatropin treatment increases cytochrome P450 (CYP450)-mediated antipyrine clearance in man. These data suggest that somatropin administration may alter the clearance of compounds metabolized by CYP450 liver enzymes. Careful monitoring is advisable when somatropin is administered in combination with other drugs known to be metabolized by CYP450 liver enzymes).

No products indexed under this heading.

Cyclobenzaprine Hydrochloride (Limited published data indicates that somatropin treatment increases cytochrome P450 (CYP450)-mediated antipyrine clearance in man. These data suggest that somatropin administration may alter the clearance of compounds metabolized by CYP450 liver enzymes. Careful monitoring is advisable when somatropin is administered in combination with other drugs known to be metabolized by CYP450 liver enzymes). Products include:

Amrix **964**

Cyclophosphamide (Limited published data indicates that somatropin treatment increases cytochrome P450 (CYP450)-mediated antipyrine clearance in man. These data suggest that somatropin administration may alter the clearance of compounds metabolized by CYP450 liver enzymes. Careful monitoring is advisable when somatropin is administered in combination with other drugs known to be metabolized by CYP450 liver enzymes).

No products indexed under this heading.

Cyclosporine (Limited published data indicates that somatropin treatment increases cytochrome P450 (CYP450)-mediated antipyrine clearance in man. These data suggest that somatropin administration may alter the clearance of compounds metabolized by CYP450 liver enzymes (eg, cyclosporine). Careful monitoring is advisable when somatropin is administered in combination with other drugs known to be metabolized by CYP450 liver enzymes). Products include:

Gengraf **440**
Neoral Oral Solution **2496**
Neoral Capsules **2496**
Restasis **605**

Desipramine Hydrochloride (Limited published data indicates that somatropin treatment increases cytochrome P450 (CYP450)-mediated antipyrine clearance in man. These data suggest that somatropin administration may alter the clearance of compounds metabolized by CYP450 liver enzymes. Careful monitoring is advisable when somatropin is administered in combination with other drugs known to be metabolized by CYP450 liver enzymes).

No products indexed under this heading.

Desogestrel (Limited published data indicates that somatropin treatment increases cytochrome P450 (CYP450)-mediated antipyrine clearance in man. These data suggest that somatropin administration may alter the clearance of compounds metabolized by CYP450 liver enzymes (eg, sex steroids). Careful monitoring is advisable when somatropin is administered in combination with other drugs known to be metabolized by CYP450 liver enzymes).

No products indexed under this heading.

Desoximetasone (Somatropin inhibits 11β-hydroxysteroid dehydrogenase type 1 (11βHSD-1) in adipose/hepatic tissue and may significantly impact the metabolism of cortisol and cortisone. Patients treated with glucocorticoid replacement therapy for previously diagnosed hypoadrenalism may require an increase in their maintenance or stress doses; this may be especially true for patients treated with cortisone acetate and prednisone. In addition, excessive glucocorticoid therapy may

attenuate the growth promoting effects of somatropin in children. Therefore, glucocorticoid replacement therapy should be carefully adjusted in children with concomitant GH and glucocorticoid deficiency to avoid both hypoadrenalism and an inhibitory effect on growth. Also, somatropin administration may alter the clearance of compounds known to be metabolized by CYP450 liver enzymes (eg, corticosteroids). Careful monitoring is advisable when somatropin is administered in combination with other drugs known to be metabolized by CYP450 liver enzymes).

No products indexed under this heading.

Dexamethasone (Somatropin inhibits 11β-hydroxysteroid dehydrogenase type 1 (11βHSD-1) in adipose/hepatic tissue and may significantly impact the metabolism of cortisol and cortisone. Patients treated with glucocorticoid replacement therapy for previously diagnosed hypoadrenalism may require an increase in their maintenance or stress doses; this may be especially true for patients treated with cortisone acetate and prednisone. In addition, excessive glucocorticoid therapy may attenuate the growth promoting effects of somatropin in children. Therefore, glucocorticoid replacement therapy should be carefully adjusted in children with concomitant GH and glucocorticoid deficiency to avoid both hypoadrenalism and an inhibitory effect on growth. Also, somatropin administration may alter the clearance of compounds known to be metabolized by CYP450 liver enzymes (eg, corticosteroids). Careful monitoring is advisable when somatropin is administered in combination with other drugs known to be metabolized by CYP450 liver enzymes). Products include:

Ciprodex **583**
Ozurdex ....⊙**223**
Tobramycin and Dexamethasone Ophthalmic Suspension ....⊙**251**

Dexamethasone Acetate (Somatropin inhibits 11β-hydroxysteroid dehydrogenase type 1 (11βHSD-1) in adipose/hepatic tissue and may significantly impact the metabolism of cortisol and cortisone. Patients treated with glucocorticoid replacement therapy for previously diagnosed hypoadrenalism may require an increase in their maintenance or stress doses; this may be especially true for patients treated with cortisone acetate and prednisone. In addition, excessive glucocorticoid therapy may attenuate the growth promoting effects of somatropin in children. Therefore, glucocorticoid replacement therapy should be carefully adjusted in children with concomitant GH and glucocorticoid deficiency to avoid both hypoadrenalism and an inhibitory effect on growth. Also, somatropin administration may alter the clearance of compounds known to be metabolized by CYP450 liver enzymes (eg, corticosteroids). Careful monitoring is advisable when somatropin is administered in combination with other drugs known to be metabolized by CYP450 liver enzymes).

No products indexed under this heading.

Dexamethasone Phosphate (Somatropin inhibits 11β-hydroxysteroid dehydrogenase type 1 (11βHSD-1) in adipose/hepatic tissue and may significantly impact the metabolism of cortisol and cortisone. Patients treated with glucocorticoid replacement therapy for previously diagnosed hypoadrenalism may require an increase in their maintenance or stress doses; this may be especially true for patients treated with cortisone acetate and prednisone. In addition, excessive glucocorticoid therapy may attenuate the growth promoting effects of somatropin in children. Therefore, glucocorticoid replacement therapy should be carefully adjusted in

children with concomitant GH and glucocorticoid deficiency to avoid both hypoadrenalism and an inhibitory effect on growth. Also, somatropin administration may alter the clearance of compounds known to be metabolized by CYP450 liver enzymes (eg, corticosteroids). Careful monitoring is advisable when somatropin is administered in combination with other drugs known to be metabolized by CYP450 liver enzymes).

No products indexed under this heading.

Dexamethasone Sodium (Somatropin inhibits 11β-hydroxysteroid dehydrogenase type 1 (11βHSD-1) in adipose/hepatic tissue and may significantly impact the metabolism of cortisol and cortisone. Patients treated with glucocorticoid replacement therapy for previously diagnosed hypoadrenalism may require an increase in their maintenance or stress doses; this may be especially true for patients treated with cortisone acetate and prednisone. In addition, excessive glucocorticoid therapy may attenuate the growth promoting effects of somatropin in children. Therefore, glucocorticoid replacement therapy should be carefully adjusted in children with concomitant GH and glucocorticoid deficiency to avoid both hypoadrenalism and an inhibitory effect on growth. Also, somatropin administration may alter the clearance of compounds known to be metabolized by CYP450 liver enzymes (eg, corticosteroids). Careful monitoring is advisable when somatropin is administered in combination with other drugs known to be metabolized by CYP450 liver enzymes).

No products indexed under this heading.

Dexamethasone Sodium Phosphate (Somatropin inhibits 11β-hydroxysteroid dehydrogenase type 1 (11βHSD-1) in adipose/hepatic tissue and may significantly impact the metabolism of cortisol and cortisone. Patients treated with glucocorticoid replacement therapy for previously diagnosed hypoadrenalism may require an increase in their maintenance or stress doses; this may be especially true for patients treated with cortisone acetate and prednisone. In addition, excessive glucocorticoid therapy may attenuate the growth promoting effects of somatropin in children. Therefore, glucocorticoid replacement therapy should be carefully adjusted in children with concomitant GH and glucocorticoid deficiency to avoid both hypoadrenalism and an inhibitory effect on growth. Also, somatropin administration may alter the clearance of compounds known to be metabolized by CYP450 liver enzymes (eg, corticosteroids). Careful monitoring is advisable when somatropin is administered in combination with other drugs known to be metabolized by CYP450 liver enzymes).

No products indexed under this heading.

Dexamethasone Sodium Phosphate Injection (Somatropin inhibits 11β-hydroxysteroid dehydrogenase type 1 (11βHSD-1) in adipose/hepatic tissue and may significantly impact the metabolism of cortisol and cortisone. Patients treated with glucocorticoid replacement therapy for previously diagnosed hypoadrenalism may require an increase in their maintenance or stress doses; this may be especially true for patients treated with cortisone acetate and prednisone. In addition, excessive glucocorticoid therapy may attenuate the growth promoting effects of somatropin in children. Therefore, glucocorticoid replacement therapy should be carefully adjusted in children with concomitant GH and glucocorticoid deficiency to avoid both hypoadrenalism and an inhibitory effect on growth. Also, somatropin administration may alter the clearance of compounds known to be

(⊙ Described in PDR® for Ophthalmic Medicines)

metabolized by CYP450 liver enzymes (eg, corticosteroids). Careful monitoring is advisable when somatropin is administered in combination with other drugs known to be metabolized by CYP450 liver enzymes).

No products indexed under this heading.

Dexfenfluramine Hydrochloride (Limited published data indicates that somatropin treatment increases cytochrome P450 (CYP450)-mediated antipyrine clearance in man. These data suggest that somatropin administration may alter the clearance of compounds metabolized by CYP450 liver enzymes. Careful monitoring is advisable when somatropin is administered in combination with other drugs known to be metabolized by CYP450 liver enzymes).

No products indexed under this heading.

Dextromethorphan (Limited published data indicates that somatropin treatment increases cytochrome P450 (CYP450)-mediated antipyrine clearance in man. These data suggest that somatropin administration may alter the clearance of compounds metabolized by CYP450 liver enzymes. Careful monitoring is advisable when somatropin is administered in combination with other drugs known to be metabolized by CYP450 liver enzymes).

No products indexed under this heading.

Dextromethorphan Hydrobromide (Limited published data indicates that somatropin treatment increases cytochrome P450 (CYP450)-mediated antipyrine clearance in man. These data suggest that somatropin administration may alter the clearance of compounds metabolized by CYP450 liver enzymes. Careful monitoring is advisable when somatropin is administered in combination with other drugs known to be metabolized by CYP450 liver enzymes).

No products indexed under this heading.

Dextromethorphan Polistirex (Limited published data indicates that somatropin treatment increases cytochrome P450 (CYP450)-mediated antipyrine clearance in man. These data suggest that somatropin administration may alter the clearance of compounds metabolized by CYP450 liver enzymes. Careful monitoring is advisable when somatropin is administered in combination with other drugs known to be metabolized by CYP450 liver enzymes).

No products indexed under this heading.

Diazepam (Limited published data indicates that somatropin treatment increases cytochrome P450 (CYP450)-mediated antipyrine clearance in man. These data suggest that somatropin administration may alter the clearance of compounds metabolized by CYP450 liver enzymes. Careful monitoring is advisable when somatropin is administered in combination with other drugs known to be metabolized by CYP450 liver enzymes). Products include:
Valium Tablets 2880

Diclofenac Potassium (Limited published data indicates that somatropin treatment increases cytochrome P450 (CYP450)-mediated antipyrine clearance in man. These data suggest that somatropin administration may alter the clearance of compounds metabolized by CYP450 liver enzymes. Careful monitoring is advisable when somatropin is administered in combination with other drugs known to be metabolized by CYP450 liver enzymes).

No products indexed under this heading.

Diclofenac Sodium (Limited published data indicates that somatropin treatment increases cytochrome P450 (CYP450)-mediated antipyrine clearance in man. These data suggest that somatropin administration may alter the clear-

ance of compounds metabolized by CYP450 liver enzymes. Careful monitoring is advisable when somatropin is administered in combination with other drugs known to be metabolized by CYP450 liver enzymes).

No products indexed under this heading.

Dienestrol (In patients on oral estrogen replacement, a larger dose of somatropin may be required to achieve the defined treatment goal).

No products indexed under this heading.

Diethylstilbestrol (In patients on oral estrogen replacement, a larger dose of somatropin may be required to achieve the defined treatment goal).

No products indexed under this heading.

Diflorasone Diacetate (Somatropin inhibits 11β-hydroxysteroid dehydrogenase type 1 (11βHSD-1) in adipose/hepatic tissue and may significantly impact the metabolism of cortisol and cortisone. Patients treated with glucocorticoid replacement therapy for previously diagnosed hypoadrenalism may require an increase in their maintenance or stress doses; this may be especially true for patients treated with cortisone acetate and prednisone. In addition, excessive glucocorticoid therapy may attenuate the growth promoting effects of somatropin in children. Therefore, glucocorticoid replacement therapy should be carefully adjusted in children with concomitant GH and glucocorticoid deficiency to avoid both hypoadrenalism and an inhibitory effect on growth. Also, somatropin administration may alter the clearance of compounds known to be metabolized by CYP450 liver enzymes (eg, corticosteroids). Careful monitoring is advisable when somatropin is administered in combination with other drugs known to be metabolized by CYP450 liver enzymes).

No products indexed under this heading.

Dihydroergotamine Mesylate (Limited published data indicates that somatropin treatment increases cytochrome P450 (CYP450)-mediated antipyrine clearance in man. These data suggest that somatropin administration may alter the clearance of compounds metabolized by CYP450 liver enzymes. Careful monitoring is advisable when somatropin is administered in combination with other drugs known to be metabolized by CYP450 liver enzymes).

No products indexed under this heading.

Diltiazem Hydrochloride (Limited published data indicates that somatropin treatment increases cytochrome P450 (CYP450)-mediated antipyrine clearance in man. These data suggest that somatropin administration may alter the clearance of compounds metabolized by CYP450 liver enzymes. Careful monitoring is advisable when somatropin is administered in combination with other drugs known to be metabolized by CYP450 liver enzymes). Products include:
Cardizem LA 423

Diltiazem Maleate (Limited published data indicates that somatropin treatment increases cytochrome P450 (CYP450)-mediated antipyrine clearance in man. These data suggest that somatropin administration may alter the clearance of compounds metabolized by CYP450 liver enzymes. Careful monitoring is advisable when somatropin is administered in combination with other drugs known to be metabolized by CYP450 liver enzymes).

No products indexed under this heading.

Disopyramide (Limited published data indicates that somatropin treatment increases cytochrome P450 (CYP450)-mediated antipyrine clearance in man. These data suggest that somatropin administration may alter the clear-

ance of compounds metabolized by CYP450 liver enzymes. Careful monitoring is advisable when somatropin is administered in combination with other drugs known to be metabolized by CYP450 liver enzymes).

No products indexed under this heading.

Disopyramide Phosphate (Limited published data indicates that somatropin treatment increases cytochrome P450 (CYP450)-mediated antipyrine clearance in man. These data suggest that somatropin administration may alter the clearance of compounds metabolized by CYP450 liver enzymes. Careful monitoring is advisable when somatropin is administered in combination with other drugs known to be metabolized by CYP450 liver enzymes).

No products indexed under this heading.

Disulfiram (Limited published data indicates that somatropin treatment increases cytochrome P450 (CYP450)-mediated antipyrine clearance in man. These data suggest that somatropin administration may alter the clearance of compounds metabolized by CYP450 liver enzymes. Careful monitoring is advisable when somatropin is administered in combination with other drugs known to be metabolized by CYP450 liver enzymes).

No products indexed under this heading.

Divalproex Sodium (Limited published data indicates that somatropin treatment increases cytochrome P450 (CYP450)-mediated antipyrine clearance in man. These data suggest that somatropin administration may alter the clearance of compounds metabolized by CYP450 liver enzymes (eg, anticonvulsants). Careful monitoring is advisable when somatropin is administered in combination with other drugs known to be metabolized by CYP450 liver enzymes). Products include:
Depakote ER 426

Docetaxel (Limited published data indicates that somatropin treatment increases cytochrome P450 (CYP450)-mediated antipyrine clearance in man. These data suggest that somatropin administration may alter the clearance of compounds metabolized by CYP450 liver enzymes. Careful monitoring is advisable when somatropin is administered in combination with other drugs known to be metabolized by CYP450 liver enzymes). Products include:
Taxotere 3035

Dolasetron Mesylate (Limited published data indicates that somatropin treatment increases cytochrome P450 (CYP450)-mediated antipyrine clearance in man. These data suggest that somatropin administration may alter the clearance of compounds metabolized by CYP450 liver enzymes. Careful monitoring is advisable when somatropin is administered in combination with other drugs known to be metabolized by CYP450 liver enzymes). Products include:
Anzemet Injection 2931
Anzemet Tablets 2934

Donepezil Hydrochloride (Limited published data indicates that somatropin treatment increases cytochrome P450 (CYP450)-mediated antipyrine clearance in man. These data suggest that somatropin administration may alter the clearance of compounds metabolized by CYP450 liver enzymes. Careful monitoring is advisable when somatropin is administered in combination with other drugs known to be metabolized by CYP450 liver enzymes). Products include:
Aricept 1045
Aricept ODT 1045

Doxepin Hydrochloride (Limited published data indicates that somatropin treatment increases cytochrome P450 (CYP450)-mediated antipyrine clearance in man. These data suggest that somatropin administration may alter the clearance of compounds metabolized by CYP450 liver enzymes. Careful monitoring is advisable when somatropin is administered in combination with other drugs known to be metabolized by CYP450 liver enzymes).

No products indexed under this heading.

Doxorubicin Hydrochloride (Limited published data indicates that somatropin treatment increases cytochrome P450 (CYP450)-mediated antipyrine clearance in man. These data suggest that somatropin administration may alter the clearance of compounds metabolized by CYP450 liver enzymes. Careful monitoring is advisable when somatropin is administered in combination with other drugs known to be metabolized by CYP450 liver enzymes).

No products indexed under this heading.

Dronabinol (Limited published data indicates that somatropin treatment increases cytochrome P450 (CYP450)-mediated antipyrine clearance in man. These data suggest that somatropin administration may alter the clearance of compounds metabolized by CYP450 liver enzymes. Careful monitoring is advisable when somatropin is administered in combination with other drugs known to be metabolized by CYP450 liver enzymes).

No products indexed under this heading.

Drugs that Undergo Biotransformation by Cytochrome P-450 Mixed Function Oxidase (Limited published data indicates that somatropin treatment increases cytochrome P450 (CYP450)-mediated antipyrine clearance in man. These data suggest that somatropin administration may alter the clearance of compounds metabolized by CYP450 liver enzymes. Careful monitoring is advisable when somatropin is administered in combination with other drugs known to be metabolized by CYP450 liver enzymes).

No products indexed under this heading.

Dyphylline (Limited published data indicates that somatropin treatment increases cytochrome P450 (CYP450)-mediated antipyrine clearance in man. These data suggest that somatropin administration may alter the clearance of compounds metabolized by CYP450 liver enzymes. Careful monitoring is advisable when somatropin is administered in combination with other drugs known to be metabolized by CYP450 liver enzymes).

No products indexed under this heading.

Encainide Hydrochloride (Limited published data indicates that somatropin treatment increases cytochrome P450 (CYP450)-mediated antipyrine clearance in man. These data suggest that somatropin administration may alter the clearance of compounds metabolized by CYP450 liver enzymes. Careful monitoring is advisable when somatropin is administered in combination with other drugs known to be metabolized by CYP450 liver enzymes).

No products indexed under this heading.

Enoxacin (Limited published data indicates that somatropin treatment increases cytochrome P450 (CYP450)-mediated antipyrine clearance in man. These data suggest that somatropin administration may alter the clearance of compounds metabolized by CYP450 liver enzymes. Careful monitoring is advisable when somatropin is administered in combination with other drugs known to be metabolized by CYP450 liver enzymes).

No products indexed under this heading.

IMPORTANT NOTE: Always consult each drug listing in the patient's regimen for possible interactions.

Genotropin Interactions Index 754

Eprosartan Mesylate (Limited published data indicates that somatropin treatment increases cytochrome P450 (CYP450)-mediated antipyrine clearance in man. These data suggest that somatropin administration may alter the clearance of compounds metabolized by CYP450 liver enzymes. Careful monitoring is advisable when somatropin is administered in combination with other drugs known to be metabolized by CYP450 liver enzymes). Products include:
Teveten 538
Teveten HCT 541

Ergotamine Tartrate (Limited published data indicates that somatropin treatment increases cytochrome P450 (CYP450)-mediated antipyrine clearance in man. These data suggest that somatropin administration may alter the clearance of compounds metabolized by CYP450 liver enzymes. Careful monitoring is advisable when somatropin is administered in combination with other drugs known to be metabolized by CYP450 liver enzymes).
No products indexed under this heading.

Erythromycin (Limited published data indicates that somatropin treatment increases cytochrome P450 (CYP450)-mediated antipyrine clearance in man. These data suggest that somatropin administration may alter the clearance of compounds metabolized by CYP450 liver enzymes. Careful monitoring is advisable when somatropin is administered in combination with other drugs known to be metabolized by CYP450 liver enzymes).
No products indexed under this heading.

Erythromycin Estolate (Limited published data indicates that somatropin treatment increases cytochrome P450 (CYP450)-mediated antipyrine clearance in man. These data suggest that somatropin administration may alter the clearance of compounds metabolized by CYP450 liver enzymes. Careful monitoring is advisable when somatropin is administered in combination with other drugs known to be metabolized by CYP450 liver enzymes).
No products indexed under this heading.

Erythromycin Ethylsuccinate (Limited published data indicates that somatropin treatment increases cytochrome P450 (CYP450)-mediated antipyrine clearance in man. These data suggest that somatropin administration may alter the clearance of compounds metabolized by CYP450 liver enzymes. Careful monitoring is advisable when somatropin is administered in combination with other drugs known to be metabolized by CYP450 liver enzymes). Products include:
E.E.S. 437
EryPed 435

Erythromycin Gluceptate (Limited published data indicates that somatropin treatment increases cytochrome P450 (CYP450)-mediated antipyrine clearance in man. These data suggest that somatropin administration may alter the clearance of compounds metabolized by CYP450 liver enzymes. Careful monitoring is advisable when somatropin is administered in combination with other drugs known to be metabolized by CYP450 liver enzymes).
No products indexed under this heading.

Erythromycin Lactobionate (Limited published data indicates that somatropin treatment increases cytochrome P450 (CYP450)-mediated antipyrine clearance in man. These data suggest that somatropin administration may alter the clearance of compounds metabolized by CYP450 liver enzymes. Careful monitoring is advisable when somatropin is administered in combination with other drugs known to be metabolized by CYP450 liver enzymes).
No products indexed under this heading.

Erythromycin Stearate (Limited published data indicates that somatropin treatment increases cytochrome P450 (CYP450)-mediated antipyrine clearance in man. These data suggest that somatropin administration may alter the clearance of compounds metabolized by CYP450 liver enzymes. Careful monitoring is advisable when somatropin is administered in combination with other drugs known to be metabolized by CYP450 liver enzymes).
No products indexed under this heading.

Esomeprazole Magnesium (Limited published data indicates that somatropin treatment increases cytochrome P450 (CYP450)-mediated antipyrine clearance in man. These data suggest that somatropin administration may alter the clearance of compounds metabolized by CYP450 liver enzymes. Careful monitoring is advisable when somatropin is administered in combination with other drugs known to be metabolized by CYP450 liver enzymes). Products include:
Nexium Capsules 704
Nexium Oral Suspension 704

Esomeprazole Sodium (Limited published data indicates that somatropin treatment increases cytochrome P450 (CYP450)-mediated antipyrine clearance in man. These data suggest that somatropin administration may alter the clearance of compounds metabolized by CYP450 liver enzymes. Careful monitoring is advisable when somatropin is administered in combination with other drugs known to be metabolized by CYP450 liver enzymes). Products include:
Nexium I.V. 712

Estradiol (Limited published data indicates that somatropin treatment increases cytochrome P450 (CYP450)-mediated antipyrine clearance in man. These data suggest that somatropin administration may alter the clearance of compounds metabolized by CYP450 liver enzymes (eg, sex steroids). Careful monitoring is advisable when somatropin is administered in combination with other drugs known to be metabolized by CYP450 liver enzymes). Products include:
Activella 2561
Angeliq 831
Climara 841
Climara Pro 847
Divigel 3467
Estrasorb 1777
Vagifem 2589

Estradiol Benzoate (Limited published data indicates that somatropin treatment increases cytochrome P450 (CYP450)-mediated antipyrine clearance in man. These data suggest that somatropin administration may alter the clearance of compounds metabolized by CYP450 liver enzymes. Careful monitoring is advisable when somatropin is administered in combination with other drugs known to be metabolized by CYP450 liver enzymes).
No products indexed under this heading.

Estradiol Cypionate (Limited published data indicates that somatropin treatment increases cytochrome P450 (CYP450)-mediated antipyrine clearance in man. These data suggest that somatropin administration may alter the clearance of compounds metabolized by CYP450 liver enzymes. Careful monitoring is advisable when somatropin is administered in combination with other drugs known to be metabolized by CYP450 liver enzymes).
No products indexed under this heading.

Estradiol Valerate (Limited published data indicates that somatropin treatment increases cytochrome P450 (CYP450)-mediated antipyrine clearance in man. These data suggest that somatropin administration may alter the clearance of compounds metabolized by CYP450 liver enzymes. Careful monitoring is advisable when somatropin is administered in combination with other drugs known to be metabolized by CYP450 liver enzymes).
No products indexed under this heading.

Estrogen (Limited published data indicates that somatropin treatment increases cytochrome P450 (CYP450)-mediated antipyrine clearance in man. These data suggest that somatropin administration may alter the clearance of compounds metabolized by CYP450 liver enzymes. Careful monitoring is advisable when somatropin is administered in combination with other drugs known to be metabolized by CYP450 liver enzymes).
No products indexed under this heading.

Estrogens, Conjugated (Limited published data indicates that somatropin treatment increases cytochrome P450 (CYP450)-mediated antipyrine clearance in man. These data suggest that somatropin administration may alter the clearance of compounds metabolized by CYP450 liver enzymes (eg, sex steroids). Careful monitoring is advisable when somatropin is administered in combination with other drugs known to be metabolized by CYP450 liver enzymes). Products include:
Premarin Intravenous 3528
Premarin Tablets 3533
Premarin Vaginal Cream 3540
Premphase 3549
Prempro 3549

Estrogens, Conjugated, Synthetic A (Limited published data indicates that somatropin treatment increases cytochrome P450 (CYP450)-mediated antipyrine clearance in man. These data suggest that somatropin administration may alter the clearance of compounds metabolized by CYP450 liver enzymes. Careful monitoring is advisable when somatropin is administered in combination with other drugs known to be metabolized by CYP450 liver enzymes).
No products indexed under this heading.

Estrogens, Esterified (In patients on oral estrogen replacement, a larger dose of somatropin may be required to achieve the defined treatment goal).
No products indexed under this heading.

Estropipate (In patients on oral estrogen replacement, a larger dose of somatropin may be required to achieve the defined treatment goal).
No products indexed under this heading.

Ethinyl Estradiol (Limited published data indicates that somatropin treatment increases cytochrome P450 (CYP450)-mediated antipyrine clearance in man. These data suggest that somatropin administration may alter the clearance of compounds metabolized by CYP450 liver enzymes (eg, sex steroids). Careful monitoring is advisable when somatropin is administered in combination with other drugs known to be metabolized by CYP450 liver enzymes). Products include:
LoSeasonique 3407
Lybrel 3514
NuvaRing 3181
Ortho Evra 2648
Ortho-Cyclen/Ortho Tri-Cyclen 2663
Ortho Tri-Cyclen Lo Tablets 2673
Seasonique 3418
Yaz 864

Ethosuximide (Limited published data indicates that somatropin treatment increases cytochrome P450 (CYP450)-mediated antipyrine clearance in man. These data suggest that somatropin administration may alter the clearance of compounds metabolized by CYP450 liver enzymes (eg, anticonvulsants). Careful monitoring is advisable when somatropin is administered in combination with other drugs known to be metabolized by CYP450 liver enzymes).
No products indexed under this heading.

Ethotoin (Limited published data indicates that somatropin treatment increases cytochrome P450 (CYP450)-mediated antipyrine clearance in man. These data suggest that somatropin administration may alter the clearance of compounds metabolized by CYP450 liver enzymes (eg, anticonvulsants). Careful monitoring is advisable when somatropin is administered in combination with other drugs known to be metabolized by CYP450 liver enzymes).
No products indexed under this heading.

Ethynodiol Diacetate (Limited published data indicates that somatropin treatment increases cytochrome P450 (CYP450)-mediated antipyrine clearance in man. These data suggest that somatropin administration may alter the clearance of compounds metabolized by CYP450 liver enzymes (eg, sex steroids). Careful monitoring is advisable when somatropin is administered in combination with other drugs known to be metabolized by CYP450 liver enzymes).
No products indexed under this heading.

Etodolac (Limited published data indicates that somatropin treatment increases cytochrome P450 (CYP450)-mediated antipyrine clearance in man. These data suggest that somatropin administration may alter the clearance of compounds metabolized by CYP450 liver enzymes. Careful monitoring is advisable when somatropin is administered in combination with other drugs known to be metabolized by CYP450 liver enzymes).
No products indexed under this heading.

Etoposide (Limited published data indicates that somatropin treatment increases cytochrome P450 (CYP450)-mediated antipyrine clearance in man. These data suggest that somatropin administration may alter the clearance of compounds metabolized by CYP450 liver enzymes. Careful monitoring is advisable when somatropin is administered in combination with other drugs known to be metabolized by CYP450 liver enzymes).
No products indexed under this heading.

Etoposide Phosphate (Limited published data indicates that somatropin treatment increases cytochrome P450 (CYP450)-mediated antipyrine clearance in man. These data suggest that somatropin administration may alter the clearance of compounds metabolized by CYP450 liver enzymes. Careful monitoring is advisable when somatropin is administered in combination with other drugs known to be metabolized by CYP450 liver enzymes).
No products indexed under this heading.

Felbamate (Limited published data indicates that somatropin treatment increases cytochrome P450 (CYP450)-mediated antipyrine clearance in man. These data suggest that somatropin administration may alter the clearance of compounds metabolized by CYP450 liver enzymes (eg, anticonvulsants). Careful monitoring is advisable when somatropin is administered in combination with other drugs known to be metabolized by CYP450 liver enzymes).
No products indexed under this heading.

Felodipine (Limited published data indicates that somatropin treatment increases cytochrome P450

(CYP450)-mediated antipyrine clearance in man. These data suggest that somatropin administration may alter the clearance of compounds metabolized by CYP450 liver enzymes. Careful monitoring is advisable when somatropin is administered in combination with other drugs known to be metabolized by CYP450 liver enzymes).
No products indexed under this heading.

Fenoprofen Calcium (Limited published data indicates that somatropin treatment increases cytochrome P450 (CYP450)-mediated antipyrine clearance in man. These data suggest that somatropin administration may alter the clearance of compounds metabolized by CYP450 liver enzymes. Careful monitoring is advisable when somatropin is administered in combination with other drugs known to be metabolized by CYP450 liver enzymes).
No products indexed under this heading.

Fentanyl (Limited published data indicates that somatropin treatment increases cytochrome P450 (CYP450)-mediated antipyrine clearance in man. These data suggest that somatropin administration may alter the clearance of compounds metabolized by CYP450 liver enzymes. Careful monitoring is advisable when somatropin is administered in combination with other drugs known to be metabolized by CYP450 liver enzymes). Products include:

Duragesic **2604**
Fentanyl Transdermal System **2346**
Onsolis **2054**

Fentanyl Citrate (Limited published data indicates that somatropin treatment increases cytochrome P450 (CYP450)-mediated antipyrine clearance in man. These data suggest that somatropin administration may alter the clearance of compounds metabolized by CYP450 liver enzymes. Careful monitoring is advisable when somatropin is administered in combination with other drugs known to be metabolized by CYP450 liver enzymes). Products include:

Fentora **966**

Flecainide Acetate (Limited published data indicates that somatropin treatment increases cytochrome P450 (CYP450)-mediated antipyrine clearance in man. These data suggest that somatropin administration may alter the clearance of compounds metabolized by CYP450 liver enzymes. Careful monitoring is advisable when somatropin is administered in combination with other drugs known to be metabolized by CYP450 liver enzymes).
No products indexed under this heading.

Fludrocortisone Acetate (Somatropin inhibits 11β-hydroxysteroid dehydrogenase type 1 (11βHSD-1) in adipose/hepatic tissue and may significantly impact the metabolism of cortisol and cortisone. Patients treated with glucocorticoid replacement therapy for previously diagnosed hypoadrenalism may require an increase in their maintenance or stress doses; this may be especially true for patients treated with cortisone acetate and prednisone. In addition, excessive glucocorticoid therapy may attenuate the growth promoting effects of somatropin in children. Therefore, glucocorticoid replacement therapy should be carefully adjusted in children with concomitant GH and glucocorticoid deficiency to avoid both hypoadrenalism and an inhibitory effect on growth. Also, somatropin administration may alter the clearance of compounds known to be metabolized by CYP450 liver enzymes (eg, corticosteroids). Careful monitoring is advisable when somatropin is administered in combination with other drugs known to be metabolized by CYP450 liver enzymes).
No products indexed under this heading.

Flumethasone Pivalate (Somatropin inhibits 11β-hydroxysteroid dehydrogenase type 1 (11βHSD-1) in adipose/hepatic tissue and may significantly impact the metabolism of cortisol and cortisone. Patients treated with glucocorticoid replacement therapy for previously diagnosed hypoadrenalism may require an increase in their maintenance or stress doses; this may be especially true for patients treated with cortisone acetate and prednisone. In addition, excessive glucocorticoid therapy may attenuate the growth promoting effects of somatropin in children. Therefore, glucocorticoid replacement therapy should be carefully adjusted in children with concomitant GH and glucocorticoid deficiency to avoid both hypoadrenalism and an inhibitory effect on growth. Also, somatropin administration may alter the clearance of compounds known to be metabolized by CYP450 liver enzymes (eg, corticosteroids). Careful monitoring is advisable when somatropin is administered in combination with other drugs known to be metabolized by CYP450 liver enzymes).
No products indexed under this heading.

Flunisolide Hemihydrate (Somatropin inhibits 11β-hydroxysteroid dehydrogenase type 1 (11βHSD-1) in adipose/hepatic tissue and may significantly impact the metabolism of cortisol and cortisone. Patients treated with glucocorticoid replacement therapy for previously diagnosed hypoadrenalism may require an increase in their maintenance or stress doses; this may be especially true for patients treated with cortisone acetate and prednisone. In addition, excessive glucocorticoid therapy may attenuate the growth promoting effects of somatropin in children. Therefore, glucocorticoid replacement therapy should be carefully adjusted in children with concomitant GH and glucocorticoid deficiency to avoid both hypoadrenalism and an inhibitory effect on growth. Also, somatropin administration may alter the clearance of compounds known to be metabolized by CYP450 liver enzymes (eg, corticosteroids). Careful monitoring is advisable when somatropin is administered in combination with other drugs known to be metabolized by CYP450 liver enzymes).
No products indexed under this heading.

Fluoxetine (Limited published data indicates that somatropin treatment increases cytochrome P450 (CYP450)-mediated antipyrine clearance in man. These data suggest that somatropin administration may alter the clearance of compounds metabolized by CYP450 liver enzymes. Careful monitoring is advisable when somatropin is administered in combination with other drugs known to be metabolized by CYP450 liver enzymes).
No products indexed under this heading.

Fluoxetine Hydrochloride (Limited published data indicates that somatropin treatment increases cytochrome P450 (CYP450)-mediated antipyrine clearance in man. These data suggest that somatropin administration may alter the clearance of compounds metabolized by CYP450 liver enzymes. Careful monitoring is advisable when somatropin is administered in combination with other drugs known to be metabolized by CYP450 liver enzymes). Products include:

Prozac Weekly **1941**
Prozac Pulvules **1941**
Symbyax **1965**

Fluoxymesterone (Limited published data indicates that somatropin treatment increases cytochrome P450 (CYP450)-mediated antipyrine clearance in man. These data suggest that somatropin administration may alter the clearance of compounds metabolized by CYP450 liver enzymes (eg, sex steroids). Careful monitoring is advisable when somatropin is administered in combination with other drugs known to be metabolized by CYP450 liver enzymes).
No products indexed under this heading.

Fluphenazine Decanoate (Limited published data indicates that somatropin treatment increases cytochrome P450 (CYP450)-mediated antipyrine clearance in man. These data suggest that somatropin administration may alter the clearance of compounds metabolized by CYP450 liver enzymes. Careful monitoring is advisable when somatropin is administered in combination with other drugs known to be metabolized by CYP450 liver enzymes).
No products indexed under this heading.

Fluphenazine Enanthate (Limited published data indicates that somatropin treatment increases cytochrome P450 (CYP450)-mediated antipyrine clearance in man. These data suggest that somatropin administration may alter the clearance of compounds metabolized by CYP450 liver enzymes. Careful monitoring is advisable when somatropin is administered in combination with other drugs known to be metabolized by CYP450 liver enzymes).
No products indexed under this heading.

Fluphenazine Hydrochloride (Limited published data indicates that somatropin treatment increases cytochrome P450 (CYP450)-mediated antipyrine clearance in man. These data suggest that somatropin administration may alter the clearance of compounds metabolized by CYP450 liver enzymes. Careful monitoring is advisable when somatropin is administered in combination with other drugs known to be metabolized by CYP450 liver enzymes).
No products indexed under this heading.

Flurbiprofen (Limited published data indicates that somatropin treatment increases cytochrome P450 (CYP450)-mediated antipyrine clearance in man. These data suggest that somatropin administration may alter the clearance of compounds metabolized by CYP450 liver enzymes. Careful monitoring is advisable when somatropin is administered in combination with other drugs known to be metabolized by CYP450 liver enzymes).
No products indexed under this heading.

Flurbiprofen Sodium (Limited published data indicates that somatropin treatment increases cytochrome P450 (CYP450)-mediated antipyrine clearance in man. These data suggest that somatropin administration may alter the clearance of compounds metabolized by CYP450 liver enzymes. Careful monitoring is advisable when somatropin is administered in combination with other drugs known to be metabolized by CYP450 liver enzymes).
No products indexed under this heading.

Flutamide (Limited published data indicates that somatropin treatment increases cytochrome P450 (CYP450)-mediated antipyrine clearance in man. These data suggest that somatropin administration may alter the clearance of compounds metabolized by CYP450 liver enzymes. Careful monitoring is advisable when somatropin is administered in combination with other drugs known to be metabolized by CYP450 liver enzymes).
No products indexed under this heading.

Fluticasone Furoate (Somatropin inhibits 11β-hydroxysteroid dehydrogenase type 1 (11βHSD-1) in adipose/hepatic tissue and may significantly impact the metabolism of cortisol and cortisone. Patients treated with glucocorticoid replacement therapy for previously diagnosed hypoadrenalism may require an increase in their maintenance or stress doses; this may be especially true for patients treated with cortisone acetate and prednisone. In addition, excessive glucocorticoid therapy may attenuate the growth promoting effects of somatropin in children. Therefore, glucocorticoid replacement therapy should be carefully adjusted in children with concomitant GH and glucocorticoid deficiency to avoid both hypoadrenalism and an inhibitory effect on growth. Also, somatropin administration may alter the clearance of compounds known to be metabolized by CYP450 liver enzymes (eg, corticosteroids). Careful monitoring is advisable when somatropin is administered in combination with other drugs known to be metabolized by CYP450 liver enzymes). Products include:

Veramyst **1713**

Fluticasone Propionate (Somatropin inhibits 11β-hydroxysteroid dehydrogenase type 1 (11βHSD-1) in adipose/hepatic tissue and may significantly impact the metabolism of cortisol and cortisone. Patients treated with glucocorticoid replacement therapy for previously diagnosed hypoadrenalism may require an increase in their maintenance or stress doses; this may be especially true for patients treated with cortisone acetate and prednisone. In addition, excessive glucocorticoid therapy may attenuate the growth promoting effects of somatropin in children. Therefore, glucocorticoid replacement therapy should be carefully adjusted in children with concomitant GH and glucocorticoid deficiency to avoid both hypoadrenalism and an inhibitory effect on growth. Also, somatropin administration may alter the clearance of compounds known to be metabolized by CYP450 liver enzymes (eg, corticosteroids). Careful monitoring is advisable when somatropin is administered in combination with other drugs known to be metabolized by CYP450 liver enzymes). Products include:

Advair 100/50 .... **1275**
Advair 250/50 .... **1275**
Advair 500/50 .... **1275**
Advair HFA 45/21 .... **1288**
Advair HFA 115/21 .... **1288**
Advair HFA 230/21 .... **1288**
Flonase **1459**
Flovent Diskus **1463**
Flovent HFA **1470**

Fluvastatin Sodium (Limited published data indicates that somatropin treatment increases cytochrome P450 (CYP450)-mediated antipyrine clearance in man. These data suggest that somatropin administration may alter the clearance of compounds metabolized by CYP450 liver enzymes. Careful monitoring is advisable when somatropin is administered in combination with other drugs known to be metabolized by CYP450 liver enzymes).
No products indexed under this heading.

Fluvoxamine Maleate (Limited published data indicates that somatropin treatment increases cytochrome P450 (CYP450)-mediated antipyrine clearance in man. These data suggest that somatropin administration may alter the clearance of compounds metabolized by CYP450 liver enzymes. Careful monitoring is advisable when somatropin is administered in combination with other drugs known to be metabolized by CYP450 liver enzymes).
No products indexed under this heading.

Formoterol Fumarate (Limited published data indicates that somatropin treatment increases cytochrome P450 (CYP450)-mediated antipyrine clearance

IMPORTANT NOTE: Always consult each drug listing in the patient's regimen for possible interactions.

Genotropin Interactions Index 756

in man. These data suggest that somatropin administration may alter the clearance of compounds metabolized by CYP450 liver enzymes. Careful monitoring is advisable when somatropin is administered in combination with other drugs known to be metabolized by CYP450 liver enzymes). Products include:
Foradil 3121
Perforomist 3634

Fosphenytoin (Limited published data indicates that somatropin treatment increases cytochrome P450 (CYP450)-mediated antipyrine clearance in man. These data suggest that somatropin administration may alter the clearance of compounds metabolized by CYP450 liver enzymes (eg, anticonvulsants). Careful monitoring is advisable when somatropin is administered in combination with other drugs known to be metabolized by CYP450 liver enzymes).
No products indexed under this heading.

Fosphenytoin Sodium (Limited published data indicates that somatropin treatment increases cytochrome P450 (CYP450)-mediated antipyrine clearance in man. These data suggest that somatropin administration may alter the clearance of compounds metabolized by CYP450 liver enzymes (eg, anticonvulsants). Careful monitoring is advisable when somatropin is administered in combination with other drugs known to be metabolized by CYP450 liver enzymes).
No products indexed under this heading.

Gabapentin (Limited published data indicates that somatropin treatment increases cytochrome P450 (CYP450)-mediated antipyrine clearance in man. These data suggest that somatropin administration may alter the clearance of compounds metabolized by CYP450 liver enzymes (eg, anticonvulsants). Careful monitoring is advisable when somatropin is administered in combination with other drugs known to be metabolized by CYP450 liver enzymes).
No products indexed under this heading.

Galantamine Hydrobromide (Limited published data indicates that somatropin treatment increases cytochrome P450 (CYP450)-mediated antipyrine clearance in man. These data suggest that somatropin administration may alter the clearance of compounds metabolized by CYP450 liver enzymes. Careful monitoring is advisable when somatropin is administered in combination with other drugs known to be metabolized by CYP450 liver enzymes).
No products indexed under this heading.

Glibenclamide (In patients with diabetes mellitus requiring drug therapy, the dose of insulin and/or oral agent may require adjustment when somatropin therapy is initiated).
No products indexed under this heading.

Glimepiride (In patients with diabetes mellitus requiring drug therapy, the dose of insulin and/or oral agent may require adjustment when somatropin therapy is initiated). Products include:
Avandaryl 1356
Duetact 3354

Glipizide (In patients with diabetes mellitus requiring drug therapy, the dose of insulin and/or oral agent may require adjustment when somatropin therapy is initiated).
No products indexed under this heading.

Glyburide (In patients with diabetes mellitus requiring drug therapy, the dose of insulin and/or oral agent may require adjustment when somatropin therapy is initiated).
No products indexed under this heading.

Grepafloxacin Hydrochloride (Limited published data indicates that somatropin treatment increases cytochrome P450 (CYP450)-mediated antipyrine clearance in man. These data suggest that somatropin administration may alter the clearance of compounds metabolized by CYP450 liver enzymes. Careful monitoring is advisable when somatropin is administered in combination with other drugs known to be metabolized by CYP450 liver enzymes).
No products indexed under this heading.

Haloperidol (Limited published data indicates that somatropin treatment increases cytochrome P450 (CYP450)-mediated antipyrine clearance in man. These data suggest that somatropin administration may alter the clearance of compounds metabolized by CYP450 liver enzymes. Careful monitoring is advisable when somatropin is administered in combination with other drugs known to be metabolized by CYP450 liver enzymes).
No products indexed under this heading.

Haloperidol Decanoate (Limited published data indicates that somatropin treatment increases cytochrome P450 (CYP450)-mediated antipyrine clearance in man. These data suggest that somatropin administration may alter the clearance of compounds metabolized by CYP450 liver enzymes. Careful monitoring is advisable when somatropin is administered in combination with other drugs known to be metabolized by CYP450 liver enzymes).
No products indexed under this heading.

Haloperidol Lactate (Limited published data indicates that somatropin treatment increases cytochrome P450 (CYP450)-mediated antipyrine clearance in man. These data suggest that somatropin administration may alter the clearance of compounds metabolized by CYP450 liver enzymes. Careful monitoring is advisable when somatropin is administered in combination with other drugs known to be metabolized by CYP450 liver enzymes).
No products indexed under this heading.

Hexobarbital (Limited published data indicates that somatropin treatment increases cytochrome P450 (CYP450)-mediated antipyrine clearance in man. These data suggest that somatropin administration may alter the clearance of compounds metabolized by CYP450 liver enzymes. Careful monitoring is advisable when somatropin is administered in combination with other drugs known to be metabolized by CYP450 liver enzymes).
No products indexed under this heading.

Hydrocodone Bitartrate (Limited published data indicates that somatropin treatment increases cytochrome P450 (CYP450)-mediated antipyrine clearance in man. These data suggest that somatropin administration may alter the clearance of compounds metabolized by CYP450 liver enzymes. Careful monitoring is advisable when somatropin is administered in combination with other drugs known to be metabolized by CYP450 liver enzymes). Products include:
Vicodin 560
Vicodin ES 561
Vicodin HP 563
Vicoprofen 564
Zydone 1138

Hydrocortisone (Somatropin inhibits 11β-hydroxysteroid dehydrogenase type 1 (11βHSD-1) in adipose/hepatic tissue and may significantly impact the metabolism of cortisol and cortisone. Patients treated with glucocorticoid replacement therapy for previously diagnosed hypoadrenalism may require an increase in their maintenance or stress doses; this may be especially true for patients treated with cortisone acetate and prednisone. In addition, excessive glucocorticoid therapy may attenuate the growth promoting effects of somatropin in children. Therefore, glucocorticoid replacement therapy should be carefully adjusted in children with concomitant GH and glucocorticoid deficiency to avoid both hypoadrenalism and an inhibitory effect on growth. Also, somatropin administration may alter the clearance of compounds known to be metabolized by CYP450 liver enzymes (eg, corticosteroids). Careful monitoring is advisable when somatropin is administered in combination with other drugs known to be metabolized by CYP450 liver enzymes).
No products indexed under this heading.

Hydrocortisone (Alcohol) (Somatropin inhibits 11β-hydroxysteroid dehydrogenase type 1 (11βHSD-1) in adipose/hepatic tissue and may significantly impact the metabolism of cortisol and cortisone. Patients treated with glucocorticoid replacement therapy for previously diagnosed hypoadrenalism may require an increase in their maintenance or stress doses; this may be especially true for patients treated with cortisone acetate and prednisone. In addition, excessive glucocorticoid therapy may attenuate the growth promoting effects of somatropin in children. Therefore, glucocorticoid replacement therapy should be carefully adjusted in children with concomitant GH and glucocorticoid deficiency to avoid both hypoadrenalism and an inhibitory effect on growth. Also, somatropin administration may alter the clearance of compounds known to be metabolized by CYP450 liver enzymes (eg, corticosteroids). Careful monitoring is advisable when somatropin is administered in combination with other drugs known to be metabolized by CYP450 liver enzymes).
No products indexed under this heading.

Hydrocortisone Acetate (Somatropin inhibits 11β-hydroxysteroid dehydrogenase type 1 (11βHSD-1) in adipose/hepatic tissue and may significantly impact the metabolism of cortisol and cortisone. Patients treated with glucocorticoid replacement therapy for previously diagnosed hypoadrenalism may require an increase in their maintenance or stress doses; this may be especially true for patients treated with cortisone acetate and prednisone. In addition, excessive glucocorticoid therapy may attenuate the growth promoting effects of somatropin in children. Therefore, glucocorticoid replacement therapy should be carefully adjusted in children with concomitant GH and glucocorticoid deficiency to avoid both hypoadrenalism and an inhibitory effect on growth. Also, somatropin administration may alter the clearance of compounds known to be metabolized by CYP450 liver enzymes (eg, corticosteroids). Careful monitoring is advisable when somatropin is administered in combination with other drugs known to be metabolized by CYP450 liver enzymes).
No products indexed under this heading.

Hydrocortisone Butyrate (Somatropin inhibits 11β-hydroxysteroid dehydrogenase type 1 (11βHSD-1) in adipose/hepatic tissue and may significantly impact the metabolism of cortisol and cortisone. Patients treated with glucocorticoid replacement therapy for previously diagnosed hypoadrenalism may require an increase in their maintenance or stress doses; this may be especially true for patients treated with cortisone acetate and prednisone. In addition, excessive glucocorticoid therapy may attenuate the growth promoting effects of somatropin in children. Therefore, glucocorticoid replacement therapy should be carefully adjusted in children with concomitant GH and glucocorticoid deficiency to avoid both hypoadrenalism and an inhibitory effect on growth. Also, somatropin administration may alter the clearance of compounds known to be metabolized by CYP450 liver enzymes (eg, corticosteroids). Careful monitoring is advisable when somatropin is administered in combination with other drugs known to be metabolized by CYP450 liver enzymes).
No products indexed under this heading.

Hydrocortisone Cypionate (Somatropin inhibits 11β-hydroxysteroid dehydrogenase type 1 (11βHSD-1) in adipose/hepatic tissue and may significantly impact the metabolism of cortisol and cortisone. Patients treated with glucocorticoid replacement therapy for previously diagnosed hypoadrenalism may require an increase in their maintenance or stress doses; this may be especially true for patients treated with cortisone acetate and prednisone. In addition, excessive glucocorticoid therapy may attenuate the growth promoting effects of somatropin in children. Therefore, glucocorticoid replacement therapy should be carefully adjusted in children with concomitant GH and glucocorticoid deficiency to avoid both hypoadrenalism and an inhibitory effect on growth. Also, somatropin administration may alter the clearance of compounds known to be metabolized by CYP450 liver enzymes (eg, corticosteroids). Careful monitoring is advisable when somatropin is administered in combination with other drugs known to be metabolized by CYP450 liver enzymes).
No products indexed under this heading.

Hydrocortisone Hemisuccinate (Somatropin inhibits 11β-hydroxysteroid dehydrogenase type 1 (11βHSD-1) in adipose/hepatic tissue and may significantly impact the metabolism of cortisol and cortisone. Patients treated with glucocorticoid replacement therapy for previously diagnosed hypoadrenalism may require an increase in their maintenance or stress doses; this may be especially true for patients treated with cortisone acetate and prednisone. In addition, excessive glucocorticoid therapy may attenuate the growth promoting effects of somatropin in children. Therefore, glucocorticoid replacement therapy should be carefully adjusted in children with concomitant GH and glucocorticoid deficiency to avoid both hypoadrenalism and an inhibitory effect on growth. Also, somatropin administration may alter the clearance of compounds known to be metabolized by CYP450 liver enzymes (eg, corticosteroids). Careful monitoring is advisable when somatropin is administered in combination with other drugs known to be metabolized by CYP450 liver enzymes).
No products indexed under this heading.

Hydrocortisone Probutate (Somatropin inhibits 11β-hydroxysteroid dehydrogenase type 1 (11βHSD-1) in adipose/hepatic tissue and may significantly impact the metabolism of cortisol and cortisone. Patients treated with glucocorticoid replacement therapy for previously diagnosed hypoadrenalism may require an increase in their maintenance or stress doses; this may be especially true for patients treated with cortisone acetate and prednisone. In addition, excessive glucocorticoid therapy may attenuate the growth promoting effects of somatropin in children. Therefore, glucocorticoid replacement therapy should be carefully adjusted in children with concomitant GH and glucocorticoid deficiency to avoid both hypoadrenalism and an inhibitory effect on growth. Also, somatropin administration may alter the clearance of compounds known to be metabolized by CYP450

liver enzymes (eg, corticosteroids). Careful monitoring is advisable when somatropin is administered in combination with other drugs known to be metabolized by CYP450 liver enzymes).
No products indexed under this heading.

Hydrocortisone Sodium Phosphate (Somatropin inhibits 11β-hydroxysteroid dehydrogenase type 1 (11βHSD-1) in adipose/hepatic tissue and may significantly impact the metabolism of cortisol and cortisone. Patients treated with glucocorticoid replacement therapy for previously diagnosed hypoadrenalism may require an increase in their maintenance or stress doses; this may be especially true for patients treated with cortisone acetate and prednisone. In addition, excessive glucocorticoid therapy may attenuate the growth promoting effects of somatropin in children. Therefore, glucocorticoid replacement therapy should be carefully adjusted in children with concomitant GH and glucocorticoid deficiency to avoid both hypoadrenalism and an inhibitory effect on growth. Also, somatropin administration may alter the clearance of compounds known to be metabolized by CYP450 liver enzymes (eg, corticosteroids). Careful monitoring is advisable when somatropin is administered in combination with other drugs known to be metabolized by CYP450 liver enzymes).
No products indexed under this heading.

Hydrocortisone Sodium Succinate (Somatropin inhibits 11β-hydroxysteroid dehydrogenase type 1 (11βHSD-1) in adipose/hepatic tissue and may significantly impact the metabolism of cortisol and cortisone. Patients treated with glucocorticoid replacement therapy for previously diagnosed hypoadrenalism may require an increase in their maintenance or stress doses; this may be especially true for patients treated with cortisone acetate and prednisone. In addition, excessive glucocorticoid therapy may attenuate the growth promoting effects of somatropin in children. Therefore, glucocorticoid replacement therapy should be carefully adjusted in children with concomitant GH and glucocorticoid deficiency to avoid both hypoadrenalism and an inhibitory effect on growth. Also, somatropin administration may alter the clearance of compounds known to be metabolized by CYP450 liver enzymes (eg, corticosteroids). Careful monitoring is advisable when somatropin is administered in combination with other drugs known to be metabolized by CYP450 liver enzymes).
No products indexed under this heading.

Hydrocortisone Valerate (Somatropin inhibits 11β-hydroxysteroid dehydrogenase type 1 (11βHSD-1) in adipose/hepatic tissue and may significantly impact the metabolism of cortisol and cortisone. Patients treated with glucocorticoid replacement therapy for previously diagnosed hypoadrenalism may require an increase in their maintenance or stress doses; this may be especially true for patients treated with cortisone acetate and prednisone. In addition, excessive glucocorticoid therapy may attenuate the growth promoting effects of somatropin in children. Therefore, glucocorticoid replacement therapy should be carefully adjusted in children with concomitant GH and glucocorticoid deficiency to avoid both hypoadrenalism and an inhibitory effect on growth. Also, somatropin administration may alter the clearance of compounds known to be metabolized by CYP450 liver enzymes (eg, corticosteroids). Careful monitoring is advisable when somatropin is administered in combination with other drugs known to be metabolized by CYP450 liver enzymes).
No products indexed under this heading.

Ibuprofen (Limited published data indicates that somatropin treatment increases cytochrome P450 (CYP450)-mediated antipyrine clearance in man. These data suggest that somatropin administration may alter the clearance of compounds metabolized by CYP450 liver enzymes. Careful monitoring is advisable when somatropin is administered in combination with other drugs known to be metabolized by CYP450 liver enzymes). Products include:
Motrin IB **2043**
Children's Motrin **2044**
Children's Motrin Non-Staining Dye-Free **2044**
Infants' Motrin **2044**
Infants' Motrin Dye-Free **2044**
Junior Strength Motrin **2044**
Vicoprofen **564**

Imipramine Hydrochloride (Limited published data indicates that somatropin treatment increases cytochrome P450 (CYP450)-mediated antipyrine clearance in man. These data suggest that somatropin administration may alter the clearance of compounds metabolized by CYP450 liver enzymes. Careful monitoring is advisable when somatropin is administered in combination with other drugs known to be metabolized by CYP450 liver enzymes).
No products indexed under this heading.

Imipramine Pamoate (Limited published data indicates that somatropin treatment increases cytochrome P450 (CYP450)-mediated antipyrine clearance in man. These data suggest that somatropin administration may alter the clearance of compounds metabolized by CYP450 liver enzymes. Careful monitoring is advisable when somatropin is administered in combination with other drugs known to be metabolized by CYP450 liver enzymes).
No products indexed under this heading.

Indinavir Sulfate (Limited published data indicates that somatropin treatment increases cytochrome P450 (CYP450)-mediated antipyrine clearance in man. These data suggest that somatropin administration may alter the clearance of compounds metabolized by CYP450 liver enzymes. Careful monitoring is advisable when somatropin is administered in combination with other drugs known to be metabolized by CYP450 liver enzymes). Products include:
Crixivan **2113**

Indomethacin (Limited published data indicates that somatropin treatment increases cytochrome P450 (CYP450)-mediated antipyrine clearance in man. These data suggest that somatropin administration may alter the clearance of compounds metabolized by CYP450 liver enzymes. Careful monitoring is advisable when somatropin is administered in combination with other drugs known to be metabolized by CYP450 liver enzymes). Products include:
Indocin **2167**

Indomethacin Sodium Trihydrate (Limited published data indicates that somatropin treatment increases cytochrome P450 (CYP450)-mediated antipyrine clearance in man. These data suggest that somatropin administration may alter the clearance of compounds metabolized by CYP450 liver enzymes. Careful monitoring is advisable when somatropin is administered in combination with other drugs known to be metabolized by CYP450 liver enzymes). Products include:
Indocin I.V. **2007**

Indoramin Hydrochloride (Limited published data indicates that somatropin treatment increases cytochrome P450 (CYP450)-mediated antipyrine clearance in man. These data suggest that somatropin administration may alter the clearance of compounds metabolized by CYP450 liver enzymes. Careful monitoring is advisable when somatropin is administered in combination with other drugs known to be metabolized by CYP450 liver enzymes).
No products indexed under this heading.

Insulin (In patients with diabetes mellitus requiring drug therapy, the dose of insulin and/or oral agent may require adjustment when somatropin therapy is initiated).
No products indexed under this heading.

Insulin, Human, Zinc Suspension (In patients with diabetes mellitus requiring drug therapy, the dose of insulin and/or oral agent may require adjustment when somatropin therapy is initiated).
No products indexed under this heading.

Insulin, Human (rDNA origin) (In patients with diabetes mellitus requiring drug therapy, the dose of insulin and/or oral agent may require adjustment when somatropin therapy is initiated). Products include:
Exubera **2717**

Insulin, Human NPH (In patients with diabetes mellitus requiring drug therapy, the dose of insulin and/or oral agent may require adjustment when somatropin therapy is initiated). Products include:
Humulin N Vial **1934**

Insulin, Human Regular (In patients with diabetes mellitus requiring drug therapy, the dose of insulin and/or oral agent may require adjustment when somatropin therapy is initiated). Products include:
Humulin R **1937**
Humulin R (U-500) **1939**

Insulin, Human Regular and Human NPH Mixture (In patients with diabetes mellitus requiring drug therapy, the dose of insulin and/or oral agent may require adjustment when somatropin therapy is initiated). Products include:
Humulin 50/50 .... **1930**
Humulin 70/30 Vial **1931**

Insulin, NPH (In patients with diabetes mellitus requiring drug therapy, the dose of insulin and/or oral agent may require adjustment when somatropin therapy is initiated).
No products indexed under this heading.

Insulin, Regular (In patients with diabetes mellitus requiring drug therapy, the dose of insulin and/or oral agent may require adjustment when somatropin therapy is initiated).
No products indexed under this heading.

Insulin, Regular and NPH mixture (In patients with diabetes mellitus requiring drug therapy, the dose of insulin and/or oral agent may require adjustment when somatropin therapy is initiated).
No products indexed under this heading.

Insulin, Zinc Crystals (In patients with diabetes mellitus requiring drug therapy, the dose of insulin and/or oral agent may require adjustment when somatropin therapy is initiated).
No products indexed under this heading.

Insulin, Zinc Suspension (In patients with diabetes mellitus requiring drug therapy, the dose of insulin and/or oral agent may require adjustment when somatropin therapy is initiated).
No products indexed under this heading.

Insulin Aspart (In patients with diabetes mellitus requiring drug therapy, the dose of insulin and/or oral agent may require adjustment when somatropin therapy is initiated).
No products indexed under this heading.

Insulin Aspart, Human (In patients with diabetes mellitus requiring drug therapy, the dose of insulin and/or oral agent may require adjustment when somatropin therapy is initiated). Products include:
NovoLog Mix 70/30 .... **2581**

Insulin Aspart, Human Regular (In patients with diabetes mellitus requiring drug therapy, the dose of insulin and/or oral agent may require adjustment when somatropin therapy is initiated). Products include:
NovoLog **2575**

Insulin Aspart Protamine, Human (In patients with diabetes mellitus requiring drug therapy, the dose of insulin and/or oral agent may require adjustment when somatropin therapy is initiated). Products include:
NovoLog Mix 70/30 .... **2581**

Insulin Detemir (rDNA Origin) (In patients with diabetes mellitus requiring drug therapy, the dose of insulin and/or oral agent may require adjustment when somatropin therapy is initiated). Products include:
Levemir **2566**

Insulin Glargine (In patients with diabetes mellitus requiring drug therapy, the dose of insulin and/or oral agent may require adjustment when somatropin therapy is initiated). Products include:
Lantus **2996**

Insulin Glulisine (In patients with diabetes mellitus requiring drug therapy, the dose of insulin and/or oral agent may require adjustment when somatropin therapy is initiated). Products include:
Apidra **2937**
Apidra SoloStar **2937**

Insulin Lispro, Human (In patients with diabetes mellitus requiring drug therapy, the dose of insulin and/or oral agent may require adjustment when somatropin therapy is initiated). Products include:
Humalog **1910**
Humalog Mix **1914**
Humalog Mix75/25 .... **1917**

Insulin Lispro Protamine, Human (In patients with diabetes mellitus requiring drug therapy, the dose of insulin and/or oral agent may require adjustment when somatropin therapy is initiated). Products include:
Humalog Mix **1914**
Humalog Mix75/25 .... **1917**

Irbesartan (Limited published data indicates that somatropin treatment increases cytochrome P450 (CYP450)-mediated antipyrine clearance in man. These data suggest that somatropin administration may alter the clearance of compounds metabolized by CYP450 liver enzymes. Careful monitoring is advisable when somatropin is administered in combination with other drugs known to be metabolized by CYP450 liver enzymes). Products include:
Avalide **2956**
Avapro **2962**

Isotretinoin (Limited published data indicates that somatropin treatment increases cytochrome P450 (CYP450)-mediated antipyrine clearance in man. These data suggest that somatropin administration may alter the clearance of compounds metabolized by CYP450 liver enzymes. Careful monitoring is advisable when somatropin is administered in combination with other drugs known to be metabolized by CYP450 liver enzymes). Products include:
Accutane **2832**

Isradipine (Limited published data indicates that somatropin treatment increases cytochrome P450

(CYP450)-mediated antipyrine clearance in man. These data suggest that somatropin administration may alter the clearance of compounds metabolized by CYP450 liver enzymes. Careful monitoring is advisable when somatropin is administered in combination with other drugs known to be metabolized by CYP450 liver enzymes). Products include:

DynaCirc CR 1432

Itraconazole (Limited published data indicates that somatropin treatment increases cytochrome P450 (CYP450)-mediated antipyrine clearance in man. These data suggest that somatropin administration may alter the clearance of compounds metabolized by CYP450 liver enzymes. Careful monitoring is advisable when somatropin is administered in combination with other drugs known to be metabolized by CYP450 liver enzymes).

No products indexed under this heading.

Ixabepilone (Limited published data indicates that somatropin treatment increases cytochrome P450 (CYP450)-mediated antipyrine clearance in man. These data suggest that somatropin administration may alter the clearance of compounds metabolized by CYP450 liver enzymes. Careful monitoring is advisable when somatropin is administered in combination with other drugs known to be metabolized by CYP450 liver enzymes).

No products indexed under this heading.

Ketoconazole (Limited published data indicates that somatropin treatment increases cytochrome P450 (CYP450)-mediated antipyrine clearance in man. These data suggest that somatropin administration may alter the clearance of compounds metabolized by CYP450 liver enzymes. Careful monitoring is advisable when somatropin is administered in combination with other drugs known to be metabolized by CYP450 liver enzymes). Products include:

Extina 3319
Xolegel 3337

Ketoprofen (Limited published data indicates that somatropin treatment increases cytochrome P450 (CYP450)-mediated antipyrine clearance in man. These data suggest that somatropin administration may alter the clearance of compounds metabolized by CYP450 liver enzymes. Careful monitoring is advisable when somatropin is administered in combination with other drugs known to be metabolized by CYP450 liver enzymes).

No products indexed under this heading.

Ketorolac Tromethamine (Limited published data indicates that somatropin treatment increases cytochrome P450 (CYP450)-mediated antipyrine clearance in man. These data suggest that somatropin administration may alter the clearance of compounds metabolized by CYP450 liver enzymes. Careful monitoring is advisable when somatropin is administered in combination with other drugs known to be metabolized by CYP450 liver enzymes). Products include:

Acuvail ....⊙ 209

Labetalol Hydrochloride (Limited published data indicates that somatropin treatment increases cytochrome P450 (CYP450)-mediated antipyrine clearance in man. These data suggest that somatropin administration may alter the clearance of compounds metabolized by CYP450 liver enzymes. Careful monitoring is advisable when somatropin is administered in combination with other drugs known to be metabolized by CYP450 liver enzymes).

No products indexed under this heading.

Lamotrigine (Limited published data indicates that somatropin treatment increases cytochrome P450 (CYP450)-mediated antipyrine clearance in man. These data suggest that somatropin administration may alter the clearance of compounds metabolized by CYP450 liver enzymes (eg, anticonvulsants). Careful monitoring is advisable when somatropin is administered in combination with other drugs known to be metabolized by CYP450 liver enzymes). Products include:

Lamictal 1522
Lamictal ODT 1522
Lamictal XR 1536

Lansoprazole (Limited published data indicates that somatropin treatment increases cytochrome P450 (CYP450)-mediated antipyrine clearance in man. These data suggest that somatropin administration may alter the clearance of compounds metabolized by CYP450 liver enzymes. Careful monitoring is advisable when somatropin is administered in combination with other drugs known to be metabolized by CYP450 liver enzymes).

No products indexed under this heading.

Levetiracetam (Limited published data indicates that somatropin treatment increases cytochrome P450 (CYP450)-mediated antipyrine clearance in man. These data suggest that somatropin administration may alter the clearance of compounds metabolized by CYP450 liver enzymes (eg, anticonvulsants). Careful monitoring is advisable when somatropin is administered in combination with other drugs known to be metabolized by CYP450 liver enzymes). Products include:

Keppra XR 3434

Levobupivacaine Hydrochloride (Limited published data indicates that somatropin treatment increases cytochrome P450 (CYP450)-mediated antipyrine clearance in man. These data suggest that somatropin administration may alter the clearance of compounds metabolized by CYP450 liver enzymes. Careful monitoring is advisable when somatropin is administered in combination with other drugs known to be metabolized by CYP450 liver enzymes).

No products indexed under this heading.

Levonorgestrel (Limited published data indicates that somatropin treatment increases cytochrome P450 (CYP450)-mediated antipyrine clearance in man. These data suggest that somatropin administration may alter the clearance of compounds metabolized by CYP450 liver enzymes (eg, sex steroids). Careful monitoring is advisable when somatropin is administered in combination with other drugs known to be metabolized by CYP450 liver enzymes). Products include:

Climara Pro 847
LoSeasonique 3407
Lybrel 3514
Mirena 854
Plan B 3416
Seasonique 3418

Lidocaine (Limited published data indicates that somatropin treatment increases cytochrome P450 (CYP450)-mediated antipyrine clearance in man. These data suggest that somatropin administration may alter the clearance of compounds metabolized by CYP450 liver enzymes. Careful monitoring is advisable when somatropin is administered in combination with other drugs known to be metabolized by CYP450 liver enzymes). Products include:

Lidoderm 1107

Lidocaine Base (Limited published data indicates that somatropin treatment increases cytochrome P450 (CYP450)-mediated antipyrine clearance

in man. These data suggest that somatropin administration may alter the clearance of compounds metabolized by CYP450 liver enzymes. Careful monitoring is advisable when somatropin is administered in combination with other drugs known to be metabolized by CYP450 liver enzymes).

No products indexed under this heading.

Lidocaine Hydrochloride (Limited published data indicates that somatropin treatment increases cytochrome P450 (CYP450)-mediated antipyrine clearance in man. These data suggest that somatropin administration may alter the clearance of compounds metabolized by CYP450 liver enzymes. Careful monitoring is advisable when somatropin is administered in combination with other drugs known to be metabolized by CYP450 liver enzymes).

No products indexed under this heading.

Lomefloxacin Hydrochloride (Limited published data indicates that somatropin treatment increases cytochrome P450 (CYP450)-mediated antipyrine clearance in man. These data suggest that somatropin administration may alter the clearance of compounds metabolized by CYP450 liver enzymes. Careful monitoring is advisable when somatropin is administered in combination with other drugs known to be metabolized by CYP450 liver enzymes).

No products indexed under this heading.

Losartan Potassium (Limited published data indicates that somatropin treatment increases cytochrome P450 (CYP450)-mediated antipyrine clearance in man. These data suggest that somatropin administration may alter the clearance of compounds metabolized by CYP450 liver enzymes. Careful monitoring is advisable when somatropin is administered in combination with other drugs known to be metabolized by CYP450 liver enzymes). Products include:

Cozaar 2106
Hyzaar 2162
Hyzaar 100-12.5 2162

Lovastatin (Limited published data indicates that somatropin treatment increases cytochrome P450 (CYP450)-mediated antipyrine clearance in man. These data suggest that somatropin administration may alter the clearance of compounds metabolized by CYP450 liver enzymes. Careful monitoring is advisable when somatropin is administered in combination with other drugs known to be metabolized by CYP450 liver enzymes). Products include:

Advicor 402
Mevacor 2212

Maprotiline Hydrochloride (Limited published data indicates that somatropin treatment increases cytochrome P450 (CYP450)-mediated antipyrine clearance in man. These data suggest that somatropin administration may alter the clearance of compounds metabolized by CYP450 liver enzymes. Careful monitoring is advisable when somatropin is administered in combination with other drugs known to be metabolized by CYP450 liver enzymes).

No products indexed under this heading.

Meclofenamate Sodium (Limited published data indicates that somatropin treatment increases cytochrome P450 (CYP450)-mediated antipyrine clearance in man. These data suggest that somatropin administration may alter the clearance of compounds metabolized by CYP450 liver enzymes. Careful monitoring is advisable when somatropin is administered in combination with other drugs known to be metabolized by CYP450 liver enzymes).

No products indexed under this heading.

Mefenamic Acid (Limited published data indicates that somatropin treatment increases cytochrome P450 (CYP450)-mediated antipyrine clearance in man. These data suggest that somatropin administration may alter the clearance of compounds metabolized by CYP450 liver enzymes. Careful monitoring is advisable when somatropin is administered in combination with other drugs known to be metabolized by CYP450 liver enzymes).

No products indexed under this heading.

Meloxicam (Limited published data indicates that somatropin treatment increases cytochrome P450 (CYP450)-mediated antipyrine clearance in man. These data suggest that somatropin administration may alter the clearance of compounds metabolized by CYP450 liver enzymes. Careful monitoring is advisable when somatropin is administered in combination with other drugs known to be metabolized by CYP450 liver enzymes).

No products indexed under this heading.

Meperidine Hydrochloride (Limited published data indicates that somatropin treatment increases cytochrome P450 (CYP450)-mediated antipyrine clearance in man. These data suggest that somatropin administration may alter the clearance of compounds metabolized by CYP450 liver enzymes. Careful monitoring is advisable when somatropin is administered in combination with other drugs known to be metabolized by CYP450 liver enzymes).

No products indexed under this heading.

Mephenytoin (Limited published data indicates that somatropin treatment increases cytochrome P450 (CYP450)-mediated antipyrine clearance in man. These data suggest that somatropin administration may alter the clearance of compounds metabolized by CYP450 liver enzymes (eg, anticonvulsants). Careful monitoring is advisable when somatropin is administered in combination with other drugs known to be metabolized by CYP450 liver enzymes).

No products indexed under this heading.

Mephobarbital (Limited published data indicates that somatropin treatment increases cytochrome P450 (CYP450)-mediated antipyrine clearance in man. These data suggest that somatropin administration may alter the clearance of compounds metabolized by CYP450 liver enzymes. Careful monitoring is advisable when somatropin is administered in combination with other drugs known to be metabolized by CYP450 liver enzymes).

No products indexed under this heading.

Meprobamate (Limited published data indicates that somatropin treatment increases cytochrome P450 (CYP450)-mediated antipyrine clearance in man. These data suggest that somatropin administration may alter the clearance of compounds metabolized by CYP450 liver enzymes. Careful monitoring is advisable when somatropin is administered in combination with other drugs known to be metabolized by CYP450 liver enzymes).

No products indexed under this heading.

Mestranol (Limited published data indicates that somatropin treatment increases cytochrome P450 (CYP450)-mediated antipyrine clearance in man. These data suggest that somatropin administration may alter the clearance of compounds metabolized by CYP450 liver enzymes (eg, sex steroids). Careful monitoring is advisable when somatropin is administered in combination with other drugs known to be metabolized by CYP450 liver enzymes).

No products indexed under this heading.

(⊙ Described in PDR® for Ophthalmic Medicines)

Metformin Hydrochloride (In patients with diabetes mellitus requiring drug therapy, the dose of insulin and/or oral agent may require adjustment when somatropin therapy is initiated). Products include:

ActoPlus 3338
Avandamet 1345
Janumet 2188

Methadone Hydrochloride (Limited published data indicates that somatropin treatment increases cytochrome P450 (CYP450)-mediated antipyrine clearance in man. These data suggest that somatropin administration may alter the clearance of compounds metabolized by CYP450 liver enzymes. Careful monitoring is advisable when somatropin is administered in combination with other drugs known to be metabolized by CYP450 liver enzymes).

No products indexed under this heading.

Methamphetamine Hydrochloride (Limited published data indicates that somatropin treatment increases cytochrome P450 (CYP450)-mediated antipyrine clearance in man. These data suggest that somatropin administration may alter the clearance of compounds metabolized by CYP450 liver enzymes. Careful monitoring is advisable when somatropin is administered in combination with other drugs known to be metabolized by CYP450 liver enzymes).

No products indexed under this heading.

Methsuximide (Limited published data indicates that somatropin treatment increases cytochrome P450 (CYP450)-mediated antipyrine clearance in man. These data suggest that somatropin administration may alter the clearance of compounds metabolized by CYP450 liver enzymes (eg, anticonvulsants). Careful monitoring is advisable when somatropin is administered in combination with other drugs known to be metabolized by CYP450 liver enzymes).

No products indexed under this heading.

Methylprednisolone (Somatropin inhibits 11β-hydroxysteroid dehydrogenase type 1 (11βHSD-1) in adipose/hepatic tissue and may significantly impact the metabolism of cortisol and cortisone. Patients treated with glucocorticoid replacement therapy for previously diagnosed hypoadrenalism may require an increase in their maintenance or stress doses; this may be especially true for patients treated with cortisone acetate and prednisone. In addition, excessive glucocorticoid therapy may attenuate the growth promoting effects of somatropin in children. Therefore, glucocorticoid replacement therapy should be carefully adjusted in children with concomitant GH and glucocorticoid deficiency to avoid both hypoadrenalism and an inhibitory effect on growth. Also, somatropin administration may alter the clearance of compounds known to be metabolized by CYP450 liver enzymes (eg, corticosteroids). Careful monitoring is advisable when somatropin is administered in combination with other drugs known to be metabolized by CYP450 liver enzymes).

No products indexed under this heading.

Methylprednisolone Acetate (Somatropin inhibits 11β-hydroxysteroid dehydrogenase type 1 (11βHSD-1) in adipose/hepatic tissue and may significantly impact the metabolism of cortisol and cortisone. Patients treated with glucocorticoid replacement therapy for previously diagnosed hypoadrenalism may require an increase in their maintenance or stress doses; this may be especially true for patients treated with cortisone acetate and prednisone. In addition, excessive glucocorticoid therapy may attenuate the growth promoting effects of somatropin in children.

Therefore, glucocorticoid replacement therapy should be carefully adjusted in children with concomitant GH and glucocorticoid deficiency to avoid both hypoadrenalism and an inhibitory effect on growth. Also, somatropin administration may alter the clearance of compounds known to be metabolized by CYP450 liver enzymes (eg, corticosteroids). Careful monitoring is advisable when somatropin is administered in combination with other drugs known to be metabolized by CYP450 liver enzymes).

No products indexed under this heading.

Methylprednisolone Sodium Succinate (Somatropin inhibits 11β-hydroxysteroid dehydrogenase type 1 (11βHSD-1) in adipose/hepatic tissue and may significantly impact the metabolism of cortisol and cortisone. Patients treated with glucocorticoid replacement therapy for previously diagnosed hypoadrenalism may require an increase in their maintenance or stress doses; this may be especially true for patients treated with cortisone acetate and prednisone. In addition, excessive glucocorticoid therapy may attenuate the growth promoting effects of somatropin in children. Therefore, glucocorticoid replacement therapy should be carefully adjusted in children with concomitant GH and glucocorticoid deficiency to avoid both hypoadrenalism and an inhibitory effect on growth. Also, somatropin administration may alter the clearance of compounds known to be metabolized by CYP450 liver enzymes (eg, corticosteroids). Careful monitoring is advisable when somatropin is administered in combination with other drugs known to be metabolized by CYP450 liver enzymes).

No products indexed under this heading.

Methyltestosterone (Limited published data indicates that somatropin treatment increases cytochrome P450 (CYP450)-mediated antipyrine clearance in man. These data suggest that somatropin administration may alter the clearance of compounds metabolized by CYP450 liver enzymes (eg, sex steroids). Careful monitoring is advisable when somatropin is administered in combination with other drugs known to be metabolized by CYP450 liver enzymes).

No products indexed under this heading.

Metoprolol Succinate (Limited published data indicates that somatropin treatment increases cytochrome P450 (CYP450)-mediated antipyrine clearance in man. These data suggest that somatropin administration may alter the clearance of compounds metabolized by CYP450 liver enzymes. Careful monitoring is advisable when somatropin is administered in combination with other drugs known to be metabolized by CYP450 liver enzymes). Products include:

Toprol XL 732

Metoprolol Tartrate (Limited published data indicates that somatropin treatment increases cytochrome P450 (CYP450)-mediated antipyrine clearance in man. These data suggest that somatropin administration may alter the clearance of compounds metabolized by CYP450 liver enzymes. Careful monitoring is advisable when somatropin is administered in combination with other drugs known to be metabolized by CYP450 liver enzymes).

No products indexed under this heading.

Mexiletine Hydrochloride (Limited published data indicates that somatropin treatment increases cytochrome P450 (CYP450)-mediated antipyrine clearance in man. These data suggest that somatropin administration may alter the clearance of compounds metabolized by CYP450 liver enzymes.

Careful monitoring is advisable when somatropin is administered in combination with other drugs known to be metabolized by CYP450 liver enzymes).

No products indexed under this heading.

Midazolam Hydrochloride (Limited published data indicates that somatropin treatment increases cytochrome P450 (CYP450)-mediated antipyrine clearance in man. These data suggest that somatropin administration may alter the clearance of compounds metabolized by CYP450 liver enzymes. Careful monitoring is advisable when somatropin is administered in combination with other drugs known to be metabolized by CYP450 liver enzymes).

No products indexed under this heading.

Miglitol (In patients with diabetes mellitus requiring drug therapy, the dose of insulin and/or oral agent may require adjustment when somatropin therapy is initiated).

No products indexed under this heading.

Mirtazapine (Limited published data indicates that somatropin treatment increases cytochrome P450 (CYP450)-mediated antipyrine clearance in man. These data suggest that somatropin administration may alter the clearance of compounds metabolized by CYP450 liver enzymes. Careful monitoring is advisable when somatropin is administered in combination with other drugs known to be metabolized by CYP450 liver enzymes). Products include:

Remeron Tablets 3214
RemeronSolTab Tablets 3219

Mometasone Furoate (Somatropin inhibits 11β-hydroxysteroid dehydrogenase type 1 (11βHSD-1) in adipose/hepatic tissue and may significantly impact the metabolism of cortisol and cortisone. Patients treated with glucocorticoid replacement therapy for previously diagnosed hypoadrenalism may require an increase in their maintenance or stress doses; this may be especially true for patients treated with cortisone acetate and prednisone. In addition, excessive glucocorticoid therapy may attenuate the growth promoting effects of somatropin in children. Therefore, glucocorticoid replacement therapy should be carefully adjusted in children with concomitant GH and glucocorticoid deficiency to avoid both hypoadrenalism and an inhibitory effect on growth. Also, somatropin administration may alter the clearance of compounds known to be metabolized by CYP450 liver enzymes (eg, corticosteroids). Careful monitoring is advisable when somatropin is administered in combination with other drugs known to be metabolized by CYP450 liver enzymes). Products include:

Asmanex 3058
Elocon Cream 3111
Elocon Lotion 3112
Elocon Ointment 3114

Mometasone Furoate Monohydrate (Somatropin inhibits 11β-hydroxysteroid dehydrogenase type 1 (11βHSD-1) in adipose/hepatic tissue and may significantly impact the metabolism of cortisol and cortisone. Patients treated with glucocorticoid replacement therapy for previously diagnosed hypoadrenalism may require an increase in their maintenance or stress doses; this may be especially true for patients treated with cortisone acetate and prednisone. In addition, excessive glucocorticoid therapy may attenuate the growth promoting effects of somatropin in children. Therefore, glucocorticoid replacement therapy should be carefully adjusted in children with concomitant GH and glucocorticoid deficiency to avoid both hypoadrenalism and an inhibitory effect on growth. Also, somatropin administration may alter the

clearance of compounds known to be metabolized by CYP450 liver enzymes (eg, corticosteroids). Careful monitoring is advisable when somatropin is administered in combination with other drugs known to be metabolized by CYP450 liver enzymes). Products include:

Nasonex 3166

Montelukast Sodium (Limited published data indicates that somatropin treatment increases cytochrome P450 (CYP450)-mediated antipyrine clearance in man. These data suggest that somatropin administration may alter the clearance of compounds metabolized by CYP450 liver enzymes. Careful monitoring is advisable when somatropin is administered in combination with other drugs known to be metabolized by CYP450 liver enzymes). Products include:

Singulair 2270

Morphine Sulfate (Limited published data indicates that somatropin treatment increases cytochrome P450 (CYP450)-mediated antipyrine clearance in man. These data suggest that somatropin administration may alter the clearance of compounds metabolized by CYP450 liver enzymes. Careful monitoring is advisable when somatropin is administered in combination with other drugs known to be metabolized by CYP450 liver enzymes). Products include:

Avinza 1822
Embeda 1831
MS Contin 2803

Moxifloxacin Hydrochloride (Limited published data indicates that somatropin treatment increases cytochrome P450 (CYP450)-mediated antipyrine clearance in man. These data suggest that somatropin administration may alter the clearance of compounds metabolized by CYP450 liver enzymes. Careful monitoring is advisable when somatropin is administered in combination with other drugs known to be metabolized by CYP450 liver enzymes). Products include:

Avelox 3064
Vigamox 589

Nabumetone (Limited published data indicates that somatropin treatment increases cytochrome P450 (CYP450)-mediated antipyrine clearance in man. These data suggest that somatropin administration may alter the clearance of compounds metabolized by CYP450 liver enzymes. Careful monitoring is advisable when somatropin is administered in combination with other drugs known to be metabolized by CYP450 liver enzymes).

No products indexed under this heading.

Nafcillin Sodium (Limited published data indicates that somatropin treatment increases cytochrome P450 (CYP450)-mediated antipyrine clearance in man. These data suggest that somatropin administration may alter the clearance of compounds metabolized by CYP450 liver enzymes. Careful monitoring is advisable when somatropin is administered in combination with other drugs known to be metabolized by CYP450 liver enzymes).

No products indexed under this heading.

Naproxen (Limited published data indicates that somatropin treatment increases cytochrome P450 (CYP450)-mediated antipyrine clearance in man. These data suggest that somatropin administration may alter the clearance of compounds metabolized by CYP450 liver enzymes. Careful monitoring is advisable when somatropin is administered in combination with other drugs known to be metabolized by CYP450 liver enzymes). Products include:

EC-Naprosyn 2850

IMPORTANT NOTE: Always consult each drug listing in the patient's regimen for possible interactions.

Naprosyn **2850**
Anaprox/Naprosyn **2850**

Naproxen Sodium (Limited published data indicates that somatropin treatment increases cytochrome P450 (CYP450)-mediated antipyrine clearance in man. These data suggest that somatropin administration may alter the clearance of compounds metabolized by CYP450 liver enzymes. Careful monitoring is advisable when somatropin is administered in combination with other drugs known to be metabolized by CYP450 liver enzymes). Products include:

Anaprox **2850**
Anaprox DS **2850**
Treximet **1681**

Nateglinide (In patients with diabetes mellitus requiring drug therapy, the dose of insulin and/or oral agent may require adjustment when somatropin therapy is initiated).
No products indexed under this heading.

Nefazodone Hydrochloride (Limited published data indicates that somatropin treatment increases cytochrome P450 (CYP450)-mediated antipyrine clearance in man. These data suggest that somatropin administration may alter the clearance of compounds metabolized by CYP450 liver enzymes. Careful monitoring is advisable when somatropin is administered in combination with other drugs known to be metabolized by CYP450 liver enzymes).
No products indexed under this heading.

Nelfinavir Mesylate (Limited published data indicates that somatropin treatment increases cytochrome P450 (CYP450)-mediated antipyrine clearance in man. These data suggest that somatropin administration may alter the clearance of compounds metabolized by CYP450 liver enzymes. Careful monitoring is advisable when somatropin is administered in combination with other drugs known to be metabolized by CYP450 liver enzymes).
No products indexed under this heading.

Nicardipine (Limited published data indicates that somatropin treatment increases cytochrome P450 (CYP450)-mediated antipyrine clearance in man. These data suggest that somatropin administration may alter the clearance of compounds metabolized by CYP450 liver enzymes. Careful monitoring is advisable when somatropin is administered in combination with other drugs known to be metabolized by CYP450 liver enzymes).
No products indexed under this heading.

Nicardipine Hydrochloride (Limited published data indicates that somatropin treatment increases cytochrome P450 (CYP450)-mediated antipyrine clearance in man. These data suggest that somatropin administration may alter the clearance of compounds metabolized by CYP450 liver enzymes. Careful monitoring is advisable when somatropin is administered in combination with other drugs known to be metabolized by CYP450 liver enzymes).
No products indexed under this heading.

Nicotine Polacrilex (Limited published data indicates that somatropin treatment increases cytochrome P450 (CYP450)-mediated antipyrine clearance in man. These data suggest that somatropin administration may alter the clearance of compounds metabolized by CYP450 liver enzymes. Careful monitoring is advisable when somatropin is administered in combination with other drugs known to be metabolized by CYP450 liver enzymes).
No products indexed under this heading.

Nicotine Salicylate (Limited published data indicates that somatropin treatment increases cytochrome P450 (CYP450)-mediated antipyrine clearance in man. These data suggest that somatropin administration may alter the clearance of compounds metabolized by CYP450 liver enzymes. Careful monitoring is advisable when somatropin is administered in combination with other drugs known to be metabolized by CYP450 liver enzymes).
No products indexed under this heading.

Nicotine Sulfate (Limited published data indicates that somatropin treatment increases cytochrome P450 (CYP450)-mediated antipyrine clearance in man. These data suggest that somatropin administration may alter the clearance of compounds metabolized by CYP450 liver enzymes. Careful monitoring is advisable when somatropin is administered in combination with other drugs known to be metabolized by CYP450 liver enzymes).
No products indexed under this heading.

Nifedipine (Limited published data indicates that somatropin treatment increases cytochrome P450 (CYP450)-mediated antipyrine clearance in man. These data suggest that somatropin administration may alter the clearance of compounds metabolized by CYP450 liver enzymes. Careful monitoring is advisable when somatropin is administered in combination with other drugs known to be metabolized by CYP450 liver enzymes).
No products indexed under this heading.

Nilutamide (Limited published data indicates that somatropin treatment increases cytochrome P450 (CYP450)-mediated antipyrine clearance in man. These data suggest that somatropin administration may alter the clearance of compounds metabolized by CYP450 liver enzymes. Careful monitoring is advisable when somatropin is administered in combination with other drugs known to be metabolized by CYP450 liver enzymes).
No products indexed under this heading.

Nimodipine (Limited published data indicates that somatropin treatment increases cytochrome P450 (CYP450)-mediated antipyrine clearance in man. These data suggest that somatropin administration may alter the clearance of compounds metabolized by CYP450 liver enzymes. Careful monitoring is advisable when somatropin is administered in combination with other drugs known to be metabolized by CYP450 liver enzymes).
No products indexed under this heading.

Nisoldipine (Limited published data indicates that somatropin treatment increases cytochrome P450 (CYP450)-mediated antipyrine clearance in man. These data suggest that somatropin administration may alter the clearance of compounds metabolized by CYP450 liver enzymes. Careful monitoring is advisable when somatropin is administered in combination with other drugs known to be metabolized by CYP450 liver enzymes).
No products indexed under this heading.

Nitrendipine (Limited published data indicates that somatropin treatment increases cytochrome P450 (CYP450)-mediated antipyrine clearance in man. These data suggest that somatropin administration may alter the clearance of compounds metabolized by CYP450 liver enzymes. Careful monitoring is advisable when somatropin is administered in combination with other drugs known to be metabolized by CYP450 liver enzymes).
No products indexed under this heading.

Norethindrone (Limited published data indicates that somatropin treatment increases cytochrome P450 (CYP450)-mediated antipyrine clearance in man. These data suggest that somatropin administration may alter the clearance of compounds metabolized by CYP450 liver enzymes (eg, sex steroids). Careful monitoring is advisable when somatropin is administered in combination with other drugs known to be metabolized by CYP450 liver enzymes). Products include:

Ortho Micronor **2660**

Norethindrone Acetate (Limited published data indicates that somatropin treatment increases cytochrome P450 (CYP450)-mediated antipyrine clearance in man. These data suggest that somatropin administration may alter the clearance of compounds metabolized by CYP450 liver enzymes (eg, sex steroids). Careful monitoring is advisable when somatropin is administered in combination with other drugs known to be metabolized by CYP450 liver enzymes). Products include:

Activella **2561**

Norfloxacin (Limited published data indicates that somatropin treatment increases cytochrome P450 (CYP450)-mediated antipyrine clearance in man. These data suggest that somatropin administration may alter the clearance of compounds metabolized by CYP450 liver enzymes. Careful monitoring is advisable when somatropin is administered in combination with other drugs known to be metabolized by CYP450 liver enzymes). Products include:

Noroxin **2220**

Norgestimate (Limited published data indicates that somatropin treatment increases cytochrome P450 (CYP450)-mediated antipyrine clearance in man. These data suggest that somatropin administration may alter the clearance of compounds metabolized by CYP450 liver enzymes (eg, sex steroids). Careful monitoring is advisable when somatropin is administered in combination with other drugs known to be metabolized by CYP450 liver enzymes). Products include:

Ortho-Cyclen/Ortho Tri-Cyclen **2663**
Ortho Tri-Cyclen Lo Tablets **2673**

Norgestrel (Limited published data indicates that somatropin treatment increases cytochrome P450 (CYP450)-mediated antipyrine clearance in man. These data suggest that somatropin administration may alter the clearance of compounds metabolized by CYP450 liver enzymes. Careful monitoring is advisable when somatropin is administered in combination with other drugs known to be metabolized by CYP450 liver enzymes).
No products indexed under this heading.

Nortriptyline Hydrochloride (Limited published data indicates that somatropin treatment increases cytochrome P450 (CYP450)-mediated antipyrine clearance in man. These data suggest that somatropin administration may alter the clearance of compounds metabolized by CYP450 liver enzymes. Careful monitoring is advisable when somatropin is administered in combination with other drugs known to be metabolized by CYP450 liver enzymes).
No products indexed under this heading.

Ofloxacin (Limited published data indicates that somatropin treatment increases cytochrome P450 (CYP450)-mediated antipyrine clearance in man. These data suggest that somatropin administration may alter the clearance of compounds metabolized by CYP450 liver enzymes. Careful monitoring is advisable when somatropin is administered in combination with other drugs known to be metabolized by CYP450 liver enzymes).
No products indexed under this heading.

Olanzapine (Limited published data indicates that somatropin treatment increases cytochrome P450 (CYP450)-mediated antipyrine clearance in man. These data suggest that somatropin administration may alter the clearance of compounds metabolized by CYP450 liver enzymes. Careful monitoring is advisable when somatropin is administered in combination with other drugs known to be metabolized by CYP450 liver enzymes). Products include:

Symbyax **1965**
Zyprexa **1984**
Zyprexa IntraMuscular **1984**
Zyprexa ZYDIS **1984**

Omeprazole (Limited published data indicates that somatropin treatment increases cytochrome P450 (CYP450)-mediated antipyrine clearance in man. These data suggest that somatropin administration may alter the clearance of compounds metabolized by CYP450 liver enzymes. Careful monitoring is advisable when somatropin is administered in combination with other drugs known to be metabolized by CYP450 liver enzymes).
No products indexed under this heading.

Omeprazole Magnesium (Limited published data indicates that somatropin treatment increases cytochrome P450 (CYP450)-mediated antipyrine clearance in man. These data suggest that somatropin administration may alter the clearance of compounds metabolized by CYP450 liver enzymes. Careful monitoring is advisable when somatropin is administered in combination with other drugs known to be metabolized by CYP450 liver enzymes).
No products indexed under this heading.

Ondansetron (Limited published data indicates that somatropin treatment increases cytochrome P450 (CYP450)-mediated antipyrine clearance in man. These data suggest that somatropin administration may alter the clearance of compounds metabolized by CYP450 liver enzymes. Careful monitoring is advisable when somatropin is administered in combination with other drugs known to be metabolized by CYP450 liver enzymes).
No products indexed under this heading.

Ondansetron Hydrochloride (Limited published data indicates that somatropin treatment increases cytochrome P450 (CYP450)-mediated antipyrine clearance in man. These data suggest that somatropin administration may alter the clearance of compounds metabolized by CYP450 liver enzymes. Careful monitoring is advisable when somatropin is administered in combination with other drugs known to be metabolized by CYP450 liver enzymes). Products include:

Zofran Injection **1750**
Zofran **1756**
Zofran ODT **1756**

Oxaprozin (Limited published data indicates that somatropin treatment increases cytochrome P450 (CYP450)-mediated antipyrine clearance in man. These data suggest that somatropin administration may alter the clearance of compounds metabolized by CYP450 liver enzymes. Careful monitoring is advisable when somatropin is administered in combination with other drugs known to be metabolized by CYP450 liver enzymes).
No products indexed under this heading.

Oxcarbazepine (Limited published data indicates that somatropin treatment increases cytochrome P450 (CYP450)-mediated antipyrine clearance in man. These data suggest that somatropin administration may alter the clearance of compounds metabolized by CYP450 liver enzymes (eg, anticonvul-

sants). Careful monitoring is advisable when somatropin is administered in combination with other drugs known to be metabolized by CYP450 liver enzymes).

No products indexed under this heading.

Oxycodone Hydrochloride (Limited published data indicates that somatropin treatment increases cytochrome P450 (CYP450)-mediated antipyrine clearance in man. These data suggest that somatropin administration may alter the clearance of compounds metabolized by CYP450 liver enzymes. Careful monitoring is advisable when somatropin is administered in combination with other drugs known to be metabolized by CYP450 liver enzymes). Products include:

OxyContin **2807**
Percocet **1121**
Percodan **1124**

Paclitaxel (Limited published data indicates that somatropin treatment increases cytochrome P450 (CYP450)-mediated antipyrine clearance in man. These data suggest that somatropin administration may alter the clearance of compounds metabolized by CYP450 liver enzymes. Careful monitoring is advisable when somatropin is administered in combination with other drugs known to be metabolized by CYP450 liver enzymes).

No products indexed under this heading.

Pantoprazole Sodium (Limited published data indicates that somatropin treatment increases cytochrome P450 (CYP450)-mediated antipyrine clearance in man. These data suggest that somatropin administration may alter the clearance of compounds metabolized by CYP450 liver enzymes. Careful monitoring is advisable when somatropin is administered in combination with other drugs known to be metabolized by CYP450 liver enzymes). Products include:

Protonix Tablets **3571**
Protonix **3575**

Paramethadione (Limited published data indicates that somatropin treatment increases cytochrome P450 (CYP450)-mediated antipyrine clearance in man. These data suggest that somatropin administration may alter the clearance of compounds metabolized by CYP450 liver enzymes (eg, anticonvulsants). Careful monitoring is advisable when somatropin is administered in combination with other drugs known to be metabolized by CYP450 liver enzymes).

No products indexed under this heading.

Paroxetine Hydrochloride (Limited published data indicates that somatropin treatment increases cytochrome P450 (CYP450)-mediated antipyrine clearance in man. These data suggest that somatropin administration may alter the clearance of compounds metabolized by CYP450 liver enzymes. Careful monitoring is advisable when somatropin is administered in combination with other drugs known to be metabolized by CYP450 liver enzymes). Products include:

Paroxetine CR **2361**
Paroxetine ER **2371**
Paxil **1586**
Paxil CR **1596**

Pentamidine Isethionate (Limited published data indicates that somatropin treatment increases cytochrome P450 (CYP450)-mediated antipyrine clearance in man. These data suggest that somatropin administration may alter the clearance of compounds metabolized by CYP450 liver enzymes. Careful monitoring is advisable when somatropin is administered in combination with other drugs known to be metabolized by CYP450 liver enzymes).

No products indexed under this heading.

Phenacemide (Limited published data indicates that somatropin treatment increases cytochrome P450 (CYP450)-mediated antipyrine clearance in man. These data suggest that somatropin administration may alter the clearance of compounds metabolized by CYP450 liver enzymes (eg, anticonvulsants). Careful monitoring is advisable when somatropin is administered in combination with other drugs known to be metabolized by CYP450 liver enzymes).

No products indexed under this heading.

Phenobarbital (Limited published data indicates that somatropin treatment increases cytochrome P450 (CYP450)-mediated antipyrine clearance in man. These data suggest that somatropin administration may alter the clearance of compounds metabolized by CYP450 liver enzymes (eg, anticonvulsants). Careful monitoring is advisable when somatropin is administered in combination with other drugs known to be metabolized by CYP450 liver enzymes). Products include:

Donnatal **2711**

Phenobarbital Sodium (Limited published data indicates that somatropin treatment increases cytochrome P450 (CYP450)-mediated antipyrine clearance in man. These data suggest that somatropin administration may alter the clearance of compounds metabolized by CYP450 liver enzymes (eg, anticonvulsants). Careful monitoring is advisable when somatropin is administered in combination with other drugs known to be metabolized by CYP450 liver enzymes).

No products indexed under this heading.

Phensuximide (Limited published data indicates that somatropin treatment increases cytochrome P450 (CYP450)-mediated antipyrine clearance in man. These data suggest that somatropin administration may alter the clearance of compounds metabolized by CYP450 liver enzymes (eg, anticonvulsants). Careful monitoring is advisable when somatropin is administered in combination with other drugs known to be metabolized by CYP450 liver enzymes).

No products indexed under this heading.

Phenylbutazone (Limited published data indicates that somatropin treatment increases cytochrome P450 (CYP450)-mediated antipyrine clearance in man. These data suggest that somatropin administration may alter the clearance of compounds metabolized by CYP450 liver enzymes. Careful monitoring is advisable when somatropin is administered in combination with other drugs known to be metabolized by CYP450 liver enzymes).

No products indexed under this heading.

Phenytoin (Limited published data indicates that somatropin treatment increases cytochrome P450 (CYP450)-mediated antipyrine clearance in man. These data suggest that somatropin administration may alter the clearance of compounds metabolized by CYP450 liver enzymes (eg, anticonvulsants). Careful monitoring is advisable when somatropin is administered in combination with other drugs known to be metabolized by CYP450 liver enzymes).

No products indexed under this heading.

Phenytoin Sodium (Limited published data indicates that somatropin treatment increases cytochrome P450 (CYP450)-mediated antipyrine clearance in man. These data suggest that somatropin administration may alter the clearance of compounds metabolized by CYP450 liver enzymes (eg, anticonvulsants). Careful monitoring is advisable when somatropin is administered in combination with other drugs known to be metabolized by CYP450 liver enzymes). Products include:

Phenytek Capsules **2380**

Pimozide (Limited published data indicates that somatropin treatment increases cytochrome P450 (CYP450)-mediated antipyrine clearance in man. These data suggest that somatropin administration may alter the clearance of compounds metabolized by CYP450 liver enzymes. Careful monitoring is advisable when somatropin is administered in combination with other drugs known to be metabolized by CYP450 liver enzymes).

No products indexed under this heading.

Pindolol (Limited published data indicates that somatropin treatment increases cytochrome P450 (CYP450)-mediated antipyrine clearance in man. These data suggest that somatropin administration may alter the clearance of compounds metabolized by CYP450 liver enzymes. Careful monitoring is advisable when somatropin is administered in combination with other drugs known to be metabolized by CYP450 liver enzymes).

No products indexed under this heading.

Pioglitazone Hydrochloride (In patients with diabetes mellitus requiring drug therapy, the dose of insulin and/or oral agent may require adjustment when somatropin therapy is initiated). Products include:

ActoPlus **3338**
Actos **3345**
Duetact **3354**

Piroxicam (Limited published data indicates that somatropin treatment increases cytochrome P450 (CYP450)-mediated antipyrine clearance in man. These data suggest that somatropin administration may alter the clearance of compounds metabolized by CYP450 liver enzymes. Careful monitoring is advisable when somatropin is administered in combination with other drugs known to be metabolized by CYP450 liver enzymes).

No products indexed under this heading.

Polyestradiol Phosphate (In patients on oral estrogen replacement, a larger dose of somatropin may be required to achieve the defined treatment goal).

No products indexed under this heading.

Prednisolone (Somatropin inhibits 11β-hydroxysteroid dehydrogenase type 1 (11βHSD-1) in adipose/hepatic tissue and may significantly impact the metabolism of cortisol and cortisone. Patients treated with glucocorticoid replacement therapy for previously diagnosed hypoadrenalism may require an increase in their maintenance or stress doses; this may be especially true for patients treated with cortisone acetate and prednisone. In addition, excessive glucocorticoid therapy may attenuate the growth promoting effects of somatropin in children. Therefore, glucocorticoid replacement therapy should be carefully adjusted in children with concomitant GH and glucocorticoid deficiency to avoid both hypoadrenalism and an inhibitory effect on growth. Also, somatropin administration may alter the clearance of compounds known to be metabolized by CYP450 liver enzymes (eg, corticosteroids). Careful monitoring is advisable when somatropin is administered in combination with other drugs known to be metabolized by CYP450 liver enzymes).

No products indexed under this heading.

Prednisolone Acetate (Somatropin inhibits 11β-hydroxysteroid dehydrogenase type 1 (11βHSD-1) in adipose/hepatic tissue and may significantly impact the metabolism of cortisol and cortisone. Patients treated with glucocorticoid replacement therapy for previously diagnosed hypoadrenalism may require an increase in their maintenance or stress doses; this may be especially true for patients treated with cortisone acetate and prednisone. In addition, excessive glucocorticoid therapy may attenuate the growth promoting effects of somatropin in children. Therefore, glucocorticoid replacement therapy should be carefully adjusted in children with concomitant GH and glucocorticoid deficiency to avoid both hypoadrenalism and an inhibitory effect on growth. Also, somatropin administration may alter the clearance of compounds known to be metabolized by CYP450 liver enzymes (eg, corticosteroids). Careful monitoring is advisable when somatropin is administered in combination with other drugs known to be metabolized by CYP450 liver enzymes). Products include:

Blephamide .... ⊙**212**, ⊙**214**
Pred Forte .... ⊙**225**
Pred Mild .... ⊙**230**
Pred-G .... ⊙**226**, ⊙**227**

Prednisolone Sodium Phosphate (Somatropin inhibits 11β-hydroxysteroid dehydrogenase type 1 (11βHSD-1) in adipose/hepatic tissue and may significantly impact the metabolism of cortisol and cortisone. Patients treated with glucocorticoid replacement therapy for previously diagnosed hypoadrenalism may require an increase in their maintenance or stress doses; this may be especially true for patients treated with cortisone acetate and prednisone. In addition, excessive glucocorticoid therapy may attenuate the growth promoting effects of somatropin in children. Therefore, glucocorticoid replacement therapy should be carefully adjusted in children with concomitant GH and glucocorticoid deficiency to avoid both hypoadrenalism and an inhibitory effect on growth. Also, somatropin administration may alter the clearance of compounds known to be metabolized by CYP450 liver enzymes (eg, corticosteroids). Careful monitoring is advisable when somatropin is administered in combination with other drugs known to be metabolized by CYP450 liver enzymes).

No products indexed under this heading.

Prednisolone Tebutate (Somatropin inhibits 11β-hydroxysteroid dehydrogenase type 1 (11βHSD-1) in adipose/hepatic tissue and may significantly impact the metabolism of cortisol and cortisone. Patients treated with glucocorticoid replacement therapy for previously diagnosed hypoadrenalism may require an increase in their maintenance or stress doses; this may be especially true for patients treated with cortisone acetate and prednisone. In addition, excessive glucocorticoid therapy may attenuate the growth promoting effects of somatropin in children. Therefore, glucocorticoid replacement therapy should be carefully adjusted in children with concomitant GH and glucocorticoid deficiency to avoid both hypoadrenalism and an inhibitory effect on growth. Also, somatropin administration may alter the clearance of compounds known to be metabolized by CYP450 liver enzymes (eg, corticosteroids). Careful monitoring is advisable when somatropin is administered in combination with other drugs known to be metabolized by CYP450 liver enzymes).

No products indexed under this heading.

Prednisone (Somatropin inhibits 11β-hydroxysteroid dehydrogenase type 1 (11βHSD-1) in adipose/hepatic tissue and may significantly impact the metabolism of cortisol and cortisone. Patients treated with glucocorticoid replacement therapy for previously

Genotropin Interactions Index 762

diagnosed hypoadrenalism may require an increase in their maintenance or stress doses; this may be especially true for patients treated with prednisone. In addition, excessive glucocorticoid therapy may attenuate the growth promoting effects of somatropin in children. Therefore, glucocorticoid replacement therapy should be carefully adjusted in children with concomitant GH and glucocorticoid deficiency to avoid both hypoadrenalism and an inhibitory effect on growth. Also, somatropin administration may alter the clearance of compounds known to be metabolized by CYP450 liver enzymes (eg, corticosteroids). Careful monitoring is advisable when somatropin is administered in combination with other drugs known to be metabolized by CYP450 liver enzymes).
No products indexed under this heading.

Prednisone sodium phosphate (Somatropin inhibits 11β-hydroxysteroid dehydrogenase type 1 (11βHSD-1) in adipose/hepatic tissue and may significantly impact the metabolism of cortisol and cortisone. Patients treated with glucocorticoid replacement therapy for previously diagnosed hypoadrenalism may require an increase in their maintenance or stress doses; this may be especially true for patients treated with prednisone. In addition, excessive glucocorticoid therapy may attenuate the growth promoting effects of somatropin in children. Therefore, glucocorticoid replacement therapy should be carefully adjusted in children with concomitant GH and glucocorticoid deficiency to avoid both hypoadrenalism and an inhibitory effect on growth. Also, somatropin administration may alter the clearance of compounds known to be metabolized by CYP450 liver enzymes (eg, corticosteroids). Careful monitoring is advisable when somatropin is administered in combination with other drugs known to be metabolized by CYP450 liver enzymes).
No products indexed under this heading.

Primidone (Limited published data indicates that somatropin treatment increases cytochrome P450 (CYP450)-mediated antipyrine clearance in man. These data suggest that somatropin administration may alter the clearance of compounds metabolized by CYP450 liver enzymes (eg, anticonvulsants). Careful monitoring is advisable when somatropin is administered in combination with other drugs known to be metabolized by CYP450 liver enzymes).
No products indexed under this heading.

Progesterone (Limited published data indicates that somatropin treatment increases cytochrome P450 (CYP450)-mediated antipyrine clearance in man. These data suggest that somatropin administration may alter the clearance of compounds metabolized by CYP450 liver enzymes. Careful monitoring is advisable when somatropin is administered in combination with other drugs known to be metabolized by CYP450 liver enzymes). Products include:
Crinone 4% 996
Crinone 8% 996
Prometrium 3307

Proguanil Hydrochloride (Limited published data indicates that somatropin treatment increases cytochrome P450 (CYP450)-mediated antipyrine clearance in man. These data suggest that somatropin administration may alter the clearance of compounds metabolized by CYP450 liver enzymes. Careful monitoring is advisable when somatropin is administered in combination with other drugs known to be metabolized by CYP450 liver enzymes). Products include:
Malarone Pediatric Tablets 1572
Malarone 1572

Propafenone Hydrochloride (Limited published data indicates that somatropin treatment increases cytochrome P450 (CYP450)-mediated antipyrine clearance in man. These data suggest that somatropin administration may alter the clearance of compounds metabolized by CYP450 liver enzymes. Careful monitoring is advisable when somatropin is administered in combination with other drugs known to be metabolized by CYP450 liver enzymes). Products include:
Rythmol 1648
Rythmol SR 1652

Propoxyphene Hydrochloride (Limited published data indicates that somatropin treatment increases cytochrome P450 (CYP450)-mediated antipyrine clearance in man. These data suggest that somatropin administration may alter the clearance of compounds metabolized by CYP450 liver enzymes. Careful monitoring is advisable when somatropin is administered in combination with other drugs known to be metabolized by CYP450 liver enzymes).
No products indexed under this heading.

Propoxyphene Napsylate (Limited published data indicates that somatropin treatment increases cytochrome P450 (CYP450)-mediated antipyrine clearance in man. These data suggest that somatropin administration may alter the clearance of compounds metabolized by CYP450 liver enzymes. Careful monitoring is advisable when somatropin is administered in combination with other drugs known to be metabolized by CYP450 liver enzymes).
No products indexed under this heading.

Propranolol Hydrochloride (Limited published data indicates that somatropin treatment increases cytochrome P450 (CYP450)-mediated antipyrine clearance in man. These data suggest that somatropin administration may alter the clearance of compounds metabolized by CYP450 liver enzymes. Careful monitoring is advisable when somatropin is administered in combination with other drugs known to be metabolized by CYP450 liver enzymes). Products include:
InnoPran XL 1517

Protriptyline Hydrochloride (Limited published data indicates that somatropin treatment increases cytochrome P450 (CYP450)-mediated antipyrine clearance in man. These data suggest that somatropin administration may alter the clearance of compounds metabolized by CYP450 liver enzymes. Careful monitoring is advisable when somatropin is administered in combination with other drugs known to be metabolized by CYP450 liver enzymes).
No products indexed under this heading.

Quetiapine Fumarate (Limited published data indicates that somatropin treatment increases cytochrome P450 (CYP450)-mediated antipyrine clearance in man. These data suggest that somatropin administration may alter the clearance of compounds metabolized by CYP450 liver enzymes. Careful monitoring is advisable when somatropin is administered in combination with other drugs known to be metabolized by CYP450 liver enzymes). Products include:
Seroquel 750
Seroquel XR 759

Quinestrol (In patients on oral estrogen replacement, a larger dose of somatropin may be required to achieve the defined treatment goal).
No products indexed under this heading.

Quinidine Gluconate (Limited published data indicates that somatropin treatment increases cytochrome P450 (CYP450)-mediated antipyrine clearance in man. These data suggest that somatropin administration may alter the clearance of compounds metabolized by CYP450 liver enzymes. Careful monitoring is advisable when somatropin is administered in combination with other drugs known to be metabolized by CYP450 liver enzymes).
No products indexed under this heading.

Quinidine Hydrochloride (Limited published data indicates that somatropin treatment increases cytochrome P450 (CYP450)-mediated antipyrine clearance in man. These data suggest that somatropin administration may alter the clearance of compounds metabolized by CYP450 liver enzymes. Careful monitoring is advisable when somatropin is administered in combination with other drugs known to be metabolized by CYP450 liver enzymes).
No products indexed under this heading.

Quinidine Polygalacturonate (Limited published data indicates that somatropin treatment increases cytochrome P450 (CYP450)-mediated antipyrine clearance in man. These data suggest that somatropin administration may alter the clearance of compounds metabolized by CYP450 liver enzymes. Careful monitoring is advisable when somatropin is administered in combination with other drugs known to be metabolized by CYP450 liver enzymes).
No products indexed under this heading.

Quinidine Sulfate (Limited published data indicates that somatropin treatment increases cytochrome P450 (CYP450)-mediated antipyrine clearance in man. These data suggest that somatropin administration may alter the clearance of compounds metabolized by CYP450 liver enzymes. Careful monitoring is advisable when somatropin is administered in combination with other drugs known to be metabolized by CYP450 liver enzymes).
No products indexed under this heading.

Quinine (Limited published data indicates that somatropin treatment increases cytochrome P450 (CYP450)-mediated antipyrine clearance in man. These data suggest that somatropin administration may alter the clearance of compounds metabolized by CYP450 liver enzymes. Careful monitoring is advisable when somatropin is administered in combination with other drugs known to be metabolized by CYP450 liver enzymes). Products include:
Hyland's Leg Cramps PM with Quinine 3315

Quinine Sulfate (Limited published data indicates that somatropin treatment increases cytochrome P450 (CYP450)-mediated antipyrine clearance in man. These data suggest that somatropin administration may alter the clearance of compounds metabolized by CYP450 liver enzymes. Careful monitoring is advisable when somatropin is administered in combination with other drugs known to be metabolized by CYP450 liver enzymes).
No products indexed under this heading.

Rabeprazole Sodium (Limited published data indicates that somatropin treatment increases cytochrome P450 (CYP450)-mediated antipyrine clearance in man. These data suggest that somatropin administration may alter the clearance of compounds metabolized by CYP450 liver enzymes. Careful monitoring is advisable when somatropin is administered in combination with other drugs known to be metabolized by CYP450 liver enzymes). Products include:
Aciphex 1035

Radiation (Intracranial tumors, in particular meningiomas, have been noted in teenagers/young adults who were treated with radiation to the head for a first neoplasm, and who subsequently received somatropin).
No products indexed under this heading.

Repaglinide (In patients with diabetes mellitus requiring drug therapy, the dose of insulin and/or oral agent may require adjustment when somatropin therapy is initiated).
No products indexed under this heading.

Rifabutin (Limited published data indicates that somatropin treatment increases cytochrome P450 (CYP450)-mediated antipyrine clearance in man. These data suggest that somatropin administration may alter the clearance of compounds metabolized by CYP450 liver enzymes. Careful monitoring is advisable when somatropin is administered in combination with other drugs known to be metabolized by CYP450 liver enzymes).
No products indexed under this heading.

Riluzole (Limited published data indicates that somatropin treatment increases cytochrome P450 (CYP450)-mediated antipyrine clearance in man. These data suggest that somatropin administration may alter the clearance of compounds metabolized by CYP450 liver enzymes. Careful monitoring is advisable when somatropin is administered in combination with other drugs known to be metabolized by CYP450 liver enzymes). Products include:
Rilutek 3032

Risperidone (Limited published data indicates that somatropin treatment increases cytochrome P450 (CYP450)-mediated antipyrine clearance in man. These data suggest that somatropin administration may alter the clearance of compounds metabolized by CYP450 liver enzymes. Careful monitoring is advisable when somatropin is administered in combination with other drugs known to be metabolized by CYP450 liver enzymes). Products include:
Risperdal Consta 2682

Ritonavir (Limited published data indicates that somatropin treatment increases cytochrome P450 (CYP450)-mediated antipyrine clearance in man. These data suggest that somatropin administration may alter the clearance of compounds metabolized by CYP450 liver enzymes. Careful monitoring is advisable when somatropin is administered in combination with other drugs known to be metabolized by CYP450 liver enzymes). Products include:
Kaletra 458
Norvir 509

Rofecoxib (Limited published data indicates that somatropin treatment increases cytochrome P450 (CYP450)-mediated antipyrine clearance in man. These data suggest that somatropin administration may alter the clearance of compounds metabolized by CYP450 liver enzymes. Careful monitoring is advisable when somatropin is administered in combination with other drugs known to be metabolized by CYP450 liver enzymes).
No products indexed under this heading.

Ropinirole Hydrochloride (Limited published data indicates that somatropin treatment increases cytochrome P450 (CYP450)-mediated antipyrine clearance in man. These data suggest that somatropin administration may alter the clearance of compounds metabolized by CYP450 liver enzymes. Careful monitoring is advisable when

somatropin is administered in combination with other drugs known to be metabolized by CYP450 liver enzymes). Products include:

Requip 1620
Requip XL 1628

Ropivacaine Hydrochloride (Limited published data indicates that somatropin treatment increases cytochrome P450 (CYP450)-mediated antipyrine clearance in man. These data suggest that somatropin administration may alter the clearance of compounds metabolized by CYP450 liver enzymes. Careful monitoring is advisable when somatropin is administered in combination with other drugs known to be metabolized by CYP450 liver enzymes).
No products indexed under this heading.

Rosiglitazone (Limited published data indicates that somatropin treatment increases cytochrome P450 (CYP450)-mediated antipyrine clearance in man. These data suggest that somatropin administration may alter the clearance of compounds metabolized by CYP450 liver enzymes. Careful monitoring is advisable when somatropin is administered in combination with other drugs known to be metabolized by CYP450 liver enzymes).
No products indexed under this heading.

Rosiglitazone Maleate (In patients with diabetes mellitus requiring drug therapy, the dose of insulin and/or oral agent may require adjustment when somatropin therapy is initiated). Products include:

Avandamet 1345
Avandaryl 1356
Avandia 1366

Rosiglitazone/Metformin (Limited published data indicates that somatropin treatment increases cytochrome P450 (CYP450)-mediated antipyrine clearance in man. These data suggest that somatropin administration may alter the clearance of compounds metabolized by CYP450 liver enzymes. Careful monitoring is advisable when somatropin is administered in combination with other drugs known to be metabolized by CYP450 liver enzymes).
No products indexed under this heading.

Rufinamide (Limited published data indicates that somatropin treatment increases cytochrome P450 (CYP450)-mediated antipyrine clearance in man. These data suggest that somatropin administration may alter the clearance of compounds metabolized by CYP450 liver enzymes (eg, anticonvulsants). Careful monitoring is advisable when somatropin is administered in combination with other drugs known to be metabolized by CYP450 liver enzymes). Products include:

Banzel 1050

Saquinavir (Limited published data indicates that somatropin treatment increases cytochrome P450 (CYP450)-mediated antipyrine clearance in man. These data suggest that somatropin administration may alter the clearance of compounds metabolized by CYP450 liver enzymes. Careful monitoring is advisable when somatropin is administered in combination with other drugs known to be metabolized by CYP450 liver enzymes).
No products indexed under this heading.

Saquinavir Mesylate (Limited published data indicates that somatropin treatment increases cytochrome P450 (CYP450)-mediated antipyrine clearance in man. These data suggest that somatropin administration may alter the clearance of compounds metabolized by CYP450 liver enzymes. Careful monitoring is advisable when somatropin is administered in combination with other drugs known to be metabolized by CYP450 liver enzymes).
No products indexed under this heading.

Sertraline Hydrochloride (Limited published data indicates that somatropin treatment increases cytochrome P450 (CYP450)-mediated antipyrine clearance in man. These data suggest that somatropin administration may alter the clearance of compounds metabolized by CYP450 liver enzymes. Careful monitoring is advisable when somatropin is administered in combination with other drugs known to be metabolized by CYP450 liver enzymes).
No products indexed under this heading.

Sildenafil Citrate (Limited published data indicates that somatropin treatment increases cytochrome P450 (CYP450)-mediated antipyrine clearance in man. These data suggest that somatropin administration may alter the clearance of compounds metabolized by CYP450 liver enzymes. Careful monitoring is advisable when somatropin is administered in combination with other drugs known to be metabolized by CYP450 liver enzymes).
No products indexed under this heading.

Simvastatin (Limited published data indicates that somatropin treatment increases cytochrome P450 (CYP450)-mediated antipyrine clearance in man. These data suggest that somatropin administration may alter the clearance of compounds metabolized by CYP450 liver enzymes. Careful monitoring is advisable when somatropin is administered in combination with other drugs known to be metabolized by CYP450 liver enzymes). Products include:

Simcor 524
Vytorin 10/10 .... 2303, 3240
Vytorin 10/20 .... 2303, 3240
Vytorin 10/40 .... 2303, 3240
Vytorin 10/80 .... 2303, 3240
Zocor 2289

Sirolimus (Limited published data indicates that somatropin treatment increases cytochrome P450 (CYP450)-mediated antipyrine clearance in man. These data suggest that somatropin administration may alter the clearance of compounds metabolized by CYP450 liver enzymes. Careful monitoring is advisable when somatropin is administered in combination with other drugs known to be metabolized by CYP450 liver enzymes). Products include:

Rapamune 3579

Sitagliptin Phosphate (In patients with diabetes mellitus requiring drug therapy, the dose of insulin and/or oral agent may require adjustment when somatropin therapy is initiated). Products include:

Janumet 2188
Januvia 2196

Sulfamethoxazole (Limited published data indicates that somatropin treatment increases cytochrome P450 (CYP450)-mediated antipyrine clearance in man. These data suggest that somatropin administration may alter the clearance of compounds metabolized by CYP450 liver enzymes. Careful monitoring is advisable when somatropin is administered in combination with other drugs known to be metabolized by CYP450 liver enzymes).
No products indexed under this heading.

Sulindac (Limited published data indicates that somatropin treatment increases cytochrome P450 (CYP450)-mediated antipyrine clearance in man. These data suggest that somatropin administration may alter the clearance of compounds metabolized by CYP450 liver enzymes. Careful monitoring is advisable when somatropin is administered in combination with other drugs known to be metabolized by CYP450 liver enzymes). Products include:

Clinoril 2098

Suprofen (Limited published data indicates that somatropin treatment increases cytochrome P450 (CYP450)-mediated antipyrine clearance in man. These data suggest that somatropin administration may alter the clearance of compounds metabolized by CYP450 liver enzymes. Careful monitoring is advisable when somatropin is administered in combination with other drugs known to be metabolized by CYP450 liver enzymes).
No products indexed under this heading.

Tacrine Hydrochloride (Limited published data indicates that somatropin treatment increases cytochrome P450 (CYP450)-mediated antipyrine clearance in man. These data suggest that somatropin administration may alter the clearance of compounds metabolized by CYP450 liver enzymes. Careful monitoring is advisable when somatropin is administered in combination with other drugs known to be metabolized by CYP450 liver enzymes).
No products indexed under this heading.

Tacrolimus (Limited published data indicates that somatropin treatment increases cytochrome P450 (CYP450)-mediated antipyrine clearance in man. These data suggest that somatropin administration may alter the clearance of compounds metabolized by CYP450 liver enzymes. Careful monitoring is advisable when somatropin is administered in combination with other drugs known to be metabolized by CYP450 liver enzymes). Products include:

Prograf Capsules 677
Prograf Injection 677
Protopic 685

Tadalafil (Limited published data indicates that somatropin treatment increases cytochrome P450 (CYP450)-mediated antipyrine clearance in man. These data suggest that somatropin administration may alter the clearance of compounds metabolized by CYP450 liver enzymes. Careful monitoring is advisable when somatropin is administered in combination with other drugs known to be metabolized by CYP450 liver enzymes). Products include:

Adcirca 3461
Cialis 1861

Tamoxifen Citrate (Limited published data indicates that somatropin treatment increases cytochrome P450 (CYP450)-mediated antipyrine clearance in man. These data suggest that somatropin administration may alter the clearance of compounds metabolized by CYP450 liver enzymes. Careful monitoring is advisable when somatropin is administered in combination with other drugs known to be metabolized by CYP450 liver enzymes).
No products indexed under this heading.

Telmisartan (Limited published data indicates that somatropin treatment increases cytochrome P450 (CYP450)-mediated antipyrine clearance in man. These data suggest that somatropin administration may alter the clearance of compounds metabolized by CYP450 liver enzymes. Careful monitoring is advisable when somatropin is administered in combination with other drugs known to be metabolized by CYP450 liver enzymes). Products include:

Micardis 887
Micardis HCT 889

Teniposide (Limited published data indicates that somatropin treatment increases cytochrome P450 (CYP450)-mediated antipyrine clearance in man. These data suggest that somatropin administration may alter the clearance of compounds metabolized by CYP450 liver enzymes. Careful monitoring is advisable when somatropin is administered in combination with other drugs known to be metabolized by CYP450 liver enzymes).
No products indexed under this heading.

Terfenadine (Limited published data indicates that somatropin treatment increases cytochrome P450 (CYP450)-mediated antipyrine clearance in man. These data suggest that somatropin administration may alter the clearance of compounds metabolized by CYP450 liver enzymes. Careful monitoring is advisable when somatropin is administered in combination with other drugs known to be metabolized by CYP450 liver enzymes).
No products indexed under this heading.

Testosterone (Limited published data indicates that somatropin treatment increases cytochrome P450 (CYP450)-mediated antipyrine clearance in man. These data suggest that somatropin administration may alter the clearance of compounds metabolized by CYP450 liver enzymes (eg, sex steroids). Careful monitoring is advisable when somatropin is administered in combination with other drugs known to be metabolized by CYP450 liver enzymes). Products include:

AndroGel 3456

Testosterone Cypionate (Limited published data indicates that somatropin treatment increases cytochrome P450 (CYP450)-mediated antipyrine clearance in man. These data suggest that somatropin administration may alter the clearance of compounds metabolized by CYP450 liver enzymes. Careful monitoring is advisable when somatropin is administered in combination with other drugs known to be metabolized by CYP450 liver enzymes).
No products indexed under this heading.

Testosterone Enanthate (Limited published data indicates that somatropin treatment increases cytochrome P450 (CYP450)-mediated antipyrine clearance in man. These data suggest that somatropin administration may alter the clearance of compounds metabolized by CYP450 liver enzymes. Careful monitoring is advisable when somatropin is administered in combination with other drugs known to be metabolized by CYP450 liver enzymes). Products include:

Delatestryl 1102

Testosterone Propionate (Limited published data indicates that somatropin treatment increases cytochrome P450 (CYP450)-mediated antipyrine clearance in man. These data suggest that somatropin administration may alter the clearance of compounds metabolized by CYP450 liver enzymes. Careful monitoring is advisable when somatropin is administered in combination with other drugs known to be metabolized by CYP450 liver enzymes).
No products indexed under this heading.

Theophylline (Limited published data indicates that somatropin treatment increases cytochrome P450 (CYP450)-mediated antipyrine clearance in man. These data suggest that somatropin administration may alter the clearance of compounds metabolized by CYP450 liver enzymes. Careful monitoring is advisable when somatropin is administered in combination with other drugs known to be metabolized by CYP450 liver enzymes).
No products indexed under this heading.

IMPORTANT NOTE: Always consult each drug listing in the patient's regimen for possible interactions.

Theophylline Anhydrous (Limited published data indicates that somatropin treatment increases cytochrome P450 (CYP450)-mediated antipyrine clearance in man. These data suggest that somatropin administration may alter the clearance of compounds metabolized by CYP450 liver enzymes. Careful monitoring is advisable when somatropin is administered in combination with other drugs known to be metabolized by CYP450 liver enzymes). Products include:

Uniphyl 2817

Theophylline Calcium Salicylate (Limited published data indicates that somatropin treatment increases cytochrome P450 (CYP450)-mediated antipyrine clearance in man. These data suggest that somatropin administration may alter the clearance of compounds metabolized by CYP450 liver enzymes. Careful monitoring is advisable when somatropin is administered in combination with other drugs known to be metabolized by CYP450 liver enzymes).

No products indexed under this heading.

Theophylline Dihydroxypropyl (Glyceryl) (Limited published data indicates that somatropin treatment increases cytochrome P450 (CYP450)-mediated antipyrine clearance in man. These data suggest that somatropin administration may alter the clearance of compounds metabolized by CYP450 liver enzymes. Careful monitoring is advisable when somatropin is administered in combination with other drugs known to be metabolized by CYP450 liver enzymes).

No products indexed under this heading.

Theophylline Ethylenediamine (Limited published data indicates that somatropin treatment increases cytochrome P450 (CYP450)-mediated antipyrine clearance in man. These data suggest that somatropin administration may alter the clearance of compounds metabolized by CYP450 liver enzymes. Careful monitoring is advisable when somatropin is administered in combination with other drugs known to be metabolized by CYP450 liver enzymes).

No products indexed under this heading.

Theophylline Sodium Glycinate (Limited published data indicates that somatropin treatment increases cytochrome P450 (CYP450)-mediated antipyrine clearance in man. These data suggest that somatropin administration may alter the clearance of compounds metabolized by CYP450 liver enzymes. Careful monitoring is advisable when somatropin is administered in combination with other drugs known to be metabolized by CYP450 liver enzymes).

No products indexed under this heading.

Thioridazine (Limited published data indicates that somatropin treatment increases cytochrome P450 (CYP450)-mediated antipyrine clearance in man. These data suggest that somatropin administration may alter the clearance of compounds metabolized by CYP450 liver enzymes. Careful monitoring is advisable when somatropin is administered in combination with other drugs known to be metabolized by CYP450 liver enzymes).

No products indexed under this heading.

Thioridazine Hydrochloride (Limited published data indicates that somatropin treatment increases cytochrome P450 (CYP450)-mediated antipyrine clearance in man. These data suggest that somatropin administration may alter the clearance of compounds metabolized by CYP450 liver enzymes. Careful monitoring is advisable when somatropin is administered in combination with other drugs known to be metabolized by CYP450 liver enzymes). Products include:

Thioridazine Hydrochloride 2384

Tiagabine Hydrochloride (Limited published data indicates that somatropin treatment increases cytochrome P450 (CYP450)-mediated antipyrine clearance in man. These data suggest that somatropin administration may alter the clearance of compounds metabolized by CYP450 liver enzymes (eg, anticonvulsants). Careful monitoring is advisable when somatropin is administered in combination with other drugs known to be metabolized by CYP450 liver enzymes). Products include:

Gabitril 972

Timolol Maleate (Limited published data indicates that somatropin treatment increases cytochrome P450 (CYP450)-mediated antipyrine clearance in man. These data suggest that somatropin administration may alter the clearance of compounds metabolized by CYP450 liver enzymes. Careful monitoring is advisable when somatropin is administered in combination with other drugs known to be metabolized by CYP450 liver enzymes). Products include:

Combigan 601
Dorzolamide
   Hydrochloride/Timolol Maleate
   Ophthalmic Solution .... ⊙ 243
Timoptic in Ocudose .... ⊙ 231

Tolazamide (In patients with diabetes mellitus requiring drug therapy, the dose of insulin and/or oral agent may require adjustment when somatropin therapy is initiated).

No products indexed under this heading.

Tolbutamide (In patients with diabetes mellitus requiring drug therapy, the dose of insulin and/or oral agent may require adjustment when somatropin therapy is initiated).

No products indexed under this heading.

Tolbutamide Sodium (Limited published data indicates that somatropin treatment increases cytochrome P450 (CYP450)-mediated antipyrine clearance in man. These data suggest that somatropin administration may alter the clearance of compounds metabolized by CYP450 liver enzymes. Careful monitoring is advisable when somatropin is administered in combination with other drugs known to be metabolized by CYP450 liver enzymes).

No products indexed under this heading.

Tolmetin Sodium (Limited published data indicates that somatropin treatment increases cytochrome P450 (CYP450)-mediated antipyrine clearance in man. These data suggest that somatropin administration may alter the clearance of compounds metabolized by CYP450 liver enzymes. Careful monitoring is advisable when somatropin is administered in combination with other drugs known to be metabolized by CYP450 liver enzymes).

No products indexed under this heading.

Tolterodine Tartrate (Limited published data indicates that somatropin treatment increases cytochrome P450 (CYP450)-mediated antipyrine clearance in man. These data suggest that somatropin administration may alter the clearance of compounds metabolized by CYP450 liver enzymes. Careful monitoring is advisable when somatropin is administered in combination with other drugs known to be metabolized by CYP450 liver enzymes).

No products indexed under this heading.

Topiramate (Limited published data indicates that somatropin treatment increases cytochrome P450 (CYP450)-mediated antipyrine clearance in man. These data suggest that somatropin administration may alter the clearance of compounds metabolized by

CYP450 liver enzymes (eg, anticonvulsants). Careful monitoring is advisable when somatropin is administered in combination with other drugs known to be metabolized by CYP450 liver enzymes).

No products indexed under this heading.

Torsemide (Limited published data indicates that somatropin treatment increases cytochrome P450 (CYP450)-mediated antipyrine clearance in man. These data suggest that somatropin administration may alter the clearance of compounds metabolized by CYP450 liver enzymes. Careful monitoring is advisable when somatropin is administered in combination with other drugs known to be metabolized by CYP450 liver enzymes).

No products indexed under this heading.

Tramadol Hydrochloride (Limited published data indicates that somatropin treatment increases cytochrome P450 (CYP450)-mediated antipyrine clearance in man. These data suggest that somatropin administration may alter the clearance of compounds metabolized by CYP450 liver enzymes. Careful monitoring is advisable when somatropin is administered in combination with other drugs known to be metabolized by CYP450 liver enzymes). Products include:

Ryzolt 2813
Ultram ER 2693

Trazodone Hydrochloride (Limited published data indicates that somatropin treatment increases cytochrome P450 (CYP450)-mediated antipyrine clearance in man. These data suggest that somatropin administration may alter the clearance of compounds metabolized by CYP450 liver enzymes. Careful monitoring is advisable when somatropin is administered in combination with other drugs known to be metabolized by CYP450 liver enzymes).

No products indexed under this heading.

Tretinoin (Limited published data indicates that somatropin treatment increases cytochrome P450 (CYP450)-mediated antipyrine clearance in man. These data suggest that somatropin administration may alter the clearance of compounds metabolized by CYP450 liver enzymes. Careful monitoring is advisable when somatropin is administered in combination with other drugs known to be metabolized by CYP450 liver enzymes).

No products indexed under this heading.

Triamcinolone (Somatropin inhibits 11β-hydroxysteroid dehydrogenase type 1 (11βHSD-1) in adipose/hepatic tissue and may significantly impact the metabolism of cortisol and cortisone. Patients treated with glucocorticoid replacement therapy for previously diagnosed hypoadrenalism may require an increase in their maintenance or stress doses; this may be especially true for patients treated with cortisone acetate and prednisone. In addition, excessive glucocorticoid therapy may attenuate the growth promoting effects of somatropin in children. Therefore, glucocorticoid replacement therapy should be carefully adjusted in children with concomitant GH and glucocorticoid deficiency to avoid both hypoadrenalism and an inhibitory effect on growth. Also, somatropin administration may alter the clearance of compounds known to be metabolized by CYP450 liver enzymes (eg, corticosteroids). Careful monitoring is advisable when somatropin is administered in combination with other drugs known to be metabolized by CYP450 liver enzymes).

No products indexed under this heading.

Triamcinolone Acetonide (Somatropin inhibits 11β-hydroxysteroid dehydrogenase type 1 (11βHSD-1) in adipose/

hepatic tissue and may significantly impact the metabolism of cortisol and cortisone. Patients treated with glucocorticoid replacement therapy for previously diagnosed hypoadrenalism may require an increase in their maintenance or stress doses; this may be especially true for patients treated with cortisone acetate and prednisone. In addition, excessive glucocorticoid therapy may attenuate the growth promoting effects of somatropin in children. Therefore, glucocorticoid replacement therapy should be carefully adjusted in children with concomitant GH and glucocorticoid deficiency to avoid both hypoadrenalism and an inhibitory effect on growth. Also, somatropin administration may alter the clearance of compounds known to be metabolized by CYP450 liver enzymes (eg, corticosteroids). Careful monitoring is advisable when somatropin is administered in combination with other drugs known to be metabolized by CYP450 liver enzymes). Products include:

Azmacort 408
Nasacort AQ 3019

Triamcinolone Diacetate (Somatropin inhibits 11β-hydroxysteroid dehydrogenase type 1 (11βHSD-1) in adipose/hepatic tissue and may significantly impact the metabolism of cortisol and cortisone. Patients treated with glucocorticoid replacement therapy for previously diagnosed hypoadrenalism may require an increase in their maintenance or stress doses; this may be especially true for patients treated with cortisone acetate and prednisone. In addition, excessive glucocorticoid therapy may attenuate the growth promoting effects of somatropin in children. Therefore, glucocorticoid replacement therapy should be carefully adjusted in children with concomitant GH and glucocorticoid deficiency to avoid both hypoadrenalism and an inhibitory effect on growth. Also, somatropin administration may alter the clearance of compounds known to be metabolized by CYP450 liver enzymes (eg, corticosteroids). Careful monitoring is advisable when somatropin is administered in combination with other drugs known to be metabolized by CYP450 liver enzymes).

No products indexed under this heading.

Triamcinolone Hexacetonide (Somatropin inhibits 11β-hydroxysteroid dehydrogenase type 1 (11βHSD-1) in adipose/hepatic tissue and may significantly impact the metabolism of cortisol and cortisone. Patients treated with glucocorticoid replacement therapy for previously diagnosed hypoadrenalism may require an increase in their maintenance or stress doses; this may be especially true for patients treated with cortisone acetate and prednisone. In addition, excessive glucocorticoid therapy may attenuate the growth promoting effects of somatropin in children. Therefore, glucocorticoid replacement therapy should be carefully adjusted in children with concomitant GH and glucocorticoid deficiency to avoid both hypoadrenalism and an inhibitory effect on growth. Also, somatropin administration may alter the clearance of compounds known to be metabolized by CYP450 liver enzymes (eg, corticosteroids). Careful monitoring is advisable when somatropin is administered in combination with other drugs known to be metabolized by CYP450 liver enzymes).

No products indexed under this heading.

Triazolam (Limited published data indicates that somatropin treatment increases cytochrome P450 (CYP450)-mediated antipyrine clearance in man. These data suggest that somatropin administration may alter the clearance of compounds metabolized by CYP450 liver enzymes. Careful monitoring is advisable when somatropin is

(⊙ Described in PDR® for Ophthalmic Medicines)

administered in combination with other drugs known to be metabolized by CYP450 liver enzymes).
No products indexed under this heading.

Trimethadione (Limited published data indicates that somatropin treatment increases cytochrome P450 (CYP450)-mediated antipyrine clearance in man. These data suggest that somatropin administration may alter the clearance of compounds metabolized by CYP450 liver enzymes (eg, anticonvulsants). Careful monitoring is advisable when somatropin is administered in combination with other drugs known to be metabolized by CYP450 liver enzymes).
No products indexed under this heading.

Trimethaphan Camsylate (Limited published data indicates that somatropin treatment increases cytochrome P450 (CYP450)-mediated antipyrine clearance in man. These data suggest that somatropin administration may alter the clearance of compounds metabolized by CYP450 liver enzymes. Careful monitoring is advisable when somatropin is administered in combination with other drugs known to be metabolized by CYP450 liver enzymes).
No products indexed under this heading.

Trimipramine Maleate (Limited published data indicates that somatropin treatment increases cytochrome P450 (CYP450)-mediated antipyrine clearance in man. These data suggest that somatropin administration may alter the clearance of compounds metabolized by CYP450 liver enzymes. Careful monitoring is advisable when somatropin is administered in combination with other drugs known to be metabolized by CYP450 liver enzymes).
No products indexed under this heading.

Troglitazone (In patients with diabetes mellitus requiring drug therapy, the dose of insulin and/or oral agent may require adjustment when somatropin therapy is initiated).
No products indexed under this heading.

Trovafloxacin Mesylate (Limited published data indicates that somatropin treatment increases cytochrome P450 (CYP450)-mediated antipyrine clearance in man. These data suggest that somatropin administration may alter the clearance of compounds metabolized by CYP450 liver enzymes. Careful monitoring is advisable when somatropin is administered in combination with other drugs known to be metabolized by CYP450 liver enzymes).
No products indexed under this heading.

Valdecoxib (Limited published data indicates that somatropin treatment increases cytochrome P450 (CYP450)-mediated antipyrine clearance in man. These data suggest that somatropin administration may alter the clearance of compounds metabolized by CYP450 liver enzymes. Careful monitoring is advisable when somatropin is administered in combination with other drugs known to be metabolized by CYP450 liver enzymes).
No products indexed under this heading.

Valproate Sodium (Limited published data indicates that somatropin treatment increases cytochrome P450 (CYP450)-mediated antipyrine clearance in man. These data suggest that somatropin administration may alter the clearance of compounds metabolized by CYP450 liver enzymes (eg, anticonvulsants). Careful monitoring is advisable when somatropin is administered in combination with other drugs known to be metabolized by CYP450 liver enzymes).
No products indexed under this heading.

Valproic Acid (Limited published data indicates that somatropin treatment increases cytochrome P450 (CYP450)-mediated antipyrine clearance in man. These data suggest that somatropin administration may alter the clearance of compounds metabolized by CYP450 liver enzymes (eg, anticonvulsants). Careful monitoring is advisable when somatropin is administered in combination with other drugs known to be metabolized by CYP450 liver enzymes).
No products indexed under this heading.

Valsartan (Limited published data indicates that somatropin treatment increases cytochrome P450 (CYP450)-mediated antipyrine clearance in man. These data suggest that somatropin administration may alter the clearance of compounds metabolized by CYP450 liver enzymes. Careful monitoring is advisable when somatropin is administered in combination with other drugs known to be metabolized by CYP450 liver enzymes). Products include:
Diovan 2413
Diovan HCT 2419
Exforge 2443
Exforge HCT 2449
Valturna 3637

Vardenafil Hydrochloride (Limited published data indicates that somatropin treatment increases cytochrome P450 (CYP450)-mediated antipyrine clearance in man. These data suggest that somatropin administration may alter the clearance of compounds metabolized by CYP450 liver enzymes. Careful monitoring is advisable when somatropin is administered in combination with other drugs known to be metabolized by CYP450 liver enzymes). Products include:
Levitra 3157

Venlafaxine Hydrochloride (Limited published data indicates that somatropin treatment increases cytochrome P450 (CYP450)-mediated antipyrine clearance in man. These data suggest that somatropin administration may alter the clearance of compounds metabolized by CYP450 liver enzymes. Careful monitoring is advisable when somatropin is administered in combination with other drugs known to be metabolized by CYP450 liver enzymes). Products include:
Effexor XR 3504
Venlafaxine Hydrochloride Tablets ... 2388

Verapamil Hydrochloride (Limited published data indicates that somatropin treatment increases cytochrome P450 (CYP450)-mediated antipyrine clearance in man. These data suggest that somatropin administration may alter the clearance of compounds metabolized by CYP450 liver enzymes. Careful monitoring is advisable when somatropin is administered in combination with other drugs known to be metabolized by CYP450 liver enzymes). Products include:
Tarka 534

Vinblastine Sulfate (Limited published data indicates that somatropin treatment increases cytochrome P450 (CYP450)-mediated antipyrine clearance in man. These data suggest that somatropin administration may alter the clearance of compounds metabolized by CYP450 liver enzymes. Careful monitoring is advisable when somatropin is administered in combination with other drugs known to be metabolized by CYP450 liver enzymes).
No products indexed under this heading.

Vincristine Sulfate (Limited published data indicates that somatropin treatment increases cytochrome P450 (CYP450)-mediated antipyrine clearance in man. These data suggest that somatropin administration may alter the clearance of compounds metabolized by CYP450 liver enzymes. Careful monitoring is advisable when somatropin is administered in combination with other drugs known to be metabolized by CYP450 liver enzymes).
No products indexed under this heading.

Vitamin A (Limited published data indicates that somatropin treatment increases cytochrome P450 (CYP450)-mediated antipyrine clearance in man. These data suggest that somatropin administration may alter the clearance of compounds metabolized by CYP450 liver enzymes. Careful monitoring is advisable when somatropin is administered in combination with other drugs known to be metabolized by CYP450 liver enzymes). Products include:
Cardio Basics 3455
Heplive 607
Norwegian Cod Liver Oil 919

Vitamin A Acetate (Limited published data indicates that somatropin treatment increases cytochrome P450 (CYP450)-mediated antipyrine clearance in man. These data suggest that somatropin administration may alter the clearance of compounds metabolized by CYP450 liver enzymes. Careful monitoring is advisable when somatropin is administered in combination with other drugs known to be metabolized by CYP450 liver enzymes).
No products indexed under this heading.

Voriconazole (Limited published data indicates that somatropin treatment increases cytochrome P450 (CYP450)-mediated antipyrine clearance in man. These data suggest that somatropin administration may alter the clearance of compounds metabolized by CYP450 liver enzymes. Careful monitoring is advisable when somatropin is administered in combination with other drugs known to be metabolized by CYP450 liver enzymes).
No products indexed under this heading.

Warfarin Sodium (Limited published data indicates that somatropin treatment increases cytochrome P450 (CYP450)-mediated antipyrine clearance in man. These data suggest that somatropin administration may alter the clearance of compounds metabolized by CYP450 liver enzymes. Careful monitoring is advisable when somatropin is administered in combination with other drugs known to be metabolized by CYP450 liver enzymes).
No products indexed under this heading.

Zafirlukast (Limited published data indicates that somatropin treatment increases cytochrome P450 (CYP450)-mediated antipyrine clearance in man. These data suggest that somatropin administration may alter the clearance of compounds metabolized by CYP450 liver enzymes. Careful monitoring is advisable when somatropin is administered in combination with other drugs known to be metabolized by CYP450 liver enzymes). Products include:
Accolate 3612

Zileuton (Limited published data indicates that somatropin treatment increases cytochrome P450 (CYP450)-mediated antipyrine clearance in man. These data suggest that somatropin administration may alter the clearance of compounds metabolized by CYP450 liver enzymes. Careful monitoring is advisable when somatropin is administered in combination with other drugs known to be metabolized by CYP450 liver enzymes).
No products indexed under this heading.

Zolmitriptan (Limited published data indicates that somatropin treatment increases cytochrome P450 (CYP450)-mediated antipyrine clearance in man. These data suggest that somatropin administration may alter the clearance of compounds metabolized by CYP450 liver enzymes. Careful monitoring is advisable when somatropin is administered in combination with other drugs known to be metabolized by CYP450 liver enzymes). Products include:
Zomig Tablets 773
Zomig Nasal Spray 768
Zomig-ZMT Tablets 773

Zonisamide (Limited published data indicates that somatropin treatment increases cytochrome P450 (CYP450)-mediated antipyrine clearance in man. These data suggest that somatropin administration may alter the clearance of compounds metabolized by CYP450 liver enzymes (eg, anticonvulsants). Careful monitoring is advisable when somatropin is administered in combination with other drugs known to be metabolized by CYP450 liver enzymes). Products include:
Zonegran 1081

Zopiclone (Limited published data indicates that somatropin treatment increases cytochrome P450 (CYP450)-mediated antipyrine clearance in man. These data suggest that somatropin administration may alter the clearance of compounds metabolized by CYP450 liver enzymes. Careful monitoring is advisable when somatropin is administered in combination with other drugs known to be metabolized by CYP450 liver enzymes).
No products indexed under this heading.

Food Interactions

Beverages, caffeine-containing (Limited published data indicates that somatropin treatment increases cytochrome P450 (CYP450)-mediated antipyrine clearance in man. These data suggest that somatropin administration may alter the clearance of compounds metabolized by CYP450 liver enzymes. Careful monitoring is advisable when somatropin is administered in combination with other drugs known to be metabolized by CYP450 liver enzymes).

Food, caffeine-containing (Limited published data indicates that somatropin treatment increases cytochrome P450 (CYP450)-mediated antipyrine clearance in man. These data suggest that somatropin administration may alter the clearance of compounds metabolized by CYP450 liver enzymes. Careful monitoring is advisable when somatropin is administered in combination with other drugs known to be metabolized by CYP450 liver enzymes).

GEODON CAPSULES

(Ziprasidone Hydrochloride) 2723
May interact with antihypertensives, centrally-acting drugs, class 1A antiarrhythmics, class III antiarrhythmics, cytochrome p450 3a4 inhibitors (selected), cytochrome p450 3a4 inhibitors, potent (selected), dopamine agonists, drugs that prolong the QT interval, quinidine, and certain other agents. Compounds in these categories include:

Acebutolol Hydrochloride (Ziprasidone may enhance the effects of certain antihypertensive agents because of its potential for inducing hypotension).
No products indexed under this heading.

Acetazolamide (Ketoconazole, a potent inhibitor of CYP3A4, at a dose of 400 mg QD for 5 days, increased the AUC and C_{max} of ziprasidone by about 35-40%. Other inhibitors of CYP3A4 would be expected to have similar effects).
No products indexed under this heading.

IMPORTANT NOTE: Always consult each drug listing in the patient's regimen for possible interactions.

Geodon Interactions Index 766

Acetazolamide Sodium (Ketoconazole, a potent inhibitor of CYP3A4, at a dose of 400 mg QD for 5 days, increased the AUC and C_{max} of ziprasidone by about 35-40%. Other inhibitors of CYP3A4 would be expected to have similar effects).
No products indexed under this heading.

Alfentanil Hydrochloride (Caution should be used when ziprasidone is taken in combination with other centrally acting drugs, given the primary CNS effects of ziprasidone).
No products indexed under this heading.

Aliskiren (Ziprasidone may enhance the effects of certain antihypertensive agents because of its potential for inducing hypotension). Products include:
Tekturna ... 2538
Tekturna HCT ... 2541
Valturna ... 3637

Alprazolam (Ziprasidone is contraindicated with drugs that have demonstrated QT prolongation as one of their pharmacodynamic effects and have this effect described in the full prescribing information as a contraindication or a boxed or bolded warning. Ziprasidone should not be used with any drug that prolongs the QT interval. An additive effect of ziprasidone and other drugs that prolong the QT interval cannot be excluded. Therefore, ziprasidone should not be given with dofetilide, sotalol, quinidine, other Class Ia and III anti-arrhythmics, mesoridazine, thioridazine, chlorpromazine, droperidol, pimozide, sparfloxacin, gatifloxacin, moxifloxacin, halofantrine, mefloquine, pentamidine, arsenic trioxide, levomethadyl acetate, dolasetron mesylate, probucol or tacrolimus).
No products indexed under this heading.

Amiodarone Hydrochloride (Ziprasidone is contraindicated with drugs that have demonstrated QT prolongation as one of their pharmacodynamic effects and have this effect described in the full prescribing information as a contraindication or a boxed or bolded warning. Ziprasidone should not be used with any drug that prolongs the QT interval. An additive effect of ziprasidone and other drugs that prolong the QT interval cannot be excluded. Therefore, ziprasidone should not be given with dofetilide, sotalol, quinidine, other Class Ia and III anti-arrhythmics, mesoridazine, thioridazine, chlorpromazine, droperidol, pimozide, sparfloxacin, gatifloxacin, moxifloxacin, halofantrine, mefloquine, pentamidine, arsenic trioxide, levomethadyl acetate, dolasetron mesylate, probucol or tacrolimus).
No products indexed under this heading.

Amitriptyline Hydrochloride (Ziprasidone is contraindicated with drugs that have demonstrated QT prolongation as one of their pharmacodynamic effects and have this effect described in the full prescribing information as a contraindication or a boxed or bolded warning. Ziprasidone should not be used with any drug that prolongs the QT interval. An additive effect of ziprasidone and other drugs that prolong the QT interval cannot be excluded. Therefore, ziprasidone should not be given with dofetilide, sotalol, quinidine, other Class Ia and III anti-arrhythmics, mesoridazine, thioridazine, chlorpromazine, droperidol, pimozide, sparfloxacin, gatifloxacin, moxifloxacin, halofantrine, mefloquine, pentamidine, arsenic trioxide, levomethadyl acetate, dolasetron mesylate, probucol or tacrolimus).
No products indexed under this heading.

Amlodipine Besylate (Ziprasidone may enhance the effects of certain antihypertensive agents because of its potential for inducing hypotension). Products include:
Azor ... 1010
Exforge ... 2443
Exforge HCT ... 2449

Amoxapine (Ziprasidone is contraindicated with drugs that have demonstrated QT prolongation as one of their pharmacodynamic effects and have this effect described in the full prescribing information as a contraindication or a boxed or bolded warning. Ziprasidone should not be used with any drug that prolongs the QT interval. An additive effect of ziprasidone and other drugs that prolong the QT interval cannot be excluded. Therefore, ziprasidone should not be given with dofetilide, sotalol, quinidine, other Class Ia and III anti-arrhythmics, mesoridazine, thioridazine, chlorpromazine, droperidol, pimozide, sparfloxacin, gatifloxacin, moxifloxacin, halofantrine, mefloquine, pentamidine, arsenic trioxide, levomethadyl acetate, dolasetron mesylate, probucol or tacrolimus).
No products indexed under this heading.

Amphetamine Aspartate (Caution should be used when ziprasidone is taken in combination with other centrally acting drugs, given the primary CNS effects of ziprasidone).
No products indexed under this heading.

Amphetamine Aspartate Monohydrate (Caution should be used when ziprasidone is taken in combination with other centrally acting drugs, given the primary CNS effects of ziprasidone).
No products indexed under this heading.

Amphetamine Resins (Caution should be used when ziprasidone is taken in combination with other centrally acting drugs, given the primary CNS effects of ziprasidone).
No products indexed under this heading.

Amphetamine Sulfate (Caution should be used when ziprasidone is taken in combination with other centrally acting drugs, given the primary CNS effects of ziprasidone).
No products indexed under this heading.

Amprenavir (Ketoconazole, a potent inhibitor of CYP3A4, at a dose of 400 mg QD for 5 days, increased the AUC and C_{max} of ziprasidone by about 35-40%. Other inhibitors of CYP3A4 would be expected to have similar effects).
No products indexed under this heading.

Anastrozole (Ketoconazole, a potent inhibitor of CYP3A4, at a dose of 400 mg QD for 5 days, increased the AUC and C_{max} of ziprasidone by about 35-40%. Other inhibitors of CYP3A4 would be expected to have similar effects).
No products indexed under this heading.

Aprepitant (Ketoconazole, a potent inhibitor of CYP3A4, at a dose of 400 mg QD for 5 days, increased the AUC and C_{max} of ziprasidone by about 35-40%. Other inhibitors of CYP3A4 would be expected to have similar effects). Products include:
Emend ... 2124

Aprobarbital (Caution should be used when ziprasidone is taken in combination with other centrally acting drugs, given the primary CNS effects of ziprasidone).
No products indexed under this heading.

Arsenic Trioxide (Ziprasidone is contraindicated with drugs that have demonstrated QT prolongation as one of their pharmacodynamic effects and have this effect described in the full prescribing information as a contraindication or a boxed or bolded warning. Ziprasidone should not be used with any drug that prolongs the QT interval. An additive effect of ziprasidone and other drugs that prolong the QT interval cannot be excluded. Therefore, ziprasidone should not be given with dofetilide, sotalol, quinidine, other Class Ia and III anti-arrhythmics, mesoridazine, thioridazine, chlorpromazine, droperidol, pimozide, sparfloxacin, gatifloxacin, moxifloxacin, halofantrine, mefloquine, pentamidine, arsenic trioxide, levomethadyl acetate, dolasetron mesylate, probucol or tacrolimus). Products include:
Trisenox ... 994

Astemizole (Ziprasidone is contraindicated with drugs that have demonstrated QT prolongation as one of their pharmacodynamic effects and have this effect described in the full prescribing information as a contraindication or a boxed or bolded warning. Ziprasidone should not be used with any drug that prolongs the QT interval. An additive effect of ziprasidone and other drugs that prolong the QT interval cannot be excluded. Therefore, ziprasidone should not be given with dofetilide, sotalol, quinidine, other Class Ia and III anti-arrhythmics, mesoridazine, thioridazine, chlorpromazine, droperidol, pimozide, sparfloxacin, gatifloxacin, moxifloxacin, halofantrine, mefloquine, pentamidine, arsenic trioxide, levomethadyl acetate, dolasetron mesylate, probucol or tacrolimus).
No products indexed under this heading.

Atazanavir (Ketoconazole, a potent inhibitor of CYP3A4, at a dose of 400 mg QD for 5 days, increased the AUC and C_{max} of ziprasidone by about 35-40%. Other inhibitors of CYP3A4 would be expected to have similar effects).
No products indexed under this heading.

Atazanavir Sulfate (Ketoconazole, a potent inhibitor of CYP3A4, at a dose of 400 mg QD for 5 days, increased the AUC and C_{max} of ziprasidone by about 35-40%. Other inhibitors of CYP3A4 would be expected to have similar effects).
No products indexed under this heading.

Atenolol (Ziprasidone may enhance the effects of certain antihypertensive agents because of its potential for inducing hypotension).
No products indexed under this heading.

Benazepril Hydrochloride (Ziprasidone may enhance the effects of certain antihypertensive agents because of its potential for inducing hypotension).
No products indexed under this heading.

Bendroflumethiazide (Ziprasidone may enhance the effects of certain antihypertensive agents because of its potential for inducing hypotension).
No products indexed under this heading.

Betaxolol Hydrochloride (Ziprasidone may enhance the effects of certain antihypertensive agents because of its potential for inducing hypotension).
No products indexed under this heading.

Bisoprolol Fumarate (Ziprasidone may enhance the effects of certain antihypertensive agents because of its potential for inducing hypotension).
No products indexed under this heading.

Bretylium Tosylate (Ziprasidone is contraindicated with drugs that have demonstrated QT prolongation as one of their pharmacodynamic effects and have this effect described in the full prescribing information as a contraindication or a boxed or bolded warning. Ziprasidone should not be used with any drug that prolongs the QT interval. An additive effect of ziprasidone and other drugs that prolong the QT interval cannot be excluded. Therefore, ziprasidone should not be given with dofetilide, sotalol, quinidine, other Class Ia and III anti-arrhythmics, mesoridazine, thioridazine, chlorpromazine, droperidol, pimozide, sparfloxacin, gatifloxacin, moxifloxacin, halofantrine, mefloquine, pentamidine, arsenic trioxide, levomethadyl acetate, dolasetron mesylate, probucol or tacrolimus).
No products indexed under this heading.

Bromocriptine Mesylate (Ziprasidone may antagonize the effects of dopamine agonists).
No products indexed under this heading.

Buprenorphine Hydrochloride (Caution should be used when ziprasidone is taken in combination with other centrally acting drugs, given the primary CNS effects of ziprasidone).
No products indexed under this heading.

Buspirone Hydrochloride (Ziprasidone is contraindicated with drugs that have demonstrated QT prolongation as one of their pharmacodynamic effects and have this effect described in the full prescribing information as a contraindication or a boxed or bolded warning. Ziprasidone should not be used with any drug that prolongs the QT interval. An additive effect of ziprasidone and other drugs that prolong the QT interval cannot be excluded. Therefore, ziprasidone should not be given with dofetilide, sotalol, quinidine, other Class Ia and III anti-arrhythmics, mesoridazine, thioridazine, chlorpromazine, droperidol, pimozide, sparfloxacin, gatifloxacin, moxifloxacin, halofantrine, mefloquine, pentamidine, arsenic trioxide, levomethadyl acetate, dolasetron mesylate, probucol or tacrolimus).
No products indexed under this heading.

Butabarbital (Caution should be used when ziprasidone is taken in combination with other centrally acting drugs, given the primary CNS effects of ziprasidone).
No products indexed under this heading.

Butalbital (Caution should be used when ziprasidone is taken in combination with other centrally acting drugs, given the primary CNS effects of ziprasidone).
No products indexed under this heading.

Candesartan Cilexetil (Ziprasidone may enhance the effects of certain antihypertensive agents because of its potential for inducing hypotension). Products include:
Atacand ... 697
Atacand HCT ... 700

Captopril (Ziprasidone may enhance the effects of certain antihypertensive agents because of its potential for inducing hypotension). Products include:
Captopril ... 2341

Carbamazepine (Carbamazepine is an inducer of CYP3A4. Administration of 200 mg of carbamazepine BID for 21 days resulted in a decrease of approximately 35% in the AUC of ziprasidone. This effect may be greater when higher doses of carbamazepine are administered). Products include:
Carbatrol ... 3280
Equetro ... 3477

Carteolol Hydrochloride (Ziprasidone may enhance the effects of certain antihypertensive agents because of its potential for inducing hypotension).
No products indexed under this heading.

Carvedilol (Ziprasidone may enhance the effects of certain antihypertensive agents because of its potential for inducing hypotension). Products include:
Coreg ... 1409

Carvedilol Phosphate (Ziprasidone may enhance the effects of certain antihypertensive agents because of its potential for inducing hypotension). Products include:
Coreg CR ... 1416

Chlordiazepoxide (Ziprasidone is contraindicated with drugs that have demonstrated QT prolongation as one

of their pharmacodynamic effects and have this effect described in the full prescribing information as a contraindication or a boxed or bolded warning. Ziprasidone should not be used with any drug that prolongs the QT interval. An additive effect of ziprasidone and other drugs that prolong the QT interval cannot be excluded. Therefore, ziprasidone should not be given with dofetilide, sotalol, quinidine, other Class la and III anti-arrhythmics, mesoridazine, thioridazine, chlorpromazine, droperidol, pimozide, sparfloxacin, gatifloxacin, moxifloxacin, halofantrine, mefloquine, pentamidine, arsenic trioxide, levomethadyl acetate, dolasetron mesylate, probucol or tacrolimus).
No products indexed under this heading.

Chlordiazepoxide Hydrochloride (Ziprasidone is contraindicated with drugs that have demonstrated QT prolongation as one of their pharmacodynamic effects and have this effect described in the full prescribing information as a contraindication or a boxed or bolded warning. Ziprasidone should not be used with any drug that prolongs the QT interval. An additive effect of ziprasidone and other drugs that prolong the QT interval cannot be excluded. Therefore, ziprasidone should not be given with dofetilide, sotalol, quinidine, other Class la and III anti-arrhythmics, mesoridazine, thioridazine, chlorpromazine, droperidol, pimozide, sparfloxacin, gatifloxacin, moxifloxacin, halofantrine, mefloquine, pentamidine, arsenic trioxide, levomethadyl acetate, dolasetron mesylate, probucol or tacrolimus).
No products indexed under this heading.

Chlorothiazide (Ziprasidone may enhance the effects of certain antihypertensive agents because of its potential for inducing hypotension).
No products indexed under this heading.

Chlorothiazide Sodium (Ziprasidone may enhance the effects of certain antihypertensive agents because of its potential for inducing hypotension). Products include:

Chlorpromazine (Ziprasidone is contraindicated with drugs that have demonstrated QT prolongation as one of their pharmacodynamic effects and have this effect described in the full prescribing information as a contraindication or a boxed or bolded warning. Ziprasidone should not be used with any drug that prolongs the QT interval. An additive effect of ziprasidone and other drugs that prolong the QT interval cannot be excluded. Therefore, ziprasidone should not be given with dofetilide, sotalol, quinidine, other Class la and III anti-arrhythmics, mesoridazine, thioridazine, chlorpromazine, droperidol, pimozide, sparfloxacin, gatifloxacin, moxifloxacin, halofantrine, mefloquine, pentamidine, arsenic trioxide, levomethadyl acetate, dolasetron mesylate, probucol or tacrolimus).
No products indexed under this heading.

Chlorpromazine Hydrochloride (Ziprasidone is contraindicated with drugs that have demonstrated QT prolongation as one of their pharmacodynamic effects and have this effect described in the full prescribing information as a contraindication or a boxed or bolded warning. Ziprasidone should not be used with any drug that prolongs the QT interval. An additive effect of ziprasidone and other drugs that prolong the QT interval cannot be excluded. Therefore, ziprasidone should not be given with dofetilide, sotalol, quinidine, other Class la and III anti-arrhythmics, mesoridazine, thioridazine, chlorpromazine, droperidol, pimozide, sparfloxacin, gatifloxacin, moxifloxacin, halofantrine,

mefloquine, pentamidine, arsenic trioxide, levomethadyl acetate, dolasetron mesylate, probucol or tacrolimus).
No products indexed under this heading.

Chlorprothixene (Ziprasidone is contraindicated with drugs that have demonstrated QT prolongation as one of their pharmacodynamic effects and have this effect described in the full prescribing information as a contraindication or a boxed or bolded warning. Ziprasidone should not be used with any drug that prolongs the QT interval. An additive effect of ziprasidone and other drugs that prolong the QT interval cannot be excluded. Therefore, ziprasidone should not be given with dofetilide, sotalol, quinidine, other Class la and III anti-arrhythmics, mesoridazine, thioridazine, chlorpromazine, droperidol, pimozide, sparfloxacin, gatifloxacin, moxifloxacin, halofantrine, mefloquine, pentamidine, arsenic trioxide, levomethadyl acetate, dolasetron mesylate, probucol or tacrolimus).
No products indexed under this heading.

Chlorprothixene Hydrochloride (Ziprasidone is contraindicated with drugs that have demonstrated QT prolongation as one of their pharmacodynamic effects and have this effect described in the full prescribing information as a contraindication or a boxed or bolded warning. Ziprasidone should not be used with any drug that prolongs the QT interval. An additive effect of ziprasidone and other drugs that prolong the QT interval cannot be excluded. Therefore, ziprasidone should not be given with dofetilide, sotalol, quinidine, other Class la and III anti-arrhythmics, mesoridazine, thioridazine, chlorpromazine, droperidol, pimozide, sparfloxacin, gatifloxacin, moxifloxacin, halofantrine, mefloquine, pentamidine, arsenic trioxide, levomethadyl acetate, dolasetron mesylate, probucol or tacrolimus).
No products indexed under this heading.

Chlorprothixene Lactate (Caution should be used when ziprasidone is taken in combination with other centrally acting drugs, given the primary CNS effects of ziprasidone).
No products indexed under this heading.

Chlorthalidone (Ziprasidone may enhance the effects of certain antihypertensive agents because of its potential for inducing hypotension). Products include:

Cimetidine (Ketoconazole, a potent inhibitor of CYP3A4, at a dose of 400 mg QD for 5 days, increased the AUC and C_{max} of ziprasidone by about 35-40%. Other inhibitors of CYP3A4 would be expected to have similar effects).
No products indexed under this heading.

Cimetidine Hydrochloride (Ketoconazole, a potent inhibitor of CYP3A4, at a dose of 400 mg QD for 5 days, increased the AUC and C_{max} of ziprasidone by about 35-40%. Other inhibitors of CYP3A4 would be expected to have similar effects).
No products indexed under this heading.

Ciprofloxacin (Ketoconazole, a potent inhibitor of CYP3A4, at a dose of 400 mg QD for 5 days, increased the AUC and C_{max} of ziprasidone by about 35-40%. Other inhibitors of CYP3A4 would be expected to have similar effects). Products include:

Clarithromycin (Ketoconazole, a potent inhibitor of CYP3A4, at a dose of 400 mg QD for 5 days, increased the AUC and C_{max} of ziprasidone by about

35-40%. Other inhibitors of CYP3A4 would be expected to have similar effects). Products include:

Clomipramine Hydrochloride (Ziprasidone is contraindicated with drugs that have demonstrated QT prolongation as one of their pharmacodynamic effects and have this effect described in the full prescribing information as a contraindication or a boxed or bolded warning. Ziprasidone should not be used with any drug that prolongs the QT interval. An additive effect of ziprasidone and other drugs that prolong the QT interval cannot be excluded. Therefore, ziprasidone should not be given with dofetilide, sotalol, quinidine, other Class la and III anti-arrhythmics, mesoridazine, thioridazine, chlorpromazine, droperidol, pimozide, sparfloxacin, gatifloxacin, moxifloxacin, halofantrine, mefloquine, pentamidine, arsenic trioxide, levomethadyl acetate, dolasetron mesylate, probucol or tacrolimus).
No products indexed under this heading.

Clonidine (Ziprasidone may enhance the effects of certain antihypertensive agents because of its potential for inducing hypotension). Products include:

Clonidine Hydrochloride (Ziprasidone may enhance the effects of certain antihypertensive agents because of its potential for inducing hypotension). Products include:

Clorazepate Dipotassium (Ziprasidone is contraindicated with drugs that have demonstrated QT prolongation as one of their pharmacodynamic effects and have this effect described in the full prescribing information as a contraindication or a boxed or bolded warning. Ziprasidone should not be used with any drug that prolongs the QT interval. An additive effect of ziprasidone and other drugs that prolong the QT interval cannot be excluded. Therefore, ziprasidone should not be given with dofetilide, sotalol, quinidine, other Class la and III anti-arrhythmics, mesoridazine, thioridazine, chlorpromazine, droperidol, pimozide, sparfloxacin, gatifloxacin, moxifloxacin, halofantrine, mefloquine, pentamidine, arsenic trioxide, levomethadyl acetate, dolasetron mesylate, probucol or tacrolimus).
No products indexed under this heading.

Clotrimazole (Ketoconazole, a potent inhibitor of CYP3A4, at a dose of 400 mg QD for 5 days, increased the AUC and C_{max} of ziprasidone by about 35-40%. Other inhibitors of CYP3A4 would be expected to have similar effects). Products include:

Clozapine (Ziprasidone is contraindicated with drugs that have demonstrated QT prolongation as one of their pharmacodynamic effects and have this effect described in the full prescribing information as a contraindication or a boxed or bolded warning. Ziprasidone should not be used with any drug that prolongs the QT interval. An additive effect of ziprasidone and other drugs that prolong the QT interval cannot be excluded. Therefore, ziprasidone should not be given with dofetilide, sotalol, quinidine, other Class la and III anti-arrhythmics, mesoridazine, thioridazine, chlorpromazine, droperidol, pimozide, sparfloxacin, gatifloxacin, moxifloxacin, halofantrine, mefloquine, pentamidine, arsenic trioxide, levomethadyl acetate, dolasetron mesylate, probucol or tacrolimus).
No products indexed under this heading.

Codeine Phosphate (Caution should be used when ziprasidone is taken in

combination with other centrally acting drugs, given the primary CNS effects of ziprasidone). Products include:

Codeine Sulfate (Caution should be used when ziprasidone is taken in combination with other centrally acting drugs, given the primary CNS effects of ziprasidone).
No products indexed under this heading.

Conivaptan Hydrochloride (Ketoconazole, a potent inhibitor of CYP3A4, at a dose of 400 mg QD for 5 days, increased the AUC and C_{max} of ziprasidone by about 35-40%. Other inhibitors of CYP3A4 would be expected to have similar effects). Products include:

Cyclosporine (Ketoconazole, a potent inhibitor of CYP3A4, at a dose of 400 mg QD for 5 days, increased the AUC and C_{max} of ziprasidone by about 35-40%. Other inhibitors of CYP3A4 would be expected to have similar effects). Products include:

Dalfopristin (Ketoconazole, a potent inhibitor of CYP3A4, at a dose of 400 mg QD for 5 days, increased the AUC and C_{max} of ziprasidone by about 35-40%. Other inhibitors of CYP3A4 would be expected to have similar effects).
No products indexed under this heading.

Danazol (Ketoconazole, a potent inhibitor of CYP3A4, at a dose of 400 mg QD for 5 days, increased the AUC and C_{max} of ziprasidone by about 35-40%. Other inhibitors of CYP3A4 would be expected to have similar effects).
No products indexed under this heading.

Darunavir (Ketoconazole, a potent inhibitor of CYP3A4, at a dose of 400 mg QD for 5 days, increased the AUC and C_{max} of ziprasidone by about 35-40%. Other inhibitors of CYP3A4 would be expected to have similar effects).
No products indexed under this heading.

Dasatinib (Ketoconazole, a potent inhibitor of CYP3A4, at a dose of 400 mg QD for 5 days, increased the AUC and C_{max} of ziprasidone by about 35-40%. Other inhibitors of CYP3A4 would be expected to have similar effects).
No products indexed under this heading.

Delavirdine Mesylate (Ketoconazole, a potent inhibitor of CYP3A4, at a dose of 400 mg QD for 5 days, increased the AUC and C_{max} of ziprasidone by about 35-40%. Other inhibitors of CYP3A4 would be expected to have similar effects).
No products indexed under this heading.

Delavirine (Ketoconazole, a potent inhibitor of CYP3A4, at a dose of 400 mg QD for 5 days, increased the AUC and C_{max} of ziprasidone by about 35-40%. Other inhibitors of CYP3A4 would be expected to have similar effects).
No products indexed under this heading.

Deserpidine (Ziprasidone may enhance the effects of certain antihypertensive agents because of its potential for inducing hypotension).
No products indexed under this heading.

Desflurane (Caution should be used when ziprasidone is taken in combination with other centrally acting drugs, given the primary CNS effects of ziprasidone).
No products indexed under this heading.

Desipramine Hydrochloride (Ziprasidone is contraindicated with drugs that have demonstrated QT pro-

Geodon Interactions Index 768

longation as one of their pharmacodynamic effects and have this effect described in the full prescribing information as a contraindication or a boxed or bolded warning. Ziprasidone should not be used with any drug that prolongs the QT interval. An additive effect of ziprasidone and other drugs that prolong the QT interval cannot be excluded. Therefore, ziprasidone should not be given with dofetilide, sotalol, quinidine, other Class Ia and III anti-arrhythmics, mesoridazine, thioridazine, chlorpromazine, droperidol, pimozide, sparfloxacin, gatifloxacin, moxifloxacin, halofantrine, mefloquine, pentamidine, arsenic trioxide, levomethadyl acetate, dolasetron mesylate, probucol or tacrolimus).
No products indexed under this heading.

Desloratadine (Ketoconazole, a potent inhibitor of CYP3A4, at a dose of 400 mg QD for 5 days, increased the AUC and C_{max} of ziprasidone by about 35-40%. Other inhibitors of CYP3A4 would be expected to have similar effects). Products include:
Clarinex Syrup 3098
Clarinex 3098
Clarinex Reditabs 3098
Clarinex-D 12-Hour 3101
Clarinex-D 3104

Dexmethylphenidate Hydrochloride (Caution should be used when ziprasidone is taken in combination with other centrally acting drugs, given the primary CNS effects of ziprasidone). Products include:
Focalin XR 2472

Dextroamphetamine (Caution should be used when ziprasidone is taken in combination with other centrally acting drugs, given the primary CNS effects of ziprasidone).
No products indexed under this heading.

Dextroamphetamine Saccharate (Caution should be used when ziprasidone is taken in combination with other centrally acting drugs, given the primary CNS effects of ziprasidone).
No products indexed under this heading.

Dextroamphetamine Sulfate (Caution should be used when ziprasidone is taken in combination with other centrally acting drugs, given the primary CNS effects of ziprasidone). Products include:
Dexedrine 1425

Dezocine (Caution should be used when ziprasidone is taken in combination with other centrally acting drugs, given the primary CNS effects of ziprasidone).
No products indexed under this heading.

Diazepam (Ziprasidone is contraindicated with drugs that have demonstrated QT prolongation as one of their pharmacodynamic effects and have this effect described in the full prescribing information as a contraindication or a boxed or bolded warning. Ziprasidone should not be used with any drug that prolongs the QT interval. An additive effect of ziprasidone and other drugs that prolong the QT interval cannot be excluded. Therefore, ziprasidone should not be given with dofetilide, sotalol, quinidine, other Class Ia and III anti-arrhythmics, mesoridazine, thioridazine, chlorpromazine, droperidol, pimozide, sparfloxacin, gatifloxacin, moxifloxacin, halofantrine, mefloquine, pentamidine, arsenic trioxide, levomethadyl acetate, dolasetron mesylate, probucol or tacrolimus). Products include:
Valium Tablets 2880

Diazoxide (Ziprasidone may enhance the effects of certain antihypertensive agents because of its potential for inducing hypotension). Products include:
Proglycem 1179
Proglycem Suspension 1179

Diltiazem Hydrochloride (Ziprasidone may enhance the effects of certain antihypertensive agents because of its potential for inducing hypotension). Products include:
Cardizem LA 423

Diltiazem Maleate (Ziprasidone may enhance the effects of certain antihypertensive agents because of its potential for inducing hypotension).
No products indexed under this heading.

Disopyramide (Ziprasidone is contraindicated with drugs that have demonstrated QT prolongation as one of their pharmacodynamic effects and have this effect described in the full prescribing information as a contraindication or a boxed or bolded warning. Ziprasidone should not be used with any drug that prolongs the QT interval. An additive effect of ziprasidone and other drugs that prolong the QT interval cannot be excluded. Therefore, ziprasidone should not be given with dofetilide, sotalol, quinidine, other Class Ia and III anti-arrhythmics, mesoridazine, thioridazine, chlorpromazine, droperidol, pimozide, sparfloxacin, gatifloxacin, moxifloxacin, halofantrine, mefloquine, pentamidine, arsenic trioxide, levomethadyl acetate, dolasetron mesylate, probucol or tacrolimus).
No products indexed under this heading.

Disopyramide Phosphate (Ziprasidone is contraindicated with drugs that have demonstrated QT prolongation as one of their pharmacodynamic effects and have this effect described in the full prescribing information as a contraindication or a boxed or bolded warning. Ziprasidone should not be used with any drug that prolongs the QT interval. An additive effect of ziprasidone and other drugs that prolong the QT interval cannot be excluded. Therefore, ziprasidone should not be given with dofetilide, sotalol, quinidine, other Class Ia and III anti-arrhythmics, mesoridazine, thioridazine, chlorpromazine, droperidol, pimozide, sparfloxacin, gatifloxacin, moxifloxacin, halofantrine, mefloquine, pentamidine, arsenic trioxide, levomethadyl acetate, dolasetron mesylate, probucol or tacrolimus).
No products indexed under this heading.

Dofetilide (Ziprasidone is contraindicated with drugs that have demonstrated QT prolongation as one of their pharmacodynamic effects and have this effect described in the full prescribing information as a contraindication or a boxed or bolded warning. Ziprasidone should not be used with any drug that prolongs the QT interval. An additive effect of ziprasidone and other drugs that prolong the QT interval cannot be excluded. Therefore, ziprasidone should not be given with dofetilide, sotalol, quinidine, other Class Ia and III anti-arrhythmics, mesoridazine, thioridazine, chlorpromazine, droperidol, pimozide, sparfloxacin, gatifloxacin, moxifloxacin, halofantrine, mefloquine, pentamidine, arsenic trioxide, levomethadyl acetate, dolasetron mesylate, probucol or tacrolimus).
No products indexed under this heading.

Dolasetron Mesylate (Ziprasidone is contraindicated with drugs that have demonstrated QT prolongation as one of their pharmacodynamic effects and have this effect described in the full prescribing information as a contraindication or a boxed or bolded warning. Ziprasidone should not be used with any drug that prolongs the QT interval. An additive effect of ziprasidone and other drugs that prolong the QT interval cannot be excluded. Therefore, ziprasidone should not be given with dofetilide, sotalol, quinidine, other Class Ia and III anti-arrhythmics, mesoridazine, thioridazine, chlorpromazine, droperidol, pimozide, sparfloxacin, gatifloxacin, moxifloxacin, halofantrine, mefloquine, pentamidine, arsenic trioxide, levomethadyl acetate, dolasetron mesylate, probucol or tacrolimus). Products include:
Anzemet Injection 2931
Anzemet Tablets 2934

Dopamine Hydrochloride (Ziprasidone may antagonize the effects of dopamine agonists).
No products indexed under this heading.

Doxazosin Mesylate (Ziprasidone may enhance the effects of certain antihypertensive agents because of its potential for inducing hypotension).
No products indexed under this heading.

Doxepin Hydrochloride (Ziprasidone is contraindicated with drugs that have demonstrated QT prolongation as one of their pharmacodynamic effects and have this effect described in the full prescribing information as a contraindication or a boxed or bolded warning. Ziprasidone should not be used with any drug that prolongs the QT interval. An additive effect of ziprasidone and other drugs that prolong the QT interval cannot be excluded. Therefore, ziprasidone should not be given with dofetilide, sotalol, quinidine, other Class Ia and III anti-arrhythmics, mesoridazine, thioridazine, chlorpromazine, droperidol, pimozide, sparfloxacin, gatifloxacin, moxifloxacin, halofantrine, mefloquine, pentamidine, arsenic trioxide, levomethadyl acetate, dolasetron mesylate, probucol or tacrolimus).
No products indexed under this heading.

Droperidol (Ziprasidone is contraindicated with drugs that have demonstrated QT prolongation as one of their pharmacodynamic effects and have this effect described in the full prescribing information as a contraindication or a boxed or bolded warning. Ziprasidone should not be used with any drug that prolongs the QT interval. An additive effect of ziprasidone and other drugs that prolong the QT interval cannot be excluded. Therefore, ziprasidone should not be given with dofetilide, sotalol, quinidine, other Class Ia and III anti-arrhythmics, mesoridazine, thioridazine, chlorpromazine, droperidol, pimozide, sparfloxacin, gatifloxacin, moxifloxacin, halofantrine, mefloquine, pentamidine, arsenic trioxide, levomethadyl acetate, dolasetron mesylate, probucol or tacrolimus).
No products indexed under this heading.

Efavirenz (Ketoconazole, a potent inhibitor of CYP3A4, at a dose of 400 mg QD for 5 days, increased the AUC and C_{max} of ziprasidone by about 35-40%. Other inhibitors of CYP3A4 would be expected to have similar effects). Products include:
Atripla 906

Enalapril Maleate (Ziprasidone may enhance the effects of certain antihypertensive agents because of its potential for inducing hypotension).
No products indexed under this heading.

Enalaprilat (Ziprasidone may enhance the effects of certain antihypertensive agents because of its potential for inducing hypotension).
No products indexed under this heading.

Enflurane (Caution should be used when ziprasidone is taken in combination with other centrally acting drugs, given the primary CNS effects of ziprasidone).
No products indexed under this heading.

Eprosartan Mesylate (Ziprasidone may enhance the effects of certain antihypertensive agents because of its potential for inducing hypotension). Products include:
Teveten 538
Teveten HCT 541

Erythromycin (Ziprasidone is contraindicated with drugs that have demonstrated QT prolongation as one of their pharmacodynamic effects and have this effect described in the full prescribing information as a contraindication or a boxed or bolded warning. Ziprasidone should not be used with any drug that prolongs the QT interval. An additive effect of ziprasidone and other drugs that prolong the QT interval cannot be excluded. Therefore, ziprasidone should not be given with dofetilide, sotalol, quinidine, other Class Ia and III anti-arrhythmics, mesoridazine, thioridazine, chlorpromazine, droperidol, pimozide, sparfloxacin, gatifloxacin, moxifloxacin, halofantrine, mefloquine, pentamidine, arsenic trioxide, levomethadyl acetate, dolasetron mesylate, probucol or tacrolimus).
No products indexed under this heading.

Erythromycin Estolate (Ziprasidone is contraindicated with drugs that have demonstrated QT prolongation as one of their pharmacodynamic effects and have this effect described in the full prescribing information as a contraindication or a boxed or bolded warning. Ziprasidone should not be used with any drug that prolongs the QT interval. An additive effect of ziprasidone and other drugs that prolong the QT interval cannot be excluded. Therefore, ziprasidone should not be given with dofetilide, sotalol, quinidine, other Class Ia and III anti-arrhythmics, mesoridazine, thioridazine, chlorpromazine, droperidol, pimozide, sparfloxacin, gatifloxacin, moxifloxacin, halofantrine, mefloquine, pentamidine, arsenic trioxide, levomethadyl acetate, dolasetron mesylate, probucol or tacrolimus).
No products indexed under this heading.

Erythromycin Ethylsuccinate (Ziprasidone is contraindicated with drugs that have demonstrated QT prolongation as one of their pharmacodynamic effects and have this effect described in the full prescribing information as a contraindication or a boxed or bolded warning. Ziprasidone should not be used with any drug that prolongs the QT interval. An additive effect of ziprasidone and other drugs that prolong the QT interval cannot be excluded. Therefore, ziprasidone should not be given with dofetilide, sotalol, quinidine, other Class Ia and III anti-arrhythmics, mesoridazine, thioridazine, chlorpromazine, droperidol, pimozide, sparfloxacin, gatifloxacin, moxifloxacin, halofantrine, mefloquine, pentamidine, arsenic trioxide, levomethadyl acetate, dolasetron mesylate, probucol or tacrolimus). Products include:
E.E.S. 437
EryPed 435

Erythromycin Gluceptate (Ziprasidone is contraindicated with drugs that have demonstrated QT prolongation as one of their pharmacodynamic effects and have this effect described in the full prescribing information as a contraindication or a boxed or bolded warning. Ziprasidone should not be used with any drug that prolongs the QT interval. An additive effect of ziprasidone and other drugs that prolong the QT interval cannot be excluded. Therefore, ziprasidone should not be given with dofetilide, sotalol, quinidine, other Class Ia and III anti-arrhythmics, mesoridazine, thioridazine, chlorpromazine, droperidol, pimozide, sparfloxacin, gatifloxacin, moxifloxacin, halofantrine, mefloquine, pentamidine, arsenic trioxide, levomethadyl acetate, dolasetron mesylate, probucol or tacrolimus).
No products indexed under this heading.

Erythromycin Lactobionate (Ziprasidone is contraindicated with

(⊙ Described in PDR® for Ophthalmic Medicines)

drugs that have demonstrated QT prolongation as one of their pharmacodynamic effects and have this effect described in the full prescribing information as a contraindication or a boxed or bolded warning. Ziprasidone should not be used with any drug that prolongs the QT interval. An additive effect of ziprasidone and other drugs that prolong the QT interval cannot be excluded. Therefore, ziprasidone should not be given with dofetilide, sotalol, quinidine, other Class la and III anti-arrhythmics, mesoridazine, thioridazine, chlorpromazine, droperidol, pimozide, sparfloxacin, gatifloxacin, moxifloxacin, halofantrine, mefloquine, pentamidine, arsenic trioxide, levomethadyl acetate, dolasetron mesylate, probucol or tacrolimus).
No products indexed under this heading.

Erythromycin Stearate (Ziprasidone is contraindicated with drugs that have demonstrated QT prolongation as one of their pharmacodynamic effects and have this effect described in the full prescribing information as a contraindication or a boxed or bolded warning. Ziprasidone should not be used with any drug that prolongs the QT interval. An additive effect of ziprasidone and other drugs that prolong the QT interval cannot be excluded. Therefore, ziprasidone should not be given with dofetilide, sotalol, quinidine, other Class la and III anti-arrhythmics, mesoridazine, thioridazine, chlorpromazine, droperidol, pimozide, sparfloxacin, gatifloxacin, moxifloxacin, halofantrine, mefloquine, pentamidine, arsenic trioxide, levomethadyl acetate, dolasetron mesylate, probucol or tacrolimus).
No products indexed under this heading.

Esmolol Hydrochloride (Ziprasidone may enhance the effects of certain antihypertensive agents because of its potential for inducing hypotension).
No products indexed under this heading.

Esomeprazole Magnesium (Ketoconazole, a potent inhibitor of CYP3A4, at a dose of 400 mg QD for 5 days, increased the AUC and C_{max} of ziprasidone by about 35-40%. Other inhibitors of CYP3A4 would be expected to have similar effects). Products include:
Nexium Capsules 704
Nexium Oral Suspension 704

Esomeprazole Sodium (Ketoconazole, a potent inhibitor of CYP3A4, at a dose of 400 mg QD for 5 days, increased the AUC and C_{max} of ziprasidone by about 35-40%. Other inhibitors of CYP3A4 would be expected to have similar effects). Products include:
Nexium I.V. 712

Estazolam (Caution should be used when ziprasidone is taken in combination with other centrally acting drugs, given the primary CNS effects of ziprasidone).
No products indexed under this heading.

Ethanol (Caution should be used when ziprasidone is taken in combination with other centrally acting drugs, given the primary CNS effects of ziprasidone).
No products indexed under this heading.

Ethchlorvynol (Caution should be used when ziprasidone is taken in combination with other centrally acting drugs, given the primary CNS effects of ziprasidone).
No products indexed under this heading.

Ethinamate (Caution should be used when ziprasidone is taken in combination with other centrally acting drugs, given the primary CNS effects of ziprasidone).
No products indexed under this heading.

Ethyl Alcohol (Caution should be used when ziprasidone is taken in combination with other centrally acting drugs, given the primary CNS effects of ziprasidone).
No products indexed under this heading.

Felodipine (Ziprasidone may enhance the effects of certain antihypertensive agents because of its potential for inducing hypotension).
No products indexed under this heading.

Fentanyl (Caution should be used when ziprasidone is taken in combination with other centrally acting drugs, given the primary CNS effects of ziprasidone). Products include:
Duragesic 2604
Fentanyl Transdermal System 2346
Onsolis 2054

Fentanyl Citrate (Caution should be used when ziprasidone is taken in combination with other centrally acting drugs, given the primary CNS effects of ziprasidone). Products include:
Fentora 966

Flecainide Acetate (Ziprasidone is contraindicated with drugs that have demonstrated QT prolongation as one of their pharmacodynamic effects and have this effect described in the full prescribing information as a contraindication or a boxed or bolded warning. Ziprasidone should not be used with any drug that prolongs the QT interval. An additive effect of ziprasidone and other drugs that prolong the QT interval cannot be excluded. Therefore, ziprasidone should not be given with dofetilide, sotalol, quinidine, other Class la and III anti-arrhythmics, mesoridazine, thioridazine, chlorpromazine, droperidol, pimozide, sparfloxacin, gatifloxacin, moxifloxacin, halofantrine, mefloquine, pentamidine, arsenic trioxide, levomethadyl acetate, dolasetron mesylate, probucol or tacrolimus).
No products indexed under this heading.

Fluconazole (Ketoconazole, a potent inhibitor of CYP3A4, at a dose of 400 mg QD for 5 days, increased the AUC and C_{max} of ziprasidone by about 35-40%. Other inhibitors of CYP3A4 would be expected to have similar effects).
No products indexed under this heading.

Fluoxetine (Ketoconazole, a potent inhibitor of CYP3A4, at a dose of 400 mg QD for 5 days, increased the AUC and C_{max} of ziprasidone by about 35-40%. Other inhibitors of CYP3A4 would be expected to have similar effects).
No products indexed under this heading.

Fluoxetine Hydrochloride (Ketoconazole, a potent inhibitor of CYP3A4, at a dose of 400 mg QD for 5 days, increased the AUC and C_{max} of ziprasidone by about 35-40%. Other inhibitors of CYP3A4 would be expected to have similar effects). Products include:
Prozac Weekly 1941
Prozac Pulvules 1941
Symbyax 1965

Fluphenazine Decanoate (Ziprasidone is contraindicated with drugs that have demonstrated QT prolongation as one of their pharmacodynamic effects and have this effect described in the full prescribing information as a contraindication or a boxed or bolded warning. Ziprasidone should not be used with any drug that prolongs the QT interval. An additive effect of ziprasidone and other drugs that prolong the QT interval cannot be excluded. Therefore, ziprasidone should not be given with dofetilide, sotalol, quinidine, other Class la and III anti-arrhythmics, mesoridazine, thioridazine, chlorpromazine, droperidol, pimozide, sparfloxacin, gatifloxacin, moxifloxacin, halofantrine, mefloquine,

pentamidine, arsenic trioxide, levomethadyl acetate, dolasetron mesylate, probucol or tacrolimus).
No products indexed under this heading.

Fluphenazine Enanthate (Ziprasidone is contraindicated with drugs that have demonstrated QT prolongation as one of their pharmacodynamic effects and have this effect described in the full prescribing information as a contraindication or a boxed or bolded warning. Ziprasidone should not be used with any drug that prolongs the QT interval. An additive effect of ziprasidone and other drugs that prolong the QT interval cannot be excluded. Therefore, ziprasidone should not be given with dofetilide, sotalol, quinidine, other Class la and III anti-arrhythmics, mesoridazine, thioridazine, chlorpromazine, droperidol, pimozide, sparfloxacin, gatifloxacin, moxifloxacin, halofantrine, mefloquine, pentamidine, arsenic trioxide, levomethadyl acetate, dolasetron mesylate, probucol or tacrolimus).
No products indexed under this heading.

Fluphenazine Hydrochloride (Ziprasidone is contraindicated with drugs that have demonstrated QT prolongation as one of their pharmacodynamic effects and have this effect described in the full prescribing information as a contraindication or a boxed or bolded warning. Ziprasidone should not be used with any drug that prolongs the QT interval. An additive effect of ziprasidone and other drugs that prolong the QT interval cannot be excluded. Therefore, ziprasidone should not be given with dofetilide, sotalol, quinidine, other Class la and III anti-arrhythmics, mesoridazine, thioridazine, chlorpromazine, droperidol, pimozide, sparfloxacin, gatifloxacin, moxifloxacin, halofantrine, mefloquine, pentamidine, arsenic trioxide, levomethadyl acetate, dolasetron mesylate, probucol or tacrolimus).
No products indexed under this heading.

Flurazepam Hydrochloride (Caution should be used when ziprasidone is taken in combination with other centrally acting drugs, given the primary CNS effects of ziprasidone).
No products indexed under this heading.

Fluvoxamine Maleate (Ketoconazole, a potent inhibitor of CYP3A4, at a dose of 400 mg QD for 5 days, increased the AUC and C_{max} of ziprasidone by about 35-40%. Other inhibitors of CYP3A4 would be expected to have similar effects).
No products indexed under this heading.

Fosamprenavir Calcium (Ketoconazole, a potent inhibitor of CYP3A4, at a dose of 400 mg QD for 5 days, increased the AUC and C_{max} of ziprasidone by about 35-40%. Other inhibitors of CYP3A4 would be expected to have similar effects). Products include:
Lexiva Oral Suspension 1558
Lexiva 1558

Fosinopril Sodium (Ziprasidone may enhance the effects of certain antihypertensive agents because of its potential for inducing hypotension).
No products indexed under this heading.

Furosemide (Ziprasidone may enhance the effects of certain antihypertensive agents because of its potential for inducing hypotension). Products include:
Furosemide 2354

Gatifloxacin (Ziprasidone is contraindicated with drugs that have demonstrated QT prolongation as one of their pharmacodynamic effects and have this effect described in the full prescribing information as a contraindication or a boxed or bolded warning. Ziprasidone should not be used with any drug that prolongs the QT interval. An additive effect of ziprasidone and other drugs

that prolong the QT interval cannot be excluded. Therefore, ziprasidone should not be given with dofetilide, sotalol, quinidine, other Class la and III anti-arrhythmics, mesoridazine, thioridazine, chlorpromazine, droperidol, pimozide, sparfloxacin, gatifloxacin, moxifloxacin, halofantrine, mefloquine, pentamidine, arsenic trioxide, levomethadyl acetate, dolasetron mesylate, probucol or tacrolimus).
No products indexed under this heading.

Glutethimide (Caution should be used when ziprasidone is taken in combination with other centrally acting drugs, given the primary CNS effects of ziprasidone).
No products indexed under this heading.

Guanabenz Acetate (Ziprasidone may enhance the effects of certain antihypertensive agents because of its potential for inducing hypotension).
No products indexed under this heading.

Guanethidine (Ziprasidone may enhance the effects of certain antihypertensive agents because of its potential for inducing hypotension).
No products indexed under this heading.

Guanethidine Monosulfate (Ziprasidone may enhance the effects of certain antihypertensive agents because of its potential for inducing hypotension).
No products indexed under this heading.

Guanethidine Sulfate (Ziprasidone may enhance the effects of certain antihypertensive agents because of its potential for inducing hypotension).
No products indexed under this heading.

Halofantrine (Ziprasidone is contraindicated with drugs that have demonstrated QT prolongation as one of their pharmacodynamic effects and have this effect described in the full prescribing information as a contraindication or a boxed or bolded warning. Ziprasidone should not be used with any drug that prolongs the QT interval. An additive effect of ziprasidone and other drugs that prolong the QT interval cannot be excluded. Therefore, ziprasidone should not be given with dofetilide, sotalol, quinidine, other Class la and III anti-arrhythmics, mesoridazine, thioridazine, chlorpromazine, droperidol, pimozide, sparfloxacin, gatifloxacin, moxifloxacin, halofantrine, mefloquine, pentamidine, arsenic trioxide, levomethadyl acetate, dolasetron mesylate, probucol or tacrolimus).
No products indexed under this heading.

Haloperidol (Ziprasidone is contraindicated with drugs that have demonstrated QT prolongation as one of their pharmacodynamic effects and have this effect described in the full prescribing information as a contraindication or a boxed or bolded warning. Ziprasidone should not be used with any drug that prolongs the QT interval. An additive effect of ziprasidone and other drugs that prolong the QT interval cannot be excluded. Therefore, ziprasidone should not be given with dofetilide, sotalol, quinidine, other Class la and III anti-arrhythmics, mesoridazine, thioridazine, chlorpromazine, droperidol, pimozide, sparfloxacin, gatifloxacin, moxifloxacin, halofantrine, mefloquine, pentamidine, arsenic trioxide, levomethadyl acetate, dolasetron mesylate, probucol or tacrolimus).
No products indexed under this heading.

Haloperidol Decanoate (Ziprasidone is contraindicated with drugs that have demonstrated QT prolongation as one of their pharmacodynamic effects and have this effect described in the full prescribing information as a contraindication or a boxed or bolded warning. Ziprasidone should not be used with any drug that prolongs the QT interval. An additive effect of ziprasidone and other

drugs that prolong the QT interval cannot be excluded. Therefore, ziprasidone should not be given with dofetilide, sotalol, quinidine, other Class Ia and III anti-arrhythmics, mesoridazine, thioridazine, chlorpromazine, droperidol, pimozide, sparfloxacin, gatifloxacin, moxifloxacin, halofantrine, mefloquine, pentamidine, arsenic trioxide, levomethadyl acetate, dolasetron mesylate, probucol or tacrolimus).
No products indexed under this heading.

Haloperidol Lactate (Ziprasidone is contraindicated with drugs that have demonstrated QT prolongation as one of their pharmacodynamic effects and have this effect described in the full prescribing information as a contraindication or a boxed or bolded warning. Ziprasidone should not be used with any drug that prolongs the QT interval. An additive effect of ziprasidone and other drugs that prolong the QT interval cannot be excluded. Therefore, ziprasidone should not be given with dofetilide, sotalol, quinidine, other Class Ia and III anti-arrhythmics, mesoridazine, thioridazine, chlorpromazine, droperidol, pimozide, sparfloxacin, gatifloxacin, moxifloxacin, halofantrine, mefloquine, pentamidine, arsenic trioxide, levomethadyl acetate, dolasetron mesylate, probucol or tacrolimus).
No products indexed under this heading.

Hydralazine Hydrochloride (Ziprasidone may enhance the effects of certain antihypertensive agents because of its potential for inducing hypotension).
No products indexed under this heading.

Hydrochlorothiazide (Ziprasidone may enhance the effects of certain antihypertensive agents because of its potential for inducing hypotension). Products include:
Atacand HCT 700
Avalide 2956
Benicar HCT 1017
Diovan HCT 2419
Dyazide 1429
Exforge HCT 2449
Hyzaar 2162
Hyzaar 100-12.5 2162
Micardis HCT 889
Prinzide 2246
Tekturna HCT 2541
Teveten HCT 541

Hydrocodone Bitartrate (Caution should be used when ziprasidone is taken in combination with other centrally acting drugs, given the primary CNS effects of ziprasidone). Products include:
Vicodin 560
Vicodin ES 561
Vicodin HP 563
Vicoprofen 564
Zydone 1138

Hydrocodone Polistirex (Caution should be used when ziprasidone is taken in combination with other centrally acting drugs, given the primary CNS effects of ziprasidone). Products include:
Tussionex 3443

Hydroflumethiazide (Ziprasidone may enhance the effects of certain antihypertensive agents because of its potential for inducing hypotension).
No products indexed under this heading.

Hydromorphone Hydrochloride (Caution should be used when ziprasidone is taken in combination with other centrally acting drugs, given the primary CNS effects of ziprasidone). Products include:
Dilaudid Injection 2800
Dilaudid Oral 2797
Dilaudid Tablets 2797
Dilaudid-HP 2800

Hydroxyamphetamine Hydrobromide (Caution should be used when ziprasidone is taken in combination with other centrally acting drugs, given the primary CNS effects of ziprasidone).
No products indexed under this heading.

Hydroxyzine Hydrochloride (Ziprasidone is contraindicated with drugs that have demonstrated QT prolongation as one of their pharmacodynamic effects and have this effect described in the full prescribing information as a contraindication or a boxed or bolded warning. Ziprasidone should not be used with any drug that prolongs the QT interval. An additive effect of ziprasidone and other drugs that prolong the QT interval cannot be excluded. Therefore, ziprasidone should not be given with dofetilide, sotalol, quinidine, other Class Ia and III anti-arrhythmics, mesoridazine, thioridazine, chlorpromazine, droperidol, pimozide, sparfloxacin, gatifloxacin, moxifloxacin, halofantrine, mefloquine, pentamidine, arsenic trioxide, levomethadyl acetate, dolasetron mesylate, probucol or tacrolimus).
No products indexed under this heading.

Imatinib Mesylate (Ketoconazole, a potent inhibitor of CYP3A4, at a dose of 400 mg QD for 5 days, increased the AUC and C_{max} of ziprasidone by about 35-40%. Other inhibitors of CYP3A4 would be expected to have similar effects). Products include:
Gleevec 2477

Imipramine Hydrochloride (Ziprasidone is contraindicated with drugs that have demonstrated QT prolongation as one of their pharmacodynamic effects and have this effect described in the full prescribing information as a contraindication or a boxed or bolded warning. Ziprasidone should not be used with any drug that prolongs the QT interval. An additive effect of ziprasidone and other drugs that prolong the QT interval cannot be excluded. Therefore, ziprasidone should not be given with dofetilide, sotalol, quinidine, other Class Ia and III anti-arrhythmics, mesoridazine, thioridazine, chlorpromazine, droperidol, pimozide, sparfloxacin, gatifloxacin, moxifloxacin, halofantrine, mefloquine, pentamidine, arsenic trioxide, levomethadyl acetate, dolasetron mesylate, probucol or tacrolimus).
No products indexed under this heading.

Imipramine Pamoate (Ziprasidone is contraindicated with drugs that have demonstrated QT prolongation as one of their pharmacodynamic effects and have this effect described in the full prescribing information as a contraindication or a boxed or bolded warning. Ziprasidone should not be used with any drug that prolongs the QT interval. An additive effect of ziprasidone and other drugs that prolong the QT interval cannot be excluded. Therefore, ziprasidone should not be given with dofetilide, sotalol, quinidine, other Class Ia and III anti-arrhythmics, mesoridazine, thioridazine, chlorpromazine, droperidol, pimozide, sparfloxacin, gatifloxacin, moxifloxacin, halofantrine, mefloquine, pentamidine, arsenic trioxide, levomethadyl acetate, dolasetron mesylate, probucol or tacrolimus).
No products indexed under this heading.

Indapamide (Ziprasidone may enhance the effects of certain antihypertensive agents because of its potential for inducing hypotension). Products include:
Indapamide 2356

Indinavir Sulfate (Ketoconazole, a potent inhibitor of CYP3A4, at a dose of 400 mg QD for 5 days, increased the AUC and C_{max} of ziprasidone by about 35-40%. Other inhibitors of CYP3A4 would be expected to have similar effects). Products include:
Crixivan 2113

Irbesartan (Ziprasidone may enhance the effects of certain antihypertensive agents because of its potential for inducing hypotension). Products include:
Avalide 2956
Avapro 2962

Isocarboxazid (Ziprasidone is contraindicated with drugs that have demonstrated QT prolongation as one of their pharmacodynamic effects and have this effect described in the full prescribing information as a contraindication or a boxed or bolded warning. Ziprasidone should not be used with any drug that prolongs the QT interval. An additive effect of ziprasidone and other drugs that prolong the QT interval cannot be excluded. Therefore, ziprasidone should not be given with dofetilide, sotalol, quinidine, other Class Ia and III anti-arrhythmics, mesoridazine, thioridazine, chlorpromazine, droperidol, pimozide, sparfloxacin, gatifloxacin, moxifloxacin, halofantrine, mefloquine, pentamidine, arsenic trioxide, levomethadyl acetate, dolasetron mesylate, probucol or tacrolimus). Products include:
Marplan 3481

Isoflurane (Caution should be used when ziprasidone is taken in combination with other centrally acting drugs, given the primary CNS effects of ziprasidone).
No products indexed under this heading.

Isoniazid (Ketoconazole, a potent inhibitor of CYP3A4, at a dose of 400 mg QD for 5 days, increased the AUC and C_{max} of ziprasidone by about 35-40%. Other inhibitors of CYP3A4 would be expected to have similar effects).
No products indexed under this heading.

Isradipine (Ziprasidone may enhance the effects of certain antihypertensive agents because of its potential for inducing hypotension). Products include:
DynaCirc CR 1432

Itraconazole (Ketoconazole, a potent inhibitor of CYP3A4, at a dose of 400 mg QD for 5 days, increased the AUC and C_{max} of ziprasidone by about 35-40%. Other inhibitors of CYP3A4 would be expected to have similar effects).
No products indexed under this heading.

Ketamine Hydrochloride (Caution should be used when ziprasidone is taken in combination with other centrally acting drugs, given the primary CNS effects of ziprasidone).
No products indexed under this heading.

Ketoconazole (Ketoconazole, a potent inhibitor of CYP3A4, at a dose of 400 mg QD for 5 days, increased the AUC and C_{max} of ziprasidone by about 35-40%. Other inhibitors of CYP3A4 would be expected to have similar effects). Products include:
Extina 3319
Xolegel 3337

Labetalol Hydrochloride (Ziprasidone may enhance the effects of certain antihypertensive agents because of its potential for inducing hypotension).
No products indexed under this heading.

Lapatinib (Ketoconazole, a potent inhibitor of CYP3A4, at a dose of 400 mg QD for 5 days, increased the AUC and C_{max} of ziprasidone by about 35-40%. Other inhibitors of CYP3A4 would be expected to have similar effects). Products include:
Tykerb 1698

Levodopa (Ziprasidone may antagonize the effects of levodopa). Products include:
Stalevo 2526

Levomethadyl Acetate Hydrochloride (Ziprasidone is contraindicated with drugs that have demonstrated QT prolongation as one of their pharmacodynamic effects and have this effect described in the full prescribing information as a contraindication or a boxed or bolded warning. Ziprasidone should not be used with any drug that prolongs the QT interval. An additive effect of ziprasidone and other drugs that prolong the QT interval cannot be excluded. Therefore, ziprasidone should not be given with dofetilide, sotalol, quinidine, other Class Ia and III anti-arrhythmics, mesoridazine, thioridazine, chlorpromazine, droperidol, pimozide, sparfloxacin, gatifloxacin, moxifloxacin, halofantrine, mefloquine, pentamidine, arsenic trioxide, levomethadyl acetate, dolasetron mesylate, probucol or tacrolimus).
No products indexed under this heading.

Levorphanol Tartrate (Caution should be used when ziprasidone is taken in combination with other centrally acting drugs, given the primary CNS effects of ziprasidone).
No products indexed under this heading.

Lidocaine (Ziprasidone is contraindicated with drugs that have demonstrated QT prolongation as one of their pharmacodynamic effects and have this effect described in the full prescribing information as a contraindication or a boxed or bolded warning. Ziprasidone should not be used with any drug that prolongs the QT interval. An additive effect of ziprasidone and other drugs that prolong the QT interval cannot be excluded. Therefore, ziprasidone should not be given with dofetilide, sotalol, quinidine, other Class Ia and III anti-arrhythmics, mesoridazine, thioridazine, chlorpromazine, droperidol, pimozide, sparfloxacin, gatifloxacin, moxifloxacin, halofantrine, mefloquine, pentamidine, arsenic trioxide, levomethadyl acetate, dolasetron mesylate, probucol or tacrolimus). Products include:
Lidoderm 1107

Lidocaine Hydrochloride (Ziprasidone is contraindicated with drugs that have demonstrated QT prolongation as one of their pharmacodynamic effects and have this effect described in the full prescribing information as a contraindication or a boxed or bolded warning. Ziprasidone should not be used with any drug that prolongs the QT interval. An additive effect of ziprasidone and other drugs that prolong the QT interval cannot be excluded. Therefore, ziprasidone should not be given with dofetilide, sotalol, quinidine, other Class Ia and III anti-arrhythmics, mesoridazine, thioridazine, chlorpromazine, droperidol, pimozide, sparfloxacin, gatifloxacin, moxifloxacin, halofantrine, mefloquine, pentamidine, arsenic trioxide, levomethadyl acetate, dolasetron mesylate, probucol or tacrolimus).
No products indexed under this heading.

Lisdexamfetamine Dimesylate (Caution should be used when ziprasidone is taken in combination with other centrally acting drugs, given the primary CNS effects of ziprasidone). Products include:
Vyvanse 3298

Lisinopril (Ziprasidone may enhance the effects of certain antihypertensive agents because of its potential for inducing hypotension). Products include:
Prinivil 2241
Prinzide 2246

Lithium Carbonate (Ziprasidone is contraindicated with drugs that have demonstrated QT prolongation as one of their pharmacodynamic effects and have this effect described in the full prescribing information as a contraindication or a boxed or bolded warning.

Ziprasidone should not be used with any drug that prolongs the QT interval. An additive effect of ziprasidone and other drugs that prolong the QT interval cannot be excluded. Therefore, ziprasidone should not be given with dofetilide, sotalol, quinidine, other Class Ia and III anti-arrhythmics, mesoridazine, thioridazine, chlorpromazine, droperidol, pimozide, sparfloxacin, gatifloxacin, moxifloxacin, halofantrine, mefloquine, pentamidine, arsenic trioxide, levomethadyl acetate, dolasetron mesylate, probucol or tacrolimus).
No products indexed under this heading.

Lithium Citrate (Ziprasidone is contraindicated with drugs that have demonstrated QT prolongation as one of their pharmacodynamic effects and have this effect described in the full prescribing information as a contraindication or a boxed or bolded warning. Ziprasidone should not be used with any drug that prolongs the QT interval. An additive effect of ziprasidone and other drugs that prolong the QT interval cannot be excluded. Therefore, ziprasidone should not be given with dofetilide, sotalol, quinidine, other Class Ia and III anti-arrhythmics, mesoridazine, thioridazine, chlorpromazine, droperidol, pimozide, sparfloxacin, gatifloxacin, moxifloxacin, halofantrine, mefloquine, pentamidine, arsenic trioxide, levomethadyl acetate, dolasetron mesylate, probucol or tacrolimus).
No products indexed under this heading.

Lopinavir (Ketoconazole, a potent inhibitor of CYP3A4, at a dose of 400 mg QD for 5 days, increased the AUC and C_{max} of ziprasidone by about 35-40%. Other inhibitors of CYP3A4 would be expected to have similar effects). Products include:
Kaletra 458

Loratadine (Ketoconazole, a potent inhibitor of CYP3A4, at a dose of 400 mg QD for 5 days, increased the AUC and C_{max} of ziprasidone by about 35-40%. Other inhibitors of CYP3A4 would be expected to have similar effects).
No products indexed under this heading.

Lorazepam (Ziprasidone is contraindicated with drugs that have demonstrated QT prolongation as one of their pharmacodynamic effects and have this effect described in the full prescribing information as a contraindication or a boxed or bolded warning. Ziprasidone should not be used with any drug that prolongs the QT interval. An additive effect of ziprasidone and other drugs that prolong the QT interval cannot be excluded. Therefore, ziprasidone should not be given with dofetilide, sotalol, quinidine, other Class Ia and III anti-arrhythmics, mesoridazine, thioridazine, chlorpromazine, droperidol, pimozide, sparfloxacin, gatifloxacin, moxifloxacin, halofantrine, mefloquine, pentamidine, arsenic trioxide, levomethadyl acetate, dolasetron mesylate, probucol or tacrolimus).
No products indexed under this heading.

Losartan Potassium (Ziprasidone may enhance the effects of certain antihypertensive agents because of its potential for inducing hypotension). Products include:
Cozaar 2106
Hyzaar 2162
Hyzaar 100-12.5 2162

Loxapine Hydrochloride (Ziprasidone is contraindicated with drugs that have demonstrated QT prolongation as one of their pharmacodynamic effects and have this effect described in the full prescribing information as a contraindication or a boxed or bolded warning. Ziprasidone should not be used with any drug that prolongs the QT interval. An additive effect of ziprasidone and other drugs that prolong the QT interval cannot be excluded. Therefore, ziprasidone should not be given with dofetilide, sotalol, quinidine, other Class Ia and III anti-arrhythmics, mesoridazine, thioridazine, chlorpromazine, droperidol, pimozide, sparfloxacin, gatifloxacin, moxifloxacin, halofantrine, mefloquine, pentamidine, arsenic trioxide, levomethadyl acetate, dolasetron mesylate, probucol or tacrolimus).
No products indexed under this heading.

Loxapine Succinate (Ziprasidone is contraindicated with drugs that have demonstrated QT prolongation as one of their pharmacodynamic effects and have this effect described in the full prescribing information as a contraindication or a boxed or bolded warning. Ziprasidone should not be used with any drug that prolongs the QT interval. An additive effect of ziprasidone and other drugs that prolong the QT interval cannot be excluded. Therefore, ziprasidone should not be given with dofetilide, sotalol, quinidine, other Class Ia and III anti-arrhythmics, mesoridazine, thioridazine, chlorpromazine, droperidol, pimozide, sparfloxacin, gatifloxacin, moxifloxacin, halofantrine, mefloquine, pentamidine, arsenic trioxide, levomethadyl acetate, dolasetron mesylate, probucol or tacrolimus).
No products indexed under this heading.

Maprotiline Hydrochloride (Ziprasidone is contraindicated with drugs that have demonstrated QT prolongation as one of their pharmacodynamic effects and have this effect described in the full prescribing information as a contraindication or a boxed or bolded warning. Ziprasidone should not be used with any drug that prolongs the QT interval. An additive effect of ziprasidone and other drugs that prolong the QT interval cannot be excluded. Therefore, ziprasidone should not be given with dofetilide, sotalol, quinidine, other Class Ia and III anti-arrhythmics, mesoridazine, thioridazine, chlorpromazine, droperidol, pimozide, sparfloxacin, gatifloxacin, moxifloxacin, halofantrine, mefloquine, pentamidine, arsenic trioxide, levomethadyl acetate, dolasetron mesylate, probucol or tacrolimus).
No products indexed under this heading.

Mecamylamine Hydrochloride (Ziprasidone may enhance the effects of certain antihypertensive agents because of its potential for inducing hypotension).
No products indexed under this heading.

Mefloquine Hydrochloride (Ziprasidone is contraindicated with drugs that have demonstrated QT prolongation as one of their pharmacodynamic effects and have this effect described in the full prescribing information as a contraindication or a boxed or bolded warning. Ziprasidone should not be used with any drug that prolongs the QT interval. An additive effect of ziprasidone and other drugs that prolong the QT interval cannot be excluded. Therefore, ziprasidone should not be given with dofetilide, sotalol, quinidine, other Class Ia and III anti-arrhythmics, mesoridazine, thioridazine, chlorpromazine, droperidol, pimozide, sparfloxacin, gatifloxacin, moxifloxacin, halofantrine, mefloquine, pentamidine, arsenic trioxide, levomethadyl acetate, dolasetron mesylate, probucol or tacrolimus).
No products indexed under this heading.

Meperidine Hydrochloride (Caution should be used when ziprasidone is taken in combination with other centrally acting drugs, given the primary CNS effects of ziprasidone).
No products indexed under this heading.

Mephobarbital (Caution should be used when ziprasidone is taken in combination with other centrally acting drugs, given the primary CNS effects of ziprasidone).
No products indexed under this heading.

Meprobamate (Ziprasidone is contraindicated with drugs that have demonstrated QT prolongation as one of their pharmacodynamic effects and have this effect described in the full prescribing information as a contraindication or a boxed or bolded warning. Ziprasidone should not be used with any drug that prolongs the QT interval. An additive effect of ziprasidone and other drugs that prolong the QT interval cannot be excluded. Therefore, ziprasidone should not be given with dofetilide, sotalol, quinidine, other Class Ia and III anti-arrhythmics, mesoridazine, thioridazine, chlorpromazine, droperidol, pimozide, sparfloxacin, gatifloxacin, moxifloxacin, halofantrine, mefloquine, pentamidine, arsenic trioxide, levomethadyl acetate, dolasetron mesylate, probucol or tacrolimus).
No products indexed under this heading.

Mesoridazine Besylate (Ziprasidone is contraindicated with drugs that have demonstrated QT prolongation as one of their pharmacodynamic effects and have this effect described in the full prescribing information as a contraindication or a boxed or bolded warning. Ziprasidone should not be used with any drug that prolongs the QT interval. An additive effect of ziprasidone and other drugs that prolong the QT interval cannot be excluded. Therefore, ziprasidone should not be given with dofetilide, sotalol, quinidine, other Class Ia and III anti-arrhythmics, mesoridazine, thioridazine, chlorpromazine, droperidol, pimozide, sparfloxacin, gatifloxacin, moxifloxacin, halofantrine, mefloquine, pentamidine, arsenic trioxide, levomethadyl acetate, dolasetron mesylate, probucol or tacrolimus).
No products indexed under this heading.

Methadone Hydrochloride (Caution should be used when ziprasidone is taken in combination with other centrally acting drugs, given the primary CNS effects of ziprasidone).
No products indexed under this heading.

Methamphetamine Hydrochloride (Caution should be used when ziprasidone is taken in combination with other centrally acting drugs, given the primary CNS effects of ziprasidone).
No products indexed under this heading.

Methohexital Sodium (Caution should be used when ziprasidone is taken in combination with other centrally acting drugs, given the primary CNS effects of ziprasidone).
No products indexed under this heading.

Methotrimeprazine (Caution should be used when ziprasidone is taken in combination with other centrally acting drugs, given the primary CNS effects of ziprasidone).
No products indexed under this heading.

Methoxyflurane (Caution should be used when ziprasidone is taken in combination with other centrally acting drugs, given the primary CNS effects of ziprasidone).
No products indexed under this heading.

Methyclothiazide (Ziprasidone may enhance the effects of certain antihypertensive agents because of its potential for inducing hypotension).
No products indexed under this heading.

Methyldopa (Ziprasidone may enhance the effects of certain antihypertensive agents because of its potential for inducing hypotension).
No products indexed under this heading.

Methyldopate Hydrochloride (Ziprasidone may enhance the effects of certain antihypertensive agents because of its potential for inducing hypotension).
No products indexed under this heading.

Methylphenidate (Caution should be used when ziprasidone is taken in combination with other centrally acting drugs, given the primary CNS effects of ziprasidone). Products include:
Daytrana 3283

Methylphenidate Hydrochloride (Caution should be used when ziprasidone is taken in combination with other centrally acting drugs, given the primary CNS effects of ziprasidone). Products include:
Concerta 2598
Metadate CD 3439

Metolazone (Ziprasidone may enhance the effects of certain antihypertensive agents because of its potential for inducing hypotension).
No products indexed under this heading.

Metoprolol Succinate (Ziprasidone may enhance the effects of certain antihypertensive agents because of its potential for inducing hypotension). Products include:
Toprol XL 732

Metoprolol Tartrate (Ziprasidone may enhance the effects of certain antihypertensive agents because of its potential for inducing hypotension).
No products indexed under this heading.

Metronidazole (Ketoconazole, a potent inhibitor of CYP3A4, at a dose of 400 mg QD for 5 days, increased the AUC and C_{max} of ziprasidone by about 35-40%. Other inhibitors of CYP3A4 would be expected to have similar effects). Products include:
Pylera 793

Metronidazole Benzoate (Ketoconazole, a potent inhibitor of CYP3A4, at a dose of 400 mg QD for 5 days, increased the AUC and C_{max} of ziprasidone by about 35-40%. Other inhibitors of CYP3A4 would be expected to have similar effects).
No products indexed under this heading.

Metronidazole Hydrochloride (Ketoconazole, a potent inhibitor of CYP3A4, at a dose of 400 mg QD for 5 days, increased the AUC and C_{max} of ziprasidone by about 35-40%. Other inhibitors of CYP3A4 would be expected to have similar effects).
No products indexed under this heading.

Metronidazole Sodium (Ketoconazole, a potent inhibitor of CYP3A4, at a dose of 400 mg QD for 5 days, increased the AUC and C_{max} of ziprasidone by about 35-40%. Other inhibitors of CYP3A4 would be expected to have similar effects).
No products indexed under this heading.

Metyrosine (Ziprasidone may enhance the effects of certain antihypertensive agents because of its potential for inducing hypotension).
No products indexed under this heading.

Mexiletine Hydrochloride (Ziprasidone is contraindicated with drugs that have demonstrated QT prolongation as one of their pharmacodynamic effects and have this effect described in the full prescribing information as a contraindication or a boxed or bolded warning. Ziprasidone should not be used with any drug that prolongs the QT interval. An additive effect of ziprasidone and other drugs that prolong the QT interval cannot be excluded. Therefore, ziprasidone should not be given with dofetilide, sotalol, quinidine, other Class Ia and III anti-arrhythmics, mesoridazine, thioridazine, chlorpromazine, droperidol, pimozide, sparfloxacin, gatifloxacin, moxifloxacin, halofantrine, mefloquine,

IMPORTANT NOTE: Always consult each drug listing in the patient's regimen for possible interactions.

Geodon Interactions Index 772

pentamidine, arsenic trioxide, levomethadyl acetate, dolasetron mesylate, probucol or tacrolimus).
No products indexed under this heading.

Mibefradil Dihydrochloride (Ziprasidone may enhance the effects of certain antihypertensive agents because of its potential for inducing hypotension).
No products indexed under this heading.

Miconazole (Ketoconazole, a potent inhibitor of CYP3A4, at a dose of 400 mg QD for 5 days, increased the AUC and C_{max} of ziprasidone by about 35-40%. Other inhibitors of CYP3A4 would be expected to have similar effects).
No products indexed under this heading.

Miconazole Nitrate (Ketoconazole, a potent inhibitor of CYP3A4, at a dose of 400 mg QD for 5 days, increased the AUC and C_{max} of ziprasidone by about 35-40%. Other inhibitors of CYP3A4 would be expected to have similar effects). Products include:
Vusion Ointment 3335

Midazolam Hydrochloride (Ziprasidone is contraindicated with drugs that have demonstrated QT prolongation as one of their pharmacodynamic effects and have this effect described in the full prescribing information as a contraindication or a boxed or bolded warning. Ziprasidone should not be used with any drug that prolongs the QT interval. An additive effect of ziprasidone and other drugs that prolong the QT interval cannot be excluded. Therefore, ziprasidone should not be given with dofetilide, sotalol, quinidine, other Class Ia and III anti-arrhythmics, mesoridazine, thioridazine, chlorpromazine, droperidol, pimozide, sparfloxacin, gatifloxacin, moxifloxacin, halofantrine, mefloquine, pentamidine, arsenic trioxide, levomethadyl acetate, dolasetron mesylate, probucol or tacrolimus).
No products indexed under this heading.

Mifepristone (Ketoconazole, a potent inhibitor of CYP3A4, at a dose of 400 mg QD for 5 days, increased the AUC and C_{max} of ziprasidone by about 35-40%. Other inhibitors of CYP3A4 would be expected to have similar effects).
No products indexed under this heading.

Minoxidil (Ziprasidone may enhance the effects of certain antihypertensive agents because of its potential for inducing hypotension).
No products indexed under this heading.

Moexipril Hydrochloride (Ziprasidone may enhance the effects of certain antihypertensive agents because of its potential for inducing hypotension).
No products indexed under this heading.

Molindone Hydrochloride (Ziprasidone is contraindicated with drugs that have demonstrated QT prolongation as one of their pharmacodynamic effects and have this effect described in the full prescribing information as a contraindication or a boxed or bolded warning. Ziprasidone should not be used with any drug that prolongs the QT interval. An additive effect of ziprasidone and other drugs that prolong the QT interval cannot be excluded. Therefore, ziprasidone should not be given with dofetilide, sotalol, quinidine, other Class Ia and III anti-arrhythmics, mesoridazine, thioridazine, chlorpromazine, droperidol, pimozide, sparfloxacin, gatifloxacin, moxifloxacin, halofantrine, mefloquine, pentamidine, arsenic trioxide, levomethadyl acetate, dolasetron mesylate, probucol or tacrolimus). Products include:
Moban 1108

Moricizine Hydrochloride (Ziprasidone is contraindicated with drugs that have demonstrated QT prolongation as one of their pharmacodynamic effects and have this effect described in the full prescribing information as a contraindication or a boxed or bolded warning. Ziprasidone should not be used with any drug that prolongs the QT interval. An additive effect of ziprasidone and other drugs that prolong the QT interval cannot be excluded. Therefore, ziprasidone should not be given with dofetilide, sotalol, quinidine, other Class Ia and III anti-arrhythmics, mesoridazine, thioridazine, chlorpromazine, droperidol, pimozide, sparfloxacin, gatifloxacin, moxifloxacin, halofantrine, mefloquine, pentamidine, arsenic trioxide, levomethadyl acetate, dolasetron mesylate, probucol or tacrolimus).
No products indexed under this heading.

Morphine Sulfate (Caution should be used when ziprasidone is taken in combination with other centrally acting drugs, given the primary CNS effects of ziprasidone). Products include:
Avinza 1822
Embeda 1831
MS Contin 2803

Moxifloxacin Hydrochloride (Ziprasidone is contraindicated with drugs that have demonstrated QT prolongation as one of their pharmacodynamic effects and have this effect described in the full prescribing information as a contraindication or a boxed or bolded warning. Ziprasidone should not be used with any drug that prolongs the QT interval. An additive effect of ziprasidone and other drugs that prolong the QT interval cannot be excluded. Therefore, ziprasidone should not be given with dofetilide, sotalol, quinidine, other Class Ia and III anti-arrhythmics, mesoridazine, thioridazine, chlorpromazine, droperidol, pimozide, sparfloxacin, gatifloxacin, moxifloxacin, halofantrine, mefloquine, pentamidine, arsenic trioxide, levomethadyl acetate, dolasetron mesylate, probucol or tacrolimus). Products include:
Avelox 3064
Vigamox 589

Nadolol (Ziprasidone may enhance the effects of certain antihypertensive agents because of its potential for inducing hypotension). Products include:
Nadolol 2359

Nebivolol (Ziprasidone may enhance the effects of certain antihypertensive agents because of its potential for inducing hypotension). Products include:
Bystolic 1147

Nefazodone Hydrochloride (Ketoconazole, a potent inhibitor of CYP3A4, at a dose of 400 mg QD for 5 days, increased the AUC and C_{max} of ziprasidone by about 35-40%. Other inhibitors of CYP3A4 would be expected to have similar effects).
No products indexed under this heading.

Nelfinavir Mesylate (Ketoconazole, a potent inhibitor of CYP3A4, at a dose of 400 mg QD for 5 days, increased the AUC and C_{max} of ziprasidone by about 35-40%. Other inhibitors of CYP3A4 would be expected to have similar effects).
No products indexed under this heading.

Nevirapine (Ketoconazole, a potent inhibitor of CYP3A4, at a dose of 400 mg QD for 5 days, increased the AUC and C_{max} of ziprasidone by about 35-40%. Other inhibitors of CYP3A4 would be expected to have similar effects). Products include:
Viramune Oral Suspension 897
Viramune Tablets 897

Niacin (Ketoconazole, a potent inhibitor of CYP3A4, at a dose of 400 mg QD for 5 days, increased the AUC and C_{max} of ziprasidone by about 35-40%. Other inhibitors of CYP3A4 would be expected to have similar effects). Products include:
Advicor 402
Cardio Basics 3455
Niaspan 497
Simcor 524

Niacinamide (Ketoconazole, a potent inhibitor of CYP3A4, at a dose of 400 mg QD for 5 days, increased the AUC and C_{max} of ziprasidone by about 35-40%. Other inhibitors of CYP3A4 would be expected to have similar effects). Products include:
CitraNatal 90 DHA Capsules 2332
CitraNatal Assure 2332
CitraNatal Rx 2332
Heplive 607

Niacinamide Hydroiodide (Ketoconazole, a potent inhibitor of CYP3A4, at a dose of 400 mg QD for 5 days, increased the AUC and C_{max} of ziprasidone by about 35-40%. Other inhibitors of CYP3A4 would be expected to have similar effects).
No products indexed under this heading.

Nicardipine Hydrochloride (Ziprasidone may enhance the effects of certain antihypertensive agents because of its potential for inducing hypotension).
No products indexed under this heading.

Nicotinamide (Ketoconazole, a potent inhibitor of CYP3A4, at a dose of 400 mg QD for 5 days, increased the AUC and C_{max} of ziprasidone by about 35-40%. Other inhibitors of CYP3A4 would be expected to have similar effects).
No products indexed under this heading.

Nifedipine (Ziprasidone may enhance the effects of certain antihypertensive agents because of its potential for inducing hypotension).
No products indexed under this heading.

Nisoldipine (Ziprasidone may enhance the effects of certain antihypertensive agents because of its potential for inducing hypotension).
No products indexed under this heading.

Nitroglycerin (Ziprasidone may enhance the effects of certain antihypertensive agents because of its potential for inducing hypotension). Products include:
Nitro-Dur 3170
Nitrolingual 3266

Norfloxacin (Ketoconazole, a potent inhibitor of CYP3A4, at a dose of 400 mg QD for 5 days, increased the AUC and C_{max} of ziprasidone by about 35-40%. Other inhibitors of CYP3A4 would be expected to have similar effects). Products include:
Noroxin 2220

Nortriptyline Hydrochloride (Ziprasidone is contraindicated with drugs that have demonstrated QT prolongation as one of their pharmacodynamic effects and have this effect described in the full prescribing information as a contraindication or a boxed or bolded warning. Ziprasidone should not be used with any drug that prolongs the QT interval. An additive effect of ziprasidone and other drugs that prolong the QT interval cannot be excluded. Therefore, ziprasidone should not be given with dofetilide, sotalol, quinidine, other Class Ia and III anti-arrhythmics, mesoridazine, thioridazine, chlorpromazine, droperidol, pimozide, sparfloxacin, gatifloxacin, moxifloxacin, halofantrine, mefloquine, pentamidine, arsenic trioxide, levomethadyl acetate, dolasetron mesylate, probucol or tacrolimus).
No products indexed under this heading.

Olanzapine (Ziprasidone is contraindicated with drugs that have demonstrated QT prolongation as one of their pharmacodynamic effects and have this effect described in the full prescribing information as a contraindication or a boxed or bolded warning. Ziprasidone should not be used with any drug that prolongs the QT interval. An additive effect of ziprasidone and other drugs that prolong the QT interval cannot be excluded. Therefore, ziprasidone should not be given with dofetilide, sotalol, quinidine, other Class Ia and III anti-arrhythmics, mesoridazine, thioridazine, chlorpromazine, droperidol, pimozide, sparfloxacin, gatifloxacin, moxifloxacin, halofantrine, mefloquine, pentamidine, arsenic trioxide, levomethadyl acetate, dolasetron mesylate, probucol or tacrolimus). Products include:
Symbyax 1965
Zyprexa 1984
Zyprexa IntraMuscular 1984
Zyprexa ZYDIS 1984

Omeprazole (Ketoconazole, a potent inhibitor of CYP3A4, at a dose of 400 mg QD for 5 days, increased the AUC and C_{max} of ziprasidone by about 35-40%. Other inhibitors of CYP3A4 would be expected to have similar effects).
No products indexed under this heading.

Oxazepam (Ziprasidone is contraindicated with drugs that have demonstrated QT prolongation as one of their pharmacodynamic effects and have this effect described in the full prescribing information as a contraindication or a boxed or bolded warning. Ziprasidone should not be used with any drug that prolongs the QT interval. An additive effect of ziprasidone and other drugs that prolong the QT interval cannot be excluded. Therefore, ziprasidone should not be given with dofetilide, sotalol, quinidine, other Class Ia and III anti-arrhythmics, mesoridazine, thioridazine, chlorpromazine, droperidol, pimozide, sparfloxacin, gatifloxacin, moxifloxacin, halofantrine, mefloquine, pentamidine, arsenic trioxide, levomethadyl acetate, dolasetron mesylate, probucol or tacrolimus).
No products indexed under this heading.

Oxycodone Hydrochloride (Caution should be used when ziprasidone is taken in combination with other centrally acting drugs, given the primary CNS effects of ziprasidone). Products include:
OxyContin 2807
Percocet 1121
Percodan 1124

Paroxetine Hydrochloride (Ketoconazole, a potent inhibitor of CYP3A4, at a dose of 400 mg QD for 5 days, increased the AUC and C_{max} of ziprasidone by about 35-40%. Other inhibitors of CYP3A4 would be expected to have similar effects). Products include:
Paroxetine CR 2361
Paroxetine ER 2371
Paxil 1586
Paxil CR 1596

Pemoline (Caution should be used when ziprasidone is taken in combination with other centrally acting drugs, given the primary CNS effects of ziprasidone).
No products indexed under this heading.

Penbutolol Sulfate (Ziprasidone may enhance the effects of certain antihypertensive agents because of its potential for inducing hypotension).
No products indexed under this heading.

Pentamidine Isethionate (Ziprasidone is contraindicated with drugs that have demonstrated QT prolongation as one of their pharmacodynamic effects and have this effect described in the full prescribing information as a contraindication or a boxed or bolded warning. Ziprasidone should not be used with any drug that prolongs the QT interval. An additive effect of ziprasidone and other drugs that prolong the QT interval cannot be excluded. Therefore, ziprasidone should not be given with dofetilide,

sotalol, quinidine, other Class la and III anti-arrhythmics, mesoridazine, thioridazine, chlorpromazine, droperidol, pimozide, sparfloxacin, gatifloxacin, moxifloxacin, halofantrine, mefloquine, pentamidine, arsenic trioxide, levomethadyl acetate, dolasetron mesylate, probucol or tacrolimus).
No products indexed under this heading.

Pentobarbital Sodium (Caution should be used when ziprasidone is taken in combination with other centrally acting drugs, given the primary CNS effects of ziprasidone). Products include:

Pergolide Mesylate (Ziprasidone may antagonize the effects of dopamine agonists).
No products indexed under this heading.

Perindopril Erbumine (Ziprasidone may enhance the effects of certain antihypertensive agents because of its potential for inducing hypotension).
No products indexed under this heading.

Perphenazine (Ziprasidone is contraindicated with drugs that have demonstrated QT prolongation as one of their pharmacodynamic effects and have this effect described in the full prescribing information as a contraindication or a boxed or bolded warning. Ziprasidone should not be used with any drug that prolongs the QT interval. An additive effect of ziprasidone and other drugs that prolong the QT interval cannot be excluded. Therefore, ziprasidone should not be given with dofetilide, sotalol, quinidine, other Class la and III anti-arrhythmics, mesoridazine, thioridazine, chlorpromazine, droperidol, pimozide, sparfloxacin, gatifloxacin, moxifloxacin, halofantrine, mefloquine, pentamidine, arsenic trioxide, levomethadyl acetate, dolasetron mesylate, probucol or tacrolimus).
No products indexed under this heading.

Phenelzine Sulfate (Ziprasidone is contraindicated with drugs that have demonstrated QT prolongation as one of their pharmacodynamic effects and have this effect described in the full prescribing information as a contraindication or a boxed or bolded warning. Ziprasidone should not be used with any drug that prolongs the QT interval. An additive effect of ziprasidone and other drugs that prolong the QT interval cannot be excluded. Therefore, ziprasidone should not be given with dofetilide, sotalol, quinidine, other Class la and III anti-arrhythmics, mesoridazine, thioridazine, chlorpromazine, droperidol, pimozide, sparfloxacin, gatifloxacin, moxifloxacin, halofantrine, mefloquine, pentamidine, arsenic trioxide, levomethadyl acetate, dolasetron mesylate, probucol or tacrolimus).
No products indexed under this heading.

Phenobarbital (Caution should be used when ziprasidone is taken in combination with other centrally acting drugs, given the primary CNS effects of ziprasidone). Products include:

Phenobarbital Sodium (Caution should be used when ziprasidone is taken in combination with other centrally acting drugs, given the primary CNS effects of ziprasidone).
No products indexed under this heading.

Phenoxybenzamine Hydrochloride (Ziprasidone may enhance the effects of certain antihypertensive agents because of its potential for inducing hypotension). Products include:

Phentolamine Mesylate (Ziprasidone may enhance the effects of certain antihypertensive agents because of its potential for inducing hypotension).
No products indexed under this heading.

Pimozide (Ziprasidone is contraindicated with drugs that have demonstrated QT prolongation as one of their pharmacodynamic effects and have this effect described in the full prescribing information as a contraindication or a boxed or bolded warning. Ziprasidone should not be used with any drug that prolongs the QT interval. An additive effect of ziprasidone and other drugs that prolong the QT interval cannot be excluded. Therefore, ziprasidone should not be given with dofetilide, sotalol, quinidine, other Class la and III anti-arrhythmics, mesoridazine, thioridazine, chlorpromazine, droperidol, pimozide, sparfloxacin, gatifloxacin, moxifloxacin, halofantrine, mefloquine, pentamidine, arsenic trioxide, levomethadyl acetate, dolasetron mesylate, probucol or tacrolimus).
No products indexed under this heading.

Pindolol (Ziprasidone may enhance the effects of certain antihypertensive agents because of its potential for inducing hypotension).
No products indexed under this heading.

Polythiazide (Ziprasidone may enhance the effects of certain antihypertensive agents because of its potential for inducing hypotension).
No products indexed under this heading.

Posaconazole (Ketoconazole, a potent inhibitor of CYP3A4, at a dose of 400 mg QD for 5 days, increased the AUC and C_{max} of ziprasidone by about 35-40%. Other inhibitors of CYP3A4 would be expected to have similar effects). Products include:

Pramipexole Dihydrochloride (Ziprasidone may antagonize the effects of dopamine agonists).
No products indexed under this heading.

Prazepam (Ziprasidone is contraindicated with drugs that have demonstrated QT prolongation as one of their pharmacodynamic effects and have this effect described in the full prescribing information as a contraindication or a boxed or bolded warning. Ziprasidone should not be used with any drug that prolongs the QT interval. An additive effect of ziprasidone and other drugs that prolong the QT interval cannot be excluded. Therefore, ziprasidone should not be given with dofetilide, sotalol, quinidine, other Class la and III anti-arrhythmics, mesoridazine, thioridazine, chlorpromazine, droperidol, pimozide, sparfloxacin, gatifloxacin, moxifloxacin, halofantrine, mefloquine, pentamidine, arsenic trioxide, levomethadyl acetate, dolasetron mesylate, probucol or tacrolimus).
No products indexed under this heading.

Prazosin Hydrochloride (Ziprasidone may enhance the effects of certain antihypertensive agents because of its potential for inducing hypotension).
No products indexed under this heading.

Probucol (Ziprasidone is contraindicated with drugs that have demonstrated QT prolongation as one of their pharmacodynamic effects and have this effect described in the full prescribing information as a contraindication or a boxed or bolded warning. Ziprasidone should not be used with any drug that prolongs the QT interval. An additive effect of ziprasidone and other drugs that prolong the QT interval cannot be excluded. Therefore, ziprasidone should not be given with dofetilide, sotalol, quinidine, other Class la and III anti-arrhythmics, mesoridazine, thioridazine, chlorpromazine, droperidol, pimozide,

sparfloxacin, gatifloxacin, moxifloxacin, halofantrine, mefloquine, pentamidine, arsenic trioxide, levomethadyl acetate, dolasetron mesylate, probucol or tacrolimus).
No products indexed under this heading.

Procainamide (Ziprasidone is contraindicated with drugs that have demonstrated QT prolongation as one of their pharmacodynamic effects and have this effect described in the full prescribing information as a contraindication or a boxed or bolded warning. Ziprasidone should not be used with any drug that prolongs the QT interval. An additive effect of ziprasidone and other drugs that prolong the QT interval cannot be excluded. Therefore, ziprasidone should not be given with dofetilide, sotalol, quinidine, other Class la and III anti-arrhythmics, mesoridazine, thioridazine, chlorpromazine, droperidol, pimozide, sparfloxacin, gatifloxacin, moxifloxacin, halofantrine, mefloquine, pentamidine, arsenic trioxide, levomethadyl acetate, dolasetron mesylate, probucol or tacrolimus).
No products indexed under this heading.

Procainamide Hydrochloride (Ziprasidone is contraindicated with drugs that have demonstrated QT prolongation as one of their pharmacodynamic effects and have this effect described in the full prescribing information as a contraindication or a boxed or bolded warning. Ziprasidone should not be used with any drug that prolongs the QT interval. An additive effect of ziprasidone and other drugs that prolong the QT interval cannot be excluded. Therefore, ziprasidone should not be given with dofetilide, sotalol, quinidine, other Class la and III anti-arrhythmics, mesoridazine, thioridazine, chlorpromazine, droperidol, pimozide, sparfloxacin, gatifloxacin, moxifloxacin, halofantrine, mefloquine, pentamidine, arsenic trioxide, levomethadyl acetate, dolasetron mesylate, probucol or tacrolimus).
No products indexed under this heading.

Prochlorperazine (Ziprasidone is contraindicated with drugs that have demonstrated QT prolongation as one of their pharmacodynamic effects and have this effect described in the full prescribing information as a contraindication or a boxed or bolded warning. Ziprasidone should not be used with any drug that prolongs the QT interval. An additive effect of ziprasidone and other drugs that prolong the QT interval cannot be excluded. Therefore, ziprasidone should not be given with dofetilide, sotalol, quinidine, other Class la and III anti-arrhythmics, mesoridazine, thioridazine, chlorpromazine, droperidol, pimozide, sparfloxacin, gatifloxacin, moxifloxacin, halofantrine, mefloquine, pentamidine, arsenic trioxide, levomethadyl acetate, dolasetron mesylate, probucol or tacrolimus).
No products indexed under this heading.

Promethazine Hydrochloride (Ziprasidone is contraindicated with drugs that have demonstrated QT prolongation as one of their pharmacodynamic effects and have this effect described in the full prescribing information as a contraindication or a boxed or bolded warning. Ziprasidone should not be used with any drug that prolongs the QT interval. An additive effect of ziprasidone and other drugs that prolong the QT interval cannot be excluded. Therefore, ziprasidone should not be given with dofetilide, sotalol, quinidine, other Class la and III anti-arrhythmics, mesoridazine, thioridazine, chlorpromazine, droperidol, pimozide, sparfloxacin, gatifloxacin, moxifloxacin, halofantrine,

mefloquine, pentamidine, arsenic trioxide, levomethadyl acetate, dolasetron mesylate, probucol or tacrolimus).
No products indexed under this heading.

Propafenone Hydrochloride (Ziprasidone is contraindicated with drugs that have demonstrated QT prolongation as one of their pharmacodynamic effects and have this effect described in the full prescribing information as a contraindication or a boxed or bolded warning. Ziprasidone should not be used with any drug that prolongs the QT interval. An additive effect of ziprasidone and other drugs that prolong the QT interval cannot be excluded. Therefore, ziprasidone should not be given with dofetilide, sotalol, quinidine, other Class la and III anti-arrhythmics, mesoridazine, thioridazine, chlorpromazine, droperidol, pimozide, sparfloxacin, gatifloxacin, moxifloxacin, halofantrine, mefloquine, pentamidine, arsenic trioxide, levomethadyl acetate, dolasetron mesylate, probucol or tacrolimus). Products include:

Propofol (Caution should be used when ziprasidone is taken in combination with other centrally acting drugs, given the primary CNS effects of ziprasidone).
No products indexed under this heading.

Propoxyphene Hydrochloride (Caution should be used when ziprasidone is taken in combination with other centrally acting drugs, given the primary CNS effects of ziprasidone).
No products indexed under this heading.

Propoxyphene Napsylate (Caution should be used when ziprasidone is taken in combination with other centrally acting drugs, given the primary CNS effects of ziprasidone).
No products indexed under this heading.

Propranolol Hydrochloride (Ziprasidone may enhance the effects of certain antihypertensive agents because of its potential for inducing hypotension). Products include:

Protriptyline Hydrochloride (Ziprasidone is contraindicated with drugs that have demonstrated QT prolongation as one of their pharmacodynamic effects and have this effect described in the full prescribing information as a contraindication or a boxed or bolded warning. Ziprasidone should not be used with any drug that prolongs the QT interval. An additive effect of ziprasidone and other drugs that prolong the QT interval cannot be excluded. Therefore, ziprasidone should not be given with dofetilide, sotalol, quinidine, other Class la and III anti-arrhythmics, mesoridazine, thioridazine, chlorpromazine, droperidol, pimozide, sparfloxacin, gatifloxacin, moxifloxacin, halofantrine, mefloquine, pentamidine, arsenic trioxide, levomethadyl acetate, dolasetron mesylate, probucol or tacrolimus).
No products indexed under this heading.

Quazepam (Caution should be used when ziprasidone is taken in combination with other centrally acting drugs, given the primary CNS effects of ziprasidone).
No products indexed under this heading.

Quetiapine Fumarate (Ziprasidone is contraindicated with drugs that have demonstrated QT prolongation as one of their pharmacodynamic effects and have this effect described in the full prescribing information as a contraindication or a boxed or bolded warning. Ziprasidone should not be used with any drug that prolongs the QT interval. An additive effect of ziprasidone and other drugs that prolong the QT interval cannot be excluded. Therefore, ziprasidone

should not be given with dofetilide, sotalol, quinidine, other Class la and III anti-arrhythmics, mesoridazine, thioridazine, chlorpromazine, droperidol, pimozide, sparfloxacin, gatifloxacin, moxifloxacin, halofantrine, mefloquine, pentamidine, arsenic trioxide, levomethadyl acetate, dolasetron mesylate, probucol or tacrolimus). Products include:

Quinapril Hydrochloride (Ziprasidone may enhance the effects of certain antihypertensive agents because of its potential for inducing hypotension).

No products indexed under this heading.

Quinidine (Ziprasidone is contraindicated with drugs that have demonstrated QT prolongation as one of their pharmacodynamic effects and have this effect described in the full prescribing information as a contraindication or a boxed or bolded warning. Ziprasidone should not be used with any drug that prolongs the QT interval. An additive effect of ziprasidone and other drugs that prolong the QT interval cannot be excluded. Therefore, ziprasidone should not be given with dofetilide, sotalol, quinidine, other Class la and III anti-arrhythmics, mesoridazine, thioridazine, chlorpromazine, droperidol, pimozide, sparfloxacin, gatifloxacin, moxifloxacin, halofantrine, mefloquine, pentamidine, arsenic trioxide, levomethadyl acetate, dolasetron mesylate, probucol or tacrolimus).

No products indexed under this heading.

Quinidine Gluconate (Ziprasidone is contraindicated with drugs that have demonstrated QT prolongation as one of their pharmacodynamic effects and have this effect described in the full prescribing information as a contraindication or a boxed or bolded warning. Ziprasidone should not be used with any drug that prolongs the QT interval. An additive effect of ziprasidone and other drugs that prolong the QT interval cannot be excluded. Therefore, ziprasidone should not be given with dofetilide, sotalol, quinidine, other Class la and III anti-arrhythmics, mesoridazine, thioridazine, chlorpromazine, droperidol, pimozide, sparfloxacin, gatifloxacin, moxifloxacin, halofantrine, mefloquine, pentamidine, arsenic trioxide, levomethadyl acetate, dolasetron mesylate, probucol or tacrolimus).

No products indexed under this heading.

Quinidine Hydrochloride (Ziprasidone is contraindicated with drugs that have demonstrated QT prolongation as one of their pharmacodynamic effects and have this effect described in the full prescribing information as a contraindication or a boxed or bolded warning. Ziprasidone should not be used with any drug that prolongs the QT interval. An additive effect of ziprasidone and other drugs that prolong the QT interval cannot be excluded. Therefore, ziprasidone should not be given with dofetilide, sotalol, quinidine, other Class la and III anti-arrhythmics, mesoridazine, thioridazine, chlorpromazine, droperidol, pimozide, sparfloxacin, gatifloxacin, moxifloxacin, halofantrine, mefloquine, pentamidine, arsenic trioxide, levomethadyl acetate, dolasetron mesylate, probucol or tacrolimus).

No products indexed under this heading.

Quinidine Polygalacturonate (Ziprasidone is contraindicated with drugs that have demonstrated QT prolongation as one of their pharmacodynamic effects and have this effect described in the full prescribing information as a contraindication or a boxed or bolded warning. Ziprasidone should not be used with any drug that prolongs the QT interval. An additive effect of ziprasi-

done and other drugs that prolong the QT interval cannot be excluded. Therefore, ziprasidone should not be given with dofetilide, sotalol, quinidine, other Class la and III anti-arrhythmics, mesoridazine, thioridazine, chlorpromazine, droperidol, pimozide, sparfloxacin, gatifloxacin, moxifloxacin, halofantrine, mefloquine, pentamidine, arsenic trioxide, levomethadyl acetate, dolasetron mesylate, probucol or tacrolimus).

No products indexed under this heading.

Quinidine Sulfate (Ziprasidone is contraindicated with drugs that have demonstrated QT prolongation as one of their pharmacodynamic effects and have this effect described in the full prescribing information as a contraindication or a boxed or bolded warning. Ziprasidone should not be used with any drug that prolongs the QT interval. An additive effect of ziprasidone and other drugs that prolong the QT interval cannot be excluded. Therefore, ziprasidone should not be given with dofetilide, sotalol, quinidine, other Class la and III anti-arrhythmics, mesoridazine, thioridazine, chlorpromazine, droperidol, pimozide, sparfloxacin, gatifloxacin, moxifloxacin, halofantrine, mefloquine, pentamidine, arsenic trioxide, levomethadyl acetate, dolasetron mesylate, probucol or tacrolimus).

No products indexed under this heading.

Quinine (Ketoconazole, a potent inhibitor of CYP3A4, at a dose of 400 mg QD for 5 days, increased the AUC and C_{max} of ziprasidone by about 35-40%. Other inhibitors of CYP3A4 would be expected to have similar effects). Products include:

Quinine Sulfate (Ketoconazole, a potent inhibitor of CYP3A4, at a dose of 400 mg QD for 5 days, increased the AUC and C_{max} of ziprasidone by about 35-40%. Other inhibitors of CYP3A4 would be expected to have similar effects).

No products indexed under this heading.

Quinupristin (Ketoconazole, a potent inhibitor of CYP3A4, at a dose of 400 mg QD for 5 days, increased the AUC and C_{max} of ziprasidone by about 35-40%. Other inhibitors of CYP3A4 would be expected to have similar effects).

No products indexed under this heading.

Ramipril (Ziprasidone may enhance the effects of certain antihypertensive agents because of its potential for inducing hypotension).

No products indexed under this heading.

Ranitidine Bismuth Citrate (Ketoconazole, a potent inhibitor of CYP3A4, at a dose of 400 mg QD for 5 days, increased the AUC and C_{max} of ziprasidone by about 35-40%. Other inhibitors of CYP3A4 would be expected to have similar effects).

No products indexed under this heading.

Ranitidine Hydrochloride (Ketoconazole, a potent inhibitor of CYP3A4, at a dose of 400 mg QD for 5 days, increased the AUC and C_{max} of ziprasidone by about 35-40%. Other inhibitors of CYP3A4 would be expected to have similar effects). Products include:

Rauwolfia Serpentina (Ziprasidone may enhance the effects of certain antihypertensive agents because of its potential for inducing hypotension).

No products indexed under this heading.

Remifentanil Hydrochloride (Caution should be used when ziprasidone is taken in combination with other centrally acting drugs, given the primary CNS effects of ziprasidone).

No products indexed under this heading.

Rescinnamine (Ziprasidone may enhance the effects of certain antihypertensive agents because of its potential for inducing hypotension).

No products indexed under this heading.

Reserpine (Ziprasidone may enhance the effects of certain antihypertensive agents because of its potential for inducing hypotension).

No products indexed under this heading.

Risperidone (Ziprasidone is contraindicated with drugs that have demonstrated QT prolongation as one of their pharmacodynamic effects and have this effect described in the full prescribing information as a contraindication or a boxed or bolded warning. Ziprasidone should not be used with any drug that prolongs the QT interval. An additive effect of ziprasidone and other drugs that prolong the QT interval cannot be excluded. Therefore, ziprasidone should not be given with dofetilide, sotalol, quinidine, other Class la and III anti-arrhythmics, mesoridazine, thioridazine, chlorpromazine, droperidol, pimozide, sparfloxacin, gatifloxacin, moxifloxacin, halofantrine, mefloquine, pentamidine, arsenic trioxide, levomethadyl acetate, dolasetron mesylate, probucol or tacrolimus). Products include:

Ritonavir (Ketoconazole, a potent inhibitor of CYP3A4, at a dose of 400 mg QD for 5 days, increased the AUC and C_{max} of ziprasidone by about 35-40%. Other inhibitors of CYP3A4 would be expected to have similar effects). Products include:

Ropinirole Hydrochloride (Ziprasidone may antagonize the effects of dopamine agonists). Products include:

Saquinavir (Ketoconazole, a potent inhibitor of CYP3A4, at a dose of 400 mg QD for 5 days, increased the AUC and C_{max} of ziprasidone by about 35-40%. Other inhibitors of CYP3A4 would be expected to have similar effects).

No products indexed under this heading.

Saquinavir Mesylate (Ketoconazole, a potent inhibitor of CYP3A4, at a dose of 400 mg QD for 5 days, increased the AUC and C_{max} of ziprasidone by about 35-40%. Other inhibitors of CYP3A4 would be expected to have similar effects).

No products indexed under this heading.

Secobarbital Sodium (Caution should be used when ziprasidone is taken in combination with other centrally acting drugs, given the primary CNS effects of ziprasidone).

No products indexed under this heading.

Sertraline Hydrochloride (Ketoconazole, a potent inhibitor of CYP3A4, at a dose of 400 mg QD for 5 days, increased the AUC and C_{max} of ziprasidone by about 35-40%. Other inhibitors of CYP3A4 would be expected to have similar effects).

No products indexed under this heading.

Sevoflurane (Caution should be used when ziprasidone is taken in combination with other centrally acting drugs, given the primary CNS effects of ziprasidone). Products include:

Sildenafil Citrate (Ketoconazole, a potent inhibitor of CYP3A4, at a dose of 400 mg QD for 5 days, increased the AUC and C_{max} of ziprasidone by about 35-40%. Other inhibitors of CYP3A4 would be expected to have similar effects).

No products indexed under this heading.

Sodium Nitroprusside (Ziprasidone may enhance the effects of certain antihypertensive agents because of its potential for inducing hypotension).

No products indexed under this heading.

Sodium Oxybate (Caution should be used when ziprasidone is taken in combination with other centrally acting drugs, given the primary CNS effects of ziprasidone).

No products indexed under this heading.

Sotalol Hydrochloride (Ziprasidone is contraindicated with drugs that have demonstrated QT prolongation as one of their pharmacodynamic effects and have this effect described in the full prescribing information as a contraindication or a boxed or bolded warning. Ziprasidone should not be used with any drug that prolongs the QT interval. An additive effect of ziprasidone and other drugs that prolong the QT interval cannot be excluded. Therefore, ziprasidone should not be given with dofetilide, sotalol, quinidine, other Class la and III anti-arrhythmics, mesoridazine, thioridazine, chlorpromazine, droperidol, pimozide, sparfloxacin, gatifloxacin, moxifloxacin, halofantrine, mefloquine, pentamidine, arsenic trioxide, levomethadyl acetate, dolasetron mesylate, probucol or tacrolimus).

No products indexed under this heading.

Sparfloxacin (Ziprasidone is contraindicated with drugs that have demonstrated QT prolongation as one of their pharmacodynamic effects and have this effect described in the full prescribing information as a contraindication or a boxed or bolded warning. Ziprasidone should not be used with any drug that prolongs the QT interval. An additive effect of ziprasidone and other drugs that prolong the QT interval cannot be excluded. Therefore, ziprasidone should not be given with dofetilide, sotalol, quinidine, other Class la and III anti-arrhythmics, mesoridazine, thioridazine, chlorpromazine, droperidol, pimozide, sparfloxacin, gatifloxacin, moxifloxacin, halofantrine, mefloquine, pentamidine, arsenic trioxide, levomethadyl acetate, dolasetron mesylate, probucol or tacrolimus).

No products indexed under this heading.

Spirapril Hydrochloride (Ziprasidone may enhance the effects of certain antihypertensive agents because of its potential for inducing hypotension).

No products indexed under this heading.

Sufentanil Citrate (Caution should be used when ziprasidone is taken in combination with other centrally acting drugs, given the primary CNS effects of ziprasidone).

No products indexed under this heading.

Tacrolimus (Ziprasidone is contraindicated with drugs that have demonstrated QT prolongation as one of their pharmacodynamic effects and have this effect described in the full prescribing information as a contraindication or a boxed or bolded warning. Ziprasidone should not be used with any drug that prolongs the QT interval. An additive effect of ziprasidone and other drugs that prolong the QT interval cannot be excluded. Therefore, ziprasidone should not be given with dofetilide, sotalol, quinidine, other Class la and III anti-arrhythmics, mesoridazine, thioridazine, chlorpromazine, droperidol, pimozide, sparfloxacin, gatifloxacin, moxifloxacin, halofantrine, mefloquine, pentamidine,

arsenic trioxide, levomethadyl acetate, dolasetron mesylate, probucol or tacrolimus). Products include:

Telithromycin (Ketoconazole, a potent inhibitor of CYP3A4, at a dose of 400 mg QD for 5 days, increased the AUC and C_{max} of ziprasidone by about 35-40%. Other inhibitors of CYP3A4 would be expected to have similar effects). Products include:

Telmisartan (Ziprasidone may enhance the effects of certain antihypertensive agents because of its potential for inducing hypotension). Products include:

Temazepam (Caution should be used when ziprasidone is taken in combination with other centrally acting drugs, given the primary CNS effects of ziprasidone).

No products indexed under this heading.

Terazosin Hydrochloride (Ziprasidone may enhance the effects of certain antihypertensive agents because of its potential for inducing hypotension).

No products indexed under this heading.

Thiamylal Sodium (Caution should be used when ziprasidone is taken in combination with other centrally acting drugs, given the primary CNS effects of ziprasidone).

No products indexed under this heading.

Thioridazine Hydrochloride (Ziprasidone is contraindicated with drugs that have demonstrated QT prolongation as one of their pharmacodynamic effects and have this effect described in the full prescribing information as a contraindication or a boxed or bolded warning. Ziprasidone should not be used with any drug that prolongs the QT interval. An additive effect of ziprasidone and other drugs that prolong the QT interval cannot be excluded. Therefore, ziprasidone should not be given with dofetilide, sotalol, quinidine, other Class Ia and III anti-arrhythmics, mesoridazine, thioridazine, chlorpromazine, droperidol, pimozide, sparfloxacin, gatifloxacin, moxifloxacin, halofantrine, mefloquine, pentamidine, arsenic trioxide, levomethadyl acetate, dolasetron mesylate, probucol or tacrolimus). Products include:

Thiothixene (Ziprasidone is contraindicated with drugs that have demonstrated QT prolongation as one of their pharmacodynamic effects and have this effect described in the full prescribing information as a contraindication or a boxed or bolded warning. Ziprasidone should not be used with any drug that prolongs the QT interval. An additive effect of ziprasidone and other drugs that prolong the QT interval cannot be excluded. Therefore, ziprasidone should not be given with dofetilide, sotalol, quinidine, other Class Ia and III anti-arrhythmics, mesoridazine, thioridazine, chlorpromazine, droperidol, pimozide, sparfloxacin, gatifloxacin, moxifloxacin, halofantrine, mefloquine, pentamidine, arsenic trioxide, levomethadyl acetate, dolasetron mesylate, probucol or tacrolimus). Products include:

Timolol Maleate (Ziprasidone may enhance the effects of certain antihypertensive agents because of its potential for inducing hypotension). Products include:

Tocainide Hydrochloride (Ziprasidone is contraindicated with drugs that have demonstrated QT prolongation as one of their pharmacodynamic effects and have this effect described in the full prescribing information as a contraindication or a boxed or bolded warning. Ziprasidone should not be used with any drug that prolongs the QT interval. An additive effect of ziprasidone and other drugs that prolong the QT interval cannot be excluded. Therefore, ziprasidone should not be given with dofetilide, sotalol, quinidine, other Class Ia and III anti-arrhythmics, mesoridazine, thioridazine, chlorpromazine, droperidol, pimozide, sparfloxacin, gatifloxacin, moxifloxacin, halofantrine, mefloquine, pentamidine, arsenic trioxide, levomethadyl acetate, dolasetron mesylate, probucol or tacrolimus).

No products indexed under this heading.

Torsemide (Ziprasidone may enhance the effects of certain antihypertensive agents because of its potential for inducing hypotension).

No products indexed under this heading.

Trandolapril (Ziprasidone may enhance the effects of certain antihypertensive agents because of its potential for inducing hypotension). Products include:

Tranylcypromine Sulfate (Ziprasidone is contraindicated with drugs that have demonstrated QT prolongation as one of their pharmacodynamic effects and have this effect described in the full prescribing information as a contraindication or a boxed or bolded warning. Ziprasidone should not be used with any drug that prolongs the QT interval. An additive effect of ziprasidone and other drugs that prolong the QT interval cannot be excluded. Therefore, ziprasidone should not be given with dofetilide, sotalol, quinidine, other Class Ia and III anti-arrhythmics, mesoridazine, thioridazine, chlorpromazine, droperidol, pimozide, sparfloxacin, gatifloxacin, moxifloxacin, halofantrine, mefloquine, pentamidine, arsenic trioxide, levomethadyl acetate, dolasetron mesylate, probucol or tacrolimus). Products include:

Triazolam (Caution should be used when ziprasidone is taken in combination with other centrally acting drugs, given the primary CNS effects of ziprasidone).

No products indexed under this heading.

Trifluoperazine Hydrochloride (Ziprasidone is contraindicated with drugs that have demonstrated QT prolongation as one of their pharmacodynamic effects and have this effect described in the full prescribing information as a contraindication or a boxed or bolded warning. Ziprasidone should not be used with any drug that prolongs the QT interval. An additive effect of ziprasidone and other drugs that prolong the QT interval cannot be excluded. Therefore, ziprasidone should not be given with dofetilide, sotalol, quinidine, other Class Ia and III anti-arrhythmics, mesoridazine, thioridazine, chlorpromazine, droperidol, pimozide, sparfloxacin, gatifloxacin, moxifloxacin, halofantrine, mefloquine, pentamidine, arsenic trioxide, levomethadyl acetate, dolasetron mesylate, probucol or tacrolimus).

No products indexed under this heading.

Trimethaphan Camsylate (Ziprasidone may enhance the effects of certain antihypertensive agents because of its potential for inducing hypotension).

No products indexed under this heading.

Trimipramine Maleate (Ziprasidone is contraindicated with drugs that have demonstrated QT prolongation as one of their pharmacodynamic effects and have this effect described in the full prescribing information as a contraindication or a boxed or bolded warning. Ziprasidone should not be used with any drug that prolongs the QT interval. An additive effect of ziprasidone and other drugs that prolong the QT interval cannot be excluded. Therefore, ziprasidone should not be given with dofetilide, sotalol, quinidine, other Class Ia and III anti-arrhythmics, mesoridazine, thioridazine, chlorpromazine, droperidol, pimozide, sparfloxacin, gatifloxacin, moxifloxacin, halofantrine, mefloquine, pentamidine, arsenic trioxide, levomethadyl acetate, dolasetron mesylate, probucol or tacrolimus).

No products indexed under this heading.

Troglitazone (Ketoconazole, a potent inhibitor of CYP3A4, at a dose of 400 mg QD for 5 days, increased the AUC and C_{max} of ziprasidone by about 35-40%. Other inhibitors of CYP3A4 would be expected to have similar effects).

No products indexed under this heading.

Troleandomycin (Ketoconazole, a potent inhibitor of CYP3A4, at a dose of 400 mg QD for 5 days, increased the AUC and C_{max} of ziprasidone by about 35-40%. Other inhibitors of CYP3A4 would be expected to have similar effects).

No products indexed under this heading.

Valproate Sodium (Ketoconazole, a potent inhibitor of CYP3A4, at a dose of 400 mg QD for 5 days, increased the AUC and C_{max} of ziprasidone by about 35-40%. Other inhibitors of CYP3A4 would be expected to have similar effects).

No products indexed under this heading.

Valsartan (Ziprasidone may enhance the effects of certain antihypertensive agents because of its potential for inducing hypotension). Products include:

Vardenafil Hydrochloride (Ketoconazole, a potent inhibitor of CYP3A4, at a dose of 400 mg QD for 5 days, increased the AUC and C_{max} of ziprasidone by about 35-40%. Other inhibitors of CYP3A4 would be expected to have similar effects). Products include:

Verapamil Hydrochloride (Ziprasidone may enhance the effects of certain antihypertensive agents because of its potential for inducing hypotension). Products include:

Voriconazole (Ketoconazole, a potent inhibitor of CYP3A4, at a dose of 400 mg QD for 5 days, increased the AUC and C_{max} of ziprasidone by about 35-40%. Other inhibitors of CYP3A4 would be expected to have similar effects).

No products indexed under this heading.

Zafirlukast (Ketoconazole, a potent inhibitor of CYP3A4, at a dose of 400 mg QD for 5 days, increased the AUC and C_{max} of ziprasidone by about 35-40%. Other inhibitors of CYP3A4 would be expected to have similar effects). Products include:

Zaleplon (Caution should be used when ziprasidone is taken in combination with other centrally acting drugs, given the primary CNS effects of ziprasidone).

No products indexed under this heading.

Zileuton (Ketoconazole, a potent inhibitor of CYP3A4, at a dose of 400 mg QD for 5 days, increased the AUC and C_{max} of ziprasidone by about 35-40%. Other inhibitors of CYP3A4 would be expected to have similar effects).

No products indexed under this heading.

Zolpidem Tartrate (Caution should be used when ziprasidone is taken in combination with other centrally acting drugs, given the primary CNS effects of ziprasidone). Products include:

Food Interactions

Alcohol (Caution should be used when ziprasidone is taken in combination with other centrally acting drugs, given the primary CNS effects of ziprasidone).

Food, unspecified (The absorption of oral ziprasidone is increased up to twofold in the presence of food).

Grapefruit (Ketoconazole, a potent inhibitor of CYP3A4, at a dose of 400 mg QD for 5 days, increased the AUC and C_{max} of ziprasidone by about 35-40%. Other inhibitors of CYP3A4 would be expected to have similar effects).

Grapefruit Juice (Ketoconazole, a potent inhibitor of CYP3A4, at a dose of 400 mg QD for 5 days, increased the AUC and C_{max} of ziprasidone by about 35-40%. Other inhibitors of CYP3A4 would be expected to have similar effects).

Meal, unspecified (The absorption of oral ziprasidone is increased up to twofold in the presence of food).

GEODON FOR INJECTION
See Geodon Capsules

GLEEVEC TABLETS
May interact with antineoplastics, calcium channel blockers that are metabolized by CYP3A4, cytochrome p450 2d6 substrates (selected), cytochrome p450 3a4 inducers (selected), cytochrome p450 3a4 inhibitors (selected), cytochrome p450 3a4 inhibitors, potent (selected), cytochrome p450 3a4 substrates (selected), dexamethasones, phenytoin, quinidine, statins that are metabolized by CYP3A4, triazolobenzodiazepines, and certain other agents. Compounds in these categories include:

Acetaminophen (*In vitro*, imatinib inhibits acetaminophen O-glucuronidation (Ki value of 58.5 uM) at therapeutic levels. Systemic exposure to acetaminophen is expected to be increased when co-administered with imatinib. No specific studies in humans have been performed and caution is recommended). Products include:

Acetaminophen-containing products (*In vitro*, imatinib inhibits acetaminophen O-glucuronidation (Ki value of 58.5 uM) at therapeutic levels. Systemic exposure to acetaminophen is expected to be increased when co-administered with imatinib. No specific studies in humans have been performed and caution is recommended).

No products indexed under this heading.

Acetazolamide (There was a significant increase in exposure to imatinib (mean C_{max} and AUC increased by 26% and 40%, respectively) in healthy subjects when imatinib was co-administered with a single dose of ketoconazole (a CYP3A4 inhibitor). Caution is recommended when administering imatinib with strong CYP3A4 inhibitors. Substances that inhibit the cytochrome P450 isoenzyme (CYP3A4) activity may decrease metabolism and increase imatinib concentrations).

No products indexed under this heading.

Acetazolamide Sodium (There was a significant increase in exposure to imatinib (mean C_{max} and AUC increased by 26% and 40%, respectively) in healthy subjects when imatinib was co-administered with a single dose of ketoconazole (a CYP3A4 inhibitor). Caution is recommended when administering imatinib with strong CYP3A4 inhibitors. Substances that inhibit the cytochrome P450 isoenzyme (CYP3A4) activity may decrease metabolism and increase imatinib concentrations).

No products indexed under this heading.

Alfentanil Hydrochloride (Imatinib increases the mean C_{max} and AUC of simvastatin (CYP3A4 substrate) 2- and 3.5-fold, respectively, suggesting an inhibition of the CYP3A4 by imatinib. Particular caution is recommended when administering imatinib with CYP3A4 substrates that have a narrow therapeutic window (eg, alfentanil). Imatinib will increase plasma concentration of other CYP3A4 metabolized drugs).

No products indexed under this heading.

Allium sativum (CYP3A4 inducers may decrease imatinib C_{max} and AUC. The use of concomitant strong CYP3A4 inducers should be avoided. If patients must be co-administered a strong CYP3A4 inducer, based on pharmacokinetic studies, the dosage of imatinib should be increased by at least 50% and clinical response should be carefully monitored).

No products indexed under this heading.

Alprazolam (Imatinib increases the mean C_{max} and AUC of simvastatin (CYP3A4 substrate) 2- and 3.5-fold, respectively, suggesting an inhibition of the CYP3A4 by imatinib. Particular caution is recommended when administering imatinib with CYP3A4 substrates that have a narrow therapeutic window. Imatinib will increase plasma concentration of other CYP3A4 metabolized drugs (eg, triazolo-benzodiazepines)).

No products indexed under this heading.

Altretamine (When imatinib is combined with chemotherapy, liver toxicity in the form of transaminase elevation and hyperbilirubinemia has been observed. Additionally, there have been reports of acute liver failure. Monitoring of hepatic function is recommended. Products include:

Hexalen 1066

Aminoglutethimide (CYP3A4 inducers may decrease imatinib C_{max} and AUC. The use of concomitant strong CYP3A4 inducers should be avoided. If patients must be co-administered a strong CYP3A4 inducer, based on pharmacokinetic studies, the dosage of imatinib should be increased by at least 50% and clinical response should be carefully monitored).

No products indexed under this heading.

Amiodarone Hydrochloride (There was a significant increase in exposure to imatinib (mean C_{max} and AUC increased by 26% and 40%, respectively) in healthy subjects when imatinib was co-administered with a single dose of ketoconazole (a CYP3A4 inhibitor). Caution is recommended when administering imatinib with strong CYP3A4 inhibitors. Substances that inhibit the cytochrome P450 isoenzyme (CYP3A4) activity may decrease metabolism and increase imatinib concentrations).

No products indexed under this heading.

Amitriptyline Hydrochloride (Imatinib increases the mean C_{max} and AUC of simvastatin (CYP3A4 substrate) 2- and 3.5-fold, respectively, suggesting an inhibition of the CYP3A4 by imatinib. Particular caution is recommended when administering imatinib with CYP3A4 substrates that have a narrow therapeutic window. Imatinib will increase plasma concentration of other CYP3A4 metabolized drugs).

No products indexed under this heading.

Amlodipine Besylate (Imatinib increases the mean C_{max} and AUC of simvastatin (CYP3A4 substrate) 2- and 3.5-fold, respectively, suggesting an inhibition of the CYP3A4 by imatinib. Particular caution is recommended when administering imatinib with CYP3A4 substrates that have a narrow therapeutic window. Imatinib will increase plasma concentration of other CYP3A4 metabolized drugs (eg, dihydropyridine calcium channel blockers)). Products include:

Azor 1010
Exforge 2443
Exforge HCT 2449

Amphetamine Aspartate (*In vitro*, imatinib inhibits the cytochrome P450 isoenzyme CYP2D6 activity at similar concentrations that affect CYP3A4 activity. Systemic exposure to substrates of CYP2D6 is expected to be increased when co-administered with imatinib. No specific studies have been performed and caution is recommended).

No products indexed under this heading.

Amphetamine Aspartate Monohydrate (*In vitro*, imatinib inhibits the cytochrome P450 isoenzyme CYP2D6 activity at similar concentrations that affect CYP3A4 activity. Systemic exposure to substrates of CYP2D6 is expected to be increased when co-administered with imatinib. No specific studies have been performed and caution is recommended).

No products indexed under this heading.

Amphetamine Sulfate (*In vitro*, imatinib inhibits the cytochrome P450 isoenzyme CYP2D6 activity at similar concentrations that affect CYP3A4 activity. Systemic exposure to substrates of CYP2D6 is expected to be increased when co-administered with imatinib. No specific studies have been performed and caution is recommended).

No products indexed under this heading.

Amprenavir (CYP3A4 inhibitors may increase imatinib C_{max} and AUC. There was a significant increase in exposure to imatinib (mean C_{max} and AUC increased by 26% and 40% respectively) in healthy subjects when imatinib was co-administered with a single dose of ketoconazole (a CYP3A4 inhibitor). Caution is recommended when administering imatinib with strong CYP3A4 inhibitors (eg, ketoconazole, itraconazole). Grapefruit juice may also increase plasma concentrations of imatinib and should be avoided. Substances that inhibit the cytochrome P450 isoenzyme (CYP3A4) activity may decrease metabolism and increase imatinib concentrations).

No products indexed under this heading.

Anastrozole (There was a significant increase in exposure to imatinib (mean C_{max} and AUC increased by 26% and 40%, respectively) in healthy subjects when imatinib was co-administered with a single dose of ketoconazole (a CYP3A4 inhibitor). Caution is recommended when administering imatinib with strong CYP3A4 inhibitors. Substances that inhibit the cytochrome P450 isoenzyme (CYP3A4) activity may decrease metabolism and increase imatinib concentrations).

No products indexed under this heading.

Aprepitant (There was a significant increase in exposure to imatinib (mean C_{max} and AUC increased by 26% and 40%, respectively) in healthy subjects when imatinib was co-administered with a single dose of ketoconazole (a CYP3A4 inhibitor). Caution is recommended when administering imatinib with strong CYP3A4 inhibitors. Substances that inhibit the cytochrome P450 isoenzyme (CYP3A4) activity may decrease metabolism and increase imatinib concentrations). Products include:

Emend 2124

Asparaginase (When imatinib is combined with chemotherapy, liver toxicity in the form of transaminase elevation and hyperbilirubinemia has been observed. Additionally, there have been reports of acute liver failure. Monitoring of hepatic function is recommended). Products include:

Elspar 2005, 2122

Astemizole (Imatinib increases the mean C_{max} and AUC of simvastatin (CYP3A4 substrate) 2- and 3.5-fold, respectively, suggesting an inhibition of the CYP3A4 by imatinib. Particular caution is recommended when administering imatinib with CYP3A4 substrates that have a narrow therapeutic window. Imatinib will increase plasma concentration of other CYP3A4 metabolized drugs).

No products indexed under this heading.

Atazanavir (There was a significant increase in exposure to imatinib (mean C_{max} and AUC increased by 26% and 40%, respectively) in healthy subjects when imatinib was co-administered with a single dose of ketoconazole (a CYP3A4 inhibitor). Caution is recommended when administering imatinib with strong CYP3A4 inhibitors (eg, atazanavir). Substances that inhibit the cytochrome P450 isoenzyme (CYP3A4) activity may decrease metabolism and increase imatinib concentrations).

No products indexed under this heading.

Atazanavir Sulfate (There was a significant increase in exposure to imatinib (mean C_{max} and AUC increased by 26% and 40%, respectively) in healthy subjects when imatinib was co-administered with a single dose of ketoconazole (a CYP3A4 inhibitor). Caution is recommended when administering imatinib with strong CYP3A4 inhibitors (eg, atazanavir). Substances that inhibit the cytochrome P450 isoenzyme (CYP3A4) activity may decrease metabolism and increase imatinib concentrations).

No products indexed under this heading.

Atomoxetine Hydrochloride (*In vitro*, imatinib inhibits the cytochrome P450 isoenzyme CYP2D6 activity at similar concentrations that affect CYP3A4 activity. Systemic exposure to substrates of CYP2D6 is expected to be increased when co-administered with imatinib. No specific studies have been performed and caution is recommended). Products include:

Strattera 1957

Atorvastatin Calcium (Imatinib increases the mean C_{max} and AUC of simvastatin (CYP3A4 substrate) 2- and 3.5-fold, respectively, suggesting an inhibition of the CYP3A4 by imatinib.

Particular caution is recommended when administering imatinib with CYP3A4 substrates that have a narrow therapeutic window. Imatinib will increase plasma concentration of other CYP3A4 metabolized drugs (eg, certain HMG-CoA reductase inhibitors)). Products include:

Lipitor 2703

Belladonna Ergotamine (Imatinib increases the mean C_{max} and AUC of simvastatin (CYP3A4 substrate) 2- and 3.5-fold, respectively, suggesting an inhibition of the CYP3A4 by imatinib. Particular caution is recommended when administering imatinib with CYP3A4 substrates that have a narrow therapeutic window. Imatinib will increase plasma concentration of other CYP3A4 metabolized drugs).

No products indexed under this heading.

Betamethasone (CYP3A4 inducers may decrease imatinib C_{max} and AUC. The use of concomitant strong CYP3A4 inducers should be avoided. If patients must be co-administered a strong CYP3A4 inducer, based on pharmacokinetic studies, the dosage of imatinib should be increased by at least 50% and clinical response should be carefully monitored).

No products indexed under this heading.

Betamethasone Acetate (CYP3A4 inducers may decrease imatinib C_{max} and AUC. The use of concomitant strong CYP3A4 inducers should be avoided. If patients must be co-administered a strong CYP3A4 inducer, based on pharmacokinetic studies, the dosage of imatinib should be increased by at least 50% and clinical response should be carefully monitored).

No products indexed under this heading.

Betamethasone Benzoate (CYP3A4 inducers may decrease imatinib C_{max} and AUC. The use of concomitant strong CYP3A4 inducers should be avoided. If patients must be co-administered a strong CYP3A4 inducer, based on pharmacokinetic studies, the dosage of imatinib should be increased by at least 50% and clinical response should be carefully monitored).

No products indexed under this heading.

Betamethasone Dipropionate (CYP3A4 inducers may decrease imatinib C_{max} and AUC. The use of concomitant strong CYP3A4 inducers should be avoided. If patients must be co-administered a strong CYP3A4 inducer, based on pharmacokinetic studies, the dosage of imatinib should be increased by at least 50% and clinical response should be carefully monitored). Products include:

Diprolene Lotion 0.05% 3108
Diprolene Ointment 0.05% 3109
Diprolene AF Cream 0.05% 3107
Lotrisone 3163

Betamethasone Sodium Phosphate (CYP3A4 inducers may decrease imatinib C_{max} and AUC. The use of concomitant strong CYP3A4 inducers should be avoided. If patients must be co-administered a strong CYP3A4 inducer, based on pharmacokinetic studies, the dosage of imatinib should be increased by at least 50% and clinical response should be carefully monitored).

No products indexed under this heading.

Betamethasone Valerate (CYP3A4 inducers may decrease imatinib C_{max} and AUC. The use of concomitant strong CYP3A4 inducers should be avoided. If patients must be co-administered a strong CYP3A4 inducer, based on pharmacokinetic studies, the dosage of imatinib should be increased by at least 50% and clinical response should be carefully monitored). Products include:

IMPORTANT NOTE: Always consult each drug listing in the patient's regimen for possible interactions.

specific studies have been performed and caution is recommended). Products include:
Tylenol with Codeine 2691

Codeine Sulfate (*In vitro*, imatinib inhibits the cytochrome P450 isoenzyme CYP2D6 activity at similar concentrations that affect CYP3A4 activity. Systemic exposure to substrates of CYP2D6 is expected to be increased when co-administered with imatinib. No specific studies have been performed and caution is recommended).
No products indexed under this heading.

Conivaptan Hydrochloride (There was a significant increase in exposure to imatinib (mean C_{max} and AUC increased by 26% and 40%, respectively) in healthy subjects when imatinib was co-administered with a single dose of ketoconazole (a CYP3A4 inhibitor). Caution is recommended when administering imatinib with strong CYP3A4 inhibitors. Substances that inhibit the cytochrome P450 isoenzyme (CYP3A4) activity may decrease metabolism and increase imatinib concentrations).
Products include:
Vaprisol 689

Cortisone Acetate (CYP3A4 inducers may decrease imatinib C_{max} and AUC. The use of concomitant strong CYP3A4 inducers should be avoided. If patients must be co-administered a strong CYP3A4 inducer, based on pharmacokinetic studies, the dosage of imatinib should be increased by at least 50% and clinical response should be carefully monitored).
No products indexed under this heading.

Cyclobenzaprine Hydrochloride (*In vitro*, imatinib inhibits the cytochrome P450 isoenzyme CYP2D6 activity at similar concentrations that affect CYP3A4 activity. Systemic exposure to substrates of CYP2D6 is expected to be increased when co-administered with imatinib. No specific studies have been performed and caution is recommended). Products include:
Amrix 964

Cyclophosphamide (When imatinib is combined with chemotherapy, liver toxicity in the form of transaminase elevation and hyperbilirubinemia has been observed. Additionally, there have been reports of acute liver failure. Monitoring of hepatic function is recommended).
No products indexed under this heading.

Cyclosporine (Imatinib increases the mean C_{max} and AUC of simvastatin (CYP3A4 substrate) 2- and 3.5-fold, respectively, suggesting an inhibition of the CYP3A4 by imatinib. Particular caution is recommended when administering imatinib with CYP3A4 substrates that have a narrow therapeutic window (eg, cyclosporine). Imatinib will increase plasma concentration of other CYP3A4 metabolized drugs). Products include:
Gengraf 440
Neoral Oral Solution 2496
Neoral Capsules 2496
Restasis 605

Dacarbazine (When imatinib is combined with chemotherapy, liver toxicity in the form of transaminase elevation and hyperbilirubinemia has been observed. Additionally, there have been reports of acute liver failure. Monitoring of hepatic function is recommended).
No products indexed under this heading.

Dalfopristin (There was a significant increase in exposure to imatinib (mean C_{max} and AUC increased by 26% and 40%, respectively) in healthy subjects when imatinib was co-administered with a single dose of ketoconazole (a CYP3A4 inhibitor). Caution is recommended when administering imatinib with strong CYP3A4 inhibitors. Substances that inhibit the cytochrome P450 isoenzyme (CYP3A4) activity may decrease metabolism and increase imatinib concentrations).
No products indexed under this heading.

Danazol (There was a significant increase in exposure to imatinib (mean C_{max} and AUC increased by 26% and 40%, respectively) in healthy subjects when imatinib was co-administered with a single dose of ketoconazole (a CYP3A4 inhibitor). Caution is recommended when administering imatinib with strong CYP3A4 inhibitors. Substances that inhibit the cytochrome P450 isoenzyme (CYP3A4) activity may decrease metabolism and increase imatinib concentrations).
No products indexed under this heading.

Darunavir (There was a significant increase in exposure to imatinib (mean C_{max} and AUC increased by 26% and 40%, respectively) in healthy subjects when imatinib was co-administered with a single dose of ketoconazole (a CYP3A4 inhibitor). Caution is recommended when administering imatinib with strong CYP3A4 inhibitors. Substances that inhibit the cytochrome P450 isoenzyme (CYP3A4) activity may decrease metabolism and increase imatinib concentrations).
No products indexed under this heading.

Dasatinib (There was a significant increase in exposure to imatinib (mean C_{max} and AUC increased by 26% and 40%, respectively) in healthy subjects when imatinib was co-administered with a single dose of ketoconazole (a CYP3A4 inhibitor). Caution is recommended when administering imatinib with strong CYP3A4 inhibitors. Substances that inhibit the cytochrome P450 isoenzyme (CYP3A4) activity may decrease metabolism and increase imatinib concentrations).
No products indexed under this heading.

Daunorubicin Citrate (When imatinib is combined with chemotherapy, liver toxicity in the form of transaminase elevation and hyperbilirubinemia has been observed. Additionally, there have been reports of acute liver failure. Monitoring of hepatic function is recommended).
No products indexed under this heading.

Daunorubicin Hydrochloride (When imatinib is combined with chemotherapy, liver toxicity in the form of transaminase elevation and hyperbilirubinemia has been observed. Additionally, there have been reports of acute liver failure. Monitoring of hepatic function is recommended).
No products indexed under this heading.

Debrisoquine (*In vitro*, imatinib inhibits the cytochrome P450 isoenzyme CYP2D6 activity at similar concentrations that affect CYP3A4 activity. Systemic exposure to substrates of CYP2D6 is expected to be increased when co-administered with imatinib. No specific studies have been performed and caution is recommended).
No products indexed under this heading.

Delavirdine Mesylate (CYP3A4 inhibitors may increase imatinib C_{max} and AUC. There was a significant increase in exposure to imatinib (mean C_{max} and AUC increased by 26% and 40% respectively) in healthy subjects when imatinib was co-administered with a single dose of ketoconazole (a CYP3A4 inhibitor). Caution is recommended when administering imatinib with strong CYP3A4 inhibitors (eg, ketoconazole, itraconazole). Grapefruit juice may also increase plasma concentrations of imatinib and should be avoided. Substances that inhibit the cytochrome P450 isoenszyme (CYP3A4) activity may decrease metabolism and increase imatinib concentrations).
No products indexed under this heading.

Delavirine (CYP3A4 inhibitors may increase imatinib C_{max} and AUC. There was a significant increase in exposure to imatinib (mean C_{max} and AUC increased by 26% and 40% respectively) in healthy subjects when imatinib was co-administered with a single dose of ketoconazole (a CYP3A4 inhibitor). Caution is recommended when administering imatinib with strong CYP3A4 inhibitors (eg, ketoconazole, itraconazole). Grapefruit juice may also increase plasma concentrations of imatinib and should be avoided. Substances that inhibit the cytochrome P450 isoenszyme (CYP3A4) activity may decrease metabolism and increase imatinib concentrations).
No products indexed under this heading.

Denileukin Diftitox (When imatinib is combined with chemotherapy, liver toxicity in the form of transaminase elevation and hyperbilirubinemia has been observed. Additionally, there have been reports of acute liver failure. Monitoring of hepatic function is recommended). Products include:
Ontak 1068

Desipramine Hydrochloride (*In vitro*, imatinib inhibits the cytochrome P450 isoenzyme CYP2D6 activity at similar concentrations that affect CYP3A4 activity. Systemic exposure to substrates of CYP2D6 is expected to be increased when co-administered with imatinib. No specific studies have been performed and caution is recommended).
No products indexed under this heading.

Desloratadine (There was a significant increase in exposure to imatinib (mean C_{max} and AUC increased by 26% and 40%, respectively) in healthy subjects when imatinib was co-administered with a single dose of ketoconazole (a CYP3A4 inhibitor). Caution is recommended when administering imatinib with strong CYP3A4 inhibitors. Substances that inhibit the cytochrome P450 isoenzyme (CYP3A4) activity may decrease metabolism and increase imatinib concentrations). Products include:
Clarinex Syrup 3098
Clarinex 3098
Clarinex Reditabs 3098
Clarinex-D 12-Hour 3101
Clarinex-D 3104

Desogestrel (Imatinib increases the mean C_{max} and AUC of simvastatin (CYP3A4 substrate) 2- and 3.5-fold, respectively, suggesting an inhibition of the CYP3A4 by imatinib. Particular caution is recommended when administering imatinib with CYP3A4 substrates that have a narrow therapeutic window. Imatinib will increase plasma concentration of other CYP3A4 metabolized drugs).
No products indexed under this heading.

Dexamethasone (CYP3A4 inducers may decrease imatinib C_{max} and AUC. The use of concomitant strong CYP3A4 inducers should be avoided (eg, dexamethasone). If patients must be co-administered a strong CYP3A4 inducer, based on pharmacokinetic studies, the dosage of imatinib should be increased by at least 50%, and clinical response should be carefully monitored).
Products include:
Ciprodex 583
Ozurdex .... ⊙ 223
Tobramycin and Dexamethasone Ophthalmic Suspension .... ⊙ 251

Dexamethasone Acetate (CYP3A4 inducers may decrease imatinib C_{max} and AUC. The use of concomitant strong CYP3A4 inducers should be avoided (eg, dexamethasone). If patients must be co-administered a strong CYP3A4 inducer, based on pharmacokinetic studies, the dosage of imatinib should be increased by at least 50%, and clinical response should be carefully monitored).
No products indexed under this heading.

Dexamethasone Phosphate (CYP3A4 inducers may decrease imatinib C_{max} and AUC. The use of concomitant strong CYP3A4 inducers should be avoided (eg, dexamethasone). If patients must be co-administered a strong CYP3A4 inducer, based on pharmacokinetic studies, the dosage of imatinib should be increased by at least 50%, and clinical response should be carefully monitored).
No products indexed under this heading.

Dexamethasone Sodium (CYP3A4 inducers may decrease imatinib C_{max} and AUC. The use of concomitant strong CYP3A4 inducers should be avoided (eg, dexamethasone). If patients must be co-administered a strong CYP3A4 inducer, based on pharmacokinetic studies, the dosage of imatinib should be increased by at least 50%, and clinical response should be carefully monitored).
No products indexed under this heading.

Dexamethasone Sodium Phosphate (CYP3A4 inducers may decrease imatinib C_{max} and AUC. The use of concomitant strong CYP3A4 inducers should be avoided (eg, dexamethasone). If patients must be co-administered a strong CYP3A4 inducer, based on pharmacokinetic studies, the dosage of imatinib should be increased by at least 50%, and clinical response should be carefully monitored).
No products indexed under this heading.

Dexamethasone Sodium Phosphate Injection (CYP3A4 inducers may decrease imatinib C_{max} and AUC. The use of concomitant strong CYP3A4 inducers should be avoided (eg, dexamethasone). If patients must be co-administered a strong CYP3A4 inducer, based on pharmacokinetic studies, the dosage of imatinib should be increased by at least 50%, and clinical response should be carefully monitored).
No products indexed under this heading.

Dexfenfluramine Hydrochloride (*In vitro*, imatinib inhibits the cytochrome P450 isoenzyme CYP2D6 activity at similar concentrations that affect CYP3A4 activity. Systemic exposure to substrates of CYP2D6 is expected to be increased when co-administered with imatinib. No specific studies have been performed and caution is recommended).
No products indexed under this heading.

Dextromethorphan Hydrobromide (*In vitro*, imatinib inhibits the cytochrome P450 isoenzyme CYP2D6 activity at similar concentrations that affect CYP3A4 activity. Systemic exposure to substrates of CYP2D6 is expected to be increased when co-administered with imatinib. No specific studies have been performed and caution is recommended).
No products indexed under this heading.

Dextromethorphan Polistirex (*In vitro*, imatinib inhibits the cytochrome P450 isoenzyme CYP2D6 activity at similar concentrations that affect CYP3A4 activity. Systemic exposure to substrates of CYP2D6 is expected to be increased when co-administered with imatinib. No specific studies have been performed and caution is recommended).
No products indexed under this heading.

Diazepam (Imatinib increases the mean C_{max} and AUC of simvastatin (CYP3A4 substrate) 2- and 3.5-fold, respectively, suggesting an inhibition of the CYP3A4 by imatinib. Particular caution is recommended when administering imatinib with CYP3A4 substrates that have a narrow therapeutic window. Imatinib will increase plasma concentration of other CYP3A4 metabolized drugs). Products include:
Valium Tablets 2880

Dihydroergotamine Mesylate (Imatinib increases the mean C_{max} and AUC of simvastatin (CYP3A4 substrate) 2- and 3.5-fold, respectively, suggesting an inhibition of the CYP3A4 by imatinib. Particular caution is recommended when administering imatinib with CYP3A4 substrates that have a narrow therapeutic window (eg, dihydroergotamine). Imatinib will increase plasma concentration of other CYP3A4 metabolized drugs).
No products indexed under this heading.

Diltiazem Hydrochloride (Imatinib increases the mean C_{max} and AUC of simvastatin (CYP3A4 substrate) 2- and 3.5-fold, respectively, suggesting an inhibition of the CYP3A4 by imatinib. Particular caution is recommended when administering imatinib with CYP3A4 substrates that have a narrow therapeutic window. Imatinib will increase plasma concentration of other CYP3A4 metabolized drugs (eg, dihydropyridine calcium channel blockers)). Products include:
Cardizem LA 423

Diltiazem Maleate (There was a significant increase in exposure to imatinib (mean C_{max} and AUC increased by 26% and 40%, respectively) in healthy subjects when imatinib was co-administered with a single dose of ketoconazole (a CYP3A4 inhibitor). Caution is recommended when administering imatinib with strong CYP3A4 inhibitors. Substances that inhibit the cytochrome P450 isoenzyme (CYP3A4) activity may decrease metabolism and increase imatinib concentrations).
No products indexed under this heading.

Disopyramide (Imatinib increases the mean C_{max} and AUC of simvastatin (CYP3A4 substrate) 2- and 3.5-fold, respectively, suggesting an inhibition of the CYP3A4 by imatinib. Particular caution is recommended when administering imatinib with CYP3A4 substrates that have a narrow therapeutic window. Imatinib will increase plasma concentration of other CYP3A4 metabolized drugs).
No products indexed under this heading.

Disopyramide Phosphate (Imatinib increases the mean C_{max} and AUC of simvastatin (CYP3A4 substrate) 2- and 3.5-fold, respectively, suggesting an inhibition of the CYP3A4 by imatinib. Particular caution is recommended when administering imatinib with CYP3A4 substrates that have a narrow therapeutic window. Imatinib will increase plasma concentration of other CYP3A4 metabolized drugs).
No products indexed under this heading.

Disulfiram (Imatinib increases the mean C_{max} and AUC of simvastatin (CYP3A4 substrate) 2- and 3.5-fold, respectively, suggesting an inhibition of the CYP3A4 by imatinib. Particular caution is recommended when administering imatinib with CYP3A4 substrates that have a narrow therapeutic window. Imatinib will increase plasma concentration of other CYP3A4 metabolized drugs).
No products indexed under this heading.

Docetaxel (When imatinib is combined with chemotherapy, liver toxicity in the form of transaminase elevation and hyperbilirubinemia has been observed. Additionally, there have been reports of acute liver failure. Monitoring of hepatic function is recommended). Products include:
Taxotere 3035

Dolasetron Mesylate (*In vitro*, imatinib inhibits the cytochrome P450 isoenzyme CYP2D6 activity at similar concentrations that affect CYP3A4 activity. Systemic exposure to substrates of CYP2D6 is expected to be increased when co-administered with imatinib. No specific studies have been performed and caution is recommended). Products include:
Anzemet Injection 2931
Anzemet Tablets 2934

Donepezil Hydrochloride (*In vitro*, imatinib inhibits the cytochrome P450 isoenzyme CYP2D6 activity at similar concentrations that affect CYP3A4 activity. Systemic exposure to substrates of CYP2D6 is expected to be increased when co-administered with imatinib. No specific studies have been performed and caution is recommended). Products include:
Aricept 1045
Aricept ODT 1045

Doxepin Hydrochloride (*In vitro*, imatinib inhibits the cytochrome P450 isoenzyme CYP2D6 activity at similar concentrations that affect CYP3A4 activity. Systemic exposure to substrates of CYP2D6 is expected to be increased when co-administered with imatinib. No specific studies have been performed and caution is recommended).
No products indexed under this heading.

Doxorubicin Hydrochloride (Imatinib increases the mean C_{max} and AUC of simvastatin (CYP3A4 substrate) 2- and 3.5-fold, respectively, suggesting an inhibition of the CYP3A4 by imatinib. Particular caution is recommended when administering imatinib with CYP3A4 substrates that have a narrow therapeutic window. Imatinib will increase plasma concentration of other CYP3A4 metabolized drugs).
No products indexed under this heading.

Dronabinol (Imatinib increases the mean C_{max} and AUC of simvastatin (CYP3A4 substrate) 2- and 3.5-fold, respectively, suggesting an inhibition of the CYP3A4 by imatinib. Particular caution is recommended when administering imatinib with CYP3A4 substrates that have a narrow therapeutic window. Imatinib will increase plasma concentration of other CYP3A4 metabolized drugs).
No products indexed under this heading.

Efavirenz (There was a significant increase in exposure to imatinib (mean C_{max} and AUC increased by 26% and 40%, respectively) in healthy subjects when imatinib was co-administered with a single dose of ketoconazole (a CYP3A4 inhibitor). Caution is recommended when administering imatinib with strong CYP3A4 inhibitors. Substances that inhibit the cytochrome P450 isoenzyme (CYP3A4) activity may decrease metabolism and increase imatinib concentrations). Products include:

Atripla 906

Encainide Hydrochloride (*In vitro*, imatinib inhibits the cytochrome P450 isoenzyme CYP2D6 activity at similar concentrations that affect CYP3A4 activity. Systemic exposure to substrates of CYP2D6 is expected to be increased when co-administered with imatinib. No specific studies have been performed and caution is recommended).
No products indexed under this heading.

Epirubicin Hydrochloride (When imatinib is combined with chemotherapy, liver toxicity in the form of transaminase elevation and hyperbilirubinemia has been observed. Additionally, there have been reports of acute liver failure. Monitoring of hepatic function is recommended).
No products indexed under this heading.

Ergotamine Tartrate (Imatinib increases the mean C_{max} and AUC of simvastatin (CYP3A4 substrate) 2- and 3.5-fold, respectively, suggesting an inhibition of the CYP3A4 by imatinib. Particular caution is recommended when administering imatinib with CYP3A4 substrates that have a narrow therapeutic window (eg, ergotamine). Imatinib will increase plasma concentration of other CYP3A4 metabolized drugs).
No products indexed under this heading.

Erythromycin (There was a significant increase in exposure to imatinib (mean C_{max} and AUC increased by 26% and 40%, respectively) in healthy subjects when imatinib was co-administered with a single dose of ketoconazole (a CYP3A4 inhibitor). Caution is recommended when administering imatinib with strong CYP3A4 inhibitors. Substances that inhibit the cytochrome P450 isoenzyme (CYP3A4) activity may decrease metabolism and increase imatinib concentrations).
No products indexed under this heading.

Erythromycin Estolate (There was a significant increase in exposure to imatinib (mean C_{max} and AUC increased by 26% and 40%, respectively) in healthy subjects when imatinib was co-administered with a single dose of ketoconazole (a CYP3A4 inhibitor). Caution is recommended when administering imatinib with strong CYP3A4 inhibitors. Substances that inhibit the cytochrome P450 isoenzyme (CYP3A4) activity may decrease metabolism and increase imatinib concentrations).
No products indexed under this heading.

Erythromycin Ethylsuccinate (There was a significant increase in exposure to imatinib (mean C_{max} and AUC increased by 26% and 40%, respectively) in healthy subjects when imatinib was co-administered with a single dose of ketoconazole (a CYP3A4 inhibitor). Caution is recommended when administering imatinib with strong CYP3A4 inhibitors. Substances that inhibit the cytochrome P450 isoenzyme (CYP3A4) activity may decrease metabolism and increase imatinib concentrations). Products include:
E.E.S. 437
EryPed 435

Erythromycin Gluceptate (There was a significant increase in exposure to imatinib (mean C_{max} and AUC increased by 26% and 40%, respectively) in healthy subjects when imatinib was co-administered with a single dose of ketoconazole (a CYP3A4 inhibitor). Caution is recommended when administering imatinib with strong CYP3A4 inhibitors. Substances that inhibit the cytochrome P450 isoenzyme (CYP3A4) activity may decrease metabolism and increase imatinib concentrations).
No products indexed under this heading.

Erythromycin Lactobionate (There was a significant increase in exposure to imatinib (mean C_{max} and AUC increased by 26% and 40%, respectively) in healthy subjects when imatinib was co-administered with a single dose of ketoconazole (a CYP3A4 inhibitor). Caution is recommended when administering imatinib with strong CYP3A4 inhibitors. Substances that inhibit the cytochrome P450 isoenzyme (CYP3A4) activity may decrease metabolism and increase imatinib concentrations).
No products indexed under this heading.

Erythromycin Stearate (There was a significant increase in exposure to imatinib (mean C_{max} and AUC increased by 26% and 40%, respectively) in healthy subjects when imatinib was co-administered with a single dose of ketoconazole (a CYP3A4 inhibitor). Caution is recommended when administering imatinib with strong CYP3A4 inhibitors. Substances that inhibit the cytochrome P450 isoenzyme (CYP3A4) activity may decrease metabolism and increase imatinib concentrations).
No products indexed under this heading.

Esomeprazole Magnesium (There was a significant increase in exposure to imatinib (mean C_{max} and AUC increased by 26% and 40%, respectively) in healthy subjects when imatinib was co-administered with a single dose of ketoconazole (a CYP3A4 inhibitor). Caution is recommended when administering imatinib with strong CYP3A4 inhibitors. Substances that inhibit the cytochrome P450 isoenzyme (CYP3A4) activity may decrease metabolism and increase imatinib concentrations). Products include:
Nexium Capsules 704
Nexium Oral Suspension 704

Esomeprazole Sodium (There was a significant increase in exposure to imatinib (mean C_{max} and AUC increased by 26% and 40%, respectively) in healthy subjects when imatinib was co-administered with a single dose of ketoconazole (a CYP3A4 inhibitor). Caution is recommended when administering imatinib with strong CYP3A4 inhibitors. Substances that inhibit the cytochrome P450 isoenzyme (CYP3A4) activity may decrease metabolism and increase imatinib concentrations). Products include:
Nexium I.V. 712

Estradiol (Imatinib increases the mean C_{max} and AUC of simvastatin (CYP3A4 substrate) 2- and 3.5-fold, respectively, suggesting an inhibition of the CYP3A4 by imatinib. Particular caution is recommended when administering imatinib with CYP3A4 substrates that have a narrow therapeutic window. Imatinib will increase plasma concentration of other CYP3A4 metabolized drugs). Products include:
Activella 2561
Angeliq 831
Climara 841
Climara Pro 847
Divigel 3467
Estrasorb 1777
Vagifem 2589

Estradiol Benzoate (Imatinib increases the mean C_{max} and AUC of simvastatin (CYP3A4 substrate) 2- and 3.5-fold, respectively, suggesting an inhibition of the CYP3A4 by imatinib. Particular caution is recommended when administering imatinib with CYP3A4 substrates that have a narrow therapeutic window. Imatinib will increase plasma concentration of other CYP3A4 metabolized drugs).
No products indexed under this heading.

Estradiol Cypionate (Imatinib increases the mean C_{max} and AUC of simvastatin (CYP3A4 substrate) 2- and 3.5-fold, respectively, suggesting an inhibition of the CYP3A4 by imatinib.

IMPORTANT NOTE: Always consult each drug listing in the patient's regimen for possible interactions.

Particular caution is recommended when administering imatinib with CYP3A4 substrates that have a narrow therapeutic window. Imatinib will increase plasma concentration of other CYP3A4 metabolized drugs).
No products indexed under this heading.

Estradiol Valerate (Imatinib increases the mean C_{max} and AUC of simvastatin (CYP3A4 substrate) 2- and 3.5-fold, respectively, suggesting an inhibition of the CYP3A4 by imatinib. Particular caution is recommended when administering imatinib with CYP3A4 substrates that have a narrow therapeutic window. Imatinib will increase plasma concentration of other CYP3A4 metabolized drugs).
No products indexed under this heading.

Estramustine Phosphate Sodium (When imatinib is combined with chemotherapy, liver toxicity in the form of transaminase elevation and hyperbilirubinemia has been observed. Additionally, there have been reports of acute liver failure. Monitoring of hepatic function is recommended).
No products indexed under this heading.

Ethinyl Estradiol (Imatinib increases the mean C_{max} and AUC of simvastatin (CYP3A4 substrate) 2- and 3.5-fold, respectively, suggesting an inhibition of the CYP3A4 by imatinib. Particular caution is recommended when administering imatinib with CYP3A4 substrates that have a narrow therapeutic window. Imatinib will increase plasma concentration of other CYP3A4 metabolized drugs). Products include:
LoSeasonique 3407
Lybrel 3514
NuvaRing 3181
Ortho Evra 2648
Ortho-Cyclen/Ortho Tri-Cyclen 2663
Ortho Tri-Cyclen Lo Tablets 2673
Seasonique 3418
Yaz 864

Ethosuximide (Imatinib increases the mean C_{max} and AUC of simvastatin (CYP3A4 substrate) 2- and 3.5-fold, respectively, suggesting an inhibition of the CYP3A4 by imatinib. Particular caution is recommended when administering imatinib with CYP3A4 substrates that have a narrow therapeutic window. Imatinib will increase plasma concentration of other CYP3A4 metabolized drugs).
No products indexed under this heading.

Ethynodiol Diacetate (Imatinib increases the mean C_{max} and AUC of simvastatin (CYP3A4 substrate) 2- and 3.5-fold, respectively, suggesting an inhibition of the CYP3A4 by imatinib. Particular caution is recommended when administering imatinib with CYP3A4 substrates that have a narrow therapeutic window. Imatinib will increase plasma concentration of other CYP3A4 metabolized drugs).
No products indexed under this heading.

Etoposide (Imatinib increases the mean C_{max} and AUC of simvastatin (CYP3A4 substrate) 2- and 3.5-fold, respectively, suggesting an inhibition of the CYP3A4 by imatinib. Particular caution is recommended when administering imatinib with CYP3A4 substrates that have a narrow therapeutic window. Imatinib will increase plasma concentration of other CYP3A4 metabolized drugs).
No products indexed under this heading.

Etoposide Phosphate (Imatinib increases the mean C_{max} and AUC of simvastatin (CYP3A4 substrate) 2- and 3.5-fold, respectively, suggesting an inhibition of the CYP3A4 by imatinib. Particular caution is recommended when administering imatinib with CYP3A4 substrates that have a narrow therapeutic window. Imatinib will increase plasma concentration of other CYP3A4 metabolized drugs).
No products indexed under this heading.

Exemestane (When imatinib is combined with chemotherapy, liver toxicity in the form of transaminase elevation and hyperbilirubinemia has been observed. Additionally, there have been reports of acute liver failure. Monitoring of hepatic function is recommended). Products include:
Aromasin 2758

Felbamate (CYP3A4 inducers may decrease imatinib C_{max} and AUC. The use of concomitant strong CYP3A4 inducers should be avoided. If patients must be co-administered a strong CYP3A4 inducer, based on pharmacokinetic studies, the dosage of imatinib should be increased by at least 50% and clinical response should be carefully monitored).
No products indexed under this heading.

Felodipine (Imatinib increases the mean C_{max} and AUC of simvastatin (CYP3A4 substrate) 2- and 3.5-fold, respectively, suggesting an inhibition of the CYP3A4 by imatinib. Particular caution is recommended when administering imatinib with CYP3A4 substrates that have a narrow therapeutic window. Imatinib will increase plasma concentration of other CYP3A4 metabolized drugs (eg, dihydropyridine calcium channel blockers)).
No products indexed under this heading.

Fentanyl (Imatinib increases the mean C_{max} and AUC of simvastatin (CYP3A4 substrate) 2- and 3.5-fold, respectively, suggesting an inhibition of the CYP3A4 by imatinib. Particular caution is recommended when administering imatinib with CYP3A4 substrates that have a narrow therapeutic window (eg, fentanyl). Imatinib will increase plasma concentration of other CYP3A4 metabolized drugs). Products include:
Duragesic 2604
Fentanyl Transdermal System 2346
Onsolis 2054

Fentanyl Citrate (Imatinib increases the mean C_{max} and AUC of simvastatin (CYP3A4 substrate) 2- and 3.5-fold, respectively, suggesting an inhibition of the CYP3A4 by imatinib. Particular caution is recommended when administering imatinib with CYP3A4 substrates that have a narrow therapeutic window (eg, fentanyl). Imatinib will increase plasma concentration of other CYP3A4 metabolized drugs). Products include:
Fentora 966

Flecainide Acetate (*In vitro*, imatinib inhibits the cytochrome P450 isoenzyme CYP2D6 activity at similar concentrations that affect CYP3A4 activity. Systemic exposure to substrates of CYP2D6 is expected to be increased when co-administered with imatinib. No specific studies have been performed and caution is recommended).
No products indexed under this heading.

Floxuridine (When imatinib is combined with chemotherapy, liver toxicity in the form of transaminase elevation and hyperbilirubinemia has been observed. Additionally, there have been reports of acute liver failure. Monitoring of hepatic function is recommended).
No products indexed under this heading.

Fluconazole (There was a significant increase in exposure to imatinib (mean C_{max} and AUC increased by 26% and 40%, respectively) in healthy subjects when imatinib was co-administered with a single dose of ketoconazole (a CYP3A4 inhibitor). Caution is recommended when administering imatinib with strong CYP3A4 inhibitors. Substances that inhibit the cytochrome P450 isoenzyme (CYP3A4) activity may decrease metabolism and increase imatinib concentrations).
No products indexed under this heading.

Fludrocortisone Acetate (CYP3A4 inducers may decrease imatinib C_{max} and AUC. The use of concomitant strong CYP3A4 inducers should be avoided. If patients must be co-administered a strong CYP3A4 inducer, based on pharmacokinetic studies, the dosage of imatinib should be increased by at least 50% and clinical response should be carefully monitored).
No products indexed under this heading.

Fluorouracil (When imatinib is combined with chemotherapy, liver toxicity in the form of transaminase elevation and hyperbilirubinemia has been observed. Additionally, there have been reports of acute liver failure. Monitoring of hepatic function is recommended). Products include:
Carac 2966

Fluoxetine (There was a significant increase in exposure to imatinib (mean C_{max} and AUC increased by 26% and 40%, respectively) in healthy subjects when imatinib was co-administered with a single dose of ketoconazole (a CYP3A4 inhibitor). Caution is recommended when administering imatinib with strong CYP3A4 inhibitors. Substances that inhibit the cytochrome P450 isoenzyme (CYP3A4) activity may decrease metabolism and increase imatinib concentrations).
No products indexed under this heading.

Fluoxetine Hydrochloride (There was a significant increase in exposure to imatinib (mean C_{max} and AUC increased by 26% and 40%, respectively) in healthy subjects when imatinib was co-administered with a single dose of ketoconazole (a CYP3A4 inhibitor). Caution is recommended when administering imatinib with strong CYP3A4 inhibitors. Substances that inhibit the cytochrome P450 isoenzyme (CYP3A4) activity may decrease metabolism and increase imatinib concentrations). Products include:
Prozac Weekly 1941
Prozac Pulvules 1941
Symbyax 1965

Fluphenazine Decanoate (*In vitro*, imatinib inhibits the cytochrome P450 isoenzyme CYP2D6 activity at similar concentrations that affect CYP3A4 activity. Systemic exposure to substrates of CYP2D6 is expected to be increased when co-administered with imatinib. No specific studies have been performed and caution is recommended).
No products indexed under this heading.

Fluphenazine Enanthate (*In vitro*, imatinib inhibits the cytochrome P450 isoenzyme CYP2D6 activity at similar concentrations that affect CYP3A4 activity. Systemic exposure to substrates of CYP2D6 is expected to be increased when co-administered with imatinib. No specific studies have been performed and caution is recommended).
No products indexed under this heading.

Fluphenazine Hydrochloride (*In vitro*, imatinib inhibits the cytochrome P450 isoenzyme CYP2D6 activity at similar concentrations that affect CYP3A4 activity. Systemic exposure to substrates of CYP2D6 is expected to be increased when co-administered with imatinib. No specific studies have been performed and caution is recommended).
No products indexed under this heading.

Flutamide (When imatinib is combined with chemotherapy, liver toxicity in the form of transaminase elevation and hyperbilirubinemia has been observed. Additionally, there have been reports of acute liver failure. Monitoring of hepatic function is recommended).
No products indexed under this heading.

Fluvoxamine Maleate (There was a significant increase in exposure to imatinib (mean C_{max} and AUC increased by 26% and 40%, respectively) in healthy subjects when imatinib was co-administered with a single dose of ketoconazole (a CYP3A4 inhibitor). Caution is recommended when administering imatinib with strong CYP3A4 inhibitors. Substances that inhibit the cytochrome P450 isoenzyme (CYP3A4) activity may decrease metabolism and increase imatinib concentrations).
No products indexed under this heading.

Formoterol Fumarate (*In vitro*, imatinib inhibits the cytochrome P450 isoenzyme CYP2D6 activity at similar concentrations that affect CYP3A4 activity. Systemic exposure to substrates of CYP2D6 is expected to be increased when co-administered with imatinib. No specific studies have been performed and caution is recommended). Products include:
Foradil 3121
Perforomist 3634

Fosamprenavir Calcium (CYP3A4 inhibitors may increase imatinib C_{max} and AUC. There was a significant increase in exposure to imatinib (mean C_{max} and AUC increased by 26% and 40% respectively) in healthy subjects when imatinib was co-administered with a single dose of ketoconazole (a CYP3A4 inhibitor). Caution is recommended when administering imatinib with strong CYP3A4 inhibitors (eg, ketoconazole, itraconazole). Grapefruit juice may also increase plasma concentrations of imatinib and should be avoided. Substances that inhibit the cytochrome P450 isoenzyme (CYP3A4) activity may decrease metabolism and increase imatinib concentrations). Products include:
Lexiva Oral Suspension 1558
Lexiva 1558

Fosphenytoin (CYP3A4 inducers may decrease imatinib C_{max} and AUC. The use of concomitant strong CYP3A4 inducers should be avoided (eg, phenytoin). If patients must be co-administered a strong CYP3A4 inducer, based on pharmacokinetic studies, the dosage of imatinib should be increased by at least 50%, and clinical response should be carefully monitored).
No products indexed under this heading.

Fosphenytoin Sodium (CYP3A4 inducers may decrease imatinib C_{max} and AUC. The use of concomitant strong CYP3A4 inducers should be avoided (eg, phenytoin). If patients must be co-administered a strong CYP3A4 inducer, based on pharmacokinetic studies, the dosage of imatinib should be increased by at least 50%, and clinical response should be carefully monitored).
No products indexed under this heading.

Galantamine Hydrobromide (*In vitro*, imatinib inhibits the cytochrome P450 isoenzyme CYP2D6 activity at similar concentrations that affect CYP3A4 activity. Systemic exposure to substrates of CYP2D6 is expected to be increased when co-administered with imatinib. No specific studies have been performed and caution is recommended).
No products indexed under this heading.

781 Interactions Index Gleevec

Garlic Extract (CYP3A4 inducers may decrease imatinib C_{max} and AUC. The use of concomitant strong CYP3A4 inducers should be avoided. If patients must be co-administered a strong CYP3A4 inducer, based on pharmacokinetic studies, the dosage of imatinib should be increased by at least 50% and clinical response should be carefully monitored).
No products indexed under this heading.

Garlic Oil (CYP3A4 inducers may decrease imatinib C_{max} and AUC. The use of concomitant strong CYP3A4 inducers should be avoided. If patients must be co-administered a strong CYP3A4 inducer, based on pharmacokinetic studies, the dosage of imatinib should be increased by at least 50% and clinical response should be carefully monitored).
No products indexed under this heading.

Gemcitabine Hydrochloride (When imatinib is combined with chemotherapy, liver toxicity in the form of transaminase elevation and hyperbilirubinemia has been observed. Additionally, there have been reports of acute liver failure. Monitoring of hepatic function is recommended). Products include:
Gemzar 1900

Haloperidol (Imatinib increases the mean C_{max} and AUC of simvastatin (CYP3A4 substrate) 2- and 3.5-fold, respectively, suggesting an inhibition of the CYP3A4 by imatinib. Particular caution is recommended when administering imatinib with CYP3A4 substrates that have a narrow therapeutic window. Imatinib will increase plasma concentration of other CYP3A4 metabolized drugs).
No products indexed under this heading.

Haloperidol Decanoate (Imatinib increases the mean C_{max} and AUC of simvastatin (CYP3A4 substrate) 2- and 3.5-fold, respectively, suggesting an inhibition of the CYP3A4 by imatinib. Particular caution is recommended when administering imatinib with CYP3A4 substrates that have a narrow therapeutic window. Imatinib will increase plasma concentration of other CYP3A4 metabolized drugs).
No products indexed under this heading.

Haloperidol Lactate (Imatinib increases the mean C_{max} and AUC of simvastatin (CYP3A4 substrate) 2- and 3.5-fold, respectively, suggesting an inhibition of the CYP3A4 by imatinib. Particular caution is recommended when administering imatinib with CYP3A4 substrates that have a narrow therapeutic window. Imatinib will increase plasma concentration of other CYP3A4 metabolized drugs).
No products indexed under this heading.

Hydrocodone Bitartrate (*In vitro*, imatinib inhibits the cytochrome P450 isoenzyme CYP2D6 activity at similar concentrations that affect CYP3A4 activity. Systemic exposure to substrates of CYP2D6 is expected to be increased when co-administered with imatinib. No specific studies have been performed and caution is recommended). Products include:
Vicodin 560
Vicodin ES 561
Vicodin HP 563
Vicoprofen 564
Zydone 1138

Hydrocortisone (CYP3A4 inducers may decrease imatinib C_{max} and AUC. The use of concomitant strong CYP3A4 inducers should be avoided. If patients must be co-administered a strong CYP3A4 inducer, based on pharmacokinetic studies, the dosage of imatinib should be increased by at least 50% and clinical response should be carefully monitored).
No products indexed under this heading.

Hydrocortisone (Alcohol) (CYP3A4 inducers may decrease imatinib C_{max} and AUC. The use of concomitant strong CYP3A4 inducers should be avoided. If patients must be co-administered a strong CYP3A4 inducer, based on pharmacokinetic studies, the dosage of imatinib should be increased by at least 50% and clinical response should be carefully monitored).
No products indexed under this heading.

Hydrocortisone Acetate (CYP3A4 inducers may decrease imatinib C_{max} and AUC. The use of concomitant strong CYP3A4 inducers should be avoided. If patients must be co-administered a strong CYP3A4 inducer, based on pharmacokinetic studies, the dosage of imatinib should be increased by at least 50% and clinical response should be carefully monitored).
No products indexed under this heading.

Hydrocortisone Butyrate (CYP3A4 inducers may decrease imatinib C_{max} and AUC. The use of concomitant strong CYP3A4 inducers should be avoided. If patients must be co-administered a strong CYP3A4 inducer, based on pharmacokinetic studies, the dosage of imatinib should be increased by at least 50% and clinical response should be carefully monitored).
No products indexed under this heading.

Hydrocortisone Cypionate (CYP3A4 inducers may decrease imatinib C_{max} and AUC. The use of concomitant strong CYP3A4 inducers should be avoided. If patients must be co-administered a strong CYP3A4 inducer, based on pharmacokinetic studies, the dosage of imatinib should be increased by at least 50% and clinical response should be carefully monitored).
No products indexed under this heading.

Hydrocortisone Hemisuccinate (CYP3A4 inducers may decrease imatinib C_{max} and AUC. The use of concomitant strong CYP3A4 inducers should be avoided. If patients must be co-administered a strong CYP3A4 inducer, based on pharmacokinetic studies, the dosage of imatinib should be increased by at least 50% and clinical response should be carefully monitored).
No products indexed under this heading.

Hydrocortisone Probutate (CYP3A4 inducers may decrease imatinib C_{max} and AUC. The use of concomitant strong CYP3A4 inducers should be avoided. If patients must be co-administered a strong CYP3A4 inducer, based on pharmacokinetic studies, the dosage of imatinib should be increased by at least 50% and clinical response should be carefully monitored).
No products indexed under this heading.

Hydrocortisone Sodium Phosphate (CYP3A4 inducers may decrease imatinib C_{max} and AUC. The use of concomitant strong CYP3A4 inducers should be avoided. If patients must be co-administered a strong CYP3A4 inducer, based on pharmacokinetic studies, the dosage of imatinib should be increased by at least 50% and clinical response should be carefully monitored).
No products indexed under this heading.

Hydrocortisone Sodium Succinate (CYP3A4 inducers may decrease imatinib C_{max} and AUC. The use of concomitant strong CYP3A4 inducers should be avoided. If patients must be co-administered a strong CYP3A4 inducer, based on pharmacokinetic studies, the dosage of imatinib should be increased by at least 50% and clinical response should be carefully monitored).
No products indexed under this heading.

Hydrocortisone Valerate (CYP3A4 inducers may decrease imatinib C_{max} and AUC. The use of concomitant strong CYP3A4 inducers should be avoided. If patients must be co-administered a strong CYP3A4 inducer, based on pharmacokinetic studies, the dosage of imatinib should be increased by at least 50% and clinical response should be carefully monitored).
No products indexed under this heading.

Hydroxyurea (When imatinib is combined with chemotherapy, liver toxicity in the form of transaminase elevation and hyperbilirubinemia has been observed. Additionally, there have been reports of acute liver failure. Monitoring of hepatic function is recommended).
No products indexed under this heading.

Hypericum (CYP3A4 inducers may decrease imatinib C_{max} and AUC. The use of concomitant strong CYP3A4 inducers should be avoided. If patients must be co-administered a strong CYP3A4 inducer, based on pharmacokinetic studies, the dosage of imatinib should be increased by at least 50% and clinical response should be carefully monitored).
No products indexed under this heading.

Hypericum Perforatum (CYP3A4 inducers may decrease imatinib C_{max} and AUC. The use of concomitant strong CYP3A4 inducers should be avoided. If patients must be co-administered a strong CYP3A4 inducer, based on pharmacokinetic studies, the dosage of imatinib should be increased by at least 50% and clinical response should be carefully monitored). Products include:
Traumeel 1800

Idarubicin Hydrochloride (When imatinib is combined with chemotherapy, liver toxicity in the form of transaminase elevation and hyperbilirubinemia has been observed. Additionally, there have been reports of acute liver failure. Monitoring of hepatic function is recommended).
No products indexed under this heading.

Ifosfamide (When imatinib is combined with chemotherapy, liver toxicity in the form of transaminase elevation and hyperbilirubinemia has been observed. Additionally, there have been reports of acute liver failure. Monitoring of hepatic function is recommended).
No products indexed under this heading.

Imipramine Hydrochloride (*In vitro*, imatinib inhibits the cytochrome P450 isoenzyme CYP2D6 activity at similar concentrations that affect CYP3A4 activity. Systemic exposure to substrates of CYP2D6 is expected to be increased when co-administered with imatinib. No specific studies have been performed and caution is recommended).
No products indexed under this heading.

Imipramine Pamoate (*In vitro*, imatinib inhibits the cytochrome P450 isoenzyme CYP2D6 activity at similar concentrations that affect CYP3A4 activity. Systemic exposure to substrates of CYP2D6 is expected to be increased when co-administered with imatinib. No specific studies have been performed and caution is recommended).
No products indexed under this heading.

Indinavir Sulfate (There was a significant increase in exposure to imatinib (mean C_{max} and AUC increased by 26% and 40%, respectively) in healthy subjects when imatinib was co-administered with a single dose of ketoconazole (a CYP3A4 inhibitor). Caution is recommended when administering imatinib with strong CYP3A4 inhibitors (eg, indinavir). Substances that inhibit the cytochrome P450 isoenzyme (CYP3A4) activity may decrease metabolism and increase imatinib concentrations). Products include:
Crixivan 2113

Indoramin Hydrochloride (*In vitro*, imatinib inhibits the cytochrome P450 isoenzyme CYP2D6 activity at similar concentrations that affect CYP3A4 activity. Systemic exposure to substrates of CYP2D6 is expected to be increased when co-administered with imatinib. No specific studies have been performed and caution is recommended).
No products indexed under this heading.

Interferon alfa-2a, Recombinant (When imatinib is combined with chemotherapy, liver toxicity in the form of transaminase elevation and hyperbilirubinemia has been observed. Additionally, there have been reports of acute liver failure. Monitoring of hepatic function is recommended).
No products indexed under this heading.

Interferon alfa-2b, Recombinant (When imatinib is combined with chemotherapy, liver toxicity in the form of transaminase elevation and hyperbilirubinemia has been observed. Additionally, there have been reports of acute liver failure. Monitoring of hepatic function is recommended). Products include:
Intron A 3140

Irinotecan Hydrochloride (When imatinib is combined with chemotherapy, liver toxicity in the form of transaminase elevation and hyperbilirubinemia has been observed. Additionally, there have been reports of acute liver failure. Monitoring of hepatic function is recommended).
No products indexed under this heading.

Isoniazid (There was a significant increase in exposure to imatinib (mean C_{max} and AUC increased by 26% and 40%, respectively) in healthy subjects when imatinib was co-administered with a single dose of ketoconazole (a CYP3A4 inhibitor). Caution is recommended when administering imatinib with strong CYP3A4 inhibitors. Substances that inhibit the cytochrome P450 isoenzyme (CYP3A4) activity may decrease metabolism and increase imatinib concentrations).
No products indexed under this heading.

Isradipine (Imatinib increases the mean C_{max} and AUC of simvastatin (CYP3A4 substrate) 2- and 3.5-fold, respectively, suggesting an inhibition of the CYP3A4 by imatinib. Particular caution is recommended when administering imatinib with CYP3A4 substrates that have a narrow therapeutic window. Imatinib will increase plasma concentration of other CYP3A4 metabolized drugs). Products include:
DynaCirc CR 1432

Itraconazole (There was a significant increase in exposure to imatinib (mean C_{max} and AUC increased by 26% and 40%, respectively) in healthy subjects when imatinib was co-administered with a single dose of ketoconazole (a CYP3A4 inhibitor). Caution is recommended when administering imatinib with strong CYP3A4 inhibitors (eg, itraconazole). Substances that inhibit the cytochrome P450 isoenzyme (CYP3A4) activity may decrease metabolism and increase imatinib concentrations).
No products indexed under this heading.

IMPORTANT NOTE: Always consult each drug listing in the patient's regimen for possible interactions.

Ixabepilone (Imatinib increases the mean C_{max} and AUC of simvastatin (CYP3A4 substrate) 2- and 3.5-fold, respectively, suggesting an inhibition of the CYP3A4 by imatinib. Particular caution is recommended when administering imatinib with CYP3A4 substrates that have a narrow therapeutic window. Imatinib will increase plasma concentration of other CYP3A4 metabolized drugs).
No products indexed under this heading.

Ketoconazole (There was a significant increase in exposure to imatinib (mean C_{max} and AUC increased by 26% and 40%, respectively) in healthy subjects when imatinib was co-administered with a single dose of ketoconazole (a CYP3A4 inhibitor). Caution is recommended when administering imatinib with strong CYP3A4 inhibitors (eg, ketoconazole). Substances that inhibit the cytochrome P450 isoenzyme (CYP3A4) activity may decrease metabolism and increase imatinib concentrations). Products include:
Extina 3319
Xolegel 3337

Labetalol Hydrochloride (*In vitro*, imatinib inhibits the cytochrome P450 isoenzyme CYP2D6 activity at similar concentrations that affect CYP3A4 activity. Systemic exposure to substrates of CYP2D6 is expected to be increased when co-administered with imatinib. No specific studies have been performed and caution is recommended).
No products indexed under this heading.

Lapatinib (There was a significant increase in exposure to imatinib (mean C_{max} and AUC increased by 26% and 40%, respectively) in healthy subjects when imatinib was co-administered with a single dose of ketoconazole (a CYP3A4 inhibitor). Caution is recommended when administering imatinib with strong CYP3A4 inhibitors. Substances that inhibit the cytochrome P450 isoenzyme (CYP3A4) activity may decrease metabolism and increase imatinib concentrations). Products include:
Tykerb 1698

Levamisole Hydrochloride (When imatinib is combined with chemotherapy, liver toxicity in the form of transaminase elevation and hyperbilirubinemia has been observed. Additionally, there have been reports of acute liver failure. Monitoring of hepatic function is recommended).
No products indexed under this heading.

Levonorgestrel (Imatinib increases the mean C_{max} and AUC of simvastatin (CYP3A4 substrate) 2- and 3.5-fold, respectively, suggesting an inhibition of the CYP3A4 by imatinib. Particular caution is recommended when administering imatinib with CYP3A4 substrates that have a narrow therapeutic window. Imatinib will increase plasma concentration of other CYP3A4 metabolized drugs). Products include:
Climara Pro 847
LoSeasonique 3407
Lybrel 3514
Mirena 854
Plan B 3416
Seasonique 3418

Lidocaine (Imatinib increases the mean C_{max} and AUC of simvastatin (CYP3A4 substrate) 2- and 3.5-fold, respectively, suggesting an inhibition of the CYP3A4 by imatinib. Particular caution is recommended when administering imatinib with CYP3A4 substrates that have a narrow therapeutic window. Imatinib will increase plasma concentration of other CYP3A4 metabolized drugs). Products include:
Lidoderm 1107

Lidocaine Hydrochloride (Imatinib increases the mean C_{max} and AUC of simvastatin (CYP3A4 substrate) 2- and 3.5-fold, respectively, suggesting an inhibition of the CYP3A4 by imatinib. Particular caution is recommended when administering imatinib with CYP3A4 substrates that have a narrow therapeutic window. Imatinib will increase plasma concentration of other CYP3A4 metabolized drugs).
No products indexed under this heading.

Lomustine (CCNU) (When imatinib is combined with chemotherapy, liver toxicity in the form of transaminase elevation and hyperbilirubinemia has been observed. Additionally, there have been reports of acute liver failure. Monitoring of hepatic function is recommended).
No products indexed under this heading.

Lopinavir (CYP3A4 inhibitors may increase imatinib C_{max} and AUC. There was a significant increase in exposure to imatinib (mean C_{max} and AUC increased by 26% and 40% respectively) in healthy subjects when imatinib was co-administered with a single dose of ketoconazole (a CYP3A4 inhibitor). Caution is recommended when administering imatinib with strong CYP3A4 inhibitors (eg, ketoconazole, itraconazole). Grapefruit juice may also increase plasma concentrations of imatinib and should be avoided. Substances that inhibit the cytochrome P450 isoenszyme (CYP3A4) activity may decrease metabolism and increase imatinib concentrations). Products include:
Kaletra 458

Loratadine (There was a significant increase in exposure to imatinib (mean C_{max} and AUC increased by 26% and 40%, respectively) in healthy subjects when imatinib was co-administered with a single dose of ketoconazole (a CYP3A4 inhibitor). Caution is recommended when administering imatinib with strong CYP3A4 inhibitors. Substances that inhibit the cytochrome P450 isoenzyme (CYP3A4) activity may decrease metabolism and increase imatinib concentrations).
No products indexed under this heading.

Lovastatin (Imatinib increases the mean C_{max} and AUC of simvastatin (CYP3A4 substrate) 2- and 3.5-fold, respectively, suggesting an inhibition of the CYP3A4 by imatinib. Particular caution is recommended when administering imatinib with CYP3A4 substrates that have a narrow therapeutic window. Imatinib will increase plasma concentration of other CYP3A4 metabolized drugs (eg, certain HMG-CoA reductase inhibitors)). Products include:
Advicor 402
Mevacor 2212

Maprotiline Hydrochloride (*In vitro*, imatinib inhibits the cytochrome P450 isoenzyme CYP2D6 activity at similar concentrations that affect CYP3A4 activity. Systemic exposure to substrates of CYP2D6 is expected to be increased when co-administered with imatinib. No specific studies have been performed and caution is recommended).
No products indexed under this heading.

Mechlorethamine Hydrochloride (When imatinib is combined with chemotherapy, liver toxicity in the form of transaminase elevation and hyperbilirubinemia has been observed. Additionally, there have been reports of acute liver failure. Monitoring of hepatic function is recommended). Products include:
Mustargen 2010

Megestrol Acetate (When imatinib is combined with chemotherapy, liver toxicity in the form of transaminase elevation and hyperbilirubinemia has been observed. Additionally, there have been reports of acute liver failure. Monitoring of hepatic function is recommended). Products include:
Megace ES 2698

Melphalan (When imatinib is combined with chemotherapy, liver toxicity in the form of transaminase elevation and hyperbilirubinemia has been observed. Additionally, there have been reports of acute liver failure. Monitoring of hepatic function is recommended). Products include:
Alkeran 1302

Meperidine Hydrochloride (*In vitro*, imatinib inhibits the cytochrome P450 isoenzyme CYP2D6 activity at similar concentrations that affect CYP3A4 activity. Systemic exposure to substrates of CYP2D6 is expected to be increased when co-administered with imatinib. No specific studies have been performed and caution is recommended).
No products indexed under this heading.

Mephenytoin (CYP3A4 inducers may decrease imatinib C_{max} and AUC. The use of concomitant strong CYP3A4 inducers should be avoided. If patients must be co-administered a strong CYP3A4 inducer, based on pharmacokinetic studies, the dosage of imatinib should be increased by at least 50% and clinical response should be carefully monitored).
No products indexed under this heading.

Mercaptopurine (When imatinib is combined with chemotherapy, liver toxicity in the form of transaminase elevation and hyperbilirubinemia has been observed. Additionally, there have been reports of acute liver failure. Monitoring of hepatic function is recommended).
No products indexed under this heading.

Mestranol (Imatinib increases the mean C_{max} and AUC of simvastatin (CYP3A4 substrate) 2- and 3.5-fold, respectively, suggesting an inhibition of the CYP3A4 by imatinib. Particular caution is recommended when administering imatinib with CYP3A4 substrates that have a narrow therapeutic window. Imatinib will increase plasma concentration of other CYP3A4 metabolized drugs).
No products indexed under this heading.

Methadone Hydrochloride (Imatinib increases the mean C_{max} and AUC of simvastatin (CYP3A4 substrate) 2- and 3.5-fold, respectively, suggesting an inhibition of the CYP3A4 by imatinib. Particular caution is recommended when administering imatinib with CYP3A4 substrates that have a narrow therapeutic window. Imatinib will increase plasma concentration of other CYP3A4 metabolized drugs).
No products indexed under this heading.

Methamphetamine Hydrochloride (*In vitro*, imatinib inhibits the cytochrome P450 isoenzyme CYP2D6 activity at similar concentrations that affect CYP3A4 activity. Systemic exposure to substrates of CYP2D6 is expected to be increased when co-administered with imatinib. No specific studies have been performed and caution is recommended).
No products indexed under this heading.

Methotrexate (When imatinib is combined with chemotherapy, liver toxicity in the form of transaminase elevation and hyperbilirubinemia has been observed. Additionally, there have been reports of acute liver failure. Monitoring of hepatic function is recommended).
No products indexed under this heading.

Methotrexate Sodium (When imatinib is combined with chemotherapy, liver toxicity in the form of transaminase elevation and hyperbilirubinemia has been observed. Additionally, there have been reports of acute liver failure. Monitoring of hepatic function is recommended).
No products indexed under this heading.

Methoxyphenamine (*In vitro*, imatinib inhibits the cytochrome P450 isoenzyme CYP2D6 activity at similar concentrations that affect CYP3A4 activity. Systemic exposure to substrates of CYP2D6 is expected to be increased when co-administered with imatinib. No specific studies have been performed and caution is recommended).
No products indexed under this heading.

Methsuximide (CYP3A4 inducers may decrease imatinib C_{max} and AUC. The use of concomitant strong CYP3A4 inducers should be avoided. If patients must be co-administered a strong CYP3A4 inducer, based on pharmacokinetic studies, the dosage of imatinib should be increased by at least 50% and clinical response should be carefully monitored).
No products indexed under this heading.

Methylprednisolone (CYP3A4 inducers may decrease imatinib C_{max} and AUC. The use of concomitant strong CYP3A4 inducers should be avoided. If patients must be co-administered a strong CYP3A4 inducer, based on pharmacokinetic studies, the dosage of imatinib should be increased by at least 50% and clinical response should be carefully monitored).
No products indexed under this heading.

Methylprednisolone Acetate (CYP3A4 inducers may decrease imatinib C_{max} and AUC. The use of concomitant strong CYP3A4 inducers should be avoided. If patients must be co-administered a strong CYP3A4 inducer, based on pharmacokinetic studies, the dosage of imatinib should be increased by at least 50% and clinical response should be carefully monitored).
No products indexed under this heading.

Methylprednisolone Sodium Succinate (CYP3A4 inducers may decrease imatinib C_{max} and AUC. The use of concomitant strong CYP3A4 inducers should be avoided. If patients must be co-administered a strong CYP3A4 inducer, based on pharmacokinetic studies, the dosage of imatinib should be increased by at least 50% and clinical response should be carefully monitored).
No products indexed under this heading.

Metoprolol Succinate (*In vitro*, imatinib inhibits the cytochrome P450 isoenzyme CYP2D6 activity at similar concentrations that affect CYP3A4 activity. Systemic exposure to substrates of CYP2D6 is expected to be increased when co-administered with imatinib. No specific studies have been performed and caution is recommended). Products include:
Toprol XL 732

Metoprolol Tartrate (*In vitro*, imatinib inhibits the cytochrome P450 isoenzyme CYP2D6 activity at similar concentrations that affect CYP3A4 activity. Systemic exposure to substrates of CYP2D6 is expected to be increased when co-administered with imatinib. No specific studies have been performed and caution is recommended).
No products indexed under this heading.

Metronidazole (There was a significant increase in exposure to imatinib (mean C_{max} and AUC increased by 26% and 40%, respectively) in healthy subjects when imatinib was co-administered with a single dose of ketoconazole (a CYP3A4 inhibitor). Caution is recom-

mended when administering imatinib with strong CYP3A4 inhibitors. Substances that inhibit the cytochrome P450 isoenzyme (CYP3A4) activity may decrease metabolism and increase imatinib concentrations). Products include:

Pylera 793

Metronidazole Benzoate (There was a significant increase in exposure to imatinib (mean C_{max} and AUC increased by 26% and 40%, respectively) in healthy subjects when imatinib was co-administered with a single dose of ketoconazole (a CYP3A4 inhibitor). Caution is recommended when administering imatinib with strong CYP3A4 inhibitors. Substances that inhibit the cytochrome P450 isoenzyme (CYP3A4) activity may decrease metabolism and increase imatinib concentrations).

No products indexed under this heading.

Metronidazole Hydrochloride (There was a significant increase in exposure to imatinib (mean C_{max} and AUC increased by 26% and 40%, respectively) in healthy subjects when imatinib was co-administered with a single dose of ketoconazole (a CYP3A4 inhibitor). Caution is recommended when administering imatinib with strong CYP3A4 inhibitors. Substances that inhibit the cytochrome P450 isoenzyme (CYP3A4) activity may decrease metabolism and increase imatinib concentrations).

No products indexed under this heading.

Metronidazole Sodium (There was a significant increase in exposure to imatinib (mean C_{max} and AUC increased by 26% and 40%, respectively) in healthy subjects when imatinib was co-administered with a single dose of ketoconazole (a CYP3A4 inhibitor). Caution is recommended when administering imatinib with strong CYP3A4 inhibitors. Substances that inhibit the cytochrome P450 isoenzyme (CYP3A4) activity may decrease metabolism and increase imatinib concentrations).

No products indexed under this heading.

Mexiletine Hydrochloride (*In vitro*, imatinib inhibits the cytochrome P450 isoenzyme CYP2D6 activity at similar concentrations that affect CYP3A4 activity. Systemic exposure to substrates of CYP2D6 is expected to be increased when co-administered with imatinib. No specific studies have been performed and caution is recommended).

No products indexed under this heading.

Miconazole (There was a significant increase in exposure to imatinib (mean C_{max} and AUC increased by 26% and 40%, respectively) in healthy subjects when imatinib was co-administered with a single dose of ketoconazole (a CYP3A4 inhibitor). Caution is recommended when administering imatinib with strong CYP3A4 inhibitors. Substances that inhibit the cytochrome P450 isoenzyme (CYP3A4) activity may decrease metabolism and increase imatinib concentrations).

No products indexed under this heading.

Miconazole Nitrate (There was a significant increase in exposure to imatinib (mean C_{max} and AUC increased by 26% and 40%, respectively) in healthy subjects when imatinib was co-administered with a single dose of ketoconazole (a CYP3A4 inhibitor). Caution is recommended when administering imatinib with strong CYP3A4 inhibitors. Substances that inhibit the cytochrome P450 isoenzyme (CYP3A4) activity may decrease metabolism and increase imatinib concentrations). Products include:

Vusion Ointment 3335

Midazolam Hydrochloride (Imatinib increases the mean C_{max} and AUC of simvastatin (CYP3A4 substrate) 2- and

3.5-fold, respectively, suggesting an inhibition of the CYP3A4 by imatinib. Particular caution is recommended when administering imatinib with CYP3A4 substrates that have a narrow therapeutic window. Imatinib will increase plasma concentration of other CYP3A4 metabolized drugs (eg, triazolo-benzodiazepines)).

No products indexed under this heading.

Mifepristone (There was a significant increase in exposure to imatinib (mean C_{max} and AUC increased by 26% and 40%, respectively) in healthy subjects when imatinib was co-administered with a single dose of ketoconazole (a CYP3A4 inhibitor). Caution is recommended when administering imatinib with strong CYP3A4 inhibitors. Substances that inhibit the cytochrome P450 isoenzyme (CYP3A4) activity may decrease metabolism and increase imatinib concentrations).

No products indexed under this heading.

Mirtazapine (*In vitro*, imatinib inhibits the cytochrome P450 isoenzyme CYP2D6 activity at similar concentrations that affect CYP3A4 activity. Systemic exposure to substrates of CYP2D6 is expected to be increased when co-administered with imatinib. No specific studies have been performed and caution is recommended). Products include:

Remeron Tablets 3214
RemeronSolTab Tablets 3219

Mitomycin (Mitomycin-C) (When imatinib is combined with chemotherapy, liver toxicity in the form of transaminase elevation and hyperbilirubinemia has been observed. Additionally, there have been reports of acute liver failure. Monitoring of hepatic function is recommended).

No products indexed under this heading.

Mitotane (When imatinib is combined with chemotherapy, liver toxicity in the form of transaminase elevation and hyperbilirubinemia has been observed. Additionally, there have been reports of acute liver failure. Monitoring of hepatic function is recommended).

No products indexed under this heading.

Mitoxantrone Hydrochloride (When imatinib is combined with chemotherapy, liver toxicity in the form of transaminase elevation and hyperbilirubinemia has been observed. Additionally, there have been reports of acute liver failure. Monitoring of hepatic function is recommended). Products include:

Novantrone 1088

Modafinil (CYP3A4 inducers may decrease imatinib C_{max} and AUC. The use of concomitant strong CYP3A4 inducers should be avoided. If patients must be co-administered a strong CYP3A4 inducer, based on pharmacokinetic studies, the dosage of imatinib should be increased by at least 50% and clinical response should be carefully monitored). Products include:

Provigil 983

Morphine Sulfate (*In vitro*, imatinib inhibits the cytochrome P450 isoenzyme CYP2D6 activity at similar concentrations that affect CYP3A4 activity. Systemic exposure to substrates of CYP2D6 is expected to be increased when co-administered with imatinib. No specific studies have been performed and caution is recommended). Products include:

Avinza 1822
Embeda 1831
MS Contin 2803

Nafcillin Sodium (CYP3A4 inducers may decrease imatinib C_{max} and AUC. The use of concomitant strong CYP3A4 inducers should be avoided. If patients must be co-administered a strong CYP3A4 inducer, based on pharmacokinetic studies, the dosage of imatinib should be increased by at least 50% and clinical response should be carefully monitored).

No products indexed under this heading.

Nefazodone Hydrochloride (There was a significant increase in exposure to imatinib (mean C_{max} and AUC increased by 26% and 40%, respectively) in healthy subjects when imatinib was co-administered with a single dose of ketoconazole (a CYP3A4 inhibitor). Caution is recommended when administering imatinib with strong CYP3A4 inhibitors (eg, nefazodone). Substances that inhibit the cytochrome P450 isoenzyme (CYP3A4) activity may decrease metabolism and increase imatinib concentrations).

No products indexed under this heading.

Nelfinavir Mesylate (There was a significant increase in exposure to imatinib (mean C_{max} and AUC increased by 26% and 40%, respectively) in healthy subjects when imatinib was co-administered with a single dose of ketoconazole (a CYP3A4 inhibitor). Caution is recommended when administering imatinib with strong CYP3A4 inhibitors (eg, nelfinavir). Substances that inhibit the cytochrome P450 isoenzyme (CYP3A4) activity may decrease metabolism and increase imatinib concentrations).

No products indexed under this heading.

Nevirapine (There was a significant increase in exposure to imatinib (mean C_{max} and AUC increased by 26% and 40%, respectively) in healthy subjects when imatinib was co-administered with a single dose of ketoconazole (a CYP3A4 inhibitor). Caution is recommended when administering imatinib with strong CYP3A4 inhibitors. Substances that inhibit the cytochrome P450 isoenzyme (CYP3A4) activity may decrease metabolism and increase imatinib concentrations). Products include:

Viramune Oral Suspension 897
Viramune Tablets 897

Niacin (There was a significant increase in exposure to imatinib (mean C_{max} and AUC increased by 26% and 40%, respectively) in healthy subjects when imatinib was co-administered with a single dose of ketoconazole (a CYP3A4 inhibitor). Caution is recommended when administering imatinib with strong CYP3A4 inhibitors. Substances that inhibit the cytochrome P450 isoenzyme (CYP3A4) activity may decrease metabolism and increase imatinib concentrations). Products include:

Advicor 402
Cardio Basics 3455
Niaspan 497
Simcor 524

Niacinamide (There was a significant increase in exposure to imatinib (mean C_{max} and AUC increased by 26% and 40%, respectively) in healthy subjects when imatinib was co-administered with a single dose of ketoconazole (a CYP3A4 inhibitor). Caution is recommended when administering imatinib with strong CYP3A4 inhibitors. Substances that inhibit the cytochrome P450 isoenzyme (CYP3A4) activity may decrease metabolism and increase imatinib concentrations). Products include:

CitraNatal 90 DHA Capsules 2332
CitraNatal Assure 2332
CitraNatal Rx 2332
Heplive 607

Niacinamide Hydroiodide (There was a significant increase in exposure to imatinib (mean C_{max} and AUC

increased by 26% and 40%, respectively) in healthy subjects when imatinib was co-administered with a single dose of ketoconazole (a CYP3A4 inhibitor). Caution is recommended when administering imatinib with strong CYP3A4 inhibitors. Substances that inhibit the cytochrome P450 isoenzyme (CYP3A4) activity may decrease metabolism and increase imatinib concentrations).

No products indexed under this heading.

Nicardipine (Imatinib increases the mean C_{max} and AUC of simvastatin (CYP3A4 substrate) 2- and 3.5-fold, respectively, suggesting an inhibition of the CYP3A4 by imatinib. Particular caution is recommended when administering imatinib with CYP3A4 substrates that have a narrow therapeutic window. Imatinib will increase plasma concentration of other CYP3A4 metabolized drugs).

No products indexed under this heading.

Nicardipine Hydrochloride (Imatinib increases the mean C_{max} and AUC of simvastatin (CYP3A4 substrate) 2- and 3.5-fold, respectively, suggesting an inhibition of the CYP3A4 by imatinib. Particular caution is recommended when administering imatinib with CYP3A4 substrates that have a narrow therapeutic window. Imatinib will increase plasma concentration of other CYP3A4 metabolized drugs).

No products indexed under this heading.

Nicotinamide (There was a significant increase in exposure to imatinib (mean C_{max} and AUC increased by 26% and 40%, respectively) in healthy subjects when imatinib was co-administered with a single dose of ketoconazole (a CYP3A4 inhibitor). Caution is recommended when administering imatinib with strong CYP3A4 inhibitors. Substances that inhibit the cytochrome P450 isoenzyme (CYP3A4) activity may decrease metabolism and increase imatinib concentrations).

No products indexed under this heading.

Nifedipine (Imatinib increases the mean C_{max} and AUC of simvastatin (CYP3A4 substrate) 2- and 3.5-fold, respectively, suggesting an inhibition of the CYP3A4 by imatinib. Particular caution is recommended when administering imatinib with CYP3A4 substrates that have a narrow therapeutic window. Imatinib will increase plasma concentration of other CYP3A4 metabolized drugs (eg, dihydropyridine calcium channel blockers)).

No products indexed under this heading.

Nimodipine (Imatinib increases the mean C_{max} and AUC of simvastatin (CYP3A4 substrate) 2- and 3.5-fold, respectively, suggesting an inhibition of the CYP3A4 by imatinib. Particular caution is recommended when administering imatinib with CYP3A4 substrates that have a narrow therapeutic window. Imatinib will increase plasma concentration of other CYP3A4 metabolized drugs).

No products indexed under this heading.

Nisoldipine (Imatinib increases the mean C_{max} and AUC of simvastatin (CYP3A4 substrate) 2- and 3.5-fold, respectively, suggesting an inhibition of the CYP3A4 by imatinib. Particular caution is recommended when administering imatinib with CYP3A4 substrates that have a narrow therapeutic window. Imatinib will increase plasma concentration of other CYP3A4 metabolized drugs (eg, dihydropyridine calcium channel blockers)).

No products indexed under this heading.

IMPORTANT NOTE: Always consult each drug listing in the patient's regimen for possible interactions.

(⊙ Described in PDR® for Ophthalmic Medicines)

IMPORTANT NOTE: Always consult each drug listing in the patient's regimen for possible interactions.

Sulfinpyrazone (CYP3A4 inducers may decrease imatinib C_{max} and AUC. The use of concomitant strong CYP3A4 inducers should be avoided. If patients must be co-administered a strong CYP3A4 inducer, based on pharmacokinetic studies, the dosage of imatinib should be increased by at least 50% and clinical response should be carefully monitored).
No products indexed under this heading.

Tacrolimus (Imatinib increases the mean C_{max} and AUC of simvastatin (CYP3A4 substrate) 2- and 3.5-fold, respectively, suggesting an inhibition of the CYP3A4 by imatinib. Particular caution is recommended when administering imatinib with CYP3A4 substrates that have a narrow therapeutic window (eg, tacrolimus). Imatinib will increase plasma concentration of other CYP3A4 metabolized drugs). Products include:
Prograf Capsules **677**
Prograf Injection **677**
Protopic **685**

Tadalafil (Imatinib increases the mean C_{max} and AUC of simvastatin (CYP3A4 substrate) 2- and 3.5-fold, respectively, suggesting an inhibition of the CYP3A4 by imatinib. Particular caution is recommended when administering imatinib with CYP3A4 substrates that have a narrow therapeutic window. Imatinib will increase plasma concentration of other CYP3A4 metabolized drugs). Products include:
Adcirca **3461**
Cialis **1861**

Tamoxifen Citrate (Imatinib increases the mean C_{max} and AUC of simvastatin (CYP3A4 substrate) 2- and 3.5-fold, respectively, suggesting an inhibition of the CYP3A4 by imatinib. Particular caution is recommended when administering imatinib with CYP3A4 substrates that have a narrow therapeutic window. Imatinib will increase plasma concentration of other CYP3A4 metabolized drugs).
No products indexed under this heading.

Telithromycin (There was a significant increase in exposure to imatinib (mean C_{max} and AUC increased by 26% and 40%, respectively) in healthy subjects when imatinib was co-administered with a single dose of ketoconazole (a CYP3A4 inhibitor). Caution is recommended when administering imatinib with strong CYP3A4 inhibitors (eg, telithromycin). Substances that inhibit the cytochrome P450 isoenzyme (CYP3A4) activity may decrease metabolism and increase imatinib concentrations). Products include:
Ketek **2991**

Teniposide (In vitro, imatinib inhibits the cytochrome P450 isoenzyme CYP2D6 activity at similar concentrations that affect CYP3A4 activity. Systemic exposure to substrates of CYP2D6 is expected to be increased when co-administered with imatinib. No specific studies have been performed and caution is recommended).
No products indexed under this heading.

Terfenadine (Imatinib increases the mean C_{max} and AUC of simvastatin (CYP3A4 substrate) 2- and 3.5-fold, respectively, suggesting an inhibition of the CYP3A4 by imatinib. Particular caution is recommended when administering imatinib with CYP3A4 substrates that have a narrow therapeutic window. Imatinib will increase plasma concentration of other CYP3A4 metabolized drugs).
No products indexed under this heading.

Testosterone (In vitro, imatinib inhibits the cytochrome P450 isoenzyme CYP2D6 activity at similar concentrations that affect CYP3A4 activity. Systemic exposure to substrates of CYP2D6 is expected to be increased

when co-administered with imatinib. No specific studies have been performed and caution is recommended). Products include:
AndroGel **3456**

Testosterone Cypionate (In vitro, imatinib inhibits the cytochrome P450 isoenzyme CYP2D6 activity at similar concentrations that affect CYP3A4 activity. Systemic exposure to substrates of CYP2D6 is expected to be increased when co-administered with imatinib. No specific studies have been performed and caution is recommended).
No products indexed under this heading.

Testosterone Enanthate (In vitro, imatinib inhibits the cytochrome P450 isoenzyme CYP2D6 activity at similar concentrations that affect CYP3A4 activity. Systemic exposure to substrates of CYP2D6 is expected to be increased when co-administered with imatinib. No specific studies have been performed and caution is recommended). Products include:
Delatestryl **1102**

Testosterone Propionate (In vitro, imatinib inhibits the cytochrome P450 isoenzyme CYP2D6 activity at similar concentrations that affect CYP3A4 activity. Systemic exposure to substrates of CYP2D6 is expected to be increased when co-administered with imatinib. No specific studies have been performed and caution is recommended).
No products indexed under this heading.

Theophyllinate (CYP3A4 inducers may decrease imatinib C_{max} and AUC. The use of concomitant strong CYP3A4 inducers should be avoided. If patients must be co-administered a strong CYP3A4 inducer, based on pharmacokinetic studies, the dosage of imatinib should be increased by at least 50% and clinical response should be carefully monitored).
No products indexed under this heading.

Theophylline (Imatinib increases the mean C_{max} and AUC of simvastatin (CYP3A4 substrate) 2- and 3.5-fold, respectively, suggesting an inhibition of the CYP3A4 by imatinib. Particular caution is recommended when administering imatinib with CYP3A4 substrates that have a narrow therapeutic window. Imatinib will increase plasma concentration of other CYP3A4 metabolized drugs).
No products indexed under this heading.

Theophylline Anhydrous (Imatinib increases the mean C_{max} and AUC of simvastatin (CYP3A4 substrate) 2- and 3.5-fold, respectively, suggesting an inhibition of the CYP3A4 by imatinib. Particular caution is recommended when administering imatinib with CYP3A4 substrates that have a narrow therapeutic window. Imatinib will increase plasma concentration of other CYP3A4 metabolized drugs). Products include:
Uniphyl **2817**

Theophylline Calcium Salicylate (Imatinib increases the mean C_{max} and AUC of simvastatin (CYP3A4 substrate) 2- and 3.5-fold, respectively, suggesting an inhibition of the CYP3A4 by imatinib. Particular caution is recommended when administering imatinib with CYP3A4 substrates that have a narrow therapeutic window. Imatinib will increase plasma concentration of other CYP3A4 metabolized drugs).
No products indexed under this heading.

Theophylline Dihydroxypropyl (Glyceryl) (Imatinib increases the mean C_{max} and AUC of simvastatin (CYP3A4 substrate) 2- and 3.5-fold, respectively, suggesting an inhibition of the CYP3A4 by imatinib. Particular cau-

tion is recommended when administering imatinib with CYP3A4 substrates that have a narrow therapeutic window. Imatinib will increase plasma concentration of other CYP3A4 metabolized drugs).
No products indexed under this heading.

Theophylline Ethylenediamine (Imatinib increases the mean C_{max} and AUC of simvastatin (CYP3A4 substrate) 2- and 3.5-fold, respectively, suggesting an inhibition of the CYP3A4 by imatinib. Particular caution is recommended when administering imatinib with CYP3A4 substrates that have a narrow therapeutic window. Imatinib will increase plasma concentration of other CYP3A4 metabolized drugs).
No products indexed under this heading.

Theophylline Sodium Glycinate (Imatinib increases the mean C_{max} and AUC of simvastatin (CYP3A4 substrate) 2- and 3.5-fold, respectively, suggesting an inhibition of the CYP3A4 by imatinib. Particular caution is recommended when administering imatinib with CYP3A4 substrates that have a narrow therapeutic window. Imatinib will increase plasma concentration of other CYP3A4 metabolized drugs).
No products indexed under this heading.

Thioguanine (When imatinib is combined with chemotherapy, liver toxicity in the form of transaminase elevation and hyperbilirubinemia has been observed. Additionally, there have been reports of acute liver failure. Monitoring of hepatic function is recommended). Products include:
Tabloid **1664**

Thioridazine (In vitro, imatinib inhibits the cytochrome P450 isoenzyme CYP2D6 activity at similar concentrations that affect CYP3A4 activity. Systemic exposure to substrates of CYP2D6 is expected to be increased when co-administered with imatinib. No specific studies have been performed and caution is recommended).
No products indexed under this heading.

Thioridazine Hydrochloride (In vitro, imatinib inhibits the cytochrome P450 isoenzyme CYP2D6 activity at similar concentrations that affect CYP3A4 activity. Systemic exposure to substrates of CYP2D6 is expected to be increased when co-administered with imatinib. No specific studies have been performed and caution is recommended). Products include:
Thioridazine Hydrochloride **2384**

Thiotepa (When imatinib is combined with chemotherapy, liver toxicity in the form of transaminase elevation and hyperbilirubinemia has been observed. Additionally, there have been reports of acute liver failure. Monitoring of hepatic function is recommended).
No products indexed under this heading.

Tiagabine Hydrochloride (Imatinib increases the mean C_{max} and AUC of simvastatin (CYP3A4 substrate) 2- and 3.5-fold, respectively, suggesting an inhibition of the CYP3A4 by imatinib. Particular caution is recommended when administering imatinib with CYP3A4 substrates that have a narrow therapeutic window. Imatinib will increase plasma concentration of other CYP3A4 metabolized drugs). Products include:
Gabitril **972**

Timolol Maleate (In vitro, imatinib inhibits the cytochrome P450 isoenzyme CYP2D6 activity at similar concentrations that affect CYP3A4 activity. Systemic exposure to substrates of CYP2D6 is expected to be increased when co-administered with imatinib. No specific studies have been performed and caution is recommended). Products include:

Combigan **601**
Dorzolamide
Hydrochloride/Timolol Maleate
Ophthalmic Solution..................... ⊙**243**
Timoptic in Ocudose .... ⊙**231**

Tolterodine Tartrate (Imatinib increases the mean C_{max} and AUC of simvastatin (CYP3A4 substrate) 2- and 3.5-fold, respectively, suggesting an inhibition of the CYP3A4 by imatinib. Particular caution is recommended when administering imatinib with CYP3A4 substrates that have a narrow therapeutic window. Imatinib will increase plasma concentration of other CYP3A4 metabolized drugs).
No products indexed under this heading.

Topotecan Hydrochloride (When imatinib is combined with chemotherapy, liver toxicity in the form of transaminase elevation and hyperbilirubinemia has been observed. Additionally, there have been reports of acute liver failure. Monitoring of hepatic function is recommended). Products include:
Hycamtin **1491**
Hycamtin Capsules **1488**

Toremifene Citrate (When imatinib is combined with chemotherapy, liver toxicity in the form of transaminase elevation and hyperbilirubinemia has been observed. Additionally, there have been reports of acute liver failure. Monitoring of hepatic function is recommended).
No products indexed under this heading.

Tramadol Hydrochloride (In vitro, imatinib inhibits the cytochrome P450 isoenzyme CYP2D6 activity at similar concentrations that affect CYP3A4 activity. Systemic exposure to substrates of CYP2D6 is expected to be increased when co-administered with imatinib. No specific studies have been performed and caution is recommended). Products include:
Ryzolt **2813**
Ultram ER **2693**

Trazodone Hydrochloride (Imatinib increases the mean C_{max} and AUC of simvastatin (CYP3A4 substrate) 2- and 3.5-fold, respectively, suggesting an inhibition of the CYP3A4 by imatinib. Particular caution is recommended when administering imatinib with CYP3A4 substrates that have a narrow therapeutic window. Imatinib will increase plasma concentration of other CYP3A4 metabolized drugs).
No products indexed under this heading.

Triamcinolone (CYP3A4 inducers may decrease imatinib C_{max} and AUC. The use of concomitant strong CYP3A4 inducers should be avoided. If patients must be co-administered a strong CYP3A4 inducer, based on pharmacokinetic studies, the dosage of imatinib should be increased by at least 50% and clinical response should be carefully monitored).
No products indexed under this heading.

Triamcinolone Acetonide (CYP3A4 inducers may decrease imatinib C_{max} and AUC. The use of concomitant strong CYP3A4 inducers should be avoided. If patients must be co-administered a strong CYP3A4 inducer, based on pharmacokinetic studies, the dosage of imatinib should be increased by at least 50% and clinical response should be carefully monitored). Products include:
Azmacort **408**
Nasacort AQ **3019**

Triamcinolone Diacetate (CYP3A4 inducers may decrease imatinib C$_{max}$ and AUC. The use of concomitant strong CYP3A4 inducers should be avoided. If patients must be co-administered a strong CYP3A4 inducer, based on pharmacokinetic studies, the dosage of imatinib should be increased by at least 50% and clinical response should be carefully monitored).
No products indexed under this heading.

Triamcinolone Hexacetonide (CYP3A4 inducers may decrease imatinib C$_{max}$ and AUC. The use of concomitant strong CYP3A4 inducers should be avoided. If patients must be co-administered a strong CYP3A4 inducer, based on pharmacokinetic studies, the dosage of imatinib should be increased by at least 50% and clinical response should be carefully monitored).
No products indexed under this heading.

Triazolam (Imatinib increases the mean C$_{max}$ and AUC of simvastatin (CYP3A4 substrate) 2- and 3.5-fold, respectively, suggesting an inhibition of the CYP3A4 by imatinib. Particular caution is recommended when administering imatinib with CYP3A4 substrates that have a narrow therapeutic window. Imatinib will increase plasma concentration of other CYP3A4 metabolized drugs (eg, triazolo-benzodiazepines)).
No products indexed under this heading.

Trimipramine Maleate (In vitro, imatinib inhibits the cytochrome P450 isoenzyme CYP2D6 activity at similar concentrations that affect CYP3A4 activity. Systemic exposure to substrates of CYP2D6 is expected to be increased when co-administered with imatinib. No specific studies have been performed and caution is recommended).
No products indexed under this heading.

Troglitazone (There was a significant increase in exposure to imatinib (mean C$_{max}$ and AUC increased by 26% and 40%, respectively) in healthy subjects when imatinib was co-administered with a single dose of ketoconazole (a CYP3A4 inhibitor). Caution is recommended when administering imatinib with strong CYP3A4 inhibitors. Substances that inhibit the cytochrome P450 isoenzyme (CYP3A4) activity may decrease metabolism and increase imatinib concentrations).
No products indexed under this heading.

Troleandomycin (CYP3A4 inhibitors may increase imatinib C$_{max}$ and AUC. There was a significant increase in exposure to imatinib (mean C$_{max}$ and AUC increased by 26% and 40% respectively) in healthy subjects when imatinib was co-administered with a single dose of ketoconazole (a CYP3A4 inhibitor). Caution is recommended when administering imatinib with strong CYP3A4 inhibitors (eg, ketoconazole, itraconazole). Grapefruit juice may also increase plasma concentrations of imatinib and should be avoided. Substances that inhibit the cytochrome P450 isoenzyme (CYP3A4) activity may decrease metabolism and increase imatinib concentrations).
No products indexed under this heading.

Valproate Sodium (There was a significant increase in exposure to imatinib (mean C$_{max}$ and AUC increased by 26% and 40%, respectively) in healthy subjects when imatinib was co-administered with a single dose of ketoconazole (a CYP3A4 inhibitor). Caution is recommended when administering imatinib with strong CYP3A4 inhibitors. Substances that inhibit the cytochrome P450 isoenzyme (CYP3A4) activity may decrease metabolism and increase imatinib concentrations).
No products indexed under this heading.

Valrubicin (When imatinib is combined with chemotherapy, liver toxicity in the

form of transaminase elevation and hyperbilirubinemia has been observed. Additionally, there have been reports of acute liver failure. Monitoring of hepatic function is recommended. Products include:
Valstar 1131

Vardenafil Hydrochloride (There was a significant increase in exposure to imatinib (mean C$_{max}$ and AUC increased by 26% and 40%, respectively) in healthy subjects when imatinib was co-administered with a single dose of ketoconazole (a CYP3A4 inhibitor). Caution is recommended when administering imatinib with strong CYP3A4 inhibitors. Substances that inhibit the cytochrome P450 isoenzyme (CYP3A4) activity may decrease metabolism and increase imatinib concentrations). Products include:
Levitra 3157

Venlafaxine Hydrochloride (In vitro, imatinib inhibits the cytochrome P450 isoenzyme CYP2D6 activity at similar concentrations that affect CYP3A4 activity. Systemic exposure to substrates of CYP2D6 is expected to be increased when co-administered with imatinib. No specific studies have been performed and caution is recommended). Products include:
Effexor XR 3504
Venlafaxine Hydrochloride Tablets ... 2388

Verapamil Hydrochloride (Imatinib increases the mean C$_{max}$ and AUC of simvastatin (CYP3A4 substrate) 2- and 3.5-fold, respectively, suggesting an inhibition of the CYP3A4 by imatinib. Particular caution is recommended when administering imatinib with CYP3A4 substrates that have a narrow therapeutic window. Imatinib will increase plasma concentration of other CYP3A4 metabolized drugs (eg, dihydropyridine calcium channel blockers)). Products include:
Tarka 534

Vinblastine Sulfate (Imatinib increases the mean C$_{max}$ and AUC of simvastatin (CYP3A4 substrate) 2- and 3.5-fold, respectively, suggesting an inhibition of the CYP3A4 by imatinib. Particular caution is recommended when administering imatinib with CYP3A4 substrates that have a narrow therapeutic window. Imatinib will increase plasma concentration of other CYP3A4 metabolized drugs).
No products indexed under this heading.

Vincristine Sulfate (Imatinib increases the mean C$_{max}$ and AUC of simvastatin (CYP3A4 substrate) 2- and 3.5-fold, respectively, suggesting an inhibition of the CYP3A4 by imatinib. Particular caution is recommended when administering imatinib with CYP3A4 substrates that have a narrow therapeutic window. Imatinib will increase plasma concentration of other CYP3A4 metabolized drugs).
No products indexed under this heading.

Vinorelbine Tartrate (When imatinib is combined with chemotherapy, liver toxicity in the form of transaminase elevation and hyperbilirubinemia has been observed. Additionally, there have been reports of acute liver failure. Monitoring of hepatic function is recommended).
No products indexed under this heading.

Voriconazole (There was a significant increase in exposure to imatinib (mean C$_{max}$ and AUC increased by 26% and 40%, respectively) in healthy subjects when imatinib was co-administered with a single dose of ketoconazole (a CYP3A4 inhibitor). Caution is recommended when administering imatinib with strong CYP3A4 inhibitors (eg, voriconazole). Substances that inhibit the

cytochrome P450 isoenzyme (CYP3A4) activity may decrease metabolism and increase imatinib concentrations).
No products indexed under this heading.

Warfarin Sodium (Imatinib will increase plasma concentration of other CYP3A4 metabolized drugs. Because warfarin is metabolized by CYP2C9 and CYP3A4, patients who require anticoagulation should receive low-molecular weight or standard heparin instead of warfarin).
No products indexed under this heading.

Zafirlukast (There was a significant increase in exposure to imatinib (mean C$_{max}$ and AUC increased by 26% and 40%, respectively) in healthy subjects when imatinib was co-administered with a single dose of ketoconazole (a CYP3A4 inhibitor). Caution is recommended when administering imatinib with strong CYP3A4 inhibitors. Substances that inhibit the cytochrome P450 isoenzyme (CYP3A4) activity may decrease metabolism and increase imatinib concentrations). Products include:
Accolate 3612

Zileuton (There was a significant increase in exposure to imatinib (mean C$_{max}$ and AUC increased by 26% and 40%, respectively) in healthy subjects when imatinib was co-administered with a single dose of ketoconazole (a CYP3A4 inhibitor). Caution is recommended when administering imatinib with strong CYP3A4 inhibitors. Substances that inhibit the cytochrome P450 isoenzyme (CYP3A4) activity may decrease metabolism and increase imatinib concentrations).
No products indexed under this heading.

Zonisamide (In vitro, imatinib inhibits the cytochrome P450 isoenzyme CYP2D6 activity at similar concentrations that affect CYP3A4 activity. Systemic exposure to substrates of CYP2D6 is expected to be increased when co-administered with imatinib. No specific studies have been performed and caution is recommended). Products include:
Zonegran 1081

Food Interactions

Grapefruit (Grapefruit juice may increase plasma concentrations of imatinib and should be avoided).

Grapefruit Juice (Grapefruit juice may increase plasma concentrations of imatinib and should be avoided).

GLIADEL WAFER
(Polifeprosan 20 with Carmustine) 1064
None cited in PDR database.

GLUCAGON FOR INJECTION VIALS AND EMERGENCY KIT
(Glucagon) 1908
None cited in PDR database.

GORDOCHOM SOLUTION
(Chloroxylenol, Undecylenic Acid) 1770
None cited in PDR database.

HAPPYCODE SPRAY
(Thymus polypeptide) 607
None cited in PDR database.

HAVRIX INJECTION VACCINE
(Hepatitis A Vaccine, Inactivated) 1485
May interact with alkylating agents, antimetabolites, corticosteroids, cytotoxic drugs, immunosuppressive agents, and certain other agents. Compounds in these categories include:

Alclometasone Dipropionate (Immunosuppressive therapies, including corticosteroids (used in greater than physiologic doses) may reduce the immune response to Hepatitis A vaccine).
No products indexed under this heading.

Azathioprine (Immunosuppressive therapies, including irradiation, antimetabolites, alkylating agents, cytotoxic drugs, and corticosteroids (used in greater than physiologic doses) may reduce the immune response to Hepatitis A vaccine).
No products indexed under this heading.

Basiliximab (Immunosuppressive therapies, including irradiation, antimetabolites, alkylating agents, cytotoxic drugs, and corticosteroids (used in greater than physiologic doses) may reduce the immune response to Hepatitis A vaccine). Products include:
Simulect 2524

Beclomethasone Dipropionate (Immunosuppressive therapies, including corticosteroids (used in greater than physiologic doses), may reduce the immune response to Hepatitis A vaccine). Products include:
Qvar 3398

Beclomethasone Dipropionate Monohydrate (Immunosuppressive therapies, including corticosteroids (used in greater than physiologic doses), may reduce the immune response to Hepatitis A vaccine). Products include:
Beconase AQ 1386

Betamethasone (Immunosuppressive therapies, including corticosteroids (used in greater than physiologic doses), may reduce the immune response to Hepatitis A vaccine).
No products indexed under this heading.

Betamethasone Acetate (Immunosuppressive therapies, including corticosteroids (used in greater than physiologic doses), may reduce the immune response to Hepatitis A vaccine).
No products indexed under this heading.

Betamethasone Benzoate (Immunosuppressive therapies, including corticosteroids (used in greater than physiologic doses), may reduce the immune response to Hepatitis A vaccine).
No products indexed under this heading.

Betamethasone Dipropionate (Immunosuppressive therapies, including corticosteroids (used in greater than physiologic doses), may reduce the immune response to Hepatitis A vaccine). Products include:
Diprolene Lotion 0.05% 3108
Diprolene Ointment 0.05% 3109
Diprolene AF Cream 0.05% 3107
Lotrisone 3163

Betamethasone Sodium Phosphate (Immunosuppressive therapies, including corticosteroids (used in greater than physiologic doses), may reduce the immune response to Hepatitis A vaccine).
No products indexed under this heading.

Betamethasone Valerate (Immunosuppressive therapies, including corticosteroids (used in greater than physiologic doses), may reduce the immune response to Hepatitis A vaccine). Products include:
Luxíq 3321

Bleomycin Sulfate (Immunosuppressive therapies, including cytotoxic drugs, may reduce the immune response to Hepatitis A vaccine).
No products indexed under this heading.

Budesonide (Immunosuppressive therapies, including corticosteroids (used in greater than physiologic doses), may reduce the immune response to Hepatitis A vaccine). Products include:

IMPORTANT NOTE: Always consult each drug listing in the patient's regimen for possible interactions.

(⊙ Described in PDR® for Ophthalmic Medicines)

Methylprednisolone Sodium Succinate (Immunosuppressive therapies, including corticosteroids (used in greater than physiologic doses), may reduce the immune response to Hepatitis A vaccine).
No products indexed under this heading.

Mitotane (Immunosuppressive therapies, including cytotoxic drugs, may reduce the immune response to Hepatitis A vaccine).
No products indexed under this heading.

Mitoxantrone Hydrochloride (Immunosuppressive therapies, including cytotoxic drugs, may reduce the immune response to Hepatitis A vaccine).
Products include:
Novantrone 1088

Mometasone Furoate (Immunosuppressive therapies, including corticosteroids (used in greater than physiologic doses), may reduce the immune response to Hepatitis A vaccine).
Products include:
Asmanex 3058
Elocon Cream 3111
Elocon Lotion 3112
Elocon Ointment 3114

Mometasone Furoate Monohydrate (Immunosuppressive therapies, including corticosteroids (used in greater than physiologic doses), may reduce the immune response to Hepatitis A vaccine). Products include:
Nasonex 3166

Muromonab-CD3 (Immunosuppressive therapies, including irradiation, antimetabolites, alkylating agents, cytotoxic drugs, and corticosteroids (used in greater than physiologic doses), may reduce the immune response to Hepatitis A vaccine). Products include:
Orthoclone OKT3 949

Mycophenolate Mofetil (Immunosuppressive therapies, including irradiation, antimetabolites, alkylating agents, cytotoxic drugs, and corticosteroids (used in greater than physiologic doses), may reduce the immune response to Hepatitis A vaccine).
No products indexed under this heading.

Pentostatin (Immunosuppressive therapies, including antimetabolites, may reduce the immune response to Hepatitis A vaccine).
No products indexed under this heading.

Pneumococcal vaccine, diphtheria conjugate (Hepatitis A vaccine (Havrix) may be given concurrently with the fourth dose of pneumococcal 7-valent conjugate vaccine in children 15 months of age (range 14 to 16 months)). Products include:
Prevnar 3557

Prednisolone (Immunosuppressive therapies, including corticosteroids (used in greater than physiologic doses), may reduce the immune response to Hepatitis A vaccine).
No products indexed under this heading.

Prednisolone Acetate (Immunosuppressive therapies, including corticosteroids (used in greater than physiologic doses), may reduce the immune response to Hepatitis A vaccine).
Products include:
Blephamide ....⊙212, ⊙214
Pred Forte .... ⊙225
Pred Mild .... ⊙230
Pred-G ....⊙226, ⊙227

Prednisolone Sodium Phosphate (Immunosuppressive therapies, including corticosteroids (used in greater than physiologic doses), may reduce the immune response to Hepatitis A vaccine).
No products indexed under this heading.

Prednisolone Tebutate (Immunosuppressive therapies, including corticosteroids (used in greater than physiologic doses), may reduce the immune response to Hepatitis A vaccine).
No products indexed under this heading.

Prednisone (Immunosuppressive therapies, including corticosteroids (used in greater than physiologic doses), may reduce the immune response to Hepatitis A vaccine).
No products indexed under this heading.

Prednisone sodium phosphate (Immunosuppressive therapies, including corticosteroids (used in greater than physiologic doses), may reduce the immune response to Hepatitis A vaccine).
No products indexed under this heading.

Procarbazine Hydrochloride (Immunosuppressive therapies, including cytotoxic drugs, may reduce the immune response to Hepatitis A vaccine).
No products indexed under this heading.

Radiation (Immunosuppressive therapies, including irradiation, may reduce the immune response to Hepatitis A vaccine).
No products indexed under this heading.

Rapamycin (Immunosuppressive therapies, including irradiation, antimetabolites, alkylating agents, cytotoxic drugs, and corticosteroids (used in greater than physiologic doses), may reduce the immune response to Hepatitis A vaccine).
No products indexed under this heading.

Sirolimus (Immunosuppressive therapies, including irradiation, antimetabolites, alkylating agents, cytotoxic drugs, and corticosteroids (used in greater than physiologic doses), may reduce the immune response to Hepatitis A vaccine). Products include:
Rapamune 3579

Tacrolimus (Immunosuppressive therapies, including irradiation, antimetabolites, alkylating agents, cytotoxic drugs, and corticosteroids (used in greater than physiologic doses), may reduce the immune response to Hepatitis A vaccine). Products include:
Prograf Capsules 677
Prograf Injection 677
Protopic 685

Tamoxifen Citrate (Immunosuppressive therapies, including cytotoxic drugs, may reduce the immune response to Hepatitis A vaccine).
No products indexed under this heading.

Thioguanine (Immunosuppressive therapies, including antimetabolites, may reduce the immune response to Hepatitis A vaccine). Products include:
Tabloid 1664

Thiotepa (Immunosuppressive therapies, including alkylating agents, may reduce the immune response to Hepatitis A vaccine).
No products indexed under this heading.

Triamcinolone (Immunosuppressive therapies, including corticosteroids (used in greater than physiologic doses), may reduce the immune response to Hepatitis A vaccine).
No products indexed under this heading.

Triamcinolone Acetonide (Immunosuppressive therapies, including corticosteroids (used in greater than physiologic doses), may reduce the immune response to Hepatitis A vaccine).
Products include:
Azmacort 408
Nasacort AQ 3019

Triamcinolone Diacetate (Immunosuppressive therapies, including corticosteroids (used in greater than physiologic doses), may reduce the immune response to Hepatitis A vaccine).
No products indexed under this heading.

Triamcinolone Hexacetonide (Immunosuppressive therapies, including corticosteroids (used in greater than physiologic doses), may reduce the immune response to Hepatitis A vaccine).
No products indexed under this heading.

Vinblastine Sulfate (Immunosuppressive therapies, including cytotoxic drugs, may reduce the immune response to Hepatitis A vaccine).
No products indexed under this heading.

Vincristine Sulfate (Immunosuppressive therapies, including cytotoxic drugs, may reduce the immune response to Hepatitis A vaccine).
No products indexed under this heading.

Vinorelbine Tartrate (Immunosuppressive therapies, including cytotoxic drugs, may reduce the immune response to Hepatitis A vaccine).
No products indexed under this heading.

HEMOFIL M
(Antihemophilic Factor (Human)) 819
None cited in PDR database.

HEP-FORTE CAPSULES
(Vitamins with Minerals) 2041
None cited in PDR database.

HEPLIVE SOFTGEL CAPSULES
(Biotin, Choline Bitartrate, Folic Acid, Inositol, Liver, Desiccated, Liver Fractions, Methionine, Niacinamide, Pantothenic Acid, Vitamin A, Vitamin B1, Vitamin B12, Vitamin B2, Vitamin B6, Vitamin C, Vitamin E, Yeast, Zinc, Zinc Sulfate) 607
None cited in PDR database.

HEPSERA TABLETS
(Adefovir dipivoxil) 1244
May interact with aminoglycosides, inhibitors of renal tubular secretion or resorption, nephrotoxic agents, and certain other agents. Compounds in these categories include:

Abacavir Sulfate (Since adefovir is eliminated by the kidney, co-administration of adefovir with drugs that reduce renal function may increase serum concentrations of either adefovir and/or these co-administered drugs). Products include:
Epzicom 1448
Trizivir 1688
Ziagen 1740

Acyclovir (Since adefovir is eliminated by the kidney, co-administration of adefovir with drugs that reduce renal function may increase serum concentrations of either adefovir and/or these co-administered drugs). Products include:
Zovirax 1760

Acyclovir Sodium (Since adefovir is eliminated by the kidney, co-administration of adefovir with drugs that reduce renal function may increase serum concentrations of either adefovir and/or these co-administered drugs).
No products indexed under this heading.

Alatrofloxacin Mesylate (Since adefovir is eliminated by the kidney, co-administration of adefovir with drugs that reduce renal function may increase serum concentrations of either adefovir and/or these co-administered drugs).
No products indexed under this heading.

Aldesleukin (Since adefovir is eliminated by the kidney, co-administration of adefovir with drugs that reduce renal function may increase serum concentra-

tions of either adefovir and/or these co-administered drugs). Products include:
Proleukin 2504

Amikacin Sulfate (Patients should be monitored closely for adverse events when adefovir dipivoxil is co-administered with other drugs that are known to affect renal function).
No products indexed under this heading.

Amoxicillin (Since adefovir is eliminated by the kidney, co-administration of adefovir with drugs that reduce renal function may increase serum concentrations of either adefovir and/or these co-administered drugs). Products include:
Amoxil Capsules 1311
Amoxil Chewable Tablets 1311
Amoxil 1311
Amoxil Powder 1311
Augmentin 1331
Augmentin Tablets 1335
Augmentin ES-600 1338
Augmentin XR 1342
Moxatag 2321

Amoxicillin Trihydrate (Since adefovir is eliminated by the kidney, co-administration of adefovir with drugs that reduce renal function may increase serum concentrations of either adefovir and/or these co-administered drugs).
No products indexed under this heading.

Amphotericin B (Since adefovir is eliminated by the kidney, co-administration of adefovir with drugs that reduce renal function may increase serum concentrations of either adefovir and/or these co-administered drugs).
No products indexed under this heading.

Amphotericin B, liposomal (Since adefovir is eliminated by the kidney, co-administration of adefovir with drugs that reduce renal function may increase serum concentrations of either adefovir and/or these co-administered drugs). Products include:
AmBisome 659

Amphotericin B Cholesteryl Sulfate (Since adefovir is eliminated by the kidney, co-administration of adefovir with drugs that reduce renal function may increase serum concentrations of either adefovir and/or these co-administered drugs).
No products indexed under this heading.

Amphotericin B Lipid Complex (Since adefovir is eliminated by the kidney, co-administration of adefovir with drugs that reduce renal function may increase serum concentrations of either adefovir and/or these co-administered drugs).
No products indexed under this heading.

Ampicillin (Since adefovir is eliminated by the kidney, co-administration of adefovir with drugs that reduce renal function may increase serum concentrations of either adefovir and/or these co-administered drugs).
No products indexed under this heading.

Ampicillin Sodium (Since adefovir is eliminated by the kidney, co-administration of adefovir with drugs that reduce renal function may increase serum concentrations of either adefovir and/or these co-administered drugs).
No products indexed under this heading.

Ampicillin Trihydrate (Since adefovir is eliminated by the kidney, co-administration of adefovir with drugs that reduce renal function may increase serum concentrations of either adefovir and/or these co-administered drugs).
No products indexed under this heading.

IMPORTANT NOTE: Always consult each drug listing in the patient's regimen for possible interactions.

Amprenavir (Since adefovir is eliminated by the kidney, co-administration of adefovir with drugs that reduce renal function may increase serum concentrations of either adefovir and/or these co-administered drugs).
No products indexed under this heading.

Aspirin (Since adefovir is eliminated by the kidney, co-administration of adefovir with drugs that reduce renal function may increase serum concentrations of either adefovir and/or these co-administered drugs). Products include:

Aggrenox	880
Bayer Aspirin	829
Percodan	1124
St. Joseph Aspirin	2045

Atazanavir (Since adefovir is eliminated by the kidney, co-administration of adefovir with drugs that reduce renal function may increase serum concentrations of either adefovir and/or these co-administered drugs).
No products indexed under this heading.

Atorvastatin Calcium (Since adefovir is eliminated by the kidney, co-administration of adefovir with drugs that reduce renal function may increase serum concentrations of either adefovir and/or these co-administered drugs). Products include:

Lipitor	2703

Azithromycin Dihydrate (Since adefovir is eliminated by the kidney, co-administration of adefovir with drugs that reduce renal function may increase serum concentrations of either adefovir and/or these co-administered drugs).
No products indexed under this heading.

Azlocillin Sodium (Since adefovir is eliminated by the kidney, co-administration of adefovir with drugs that reduce renal function may increase serum concentrations of either adefovir and/or these co-administered drugs).
No products indexed under this heading.

Aztreonam (Since adefovir is eliminated by the kidney, co-administration of adefovir with drugs that reduce renal function may increase serum concentrations of either adefovir and/or these co-administered drugs).
No products indexed under this heading.

Bacampicillin Hydrochloride (Since adefovir is eliminated by the kidney, co-administration of adefovir with drugs that reduce renal function may increase serum concentrations of either adefovir and/or these co-administered drugs).
No products indexed under this heading.

Bacitracin (Since adefovir is eliminated by the kidney, co-administration of adefovir with drugs that reduce renal function may increase serum concentrations of either adefovir and/or these co-administered drugs).
No products indexed under this heading.

Bacitracin Zinc (Since adefovir is eliminated by the kidney, co-administration of adefovir with drugs that reduce renal function may increase serum concentrations of either adefovir and/or these co-administered drugs).
No products indexed under this heading.

Balsalazide Disodium (Since adefovir is eliminated by the kidney, co-administration of adefovir with drugs that reduce renal function may increase serum concentrations of either adefovir and/or these co-administered drugs).
No products indexed under this heading.

Benazepril Hydrochloride (Since adefovir is eliminated by the kidney, co-administration of adefovir with drugs that reduce renal function may increase serum concentrations of either adefovir and/or these co-administered drugs).
No products indexed under this heading.

Bendroflumethiazide (Since adefovir is eliminated by the kidney, co-administration of adefovir with drugs that reduce renal function may increase serum concentrations of either adefovir and/or these co-administered drugs).
No products indexed under this heading.

Caffeine (Since adefovir is eliminated by the kidney, co-administration of adefovir with drugs that reduce renal function may increase serum concentrations of either adefovir and/or these co-administered drugs).
No products indexed under this heading.

Captopril (Since adefovir is eliminated by the kidney, co-administration of adefovir with drugs that reduce renal function may increase serum concentrations of either adefovir and/or these co-administered drugs). Products include:

Captopril	2341

Carbenicillin Disodium (Since adefovir is eliminated by the kidney, co-administration of adefovir with drugs that reduce renal function may increase serum concentrations of either adefovir and/or these co-administered drugs).
No products indexed under this heading.

Carbenicillin Indanyl Sodium (Since adefovir is eliminated by the kidney, co-administration of adefovir with drugs that reduce renal function may increase serum concentrations of either adefovir and/or these co-administered drugs).
No products indexed under this heading.

Carboplatin (Since adefovir is eliminated by the kidney, co-administration of adefovir with drugs that reduce renal function may increase serum concentrations of either adefovir and/or these co-administered drugs).
No products indexed under this heading.

Carmustine (BCNU) (Since adefovir is eliminated by the kidney, co-administration of adefovir with drugs that reduce renal function may increase serum concentrations of either adefovir and/or these co-administered drugs).
No products indexed under this heading.

Cefaclor (Since adefovir is eliminated by the kidney, co-administration of adefovir with drugs that reduce renal function may increase serum concentrations of either adefovir and/or these co-administered drugs).
No products indexed under this heading.

Cefadroxil (Since adefovir is eliminated by the kidney, co-administration of adefovir with drugs that reduce renal function may increase serum concentrations of either adefovir and/or these co-administered drugs).
No products indexed under this heading.

Cefamandole Nafate (Since adefovir is eliminated by the kidney, co-administration of adefovir with drugs that reduce renal function may increase serum concentrations of either adefovir and/or these co-administered drugs).
No products indexed under this heading.

Cefazolin Sodium (Since adefovir is eliminated by the kidney, co-administration of adefovir with drugs that reduce renal function may increase serum concentrations of either adefovir and/or these co-administered drugs).
No products indexed under this heading.

Cefdinir (Since adefovir is eliminated by the kidney, co-administration of adefovir with drugs that reduce renal function may increase serum concentrations of either adefovir and/or these co-administered drugs). Products include:

Omnicef Capsules	518
Omnicef Oral Suspension	518

Cefepime Hydrochloride (Since adefovir is eliminated by the kidney, co-administration of adefovir with drugs that reduce renal function may increase serum concentrations of either adefovir and/or these co-administered drugs).
No products indexed under this heading.

Cefixime (Since adefovir is eliminated by the kidney, co-administration of adefovir with drugs that reduce renal function may increase serum concentrations of either adefovir and/or these co-administered drugs). Products include:

Suprax for Oral Suspension	2038
Suprax Tablets	2038

Cefmetazole Sodium (Since adefovir is eliminated by the kidney, co-administration of adefovir with drugs that reduce renal function may increase serum concentrations of either adefovir and/or these co-administered drugs).
No products indexed under this heading.

Cefonicid Sodium (Since adefovir is eliminated by the kidney, co-administration of adefovir with drugs that reduce renal function may increase serum concentrations of either adefovir and/or these co-administered drugs).
No products indexed under this heading.

Cefoperazone Sodium (Since adefovir is eliminated by the kidney, co-administration of adefovir with drugs that reduce renal function may increase serum concentrations of either adefovir and/or these co-administered drugs).
No products indexed under this heading.

Ceforanide (Since adefovir is eliminated by the kidney, co-administration of adefovir with drugs that reduce renal function may increase serum concentrations of either adefovir and/or these co-administered drugs).
No products indexed under this heading.

Cefotaxime Sodium (Since adefovir is eliminated by the kidney, co-administration of adefovir with drugs that reduce renal function may increase serum concentrations of either adefovir and/or these co-administered drugs).
No products indexed under this heading.

Cefotetan (Since adefovir is eliminated by the kidney, co-administration of adefovir with drugs that reduce renal function may increase serum concentrations of either adefovir and/or these co-administered drugs).
No products indexed under this heading.

Cefoxitin Sodium (Since adefovir is eliminated by the kidney, co-administration of adefovir with drugs that reduce renal function may increase serum concentrations of either adefovir and/or these co-administered drugs).
No products indexed under this heading.

Cefpodoxime Proxetil (Since adefovir is eliminated by the kidney, co-administration of adefovir with drugs that reduce renal function may increase serum concentrations of either adefovir and/or these co-administered drugs).
No products indexed under this heading.

Cefprozil (Since adefovir is eliminated by the kidney, co-administration of adefovir with drugs that reduce renal function may increase serum concentrations of either adefovir and/or these co-administered drugs).
No products indexed under this heading.

Ceftazidime (Since adefovir is eliminated by the kidney, co-administration of adefovir with drugs that reduce renal function may increase serum concentrations of either adefovir and/or these co-administered drugs). Products include:

Fortaz	1481

Ceftizoxime Sodium (Since adefovir is eliminated by the kidney, co-administration of adefovir with drugs that reduce renal function may increase serum concentrations of either adefovir and/or these co-administered drugs).
No products indexed under this heading.

Ceftriaxone Sodium (Since adefovir is eliminated by the kidney, co-administration of adefovir with drugs that reduce renal function may increase serum concentrations of either adefovir and/or these co-administered drugs). Products include:

Rocephin	2859

Cefuroxime Axetil (Since adefovir is eliminated by the kidney, co-administration of adefovir with drugs that reduce renal function may increase serum concentrations of either adefovir and/or these co-administered drugs). Products include:

Ceftin	1399

Cefuroxime Sodium (Since adefovir is eliminated by the kidney, co-administration of adefovir with drugs that reduce renal function may increase serum concentrations of either adefovir and/or these co-administered drugs).
No products indexed under this heading.

Celecoxib (Since adefovir is eliminated by the kidney, co-administration of adefovir with drugs that reduce renal function may increase serum concentrations of either adefovir and/or these co-administered drugs). Products include:

Celebrex	3272

Cephalexin (Since adefovir is eliminated by the kidney, co-administration of adefovir with drugs that reduce renal function may increase serum concentrations of either adefovir and/or these co-administered drugs).
No products indexed under this heading.

Cephalothin Sodium (Since adefovir is eliminated by the kidney, co-administration of adefovir with drugs that reduce renal function may increase serum concentrations of either adefovir and/or these co-administered drugs).
No products indexed under this heading.

Cephapirin Sodium (Since adefovir is eliminated by the kidney, co-administration of adefovir with drugs that reduce renal function may increase serum concentrations of either adefovir and/or these co-administered drugs).
No products indexed under this heading.

Cephradine (Since adefovir is eliminated by the kidney, co-administration of adefovir with drugs that reduce renal function may increase serum concentrations of either adefovir and/or these co-administered drugs).
No products indexed under this heading.

Cerivastatin Sodium (Since adefovir is eliminated by the kidney, co-administration of adefovir with drugs that reduce renal function may increase serum concentrations of either adefovir and/or these co-administered drugs).
No products indexed under this heading.

Chlorothiazide (Since adefovir is eliminated by the kidney, co-administration of adefovir with drugs that reduce renal function may increase serum concentrations of either adefovir and/or these co-administered drugs).
No products indexed under this heading.

Chlorothiazide Sodium (Since adefovir is eliminated by the kidney, co-administration of adefovir with drugs that reduce renal function may increase serum concentrations of either adefovir and/or these co-administered drugs). Products include:

Diuril Intravenous	2009

(⊙ Described in PDR® for Ophthalmic Medicines)

IMPORTANT NOTE: Always consult each drug listing in the patient's regimen for possible interactions.

(⊙ Described in PDR® for Ophthalmic Medicines)

793 **Interactions Index** **Hepsera**

Treximet **1681**

Nelfinavir Mesylate (Since adefovir is eliminated by the kidney, co-administration of adefovir with drugs that reduce renal function may increase serum concentrations of either adefovir and/or these co-administered drugs).
No products indexed under this heading.

Neomycin (Patients should be monitored closely for adverse events when adefovir dipivoxil is co-administered with other drugs that are known to affect renal function).
No products indexed under this heading.

Neomycin, oral (Patients should be monitored closely for adverse events when adefovir dipivoxil is co-administered with other drugs that are known to affect renal function).
No products indexed under this heading.

Neomycin Sulfate (Patients should be monitored closely for adverse events when adefovir dipivoxil is co-administered with other drugs that are known to affect renal function).
No products indexed under this heading.

Nevirapine (Since adefovir is eliminated by the kidney, co-administration of adefovir with drugs that reduce renal function may increase serum concentrations of either adefovir and/or these co-administered drugs). Products include:
Viramune Oral Suspension **897**
Viramune Tablets **897**

Norfloxacin (Since adefovir is eliminated by the kidney, co-administration of adefovir with drugs that reduce renal function may increase serum concentrations of either adefovir and/or these co-administered drugs). Products include:
Noroxin **2220**

Olsalazine Sodium (Since adefovir is eliminated by the kidney, co-administration of adefovir with drugs that reduce renal function may increase serum concentrations of either adefovir and/or these co-administered drugs).
No products indexed under this heading.

Omeprazole (Since adefovir is eliminated by the kidney, co-administration of adefovir with drugs that reduce renal function may increase serum concentrations of either adefovir and/or these co-administered drugs).
No products indexed under this heading.

Oxaprozin (Since adefovir is eliminated by the kidney, co-administration of adefovir with drugs that reduce renal function may increase serum concentrations of either adefovir and/or these co-administered drugs).
No products indexed under this heading.

Pamidronate Disodium (Since adefovir is eliminated by the kidney, co-administration of adefovir with drugs that reduce renal function may increase serum concentrations of either adefovir and/or these co-administered drugs).
No products indexed under this heading.

Paroxetine Hydrochloride (Since adefovir is eliminated by the kidney, co-administration of adefovir with drugs that reduce renal function may increase serum concentrations of either adefovir and/or these co-administered drugs). Products include:
Paroxetine CR **2361**
Paroxetine ER **2371**
Paxil **1586**
Paxil CR **1596**

Penicillamine (Since adefovir is eliminated by the kidney, co-administration of adefovir with drugs that reduce renal function may increase serum concentrations of either adefovir and/or these co-administered drugs).
No products indexed under this heading.

Penicillin G Benzathine (Since adefovir is eliminated by the kidney, co-administration of adefovir with drugs that reduce renal function may increase serum concentrations of either adefovir and/or these co-administered drugs). Products include:
Bicillin C-R Injectable Suspension **1826**
Bicillin L-A **1828**

Penicillin G Potassium (Since adefovir is eliminated by the kidney, co-administration of adefovir with drugs that reduce renal function may increase serum concentrations of either adefovir and/or these co-administered drugs).
No products indexed under this heading.

Penicillin G Procaine (Since adefovir is eliminated by the kidney, co-administration of adefovir with drugs that reduce renal function may increase serum concentrations of either adefovir and/or these co-administered drugs). Products include:
Bicillin C-R Injectable Suspension **1826**
Bicillin L-A **1828**

Penicillin G Sodium (Since adefovir is eliminated by the kidney, co-administration of adefovir with drugs that reduce renal function may increase serum concentrations of either adefovir and/or these co-administered drugs).
No products indexed under this heading.

Penicillin V Potassium (Since adefovir is eliminated by the kidney, co-administration of adefovir with drugs that reduce renal function may increase serum concentrations of either adefovir and/or these co-administered drugs).
No products indexed under this heading.

Pentamidine Isethionate (Since adefovir is eliminated by the kidney, co-administration of adefovir with drugs that reduce renal function may increase serum concentrations of either adefovir and/or these co-administered drugs).
No products indexed under this heading.

Perindopril Erbumine (Since adefovir is eliminated by the kidney, co-administration of adefovir with drugs that reduce renal function may increase serum concentrations of either adefovir and/or these co-administered drugs).
No products indexed under this heading.

Phenylbutazone (Since adefovir is eliminated by the kidney, co-administration of adefovir with drugs that reduce renal function may increase serum concentrations of either adefovir and/or these co-administered drugs).
No products indexed under this heading.

Piroxicam (Since adefovir is eliminated by the kidney, co-administration of adefovir with drugs that reduce renal function may increase serum concentrations of either adefovir and/or these co-administered drugs).
No products indexed under this heading.

Plicamycin (Since adefovir is eliminated by the kidney, co-administration of adefovir with drugs that reduce renal function may increase serum concentrations of either adefovir and/or these co-administered drugs).
No products indexed under this heading.

Polymyxin (Since adefovir is eliminated by the kidney, co-administration of adefovir with drugs that reduce renal function may increase serum concentrations of either adefovir and/or these co-administered drugs).
No products indexed under this heading.

Polymyxin B Sulfate (Since adefovir is eliminated by the kidney, co-administration of adefovir with drugs that reduce renal function may increase serum concentrations of either adefovir and/or these co-administered drugs).
No products indexed under this heading.

Polythiazide (Since adefovir is eliminated by the kidney, co-administration of adefovir with drugs that reduce renal function may increase serum concentrations of either adefovir and/or these co-administered drugs).
No products indexed under this heading.

Pravastatin Sodium (Since adefovir is eliminated by the kidney, co-administration of adefovir with drugs that reduce renal function may increase serum concentrations of either adefovir and/or these co-administered drugs).
No products indexed under this heading.

Probenecid (Since adefovir is eliminated by the kidney, co-administration of adefovir with drugs that compete for active tubular secretion may increase serum concentrations of either adefovir and/or these co-administered drugs).
No products indexed under this heading.

Quinapril Hydrochloride (Since adefovir is eliminated by the kidney, co-administration of adefovir with drugs that reduce renal function may increase serum concentrations of either adefovir and/or these co-administered drugs).
No products indexed under this heading.

Rabeprazole Sodium (Since adefovir is eliminated by the kidney, co-administration of adefovir with drugs that reduce renal function may increase serum concentrations of either adefovir and/or these co-administered drugs). Products include:
Aciphex **1035**

Ramipril (Since adefovir is eliminated by the kidney, co-administration of adefovir with drugs that reduce renal function may increase serum concentrations of either adefovir and/or these co-administered drugs).
No products indexed under this heading.

Rifampin (Since adefovir is eliminated by the kidney, co-administration of adefovir with drugs that reduce renal function may increase serum concentrations of either adefovir and/or these co-administered drugs).
No products indexed under this heading.

Riluzole (Since adefovir is eliminated by the kidney, co-administration of adefovir with drugs that reduce renal function may increase serum concentrations of either adefovir and/or these co-administered drugs). Products include:
Rilutek **3032**

Ritonavir (Since adefovir is eliminated by the kidney, co-administration of adefovir with drugs that reduce renal function may increase serum concentrations of either adefovir and/or these co-administered drugs). Products include:
Kaletra **458**
Norvir **509**

Rofecoxib (Since adefovir is eliminated by the kidney, co-administration of adefovir with drugs that reduce renal function may increase serum concentrations of either adefovir and/or these co-administered drugs).
No products indexed under this heading.

Saquinavir (Since adefovir is eliminated by the kidney, co-administration of adefovir with drugs that reduce renal function may increase serum concentrations of either adefovir and/or these co-administered drugs).
No products indexed under this heading.

Sibutramine Hydrochloride Monohydrate (Since adefovir is eliminated by the kidney, co-administration of adefovir with drugs that reduce renal function may increase serum concentrations of either adefovir and/or these co-administered drugs). Products include:
Meridia **492**

Simvastatin (Since adefovir is eliminated by the kidney, co-administration of adefovir with drugs that reduce renal function may increase serum concentrations of either adefovir and/or these co-administered drugs). Products include:
Simcor **524**
Vytorin 10/10 .... **2303, 3240**
Vytorin 10/20 .... **2303, 3240**
Vytorin 10/40 .... **2303, 3240**
Vytorin 10/80 .... **2303, 3240**
Zocor **2289**

Spirapril Hydrochloride (Since adefovir is eliminated by the kidney, co-administration of adefovir with drugs that reduce renal function may increase serum concentrations of either adefovir and/or these co-administered drugs).
No products indexed under this heading.

Stavudine (Since adefovir is eliminated by the kidney, co-administration of adefovir with drugs that reduce renal function may increase serum concentrations of either adefovir and/or these co-administered drugs).
No products indexed under this heading.

Streptomycin Sulfate (Patients should be monitored closely for adverse events when adefovir dipivoxil is co-administered with other drugs that are known to affect renal function).
No products indexed under this heading.

Streptozocin (Since adefovir is eliminated by the kidney, co-administration of adefovir with drugs that reduce renal function may increase serum concentrations of either adefovir and/or these co-administered drugs).
No products indexed under this heading.

Sulfacytine (Since adefovir is eliminated by the kidney, co-administration of adefovir with drugs that reduce renal function may increase serum concentrations of either adefovir and/or these co-administered drugs).
No products indexed under this heading.

Sulfamethizole (Since adefovir is eliminated by the kidney, co-administration of adefovir with drugs that reduce renal function may increase serum concentrations of either adefovir and/or these co-administered drugs).
No products indexed under this heading.

Sulfamethoxazole (Since adefovir is eliminated by the kidney, co-administration of adefovir with drugs that reduce renal function may increase serum concentrations of either adefovir and/or these co-administered drugs).
No products indexed under this heading.

Sulfasalazine (Since adefovir is eliminated by the kidney, co-administration of adefovir with drugs that reduce renal function may increase serum concentrations of either adefovir and/or these co-administered drugs).
No products indexed under this heading.

Sulfinpyrazone (Since adefovir is eliminated by the kidney, co-administration of adefovir with drugs that reduce renal function may increase serum concentrations of either adefovir and/or these co-administered drugs).
No products indexed under this heading.

Sulfisoxazole Acetyl (Since adefovir is eliminated by the kidney, co-administration of adefovir with drugs that reduce renal function may increase serum concentrations of either adefovir and/or these co-administered drugs).
No products indexed under this heading.

Sulfisoxazole Diolamine (Since adefovir is eliminated by the kidney, co-administration of adefovir with drugs that reduce renal function may increase serum concentrations of either adefovir and/or these co-administered drugs).
No products indexed under this heading.

Sulindac (Since adefovir is eliminated by the kidney, co-administration of adefovir with drugs that reduce renal function may increase serum concentrations of either adefovir and/or these co-administered drugs). Products include:

IMPORTANT NOTE: Always consult each drug listing in the patient's regimen for possible interactions.

(⊙ Described in PDR® for Ophthalmic Medicines)

Aspirin Buffered (Co-administration with drugs with hypoglycemic activity, such as salicylates, may result in decreased insulin requirements).
No products indexed under this heading.

Atenolol (Co-administration with drugs with hypoglycemic activity, such as beta blockers, may result in decreased insulin requirements; beta blockers may mask the symptoms of hypoglycemia in some patients).
No products indexed under this heading.

Beclomethasone Dipropionate (Co-administration may result in increased insulin requirements).
Products include:
Qvar ... **3398**

Beclomethasone Dipropionate Monohydrate (Co-administration may result in increased insulin requirements).
Products include:
Beconase AQ ... **1386**

Benazepril Hydrochloride (Co-administration with drugs with hypoglycemic activity, such as certain ACE inhibitors, may result in decreased insulin requirements).
No products indexed under this heading.

Betamethasone (Co-administration may result in increased insulin requirements).
No products indexed under this heading.

Betamethasone Acetate (Co-administration may result in increased insulin requirements).
No products indexed under this heading.

Betamethasone Benzoate (Co-administration may result in increased insulin requirements).
No products indexed under this heading.

Betamethasone Dipropionate (Co-administration may result in increased insulin requirements). Products include:
Diprolene Lotion 0.05% ... **3108**
Diprolene Ointment 0.05% ... **3109**
Diprolene AF Cream 0.05% ... **3107**
Lotrisone ... **3163**

Betamethasone Sodium Phosphate (Co-administration may result in increased insulin requirements).
No products indexed under this heading.

Betamethasone Valerate (Co-administration may result in increased insulin requirements). Products include:
Luxíq ... **3321**

Betaxolol Hydrochloride (Co-administration with drugs with hypoglycemic activity, such as beta blockers, may result in decreased insulin requirements; beta blockers may mask the symptoms of hypoglycemia in some patients).
No products indexed under this heading.

Bisoprolol Fumarate (Co-administration with drugs with hypoglycemic activity, such as beta blockers, may result in decreased insulin requirements; beta blockers may mask the symptoms of hypoglycemia in some patients).
No products indexed under this heading.

Budesonide (Co-administration may result in increased insulin requirements).
Products include:
Pulmicort Flexhaler ... **714**
Symbicort 80/4.5 ... **720**
Symbicort 160/4.5 ... **720**

Candesartan Cilexetil (Insulin requirements may be decreased in the presence of drugs with hypoglycemicartivity, such as angiotension II receptor blocking agents). Products include:
Atacand ... **697**
Atacand HCT ... **700**

Captopril (Co-administration with drugs with hypoglycemic activity, such as certain ACE inhibitors, may result in decreased insulin requirements).
Products include:
Captopril ... **2341**

Carteolol Hydrochloride (Co-administration with drugs with hypoglycemic activity, such as beta blockers, may result in decreased insulin requirements; beta blockers may mask the symptoms of hypoglycemia in some patients).
No products indexed under this heading.

Carvedilol (Co-administration with drugs with hypoglycemic activity, such as beta blockers, may result in decreased insulin requirements; beta blockers may mask the symptoms of hypoglycemia in some patients).
Products include:
Coreg ... **1409**

Carvedilol Phosphate (Co-administration with drugs with hypoglycemic activity, such as beta blockers, may result in decreased insulin requirements; beta blockers may mask the symptoms of hypoglycemia in some patients). Products include:
Coreg CR ... **1416**

Chlorotrianisene (Co-administration may result in increased insulin requirements).
No products indexed under this heading.

Chlorpromazine (Co-administration with phenothiazines may result in increased insulin requirements).
No products indexed under this heading.

Chlorpromazine Hydrochloride (Co-administration with phenothiazines may result in increased insulin requirements).
No products indexed under this heading.

Chlorpropamide (Co-administration with drugs with hypoglycemic activity, such as oral hypoglycemic agents, may result in decreased insulin requirements).
No products indexed under this heading.

Choline Magnesium Trisalicylate (Co-administration with drugs with hypoglycemic activity, such as salicylates, may result in decreased insulin requirements).
No products indexed under this heading.

Ciclesonide (Co-administration may result in increased insulin requirements).
No products indexed under this heading.

Cortisone Acetate (Co-administration may result in increased insulin requirements).
No products indexed under this heading.

Desogestrel (Co-admininstration with oral contraceptives may result in increased insulin requirements).
No products indexed under this heading.

Desoximetasone (Co-administration may result in increased insulin requirements).
No products indexed under this heading.

Dexamethasone (Co-administration may result in increased insulin requirements). Products include:
Ciprodex ... **583**
Ozurdex ... ⊙**223**
Tobramycin and Dexamethasone Ophthalmic Suspension ... ⊙**251**

Dexamethasone Acetate (Co-administration may result in increased insulin requirements).
No products indexed under this heading.

Dexamethasone Phosphate (Co-administration may result in increased insulin requirements).
No products indexed under this heading.

Dexamethasone Sodium (Co-administration may result in increased insulin requirements).
No products indexed under this heading.

Dexamethasone Sodium Phosphate (Co-administration may result in increased insulin requirements).
No products indexed under this heading.

Dexamethasone Sodium Phosphate Injection (Co-administration may result in increased insulin requirements).
No products indexed under this heading.

Dienestrol (Co-administration may result in increased insulin requirements).
No products indexed under this heading.

Diethylstilbestrol (Co-administration may result in increased insulin requirements).
No products indexed under this heading.

Diflorasone Diacetate (Co-administration may result in increased insulin requirements).
No products indexed under this heading.

Diflunisal (Co-administration with drugs with hypoglycemic activity, such as salicylates, may result in decreased insulin requirements).
No products indexed under this heading.

Enalapril Maleate (Co-administration with drugs with hypoglycemic activity, such as certain ACE inhibitors, may result in decreased insulin requirements).
No products indexed under this heading.

Enalaprilat (Co-administration with drugs with hypoglycemic activity, such as certain ACE inhibitors, may result in decreased insulin requirements).
No products indexed under this heading.

Eprosartan Mesylate (Insulin requirements may be decreased in the presence of drugs with hypoglycemicartivity, such as angiotension II receptor blocking agents). Products include:
Teveten ... **538**
Teveten HCT ... **541**

Esmolol Hydrochloride (Co-administration with drugs with hypoglycemic activity, such as beta blockers, may result in decreased insulin requirements; beta blockers may mask the symptoms of hypoglycemia in some patients).
No products indexed under this heading.

Estradiol (Co-administration may result in increased insulin requirements).
Products include:
Activella ... **2561**
Angeliq ... **831**
Climara ... **841**
Climara Pro ... **847**
Divigel ... **3467**
Estrasorb ... **1777**
Vagifem ... **2589**

Estrogens, Conjugated (Co-administration may result in increased insulin requirements). Products include:
Premarin Intravenous ... **3528**
Premarin Tablets ... **3533**
Premarin Vaginal Cream ... **3540**
Premphase ... **3549**
Prempro ... **3549**

Estrogens, Esterified (Co-administration may result in increased insulin requirements).
No products indexed under this heading.

Estropipate (Co-administration may result in increased insulin requirements).
No products indexed under this heading.

Ethanol (Co-administration with drugs with hypoglycemic activity may result in decreased insulin requirements).
No products indexed under this heading.

Ethinyl Estradiol (Co-administration may result in increased insulin requirements). Products include:
LoSeasonique ... **3407**
Lybrel ... **3514**
NuvaRing ... **3181**
Ortho Evra ... **2648**
Ortho-Cyclen/Ortho Tri-Cyclen ... **2663**
Ortho Tri-Cyclen Lo Tablets ... **2673**
Seasonique ... **3418**
Yaz ... **864**

Ethyl Alcohol (Co-administration with drugs with hypoglycemic activity may result in decreased insulin requirements).
No products indexed under this heading.

Ethynodiol Diacetate (Co-admininstration with oral contraceptives may result in increased insulin requirements).
No products indexed under this heading.

Fludrocortisone Acetate (Co-administration may result in increased insulin requirements).
No products indexed under this heading.

Flumethasone Pivalate (Co-administration may result in increased insulin requirements).
No products indexed under this heading.

Flunisolide Hemihydrate (Co-administration may result in increased insulin requirements).
No products indexed under this heading.

Fluphenazine Decanoate (Co-administration with phenothiazines may result in increased insulin requirements).
No products indexed under this heading.

Fluphenazine Enanthate (Co-administration with phenothiazines may result in increased insulin requirements).
No products indexed under this heading.

Fluphenazine Hydrochloride (Co-administration with phenothiazines may result in increased insulin requirements).
No products indexed under this heading.

Fluticasone Furoate (Co-administration may result in increased insulin requirements). Products include:
Veramyst ... **1713**

Fluticasone Propionate (Co-administration may result in increased insulin requirements). Products include:
Advair 100/50 ... **1275**
Advair 250/50 ... **1275**
Advair 500/50 ... **1275**
Advair HFA 45/21 ... **1288**
Advair HFA 115/21 ... **1288**
Advair HFA 230/21 ... **1288**
Flonase ... **1459**
Flovent Diskus ... **1463**
Flovent HFA ... **1470**

Fosinopril Sodium (Co-administration with drugs with hypoglycemic activity, such as certain ACE inhibitors, may result in decreased insulin requirements).
No products indexed under this heading.

Glibenclamide (Co-administration with drugs with hypoglycemic activity, such as oral hypoglycemic agents, may result in decreased insulin requirements).
No products indexed under this heading.

Glimepiride (Co-administration with drugs with hypoglycemic activity, such as oral hypoglycemic agents, may result in decreased insulin requirements). Products include:
Avandaryl ... **1356**
Duetact ... **3354**

Glipizide (Co-administration with drugs with hypoglycemic activity, such as oral hypoglycemic agents, may result in decreased insulin requirements).
No products indexed under this heading.

Glyburide (Co-administration with drugs with hypoglycemic activity, such as oral hypoglycemic agents, may result in decreased insulin requirements).
No products indexed under this heading.

Hydrocortisone (Co-administration may result in increased insulin requirements).
No products indexed under this heading.

Hydrocortisone (Alcohol) (Co-administration may result in increased insulin requirements).
No products indexed under this heading.

IMPORTANT NOTE: Always consult each drug listing in the patient's regimen for possible interactions.

Hydrocortisone Acetate (Co-administration may result in increased insulin requirements).
No products indexed under this heading.

Hydrocortisone Butyrate (Co-administration may result in increased insulin requirements).
No products indexed under this heading.

Hydrocortisone Cypionate (Co-administration may result in increased insulin requirements).
No products indexed under this heading.

Hydrocortisone Hemisuccinate (Co-administration may result in increased insulin requirements).
No products indexed under this heading.

Hydrocortisone Probutate (Co-administration may result in increased insulin requirements).
No products indexed under this heading.

Hydrocortisone Sodium Phosphate (Co-administration may result in increased insulin requirements).
No products indexed under this heading.

Hydrocortisone Sodium Succinate (Co-administration may result in increased insulin requirements).
No products indexed under this heading.

Hydrocortisone Valerate (Co-administration may result in increased insulin requirements).
No products indexed under this heading.

Irbesartan (Insulin requirements may be decreased in the presence of drugs with hypoglycemicartivity, such as angiotension II receptor blocking agents). Products include:

Isoniazid (Co-administration may result in increased insulin requirements).
No products indexed under this heading.

Labetalol Hydrochloride (Co-administration with drugs with hypoglycemic activity, such as beta blockers, may result in decreased insulin requirements; beta blockers may mask the symptoms of hypoglycemia in some patients).
No products indexed under this heading.

Levobunolol Hydrochloride (Co-administration with drugs with hypoglycemic activity, such as beta blockers, may result in decreased insulin requirements; beta blockers may mask the symptoms of hypoglycemia in some patients).
No products indexed under this heading.

Levonorgestrel (Co-admininstration with oral contraceptives may result in increased insulin requirements). Products include:

Levothyroxine Sodium (Co-administration with thyroid replacement therapy may result in increased insulin requirements). Products include:

Liothyronine Sodium (Co-administration with thyroid replacement therapy may result in increased insulin requirements). Products include:

Liotrix (Co-administration with thyroid replacement therapy may result in increased insulin requirements).
No products indexed under this heading.

Lisinopril (Co-administration with drugs with hypoglycemic activity, such as certain ACE inhibitors, may result in decreased insulin requirements). Products include:

Losartan Potassium (Insulin requirements may be decreased in the presence of drugs with hypoglycemicartivity, such as angiotension II receptor blocking agents). Products include:

Magnesium Salicylate (Co-administration with drugs with hypoglycemic activity, such as salicylates, may result in decreased insulin requirements).
No products indexed under this heading.

Mesoridazine Besylate (Co-administration with phenothiazines may result in increased insulin requirements).
No products indexed under this heading.

Mestranol (Co-admininstration with oral contraceptives may result in increased insulin requirements).
No products indexed under this heading.

Metformin Hydrochloride (Co-administration with drugs with hypoglycemic activity, such as oral hypoglycemic agents, may result in decreased insulin requirements). Products include:

Methotrimeprazine (Co-administration with phenothiazines may result in increased insulin requirements).
No products indexed under this heading.

Methylprednisolone (Co-administration may result in increased insulin requirements).
No products indexed under this heading.

Methylprednisolone Acetate (Co-administration may result in increased insulin requirements).
No products indexed under this heading.

Methylprednisolone Sodium Succinate (Co-admininstration may result in increased insulin requirements).
No products indexed under this heading.

Metipranolol Hydrochloride (Co-administration with drugs with hypoglycemic activity, such as beta blockers, may result in decreased insulin requirements; beta blockers may mask the symptoms of hypoglycemia in some patients).
No products indexed under this heading.

Metoprolol Succinate (Co-administration with drugs with hypoglycemic activity, such as beta blockers, may result in decreased insulin requirements; beta blockers may mask the symptoms of hypoglycemia in some patients). Products include:

Metoprolol Tartrate (Co-administration with drugs with hypoglycemic activity, such as beta blockers, may result in decreased insulin requirements; beta blockers may mask the symptoms of hypoglycemia in some patients).
No products indexed under this heading.

Miglitol (Co-administration with drugs with hypoglycemic activity, such as oral hypoglycemic agents, may result in decreased insulin requirements).
No products indexed under this heading.

Moexipril Hydrochloride (Co-administration with drugs with hypoglycemic activity, such as certain ACE inhibitors, may result in decreased insulin requirements).
No products indexed under this heading.

Mometasone Furoate (Co-administration may result in increased insulin requirements). Products include:

Mometasone Furoate Monohydrate (Co-administration may result in increased insulin requirements). Products include:

Nadolol (Co-administration with drugs with hypoglycemic activity, such as beta blockers, may result in decreased insulin requirements; beta blockers may mask the symptoms of hypoglycemia in some patients). Products include:

Nateglinide (Co-administration with drugs with hypoglycemic activity, such as oral hypoglycemic agents, may result in decreased insulin requirements).
No products indexed under this heading.

Nebivolol (Co-administration with drugs with hypoglycemic activity, such as beta blockers, may result in decreased insulin requirements; beta blockers may mask the symptoms of hypoglycemia in some patients). Products include:

Niacin (Co-administration may result in increased insulin requirements). Products include:

Norethindrone (Co-admininstration with oral contraceptives may result in increased insulin requirements). Products include:

Norethynodrel (Co-administration with oral contraceptives may result in increased insulin requirements).
No products indexed under this heading.

Norgestimate (Co-admininstration with oral contraceptives may result in increased insulin requirements). Products include:

Norgestrel (Co-admininstration with oral contraceptives may result in increased insulin requirements).
No products indexed under this heading.

Octreotide Acetate (Co-administration with drugs with hypoglycemic activity, such as inhibitors of pancreatic function, may result in decreased insulin requirements). Products include:

Penbutolol Sulfate (Co-administration with drugs with hypoglycemic activity, such as beta blockers, may result in decreased insulin requirements; beta blockers may mask the symptoms of hypoglycemia in some patients).
No products indexed under this heading.

Perindopril Erbumine (Co-administration with drugs with hypoglycemic activity, such as certain ACE inhibitors, may result in decreased insulin requirements).
No products indexed under this heading.

Perphenazine (Co-administration with phenothiazines may result in increased insulin requirements).
No products indexed under this heading.

Phenelzine Sulfate (Co-administration with drugs with hypoglycemic activity, such as certain MAO inhibitor antidepressants, may result in decreased insulin requirements).
No products indexed under this heading.

Phenothiazine Derivatives (Co-administration with phenothiazines may result in increased insulin requirements).
No products indexed under this heading.

Phenothiazines (Co-administration with phenothiazines may result in increased insulin requirements).
No products indexed under this heading.

Pindolol (Co-administration with drugs with hypoglycemic activity, such as beta blockers, may result in decreased insulin requirements; beta blockers may mask the symptoms of hypoglycemia in some patients).
No products indexed under this heading.

Pioglitazone Hydrochloride (Co-administration with drugs with hypoglycemic activity, such as oral hypoglycemic agents, may result in decreased insulin requirements). Products include:

Polyestradiol Phosphate (Co-administration may result in increased insulin requirements).
No products indexed under this heading.

Prednisolone (Co-administration may result in increased insulin requirements).
No products indexed under this heading.

Prednisolone Acetate (Co-administration may result in increased insulin requirements). Products include:

Prednisolone Sodium Phosphate (Co-administration may result in increased insulin requirements).
No products indexed under this heading.

Prednisolone Tebutate (Co-administration may result in increased insulin requirements).
No products indexed under this heading.

Prednisone (Co-administration may result in increased insulin requirements).
No products indexed under this heading.

Prednisone sodium phosphate (Co-administration may result in increased insulin requirements).
No products indexed under this heading.

Prochlorperazine (Co-administration with phenothiazines may result in increased insulin requirements).
No products indexed under this heading.

Prochlorperazine Edisylate (Co-administration with phenothiazines may result in increased insulin requirements).
No products indexed under this heading.

Prochlorperazine Maleate (Co-administration with phenothiazines may result in increased insulin requirements).
No products indexed under this heading.

Promethazine (Co-administration with phenothiazines may result in increased insulin requirements).
No products indexed under this heading.

Promethazine Hydrochloride (Co-administration with phenothiazines may result in increased insulin requirements).
No products indexed under this heading.

Propranolol Hydrochloride (Co-administration with drugs with hypoglycemic activity, such as beta blockers, may result in decreased insulin requirements; beta blockers may mask the symptoms of hypoglycemia in some patients). Products include:

Quinapril Hydrochloride (Co-administration with drugs with hypoglycemic activity, such as certain ACE inhibitors, may result in decreased insulin requirements).
No products indexed under this heading.

Quinestrol (Co-administration may result in increased insulin requirements).
No products indexed under this heading.

Ramipril (Co-administration with drugs with hypoglycemic activity, such as certain ACE inhibitors, may result in decreased insulin requirements).
No products indexed under this heading.

Repaglinide (Co-administration with drugs with hypoglycemic activity, such as oral hypoglycemic agents, may result in decreased insulin requirements).
No products indexed under this heading.

Rosiglitazone Maleate (Co-administration with drugs with hypoglycemic activity, such as oral hypoglycemic agents, may result in decreased insulin requirements). Products include:
Avandamet 1345
Avandaryl 1356
Avandia 1366

Salsalate (Co-administration with drugs with hypoglycemic activity, such as salicylates, may result in decreased insulin requirements).
No products indexed under this heading.

Sitagliptin Phosphate (Co-administration with drugs with hypoglycemic activity, such as oral hypoglycemic agents, may result in decreased insulin requirements). Products include:
Janumet 2188
Januvia 2196

Sotalol Hydrochloride (Co-administration with drugs with hypoglycemic activity, such as beta blockers, may result in decreased insulin requirements; beta blockers may mask the symptoms of hypoglycemia in some patients).
No products indexed under this heading.

Spirapril Hydrochloride (Co-administration with drugs with hypoglycemic activity, such as certain ACE inhibitors, may result in decreased insulin requirements).
No products indexed under this heading.

Sulfacytine (Co-administration with drugs with hypoglycemic activity, such as sulfa antibiotics, may result in decreased insulin requirements).
No products indexed under this heading.

Sulfamethizole (Co-administration with drugs with hypoglycemic activity, such as sulfa antibiotics, may result in decreased insulin requirements).
No products indexed under this heading.

Sulfamethoxazole (Co-administration with drugs with hypoglycemic activity, such as sulfa antibiotics, may result in decreased insulin requirements).
No products indexed under this heading.

Sulfasalazine (Co-administration with drugs with hypoglycemic activity, such as sulfa antibiotics, may result in decreased insulin requirements).
No products indexed under this heading.

Telmisartan (Insulin requirements may be decreased in the presence of drugs with hypoglycemicartivity, such as angiotension II receptor blocking agents). Products include:
Micardis 887
Micardis HCT 889

Thioridazine (Co-administration with phenothiazines may result in increased insulin requirements).
No products indexed under this heading.

Thioridazine Hydrochloride (Co-administration with phenothiazines may result in increased insulin requirements). Products include:
Thioridazine Hydrochloride 2384

Thyroglobulin (Co-administration with thyroid replacement therapy may result in increased insulin requirements).
No products indexed under this heading.

Thyroid (Co-administration with thyroid replacement therapy may result in increased insulin requirements). Products include:
Naturethroid 2830

Thyroxine (Co-administration with thyroid replacement therapy may result in increased insulin requirements).
No products indexed under this heading.

Thyroxine Sodium (Co-administration with thyroid replacement therapy may result in increased insulin requirements).
No products indexed under this heading.

Timolol Hemihydrate (Co-administration with drugs with hypoglycemic activity, such as beta blockers, may result in decreased insulin requirements; beta blockers may mask the symptoms of hypoglycemia in some patients). Products include:
Betimol 3490

Timolol Maleate (Co-administration with drugs with hypoglycemic activity, such as beta blockers, may result in decreased insulin requirements; beta blockers may mask the symptoms of hypoglycemia in some patients). Products include:
Combigan 601
Dorzolamide Hydrochloride/Timolol Maleate Ophthalmic Solution .... ⊙ 243
Timoptic in Ocudose .... ⊙ 231

Tolazamide (Co-administration with drugs with hypoglycemic activity, such as oral hypoglycemic agents, may result in decreased insulin requirements).
No products indexed under this heading.

Tolbutamide (Co-administration with drugs with hypoglycemic activity, such as oral hypoglycemic agents, may result in decreased insulin requirements).
No products indexed under this heading.

Trandolapril (Co-administration with drugs with hypoglycemic activity, such as certain ACE inhibitors, may result in decreased insulin requirements). Products include:
Mavik 489
Tarka 534

Tranylcypromine Sulfate (Co-administration with drugs with hypoglycemic activity, such as certain MAO inhibitor antidepressants, may result in decreased insulin requirements). Products include:
Parnate 1584

Triamcinolone (Co-administration may result in increased insulin requirements).
No products indexed under this heading.

Triamcinolone Acetonide (Co-administration may result in increased insulin requirements). Products include:
Azmacort 408
Nasacort AQ 3019

Triamcinolone Diacetate (Co-administration may result in increased insulin requirements).
No products indexed under this heading.

Triamcinolone Hexacetonide (Co-administration may result in increased insulin requirements).
No products indexed under this heading.

Trifluoperazine Hydrochloride (Co-administration with phenothiazines may result in increased insulin requirements).
No products indexed under this heading.

Troglitazone (Co-administration with drugs with hypoglycemic activity, such as oral hypoglycemic agents, may result in decreased insulin requirements).
No products indexed under this heading.

Valsartan (Insulin requirements may be decreased in the presence of drugs with hypoglycemicartivity, such as angiotension II receptor blocking agents). Products include:
Diovan 2413
Diovan HCT 2419
Exforge 2443
Exforge HCT 2449
Valturna 3637

Food Interactions

Alcohol (Co-administration with drugs with hypoglycemic activity may result in decreased insulin requirements).

Beer, reduced-alcohol (Co-administration with drugs with hypoglycemic activity may result in decreased insulin requirements).

Beer, unspecified (Co-administration with drugs with hypoglycemic activity may result in decreased insulin requirements).

Wine, Chianti (Co-administration with drugs with hypoglycemic activity may result in decreased insulin requirements).

Wine, Red (Co-administration with drugs with hypoglycemic activity may result in decreased insulin requirements).

Wine, unspecified (Co-administration with drugs with hypoglycemic activity may result in decreased insulin requirements).

Wine products (Co-administration with drugs with hypoglycemic activity may result in decreased insulin requirements).

HUMALOG MIX 50/50-PEN AND KWIKPEN

(Insulin Lispro, Human, Insulin Lispro Protamine, Human) 1914
May interact with ACE inhibitors, alcohols, beta-blockers, corticosteroids, estrogens, monoamine oxidase inhibitors, oral contraceptives, oral hypoglycemic agents, phenothiazines, salicylates, thyroid preparations, and certain other agents. Compounds in these categories include:

Acarbose (Insulin requirements may be decreased in the presence of drugs with with hypoglycemic activity, such as oral antidiabetic agents).
No products indexed under this heading.

Acebutolol Hydrochloride (Beta-adrenergic blockers may mask the symptoms of hypoglycemia in some patients).
No products indexed under this heading.

Alclometasone Dipropionate (Insulin requirements may be increased by medications with hypoglycemic activity, such as corticosteroids).
No products indexed under this heading.

Aspirin (Insulin requirements may be decreased in the presence of drugs with hypoglycemic activity, such as salicylates). Products include:
Aggrenox 880
Bayer Aspirin 829
Percodan 1124
St. Joseph Aspirin 2045

Aspirin, Enteric Coated (Insulin requirements may be decreased in the presence of drugs with hypoglycemic activity, such as salicylates).
No products indexed under this heading.

Aspirin Buffered (Insulin requirements may be decreased in the presence of drugs with hypoglycemic activity, such as salicylates).
No products indexed under this heading.

Atenolol (Beta-adrenergic blockers may mask the symptoms of hypoglycemia in some patients).
No products indexed under this heading.

Beclomethasone Dipropionate (Insulin requirements may be increased by medications with hypoglycemic activity, such as corticosteroids). Products include:
Qvar 3398

Beclomethasone Dipropionate Monohydrate (Insulin requirements may be increased by medications with hypoglycemic activity, such as corticosteroids). Products include:
Beconase AQ 1386

Benazepril Hydrochloride (Insulin requirements may be decreased in the presence of drugs with hypoglycemic activity, such as certain angiotensin converting enzyme inhibitors).
No products indexed under this heading.

Betamethasone (Insulin requirements may be increased by medications with hypoglycemic activity, such as corticosteroids).
No products indexed under this heading.

Betamethasone Acetate (Insulin requirements may be increased by medications with hypoglycemic activity, such as corticosteroids).
No products indexed under this heading.

Betamethasone Benzoate (Insulin requirements may be increased by medications with hypoglycemic activity, such as corticosteroids).
No products indexed under this heading.

Betamethasone Dipropionate (Insulin requirements may be increased by medications with hypoglycemic activity, such as corticosteroids). Products include:
Diprolene Lotion 0.05% 3108
Diprolene Ointment 0.05% 3109
Diprolene AF Cream 0.05% 3107
Lotrisone 3163

Betamethasone Sodium Phosphate (Insulin requirements may be increased by medications with hypoglycemic activity, such as corticosteroids).
No products indexed under this heading.

Betamethasone Valerate (Insulin requirements may be increased by medications with hypoglycemic activity, such as corticosteroids). Products include:
Luxiq 3321

Betaxolol Hydrochloride (Beta-adrenergic blockers may mask the symptoms of hypoglycemia in some patients).
No products indexed under this heading.

Bisoprolol Fumarate (Beta-adrenergic blockers may mask the symptoms of hypoglycemia in some patients).
No products indexed under this heading.

Budesonide (Insulin requirements may be increased by medications with hypoglycemic activity, such as corticosteroids). Products include:
Pulmicort Flexhaler 714
Symbicort 80/4.5 720
Symbicort 160/4.5 720

Captopril (Insulin requirements may be decreased in the presence of drugs with hypoglycemic activity, such as certain angiotensin converting enzyme inhibitors). Products include:
Captopril 2341

Carteolol Hydrochloride (Beta-adrenergic blockers may mask the symptoms of hypoglycemia in some patients).
No products indexed under this heading.

Carvedilol (Beta-adrenergic blockers may mask the symptoms of hypoglycemia in some patients). Products include:
Coreg 1409

Carvedilol Phosphate (Beta-adrenergic blockers may mask the symptoms of hypoglycemia in some patients). Products include:
Coreg CR 1416

Chlorotrianisene (Insulin requirements may be increased by medications with hypoglycemic activity, such as estrogens).
No products indexed under this heading.

IMPORTANT NOTE: Always consult each drug listing in the patient's regimen for possible interactions.

Chlorpromazine (Insulin requirements may be increased by medications with hypoglycemic activity, such as phenothiazines).
No products indexed under this heading.

Chlorpromazine Hydrochloride (Insulin requirements may be increased by medications with hypoglycemic activity, such as phenothiazines).
No products indexed under this heading.

Chlorpropamide (Insulin requirements may be decreased in the presence of drugs with with hypoglycemic activity, such as oral antidiabetic agents).
No products indexed under this heading.

Choline Magnesium Trisalicylate (Insulin requirements may be decreased in the presence of drugs with hypoglycemic activity, such as salicylates).
No products indexed under this heading.

Ciclesonide (Insulin requirements may be increased by medications with hypoglycemic activity, such as corticosteroids).
No products indexed under this heading.

Cortisone Acetate (Insulin requirements may be increased by medications with hypoglycemic activity, such as corticosteroids).
No products indexed under this heading.

Desogestrel (Insulin requirements may be increased by medications with hypoglycemic activity, such as oral contraceptives).
No products indexed under this heading.

Desoximetasone (Insulin requirements may be increased by medications with hypoglycemic activity, such as corticosteroids).
No products indexed under this heading.

Dexamethasone (Insulin requirements may be increased by medications with hypoglycemic activity, such as corticosteroids). Products include:
Ciprodex 583
Ozurdex .... ⊙ 223
Tobramycin and Dexamethasone Ophthalmic Suspension .... ⊙ 251

Dexamethasone Acetate (Insulin requirements may be increased by medications with hypoglycemic activity, such as corticosteroids).
No products indexed under this heading.

Dexamethasone Phosphate (Insulin requirements may be increased by medications with hypoglycemic activity, such as corticosteroids).
No products indexed under this heading.

Dexamethasone Sodium (Insulin requirements may be increased by medications with hypoglycemic activity, such as corticosteroids).
No products indexed under this heading.

Dexamethasone Sodium Phosphate (Insulin requirements may be increased by medications with hypoglycemic activity, such as corticosteroids).
No products indexed under this heading.

Dexamethasone Sodium Phosphate Injection (Insulin requirements may be increased by medications with hypoglycemic activity, such as corticosteroids).
No products indexed under this heading.

Dienestrol (Insulin requirements may be increased by medications with hypoglycemic activity, such as estrogens).
No products indexed under this heading.

Diethylstilbestrol (Insulin requirements may be increased by medications with hypoglycemic activity, such as estrogens).
No products indexed under this heading.

Diflorasone Diacetate (Insulin requirements may be increased by medications with hypoglycemic activity, such as corticosteroids).
No products indexed under this heading.

Diflunisal (Insulin requirements may be decreased in the presence of drugs with hypoglycemic activity, such as salicylates).
No products indexed under this heading.

Enalapril Maleate (Insulin requirements may be decreased in the presence of drugs with hypoglycemic activity, such as certain angiotensin converting enzyme inhibitors).
No products indexed under this heading.

Enalaprilat (Insulin requirements may be decreased in the presence of drugs with hypoglycemic activity, such as certain angiotensin converting enzyme inhibitors).
No products indexed under this heading.

Esmolol Hydrochloride (Beta-adrenergic blockers may mask the symptoms of hypoglycemia in some patients).
No products indexed under this heading.

Estradiol (Insulin requirements may be increased by medications with hypoglycemic activity, such as estrogens). Products include:
Activella 2561
Angeliq 831
Climara 841
Climara Pro 847
Divigel 3467
Estrasorb 1777
Vagifem 2589

Estrogens, Conjugated (Insulin requirements may be increased by medications with hypoglycemic activity, such as estrogens). Products include:
Premarin Intravenous 3528
Premarin Tablets 3533
Premarin Vaginal Cream 3540
Premphase 3549
Prempro 3549

Estrogens, Esterified (Insulin requirements may be increased by medications with hypoglycemic activity, such as estrogens).
No products indexed under this heading.

Estropipate (Insulin requirements may be increased by medications with hypoglycemic activity, such as estrogens).
No products indexed under this heading.

Ethanol (Insulin requirements may be decreased in the presence of drugs with hypoglycemic activity, such as alcohol).
No products indexed under this heading.

Ethinyl Estradiol (Insulin requirements may be increased by medications with hypoglycemic activity, such as oral contraceptives). Products include:
LoSeasonique 3407
Lybrel 3514
NuvaRing 3181
Ortho Evra 2648
Ortho-Cyclen/Ortho Tri-Cyclen 2663
Ortho Tri-Cyclen Lo Tablets 2673
Seasonique 3418
Yaz 864

Ethyl Alcohol (Insulin requirements may be decreased in the presence of drugs with hypoglycemic activity, such as alcohol).
No products indexed under this heading.

Ethynodiol Diacetate (Insulin requirements may be increased by medications with hypoglycemic activity, such as oral contraceptives).
No products indexed under this heading.

Fludrocortisone Acetate (Insulin requirements may be increased by medications with hypoglycemic activity, such as corticosteroids).
No products indexed under this heading.

Flumethasone Pivalate (Insulin requirements may be increased by medications with hypoglycemic activity, such as corticosteroids).
No products indexed under this heading.

Flunisolide Hemihydrate (Insulin requirements may be increased by medications with hypoglycemic activity, such as corticosteroids).
No products indexed under this heading.

Fluphenazine Decanoate (Insulin requirements may be increased by medications with hypoglycemic activity, such as phenothiazines).
No products indexed under this heading.

Fluphenazine Enanthate (Insulin requirements may be increased by medications with hypoglycemic activity, such as phenothiazines).
No products indexed under this heading.

Fluphenazine Hydrochloride (Insulin requirements may be increased by medications with hypoglycemic activity, such as phenothiazines).
No products indexed under this heading.

Fluticasone Furoate (Insulin requirements may be increased by medications with hypoglycemic activity, such as corticosteroids). Products include:
Veramyst 1713

Fluticasone Propionate (Insulin requirements may be increased by medications with hypoglycemic activity, such as corticosteroids). Products include:
Advair 100/50 1275
Advair 250/50 1275
Advair 500/50 1275
Advair HFA 45/21 1288
Advair HFA 115/21 1288
Advair HFA 230/21 1288
Flonase 1459
Flovent Diskus 1463
Flovent HFA 1470

Fosinopril Sodium (Insulin requirements may be decreased in the presence of drugs with hypoglycemic activity, such as certain angiotensin converting enzyme inhibitors).
No products indexed under this heading.

Glibenclamide (Insulin requirements may be decreased in the presence of drugs with with hypoglycemic activity, such as oral antidiabetic agents).
No products indexed under this heading.

Glimepiride (Insulin requirements may be decreased in the presence of drugs with with hypoglycemic activity, such as oral antidiabetic agents). Products include:
Avandaryl 1356
Duetact 3354

Glipizide (Insulin requirements may be decreased in the presence of drugs with with hypoglycemic activity, such as oral antidiabetic agents).
No products indexed under this heading.

Glyburide (Insulin requirements may be decreased in the presence of drugs with with hypoglycemic activity, such as oral antidiabetic agents).
No products indexed under this heading.

Hydrocortisone (Insulin requirements may be increased by medications with hypoglycemic activity, such as corticosteroids).
No products indexed under this heading.

Hydrocortisone (Alcohol) (Insulin requirements may be increased by medications with hypoglycemic activity, such as corticosteroids).
No products indexed under this heading.

Hydrocortisone Acetate (Insulin requirements may be increased by medications with hypoglycemic activity, such as corticosteroids).
No products indexed under this heading.

Hydrocortisone Butyrate (Insulin requirements may be increased by medications with hypoglycemic activity, such as corticosteroids).
No products indexed under this heading.

Hydrocortisone Cypionate (Insulin requirements may be increased by medications with hypoglycemic activity, such as corticosteroids).
No products indexed under this heading.

Hydrocortisone Hemisuccinate (Insulin requirements may be increased by medications with hypoglycemic activity, such as corticosteroids).
No products indexed under this heading.

Hydrocortisone Probutate (Insulin requirements may be increased by medications with hypoglycemic activity, such as corticosteroids).
No products indexed under this heading.

Hydrocortisone Sodium Phosphate (Insulin requirements may be increased by medications with hypoglycemic activity, such as corticosteroids).
No products indexed under this heading.

Hydrocortisone Sodium Succinate (Insulin requirements may be increased by medications with hypoglycemic activity, such as corticosteroids).
No products indexed under this heading.

Hydrocortisone Valerate (Insulin requirements may be increased by medications with hypoglycemic activity, such as corticosteroids).
No products indexed under this heading.

Isocarboxazid (Insulin requirements may be decreased in the presence of drugs with hypoglycemic activity, such as monoamine oxidase inhibitors). Products include:
Marplan 3481

Isoniazid (Insulin requirements may be increased by medications with hypoglycemic activity, such as isoniazid).
No products indexed under this heading.

Labetalol Hydrochloride (Beta-adrenergic blockers may mask the symptoms of hypoglycemia in some patients).
No products indexed under this heading.

Levobunolol Hydrochloride (Beta-adrenergic blockers may mask the symptoms of hypoglycemia in some patients).
No products indexed under this heading.

Levonorgestrel (Insulin requirements may be increased by medications with hypoglycemic activity, such as oral contraceptives). Products include:
Climara Pro 847
LoSeasonique 3407
Lybrel 3514
Mirena 854
Plan B 3416
Seasonique 3418

Levothyroxine Sodium (Insulin requirements may be increased by medications with hypoglycemic activity, such as thyroid replacement therapy). Products include:
Levoxyl Tablets 1843
Synthroid 529

Liothyronine Sodium (Insulin requirements may be increased by medications with hypoglycemic activity, such as thyroid replacement therapy). Products include:
Cytomel 1830

Liotrix (Insulin requirements may be increased by medications with hypoglycemic activity, such as thyroid replacement therapy).
No products indexed under this heading.

Lisinopril (Insulin requirements may be decreased in the presence of drugs with hypoglycemic activity, such as certain angiotensin converting enzyme inhibitors). Products include:
Prinivil 2241
Prinzide 2246

(⊙ Described in PDR® for Ophthalmic Medicines)

IMPORTANT NOTE: Always consult each drug listing in the patient's regimen for possible interactions.

Food Interactions

Alcohol (Insulin requirements may be decreased in the presence of drugs with hypoglycemic activity, such as alcohol).

Beer, reduced-alcohol (Insulin requirements may be decreased in the presence of drugs with hypoglycemic activity, such as alcohol).

Beer, unspecified (Insulin requirements may be decreased in the presence of drugs with hypoglycemic activity, such as alcohol).

Wine, Chianti (Insulin requirements may be decreased in the presence of drugs with hypoglycemic activity, such as alcohol).

Wine, Red (Insulin requirements may be decreased in the presence of drugs with hypoglycemic activity, such as alcohol).

Wine, unspecified (Insulin requirements may be decreased in the presence of drugs with hypoglycemic activity, such as alcohol).

Wine products (Insulin requirements may be decreased in the presence of drugs with hypoglycemic activity, such as alcohol).

HUMALOG MIX75/25-PEN AND KWIKPEN

See Humalog-Pen and KwikPen

HUMATROPE VIALS AND CARTRIDGES

May interact with anticonvulsants, corticosteroids, drugs which undergo biotransformation by cytochrome p-450 mixed function oxidase, estrogens, glucocorticoids, insulin, oral hypoglycemic agents, sex steroids, and certain other agents. Compounds in these categories include:

Alatrofloxacin Mesylate (Limited published data indicates that somatropin treatment increases cytochrome P450 (CP450)-mediated antipyrine clearance in man. These data suggest that somatropin administration may alter the clearance of compounds metabolized by CP450 liver enzymes. Therefore, careful monitoring is advised when somatropin is administered in combination with drugs metabolized by CP450 liver enzymes).
No products indexed under this heading.

Alclometasone Dipropionate (Introduction of somatropin treatment may result in inhibition of 11βHSD-1 and reduced serum cortisol concentrations. As a consequence, patients treated with glucocorticoid replacement therapy for previously diagnosed hypoadrenalism may require an increase in their maintenance or stress doses; this may be especially true for patients treated with cortisone acetate and prednisone. In addition, excessive glucocorticoid therapy may attenuate the growth promoting effects of somatropin in children. Therefore, glucocorticoid replacement therapy should be carefully adjusted in children with concomitant GH and glucocorticoid deficiency to avoid both hypoadrenalism and an inhibitory effect on growth. Also, somatropin administration may alter the clearance of compounds known to be metabolized by CYP450 liver enzymes (eg, corticosteroids). Careful monitoring is advisable when somatropin is administered in combination with other drugs known to be metabolized by CYP450 liver enzymes).
No products indexed under this heading.

Alfentanil Hydrochloride (Limited published data indicates that somatropin treatment increases cytochrome P450 (CP450)-mediated antipyrine clearance in man. These data suggest that somatropin administration may alter the clearance of compounds metabolized by CP450 liver enzymes. Therefore, careful monitoring is advised when somatropin is administered in combination with drugs metabolized by CP450 liver enzymes).
No products indexed under this heading.

Alprazolam (Limited published data indicates that somatropin treatment increases cytochrome P450 (CP450)-mediated antipyrine clearance in man. These data suggest that somatropin administration may alter the clearance of compounds metabolized by CP450 liver enzymes. Therefore, careful monitoring is advised when somatropin is administered in combination with drugs metabolized by CP450 liver enzymes).
No products indexed under this heading.

Aminophylline (Limited published data indicates that somatropin treatment increases cytochrome P450 (CP450)-mediated antipyrine clearance in man. These data suggest that somatropin administration may alter the clearance of compounds metabolized by CP450 liver enzymes. Therefore, careful monitoring is advised when somatropin is administered in combination with drugs metabolized by CP450 liver enzymes).
No products indexed under this heading.

Amiodarone Hydrochloride (Limited published data indicates that somatropin treatment increases cytochrome P450 (CP450)-mediated antipyrine clearance in man. These data suggest that somatropin administration may alter the clearance of compounds metabolized by CP450 liver enzymes. Therefore, careful monitoring is advised when somatropin is administered in combination with drugs metabolized by CP450 liver enzymes).
No products indexed under this heading.

Amitriptyline Hydrochloride (Limited published data indicates that somatropin treatment increases cytochrome P450 (CP450)-mediated antipyrine clearance in man. These data suggest that somatropin administration may

alter the clearance of compounds metabolized by CP450 liver enzymes. Therefore, careful monitoring is advised when somatropin is administered in combination with drugs metabolized by CP450 liver enzymes).
No products indexed under this heading.

Alclometasone Dipropionate (Introduction of somatropin treatment may result in inhibition of 11βHSD-1 and reduced serum cortisol concentrations. As a consequence, patients treated with glucocorticoid replacement therapy for previously diagnosed hypoadrenalism may require an increase in their maintenance or stress doses; this may be especially true for patients treated with cortisone acetate and prednisone. In addition, excessive glucocorticoid therapy may attenuate the growth promoting effects of somatropin in children. Therefore, glucocorticoid replacement therapy should be carefully adjusted in children with concomitant GH and glucocorticoid deficiency to avoid both hypoadrenalism and an inhibitory effect on growth. Also, somatropin administration may alter the clearance of compounds known to be metabolized by CYP450 liver enzymes (eg, corticosteroids). Careful monitoring is advisable when somatropin is administered in combination with other drugs known to be metabolized by CYP450 liver enzymes).
No products indexed under this heading.

Amlodipine Besylate (Limited published data indicates that somatropin treatment increases cytochrome P450 (CP450)-mediated antipyrine clearance in man. These data suggest that somatropin administration may alter the clearance of compounds metabolized by CP450 liver enzymes. Therefore, careful monitoring is advised when somatropin is administered in combination with drugs metabolized by CP450 liver enzymes). Products include:
Azor 1010
Exforge 2443
Exforge HCT 2449

Amoxapine (Limited published data indicates that somatropin treatment increases cytochrome P450 (CP450)-mediated antipyrine clearance in man. These data suggest that somatropin administration may alter the clearance of compounds metabolized by CP450 liver enzymes. Therefore, careful monitoring is advised when somatropin is administered in combination with drugs metabolized by CP450 liver enzymes).
No products indexed under this heading.

Amphetamine Aspartate (Limited published data indicates that somatropin treatment increases cytochrome P450 (CP450)-mediated antipyrine clearance in man. These data suggest that somatropin administration may alter the clearance of compounds metabolized by CP450 liver enzymes. Therefore, careful monitoring is advised when somatropin is administered in combination with drugs metabolized by CP450 liver enzymes).
No products indexed under this heading.

Amphetamine Aspartate Monohydrate (Limited published data indicates that somatropin treatment increases cytochrome P450 (CP450)-mediated antipyrine clearance in man. These data suggest that somatropin administration may alter the clearance of compounds metabolized by CP450 liver enzymes. Therefore, careful monitoring is advised when somatropin is administered in combination with drugs metabolized by CP450 liver enzymes).
No products indexed under this heading.

Amphetamine Sulfate (Limited published data indicates that somatropin treatment increases cytochrome P450 (CP450)-mediated antipyrine clearance in man. These data suggest that somatropin administration may alter the clearance of compounds metabolized by CP450 liver enzymes. Therefore, careful monitoring is advised when somatropin is administered in combination with drugs metabolized by CP450 liver enzymes).
No products indexed under this heading.

Anagrelide Hydrochloride (Limited published data indicates that somatropin treatment increases cytochrome P450 (CP450)-mediated antipyrine clearance in man. These data suggest that somatropin administration may alter the clearance of compounds metabolized by CP450 liver enzymes. Therefore, careful monitoring is advised when somatropin is administered in combination with drugs metabolized by CP450 liver enzymes).
No products indexed under this heading.

Antipyrine (Limited published data indicates that somatropin treatment increases cytochrome P450 (CP450)-mediated antipyrine clearance in man. These data suggest that somat-

ropin administration may alter the clearance of compounds metabolized by CP450 liver enzymes. Therefore, careful monitoring is advised when somatropin is administered in combination with drugs metabolized by CP450 liver enzymes).

No products indexed under this heading.

Aprepitant (Limited published data indicates that somatropin treatment increases cytochrome P450 (CP450)-mediated antipyrine clearance in man. These data suggest that somatropin administration may alter the clearance of compounds metabolized by CP450 liver enzymes. Therefore, careful monitoring is advised when somatropin is administered in combination with drugs metabolized by CP450 liver enzymes). Products include:

Emend **2124**

Astemizole (Limited published data indicates that somatropin treatment increases cytochrome P450 (CP450)-mediated antipyrine clearance in man. These data suggest that somatropin administration may alter the clearance of compounds metabolized by CP450 liver enzymes. Therefore, careful monitoring is advised when somatropin is administered in combination with drugs metabolized by CP450 liver enzymes).

No products indexed under this heading.

Atomoxetine Hydrochloride (Limited published data indicates that somatropin treatment increases cytochrome P450 (CP450)-mediated antipyrine clearance in man. These data suggest that somatropin administration may alter the clearance of compounds metabolized by CP450 liver enzymes. Therefore, careful monitoring is advised when somatropin is administered in combination with drugs metabolized by CP450 liver enzymes). Products include:

Strattera **1957**

Atorvastatin Calcium (Limited published data indicates that somatropin treatment increases cytochrome P450 (CP450)-mediated antipyrine clearance in man. These data suggest that somatropin administration may alter the clearance of compounds metabolized by CP450 liver enzymes. Therefore, careful monitoring is advised when somatropin is administered in combination with drugs metabolized by CP450 liver enzymes). Products include:

Lipitor **2703**

Beclomethasone Dipropionate (Introduction of somatropin treatment may result in inhibition of 11βHSD-1 and reduced serum cortisol concentrations. As a consequence, patients treated with glucocorticoid replacement therapy for previously diagnosed hypoadrenalism may require an increase in their maintenance or stress doses; this may be especially true for patients treated with cortisone acetate and prednisone. In addition, excessive glucocorticoid therapy may attenuate the growth promoting effects of somatropin in children. Therefore, glucocorticoid replacement therapy should be carefully adjusted in children with concomitant GH and glucocorticoid deficiency to avoid both hypoadrenalism and an inhibitory effect on growth. Also, somatropin administration may alter the clearance of compounds known to be metabolized by CYP450 liver enzymes (eg, corticosteroids). Careful monitoring is advisable when somatropin is administered in combination with other drugs known to be metabolized by CYP450 liver enzymes). Products include:

Qvar **3398**

Beclomethasone Dipropionate Monohydrate (Introduction of somatropin treatment may result in inhibition of 11βHSD-1 and reduced serum cortisol concentrations. As a consequence, patients treated with glucocorticoid replacement therapy for previously diagnosed hypoadrenalism may require an increase in their maintenance or stress doses; this may be especially true for patients treated with cortisone acetate and prednisone. In addition, excessive glucocorticoid therapy may attenuate the growth promoting effects of somatropin in children. Therefore, glucocorticoid replacement therapy should be carefully adjusted in children with concomitant GH and glucocorticoid deficiency to avoid both hypoadrenalism and an inhibitory effect on growth. Also, somatropin administration may alter the clearance of compounds known to be metabolized by CYP450 liver enzymes (eg, corticosteroids). Careful monitoring is advisable when somatropin is administered in combination with other drugs known to be metabolized by CYP450 liver enzymes). Products include:

Beconase AQ **1386**

Belladonna Ergotamine (Limited published data indicates that somatropin treatment increases cytochrome P450 (CP450)-mediated antipyrine clearance in man. These data suggest that somatropin administration may alter the clearance of compounds metabolized by CP450 liver enzymes. Therefore, careful monitoring is advised when somatropin is administered in combination with drugs metabolized by CP450 liver enzymes).

No products indexed under this heading.

Benzphetamine Hydrochloride (Limited published data indicates that somatropin treatment increases cytochrome P450 (CP450)-mediated antipyrine clearance in man. These data suggest that somatropin administration may alter the clearance of compounds metabolized by CP450 liver enzymes. Therefore, careful monitoring is advised when somatropin is administered in combination with drugs metabolized by CP450 liver enzymes).

No products indexed under this heading.

Betamethasone (Introduction of somatropin treatment may result in inhibition of 11βHSD-1 and reduced serum cortisol concentrations. As a consequence, patients treated with glucocorticoid replacement therapy for previously diagnosed hypoadrenalism may require an increase in their maintenance or stress doses; this may be especially true for patients treated with cortisone acetate and prednisone. In addition, excessive glucocorticoid therapy may attenuate the growth promoting effects of somatropin in children. Therefore, glucocorticoid replacement therapy should be carefully adjusted in children with concomitant GH and glucocorticoid deficiency to avoid both hypoadrenalism and an inhibitory effect on growth. Also, somatropin administration may alter the clearance of compounds known to be metabolized by CYP450 liver enzymes (eg, corticosteroids). Careful monitoring is advisable when somatropin is administered in combination with other drugs known to be metabolized by CYP450 liver enzymes).

No products indexed under this heading.

Betamethasone Acetate (Introduction of somatropin treatment may result in inhibition of 11βHSD-1 and reduced serum cortisol concentrations. As a consequence, patients treated with glucocorticoid replacement therapy for previously diagnosed hypoadrenalism may require an increase in their maintenance or stress doses; this may be especially true for patients treated with cortisone acetate and prednisone. In addition, excessive glucocorticoid therapy may attenuate the growth promoting effects of somatropin in children. Therefore, glucocorticoid replacement therapy should be carefully adjusted in children with concomitant GH and glucocorticoid deficiency to avoid both hypoadrenalism and an inhibitory effect on growth. Also, somatropin administration may alter the clearance of compounds known to be metabolized by CYP450 liver enzymes (eg, corticosteroids). Careful monitoring is advisable when somatropin is administered in combination with other drugs known to be metabolized by CYP450 liver enzymes).

No products indexed under this heading.

Betamethasone Benzoate (Introduction of somatropin treatment may result in inhibition of 11βHSD-1 and reduced serum cortisol concentrations. As a consequence, patients treated with glucocorticoid replacement therapy for previously diagnosed hypoadrenalism may require an increase in their maintenance or stress doses; this may be especially true for patients treated with cortisone acetate and prednisone. In addition, excessive glucocorticoid therapy may attenuate the growth promoting effects of somatropin in children. Therefore, glucocorticoid replacement therapy should be carefully adjusted in children with concomitant GH and glucocorticoid deficiency to avoid both hypoadrenalism and an inhibitory effect on growth. Also, somatropin administration may alter the clearance of compounds known to be metabolized by CYP450 liver enzymes (eg, corticosteroids). Careful monitoring is advisable when somatropin is administered in combination with other drugs known to be metabolized by CYP450 liver enzymes).

No products indexed under this heading.

Betamethasone Dipropionate (Introduction of somatropin treatment may result in inhibition of 11βHSD-1 and reduced serum cortisol concentrations. As a consequence, patients treated with glucocorticoid replacement therapy for previously diagnosed hypoadrenalism may require an increase in their maintenance or stress doses; this may be especially true for patients treated with cortisone acetate and prednisone. In addition, excessive glucocorticoid therapy may attenuate the growth promoting effects of somatropin in children. Therefore, glucocorticoid replacement therapy should be carefully adjusted in children with concomitant GH and glucocorticoid deficiency to avoid both hypoadrenalism and an inhibitory effect on growth. Also, somatropin administration may alter the clearance of compounds known to be metabolized by CYP450 liver enzymes (eg, corticosteroids). Careful monitoring is advisable when somatropin is administered in combination with other drugs known to be metabolized by CYP450 liver enzymes). Products include:

Diprolene Lotion 0.05% **3108**
Diprolene Ointment 0.05% **3109**
Diprolene AF Cream 0.05% **3107**
Lotrisone **3163**

Betamethasone Sodium Phosphate (Introduction of somatropin treatment may result in inhibition of 11βHSD-1 and reduced serum cortisol concentrations. As a consequence, patients treated with glucocorticoid replacement therapy for previously diagnosed hypoadrenalism may require an increase in their maintenance or stress doses; this may be especially true for patients treated with cortisone acetate and prednisone. In addition, excessive glucocorticoid therapy may attenuate the growth promoting effects of somatropin in children. Therefore, glucocorticoid replacement therapy should be carefully adjusted in children with concomitant GH and glucocorticoid deficiency to avoid both hypoadrenalism and an inhibitory effect on growth. Also, somatropin administration may alter the clearance of compounds known to be metabolized by CYP450 liver enzymes (eg, corticosteroids). Careful monitoring is advisable when somatropin is administered in combination with other drugs known to be metabolized by CYP450 liver enzymes).

No products indexed under this heading.

Betamethasone Valerate (Introduction of somatropin treatment may result in inhibition of 11βHSD-1 and reduced serum cortisol concentrations. As a consequence, patients treated with glucocorticoid replacement therapy for previously diagnosed hypoadrenalism may require an increase in their maintenance or stress doses; this may be especially true for patients treated with cortisone acetate and prednisone. In addition, excessive glucocorticoid therapy may attenuate the growth promoting effects of somatropin in children. Therefore, glucocorticoid replacement therapy should be carefully adjusted in children with concomitant GH and glucocorticoid deficiency to avoid both hypoadrenalism and an inhibitory effect on growth. Also, somatropin administration may alter the clearance of compounds known to be metabolized by CYP450 liver enzymes (eg, corticosteroids). Careful monitoring is advisable when somatropin is administered in combination with other drugs known to be metabolized by CYP450 liver enzymes). Products include:

Luxíq **3321**

Bisoprolol Fumarate (Limited published data indicates that somatropin treatment increases cytochrome P450 (CP450)-mediated antipyrine clearance in man. These data suggest that somatropin administration may alter the clearance of compounds metabolized by CP450 liver enzymes. Therefore, careful monitoring is advised when somatropin is administered in combination with drugs metabolized by CP450 liver enzymes).

No products indexed under this heading.

Bromocriptine Mesylate (Limited published data indicates that somatropin treatment increases cytochrome P450 (CP450)-mediated antipyrine clearance in man. These data suggest that somatropin administration may alter the clearance of compounds metabolized by CP450 liver enzymes. Therefore, careful monitoring is advised when somatropin is administered in combination with drugs metabolized by CP450 liver enzymes).

No products indexed under this heading.

Budesonide (Introduction of somatropin treatment may result in inhibition of 11βHSD-1 and reduced serum cortisol concentrations. As a consequence, patients treated with glucocorticoid replacement therapy for previously diagnosed hypoadrenalism may require an increase in their maintenance or stress doses; this may be especially true for patients treated with cortisone acetate and prednisone. In addition, excessive glucocorticoid therapy may attenuate the growth promoting effects of somatropin in children. Therefore, glucocorticoid replacement therapy should be carefully adjusted in children with concomitant GH and glucocorticoid deficiency to avoid both hypoadrenalism and an inhibitory effect on growth. Also, somatropin administration may alter the clearance of compounds known to be metabolized by CYP450 liver enzymes (eg, corticosteroids). Careful monitoring is advisable when somatropin is administered in combination with other drugs known to be metabolized by CYP450 liver enzymes). Products include:

Pulmicort Flexhaler **714**

IMPORTANT NOTE: Always consult each drug listing in the patient's regimen for possible interactions.

Symbicort 80/4.5 720
Symbicort 160/4.5 720

Buspirone Hydrochloride (Limited published data indicates that somatropin treatment increases cytochrome P450 (CP450)-mediated antipyrine clearance in man. These data suggest that somatropin administration may alter the clearance of compounds metabolized by CP450 liver enzymes. Therefore, careful monitoring is advised when somatropin is administered in combination with drugs metabolized by CP450 liver enzymes).

No products indexed under this heading.

Busulfan (Limited published data indicates that somatropin treatment increases cytochrome P450 (CP450)-mediated antipyrine clearance in man. These data suggest that somatropin administration may alter the clearance of compounds metabolized by CP450 liver enzymes. Therefore, careful monitoring is advised when somatropin is administered in combination with drugs metabolized by CP450 liver enzymes). Products include:
Myleran 1581

Caffeine (Limited published data indicates that somatropin treatment increases cytochrome P450 (CP450)-mediated antipyrine clearance in man. These data suggest that somatropin administration may alter the clearance of compounds metabolized by CP450 liver enzymes. Therefore, careful monitoring is advised when somatropin is administered in combination with drugs metabolized by CP450 liver enzymes).

No products indexed under this heading.

Caffeine Anhydrous (Limited published data indicates that somatropin treatment increases cytochrome P450 (CP450)-mediated antipyrine clearance in man. These data suggest that somatropin administration may alter the clearance of compounds metabolized by CP450 liver enzymes. Therefore, careful monitoring is advised when somatropin is administered in combination with drugs metabolized by CP450 liver enzymes).

No products indexed under this heading.

Caffeine Citrate (Limited published data indicates that somatropin treatment increases cytochrome P450 (CP450)-mediated antipyrine clearance in man. These data suggest that somatropin administration may alter the clearance of compounds metabolized by CP450 liver enzymes. Therefore, careful monitoring is advised when somatropin is administered in combination with drugs metabolized by CP450 liver enzymes).

No products indexed under this heading.

Caffeine-containing medications (Limited published data indicates that somatropin treatment increases cytochrome P450 (CP450)-mediated antipyrine clearance in man. These data suggest that somatropin administration may alter the clearance of compounds metabolized by CP450 liver enzymes. Therefore, careful monitoring is advised when somatropin is administered in combination with drugs metabolized by CP450 liver enzymes).

No products indexed under this heading.

Caffeine Sodium Benzoate (Limited published data indicates that somatropin treatment increases cytochrome P450 (CP450)-mediated antipyrine clearance in man. These data suggest that somatropin administration may alter the clearance of compounds metabolized by CP450 liver enzymes. Therefore, careful monitoring is advised when somatropin is administered in combination with drugs metabolized by CP450 liver enzymes).

No products indexed under this heading.

Candesartan Cilexetil (Limited published data indicates that somatropin treatment increases cytochrome P450 (CP450)-mediated antipyrine clearance in man. These data suggest that somatropin administration may alter the clearance of compounds metabolized by CP450 liver enzymes. Therefore, careful monitoring is advised when somatropin is administered in combination with drugs metabolized by CP450 liver enzymes). Products include:
Atacand 697
Atacand HCT 700

Captopril (Limited published data indicates that somatropin treatment increases cytochrome P450 (CP450)-mediated antipyrine clearance in man. These data suggest that somatropin administration may alter the clearance of compounds metabolized by CP450 liver enzymes. Therefore, careful monitoring is advised when somatropin is administered in combination with drugs metabolized by CP450 liver enzymes). Products include:
Captopril 2341

Carbamazepine (Limited published data indicates that somatropin treatment increases cytochrome P450 (CP450)-mediated antipyrine clearance in man. These data suggest that somatropin administration may alter the clearance of compounds metabolized by CP450 liver enzymes (eg, anticonvulsants). Therefore, careful monitoring is advised when somatropin is administered in combination with drugs metabolized by CP450 liver enzymes). Products include:
Carbatrol 3280
Equetro 3477

Carisoprodol (Limited published data indicates that somatropin treatment increases cytochrome P450 (CP450)-mediated antipyrine clearance in man. These data suggest that somatropin administration may alter the clearance of compounds metabolized by CP450 liver enzymes. Therefore, careful monitoring is advised when somatropin is administered in combination with drugs metabolized by CP450 liver enzymes).

No products indexed under this heading.

Carvedilol (Limited published data indicates that somatropin treatment increases cytochrome P450 (CP450)-mediated antipyrine clearance in man. These data suggest that somatropin administration may alter the clearance of compounds metabolized by CP450 liver enzymes. Therefore, careful monitoring is advised when somatropin is administered in combination with drugs metabolized by CP450 liver enzymes). Products include:
Coreg 1409

Celecoxib (Limited published data indicates that somatropin treatment increases cytochrome P450 (CP450)-mediated antipyrine clearance in man. These data suggest that somatropin administration may alter the clearance of compounds metabolized by CP450 liver enzymes. Therefore, careful monitoring is advised when somatropin is administered in combination with drugs metabolized by CP450 liver enzymes). Products include:
Celebrex 3272

Cerivastatin Sodium (Limited published data indicates that somatropin treatment increases cytochrome P450 (CP450)-mediated antipyrine clearance in man. These data suggest that somatropin administration may alter the clearance of compounds metabolized by CP450 liver enzymes. Therefore, careful monitoring is advised when somatro-

pin is administered in combination with drugs metabolized by CP450 liver enzymes.

No products indexed under this heading.

Cevimeline Hydrochloride (Limited published data indicates that somatropin treatment increases cytochrome P450 (CP450)-mediated antipyrine clearance in man. These data suggest that somatropin administration may alter the clearance of compounds metabolized by CP450 liver enzymes. Therefore, careful monitoring is advised when somatropin is administered in combination with drugs metabolized by CP450 liver enzymes). Products include:
Evoxac 1027

Chlordiazepoxide (Limited published data indicates that somatropin treatment increases cytochrome P450 (CP450)-mediated antipyrine clearance in man. These data suggest that somatropin administration may alter the clearance of compounds metabolized by CP450 liver enzymes. Therefore, careful monitoring is advised when somatropin is administered in combination with drugs metabolized by CP450 liver enzymes).

No products indexed under this heading.

Chlordiazepoxide Hydrochloride (Limited published data indicates that somatropin treatment increases cytochrome P450 (CP450)-mediated antipyrine clearance in man. These data suggest that somatropin administration may alter the clearance of compounds metabolized by CP450 liver enzymes. Therefore, careful monitoring is advised when somatropin is administered in combination with drugs metabolized by CP450 liver enzymes).

No products indexed under this heading.

Chlorotrianisene (Because oral estrogens may reduce the serum insulin-like growth factor I (IGF-I) response to somatropin treatment, girls and women receiving oral estrogen replacement may require greater somatropin dosages).

No products indexed under this heading.

Chlorpheniramine (Limited published data indicates that somatropin treatment increases cytochrome P450 (CP450)-mediated antipyrine clearance in man. These data suggest that somatropin administration may alter the clearance of compounds metabolized by CP450 liver enzymes. Therefore, careful monitoring is advised when somatropin is administered in combination with drugs metabolized by CP450 liver enzymes).

No products indexed under this heading.

Chlorpheniramine Maleate (Limited published data indicates that somatropin treatment increases cytochrome P450 (CP450)-mediated antipyrine clearance in man. These data suggest that somatropin administration may alter the clearance of compounds metabolized by CP450 liver enzymes. Therefore, careful monitoring is advised when somatropin is administered in combination with drugs metabolized by CP450 liver enzymes).

No products indexed under this heading.

Chlorpheniramine Polistirex (Limited published data indicates that somatropin treatment increases cytochrome P450 (CP450)-mediated antipyrine clearance in man. These data suggest that somatropin administration may alter the clearance of compounds metabolized by CP450 liver enzymes. Therefore, careful monitoring is advised when somatropin is administered in combination with drugs metabolized by CP450 liver enzymes). Products include:
Tussionex 3443

Chlorpheniramine Tannate (Limited published data indicates that somatropin treatment increases cytochrome P450 (CP450)-mediated antipyrine clearance in man. These data suggest that somatropin administration may alter the clearance of compounds metabolized by CP450 liver enzymes. Therefore, careful monitoring is advised when somatropin is administered in combination with drugs metabolized by CP450 liver enzymes).

No products indexed under this heading.

Chlorpromazine (Limited published data indicates that somatropin treatment increases cytochrome P450 (CP450)-mediated antipyrine clearance in man. These data suggest that somatropin administration may alter the clearance of compounds metabolized by CP450 liver enzymes. Therefore, careful monitoring is advised when somatropin is administered in combination with drugs metabolized by CP450 liver enzymes).

No products indexed under this heading.

Chlorpromazine Hydrochloride (Limited published data indicates that somatropin treatment increases cytochrome P450 (CP450)-mediated antipyrine clearance in man. These data suggest that somatropin administration may alter the clearance of compounds metabolized by CP450 liver enzymes. Therefore, careful monitoring is advised when somatropin is administered in combination with drugs metabolized by CP450 liver enzymes).

No products indexed under this heading.

Chlorpropamide (Patients with diabetes mellitus who receive concomitant treatment with somatropin may require adjustment of their doses of insulin and/or other hypoglycemic agents).

No products indexed under this heading.

Ciclesonide (Introduction of somatropin treatment may result in inhibition of 11βHSD-1 and reduced serum cortisol concentrations. As a consequence, patients treated with glucocorticoid replacement therapy for previously diagnosed hypoadrenalism may require an increase in their maintenance or stress doses; this may be especially true for patients treated with cortisone acetate and prednisone. In addition, excessive glucocorticoid therapy may attenuate the growth promoting effects of somatropin in children. Therefore, glucocorticoid replacement therapy should be carefully adjusted in children with concomitant GH and glucocorticoid deficiency to avoid both hypoadrenalism and an inhibitory effect on growth. Also, somatropin administration may alter the clearance of compounds known to be metabolized by CYP450 liver enzymes (eg, corticosteroids). Careful monitoring is advisable when somatropin is administered in combination with other drugs known to be metabolized by CYP450 liver enzymes).

No products indexed under this heading.

Cilostazol (Limited published data indicates that somatropin treatment increases cytochrome P450 (CP450)-mediated antipyrine clearance in man. These data suggest that somatropin administration may alter the clearance of compounds metabolized by CP450 liver enzymes. Therefore, careful monitoring is advised when somatropin is administered in combination with drugs metabolized by CP450 liver enzymes).

No products indexed under this heading.

Cimetidine Hydrochloride (Limited published data indicates that somatropin treatment increases cytochrome P450 (CP450)-mediated antipyrine clearance in man. These data suggest that somatropin administration may alter the clearance of compounds

803 Interactions Index Humatrope

metabolized by CP450 liver enzymes. Therefore, careful monitoring is advised when somatropin is administered in combination with drugs metabolized by CP450 liver enzymes).
No products indexed under this heading.

Ciprofloxacin (Limited published data indicates that somatropin treatment increases cytochrome P450 (CP450)-mediated antipyrine clearance in man. These data suggest that somatropin administration may alter the clearance of compounds metabolized by CP450 liver enzymes. Therefore, careful monitoring is advised when somatropin is administered in combination with drugs metabolized by CP450 liver enzymes). Products include:
Cipro I.V. 3082
Cipro 3073
Cipro XR 3091
Ciprodex 583

Ciprofloxacin Hydrochloride (Limited published data indicates that somatropin treatment increases cytochrome P450 (CP450)-mediated antipyrine clearance in man. These data suggest that somatropin administration may alter the clearance of compounds metabolized by CP450 liver enzymes. Therefore, careful monitoring is advised when somatropin is administered in combination with drugs metabolized by CP450 liver enzymes). Products include:
Cipro 3073

Cisapride (Limited published data indicates that somatropin treatment increases cytochrome P450 (CP450)-mediated antipyrine clearance in man. These data suggest that somatropin administration may alter the clearance of compounds metabolized by CP450 liver enzymes. Therefore, careful monitoring is advised when somatropin is administered in combination with drugs metabolized by CP450 liver enzymes).
No products indexed under this heading.

Citalopram Hydrobromide (Limited published data indicates that somatropin treatment increases cytochrome P450 (CP450)-mediated antipyrine clearance in man. These data suggest that somatropin administration may alter the clearance of compounds metabolized by CP450 liver enzymes. Therefore, careful monitoring is advised when somatropin is administered in combination with drugs metabolized by CP450 liver enzymes). Products include:
Celexa 1153

Clarithromycin (Limited published data indicates that somatropin treatment increases cytochrome P450 (CP450)-mediated antipyrine clearance in man. These data suggest that somatropin administration may alter the clearance of compounds metabolized by CP450 liver enzymes. Therefore, careful monitoring is advised when somatropin is administered in combination with drugs metabolized by CP450 liver enzymes). Products include:
Biaxin/Biaxin XL 412

Clomipramine Hydrochloride (Limited published data indicates that somatropin treatment increases cytochrome P450 (CP450)-mediated antipyrine clearance in man. These data suggest that somatropin administration may alter the clearance of compounds metabolized by CP450 liver enzymes. Therefore, careful monitoring is advised when somatropin is administered in combination with drugs metabolized by CP450 liver enzymes).
No products indexed under this heading.

Clopidogrel Bisulfate (Limited published data indicates that somatropin treatment increases cytochrome P450 (CP450)-mediated antipyrine clearance in man. These data suggest that somatropin administration may alter the clearance of compounds metabolized by CP450 liver enzymes. Therefore, careful monitoring is advised when somatropin is administered in combination with drugs metabolized by CP450 liver enzymes). Products include:
Plavix 3027

Clopidogrel Hydrogen Sulfate (Limited published data indicates that somatropin treatment increases cytochrome P450 (CP450)-mediated antipyrine clearance in man. These data suggest that somatropin administration may alter the clearance of compounds metabolized by CP450 liver enzymes. Therefore, careful monitoring is advised when somatropin is administered in combination with drugs metabolized by CP450 liver enzymes).
No products indexed under this heading.

Clozapine (Limited published data indicates that somatropin treatment increases cytochrome P450 (CP450)-mediated antipyrine clearance in man. These data suggest that somatropin administration may alter the clearance of compounds metabolized by CP450 liver enzymes. Therefore, careful monitoring is advised when somatropin is administered in combination with drugs metabolized by CP450 liver enzymes).
No products indexed under this heading.

Codeine Phosphate (Limited published data indicates that somatropin treatment increases cytochrome P450 (CP450)-mediated antipyrine clearance in man. These data suggest that somatropin administration may alter the clearance of compounds metabolized by CP450 liver enzymes. Therefore, careful monitoring is advised when somatropin is administered in combination with drugs metabolized by CP450 liver enzymes). Products include:
Tylenol with Codeine 2691

Codeine Sulfate (Limited published data indicates that somatropin treatment increases cytochrome P450 (CP450)-mediated antipyrine clearance in man. These data suggest that somatropin administration may alter the clearance of compounds metabolized by CP450 liver enzymes. Therefore, careful monitoring is advised when somatropin is administered in combination with drugs metabolized by CP450 liver enzymes).
No products indexed under this heading.

Cortisol (Introduction of somatropin treatment may result in inhibition of 11βHSD-1 and reduced serum cortisol concentrations. As a consequence, patients treated with glucocorticoid replacement therapy for previously diagnosed hypoadrenalism may require an increase in their maintenance or stress doses; this may be especially true for patients treated with cortisone acetate and prednisone. In addition, excessive glucocorticoid therapy may attenuate the growth promoting effects of somatropin in children. Therefore, glucocorticoid replacement therapy should be carefully adjusted in children with concomitant GH and glucocorticoid deficiency to avoid both hypoadrenalism and an inhibitory effect on growth. Also, somatropin administration may alter the clearance of compounds known to be metabolized by CYP450 liver enzymes (eg, corticosteroids). Careful monitoring is advisable when somatropin is administered in combination with other drugs known to be metabolized by CYP450 liver enzymes 1).
No products indexed under this heading.

Cortisone Acetate (Introduction of somatropin treatment may result in inhibition of 11βHSD-1 and reduced serum cortisol concentrations.As a consequence, patients treated with glucocorticoid replacement therapy for previously diagnosed hypoadrenalism may require an increase in their maintenance or stress doses; this may be especially true for patients treated with cortisone acetate and prednisone. In addition, excessive glucocorticoid therapy may attenuate the growth promoting effects of somatropin in children. Therefore, glucocorticoid replacement therapy should be carefully adjusted in children with concomitant GH and glucocorticoid deficiency to avoid both hypoadrenalism and an inhibitory effect on growth. Also, somatropin administration may alter the clearance of compounds known to be metabolized by CYP450 liver enzymes (eg, corticosteroids). Careful monitoring is advisable when somatropin is administered in combination with other drugs known to be metabolized by CYP450 liver enzymes).
No products indexed under this heading.

Cyclobenzaprine (Limited published data indicates that somatropin treatment increases cytochrome P450 (CP450)-mediated antipyrine clearance in man. These data suggest that somatropin administration may alter the clearance of compounds metabolized by CP450 liver enzymes. Therefore, careful monitoring is advised when somatropin is administered in combination with drugs metabolized by CP450 liver enzymes).
No products indexed under this heading.

Cyclobenzaprine Hydrochloride (Limited published data indicates that somatropin treatment increases cytochrome P450 (CP450)-mediated antipyrine clearance in man. These data suggest that somatropin administration may alter the clearance of compounds metabolized by CP450 liver enzymes. Therefore, careful monitoring is advised when somatropin is administered in combination with drugs metabolized by CP450 liver enzymes). Products include:
Amrix 964

Cyclophosphamide (Limited published data indicates that somatropin treatment increases cytochrome P450 (CP450)-mediated antipyrine clearance in man. These data suggest that somatropin administration may alter the clearance of compounds metabolized by CP450 liver enzymes. Therefore, careful monitoring is advised when somatropin is administered in combination with drugs metabolized by CP450 liver enzymes).
No products indexed under this heading.

Cyclosporine (Limited published data indicates that somatropin treatment increases cytochrome P450 (CP450)-mediated antipyrine clearance in man. These data suggest that somatropin administration may alter the clearance of compounds metabolized by CP450 liver enzymes (eg, corticosteroids, sex steroids, anticonvulsants, cyclosporine). Therefore, careful monitoring is advised when somatropin is administered in combination with drugs metabolized by CP450 liver enzymes). Products include:
Gengraf 440
Neoral Oral Solution 2496
Neoral Capsules 2496
Restasis 605

Desipramine Hydrochloride (Limited published data indicates that somatropin treatment increases cytochrome P450 (CP450)-mediated antipyrine clearance in man. These data suggest that somatropin administration may alter the clearance of compounds metabolized by CP450 liver enzymes. Therefore, careful monitoring is advised when somatropin is administered in combination with drugs metabolized by CP450 liver enzymes).
No products indexed under this heading.

Desogestrel (Limited published data indicates that somatropin treatment increases cytochrome P450 (CP450)-mediated antipyrine clearance in man. These data suggest that somatropin administration may alter the clearance of compounds metabolized by CP450 liver enzymes (eg, sex steroids). Therefore, careful monitoring is advised when somatropin is administered in combination with drugs metabolized by CP450 liver enzymes).
No products indexed under this heading.

Desoximetasone (Introduction of somatropin treatment may result in inhibition of 11βHSD-1 and reduced serum cortisol concentrations. As a consequence, patients treated with glucocorticoid replacement therapy for previously diagnosed hypoadrenalism may require an increase in their maintenance or stress doses; this may be especially true for patients treated with cortisone acetate and prednisone. In addition, excessive glucocorticoid therapy may attenuate the growth promoting effects of somatropin in children. Therefore, glucocorticoid replacement therapy should be carefully adjusted in children with concomitant GH and glucocorticoid deficiency to avoid both hypoadrenalism and an inhibitory effect on growth. Also, somatropin administration may alter the clearance of compounds known to be metabolized by CYP450 liver enzymes (eg, corticosteroids). Careful monitoring is advisable when somatropin is administered in combination with other drugs known to be metabolized by CYP450 liver enzymes).
No products indexed under this heading.

Dexamethasone (Introduction of somatropin treatment may result in inhibition of 11βHSD-1 and reduced serum cortisol concentrations. As a consequence, patients treated with glucocorticoid replacement therapy for previously diagnosed hypoadrenalism may require an increase in their maintenance or stress doses; this may be especially true for patients treated with cortisone acetate and prednisone. In addition, excessive glucocorticoid therapy may attenuate the growth promoting effects of somatropin in children. Therefore, glucocorticoid replacement therapy should be carefully adjusted in children with concomitant GH and glucocorticoid deficiency to avoid both hypoadrenalism and an inhibitory effect on growth. Also, somatropin administration may alter the clearance of compounds known to be metabolized by CYP450 liver enzymes (eg, corticosteroids). Careful monitoring is advisable when somatropin is administered in combination with other drugs known to be metabolized by CYP450 liver enzymes). Products include:
Ciprodex 583
Ozurdex .... ⊙ 223
Tobramycin and Dexamethasone Ophthalmic Suspension .... ⊙ 251

Dexamethasone Acetate (Introduction of somatropin treatment may result in inhibition of 11βHSD-1 and reduced serum cortisol concentrations. As a consequence, patients treated with glucocorticoid replacement therapy for previously diagnosed hypoadrenalism may require an increase in their maintenance or stress doses; this may be especially true for patients treated with cortisone acetate and prednisone. In addition, excessive glucocorticoid therapy may attenuate the growth promoting effects of somatropin in children. Therefore, glucocorticoid replacement therapy should be carefully adjusted in children with concomitant GH and gluco-

IMPORTANT NOTE: Always consult each drug listing in the patient's regimen for possible interactions.

corticoid deficiency to avoid both hypoadrenalism and an inhibitory effect on growth. Also, somatropin administration may alter the clearance of compounds known to be metabolized by CYP450 liver enzymes (eg, corticosteroids). Careful monitoring is advisable when somatropin is administered in combination with other drugs known to be metabolized by CYP450 liver enzymes).
No products indexed under this heading.

Dexamethasone Phosphate (Introduction of somatropin treatment may result in inhibition of 11βHSD-1 and reduced serum cortisol concentrations. As a consequence, patients treated with glucocorticoid replacement therapy for previously diagnosed hypoadrenalism may require an increase in their maintenance or stress doses; this may be especially true for patients treated with cortisone acetate and prednisone. In addition, excessive glucocorticoid therapy may attenuate the growth promoting effects of somatropin in children. Therefore, glucocorticoid replacement therapy should be carefully adjusted in children with concomitant GH and glucocorticoid deficiency to avoid both hypoadrenalism and an inhibitory effect on growth. Also, somatropin administration may alter the clearance of compounds known to be metabolized by CYP450 liver enzymes (eg, corticosteroids). Careful monitoring is advisable when somatropin is administered in combination with other drugs known to be metabolized by CYP450 liver enzymes).
No products indexed under this heading.

Dexamethasone Sodium (Introduction of somatropin treatment may result in inhibition of 11βHSD-1 and reduced serum cortisol concentrations. As a consequence, patients treated with glucocorticoid replacement therapy for previously diagnosed hypoadrenalism may require an increase in their maintenance or stress doses; this may be especially true for patients treated with cortisone acetate and prednisone. In addition, excessive glucocorticoid therapy may attenuate the growth promoting effects of somatropin in children. Therefore, glucocorticoid replacement therapy should be carefully adjusted in children with concomitant GH and glucocorticoid deficiency to avoid both hypoadrenalism and an inhibitory effect on growth. Also, somatropin administration may alter the clearance of compounds known to be metabolized by CYP450 liver enzymes (eg, corticosteroids). Careful monitoring is advisable when somatropin is administered in combination with other drugs known to be metabolized by CYP450 liver enzymes).
No products indexed under this heading.

Dexamethasone Sodium Phosphate (Introduction of somatropin treatment may result in inhibition of 11βHSD-1 and reduced serum cortisol concentrations. As a consequence, patients treated with glucocorticoid replacement therapy for previously diagnosed hypoadrenalism may require an increase in their maintenance or stress doses; this may be especially true for patients treated with cortisone acetate and prednisone. In addition, excessive glucocorticoid therapy may attenuate the growth promoting effects of somatropin in children. Therefore, glucocorticoid replacement therapy should be carefully adjusted in children with concomitant GH and glucocorticoid deficiency to avoid both hypoadrenalism and an inhibitory effect on growth. Also, somatropin administration may alter the clearance of compounds known to be metabolized by CYP450 liver enzymes (eg, corticosteroids). Careful monitoring is advisable when somatropin is administered in combination with other drugs known to be metabolized by CYP450 liver enzymes).
No products indexed under this heading.

Dexamethasone Sodium Phosphate Injection (Introduction of somatropin treatment may result in inhibition of 11βHSD-1 and reduced serum cortisol concentrations. As a consequence, patients treated with glucocorticoid replacement therapy for previously diagnosed hypoadrenalism may require an increase in their maintenance or stress doses; this may be especially true for patients treated with cortisone acetate and prednisone. In addition, excessive glucocorticoid therapy may attenuate the growth promoting effects of somatropin in children. Therefore, glucocorticoid replacement therapy should be carefully adjusted in children with concomitant GH and glucocorticoid deficiency to avoid both hypoadrenalism and an inhibitory effect on growth. Also, somatropin administration may alter the clearance of compounds known to be metabolized by CYP450 liver enzymes (eg, corticosteroids). Careful monitoring is advisable when somatropin is administered in combination with other drugs known to be metabolized by CYP450 liver enzymes).
No products indexed under this heading.

Dexfenfluramine Hydrochloride (Limited published data indicates that somatropin treatment increases cytochrome P450 (CP450)-mediated antipyrine clearance in man. These data suggest that somatropin administration may alter the clearance of compounds metabolized by CP450 liver enzymes. Therefore, careful monitoring is advised when somatropin is administered in combination with drugs metabolized by CP450 liver enzymes).
No products indexed under this heading.

Dextromethorphan (Limited published data indicates that somatropin treatment increases cytochrome P450 (CP450)-mediated antipyrine clearance in man. These data suggest that somatropin administration may alter the clearance of compounds metabolized by CP450 liver enzymes. Therefore, careful monitoring is advised when somatropin is administered in combination with drugs metabolized by CP450 liver enzymes).
No products indexed under this heading.

Dextromethorphan Hydrobromide (Limited published data indicates that somatropin treatment increases cytochrome P450 (CP450)-mediated antipyrine clearance in man. These data suggest that somatropin administration may alter the clearance of compounds metabolized by CP450 liver enzymes. Therefore, careful monitoring is advised when somatropin is administered in combination with drugs metabolized by CP450 liver enzymes).
No products indexed under this heading.

Dextromethorphan Polistirex (Limited published data indicates that somatropin treatment increases cytochrome P450 (CP450)-mediated antipyrine clearance in man. These data suggest that somatropin administration may alter the clearance of compounds metabolized by CP450 liver enzymes. Therefore, careful monitoring is advised when somatropin is administered in combination with drugs metabolized by CP450 liver enzymes).
No products indexed under this heading.

Diazepam (Limited published data indicates that somatropin treatment increases cytochrome P450 (CP450)-mediated antipyrine clearance in man. These data suggest that somatropin administration may alter the clearance of compounds metabolized by CP450 liver enzymes. Therefore, careful monitoring is advised when somatropin is administered in combination with drugs metabolized by CP450 liver enzymes). Products include:
Valium Tablets **2880**

Diclofenac Potassium (Limited published data indicates that somatropin treatment increases cytochrome P450 (CP450)-mediated antipyrine clearance in man. These data suggest that somatropin administration may alter the clearance of compounds metabolized by CP450 liver enzymes. Therefore, careful monitoring is advised when somatropin is administered in combination with drugs metabolized by CP450 liver enzymes).
No products indexed under this heading.

Diclofenac Sodium (Limited published data indicates that somatropin treatment increases cytochrome P450 (CP450)-mediated antipyrine clearance in man. These data suggest that somatropin administration may alter the clearance of compounds metabolized by CP450 liver enzymes. Therefore, careful monitoring is advised when somatropin is administered in combination with drugs metabolized by CP450 liver enzymes).
No products indexed under this heading.

Dienestrol (Because oral estrogens may reduce the serum insulin-like growth factor I (IGF-I) response to somatropin treatment, girls and women receiving oral estrogen replacement may require greater somatropin dosages).
No products indexed under this heading.

Diethylstilbestrol (Because oral estrogens may reduce the serum insulin-like growth factor I (IGF-I) response to somatropin treatment, girls and women receiving oral estrogen replacement may require greater somatropin dosages).
No products indexed under this heading.

Diflorasone Diacetate (Introduction of somatropin treatment may result in inhibition of 11βHSD-1 and reduced serum cortisol concentrations. As a consequence, patients treated with glucocorticoid replacement therapy for previously diagnosed hypoadrenalism may require an increase in their maintenance or stress doses; this may be especially true for patients treated with cortisone acetate and prednisone. In addition, excessive glucocorticoid therapy may attenuate the growth promoting effects of somatropin in children. Therefore, glucocorticoid replacement therapy should be carefully adjusted in children with concomitant GH and glucocorticoid deficiency to avoid both hypoadrenalism and an inhibitory effect on growth. Also, somatropin administration may alter the clearance of compounds known to be metabolized by CYP450 liver enzymes (eg, corticosteroids). Careful monitoring is advisable when somatropin is administered in combination with other drugs known to be metabolized by CYP450 liver enzymes).
No products indexed under this heading.

Dihydroergotamine Mesylate (Limited published data indicates that somatropin treatment increases cytochrome P450 (CP450)-mediated antipyrine clearance in man. These data suggest that somatropin administration may alter the clearance of compounds metabolized by CP450 liver enzymes. Therefore, careful monitoring is advised when somatropin is administered in combination with drugs metabolized by CP450 liver enzymes).
No products indexed under this heading.

Diltiazem Hydrochloride (Limited published data indicates that somatropin treatment increases cytochrome P450 (CP450)-mediated antipyrine clearance in man. These data suggest that somatropin administration may alter the clearance of compounds metabolized by CP450 liver enzymes. Therefore, careful monitoring is advised when somatropin is administered in combination with drugs metabolized by CP450 liver enzymes). Products include:
Cardizem LA **423**

Diltiazem Maleate (Limited published data indicates that somatropin treatment increases cytochrome P450 (CP450)-mediated antipyrine clearance in man. These data suggest that somatropin administration may alter the clearance of compounds metabolized by CP450 liver enzymes. Therefore, careful monitoring is advised when somatropin is administered in combination with drugs metabolized by CP450 liver enzymes).
No products indexed under this heading.

Disopyramide (Limited published data indicates that somatropin treatment increases cytochrome P450 (CP450)-mediated antipyrine clearance in man. These data suggest that somatropin administration may alter the clearance of compounds metabolized by CP450 liver enzymes. Therefore, careful monitoring is advised when somatropin is administered in combination with drugs metabolized by CP450 liver enzymes).
No products indexed under this heading.

Disopyramide Phosphate (Limited published data indicates that somatropin treatment increases cytochrome P450 (CP450)-mediated antipyrine clearance in man. These data suggest that somatropin administration may alter the clearance of compounds metabolized by CP450 liver enzymes. Therefore, careful monitoring is advised when somatropin is administered in combination with drugs metabolized by CP450 liver enzymes).
No products indexed under this heading.

Disulfiram (Limited published data indicates that somatropin treatment increases cytochrome P450 (CP450)-mediated antipyrine clearance in man. These data suggest that somatropin administration may alter the clearance of compounds metabolized by CP450 liver enzymes. Therefore, careful monitoring is advised when somatropin is administered in combination with drugs metabolized by CP450 liver enzymes).
No products indexed under this heading.

Divalproex Sodium (Limited published data indicates that somatropin treatment increases cytochrome P450 (CP450)-mediated antipyrine clearance in man. These data suggest that somatropin administration may alter the clearance of compounds metabolized by CP450 liver enzymes (eg, anticonvulsants). Therefore, careful monitoring is advised when somatropin is administered in combination with drugs metabolized by CP450 liver enzymes). Products include:
Depakote ER **426**

Docetaxel (Limited published data indicates that somatropin treatment increases cytochrome P450 (CP450)-mediated antipyrine clearance in man. These data suggest that somatropin administration may alter the clearance of compounds metabolized by CP450 liver enzymes. Therefore, careful monitoring is advised when somatropin is administered in combination with drugs metabolized by CP450 liver enzymes). Products include:
Taxotere **3035**

Dolasetron Mesylate (Limited published data indicates that somatropin treatment increases cytochrome P450 (CP450)-mediated antipyrine clearance

in man. These data suggest that somatropin administration may alter the clearance of compounds metabolized by CP450 liver enzymes. Therefore, careful monitoring is advised when somatropin is administered in combination with drugs metabolized by CP450 liver enzymes. Products include:

Donepezil Hydrochloride (Limited published data indicates that somatropin treatment increases cytochrome P450 (CP450)-mediated antipyrine clearance in man. These data suggest that somatropin administration may alter the clearance of compounds metabolized by CP450 liver enzymes. Therefore, careful monitoring is advised when somatropin is administered in combination with drugs metabolized by CP450 liver enzymes. Products include:

Doxepin Hydrochloride (Limited published data indicates that somatropin treatment increases cytochrome P450 (CP450)-mediated antipyrine clearance in man. These data suggest that somatropin administration may alter the clearance of compounds metabolized by CP450 liver enzymes. Therefore, careful monitoring is advised when somatropin is administered in combination with drugs metabolized by CP450 liver enzymes.)

No products indexed under this heading.

Doxorubicin Hydrochloride (Limited published data indicates that somatropin treatment increases cytochrome P450 (CP450)-mediated antipyrine clearance in man. These data suggest that somatropin administration may alter the clearance of compounds metabolized by CP450 liver enzymes. Therefore, careful monitoring is advised when somatropin is administered in combination with drugs metabolized by CP450 liver enzymes.)

No products indexed under this heading.

Dronabinol (Limited published data indicates that somatropin treatment increases cytochrome P450 (CP450)-mediated antipyrine clearance in man. These data suggest that somatropin administration may alter the clearance of compounds metabolized by CP450 liver enzymes. Therefore, careful monitoring is advised when somatropin is administered in combination with drugs metabolized by CP450 liver enzymes.)

No products indexed under this heading.

Drugs that Undergo Biotransformation by Cytochrome P-450 Mixed Function Oxidase (Limited published data indicates that somatropin treatment increases cytochrome P450 (CP450)-mediated antipyrine clearance in man. These data suggest that somatropin administration may alter the clearance of compounds metabolized by CP450 liver enzymes. Therefore, careful monitoring is advised when somatropin is administered in combination with drugs metabolized by CP450 liver enzymes.)

No products indexed under this heading.

Dyphylline (Limited published data indicates that somatropin treatment increases cytochrome P450 (CP450)-mediated antipyrine clearance in man. These data suggest that somatropin administration may alter the clearance of compounds metabolized by CP450 liver enzymes. Therefore, careful monitoring is advised when somatropin is administered in combination with drugs metabolized by CP450 liver enzymes.)

No products indexed under this heading.

Encainide Hydrochloride (Limited published data indicates that somatropin treatment increases cytochrome P450 (CP450)-mediated antipyrine clearance in man. These data suggest that somatropin administration may alter the clearance of compounds metabolized by CP450 liver enzymes. Therefore, careful monitoring is advised when somatropin is administered in combination with drugs metabolized by CP450 liver enzymes.)

No products indexed under this heading.

Enoxacin (Limited published data indicates that somatropin treatment increases cytochrome P450 (CP450)-mediated antipyrine clearance in man. These data suggest that somatropin administration may alter the clearance of compounds metabolized by CP450 liver enzymes. Therefore, careful monitoring is advised when somatropin is administered in combination with drugs metabolized by CP450 liver enzymes.)

No products indexed under this heading.

Eprosartan Mesylate (Limited published data indicates that somatropin treatment increases cytochrome P450 (CP450)-mediated antipyrine clearance in man. These data suggest that somatropin administration may alter the clearance of compounds metabolized by CP450 liver enzymes. Therefore, careful monitoring is advised when somatropin is administered in combination with drugs metabolized by CP450 liver enzymes. Products include:

Ergotamine Tartrate (Limited published data indicates that somatropin treatment increases cytochrome P450 (CP450)-mediated antipyrine clearance in man. These data suggest that somatropin administration may alter the clearance of compounds metabolized by CP450 liver enzymes. Therefore, careful monitoring is advised when somatropin is administered in combination with drugs metabolized by CP450 liver enzymes.)

No products indexed under this heading.

Erythromycin (Limited published data indicates that somatropin treatment increases cytochrome P450 (CP450)-mediated antipyrine clearance in man. These data suggest that somatropin administration may alter the clearance of compounds metabolized by CP450 liver enzymes. Therefore, careful monitoring is advised when somatropin is administered in combination with drugs metabolized by CP450 liver enzymes.)

No products indexed under this heading.

Erythromycin Estolate (Limited published data indicates that somatropin treatment increases cytochrome P450 (CP450)-mediated antipyrine clearance in man. These data suggest that somatropin administration may alter the clearance of compounds metabolized by CP450 liver enzymes. Therefore, careful monitoring is advised when somatropin is administered in combination with drugs metabolized by CP450 liver enzymes.)

No products indexed under this heading.

Erythromycin Ethylsuccinate (Limited published data indicates that somatropin treatment increases cytochrome P450 (CP450)-mediated antipyrine clearance in man. These data suggest that somatropin administration may alter the clearance of compounds metabolized by CP450 liver enzymes. Therefore, careful monitoring is advised when somatropin is administered in combination with drugs metabolized by CP450 liver enzymes. Products include:

Erythromycin Gluceptate (Limited published data indicates that somatropin treatment increases cytochrome P450 (CP450)-mediated antipyrine clearance in man. These data suggest that somatropin administration may alter the clearance of compounds metabolized by CP450 liver enzymes. Therefore, careful monitoring is advised when somatropin is administered in combination with drugs metabolized by CP450 liver enzymes.)

No products indexed under this heading.

Erythromycin Lactobionate (Limited published data indicates that somatropin treatment increases cytochrome P450 (CP450)-mediated antipyrine clearance in man. These data suggest that somatropin administration may alter the clearance of compounds metabolized by CP450 liver enzymes. Therefore, careful monitoring is advised when somatropin is administered in combination with drugs metabolized by CP450 liver enzymes.)

No products indexed under this heading.

Erythromycin Stearate (Limited published data indicates that somatropin treatment increases cytochrome P450 (CP450)-mediated antipyrine clearance in man. These data suggest that somatropin administration may alter the clearance of compounds metabolized by CP450 liver enzymes. Therefore, careful monitoring is advised when somatropin is administered in combination with drugs metabolized by CP450 liver enzymes.)

No products indexed under this heading.

Esomeprazole Magnesium (Limited published data indicates that somatropin treatment increases cytochrome P450 (CP450)-mediated antipyrine clearance in man. These data suggest that somatropin administration may alter the clearance of compounds metabolized by CP450 liver enzymes. Therefore, careful monitoring is advised when somatropin is administered in combination with drugs metabolized by CP450 liver enzymes. Products include:

Esomeprazole Sodium (Limited published data indicates that somatropin treatment increases cytochrome P450 (CP450)-mediated antipyrine clearance in man. These data suggest that somatropin administration may alter the clearance of compounds metabolized by CP450 liver enzymes. Therefore, careful monitoring is advised when somatropin is administered in combination with drugs metabolized by CP450 liver enzymes. Products include:

Estradiol (Limited published data indicates that somatropin treatment increases cytochrome P450 (CP450)-mediated antipyrine clearance in man. These data suggest that somatropin administration may alter the clearance of compounds metabolized by CP450 liver enzymes (eg, sex steroids). Therefore, careful monitoring is advised when somatropin is administered in combination with drugs metabolized by CP450 liver enzymes. Products include:

Estradiol Benzoate (Limited published data indicates that somatropin treatment increases cytochrome P450

(CP450)-mediated antipyrine clearance in man. These data suggest that somatropin administration may alter the clearance of compounds metabolized by CP450 liver enzymes. Therefore, careful monitoring is advised when somatropin is administered in combination with drugs metabolized by CP450 liver enzymes.)

No products indexed under this heading.

Estradiol Cypionate (Limited published data indicates that somatropin treatment increases cytochrome P450 (CP450)-mediated antipyrine clearance in man. These data suggest that somatropin administration may alter the clearance of compounds metabolized by CP450 liver enzymes. Therefore, careful monitoring is advised when somatropin is administered in combination with drugs metabolized by CP450 liver enzymes.)

No products indexed under this heading.

Estradiol Valerate (Limited published data indicates that somatropin treatment increases cytochrome P450 (CP450)-mediated antipyrine clearance in man. These data suggest that somatropin administration may alter the clearance of compounds metabolized by CP450 liver enzymes. Therefore, careful monitoring is advised when somatropin is administered in combination with drugs metabolized by CP450 liver enzymes.)

No products indexed under this heading.

Estrogen (Limited published data indicates that somatropin treatment increases cytochrome P450 (CP450)-mediated antipyrine clearance in man. These data suggest that somatropin administration may alter the clearance of compounds metabolized by CP450 liver enzymes. Therefore, careful monitoring is advised when somatropin is administered in combination with drugs metabolized by CP450 liver enzymes.)

No products indexed under this heading.

Estrogens, Conjugated (Limited published data indicates that somatropin treatment increases cytochrome P450 (CP450)-mediated antipyrine clearance in man. These data suggest that somatropin administration may alter the clearance of compounds metabolized by CP450 liver enzymes (eg, sex steroids). Therefore, careful monitoring is advised when somatropin is administered in combination with drugs metabolized by CP450 liver enzymes. Products include:

Estrogens, Conjugated, Synthetic A (Limited published data indicates that somatropin treatment increases cytochrome P450 (CP450)-mediated antipyrine clearance in man. These data suggest that somatropin administration may alter the clearance of compounds metabolized by CP450 liver enzymes. Therefore, careful monitoring is advised when somatropin is administered in combination with drugs metabolized by CP450 liver enzymes.)

No products indexed under this heading.

Estrogens, Esterified (Because oral estrogens may reduce the serum insulin-like growth factor I (IGF-I) response to somatropin treatment, girls and women receiving oral estrogen replacement may require greater somatropin dosages).

No products indexed under this heading.

Estropipate (Because oral estrogens may reduce the serum insulin-like growth factor I (IGF-I) response to somatropin treatment, girls and women receiving oral estrogen replacement may require greater somatropin dosages).
No products indexed under this heading.

Ethinyl Estradiol (Limited published data indicates that somatropin treatment increases cytochrome P450 (CP450)-mediated antipyrine clearance in man. These data suggest that somatropin administration may alter the clearance of compounds metabolized by CP450 liver enzymes (eg, sex steroids). Therefore, careful monitoring is advised when somatropin is administered in combination with drugs metabolized by CP450 liver enzymes). Products include:
LoSeasonique 3407
Lybrel 3514
NuvaRing 3181
Ortho Evra 2648
Ortho-Cyclen/Ortho Tri-Cyclen 2663
Ortho Tri-Cyclen Lo Tablets 2673
Seasonique 3418
Yaz 864

Ethosuximide (Limited published data indicates that somatropin treatment increases cytochrome P450 (CP450)-mediated antipyrine clearance in man. These data suggest that somatropin administration may alter the clearance of compounds metabolized by CP450 liver enzymes (eg, anticonvulsants). Therefore, careful monitoring is advised when somatropin is administered in combination with drugs metabolized by CP450 liver enzymes).
No products indexed under this heading.

Ethotoin (Limited published data indicates that somatropin treatment increases cytochrome P450 (CP450)-mediated antipyrine clearance in man. These data suggest that somatropin administration may alter the clearance of compounds metabolized by CP450 liver enzymes (eg, anticonvulsants). Therefore, careful monitoring is advised when somatropin is administered in combination with drugs metabolized by CP450 liver enzymes).
No products indexed under this heading.

Ethynodiol Diacetate (Limited published data indicates that somatropin treatment increases cytochrome P450 (CP450)-mediated antipyrine clearance in man. These data suggest that somatropin administration may alter the clearance of compounds metabolized by CP450 liver enzymes (eg, sex steroids). Therefore, careful monitoring is advised when somatropin is administered in combination with drugs metabolized by CP450 liver enzymes).
No products indexed under this heading.

Etodolac (Limited published data indicates that somatropin treatment increases cytochrome P450 (CP450)-mediated antipyrine clearance in man. These data suggest that somatropin administration may alter the clearance of compounds metabolized by CP450 liver enzymes. Therefore, careful monitoring is advised when somatropin is administered in combination with drugs metabolized by CP450 liver enzymes).
No products indexed under this heading.

Etoposide (Limited published data indicates that somatropin treatment increases cytochrome P450 (CP450)-mediated antipyrine clearance in man. These data suggest that somatropin administration may alter the clearance of compounds metabolized by CP450 liver enzymes. Therefore, careful monitoring is advised when somatropin is administered in combination with drugs metabolized by CP450 liver enzymes).
No products indexed under this heading.

Etoposide Phosphate (Limited published data indicates that somatropin treatment increases cytochrome P450 (CP450)-mediated antipyrine clearance in man. These data suggest that somatropin administration may alter the clearance of compounds metabolized by CP450 liver enzymes. Therefore, careful monitoring is advised when somatropin is administered in combination with drugs metabolized by CP450 liver enzymes).
No products indexed under this heading.

Felbamate (Limited published data indicates that somatropin treatment increases cytochrome P450 (CP450)-mediated antipyrine clearance in man. These data suggest that somatropin administration may alter the clearance of compounds metabolized by CP450 liver enzymes (eg, anticonvulsants). Therefore, careful monitoring is advised when somatropin is administered in combination with drugs metabolized by CP450 liver enzymes).
No products indexed under this heading.

Felodipine (Limited published data indicates that somatropin treatment increases cytochrome P450 (CP450)-mediated antipyrine clearance in man. These data suggest that somatropin administration may alter the clearance of compounds metabolized by CP450 liver enzymes. Therefore, careful monitoring is advised when somatropin is administered in combination with drugs metabolized by CP450 liver enzymes).
No products indexed under this heading.

Fenoprofen Calcium (Limited published data indicates that somatropin treatment increases cytochrome P450 (CP450)-mediated antipyrine clearance in man. These data suggest that somatropin administration may alter the clearance of compounds metabolized by CP450 liver enzymes. Therefore, careful monitoring is advised when somatropin is administered in combination with drugs metabolized by CP450 liver enzymes).
No products indexed under this heading.

Fentanyl (Limited published data indicates that somatropin treatment increases cytochrome P450 (CP450)-mediated antipyrine clearance in man. These data suggest that somatropin administration may alter the clearance of compounds metabolized by CP450 liver enzymes. Therefore, careful monitoring is advised when somatropin is administered in combination with drugs metabolized by CP450 liver enzymes). Products include:
Duragesic 2604
Fentanyl Transdermal System 2346
Onsolis 2054

Fentanyl Citrate (Limited published data indicates that somatropin treatment increases cytochrome P450 (CP450)-mediated antipyrine clearance in man. These data suggest that somatropin administration may alter the clearance of compounds metabolized by CP450 liver enzymes. Therefore, careful monitoring is advised when somatropin is administered in combination with drugs metabolized by CP450 liver enzymes). Products include:
Fentora 966

Flecainide Acetate (Limited published data indicates that somatropin treatment increases cytochrome P450 (CP450)-mediated antipyrine clearance in man. These data suggest that somatropin administration may alter the clearance of compounds metabolized by CP450 liver enzymes. Therefore, careful monitoring is advised when somatropin is administered in combination with drugs metabolized by CP450 liver enzymes).
No products indexed under this heading.

Fludrocortisone Acetate (Introduction of somatropin treatment may result in inhibition of 11βHSD-1 and reduced serum cortisol concentrations. As a consequence, patients treated with glucocorticoid replacement therapy for previously diagnosed hypoadrenalism may require an increase in their maintenance or stress doses; this may be especially true for patients treated with cortisone acetate and prednisone. In addition, excessive glucocorticoid therapy may attenuate the growth promoting effects of somatropin in children. Therefore, glucocorticoid replacement therapy should be carefully adjusted in children with concomitant GH and glucocorticoid deficiency to avoid both hypoadrenalism and an inhibitory effect on growth. Also, somatropin administration may alter the clearance of compounds known to be metabolized by CYP450 liver enzymes (eg, corticosteroids). Careful monitoring is advisable when somatropin is administered in combination with other drugs known to be metabolized by CYP450 liver enzymes).
No products indexed under this heading.

Flumethasone Pivalate (Introduction of somatropin treatment may result in inhibition of 11βHSD-1 and reduced serum cortisol concentrations. As a consequence, patients treated with glucocorticoid replacement therapy for previously diagnosed hypoadrenalism may require an increase in their maintenance or stress doses; this may be especially true for patients treated with cortisone acetate and prednisone. In addition, excessive glucocorticoid therapy may attenuate the growth promoting effects of somatropin in children. Therefore, glucocorticoid replacement therapy should be carefully adjusted in children with concomitant GH and glucocorticoid deficiency to avoid both hypoadrenalism and an inhibitory effect on growth. Also, somatropin administration may alter the clearance of compounds known to be metabolized by CYP450 liver enzymes (eg, corticosteroids). Careful monitoring is advisable when somatropin is administered in combination with other drugs known to be metabolized by CYP450 liver enzymes).
No products indexed under this heading.

Flunisolide Hemihydrate (Introduction of somatropin treatment may result in inhibition of 11βHSD-1 and reduced serum cortisol concentrations. As a consequence, patients treated with glucocorticoid replacement therapy for previously diagnosed hypoadrenalism may require an increase in their maintenance or stress doses; this may be especially true for patients treated with cortisone acetate and prednisone. In addition, excessive glucocorticoid therapy may attenuate the growth promoting effects of somatropin in children. Therefore, glucocorticoid replacement therapy should be carefully adjusted in children with concomitant GH and glucocorticoid deficiency to avoid both hypoadrenalism and an inhibitory effect on growth. Also, somatropin administration may alter the clearance of compounds known to be metabolized by CYP450 liver enzymes (eg, corticosteroids). Careful monitoring is advisable when somatropin is administered in combination with other drugs known to be metabolized by CYP450 liver enzymes).
No products indexed under this heading.

Fluoxetine (Limited published data indicates that somatropin treatment increases cytochrome P450 (CP450)-mediated antipyrine clearance in man. These data suggest that somatropin administration may alter the clearance of compounds metabolized by CP450 liver enzymes. Therefore, careful monitoring is advised when somatropin is administered in combination with drugs metabolized by CP450 liver enzymes).
No products indexed under this heading.

Fluoxetine Hydrochloride (Limited published data indicates that somatropin treatment increases cytochrome P450 (CP450)-mediated antipyrine clearance in man. These data suggest that somatropin administration may alter the clearance of compounds metabolized by CP450 liver enzymes. Therefore, careful monitoring is advised when somatropin is administered in combination with drugs metabolized by CP450 liver enzymes). Products include:
Prozac Weekly 1941
Prozac Pulvules 1941
Symbyax 1965

Fluoxymesterone (Limited published data indicates that somatropin treatment increases cytochrome P450 (CP450)-mediated antipyrine clearance in man. These data suggest that somatropin administration may alter the clearance of compounds metabolized by CP450 liver enzymes (eg, sex steroids). Therefore, careful monitoring is advised when somatropin is administered in combination with drugs metabolized by CP450 liver enzymes).
No products indexed under this heading.

Fluphenazine Decanoate (Limited published data indicates that somatropin treatment increases cytochrome P450 (CP450)-mediated antipyrine clearance in man. These data suggest that somatropin administration may alter the clearance of compounds metabolized by CP450 liver enzymes. Therefore, careful monitoring is advised when somatropin is administered in combination with drugs metabolized by CP450 liver enzymes).
No products indexed under this heading.

Fluphenazine Enanthate (Limited published data indicates that somatropin treatment increases cytochrome P450 (CP450)-mediated antipyrine clearance in man. These data suggest that somatropin administration may alter the clearance of compounds metabolized by CP450 liver enzymes. Therefore, careful monitoring is advised when somatropin is administered in combination with drugs metabolized by CP450 liver enzymes).
No products indexed under this heading.

Fluphenazine Hydrochloride (Limited published data indicates that somatropin treatment increases cytochrome P450 (CP450)-mediated antipyrine clearance in man. These data suggest that somatropin administration may alter the clearance of compounds metabolized by CP450 liver enzymes. Therefore, careful monitoring is advised when somatropin is administered in combination with drugs metabolized by CP450 liver enzymes).
No products indexed under this heading.

Flurbiprofen (Limited published data indicates that somatropin treatment increases cytochrome P450 (CP450)-mediated antipyrine clearance in man. These data suggest that somatropin administration may alter the clearance of compounds metabolized by CP450 liver enzymes. Therefore, careful monitoring is advised when somatropin is administered in combination with drugs metabolized by CP450 liver enzymes).
No products indexed under this heading.

Flurbiprofen Sodium (Limited published data indicates that somatropin

treatment increases cytochrome P450 (CP450)-mediated antipyrine clearance in man. These data suggest that somatropin administration may alter the clearance of compounds metabolized by CP450 liver enzymes. Therefore, careful monitoring is advised when somatropin is administered in combination with drugs metabolized by CP450 liver enzymes).
No products indexed under this heading.

Flutamide (Limited published data indicates that somatropin treatment increases cytochrome P450 (CP450)-mediated antipyrine clearance in man. These data suggest that somatropin administration may alter the clearance of compounds metabolized by CP450 liver enzymes. Therefore, careful monitoring is advised when somatropin is administered in combination with drugs metabolized by CP450 liver enzymes).
No products indexed under this heading.

Fluticasone Furoate (Introduction of somatropin treatment may result in inhibition of 11βHSD-1 and reduced serum cortisol concentrations. As a consequence, patients treated with glucocorticoid replacement therapy for previously diagnosed hypoadrenalism may require an increase in their maintenance or stress doses; this may be especially true for patients treated with cortisone acetate and prednisone. In addition, excessive glucocorticoid therapy may attenuate the growth promoting effects of somatropin in children. Therefore, glucocorticoid replacement therapy should be carefully adjusted in children with concomitant GH and glucocorticoid deficiency to avoid both hypoadrenalism and an inhibitory effect on growth. Also, somatropin administration may alter the clearance of compounds known to be metabolized by CYP450 liver enzymes (eg, corticosteroids). Careful monitoring is advisable when somatropin is administered in combination with other drugs known to be metabolized by CYP450 liver enzymes). Products include:
Veramyst 1713

Fluticasone Propionate (Introduction of somatropin treatment may result in inhibition of 11βHSD-1 and reduced serum cortisol concentrations. As a consequence, patients treated with glucocorticoid replacement therapy for previously diagnosed hypoadrenalism may require an increase in their maintenance or stress doses; this may be especially true for patients treated with cortisone acetate and prednisone. In addition, excessive glucocorticoid therapy may attenuate the growth promoting effects of somatropin in children. Therefore, glucocorticoid replacement therapy should be carefully adjusted in children with concomitant GH and glucocorticoid deficiency to avoid both hypoadrenalism and an inhibitory effect on growth. Also, somatropin administration may alter the clearance of compounds known to be metabolized by CYP450 liver enzymes (eg, corticosteroids). Careful monitoring is advisable when somatropin is administered in combination with other drugs known to be metabolized by CYP450 liver enzymes). Products include:
Advair 100/50 1275
Advair 250/50 1275
Advair 500/50 1275
Advair HFA 45/21 1288
Advair HFA 115/21 1288
Advair HFA 230/21 1288
Flonase 1459
Flovent Diskus 1463
Flovent HFA 1470

Fluvastatin Sodium (Limited published data indicates that somatropin treatment increases cytochrome P450 (CP450)-mediated antipyrine clearance in man. These data suggest that somatropin administration may alter the clearance of compounds metabolized by CP450 liver enzymes. Therefore, careful monitoring is advised when somatropin is administered in combination with drugs metabolized by CP450 liver enzymes).
No products indexed under this heading.

Fluvoxamine Maleate (Limited published data indicates that somatropin treatment increases cytochrome P450 (CP450)-mediated antipyrine clearance in man. These data suggest that somatropin administration may alter the clearance of compounds metabolized by CP450 liver enzymes. Therefore, careful monitoring is advised when somatropin is administered in combination with drugs metabolized by CP450 liver enzymes).
No products indexed under this heading.

Formoterol Fumarate (Limited published data indicates that somatropin treatment increases cytochrome P450 (CP450)-mediated antipyrine clearance in man. These data suggest that somatropin administration may alter the clearance of compounds metabolized by CP450 liver enzymes. Therefore, careful monitoring is advised when somatropin is administered in combination with drugs metabolized by CP450 liver enzymes). Products include:
Foradil 3121
Perforomist 3634

Fosphenytoin (Limited published data indicates that somatropin treatment increases cytochrome P450 (CP450)-mediated antipyrine clearance in man. These data suggest that somatropin administration may alter the clearance of compounds metabolized by CP450 liver enzymes (eg, anticonvulsants). Therefore, careful monitoring is advised when somatropin is administered in combination with drugs metabolized by CP450 liver enzymes).
No products indexed under this heading.

Fosphenytoin Sodium (Limited published data indicates that somatropin treatment increases cytochrome P450 (CP450)-mediated antipyrine clearance in man. These data suggest that somatropin administration may alter the clearance of compounds metabolized by CP450 liver enzymes (eg, anticonvulsants). Therefore, careful monitoring is advised when somatropin is administered in combination with drugs metabolized by CP450 liver enzymes).
No products indexed under this heading.

Gabapentin (Limited published data indicates that somatropin treatment increases cytochrome P450 (CP450)-mediated antipyrine clearance in man. These data suggest that somatropin administration may alter the clearance of compounds metabolized by CP450 liver enzymes (eg, anticonvulsants). Therefore, careful monitoring is advised when somatropin is administered in combination with drugs metabolized by CP450 liver enzymes).
No products indexed under this heading.

Galantamine Hydrobromide (Limited published data indicates that somatropin treatment increases cytochrome P450 (CP450)-mediated antipyrine clearance in man. These data suggest that somatropin administration may alter the clearance of compounds metabolized by CP450 liver enzymes. Therefore, careful monitoring is advised when somatropin is administered in combination with drugs metabolized by CP450 liver enzymes).
No products indexed under this heading.

Glibenclamide (Patients with diabetes mellitus who receive concomitant treatment with somatropin may require adjustment of their doses of insulin and/or other hypoglycemic agents).
No products indexed under this heading.

Glimepiride (Patients with diabetes mellitus who receive concomitant treatment with somatropin may require adjustment of their doses of insulin and/or other hypoglycemic agents). Products include:
Avandaryl 1356
Duetact 3354

Glipizide (Patients with diabetes mellitus who receive concomitant treatment with somatropin may require adjustment of their doses of insulin and/or other hypoglycemic agents).
No products indexed under this heading.

Glyburide (Patients with diabetes mellitus who receive concomitant treatment with somatropin may require adjustment of their doses of insulin and/or other hypoglycemic agents).
No products indexed under this heading.

Grepafloxacin Hydrochloride (Limited published data indicates that somatropin treatment increases cytochrome P450 (CP450)-mediated antipyrine clearance in man. These data suggest that somatropin administration may alter the clearance of compounds metabolized by CP450 liver enzymes. Therefore, careful monitoring is advised when somatropin is administered in combination with drugs metabolized by CP450 liver enzymes).
No products indexed under this heading.

Haloperidol (Limited published data indicates that somatropin treatment increases cytochrome P450 (CP450)-mediated antipyrine clearance in man. These data suggest that somatropin administration may alter the clearance of compounds metabolized by CP450 liver enzymes. Therefore, careful monitoring is advised when somatropin is administered in combination with drugs metabolized by CP450 liver enzymes).
No products indexed under this heading.

Haloperidol Decanoate (Limited published data indicates that somatropin treatment increases cytochrome P450 (CP450)-mediated antipyrine clearance in man. These data suggest that somatropin administration may alter the clearance of compounds metabolized by CP450 liver enzymes. Therefore, careful monitoring is advised when somatropin is administered in combination with drugs metabolized by CP450 liver enzymes).
No products indexed under this heading.

Haloperidol Lactate (Limited published data indicates that somatropin treatment increases cytochrome P450 (CP450)-mediated antipyrine clearance in man. These data suggest that somatropin administration may alter the clearance of compounds metabolized by CP450 liver enzymes. Therefore, careful monitoring is advised when somatropin is administered in combination with drugs metabolized by CP450 liver enzymes).
No products indexed under this heading.

Hexobarbital (Limited published data indicates that somatropin treatment increases cytochrome P450 (CP450)-mediated antipyrine clearance in man. These data suggest that somatropin administration may alter the clearance of compounds metabolized by CP450 liver enzymes. Therefore, careful monitoring is advised when somatropin is administered in combination with drugs metabolized by CP450 liver enzymes).
No products indexed under this heading.

Hydrocodone Bitartrate (Limited published data indicates that somatropin treatment increases cytochrome P450 (CP450)-mediated antipyrine clearance in man. These data suggest that somatropin administration may alter the clearance of compounds metabolized by CP450 liver enzymes. Therefore, careful monitoring is advised when somatropin is administered in combination with drugs metabolized by CP450 liver enzymes). Products include:
Vicodin 560
Vicodin ES 561
Vicodin HP 563
Vicoprofen 564
Zydone 1138

Hydrocortisone (Introduction of somatropin treatment may result in inhibition of 11βHSD-1 and reduced serum cortisol concentrations. As a consequence, patients treated with glucocorticoid replacement therapy for previously diagnosed hypoadrenalism may require an increase in their maintenance or stress doses; this may be especially true for patients treated with cortisone acetate and prednisone. In addition, excessive glucocorticoid therapy may attenuate the growth promoting effects of somatropin in children. Therefore, glucocorticoid replacement therapy should be carefully adjusted in children with concomitant GH and glucocorticoid deficiency to avoid both hypoadrenalism and an inhibitory effect on growth. Also, somatropin administration may alter the clearance of compounds known to be metabolized by CYP450 liver enzymes (eg, corticosteroids). Careful monitoring is advisable when somatropin is administered in combination with other drugs known to be metabolized by CYP450 liver enzymes).
No products indexed under this heading.

Hydrocortisone (Alcohol) (Introduction of somatropin treatment may result in inhibition of 11βHSD-1 and reduced serum cortisol concentrations. As a consequence, patients treated with glucocorticoid replacement therapy for previously diagnosed hypoadrenalism may require an increase in their maintenance or stress doses; this may be especially true for patients treated with cortisone acetate and prednisone. In addition, excessive glucocorticoid therapy may attenuate the growth promoting effects of somatropin in children. Therefore, glucocorticoid replacement therapy should be carefully adjusted in children with concomitant GH and glucocorticoid deficiency to avoid both hypoadrenalism and an inhibitory effect on growth. Also, somatropin administration may alter the clearance of compounds known to be metabolized by CYP450 liver enzymes (eg, corticosteroids). Careful monitoring is advisable when somatropin is administered in combination with other drugs known to be metabolized by CYP450 liver enzymes).
No products indexed under this heading.

Hydrocortisone Acetate (Introduction of somatropin treatment may result in inhibition of 11βHSD-1 and reduced serum cortisol concentrations. As a consequence, patients treated with glucocorticoid replacement therapy for previously diagnosed hypoadrenalism may require an increase in their maintenance or stress doses; this may be especially true for patients treated with cortisone acetate and prednisone. In addition, excessive glucocorticoid therapy may attenuate the growth promoting effects of somatropin in children. Therefore, glucocorticoid replacement therapy should be carefully adjusted in children with concomitant GH and glucocorticoid deficiency to avoid both hypoadrenalism and an inhibitory effect on growth. Also, somatropin administration

IMPORTANT NOTE: Always consult each drug listing in the patient's regimen for possible interactions.

may alter the clearance of compounds known to be metabolized by CYP450 liver enzymes (eg, corticosteroids). Careful monitoring is advisable when somatropin is administered in combination with other drugs known to be metabolized by CYP450 liver enzymes).

No products indexed under this heading.

Hydrocortisone Butyrate (Introduction of somatropin treatment may result in inhibition of 11βHSD-1 and reduced serum cortisol concentrations. As a consequence, patients treated with glucocorticoid replacement therapy for previously diagnosed hypoadrenalism may require an increase in their maintenance or stress doses; this may be especially true for patients treated with cortisone acetate and prednisone. In addition, excessive glucocorticoid therapy may attenuate the growth promoting effects of somatropin in children. Therefore, glucocorticoid replacement therapy should be carefully adjusted in children with concomitant GH and glucocorticoid deficiency to avoid both hypoadrenalism and an inhibitory effect on growth. Also, somatropin administration may alter the clearance of compounds known to be metabolized by CYP450 liver enzymes (eg, corticosteroids). Careful monitoring is advisable when somatropin is administered in combination with other drugs known to be metabolized by CYP450 liver enzymes).

No products indexed under this heading.

Hydrocortisone Cypionate (Introduction of somatropin treatment may result in inhibition of 11βHSD-1 and reduced serum cortisol concentrations. As a consequence, patients treated with glucocorticoid replacement therapy for previously diagnosed hypoadrenalism may require an increase in their maintenance or stress doses; this may be especially true for patients treated with cortisone acetate and prednisone. In addition, excessive glucocorticoid therapy may attenuate the growth promoting effects of somatropin in children. Therefore, glucocorticoid replacement therapy should be carefully adjusted in children with concomitant GH and glucocorticoid deficiency to avoid both hypoadrenalism and an inhibitory effect on growth. Also, somatropin administration may alter the clearance of compounds known to be metabolized by CYP450 liver enzymes (eg, corticosteroids). Careful monitoring is advisable when somatropin is administered in combination with other drugs known to be metabolized by CYP450 liver enzymes).

No products indexed under this heading.

Hydrocortisone Hemisuccinate (Introduction of somatropin treatment may result in inhibition of 11βHSD-1 and reduced serum cortisol concentrations. As a consequence, patients treated with glucocorticoid replacement therapy for previously diagnosed hypoadrenalism may require an increase in their maintenance or stress doses; this may be especially true for patients treated with cortisone acetate and prednisone. In addition, excessive glucocorticoid therapy may attenuate the growth promoting effects of somatropin in children. Therefore, glucocorticoid replacement therapy should be carefully adjusted in children with concomitant GH and glucocorticoid deficiency to avoid both hypoadrenalism and an inhibitory effect on growth. Also, somatropin administration may alter the clearance of compounds known to be metabolized by CYP450 liver enzymes (eg, corticosteroids). Careful monitoring is advisable when somatropin is administered in combination with other drugs known to be metabolized by CYP450 liver enzymes).

No products indexed under this heading.

Hydrocortisone Probutate (Introduction of somatropin treatment may result in inhibition of 11βHSD-1 and reduced serum cortisol concentrations. As a consequence, patients treated with glucocorticoid replacement therapy for previously diagnosed hypoadrenalism may require an increase in their maintenance or stress doses; this may be especially true for patients treated with cortisone acetate and prednisone. In addition, excessive glucocorticoid therapy may attenuate the growth promoting effects of somatropin in children. Therefore, glucocorticoid replacement therapy should be carefully adjusted in children with concomitant GH and glucocorticoid deficiency to avoid both hypoadrenalism and an inhibitory effect on growth. Also, somatropin administration may alter the clearance of compounds known to be metabolized by CYP450 liver enzymes (eg, corticosteroids). Careful monitoring is advisable when somatropin is administered in combination with other drugs known to be metabolized by CYP450 liver enzymes).

No products indexed under this heading.

Hydrocortisone Sodium Phosphate (Introduction of somatropin treatment may result in inhibition of 11βHSD-1 and reduced serum cortisol concentrations. As a consequence, patients treated with glucocorticoid replacement therapy for previously diagnosed hypoadrenalism may require an increase in their maintenance or stress doses; this may be especially true for patients treated with cortisone acetate and prednisone. In addition, excessive glucocorticoid therapy may attenuate the growth promoting effects of somatropin in children. Therefore, glucocorticoid replacement therapy should be carefully adjusted in children with concomitant GH and glucocorticoid deficiency to avoid both hypoadrenalism and an inhibitory effect on growth. Also, somatropin administration may alter the clearance of compounds known to be metabolized by CYP450 liver enzymes (eg, corticosteroids). Careful monitoring is advisable when somatropin is administered in combination with other drugs known to be metabolized by CYP450 liver enzymes).

No products indexed under this heading.

Hydrocortisone Sodium Succinate (Introduction of somatropin treatment may result in inhibition of 11βHSD-1 and reduced serum cortisol concentrations. As a consequence, patients treated with glucocorticoid replacement therapy for previously diagnosed hypoadrenalism may require an increase in their maintenance or stress doses; this may be especially true for patients treated with cortisone acetate and prednisone. In addition, excessive glucocorticoid therapy may attenuate the growth promoting effects of somatropin in children. Therefore, glucocorticoid replacement therapy should be carefully adjusted in children with concomitant GH and glucocorticoid deficiency to avoid both hypoadrenalism and an inhibitory effect on growth. Also, somatropin administration may alter the clearance of compounds known to be metabolized by CYP450 liver enzymes (eg, corticosteroids). Careful monitoring is advisable when somatropin is administered in combination with other drugs known to be metabolized by CYP450 liver enzymes).

No products indexed under this heading.

Hydrocortisone Valerate (Introduction of somatropin treatment may result in inhibition of 11βHSD-1 and reduced serum cortisol concentrations. As a consequence, patients treated with glucocorticoid replacement therapy for previously diagnosed hypoadrenalism may require an increase in their mainte-

nance or stress doses; this may be especially true for patients treated with cortisone acetate and prednisone. In addition, excessive glucocorticoid therapy may attenuate the growth promoting effects of somatropin in children. Therefore, glucocorticoid replacement therapy should be carefully adjusted in children with concomitant GH and glucocorticoid deficiency to avoid both hypoadrenalism and an inhibitory effect on growth. Also, somatropin administration may alter the clearance of compounds known to be metabolized by CYP450 liver enzymes (eg, corticosteroids). Careful monitoring is advisable when somatropin is administered in combination with other drugs known to be metabolized by CYP450 liver enzymes).

No products indexed under this heading.

Ibuprofen (Limited published data indicates that somatropin treatment increases cytochrome P450 (CP450)-mediated antipyrine clearance in man. These data suggest that somatropin administration may alter the clearance of compounds metabolized by CP450 liver enzymes. Therefore, careful monitoring is advised when somatropin is administered in combination with drugs metabolized by CP450 liver enzymes). Products include:

Motrin IB **2043**
Children's Motrin **2044**
Children's Motrin Non-Staining
Dye-Free **2044**
Infants' Motrin **2044**
Infants' Motrin Dye-Free **2044**
Junior Strength Motrin **2044**
Vicoprofen **564**

Imipramine Hydrochloride (Limited published data indicates that somatropin treatment increases cytochrome P450 (CP450)-mediated antipyrine clearance in man. These data suggest that somatropin administration may alter the clearance of compounds metabolized by CP450 liver enzymes. Therefore, careful monitoring is advised when somatropin is administered in combination with drugs metabolized by CP450 liver enzymes).

No products indexed under this heading.

Imipramine Pamoate (Limited published data indicates that somatropin treatment increases cytochrome P450 (CP450)-mediated antipyrine clearance in man. These data suggest that somatropin administration may alter the clearance of compounds metabolized by CP450 liver enzymes. Therefore, careful monitoring is advised when somatropin is administered in combination with drugs metabolized by CP450 liver enzymes).

No products indexed under this heading.

Indinavir Sulfate (Limited published data indicates that somatropin treatment increases cytochrome P450 (CP450)-mediated antipyrine clearance in man. These data suggest that somatropin administration may alter the clearance of compounds metabolized by CP450 liver enzymes. Therefore, careful monitoring is advised when somatropin is administered in combination with drugs metabolized by CP450 liver enzymes). Products include:

Crixivan **2113**

Indomethacin (Limited published data indicates that somatropin treatment increases cytochrome P450 (CP450)-mediated antipyrine clearance in man. These data suggest that somatropin administration may alter the clearance of compounds metabolized by CP450 liver enzymes. Therefore, careful monitoring is advised when somatropin is administered in combination with drugs metabolized by CP450 liver enzymes). Products include:

Indocin **2167**

Indomethacin Sodium Trihydrate (Limited published data indicates that somatropin treatment increases cytochrome P450 (CP450)-mediated antipyrine clearance in man. These data suggest that somatropin administration may alter the clearance of compounds metabolized by CP450 liver enzymes. Therefore, careful monitoring is advised when somatropin is administered in combination with drugs metabolized by CP450 liver enzymes). Products include:

Indocin I.V. **2007**

Indoramin Hydrochloride (Limited published data indicates that somatropin treatment increases cytochrome P450 (CP450)-mediated antipyrine clearance in man. These data suggest that somatropin administration may alter the clearance of compounds metabolized by CP450 liver enzymes. Therefore, careful monitoring is advised when somatropin is administered in combination with drugs metabolized by CP450 liver enzymes).

No products indexed under this heading.

Insulin (Patients with diabetes mellitus who receive concomitant treatment with somatropin may require adjustment of their doses of insulin and/or other hypoglycemic agents).

No products indexed under this heading.

Insulin, Human, Zinc Suspension (Patients with diabetes mellitus who receive concomitant treatment with somatropin may require adjustment of their doses of insulin and/or other hypoglycemic agents).

No products indexed under this heading.

Insulin, Human (rDNA origin) (Patients with diabetes mellitus who receive concomitant treatment with somatropin may require adjustment of their doses of insulin and/or other hypoglycemic agents). Products include:

Exubera **2717**

Insulin, Human NPH (Patients with diabetes mellitus who receive concomitant treatment with somatropin may require adjustment of their doses of insulin and/or other hypoglycemic agents). Products include:

Humulin N Vial **1934**

Insulin, Human Regular (Patients with diabetes mellitus who receive concomitant treatment with somatropin may require adjustment of their doses of insulin and/or other hypoglycemic agents). Products include:

Humulin R **1937**
Humulin R (U-500) **1939**

Insulin, Human Regular and Human NPH Mixture (Patients with diabetes mellitus who receive concomitant treatment with somatropin may require adjustment of their doses of insulin and/or other hypoglycemic agents). Products include:

Humulin 50/50 .... **1930**
Humulin 70/30 Vial **1931**

Insulin, NPH (Patients with diabetes mellitus who receive concomitant treatment with somatropin may require adjustment of their doses of insulin and/or other hypoglycemic agents).

No products indexed under this heading.

Insulin, Regular (Patients with diabetes mellitus who receive concomitant treatment with somatropin may require adjustment of their doses of insulin and/or other hypoglycemic agents).

No products indexed under this heading.

Insulin, Regular and NPH mixture (Patients with diabetes mellitus who receive concomitant treatment with somatropin may require adjustment of their doses of insulin and/or other hypoglycemic agents).

No products indexed under this heading.

Insulin, Zinc Crystals (Patients with diabetes mellitus who receive concomitant treatment with somatropin may require adjustment of their doses of insulin and/or other hypoglycemic agents).
No products indexed under this heading.

Insulin, Zinc Suspension (Patients with diabetes mellitus who receive concomitant treatment with somatropin may require adjustment of their doses of insulin and/or other hypoglycemic agents).
No products indexed under this heading.

Insulin Aspart (Patients with diabetes mellitus who receive concomitant treatment with somatropin may require adjustment of their doses of insulin and/or other hypoglycemic agents).
No products indexed under this heading.

Insulin Aspart, Human (Patients with diabetes mellitus who receive concomitant treatment with somatropin may require adjustment of their doses of insulin and/or other hypoglycemic agents). Products include:
NovoLog Mix 70/30 2581

Insulin Aspart, Human Regular (Patients with diabetes mellitus who receive concomitant treatment with somatropin may require adjustment of their doses of insulin and/or other hypoglycemic agents). Products include:
NovoLog 2575

Insulin Aspart Protamine, Human (Patients with diabetes mellitus who receive concomitant treatment with somatropin may require adjustment of their doses of insulin and/or other hypoglycemic agents). Products include:
NovoLog Mix 70/30 2581

Insulin Detemir (rDNA Origin) (Patients with diabetes mellitus who receive concomitant treatment with somatropin may require adjustment of their doses of insulin and/or other hypoglycemic agents). Products include:
Levemir 2566

Insulin Glargine (Patients with diabetes mellitus who receive concomitant treatment with somatropin may require adjustment of their doses of insulin and/or other hypoglycemic agents). Products include:
Lantus 2996

Insulin Glulisine (Patients with diabetes mellitus who receive concomitant treatment with somatropin may require adjustment of their doses of insulin and/or other hypoglycemic agents). Products include:
Apidra 2937
Apidra SoloStar 2937

Insulin Lispro, Human (Patients with diabetes mellitus who receive concomitant treatment with somatropin may require adjustment of their doses of insulin and/or other hypoglycemic agents). Products include:
Humalog 1910
Humalog Mix 1914
Humalog Mix75/25 1917

Insulin Lispro Protamine, Human (Patients with diabetes mellitus who receive concomitant treatment with somatropin may require adjustment of their doses of insulin and/or other hypoglycemic agents). Products include:
Humalog Mix 1914
Humalog Mix75/25 1917

Irbesartan (Limited published data indicates that somatropin treatment increases cytochrome P450 (CP450)-mediated antipyrine clearance in man. These data suggest that somatropin administration may alter the clearance of compounds metabolized by CP450 liver enzymes. Therefore, careful monitoring is advised when somatro-

pin is administered in combination with drugs metabolized by CP450 liver enzymes). Products include:
Avalide 2956
Avapro 2962

Isotretinoin (Limited published data indicates that somatropin treatment increases cytochrome P450 (CP450)-mediated antipyrine clearance in man. These data suggest that somatropin administration may alter the clearance of compounds metabolized by CP450 liver enzymes. Therefore, careful monitoring is advised when somatropin is administered in combination with drugs metabolized by CP450 liver enzymes). Products include:
Accutane 2832

Isradipine (Limited published data indicates that somatropin treatment increases cytochrome P450 (CP450)-mediated antipyrine clearance in man. These data suggest that somatropin administration may alter the clearance of compounds metabolized by CP450 liver enzymes. Therefore, careful monitoring is advised when somatropin is administered in combination with drugs metabolized by CP450 liver enzymes). Products include:
DynaCirc CR 1432

Itraconazole (Limited published data indicates that somatropin treatment increases cytochrome P450 (CP450)-mediated antipyrine clearance in man. These data suggest that somatropin administration may alter the clearance of compounds metabolized by CP450 liver enzymes. Therefore, careful monitoring is advised when somatropin is administered in combination with drugs metabolized by CP450 liver enzymes).
No products indexed under this heading.

Ixabepilone (Limited published data indicates that somatropin treatment increases cytochrome P450 (CP450)-mediated antipyrine clearance in man. These data suggest that somatropin administration may alter the clearance of compounds metabolized by CP450 liver enzymes. Therefore, careful monitoring is advised when somatropin is administered in combination with drugs metabolized by CP450 liver enzymes).
No products indexed under this heading.

Ketoconazole (Limited published data indicates that somatropin treatment increases cytochrome P450 (CP450)-mediated antipyrine clearance in man. These data suggest that somatropin administration may alter the clearance of compounds metabolized by CP450 liver enzymes. Therefore, careful monitoring is advised when somatropin is administered in combination with drugs metabolized by CP450 liver enzymes). Products include:
Extina 3319
Xolegel 3337

Ketoprofen (Limited published data indicates that somatropin treatment increases cytochrome P450 (CP450)-mediated antipyrine clearance in man. These data suggest that somatropin administration may alter the clearance of compounds metabolized by CP450 liver enzymes. Therefore, careful monitoring is advised when somatropin is administered in combination with drugs metabolized by CP450 liver enzymes).
No products indexed under this heading.

Ketorolac Tromethamine (Limited published data indicates that somatropin treatment increases cytochrome P450 (CP450)-mediated antipyrine clearance in man. These data suggest that somatropin administration may alter the clearance of compounds metabolized by CP450 liver enzymes. Therefore, careful monitoring is advised

when somatropin is administered in combination with drugs metabolized by CP450 liver enzymes). Products include:
Acuvail .... ⊙209

Labetalol Hydrochloride (Limited published data indicates that somatropin treatment increases cytochrome P450 (CP450)-mediated antipyrine clearance in man. These data suggest that somatropin administration may alter the clearance of compounds metabolized by CP450 liver enzymes. Therefore, careful monitoring is advised when somatropin is administered in combination with drugs metabolized by CP450 liver enzymes).
No products indexed under this heading.

Lamotrigine (Limited published data indicates that somatropin treatment increases cytochrome P450 (CP450)-mediated antipyrine clearance in man. These data suggest that somatropin administration may alter the clearance of compounds metabolized by CP450 liver enzymes (eg, anticonvulsants). Therefore, careful monitoring is advised when somatropin is administered in combination with drugs metabolized by CP450 liver enzymes). Products include:
Lamictal 1522
Lamictal ODT 1522
Lamictal XR 1536

Lansoprazole (Limited published data indicates that somatropin treatment increases cytochrome P450 (CP450)-mediated antipyrine clearance in man. These data suggest that somatropin administration may alter the clearance of compounds metabolized by CP450 liver enzymes. Therefore, careful monitoring is advised when somatropin is administered in combination with drugs metabolized by CP450 liver enzymes).
No products indexed under this heading.

Levetiracetam (Limited published data indicates that somatropin treatment increases cytochrome P450 (CP450)-mediated antipyrine clearance in man. These data suggest that somatropin administration may alter the clearance of compounds metabolized by CP450 liver enzymes (eg, anticonvulsants). Therefore, careful monitoring is advised when somatropin is administered in combination with drugs metabolized by CP450 liver enzymes). Products include:
Keppra XR 3434

Levobupivacaine Hydrochloride (Limited published data indicates that somatropin treatment increases cytochrome P450 (CP450)-mediated antipyrine clearance in man. These data suggest that somatropin administration may alter the clearance of compounds metabolized by CP450 liver enzymes. Therefore, careful monitoring is advised when somatropin is administered in combination with drugs metabolized by CP450 liver enzymes).
No products indexed under this heading.

Levonorgestrel (Limited published data indicates that somatropin treatment increases cytochrome P450 (CP450)-mediated antipyrine clearance in man. These data suggest that somatropin administration may alter the clearance of compounds metabolized by CP450 liver enzymes (eg, sex steroids). Therefore, careful monitoring is advised when somatropin is administered in combination with drugs metabolized by CP450 liver enzymes). Products include:
Climara Pro 847
LoSeasonique 3407
Lybrel 3514
Mirena 854
Plan B 3416

Seasonique 3418

Lidocaine (Limited published data indicates that somatropin treatment increases cytochrome P450 (CP450)-mediated antipyrine clearance in man. These data suggest that somatropin administration may alter the clearance of compounds metabolized by CP450 liver enzymes. Therefore, careful monitoring is advised when somatropin is administered in combination with drugs metabolized by CP450 liver enzymes). Products include:
Lidoderm 1107

Lidocaine Base (Limited published data indicates that somatropin treatment increases cytochrome P450 (CP450)-mediated antipyrine clearance in man. These data suggest that somatropin administration may alter the clearance of compounds metabolized by CP450 liver enzymes. Therefore, careful monitoring is advised when somatropin is administered in combination with drugs metabolized by CP450 liver enzymes).
No products indexed under this heading.

Lidocaine Hydrochloride (Limited published data indicates that somatropin treatment increases cytochrome P450 (CP450)-mediated antipyrine clearance in man. These data suggest that somatropin administration may alter the clearance of compounds metabolized by CP450 liver enzymes. Therefore, careful monitoring is advised when somatropin is administered in combination with drugs metabolized by CP450 liver enzymes).
No products indexed under this heading.

Lomefloxacin Hydrochloride (Limited published data indicates that somatropin treatment increases cytochrome P450 (CP450)-mediated antipyrine clearance in man. These data suggest that somatropin administration may alter the clearance of compounds metabolized by CP450 liver enzymes. Therefore, careful monitoring is advised when somatropin is administered in combination with drugs metabolized by CP450 liver enzymes).
No products indexed under this heading.

Losartan Potassium (Limited published data indicates that somatropin treatment increases cytochrome P450 (CP450)-mediated antipyrine clearance in man. These data suggest that somatropin administration may alter the clearance of compounds metabolized by CP450 liver enzymes. Therefore, careful monitoring is advised when somatropin is administered in combination with drugs metabolized by CP450 liver enzymes). Products include:
Cozaar 2106
Hyzaar 2162
Hyzaar 100-12.5 2162

Lovastatin (Limited published data indicates that somatropin treatment increases cytochrome P450 (CP450)-mediated antipyrine clearance in man. These data suggest that somatropin administration may alter the clearance of compounds metabolized by CP450 liver enzymes. Therefore, careful monitoring is advised when somatropin is administered in combination with drugs metabolized by CP450 liver enzymes). Products include:
Advicor 402
Mevacor 2212

Maprotiline Hydrochloride (Limited published data indicates that somatropin treatment increases cytochrome P450 (CP450)-mediated antipyrine clearance in man. These data suggest that somatropin administration may alter the clearance of compounds metabolized by CP450 liver enzymes. Therefore, careful monitoring is advised

IMPORTANT NOTE: Always consult each drug listing in the patient's regimen for possible interactions.

when somatropin is administered in combination with drugs metabolized by CP450 liver enzymes).
No products indexed under this heading.

Meclofenamate Sodium (Limited published data indicates that somatropin treatment increases cytochrome P450 (CP450)-mediated antipyrine clearance in man. These data suggest that somatropin administration may alter the clearance of compounds metabolized by CP450 liver enzymes. Therefore, careful monitoring is advised when somatropin is administered in combination with drugs metabolized by CP450 liver enzymes).
No products indexed under this heading.

Mefenamic Acid (Limited published data indicates that somatropin treatment increases cytochrome P450 (CP450)-mediated antipyrine clearance in man. These data suggest that somatropin administration may alter the clearance of compounds metabolized by CP450 liver enzymes. Therefore, careful monitoring is advised when somatropin is administered in combination with drugs metabolized by CP450 liver enzymes).
No products indexed under this heading.

Meloxicam (Limited published data indicates that somatropin treatment increases cytochrome P450 (CP450)-mediated antipyrine clearance in man. These data suggest that somatropin administration may alter the clearance of compounds metabolized by CP450 liver enzymes. Therefore, careful monitoring is advised when somatropin is administered in combination with drugs metabolized by CP450 liver enzymes).
No products indexed under this heading.

Meperidine Hydrochloride (Limited published data indicates that somatropin treatment increases cytochrome P450 (CP450)-mediated antipyrine clearance in man. These data suggest that somatropin administration may alter the clearance of compounds metabolized by CP450 liver enzymes. Therefore, careful monitoring is advised when somatropin is administered in combination with drugs metabolized by CP450 liver enzymes).
No products indexed under this heading.

Mephenytoin (Limited published data indicates that somatropin treatment increases cytochrome P450 (CP450)-mediated antipyrine clearance in man. These data suggest that somatropin administration may alter the clearance of compounds metabolized by CP450 liver enzymes (eg, anticonvulsants). Therefore, careful monitoring is advised when somatropin is administered in combination with drugs metabolized by CP450 liver enzymes).
No products indexed under this heading.

Mephobarbital (Limited published data indicates that somatropin treatment increases cytochrome P450 (CP450)-mediated antipyrine clearance in man. These data suggest that somatropin administration may alter the clearance of compounds metabolized by CP450 liver enzymes. Therefore, careful monitoring is advised when somatropin is administered in combination with drugs metabolized by CP450 liver enzymes).
No products indexed under this heading.

Meprobamate (Limited published data indicates that somatropin treatment increases cytochrome P450 (CP450)-mediated antipyrine clearance in man. These data suggest that somatropin administration may alter the clearance of compounds metabolized by CP450 liver enzymes. Therefore, careful monitoring is advised when somatropin is administered in combination with drugs metabolized by CP450 liver enzymes).
No products indexed under this heading.

Mestranol (Limited published data indicates that somatropin treatment increases cytochrome P450 (CP450)-mediated antipyrine clearance in man. These data suggest that somatropin administration may alter the clearance of compounds metabolized by CP450 liver enzymes (eg, sex steroids). Therefore, careful monitoring is advised when somatropin is administered in combination with drugs metabolized by CP450 liver enzymes).
No products indexed under this heading.

Metformin Hydrochloride (Patients with diabetes mellitus who receive concomitant treatment with somatropin may require adjustment of their doses of insulin and/or other hypoglycemic agents). Products include:
ActoPlus **3338**
Avandamet **1345**
Janumet **2188**

Methadone Hydrochloride (Limited published data indicates that somatropin treatment increases cytochrome P450 (CP450)-mediated antipyrine clearance in man. These data suggest that somatropin administration may alter the clearance of compounds metabolized by CP450 liver enzymes. Therefore, careful monitoring is advised when somatropin is administered in combination with drugs metabolized by CP450 liver enzymes).
No products indexed under this heading.

Methamphetamine Hydrochloride (Limited published data indicates that somatropin treatment increases cytochrome P450 (CP450)-mediated antipyrine clearance in man. These data suggest that somatropin administration may alter the clearance of compounds metabolized by CP450 liver enzymes. Therefore, careful monitoring is advised when somatropin is administered in combination with drugs metabolized by CP450 liver enzymes).
No products indexed under this heading.

Methsuximide (Limited published data indicates that somatropin treatment increases cytochrome P450 (CP450)-mediated antipyrine clearance in man. These data suggest that somatropin administration may alter the clearance of compounds metabolized by CP450 liver enzymes (eg, anticonvulsants). Therefore, careful monitoring is advised when somatropin is administered in combination with drugs metabolized by CP450 liver enzymes).
No products indexed under this heading.

Methylprednisolone (Introduction of somatropin treatment may result in inhibition of 11βHSD-1 and reduced serum cortisol concentrations. As a consequence, patients treated with glucocorticoid replacement therapy for previously diagnosed hypoadrenalism may require an increase in their maintenance or stress doses; this may be especially true for patients treated with cortisone acetate and prednisone. In addition, excessive glucocorticoid therapy may attenuate the growth promoting effects of somatropin in children. Therefore, glucocorticoid replacement therapy should be carefully adjusted in children with concomitant GH and glucocorticoid deficiency to avoid both hypoadrenalism and an inhibitory effect on growth. Also, somatropin administration may alter the clearance of compounds known to be metabolized by CYP450 liver enzymes (eg, corticosteroids). Careful monitoring is advisable when somatropin is administered in combination with other drugs known to be metabolized by CYP450 liver enzymes).
No products indexed under this heading.

Methylprednisolone Acetate (Introduction of somatropin treatment may result in inhibition of 11βHSD-1 and reduced serum cortisol concentrations. As a consequence, patients treated with glucocorticoid replacement therapy for previously diagnosed hypoadrenalism may require an increase in their maintenance or stress doses; this may be especially true for patients treated with cortisone acetate and prednisone. In addition, excessive glucocorticoid therapy may attenuate the growth promoting effects of somatropin in children. Therefore, glucocorticoid replacement therapy should be carefully adjusted in children with concomitant GH and glucocorticoid deficiency to avoid both hypoadrenalism and an inhibitory effect on growth. Also, somatropin administration may alter the clearance of compounds known to be metabolized by CYP450 liver enzymes (eg, corticosteroids). Careful monitoring is advisable when somatropin is administered in combination with other drugs known to be metabolized by CYP450 liver enzymes).
No products indexed under this heading.

Methylprednisolone Sodium Succinate (Introduction of somatropin treatment may result in inhibition of 11βHSD-1 and reduced serum cortisol concentrations. As a consequence, patients treated with glucocorticoid replacement therapy for previously diagnosed hypoadrenalism may require an increase in their maintenance or stress doses; this may be especially true for patients treated with cortisone acetate and prednisone. In addition, excessive glucocorticoid therapy may attenuate the growth promoting effects of somatropin in children. Therefore, glucocorticoid replacement therapy should be carefully adjusted in children with concomitant GH and glucocorticoid deficiency to avoid both hypoadrenalism and an inhibitory effect on growth. Also, somatropin administration may alter the clearance of compounds known to be metabolized by CYP450 liver enzymes (eg, corticosteroids). Careful monitoring is advisable when somatropin is administered in combination with other drugs known to be metabolized by CYP450 liver enzymes).
No products indexed under this heading.

Methyltestosterone (Limited published data indicates that somatropin treatment increases cytochrome P450 (CP450)-mediated antipyrine clearance in man. These data suggest that somatropin administration may alter the clearance of compounds metabolized by CP450 liver enzymes (eg, sex steroids). Therefore, careful monitoring is advised when somatropin is administered in combination with drugs metabolized by CP450 liver enzymes).
No products indexed under this heading.

Metoprolol Succinate (Limited published data indicates that somatropin treatment increases cytochrome P450 (CP450)-mediated antipyrine clearance in man. These data suggest that somatropin administration may alter the clearance of compounds metabolized by CP450 liver enzymes. Therefore, careful monitoring is advised when somatropin is administered in combination with drugs metabolized by CP450 liver enzymes). Products include:
Toprol XL **732**

Metoprolol Tartrate (Limited published data indicates that somatropin treatment increases cytochrome P450 (CP450)-mediated antipyrine clearance in man. These data suggest that somatropin administration may alter the clearance of compounds metabolized by CP450 liver enzymes. Therefore, careful monitoring is advised when somatropin is administered in combination with drugs metabolized by CP450 liver enzymes).
No products indexed under this heading.

Mexiletine Hydrochloride (Limited published data indicates that somatropin treatment increases cytochrome P450 (CP450)-mediated antipyrine clearance in man. These data suggest that somatropin administration may alter the clearance of compounds metabolized by CP450 liver enzymes. Therefore, careful monitoring is advised when somatropin is administered in combination with drugs metabolized by CP450 liver enzymes).
No products indexed under this heading.

Midazolam Hydrochloride (Limited published data indicates that somatropin treatment increases cytochrome P450 (CP450)-mediated antipyrine clearance in man. These data suggest that somatropin administration may alter the clearance of compounds metabolized by CP450 liver enzymes. Therefore, careful monitoring is advised when somatropin is administered in combination with drugs metabolized by CP450 liver enzymes).
No products indexed under this heading.

Miglitol (Patients with diabetes mellitus who receive concomitant treatment with somatropin may require adjustment of their doses of insulin and/or other hypoglycemic agents).
No products indexed under this heading.

Mirtazapine (Limited published data indicates that somatropin treatment increases cytochrome P450 (CP450)-mediated antipyrine clearance in man. These data suggest that somatropin administration may alter the clearance of compounds metabolized by CP450 liver enzymes. Therefore, careful monitoring is advised when somatropin is administered in combination with drugs metabolized by CP450 liver enzymes). Products include:
Remeron Tablets **3214**
RemeronSolTab Tablets **3219**

Mometasone Furoate (Introduction of somatropin treatment may result in inhibition of 11βHSD-1 and reduced serum cortisol concentrations. As a consequence, patients treated with glucocorticoid replacement therapy for previously diagnosed hypoadrenalism may require an increase in their maintenance or stress doses; this may be especially true for patients treated with cortisone acetate and prednisone. In addition, excessive glucocorticoid therapy may attenuate the growth promoting effects of somatropin in children. Therefore, glucocorticoid replacement therapy should be carefully adjusted in children with concomitant GH and glucocorticoid deficiency to avoid both hypoadrenalism and an inhibitory effect on growth. Also, somatropin administration may alter the clearance of compounds known to be metabolized by CYP450 liver enzymes (eg, corticosteroids). Careful monitoring is advisable when somatropin is administered in combination with other drugs known to be metabolized by CYP450 liver enzymes). Products include:
Asmanex **3058**
Elocon Cream **3111**
Elocon Lotion **3112**
Elocon Ointment **3114**

Mometasone Furoate Monohydrate (Introduction of somatropin treatment may result in inhibition of 11βHSD-1 and reduced serum cortisol concentrations. As a consequence, patients treated with glucocorticoid replacement therapy for previously diagnosed hypoadrenalism may require an increase in their maintenance or stress doses; this may be especially

true for patients treated with cortisone acetate and prednisone. In addition, excessive glucocorticoid therapy may attenuate the growth promoting effects of somatropin in children. Therefore, glucocorticoid replacement therapy should be carefully adjusted in children with concomitant GH and glucocorticoid deficiency to avoid both hypoadrenalism and an inhibitory effect on growth. Also, somatropin administration may alter the clearance of compounds known to be metabolized by CYP450 liver enzymes (eg, corticosteroids). Careful monitoring is advisable when somatropin is administered in combination with other drugs known to be metabolized by CYP450 liver enzymes). Products include:
Nasonex 3166

Montelukast Sodium (Limited published data indicates that somatropin treatment increases cytochrome P450 (CP450)-mediated antipyrine clearance in man. These data suggest that somatropin administration may alter the clearance of compounds metabolized by CP450 liver enzymes. Therefore, careful monitoring is advised when somatropin is administered in combination with drugs metabolized by CP450 liver enzymes). Products include:
Singulair 2270

Morphine Sulfate (Limited published data indicates that somatropin treatment increases cytochrome P450 (CP450)-mediated antipyrine clearance in man. These data suggest that somatropin administration may alter the clearance of compounds metabolized by CP450 liver enzymes. Therefore, careful monitoring is advised when somatropin is administered in combination with drugs metabolized by CP450 liver enzymes). Products include:
Avinza 1822
Embeda 1831
MS Contin 2803

Moxifloxacin Hydrochloride (Limited published data indicates that somatropin treatment increases cytochrome P450 (CP450)-mediated antipyrine clearance in man. These data suggest that somatropin administration may alter the clearance of compounds metabolized by CP450 liver enzymes. Therefore, careful monitoring is advised when somatropin is administered in combination with drugs metabolized by CP450 liver enzymes). Products include:
Avelox 3064
Vigamox 589

Nabumetone (Limited published data indicates that somatropin treatment increases cytochrome P450 (CP450)-mediated antipyrine clearance in man. These data suggest that somatropin administration may alter the clearance of compounds metabolized by CP450 liver enzymes. Therefore, careful monitoring is advised when somatropin is administered in combination with drugs metabolized by CP450 liver enzymes).
No products indexed under this heading.

Nafcillin Sodium (Limited published data indicates that somatropin treatment increases cytochrome P450 (CP450)-mediated antipyrine clearance in man. These data suggest that somatropin administration may alter the clearance of compounds metabolized by CP450 liver enzymes. Therefore, careful monitoring is advised when somatropin is administered in combination with drugs metabolized by CP450 liver enzymes).
No products indexed under this heading.

Naproxen (Limited published data indicates that somatropin treatment increases cytochrome P450 (CP450)-mediated antipyrine clearance in man. These data suggest that somat-

ropin administration may alter the clearance of compounds metabolized by CP450 liver enzymes. Therefore, careful monitoring is advised when somatropin is administered in combination with drugs metabolized by CP450 liver enzymes). Products include:
EC-Naprosyn 2850
Naprosyn 2850
Anaprox/Naprosyn 2850

Naproxen Sodium (Limited published data indicates that somatropin treatment increases cytochrome P450 (CP450)-mediated antipyrine clearance in man. These data suggest that somatropin administration may alter the clearance of compounds metabolized by CP450 liver enzymes. Therefore, careful monitoring is advised when somatropin is administered in combination with drugs metabolized by CP450 liver enzymes). Products include:
Anaprox 2850
Anaprox DS 2850
Treximet 1681

Nateglinide (Patients with diabetes mellitus who receive concomitant treatment with somatropin may require adjustment of their doses of insulin and/or other hypoglycemic agents).
No products indexed under this heading.

Nefazodone Hydrochloride (Limited published data indicates that somatropin treatment increases cytochrome P450 (CP450)-mediated antipyrine clearance in man. These data suggest that somatropin administration may alter the clearance of compounds metabolized by CP450 liver enzymes. Therefore, careful monitoring is advised when somatropin is administered in combination with drugs metabolized by CP450 liver enzymes).
No products indexed under this heading.

Nelfinavir Mesylate (Limited published data indicates that somatropin treatment increases cytochrome P450 (CP450)-mediated antipyrine clearance in man. These data suggest that somatropin administration may alter the clearance of compounds metabolized by CP450 liver enzymes. Therefore, careful monitoring is advised when somatropin is administered in combination with drugs metabolized by CP450 liver enzymes).
No products indexed under this heading.

Nicardipine (Limited published data indicates that somatropin treatment increases cytochrome P450 (CP450)-mediated antipyrine clearance in man. These data suggest that somatropin administration may alter the clearance of compounds metabolized by CP450 liver enzymes. Therefore, careful monitoring is advised when somatropin is administered in combination with drugs metabolized by CP450 liver enzymes).
No products indexed under this heading.

Nicardipine Hydrochloride (Limited published data indicates that somatropin treatment increases cytochrome P450 (CP450)-mediated antipyrine clearance in man. These data suggest that somatropin administration may alter the clearance of compounds metabolized by CP450 liver enzymes. Therefore, careful monitoring is advised when somatropin is administered in combination with drugs metabolized by CP450 liver enzymes).
No products indexed under this heading.

Nicotine Polacrilex (Limited published data indicates that somatropin treatment increases cytochrome P450 (CP450)-mediated antipyrine clearance in man. These data suggest that somatropin administration may alter the clearance of compounds metabolized by CP450 liver enzymes. Therefore, careful monitoring is advised when somatro-

pin is administered in combination with drugs metabolized by CP450 liver enzymes).
No products indexed under this heading.

Nicotine Salicylate (Limited published data indicates that somatropin treatment increases cytochrome P450 (CP450)-mediated antipyrine clearance in man. These data suggest that somatropin administration may alter the clearance of compounds metabolized by CP450 liver enzymes. Therefore, careful monitoring is advised when somatropin is administered in combination with drugs metabolized by CP450 liver enzymes).
No products indexed under this heading.

Nicotine Sulfate (Limited published data indicates that somatropin treatment increases cytochrome P450 (CP450)-mediated antipyrine clearance in man. These data suggest that somatropin administration may alter the clearance of compounds metabolized by CP450 liver enzymes. Therefore, careful monitoring is advised when somatropin is administered in combination with drugs metabolized by CP450 liver enzymes).
No products indexed under this heading.

Nifedipine (Limited published data indicates that somatropin treatment increases cytochrome P450 (CP450)-mediated antipyrine clearance in man. These data suggest that somatropin administration may alter the clearance of compounds metabolized by CP450 liver enzymes. Therefore, careful monitoring is advised when somatropin is administered in combination with drugs metabolized by CP450 liver enzymes).
No products indexed under this heading.

Nilutamide (Limited published data indicates that somatropin treatment increases cytochrome P450 (CP450)-mediated antipyrine clearance in man. These data suggest that somatropin administration may alter the clearance of compounds metabolized by CP450 liver enzymes. Therefore, careful monitoring is advised when somatropin is administered in combination with drugs metabolized by CP450 liver enzymes).
No products indexed under this heading.

Nimodipine (Limited published data indicates that somatropin treatment increases cytochrome P450 (CP450)-mediated antipyrine clearance in man. These data suggest that somatropin administration may alter the clearance of compounds metabolized by CP450 liver enzymes. Therefore, careful monitoring is advised when somatropin is administered in combination with drugs metabolized by CP450 liver enzymes).
No products indexed under this heading.

Nisoldipine (Limited published data indicates that somatropin treatment increases cytochrome P450 (CP450)-mediated antipyrine clearance in man. These data suggest that somatropin administration may alter the clearance of compounds metabolized by CP450 liver enzymes. Therefore, careful monitoring is advised when somatropin is administered in combination with drugs metabolized by CP450 liver enzymes).
No products indexed under this heading.

Nitrendipine (Limited published data indicates that somatropin treatment increases cytochrome P450 (CP450)-mediated antipyrine clearance in man. These data suggest that somatropin administration may alter the clearance of compounds metabolized by CP450 liver enzymes. Therefore, careful monitoring is advised when somatro-

pin is administered in combination with drugs metabolized by CP450 liver enzymes).
No products indexed under this heading.

Norethindrone (Limited published data indicates that somatropin treatment increases cytochrome P450 (CP450)-mediated antipyrine clearance in man. These data suggest that somatropin administration may alter the clearance of compounds metabolized by CP450 liver enzymes (eg, sex steroids). Therefore, careful monitoring is advised when somatropin is administered in combination with drugs metabolized by CP450 liver enzymes). Products include:
Ortho Micronor 2660

Norethindrone Acetate (Limited published data indicates that somatropin treatment increases cytochrome P450 (CP450)-mediated antipyrine clearance in man. These data suggest that somatropin administration may alter the clearance of compounds metabolized by CP450 liver enzymes (eg, sex steroids). Therefore, careful monitoring is advised when somatropin is administered in combination with drugs metabolized by CP450 liver enzymes). Products include:
Activella 2561

Norfloxacin (Limited published data indicates that somatropin treatment increases cytochrome P450 (CP450)-mediated antipyrine clearance in man. These data suggest that somatropin administration may alter the clearance of compounds metabolized by CP450 liver enzymes. Therefore, careful monitoring is advised when somatropin is administered in combination with drugs metabolized by CP450 liver enzymes). Products include:
Noroxin 2220

Norgestimate (Limited published data indicates that somatropin treatment increases cytochrome P450 (CP450)-mediated antipyrine clearance in man. These data suggest that somatropin administration may alter the clearance of compounds metabolized by CP450 liver enzymes (eg, sex steroids). Therefore, careful monitoring is advised when somatropin is administered in combination with drugs metabolized by CP450 liver enzymes). Products include:
Ortho-Cyclen/Ortho Tri-Cyclen 2663
Ortho Tri-Cyclen Lo Tablets 2673

Norgestrel (Limited published data indicates that somatropin treatment increases cytochrome P450 (CP450)-mediated antipyrine clearance in man. These data suggest that somatropin administration may alter the clearance of compounds metabolized by CP450 liver enzymes. Therefore, careful monitoring is advised when somatropin is administered in combination with drugs metabolized by CP450 liver enzymes).
No products indexed under this heading.

Nortriptyline Hydrochloride (Limited published data indicates that somatropin treatment increases cytochrome P450 (CP450)-mediated antipyrine clearance in man. These data suggest that somatropin administration may alter the clearance of compounds metabolized by CP450 liver enzymes. Therefore, careful monitoring is advised when somatropin is administered in combination with drugs metabolized by CP450 liver enzymes).
No products indexed under this heading.

Ofloxacin (Limited published data indicates that somatropin treatment increases cytochrome P450 (CP450)-mediated antipyrine clearance in man. These data suggest that somatropin administration may alter the clearance of compounds metabolized by

---

IMPORTANT NOTE: Always consult each drug listing in the patient's regimen for possible interactions.

Humatrope Interactions Index 812

CP450 liver enzymes. Therefore, careful monitoring is advised when somatropin is administered in combination with drugs metabolized by CP450 liver enzymes).
No products indexed under this heading.

Olanzapine (Limited published data indicates that somatropin treatment increases cytochrome P450 (CP450)-mediated antipyrine clearance in man. These data suggest that somatropin administration may alter the clearance of compounds metabolized by CP450 liver enzymes. Therefore, careful monitoring is advised when somatropin is administered in combination with drugs metabolized by CP450 liver enzymes). Products include:
Symbyax 1965
Zyprexa 1984
Zyprexa IntraMuscular 1984
Zyprexa ZYDIS 1984

Omeprazole (Limited published data indicates that somatropin treatment increases cytochrome P450 (CP450)-mediated antipyrine clearance in man. These data suggest that somatropin administration may alter the clearance of compounds metabolized by CP450 liver enzymes. Therefore, careful monitoring is advised when somatropin is administered in combination with drugs metabolized by CP450 liver enzymes).
No products indexed under this heading.

Omeprazole Magnesium (Limited published data indicates that somatropin treatment increases cytochrome P450 (CP450)-mediated antipyrine clearance in man. These data suggest that somatropin administration may alter the clearance of compounds metabolized by CP450 liver enzymes. Therefore, careful monitoring is advised when somatropin is administered in combination with drugs metabolized by CP450 liver enzymes).
No products indexed under this heading.

Ondansetron (Limited published data indicates that somatropin treatment increases cytochrome P450 (CP450)-mediated antipyrine clearance in man. These data suggest that somatropin administration may alter the clearance of compounds metabolized by CP450 liver enzymes. Therefore, careful monitoring is advised when somatropin is administered in combination with drugs metabolized by CP450 liver enzymes).
No products indexed under this heading.

Ondansetron Hydrochloride (Limited published data indicates that somatropin treatment increases cytochrome P450 (CP450)-mediated antipyrine clearance in man. These data suggest that somatropin administration may alter the clearance of compounds metabolized by CP450 liver enzymes. Therefore, careful monitoring is advised when somatropin is administered in combination with drugs metabolized by CP450 liver enzymes). Products include:
Zofran Injection 1750
Zofran 1756
Zofran ODT 1756

Oxaprozin (Limited published data indicates that somatropin treatment increases cytochrome P450 (CP450)-mediated antipyrine clearance in man. These data suggest that somatropin administration may alter the clearance of compounds metabolized by CP450 liver enzymes. Therefore, careful monitoring is advised when somatropin is administered in combination with drugs metabolized by CP450 liver enzymes).
No products indexed under this heading.

Oxcarbazepine (Limited published data indicates that somatropin treatment increases cytochrome P450 (CP450)-mediated antipyrine clearance in man. These data suggest that somatropin administration may alter the clearance of compounds metabolized by CP450 liver enzymes (eg, anticonvulsants). Therefore, careful monitoring is advised when somatropin is administered in combination with drugs metabolized by CP450 liver enzymes).
No products indexed under this heading.

Oxycodone Hydrochloride (Limited published data indicates that somatropin treatment increases cytochrome P450 (CP450)-mediated antipyrine clearance in man. These data suggest that somatropin administration may alter the clearance of compounds metabolized by CP450 liver enzymes. Therefore, careful monitoring is advised when somatropin is administered in combination with drugs metabolized by CP450 liver enzymes). Products include:
OxyContin 2807
Percocet 1121
Percodan 1124

Paclitaxel (Limited published data indicates that somatropin treatment increases cytochrome P450 (CP450)-mediated antipyrine clearance in man. These data suggest that somatropin administration may alter the clearance of compounds metabolized by CP450 liver enzymes. Therefore, careful monitoring is advised when somatropin is administered in combination with drugs metabolized by CP450 liver enzymes).
No products indexed under this heading.

Pantoprazole Sodium (Limited published data indicates that somatropin treatment increases cytochrome P450 (CP450)-mediated antipyrine clearance in man. These data suggest that somatropin administration may alter the clearance of compounds metabolized by CP450 liver enzymes. Therefore, careful monitoring is advised when somatropin is administered in combination with drugs metabolized by CP450 liver enzymes). Products include:
Protonix Tablets 3571
Protonix 3575

Paramethadione (Limited published data indicates that somatropin treatment increases cytochrome P450 (CP450)-mediated antipyrine clearance in man. These data suggest that somatropin administration may alter the clearance of compounds metabolized by CP450 liver enzymes (eg, anticonvulsants). Therefore, careful monitoring is advised when somatropin is administered in combination with drugs metabolized by CP450 liver enzymes).
No products indexed under this heading.

Paroxetine Hydrochloride (Limited published data indicates that somatropin treatment increases cytochrome P450 (CP450)-mediated antipyrine clearance in man. These data suggest that somatropin administration may alter the clearance of compounds metabolized by CP450 liver enzymes. Therefore, careful monitoring is advised when somatropin is administered in combination with drugs metabolized by CP450 liver enzymes). Products include:
Paroxetine CR 2361
Paroxetine ER 2371
Paxil 1586
Paxil CR 1596

Pentamidine Isethionate (Limited published data indicates that somatropin treatment increases cytochrome P450 (CP450)-mediated antipyrine clearance in man. These data suggest that somatropin administration may alter the clearance of compounds metabolized by CP450 liver enzymes. Therefore, careful monitoring is advised when somatropin is administered in combination with drugs metabolized by CP450 liver enzymes).
No products indexed under this heading.

Phenacemide (Limited published data indicates that somatropin treatment increases cytochrome P450 (CP450)-mediated antipyrine clearance in man. These data suggest that somatropin administration may alter the clearance of compounds metabolized by CP450 liver enzymes (eg, anticonvulsants). Therefore, careful monitoring is advised when somatropin is administered in combination with drugs metabolized by CP450 liver enzymes).
No products indexed under this heading.

Phenobarbital (Limited published data indicates that somatropin treatment increases cytochrome P450 (CP450)-mediated antipyrine clearance in man. These data suggest that somatropin administration may alter the clearance of compounds metabolized by CP450 liver enzymes (eg, anticonvulsants). Therefore, careful monitoring is advised when somatropin is administered in combination with drugs metabolized by CP450 liver enzymes). Products include:
Donnatal 2711

Phenobarbital Sodium (Limited published data indicates that somatropin treatment increases cytochrome P450 (CP450)-mediated antipyrine clearance in man. These data suggest that somatropin administration may alter the clearance of compounds metabolized by CP450 liver enzymes (eg, anticonvulsants). Therefore, careful monitoring is advised when somatropin is administered in combination with drugs metabolized by CP450 liver enzymes).
No products indexed under this heading.

Phensuximide (Limited published data indicates that somatropin treatment increases cytochrome P450 (CP450)-mediated antipyrine clearance in man. These data suggest that somatropin administration may alter the clearance of compounds metabolized by CP450 liver enzymes (eg, anticonvulsants). Therefore, careful monitoring is advised when somatropin is administered in combination with drugs metabolized by CP450 liver enzymes).
No products indexed under this heading.

Phenylbutazone (Limited published data indicates that somatropin treatment increases cytochrome P450 (CP450)-mediated antipyrine clearance in man. These data suggest that somatropin administration may alter the clearance of compounds metabolized by CP450 liver enzymes. Therefore, careful monitoring is advised when somatropin is administered in combination with drugs metabolized by CP450 liver enzymes).
No products indexed under this heading.

Phenytoin (Limited published data indicates that somatropin treatment increases cytochrome P450 (CP450)-mediated antipyrine clearance in man. These data suggest that somatropin administration may alter the clearance of compounds metabolized by CP450 liver enzymes (eg, anticonvulsants). Therefore, careful monitoring is advised when somatropin is administered in combination with drugs metabolized by CP450 liver enzymes).
No products indexed under this heading.

Phenytoin Sodium (Limited published data indicates that somatropin treatment increases cytochrome P450 (CP450)-mediated antipyrine clearance in man. These data suggest that somatropin administration may alter the clearance of compounds metabolized by CP450 liver enzymes (eg, anticonvulsants). Therefore, careful monitoring is advised when somatropin is administered in combination with drugs metabolized by CP450 liver enzymes). Products include:
Phenytek Capsules 2380

Pimozide (Limited published data indicates that somatropin treatment increases cytochrome P450 (CP450)-mediated antipyrine clearance in man. These data suggest that somatropin administration may alter the clearance of compounds metabolized by CP450 liver enzymes. Therefore, careful monitoring is advised when somatropin is administered in combination with drugs metabolized by CP450 liver enzymes).
No products indexed under this heading.

Pindolol (Limited published data indicates that somatropin treatment increases cytochrome P450 (CP450)-mediated antipyrine clearance in man. These data suggest that somatropin administration may alter the clearance of compounds metabolized by CP450 liver enzymes. Therefore, careful monitoring is advised when somatropin is administered in combination with drugs metabolized by CP450 liver enzymes).
No products indexed under this heading.

Pioglitazone Hydrochloride (Patients with diabetes mellitus who receive concomitant treatment with somatropin may require adjustment of their doses of insulin and/or other hypoglycemic agents). Products include:
ActoPlus 3338
Actos 3345
Duetact 3354

Piroxicam (Limited published data indicates that somatropin treatment increases cytochrome P450 (CP450)-mediated antipyrine clearance in man. These data suggest that somatropin administration may alter the clearance of compounds metabolized by CP450 liver enzymes. Therefore, careful monitoring is advised when somatropin is administered in combination with drugs metabolized by CP450 liver enzymes).
No products indexed under this heading.

Polyestradiol Phosphate (Because oral estrogens may reduce the serum insulin-like growth factor I (IGF-I) response to somatropin treatment, girls and women receiving oral estrogen replacement may require greater somatropin dosages).
No products indexed under this heading.

Prednisolone (Introduction of somatropin treatment may result in inhibition of 11βHSD-1 and reduced serum cortisol concentrations. As a consequence, patients treated with glucocorticoid replacement therapy for previously diagnosed hypoadrenalism may require an increase in their maintenance or stress doses; this may be especially true for patients treated with cortisone acetate and prednisone. In addition, excessive glucocorticoid therapy may attenuate the growth promoting effects of somatropin in children. Therefore, glucocorticoid replacement therapy should be carefully adjusted in children with concomitant GH and glucocorticoid deficiency to avoid both hypoadrenalism and an inhibitory effect on growth. Also, somatropin administration may alter the clearance of compounds known to be metabolized by CYP450 liver enzymes (eg, corticosteroids). Careful monitoring is advisable when somatropin is administered in combination with other drugs known to be metabolized by CYP450 liver enzymes).
No products indexed under this heading.

Prednisolone Acetate (Introduction of somatropin treatment may result in inhibition of 11βHSD-1 and reduced serum cortisol concentrations. As a

consequence, patients treated with glucocorticoid replacement therapy for previously diagnosed hypoadrenalism may require an increase in their maintenance or stress doses; this may be especially true for patients treated with cortisone acetate and prednisone. In addition, excessive glucocorticoid therapy may attenuate the growth promoting effects of somatropin in children. Therefore, glucocorticoid replacement therapy should be carefully adjusted in children with concomitant GH and glucocorticoid deficiency to avoid both hypoadrenalism and an inhibitory effect on growth. Also, somatropin administration may alter the clearance of compounds known to be metabolized by CYP450 liver enzymes (eg, corticosteroids). Careful monitoring is advisable when somatropin is administered in combination with other drugs known to be metabolized by CYP450 liver enzymes). Products include:

Blephamide .... ⊙**212**, ⊙**214**
Pred Forte .... ⊙**225**
Pred Mild .... ⊙**230**
Pred-G .... ⊙**226**, ⊙**227**

Prednisolone Sodium Phosphate (Introduction of somatropin treatment may result in inhibition of 11βHSD-1 and reduced serum cortisol concentrations. As a consequence, patients treated with glucocorticoid replacement therapy for previously diagnosed hypoadrenalism may require an increase in their maintenance or stress doses; this may be especially true for patients treated with cortisone acetate and prednisone. In addition, excessive glucocorticoid therapy may attenuate the growth promoting effects of somatropin in children. Therefore, glucocorticoid replacement therapy should be carefully adjusted in children with concomitant GH and glucocorticoid deficiency to avoid both hypoadrenalism and an inhibitory effect on growth. Also, somatropin administration may alter the clearance of compounds known to be metabolized by CYP450 liver enzymes (eg, corticosteroids). Careful monitoring is advisable when somatropin is administered in combination with other drugs known to be metabolized by CYP450 liver enzymes).
No products indexed under this heading.

Prednisolone Tebutate (Introduction of somatropin treatment may result in inhibition of 11βHSD-1 and reduced serum cortisol concentrations. As a consequence, patients treated with glucocorticoid replacement therapy for previously diagnosed hypoadrenalism may require an increase in their maintenance or stress doses; this may be especially true for patients treated with cortisone acetate and prednisone. In addition, excessive glucocorticoid therapy may attenuate the growth promoting effects of somatropin in children. Therefore, glucocorticoid replacement therapy should be carefully adjusted in children with concomitant GH and glucocorticoid deficiency to avoid both hypoadrenalism and an inhibitory effect on growth. Also, somatropin administration may alter the clearance of compounds known to be metabolized by CYP450 liver enzymes (eg, corticosteroids). Careful monitoring is advisable when somatropin is administered in combination with other drugs known to be metabolized by CYP450 liver enzymes).
No products indexed under this heading.

Prednisone (Introduction of somatropin treatment may result in inhibition of 11βHSD-1 and reduced serum cortisol concentrations. As a consequence, patients treated with glucocorticoid replacement therapy for previously diagnosed hypoadrenalism may require an increase in their maintenance or stress doses; this may be especially true for patients treated with cortisone acetate and prednisone. In addition, excessive glucocorticoid therapy may attenuate the growth promoting effects of somatropin in children. Therefore, glucocorticoid replacement therapy should be carefully adjusted in children with concomitant GH and glucocorticoid deficiency to avoid both hypoadrenalism and an inhibitory effect on growth. Also, somatropin administration may alter the clearance of compounds known to be metabolized by CYP450 liver enzymes (eg, corticosteroids). Careful monitoring is advisable when somatropin is administered in combination with other drugs known to be metabolized by CYP450 liver enzymes 1).
No products indexed under this heading.

Prednisone sodium phosphate (Introduction of somatropin treatment may result in inhibition of 11βHSD-1 and reduced serum cortisol concentrations. As a consequence, patients treated with glucocorticoid replacement therapy for previously diagnosed hypoadrenalism may require an increase in their maintenance or stress doses; this may be especially true for patients treated with cortisone acetate and prednisone. In addition, excessive glucocorticoid therapy may attenuate the growth promoting effects of somatropin in children. Therefore, glucocorticoid replacement therapy should be carefully adjusted in children with concomitant GH and glucocorticoid deficiency to avoid both hypoadrenalism and an inhibitory effect on growth. Also, somatropin administration may alter the clearance of compounds known to be metabolized by CYP450 liver enzymes (eg, corticosteroids). Careful monitoring is advisable when somatropin is administered in combination with other drugs known to be metabolized by CYP450 liver enzymes 1).
No products indexed under this heading.

Primidone (Limited published data indicates that somatropin treatment increases cytochrome P450 (CP450)-mediated antipyrine clearance in man. These data suggest that somatropin administration may alter the clearance of compounds metabolized by CP450 liver enzymes (eg, anticonvulsants). Therefore, careful monitoring is advised when somatropin is administered in combination with drugs metabolized by CP450 liver enzymes).
No products indexed under this heading.

Progesterone (Limited published data indicates that somatropin treatment increases cytochrome P450 (CP450)-mediated antipyrine clearance in man. These data suggest that somatropin administration may alter the clearance of compounds metabolized by CP450 liver enzymes. Therefore, careful monitoring is advised when somatropin is administered in combination with drugs metabolized by CP450 liver enzymes). Products include:

Crinone 4% **996**
Crinone 8% **996**
Prometrium **3307**

Proguanil Hydrochloride (Limited published data indicates that somatropin treatment increases cytochrome P450 (CP450)-mediated antipyrine clearance in man. These data suggest that somatropin administration may alter the clearance of compounds metabolized by CP450 liver enzymes. Therefore, careful monitoring is advised when somatropin is administered in combination with drugs metabolized by CP450 liver enzymes). Products include:

Malarone Pediatric Tablets **1572**
Malarone **1572**

Propafenone Hydrochloride (Limited published data indicates that somatropin treatment increases cytochrome P450 (CP450)-mediated antipyrine clearance in man. These data suggest that somatropin administration may alter the clearance of compounds metabolized by CP450 liver enzymes. Therefore, careful monitoring is advised when somatropin is administered in combination with drugs metabolized by CP450 liver enzymes). Products include:

Rythmol **1648**
Rythmol SR **1652**

Propoxyphene Hydrochloride (Limited published data indicates that somatropin treatment increases cytochrome P450 (CP450)-mediated antipyrine clearance in man. These data suggest that somatropin administration may alter the clearance of compounds metabolized by CP450 liver enzymes. Therefore, careful monitoring is advised when somatropin is administered in combination with drugs metabolized by CP450 liver enzymes).
No products indexed under this heading.

Propoxyphene Napsylate (Limited published data indicates that somatropin treatment increases cytochrome P450 (CP450)-mediated antipyrine clearance in man. These data suggest that somatropin administration may alter the clearance of compounds metabolized by CP450 liver enzymes. Therefore, careful monitoring is advised when somatropin is administered in combination with drugs metabolized by CP450 liver enzymes).
No products indexed under this heading.

Propranolol Hydrochloride (Limited published data indicates that somatropin treatment increases cytochrome P450 (CP450)-mediated antipyrine clearance in man. These data suggest that somatropin administration may alter the clearance of compounds metabolized by CP450 liver enzymes. Therefore, careful monitoring is advised when somatropin is administered in combination with drugs metabolized by CP450 liver enzymes). Products include:

InnoPran XL **1517**

Protriptyline Hydrochloride (Limited published data indicates that somatropin treatment increases cytochrome P450 (CP450)-mediated antipyrine clearance in man. These data suggest that somatropin administration may alter the clearance of compounds metabolized by CP450 liver enzymes. Therefore, careful monitoring is advised when somatropin is administered in combination with drugs metabolized by CP450 liver enzymes).
No products indexed under this heading.

Quetiapine Fumarate (Limited published data indicates that somatropin treatment increases cytochrome P450 (CP450)-mediated antipyrine clearance in man. These data suggest that somatropin administration may alter the clearance of compounds metabolized by CP450 liver enzymes. Therefore, careful monitoring is advised when somatropin is administered in combination with drugs metabolized by CP450 liver enzymes). Products include:

Seroquel **750**
Seroquel XR **759**

Quinestrol (Because oral estrogens may reduce the serum insulin-like growth factor I (IGF-I) response to somatropin treatment, girls and women receiving oral estrogen replacement may require greater somatropin dosages).
No products indexed under this heading.

Quinidine Gluconate (Limited published data indicates that somatropin treatment increases cytochrome P450 (CP450)-mediated antipyrine clearance in man. These data suggest that somatropin administration may alter the clearance of compounds metabolized by CP450 liver enzymes. Therefore, careful monitoring is advised when somatropin is administered in combination with drugs metabolized by CP450 liver enzymes).
No products indexed under this heading.

Quinidine Hydrochloride (Limited published data indicates that somatropin treatment increases cytochrome P450 (CP450)-mediated antipyrine clearance in man. These data suggest that somatropin administration may alter the clearance of compounds metabolized by CP450 liver enzymes. Therefore, careful monitoring is advised when somatropin is administered in combination with drugs metabolized by CP450 liver enzymes).
No products indexed under this heading.

Quinidine Polygalacturonate (Limited published data indicates that somatropin treatment increases cytochrome P450 (CP450)-mediated antipyrine clearance in man. These data suggest that somatropin administration may alter the clearance of compounds metabolized by CP450 liver enzymes. Therefore, careful monitoring is advised when somatropin is administered in combination with drugs metabolized by CP450 liver enzymes).
No products indexed under this heading.

Quinidine Sulfate (Limited published data indicates that somatropin treatment increases cytochrome P450 (CP450)-mediated antipyrine clearance in man. These data suggest that somatropin administration may alter the clearance of compounds metabolized by CP450 liver enzymes. Therefore, careful monitoring is advised when somatropin is administered in combination with drugs metabolized by CP450 liver enzymes).
No products indexed under this heading.

Quinine (Limited published data indicates that somatropin treatment increases cytochrome P450 (CP450)-mediated antipyrine clearance in man. These data suggest that somatropin administration may alter the clearance of compounds metabolized by CP450 liver enzymes. Therefore, careful monitoring is advised when somatropin is administered in combination with drugs metabolized by CP450 liver enzymes). Products include:

Hyland's Leg Cramps PM with
Quinine **3315**

Quinine Sulfate (Limited published data indicates that somatropin treatment increases cytochrome P450 (CP450)-mediated antipyrine clearance in man. These data suggest that somatropin administration may alter the clearance of compounds metabolized by CP450 liver enzymes. Therefore, careful monitoring is advised when somatropin is administered in combination with drugs metabolized by CP450 liver enzymes).
No products indexed under this heading.

Rabeprazole Sodium (Limited published data indicates that somatropin treatment increases cytochrome P450 (CP450)-mediated antipyrine clearance in man. These data suggest that somatropin administration may alter the clearance of compounds metabolized by CP450 liver enzymes. Therefore, careful monitoring is advised when somatropin is administered in combination with drugs metabolized by CP450 liver enzymes). Products include:

Aciphex **1035**

IMPORTANT NOTE: Always consult each drug listing in the patient's regimen for possible interactions.

increases cytochrome P450 (CP450)-mediated antipyrine clearance in man. These data suggest that somatropin administration may alter the clearance of compounds metabolized by CP450 liver enzymes. Therefore, careful monitoring is advised when somatropin is administered in combination with drugs metabolized by CP450 liver enzymes).
No products indexed under this heading.

Testosterone (Limited published data indicates that somatropin treatment increases cytochrome P450 (CP450)-mediated antipyrine clearance in man. These data suggest that somatropin administration may alter the clearance of compounds metabolized by CP450 liver enzymes (eg, sex steroids). Therefore, careful monitoring is advised when somatropin is administered in combination with drugs metabolized by CP450 liver enzymes). Products include:
AndroGel **3456**

Testosterone Cypionate (Limited published data indicates that somatropin treatment increases cytochrome P450 (CP450)-mediated antipyrine clearance in man. These data suggest that somatropin administration may alter the clearance of compounds metabolized by CP450 liver enzymes. Therefore, careful monitoring is advised when somatropin is administered in combination with drugs metabolized by CP450 liver enzymes).
No products indexed under this heading.

Testosterone Enanthate (Limited published data indicates that somatropin treatment increases cytochrome P450 (CP450)-mediated antipyrine clearance in man. These data suggest that somatropin administration may alter the clearance of compounds metabolized by CP450 liver enzymes. Therefore, careful monitoring is advised when somatropin is administered in combination with drugs metabolized by CP450 liver enzymes). Products include:
Delatestryl **1102**

Testosterone Propionate (Limited published data indicates that somatropin treatment increases cytochrome P450 (CP450)-mediated antipyrine clearance in man. These data suggest that somatropin administration may alter the clearance of compounds metabolized by CP450 liver enzymes. Therefore, careful monitoring is advised when somatropin is administered in combination with drugs metabolized by CP450 liver enzymes).
No products indexed under this heading.

Theophylline (Limited published data indicates that somatropin treatment increases cytochrome P450 (CP450)-mediated antipyrine clearance in man. These data suggest that somatropin administration may alter the clearance of compounds metabolized by CP450 liver enzymes. Therefore, careful monitoring is advised when somatropin is administered in combination with drugs metabolized by CP450 liver enzymes).
No products indexed under this heading.

Theophylline Anhydrous (Limited published data indicates that somatropin treatment increases cytochrome P450 (CP450)-mediated antipyrine clearance in man. These data suggest that somatropin administration may alter the clearance of compounds metabolized by CP450 liver enzymes. Therefore, careful monitoring is advised when somatropin is administered in combination with drugs metabolized by CP450 liver enzymes). Products include:
Uniphyl **2817**

Theophylline Calcium Salicylate (Limited published data indicates that somatropin treatment increases cytochrome P450 (CP450)-mediated antipyrine clearance in man. These data suggest that somatropin administration may alter the clearance of compounds metabolized by CP450 liver enzymes. Therefore, careful monitoring is advised when somatropin is administered in combination with drugs metabolized by CP450 liver enzymes).
No products indexed under this heading.

Theophylline Dihydroxypropyl (Glyceryl) (Limited published data indicates that somatropin treatment increases cytochrome P450 (CP450)-mediated antipyrine clearance in man. These data suggest that somatropin administration may alter the clearance of compounds metabolized by CP450 liver enzymes. Therefore, careful monitoring is advised when somatropin is administered in combination with drugs metabolized by CP450 liver enzymes).
No products indexed under this heading.

Theophylline Ethylenediamine (Limited published data indicates that somatropin treatment increases cytochrome P450 (CP450)-mediated antipyrine clearance in man. These data suggest that somatropin administration may alter the clearance of compounds metabolized by CP450 liver enzymes. Therefore, careful monitoring is advised when somatropin is administered in combination with drugs metabolized by CP450 liver enzymes).
No products indexed under this heading.

Theophylline Sodium Glycinate (Limited published data indicates that somatropin treatment increases cytochrome P450 (CP450)-mediated antipyrine clearance in man. These data suggest that somatropin administration may alter the clearance of compounds metabolized by CP450 liver enzymes. Therefore, careful monitoring is advised when somatropin is administered in combination with drugs metabolized by CP450 liver enzymes).
No products indexed under this heading.

Thioridazine (Limited published data indicates that somatropin treatment increases cytochrome P450 (CP450)-mediated antipyrine clearance in man. These data suggest that somatropin administration may alter the clearance of compounds metabolized by CP450 liver enzymes. Therefore, careful monitoring is advised when somatropin is administered in combination with drugs metabolized by CP450 liver enzymes).
No products indexed under this heading.

Thioridazine Hydrochloride (Limited published data indicates that somatropin treatment increases cytochrome P450 (CP450)-mediated antipyrine clearance in man. These data suggest that somatropin administration may alter the clearance of compounds metabolized by CP450 liver enzymes. Therefore, careful monitoring is advised when somatropin is administered in combination with drugs metabolized by CP450 liver enzymes). Products include:
Thioridazine Hydrochloride **2384**

Tiagabine Hydrochloride (Limited published data indicates that somatropin treatment increases cytochrome P450 (CP450)-mediated antipyrine clearance in man. These data suggest that somatropin administration may alter the clearance of compounds metabolized by CP450 liver enzymes (eg, anticonvulsants). Therefore, careful monitoring is advised when somatropin is administered in combination with drugs metabolized by CP450 liver enzymes). Products include:
Gabitril **972**

Timolol Maleate (Limited published data indicates that somatropin treatment increases cytochrome P450 (CP450)-mediated antipyrine clearance in man. These data suggest that somatropin administration may alter the clearance of compounds metabolized by CP450 liver enzymes. Therefore, careful monitoring is advised when somatropin is administered in combination with drugs metabolized by CP450 liver enzymes). Products include:
Combigan **601**
Dorzolamide Hydrochloride/Timolol Maleate Ophthalmic Solution........ ⊙ **243**
Timoptic in Ocudose .... ⊙ **231**

Tolazamide (Patients with diabetes mellitus who receive concomitant treatment with somatropin may require adjustment of their doses of insulin and/or other hypoglycemic agents).
No products indexed under this heading.

Tolbutamide (Patients with diabetes mellitus who receive concomitant treatment with somatropin may require adjustment of their doses of insulin and/or other hypoglycemic agents).
No products indexed under this heading.

Tolbutamide Sodium (Limited published data indicates that somatropin treatment increases cytochrome P450 (CP450)-mediated antipyrine clearance in man. These data suggest that somatropin administration may alter the clearance of compounds metabolized by CP450 liver enzymes. Therefore, careful monitoring is advised when somatropin is administered in combination with drugs metabolized by CP450 liver enzymes).
No products indexed under this heading.

Tolmetin Sodium (Limited published data indicates that somatropin treatment increases cytochrome P450 (CP450)-mediated antipyrine clearance in man. These data suggest that somatropin administration may alter the clearance of compounds metabolized by CP450 liver enzymes. Therefore, careful monitoring is advised when somatropin is administered in combination with drugs metabolized by CP450 liver enzymes).
No products indexed under this heading.

Tolterodine Tartrate (Limited published data indicates that somatropin treatment increases cytochrome P450 (CP450)-mediated antipyrine clearance in man. These data suggest that somatropin administration may alter the clearance of compounds metabolized by CP450 liver enzymes. Therefore, careful monitoring is advised when somatropin is administered in combination with drugs metabolized by CP450 liver enzymes).
No products indexed under this heading.

Topiramate (Limited published data indicates that somatropin treatment increases cytochrome P450 (CP450)-mediated antipyrine clearance in man. These data suggest that somatropin administration may alter the clearance of compounds metabolized by CP450 liver enzymes (eg, anticonvulsants). Therefore, careful monitoring is advised when somatropin is administered in combination with drugs metabolized by CP450 liver enzymes).
No products indexed under this heading.

Torsemide (Limited published data indicates that somatropin treatment increases cytochrome P450 (CP450)-mediated antipyrine clearance in man. These data suggest that somatropin administration may alter the clearance of compounds metabolized by CP450 liver enzymes. Therefore, careful monitoring is advised when somatropin is administered in combination with drugs metabolized by CP450 liver enzymes).
No products indexed under this heading.

Tramadol Hydrochloride (Limited published data indicates that somatropin treatment increases cytochrome P450 (CP450)-mediated antipyrine clearance in man. These data suggest that somatropin administration may alter the clearance of compounds metabolized by CP450 liver enzymes. Therefore, careful monitoring is advised when somatropin is administered in combination with drugs metabolized by CP450 liver enzymes). Products include:
Ryzolt **2813**
Ultram ER **2693**

Trazodone Hydrochloride (Limited published data indicates that somatropin treatment increases cytochrome P450 (CP450)-mediated antipyrine clearance in man. These data suggest that somatropin administration may alter the clearance of compounds metabolized by CP450 liver enzymes. Therefore, careful monitoring is advised when somatropin is administered in combination with drugs metabolized by CP450 liver enzymes).
No products indexed under this heading.

Tretinoin (Limited published data indicates that somatropin treatment increases cytochrome P450 (CP450)-mediated antipyrine clearance in man. These data suggest that somatropin administration may alter the clearance of compounds metabolized by CP450 liver enzymes. Therefore, careful monitoring is advised when somatropin is administered in combination with drugs metabolized by CP450 liver enzymes).
No products indexed under this heading.

Triamcinolone (Introduction of somatropin treatment may result in inhibition of 11βHSD-1 and reduced serum cortisol concentrations. As a consequence, patients treated with glucocorticoid replacement therapy for previously diagnosed hypoadrenalism may require an increase in their maintenance or stress doses; this may be especially true for patients treated with cortisone acetate and prednisone. In addition, excessive glucocorticoid therapy may attenuate the growth promoting effects of somatropin in children. Therefore, glucocorticoid replacement therapy should be carefully adjusted in children with concomitant GH and glucocorticoid deficiency to avoid both hypoadrenalism and an inhibitory effect on growth. Also, somatropin administration may alter the clearance of compounds known to be metabolized by CYP450 liver enzymes (eg, corticosteroids). Careful monitoring is advisable when somatropin is administered in combination with other drugs known to be metabolized by CYP450 liver enzymes).
No products indexed under this heading.

Triamcinolone Acetonide (Introduction of somatropin treatment may result in inhibition of 11βHSD-1 and reduced serum cortisol concentrations. As a consequence, patients treated with glucocorticoid replacement therapy for previously diagnosed hypoadrenalism may require an increase in their maintenance or stress doses; this may be especially true for patients treated with cortisone acetate and prednisone. In addition, excessive glucocorticoid therapy may attenuate the growth promoting effects of somatropin in children. Therefore, glucocorticoid replacement therapy should be carefully adjusted in children with concomitant GH and glucocorticoid deficiency to avoid both hypoadrenalism and an inhibitory effect on growth. Also, somatropin administration

Humatrope Interactions Index 816

may alter the clearance of compounds known to be metabolized by CYP450 liver enzymes (eg, corticosteroids). Careful monitoring is advisable when somatropin is administered in combination with other drugs known to be metabolized by CYP450 liver enzymes). Products include:
Azmacort 408
Nasacort AQ 3019

Triamcinolone Diacetate (Introduction of somatropin treatment may result in inhibition of 11βHSD-1 and reduced serum cortisol concentrations. As a consequence, patients treated with glucocorticoid replacement therapy for previously diagnosed hypoadrenalism may require an increase in their maintenance or stress doses; this may be especially true for patients treated with cortisone acetate and prednisone. In addition, excessive glucocorticoid therapy may attenuate the growth promoting effects of somatropin in children. Therefore, glucocorticoid replacement therapy should be carefully adjusted in children with concomitant GH and glucocorticoid deficiency to avoid both hypoadrenalism and an inhibitory effect on growth. Also, somatropin administration may alter the clearance of compounds known to be metabolized by CYP450 liver enzymes (eg, corticosteroids). Careful monitoring is advisable when somatropin is administered in combination with other drugs known to be metabolized by CYP450 liver enzymes).
No products indexed under this heading.

Triamcinolone Hexacetonide (Introduction of somatropin treatment may result in inhibition of 11βHSD-1 and reduced serum cortisol concentrations. As a consequence, patients treated with glucocorticoid replacement therapy for previously diagnosed hypoadrenalism may require an increase in their maintenance or stress doses; this may be especially true for patients treated with cortisone acetate and prednisone. In addition, excessive glucocorticoid therapy may attenuate the growth promoting effects of somatropin in children. Therefore, glucocorticoid replacement therapy should be carefully adjusted in children with concomitant GH and glucocorticoid deficiency to avoid both hypoadrenalism and an inhibitory effect on growth. Also, somatropin administration may alter the clearance of compounds known to be metabolized by CYP450 liver enzymes (eg, corticosteroids). Careful monitoring is advisable when somatropin is administered in combination with other drugs known to be metabolized by CYP450 liver enzymes).
No products indexed under this heading.

Triazolam (Limited published data indicates that somatropin treatment increases cytochrome P450 (CP450)-mediated antipyrine clearance in man. These data suggest that somatropin administration may alter the clearance of compounds metabolized by CP450 liver enzymes. Therefore, careful monitoring is advised when somatropin is administered in combination with drugs metabolized by CP450 liver enzymes).
No products indexed under this heading.

Trimethadione (Limited published data indicates that somatropin treatment increases cytochrome P450 (CP450)-mediated antipyrine clearance in man. These data suggest that somatropin administration may alter the clearance of compounds metabolized by CP450 liver enzymes (eg, anticonvulsants). Therefore, careful monitoring is advised when somatropin is administered in combination with drugs metabolized by CP450 liver enzymes).
No products indexed under this heading.

Trimethaphan Camsylate (Limited published data indicates that somatropin treatment increases cytochrome P450 (CP450)-mediated antipyrine clearance in man. These data suggest that somatropin administration may alter the clearance of compounds metabolized by CP450 liver enzymes. Therefore, careful monitoring is advised when somatropin is administered in combination with drugs metabolized by CP450 liver enzymes).
No products indexed under this heading.

Trimipramine Maleate (Limited published data indicates that somatropin treatment increases cytochrome P450 (CP450)-mediated antipyrine clearance in man. These data suggest that somatropin administration may alter the clearance of compounds metabolized by CP450 liver enzymes. Therefore, careful monitoring is advised when somatropin is administered in combination with drugs metabolized by CP450 liver enzymes).
No products indexed under this heading.

Troglitazone (Patients with diabetes mellitus who receive concomitant treatment with somatropin may require adjustment of their doses of insulin and/or other hypoglycemic agents).
No products indexed under this heading.

Trovafloxacin Mesylate (Limited published data indicates that somatropin treatment increases cytochrome P450 (CP450)-mediated antipyrine clearance in man. These data suggest that somatropin administration may alter the clearance of compounds metabolized by CP450 liver enzymes. Therefore, careful monitoring is advised when somatropin is administered in combination with drugs metabolized by CP450 liver enzymes).
No products indexed under this heading.

Valdecoxib (Limited published data indicates that somatropin treatment increases cytochrome P450 (CP450)-mediated antipyrine clearance in man. These data suggest that somatropin administration may alter the clearance of compounds metabolized by CP450 liver enzymes. Therefore, careful monitoring is advised when somatropin is administered in combination with drugs metabolized by CP450 liver enzymes).
No products indexed under this heading.

Valproate Sodium (Limited published data indicates that somatropin treatment increases cytochrome P450 (CP450)-mediated antipyrine clearance in man. These data suggest that somatropin administration may alter the clearance of compounds metabolized by CP450 liver enzymes (eg, anticonvulsants). Therefore, careful monitoring is advised when somatropin is administered in combination with drugs metabolized by CP450 liver enzymes).
No products indexed under this heading.

Valproic Acid (Limited published data indicates that somatropin treatment increases cytochrome P450 (CP450)-mediated antipyrine clearance in man. These data suggest that somatropin administration may alter the clearance of compounds metabolized by CP450 liver enzymes (eg, anticonvulsants). Therefore, careful monitoring is advised when somatropin is administered in combination with drugs metabolized by CP450 liver enzymes).
No products indexed under this heading.

Valsartan (Limited published data indicates that somatropin treatment increases cytochrome P450 (CP450)-mediated antipyrine clearance in man. These data suggest that somatropin administration may alter the clearance of compounds metabolized by CP450 liver enzymes. Therefore, careful monitoring is advised when somatropin is administered in combination with drugs metabolized by CP450 liver enzymes). Products include:
Diovan 2413
Diovan HCT 2419
Exforge 2443
Exforge HCT 2449
Valturna 3637

Vardenafil Hydrochloride (Limited published data indicates that somatropin treatment increases cytochrome P450 (CP450)-mediated antipyrine clearance in man. These data suggest that somatropin administration may alter the clearance of compounds metabolized by CP450 liver enzymes. Therefore, careful monitoring is advised when somatropin is administered in combination with drugs metabolized by CP450 liver enzymes). Products include:
Levitra 3157

Venlafaxine Hydrochloride (Limited published data indicates that somatropin treatment increases cytochrome P450 (CP450)-mediated antipyrine clearance in man. These data suggest that somatropin administration may alter the clearance of compounds metabolized by CP450 liver enzymes. Therefore, careful monitoring is advised when somatropin is administered in combination with drugs metabolized by CP450 liver enzymes). Products include:
Effexor XR 3504
Venlafaxine Hydrochloride Tablets ... 2388

Verapamil Hydrochloride (Limited published data indicates that somatropin treatment increases cytochrome P450 (CP450)-mediated antipyrine clearance in man. These data suggest that somatropin administration may alter the clearance of compounds metabolized by CP450 liver enzymes. Therefore, careful monitoring is advised when somatropin is administered in combination with drugs metabolized by CP450 liver enzymes). Products include:
Tarka 534

Vinblastine Sulfate (Limited published data indicates that somatropin treatment increases cytochrome P450 (CP450)-mediated antipyrine clearance in man. These data suggest that somatropin administration may alter the clearance of compounds metabolized by CP450 liver enzymes. Therefore, careful monitoring is advised when somatropin is administered in combination with drugs metabolized by CP450 liver enzymes).
No products indexed under this heading.

Vincristine Sulfate (Limited published data indicates that somatropin treatment increases cytochrome P450 (CP450)-mediated antipyrine clearance in man. These data suggest that somatropin administration may alter the clearance of compounds metabolized by CP450 liver enzymes. Therefore, careful monitoring is advised when somatropin is administered in combination with drugs metabolized by CP450 liver enzymes).
No products indexed under this heading.

Vitamin A (Limited published data indicates that somatropin treatment increases cytochrome P450 (CP450)-mediated antipyrine clearance in man. These data suggest that somatropin administration may alter the clearance of compounds metabolized by CP450 liver enzymes. Therefore, careful monitoring is advised when somatropin is administered in combination with drugs metabolized by CP450 liver enzymes). Products include:
Cardio Basics 3455
Heplive 607
Norwegian Cod Liver Oil 919

Vitamin A Acetate (Limited published data indicates that somatropin treatment increases cytochrome P450 (CP450)-mediated antipyrine clearance in man. These data suggest that somatropin administration may alter the clearance of compounds metabolized by CP450 liver enzymes. Therefore, careful monitoring is advised when somatropin is administered in combination with drugs metabolized by CP450 liver enzymes).
No products indexed under this heading.

Voriconazole (Limited published data indicates that somatropin treatment increases cytochrome P450 (CP450)-mediated antipyrine clearance in man. These data suggest that somatropin administration may alter the clearance of compounds metabolized by CP450 liver enzymes. Therefore, careful monitoring is advised when somatropin is administered in combination with drugs metabolized by CP450 liver enzymes).
No products indexed under this heading.

Warfarin Sodium (Limited published data indicates that somatropin treatment increases cytochrome P450 (CP450)-mediated antipyrine clearance in man. These data suggest that somatropin administration may alter the clearance of compounds metabolized by CP450 liver enzymes. Therefore, careful monitoring is advised when somatropin is administered in combination with drugs metabolized by CP450 liver enzymes).
No products indexed under this heading.

Zafirlukast (Limited published data indicates that somatropin treatment increases cytochrome P450 (CP450)-mediated antipyrine clearance in man. These data suggest that somatropin administration may alter the clearance of compounds metabolized by CP450 liver enzymes. Therefore, careful monitoring is advised when somatropin is administered in combination with drugs metabolized by CP450 liver enzymes). Products include:
Accolate 3612

Zileuton (Limited published data indicates that somatropin treatment increases cytochrome P450 (CP450)-mediated antipyrine clearance in man. These data suggest that somatropin administration may alter the clearance of compounds metabolized by CP450 liver enzymes. Therefore, careful monitoring is advised when somatropin is administered in combination with drugs metabolized by CP450 liver enzymes).
No products indexed under this heading.

Zolmitriptan (Limited published data indicates that somatropin treatment increases cytochrome P450 (CP450)-mediated antipyrine clearance in man. These data suggest that somatropin administration may alter the clearance of compounds metabolized by CP450 liver enzymes. Therefore, careful monitoring is advised when somatropin is administered in combination with drugs metabolized by CP450 liver enzymes). Products include:
Zomig Tablets 773
Zomig Nasal Spray 768
Zomig-ZMT Tablets 773

Zonisamide (Limited published data indicates that somatropin treatment increases cytochrome P450 (CP450)-mediated antipyrine clearance in man. These data suggest that somatropin administration may alter the clearance of compounds metabolized by CP450 liver enzymes (eg, anticonvulsants). Therefore, careful monitoring is advised when somatropin is administered in combination with drugs metabolized by CP450 liver enzymes). Products include:

Zopiclone (Limited published data indicates that somatropin treatment increases cytochrome P450 (CP450)-mediated antipyrine clearance in man. These data suggest that somatropin administration may alter the clearance of compounds metabolized by CP450 liver enzymes. Therefore, careful monitoring is advised when somatropin is administered in combination with drugs metabolized by CP450 liver enzymes).
No products indexed under this heading.

Food Interactions

Beverages, caffeine-containing (Limited published data indicates that somatropin treatment increases cytochrome P450 (CP450)-mediated antipyrine clearance in man. These data suggest that somatropin administration may alter the clearance of compounds metabolized by CP450 liver enzymes. Therefore, careful monitoring is advised when somatropin is administered in combination with drugs metabolized by CP450 liver enzymes).

Food, caffeine-containing (Limited published data indicates that somatropin treatment increases cytochrome P450 (CP450)-mediated antipyrine clearance in man. These data suggest that somatropin administration may alter the clearance of compounds metabolized by CP450 liver enzymes. Therefore, careful monitoring is advised when somatropin is administered in combination with drugs metabolized by CP450 liver enzymes).

HUMIRA INJECTION SYRINGE AND PEN

May interact with corticosteroids, immunosuppressive agents, vaccines, live, and certain other agents. Compounds in these categories include:

Alclometasone Dipropionate (Patients treated with adalimumab are at increased risk for developing serious infections that may lead to hospitalization or death. Most patients who developed these infections were taking concomitant immunosuppressants, such as corticosteroids).
No products indexed under this heading.

Anakinra (Concurrent administration of anakinra (an interleukin-1 antagonist) and another TNF-blocking agent has been associated with an increased risk of serious infections, an increased risk of neutropenia and no additional benefit compared to these medicinal products alone. Therefore, the combination of anakinra with other TNF-blocking agents, including adalimumab, may also result in similar toxicities). Products include:

Azathioprine (Patients treated with adalimumab are at increased risk for developing serious infections that may lead to hospitalization or death. Most patients who developed these infections were taking concomitant immunosuppressants, such as methotrexate or corticosteroids).
No products indexed under this heading.

Basiliximab (Patients treated with adalimumab are at increased risk for developing serious infections that may lead to hospitalization or death. Most patients who developed these infections were taking concomitant immunosuppressants, such as methotrexate or corticosteroids). Products include:

BCG Vaccine (Live vaccines should not be given concurrently with adalimumab).
No products indexed under this heading.

Beclomethasone Dipropionate (Patients treated with adalimumab are at increased risk for developing serious infections that may lead to hospitalization or death. Most patients who developed these infections were taking concomitant immunosuppressants, such as corticosteroids). Products include:

Beclomethasone Dipropionate Monohydrate (Patients treated with adalimumab are at increased risk for developing serious infections that may lead to hospitalization or death. Most patients who developed these infections were taking concomitant immunosuppressants, such as corticosteroids). Products include:

Betamethasone (Patients treated with adalimumab are at increased risk for developing serious infections that may lead to hospitalization or death. Most patients who developed these infections were taking concomitant immunosuppressants, such as corticosteroids).
No products indexed under this heading.

Betamethasone Acetate (Patients treated with adalimumab are at increased risk for developing serious infections that may lead to hospitalization or death. Most patients who developed these infections were taking concomitant immunosuppressants, such as corticosteroids).
No products indexed under this heading.

Betamethasone Benzoate (Patients treated with adalimumab are at increased risk for developing serious infections that may lead to hospitalization or death. Most patients who developed these infections were taking concomitant immunosuppressants, such as corticosteroids).
No products indexed under this heading.

Betamethasone Dipropionate (Patients treated with adalimumab are at increased risk for developing serious infections that may lead to hospitalization or death. Most patients who developed these infections were taking concomitant immunosuppressants, such as corticosteroids). Products include:

Betamethasone Sodium Phosphate (Patients treated with adalimumab are at increased risk for developing serious infections that may lead to hospitalization or death. Most patients who developed these infections were taking concomitant immunosuppressants, such as corticosteroids).
No products indexed under this heading.

Betamethasone Valerate (Patients treated with adalimumab are at increased risk for developing serious infections that may lead to hospitalization or death. Most patients who developed these infections were taking concomitant immunosuppressants, such as corticosteroids). Products include:

Budesonide (Patients treated with adalimumab are at increased risk for developing serious infections that may lead to hospitalization or death. Most patients who developed these infections were taking concomitant immunosuppressants, such as corticosteroids). Products include:

Ciclesonide (Patients treated with adalimumab are at increased risk for developing serious infections that may lead to hospitalization or death. Most patients who developed these infections were taking concomitant immunosuppressants, such as corticosteroids).
No products indexed under this heading.

Cortisone Acetate (Patients treated with adalimumab are at increased risk for developing serious infections that may lead to hospitalization or death. Most patients who developed these infections were taking concomitant immunosuppressants, such as corticosteroids).
No products indexed under this heading.

Cyclosporine (Patients treated with adalimumab are at increased risk for developing serious infections that may lead to hospitalization or death. Most patients who developed these infections were taking concomitant immunosuppressants, such as methotrexate or corticosteroids). Products include:

Desoximetasone (Patients treated with adalimumab are at increased risk for developing serious infections that may lead to hospitalization or death. Most patients who developed these infections were taking concomitant immunosuppressants, such as corticosteroids).
No products indexed under this heading.

Dexamethasone (Patients treated with adalimumab are at increased risk for developing serious infections that may lead to hospitalization or death. Most patients who developed these infections were taking concomitant immunosuppressants, such as corticosteroids). Products include:

Dexamethasone Acetate (Patients treated with adalimumab are at increased risk for developing serious infections that may lead to hospitalization or death. Most patients who developed these infections were taking concomitant immunosuppressants, such as corticosteroids).
No products indexed under this heading.

Dexamethasone Phosphate (Patients treated with adalimumab are at increased risk for developing serious infections that may lead to hospitalization or death. Most patients who developed these infections were taking concomitant immunosuppressants, such as corticosteroids).
No products indexed under this heading.

Dexamethasone Sodium (Patients treated with adalimumab are at increased risk for developing serious infections that may lead to hospitalization or death. Most patients who developed these infections were taking concomitant immunosuppressants, such as corticosteroids).
No products indexed under this heading.

Dexamethasone Sodium Phosphate (Patients treated with adalimumab are at increased risk for developing serious infections that may lead to hospitalization or death. Most patients who developed these infections were taking concomitant immunosuppressants, such as corticosteroids).
No products indexed under this heading.

Dexamethasone Sodium Phosphate Injection (Patients treated with adalimumab are at increased risk for developing serious infections that may lead to hospitalization or death. Most patients who developed these infections were taking concomitant immunosuppressants, such as corticosteroids).
No products indexed under this heading.

Diflorasone Diacetate (Patients treated with adalimumab are at increased risk for developing serious infections that may lead to hospitalization or death. Most patients who developed these infections were taking concomitant immunosuppressants, such as corticosteroids).
No products indexed under this heading.

Fludrocortisone Acetate (Patients treated with adalimumab are at increased risk for developing serious infections that may lead to hospitalization or death. Most patients who developed these infections were taking concomitant immunosuppressants, such as corticosteroids).
No products indexed under this heading.

Flumethasone Pivalate (Patients treated with adalimumab are at increased risk for developing serious infections that may lead to hospitalization or death. Most patients who developed these infections were taking concomitant immunosuppressants, such as corticosteroids).
No products indexed under this heading.

Flunisolide Hemihydrate (Patients treated with adalimumab are at increased risk for developing serious infections that may lead to hospitalization or death. Most patients who developed these infections were taking concomitant immunosuppressants, such as corticosteroids).
No products indexed under this heading.

Fluticasone Furoate (Patients treated with adalimumab are at increased risk for developing serious infections that may lead to hospitalization or death. Most patients who developed these infections were taking concomitant immunosuppressants, such as corticosteroids). Products include:

Fluticasone Propionate (Patients treated with adalimumab are at increased risk for developing serious infections that may lead to hospitalization or death. Most patients who developed these infections were taking concomitant immunosuppressants, such as corticosteroids). Products include:

Hydrocortisone (Patients treated with adalimumab are at increased risk for developing serious infections that may lead to hospitalization or death. Most patients who developed these infections were taking concomitant immunosuppressants, such as corticosteroids).
No products indexed under this heading.

Hydrocortisone (Alcohol) (Patients treated with adalimumab are at increased risk for developing serious infections that may lead to hospitalization or death. Most patients who developed these infections were taking concomitant immunosuppressants, such as corticosteroids).
No products indexed under this heading.

(⊙ Described in PDR® for Ophthalmic Medicines)

May interact with alcohols, antihypertensives, corticosteroids, oral contraceptives, oral hypoglycemic agents, salicylates, sulfonamides, thyroid preparations, and certain other agents. Compounds in these categories include:

Acarbose (Co-administration with drugs with hypoglycemic activity, such as oral hypoglycemic agents, may result in decreased insulin requirements).
No products indexed under this heading.

Acebutolol Hydrochloride (Insulin requirements may be reduced in the presence of drugs that lower blood glucose or affect how the body responds to insulin).
No products indexed under this heading.

Alclometasone Dipropionate (Co-administration may result in increased insulin requirements).
No products indexed under this heading.

Aliskiren (Insulin requirements may be reduced in the presence of drugs that lower blood glucose or affect how the body responds to insulin). Products include:

Amlodipine Besylate (Insulin requirements may be reduced in the presence of drugs that lower blood glucose or affect how the body responds to insulin). Products include:

Aspirin (Co-administration with drugs with hypoglycemic activity, such as salicylates, may result in decreased insulin requirements). Products include:

Aspirin, Enteric Coated (Co-administration with drugs with hypoglycemic activity, such as salicylates, may result in decreased insulin requirements).
No products indexed under this heading.

Aspirin Buffered (Co-administration with drugs with hypoglycemic activity, such as salicylates, may result in decreased insulin requirements).
No products indexed under this heading.

Atenolol (Insulin requirements may be reduced in the presence of drugs that lower blood glucose or affect how the body responds to insulin).
No products indexed under this heading.

Beclomethasone Dipropionate (Co-administration may result in increased insulin requirements). Products include:

Beclomethasone Dipropionate Monohydrate (Co-administration may result in increased insulin requirements). Products include:

Benazepril Hydrochloride (Insulin requirements may be reduced in the presence of drugs that lower blood glucose or affect how the body responds to insulin).
No products indexed under this heading.

Bendroflumethiazide (Insulin requirements may be reduced in the presence of drugs that lower blood glucose or affect how the body responds to insulin).
No products indexed under this heading.

Betamethasone (Co-administration may result in increased insulin requirements).
No products indexed under this heading.

Betamethasone Acetate (Co-administration may result in increased insulin requirements).
No products indexed under this heading.

Betamethasone Benzoate (Co-administration may result in increased insulin requirements).
No products indexed under this heading.

Betamethasone Dipropionate (Co-administration may result in increased insulin requirements). Products include:

Betamethasone Sodium Phosphate (Co-administration may result in increased insulin requirements).
No products indexed under this heading.

Betamethasone Valerate (Co-administration may result in increased insulin requirements). Products include:

Betaxolol Hydrochloride (Insulin requirements may be reduced in the presence of drugs that lower blood glucose or affect how the body responds to insulin).
No products indexed under this heading.

Bisoprolol Fumarate (Insulin requirements may be reduced in the presence of drugs that lower blood glucose or affect how the body responds to insulin).
No products indexed under this heading.

Budesonide (Co-administration may result in increased insulin requirements). Products include:

Candesartan Cilexetil (Insulin requirements may be reduced in the presence of drugs that lower blood glucose or affect how the body responds to insulin). Products include:

Captopril (Insulin requirements may be reduced in the presence of drugs that lower blood glucose or affect how the body responds to insulin). Products include:

Carteolol Hydrochloride (Insulin requirements may be reduced in the presence of drugs that lower blood glucose or affect how the body responds to insulin).
No products indexed under this heading.

Carvedilol (Insulin requirements may be reduced in the presence of drugs that lower blood glucose or affect how the body responds to insulin). Products include:

Carvedilol Phosphate (Insulin requirements may be reduced in the presence of drugs that lower blood glucose or affect how the body responds to insulin). Products include:

Chlorothiazide (Insulin requirements may be reduced in the presence of drugs that lower blood glucose or affect how the body responds to insulin).
No products indexed under this heading.

Chlorothiazide Sodium (Insulin requirements may be reduced in the presence of drugs that lower blood glucose or affect how the body responds to insulin). Products include:

Chlorpropamide (Co-administration with drugs with hypoglycemic activity, such as oral hypoglycemic agents, may result in decreased insulin requirements).
No products indexed under this heading.

Chlorthalidone (Insulin requirements may be reduced in the presence of drugs that lower blood glucose or affect how the body responds to insulin). Products include:

Choline Magnesium Trisalicylate (Co-administration with drugs with hypoglycemic activity, such as salicylates, may result in decreased insulin requirements).
No products indexed under this heading.

Ciclesonide (Co-administration may result in increased insulin requirements).
No products indexed under this heading.

Clonidine (Insulin requirements may be reduced in the presence of drugs that lower blood glucose or affect how the body responds to insulin). Products include:

Clonidine Hydrochloride (Insulin requirements may be reduced in the presence of drugs that lower blood glucose or affect how the body responds to insulin). Products include:

Cortisone Acetate (Co-administration may result in increased insulin requirements).
No products indexed under this heading.

Deserpidine (Insulin requirements may be reduced in the presence of drugs that lower blood glucose or affect how the body responds to insulin).
No products indexed under this heading.

Desogestrel (Co-administration with oral contraceptives may result in increased insulin requirements).
No products indexed under this heading.

Desoximetasone (Co-administration may result in increased insulin requirements).
No products indexed under this heading.

Dexamethasone (Co-administration may result in increased insulin requirements). Products include:

Dexamethasone Acetate (Co-administration may result in increased insulin requirements).
No products indexed under this heading.

Dexamethasone Phosphate (Co-administration may result in increased insulin requirements).
No products indexed under this heading.

Dexamethasone Sodium (Co-administration may result in increased insulin requirements).
No products indexed under this heading.

Dexamethasone Sodium Phosphate (Co-administration may result in increased insulin requirements).
No products indexed under this heading.

Dexamethasone Sodium Phosphate Injection (Co-administration may result in increased insulin requirements).
No products indexed under this heading.

Diazoxide (Insulin requirements may be reduced in the presence of drugs that lower blood glucose or affect how the body responds to insulin). Products include:

Diflorasone Diacetate (Co-administration may result in increased insulin requirements).
No products indexed under this heading.

Diflunisal (Co-administration with drugs with hypoglycemic activity, such as salicylates, may result in decreased insulin requirements).
No products indexed under this heading.

Diltiazem Hydrochloride (Insulin requirements may be reduced in the presence of drugs that lower blood glucose or affect how the body responds to insulin). Products include:

Diltiazem Maleate (Insulin requirements may be reduced in the presence of drugs that lower blood glucose or affect how the body responds to insulin).
No products indexed under this heading.

Doxazosin Mesylate (Insulin requirements may be reduced in the presence of drugs that lower blood glucose or affect how the body responds to insulin).
No products indexed under this heading.

Enalapril Maleate (Insulin requirements may be reduced in the presence of drugs that lower blood glucose or affect how the body responds to insulin).
No products indexed under this heading.

Enalaprilat (Insulin requirements may be reduced in the presence of drugs that lower blood glucose or affect how the body responds to insulin).
No products indexed under this heading.

Eprosartan Mesylate (Insulin requirements may be reduced in the presence of drugs that lower blood glucose or affect how the body responds to insulin). Products include:

Esmolol Hydrochloride (Insulin requirements may be reduced in the presence of drugs that lower blood glucose or affect how the body responds to insulin).
No products indexed under this heading.

Ethanol (Insulin requirements may be reduced in the presence of drugs that lower blood glucose or affect how the body responds to insulin).
No products indexed under this heading.

Ethinyl Estradiol (Co-administration with oral contraceptives may result in increased insulin requirements). Products include:

Ethyl Alcohol (Insulin requirements may be reduced in the presence of drugs that lower blood glucose or affect how the body responds to insulin).
No products indexed under this heading.

Ethynodiol Diacetate (Co-administration with oral contraceptives may result in increased insulin requirements).
No products indexed under this heading.

Felodipine (Insulin requirements may be reduced in the presence of drugs that lower blood glucose or affect how the body responds to insulin).
No products indexed under this heading.

Fludrocortisone Acetate (Co-administration may result in increased insulin requirements).
No products indexed under this heading.

Flumethasone Pivalate (Co-administration may result in increased insulin requirements).
No products indexed under this heading.

Flunisolide Hemihydrate (Co-administration may result in increased insulin requirements).
No products indexed under this heading.

Fluticasone Furoate (Co-administration may result in increased insulin requirements). Products include:

(⊙ Described in PDR® for Ophthalmic Medicines)

Nitrolingual **3266**

Norethindrone (Co-administration with oral contraceptives may result in increased insulin requirements). Products include:
Ortho Micronor **2660**

Norethynodrel (Co-administration with oral contraceptives may result in increased insulin requirements).
No products indexed under this heading.

Norgestimate (Co-administration with oral contraceptives may result in increased insulin requirements). Products include:
Ortho-Cyclen/Ortho Tri-Cyclen **2663**
Ortho Tri-Cyclen Lo Tablets **2673**

Norgestrel (Co-administration with oral contraceptives may result in increased insulin requirements).
No products indexed under this heading.

Penbutolol Sulfate (Insulin requirements may be reduced in the presence of drugs that lower blood glucose or affect how the body responds to insulin).
No products indexed under this heading.

Perindopril Erbumine (Insulin requirements may be reduced in the presence of drugs that lower blood glucose or affect how the body responds to insulin).
No products indexed under this heading.

Phenelzine Sulfate (Co-administration with drugs with hypoglycemic activity, such as certain MAO inhibitor antidepressants, may result in decreased insulin requirements).
No products indexed under this heading.

Phenoxybenzamine Hydrochloride (Insulin requirements may be reduced in the presence of drugs that lower blood glucose or affect how the body responds to insulin). Products include:
Dibenzyline **3495**

Phentolamine Mesylate (Insulin requirements may be reduced in the presence of drugs that lower blood glucose or affect how the body responds to insulin).
No products indexed under this heading.

Pindolol (Insulin requirements may be reduced in the presence of drugs that lower blood glucose or affect how the body responds to insulin).
No products indexed under this heading.

Pioglitazone Hydrochloride (Co-administration with drugs with hypoglycemic activity, such as oral hypoglycemic agents, may result in decreased insulin requirements). Products include:
ActoPlus **3338**
Actos **3345**
Duetact **3354**

Polythiazide (Insulin requirements may be reduced in the presence of drugs that lower blood glucose or affect how the body responds to insulin).
No products indexed under this heading.

Prazosin Hydrochloride (Insulin requirements may be reduced in the presence of drugs that lower blood glucose or affect how the body responds to insulin).
No products indexed under this heading.

Prednisolone (Co-administration may result in increased insulin requirements).
No products indexed under this heading.

Prednisolone Acetate (Co-administration may result in increased insulin requirements). Products include:
Blephamide .... ⊙**212**, ⊙**214**
Pred Forte .... ⊙**225**
Pred Mild .... ⊙**230**
Pred-G .... ⊙**226**, ⊙**227**

Prednisolone Sodium Phosphate (Co-administration may result in increased insulin requirements).
No products indexed under this heading.

Prednisolone Tebutate (Co-administration may result in increased insulin requirements).
No products indexed under this heading.

Prednisone (Co-administration may result in increased insulin requirements).
No products indexed under this heading.

Prednisone sodium phosphate (Co-administration may result in increased insulin requirements).
No products indexed under this heading.

Propranolol Hydrochloride (Insulin requirements may be reduced in the presence of drugs that lower blood glucose or affect how the body responds to insulin). Products include:
InnoPran XL **1517**

Quinapril Hydrochloride (Insulin requirements may be reduced in the presence of drugs that lower blood glucose or affect how the body responds to insulin).
No products indexed under this heading.

Ramipril (Insulin requirements may be reduced in the presence of drugs that lower blood glucose or affect how the body responds to insulin).
No products indexed under this heading.

Rauwolfia Serpentina (Insulin requirements may be reduced in the presence of drugs that lower blood glucose or affect how the body responds to insulin).
No products indexed under this heading.

Repaglinide (Co-administration with drugs with hypoglycemic activity, such as oral hypoglycemic agents, may result in decreased insulin requirements).
No products indexed under this heading.

Rescinnamine (Insulin requirements may be reduced in the presence of drugs that lower blood glucose or affect how the body responds to insulin).
No products indexed under this heading.

Reserpine (Insulin requirements may be reduced in the presence of drugs that lower blood glucose or affect how the body responds to insulin).
No products indexed under this heading.

Rosiglitazone Maleate (Co-administration with drugs with hypoglycemic activity, such as oral hypoglycemic agents, may result in decreased insulin requirements). Products include:
Avandamet **1345**
Avandaryl **1356**
Avandia **1366**

Salsalate (Co-administration with drugs with hypoglycemic activity, such as salicylates, may result in decreased insulin requirements).
No products indexed under this heading.

Sitagliptin Phosphate (Co-administration with drugs with hypoglycemic activity, such as oral hypoglycemic agents, may result in decreased insulin requirements). Products include:
Janumet **2188**
Januvia **2196**

Sodium Nitroprusside (Insulin requirements may be reduced in the presence of drugs that lower blood glucose or affect how the body responds to insulin).
No products indexed under this heading.

Sotalol Hydrochloride (Insulin requirements may be reduced in the presence of drugs that lower blood glucose or affect how the body responds to insulin).
No products indexed under this heading.

Spirapril Hydrochloride (Insulin requirements may be reduced in the presence of drugs that lower blood glucose or affect how the body responds to insulin).
No products indexed under this heading.

Sulfacytine (Co-administration with drugs with hypoglycemic activity, such as sulfa antibiotics, may result in decreased insulin requirements).
No products indexed under this heading.

Sulfamethizole (Co-administration with drugs with hypoglycemic activity, such as sulfa antibiotics, may result in decreased insulin requirements).
No products indexed under this heading.

Sulfamethoxazole (Co-administration with drugs with hypoglycemic activity, such as sulfa antibiotics, may result in decreased insulin requirements).
No products indexed under this heading.

Sulfasalazine (Co-administration with drugs with hypoglycemic activity, such as sulfa antibiotics, may result in decreased insulin requirements).
No products indexed under this heading.

Sulfinpyrazone (Insulin requirements may be reduced in the presence of drugs that lower blood glucose or affect how the body responds to insulin).
No products indexed under this heading.

Sulfisoxazole Acetyl (Insulin requirements may be reduced in the presence of drugs that lower blood glucose or affect how the body responds to insulin).
No products indexed under this heading.

Sulfisoxazole Diolamine (Insulin requirements may be reduced in the presence of drugs that lower blood glucose or affect how the body responds to insulin).
No products indexed under this heading.

Telmisartan (Insulin requirements may be reduced in the presence of drugs that lower blood glucose or affect how the body responds to insulin). Products include:
Micardis **887**
Micardis HCT **889**

Terazosin Hydrochloride (Insulin requirements may be reduced in the presence of drugs that lower blood glucose or affect how the body responds to insulin).
No products indexed under this heading.

Thyroglobulin (Co-administration with thyroid replacement therapy may result in increased insulin requirements).
No products indexed under this heading.

Thyroid (Co-administration with thyroid replacement therapy may result in increased insulin requirements). Products include:
Naturethroid **2830**

Thyroxine (Co-administration with thyroid replacement therapy may result in increased insulin requirements).
No products indexed under this heading.

Thyroxine Sodium (Co-administration with thyroid replacement therapy may result in increased insulin requirements).
No products indexed under this heading.

Timolol Maleate (Insulin requirements may be reduced in the presence of drugs that lower blood glucose or affect how the body responds to insulin). Products include:
Combigan **601**
Dorzolamide
Hydrochloride/Timolol Maleate
Ophthalmic Solution .... ⊙**243**
Timoptic in Ocudose .... ⊙**231**

Tolazamide (Co-administration with drugs with hypoglycemic activity, such as oral hypoglycemic agents, may result in decreased insulin requirements).
No products indexed under this heading.

Tolbutamide (Co-administration with drugs with hypoglycemic activity, such as oral hypoglycemic agents, may result in decreased insulin requirements).
No products indexed under this heading.

Torsemide (Insulin requirements may be reduced in the presence of drugs that lower blood glucose or affect how the body responds to insulin).
No products indexed under this heading.

Trandolapril (Insulin requirements may be reduced in the presence of drugs that lower blood glucose or affect how the body responds to insulin). Products include:
Mavik **489**
Tarka **534**

Tranylcypromine Sulfate (Co-administration with drugs with hypoglycemic activity, such as certain MAO inhibitor antidepressants, may result in decreased insulin requirements). Products include:
Parnate **1584**

Triamcinolone (Co-administration may result in increased insulin requirements).
No products indexed under this heading.

Triamcinolone Acetonide (Co-administration may result in increased insulin requirements). Products include:
Azmacort **408**
Nasacort AQ **3019**

Triamcinolone Diacetate (Co-administration may result in increased insulin requirements).
No products indexed under this heading.

Triamcinolone Hexacetonide (Co-administration may result in increased insulin requirements).
No products indexed under this heading.

Trimethaphan Camsylate (Insulin requirements may be reduced in the presence of drugs that lower blood glucose or affect how the body responds to insulin).
No products indexed under this heading.

Troglitazone (Co-administration with drugs with hypoglycemic activity, such as oral hypoglycemic agents, may result in decreased insulin requirements).
No products indexed under this heading.

Valsartan (Insulin requirements may be reduced in the presence of drugs that lower blood glucose or affect how the body responds to insulin). Products include:
Diovan **2413**
Diovan HCT **2419**
Exforge **2443**
Exforge HCT **2449**
Valturna **3637**

Verapamil Hydrochloride (Insulin requirements may be reduced in the presence of drugs that lower blood glucose or affect how the body responds to insulin). Products include:
Tarka **534**

Food Interactions

Alcohol (Insulin requirements may be reduced in the presence of drugs that lower blood glucose or affect how the body responds to insulin).

Beer, reduced-alcohol (Insulin requirements may be reduced in the presence of drugs that lower blood glucose or affect how the body responds to insulin).

Beer, unspecified (Insulin requirements may be reduced in the presence of drugs that lower blood glucose or affect how the body responds to insulin).

Wine, Chianti (Insulin requirements may be reduced in the presence of drugs that lower blood glucose or affect how the body responds to insulin).

IMPORTANT NOTE: Always consult each drug listing in the patient's regimen for possible interactions.

Humulin N Interactions Index 822

Wine, Red (Insulin requirements may be reduced in the presence of drugs that lower blood glucose or affect how the body responds to insulin).

Wine, unspecified (Insulin requirements may be reduced in the presence of drugs that lower blood glucose or affect how the body responds to insulin).

Wine products (Insulin requirements may be reduced in the presence of drugs that lower blood glucose or affect how the body responds to insulin).

HUMULIN R

(Insulin, Human Regular) 1937
May interact with oral hypoglycemic agents. Compounds in these categories include:

Acarbose (The concurrent use of oral hypoglycemic agents with regular human insulin is not recommended).
No products indexed under this heading.

Chlorpropamide (The concurrent use of oral hypoglycemic agents with regular human insulin is not recommended).
No products indexed under this heading.

Glibenclamide (The concurrent use of oral hypoglycemic agents with regular human insulin is not recommended).
No products indexed under this heading.

Glimepiride (The concurrent use of oral hypoglycemic agents with regular human insulin is not recommended). Products include:
Avandaryl 1356
Duetact 3354

Glipizide (The concurrent use of oral hypoglycemic agents with regular human insulin is not recommended).
No products indexed under this heading.

Glyburide (The concurrent use of oral hypoglycemic agents with regular human insulin is not recommended).
No products indexed under this heading.

Metformin Hydrochloride (The concurrent use of oral hypoglycemic agents with regular human insulin is not recommended). Products include:
ActoPlus 3338
Avandamet 1345
Janumet 2188

Miglitol (The concurrent use of oral hypoglycemic agents with regular human insulin is not recommended).
No products indexed under this heading.

Nateglinide (The concurrent use of oral hypoglycemic agents with regular human insulin is not recommended).
No products indexed under this heading.

Pioglitazone Hydrochloride (The concurrent use of oral hypoglycemic agents with regular human insulin is not recommended). Products include:
ActoPlus 3338
Actos 3345
Duetact 3354

Repaglinide (The concurrent use of oral hypoglycemic agents with regular human insulin is not recommended).
No products indexed under this heading.

Rosiglitazone Maleate (The concurrent use of oral hypoglycemic agents with regular human insulin is not recommended). Products include:
Avandamet 1345
Avandaryl 1356
Avandia 1366

Sitagliptin Phosphate (The concurrent use of oral hypoglycemic agents with regular human insulin is not recommended). Products include:
Janumet 2188
Januvia 2196

Tolazamide (The concurrent use of oral hypoglycemic agents with regular human insulin is not recommended).
No products indexed under this heading.

Tolbutamide (The concurrent use of oral hypoglycemic agents with regular human insulin is not recommended).
No products indexed under this heading.

Troglitazone (The concurrent use of oral hypoglycemic agents with regular human insulin is not recommended).
No products indexed under this heading.

HUMULIN R (U-500)

(Insulin, Human Regular) 1939
May interact with ACE inhibitors, alcohols, angiotensin-II receptor antagonists, beta-blockers, corticosteroids, estrogens, monoamine oxidase inhibitors, oral contraceptives, oral hypoglycemic agents, phenothiazines, salicylates, sulfonamides, thyroid preparations, and certain other agents. Compounds in these categories include:

Acarbose (Insulin requirements may be decreased in the presence of drugs that increase insulin sensitivity or have hypoglycemic activity, such as oral hypoglycemic agents).
No products indexed under this heading.

Acebutolol Hydrochloride (Insulin requirements may be decreased in the presence of drugs that increase insulin sensitivity or have hypoglycemic activity, such as beta-adrenergic blockers. Beta-adrenergic blockers may mask the symptoms of hypoglycemia in some patients).
No products indexed under this heading.

Alclometasone Dipropionate (Insulin requirements may be increased by medications with hyperglycemic activity such as corticosteroids).
No products indexed under this heading.

Aspirin (Insulin requirements may be decreased in the presence of drugs that increase insulin sensitivity or have hypoglycemic activity, such as salicylates). Products include:
Aggrenox 880
Bayer Aspirin 829
Percodan 1124
St. Joseph Aspirin 2045

Aspirin, Enteric Coated (Insulin requirements may be decreased in the presence of drugs that increase insulin sensitivity or have hypoglycemic activity, such as salicylates).
No products indexed under this heading.

Aspirin Buffered (Insulin requirements may be decreased in the presence of drugs that increase insulin sensitivity or have hypoglycemic activity, such as salicylates).
No products indexed under this heading.

Atenolol (Insulin requirements may be decreased in the presence of drugs that increase insulin sensitivity or have hypoglycemic activity, such as beta-adrenergic blockers. Beta-adrenergic blockers may mask the symptoms of hypoglycemia in some patients).
No products indexed under this heading.

Beclomethasone Dipropionate (Insulin requirements may be increased by medications with hyperglycemic activity such as corticosteroids). Products include:
Qvar 3398

Beclomethasone Dipropionate Monohydrate (Insulin requirements may be increased by medications with hyperglycemic activity such as corticosteroids). Products include:
Beconase AQ 1386

Benazepril Hydrochloride (Insulin requirements may be decreased in the presence of drugs that increase insulin sensitivity or have hypoglycemic activity, such as ACE inhibitors).
No products indexed under this heading.

Bendroflumethiazide (Insulin requirements may be decreased in the presence of drugs that increase insulin sensitivity or have hypoglycemic activity, such as sulfa antibiotics).
No products indexed under this heading.

Betamethasone (Insulin requirements may be increased by medications with hyperglycemic activity such as corticosteroids).
No products indexed under this heading.

Betamethasone Acetate (Insulin requirements may be increased by medications with hyperglycemic activity such as corticosteroids).
No products indexed under this heading.

Betamethasone Benzoate (Insulin requirements may be increased by medications with hyperglycemic activity such as corticosteroids).
No products indexed under this heading.

Betamethasone Dipropionate (Insulin requirements may be increased by medications with hyperglycemic activity such as corticosteroids). Products include:
Diprolene Lotion 0.05% 3108
Diprolene Ointment 0.05% 3109
Diprolene AF Cream 0.05% 3107
Lotrisone 3163

Betamethasone Sodium Phosphate (Insulin requirements may be increased by medications with hyperglycemic activity such as corticosteroids).
No products indexed under this heading.

Betamethasone Valerate (Insulin requirements may be increased by medications with hyperglycemic activity such as corticosteroids). Products include:
Luxíq 3321

Betaxolol Hydrochloride (Insulin requirements may be decreased in the presence of drugs that increase insulin sensitivity or have hypoglycemic activity, such as beta-adrenergic blockers. Beta-adrenergic blockers may mask the symptoms of hypoglycemia in some patients).
No products indexed under this heading.

Bisoprolol Fumarate (Insulin requirements may be decreased in the presence of drugs that increase insulin sensitivity or have hypoglycemic activity, such as beta-adrenergic blockers. Beta-adrenergic blockers may mask the symptoms of hypoglycemia in some patients).
No products indexed under this heading.

Budesonide (Insulin requirements may be increased by medications with hyperglycemic activity such as corticosteroids). Products include:
Pulmicort Flexhaler 714
Symbicort 80/4.5 720
Symbicort 160/4.5 720

Candesartan Cilexetil (Insulin requirements may be decreased in the presence of drugs that increase insulin sensitivity or have hypoglycemic activity, such as angiotensin-II receptor antagonists). Products include:
Atacand 697
Atacand HCT 700

Captopril (Insulin requirements may be decreased in the presence of drugs that increase insulin sensitivity or have hypoglycemic activity, such as ACE inhibitors). Products include:
Captopril 2341

Carteolol Hydrochloride (Insulin requirements may be decreased in the presence of drugs that increase insulin sensitivity or have hypoglycemic activity, such as beta-adrenergic blockers. Beta-adrenergic blockers may mask the symptoms of hypoglycemia in some patients).
No products indexed under this heading.

Carvedilol (Insulin requirements may be decreased in the presence of drugs that increase insulin sensitivity or have hypoglycemic activity, such as beta-adrenergic blockers. Beta-adrenergic blockers may mask the symptoms of hypoglycemia in some patients).
Products include:
Coreg 1409

Carvedilol Phosphate (Insulin requirements may be decreased in the presence of drugs that increase insulin sensitivity or have hypoglycemic activity, such as beta-adrenergic blockers. Beta-adrenergic blockers may mask the symptoms of hypoglycemia in some patients). Products include:
Coreg CR 1416

Chlorothiazide (Insulin requirements may be decreased in the presence of drugs that increase insulin sensitivity or have hypoglycemic activity, such as sulfa antibiotics).
No products indexed under this heading.

Chlorothiazide Sodium (Insulin requirements may be decreased in the presence of drugs that increase insulin sensitivity or have hypoglycemic activity, such as sulfa antibiotics). Products include:
Diuril Intravenous 2009

Chlorotrianisene (Insulin requirements may increase by estrogens).
No products indexed under this heading.

Chlorpromazine (Insulin requirements may be increased by phenothiazines).
No products indexed under this heading.

Chlorpromazine Hydrochloride (Insulin requirements may be increased by phenothiazines).
No products indexed under this heading.

Chlorpropamide (Insulin requirements may be decreased in the presence of drugs that increase insulin sensitivity or have hypoglycemic activity, such as oral hypoglycemic agents).
No products indexed under this heading.

Choline Magnesium Trisalicylate (Insulin requirements may be decreased in the presence of drugs that increase insulin sensitivity or have hypoglycemic activity, such as salicylates).
No products indexed under this heading.

Ciclesonide (Insulin requirements may be increased by medications with hyperglycemic activity such as corticosteroids).
No products indexed under this heading.

Cortisone Acetate (Insulin requirements may be increased by medications with hyperglycemic activity such as corticosteroids).
No products indexed under this heading.

Desogestrel (Insulin requirements may be increased by oral contraceptives).
No products indexed under this heading.

Desoximetasone (Insulin requirements may be increased by medications with hyperglycemic activity such as corticosteroids).
No products indexed under this heading.

Dexamethasone (Insulin requirements may be increased by medications with hyperglycemic activity such as corticosteroids). Products include:
Ciprodex 583
Ozurdex .... ⊙ 223
Tobramycin and Dexamethasone Ophthalmic Suspension .... ⊙ 251

Dexamethasone Acetate (Insulin requirements may be increased by medications with hyperglycemic activity such as corticosteroids).
No products indexed under this heading.

Dexamethasone Phosphate (Insulin requirements may be increased by medications with hyperglycemic activity such as corticosteroids).
No products indexed under this heading.

(⊙ Described in PDR® for Ophthalmic Medicines)

IMPORTANT NOTE: Always consult each drug listing in the patient's regimen for possible interactions.

(⊙ Described in PDR® for Ophthalmic Medicines)

Spirapril Hydrochloride (Insulin requirements may be decreased in the presence of drugs that increase insulin sensitivity or have hypoglycemic activity, such as ACE inhibitors).
No products indexed under this heading.

Sulfacytine (Insulin requirements may be decreased in the presence of drugs that increase insulin sensitivity or have hypoglycemic activity, such as sulfa antibiotics).
No products indexed under this heading.

Sulfamethizole (Insulin requirements may be decreased in the presence of drugs that increase insulin sensitivity or have hypoglycemic activity, such as sulfa antibiotics).
No products indexed under this heading.

Sulfamethoxazole (Insulin requirements may be decreased in the presence of drugs that increase insulin sensitivity or have hypoglycemic activity, such as sulfa antibiotics).
No products indexed under this heading.

Sulfasalazine (Insulin requirements may be decreased in the presence of drugs that increase insulin sensitivity or have hypoglycemic activity, such as sulfa antibiotics).
No products indexed under this heading.

Sulfinpyrazone (Insulin requirements may be decreased in the presence of drugs that increase insulin sensitivity or have hypoglycemic activity, such as sulfa antibiotics).
No products indexed under this heading.

Sulfisoxazole Acetyl (Insulin requirements may be decreased in the presence of drugs that increase insulin sensitivity or have hypoglycemic activity, such as sulfa antibiotics).
No products indexed under this heading.

Sulfisoxazole Diolamine (Insulin requirements may be decreased in the presence of drugs that increase insulin sensitivity or have hypoglycemic activity, such as sulfa antibiotics).
No products indexed under this heading.

Telmisartan (Insulin requirements may be decreased in the presence of drugs that increase insulin sensitivity or have hypoglycemic activity, such as angiotensin-II receptor antagonists). Products include:

Thioridazine (Insulin requirements may be increased by phenothiazines).
No products indexed under this heading.

Thioridazine Hydrochloride (Insulin requirements may be increased by phenothiazines). Products include:

Thyroglobulin (Insulin requirements may increase by thyroid replacement therapy/thyroid preparations).
No products indexed under this heading.

Thyroid (Insulin requirements may increase by thyroid replacement therapy/thyroid preparations). Products include:

Thyroxine (Insulin requirements may increase by thyroid replacement therapy/thyroid preparations).
No products indexed under this heading.

Thyroxine Sodium (Insulin requirements may increase by thyroid replacement therapy/thyroid preparations).
No products indexed under this heading.

Timolol Hemihydrate (Insulin requirements may be decreased in the presence of drugs that increase insulin sensitivity or have hypoglycemic activity, such as beta-adrenergic blockers. Beta-adrenergic blockers may mask the symptoms of hypoglycemia in some patients). Products include:

Timolol Maleate (Insulin requirements may be decreased in the presence of drugs that increase insulin sensitivity or have hypoglycemic activity, such as beta-adrenergic blockers. Beta-adrenergic blockers may mask the symptoms of hypoglycemia in some patients). Products include:

Tolazamide (Insulin requirements may be decreased in the presence of drugs that increase insulin sensitivity or have hypoglycemic activity, such as oral hypoglycemic agents).
No products indexed under this heading.

Tolbutamide (Insulin requirements may be decreased in the presence of drugs that increase insulin sensitivity or have hypoglycemic activity, such as oral hypoglycemic agents).
No products indexed under this heading.

Trandolapril (Insulin requirements may be decreased in the presence of drugs that increase insulin sensitivity or have hypoglycemic activity, such as ACE inhibitors). Products include:

Tranylcypromine Sulfate (Insulin requirements may be decreased in the presence of drugs that increase insulin sensitivity or have hypoglycemic activity, such as monoamine oxidase inhibitors). Products include:

Triamcinolone (Insulin requirements may be increased by medications with hyperglycemic activity such as corticosteroids).
No products indexed under this heading.

Triamcinolone Acetonide (Insulin requirements may be increased by medications with hyperglycemic activity such as corticosteroids). Products include:

Triamcinolone Diacetate (Insulin requirements may be increased by medications with hyperglycemic activity such as corticosteroids).
No products indexed under this heading.

Triamcinolone Hexacetonide (Insulin requirements may be increased by medications with hyperglycemic activity such as corticosteroids).
No products indexed under this heading.

Trifluoperazine Hydrochloride (Insulin requirements may be increased by phenothiazines).
No products indexed under this heading.

Troglitazone (Insulin requirements may be decreased in the presence of drugs that increase insulin sensitivity or have hypoglycemic activity, such as oral hypoglycemic agents).
No products indexed under this heading.

Valsartan (Insulin requirements may be decreased in the presence of drugs that increase insulin sensitivity or have hypoglycemic activity, such as angiotensin-II receptor antagonists). Products include:

Food Interactions

Alcohol (Insulin requirements may be decreased in the presence of drugs that increase insulin sensitivity or have hypoglycemic activity, such as alcohol).

Beer, reduced-alcohol (Insulin requirements may be decreased in the presence of drugs that increase insulin sensitivity or have hypoglycemic activity, such as alcohol).

Beer, unspecified (Insulin requirements may be decreased in the presence of drugs that increase insulin sensitivity or have hypoglycemic activity, such as alcohol).

Wine, Chianti (Insulin requirements may be decreased in the presence of drugs that increase insulin sensitivity or have hypoglycemic activity, such as alcohol).

Wine, Red (Insulin requirements may be decreased in the presence of drugs that increase insulin sensitivity or have hypoglycemic activity, such as alcohol).

Wine, unspecified (Insulin requirements may be decreased in the presence of drugs that increase insulin sensitivity or have hypoglycemic activity, such as alcohol).

Wine products (Insulin requirements may be decreased in the presence of drugs that increase insulin sensitivity or have hypoglycemic activity, such as alcohol).

HYALGAN SOLUTION

Food Interactions

Egg Product (Use caution when injecting sodium hyaluronate into patients who are allergic to avian proteins, feathers, and egg products).

HYCAMTIN FOR INJECTION
May interact with cytotoxic drugs, and certain other agents. Compounds in these categories include:

Bleomycin Sulfate (Greater myelosuppression is likely to be seen when topotecan hydrochloride is used in combination with other cytotoxic agents, thereby necessitating a dose reduction).
No products indexed under this heading.

Carboplatin (Greater myelosuppression is likely to be seen when topotecan hydrochloride is used in combination with other cytotoxic agents, thereby necessitating a dose reduction. However, when combining topotecan hydrochloride with platinum agents (eg, carboplatin), a distinct sequence dependent interaction on myelosuppression has been reported. Co-administration of a platinum agent on day one of topotecan hydrochloride dosing required lower doses of each agent compared to co-administration on day five of the topotecan hydrochloride dosing schedule).
No products indexed under this heading.

Cisplatin (Greater myelosuppression is likely to be seen when topotecan hydrochloride is used in combination with other cytotoxic agents, thereby necessitating a dose reduction. However, when combining topotecan hydrochloride with plainum agents (eg, cisplatin), a distinct sequence dependent interaction on myelosuppression has been reported. Co-administration of a platinum agent on day one of topotecan hydrochloride dosing required lower doses of each agent compared to co-administration on day five of the topotecan hydrochloride dosing schedule).
No products indexed under this heading.

Cyclophosphamide (Greater myelosuppression is likely to be seen when topotecan hydrochloride is used in combination with other cytotoxic agents, thereby necessitating a dose reduction).
No products indexed under this heading.

Daunorubicin Hydrochloride (Greater myelosuppression is likely to be seen when topotecan hydrochloride is used in combination with other cytotoxic agents, thereby necessitating a dose reduction).
No products indexed under this heading.

Doxorubicin Hydrochloride (Greater myelosuppression is likely to be seen when topotecan hydrochloride is used in combination with other cytotoxic agents, thereby necessitating a dose reduction).
No products indexed under this heading.

Epirubicin Hydrochloride (Greater myelosuppression is likely to be seen when topotecan hydrochloride is used in combination with other cytotoxic agents, thereby necessitating a dose reduction).
No products indexed under this heading.

Filgrastim (Concomitant administration of granulocyte colony stimulating factor (G-CSF) can prolong the duration of neutropenia, so if G-CSF is to be used, it should not be initiated until day 6 of the course of therapy, 24 hours after completion of treatment with topotecan hydrochloride). Products include:

Fluorouracil (Greater myelosuppression is likely to be seen when topotecan hydrochloride is used in combination with other cytotoxic agents, thereby necessitating a dose reduction). Products include:

Hydroxyurea (Greater myelosuppression is likely to be seen when topotecan hydrochloride is used in combination with other cytotoxic agents, thereby necessitating a dose reduction).
No products indexed under this heading.

Methotrexate Sodium (Greater myelosuppression is likely to be seen when topotecan hydrochloride is used in combination with other cytotoxic agents, thereby necessitating a dose reduction).
No products indexed under this heading.

Mitotane (Greater myelosuppression is likely to be seen when topotecan hydrochloride is used in combination with other cytotoxic agents, thereby necessitating a dose reduction).
No products indexed under this heading.

Mitoxantrone Hydrochloride (Greater myelosuppression is likely to be seen when topotecan hydrochloride is used in combination with other cytotoxic agents, thereby necessitating a dose reduction). Products include:

Procarbazine Hydrochloride (Greater myelosuppression is likely to be seen when topotecan hydrochloride is used in combination with other cytotoxic agents, thereby necessitating a dose reduction).
No products indexed under this heading.

Tamoxifen Citrate (Greater myelosuppression is likely to be seen when topotecan hydrochloride is used in combination with other cytotoxic agents, thereby necessitating a dose reduction).
No products indexed under this heading.

Vinblastine Sulfate (Greater myelosuppression is likely to be seen when topotecan hydrochloride is used in combination with other cytotoxic agents, thereby necessitating a dose reduction).
No products indexed under this heading.

IMPORTANT NOTE: Always consult each drug listing in the patient's regimen for possible interactions.

Vincristine Sulfate (Greater myelo-suppression is likely to be seen when topotecan hydrochloride is used in combination with other cytotoxic agents, thereby necessitating a dose reduction).

No products indexed under this heading.

Vinorelbine Tartrate (Greater myelo-suppression is likely to be seen when topotecan hydrochloride is used in combination with other cytotoxic agents, thereby necessitating a dose reduction).

No products indexed under this heading.

HYCAMTIN CAPSULES

(Topotecan Hydrochloride) **1488**
May interact with P-glycoprotein inhibitors, and certain other agents. Compounds in these categories include:

Amiodarone Hydrochloride
(P-glycoprotein inhibitors (eg, cyclosporine A, elacridar, ketoconazole, ritonavir, saquinavir) can cause significant increases in topotecan exposure. The concomitant use of P-glycoprotein inhibitors with topotecan capsules should be avoided).

No products indexed under this heading.

Amlodipine Besylate (P-glycoprotein inhibitors (eg, cyclosporine A, elacridar, ketoconazole, ritonavir, saquinavir) can cause significant increases in topotecan exposure. The concomitant use of P-glycoprotein inhibitors with topotecan capsules should be avoided). Products include:

Azor **1010**
Exforge **2443**
Exforge HCT **2449**

Atenolol (P-glycoprotein inhibitors (eg, cyclosporine A, elacridar, ketoconazole, ritonavir, saquinavir) can cause significant increases in topotecan exposure. The concomitant use of P-glycoprotein inhibitors with topotecan capsules should be avoided).

No products indexed under this heading.

Atorvastatin Calcium (P-glycoprotein inhibitors (eg, cyclosporine A, elacridar, ketoconazole, ritonavir, saquinavir) can cause significant increases in topotecan exposure. The concomitant use of P-glycoprotein inhibitors with topotecan capsules should be avoided). Products include:

Lipitor **2703**

Azithromycin Dihydrate
(P-glycoprotein inhibitors (eg, cyclosporine A, elacridar, ketoconazole, ritonavir, saquinavir) can cause significant increases in topotecan exposure. The concomitant use of P-glycoprotein inhibitors with topotecan capsules should be avoided).

No products indexed under this heading.

Carvedilol (P-glycoprotein inhibitors (eg, cyclosporine A, elacridar, ketoconazole, ritonavir, saquinavir) can cause significant increases in topotecan exposure. The concomitant use of P-glycoprotein inhibitors with topotecan capsules should be avoided). Products include:

Coreg **1409**

Carvedilol Phosphate
(P-glycoprotein inhibitors (eg, cyclosporine A, elacridar, ketoconazole, ritonavir, saquinavir) can cause significant increases in topotecan exposure. The concomitant use of P-glycoprotein inhibitors with topotecan capsules should be avoided). Products include:

Coreg CR **1416**

Clarithromycin (P-glycoprotein inhibitors (eg, cyclosporine A, elacridar, ketoconazole, ritonavir, saquinavir) can cause significant increases in topotecan exposure. The concomitant use of

P-glycoprotein inhibitors with topotecan capsules should be avoided). Products include:

Biaxin/Biaxin XL **412**

Cyclosporine (Topotecan is a substrate for both ABCB1 [P-glycoprotein (P-gp)] and ABCG2 (BCRP). Cyclosporine A (inhibitor of ABCB1, ABCC1 [MRP-1], and CYP3A4) with topotecan capsules increased topotecan exposure to 2- to 3-fold of control. Patients should be carefully monitored for adverse reactions when topotecan capsules are administered with a drug known to inhibit these transporters). Products include:

Gengraf **440**
Neoral Oral Solution **2496**
Neoral Capsules **2496**
Restasis **605**

Digoxin (P-glycoprotein inhibitors (eg, cyclosporine A, elacridar, ketoconazole, ritonavir, saquinavir) can cause significant increases in topotecan exposure. The concomitant use of P-glycoprotein inhibitors with topotecan capsules should be avoided). Products include:

Lanoxin Injection **1546**
Lanoxin Injection Pediatric **1549**
Lanoxin Tablets **1553**

Diltiazem Hydrochloride
(P-glycoprotein inhibitors (eg, cyclosporine A, elacridar, ketoconazole, ritonavir, saquinavir) can cause significant increases in topotecan exposure. The concomitant use of P-glycoprotein inhibitors with topotecan capsules should be avoided). Products include:

Cardizem LA **423**

Diltiazem Maleate (P-glycoprotein inhibitors (eg, cyclosporine A, elacridar, ketoconazole, ritonavir, saquinavir) can cause significant increases in topotecan exposure. The concomitant use of P-glycoprotein inhibitors with topotecan capsules should be avoided).

No products indexed under this heading.

Dirithromycin (P-glycoprotein inhibitors (eg, cyclosporine A, elacridar, ketoconazole, ritonavir, saquinavir) can cause significant increases in topotecan exposure. The concomitant use of P-glycoprotein inhibitors with topotecan capsules should be avoided).

No products indexed under this heading.

Elacridar (Topotecan is a substrate for both ABCB1 [P-glycoprotein (P-gp)] and ABCG2 (BCRP). Elacridar (inhibitor of ABCB1 and ABCG2) administered with topotecan capsules increased topotecan exposure to approximately 2.5-fold of control. Patients should be carefully monitored for adverse reactions when topotecan capsules are administered with a drug known to inhibit these transporters).

No products indexed under this heading.

Erythromycin (P-glycoprotein inhibitors (eg, cyclosporine A, elacridar, ketoconazole, ritonavir, saquinavir) can cause significant increases in topotecan exposure. The concomitant use of P-glycoprotein inhibitors with topotecan capsules should be avoided).

No products indexed under this heading.

Erythromycin, Topical
(P-glycoprotein inhibitors (eg, cyclosporine A, elacridar, ketoconazole, ritonavir, saquinavir) can cause significant increases in topotecan exposure. The concomitant use of P-glycoprotein inhibitors with topotecan capsules should be avoided).

No products indexed under this heading.

Erythromycin Estolate
(P-glycoprotein inhibitors (eg, cyclosporine A, elacridar, ketoconazole, ritonavir, saquinavir) can cause significant increases in topotecan exposure. The concomitant use of P-glycoprotein inhibitors with topotecan capsules should be avoided).

No products indexed under this heading.

Erythromycin Ethylsuccinate
(P-glycoprotein inhibitors (eg, cyclosporine A, elacridar, ketoconazole, ritonavir, saquinavir) can cause significant increases in topotecan exposure. The concomitant use of P-glycoprotein inhibitors with topotecan capsules should be avoided). Products include:

E.E.S. **437**
EryPed **435**

Erythromycin Gluceptate
(P-glycoprotein inhibitors (eg, cyclosporine A, elacridar, ketoconazole, ritonavir, saquinavir) can cause significant increases in topotecan exposure. The concomitant use of P-glycoprotein inhibitors with topotecan capsules should be avoided).

No products indexed under this heading.

Erythromycin Lactobionate
(P-glycoprotein inhibitors (eg, cyclosporine A, elacridar, ketoconazole, ritonavir, saquinavir) can cause significant increases in topotecan exposure. The concomitant use of P-glycoprotein inhibitors with topotecan capsules should be avoided).

No products indexed under this heading.

Erythromycin Stearate
(P-glycoprotein inhibitors (eg, cyclosporine A, elacridar, ketoconazole, ritonavir, saquinavir) can cause significant increases in topotecan exposure. The concomitant use of P-glycoprotein inhibitors with topotecan capsules should be avoided).

No products indexed under this heading.

Itraconazole (P-glycoprotein inhibitors (eg, cyclosporine A, elacridar, ketoconazole, ritonavir, saquinavir) can cause significant increases in topotecan exposure. The concomitant use of P-glycoprotein inhibitors with topotecan capsules should be avoided).

No products indexed under this heading.

Ketoconazole (P-glycoprotein inhibitors (eg, ketoconazole) can cause significant increases in topotecan exposure. The concomitant use of P-glycoprotein inhibitors with topotecan capsules should be avoided). Products include:

Extina **3319**
Xolegel **3337**

Mibefradil Dihydrochloride
(P-glycoprotein inhibitors (eg, cyclosporine A, elacridar, ketoconazole, ritonavir, saquinavir) can cause significant increases in topotecan exposure. The concomitant use of P-glycoprotein inhibitors with topotecan capsules should be avoided).

No products indexed under this heading.

Quinidine (P-glycoprotein inhibitors (eg, cyclosporine A, elacridar, ketoconazole, ritonavir, saquinavir) can cause significant increases in topotecan exposure. The concomitant use of P-glycoprotein inhibitors with topotecan capsules should be avoided).

No products indexed under this heading.

Quinidine Gluconate (P-glycoprotein inhibitors (eg, cyclosporine A, elacridar, ketoconazole, ritonavir, saquinavir) can cause significant increases in topotecan exposure. The concomitant use of P-glycoprotein inhibitors with topotecan capsules should be avoided).

No products indexed under this heading.

Quinidine Hydrochloride
(P-glycoprotein inhibitors (eg, cyclosporine A, elacridar, ketoconazole, ritonavir, saquinavir) can cause significant increases in topotecan exposure. The concomitant use of P-glycoprotein inhibitors with topotecan capsules should be avoided).

No products indexed under this heading.

Quinidine Polygalacturonate
(P-glycoprotein inhibitors (eg, cyclosporine A, elacridar, ketoconazole, ritonavir, saquinavir) can cause significant increases in topotecan exposure. The concomitant use of P-glycoprotein inhibitors with topotecan capsules should be avoided).

No products indexed under this heading.

Quinidine Sulfate (P-glycoprotein inhibitors (eg, cyclosporine A, elacridar, ketoconazole, ritonavir, saquinavir) can cause significant increases in topotecan exposure. The concomitant use of P-glycoprotein inhibitors with topotecan capsules should be avoided).

No products indexed under this heading.

Ritonavir (P-glycoprotein inhibitors (eg, ritonavir) can cause significant increases in topotecan exposure. The concomitant use of P-glycoprotein inhibitors with topotecan capsules should be avoided). Products include:

Kaletra **458**
Norvir **509**

Saquinavir (P-glycoprotein inhibitors (eg, saquinavir) can cause significant increases in topotecan exposure. The concomitant use of P-glycoprotein inhibitors with topotecan capsules should be avoided).

No products indexed under this heading.

Saquinavir Mesylate (P-glycoprotein inhibitors (eg, saquinavir) can cause significant increases in topotecan exposure. The concomitant use of P-glycoprotein inhibitors with topotecan capsules should be avoided).

No products indexed under this heading.

Tamoxifen Citrate (P-glycoprotein inhibitors (eg, cyclosporine A, elacridar, ketoconazole, ritonavir, saquinavir) can cause significant increases in topotecan exposure. The concomitant use of P-glycoprotein inhibitors with topotecan capsules should be avoided).

No products indexed under this heading.

Troleandomycin (P-glycoprotein inhibitors (eg, cyclosporine A, elacridar, ketoconazole, ritonavir, saquinavir) can cause significant increases in topotecan exposure. The concomitant use of P-glycoprotein inhibitors with topotecan capsules should be avoided).

No products indexed under this heading.

Verapamil Hydrochloride
(P-glycoprotein inhibitors (eg, cyclosporine A, elacridar, ketoconazole, ritonavir, saquinavir) can cause significant increases in topotecan exposure. The concomitant use of P-glycoprotein inhibitors with topotecan capsules should be avoided). Products include:

Tarka **534**

HYLAND'S CALMS FORTÉ 4 KIDS TABLETS

(Homeopathic Formulations, Sulfur) **3314**
None cited in PDR database.

HYLAND'S CALMS FORTÉ CAPLETS

(Homeopathic Formulations) **3314**
None cited in PDR database.

HYLAND'S CALMS FORTÉ TABLETS

(Homeopathic Formulations) **3314**
None cited in PDR database.

HYLAND'S COLD 'N COUGH 4 KIDS

(Allium cepa, Hydrastis canadensis, Phosphorus, Pulsatilla pratensis, Sulfur)..................................3314
None cited in PDR database.

HYLAND'S COLIC TABLETS

(Chamomilla, Colocynthis, Disocorea, Homeopathic Formulations)..........................3314
None cited in PDR database.

HYLAND'S COUGH SYRUP WITH 100% NATURAL HONEY 4 KIDS

(Aconitum napellus, Cephaelis ipecacuanha)........................3315
None cited in PDR database.

HYLAND'S EARACHE DROPS

(Herbals, Multiple) 3315
None cited in PDR database.

HYLAND'S LEG CRAMPS PM WITH QUININE TABLETS

(Chamomilla, Herbals with Minerals, Lycopodium Clavatum, Quinine, Rhus Toxicodendron, Silicea, Silicea-Don Not Use, Sulfur) 3315
None cited in PDR database.

HYLAND'S LEG CRAMPS WITH QUININE CAPLETS

(Homeopathic Formulations) 3315
None cited in PDR database.

HYLAND'S LEG CRAMPS WITH QUININE TABLETS

(Homeopathic Formulations) 3315
None cited in PDR database.

HYLAND'S NERVE TONIC CAPLETS

(Homeopathic Formulations) 3315
None cited in PDR database.

HYLAND'S NERVE TONIC TABLETS

(Homeopathic Formulations) 3315
None cited in PDR database.

HYLAND'S RESTFUL LEGS TABLETS

(Homeopathic Formulations) 3315
None cited in PDR database.

HYLAND'S SNIFFLES 'N SNEEZES 4 KIDS TABLETS

(Dietary Supplement) 3315
None cited in PDR database.

HYLAND'S TEETHING GEL

(Homeopathic Formulations) 3316
None cited in PDR database.

HYLAND'S TEETHING TABLETS

(Belladonna Alkaloids, Homeopathic Formulations) 3316
None cited in PDR database.

HYZAAR 50-12.5 TABLETS

(Hydrochlorothiazide, Losartan Potassium) 2162
May interact with alcohols, antihypertensives, barbiturates, corticosteroids, erythromycin, insulin, lithium preparations, narcotic analgesics, non-steroidal anti-inflammatory agents, nondepolarizing neuromuscular blocking agents, oral hypoglycemic agents, potassium preparations, potassium sparing diuretics, vasopressors, and certain other agents. Compounds in these categories include:

Acarbose (Hyperglycemia may occur with thiazide diuretics; dosage adjustment of the antidiabetic drug may be required).
No products indexed under this heading.

Acebutolol Hydrochloride (Additive effect or potentiation of other antihypertensives).
No products indexed under this heading.

ACTH (Potential for intensified electrolyte depletion, particularly hypokalemia).
No products indexed under this heading.

Alclometasone Dipropionate (Potential for intensified electrolyte depletion, particularly hypokalemia).
No products indexed under this heading.

Alfentanil Hydrochloride (Potentiation of orthostatic hypotension may occur).
No products indexed under this heading.

Aliskiren (Additive effect or potentiation of other antihypertensives). Products include:
Tekturna 2538
Tekturna HCT 2541
Valturna 3637

Amiloride Hydrochloride (Concomitant use with potassium-sparing diuretics may lead to hyperkalemia).
No products indexed under this heading.

Amlodipine Besylate (Additive effect or potentiation of other antihypertensives). Products include:
Azor 1010
Exforge 2443
Exforge HCT 2449

Amobarbital (Potentiation of orthostatic hypotension may occur).
No products indexed under this heading.

Amobarbital Sodium (Potentiation of orthostatic hypotension may occur).
No products indexed under this heading.

Apomorphine (Potentiation of orthostatic hypotension may occur).
No products indexed under this heading.

Apomorphine Hydrochloride (Potentiation of orthostatic hypotension may occur).
No products indexed under this heading.

Aprobarbital (Potentiation of orthostatic hypotension may occur).
No products indexed under this heading.

Atenolol (Additive effect or potentiation of other antihypertensives).
No products indexed under this heading.

Atracurium Besylate (Possible increased responsiveness to the muscle relaxant).
No products indexed under this heading.

Beclomethasone Dipropionate (Potential for intensified electrolyte depletion, particularly hypokalemia). Products include:
Qvar 3398

Beclomethasone Dipropionate Monohydrate (Potential for intensified electrolyte depletion, particularly hypokalemia). Products include:
Beconase AQ 1386

Benazepril Hydrochloride (Additive effect or potentiation of other antihypertensives).
No products indexed under this heading.

Bendroflumethiazide (Additive effect or potentiation of other antihypertensives).
No products indexed under this heading.

Betamethasone (Potential for intensified electrolyte depletion, particularly hypokalemia).
No products indexed under this heading.

Betamethasone Acetate (Potential for intensified electrolyte depletion, particularly hypokalemia).
No products indexed under this heading.

Betamethasone Benzoate (Potential for intensified electrolyte depletion, particularly hypokalemia).
No products indexed under this heading.

Betamethasone Dipropionate (Potential for intensified electrolyte depletion, particularly hypokalemia). Products include:
Diprolene Lotion 0.05% 3108
Diprolene Ointment 0.05% 3109
Diprolene AF Cream 0.05% 3107
Lotrisone 3163

Betamethasone Sodium Phosphate (Potential for intensified electrolyte depletion, particularly hypokalemia).
No products indexed under this heading.

Betamethasone Valerate (Potential for intensified electrolyte depletion, particularly hypokalemia). Products include:
Luxiq 3321

Betaxolol Hydrochloride (Additive effect or potentiation of other antihypertensives).
No products indexed under this heading.

Bisoprolol Fumarate (Additive effect or potentiation of other antihypertensives).
No products indexed under this heading.

Budesonide (Potential for intensified electrolyte depletion, particularly hypokalemia). Products include:
Pulmicort Flexhaler 714
Symbicort 80/4.5 720
Symbicort 160/4.5 720

Buprenorphine Hydrochloride (Potentiation of orthostatic hypotension may occur).
No products indexed under this heading.

Butabarbital (Potentiation of orthostatic hypotension may occur).
No products indexed under this heading.

Butabarbital Sodium (Potentiation of orthostatic hypotension may occur).
No products indexed under this heading.

Butalbital (Potentiation of orthostatic hypotension may occur).
No products indexed under this heading.

Candesartan Cilexetil (Additive effect or potentiation of other antihypertensives). Products include:
Atacand 697
Atacand HCT 700

Captopril (Additive effect or potentiation of other antihypertensives). Products include:
Captopril 2341

Carteolol Hydrochloride (Additive effect or potentiation of other antihypertensives).
No products indexed under this heading.

Carvedilol (Additive effect or potentiation of other antihypertensives). Products include:
Coreg 1409

Carvedilol Phosphate (Additive effect or potentiation of other antihypertensives). Products include:
Coreg CR 1416

Celecoxib (In some patients with compromised renal function who are being treated with non-steroidal anti-inflammatory drugs (NSAIDs), including those that selectively inhibit cyclooxygenase-2 inhibitors (COX-2 inhibitors), the co-administration of angiotensin II receptor antagonists including losartan may result in a further deterioration of renal function. These effects are usually reversible. Reports suggest that NSAIDs, including selective COX-2 inhibitors, may diminish the antihypertensive effect of angiotensin II receptor antagonists, including losartan. This interaction should be given consideration in patients taking NSAIDs, including selective COX-2 inhibitors, concomitantly with angiotensin II receptor antagonists). Products include:

Celebrex 3272

Chlorothiazide (Additive effect or potentiation of other antihypertensives).
No products indexed under this heading.

Chlorothiazide Sodium (Additive effect or potentiation of other antihypertensives). Products include:
Diuril Intravenous 2009

Chlorpropamide (Hyperglycemia may occur with thiazide diuretics; dosage adjustment of the antidiabetic drug may be required).
No products indexed under this heading.

Chlorthalidone (Additive effect or potentiation of other antihypertensives). Products include:
Clorpres 2344

Cholestyramine (Absorption of hydryochlorthiazide is impaired in the presence of anionic exchange resins. Single doses of either cholestyramine or colestipol resins bind the hydrochlorthiazide and reduce its absorption from the gastrointestinal track by up to 85% and 43%, respectively).
No products indexed under this heading.

Ciclesonide (Potential for intensified electrolyte depletion, particularly hypokalemia).
No products indexed under this heading.

Cisatracurium Besylate (Possible increased responsiveness to the muscle relaxant). Products include:
Nimbex 503

Clonidine (Additive effect or potentiation of other antihypertensives). Products include:
Catapres-TTS 884

Clonidine Hydrochloride (Additive effect or potentiation of other antihypertensives). Products include:
Clorpres 2344

Codeine Phosphate (Potentiation of orthostatic hypotension may occur). Products include:
Tylenol with Codeine 2691

Codeine Sulfate (Potentiation of orthostatic hypotension may occur).
No products indexed under this heading.

Colestipol (Absorption of hydryochlorthiazide is impaired in the presence of anionic exchange resins. Single doses of either cholestryramine or colestipol resins bind the hydrochlorthiazide and reduce its absorption from the gastrointestinal track by up to 85% and 43%, respectively).
No products indexed under this heading.

Colestipol Hydrochloride (Absorption of hydryochlorthiazide is impaired in the presence of anionic exchange resins. Single doses of either cholestryramine or colestipol resins bind the hydrochlorthiazide and reduce its absorption from the gastrointestinal track by up to 85% and 43%, respectively).
No products indexed under this heading.

Cortisone Acetate (Potential for intensified electrolyte depletion, particularly hypokalemia).
No products indexed under this heading.

Deserpidine (Additive effect or potentiation of other antihypertensives).
No products indexed under this heading.

Desoximetasone (Potential for intensified electrolyte depletion, particularly hypokalemia).
No products indexed under this heading.

Dexamethasone (Potential for intensified electrolyte depletion, particularly hypokalemia). Products include:
Ciprodex 583
Ozurdex ....⊙223
Tobramycin and Dexamethasone Ophthalmic Suspension ....⊙251

IMPORTANT NOTE: Always consult each drug listing in the patient's regimen for possible interactions.

Hyzaar Interactions Index 828

Dexamethasone Acetate (Potential for intensified electrolyte depletion, particularly hypokalemia).
No products indexed under this heading.

Dexamethasone Phosphate (Potential for intensified electrolyte depletion, particularly hypokalemia).
No products indexed under this heading.

Dexamethasone Sodium (Potential for intensified electrolyte depletion, particularly hypokalemia).
No products indexed under this heading.

Dexamethasone Sodium Phosphate (Potential for intensified electrolyte depletion, particularly hypokalemia).
No products indexed under this heading.

Dexamethasone Sodium Phosphate Injection (Potential for intensified electrolyte depletion, particularly hypokalemia).
No products indexed under this heading.

Dezocine (Potentiation of orthostatic hypotension may occur).
No products indexed under this heading.

Diazoxide (Additive effect or potentiation of other antihypertensives). Products include:
Proglycem 1179
Proglycem Suspension 1179

Diclofenac Epolamine (In some patients with compromised renal function who are being treated with non-steroidal anti-inflammatory drugs (NSAIDs), including those that selectively inhibit cyclooxygenase-2 inhibitors (COX-2 inhibitors), the co-administration of angiotensin II receptor antagonists including losartan may result in a further deterioration of renal function. These effects are usually reversible. Reports suggest that NSAIDs, including selective COX-2 inhibitors, may diminish the antihypertensive effect of angiotensin II receptor antagonists, including losartan. This interaction should be given consideration in patients taking NSAIDs, including selective COX-2 inhibitors, concomitantly with angiotensin II receptor antagonists). Products include:
Flector 1839

Diclofenac Potassium (In some patients with compromised renal function who are being treated with non-steroidal anti-inflammatory drugs (NSAIDs), including those that selectively inhibit cyclooxygenase-2 inhibitors (COX-2 inhibitors), the co-administration of angiotensin II receptor antagonists including losartan may result in a further deterioration of renal function. These effects are usually reversible. Reports suggest that NSAIDs, including selective COX-2 inhibitors, may diminish the antihypertensive effect of angiotensin II receptor antagonists, including losartan. This interaction should be given consideration in patients taking NSAIDs, including selective COX-2 inhibitors, concomitantly with angiotensin II receptor antagonists).
No products indexed under this heading.

Diclofenac Sodium (In some patients with compromised renal function who are being treated with non-steroidal anti-inflammatory drugs (NSAIDs), including those that selectively inhibit cyclooxygenase-2 inhibitors (COX-2 inhibitors), the co-administration of angiotensin II receptor antagonists including losartan may result in a further deterioration of renal function. These effects are usually reversible. Reports suggest that NSAIDs, including selective COX-2 inhibitors, may diminish the antihypertensive effect of angiotensin II receptor antagonists, including losartan. This interaction should be given consideration in patients taking NSAIDs, including selective COX-2 inhibitors, concomitantly with angiotensin II receptor antagonists).
No products indexed under this heading.

Diflorasone Diacetate (Potential for intensified electrolyte depletion, particularly hypokalemia).
No products indexed under this heading.

Dihydrocodeine Bitartrate (Potentiation of orthostatic hypotension may occur).
No products indexed under this heading.

Dihydrocodeinone Bitartrate (Potentiation of orthostatic hypotension may occur).
No products indexed under this heading.

Diltiazem Hydrochloride (Additive effect or potentiation of other antihypertensives). Products include:
Cardizem LA 423

Diltiazem Maleate (Additive effect or potentiation of other antihypertensives).
No products indexed under this heading.

Dobutamine (Possible decreased response to vasopressor amines).
No products indexed under this heading.

Dobutamine Hydrochloride (Possible decreased response to vasopressor amines).
No products indexed under this heading.

Dopamine Hydrochloride (Possible decreased response to vasopressor amines).
No products indexed under this heading.

Doxacurium Chloride (Possible increased responsiveness to the muscle relaxant).
No products indexed under this heading.

Doxazosin Mesylate (Additive effect or potentiation of other antihypertensives).
No products indexed under this heading.

d-Tubocurarine (Possible increased responsiveness to the muscle relaxant).
No products indexed under this heading.

Enalapril Maleate (Additive effect or potentiation of other antihypertensives).
No products indexed under this heading.

Enalaprilat (Additive effect or potentiation of other antihypertensives).
No products indexed under this heading.

Ephedrine Sulfate (Possible decreased response to vasopressor amines).
No products indexed under this heading.

Epinephrine Bitartrate (Possible decreased response to vasopressor amines).
No products indexed under this heading.

Epinephrine Hydrochloride (Possible decreased response to vasopressor amines).
No products indexed under this heading.

Eprosartan Mesylate (Additive effect or potentiation of other antihypertensives). Products include:
Teveten 538
Teveten HCT 541

Erythromycin (Erythromycin increased the AUC of losartan by 30%).
No products indexed under this heading.

Erythromycin, Topical (Erythromycin increased the AUC of losartan by 30%).
No products indexed under this heading.

Erythromycin Estolate (Erythromycin increased the AUC of losartan by 30%).
No products indexed under this heading.

Erythromycin Ethylsuccinate (Erythromycin increased the AUC of losartan by 30%). Products include:
E.E.S. 437
EryPed 435

Erythromycin Gluceptate (Erythromycin increased the AUC of losartan by 30%).
No products indexed under this heading.

Erythromycin Lactobionate (Erythromycin increased the AUC of losartan by 30%).
No products indexed under this heading.

Erythromycin Stearate (Erythromycin increased the AUC of losartan by 30%).
No products indexed under this heading.

Esmolol Hydrochloride (Additive effect or potentiation of other antihypertensives).
No products indexed under this heading.

Ethanol (Potentiation of orthostatic hypotension may occur).
No products indexed under this heading.

Ethyl Alcohol (Potentiation of orthostatic hypotension may occur).
No products indexed under this heading.

Etodolac (In some patients with compromised renal function who are being treated with non-steroidal anti-inflammatory drugs (NSAIDs), including those that selectively inhibit cyclooxygenase-2 inhibitors (COX-2 inhibitors), the co-administration of angiotensin II receptor antagonists including losartan may result in a further deterioration of renal function. These effects are usually reversible. Reports suggest that NSAIDs, including selective COX-2 inhibitors, may diminish the antihypertensive effect of angiotensin II receptor antagonists, including losartan. This interaction should be given consideration in patients taking NSAIDs, including selective COX-2 inhibitors, concomitantly with angiotensin II receptor antagonists).
No products indexed under this heading.

Felodipine (Additive effect or potentiation of other antihypertensives).
No products indexed under this heading.

Fenoprofen Calcium (In some patients with compromised renal function who are being treated with non-steroidal anti-inflammatory drugs (NSAIDs), including those that selectively inhibit cyclooxygenase-2 inhibitors (COX-2 inhibitors), the co-administration of angiotensin II receptor antagonists including losartan may result in a further deterioration of renal function. These effects are usually reversible. Reports suggest that NSAIDs, including selective COX-2 inhibitors, may diminish the antihypertensive effect of angiotensin II receptor antagonists, including losartan. This interaction should be given consideration in patients taking NSAIDs, including selective COX-2 inhibitors, concomitantly with angiotensin II receptor antagonists).
No products indexed under this heading.

Fentanyl (Potentiation of orthostatic hypotension may occur). Products include:
Duragesic 2604
Fentanyl Transdermal System 2346
Onsolis 2054

Fentanyl Citrate (Potentiation of orthostatic hypotension may occur). Products include:
Fentora 966

Fluconazole (Fluconazole decreased the AUC of the active metabolite of losartan by approximately 40%, but increased the AUC of losartan by 70%).
No products indexed under this heading.

Fludrocortisone Acetate (Potential for intensified electrolyte depletion, particularly hypokalemia).
No products indexed under this heading.

Flumethasone Pivalate (Potential for intensified electrolyte depletion, particularly hypokalemia).
No products indexed under this heading.

Flunisolide Hemihydrate (Potential for intensified electrolyte depletion, particularly hypokalemia).
No products indexed under this heading.

Flurbiprofen (In some patients with compromised renal function who are being treated with non-steroidal anti-inflammatory drugs (NSAIDs), including those that selectively inhibit cyclooxygenase-2 inhibitors (COX-2 inhibitors), the co-administration of angiotensin II receptor antagonists including losartan may result in a further deterioration of renal function. These effects are usually reversible. Reports suggest that NSAIDs, including selective COX-2 inhibitors, may diminish the antihypertensive effect of angiotensin II receptor antagonists, including losartan. This interaction should be given consideration in patients taking NSAIDs, including selective COX-2 inhibitors, concomitantly with angiotensin II receptor antagonists).
No products indexed under this heading.

Fluticasone Furoate (Potential for intensified electrolyte depletion, particularly hypokalemia). Products include:
Veramyst 1713

Fluticasone Propionate (Potential for intensified electrolyte depletion, particularly hypokalemia). Products include:
Advair 100/50 1275
Advair 250/50 1275
Advair 500/50 1275
Advair HFA 45/21 1288
Advair HFA 115/21 1288
Advair HFA 230/21 1288
Flonase 1459
Flovent Diskus 1463
Flovent HFA 1470

Fosinopril Sodium (Additive effect or potentiation of other antihypertensives).
No products indexed under this heading.

Furosemide (Additive effect or potentiation of other antihypertensives). Products include:
Furosemide 2354

Gallamine (Possible increased responsiveness to the muscle relaxant).
No products indexed under this heading.

Gallamine Triethiodide (Possible increased responsiveness to the muscle relaxant).
No products indexed under this heading.

Glibenclamide (Hyperglycemia may occur with thiazide diuretics; dosage adjustment of the antidiabetic drug may be required).
No products indexed under this heading.

Glimepiride (Hyperglycemia may occur with thiazide diuretics; dosage adjustment of the antidiabetic drug may be required). Products include:
Avandaryl 1356
Duetact 3354

Glipizide (Hyperglycemia may occur with thiazide diuretics; dosage adjustment of the antidiabetic drug may be required).
No products indexed under this heading.

Glyburide (Hyperglycemia may occur with thiazide diuretics; dosage adjustment of the antidiabetic drug may be required).
No products indexed under this heading.

Guanabenz Acetate (Additive effect or potentiation of other antihypertensives).
No products indexed under this heading.

Guanethidine (Additive effect or potentiation of other antihypertensives).
No products indexed under this heading.

Guanethidine Monosulfate (Additive effect or potentiation of other antihypertensives).
No products indexed under this heading.

Guanethidine Sulfate (Additive effect or potentiation of other antihypertensives).
No products indexed under this heading.

Hexobarbital (Potentiation of orthostatic hypotension may occur).
No products indexed under this heading.

(⊙ Described in PDR® for Ophthalmic Medicines)

829 Interactions Index Hyzaar

Hydralazine Hydrochloride (Additive effect or potentiation of other antihypertensives).
No products indexed under this heading.

Hydrocodone Bitartrate (Potentiation of orthostatic hypotension may occur). Products include:
Vicodin ... 560
Vicodin ES ... 561
Vicodin HP ... 563
Vicoprofen ... 564
Zydone ... 1138

Hydrocodone Polistirex (Potentiation of orthostatic hypotension may occur). Products include:
Tussionex ... 3443

Hydrocortisone (Potential for intensified electrolyte depletion, particularly hypokalemia).
No products indexed under this heading.

Hydrocortisone (Alcohol) (Potential for intensified electrolyte depletion, particularly hypokalemia).
No products indexed under this heading.

Hydrocortisone Acetate (Potential for intensified electrolyte depletion, particularly hypokalemia).
No products indexed under this heading.

Hydrocortisone Butyrate (Potential for intensified electrolyte depletion, particularly hypokalemia).
No products indexed under this heading.

Hydrocortisone Cypionate (Potential for intensified electrolyte depletion, particularly hypokalemia).
No products indexed under this heading.

Hydrocortisone Hemisuccinate (Potential for intensified electrolyte depletion, particularly hypokalemia).
No products indexed under this heading.

Hydrocortisone Probutate (Potential for intensified electrolyte depletion, particularly hypokalemia).
No products indexed under this heading.

Hydrocortisone Sodium Phosphate (Potential for intensified electrolyte depletion, particularly hypokalemia).
No products indexed under this heading.

Hydrocortisone Sodium Succinate (Potential for intensified electrolyte depletion, particularly hypokalemia).
No products indexed under this heading.

Hydrocortisone Valerate (Potential for intensified electrolyte depletion, particularly hypokalemia).
No products indexed under this heading.

Hydroflumethiazide (Additive effect or potentiation of other antihypertensives).
No products indexed under this heading.

Hydromorphone (Potentiation of orthostatic hypotension may occur).
No products indexed under this heading.

Hydromorphone Hydrochloride (Potentiation of orthostatic hypotension may occur). Products include:
Dilaudid Injection ... 2800
Dilaudid Oral ... 2797
Dilaudid Tablets ... 2797
Dilaudid-HP ... 2800

Ibuprofen (In some patients with compromised renal function who are being treated with non-steroidal anti-inflammatory drugs (NSAIDs), including those that selectively inhibit cyclooxygenase-2 inhibitors (COX-2 inhibitors), the co-administration of angiotensin II receptor antagonists including losartan may result in a further deterioration of renal function. These effects are usually reversible. Reports suggest that NSAIDs, including selective COX-2 inhibitors, may diminish the antihypertensive effect of angiotensin II receptor antagonists, including losartan. This interaction should be given consideration in patients taking NSAIDs, including selective COX-2 inhibitors, concomitantly with angiotensin II receptor antagonists). Products include:
Motrin IB ... 2043
Children's Motrin ... 2044
Children's Motrin Non-Staining Dye-Free ... 2044
Infants' Motrin ... 2044
Infants' Motrin Dye-Free ... 2044
Junior Strength Motrin ... 2044
Vicoprofen ... 564

Indapamide (Additive effect or potentiation of other antihypertensives). Products include:
Indapamide ... 2356

Indomethacin (In some patients with compromised renal function who are being treated with non-steroidal anti-inflammatory drugs (NSAIDs), including those that selectively inhibit cyclooxygenase-2 inhibitors (COX-2 inhibitors), the co-administration of angiotensin II receptor antagonists including losartan may result in a further deterioration of renal function. These effects are usually reversible. Reports suggest that NSAIDs, including selective COX-2 inhibitors, may diminish the antihypertensive effect of angiotensin II receptor antagonists, including losartan. This interaction should be given consideration in patients taking NSAIDs, including selective COX-2 inhibitors, concomitantly with angiotensin II receptor antagonists). Products include:
Indocin ... 2167

Indomethacin Sodium Trihydrate (In some patients with compromised renal function who are being treated with non-steroidal anti-inflammatory drugs (NSAIDs), including those that selectively inhibit cyclooxygenase-2 inhibitors (COX-2 inhibitors), the co-administration of angiotensin II receptor antagonists including losartan may result in a further deterioration of renal function. These effects are usually reversible. Reports suggest that NSAIDs, including selective COX-2 inhibitors, may diminish the antihypertensive effect of angiotensin II receptor antagonists, including losartan. This interaction should be given consideration in patients taking NSAIDs, including selective COX-2 inhibitors, concomitantly with angiotensin II receptor antagonists). Products include:
Indocin I.V. ... 2007

Insulin (Hyperglycemia may occur with thiazide diuretics; dosage adjustment of the antidiabetic drug may be required).
No products indexed under this heading.

Insulin, Human, Zinc Suspension (Hyperglycemia may occur with thiazide diuretics; dosage adjustment of the antidiabetic drug may be required).
No products indexed under this heading.

Insulin, Human (rDNA origin) (Hyperglycemia may occur with thiazide diuretics; dosage adjustment of the antidiabetic drug may be required). Products include:
Exubera ... 2717

Insulin, Human NPH (Hyperglycemia may occur with thiazide diuretics; dosage adjustment of the antidiabetic drug may be required). Products include:
Humulin N Vial ... 1934

Insulin, Human Regular (Hyperglycemia may occur with thiazide diuretics; dosage adjustment of the antidiabetic drug may be required). Products include:
Humulin R ... 1937
Humulin R (U-500) ... 1939

Insulin, Human Regular and Human NPH Mixture (Hyperglycemia may occur with thiazide diuretics; dosage adjustment of the antidiabetic drug may be required). Products include:
Humulin 50/50 ... 1930
Humulin 70/30 Vial ... 1931

Insulin, NPH (Hyperglycemia may occur with thiazide diuretics; dosage adjustment of the antidiabetic drug may be required).
No products indexed under this heading.

Insulin, Regular (Hyperglycemia may occur with thiazide diuretics; dosage adjustment of the antidiabetic drug may be required).
No products indexed under this heading.

Insulin, Regular and NPH mixture (Hyperglycemia may occur with thiazide diuretics; dosage adjustment of the antidiabetic drug may be required).
No products indexed under this heading.

Insulin, Zinc Crystals (Hyperglycemia may occur with thiazide diuretics; dosage adjustment of the antidiabetic drug may be required).
No products indexed under this heading.

Insulin, Zinc Suspension (Hyperglycemia may occur with thiazide diuretics; dosage adjustment of the antidiabetic drug may be required).
No products indexed under this heading.

Insulin Aspart (Hyperglycemia may occur with thiazide diuretics; dosage adjustment of the antidiabetic drug may be required).
No products indexed under this heading.

Insulin Aspart, Human (Hyperglycemia may occur with thiazide diuretics; dosage adjustment of the antidiabetic drug may be required). Products include:
NovoLog Mix 70/30 ... 2581

Insulin Aspart, Human Regular (Hyperglycemia may occur with thiazide diuretics; dosage adjustment of the antidiabetic drug may be required). Products include:
NovoLog ... 2575

Insulin Aspart Protamine, Human (Hyperglycemia may occur with thiazide diuretics; dosage adjustment of the antidiabetic drug may be required). Products include:
NovoLog Mix 70/30 ... 2581

Insulin Detemir (rDNA Origin) (Hyperglycemia may occur with thiazide diuretics; dosage adjustment of the antidiabetic drug may be required). Products include:
Levemir ... 2566

Insulin Glargine (Hyperglycemia may occur with thiazide diuretics; dosage adjustment of the antidiabetic drug may be required). Products include:
Lantus ... 2996

Insulin Glulisine (Hyperglycemia may occur with thiazide diuretics; dosage adjustment of the antidiabetic drug may be required). Products include:
Apidra ... 2937
Apidra SoloStar ... 2937

Insulin Lispro, Human (Hyperglycemia may occur with thiazide diuretics; dosage adjustment of the antidiabetic drug may be required). Products include:
Humalog ... 1910
Humalog Mix ... 1914
Humalog Mix75/25 ... 1917

Insulin Lispro Protamine, Human (Hyperglycemia may occur with thiazide diuretics; dosage adjustment of the antidiabetic drug may be required). Products include:
Humalog Mix ... 1914
Humalog Mix75/25 ... 1917

Irbesartan (Additive effect or potentiation of other antihypertensives). Products include:
Avalide ... 2956
Avapro ... 2962

Isoproterenol Hydrochloride (Possible decreased response to vasopressor amines).
No products indexed under this heading.

Isoproterenol Sulfate (Possible decreased response to vasopressor amines).
No products indexed under this heading.

Isradipine (Additive effect or potentiation of other antihypertensives). Products include:
DynaCirc CR ... 1432

Ketoprofen (In some patients with compromised renal function who are being treated with non-steroidal anti-inflammatory drugs (NSAIDs), including those that selectively inhibit cyclooxygenase-2 inhibitors (COX-2 inhibitors), the co-administration of angiotensin II receptor antagonists including losartan may result in a further deterioration of renal function. These effects are usually reversible. Reports suggest that NSAIDs, including selective COX-2 inhibitors, may diminish the antihypertensive effect of angiotensin II receptor antagonists, including losartan. This interaction should be given consideration in patients taking NSAIDs, including selective COX-2 inhibitors, concomitantly with angiotensin II receptor antagonists).
No products indexed under this heading.

Ketorolac Tromethamine (In some patients with compromised renal function who are being treated with non-steroidal anti-inflammatory drugs (NSAIDs), including those that selectively inhibit cyclooxygenase-2 inhibitors (COX-2 inhibitors), the co-administration of angiotensin II receptor antagonists including losartan may result in a further deterioration of renal function. These effects are usually reversible. Reports suggest that NSAIDs, including selective COX-2 inhibitors, may diminish the antihypertensive effect of angiotensin II receptor antagonists, including losartan. This interaction should be given consideration in patients taking NSAIDs, including selective COX-2 inhibitors, concomitantly with angiotensin II receptor antagonists). Products include:
Acuvail ... ⊙ 209

Labetalol Hydrochloride (Additive effect or potentiation of other antihypertensives).
No products indexed under this heading.

Levorphanol Tartrate (Potentiation of orthostatic hypotension may occur).
No products indexed under this heading.

Lisinopril (Additive effect or potentiation of other antihypertensives). Products include:
Prinivil ... 2241
Prinzide ... 2246

Lithium (Diuretics reduce the renal clearance of lithium and add a high risk of lithium toxicity; serum lithium levels should be monitored if lithium salts are co-administered).
No products indexed under this heading.

Lithium Carbonate (Diuretics reduce the renal clearance of lithium and add a high risk of lithium toxicity; serum lithium levels should be monitored if lithium salts are co-administered).
No products indexed under this heading.

Lithium Citrate (Diuretics reduce the renal clearance of lithium and add a high risk of lithium toxicity; serum lithium levels should be monitored if lithium salts are co-administered).
No products indexed under this heading.

Mecamylamine Hydrochloride (Additive effect or potentiation of other antihypertensives).
No products indexed under this heading.

Meclofenamate Sodium (In some patients with compromised renal function who are being treated with non-steroidal anti-inflammatory drugs (NSAIDs), including those that selectively inhibit cyclooxygenase-2 inhibitors (COX-2 inhibitors), the co-administration

IMPORTANT NOTE: Always consult each drug listing in the patient's regimen for possible interactions.

IMPORTANT NOTE: Always consult each drug listing in the patient's regimen for possible interactions.

consideration in patients taking NSAIDs, including selective COX-2 inhibitors, concomitantly with angiotensin II receptor antagonists).
No products indexed under this heading.

Valsartan (Additive effect or potentiation of other antihypertensives).
Products include:
Diovan 2413
Diovan HCT 2419
Exforge 2443
Exforge HCT 2449
Valturna 3637

Vecuronium Bromide (Possible increased responsiveness to the muscle relaxant).
No products indexed under this heading.

Verapamil Hydrochloride (Additive effect or potentiation of other antihypertensives). Products include:
Tarka 534

Food Interactions

Alcohol (Potentiation of orthostatic hypotension may occur).

Beer, reduced-alcohol (Potentiation of orthostatic hypotension may occur).

Beer, unspecified (Potentiation of orthostatic hypotension may occur).

Meal, unspecified (Meal slows absorption and decreases C_{max}, but has minor effects on losartan AUC or on the AUC of the metabolite).

Wine, Chianti (Potentiation of orthostatic hypotension may occur).

Wine, Red (Potentiation of orthostatic hypotension may occur).

Wine, unspecified (Potentiation of orthostatic hypotension may occur).

Wine products (Potentiation of orthostatic hypotension may occur).

HYZAAR 100-12.5 TABLETS

(Hydrochlorothiazide, Losartan Potassium) 2162
See Hyzaar 50-12.5 Tablets

HYZAAR 100-25 TABLETS

(Hydrochlorothiazide, Losartan Potassium) 2162
See Hyzaar 50-12.5 Tablets

ILARIS INJECTION

(Canakinumab) 2488
May interact with drugs which undergo biotransformation by cytochrome p-450 mixed function oxidase, TNF antagonists, vaccines, live. Compounds in these categories include:

Acarbose (The formation of CYP450 enzymes is suppressed by increased levels of cytokines (eg, IL-1) during chronic inflammation. Thus it is expected that for a molecule that binds to IL-1, such as canakinumab, the formation of CYP450 enzymes could be normalized. This is clinically relevant for CYP450 substrates with a narrow therapeutic index, where the dose is individually adjusted (eg, warfarin). Upon initiation of canakinumab, in patients being treated with these types of medicinal products, therapeutic monitoring of the effect or drug concentration should be performed and the individual dose of the medicinal product may need to be adjusted as needed).
No products indexed under this heading.

Acetaminophen (The formation of CYP450 enzymes is suppressed by increased levels of cytokines (eg, IL-1) during chronic inflammation. Thus it is expected that for a molecule that binds to IL-1, such as canakinumab, the formation of CYP450 enzymes could be normalized. This is clinically relevant for CYP450 substrates with a narrow therapeutic index, where the dose is individually adjusted (eg, warfarin). Upon initiation of canakinumab, in patients being treated with these types of medicinal products, therapeutic monitoring of the effect or drug concentration should be performed and the individual dose of the medicinal product may need to be adjusted as needed). Products include:
Percocet 1121
Tylenol 2049
Tylenol 8 Hour 2049
Extra Strength Tylenol Caplets, Cool Caplets, and EZ Tabs 2049
Extra Strength Tylenol Adult Rapid Blast Liquid 2049
Extra Strength Tylenol Rapid Release 2049
Tylenol with Codeine 2691
Tylenol Arthritis Pain Extended Release Geltabs/Caplets 2049
Children's Tylenol Suspension Liquid 2048
Children's Tylenol Meltaways 2048
Tylenol, Infants' Drops 2048
Junior Tylenol 2048
Vicodin 560
Vicodin ES 561
Vicodin HP 563
Zydone 1138

Adalimumab (An increased incidence of serious infections and an increased risk of neutropenia have been associated with administration of another IL-1 blocker in combination with TNF inhibitors in another patient population. Use of canakinumab with TNF inhibitors may also result in similar toxicities and is not recommended because this may increase the risk of serious infection). Products include:
Humira 448

Alatrofloxacin Mesylate (The formation of CYP450 enzymes is suppressed by increased levels of cytokines (eg, IL-1) during chronic inflammation. Thus it is expected that for a molecule that binds to IL-1, such as canakinumab, the formation of CYP450 enzymes could be normalized. This is clinically relevant for CYP450 substrates with a narrow therapeutic index, where the dose is individually adjusted (eg, warfarin). Upon initiation of canakinumab, in patients being treated with these types of medicinal products, therapeutic monitoring of the effect or drug concentration should be performed and the individual dose of the medicinal product may need to be adjusted as needed).
No products indexed under this heading.

Alfentanil Hydrochloride (The formation of CYP450 enzymes is suppressed by increased levels of cytokines (eg, IL-1) during chronic inflammation. Thus it is expected that for a molecule that binds to IL-1, such as canakinumab, the formation of CYP450 enzymes could be normalized. This is clinically relevant for CYP450 substrates with a narrow therapeutic index, where the dose is individually adjusted (eg, warfarin). Upon initiation of canakinumab, in patients being treated with these types of medicinal products, therapeutic monitoring of the effect or drug concentration should be performed and the individual dose of the medicinal product may need to be adjusted as needed).
No products indexed under this heading.

Alprazolam (The formation of CYP450 enzymes is suppressed by increased levels of cytokines (eg, IL-1) during chronic inflammation. Thus it is expected that for a molecule that binds to IL-1, such as canakinumab, the formation of CYP450 enzymes could be normalized. This is clinically relevant for CYP450 substrates with a narrow therapeutic index, where the dose is individually adjusted (eg, warfarin). Upon initiation of canakinumab, in patients being treated with these types of medicinal products, therapeutic monitoring of the effect or drug concentration should be performed and the individual dose of the medicinal product may need to be adjusted as needed).
No products indexed under this heading.

Aminophylline (The formation of CYP450 enzymes is suppressed by increased levels of cytokines (eg, IL-1) during chronic inflammation. Thus it is expected that for a molecule that binds to IL-1, such as canakinumab, the formation of CYP450 enzymes could be normalized. This is clinically relevant for CYP450 substrates with a narrow therapeutic index, where the dose is individually adjusted (eg, warfarin). Upon initiation of canakinumab, in patients being treated with these types of medicinal products, therapeutic monitoring of the effect or drug concentration should be performed and the individual dose of the medicinal product may need to be adjusted as needed).
No products indexed under this heading.

Amiodarone Hydrochloride (The formation of CYP450 enzymes is suppressed by increased levels of cytokines (eg, IL-1) during chronic inflammation. Thus it is expected that for a molecule that binds to IL-1, such as canakinumab, the formation of CYP450 enzymes could be normalized. This is clinically relevant for CYP450 substrates with a narrow therapeutic index, where the dose is individually adjusted (eg, warfarin). Upon initiation of canakinumab, in patients being treated with these types of medicinal products, therapeutic monitoring of the effect or drug concentration should be performed and the individual dose of the medicinal product may need to be adjusted as needed).
No products indexed under this heading.

Amitriptyline Hydrochloride (The formation of CYP450 enzymes is suppressed by increased levels of cytokines (eg, IL-1) during chronic inflammation. Thus it is expected that for a molecule that binds to IL-1, such as canakinumab, the formation of CYP450 enzymes could be normalized. This is clinically relevant for CYP450 substrates with a narrow therapeutic index, where the dose is individually adjusted (eg, warfarin). Upon initiation of canakinumab, in patients being treated with these types of medicinal products, therapeutic monitoring of the effect or drug concentration should be performed and the individual dose of the medicinal product may need to be adjusted as needed).
No products indexed under this heading.

Amlodipine Besylate (The formation of CYP450 enzymes is suppressed by increased levels of cytokines (eg, IL-1) during chronic inflammation. Thus it is expected that for a molecule that binds to IL-1, such as canakinumab, the formation of CYP450 enzymes could be normalized. This is clinically relevant for CYP450 substrates with a narrow therapeutic index, where the dose is individually adjusted (eg, warfarin). Upon initiation of canakinumab, in patients being treated with these types of medicinal products, therapeutic monitoring of the effect or drug concentration should be performed and the individual dose of the medicinal product may need to be adjusted as needed). Products include:
Azor 1010
Exforge 2443
Exforge HCT 2449

Amoxapine (The formation of CYP450 enzymes is suppressed by increased levels of cytokines (eg, IL-1) during chronic inflammation. Thus it is expected that for a molecule that binds to IL-1, such as canakinumab, the formation of CYP450 enzymes could be normalized. This is clinically relevant for CYP450 substrates with a narrow therapeutic index, where the dose is individually adjusted (eg, warfarin). Upon initiation of canakinumab, in patients being treated with these types of medicinal products, therapeutic monitoring of the effect or drug concentration should be performed and the individual dose of the medicinal product may need to be adjusted as needed).
No products indexed under this heading.

Amphetamine Aspartate (The formation of CYP450 enzymes is suppressed by increased levels of cytokines (eg, IL-1) during chronic inflammation. Thus it is expected that for a molecule that binds to IL-1, such as canakinumab, the formation of CYP450 enzymes could be normalized. This is clinically relevant for CYP450 substrates with a narrow therapeutic index, where the dose is individually adjusted (eg, warfarin). Upon initiation of canakinumab, in patients being treated with these types of medicinal products, therapeutic monitoring of the effect or drug concentration should be performed and the individual dose of the medicinal product may need to be adjusted as needed).
No products indexed under this heading.

Amphetamine Aspartate Monohydrate (The formation of CYP450 enzymes is suppressed by increased levels of cytokines (eg, IL-1) during chronic inflammation. Thus it is expected that for a molecule that binds to IL-1, such as canakinumab, the formation of CYP450 enzymes could be normalized. This is clinically relevant for CYP450 substrates with a narrow therapeutic index, where the dose is individually adjusted (eg, warfarin). Upon initiation of canakinumab, in patients being treated with these types of medicinal products, therapeutic monitoring of the effect or drug concentration should be performed and the individual dose of the medicinal product may need to be adjusted as needed).
No products indexed under this heading.

Amphetamine Sulfate (The formation of CYP450 enzymes is suppressed by increased levels of cytokines (eg, IL-1) during chronic inflammation. Thus it is expected that for a molecule that binds to IL-1, such as canakinumab, the formation of CYP450 enzymes could be normalized. This is clinically relevant for CYP450 substrates with a narrow therapeutic index, where the dose is individually adjusted (eg, warfarin). Upon initiation of canakinumab, in patients being treated with these types of medicinal products, therapeutic monitoring of the effect or drug concentration should be performed and the individual dose of the medicinal product may need to be adjusted as needed).
No products indexed under this heading.

Anagrelide Hydrochloride (The formation of CYP450 enzymes is suppressed by increased levels of cytokines (eg, IL-1) during chronic inflammation. Thus it is expected that for a molecule that binds to IL-1, such as canakinumab, the formation of CYP450 enzymes could be normalized. This is clinically relevant for CYP450 substrates with a narrow therapeutic index, where the dose is individually adjusted (eg, warfarin). Upon initiation of canakinumab, in patients being treated with these types of medicinal products, therapeutic monitoring of the effect or drug concentration should be performed and the individual dose of the medicinal product may need to be adjusted as needed).
No products indexed under this heading.

Aprepitant (The formation of CYP450 enzymes is suppressed by increased levels of cytokines (eg, IL-1) during

effect or drug concentration should be performed and the individual dose of the medicinal product may need to be adjusted as needed.

No products indexed under this heading.

Carvedilol (The formation of CYP450 enzymes is suppressed by increased levels of cytokines (eg, IL-1) during chronic inflammation. Thus it is expected that for a molecule that binds to IL-1, such as canakinumab, the formation of CYP450 enzymes could be normalized. This is clinically relevant for CYP450 substrates with a narrow therapeutic index, where the dose is individually adjusted (eg, warfarin). Upon initiation of canakinumab, in patients being treated with these types of medicinal products, therapeutic monitoring of the effect or drug concentration should be performed and the individual dose of the medicinal product may need to be adjusted as needed). Products include:
Coreg 1409

Celecoxib (The formation of CYP450 enzymes is suppressed by increased levels of cytokines (eg, IL-1) during chronic inflammation. Thus it is expected that for a molecule that binds to IL-1, such as canakinumab, the formation of CYP450 enzymes could be normalized. This is clinically relevant for CYP450 substrates with a narrow therapeutic index, where the dose is individually adjusted (eg, warfarin). Upon initiation of canakinumab, in patients being treated with these types of medicinal products, therapeutic monitoring of the effect or drug concentration should be performed and the individual dose of the medicinal product may need to be adjusted as needed). Products include:
Celebrex 3272

Cerivastatin Sodium (The formation of CYP450 enzymes is suppressed by increased levels of cytokines (eg, IL-1) during chronic inflammation. Thus it is expected that for a molecule that binds to IL-1, such as canakinumab, the formation of CYP450 enzymes could be normalized. This is clinically relevant for CYP450 substrates with a narrow therapeutic index, where the dose is individually adjusted (eg, warfarin). Upon initiation of canakinumab, in patients being treated with these types of medicinal products, therapeutic monitoring of the effect or drug concentration should be performed and the individual dose of the medicinal product may need to be adjusted as needed).

No products indexed under this heading.

Cevimeline Hydrochloride (The formation of CYP450 enzymes is suppressed by increased levels of cytokines (eg, IL-1) during chronic inflammation. Thus it is expected that for a molecule that binds to IL-1, such as canakinumab, the formation of CYP450 enzymes could be normalized. This is clinically relevant for CYP450 substrates with a narrow therapeutic index, where the dose is individually adjusted (eg, warfarin). Upon initiation of canakinumab, in patients being treated with these types of medicinal products, therapeutic monitoring of the effect or drug concentration should be performed and the individual dose of the medicinal product may need to be adjusted as needed). Products include:
Evoxac 1027

Chlordiazepoxide (The formation of CYP450 enzymes is suppressed by increased levels of cytokines (eg, IL-1) during chronic inflammation. Thus it is expected that for a molecule that binds to IL-1, such as canakinumab, the formation of CYP450 enzymes could be normalized. This is clinically relevant for CYP450 substrates with a narrow therapeutic index, where the dose is individually adjusted (eg, warfarin). Upon initia-

tion of canakinumab, in patients being treated with these types of medicinal products, therapeutic monitoring of the effect or drug concentration should be performed and the individual dose of the medicinal product may need to be adjusted as needed).

No products indexed under this heading.

Chlordiazepoxide Hydrochloride (The formation of CYP450 enzymes is suppressed by increased levels of cytokines (eg, IL-1) during chronic inflammation. Thus it is expected that for a molecule that binds to IL-1, such as canakinumab, the formation of CYP450 enzymes could be normalized. This is clinically relevant for CYP450 substrates with a narrow therapeutic index, where the dose is individually adjusted (eg, warfarin). Upon initiation of canakinumab, in patients being treated with these types of medicinal products, therapeutic monitoring of the effect or drug concentration should be performed and the individual dose of the medicinal product may need to be adjusted as needed).

No products indexed under this heading.

Chlorpheniramine (The formation of CYP450 enzymes is suppressed by increased levels of cytokines (eg, IL-1) during chronic inflammation. Thus it is expected that for a molecule that binds to IL-1, such as canakinumab, the formation of CYP450 enzymes could be normalized. This is clinically relevant for CYP450 substrates with a narrow therapeutic index, where the dose is individually adjusted (eg, warfarin). Upon initiation of canakinumab, in patients being treated with these types of medicinal products, therapeutic monitoring of the effect or drug concentration should be performed and the individual dose of the medicinal product may need to be adjusted as needed).

No products indexed under this heading.

Chlorpheniramine Maleate (The formation of CYP450 enzymes is suppressed by increased levels of cytokines (eg, IL-1) during chronic inflammation. Thus it is expected that for a molecule that binds to IL-1, such as canakinumab, the formation of CYP450 enzymes could be normalized. This is clinically relevant for CYP450 substrates with a narrow therapeutic index, where the dose is individually adjusted (eg, warfarin). Upon initiation of canakinumab, in patients being treated with these types of medicinal products, therapeutic monitoring of the effect or drug concentration should be performed and the individual dose of the medicinal product may need to be adjusted as needed).

No products indexed under this heading.

Chlorpheniramine Polistirex (The formation of CYP450 enzymes is suppressed by increased levels of cytokines (eg, IL-1) during chronic inflammation. Thus it is expected that for a molecule that binds to IL-1, such as canakinumab, the formation of CYP450 enzymes could be normalized. This is clinically relevant for CYP450 substrates with a narrow therapeutic index, where the dose is individually adjusted (eg, warfarin). Upon initiation of canakinumab, in patients being treated with these types of medicinal products, therapeutic monitoring of the effect or drug concentration should be performed and the individual dose of the medicinal product may need to be adjusted as needed). Products include:
Tussionex 3443

Chlorpheniramine Tannate (The formation of CYP450 enzymes is suppressed by increased levels of cytokines (eg, IL-1) during chronic inflammation. Thus it is expected that for a molecule that binds to IL-1, such as

canakinumab, the formation of CYP450 enzymes could be normalized. This is clinically relevant for CYP450 substrates with a narrow therapeutic index, where the dose is individually adjusted (eg, warfarin). Upon initiation of canakinumab, in patients being treated with these types of medicinal products, therapeutic monitoring of the effect or drug concentration should be performed and the individual dose of the medicinal product may need to be adjusted as needed).

No products indexed under this heading.

Chlorpromazine (The formation of CYP450 enzymes is suppressed by increased levels of cytokines (eg, IL-1) during chronic inflammation. Thus it is expected that for a molecule that binds to IL-1, such as canakinumab, the formation of CYP450 enzymes could be normalized. This is clinically relevant for CYP450 substrates with a narrow therapeutic index, where the dose is individually adjusted (eg, warfarin). Upon initiation of canakinumab, in patients being treated with these types of medicinal products, therapeutic monitoring of the effect or drug concentration should be performed and the individual dose of the medicinal product may need to be adjusted as needed).

No products indexed under this heading.

Chlorpromazine Hydrochloride (The formation of CYP450 enzymes is suppressed by increased levels of cytokines (eg, IL-1) during chronic inflammation. Thus it is expected that for a molecule that binds to IL-1, such as canakinumab, the formation of CYP450 enzymes could be normalized. This is clinically relevant for CYP450 substrates with a narrow therapeutic index, where the dose is individually adjusted (eg, warfarin). Upon initiation of canakinumab, in patients being treated with these types of medicinal products, therapeutic monitoring of the effect or drug concentration should be performed and the individual dose of the medicinal product may need to be adjusted as needed).

No products indexed under this heading.

Chlorpropamide (The formation of CYP450 enzymes is suppressed by increased levels of cytokines (eg, IL-1) during chronic inflammation. Thus it is expected that for a molecule that binds to IL-1, such as canakinumab, the formation of CYP450 enzymes could be normalized. This is clinically relevant for CYP450 substrates with a narrow therapeutic index, where the dose is individually adjusted (eg, warfarin). Upon initiation of canakinumab, in patients being treated with these types of medicinal products, therapeutic monitoring of the effect or drug concentration should be performed and the individual dose of the medicinal product may need to be adjusted as needed).

No products indexed under this heading.

Cilostazol (The formation of CYP450 enzymes is suppressed by increased levels of cytokines (eg, IL-1) during chronic inflammation. Thus it is expected that for a molecule that binds to IL-1, such as canakinumab, the formation of CYP450 enzymes could be normalized. This is clinically relevant for CYP450 substrates with a narrow therapeutic index, where the dose is individually adjusted (eg, warfarin). Upon initiation of canakinumab, in patients being treated with these types of medicinal products, therapeutic monitoring of the effect or drug concentration should be performed and the individual dose of the medicinal product may need to be adjusted as needed).

No products indexed under this heading.

Cimetidine Hydrochloride (The formation of CYP450 enzymes is sup-

pressed by increased levels of cytokines (eg, IL-1) during chronic inflammation. Thus it is expected that for a molecule that binds to IL-1, such as canakinumab, the formation of CYP450 enzymes could be normalized. This is clinically relevant for CYP450 substrates with a narrow therapeutic index, where the dose is individually adjusted (eg, warfarin). Upon initiation of canakinumab, in patients being treated with these types of medicinal products, therapeutic monitoring of the effect or drug concentration should be performed and the individual dose of the medicinal product may need to be adjusted as needed).

No products indexed under this heading.

Ciprofloxacin (The formation of CYP450 enzymes is suppressed by increased levels of cytokines (eg, IL-1) during chronic inflammation. Thus it is expected that for a molecule that binds to IL-1, such as canakinumab, the formation of CYP450 enzymes could be normalized. This is clinically relevant for CYP450 substrates with a narrow therapeutic index, where the dose is individually adjusted (eg, warfarin). Upon initiation of canakinumab, in patients being treated with these types of medicinal products, therapeutic monitoring of the effect or drug concentration should be performed and the individual dose of the medicinal product may need to be adjusted as needed). Products include:
Cipro I.V. 3082
Cipro 3073
Cipro XR 3091
Ciprodex 583

Ciprofloxacin Hydrochloride (The formation of CYP450 enzymes is suppressed by increased levels of cytokines (eg, IL-1) during chronic inflammation. Thus it is expected that for a molecule that binds to IL-1, such as canakinumab, the formation of CYP450 enzymes could be normalized. This is clinically relevant for CYP450 substrates with a narrow therapeutic index, where the dose is individually adjusted (eg, warfarin). Upon initiation of canakinumab, in patients being treated with these types of medicinal products, therapeutic monitoring of the effect or drug concentration should be performed and the individual dose of the medicinal product may need to be adjusted as needed). Products include:
Cipro 3073

Cisapride (The formation of CYP450 enzymes is suppressed by increased levels of cytokines (eg, IL-1) during chronic inflammation. Thus it is expected that for a molecule that binds to IL-1, such as canakinumab, the formation of CYP450 enzymes could be normalized. This is clinically relevant for CYP450 substrates with a narrow therapeutic index, where the dose is individually adjusted (eg, warfarin). Upon initiation of canakinumab, in patients being treated with these types of medicinal products, therapeutic monitoring of the effect or drug concentration should be performed and the individual dose of the medicinal product may need to be adjusted as needed).

No products indexed under this heading.

Citalopram Hydrobromide (The formation of CYP450 enzymes is suppressed by increased levels of cytokines (eg, IL-1) during chronic inflammation. Thus it is expected that for a molecule that binds to IL-1, such as canakinumab, the formation of CYP450 enzymes could be normalized. This is clinically relevant for CYP450 substrates with a narrow therapeutic index, where the dose is individually adjusted (eg, warfarin). Upon initiation of canakinumab, in patients being treated with these types of medicinal products, ther-

apeutic monitoring of the effect or drug concentration should be performed and the individual dose of the medicinal product may need to be adjusted as needed). Products include:

Celexa 1153

Clarithromycin (The formation of CYP450 enzymes is suppressed by increased levels of cytokines (eg, IL-1) during chronic inflammation. Thus it is expected that for a molecule that binds to IL-1, such as canakinumab, the formation of CYP450 enzymes could be normalized. This is clinically relevant for CYP450 substrates with a narrow therapeutic index, where the dose is individually adjusted (eg, warfarin). Upon initiation of canakinumab, in patients being treated with these types of medicinal products, therapeutic monitoring of the effect or drug concentration should be performed and the individual dose of the medicinal product may need to be adjusted as needed). Products include:

Biaxin/Biaxin XL 412

Clomipramine Hydrochloride (The formation of CYP450 enzymes is suppressed by increased levels of cytokines (eg, IL-1) during chronic inflammation. Thus it is expected that for a molecule that binds to IL-1, such as canakinumab, the formation of CYP450 enzymes could be normalized. This is clinically relevant for CYP450 substrates with a narrow therapeutic index, where the dose is individually adjusted (eg, warfarin). Upon initiation of canakinumab, in patients being treated with these types of medicinal products, therapeutic monitoring of the effect or drug concentration should be performed and the individual dose of the medicinal product may need to be adjusted as needed).

No products indexed under this heading.

Clopidogrel Bisulfate (The formation of CYP450 enzymes is suppressed by increased levels of cytokines (eg, IL-1) during chronic inflammation. Thus it is expected that for a molecule that binds to IL-1, such as canakinumab, the formation of CYP450 enzymes could be normalized. This is clinically relevant for CYP450 substrates with a narrow therapeutic index, where the dose is individually adjusted (eg, warfarin). Upon initiation of canakinumab, in patients being treated with these types of medicinal products, therapeutic monitoring of the effect or drug concentration should be performed and the individual dose of the medicinal product may need to be adjusted as needed). Products include:

Plavix 3027

Clopidogrel Hydrogen Sulfate (The formation of CYP450 enzymes is suppressed by increased levels of cytokines (eg, IL-1) during chronic inflammation. Thus it is expected that for a molecule that binds to IL-1, such as canakinumab, the formation of CYP450 enzymes could be normalized. This is clinically relevant for CYP450 substrates with a narrow therapeutic index, where the dose is individually adjusted (eg, warfarin). Upon initiation of canakinumab, in patients being treated with these types of medicinal products, therapeutic monitoring of the effect or drug concentration should be performed and the individual dose of the medicinal product may need to be adjusted as needed).

No products indexed under this heading.

Clozapine (The formation of CYP450 enzymes is suppressed by increased levels of cytokines (eg, IL-1) during chronic inflammation. Thus it is expected that for a molecule that binds to IL-1, such as canakinumab, the formation of CYP450 enzymes could be normalized. This is clinically relevant for CYP450 substrates with a narrow thera-

peutic index, where the dose is individually adjusted (eg, warfarin). Upon initiation of canakinumab, in patients being treated with these types of medicinal products, therapeutic monitoring of the effect or drug concentration should be performed and the individual dose of the medicinal product may need to be adjusted as needed).

No products indexed under this heading.

Codeine Phosphate (The formation of CYP450 enzymes is suppressed by increased levels of cytokines (eg, IL-1) during chronic inflammation. Thus it is expected that for a molecule that binds to IL-1, such as canakinumab, the formation of CYP450 enzymes could be normalized. This is clinically relevant for CYP450 substrates with a narrow therapeutic index, where the dose is individually adjusted (eg, warfarin). Upon initiation of canakinumab, in patients being treated with these types of medicinal products, therapeutic monitoring of the effect or drug concentration should be performed and the individual dose of the medicinal product may need to be adjusted as needed). Products include:

Tylenol with Codeine 2691

Codeine Sulfate (The formation of CYP450 enzymes is suppressed by increased levels of cytokines (eg, IL-1) during chronic inflammation. Thus it is expected that for a molecule that binds to IL-1, such as canakinumab, the formation of CYP450 enzymes could be normalized. This is clinically relevant for CYP450 substrates with a narrow therapeutic index, where the dose is individually adjusted (eg, warfarin). Upon initiation of canakinumab, in patients being treated with these types of medicinal products, therapeutic monitoring of the effect or drug concentration should be performed and the individual dose of the medicinal product may need to be adjusted as needed).

No products indexed under this heading.

Cyclobenzaprine (The formation of CYP450 enzymes is suppressed by increased levels of cytokines (eg, IL-1) during chronic inflammation. Thus it is expected that for a molecule that binds to IL-1, such as canakinumab, the formation of CYP450 enzymes could be normalized. This is clinically relevant for CYP450 substrates with a narrow therapeutic index, where the dose is individually adjusted (eg, warfarin). Upon initiation of canakinumab, in patients being treated with these types of medicinal products, therapeutic monitoring of the effect or drug concentration should be performed and the individual dose of the medicinal product may need to be adjusted as needed).

No products indexed under this heading.

Cyclobenzaprine Hydrochloride (The formation of CYP450 enzymes is suppressed by increased levels of cytokines (eg, IL-1) during chronic inflammation. Thus it is expected that for a molecule that binds to IL-1, such as canakinumab, the formation of CYP450 enzymes could be normalized. This is clinically relevant for CYP450 substrates with a narrow therapeutic index, where the dose is individually adjusted (eg, warfarin). Upon initiation of canakinumab, in patients being treated with these types of medicinal products, therapeutic monitoring of the effect or drug concentration should be performed and the individual dose of the medicinal product may need to be adjusted as needed). Products include:

Amrix 964

Cyclophosphamide (The formation of CYP450 enzymes is suppressed by increased levels of cytokines (eg, IL-1) during chronic inflammation. Thus it is expected that for a molecule that binds to IL-1, such as canakinumab, the for-

mation of CYP450 enzymes could be normalized. This is clinically relevant for CYP450 substrates with a narrow therapeutic index, where the dose is individually adjusted (eg, warfarin). Upon initiation of canakinumab, in patients being treated with these types of medicinal products, therapeutic monitoring of the effect or drug concentration should be performed and the individual dose of the medicinal product may need to be adjusted as needed).

No products indexed under this heading.

Cyclosporine (The formation of CYP450 enzymes is suppressed by increased levels of cytokines (eg, IL-1) during chronic inflammation. Thus it is expected that for a molecule that binds to IL-1, such as canakinumab, the formation of CYP450 enzymes could be normalized. This is clinically relevant for CYP450 substrates with a narrow therapeutic index, where the dose is individually adjusted (eg, warfarin). Upon initiation of canakinumab, in patients being treated with these types of medicinal products, therapeutic monitoring of the effect or drug concentration should be performed and the individual dose of the medicinal product may need to be adjusted as needed). Products include:

Gengraf 440
Neoral Oral Solution 2496
Neoral Capsules 2496
Restasis 605

Desipramine Hydrochloride (The formation of CYP450 enzymes is suppressed by increased levels of cytokines (eg, IL-1) during chronic inflammation. Thus it is expected that for a molecule that binds to IL-1, such as canakinumab, the formation of CYP450 enzymes could be normalized. This is clinically relevant for CYP450 substrates with a narrow therapeutic index, where the dose is individually adjusted (eg, warfarin). Upon initiation of canakinumab, in patients being treated with these types of medicinal products, therapeutic monitoring of the effect or drug concentration should be performed and the individual dose of the medicinal product may need to be adjusted as needed).

No products indexed under this heading.

Desogestrel (The formation of CYP450 enzymes is suppressed by increased levels of cytokines (eg, IL-1) during chronic inflammation. Thus it is expected that for a molecule that binds to IL-1, such as canakinumab, the formation of CYP450 enzymes could be normalized. This is clinically relevant for CYP450 substrates with a narrow therapeutic index, where the dose is individually adjusted (eg, warfarin). Upon initiation of canakinumab, in patients being treated with these types of medicinal products, therapeutic monitoring of the effect or drug concentration should be performed and the individual dose of the medicinal product may need to be adjusted as needed).

No products indexed under this heading.

Dexamethasone (The formation of CYP450 enzymes is suppressed by increased levels of cytokines (eg, IL-1) during chronic inflammation. Thus it is expected that for a molecule that binds to IL-1, such as canakinumab, the formation of CYP450 enzymes could be normalized. This is clinically relevant for CYP450 substrates with a narrow therapeutic index, where the dose is individually adjusted (eg, warfarin). Upon initiation of canakinumab, in patients being treated with these types of medicinal products, therapeutic monitoring of the effect or drug concentration should be performed and the individual dose of the medicinal product may need to be adjusted as needed). Products include:

Ciprodex 583

Ozurdex .... ⊙223
Tobramycin and Dexamethasone
Ophthalmic Suspension............... ⊙251

Dexamethasone Acetate (The formation of CYP450 enzymes is suppressed by increased levels of cytokines (eg, IL-1) during chronic inflammation. Thus it is expected that for a molecule that binds to IL-1, such as canakinumab, the formation of CYP450 enzymes could be normalized. This is clinically relevant for CYP450 substrates with a narrow therapeutic index, where the dose is individually adjusted (eg, warfarin). Upon initiation of canakinumab, in patients being treated with these types of medicinal products, therapeutic monitoring of the effect or drug concentration should be performed and the individual dose of the medicinal product may need to be adjusted as needed).

No products indexed under this heading.

Dexamethasone Phosphate (The formation of CYP450 enzymes is suppressed by increased levels of cytokines (eg, IL-1) during chronic inflammation. Thus it is expected that for a molecule that binds to IL-1, such as canakinumab, the formation of CYP450 enzymes could be normalized. This is clinically relevant for CYP450 substrates with a narrow therapeutic index, where the dose is individually adjusted (eg, warfarin). Upon initiation of canakinumab, in patients being treated with these types of medicinal products, therapeutic monitoring of the effect or drug concentration should be performed and the individual dose of the medicinal product may need to be adjusted as needed).

No products indexed under this heading.

Dexamethasone Sodium (The formation of CYP450 enzymes is suppressed by increased levels of cytokines (eg, IL-1) during chronic inflammation. Thus it is expected that for a molecule that binds to IL-1, such as canakinumab, the formation of CYP450 enzymes could be normalized. This is clinically relevant for CYP450 substrates with a narrow therapeutic index, where the dose is individually adjusted (eg, warfarin). Upon initiation of canakinumab, in patients being treated with these types of medicinal products, therapeutic monitoring of the effect or drug concentration should be performed and the individual dose of the medicinal product may need to be adjusted as needed).

No products indexed under this heading.

Dexamethasone Sodium Phosphate (The formation of CYP450 enzymes is suppressed by increased levels of cytokines (eg, IL-1) during chronic inflammation. Thus it is expected that for a molecule that binds to IL-1, such as canakinumab, the formation of CYP450 enzymes could be normalized. This is clinically relevant for CYP450 substrates with a narrow therapeutic index, where the dose is individually adjusted (eg, warfarin). Upon initiation of canakinumab, in patients being treated with these types of medicinal products, therapeutic monitoring of the effect or drug concentration should be performed and the individual dose of the medicinal product may need to be adjusted as needed).

No products indexed under this heading.

Dexfenfluramine Hydrochloride (The formation of CYP450 enzymes is suppressed by increased levels of cytokines (eg, IL-1) during chronic inflammation. Thus it is expected that for a molecule that binds to IL-1, such as canakinumab, the formation of CYP450 enzymes could be normalized. This is clinically relevant for CYP450 substrates with a narrow therapeutic

index, where the dose is individually adjusted (eg, warfarin). Upon initiation of canakinumab, in patients being treated with these types of medicinal products, therapeutic monitoring of the effect or drug concentration should be performed and the individual dose of the medicinal product may need to be adjusted as needed).

No products indexed under this heading.

Dextromethorphan (The formation of CYP450 enzymes is suppressed by increased levels of cytokines (eg, IL-1) during chronic inflammation. Thus it is expected that for a molecule that binds to IL-1, such as canakinumab, the formation of CYP450 enzymes could be normalized. This is clinically relevant for CYP450 substrates with a narrow therapeutic index, where the dose is individually adjusted (eg, warfarin). Upon initiation of canakinumab, in patients being treated with these types of medicinal products, therapeutic monitoring of the effect or drug concentration should be performed and the individual dose of the medicinal product may need to be adjusted as needed).

No products indexed under this heading.

Dextromethorphan Hydrobromide (The formation of CYP450 enzymes is suppressed by increased levels of cytokines (eg, IL-1) during chronic inflammation. Thus it is expected that for a molecule that binds to IL-1, such as canakinumab, the formation of CYP450 enzymes could be normalized. This is clinically relevant for CYP450 substrates with a narrow therapeutic index, where the dose is individually adjusted (eg, warfarin). Upon initiation of canakinumab, in patients being treated with these types of medicinal products, therapeutic monitoring of the effect or drug concentration should be performed and the individual dose of the medicinal product may need to be adjusted as needed).

No products indexed under this heading.

Dextromethorphan Polistirex (The formation of CYP450 enzymes is suppressed by increased levels of cytokines (eg, IL-1) during chronic inflammation. Thus it is expected that for a molecule that binds to IL-1, such as canakinumab, the formation of CYP450 enzymes could be normalized. This is clinically relevant for CYP450 substrates with a narrow therapeutic index, where the dose is individually adjusted (eg, warfarin). Upon initiation of canakinumab, in patients being treated with these types of medicinal products, therapeutic monitoring of the effect or drug concentration should be performed and the individual dose of the medicinal product may need to be adjusted as needed).

No products indexed under this heading.

Diazepam (The formation of CYP450 enzymes is suppressed by increased levels of cytokines (eg, IL-1) during chronic inflammation. Thus it is expected that for a molecule that binds to IL-1, such as canakinumab, the formation of CYP450 enzymes could be normalized. This is clinically relevant for CYP450 substrates with a narrow therapeutic index, where the dose is individually adjusted (eg, warfarin). Upon initiation of canakinumab, in patients being treated with these types of medicinal products, therapeutic monitoring of the effect or drug concentration should be performed and the individual dose of the medicinal product may need to be adjusted as needed). Products include:

Valium Tablets **2880**

Diclofenac Potassium (The formation of CYP450 enzymes is suppressed by increased levels of cytokines (eg, IL-1) during chronic inflammation. Thus it is expected that for a molecule that binds to IL-1, such as canakinumab, the formation of CYP450 enzymes could be normalized. This is clinically relevant for CYP450 substrates with a narrow therapeutic index, where the dose is individually adjusted (eg, warfarin). Upon initiation of canakinumab, in patients being treated with these types of medicinal products, therapeutic monitoring of the effect or drug concentration should be performed and the individual dose of the medicinal product may need to be adjusted as needed).

No products indexed under this heading.

Diclofenac Sodium (The formation of CYP450 enzymes is suppressed by increased levels of cytokines (eg, IL-1) during chronic inflammation. Thus it is expected that for a molecule that binds to IL-1, such as canakinumab, the formation of CYP450 enzymes could be normalized. This is clinically relevant for CYP450 substrates with a narrow therapeutic index, where the dose is individually adjusted (eg, warfarin). Upon initiation of canakinumab, in patients being treated with these types of medicinal products, therapeutic monitoring of the effect or drug concentration should be performed and the individual dose of the medicinal product may need to be adjusted as needed).

No products indexed under this heading.

Dihydroergotamine Mesylate (The formation of CYP450 enzymes is suppressed by increased levels of cytokines (eg, IL-1) during chronic inflammation. Thus it is expected that for a molecule that binds to IL-1, such as canakinumab, the formation of CYP450 enzymes could be normalized. This is clinically relevant for CYP450 substrates with a narrow therapeutic index, where the dose is individually adjusted (eg, warfarin). Upon initiation of canakinumab, in patients being treated with these types of medicinal products, therapeutic monitoring of the effect or drug concentration should be performed and the individual dose of the medicinal product may need to be adjusted as needed).

No products indexed under this heading.

Diltiazem Hydrochloride (The formation of CYP450 enzymes is suppressed by increased levels of cytokines (eg, IL-1) during chronic inflammation. Thus it is expected that for a molecule that binds to IL-1, such as canakinumab, the formation of CYP450 enzymes could be normalized. This is clinically relevant for CYP450 substrates with a narrow therapeutic index, where the dose is individually adjusted (eg, warfarin). Upon initiation of canakinumab, in patients being treated with these types of medicinal products, therapeutic monitoring of the effect or drug concentration should be performed and the individual dose of the medicinal product may need to be adjusted as needed). Products include:

Cardizem LA **423**

Diltiazem Maleate (The formation of CYP450 enzymes is suppressed by increased levels of cytokines (eg, IL-1) during chronic inflammation. Thus it is expected that for a molecule that binds to IL-1, such as canakinumab, the formation of CYP450 enzymes could be normalized. This is clinically relevant for CYP450 substrates with a narrow therapeutic index, where the dose is individually adjusted (eg, warfarin). Upon initiation of canakinumab, in patients being treated with these types of medicinal products, therapeutic monitoring of the effect or drug concentration should be performed and the individual dose of the medicinal product may need to be adjusted as needed).

No products indexed under this heading.

Disopyramide (The formation of CYP450 enzymes is suppressed by increased levels of cytokines (eg, IL-1) during chronic inflammation. Thus it is expected that for a molecule that binds to IL-1, such as canakinumab, the formation of CYP450 enzymes could be normalized. This is clinically relevant for CYP450 substrates with a narrow therapeutic index, where the dose is individually adjusted (eg, warfarin). Upon initiation of canakinumab, in patients being treated with these types of medicinal products, therapeutic monitoring of the effect or drug concentration should be performed and the individual dose of the medicinal product may need to be adjusted as needed).

No products indexed under this heading.

Disopyramide Phosphate (The formation of CYP450 enzymes is suppressed by increased levels of cytokines (eg, IL-1) during chronic inflammation. Thus it is expected that for a molecule that binds to IL-1, such as canakinumab, the formation of CYP450 enzymes could be normalized. This is clinically relevant for CYP450 substrates with a narrow therapeutic index, where the dose is individually adjusted (eg, warfarin). Upon initiation of canakinumab, in patients being treated with these types of medicinal products, therapeutic monitoring of the effect or drug concentration should be performed and the individual dose of the medicinal product may need to be adjusted as needed).

No products indexed under this heading.

Disulfiram (The formation of CYP450 enzymes is suppressed by increased levels of cytokines (eg, IL-1) during chronic inflammation. Thus it is expected that for a molecule that binds to IL-1, such as canakinumab, the formation of CYP450 enzymes could be normalized. This is clinically relevant for CYP450 substrates with a narrow therapeutic index, where the dose is individually adjusted (eg, warfarin). Upon initiation of canakinumab, in patients being treated with these types of medicinal products, therapeutic monitoring of the effect or drug concentration should be performed and the individual dose of the medicinal product may need to be adjusted as needed).

No products indexed under this heading.

Divalproex Sodium (The formation of CYP450 enzymes is suppressed by increased levels of cytokines (eg, IL-1) during chronic inflammation. Thus it is expected that for a molecule that binds to IL-1, such as canakinumab, the formation of CYP450 enzymes could be normalized. This is clinically relevant for CYP450 substrates with a narrow therapeutic index, where the dose is individually adjusted (eg, warfarin). Upon initiation of canakinumab, in patients being treated with these types of medicinal products, therapeutic monitoring of the effect or drug concentration should be performed and the individual dose of the medicinal product may need to be adjusted as needed). Products include:

Depakote ER **426**

Docetaxel (The formation of CYP450 enzymes is suppressed by increased levels of cytokines (eg, IL-1) during chronic inflammation. Thus it is expected that for a molecule that binds to IL-1, such as canakinumab, the formation of CYP450 enzymes could be normalized. This is clinically relevant for CYP450 substrates with a narrow therapeutic index, where the dose is individually adjusted (eg, warfarin). Upon initiation of canakinumab, in patients being treated with these types of medicinal products, therapeutic monitoring of the effect or drug concentration should be performed and the individual dose of the medicinal product may need to be adjusted as needed). Products include:

Taxotere **3035**

Dolasetron Mesylate (The formation of CYP450 enzymes is suppressed by increased levels of cytokines (eg, IL-1) during chronic inflammation. Thus it is expected that for a molecule that binds to IL-1, such as canakinumab, the formation of CYP450 enzymes could be normalized. This is clinically relevant for CYP450 substrates with a narrow therapeutic index, where the dose is individually adjusted (eg, warfarin). Upon initiation of canakinumab, in patients being treated with these types of medicinal products, therapeutic monitoring of the effect or drug concentration should be performed and the individual dose of the medicinal product may need to be adjusted as needed). Products include:

Anzemet Injection **2931**
Anzemet Tablets **2934**

Donepezil Hydrochloride (The formation of CYP450 enzymes is suppressed by increased levels of cytokines (eg, IL-1) during chronic inflammation. Thus it is expected that for a molecule that binds to IL-1, such as canakinumab, the formation of CYP450 enzymes could be normalized. This is clinically relevant for CYP450 substrates with a narrow therapeutic index, where the dose is individually adjusted (eg, warfarin). Upon initiation of canakinumab, in patients being treated with these types of medicinal products, therapeutic monitoring of the effect or drug concentration should be performed and the individual dose of the medicinal product may need to be adjusted as needed). Products include:

Aricept **1045**
Aricept ODT **1045**

Doxepin Hydrochloride (The formation of CYP450 enzymes is suppressed by increased levels of cytokines (eg, IL-1) during chronic inflammation. Thus it is expected that for a molecule that binds to IL-1, such as canakinumab, the formation of CYP450 enzymes could be normalized. This is clinically relevant for CYP450 substrates with a narrow therapeutic index, where the dose is individually adjusted (eg, warfarin). Upon initiation of canakinumab, in patients being treated with these types of medicinal products, therapeutic monitoring of the effect or drug concentration should be performed and the individual dose of the medicinal product may need to be adjusted as needed).

No products indexed under this heading.

Doxorubicin Hydrochloride (The formation of CYP450 enzymes is suppressed by increased levels of cytokines (eg, IL-1) during chronic inflammation. Thus it is expected that for a molecule that binds to IL-1, such as canakinumab, the formation of CYP450 enzymes could be normalized. This is clinically relevant for CYP450 substrates with a narrow therapeutic index, where the dose is individually adjusted (eg, warfarin). Upon initiation of canakinumab, in patients being treated with these types of medicinal products, therapeutic monitoring of the effect or drug concentration should be performed and the individual dose of the medicinal product may need to be adjusted as needed).

No products indexed under this heading.

Dronabinol (The formation of CYP450 enzymes is suppressed by increased levels of cytokines (eg, IL-1) during chronic inflammation. Thus it is expected that for a molecule that binds to IL-1, such as canakinumab, the formation of CYP450 enzymes could be normalized. This is clinically relevant for CYP450 substrates with a narrow therapeutic index, where the dose is individu-

ally adjusted (eg, warfarin). Upon initiation of canakinumab, in patients being treated with these types of medicinal products, therapeutic monitoring of the effect or drug concentration should be performed and the individual dose of the medicinal product may need to be adjusted as needed).

No products indexed under this heading.

Drugs that Undergo Biotransformation by Cytochrome P-450 Mixed Function Oxidase (The formation of CYP450 enzymes is suppressed by increased levels of cytokines (eg, IL-1) during chronic inflammation. Thus it is expected that for a molecule that binds to IL-1, such as canakinumab, the formation of CYP450 enzymes could be normalized. This is clinically relevant for CYP450 substrates with a narrow therapeutic index, where the dose is individually adjusted (eg, warfarin). Upon initiation of canakinumab, in patients being treated with these types of medicinal products, therapeutic monitoring of the effect or drug concentration should be performed and the individual dose of the medicinal product may need to be adjusted as needed).

No products indexed under this heading.

Dyphylline (The formation of CYP450 enzymes is suppressed by increased levels of cytokines (eg, IL-1) during chronic inflammation. Thus it is expected that for a molecule that binds to IL-1, such as canakinumab, the formation of CYP450 enzymes could be normalized. This is clinically relevant for CYP450 substrates with a narrow therapeutic index, where the dose is individually adjusted (eg, warfarin). Upon initiation of canakinumab, in patients being treated with these types of medicinal products, therapeutic monitoring of the effect or drug concentration should be performed and the individual dose of the medicinal product may need to be adjusted as needed).

No products indexed under this heading.

Encainide Hydrochloride (The formation of CYP450 enzymes is suppressed by increased levels of cytokines (eg, IL-1) during chronic inflammation. Thus it is expected that for a molecule that binds to IL-1, such as canakinumab, the formation of CYP450 enzymes could be normalized. This is clinically relevant for CYP450 substrates with a narrow therapeutic index, where the dose is individually adjusted (eg, warfarin). Upon initiation of canakinumab, in patients being treated with these types of medicinal products, therapeutic monitoring of the effect or drug concentration should be performed and the individual dose of the medicinal product may need to be adjusted as needed).

No products indexed under this heading.

Enoxacin (The formation of CYP450 enzymes is suppressed by increased levels of cytokines (eg, IL-1) during chronic inflammation. Thus it is expected that for a molecule that binds to IL-1, such as canakinumab, the formation of CYP450 enzymes could be normalized. This is clinically relevant for CYP450 substrates with a narrow therapeutic index, where the dose is individually adjusted (eg, warfarin). Upon initiation of canakinumab, in patients being treated with these types of medicinal products, therapeutic monitoring of the effect or drug concentration should be performed and the individual dose of the medicinal product may need to be adjusted as needed).

No products indexed under this heading.

Eprosartan Mesylate (The formation of CYP450 enzymes is suppressed by increased levels of cytokines (eg, IL-1) during chronic inflammation. Thus it is expected that for a molecule that binds

to IL-1, such as canakinumab, the formation of CYP450 enzymes could be normalized. This is clinically relevant for CYP450 substrates with a narrow therapeutic index, where the dose is individually adjusted (eg, warfarin). Upon initiation of canakinumab, in patients being treated with these types of medicinal products, therapeutic monitoring of the effect or drug concentration should be performed and the individual dose of the medicinal product may need to be adjusted as needed). Products include:

Teveten 538
Teveten HCT 541

Ergotamine Tartrate (The formation of CYP450 enzymes is suppressed by increased levels of cytokines (eg, IL-1) during chronic inflammation. Thus it is expected that for a molecule that binds to IL-1, such as canakinumab, the formation of CYP450 enzymes could be normalized. This is clinically relevant for CYP450 substrates with a narrow therapeutic index, where the dose is individually adjusted (eg, warfarin). Upon initiation of canakinumab, in patients being treated with these types of medicinal products, therapeutic monitoring of the effect or drug concentration should be performed and the individual dose of the medicinal product may need to be adjusted as needed).

No products indexed under this heading.

Erythromycin (The formation of CYP450 enzymes is suppressed by increased levels of cytokines (eg, IL-1) during chronic inflammation. Thus it is expected that for a molecule that binds to IL-1, such as canakinumab, the formation of CYP450 enzymes could be normalized. This is clinically relevant for CYP450 substrates with a narrow therapeutic index, where the dose is individually adjusted (eg, warfarin). Upon initiation of canakinumab, in patients being treated with these types of medicinal products, therapeutic monitoring of the effect or drug concentration should be performed and the individual dose of the medicinal product may need to be adjusted as needed).

No products indexed under this heading.

Erythromycin Estolate (The formation of CYP450 enzymes is suppressed by increased levels of cytokines (eg, IL-1) during chronic inflammation. Thus it is expected that for a molecule that binds to IL-1, such as canakinumab, the formation of CYP450 enzymes could be normalized. This is clinically relevant for CYP450 substrates with a narrow therapeutic index, where the dose is individually adjusted (eg, warfarin). Upon initiation of canakinumab, in patients being treated with these types of medicinal products, therapeutic monitoring of the effect or drug concentration should be performed and the individual dose of the medicinal product may need to be adjusted as needed).

No products indexed under this heading.

Erythromycin Ethylsuccinate (The formation of CYP450 enzymes is suppressed by increased levels of cytokines (eg, IL-1) during chronic inflammation. Thus it is expected that for a molecule that binds to IL-1, such as canakinumab, the formation of CYP450 enzymes could be normalized. This is clinically relevant for CYP450 substrates with a narrow therapeutic index, where the dose is individually adjusted (eg, warfarin). Upon initiation of canakinumab, in patients being treated with these types of medicinal products, therapeutic monitoring of the effect or drug concentration should be performed and the individual dose of the medicinal product may need to be adjusted as needed). Products include:

E.E.S. 437
EryPed 435

Erythromycin Gluceptate (The formation of CYP450 enzymes is suppressed by increased levels of cytokines (eg, IL-1) during chronic inflammation. Thus it is expected that for a molecule that binds to IL-1, such as canakinumab, the formation of CYP450 enzymes could be normalized. This is clinically relevant for CYP450 substrates with a narrow therapeutic index, where the dose is individually adjusted (eg, warfarin). Upon initiation of canakinumab, in patients being treated with these types of medicinal products, therapeutic monitoring of the effect or drug concentration should be performed and the individual dose of the medicinal product may need to be adjusted as needed).

No products indexed under this heading.

Erythromycin Lactobionate (The formation of CYP450 enzymes is suppressed by increased levels of cytokines (eg, IL-1) during chronic inflammation. Thus it is expected that for a molecule that binds to IL-1, such as canakinumab, the formation of CYP450 enzymes could be normalized. This is clinically relevant for CYP450 substrates with a narrow therapeutic index, where the dose is individually adjusted (eg, warfarin). Upon initiation of canakinumab, in patients being treated with these types of medicinal products, therapeutic monitoring of the effect or drug concentration should be performed and the individual dose of the medicinal product may need to be adjusted as needed).

No products indexed under this heading.

Erythromycin Stearate (The formation of CYP450 enzymes is suppressed by increased levels of cytokines (eg, IL-1) during chronic inflammation. Thus it is expected that for a molecule that binds to IL-1, such as canakinumab, the formation of CYP450 enzymes could be normalized. This is clinically relevant for CYP450 substrates with a narrow therapeutic index, where the dose is individually adjusted (eg, warfarin). Upon initiation of canakinumab, in patients being treated with these types of medicinal products, therapeutic monitoring of the effect or drug concentration should be performed and the individual dose of the medicinal product may need to be adjusted as needed).

No products indexed under this heading.

Esomeprazole Magnesium (The formation of CYP450 enzymes is suppressed by increased levels of cytokines (eg, IL-1) during chronic inflammation. Thus it is expected that for a molecule that binds to IL-1, such as canakinumab, the formation of CYP450 enzymes could be normalized. This is clinically relevant for CYP450 substrates with a narrow therapeutic index, where the dose is individually adjusted (eg, warfarin). Upon initiation of canakinumab, in patients being treated with these types of medicinal products, therapeutic monitoring of the effect or drug concentration should be performed and the individual dose of the medicinal product may need to be adjusted as needed). Products include:

Nexium Capsules 704
Nexium Oral Suspension 704

Esomeprazole Sodium (The formation of CYP450 enzymes is suppressed by increased levels of cytokines (eg, IL-1) during chronic inflammation. Thus it is expected that for a molecule that binds to IL-1, such as canakinumab, the formation of CYP450 enzymes could be normalized. This is clinically relevant for CYP450 substrates with a narrow therapeutic index, where the dose is individually adjusted (eg, warfarin). Upon initiation of canakinumab, in patients being treated with these types of medicinal

products, therapeutic monitoring of the effect or drug concentration should be performed and the individual dose of the medicinal product may need to be adjusted as needed). Products include:

Nexium I.V. 712

Estradiol (The formation of CYP450 enzymes is suppressed by increased levels of cytokines (eg, IL-1) during chronic inflammation. Thus it is expected that for a molecule that binds to IL-1, such as canakinumab, the formation of CYP450 enzymes could be normalized. This is clinically relevant for CYP450 substrates with a narrow therapeutic index, where the dose is individually adjusted (eg, warfarin). Upon initiation of canakinumab, in patients being treated with these types of medicinal products, therapeutic monitoring of the effect or drug concentration should be performed and the individual dose of the medicinal product may need to be adjusted as needed). Products include:

Activella 2561
Angeliq 831
Climara 841
Climara Pro 847
Divigel 3467
Estrasorb 1777
Vagifem 2589

Estradiol Benzoate (The formation of CYP450 enzymes is suppressed by increased levels of cytokines (eg, IL-1) during chronic inflammation. Thus it is expected that for a molecule that binds to IL-1, such as canakinumab, the formation of CYP450 enzymes could be normalized. This is clinically relevant for CYP450 substrates with a narrow therapeutic index, where the dose is individually adjusted (eg, warfarin). Upon initiation of canakinumab, in patients being treated with these types of medicinal products, therapeutic monitoring of the effect or drug concentration should be performed and the individual dose of the medicinal product may need to be adjusted as needed).

No products indexed under this heading.

Estradiol Cypionate (The formation of CYP450 enzymes is suppressed by increased levels of cytokines (eg, IL-1) during chronic inflammation. Thus it is expected that for a molecule that binds to IL-1, such as canakinumab, the formation of CYP450 enzymes could be normalized. This is clinically relevant for CYP450 substrates with a narrow therapeutic index, where the dose is individually adjusted (eg, warfarin). Upon initiation of canakinumab, in patients being treated with these types of medicinal products, therapeutic monitoring of the effect or drug concentration should be performed and the individual dose of the medicinal product may need to be adjusted as needed).

No products indexed under this heading.

Estradiol Valerate (The formation of CYP450 enzymes is suppressed by increased levels of cytokines (eg, IL-1) during chronic inflammation. Thus it is expected that for a molecule that binds to IL-1, such as canakinumab, the formation of CYP450 enzymes could be normalized. This is clinically relevant for CYP450 substrates with a narrow therapeutic index, where the dose is individually adjusted (eg, warfarin). Upon initiation of canakinumab, in patients being treated with these types of medicinal products, therapeutic monitoring of the effect or drug concentration should be performed and the individual dose of the medicinal product may need to be adjusted as needed).

No products indexed under this heading.

Estrogen (The formation of CYP450 enzymes is suppressed by increased levels of cytokines (eg, IL-1) during chronic inflammation. Thus it is expected that for a molecule that binds

---

IMPORTANT NOTE: Always consult each drug listing in the patient's regimen for possible interactions.

to IL-1, such as canakinumab, the formation of CYP450 enzymes could be normalized. This is clinically relevant for CYP450 substrates with a narrow therapeutic index, where the dose is individually adjusted (eg, warfarin). Upon initiation of canakinumab, in patients being treated with these types of medicinal products, therapeutic monitoring of the effect or drug concentration should be performed and the individual dose of the medicinal product may need to be adjusted as needed).

No products indexed under this heading.

Estrogens, Conjugated (The formation of CYP450 enzymes is suppressed by increased levels of cytokines (eg, IL-1) during chronic inflammation. Thus it is expected that for a molecule that binds to IL-1, such as canakinumab, the formation of CYP450 enzymes could be normalized. This is clinically relevant for CYP450 substrates with a narrow therapeutic index, where the dose is individually adjusted (eg, warfarin). Upon initiation of canakinumab, in patients being treated with these types of medicinal products, therapeutic monitoring of the effect or drug concentration should be performed and the individual dose of the medicinal product may need to be adjusted as needed). Products include:

Premarin Intravenous **3528**
Premarin Tablets **3533**
Premarin Vaginal Cream **3540**
Premphase **3549**
Prempro **3549**

Estrogens, Conjugated, Synthetic A (The formation of CYP450 enzymes is suppressed by increased levels of cytokines (eg, IL-1) during chronic inflammation. Thus it is expected that for a molecule that binds to IL-1, such as canakinumab, the formation of CYP450 enzymes could be normalized. This is clinically relevant for CYP450 substrates with a narrow therapeutic index, where the dose is individually adjusted (eg, warfarin). Upon initiation of canakinumab, in patients being treated with these types of medicinal products, therapeutic monitoring of the effect or drug concentration should be performed and the individual dose of the medicinal product may need to be adjusted as needed).

No products indexed under this heading.

Estrogens, Esterified (The formation of CYP450 enzymes is suppressed by increased levels of cytokines (eg, IL-1) during chronic inflammation. Thus it is expected that for a molecule that binds to IL-1, such as canakinumab, the formation of CYP450 enzymes could be normalized. This is clinically relevant for CYP450 substrates with a narrow therapeutic index, where the dose is individually adjusted (eg, warfarin). Upon initiation of canakinumab, in patients being treated with these types of medicinal products, therapeutic monitoring of the effect or drug concentration should be performed and the individual dose of the medicinal product may need to be adjusted as needed).

No products indexed under this heading.

Etanercept (An increased incidence of serious infections and an increased risk of neutropenia have been associated with administration of another IL-1 blocker in combination with TNF inhibitors in another patient population. Use of canakinumab with TNF inhibitors may also result in similar toxicities and is not recommended because this may increase the risk of serious infection). Products include:

Enbrel **613**

Ethinyl Estradiol (The formation of CYP450 enzymes is suppressed by increased levels of cytokines (eg, IL-1) during chronic inflammation. Thus it is expected that for a molecule that binds to IL-1, such as canakinumab, the formation of CYP450 enzymes could be normalized. This is clinically relevant for CYP450 substrates with a narrow therapeutic index, where the dose is individually adjusted (eg, warfarin). Upon initiation of canakinumab, in patients being treated with these types of medicinal products, therapeutic monitoring of the effect or drug concentration should be performed and the individual dose of the medicinal product may need to be adjusted as needed). Products include:

LoSeasonique **3407**
Lybrel **3514**
NuvaRing **3181**
Ortho Evra **2648**
Ortho-Cyclen/Ortho Tri-Cyclen **2663**
Ortho Tri-Cyclen Lo Tablets **2673**
Seasonique **3418**
Yaz **864**

Ethosuximide (The formation of CYP450 enzymes is suppressed by increased levels of cytokines (eg, IL-1) during chronic inflammation. Thus it is expected that for a molecule that binds to IL-1, such as canakinumab, the formation of CYP450 enzymes could be normalized. This is clinically relevant for CYP450 substrates with a narrow therapeutic index, where the dose is individually adjusted (eg, warfarin). Upon initiation of canakinumab, in patients being treated with these types of medicinal products, therapeutic monitoring of the effect or drug concentration should be performed and the individual dose of the medicinal product may need to be adjusted as needed).

No products indexed under this heading.

Ethotoin (The formation of CYP450 enzymes is suppressed by increased levels of cytokines (eg, IL-1) during chronic inflammation. Thus it is expected that for a molecule that binds to IL-1, such as canakinumab, the formation of CYP450 enzymes could be normalized. This is clinically relevant for CYP450 substrates with a narrow therapeutic index, where the dose is individually adjusted (eg, warfarin). Upon initiation of canakinumab, in patients being treated with these types of medicinal products, therapeutic monitoring of the effect or drug concentration should be performed and the individual dose of the medicinal product may need to be adjusted as needed).

No products indexed under this heading.

Ethynodiol Diacetate (The formation of CYP450 enzymes is suppressed by increased levels of cytokines (eg, IL-1) during chronic inflammation. Thus it is expected that for a molecule that binds to IL-1, such as canakinumab, the formation of CYP450 enzymes could be normalized. This is clinically relevant for CYP450 substrates with a narrow therapeutic index, where the dose is individually adjusted (eg, warfarin). Upon initiation of canakinumab, in patients being treated with these types of medicinal products, therapeutic monitoring of the effect or drug concentration should be performed and the individual dose of the medicinal product may need to be adjusted as needed).

No products indexed under this heading.

Etodolac (The formation of CYP450 enzymes is suppressed by increased levels of cytokines (eg, IL-1) during chronic inflammation. Thus it is expected that for a molecule that binds to IL-1, such as canakinumab, the formation of CYP450 enzymes could be normalized. This is clinically relevant for CYP450 substrates with a narrow therapeutic index, where the dose is individually adjusted (eg, warfarin). Upon initiation of canakinumab, in patients being treated with these types of medicinal products, therapeutic monitoring of the effect or drug concentration should be performed and the individual dose of the medicinal product may need to be adjusted as needed).

No products indexed under this heading.

Etoposide (The formation of CYP450 enzymes is suppressed by increased levels of cytokines (eg, IL-1) during chronic inflammation. Thus it is expected that for a molecule that binds to IL-1, such as canakinumab, the formation of CYP450 enzymes could be normalized. This is clinically relevant for CYP450 substrates with a narrow therapeutic index, where the dose is individually adjusted (eg, warfarin). Upon initiation of canakinumab, in patients being treated with these types of medicinal products, therapeutic monitoring of the effect or drug concentration should be performed and the individual dose of the medicinal product may need to be adjusted as needed).

No products indexed under this heading.

Etoposide Phosphate (The formation of CYP450 enzymes is suppressed by increased levels of cytokines (eg, IL-1) during chronic inflammation. Thus it is expected that for a molecule that binds to IL-1, such as canakinumab, the formation of CYP450 enzymes could be normalized. This is clinically relevant for CYP450 substrates with a narrow therapeutic index, where the dose is individually adjusted (eg, warfarin). Upon initiation of canakinumab, in patients being treated with these types of medicinal products, therapeutic monitoring of the effect or drug concentration should be performed and the individual dose of the medicinal product may need to be adjusted as needed).

No products indexed under this heading.

Felbamate (The formation of CYP450 enzymes is suppressed by increased levels of cytokines (eg, IL-1) during chronic inflammation. Thus it is expected that for a molecule that binds to IL-1, such as canakinumab, the formation of CYP450 enzymes could be normalized. This is clinically relevant for CYP450 substrates with a narrow therapeutic index, where the dose is individually adjusted (eg, warfarin). Upon initiation of canakinumab, in patients being treated with these types of medicinal products, therapeutic monitoring of the effect or drug concentration should be performed and the individual dose of the medicinal product may need to be adjusted as needed).

No products indexed under this heading.

Felodipine (The formation of CYP450 enzymes is suppressed by increased levels of cytokines (eg, IL-1) during chronic inflammation. Thus it is expected that for a molecule that binds to IL-1, such as canakinumab, the formation of CYP450 enzymes could be normalized. This is clinically relevant for CYP450 substrates with a narrow therapeutic index, where the dose is individually adjusted (eg, warfarin). Upon initiation of canakinumab, in patients being treated with these types of medicinal products, therapeutic monitoring of the effect or drug concentration should be performed and the individual dose of the medicinal product may need to be adjusted as needed).

No products indexed under this heading.

Fenoprofen Calcium (The formation of CYP450 enzymes is suppressed by increased levels of cytokines (eg, IL-1) during chronic inflammation. Thus it is expected that for a molecule that binds to IL-1, such as canakinumab, the formation of CYP450 enzymes could be normalized. This is clinically relevant for CYP450 substrates with a narrow therapeutic index, where the dose is individually adjusted (eg, warfarin). Upon initiation of canakinumab, in patients being treated with these types of medicinal products, therapeutic monitoring of the effect or drug concentration should be performed and the individual dose of the medicinal product may need to be adjusted as needed).

No products indexed under this heading.

Fentanyl (The formation of CYP450 enzymes is suppressed by increased levels of cytokines (eg, IL-1) during chronic inflammation. Thus it is expected that for a molecule that binds to IL-1, such as canakinumab, the formation of CYP450 enzymes could be normalized. This is clinically relevant for CYP450 substrates with a narrow therapeutic index, where the dose is individually adjusted (eg, warfarin). Upon initiation of canakinumab, in patients being treated with these types of medicinal products, therapeutic monitoring of the effect or drug concentration should be performed and the individual dose of the medicinal product may need to be adjusted as needed). Products include:

Duragesic **2604**
Fentanyl Transdermal System **2346**
Onsolis **2054**

Fentanyl Citrate (The formation of CYP450 enzymes is suppressed by increased levels of cytokines (eg, IL-1) during chronic inflammation. Thus it is expected that for a molecule that binds to IL-1, such as canakinumab, the formation of CYP450 enzymes could be normalized. This is clinically relevant for CYP450 substrates with a narrow therapeutic index, where the dose is individually adjusted (eg, warfarin). Upon initiation of canakinumab, in patients being treated with these types of medicinal products, therapeutic monitoring of the effect or drug concentration should be performed and the individual dose of the medicinal product may need to be adjusted as needed). Products include:

Fentora **966**

Flecainide Acetate (The formation of CYP450 enzymes is suppressed by increased levels of cytokines (eg, IL-1) during chronic inflammation. Thus it is expected that for a molecule that binds to IL-1, such as canakinumab, the formation of CYP450 enzymes could be normalized. This is clinically relevant for CYP450 substrates with a narrow therapeutic index, where the dose is individually adjusted (eg, warfarin). Upon initiation of canakinumab, in patients being treated with these types of medicinal products, therapeutic monitoring of the effect or drug concentration should be performed and the individual dose of the medicinal product may need to be adjusted as needed).

No products indexed under this heading.

Fluoxetine (The formation of CYP450 enzymes is suppressed by increased levels of cytokines (eg, IL-1) during chronic inflammation. Thus it is expected that for a molecule that binds to IL-1, such as canakinumab, the formation of CYP450 enzymes could be normalized. This is clinically relevant for CYP450 substrates with a narrow therapeutic index, where the dose is individually adjusted (eg, warfarin). Upon initiation of canakinumab, in patients being treated with these types of medicinal products, therapeutic monitoring of the effect or drug concentration should be performed and the individual dose of the medicinal product may need to be adjusted as needed).

No products indexed under this heading.

Fluoxetine Hydrochloride (The formation of CYP450 enzymes is suppressed by increased levels of cytokines (eg, IL-1) during chronic inflammation. Thus it is expected that for a molecule that binds to IL-1, such as canakinumab, the formation of CYP450 enzymes could be normalized. This is clinically relevant for CYP450

839 Interactions Index Ilaris

substrates with a narrow therapeutic index, where the dose is individually adjusted (eg, warfarin). Upon initiation of canakinumab, in patients being treated with these types of medicinal products, therapeutic monitoring of the effect or drug concentration should be performed and the individual dose of the medicinal product may need to be adjusted as needed). Products include:

Prozac Weekly **1941**
Prozac Pulvules **1941**
Symbyax **1965**

Fluphenazine Decanoate (The formation of CYP450 enzymes is suppressed by increased levels of cytokines (eg, IL-1) during chronic inflammation. Thus it is expected that for a molecule that binds to IL-1, such as canakinumab, the formation of CYP450 enzymes could be normalized. This is clinically relevant for CYP450 substrates with a narrow therapeutic index, where the dose is individually adjusted (eg, warfarin). Upon initiation of canakinumab, in patients being treated with these types of medicinal products, therapeutic monitoring of the effect or drug concentration should be performed and the individual dose of the medicinal product may need to be adjusted as needed).

No products indexed under this heading.

Fluphenazine Enanthate (The formation of CYP450 enzymes is suppressed by increased levels of cytokines (eg, IL-1) during chronic inflammation. Thus it is expected that for a molecule that binds to IL-1, such as canakinumab, the formation of CYP450 enzymes could be normalized. This is clinically relevant for CYP450 substrates with a narrow therapeutic index, where the dose is individually adjusted (eg, warfarin). Upon initiation of canakinumab, in patients being treated with these types of medicinal products, therapeutic monitoring of the effect or drug concentration should be performed and the individual dose of the medicinal product may need to be adjusted as needed).

No products indexed under this heading.

Fluphenazine Hydrochloride (The formation of CYP450 enzymes is suppressed by increased levels of cytokines (eg, IL-1) during chronic inflammation. Thus it is expected that for a molecule that binds to IL-1, such as canakinumab, the formation of CYP450 enzymes could be normalized. This is clinically relevant for CYP450 substrates with a narrow therapeutic index, where the dose is individually adjusted (eg, warfarin). Upon initiation of canakinumab, in patients being treated with these types of medicinal products, therapeutic monitoring of the effect or drug concentration should be performed and the individual dose of the medicinal product may need to be adjusted as needed).

No products indexed under this heading.

Flurbiprofen (The formation of CYP450 enzymes is suppressed by increased levels of cytokines (eg, IL-1) during chronic inflammation. Thus it is expected that for a molecule that binds to IL-1, such as canakinumab, the formation of CYP450 enzymes could be normalized. This is clinically relevant for CYP450 substrates with a narrow therapeutic index, where the dose is individually adjusted (eg, warfarin). Upon initiation of canakinumab, in patients being treated with these types of medicinal products, therapeutic monitoring of the effect or drug concentration should be performed and the individual dose of the medicinal product may need to be adjusted as needed).

No products indexed under this heading.

Flurbiprofen Sodium (The formation of CYP450 enzymes is suppressed by increased levels of cytokines (eg, IL-1) during chronic inflammation. Thus it is expected that for a molecule that binds to IL-1, such as canakinumab, the formation of CYP450 enzymes could be normalized. This is clinically relevant for CYP450 substrates with a narrow therapeutic index, where the dose is individually adjusted (eg, warfarin). Upon initiation of canakinumab, in patients being treated with these types of medicinal products, therapeutic monitoring of the effect or drug concentration should be performed and the individual dose of the medicinal product may need to be adjusted as needed).

No products indexed under this heading.

Flutamide (The formation of CYP450 enzymes is suppressed by increased levels of cytokines (eg, IL-1) during chronic inflammation. Thus it is expected that for a molecule that binds to IL-1, such as canakinumab, the formation of CYP450 enzymes could be normalized. This is clinically relevant for CYP450 substrates with a narrow therapeutic index, where the dose is individually adjusted (eg, warfarin). Upon initiation of canakinumab, in patients being treated with these types of medicinal products, therapeutic monitoring of the effect or drug concentration should be performed and the individual dose of the medicinal product may need to be adjusted as needed).

No products indexed under this heading.

Fluticasone Propionate (The formation of CYP450 enzymes is suppressed by increased levels of cytokines (eg, IL-1) during chronic inflammation. Thus it is expected that for a molecule that binds to IL-1, such as canakinumab, the formation of CYP450 enzymes could be normalized. This is clinically relevant for CYP450 substrates with a narrow therapeutic index, where the dose is individually adjusted (eg, warfarin). Upon initiation of canakinumab, in patients being treated with these types of medicinal products, therapeutic monitoring of the effect or drug concentration should be performed and the individual dose of the medicinal product may need to be adjusted as needed). Products include:

Advair 100/50 .... **1275**
Advair 250/50 .... **1275**
Advair 500/50 .... **1275**
Advair HFA 45/21 .... **1288**
Advair HFA 115/21 .... **1288**
Advair HFA 230/21 .... **1288**
Flonase **1459**
Flovent Diskus **1463**
Flovent HFA **1470**

Fluvastatin Sodium (The formation of CYP450 enzymes is suppressed by increased levels of cytokines (eg, IL-1) during chronic inflammation. Thus it is expected that for a molecule that binds to IL-1, such as canakinumab, the formation of CYP450 enzymes could be normalized. This is clinically relevant for CYP450 substrates with a narrow therapeutic index, where the dose is individually adjusted (eg, warfarin). Upon initiation of canakinumab, in patients being treated with these types of medicinal products, therapeutic monitoring of the effect or drug concentration should be performed and the individual dose of the medicinal product may need to be adjusted as needed).

No products indexed under this heading.

Fluvoxamine Maleate (The formation of CYP450 enzymes is suppressed by increased levels of cytokines (eg, IL-1) during chronic inflammation. Thus it is expected that for a molecule that binds to IL-1, such as canakinumab, the formation of CYP450 enzymes could be normalized. This is clinically relevant for CYP450 substrates with a narrow therapeutic index, where the dose is individually adjusted (eg, warfarin). Upon initiation of canakinumab, in patients being treated with these types of medicinal products, therapeutic monitoring of the effect or drug concentration should be performed and the individual dose of the medicinal product may need to be adjusted as needed).

No products indexed under this heading.

Formoterol Fumarate (The formation of CYP450 enzymes is suppressed by increased levels of cytokines (eg, IL-1) during chronic inflammation. Thus it is expected that for a molecule that binds to IL-1, such as canakinumab, the formation of CYP450 enzymes could be normalized. This is clinically relevant for CYP450 substrates with a narrow therapeutic index, where the dose is individually adjusted (eg, warfarin). Upon initiation of canakinumab, in patients being treated with these types of medicinal products, therapeutic monitoring of the effect or drug concentration should be performed and the individual dose of the medicinal product may need to be adjusted as needed). Products include:

Foradil **3121**
Perforomist **3634**

Fosphenytoin (The formation of CYP450 enzymes is suppressed by increased levels of cytokines (eg, IL-1) during chronic inflammation. Thus it is expected that for a molecule that binds to IL-1, such as canakinumab, the formation of CYP450 enzymes could be normalized. This is clinically relevant for CYP450 substrates with a narrow therapeutic index, where the dose is individually adjusted (eg, warfarin). Upon initiation of canakinumab, in patients being treated with these types of medicinal products, therapeutic monitoring of the effect or drug concentration should be performed and the individual dose of the medicinal product may need to be adjusted as needed).

No products indexed under this heading.

Fosphenytoin Sodium (The formation of CYP450 enzymes is suppressed by increased levels of cytokines (eg, IL-1) during chronic inflammation. Thus it is expected that for a molecule that binds to IL-1, such as canakinumab, the formation of CYP450 enzymes could be normalized. This is clinically relevant for CYP450 substrates with a narrow therapeutic index, where the dose is individually adjusted (eg, warfarin). Upon initiation of canakinumab, in patients being treated with these types of medicinal products, therapeutic monitoring of the effect or drug concentration should be performed and the individual dose of the medicinal product may need to be adjusted as needed).

No products indexed under this heading.

Gabapentin (The formation of CYP450 enzymes is suppressed by increased levels of cytokines (eg, IL-1) during chronic inflammation. Thus it is expected that for a molecule that binds to IL-1, such as canakinumab, the formation of CYP450 enzymes could be normalized. This is clinically relevant for CYP450 substrates with a narrow therapeutic index, where the dose is individually adjusted (eg, warfarin). Upon initiation of canakinumab, in patients being treated with these types of medicinal products, therapeutic monitoring of the effect or drug concentration should be performed and the individual dose of the medicinal product may need to be adjusted as needed).

No products indexed under this heading.

Galantamine Hydrobromide (The formation of CYP450 enzymes is suppressed by increased levels of cytokines (eg, IL-1) during chronic inflammation. Thus it is expected that for a molecule that binds to IL-1, such as canakinumab, the formation of CYP450 enzymes could be normalized. This is clinically relevant for CYP450 substrates with a narrow therapeutic index, where the dose is individually adjusted (eg, warfarin). Upon initiation of canakinumab, in patients being treated with these types of medicinal products, therapeutic monitoring of the effect or drug concentration should be performed and the individual dose of the medicinal product may need to be adjusted as needed).

No products indexed under this heading.

Glimepiride (The formation of CYP450 enzymes is suppressed by increased levels of cytokines (eg, IL-1) during chronic inflammation. Thus it is expected that for a molecule that binds to IL-1, such as canakinumab, the formation of CYP450 enzymes could be normalized. This is clinically relevant for CYP450 substrates with a narrow therapeutic index, where the dose is individually adjusted (eg, warfarin). Upon initiation of canakinumab, in patients being treated with these types of medicinal products, therapeutic monitoring of the effect or drug concentration should be performed and the individual dose of the medicinal product may need to be adjusted as needed). Products include:

Avandaryl **1356**
Duetact **3354**

Glipizide (The formation of CYP450 enzymes is suppressed by increased levels of cytokines (eg, IL-1) during chronic inflammation. Thus it is expected that for a molecule that binds to IL-1, such as canakinumab, the formation of CYP450 enzymes could be normalized. This is clinically relevant for CYP450 substrates with a narrow therapeutic index, where the dose is individually adjusted (eg, warfarin). Upon initiation of canakinumab, in patients being treated with these types of medicinal products, therapeutic monitoring of the effect or drug concentration should be performed and the individual dose of the medicinal product may need to be adjusted as needed).

No products indexed under this heading.

Glyburide (The formation of CYP450 enzymes is suppressed by increased levels of cytokines (eg, IL-1) during chronic inflammation. Thus it is expected that for a molecule that binds to IL-1, such as canakinumab, the formation of CYP450 enzymes could be normalized. This is clinically relevant for CYP450 substrates with a narrow therapeutic index, where the dose is individually adjusted (eg, warfarin). Upon initiation of canakinumab, in patients being treated with these types of medicinal products, therapeutic monitoring of the effect or drug concentration should be performed and the individual dose of the medicinal product may need to be adjusted as needed).

No products indexed under this heading.

Grepafloxacin Hydrochloride (The formation of CYP450 enzymes is suppressed by increased levels of cytokines (eg, IL-1) during chronic inflammation. Thus it is expected that for a molecule that binds to IL-1, such as canakinumab, the formation of CYP450 enzymes could be normalized. This is clinically relevant for CYP450 substrates with a narrow therapeutic index, where the dose is individually adjusted (eg, warfarin). Upon initiation of canakinumab, in patients being treated with these types of medicinal products, therapeutic monitoring of the effect or drug concentration should be performed and the individual dose of the medicinal product may need to be adjusted as needed).

No products indexed under this heading.

IMPORTANT NOTE: Always consult each drug listing in the patient's regimen for possible interactions.

Ilaris
Interactions Index
840

Haloperidol (The formation of CYP450 enzymes is suppressed by increased levels of cytokines (eg, IL-1) during chronic inflammation. Thus it is expected that for a molecule that binds to IL-1, such as canakinumab, the formation of CYP450 enzymes could be normalized. This is clinically relevant for CYP450 substrates with a narrow therapeutic index, where the dose is individually adjusted (eg, warfarin). Upon initiation of canakinumab, in patients being treated with these types of medicinal products, therapeutic monitoring of the effect or drug concentration should be performed and the individual dose of the medicinal product may need to be adjusted as needed).
No products indexed under this heading.

Haloperidol Decanoate (The formation of CYP450 enzymes is suppressed by increased levels of cytokines (eg, IL-1) during chronic inflammation. Thus it is expected that for a molecule that binds to IL-1, such as canakinumab, the formation of CYP450 enzymes could be normalized. This is clinically relevant for CYP450 substrates with a narrow therapeutic index, where the dose is individually adjusted (eg, warfarin). Upon initiation of canakinumab, in patients being treated with these types of medicinal products, therapeutic monitoring of the effect or drug concentration should be performed and the individual dose of the medicinal product may need to be adjusted as needed).
No products indexed under this heading.

Haloperidol Lactate (The formation of CYP450 enzymes is suppressed by increased levels of cytokines (eg, IL-1) during chronic inflammation. Thus it is expected that for a molecule that binds to IL-1, such as canakinumab, the formation of CYP450 enzymes could be normalized. This is clinically relevant for CYP450 substrates with a narrow therapeutic index, where the dose is individually adjusted (eg, warfarin). Upon initiation of canakinumab, in patients being treated with these types of medicinal products, therapeutic monitoring of the effect or drug concentration should be performed and the individual dose of the medicinal product may need to be adjusted as needed).
No products indexed under this heading.

Hexobarbital (The formation of CYP450 enzymes is suppressed by increased levels of cytokines (eg, IL-1) during chronic inflammation. Thus it is expected that for a molecule that binds to IL-1, such as canakinumab, the formation of CYP450 enzymes could be normalized. This is clinically relevant for CYP450 substrates with a narrow therapeutic index, where the dose is individually adjusted (eg, warfarin). Upon initiation of canakinumab, in patients being treated with these types of medicinal products, therapeutic monitoring of the effect or drug concentration should be performed and the individual dose of the medicinal product may need to be adjusted as needed).
No products indexed under this heading.

Hydrocodone Bitartrate (The formation of CYP450 enzymes is suppressed by increased levels of cytokines (eg, IL-1) during chronic inflammation. Thus it is expected that for a molecule that binds to IL-1, such as canakinumab, the formation of CYP450 enzymes could be normalized. This is clinically relevant for CYP450 substrates with a narrow therapeutic index, where the dose is individually adjusted (eg, warfarin). Upon initiation of canakinumab, in patients being treated with these types of medicinal products, therapeutic monitoring of the effect or drug concentration should be performed and the individual dose of the medicinal product may need to be adjusted as needed). Products include:
Vicodin 560
Vicodin ES 561
Vicodin HP 563
Vicoprofen 564
Zydone 1138

Ibuprofen (The formation of CYP450 enzymes is suppressed by increased levels of cytokines (eg, IL-1) during chronic inflammation. Thus it is expected that for a molecule that binds to IL-1, such as canakinumab, the formation of CYP450 enzymes could be normalized. This is clinically relevant for CYP450 substrates with a narrow therapeutic index, where the dose is individually adjusted (eg, warfarin). Upon initiation of canakinumab, in patients being treated with these types of medicinal products, therapeutic monitoring of the effect or drug concentration should be performed and the individual dose of the medicinal product may need to be adjusted as needed). Products include:
Motrin IB 2043
Children's Motrin 2044
Children's Motrin Non-Staining Dye-Free 2044
Infants' Motrin 2044
Infants' Motrin Dye-Free 2044
Junior Strength Motrin 2044
Vicoprofen 564

Imipramine Hydrochloride (The formation of CYP450 enzymes is suppressed by increased levels of cytokines (eg, IL-1) during chronic inflammation. Thus it is expected that for a molecule that binds to IL-1, such as canakinumab, the formation of CYP450 enzymes could be normalized. This is clinically relevant for CYP450 substrates with a narrow therapeutic index, where the dose is individually adjusted (eg, warfarin). Upon initiation of canakinumab, in patients being treated with these types of medicinal products, therapeutic monitoring of the effect or drug concentration should be performed and the individual dose of the medicinal product may need to be adjusted as needed).
No products indexed under this heading.

Imipramine Pamoate (The formation of CYP450 enzymes is suppressed by increased levels of cytokines (eg, IL-1) during chronic inflammation. Thus it is expected that for a molecule that binds to IL-1, such as canakinumab, the formation of CYP450 enzymes could be normalized. This is clinically relevant for CYP450 substrates with a narrow therapeutic index, where the dose is individually adjusted (eg, warfarin). Upon initiation of canakinumab, in patients being treated with these types of medicinal products, therapeutic monitoring of the effect or drug concentration should be performed and the individual dose of the medicinal product may need to be adjusted as needed).
No products indexed under this heading.

Indinavir Sulfate (The formation of CYP450 enzymes is suppressed by increased levels of cytokines (eg, IL-1) during chronic inflammation. Thus it is expected that for a molecule that binds to IL-1, such as canakinumab, the formation of CYP450 enzymes could be normalized. This is clinically relevant for CYP450 substrates with a narrow therapeutic index, where the dose is individually adjusted (eg, warfarin). Upon initiation of canakinumab, in patients being treated with these types of medicinal products, therapeutic monitoring of the effect or drug concentration should be performed and the individual dose of the medicinal product may need to be adjusted as needed). Products include:
Crixivan 2113

Indomethacin (The formation of CYP450 enzymes is suppressed by increased levels of cytokines (eg, IL-1) during chronic inflammation. Thus it is expected that for a molecule that binds to IL-1, such as canakinumab, the formation of CYP450 enzymes could be normalized. This is clinically relevant for CYP450 substrates with a narrow therapeutic index, where the dose is individually adjusted (eg, warfarin). Upon initiation of canakinumab, in patients being treated with these types of medicinal products, therapeutic monitoring of the effect or drug concentration should be performed and the individual dose of the medicinal product may need to be adjusted as needed). Products include:
Indocin 2167

Indomethacin Sodium Trihydrate (The formation of CYP450 enzymes is suppressed by increased levels of cytokines (eg, IL-1) during chronic inflammation. Thus it is expected that for a molecule that binds to IL-1, such as canakinumab, the formation of CYP450 enzymes could be normalized. This is clinically relevant for CYP450 substrates with a narrow therapeutic index, where the dose is individually adjusted (eg, warfarin). Upon initiation of canakinumab, in patients being treated with these types of medicinal products, therapeutic monitoring of the effect or drug concentration should be performed and the individual dose of the medicinal product may need to be adjusted as needed). Products include:
Indocin I.V. 2007

Indoramin Hydrochloride (The formation of CYP450 enzymes is suppressed by increased levels of cytokines (eg, IL-1) during chronic inflammation. Thus it is expected that for a molecule that binds to IL-1, such as canakinumab, the formation of CYP450 enzymes could be normalized. This is clinically relevant for CYP450 substrates with a narrow therapeutic index, where the dose is individually adjusted (eg, warfarin). Upon initiation of canakinumab, in patients being treated with these types of medicinal products, therapeutic monitoring of the effect or drug concentration should be performed and the individual dose of the medicinal product may need to be adjusted as needed).
No products indexed under this heading.

Infliximab (An increased incidence of serious infections and an increased risk of neutropenia have been associated with administration of another IL-1 blocker in combination with TNF inhibitors in another patient population. Use of canakinumab with TNF inhibitors may also result in similar toxicities and is not recommended because this may increase the risk of serious infection). Products include:
Remicade 919

Influenza Vaccine, Live Attenuated (No data are available on either the effects of live vaccination or the secondary transmission of infection by live vaccines in patients receiving canakinumab. Therefore, live vaccines should not be given concurrently with canakinumab. It is recommended that, if possible, pediatric and adult patients should complete all immunizations in accordance with current immunization guidelines prior to initiating canakinumab therapy).
No products indexed under this heading.

Influenza Virus Vaccine Live, Intranasal (No data are available on either the effects of live vaccination or the secondary transmission of infection by live vaccines in patients receiving canakinumab. Therefore, live vaccines should not be given concurrently with canakinumab. It is recommended that, if possible, pediatric and adult patients should complete all immunizations in accordance with current immunization guidelines prior to initiating canakinumab therapy). Products include:
FluMist 2078

Irbesartan (The formation of CYP450 enzymes is suppressed by increased levels of cytokines (eg, IL-1) during chronic inflammation. Thus it is expected that for a molecule that binds to IL-1, such as canakinumab, the formation of CYP450 enzymes could be normalized. This is clinically relevant for CYP450 substrates with a narrow therapeutic index, where the dose is individually adjusted (eg, warfarin). Upon initiation of canakinumab, in patients being treated with these types of medicinal products, therapeutic monitoring of the effect or drug concentration should be performed and the individual dose of the medicinal product may need to be adjusted as needed). Products include:
Avalide 2956
Avapro 2962

Isotretinoin (The formation of CYP450 enzymes is suppressed by increased levels of cytokines (eg, IL-1) during chronic inflammation. Thus it is expected that for a molecule that binds to IL-1, such as canakinumab, the formation of CYP450 enzymes could be normalized. This is clinically relevant for CYP450 substrates with a narrow therapeutic index, where the dose is individually adjusted (eg, warfarin). Upon initiation of canakinumab, in patients being treated with these types of medicinal products, therapeutic monitoring of the effect or drug concentration should be performed and the individual dose of the medicinal product may need to be adjusted as needed). Products include:
Accutane 2832

Isradipine (The formation of CYP450 enzymes is suppressed by increased levels of cytokines (eg, IL-1) during chronic inflammation. Thus it is expected that for a molecule that binds to IL-1, such as canakinumab, the formation of CYP450 enzymes could be normalized. This is clinically relevant for CYP450 substrates with a narrow therapeutic index, where the dose is individually adjusted (eg, warfarin). Upon initiation of canakinumab, in patients being treated with these types of medicinal products, therapeutic monitoring of the effect or drug concentration should be performed and the individual dose of the medicinal product may need to be adjusted as needed). Products include:
DynaCirc CR 1432

Itraconazole (The formation of CYP450 enzymes is suppressed by increased levels of cytokines (eg, IL-1) during chronic inflammation. Thus it is expected that for a molecule that binds to IL-1, such as canakinumab, the formation of CYP450 enzymes could be normalized. This is clinically relevant for CYP450 substrates with a narrow therapeutic index, where the dose is individually adjusted (eg, warfarin). Upon initiation of canakinumab, in patients being treated with these types of medicinal products, therapeutic monitoring of the effect or drug concentration should be performed and the individual dose of the medicinal product may need to be adjusted as needed).
No products indexed under this heading.

Ixabepilone (The formation of CYP450 enzymes is suppressed by increased levels of cytokines (eg, IL-1) during chronic inflammation. Thus it is expected that for a molecule that binds to IL-1, such as canakinumab, the formation of CYP450 enzymes could be normalized. This is clinically relevant for CYP450 substrates with a narrow therapeutic index, where the dose is individually adjusted (eg, warfarin). Upon initiation of canakinumab, in patients being

IMPORTANT NOTE: Always consult each drug listing in the patient's regimen for possible interactions.

Ilaris Interactions Index 842

Measles Virus Vaccine Live (No data are available on either the effects of live vaccination or the secondary transmission of infection by live vaccines in patients receiving canakinumab. Therefore, live vaccines should not be given concurrently with canakinumab. It is recommended that, if possible, pediatric and adult patients should complete all immunizations in accordance with current immunization guidelines prior to initiating canakinumab therapy). Products include:
Attenuvax 2086

Meclofenamate Sodium (The formation of CYP450 enzymes is suppressed by increased levels of cytokines (eg, IL-1) during chronic inflammation. Thus it is expected that for a molecule that binds to IL-1, such as canakinumab, the formation of CYP450 enzymes could be normalized. This is clinically relevant for CYP450 substrates with a narrow therapeutic index, where the dose is individually adjusted (eg, warfarin). Upon initiation of canakinumab, in patients being treated with these types of medicinal products, therapeutic monitoring of the effect or drug concentration should be performed and the individual dose of the medicinal product may need to be adjusted as needed).
No products indexed under this heading.

Mefenamic Acid (The formation of CYP450 enzymes is suppressed by increased levels of cytokines (eg, IL-1) during chronic inflammation. Thus it is expected that for a molecule that binds to IL-1, such as canakinumab, the formation of CYP450 enzymes could be normalized. This is clinically relevant for CYP450 substrates with a narrow therapeutic index, where the dose is individually adjusted (eg, warfarin). Upon initiation of canakinumab, in patients being treated with these types of medicinal products, therapeutic monitoring of the effect or drug concentration should be performed and the individual dose of the medicinal product may need to be adjusted as needed).
No products indexed under this heading.

Meloxicam (The formation of CYP450 enzymes is suppressed by increased levels of cytokines (eg, IL-1) during chronic inflammation. Thus it is expected that for a molecule that binds to IL-1, such as canakinumab, the formation of CYP450 enzymes could be normalized. This is clinically relevant for CYP450 substrates with a narrow therapeutic index, where the dose is individually adjusted (eg, warfarin). Upon initiation of canakinumab, in patients being treated with these types of medicinal products, therapeutic monitoring of the effect or drug concentration should be performed and the individual dose of the medicinal product may need to be adjusted as needed).
No products indexed under this heading.

Meperidine Hydrochloride (The formation of CYP450 enzymes is suppressed by increased levels of cytokines (eg, IL-1) during chronic inflammation. Thus it is expected that for a molecule that binds to IL-1, such as canakinumab, the formation of CYP450 enzymes could be normalized. This is clinically relevant for CYP450 substrates with a narrow therapeutic index, where the dose is individually adjusted (eg, warfarin). Upon initiation of canakinumab, in patients being treated with these types of medicinal products, therapeutic monitoring of the effect or drug concentration should be performed and the individual dose of the medicinal product may need to be adjusted as needed).
No products indexed under this heading.

Mephenytoin (The formation of CYP450 enzymes is suppressed by increased levels of cytokines (eg, IL-1) during chronic inflammation. Thus it is expected that for a molecule that binds to IL-1, such as canakinumab, the formation of CYP450 enzymes could be normalized. This is clinically relevant for CYP450 substrates with a narrow therapeutic index, where the dose is individually adjusted (eg, warfarin). Upon initiation of canakinumab, in patients being treated with these types of medicinal products, therapeutic monitoring of the effect or drug concentration should be performed and the individual dose of the medicinal product may need to be adjusted as needed).
No products indexed under this heading.

Mephobarbital (The formation of CYP450 enzymes is suppressed by increased levels of cytokines (eg, IL-1) during chronic inflammation. Thus it is expected that for a molecule that binds to IL-1, such as canakinumab, the formation of CYP450 enzymes could be normalized. This is clinically relevant for CYP450 substrates with a narrow therapeutic index, where the dose is individually adjusted (eg, warfarin). Upon initiation of canakinumab, in patients being treated with these types of medicinal products, therapeutic monitoring of the effect or drug concentration should be performed and the individual dose of the medicinal product may need to be adjusted as needed).
No products indexed under this heading.

Meprobamate (The formation of CYP450 enzymes is suppressed by increased levels of cytokines (eg, IL-1) during chronic inflammation. Thus it is expected that for a molecule that binds to IL-1, such as canakinumab, the formation of CYP450 enzymes could be normalized. This is clinically relevant for CYP450 substrates with a narrow therapeutic index, where the dose is individually adjusted (eg, warfarin). Upon initiation of canakinumab, in patients being treated with these types of medicinal products, therapeutic monitoring of the effect or drug concentration should be performed and the individual dose of the medicinal product may need to be adjusted as needed).
No products indexed under this heading.

Mestranol (The formation of CYP450 enzymes is suppressed by increased levels of cytokines (eg, IL-1) during chronic inflammation. Thus it is expected that for a molecule that binds to IL-1, such as canakinumab, the formation of CYP450 enzymes could be normalized. This is clinically relevant for CYP450 substrates with a narrow therapeutic index, where the dose is individually adjusted (eg, warfarin). Upon initiation of canakinumab, in patients being treated with these types of medicinal products, therapeutic monitoring of the effect or drug concentration should be performed and the individual dose of the medicinal product may need to be adjusted as needed).
No products indexed under this heading.

Metformin Hydrochloride (The formation of CYP450 enzymes is suppressed by increased levels of cytokines (eg, IL-1) during chronic inflammation. Thus it is expected that for a molecule that binds to IL-1, such as canakinumab, the formation of CYP450 enzymes could be normalized. This is clinically relevant for CYP450 substrates with a narrow therapeutic index, where the dose is individually adjusted (eg, warfarin). Upon initiation of canakinumab, in patients being treated with these types of medicinal products, therapeutic monitoring of the effect or drug concentration should be performed and the individual dose of the medicinal product may need to be adjusted as needed). Products include:
ActoPlus 3338
Avandamet 1345
Janumet 2188

Methadone Hydrochloride (The formation of CYP450 enzymes is suppressed by increased levels of cytokines (eg, IL-1) during chronic inflammation. Thus it is expected that for a molecule that binds to IL-1, such as canakinumab, the formation of CYP450 enzymes could be normalized. This is clinically relevant for CYP450 substrates with a narrow therapeutic index, where the dose is individually adjusted (eg, warfarin). Upon initiation of canakinumab, in patients being treated with these types of medicinal products, therapeutic monitoring of the effect or drug concentration should be performed and the individual dose of the medicinal product may need to be adjusted as needed).
No products indexed under this heading.

Methamphetamine Hydrochloride (The formation of CYP450 enzymes is suppressed by increased levels of cytokines (eg, IL-1) during chronic inflammation. Thus it is expected that for a molecule that binds to IL-1, such as canakinumab, the formation of CYP450 enzymes could be normalized. This is clinically relevant for CYP450 substrates with a narrow therapeutic index, where the dose is individually adjusted (eg, warfarin). Upon initiation of canakinumab, in patients being treated with these types of medicinal products, therapeutic monitoring of the effect or drug concentration should be performed and the individual dose of the medicinal product may need to be adjusted as needed).
No products indexed under this heading.

Methsuximide (The formation of CYP450 enzymes is suppressed by increased levels of cytokines (eg, IL-1) during chronic inflammation. Thus it is expected that for a molecule that binds to IL-1, such as canakinumab, the formation of CYP450 enzymes could be normalized. This is clinically relevant for CYP450 substrates with a narrow therapeutic index, where the dose is individually adjusted (eg, warfarin). Upon initiation of canakinumab, in patients being treated with these types of medicinal products, therapeutic monitoring of the effect or drug concentration should be performed and the individual dose of the medicinal product may need to be adjusted as needed).
No products indexed under this heading.

Metoprolol Succinate (The formation of CYP450 enzymes is suppressed by increased levels of cytokines (eg, IL-1) during chronic inflammation. Thus it is expected that for a molecule that binds to IL-1, such as canakinumab, the formation of CYP450 enzymes could be normalized. This is clinically relevant for CYP450 substrates with a narrow therapeutic index, where the dose is individually adjusted (eg, warfarin). Upon initiation of canakinumab, in patients being treated with these types of medicinal products, therapeutic monitoring of the effect or drug concentration should be performed and the individual dose of the medicinal product may need to be adjusted as needed). Products include:
Toprol XL 732

Metoprolol Tartrate (The formation of CYP450 enzymes is suppressed by increased levels of cytokines (eg, IL-1) during chronic inflammation. Thus it is expected that for a molecule that binds to IL-1, such as canakinumab, the formation of CYP450 enzymes could be normalized. This is clinically relevant for CYP450 substrates with a narrow therapeutic index, where the dose is individually adjusted (eg, warfarin). Upon initiation of canakinumab, in patients being treated with these types of medicinal products, therapeutic monitoring of the effect or drug concentration should be performed and the individual dose of the medicinal product may need to be adjusted as needed).
No products indexed under this heading.

Mexiletine Hydrochloride (The formation of CYP450 enzymes is suppressed by increased levels of cytokines (eg, IL-1) during chronic inflammation. Thus it is expected that for a molecule that binds to IL-1, such as canakinumab, the formation of CYP450 enzymes could be normalized. This is clinically relevant for CYP450 substrates with a narrow therapeutic index, where the dose is individually adjusted (eg, warfarin). Upon initiation of canakinumab, in patients being treated with these types of medicinal products, therapeutic monitoring of the effect or drug concentration should be performed and the individual dose of the medicinal product may need to be adjusted as needed).
No products indexed under this heading.

Midazolam Hydrochloride (The formation of CYP450 enzymes is suppressed by increased levels of cytokines (eg, IL-1) during chronic inflammation. Thus it is expected that for a molecule that binds to IL-1, such as canakinumab, the formation of CYP450 enzymes could be normalized. This is clinically relevant for CYP450 substrates with a narrow therapeutic index, where the dose is individually adjusted (eg, warfarin). Upon initiation of canakinumab, in patients being treated with these types of medicinal products, therapeutic monitoring of the effect or drug concentration should be performed and the individual dose of the medicinal product may need to be adjusted as needed).
No products indexed under this heading.

Miglitol (The formation of CYP450 enzymes is suppressed by increased levels of cytokines (eg, IL-1) during chronic inflammation. Thus it is expected that for a molecule that binds to IL-1, such as canakinumab, the formation of CYP450 enzymes could be normalized. This is clinically relevant for CYP450 substrates with a narrow therapeutic index, where the dose is individually adjusted (eg, warfarin). Upon initiation of canakinumab, in patients being treated with these types of medicinal products, therapeutic monitoring of the effect or drug concentration should be performed and the individual dose of the medicinal product may need to be adjusted as needed).
No products indexed under this heading.

Mirtazapine (The formation of CYP450 enzymes is suppressed by increased levels of cytokines (eg, IL-1) during chronic inflammation. Thus it is expected that for a molecule that binds to IL-1, such as canakinumab, the formation of CYP450 enzymes could be normalized. This is clinically relevant for CYP450 substrates with a narrow therapeutic index, where the dose is individually adjusted (eg, warfarin). Upon initiation of canakinumab, in patients being treated with these types of medicinal products, therapeutic monitoring of the effect or drug concentration should be performed and the individual dose of the medicinal product may need to be adjusted as needed). Products include:
Remeron Tablets 3214
RemeronSolTab Tablets 3219

Montelukast Sodium (The formation of CYP450 enzymes is suppressed by increased levels of cytokines (eg, IL-1) during chronic inflammation. Thus it is expected that for a molecule that binds to IL-1, such as canakinumab, the formation of CYP450 enzymes could be

843 Interactions Index Ilaris

normalized. This is clinically relevant for CYP450 substrates with a narrow therapeutic index, where the dose is individually adjusted (eg, warfarin). Upon initiation of canakinumab, in patients being treated with these types of medicinal products, therapeutic monitoring of the effect or drug concentration should be performed and the individual dose of the medicinal product may need to be adjusted as needed). Products include:

Singulair 2270

Morphine Sulfate (The formation of CYP450 enzymes is suppressed by increased levels of cytokines (eg, IL-1) during chronic inflammation. Thus it is expected that for a molecule that binds to IL-1, such as canakinumab, the formation of CYP450 enzymes could be normalized. This is clinically relevant for CYP450 substrates with a narrow therapeutic index, where the dose is individually adjusted (eg, warfarin). Upon initiation of canakinumab, in patients being treated with these types of medicinal products, therapeutic monitoring of the effect or drug concentration should be performed and the individual dose of the medicinal product may need to be adjusted as needed). Products include:

Avinza 1822
Embeda 1831
MS Contin 2803

Moxifloxacin Hydrochloride (The formation of CYP450 enzymes is suppressed by increased levels of cytokines (eg, IL-1) during chronic inflammation. Thus it is expected that for a molecule that binds to IL-1, such as canakinumab, the formation of CYP450 enzymes could be normalized. This is clinically relevant for CYP450 substrates with a narrow therapeutic index, where the dose is individually adjusted (eg, warfarin). Upon initiation of canakinumab, in patients being treated with these types of medicinal products, therapeutic monitoring of the effect or drug concentration should be performed and the individual dose of the medicinal product may need to be adjusted as needed). Products include:

Avelox 3064
Vigamox 589

Mumps Virus Vaccine, Live (No data are available on either the effects of live vaccination or the secondary transmission of infection by live vaccines in patients receiving canakinumab. Therefore, live vaccines should not be given concurrently with canakinumab. It is recommended that, if possible, pediatric and adult patients should complete all immunizations in accordance with current immunization guidelines prior to initiating canakinumab therapy). Products include:

Mumpsvax 2218

Nabumetone (The formation of CYP450 enzymes is suppressed by increased levels of cytokines (eg, IL-1) during chronic inflammation. Thus it is expected that for a molecule that binds to IL-1, such as canakinumab, the formation of CYP450 enzymes could be normalized. This is clinically relevant for CYP450 substrates with a narrow therapeutic index, where the dose is individually adjusted (eg, warfarin). Upon initiation of canakinumab, in patients being treated with these types of medicinal products, therapeutic monitoring of the effect or drug concentration should be performed and the individual dose of the medicinal product may need to be adjusted as needed).

No products indexed under this heading.

Nafcillin Sodium (The formation of CYP450 enzymes is suppressed by increased levels of cytokines (eg, IL-1) during chronic inflammation. Thus it is expected that for a molecule that binds to IL-1, such as canakinumab, the formation of CYP450 enzymes could be normalized. This is clinically relevant for CYP450 substrates with a narrow therapeutic index, where the dose is individually adjusted (eg, warfarin). Upon initiation of canakinumab, in patients being treated with these types of medicinal products, therapeutic monitoring of the effect or drug concentration should be performed and the individual dose of the medicinal product may need to be adjusted as needed).

No products indexed under this heading.

Naproxen (The formation of CYP450 enzymes is suppressed by increased levels of cytokines (eg, IL-1) during chronic inflammation. Thus it is expected that for a molecule that binds to IL-1, such as canakinumab, the formation of CYP450 enzymes could be normalized. This is clinically relevant for CYP450 substrates with a narrow therapeutic index, where the dose is individually adjusted (eg, warfarin). Upon initiation of canakinumab, in patients being treated with these types of medicinal products, therapeutic monitoring of the effect or drug concentration should be performed and the individual dose of the medicinal product may need to be adjusted as needed). Products include:

EC-Naprosyn 2850
Naprosyn 2850
Anaprox/Naprosyn 2850

Naproxen Sodium (The formation of CYP450 enzymes is suppressed by increased levels of cytokines (eg, IL-1) during chronic inflammation. Thus it is expected that for a molecule that binds to IL-1, such as canakinumab, the formation of CYP450 enzymes could be normalized. This is clinically relevant for CYP450 substrates with a narrow therapeutic index, where the dose is individually adjusted (eg, warfarin). Upon initiation of canakinumab, in patients being treated with these types of medicinal products, therapeutic monitoring of the effect or drug concentration should be performed and the individual dose of the medicinal product may need to be adjusted as needed). Products include:

Anaprox 2850
Anaprox DS 2850
Treximet 1681

Nateglinide (The formation of CYP450 enzymes is suppressed by increased levels of cytokines (eg, IL-1) during chronic inflammation. Thus it is expected that for a molecule that binds to IL-1, such as canakinumab, the formation of CYP450 enzymes could be normalized. This is clinically relevant for CYP450 substrates with a narrow therapeutic index, where the dose is individually adjusted (eg, warfarin). Upon initiation of canakinumab, in patients being treated with these types of medicinal products, therapeutic monitoring of the effect or drug concentration should be performed and the individual dose of the medicinal product may need to be adjusted as needed).

No products indexed under this heading.

Nefazodone Hydrochloride (The formation of CYP450 enzymes is suppressed by increased levels of cytokines (eg, IL-1) during chronic inflammation. Thus it is expected that for a molecule that binds to IL-1, such as canakinumab, the formation of CYP450 enzymes could be normalized. This is clinically relevant for CYP450 substrates with a narrow therapeutic index, where the dose is individually adjusted (eg, warfarin). Upon initiation of canakinumab, in patients being treated with these types of medicinal products, therapeutic monitoring of the effect or drug concentration should be performed and the individual dose of the medicinal product may need to be adjusted as needed).

No products indexed under this heading.

Nelfinavir Mesylate (The formation of CYP450 enzymes is suppressed by increased levels of cytokines (eg, IL-1) during chronic inflammation. Thus it is expected that for a molecule that binds to IL-1, such as canakinumab, the formation of CYP450 enzymes could be normalized. This is clinically relevant for CYP450 substrates with a narrow therapeutic index, where the dose is individually adjusted (eg, warfarin). Upon initiation of canakinumab, in patients being treated with these types of medicinal products, therapeutic monitoring of the effect or drug concentration should be performed and the individual dose of the medicinal product may need to be adjusted as needed).

No products indexed under this heading.

Nicardipine (The formation of CYP450 enzymes is suppressed by increased levels of cytokines (eg, IL-1) during chronic inflammation. Thus it is expected that for a molecule that binds to IL-1, such as canakinumab, the formation of CYP450 enzymes could be normalized. This is clinically relevant for CYP450 substrates with a narrow therapeutic index, where the dose is individually adjusted (eg, warfarin). Upon initiation of canakinumab, in patients being treated with these types of medicinal products, therapeutic monitoring of the effect or drug concentration should be performed and the individual dose of the medicinal product may need to be adjusted as needed).

No products indexed under this heading.

Nicardipine Hydrochloride (The formation of CYP450 enzymes is suppressed by increased levels of cytokines (eg, IL-1) during chronic inflammation. Thus it is expected that for a molecule that binds to IL-1, such as canakinumab, the formation of CYP450 enzymes could be normalized. This is clinically relevant for CYP450 substrates with a narrow therapeutic index, where the dose is individually adjusted (eg, warfarin). Upon initiation of canakinumab, in patients being treated with these types of medicinal products, therapeutic monitoring of the effect or drug concentration should be performed and the individual dose of the medicinal product may need to be adjusted as needed).

No products indexed under this heading.

Nicotine Polacrilex (The formation of CYP450 enzymes is suppressed by increased levels of cytokines (eg, IL-1) during chronic inflammation. Thus it is expected that for a molecule that binds to IL-1, such as canakinumab, the formation of CYP450 enzymes could be normalized. This is clinically relevant for CYP450 substrates with a narrow therapeutic index, where the dose is individually adjusted (eg, warfarin). Upon initiation of canakinumab, in patients being treated with these types of medicinal products, therapeutic monitoring of the effect or drug concentration should be performed and the individual dose of the medicinal product may need to be adjusted as needed).

No products indexed under this heading.

Nicotine Salicylate (The formation of CYP450 enzymes is suppressed by increased levels of cytokines (eg, IL-1) during chronic inflammation. Thus it is expected that for a molecule that binds to IL-1, such as canakinumab, the formation of CYP450 enzymes could be normalized. This is clinically relevant for CYP450 substrates with a narrow therapeutic index, where the dose is individually adjusted (eg, warfarin). Upon initiation of canakinumab, in patients being treated with these types of medicinal products, therapeutic monitoring of the effect or drug concentration should be performed and the individual dose of the medicinal product may need to be adjusted as needed).

No products indexed under this heading.

Nicotine Sulfate (The formation of CYP450 enzymes is suppressed by increased levels of cytokines (eg, IL-1) during chronic inflammation. Thus it is expected that for a molecule that binds to IL-1, such as canakinumab, the formation of CYP450 enzymes could be normalized. This is clinically relevant for CYP450 substrates with a narrow therapeutic index, where the dose is individually adjusted (eg, warfarin). Upon initiation of canakinumab, in patients being treated with these types of medicinal products, therapeutic monitoring of the effect or drug concentration should be performed and the individual dose of the medicinal product may need to be adjusted as needed).

No products indexed under this heading.

Nifedipine (The formation of CYP450 enzymes is suppressed by increased levels of cytokines (eg, IL-1) during chronic inflammation. Thus it is expected that for a molecule that binds to IL-1, such as canakinumab, the formation of CYP450 enzymes could be normalized. This is clinically relevant for CYP450 substrates with a narrow therapeutic index, where the dose is individually adjusted (eg, warfarin). Upon initiation of canakinumab, in patients being treated with these types of medicinal products, therapeutic monitoring of the effect or drug concentration should be performed and the individual dose of the medicinal product may need to be adjusted as needed).

No products indexed under this heading.

Nilutamide (The formation of CYP450 enzymes is suppressed by increased levels of cytokines (eg, IL-1) during chronic inflammation. Thus it is expected that for a molecule that binds to IL-1, such as canakinumab, the formation of CYP450 enzymes could be normalized. This is clinically relevant for CYP450 substrates with a narrow therapeutic index, where the dose is individually adjusted (eg, warfarin). Upon initiation of canakinumab, in patients being treated with these types of medicinal products, therapeutic monitoring of the effect or drug concentration should be performed and the individual dose of the medicinal product may need to be adjusted as needed).

No products indexed under this heading.

Nimodipine (The formation of CYP450 enzymes is suppressed by increased levels of cytokines (eg, IL-1) during chronic inflammation. Thus it is expected that for a molecule that binds to IL-1, such as canakinumab, the formation of CYP450 enzymes could be normalized. This is clinically relevant for CYP450 substrates with a narrow therapeutic index, where the dose is individually adjusted (eg, warfarin). Upon initiation of canakinumab, in patients being treated with these types of medicinal products, therapeutic monitoring of the effect or drug concentration should be performed and the individual dose of the medicinal product may need to be adjusted as needed).

No products indexed under this heading.

Nisoldipine (The formation of CYP450 enzymes is suppressed by increased levels of cytokines (eg, IL-1) during chronic inflammation. Thus it is expected that for a molecule that binds to IL-1, such as canakinumab, the formation of CYP450 enzymes could be normalized. This is clinically relevant for CYP450 substrates with a narrow therapeutic index, where the dose is individually adjusted (eg, warfarin). Upon initiation of canakinumab, in patients being treated with these types of medicinal

Ilaris Interactions Index 844

products, therapeutic monitoring of the effect or drug concentration should be performed and the individual dose of the medicinal product may need to be adjusted as needed).
No products indexed under this heading.

Nitrendipine (The formation of CYP450 enzymes is suppressed by increased levels of cytokines (eg, IL-1) during chronic inflammation. Thus it is expected that for a molecule that binds to IL-1, such as canakinumab, the formation of CYP450 enzymes could be normalized. This is clinically relevant for CYP450 substrates with a narrow therapeutic index, where the dose is individually adjusted (eg, warfarin). Upon initiation of canakinumab, in patients being treated with these types of medicinal products, therapeutic monitoring of the effect or drug concentration should be performed and the individual dose of the medicinal product may need to be adjusted as needed).
No products indexed under this heading.

Norethindrone (The formation of CYP450 enzymes is suppressed by increased levels of cytokines (eg, IL-1) during chronic inflammation. Thus it is expected that for a molecule that binds to IL-1, such as canakinumab, the formation of CYP450 enzymes could be normalized. This is clinically relevant for CYP450 substrates with a narrow therapeutic index, where the dose is individually adjusted (eg, warfarin). Upon initiation of canakinumab, in patients being treated with these types of medicinal products, therapeutic monitoring of the effect or drug concentration should be performed and the individual dose of the medicinal product may need to be adjusted as needed). Products include:
Ortho Micronor 2660

Norethindrone Acetate (The formation of CYP450 enzymes is suppressed by increased levels of cytokines (eg, IL-1) during chronic inflammation. Thus it is expected that for a molecule that binds to IL-1, such as canakinumab, the formation of CYP450 enzymes could be normalized. This is clinically relevant for CYP450 substrates with a narrow therapeutic index, where the dose is individually adjusted (eg, warfarin). Upon initiation of canakinumab, in patients being treated with these types of medicinal products, therapeutic monitoring of the effect or drug concentration should be performed and the individual dose of the medicinal product may need to be adjusted as needed). Products include:
Activella 2561

Norfloxacin (The formation of CYP450 enzymes is suppressed by increased levels of cytokines (eg, IL-1) during chronic inflammation. Thus it is expected that for a molecule that binds to IL-1, such as canakinumab, the formation of CYP450 enzymes could be normalized. This is clinically relevant for CYP450 substrates with a narrow therapeutic index, where the dose is individually adjusted (eg, warfarin). Upon initiation of canakinumab, in patients being treated with these types of medicinal products, therapeutic monitoring of the effect or drug concentration should be performed and the individual dose of the medicinal product may need to be adjusted as needed). Products include:
Noroxin 2220

Norgestrel (The formation of CYP450 enzymes is suppressed by increased levels of cytokines (eg, IL-1) during chronic inflammation. Thus it is expected that for a molecule that binds to IL-1, such as canakinumab, the formation of CYP450 enzymes could be normalized. This is clinically relevant for CYP450 substrates with a narrow therapeutic index, where the dose is individually adjusted (eg, warfarin). Upon initiation of canakinumab, in patients being treated with these types of medicinal products, therapeutic monitoring of the effect or drug concentration should be performed and the individual dose of the medicinal product may need to be adjusted as needed).
No products indexed under this heading.

Nortriptyline Hydrochloride (The formation of CYP450 enzymes is suppressed by increased levels of cytokines (eg, IL-1) during chronic inflammation. Thus it is expected that for a molecule that binds to IL-1, such as canakinumab, the formation of CYP450 enzymes could be normalized. This is clinically relevant for CYP450 substrates with a narrow therapeutic index, where the dose is individually adjusted (eg, warfarin). Upon initiation of canakinumab, in patients being treated with these types of medicinal products, therapeutic monitoring of the effect or drug concentration should be performed and the individual dose of the medicinal product may need to be adjusted as needed).
No products indexed under this heading.

Ofloxacin (The formation of CYP450 enzymes is suppressed by increased levels of cytokines (eg, IL-1) during chronic inflammation. Thus it is expected that for a molecule that binds to IL-1, such as canakinumab, the formation of CYP450 enzymes could be normalized. This is clinically relevant for CYP450 substrates with a narrow therapeutic index, where the dose is individually adjusted (eg, warfarin). Upon initiation of canakinumab, in patients being treated with these types of medicinal products, therapeutic monitoring of the effect or drug concentration should be performed and the individual dose of the medicinal product may need to be adjusted as needed).
No products indexed under this heading.

Olanzapine (The formation of CYP450 enzymes is suppressed by increased levels of cytokines (eg, IL-1) during chronic inflammation. Thus it is expected that for a molecule that binds to IL-1, such as canakinumab, the formation of CYP450 enzymes could be normalized. This is clinically relevant for CYP450 substrates with a narrow therapeutic index, where the dose is individually adjusted (eg, warfarin). Upon initiation of canakinumab, in patients being treated with these types of medicinal products, therapeutic monitoring of the effect or drug concentration should be performed and the individual dose of the medicinal product may need to be adjusted as needed). Products include:
Symbyax 1965
Zyprexa 1984
Zyprexa IntraMuscular 1984
Zyprexa ZYDIS 1984

Omeprazole (The formation of CYP450 enzymes is suppressed by increased levels of cytokines (eg, IL-1) during chronic inflammation. Thus it is expected that for a molecule that binds to IL-1, such as canakinumab, the formation of CYP450 enzymes could be normalized. This is clinically relevant for CYP450 substrates with a narrow therapeutic index, where the dose is individually adjusted (eg, warfarin). Upon initiation of canakinumab, in patients being treated with these types of medicinal products, therapeutic monitoring of the effect or drug concentration should be performed and the individual dose of the medicinal product may need to be adjusted as needed).
No products indexed under this heading.

Omeprazole Magnesium (The formation of CYP450 enzymes is suppressed by increased levels of cytokines (eg, IL-1) during chronic inflammation. Thus it is expected that for a molecule that binds to IL-1, such as canakinumab, the formation of CYP450 enzymes could be normalized. This is clinically relevant for CYP450 substrates with a narrow therapeutic index, where the dose is individually adjusted (eg, warfarin). Upon initiation of canakinumab, in patients being treated with these types of medicinal products, therapeutic monitoring of the effect or drug concentration should be performed and the individual dose of the medicinal product may need to be adjusted as needed).
No products indexed under this heading.

Ondansetron (The formation of CYP450 enzymes is suppressed by increased levels of cytokines (eg, IL-1) during chronic inflammation. Thus it is expected that for a molecule that binds to IL-1, such as canakinumab, the formation of CYP450 enzymes could be normalized. This is clinically relevant for CYP450 substrates with a narrow therapeutic index, where the dose is individually adjusted (eg, warfarin). Upon initiation of canakinumab, in patients being treated with these types of medicinal products, therapeutic monitoring of the effect or drug concentration should be performed and the individual dose of the medicinal product may need to be adjusted as needed).
No products indexed under this heading.

Ondansetron Hydrochloride (The formation of CYP450 enzymes is suppressed by increased levels of cytokines (eg, IL-1) during chronic inflammation. Thus it is expected that for a molecule that binds to IL-1, such as canakinumab, the formation of CYP450 enzymes could be normalized. This is clinically relevant for CYP450 substrates with a narrow therapeutic index, where the dose is individually adjusted (eg, warfarin). Upon initiation of canakinumab, in patients being treated with these types of medicinal products, therapeutic monitoring of the effect or drug concentration should be performed and the individual dose of the medicinal product may need to be adjusted as needed). Products include:
Zofran Injection 1750
Zofran 1756
Zofran ODT 1756

Oxaprozin (The formation of CYP450 enzymes is suppressed by increased levels of cytokines (eg, IL-1) during chronic inflammation. Thus it is expected that for a molecule that binds to IL-1, such as canakinumab, the formation of CYP450 enzymes could be normalized. This is clinically relevant for CYP450 substrates with a narrow therapeutic index, where the dose is individually adjusted (eg, warfarin). Upon initiation of canakinumab, in patients being treated with these types of medicinal products, therapeutic monitoring of the effect or drug concentration should be performed and the individual dose of the medicinal product may need to be adjusted as needed).
No products indexed under this heading.

Oxcarbazepine (The formation of CYP450 enzymes is suppressed by increased levels of cytokines (eg, IL-1) during chronic inflammation. Thus it is expected that for a molecule that binds to IL-1, such as canakinumab, the formation of CYP450 enzymes could be normalized. This is clinically relevant for CYP450 substrates with a narrow therapeutic index, where the dose is individually adjusted (eg, warfarin). Upon initiation of canakinumab, in patients being treated with these types of medicinal products, therapeutic monitoring of the effect or drug concentration should be performed and the individual dose of the medicinal product may need to be adjusted as needed).
No products indexed under this heading.

Oxycodone Hydrochloride (The formation of CYP450 enzymes is suppressed by increased levels of cytokines (eg, IL-1) during chronic inflammation. Thus it is expected that for a molecule that binds to IL-1, such as canakinumab, the formation of CYP450 enzymes could be normalized. This is clinically relevant for CYP450 substrates with a narrow therapeutic index, where the dose is individually adjusted (eg, warfarin). Upon initiation of canakinumab, in patients being treated with these types of medicinal products, therapeutic monitoring of the effect or drug concentration should be performed and the individual dose of the medicinal product may need to be adjusted as needed). Products include:
OxyContin 2807
Percocet 1121
Percodan 1124

Paclitaxel (The formation of CYP450 enzymes is suppressed by increased levels of cytokines (eg, IL-1) during chronic inflammation. Thus it is expected that for a molecule that binds to IL-1, such as canakinumab, the formation of CYP450 enzymes could be normalized. This is clinically relevant for CYP450 substrates with a narrow therapeutic index, where the dose is individually adjusted (eg, warfarin). Upon initiation of canakinumab, in patients being treated with these types of medicinal products, therapeutic monitoring of the effect or drug concentration should be performed and the individual dose of the medicinal product may need to be adjusted as needed).
No products indexed under this heading.

Pantoprazole Sodium (The formation of CYP450 enzymes is suppressed by increased levels of cytokines (eg, IL-1) during chronic inflammation. Thus it is expected that for a molecule that binds to IL-1, such as canakinumab, the formation of CYP450 enzymes could be normalized. This is clinically relevant for CYP450 substrates with a narrow therapeutic index, where the dose is individually adjusted (eg, warfarin). Upon initiation of canakinumab, in patients being treated with these types of medicinal products, therapeutic monitoring of the effect or drug concentration should be performed and the individual dose of the medicinal product may need to be adjusted as needed). Products include:
Protonix Tablets 3571
Protonix 3575

Paramethadione (The formation of CYP450 enzymes is suppressed by increased levels of cytokines (eg, IL-1) during chronic inflammation. Thus it is expected that for a molecule that binds to IL-1, such as canakinumab, the formation of CYP450 enzymes could be normalized. This is clinically relevant for CYP450 substrates with a narrow therapeutic index, where the dose is individually adjusted (eg, warfarin). Upon initiation of canakinumab, in patients being treated with these types of medicinal products, therapeutic monitoring of the effect or drug concentration should be performed and the individual dose of the medicinal product may need to be adjusted as needed).
No products indexed under this heading.

Paroxetine Hydrochloride (The formation of CYP450 enzymes is suppressed by increased levels of cytokines (eg, IL-1) during chronic inflammation. Thus it is expected that for a molecule that binds to IL-1, such as canakinumab, the formation of CYP450 enzymes could be normalized. This is clinically relevant for CYP450

845 Interactions Index Ilaris

substrates with a narrow therapeutic index, where the dose is individually adjusted (eg, warfarin). Upon initiation of canakinumab, in patients being treated with these types of medicinal products, therapeutic monitoring of the effect or drug concentration should be performed and the individual dose of the medicinal product may need to be adjusted as needed). Products include:

Paroxetine CR 2361
Paroxetine ER 2371
Paxil 1586
Paxil CR 1596

Pentamidine Isethionate (The formation of CYP450 enzymes is suppressed by increased levels of cytokines (eg, IL-1) during chronic inflammation. Thus it is expected that for a molecule that binds to IL-1, such as canakinumab, the formation of CYP450 enzymes could be normalized. This is clinically relevant for CYP450 substrates with a narrow therapeutic index, where the dose is individually adjusted (eg, warfarin). Upon initiation of canakinumab, in patients being treated with these types of medicinal products, therapeutic monitoring of the effect or drug concentration should be performed and the individual dose of the medicinal product may need to be adjusted as needed).

No products indexed under this heading.

Phenacemide (The formation of CYP450 enzymes is suppressed by increased levels of cytokines (eg, IL-1) during chronic inflammation. Thus it is expected that for a molecule that binds to IL-1, such as canakinumab, the formation of CYP450 enzymes could be normalized. This is clinically relevant for CYP450 substrates with a narrow therapeutic index, where the dose is individually adjusted (eg, warfarin). Upon initiation of canakinumab, in patients being treated with these types of medicinal products, therapeutic monitoring of the effect or drug concentration should be performed and the individual dose of the medicinal product may need to be adjusted as needed).

No products indexed under this heading.

Phenobarbital (The formation of CYP450 enzymes is suppressed by increased levels of cytokines (eg, IL-1) during chronic inflammation. Thus it is expected that for a molecule that binds to IL-1, such as canakinumab, the formation of CYP450 enzymes could be normalized. This is clinically relevant for CYP450 substrates with a narrow therapeutic index, where the dose is individually adjusted (eg, warfarin). Upon initiation of canakinumab, in patients being treated with these types of medicinal products, therapeutic monitoring of the effect or drug concentration should be performed and the individual dose of the medicinal product may need to be adjusted as needed). Products include:

Donnatal 2711

Phenobarbital Sodium (The formation of CYP450 enzymes is suppressed by increased levels of cytokines (eg, IL-1) during chronic inflammation. Thus it is expected that for a molecule that binds to IL-1, the formation of CYP450 enzymes could be normalized. This is clinically relevant for CYP450 substrates with a narrow therapeutic index, where the dose is individually adjusted (eg, warfarin). Upon initiation of canakinumab, in patients being treated with these types of medicinal products, therapeutic monitoring of the effect or drug concentration should be performed and the individual dose of the medicinal product may need to be adjusted as needed).

No products indexed under this heading.

Phensuximide (The formation of CYP450 enzymes is suppressed by increased levels of cytokines (eg, IL-1) during chronic inflammation. Thus it is expected that for a molecule that binds to IL-1, such as canakinumab, the formation of CYP450 enzymes could be normalized. This is clinically relevant for CYP450 substrates with a narrow therapeutic index, where the dose is individually adjusted (eg, warfarin). Upon initiation of canakinumab, in patients being treated with these types of medicinal products, therapeutic monitoring of the effect or drug concentration should be performed and the individual dose of the medicinal product may need to be adjusted as needed).

No products indexed under this heading.

Phenylbutazone (The formation of CYP450 enzymes is suppressed by increased levels of cytokines (eg, IL-1) during chronic inflammation. Thus it is expected that for a molecule that binds to IL-1, such as canakinumab, the formation of CYP450 enzymes could be normalized. This is clinically relevant for CYP450 substrates with a narrow therapeutic index, where the dose is individually adjusted (eg, warfarin). Upon initiation of canakinumab, in patients being treated with these types of medicinal products, therapeutic monitoring of the effect or drug concentration should be performed and the individual dose of the medicinal product may need to be adjusted as needed).

No products indexed under this heading.

Phenytoin (The formation of CYP450 enzymes is suppressed by increased levels of cytokines (eg, IL-1) during chronic inflammation. Thus it is expected that for a molecule that binds to IL-1, such as canakinumab, the formation of CYP450 enzymes could be normalized. This is clinically relevant for CYP450 substrates with a narrow therapeutic index, where the dose is individually adjusted (eg, warfarin). Upon initiation of canakinumab, in patients being treated with these types of medicinal products, therapeutic monitoring of the effect or drug concentration should be performed and the individual dose of the medicinal product may need to be adjusted as needed).

No products indexed under this heading.

Phenytoin Sodium (The formation of CYP450 enzymes is suppressed by increased levels of cytokines (eg, IL-1) during chronic inflammation. Thus it is expected that for a molecule that binds to IL-1, such as canakinumab, the formation of CYP450 enzymes could be normalized. This is clinically relevant for CYP450 substrates with a narrow therapeutic index, where the dose is individually adjusted (eg, warfarin). Upon initiation of canakinumab, in patients being treated with these types of medicinal products, therapeutic monitoring of the effect or drug concentration should be performed and the individual dose of the medicinal product may need to be adjusted as needed). Products include:

Phenytek Capsules 2380

Pimozide (The formation of CYP450 enzymes is suppressed by increased levels of cytokines (eg, IL-1) during chronic inflammation. Thus it is expected that for a molecule that binds to IL-1, such as canakinumab, the formation of CYP450 enzymes could be normalized. This is clinically relevant for CYP450 substrates with a narrow therapeutic index, where the dose is individually adjusted (eg, warfarin). Upon initiation of canakinumab, in patients being treated with these types of medicinal products, therapeutic monitoring of the effect or drug concentration should be performed and the individual dose of the medicinal product may need to be adjusted as needed).

No products indexed under this heading.

Pindolol (The formation of CYP450 enzymes is suppressed by increased levels of cytokines (eg, IL-1) during chronic inflammation. Thus it is expected that for a molecule that binds to IL-1, such as canakinumab, the formation of CYP450 enzymes could be normalized. This is clinically relevant for CYP450 substrates with a narrow therapeutic index, where the dose is individually adjusted (eg, warfarin). Upon initiation of canakinumab, in patients being treated with these types of medicinal products, therapeutic monitoring of the effect or drug concentration should be performed and the individual dose of the medicinal product may need to be adjusted as needed).

No products indexed under this heading.

Pioglitazone Hydrochloride (The formation of CYP450 enzymes is suppressed by increased levels of cytokines (eg, IL-1) during chronic inflammation. Thus it is expected that for a molecule that binds to IL-1, such as canakinumab, the formation of CYP450 enzymes could be normalized. This is clinically relevant for CYP450 substrates with a narrow therapeutic index, where the dose is individually adjusted (eg, warfarin). Upon initiation of canakinumab, in patients being treated with these types of medicinal products, therapeutic monitoring of the effect or drug concentration should be performed and the individual dose of the medicinal product may need to be adjusted as needed). Products include:

ActoPlus 3338
Actos 3345
Duetact 3354

Piroxicam (The formation of CYP450 enzymes is suppressed by increased levels of cytokines (eg, IL-1) during chronic inflammation. Thus it is expected that for a molecule that binds to IL-1, such as canakinumab, the formation of CYP450 enzymes could be normalized. This is clinically relevant for CYP450 substrates with a narrow therapeutic index, where the dose is individually adjusted (eg, warfarin). Upon initiation of canakinumab, in patients being treated with these types of medicinal products, therapeutic monitoring of the effect or drug concentration should be performed and the individual dose of the medicinal product may need to be adjusted as needed).

No products indexed under this heading.

Poliovirus Vaccine, Live, Oral, Trivalent, Types 1,2,3 (Sabin) (No data are available on either the effects of live vaccination or the secondary transmission of infection by live vaccines in patients receiving canakinumab. Therefore, live vaccines should not be given concurrently with canakinumab. It is recommended that, if possible, pediatric and adult patients should complete all immunizations in accordance with current immunization guidelines prior to initiating canakinumab therapy).

No products indexed under this heading.

Polyestradiol Phosphate (The formation of CYP450 enzymes is suppressed by increased levels of cytokines (eg, IL-1) during chronic inflammation. Thus it is expected that for a molecule that binds to IL-1, such as canakinumab, the formation of CYP450 enzymes could be normalized. This is clinically relevant for CYP450 substrates with a narrow therapeutic index, where the dose is individually adjusted (eg, warfarin). Upon initiation of canakinumab, in patients being treated with these types of medicinal products, therapeutic monitoring of the effect or drug concentration should be performed and the individual dose of the medicinal product may need to be adjusted as needed).

No products indexed under this heading.

Primidone (The formation of CYP450 enzymes is suppressed by increased levels of cytokines (eg, IL-1) during chronic inflammation. Thus it is expected that for a molecule that binds to IL-1, such as canakinumab, the formation of CYP450 enzymes could be normalized. This is clinically relevant for CYP450 substrates with a narrow therapeutic index, where the dose is individually adjusted (eg, warfarin). Upon initiation of canakinumab, in patients being treated with these types of medicinal products, therapeutic monitoring of the effect or drug concentration should be performed and the individual dose of the medicinal product may need to be adjusted as needed).

No products indexed under this heading.

Progesterone (The formation of CYP450 enzymes is suppressed by increased levels of cytokines (eg, IL-1) during chronic inflammation. Thus it is expected that for a molecule that binds to IL-1, such as canakinumab, the formation of CYP450 enzymes could be normalized. This is clinically relevant for CYP450 substrates with a narrow therapeutic index, where the dose is individually adjusted (eg, warfarin). Upon initiation of canakinumab, in patients being treated with these types of medicinal products, therapeutic monitoring of the effect or drug concentration should be performed and the individual dose of the medicinal product may need to be adjusted as needed). Products include:

Crinone 4% 996
Crinone 8% 996
Prometrium 3307

Proguanil Hydrochloride (The formation of CYP450 enzymes is suppressed by increased levels of cytokines (eg, IL-1) during chronic inflammation. Thus it is expected that for a molecule that binds to IL-1, such as canakinumab, the formation of CYP450 enzymes could be normalized. This is clinically relevant for CYP450 substrates with a narrow therapeutic index, where the dose is individually adjusted (eg, warfarin). Upon initiation of canakinumab, in patients being treated with these types of medicinal products, therapeutic monitoring of the effect or drug concentration should be performed and the individual dose of the medicinal product may need to be adjusted as needed). Products include:

Malarone Pediatric Tablets 1572
Malarone 1572

Propafenone Hydrochloride (The formation of CYP450 enzymes is suppressed by increased levels of cytokines (eg, IL-1) during chronic inflammation. Thus it is expected that for a molecule that binds to IL-1, such as canakinumab, the formation of CYP450 enzymes could be normalized. This is clinically relevant for CYP450 substrates with a narrow therapeutic index, where the dose is individually adjusted (eg, warfarin). Upon initiation of canakinumab, in patients being treated with these types of medicinal products, therapeutic monitoring of the effect or drug concentration should be performed and the individual dose of the medicinal product may need to be adjusted as needed). Products include:

Rythmol 1648
Rythmol SR 1652

Propoxyphene Hydrochloride (The formation of CYP450 enzymes is suppressed by increased levels of cytokines (eg, IL-1) during chronic inflammation. Thus it is expected that for a molecule that binds to IL-1, such as canakinumab, the formation of CYP450

enzymes could be normalized. This is clinically relevant for CYP450 substrates with a narrow therapeutic index, where the dose is individually adjusted (eg, warfarin). Upon initiation of canakinumab, in patients being treated with these types of medicinal products, therapeutic monitoring of the effect or drug concentration should be performed and the individual dose of the medicinal product may need to be adjusted as needed).
No products indexed under this heading.

Propoxyphene Napsylate (The formation of CYP450 enzymes is suppressed by increased levels of cytokines (eg, IL-1) during chronic inflammation. Thus it is expected that for a molecule that binds to IL-1, such as canakinumab, the formation of CYP450 enzymes could be normalized. This is clinically relevant for CYP450 substrates with a narrow therapeutic index, where the dose is individually adjusted (eg, warfarin). Upon initiation of canakinumab, in patients being treated with these types of medicinal products, therapeutic monitoring of the effect or drug concentration should be performed and the individual dose of the medicinal product may need to be adjusted as needed).
No products indexed under this heading.

Propranolol Hydrochloride (The formation of CYP450 enzymes is suppressed by increased levels of cytokines (eg, IL-1) during chronic inflammation. Thus it is expected that for a molecule that binds to IL-1, such as canakinumab, the formation of CYP450 enzymes could be normalized. This is clinically relevant for CYP450 substrates with a narrow therapeutic index, where the dose is individually adjusted (eg, warfarin). Upon initiation of canakinumab, in patients being treated with these types of medicinal products, therapeutic monitoring of the effect or drug concentration should be performed and the individual dose of the medicinal product may need to be adjusted as needed). Products include:
InnoPran XL **1517**

Protriptyline Hydrochloride (The formation of CYP450 enzymes is suppressed by increased levels of cytokines (eg, IL-1) during chronic inflammation. Thus it is expected that for a molecule that binds to IL-1, such as canakinumab, the formation of CYP450 enzymes could be normalized. This is clinically relevant for CYP450 substrates with a narrow therapeutic index, where the dose is individually adjusted (eg, warfarin). Upon initiation of canakinumab, in patients being treated with these types of medicinal products, therapeutic monitoring of the effect or drug concentration should be performed and the individual dose of the medicinal product may need to be adjusted as needed).
No products indexed under this heading.

Quetiapine Fumarate (The formation of CYP450 enzymes is suppressed by increased levels of cytokines (eg, IL-1) during chronic inflammation. Thus it is expected that for a molecule that binds to IL-1, such as canakinumab, the formation of CYP450 enzymes could be normalized. This is clinically relevant for CYP450 substrates with a narrow therapeutic index, where the dose is individually adjusted (eg, warfarin). Upon initiation of canakinumab, in patients being treated with these types of medicinal products, therapeutic monitoring of the effect or drug concentration should be performed and the individual dose of the medicinal product may need to be adjusted as needed). Products include:
Seroquel **750**
Seroquel XR **759**

Quinidine Gluconate (The formation of CYP450 enzymes is suppressed by increased levels of cytokines (eg, IL-1) during chronic inflammation. Thus it is expected that for a molecule that binds to IL-1, such as canakinumab, the formation of CYP450 enzymes could be normalized. This is clinically relevant for CYP450 substrates with a narrow therapeutic index, where the dose is individually adjusted (eg, warfarin). Upon initiation of canakinumab, in patients being treated with these types of medicinal products, therapeutic monitoring of the effect or drug concentration should be performed and the individual dose of the medicinal product may need to be adjusted as needed).
No products indexed under this heading.

Quinidine Hydrochloride (The formation of CYP450 enzymes is suppressed by increased levels of cytokines (eg, IL-1) during chronic inflammation. Thus it is expected that for a molecule that binds to IL-1, such as canakinumab, the formation of CYP450 enzymes could be normalized. This is clinically relevant for CYP450 substrates with a narrow therapeutic index, where the dose is individually adjusted (eg, warfarin). Upon initiation of canakinumab, in patients being treated with these types of medicinal products, therapeutic monitoring of the effect or drug concentration should be performed and the individual dose of the medicinal product may need to be adjusted as needed).
No products indexed under this heading.

Quinidine Polygalacturonate (The formation of CYP450 enzymes is suppressed by increased levels of cytokines (eg, IL-1) during chronic inflammation. Thus it is expected that for a molecule that binds to IL-1, such as canakinumab, the formation of CYP450 enzymes could be normalized. This is clinically relevant for CYP450 substrates with a narrow therapeutic index, where the dose is individually adjusted (eg, warfarin). Upon initiation of canakinumab, in patients being treated with these types of medicinal products, therapeutic monitoring of the effect or drug concentration should be performed and the individual dose of the medicinal product may need to be adjusted as needed).
No products indexed under this heading.

Quinidine Sulfate (The formation of CYP450 enzymes is suppressed by increased levels of cytokines (eg, IL-1) during chronic inflammation. Thus it is expected that for a molecule that binds to IL-1, such as canakinumab, the formation of CYP450 enzymes could be normalized. This is clinically relevant for CYP450 substrates with a narrow therapeutic index, where the dose is individually adjusted (eg, warfarin). Upon initiation of canakinumab, in patients being treated with these types of medicinal products, therapeutic monitoring of the effect or drug concentration should be performed and the individual dose of the medicinal product may need to be adjusted as needed).
No products indexed under this heading.

Quinine (The formation of CYP450 enzymes is suppressed by increased levels of cytokines (eg, IL-1) during chronic inflammation. Thus it is expected that for a molecule that binds to IL-1, such as canakinumab, the formation of CYP450 enzymes could be normalized. This is clinically relevant for CYP450 substrates with a narrow therapeutic index, where the dose is individually adjusted (eg, warfarin). Upon initiation of canakinumab, in patients being treated with these types of medicinal products, therapeutic monitoring of the effect or drug concentration should be performed and the individual dose of the medicinal product may need to be adjusted as needed). Products include:
Hyland's Leg Cramps PM with Quinine **3315**

Quinine Sulfate (The formation of CYP450 enzymes is suppressed by increased levels of cytokines (eg, IL-1) during chronic inflammation. Thus it is expected that for a molecule that binds to IL-1, such as canakinumab, the formation of CYP450 enzymes could be normalized. This is clinically relevant for CYP450 substrates with a narrow therapeutic index, where the dose is individually adjusted (eg, warfarin). Upon initiation of canakinumab, in patients being treated with these types of medicinal products, therapeutic monitoring of the effect or drug concentration should be performed and the individual dose of the medicinal product may need to be adjusted as needed).
No products indexed under this heading.

Rabeprazole Sodium (The formation of CYP450 enzymes is suppressed by increased levels of cytokines (eg, IL-1) during chronic inflammation. Thus it is expected that for a molecule that binds to IL-1, such as canakinumab, the formation of CYP450 enzymes could be normalized. This is clinically relevant for CYP450 substrates with a narrow therapeutic index, where the dose is individually adjusted (eg, warfarin). Upon initiation of canakinumab, in patients being treated with these types of medicinal products, therapeutic monitoring of the effect or drug concentration should be performed and the individual dose of the medicinal product may need to be adjusted as needed). Products include:
Aciphex **1035**

Repaglinide (The formation of CYP450 enzymes is suppressed by increased levels of cytokines (eg, IL-1) during chronic inflammation. Thus it is expected that for a molecule that binds to IL-1, such as canakinumab, the formation of CYP450 enzymes could be normalized. This is clinically relevant for CYP450 substrates with a narrow therapeutic index, where the dose is individually adjusted (eg, warfarin). Upon initiation of canakinumab, in patients being treated with these types of medicinal products, therapeutic monitoring of the effect or drug concentration should be performed and the individual dose of the medicinal product may need to be adjusted as needed).
No products indexed under this heading.

Rifabutin (The formation of CYP450 enzymes is suppressed by increased levels of cytokines (eg, IL-1) during chronic inflammation. Thus it is expected that for a molecule that binds to IL-1, such as canakinumab, the formation of CYP450 enzymes could be normalized. This is clinically relevant for CYP450 substrates with a narrow therapeutic index, where the dose is individually adjusted (eg, warfarin). Upon initiation of canakinumab, in patients being treated with these types of medicinal products, therapeutic monitoring of the effect or drug concentration should be performed and the individual dose of the medicinal product may need to be adjusted as needed).
No products indexed under this heading.

Riluzole (The formation of CYP450 enzymes is suppressed by increased levels of cytokines (eg, IL-1) during chronic inflammation. Thus it is expected that for a molecule that binds to IL-1, such as canakinumab, the formation of CYP450 enzymes could be normalized. This is clinically relevant for CYP450 substrates with a narrow therapeutic index, where the dose is individually adjusted (eg, warfarin). Upon initiation of canakinumab, in patients being treated with these types of medicinal products, therapeutic monitoring of the effect or drug concentration should be performed and the individual dose of the medicinal product may need to be adjusted as needed). Products include:
Rilutek **3032**

Risperidone (The formation of CYP450 enzymes is suppressed by increased levels of cytokines (eg, IL-1) during chronic inflammation. Thus it is expected that for a molecule that binds to IL-1, such as canakinumab, the formation of CYP450 enzymes could be normalized. This is clinically relevant for CYP450 substrates with a narrow therapeutic index, where the dose is individually adjusted (eg, warfarin). Upon initiation of canakinumab, in patients being treated with these types of medicinal products, therapeutic monitoring of the effect or drug concentration should be performed and the individual dose of the medicinal product may need to be adjusted as needed). Products include:
Risperdal Consta **2682**

Ritonavir (The formation of CYP450 enzymes is suppressed by increased levels of cytokines (eg, IL-1) during chronic inflammation. Thus it is expected that for a molecule that binds to IL-1, such as canakinumab, the formation of CYP450 enzymes could be normalized. This is clinically relevant for CYP450 substrates with a narrow therapeutic index, where the dose is individually adjusted (eg, warfarin). Upon initiation of canakinumab, in patients being treated with these types of medicinal products, therapeutic monitoring of the effect or drug concentration should be performed and the individual dose of the medicinal product may need to be adjusted as needed). Products include:
Kaletra **458**
Norvir **509**

Rofecoxib (The formation of CYP450 enzymes is suppressed by increased levels of cytokines (eg, IL-1) during chronic inflammation. Thus it is expected that for a molecule that binds to IL-1, such as canakinumab, the formation of CYP450 enzymes could be normalized. This is clinically relevant for CYP450 substrates with a narrow therapeutic index, where the dose is individually adjusted (eg, warfarin). Upon initiation of canakinumab, in patients being treated with these types of medicinal products, therapeutic monitoring of the effect or drug concentration should be performed and the individual dose of the medicinal product may need to be adjusted as needed).
No products indexed under this heading.

Ropinirole Hydrochloride (The formation of CYP450 enzymes is suppressed by increased levels of cytokines (eg, IL-1) during chronic inflammation. Thus it is expected that for a molecule that binds to IL-1, such as canakinumab, the formation of CYP450 enzymes could be normalized. This is clinically relevant for CYP450 substrates with a narrow therapeutic index, where the dose is individually adjusted (eg, warfarin). Upon initiation of canakinumab, in patients being treated with these types of medicinal products, therapeutic monitoring of the effect or drug concentration should be performed and the individual dose of the medicinal product may need to be adjusted as needed). Products include:
Requip **1620**
Requip XL **1628**

Ropivacaine Hydrochloride (The formation of CYP450 enzymes is suppressed by increased levels of cytokines (eg, IL-1) during chronic inflammation. Thus it is expected that for a molecule that binds to IL-1, such as canakinumab, the formation of CYP450

847 **Interactions Index** **Ilaris**

enzymes could be normalized. This is clinically relevant for CYP450 substrates with a narrow therapeutic index, where the dose is individually adjusted (eg, warfarin). Upon initiation of canakinumab, in patients being treated with these types of medicinal products, therapeutic monitoring of the effect or drug concentration should be performed and the individual dose of the medicinal product may need to be adjusted as needed).
No products indexed under this heading.

Rosiglitazone (The formation of CYP450 enzymes is suppressed by increased levels of cytokines (eg, IL-1) during chronic inflammation. Thus it is expected that for a molecule that binds to IL-1, such as canakinumab, the formation of CYP450 enzymes could be normalized. This is clinically relevant for CYP450 substrates with a narrow therapeutic index, where the dose is individually adjusted (eg, warfarin). Upon initiation of canakinumab, in patients being treated with these types of medicinal products, therapeutic monitoring of the effect or drug concentration should be performed and the individual dose of the medicinal product may need to be adjusted as needed).
No products indexed under this heading.

Rosiglitazone Maleate (The formation of CYP450 enzymes is suppressed by increased levels of cytokines (eg, IL-1) during chronic inflammation. Thus it is expected that for a molecule that binds to IL-1, such as canakinumab, the formation of CYP450 enzymes could be normalized. This is clinically relevant for CYP450 substrates with a narrow therapeutic index, where the dose is individually adjusted (eg, warfarin). Upon initiation of canakinumab, in patients being treated with these types of medicinal products, therapeutic monitoring of the effect or drug concentration should be performed and the individual dose of the medicinal product may need to be adjusted as needed). Products include:
Avandamet **1345**
Avandaryl **1356**
Avandia **1366**

Rosiglitazone/Metformin (The formation of CYP450 enzymes is suppressed by increased levels of cytokines (eg, IL-1) during chronic inflammation. Thus it is expected that for a molecule that binds to IL-1, such as canakinumab, the formation of CYP450 enzymes could be normalized. This is clinically relevant for CYP450 substrates with a narrow therapeutic index, where the dose is individually adjusted (eg, warfarin). Upon initiation of canakinumab, in patients being treated with these types of medicinal products, therapeutic monitoring of the effect or drug concentration should be performed and the individual dose of the medicinal product may need to be adjusted as needed).
No products indexed under this heading.

Rotavirus Vaccine, Live, Oral, Tetravalent (No data are available on either the effects of live vaccination or the secondary transmission of infection by live vaccines in patients receiving canakinumab. Therefore, live vaccines should not be given concurrently with canakinumab. It is recommended that, if possible, pediatric and adult patients should complete all immunizations in accordance with current immunization guidelines prior to initiating canakinumab therapy).
No products indexed under this heading.

Rubella & Mumps Virus Vaccine Live (No data are available on either the effects of live vaccination or the secondary transmission of infection by live vaccines in patients receiving canakinumab. Therefore, live vaccines should not be given concurrently with canakinumab. It is recommended that, if possible, pediatric and adult patients should complete all immunizations in accordance with current immunization guidelines prior to initiating canakinumab therapy).
No products indexed under this heading.

Rubella Virus Vaccine Live (No data are available on either the effects of live vaccination or the secondary transmission of infection by live vaccines in patients receiving canakinumab. Therefore, live vaccines should not be given concurrently with canakinumab. It is recommended that, if possible, pediatric and adult patients should complete all immunizations in accordance with current immunization guidelines prior to initiating canakinumab therapy). Products include:
Meruvax II **2210**

Saquinavir (The formation of CYP450 enzymes is suppressed by increased levels of cytokines (eg, IL-1) during chronic inflammation. Thus it is expected that for a molecule that binds to IL-1, such as canakinumab, the formation of CYP450 enzymes could be normalized. This is clinically relevant for CYP450 substrates with a narrow therapeutic index, where the dose is individually adjusted (eg, warfarin). Upon initiation of canakinumab, in patients being treated with these types of medicinal products, therapeutic monitoring of the effect or drug concentration should be performed and the individual dose of the medicinal product may need to be adjusted as needed).
No products indexed under this heading.

Saquinavir Mesylate (The formation of CYP450 enzymes is suppressed by increased levels of cytokines (eg, IL-1) during chronic inflammation. Thus it is expected that for a molecule that binds to IL-1, such as canakinumab, the formation of CYP450 enzymes could be normalized. This is clinically relevant for CYP450 substrates with a narrow therapeutic index, where the dose is individually adjusted (eg, warfarin). Upon initiation of canakinumab, in patients being treated with these types of medicinal products, therapeutic monitoring of the effect or drug concentration should be performed and the individual dose of the medicinal product may need to be adjusted as needed).
No products indexed under this heading.

Sertraline Hydrochloride (The formation of CYP450 enzymes is suppressed by increased levels of cytokines (eg, IL-1) during chronic inflammation. Thus it is expected that for a molecule that binds to IL-1, such as canakinumab, the formation of CYP450 enzymes could be normalized. This is clinically relevant for CYP450 substrates with a narrow therapeutic index, where the dose is individually adjusted (eg, warfarin). Upon initiation of canakinumab, in patients being treated with these types of medicinal products, therapeutic monitoring of the effect or drug concentration should be performed and the individual dose of the medicinal product may need to be adjusted as needed).
No products indexed under this heading.

Sildenafil Citrate (The formation of CYP450 enzymes is suppressed by increased levels of cytokines (eg, IL-1) during chronic inflammation. Thus it is expected that for a molecule that binds to IL-1, such as canakinumab, the formation of CYP450 enzymes could be normalized. This is clinically relevant for CYP450 substrates with a narrow therapeutic index, where the dose is individually adjusted (eg, warfarin). Upon initiation of canakinumab, in patients being treated with these types of medicinal products, therapeutic monitoring of the effect or drug concentration should be performed and the individual dose of the medicinal product may need to be adjusted as needed).
No products indexed under this heading.

Simvastatin (The formation of CYP450 enzymes is suppressed by increased levels of cytokines (eg, IL-1) during chronic inflammation. Thus it is expected that for a molecule that binds to IL-1, such as canakinumab, the formation of CYP450 enzymes could be normalized. This is clinically relevant for CYP450 substrates with a narrow therapeutic index, where the dose is individually adjusted (eg, warfarin). Upon initiation of canakinumab, in patients being treated with these types of medicinal products, therapeutic monitoring of the effect or drug concentration should be performed and the individual dose of the medicinal product may need to be adjusted as needed). Products include:
Simcor **524**
Vytorin 10/10 .... **2303, 3240**
Vytorin 10/20 .... **2303, 3240**
Vytorin 10/40 .... **2303, 3240**
Vytorin 10/80 .... **2303, 3240**
Zocor **2289**

Sirolimus (The formation of CYP450 enzymes is suppressed by increased levels of cytokines (eg, IL-1) during chronic inflammation. Thus it is expected that for a molecule that binds to IL-1, such as canakinumab, the formation of CYP450 enzymes could be normalized. This is clinically relevant for CYP450 substrates with a narrow therapeutic index, where the dose is individually adjusted (eg, warfarin). Upon initiation of canakinumab, in patients being treated with these types of medicinal products, therapeutic monitoring of the effect or drug concentration should be performed and the individual dose of the medicinal product may need to be adjusted as needed). Products include:
Rapamune **3579**

Smallpox Vaccine (No data are available on either the effects of live vaccination or the secondary transmission of infection by live vaccines in patients receiving canakinumab. Therefore, live vaccines should not be given concurrently with canakinumab. It is recommended that, if possible, pediatric and adult patients should complete all immunizations in accordance with current immunization guidelines prior to initiating canakinumab therapy).
No products indexed under this heading.

Sulfamethoxazole (The formation of CYP450 enzymes is suppressed by increased levels of cytokines (eg, IL-1) during chronic inflammation. Thus it is expected that for a molecule that binds to IL-1, such as canakinumab, the formation of CYP450 enzymes could be normalized. This is clinically relevant for CYP450 substrates with a narrow therapeutic index, where the dose is individually adjusted (eg, warfarin). Upon initiation of canakinumab, in patients being treated with these types of medicinal products, therapeutic monitoring of the effect or drug concentration should be performed and the individual dose of the medicinal product may need to be adjusted as needed).
No products indexed under this heading.

Sulindac (The formation of CYP450 enzymes is suppressed by increased levels of cytokines (eg, IL-1) during chronic inflammation. Thus it is expected that for a molecule that binds to IL-1, such as canakinumab, the formation of CYP450 enzymes could be normalized. This is clinically relevant for CYP450 substrates with a narrow therapeutic index, where the dose is individually adjusted (eg, warfarin). Upon initiation of canakinumab, in patients being treated with these types of medicinal products, therapeutic monitoring of the effect or drug concentration should be performed and the individual dose of the medicinal product may need to be adjusted as needed). Products include:
Clinoril **2098**

Suprofen (The formation of CYP450 enzymes is suppressed by increased levels of cytokines (eg, IL-1) during chronic inflammation. Thus it is expected that for a molecule that binds to IL-1, such as canakinumab, the formation of CYP450 enzymes could be normalized. This is clinically relevant for CYP450 substrates with a narrow therapeutic index, where the dose is individually adjusted (eg, warfarin). Upon initiation of canakinumab, in patients being treated with these types of medicinal products, therapeutic monitoring of the effect or drug concentration should be performed and the individual dose of the medicinal product may need to be adjusted as needed).
No products indexed under this heading.

Tacrine Hydrochloride (The formation of CYP450 enzymes is suppressed by increased levels of cytokines (eg, IL-1) during chronic inflammation. Thus it is expected that for a molecule that binds to IL-1, such as canakinumab, the formation of CYP450 enzymes could be normalized. This is clinically relevant for CYP450 substrates with a narrow therapeutic index, where the dose is individually adjusted (eg, warfarin). Upon initiation of canakinumab, in patients being treated with these types of medicinal products, therapeutic monitoring of the effect or drug concentration should be performed and the individual dose of the medicinal product may need to be adjusted as needed).
No products indexed under this heading.

Tacrolimus (The formation of CYP450 enzymes is suppressed by increased levels of cytokines (eg, IL-1) during chronic inflammation. Thus it is expected that for a molecule that binds to IL-1, such as canakinumab, the formation of CYP450 enzymes could be normalized. This is clinically relevant for CYP450 substrates with a narrow therapeutic index, where the dose is individually adjusted (eg, warfarin). Upon initiation of canakinumab, in patients being treated with these types of medicinal products, therapeutic monitoring of the effect or drug concentration should be performed and the individual dose of the medicinal product may need to be adjusted as needed). Products include:
Prograf Capsules **677**
Prograf Injection **677**
Protopic **685**

Tadalafil (The formation of CYP450 enzymes is suppressed by increased levels of cytokines (eg, IL-1) during chronic inflammation. Thus it is expected that for a molecule that binds to IL-1, such as canakinumab, the formation of CYP450 enzymes could be normalized. This is clinically relevant for CYP450 substrates with a narrow therapeutic index, where the dose is individually adjusted (eg, warfarin). Upon initiation of canakinumab, in patients being treated with these types of medicinal products, therapeutic monitoring of the effect or drug concentration should be performed and the individual dose of the medicinal product may need to be adjusted as needed). Products include:
Adcirca **3461**
Cialis **1861**

Tamoxifen Citrate (The formation of CYP450 enzymes is suppressed by increased levels of cytokines (eg, IL-1) during chronic inflammation. Thus it is expected that for a molecule that binds to IL-1, such as canakinumab, the formation of CYP450 enzymes could be

normalized. This is clinically relevant for CYP450 substrates with a narrow therapeutic index, where the dose is individually adjusted (eg, warfarin). Upon initiation of canakinumab, in patients being treated with these types of medicinal products, therapeutic monitoring of the effect or drug concentration should be performed and the individual dose of the medicinal product may need to be adjusted as needed).

No products indexed under this heading.

Telmisartan (The formation of CYP450 enzymes is suppressed by increased levels of cytokines (eg, IL-1) during chronic inflammation. Thus it is expected that for a molecule that binds to IL-1, such as canakinumab, the formation of CYP450 enzymes could be normalized. This is clinically relevant for CYP450 substrates with a narrow therapeutic index, where the dose is individually adjusted (eg, warfarin). Upon initiation of canakinumab, in patients being treated with these types of medicinal products, therapeutic monitoring of the effect or drug concentration should be performed and the individual dose of the medicinal product may need to be adjusted as needed). Products include:

Teniposide (The formation of CYP450 enzymes is suppressed by increased levels of cytokines (eg, IL-1) during chronic inflammation. Thus it is expected that for a molecule that binds to IL-1, such as canakinumab, the formation of CYP450 enzymes could be normalized. This is clinically relevant for CYP450 substrates with a narrow therapeutic index, where the dose is individually adjusted (eg, warfarin). Upon initiation of canakinumab, in patients being treated with these types of medicinal products, therapeutic monitoring of the effect or drug concentration should be performed and the individual dose of the medicinal product may need to be adjusted as needed).

No products indexed under this heading.

Terfenadine (The formation of CYP450 enzymes is suppressed by increased levels of cytokines (eg, IL-1) during chronic inflammation. Thus it is expected that for a molecule that binds to IL-1, such as canakinumab, the formation of CYP450 enzymes could be normalized. This is clinically relevant for CYP450 substrates with a narrow therapeutic index, where the dose is individually adjusted (eg, warfarin). Upon initiation of canakinumab, in patients being treated with these types of medicinal products, therapeutic monitoring of the effect or drug concentration should be performed and the individual dose of the medicinal product may need to be adjusted as needed).

No products indexed under this heading.

Testosterone (The formation of CYP450 enzymes is suppressed by increased levels of cytokines (eg, IL-1) during chronic inflammation. Thus it is expected that for a molecule that binds to IL-1, such as canakinumab, the formation of CYP450 enzymes could be normalized. This is clinically relevant for CYP450 substrates with a narrow therapeutic index, where the dose is individually adjusted (eg, warfarin). Upon initiation of canakinumab, in patients being treated with these types of medicinal products, therapeutic monitoring of the effect or drug concentration should be performed and the individual dose of the medicinal product may need to be adjusted as needed). Products include:

Testosterone Cypionate (The formation of CYP450 enzymes is suppressed by increased levels of cytokines (eg, IL-1) during chronic inflammation. Thus

it is expected that for a molecule that binds to IL-1, such as canakinumab, the formation of CYP450 enzymes could be normalized. This is clinically relevant for CYP450 substrates with a narrow therapeutic index, where the dose is individually adjusted (eg, warfarin). Upon initiation of canakinumab, in patients being treated with these types of medicinal products, therapeutic monitoring of the effect or drug concentration should be performed and the individual dose of the medicinal product may need to be adjusted as needed).

No products indexed under this heading.

Testosterone Enanthate (The formation of CYP450 enzymes is suppressed by increased levels of cytokines (eg, IL-1) during chronic inflammation. Thus it is expected that for a molecule that binds to IL-1, such as canakinumab, the formation of CYP450 enzymes could be normalized. This is clinically relevant for CYP450 substrates with a narrow therapeutic index, where the dose is individually adjusted (eg, warfarin). Upon initiation of canakinumab, in patients being treated with these types of medicinal products, therapeutic monitoring of the effect or drug concentration should be performed and the individual dose of the medicinal product may need to be adjusted as needed). Products include:

Testosterone Propionate (The formation of CYP450 enzymes is suppressed by increased levels of cytokines (eg, IL-1) during chronic inflammation. Thus it is expected that for a molecule that binds to IL-1, such as canakinumab, the formation of CYP450 enzymes could be normalized. This is clinically relevant for CYP450 substrates with a narrow therapeutic index, where the dose is individually adjusted (eg, warfarin). Upon initiation of canakinumab, in patients being treated with these types of medicinal products, therapeutic monitoring of the effect or drug concentration should be performed and the individual dose of the medicinal product may need to be adjusted as needed).

No products indexed under this heading.

Theophylline (The formation of CYP450 enzymes is suppressed by increased levels of cytokines (eg, IL-1) during chronic inflammation. Thus it is expected that for a molecule that binds to IL-1, such as canakinumab, the formation of CYP450 enzymes could be normalized. This is clinically relevant for CYP450 substrates with a narrow therapeutic index, where the dose is individually adjusted (eg, warfarin). Upon initiation of canakinumab, in patients being treated with these types of medicinal products, therapeutic monitoring of the effect or drug concentration should be performed and the individual dose of the medicinal product may need to be adjusted as needed).

No products indexed under this heading.

Theophylline Anhydrous (The formation of CYP450 enzymes is suppressed by increased levels of cytokines (eg, IL-1) during chronic inflammation. Thus it is expected that for a molecule that binds to IL-1, such as canakinumab, the formation of CYP450 enzymes could be normalized. This is clinically relevant for CYP450 substrates with a narrow therapeutic index, where the dose is individually adjusted (eg, warfarin). Upon initiation of canakinumab, in patients being treated with these types of medicinal products, therapeutic monitoring of the effect or drug concentration should be performed and the individual dose of the medicinal product may need to be adjusted as needed). Products include:

Theophylline Calcium Salicylate (The formation of CYP450 enzymes is suppressed by increased levels of cytokines (eg, IL-1) during chronic inflammation. Thus it is expected that for a molecule that binds to IL-1, such as canakinumab, the formation of CYP450 enzymes could be normalized. This is clinically relevant for CYP450 substrates with a narrow therapeutic index, where the dose is individually adjusted (eg, warfarin). Upon initiation of canakinumab, in patients being treated with these types of medicinal products, therapeutic monitoring of the effect or drug concentration should be performed and the individual dose of the medicinal product may need to be adjusted as needed).

No products indexed under this heading.

Theophylline Dihydroxypropyl (Glyceryl) (The formation of CYP450 enzymes is suppressed by increased levels of cytokines (eg, IL-1) during chronic inflammation. Thus it is expected that for a molecule that binds to IL-1, such as canakinumab, the formation of CYP450 enzymes could be normalized. This is clinically relevant for CYP450 substrates with a narrow therapeutic index, where the dose is individually adjusted (eg, warfarin). Upon initiation of canakinumab, in patients being treated with these types of medicinal products, therapeutic monitoring of the effect or drug concentration should be performed and the individual dose of the medicinal product may need to be adjusted as needed).

No products indexed under this heading.

Theophylline Ethylenediamine (The formation of CYP450 enzymes is suppressed by increased levels of cytokines (eg, IL-1) during chronic inflammation. Thus it is expected that for a molecule that binds to IL-1, such as canakinumab, the formation of CYP450 enzymes could be normalized. This is clinically relevant for CYP450 substrates with a narrow therapeutic index, where the dose is individually adjusted (eg, warfarin). Upon initiation of canakinumab, in patients being treated with these types of medicinal products, therapeutic monitoring of the effect or drug concentration should be performed and the individual dose of the medicinal product may need to be adjusted as needed).

No products indexed under this heading.

Theophylline Sodium Glycinate (The formation of CYP450 enzymes is suppressed by increased levels of cytokines (eg, IL-1) during chronic inflammation. Thus it is expected that for a molecule that binds to IL-1, such as canakinumab, the formation of CYP450 enzymes could be normalized. This is clinically relevant for CYP450 substrates with a narrow therapeutic index, where the dose is individually adjusted (eg, warfarin). Upon initiation of canakinumab, in patients being treated with these types of medicinal products, therapeutic monitoring of the effect or drug concentration should be performed and the individual dose of the medicinal product may need to be adjusted as needed).

No products indexed under this heading.

Thioridazine (The formation of CYP450 enzymes is suppressed by increased levels of cytokines (eg, IL-1) during chronic inflammation. Thus it is expected that for a molecule that binds to IL-1, such as canakinumab, the formation of CYP450 enzymes could be normalized. This is clinically relevant for CYP450 substrates with a narrow therapeutic index, where the dose is individually adjusted (eg, warfarin). Upon initiation of canakinumab, in patients being treated with these types of medicinal

products, therapeutic monitoring of the effect or drug concentration should be performed and the individual dose of the medicinal product may need to be adjusted as needed).

No products indexed under this heading.

Thioridazine Hydrochloride (The formation of CYP450 enzymes is suppressed by increased levels of cytokines (eg, IL-1) during chronic inflammation. Thus it is expected that for a molecule that binds to IL-1, such as canakinumab, the formation of CYP450 enzymes could be normalized. This is clinically relevant for CYP450 substrates with a narrow therapeutic index, where the dose is individually adjusted (eg, warfarin). Upon initiation of canakinumab, in patients being treated with these types of medicinal products, therapeutic monitoring of the effect or drug concentration should be performed and the individual dose of the medicinal product may need to be adjusted as needed). Products include:

Tiagabine Hydrochloride (The formation of CYP450 enzymes is suppressed by increased levels of cytokines (eg, IL-1) during chronic inflammation. Thus it is expected that for a molecule that binds to IL-1, such as canakinumab, the formation of CYP450 enzymes could be normalized. This is clinically relevant for CYP450 substrates with a narrow therapeutic index, where the dose is individually adjusted (eg, warfarin). Upon initiation of canakinumab, in patients being treated with these types of medicinal products, therapeutic monitoring of the effect or drug concentration should be performed and the individual dose of the medicinal product may need to be adjusted as needed). Products include:

Timolol Maleate (The formation of CYP450 enzymes is suppressed by increased levels of cytokines (eg, IL-1) during chronic inflammation. Thus it is expected that for a molecule that binds to IL-1, such as canakinumab, the formation of CYP450 enzymes could be normalized. This is clinically relevant for CYP450 substrates with a narrow therapeutic index, where the dose is individually adjusted (eg, warfarin). Upon initiation of canakinumab, in patients being treated with these types of medicinal products, therapeutic monitoring of the effect or drug concentration should be performed and the individual dose of the medicinal product may need to be adjusted as needed). Products include:

Tolazamide (The formation of CYP450 enzymes is suppressed by increased levels of cytokines (eg, IL-1) during chronic inflammation. Thus it is expected that for a molecule that binds to IL-1, such as canakinumab, the formation of CYP450 enzymes could be normalized. This is clinically relevant for CYP450 substrates with a narrow therapeutic index, where the dose is individually adjusted (eg, warfarin). Upon initiation of canakinumab, in patients being treated with these types of medicinal products, therapeutic monitoring of the effect or drug concentration should be performed and the individual dose of the medicinal product may need to be adjusted as needed).

No products indexed under this heading.

Tolbutamide (The formation of CYP450 enzymes is suppressed by increased levels of cytokines (eg, IL-1) during chronic inflammation. Thus it is expected that for a molecule that binds

to IL-1, such as canakinumab, the formation of CYP450 enzymes could be normalized. This is clinically relevant for CYP450 substrates with a narrow therapeutic index, where the dose is individually adjusted (eg, warfarin). Upon initiation of canakinumab, in patients being treated with these types of medicinal products, therapeutic monitoring of the effect or drug concentration should be performed and the individual dose of the medicinal product may need to be adjusted as needed).
No products indexed under this heading.

Tolbutamide Sodium (The formation of CYP450 enzymes is suppressed by increased levels of cytokines (eg, IL-1) during chronic inflammation. Thus it is expected that for a molecule that binds to IL-1, such as canakinumab, the formation of CYP450 enzymes could be normalized. This is clinically relevant for CYP450 substrates with a narrow therapeutic index, where the dose is individually adjusted (eg, warfarin). Upon initiation of canakinumab, in patients being treated with these types of medicinal products, therapeutic monitoring of the effect or drug concentration should be performed and the individual dose of the medicinal product may need to be adjusted as needed).
No products indexed under this heading.

Tolmetin Sodium (The formation of CYP450 enzymes is suppressed by increased levels of cytokines (eg, IL-1) during chronic inflammation. Thus it is expected that for a molecule that binds to IL-1, such as canakinumab, the formation of CYP450 enzymes could be normalized. This is clinically relevant for CYP450 substrates with a narrow therapeutic index, where the dose is individually adjusted (eg, warfarin). Upon initiation of canakinumab, in patients being treated with these types of medicinal products, therapeutic monitoring of the effect or drug concentration should be performed and the individual dose of the medicinal product may need to be adjusted as needed).
No products indexed under this heading.

Tolterodine Tartrate (The formation of CYP450 enzymes is suppressed by increased levels of cytokines (eg, IL-1) during chronic inflammation. Thus it is expected that for a molecule that binds to IL-1, such as canakinumab, the formation of CYP450 enzymes could be normalized. This is clinically relevant for CYP450 substrates with a narrow therapeutic index, where the dose is individually adjusted (eg, warfarin). Upon initiation of canakinumab, in patients being treated with these types of medicinal products, therapeutic monitoring of the effect or drug concentration should be performed and the individual dose of the medicinal product may need to be adjusted as needed).
No products indexed under this heading.

Topiramate (The formation of CYP450 enzymes is suppressed by increased levels of cytokines (eg, IL-1) during chronic inflammation. Thus it is expected that for a molecule that binds to IL-1, such as canakinumab, the formation of CYP450 enzymes could be normalized. This is clinically relevant for CYP450 substrates with a narrow therapeutic index, where the dose is individually adjusted (eg, warfarin). Upon initiation of canakinumab, in patients being treated with these types of medicinal products, therapeutic monitoring of the effect or drug concentration should be performed and the individual dose of the medicinal product may need to be adjusted as needed).
No products indexed under this heading.

Torsemide (The formation of CYP450 enzymes is suppressed by increased levels of cytokines (eg, IL-1) during

chronic inflammation. Thus it is expected that for a molecule that binds to IL-1, such as canakinumab, the formation of CYP450 enzymes could be normalized. This is clinically relevant for CYP450 substrates with a narrow therapeutic index, where the dose is individually adjusted (eg, warfarin). Upon initiation of canakinumab, in patients being treated with these types of medicinal products, therapeutic monitoring of the effect or drug concentration should be performed and the individual dose of the medicinal product may need to be adjusted as needed).
No products indexed under this heading.

Tramadol Hydrochloride (The formation of CYP450 enzymes is suppressed by increased levels of cytokines (eg, IL-1) during chronic inflammation. Thus it is expected that for a molecule that binds to IL-1, such as canakinumab, the formation of CYP450 enzymes could be normalized. This is clinically relevant for CYP450 substrates with a narrow therapeutic index, where the dose is individually adjusted (eg, warfarin). Upon initiation of canakinumab, in patients being treated with these types of medicinal products, therapeutic monitoring of the effect or drug concentration should be performed and the individual dose of the medicinal product may need to be adjusted as needed). Products include:

Trazodone Hydrochloride (The formation of CYP450 enzymes is suppressed by increased levels of cytokines (eg, IL-1) during chronic inflammation. Thus it is expected that for a molecule that binds to IL-1, such as canakinumab, the formation of CYP450 enzymes could be normalized. This is clinically relevant for CYP450 substrates with a narrow therapeutic index, where the dose is individually adjusted (eg, warfarin). Upon initiation of canakinumab, in patients being treated with these types of medicinal products, therapeutic monitoring of the effect or drug concentration should be performed and the individual dose of the medicinal product may need to be adjusted as needed).
No products indexed under this heading.

Tretinoin (The formation of CYP450 enzymes is suppressed by increased levels of cytokines (eg, IL-1) during chronic inflammation. Thus it is expected that for a molecule that binds to IL-1, such as canakinumab, the formation of CYP450 enzymes could be normalized. This is clinically relevant for CYP450 substrates with a narrow therapeutic index, where the dose is individually adjusted (eg, warfarin). Upon initiation of canakinumab, in patients being treated with these types of medicinal products, therapeutic monitoring of the effect or drug concentration should be performed and the individual dose of the medicinal product may need to be adjusted as needed).
No products indexed under this heading.

Triazolam (The formation of CYP450 enzymes is suppressed by increased levels of cytokines (eg, IL-1) during chronic inflammation. Thus it is expected that for a molecule that binds to IL-1, such as canakinumab, the formation of CYP450 enzymes could be normalized. This is clinically relevant for CYP450 substrates with a narrow therapeutic index, where the dose is individually adjusted (eg, warfarin). Upon initiation of canakinumab, in patients being treated with these types of medicinal products, therapeutic monitoring of the effect or drug concentration should be

performed and the individual dose of the medicinal product may need to be adjusted as needed).
No products indexed under this heading.

Trimethadione (The formation of CYP450 enzymes is suppressed by increased levels of cytokines (eg, IL-1) during chronic inflammation. Thus it is expected that for a molecule that binds to IL-1, such as canakinumab, the formation of CYP450 enzymes could be normalized. This is clinically relevant for CYP450 substrates with a narrow therapeutic index, where the dose is individually adjusted (eg, warfarin). Upon initiation of canakinumab, in patients being treated with these types of medicinal products, therapeutic monitoring of the effect or drug concentration should be performed and the individual dose of the medicinal product may need to be adjusted as needed).
No products indexed under this heading.

Trimethaphan Camsylate (The formation of CYP450 enzymes is suppressed by increased levels of cytokines (eg, IL-1) during chronic inflammation. Thus it is expected that for a molecule that binds to IL-1, such as canakinumab, the formation of CYP450 enzymes could be normalized. This is clinically relevant for CYP450 substrates with a narrow therapeutic index, where the dose is individually adjusted (eg, warfarin). Upon initiation of canakinumab, in patients being treated with these types of medicinal products, therapeutic monitoring of the effect or drug concentration should be performed and the individual dose of the medicinal product may need to be adjusted as needed).
No products indexed under this heading.

Trimipramine Maleate (The formation of CYP450 enzymes is suppressed by increased levels of cytokines (eg, IL-1) during chronic inflammation. Thus it is expected that for a molecule that binds to IL-1, such as canakinumab, the formation of CYP450 enzymes could be normalized. This is clinically relevant for CYP450 substrates with a narrow therapeutic index, where the dose is individually adjusted (eg, warfarin). Upon initiation of canakinumab, in patients being treated with these types of medicinal products, therapeutic monitoring of the effect or drug concentration should be performed and the individual dose of the medicinal product may need to be adjusted as needed).
No products indexed under this heading.

Troglitazone (The formation of CYP450 enzymes is suppressed by increased levels of cytokines (eg, IL-1) during chronic inflammation. Thus it is expected that for a molecule that binds to IL-1, such as canakinumab, the formation of CYP450 enzymes could be normalized. This is clinically relevant for CYP450 substrates with a narrow therapeutic index, where the dose is individually adjusted (eg, warfarin). Upon initiation of canakinumab, in patients being treated with these types of medicinal products, therapeutic monitoring of the effect or drug concentration should be performed and the individual dose of the medicinal product may need to be adjusted as needed).
No products indexed under this heading.

Trovafloxacin Mesylate (The formation of CYP450 enzymes is suppressed by increased levels of cytokines (eg, IL-1) during chronic inflammation. Thus it is expected that for a molecule that binds to IL-1, such as canakinumab, the formation of CYP450 enzymes could be normalized. This is clinically relevant for CYP450 substrates with a narrow therapeutic index, where the dose is individually adjusted (eg, warfarin). Upon initiation of canakinumab, in patients being

treated with these types of medicinal products, therapeutic monitoring of the effect or drug concentration should be performed and the individual dose of the medicinal product may need to be adjusted as needed).
No products indexed under this heading.

Typhoid Vaccine (No data are available on either the effects of live vaccination or the secondary transmission of infection by live vaccines in patients receiving canakinumab. Therefore, live vaccines should not be given concurrently with canakinumab. It is recommended that, if possible, pediatric and adult patients should complete all immunizations in accordance with current immunization guidelines prior to initiating canakinumab therapy).
No products indexed under this heading.

Valdecoxib (The formation of CYP450 enzymes is suppressed by increased levels of cytokines (eg, IL-1) during chronic inflammation. Thus it is expected that for a molecule that binds to IL-1, such as canakinumab, the formation of CYP450 enzymes could be normalized. This is clinically relevant for CYP450 substrates with a narrow therapeutic index, where the dose is individually adjusted (eg, warfarin). Upon initiation of canakinumab, in patients being treated with these types of medicinal products, therapeutic monitoring of the effect or drug concentration should be performed and the individual dose of the medicinal product may need to be adjusted as needed).
No products indexed under this heading.

Valproate Sodium (The formation of CYP450 enzymes is suppressed by increased levels of cytokines (eg, IL-1) during chronic inflammation. Thus it is expected that for a molecule that binds to IL-1, such as canakinumab, the formation of CYP450 enzymes could be normalized. This is clinically relevant for CYP450 substrates with a narrow therapeutic index, where the dose is individually adjusted (eg, warfarin). Upon initiation of canakinumab, in patients being treated with these types of medicinal products, therapeutic monitoring of the effect or drug concentration should be performed and the individual dose of the medicinal product may need to be adjusted as needed).
No products indexed under this heading.

Valproic Acid (The formation of CYP450 enzymes is suppressed by increased levels of cytokines (eg, IL-1) during chronic inflammation. Thus it is expected that for a molecule that binds to IL-1, such as canakinumab, the formation of CYP450 enzymes could be normalized. This is clinically relevant for CYP450 substrates with a narrow therapeutic index, where the dose is individually adjusted (eg, warfarin). Upon initiation of canakinumab, in patients being treated with these types of medicinal products, therapeutic monitoring of the effect or drug concentration should be performed and the individual dose of the medicinal product may need to be adjusted as needed).
No products indexed under this heading.

Valsartan (The formation of CYP450 enzymes is suppressed by increased levels of cytokines (eg, IL-1) during chronic inflammation. Thus it is expected that for a molecule that binds to IL-1, such as canakinumab, the formation of CYP450 enzymes could be normalized. This is clinically relevant for CYP450 substrates with a narrow therapeutic index, where the dose is individually adjusted (eg, warfarin). Upon initiation of canakinumab, in patients being treated with these types of medicinal products, therapeutic monitoring of the effect or drug concentration should be performed and the individual dose of

Ilaris Interactions Index 850

the medicinal product may need to be adjusted as needed). Products include:
Diovan 2413
Diovan HCT 2419
Exforge 2443
Exforge HCT 2449
Valturna 3637

Vardenafil Hydrochloride (The formation of CYP450 enzymes is suppressed by increased levels of cytokines (eg, IL-1) during chronic inflammation. Thus it is expected that for a molecule that binds to IL-1, such as canakinumab, the formation of CYP450 enzymes could be normalized. This is clinically relevant for CYP450 substrates with a narrow therapeutic index, where the dose is individually adjusted (eg, warfarin). Upon initiation of canakinumab, in patients being treated with these types of medicinal products, therapeutic monitoring of the effect or drug concentration should be performed and the individual dose of the medicinal product may need to be adjusted as needed). Products include:
Levitra 3157

Varicella Virus Vaccine, Live (No data are available on either the effects of live vaccination or the secondary transmission of infection by live vaccines in patients receiving canakinumab. Therefore, live vaccines should not be given concurrently with canakinumab. It is recommended that, if possible, pediatric and adult patients should complete all immunizations in accordance with current immunization guidelines prior to initiating canakinumab therapy). Products include:
Varivax 2285

Venlafaxine Hydrochloride (The formation of CYP450 enzymes is suppressed by increased levels of cytokines (eg, IL-1) during chronic inflammation. Thus it is expected that for a molecule that binds to IL-1, such as canakinumab, the formation of CYP450 enzymes could be normalized. This is clinically relevant for CYP450 substrates with a narrow therapeutic index, where the dose is individually adjusted (eg, warfarin). Upon initiation of canakinumab, in patients being treated with these types of medicinal products, therapeutic monitoring of the effect or drug concentration should be performed and the individual dose of the medicinal product may need to be adjusted as needed). Products include:
Effexor XR 3504
Venlafaxine Hydrochloride Tablets 2388

Verapamil Hydrochloride (The formation of CYP450 enzymes is suppressed by increased levels of cytokines (eg, IL-1) during chronic inflammation. Thus it is expected that for a molecule that binds to IL-1, such as canakinumab, the formation of CYP450 enzymes could be normalized. This is clinically relevant for CYP450 substrates with a narrow therapeutic index, where the dose is individually adjusted (eg, warfarin). Upon initiation of canakinumab, in patients being treated with these types of medicinal products, therapeutic monitoring of the effect or drug concentration should be performed and the individual dose of the medicinal product may need to be adjusted as needed). Products include:
Tarka 534

Vinblastine Sulfate (The formation of CYP450 enzymes is suppressed by increased levels of cytokines (eg, IL-1) during chronic inflammation. Thus it is expected that for a molecule that binds to IL-1, such as canakinumab, the formation of CYP450 enzymes could be normalized. This is clinically relevant for CYP450 substrates with a narrow therapeutic index, where the dose is individually adjusted (eg, warfarin). Upon initiation of canakinumab, in patients being treated with these types of medicinal products, therapeutic monitoring of the effect or drug concentration should be performed and the individual dose of the medicinal product may need to be adjusted as needed).
No products indexed under this heading.

Vincristine Sulfate (The formation of CYP450 enzymes is suppressed by increased levels of cytokines (eg, IL-1) during chronic inflammation. Thus it is expected that for a molecule that binds to IL-1, such as canakinumab, the formation of CYP450 enzymes could be normalized. This is clinically relevant for CYP450 substrates with a narrow therapeutic index, where the dose is individually adjusted (eg, warfarin). Upon initiation of canakinumab, in patients being treated with these types of medicinal products, therapeutic monitoring of the effect or drug concentration should be performed and the individual dose of the medicinal product may need to be adjusted as needed).
No products indexed under this heading.

Vitamin A (The formation of CYP450 enzymes is suppressed by increased levels of cytokines (eg, IL-1) during chronic inflammation. Thus it is expected that for a molecule that binds to IL-1, such as canakinumab, the formation of CYP450 enzymes could be normalized. This is clinically relevant for CYP450 substrates with a narrow therapeutic index, where the dose is individually adjusted (eg, warfarin). Upon initiation of canakinumab, in patients being treated with these types of medicinal products, therapeutic monitoring of the effect or drug concentration should be performed and the individual dose of the medicinal product may need to be adjusted as needed). Products include:
Cardio Basics 3455
Heplive 607
Norwegian Cod Liver Oil 919

Vitamin A Acetate (The formation of CYP450 enzymes is suppressed by increased levels of cytokines (eg, IL-1) during chronic inflammation. Thus it is expected that for a molecule that binds to IL-1, such as canakinumab, the formation of CYP450 enzymes could be normalized. This is clinically relevant for CYP450 substrates with a narrow therapeutic index, where the dose is individually adjusted (eg, warfarin). Upon initiation of canakinumab, in patients being treated with these types of medicinal products, therapeutic monitoring of the effect or drug concentration should be performed and the individual dose of the medicinal product may need to be adjusted as needed).
No products indexed under this heading.

Voriconazole (The formation of CYP450 enzymes is suppressed by increased levels of cytokines (eg, IL-1) during chronic inflammation. Thus it is expected that for a molecule that binds to IL-1, such as canakinumab, the formation of CYP450 enzymes could be normalized. This is clinically relevant for CYP450 substrates with a narrow therapeutic index, where the dose is individually adjusted (eg, warfarin). Upon initiation of canakinumab, in patients being treated with these types of medicinal products, therapeutic monitoring of the effect or drug concentration should be performed and the individual dose of the medicinal product may need to be adjusted as needed).
No products indexed under this heading.

Warfarin Sodium (The formation of CYP450 enzymes is suppressed by increased levels of cytokines (eg, IL-1) during chronic inflammation. Thus it is expected that for a molecule that binds to IL-1, such as canakinumab, the formation of CYP450 enzymes could be normalized. This is clinically relevant for CYP450 substrates with a narrow therapeutic index, where the dose is individually adjusted (eg, warfarin). Upon initiation of canakinumab, in patients being treated with these types of medicinal products, therapeutic monitoring of the effect or drug concentration should be performed and the individual dose of the medicinal product may need to be adjusted as needed).
No products indexed under this heading.

Yellow Fever Vaccine (No data are available on either the effects of live vaccination or the secondary transmission of infection by live vaccines in patients receiving canakinumab. Therefore, live vaccines should not be given concurrently with canakinumab. It is recommended that, if possible, pediatric and adult patients should complete all immunizations in accordance with current immunization guidelines prior to initiating canakinumab therapy).
No products indexed under this heading.

Zafirlukast (The formation of CYP450 enzymes is suppressed by increased levels of cytokines (eg, IL-1) during chronic inflammation. Thus it is expected that for a molecule that binds to IL-1, such as canakinumab, the formation of CYP450 enzymes could be normalized. This is clinically relevant for CYP450 substrates with a narrow therapeutic index, where the dose is individually adjusted (eg, warfarin). Upon initiation of canakinumab, in patients being treated with these types of medicinal products, therapeutic monitoring of the effect or drug concentration should be performed and the individual dose of the medicinal product may need to be adjusted as needed). Products include:
Accolate 3612

Zileuton (The formation of CYP450 enzymes is suppressed by increased levels of cytokines (eg, IL-1) during chronic inflammation. Thus it is expected that for a molecule that binds to IL-1, such as canakinumab, the formation of CYP450 enzymes could be normalized. This is clinically relevant for CYP450 substrates with a narrow therapeutic index, where the dose is individually adjusted (eg, warfarin). Upon initiation of canakinumab, in patients being treated with these types of medicinal products, therapeutic monitoring of the effect or drug concentration should be performed and the individual dose of the medicinal product may need to be adjusted as needed).
No products indexed under this heading.

Zolmitriptan (The formation of CYP450 enzymes is suppressed by increased levels of cytokines (eg, IL-1) during chronic inflammation. Thus it is expected that for a molecule that binds to IL-1, such as canakinumab, the formation of CYP450 enzymes could be normalized. This is clinically relevant for CYP450 substrates with a narrow therapeutic index, where the dose is individually adjusted (eg, warfarin). Upon initiation of canakinumab, in patients being treated with these types of medicinal products, therapeutic monitoring of the effect or drug concentration should be performed and the individual dose of the medicinal product may need to be adjusted as needed). Products include:
Zomig Tablets 773
Zomig Nasal Spray 768
Zomig-ZMT Tablets 773

Zonisamide (The formation of CYP450 enzymes is suppressed by increased levels of cytokines (eg, IL-1) during chronic inflammation. Thus it is expected that for a molecule that binds to IL-1, such as canakinumab, the formation of CYP450 enzymes could be normalized. This is clinically relevant for CYP450 substrates with a narrow therapeutic index, where the dose is individually adjusted (eg, warfarin). Upon initiation of canakinumab, in patients being treated with these types of medicinal products, therapeutic monitoring of the effect or drug concentration should be performed and the individual dose of the medicinal product may need to be adjusted as needed). Products include:
Zonegran 1081

Zopiclone (The formation of CYP450 enzymes is suppressed by increased levels of cytokines (eg, IL-1) during chronic inflammation. Thus it is expected that for a molecule that binds to IL-1, such as canakinumab, the formation of CYP450 enzymes could be normalized. This is clinically relevant for CYP450 substrates with a narrow therapeutic index, where the dose is individually adjusted (eg, warfarin). Upon initiation of canakinumab, in patients being treated with these types of medicinal products, therapeutic monitoring of the effect or drug concentration should be performed and the individual dose of the medicinal product may need to be adjusted as needed).
No products indexed under this heading.

Zoster Vaccine Live (No data are available on either the effects of live vaccination or the secondary transmission of infection by live vaccines in patients receiving canakinumab. Therefore, live vaccines should not be given concurrently with canakinumab. It is recommended that, if possible, pediatric and adult patients should complete all immunizations in accordance with current immunization guidelines prior to initiating canakinumab therapy).
Products include:
Zostavax 2299

Food Interactions

Beverages, caffeine-containing (The formation of CYP450 enzymes is suppressed by increased levels of cytokines (eg, IL-1) during chronic inflammation. Thus it is expected that for a molecule that binds to IL-1, such as canakinumab, the formation of CYP450 enzymes could be normalized. This is clinically relevant for CYP450 substrates with a narrow therapeutic index, where the dose is individually adjusted (eg, warfarin). Upon initiation of canakinumab, in patients being treated with these types of medicinal products, therapeutic monitoring of the effect or drug concentration should be performed and the individual dose of the medicinal product may need to be adjusted as needed).

Food, caffeine-containing (The formation of CYP450 enzymes is suppressed by increased levels of cytokines (eg, IL-1) during chronic inflammation. Thus it is expected that for a molecule that binds to IL-1, such as canakinumab, the formation of CYP450 enzymes could be normalized. This is clinically relevant for CYP450 substrates with a narrow therapeutic index, where the dose is individually adjusted (eg, warfarin). Upon initiation of canakinumab, in patients being treated with these types of medicinal products, therapeutic monitoring of the effect or drug concentration should be performed and the individual dose of the medicinal product may need to be adjusted as needed).

IMITREX INJECTION

(Sumatriptan Succinate) 1497
May interact with 5HT1-receptor agonists, ergot-containing drugs, nonselective MAO inhibitors, selective serotonin reuptake inhibitors, serotonin and norepinephrine reuptake inhibitors, and certain other agents. Compounds in these categories include:

Almotriptan Malate (Sumatriptan succinate injection and any ergotamine-

851 Interactions Index Imitrex

containing or ergot-type medication (like dihydroergotamine or methysergide) should not be used within 24 hours of each other, nor should sumatriptan succinate injection and another 5-HT_1 agonist). Products include:
Axert 2593

Citalopram Hydrobromide (The development of a potentially life-threatening serotonin syndrome may occur with triptans, including treatment with sumatriptan succinate, particularly during combined use with selective serotonin reuptake inhibitors (SSRIs) or serotonin norepinephrine reuptake inhibitors (SNRIs). If concomitant treatment with sumatriptan and an SSRI (eg, fluoxetine,paroxetine, sertraline, fluvoxamine, citalopram, escitalopram) or SNRI (eg, venlafaxine, duloxetine) is clinically warranted, careful observation of the patient is advised, particularly during treatment initiation and dose increases). Products include:
Celexa 1153

Desvenlafaxine Succinate (The development of a potentially life-threatening serotonin syndrome may occur with triptans, including sumatriptan treatment, particularly during combined use with selective serotonin reuptake inhibitors (SSRIs) or serotonin norepinephrine reuptake inhibitors (SNRIs). If concomitant treatment with sumatriptan and an SSRI (eg, fluoxetine, paroxetine, sertraline, fluvoxamine, citalopram, escitalopram) or SNRI (eg, venlafaxine, duloxetine) is clinically warranted, careful observation of the patient is advised, particularly during treatment initiation and dose increases). Products include:
Pristiq 3564

Dihydroergotamine Mesylate (Ergot-containing drugs have been reported to cause prolonged vasospastic reactions; because there is a theoretical basis that these effects may be additive, use of ergot-type agents and sumatriptan within 24 hours is contraindicated).
No products indexed under this heading.

Duloxetine Hydrochloride (The development of a potentially life-threatening serotonin syndrome may occur with triptans, including treatment with sumatriptan succinate, particularly during combined use with selective serotonin reuptake inhibitors (SSRIs) or serotonin norepinephrine reuptake inhibitors (SNRIs). If concomitant treatment with sumatriptan and an SSRI (eg, fluoxetine,paroxetine, sertraline, fluvoxamine, citalopram, escitalopram) or SNRI (eg, venlafaxine, duloxetine) is clinically warranted, careful observation of the patient is advised, particularly during treatment initiation and dose increases). Products include:
Cymbalta 1871

Eletriptan Hydrobromide (Sumatriptan succinate injection and any ergotamine-containing or ergot-type medication (like dihydroergotamine or methysergide) should not be used within 24 hours of each other, nor should sumatriptan succinate injection and another 5-HT_1 agonist).
No products indexed under this heading.

Ergonovine Maleate (Ergot-containing drugs have been reported to cause prolonged vasospastic reactions; because there is a theoretical basis that these effects may be additive, use of ergot-type agents and sumatriptan within 24 hours is contraindicated).
No products indexed under this heading.

Ergotamine Tartrate (Ergot-containing drugs have been reported to cause prolonged vasospastic reactions; because there is a theoretical basis that these effects may be additive, use of ergot-type agents and sumatriptan within 24 hours is contraindicated).
No products indexed under this heading.

Escitalopram Oxalate (The development of a potentially life-threatening serotonin syndrome may occur with triptans, including treatment with sumatriptan succinate, particularly during combined use with selective serotonin reuptake inhibitors (SSRIs) or serotonin norepinephrine reuptake inhibitors (SNRIs). If concomitant treatment with sumatriptan and an SSRI (eg, fluoxetine,paroxetine, sertraline, fluvoxamine, citalopram, escitalopram) or SNRI (eg, venlafaxine, duloxetine) is clinically warranted, careful observation of the patient is advised, particularly during treatment initiation and dose increases). Products include:
Lexapro Oral Suspension 1160
Lexapro Tablets 1160

Fluoxetine (The development of a potentially life-threatening serotonin syndrome may occur with triptans, including treatment with sumatriptan succinate, particularly during combined use with selective serotonin reuptake inhibitors (SSRIs) or serotonin norepinephrine reuptake inhibitors (SNRIs). If concomitant treatment with sumatriptan and an SSRI (eg, fluoxetine,paroxetine, sertraline, fluvoxamine, citalopram, escitalopram) or SNRI (eg, venlafaxine, duloxetine) is clinically warranted, careful observation of the patient is advised, particularly during treatment initiation and dose increases).
No products indexed under this heading.

Fluoxetine Hydrochloride (The development of a potentially life-threatening serotonin syndrome may occur with triptans, including treatment with sumatriptan succinate, particularly during combined use with selective serotonin reuptake inhibitors (SSRIs) or serotonin norepinephrine reuptake inhibitors (SNRIs). If concomitant treatment with sumatriptan and an SSRI (eg, fluoxetine,paroxetine, sertraline, fluvoxamine, citalopram, escitalopram) or SNRI (eg, venlafaxine, duloxetine) is clinically warranted, careful observation of the patient is advised, particularly during treatment initiation and dose increases). Products include:
Prozac Weekly 1941
Prozac Pulvules 1941
Symbyax 1965

Fluvoxamine (The development of a potentially life-threatening serotonin syndrome may occur with triptans, including treatment with sumatriptan succinate, particularly during combined use with selective serotonin reuptake inhibitors (SSRIs) or serotonin norepinephrine reuptake inhibitors (SNRIs). If concomitant treatment with sumatriptan and an SSRI (eg, fluoxetine,paroxetine, sertraline, fluvoxamine, citalopram, escitalopram) or SNRI (eg, venlafaxine, duloxetine) is clinically warranted, careful observation of the patient is advised, particularly during treatment initiation and dose increases).
No products indexed under this heading.

Fluvoxamine Maleate (The development of a potentially life-threatening serotonin syndrome may occur with triptans, including treatment with sumatriptan succinate, particularly during combined use with selective serotonin reuptake inhibitors (SSRIs) or serotonin norepinephrine reuptake inhibitors (SNRIs). If concomitant treatment with sumatriptan and an SSRI (eg, fluoxetine,paroxetine, sertraline, fluvoxamine, citalopram, escitalopram) or SNRI (eg, venlafaxine, duloxetine) is clinically warranted, careful observation of the patient is advised, particularly during treatment initiation and dose increases).
No products indexed under this heading.

Frovatriptan Succinate (Sumatriptan succinate injection and any ergotamine-containing or ergot-type medication (like dihydroergotamine or methysergide) should not be used within 24 hours of each other, nor should sumatriptan succinate injection and another 5-HT_1 agonist). Products include:
Frova 1103

Isocarboxazid (*In vitro* studies with human microsomes suggest that sumatriptan is metabolized by monoamine oxidase (MAO), predominantly the A isoenzyme. In a study of 14 healthy females, pretreatment with MAO-A inhibitor decreased the clearance of sumatriptan. Under the conditions of this experiment, the result was a 2-fold increase in the area under the sumatriptan plasma concentration x time curve (AUC), corresponding to a 40% increase in elimination half-life. No significant effect was seen with an MAO-B inhibitor). Products include:
Marplan 3481

Methylergonovine Maleate (Ergot-containing drugs have been reported to cause prolonged vasospastic reactions; because there is a theoretical basis that these effects may be additive, use of ergot-type agents and sumatriptan within 24 hours is contraindicated).
No products indexed under this heading.

Methysergide Maleate (Ergot-containing drugs have been reported to cause prolonged vasospastic reactions; because there is a theoretical basis that these effects may be additive, use of ergot-type agents and sumatriptan within 24 hours is contraindicated).
No products indexed under this heading.

Naratriptan Hydrochloride (Sumatriptan succinate injection and any ergotamine-containing or ergot-type medication (like dihydroergotamine or methysergide) should not be used within 24 hours of each other, nor should sumatriptan succinate injection and another 5-HT_1 agonist). Products include:
Amerge 1306

Nefazodone Hydrochloride (The development of a potentially life-threatening serotonin syndrome may occur with triptans, including sumatriptan treatment, particularly during combined use with selective serotonin reuptake inhibitors (SSRIs) or serotonin norepinephrine reuptake inhibitors (SNRIs). If concomitant treatment with sumatriptan and an SSRI (eg, fluoxetine, paroxetine, sertraline, fluvoxamine, citalopram, escitalopram) or SNRI (eg, venlafaxine, duloxetine) is clinically warranted, careful observation of the patient is advised, particularly during treatment initiation and dose increases).
No products indexed under this heading.

Pargyline Hydrochloride (*In vitro* studies with human microsomes suggest that sumatriptan is metabolized by monoamine oxidase (MAO), predominantly the A isoenzyme. In a study of 14 healthy females, pretreatment with MAO-A inhibitor decreased the clearance of sumatriptan. Under the conditions of this experiment, the result was a 2-fold increase in the area under the sumatriptan plasma concentration x time curve (AUC), corresponding to a 40% increase in elimination half-life. No significant effect was seen with an MAO-B inhibitor).
No products indexed under this heading.

Paroxetine (The development of a potentially life-threatening serotonin syndrome may occur with triptans, including treatment with sumatriptan succinate, particularly during combined use with selective serotonin reuptake inhibitors (SSRIs) or serotonin norepinephrine reuptake inhibitors (SNRIs). If concomitant treatment with sumatriptan and an SSRI (eg, fluoxetine,paroxetine, sertraline, fluvoxamine, citalopram, escitalopram) or SNRI (eg, venlafaxine, duloxetine) is clinically warranted, careful observation of the patient is advised, particularly during treatment initiation and dose increases).
No products indexed under this heading.

Paroxetine Hydrochloride (The development of a potentially life-threatening serotonin syndrome may occur with triptans, including treatment with sumatriptan succinate, particularly during combined use with selective serotonin reuptake inhibitors (SSRIs) or serotonin norepinephrine reuptake inhibitors (SNRIs). If concomitant treatment with sumatriptan and an SSRI (eg, fluoxetine,paroxetine, sertraline, fluvoxamine, citalopram, escitalopram) or SNRI (eg, venlafaxine, duloxetine) is clinically warranted, careful observation of the patient is advised, particularly during treatment initiation and dose increases). Products include:
Paroxetine CR 2361
Paroxetine ER 2371
Paxil 1586
Paxil CR 1596

Paroxetine Mesylate (The development of a potentially life-threatening serotonin syndrome may occur with triptans, including sumatriptan treatment, particularly during combined use with selective serotonin reuptake inhibitors (SSRIs) or serotonin norepinephrine reuptake inhibitors (SNRIs). If concomitant treatment with sumatriptan and an SSRI (eg, fluoxetine, paroxetine, sertraline, fluvoxamine, citalopram, escitalopram) or SNRI (eg, venlafaxine, duloxetine) is clinically warranted, careful observation of the patient is advised, particularly during treatment initiation and dose increases).
No products indexed under this heading.

Phenelzine Sulfate (*In vitro* studies with human microsomes suggest that sumatriptan is metabolized by monoamine oxidase (MAO), predominantly the A isoenzyme. In a study of 14 healthy females, pretreatment with MAO-A inhibitor decreased the clearance of sumatriptan. Under the conditions of this experiment, the result was a 2-fold increase in the area under the sumatriptan plasma concentration x time curve (AUC), corresponding to a 40% increase in elimination half-life. No significant effect was seen with an MAO-B inhibitor).
No products indexed under this heading.

Procarbazine Hydrochloride (*In vitro* studies with human microsomes suggest that sumatriptan is metabolized by monoamine oxidase (MAO), predominantly the A isoenzyme. In a study of 14 healthy females, pretreatment with MAO-A inhibitor decreased the clearance of sumatriptan. Under the conditions of this experiment, the result was a 2-fold increase in the area under the sumatriptan plasma concentration x time curve (AUC), corresponding to a 40% increase in elimination half-life. No significant effect was seen with an MAO-B inhibitor).
No products indexed under this heading.

Rizatriptan Benzoate (Sumatriptan succinate injection and any ergotamine-containing or ergot-type medication (like dihydroergotamine or methysergide) should not be used within 24 hours of each other, nor should sumatriptan succinate injection and another 5-HT_1 agonist). Products include:
Maxalt 2206

IMPORTANT NOTE: Always consult each drug listing in the patient's regimen for possible interactions.

Sertraline Hydrochloride (The development of a potentially life-threatening serotonin syndrome may occur with triptans, including treatment with sumatriptan succinate, particularly during combined use with selective serotonin reuptake inhibitors (SSRIs) or serotonin norepinephrine reuptake inhibitors (SNRIs). If concomitant treatment with sumatriptan and an SSRI (eg, fluoxetine, paroxetine, sertraline, fluvoxamine, citalopram, escitalopram) or SNRI (eg, venlafaxine, duloxetine) is clinically warranted, careful observation of the patient is advised, particularly during treatment initiation and dose increases).

No products indexed under this heading.

Sumatriptan (Sumatriptan succinate injection and any ergotamine-containing or ergot-type medication (like dihydroergotamine or methysergide) should not be used within 24 hours of each other, nor should sumatriptan succinate injection and another 5-HT$_1$ agonist).
Products include:

Tranylcypromine Sulfate (In vitro studies with human microsomes suggest that sumatriptan is metabolized by monoamine oxidase (MAO), predominantly the A isoenzyme. In a study of 14 healthy females, pretreatment with MAO-A inhibitor decreased the clearance of sumatriptan. Under the conditions of this experiment, the result was a 2-fold increase in the area under the sumatriptan plasma concentration x time curve (AUC), corresponding to a 40% increase in elimination half-life. No significant effect was seen with an MAO-B inhibitor). Products include:

Venlafaxine Hydrochloride (The development of a potentially life-threatening serotonin syndrome may occur with triptans, including treatment with sumatriptan succinate, particularly during combined use with selective serotonin reuptake inhibitors (SSRIs) or serotonin norepinephrine reuptake inhibitors (SNRIs). If concomitant treatment with sumatriptan and an SSRI (eg, fluoxetine, paroxetine, sertraline, fluvoxamine, citalopram, escitalopram) or SNRI (eg, venlafaxine, duloxetine) is clinically warranted, careful observation of the patient is advised, particularly during treatment initiation and dose increases). Products include:

Zolmitriptan (Sumatriptan succinate injection and any ergotamine-containing or ergot-type medication (like dihydroergotamine or methysergide) should not be used within 24 hours of each other, nor should sumatriptan succinate injection and another 5-HT$_1$ agonist). Products include:

IMITREX NASAL SPRAY

(Sumatriptan) 1503
See Imitrex Tablets

IMITREX TABLETS

(Sumatriptan Succinate) 1508
May interact with 5HT1-receptor agonists, ergot-containing drugs, nonselective MAO inhibitors, selective serotonin reuptake inhibitors, serotonin and norepinephrine reuptake inhibitors, and certain other agents. Compounds in these categories include:

Almotriptan Malate (Co-administration with other 5-HT1 agonists within 24 hours of each other is contraindicated because the vasospastic effects may be additive). Products include:

Citalopram Hydrobromide (The development of a potentially life-threatening serotonin syndrome may occur with triptans, including sumatriptan treatment, particularly during combined use with selective serotonin reuptake inhibitors (SSRIs) or serotonin norepinephrine reuptake inhibitors (SNRIs). If concomitant treatment with sumatriptan and an SSRI (eg, fluoxetine, paroxetine, sertraline, fluvoxamine, citalopram, escitalopram) or SNRI (eg, venlafaxine, duloxetine) is clinically warranted, careful observation of the patient is advised, particularly during treatment initiation and dose increases). Products include:

Desvenlafaxine Succinate (The development of a potentially life-threatening serotonin syndrome may occur with triptans, including sumatriptan treatment, particularly during combined use with selective serotonin reuptake inhibitors (SSRIs) or serotonin norepinephrine reuptake inhibitors (SNRIs). If concomitant treatment with sumatriptan and an SSRI (eg, fluoxetine, paroxetine, sertraline, fluvoxamine, citalopram, escitalopram) or SNRI (eg, venlafaxine, duloxetine) is clinically warranted, careful observation of the patient is advised, particularly during treatment initiation and dose increases). Products include:

Dihydroergotamine Mesylate (Ergot-containing drugs have been reported to cause prolonged vasospastic reactions; because there is a theoretical basis that these effects may be additive, use of ergot-type agents and sumatriptan within 24 hours is contraindicated).

No products indexed under this heading.

Duloxetine Hydrochloride (Cases of life-threatening serotonin syndrome have been reported during combined use of serotonin and norepinephrine reuptake inhibitors (SNRIs) and triptans. If concomitant treatment with sumatriptan succinate is clinically warranted, careful observation of the patient is advised, particularly during treatment initiation and dose increases. Serotonin syndrome symptoms may include mental status changes, autonomic instability, neuromuscular aberrations and/or gastrointestinal symptoms). Products include:

Eletriptan Hydrobromide (Co-administration with other 5-HT1 agonists within 24 hours of each other is contraindicated because the vasospastic effects may be additive).

No products indexed under this heading.

Ergonovine Maleate (Ergot-containing drugs have been reported to cause prolonged vasospastic reactions; because there is a theoretical basis that these effects may be additive, use of ergot-type agents and sumatriptan within 24 hours is contraindicated).

No products indexed under this heading.

Ergotamine Tartrate (Ergot-containing drugs have been reported to cause prolonged vasospastic reactions; because there is a theoretical basis that these effects may be additive, use of ergot-type agents and sumatriptan within 24 hours is contraindicated).

No products indexed under this heading.

Escitalopram Oxalate (The development of a potentially life-threatening serotonin syndrome may occur with triptans, including sumatriptan treatment, particularly during combined use with selective serotonin reuptake inhibitors (SSRIs) or serotonin norepinephrine reuptake inhibitors (SNRIs). If concomi-

---

tant treatment with sumatriptan and an SSRI (eg, fluoxetine, paroxetine, sertraline, fluvoxamine, citalopram, escitalopram) or SNRI (eg, venlafaxine, duloxetine) is clinically warranted, careful observation of the patient is advised, particularly during treatment initiation and dose increases). Products include:

Fluoxetine (The development of a potentially life-threatening serotonin syndrome may occur with triptans, including sumatriptan treatment, particularly during combined use with selective serotonin reuptake inhibitors (SSRIs) or serotonin norepinephrine reuptake inhibitors (SNRIs). If concomitant treatment with sumatriptan and an SSRI (eg, fluoxetine, paroxetine, sertraline, fluvoxamine, citalopram, escitalopram) or SNRI (eg, venlafaxine, duloxetine) is clinically warranted, careful observation of the patient is advised, particularly during treatment initiation and dose increases).

No products indexed under this heading.

Fluoxetine Hydrochloride (The development of a potentially life-threatening serotonin syndrome may occur with triptans, including sumatriptan treatment, particularly during combined use with selective serotonin reuptake inhibitors (SSRIs) or serotonin norepinephrine reuptake inhibitors (SNRIs). If concomitant treatment with sumatriptan and an SSRI (eg, fluoxetine, paroxetine, sertraline, fluvoxamine, citalopram, escitalopram) or SNRI (eg, venlafaxine, duloxetine) is clinically warranted, careful observation of the patient is advised, particularly during treatment initiation and dose increases). Products include:

Fluvoxamine (The development of a potentially life-threatening serotonin syndrome may occur with triptans, including sumatriptan treatment, particularly during combined use with selective serotonin reuptake inhibitors (SSRIs) or serotonin norepinephrine reuptake inhibitors (SNRIs). If concomitant treatment with sumatriptan and an SSRI (eg, fluoxetine, paroxetine, sertraline, fluvoxamine, citalopram, escitalopram) or SNRI (eg, venlafaxine, duloxetine) is clinically warranted, careful observation of the patient is advised, particularly during treatment initiation and dose increases).

No products indexed under this heading.

Fluvoxamine Maleate (The development of a potentially life-threatening serotonin syndrome may occur with triptans, including sumatriptan treatment, particularly during combined use with selective serotonin reuptake inhibitors (SSRIs) or serotonin norepinephrine reuptake inhibitors (SNRIs). If concomitant treatment with sumatriptan and an SSRI (eg, fluoxetine, paroxetine, sertraline, fluvoxamine, citalopram, escitalopram) or SNRI (eg, venlafaxine, duloxetine) is clinically warranted, careful observation of the patient is advised, particularly during treatment initiation and dose increases).

No products indexed under this heading.

Frovatriptan Succinate (Co-administration with other 5-HT1 agonists within 24 hours of each other is contraindicated because the vasospastic effects may be additive). Products include:

Isocarboxazid (MAO-A inhibitors reduce sumatriptan clearance and significantly increasing systemic exposure; concurrent and/or sequential use is contraindicated). Products include:

Methylergonovine Maleate (Ergot-containing drugs have been reported to cause prolonged vasospastic reactions; because there is a theoretical basis that these effects may be additive, use of ergot-type agents and sumatriptan within 24 hours is contraindicated).

No products indexed under this heading.

Methysergide Maleate (Ergot-containing drugs have been reported to cause prolonged vasospastic reactions; because there is a theoretical basis that these effects may be additive, use of ergot-type agents and sumatriptan within 24 hours is contraindicated).

No products indexed under this heading.

Naratriptan Hydrochloride (Co-administration with other 5-HT1 agonists within 24 hours of each other is contraindicated because the vasospastic effects may be additive). Products include:

Nefazodone Hydrochloride (Cases of life-threatening serotonin syndrome have been reported during combined use of serotonin and norepinephrine reuptake inhibitors (SNRIs) and triptans. If concomitant treatment with sumatriptan succinate is clinically warranted, careful observation of the patient is advised, particularly during treatment initiation and dose increases. Serotonin syndrome symptoms may include mental status changes, autonomic instability, neuromuscular aberrations and/or gastrointestinal symptoms).

No products indexed under this heading.

Pargyline Hydrochloride (MAO-A inhibitors reduce sumatriptan clearance and significantly increasing systemic exposure; concurrent and/or sequential use is contraindicated).

No products indexed under this heading.

Paroxetine (The development of a potentially life-threatening serotonin syndrome may occur with triptans, including sumatriptan treatment, particularly during combined use with selective serotonin reuptake inhibitors (SSRIs) or serotonin norepinephrine reuptake inhibitors (SNRIs). If concomitant treatment with sumatriptan and an SSRI (eg, fluoxetine, paroxetine, sertraline, fluvoxamine, citalopram, escitalopram) or SNRI (eg, venlafaxine, duloxetine) is clinically warranted, careful observation of the patient is advised, particularly during treatment initiation and dose increases).

No products indexed under this heading.

Paroxetine Hydrochloride (The development of a potentially life-threatening serotonin syndrome may occur with triptans, including sumatriptan treatment, particularly during combined use with selective serotonin reuptake inhibitors (SSRIs) or serotonin norepinephrine reuptake inhibitors (SNRIs). If concomitant treatment with sumatriptan and an SSRI (eg, fluoxetine, paroxetine, sertraline, fluvoxamine, citalopram, escitalopram) or SNRI (eg, venlafaxine, duloxetine) is clinically warranted, careful observation of the patient is advised, particularly during treatment initiation and dose increases). Products include:

Paroxetine Mesylate (The development of a potentially life-threatening serotonin syndrome may occur with triptans, including sumatriptan treatment, particularly during combined use with selective serotonin reuptake inhibitors (SSRIs) or serotonin norepinephrine reuptake inhibitors (SNRIs). If concomitant treatment with sumatriptan and an

---

SSRI (eg, fluoxetine, paroxetine, sertraline, fluvoxamine, citalopram, escitalopram) or SNRI (eg, venlafaxine, duloxetine) is clinically warranted, careful observation of the patient is advised, particularly during treatment initiation and dose increases.

No products indexed under this heading.

Phenelzine Sulfate (MAO-A inhibitors reduce sumatriptan clearance and significantly increasing systemic exposure; concurrent and/or sequential use is contraindicated).

No products indexed under this heading.

Procarbazine Hydrochloride (MAO-A inhibitors reduce sumatriptan clearance and significantly increasing systemic exposure; concurrent and/or sequential use is contraindicated).

No products indexed under this heading.

Rizatriptan Benzoate (Co-administration with other 5-HT1 agonists within 24 hours of each other is contraindicated because the vasospastic effects may be additive). Products include:

Sertraline Hydrochloride (The development of a potentially life-threatening serotonin syndrome may occur with triptans, including sumatriptan treatment, particularly during combined use with selective serotonin reuptake inhibitors (SSRIs) or serotonin norepinephrine reuptake inhibitors (SNRIs). If concomitant treatment with sumatriptan and an SSRI (eg, fluoxetine, paroxetine, sertraline, fluvoxamine, citalopram, escitalopram) or SNRI (eg, venlafaxine, duloxetine) is clinically warranted, careful observation of the patient is advised, particularly during treatment initiation and dose increases.

No products indexed under this heading.

Sumatriptan (Co-administration with other 5-HT1 agonists within 24 hours of each other is contraindicated because the vasospastic effects may be additive). Products include:

Tranylcypromine Sulfate (MAO-A inhibitors reduce sumatriptan clearance and significantly increasing systemic exposure; concurrent and/or sequential use is contraindicated). Products include:

Venlafaxine Hydrochloride (Cases of life-threatening serotonin syndrome have been reported during combined use of serotonin and norepinephrine reuptake inhibitors (SNRIs) and triptans. If concomitant treatment with sumatriptan succinate is clinically warranted, careful observation of the patient is advised, particularly during treatment initiation and dose increases. Serotonin syndrome symptoms may include mental status changes, autonomic instability, neuromuscular aberrations and/or gastrointestinal symptoms). Products include:

Zolmitriptan (Co-administration with other 5-HT1 agonists within 24 hours of each other is contraindicated because the vasospastic effects may be additive). Products include:

Food Interactions

Food, unspecified (Delays the T_{max} slightly by about 0.5 hour with no significant effect on the bioavailability).

IMMUNIZEN CAPSULES

(Colostrum, Dietary Supplement, Yeast) 3455
None cited in PDR database.

IMMUNOCAL POWDER SACHETS

(Cysteine) 1805
May interact with immunosuppressive agents, and certain other agents. Compounds in these categories include:

Azathioprine (Patients undergoing immunosuppressive therapy should discuss the concomitant use of this bonded cysteine supplement with their doctor).

No products indexed under this heading.

Basiliximab (Patients undergoing immunosuppressive therapy should discuss the concomitant use of this bonded cysteine supplement with their doctor). Products include:

Cyclosporine (Patients undergoing immunosuppressive therapy should discuss the concomitant use of this bonded cysteine supplement with their doctor). Products include:

Muromonab-CD3 (Patients undergoing immunosuppressive therapy should discuss the concomitant use of this bonded cysteine supplement with their doctor). Products include:

Mycophenolate Mofetil (Patients undergoing immunosuppressive therapy should discuss the concomitant use of this bonded cysteine supplement with their doctor).

No products indexed under this heading.

Protein Preparations (Concomitant intake of another high protein load may adversely affect absorption).

No products indexed under this heading.

Rapamycin (Patients undergoing immunosuppressive therapy should discuss the concomitant use of this bonded cysteine supplement with their doctor).

No products indexed under this heading.

Sirolimus (Patients undergoing immunosuppressive therapy should discuss the concomitant use of this bonded cysteine supplement with their doctor). Products include:

Tacrolimus (Patients undergoing immunosuppressive therapy should discuss the concomitant use of this bonded cysteine supplement with their doctor). Products include:

IMODIUM A-D LIQUID, CAPLETS, AND EZ CHEWS

(Loperamide Hydrochloride) 2042
None cited in PDR database.

IMODIUM MULTI-SYMPTOM RELIEF CAPLETS AND CHEWABLE TABLETS

(Loperamide Hydrochloride, Simethicone) 2043
None cited in PDR database.

IMPLANON IMPLANT

(Etonogestrel) 3128
May interact with antibiotics, anticonvulsants, antifungals, barbiturates, cytochrome p450 inhibitors (selected), hepatic microsomal enzyme inducers, phenytoin, protease inhibitors, and certain other agents. Compounds in these categories include:

Acetazolamide (Inhibitors of hepatic enzymes may increase plasma hormone levels).

No products indexed under this heading.

Acetazolamide Sodium (Inhibitors of hepatic enzymes may increase plasma hormone levels).

No products indexed under this heading.

Alatrofloxacin Mesylate (Contraceptive effectiveness may be reduced when hormonal contraceptives are co-administered with some antibiotics, antifungals, anticonvulsants, and other drugs that increase the metabolism of contraceptive steroids. This could result in an unintended pregnancy or breakthrough bleeding. Patients should use an additional nonhormonal contraceptive method when taking medications that may decrease the efficacy of hormonal contraceptives).

No products indexed under this heading.

Allium sativum (Etonogestrel implant is not recommended for women who require chronic use of drugs that are potent inducers of hepatic enzymes because etonogestrel implant is likely to be less effective for these women).

No products indexed under this heading.

Amikacin Sulfate (Contraceptive effectiveness may be reduced when hormonal contraceptives are co-administered with some antibiotics, antifungals, anticonvulsants, and other drugs that increase the metabolism of contraceptive steroids. This could result in an unintended pregnancy or breakthrough bleeding. Patients should use an additional nonhormonal contraceptive method when taking medications that may decrease the efficacy of hormonal contraceptives).

No products indexed under this heading.

Aminoglutethimide (Etonogestrel implant is not recommended for women who require chronic use of drugs that are potent inducers of hepatic enzymes because etonogestrel implant is likely to be less effective for these women).

No products indexed under this heading.

Amiodarone Hydrochloride (Inhibitors of hepatic enzymes may increase plasma hormone levels).

No products indexed under this heading.

Amitriptyline Hydrochloride (Inhibitors of hepatic enzymes may increase plasma hormone levels).

No products indexed under this heading.

Amobarbital (Contraceptive effectiveness may be reduced when hormonal contraceptives are co-administered with barbiturates. This could result in an unintended pregnancy or breakthrough bleeding. Patients should use an additional nonhormonal contraceptive method when taking medications that may decrease the efficacy of hormonal contraceptives).

No products indexed under this heading.

Amobarbital Sodium (Contraceptive effectiveness may be reduced when hormonal contraceptives are co-administered with barbiturates. This could result in an unintended pregnancy or breakthrough bleeding. Patients should use an additional nonhormonal contraceptive method when taking medications that may decrease the efficacy of hormonal contraceptives).

No products indexed under this heading.

Amoxapine (Inhibitors of hepatic enzymes may increase plasma hormone levels).

No products indexed under this heading.

Amoxicillin (Contraceptive effectiveness may be reduced when hormonal contraceptives are co-administered with some antibiotics, antifungals, anticonvulsants, and other drugs that increase the metabolism of contraceptive steroids. This could result in an unintended pregnancy or breakthrough bleeding. Patients should use an additional nonhormonal contraceptive method when taking medications that may decrease the efficacy of hormonal contraceptives). Products include:

Amoxicillin Trihydrate (Contraceptive effectiveness may be reduced when hormonal contraceptives are co-administered with some antibiotics, antifungals, anticonvulsants, and other drugs that increase the metabolism of contraceptive steroids. This could result in an unintended pregnancy or breakthrough bleeding. Patients should use an additional nonhormonal contraceptive method when taking medications that may decrease the efficacy of hormonal contraceptives).

No products indexed under this heading.

Amphotericin B (Contraceptive effectiveness may be reduced when hormonal contraceptives are co-administered with some antibiotics, antifungals, anticonvulsants, and other drugs that increase the metabolism of contraceptive steroids. This could result in an unintended pregnancy or breakthrough bleeding. Patients should use an additional nonhormonal contraceptive method when taking medications that may decrease the efficacy of hormonal contraceptives).

No products indexed under this heading.

Amphotericin B, liposomal (Contraceptive effectiveness may be reduced when hormonal contraceptives are co-administered with some antibiotics, antifungals, anticonvulsants, and other drugs that increase the metabolism of contraceptive steroids. This could result in an unintended pregnancy or breakthrough bleeding. Patients should use an additional nonhormonal contraceptive method when taking medications that may decrease the efficacy of hormonal contraceptives). Products include:

Amphotericin B Cholesteryl Sulfate (Contraceptive effectiveness may be reduced when hormonal contraceptives are co-administered with some antibiotics, antifungals, anticonvulsants, and other drugs that increase the metabolism of contraceptive steroids. This could result in an unintended pregnancy or breakthrough bleeding. Patients should use an additional nonhormonal contraceptive method when taking medications that may decrease the efficacy of hormonal contraceptives).

No products indexed under this heading.

Amphotericin B Lipid Complex (Contraceptive effectiveness may be reduced when hormonal contraceptives are co-administered with some antibiotics, antifungals, anticonvulsants, and other drugs that increase the metabolism of contraceptive steroids. This could result in an unintended pregnancy or breakthrough bleeding. Patients should use an additional nonhormonal contraceptive method when taking medications that may decrease the efficacy of hormonal contraceptives).

No products indexed under this heading.

Ampicillin (Contraceptive effectiveness may be reduced when hormonal contraceptives are co-administered with some antibiotics, antifungals, anticonvulsants, and other drugs that increase the metabolism of contraceptive steroids. This could result in an unintended pregnancy or breakthrough bleeding. Patients should use an additional non-

IMPORTANT NOTE: Always consult each drug listing in the patient's regimen for possible interactions.

Implanon Interactions Index 854

hormonal contraceptive method when taking medications that may decrease the efficacy of hormonal contraceptives).
No products indexed under this heading.

Ampicillin Sodium (Contraceptive effectiveness may be reduced when hormonal contraceptives are co-administered with some antibiotics, antifungals, anticonvulsants, and other drugs that increase the metabolism of contraceptive steroids. This could result in an unintended pregnancy or breakthrough bleeding. Patients should use an additional nonhormonal contraceptive method when taking medications that may decrease the efficacy of hormonal contraceptives).
No products indexed under this heading.

Ampicillin Trihydrate (Contraceptive effectiveness may be reduced when hormonal contraceptives are co-administered with some antibiotics, antifungals, anticonvulsants, and other drugs that increase the metabolism of contraceptive steroids. This could result in an unintended pregnancy or breakthrough bleeding. Patients should use an additional nonhormonal contraceptive method when taking medications that may decrease the efficacy of hormonal contraceptives).
No products indexed under this heading.

Amprenavir (Several of the anti-HIV protease inhibitors have been studied with co-administration of combination oral contraceptives; significant changes (increase and decrease) in the mean area under the curve (AUC) of the estrogen and progestin have been noted in some cases. The efficacy and safety of combination oral contraceptive products may be affected with co-administration of anti-HIV protease inhibitors; it is unknown whether this applies to etonogestrel implant).
No products indexed under this heading.

Anastrozole (Inhibitors of hepatic enzymes may increase plasma hormone levels).
No products indexed under this heading.

Anidulafungin (Contraceptive effectiveness may be reduced when hormonal contraceptives are co-administered with some antibiotics, antifungals, anticonvulsants, and other drugs that increase the metabolism of contraceptive steroids. This could result in an unintended pregnancy or breakthrough bleeding. Patients should use an additional nonhormonal contraceptive method when taking medications that may decrease the efficacy of hormonal contraceptives).
No products indexed under this heading.

Antibiotics, non-penicillin, unspecified (Contraceptive effectiveness may be reduced when hormonal contraceptives are co-administered with some antibiotics, antifungals, anticonvulsants, and other drugs that increase the metabolism of contraceptive steroids. This could result in an unintended pregnancy or breakthrough bleeding. Patients should use an additional nonhormonal contraceptive method when taking medications that may decrease the efficacy of hormonal contraceptives).
No products indexed under this heading.

Aprepitant (Etonogestrel implant is not recommended for women who require chronic use of drugs that are potent inducers of hepatic enzymes because etonogestrel implant is likely to be less effective for these women). Products include:
Emend **2124**

Aprobarbital (Contraceptive effectiveness may be reduced when hormonal contraceptives are co-administered with barbiturates. This could result in an unintended pregnancy or breakthrough bleeding. Patients should use an additional nonhormonal contraceptive method when taking medications that may decrease the efficacy of hormonal contraceptives).
No products indexed under this heading.

Atazanavir (Several of the anti-HIV protease inhibitors have been studied with co-administration of combination oral contraceptives; significant changes (increase and decrease) in the mean area under the curve (AUC) of the estrogen and progestin have been noted in some cases. The efficacy and safety of combination oral contraceptive products may be affected with co-administration of anti-HIV protease inhibitors; it is unknown whether this applies to etonogestrel implant).
No products indexed under this heading.

Atazanavir Sulfate (Several of the anti-HIV protease inhibitors have been studied with co-administration of combination oral contraceptives; significant changes (increase and decrease) in the mean area under the curve (AUC) of the estrogen and progestin have been noted in some cases. The efficacy and safety of combination oral contraceptive products may be affected with co-administration of anti-HIV protease inhibitors; it is unknown whether this applies to etonogestrel implant).
No products indexed under this heading.

Azithromycin Dihydrate (Contraceptive effectiveness may be reduced when hormonal contraceptives are co-administered with some antibiotics, antifungals, anticonvulsants, and other drugs that increase the metabolism of contraceptive steroids. This could result in an unintended pregnancy or breakthrough bleeding. Patients should use an additional nonhormonal contraceptive method when taking medications that may decrease the efficacy of hormonal contraceptives).
No products indexed under this heading.

Azlocillin Sodium (Contraceptive effectiveness may be reduced when hormonal contraceptives are co-administered with some antibiotics, antifungals, anticonvulsants, and other drugs that increase the metabolism of contraceptive steroids. This could result in an unintended pregnancy or breakthrough bleeding. Patients should use an additional nonhormonal contraceptive method when taking medications that may decrease the efficacy of hormonal contraceptives).
No products indexed under this heading.

Azosulfisoxazole (Inhibitors of hepatic enzymes may increase plasma hormone levels).
No products indexed under this heading.

Aztreonam (Contraceptive effectiveness may be reduced when hormonal contraceptives are co-administered with some antibiotics, antifungals, anticonvulsants, and other drugs that increase the metabolism of contraceptive steroids. This could result in an unintended pregnancy or breakthrough bleeding. Patients should use an additional nonhormonal contraceptive method when taking medications that may decrease the efficacy of hormonal contraceptives).
No products indexed under this heading.

Bacampicillin Hydrochloride (Contraceptive effectiveness may be reduced when hormonal contraceptives are co-administered with some antibiotics, antifungals, anticonvulsants, and other drugs that increase the metabolism of contraceptive steroids. This could result in an unintended pregnancy or breakthrough bleeding. Patients should use an additional nonhormonal contraceptive method when taking medications that may decrease the efficacy of hormonal contraceptives).
No products indexed under this heading.

Bendroflumethiazide (Inhibitors of hepatic enzymes may increase plasma hormone levels).
No products indexed under this heading.

Betamethasone (Etonogestrel implant is not recommended for women who require chronic use of drugs that are potent inducers of hepatic enzymes because etonogestrel implant is likely to be less effective for these women).
No products indexed under this heading.

Betamethasone Sodium Phosphate (Etonogestrel implant is not recommended for women who require chronic use of drugs that are potent inducers of hepatic enzymes because etonogestrel implant is likely to be less effective for these women).
No products indexed under this heading.

Bosentan (Etonogestrel implant is not recommended for women who require chronic use of drugs that are potent inducers of hepatic enzymes because etonogestrel implant is likely to be less effective for these women). Products include:
Tracleer **573**

Bupropion Hydrochloride (Inhibitors of hepatic enzymes may increase plasma hormone levels). Products include:
Aplenzin **2948**
Wellbutrin **1719**
Wellbutrin SR **1725**
Zyban **1762**

Butabarbital (Contraceptive effectiveness may be reduced when hormonal contraceptives are co-administered with barbiturates. This could result in an unintended pregnancy or breakthrough bleeding. Patients should use an additional nonhormonal contraceptive method when taking medications that may decrease the efficacy of hormonal contraceptives).
No products indexed under this heading.

Butabarbital Sodium (Contraceptive effectiveness may be reduced when hormonal contraceptives are co-administered with barbiturates. This could result in an unintended pregnancy or breakthrough bleeding. Patients should use an additional nonhormonal contraceptive method when taking medications that may decrease the efficacy of hormonal contraceptives).
No products indexed under this heading.

Butalbital (Contraceptive effectiveness may be reduced when hormonal contraceptives are co-administered with barbiturates. This could result in an unintended pregnancy or breakthrough bleeding. Patients should use an additional nonhormonal contraceptive method when taking medications that may decrease the efficacy of hormonal contraceptives).
No products indexed under this heading.

Butoconazole Nitrate (Contraceptive effectiveness may be reduced when hormonal contraceptives are co-administered with some antibiotics, antifungals, anticonvulsants, and other drugs that increase the metabolism of contraceptive steroids. This could result in an unintended pregnancy or breakthrough bleeding. Patients should use an additional nonhormonal contraceptive method when taking medications that may decrease the efficacy of hormonal contraceptives).
No products indexed under this heading.

Carbamazepine (Contraceptive effectiveness may be reduced when hormonal contraceptives are co-administered with anticonvulsants such as carbamazepine. This could result in an unintended pregnancy or breakthrough bleeding. Patients should use an additional nonhormonal contraceptive method when taking medications that may decrease the efficacy of hormonal contraceptives). Products include:
Carbatrol **3280**
Equetro **3477**

Carbenicillin Disodium (Contraceptive effectiveness may be reduced when hormonal contraceptives are co-administered with some antibiotics, antifungals, anticonvulsants, and other drugs that increase the metabolism of contraceptive steroids. This could result in an unintended pregnancy or breakthrough bleeding. Patients should use an additional nonhormonal contraceptive method when taking medications that may decrease the efficacy of hormonal contraceptives).
No products indexed under this heading.

Carbenicillin Indanyl Sodium (Contraceptive effectiveness may be reduced when hormonal contraceptives are co-administered with some antibiotics, antifungals, anticonvulsants, and other drugs that increase the metabolism of contraceptive steroids. This could result in an unintended pregnancy or breakthrough bleeding. Patients should use an additional nonhormonal contraceptive method when taking medications that may decrease the efficacy of hormonal contraceptives).
No products indexed under this heading.

Caspofungin acetate (Contraceptive effectiveness may be reduced when hormonal contraceptives are co-administered with some antibiotics, antifungals, anticonvulsants, and other drugs that increase the metabolism of contraceptive steroids. This could result in an unintended pregnancy or breakthrough bleeding. Patients should use an additional nonhormonal contraceptive method when taking medications that may decrease the efficacy of hormonal contraceptives). Products include:
Cancidas **2088**

Cefaclor (Contraceptive effectiveness may be reduced when hormonal contraceptives are co-administered with some antibiotics, antifungals, anticonvulsants, and other drugs that increase the metabolism of contraceptive steroids. This could result in an unintended pregnancy or breakthrough bleeding. Patients should use an additional nonhormonal contraceptive method when taking medications that may decrease the efficacy of hormonal contraceptives).
No products indexed under this heading.

Cefadroxil (Contraceptive effectiveness may be reduced when hormonal contraceptives are co-administered with some antibiotics, antifungals, anticonvulsants, and other drugs that increase the metabolism of contraceptive steroids. This could result in an unintended pregnancy or breakthrough bleeding. Patients should use an additional nonhormonal contraceptive method when taking medications that may decrease the efficacy of hormonal contraceptives).
No products indexed under this heading.

Cefamandole Nafate (Contraceptive effectiveness may be reduced when hormonal contraceptives are co-administered with some antibiotics, antifungals, anticonvulsants, and other drugs that increase the metabolism of contraceptive steroids. This could result in an unintended pregnancy or breakthrough bleeding. Patients should use an additional nonhormonal contraceptive-

855 **Interactions Index** **Implanon**

tive method when taking medications that may decrease the efficacy of hormonal contraceptives).
No products indexed under this heading.

Cefazolin Sodium (Contraceptive effectiveness may be reduced when hormonal contraceptives are co-administered with some antibiotics, antifungals, anticonvulsants, and other drugs that increase the metabolism of contraceptive steroids. This could result in an unintended pregnancy or breakthrough bleeding. Patients should use an additional nonhormonal contraceptive method when taking medications that may decrease the efficacy of hormonal contraceptives).
No products indexed under this heading.

Cefixime (Contraceptive effectiveness may be reduced when hormonal contraceptives are co-administered with some antibiotics, antifungals, anticonvulsants, and other drugs that increase the metabolism of contraceptive steroids. This could result in an unintended pregnancy or breakthrough bleeding. Patients should use an additional nonhormonal contraceptive method when taking medications that may decrease the efficacy of hormonal contraceptives). Products include:
Suprax for Oral Suspension **2038**
Suprax Tablets **2038**

Cefmetazole Sodium (Contraceptive effectiveness may be reduced when hormonal contraceptives are co-administered with some antibiotics, antifungals, anticonvulsants, and other drugs that increase the metabolism of contraceptive steroids. This could result in an unintended pregnancy or breakthrough bleeding. Patients should use an additional nonhormonal contraceptive method when taking medications that may decrease the efficacy of hormonal contraceptives).
No products indexed under this heading.

Cefonicid Sodium (Contraceptive effectiveness may be reduced when hormonal contraceptives are co-administered with some antibiotics, antifungals, anticonvulsants, and other drugs that increase the metabolism of contraceptive steroids. This could result in an unintended pregnancy or breakthrough bleeding. Patients should use an additional nonhormonal contraceptive method when taking medications that may decrease the efficacy of hormonal contraceptives).
No products indexed under this heading.

Cefoperazone Sodium (Contraceptive effectiveness may be reduced when hormonal contraceptives are co-administered with some antibiotics, antifungals, anticonvulsants, and other drugs that increase the metabolism of contraceptive steroids. This could result in an unintended pregnancy or breakthrough bleeding. Patients should use an additional nonhormonal contraceptive method when taking medications that may decrease the efficacy of hormonal contraceptives).
No products indexed under this heading.

Ceforanide (Contraceptive effectiveness may be reduced when hormonal contraceptives are co-administered with some antibiotics, antifungals, anticonvulsants, and other drugs that increase the metabolism of contraceptive steroids. This could result in an unintended pregnancy or breakthrough bleeding. Patients should use an additional nonhormonal contraceptive method when taking medications that may decrease the efficacy of hormonal contraceptives).
No products indexed under this heading.

Cefotaxime Sodium (Contraceptive effectiveness may be reduced when hormonal contraceptives are co-administered with some antibiotics, antifungals, anticonvulsants, and other drugs that increase the metabolism of contraceptive steroids. This could result in an unintended pregnancy or breakthrough bleeding. Patients should use an additional nonhormonal contraceptive method when taking medications that may decrease the efficacy of hormonal contraceptives).
No products indexed under this heading.

Cefotetan (Contraceptive effectiveness may be reduced when hormonal contraceptives are co-administered with some antibiotics, antifungals, anticonvulsants, and other drugs that increase the metabolism of contraceptive steroids. This could result in an unintended pregnancy or breakthrough bleeding. Patients should use an additional nonhormonal contraceptive method when taking medications that may decrease the efficacy of hormonal contraceptives).
No products indexed under this heading.

Cefoxitin Sodium (Contraceptive effectiveness may be reduced when hormonal contraceptives are co-administered with some antibiotics, antifungals, anticonvulsants, and other drugs that increase the metabolism of contraceptive steroids. This could result in an unintended pregnancy or breakthrough bleeding. Patients should use an additional nonhormonal contraceptive method when taking medications that may decrease the efficacy of hormonal contraceptives).
No products indexed under this heading.

Cefpodoxime Proxetil (Contraceptive effectiveness may be reduced when hormonal contraceptives are co-administered with some antibiotics, antifungals, anticonvulsants, and other drugs that increase the metabolism of contraceptive steroids. This could result in an unintended pregnancy or breakthrough bleeding. Patients should use an additional nonhormonal contraceptive method when taking medications that may decrease the efficacy of hormonal contraceptives).
No products indexed under this heading.

Cefprozil (Contraceptive effectiveness may be reduced when hormonal contraceptives are co-administered with some antibiotics, antifungals, anticonvulsants, and other drugs that increase the metabolism of contraceptive steroids. This could result in an unintended pregnancy or breakthrough bleeding. Patients should use an additional nonhormonal contraceptive method when taking medications that may decrease the efficacy of hormonal contraceptives).
No products indexed under this heading.

Ceftazidime (Contraceptive effectiveness may be reduced when hormonal contraceptives are co-administered with some antibiotics, antifungals, anticonvulsants, and other drugs that increase the metabolism of contraceptive steroids. This could result in an unintended pregnancy or breakthrough bleeding. Patients should use an additional nonhormonal contraceptive method when taking medications that may decrease the efficacy of hormonal contraceptives). Products include:
Fortaz **1481**

Ceftizoxime Sodium (Contraceptive effectiveness may be reduced when hormonal contraceptives are co-administered with some antibiotics, antifungals, anticonvulsants, and other drugs that increase the metabolism of contraceptive steroids. This could result in an unintended pregnancy or breakthrough bleeding. Patients should use an additional nonhormonal contraceptive method when taking medications that may decrease the efficacy of hormonal contraceptives).
No products indexed under this heading.

Ceftriaxone Sodium (Contraceptive effectiveness may be reduced when hormonal contraceptives are co-administered with some antibiotics, antifungals, anticonvulsants, and other drugs that increase the metabolism of contraceptive steroids. This could result in an unintended pregnancy or breakthrough bleeding. Patients should use an additional nonhormonal contraceptive method when taking medications that may decrease the efficacy of hormonal contraceptives). Products include:
Rocephin **2859**

Cefuroxime Axetil (Contraceptive effectiveness may be reduced when hormonal contraceptives are co-administered with some antibiotics, antifungals, anticonvulsants, and other drugs that increase the metabolism of contraceptive steroids. This could result in an unintended pregnancy or breakthrough bleeding. Patients should use an additional nonhormonal contraceptive method when taking medications that may decrease the efficacy of hormonal contraceptives). Products include:
Ceftin **1399**

Cefuroxime Sodium (Contraceptive effectiveness may be reduced when hormonal contraceptives are co-administered with some antibiotics, antifungals, anticonvulsants, and other drugs that increase the metabolism of contraceptive steroids. This could result in an unintended pregnancy or breakthrough bleeding. Patients should use an additional nonhormonal contraceptive method when taking medications that may decrease the efficacy of hormonal contraceptives).
No products indexed under this heading.

Celecoxib (Inhibitors of hepatic enzymes may increase plasma hormone levels). Products include:
Celebrex **3272**

Cephalexin (Contraceptive effectiveness may be reduced when hormonal contraceptives are co-administered with some antibiotics, antifungals, anticonvulsants, and other drugs that increase the metabolism of contraceptive steroids. This could result in an unintended pregnancy or breakthrough bleeding. Patients should use an additional nonhormonal contraceptive method when taking medications that may decrease the efficacy of hormonal contraceptives).
No products indexed under this heading.

Cephalothin Sodium (Contraceptive effectiveness may be reduced when hormonal contraceptives are co-administered with some antibiotics, antifungals, anticonvulsants, and other drugs that increase the metabolism of contraceptive steroids. This could result in an unintended pregnancy or breakthrough bleeding. Patients should use an additional nonhormonal contraceptive method when taking medications that may decrease the efficacy of hormonal contraceptives).
No products indexed under this heading.

Cephapirin Sodium (Contraceptive effectiveness may be reduced when hormonal contraceptives are co-administered with some antibiotics, antifungals, anticonvulsants, and other drugs that increase the metabolism of contraceptive steroids. This could result in an unintended pregnancy or breakthrough bleeding. Patients should use an additional nonhormonal contraceptive method when taking medications that may decrease the efficacy of hormonal contraceptives).
No products indexed under this heading.

Cephradine (Contraceptive effectiveness may be reduced when hormonal contraceptives are co-administered with some antibiotics, antifungals, anticonvulsants, and other drugs that increase the metabolism of contraceptive steroids. This could result in an unintended pregnancy or breakthrough bleeding. Patients should use an additional nonhormonal contraceptive method when taking medications that may decrease the efficacy of hormonal contraceptives).
No products indexed under this heading.

Chloramphenicol (Contraceptive effectiveness may be reduced when hormonal contraceptives are co-administered with some antibiotics, antifungals, anticonvulsants, and other drugs that increase the metabolism of contraceptive steroids. This could result in an unintended pregnancy or breakthrough bleeding. Patients should use an additional nonhormonal contraceptive method when taking medications that may decrease the efficacy of hormonal contraceptives).
No products indexed under this heading.

Chloramphenicol Palmitate (Contraceptive effectiveness may be reduced when hormonal contraceptives are co-administered with some antibiotics, antifungals, anticonvulsants, and other drugs that increase the metabolism of contraceptive steroids. This could result in an unintended pregnancy or breakthrough bleeding. Patients should use an additional nonhormonal contraceptive method when taking medications that may decrease the efficacy of hormonal contraceptives).
No products indexed under this heading.

Chloramphenicol Sodium Succinate (Contraceptive effectiveness may be reduced when hormonal contraceptives are co-administered with some antibiotics, antifungals, anticonvulsants, and other drugs that increase the metabolism of contraceptive steroids. This could result in an unintended pregnancy or breakthrough bleeding. Patients should use an additional nonhormonal contraceptive method when taking medications that may decrease the efficacy of hormonal contraceptives).
No products indexed under this heading.

Chloroquine (Inhibitors of hepatic enzymes may increase plasma hormone levels).
No products indexed under this heading.

Chloroquine Hydrochloride (Inhibitors of hepatic enzymes may increase plasma hormone levels).
No products indexed under this heading.

Chloroquine Phosphate (Inhibitors of hepatic enzymes may increase plasma hormone levels).
No products indexed under this heading.

Chlorothiazide (Inhibitors of hepatic enzymes may increase plasma hormone levels).
No products indexed under this heading.

Chlorothiazide Sodium (Inhibitors of hepatic enzymes may increase plasma hormone levels). Products include:
Diuril Intravenous **2009**

Chlorpheniramine (Inhibitors of hepatic enzymes may increase plasma hormone levels).
No products indexed under this heading.

Chlorpheniramine Maleate (Inhibitors of hepatic enzymes may increase plasma hormone levels).
No products indexed under this heading.

IMPORTANT NOTE: Always consult each drug listing in the patient's regimen for possible interactions.

(⊙ Described in PDR® for Ophthalmic Medicines)

857 Interactions Index Implanon

Diltiazem Hydrochloride (Etonogestrel implant is not recommended for women who require chronic use of drugs that are potent inducers of hepatic enzymes because etonogestrel implant is likely to be less effective for these women). Products include:
Cardizem LA 423

Diltiazem Maleate (Etonogestrel implant is not recommended for women who require chronic use of drugs that are potent inducers of hepatic enzymes because etonogestrel implant is likely to be less effective for these women).
No products indexed under this heading.

Diphenhydramine (Inhibitors of hepatic enzymes may increase plasma hormone levels).
No products indexed under this heading.

Diphenhydramine Hydrochloride (Inhibitors of hepatic enzymes may increase plasma hormone levels). Products include:
Benadryl Allergy Ultratab 2042
Children's Benadryl Allergy Liquid 2042

Dirithromycin (Contraceptive effectiveness may be reduced when hormonal contraceptives are co-administered with some antibiotics, antifungals, anticonvulsants, and other drugs that increase the metabolism of contraceptive steroids. This could result in an unintended pregnancy or breakthrough bleeding. Patients should use an additional nonhormonal contraceptive method when taking medications that may decrease the efficacy of hormonal contraceptives).
No products indexed under this heading.

Disodium Carbenicillin (Contraceptive effectiveness may be reduced when hormonal contraceptives are co-administered with some antibiotics, antifungals, anticonvulsants, and other drugs that increase the metabolism of contraceptive steroids. This could result in an unintended pregnancy or breakthrough bleeding. Patients should use an additional nonhormonal contraceptive method when taking medications that may decrease the efficacy of hormonal contraceptives).
No products indexed under this heading.

Disulfiram (Inhibitors of hepatic enzymes may increase plasma hormone levels).
No products indexed under this heading.

Divalproex Sodium (Contraceptive effectiveness may be reduced when hormonal contraceptives are co-administered with some antibiotics, antifungals, anticonvulsants, and other drugs that increase the metabolism of contraceptive steroids. This could result in an unintended pregnancy or breakthrough bleeding. Patients should use an additional nonhormonal contraceptive method when taking medications that may decrease the efficacy of hormonal contraceptives). Products include:
Depakote ER 426

Doxepin Hydrochloride (Inhibitors of hepatic enzymes may increase plasma hormone levels).
No products indexed under this heading.

Doxorubicin Hydrochloride (Etonogestrel implant is not recommended for women who require chronic use of drugs that are potent inducers of hepatic enzymes because etonogestrel implant is likely to be less effective for these women).
No products indexed under this heading.

Doxycycline Calcium (Contraceptive effectiveness may be reduced when hormonal contraceptives are co-administered with some antibiotics, antifungals, anticonvulsants, and other drugs that increase the metabolism of contraceptive steroids. This could result in an unintended pregnancy or breakthrough bleeding. Patients should use an additional nonhormonal contraceptive method when taking medications that may decrease the efficacy of hormonal contraceptives).
No products indexed under this heading.

Doxycycline Hyclate (Contraceptive effectiveness may be reduced when hormonal contraceptives are co-administered with some antibiotics, antifungals, anticonvulsants, and other drugs that increase the metabolism of contraceptive steroids. This could result in an unintended pregnancy or breakthrough bleeding. Patients should use an additional nonhormonal contraceptive method when taking medications that may decrease the efficacy of hormonal contraceptives).
No products indexed under this heading.

Doxycycline Monohydrate (Contraceptive effectiveness may be reduced when hormonal contraceptives are co-administered with some antibiotics, antifungals, anticonvulsants, and other drugs that increase the metabolism of contraceptive steroids. This could result in an unintended pregnancy or breakthrough bleeding. Patients should use an additional nonhormonal contraceptive method when taking medications that may decrease the efficacy of hormonal contraceptives).
No products indexed under this heading.

Econazole Nitrate (Contraceptive effectiveness may be reduced when hormonal contraceptives are co-administered with some antibiotics, antifungals, anticonvulsants, and other drugs that increase the metabolism of contraceptive steroids. This could result in an unintended pregnancy or breakthrough bleeding. Patients should use an additional nonhormonal contraceptive method when taking medications that may decrease the efficacy of hormonal contraceptives).
No products indexed under this heading.

Efavirenz (Etonogestrel implant is not recommended for women who require chronic use of drugs that are potent inducers of hepatic enzymes because etonogestrel implant is likely to be less effective for these women). Products include:
Atripla 906

Enoxacin (Contraceptive effectiveness may be reduced when hormonal contraceptives are co-administered with some antibiotics, antifungals, anticonvulsants, and other drugs that increase the metabolism of contraceptive steroids. This could result in an unintended pregnancy or breakthrough bleeding. Patients should use an additional nonhormonal contraceptive method when taking medications that may decrease the efficacy of hormonal contraceptives).
No products indexed under this heading.

Epirubicin Hydrochloride (Contraceptive effectiveness may be reduced when hormonal contraceptives are co-administered with some antibiotics, antifungals, anticonvulsants, and other drugs that increase the metabolism of contraceptive steroids. This could result in an unintended pregnancy or breakthrough bleeding. Patients should use an additional nonhormonal contraceptive method when taking medications that may decrease the efficacy of hormonal contraceptives).
No products indexed under this heading.

Erythromycin (Contraceptive effectiveness may be reduced when hormonal contraceptives are co-administered with some antibiotics, antifungals, anticonvulsants, and other drugs that increase the metabolism of contraceptive steroids. This could result in an unintended pregnancy or breakthrough bleeding. Patients should use an additional nonhormonal contraceptive method when taking medications that may decrease the efficacy of hormonal contraceptives).
No products indexed under this heading.

Erythromycin, Topical (Contraceptive effectiveness may be reduced when hormonal contraceptives are co-administered with some antibiotics, antifungals, anticonvulsants, and other drugs that increase the metabolism of contraceptive steroids. This could result in an unintended pregnancy or breakthrough bleeding. Patients should use an additional nonhormonal contraceptive method when taking medications that may decrease the efficacy of hormonal contraceptives).
No products indexed under this heading.

Erythromycin Estolate (Contraceptive effectiveness may be reduced when hormonal contraceptives are co-administered with some antibiotics, antifungals, anticonvulsants, and other drugs that increase the metabolism of contraceptive steroids. This could result in an unintended pregnancy or breakthrough bleeding. Patients should use an additional nonhormonal contraceptive method when taking medications that may decrease the efficacy of hormonal contraceptives).
No products indexed under this heading.

Erythromycin Ethylsuccinate (Contraceptive effectiveness may be reduced when hormonal contraceptives are co-administered with some antibiotics, antifungals, anticonvulsants, and other drugs that increase the metabolism of contraceptive steroids. This could result in an unintended pregnancy or breakthrough bleeding. Patients should use an additional nonhormonal contraceptive method when taking medications that may decrease the efficacy of hormonal contraceptives). Products include:
E.E.S. 437
EryPed 435

Erythromycin Gluceptate (Contraceptive effectiveness may be reduced when hormonal contraceptives are co-administered with some antibiotics, antifungals, anticonvulsants, and other drugs that increase the metabolism of contraceptive steroids. This could result in an unintended pregnancy or breakthrough bleeding. Patients should use an additional nonhormonal contraceptive method when taking medications that may decrease the efficacy of hormonal contraceptives).
No products indexed under this heading.

Erythromycin Lactobionate (Contraceptive effectiveness may be reduced when hormonal contraceptives are co-administered with some antibiotics, antifungals, anticonvulsants, and other drugs that increase the metabolism of contraceptive steroids. This could result in an unintended pregnancy or breakthrough bleeding. Patients should use an additional nonhormonal contraceptive method when taking medications that may decrease the efficacy of hormonal contraceptives).
No products indexed under this heading.

Erythromycin Stearate (Contraceptive effectiveness may be reduced when hormonal contraceptives are co-administered with some antibiotics, antifungals, anticonvulsants, and other drugs that increase the metabolism of contraceptive steroids. This could result in an unintended pregnancy or breakthrough bleeding. Patients should use an additional nonhormonal contraceptive method when taking medications that may decrease the efficacy of hormonal contraceptives).
No products indexed under this heading.

Escitalopram Oxalate (Etonogestrel implant is not recommended for women who require chronic use of drugs that are potent inducers of hepatic enzymes because etonogestrel implant is likely to be less effective for these women). Products include:
Lexapro Oral Suspension 1160
Lexapro Tablets 1160

Esomeprazole Magnesium (Etonogestrel implant is not recommended for women who require chronic use of drugs that are potent inducers of hepatic enzymes because etonogestrel implant is likely to be less effective for these women). Products include:
Nexium Capsules 704
Nexium Oral Suspension 704

Esomeprazole Sodium (Etonogestrel implant is not recommended for women who require chronic use of drugs that are potent inducers of hepatic enzymes because etonogestrel implant is likely to be less effective for these women). Products include:
Nexium I.V. 712

Ethanol (Etonogestrel implant is not recommended for women who require chronic use of drugs that are potent inducers of hepatic enzymes because etonogestrel implant is likely to be less effective for these women).
No products indexed under this heading.

Ethinyl Estradiol (Inhibitors of hepatic enzymes may increase plasma hormone levels). Products include:
LoSeasonique 3407
Lybrel 3514
NuvaRing 3181
Ortho Evra 2648
Ortho-Cyclen/Ortho Tri-Cyclen 2663
Ortho Tri-Cyclen Lo Tablets 2673
Seasonique 3418
Yaz 864

Ethosuximide (Contraceptive effectiveness may be reduced when hormonal contraceptives are co-administered with some antibiotics, antifungals, anticonvulsants, and other drugs that increase the metabolism of contraceptive steroids. This could result in an unintended pregnancy or breakthrough bleeding. Patients should use an additional nonhormonal contraceptive method when taking medications that may decrease the efficacy of hormonal contraceptives).
No products indexed under this heading.

Ethotoin (Contraceptive effectiveness may be reduced when hormonal contraceptives are co-administered with some antibiotics, antifungals, anticonvulsants, and other drugs that increase the metabolism of contraceptive steroids. This could result in an unintended pregnancy or breakthrough bleeding. Patients should use an additional nonhormonal contraceptive method when taking medications that may decrease the efficacy of hormonal contraceptives).
No products indexed under this heading.

Ethyl Alcohol (Etonogestrel implant is not recommended for women who require chronic use of drugs that are potent inducers of hepatic enzymes because etonogestrel implant is likely to be less effective for these women).
No products indexed under this heading.

Ethynodiol Diacetate (Inhibitors of hepatic enzymes may increase plasma hormone levels).
No products indexed under this heading.

IMPORTANT NOTE: Always consult each drug listing in the patient's regimen for possible interactions.

Felbamate (Contraceptive effectiveness may be reduced when hormonal contraceptives are co-administered with felbamate. This could result in an unintended pregnancy or breakthrough bleeding. Patients should use an additional nonhormonal contraceptive method when taking medications that may decrease the efficacy of hormonal contraceptives).

No products indexed under this heading.

Fenofibrate (Inhibitors of hepatic enzymes may increase plasma hormone levels). Products include:

Fenoglide	3263
Tricor	544
Trilipix	548

Fluconazole (Contraceptive effectiveness may be reduced when hormonal contraceptives are co-administered with some antibiotics, antifungals, anticonvulsants, and other drugs that increase the metabolism of contraceptive steroids. This could result in an unintended pregnancy or breakthrough bleeding. Patients should use an additional nonhormonal contraceptive method when taking medications that may decrease the efficacy of hormonal contraceptives).

No products indexed under this heading.

Flucytosine (Contraceptive effectiveness may be reduced when hormonal contraceptives are co-administered with some antibiotics, antifungals, anticonvulsants, and other drugs that increase the metabolism of contraceptive steroids. This could result in an unintended pregnancy or breakthrough bleeding. Patients should use an additional nonhormonal contraceptive method when taking medications that may decrease the efficacy of hormonal contraceptives).

No products indexed under this heading.

Fludrocortisone Acetate (Etonogestrel implant is not recommended for women who require chronic use of drugs that are potent inducers of hepatic enzymes because etonogestrel implant is likely to be less effective for these women).

No products indexed under this heading.

Fluorouracil (Inhibitors of hepatic enzymes may increase plasma hormone levels). Products include:

Carac	2966

Fluoxetine (Inhibitors of hepatic enzymes may increase plasma hormone levels).

No products indexed under this heading.

Fluoxetine Hydrochloride (Inhibitors of hepatic enzymes may increase plasma hormone levels). Products include:

Prozac Weekly	1941
Prozac Pulvules	1941
Symbyax	1965

Fluphenazine Decanoate (Inhibitors of hepatic enzymes may increase plasma hormone levels).

No products indexed under this heading.

Fluphenazine Enanthate (Inhibitors of hepatic enzymes may increase plasma hormone levels).

No products indexed under this heading.

Fluphenazine Hydrochloride (Inhibitors of hepatic enzymes may increase plasma hormone levels).

No products indexed under this heading.

Flurbiprofen (Inhibitors of hepatic enzymes may increase plasma hormone levels).

No products indexed under this heading.

Flurbiprofen Sodium (Inhibitors of hepatic enzymes may increase plasma hormone levels).

No products indexed under this heading.

Fluvastatin Sodium (Inhibitors of hepatic enzymes may increase plasma hormone levels).

No products indexed under this heading.

Fluvoxamine (Etonogestrel implant is not recommended for women who require chronic use of drugs that are potent inducers of hepatic enzymes because etonogestrel implant is likely to be less effective for these women).

No products indexed under this heading.

Fluvoxamine Maleate (Etonogestrel implant is not recommended for women who require chronic use of drugs that are potent inducers of hepatic enzymes because etonogestrel implant is likely to be less effective for these women).

No products indexed under this heading.

Fosamprenavir Calcium (Several of the anti-HIV protease inhibitors have been studied with co-administration of combination oral contraceptives; significant changes (increase and decrease) in the mean area under the curve (AUC) of the estrogen and progestin have been noted in some cases. The efficacy and safety of combination oral contraceptive products may be affected with co-administration of anti-HIV protease inhibitors; it is unknown whether this applies to etonogestrel implant). Products include:

Lexiva Oral Suspension	1558
Lexiva	1558

Fosphenytoin (Contraceptive effectiveness may be reduced when hormonal contraceptives are co-administered with phenytoin. This could result in an unintended pregnancy or breakthrough bleeding. Patients should use an additional nonhormonal contraceptive method when taking medications that may decrease the efficacy of hormonal contraceptives).

No products indexed under this heading.

Fosphenytoin Sodium (Contraceptive effectiveness may be reduced when hormonal contraceptives are co-administered with phenytoin. This could result in an unintended pregnancy or breakthrough bleeding. Patients should use an additional nonhormonal contraceptive method when taking medications that may decrease the efficacy of hormonal contraceptives).

No products indexed under this heading.

Gabapentin (Contraceptive effectiveness may be reduced when hormonal contraceptives are co-administered with some antibiotics, antifungals, anticonvulsants, and other drugs that increase the metabolism of contraceptive steroids. This could result in an unintended pregnancy or breakthrough bleeding. Patients should use an additional nonhormonal contraceptive method when taking medications that may decrease the efficacy of hormonal contraceptives).

No products indexed under this heading.

Garlic Extract (Etonogestrel implant is not recommended for women who require chronic use of drugs that are potent inducers of hepatic enzymes because etonogestrel implant is likely to be less effective for these women).

No products indexed under this heading.

Garlic Oil (Etonogestrel implant is not recommended for women who require chronic use of drugs that are potent inducers of hepatic enzymes because etonogestrel implant is likely to be less effective for these women).

No products indexed under this heading.

Gatifloxacin (Contraceptive effectiveness may be reduced when hormonal contraceptives are co-administered with some antibiotics, antifungals, anticonvulsants, and other drugs that increase the metabolism of contraceptive steroids. This could result in an unintended pregnancy or breakthrough bleeding. Patients should use an additional nonhormonal contraceptive method when

taking medications that may decrease the efficacy of hormonal contraceptives).

No products indexed under this heading.

Gemfibrozil (Inhibitors of hepatic enzymes may increase plasma hormone levels).

No products indexed under this heading.

Gemifloxacin Mesylate (Contraceptive effectiveness may be reduced when hormonal contraceptives are co-administered with some antibiotics, antifungals, anticonvulsants, and other drugs that increase the metabolism of contraceptive steroids. This could result in an unintended pregnancy or breakthrough bleeding. Patients should use an additional nonhormonal contraceptive method when taking medications that may decrease the efficacy of hormonal contraceptives).

No products indexed under this heading.

Gentamicin Sulfate (Contraceptive effectiveness may be reduced when hormonal contraceptives are co-administered with some antibiotics, antifungals, anticonvulsants, and other drugs that increase the metabolism of contraceptive steroids. This could result in an unintended pregnancy or breakthrough bleeding. Patients should use an additional nonhormonal contraceptive method when taking medications that may decrease the efficacy of hormonal contraceptives). Products include:

Pred-G	⊙ 226, ⊙ 227

Glipizide (Etonogestrel implant is not recommended for women who require chronic use of drugs that are potent inducers of hepatic enzymes because etonogestrel implant is likely to be less effective for these women).

No products indexed under this heading.

Glyburide (Etonogestrel implant is not recommended for women who require chronic use of drugs that are potent inducers of hepatic enzymes because etonogestrel implant is likely to be less effective for these women).

No products indexed under this heading.

Grepafloxacin Hydrochloride (Contraceptive effectiveness may be reduced when hormonal contraceptives are co-administered with some antibiotics, antifungals, anticonvulsants, and other drugs that increase the metabolism of contraceptive steroids. This could result in an unintended pregnancy or breakthrough bleeding. Patients should use an additional nonhormonal contraceptive method when taking medications that may decrease the efficacy of hormonal contraceptives).

No products indexed under this heading.

Griseofulvin (Contraceptive effectiveness may be reduced when hormonal contraceptives are co-administered with griseofulvin. This could result in an unintended pregnancy or breakthrough bleeding. Patients should use an additional nonhormonal contraceptive method when taking medications that may decrease the efficacy of hormonal contraceptives).

No products indexed under this heading.

Halofantrine Hydrochloride (Inhibitors of hepatic enzymes may increase plasma hormone levels).

No products indexed under this heading.

Haloperidol (Inhibitors of hepatic enzymes may increase plasma hormone levels).

No products indexed under this heading.

Haloperidol Decanoate (Inhibitors of hepatic enzymes may increase plasma hormone levels).

No products indexed under this heading.

Haloperidol Lactate (Inhibitors of hepatic enzymes may increase plasma hormone levels).

No products indexed under this heading.

Hepatic Enzyme-Inducing Agents (Etonogestrel implant is not recommended for women who require chronic use of drugs that are potent inducers of hepatic enzymes because etonogestrel implant is likely to be less effective for these women).

No products indexed under this heading.

Hexobarbital (Contraceptive effectiveness may be reduced when hormonal contraceptives are co-administered with barbiturates. This could result in an unintended pregnancy or breakthrough bleeding. Patients should use an additional nonhormonal contraceptive method when taking medications that may decrease the efficacy of hormonal contraceptives).

No products indexed under this heading.

Hydrochlorothiazide (Inhibitors of hepatic enzymes may increase plasma hormone levels). Products include:

Atacand HCT	700
Avalide	2956
Benicar HCT	1017
Diovan HCT	2419
Dyazide	1429
Exforge HCT	2449
Hyzaar	2162
Hyzaar 100-12.5	2162
Micardis HCT	889
Prinzide	2246
Tekturna HCT	2541
Teveten HCT	541

Hydrochlorothiazide Hydrochloride (Inhibitors of hepatic enzymes may increase plasma hormone levels).

No products indexed under this heading.

Hydrocortisone (Alcohol) (Etonogestrel implant is not recommended for women who require chronic use of drugs that are potent inducers of hepatic enzymes because etonogestrel implant is likely to be less effective for these women).

No products indexed under this heading.

Hydrocortisone Acetate (Etonogestrel implant is not recommended for women who require chronic use of drugs that are potent inducers of hepatic enzymes because etonogestrel implant is likely to be less effective for these women).

No products indexed under this heading.

Hydrocortisone Butyrate (Etonogestrel implant is not recommended for women who require chronic use of drugs that are potent inducers of hepatic enzymes because etonogestrel implant is likely to be less effective for these women).

No products indexed under this heading.

Hydrocortisone Cypionate (Etonogestrel implant is not recommended for women who require chronic use of drugs that are potent inducers of hepatic enzymes because etonogestrel implant is likely to be less effective for these women).

No products indexed under this heading.

Hydrocortisone Hemisuccinate (Etonogestrel implant is not recommended for women who require chronic use of drugs that are potent inducers of hepatic enzymes because etonogestrel implant is likely to be less effective for these women).

No products indexed under this heading.

Hydrocortisone Probutate (Etonogestrel implant is not recommended for women who require chronic use of drugs that are potent inducers of hepatic enzymes because etonogestrel implant is likely to be less effective for these women).

No products indexed under this heading.

(⊙ Described in PDR® for Ophthalmic Medicines)

IMPORTANT NOTE: Always consult each drug listing in the patient's regimen for possible interactions.

some antibiotics, antifungals, anticonvulsants, and other drugs that increase the metabolism of contraceptive steroids. This could result in an unintended pregnancy or breakthrough bleeding. Patients should use an additional nonhormonal contraceptive method when taking medications that may decrease the efficacy of hormonal contraceptives). Products include:

Levonorgestrel (Inhibitors of hepatic enzymes may increase plasma hormone levels). Products include:

Lomefloxacin Hydrochloride (Contraceptive effectiveness may be reduced when hormonal contraceptives are co-administered with some antibiotics, antifungals, anticonvulsants, and other drugs that increase the metabolism of contraceptive steroids. This could result in an unintended pregnancy or breakthrough bleeding. Patients should use an additional nonhormonal contraceptive method when taking medications that may decrease the efficacy of hormonal contraceptives).
No products indexed under this heading.

Lopinavir (Several of the anti-HIV protease inhibitors have been studied with co-administration of combination oral contraceptives; significant changes (increase and decrease) in the mean area under the curve (AUC) of the estrogen and progestin have been noted in some cases. The efficacy and safety of combination oral contraceptive products may be affected with co-administration of anti-HIV protease inhibitors; it is unknown whether this applies to etonogestrel implant). Products include:

Loracarbef (Contraceptive effectiveness may be reduced when hormonal contraceptives are co-administered with some antibiotics, antifungals, anticonvulsants, and other drugs that increase the metabolism of contraceptive steroids. This could result in an unintended pregnancy or breakthrough bleeding. Patients should use an additional nonhormonal contraceptive method when taking medications that may decrease the efficacy of hormonal contraceptives).
No products indexed under this heading.

Loratadine (Inhibitors of hepatic enzymes may increase plasma hormone levels).
No products indexed under this heading.

Lovastatin (Inhibitors of hepatic enzymes may increase plasma hormone levels). Products include:

Maprotiline Hydrochloride (Inhibitors of hepatic enzymes may increase plasma hormone levels).
No products indexed under this heading.

Mephenytoin (Contraceptive effectiveness may be reduced when hormonal contraceptives are co-administered with some antibiotics, antifungals, anticonvulsants, and other drugs that increase the metabolism of contraceptive steroids. This could result in an unintended pregnancy or breakthrough bleeding. Patients should use an additional nonhormonal contraceptive method when

taking medications that may decrease the efficacy of hormonal contraceptives).
No products indexed under this heading.

Mephobarbital (Contraceptive effectiveness may be reduced when hormonal contraceptives are co-administered with barbiturates. This could result in an unintended pregnancy or breakthrough bleeding. Patients should use an additional nonhormonal contraceptive method when taking medications that may decrease the efficacy of hormonal contraceptives).
No products indexed under this heading.

Mestranol (Inhibitors of hepatic enzymes may increase plasma hormone levels).
No products indexed under this heading.

Methacycline Hydrochloride (Contraceptive effectiveness may be reduced when hormonal contraceptives are co-administered with some antibiotics, antifungals, anticonvulsants, and other drugs that increase the metabolism of contraceptive steroids. This could result in an unintended pregnancy or breakthrough bleeding. Patients should use an additional nonhormonal contraceptive method when taking medications that may decrease the efficacy of hormonal contraceptives).
No products indexed under this heading.

Methadone Hydrochloride (Inhibitors of hepatic enzymes may increase plasma hormone levels).
No products indexed under this heading.

Methicillin Sodium (Contraceptive effectiveness may be reduced when hormonal contraceptives are co-administered with some antibiotics, antifungals, anticonvulsants, and other drugs that increase the metabolism of contraceptive steroids. This could result in an unintended pregnancy or breakthrough bleeding. Patients should use an additional nonhormonal contraceptive method when taking medications that may decrease the efficacy of hormonal contraceptives).
No products indexed under this heading.

Methoxsalen (Inhibitors of hepatic enzymes may increase plasma hormone levels).
No products indexed under this heading.

Methsuximide (Contraceptive effectiveness may be reduced when hormonal contraceptives are co-administered with some antibiotics, antifungals, anticonvulsants, and other drugs that increase the metabolism of contraceptive steroids. This could result in an unintended pregnancy or breakthrough bleeding. Patients should use an additional nonhormonal contraceptive method when taking medications that may decrease the efficacy of hormonal contraceptives).
No products indexed under this heading.

Methyclothiazide (Inhibitors of hepatic enzymes may increase plasma hormone levels).
No products indexed under this heading.

Methylprednisolone (Etonogestrel implant is not recommended for women who require chronic use of drugs that are potent inducers of hepatic enzymes because etonogestrel implant is likely to be less effective for these women).
No products indexed under this heading.

Methylprednisolone Acetate (Etonogestrel implant is not recommended for women who require chronic use of drugs that are potent inducers of hepatic enzymes because etonogestrel implant is likely to be less effective for these women).
No products indexed under this heading.

Methylprednisolone Sodium Succinate (Etonogestrel implant is not recommended for women who require chronic use of drugs that are potent inducers of hepatic enzymes because etonogestrel implant is likely to be less effective for these women).
No products indexed under this heading.

Metronidazole (Inhibitors of hepatic enzymes may increase plasma hormone levels). Products include:

Metronidazole Benzoate (Inhibitors of hepatic enzymes may increase plasma hormone levels).
No products indexed under this heading.

Metronidazole Hydrochloride (Inhibitors of hepatic enzymes may increase plasma hormone levels).
No products indexed under this heading.

Metronidazole Sodium (Inhibitors of hepatic enzymes may increase plasma hormone levels).
No products indexed under this heading.

Mexiletine Hydrochloride (Inhibitors of hepatic enzymes may increase plasma hormone levels).
No products indexed under this heading.

Mezlocillin Sodium (Contraceptive effectiveness may be reduced when hormonal contraceptives are co-administered with some antibiotics, antifungals, anticonvulsants, and other drugs that increase the metabolism of contraceptive steroids. This could result in an unintended pregnancy or breakthrough bleeding. Patients should use an additional nonhormonal contraceptive method when taking medications that may decrease the efficacy of hormonal contraceptives).
No products indexed under this heading.

Mibefradil Dihydrochloride (Inhibitors of hepatic enzymes may increase plasma hormone levels).
No products indexed under this heading.

Micafungin Sodium (Contraceptive effectiveness may be reduced when hormonal contraceptives are co-administered with some antibiotics, antifungals, anticonvulsants, and other drugs that increase the metabolism of contraceptive steroids. This could result in an unintended pregnancy or breakthrough bleeding. Patients should use an additional nonhormonal contraceptive method when taking medications that may decrease the efficacy of hormonal contraceptives). Products include:

Miconazole (Contraceptive effectiveness may be reduced when hormonal contraceptives are co-administered with some antibiotics, antifungals, anticonvulsants, and other drugs that increase the metabolism of contraceptive steroids. This could result in an unintended pregnancy or breakthrough bleeding. Patients should use an additional nonhormonal contraceptive method when taking medications that may decrease the efficacy of hormonal contraceptives).
No products indexed under this heading.

Miconazole Nitrate (Inhibitors of hepatic enzymes may increase plasma hormone levels). Products include:

Mifepristone (Inhibitors of hepatic enzymes may increase plasma hormone levels).
No products indexed under this heading.

Minocycline Hydrochloride (Contraceptive effectiveness may be reduced when hormonal contraceptives are co-administered with some antibiotics, antifungals, anticonvulsants, and other drugs that increase the metabolism of contraceptive steroids. This could result in an unintended pregnancy or break-

through bleeding. Patients should use an additional nonhormonal contraceptive method when taking medications that may decrease the efficacy of hormonal contraceptives). Products include:

Moclobemide (Inhibitors of hepatic enzymes may increase plasma hormone levels).
No products indexed under this heading.

Modafinil (Contraceptive effectiveness may be reduced when hormonal contraceptives are co-administered with modafinil. This could result in an unintended pregnancy or breakthrough bleeding. Patients should use an additional nonhormonal contraceptive method when taking medications that may decrease the efficacy of hormonal contraceptives). Products include:

Moxifloxacin Hydrochloride (Contraceptive effectiveness may be reduced when hormonal contraceptives are co-administered with some antibiotics, antifungals, anticonvulsants, and other drugs that increase the metabolism of contraceptive steroids. This could result in an unintended pregnancy or breakthrough bleeding. Patients should use an additional nonhormonal contraceptive method when taking medications that may decrease the efficacy of hormonal contraceptives). Products include:

Nafcillin Sodium (Contraceptive effectiveness may be reduced when hormonal contraceptives are co-administered with some antibiotics, antifungals, anticonvulsants, and other drugs that increase the metabolism of contraceptive steroids. This could result in an unintended pregnancy or breakthrough bleeding. Patients should use an additional nonhormonal contraceptive method when taking medications that may decrease the efficacy of hormonal contraceptives).
No products indexed under this heading.

Nalidixic Acid (Inhibitors of hepatic enzymes may increase plasma hormone levels).
No products indexed under this heading.

Nefazodone Hydrochloride (Inhibitors of hepatic enzymes may increase plasma hormone levels).
No products indexed under this heading.

Nelfinavir Mesylate (Several of the anti-HIV protease inhibitors have been studied with co-administration of combination oral contraceptives; significant changes (increase and decrease) in the mean area under the curve (AUC) of the estrogen and progestin have been noted in some cases. The efficacy and safety of combination oral contraceptive products may be affected with co-administration of anti-HIV protease inhibitors; it is unknown whether this applies to etonogestrel implant).
No products indexed under this heading.

Nevirapine (Etonogestrel implant is not recommended for women who require chronic use of drugs that are potent inducers of hepatic enzymes because etonogestrel implant is likely to be less effective for these women). Products include:

Niacinamide (Inhibitors of hepatic enzymes may increase plasma hormone levels). Products include:

Niacinamide Hydroiodide (Inhibitors of hepatic enzymes may increase plasma hormone levels).
No products indexed under this heading.

Nicardipine (Inhibitors of hepatic enzymes may increase plasma hormone levels).
No products indexed under this heading.

Nicardipine Hydrochloride (Inhibitors of hepatic enzymes may increase plasma hormone levels).
No products indexed under this heading.

Nicotinamide (Inhibitors of hepatic enzymes may increase plasma hormone levels).
No products indexed under this heading.

Nicotine (Etonogestrel implant is not recommended for women who require chronic use of drugs that are potent inducers of hepatic enzymes because etonogestrel implant is likely to be less effective for these women).
No products indexed under this heading.

Nicotine Polacrilex (Etonogestrel implant is not recommended for women who require chronic use of drugs that are potent inducers of hepatic enzymes because etonogestrel implant is likely to be less effective for these women).
No products indexed under this heading.

Nicotine Salicylate (Etonogestrel implant is not recommended for women who require chronic use of drugs that are potent inducers of hepatic enzymes because etonogestrel implant is likely to be less effective for these women).
No products indexed under this heading.

Nicotine Sulfate (Etonogestrel implant is not recommended for women who require chronic use of drugs that are potent inducers of hepatic enzymes because etonogestrel implant is likely to be less effective for these women).
No products indexed under this heading.

Nifedipine (Inhibitors of hepatic enzymes may increase plasma hormone levels).
No products indexed under this heading.

Norethindrone (Etonogestrel implant is not recommended for women who require chronic use of drugs that are potent inducers of hepatic enzymes because etonogestrel implant is likely to be less effective for these women). Products include:
Ortho Micronor **2660**

Norethindrone Acetate (Etonogestrel implant is not recommended for women who require chronic use of drugs that are potent inducers of hepatic enzymes because etonogestrel implant is likely to be less effective for these women). Products include:
Activella **2561**

Norethynodrel (Inhibitors of hepatic enzymes may increase plasma hormone levels).
No products indexed under this heading.

Norfloxacin (Contraceptive effectiveness may be reduced when hormonal contraceptives are co-administered with some antibiotics, antifungals, anticonvulsants, and other drugs that increase the metabolism of contraceptive steroids. This could result in an unintended pregnancy or breakthrough bleeding. Patients should use an additional nonhormonal contraceptive method when taking medications that may decrease the efficacy of hormonal contraceptives). Products include:
Noroxin **2220**

Norgestimate (Inhibitors of hepatic enzymes may increase plasma hormone levels). Products include:
Ortho-Cyclen/Ortho Tri-Cyclen **2663**
Ortho Tri-Cyclen Lo Tablets **2673**

Norgestrel (Inhibitors of hepatic enzymes may increase plasma hormone levels).
No products indexed under this heading.

Nortriptyline Hydrochloride (Inhibitors of hepatic enzymes may increase plasma hormone levels).
No products indexed under this heading.

Ofloxacin (Contraceptive effectiveness may be reduced when hormonal contraceptives are co-administered with some antibiotics, antifungals, anticonvulsants, and other drugs that increase the metabolism of contraceptive steroids. This could result in an unintended pregnancy or breakthrough bleeding. Patients should use an additional nonhormonal contraceptive method when taking medications that may decrease the efficacy of hormonal contraceptives).
No products indexed under this heading.

Omeprazole (Etonogestrel implant is not recommended for women who require chronic use of drugs that are potent inducers of hepatic enzymes because etonogestrel implant is likely to be less effective for these women).
No products indexed under this heading.

Omeprazole Magnesium (Etonogestrel implant is not recommended for women who require chronic use of drugs that are potent inducers of hepatic enzymes because etonogestrel implant is likely to be less effective for these women).
No products indexed under this heading.

Oxacillin (Contraceptive effectiveness may be reduced when hormonal contraceptives are co-administered with some antibiotics, antifungals, anticonvulsants, and other drugs that increase the metabolism of contraceptive steroids. This could result in an unintended pregnancy or breakthrough bleeding. Patients should use an additional nonhormonal contraceptive method when taking medications that may decrease the efficacy of hormonal contraceptives).
No products indexed under this heading.

Oxacillin Sodium (Contraceptive effectiveness may be reduced when hormonal contraceptives are co-administered with some antibiotics, antifungals, anticonvulsants, and other drugs that increase the metabolism of contraceptive steroids. This could result in an unintended pregnancy or breakthrough bleeding. Patients should use an additional nonhormonal contraceptive method when taking medications that may decrease the efficacy of hormonal contraceptives).
No products indexed under this heading.

Oxcarbazepine (Contraceptive effectiveness may be reduced when hormonal contraceptives are co-administered with oxcarbazepine. This could result in an unintended pregnancy or breakthrough bleeding. Patients should use an additional nonhormonal contraceptive method when taking medications that may decrease the efficacy of hormonal contraceptives).
No products indexed under this heading.

Oxiconazole Nitrate (Contraceptive effectiveness may be reduced when hormonal contraceptives are co-administered with some antibiotics, antifungals, anticonvulsants, and other drugs that increase the metabolism of contraceptive steroids. This could result in an unintended pregnancy or breakthrough bleeding. Patients should use an additional nonhormonal contraceptive method when taking medications that may decrease the efficacy of hormonal contraceptives).
No products indexed under this heading.

Oxytetracycline Hydrochloride (Contraceptive effectiveness may be reduced when hormonal contraceptives are co-administered with some antibiotics, antifungals, anticonvulsants, and other drugs that increase the metabolism of contraceptive steroids. This could result in an unintended pregnancy or breakthrough bleeding. Patients should use an additional nonhormonal contraceptive method when taking medications that may decrease the efficacy of hormonal contraceptives).
No products indexed under this heading.

Paramethadione (Contraceptive effectiveness may be reduced when hormonal contraceptives are co-administered with some antibiotics, antifungals, anticonvulsants, and other drugs that increase the metabolism of contraceptive steroids. This could result in an unintended pregnancy or breakthrough bleeding. Patients should use an additional nonhormonal contraceptive method when taking medications that may decrease the efficacy of hormonal contraceptives).
No products indexed under this heading.

Paroxetine (Inhibitors of hepatic enzymes may increase plasma hormone levels).
No products indexed under this heading.

Paroxetine Hydrochloride (Inhibitors of hepatic enzymes may increase plasma hormone levels). Products include:
Paroxetine CR **2361**
Paroxetine ER **2371**
Paxil **1586**
Paxil CR **1596**

Paroxetine Mesylate (Inhibitors of hepatic enzymes may increase plasma hormone levels).
No products indexed under this heading.

Penicillin, Potassium Phenoxymethyl (Contraceptive effectiveness may be reduced when hormonal contraceptives are co-administered with some antibiotics, antifungals, anticonvulsants, and other drugs that increase the metabolism of contraceptive steroids. This could result in an unintended pregnancy or breakthrough bleeding. Patients should use an additional nonhormonal contraceptive method when taking medications that may decrease the efficacy of hormonal contraceptives).
No products indexed under this heading.

Penicillin G Benzathine (Contraceptive effectiveness may be reduced when hormonal contraceptives are co-administered with some antibiotics, antifungals, anticonvulsants, and other drugs that increase the metabolism of contraceptive steroids. This could result in an unintended pregnancy or breakthrough bleeding. Patients should use an additional nonhormonal contraceptive method when taking medications that may decrease the efficacy of hormonal contraceptives). Products include:
Bicillin C-R Injectable Suspension **1826**
Bicillin L-A **1828**

Penicillin G Dibenzylethyenediamine (Contraceptive effectiveness may be reduced when hormonal contraceptives are co-administered with some antibiotics, antifungals, anticonvulsants, and other drugs that increase the metabolism of contraceptive steroids. This could result in an unintended pregnancy or breakthrough bleeding. Patients should use an additional nonhormonal contraceptive method when taking medications that may decrease the efficacy of hormonal contraceptives).
No products indexed under this heading.

Penicillin G Potassium (Contraceptive effectiveness may be reduced when hormonal contraceptives are co-administered with some antibiotics, antifungals, anticonvulsants, and other drugs that increase the metabolism of contraceptive steroids. This could result in an unintended pregnancy or breakthrough bleeding. Patients should use an additional nonhormonal contraceptive method when taking medications that may decrease the efficacy of hormonal contraceptives).
No products indexed under this heading.

Penicillin G Procaine (Contraceptive effectiveness may be reduced when hormonal contraceptives are co-administered with some antibiotics, antifungals, anticonvulsants, and other drugs that increase the metabolism of contraceptive steroids. This could result in an unintended pregnancy or breakthrough bleeding. Patients should use an additional nonhormonal contraceptive method when taking medications that may decrease the efficacy of hormonal contraceptives). Products include:
Bicillin C-R Injectable Suspension **1826**
Bicillin L-A **1828**

Penicillin G Sodium (Contraceptive effectiveness may be reduced when hormonal contraceptives are co-administered with some antibiotics, antifungals, anticonvulsants, and other drugs that increase the metabolism of contraceptive steroids. This could result in an unintended pregnancy or breakthrough bleeding. Patients should use an additional nonhormonal contraceptive method when taking medications that may decrease the efficacy of hormonal contraceptives).
No products indexed under this heading.

Penicillin V (Contraceptive effectiveness may be reduced when hormonal contraceptives are co-administered with some antibiotics, antifungals, anticonvulsants, and other drugs that increase the metabolism of contraceptive steroids. This could result in an unintended pregnancy or breakthrough bleeding. Patients should use an additional nonhormonal contraceptive method when taking medications that may decrease the efficacy of hormonal contraceptives).
No products indexed under this heading.

Penicillin V Potassium (Contraceptive effectiveness may be reduced when hormonal contraceptives are co-administered with some antibiotics, antifungals, anticonvulsants, and other drugs that increase the metabolism of contraceptive steroids. This could result in an unintended pregnancy or breakthrough bleeding. Patients should use an additional nonhormonal contraceptive method when taking medications that may decrease the efficacy of hormonal contraceptives).
No products indexed under this heading.

Penicillins (Contraceptive effectiveness may be reduced when hormonal contraceptives are co-administered with some antibiotics, antifungals, anticonvulsants, and other drugs that increase the metabolism of contraceptive steroids. This could result in an unintended pregnancy or breakthrough bleeding. Patients should use an additional nonhormonal contraceptive method when taking medications that may decrease the efficacy of hormonal contraceptives).
No products indexed under this heading.

Pentobarbital (Contraceptive effectiveness may be reduced when hormonal contraceptives are co-administered with barbiturates. This could result in an unintended pregnancy or breakthrough bleeding. Patients should use an additional nonhormonal contraceptive method when taking medications that may decrease the efficacy of hormonal contraceptives).
No products indexed under this heading.

Pentobarbital Sodium (Contraceptive effectiveness may be reduced when hormonal contraceptives are co-administered with barbiturates. This could result in an unintended pregnancy or breakthrough bleeding. Patients should use an additional nonhormonal contraceptive method when taking medications that may decrease the efficacy of hormonal contraceptives). Products include:
Nembutal 2012

Perphenazine (Inhibitors of hepatic enzymes may increase plasma hormone levels).
No products indexed under this heading.

Phenacemide (Contraceptive effectiveness may be reduced when hormonal contraceptives are co-administered with some antibiotics, antifungals, anticonvulsants, and other drugs that increase the metabolism of contraceptive steroids. This could result in an unintended pregnancy or breakthrough bleeding. Patients should use an additional nonhormonal contraceptive method when taking medications that may decrease the efficacy of hormonal contraceptives).
No products indexed under this heading.

Phenobarbital (Contraceptive effectiveness may be reduced when hormonal contraceptives are co-administered with barbiturates. This could result in an unintended pregnancy or breakthrough bleeding. Patients should use an additional nonhormonal contraceptive method when taking medications that may decrease the efficacy of hormonal contraceptives). Products include:
Donnatal 2711

Phenobarbital Sodium (Contraceptive effectiveness may be reduced when hormonal contraceptives are co-administered with barbiturates. This could result in an unintended pregnancy or breakthrough bleeding. Patients should use an additional nonhormonal contraceptive method when taking medications that may decrease the efficacy of hormonal contraceptives).
No products indexed under this heading.

Phensuximide (Contraceptive effectiveness may be reduced when hormonal contraceptives are co-administered with some antibiotics, antifungals, anticonvulsants, and other drugs that increase the metabolism of contraceptive steroids. This could result in an unintended pregnancy or breakthrough bleeding. Patients should use an additional nonhormonal contraceptive method when taking medications that may decrease the efficacy of hormonal contraceptives).
No products indexed under this heading.

Phenylbutazone (Contraceptive effectiveness may be reduced when hormonal contraceptives are co-administered with phenylbutazone. This could result in an unintended pregnancy or breakthrough bleeding. Patients should use an additional nonhormonal contraceptive method when taking medications that may decrease the efficacy of hormonal contraceptives).
No products indexed under this heading.

Phenytoin (Contraceptive effectiveness may be reduced when hormonal contraceptives are co-administered with phenytoin. This could result in an unintended pregnancy or breakthrough bleeding. Patients should use an additional nonhormonal contraceptive method when taking medications that may decrease the efficacy of hormonal contraceptives).
No products indexed under this heading.

Phenytoin Sodium (Contraceptive effectiveness may be reduced when hormonal contraceptives are co-administered with phenytoin. This could

result in an unintended pregnancy or breakthrough bleeding. Patients should use an additional nonhormonal contraceptive method when taking medications that may decrease the efficacy of hormonal contraceptives). Products include:
Phenytek Capsules 2380

Piperacillin Sodium (Contraceptive effectiveness may be reduced when hormonal contraceptives are co-administered with some antibiotics, antifungals, anticonvulsants, and other drugs that increase the metabolism of contraceptive steroids. This could result in an unintended pregnancy or breakthrough bleeding. Patients should use an additional nonhormonal contraceptive method when taking medications that may decrease the efficacy of hormonal contraceptives). Products include:
Zosyn 3607

Polythiazide (Inhibitors of hepatic enzymes may increase plasma hormone levels).
No products indexed under this heading.

Posaconazole (Contraceptive effectiveness may be reduced when hormonal contraceptives are co-administered with some antibiotics, antifungals, anticonvulsants, and other drugs that increase the metabolism of contraceptive steroids. This could result in an unintended pregnancy or breakthrough bleeding. Patients should use an additional nonhormonal contraceptive method when taking medications that may decrease the efficacy of hormonal contraceptives). Products include:
Noxafil 3172

Prednisolone (Etonogestrel implant is not recommended for women who require chronic use of drugs that are potent inducers of hepatic enzymes because etonogestrel implant is likely to be less effective for these women).
No products indexed under this heading.

Prednisolone Acetate (Etonogestrel implant is not recommended for women who require chronic use of drugs that are potent inducers of hepatic enzymes because etonogestrel implant is likely to be less effective for these women). Products include:
Blephamide .... ⊙ 212, ⊙ 214
Pred Forte .... ⊙ 225
Pred Mild .... ⊙ 230
Pred-G .... ⊙ 226, ⊙ 227

Prednisolone Sodium Phosphate (Etonogestrel implant is not recommended for women who require chronic use of drugs that are potent inducers of hepatic enzymes because etonogestrel implant is likely to be less effective for these women).
No products indexed under this heading.

Prednisolone Tebutate (Etonogestrel implant is not recommended for women who require chronic use of drugs that are potent inducers of hepatic enzymes because etonogestrel implant is likely to be less effective for these women).
No products indexed under this heading.

Prednisone (Etonogestrel implant is not recommended for women who require chronic use of drugs that are potent inducers of hepatic enzymes because etonogestrel implant is likely to be less effective for these women).
No products indexed under this heading.

Prednisone sodium phosphate (Etonogestrel implant is not recommended for women who require chronic use of drugs that are potent inducers of hepatic enzymes because etonogestrel implant is likely to be less effective for these women).
No products indexed under this heading.

Primidone (Contraceptive effectiveness may be reduced when hormonal

contraceptives are co-administered with some antibiotics, antifungals, anticonvulsants, and other drugs that increase the metabolism of contraceptive steroids. This could result in an unintended pregnancy or breakthrough bleeding. Patients should use an additional nonhormonal contraceptive method when taking medications that may decrease the efficacy of hormonal contraceptives).
No products indexed under this heading.

Propafenone Hydrochloride (Inhibitors of hepatic enzymes may increase plasma hormone levels). Products include:
Rythmol 1648
Rythmol SR 1652

Propoxyphene Hydrochloride (Inhibitors of hepatic enzymes may increase plasma hormone levels).
No products indexed under this heading.

Propoxyphene Napsylate (Inhibitors of hepatic enzymes may increase plasma hormone levels).
No products indexed under this heading.

Protriptyline Hydrochloride (Inhibitors of hepatic enzymes may increase plasma hormone levels).
No products indexed under this heading.

Quercetin (Inhibitors of hepatic enzymes may increase plasma hormone levels).
No products indexed under this heading.

Quinacrine Hydrochloride (Inhibitors of hepatic enzymes may increase plasma hormone levels).
No products indexed under this heading.

Quinidine (Inhibitors of hepatic enzymes may increase plasma hormone levels).
No products indexed under this heading.

Quinidine Gluconate (Inhibitors of hepatic enzymes may increase plasma hormone levels).
No products indexed under this heading.

Quinidine Hydrochloride (Inhibitors of hepatic enzymes may increase plasma hormone levels).
No products indexed under this heading.

Quinidine Polygalacturonate (Inhibitors of hepatic enzymes may increase plasma hormone levels).
No products indexed under this heading.

Quinidine Sulfate (Inhibitors of hepatic enzymes may increase plasma hormone levels).
No products indexed under this heading.

Quinine (Inhibitors of hepatic enzymes may increase plasma hormone levels). Products include:
Hyland's Leg Cramps PM with
   Quinine 3315

Quinine Sulfate (Inhibitors of hepatic enzymes may increase plasma hormone levels).
No products indexed under this heading.

Quinupristin (Inhibitors of hepatic enzymes may increase plasma hormone levels).
No products indexed under this heading.

Ranitidine Bismuth Citrate (Inhibitors of hepatic enzymes may increase plasma hormone levels).
No products indexed under this heading.

Ranitidine Hydrochloride (Inhibitors of hepatic enzymes may increase plasma hormone levels). Products include:
Zantac 1737
Zantac Injection 1732
Zantac Pharmacy 1735

Rifabutin (Etonogestrel implant is not recommended for women who require chronic use of drugs that are potent inducers of hepatic enzymes because etonogestrel implant is likely to be less effective for these women).
No products indexed under this heading.

Rifampicin (Etonogestrel implant is not recommended for women who require chronic use of drugs that are potent inducers of hepatic enzymes because etonogestrel implant is likely to be less effective for these women).
No products indexed under this heading.

Rifampin (Contraceptive effectiveness may be reduced when hormonal contraceptives are co-administered with rifampin. This could result in an unintended pregnancy or breakthrough bleeding. Patients should use an additional nonhormonal contraceptive method when taking medications that may decrease the efficacy of hormonal contraceptives).
No products indexed under this heading.

Rifapentine (Etonogestrel implant is not recommended for women who require chronic use of drugs that are potent inducers of hepatic enzymes because etonogestrel implant is likely to be less effective for these women).
No products indexed under this heading.

Ritonavir (Several of the anti-HIV protease inhibitors have been studied with co-administration of combination oral contraceptives; significant changes (increase and decrease) in the mean area under the curve (AUC) of the estrogen and progestin have been noted in some cases. The efficacy and safety of combination oral contraceptive products may be affected with co-administration of anti-HIV protease inhibitors; it is unknown whether this applies to etonogestrel implant). Products include:
Kaletra 458
Norvir 509

Rufinamide (Contraceptive effectiveness may be reduced when hormonal contraceptives are co-administered with some antibiotics, antifungals, anticonvulsants, and other drugs that increase the metabolism of contraceptive steroids. This could result in an unintended pregnancy or breakthrough bleeding. Patients should use an additional nonhormonal contraceptive method when taking medications that may decrease the efficacy of hormonal contraceptives). Products include:
Banzel 1050

Saquinavir (Several of the anti-HIV protease inhibitors have been studied with co-administration of combination oral contraceptives; significant changes (increase and decrease) in the mean area under the curve (AUC) of the estrogen and progestin have been noted in some cases. The efficacy and safety of combination oral contraceptive products may be affected with co-administration of anti-HIV protease inhibitors; it is unknown whether this applies to etonogestrel implant).
No products indexed under this heading.

Saquinavir Mesylate (Several of the anti-HIV protease inhibitors have been studied with co-administration of combination oral contraceptives; significant changes (increase and decrease) in the mean area under the curve (AUC) of the estrogen and progestin have been noted in some cases. The efficacy and safety of combination oral contraceptive products may be affected with co-administration of anti-HIV protease inhibitors; it is unknown whether this applies to etonogestrel implant).
No products indexed under this heading.

Secobarbital Sodium (Contraceptive effectiveness may be reduced when hormonal contraceptives are co-administered with barbiturates. This could result in an unintended pregnancy or breakthrough bleeding. Patients should use an additional nonhormonal contraceptive method when taking medications that may decrease the efficacy of hormonal contraceptives).
No products indexed under this heading.

Sertaconazole Nitrate (Contraceptive effectiveness may be reduced when hormonal contraceptives are co-administered with some antibiotics, antifungals, anticonvulsants, and other drugs that increase the metabolism of contraceptive steroids. This could result in an unintended pregnancy or breakthrough bleeding. Patients should use an additional nonhormonal contraceptive method when taking medications that may decrease the efficacy of hormonal contraceptives).
No products indexed under this heading.

Sertraline Hydrochloride (Inhibitors of hepatic enzymes may increase plasma hormone levels).
No products indexed under this heading.

Sildenafil Citrate (Inhibitors of hepatic enzymes may increase plasma hormone levels).
No products indexed under this heading.

Sodium Butabarbital (Contraceptive effectiveness may be reduced when hormonal contraceptives are co-administered with barbiturates. This could result in an unintended pregnancy or breakthrough bleeding. Patients should use an additional nonhormonal contraceptive method when taking medications that may decrease the efficacy of hormonal contraceptives).
No products indexed under this heading.

Sodium Cloxacillin Monohydrate (Contraceptive effectiveness may be reduced when hormonal contraceptives are co-administered with some antibiotics, antifungals, anticonvulsants, and other drugs that increase the metabolism of contraceptive steroids. This could result in an unintended pregnancy or breakthrough bleeding. Patients should use an additional nonhormonal contraceptive method when taking medications that may decrease the efficacy of hormonal contraceptives).
No products indexed under this heading.

Sodium Pentobarbital (Contraceptive effectiveness may be reduced when hormonal contraceptives are co-administered with barbiturates. This could result in an unintended pregnancy or breakthrough bleeding. Patients should use an additional nonhormonal contraceptive method when taking medications that may decrease the efficacy of hormonal contraceptives).
No products indexed under this heading.

Sparfloxacin (Contraceptive effectiveness may be reduced when hormonal contraceptives are co-administered with some antibiotics, antifungals, anticonvulsants, and other drugs that increase the metabolism of contraceptive steroids. This could result in an unintended pregnancy or breakthrough bleeding. Patients should use an additional nonhormonal contraceptive method when taking medications that may decrease the efficacy of hormonal contraceptives).
No products indexed under this heading.

Streptomycin Sulfate (Contraceptive effectiveness may be reduced when hormonal contraceptives are co-administered with some antibiotics, antifungals, anticonvulsants, and other drugs that increase the metabolism of contraceptive steroids. This could result in an unintended pregnancy or breakthrough bleeding. Patients should use an additional nonhormonal contraceptive method when taking medications that may decrease the efficacy of hormonal contraceptives).
No products indexed under this heading.

Sulfacytine (Inhibitors of hepatic enzymes may increase plasma hormone levels).
No products indexed under this heading.

Sulfamethizole (Contraceptive effectiveness may be reduced when hormonal contraceptives are co-administered with some antibiotics, antifungals, anticonvulsants, and other drugs that increase the metabolism of contraceptive steroids. This could result in an unintended pregnancy or breakthrough bleeding. Patients should use an additional nonhormonal contraceptive method when taking medications that may decrease the efficacy of hormonal contraceptives).
No products indexed under this heading.

Sulfamethoxazole (Contraceptive effectiveness may be reduced when hormonal contraceptives are co-administered with some antibiotics, antifungals, anticonvulsants, and other drugs that increase the metabolism of contraceptive steroids. This could result in an unintended pregnancy or breakthrough bleeding. Patients should use an additional nonhormonal contraceptive method when taking medications that may decrease the efficacy of hormonal contraceptives).
No products indexed under this heading.

Sulfaphenazole (Inhibitors of hepatic enzymes may increase plasma hormone levels).
No products indexed under this heading.

Sulfasalazine (Inhibitors of hepatic enzymes may increase plasma hormone levels).
No products indexed under this heading.

Sulfinpyrazone (Inhibitors of hepatic enzymes may increase plasma hormone levels).
No products indexed under this heading.

Sulfisoxazole Acetyl (Contraceptive effectiveness may be reduced when hormonal contraceptives are co-administered with some antibiotics, antifungals, anticonvulsants, and other drugs that increase the metabolism of contraceptive steroids. This could result in an unintended pregnancy or breakthrough bleeding. Patients should use an additional nonhormonal contraceptive method when taking medications that may decrease the efficacy of hormonal contraceptives).
No products indexed under this heading.

Sulfisoxazole Diolamine (Contraceptive effectiveness may be reduced when hormonal contraceptives are co-administered with some antibiotics, antifungals, anticonvulsants, and other drugs that increase the metabolism of contraceptive steroids. This could result in an unintended pregnancy or breakthrough bleeding. Patients should use an additional nonhormonal contraceptive method when taking medications that may decrease the efficacy of hormonal contraceptives).
No products indexed under this heading.

Tacrine Hydrochloride (Inhibitors of hepatic enzymes may increase plasma hormone levels).
No products indexed under this heading.

Telithromycin (Inhibitors of hepatic enzymes may increase plasma hormone levels). Products include:
Ketek 2991

Telmisartan (Inhibitors of hepatic enzymes may increase plasma hormone levels). Products include:
Micardis 887
Micardis HCT 889

Terbinafine Hydrochloride (Contraceptive effectiveness may be reduced when hormonal contraceptives are co-administered with some antibiotics, antifungals, anticonvulsants, and other drugs that increase the metabolism of contraceptive steroids. This could result in an unintended pregnancy or breakthrough bleeding. Patients should use an additional nonhormonal contraceptive method when taking medications that may decrease the efficacy of hormonal contraceptives).
No products indexed under this heading.

Terconazole (Contraceptive effectiveness may be reduced when hormonal contraceptives are co-administered with some antibiotics, antifungals, anticonvulsants, and other drugs that increase the metabolism of contraceptive steroids. This could result in an unintended pregnancy or breakthrough bleeding. Patients should use an additional nonhormonal contraceptive method when taking medications that may decrease the efficacy of hormonal contraceptives).
No products indexed under this heading.

Tetracycline Hydrochloride (Contraceptive effectiveness may be reduced when hormonal contraceptives are co-administered with some antibiotics, antifungals, anticonvulsants, and other drugs that increase the metabolism of contraceptive steroids. This could result in an unintended pregnancy or breakthrough bleeding. Patients should use an additional nonhormonal contraceptive method when taking medications that may decrease the efficacy of hormonal contraceptives). Products include:
Pylera 793

Theophylline (Etonogestrel implant is not recommended for women who require chronic use of drugs that are potent inducers of hepatic enzymes because etonogestrel implant is likely to be less effective for these women).
No products indexed under this heading.

Theophylline Anhydrous (Etonogestrel implant is not recommended for women who require chronic use of drugs that are potent inducers of hepatic enzymes because etonogestrel implant is likely to be less effective for these women). Products include:
Uniphyl 2817

Theophylline Calcium Salicylate (Etonogestrel implant is not recommended for women who require chronic use of drugs that are potent inducers of hepatic enzymes because etonogestrel implant is likely to be less effective for these women).
No products indexed under this heading.

Theophylline Dihydroxypropyl (Glyceryl) (Etonogestrel implant is not recommended for women who require chronic use of drugs that are potent inducers of hepatic enzymes because etonogestrel implant is likely to be less effective for these women).
No products indexed under this heading.

Theophylline Ethylenediamine (Etonogestrel implant is not recommended for women who require chronic use of drugs that are potent inducers of hepatic enzymes because etonogestrel implant is likely to be less effective for these women).
No products indexed under this heading.

Theophylline Sodium Glycinate (Etonogestrel implant is not recommended for women who require chronic use of drugs that are potent inducers of hepatic enzymes because etonogestrel implant is likely to be less effective for these women).
No products indexed under this heading.

Thiamylal Sodium (Contraceptive effectiveness may be reduced when hormonal contraceptives are co-administered with barbiturates. This could result in an unintended pregnancy or breakthrough bleeding. Patients should use an additional nonhormonal contraceptive method when taking medications that may decrease the efficacy of hormonal contraceptives).
No products indexed under this heading.

Thioridazine Hydrochloride (Inhibitors of hepatic enzymes may increase plasma hormone levels). Products include:
Thioridazine Hydrochloride 2384

Tiagabine Hydrochloride (Contraceptive effectiveness may be reduced when hormonal contraceptives are co-administered with some antibiotics, antifungals, anticonvulsants, and other drugs that increase the metabolism of contraceptive steroids. This could result in an unintended pregnancy or breakthrough bleeding. Patients should use an additional nonhormonal contraceptive method when taking medications that may decrease the efficacy of hormonal contraceptives). Products include:
Gabitril 972

Ticarcillin Disodium (Contraceptive effectiveness may be reduced when hormonal contraceptives are co-administered with some antibiotics, antifungals, anticonvulsants, and other drugs that increase the metabolism of contraceptive steroids. This could result in an unintended pregnancy or breakthrough bleeding. Patients should use an additional nonhormonal contraceptive method when taking medications that may decrease the efficacy of hormonal contraceptives). Products include:
Timentin ADD-Vantage 1670
Timentin Galaxy 1674
Timentin 1666
Timentin Pharmacy 1678

Ticlopidine Hydrochloride (Inhibitors of hepatic enzymes may increase plasma hormone levels).
No products indexed under this heading.

Tipranavir (Several of the anti-HIV protease inhibitors have been studied with co-administration of combination oral contraceptives; significant changes (increase and decrease) in the mean area under the curve (AUC) of the estrogen and progestin have been noted in some cases. The efficacy and safety of combination oral contraceptive products may be affected with co-administration of anti-HIV protease inhibitors; it is unknown whether this applies to etonogestrel implant).
No products indexed under this heading.

Tobacco (Cigarette smoking increases the risk of serious cardiovascular side effects from the use of combination hormonal contraceptives. This risk increases with age and with heavy smoking (15 or more cigarettes per day) and is quite marked in women over 35 years old who smoke).
No products indexed under this heading.

Tobramycin (Contraceptive effectiveness may be reduced when hormonal contraceptives are co-administered with some antibiotics, antifungals, anticonvulsants, and other drugs that increase the metabolism of contraceptive steroids. This could result in an unintended pregnancy or breakthrough bleeding. Patients should use an additional nonhormonal contraceptive method when taking medications that may decrease the efficacy of hormonal contraceptives). Products include:
Tobi Nebulizer 2546
Tobramycin and Dexamethasone Ophthalmic Suspension .... ⊙ 251

IMPORTANT NOTE: Always consult each drug listing in the patient's regimen for possible interactions.

Tobramycin Sulfate (Contraceptive effectiveness may be reduced when hormonal contraceptives are co-administered with some antibiotics, antifungals, anticonvulsants, and other drugs that increase the metabolism of contraceptive steroids. This could result in an unintended pregnancy or breakthrough bleeding. Patients should use an additional nonhormonal contraceptive method when taking medications that may decrease the efficacy of hormonal contraceptives).
    No products indexed under this heading.

Tolazamide (Etonogestrel implant is not recommended for women who require chronic use of drugs that are potent inducers of hepatic enzymes because etonogestrel implant is likely to be less effective for these women).
    No products indexed under this heading.

Tolbutamide (Etonogestrel implant is not recommended for women who require chronic use of drugs that are potent inducers of hepatic enzymes because etonogestrel implant is likely to be less effective for these women).
    No products indexed under this heading.

Tolbutamide Sodium (Inhibitors of hepatic enzymes may increase plasma hormone levels).
    No products indexed under this heading.

Topiramate (Contraceptive effectiveness may be reduced when hormonal contraceptives are co-administered with topiramate. This could result in an unintended pregnancy or breakthrough bleeding. Patients should use an additional nonhormonal contraceptive method when taking medications that may decrease the efficacy of hormonal contraceptives).
    No products indexed under this heading.

Triamcinolone (Etonogestrel implant is not recommended for women who require chronic use of drugs that are potent inducers of hepatic enzymes because etonogestrel implant is likely to be less effective for these women).
    No products indexed under this heading.

Triamcinolone Acetonide (Etonogestrel implant is not recommended for women who require chronic use of drugs that are potent inducers of hepatic enzymes because etonogestrel implant is likely to be less effective for these women). Products include:

Triamcinolone Diacetate (Etonogestrel implant is not recommended for women who require chronic use of drugs that are potent inducers of hepatic enzymes because etonogestrel implant is likely to be less effective for these women).
    No products indexed under this heading.

Triamcinolone Hexacetonide (Etonogestrel implant is not recommended for women who require chronic use of drugs that are potent inducers of hepatic enzymes because etonogestrel implant is likely to be less effective for these women).
    No products indexed under this heading.

Trimethadione (Contraceptive effectiveness may be reduced when hormonal contraceptives are co-administered with some antibiotics, antifungals, anticonvulsants, and other drugs that increase the metabolism of contraceptive steroids. This could result in an unintended pregnancy or breakthrough bleeding. Patients should use an additional nonhormonal contraceptive method when taking medications that may decrease the efficacy of hormonal contraceptives).
    No products indexed under this heading.

Trimethoprim (Inhibitors of hepatic enzymes may increase plasma hormone levels).
    No products indexed under this heading.

Trimethoprim Hydrochloride (Inhibitors of hepatic enzymes may increase plasma hormone levels).
    No products indexed under this heading.

Trimethoprim Sulfate (Inhibitors of hepatic enzymes may increase plasma hormone levels).
    No products indexed under this heading.

Trimipramine Maleate (Inhibitors of hepatic enzymes may increase plasma hormone levels).
    No products indexed under this heading.

Troglitazone (Etonogestrel implant is not recommended for women who require chronic use of drugs that are potent inducers of hepatic enzymes because etonogestrel implant is likely to be less effective for these women).
    No products indexed under this heading.

Troleandomycin (Contraceptive effectiveness may be reduced when hormonal contraceptives are co-administered with some antibiotics, antifungals, anticonvulsants, and other drugs that increase the metabolism of contraceptive steroids. This could result in an unintended pregnancy or breakthrough bleeding. Patients should use an additional nonhormonal contraceptive method when taking medications that may decrease the efficacy of hormonal contraceptives).
    No products indexed under this heading.

Trovafloxacin Mesylate (Contraceptive effectiveness may be reduced when hormonal contraceptives are co-administered with some antibiotics, antifungals, anticonvulsants, and other drugs that increase the metabolism of contraceptive steroids. This could result in an unintended pregnancy or breakthrough bleeding. Patients should use an additional nonhormonal contraceptive method when taking medications that may decrease the efficacy of hormonal contraceptives).
    No products indexed under this heading.

Valproate Sodium (Contraceptive effectiveness may be reduced when hormonal contraceptives are co-administered with some antibiotics, antifungals, anticonvulsants, and other drugs that increase the metabolism of contraceptive steroids. This could result in an unintended pregnancy or breakthrough bleeding. Patients should use an additional nonhormonal contraceptive method when taking medications that may decrease the efficacy of hormonal contraceptives).
    No products indexed under this heading.

Valproic Acid (Contraceptive effectiveness may be reduced when hormonal contraceptives are co-administered with some antibiotics, antifungals, anticonvulsants, and other drugs that increase the metabolism of contraceptive steroids. This could result in an unintended pregnancy or breakthrough bleeding. Patients should use an additional nonhormonal contraceptive method when taking medications that may decrease the efficacy of hormonal contraceptives).
    No products indexed under this heading.

Vardenafil Hydrochloride (Inhibitors of hepatic enzymes may increase plasma hormone levels). Products include:

Venlafaxine Hydrochloride (Inhibitors of hepatic enzymes may increase plasma hormone levels). Products include:

Verapamil Hydrochloride (Inhibitors of hepatic enzymes may increase plasma hormone levels). Products include:

Voriconazole (Contraceptive effectiveness may be reduced when hormonal contraceptives are co-administered with some antibiotics, antifungals, anticonvulsants, and other drugs that increase the metabolism of contraceptive steroids. This could result in an unintended pregnancy or breakthrough bleeding. Patients should use an additional nonhormonal contraceptive method when taking medications that may decrease the efficacy of hormonal contraceptives).
    No products indexed under this heading.

Zafirlukast (Inhibitors of hepatic enzymes may increase plasma hormone levels). Products include:

Zileuton (Inhibitors of hepatic enzymes may increase plasma hormone levels).
    No products indexed under this heading.

Zonisamide (Contraceptive effectiveness may be reduced when hormonal contraceptives are co-administered with some antibiotics, antifungals, anticonvulsants, and other drugs that increase the metabolism of contraceptive steroids. This could result in an unintended pregnancy or breakthrough bleeding. Patients should use an additional nonhormonal contraceptive method when taking medications that may decrease the efficacy of hormonal contraceptives). Products include:

Food Interactions

Broccoli (Etonogestrel implant is not recommended for women who require chronic use of drugs that are potent inducers of hepatic enzymes because etonogestrel implant is likely to be less effective for these women).

Brussel Sprouts (Etonogestrel implant is not recommended for women who require chronic use of drugs that are potent inducers of hepatic enzymes because etonogestrel implant is likely to be less effective for these women).

Charbroiled Food (Etonogestrel implant is not recommended for women who require chronic use of drugs that are potent inducers of hepatic enzymes because etonogestrel implant is likely to be less effective for these women).

Grapefruit (Inhibitors of hepatic enzymes may increase plasma hormone levels).

Grapefruit Juice (Inhibitors of hepatic enzymes may increase plasma hormone levels).

INDAPAMIDE TABLETS
May interact with alcohols, antihypertensives, barbiturates, cardiac glycosides, corticosteroids, insulin, lithium preparations, narcotic analgesics, and certain other agents. Compounds in these categories include:

Acebutolol Hydrochloride (Indapamide may add to or potentiate the therapeutic effect of other antihypertensive drugs).
    No products indexed under this heading.

ACTH (Co-administration with ACTH may increase the risk of hypokalemia).
    No products indexed under this heading.

Alclometasone Dipropionate (Co-administration with corticosteroids may increase the risk of hypokalemia).
    No products indexed under this heading.

Alfentanil Hydrochloride (Aggravates orthostatic hypotension).
    No products indexed under this heading.

Aliskiren (Indapamide may add to or potentiate the therapeutic effect of other antihypertensive drugs). Products include:

Amlodipine Besylate (Indapamide may add to or potentiate the therapeutic effect of other antihypertensive drugs). Products include:

Amobarbital (Aggravates orthostatic hypotension).
    No products indexed under this heading.

Amobarbital Sodium (Aggravates orthostatic hypotension).
    No products indexed under this heading.

Apomorphine (Aggravates orthostatic hypotension).
    No products indexed under this heading.

Apomorphine Hydrochloride (Aggravates orthostatic hypotension).
    No products indexed under this heading.

Aprobarbital (Aggravates orthostatic hypotension).
    No products indexed under this heading.

Atenolol (Indapamide may add to or potentiate the therapeutic effect of other antihypertensive drugs).
    No products indexed under this heading.

Beclomethasone Dipropionate (Co-administration with corticosteroids may increase the risk of hypokalemia). Products include:

Beclomethasone Dipropionate Monohydrate (Co-administration with corticosteroids may increase the risk of hypokalemia). Products include:

Benazepril Hydrochloride (Indapamide may add to or potentiate the therapeutic effect of other antihypertensive drugs).
    No products indexed under this heading.

Bendroflumethiazide (Indapamide may add to or potentiate the therapeutic effect of other antihypertensive drugs).
    No products indexed under this heading.

Betamethasone (Co-administration with corticosteroids may increase the risk of hypokalemia).
    No products indexed under this heading.

Betamethasone Acetate (Co-administration with corticosteroids may increase the risk of hypokalemia).
    No products indexed under this heading.

Betamethasone Benzoate (Co-administration with corticosteroids may increase the risk of hypokalemia).
    No products indexed under this heading.

Betamethasone Dipropionate (Co-administration with corticosteroids may increase the risk of hypokalemia). Products include:

Betamethasone Sodium Phosphate (Co-administration with corticosteroids may increase the risk of hypokalemia).
    No products indexed under this heading.

Betamethasone Valerate (Co-administration with corticosteroids may increase the risk of hypokalemia). Products include:

Betaxolol Hydrochloride (Indapamide may add to or potentiate the therapeutic effect of other antihypertensive drugs).
    No products indexed under this heading.

865 **Interactions Index** **Indapamide**

Bisoprolol Fumarate (Indapamide may add to or potentiate the therapeutic effect of other antihypertensive drugs).
No products indexed under this heading.

Budesonide (Co-administration with corticosteroids may increase the risk of hypokalemia). Products include:
Pulmicort Flexhaler 714
Symbicort 80/4.5 720
Symbicort 160/4.5 720

Buprenorphine Hydrochloride (Aggravates orthostatic hypotension).
No products indexed under this heading.

Butabarbital (Aggravates orthostatic hypotension).
No products indexed under this heading.

Butabarbital Sodium (Aggravates orthostatic hypotension).
No products indexed under this heading.

Butalbital (Aggravates orthostatic hypotension).
No products indexed under this heading.

Candesartan Cilexetil (Indapamide may add to or potentiate the therapeutic effect of other antihypertensive drugs). Products include:
Atacand 697
Atacand HCT 700

Captopril (Indapamide may add to or potentiate the therapeutic effect of other antihypertensive drugs). Products include:
Captopril 2341

Carteolol Hydrochloride (Indapamide may add to or potentiate the therapeutic effect of other antihypertensive drugs).
No products indexed under this heading.

Carvedilol (Indapamide may add to or potentiate the therapeutic effect of other antihypertensive drugs). Products include:
Coreg 1409

Carvedilol Phosphate (Indapamide may add to or potentiate the therapeutic effect of other antihypertensive drugs). Products include:
Coreg CR 1416

Chlorothiazide (Indapamide may add to or potentiate the therapeutic effect of other antihypertensive drugs).
No products indexed under this heading.

Chlorothiazide Sodium (Indapamide may add to or potentiate the therapeutic effect of other antihypertensive drugs). Products include:
Diuril Intravenous 2009

Chlorthalidone (Indapamide may add to or potentiate the therapeutic effect of other antihypertensive drugs). Products include:
Clorpres 2344

Ciclesonide (Co-administration with corticosteroids may increase the risk of hypokalemia).
No products indexed under this heading.

Clonidine (Indapamide may add to or potentiate the therapeutic effect of other antihypertensive drugs). Products include:
Catapres-TTS 884

Clonidine Hydrochloride (Indapamide may add to or potentiate the therapeutic effect of other antihypertensive drugs). Products include:
Clorpres 2344

Codeine Phosphate (Aggravates orthostatic hypotension). Products include:
Tylenol with Codeine 2691

Codeine Sulfate (Aggravates orthostatic hypotension).
No products indexed under this heading.

Cortisone Acetate (Co-administration with corticosteroids may increase the risk of hypokalemia).
No products indexed under this heading.

Deserpidine (Indapamide may add to or potentiate the therapeutic effect of other antihypertensive drugs).
No products indexed under this heading.

Deslanoside (Concurrent digitalis therapy may exaggerate metabolic effects of hypokalemia; especially myocardial effects such as increase ventricular irritability).
No products indexed under this heading.

Desoximetasone (Co-administration with corticosteroids may increase the risk of hypokalemia).
No products indexed under this heading.

Dexamethasone (Co-administration with corticosteroids may increase the risk of hypokalemia). Products include:
Ciprodex 583
Ozurdex .... ⊙ 223
Tobramycin and Dexamethasone Ophthalmic Suspension .... ⊙ 251

Dexamethasone Acetate (Co-administration with corticosteroids may increase the risk of hypokalemia).
No products indexed under this heading.

Dexamethasone Phosphate (Co-administration with corticosteroids may increase the risk of hypokalemia).
No products indexed under this heading.

Dexamethasone Sodium (Co-administration with corticosteroids may increase the risk of hypokalemia).
No products indexed under this heading.

Dexamethasone Sodium Phosphate (Co-administration with corticosteroids may increase the risk of hypokalemia).
No products indexed under this heading.

Dexamethasone Sodium Phosphate Injection (Co-administration with corticosteroids may increase the risk of hypokalemia).
No products indexed under this heading.

Dezocine (Aggravates orthostatic hypotension).
No products indexed under this heading.

Diazoxide (Indapamide may add to or potentiate the therapeutic effect of other antihypertensive drugs). Products include:
Proglycem 1179
Proglycem Suspension 1179

Diflorasone Diacetate (Co-administration with corticosteroids may increase the risk of hypokalemia).
No products indexed under this heading.

Digitalis Glycoside Preparations (Concurrent digitalis therapy may exaggerate metabolic effects of hypokalemia; especially myocardial effects such as increase ventricular irritability).
No products indexed under this heading.

Digitalis Lanata (Concurrent digitalis therapy may exaggerate metabolic effects of hypokalemia; especially myocardial effects such as increase ventricular irritability).
No products indexed under this heading.

Digitalis Purpurea (Concurrent digitalis therapy may exaggerate metabolic effects of hypokalemia; especially myocardial effects such as increase ventricular irritability).
No products indexed under this heading.

Digitoxin (Concurrent digitalis therapy may exaggerate metabolic effects of hypokalemia; especially myocardial effects such as increase ventricular irritability).
No products indexed under this heading.

Digoxin (Concurrent digitalis therapy may exaggerate metabolic effects of hypokalemia; especially myocardial effects such as increase ventricular irritability). Products include:
Lanoxin Injection 1546
Lanoxin Injection Pediatric 1549
Lanoxin Tablets 1553

Dihydrocodeine Bitartrate (Aggravates orthostatic hypotension).
No products indexed under this heading.

Dihydrocodeinone Bitartrate (Aggravates orthostatic hypotension).
No products indexed under this heading.

Diltiazem Hydrochloride (Indapamide may add to or potentiate the therapeutic effect of other antihypertensive drugs). Products include:
Cardizem LA 423

Diltiazem Maleate (Indapamide may add to or potentiate the therapeutic effect of other antihypertensive drugs).
No products indexed under this heading.

Doxazosin Mesylate (Indapamide may add to or potentiate the therapeutic effect of other antihypertensive drugs).
No products indexed under this heading.

Enalapril Maleate (Indapamide may add to or potentiate the therapeutic effect of other antihypertensive drugs).
No products indexed under this heading.

Enalaprilat (Indapamide may add to or potentiate the therapeutic effect of other antihypertensive drugs).
No products indexed under this heading.

Eprosartan Mesylate (Indapamide may add to or potentiate the therapeutic effect of other antihypertensive drugs). Products include:
Teveten 538
Teveten HCT 541

Esmolol Hydrochloride (Indapamide may add to or potentiate the therapeutic effect of other antihypertensive drugs).
No products indexed under this heading.

Ethanol (Aggravates orthostatic hypotension).
No products indexed under this heading.

Ethyl Alcohol (Aggravates orthostatic hypotension).
No products indexed under this heading.

Felodipine (Indapamide may add to or potentiate the therapeutic effect of other antihypertensive drugs).
No products indexed under this heading.

Fentanyl (Aggravates orthostatic hypotension). Products include:
Duragesic 2604
Fentanyl Transdermal System 2346
Onsolis 2054

Fentanyl Citrate (Aggravates orthostatic hypotension). Products include:
Fentora 966

Fludrocortisone Acetate (Co-administration with corticosteroids may increase the risk of hypokalemia).
No products indexed under this heading.

Flumethasone Pivalate (Co-administration with corticosteroids may increase the risk of hypokalemia).
No products indexed under this heading.

Flunisolide Hemihydrate (Co-administration with corticosteroids may increase the risk of hypokalemia).
No products indexed under this heading.

Fluticasone Furoate (Co-administration with corticosteroids may increase the risk of hypokalemia). Products include:
Veramyst 1713

Fluticasone Propionate (Co-administration with corticosteroids may increase the risk of hypokalemia). Products include:
Advair 100/50 1275
Advair 250/50 1275
Advair 500/50 1275
Advair HFA 45/21 1288
Advair HFA 115/21 1288
Advair HFA 230/21 1288
Flonase 1459
Flovent Diskus 1463
Flovent HFA 1470

Fosinopril Sodium (Indapamide may add to or potentiate the therapeutic effect of other antihypertensive drugs).
No products indexed under this heading.

Furosemide (Indapamide may add to or potentiate the therapeutic effect of other antihypertensive drugs). Products include:
Furosemide 2354

Guanabenz Acetate (Indapamide may add to or potentiate the therapeutic effect of other antihypertensive drugs).
No products indexed under this heading.

Guanethidine (Indapamide may add to or potentiate the therapeutic effect of other antihypertensive drugs).
No products indexed under this heading.

Guanethidine Monosulfate (Indapamide may add to or potentiate the therapeutic effect of other antihypertensive drugs).
No products indexed under this heading.

Guanethidine Sulfate (Indapamide may add to or potentiate the therapeutic effect of other antihypertensive drugs).
No products indexed under this heading.

Hexobarbital (Aggravates orthostatic hypotension).
No products indexed under this heading.

Hydralazine Hydrochloride (Indapamide may add to or potentiate the therapeutic effect of other antihypertensive drugs).
No products indexed under this heading.

Hydrochlorothiazide (Indapamide may add to or potentiate the therapeutic effect of other antihypertensive drugs). Products include:
Atacand HCT 700
Avalide 2956
Benicar HCT 1017
Diovan HCT 2419
Dyazide 1429
Exforge HCT 2449
Hyzaar 2162
Hyzaar 100-12.5 2162
Micardis HCT 889
Prinzide 2246
Tekturna HCT 2541
Teveten HCT 541

Hydrocodone Bitartrate (Aggravates orthostatic hypotension). Products include:
Vicodin 560
Vicodin ES 561
Vicodin HP 563
Vicoprofen 564
Zydone 1138

Hydrocodone Polistirex (Aggravates orthostatic hypotension). Products include:
Tussionex 3443

Hydrocortisone (Co-administration with corticosteroids may increase the risk of hypokalemia).
No products indexed under this heading.

Hydrocortisone (Alcohol) (Co-administration with corticosteroids may increase the risk of hypokalemia).
No products indexed under this heading.

Hydrocortisone Acetate (Co-administration with corticosteroids may increase the risk of hypokalemia).
No products indexed under this heading.

Hydrocortisone Butyrate (Co-administration with corticosteroids may increase the risk of hypokalemia).
No products indexed under this heading.

Hydrocortisone Cypionate (Co-administration with corticosteroids may increase the risk of hypokalemia).
No products indexed under this heading.

Hydrocortisone Hemisuccinate (Co-administration with corticosteroids may increase the risk of hypokalemia).
No products indexed under this heading.

IMPORTANT NOTE: Always consult each drug listing in the patient's regimen for possible interactions.

Hydrocortisone Probutate (Co-administration with corticosteroids may increase the risk of hypokalemia).
No products indexed under this heading.

Hydrocortisone Sodium Phosphate (Co-administration with corticosteroids may increase the risk of hypokalemia).
No products indexed under this heading.

Hydrocortisone Sodium Succinate (Co-administration with corticosteroids may increase the risk of hypokalemia).
No products indexed under this heading.

Hydrocortisone Valerate (Co-administration with corticosteroids may increase the risk of hypokalemia).
No products indexed under this heading.

Hydroflumethiazide (Indapamide may add to or potentiate the therapeutic effect of other antihypertensive drugs).
No products indexed under this heading.

Hydromorphone (Aggravates orthostatic hypotension).
No products indexed under this heading.

Hydromorphone Hydrochloride (Aggravates orthostatic hypotension). Products include:
Dilaudid Injection 2800
Dilaudid Oral 2797
Dilaudid Tablets 2797
Dilaudid-HP 2800

Insulin (Hyperglycemia has been reported with the use of indapamide; co-administration may require adjustment in insulin dosage in diabetic patients).
No products indexed under this heading.

Insulin, Human, Zinc Suspension (Hyperglycemia has been reported with the use of indapamide; co-administration may require adjustment in insulin dosage in diabetic patients).
No products indexed under this heading.

Insulin, Human (rDNA origin) (Hyperglycemia has been reported with the use of indapamide; co-administration may require adjustment in insulin dosage in diabetic patients). Products include:
Exubera 2717

Insulin, Human NPH (Hyperglycemia has been reported with the use of indapamide; co-administration may require adjustment in insulin dosage in diabetic patients). Products include:
Humulin N Vial 1934

Insulin, Human Regular (Hyperglycemia has been reported with the use of indapamide; co-administration may require adjustment in insulin dosage in diabetic patients). Products include:
Humulin R 1937
Humulin R (U-500) 1939

Insulin, Human Regular and Human NPH Mixture (Hyperglycemia has been reported with the use of indapamide; co-administration may require adjustment in insulin dosage in diabetic patients). Products include:
Humulin 50/50 1930
Humulin 70/30 Vial 1931

Insulin, NPH (Hyperglycemia has been reported with the use of indapamide; co-administration may require adjustment in insulin dosage in diabetic patients).
No products indexed under this heading.

Insulin, Regular (Hyperglycemia has been reported with the use of indapamide; co-administration may require adjustment in insulin dosage in diabetic patients).
No products indexed under this heading.

Insulin, Regular and NPH mixture (Hyperglycemia has been reported with the use of indapamide; co-administration may require adjustment in insulin dosage in diabetic patients).
No products indexed under this heading.

Insulin, Zinc Crystals (Hyperglycemia has been reported with the use of indapamide; co-administration may require adjustment in insulin dosage in diabetic patients).
No products indexed under this heading.

Insulin, Zinc Suspension (Hyperglycemia has been reported with the use of indapamide; co-administration may require adjustment in insulin dosage in diabetic patients).
No products indexed under this heading.

Insulin Aspart (Hyperglycemia has been reported with the use of indapamide; co-administration may require adjustment in insulin dosage in diabetic patients).
No products indexed under this heading.

Insulin Aspart, Human (Hyperglycemia has been reported with the use of indapamide; co-administration may require adjustment in insulin dosage in diabetic patients). Products include:
NovoLog Mix 70/30 2581

Insulin Aspart, Human Regular (Hyperglycemia has been reported with the use of indapamide; co-administration may require adjustment in insulin dosage in diabetic patients). Products include:
NovoLog 2575

Insulin Aspart Protamine, Human (Hyperglycemia has been reported with the use of indapamide; co-administration may require adjustment in insulin dosage in diabetic patients). Products include:
NovoLog Mix 70/30 2581

Insulin Detemir (rDNA Origin) (Hyperglycemia has been reported with the use of indapamide; co-administration may require adjustment in insulin dosage in diabetic patients). Products include:
Levemir 2566

Insulin Glargine (Hyperglycemia has been reported with the use of indapamide; co-administration may require adjustment in insulin dosage in diabetic patients). Products include:
Lantus 2996

Insulin Glulisine (Hyperglycemia has been reported with the use of indapamide; co-administration may require adjustment in insulin dosage in diabetic patients). Products include:
Apidra 2937
Apidra SoloStar 2937

Insulin Lispro, Human (Hyperglycemia has been reported with the use of indapamide; co-administration may require adjustment in insulin dosage in diabetic patients). Products include:
Humalog 1910
Humalog Mix 1914
Humalog Mix75/25 1917

Insulin Lispro Protamine, Human (Hyperglycemia has been reported with the use of indapamide; co-administration may require adjustment in insulin dosage in diabetic patients). Products include:
Humalog Mix 1914
Humalog Mix75/25 1917

Irbesartan (Indapamide may add to or potentiate the therapeutic effect of other antihypertensive drugs). Products include:
Avalide 2956
Avapro 2962

Isradipine (Indapamide may add to or potentiate the therapeutic effect of other antihypertensive drugs). Products include:
DynaCirc CR 1432

Labetalol Hydrochloride (Indapamide may add to or potentiate the therapeutic effect of other antihypertensive drugs).
No products indexed under this heading.

Levorphanol Tartrate (Aggravates orthostatic hypotension).
No products indexed under this heading.

Lisinopril (Indapamide may add to or potentiate the therapeutic effect of other antihypertensive drugs). Products include:
Prinivil 2241
Prinzide 2246

Lithium (Diuretics reduce lithium's renal clearance and add a high risk of lithium toxicity).
No products indexed under this heading.

Lithium Carbonate (Diuretics reduce lithium's renal clearance and add a high risk of lithium toxicity).
No products indexed under this heading.

Lithium Citrate (Diuretics reduce lithium's renal clearance and add a high risk of lithium toxicity).
No products indexed under this heading.

Losartan Potassium (Indapamide may add to or potentiate the therapeutic effect of other antihypertensive drugs). Products include:
Cozaar 2106
Hyzaar 2162
Hyzaar 100-12.5 2162

Mecamylamine Hydrochloride (Indapamide may add to or potentiate the therapeutic effect of other antihypertensive drugs).
No products indexed under this heading.

Meperidine Hydrochloride (Aggravates orthostatic hypotension).
No products indexed under this heading.

Mephobarbital (Aggravates orthostatic hypotension).
No products indexed under this heading.

Methadone Hydrochloride (Aggravates orthostatic hypotension).
No products indexed under this heading.

Methyclothiazide (Indapamide may add to or potentiate the therapeutic effect of other antihypertensive drugs).
No products indexed under this heading.

Methyldopa (Indapamide may add to or potentiate the therapeutic effect of other antihypertensive drugs).
No products indexed under this heading.

Methyldopate Hydrochloride (Indapamide may add to or potentiate the therapeutic effect of other antihypertensive drugs).
No products indexed under this heading.

Methylprednisolone (Co-administration with corticosteroids may increase the risk of hypokalemia).
No products indexed under this heading.

Methylprednisolone Acetate (Co-administration with corticosteroids may increase the risk of hypokalemia).
No products indexed under this heading.

Methylprednisolone Sodium Succinate (Co-administration with corticosteroids may increase the risk of hypokalemia).
No products indexed under this heading.

Metolazone (Indapamide may add to or potentiate the therapeutic effect of other antihypertensive drugs).
No products indexed under this heading.

Metoprolol Succinate (Indapamide may add to or potentiate the therapeutic effect of other antihypertensive drugs). Products include:
Toprol XL 732

Metoprolol Tartrate (Indapamide may add to or potentiate the therapeutic effect of other antihypertensive drugs).
No products indexed under this heading.

Metyrosine (Indapamide may add to or potentiate the therapeutic effect of other antihypertensive drugs).
No products indexed under this heading.

Mibefradil Dihydrochloride (Indapamide may add to or potentiate the therapeutic effect of other antihypertensive drugs).
No products indexed under this heading.

Minoxidil (Indapamide may add to or potentiate the therapeutic effect of other antihypertensive drugs).
No products indexed under this heading.

Moexipril Hydrochloride (Indapamide may add to or potentiate the therapeutic effect of other antihypertensive drugs).
No products indexed under this heading.

Mometasone Furoate (Co-administration with corticosteroids may increase the risk of hypokalemia). Products include:
Asmanex 3058
Elocon Cream 3111
Elocon Lotion 3112
Elocon Ointment 3114

Mometasone Furoate Monohydrate (Co-administration with corticosteroids may increase the risk of hypokalemia). Products include:
Nasonex 3166

Morphine Sulfate (Aggravates orthostatic hypotension). Products include:
Avinza 1822
Embeda 1831
MS Contin 2803

Morphine Sulfate, Liposomal (Aggravates orthostatic hypotension).
No products indexed under this heading.

Nadolol (Indapamide may add to or potentiate the therapeutic effect of other antihypertensive drugs). Products include:
Nadolol 2359

Nebivolol (Indapamide may add to or potentiate the therapeutic effect of other antihypertensive drugs). Products include:
Bystolic 1147

Nicardipine Hydrochloride (Indapamide may add to or potentiate the therapeutic effect of other antihypertensive drugs).
No products indexed under this heading.

Nifedipine (Indapamide may add to or potentiate the therapeutic effect of other antihypertensive drugs).
No products indexed under this heading.

Nisoldipine (Indapamide may add to or potentiate the therapeutic effect of other antihypertensive drugs).
No products indexed under this heading.

Nitroglycerin (Indapamide may add to or potentiate the therapeutic effect of other antihypertensive drugs). Products include:
Nitro-Dur 3170
Nitrolingual 3266

Norepinephrine Bitartrate (Indapamide may decrease arterial responsiveness to norepinephrine).
No products indexed under this heading.

Oxycodone Hydrochloride (Aggravates orthostatic hypotension). Products include:
OxyContin 2807
Percocet 1121
Percodan 1124

Oxycodone Terephthalate (Aggravates orthostatic hypotension).
No products indexed under this heading.

Oxymorphone Hydrochloride (Aggravates orthostatic hypotension). Products include:
Opana 1110
Opana ER 1114

Penbutolol Sulfate (Indapamide may add to or potentiate the therapeutic effect of other antihypertensive drugs).
No products indexed under this heading.

Pentobarbital (Aggravates orthostatic hypotension).
No products indexed under this heading.

Food Interactions

Alcohol (Aggravates orthostatic hypotension).

Beer, reduced-alcohol (Aggravates orthostatic hypotension).

Beer, unspecified (Aggravates orthostatic hypotension).

Wine, Chianti (Aggravates orthostatic hypotension).

Wine, Red (Aggravates orthostatic hypotension).

Wine, unspecified (Aggravates orthostatic hypotension).

Wine products (Aggravates orthostatic hypotension).

INDOCIN CAPSULES
May interact with ACE inhibitors, angiotensin-II receptor antagonists, anticoagulants, beta-blockers, lithium preparations, loop diuretics, non-steroidal anti-inflammatory agents, potassium sparing diuretics, thiazides, and certain other agents. Compounds in these categories include:

Metoprolol Tartrate (Blunting of antihypertensive effect of beta blockers). No products indexed under this heading.

Moexipril Hydrochloride (Reports suggest that NSAIDs may diminish the antihypertensive effect of ACE-inhibitors and angiotensin II antagonists. These interactions should be given consideration in patients taking NSAIDs concomitantly with ACE-inhibitors or angiotensin II antagonists. In some patients with compromised renal function, the co-administration of an NSAID and an ACE-inhibitor or an angiotensin II antagonist may result in further deterioration of renal funchtion, including possible acute renal failure, which is usually reversible). No products indexed under this heading.

Nabumetone (Concomitant use is not recommended due to the increased possibility of gastrointestinal toxicity, with little or no increase in efficacy). No products indexed under this heading.

Nadolol (Blunting of antihypertensive effect of beta blockers). Products include:
Nadolol 2359

Naproxen (Concomitant use is not recommended due to the increased possibility of gastrointestinal toxicity, with little or no increase in efficacy). Products include:
EC-Naprosyn 2850
Naprosyn 2850
Anaprox/Naprosyn 2850

Naproxen Sodium (Concomitant use is not recommended due to the increased possibility of gastrointestinal toxicity, with little or no increase in efficacy). Products include:
Anaprox 2850
Anaprox DS 2850
Treximet 1681

Nebivolol (Blunting of antihypertensive effect of beta blockers). Products include:
Bystolic 1147

Nephrotoxic Drugs (Overt renal decompensation). No products indexed under this heading.

Oxaprozin (Concomitant use is not recommended due to the increased possibility of gastrointestinal toxicity, with little or no increase in efficacy). No products indexed under this heading.

Penbutolol Sulfate (Blunting of antihypertensive effect of beta blockers). No products indexed under this heading.

Perindopril Erbumine (Reports suggest that NSAIDs may diminish the antihypertensive effect of ACE-inhibitors and angiotensin II antagonists. These interactions should be given consideration in patients taking NSAIDs concomitantly with ACE-inhibitors or angiotensin II antagonists. In some patients with compromised renal function, the co-administration of an NSAID and an ACE-inhibitor or an angiotensin II antagonist may result in further deterioration of renal funchtion, including possible acute renal failure, which is usually reversible). No products indexed under this heading.

Phenylbutazone (Concomitant use is not recommended due to the increased possibility of gastrointestinal toxicity, with little or no increase in efficacy). No products indexed under this heading.

Pindolol (Blunting of antihypertensive effect of beta blockers). No products indexed under this heading.

Piroxicam (Concomitant use is not recommended due to the increased possibility of gastrointestinal toxicity, with little or no increase in efficacy). No products indexed under this heading.

Polythiazide (Reduced diuretic, natriuretic, and antihypertensive effects of thiazide diuretics). No products indexed under this heading.

Probenecid (Increased plasma levels of indomethacin). No products indexed under this heading.

Propranolol Hydrochloride (Blunting of antihypertensive effect of beta blockers). Products include:
InnoPran XL 1517

Quinapril Hydrochloride (Reports suggest that NSAIDs may diminish the antihypertensive effect of ACE-inhibitors and angiotensin II antagonists. These interactions should be given consideration in patients taking NSAIDs concomitantly with ACE-inhibitors or angiotensin II antagonists. In some patients with compromised renal function, the co-administration of an NSAID and an ACE-inhibitor or an angiotensin II antagonist may result in further deterioration of renal funchtion, including possible acute renal failure, which is usually reversible). No products indexed under this heading.

Ramipril (Reports suggest that NSAIDs may diminish the antihypertensive effect of ACE-inhibitors and angiotensin II antagonists. These interactions should be given consideration in patients taking NSAIDs concomitantly with ACE-inhibitors or angiotensin II antagonists. In some patients with compromised renal function, the co-administration of an NSAID and an ACE-inhibitor or an angiotensin II antagonist may result in further deterioration of renal funchtion, including possible acute renal failure, which is usually reversible). No products indexed under this heading.

Rofecoxib (Concomitant use is not recommended due to the increased possibility of gastrointestinal toxicity, with little or no increase in efficacy). No products indexed under this heading.

Sotalol Hydrochloride (Blunting of antihypertensive effect of beta blockers). No products indexed under this heading.

Spirapril Hydrochloride (Reports suggest that NSAIDs may diminish the antihypertensive effect of ACE-inhibitors and angiotensin II antagonists. These interactions should be given consideration in patients taking NSAIDs concomitantly with ACE-inhibitors or angiotensin II antagonists. In some patients with compromised renal function, the co-administration of an NSAID and an ACE-inhibitor or an angiotensin II antagonist may result in further deterioration of renal funchtion, including possible acute renal failure, which is usually reversible). No products indexed under this heading.

Spironolactone (Reduced diuretic, natriuretic and antihypertensive effects of increased serum potassium levels). No products indexed under this heading.

Sulindac (Concomitant use is not recommended due to the increased possibility of gastrointestinal toxicity, with little or no increase in efficacy). Products include:
Clinoril 2098

Telmisartan (Reports suggest that NSAIDs may diminish the antihypertensive effect of ACE-inhibitors and angiotensin II antagonists. These interactions should be given consideration in patients taking NSAIDs concomitantly with ACE-inhibitors or angiotensin II antagonists. In some patients with compromised renal function, the co-administration of an NSAID and an ACE-inhibitor or an angiotensin II antagonist may result in further deterioration of renal funchtion, including possible acute renal failure, which is usually reversible). Products include:
Micardis 887
Micardis HCT 889

Timolol Hemihydrate (Blunting of antihypertensive effect of beta blockers). Products include:

Betimol 3490

Timolol Maleate (Blunting of antihypertensive effect of beta blockers). Products include:
Combigan 601
Dorzolamide
Hydrochloride/Timolol Maleate
Ophthalmic Solution .... ⊙243
Timoptic in Ocudose .... ⊙231

Tinzaparin Sodium (Bleeding has been reported in patients on concomitant treatment with anticoagulants and indomethacin. Caution should be exercised when indomethacin and anticoagulants are administered concomitantly). No products indexed under this heading.

Tolmetin Sodium (Concomitant use is not recommended due to the increased possibility of gastrointestinal toxicity, with little or no increase in efficacy). No products indexed under this heading.

Torsemide (Reduced diuretic, natriuretic, and antihypertensive effects of loop diuretics). No products indexed under this heading.

Trandolapril (Reports suggest that NSAIDs may diminish the antihypertensive effect of ACE-inhibitors and angiotensin II antagonists. These interactions should be given consideration in patients taking NSAIDs concomitantly with ACE-inhibitors or angiotensin II antagonists. In some patients with compromised renal function, the co-administration of an NSAID and an ACE-inhibitor or an angiotensin II antagonist may result in further deterioration of renal funchtion, including possible acute renal failure, which is usually reversible). Products include:
Mavik 489
Tarka 534

Triamterene (The addition of triamterene to maintenance schedule of indomethacin has resulted in reversible acute renal failure; potential for increased hyperkalemia; concurrent therapy should be avoided). Products include:
Dyazide 1429
Dyrenium 3495

Valdecoxib (Concomitant use is not recommended due to the increased possibility of gastrointestinal toxicity, with little or no increase in efficacy). No products indexed under this heading.

Valsartan (Reports suggest that NSAIDs may diminish the antihypertensive effect of ACE-inhibitors and angiotensin II antagonists. These interactions should be given consideration in patients taking NSAIDs concomitantly with ACE-inhibitors or angiotensin II antagonists. In some patients with compromised renal function, the co-administration of an NSAID and an ACE-inhibitor or an angiotensin II antagonist may result in further deterioration of renal funchtion, including possible acute renal failure, which is usually reversible). Products include:
Diovan 2413
Diovan HCT 2419
Exforge 2443
Exforge HCT 2449
Valturna 3637

Warfarin Sodium (Bleeding has been reported in patients on concomitant treatment with anticoagulants and indomethacin. Caution should be exercised when indomethacin and anticoagulants are administered concomitantly). No products indexed under this heading.

INDOCIN I.V.
(Indomethacin Sodium Trihydrate) 2007
May interact with ACE inhibitors, angiotensin-II receptor antagonists, anticoagulants, cardiac glycosides, and certain other agents. Compounds in these categories include:

Amikacin Sulfate (Serum levels of amikacin significantly elevated). No products indexed under this heading.

Anisindione (Bleeding has been reported in patients on concomitant treatment with anticoagulants and indomethacin, therefore they should be co-administered with caution). No products indexed under this heading.

Ardeparin Sodium (Bleeding has been reported in patients on concomitant treatment with anticoagulants and indomethacin, therefore they should be co-administered with caution). No products indexed under this heading.

Benazepril Hydrochloride (In patients with compromised renal function, the co-administration of an NSAID and an ACE inhibitor may result in further deterioration of renal function, including possible acute renal failure, which is usually reversible). No products indexed under this heading.

Candesartan Cilexetil (In patients with compromised renal function, the co-administration of an NSAID and an angiotensin II antagonist may result in further deterioration of renal function, including possible acute renal failure, which is usually reversible). Products include:
Atacand 697
Atacand HCT 700

Captopril (In patients with compromised renal function, the co-administration of an NSAID and an ACE inhibitor may result in further deterioration of renal function, including possible acute renal failure, which is usually reversible). Products include:
Captopril 2341

Dalteparin Sodium (Bleeding has been reported in patients on concomitant treatment with anticoagulants and indomethacin, therefore they should be co-administered with caution). Products include:
Fragmin 1058

Danaparoid Sodium (Bleeding has been reported in patients on concomitant treatment with anticoagulants and indomethacin, therefore they should be co-administered with caution). No products indexed under this heading.

Deslanoside (Half-life of digitalis may be prolonged when given concomitantly). No products indexed under this heading.

Dicumarol (Bleeding has been reported in patients on concomitant treatment with anticoagulants and indomethacin, therefore they should be co-administered with caution). No products indexed under this heading.

Digitalis Glycoside Preparations (Half-life of digitalis may be prolonged when given concomitantly). No products indexed under this heading.

Digitalis Lanata (Half-life of digitalis may be prolonged when given concomitantly). No products indexed under this heading.

Digitalis Purpurea (Half-life of digitalis may be prolonged when given concomitantly). No products indexed under this heading.

Digitoxin (Half-life of digitalis may be prolonged when given concomitantly). No products indexed under this heading.

Digoxin (Half-life of digitalis may be prolonged when given concomitantly). Products include:
Lanoxin Injection 1546
Lanoxin Injection Pediatric 1549
Lanoxin Tablets 1553

IMPORTANT NOTE: Always consult each drug listing in the patient's regimen for possible interactions.

(⊙ Described in PDR® for Ophthalmic Medicines)

IMPORTANT NOTE: Always consult each drug listing in the patient's regimen for possible interactions.

lites, alkylating agents, cytotoxic drugs, and corticosteroids (used in greater than physiologic doses), may reduce the immune response to vaccines). Products include:

Tacrolimus (Immunosuppressive therapies, including irradiation, antimetabolites, alkylating agents, cytotoxic drugs, and corticosteroids (used in greater than physiologic doses), may reduce the immune response to vaccines). Products include:

Tamoxifen Citrate (Immunosuppressive therapies, including cytotoxic drugs, may reduce the immune response to vaccines).

No products indexed under this heading.

Thioguanine (Immunosuppressive therapies, including antimetabolites, may reduce the immune response to vaccines). Products include:

Thiotepa (Immunosuppressive therapies, including alkylating agents, may reduce the immune response to vaccines).

No products indexed under this heading.

Triamcinolone (Immunosuppressive therapies, including corticosteroids (used in greater than physiologic doses), may reduce the immune response to vaccines).

No products indexed under this heading.

Triamcinolone Acetonide (Immunosuppressive therapies, including corticosteroids (used in greater than physiologic doses), may reduce the immune response to vaccines). Products include:

Triamcinolone Diacetate (Immunosuppressive therapies, including corticosteroids (used in greater than physiologic doses), may reduce the immune response to vaccines).

No products indexed under this heading.

Triamcinolone Hexacetonide (Immunosuppressive therapies, including corticosteroids (used in greater than physiologic doses), may reduce the immune response to vaccines).

No products indexed under this heading.

Vinblastine Sulfate (Immunosuppressive therapies, including cytotoxic drugs, may reduce the immune response to vaccines).

No products indexed under this heading.

Vincristine Sulfate (Immunosuppressive therapies, including cytotoxic drugs, may reduce the immune response to vaccines).

No products indexed under this heading.

Vinorelbine Tartrate (Immunosuppressive therapies, including cytotoxic drugs, may reduce the immune response to vaccines).

No products indexed under this heading.

INNOPRAN XL EXTENDED RELEASE CAPSULES

(Propranolol Hydrochloride) 1517
May interact with ACE inhibitors, calcium channel blockers, cardiac glycosides, catecholamine-depleting drugs, cytochrome p450 1a2 inhibitors (selected), cytochrome p450 1a2 substrates (selected), cytochrome p450 2c19 inhibitors (selected), cytochrome p450 2c19 substrates (selected), cytochrome p450 2d6 inhibitors (selected), cytochrome p450 2d6 substrates (selected), epinephrine-containing products, haloperidols, hepatic microsomal enzyme inducers, insulin, monoamine oxidase inhibitors, non-steroidal anti-inflammatory agents, quinidine, theophyllines, tricyclic antidepressants, and certain other agents. Compounds in these categories include:

Acetaminophen (Blood levels and/or toxicity of propranolol may be increased by administration of propranolol with substrates of CYP1A2). Products include:

Alatrofloxacin Mesylate (Blood levels and/or toxicity of propranolol may be increased by administration of propranolol with inhibitors of CYP1A2).

No products indexed under this heading.

Allium sativum (Blood levels of propranolol may be decreased by administration of propranolol with inducers of hepatic drug metabolism).

No products indexed under this heading.

Aluminum Hydroxide (Co-administration of propranolol with aluminum hydroxide gel (1,200 mg) resulted in a 50% decrease in propranolol concentrations).

No products indexed under this heading.

Aminoglutethimide (Blood levels of propranolol may be decreased by administration of propranolol with inducers of hepatic drug metabolism).

No products indexed under this heading.

Aminophylline (Blood levels and/or toxicity of propranolol may be increased by administration of propranolol with substrates of CYP1A2).

No products indexed under this heading.

Amiodarone Hydrochloride (Amiodarone is an antiarrhythmic agent with negative chronotropic properties that may be additive to those seen with propranolol. Blood levels and/or toxicity of propranolol may be increased by administration of substrates or inhibitors of CYP2D6, such as amiodarone).

No products indexed under this heading.

Amitriptyline Hydrochloride (The hypotensive effects of tricyclic antidepressants may be exacerbated when administered with β-blockers by interfering with the β-blocking activity of propranolol).

No products indexed under this heading.

Amlodipine Besylate (Caution should be exercised when patients receiving a β-blocker are administered a calcium-channel-blocking drug with negative inotropic and/or chronotropic effects. Both agents may depress myocardial contractility or atrioventricular conduction). Products include:

Amoxapine (The hypotensive effects of tricyclic antidepressants may be exacerbated when administered with β-blockers by interfering with the β-blocking activity of propranolol).

No products indexed under this heading.

Amphetamine Aspartate (Blood levels and/or toxicity of propranolol may be increased by administration of propranolol with substrates of CYP2D6).

No products indexed under this heading.

Amphetamine Aspartate Monohydrate (Blood levels and/or toxicity of propranolol may be increased by administration of propranolol with substrates of CYP2D6).

No products indexed under this heading.

Amphetamine Sulfate (Blood levels and/or toxicity of propranolol may be increased by administration of propranolol with substrates of CYP2D6).

No products indexed under this heading.

Anagrelide Hydrochloride (Blood levels and/or toxicity of propranolol may be increased by administration of propranolol with substrates of CYP1A2).

No products indexed under this heading.

Anastrozole (Blood levels and/or toxicity of propranolol may be increased by administration of propranolol with inhibitors of CYP1A2).

No products indexed under this heading.

Aprepitant (Blood levels of propranolol may be decreased by administration of propranolol with inducers of hepatic drug metabolism). Products include:

Atomoxetine Hydrochloride (Blood levels and/or toxicity of propranolol may be increased by administration of propranolol with substrates of CYP2D6). Products include:

Benazepril Hydrochloride (When combined with β-blockers, ACE inhibitors can cause hypotension, particularly in the setting of acute myocardial infarction. Certain ACE inhibitors have been reported to increase bronchial hyper-reactivity when administered with propranolol).

No products indexed under this heading.

Bepridil Hydrochloride (Caution should be exercised when patients receiving a β-blocker are administered a calcium-channel-blocking drug with negative inotropic and/or chronotropic effects. Both agents may depress myocardial contractility or atrioventricular conduction).

No products indexed under this heading.

Betamethasone (Blood levels of propranolol may be decreased by administration of propranolol with inducers of hepatic drug metabolism).

No products indexed under this heading.

Betamethasone Sodium Phosphate (Blood levels of propranolol may be decreased by administration of propranolol with inducers of hepatic drug metabolism).

No products indexed under this heading.

Bisoprolol Fumarate (Blood levels and/or toxicity of propranolol may be increased by administration of propranolol with substrates of CYP2D6).

No products indexed under this heading.

Bosentan (Blood levels of propranolol may be decreased by administration of propranolol with inducers of hepatic drug metabolism). Products include:

Bupivacaine Hydrochloride (Concomitant administration of bupivacaine with propranolol has been reported to decrease the clearance of these amide anesthetics significantly, resulting in higher concentrations of the anesthetic. Bupivacaine toxicity has been reported following co-administration. Caution should be exercised when amide anesthetic agents are administered concomitantly with propranolol).

No products indexed under this heading.

Bupropion Hydrochloride (Blood levels and/or toxicity of propranolol may be increased by administration of propranolol with inhibitors of CYP2D6). Products include:

Caffeine (Blood levels and/or toxicity of propranolol may be increased by administration of propranolol with substrates of CYP1A2).

No products indexed under this heading.

Caffeine Anhydrous (Blood levels and/or toxicity of propranolol may be increased by administration of propranolol with substrates of CYP1A2).

No products indexed under this heading.

Caffeine Citrate (Blood levels and/or toxicity of propranolol may be increased by administration of propranolol with substrates of CYP1A2).

No products indexed under this heading.

Caffeine-containing medications (Blood levels and/or toxicity of propranolol may be increased by administration of propranolol with substrates of CYP1A2).

No products indexed under this heading.

Caffeine Sodium Benzoate (Blood levels and/or toxicity of propranolol may be increased by administration of propranolol with substrates of CYP1A2).

No products indexed under this heading.

Captopril (When combined with β-blockers, ACE inhibitors can cause hypotension, particularly in the setting of acute myocardial infarction. Certain ACE inhibitors have been reported to increase bronchial hyper-reactivity when administered with propranolol). Products include:

Carbamazepine (Blood levels of propranolol may be decreased by administration of propranolol with inducers of hepatic drug metabolism). Products include:

Carisoprodol (Blood levels and/or toxicity of propranolol may be increased by administration of propranolol with substrates of CYP2C19).

No products indexed under this heading.

Carvedilol (Blood levels and/or toxicity of propranolol may be increased by administration of propranolol with substrates of CYP2D6). Products include:

Celecoxib (Non-steroidal anti-inflammatory drugs (NSAIDs) have been reported to blunt the antihypertensive effects of β-adreno receptor blocking agents). Products include:

Cevimeline Hydrochloride (Blood levels and/or toxicity of propranolol may be increased by administration of propranolol with substrates of CYP2D6). Products include:

Chlordiazepoxide (Blood levels and/or toxicity of propranolol may be increased by administration of propranolol with substrates of CYP1A2).

No products indexed under this heading.

Chlordiazepoxide Hydrochloride (Blood levels and/or toxicity of propranolol may be increased by administration of propranolol with substrates of CYP1A2).

No products indexed under this heading.

Chloroquine (Blood levels and/or toxicity of propranolol may be increased by administration of propranolol with inhibitors of CYP2D6).

No products indexed under this heading.

Chloroquine Hydrochloride (Blood levels and/or toxicity of propranolol may be increased by administration of propranolol with inhibitors of CYP2D6).

No products indexed under this heading.

Chloroquine Phosphate (Blood levels and/or toxicity of propranolol may be increased by administration of propranolol with inhibitors of CYP2D6).
No products indexed under this heading.

Chlorpheniramine (Blood levels and/or toxicity of propranolol may be increased by administration of propranolol with inhibitors of CYP2D6).
No products indexed under this heading.

Chlorpheniramine Maleate (Blood levels and/or toxicity of propranolol may be increased by administration of propranolol with inhibitors of CYP2D6).
No products indexed under this heading.

Chlorpheniramine Polistirex (Blood levels and/or toxicity of propranolol may be increased by administration of propranolol with inhibitors of CYP2D6). Products include:

Chlorpheniramine Tannate (Blood levels and/or toxicity of propranolol may be increased by administration of propranolol with inhibitors of CYP2D6).
No products indexed under this heading.

Chlorpromazine (Co-administration of chlorpromazine with propranolol resulted in increased plasma levels of both drugs (70% increase in propranolol concentrations)).
No products indexed under this heading.

Chlorpromazine Hydrochloride (Co-administration of chlorpromazine with propranolol resulted in increased plasma levels of both drugs (70% increase in propranolol concentrations)).
No products indexed under this heading.

Chlorpropamide (Blood levels and/or toxicity of propranolol may be increased by administration of propranolol with substrates of CYP2D6).
No products indexed under this heading.

Cholestyramine (Co-administration of cholestyramine with propranolol resulted in up to 50% decrease in propranolol concentrations).
No products indexed under this heading.

Cilostazol (Blood levels and/or toxicity of propranolol may be increased by administration of propranolol with substrates of CYP2C19).
No products indexed under this heading.

Cimetidine (Co-administration of propranolol with cimetidine, a non-specific CYP450 inhibitor, increased propranolol concentrations by about 40%).
No products indexed under this heading.

Cimetidine Hydrochloride (Co-administration of propranolol with cimetidine, a non-specific CYP450 inhibitor, increased propranolol concentrations by about 40%).
No products indexed under this heading.

Ciprofloxacin (Blood levels and/or toxicity of propranolol may be increased by administration of propranolol with inhibitors of CYP1A2). Products include:

Ciprofloxacin Hydrochloride (Blood levels and/or toxicity of propranolol may be increased by administration of propranolol with inhibitors of CYP1A2). Products include:

Cisplatin (Blood levels of propranolol may be decreased by administration of propranolol with inducers of hepatic drug metabolism).
No products indexed under this heading.

Citalopram Hydrobromide (Blood levels and/or toxicity of propranolol may be increased by administration of propranolol with inhibitors of CYP2D6). Products include:

Clarithromycin (Blood levels and/or toxicity of propranolol may be increased by administration of propranolol with inhibitors of CYP1A2). Products include:

Clomipramine Hydrochloride (The hypotensive effects of tricyclic antidepressants may be exacerbated when administered with β-blockers by interfering with the β-blocking activity of propranolol).
No products indexed under this heading.

Clonidine (The antihypertensive effects of clonidine may be antagonized by β-blockers. Propranolol extended-release capsules should be administered cautiously to patients withdrawing from clonidine). Products include:

Clonidine Hydrochloride (The antihypertensive effects of clonidine may be antagonized by β-blockers. Propranolol extended-release capsules should be administered cautiously to patients withdrawing from clonidine). Products include:

Clopidogrel Bisulfate (Blood levels and/or toxicity of propranolol may be increased by administration of propranolol with substrates of CYP1A2). Products include:

Clozapine (Blood levels and/or toxicity of propranolol may be increased by administration of propranolol with substrates of CYP1A2).
No products indexed under this heading.

Cocaine Hydrochloride (Blood levels and/or toxicity of propranolol may be increased by administration of propranolol with inhibitors of CYP2D6).
No products indexed under this heading.

Codeine Phosphate (Blood levels and/or toxicity of propranolol may be increased by administration of propranolol with substrates of CYP2D6). Products include:

Codeine Sulfate (Blood levels and/or toxicity of propranolol may be increased by administration of propranolol with substrates of CYP2D6).
No products indexed under this heading.

Colestipol (Co-administration of colestipol with propranolol resulted in up to 50% decrease in propranolol concentrations).
No products indexed under this heading.

Colestipol Hydrochloride (Co-administration of colestipol with propranolol resulted in up to 50% decrease in propranolol concentrations).
No products indexed under this heading.

Cortisone Acetate (Blood levels of propranolol may be decreased by administration of propranolol with inducers of hepatic drug metabolism).
No products indexed under this heading.

Cyclobenzaprine (Blood levels and/or toxicity of propranolol may be increased by administration of propranolol with substrates of CYP1A2).
No products indexed under this heading.

Cyclobenzaprine Hydrochloride (Blood levels and/or toxicity of propranolol may be increased by administration of propranolol with substrates of CYP1A2). Products include:

Cyclophosphamide (Blood levels and/or toxicity of propranolol may be increased by administration of propranolol with substrates of CYP2C19).
No products indexed under this heading.

Debrisoquine (Blood levels and/or toxicity of propranolol may be increased by administration of propranolol with substrates of CYP2D6).
No products indexed under this heading.

Delavirdine Mesylate (Blood levels and/or toxicity of propranolol may be increased by administration of propranolol with inhibitors of CYP2C19).
No products indexed under this heading.

Deserpidine (Patients receiving catecholamine-depleting drugs, (eg, reserpine) and propranolol should be closely observed for excessive reduction of resting sympathetic nervous activity, which may result in hypotension, marked bradycardia, vertigo, syncopal attacks, or orthostatic hypotension).
No products indexed under this heading.

Desipramine Hydrochloride (The hypotensive effects of tricyclic antidepressants may be exacerbated when administered with β-blockers by interfering with the β-blocking activity of propranolol).
No products indexed under this heading.

Deslanoside (Both digitalis glycosides and β-blockers slow atrioventricular conduction and decrease heart rate. Concomitant use can increase the risk of bradycardia).
No products indexed under this heading.

Desogestrel (Blood levels and/or toxicity of propranolol may be increased by administration of propranolol with inhibitors of CYP1A2).
No products indexed under this heading.

Dexamethasone (Blood levels of propranolol may be decreased by administration of propranolol with inducers of hepatic drug metabolism). Products include:

Dexamethasone Acetate (Blood levels of propranolol may be decreased by administration of propranolol with inducers of hepatic drug metabolism).
No products indexed under this heading.

Dexamethasone Phosphate (Blood levels of propranolol may be decreased by administration of propranolol with inducers of hepatic drug metabolism).
No products indexed under this heading.

Dexamethasone Sodium (Blood levels of propranolol may be decreased by administration of propranolol with inducers of hepatic drug metabolism).
No products indexed under this heading.

Dexamethasone Sodium Phosphate (Blood levels of propranolol may be decreased by administration of propranolol with inducers of hepatic drug metabolism).
No products indexed under this heading.

Dexfenfluramine Hydrochloride (Blood levels and/or toxicity of propranolol may be increased by administration of propranolol with substrates of CYP2D6).
No products indexed under this heading.

Dextromethorphan (Blood levels and/or toxicity of propranolol may be increased by administration of propranolol with substrates of CYP2C19).
No products indexed under this heading.

Dextromethorphan Hydrobromide (Blood levels and/or toxicity of propranolol may be increased by administration of propranolol with substrates of CYP2D6).
No products indexed under this heading.

Dextromethorphan Polistirex (Blood levels and/or toxicity of propranolol may be increased by administration of propranolol with substrates of CYP2D6).
No products indexed under this heading.

Diazepam (Propranolol can inhibit the metabolism of diazepam, resulting in increased concentrations of diazepam and its metabolites. Diazepam does not alter the pharmacokinetics of propranolol). Products include:

Diclofenac Epolamine (Non-steroidal anti-inflammatory drugs (NSAIDs) have been reported to blunt the antihypertensive effects of β-adreno receptor blocking agents). Products include:

Diclofenac Potassium (Non-steroidal anti-inflammatory drugs (NSAIDs) have been reported to blunt the antihypertensive effects of β-adreno receptor blocking agents).
No products indexed under this heading.

Diclofenac Sodium (Non-steroidal anti-inflammatory drugs (NSAIDs) have been reported to blunt the antihypertensive effects of β-adreno receptor blocking agents).
No products indexed under this heading.

Digitalis Glycoside Preparations (Both digitalis glycosides and β-blockers slow atrioventricular conduction and decrease heart rate. Concomitant use can increase the risk of bradycardia).
No products indexed under this heading.

Digitalis Lanata (Both digitalis glycosides and β-blockers slow atrioventricular conduction and decrease heart rate. Concomitant use can increase the risk of bradycardia).
No products indexed under this heading.

Digitalis Purpurea (Both digitalis glycosides and β-blockers slow atrioventricular conduction and decrease heart rate. Concomitant use can increase the risk of bradycardia).
No products indexed under this heading.

Digitoxin (Both digitalis glycosides and β-blockers slow atrioventricular conduction and decrease heart rate. Concomitant use can increase the risk of bradycardia).
No products indexed under this heading.

Digoxin (Both digitalis glycosides and β-blockers slow atrioventricular conduction and decrease heart rate. Concomitant use can increase the risk of bradycardia). Products include:

Diltiazem Hydrochloride (Co-administration of propranolol and diltiazem in patients with cardiac disease has been associated with bradycardia, hypotension, high degree heart block, and heart failure). Products include:

Diltiazem Maleate (Co-administration of propranolol and diltiazem in patients with cardiac disease has been associated with bradycardia, hypotension, high degree heart block, and heart failure).
No products indexed under this heading.

Diphenhydramine (Blood levels and/or toxicity of propranolol may be increased by administration of propranolol with inhibitors of CYP2D6).
No products indexed under this heading.

Diphenhydramine Hydrochloride (Blood levels and/or toxicity of propranolol may be increased by administration of propranolol with inhibitors of CYP2D6). Products include:

IMPORTANT NOTE: Always consult each drug listing in the patient's regimen for possible interactions.

Disopyramide (Disopyramide is a Type I antiarrhythmic drug with potent negative inotropic and chronotropic effects and has been associated with severe bradycardia, asystole, and heart failure when administered with propranolol).
No products indexed under this heading.

Disopyramide Phosphate (Disopyramide is a Type I antiarrhythmic drug with potent negative inotropic and chronotropic effects and has been associated with severe bradycardia, asystole, and heart failure when administered with propranolol).
No products indexed under this heading.

Divalproex Sodium (Blood levels and/or toxicity of propranolol may be increased by administration of propranolol with substrates of CYP2C19).
Products include:
Depakote ER 426

Dobutamine (Propranolol is a competitive inhibitor of β-receptor agonists, and its effects can be reversed by administration of such agents, (eg, dobutamine). Also, propranolol may reduce sensitivity to dobutamine stress echocardiography in patients undergoing evaluation for myocardial ischemia).
No products indexed under this heading.

Dobutamine Hydrochloride (Propranolol is a competitive inhibitor of β-receptor agonists, and its effects can be reversed by administration of such agents, (eg, dobutamine). Also, propranolol may reduce sensitivity to dobutamine stress echocardiography in patients undergoing evaluation for myocardial ischemia).
No products indexed under this heading.

Dolasetron Mesylate (Blood levels and/or toxicity of propranolol may be increased by administration of propranolol with substrates of CYP2D6).
Products include:
Anzemet Injection 2931
Anzemet Tablets 2934

Donepezil Hydrochloride (Blood levels and/or toxicity of propranolol may be increased by administration of propranolol with substrates of CYP2D6). Products include:
Aricept 1045
Aricept ODT 1045

Doxazosin Mesylate (Postural hypotension has been reported in patients taking both β-blockers and doxazosin).
No products indexed under this heading.

Doxepin Hydrochloride (The hypotensive effects of tricyclic antidepressants may be exacerbated when administered with β-blockers by interfering with the β-blocking activity of propranolol).
No products indexed under this heading.

Doxorubicin Hydrochloride (Blood levels of propranolol may be decreased by administration of propranolol with inducers of hepatic drug metabolism).
No products indexed under this heading.

Efavirenz (Blood levels and/or toxicity of propranolol may be increased by administration of propranolol with inhibitors of CYP2C19). Products include:
Atripla 906

Enalapril Maleate (When combined with β-blockers, ACE inhibitors can cause hypotension, particularly in the setting of acute myocardial infarction. Certain ACE inhibitors have been reported to increase bronchial hyper-reactivity when administered with propranolol).
No products indexed under this heading.

Enalaprilat (When combined with β-blockers, ACE inhibitors can cause hypotension, particularly in the setting of acute myocardial infarction. Certain ACE inhibitors have been reported to increase bronchial hyper-reactivity when administered with propranolol).
No products indexed under this heading.

Encainide Hydrochloride (Blood levels and/or toxicity of propranolol may be increased by administration of propranolol with substrates of CYP2D6).
No products indexed under this heading.

Enoxacin (Blood levels and/or toxicity of propranolol may be increased by administration of propranolol with inhibitors of CYP1A2).
No products indexed under this heading.

Epinephrine (Patients on long term therapy with propranolol may experience uncontrolled hypertension if administered epinephrine as a consequence of unopposed α-receptor stimulation. Epinephrine is therefore not indicated in the treatment of propranolol overdose). Products include:
EpiPen 3631
Twinject 3268

Epinephrine, Racemic (Patients on long term therapy with propranolol may experience uncontrolled hypertension if administered epinephrine as a consequence of unopposed α-receptor stimulation. Epinephrine is therefore not indicated in the treatment of propranolol overdose).
No products indexed under this heading.

Epinephrine Bitartrate (Patients on long term therapy with propranolol may experience uncontrolled hypertension if administered epinephrine as a consequence of unopposed α-receptor stimulation. Epinephrine is therefore not indicated in the treatment of propranolol overdose).
No products indexed under this heading.

Epinephrine Hydrochloride (Patients on long term therapy with propranolol may experience uncontrolled hypertension if administered epinephrine as a consequence of unopposed α-receptor stimulation. Epinephrine is therefore not indicated in the treatment of propranolol overdose).
No products indexed under this heading.

Erythromycin (Blood levels and/or toxicity of propranolol may be increased by administration of propranolol with substrates of CYP1A2).
No products indexed under this heading.

Erythromycin, Topical (Blood levels of propranolol may be decreased by administration of propranolol with inducers of hepatic drug metabolism).
No products indexed under this heading.

Erythromycin Estolate (Blood levels and/or toxicity of propranolol may be increased by administration of propranolol with substrates of CYP1A2).
No products indexed under this heading.

Erythromycin Ethylsuccinate (Blood levels and/or toxicity of propranolol may be increased by administration of propranolol with substrates of CYP1A2). Products include:
E.E.S. 437
EryPed 435

Erythromycin Gluceptate (Blood levels and/or toxicity of propranolol may be increased by administration of propranolol with substrates of CYP1A2).
No products indexed under this heading.

Erythromycin Lactobionate (Blood levels and/or toxicity of propranolol may be increased by administration of propranolol with substrates of CYP1A2).
No products indexed under this heading.

Erythromycin Stearate (Blood levels and/or toxicity of propranolol may be increased by administration of propranolol with substrates of CYP1A2).
No products indexed under this heading.

Escitalopram Oxalate (Blood levels and/or toxicity of propranolol may be increased by administration of propranolol with inhibitors of CYP2D6). Products include:
Lexapro Oral Suspension 1160
Lexapro Tablets 1160

Esomeprazole Magnesium (Blood levels and/or toxicity of propranolol may be increased by administration of propranolol with inhibitors of CYP1A2). Products include:
Nexium Capsules 704
Nexium Oral Suspension 704

Esomeprazole Sodium (Blood levels and/or toxicity of propranolol may be increased by administration of propranolol with inhibitors of CYP1A2). Products include:
Nexium I.V. 712

Estradiol (Blood levels and/or toxicity of propranolol may be increased by administration of propranolol with substrates of CYP1A2). Products include:
Activella 2561
Angeliq 831
Climara 841
Climara Pro 847
Divigel 3467
Estrasorb 1777
Vagifem 2589

Estradiol Benzoate (Blood levels and/or toxicity of propranolol may be increased by administration of propranolol with substrates of CYP1A2).
No products indexed under this heading.

Estradiol Cypionate (Blood levels and/or toxicity of propranolol may be increased by administration of propranolol with substrates of CYP1A2).
No products indexed under this heading.

Ethanol (Blood levels of propranolol may be decreased by administration of propranolol with inducers of hepatic drug metabolism).
No products indexed under this heading.

Ethinyl Estradiol (Blood levels and/or toxicity of propranolol may be increased by administration of propranolol with inhibitors of CYP1A2). Products include:
LoSeasonique 3407
Lybrel 3514
NuvaRing 3181
Ortho Evra 2648
Ortho-Cyclen/Ortho Tri-Cyclen 2663
Ortho Tri-Cyclen Lo Tablets 2673
Seasonique 3418
Yaz 864

Ethosuximide (Blood levels and/or toxicity of propranolol may be increased by administration of propranolol with substrates of CYP2C19).
No products indexed under this heading.

Ethotoin (Blood levels and/or toxicity of propranolol may be increased by administration of propranolol with substrates of CYP2C19).
No products indexed under this heading.

Ethyl Alcohol (Blood levels of propranolol may be decreased by administration of propranolol with inducers of hepatic drug metabolism).
No products indexed under this heading.

Ethynodiol Diacetate (Blood levels and/or toxicity of propranolol may be increased by administration of propranolol with inhibitors of CYP2C19).
No products indexed under this heading.

Etodolac (Non-steroidal anti-inflammatory drugs (NSAIDs) have been reported to blunt the antihypertensive effects of β-adreno receptor blocking agents).
No products indexed under this heading.

Felbamate (Blood levels and/or toxicity of propranolol may be increased by administration of propranolol with substrates of CYP2C19).
No products indexed under this heading.

Felodipine (Caution should be exercised when patients receiving a β-blocker are administered a calcium-channel-blocking drug with negative inotropic and/or chronotropic effects. Both agents may depress myocardial contractility or atrioventricular conduction).
No products indexed under this heading.

Fenoprofen Calcium (Non-steroidal anti-inflammatory drugs (NSAIDs) have been reported to blunt the antihypertensive effects of β-adreno receptor blocking agents).
No products indexed under this heading.

Fentanyl (Blood levels and/or toxicity of propranolol may be increased by administration of propranolol with substrates of CYP2D6). Products include:
Duragesic 2604
Fentanyl Transdermal System 2346
Onsolis 2054

Fentanyl Citrate (Blood levels and/or toxicity of propranolol may be increased by administration of propranolol with substrates of CYP2D6). Products include:
Fentora 966

Flecainide Acetate (Blood levels and/or toxicity of propranolol may be increased by administration of propranolol with substrates of CYP2D6).
No products indexed under this heading.

Fluconazole (Blood levels and/or toxicity of propranolol may be increased by administration of propranolol extended release capsules with inhibitors of CYP2C19 such as fluconazole).
No products indexed under this heading.

Fludrocortisone Acetate (Blood levels of propranolol may be decreased by administration of propranolol with inducers of hepatic drug metabolism).
No products indexed under this heading.

Fluoxetine (Blood levels and/or toxicity of propranolol may be increased by administration of propranolol with substrates or inhibitors of CYP2D6 and CYP2C19).
No products indexed under this heading.

Fluoxetine Hydrochloride (Blood levels and/or toxicity of propranolol may be increased by administration of propranolol with substrates or inhibitors of CYP2D6 and CYP2C19). Products include:
Prozac Weekly 1941
Prozac Pulvules 1941
Symbyax 1965

Fluphenazine Decanoate (Blood levels and/or toxicity of propranolol may be increased by administration of propranolol with inhibitors of CYP2D6).
No products indexed under this heading.

Fluphenazine Enanthate (Blood levels and/or toxicity of propranolol may be increased by administration of propranolol with inhibitors of CYP2D6).
No products indexed under this heading.

Fluphenazine Hydrochloride (Blood levels and/or toxicity of propranolol may be increased by administration of propranolol with inhibitors of CYP2D6).
No products indexed under this heading.

Flurbiprofen (Non-steroidal anti-inflammatory drugs (NSAIDs) have been reported to blunt the antihypertensive effects of β-adreno receptor blocking agents).
No products indexed under this heading.

Flutamide (Blood levels and/or toxicity of propranolol may be increased by administration of propranolol with substrates of CYP1A2).
No products indexed under this heading.

Fluticasone Propionate (Blood levels and/or toxicity of propranolol may be increased by administration of propranolol with substrates of CYP1A2). Products include:

Fluvastatin Sodium (Blood levels and/or toxicity of propranolol may be increased by administration of propranolol with inhibitors of CYP2C19).
No products indexed under this heading.

Fluvoxamine (Blood levels and/or toxicity of propranolol may be increased by administration of propranolol with inhibitors of CYP1A2).
No products indexed under this heading.

Fluvoxamine Maleate (Blood levels and/or toxicity of propranolol may be increased by administration of propranolol with inhibitors of CYP1A2).
No products indexed under this heading.

Formoterol Fumarate (Blood levels and/or toxicity of propranolol may be increased by administration of propranolol with substrates of CYP2D6). Products include:

Fosinopril Sodium (When combined with β-blockers, ACE inhibitors can cause hypotension, particularly in the setting of acute myocardial infarction. Certain ACE inhibitors have been reported to increase bronchial hyper-reactivity when administered with propranolol).
No products indexed under this heading.

Fosphenytoin (Blood levels and/or toxicity of propranolol may be increased by administration of propranolol with substrates of CYP2C19).
No products indexed under this heading.

Fosphenytoin Sodium (Blood levels and/or toxicity of propranolol may be increased by administration of propranolol with substrates of CYP2C19).
No products indexed under this heading.

Gabapentin (Blood levels and/or toxicity of propranolol may be increased by administration of propranolol with substrates of CYP2C19).
No products indexed under this heading.

Galantamine Hydrobromide (Blood levels and/or toxicity of propranolol may be increased by administration of propranolol with substrates of CYP2D6).
No products indexed under this heading.

Garlic Extract (Blood levels of propranolol may be decreased by administration of propranolol with inducers of hepatic drug metabolism).
No products indexed under this heading.

Garlic Oil (Blood levels of propranolol may be decreased by administration of propranolol with inducers of hepatic drug metabolism).
No products indexed under this heading.

Gatifloxacin (Blood levels and/or toxicity of propranolol may be increased by administration of propranolol with inhibitors of CYP1A2).
No products indexed under this heading.

Gemifloxacin Mesylate (Blood levels and/or toxicity of propranolol may be increased by administration of propranolol with inhibitors of CYP1A2).
No products indexed under this heading.

Glipizide (Blood levels of propranolol may be decreased by administration of propranolol with inducers of hepatic drug metabolism).
No products indexed under this heading.

Glyburide (Blood levels of propranolol may be decreased by administration of propranolol with inducers of hepatic drug metabolism).
No products indexed under this heading.

Grepafloxacin Hydrochloride (Blood levels and/or toxicity of propranolol may be increased by administration of propranolol with inhibitors of CYP1A2).
No products indexed under this heading.

Guanethidine (Patients receiving catecholamine-depleting drugs, (eg, reserpine) and propranolol should be closely observed for excessive reduction of resting sympathetic nervous activity, which may result in hypotension, marked bradycardia, vertigo, syncopal attacks, or orthostatic hypotension).
No products indexed under this heading.

Guanethidine Monosulfate (Patients receiving catecholamine-depleting drugs, (eg, reserpine) and propranolol should be closely observed for excessive reduction of resting sympathetic nervous activity, which may result in hypotension, marked bradycardia, vertigo, syncopal attacks, or orthostatic hypotension).
No products indexed under this heading.

Guanethidine Sulfate (Patients receiving catecholamine-depleting drugs, (eg, reserpine) and propranolol should be closely observed for excessive reduction of resting sympathetic nervous activity, which may result in hypotension, marked bradycardia, vertigo, syncopal attacks, or orthostatic hypotension).
No products indexed under this heading.

Halofantrine Hydrochloride (Blood levels and/or toxicity of propranolol may be increased by administration of propranolol with inhibitors of CYP2D6).
No products indexed under this heading.

Haloperidol (Hypotension and cardiac arrest have been reported with the concomitant use of propranolol and haloperidol).
No products indexed under this heading.

Haloperidol Decanoate (Hypotension and cardiac arrest have been reported with the concomitant use of propranolol and haloperidol).
No products indexed under this heading.

Haloperidol Lactate (Hypotension and cardiac arrest have been reported with the concomitant use of propranolol and haloperidol).
No products indexed under this heading.

Hepatic Enzyme-Inducing Agents (Blood levels of propranolol may be decreased by administration of propranolol with inducers of hepatic drug metabolism).
No products indexed under this heading.

Hydrocodone Bitartrate (Blood levels and/or toxicity of propranolol may be increased by administration of propranolol with substrates of CYP2D6). Products include:

Hydrocortisone (Alcohol) (Blood levels of propranolol may be decreased by administration of propranolol with inducers of hepatic drug metabolism).
No products indexed under this heading.

Hydrocortisone Acetate (Blood levels of propranolol may be decreased by administration of propranolol with inducers of hepatic drug metabolism).
No products indexed under this heading.

Hydrocortisone Butyrate (Blood levels of propranolol may be decreased by administration of propranolol with inducers of hepatic drug metabolism).
No products indexed under this heading.

Hydrocortisone Cypionate (Blood levels of propranolol may be decreased by administration of propranolol with inducers of hepatic drug metabolism).
No products indexed under this heading.

Hydrocortisone Hemisuccinate (Blood levels of propranolol may be decreased by administration of propranolol with inducers of hepatic drug metabolism).
No products indexed under this heading.

Hydrocortisone Probutate (Blood levels of propranolol may be decreased by administration of propranolol with inducers of hepatic drug metabolism).
No products indexed under this heading.

Hydrocortisone Sodium Phosphate (Blood levels of propranolol may be decreased by administration of propranolol with inducers of hepatic drug metabolism).
No products indexed under this heading.

Hydrocortisone Sodium Succinate (Blood levels of propranolol may be decreased by administration of propranolol with inducers of hepatic drug metabolism).
No products indexed under this heading.

Hydrocortisone Valerate (Blood levels of propranolol may be decreased by administration of propranolol with inducers of hepatic drug metabolism).
No products indexed under this heading.

Hydroxychloroquine Sulfate (Blood levels and/or toxicity of propranolol may be increased by administration of propranolol with inhibitors of CYP2D6).
No products indexed under this heading.

Hypericum (Blood levels of propranolol may be decreased by administration of propranolol with inducers of hepatic drug metabolism).
No products indexed under this heading.

Hypericum Perforatum (Blood levels of propranolol may be decreased by administration of propranolol with inducers of hepatic drug metabolism). Products include:

Ibuprofen (Non-steroidal anti-inflammatory drugs (NSAIDs) have been reported to blunt the antihypertensive effects of β-adreno receptor blocking agents). Products include:

Imatinib Mesylate (Blood levels and/or toxicity of propranolol may be increased by administration of propranolol with inhibitors of CYP2D6). Products include:

Imipramine Hydrochloride (The hypotensive effects of tricyclic antidepressants may be exacerbated when administered with β-blockers by interfering with the β-blocking activity of propranolol. Blood levels and/or toxicity of propranolol may be increased by administration of propranolol with substrates or inhibitors of CYP1A2).
No products indexed under this heading.

Imipramine Pamoate (The hypotensive effects of tricyclic antidepressants may be exacerbated when administered with β-blockers by interfering with the β-blocking activity of propranolol. Blood levels and/or toxicity of propranolol may be increased by administration of propranolol with substrates or inhibitors of CYP1A2).
No products indexed under this heading.

Indomethacin (Administration of indomethacin with propranolol may reduce the efficacy of propranolol in reducing blood pressure and heart rate). Products include:

Indomethacin Sodium Trihydrate (Administration of indomethacin with propranolol may reduce the efficacy of propranolol in reducing blood pressure and heart rate). Products include:

Indoramin Hydrochloride (Blood levels and/or toxicity of propranolol may be increased by administration of propranolol with substrates of CYP2D6).
No products indexed under this heading.

Insulin (β-adrenergic blockade may prevent the appearance of certain premonitory signs and symptoms (pulse rate and blood pressure changes) of acute hypoglycemia, especially in labile insulin-dependent diabetics. In these patients, it may be more difficult to adjust the dosage of insulin).
No products indexed under this heading.

Insulin, Human, Zinc Suspension (β-adrenergic blockade may prevent the appearance of certain premonitory signs and symptoms (pulse rate and blood pressure changes) of acute hypoglycemia, especially in labile insulin-dependent diabetics. In these patients, it may be more difficult to adjust the dosage of insulin).
No products indexed under this heading.

Insulin, Human (rDNA origin) (β-adrenergic blockade may prevent the appearance of certain premonitory signs and symptoms (pulse rate and blood pressure changes) of acute hypoglycemia, especially in labile insulin-dependent diabetics. In these patients, it may be more difficult to adjust the dosage of insulin). Products include:

Insulin, Human NPH (β-adrenergic blockade may prevent the appearance of certain premonitory signs and symptoms (pulse rate and blood pressure changes) of acute hypoglycemia, especially in labile insulin-dependent diabetics. In these patients, it may be more difficult to adjust the dosage of insulin). Products include:

Insulin, Human Regular (β-adrenergic blockade may prevent the appearance of certain premonitory signs and symptoms (pulse rate and blood pressure changes) of acute hypoglycemia, especially in labile insulin-dependent diabetics. In these patients, it may be more difficult to adjust the dosage of insulin). Products include:

Insulin, Human Regular and Human NPH Mixture (β-adrenergic blockade may prevent the appearance of certain premonitory signs and symptoms (pulse rate and blood pressure changes) of acute hypoglycemia, especially in labile insulin-dependent diabetics. In these patients, it may be more difficult to adjust the dosage of insulin). Products include:

IMPORTANT NOTE: Always consult each drug listing in the patient's regimen for possible interactions.

Insulin, NPH (β-adrenergic blockade may prevent the appearance of certain premonitory signs and symptoms (pulse rate and blood pressure changes) of acute hypoglycemia, especially in labile insulin-dependent diabetics. In these patients, it may be more difficult to adjust the dosage of insulin).
No products indexed under this heading.

Insulin, Regular (β-adrenergic blockade may prevent the appearance of certain premonitory signs and symptoms (pulse rate and blood pressure changes) of acute hypoglycemia, especially in labile insulin-dependent diabetics. In these patients, it may be more difficult to adjust the dosage of insulin).
No products indexed under this heading.

Insulin, Regular and NPH mixture (β-adrenergic blockade may prevent the appearance of certain premonitory signs and symptoms (pulse rate and blood pressure changes) of acute hypoglycemia, especially in labile insulin-dependent diabetics. In these patients, it may be more difficult to adjust the dosage of insulin).
No products indexed under this heading.

Insulin, Zinc Crystals (β-adrenergic blockade may prevent the appearance of certain premonitory signs and symptoms (pulse rate and blood pressure changes) of acute hypoglycemia, especially in labile insulin-dependent diabetics. In these patients, it may be more difficult to adjust the dosage of insulin).
No products indexed under this heading.

Insulin, Zinc Suspension (β-adrenergic blockade may prevent the appearance of certain premonitory signs and symptoms (pulse rate and blood pressure changes) of acute hypoglycemia, especially in labile insulin-dependent diabetics. In these patients, it may be more difficult to adjust the dosage of insulin).
No products indexed under this heading.

Insulin Aspart (β-adrenergic blockade may prevent the appearance of certain premonitory signs and symptoms (pulse rate and blood pressure changes) of acute hypoglycemia, especially in labile insulin-dependent diabetics. In these patients, it may be more difficult to adjust the dosage of insulin).
No products indexed under this heading.

Insulin Aspart, Human (β-adrenergic blockade may prevent the appearance of certain premonitory signs and symptoms (pulse rate and blood pressure changes) of acute hypoglycemia, especially in labile insulin-dependent diabetics. In these patients, it may be more difficult to adjust the dosage of insulin). Products include:

Insulin Aspart, Human Regular (β-adrenergic blockade may prevent the appearance of certain premonitory signs and symptoms (pulse rate and blood pressure changes) of acute hypoglycemia, especially in labile insulin-dependent diabetics. In these patients, it may be more difficult to adjust the dosage of insulin). Products include:

Insulin Aspart Protamine, Human (β-adrenergic blockade may prevent the appearance of certain premonitory signs and symptoms (pulse rate and blood pressure changes) of acute hypoglycemia, especially in labile insulin-dependent diabetics. In these patients, it may be more difficult to adjust the dosage of insulin). Products include:

Insulin Detemir (rDNA Origin) (β-adrenergic blockade may prevent the appearance of certain premonitory signs and symptoms (pulse rate and blood pressure changes) of acute hypoglycemia, especially in labile insulin-

dependent diabetics. In these patients, it may be more difficult to adjust the dosage of insulin). Products include:

Insulin Glargine (β-adrenergic blockade may prevent the appearance of certain premonitory signs and symptoms (pulse rate and blood pressure changes) of acute hypoglycemia, especially in labile insulin-dependent diabetics. In these patients, it may be more difficult to adjust the dosage of insulin). Products include:

Insulin Glulisine (β-adrenergic blockade may prevent the appearance of certain premonitory signs and symptoms (pulse rate and blood pressure changes) of acute hypoglycemia, especially in labile insulin-dependent diabetics. In these patients, it may be more difficult to adjust the dosage of insulin). Products include:

Insulin Lispro, Human (β-adrenergic blockade may prevent the appearance of certain premonitory signs and symptoms (pulse rate and blood pressure changes) of acute hypoglycemia, especially in labile insulin-dependent diabetics. In these patients, it may be more difficult to adjust the dosage of insulin). Products include:

Insulin Lispro Protamine, Human (β-adrenergic blockade may prevent the appearance of certain premonitory signs and symptoms (pulse rate and blood pressure changes) of acute hypoglycemia, especially in labile insulin-dependent diabetics. In these patients, it may be more difficult to adjust the dosage of insulin). Products include:

Isocarboxazid (The hypotensive effects of MAO inhibitors may be exacerbated when administered with β-blockers by interfering with the β-blocking activity of propranolol). Products include:

Isoniazid (Blood levels and/or toxicity of propranolol may be increased by administration of propranolol with inhibitors of CYP1A2).
No products indexed under this heading.

Isoproterenol Hydrochloride (Propranolol is a competitive inhibitor of β-receptor agonists, and its effects can be reversed by administration of such agents, (eg, isoproterenol)).
No products indexed under this heading.

Isoproterenol Sulfate (Propranolol is a competitive inhibitor of β-receptor agonists, and its effects can be reversed by administration of such agents, (eg, isoproterenol)).
No products indexed under this heading.

Isradipine (Caution should be exercised when patients receiving a β-blocker are administered a calcium-channel-blocking drug with negative inotropic and/or chronotropic effects. Both agents may depress myocardial contractility or atrioventricular conduction). Products include:

Ketoconazole (Blood levels and/or toxicity of propranolol may be increased by administration of propranolol with inhibitors of CYP1A2). Products include:

Ketoprofen (Non-steroidal anti-inflammatory drugs (NSAIDs) have been reported to blunt the antihypertensive effects of β-adreno receptor blocking agents).
No products indexed under this heading.

Ketorolac Tromethamine (Non-steroidal anti-inflammatory drugs (NSAIDs) have been reported to blunt the antihypertensive effects of β-adreno receptor blocking agents). Products include:

Labetalol Hydrochloride (Blood levels and/or toxicity of propranolol may be increased by administration of propranolol with substrates of CYP2D6).
No products indexed under this heading.

Lamotrigine (Blood levels and/or toxicity of propranolol may be increased by administration of propranolol with substrates of CYP2C19). Products include:

Lansoprazole (Blood levels and/or toxicity of propranolol may be increased by administration of propranolol with substrates of CYP2C19).
No products indexed under this heading.

Letrozole (Blood levels and/or toxicity of propranolol may be increased by administration of propranolol with inhibitors of CYP2C19). Products include:

Levetiracetam (Blood levels and/or toxicity of propranolol may be increased by administration of propranolol with substrates of CYP2C19). Products include:

Levobupivacaine Hydrochloride (Blood levels and/or toxicity of propranolol may be increased by administration of propranolol with substrates of CYP1A2).
No products indexed under this heading.

Levofloxacin (Blood levels and/or toxicity of propranolol may be increased by administration of propranolol with inhibitors of CYP1A2). Products include:

Levonorgestrel (Blood levels and/or toxicity of propranolol may be increased by administration of propranolol with inhibitors of CYP1A2). Products include:

Lidocaine (The metabolism of lidocaine is inhibited by co-administration of propranolol, resulting in a 25% increase in lidocaine concentrations. Concomitant administration of propranolol with lidocaine has been reported to decrease the clearance of these amide anesthetics significantly, resulting in higher serum concentrations of anesthetic. Lidocaine toxicity has been reported following co-administration with propranolol. Caution should be exercised when administering propranolol with drugs that slow A-V nodal conduction (eg, lidocaine)). Products include:

Lidocaine Base (The metabolism of lidocaine is inhibited by co-administration of propranolol, resulting in a 25% increase in lidocaine concentrations. Concomitant administration of propranolol with lidocaine has been reported to decrease the clearance of these amide anesthetics significantly, resulting in higher serum concentra-

tions of anesthetic. Lidocaine toxicity has been reported following co-administration with propranolol. Caution should be exercised when administering propranolol with drugs that slow A-V nodal conduction (eg, lidocaine)).
No products indexed under this heading.

Lidocaine Hydrochloride (The metabolism of lidocaine is inhibited by co-administration of propranolol, resulting in a 25% increase in lidocaine concentrations. Concomitant administration of propranolol with lidocaine has been reported to decrease the clearance of these amide anesthetics significantly, resulting in higher serum concentrations of anesthetic. Lidocaine toxicity has been reported following co-administration with propranolol. Caution should be exercised when administering propranolol with drugs that slow A-V nodal conduction (eg, lidocaine)).
No products indexed under this heading.

Lisinopril (When combined with β-blockers, ACE inhibitors can cause hypotension, particularly in the setting of acute myocardial infarction. Certain ACE inhibitors have been reported to increase bronchial hyper-reactivity when administered with propranolol). Products include:

Lomefloxacin Hydrochloride (Blood levels and/or toxicity of propranolol may be increased by administration of propranolol with inhibitors of CYP1A2).
No products indexed under this heading.

Lovastatin (Co-administration of propranolol with lovastatin decreased the AUC of lovastatin by 20% to 25% but did not alter its pharmacodynamics). Products include:

Maprotiline Hydrochloride (The hypotensive effects of tricyclic antidepressants may be exacerbated when administered with β-blockers by interfering with the β-blocking activity of propranolol).
No products indexed under this heading.

Meclofenamate Sodium (Non-steroidal anti-inflammatory drugs (NSAIDs) have been reported to blunt the antihypertensive effects of β-adreno receptor blocking agents).
No products indexed under this heading.

Mefenamic Acid (Non-steroidal anti-inflammatory drugs (NSAIDs) have been reported to blunt the antihypertensive effects of β-adreno receptor blocking agents).
No products indexed under this heading.

Meloxicam (Non-steroidal anti-inflammatory drugs (NSAIDs) have been reported to blunt the antihypertensive effects of β-adreno receptor blocking agents).
No products indexed under this heading.

Meperidine Hydrochloride (Blood levels and/or toxicity of propranolol may be increased by administration of propranolol with substrates of CYP2D6).
No products indexed under this heading.

Mephenytoin (Blood levels and/or toxicity of propranolol may be increased by administration of propranolol with substrates of CYP2C19).
No products indexed under this heading.

Mephobarbital (Blood levels and/or toxicity of propranolol may be increased by administration of propranolol with substrates of CYP2C19).
No products indexed under this heading.

Mepivacaine Hydrochloride (Concomitant administration of mepivacaine with propranolol has been reported to decrease the clearance of these amide anesthetics significantly, resulting in higher concentrations of the anesthetic. Caution should be exercised when amide anesthetic agents are administered concomitantly with propranolol).
No products indexed under this heading.

Meprobamate (Blood levels and/or toxicity of propranolol may be increased by administration of propranolol with substrates of CYP2C19).
No products indexed under this heading.

Mestranol (Blood levels and/or toxicity of propranolol may be increased by administration of propranolol with inhibitors of CYP1A2).
No products indexed under this heading.

Methadone Hydrochloride (Blood levels and/or toxicity of propranolol may be increased by administration of propranolol with substrates of CYP1A2).
No products indexed under this heading.

Methamphetamine Hydrochloride (Blood levels and/or toxicity of propranolol may be increased by administration of propranolol with substrates of CYP2D6).
No products indexed under this heading.

Methoxsalen (Blood levels and/or toxicity of propranolol may be increased by administration of propranolol with inhibitors of CYP1A2).
No products indexed under this heading.

Methoxyflurane (Methoxyflurane may depress myocardial contractility when administered with propranolol).
No products indexed under this heading.

Methoxyphenamine (Blood levels and/or toxicity of propranolol may be increased by administration of propranolol with substrates of CYP2D6).
No products indexed under this heading.

Methsuximide (Blood levels and/or toxicity of propranolol may be increased by administration of propranolol with substrates of CYP2C19).
No products indexed under this heading.

Methylprednisolone (Blood levels of propranolol may be decreased by administration of propranolol with inducers of hepatic drug metabolism).
No products indexed under this heading.

Methylprednisolone Acetate (Blood levels of propranolol may be decreased by administration of propranolol with inducers of hepatic drug metabolism).
No products indexed under this heading.

Methylprednisolone Sodium Succinate (Blood levels of propranolol may be decreased by administration of propranolol with inducers of hepatic drug metabolism).
No products indexed under this heading.

Metoprolol Succinate (Blood levels and/or toxicity of propranolol may be increased by administration of propranolol with substrates of CYP2D6). Products include:
Toprol XL 732

Metoprolol Tartrate (Blood levels and/or toxicity of propranolol may be increased by administration of propranolol with substrates of CYP2D6).
No products indexed under this heading.

Mexiletine Hydrochloride (Blood levels and/or toxicity of propranolol may be increased by administration of propranolol with inhibitors of CYP1A2).
No products indexed under this heading.

Mibefradil Dihydrochloride (Caution should be exercised when patients receiving a β-blocker are administered a calcium-channel-blocking drug with negative inotropic and/or chronotropic effects. Both agents may depress myocardial contractility or atrioventricular conduction).
No products indexed under this heading.

Midazolam Hydrochloride (Blood levels and/or toxicity of propranolol may be increased by administration of propranolol with substrates of CYP2C19).
No products indexed under this heading.

Mirtazapine (Blood levels and/or toxicity of propranolol may be increased by administration of propranolol with substrates of CYP1A2). Products include:
Remeron Tablets 3214
RemeronSolTab Tablets 3219

Moclobemide (The hypotensive effects of MAO inhibitors may be exacerbated when administered with β-blockers by interfering with the β-blocking activity of propranolol).
No products indexed under this heading.

Modafinil (Blood levels and/or toxicity of propranolol may be increased by administration of propranolol with inhibitors of CYP2C19). Products include:
Provigil 983

Moexipril Hydrochloride (When combined with β-blockers, ACE inhibitors can cause hypotension, particularly in the setting of acute myocardial infarction. Certain ACE inhibitors have been reported to increase bronchial hyperreactivity when administered with propranolol).
No products indexed under this heading.

Morphine Sulfate (Blood levels and/or toxicity of propranolol may be increased by administration of propranolol with substrates of CYP2D6). Products include:
Avinza 1822
Embeda 1831
MS Contin 2803

Moxifloxacin Hydrochloride (Blood levels and/or toxicity of propranolol may be increased by administration of propranolol with inhibitors of CYP1A2). Products include:
Avelox 3064
Vigamox 589

Nabumetone (Non-steroidal anti-inflammatory drugs (NSAIDs) have been reported to blunt the antihypertensive effects of β-adreno receptor blocking agents).
No products indexed under this heading.

Nafcillin Sodium (Blood levels and/or toxicity of propranolol may be increased by administration of propranolol with substrates of CYP1A2).
No products indexed under this heading.

Nalidixic Acid (Blood levels and/or toxicity of propranolol may be increased by administration of propranolol with inhibitors of CYP1A2).
No products indexed under this heading.

Naproxen (Non-steroidal anti-inflammatory drugs (NSAIDs) have been reported to blunt the antihypertensive effects of β-adreno receptor blocking agents). Products include:
EC-Naprosyn 2850
Naprosyn 2850
Anaprox/Naprosyn 2850

Naproxen Sodium (Non-steroidal anti-inflammatory drugs (NSAIDs) have been reported to blunt the antihypertensive effects of β-adreno receptor blocking agents). Products include:
Anaprox 2850
Anaprox DS 2850
Treximet 1681

Nelfinavir Mesylate (Blood levels and/or toxicity of propranolol may be increased by administration of propranolol with substrates of CYP2D6).
No products indexed under this heading.

Nevirapine (Blood levels of propranolol may be decreased by administration of propranolol with inducers of hepatic drug metabolism). Products include:
Viramune Oral Suspension 897
Viramune Tablets 897

Nicardipine (The mean C_{max} and AUC of propranolol are increased respectively, by 80% and 47% by co-administration of nicardipine).
No products indexed under this heading.

Nicardipine Hydrochloride (The mean C_{max} and AUC of propranolol are increased respectively, by 80% and 47% by co-administration of nicardipine).
No products indexed under this heading.

Nicotine (Blood levels of propranolol may be decreased by administration of propranolol with inducers of hepatic drug metabolism).
No products indexed under this heading.

Nicotine Polacrilex (Blood levels and/or toxicity of propranolol may be increased by administration of propranolol with substrates of CYP1A2).
No products indexed under this heading.

Nicotine Salicylate (Blood levels and/or toxicity of propranolol may be increased by administration of propranolol with substrates of CYP1A2).
No products indexed under this heading.

Nicotine Sulfate (Blood levels and/or toxicity of propranolol may be increased by administration of propranolol with substrates of CYP1A2).
No products indexed under this heading.

Nifedipine (The mean C_{max} and AUC of nifedipine are increased by 64% and 79% respectively, by co-administration of propranolol).
No products indexed under this heading.

Nilutamide (Blood levels and/or toxicity of propranolol may be increased by administration of propranolol with substrates of CYP2C19).
No products indexed under this heading.

Nimodipine (Caution should be exercised when patients receiving a β-blocker are administered a calcium-channel-blocking drug with negative inotropic and/or chronotropic effects. Both agents may depress myocardial contractility or atrioventricular conduction).
No products indexed under this heading.

Nisoldipine (The mean C_{max} and AUC of propranolol are increased respectively, by 50% and 30% by co-administration of nisoldipine).
No products indexed under this heading.

Norepinephrine Bitartrate (Patients on long term therapy with propranolol may experience uncontrolled hypertension if administered epinephrine as a consequence of unopposed α-receptor stimulation. Epinephrine is therefore not indicated in the treatment of propranolol overdose).
No products indexed under this heading.

Norepinephrine Hydrochloride (Patients on long term therapy with propranolol may experience uncontrolled hypertension if administered epinephrine as a consequence of unopposed α-receptor stimulation. Epinephrine is therefore not indicated in the treatment of propranolol overdose).
No products indexed under this heading.

Norethindrone (Blood levels and/or toxicity of propranolol may be increased by administration of propranolol with inhibitors of CYP1A2). Products include:
Ortho Micronor 2660

Norethindrone Acetate (Blood levels and/or toxicity of propranolol may be increased by administration of propranolol with inhibitors of CYP1A2). Products include:
Activella 2561

Norethynodrel (Blood levels and/or toxicity of propranolol may be increased by administration of propranolol with inhibitors of CYP2C19).
No products indexed under this heading.

Norfloxacin (Blood levels and/or toxicity of propranolol may be increased by administration of propranolol with inhibitors of CYP1A2). Products include:
Noroxin 2220

Norgestimate (Blood levels and/or toxicity of propranolol may be increased by administration of propranolol with inhibitors of CYP2C19). Products include:
Ortho-Cyclen/Ortho Tri-Cyclen 2663
Ortho Tri-Cyclen Lo Tablets 2673

Norgestrel (Blood levels and/or toxicity of propranolol may be increased by administration of propranolol with inhibitors of CYP1A2).
No products indexed under this heading.

Nortriptyline Hydrochloride (The hypotensive effects of tricyclic antidepressants may be exacerbated when administered with β-blockers by interfering with the β-blocking activity of propranolol).
No products indexed under this heading.

Ofloxacin (Blood levels and/or toxicity of propranolol may be increased by administration of propranolol with inhibitors of CYP1A2).
No products indexed under this heading.

Olanzapine (Blood levels and/or toxicity of propranolol may be increased by administration of propranolol with substrates of CYP1A2). Products include:
Symbyax 1965
Zyprexa 1984
Zyprexa IntraMuscular 1984
Zyprexa ZYDIS 1984

Omeprazole (Blood levels and/or toxicity of propranolol may be increased by administration of propranolol with inhibitors of CYP1A2).
No products indexed under this heading.

Omeprazole Magnesium (Blood levels and/or toxicity of propranolol may be increased by administration of propranolol with inhibitors of CYP1A2).
No products indexed under this heading.

Ondansetron (Blood levels and/or toxicity of propranolol may be increased by administration of propranolol with substrates of CYP1A2).
No products indexed under this heading.

Ondansetron Hydrochloride (Blood levels and/or toxicity of propranolol may be increased by administration of propranolol with substrates of CYP1A2). Products include:
Zofran Injection 1750
Zofran 1756
Zofran ODT 1756

Oxaprozin (Non-steroidal anti-inflammatory drugs (NSAIDs) have been reported to blunt the antihypertensive effects of β-adreno receptor blocking agents).
No products indexed under this heading.

Oxcarbazepine (Blood levels and/or toxicity of propranolol may be increased by administration of propranolol with substrates of CYP2C19).
No products indexed under this heading.

Oxycodone Hydrochloride (Blood levels and/or toxicity of propranolol may be increased by administration of propranolol with substrates of CYP2D6). Products include:
OxyContin 2807
Percocet 1121
Percodan 1124

IMPORTANT NOTE: Always consult each drug listing in the patient's regimen for possible interactions.

Paclitaxel (Blood levels and/or toxicity of propranolol may be increased by administration of propranolol with substrates of CYP2D6).
No products indexed under this heading.

Pantoprazole Sodium (Blood levels and/or toxicity of propranolol may be increased by administration of propranolol with substrates of CYP2C19). Products include:

Paramethadione (Blood levels and/or toxicity of propranolol may be increased by administration of propranolol with substrates of CYP2C19).
No products indexed under this heading.

Pargyline Hydrochloride (The hypotensive effects of MAO inhibitors may be exacerbated when administered with β-blockers by interfering with the β-blocking activity of propranolol).
No products indexed under this heading.

Paroxetine (Blood levels and/or toxicity of propranolol may be increased by administration of propranolol with inhibitors of CYP1A2).
No products indexed under this heading.

Paroxetine Hydrochloride (Blood levels and/or toxicity of propranolol may be increased by administration of propranolol with inhibitors of CYP1A2). Products include:

Paroxetine Mesylate (Blood levels and/or toxicity of propranolol may be increased by administration of propranolol with inhibitors of CYP1A2).
No products indexed under this heading.

Pentamidine Isethionate (Blood levels and/or toxicity of propranolol may be increased by administration of propranolol with substrates of CYP2C19).
No products indexed under this heading.

Perindopril Erbumine (When combined with β-blockers, ACE inhibitors can cause hypotension, particularly in the setting of acute myocardial infarction. Certain ACE inhibitors have been reported to increase bronchial hyper-reactivity when administered with propranolol).
No products indexed under this heading.

Perphenazine (Blood levels and/or toxicity of propranolol may be increased by administration of propranolol with inhibitors of CYP2D6).
No products indexed under this heading.

Phenacemide (Blood levels and/or toxicity of propranolol may be increased by administration of propranolol with substrates of CYP2C19).
No products indexed under this heading.

Phenelzine Sulfate (The hypotensive effects of MAO inhibitors may be exacerbated when administered with β-blockers by interfering with the β-blocking activity of propranolol).
No products indexed under this heading.

Phenobarbital (Blood levels and/or toxicity of propranolol may be increased by administration of propranolol with substrates of CYP1A2). Products include:

Phenobarbital Sodium (Blood levels and/or toxicity of propranolol may be increased by administration of propranolol with substrates of CYP1A2).
No products indexed under this heading.

Phensuximide (Blood levels and/or toxicity of propranolol may be increased by administration of propranolol with substrates of CYP2C19).
No products indexed under this heading.

Phenylbutazone (Non-steroidal anti-inflammatory drugs (NSAIDs) have been reported to blunt the antihypertensive effects of β-adreno receptor blocking agents).
No products indexed under this heading.

Phenytoin (Blood levels and/or toxicity of propranolol may be increased by administration of propranolol with substrates of CYP1A2).
No products indexed under this heading.

Phenytoin Sodium (Blood levels and/or toxicity of propranolol may be increased by administration of propranolol with substrates of CYP1A2). Products include:

Pindolol (Blood levels and/or toxicity of propranolol may be increased by administration of propranolol with substrates of CYP2D6).
No products indexed under this heading.

Piroxicam (Non-steroidal anti-inflammatory drugs (NSAIDs) have been reported to blunt the antihypertensive effects of β-adreno receptor blocking agents).
No products indexed under this heading.

Pravastatin Sodium (Co-administration of propranolol with pravastatin decreased the AUC of pravastatin by 20% to 25% but did not alter its pharmacodynamics).
No products indexed under this heading.

Prazosin Hydrochloride (Prazosin has been associated with prolongation of first dose hypotension in the presence of β-blockers).
No products indexed under this heading.

Prednisolone (Blood levels of propranolol may be decreased by administration of propranolol with inducers of hepatic drug metabolism).
No products indexed under this heading.

Prednisolone Acetate (Blood levels of propranolol may be decreased by administration of propranolol with inducers of hepatic drug metabolism). Products include:

Prednisolone Sodium Phosphate (Blood levels of propranolol may be decreased by administration of propranolol with inducers of hepatic drug metabolism).
No products indexed under this heading.

Prednisolone Tebutate (Blood levels of propranolol may be decreased by administration of propranolol with inducers of hepatic drug metabolism).
No products indexed under this heading.

Prednisone (Blood levels of propranolol may be decreased by administration of propranolol with inducers of hepatic drug metabolism).
No products indexed under this heading.

Prednisone sodium phosphate (Blood levels of propranolol may be decreased by administration of propranolol with inducers of hepatic drug metabolism).
No products indexed under this heading.

Primidone (Blood levels and/or toxicity of propranolol may be increased by administration of propranolol with substrates of CYP2C19).
No products indexed under this heading.

Procarbazine Hydrochloride (The hypotensive effects of MAO inhibitors may be exacerbated when administered with β-blockers by interfering with the β-blocking activity of propranolol).
No products indexed under this heading.

Progesterone (Blood levels and/or toxicity of propranolol may be increased by administration of propranolol with substrates of CYP2C19). Products include:

Proguanil Hydrochloride (Blood levels and/or toxicity of propranolol may be increased by administration of propranolol with substrates of CYP2C19). Products include:

Propafenone Hydrochloride (Propafenone has negative inotropic and β-blocking properties that can be additive to those of propranolol. Concomitant administration of propranolol and propafenone increased propranolol average steady-state plasma concentrations (213%), AUC (113%), C_{max} (83%), T_{max} (55%), and undefined $T_{1/2}$(30%), and significantly decreased plasma levels of 4-hydroxy-propranolol. Co-administration of propranolol and propafenone did not produce any significant change in propafenone pharmacokinetics. While the therapeutic range for propranolol is wide, a reduction in dosage may be necessary during concomitant administration with propafenone). Products include:

Propoxyphene Hydrochloride (Blood levels and/or toxicity of propranolol may be increased by administration of propranolol with inhibitors of CYP2D6).
No products indexed under this heading.

Propoxyphene Napsylate (Blood levels and/or toxicity of propranolol may be increased by administration of propranolol with inhibitors of CYP2D6).
No products indexed under this heading.

Protriptyline Hydrochloride (The hypotensive effects of tricyclic antidepressants may be exacerbated when administered with β-blockers by interfering with the β-blocking activity of propranolol).
No products indexed under this heading.

Quetiapine Fumarate (Blood levels and/or toxicity of propranolol may be increased by administration of propranolol with substrates of CYP2D6). Products include:

Quinacrine Hydrochloride (Blood levels and/or toxicity of propranolol may be increased by administration of propranolol with inhibitors of CYP2D6).
No products indexed under this heading.

Quinapril Hydrochloride (When combined with β-blockers, ACE inhibitors can cause hypotension, particularly in the setting of acute myocardial infarction. Certain ACE inhibitors have been reported to increase bronchial hyper-reactivity when administered with propranolol).
No products indexed under this heading.

Quinidine (Blood levels and/or toxicity of propranolol may be increased by administration of propranolol with substrates or inhibitors of CYP2D6, such as quinidine. The metabolism of propranolol is reduced by co-administration of quinidine, leading to a 2- to 3-fold increase in blood concentrations and greater degrees of clinical β-blockade. Concurrent use my cause postural hypotension).
No products indexed under this heading.

Quinidine Gluconate (Blood levels and/or toxicity of propranolol may be increased by administration of propranolol with substrates or inhibitors of CYP2D6, such as quinidine. The metabolism of propranolol is reduced by co-administration of quinidine, leading to a 2- to 3-fold increase in blood concentrations and greater degrees of clinical β-blockade. Concurrent use my cause postural hypotension).
No products indexed under this heading.

Quinidine Hydrochloride (Blood levels and/or toxicity of propranolol may be increased by administration of propranolol with substrates or inhibitors of CYP2D6, such as quinidine. The metabolism of propranolol is reduced by co-administration of quinidine, leading to a 2- to 3-fold increase in blood concentrations and greater degrees of clinical β-blockade. Concurrent use my cause postural hypotension).
No products indexed under this heading.

Quinidine Polygalacturonate (Blood levels and/or toxicity of propranolol may be increased by administration of propranolol with substrates or inhibitors of CYP2D6, such as quinidine. The metabolism of propranolol is reduced by co-administration of quinidine, leading to a 2- to 3-fold increase in blood concentrations and greater degrees of clinical β-blockade. Concurrent use my cause postural hypotension).
No products indexed under this heading.

Quinidine Sulfate (Blood levels and/or toxicity of propranolol may be increased by administration of propranolol with substrates or inhibitors of CYP2D6, such as quinidine. The metabolism of propranolol is reduced by co-administration of quinidine, leading to a 2- to 3-fold increase in blood concentrations and greater degrees of clinical β-blockade. Concurrent use my cause postural hypotension).
No products indexed under this heading.

Rabeprazole Sodium (Blood levels and/or toxicity of propranolol may be increased by administration of propranolol with substrates of CYP2C19). Products include:

Ramipril (When combined with β-blockers, ACE inhibitors can cause hypotension, particularly in the setting of acute myocardial infarction. Certain ACE inhibitors have been reported to increase bronchial hyper-reactivity when administered with propranolol).
No products indexed under this heading.

Ranitidine Bismuth Citrate (Blood levels and/or toxicity of propranolol may be increased by administration of propranolol with inhibitors of CYP1A2).
No products indexed under this heading.

Ranitidine Hydrochloride (Blood levels and/or toxicity of propranolol may be increased by administration of propranolol with inhibitors of CYP1A2). Products include:

Rasagiline Mesylate (The hypotensive effects of MAO inhibitors may be exacerbated when administered with β-blockers by interfering with the β-blocking activity of propranolol). Products include:

Rauwolfia Serpentina (Patients receiving catecholamine-depleting drugs, (eg, reserpine) and propranolol should be closely observed for excessive reduction of resting sympathetic nervous activity, which may result in hypotension, marked bradycardia, vertigo, syncopal attacks, or orthostatic hypotension).
No products indexed under this heading.

(⊙ Described in PDR® for Ophthalmic Medicines)

Rescinnamine (Patients receiving catecholamine-depleting drugs, (eg, reserpine) and propranolol should be closely observed for excessive reduction of resting sympathetic nervous activity, which may result in hypotension, marked bradycardia,vertigo, syncopal attacks, or orthostatic hypotension).
No products indexed under this heading.

Reserpine (Patients receiving catecholamine-depleting drugs such as reserpine and propranolol hydrochloride extended-release capsules should be observed closely for excessive reduction of resting sympathetic nervous activity, which may result in hypotension, marked bradycardia, vertigo, syncopal attacks, or orthostatic hypotension. Administration of reserpine with propranolol may also potentiate depression).
No products indexed under this heading.

Rifabutin (Blood levels of propranolol may be decreased by administration of propranolol with inducers of hepatic drug metabolism).
No products indexed under this heading.

Rifampicin (Blood levels of propranolol may be decreased by administration of propranolol with inducers of hepatic drug metabolism).
No products indexed under this heading.

Rifampin (Blood levels of propranolol may be decreased by administration of propranolol with inducers of hepatic drug metabolism).
No products indexed under this heading.

Rifapentine (Blood levels of propranolol may be decreased by administration of propranolol with inducers of hepatic drug metabolism).
No products indexed under this heading.

Riluzole (Blood levels and/or toxicity of propranolol may be increased by administration of propranolol with substrates of CYP1A2). Products include:
Rilutek 3032

Risperidone (Blood levels and/or toxicity of propranolol may be increased by administration of propranolol with substrates of CYP2D6). Products include:
Risperdal Consta 2682

Ritonavir (Blood levels and/or toxicity of propranolol may be increased by administration of propranolol with inhibitors of CYP1A2). Products include:
Kaletra 458
Norvir 509

Rizatriptan Benzoate (Administration of rizatriptan with propranolol resulted in increased concentrations of rizatriptan (the AUC and C_{max} were increased by 67% and 75%, respectively)). Products include:
Maxalt 2206
Maxalt-MLT 2206

Rofecoxib (Non-steroidal anti-inflammatory drugs (NSAIDs) have been reported to blunt the antihypertensive effects of β-adreno receptor blocking agents).
No products indexed under this heading.

Ropinirole Hydrochloride (Blood levels and/or toxicity of propranolol may be increased by administration of propranolol with substrates of CYP1A2). Products include:
Requip 1620
Requip XL 1628

Ropivacaine Hydrochloride (Blood levels and/or toxicity of propranolol may be increased by administration of propranolol with substrates of CYP1A2).
No products indexed under this heading.

Secobarbital Sodium (Blood levels of propranolol may be decreased by administration of propranolol with inducers of hepatic drug metabolism).
No products indexed under this heading.

Selegiline (The hypotensive effects of MAO inhibitors may be exacerbated when administered with β-blockers by interfering with the β-blocking activity of propranolol). Products include:
Emsam 3623

Selegiline Hydrochloride (The hypotensive effects of MAO inhibitors may be exacerbated when administered with β-blockers by interfering with the β-blocking activity of propranolol). Products include:
Eldepryl 3312

Sertraline Hydrochloride (Blood levels and/or toxicity of propranolol may be increased by administration of propranolol with inhibitors of CYP2D6).
No products indexed under this heading.

Sildenafil Citrate (Blood levels and/or toxicity of propranolol may be increased by administration of propranolol with inhibitors of CYP1A2).
No products indexed under this heading.

Sparfloxacin (Blood levels and/or toxicity of propranolol may be increased by administration of propranolol with inhibitors of CYP1A2).
No products indexed under this heading.

Spirapril Hydrochloride (When combined with β-blockers, ACE inhibitors can cause hypotension, particularly in the setting of acute myocardial infarction. Certain ACE inhibitors have been reported to increase bronchial hyperreactivity when administered with propranolol).
No products indexed under this heading.

Sulfaphenazole (Blood levels and/or toxicity of propranolol may be increased by administration of propranolol with inhibitors of CYP2C19).
No products indexed under this heading.

Sulindac (Non-steroidal anti-inflammatory drugs (NSAIDs) have been reported to blunt the antihypertensive effects of β-adreno receptor blocking agents). Products include:
Clinoril 2098

Tacrine Hydrochloride (Blood levels and/or toxicity of propranolol may be increased by administration of propranolol with inhibitors of CYP1A2).
No products indexed under this heading.

Tamoxifen Citrate (Blood levels and/or toxicity of propranolol may be increased by administration of propranolol with substrates of CYP1A2).
No products indexed under this heading.

Telmisartan (Blood levels and/or toxicity of propranolol may be increased by administration of propranolol with inhibitors of CYP2C19). Products include:
Micardis 887
Micardis HCT 889

Teniposide (Blood levels and/or toxicity of propranolol may be increased by administration of propranolol with substrates of CYP2D6).
No products indexed under this heading.

Terazosin Hydrochloride (Postural hypotension has been reported in patients taking both β-blockers and terazosin).
No products indexed under this heading.

Terbinafine Hydrochloride (Blood levels and/or toxicity of propranolol may be increased by administration of propranolol with inhibitors of CYP2D6).
No products indexed under this heading.

Testosterone (Blood levels and/or toxicity of propranolol may be increased by administration of propranolol with substrates of CYP2D6). Products include:
AndroGel 3456

Testosterone Cypionate (Blood levels and/or toxicity of propranolol may be increased by administration of propranolol with substrates of CYP2D6).
No products indexed under this heading.

Testosterone Enanthate (Blood levels and/or toxicity of propranolol may be increased by administration of propranolol with substrates of CYP2D6). Products include:
Delatestryl 1102

Testosterone Propionate (Blood levels and/or toxicity of propranolol may be increased by administration of propranolol with substrates of CYP2D6).
No products indexed under this heading.

Theobromine (Blood levels and/or toxicity of propranolol may be increased by administration of propranolol with substrates of CYP1A2).
No products indexed under this heading.

Theophylline (Blood levels and/or toxicity of propranolol may be increased by administration of propranolol with substrates or inhibitors of CYP1A2 such as theophylline. Co-administration of theophylline with propranolol decreases theophylline oral clearance by 33% to 52%).
No products indexed under this heading.

Theophylline Anhydrous (Blood levels and/or toxicity of propranolol may be increased by administration of propranolol with substrates or inhibitors of CYP1A2 such as theophylline. Co-administration of theophylline with propranolol decreases theophylline oral clearance by 33% to 52%). Products include:
Uniphyl 2817

Theophylline Calcium Salicylate (Blood levels and/or toxicity of propranolol may be increased by administration of propranolol with substrates or inhibitors of CYP1A2 such as theophylline. Co-administration of theophylline with propranolol decreases theophylline oral clearance by 33% to 52%).
No products indexed under this heading.

Theophylline Dihydroxypropyl (Glyceryl) (Blood levels and/or toxicity of propranolol may be increased by administration of propranolol with substrates or inhibitors of CYP1A2 such as theophylline. Co-administration of theophylline with propranolol decreases theophylline oral clearance by 33% to 52%).
No products indexed under this heading.

Theophylline Ethylenediamine (Blood levels and/or toxicity of propranolol may be increased by administration of propranolol with substrates or inhibitors of CYP1A2 such as theophylline. Co-administration of theophylline with propranolol decreases theophylline oral clearance by 33% to 52%).
No products indexed under this heading.

Theophylline Sodium Glycinate (Blood levels and/or toxicity of propranolol may be increased by administration of propranolol with substrates or inhibitors of CYP1A2 such as theophylline. Co-administration of theophylline with propranolol decreases theophylline oral clearance by 33% to 52%).
No products indexed under this heading.

Thioridazine (Co-administration of propranolol at doses greater than or equal to 160 mg/day resulted in increased thioridazine plasma concentrations, ranging from 50% to 370% and increased thioridazine metabolites concentrations ranging from 33% to 210%).
No products indexed under this heading.

Thioridazine Hydrochloride (Co-administration of propranolol at doses greater than or equal to 160 mg/day resulted in increased thioridazine plasma concentrations, ranging from 50% to 370% and increased thioridazine metabolites concentrations ranging from 33% to 210%). Products include:
Thioridazine Hydrochloride 2384

Thyroxine (Thyroxine may result in a lower than expected T_3 concentration when used concomitantly with propranolol).
No products indexed under this heading.

Thyroxine Sodium (Thyroxine may result in a lower than expected T_3 concentration when used concomitantly with propranolol).
No products indexed under this heading.

Tiagabine Hydrochloride (Blood levels and/or toxicity of propranolol may be increased by administration of propranolol with substrates of CYP2C19). Products include:
Gabitril 972

Ticlopidine Hydrochloride (Blood levels and/or toxicity of propranolol may be increased by administration of propranolol with inhibitors of CYP1A2).
No products indexed under this heading.

Timolol Maleate (Blood levels and/or toxicity of propranolol may be increased by administration of propranolol with substrates of CYP2D6). Products include:
Combigan 601
Dorzolamide Hydrochloride/Timolol Maleate Ophthalmic Solution .... ⊙243
Timoptic in Ocudose .... ⊙231

Tizanidine (Blood levels and/or toxicity of propranolol may be increased by administration of propranolol with substrates of CYP1A2).
No products indexed under this heading.

Tizanidine Hydrochloride (Blood levels and/or toxicity of propranolol may be increased by administration of propranolol with substrates of CYP1A2).
No products indexed under this heading.

Tobacco (Cigarette smoking induces hepatic metabolism and has been shown to increase up to 100% the clearance of propranolol, resulting in decreased plasma concentrations).
No products indexed under this heading.

Tolazamide (Blood levels of propranolol may be decreased by administration of propranolol with inducers of hepatic drug metabolism).
No products indexed under this heading.

Tolbutamide (Blood levels and/or toxicity of propranolol may be increased by administration of propranolol with substrates of CYP2C19).
No products indexed under this heading.

Tolbutamide Sodium (Blood levels and/or toxicity of propranolol may be increased by administration of propranolol with substrates of CYP2C19).
No products indexed under this heading.

Tolmetin Sodium (Non-steroidal anti-inflammatory drugs (NSAIDs) have been reported to blunt the antihypertensive effects of β-adreno receptor blocking agents).
No products indexed under this heading.

Tolterodine Tartrate (Blood levels and/or toxicity of propranolol may be increased by administration of propranolol with substrates of CYP2D6).
No products indexed under this heading.

Topiramate (Blood levels and/or toxicity of propranolol may be increased by administration of propranolol with substrates of CYP2C19).
No products indexed under this heading.

Tramadol Hydrochloride (Blood levels and/or toxicity of propranolol may be increased by administration of propranolol with substrates of CYP2D6). Products include:
Ryzolt 2813
Ultram ER 2693

Trandolapril (When combined with β-blockers, ACE inhibitors can cause hypotension, particularly in the setting of acute myocardial infarction. Certain ACE inhibitors have been reported to

IMPORTANT NOTE: Always consult each drug listing in the patient's regimen for possible interactions.

increase bronchial hyper-reactivity when administered with propranolol). Products include:

Tranylcypromine Sulfate (The hypotensive effects of MAO inhibitors may be exacerbated when administered with β-blockers by interfering with the β-blocking activity of propranolol). Products include:

Trazodone Hydrochloride (Blood levels and/or toxicity of propranolol may be increased by administration of propranolol with substrates of CYP2D6).
No products indexed under this heading.

Triamcinolone (Blood levels of propranolol may be decreased by administration of propranolol with inducers of hepatic drug metabolism).
No products indexed under this heading.

Triamcinolone Acetonide (Blood levels of propranolol may be decreased by administration of propranolol with inducers of hepatic drug metabolism). Products include:

Triamcinolone Diacetate (Blood levels of propranolol may be decreased by administration of propranolol with inducers of hepatic drug metabolism).
No products indexed under this heading.

Triamcinolone Hexacetonide (Blood levels of propranolol may be decreased by administration of propranolol with inducers of hepatic drug metabolism).
No products indexed under this heading.

Triazolam (Blood levels and/or toxicity of propranolol may be increased by administration of propranolol with substrates of CYP2D6).
No products indexed under this heading.

Trichloroethylene (Trichloroethylene may depress myocardial contractility when administered with propranolol).
No products indexed under this heading.

Trimethadione (Blood levels and/or toxicity of propranolol may be increased by administration of propranolol with substrates of CYP2C19).
No products indexed under this heading.

Trimethaphan Camsylate (Blood levels and/or toxicity of propranolol may be increased by administration of propranolol with substrates of CYP1A2).
No products indexed under this heading.

Trimipramine Maleate (The hypotensive effects of tricyclic antidepressants may be exacerbated when administered with β-blockers by interfering with the β-blocking activity of propranolol).
No products indexed under this heading.

Troglitazone (Blood levels of propranolol may be decreased by administration of propranolol with inducers of hepatic drug metabolism).
No products indexed under this heading.

Troleandomycin (Blood levels and/or toxicity of propranolol may be increased by administration of propranolol with inhibitors of CYP1A2).
No products indexed under this heading.

Trovafloxacin Mesylate (Blood levels and/or toxicity of propranolol may be increased by administration of propranolol with inhibitors of CYP1A2).
No products indexed under this heading.

Valdecoxib (Non-steroidal anti-inflammatory drugs (NSAIDs) have been reported to blunt the antihypertensive effects of β-adreno receptor blocking agents).
No products indexed under this heading.

Valproate Sodium (Blood levels and/or toxicity of propranolol may be increased by administration of propranolol with substrates of CYP2C19).
No products indexed under this heading.

Valproic Acid (Blood levels and/or toxicity of propranolol may be increased by administration of propranolol with substrates of CYP2C19).
No products indexed under this heading.

Vardenafil Hydrochloride (Blood levels and/or toxicity of propranolol may be increased by administration of propranolol with inhibitors of CYP1A2). Products include:

Venlafaxine Hydrochloride (Blood levels and/or toxicity of propranolol may be increased by administration of propranolol with substrates of CYP2D6). Products include:

Verapamil Hydrochloride (There have been reports of significant bradycardia, heart failure, and cardiovascular collapse with concurrent use of verapamil and β-blockers). Products include:

Vinblastine Sulfate (Blood levels and/or toxicity of propranolol may be increased by administration of propranolol with substrates of CYP2D6).
No products indexed under this heading.

Voriconazole (Blood levels and/or toxicity of propranolol may be increased by administration of propranolol with substrates of CYP2C19).
No products indexed under this heading.

Warfarin Sodium (Propranolol when administered with warfarin increases the concentration of warfarin. Prothrombin time, therefore, should be monitored).
No products indexed under this heading.

Zileuton (Blood levels and/or toxicity of propranolol may be increased by administration of propranolol with inhibitors of CYP1A2).
No products indexed under this heading.

Zolmitriptan (Administration of zolmitriptan with propranolol resulted in increased concentrations of zolmitriptan (AUC increased by 56% and C_{max} by 37%)). Products include:

Zonisamide (Blood levels and/or toxicity of propranolol may be increased by administration of propranolol with substrates of CYP2D6). Products include:

Food Interactions

Broccoli (Blood levels of propranolol may be decreased by administration of propranolol with inducers of hepatic drug metabolism).

Brussel Sprouts (Blood levels of propranolol may be decreased by administration of propranolol with inducers of hepatic drug metabolism).

Charbroiled Food (Blood levels of propranolol may be decreased by administration of propranolol with inducers of hepatic drug metabolism).

Food, caffeine-containing (Blood levels and/or toxicity of propranolol may be increased by administration of propranolol with substrates of CYP1A2).

Grapefruit (Blood levels and/or toxicity of propranolol may be increased by administration of propranolol with inhibitors of CYP1A2).

Grapefruit Juice (Blood levels and/or toxicity of propranolol may be increased by administration of propranolol with inhibitors of CYP1A2).

INTEGRILIN INJECTION

May interact with anticoagulants, glycoprotein (GP) IIb/IIIa inhibitors, non-steroidal anti-inflammatory agents, oral anticoagulants, platelet inhibitors, thrombolytics, and certain other agents. Compounds in these categories include:

Abciximab (Current or planned administration of another parenteral GP IIb/IIIa inhibitor is contraindicated). Products include:

Alteplase (Potential for additive pharmacologic effects because eptifibatide inhibits platelet aggregation; concurrent use requires caution). Products include:

Anisindione (Potential for additive pharmacologic effects because eptifibatide inhibits platelet aggregation; concurrent use requires caution).
No products indexed under this heading.

Anistreplase (Potential for additive pharmacologic effects because eptifibatide inhibits platelet aggregation; concurrent use requires caution).
No products indexed under this heading.

Ardeparin Sodium (Because eptifibatide inhibits platelet aggregation, caution should be employed when it is used with other drugs that affect hemostasis).
No products indexed under this heading.

Aspirin (Co-administration of eptifibatide with heparin and aspirin has resulted in some cases of cerebral, GI and pulmonary hemorrhage). Products include:

Aspirin, Enteric Coated (Because eptifibatide inhibits platelet aggregation, caution should be employed when it is used with other drugs that affect hemostasis).
No products indexed under this heading.

Aspirin Buffered (Because eptifibatide inhibits platelet aggregation, caution should be employed when it is used with other drugs that affect hemostasis).
No products indexed under this heading.

Azlocillin Sodium (Because eptifibatide inhibits platelet aggregation, caution should be employed when it is used with other drugs that affect hemostasis).
No products indexed under this heading.

Bivalirudin (Potential for additive pharmacologic effects because eptifibatide inhibits platelet aggregation; concurrent use requires caution). Products include:

Carbenicillin Indanyl Sodium (Because eptifibatide inhibits platelet aggregation, caution should be employed when it is used with other drugs that affect hemostasis).
No products indexed under this heading.

Celecoxib (Potential for additive pharmacologic effects because eptifibatide inhibits platelet aggregation; concurrent use requires caution). Products include:

Choline Magnesium Trisalicylate (Because eptifibatide inhibits platelet aggregation, caution should be employed when it is used with other drugs that affect hemostasis).
No products indexed under this heading.

Clopidogrel Bisulfate (Potential for additive pharmacologic effects because eptifibatide inhibits platelet aggregation; concurrent use requires caution). Products include:

Dalteparin Sodium (Because eptifibatide inhibits platelet aggregation, caution should be employed when it is used with other drugs that affect hemostasis). Products include:

Danaparoid Sodium (Because eptifibatide inhibits platelet aggregation, caution should be employed when it is used with other drugs that affect hemostasis).
No products indexed under this heading.

Dextran (Because eptifibatide inhibits platelet aggregation, caution should be employed when it is used with other drugs that affect hemostasis).
No products indexed under this heading.

Dextran 40 (Because eptifibatide inhibits platelet aggregation, caution should be employed when it is used with other drugs that affect hemostasis).
No products indexed under this heading.

Dextran 70 (Because eptifibatide inhibits platelet aggregation, caution should be employed when it is used with other drugs that affect hemostasis).
No products indexed under this heading.

Dextran I (Because eptifibatide inhibits platelet aggregation, caution should be employed when it is used with other drugs that affect hemostasis).
No products indexed under this heading.

Dextrans (Low Molecular Weight) (Because eptifibatide inhibits platelet aggregation, caution should be employed when it is used with other drugs that affect hemostasis).
No products indexed under this heading.

Diclofenac Epolamine (Potential for additive pharmacologic effects because eptifibatide inhibits platelet aggregation; concurrent use requires caution). Products include:

Diclofenac Potassium (Potential for additive pharmacologic effects because eptifibatide inhibits platelet aggregation; concurrent use requires caution).
No products indexed under this heading.

Diclofenac Sodium (Potential for additive pharmacologic effects because eptifibatide inhibits platelet aggregation; concurrent use requires caution).
No products indexed under this heading.

Dicumarol (Potential for additive pharmacologic effects because eptifibatide inhibits platelet aggregation; concurrent use requires caution).
No products indexed under this heading.

Diflunisal (Because eptifibatide inhibits platelet aggregation, caution should be employed when it is used with other drugs that affect hemostasis).
No products indexed under this heading.

Dipyridamole (Potential for additive pharmacologic effects because eptifibatide inhibits platelet aggregation; concurrent use requires caution). Products include:

Enoxaparin Sodium (Because eptifibatide inhibits platelet aggregation, caution should be employed when it is used with other drugs that affect hemostasis). Products include:

Etodolac (Potential for additive pharmacologic effects because eptifibatide inhibits platelet aggregation; concurrent use requires caution).
No products indexed under this heading.

Fenoprofen Calcium (Potential for additive pharmacologic effects because eptifibatide inhibits platelet aggregation; concurrent use requires caution).
No products indexed under this heading.

(☉ Described in PDR® for Ophthalmic Medicines)

INTRAVENOUS SODIUM DIURIL

May interact with alcohols, antihypertensives, barbiturates, cardiac glycosides, corticosteroids, insulin, lithium preparations, narcotic analgesics, nonsteroidal anti-inflammatory agents, nondepolarizing neuromuscular blocking agents, oral hypoglycemic agents, vasopressors, and certain other agents. Compounds in these categories include:

IMPORTANT NOTE: Always consult each drug listing in the patient's regimen for possible interactions.

883 Interactions Index Intravenous Diuril

Dobutamine (Co-administration of pressor amines and chlorothiazide may lead to possible decreased response to pressor amines but not sufficient to preclude their use).
No products indexed under this heading.

Dobutamine Hydrochloride (Co-administration of pressor amines and chlorothiazide may lead to possible decreased response to pressor amines but not sufficient to preclude their use).
No products indexed under this heading.

Dopamine Hydrochloride (Co-administration of pressor amines and chlorothiazide may lead to possible decreased response to pressor amines but not sufficient to preclude their use).
No products indexed under this heading.

Doxacurium Chloride (Co-administration of nondepolarizing skeletal muscle relaxants and chlorothiazide may lead to possible increased responsiveness to the muscle relaxant).
No products indexed under this heading.

Doxazosin Mesylate (Thiazides may add to or potentiate the action of other antihypertensive drugs; hypotension including orthostatic hypotension may be aggravated with concomitant use).
No products indexed under this heading.

d-Tubocurarine (Co-administration of nondepolarizing skeletal muscle relaxants and chlorothiazide may lead to possible increased responsiveness to the muscle relaxant).
No products indexed under this heading.

Enalapril Maleate (Thiazides may add to or potentiate the action of other antihypertensive drugs; hypotension including orthostatic hypotension may be aggravated with concomitant use).
No products indexed under this heading.

Enalaprilat (Thiazides may add to or potentiate the action of other antihypertensive drugs; hypotension including orthostatic hypotension may be aggravated with concomitant use).
No products indexed under this heading.

Ephedrine Sulfate (Co-administration of pressor amines and chlorothiazide may lead to possible decreased response to pressor amines but not sufficient to preclude their use).
No products indexed under this heading.

Epinephrine Bitartrate (Co-administration of pressor amines and chlorothiazide may lead to possible decreased response to pressor amines but not sufficient to preclude their use).
No products indexed under this heading.

Epinephrine Hydrochloride (Co-administration of pressor amines and chlorothiazide may lead to possible decreased response to pressor amines but not sufficient to preclude their use).
No products indexed under this heading.

Eprosartan Mesylate (Thiazides may add to or potentiate the action of other antihypertensive drugs; hypotension including orthostatic hypotension may be aggravated with concomitant use).
Products include:
Teveten 538
Teveten HCT 541

Esmolol Hydrochloride (Thiazides may add to or potentiate the action of other antihypertensive drugs; hypotension including orthostatic hypotension may be aggravated with concomitant use).
No products indexed under this heading.

Ethanol (Hypotension including orthostatic hypotension may be aggravated or potentiated by alcohol when co-administered with chlorothiazide).
No products indexed under this heading.

Ethyl Alcohol (Hypotension including orthostatic hypotension may be aggravated or potentiated by alcohol when co-administered with chlorothiazide).
No products indexed under this heading.

Etodolac (In some patients, the administration of a non-steroidal anti-inflammatory agent can reduce the diuretic, natriuretic, and antihypertensive effects of loop, potassium sparing and thiazide diuretics. Therefore, when chlorothiazide and NSAIDs are used concomitantly, the patient should be observed closely to determine if the desired effect of the diuretic is obtained).
No products indexed under this heading.

Felodipine (Thiazides may add to or potentiate the action of other antihypertensive drugs; hypotension including orthostatic hypotension may be aggravated with concomitant use).
No products indexed under this heading.

Fenoprofen Calcium (In some patients, the administration of a non-steroidal anti-inflammatory agent can reduce the diuretic, natriuretic, and antihypertensive effects of loop, potassium sparing and thiazide diuretics. Therefore, when chlorothiazide and NSAIDs are used concomitantly, the patient should be observed closely to determine if the desired effect of the diuretic is obtained).
No products indexed under this heading.

Fentanyl (Hypotension including orthostatic hypotension may be aggravated or potentiated by narcotics when co-administered with chlorothiazide).
Products include:
Duragesic 2604
Fentanyl Transdermal System 2346
Onsolis 2054

Fentanyl Citrate (Hypotension including orthostatic hypotension may be aggravated or potentiated by narcotics when co-administered with chlorothiazide). Products include:
Fentora 966

Fludrocortisone Acetate (Co-administration of corticosteroids and chlorothiazide may lead to intensified electrolyte depletion, particularly hypokalemia).
No products indexed under this heading.

Flumethasone Pivalate (Co-administration of corticosteroids and chlorothiazide may lead to intensified electrolyte depletion, particularly hypokalemia).
No products indexed under this heading.

Flunisolide Hemihydrate (Co-administration of corticosteroids and chlorothiazide may lead to intensified electrolyte depletion, particularly hypokalemia).
No products indexed under this heading.

Flurbiprofen (In some patients, the administration of a non-steroidal anti-inflammatory agent can reduce the diuretic, natriuretic, and antihypertensive effects of loop, potassium sparing and thiazide diuretics. Therefore, when chlorothiazide and NSAIDs are used concomitantly, the patient should be observed closely to determine if the desired effect of the diuretic is obtained).
No products indexed under this heading.

Fluticasone Furoate (Co-administration of corticosteroids and chlorothiazide may lead to intensified electrolyte depletion, particularly hypokalemia). Products include:
Veramyst 1713

Fluticasone Propionate (Co-administration of corticosteroids and chlorothiazide may lead to intensified electrolyte depletion, particularly hypokalemia). Products include:
Advair 100/50 1275
Advair 250/50 1275
Advair 500/50 1275
Advair HFA 45/21 1288
Advair HFA 115/21 1288
Advair HFA 230/21 1288
Flonase 1459
Flovent Diskus 1463
Flovent HFA 1470

Fosinopril Sodium (Thiazides may add to or potentiate the action of other antihypertensive drugs; hypotension including orthostatic hypotension may be aggravated with concomitant use).
No products indexed under this heading.

Furosemide (Thiazides may add to or potentiate the action of other antihypertensive drugs; hypotension including orthostatic hypotension may be aggravated with concomitant use). Products include:
Furosemide 2354

Gallamine (Co-administration of nondepolarizing skeletal muscle relaxants and chlorothiazide may lead to possible increased responsiveness to the muscle relaxant).
No products indexed under this heading.

Gallamine Triethiodide (Co-administration of nondepolarizing skeletal muscle relaxants and chlorothiazide may lead to possible increased responsiveness to the muscle relaxant).
No products indexed under this heading.

Glibenclamide (Dosage adjustment of the antidiabetic drug may be required when anti-diabetic drugs (eg, oral agents, insulin) and chlorothiazide are used concomitantly).
No products indexed under this heading.

Glimepiride (Dosage adjustment of the antidiabetic drug may be required when anti-diabetic drugs (eg, oral agents, insulin) and chlorothiazide are used concomitantly). Products include:
Avandaryl 1356
Duetact 3354

Glipizide (Dosage adjustment of the antidiabetic drug may be required when anti-diabetic drugs (eg, oral agents, insulin) and chlorothiazide are used concomitantly).
No products indexed under this heading.

Glyburide (Dosage adjustment of the antidiabetic drug may be required when anti-diabetic drugs (eg, oral agents, insulin) and chlorothiazide are used concomitantly).
No products indexed under this heading.

Guanabenz Acetate (Thiazides may add to or potentiate the action of other antihypertensive drugs; hypotension including orthostatic hypotension may be aggravated with concomitant use).
No products indexed under this heading.

Guanethidine (Thiazides may add to or potentiate the action of other antihypertensive drugs; hypotension including orthostatic hypotension may be aggravated with concomitant use).
No products indexed under this heading.

Guanethidine Monosulfate (Thiazides may add to or potentiate the action of other antihypertensive drugs; hypotension including orthostatic hypotension may be aggravated with concomitant use).
No products indexed under this heading.

Guanethidine Sulfate (Thiazides may add to or potentiate the action of other antihypertensive drugs; hypotension including orthostatic hypotension may be aggravated with concomitant use).
No products indexed under this heading.

Hexobarbital (Hypotension including orthostatic hypotension may be aggravated or potentiated by barbiturates when co-administered with chlorothiazide).
No products indexed under this heading.

Hydralazine Hydrochloride (Thiazides may add to or potentiate the action of other antihypertensive drugs; hypotension including orthostatic hypotension may be aggravated with concomitant use).
No products indexed under this heading.

Hydrochlorothiazide (Thiazides may add to or potentiate the action of other antihypertensive drugs; hypotension including orthostatic hypotension may be aggravated with concomitant use).
Products include:
Atacand HCT 700
Avalide 2956
Benicar HCT 1017
Diovan HCT 2419
Dyazide 1429
Exforge HCT 2449
Hyzaar 2162
Hyzaar 100-12.5 2162
Micardis HCT 889
Prinzide 2246
Tekturna HCT 2541
Teveten HCT 541

Hydrocodone Bitartrate (Hypotension including orthostatic hypotension may be aggravated or potentiated by narcotics when co-administered with chlorothiazide). Products include:
Vicodin 560
Vicodin ES 561
Vicodin HP 563
Vicoprofen 564
Zydone 1138

Hydrocodone Polistirex (Hypotension including orthostatic hypotension may be aggravated or potentiated by narcotics when co-administered with chlorothiazide). Products include:
Tussionex 3443

Hydrocortisone (Co-administration of corticosteroids and chlorothiazide may lead to intensified electrolyte depletion, particularly hypokalemia).
No products indexed under this heading.

Hydrocortisone (Alcohol) (Co-administration of corticosteroids and chlorothiazide may lead to intensified electrolyte depletion, particularly hypokalemia).
No products indexed under this heading.

Hydrocortisone Acetate (Co-administration of corticosteroids and chlorothiazide may lead to intensified electrolyte depletion, particularly hypokalemia).
No products indexed under this heading.

Hydrocortisone Butyrate (Co-administration of corticosteroids and chlorothiazide may lead to intensified electrolyte depletion, particularly hypokalemia).
No products indexed under this heading.

Hydrocortisone Cypionate (Co-administration of corticosteroids and chlorothiazide may lead to intensified electrolyte depletion, particularly hypokalemia).
No products indexed under this heading.

Hydrocortisone Hemisuccinate (Co-administration of corticosteroids and chlorothiazide may lead to intensified electrolyte depletion, particularly hypokalemia).
No products indexed under this heading.

Hydrocortisone Probutate (Co-administration of corticosteroids and chlorothiazide may lead to intensified electrolyte depletion, particularly hypokalemia).
No products indexed under this heading.

Hydrocortisone Sodium Phosphate (Co-administration of corticosteroids and chlorothiazide may lead to intensified electrolyte depletion, particularly hypokalemia).
No products indexed under this heading.

IMPORTANT NOTE: Always consult each drug listing in the patient's regimen for possible interactions.

Intravenous Diuril Interactions Index 884

Hydrocortisone Sodium Succinate (Co-administration of corticosteroids and chlorothiazide may lead to intensified electrolyte depletion, particularly hypokalemia).
No products indexed under this heading.

Hydrocortisone Valerate (Co-administration of corticosteroids and chlorothiazide may lead to intensified electrolyte depletion, particularly hypokalemia).
No products indexed under this heading.

Hydroflumethiazide (Thiazides may add to or potentiate the action of other antihypertensive drugs; hypotension including orthostatic hypotension may be aggravated with concomitant use).
No products indexed under this heading.

Hydromorphone (Hypotension including orthostatic hypotension may be aggravated or potentiated by narcotics when co-administered with chlorothiazide).
No products indexed under this heading.

Hydromorphone Hydrochloride (Hypotension including orthostatic hypotension may be aggravated or potentiated by narcotics when co-administered with chlorothiazide). Products include:
Dilaudid Injection ... 2800
Dilaudid Oral ... 2797
Dilaudid Tablets ... 2797
Dilaudid-HP ... 2800

Ibuprofen (In some patients, the administration of a non-steroidal anti-inflammatory agent can reduce the diuretic, natriuretic, and antihypertensive effects of loop, potassium sparing and thiazide diuretics. Therefore, when chlorothiazide and NSAIDs are used concomitantly, the patient should be observed closely to determine if the desired effect of the diuretic is obtained). Products include:
Motrin IB ... 2043
Children's Motrin ... 2044
Children's Motrin Non-Staining Dye-Free ... 2044
Infants' Motrin ... 2044
Infants' Motrin Dye-Free ... 2044
Junior Strength Motrin ... 2044
Vicoprofen ... 564

Indapamide (Thiazides may add to or potentiate the action of other antihypertensive drugs; hypotension including orthostatic hypotension may be aggravated with concomitant use). Products include:
Indapamide ... 2356

Indomethacin (In some patients, the administration of a non-steroidal anti-inflammatory agent can reduce the diuretic, natriuretic, and antihypertensive effects of loop, potassium sparing and thiazide diuretics. Therefore, when chlorothiazide and NSAIDs are used concomitantly, the patient should be observed closely to determine if the desired effect of the diuretic is obtained). Products include:
Indocin ... 2167

Indomethacin Sodium Trihydrate (In some patients, the administration of a non-steroidal anti-inflammatory agent can reduce the diuretic, natriuretic, and antihypertensive effects of loop, potassium sparing and thiazide diuretics. Therefore, when chlorothiazide and NSAIDs are used concomitantly, the patient should be observed closely to determine if the desired effect of the diuretic is obtained). Products include:
Indocin I.V. ... 2007

Insulin (Dosage adjustment of the antidiabetic drug may be required when anti-diabetic drugs (eg, oral agents, insulin) and chlorothiazide are used concomitantly).
No products indexed under this heading.

Insulin, Human, Zinc Suspension (Dosage adjustment of the antidiabetic drug may be required when anti-diabetic drugs (eg, oral agents, insulin) and chlorothiazide are used concomitantly).
No products indexed under this heading.

Insulin, Human (rDNA origin) (Dosage adjustment of the antidiabetic drug may be required when anti-diabetic drugs (eg, oral agents, insulin) and chlorothiazide are used concomitantly). Products include:
Exubera ... 2717

Insulin, Human NPH (Dosage adjustment of the antidiabetic drug may be required when anti-diabetic drugs (eg, oral agents, insulin) and chlorothiazide are used concomitantly). Products include:
Humulin N Vial ... 1934

Insulin, Human Regular (Dosage adjustment of the antidiabetic drug may be required when anti-diabetic drugs (eg, oral agents, insulin) and chlorothiazide are used concomitantly). Products include:
Humulin R ... 1937
Humulin R (U-500) ... 1939

Insulin, Human Regular and Human NPH Mixture (Dosage adjustment of the antidiabetic drug may be required when anti-diabetic drugs (eg, oral agents, insulin) and chlorothiazide are used concomitantly). Products include:
Humulin 50/50 ... 1930
Humulin 70/30 Vial ... 1931

Insulin, NPH (Dosage adjustment of the antidiabetic drug may be required when anti-diabetic drugs (eg, oral agents, insulin) and chlorothiazide are used concomitantly).
No products indexed under this heading.

Insulin, Regular (Dosage adjustment of the antidiabetic drug may be required when anti-diabetic drugs (eg, oral agents, insulin) and chlorothiazide are used concomitantly).
No products indexed under this heading.

Insulin, Regular and NPH mixture (Dosage adjustment of the antidiabetic drug may be required when anti-diabetic drugs (eg, oral agents, insulin) and chlorothiazide are used concomitantly).
No products indexed under this heading.

Insulin, Zinc Crystals (Dosage adjustment of the antidiabetic drug may be required when anti-diabetic drugs (eg, oral agents, insulin) and chlorothiazide are used concomitantly).
No products indexed under this heading.

Insulin, Zinc Suspension (Dosage adjustment of the antidiabetic drug may be required when anti-diabetic drugs (eg, oral agents, insulin) and chlorothiazide are used concomitantly).
No products indexed under this heading.

Insulin Aspart (Dosage adjustment of the antidiabetic drug may be required when anti-diabetic drugs (eg, oral agents, insulin) and chlorothiazide are used concomitantly).
No products indexed under this heading.

Insulin Aspart, Human (Dosage adjustment of the antidiabetic drug may be required when anti-diabetic drugs (eg, oral agents, insulin) and chlorothiazide are used concomitantly). Products include:
NovoLog Mix 70/30 ... 2581

Insulin Aspart, Human Regular (Dosage adjustment of the antidiabetic drug may be required when anti-diabetic drugs (eg, oral agents, insulin) and chlorothiazide are used concomitantly). Products include:
NovoLog ... 2575

Insulin Aspart Protamine, Human (Dosage adjustment of the antidiabetic drug may be required when anti-diabetic drugs (eg, oral agents, insulin) and chlorothiazide are used concomitantly). Products include:
NovoLog Mix 70/30 ... 2581

Insulin Detemir (rDNA Origin) (Dosage adjustment of the antidiabetic drug may be required when anti-diabetic drugs (eg, oral agents, insulin) and chlorothiazide are used concomitantly). Products include:
Levemir ... 2566

Insulin Glargine (Dosage adjustment of the antidiabetic drug may be required when anti-diabetic drugs (eg, oral agents, insulin) and chlorothiazide are used concomitantly). Products include:
Lantus ... 2996

Insulin Glulisine (Dosage adjustment of the antidiabetic drug may be required when anti-diabetic drugs (eg, oral agents, insulin) and chlorothiazide are used concomitantly). Products include:
Apidra ... 2937
Apidra SoloStar ... 2937

Insulin Lispro, Human (Dosage adjustment of the antidiabetic drug may be required when anti-diabetic drugs (eg, oral agents, insulin) and chlorothiazide are used concomitantly). Products include:
Humalog ... 1910
Humalog Mix ... 1914
Humalog Mix75/25 ... 1917

Insulin Lispro Protamine, Human (Dosage adjustment of the antidiabetic drug may be required when anti-diabetic drugs (eg, oral agents, insulin) and chlorothiazide are used concomitantly). Products include:
Humalog Mix ... 1914
Humalog Mix75/25 ... 1917

Irbesartan (Thiazides may add to or potentiate the action of other antihypertensive drugs; hypotension including orthostatic hypotension may be aggravated with concomitant use). Products include:
Avalide ... 2956
Avapro ... 2962

Isoproterenol Hydrochloride (Co-administration of pressor amines and chlorothiazide may lead to possible decreased response to pressor amines but not sufficient to preclude their use).
No products indexed under this heading.

Isoproterenol Sulfate (Co-administration of pressor amines and chlorothiazide may lead to possible decreased response to pressor amines but not sufficient to preclude their use).
No products indexed under this heading.

Isradipine (Thiazides may add to or potentiate the action of other antihypertensive drugs; hypotension including orthostatic hypotension may be aggravated with concomitant use). Products include:
DynaCirc CR ... 1432

Ketoprofen (In some patients, the administration of a non-steroidal anti-inflammatory agent can reduce the diuretic, natriuretic, and antihypertensive effects of loop, potassium sparing and thiazide diuretics. Therefore, when chlorothiazide and NSAIDs are used concomitantly, the patient should be observed closely to determine if the desired effect of the diuretic is obtained).
No products indexed under this heading.

Ketorolac Tromethamine (In some patients, the administration of a non-steroidal anti-inflammatory agent can reduce the diuretic, natriuretic, and antihypertensive effects of loop, potassium sparing and thiazide diuretics. Therefore, when chlorothiazide and NSAIDs are used concomitantly, the patient should be observed closely to determine if the desired effect of the diuretic is obtained). Products include:
Acuvail ... ⊙ 209

Labetalol Hydrochloride (Thiazides may add to or potentiate the action of other antihypertensive drugs; hypotension including orthostatic hypotension may be aggravated with concomitant use).
No products indexed under this heading.

Levorphanol Tartrate (Hypotension including orthostatic hypotension may be aggravated or potentiated by narcotics when co-administered with chlorothiazide).
No products indexed under this heading.

Lisinopril (Thiazides may add to or potentiate the action of other antihypertensive drugs; hypotension including orthostatic hypotension may be aggravated with concomitant use). Products include:
Prinivil ... 2241
Prinzide ... 2246

Lithium (Lithium, generally should not be given with diuretics. Diuretic agents reduce the renal clearance of lithium and add a high risk of lithium toxicity).
No products indexed under this heading.

Lithium Carbonate (Lithium, generally should not be given with diuretics. Diuretic agents reduce the renal clearance of lithium and add a high risk of lithium toxicity).
No products indexed under this heading.

Lithium Citrate (Lithium, generally should not be given with diuretics. Diuretic agents reduce the renal clearance of lithium and add a high risk of lithium toxicity).
No products indexed under this heading.

Losartan Potassium (Thiazides may add to or potentiate the action of other antihypertensive drugs; hypotension including orthostatic hypotension may be aggravated with concomitant use). Products include:
Cozaar ... 2106
Hyzaar ... 2162
Hyzaar 100-12.5 ... 2162

Mecamylamine Hydrochloride (Thiazides may add to or potentiate the action of other antihypertensive drugs; hypotension including orthostatic hypotension may be aggravated with concomitant use).
No products indexed under this heading.

Meclofenamate Sodium (In some patients, the administration of a non-steroidal anti-inflammatory agent can reduce the diuretic, natriuretic, and antihypertensive effects of loop, potassium sparing and thiazide diuretics. Therefore, when chlorothiazide and NSAIDs are used concomitantly, the patient should be observed closely to determine if the desired effect of the diuretic is obtained).
No products indexed under this heading.

Mefenamic Acid (In some patients, the administration of a non-steroidal anti-inflammatory agent can reduce the diuretic, natriuretic, and antihypertensive effects of loop, potassium sparing and thiazide diuretics. Therefore, when chlorothiazide and NSAIDs are used concomitantly, the patient should be observed closely to determine if the desired effect of the diuretic is obtained).
No products indexed under this heading.

Meloxicam (In some patients, the administration of a non-steroidal anti-inflammatory agent can reduce the diuretic, natriuretic, and antihypertensive effects of loop, potassium sparing and thiazide diuretics. Therefore, when chlorothiazide and NSAIDs are used concomitantly, the patient should be observed closely to determine if the desired effect of the diuretic is obtained).
No products indexed under this heading.

IMPORTANT NOTE: Always consult each drug listing in the patient's regimen for possible interactions.

Triamcinolone Diacetate (Co-administration of corticosteroids and chlorothiazide may lead to intensified electrolyte depletion, particularly hypokalemia).
No products indexed under this heading.

Triamcinolone Hexacetonide (Co-administration of corticosteroids and chlorothiazide may lead to intensified electrolyte depletion, particularly hypokalemia).
No products indexed under this heading.

Trimethaphan Camsylate (Thiazides may add to or potentiate the action of other antihypertensive drugs; hypotension including orthostatic hypotension may be aggravated with concomitant use).
No products indexed under this heading.

Troglitazone (Dosage adjustment of the antidiabetic drug may be required when anti-diabetic drugs (eg, oral agents, insulin) and chlorothiazide are used concomitantly).
No products indexed under this heading.

Tubocurarine Chloride (Co-administration of nondepolarizing skeletal muscle relaxants (eg, tubocurarine) and chlorothiazide may lead to possible increased responsiveness to the muscle relaxant).
No products indexed under this heading.

Valdecoxib (In some patients, the administration of a non-steroidal anti-inflammatory agent can reduce the diuretic, natriuretic, and antihypertensive effects of loop, potassium sparing and thiazide diuretics. Therefore, when chlorothiazide and NSAIDs are used concomitantly, the patient should be observed closely to determine if the desired effect of the diuretic is obtained).
No products indexed under this heading.

Valsartan (Thiazides may add to or potentiate the action of other antihypertensive drugs; hypotension including orthostatic hypotension may be aggravated with concomitant use). Products include:

Diovan	2413
Diovan HCT	2419
Exforge	2443
Exforge HCT	2449
Valturna	3637

Vecuronium Bromide (Co-administration of nondepolarizing skeletal muscle relaxants and chlorothiazide may lead to possible increased responsiveness to the muscle relaxant).
No products indexed under this heading.

Verapamil Hydrochloride (Thiazides may add to or potentiate the action of other antihypertensive drugs; hypotension including orthostatic hypotension may be aggravated with concomitant use). Products include:

Tarka	534

Food Interactions

Alcohol (Hypotension including orthostatic hypotension may be aggravated or potentiated by alcohol when co-administered with chlorothiazide).

Beer, reduced-alcohol (Hypotension including orthostatic hypotension may be aggravated or potentiated by alcohol when co-administered with chlorothiazide).

Beer, unspecified (Hypotension including orthostatic hypotension may be aggravated or potentiated by alcohol when co-administered with chlorothiazide).

Wine, Chianti (Hypotension including orthostatic hypotension may be aggravated or potentiated by alcohol when co-administered with chlorothiazide).

Wine, Red (Hypotension including orthostatic hypotension may be aggravated or potentiated by alcohol when co-administered with chlorothiazide).

Wine, unspecified (Hypotension including orthostatic hypotension may be aggravated or potentiated by alcohol when co-administered with chlorothiazide).

Wine products (Hypotension including orthostatic hypotension may be aggravated or potentiated by alcohol when co-administered with chlorothiazide).

INTRON A FOR INJECTION

(Interferon alfa-2b, Recombinant) 3140
May interact with xanthines, and certain other agents. Compounds in these categories include:

Aminophylline (Co-administration results in decreased theophylline clearance resulting in a 100% increase in serum theophylline levels).
No products indexed under this heading.

Bone Marrow Depressants, unspecified (Careful monitoring of the WBC count is indicated).
No products indexed under this heading.

Dyphylline (Co-administration results in decreased theophylline clearance resulting in a 100% increase in serum theophylline levels).
No products indexed under this heading.

Theophylline (Co-administration results in decreased theophylline clearance resulting in a 100% increase in serum theophylline levels).
No products indexed under this heading.

Theophylline Anhydrous (Co-administration results in decreased theophylline clearance resulting in a 100% increase in serum theophylline levels). Products include:

Uniphyl	2817

Theophylline Calcium Salicylate (Co-administration results in decreased theophylline clearance resulting in a 100% increase in serum theophylline levels).
No products indexed under this heading.

Theophylline Dihydroxypropyl (Glyceryl) (Co-administration results in decreased theophylline clearance resulting in a 100% increase in serum theophylline levels).
No products indexed under this heading.

Theophylline Ethylenediamine (Co-administration results in decreased theophylline clearance resulting in a 100% increase in serum theophylline levels).
No products indexed under this heading.

Theophylline Sodium Glycinate (Co-administration results in decreased theophylline clearance resulting in a 100% increase in serum theophylline levels).
No products indexed under this heading.

Zidovudine (Concomitant administration may result in a higher incidence of neutropenia). Products include:

Combivir	1404
Retrovir	1634
Retrovir IV	1640
Trizivir	1688

INTUNIV EXTENDED-RELEASE TABLETS

(Guanfacine Hydrochloride) 3291
May interact with alcohols, antihypertensives, antipsychotic agents, barbiturates, benzodiazepines, central nervous system depressants, cytochrome p450 3a4 inducers (selected), cytochrome p450 3a4 inhibitors, potent (selected), hypnotics and sedatives, valproate, and certain other agents. Compounds in these categories include:

Acebutolol Hydrochloride (Caution should be exercised when guanfacine is administered concomitantly with antihypertensive drugs, due to the potential for additive pharmacodynamic effects).
No products indexed under this heading.

Alfentanil Hydrochloride (Caution should be exercised when guanfacine is administered concomitantly with CNS depressant drugs (eg, alcohol, sedative/hypnotics, benzodiazepines, barbiturates, and antipsychotics) due to the potential for additive pharmacodynamic effects).
No products indexed under this heading.

Aliskiren (Caution should be exercised when guanfacine is administered concomitantly with antihypertensive drugs, due to the potential for additive pharmacodynamic effects). Products include:

Tekturna	2538
Tekturna HCT	2541
Valturna	3637

Allium sativum (Significant decrease in the rate and extent of guanfacine exposure when co-administered with a CYP3A4 inducer).
No products indexed under this heading.

Alprazolam (Caution should be exercised when guanfacine is administered concomitantly with benzodiazepines due to the potential for additive pharmacodynamic effects).
No products indexed under this heading.

Aminoglutethimide (Significant decrease in the rate and extent of guanfacine exposure when co-administered with a CYP3A4 inducer).
No products indexed under this heading.

Amlodipine Besylate (Caution should be exercised when guanfacine is administered concomitantly with antihypertensive drugs, due to the potential for additive pharmacodynamic effects). Products include:

Azor	1010
Exforge	2443
Exforge HCT	2449

Amobarbital (Caution should be exercised when guanfacine is administered concomitantly with barbiturates due to the potential for additive pharmacodynamic effects).
No products indexed under this heading.

Amobarbital Sodium (Caution should be exercised when guanfacine is administered concomitantly with barbiturates due to the potential for additive pharmacodynamic effects).
No products indexed under this heading.

Amprenavir (Caution should be exercised when guanfacine is administered to patients taking other strong CYP3A4 inhibitors, since elevation of plasma guanfacine concentration increases the risk of adverse events such as hypotension, bradycardia, and sedation).
No products indexed under this heading.

Aprepitant (Significant decrease in the rate and extent of guanfacine exposure when co-administered with a CYP3A4 inducer). Products include:

Emend	2124

Aprobarbital (Caution should be exercised when guanfacine is administered concomitantly with barbiturates due to the potential for additive pharmacodynamic effects).
No products indexed under this heading.

Aripiprazole (Caution should be exercised when guanfacine is administered concomitantly with antipsychotics due to the potential for additive pharmacodynamic effects).
No products indexed under this heading.

Atazanavir (Caution should be exercised when guanfacine is administered to patients taking other strong CYP3A4 inhibitors, since elevation of plasma guanfacine concentration increases the risk of adverse events such as hypotension, bradycardia, and sedation).
No products indexed under this heading.

Atazanavir Sulfate (Caution should be exercised when guanfacine is administered to patients taking other strong CYP3A4 inhibitors, since elevation of plasma guanfacine concentration increases the risk of adverse events such as hypotension, bradycardia, and sedation).
No products indexed under this heading.

Atenolol (Caution should be exercised when guanfacine is administered concomitantly with antihypertensive drugs, due to the potential for additive pharmacodynamic effects).
No products indexed under this heading.

Benazepril Hydrochloride (Caution should be exercised when guanfacine is administered concomitantly with antihypertensive drugs, due to the potential for additive pharmacodynamic effects).
No products indexed under this heading.

Bendroflumethiazide (Caution should be exercised when guanfacine is administered concomitantly with antihypertensive drugs, due to the potential for additive pharmacodynamic effects).
No products indexed under this heading.

Betamethasone (Significant decrease in the rate and extent of guanfacine exposure when co-administered with a CYP3A4 inducer).
No products indexed under this heading.

Betamethasone Acetate (Significant decrease in the rate and extent of guanfacine exposure when co-administered with a CYP3A4 inducer).
No products indexed under this heading.

Betamethasone Benzoate (Significant decrease in the rate and extent of guanfacine exposure when co-administered with a CYP3A4 inducer).
No products indexed under this heading.

Betamethasone Dipropionate (Significant decrease in the rate and extent of guanfacine exposure when co-administered with a CYP3A4 inducer). Products include:

Diprolene Lotion 0.05%	3108
Diprolene Ointment 0.05%	3109
Diprolene AF Cream 0.05%	3107
Lotrisone	3163

Betamethasone Sodium Phosphate (Significant decrease in the rate and extent of guanfacine exposure when co-administered with a CYP3A4 inducer).
No products indexed under this heading.

Betamethasone Valerate (Significant decrease in the rate and extent of guanfacine exposure when co-administered with a CYP3A4 inducer). Products include:

Luxíq	3321

Betaxolol Hydrochloride (Caution should be exercised when guanfacine is administered concomitantly with antihypertensive drugs, due to the potential for additive pharmacodynamic effects).
No products indexed under this heading.

Bisoprolol Fumarate (Caution should be exercised when guanfacine is administered concomitantly with antihypertensive drugs, due to the potential for additive pharmacodynamic effects).
No products indexed under this heading.

Bosentan (Significant decrease in the rate and extent of guanfacine exposure when co-administered with a CYP3A4 inducer). Products include:

Tracleer	573

IMPORTANT NOTE: Always consult each drug listing in the patient's regimen for possible interactions.

Buprenorphine Hydrochloride
(Caution should be exercised when guanfacine is administered concomitantly with CNS depressant drugs (eg, alcohol, sedative/hypnotics, benzodiazepines, barbiturates, and antipsychotics) due to the potential for additive pharmacodynamic effects).
No products indexed under this heading.

Buspirone Hydrochloride (Caution should be exercised when guanfacine is administered concomitantly with CNS depressant drugs (eg, alcohol, sedative/hypnotics, benzodiazepines, barbiturates, and antipsychotics) due to the potential for additive pharmacodynamic effects).
No products indexed under this heading.

Butabarbital (Caution should be exercised when guanfacine is administered concomitantly with barbiturates due to the potential for additive pharmacodynamic effects).
No products indexed under this heading.

Butabarbital Sodium (Caution should be exercised when guanfacine is administered concomitantly with barbiturates due to the potential for additive pharmacodynamic effects).
No products indexed under this heading.

Butalbital (Caution should be exercised when guanfacine is administered concomitantly with barbiturates due to the potential for additive pharmacodynamic effects).
No products indexed under this heading.

Candesartan Cilexetil (Caution should be exercised when guanfacine is administered concomitantly with antihypertensive drugs, due to the potential for additive pharmacodynamic effects). Products include:

Captopril (Caution should be exercised when guanfacine is administered concomitantly with antihypertensive drugs, due to the potential for additive pharmacodynamic effects). Products include:

Carbamazepine (Co-administration with carbamazepine may lead to symptomatic hyponatremia). Products include:

Carteolol Hydrochloride (Caution should be exercised when guanfacine is administered concomitantly with antihypertensive drugs, due to the potential for additive pharmacodynamic effects).
No products indexed under this heading.

Carvedilol (Caution should be exercised when guanfacine is administered concomitantly with antihypertensive drugs, due to the potential for additive pharmacodynamic effects). Products include:

Carvedilol Phosphate (Caution should be exercised when guanfacine is administered concomitantly with antihypertensive drugs, due to the potential for additive pharmacodynamic effects). Products include:

Chloral Hydrate (Caution should be exercised concomitantly with hypnotics and sedatives due to the potential for additive pharmacodynamic effects).
No products indexed under this heading.

Chlordiazepoxide (Caution should be exercised when guanfacine is administered concomitantly with benzodiazepines due to the potential for additive pharmacodynamic effects).

Chlordiazepoxide Hydrochloride
(Caution should be exercised when guanfacine is administered concomitantly with benzodiazepines due to the potential for additive pharmacodynamic effects).
No products indexed under this heading.

Chlorothiazide (Caution should be exercised when guanfacine is administered concomitantly with antihypertensive drugs, due to the potential for additive pharmacodynamic effects).
No products indexed under this heading.

Chlorothiazide Sodium (Caution should be exercised when guanfacine is administered concomitantly with antihypertensive drugs, due to the potential for additive pharmacodynamic effects). Products include:

Chlorpromazine (Caution should be exercised when guanfacine is administered concomitantly with antipsychotics due to the potential for additive pharmacodynamic effects).
No products indexed under this heading.

Chlorpromazine Hydrochloride
(Caution should be exercised when guanfacine is administered concomitantly with antipsychotics due to the potential for additive pharmacodynamic effects).
No products indexed under this heading.

Chlorprothixene (Caution should be exercised when guanfacine is administered concomitantly with antipsychotics due to the potential for additive pharmacodynamic effects).
No products indexed under this heading.

Chlorprothixene Hydrochloride
(Caution should be exercised when guanfacine is administered concomitantly with antipsychotics due to the potential for additive pharmacodynamic effects).
No products indexed under this heading.

Chlorprothixene Lactate (Caution should be exercised when guanfacine is administered concomitantly with antipsychotics due to the potential for additive pharmacodynamic effects).
No products indexed under this heading.

Chlorthalidone (Caution should be exercised when guanfacine is administered concomitantly with antihypertensive drugs, due to the potential for additive pharmacodynamic effects). Products include:

Ciprofloxacin (Significant decrease in the rate and extent of guanfacine exposure when co-administered with a CYP3A4 inducer). Products include:

Ciprofloxacin Hydrochloride (Significant decrease in the rate and extent of guanfacine exposure when co-administered with a CYP3A4 inducer). Products include:

Cisplatin (Significant decrease in the rate and extent of guanfacine exposure when co-administered with a CYP3A4 inducer).
No products indexed under this heading.

Clarithromycin (Caution should be exercised to patients taking other strong CYP3A4 inhibitors, since elevation of plasma guanfacine concentration increases the risk of adverse events such as hypotension, bradycardia, and sedation). Products include:

Clonazepam (Caution should be exercised when guanfacine is administered concomitantly with CNS depressant

drugs (eg, alcohol, sedative/hypnotics, benzodiazepines, barbiturates, and antipsychotics) due to the potential for additive pharmacodynamic effects).
Products include:

Clonidine (Caution should be exercised when guanfacine is administered concomitantly with antihypertensive drugs, due to the potential for additive pharmacodynamic effects). Products include:

Clonidine Hydrochloride (Caution should be exercised when guanfacine is administered concomitantly with antihypertensive drugs, due to the potential for additive pharmacodynamic effects). Products include:

Clorazepate Dipotassium (Caution should be exercised when guanfacine is administered concomitantly with benzodiazepines due to the potential for additive pharmacodynamic effects).
No products indexed under this heading.

Clozapine (Caution should be exercised when guanfacine is administered concomitantly with antipsychotics due to the potential for additive pharmacodynamic effects).
No products indexed under this heading.

Codeine Phosphate (Caution should be exercised when guanfacine is administered concomitantly with CNS depressant drugs (eg, alcohol, sedative/hypnotics, benzodiazepines, barbiturates, and antipsychotics) due to the potential for additive pharmacodynamic effects). Products include:

Codeine Sulfate (Caution should be exercised when guanfacine is administered concomitantly with CNS depressant drugs (eg, alcohol, sedative/hypnotics, benzodiazepines, barbiturates, and antipsychotics) due to the potential for additive pharmacodynamic effects).
No products indexed under this heading.

Cortisone Acetate (Significant decrease in the rate and extent of guanfacine exposure when co-administered with a CYP3A4 inducer).
No products indexed under this heading.

Delavirdine Mesylate (Caution should be exercised when guanfacine is administered to patients taking other strong CYP3A4 inhibitors, since elevation of plasma guanfacine concentration increases the risk of adverse events such as hypotension, bradycardia, and sedation).
No products indexed under this heading.

Delavirine (Caution should be exercised when guanfacine is administered to patients taking other strong CYP3A4 inhibitors, since elevation of plasma guanfacine concentration increases the risk of adverse events such as hypotension, bradycardia, and sedation).
No products indexed under this heading.

Deserpidine (Caution should be exercised when guanfacine is administered concomitantly with antihypertensive drugs, due to the potential for additive pharmacodynamic effects).
No products indexed under this heading.

Desflurane (Caution should be exercised when guanfacine is administered concomitantly with CNS depressant drugs (eg, alcohol, sedative/hypnotics, benzodiazepines, barbiturates, and antipsychotics) due to the potential for additive pharmacodynamic effects).
No products indexed under this heading.

Dexamethasone (Significant decrease in the rate and extent of guanfacine exposure when co-administered with a CYP3A4 inducer). Products include:

Dexamethasone Acetate (Significant decrease in the rate and extent of guanfacine exposure when co-administered with a CYP3A4 inducer).
No products indexed under this heading.

Dexamethasone Phosphate (Significant decrease in the rate and extent of guanfacine exposure when co-administered with a CYP3A4 inducer).
No products indexed under this heading.

Dexamethasone Sodium (Significant decrease in the rate and extent of guanfacine exposure when co-administered with a CYP3A4 inducer).
No products indexed under this heading.

Dexamethasone Sodium Phosphate (Significant decrease in the rate and extent of guanfacine exposure when co-administered with a CYP3A4 inducer).
No products indexed under this heading.

Dexamethasone Sodium Phosphate Injection (Significant decrease in the rate and extent of guanfacine exposure when co-administered with a CYP3A4 inducer).
No products indexed under this heading.

Dezocine (Caution should be exercised when guanfacine is administered concomitantly with CNS depressant drugs (eg, alcohol, sedative/hypnotics, benzodiazepines, barbiturates, and antipsychotics) due to the potential for additive pharmacodynamic effects).
No products indexed under this heading.

Diazepam (Caution should be exercised when guanfacine is administered concomitantly with benzodiazepines due to the potential for additive pharmacodynamic effects). Products include:

Diazoxide (Caution should be exercised when guanfacine is administered concomitantly with antihypertensive drugs, due to the potential for additive pharmacodynamic effects). Products include:

Diltiazem Hydrochloride (Caution should be exercised when guanfacine is administered concomitantly with antihypertensive drugs, due to the potential for additive pharmacodynamic effects). Products include:

Diltiazem Maleate (Caution should be exercised when guanfacine is administered concomitantly with antihypertensive drugs, due to the potential for additive pharmacodynamic effects).
No products indexed under this heading.

Divalproex Sodium (Co-administration of guanfacine and valproic acid may result in increased concentrations of valproic acid; adjustments in the dose of valproic acid may be indicated). Products include:

Doxazosin Mesylate (Caution should be exercised when guanfacine is administered concomitantly with antihypertensive drugs, due to the potential for additive pharmacodynamic effects).
No products indexed under this heading.

Doxorubicin Hydrochloride (Significant decrease in the rate and extent of guanfacine exposure when co-administered with a CYP3A4 inducer).
No products indexed under this heading.

Droperidol (Caution should be exercised when guanfacine is administered concomitantly with CNS depressant drugs (eg, alcohol, sedative/hypnotics, benzodiazepines, barbiturates, and antipsychotics) due to the potential for additive pharmacodynamic effects).
No products indexed under this heading.

Efavirenz (Significant decrease in the rate and extent of guanfacine exposure when co-administered with a CYP3A4 inducer). Products include:
Atripla 906

Enalapril Maleate (Caution should be exercised when guanfacine is administered concomitantly with antihypertensive drugs, due to the potential for additive pharmacodynamic effects).
No products indexed under this heading.

Enalaprilat (Caution should be exercised when guanfacine is administered concomitantly with antihypertensive drugs, due to the potential for additive pharmacodynamic effects).
No products indexed under this heading.

Enflurane (Caution should be exercised when guanfacine is administered concomitantly with CNS depressant drugs (eg, alcohol, sedative/hypnotics, benzodiazepines, barbiturates, and antipsychotics) due to the potential for additive pharmacodynamic effects).
No products indexed under this heading.

Eprosartan Mesylate (Caution should be exercised when guanfacine is administered concomitantly with antihypertensive drugs, due to the potential for additive pharmacodynamic effects). Products include:
Teveten 538
Teveten HCT 541

Esmolol Hydrochloride (Caution should be exercised when guanfacine is administered concomitantly with antihypertensive drugs, due to the potential for additive pharmacodynamic effects).
No products indexed under this heading.

Estazolam (Caution should be exercised when guanfacine is administered concomitantly with benzodiazepines due to the potential for additive pharmacodynamic effects).
No products indexed under this heading.

Ethanol (Caution should be exercised when guanfacine is administered concomitantly with alcohol due to the potential for additive pharmacodynamic effects).
No products indexed under this heading.

Ethchlorvynol (Caution should be exercised when guanfacine is administered concomitantly with hypnotics and sedatives due to the potential for additive pharmacodynamic effects).
No products indexed under this heading.

Ethinamate (Caution should be exercised when guanfacine is administered concomitantly with hypnotics and sedatives due to the potential for additive pharmacodynamic effects).
No products indexed under this heading.

Ethosuximide (Significant decrease in the rate and extent of guanfacine exposure when co-administered with a CYP3A4 inducer).
No products indexed under this heading.

Ethyl Alcohol (Caution should be exercised when guanfacine is administered concomitantly with alcohol due to the potential for additive pharmacodynamic effects).
No products indexed under this heading.

Fat (High-fat meals increase exposure of guanfacine).
No products indexed under this heading.

Felbamate (Significant decrease in the rate and extent of guanfacine exposure when co-administered with a CYP3A4 inducer).
No products indexed under this heading.

Felodipine (Caution should be exercised when guanfacine is administered concomitantly with antihypertensive drugs, due to the potential for additive pharmacodynamic effects).
No products indexed under this heading.

Fentanyl (Caution should be exercised when guanfacine is administered concomitantly with CNS depressant drugs (eg, alcohol, sedative/hypnotics, benzodiazepines, barbiturates, and antipsychotics) due to the potential for additive pharmacodynamic effects). Products include:
Duragesic 2604
Fentanyl Transdermal System 2346
Onsolis 2054

Fentanyl Citrate (Caution should be exercised when guanfacine is administered concomitantly with CNS depressant drugs (eg, alcohol, sedative/hypnotics, benzodiazepines, barbiturates, and antipsychotics) due to the potential for additive pharmacodynamic effects). Products include:
Fentora 966

Fludrocortisone Acetate (Significant decrease in the rate and extent of guanfacine exposure when co-administered with a CYP3A4 inducer).
No products indexed under this heading.

Fluphenazine Decanoate (Caution should be exercised when guanfacine is administered concomitantly with antipsychotics due to the potential for additive pharmacodynamic effects).
No products indexed under this heading.

Fluphenazine Enanthate (Caution should be exercised when guanfacine is administered concomitantly with antipsychotics due to the potential for additive pharmacodynamic effects).
No products indexed under this heading.

Fluphenazine Hydrochloride (Caution should be exercised when guanfacine is administered concomitantly with antipsychotics due to the potential for additive pharmacodynamic effects).
No products indexed under this heading.

Flurazepam Hydrochloride (Caution should be exercised when guanfacine is administered concomitantly with benzodiazepines due to the potential for additive pharmacodynamic effects).
No products indexed under this heading.

Fosamprenavir Calcium (Caution should be exercised when guanfacine is administered to patients taking other strong CYP3A4 inhibitors, since elevation of plasma guanfacine concentration increases the risk of adverse events such as hypotension, bradycardia, and sedation). Products include:
Lexiva Oral Suspension 1558
Lexiva 1558

Fosinopril Sodium (Caution should be exercised when guanfacine is administered concomitantly with antihypertensive drugs, due to the potential for additive pharmacodynamic effects).
No products indexed under this heading.

Fosphenytoin Sodium (Significant decrease in the rate and extent of guanfacine exposure when co-administered with a CYP3A4 inducer).
No products indexed under this heading.

Furosemide (Caution should be exercised when guanfacine is administered concomitantly with antihypertensive drugs, due to the potential for additive pharmacodynamic effects). Products include:
Furosemide 2354

Garlic Extract (Significant decrease in the rate and extent of guanfacine exposure when co-administered with a CYP3A4 inducer).
No products indexed under this heading.

Garlic Oil (Significant decrease in the rate and extent of guanfacine exposure when co-administered with a CYP3A4 inducer).
No products indexed under this heading.

Glutethimide (Caution should be exercised when guanfacine is administered concomitantly with hypnotics and sedatives due to the potential for additive pharmacodynamic effects).
No products indexed under this heading.

Guanabenz Acetate (Caution should be exercised when guanfacine is administered concomitantly with antihypertensive drugs, due to the potential for additive pharmacodynamic effects).
No products indexed under this heading.

Guanethidine (Caution should be exercised when guanfacine is administered concomitantly with antihypertensive drugs, due to the potential for additive pharmacodynamic effects).
No products indexed under this heading.

Guanethidine Monosulfate (Caution should be exercised when guanfacine is administered concomitantly with antihypertensive drugs, due to the potential for additive pharmacodynamic effects).
No products indexed under this heading.

Guanethidine Sulfate (Caution should be exercised when guanfacine is administered concomitantly with antihypertensive drugs, due to the potential for additive pharmacodynamic effects).
No products indexed under this heading.

Halazepam (Caution should be exercised when guanfacine is administered concomitantly with benzodiazepines due to the potential for additive pharmacodynamic effects).
No products indexed under this heading.

Haloperidol (Caution should be exercised when guanfacine is administered concomitantly with antipsychotics due to the potential for additive pharmacodynamic effects).
No products indexed under this heading.

Haloperidol Decanoate (Caution should be exercised when guanfacine is administered concomitantly with antipsychotics due to the potential for additive pharmacodynamic effects).
No products indexed under this heading.

Haloperidol Lactate (Caution should be exercised when guanfacine is administered concomitantly with antipsychotics due to the potential for additive pharmacodynamic effects).
No products indexed under this heading.

Hexobarbital (Caution should be exercised when guanfacine is administered concomitantly with barbiturates due to the potential for additive pharmacodynamic effects).
No products indexed under this heading.

Hydralazine Hydrochloride (Caution should be exercised when guanfacine is administered concomitantly with antihypertensive drugs, due to the potential for additive pharmacodynamic effects).
No products indexed under this heading.

Hydrochlorothiazide (Caution should be exercised when guanfacine is administered concomitantly with antihypertensive drugs, due to the potential for additive pharmacodynamic effects). Products include:
Atacand HCT 700
Avalide 2956
Benicar HCT 1017
Diovan HCT 2419
Dyazide 1429
Exforge HCT 2449
Hyzaar 2162
Hyzaar 100-12.5 2162
Micardis HCT 889
Prinzide 2246
Tekturna HCT 2541
Teveten HCT 541

Hydrocodone Bitartrate (Caution should be exercised when guanfacine is administered concomitantly with CNS depressant drugs (eg, alcohol, sedative/hypnotics, benzodiazepines, barbiturates, and antipsychotics) due to the potential for additive pharmacodynamic effects). Products include:
Vicodin 560
Vicodin ES 561
Vicodin HP 563
Vicoprofen 564
Zydone 1138

Hydrocodone Polistirex (Caution should be exercised when guanfacine is administered concomitantly with CNS depressant drugs (eg, alcohol, sedative/hypnotics, benzodiazepines, barbiturates, and antipsychotics) due to the potential for additive pharmacodynamic effects). Products include:
Tussionex 3443

Hydrocortisone (Significant decrease in the rate and extent of guanfacine exposure when co-administered with a CYP3A4 inducer).
No products indexed under this heading.

Hydrocortisone (Alcohol) (Significant decrease in the rate and extent of guanfacine exposure when co-administered with a CYP3A4 inducer).
No products indexed under this heading.

Hydrocortisone Acetate (Significant decrease in the rate and extent of guanfacine exposure when co-administered with a CYP3A4 inducer).
No products indexed under this heading.

Hydrocortisone Butyrate (Significant decrease in the rate and extent of guanfacine exposure when co-administered with a CYP3A4 inducer).
No products indexed under this heading.

Hydrocortisone Cypionate (Significant decrease in the rate and extent of guanfacine exposure when co-administered with a CYP3A4 inducer).
No products indexed under this heading.

Hydrocortisone Hemisuccinate (Significant decrease in the rate and extent of guanfacine exposure when co-administered with a CYP3A4 inducer).
No products indexed under this heading.

Hydrocortisone Probutate (Significant decrease in the rate and extent of guanfacine exposure when co-administered with a CYP3A4 inducer).
No products indexed under this heading.

Hydrocortisone Sodium Phosphate (Significant decrease in the rate and extent of guanfacine exposure when co-administered with a CYP3A4 inducer).
No products indexed under this heading.

Hydrocortisone Sodium Succinate (Significant decrease in the rate and extent of guanfacine exposure when co-administered with a CYP3A4 inducer).
No products indexed under this heading.

Hydrocortisone Valerate (Significant decrease in the rate and extent of guanfacine exposure when co-administered with a CYP3A4 inducer).
No products indexed under this heading.

Hydroflumethiazide (Caution should be exercised when guanfacine is administered concomitantly with antihypertensive drugs, due to the potential for additive pharmacodynamic effects).
No products indexed under this heading.

Hydromorphone (Caution should be exercised when guanfacine is administered concomitantly with CNS depressant drugs (eg, alcohol, sedative/hypnotics, benzodiazepines, barbiturates, and antipsychotics) due to the potential for additive pharmacodynamic effects).
No products indexed under this heading.

IMPORTANT NOTE: Always consult each drug listing in the patient's regimen for possible interactions.

891 **Interactions Index** **Intuniv**

Molindone Hydrochloride (Caution should be exercised when guanfacine is administered concomitantly with antipsychotics due to the potential for additive pharmacodynamic effects). Products include:
Moban 1108

Morphine Sulfate (Caution should be exercised when guanfacine is administered concomitantly with CNS depressant drugs (eg, alcohol, sedative/hypnotics, benzodiazepines, barbiturates, and antipsychotics) due to the potential for additive pharmacodynamic effects). Products include:
Avinza 1822
Embeda 1831
MS Contin 2803

Morphine Sulfate, Liposomal (Caution should be exercised when guanfacine is administered concomitantly with CNS depressant drugs (eg, alcohol, sedative/hypnotics, benzodiazepines, barbiturates, and antipsychotics) due to the potential for additive pharmacodynamic effects).
No products indexed under this heading.

Nadolol (Caution should be exercised when guanfacine is administered concomitantly with antihypertensive drugs, due to the potential for additive pharmacodynamic effects). Products include:
Nadolol 2359

Nafcillin Sodium (Significant decrease in the rate and extent of guanfacine exposure when co-administered with a CYP3A4 inducer).
No products indexed under this heading.

Nebivolol (Caution should be exercised when guanfacine is administered concomitantly with antihypertensive drugs, due to the potential for additive pharmacodynamic effects). Products include:
Bystolic 1147

Nefazodone Hydrochloride (Caution should be exercised when guanfacine is administered to patients taking other strong CYP3A4 inhibitors, since elevation of plasma guanfacine concentration increases the risk of adverse events such as hypotension, bradycardia, and sedation).
No products indexed under this heading.

Nelfinavir Mesylate (Caution should be exercised when guanfacine is administered to patients taking other strong CYP3A4 inhibitors, since elevation of plasma guanfacine concentration increases the risk of adverse events such as hypotension, bradycardia, and sedation).
No products indexed under this heading.

Nevirapine (Significant decrease in the rate and extent of guanfacine exposure when co-administered with a CYP3A4 inducer). Products include:
Viramune Oral Suspension 897
Viramune Tablets 897

Nicardipine Hydrochloride (Caution should be exercised when guanfacine is administered concomitantly with antihypertensive drugs, due to the potential for additive pharmacodynamic effects).
No products indexed under this heading.

Nifedipine (Caution should be exercised when guanfacine is administered concomitantly with antihypertensive drugs, due to the potential for additive pharmacodynamic effects).
No products indexed under this heading.

Nisoldipine (Caution should be exercised when guanfacine is administered concomitantly with antihypertensive drugs, due to the potential for additive pharmacodynamic effects).
No products indexed under this heading.

Nitroglycerin (Caution should be exercised when guanfacine is administered concomitantly with antihypertensive drugs, due to the potential for additive pharmacodynamic effects). Products include:
Nitro-Dur 3170
Nitrolingual 3266

Olanzapine (Caution should be exercised when guanfacine is administered concomitantly with antipsychotics due to the potential for additive pharmacodynamic effects). Products include:
Symbyax 1965
Zyprexa 1984
Zyprexa IntraMuscular 1984
Zyprexa ZYDIS 1984

Oxazepam (Caution should be exercised when guanfacine is administered concomitantly with benzodiazepines due to the potential for additive pharmacodynamic effects).
No products indexed under this heading.

Oxcarbazepine (Significant decrease in the rate and extent of guanfacine exposure when co-administered with a CYP3A4 inducer).
No products indexed under this heading.

Oxycodone Hydrochloride (Caution should be exercised when guanfacine is administered concomitantly with CNS depressant drugs (eg, alcohol, sedative/hypnotics, benzodiazepines, barbiturates, and antipsychotics) due to the potential for additive pharmacodynamic effects). Products include:
OxyContin 2807
Percocet 1121
Percodan 1124

Oxycodone Terephthalate (Caution should be exercised when guanfacine is administered concomitantly with CNS depressant drugs (eg, alcohol, sedative/hypnotics, benzodiazepines, barbiturates, and antipsychotics) due to the potential for additive pharmacodynamic effects).
No products indexed under this heading.

Oxymorphone Hydrochloride (Caution should be exercised when guanfacine is administered concomitantly with CNS depressant drugs (eg, alcohol, sedative/hypnotics, benzodiazepines, barbiturates, and antipsychotics) due to the potential for additive pharmacodynamic effects). Products include:
Opana 1110
Opana ER 1114

Paliperidone (Caution should be exercised when guanfacine is administered concomitantly with antipsychotics due to the potential for additive pharmacodynamic effects). Products include:
Invega 2613
Invega Sustenna 2621

Penbutolol Sulfate (Caution should be exercised when guanfacine is administered concomitantly with antihypertensive drugs, due to the potential for additive pharmacodynamic effects).
No products indexed under this heading.

Pentobarbital (Caution should be exercised when guanfacine is administered concomitantly with barbiturates due to the potential for additive pharmacodynamic effects).
No products indexed under this heading.

Pentobarbital Sodium (Caution should be exercised when guanfacine is administered concomitantly with barbiturates due to the potential for additive pharmacodynamic effects). Products include:
Nembutal 2012

Perindopril Erbumine (Caution should be exercised when guanfacine is administered concomitantly with antihypertensive drugs, due to the potential for additive pharmacodynamic effects).
No products indexed under this heading.

Perphenazine (Caution should be exercised when guanfacine is administered concomitantly with antipsychotics due to the potential for additive pharmacodynamic effects).
No products indexed under this heading.

Phenobarbital (Caution should be exercised when guanfacine is administered concomitantly with barbiturates due to the potential for additive pharmacodynamic effects). Products include:
Donnatal 2711

Phenobarbital Sodium (Caution should be exercised when guanfacine is administered concomitantly with barbiturates due to the potential for additive pharmacodynamic effects).
No products indexed under this heading.

Phenoxybenzamine Hydrochloride (Caution should be exercised when guanfacine is administered concomitantly with antihypertensive drugs, due to the potential for additive pharmacodynamic effects). Products include:
Dibenzyline 3495

Phentolamine Mesylate (Caution should be exercised when guanfacine is administered concomitantly with antihypertensive drugs, due to the potential for additive pharmacodynamic effects).
No products indexed under this heading.

Phenytoin (Significant decrease in the rate and extent of guanfacine exposure when co-administered with a CYP3A4 inducer).
No products indexed under this heading.

Phenytoin Sodium (Significant decrease in the rate and extent of guanfacine exposure when co-administered with a CYP3A4 inducer). Products include:
Phenytek Capsules 2380

Pimozide (Caution should be exercised when guanfacine is administered concomitantly with antipsychotics due to the potential for additive pharmacodynamic effects).
No products indexed under this heading.

Pindolol (Caution should be exercised when guanfacine is administered concomitantly with antihypertensive drugs, due to the potential for additive pharmacodynamic effects).
No products indexed under this heading.

Polythiazide (Caution should be exercised when guanfacine is administered concomitantly with antihypertensive drugs, due to the potential for additive pharmacodynamic effects).
No products indexed under this heading.

Prazepam (Caution should be exercised when guanfacine is administered concomitantly with benzodiazepines due to the potential for additive pharmacodynamic effects).
No products indexed under this heading.

Prazosin Hydrochloride (Caution should be exercised when guanfacine is administered concomitantly with antihypertensive drugs, due to the potential for additive pharmacodynamic effects).
No products indexed under this heading.

Prednisolone (Significant decrease in the rate and extent of guanfacine exposure when co-administered with a CYP3A4 inducer).
No products indexed under this heading.

Prednisolone Acetate (Significant decrease in the rate and extent of guanfacine exposure when co-administered with a CYP3A4 inducer). Products include:
Blephamide .... ⊙212, ⊙214
Pred Forte .... ⊙225
Pred Mild .... ⊙230
Pred-G .... ⊙226, ⊙227

Prednisolone Sodium Phosphate (Significant decrease in the rate and extent of guanfacine exposure when co-administered with a CYP3A4 inducer).
No products indexed under this heading.

Prednisolone Tebutate (Significant decrease in the rate and extent of guanfacine exposure when co-administered with a CYP3A4 inducer).
No products indexed under this heading.

Prednisone (Significant decrease in the rate and extent of guanfacine exposure when co-administered with a CYP3A4 inducer).
No products indexed under this heading.

Prednisone sodium phosphate (Significant decrease in the rate and extent of guanfacine exposure when co-administered with a CYP3A4 inducer).
No products indexed under this heading.

Primidone (Significant decrease in the rate and extent of guanfacine exposure when co-administered with a CYP3A4 inducer).
No products indexed under this heading.

Prochlorperazine (Caution should be exercised when guanfacine is administered concomitantly with antipsychotics due to the potential for additive pharmacodynamic effects).
No products indexed under this heading.

Prochlorperazine Edisylate (Caution should be exercised when guanfacine is administered concomitantly with CNS depressant drugs (eg, alcohol, sedative/hypnotics, benzodiazepines, barbiturates, and antipsychotics) due to the potential for additive pharmacodynamic effects).
No products indexed under this heading.

Prochlorperazine Maleate (Caution should be exercised when guanfacine is administered concomitantly with CNS depressant drugs (eg, alcohol, sedative/hypnotics, benzodiazepines, barbiturates, and antipsychotics) due to the potential for additive pharmacodynamic effects).
No products indexed under this heading.

Promethazine (Caution should be exercised when guanfacine is administered concomitantly with CNS depressant drugs (eg, alcohol, sedative/hypnotics, benzodiazepines, barbiturates, and antipsychotics) due to the potential for additive pharmacodynamic effects).
No products indexed under this heading.

Promethazine Hydrochloride (Caution should be exercised when guanfacine is administered concomitantly with CNS depressant drugs (eg, alcohol, sedative/hypnotics, benzodiazepines, barbiturates, and antipsychotics) due to the potential for additive pharmacodynamic effects).
No products indexed under this heading.

Propofol (Caution should be exercised when guanfacine is administered concomitantly with hypnotics and sedatives due to the potential for additive pharmacodynamic effects).
No products indexed under this heading.

Propoxyphene Hydrochloride (Caution should be exercised when guanfacine is administered concomitantly with CNS depressant drugs (eg, alcohol, sedative/hypnotics, benzodiazepines, barbiturates, and antipsychotics) due to the potential for additive pharmacodynamic effects).
No products indexed under this heading.

IMPORTANT NOTE: Always consult each drug listing in the patient's regimen for possible interactions.

Propoxyphene Napsylate (Caution should be exercised when guanfacine is administered concomitantly with CNS depressant drugs (eg, alcohol, sedative/hypnotics, benzodiazepines, barbiturates, and antipsychotics) due to the potential for additive pharmacodynamic effects).
No products indexed under this heading.

Propranolol Hydrochloride (Caution should be exercised when guanfacine is administered concomitantly with antihypertensive drugs, due to the potential for additive pharmacodynamic effects). Products include:
InnoPran XL 1517

Quazepam (Caution should be exercised when guanfacine is administered concomitantly with benzodiazepines due to the potential for additive pharmacodynamic effects).
No products indexed under this heading.

Quetiapine Fumarate (Caution should be exercised when guanfacine is administered concomitantly with antipsychotics due to the potential for additive pharmacodynamic effects). Products include:
Seroquel 750
Seroquel XR 759

Quinapril Hydrochloride (Caution should be exercised when guanfacine is administered concomitantly with antihypertensive drugs, due to the potential for additive pharmacodynamic effects).
No products indexed under this heading.

Ramelteon (Caution should be exercised when guanfacine is administered concomitantly with hypnotics and sedatives due to the potential for additive pharmacodynamic effects). Products include:
Rozerem 3366

Ramipril (Caution should be exercised when guanfacine is administered concomitantly with antihypertensive drugs, due to the potential for additive pharmacodynamic effects).
No products indexed under this heading.

Rauwolfia Serpentina (Caution should be exercised when guanfacine is administered concomitantly with antihypertensive drugs, due to the potential for additive pharmacodynamic effects).
No products indexed under this heading.

Remifentanil Hydrochloride (Caution should be exercised when guanfacine is administered concomitantly with CNS depressant drugs (eg, alcohol, sedative/hypnotics, benzodiazepines, barbiturates, and antipsychotics) due to the potential for additive pharmacodynamic effects).
No products indexed under this heading.

Rescinnamine (Caution should be exercised when guanfacine is administered concomitantly with antihypertensive drugs, due to the potential for additive pharmacodynamic effects).
No products indexed under this heading.

Reserpine (Caution should be exercised when guanfacine is administered concomitantly with antihypertensive drugs, due to the potential for additive pharmacodynamic effects).
No products indexed under this heading.

Rifabutin (Significant decrease in the rate and extent of guanfacine exposure when co-administered with a CYP3A4 inducer).
No products indexed under this heading.

Rifampicin (Significant decrease in the rate and extent of guanfacine exposure when co-administered with a CYP3A4 inducer).
No products indexed under this heading.

Rifampin (Significant decrease in the rate and extent of guanfacine exposure when co-administered with rifampin, A CYP3A4 inducer. The exposure to guanfacine decreased by 70% (AUC)).
No products indexed under this heading.

Rifapentine (Significant decrease in the rate and extent of guanfacine exposure when co-administered with a CYP3A4 inducer).
No products indexed under this heading.

Risperidone (Caution should be exercised when guanfacine is administered concomitantly with antipsychotics due to the potential for additive pharmacodynamic effects). Products include:
Risperdal Consta 2682

Ritonavir (Caution should be exercised when guanfacine is administered to patients taking other strong CYP3A4 inhibitors, since elevation of plasma guanfacine concentration increases the risk of adverse events such as hypotension, bradycardia, and sedation). Products include:
Kaletra 458
Norvir 509

Saquinavir (Caution should be exercised when guanfacine is administered to patients taking other strong CYP3A4 inhibitors, since elevation of plasma guanfacine concentration increases the risk of adverse events such as hypotension, bradycardia, and sedation).
No products indexed under this heading.

Saquinavir Mesylate (Caution should be exercised when guanfacine is administered to patients taking other strong CYP3A4 inhibitors, since elevation of plasma guanfacine concentration increases the risk of adverse events such as hypotension, bradycardia, and sedation).
No products indexed under this heading.

Secobarbital Sodium (Caution should be exercised when guanfacine is administered concomitantly with barbiturates due to the potential for additive pharmacodynamic effects).
No products indexed under this heading.

Sevoflurane (Caution should be exercised when guanfacine is administered concomitantly with CNS depressant drugs (eg, alcohol, sedative/hypnotics, benzodiazepines, barbiturates, and antipsychotics) due to the potential for additive pharmacodynamic effects). Products include:
Ultane 554

Sodium Butabarbital (Caution should be exercised when guanfacine is administered concomitantly with barbiturates due to the potential for additive pharmacodynamic effects).
No products indexed under this heading.

Sodium Nitroprusside (Caution should be exercised when guanfacine is administered concomitantly with antihypertensive drugs, due to the potential for additive pharmacodynamic effects).
No products indexed under this heading.

Sodium Oxybate (Caution should be exercised when guanfacine is administered concomitantly with CNS depressant drugs (eg, alcohol, sedative/hypnotics, benzodiazepines, barbiturates, and antipsychotics) due to the potential for additive pharmacodynamic effects).
No products indexed under this heading.

Sodium Pentobarbital (Caution should be exercised when guanfacine is administered concomitantly with barbiturates due to the potential for additive pharmacodynamic effects).
No products indexed under this heading.

Sotalol Hydrochloride (Caution should be exercised when guanfacine is administered concomitantly with antihypertensive drugs, due to the potential for additive pharmacodynamic effects).
No products indexed under this heading.

Spirapril Hydrochloride (Caution should be exercised when guanfacine is administered concomitantly with antihypertensive drugs, due to the potential for additive pharmacodynamic effects).
No products indexed under this heading.

Sufentanil Citrate (Caution should be exercised when guanfacine is administered concomitantly with CNS depressant drugs (eg, alcohol, sedative/hypnotics, benzodiazepines, barbiturates, and antipsychotics) due to the potential for additive pharmacodynamic effects).
No products indexed under this heading.

Sulfinpyrazone (Significant decrease in the rate and extent of guanfacine exposure when co-administered with a CYP3A4 inducer).
No products indexed under this heading.

Talbutal (Caution should be exercised when guanfacine is administered concomitantly with CNS depressant drugs (eg, alcohol, sedative/hypnotics, benzodiazepines, barbiturates, and antipsychotics) due to the potential for additive pharmacodynamic effects).
No products indexed under this heading.

Telithromycin (Caution should be exercised when guanfacine is administered to patients taking other strong CYP3A4 inhibitors, since elevation of plasma guanfacine concentration increases the risk of adverse events such as hypotension, bradycardia, and sedation). Products include:
Ketek 2991

Telmisartan (Caution should be exercised when guanfacine is administered concomitantly with antihypertensive drugs, due to the potential for additive pharmacodynamic effects). Products include:
Micardis 887
Micardis HCT 889

Temazepam (Caution should be exercised when guanfacine is administered concomitantly with benzodiazepines due to the potential for additive pharmacodynamic effects).
No products indexed under this heading.

Terazosin Hydrochloride (Caution should be exercised when guanfacine is administered concomitantly with antihypertensive drugs, due to the potential for additive pharmacodynamic effects).
No products indexed under this heading.

Theophyllinate (Significant decrease in the rate and extent of guanfacine exposure when co-administered with a CYP3A4 inducer).
No products indexed under this heading.

Theophylline (Significant decrease in the rate and extent of guanfacine exposure when co-administered with a CYP3A4 inducer).
No products indexed under this heading.

Theophylline Anhydrous (Significant decrease in the rate and extent of guanfacine exposure when co-administered with a CYP3A4 inducer). Products include:
Uniphyl 2817

Theophylline Calcium Salicylate (Significant decrease in the rate and extent of guanfacine exposure when co-administered with a CYP3A4 inducer).
No products indexed under this heading.

Theophylline Dihydroxypropyl (Glyceryl) (Significant decrease in the rate and extent of guanfacine exposure when co-administered with a CYP3A4 inducer).
No products indexed under this heading.

Theophylline Ethylenediamine (Significant decrease in the rate and extent of guanfacine exposure when co-administered with a CYP3A4 inducer).
No products indexed under this heading.

Theophylline Sodium Glycinate (Significant decrease in the rate and extent of guanfacine exposure when co-administered with a CYP3A4 inducer).
No products indexed under this heading.

Thiamylal Sodium (Caution should be exercised when guanfacine is administered concomitantly with barbiturates due to the potential for additive pharmacodynamic effects).
No products indexed under this heading.

Thioridazine (Caution should be exercised when guanfacine is administered concomitantly with CNS depressant drugs (eg, alcohol, sedative/hypnotics, benzodiazepines, barbiturates, and antipsychotics) due to the potential for additive pharmacodynamic effects).
No products indexed under this heading.

Thioridazine Hydrochloride (Caution should be exercised when guanfacine is administered concomitantly with antipsychotics due to the potential for additive pharmacodynamic effects). Products include:
Thioridazine Hydrochloride 2384

Thiothixene (Caution should be exercised when guanfacine is administered concomitantly with antipsychotics due to the potential for additive pharmacodynamic effects). Products include:
Thiothixene 2386

Thiothixene Hydrochloride (Caution should be exercised when guanfacine is administered concomitantly with CNS depressant drugs (eg, alcohol, sedative/hypnotics, benzodiazepines, barbiturates, and antipsychotics) due to the potential for additive pharmacodynamic effects).
No products indexed under this heading.

Timolol Maleate (Caution should be exercised when guanfacine is administered concomitantly with antihypertensive drugs, due to the potential for additive pharmacodynamic effects). Products include:
Combigan 601
Dorzolamide Hydrochloride/Timolol Maleate Ophthalmic Solution .... ⊙ 243
Timoptic in Ocudose .... ⊙ 231

Torsemide (Caution should be exercised when guanfacine is administered concomitantly with antihypertensive drugs, due to the potential for additive pharmacodynamic effects).
No products indexed under this heading.

Trandolapril (Caution should be exercised when guanfacine is administered concomitantly with antihypertensive drugs, due to the potential for additive pharmacodynamic effects). Products include:
Mavik 489
Tarka 534

Triamcinolone (Significant decrease in the rate and extent of guanfacine exposure when co-administered with a CYP3A4 inducer).
No products indexed under this heading.

Triamcinolone Acetonide (Significant decrease in the rate and extent of guanfacine exposure when co-administered with a CYP3A4 inducer). Products include:
Azmacort 408
Nasacort AQ 3019

Triamcinolone Diacetate (Significant decrease in the rate and extent of guanfacine exposure when co-administered with a CYP3A4 inducer).
No products indexed under this heading.

(⊙ Described in PDR® for Ophthalmic Medicines)

Triamcinolone Hexacetonide (Significant decrease in the rate and extent of guanfacine exposure when co-administered with a CYP3A4 inducer).
No products indexed under this heading.

Triazolam (Caution should be exercised when guanfacine is administered concomitantly with benzodiazepines due to the potential for additive pharmacodynamic effects).
No products indexed under this heading.

Trifluoperazine Hydrochloride (Caution should be exercised when guanfacine is administered concomitantly with antipsychotics due to the potential for additive pharmacodynamic effects).
No products indexed under this heading.

Trimethaphan Camsylate (Caution should be exercised when guanfacine is administered concomitantly with antihypertensive drugs, due to the potential for additive pharmacodynamic effects).
No products indexed under this heading.

Troglitazone (Significant decrease in the rate and extent of guanfacine exposure when co-administered with a CYP3A4 inducer).
No products indexed under this heading.

Troleandomycin (Caution should be exercised when guanfacine is administered to patients taking other strong CYP3A4 inhibitors, since elevation of plasma guanfacine concentration increases the risk of adverse events such as hypotension, bradycardia, and sedation).
No products indexed under this heading.

Valproate Sodium (Co-administration of guanfacine and valproic acid may result in increased concentrations of valproic acid; adjustments in the dose of valproic acid may be indicated).
No products indexed under this heading.

Valproic Acid (Co-administration of guanfacine and valproic acid may result in increased concentrations of valproic acid; adjustments in the dose of valproic acid may be indicated).
No products indexed under this heading.

Valsartan (Caution should be exercised when guanfacine is administered concomitantly with antihypertensive drugs, due to the potential for additive pharmacodynamic effects). Products include:
Diovan **2413**
Diovan HCT **2419**
Exforge **2443**
Exforge HCT **2449**
Valturna **3637**

Verapamil Hydrochloride (Caution should be exercised when guanfacine is administered concomitantly with antihypertensive drugs, due to the potential for additive pharmacodynamic effects). Products include:
Tarka **534**

Voriconazole (Caution should be exercised when guanfacine is administered to patients taking other strong CYP3A4 inhibitors, since elevation of plasma guanfacine concentration increases the risk of adverse events such as hypotension, bradycardia, and sedation).
No products indexed under this heading.

Zaleplon (Caution should be exercised when guanfacine is administered concomitantly with hypnotics and sedatives due to the potential for additive pharmacodynamic effects).
No products indexed under this heading.

Ziprasidone Hydrochloride (Caution should be exercised when guanfacine is administered concomitantly with antipsychotics due to the potential for additive pharmacodynamic effects). Products include:
Geodon **2723**

Zolpidem Tartrate (Caution should be exercised when guanfacine is administered concomitantly with hypnotics and sedatives due to the potential for additive pharmacodynamic effects). Products include:
Ambien **2920**
Ambien CR **2925**

Food Interactions

Alcohol (Caution should be exercised when guanfacine is administered concomitantly with alcohol due to the potential for additive pharmacodynamic effects).

Beer, reduced-alcohol (Caution should be exercised when guanfacine is administered concomitantly with alcohol due to the potential for additive pharmacodynamic effects).

Beer, unspecified (Caution should be exercised when guanfacine is administered concomitantly with alcohol due to the potential for additive pharmacodynamic effects).

Food, unspecified (High-fat meals increase exposure of guanfacine).

Meal, unspecified (High-fat meals increase exposure of guanfacine).

Wine, Chianti (Caution should be exercised when guanfacine is administered concomitantly with alcohol due to the potential for additive pharmacodynamic effects).

Wine, Red (Caution should be exercised when guanfacine is administered concomitantly with alcohol due to the potential for additive pharmacodynamic effects).

Wine, unspecified (Caution should be exercised when guanfacine is administered concomitantly with alcohol due to the potential for additive pharmacodynamic effects).

Wine products (Caution should be exercised when guanfacine is administered concomitantly with alcohol due to the potential for additive pharmacodynamic effects).

INVANZ FOR INJECTION

(Ertapenem) **2172**
May interact with valproate, and certain other agents. Compounds in these categories include:

Divalproex Sodium (Carbapenems, including ertapenem, may reduce serum valproic acid concentrations to subtherapeutic levels, resulting in loss of seizure control. Serum valproic acid concentrations should be monitored frequently after initiating carbapenem therapy. Alternative antibacterial or anticonvulsant therapy should be considered if serum valproic acid concentrations drop below the therapeutic range or seizure occurs). Products include:
Depakote ER **426**

Probenecid (When ertapenem is co-administered with probenecid (500 mg p.o. every 6 hours), probenecid competes for active tubular secretion and reduces the renal clearance of ertapenem. Based on total ertapenem concentrations, probenecid increased the AUC by 25% and reduced the plasma and renal clearances by 20% and 35%, respectively. The half-life increased from 4.0 to 4.8 hours. Because of the small effect on half-life, the co-administration with probenecid to extend the half-life of ertapenem is not recommended).
No products indexed under this heading.

Valproate Sodium (Carbapenems, including ertapenem, may reduce serum valproic acid concentrations to subtherapeutic levels, resulting in loss of seizure control. Serum valproic acid concentrations should be monitored frequently after initiating carbapenem therapy. Alternative antibacterial or anticonvulsant therapy should be considered if serum valproic acid concentrations drop below the therapeutic range or seizure occurs).
No products indexed under this heading.

Valproic Acid (Carbapenems, including ertapenem, may reduce serum valproic acid concentrations to subtherapeutic levels, resulting in loss of seizure control. Serum valproic acid concentrations should be monitored frequently after initiating carbapenem therapy. Alternative antibacterial or anticonvulsant therapy should be considered if serum valproic acid concentrations drop below the therapeutic range or seizure occurs).
No products indexed under this heading.

INVEGA EXTENDED-RELEASE TABLETS

(Paliperidone) **2613**
May interact with alcohols, alpha adrenergic blockers, alpha adrenergic stimulants, antibiotics, antihypertensives, antipsychotic agents, centrally-acting drugs, class 1A antiarrhythmics, class III antiarrhythmics, cytochrome p450 2d6 inhibitors (selected), dopamine agonists, drugs that prolong the QT interval, monoamine oxidase inhibitors, quinidine, tricyclic antidepressants, and certain other agents. Compounds in these categories include:

Acebutolol Hydrochloride (Because of its potential for inducing orthostatic hypotension, an additive effect may be observed when paliperidone is administered with other therapeutic agents that have this potential).
No products indexed under this heading.

Alatrofloxacin Mesylate (Paliperidone causes a modest increase in the corrected QT (QTc) interval. The use of paliperidone should be avoided in combination with other drugs that are known to prolong QTc including antibiotics (eg, gatifloxacin, moxifloxacin), or any other class of medications known to prolong the QTc interval. Paliperidone should also be avoided in patients with congenital long QT syndrome and in patients with a history of cardiac arrhythmias).
No products indexed under this heading.

Alfentanil Hydrochloride (Given the primary CNS effects of paliperidone, paliperidone should be used with caution in combination with other centrally acting drugs and alcohol).
No products indexed under this heading.

Alfuzosin Hydrochloride (Because of its potential for inducing orthostatic hypotension, an additive effect may be observed when paliperidone is administered with other therapeutic agents that have this potential). Products include:
Uroxatral **3050**

Aliskiren (Because of its potential for inducing orthostatic hypotension, an additive effect may be observed when paliperidone is administered with other therapeutic agents that have this potential). Products include:
Tekturna **2538**
Tekturna HCT **2541**
Valturna **3637**

Alprazolam (Paliperidone causes a modest increase in the corrected QT (QTc) interval. The use of paliperidone should be avoided in combination with other drugs that are known to prolong QTc including Class 1A (eg, quinidine, procainamide) or Class III (eg, amiodarone, sotalol) antiarrhythmic medications, antipsychotic medications (eg, chlorpromazine, thioridazine), antibiotics (eg, gatifloxacin, moxifloxacin), or any other class of medications known to prolong the QTc interval. Paliperidone should also be avoided in patients with congenital long QT syndrome and in patients with a history of cardiac arrhythmias).
No products indexed under this heading.

Amikacin Sulfate (Paliperidone causes a modest increase in the corrected QT (QTc) interval. The use of paliperidone should be avoided in combination with other drugs that are known to prolong QTc including antibiotics (eg, gatifloxacin, moxifloxacin), or any other class of medications known to prolong the QTc interval. Paliperidone should also be avoided in patients with congenital long QT syndrome and in patients with a history of cardiac arrhythmias).
No products indexed under this heading.

Amiodarone Hydrochloride (Paliperidone causes a modest increase in the corrected QT (QTc) interval. The use of paliperidone should be avoided in combination with other drugs that are known to prolong QTc including Class III (eg, amiodarone, sotalol) antiarrhythmic medications, or any other class of medications known to prolong the QTc interval. Paliperidone should also be avoided in patients with congenital long QT syndrome and in patients with a history of cardiac arrhythmias).
No products indexed under this heading.

Amitriptyline Hydrochloride (Paliperidone causes a modest increase in the corrected QT (QTc) interval. The use of paliperidone should be avoided in combination with other drugs that are known to prolong QTc including Class 1A (eg, quinidine, procainamide) or Class III (eg, amiodarone, sotalol) antiarrhythmic medications, antipsychotic medications (eg, chlorpromazine, thioridazine), antibiotics (eg, gatifloxacin, moxifloxacin), or any other class of medications known to prolong the QTc interval. Paliperidone should also be avoided in patients with congenital long QT syndrome and in patients with a history of cardiac arrhythmias).
No products indexed under this heading.

Amlodipine Besylate (Because of its potential for inducing orthostatic hypotension, an additive effect may be observed when paliperidone is administered with other therapeutic agents that have this potential). Products include:
Azor **1010**
Exforge **2443**
Exforge HCT **2449**

Amoxapine (Paliperidone causes a modest increase in the corrected QT (QTc) interval. The use of paliperidone should be avoided in combination with other drugs that are known to prolong QTc including Class 1A (eg, quinidine, procainamide) or Class III (eg, amiodarone, sotalol) antiarrhythmic medications, antipsychotic medications (eg, chlorpromazine, thioridazine), antibiotics (eg, gatifloxacin, moxifloxacin), or any other class of medications known to prolong the QTc interval. Paliperidone should also be avoided in patients with congenital long QT syndrome and in patients with a history of cardiac arrhythmias).
No products indexed under this heading.

Amoxicillin (Paliperidone causes a modest increase in the corrected QT (QTc) interval. The use of paliperidone should be avoided in combination with other drugs that are known to prolong QTc including antibiotics (eg, gatifloxacin, moxifloxacin), or any other class of medications known to prolong the QTc interval. Paliperidone should also be avoided in patients with congenital long QT syndrome and in patients with a history of cardiac arrhythmias). Products include:
Amoxil Capsules **1311**
Amoxil Chewable Tablets **1311**
Amoxil **1311**

Amoxicillin Trihydrate (Paliperidone causes a modest increase in the corrected QT (QTc) interval. The use of paliperidone should be avoided in combination with other drugs that are known to prolong QTc including antibiotics (eg, gatifloxacin, moxifloxacin), or any other class of medications known to prolong the QTc interval. Paliperidone should also be avoided in patients with congenital long QT syndrome and in patients with a history of cardiac arrhythmias).

No products indexed under this heading.

Amphetamine Aspartate (Given the primary CNS effects of paliperidone, paliperidone should be used with caution in combination with other centrally acting drugs and alcohol).

No products indexed under this heading.

Amphetamine Aspartate Monohydrate (Given the primary CNS effects of paliperidone, paliperidone should be used with caution in combination with other centrally acting drugs and alcohol).

No products indexed under this heading.

Amphetamine Resins (Given the primary CNS effects of paliperidone, paliperidone should be used with caution in combination with other centrally acting drugs and alcohol).

No products indexed under this heading.

Amphetamine Sulfate (Given the primary CNS effects of paliperidone, paliperidone should be used with caution in combination with other centrally acting drugs and alcohol).

No products indexed under this heading.

Ampicillin (Paliperidone causes a modest increase in the corrected QT (QTc) interval. The use of paliperidone should be avoided in combination with other drugs that are known to prolong QTc including antibiotics (eg, gatifloxacin, moxifloxacin), or any other class of medications known to prolong the QTc interval. Paliperidone should also be avoided in patients with congenital long QT syndrome and in patients with a history of cardiac arrhythmias).

No products indexed under this heading.

Ampicillin Sodium (Paliperidone causes a modest increase in the corrected QT (QTc) interval. The use of paliperidone should be avoided in combination with other drugs that are known to prolong QTc including antibiotics (eg, gatifloxacin, moxifloxacin), or any other class of medications known to prolong the QTc interval. Paliperidone should also be avoided in patients with congenital long QT syndrome and in patients with a history of cardiac arrhythmias).

No products indexed under this heading.

Ampicillin Trihydrate (Paliperidone causes a modest increase in the corrected QT (QTc) interval. The use of paliperidone should be avoided in combination with other drugs that are known to prolong QTc including antibiotics (eg, gatifloxacin, moxifloxacin), or any other class of medications known to prolong the QTc interval. Paliperidone should also be avoided in patients with congenital long QT syndrome and in patients with a history of cardiac arrhythmias).

No products indexed under this heading.

Antibiotics, non-penicillin, unspecified (Paliperidone causes a modest increase in the corrected QT (QTc) interval. The use of paliperidone should be avoided in combination with other drugs that are known to prolong QTc including antibiotics (eg, gatifloxacin, moxifloxacin), or any other class of

medications known to prolong the QTc interval. Paliperidone should also be avoided in patients with congenital long QT syndrome and in patients with a history of cardiac arrhythmias).

No products indexed under this heading.

Apraclonidine Hydrochloride (Because of its potential for inducing orthostatic hypotension, an additive effect may be observed when paliperidone is administered with other therapeutic agents that have this potential).

No products indexed under this heading.

Aprobarbital (Given the primary CNS effects of paliperidone, paliperidone should be used with caution in combination with other centrally acting drugs and alcohol).

No products indexed under this heading.

Aripiprazole (Paliperidone causes a modest increase in the corrected QT (QTc) interval. The use of paliperidone should be avoided in combination with other drugs that are known to prolong QTc including antipsychotic medications (eg, chlorpromazine, thioridazine) or any other class of medications known to prolong the QTc interval. Paliperidone should also be avoided in patients with congenital long QT syndrome and in patients with a history of cardiac arrhythmias).

No products indexed under this heading.

Astemizole (Paliperidone causes a modest increase in the corrected QT (QTc) interval. The use of paliperidone should be avoided in combination with other drugs that are known to prolong QTc including Class 1A (eg, quinidine, procainamide) or Class III (eg, amiodarone, sotalol) antiarrhythmic medications, antipsychotic medications (eg, chlorpromazine, thioridazine), antibiotics (eg, gatifloxacin, moxifloxacin), or any other class of medications known to prolong the QTc interval. Paliperidone should also be avoided in patients with congenital long QT syndrome and in patients with a history of cardiac arrhythmias).

No products indexed under this heading.

Atenolol (Because of its potential for inducing orthostatic hypotension, an additive effect may be observed when paliperidone is administered with other therapeutic agents that have this potential).

No products indexed under this heading.

Azithromycin Dihydrate (Paliperidone causes a modest increase in the corrected QT (QTc) interval. The use of paliperidone should be avoided in combination with other drugs that are known to prolong QTc including antibiotics (eg, gatifloxacin, moxifloxacin), or any other class of medications known to prolong the QTc interval. Paliperidone should also be avoided in patients with congenital long QT syndrome and in patients with a history of cardiac arrhythmias).

No products indexed under this heading.

Azlocillin Sodium (Paliperidone causes a modest increase in the corrected QT (QTc) interval. The use of paliperidone should be avoided in combination with other drugs that are known to prolong QTc including antibiotics (eg, gatifloxacin, moxifloxacin), or any other class of medications known to prolong the QTc interval. Paliperidone should also be avoided in patients with congenital long QT syndrome and in patients with a history of cardiac arrhythmias).

No products indexed under this heading.

Aztreonam (Paliperidone causes a modest increase in the corrected QT (QTc) interval. The use of paliperidone should be avoided in combination with other drugs that are known to prolong QTc including antibiotics (eg, gatifloxacin, moxifloxacin), or any other class of medications known to prolong the QTc

interval. Paliperidone should also be avoided in patients with congenital long QT syndrome and in patients with a history of cardiac arrhythmias).

No products indexed under this heading.

Bacampicillin Hydrochloride (Paliperidone causes a modest increase in the corrected QT (QTc) interval. The use of paliperidone should be avoided in combination with other drugs that are known to prolong QTc including antibiotics (eg, gatifloxacin, moxifloxacin), or any other class of medications known to prolong the QTc interval. Paliperidone should also be avoided in patients with congenital long QT syndrome and in patients with a history of cardiac arrhythmias).

No products indexed under this heading.

Benazepril Hydrochloride (Because of its potential for inducing orthostatic hypotension, an additive effect may be observed when paliperidone is administered with other therapeutic agents that have this potential).

No products indexed under this heading.

Bendroflumethiazide (Because of its potential for inducing orthostatic hypotension, an additive effect may be observed when paliperidone is administered with other therapeutic agents that have this potential).

No products indexed under this heading.

Betaxolol Hydrochloride (Because of its potential for inducing orthostatic hypotension, an additive effect may be observed when paliperidone is administered with other therapeutic agents that have this potential).

No products indexed under this heading.

Bisoprolol Fumarate (Because of its potential for inducing orthostatic hypotension, an additive effect may be observed when paliperidone is administered with other therapeutic agents that have this potential).

No products indexed under this heading.

Bretylium Tosylate (Paliperidone causes a modest increase in the corrected QT (QTc) interval. The use of paliperidone should be avoided in combination with other drugs that are known to prolong QTc including Class 1A (eg, quinidine, procainamide) or Class III (eg, amiodarone, sotalol) antiarrhythmic medications, antipsychotic medications (eg, chlorpromazine, thioridazine), antibiotics (eg, gatifloxacin, moxifloxacin), or any other class of medications known to prolong the QTc interval. Paliperidone should also be avoided in patients with congenital long QT syndrome and in patients with a history of cardiac arrhythmias).

No products indexed under this heading.

Bromocriptine Mesylate (Given the primary CNS effects of paliperidone, paliperidone should be used with caution in combination with other centrally acting drugs and alcohol. Paliperidone may antagonize the effect of levodopa and other dopamine agonists).

No products indexed under this heading.

Buprenorphine Hydrochloride (Given the primary CNS effects of paliperidone, paliperidone should be used with caution in combination with other centrally acting drugs and alcohol).

No products indexed under this heading.

Bupropion Hydrochloride (Paliperidone is metabolized to a limited extent by CYP2D6. In an interaction study in healthy subjects in which a single 3 mg dose of paliperidone was administered concomitantly with 20 mg per day of paroxetine (a potent CYP2D6 inhibitor), paliperidone exposures were on average 16% (90% CI: 4, 30) higher in CYP2D6 extensive metabolizers. Higher doses of paroxetine have not been studied. The clinical relevance is unknown). Products include:

Buspirone Hydrochloride (Paliperidone causes a modest increase in the corrected QT (QTc) interval. The use of paliperidone should be avoided in combination with other drugs that are known to prolong QTc including Class 1A (eg, quinidine, procainamide) or Class III (eg, amiodarone, sotalol) antiarrhythmic medications, antipsychotic medications (eg, chlorpromazine, thioridazine), antibiotics (eg, gatifloxacin, moxifloxacin), or any other class of medications known to prolong the QTc interval. Paliperidone should also be avoided in patients with congenital long QT syndrome and in patients with a history of cardiac arrhythmias).

No products indexed under this heading.

Butabarbital (Given the primary CNS effects of paliperidone, paliperidone should be used with caution in combination with other centrally acting drugs and alcohol).

No products indexed under this heading.

Butalbital (Given the primary CNS effects of paliperidone, paliperidone should be used with caution in combination with other centrally acting drugs and alcohol).

No products indexed under this heading.

Candesartan Cilexetil (Because of its potential for inducing orthostatic hypotension, an additive effect may be observed when paliperidone is administered with other therapeutic agents that have this potential). Products include:

Cannabis sativa (Because of its potential for inducing orthostatic hypotension, an additive effect may be observed when paliperidone is administered with other therapeutic agents that have this potential).

No products indexed under this heading.

Captopril (Because of its potential for inducing orthostatic hypotension, an additive effect may be observed when paliperidone is administered with other therapeutic agents that have this potential). Products include:

Carbamazepine (Co-administration of paliperidone 6 mg once daily with carbamazepine 200 mg twice daily caused a decrease of approximately 37% in the mean steady-state C_{max} and AUC of paliperidone. This decrease is caused, to a substantial degree, by a 35% increase in renal clearance of paliperidone. A minor decrease in the amount of drug excreted unchanged in the urine suggests that there was little effect on the CYP metabolism or bioavailability of paliperidone during carbamazepine co-administration. On initiation of carbamazepine, the dose of paliperidone should be re-evaluated and increased if necessary. Conversely, on discontinuation of carbamazepine, the dose of paliperidone should be re-evaluated and decreased if necessary). Products include:

Carbenicillin Disodium (Paliperidone causes a modest increase in the corrected QT (QTc) interval. The use of paliperidone should be avoided in combination with other drugs that are known to prolong QTc including antibiotics (eg, gatifloxacin, moxifloxacin), or any other class of medications known to prolong the QTc interval. Paliperidone should also be avoided in patients with congenital long QT syndrome and in patients with a history of cardiac arrhythmias).

No products indexed under this heading.

Carbenicillin Indanyl Sodium (Paliperidone causes a modest increase in the corrected QT (QTc) interval. The use of paliperidone should be avoided in combination with other drugs that are known to prolong QTc including antibiotics (eg, gatifloxacin, moxifloxacin), or any other class of medications known to prolong the QTc interval. Paliperidone should also be avoided in patients with congenital long QT syndrome and in patients with a history of cardiac arrhythmias).
No products indexed under this heading.

Carteolol Hydrochloride (Because of its potential for inducing orthostatic hypotension, an additive effect may be observed when paliperidone is administered with other therapeutic agents that have this potential).
No products indexed under this heading.

Carvedilol (Because of its potential for inducing orthostatic hypotension, an additive effect may be observed when paliperidone is administered with other therapeutic agents that have this potential). Products include:
Coreg **1409**

Carvedilol Phosphate (Because of its potential for inducing orthostatic hypotension, an additive effect may be observed when paliperidone is administered with other therapeutic agents that have this potential). Products include:
Coreg CR **1416**

Cefaclor (Paliperidone causes a modest increase in the corrected QT (QTc) interval. The use of paliperidone should be avoided in combination with other drugs that are known to prolong QTc including antibiotics (eg, gatifloxacin, moxifloxacin), or any other class of medications known to prolong the QTc interval. Paliperidone should also be avoided in patients with congenital long QT syndrome and in patients with a history of cardiac arrhythmias).
No products indexed under this heading.

Cefadroxil (Paliperidone causes a modest increase in the corrected QT (QTc) interval. The use of paliperidone should be avoided in combination with other drugs that are known to prolong QTc including antibiotics (eg, gatifloxacin, moxifloxacin), or any other class of medications known to prolong the QTc interval. Paliperidone should also be avoided in patients with congenital long QT syndrome and in patients with a history of cardiac arrhythmias).
No products indexed under this heading.

Cefamandole Nafate (Paliperidone causes a modest increase in the corrected QT (QTc) interval. The use of paliperidone should be avoided in combination with other drugs that are known to prolong QTc including antibiotics (eg, gatifloxacin, moxifloxacin), or any other class of medications known to prolong the QTc interval. Paliperidone should also be avoided in patients with congenital long QT syndrome and in patients with a history of cardiac arrhythmias).
No products indexed under this heading.

Cefazolin Sodium (Paliperidone causes a modest increase in the corrected QT (QTc) interval. The use of paliperidone should be avoided in combination with other drugs that are known to prolong QTc including antibiotics (eg, gatifloxacin, moxifloxacin), or any other class of medications known to prolong the QTc interval. Paliperidone should also be avoided in patients with congenital long QT syndrome and in patients with a history of cardiac arrhythmias).
No products indexed under this heading.

Cefixime (Paliperidone causes a modest increase in the corrected QT (QTc) interval. The use of paliperidone should be avoided in combination with other drugs that are known to prolong QTc including antibiotics (eg, gatifloxacin, moxifloxacin), or any other class of medications known to prolong the QTc interval. Paliperidone should also be avoided in patients with congenital long QT syndrome and in patients with a history of cardiac arrhythmias). Products include:
Suprax for Oral Suspension **2038**
Suprax Tablets **2038**

Cefmetazole Sodium (Paliperidone causes a modest increase in the corrected QT (QTc) interval. The use of paliperidone should be avoided in combination with other drugs that are known to prolong QTc including antibiotics (eg, gatifloxacin, moxifloxacin), or any other class of medications known to prolong the QTc interval. Paliperidone should also be avoided in patients with congenital long QT syndrome and in patients with a history of cardiac arrhythmias).
No products indexed under this heading.

Cefonicid Sodium (Paliperidone causes a modest increase in the corrected QT (QTc) interval. The use of paliperidone should be avoided in combination with other drugs that are known to prolong QTc including antibiotics (eg, gatifloxacin, moxifloxacin), or any other class of medications known to prolong the QTc interval. Paliperidone should also be avoided in patients with congenital long QT syndrome and in patients with a history of cardiac arrhythmias).
No products indexed under this heading.

Cefoperazone Sodium (Paliperidone causes a modest increase in the corrected QT (QTc) interval. The use of paliperidone should be avoided in combination with other drugs that are known to prolong QTc including antibiotics (eg, gatifloxacin, moxifloxacin), or any other class of medications known to prolong the QTc interval. Paliperidone should also be avoided in patients with congenital long QT syndrome and in patients with a history of cardiac arrhythmias).
No products indexed under this heading.

Ceforanide (Paliperidone causes a modest increase in the corrected QT (QTc) interval. The use of paliperidone should be avoided in combination with other drugs that are known to prolong QTc including antibiotics (eg, gatifloxacin, moxifloxacin), or any other class of medications known to prolong the QTc interval. Paliperidone should also be avoided in patients with congenital long QT syndrome and in patients with a history of cardiac arrhythmias).
No products indexed under this heading.

Cefotaxime Sodium (Paliperidone causes a modest increase in the corrected QT (QTc) interval. The use of paliperidone should be avoided in combination with other drugs that are known to prolong QTc including antibiotics (eg, gatifloxacin, moxifloxacin), or any other class of medications known to prolong the QTc interval. Paliperidone should also be avoided in patients with congenital long QT syndrome and in patients with a history of cardiac arrhythmias).
No products indexed under this heading.

Cefotetan (Paliperidone causes a modest increase in the corrected QT (QTc) interval. The use of paliperidone should be avoided in combination with other drugs that are known to prolong QTc including antibiotics (eg, gatifloxacin, moxifloxacin), or any other class of medications known to prolong the QTc interval. Paliperidone should also be avoided in patients with congenital long QT syndrome and in patients with a history of cardiac arrhythmias).
No products indexed under this heading.

Cefoxitin Sodium (Paliperidone causes a modest increase in the corrected QT (QTc) interval. The use of paliperidone should be avoided in combination with other drugs that are known to prolong QTc including antibiotics (eg, gatifloxacin, moxifloxacin), or any other class of medications known to prolong the QTc interval. Paliperidone should also be avoided in patients with congenital long QT syndrome and in patients with a history of cardiac arrhythmias).
No products indexed under this heading.

Cefpodoxime Proxetil (Paliperidone causes a modest increase in the corrected QT (QTc) interval. The use of paliperidone should be avoided in combination with other drugs that are known to prolong QTc including antibiotics (eg, gatifloxacin, moxifloxacin), or any other class of medications known to prolong the QTc interval. Paliperidone should also be avoided in patients with congenital long QT syndrome and in patients with a history of cardiac arrhythmias).
No products indexed under this heading.

Cefprozil (Paliperidone causes a modest increase in the corrected QT (QTc) interval. The use of paliperidone should be avoided in combination with other drugs that are known to prolong QTc including antibiotics (eg, gatifloxacin, moxifloxacin), or any other class of medications known to prolong the QTc interval. Paliperidone should also be avoided in patients with congenital long QT syndrome and in patients with a history of cardiac arrhythmias).
No products indexed under this heading.

Ceftazidime (Paliperidone causes a modest increase in the corrected QT (QTc) interval. The use of paliperidone should be avoided in combination with other drugs that are known to prolong QTc including antibiotics (eg, gatifloxacin, moxifloxacin), or any other class of medications known to prolong the QTc interval. Paliperidone should also be avoided in patients with congenital long QT syndrome and in patients with a history of cardiac arrhythmias). Products include:
Fortaz **1481**

Ceftizoxime Sodium (Paliperidone causes a modest increase in the corrected QT (QTc) interval. The use of paliperidone should be avoided in combination with other drugs that are known to prolong QTc including antibiotics (eg, gatifloxacin, moxifloxacin), or any other class of medications known to prolong the QTc interval. Paliperidone should also be avoided in patients with congenital long QT syndrome and in patients with a history of cardiac arrhythmias).
No products indexed under this heading.

Ceftriaxone Sodium (Paliperidone causes a modest increase in the corrected QT (QTc) interval. The use of paliperidone should be avoided in combination with other drugs that are known to prolong QTc including antibiotics (eg, gatifloxacin, moxifloxacin), or any other class of medications known to prolong the QTc interval. Paliperidone should also be avoided in patients with congenital long QT syndrome and in patients with a history of cardiac arrhythmias). Products include:
Rocephin **2859**

Cefuroxime Axetil (Paliperidone causes a modest increase in the corrected QT (QTc) interval. The use of paliperidone should be avoided in combination with other drugs that are known to prolong QTc including antibiotics (eg, gatifloxacin, moxifloxacin), or any other class of medications known to prolong the QTc interval. Paliperidone should also be avoided in patients with congenital long QT syndrome and in patients with a history of cardiac arrhythmias). Products include:
Ceftin **1399**

Cefuroxime Sodium (Paliperidone causes a modest increase in the corrected QT (QTc) interval. The use of paliperidone should be avoided in combination with other drugs that are known to prolong QTc including antibiotics (eg, gatifloxacin, moxifloxacin), or any other class of medications known to prolong the QTc interval. Paliperidone should also be avoided in patients with congenital long QT syndrome and in patients with a history of cardiac arrhythmias).
No products indexed under this heading.

Celecoxib (Paliperidone is metabolized to a limited extent by CYP2D6. In an interaction study in healthy subjects in which a single 3 mg dose of paliperidone was administered concomitantly with 20 mg per day of paroxetine (a potent CYP2D6 inhibitor), paliperidone exposures were on average 16% (90% CI: 4, 30) higher in CYP2D6 extensive metabolizers. Higher doses of paroxetine have not been studied. The clinical relevance is unknown). Products include:
Celebrex **3272**

Cephalexin (Paliperidone causes a modest increase in the corrected QT (QTc) interval. The use of paliperidone should be avoided in combination with other drugs that are known to prolong QTc including antibiotics (eg, gatifloxacin, moxifloxacin), or any other class of medications known to prolong the QTc interval. Paliperidone should also be avoided in patients with congenital long QT syndrome and in patients with a history of cardiac arrhythmias).
No products indexed under this heading.

Cephalothin Sodium (Paliperidone causes a modest increase in the corrected QT (QTc) interval. The use of paliperidone should be avoided in combination with other drugs that are known to prolong QTc including antibiotics (eg, gatifloxacin, moxifloxacin), or any other class of medications known to prolong the QTc interval. Paliperidone should also be avoided in patients with congenital long QT syndrome and in patients with a history of cardiac arrhythmias).
No products indexed under this heading.

Cephapirin Sodium (Paliperidone causes a modest increase in the corrected QT (QTc) interval. The use of paliperidone should be avoided in combination with other drugs that are known to prolong QTc including antibiotics (eg, gatifloxacin, moxifloxacin), or any other class of medications known to prolong the QTc interval. Paliperidone should also be avoided in patients with congenital long QT syndrome and in patients with a history of cardiac arrhythmias).
No products indexed under this heading.

Cephradine (Paliperidone causes a modest increase in the corrected QT (QTc) interval. The use of paliperidone should be avoided in combination with other drugs that are known to prolong QTc including antibiotics (eg, gatifloxacin, moxifloxacin), or any other class of medications known to prolong the QTc interval. Paliperidone should also be avoided in patients with congenital long QT syndrome and in patients with a history of cardiac arrhythmias).
No products indexed under this heading.

Chloramphenicol (Paliperidone causes a modest increase in the corrected QT (QTc) interval. The use of paliperidone should be avoided in combination with other drugs that are known to prolong QTc including antibiotics (eg, gatifloxacin, moxifloxacin), or any other class of medications known to prolong the QTc interval. Paliperidone should also be avoided in patients with congenital long QT syndrome and in patients with a history of cardiac arrhythmias).
No products indexed under this heading.

Chloramphenicol Palmitate (Paliperidone causes a modest increase in the corrected QT (QTc) interval. The use

of paliperidone should be avoided in combination with other drugs that are known to prolong QTc including antibiotics (eg, gatifloxacin, moxifloxacin), or any other class of medications known to prolong the QTc interval. Paliperidone should also be avoided in patients with congenital long QT syndrome and in patients with a history of cardiac arrhythmias).
No products indexed under this heading.

Chloramphenicol Sodium Succinate (Paliperidone causes a modest increase in the corrected QT (QTc) interval. The use of paliperidone should be avoided in combination with other drugs that are known to prolong QTc including antibiotics (eg, gatifloxacin, moxifloxacin), or any other class of medications known to prolong the QTc interval. Paliperidone should also be avoided in patients with congenital long QT syndrome and in patients with a history of cardiac arrhythmias).
No products indexed under this heading.

Chlordiazepoxide (Paliperidone causes a modest increase in the corrected QT (QTc) interval. The use of paliperidone should be avoided in combination with other drugs that are known to prolong QTc including Class 1A (eg, quinidine, procainamide) or Class III (eg, amiodarone, sotalol) antiarrhythmic medications, antipsychotic medications (eg, chlorpromazine, thioridazine), antibiotics (eg, gatifloxacin, moxifloxacin), or any other class of medications known to prolong the QTc interval. Paliperidone should also be avoided in patients with congenital long QT syndrome and in patients with a history of cardiac arrhythmias).
No products indexed under this heading.

Chlordiazepoxide Hydrochloride (Paliperidone causes a modest increase in the corrected QT (QTc) interval. The use of paliperidone should be avoided in combination with other drugs that are known to prolong QTc including Class 1A (eg, quinidine, procainamide) or Class III (eg, amiodarone, sotalol) antiarrhythmic medications, antipsychotic medications (eg, chlorpromazine, thioridazine), antibiotics (eg, gatifloxacin, moxifloxacin), or any other class of medications known to prolong the QTc interval. Paliperidone should also be avoided in patients with congenital long QT syndrome and in patients with a history of cardiac arrhythmias).
No products indexed under this heading.

Chloroquine (Paliperidone is metabolized to a limited extent by CYP2D6. In an interaction study in healthy subjects in which a single 3 mg dose of paliperidone was administered concomitantly with 20 mg per day of paroxetine (a potent CYP2D6 inhibitor), paliperidone exposures were on average 16% (90% CI: 4, 30) higher in CYP2D6 extensive metabolizers. Higher doses of paroxetine have not been studied. The clinical relevance is unknown).
No products indexed under this heading.

Chloroquine Hydrochloride (Paliperidone is metabolized to a limited extent by CYP2D6. In an interaction study in healthy subjects in which a single 3 mg dose of paliperidone was administered concomitantly with 20 mg per day of paroxetine (a potent CYP2D6 inhibitor), paliperidone exposures were on average 16% (90% CI: 4, 30) higher in CYP2D6 extensive metabolizers. Higher doses of paroxetine have not been studied. The clinical relevance is unknown).
No products indexed under this heading.

Chloroquine Phosphate (Paliperidone is metabolized to a limited extent by CYP2D6. In an interaction study in healthy subjects in which a single 3 mg dose of paliperidone was administered concomitantly with 20 mg per day of paroxetine (a potent CYP2D6 inhibitor), paliperidone exposures were on average 16% (90% CI: 4, 30) higher in CYP2D6 extensive metabolizers. Higher doses of paroxetine have not been studied. The clinical relevance is unknown).
No products indexed under this heading.

Chlorothiazide (Because of its potential for inducing orthostatic hypotension, an additive effect may be observed when paliperidone is administered with other therapeutic agents that have this potential).
No products indexed under this heading.

Chlorothiazide Sodium (Because of its potential for inducing orthostatic hypotension, an additive effect may be observed when paliperidone is administered with other therapeutic agents that have this potential). Products include:
Diuril Intravenous 2009

Chlorpheniramine (Paliperidone is metabolized to a limited extent by CYP2D6. In an interaction study in healthy subjects in which a single 3 mg dose of paliperidone was administered concomitantly with 20 mg per day of paroxetine (a potent CYP2D6 inhibitor), paliperidone exposures were on average 16% (90% CI: 4, 30) higher in CYP2D6 extensive metabolizers. Higher doses of paroxetine have not been studied. The clinical relevance is unknown).
No products indexed under this heading.

Chlorpheniramine Maleate (Paliperidone is metabolized to a limited extent by CYP2D6. In an interaction study in healthy subjects in which a single 3 mg dose of paliperidone was administered concomitantly with 20 mg per day of paroxetine (a potent CYP2D6 inhibitor), paliperidone exposures were on average 16% (90% CI: 4, 30) higher in CYP2D6 extensive metabolizers. Higher doses of paroxetine have not been studied. The clinical relevance is unknown).
No products indexed under this heading.

Chlorpheniramine Polistirex (Paliperidone is metabolized to a limited extent by CYP2D6. In an interaction study in healthy subjects in which a single 3 mg dose of paliperidone was administered concomitantly with 20 mg per day of paroxetine (a potent CYP2D6 inhibitor), paliperidone exposures were on average 16% (90% CI: 4, 30) higher in CYP2D6 extensive metabolizers. Higher doses of paroxetine have not been studied. The clinical relevance is unknown). Products include:
Tussionex 3443

Chlorpheniramine Tannate (Paliperidone is metabolized to a limited extent by CYP2D6. In an interaction study in healthy subjects in which a single 3 mg dose of paliperidone was administered concomitantly with 20 mg per day of paroxetine (a potent CYP2D6 inhibitor), paliperidone exposures were on average 16% (90% CI: 4, 30) higher in CYP2D6 extensive metabolizers. Higher doses of paroxetine have not been studied. The clinical relevance is unknown).
No products indexed under this heading.

Chlorpromazine (Paliperidone causes a modest increase in the corrected QT (QTc) interval. The use of paliperidone should be avoided in combination with other drugs that are known to prolong QTc including antipsychotic medications (eg, chlorpromazine, thioridazine), or any other class of medications known to prolong the QTc interval. Paliperidone should also be avoided in patients with congenital long QT syndrome and in patients with a history of cardiac arrhythmias).
No products indexed under this heading.

Chlorpromazine Hydrochloride (Paliperidone causes a modest increase in the corrected QT (QTc) interval. The use of paliperidone should be avoided in combination with other drugs that are known to prolong QTc including antipsychotic medications (eg, chlorpromazine, thioridazine), or any other class of medications known to prolong the QTc interval. Paliperidone should also be avoided in patients with congenital long QT syndrome and in patients with a history of cardiac arrhythmias).
No products indexed under this heading.

Chlorprothixene (Paliperidone causes a modest increase in the corrected QT (QTc) interval. The use of paliperidone should be avoided in combination with other drugs that are known to prolong QTc including Class 1A (eg, quinidine, procainamide) or Class III (eg, amiodarone, sotalol) antiarrhythmic medications, antipsychotic medications (eg, chlorpromazine, thioridazine), antibiotics (eg, gatifloxacin, moxifloxacin), or any other class of medications known to prolong the QTc interval. Paliperidone should also be avoided in patients with congenital long QT syndrome and in patients with a history of cardiac arrhythmias).
No products indexed under this heading.

Chlorprothixene Hydrochloride (Paliperidone causes a modest increase in the corrected QT (QTc) interval. The use of paliperidone should be avoided in combination with other drugs that are known to prolong QTc including Class 1A (eg, quinidine, procainamide) or Class III (eg, amiodarone, sotalol) antiarrhythmic medications, antipsychotic medications (eg, chlorpromazine, thioridazine), antibiotics (eg, gatifloxacin, moxifloxacin), or any other class of medications known to prolong the QTc interval. Paliperidone should also be avoided in patients with congenital long QT syndrome and in patients with a history of cardiac arrhythmias).
No products indexed under this heading.

Chlorprothixene Lactate (Given the primary CNS effects of paliperidone, paliperidone should be used with caution in combination with other centrally acting drugs and alcohol).
No products indexed under this heading.

Chlorthalidone (Because of its potential for inducing orthostatic hypotension, an additive effect may be observed when paliperidone is administered with other therapeutic agents that have this potential). Products include:
Clorpres 2344

Cilastatin Sodium (Paliperidone causes a modest increase in the corrected QT (QTc) interval. The use of paliperidone should be avoided in combination with other drugs that are known to prolong QTc including antibiotics (eg, gatifloxacin, moxifloxacin), or any other class of medications known to prolong the QTc interval. Paliperidone should also be avoided in patients with congenital long QT syndrome and in patients with a history of cardiac arrhythmias). Products include:
Primaxin I.M. 2232
Primaxin I.V. 2235

Cimetidine (Paliperidone is metabolized to a limited extent by CYP2D6. In an interaction study in healthy subjects in which a single 3 mg dose of paliperidone was administered concomitantly with 20 mg per day of paroxetine (a potent CYP2D6 inhibitor), paliperidone exposures were on average 16% (90% CI: 4, 30) higher in CYP2D6 extensive metabolizers. Higher doses of paroxetine have not been studied. The clinical relevance is unknown).
No products indexed under this heading.

Cimetidine Hydrochloride (Paliperidone is metabolized to a limited extent by CYP2D6. In an interaction study in healthy subjects in which a single 3 mg dose of paliperidone was administered concomitantly with 20 mg per day of paroxetine (a potent CYP2D6 inhibitor), paliperidone exposures were on average 16% (90% CI: 4, 30) higher in CYP2D6 extensive metabolizers. Higher doses of paroxetine have not been studied. The clinical relevance is unknown).
No products indexed under this heading.

Ciprofloxacin (Paliperidone causes a modest increase in the corrected QT (QTc) interval. The use of paliperidone should be avoided in combination with other drugs that are known to prolong QTc including antibiotics (eg, gatifloxacin, moxifloxacin), or any other class of medications known to prolong the QTc interval. Paliperidone should also be avoided in patients with congenital long QT syndrome and in patients with a history of cardiac arrhythmias). Products include:
Cipro I.V. 3082
Cipro 3073
Cipro XR 3091
Ciprodex 583

Ciprofloxacin Hydrochloride (Paliperidone causes a modest increase in the corrected QT (QTc) interval. The use of paliperidone should be avoided in combination with other drugs that are known to prolong QTc including antibiotics (eg, gatifloxacin, moxifloxacin), or any other class of medications known to prolong the QTc interval. Paliperidone should also be avoided in patients with congenital long QT syndrome and in patients with a history of cardiac arrhythmias). Products include:
Cipro 3073

Citalopram Hydrobromide (Paliperidone is metabolized to a limited extent by CYP2D6. In an interaction study in healthy subjects in which a single 3 mg dose of paliperidone was administered concomitantly with 20 mg per day of paroxetine (a potent CYP2D6 inhibitor), paliperidone exposures were on average 16% (90% CI: 4, 30) higher in CYP2D6 extensive metabolizers. Higher doses of paroxetine have not been studied. The clinical relevance is unknown). Products include:
Celexa 1153

Clarithromycin (Paliperidone causes a modest increase in the corrected QT (QTc) interval. The use of paliperidone should be avoided in combination with other drugs that are known to prolong QTc including antibiotics (eg, gatifloxacin, moxifloxacin), or any other class of medications known to prolong the QTc interval. Paliperidone should also be avoided in patients with congenital long QT syndrome and in patients with a history of cardiac arrhythmias). Products include:
Biaxin/Biaxin XL 412

Clomipramine Hydrochloride (Paliperidone causes a modest increase in the corrected QT (QTc) interval. The use of paliperidone should be avoided in combination with other drugs that are known to prolong QTc including Class 1A (eg, quinidine, procainamide) or Class III (eg, amiodarone, sotalol) antiarrhythmic medications, antipsychotic medications (eg, chlorpromazine, thioridazine), antibiotics (eg, gatifloxacin, moxifloxacin), or any other class of medications known to prolong the QTc interval. Paliperidone should also be avoided in patients with congenital long QT syndrome and in patients with a history of cardiac arrhythmias).
No products indexed under this heading.

Clonidine (Because of its potential for inducing orthostatic hypotension, an additive effect may be observed when

paliperidone is administered with other therapeutic agents that have this potential). Products include:

Catapres-TTS 884

Clonidine Hydrochloride (Because of its potential for inducing orthostatic hypotension, an additive effect may be observed when paliperidone is administered with other therapeutic agents that have this potential). Products include:

Clorpres 2344

Clorazepate Dipotassium (Paliperidone causes a modest increase in the corrected QT (QTc) interval. The use of paliperidone should be avoided in combination with other drugs that are known to prolong QTc including Class 1A (eg, quinidine, procainamide) or Class III (eg, amiodarone, sotalol) antiarrhythmic medications, antipsychotic medications (eg, chlorpromazine, thioridazine), antibiotics (eg, gatifloxacin, moxifloxacin), or any other class of medications known to prolong the QTc interval. Paliperidone should also be avoided in patients with congenital long QT syndrome and in patients with a history of cardiac arrhythmias).

No products indexed under this heading.

Clotrimazole (Paliperidone causes a modest increase in the corrected QT (QTc) interval. The use of paliperidone should be avoided in combination with other drugs that are known to prolong QTc including antibiotics (eg, gatifloxacin, moxifloxacin), or any other class of medications known to prolong the QTc interval. Paliperidone should also be avoided in patients with congenital long QT syndrome and in patients with a history of cardiac arrhythmias). Products include:

Lotrisone 3163

Cloxacillin (Paliperidone causes a modest increase in the corrected QT (QTc) interval. The use of paliperidone should be avoided in combination with other drugs that are known to prolong QTc including antibiotics (eg, gatifloxacin, moxifloxacin), or any other class of medications known to prolong the QTc interval. Paliperidone should also be avoided in patients with congenital long QT syndrome and in patients with a history of cardiac arrhythmias).

No products indexed under this heading.

Cloxacillin Sodium (Paliperidone causes a modest increase in the corrected QT (QTc) interval. The use of paliperidone should be avoided in combination with other drugs that are known to prolong QTc including antibiotics (eg, gatifloxacin, moxifloxacin), or any other class of medications known to prolong the QTc interval. Paliperidone should also be avoided in patients with congenital long QT syndrome and in patients with a history of cardiac arrhythmias).

No products indexed under this heading.

Cloxacillin Sodium Monohydrate (Paliperidone causes a modest increase in the corrected QT (QTc) interval. The use of paliperidone should be avoided in combination with other drugs that are known to prolong QTc including antibiotics (eg, gatifloxacin, moxifloxacin), or any other class of medications known to prolong the QTc interval. Paliperidone should also be avoided in patients with congenital long QT syndrome and in patients with a history of cardiac arrhythmias).

No products indexed under this heading.

Clozapine (Paliperidone causes a modest increase in the corrected QT (QTc) interval. The use of paliperidone should be avoided in combination with other drugs that are known to prolong QTc including Class 1A (eg, quinidine, procainamide) or Class III (eg, amiodarone, sotalol) antiarrhythmic medications, antipsychotic medications (eg, chlorpromazine, thioridazine), antibiotics (eg, gatifloxacin, moxifloxacin), or any other class of medications known to prolong the QTc interval. Paliperidone should also be avoided in patients with congenital long QT syndrome and in patients with a history of cardiac arrhythmias).

No products indexed under this heading.

Cocaine Hydrochloride (Paliperidone is metabolized to a limited extent by CYP2D6. In an interaction study in healthy subjects in which a single 3 mg dose of paliperidone was administered concomitantly with 20 mg per day of paroxetine (a potent CYP2D6 inhibitor), paliperidone exposures were on average 16% (90% CI: 4, 30) higher in CYP2D6 extensive metabolizers. Higher doses of paroxetine have not been studied. The clinical relevance is unknown).

No products indexed under this heading.

Codeine Phosphate (Given the primary CNS effects of paliperidone, paliperidone should be used with caution in combination with other centrally acting drugs and alcohol). Products include:

Tylenol with Codeine 2691

Codeine Sulfate (Given the primary CNS effects of paliperidone, paliperidone should be used with caution in combination with other centrally acting drugs and alcohol).

No products indexed under this heading.

Daunorubicin Hydrochloride (Paliperidone causes a modest increase in the corrected QT (QTc) interval. The use of paliperidone should be avoided in combination with other drugs that are known to prolong QTc including antibiotics (eg, gatifloxacin, moxifloxacin), or any other class of medications known to prolong the QTc interval. Paliperidone should also be avoided in patients with congenital long QT syndrome and in patients with a history of cardiac arrhythmias).

No products indexed under this heading.

Demeclocycline Hydrochloride (Paliperidone causes a modest increase in the corrected QT (QTc) interval. The use of paliperidone should be avoided in combination with other drugs that are known to prolong QTc including antibiotics (eg, gatifloxacin, moxifloxacin), or any other class of medications known to prolong the QTc interval. Paliperidone should also be avoided in patients with congenital long QT syndrome and in patients with a history of cardiac arrhythmias).

No products indexed under this heading.

Deserpidine (Because of its potential for inducing orthostatic hypotension, an additive effect may be observed when paliperidone is administered with other therapeutic agents that have this potential).

No products indexed under this heading.

Desflurane (Given the primary CNS effects of paliperidone, paliperidone should be used with caution in combination with other centrally acting drugs and alcohol).

No products indexed under this heading.

Desipramine Hydrochloride (Paliperidone causes a modest increase in the corrected QT (QTc) interval. The use of paliperidone should be avoided in combination with other drugs that are known to prolong QTc including Class 1A (eg, quinidine, procainamide) or Class III (eg, amiodarone, sotalol) antiarrhythmic medications, antipsychotic medications (eg, chlorpromazine, thioridazine), antibiotics (eg, gatifloxacin, moxifloxacin), or any other class of medications known to prolong the QTc interval. Paliperidone should also be avoided in patients with congenital long QT syndrome and in patients with a history of cardiac arrhythmias).

No products indexed under this heading.

Dexmethylphenidate Hydrochloride (Given the primary CNS effects of paliperidone, paliperidone should be used with caution in combination with other centrally acting drugs and alcohol). Products include:

Focalin XR 2472

Dextroamphetamine (Given the primary CNS effects of paliperidone, paliperidone should be used with caution in combination with other centrally acting drugs and alcohol).

No products indexed under this heading.

Dextroamphetamine Saccharate (Given the primary CNS effects of paliperidone, paliperidone should be used with caution in combination with other centrally acting drugs and alcohol).

No products indexed under this heading.

Dextroamphetamine Sulfate (Given the primary CNS effects of paliperidone, paliperidone should be used with caution in combination with other centrally acting drugs and alcohol). Products include:

Dexedrine 1425

Dezocine (Given the primary CNS effects of paliperidone, paliperidone should be used with caution in combination with other centrally acting drugs and alcohol).

No products indexed under this heading.

Diazepam (Paliperidone causes a modest increase in the corrected QT (QTc) interval. The use of paliperidone should be avoided in combination with other drugs that are known to prolong QTc including Class 1A (eg, quinidine, procainamide) or Class III (eg, amiodarone, sotalol) antiarrhythmic medications, antipsychotic medications (eg, chlorpromazine, thioridazine), antibiotics (eg, gatifloxacin, moxifloxacin), or any other class of medications known to prolong the QTc interval. Paliperidone should also be avoided in patients with congenital long QT syndrome and in patients with a history of cardiac arrhythmias). Products include:

Valium Tablets 2880

Diazoxide (Because of its potential for inducing orthostatic hypotension, an additive effect may be observed when paliperidone is administered with other therapeutic agents that have this potential). Products include:

Proglycem 1179
Proglycem Suspension 1179

Dicloxacillin (Paliperidone causes a modest increase in the corrected QT (QTc) interval. The use of paliperidone should be avoided in combination with other drugs that are known to prolong QTc including antibiotics (eg, gatifloxacin, moxifloxacin), or any other class of medications known to prolong the QTc interval. Paliperidone should also be avoided in patients with congenital long QT syndrome and in patients with a history of cardiac arrhythmias).

No products indexed under this heading.

Dicloxacillin Sodium (Paliperidone causes a modest increase in the corrected QT (QTc) interval. The use of paliperidone should be avoided in combination with other drugs that are known to prolong QTc including antibiotics (eg, gatifloxacin, moxifloxacin), or any other class of medications known to prolong the QTc interval. Paliperidone should also be avoided in patients with congenital long QT syndrome and in patients with a history of cardiac arrhythmias).

No products indexed under this heading.

Diltiazem Hydrochloride (Because of its potential for inducing orthostatic hypotension, an additive effect may be observed when paliperidone is administered with other therapeutic agents that have this potential). Products include:

Cardizem LA 423

Diltiazem Maleate (Because of its potential for inducing orthostatic hypotension, an additive effect may be observed when paliperidone is administered with other therapeutic agents that have this potential).

No products indexed under this heading.

Diphenhydramine (Paliperidone is metabolized to a limited extent by CYP2D6. In an interaction study in healthy subjects in which a single 3 mg dose of paliperidone was administered concomitantly with 20 mg per day of paroxetine (a potent CYP2D6 inhibitor), paliperidone exposures were on average 16% (90% CI: 4, 30) higher in CYP2D6 extensive metabolizers. Higher doses of paroxetine have not been studied. The clinical relevance is unknown).

No products indexed under this heading.

Diphenhydramine Hydrochloride (Paliperidone is metabolized to a limited extent by CYP2D6. In an interaction study in healthy subjects in which a single 3 mg dose of paliperidone was administered concomitantly with 20 mg per day of paroxetine (a potent CYP2D6 inhibitor), paliperidone exposures were on average 16% (90% CI: 4, 30) higher in CYP2D6 extensive metabolizers. Higher doses of paroxetine have not been studied. The clinical relevance is unknown). Products include:

Benadryl Allergy Ultratab 2042
Children's Benadryl Allergy Liquid 2042

Dirithromycin (Paliperidone causes a modest increase in the corrected QT (QTc) interval. The use of paliperidone should be avoided in combination with other drugs that are known to prolong QTc including antibiotics (eg, gatifloxacin, moxifloxacin), or any other class of medications known to prolong the QTc interval. Paliperidone should also be avoided in patients with congenital long QT syndrome and in patients with a history of cardiac arrhythmias).

No products indexed under this heading.

Disodium Carbenicillin (Paliperidone causes a modest increase in the corrected QT (QTc) interval. The use of paliperidone should be avoided in combination with other drugs that are known to prolong QTc including antibiotics (eg, gatifloxacin, moxifloxacin), or any other class of medications known to prolong the QTc interval. Paliperidone should also be avoided in patients with congenital long QT syndrome and in patients with a history of cardiac arrhythmias).

No products indexed under this heading.

Disopyramide (Paliperidone causes a modest increase in the corrected QT (QTc) interval. The use of paliperidone should be avoided in combination with other drugs that are known to prolong QTc including Class 1A (eg, quinidine, procainamide) or Class III (eg, amiodarone, sotalol) antiarrhythmic medications, antipsychotic medications (eg, chlorpromazine, thioridazine), antibiotics (eg, gatifloxacin, moxifloxacin), or any other class of medications known to prolong the QTc interval. Paliperidone should also be avoided in patients with congenital long QT syndrome and in patients with a history of cardiac arrhythmias).

No products indexed under this heading.

Disopyramide Phosphate (Paliperidone causes a modest increase in the corrected QT (QTc) interval. The use of paliperidone should be avoided in combination with other drugs that are known to prolong QTc including Class 1A (eg, quinidine, procainamide) or Class III (eg, amiodarone, sotalol) antiarrhythmic medications, antipsychotic medications (eg, chlorpromazine, thioridazine), antibiotics (eg, gatifloxacin, moxifloxacin), or any other class of medications known to prolong the QTc interval. Paliperidone should also be avoided in

IMPORTANT NOTE: Always consult each drug listing in the patient's regimen for possible interactions.

patients with congenital long QT syndrome and in patients with a history of cardiac arrhythmias).
No products indexed under this heading.

Dofetilide (Paliperidone causes a modest increase in the corrected QT (QTc) interval. The use of paliperidone should be avoided in combination with other drugs that are known to prolong QTc including Class 1A (eg, quinidine, procainamide) or Class III (eg, amiodarone, sotalol) antiarrhythmic medications, antipsychotic medications (eg, chlorpromazine, thioridazine), antibiotics (eg, gatifloxacin, moxifloxacin), or any other class of medications known to prolong the QTc interval. Paliperidone should also be avoided in patients with congenital long QT syndrome and in patients with a history of cardiac arrhythmias).
No products indexed under this heading.

Dopamine Hydrochloride (Given the primary CNS effects of paliperidone, paliperidone should be used with caution in combination with other centrally acting drugs and alcohol. Paliperidone may antagonize the effect of levodopa and other dopamine agonists).
No products indexed under this heading.

Doxazosin Mesylate (Because of its potential for inducing orthostatic hypotension, an additive effect may be observed when paliperidone is administered with other therapeutic agents that have this potential).
No products indexed under this heading.

Doxepin Hydrochloride (Paliperidone causes a modest increase in the corrected QT (QTc) interval. The use of paliperidone should be avoided in combination with other drugs that are known to prolong QTc including Class 1A (eg, quinidine, procainamide) or Class III (eg, amiodarone, sotalol) antiarrhythmic medications, antipsychotic medications (eg, chlorpromazine, thioridazine), antibiotics (eg, gatifloxacin, moxifloxacin), or any other class of medications known to prolong the QTc interval. Paliperidone should also be avoided in patients with congenital long QT syndrome and in patients with a history of cardiac arrhythmias).
No products indexed under this heading.

Doxycycline Calcium (Paliperidone causes a modest increase in the corrected QT (QTc) interval. The use of paliperidone should be avoided in combination with other drugs that are known to prolong QTc including antibiotics (eg, gatifloxacin, moxifloxacin), or any other class of medications known to prolong the QTc interval. Paliperidone should also be avoided in patients with congenital long QT syndrome and in patients with a history of cardiac arrhythmias).
No products indexed under this heading.

Doxycycline Hyclate (Paliperidone causes a modest increase in the corrected QT (QTc) interval. The use of paliperidone should be avoided in combination with other drugs that are known to prolong QTc including antibiotics (eg, gatifloxacin, moxifloxacin), or any other class of medications known to prolong the QTc interval. Paliperidone should also be avoided in patients with congenital long QT syndrome and in patients with a history of cardiac arrhythmias).
No products indexed under this heading.

Doxycycline Monohydrate (Paliperidone causes a modest increase in the corrected QT (QTc) interval. The use of paliperidone should be avoided in combination with other drugs that are known to prolong QTc including antibiotics (eg, gatifloxacin, moxifloxacin), or any other class of medications known to prolong the QTc interval. Paliperidone should also be avoided in patients with congenital long QT syndrome and in patients with a history of cardiac arrhythmias).
No products indexed under this heading.

Droperidol (Paliperidone causes a modest increase in the corrected QT (QTc) interval. The use of paliperidone should be avoided in combination with other drugs that are known to prolong QTc including Class 1A (eg, quinidine, procainamide) or Class III (eg, amiodarone, sotalol) antiarrhythmic medications, antipsychotic medications (eg, chlorpromazine, thioridazine), antibiotics (eg, gatifloxacin, moxifloxacin), or any other class of medications known to prolong the QTc interval. Paliperidone should also be avoided in patients with congenital long QT syndrome and in patients with a history of cardiac arrhythmias).
No products indexed under this heading.

Enalapril Maleate (Because of its potential for inducing orthostatic hypotension, an additive effect may be observed when paliperidone is administered with other therapeutic agents that have this potential).
No products indexed under this heading.

Enalaprilat (Because of its potential for inducing orthostatic hypotension, an additive effect may be observed when paliperidone is administered with other therapeutic agents that have this potential).
No products indexed under this heading.

Enflurane (Given the primary CNS effects of paliperidone, paliperidone should be used with caution in combination with other centrally acting drugs and alcohol).
No products indexed under this heading.

Enoxacin (Paliperidone causes a modest increase in the corrected QT (QTc) interval. The use of paliperidone should be avoided in combination with other drugs that are known to prolong QTc including antibiotics (eg, gatifloxacin, moxifloxacin), or any other class of medications known to prolong the QTc interval. Paliperidone should also be avoided in patients with congenital long QT syndrome and in patients with a history of cardiac arrhythmias).
No products indexed under this heading.

Epirubicin Hydrochloride (Paliperidone causes a modest increase in the corrected QT (QTc) interval. The use of paliperidone should be avoided in combination with other drugs that are known to prolong QTc including antibiotics (eg, gatifloxacin, moxifloxacin), or any other class of medications known to prolong the QTc interval. Paliperidone should also be avoided in patients with congenital long QT syndrome and in patients with a history of cardiac arrhythmias).
No products indexed under this heading.

Eprosartan Mesylate (Because of its potential for inducing orthostatic hypotension, an additive effect may be observed when paliperidone is administered with other therapeutic agents that have this potential). Products include:
Teveten 538
Teveten HCT 541

Erythromycin (Paliperidone causes a modest increase in the corrected QT (QTc) interval. The use of paliperidone should be avoided in combination with other drugs that are known to prolong QTc including Class 1A (eg, quinidine, procainamide) or Class III (eg, amiodarone, sotalol) antiarrhythmic medications, antipsychotic medications (eg, chlorpromazine, thioridazine), antibiotics (eg, gatifloxacin, moxifloxacin), or any other class of medications known to prolong the QTc interval. Paliperidone should also be avoided in patients with congenital long QT syndrome and in patients with a history of cardiac arrhythmias).
No products indexed under this heading.

Erythromycin, Topical (Paliperidone causes a modest increase in the corrected QT (QTc) interval. The use of paliperidone should be avoided in combination with other drugs that are known to prolong QTc including antibiotics (eg, gatifloxacin, moxifloxacin), or any other class of medications known to prolong the QTc interval. Paliperidone should also be avoided in patients with congenital long QT syndrome and in patients with a history of cardiac arrhythmias).
No products indexed under this heading.

Erythromycin Estolate (Paliperidone causes a modest increase in the corrected QT (QTc) interval. The use of paliperidone should be avoided in combination with other drugs that are known to prolong QTc including Class 1A (eg, quinidine, procainamide) or Class III (eg, amiodarone, sotalol) antiarrhythmic medications, antipsychotic medications (eg, chlorpromazine, thioridazine), antibiotics (eg, gatifloxacin, moxifloxacin), or any other class of medications known to prolong the QTc interval. Paliperidone should also be avoided in patients with congenital long QT syndrome and in patients with a history of cardiac arrhythmias).
No products indexed under this heading.

Erythromycin Ethylsuccinate (Paliperidone causes a modest increase in the corrected QT (QTc) interval. The use of paliperidone should be avoided in combination with other drugs that are known to prolong QTc including Class 1A (eg, quinidine, procainamide) or Class III (eg, amiodarone, sotalol) antiarrhythmic medications, antipsychotic medications (eg, chlorpromazine, thioridazine), antibiotics (eg, gatifloxacin, moxifloxacin), or any other class of medications known to prolong the QTc interval. Paliperidone should also be avoided in patients with congenital long QT syndrome and in patients with a history of cardiac arrhythmias). Products include:
E.E.S. 437
EryPed 435

Erythromycin Gluceptate (Paliperidone causes a modest increase in the corrected QT (QTc) interval. The use of paliperidone should be avoided in combination with other drugs that are known to prolong QTc including Class 1A (eg, quinidine, procainamide) or Class III (eg, amiodarone, sotalol) antiarrhythmic medications, antipsychotic medications (eg, chlorpromazine, thioridazine), antibiotics (eg, gatifloxacin, moxifloxacin), or any other class of medications known to prolong the QTc interval. Paliperidone should also be avoided in patients with congenital long QT syndrome and in patients with a history of cardiac arrhythmias).
No products indexed under this heading.

Erythromycin Lactobionate (Paliperidone causes a modest increase in the corrected QT (QTc) interval. The use of paliperidone should be avoided in combination with other drugs that are known to prolong QTc including Class 1A (eg, quinidine, procainamide) or Class III (eg, amiodarone, sotalol) antiarrhythmic medications, antipsychotic medications (eg, chlorpromazine, thioridazine), antibiotics (eg, gatifloxacin, moxifloxacin), or any other class of medications known to prolong the QTc interval. Paliperidone should also be avoided in patients with congenital long QT syndrome and in patients with a history of cardiac arrhythmias).
No products indexed under this heading.

Erythromycin Stearate (Paliperidone causes a modest increase in the corrected QT (QTc) interval. The use of paliperidone should be avoided in combination with other drugs that are known to prolong QTc including Class 1A (eg, quinidine, procainamide) or Class III (eg, amiodarone, sotalol) antiarrhythmic medications, antipsychotic medications (eg, chlorpromazine, thioridazine), antibiotics (eg, gatifloxacin, moxifloxacin), or any other class of medications known to prolong the QTc interval. Paliperidone should also be avoided in patients with congenital long QT syndrome and in patients with a history of cardiac arrhythmias).
No products indexed under this heading.

Escitalopram Oxalate (Paliperidone is metabolized to a limited extent by CYP2D6. In an interaction study in healthy subjects in which a single 3 mg dose of paliperidone was administered concomitantly with 20 mg per day of paroxetine (a potent CYP2D6 inhibitor), paliperidone exposures were on average 16% (90% CI: 4, 30) higher in CYP2D6 extensive metabolizers. Higher doses of paroxetine have not been studied. The clinical relevance is unknown). Products include:
Lexapro Oral Suspension 1160
Lexapro Tablets 1160

Esmolol Hydrochloride (Because of its potential for inducing orthostatic hypotension, an additive effect may be observed when paliperidone is administered with other therapeutic agents that have this potential).
No products indexed under this heading.

Estazolam (Given the primary CNS effects of paliperidone, paliperidone should be used with caution in combination with other centrally acting drugs and alcohol).
No products indexed under this heading.

Ethanol (Given the primary CNS effects of paliperidone, paliperidone should be used with caution in combination with other centrally acting drugs and alcohol).
No products indexed under this heading.

Ethchlorvynol (Given the primary CNS effects of paliperidone, paliperidone should be used with caution in combination with other centrally acting drugs and alcohol).
No products indexed under this heading.

Ethinamate (Given the primary CNS effects of paliperidone, paliperidone should be used with caution in combination with other centrally acting drugs and alcohol).
No products indexed under this heading.

Ethyl Alcohol (Given the primary CNS effects of paliperidone, paliperidone should be used with caution in combination with other centrally acting drugs and alcohol).
No products indexed under this heading.

Fat (Administration of a 12 mg paliperidone extended-release tablet to healthy ambulatory subjects with a standard high-fat/high-caloric meal gave mean C_{max} and AUC values of paliperidone that were increased by 60% and 54%, respectively, compared with administration under fasting conditions. Clinical trials establishing the safety and efficacy of paliperidone were carried out in subjects without regard to the timing of meals. While paliperidone can be taken without regard to food, the presence of food at the time of paliperidone administration may increase exposure to paliperidone).
No products indexed under this heading.

Felodipine (Because of its potential for inducing orthostatic hypotension, an additive effect may be observed when paliperidone is administered with other therapeutic agents that have this potential).
No products indexed under this heading.

Fentanyl (Given the primary CNS effects of paliperidone, paliperidone should be used with caution in combination with other centrally acting drugs and alcohol). Products include:

Duragesic 2604
Fentanyl Transdermal System 2346
Onsolis 2054

Fentanyl Citrate (Given the primary CNS effects of paliperidone, paliperidone should be used with caution in combination with other centrally acting drugs and alcohol). Products include:
Fentora 966

Flecainide Acetate (Paliperidone causes a modest increase in the corrected QT (QTc) interval. The use of paliperidone should be avoided in combination with other drugs that are known to prolong QTc including Class 1A (eg, quinidine, procainamide) or Class III (eg, amiodarone, sotalol) antiarrhythmic medications, antipsychotic medications (eg, chlorpromazine, thioridazine), antibiotics (eg, gatifloxacin, moxifloxacin), or any other class of medications known to prolong the QTc interval. Paliperidone should also be avoided in patients with congenital long QT syndrome and in patients with a history of cardiac arrhythmias).
No products indexed under this heading.

Fluoxetine (Paliperidone is metabolized to a limited extent by CYP2D6. In an interaction study in healthy subjects in which a single 3 mg dose of paliperidone was administered concomitantly with 20 mg per day of paroxetine (a potent CYP2D6 inhibitor), paliperidone exposures were on average 16% (90% CI: 4, 30) higher in CYP2D6 extensive metabolizers. Higher doses of paroxetine have not been studied. The clinical relevance is unknown).
No products indexed under this heading.

Fluoxetine Hydrochloride (Paliperidone is metabolized to a limited extent by CYP2D6. In an interaction study in healthy subjects in which a single 3 mg dose of paliperidone was administered concomitantly with 20 mg per day of paroxetine (a potent CYP2D6 inhibitor), paliperidone exposures were on average 16% (90% CI: 4, 30) higher in CYP2D6 extensive metabolizers. Higher doses of paroxetine have not been studied. The clinical relevance is unknown). Products include:
Prozac Weekly 1941
Prozac Pulvules 1941
Symbyax 1965

Fluphenazine Decanoate (Paliperidone causes a modest increase in the corrected QT (QTc) interval. The use of paliperidone should be avoided in combination with other drugs that are known to prolong QTc including Class 1A (eg, quinidine, procainamide) or Class III (eg, amiodarone, sotalol) antiarrhythmic medications, antipsychotic medications (eg, chlorpromazine, thioridazine), antibiotics (eg, gatifloxacin, moxifloxacin), or any other class of medications known to prolong the QTc interval. Paliperidone should also be avoided in patients with congenital long QT syndrome and in patients with a history of cardiac arrhythmias).
No products indexed under this heading.

Fluphenazine Enanthate (Paliperidone causes a modest increase in the corrected QT (QTc) interval. The use of paliperidone should be avoided in combination with other drugs that are known to prolong QTc including Class 1A (eg, quinidine, procainamide) or Class III (eg, amiodarone, sotalol) antiarrhythmic medications, antipsychotic medications (eg, chlorpromazine, thioridazine), antibiotics (eg, gatifloxacin, moxifloxacin), or any other class of medications known to prolong the QTc interval. Paliperidone should also be avoided in patients with congenital long QT syndrome and in patients with a history of cardiac arrhythmias).
No products indexed under this heading.

Fluphenazine Hydrochloride (Paliperidone causes a modest increase in the corrected QT (QTc) interval. The use of paliperidone should be avoided in combination with other drugs that are known to prolong QTc including Class 1A (eg, quinidine, procainamide) or Class III (eg, amiodarone, sotalol) antiarrhythmic medications, antipsychotic medications (eg, chlorpromazine, thioridazine), antibiotics (eg, gatifloxacin, moxifloxacin), or any other class of medications known to prolong the QTc interval. Paliperidone should also be avoided in patients with congenital long QT syndrome and in patients with a history of cardiac arrhythmias).
No products indexed under this heading.

Flurazepam Hydrochloride (Given the primary CNS effects of paliperidone, paliperidone should be used with caution in combination with other centrally acting drugs and alcohol).
No products indexed under this heading.

Fluvoxamine Maleate (Paliperidone is metabolized to a limited extent by CYP2D6. In an interaction study in healthy subjects in which a single 3 mg dose of paliperidone was administered concomitantly with 20 mg per day of paroxetine (a potent CYP2D6 inhibitor), paliperidone exposures were on average 16% (90% CI: 4, 30) higher in CYP2D6 extensive metabolizers. Higher doses of paroxetine have not been studied. The clinical relevance is unknown).
No products indexed under this heading.

Fosinopril Sodium (Because of its potential for inducing orthostatic hypotension, an additive effect may be observed when paliperidone is administered with other therapeutic agents that have this potential).
No products indexed under this heading.

Furosemide (Because of its potential for inducing orthostatic hypotension, an additive effect may be observed when paliperidone is administered with other therapeutic agents that have this potential). Products include:
Furosemide 2354

Gatifloxacin (Paliperidone causes a modest increase in the corrected QT (QTc) interval. The use of paliperidone should be avoided in combination with other drugs that are known to prolong QTc including antibiotics (eg, gatifloxacin, moxifloxacin), or any other class of medications known to prolong the QTc interval. Paliperidone should also be avoided in patients with congenital long QT syndrome and in patients with a history of cardiac arrhythmias).
No products indexed under this heading.

Gemifloxacin Mesylate (Paliperidone causes a modest increase in the corrected QT (QTc) interval. The use of paliperidone should be avoided in combination with other drugs that are known to prolong QTc including antibiotics (eg, gatifloxacin, moxifloxacin), or any other class of medications known to prolong the QTc interval. Paliperidone should also be avoided in patients with congenital long QT syndrome and in patients with a history of cardiac arrhythmias).
No products indexed under this heading.

Gentamicin Sulfate (Paliperidone causes a modest increase in the corrected QT (QTc) interval. The use of paliperidone should be avoided in combination with other drugs that are known to prolong QTc including antibiotics (eg, gatifloxacin, moxifloxacin), or any other class of medications known to prolong the QTc interval. Paliperidone should also be avoided in patients with congenital long QT syndrome and in patients with a history of cardiac arrhythmias). Products include:
Pred-G .... ⊙226, ⊙227

Glutethimide (Given the primary CNS effects of paliperidone, paliperidone should be used with caution in combination with other centrally acting drugs and alcohol).
No products indexed under this heading.

Grepafloxacin Hydrochloride (Paliperidone causes a modest increase in the corrected QT (QTc) interval. The use of paliperidone should be avoided in combination with other drugs that are known to prolong QTc including antibiotics (eg, gatifloxacin, moxifloxacin), or any other class of medications known to prolong the QTc interval. Paliperidone should also be avoided in patients with congenital long QT syndrome and in patients with a history of cardiac arrhythmias).
No products indexed under this heading.

Griseofulvin (Paliperidone causes a modest increase in the corrected QT (QTc) interval. The use of paliperidone should be avoided in combination with other drugs that are known to prolong QTc including antibiotics (eg, gatifloxacin, moxifloxacin), or any other class of medications known to prolong the QTc interval. Paliperidone should also be avoided in patients with congenital long QT syndrome and in patients with a history of cardiac arrhythmias).
No products indexed under this heading.

Guanabenz Acetate (Because of its potential for inducing orthostatic hypotension, an additive effect may be observed when paliperidone is administered with other therapeutic agents that have this potential).
No products indexed under this heading.

Guanethidine (Because of its potential for inducing orthostatic hypotension, an additive effect may be observed when paliperidone is administered with other therapeutic agents that have this potential).
No products indexed under this heading.

Guanethidine Monosulfate (Because of its potential for inducing orthostatic hypotension, an additive effect may be observed when paliperidone is administered with other therapeutic agents that have this potential).
No products indexed under this heading.

Guanethidine Sulfate (Because of its potential for inducing orthostatic hypotension, an additive effect may be observed when paliperidone is administered with other therapeutic agents that have this potential).
No products indexed under this heading.

Halofantrine Hydrochloride (Paliperidone is metabolized to a limited extent by CYP2D6. In an interaction study in healthy subjects in which a single 3 mg dose of paliperidone was administered concomitantly with 20 mg per day of paroxetine (a potent CYP2D6 inhibitor), paliperidone exposures were on average 16% (90% CI: 4, 30) higher in CYP2D6 extensive metabolizers. Higher doses of paroxetine have not been studied. The clinical relevance is unknown).
No products indexed under this heading.

Haloperidol (Paliperidone causes a modest increase in the corrected QT (QTc) interval. The use of paliperidone should be avoided in combination with other drugs that are known to prolong QTc including Class 1A (eg, quinidine, procainamide) or Class III (eg, amiodarone, sotalol) antiarrhythmic medications, antipsychotic medications (eg, chlorpromazine, thioridazine), antibiotics (eg, gatifloxacin, moxifloxacin), or any other class of medications known to prolong the QTc interval. Paliperidone should also be avoided in patients with congenital long QT syndrome and in patients with a history of cardiac arrhythmias).
No products indexed under this heading.

Haloperidol Decanoate (Paliperidone causes a modest increase in the corrected QT (QTc) interval. The use of paliperidone should be avoided in combination with other drugs that are known to prolong QTc including Class 1A (eg, quinidine, procainamide) or Class III (eg, amiodarone, sotalol) antiarrhythmic medications, antipsychotic medications (eg, chlorpromazine, thioridazine), antibiotics (eg, gatifloxacin, moxifloxacin), or any other class of medications known to prolong the QTc interval. Paliperidone should also be avoided in patients with congenital long QT syndrome and in patients with a history of cardiac arrhythmias).
No products indexed under this heading.

Haloperidol Lactate (Paliperidone causes a modest increase in the corrected QT (QTc) interval. The use of paliperidone should be avoided in combination with other drugs that are known to prolong QTc including Class 1A (eg, quinidine, procainamide) or Class III (eg, amiodarone, sotalol) antiarrhythmic medications, antipsychotic medications (eg, chlorpromazine, thioridazine), antibiotics (eg, gatifloxacin, moxifloxacin), or any other class of medications known to prolong the QTc interval. Paliperidone should also be avoided in patients with congenital long QT syndrome and in patients with a history of cardiac arrhythmias).
No products indexed under this heading.

Hydralazine Hydrochloride (Because of its potential for inducing orthostatic hypotension, an additive effect may be observed when paliperidone is administered with other therapeutic agents that have this potential).
No products indexed under this heading.

Hydrochlorothiazide (Because of its potential for inducing orthostatic hypotension, an additive effect may be observed when paliperidone is administered with other therapeutic agents that have this potential). Products include:
Atacand HCT 700
Avalide 2956
Benicar HCT 1017
Diovan HCT 2419
Dyazide 1429
Exforge HCT 2449
Hyzaar 2162
Hyzaar 100-12.5 2162
Micardis HCT 889
Prinzide 2246
Tekturna HCT 2541
Teveten HCT 541

Hydrocodone Bitartrate (Given the primary CNS effects of paliperidone, paliperidone should be used with caution in combination with other centrally acting drugs and alcohol). Products include:
Vicodin 560
Vicodin ES 561
Vicodin HP 563
Vicoprofen 564
Zydone 1138

Hydrocodone Polistirex (Given the primary CNS effects of paliperidone, paliperidone should be used with caution in combination with other centrally acting drugs and alcohol). Products include:
Tussionex 3443

Hydroflumethiazide (Because of its potential for inducing orthostatic hypotension, an additive effect may be observed when paliperidone is administered with other therapeutic agents that have this potential).
No products indexed under this heading.

Hydromorphone Hydrochloride (Given the primary CNS effects of pali-

peridone, paliperidone should be used with caution in combination with other centrally acting drugs and alcohol). Products include:

Hydroxyamphetamine Hydrobromide (Given the primary CNS effects of paliperidone, paliperidone should be used with caution in combination with other centrally acting drugs and alcohol).

No products indexed under this heading.

Hydroxychloroquine Sulfate (Paliperidone is metabolized to a limited extent by CYP2D6. In an interaction study in healthy subjects in which a single 3 mg dose of paliperidone was administered concomitantly with 20 mg per day of paroxetine (a potent CYP2D6 inhibitor), paliperidone exposures were on average 16% (90% CI: 4, 30) higher in CYP2D6 extensive metabolizers. Higher doses of paroxetine have not been studied. The clinical relevance is unknown).

No products indexed under this heading.

Hydroxyzine Hydrochloride (Paliperidone causes a modest increase in the corrected QT (QTc) interval. The use of paliperidone should be avoided in combination with other drugs that are known to prolong QTc including Class 1A (eg, quinidine, procainamide) or Class III (eg, amiodarone, sotalol) antiarrhythmic medications, antipsychotic medications (eg, chlorpromazine, thioridazine), antibiotics (eg, gatifloxacin, moxifloxacin), or any other class of medications known to prolong the QTc interval. Paliperidone should also be avoided in patients with congenital long QT syndrome and in patients with a history of cardiac arrhythmias).

No products indexed under this heading.

Idarubicin Hydrochloride (Paliperidone causes a modest increase in the corrected QT (QTc) interval. The use of paliperidone should be avoided in combination with other drugs that are known to prolong QTc including antibiotics (eg, gatifloxacin, moxifloxacin), or any other class of medications known to prolong the QTc interval. Paliperidone should also be avoided in patients with congenital long QT syndrome and in patients with a history of cardiac arrhythmias).

No products indexed under this heading.

Imatinib Mesylate (Paliperidone is metabolized to a limited extent by CYP2D6. In an interaction study in healthy subjects in which a single 3 mg dose of paliperidone was administered concomitantly with 20 mg per day of paroxetine (a potent CYP2D6 inhibitor), paliperidone exposures were on average 16% (90% CI: 4, 30) higher in CYP2D6 extensive metabolizers. Higher doses of paroxetine have not been studied. The clinical relevance is unknown). Products include:

Imipenem (Paliperidone causes a modest increase in the corrected QT (QTc) interval. The use of paliperidone should be avoided in combination with other drugs that are known to prolong QTc including antibiotics (eg, gatifloxacin, moxifloxacin), or any other class of medications known to prolong the QTc interval. Paliperidone should also be avoided in patients with congenital long QT syndrome and in patients with a history of cardiac arrhythmias). Products include:

Imipramine Hydrochloride (Paliperidone causes a modest increase in the corrected QT (QTc) interval. The use of paliperidone should be avoided in com-

bination with other drugs that are known to prolong QTc including Class 1A (eg, quinidine, procainamide) or Class III (eg, amiodarone, sotalol) antiarrhythmic medications, antipsychotic medications (eg, chlorpromazine, thioridazine), antibiotics (eg, gatifloxacin, moxifloxacin), or any other class of medications known to prolong the QTc interval. Paliperidone should also be avoided in patients with congenital long QT syndrome and in patients with a history of cardiac arrhythmias).

No products indexed under this heading.

Imipramine Pamoate (Paliperidone causes a modest increase in the corrected QT (QTc) interval. The use of paliperidone should be avoided in combination with other drugs that are known to prolong QTc including Class 1A (eg, quinidine, procainamide) or Class III (eg, amiodarone, sotalol) antiarrhythmic medications, antipsychotic medications (eg, chlorpromazine, thioridazine), antibiotics (eg, gatifloxacin, moxifloxacin), or any other class of medications known to prolong the QTc interval. Paliperidone should also be avoided in patients with congenital long QT syndrome and in patients with a history of cardiac arrhythmias).

No products indexed under this heading.

Indapamide (Because of its potential for inducing orthostatic hypotension, an additive effect may be observed when paliperidone is administered with other therapeutic agents that have this potential). Products include:

Irbesartan (Because of its potential for inducing orthostatic hypotension, an additive effect may be observed when paliperidone is administered with other therapeutic agents that have this potential). Products include:

Isocarboxazid (Paliperidone causes a modest increase in the corrected QT (QTc) interval. The use of paliperidone should be avoided in combination with other drugs that are known to prolong QTc including Class 1A (eg, quinidine, procainamide) or Class III (eg, amiodarone, sotalol) antiarrhythmic medications, antipsychotic medications (eg, chlorpromazine, thioridazine), antibiotics (eg, gatifloxacin, moxifloxacin), or any other class of medications known to prolong the QTc interval. Paliperidone should also be avoided in patients with congenital long QT syndrome and in patients with a history of cardiac arrhythmias). Products include:

Isoflurane (Given the primary CNS effects of paliperidone, paliperidone should be used with caution in combination with other centrally acting drugs and alcohol).

No products indexed under this heading.

Isradipine (Because of its potential for inducing orthostatic hypotension, an additive effect may be observed when paliperidone is administered with other therapeutic agents that have this potential). Products include:

Kanamycin Sulfate (Paliperidone causes a modest increase in the corrected QT (QTc) interval. The use of paliperidone should be avoided in combination with other drugs that are known to prolong QTc including antibiotics (eg, gatifloxacin, moxifloxacin), or any other class of medications known to prolong the QTc interval. Paliperidone should also be avoided in patients with congenital long QT syndrome and in patients with a history of cardiac arrhythmias).

No products indexed under this heading.

Ketamine Hydrochloride (Given the primary CNS effects of paliperidone, paliperidone should be used with caution in combination with other centrally acting drugs and alcohol).

No products indexed under this heading.

Labetalol Hydrochloride (Because of its potential for inducing orthostatic hypotension, an additive effect may be observed when paliperidone is administered with other therapeutic agents that have this potential).

No products indexed under this heading.

Levodopa (Given the primary CNS effects of paliperidone, paliperidone should be used with caution in combination with other centrally acting drugs and alcohol. Paliperidone may antagonize the effect of levodopa and other dopamine agonists). Products include:

Levofloxacin (Paliperidone causes a modest increase in the corrected QT (QTc) interval. The use of paliperidone should be avoided in combination with other drugs that are known to prolong QTc including antibiotics (eg, gatifloxacin, moxifloxacin), or any other class of medications known to prolong the QTc interval. Paliperidone should also be avoided in patients with congenital long QT syndrome and in patients with a history of cardiac arrhythmias). Products include:

Levomethadyl Acetate Hydrochloride (Given the primary CNS effects of paliperidone, paliperidone should be used with caution in combination with other centrally acting drugs and alcohol).

No products indexed under this heading.

Levorphanol Tartrate (Given the primary CNS effects of paliperidone, paliperidone should be used with caution in combination with other centrally acting drugs and alcohol).

No products indexed under this heading.

Lidocaine (Paliperidone causes a modest increase in the corrected QT (QTc) interval. The use of paliperidone should be avoided in combination with other drugs that are known to prolong QTc including Class 1A (eg, quinidine, procainamide) or Class III (eg, amiodarone, sotalol) antiarrhythmic medications, antipsychotic medications (eg, chlorpromazine, thioridazine), antibiotics (eg, gatifloxacin, moxifloxacin), or any other class of medications known to prolong the QTc interval. Paliperidone should also be avoided in patients with congenital long QT syndrome and in patients with a history of cardiac arrhythmias). Products include:

Lidocaine Hydrochloride (Paliperidone causes a modest increase in the corrected QT (QTc) interval. The use of paliperidone should be avoided in combination with other drugs that are known to prolong QTc including Class 1A (eg, quinidine, procainamide) or Class III (eg, amiodarone, sotalol) antiarrhythmic medications, antipsychotic medications (eg, chlorpromazine, thioridazine), antibiotics (eg, gatifloxacin, moxifloxacin), or any other class of medications known to prolong the QTc interval. Paliperidone should also be avoided in patients with congenital long QT syndrome and in patients with a history of cardiac arrhythmias).

No products indexed under this heading.

Lisdexamfetamine Dimesylate (Given the primary CNS effects of paliperidone, paliperidone should be used

with caution in combination with other centrally acting drugs and alcohol). Products include:

Lisinopril (Because of its potential for inducing orthostatic hypotension, an additive effect may be observed when paliperidone is administered with other therapeutic agents that have this potential). Products include:

Lithium (Paliperidone causes a modest increase in the corrected QT (QTc) interval. The use of paliperidone should be avoided in combination with other drugs that are known to prolong QTc including antipsychotic medications (eg, chlorpromazine, thioridazine) or any other class of medications known to prolong the QTc interval. Paliperidone should also be avoided in patients with congenital long QT syndrome and in patients with a history of cardiac arrhythmias).

No products indexed under this heading.

Lithium Carbonate (Paliperidone causes a modest increase in the corrected QT (QTc) interval. The use of paliperidone should be avoided in combination with other drugs that are known to prolong QTc including Class 1A (eg, quinidine, procainamide) or Class III (eg, amiodarone, sotalol) antiarrhythmic medications, antipsychotic medications (eg, chlorpromazine, thioridazine), antibiotics (eg, gatifloxacin, moxifloxacin), or any other class of medications known to prolong the QTc interval. Paliperidone should also be avoided in patients with congenital long QT syndrome and in patients with a history of cardiac arrhythmias).

No products indexed under this heading.

Lithium Citrate (Paliperidone causes a modest increase in the corrected QT (QTc) interval. The use of paliperidone should be avoided in combination with other drugs that are known to prolong QTc including Class 1A (eg, quinidine, procainamide) or Class III (eg, amiodarone, sotalol) antiarrhythmic medications, antipsychotic medications (eg, chlorpromazine, thioridazine), antibiotics (eg, gatifloxacin, moxifloxacin), or any other class of medications known to prolong the QTc interval. Paliperidone should also be avoided in patients with congenital long QT syndrome and in patients with a history of cardiac arrhythmias).

No products indexed under this heading.

Lomefloxacin Hydrochloride (Paliperidone causes a modest increase in the corrected QT (QTc) interval. The use of paliperidone should be avoided in combination with other drugs that are known to prolong QTc including antibiotics (eg, gatifloxacin, moxifloxacin), or any other class of medications known to prolong the QTc interval. Paliperidone should also be avoided in patients with congenital long QT syndrome and in patients with a history of cardiac arrhythmias).

No products indexed under this heading.

Loracarbef (Paliperidone causes a modest increase in the corrected QT (QTc) interval. The use of paliperidone should be avoided in combination with other drugs that are known to prolong QTc including antibiotics (eg, gatifloxacin, moxifloxacin), or any other class of medications known to prolong the QTc interval. Paliperidone should also be avoided in patients with congenital long QT syndrome and in patients with a history of cardiac arrhythmias).

No products indexed under this heading.

Lorazepam (Paliperidone causes a modest increase in the corrected QT (QTc) interval. The use of paliperidone should be avoided in combination with

other drugs that are known to prolong QTc including Class 1A (eg, quinidine, procainamide) or Class III (eg, amiodarone, sotalol) antiarrhythmic medications, antipsychotic medications (eg, chlorpromazine, thioridazine), antibiotics (eg, gatifloxacin, moxifloxacin), or any other class of medications known to prolong the QTc interval. Paliperidone should also be avoided in patients with congenital long QT syndrome and in patients with a history of cardiac arrhythmias).
No products indexed under this heading.

Losartan Potassium (Because of its potential for inducing orthostatic hypotension, an additive effect may be observed when paliperidone is administered with other therapeutic agents that have this potential). Products include:
Cozaar ... **2106**
Hyzaar ... **2162**
Hyzaar 100-12.5 ... **2162**

Loxapine Hydrochloride (Paliperidone causes a modest increase in the corrected QT (QTc) interval. The use of paliperidone should be avoided in combination with other drugs that are known to prolong QTc including Class 1A (eg, quinidine, procainamide) or Class III (eg, amiodarone, sotalol) antiarrhythmic medications, antipsychotic medications (eg, chlorpromazine, thioridazine), antibiotics (eg, gatifloxacin, moxifloxacin), or any other class of medications known to prolong the QTc interval. Paliperidone should also be avoided in patients with congenital long QT syndrome and in patients with a history of cardiac arrhythmias).
No products indexed under this heading.

Loxapine Succinate (Paliperidone causes a modest increase in the corrected QT (QTc) interval. The use of paliperidone should be avoided in combination with other drugs that are known to prolong QTc including Class 1A (eg, quinidine, procainamide) or Class III (eg, amiodarone, sotalol) antiarrhythmic medications, antipsychotic medications (eg, chlorpromazine, thioridazine), antibiotics (eg, gatifloxacin, moxifloxacin), or any other class of medications known to prolong the QTc interval. Paliperidone should also be avoided in patients with congenital long QT syndrome and in patients with a history of cardiac arrhythmias).
No products indexed under this heading.

Maprotiline Hydrochloride (Paliperidone causes a modest increase in the corrected QT (QTc) interval. The use of paliperidone should be avoided in combination with other drugs that are known to prolong QTc including Class 1A (eg, quinidine, procainamide) or Class III (eg, amiodarone, sotalol) antiarrhythmic medications, antipsychotic medications (eg, chlorpromazine, thioridazine), antibiotics (eg, gatifloxacin, moxifloxacin), or any other class of medications known to prolong the QTc interval. Paliperidone should also be avoided in patients with congenital long QT syndrome and in patients with a history of cardiac arrhythmias).
No products indexed under this heading.

Mecamylamine Hydrochloride (Because of its potential for inducing orthostatic hypotension, an additive effect may be observed when paliperidone is administered with other therapeutic agents that have this potential).
No products indexed under this heading.

Meperidine Hydrochloride (Given the primary CNS effects of paliperidone, paliperidone should be used with caution in combination with other centrally acting drugs and alcohol).
No products indexed under this heading.

Mephobarbital (Given the primary CNS effects of paliperidone, paliperidone should be used with caution in combination with other centrally acting drugs and alcohol).
No products indexed under this heading.

Meprobamate (Paliperidone causes a modest increase in the corrected QT (QTc) interval. The use of paliperidone should be avoided in combination with other drugs that are known to prolong QTc including Class 1A (eg, quinidine, procainamide) or Class III (eg, amiodarone, sotalol) antiarrhythmic medications, antipsychotic medications (eg, chlorpromazine, thioridazine), antibiotics (eg, gatifloxacin, moxifloxacin), or any other class of medications known to prolong the QTc interval. Paliperidone should also be avoided in patients with congenital long QT syndrome and in patients with a history of cardiac arrhythmias).
No products indexed under this heading.

Mesoridazine Besylate (Paliperidone causes a modest increase in the corrected QT (QTc) interval. The use of paliperidone should be avoided in combination with other drugs that are known to prolong QTc including Class 1A (eg, quinidine, procainamide) or Class III (eg, amiodarone, sotalol) antiarrhythmic medications, antipsychotic medications (eg, chlorpromazine, thioridazine), antibiotics (eg, gatifloxacin, moxifloxacin), or any other class of medications known to prolong the QTc interval. Paliperidone should also be avoided in patients with congenital long QT syndrome and in patients with a history of cardiac arrhythmias).
No products indexed under this heading.

Methacycline Hydrochloride (Paliperidone causes a modest increase in the corrected QT (QTc) interval. The use of paliperidone should be avoided in combination with other drugs that are known to prolong QTc including antibiotics (eg, gatifloxacin, moxifloxacin), or any other class of medications known to prolong the QTc interval. Paliperidone should also be avoided in patients with congenital long QT syndrome and in patients with a history of cardiac arrhythmias).
No products indexed under this heading.

Methadone Hydrochloride (Given the primary CNS effects of paliperidone, paliperidone should be used with caution in combination with other centrally acting drugs and alcohol).
No products indexed under this heading.

Methamphetamine Hydrochloride (Given the primary CNS effects of paliperidone, paliperidone should be used with caution in combination with other centrally acting drugs and alcohol).
No products indexed under this heading.

Methicillin Sodium (Paliperidone causes a modest increase in the corrected QT (QTc) interval. The use of paliperidone should be avoided in combination with other drugs that are known to prolong QTc including antibiotics (eg, gatifloxacin, moxifloxacin), or any other class of medications known to prolong the QTc interval. Paliperidone should also be avoided in patients with congenital long QT syndrome and in patients with a history of cardiac arrhythmias).
No products indexed under this heading.

Methohexital Sodium (Given the primary CNS effects of paliperidone, paliperidone should be used with caution in combination with other centrally acting drugs and alcohol).
No products indexed under this heading.

Methotrimeprazine (Given the primary CNS effects of paliperidone, paliperidone should be used with caution in combination with other centrally acting drugs and alcohol).
No products indexed under this heading.

Methoxyflurane (Given the primary CNS effects of paliperidone, paliperidone should be used with caution in combination with other centrally acting drugs and alcohol).
No products indexed under this heading.

Methyclothiazide (Because of its potential for inducing orthostatic hypotension, an additive effect may be observed when paliperidone is administered with other therapeutic agents that have this potential).
No products indexed under this heading.

Methyldopa (Because of its potential for inducing orthostatic hypotension, an additive effect may be observed when paliperidone is administered with other therapeutic agents that have this potential).
No products indexed under this heading.

Methyldopate Hydrochloride (Because of its potential for inducing orthostatic hypotension, an additive effect may be observed when paliperidone is administered with other therapeutic agents that have this potential).
No products indexed under this heading.

Methylphenidate (Given the primary CNS effects of paliperidone, paliperidone should be used with caution in combination with other centrally acting drugs and alcohol). Products include:
Daytrana ... **3283**

Methylphenidate Hydrochloride (Given the primary CNS effects of paliperidone, paliperidone should be used with caution in combination with other centrally acting drugs and alcohol). Products include:
Concerta ... **2598**
Metadate CD ... **3439**

Metolazone (Because of its potential for inducing orthostatic hypotension, an additive effect may be observed when paliperidone is administered with other therapeutic agents that have this potential).
No products indexed under this heading.

Metoprolol Succinate (Because of its potential for inducing orthostatic hypotension, an additive effect may be observed when paliperidone is administered with other therapeutic agents that have this potential). Products include:
Toprol XL ... **732**

Metoprolol Tartrate (Because of its potential for inducing orthostatic hypotension, an additive effect may be observed when paliperidone is administered with other therapeutic agents that have this potential).
No products indexed under this heading.

Metyrosine (Because of its potential for inducing orthostatic hypotension, an additive effect may be observed when paliperidone is administered with other therapeutic agents that have this potential).
No products indexed under this heading.

Mexiletine Hydrochloride (Paliperidone causes a modest increase in the corrected QT (QTc) interval. The use of paliperidone should be avoided in combination with other drugs that are known to prolong QTc including Class 1A (eg, quinidine, procainamide) or Class III (eg, amiodarone, sotalol) antiarrhythmic medications, antipsychotic medications (eg, chlorpromazine, thioridazine), antibiotics (eg, gatifloxacin, moxifloxacin), or any other class of medications known to prolong the QTc interval. Paliperidone should also be avoided in patients with congenital long QT syndrome and in patients with a history of cardiac arrhythmias).
No products indexed under this heading.

Mezlocillin Sodium (Paliperidone causes a modest increase in the corrected QT (QTc) interval. The use of paliperidone should be avoided in combination with other drugs that are known to prolong QTc including antibiotics (eg, gatifloxacin, moxifloxacin), or any other class of medications known to prolong the QTc interval. Paliperidone should also be avoided in patients with congenital long QT syndrome and in patients with a history of cardiac arrhythmias).
No products indexed under this heading.

Mibefradil Dihydrochloride (Because of its potential for inducing orthostatic hypotension, an additive effect may be observed when paliperidone is administered with other therapeutic agents that have this potential).
No products indexed under this heading.

Midazolam Hydrochloride (Paliperidone causes a modest increase in the corrected QT (QTc) interval. The use of paliperidone should be avoided in combination with other drugs that are known to prolong QTc including Class 1A (eg, quinidine, procainamide) or Class III (eg, amiodarone, sotalol) antiarrhythmic medications, antipsychotic medications (eg, chlorpromazine, thioridazine), antibiotics (eg, gatifloxacin, moxifloxacin), or any other class of medications known to prolong the QTc interval. Paliperidone should also be avoided in patients with congenital long QT syndrome and in patients with a history of cardiac arrhythmias).
No products indexed under this heading.

Minocycline Hydrochloride (Paliperidone causes a modest increase in the corrected QT (QTc) interval. The use of paliperidone should be avoided in combination with other drugs that are known to prolong QTc including antibiotics (eg, gatifloxacin, moxifloxacin), or any other class of medications known to prolong the QTc interval. Paliperidone should also be avoided in patients with congenital long QT syndrome and in patients with a history of cardiac arrhythmias). Products include:
Solodyn ... **2073**

Minoxidil (Because of its potential for inducing orthostatic hypotension, an additive effect may be observed when paliperidone is administered with other therapeutic agents that have this potential).
No products indexed under this heading.

Moclobemide (Because of its potential for inducing orthostatic hypotension, an additive effect may be observed when paliperidone is administered with other therapeutic agents that have this potential).
No products indexed under this heading.

Moexipril Hydrochloride (Because of its potential for inducing orthostatic hypotension, an additive effect may be observed when paliperidone is administered with other therapeutic agents that have this potential).
No products indexed under this heading.

Molindone Hydrochloride (Paliperidone causes a modest increase in the corrected QT (QTc) interval. The use of paliperidone should be avoided in combination with other drugs that are known to prolong QTc including Class 1A (eg, quinidine, procainamide) or Class III (eg, amiodarone, sotalol) antiarrhythmic medications, antipsychotic medications (eg, chlorpromazine, thioridazine), antibiotics (eg, gatifloxacin, moxifloxacin), or any other class of medications known to prolong the QTc interval. Paliperidone should also be avoided in patients with congenital long QT syn-

IMPORTANT NOTE: Always consult each drug listing in the patient's regimen for possible interactions.

drome and in patients with a history of cardiac arrhythmias). Products include:

Moban 1108

Moricizine Hydrochloride (Paliperidone causes a modest increase in the corrected QT (QTc) interval. The use of paliperidone should be avoided in combination with other drugs that are known to prolong QTc including Class 1A (eg, quinidine, procainamide) or any other class of medications known to prolong the QTc interval. Paliperidone should also be avoided in patients with congenital long QT syndrome and in patients with a history of cardiac arrhythmias).
No products indexed under this heading.

Morphine Sulfate (Given the primary CNS effects of paliperidone, paliperidone should be used with caution in combination with other centrally acting drugs and alcohol). Products include:

Avinza 1822
Embeda 1831
MS Contin 2803

Moxifloxacin Hydrochloride (Paliperidone causes a modest increase in the corrected QT (QTc) interval. The use of paliperidone should be avoided in combination with other drugs that are known to prolong QTc including antibiotics (eg, gatifloxacin, moxifloxacin), or any other class of medications known to prolong the QTc interval. Paliperidone should also be avoided in patients with congenital long QT syndrome and in patients with a history of cardiac arrhythmias). Products include:

Avelox 3064
Vigamox 589

Nadolol (Because of its potential for inducing orthostatic hypotension, an additive effect may be observed when paliperidone is administered with other therapeutic agents that have this potential). Products include:

Nadolol 2359

Nafcillin Sodium (Paliperidone causes a modest increase in the corrected QT (QTc) interval. The use of paliperidone should be avoided in combination with other drugs that are known to prolong QTc including antibiotics (eg, gatifloxacin, moxifloxacin), or any other class of medications known to prolong the QTc interval. Paliperidone should also be avoided in patients with congenital long QT syndrome and in patients with a history of cardiac arrhythmias).
No products indexed under this heading.

Naphazoline Hydrochloride (Because of its potential for inducing orthostatic hypotension, an additive effect may be observed when paliperidone is administered with other therapeutic agents that have this potential). Products include:

Visine-A .... ⊙ 257

Nebivolol (Because of its potential for inducing orthostatic hypotension, an additive effect may be observed when paliperidone is administered with other therapeutic agents that have this potential). Products include:

Bystolic 1147

Nicardipine Hydrochloride (Because of its potential for inducing orthostatic hypotension, an additive effect may be observed when paliperidone is administered with other therapeutic agents that have this potential).
No products indexed under this heading.

Nifedipine (Because of its potential for inducing orthostatic hypotension, an additive effect may be observed when paliperidone is administered with other therapeutic agents that have this potential).
No products indexed under this heading.

Nisoldipine (Because of its potential for inducing orthostatic hypotension, an additive effect may be observed when paliperidone is administered with other therapeutic agents that have this potential).
No products indexed under this heading.

Nitroglycerin (Because of its potential for inducing orthostatic hypotension, an additive effect may be observed when paliperidone is administered with other therapeutic agents that have this potential). Products include:

Nitro-Dur 3170
Nitrolingual 3266

Norfloxacin (Paliperidone causes a modest increase in the corrected QT (QTc) interval. The use of paliperidone should be avoided in combination with other drugs that are known to prolong QTc including antibiotics (eg, gatifloxacin, moxifloxacin), or any other class of medications known to prolong the QTc interval. Paliperidone should also be avoided in patients with congenital long QT syndrome and in patients with a history of cardiac arrhythmias). Products include:

Noroxin 2220

Nortriptyline Hydrochloride (Paliperidone causes a modest increase in the corrected QT (QTc) interval. The use of paliperidone should be avoided in combination with other drugs that are known to prolong QTc including Class 1A (eg, quinidine, procainamide) or Class III (eg, amiodarone, sotalol) antiarrhythmic medications, antipsychotic medications (eg, chlorpromazine, thioridazine), antibiotics (eg, gatifloxacin, moxifloxacin), or any other class of medications known to prolong the QTc interval. Paliperidone should also be avoided in patients with congenital long QT syndrome and in patients with a history of cardiac arrhythmias).
No products indexed under this heading.

Ofloxacin (Paliperidone causes a modest increase in the corrected QT (QTc) interval. The use of paliperidone should be avoided in combination with other drugs that are known to prolong QTc including antibiotics (eg, gatifloxacin, moxifloxacin), or any other class of medications known to prolong the QTc interval. Paliperidone should also be avoided in patients with congenital long QT syndrome and in patients with a history of cardiac arrhythmias).
No products indexed under this heading.

Olanzapine (Paliperidone causes a modest increase in the corrected QT (QTc) interval. The use of paliperidone should be avoided in combination with other drugs that are known to prolong QTc including Class 1A (eg, quinidine, procainamide) or Class III (eg, amiodarone, sotalol) antiarrhythmic medications, antipsychotic medications (eg, chlorpromazine, thioridazine), antibiotics (eg, gatifloxacin, moxifloxacin), or any other class of medications known to prolong the QTc interval. Paliperidone should also be avoided in patients with congenital long QT syndrome and in patients with a history of cardiac arrhythmias). Products include:

Symbyax 1965
Zyprexa 1984
Zyprexa IntraMuscular 1984
Zyprexa ZYDIS 1984

Oxacillin (Paliperidone causes a modest increase in the corrected QT (QTc) interval. The use of paliperidone should be avoided in combination with other drugs that are known to prolong QTc including antibiotics (eg, gatifloxacin, moxifloxacin), or any other class of medications known to prolong the QTc interval. Paliperidone should also be avoided in patients with congenital long QT syndrome and in patients with a history of cardiac arrhythmias).
No products indexed under this heading.

Oxacillin Sodium (Paliperidone causes a modest increase in the corrected QT (QTc) interval. The use of paliperidone should be avoided in combination with other drugs that are known to prolong QTc including antibiotics (eg, gatifloxacin, moxifloxacin), or any other class of medications known to prolong the QTc interval. Paliperidone should also be avoided in patients with congenital long QT syndrome and in patients with a history of cardiac arrhythmias).
No products indexed under this heading.

Oxazepam (Paliperidone causes a modest increase in the corrected QT (QTc) interval. The use of paliperidone should be avoided in combination with other drugs that are known to prolong QTc including Class 1A (eg, quinidine, procainamide) or Class III (eg, amiodarone, sotalol) antiarrhythmic medications, antipsychotic medications (eg, chlorpromazine, thioridazine), antibiotics (eg, gatifloxacin, moxifloxacin), or any other class of medications known to prolong the QTc interval. Paliperidone should also be avoided in patients with congenital long QT syndrome and in patients with a history of cardiac arrhythmias).
No products indexed under this heading.

Oxycodone Hydrochloride (Given the primary CNS effects of paliperidone, paliperidone should be used with caution in combination with other centrally acting drugs and alcohol). Products include:

OxyContin 2807
Percocet 1121
Percodan 1124

Oxymetazoline Hydrochloride (Because of its potential for inducing orthostatic hypotension, an additive effect may be observed when paliperidone is administered with other therapeutic agents that have this potential). Products include:

Sudafed OM Sinus Congestion 2048

Oxytetracycline Hydrochloride (Paliperidone causes a modest increase in the corrected QT (QTc) interval. The use of paliperidone should be avoided in combination with other drugs that are known to prolong QTc including antibiotics (eg, gatifloxacin, moxifloxacin), or any other class of medications known to prolong the QTc interval. Paliperidone should also be avoided in patients with congenital long QT syndrome and in patients with a history of cardiac arrhythmias).
No products indexed under this heading.

Pargyline Hydrochloride (Because of its potential for inducing orthostatic hypotension, an additive effect may be observed when paliperidone is administered with other therapeutic agents that have this potential).
No products indexed under this heading.

Paroxetine (Paliperidone is metabolized to a limited extent by CYP2D6. In an interaction study in healthy subjects in which a single 3 mg dose of paliperidone was administered concomitantly with 20 mg per day of paroxetine (a potent CYP2D6 inhibitor), paliperidone exposures were on average 16% (90% CI: 4, 30) higher in CYP2D6 extensive metabolizers. Higher doses of paroxetine have not been studied. The clinical relevance is unknown).
No products indexed under this heading.

Paroxetine Hydrochloride (Paliperidone is metabolized to a limited extent by CYP2D6. In an interaction study in healthy subjects in which a single 3 mg dose of paliperidone was administered concomitantly with 20 mg per day of paroxetine (a potent CYP2D6 inhibitor), paliperidone exposures were on average 16% (90% CI: 4, 30) higher in CYP2D6 extensive metabolizers. Higher doses of paroxetine have not been studied. The clinical relevance is unknown). Products include:

Paroxetine CR 2361
Paroxetine ER 2371
Paxil 1586
Paxil CR 1596

Paroxetine Mesylate (Paliperidone is metabolized to a limited extent by CYP2D6. In an interaction study in healthy subjects in which a single 3 mg dose of paliperidone was administered concomitantly with 20 mg per day of paroxetine (a potent CYP2D6 inhibitor), paliperidone exposures were on average 16% (90% CI: 4, 30) higher in CYP2D6 extensive metabolizers. Higher doses of paroxetine have not been studied. The clinical relevance is unknown).
No products indexed under this heading.

Pemoline (Given the primary CNS effects of paliperidone, paliperidone should be used with caution in combination with other centrally acting drugs and alcohol).
No products indexed under this heading.

Penbutolol Sulfate (Because of its potential for inducing orthostatic hypotension, an additive effect may be observed when paliperidone is administered with other therapeutic agents that have this potential).
No products indexed under this heading.

Penicillin, Potassium Phenoxymethyl (Paliperidone causes a modest increase in the corrected QT (QTc) interval. The use of paliperidone should be avoided in combination with other drugs that are known to prolong QTc including antibiotics (eg, gatifloxacin, moxifloxacin), or any other class of medications known to prolong the QTc interval. Paliperidone should also be avoided in patients with congenital long QT syndrome and in patients with a history of cardiac arrhythmias).
No products indexed under this heading.

Penicillin G Benzathine (Paliperidone causes a modest increase in the corrected QT (QTc) interval. The use of paliperidone should be avoided in combination with other drugs that are known to prolong QTc including antibiotics (eg, gatifloxacin, moxifloxacin), or any other class of medications known to prolong the QTc interval. Paliperidone should also be avoided in patients with congenital long QT syndrome and in patients with a history of cardiac arrhythmias). Products include:

Bicillin C-R Injectable Suspension 1826
Bicillin L-A 1828

Penicillin G Dibenzylethyenediamine (Paliperidone causes a modest increase in the corrected QT (QTc) interval. The use of paliperidone should be avoided in combination with other drugs that are known to prolong QTc including antibiotics (eg, gatifloxacin, moxifloxacin), or any other class of medications known to prolong the QTc interval. Paliperidone should also be avoided in patients with congenital long QT syndrome and in patients with a history of cardiac arrhythmias).
No products indexed under this heading.

Penicillin G Potassium (Paliperidone causes a modest increase in the corrected QT (QTc) interval. The use of paliperidone should be avoided in combination with other drugs that are known to prolong QTc including antibiotics (eg, gatifloxacin, moxifloxacin), or any other class of medications known to prolong the QTc interval. Paliperidone should also be avoided in patients with congenital long QT syndrome and in patients with a history of cardiac arrhythmias).
No products indexed under this heading.

903 **Interactions Index** **Invega**

Penicillin G Procaine (Paliperidone causes a modest increase in the corrected QT (QTc) interval. The use of paliperidone should be avoided in combination with other drugs that are known to prolong QTc including antibiotics (eg, gatifloxacin, moxifloxacin), or any other class of medications known to prolong the QTc interval. Paliperidone should also be avoided in patients with congenital long QT syndrome and in patients with a history of cardiac arrhythmias). Products include:

Bicillin C-R Injectable Suspension 1826
Bicillin L-A 1828

Penicillin G Sodium (Paliperidone causes a modest increase in the corrected QT (QTc) interval. The use of paliperidone should be avoided in combination with other drugs that are known to prolong QTc including antibiotics (eg, gatifloxacin, moxifloxacin), or any other class of medications known to prolong the QTc interval. Paliperidone should also be avoided in patients with congenital long QT syndrome and in patients with a history of cardiac arrhythmias).

No products indexed under this heading.

Penicillin V (Paliperidone causes a modest increase in the corrected QT (QTc) interval. The use of paliperidone should be avoided in combination with other drugs that are known to prolong QTc including antibiotics (eg, gatifloxacin, moxifloxacin), or any other class of medications known to prolong the QTc interval. Paliperidone should also be avoided in patients with congenital long QT syndrome and in patients with a history of cardiac arrhythmias).

No products indexed under this heading.

Penicillin V Potassium (Paliperidone causes a modest increase in the corrected QT (QTc) interval. The use of paliperidone should be avoided in combination with other drugs that are known to prolong QTc including antibiotics (eg, gatifloxacin, moxifloxacin), or any other class of medications known to prolong the QTc interval. Paliperidone should also be avoided in patients with congenital long QT syndrome and in patients with a history of cardiac arrhythmias).

No products indexed under this heading.

Penicillins (Paliperidone causes a modest increase in the corrected QT (QTc) interval. The use of paliperidone should be avoided in combination with other drugs that are known to prolong QTc including antibiotics (eg, gatifloxacin, moxifloxacin), or any other class of medications known to prolong the QTc interval. Paliperidone should also be avoided in patients with congenital long QT syndrome and in patients with a history of cardiac arrhythmias).

No products indexed under this heading.

Pentobarbital Sodium (Given the primary CNS effects of paliperidone, paliperidone should be used with caution in combination with other centrally acting drugs and alcohol). Products include:

Nembutal 2012

Pergolide Mesylate (Given the primary CNS effects of paliperidone, paliperidone should be used with caution in combination with other centrally acting drugs and alcohol. Paliperidone may antagonize the effect of levodopa and other dopamine agonists).

No products indexed under this heading.

Perindopril Erbumine (Because of its potential for inducing orthostatic hypotension, an additive effect may be observed when paliperidone is administered with other therapeutic agents that have this potential).

No products indexed under this heading.

Perphenazine (Paliperidone causes a modest increase in the corrected QT (QTc) interval. The use of paliperidone should be avoided in combination with other drugs that are known to prolong QTc including Class 1A (eg, quinidine, procainamide) or Class III (eg, amiodarone, sotalol) antiarrhythmic medications, antipsychotic medications (eg, chlorpromazine, thioridazine), antibiotics (eg, gatifloxacin, moxifloxacin), or any other class of medications known to prolong the QTc interval. Paliperidone should also be avoided in patients with congenital long QT syndrome and in patients with a history of cardiac arrhythmias).

No products indexed under this heading.

Phenelzine Sulfate (Paliperidone causes a modest increase in the corrected QT (QTc) interval. The use of paliperidone should be avoided in combination with other drugs that are known to prolong QTc including Class 1A (eg, quinidine, procainamide) or Class III (eg, amiodarone, sotalol) antiarrhythmic medications, antipsychotic medications (eg, chlorpromazine, thioridazine), antibiotics (eg, gatifloxacin, moxifloxacin), or any other class of medications known to prolong the QTc interval. Paliperidone should also be avoided in patients with congenital long QT syndrome and in patients with a history of cardiac arrhythmias).

No products indexed under this heading.

Phenobarbital (Given the primary CNS effects of paliperidone, paliperidone should be used with caution in combination with other centrally acting drugs and alcohol). Products include:

Donnatal 2711

Phenobarbital Sodium (Given the primary CNS effects of paliperidone, paliperidone should be used with caution in combination with other centrally acting drugs and alcohol).

No products indexed under this heading.

Phenoxybenzamine Hydrochloride (Because of its potential for inducing orthostatic hypotension, an additive effect may be observed when paliperidone is administered with other therapeutic agents that have this potential). Products include:

Dibenzyline 3495

Phentolamine Mesylate (Because of its potential for inducing orthostatic hypotension, an additive effect may be observed when paliperidone is administered with other therapeutic agents that have this potential).

No products indexed under this heading.

Phenylephrine Hydrochloride (Because of its potential for inducing orthostatic hypotension, an additive effect may be observed when paliperidone is administered with other therapeutic agents that have this potential). Products include:

Sudafed PE Nasal Decongestant 2048
Children's Sudafed PE Nasal Decongestant 2047

Phenylpropanolamine Hydrochloride (Because of its potential for inducing orthostatic hypotension, an additive effect may be observed when paliperidone is administered with other therapeutic agents that have this potential).

No products indexed under this heading.

Pimozide (Paliperidone causes a modest increase in the corrected QT (QTc) interval. The use of paliperidone should be avoided in combination with other drugs that are known to prolong QTc including antipsychotic medications (eg, chlorpromazine, thioridazine) or any other class of medications known to prolong the QTc interval. Paliperidone should also be avoided in patients with congenital long QT syndrome and in patients with a history of cardiac arrhythmias).

No products indexed under this heading.

Pindolol (Because of its potential for inducing orthostatic hypotension, an additive effect may be observed when paliperidone is administered with other therapeutic agents that have this potential).

No products indexed under this heading.

Piperacillin Sodium (Paliperidone causes a modest increase in the corrected QT (QTc) interval. The use of paliperidone should be avoided in combination with other drugs that are known to prolong QTc including antibiotics (eg, gatifloxacin, moxifloxacin), or any other class of medications known to prolong the QTc interval. Paliperidone should also be avoided in patients with congenital long QT syndrome and in patients with a history of cardiac arrhythmias). Products include:

Zosyn 3607

Polythiazide (Because of its potential for inducing orthostatic hypotension, an additive effect may be observed when paliperidone is administered with other therapeutic agents that have this potential).

No products indexed under this heading.

Pramipexole Dihydrochloride (Given the primary CNS effects of paliperidone, paliperidone should be used with caution in combination with other centrally acting drugs and alcohol. Paliperidone may antagonize the effect of levodopa and other dopamine agonists).

No products indexed under this heading.

Prazepam (Paliperidone causes a modest increase in the corrected QT (QTc) interval. The use of paliperidone should be avoided in combination with other drugs that are known to prolong QTc including Class 1A (eg, quinidine, procainamide) or Class III (eg, amiodarone, sotalol) antiarrhythmic medications, antipsychotic medications (eg, chlorpromazine, thioridazine), antibiotics (eg, gatifloxacin, moxifloxacin), or any other class of medications known to prolong the QTc interval. Paliperidone should also be avoided in patients with congenital long QT syndrome and in patients with a history of cardiac arrhythmias).

No products indexed under this heading.

Prazosin Hydrochloride (Because of its potential for inducing orthostatic hypotension, an additive effect may be observed when paliperidone is administered with other therapeutic agents that have this potential).

No products indexed under this heading.

Procainamide (Paliperidone causes a modest increase in the corrected QT (QTc) interval. The use of paliperidone should be avoided in combination with other drugs that are known to prolong QTc including Class 1A (eg, quinidine, procainamide), or any other class of medications known to prolong the QTc interval. Paliperidone should also be avoided in patients with congenital long QT syndrome and in patients with a history of cardiac arrhythmias).

No products indexed under this heading.

Procainamide Hydrochloride (Paliperidone causes a modest increase in the corrected QT (QTc) interval. The use of paliperidone should be avoided in combination with other drugs that are known to prolong QTc including Class 1A (eg, quinidine, procainamide), or any other class of medications known to prolong the QTc interval. Paliperidone should also be avoided in patients with congenital long QT syndrome and in patients with a history of cardiac arrhythmias).

No products indexed under this heading.

Procarbazine Hydrochloride (Because of its potential for inducing orthostatic hypotension, an additive effect may be observed when paliperidone is administered with other therapeutic agents that have this potential).

No products indexed under this heading.

Prochlorperazine (Paliperidone causes a modest increase in the corrected QT (QTc) interval. The use of paliperidone should be avoided in combination with other drugs that are known to prolong QTc including Class 1A (eg, quinidine, procainamide) or Class III (eg, amiodarone, sotalol) antiarrhythmic medications, antipsychotic medications (eg, chlorpromazine, thioridazine), antibiotics (eg, gatifloxacin, moxifloxacin), or any other class of medications known to prolong the QTc interval. Paliperidone should also be avoided in patients with congenital long QT syndrome and in patients with a history of cardiac arrhythmias).

No products indexed under this heading.

Promethazine Hydrochloride (Paliperidone causes a modest increase in the corrected QT (QTc) interval. The use of paliperidone should be avoided in combination with other drugs that are known to prolong QTc including Class 1A (eg, quinidine, procainamide) or Class III (eg, amiodarone, sotalol) antiarrhythmic medications, antipsychotic medications (eg, chlorpromazine, thioridazine), antibiotics (eg, gatifloxacin, moxifloxacin), or any other class of medications known to prolong the QTc interval. Paliperidone should also be avoided in patients with congenital long QT syndrome and in patients with a history of cardiac arrhythmias).

No products indexed under this heading.

Propafenone Hydrochloride (Paliperidone causes a modest increase in the corrected QT (QTc) interval. The use of paliperidone should be avoided in combination with other drugs that are known to prolong QTc including Class 1A (eg, quinidine, procainamide) or Class III (eg, amiodarone, sotalol) antiarrhythmic medications, antipsychotic medications (eg, chlorpromazine, thioridazine), antibiotics (eg, gatifloxacin, moxifloxacin), or any other class of medications known to prolong the QTc interval. Paliperidone should also be avoided in patients with congenital long QT syndrome and in patients with a history of cardiac arrhythmias). Products include:

Rythmol 1648
Rythmol SR 1652

Propofol (Given the primary CNS effects of paliperidone, paliperidone should be used with caution in combination with other centrally acting drugs and alcohol).

No products indexed under this heading.

Propoxyphene Hydrochloride (Given the primary CNS effects of paliperidone, paliperidone should be used with caution in combination with other centrally acting drugs and alcohol).

No products indexed under this heading.

Propoxyphene Napsylate (Given the primary CNS effects of paliperidone, paliperidone should be used with caution in combination with other centrally acting drugs and alcohol).

No products indexed under this heading.

Propranolol Hydrochloride (Because of its potential for inducing orthostatic hypotension, an additive effect may be observed when paliperidone is administered with other therapeutic agents that have this potential). Products include:

InnoPran XL 1517

Protriptyline Hydrochloride (Paliperidone causes a modest increase in the corrected QT (QTc) interval. The use

Invega Interactions Index 904

of paliperidone should be avoided in combination with other drugs that are known to prolong QTc including Class 1A (eg, quinidine, procainamide) or Class III (eg, amiodarone, sotalol) antiarrhythmic medications, antipsychotic medications (eg, chlorpromazine, thioridazine), antibiotics (eg, gatifloxacin, moxifloxacin), or any other class of medications known to prolong the QTc interval. Paliperidone should also be avoided in patients with congenital long QT syndrome and in patients with a history of cardiac arrhythmias).
No products indexed under this heading.

Pseudoephedrine Hydrochloride (Because of its potential for inducing orthostatic hypotension, an additive effect may be observed when paliperidone is administered with other therapeutic agents that have this potential). Products include:
Allegra-D 2915
Allegra-D 24 2918
Sudafed 12 Hour Nasal Decongestant Non-Drowsy 2048
Sudafed 24 Hour 2048
Sudafed Nasal Decongestant 2047
Children's Sudafed Nasal Decongestant Liquid 2047
Zyrtec-D Allergy & Congestion 2054

Quazepam (Given the primary CNS effects of paliperidone, paliperidone should be used with caution in combination with other centrally acting drugs and alcohol).
No products indexed under this heading.

Quetiapine Fumarate (Paliperidone causes a modest increase in the corrected QT (QTc) interval. The use of paliperidone should be avoided in combination with other drugs that are known to prolong QTc including Class 1A (eg, quinidine, procainamide) or Class III (eg, amiodarone, sotalol) antiarrhythmic medications, antipsychotic medications (eg, chlorpromazine, thioridazine), antibiotics (eg, gatifloxacin, moxifloxacin), or any other class of medications known to prolong the QTc interval. Paliperidone should also be avoided in patients with congenital long QT syndrome and in patients with a history of cardiac arrhythmias). Products include:
Seroquel 750
Seroquel XR 759

Quinacrine Hydrochloride (Paliperidone is metabolized to a limited extent by CYP2D6. In an interaction study in healthy subjects in which a single 3 mg dose of paliperidone was administered concomitantly with 20 mg per day of paroxetine (a potent CYP2D6 inhibitor), paliperidone exposures were on average 16% (90% CI: 4, 30) higher in CYP2D6 extensive metabolizers. Higher doses of paroxetine have not been studied. The clinical relevance is unknown).
No products indexed under this heading.

Quinapril Hydrochloride (Because of its potential for inducing orthostatic hypotension, an additive effect may be observed when paliperidone is administered with other therapeutic agents that have this potential).
No products indexed under this heading.

Quinidine (Paliperidone causes a modest increase in the corrected QT (QTc) interval. The use of paliperidone should be avoided in combination with other drugs that are known to prolong QTc including Class 1A (eg, quinidine, procainamide) or Class III (eg, amiodarone, sotalol) antiarrhythmic medications, antipsychotic medications (eg, chlorpromazine, thioridazine), antibiotics (eg, gatifloxacin, moxifloxacin), or any other class of medications known to prolong the QTc interval. Paliperidone should also be avoided in patients with congenital long QT syndrome and in patients with a history of cardiac arrhythmias).
No products indexed under this heading.

Quinidine Gluconate (Paliperidone causes a modest increase in the corrected QT (QTc) interval. The use of paliperidone should be avoided in combination with other drugs that are known to prolong QTc including Class 1A (eg, quinidine, procainamide) or Class III (eg, amiodarone, sotalol) antiarrhythmic medications, antipsychotic medications (eg, chlorpromazine, thioridazine), antibiotics (eg, gatifloxacin, moxifloxacin), or any other class of medications known to prolong the QTc interval. Paliperidone should also be avoided in patients with congenital long QT syndrome and in patients with a history of cardiac arrhythmias).
No products indexed under this heading.

Quinidine Hydrochloride (Paliperidone causes a modest increase in the corrected QT (QTc) interval. The use of paliperidone should be avoided in combination with other drugs that are known to prolong QTc including Class 1A (eg, quinidine, procainamide) or Class III (eg, amiodarone, sotalol) antiarrhythmic medications, antipsychotic medications (eg, chlorpromazine, thioridazine), antibiotics (eg, gatifloxacin, moxifloxacin), or any other class of medications known to prolong the QTc interval. Paliperidone should also be avoided in patients with congenital long QT syndrome and in patients with a history of cardiac arrhythmias).
No products indexed under this heading.

Quinidine Polygalacturonate (Paliperidone causes a modest increase in the corrected QT (QTc) interval. The use of paliperidone should be avoided in combination with other drugs that are known to prolong QTc including Class 1A (eg, quinidine, procainamide) or Class III (eg, amiodarone, sotalol) antiarrhythmic medications, antipsychotic medications (eg, chlorpromazine, thioridazine), antibiotics (eg, gatifloxacin, moxifloxacin), or any other class of medications known to prolong the QTc interval. Paliperidone should also be avoided in patients with congenital long QT syndrome and in patients with a history of cardiac arrhythmias).
No products indexed under this heading.

Quinidine Sulfate (Paliperidone causes a modest increase in the corrected QT (QTc) interval. The use of paliperidone should be avoided in combination with other drugs that are known to prolong QTc including Class 1A (eg, quinidine, procainamide) or Class III (eg, amiodarone, sotalol) antiarrhythmic medications, antipsychotic medications (eg, chlorpromazine, thioridazine), antibiotics (eg, gatifloxacin, moxifloxacin), or any other class of medications known to prolong the QTc interval. Paliperidone should also be avoided in patients with congenital long QT syndrome and in patients with a history of cardiac arrhythmias).
No products indexed under this heading.

Ramipril (Because of its potential for inducing orthostatic hypotension, an additive effect may be observed when paliperidone is administered with other therapeutic agents that have this potential).
No products indexed under this heading.

Ranitidine Bismuth Citrate (Paliperidone is metabolized to a limited extent by CYP2D6. In an interaction study in healthy subjects in which a single 3 mg dose of paliperidone was administered concomitantly with 20 mg per day of paroxetine (a potent CYP2D6 inhibitor), paliperidone exposures were on average 16% (90% CI: 4, 30) higher in CYP2D6 extensive metabolizers. Higher doses of paroxetine have not been studied. The clinical relevance is unknown).
No products indexed under this heading.

Ranitidine Hydrochloride (Paliperidone is metabolized to a limited extent by CYP2D6. In an interaction study in healthy subjects in which a single 3 mg dose of paliperidone was administered concomitantly with 20 mg per day of paroxetine (a potent CYP2D6 inhibitor), paliperidone exposures were on average 16% (90% CI: 4, 30) higher in CYP2D6 extensive metabolizers. Higher doses of paroxetine have not been studied. The clinical relevance is unknown). Products include:
Zantac 1737
Zantac Injection 1732
Zantac Pharmacy 1735

Rasagiline Mesylate (Because of its potential for inducing orthostatic hypotension, an additive effect may be observed when paliperidone is administered with other therapeutic agents that have this potential). Products include:
Azilect 3383

Rauwolfia Serpentina (Because of its potential for inducing orthostatic hypotension, an additive effect may be observed when paliperidone is administered with other therapeutic agents that have this potential).
No products indexed under this heading.

Remifentanil Hydrochloride (Given the primary CNS effects of paliperidone, paliperidone should be used with caution in combination with other centrally acting drugs and alcohol).
No products indexed under this heading.

Rescinnamine (Because of its potential for inducing orthostatic hypotension, an additive effect may be observed when paliperidone is administered with other therapeutic agents that have this potential).
No products indexed under this heading.

Reserpine (Because of its potential for inducing orthostatic hypotension, an additive effect may be observed when paliperidone is administered with other therapeutic agents that have this potential).
No products indexed under this heading.

Risperidone (Concomitant use of paliperidone with risperidone has not been studied. Since paliperidone is the major active metabolite of risperidone, consideration should be given to the additive paliperidone exposure if risperidone is co-administered with paliperidone). Products include:
Risperdal Consta 2682

Ritonavir (Paliperidone is metabolized to a limited extent by CYP2D6. In an interaction study in healthy subjects in which a single 3 mg dose of paliperidone was administered concomitantly with 20 mg per day of paroxetine (a potent CYP2D6 inhibitor), paliperidone exposures were on average 16% (90% CI: 4, 30) higher in CYP2D6 extensive metabolizers. Higher doses of paroxetine have not been studied. The clinical relevance is unknown). Products include:
Kaletra 458
Norvir 509

Ropinirole Hydrochloride (Given the primary CNS effects of paliperidone, paliperidone should be used with caution in combination with other centrally acting drugs and alcohol. Paliperidone may antagonize the effect of levodopa and other dopamine agonists). Products include:
Requip 1620
Requip XL 1628

Secobarbital Sodium (Given the primary CNS effects of paliperidone, paliperidone should be used with caution in combination with other centrally acting drugs and alcohol).
No products indexed under this heading.

Selegiline (Because of its potential for inducing orthostatic hypotension, an additive effect may be observed when paliperidone is administered with other therapeutic agents that have this potential). Products include:
Emsam 3623

Selegiline Hydrochloride (Because of its potential for inducing orthostatic hypotension, an additive effect may be observed when paliperidone is administered with other therapeutic agents that have this potential). Products include:
Eldepryl 3312

Sertraline Hydrochloride (Paliperidone is metabolized to a limited extent by CYP2D6. In an interaction study in healthy subjects in which a single 3 mg dose of paliperidone was administered concomitantly with 20 mg per day of paroxetine (a potent CYP2D6 inhibitor), paliperidone exposures were on average 16% (90% CI: 4, 30) higher in CYP2D6 extensive metabolizers. Higher doses of paroxetine have not been studied. The clinical relevance is unknown).
No products indexed under this heading.

Sevoflurane (Given the primary CNS effects of paliperidone, paliperidone should be used with caution in combination with other centrally acting drugs and alcohol). Products include:
Ultane 554

Sildenafil Citrate (Paliperidone is metabolized to a limited extent by CYP2D6. In an interaction study in healthy subjects in which a single 3 mg dose of paliperidone was administered concomitantly with 20 mg per day of paroxetine (a potent CYP2D6 inhibitor), paliperidone exposures were on average 16% (90% CI: 4, 30) higher in CYP2D6 extensive metabolizers. Higher doses of paroxetine have not been studied. The clinical relevance is unknown).
No products indexed under this heading.

Sodium Cloxacillin Monohydrate (Paliperidone causes a modest increase in the corrected QT (QTc) interval. The use of paliperidone should be avoided in combination with other drugs that are known to prolong QTc including antibiotics (eg, gatifloxacin, moxifloxacin), or any other class of medications known to prolong the QTc interval. Paliperidone should also be avoided in patients with congenital long QT syndrome and in patients with a history of cardiac arrhythmias).
No products indexed under this heading.

Sodium Nitroprusside (Because of its potential for inducing orthostatic hypotension, an additive effect may be observed when paliperidone is administered with other therapeutic agents that have this potential).
No products indexed under this heading.

Sodium Oxybate (Given the primary CNS effects of paliperidone, paliperidone should be used with caution in combination with other centrally acting drugs and alcohol).
No products indexed under this heading.

Sotalol Hydrochloride (Paliperidone causes a modest increase in the corrected QT (QTc) interval. The use of paliperidone should be avoided in combination with other drugs that are known to prolong QTc including Class III (eg, amiodarone, sotalol) antiarrhythmic medications, or any other class of medications known to prolong the QTc interval. Paliperidone should also be avoided in patients with congenital long QT syndrome and in patients with a history of cardiac arrhythmias).
No products indexed under this heading.

Sparfloxacin (Paliperidone causes a modest increase in the corrected QT (QTc) interval. The use of paliperidone should be avoided in combination with other drugs that are known to prolong QTc including antibiotics (eg, gatifloxacin, moxifloxacin), or any other class of

medications known to prolong the QTc interval. Paliperidone should also be avoided in patients with congenital long QT syndrome and in patients with a history of cardiac arrhythmias).
No products indexed under this heading.

Spirapril Hydrochloride (Because of its potential for inducing orthostatic hypotension, an additive effect may be observed when paliperidone is administered with other therapeutic agents that have this potential).
No products indexed under this heading.

Streptomycin Sulfate (Paliperidone causes a modest increase in the corrected QT (QTc) interval. The use of paliperidone should be avoided in combination with other drugs that are known to prolong QTc including antibiotics (eg, gatifloxacin, moxifloxacin), or any other class of medications known to prolong the QTc interval. Paliperidone should also be avoided in patients with congenital long QT syndrome and in patients with a history of cardiac arrhythmias).
No products indexed under this heading.

Sufentanil Citrate (Given the primary CNS effects of paliperidone, paliperidone should be used with caution in combination with other centrally acting drugs and alcohol).
No products indexed under this heading.

Sulfamethizole (Paliperidone causes a modest increase in the corrected QT (QTc) interval. The use of paliperidone should be avoided in combination with other drugs that are known to prolong QTc including antibiotics (eg, gatifloxacin, moxifloxacin), or any other class of medications known to prolong the QTc interval. Paliperidone should also be avoided in patients with congenital long QT syndrome and in patients with a history of cardiac arrhythmias).
No products indexed under this heading.

Sulfamethoxazole (Paliperidone causes a modest increase in the corrected QT (QTc) interval. The use of paliperidone should be avoided in combination with other drugs that are known to prolong QTc including antibiotics (eg, gatifloxacin, moxifloxacin), or any other class of medications known to prolong the QTc interval. Paliperidone should also be avoided in patients with congenital long QT syndrome and in patients with a history of cardiac arrhythmias).
No products indexed under this heading.

Sulfisoxazole Acetyl (Paliperidone causes a modest increase in the corrected QT (QTc) interval. The use of paliperidone should be avoided in combination with other drugs that are known to prolong QTc including antibiotics (eg, gatifloxacin, moxifloxacin), or any other class of medications known to prolong the QTc interval. Paliperidone should also be avoided in patients with congenital long QT syndrome and in patients with a history of cardiac arrhythmias).
No products indexed under this heading.

Sulfisoxazole Diolamine (Paliperidone causes a modest increase in the corrected QT (QTc) interval. The use of paliperidone should be avoided in combination with other drugs that are known to prolong QTc including antibiotics (eg, gatifloxacin, moxifloxacin), or any other class of medications known to prolong the QTc interval. Paliperidone should also be avoided in patients with congenital long QT syndrome and in patients with a history of cardiac arrhythmias).
No products indexed under this heading.

Tamsulosin Hydrochloride (Because of its potential for inducing orthostatic hypotension, an additive effect may be observed when paliperidone is administered with other therapeutic agents that have this potential).
No products indexed under this heading.

Telmisartan (Because of its potential for inducing orthostatic hypotension, an additive effect may be observed when paliperidone is administered with other therapeutic agents that have this potential). Products include:
Micardis **887**
Micardis HCT **889**

Temazepam (Given the primary CNS effects of paliperidone, paliperidone should be used with caution in combination with other centrally acting drugs and alcohol).
No products indexed under this heading.

Terazosin Hydrochloride (Because of its potential for inducing orthostatic hypotension, an additive effect may be observed when paliperidone is administered with other therapeutic agents that have this potential).
No products indexed under this heading.

Terbinafine Hydrochloride (Paliperidone is metabolized to a limited extent by CYP2D6. In an interaction study in healthy subjects in which a single 3 mg dose of paliperidone was administered concomitantly with 20 mg per day of paroxetine (a potent CYP2D6 inhibitor), paliperidone exposures were on average 16% (90% CI: 4, 30) higher in CYP2D6 extensive metabolizers. Higher doses of paroxetine have not been studied. The clinical relevance is unknown).
No products indexed under this heading.

Tetracycline Hydrochloride (Paliperidone causes a modest increase in the corrected QT (QTc) interval. The use of paliperidone should be avoided in combination with other drugs that are known to prolong QTc including antibiotics (eg, gatifloxacin, moxifloxacin), or any other class of medications known to prolong the QTc interval. Paliperidone should also be avoided in patients with congenital long QT syndrome and in patients with a history of cardiac arrhythmias). Products include:
Pylera **793**

Tetrahydrozoline Hydrochloride (Because of its potential for inducing orthostatic hypotension, an additive effect may be observed when paliperidone is administered with other therapeutic agents that have this potential).
No products indexed under this heading.

Thiamylal Sodium (Given the primary CNS effects of paliperidone, paliperidone should be used with caution in combination with other centrally acting drugs and alcohol).
No products indexed under this heading.

Thioridazine (Paliperidone causes a modest increase in the corrected QT (QTc) interval. The use of paliperidone should be avoided in combination with other drugs that are known to prolong QTc including antipsychotic medications (eg, chlorpromazine, thioridazine), or any other class of medications known to prolong the QTc interval. Paliperidone should also be avoided in patients with congenital long QT syndrome and in patients with a history of cardiac arrhythmias).
No products indexed under this heading.

Thioridazine Hydrochloride (Paliperidone causes a modest increase in the corrected QT (QTc) interval. The use of paliperidone should be avoided in combination with other drugs that are known to prolong QTc including antipsychotic medications (eg, chlorpromazine, thioridazine), or any other class of medications known to prolong the QTc interval. Paliperidone should also be avoided in patients with congenital long QT syndrome and in patients with a history of cardiac arrhythmias). Products include:
Thioridazine Hydrochloride **2384**

Thiothixene (Paliperidone causes a modest increase in the corrected QT (QTc) interval. The use of paliperidone should be avoided in combination with other drugs that are known to prolong QTc including Class 1A (eg, quinidine, procainamide) or Class III (eg, amiodarone, sotalol) antiarrhythmic medications, antipsychotic medications (eg, chlorpromazine, thioridazine), antibiotics (eg, gatifloxacin, moxifloxacin), or any other class of medications known to prolong the QTc interval. Paliperidone should also be avoided in patients with congenital long QT syndrome and in patients with a history of cardiac arrhythmias). Products include:
Thiothixene **2386**

Ticarcillin Disodium (Paliperidone causes a modest increase in the corrected QT (QTc) interval. The use of paliperidone should be avoided in combination with other drugs that are known to prolong QTc including antibiotics (eg, gatifloxacin, moxifloxacin), or any other class of medications known to prolong the QTc interval. Paliperidone should also be avoided in patients with congenital long QT syndrome and in patients with a history of cardiac arrhythmias). Products include:
Timentin ADD-Vantage **1670**
Timentin Galaxy **1674**
Timentin **1666**
Timentin Pharmacy **1678**

Timolol Maleate (Because of its potential for inducing orthostatic hypotension, an additive effect may be observed when paliperidone is administered with other therapeutic agents that have this potential). Products include:
Combigan **601**
Dorzolamide Hydrochloride/Timolol Maleate Ophthalmic Solution .... ⊙**243**
Timoptic in Ocudose .... ⊙**231**

Tobramycin (Paliperidone causes a modest increase in the corrected QT (QTc) interval. The use of paliperidone should be avoided in combination with other drugs that are known to prolong QTc including antibiotics (eg, gatifloxacin, moxifloxacin), or any other class of medications known to prolong the QTc interval. Paliperidone should also be avoided in patients with congenital long QT syndrome and in patients with a history of cardiac arrhythmias). Products include:
Tobi Nebulizer **2546**
Tobramycin and Dexamethasone Ophthalmic Suspension .... ⊙**251**
Zylet .... ⊙**252**

Tobramycin Sulfate (Paliperidone causes a modest increase in the corrected QT (QTc) interval. The use of paliperidone should be avoided in combination with other drugs that are known to prolong QTc including antibiotics (eg, gatifloxacin, moxifloxacin), or any other class of medications known to prolong the QTc interval. Paliperidone should also be avoided in patients with congenital long QT syndrome and in patients with a history of cardiac arrhythmias).
No products indexed under this heading.

Tocainide Hydrochloride (Paliperidone causes a modest increase in the corrected QT (QTc) interval. The use of paliperidone should be avoided in combination with other drugs that are known to prolong QTc including Class 1A (eg, quinidine, procainamide) or Class III (eg, amiodarone, sotalol) antiarrhythmic medications, antipsychotic medications (eg, chlorpromazine, thioridazine), antibiotics (eg, gatifloxacin, moxifloxacin), or any other class of medications known to prolong the QTc interval. Paliperidone should also be avoided in patients with congenital long QT syndrome and in patients with a history of cardiac arrhythmias).
No products indexed under this heading.

Torsemide (Because of its potential for inducing orthostatic hypotension, an additive effect may be observed when paliperidone is administered with other therapeutic agents that have this potential).
No products indexed under this heading.

Trandolapril (Because of its potential for inducing orthostatic hypotension, an additive effect may be observed when paliperidone is administered with other therapeutic agents that have this potential). Products include:
Mavik **489**
Tarka **534**

Tranylcypromine Sulfate (Paliperidone causes a modest increase in the corrected QT (QTc) interval. The use of paliperidone should be avoided in combination with other drugs that are known to prolong QTc including Class 1A (eg, quinidine, procainamide) or Class III (eg, amiodarone, sotalol) antiarrhythmic medications, antipsychotic medications (eg, chlorpromazine, thioridazine), antibiotics (eg, gatifloxacin, moxifloxacin), or any other class of medications known to prolong the QTc interval. Paliperidone should also be avoided in patients with congenital long QT syndrome and in patients with a history of cardiac arrhythmias). Products include:
Parnate **1584**

Triazolam (Given the primary CNS effects of paliperidone, paliperidone should be used with caution in combination with other centrally acting drugs and alcohol).
No products indexed under this heading.

Trifluoperazine Hydrochloride (Paliperidone causes a modest increase in the corrected QT (QTc) interval. The use of paliperidone should be avoided in combination with other drugs that are known to prolong QTc including Class 1A (eg, quinidine, procainamide) or Class III (eg, amiodarone, sotalol) antiarrhythmic medications, antipsychotic medications (eg, chlorpromazine, thioridazine), antibiotics (eg, gatifloxacin, moxifloxacin), or any other class of medications known to prolong the QTc interval. Paliperidone should also be avoided in patients with congenital long QT syndrome and in patients with a history of cardiac arrhythmias).
No products indexed under this heading.

Trimethaphan Camsylate (Because of its potential for inducing orthostatic hypotension, an additive effect may be observed when paliperidone is administered with other therapeutic agents that have this potential).
No products indexed under this heading.

Trimipramine Maleate (Paliperidone causes a modest increase in the corrected QT (QTc) interval. The use of paliperidone should be avoided in combination with other drugs that are known to prolong QTc including Class 1A (eg, quinidine, procainamide) or Class III (eg, amiodarone, sotalol) antiarrhythmic medications, antipsychotic medications (eg, chlorpromazine, thioridazine), antibiotics (eg, gatifloxacin, moxifloxacin), or any other class of medications known to prolong the QTc interval. Paliperidone should also be avoided in patients with congenital long QT syndrome and in patients with a history of cardiac arrhythmias).
No products indexed under this heading.

Troleandomycin (Paliperidone causes a modest increase in the corrected QT (QTc) interval. The use of paliperidone should be avoided in combination with other drugs that are known to prolong QTc including antibiotics (eg, gatifloxacin, moxifloxacin), or any other class of medications known to prolong the QTc interval. Paliperidone should also be

Invega Interactions Index 906

avoided in patients with congenital long QT syndrome and in patients with a history of cardiac arrhythmias).
No products indexed under this heading.

Trovafloxacin Mesylate (Paliperidone causes a modest increase in the corrected QT (QTc) interval. The use of paliperidone should be avoided in combination with other drugs that are known to prolong QTc including antibiotics (eg, gatifloxacin, moxifloxacin), or any other class of medications known to prolong the QTc interval. Paliperidone should also be avoided in patients with congenital long QT syndrome and in patients with a history of cardiac arrhythmias).
No products indexed under this heading.

Valsartan (Because of its potential for inducing orthostatic hypotension, an additive effect may be observed when paliperidone is administered with other therapeutic agents that have this potential). Products include:
Diovan **2413**
Diovan HCT **2419**
Exforge **2443**
Exforge HCT **2449**
Valturna **3637**

Vardenafil Hydrochloride (Paliperidone is metabolized to a limited extent by CYP2D6. In an interaction study in healthy subjects in which a single 3 mg dose of paliperidone was administered concomitantly with 20 mg per day of paroxetine (a potent CYP2D6 inhibitor), paliperidone exposures were on average 16% (90% CI: 4, 30) higher in CYP2D6 extensive metabolizers. Higher doses of paroxetine have not been studied. The clinical relevance is unknown). Products include:
Levitra **3157**

Verapamil Hydrochloride (Because of its potential for inducing orthostatic hypotension, an additive effect may be observed when paliperidone is administered with other therapeutic agents that have this potential). Products include:
Tarka **534**

Zaleplon (Given the primary CNS effects of paliperidone, paliperidone should be used with caution in combination with other centrally acting drugs and alcohol).
No products indexed under this heading.

Ziprasidone Hydrochloride (Paliperidone causes a modest increase in the corrected QT (QTc) interval. The use of paliperidone should be avoided in combination with other drugs that are known to prolong QTc including Class 1A (eg, quinidine, procainamide) or Class III (eg, amiodarone, sotalol) antiarrhythmic medications, antipsychotic medications (eg, chlorpromazine, thioridazine), antibiotics (eg, gatifloxacin, moxifloxacin), or any other class of medications known to prolong the QTc interval. Paliperidone should also be avoided in patients with congenital long QT syndrome and in patients with a history of cardiac arrhythmias). Products include:
Geodon **2723**

Zolpidem Tartrate (Given the primary CNS effects of paliperidone, paliperidone should be used with caution in combination with other centrally acting drugs and alcohol). Products include:
Ambien **2920**
Ambien CR **2925**

Food Interactions

Alcohol (Given the primary CNS effects of paliperidone, paliperidone should be used with caution in combination with other centrally acting drugs and alcohol).

Beer, reduced-alcohol (Given the primary CNS effects of paliperidone, paliperidone should be used with caution in combination with other centrally acting drugs and alcohol).

Beer, unspecified (Given the primary CNS effects of paliperidone, paliperidone should be used with caution in combination with other centrally acting drugs and alcohol).

Food, unspecified (Administration of a 12 mg paliperidone extended-release tablet to healthy ambulatory subjects with a standard high-fat/high-caloric meal gave mean C_{max} and AUC values of paliperidone that were increased by 60% and 54%, respectively, compared with administration under fasting conditions. Clinical trials establishing the safety and efficacy of paliperidone were carried out in subjects without regard to the timing of meals. While paliperidone can be taken without regard to food, the presence of food at the time of paliperidone administration may increase exposure to paliperidone).

Meal, unspecified (Administration of a 12 mg paliperidone extended-release tablet to healthy ambulatory subjects with a standard high-fat/high-caloric meal gave mean C_{max} and AUC values of paliperidone that were increased by 60% and 54%, respectively, compared with administration under fasting conditions. Clinical trials establishing the safety and efficacy of paliperidone were carried out in subjects without regard to the timing of meals. While paliperidone can be taken without regard to food, the presence of food at the time of paliperidone administration may increase exposure to paliperidone).

Wine, Chianti (Given the primary CNS effects of paliperidone, paliperidone should be used with caution in combination with other centrally acting drugs and alcohol).

Wine, Red (Given the primary CNS effects of paliperidone, paliperidone should be used with caution in combination with other centrally acting drugs and alcohol).

Wine, unspecified (Given the primary CNS effects of paliperidone, paliperidone should be used with caution in combination with other centrally acting drugs and alcohol).

Wine products (Given the primary CNS effects of paliperidone, paliperidone should be used with caution in combination with other centrally acting drugs and alcohol).

INVEGA SUSTENNA EXTENDED-RELEASE INJECTABLE SUSPENSION

(Paliperidone) **2621**
May interact with alcohols, antiarrhythmics, antibiotics, antihypertensives, antipsychotic agents, centrally-acting drugs, class I antiarrhythmics, class III antiarrhythmics, drugs that prolong the QT interval, quinidine, and certain other agents. Compounds in these categories include:

Acebutolol Hydrochloride (Paliperidone causes a modest increase in the corrected QT (QTc) interval. The use of paliperidone should be avoided in combination with drugs that are known to prolong QTc including Class 1A (eg, quinidine, procainamide) or Class III (eg, amiodarone, sotalol) antiarrhythmic medications or any other class of medications known to prolong QTc interval. Paliperidone should also be avoided in patients with congenital long QT syndrome and in patients with a history of cardiac arrhythmias).
No products indexed under this heading.

Adenosine (Paliperidone causes a modest increase in the corrected QT (QTc) interval. The use of paliperidone should be avoided in combination with drugs that are known to prolong QTc including Class 1A (eg, quinidine, procainamide) or Class III (eg, amiodarone, sotalol) antiarrhythmic medications or any other class of medications known to prolong QTc interval. Paliperidone should also be avoided in patients with congenital long QT syndrome and in patients with a history of cardiac arrhythmias). Products include:
Adenocard **656**
Adenoscan **657**

Alatrofloxacin Mesylate (Paliperidone causes a modest increase in the corrected QT (QTc) interval. The use of paliperidone should be avoided in combination with drugs that are known to prolong QTc including antibiotics (eg, gatifloxacin, moxifloxacin), or any other class of medications known to prolong QTc interval. Paliperidone should also be avoided in patients with congenital long QT syndrome and in patients with a history of cardiac arrhythmias).
No products indexed under this heading.

Alfentanil Hydrochloride (Given the primary CNS effects paliperidone should be used with caution in combination with other centrally acting drugs and alcohol. Paliperidone may antagonize the effect of levodopa and other dopamine antagonists).
No products indexed under this heading.

Aliskiren (Because of its potential for inducing orthostatic hypotension, an additive effect may be observed when paliperidone is administered with other therapeutic agents that have this potential). Products include:
Tekturna **2538**
Tekturna HCT **2541**
Valturna **3637**

Alprazolam (Given the primary CNS effects paliperidone should be used with caution in combination with other centrally acting drugs and alcohol. Paliperidone may antagonize the effect of levodopa and other dopamine antagonists).
No products indexed under this heading.

Amikacin Sulfate (Paliperidone causes a modest increase in the corrected QT (QTc) interval. The use of paliperidone should be avoided in combination with drugs that are known to prolong QTc including antibiotics (eg, gatifloxacin, moxifloxacin), or any other class of medications known to prolong QTc interval. Paliperidone should also be avoided in patients with congenital long QT syndrome and in patients with a history of cardiac arrhythmias).
No products indexed under this heading.

Amiodarone Hydrochloride (Paliperidone causes a modest increase in the corrected QT (QTc) interval. The use of paliperidone should be avoided in combination with drugs that are known to prolong QTc including Class 1A (eg, quinidine, procainamide) or Class III (eg, amiodarone, sotalol) antiarrhythmic medications, antipsychotic medications (eg, chlorpromazine, thioridazine), antibiotics (eg, gatifloxacin, moxifloxacin), or any other class of medications known to prolong QTc interval. Paliperidone should also be avoided in patients with congenital long QT syndrome and in patients with a history of cardiac arrhythmias).
No products indexed under this heading.

Amitriptyline Hydrochloride (Paliperidone causes a modest increase in the corrected QT (QTc) interval. The use of paliperidone should be avoided in combination with drugs that are known to prolong QTc including Class 1A (eg, quinidine, procainamide) or Class III (eg, amiodarone, sotalol) antiarrhythmic medications, antipsychotic medications (eg, chlorpromazine, thioridazine), antibiotics (eg, gatifloxacin, moxifloxacin), or any other class of medications known to prolong QTc interval. Paliperidone should also be avoided in patients with congenital long QT syndrome and in patients with a history of cardiac arrhythmias).
No products indexed under this heading.

Amlodipine Besylate (Because of its potential for inducing orthostatic hypotension, an additive effect may be observed when paliperidone is administered with other therapeutic agents that have this potential). Products include:
Azor **1010**
Exforge **2443**
Exforge HCT **2449**

Amoxapine (Paliperidone causes a modest increase in the corrected QT (QTc) interval. The use of paliperidone should be avoided in combination with drugs that are known to prolong QTc including Class 1A (eg, quinidine, procainamide) or Class III (eg, amiodarone, sotalol) antiarrhythmic medications, antipsychotic medications (eg, chlorpromazine, thioridazine), antibiotics (eg, gatifloxacin, moxifloxacin), or any other class of medications known to prolong QTc interval. Paliperidone should also be avoided in patients with congenital long QT syndrome and in patients with a history of cardiac arrhythmias).
No products indexed under this heading.

Amoxicillin (Paliperidone causes a modest increase in the corrected QT (QTc) interval. The use of paliperidone should be avoided in combination with drugs that are known to prolong QTc including antibiotics (eg, gatifloxacin, moxifloxacin), or any other class of medications known to prolong QTc interval. Paliperidone should also be avoided in patients with congenital long QT syndrome and in patients with a history of cardiac arrhythmias). Products include:
Amoxil Capsules **1311**
Amoxil Chewable Tablets **1311**
Amoxil **1311**
Amoxil Powder **1311**
Augmentin **1331**
Augmentin Tablets **1335**
Augmentin ES-600 .... **1338**
Augmentin XR **1342**
Moxatag **2321**

Amoxicillin Trihydrate (Paliperidone causes a modest increase in the corrected QT (QTc) interval. The use of paliperidone should be avoided in combination with drugs that are known to prolong QTc including antibiotics (eg, gatifloxacin, moxifloxacin), or any other class of medications known to prolong QTc interval. Paliperidone should also be avoided in patients with congenital long QT syndrome and in patients with a history of cardiac arrhythmias).
No products indexed under this heading.

Amphetamine Aspartate (Given the primary CNS effects paliperidone should be used with caution in combination with other centrally acting drugs and alcohol. Paliperidone may antagonize the effect of levodopa and other dopamine antagonists).
No products indexed under this heading.

Amphetamine Aspartate Monohydrate (Given the primary CNS effects paliperidone should be used with caution in combination with other centrally acting drugs and alcohol. Paliperidone may antagonize the effect of levodopa and other dopamine antagonists).
No products indexed under this heading.

Amphetamine Resins (Given the primary CNS effects paliperidone should be used with caution in combination with other centrally acting drugs and alcohol. Paliperidone may antagonize the effect of levodopa and other dopamine antagonists).
No products indexed under this heading.

Amphetamine Sulfate (Given the primary CNS effects paliperidone should be used with caution in combination with other centrally acting drugs and alcohol. Paliperidone may antagonize the effect of levodopa and other dopamine antagonists).
No products indexed under this heading.

Ampicillin (Paliperidone causes a modest increase in the corrected QT (QTc) interval. The use of paliperidone should be avoided in combination with drugs that are known to prolong QTc including antibiotics (eg, gatifloxacin, moxifloxacin), or any other class of medications known to prolong QTc interval. Paliperidone should also be avoided in patients with congenital long QT syndrome and in patients with a history of cardiac arrhythmias).
No products indexed under this heading.

Ampicillin Sodium (Paliperidone causes a modest increase in the corrected QT (QTc) interval. The use of paliperidone should be avoided in combination with drugs that are known to prolong QTc including antibiotics (eg, gatifloxacin, moxifloxacin), or any other class of medications known to prolong QTc interval. Paliperidone should also be avoided in patients with congenital long QT syndrome and in patients with a history of cardiac arrhythmias).
No products indexed under this heading.

Ampicillin Trihydrate (Paliperidone causes a modest increase in the corrected QT (QTc) interval. The use of paliperidone should be avoided in combination with drugs that are known to prolong QTc including antibiotics (eg, gatifloxacin, moxifloxacin), or any other class of medications known to prolong QTc interval. Paliperidone should also be avoided in patients with congenital long QT syndrome and in patients with a history of cardiac arrhythmias).
No products indexed under this heading.

Antibiotics, non-penicillin, unspecified (Paliperidone causes a modest increase in the corrected QT (QTc) interval. The use of paliperidone should be avoided in combination with drugs that are known to prolong QTc including antibiotics (eg, gatifloxacin, moxifloxacin), or any other class of medications known to prolong QTc interval. Paliperidone should also be avoided in patients with congenital long QT syndrome and in patients with a history of cardiac arrhythmias).
No products indexed under this heading.

Aprobarbital (Given the primary CNS effects paliperidone should be used with caution in combination with other centrally acting drugs and alcohol. Paliperidone may antagonize the effect of levodopa and other dopamine antagonists).
No products indexed under this heading.

Aripiprazole (Paliperidone causes a modest increase in the corrected QT (QTc) interval. The use of paliperidone should be avoided in combination with drugs that are known to prolong QTc including antipsychotic medications (eg, chlorpromazine, thioridazine) or any other class of medications known to prolong QTc interval. Paliperidone should also be avoided in patients with congenital long QT syndrome and in patients with a history of cardiac arrhythmias).
No products indexed under this heading.

Astemizole (Paliperidone causes a modest increase in the corrected QT (QTc) interval. The use of paliperidone should be avoided in combination with drugs that are known to prolong QTc including Class 1A (eg, quinidine, procainamide) or Class III (eg, amiodarone, sotalol) antiarrhythmic medications, antipsychotic medications (eg, chlorpromazine, thioridazine), antibiotics (eg, gatifloxacin, moxifloxacin), or any other class of medications known to prolong QTc interval. Paliperidone should also be avoided in patients with congenital long QT syndrome and in patients with a history of cardiac arrhythmias).
No products indexed under this heading.

Atenolol (Because of its potential for inducing orthostatic hypotension, an additive effect may be observed when paliperidone is administered with other therapeutic agents that have this potential).
No products indexed under this heading.

Azithromycin Dihydrate (Paliperidone causes a modest increase in the corrected QT (QTc) interval. The use of paliperidone should be avoided in combination with drugs that are known to prolong QTc including antibiotics (eg, gatifloxacin, moxifloxacin), or any other class of medications known to prolong QTc interval. Paliperidone should also be avoided in patients with congenital long QT syndrome and in patients with a history of cardiac arrhythmias).
No products indexed under this heading.

Azlocillin Sodium (Paliperidone causes a modest increase in the corrected QT (QTc) interval. The use of paliperidone should be avoided in combination with drugs that are known to prolong QTc including antibiotics (eg, gatifloxacin, moxifloxacin), or any other class of medications known to prolong QTc interval. Paliperidone should also be avoided in patients with congenital long QT syndrome and in patients with a history of cardiac arrhythmias).
No products indexed under this heading.

Aztreonam (Paliperidone causes a modest increase in the corrected QT (QTc) interval. The use of paliperidone should be avoided in combination with drugs that are known to prolong QTc including antibiotics (eg, gatifloxacin, moxifloxacin), or any other class of medications known to prolong QTc interval. Paliperidone should also be avoided in patients with congenital long QT syndrome and in patients with a history of cardiac arrhythmias).
No products indexed under this heading.

Bacampicillin Hydrochloride (Paliperidone causes a modest increase in the corrected QT (QTc) interval. The use of paliperidone should be avoided in combination with drugs that are known to prolong QTc including antibiotics (eg, gatifloxacin, moxifloxacin), or any other class of medications known to prolong QTc interval. Paliperidone should also be avoided in patients with congenital long QT syndrome and in patients with a history of cardiac arrhythmias).
No products indexed under this heading.

Benazepril Hydrochloride (Because of its potential for inducing orthostatic hypotension, an additive effect may be observed when paliperidone is administered with other therapeutic agents that have this potential).
No products indexed under this heading.

Bendroflumethiazide (Because of its potential for inducing orthostatic hypotension, an additive effect may be observed when paliperidone is administered with other therapeutic agents that have this potential).
No products indexed under this heading.

Betaxolol Hydrochloride (Because of its potential for inducing orthostatic hypotension, an additive effect may be observed when paliperidone is administered with other therapeutic agents that have this potential).
No products indexed under this heading.

Bisoprolol Fumarate (Because of its potential for inducing orthostatic hypotension, an additive effect may be observed when paliperidone is administered with other therapeutic agents that have this potential).
No products indexed under this heading.

Bretylium Tosylate (Paliperidone causes a modest increase in the corrected QT (QTc) interval. The use of paliperidone should be avoided in combination with drugs that are known to prolong QTc including Class 1A (eg, quinidine, procainamide) or Class III (eg, amiodarone, sotalol) antiarrhythmic medications, antipsychotic medications (eg, chlorpromazine, thioridazine), antibiotics (eg, gatifloxacin, moxifloxacin), or any other class of medications known to prolong QTc interval. Paliperidone should also be avoided in patients with congenital long QT syndrome and in patients with a history of cardiac arrhythmias).
No products indexed under this heading.

Buprenorphine Hydrochloride (Given the primary CNS effects paliperidone should be used with caution in combination with other centrally acting drugs and alcohol. Paliperidone may antagonize the effect of levodopa and other dopamine antagonists).
No products indexed under this heading.

Buspirone Hydrochloride (Given the primary CNS effects paliperidone should be used with caution in combination with other centrally acting drugs and alcohol. Paliperidone may antagonize the effect of levodopa and other dopamine antagonists).
No products indexed under this heading.

Butabarbital (Given the primary CNS effects paliperidone should be used with caution in combination with other centrally acting drugs and alcohol. Paliperidone may antagonize the effect of levodopa and other dopamine antagonists).
No products indexed under this heading.

Butalbital (Given the primary CNS effects paliperidone should be used with caution in combination with other centrally acting drugs and alcohol. Paliperidone may antagonize the effect of levodopa and other dopamine antagonists).
No products indexed under this heading.

Candesartan Cilexetil (Because of its potential for inducing orthostatic hypotension, an additive effect may be observed when paliperidone is administered with other therapeutic agents that have this potential). Products include:
Atacand **697**
Atacand HCT **700**

Captopril (Because of its potential for inducing orthostatic hypotension, an additive effect may be observed when paliperidone is administered with other therapeutic agents that have this potential). Products include:
Captopril **2341**

Carbamazepine (Co-administration of oral paliperidone extended release once daily with carbamazepine 200 mg twice daily caused a decrease of approximately 37% in the mean steady state C_{max} and AUC of paliperidone. This decrease is caused, to a substantial degree, by a 35% increase in renal clearance of paliperidone. A minor decrease in the amount of drug excreted unchanged in the urine suggests that there was a little effect on the CYP metabolism or bioavailability of paliperidone during carbamazepine co-administration. On initiation of carbamazepine, the dose of paliperidone should be re-evaluated and increased if necessary. Conversely, on discontinuation of carbamazepine, the dose of paliperidone should be re-evaluated and decreased if necessary). Products include:
Carbatrol **3280**
Equetro **3477**

Carbenicillin Disodium (Paliperidone causes a modest increase in the corrected QT (QTc) interval. The use of paliperidone should be avoided in combination with drugs that are known to prolong QTc including antibiotics (eg, gatifloxacin, moxifloxacin), or any other class of medications known to prolong QTc interval. Paliperidone should also be avoided in patients with congenital long QT syndrome and in patients with a history of cardiac arrhythmias).
No products indexed under this heading.

Carbenicillin Indanyl Sodium (Paliperidone causes a modest increase in the corrected QT (QTc) interval. The use of paliperidone should be avoided in combination with drugs that are known to prolong QTc including antibiotics (eg, gatifloxacin, moxifloxacin), or any other class of medications known to prolong QTc interval. Paliperidone should also be avoided in patients with congenital long QT syndrome and in patients with a history of cardiac arrhythmias).
No products indexed under this heading.

Carteolol Hydrochloride (Because of its potential for inducing orthostatic hypotension, an additive effect may be observed when paliperidone is administered with other therapeutic agents that have this potential).
No products indexed under this heading.

Carvedilol (Because of its potential for inducing orthostatic hypotension, an additive effect may be observed when paliperidone is administered with other therapeutic agents that have this potential). Products include:
Coreg **1409**

Carvedilol Phosphate (Because of its potential for inducing orthostatic hypotension, an additive effect may be observed when paliperidone is administered with other therapeutic agents that have this potential). Products include:
Coreg CR **1416**

Cefaclor (Paliperidone causes a modest increase in the corrected QT (QTc) interval. The use of paliperidone should be avoided in combination with drugs that are known to prolong QTc including antibiotics (eg, gatifloxacin, moxifloxacin), or any other class of medications known to prolong QTc interval. Paliperidone should also be avoided in patients with congenital long QT syndrome and in patients with a history of cardiac arrhythmias).
No products indexed under this heading.

Cefadroxil (Paliperidone causes a modest increase in the corrected QT (QTc) interval. The use of paliperidone should be avoided in combination with drugs that are known to prolong QTc including antibiotics (eg, gatifloxacin, moxifloxacin), or any other class of medications known to prolong QTc interval. Paliperidone should also be avoided in patients with congenital long QT syndrome and in patients with a history of cardiac arrhythmias).
No products indexed under this heading.

Cefamandole Nafate (Paliperidone causes a modest increase in the corrected QT (QTc) interval. The use of paliperidone should be avoided in combination with drugs that are known to prolong QTc including antibiotics (eg, gatifloxacin, moxifloxacin), or any other class of medications known to prolong QTc interval. Paliperidone should also be avoided in patients with congenital long QT syndrome and in patients with a history of cardiac arrhythmias).
No products indexed under this heading.

Chlorprothixene Lactate (Given the primary CNS effects paliperidone should be used with caution in combination with other centrally acting drugs and alcohol. Paliperidone may antagonize the effect of levodopa and other dopamine antagonists).

No products indexed under this heading.

Chlorthalidone (Because of its potential for inducing orthostatic hypotension, an additive effect may be observed when paliperidone is administered with other therapeutic agents that have this potential). Products include:

Cilastatin Sodium (Paliperidone causes a modest increase in the corrected QT (QTc) interval. The use of paliperidone should be avoided in combination with drugs that are known to prolong QTc including antibiotics (eg, gatifloxacin, moxifloxacin), or any other class of medications known to prolong QTc interval. Paliperidone should also be avoided in patients with congenital long QT syndrome and in patients with a history of cardiac arrhythmias). Products include:

Ciprofloxacin (Paliperidone causes a modest increase in the corrected QT (QTc) interval. The use of paliperidone should be avoided in combination with drugs that are known to prolong QTc including antibiotics (eg, gatifloxacin, moxifloxacin), or any other class of medications known to prolong QTc interval. Paliperidone should also be avoided in patients with congenital long QT syndrome and in patients with a history of cardiac arrhythmias). Products include:

Ciprofloxacin Hydrochloride (Paliperidone causes a modest increase in the corrected QT (QTc) interval. The use of paliperidone should be avoided in combination with drugs that are known to prolong QTc including antibiotics (eg, gatifloxacin, moxifloxacin), or any other class of medications known to prolong QTc interval. Paliperidone should also be avoided in patients with congenital long QT syndrome and in patients with a history of cardiac arrhythmias). Products include:

Clarithromycin (Paliperidone causes a modest increase in the corrected QT (QTc) interval. The use of paliperidone should be avoided in combination with drugs that are known to prolong QTc including antibiotics (eg, gatifloxacin, moxifloxacin), or any other class of medications known to prolong QTc interval. Paliperidone should also be avoided in patients with congenital long QT syndrome and in patients with a history of cardiac arrhythmias). Products include:

Clomipramine Hydrochloride (Paliperidone causes a modest increase in the corrected QT (QTc) interval. The use of paliperidone should be avoided in combination with drugs that are known to prolong QTc including Class 1A (eg, quinidine, procainamide) or Class III (eg, amiodarone, sotalol) antiarrhythmic medications, antipsychotic medications (eg, chlorpromazine, thioridazine), antibiotics (eg, gatifloxacin, moxifloxacin), or any other class of medications known to prolong QTc interval. Paliperidone should also be avoided in patients with congenital long QT syndrome and in patients with a history of cardiac arrhythmias).

No products indexed under this heading.

Clonidine (Because of its potential for inducing orthostatic hypotension, an additive effect may be observed when paliperidone is administered with other therapeutic agents that have this potential). Products include:

Clonidine Hydrochloride (Because of its potential for inducing orthostatic hypotension, an additive effect may be observed when paliperidone is administered with other therapeutic agents that have this potential). Products include:

Clorazepate Dipotassium (Given the primary CNS effects paliperidone should be used with caution in combination with other centrally acting drugs and alcohol. Paliperidone may antagonize the effect of levodopa and other dopamine antagonists).

No products indexed under this heading.

Clotrimazole (Paliperidone causes a modest increase in the corrected QT (QTc) interval. The use of paliperidone should be avoided in combination with drugs that are known to prolong QTc including antibiotics (eg, gatifloxacin, moxifloxacin), or any other class of medications known to prolong QTc interval. Paliperidone should also be avoided in patients with congenital long QT syndrome and in patients with a history of cardiac arrhythmias). Products include:

Cloxacillin (Paliperidone causes a modest increase in the corrected QT (QTc) interval. The use of paliperidone should be avoided in combination with drugs that are known to prolong QTc including antibiotics (eg, gatifloxacin, moxifloxacin), or any other class of medications known to prolong QTc interval. Paliperidone should also be avoided in patients with congenital long QT syndrome and in patients with a history of cardiac arrhythmias).

No products indexed under this heading.

Cloxacillin Sodium (Paliperidone causes a modest increase in the corrected QT (QTc) interval. The use of paliperidone should be avoided in combination with drugs that are known to prolong QTc including antibiotics (eg, gatifloxacin, moxifloxacin), or any other class of medications known to prolong QTc interval. Paliperidone should also be avoided in patients with congenital long QT syndrome and in patients with a history of cardiac arrhythmias).

No products indexed under this heading.

Cloxacillin Sodium Monohydrate (Paliperidone causes a modest increase in the corrected QT (QTc) interval. The use of paliperidone should be avoided in combination with drugs that are known to prolong QTc including antibiotics (eg, gatifloxacin, moxifloxacin), or any other class of medications known to prolong QTc interval. Paliperidone should also be avoided in patients with congenital long QT syndrome and in patients with a history of cardiac arrhythmias).

No products indexed under this heading.

Clozapine (Given the primary CNS effects paliperidone should be used with caution in combination with other centrally acting drugs and alcohol. Paliperidone may antagonize the effect of levodopa and other dopamine antagonists).

No products indexed under this heading.

Codeine Phosphate (Given the primary CNS effects paliperidone should be used with caution in combination with other centrally acting drugs and alcohol. Paliperidone may antagonize the effect of levodopa and other dopamine antagonists). Products include:

Codeine Sulfate (Given the primary CNS effects paliperidone should be used with caution in combination with other centrally acting drugs and alcohol. Paliperidone may antagonize the effect of levodopa and other dopamine antagonists).

No products indexed under this heading.

Daunorubicin Hydrochloride (Paliperidone causes a modest increase in the corrected QT (QTc) interval. The use of paliperidone should be avoided in combination with drugs that are known to prolong QTc including antibiotics (eg, gatifloxacin, moxifloxacin), or any other class of medications known to prolong QTc interval. Paliperidone should also be avoided in patients with congenital long QT syndrome and in patients with a history of cardiac arrhythmias).

No products indexed under this heading.

Demeclocycline Hydrochloride (Paliperidone causes a modest increase in the corrected QT (QTc) interval. The use of paliperidone should be avoided in combination with drugs that are known to prolong QTc including antibiotics (eg, gatifloxacin, moxifloxacin), or any other class of medications known to prolong QTc interval. Paliperidone should also be avoided in patients with congenital long QT syndrome and in patients with a history of cardiac arrhythmias).

No products indexed under this heading.

Deserpidine (Because of its potential for inducing orthostatic hypotension, an additive effect may be observed when paliperidone is administered with other therapeutic agents that have this potential).

No products indexed under this heading.

Desflurane (Given the primary CNS effects paliperidone should be used with caution in combination with other centrally acting drugs and alcohol. Paliperidone may antagonize the effect of levodopa and other dopamine antagonists).

No products indexed under this heading.

Desipramine Hydrochloride (Paliperidone causes a modest increase in the corrected QT (QTc) interval. The use of paliperidone should be avoided in combination with drugs that are known to prolong QTc including Class 1A (eg, quinidine, procainamide) or Class III (eg, amiodarone, sotalol) antiarrhythmic medications, antipsychotic medications (eg, chlorpromazine, thioridazine), antibiotics (eg, gatifloxacin, moxifloxacin), or any other class of medications known to prolong QTc interval. Paliperidone should also be avoided in patients with congenital long QT syndrome and in patients with a history of cardiac arrhythmias).

No products indexed under this heading.

Dexmethylphenidate Hydrochloride (Given the primary CNS effects paliperidone should be used with caution in combination with other centrally acting drugs and alcohol. Paliperidone may antagonize the effect of levodopa and other dopamine antagonists). Products include:

Dextroamphetamine (Given the primary CNS effects paliperidone should be used with caution in combination with other centrally acting drugs and alcohol. Paliperidone may antagonize the effect of levodopa and other dopamine antagonists).

No products indexed under this heading.

Dextroamphetamine Saccharate (Given the primary CNS effects paliperidone should be used with caution in combination with other centrally acting drugs and alcohol. Paliperidone may antagonize the effect of levodopa and other dopamine antagonists).

No products indexed under this heading.

Dextroamphetamine Sulfate (Given the primary CNS effects paliperidone should be used with caution in combination with other centrally acting drugs and alcohol. Paliperidone may antagonize the effect of levodopa and other dopamine antagonists). Products include:

Dezocine (Given the primary CNS effects paliperidone should be used with caution in combination with other centrally acting drugs and alcohol. Paliperidone may antagonize the effect of levodopa and other dopamine antagonists).

No products indexed under this heading.

Diazepam (Given the primary CNS effects paliperidone should be used with caution in combination with other centrally acting drugs and alcohol. Paliperidone may antagonize the effect of levodopa and other dopamine antagonists). Products include:

Diazoxide (Because of its potential for inducing orthostatic hypotension, an additive effect may be observed when paliperidone is administered with other therapeutic agents that have this potential). Products include:

Dicloxacillin (Paliperidone causes a modest increase in the corrected QT (QTc) interval. The use of paliperidone should be avoided in combination with drugs that are known to prolong QTc including antibiotics (eg, gatifloxacin, moxifloxacin), or any other class of medications known to prolong QTc interval. Paliperidone should also be avoided in patients with congenital long QT syndrome and in patients with a history of cardiac arrhythmias).

No products indexed under this heading.

Dicloxacillin Sodium (Paliperidone causes a modest increase in the corrected QT (QTc) interval. The use of paliperidone should be avoided in combination with drugs that are known to prolong QTc including antibiotics (eg, gatifloxacin, moxifloxacin), or any other class of medications known to prolong QTc interval. Paliperidone should also be avoided in patients with congenital long QT syndrome and in patients with a history of cardiac arrhythmias).

No products indexed under this heading.

Diltiazem Hydrochloride (Because of its potential for inducing orthostatic hypotension, an additive effect may be observed when paliperidone is administered with other therapeutic agents that have this potential). Products include:

Diltiazem Maleate (Because of its potential for inducing orthostatic hypotension, an additive effect may be observed when paliperidone is administered with other therapeutic agents that have this potential).

No products indexed under this heading.

Dirithromycin (Paliperidone causes a modest increase in the corrected QT (QTc) interval. The use of paliperidone should be avoided in combination with drugs that are known to prolong QTc including antibiotics (eg, gatifloxacin, moxifloxacin), or any other class of medications known to prolong QTc interval. Paliperidone should also be avoided in patients with congenital long QT syndrome and in patients with a history of cardiac arrhythmias).

No products indexed under this heading.

Disodium Carbenicillin (Paliperidone causes a modest increase in the corrected QT (QTc) interval. The use of paliperidone should be avoided in combination with drugs that are known to prolong QTc including antibiotics (eg,

---

IMPORTANT NOTE: Always consult each drug listing in the patient's regimen for possible interactions.

gatifloxacin, moxifloxacin), or any other class of medications known to prolong QTc interval. Paliperidone should also be avoided in patients with congenital long QT syndrome and in patients with a history of cardiac arrhythmias).
No products indexed under this heading.

Disopyramide (Paliperidone causes a modest increase in the corrected QT (QTc) interval. The use of paliperidone should be avoided in combination with drugs that are known to prolong QTc including Class 1A (eg, quinidine, procainamide) or Class III (eg, amiodarone, sotalol) antiarrhythmic medications, antipsychotic medications (eg, chlorpromazine, thioridazine), antibiotics (eg, gatifloxacin, moxifloxacin), or any other class of medications known to prolong QTc interval. Paliperidone should also be avoided in patients with congenital long QT syndrome and in patients with a history of cardiac arrhythmias).
No products indexed under this heading.

Disopyramide Phosphate (Paliperidone causes a modest increase in the corrected QT (QTc) interval. The use of paliperidone should be avoided in combination with drugs that are known to prolong QTc including Class 1A (eg, quinidine, procainamide) or Class III (eg, amiodarone, sotalol) antiarrhythmic medications, antipsychotic medications (eg, chlorpromazine, thioridazine), antibiotics (eg, gatifloxacin, moxifloxacin), or any other class of medications known to prolong QTc interval. Paliperidone should also be avoided in patients with congenital long QT syndrome and in patients with a history of cardiac arrhythmias).
No products indexed under this heading.

Divalproex Sodium (Coadministration of a single dose of an oral paliperidone extended release 12 mg tablet with divalproex sodium extended tablets (two 500 mg tablets once daily at steady state) resulted in an increase of approximately 50% in the C_{max} and AUC of paliperidone. Although this interaction has not been studied with paliperidone, a clinically significant interaction would not be expected between divalproex sodium and paliperidone intramuscular injection). Products include:
Depakote ER 426

Dofetilide (Paliperidone causes a modest increase in the corrected QT (QTc) interval. The use of paliperidone should be avoided in combination with drugs that are known to prolong QTc including Class 1A (eg, quinidine, procainamide) or Class III (eg, amiodarone, sotalol) antiarrhythmic medications, antipsychotic medications (eg, chlorpromazine, thioridazine), antibiotics (eg, gatifloxacin, moxifloxacin), or any other class of medications known to prolong QTc interval. Paliperidone should also be avoided in patients with congenital long QT syndrome and in patients with a history of cardiac arrhythmias).
No products indexed under this heading.

Doxazosin Mesylate (Because of its potential for inducing orthostatic hypotension, an additive effect may be observed when paliperidone is administered with other therapeutic agents that have this potential).
No products indexed under this heading.

Doxepin Hydrochloride (Paliperidone causes a modest increase in the corrected QT (QTc) interval. The use of paliperidone should be avoided in combination with drugs that are known to prolong QTc including Class 1A (eg, quinidine, procainamide) or Class III (eg, amiodarone, sotalol) antiarrhythmic medications, antipsychotic medications (eg, chlorpromazine, thioridazine), antibiotics (eg, gatifloxacin, moxifloxacin), or any other class of medications known to prolong QTc interval. Paliperidone should also be avoided in patients with congenital long QT syndrome and in patients with a history of cardiac arrhythmias).
No products indexed under this heading.

Doxycycline Calcium (Paliperidone causes a modest increase in the corrected QT (QTc) interval. The use of paliperidone should be avoided in combination with drugs that are known to prolong QTc including antibiotics (eg, gatifloxacin, moxifloxacin), or any other class of medications known to prolong QTc interval. Paliperidone should also be avoided in patients with congenital long QT syndrome and in patients with a history of cardiac arrhythmias).
No products indexed under this heading.

Doxycycline Hyclate (Paliperidone causes a modest increase in the corrected QT (QTc) interval. The use of paliperidone should be avoided in combination with drugs that are known to prolong QTc including antibiotics (eg, gatifloxacin, moxifloxacin), or any other class of medications known to prolong QTc interval. Paliperidone should also be avoided in patients with congenital long QT syndrome and in patients with a history of cardiac arrhythmias).
No products indexed under this heading.

Doxycycline Monohydrate (Paliperidone causes a modest increase in the corrected QT (QTc) interval. The use of paliperidone should be avoided in combination with drugs that are known to prolong QTc including antibiotics (eg, gatifloxacin, moxifloxacin), or any other class of medications known to prolong QTc interval. Paliperidone should also be avoided in patients with congenital long QT syndrome and in patients with a history of cardiac arrhythmias).
No products indexed under this heading.

Droperidol (Given the primary CNS effects paliperidone should be used with caution in combination with other centrally acting drugs and alcohol. Paliperidone may antagonize the effect of levodopa and other dopamine antagonists).
No products indexed under this heading.

Enalapril Maleate (Because of its potential for inducing orthostatic hypotension, an additive effect may be observed when paliperidone is administered with other therapeutic agents that have this potential).
No products indexed under this heading.

Enalaprilat (Because of its potential for inducing orthostatic hypotension, an additive effect may be observed when paliperidone is administered with other therapeutic agents that have this potential).
No products indexed under this heading.

Enflurane (Given the primary CNS effects paliperidone should be used with caution in combination with other centrally acting drugs and alcohol. Paliperidone may antagonize the effect of levodopa and other dopamine antagonists).
No products indexed under this heading.

Enoxacin (Paliperidone causes a modest increase in the corrected QT (QTc) interval. The use of paliperidone should be avoided in combination with drugs that are known to prolong QTc including antibiotics (eg, gatifloxacin, moxifloxacin), or any other class of medications known to prolong QTc interval. Paliperidone should also be avoided in patients with congenital long QT syndrome and in patients with a history of cardiac arrhythmias).
No products indexed under this heading.

Epirubicin Hydrochloride (Paliperidone causes a modest increase in the corrected QT (QTc) interval. The use of paliperidone should be avoided in combination with drugs that are known to prolong QTc including antibiotics (eg, gatifloxacin, moxifloxacin), or any other class of medications known to prolong QTc interval. Paliperidone should also be avoided in patients with congenital long QT syndrome and in patients with a history of cardiac arrhythmias).
No products indexed under this heading.

Eprosartan Mesylate (Because of its potential for inducing orthostatic hypotension, an additive effect may be observed when paliperidone is administered with other therapeutic agents that have this potential). Products include:
Teveten 538
Teveten HCT 541

Erythromycin (Paliperidone causes a modest increase in the corrected QT (QTc) interval. The use of paliperidone should be avoided in combination with drugs that are known to prolong QTc including Class 1A (eg, quinidine, procainamide) or Class III (eg, amiodarone, sotalol) antiarrhythmic medications, antipsychotic medications (eg, chlorpromazine, thioridazine), antibiotics (eg, gatifloxacin, moxifloxacin), or any other class of medications known to prolong QTc interval. Paliperidone should also be avoided in patients with congenital long QT syndrome and in patients with a history of cardiac arrhythmias).
No products indexed under this heading.

Erythromycin, Topical (Paliperidone causes a modest increase in the corrected QT (QTc) interval. The use of paliperidone should be avoided in combination with drugs that are known to prolong QTc including antibiotics (eg, gatifloxacin, moxifloxacin), or any other class of medications known to prolong QTc interval. Paliperidone should also be avoided in patients with congenital long QT syndrome and in patients with a history of cardiac arrhythmias).
No products indexed under this heading.

Erythromycin Estolate (Paliperidone causes a modest increase in the corrected QT (QTc) interval. The use of paliperidone should be avoided in combination with drugs that are known to prolong QTc including Class 1A (eg, quinidine, procainamide) or Class III (eg, amiodarone, sotalol) antiarrhythmic medications, antipsychotic medications (eg, chlorpromazine, thioridazine), antibiotics (eg, gatifloxacin, moxifloxacin), or any other class of medications known to prolong QTc interval. Paliperidone should also be avoided in patients with congenital long QT syndrome and in patients with a history of cardiac arrhythmias).
No products indexed under this heading.

Erythromycin Ethylsuccinate (Paliperidone causes a modest increase in the corrected QT (QTc) interval. The use of paliperidone should be avoided in combination with drugs that are known to prolong QTc including Class 1A (eg, quinidine, procainamide) or Class III (eg, amiodarone, sotalol) antiarrhythmic medications, antipsychotic medications (eg, chlorpromazine, thioridazine), antibiotics (eg, gatifloxacin, moxifloxacin), or any other class of medications known to prolong QTc interval. Paliperidone should also be avoided in patients with congenital long QT syndrome and in patients with a history of cardiac arrhythmias). Products include:
E.E.S. 437
EryPed 435

Erythromycin Gluceptate (Paliperidone causes a modest increase in the corrected QT (QTc) interval. The use of paliperidone should be avoided in combination with drugs that are known to prolong QTc including Class 1A (eg, quinidine, procainamide) or Class III (eg, amiodarone, sotalol) antiarrhythmic medications, antipsychotic medications (eg, chlorpromazine, thioridazine), antibiotics (eg, gatifloxacin, moxifloxacin), or any other class of medications known to prolong QTc interval. Paliperidone should also be avoided in patients with congenital long QT syndrome and in patients with a history of cardiac arrhythmias).
No products indexed under this heading.

Erythromycin Lactobionate (Paliperidone causes a modest increase in the corrected QT (QTc) interval. The use of paliperidone should be avoided in combination with drugs that are known to prolong QTc including Class 1A (eg, quinidine, procainamide) or Class III (eg, amiodarone, sotalol) antiarrhythmic medications, antipsychotic medications (eg, chlorpromazine, thioridazine), antibiotics (eg, gatifloxacin, moxifloxacin), or any other class of medications known to prolong QTc interval. Paliperidone should also be avoided in patients with congenital long QT syndrome and in patients with a history of cardiac arrhythmias).
No products indexed under this heading.

Erythromycin Stearate (Paliperidone causes a modest increase in the corrected QT (QTc) interval. The use of paliperidone should be avoided in combination with drugs that are known to prolong QTc including Class 1A (eg, quinidine, procainamide) or Class III (eg, amiodarone, sotalol) antiarrhythmic medications, antipsychotic medications (eg, chlorpromazine, thioridazine), antibiotics (eg, gatifloxacin, moxifloxacin), or any other class of medications known to prolong QTc interval. Paliperidone should also be avoided in patients with congenital long QT syndrome and in patients with a history of cardiac arrhythmias).
No products indexed under this heading.

Esmolol Hydrochloride (Because of its potential for inducing orthostatic hypotension, an additive effect may be observed when paliperidone is administered with other therapeutic agents that have this potential).
No products indexed under this heading.

Estazolam (Given the primary CNS effects paliperidone should be used with caution in combination with other centrally acting drugs and alcohol. Paliperidone may antagonize the effect of levodopa and other dopamine antagonists).
No products indexed under this heading.

Ethanol (Given the primary CNS effects paliperidone should be used with caution in combination with other centrally acting drugs and alcohol. Paliperidone may antagonize the effect of levodopa and other dopamine antagonists).
No products indexed under this heading.

Ethchlorvynol (Given the primary CNS effects paliperidone should be used with caution in combination with other centrally acting drugs and alcohol. Paliperidone may antagonize the effect of levodopa and other dopamine antagonists).
No products indexed under this heading.

Ethinamate (Given the primary CNS effects paliperidone should be used with caution in combination with other centrally acting drugs and alcohol. Paliperidone may antagonize the effect of levodopa and other dopamine antagonists).
No products indexed under this heading.

Ethyl Alcohol (Given the primary CNS effects paliperidone should be used with caution in combination with other centrally acting drugs and alcohol. Paliperidone may antagonize the effect of levodopa and other dopamine antagonists).
No products indexed under this heading.

Felodipine (Because of its potential for inducing orthostatic hypotension, an additive effect may be observed when paliperidone is administered with other therapeutic agents that have this potential).
No products indexed under this heading.

Fentanyl (Given the primary CNS effects paliperidone should be used with caution in combination with other centrally acting drugs and alcohol. Paliperidone may antagonize the effect of levodopa and other dopamine antagonists). Products include:
Duragesic 2604
Fentanyl Transdermal System 2346
Onsolis 2054

Fentanyl Citrate (Given the primary CNS effects paliperidone should be used with caution in combination with other centrally acting drugs and alcohol. Paliperidone may antagonize the effect of levodopa and other dopamine antagonists). Products include:
Fentora 966

Flecainide Acetate (Paliperidone causes a modest increase in the corrected QT (QTc) interval. The use of paliperidone should be avoided in combination with drugs that are known to prolong QTc including Class 1A (eg, quinidine, procainamide) or Class III (eg, amiodarone, sotalol) antiarrhythmic medications, antipsychotic medications (eg, chlorpromazine, thioridazine), antibiotics (eg, gatifloxacin, moxifloxacin), or any other class of medications known to prolong QTc interval. Paliperidone should also be avoided in patients with congenital long QT syndrome and in patients with a history of cardiac arrhythmias).
No products indexed under this heading.

Fluphenazine Decanoate (Given the primary CNS effects paliperidone should be used with caution in combination with other centrally acting drugs and alcohol. Paliperidone may antagonize the effect of levodopa and other dopamine antagonists).
No products indexed under this heading.

Fluphenazine Enanthate (Given the primary CNS effects paliperidone should be used with caution in combination with other centrally acting drugs and alcohol. Paliperidone may antagonize the effect of levodopa and other dopamine antagonists).
No products indexed under this heading.

Fluphenazine Hydrochloride (Given the primary CNS effects paliperidone should be used with caution in combination with other centrally acting drugs and alcohol. Paliperidone may antagonize the effect of levodopa and other dopamine antagonists).
No products indexed under this heading.

Flurazepam Hydrochloride (Given the primary CNS effects paliperidone should be used with caution in combination with other centrally acting drugs and alcohol. Paliperidone may antagonize the effect of levodopa and other dopamine antagonists).
No products indexed under this heading.

Fosinopril Sodium (Because of its potential for inducing orthostatic hypotension, an additive effect may be observed when paliperidone is administered with other therapeutic agents that have this potential).
No products indexed under this heading.

Furosemide (Because of its potential for inducing orthostatic hypotension, an additive effect may be observed when paliperidone is administered with other therapeutic agents that have this potential). Products include:
Furosemide 2354

Gatifloxacin (Paliperidone causes a modest increase in the corrected QT (QTc) interval. The use of paliperidone should be avoided in combination with drugs that are known to prolong QTc including antibiotics (eg, gatifloxacin, moxifloxacin), or any other class of medications known to prolong QTc interval. Paliperidone should also be avoided in patients with congenital long QT syndrome and in patients with a history of cardiac arrhythmias).
No products indexed under this heading.

Gemifloxacin Mesylate (Paliperidone causes a modest increase in the corrected QT (QTc) interval. The use of paliperidone should be avoided in combination with drugs that are known to prolong QTc including antibiotics (eg, gatifloxacin, moxifloxacin), or any other class of medications known to prolong QTc interval. Paliperidone should also be avoided in patients with congenital long QT syndrome and in patients with a history of cardiac arrhythmias).
No products indexed under this heading.

Gentamicin Sulfate (Paliperidone causes a modest increase in the corrected QT (QTc) interval. The use of paliperidone should be avoided in combination with drugs that are known to prolong QTc including antibiotics (eg, gatifloxacin, moxifloxacin), or any other class of medications known to prolong QTc interval. Paliperidone should also be avoided in patients with congenital long QT syndrome and in patients with a history of cardiac arrhythmias). Products include:
Pred-G .... ⊙226, ⊙227

Glutethimide (Given the primary CNS effects paliperidone should be used with caution in combination with other centrally acting drugs and alcohol. Paliperidone may antagonize the effect of levodopa and other dopamine antagonists).
No products indexed under this heading.

Grepafloxacin Hydrochloride (Paliperidone causes a modest increase in the corrected QT (QTc) interval. The use of paliperidone should be avoided in combination with drugs that are known to prolong QTc including antibiotics (eg, gatifloxacin, moxifloxacin), or any other class of medications known to prolong QTc interval. Paliperidone should also be avoided in patients with congenital long QT syndrome and in patients with a history of cardiac arrhythmias).
No products indexed under this heading.

Griseofulvin (Paliperidone causes a modest increase in the corrected QT (QTc) interval. The use of paliperidone should be avoided in combination with drugs that are known to prolong QTc including antibiotics (eg, gatifloxacin, moxifloxacin), or any other class of medications known to prolong QTc interval. Paliperidone should also be avoided in patients with congenital long QT syndrome and in patients with a history of cardiac arrhythmias).
No products indexed under this heading.

Guanabenz Acetate (Because of its potential for inducing orthostatic hypotension, an additive effect may be observed when paliperidone is administered with other therapeutic agents that have this potential).
No products indexed under this heading.

Guanethidine (Because of its potential for inducing orthostatic hypotension, an additive effect may be observed when paliperidone is administered with other therapeutic agents that have this potential).
No products indexed under this heading.

Guanethidine Monosulfate (Because of its potential for inducing orthostatic hypotension, an additive effect may be observed when paliperidone is administered with other therapeutic agents that have this potential).
No products indexed under this heading.

Guanethidine Sulfate (Because of its potential for inducing orthostatic hypotension, an additive effect may be observed when paliperidone is administered with other therapeutic agents that have this potential).
No products indexed under this heading.

Haloperidol (Given the primary CNS effects paliperidone should be used with caution in combination with other centrally acting drugs and alcohol. Paliperidone may antagonize the effect of levodopa and other dopamine antagonists).
No products indexed under this heading.

Haloperidol Decanoate (Given the primary CNS effects paliperidone should be used with caution in combination with other centrally acting drugs and alcohol. Paliperidone may antagonize the effect of levodopa and other dopamine antagonists).
No products indexed under this heading.

Haloperidol Lactate (Paliperidone causes a modest increase in the corrected QT (QTc) interval. The use of paliperidone should be avoided in combination with drugs that are known to prolong QTc including Class 1A (eg, quinidine, procainamide) or Class III (eg, amiodarone, sotalol) antiarrhythmic medications, antipsychotic medications (eg, chlorpromazine, thioridazine), antibiotics (eg, gatifloxacin, moxifloxacin), or any other class of medications known to prolong QTc interval. Paliperidone should also be avoided in patients with congenital long QT syndrome and in patients with a history of cardiac arrhythmias).
No products indexed under this heading.

Hydralazine Hydrochloride (Because of its potential for inducing orthostatic hypotension, an additive effect may be observed when paliperidone is administered with other therapeutic agents that have this potential).
No products indexed under this heading.

Hydrochlorothiazide (Because of its potential for inducing orthostatic hypotension, an additive effect may be observed when paliperidone is administered with other therapeutic agents that have this potential). Products include:
Atacand HCT 700
Avalide 2956
Benicar HCT 1017
Diovan HCT 2419
Dyazide 1429
Exforge HCT 2449
Hyzaar 2162
Hyzaar 100-12.5 2162
Micardis HCT 889
Prinzide 2246
Tekturna HCT 2541
Teveten HCT 541

Hydrocodone Bitartrate (Given the primary CNS effects paliperidone should be used with caution in combination with other centrally acting drugs and alcohol. Paliperidone may antagonize the effect of levodopa and other dopamine antagonists). Products include:
Vicodin 560
Vicodin ES 561
Vicodin HP 563
Vicoprofen 564
Zydone 1138

Hydrocodone Polistirex (Given the primary CNS effects paliperidone should be used with caution in combination with other centrally acting drugs and alcohol. Paliperidone may antagonize the effect of levodopa and other dopamine antagonists). Products include:
Tussionex 3443

Hydroflumethiazide (Because of its potential for inducing orthostatic hypotension, an additive effect may be observed when paliperidone is administered with other therapeutic agents that have this potential).
No products indexed under this heading.

Hydromorphone Hydrochloride (Given the primary CNS effects paliperidone should be used with caution in combination with other centrally acting drugs and alcohol. Paliperidone may antagonize the effect of levodopa and other dopamine antagonists). Products include:
Dilaudid Injection 2800
Dilaudid Oral 2797
Dilaudid Tablets 2797
Dilaudid-HP 2800

Hydroxyamphetamine Hydrobromide (Given the primary CNS effects paliperidone should be used with caution in combination with other centrally acting drugs and alcohol. Paliperidone may antagonize the effect of levodopa and other dopamine antagonists).
No products indexed under this heading.

Hydroxyzine Hydrochloride (Given the primary CNS effects paliperidone should be used with caution in combination with other centrally acting drugs and alcohol. Paliperidone may antagonize the effect of levodopa and other dopamine antagonists).
No products indexed under this heading.

Idarubicin Hydrochloride (Paliperidone causes a modest increase in the corrected QT (QTc) interval. The use of paliperidone should be avoided in combination with drugs that are known to prolong QTc including antibiotics (eg, gatifloxacin, moxifloxacin), or any other class of medications known to prolong QTc interval. Paliperidone should also be avoided in patients with congenital long QT syndrome and in patients with a history of cardiac arrhythmias).
No products indexed under this heading.

Imipenem (Paliperidone causes a modest increase in the corrected QT (QTc) interval. The use of paliperidone should be avoided in combination with drugs that are known to prolong QTc including antibiotics (eg, gatifloxacin, moxifloxacin), or any other class of medications known to prolong QTc interval. Paliperidone should also be avoided in patients with congenital long QT syndrome and in patients with a history of cardiac arrhythmias). Products include:
Primaxin I.M. 2232
Primaxin I.V. 2235

Imipramine Hydrochloride (Paliperidone causes a modest increase in the corrected QT (QTc) interval. The use of paliperidone should be avoided in combination with drugs that are known to prolong QTc including Class 1A (eg, quinidine, procainamide) or Class III (eg, amiodarone, sotalol) antiarrhythmic medications, antipsychotic medications (eg, chlorpromazine, thioridazine), antibiotics (eg, gatifloxacin, moxifloxacin), or any other class of medications known to prolong QTc interval. Paliperidone should also be avoided in patients with congenital long QT syndrome and in patients with a history of cardiac arrhythmias).
No products indexed under this heading.

Invega Interactions Index 912

Imipramine Pamoate (Paliperidone causes a modest increase in the corrected QT (QTc) interval. The use of paliperidone should be avoided in combination with drugs that are known to prolong QTc including Class 1A (eg, quinidine, procainamide) or Class III (eg, amiodarone, sotalol) antiarrhythmic medications, antipsychotic medications (eg, chlorpromazine, thioridazine), antibiotics (eg, gatifloxacin, moxifloxacin), or any other class of medications known to prolong QTc interval. Paliperidone should also be avoided in patients with congenital long QT syndrome and in patients with a history of cardiac arrhythmias).
No products indexed under this heading.

Indapamide (Because of its potential for inducing orthostatic hypotension, an additive effect may be observed when paliperidone is administered with other therapeutic agents that have this potential). Products include:
Indapamide 2356

Irbesartan (Because of its potential for inducing orthostatic hypotension, an additive effect may be observed when paliperidone is administered with other therapeutic agents that have this potential). Products include:
Avalide 2956
Avapro 2962

Isocarboxazid (Paliperidone causes a modest increase in the corrected QT (QTc) interval. The use of paliperidone should be avoided in combination with drugs that are known to prolong QTc including Class 1A (eg, quinidine, procainamide) or Class III (eg, amiodarone, sotalol) antiarrhythmic medications, antipsychotic medications (eg, chlorpromazine, thioridazine), antibiotics (eg, gatifloxacin, moxifloxacin), or any other class of medications known to prolong QTc interval. Paliperidone should also be avoided in patients with congenital long QT syndrome and in patients with a history of cardiac arrhythmias). Products include:
Marplan 3481

Isoflurane (Given the primary CNS effects paliperidone should be used with caution in combination with other centrally acting drugs and alcohol. Paliperidone may antagonize the effect of levodopa and other dopamine antagonists).
No products indexed under this heading.

Isradipine (Because of its potential for inducing orthostatic hypotension, an additive effect may be observed when paliperidone is administered with other therapeutic agents that have this potential). Products include:
DynaCirc CR 1432

Kanamycin Sulfate (Paliperidone causes a modest increase in the corrected QT (QTc) interval. The use of paliperidone should be avoided in combination with drugs that are known to prolong QTc including antibiotics (eg, gatifloxacin, moxifloxacin), or any other class of medications known to prolong QTc interval. Paliperidone should also be avoided in patients with congenital long QT syndrome and in patients with a history of cardiac arrhythmias).
No products indexed under this heading.

Ketamine Hydrochloride (Given the primary CNS effects paliperidone should be used with caution in combination with other centrally acting drugs and alcohol. Paliperidone may antagonize the effect of levodopa and other dopamine antagonists).
No products indexed under this heading.

Labetalol Hydrochloride (Because of its potential for inducing orthostatic hypotension, an additive effect may be observed when paliperidone is administered with other therapeutic agents that have this potential).
No products indexed under this heading.

Levofloxacin (Paliperidone causes a modest increase in the corrected QT (QTc) interval. The use of paliperidone should be avoided in combination with drugs that are known to prolong QTc including antibiotics (eg, gatifloxacin, moxifloxacin), or any other class of medications known to prolong QTc interval. Paliperidone should also be avoided in patients with congenital long QT syndrome and in patients with a history of cardiac arrhythmias). Products include:
Iquix 3492
Levaquin 2629
Levaquin in 5% Dextrose 2629
Quixin 3493

Levomethadyl Acetate Hydrochloride (Given the primary CNS effects paliperidone should be used with caution in combination with other centrally acting drugs and alcohol. Paliperidone may antagonize the effect of levodopa and other dopamine antagonists).
No products indexed under this heading.

Levorphanol Tartrate (Given the primary CNS effects paliperidone should be used with caution in combination with other centrally acting drugs and alcohol. Paliperidone may antagonize the effect of levodopa and other dopamine antagonists).
No products indexed under this heading.

Lidocaine (Paliperidone causes a modest increase in the corrected QT (QTc) interval. The use of paliperidone should be avoided in combination with drugs that are known to prolong QTc including Class 1A (eg, quinidine, procainamide) or Class III (eg, amiodarone, sotalol) antiarrhythmic medications, antipsychotic medications (eg, chlorpromazine, thioridazine), antibiotics (eg, gatifloxacin, moxifloxacin), or any other class of medications known to prolong QTc interval. Paliperidone should also be avoided in patients with congenital long QT syndrome and in patients with a history of cardiac arrhythmias). Products include:
Lidoderm 1107

Lidocaine Hydrochloride (Paliperidone causes a modest increase in the corrected QT (QTc) interval. The use of paliperidone should be avoided in combination with drugs that are known to prolong QTc including Class 1A (eg, quinidine, procainamide) or Class III (eg, amiodarone, sotalol) antiarrhythmic medications, antipsychotic medications (eg, chlorpromazine, thioridazine), antibiotics (eg, gatifloxacin, moxifloxacin), or any other class of medications known to prolong QTc interval. Paliperidone should also be avoided in patients with congenital long QT syndrome and in patients with a history of cardiac arrhythmias).
No products indexed under this heading.

Lisdexamfetamine Dimesylate (Given the primary CNS effects paliperidone should be used with caution in combination with other centrally acting drugs and alcohol. Paliperidone may antagonize the effect of levodopa and other dopamine antagonists). Products include:
Vyvanse 3298

Lisinopril (Because of its potential for inducing orthostatic hypotension, an additive effect may be observed when paliperidone is administered with other therapeutic agents that have this potential). Products include:
Prinivil 2241
Prinzide 2246

Lithium (Paliperidone causes a modest increase in the corrected QT (QTc) interval. The use of paliperidone should be avoided in combination with drugs that are known to prolong QTc including antipsychotic medications (eg, chlorpromazine, thioridazine) or any other class of medications known to prolong QTc interval. Paliperidone should also be avoided in patients with congenital long QT syndrome and in patients with a history of cardiac arrhythmias).
No products indexed under this heading.

Lithium Carbonate (Paliperidone causes a modest increase in the corrected QT (QTc) interval. The use of paliperidone should be avoided in combination with drugs that are known to prolong QTc including Class 1A (eg, quinidine, procainamide) or Class III (eg, amiodarone, sotalol) antiarrhythmic medications, antipsychotic medications (eg, chlorpromazine, thioridazine), antibiotics (eg, gatifloxacin, moxifloxacin), or any other class of medications known to prolong QTc interval. Paliperidone should also be avoided in patients with congenital long QT syndrome and in patients with a history of cardiac arrhythmias).
No products indexed under this heading.

Lithium Citrate (Paliperidone causes a modest increase in the corrected QT (QTc) interval. The use of paliperidone should be avoided in combination with drugs that are known to prolong QTc including Class 1A (eg, quinidine, procainamide) or Class III (eg, amiodarone, sotalol) antiarrhythmic medications, antipsychotic medications (eg, chlorpromazine, thioridazine), antibiotics (eg, gatifloxacin, moxifloxacin), or any other class of medications known to prolong QTc interval. Paliperidone should also be avoided in patients with congenital long QT syndrome and in patients with a history of cardiac arrhythmias).
No products indexed under this heading.

Lomefloxacin Hydrochloride (Paliperidone causes a modest increase in the corrected QT (QTc) interval. The use of paliperidone should be avoided in combination with drugs that are known to prolong QTc including antibiotics (eg, gatifloxacin, moxifloxacin), or any other class of medications known to prolong QTc interval. Paliperidone should also be avoided in patients with congenital long QT syndrome and in patients with a history of cardiac arrhythmias).
No products indexed under this heading.

Loracarbef (Paliperidone causes a modest increase in the corrected QT (QTc) interval. The use of paliperidone should be avoided in combination with drugs that are known to prolong QTc including antibiotics (eg, gatifloxacin, moxifloxacin), or any other class of medications known to prolong QTc interval. Paliperidone should also be avoided in patients with congenital long QT syndrome and in patients with a history of cardiac arrhythmias).
No products indexed under this heading.

Lorazepam (Given the primary CNS effects paliperidone should be used with caution in combination with other centrally acting drugs and alcohol. Paliperidone may antagonize the effect of levodopa and other dopamine antagonists).
No products indexed under this heading.

Losartan Potassium (Because of its potential for inducing orthostatic hypotension, an additive effect may be observed when paliperidone is administered with other therapeutic agents that have this potential). Products include:
Cozaar 2106
Hyzaar 2162
Hyzaar 100-12.5 2162

Loxapine Hydrochloride (Given the primary CNS effects paliperidone should be used with caution in combination with other centrally acting drugs and alcohol. Paliperidone may antagonize the effect of levodopa and other dopamine antagonists).
No products indexed under this heading.

Loxapine Succinate (Given the primary CNS effects paliperidone should be used with caution in combination with other centrally acting drugs and alcohol. Paliperidone may antagonize the effect of levodopa and other dopamine antagonists).
No products indexed under this heading.

Maprotiline Hydrochloride (Paliperidone causes a modest increase in the corrected QT (QTc) interval. The use of paliperidone should be avoided in combination with drugs that are known to prolong QTc including Class 1A (eg, quinidine, procainamide) or Class III (eg, amiodarone, sotalol) antiarrhythmic medications, antipsychotic medications (eg, chlorpromazine, thioridazine), antibiotics (eg, gatifloxacin, moxifloxacin), or any other class of medications known to prolong QTc interval. Paliperidone should also be avoided in patients with congenital long QT syndrome and in patients with a history of cardiac arrhythmias).
No products indexed under this heading.

Mecamylamine Hydrochloride (Because of its potential for inducing orthostatic hypotension, an additive effect may be observed when paliperidone is administered with other therapeutic agents that have this potential).
No products indexed under this heading.

Meperidine Hydrochloride (Given the primary CNS effects paliperidone should be used with caution in combination with other centrally acting drugs and alcohol. Paliperidone may antagonize the effect of levodopa and other dopamine antagonists).
No products indexed under this heading.

Mephobarbital (Given the primary CNS effects paliperidone should be used with caution in combination with other centrally acting drugs and alcohol. Paliperidone may antagonize the effect of levodopa and other dopamine antagonists).
No products indexed under this heading.

Meprobamate (Given the primary CNS effects paliperidone should be used with caution in combination with other centrally acting drugs and alcohol. Paliperidone may antagonize the effect of levodopa and other dopamine antagonists).
No products indexed under this heading.

Mesoridazine Besylate (Given the primary CNS effects paliperidone should be used with caution in combination with other centrally acting drugs and alcohol. Paliperidone may antagonize the effect of levodopa and other dopamine antagonists).
No products indexed under this heading.

Methacycline Hydrochloride (Paliperidone causes a modest increase in the corrected QT (QTc) interval. The use of paliperidone should be avoided in combination with drugs that are known to prolong QTc including antibiotics (eg, gatifloxacin, moxifloxacin), or any other class of medications known to prolong QTc interval. Paliperidone should also be avoided in patients with congenital long QT syndrome and in patients with a history of cardiac arrhythmias).
No products indexed under this heading.

913 Interactions Index Invega

Methadone Hydrochloride (Given the primary CNS effects paliperidone should be used with caution in combination with other centrally acting drugs and alcohol. Paliperidone may antagonize the effect of levodopa and other dopamine antagonists).
No products indexed under this heading.

Methamphetamine Hydrochloride (Given the primary CNS effects paliperidone should be used with caution in combination with other centrally acting drugs and alcohol. Paliperidone may antagonize the effect of levodopa and other dopamine antagonists).
No products indexed under this heading.

Methicillin Sodium (Paliperidone causes a modest increase in the corrected QT (QTc) interval. The use of paliperidone should be avoided in combination with drugs that are known to prolong QTc including antibiotics (eg, gatifloxacin, moxifloxacin), or any other class of medications known to prolong QTc interval. Paliperidone should also be avoided in patients with congenital long QT syndrome and in patients with a history of cardiac arrhythmias).
No products indexed under this heading.

Methohexital Sodium (Given the primary CNS effects paliperidone should be used with caution in combination with other centrally acting drugs and alcohol. Paliperidone may antagonize the effect of levodopa and other dopamine antagonists).
No products indexed under this heading.

Methotrimeprazine (Given the primary CNS effects paliperidone should be used with caution in combination with other centrally acting drugs and alcohol. Paliperidone may antagonize the effect of levodopa and other dopamine antagonists).
No products indexed under this heading.

Methoxyflurane (Given the primary CNS effects paliperidone should be used with caution in combination with other centrally acting drugs and alcohol. Paliperidone may antagonize the effect of levodopa and other dopamine antagonists).
No products indexed under this heading.

Methyclothiazide (Because of its potential for inducing orthostatic hypotension, an additive effect may be observed when paliperidone is administered with other therapeutic agents that have this potential).
No products indexed under this heading.

Methyldopa (Because of its potential for inducing orthostatic hypotension, an additive effect may be observed when paliperidone is administered with other therapeutic agents that have this potential).
No products indexed under this heading.

Methyldopate Hydrochloride (Because of its potential for inducing orthostatic hypotension, an additive effect may be observed when paliperidone is administered with other therapeutic agents that have this potential).
No products indexed under this heading.

Methylphenidate (Given the primary CNS effects paliperidone should be used with caution in combination with other centrally acting drugs and alcohol. Paliperidone may antagonize the effect of levodopa and other dopamine antagonists). Products include:
Daytrana 3283

Methylphenidate Hydrochloride (Given the primary CNS effects paliperidone should be used with caution in combination with other centrally acting drugs and alcohol. Paliperidone may antagonize the effect of levodopa and other dopamine antagonists). Products include:
Concerta 2598
Metadate CD 3439

Metolazone (Because of its potential for inducing orthostatic hypotension, an additive effect may be observed when paliperidone is administered with other therapeutic agents that have this potential).
No products indexed under this heading.

Metoprolol Succinate (Because of its potential for inducing orthostatic hypotension, an additive effect may be observed when paliperidone is administered with other therapeutic agents that have this potential). Products include:
Toprol XL 732

Metoprolol Tartrate (Because of its potential for inducing orthostatic hypotension, an additive effect may be observed when paliperidone is administered with other therapeutic agents that have this potential).
No products indexed under this heading.

Metyrosine (Because of its potential for inducing orthostatic hypotension, an additive effect may be observed when paliperidone is administered with other therapeutic agents that have this potential).
No products indexed under this heading.

Mexiletine Hydrochloride (Paliperidone causes a modest increase in the corrected QT (QTc) interval. The use of paliperidone should be avoided in combination with drugs that are known to prolong QTc including Class 1A (eg, quinidine, procainamide) or Class III (eg, amiodarone, sotalol) antiarrhythmic medications, antipsychotic medications (eg, chlorpromazine, thioridazine), antibiotics (eg, gatifloxacin, moxifloxacin), or any other class of medications known to prolong QTc interval. Paliperidone should also be avoided in patients with congenital long QT syndrome and in patients with a history of cardiac arrhythmias).
No products indexed under this heading.

Mezlocillin Sodium (Paliperidone causes a modest increase in the corrected QT (QTc) interval. The use of paliperidone should be avoided in combination with drugs that are known to prolong QTc including antibiotics (eg, gatifloxacin, moxifloxacin), or any other class of medications known to prolong QTc interval. Paliperidone should also be avoided in patients with congenital long QT syndrome and in patients with a history of cardiac arrhythmias).
No products indexed under this heading.

Mibefradil Dihydrochloride (Because of its potential for inducing orthostatic hypotension, an additive effect may be observed when paliperidone is administered with other therapeutic agents that have this potential).
No products indexed under this heading.

Midazolam Hydrochloride (Given the primary CNS effects paliperidone should be used with caution in combination with other centrally acting drugs and alcohol. Paliperidone may antagonize the effect of levodopa and other dopamine antagonists).
No products indexed under this heading.

Minocycline Hydrochloride (Paliperidone causes a modest increase in the corrected QT (QTc) interval. The use of paliperidone should be avoided in combination with drugs that are known to prolong QTc including antibiotics (eg, gatifloxacin, moxifloxacin), or any other class of medications known to prolong QTc interval. Paliperidone should also be avoided in patients with congenital long QT syndrome and in patients with a history of cardiac arrhythmias). Products include:
Solodyn 2073

Minoxidil (Because of its potential for inducing orthostatic hypotension, an additive effect may be observed when paliperidone is administered with other therapeutic agents that have this potential).
No products indexed under this heading.

Moexipril Hydrochloride (Because of its potential for inducing orthostatic hypotension, an additive effect may be observed when paliperidone is administered with other therapeutic agents that have this potential).
No products indexed under this heading.

Molindone Hydrochloride (Given the primary CNS effects paliperidone should be used with caution in combination with other centrally acting drugs and alcohol. Paliperidone may antagonize the effect of levodopa and other dopamine antagonists). Products include:
Moban 1108

Moricizine Hydrochloride (Paliperidone causes a modest increase in the corrected QT (QTc) interval. The use of paliperidone should be avoided in combination with drugs that are known to prolong QTc including Class 1A (eg, quinidine, procainamide) or Class III (eg, amiodarone, sotalol) antiarrhythmic medications or any other class of medications known to prolong QTc interval. Paliperidone should also be avoided in patients with congenital long QT syndrome and in patients with a history of cardiac arrhythmias).
No products indexed under this heading.

Morphine Sulfate (Given the primary CNS effects paliperidone should be used with caution in combination with other centrally acting drugs and alcohol. Paliperidone may antagonize the effect of levodopa and other dopamine antagonists). Products include:
Avinza 1822
Embeda 1831
MS Contin 2803

Moxifloxacin Hydrochloride (Paliperidone causes a modest increase in the corrected QT (QTc) interval. The use of paliperidone should be avoided in combination with drugs that are known to prolong QTc including antibiotics (eg, gatifloxacin, moxifloxacin), or any other class of medications known to prolong QTc interval. Paliperidone should also be avoided in patients with congenital long QT syndrome and in patients with a history of cardiac arrhythmias). Products include:
Avelox 3064
Vigamox 589

Nadolol (Because of its potential for inducing orthostatic hypotension, an additive effect may be observed when paliperidone is administered with other therapeutic agents that have this potential). Products include:
Nadolol 2359

Nafcillin Sodium (Paliperidone causes a modest increase in the corrected QT (QTc) interval. The use of paliperidone should be avoided in combination with drugs that are known to prolong QTc including antibiotics (eg, gatifloxacin, moxifloxacin), or any other class of medications known to prolong QTc interval. Paliperidone should also be avoided in patients with congenital long QT syndrome and in patients with a history of cardiac arrhythmias).
No products indexed under this heading.

Nebivolol (Because of its potential for inducing orthostatic hypotension, an additive effect may be observed when paliperidone is administered with other therapeutic agents that have this potential). Products include:
Bystolic 1147

Nicardipine Hydrochloride (Because of its potential for inducing orthostatic hypotension, an additive effect may be observed when paliperidone is administered with other therapeutic agents that have this potential).
No products indexed under this heading.

Nifedipine (Because of its potential for inducing orthostatic hypotension, an additive effect may be observed when paliperidone is administered with other therapeutic agents that have this potential).
No products indexed under this heading.

Nisoldipine (Because of its potential for inducing orthostatic hypotension, an additive effect may be observed when paliperidone is administered with other therapeutic agents that have this potential).
No products indexed under this heading.

Nitroglycerin (Because of its potential for inducing orthostatic hypotension, an additive effect may be observed when paliperidone is administered with other therapeutic agents that have this potential). Products include:
Nitro-Dur 3170
Nitrolingual 3266

Norfloxacin (Paliperidone causes a modest increase in the corrected QT (QTc) interval. The use of paliperidone should be avoided in combination with drugs that are known to prolong QTc including antibiotics (eg, gatifloxacin, moxifloxacin), or any other class of medications known to prolong QTc interval. Paliperidone should also be avoided in patients with congenital long QT syndrome and in patients with a history of cardiac arrhythmias). Products include:
Noroxin 2220

Nortriptyline Hydrochloride (Paliperidone causes a modest increase in the corrected QT (QTc) interval. The use of paliperidone should be avoided in combination with drugs that are known to prolong QTc including Class 1A (eg, quinidine, procainamide) or Class III (eg, amiodarone, sotalol) antiarrhythmic medications, antipsychotic medications (eg, chlorpromazine, thioridazine), antibiotics (eg, gatifloxacin, moxifloxacin), or any other class of medications known to prolong QTc interval. Paliperidone should also be avoided in patients with congenital long QT syndrome and in patients with a history of cardiac arrhythmias).
No products indexed under this heading.

Ofloxacin (Paliperidone causes a modest increase in the corrected QT (QTc) interval. The use of paliperidone should be avoided in combination with drugs that are known to prolong QTc including antibiotics (eg, gatifloxacin, moxifloxacin), or any other class of medications known to prolong QTc interval. Paliperidone should also be avoided in patients with congenital long QT syndrome and in patients with a history of cardiac arrhythmias).
No products indexed under this heading.

Olanzapine (Given the primary CNS effects paliperidone should be used with caution in combination with other centrally acting drugs and alcohol. Paliperidone may antagonize the effect of levodopa and other dopamine antagonists). Products include:
Symbyax 1965
Zyprexa 1984
Zyprexa IntraMuscular 1984
Zyprexa ZYDIS 1984

Oxacillin (Paliperidone causes a modest increase in the corrected QT (QTc) interval. The use of paliperidone should be avoided in combination with drugs that are known to prolong QTc including antibiotics (eg, gatifloxacin, moxifloxacin), or any other class of medications known to prolong QTc interval. Paliperi-

Invega Interactions Index 914

done should also be avoided in patients with congenital long QT syndrome and in patients with a history of cardiac arrhythmias).
No products indexed under this heading.

Oxacillin Sodium (Paliperidone causes a modest increase in the corrected QT (QTc) interval. The use of paliperidone should be avoided in combination with drugs that are known to prolong QTc including antibiotics (eg, gatifloxacin, moxifloxacin), or any other class of medications known to prolong QTc interval. Paliperidone should also be avoided in patients with congenital long QT syndrome and in patients with a history of cardiac arrhythmias).
No products indexed under this heading.

Oxazepam (Given the primary CNS effects paliperidone should be used with caution in combination with other centrally acting drugs and alcohol. Paliperidone may antagonize the effect of levodopa and other dopamine antagonists).
No products indexed under this heading.

Oxycodone Hydrochloride (Given the primary CNS effects paliperidone should be used with caution in combination with other centrally acting drugs and alcohol. Paliperidone may antagonize the effect of levodopa and other dopamine antagonists). Products include:
OxyContin **2807**
Percocet **1121**
Percodan **1124**

Oxytetracycline Hydrochloride (Paliperidone causes a modest increase in the corrected QT (QTc) interval. The use of paliperidone should be avoided in combination with drugs that are known to prolong QTc including antibiotics (eg, gatifloxacin, moxifloxacin), or any other class of medications known to prolong QTc interval. Paliperidone should also be avoided in patients with congenital long QT syndrome and in patients with a history of cardiac arrhythmias).
No products indexed under this heading.

Paroxetine (Paliperidone is metabolized to a limited extent by CYP2D6. In an interaction study in healthy subjects in which a single 3 mg dose of oral paliperidone extended release was administered concomitantly with 20 mg per day of paroxetine (a potent CYP2D6 inhibitor), paliperidone exposures were on average 16% (90% CI: 4, 30) higher in CYP2D6 extensive metabolizers. Higher doses of paroxetine have not been studied. The clinical relevance is unknown).
No products indexed under this heading.

Paroxetine Hydrochloride (Paliperidone is metabolized to a limited extent by CYP2D6. In an interaction study in healthy subjects in which a single 3 mg dose of oral paliperidone extended release was administered concomitantly with 20 mg per day of paroxetine (a potent CYP2D6 inhibitor), paliperidone exposures were on average 16% (90% CI: 4, 30) higher in CYP2D6 extensive metabolizers. Higher doses of paroxetine have not been studied. The clinical relevance is unknown). Products include:
Paroxetine CR **2361**
Paroxetine ER **2371**
Paxil **1586**
Paxil CR **1596**

Paroxetine Mesylate (Paliperidone is metabolized to a limited extent by CYP2D6. In an interaction study in healthy subjects in which a single 3 mg dose of oral paliperidone extended release was administered concomitantly with 20 mg per day of paroxetine (a potent CYP2D6 inhibitor), paliperidone exposures were on average 16% (90% CI: 4, 30) higher in CYP2D6 extensive metabolizers. Higher doses of paroxetine have not been studied. The clinical relevance is unknown).
No products indexed under this heading.

Pemoline (Given the primary CNS effects paliperidone should be used with caution in combination with other centrally acting drugs and alcohol. Paliperidone may antagonize the effect of levodopa and other dopamine antagonists).
No products indexed under this heading.

Penbutolol Sulfate (Because of its potential for inducing orthostatic hypotension, an additive effect may be observed when paliperidone is administered with other therapeutic agents that have this potential).
No products indexed under this heading.

Penicillin, Potassium Phenoxymethyl (Paliperidone causes a modest increase in the corrected QT (QTc) interval. The use of paliperidone should be avoided in combination with drugs that are known to prolong QTc including antibiotics (eg, gatifloxacin, moxifloxacin), or any other class of medications known to prolong QTc interval. Paliperidone should also be avoided in patients with congenital long QT syndrome and in patients with a history of cardiac arrhythmias).
No products indexed under this heading.

Penicillin G Benzathine (Paliperidone causes a modest increase in the corrected QT (QTc) interval. The use of paliperidone should be avoided in combination with drugs that are known to prolong QTc including antibiotics (eg, gatifloxacin, moxifloxacin), or any other class of medications known to prolong QTc interval. Paliperidone should also be avoided in patients with congenital long QT syndrome and in patients with a history of cardiac arrhythmias). Products include:
Bicillin C-R Injectable Suspension **1826**
Bicillin L-A **1828**

Penicillin G Dibenzylethyenediamine (Paliperidone causes a modest increase in the corrected QT (QTc) interval. The use of paliperidone should be avoided in combination with drugs that are known to prolong QTc including antibiotics (eg, gatifloxacin, moxifloxacin), or any other class of medications known to prolong QTc interval. Paliperidone should also be avoided in patients with congenital long QT syndrome and in patients with a history of cardiac arrhythmias).
No products indexed under this heading.

Penicillin G Potassium (Paliperidone causes a modest increase in the corrected QT (QTc) interval. The use of paliperidone should be avoided in combination with drugs that are known to prolong QTc including antibiotics (eg, gatifloxacin, moxifloxacin), or any other class of medications known to prolong QTc interval. Paliperidone should also be avoided in patients with congenital long QT syndrome and in patients with a history of cardiac arrhythmias).
No products indexed under this heading.

Penicillin G Procaine (Paliperidone causes a modest increase in the corrected QT (QTc) interval. The use of paliperidone should be avoided in combination with drugs that are known to prolong QTc including antibiotics (eg, gatifloxacin, moxifloxacin), or any other class of medications known to prolong QTc interval. Paliperidone should also be avoided in patients with congenital long QT syndrome and in patients with a history of cardiac arrhythmias). Products include:
Bicillin C-R Injectable Suspension **1826**
Bicillin L-A **1828**

Penicillin G Sodium (Paliperidone causes a modest increase in the corrected QT (QTc) interval. The use of paliperidone should be avoided in combination with drugs that are known to prolong QTc including antibiotics (eg, gatifloxacin, moxifloxacin), or any other class of medications known to prolong QTc interval. Paliperidone should also be avoided in patients with congenital long QT syndrome and in patients with a history of cardiac arrhythmias).
No products indexed under this heading.

Penicillin V (Paliperidone causes a modest increase in the corrected QT (QTc) interval. The use of paliperidone should be avoided in combination with drugs that are known to prolong QTc including antibiotics (eg, gatifloxacin, moxifloxacin), or any other class of medications known to prolong QTc interval. Paliperidone should also be avoided in patients with congenital long QT syndrome and in patients with a history of cardiac arrhythmias).
No products indexed under this heading.

Penicillin V Potassium (Paliperidone causes a modest increase in the corrected QT (QTc) interval. The use of paliperidone should be avoided in combination with drugs that are known to prolong QTc including antibiotics (eg, gatifloxacin, moxifloxacin), or any other class of medications known to prolong QTc interval. Paliperidone should also be avoided in patients with congenital long QT syndrome and in patients with a history of cardiac arrhythmias).
No products indexed under this heading.

Penicillins (Paliperidone causes a modest increase in the corrected QT (QTc) interval. The use of paliperidone should be avoided in combination with drugs that are known to prolong QTc including antibiotics (eg, gatifloxacin, moxifloxacin), or any other class of medications known to prolong QTc interval. Paliperidone should also be avoided in patients with congenital long QT syndrome and in patients with a history of cardiac arrhythmias).
No products indexed under this heading.

Pentobarbital Sodium (Given the primary CNS effects paliperidone should be used with caution in combination with other centrally acting drugs and alcohol. Paliperidone may antagonize the effect of levodopa and other dopamine antagonists). Products include:
Nembutal **2012**

Perindopril Erbumine (Because of its potential for inducing orthostatic hypotension, an additive effect may be observed when paliperidone is administered with other therapeutic agents that have this potential).
No products indexed under this heading.

Perphenazine (Given the primary CNS effects paliperidone should be used with caution in combination with other centrally acting drugs and alcohol. Paliperidone may antagonize the effect of levodopa and other dopamine antagonists).
No products indexed under this heading.

Phenelzine Sulfate (Paliperidone causes a modest increase in the corrected QT (QTc) interval. The use of paliperidone should be avoided in combination with drugs that are known to prolong QTc including Class 1A (eg, quinidine, procainamide) or Class III (eg, amiodarone, sotalol) antiarrhythmic medications, antipsychotic medications (eg, chlorpromazine, thioridazine), antibiotics (eg, gatifloxacin, moxifloxacin), or any other class of medications known to prolong QTc interval. Paliperidone should also be avoided in patients with congenital long QT syndrome and in patients with a history of cardiac arrhythmias).
No products indexed under this heading.

Phenobarbital (Given the primary CNS effects paliperidone should be used with caution in combination with other centrally acting drugs and alcohol. Paliperidone may antagonize the effect of levodopa and other dopamine antagonists). Products include:
Donnatal **2711**

Phenobarbital Sodium (Given the primary CNS effects paliperidone should be used with caution in combination with other centrally acting drugs and alcohol. Paliperidone may antagonize the effect of levodopa and other dopamine antagonists).
No products indexed under this heading.

Phenoxybenzamine Hydrochloride (Because of its potential for inducing orthostatic hypotension, an additive effect may be observed when paliperidone is administered with other therapeutic agents that have this potential). Products include:
Dibenzyline **3495**

Phentolamine Mesylate (Because of its potential for inducing orthostatic hypotension, an additive effect may be observed when paliperidone is administered with other therapeutic agents that have this potential).
No products indexed under this heading.

Pimozide (Paliperidone causes a modest increase in the corrected QT (QTc) interval. The use of paliperidone should be avoided in combination with drugs that are known to prolong QTc including antipsychotic medications (eg, chlorpromazine, thioridazine) or any other class of medications known to prolong QTc interval. Paliperidone should also be avoided in patients with congenital long QT syndrome and in patients with a history of cardiac arrhythmias).
No products indexed under this heading.

Pindolol (Because of its potential for inducing orthostatic hypotension, an additive effect may be observed when paliperidone is administered with other therapeutic agents that have this potential).
No products indexed under this heading.

Piperacillin Sodium (Paliperidone causes a modest increase in the corrected QT (QTc) interval. The use of paliperidone should be avoided in combination with drugs that are known to prolong QTc including antibiotics (eg, gatifloxacin, moxifloxacin), or any other class of medications known to prolong QTc interval. Paliperidone should also be avoided in patients with congenital long QT syndrome and in patients with a history of cardiac arrhythmias). Products include:
Zosyn **3607**

Polythiazide (Because of its potential for inducing orthostatic hypotension, an additive effect may be observed when paliperidone is administered with other therapeutic agents that have this potential).
No products indexed under this heading.

Prazepam (Given the primary CNS effects paliperidone should be used with caution in combination with other centrally acting drugs and alcohol. Paliperidone may antagonize the effect of levodopa and other dopamine antagonists).
No products indexed under this heading.

Prazosin Hydrochloride (Because of its potential for inducing orthostatic hypotension, an additive effect may be observed when paliperidone is administered with other therapeutic agents that have this potential).
No products indexed under this heading.

Procainamide (Paliperidone causes a modest increase in the corrected QT (QTc) interval. The use of paliperidone should be avoided in combination with

915 Interactions Index Invega

drugs that are known to prolong QTc including Class 1A (eg, quinidine, procainamide) or Class III (eg, amiodarone, sotalol) antiarrhythmic medications or any other class of medications known to prolong QTc interval. Paliperidone should also be avoided in patients with congenital long QT syndrome and in patients with a history of cardiac arrhythmias).
No products indexed under this heading.

Procainamide Hydrochloride (Paliperidone causes a modest increase in the corrected QT (QTc) interval. The use of paliperidone should be avoided in combination with drugs that are known to prolong QTc including Class 1A (eg, quinidine, procainamide) or Class III (eg, amiodarone, sotalol) antiarrhythmic medications, antipsychotic medications (eg, chlorpromazine, thioridazine), antibiotics (eg, gatifloxacin, moxifloxacin), or any other class of medications known to prolong QTc interval. Paliperidone should also be avoided in patients with congenital long QT syndrome and in patients with a history of cardiac arrhythmias).
No products indexed under this heading.

Prochlorperazine (Given the primary CNS effects paliperidone should be used with caution in combination with other centrally acting drugs and alcohol. Paliperidone may antagonize the effect of levodopa and other dopamine antagonists).
No products indexed under this heading.

Promethazine Hydrochloride (Given the primary CNS effects paliperidone should be used with caution in combination with other centrally acting drugs and alcohol. Paliperidone may antagonize the effect of levodopa and other dopamine antagonists).
No products indexed under this heading.

Propafenone Hydrochloride (Paliperidone causes a modest increase in the corrected QT (QTc) interval. The use of paliperidone should be avoided in combination with drugs that are known to prolong QTc including Class 1A (eg, quinidine, procainamide) or Class III (eg, amiodarone, sotalol) antiarrhythmic medications, antipsychotic medications (eg, chlorpromazine, thioridazine), antibiotics (eg, gatifloxacin, moxifloxacin), or any other class of medications known to prolong QTc interval. Paliperidone should also be avoided in patients with congenital long QT syndrome and in patients with a history of cardiac arrhythmias). Products include:
Rythmol 1648
Rythmol SR 1652

Propofol (Given the primary CNS effects paliperidone should be used with caution in combination with other centrally acting drugs and alcohol. Paliperidone may antagonize the effect of levodopa and other dopamine antagonists).
No products indexed under this heading.

Propoxyphene Hydrochloride (Given the primary CNS effects paliperidone should be used with caution in combination with other centrally acting drugs and alcohol. Paliperidone may antagonize the effect of levodopa and other dopamine antagonists).
No products indexed under this heading.

Propoxyphene Napsylate (Given the primary CNS effects paliperidone should be used with caution in combination with other centrally acting drugs and alcohol. Paliperidone may antagonize the effect of levodopa and other dopamine antagonists).
No products indexed under this heading.

Propranolol Hydrochloride (Paliperidone causes a modest increase in the corrected QT (QTc) interval. The use of paliperidone should be avoided in combination with drugs that are known to prolong QTc including Class 1A (eg, quinidine, procainamide) or Class III (eg, amiodarone, sotalol) antiarrhythmic medications or any other class of medications known to prolong QTc interval. Paliperidone should also be avoided in patients with congenital long QT syndrome and in patients with a history of cardiac arrhythmias). Products include:
InnoPran XL 1517

Protriptyline Hydrochloride (Paliperidone causes a modest increase in the corrected QT (QTc) interval. The use of paliperidone should be avoided in combination with drugs that are known to prolong QTc including Class 1A (eg, quinidine, procainamide) or Class III (eg, amiodarone, sotalol) antiarrhythmic medications, antipsychotic medications (eg, chlorpromazine, thioridazine), antibiotics (eg, gatifloxacin, moxifloxacin), or any other class of medications known to prolong QTc interval. Paliperidone should also be avoided in patients with congenital long QT syndrome and in patients with a history of cardiac arrhythmias).
No products indexed under this heading.

Quazepam (Given the primary CNS effects paliperidone should be used with caution in combination with other centrally acting drugs and alcohol. Paliperidone may antagonize the effect of levodopa and other dopamine antagonists).
No products indexed under this heading.

Quetiapine Fumarate (Given the primary CNS effects paliperidone should be used with caution in combination with other centrally acting drugs and alcohol. Paliperidone may antagonize the effect of levodopa and other dopamine antagonists). Products include:
Seroquel 750
Seroquel XR 759

Quinapril Hydrochloride (Because of its potential for inducing orthostatic hypotension, an additive effect may be observed when paliperidone is administered with other therapeutic agents that have this potential).
No products indexed under this heading.

Quinidine (Paliperidone causes a modest increase in the corrected QT (QTc) interval. The use of paliperidone should be avoided in combination with drugs that are known to prolong QTc including Class 1A (eg, quinidine, procainamide) or Class III (eg, amiodarone, sotalol) antiarrhythmic medications, antipsychotic medications (eg, chlorpromazine, thioridazine), antibiotics (eg, gatifloxacin, moxifloxacin), or any other class of medications known to prolong QTc interval. Paliperidone should also be avoided in patients with congenital long QT syndrome and in patients with a history of cardiac arrhythmias).
No products indexed under this heading.

Quinidine Gluconate (Paliperidone causes a modest increase in the corrected QT (QTc) interval. The use of paliperidone should be avoided in combination with drugs that are known to prolong QTc including Class 1A (eg, quinidine, procainamide) or Class III (eg, amiodarone, sotalol) antiarrhythmic medications, antipsychotic medications (eg, chlorpromazine, thioridazine), antibiotics (eg, gatifloxacin, moxifloxacin), or any other class of medications known to prolong QTc interval. Paliperidone should also be avoided in patients with congenital long QT syndrome and in patients with a history of cardiac arrhythmias).
No products indexed under this heading.

Quinidine Hydrochloride (Paliperidone causes a modest increase in the corrected QT (QTc) interval. The use of paliperidone should be avoided in combination with drugs that are known to prolong QTc including Class 1A (eg, quinidine, procainamide) or Class III (eg, amiodarone, sotalol) antiarrhythmic medications, antipsychotic medications (eg, chlorpromazine, thioridazine), antibiotics (eg, gatifloxacin, moxifloxacin), or any other class of medications known to prolong QTc interval. Paliperidone should also be avoided in patients with congenital long QT syndrome and in patients with a history of cardiac arrhythmias).
No products indexed under this heading.

Quinidine Polygalacturonate (Paliperidone causes a modest increase in the corrected QT (QTc) interval. The use of paliperidone should be avoided in combination with drugs that are known to prolong QTc including Class 1A (eg, quinidine, procainamide) or Class III (eg, amiodarone, sotalol) antiarrhythmic medications, antipsychotic medications (eg, chlorpromazine, thioridazine), antibiotics (eg, gatifloxacin, moxifloxacin), or any other class of medications known to prolong QTc interval. Paliperidone should also be avoided in patients with congenital long QT syndrome and in patients with a history of cardiac arrhythmias).
No products indexed under this heading.

Quinidine Sulfate (Paliperidone causes a modest increase in the corrected QT (QTc) interval. The use of paliperidone should be avoided in combination with drugs that are known to prolong QTc including Class 1A (eg, quinidine, procainamide) or Class III (eg, amiodarone, sotalol) antiarrhythmic medications, antipsychotic medications (eg, chlorpromazine, thioridazine), antibiotics (eg, gatifloxacin, moxifloxacin), or any other class of medications known to prolong QTc interval. Paliperidone should also be avoided in patients with congenital long QT syndrome and in patients with a history of cardiac arrhythmias).
No products indexed under this heading.

Ramipril (Because of its potential for inducing orthostatic hypotension, an additive effect may be observed when paliperidone is administered with other therapeutic agents that have this potential).
No products indexed under this heading.

Rauwolfia Serpentina (Because of its potential for inducing orthostatic hypotension, an additive effect may be observed when paliperidone is administered with other therapeutic agents that have this potential).
No products indexed under this heading.

Remifentanil Hydrochloride (Given the primary CNS effects paliperidone should be used with caution in combination with other centrally acting drugs and alcohol. Paliperidone may antagonize the effect of levodopa and other dopamine antagonists).
No products indexed under this heading.

Rescinnamine (Because of its potential for inducing orthostatic hypotension, an additive effect may be observed when paliperidone is administered with other therapeutic agents that have this potential).
No products indexed under this heading.

Reserpine (Because of its potential for inducing orthostatic hypotension, an additive effect may be observed when paliperidone is administered with other therapeutic agents that have this potential).
No products indexed under this heading.

Risperidone (Given the primary CNS effects paliperidone should be used with caution in combination with other centrally acting drugs and alcohol. Paliperidone may antagonize the effect of levodopa and other dopamine antagonists). Products include:
Risperdal Consta 2682

Secobarbital Sodium (Given the primary CNS effects paliperidone should be used with caution in combination with other centrally acting drugs and alcohol. Paliperidone may antagonize the effect of levodopa and other dopamine antagonists).
No products indexed under this heading.

Sevoflurane (Given the primary CNS effects paliperidone should be used with caution in combination with other centrally acting drugs and alcohol. Paliperidone may antagonize the effect of levodopa and other dopamine antagonists). Products include:
Ultane 554

Sodium Cloxacillin Monohydrate (Paliperidone causes a modest increase in the corrected QT (QTc) interval. The use of paliperidone should be avoided in combination with drugs that are known to prolong QTc including antibiotics (eg, gatifloxacin, moxifloxacin), or any other class of medications known to prolong QTc interval. Paliperidone should also be avoided in patients with congenital long QT syndrome and in patients with a history of cardiac arrhythmias).
No products indexed under this heading.

Sodium Nitroprusside (Because of its potential for inducing orthostatic hypotension, an additive effect may be observed when paliperidone is administered with other therapeutic agents that have this potential).
No products indexed under this heading.

Sodium Oxybate (Given the primary CNS effects paliperidone should be used with caution in combination with other centrally acting drugs and alcohol. Paliperidone may antagonize the effect of levodopa and other dopamine antagonists).
No products indexed under this heading.

Sotalol Hydrochloride (Paliperidone causes a modest increase in the corrected QT (QTc) interval. The use of paliperidone should be avoided in combination with drugs that are known to prolong QTc including Class 1A (eg, quinidine, procainamide) or Class III (eg, amiodarone, sotalol) antiarrhythmic medications or any other class of medications known to prolong QTc interval. Paliperidone should also be avoided in patients with congenital long QT syndrome and in patients with a history of cardiac arrhythmias).
No products indexed under this heading.

Sparfloxacin (Paliperidone causes a modest increase in the corrected QT (QTc) interval. The use of paliperidone should be avoided in combination with drugs that are known to prolong QTc including antibiotics (eg, gatifloxacin, moxifloxacin), or any other class of medications known to prolong QTc interval. Paliperidone should also be avoided in patients with congenital long QT syndrome and in patients with a history of cardiac arrhythmias).
No products indexed under this heading.

Spirapril Hydrochloride (Because of its potential for inducing orthostatic hypotension, an additive effect may be observed when paliperidone is administered with other therapeutic agents that have this potential).
No products indexed under this heading.

Streptomycin Sulfate (Paliperidone causes a modest increase in the corrected QT (QTc) interval. The use of paliperidone should be avoided in combination with drugs that are known to prolong QTc including antibiotics (eg, gatifloxacin, moxifloxacin), or any other class of medications known to prolong QTc interval. Paliperidone should also

(⊙ Described in PDR® for Ophthalmic Medicines)

917 Interactions Index Isentress

Food Interactions

Alcohol (Given the primary CNS effects paliperidone should be used with caution in combination with other centrally acting drugs and alcohol. Paliperidone may antagonize the effect of levodopa and other dopamine antagonists).

Beer, reduced-alcohol (Given the primary CNS effects paliperidone should be used with caution in combination with other centrally acting drugs and alcohol. Paliperidone may antagonize the effect of levodopa and other dopamine antagonists).

Beer, unspecified (Given the primary CNS effects paliperidone should be used with caution in combination with other centrally acting drugs and alcohol. Paliperidone may antagonize the effect of levodopa and other dopamine antagonists).

Wine, Chianti (Given the primary CNS effects paliperidone should be used with caution in combination with other centrally acting drugs and alcohol. Paliperidone may antagonize the effect of levodopa and other dopamine antagonists).

Wine, Red (Given the primary CNS effects paliperidone should be used with caution in combination with other centrally acting drugs and alcohol. Paliperidone may antagonize the effect of levodopa and other dopamine antagonists).

Wine, unspecified (Given the primary CNS effects paliperidone should be used with caution in combination with other centrally acting drugs and alcohol. Paliperidone may antagonize the effect of levodopa and other dopamine antagonists).

Wine products (Given the primary CNS effects paliperidone should be used with caution in combination with other centrally acting drugs and alcohol. Paliperidone may antagonize the effect of levodopa and other dopamine antagonists).

IQUIX OPHTHALMIC SOLUTION

(Levofloxacin) 3492
May interact with xanthines, and certain other agents. Compounds in these categories include:

Aminophylline (Systemic administration of some quinolones has been shown to elevate plasma concentrations of theophylline).
No products indexed under this heading.

Caffeine (Systemic administration of some quinolones has been shown to interfere with the metabolism of caffeine).
No products indexed under this heading.

Caffeine Anhydrous (Systemic administration of some quinolones has been shown to interfere with the metabolism of caffeine).
No products indexed under this heading.

Caffeine Citrate (Systemic administration of some quinolones has been shown to interfere with the metabolism of caffeine).
No products indexed under this heading.

Caffeine-containing medications (Systemic administration of some quinolones has been shown to interfere with the metabolism of caffeine).
No products indexed under this heading.

Caffeine Sodium Benzoate (Systemic administration of some quinolones has been shown to interfere with the metabolism of caffeine).
No products indexed under this heading.

Cyclosporine (Systemic administration of some quinolones has been associated with transient elevations in serum creatinine in patients receiving systemic cyclosporine concomitantly). Products include:
Gengraf 440
Neoral Oral Solution 2496
Neoral Capsules 2496
Restasis 605

Dyphylline (Systemic administration of some quinolones has been shown to elevate plasma concentrations of theophylline).
No products indexed under this heading.

Theophylline (Systemic administration of some quinolones has been shown to elevate plasma concentrations of theophylline).
No products indexed under this heading.

Theophylline Anhydrous (Systemic administration of some quinolones has been shown to elevate plasma concentrations of theophylline). Products include:
Uniphyl 2817

Theophylline Calcium Salicylate (Systemic administration of some quinolones has been shown to elevate plasma concentrations of theophylline).
No products indexed under this heading.

Theophylline Dihydroxypropyl (Glyceryl) (Systemic administration of some quinolones has been shown to elevate plasma concentrations of theophylline).
No products indexed under this heading.

Theophylline Ethylenediamine (Systemic administration of some quinolones has been shown to elevate plasma concentrations of theophylline).
No products indexed under this heading.

Theophylline Sodium Glycinate (Systemic administration of some quinolones has been shown to elevate plasma concentrations of theophylline).
No products indexed under this heading.

Warfarin Sodium (Systemic administration of some quinolones has been shown to enhance the effects of warfarin).
No products indexed under this heading.

Food Interactions

Beverages, caffeine-containing (Systemic administration of some quinolones has been shown to interfere with the metabolism of caffeine).

Food, caffeine-containing (Systemic administration of some quinolones has been shown to interfere with the metabolism of caffeine).

ISENTRESS TABLETS

(Raltegravir) 2180
May interact with HMG-CoA reductase inhibitors, UDP-glucuronosyltransferase (UGT) inducers (selected), and certain other agents. Compounds in these categories include:

Atazanavir (Co-administration of raltegravir with drugs that inhibit UGT1A1 may increase plasma levels of raltegravir. Concomitant use with atazanavir, a strong inhibitor of UGT1A1 and atazanavir/ritonavir was shown to increase the plasma concentrations of raltegravir. However, since concomitant use of raltegravir with atazanavir or atazanavir/ritonavir did not result in a unique safety signal in Phase 3 studies, no dose adjustment is recommended).
No products indexed under this heading.

Atazanavir Sulfate (Co-administration of raltegravir with drugs that inhibit UGT1A1 may increase plasma levels of raltegravir. Concomitant use with atazanavir, a strong inhibitor of UGT1A1 and atazanavir/ritonavir was shown to increase the plasma concentrations of raltegravir. However, since concomitant use of raltegravir with atazanavir or atazanavir/ritonavir did not result in a unique safety signal in Phase 3 studies, no dose adjustment is recommended).
No products indexed under this heading.

Atorvastatin Calcium (Myopathy and rhabdomyolysis have been reported; however, the relationship of raltegravir to these events is not known. Use with caution in patients at increased risk of myopathy or rhabdomyolysis, such as patients receiving concomitant medications known to cause these conditions). Products include:
Lipitor 2703

Cerivastatin Sodium (Myopathy and rhabdomyolysis have been reported; however, the relationship of raltegravir to these events is not known. Use with caution in patients at increased risk of myopathy or rhabdomyolysis, such as patients receiving concomitant medications known to cause these conditions).
No products indexed under this heading.

Efavirenz (Efavirenz reduces plasma concentrations of raltegravir. The clinical significance of this interaction has not been directly assessed). Products include:
Atripla 906

Etravirine (Etravirine reduces plasma concentrations of raltegravir. The clinical significance of this interaction has not been directly assessed).
No products indexed under this heading.

Fat (Raltegravir may be administered with or without food. Administration of multiple doses of raltegravir following a moderate-fat meal (600 Kcal, 21 g fat) did not affect raltegravir AUC to a clinically meaningful degree with an increase of 13% relative to fasting. Raltegravir C_{12hr} was 66% higher and C_{max} was 5% higher following a moderate-fat meal compared to fasting. Administration of raltegravir following a high-fat meal (825 Kcal, 52 g fat) increased AUC and C_{max} by approximately 2-fold and increased C_{12hr} by 4.1-fold. Administration of raltegravir following a low-fat meal (300 Kcal, 2.5 g fat) decreased AUC and C_{max} by 46% and 52%, respectively; C_{12hr} was essentially unchanged. Food appears to increase pharmacokinetic variability relative to fasting).
No products indexed under this heading.

Fluvastatin Sodium (Myopathy and rhabdomyolysis have been reported; however, the relationship of raltegravir to these events is not known. Use with caution in patients at increased risk of myopathy or rhabdomyolysis, such as patients receiving concomitant medications known to cause these conditions).
No products indexed under this heading.

Fosphenytoin (Co-administration of raltegravir with drugs that are strong inducers of UGT1A1 may result in reduced plasma concentrations of raltegravir).
No products indexed under this heading.

Fosphenytoin Sodium (Co-administration of raltegravir with drugs that are strong inducers of UGT1A1 may result in reduced plasma concentrations of raltegravir).
No products indexed under this heading.

Lovastatin (Myopathy and rhabdomyolysis have been reported; however, the relationship of raltegravir to these events is not known. Use with caution in patients at increased risk of myopathy or rhabdomyolysis, such as patients receiving concomitant medications known to cause these conditions). Products include:
Advicor 402
Mevacor 2212

Mephenytoin (Co-administration of raltegravir with drugs that are strong inducers of UGT1A1 may result in reduced plasma concentrations of raltegravir).
No products indexed under this heading.

Omeprazole (Co-administration of medicinal products that increase gastric pH (eg, omeprazole) may increase raltegravir levels based on increased raltegravir solubility at higher pH. However, since concomitant use of raltegravir with proton pump inhibitors and H_2 blockers did not result in a unique safety signal in Phase 3 studies, no dose adjustment is recommended).
No products indexed under this heading.

Omeprazole Magnesium (Co-administration of medicinal products that increase gastric pH (eg, omeprazole) may increase raltegravir levels based on increased raltegravir solubility at higher pH. However, since concomitant use of raltegravir with proton pump inhibitors and H_2 blockers did not result in a unique safety signal in Phase 3 studies, no dose adjustment is recommended).
No products indexed under this heading.

Phenobarbital (Co-administration of raltegravir with drugs that are strong inducers of UGT1A1 may result in reduced plasma concentrations of raltegravir). Products include:
Donnatal 2711

Phenobarbital Sodium (Co-administration of raltegravir with drugs that are strong inducers of UGT1A1 may result in reduced plasma concentrations of raltegravir).
No products indexed under this heading.

Phenytoin (Co-administration of raltegravir with drugs that are strong inducers of UGT1A1 may result in reduced plasma concentrations of raltegravir).
No products indexed under this heading.

Phenytoin Sodium (Co-administration of raltegravir with drugs that are strong inducers of UGT1A1 may result in reduced plasma concentrations of raltegravir). Products include:
Phenytek Capsules 2380

Pravastatin Sodium (Myopathy and rhabdomyolysis have been reported; however, the relationship of raltegravir to these events is not known. Use with caution in patients at increased risk of myopathy or rhabdomyolysis, such as patients receiving concomitant medications known to cause these conditions).
No products indexed under this heading.

Rifampicin (Co-administration of raltegravir with drugs that are strong inducers of UGT1A1 may result in reduced plasma concentrations of raltegravir).
No products indexed under this heading.

Rifampin (Rifampin, a strong inducer of UGT1A1, reduces plasma concentrations of raltegravir. The recommended dosage of raltegravir is 800 mg twice daily during co-administration with rifampin).
No products indexed under this heading.

Ritonavir (Atazanavir/ritonavir increases plasma concentrations of raltegravir. However, since concomitant use of raltegravir with atazanavir/ritonavir did not result in a unique safety signal in Phase 3 studies, no dose adjustment is recommended. In addition, tipranavir/ritonavir reduces plasma concentrations of raltegravir. However, since comparable efficacy was observed for this combination relative to other raltegravir- containing regimens in Phase 3 studies 018 and 019, no dose adjustment is recommended). Products include:
Kaletra 458
Norvir 509

IMPORTANT NOTE: Always consult each drug listing in the patient's regimen for possible interactions.

Isentress Interactions Index 918

Rosuvastatin Calcium (Myopathy and rhabdomyolysis have been reported; however, the relationship of raltegravir to these events is not known. Use with caution in patients at increased risk of myopathy or rhabdomyolysis, such as patients receiving concomitant medications known to cause these conditions). Products include:
Crestor 736

Simvastatin (Myopathy and rhabdomyolysis have been reported; however, the relationship of raltegravir to these events is not known. Use with caution in patients at increased risk of myopathy or rhabdomyolysis, such as patients receiving concomitant medications known to cause these conditions). Products include:
Simcor 524
Vytorin 10/10 .... 2303, 3240
Vytorin 10/20 .... 2303, 3240
Vytorin 10/40 .... 2303, 3240
Vytorin 10/80 .... 2303, 3240
Zocor 2289

Tipranavir (Tipranavir/ritonavir reduces plasma concentrations of raltegravir. However, since comparable efficacy was observed for this combination relative to other raltegravir- containing regimens in Phase 3 studies 018 and 019, no dose adjustment is recommended).
No products indexed under this heading.

Food Interactions

Food, unspecified (Raltegravir may be administered with or without food. Administration of multiple doses of raltegravir following a moderate-fat meal (600 Kcal, 21 g fat) did not affect raltegravir AUC to a clinically meaningful degree with an increase of 13% relative to fasting. Raltegravir C_{12hr} was 66% higher and C_{max} was 5% higher following a moderate-fat meal compared to fasting. Administration of raltegravir following a high-fat meal (825 Kcal, 52 g fat) increased AUC and C_{max} by approximately 2-fold and increased C_{12hr} by 4.1-fold. Administration of raltegravir following a low-fat meal (300 Kcal, 2.5 g fat) decreased AUC and C_{max} by 46% and 52%, respectively; C_{12hr} was essentially unchanged. Food appears to increase pharmacokinetic variability relative to fasting).

Meal, unspecified (Raltegravir may be administered with or without food. Administration of multiple doses of raltegravir following a moderate-fat meal (600 Kcal, 21 g fat) did not affect raltegravir AUC to a clinically meaningful degree with an increase of 13% relative to fasting. Raltegravir C_{12hr} was 66% higher and C_{max} was 5% higher following a moderate-fat meal compared to fasting. Administration of raltegravir following a high-fat meal (825 Kcal, 52 g fat) increased AUC and C_{max} by approximately 2-fold and increased C_{12hr} by 4.1-fold. Administration of raltegravir following a low-fat meal (300 Kcal, 2.5 g fat) decreased AUC and C_{max} by 46% and 52%, respectively; C_{12hr} was essentially unchanged. Food appears to increase pharmacokinetic variability relative to fasting).

IVY BLOCK
(Bentoquatam) 3316
None cited in PDR database.

JANUMET TABLETS
(Metformin Hydrochloride, Sitagliptin Phosphate) 2188
May interact with alcohols, calcium channel blockers, cationic drugs that are eliminated by renal tubular, corticosteroids, diuretics, estrogens, oral contraceptives, oral hypoglycemic agents, phenothiazines, phenytoin, radiographic iodinated contrast media, sympathomimetics, thiazides, thyroid preparations, and certain other agents. Compounds in these categories include:

Acarbose (Patients also receiving an insulin secretagogue (eg, sulfonylurea, meglitinide) may require a lower dose of the insulin secretagogue to reduce the risk of hypoglycemia).
No products indexed under this heading.

Albuterol (Sympathomimetics tend to produce hyperglycemia and may lead to loss of glycemic control. When sympathomimetics are administered to a patient receiving Janumet, the patient should be closely observed to maintain adequate glycemic control).
No products indexed under this heading.

Albuterol Sulfate (Sympathomimetics tend to produce hyperglycemia and may lead to loss of glycemic control. When sympathomimetics are administered to a patient receiving Janumet, the patient should be closely observed to maintain adequate glycemic control). Products include:
ProAir HFA 3393
Proventil HFA 3204
Ventolin HFA 1708

Alclometasone Dipropionate (Corticosteroids tend to produce hyperglycemia and may lead to loss of glycemic control. When corticosteroids are administered to a patient receiving Janumet, the patient should be closely observed to maintain adequate glycemic control).
No products indexed under this heading.

Amiloride Hydrochloride (Diuretics tend to produce hyperglycemia and may lead to loss of glycemic control. When diuretics are administered to a patient receiving Janumet, the patient should be closely observed to maintain adequate glycemic control).
No products indexed under this heading.

Amlodipine Besylate (Calcium channel blocking agents tend to produce hyperglycemia and may lead to loss of glycemic control. When calcium channel blocking agents are administered to a patient receiving Janumet, the patient should be closely observed to maintain adequate glycemic control). Products include:
Azor 1010
Exforge 2443
Exforge HCT 2449

Beclomethasone Dipropionate (Corticosteroids tend to produce hyperglycemia and may lead to loss of glycemic control. When corticosteroids are administered to a patient receiving Janumet, the patient should be closely observed to maintain adequate glycemic control). Products include:
Qvar 3398

Beclomethasone Dipropionate Monohydrate (Corticosteroids tend to produce hyperglycemia and may lead to loss of glycemic control. When corticosteroids are administered to a patient receiving Janumet, the patient should be closely observed to maintain adequate glycemic control). Products include:
Beconase AQ 1386

Bendroflumethiazide (Thiazides tend to produce hyperglycemia and may lead to loss of glycemic control. When thiazides are administered to a patient receiving Janumet, the patient should be closely observed to maintain adequate glycemic control).
No products indexed under this heading.

Bepridil Hydrochloride (Calcium channel blocking agents tend to produce hyperglycemia and may lead to loss of glycemic control. When calcium channel blocking agents are administered to a patient receiving Janumet, the patient should be closely observed to maintain adequate glycemic control).
No products indexed under this heading.

Betamethasone (Corticosteroids tend to produce hyperglycemia and may lead to loss of glycemic control. When corticosteroids are administered to a patient receiving Janumet, the patient should be closely observed to maintain adequate glycemic control).
No products indexed under this heading.

Betamethasone Acetate (Corticosteroids tend to produce hyperglycemia and may lead to loss of glycemic control. When corticosteroids are administered to a patient receiving Janumet, the patient should be closely observed to maintain adequate glycemic control).
No products indexed under this heading.

Betamethasone Benzoate (Corticosteroids tend to produce hyperglycemia and may lead to loss of glycemic control. When corticosteroids are administered to a patient receiving Janumet, the patient should be closely observed to maintain adequate glycemic control).
No products indexed under this heading.

Betamethasone Dipropionate (Corticosteroids tend to produce hyperglycemia and may lead to loss of glycemic control. When corticosteroids are administered to a patient receiving Janumet, the patient should be closely observed to maintain adequate glycemic control). Products include:
Diprolene Lotion 0.05% 3108
Diprolene Ointment 0.05% 3109
Diprolene AF Cream 0.05% 3107
Lotrisone 3163

Betamethasone Sodium Phosphate (Corticosteroids tend to produce hyperglycemia and may lead to loss of glycemic control. When corticosteroids are administered to a patient receiving Janumet, the patient should be closely observed to maintain adequate glycemic control).
No products indexed under this heading.

Betamethasone Valerate (Corticosteroids tend to produce hyperglycemia and may lead to loss of glycemic control. When corticosteroids are administered to a patient receiving Janumet, the patient should be closely observed to maintain adequate glycemic control). Products include:
Luxíq 3321

Budesonide (Corticosteroids tend to produce hyperglycemia and may lead to loss of glycemic control. When corticosteroids are administered to a patient receiving Janumet, the patient should be closely observed to maintain adequate glycemic control). Products include:
Pulmicort Flexhaler 714
Symbicort 80/4.5 720
Symbicort 160/4.5 720

Bumetanide (Diuretics tend to produce hyperglycemia and may lead to loss of glycemic control. When diuretics are administered to a patient receiving Janumet, the patient should be closely observed to maintain adequate glycemic control).
No products indexed under this heading.

Chlorothiazide (Thiazides tend to produce hyperglycemia and may lead to loss of glycemic control. When thiazides are administered to a patient receiving Janumet, the patient should be closely observed to maintain adequate glycemic control).
No products indexed under this heading.

Chlorothiazide Sodium (Thiazides tend to produce hyperglycemia and may lead to loss of glycemic control. When thiazides are administered to a patient receiving Janumet, the patient should be closely observed to maintain adequate glycemic control). Products include:
Diuril Intravenous 2009

Chlorotrianisene (Estrogens tend to produce hyperglycemia and may lead to loss of glycemic control. When estrogens are administered to a patient receiving Janumet, the patient should be closely observed to maintain adequate glycemic control).
No products indexed under this heading.

Chlorpromazine (Phenothiazines tend to produce hyperglycemia and may lead to loss of glycemic control. When phenothiazines are administered to a patient receiving Janumet, the patient should be closely observed to maintain adequate glycemic control).
No products indexed under this heading.

Chlorpromazine Hydrochloride (Phenothiazines tend to produce hyperglycemia and may lead to loss of glycemic control. When phenothiazines are administered to a patient receiving Janumet, the patient should be closely observed to maintain adequate glycemic control).
No products indexed under this heading.

Chlorpropamide (Patients also receiving an insulin secretagogue (eg, sulfonylurea, meglitinide) may require a lower dose of the insulin secretagogue to reduce the risk of hypoglycemia).
No products indexed under this heading.

Chlorthalidone (Diuretics tend to produce hyperglycemia and may lead to loss of glycemic control. When diuretics are administered to a patient receiving Janumet, the patient should be closely observed to maintain adequate glycemic control). Products include:
Clorpres 2344

Ciclesonide (Corticosteroids tend to produce hyperglycemia and may lead to loss of glycemic control. When corticosteroids are administered to a patient receiving Janumet, the patient should be closely observed to maintain adequate glycemic control).
No products indexed under this heading.

Cimetidine (Drugs that are eliminated by renal tubular secretion theoretically have the potential for interaction with metformin by competing for common renal tubular transport systems. Drug interaction studies between metformin and oral cimetidine has been observed with a 60% increase in peak metformin plasma and whole blood concentrations and a 40% increase in plasma and whole blood metformin AUC. Careful patient monitoring and dose adjustment of Janumet and/or the interfering drug is recommended in patients who are taking cationic medications that are excreted via the proximal renal tubular secretory system).
No products indexed under this heading.

Cimetidine Hydrochloride (Drugs that are eliminated by renal tubular secretion theoretically have the potential for interaction with metformin by competing for common renal tubular transport systems. Drug interaction studies between metformin and oral cimetidine has been observed with a 60% increase in peak metformin plasma and whole blood concentrations and a 40% increase in plasma and whole blood metformin AUC. Careful patient monitoring and dose adjustment of Janumet and/or the interfering drug is recommended in patients who are tak-

ing cationic medications that are excreted via the proximal renal tubular secretory system).

No products indexed under this heading.

Cortisone Acetate (Corticosteroids tend to produce hyperglycemia and may lead to loss of glycemic control. When corticosteroids are administered to a patient receiving Janumet, the patient should be closely observed to maintain adequate glycemic control).

No products indexed under this heading.

Cyclosporine (Cyclosporine is a potent inhibitor of p-glycoprotein. Co-administration of 600 mg oral dose of cyclosprone with 100 mg of sitagliptin shows an increase in area under the curve (AUC) and maximum concentration (C_{max}) of sitagliptin). Products include:

Desogestrel (Oral contraceptives tend to produce hyperglycemia and may lead to loss of glycemic control. When oral contraceptives are administered to a patient receiving Janumet, the patient should be closely observed to maintain adequate glycemic control).

No products indexed under this heading.

Desoximetasone (Corticosteroids tend to produce hyperglycemia and may lead to loss of glycemic control. When corticosteroids are administered to a patient receiving Janumet, the patient should be closely observed to maintain adequate glycemic control).

No products indexed under this heading.

Dexamethasone (Corticosteroids tend to produce hyperglycemia and may lead to loss of glycemic control. When corticosteroids are administered to a patient receiving Janumet, the patient should be closely observed to maintain adequate glycemic control). Products include:

Dexamethasone Acetate (Corticosteroids tend to produce hyperglycemia and may lead to loss of glycemic control. When corticosteroids are administered to a patient receiving Janumet, the patient should be closely observed to maintain adequate glycemic control).

No products indexed under this heading.

Dexamethasone Phosphate (Corticosteroids tend to produce hyperglycemia and may lead to loss of glycemic control. When corticosteroids are administered to a patient receiving Janumet, the patient should be closely observed to maintain adequate glycemic control).

No products indexed under this heading.

Dexamethasone Sodium (Corticosteroids tend to produce hyperglycemia and may lead to loss of glycemic control. When corticosteroids are administered to a patient receiving Janumet, the patient should be closely observed to maintain adequate glycemic control).

No products indexed under this heading.

Dexamethasone Sodium Phosphate (Corticosteroids tend to produce hyperglycemia and may lead to loss of glycemic control. When corticosteroids are administered to a patient receiving Janumet, the patient should be closely observed to maintain adequate glycemic control).

No products indexed under this heading.

Dexamethasone Sodium Phosphate Injection (Corticosteroids tend to produce hyperglycemia and may lead to loss of glycemic control. When corticosteroids are administered to a patient receiving Janumet, the patient should be closely observed to maintain adequate glycemic control).

No products indexed under this heading.

Diatrizoate Meglumine (Intravascular contrast studies with iodinated materials (for example, intravenous urogram, intravenous cholangiography, angiography, and computed tomography (CT) scans with intravascular contrast materials) can lead to acute alteration of renal function and have been associated with lactic acidosis in patients receiving metformin. Therefore, in patients in whom any such study is planned, Janumet should be temporarily discontinued at the time of or prior to the procedure, and withheld for 48 hours subsequent to the procedure and reinstituted only after renal function has been re-evaluated and found to be normal).

No products indexed under this heading.

Diatrizoate Sodium (Intravascular contrast studies with iodinated materials (for example, intravenous urogram, intravenous cholangiography, angiography, and computed tomography (CT) scans with intravascular contrast materials) can lead to acute alteration of renal function and have been associated with lactic acidosis in patients receiving metformin. Therefore, in patients in whom any such study is planned, Janumet should be temporarily discontinued at the time of or prior to the procedure, and withheld for 48 hours subsequent to the procedure and reinstituted only after renal function has been re-evaluated and found to be normal).

No products indexed under this heading.

Dienestrol (Estrogens tend to produce hyperglycemia and may lead to loss of glycemic control. When estrogens are administered to a patient receiving Janumet, the patient should be closely observed to maintain adequate glycemic control).

No products indexed under this heading.

Diethylstilbestrol (Estrogens tend to produce hyperglycemia and may lead to loss of glycemic control. When estrogens are administered to a patient receiving Janumet, the patient should be closely observed to maintain adequate glycemic control).

No products indexed under this heading.

Diflorasone Diacetate (Corticosteroids tend to produce hyperglycemia and may lead to loss of glycemic control. When corticosteroids are administered to a patient receiving Janumet, the patient should be closely observed to maintain adequate glycemic control).

No products indexed under this heading.

Digoxin (Digoxin, a cationic drug, has the potential to compete with metformin for common renal tubular transport systems, thus affecting the serum concentrations of either digoxin, metformin or both. Patients receiving digoxin should be monitored appropriately. No dosage adjustment if digoxin or Janumet is recommended. There was a slight increase in the area under the curve (AUC, 11%) and mean peak drug concentration (C_{max}, 18%) of digoxin with the co-administration of 100 mg sitagliptin for 10 days). Products include:

Diltiazem Hydrochloride (Calcium channel blocking agents tend to produce hyperglycemia and may lead to loss of glycemic control. When calcium channel blocking agents are administered to a patient receiving Janumet, the patient should be closely observed to maintain adequate glycemic control). Products include:

Dobutamine Hydrochloride (Sympathomimetics tend to produce hyperglycemia and may lead to loss of glycemic control. When sympathomimetics are administered to a patient receiving Janumet, the patient should be closely observed to maintain adequate glycemic control).

No products indexed under this heading.

Dopamine Hydrochloride (Sympathomimetics tend to produce hyperglycemia and may lead to loss of glycemic control. When sympathomimetics are administered to a patient receiving Janumet, the patient should be closely observed to maintain adequate glycemic control).

No products indexed under this heading.

Ephedrine Hydrochloride (Sympathomimetics tend to produce hyperglycemia and may lead to loss of glycemic control. When sympathomimetics are administered to a patient receiving Janumet, the patient should be closely observed to maintain adequate glycemic control).

No products indexed under this heading.

Ephedrine Sulfate (Sympathomimetics tend to produce hyperglycemia and may lead to loss of glycemic control. When sympathomimetics are administered to a patient receiving Janumet, the patient should be closely observed to maintain adequate glycemic control).

No products indexed under this heading.

Ephedrine Tannate (Sympathomimetics tend to produce hyperglycemia and may lead to loss of glycemic control. When sympathomimetics are administered to a patient receiving Janumet, the patient should be closely observed to maintain adequate glycemic control).

No products indexed under this heading.

Epinephrine (Sympathomimetics tend to produce hyperglycemia and may lead to loss of glycemic control. When sympathomimetics are administered to a patient receiving Janumet, the patient should be closely observed to maintain adequate glycemic control). Products include:

Epinephrine Bitartrate (Sympathomimetics tend to produce hyperglycemia and may lead to loss of glycemic control. When sympathomimetics are administered to a patient receiving Janumet, the patient should be closely observed to maintain adequate glycemic control).

No products indexed under this heading.

Epinephrine Hydrochloride (Sympathomimetics tend to produce hyperglycemia and may lead to loss of glycemic control. When sympathomimetics are administered to a patient receiving Janumet, the patient should be closely observed to maintain adequate glycemic control).

No products indexed under this heading.

Estradiol (Estrogens tend to produce hyperglycemia and may lead to loss of glycemic control. When estrogens are administered to a patient receiving Janumet, the patient should be closely observed to maintain adequate glycemic control). Products include:

Estrogens, Conjugated (Estrogens tend to produce hyperglycemia and may lead to loss of glycemic control. When estrogens are administered to a patient receiving Janumet, the patient should be closely observed to maintain adequate glycemic control). Products include:

Estrogens, Esterified (Estrogens tend to produce hyperglycemia and may lead to loss of glycemic control. When estrogens are administered to a patient receiving Janumet, the patient should be closely observed to maintain adequate glycemic control).

No products indexed under this heading.

Estropipate (Estrogens tend to produce hyperglycemia and may lead to loss of glycemic control. When estrogens are administered to a patient receiving Janumet, the patient should be closely observed to maintain adequate glycemic control).

No products indexed under this heading.

Ethacrynic Acid (Diuretics tend to produce hyperglycemia and may lead to loss of glycemic control. When diuretics are administered to a patient receiving Janumet, the patient should be closely observed to maintain adequate glycemic control).

No products indexed under this heading.

Ethanol (Alcohol is known to potentiate the effect of metformin on lactate metabolism. Patients, therefore, should be warned against excessive alcohol intake, acute or chronic, while receiving Janumet).

No products indexed under this heading.

Ethinyl Estradiol (Estrogens tend to produce hyperglycemia and may lead to loss of glycemic control. When estrogens are administered to a patient receiving Janumet, the patient should be closely observed to maintain adequate glycemic control). Products include:

Ethiodized Oil (Intravascular contrast studies with iodinated materials (for example, intravenous urogram, intravenous cholangiography, angiography, and computed tomography (CT) scans with intravascular contrast materials) can lead to acute alteration of renal function and have been associated with lactic acidosis in patients receiving metformin. Therefore, in patients in whom any such study is planned, Janumet should be temporarily discontinued at the time of or prior to the procedure, and withheld for 48 hours subsequent to the procedure and reinstituted only after renal function has been re-evaluated and found to be normal).

No products indexed under this heading.

Ethyl Alcohol (Alcohol is known to potentiate the effect of metformin on lactate metabolism. Patients, therefore, should be warned against excessive alcohol intake, acute or chronic, while receiving Janumet).

No products indexed under this heading.

Ethynodiol Diacetate (Oral contraceptives tend to produce hyperglycemia and may lead to loss of glycemic control. When oral contraceptives are administered to a patient receiving Janumet, the patient should be closely observed to maintain adequate glycemic control).

No products indexed under this heading.

IMPORTANT NOTE: Always consult each drug listing in the patient's regimen for possible interactions.

Janumet Interactions Index 920

Felodipine (Calcium channel blocking agents tend to produce hyperglycemia and may lead to loss of glycemic control. When calcium channel blocking agents are administered to a patient receiving Janumet, the patient should be closely observed to maintain adequate glycemic control).
No products indexed under this heading.

Fludrocortisone Acetate (Corticosteroids tend to produce hyperglycemia and may lead to loss of glycemic control. When corticosteroids are administered to a patient receiving Janumet, the patient should be closely observed to maintain adequate glycemic control).
No products indexed under this heading.

Flumethasone Pivalate (Corticosteroids tend to produce hyperglycemia and may lead to loss of glycemic control. When corticosteroids are administered to a patient receiving Janumet, the patient should be closely observed to maintain adequate glycemic control).
No products indexed under this heading.

Flunisolide Hemihydrate (Corticosteroids tend to produce hyperglycemia and may lead to loss of glycemic control. When corticosteroids are administered to a patient receiving Janumet, the patient should be closely observed to maintain adequate glycemic control).
No products indexed under this heading.

Fluphenazine Decanoate (Phenothiazines tend to produce hyperglycemia and may lead to loss of glycemic control. When phenothiazines are administered to a patient receiving Janumet, the patient should be closely observed to maintain adequate glycemic control).
No products indexed under this heading.

Fluphenazine Enanthate (Phenothiazines tend to produce hyperglycemia and may lead to loss of glycemic control. When phenothiazines are administered to a patient receiving Janumet, the patient should be closely observed to maintain adequate glycemic control).
No products indexed under this heading.

Fluphenazine Hydrochloride (Phenothiazines tend to produce hyperglycemia and may lead to loss of glycemic control. When phenothiazines are administered to a patient receiving Janumet, the patient should be closely observed to maintain adequate glycemic control).
No products indexed under this heading.

Fluticasone Furoate (Corticosteroids tend to produce hyperglycemia and may lead to loss of glycemic control. When corticosteroids are administered to a patient receiving Janumet, the patient should be closely observed to maintain adequate glycemic control). Products include:
Veramyst 1713

Fluticasone Propionate (Corticosteroids tend to produce hyperglycemia and may lead to loss of glycemic control. When corticosteroids are administered to a patient receiving Janumet, the patient should be closely observed to maintain adequate glycemic control). Products include:
Advair 100/50 1275
Advair 250/50 1275
Advair 500/50 1275
Advair HFA 45/21 1288
Advair HFA 115/21 1288
Advair HFA 230/21 1288
Flonase 1459
Flovent Diskus 1463
Flovent HFA 1470

Fosphenytoin (Phenytoin tends to produce hyperglycemia and may lead to loss of glycemic control. When phenytoin is administered to a patient receiving Janumet, the patient should be closely observed to maintain adequate glycemic control).
No products indexed under this heading.

Fosphenytoin Sodium (Phenytoin tends to produce hyperglycemia and may lead to loss of glycemic control. When phenytoin is administered to a patient receiving Janumet, the patient should be closely observed to maintain adequate glycemic control).
No products indexed under this heading.

Furosemide (Furosemide has been shown to increase the metformin plasma and blood C_{max} by 22% and blood AUC by 15%, without any significant change in metformin renal clearance. When administered with metformin, there may be a decrease in C_{max} and AUC of furosemide than when administered alone, and the terminal half-life of metformin may be decreased without any significant change in furosemide renal clearance. Diuretics tend to produce hyperglycemia and may lead to loss of glycemic control. When diuretics are administered to a patient receiving sitagliptin/metformin HCL, the patient should be closely observed to maintain adequate glycemic control). Products include:
Furosemide 2354

Gadopentetate Dimeglumine (Intravascular contrast studies with iodinated materials (for example, intravenous urogram, intravenous cholangiography, angiography, and computed tomography (CT) scans with intravascular contrast materials) can lead to acute alteration of renal function and have been associated with lactic acidosis in patients receiving metformin. Therefore, in patients in whom any such study is planned, Janumet should be temporarily discontinued at the time of or prior to the procedure, and withheld for 48 hours subsequent to the procedure and reinstituted only after renal function has been re-evaluated and found to be normal).
No products indexed under this heading.

Glibenclamide (Patients also receiving an insulin secretagogue (eg, sulfonylurea, meglitinide) may require a lower dose of the insulin secretagogue to reduce the risk of hypoglycemia).
No products indexed under this heading.

Glimepiride (Patients also receiving an insulin secretagogue (eg, sulfonylurea, meglitinide) may require a lower dose of the insulin secretagogue to reduce the risk of hypoglycemia). Products include:
Avandaryl 1356
Duetact 3354

Glipizide (Patients also receiving an insulin secretagogue (eg, sulfonylurea, meglitinide) may require a lower dose of the insulin secretagogue to reduce the risk of hypoglycemia).
No products indexed under this heading.

Glyburide (A decrease in glyburide area under the curve (AUC) and mean peak drug concentration (C_{max}) were observed but were highly variable in a single-dose interaction study in type 2 diabetes patients when co-administering metformin with glyburide).
No products indexed under this heading.

Hydrochlorothiazide (Thiazides tend to produce hyperglycemia and may lead to loss of glycemic control. When thiazides are administered to a patient receiving Janumet, the patient should be closely observed to maintain adequate glycemic control). Products include:
Atacand HCT 700
Avalide 2956
Benicar HCT 1017
Diovan HCT 2419
Dyazide 1429
Exforge HCT 2449
Hyzaar 2162
Hyzaar 100-12.5 2162
Micardis HCT 889
Prinzide 2246
Tekturna HCT 2541
Teveten HCT 541

Hydrocortisone (Corticosteroids tend to produce hyperglycemia and may lead to loss of glycemic control. When corticosteroids are administered to a patient receiving Janumet, the patient should be closely observed to maintain adequate glycemic control).
No products indexed under this heading.

Hydrocortisone (Alcohol) (Corticosteroids tend to produce hyperglycemia and may lead to loss of glycemic control. When corticosteroids are administered to a patient receiving Janumet, the patient should be closely observed to maintain adequate glycemic control).
No products indexed under this heading.

Hydrocortisone Acetate (Corticosteroids tend to produce hyperglycemia and may lead to loss of glycemic control. When corticosteroids are administered to a patient receiving Janumet, the patient should be closely observed to maintain adequate glycemic control).
No products indexed under this heading.

Hydrocortisone Butyrate (Corticosteroids tend to produce hyperglycemia and may lead to loss of glycemic control. When corticosteroids are administered to a patient receiving Janumet, the patient should be closely observed to maintain adequate glycemic control).
No products indexed under this heading.

Hydrocortisone Cypionate (Corticosteroids tend to produce hyperglycemia and may lead to loss of glycemic control. When corticosteroids are administered to a patient receiving Janumet, the patient should be closely observed to maintain adequate glycemic control).
No products indexed under this heading.

Hydrocortisone Hemisuccinate (Corticosteroids tend to produce hyperglycemia and may lead to loss of glycemic control. When corticosteroids are administered to a patient receiving Janumet, the patient should be closely observed to maintain adequate glycemic control).
No products indexed under this heading.

Hydrocortisone Probutate (Corticosteroids tend to produce hyperglycemia and may lead to loss of glycemic control. When corticosteroids are administered to a patient receiving Janumet, the patient should be closely observed to maintain adequate glycemic control).
No products indexed under this heading.

Hydrocortisone Sodium Phosphate (Corticosteroids tend to produce hyperglycemia and may lead to loss of glycemic control. When corticosteroids are administered to a patient receiving Janumet, the patient should be closely observed to maintain adequate glycemic control).
No products indexed under this heading.

Hydrocortisone Sodium Succinate (Corticosteroids tend to produce hyperglycemia and may lead to loss of glycemic control. When corticosteroids are administered to a patient receiving Janumet, the patient should be closely observed to maintain adequate glycemic control).
No products indexed under this heading.

Hydrocortisone Valerate (Corticosteroids tend to produce hyperglycemia and may lead to loss of glycemic control. When corticosteroids are administered to a patient receiving Janumet, the patient should be closely observed to maintain adequate glycemic control).
No products indexed under this heading.

Hydroflumethiazide (Thiazides tend to produce hyperglycemia and may lead to loss of glycemic control. When thiazides are administered to a patient receiving Janumet, the patient should be closely observed to maintain adequate glycemic control).
No products indexed under this heading.

Indapamide (Diuretics tend to produce hyperglycemia and may lead to loss of glycemic control. When diuretics are administered to a patient receiving Janumet, the patient should be closely observed to maintain adequate glycemic control). Products include:
Indapamide 2356

Iodamide Meglumine (Intravascular contrast studies with iodinated materials (for example, intravenous urogram, intravenous cholangiography, angiography, and computed tomography (CT) scans with intravascular contrast materials) can lead to acute alteration of renal function and have been associated with lactic acidosis in patients receiving metformin. Therefore, in patients in whom any such study is planned, Janumet should be temporarily discontinued at the time of or prior to the procedure, and withheld for 48 hours subsequent to the procedure and reinstituted only after renal function has been re-evaluated and found to be normal).
No products indexed under this heading.

Iohexol (Intravascular contrast studies with iodinated materials (for example, intravenous urogram, intravenous cholangiography, angiography, and computed tomography (CT) scans with intravascular contrast materials) can lead to acute alteration of renal function and have been associated with lactic acidosis in patients receiving metformin. Therefore, in patients in whom any such study is planned, Janumet should be temporarily discontinued at the time of or prior to the procedure, and withheld for 48 hours subsequent to the procedure and reinstituted only after renal function has been re-evaluated and found to be normal).
No products indexed under this heading.

Iopamidol (Intravascular contrast studies with iodinated materials (for example, intravenous urogram, intravenous cholangiography, angiography, and computed tomography (CT) scans with intravascular contrast materials) can lead to acute alteration of renal function and have been associated with lactic acidosis in patients receiving metformin. Therefore, in patients in whom any such study is planned, Janumet should be temporarily discontinued at the time of or prior to the procedure, and withheld for 48 hours subsequent to the procedure and reinstituted only after renal function has been re-evaluated and found to be normal).
No products indexed under this heading.

Iopanoic Acid (Intravascular contrast studies with iodinated materials (for example, intravenous urogram, intravenous cholangiography, angiography, and computed tomography (CT) scans with intravascular contrast materials) can lead to acute alteration of renal function and have been associated with lactic acidosis in patients receiving metformin. Therefore, in patients in whom any such study is planned, Janumet should be temporarily discontinued at the time of or prior to the procedure, and withheld for 48 hours subsequent

(⊙ Described in PDR® for Ophthalmic Medicines)

921 Interactions Index Janumet

to the procedure and reinstituted only after renal function has been re-evaluated and found to be normal).
No products indexed under this heading.

Iothalamate Meglumine (Intravascular contrast studies with iodinated materials (for example, intravenous urogram, intravenous cholangiography, angiography, and computed tomography (CT) scans with intravascular contrast materials) can lead to acute alteration of renal function and have been associated with lactic acidosis in patients receiving metformin. Therefore, in patients in whom any such study is planned, Janumet should be temporarily discontinued at the time of or prior to the procedure, and withheld for 48 hours subsequent to the procedure and reinstituted only after renal function has been re-evaluated and found to be normal).
No products indexed under this heading.

Ioxaglate Meglumine (Intravascular contrast studies with iodinated materials (for example, intravenous urogram, intravenous cholangiography, angiography, and computed tomography (CT) scans with intravascular contrast materials) can lead to acute alteration of renal function and have been associated with lactic acidosis in patients receiving metformin. Therefore, in patients in whom any such study is planned, Janumet should be temporarily discontinued at the time of or prior to the procedure, and withheld for 48 hours subsequent to the procedure and reinstituted only after renal function has been re-evaluated and found to be normal).
No products indexed under this heading.

Ioxaglate Sodium (Intravascular contrast studies with iodinated materials (for example, intravenous urogram, intravenous cholangiography, angiography, and computed tomography (CT) scans with intravascular contrast materials) can lead to acute alteration of renal function and have been associated with lactic acidosis in patients receiving metformin. Therefore, in patients in whom any such study is planned, Janumet should be temporarily discontinued at the time of or prior to the procedure, and withheld for 48 hours subsequent to the procedure and reinstituted only after renal function has been re-evaluated and found to be normal).
No products indexed under this heading.

Isoniazid (Isoniazides tend to produce hyperglycemia and may lead to loss of glycemic control. When isoniazides are administered to a patient receiving Janumet, the patient should be closely observed to maintain adequate glycemic control).
No products indexed under this heading.

Isoproterenol Hydrochloride (Sympathomimetics tend to produce hyperglycemia and may lead to loss of glycemic control. When sympathomimetics are administered to a patient receiving Janumet, the patient should be closely observed to maintain adequate glycemic control).
No products indexed under this heading.

Isoproterenol Sulfate (Sympathomimetics tend to produce hyperglycemia and may lead to loss of glycemic control. When sympathomimetics are administered to a patient receiving Janumet, the patient should be closely observed to maintain adequate glycemic control).
No products indexed under this heading.

Isradipine (Calcium channel blocking agents tend to produce hyperglycemia and may lead to loss of glycemic control. When calcium channel blocking agents are administered to a patient receiving Janumet, the patient should be closely observed to maintain adequate glycemic control). Products include:
DynaCirc CR 1432

Levalbuterol Hydrochloride (Sympathomimetics tend to produce hyperglycemia and may lead to loss of glycemic control. When sympathomimetics are administered to a patient receiving Janumet, the patient should be closely observed to maintain adequate glycemic control).
No products indexed under this heading.

Levonorgestrel (Oral contraceptives tend to produce hyperglycemia and may lead to loss of glycemic control. When oral contraceptives are administered to a patient receiving Janumet, the patient should be closely observed to maintain adequate glycemic control). Products include:
Climara Pro 847
LoSeasonique 3407
Lybrel 3514
Mirena 854
Plan B 3416
Seasonique 3418

Levothyroxine Sodium (Thyroid products tend to produce hyperglycemia and may lead to loss of glycemic control. When thyroid products are administered to a patient receiving Janumet, the patient should be closely observed to maintain adequate glycemic control). Products include:
Levoxyl Tablets 1843
Synthroid 529

Liothyronine Sodium (Thyroid products tend to produce hyperglycemia and may lead to loss of glycemic control. When thyroid products are administered to a patient receiving Janumet, the patient should be closely observed to maintain adequate glycemic control). Products include:
Cytomel 1830

Liotrix (Thyroid products tend to produce hyperglycemia and may lead to loss of glycemic control. When thyroid products are administered to a patient receiving Janumet, the patient should be closely observed to maintain adequate glycemic control).
No products indexed under this heading.

Mesoridazine Besylate (Phenothiazines tend to produce hyperglycemia and may lead to loss of glycemic control. When phenothiazines are administered to a patient receiving Janumet, the patient should be closely observed to maintain adequate glycemic control).
No products indexed under this heading.

Mestranol (Oral contraceptives tend to produce hyperglycemia and may lead to loss of glycemic control. When oral contraceptives are administered to a patient receiving Janumet, the patient should be closely observed to maintain adequate glycemic control).
No products indexed under this heading.

Metaproterenol Sulfate (Sympathomimetics tend to produce hyperglycemia and may lead to loss of glycemic control. When sympathomimetics are administered to a patient receiving Janumet, the patient should be closely observed to maintain adequate glycemic control).
No products indexed under this heading.

Metaraminol Bitartrate (Sympathomimetics tend to produce hyperglycemia and may lead to loss of glycemic control. When sympathomimetics are administered to a patient receiving Janumet, the patient should be closely observed to maintain adequate glycemic control).
No products indexed under this heading.

Methotrimeprazine (Phenothiazines tend to produce hyperglycemia and may lead to loss of glycemic control. When phenothiazines are administered to a patient receiving Janumet, the patient should be closely observed to maintain adequate glycemic control).
No products indexed under this heading.

Methoxamine Hydrochloride (Sympathomimetics tend to produce hyperglycemia and may lead to loss of glycemic control. When sympathomimetics are administered to a patient receiving Janumet, the patient should be closely observed to maintain adequate glycemic control).
No products indexed under this heading.

Methyclothiazide (Thiazides tend to produce hyperglycemia and may lead to loss of glycemic control. When thiazides are administered to a patient receiving Janumet, the patient should be closely observed to maintain adequate glycemic control).
No products indexed under this heading.

Methylprednisolone (Corticosteroids tend to produce hyperglycemia and may lead to loss of glycemic control. When corticosteroids are administered to a patient receiving Janumet, the patient should be closely observed to maintain adequate glycemic control).
No products indexed under this heading.

Methylprednisolone Acetate (Corticosteroids tend to produce hyperglycemia and may lead to loss of glycemic control. When corticosteroids are administered to a patient receiving Janumet, the patient should be closely observed to maintain adequate glycemic control).
No products indexed under this heading.

Methylprednisolone Sodium Succinate (Corticosteroids tend to produce hyperglycemia and may lead to loss of glycemic control. When corticosteroids are administered to a patient receiving Janumet, the patient should be closely observed to maintain adequate glycemic control).
No products indexed under this heading.

Metolazone (Diuretics tend to produce hyperglycemia and may lead to loss of glycemic control. When diuretics are administered to a patient receiving Janumet, the patient should be closely observed to maintain adequate glycemic control).
No products indexed under this heading.

Mibefradil Dihydrochloride (Calcium channel blocking agents tend to produce hyperglycemia and may lead to loss of glycemic control. When calcium channel blocking agents are administered to a patient receiving Janumet, the patient should be closely observed to maintain adequate glycemic control).
No products indexed under this heading.

Miglitol (Patients also receiving an insulin secretagogue (eg, sulfonylurea, meglitinide) may require a lower dose of the insulin secretagogue to reduce the risk of hypoglycemia).
No products indexed under this heading.

Mometasone Furoate (Corticosteroids tend to produce hyperglycemia and may lead to loss of glycemic control. When corticosteroids are administered to a patient receiving Janumet, the patient should be closely observed to maintain adequate glycemic control). Products include:
Asmanex 3058
Elocon Cream 3111
Elocon Lotion 3112
Elocon Ointment 3114

Mometasone Furoate Monohydrate (Corticosteroids tend to produce hyperglycemia and may lead to loss of glycemic control. When corticosteroids are administered to a patient receiving Janumet, the patient should be closely observed to maintain adequate glycemic control). Products include:
Nasonex 3166

Morphine Sulfate (Cationic drugs that are eliminated by renal tubular secretion theoretically have the potential for interaction with metformin by competing for common renal tubular transport systems. Careful patient monitoring and dose adjustment of Janumet and/or interfering drug is recommended in patients taking cationic medications that are excreted via the proximal renal tubular secretory system). Products include:
Avinza 1822
Embeda 1831
MS Contin 2803

Nateglinide (Patients also receiving an insulin secretagogue (eg, sulfonylurea, meglitinide) may require a lower dose of the insulin secretagogue to reduce the risk of hypoglycemia).
No products indexed under this heading.

Nicardipine (Calcium channel blocking agents tend to produce hyperglycemia and may lead to loss of glycemic control. When calcium channel blocking agents are administered to a patient receiving Janumet, the patient should be closely observed to maintain adequate glycemic control).
No products indexed under this heading.

Nicardipine Hydrochloride (Calcium channel blocking agents tend to produce hyperglycemia and may lead to loss of glycemic control. When calcium channel blocking agents are administered to a patient receiving Janumet, the patient should be closely observed to maintain adequate glycemic control).
No products indexed under this heading.

Nicotinic Acid (Nicotinic acid tends to produce hyperglycemia and may lead to loss of glycemic control. When nicotinic acid is administered to a patient receiving Janumet, the patient should be closely observed to maintain adequate glycemic control).
No products indexed under this heading.

Nifedipine (A single-dose, metformin-nifedipine drug interaction study in normal healthy volunteers demonstrated an increase in plasma metformin C_{max} and AUC by 10% to 9%, respectively in co-administering metformin with nifedipine and increased the amount excreted in the urine. Nifedipine appears to enhance the absorption of metformin. Metformin had minimal effects on nifedipine).
No products indexed under this heading.

Nimodipine (Calcium channel blocking agents tend to produce hyperglycemia and may lead to loss of glycemic control. When calcium channel blocking agents are administered to a patient receiving Janumet, the patient should be closely observed to maintain adequate glycemic control).
No products indexed under this heading.

Nisoldipine (Calcium channel blocking agents tend to produce hyperglycemia and may lead to loss of glycemic control. When calcium channel blocking agents are administered to a patient receiving Janumet, the patient should be closely observed to maintain adequate glycemic control).
No products indexed under this heading.

Norepinephrine Bitartrate (Sympathomimetics tend to produce hyperglycemia and may lead to loss of glycemic control. When sympathomimetics are administered to a patient receiving Janumet, the patient should be closely observed to maintain adequate glycemic control).
No products indexed under this heading.

Norethindrone (Oral contraceptives tend to produce hyperglycemia and may

lead to loss of glycemic control. When oral contraceptives are administered to a patient receiving Janumet, the patient should be closely observed to maintain adequate glycemic control). Products include:

Norethynodrel (Oral contraceptives tend to produce hyperglycemia and may lead to loss of glycemic control. When oral contraceptives are administered to a patient receiving Janumet, the patient should be closely observed to maintain adequate glycemic control).
No products indexed under this heading.

Norgestimate (Oral contraceptives tend to produce hyperglycemia and may lead to loss of glycemic control. When oral contraceptives are administered to a patient receiving Janumet, the patient should be closely observed to maintain adequate glycemic control). Products include:

Norgestrel (Oral contraceptives tend to produce hyperglycemia and may lead to loss of glycemic control. When oral contraceptives are administered to a patient receiving Janumet, the patient should be closely observed to maintain adequate glycemic control).
No products indexed under this heading.

Perphenazine (Phenothiazines tend to produce hyperglycemia and may lead to loss of glycemic control. When phenothiazines are administered to a patient receiving Janumet, the patient should be closely observed to maintain adequate glycemic control).
No products indexed under this heading.

Phenothiazine Derivatives (Phenothiazines tend to produce hyperglycemia and may lead to loss of glycemic control. When phenothiazines are administered to a patient receiving Janumet, the patient should be closely observed to maintain adequate glycemic control).
No products indexed under this heading.

Phenothiazines (Phenothiazines tend to produce hyperglycemia and may lead to loss of glycemic control. When phenothiazines are administered to a patient receiving Janumet, the patient should be closely observed to maintain adequate glycemic control).
No products indexed under this heading.

Phenylephrine Bitartrate (Sympathomimetics tend to produce hyperglycemia and may lead to loss of glycemic control. When sympathomimetics are administered to a patient receiving Janumet, the patient should be closely observed to maintain adequate glycemic control).
No products indexed under this heading.

Phenylephrine Hydrochloride (Sympathomimetics tend to produce hyperglycemia and may lead to loss of glycemic control. When sympathomimetics are administered to a patient receiving Janumet, the patient should be closely observed to maintain adequate glycemic control). Products include:

Phenylephrine Tannate (Sympathomimetics tend to produce hyperglycemia and may lead to loss of glycemic control. When sympathomimetics are administered to a patient receiving Janumet, the patient should be closely observed to maintain adequate glycemic control).
No products indexed under this heading.

Phenylpropanolamine Hydrochloride (Sympathomimetics tend to produce hyperglycemia and may lead to loss of glycemic control. When sympathomimetics are administered to a patient receiving Janumet, the patient should be closely observed to maintain adequate glycemic control).
No products indexed under this heading.

Phenytoin (Phenytoin tends to produce hyperglycemia and may lead to loss of glycemic control. When phenytoin is administered to a patient receiving Janumet, the patient should be closely observed to maintain adequate glycemic control).
No products indexed under this heading.

Phenytoin Sodium (Phenytoin tends to produce hyperglycemia and may lead to loss of glycemic control. When phenytoin is administered to a patient receiving Janumet, the patient should be closely observed to maintain adequate glycemic control). Products include:

Pioglitazone Hydrochloride (Patients also receiving an insulin secretagogue (eg, sulfonylurea, meglitinide) may require a lower dose of the insulin secretagogue to reduce the risk of hypoglycemia). Products include:

Pirbuterol Acetate (Sympathomimetics tend to produce hyperglycemia and may lead to loss of glycemic control. When sympathomimetics are administered to a patient receiving Janumet, the patient should be closely observed to maintain adequate glycemic control). Products include:

Polyestradiol Phosphate (Estrogens tend to produce hyperglycemia and may lead to loss of glycemic control. When estrogens are administered to a patient receiving Janumet, the patient should be closely observed to maintain adequate glycemic control).
No products indexed under this heading.

Polythiazide (Thiazides tend to produce hyperglycemia and may lead to loss of glycemic control. When thiazides are administered to a patient receiving Janumet, the patient should be closely observed to maintain adequate glycemic control).
No products indexed under this heading.

Prednisolone (Corticosteroids tend to produce hyperglycemia and may lead to loss of glycemic control. When corticosteroids are administered to a patient receiving Janumet, the patient should be closely observed to maintain adequate glycemic control).
No products indexed under this heading.

Prednisolone Acetate (Corticosteroids tend to produce hyperglycemia and may lead to loss of glycemic control. When corticosteroids are administered to a patient receiving Janumet, the patient should be closely observed to maintain adequate glycemic control). Products include:

Prednisolone Sodium Phosphate (Corticosteroids tend to produce hyperglycemia and may lead to loss of glycemic control. When corticosteroids are administered to a patient receiving Janumet, the patient should be closely observed to maintain adequate glycemic control).
No products indexed under this heading.

Prednisolone Tebutate (Corticosteroids tend to produce hyperglycemia and may lead to loss of glycemic control. When corticosteroids are administered to a patient receiving Janumet, the patient should be closely observed to maintain adequate glycemic control).
No products indexed under this heading.

Prednisone (Corticosteroids tend to produce hyperglycemia and may lead to loss of glycemic control. When corticosteroids are administered to a patient receiving Janumet, the patient should be closely observed to maintain adequate glycemic control).
No products indexed under this heading.

Prednisone sodium phosphate (Corticosteroids tend to produce hyperglycemia and may lead to loss of glycemic control. When corticosteroids are administered to a patient receiving Janumet, the patient should be closely observed to maintain adequate glycemic control).
No products indexed under this heading.

Procainamide Hydrochloride (Cationic drugs that are eliminated by renal tubular secretion theoretically have the potential for interaction with metformin by competing for common renal tubular transport systems. Careful patient monitoring and dose adjustment of Janumet and/or interfering drug is recommended in patients taking cationic medications that are excreted via the proximal renal tubular secretory system).
No products indexed under this heading.

Prochlorperazine (Phenothiazines tend to produce hyperglycemia and may lead to loss of glycemic control. When phenothiazines are administered to a patient receiving Janumet, the patient should be closely observed to maintain adequate glycemic control).
No products indexed under this heading.

Prochlorperazine Edisylate (Phenothiazines tend to produce hyperglycemia and may lead to loss of glycemic control. When phenothiazines are administered to a patient receiving Janumet, the patient should be closely observed to maintain adequate glycemic control).
No products indexed under this heading.

Prochlorperazine Maleate (Phenothiazines tend to produce hyperglycemia and may lead to loss of glycemic control. When phenothiazines are administered to a patient receiving Janumet, the patient should be closely observed to maintain adequate glycemic control).
No products indexed under this heading.

Promethazine (Phenothiazines tend to produce hyperglycemia and may lead to loss of glycemic control. When phenothiazines are administered to a patient receiving Janumet, the patient should be closely observed to maintain adequate glycemic control).
No products indexed under this heading.

Promethazine Hydrochloride (Phenothiazines tend to produce hyperglycemia and may lead to loss of glycemic control. When phenothiazines are administered to a patient receiving Janumet, the patient should be closely observed to maintain adequate glycemic control).
No products indexed under this heading.

Pseudoephedrine Hydrochloride (Sympathomimetics tend to produce hyperglycemia and may lead to loss of glycemic control. When sympathomimetics are administered to a patient receiving Janumet, the patient should be closely observed to maintain adequate glycemic control). Products include:

Pseudoephedrine Sulfate (Sympathomimetics tend to produce hyperglycemic control. When sympathomimetics are administered to a patient receiving Janumet, the patient should be closely observed to maintain adequate glycemic control). Products include:

Quinestrol (Estrogens tend to produce hyperglycemia and may lead to loss of glycemic control. When estrogens are administered to a patient receiving Janumet, the patient should be closely observed to maintain adequate glycemic control).
No products indexed under this heading.

Quinidine Gluconate (Cationic drugs that are eliminated by renal tubular secretion theoretically have the potential for interaction with metformin by competing for common renal tubular transport systems. Careful patient monitoring and dose adjustment of Janumet and/or interfering drug is recommended in patients taking cationic medications that are excreted via the proximal renal tubular secretory system).
No products indexed under this heading.

Quinidine Polygalacturonate (Cationic drugs that are eliminated by renal tubular secretion theoretically have the potential for interaction with metformin by competing for common renal tubular transport systems. Careful patient monitoring and dose adjustment of Janumet and/or interfering drug is recommended in patients taking cationic medications that are excreted via the proximal renal tubular secretory system).
No products indexed under this heading.

Quinidine Sulfate (Cationic drugs that are eliminated by renal tubular secretion theoretically have the potential for interaction with metformin by competing for common renal tubular transport systems. Careful patient monitoring and dose adjustment of Janumet and/or interfering drug is recommended in patients taking cationic medications that are excreted via the proximal renal tubular secretory system).
No products indexed under this heading.

Quinine Sulfate (Cationic drugs that are eliminated by renal tubular secretion theoretically have the potential for interaction with metformin by competing for common renal tubular transport systems. Careful patient monitoring and dose adjustment of Janumet and/or interfering drug is recommended in patients taking cationic medications that are excreted via the proximal renal tubular secretory system).
No products indexed under this heading.

Ranitidine Hydrochloride (Cationic drugs that are eliminated by renal tubular secretion theoretically have the potential for interaction with metformin by competing for common renal tubular transport systems. Careful patient monitoring and dose adjustment of Janumet and/or interfering drug is recommended in patients taking cationic medications that are excreted via the proximal renal tubular secretory system). Products include:

Food Interactions

JANUVIA TABLETS

Januvia Interactions Index 924

tolbutamide, and glimepiride) which, like glyburide, are primarily eliminated by CYP2C9).
No products indexed under this heading.

Glyburide (When sitagliptin is used in combination with a sulfonylurea, a lower dose of sulfonylurea may be required to reduce the risk of hypoglycemia. Single-dose pharmacokinetics of glyburide, a CYP2C9 substrate, was not meaningfully altered in subjects receiving multiple doses of sitagliptin. Clinically meaningful interactions would not be expected with other sulfonylureas (eg, glipizide, tolbutamide, and glimepiride) which, like glyburide, are primarily eliminated by CYP2C9).
No products indexed under this heading.

Tolazamide (When sitagliptin is used in combination with a sulfonylurea, a lower dose of sulfonylurea may be required to reduce the risk of hypoglycemia. Single-dose pharmacokinetics of glyburide, a CYP2C9 substrate, was not meaningfully altered in subjects receiving multiple doses of sitagliptin. Clinically meaningful interactions would not be expected with other sulfonylureas (eg, glipizide, tolbutamide, and glimepiride) which, like glyburide, are primarily eliminated by CYP2C9).
No products indexed under this heading.

Tolbutamide (When sitagliptin is used in combination with a sulfonylurea, a lower dose of sulfonylurea may be required to reduce the risk of hypoglycemia. Single-dose pharmacokinetics of glyburide, a CYP2C9 substrate, was not meaningfully altered in subjects receiving multiple doses of sitagliptin. Clinically meaningful interactions would not be expected with other sulfonylureas (eg, glipizide, tolbutamide, and glimepiride) which, like glyburide, are primarily eliminated by CYP2C9).
No products indexed under this heading.

KALETRA ORAL SOLUTION
(Lopinavir, Ritonavir) 458
See Kaletra Tablets

KALETRA TABLETS
(Lopinavir, Ritonavir) 458
May interact with beta-blockers, calcium channel blockers, cytochrome p450 3a inducers (selected), cytochrome p450 3a inhibitors (selected), cytochrome p450 3a substrates (selected), dexamethasones, dihydropyridine calcium channel blockers, drugs that prolong the PR interval, drugs that prolong the QT interval, ergot-containing drugs, insulin, oral contraceptives, oral hypoglycemic agents, phenytoin, quinidine, and certain other agents. Compounds in these categories include:

Abacavir Sulfate (Kaletra induces glucuronidation; therefore, Kaletra has the potential to reduce abacavir plasma concentrations; the clinical significance is unknown). Products include:
Epzicom 1448
Trizivir 1688
Ziagen 1740

Acarbose (New onset diabetes mellitus, exacerbation of pre-existing diabetes mellitus, and hyperglycemia have been reported during post-marketing surveillance in HIV-1 infected patients receiving protease inhibitor therapy. Some patients required either initiation or dose adjustments of oral hypoglycemic agents for treatment of these events).
No products indexed under this heading.

Acebutolol Hydrochloride (PR interval prolongation may occur in some patients. Cases of second and third degree heart block have been reported. Caution must be used in patients with pre-existing conduction system disease, ischemic heart disease, cardiomyopathy, underlying structural heart disease or when administering with other drugs that may prolong the PR interval including β-adrenergic blockers).
No products indexed under this heading.

Alfentanil Hydrochloride (Kaletra is an inhibitor of CYP3A and may increase plasma concentrations of agents that are primarily metabolized by CYP3A. Agents that are extensively metabolized by CYP3A and have high first pass metabolism appear to be the most susceptible to large increases in AUC (> 3-fold) when co-administered with Kaletra. Thus, co-administration of Kaletra with drugs highly dependent on CYP3A for clearance and for which elevated plasma concentrations are associated with serious and/or life-threatening events is contraindicated. Co-administration with other CYP3A substrates may require a dose adjustment or additional monitoring).
No products indexed under this heading.

Allium sativum (Co-administration of Kaletra is contraindicated with potent CYP3A inducers where significantly reduced lopinavir plasma concentrations may be associated with the potential for loss of virologic response and possible resistance and cross-resistance).
No products indexed under this heading.

Alprazolam (Cases of QT interval prolongation and torsade de pointes have been reported although causality of Kaletra could not be established. Avoid use in patients with congenital long QT syndrome, those with hypokalemia, and with other drugs that prolong the QT interval).
No products indexed under this heading.

Aminophylline (Kaletra is an inhibitor of CYP3A and may increase plasma concentrations of agents that are primarily metabolized by CYP3A. Agents that are extensively metabolized by CYP3A and have high first pass metabolism appear to be the most susceptible to large increases in AUC (> 3-fold) when co-administered with Kaletra. Thus, co-administration of Kaletra with drugs highly dependent on CYP3A for clearance and for which elevated plasma concentrations are associated with serious and/or life-threatening events is contraindicated. Co-administration with other CYP3A substrates may require a dose adjustment or additional monitoring).
No products indexed under this heading.

Amiodarone Hydrochloride (Co-administration can result in increased amiodarone plasma concentrations. Caution is warranted and therapeutic concentration monitoring is recommended when co-administered with Kaletra).
No products indexed under this heading.

Amitriptyline Hydrochloride (Cases of QT interval prolongation and torsade de pointes have been reported although causality of Kaletra could not be established. Avoid use in patients with congenital long QT syndrome, those with hypokalemia, and with other drugs that prolong the QT interval).
No products indexed under this heading.

Amlodipine Besylate (Increased plasma concentrations of dihydropyridine calcium channel blockers. Caution is warranted and clinical monitoring of patients is recommended). Products include:
Azor 1010
Exforge 2443
Exforge HCT 2449

Amoxapine (Cases of QT interval prolongation and torsade de pointes have been reported although causality of Kaletra could not be established. Avoid use in patients with congenital long QT syndrome, those with hypokalemia, and with other drugs that prolong the QT interval).
No products indexed under this heading.

Amprenavir (Co-administration may result in increased amprenavir plasma concentration. Kaletra should not be administered once-daily in combination with amprenavir).
No products indexed under this heading.

Aprepitant (Co-administration of Kaletra is contraindicated with potent CYP3A inducers where significantly reduced lopinavir plasma concentrations may be associated with the potential for loss of virologic response and possible resistance and cross-resistance). Products include:
Emend 2124

Astemizole (Kaletra is an inhibitor of the CYP450 3A. Co-administration with drugs that are highly dependent on CYP450 3A for clearance and for which elevated plasma concentrations are associated with serious and/or life threatening events, such as astemizole, is contraindicated).
No products indexed under this heading.

Atazanavir (The impact on the PR interval of co-administration of Kaletra with other drugs that prolong the PR interval (including atanazavir) has not been evaluated. As a result, co-administration of Kaletra with these drugs should be undertaken with caution, particularly with those drugs metabolized by CYP3A. Clinical monitoring is recommended).
No products indexed under this heading.

Atazanavir Sulfate (The impact on the PR interval of co-administration of Kaletra with other drugs that prolong the PR interval (including digoxin) has not been evaluated. As a result, co-administration of Kaletra with these drugs should be undertaken with caution, particularly with those drugs metabolized by CYP3A. Clinical monitoring is recommended).
No products indexed under this heading.

Atenolol (PR interval prolongation may occur in some patients. Cases of second and third degree heart block have been reported. Caution must be used in patients with pre-existing conduction system disease, ischemic heart disease, cardiomyopathy, underlying structural heart disease or when administering with other drugs that may prolong the PR interval including β-adrenergic blockers).
No products indexed under this heading.

Atorvastatin Calcium (Use lowest possible dose of atorvastatin with careful monitoring, or consider other HMG-CoA reductase inhibitors such as pravastatin or fluvastatin in combination with Kaletra). Products include:
Lipitor 2703

Atovaquone (Co-administration can result in decreased atovaquone plasma concentrations; clinical significance is unknown; however, increase in atovaquone doses may be needed). Products include:
Malarone Pediatric Tablets 1572
Malarone 1572
Mepron Suspension 1576

Bepridil Hydrochloride (Co-administration can result in increased bepridil plasma concentrations; caution and monitoring is recommended).
No products indexed under this heading.

Betaxolol Hydrochloride (PR interval prolongation may occur in some patients. Cases of second and third degree heart block have been reported. Caution must be used in patients with pre-existing conduction system disease, ischemic heart disease, cardiomyopathy, underlying structural heart disease or when administering with other drugs that may prolong the PR interval including β-adrenergic blockers).
No products indexed under this heading.

Bisoprolol Fumarate (PR interval prolongation may occur in some patients. Cases of second and third degree heart block have been reported. Caution must be used in patients with pre-existing conduction system disease, ischemic heart disease, cardiomyopathy, underlying structural heart disease or when administering with other drugs that may prolong the PR interval including β-adrenergic blockers).
No products indexed under this heading.

Bretylium Tosylate (Cases of QT interval prolongation and torsade de pointes have been reported although causality of Kaletra could not be established. Avoid use in patients with congenital long QT syndrome, those with hypokalemia, and with other drugs that prolong the QT interval).
No products indexed under this heading.

Bromocriptine Mesylate (Kaletra is an inhibitor of CYP3A and may increase plasma concentrations of agents that are primarily metabolized by CYP3A. Agents that are extensively metabolized by CYP3A and have high first pass metabolism appear to be the most susceptible to large increases in AUC (> 3-fold) when co-administered with Kaletra. Thus, co-administration of Kaletra with drugs highly dependent on CYP3A for clearance and for which elevated plasma concentrations are associated with serious and/or life-threatening events is contraindicated. Co-administration with other CYP3A substrates may require a dose adjustment or additional monitoring).
No products indexed under this heading.

Buspirone Hydrochloride (Cases of QT interval prolongation and torsade de pointes have been reported although causality of Kaletra could not be established. Avoid use in patients with congenital long QT syndrome, those with hypokalemia, and with other drugs that prolong the QT interval).
No products indexed under this heading.

Busulfan (Kaletra is an inhibitor of CYP3A and may increase plasma concentrations of agents that are primarily metabolized by CYP3A. Agents that are extensively metabolized by CYP3A and have high first pass metabolism appear to be the most susceptible to large increases in AUC (> 3-fold) when co-administered with Kaletra. Thus, co-administration of Kaletra with drugs highly dependent on CYP3A for clearance and for which elevated plasma concentrations are associated with serious and/or life-threatening events is contraindicated. Co-administration with other CYP3A substrates may require a dose adjustment or additional monitoring). Products include:
Myleran 1581

Carbamazepine (Kaletra may be less effective due to decreased lopinavir plasma concentrations in patients taking carbamazepine concomitantly and should be used with caution. Kaletra should not be administered once daily in combination with carbamazepine). Products include:
Carbatrol 3280
Equetro 3477

Carteolol Hydrochloride (PR interval prolongation may occur in some patients. Cases of second and third degree heart block have been reported. Caution must be used in patients with pre-existing conduction system disease,

ischemic heart disease, cardiomyopathy, underlying structural heart disease or when administering with other drugs that may prolong the PR interval including β-adrenergic blockers).
No products indexed under this heading.

Carvedilol (PR interval prolongation may occur in some patients. Cases of second and third degree heart block have been reported. Caution must be used in patients with pre-existing conduction system disease, ischemic heart disease, cardiomyopathy, underlying structural heart disease or when administering with other drugs that may prolong the PR interval including β-adrenergic blockers). Products include:
Coreg **1409**

Carvedilol Phosphate (PR interval prolongation may occur in some patients. Cases of second and third degree heart block have been reported. Caution must be used in patients with pre-existing conduction system disease, ischemic heart disease, cardiomyopathy, underlying structural heart disease or when administering with other drugs that may prolong the PR interval including β-adrenergic blockers). Products include:
Coreg CR **1416**

Cerivastatin Sodium (Kaletra is an inhibitor of CYP3A and may increase plasma concentrations of agents that are primarily metabolized by CYP3A. Agents that are extensively metabolized by CYP3A and have high first pass metabolism appear to be the most susceptible to large increases in AUC (> 3-fold) when co-administered with Kaletra. Thus, co-administration of Kaletra with drugs highly dependent on CYP3A for clearance and for which elevated plasma concentrations are associated with serious and/or life-threatening events is contraindicated. Co-administration with other CYP3A substrates may require a dose adjustment or additional monitoring).
No products indexed under this heading.

Chlordiazepoxide (Cases of QT interval prolongation and torsade de pointes have been reported although causality of Kaletra could not be established. Avoid use in patients with congenital long QT syndrome, those with hypokalemia, and with other drugs that prolong the QT interval).
No products indexed under this heading.

Chlordiazepoxide Hydrochloride (Cases of QT interval prolongation and torsade de pointes have been reported although causality of Kaletra could not be established. Avoid use in patients with congenital long QT syndrome, those with hypokalemia, and with other drugs that prolong the QT interval).
No products indexed under this heading.

Chlorpheniramine (Kaletra is an inhibitor of CYP3A and may increase plasma concentrations of agents that are primarily metabolized by CYP3A. Agents that are extensively metabolized by CYP3A and have high first pass metabolism appear to be the most susceptible to large increases in AUC (> 3-fold) when co-administered with Kaletra. Thus, co-administration of Kaletra with drugs highly dependent on CYP3A for clearance and for which elevated plasma concentrations are associated with serious and/or life-threatening events is contraindicated. Co-administration with other CYP3A substrates may require a dose adjustment or additional monitoring).
No products indexed under this heading.

Chlorpheniramine Maleate (Kaletra is an inhibitor of CYP3A and may increase plasma concentrations of agents that are primarily metabolized by CYP3A. Agents that are extensively metabolized by CYP3A and have high first pass metabolism appear to be the most susceptible to large increases in AUC (> 3-fold) when co-administered with Kaletra. Thus, co-administration of Kaletra with drugs highly dependent on CYP3A for clearance and for which elevated plasma concentrations are associated with serious and/or life-threatening events is contraindicated. Co-administration with other CYP3A substrates may require a dose adjustment or additional monitoring).
No products indexed under this heading.

Chlorpheniramine Polistirex (Kaletra is an inhibitor of CYP3A and may increase plasma concentrations of agents that are primarily metabolized by CYP3A. Agents that are extensively metabolized by CYP3A and have high first pass metabolism appear to be the most susceptible to large increases in AUC (> 3-fold) when co-administered with Kaletra. Thus, co-administration of Kaletra with drugs highly dependent on CYP3A for clearance and for which elevated plasma concentrations are associated with serious and/or life-threatening events is contraindicated. Co-administration with other CYP3A substrates may require a dose adjustment or additional monitoring). Products include:
Tussionex **3443**

Chlorpheniramine Tannate (Kaletra is an inhibitor of CYP3A and may increase plasma concentrations of agents that are primarily metabolized by CYP3A. Agents that are extensively metabolized by CYP3A and have high first pass metabolism appear to be the most susceptible to large increases in AUC (> 3-fold) when co-administered with Kaletra. Thus, co-administration of Kaletra with drugs highly dependent on CYP3A for clearance and for which elevated plasma concentrations are associated with serious and/or life-threatening events is contraindicated. Co-administration with other CYP3A substrates may require a dose adjustment or additional monitoring).
No products indexed under this heading.

Chlorpromazine (Cases of QT interval prolongation and torsade de pointes have been reported although causality of Kaletra could not be established. Avoid use in patients with congenital long QT syndrome, those with hypokalemia, and with other drugs that prolong the QT interval).
No products indexed under this heading.

Chlorpromazine Hydrochloride (Cases of QT interval prolongation and torsade de pointes have been reported although causality of Kaletra could not be established. Avoid use in patients with congenital long QT syndrome, those with hypokalemia, and with other drugs that prolong the QT interval).
No products indexed under this heading.

Chlorpropamide (New onset diabetes mellitus, exacerbation of pre-existing diabetes mellitus, and hyperglycemia have been reported during post-marketing surveillance in HIV-1 infected patients receiving protease inhibitor therapy. Some patients required either initiation or dose adjustments of oral hypoglycemic agents for treatment of these events).
No products indexed under this heading.

Chlorprothixene (Cases of QT interval prolongation and torsade de pointes have been reported although causality of Kaletra could not be established. Avoid use in patients with congenital long QT syndrome, those with hypokalemia, and with other drugs that prolong the QT interval).
No products indexed under this heading.

Chlorprothixene Hydrochloride (Cases of QT interval prolongation and torsade de pointes have been reported although causality of Kaletra could not be established. Avoid use in patients with congenital long QT syndrome, those with hypokalemia, and with other drugs that prolong the QT interval).
No products indexed under this heading.

Cilostazol (Kaletra is an inhibitor of CYP3A and may increase plasma concentrations of agents that are primarily metabolized by CYP3A. Agents that are extensively metabolized by CYP3A and have high first pass metabolism appear to be the most susceptible to large increases in AUC (> 3-fold) when co-administered with Kaletra. Thus, co-administration of Kaletra with drugs highly dependent on CYP3A for clearance and for which elevated plasma concentrations are associated with serious and/or life-threatening events is contraindicated. Co-administration with other CYP3A substrates may require a dose adjustment or additional monitoring).
No products indexed under this heading.

Cimetidine (Although not noted with concurrent ketoconazole, co-administration of Kaletra and other drugs that inhibit CYP3A may increase lopinavir plasma concentrations).
No products indexed under this heading.

Cimetidine Hydrochloride (Although not noted with concurrent ketoconazole, co-administration of Kaletra and other drugs that inhibit CYP3A may increase lopinavir plasma concentrations).
No products indexed under this heading.

Ciprofloxacin (Although not noted with concurrent ketoconazole, co-administration of Kaletra and other drugs that inhibit CYP3A may increase lopinavir plasma concentrations). Products include:
Cipro I.V. **3082**
Cipro **3073**
Cipro XR **3091**
Ciprodex **583**

Ciprofloxacin Hydrochloride (Although not noted with concurrent ketoconazole, co-administration of Kaletra and other drugs that inhibit CYP3A may increase lopinavir plasma concentrations). Products include:
Cipro **3073**

Cisapride (Kaletra is an inhibitor of the CYP450 3A. Co-administration with drugs that are highly dependent on CYP450 3A for clearance and for which elevated plasma concentrations are associated with serious and/or life threatening events, such as cisapride, is contraindicated. Co-administration of Kaletra and cisapride may lead to cardiac arrhythmias).
No products indexed under this heading.

Clarithromycin (Co-administration can result in increased clarithromycin plasma concentrations. For patients with renal impairment, the following dosage adjustments should be considered: For patients with CLCR < 30 to 60 mL/min the dose of clarithromycin should be reduced by 50%. For patients with CLCR < 30mL/min the dose of clarithromycin should be decreased by 75%). Products include:
Biaxin/Biaxin XL **412**

Clomipramine Hydrochloride (Cases of QT interval prolongation and torsade de pointes have been reported although causality of Kaletra could not be established. Avoid use in patients with congenital long QT syndrome, those with hypokalemia, and with other drugs that prolong the QT interval).
No products indexed under this heading.

Clorazepate Dipotassium (Cases of QT interval prolongation and torsade de pointes have been reported although causality of Kaletra could not be established. Avoid use in patients with congenital long QT syndrome, those with hypokalemia, and with other drugs that prolong the QT interval).
No products indexed under this heading.

Clozapine (Cases of QT interval prolongation and torsade de pointes have been reported although causality of Kaletra could not be established. Avoid use in patients with congenital long QT syndrome, those with hypokalemia, and with other drugs that prolong the QT interval).
No products indexed under this heading.

Cyclosporine (Co-administration results in increased plasma concentrations of immunosuppressants. Therapeutic concentration monitoring is recommended for immunosuppressant agents when co-administered with Kaletra). Products include:
Gengraf **440**
Neoral Oral Solution **2496**
Neoral Capsules **2496**
Restasis **605**

Delavirdine Mesylate (Co-administration has a potential to increase lopinavir plasma concentrations).
No products indexed under this heading.

Desipramine Hydrochloride (Cases of QT interval prolongation and torsade de pointes have been reported although causality of Kaletra could not be established. Avoid use in patients with congenital long QT syndrome, those with hypokalemia, and with other drugs that prolong the QT interval).
No products indexed under this heading.

Desogestrel (Because contraceptive steroid concentrations may be altered when Kaletra is co-administered with oral contraceptives or with the contraceptive patch, alternative methods of nonhormonal contraception are recommended).
No products indexed under this heading.

Dexamethasone (Co-administration can result in decreased lopinavir plasma concentrations. Kaletra may be less effective due to decreased lopinavir plasma concentrations in patients taking these agents concomitantly. Co-administer with caution). Products include:
Ciprodex **583**
Ozurdex .... **⊙ 223**
Tobramycin and Dexamethasone Ophthalmic Suspension .... **⊙ 251**

Dexamethasone Acetate (Co-administration can result in decreased lopinavir plasma concentrations. Kaletra may be less effective due to decreased lopinavir plasma concentrations in patients taking these agents concomitantly. Co-administer with caution).
No products indexed under this heading.

Dexamethasone Phosphate (Co-administration can result in decreased lopinavir plasma concentrations. Kaletra may be less effective due to decreased lopinavir plasma concentrations in patients taking these agents concomitantly. Co-administer with caution).
No products indexed under this heading.

Dexamethasone Sodium (Co-administration can result in decreased lopinavir plasma concentrations. Kaletra may be less effective due to decreased lopinavir plasma concentrations in patients taking these agents concomitantly. Co-administer with caution).
No products indexed under this heading.

Dexamethasone Sodium Phosphate (Co-administration can result in decreased lopinavir plasma concentrations. Kaletra may be less effective due to decreased lopinavir plasma concentrations in patients taking these agents concomitantly. Co-administer with caution).
No products indexed under this heading.

Dexamethasone Sodium Phosphate Injection (Co-administration can result in decreased lopinavir plasma concentrations. Kaletra may be less effective due to decreased lopinavir plasma concentrations in patients taking these agents concomitantly. Co-administer with caution).
No products indexed under this heading.

Diazepam (Cases of QT interval prolongation and torsade de pointes have been reported although causality of Kaletra could not be established. Avoid use in patients with congenital long QT syndrome, those with hypokalemia, and with other drugs that prolong the QT interval). Products include:
Valium Tablets 2880

Didanosine (Kaletra tablets can be administered simultaneously with didanosine without food. For Kaletra oral solution, it is recommended that didanosine be administered on an empty stomach; therefore, didanosine should be given one hour before or two hours after Kaletra oral solution (given with food)).
No products indexed under this heading.

Digoxin (PR interval prolongation may occur in some patients. Cases of second and third degree heart block have been reported. Caution must be use in patients with pre-existing conduction system disease, ischemic heart disease, cardiomyopathy, underlying structural heart disease or when administering with other drugs that may prolong the PR interval including digoxin). Products include:
Lanoxin Injection 1546
Lanoxin Injection Pediatric 1549
Lanoxin Tablets 1553

Digoxin Immune Fab (Ovine) (The impact on the PR interval of co-administration of Kaletra with other drugs that prolong the PR interval (including digoxin) has not been evaluated. As a result, co-administration of Kaletra with these drugs should be undertaken with caution, particularly with those drugs metabolized by CYP3A. Clinical monitoring is recommended). Products include:
Digibind 1427

Dihydroergotamine Mesylate (Co-administration of Kaletra is contraindicated with potent CYP3A4 inducers where significantly reduced lopinavir plasma concentrations may be associated with the potential for loss of virologic response and possible resistance and cross-resistance. Co-administration may lead to the potential for causing acute ergot toxicity characterized by peripheral vasospasm and ischemia of the extremities and other tissues).
No products indexed under this heading.

Diltiazem Hydrochloride (PR interval prolongation may occur in some patients. Cases of second and third degree heart block have been reported. Caution must be used in patients with pre-existing conduction system disease, ischemic heart disease, cardiomyopathy, underlying structural heart disease or when administering with other drugs that may prolong the PR interval including calcium channel blockers). Products include:
Cardizem LA 423

Diltiazem Maleate (The impact on the PR interval of co-administration of Kaletra with other drugs that prolong the PR interval (including calcium channel blockers, β-adrenergic blockers, digoxin and atazanavir) has not been evaluated. As a result, co-administration of Kaletra with these drugs should be undertaken with caution, particularly with those drugs metabolized by CYP3A. Clinical monitoring is recommended).
No products indexed under this heading.

Disopyramide (Cases of QT interval prolongation and torsade de pointes have been reported although causality of Kaletra could not be established. Avoid use in patients with congenital long QT syndrome, those with hypokalemia, and with other drugs that prolong the QT interval).
No products indexed under this heading.

Disopyramide Phosphate (Cases of QT interval prolongation and torsade de pointes have been reported although causality of Kaletra could not be established. Avoid use in patients with congenital long QT syndrome, those with hypokalemia, and with other drugs that prolong the QT interval).
No products indexed under this heading.

Disulfiram (Kaletra oral solution contains alcohol which can produce disulfiram-like reactions when co-administered with disulfiram).
No products indexed under this heading.

Dofetilide (Cases of QT interval prolongation and torsade de pointes have been reported although causality of Kaletra could not be established. Avoid use in patients with congenital long QT syndrome, those with hypokalemia, and with other drugs that prolong the QT interval).
No products indexed under this heading.

Doxepin Hydrochloride (Cases of QT interval prolongation and torsade de pointes have been reported although causality of Kaletra could not be established. Avoid use in patients with congenital long QT syndrome, those with hypokalemia, and with other drugs that prolong the QT interval).
No products indexed under this heading.

Doxorubicin Hydrochloride (Kaletra is an inhibitor of CYP3A and may increase plasma concentrations of agents that are primarily metabolized by CYP3A. Agents that are extensively metabolized by CYP3A and have high first pass metabolism appear to be the most susceptible to large increases in AUC (> 3-fold) when co-administered with Kaletra. Thus, co-administration of Kaletra with drugs highly dependent on CYP3A for clearance and for which elevated plasma concentrations are associated with serious and/or life-threatening events is contraindicated. Co-administration with other CYP3A substrates may require a dose adjustment or additional monitoring).
No products indexed under this heading.

Dronabinol (Kaletra is an inhibitor of CYP3A and may increase plasma concentrations of agents that are primarily metabolized by CYP3A. Agents that are extensively metabolized by CYP3A and have high first pass metabolism appear to be the most susceptible to large increases in AUC (> 3-fold) when co-administered with Kaletra. Thus, co-administration of Kaletra with drugs highly dependent on CYP3A for clearance and for which elevated plasma concentrations are associated with serious and/or life-threatening events is contraindicated. Co-administration with other CYP3A substrates may require a dose adjustment or additional monitoring).
No products indexed under this heading.

Droperidol (Cases of QT interval prolongation and torsade de pointes have been reported although causality of Kaletra could not be established. Avoid use in patients with congenital long QT syndrome, those with hypokalemia, and with other drugs that prolong the QT interval).
No products indexed under this heading.

Dyphylline (Kaletra is an inhibitor of CYP3A and may increase plasma concentrations of agents that are primarily metabolized by CYP3A. Agents that are extensively metabolized by CYP3A and have high first pass metabolism appear to be the most susceptible to large increases in AUC (> 3-fold) when co-administered with Kaletra. Thus, co-administration of Kaletra with drugs highly dependent on CYP3A for clearance and for which elevated plasma concentrations are associated with serious and/or life-threatening events is contraindicated. Co-administration with other CYP3A substrates may require a dose adjustment or additional monitoring).
No products indexed under this heading.

Efavirenz (Efavirenz may decrease the serum concentration of lopinavir. The dose of kaletra may need to be adjusted to maintain efficacy). Products include:
Atripla 906

Ergonovine Maleate (Co-administration of Kaletra is contraindicated with potent CYP3A4 inducers where significantly reduced lopinavir plasma concentrations may be associated with the potential for loss of virologic response and possible resistance and cross-resistance. Co-administration may lead to the potential for causing acute ergot toxicity characterized by peripheral vasospam and ischemia of the extremities and other tissues).
No products indexed under this heading.

Ergotamine Tartrate (Co-administration of Kaletra is contraindicated with potent CYP3A4 inducers where significantly reduced lopinavir plasma concentrations may be associated with the potential for loss of virologic response and possible resistance and cross-resistance. Co-administration may lead to the potential for causing acute ergot toxicity characterized by peripheral vasospam and ischemia of the extremities and other tissues).
No products indexed under this heading.

Erythromycin (Cases of QT interval prolongation and torsade de pointes have been reported although causality of Kaletra could not be established. Avoid use in patients with congenital long QT syndrome, those with hypokalemia, and with other drugs that prolong the QT interval).
No products indexed under this heading.

Erythromycin Estolate (Cases of QT interval prolongation and torsade de pointes have been reported although causality of Kaletra could not be established. Avoid use in patients with congenital long QT syndrome, those with hypokalemia, and with other drugs that prolong the QT interval).
No products indexed under this heading.

Erythromycin Ethylsuccinate (Cases of QT interval prolongation and torsade de pointes have been reported although causality of Kaletra could not be established. Avoid use in patients with congenital long QT syndrome, those with hypokalemia, and with other drugs that prolong the QT interval). Products include:
E.E.S. 437
EryPed 435

Erythromycin Gluceptate (Cases of QT interval prolongation and torsade de pointes have been reported although causality of Kaletra could not be established. Avoid use in patients with congenital long QT syndrome, those with hypokalemia, and with other drugs that prolong the QT interval).
No products indexed under this heading.

Erythromycin Lactobionate (Cases of QT interval prolongation and torsade de pointes have been reported although causality of Kaletra could not be established. Avoid use in patients with congenital long QT syndrome, those with hypokalemia, and with other drugs that prolong the QT interval).
No products indexed under this heading.

Erythromycin Stearate (Cases of QT interval prolongation and torsade de pointes have been reported although causality of Kaletra could not be established. Avoid use in patients with congenital long QT syndrome, those with hypokalemia, and with other drugs that prolong the QT interval).
No products indexed under this heading.

Esmolol Hydrochloride (PR interval prolongation may occur in some patients. Cases of second and third degree heart block have been reported. Caution must be used in patients with pre-existing conduction system disease, ischemic heart disease, cardiomyopathy, underlying structural heart disease or when administering with other drugs that may prolong the PR interval including β-adrenergic blockers).
No products indexed under this heading.

Estrogen (Kaletra is an inhibitor of CYP3A and may increase plasma concentrations of agents that are primarily metabolized by CYP3A. Agents that are extensively metabolized by CYP3A and have high first pass metabolism appear to be the most susceptible to large increases in AUC (> 3-fold) when co-administered with Kaletra. Thus, co-administration of Kaletra with drugs highly dependent on CYP3A for clearance and for which elevated plasma concentrations are associated with serious and/or life-threatening events is contraindicated. Co-administration with other CYP3A substrates may require a dose adjustment or additional monitoring).
No products indexed under this heading.

Estrogens, Conjugated (Kaletra is an inhibitor of CYP3A and may increase plasma concentrations of agents that are primarily metabolized by CYP3A. Agents that are extensively metabolized by CYP3A and have high first pass metabolism appear to be the most susceptible to large increases in AUC (> 3-fold) when co-administered with Kaletra. Thus, co-administration of Kaletra with drugs highly dependent on CYP3A for clearance and for which elevated plasma concentrations are associated with serious and/or life-threatening events is contraindicated. Co-administration with other CYP3A substrates may require a dose adjustment or additional monitoring). Products include:
Premarin Intravenous 3528
Premarin Tablets 3533
Premarin Vaginal Cream 3540
Premphase 3549
Prempro 3549

Estrogens, Conjugated, Synthetic A (Kaletra is an inhibitor of CYP3A and may increase plasma concentrations of agents that are primarily metabolized by CYP3A. Agents that are extensively metabolized by CYP3A and have high first pass metabolism appear to be the most susceptible to large increases in AUC (> 3-fold) when co-administered with Kaletra. Thus, co-administration of

Kaletra with drugs highly dependent on CYP3A for clearance and for which elevated plasma concentrations are associated with serious and/or life-threatening events is contraindicated. Co-administration with other CYP3A substrates may require a dose adjustment or additional monitoring).

No products indexed under this heading.

Estrogens, Esterified (Kaletra is an inhibitor of CYP3A and may increase plasma concentrations of agents that are primarily metabolized by CYP3A. Agents that are extensively metabolized by CYP3A and have high first pass metabolism appear to be the most susceptible to large increases in AUC (> 3-fold) when co-administered with Kaletra. Thus, co-administration of Kaletra with drugs highly dependent on CYP3A for clearance and for which elevated plasma concentrations are associated with serious and/or life-threatening events is contraindicated. Co-administration with other CYP3A substrates may require a dose adjustment or additional monitoring).

No products indexed under this heading.

Ethinyl Estradiol (Co-administration results in decreased plasma concentrations of ethinyl estradiol; alternative methods of non-hormonal contraception should be used when estrogen-based oral contraceptives and Kaletra are co-administered). Products include:

Ethosuximide (Co-administration of Kaletra is contraindicated with potent CYP3A inducers where significantly reduced lopinavir plasma concentrations may be associated with the potential for loss of virologic response and possible resistance and cross-resistance).

No products indexed under this heading.

Ethynodiol Diacetate (Because contraceptive steroid concentrations may be altered when Kaletra is co-administered with oral contraceptives or with the contraceptive patch, alternative methods of nonhormonal contraception are recommended).

No products indexed under this heading.

Etoposide (Kaletra is an inhibitor of CYP3A and may increase plasma concentrations of agents that are primarily metabolized by CYP3A. Agents that are extensively metabolized by CYP3A and have high first pass metabolism appear to be the most susceptible to large increases in AUC (> 3-fold) when co-administered with Kaletra. Thus, co-administration of Kaletra with drugs highly dependent on CYP3A for clearance and for which elevated plasma concentrations are associated with serious and/or life-threatening events is contraindicated. Co-administration with other CYP3A substrates may require a dose adjustment or additional monitoring).

No products indexed under this heading.

Etoposide Phosphate (Kaletra is an inhibitor of CYP3A and may increase plasma concentrations of agents that are primarily metabolized by CYP3A. Agents that are extensively metabolized by CYP3A and have high first pass metabolism appear to be the most susceptible to large increases in AUC (> 3-fold) when co-administered with Kaletra. Thus, co-administration of Kaletra with drugs highly dependent on CYP3A for clearance and for which elevated plasma concentrations are associated with serious and/or life-threatening

events is contraindicated. Co-administration with other CYP3A substrates may require a dose adjustment or additional monitoring).

No products indexed under this heading.

Fat (Relative to fasting, administration of Kaletra tablets with a moderate fat meal (500 - 682 Kcal, 23 to 25% calories from fat) increased lopinavir AUC and C_{max} by 26.9% and 17.6%, respectively. Relative to fasting, administration of Kaletra tablets with a high fat meal (872 Kcal, 56% from fat) increased lopinavir AUC by 18.9% but not C_{max}. Therefore, Kaletra tablets may be taken with or without food).

No products indexed under this heading.

Felodipine (Increased plasma concentrations of dihydropyridine calcium channel blockers. Caution is warranted and clinical monitoring of patients is recommended).

No products indexed under this heading.

Fentanyl (Kaletra is an inhibitor of CYP3A and may increase plasma concentrations of agents that are primarily metabolized by CYP3A. Agents that are extensively metabolized by CYP3A and have high first pass metabolism appear to be the most susceptible to large increases in AUC (> 3-fold) when co-administered with Kaletra. Thus, co-administration of Kaletra with drugs highly dependent on CYP3A for clearance and for which elevated plasma concentrations are associated with serious and/or life-threatening events is contraindicated. Co-administration with other CYP3A substrates may require a dose adjustment or additional monitoring). Products include:

Fentanyl Citrate (Kaletra is an inhibitor of CYP3A and may increase plasma concentrations of agents that are primarily metabolized by CYP3A. Agents that are extensively metabolized by CYP3A and have high first pass metabolism appear to be the most susceptible to large increases in AUC (> 3-fold) when co-administered with Kaletra. Thus, co-administration of Kaletra with drugs highly dependent on CYP3A for clearance and for which elevated plasma concentrations are associated with serious and/or life-threatening events is contraindicated. Co-administration with other CYP3A substrates may require a dose adjustment or additional monitoring). Products include:

Flecainide Acetate (Kaletra is an *in vitro* inhibitor of the CYP450 3A and inhibits CYP2D6 to a lesser extent; co-administration with drugs that are highly dependent on these isoforms for clearance and for which elevated plasma concentrations are associated with serious and/or life threatening events, such as flecainide, is contraindicated).

No products indexed under this heading.

Fluconazole (Although not noted with concurrent ketoconazole, co-administration of Kaletra and other drugs that inhibit CYP3A may increase lopinavir plasma concentrations).

No products indexed under this heading.

Fluoxetine (Although not noted with concurrent ketoconazole, co-administration of Kaletra and other drugs that inhibit CYP3A may increase lopinavir plasma concentrations).

No products indexed under this heading.

Fluoxetine Hydrochloride (Although not noted with concurrent ketoconazole, co-administration of Kaletra and other drugs that inhibit CYP3A may increase lopinavir plasma concentrations). Products include:

Fluphenazine Decanoate (Cases of QT interval prolongation and torsade de pointes have been reported although causality of Kaletra could not be established. Avoid use in patients with congenital long QT syndrome, those with hypokalemia, and with other drugs that prolong the QT interval).

No products indexed under this heading.

Fluphenazine Enanthate (Cases of QT interval prolongation and torsade de pointes have been reported although causality of Kaletra could not be established. Avoid use in patients with congenital long QT syndrome, those with hypokalemia, and with other drugs that prolong the QT interval).

No products indexed under this heading.

Fluphenazine Hydrochloride (Cases of QT interval prolongation and torsade de pointes have been reported although causality of Kaletra could not be established. Avoid use in patients with congenital long QT syndrome, those with hypokalemia, and with other drugs that prolong the QT interval).

No products indexed under this heading.

Fluticasone Propionate (Concomitant use of fluticasone propionate and Kaletra may increase plasma concentrations of fluticasone propionate, resulting in significantly reduced serum cortisol concentrations. Co-administration of fluticasone propionate and Kaletra is not recommended unless the potential benefit to the patient outweighs the risk of system corticosteroid side effect). Products include:

Fluvoxamine Maleate (Although not noted with concurrent ketoconazole, co-administration of Kaletra and other drugs that inhibit CYP3A may increase lopinavir plasma concentrations).

No products indexed under this heading.

Fosamprenavir Calcium (Co-administration may result in decreased levels of amprenavir and/or lopinavir. An increased rate of adverse effects has also been observed with co-administration of these medications). Products include:

Fosphenytoin (Kaletra may be less effective due to decreased lopinavir concentrations in patients taking phenytoin concomitantly and should be used with caution. Kaletra should not be administered once daily in combination with phenytoin. In addition, co-administration of phenytoin and Kaletra may cause decreases in steadystate phenytoin concentrations. Phenytoin levels should be monitored when co-administering with Kaletra).

No products indexed under this heading.

Fosphenytoin Sodium (Kaletra may be less effective due to decreased lopinavir concentrations in patients taking phenytoin concomitantly and should be used with caution. Kaletra should not be administered once daily in combination with phenytoin. In addition, co-administration of phenytoin and Kaletra may cause decreases in steadystate phenytoin concentrations. Phenytoin levels should be monitored when co-administering with Kaletra).

No products indexed under this heading.

Glibenclamide (New onset diabetes mellitus, exacerbation of pre-existing diabetes mellitus, and hyperglycemia have been reported during post-marketing surveillance in HIV-1 infected patients receiving protease inhibitor therapy. Some patients required either initiation or dose adjustments of oral hypoglycemic agents for treatment of these events).

No products indexed under this heading.

Glimepiride (New onset diabetes mellitus, exacerbation of pre-existing diabetes mellitus, and hyperglycemia have been reported during post-marketing surveillance in HIV-1 infected patients receiving protease inhibitor therapy. Some patients required either initiation or dose adjustments of oral hypoglycemic agents for treatment of these events). Products include:

Glipizide (New onset diabetes mellitus, exacerbation of pre-existing diabetes mellitus, and hyperglycemia have been reported during post-marketing surveillance in HIV-1 infected patients receiving protease inhibitor therapy. Some patients required either initiation or dose adjustments of oral hypoglycemic agents for treatment of these events).

No products indexed under this heading.

Glyburide (New onset diabetes mellitus, exacerbation of pre-existing diabetes mellitus, and hyperglycemia have been reported during post-marketing surveillance in HIV-1 infected patients receiving protease inhibitor therapy. Some patients required either initiation or dose adjustments of oral hypoglycemic agents for treatment of these events).

No products indexed under this heading.

Haloperidol (Cases of QT interval prolongation and torsade de pointes have been reported although causality of Kaletra could not be established. Avoid use in patients with congenital long QT syndrome, those with hypokalemia, and with other drugs that prolong the QT interval).

No products indexed under this heading.

Haloperidol Decanoate (Cases of QT interval prolongation and torsade de pointes have been reported although causality of Kaletra could not be established. Avoid use in patients with congenital long QT syndrome, those with hypokalemia, and with other drugs that prolong the QT interval).

No products indexed under this heading.

Haloperidol Lactate (Cases of QT interval prolongation and torsade de pointes have been reported although causality of Kaletra could not be established. Avoid use in patients with congenital long QT syndrome, those with hypokalemia, and with other drugs that prolong the QT interval).

No products indexed under this heading.

Hydroxyzine Hydrochloride (Cases of QT interval prolongation and torsade de pointes have been reported although causality of Kaletra could not be established. Avoid use in patients with congenital long QT syndrome, those with hypokalemia, and with other drugs that prolong the QT interval).

No products indexed under this heading.

Hypericum Perforatum (Co-administration of Kaletra is contraindicated with potent CYP3A4 inducers where significantly reduced lopinavir plasma concentrations may be associated with the potential for loss of virologic response and possible resistance and cross-resistance. Co-administration may lead to loss of virologic response

IMPORTANT NOTE: Always consult each drug listing in the patient's regimen for possible interactions.

Kaletra Interactions Index 928

and possible resistance to Kaletra or to the class of protease inhibitors). Products include:
Traumeel 1800

Imipramine Hydrochloride (Cases of QT interval prolongation and torsade de pointes have been reported although causality of Kaletra could not be established. Avoid use in patients with congenital long QT syndrome, those with hypokalemia, and with other drugs that prolong the QT interval).
No products indexed under this heading.

Imipramine Pamoate (Cases of QT interval prolongation and torsade de pointes have been reported although causality of Kaletra could not be established. Avoid use in patients with congenital long QT syndrome, those with hypokalemia, and with other drugs that prolong the QT interval).
No products indexed under this heading.

Indinavir Sulfate (Co-administration may result in increased indinavir concentrations. Decrease indinavir dose to 600 mg twice daily, when co-administered with Kaletra 400/100 mg twice daily). Products include:
Crixivan 2113

Insulin (New onset diabetes mellitus, exacerbation of pre-existing diabetes mellitus, and hyperglycemia have been reported during post-marketing surveillance in HIV-1 infected patients receiving protease inhibitor therapy. Some patients required either initiation or dose adjustments of insulin for treatment of these events).
No products indexed under this heading.

Insulin, Human, Zinc Suspension (New onset diabetes mellitus, exacerbation of pre-existing diabetes mellitus, and hyperglycemia have been reported during post-marketing surveillance in HIV-1 infected patients receiving protease inhibitor therapy. Some patients required either initiation or dose adjustments of insulin for treatment of these events).
No products indexed under this heading.

Insulin, Human (rDNA origin) (New onset diabetes mellitus, exacerbation of pre-existing diabetes mellitus, and hyperglycemia have been reported during post-marketing surveillance in HIV-1 infected patients receiving protease inhibitor therapy. Some patients required either initiation or dose adjustments of insulin for treatment of these events). Products include:
Exubera 2717

Insulin, Human NPH (New onset diabetes mellitus, exacerbation of pre-existing diabetes mellitus, and hyperglycemia have been reported during post-marketing surveillance in HIV-1 infected patients receiving protease inhibitor therapy. Some patients required either initiation or dose adjustments of insulin for treatment of these events). Products include:
Humulin N Vial 1934

Insulin, Human Regular (New onset diabetes mellitus, exacerbation of pre-existing diabetes mellitus, and hyperglycemia have been reported during post-marketing surveillance in HIV-1 infected patients receiving protease inhibitor therapy. Some patients required either initiation or dose adjustments of insulin for treatment of these events). Products include:
Humulin R 1937
Humulin R (U-500) 1939

Insulin, Human Regular and Human NPH Mixture (New onset diabetes mellitus, exacerbation of pre-existing diabetes mellitus, and hyperglycemia have been reported during post-marketing surveillance in HIV-1 infected patients receiving protease inhibitor therapy. Some patients required either initiation or dose adjustments of insulin for treatment of these events). Products include:
Humulin 50/50 1930
Humulin 70/30 Vial 1931

Insulin, NPH (New onset diabetes mellitus, exacerbation of pre-existing diabetes mellitus, and hyperglycemia have been reported during post-marketing surveillance in HIV-1 infected patients receiving protease inhibitor therapy. Some patients required either initiation or dose adjustments of insulin for treatment of these events).
No products indexed under this heading.

Insulin, Regular (New onset diabetes mellitus, exacerbation of pre-existing diabetes mellitus, and hyperglycemia have been reported during post-marketing surveillance in HIV-1 infected patients receiving protease inhibitor therapy. Some patients required either initiation or dose adjustments of insulin for treatment of these events).
No products indexed under this heading.

Insulin, Regular and NPH mixture (New onset diabetes mellitus, exacerbation of pre-existing diabetes mellitus, and hyperglycemia have been reported during post-marketing surveillance in HIV-1 infected patients receiving protease inhibitor therapy. Some patients required either initiation or dose adjustments of insulin for treatment of these events).
No products indexed under this heading.

Insulin, Zinc Crystals (New onset diabetes mellitus, exacerbation of pre-existing diabetes mellitus, and hyperglycemia have been reported during post-marketing surveillance in HIV-1 infected patients receiving protease inhibitor therapy. Some patients required either initiation or dose adjustments of insulin for treatment of these events).
No products indexed under this heading.

Insulin, Zinc Suspension (New onset diabetes mellitus, exacerbation of pre-existing diabetes mellitus, and hyperglycemia have been reported during post-marketing surveillance in HIV-1 infected patients receiving protease inhibitor therapy. Some patients required either initiation or dose adjustments of insulin for treatment of these events).
No products indexed under this heading.

Insulin Aspart (New onset diabetes mellitus, exacerbation of pre-existing diabetes mellitus, and hyperglycemia have been reported during post-marketing surveillance in HIV-1 infected patients receiving protease inhibitor therapy. Some patients required either initiation or dose adjustments of insulin for treatment of these events).
No products indexed under this heading.

Insulin Aspart, Human (New onset diabetes mellitus, exacerbation of pre-existing diabetes mellitus, and hyperglycemia have been reported during post-marketing surveillance in HIV-1 infected patients receiving protease inhibitor therapy. Some patients required either initiation or dose adjustments of insulin for treatment of these events). Products include:
NovoLog Mix 70/30 2581

Insulin Aspart, Human Regular (New onset diabetes mellitus, exacerbation of pre-existing diabetes mellitus, and hyperglycemia have been reported during post-marketing surveillance in HIV-1 infected patients receiving protease inhibitor therapy. Some patients required either initiation or dose adjustments of insulin for treatment of these events). Products include:
NovoLog 2575

Insulin Aspart Protamine, Human (New onset diabetes mellitus, exacerbation of pre-existing diabetes mellitus, and hyperglycemia have been reported during post-marketing surveillance in HIV-1 infected patients receiving protease inhibitor therapy. Some patients required either initiation or dose adjustments of insulin for treatment of these events). Products include:
NovoLog Mix 70/30 2581

Insulin Detemir (rDNA Origin) (New onset diabetes mellitus, exacerbation of pre-existing diabetes mellitus, and hyperglycemia have been reported during post-marketing surveillance in HIV-1 infected patients receiving protease inhibitor therapy. Some patients required either initiation or dose adjustments of insulin for treatment of these events). Products include:
Levemir 2566

Insulin Glargine (New onset diabetes mellitus, exacerbation of pre-existing diabetes mellitus, and hyperglycemia have been reported during post-marketing surveillance in HIV-1 infected patients receiving protease inhibitor therapy. Some patients required either initiation or dose adjustments of insulin for treatment of these events). Products include:
Lantus 2996

Insulin Glulisine (New onset diabetes mellitus, exacerbation of pre-existing diabetes mellitus, and hyperglycemia have been reported during post-marketing surveillance in HIV-1 infected patients receiving protease inhibitor therapy. Some patients required either initiation or dose adjustments of insulin for treatment of these events). Products include:
Apidra 2937
Apidra SoloStar 2937

Insulin Lispro, Human (New onset diabetes mellitus, exacerbation of pre-existing diabetes mellitus, and hyperglycemia have been reported during post-marketing surveillance in HIV-1 infected patients receiving protease inhibitor therapy. Some patients required either initiation or dose adjustments of insulin for treatment of these events). Products include:
Humalog 1910
Humalog Mix 1914
Humalog Mix75/25 1917

Insulin Lispro Protamine, Human (New onset diabetes mellitus, exacerbation of pre-existing diabetes mellitus, and hyperglycemia have been reported during post-marketing surveillance in HIV-1 infected patients receiving protease inhibitor therapy. Some patients required either initiation or dose adjustments of insulin for treatment of these events). Products include:
Humalog Mix 1914
Humalog Mix75/25 1917

Isocarboxazid (Cases of QT interval prolongation and torsade de pointes have been reported although causality of Kaletra could not be established. Avoid use in patients with congenital long QT syndrome, those with hypokalemia, and with other drugs that prolong the QT interval). Products include:
Marplan 3481

Isoniazid (Although not noted with concurrent ketoconazole, co-administration of Kaletra and other drugs that inhibit CYP3A may increase lopinavir plasma concentrations).
No products indexed under this heading.

Isradipine (Increased plasma concentrations of dihydropyridine calcium channel blockers. Caution is warranted and clinical monitoring of patients is recommended). Products include:
DynaCirc CR 1432

Itraconazole (Co-administration can result in increased itraconazole plasma concentrations. High doses of itraconazole (>200 mg/day) is not recommended).
No products indexed under this heading.

Ketoconazole (Co-administration can result in increased ketoconazole plasma concentrations. High doses of ketoconazole (>200 mg/day) is not recommended). Products include:
Extina 3319
Xolegel 3337

Labetalol Hydrochloride (PR interval prolongation may occur in some patients. Cases of second and third degree heart block have been reported. Caution must be used in patients with pre-existing conduction system disease, ischemic heart disease, cardiomyopathy, underlying structural heart disease or when administering with other drugs that may prolong the PR interval including β-adrenergic blockers).
No products indexed under this heading.

Levobunolol Hydrochloride (PR interval prolongation may occur in some patients. Cases of second and third degree heart block have been reported. Caution must be used in patients with pre-existing conduction system disease, ischemic heart disease, cardiomyopathy, underlying structural heart disease or when administering with other drugs that may prolong the PR interval including β-adrenergic blockers).
No products indexed under this heading.

Levonorgestrel (Because contraceptive steroid concentrations may be altered when Kaletra is co-administered with oral contraceptives or with the contraceptive patch, alternative methods of nonhormonal contraception are recommended). Products include:
Climara Pro 847
LoSeasonique 3407
Lybrel 3514
Mirena 854
Plan B 3416
Seasonique 3418

Lidocaine (Cases of QT interval prolongation and torsade de pointes have been reported although causality of Kaletra could not be established. Avoid use in patients with congenital long QT syndrome, those with hypokalemia, and with other drugs that prolong the QT interval). Products include:
Lidoderm 1107

Lidocaine Hydrochloride (Co-administration with systemic lidocaine can result in increased lidocaine plasma concentrations; caution and monitoring is recommended).
No products indexed under this heading.

Lithium Carbonate (Cases of QT interval prolongation and torsade de pointes have been reported although causality of Kaletra could not be established. Avoid use in patients with congenital long QT syndrome, those with hypokalemia, and with other drugs that prolong the QT interval).
No products indexed under this heading.

Lithium Citrate (Cases of QT interval prolongation and torsade de pointes have been reported although causality of Kaletra could not be established. Avoid use in patients with congenital long QT syndrome, those with hypokalemia, and with other drugs that prolong the QT interval).
No products indexed under this heading.

Lorazepam (Cases of QT interval prolongation and torsade de pointes have been reported although causality of Kaletra could not be established. Avoid use in patients with congenital long QT syndrome, those with hypokalemia, and with other drugs that prolong the QT interval).
No products indexed under this heading.

Lovastatin (Concurrent use of kaletra and lovastatin metabolised by CYP 3A may increase the risk of myopathy including rhabdomyolysis). Products include:

Advicor **402**
Mevacor **2212**

Loxapine Hydrochloride (Cases of QT interval prolongation and torsade de pointes have been reported although causality of Kaletra could not be established. Avoid use in patients with congenital long QT syndrome, those with hypokalemia, and with other drugs that prolong the QT interval).
No products indexed under this heading.

Loxapine Succinate (Cases of QT interval prolongation and torsade de pointes have been reported although causality of Kaletra could not be established. Avoid use in patients with congenital long QT syndrome, those with hypokalemia, and with other drugs that prolong the QT interval).
No products indexed under this heading.

Maprotiline Hydrochloride (Cases of QT interval prolongation and torsade de pointes have been reported although causality of Kaletra could not be established. Avoid use in patients with congenital long QT syndrome, those with hypokalemia, and with other drugs that prolong the QT interval).
No products indexed under this heading.

Maraviroc (Concurrent administration of maraviroc with Kaletra will increase plasma levels of maraviroc. When co-administered, patients should receive 150 mg twice daily of maraviroc). Products include:

Selzentry **2740**

Meprobamate (Cases of QT interval prolongation and torsade de pointes have been reported although causality of Kaletra could not be established. Avoid use in patients with congenital long QT syndrome, those with hypokalemia, and with other drugs that prolong the QT interval).
No products indexed under this heading.

Mesoridazine Besylate (Cases of QT interval prolongation and torsade de pointes have been reported although causality of Kaletra could not be established. Avoid use in patients with congenital long QT syndrome, those with hypokalemia, and with other drugs that prolong the QT interval).
No products indexed under this heading.

Mestranol (Because contraceptive steroid concentrations may be altered when Kaletra is co-administered with oral contraceptives or with the contraceptive patch, alternative methods of nonhormonal contraception are recommended).
No products indexed under this heading.

Metformin Hydrochloride (New onset diabetes mellitus, exacerbation of pre-existing diabetes mellitus, and hyperglycemia have been reported during post-marketing surveillance in HIV-1 infected patients receiving protease inhibitor therapy. Some patients required either initiation or dose adjustments of oral hypoglycemic agents for treatment of these events). Products include:

ActoPlus **3338**
Avandamet **1345**
Janumet **2188**

Methadone Hydrochloride (Co-administration results in decreased plasma concentrations of methadone. Dosage of methadone may need to be increased when co-administered).
No products indexed under this heading.

Methylergonovine Maleate (Co-administration of Kaletra is contraindicated with potent CYP3A4 inducers where significantly reduced lopinavir plasma concentrations may be associated with the potential for loss of virologic response and possible resistance and cross-resistance. Co-administration may lead to the potential for causing acute ergot toxicity characterized by peripheral vasospam and ischemia of the extremities and other tissues).
No products indexed under this heading.

Methylprednisolone (Kaletra is an inhibitor of CYP3A and may increase plasma concentrations of agents that are primarily metabolized by CYP3A. Agents that are extensively metabolized by CYP3A and have high first pass metabolism appear to be the most susceptible to large increases in AUC (> 3-fold) when co-administered with Kaletra. Thus, co-administration of Kaletra with drugs highly dependent on CYP3A for clearance and for which elevated plasma concentrations are associated with serious and/or life-threatening events is contraindicated. Co-administration with other CYP3A substrates may require a dose adjustment or additional monitoring).
No products indexed under this heading.

Methylprednisolone Acetate (Kaletra is an inhibitor of CYP3A and may increase plasma concentrations of agents that are primarily metabolized by CYP3A. Agents that are extensively metabolized by CYP3A and have high first pass metabolism appear to be the most susceptible to large increases in AUC (> 3-fold) when co-administered with Kaletra. Thus, co-administration of Kaletra with drugs highly dependent on CYP3A for clearance and for which elevated plasma concentrations are associated with serious and/or life-threatening events is contraindicated. Co-administration with other CYP3A substrates may require a dose adjustment or additional monitoring).
No products indexed under this heading.

Methylprednisolone Sodium Succinate (Kaletra is an inhibitor of CYP3A and may increase plasma concentrations of agents that are primarily metabolized by CYP3A. Agents that are extensively metabolized by CYP3A and have high first pass metabolism appear to be the most susceptible to large increases in AUC (> 3-fold) when co-administered with Kaletra. Thus, co-administration of Kaletra with drugs highly dependent on CYP3A for clearance and for which elevated plasma concentrations are associated with serious and/or life-threatening events is contraindicated. Co-administration with other CYP3A substrates may require a dose adjustment or additional monitoring).
No products indexed under this heading.

Methysergide Maleate (Co-administration of Kaletra and the ergot derivatives dihydroergotamine, ergonovine, ergotamine, or methylergonovine is contraindicated due to potential for serious and/or life-threatening reactions, such as acute ergot toxicity characterized by vasospasm and ischemia of the extremities and other tissues).
No products indexed under this heading.

Metipranolol Hydrochloride (PR interval prolongation may occur in some patients. Cases of second and third degree heart block have been reported. Caution must be used in patients with pre-existing conduction system disease, ischemic heart disease, cardiomyopathy, underlying structural heart disease or when administering with other drugs that may prolong the PR interval including β-adrenergic blockers).
No products indexed under this heading.

Metoprolol Succinate (PR interval prolongation may occur in some patients. Cases of second and third degree heart block have been reported. Caution must be used in patients with pre-existing conduction system disease, ischemic heart disease, cardiomyopathy, underlying structural heart disease or when administering with other drugs that may prolong the PR interval including β-adrenergic blockers). Products include:

Toprol XL **732**

Metoprolol Tartrate (PR interval prolongation may occur in some patients. Cases of second and third degree heart block have been reported. Caution must be used in patients with pre-existing conduction system disease, ischemic heart disease, cardiomyopathy, underlying structural heart disease or when administering with other drugs that may prolong the PR interval including β-adrenergic blockers).
No products indexed under this heading.

Metronidazole (Kaletra oral solution contains alcohol, which can produce disulfiram-like reactions when co-administered with disulfiram or other drugs that produce this reaction, such as metronidazole). Products include:

Pylera **793**

Metronidazole Benzoate (Although not noted with concurrent ketoconazole, co-administration of Kaletra and other drugs that inhibit CYP3A may increase lopinavir plasma concentrations).
No products indexed under this heading.

Metronidazole Hydrochloride (Kaletra oral solution contains alcohol, which can produce disulfiram-like reactions when co-administered with disulfiram or other drugs that produce this reaction, such as metronidazole).
No products indexed under this heading.

Mexiletine Hydrochloride (Cases of QT interval prolongation and torsade de pointes have been reported although causality of Kaletra could not be established. Avoid use in patients with congenital long QT syndrome, those with hypokalemia, and with other drugs that prolong the QT interval).
No products indexed under this heading.

Mibefradil Dihydrochloride (PR interval prolongation may occur in some patients. Cases of second and third degree heart block have been reported. Caution must be used in patients with pre-existing conduction system disease, ischemic heart disease, cardiomyopathy, underlying structural heart disease or when administering with other drugs that may prolong the PR interval including calcium channel blockers).
No products indexed under this heading.

Miconazole (Although not noted with concurrent ketoconazole, co-administration of Kaletra and other drugs that inhibit CYP3A may increase lopinavir plasma concentrations).
No products indexed under this heading.

Midazolam Hydrochloride (Kaletra is an inhibitor of CYP3A and may increase plasma concentrations of agents that are primarily metabolized by CYP3A such as midazolam. Concurrent administration of kaletra and midazolam may result to prolonged or increased sedation or respiratory depression).
No products indexed under this heading.

Miglitol (New onset diabetes mellitus, exacerbation of pre-existing diabetes mellitus, and hyperglycemia have been reported during post-marketing surveillance in HIV-1 infected patients receiving protease inhibitor therapy. Some patients required either initiation or dose adjustments of oral hypoglycemic agents for treatment of these events).
No products indexed under this heading.

Modafinil (Co-administration of Kaletra is contraindicated with potent CYP3A inducers where significantly reduced lopinavir plasma concentrations may be associated with the potential for loss of virologic response and possible resistance and cross-resistance). Products include:

Provigil **983**

Molindone Hydrochloride (Cases of QT interval prolongation and torsade de pointes have been reported although causality of Kaletra could not be established. Avoid use in patients with congenital long QT syndrome, those with hypokalemia, and with other drugs that prolong the QT interval). Products include:

Moban **1108**

Nadolol (PR interval prolongation may occur in some patients. Cases of second and third degree heart block have been reported. Caution must be used in patients with pre-existing conduction system disease, ischemic heart disease, cardiomyopathy, underlying structural heart disease or when administering with other drugs that may prolong the PR interval including β-adrenergic blockers). Products include:

Nadolol **2359**

Nateglinide (New onset diabetes mellitus, exacerbation of pre-existing diabetes mellitus, and hyperglycemia have been reported during post-marketing surveillance in HIV-1 infected patients receiving protease inhibitor therapy. Some patients required either initiation or dose adjustments of oral hypoglycemic agents for treatment of these events).
No products indexed under this heading.

Nebivolol (PR interval prolongation may occur in some patients. Cases of second and third degree heart block have been reported. Caution must be used in patients with pre-existing conduction system disease, ischemic heart disease, cardiomyopathy, underlying structural heart disease or when administering with other drugs that may prolong the PR interval including β-adrenergic blockers). Products include:

Bystolic **1147**

Nefazodone Hydrochloride (Kaletra is an inhibitor of CYP3A and may increase plasma concentrations of agents that are primarily metabolized by CYP3A. Agents that are extensively metabolized by CYP3A and have high first pass metabolism appear to be the most susceptible to large increases in AUC (> 3-fold) when co-administered with Kaletra. Thus, co-administration of Kaletra with drugs highly dependent on CYP3A for clearance and for which elevated plasma concentrations are associated with serious and/or life-threatening events is contraindicated. Co-administration with other CYP3A substrates may require a dose adjustment or additional monitoring).
No products indexed under this heading.

Nelfinavir Mesylate (Co-administration may result in increased nelfinavir plasma concentration. Kaletra should not be administered once-daily in combination with nelfinavir).
No products indexed under this heading.

Nevirapine (Nevirapine may decrease concentration of lopinavir. Dose adjustment may be needed). Products include:

Viramune Oral Suspension **897**
Viramune Tablets **897**

Nicardipine (PR interval prolongation may occur in some patients. Cases of second and third degree heart block have been reported. Caution must be used in patients with pre-existing conduction system disease, ischemic heart disease, cardiomyopathy, underlying structural heart disease or when admin-

istering with other drugs that may pro-long the PR interval including calcium channel blockers).

No products indexed under this heading.

Nicardipine Hydrochloride (Increased plasma concentrations of dihydropyridine calcium channel blockers. Caution is warranted and clinical monitoring of patients is recommended).

No products indexed under this heading.

Nifedipine (Increased plasma concentrations of dihydropyridine calcium channel blockers. Caution is warranted and clinical monitoring of patients is recommended).

No products indexed under this heading.

Nimodipine (Increased plasma concentrations of dihydropyridine calcium channel blockers. Caution is warranted and clinical monitoring of patients is recommended).

No products indexed under this heading.

Nisoldipine (PR interval prolongation may occur in some patients. Cases of second and third degree heart block have been reported. Caution must be used in patients with pre-existing conduction system disease, ischemic heart disease, cardiomyopathy, underlying structural heart disease or when administering with other drugs that may prolong the PR interval including calcium channel blockers).

No products indexed under this heading.

Norethindrone (Because contraceptive steroid concentrations may be altered when Kaletra is co-administered with oral contraceptives or with the contraceptive patch, alternative methods of nonhormonal contraception are recommended). Products include:

Norethynodrel (Because contraceptive steroid concentrations may be altered when Kaletra is co-administered with oral contraceptives or with the contraceptive patch, alternative methods of nonhormonal contraception are recommended).

No products indexed under this heading.

Norfloxacin (Although not noted with concurrent ketoconazole, co-administration of Kaletra and other drugs that inhibit CYP3A may increase lopinavir plasma concentrations). Products include:

Norgestimate (Because contraceptive steroid concentrations may be altered when Kaletra is co-administered with oral contraceptives or with the contraceptive patch, alternative methods of nonhormonal contraception are recommended). Products include:

Norgestrel (Because contraceptive steroid concentrations may be altered when Kaletra is co-administered with oral contraceptives or with the contraceptive patch, alternative methods of nonhormonal contraception are recommended).

No products indexed under this heading.

Nortriptyline Hydrochloride (Cases of QT interval prolongation and torsade de pointes have been reported although causality of Kaletra could not be established. Avoid use in patients with congenital long QT syndrome, those with hypokalemia, and with other drugs that prolong the QT interval).

No products indexed under this heading.

Olanzapine (Cases of QT interval prolongation and torsade de pointes have been reported although causality of Kaletra could not be established. Avoid use in patients with congenital long QT

syndrome, those with hypokalemia, and with other drugs that prolong the QT interval). Products include:

Ondansetron Hydrochloride (Kaletra is an inhibitor of CYP3A and may increase plasma concentrations of agents that are primarily metabolized by CYP3A. Agents that are extensively metabolized by CYP3A and have high first pass metabolism appear to be the most susceptible to large increases in AUC (> 3-fold) when co-administered with Kaletra. Thus, co-administration of Kaletra with drugs highly dependent on CYP3A for clearance and for which elevated plasma concentrations are associated with serious and/or life-threatening events is contraindicated. Co-administration with other CYP3A substrates may require a dose adjustment or additional monitoring). Products include:

Oxazepam (Cases of QT interval prolongation and torsade de pointes have been reported although causality of Kaletra could not be established. Avoid use in patients with congenital long QT syndrome, those with hypokalemia, and with other drugs that prolong the QT interval).

No products indexed under this heading.

Paclitaxel (Kaletra is an inhibitor of CYP3A and may increase plasma concentrations of agents that are primarily metabolized by CYP3A. Agents that are extensively metabolized by CYP3A and have high first pass metabolism appear to be the most susceptible to large increases in AUC (> 3-fold) when co-administered with Kaletra. Thus, co-administration of Kaletra with drugs highly dependent on CYP3A for clearance and for which elevated plasma concentrations are associated with serious and/or life-threatening events is contraindicated. Co-administration with other CYP3A substrates may require a dose adjustment or additional monitoring).

No products indexed under this heading.

Paroxetine Hydrochloride (Although not noted with concurrent ketoconazole, co-administration of Kaletra and other drugs that inhibit CYP3A may increase lopinavir plasma concentrations). Products include:

Penbutolol Sulfate (PR interval prolongation may occur in some patients. Cases of second and third degree heart block have been reported. Caution must be used in patients with pre-existing conduction system disease, ischemic heart disease, cardiomyopathy, underlying structural heart disease or when administering with other drugs that may prolong the PR interval including β-adrenergic blockers).

No products indexed under this heading.

Perphenazine (Cases of QT interval prolongation and torsade de pointes have been reported although causality of Kaletra could not be established. Avoid use in patients with congenital long QT syndrome, those with hypokalemia, and with other drugs that prolong the QT interval).

No products indexed under this heading.

Phenelzine Sulfate (Cases of QT interval prolongation and torsade de pointes have been reported although causality of Kaletra could not be established. Avoid use in patients with congenital long QT syndrome, those with hypokalemia, and with other drugs that prolong the QT interval).

No products indexed under this heading.

Phenobarbital (Co-administration can result in decreased lopinavir plasma concentrations; Kaletra may be less effective due to decreased lopinavir plasma concentrations. Co-administer with caution). Products include:

Phenobarbital Sodium (Kaletra may be less effective due to decreased lopinavir plasma concentrations in patients taking phenobarbital concomitantly and should be used with caution. Kaletra should not be administered once daily in combination with phenobarbital).

No products indexed under this heading.

Phenytoin (Kaletra may be less effective due to decreased lopinavir concentrations in patients taking phenytoin concomitantly and should be used with caution. Kaletra should not be administered once daily in combination with phenytoin. In addition, co-administration of phenytoin and Kaletra may cause decreases in steadystate phenytoin concentrations. Phenytoin levels should be monitored when co-administering with Kaletra).

No products indexed under this heading.

Phenytoin Sodium (Kaletra may be less effective due to decreased lopinavir concentrations in patients taking phenytoin concomitantly and should be used with caution. Kaletra should not be administered once daily in combination with phenytoin. In addition, co-administration of phenytoin and Kaletra may cause decreases in steadystate phenytoin concentrations. Phenytoin levels should be monitored when co-administering with Kaletra). Products include:

Pimozide (Kaletra is an inhibitor of CYP3A and may increase plasma concentrations of agents that are primarily metabolized by CYP3A such as pimozide. Concurrent administration of kaletra and pimozide may increase the risk of cardiac arrhythmias).

No products indexed under this heading.

Pindolol (PR interval prolongation may occur in some patients. Cases of second and third degree heart block have been reported. Caution must be used in patients with pre-existing conduction system disease, ischemic heart disease, cardiomyopathy, underlying structural heart disease or when administering with other drugs that may prolong the PR interval including β-adrenergic blockers).

No products indexed under this heading.

Pioglitazone Hydrochloride (New onset diabetes mellitus, exacerbation of pre-existing diabetes mellitus, and hyperglycemia have been reported during post-marketing surveillance in HIV-1 infected patients receiving protease inhibitor therapy. Some patients required either initiation or dose adjustments of oral hypoglycemic agents for treatment of these events). Products include:

Prazepam (Cases of QT interval prolongation and torsade de pointes have been reported although causality of Kaletra could not be established. Avoid use in patients with congenital long QT syndrome, those with hypokalemia, and with other drugs that prolong the QT interval).

No products indexed under this heading.

Procainamide Hydrochloride (Cases of QT interval prolongation and torsade de pointes have been reported although causality of Kaletra could not be established. Avoid use in patients with congenital long QT syndrome, those with hypokalemia, and with other drugs that prolong the QT interval).

No products indexed under this heading.

Prochlorperazine (Cases of QT interval prolongation and torsade de pointes have been reported although causality of Kaletra could not be established. Avoid use in patients with congenital long QT syndrome, those with hypokalemia, and with other drugs that prolong the QT interval).

No products indexed under this heading.

Promethazine Hydrochloride (Cases of QT interval prolongation and torsade de pointes have been reported although causality of Kaletra could not be established. Avoid use in patients with congenital long QT syndrome, those with hypokalemia, and with other drugs that prolong the QT interval).

No products indexed under this heading.

Propafenone Hydrochloride (Kaletra is an inhibitor of CYP450 3A. Co-administration with drugs that are highly dependent on CYP450 3A for clearance and for which elevated plasma concentrations are associated with serious and/or life threatening events, such as propafenone, is contraindicated). Products include:

Propranolol Hydrochloride (PR interval prolongation may occur in some patients. Cases of second and third degree heart block have been reported. Caution must be used in patients with pre-existing conduction system disease, ischemic heart disease, cardiomyopathy, underlying structural heart disease or when administering with other drugs that may prolong the PR interval including β-adrenergic blockers). Products include:

Protriptyline Hydrochloride (Cases of QT interval prolongation and torsade de pointes have been reported although causality of Kaletra could not be established. Avoid use in patients with congenital long QT syndrome, those with hypokalemia, and with other drugs that prolong the QT interval).

No products indexed under this heading.

Quetiapine Fumarate (Cases of QT interval prolongation and torsade de pointes have been reported although causality of Kaletra could not be established. Avoid use in patients with congenital long QT syndrome, those with hypokalemia, and with other drugs that prolong the QT interval). Products include:

Quinidine (Co-administration can result in increased quinidine plasma concentrations. Caution is warranted and therapeutic concentration monitoring (if available) is recommended for antiarrhythmics when co-administered with Kaletra).

No products indexed under this heading.

931 Interactions Index Kaletra

Quinidine Gluconate (Co-administration can result in increased quinidine plasma concentrations. Caution is warranted and therapeutic concentration monitoring (if available) is recommended for antiarrhythmics when co-administered with Kaletra).
No products indexed under this heading.

Quinidine Hydrochloride (Co-administration can result in increased quinidine plasma concentrations. Caution is warranted and therapeutic concentration monitoring (if available) is recommended for antiarrhythmics when co-administered with Kaletra).
No products indexed under this heading.

Quinidine Polygalacturonate (Co-administration can result in increased quinidine plasma concentrations. Caution is warranted and therapeutic concentration monitoring (if available) is recommended for antiarrhythmics when co-administered with Kaletra).
No products indexed under this heading.

Quinidine Sulfate (Co-administration can result in increased quinidine plasma concentrations. Caution is warranted and therapeutic concentration monitoring (if available) is recommended for antiarrhythmics when co-administered with Kaletra).
No products indexed under this heading.

Quinine (Kaletra is an inhibitor of CYP3A and may increase plasma concentrations of agents that are primarily metabolized by CYP3A. Agents that are extensively metabolized by CYP3A and have high first pass metabolism appear to be the most susceptible to large increases in AUC (> 3-fold) when co-administered with Kaletra. Thus, co-administration of Kaletra with drugs highly dependent on CYP3A for clearance and for which elevated plasma concentrations are associated with serious and/or life-threatening events is contraindicated. Co-administration with other CYP3A substrates may require a dose adjustment or additional monitoring). Products include:
Hyland's Leg Cramps PM with Quinine 3315

Quinine Sulfate (Kaletra is an inhibitor of CYP3A and may increase plasma concentrations of agents that are primarily metabolized by CYP3A. Agents that are extensively metabolized by CYP3A and have high first pass metabolism appear to be the most susceptible to large increases in AUC (> 3-fold) when co-administered with Kaletra. Thus, co-administration of Kaletra with drugs highly dependent on CYP3A for clearance and for which elevated plasma concentrations are associated with serious and/or life-threatening events is contraindicated. Co-administration with other CYP3A substrates may require a dose adjustment or additional monitoring).
No products indexed under this heading.

Rapamycin (Co-administration results in increased plasma concentrations of immunosuppressants. Therapeutic concentration monitoring is recommended for immunosuppressant agents when co-administered with Kaletra).
No products indexed under this heading.

Repaglinide (New onset diabetes mellitus, exacerbation of pre-existing diabetes mellitus, and hyperglycemia have been reported during post-marketing surveillance in HIV-1 infected patients receiving protease inhibitor therapy. Some patients required either initiation or dose adjustments of oral hypoglycemic agents for treatment of these events).
No products indexed under this heading.

Rifabutin (Co-administration can result in increased rifabutin and rifabutin metabolite plasma concentrations. Dosage reduction of rifabutin by at least 75% of the usual dose of 300 mg/day is recommended (ie, a maximum dose of 150 mg every other day or three times per week). Increased monitoring for adverse reactions is warranted in patients receiving the combination. Further dosage reduction of rifabutin may be necessary).
No products indexed under this heading.

Rifampicin (Co-administration of Kaletra is contraindicated with potent CYP3A inducers where significantly reduced lopinavir plasma concentrations may be associated with the potential for loss of virologic response and possible resistance and cross-resistance).
No products indexed under this heading.

Rifampin (Co-administration of Kaletra is contraindicated with rifampin, a potent CYP 3a inducer, where significantly reduced lopinavir plasma concentrations may be associated with the potential for loss of virologic response and possible resistance).
No products indexed under this heading.

Rifapentine (Co-administration of Kaletra is contraindicated with potent CYP3A inducers where significantly reduced lopinavir plasma concentrations may be associated with the potential for loss of virologic response and possible resistance and cross-resistance).
No products indexed under this heading.

Risperidone (Cases of QT interval prolongation and torsade de pointes have been reported although causality of Kaletra could not be established. Avoid use in patients with congenital long QT syndrome, those with hypokalemia, and with other drugs that prolong the QT interval). Products include:
Risperdal Consta 2682

Rosiglitazone Maleate (New onset diabetes mellitus, exacerbation of pre-existing diabetes mellitus, and hyperglycemia have been reported during post-marketing surveillance in HIV-1 infected patients receiving protease inhibitor therapy. Some patients required either initiation or dose adjustments of oral hypoglycemic agents for treatment of these events). Products include:
Avandamet 1345
Avandaryl 1356
Avandia 1366

Rosuvastatin Calcium (Use lowest possible dose of rosuvastatin with careful monitoring, or consider other HMG-CoA reductase inhibitors, such as pravastatin or fluvastatin in combination with Kaletra). Products include:
Crestor 736

Saquinavir (Co-administration may increase saquinavir concentrations. The saquinavir dose is 1000 mg BID, when co-administered with Kaletra 400/100 mg. Kaletra once-daily has not been studied in combination with saquinavir).
No products indexed under this heading.

Saquinavir Mesylate (Co-administration may increase saquinavir concentrations. The saquinavir dose is 1000 mg BID, when co-administered with Kaletra 400/100 mg. Kaletra once-daily has not been studied in combination with saquinavir).
No products indexed under this heading.

Sertraline Hydrochloride (Kaletra is an inhibitor of CYP3A and may increase plasma concentrations of agents that are primarily metabolized by CYP3A. Agents that are extensively metabolized by CYP3A and have high first pass metabolism appear to be the most susceptible to large increases in AUC (> 3-fold) when co-administered with Kaletra. Thus, co-administration of Kaletra with drugs highly dependent on CYP3A for clearance and for which elevated plasma concentrations are associated with serious and/or life-threatening events is contraindicated. Co-administration with other CYP3A substrates may require a dose adjustment or additional monitoring).
No products indexed under this heading.

Sildenafil Citrate (Particular caution should be used when prescribing sildenafil in patients receiving Kaletra. Co-administration of Kaletra with these drugs is expected to substantially increase their concentrations and may result in an increase in associated adverse reactions including hypotension, syncope, visual changes and prolonged erection. It is recommended not to exceed the following dose of 25 mg every 48 hours).
No products indexed under this heading.

Simvastatin (Concurrent use of kaletra and lovastatin metabolised by CYP 3A may increase the risk of myopathy including rhabdomyolysis). Products include:
Simcor 524
Vytorin 10/10 .... 2303, 3240
Vytorin 10/20 .... 2303, 3240
Vytorin 10/40 .... 2303, 3240
Vytorin 10/80 .... 2303, 3240
Zocor 2289

Sirolimus (Kaletra is an inhibitor of CYP3A and may increase plasma concentrations of agents that are primarily metabolized by CYP3A. Agents that are extensively metabolized by CYP3A and have high first pass metabolism appear to be the most susceptible to large increases in AUC (> 3-fold) when co-administered with Kaletra. Thus, co-administration of Kaletra with drugs highly dependent on CYP3A for clearance and for which elevated plasma concentrations are associated with serious and/or life-threatening events is contraindicated. Co-administration with other CYP3A substrates may require a dose adjustment or additional monitoring). Products include:
Rapamune 3579

Sitagliptin Phosphate (New onset diabetes mellitus, exacerbation of pre-existing diabetes mellitus, and hyperglycemia have been reported during post-marketing surveillance in HIV-1 infected patients receiving protease inhibitor therapy. Some patients required either initiation or dose adjustments of oral hypoglycemic agents for treatment of these events). Products include:
Janumet 2188
Januvia 2196

Sotalol Hydrochloride (PR interval prolongation may occur in some patients. Cases of second and third degree heart block have been reported. Caution must be used in patients with pre-existing conduction system disease, ischemic heart disease, cardiomyopathy, underlying structural heart disease or when administering with other drugs that may prolong the PR interval including β-adrenergic blockers).
No products indexed under this heading.

Tacrolimus (Co-administration results in increased plasma concentrations of immunosuppressants; monitoring is recommended). Products include:
Prograf Capsules 677
Prograf Injection 677
Protopic 685

Tadalafil (Particular caution should be used when prescribing tadalafil in patients receiving Kaletra. Co-administration of Kaletra with these drugs is expected to substantially increase their concentrations and may result in an increase in associated adverse reactions including hypotension, syncope, visual changes and prolonged erection. It is recommended not to exceed the following dose of 10 mg every 72 hours). Products include:
Adcirca 3461
Cialis 1861

Tamoxifen Citrate (Kaletra is an inhibitor of CYP3A and may increase plasma concentrations of agents that are primarily metabolized by CYP3A. Agents that are extensively metabolized by CYP3A and have high first pass metabolism appear to be the most susceptible to large increases in AUC (> 3-fold) when co-administered with Kaletra. Thus, co-administration of Kaletra with drugs highly dependent on CYP3A for clearance and for which elevated plasma concentrations are associated with serious and/or life-threatening events is contraindicated. Co-administration with other CYP3A substrates may require a dose adjustment or additional monitoring).
No products indexed under this heading.

Tenofovir Disoproxil Fumarate (Kaletra increases tenofovir concentrations. Patients receiving Kaletra and tenofovir should be monitored for adverse reactions associated with tenofovir). Products include:
Atripla 906
Truvada 1258
Viread 1266

Terfenadine (Kaletra is an inhibitor of CYP450 3A. Co-administration with drugs that are highly dependent on CYP450 3A for clearance and for which elevated plasma concentrations are associated with serious and/or life threatening events, such as terfenadine, is contraindicated).
No products indexed under this heading.

Testosterone (Kaletra is an inhibitor of CYP3A and may increase plasma concentrations of agents that are primarily metabolized by CYP3A. Agents that are extensively metabolized by CYP3A and have high first pass metabolism appear to be the most susceptible to large increases in AUC (> 3-fold) when co-administered with Kaletra. Thus, co-administration of Kaletra with drugs highly dependent on CYP3A for clearance and for which elevated plasma concentrations are associated with serious and/or life-threatening events is contraindicated. Co-administration with other CYP3A substrates may require a dose adjustment or additional monitoring). Products include:
AndroGel 3456

Testosterone Cypionate (Kaletra is an inhibitor of CYP3A and may increase plasma concentrations of agents that are primarily metabolized by CYP3A. Agents that are extensively metabolized by CYP3A and have high first pass metabolism appear to be the most susceptible to large increases in AUC (> 3-fold) when co-administered with Kaletra. Thus, co-administration of Kaletra with drugs highly dependent on CYP3A for clearance and for which elevated plasma concentrations are associated with serious and/or life-threatening events is contraindicated. Co-administration with other CYP3A substrates may require a dose adjustment or additional monitoring).
No products indexed under this heading.

Testosterone Enanthate (Kaletra is an inhibitor of CYP3A and may increase plasma concentrations of agents that are primarily metabolized by CYP3A. Agents that are extensively metabolized by CYP3A and have high first pass metabolism appear to be the most susceptible to large increases in AUC (> 3-fold) when co-administered with Kaletra. Thus, co-administration of Kaletra with drugs highly dependent on CYP3A for clearance and for which elevated plasma concentrations are associated

IMPORTANT NOTE: Always consult each drug listing in the patient's regimen for possible interactions.

Kaletra Interactions Index 932

with serious and/or life-threatening events is contraindicated. Co-administration with other CYP3A substrates may require a dose adjustment or additional monitoring). Products include:

Delatestryl 1102

Testosterone Propionate (Kaletra is an inhibitor of CYP3A and may increase plasma concentrations of agents that are primarily metabolized by CYP3A. Agents that are extensively metabolized by CYP3A and have high first pass metabolism appear to be the most susceptible to large increases in AUC (> 3-fold) when co-administered with Kaletra. Thus, co-administration of Kaletra with drugs highly dependent on CYP3A for clearance and for which elevated plasma concentrations are associated with serious and/or life-threatening events is contraindicated. Co-administration with other CYP3A substrates may require a dose adjustment or additional monitoring).

No products indexed under this heading.

Theophylline (Kaletra is an inhibitor of CYP3A and may increase plasma concentrations of agents that are primarily metabolized by CYP3A. Agents that are extensively metabolized by CYP3A and have high first pass metabolism appear to be the most susceptible to large increases in AUC (> 3-fold) when co-administered with Kaletra. Thus, co-administration of Kaletra with drugs highly dependent on CYP3A for clearance and for which elevated plasma concentrations are associated with serious and/or life-threatening events is contraindicated. Co-administration with other CYP3A substrates may require a dose adjustment or additional monitoring).

No products indexed under this heading.

Theophylline Anhydrous (Kaletra is an inhibitor of CYP3A and may increase plasma concentrations of agents that are primarily metabolized by CYP3A. Agents that are extensively metabolized by CYP3A and have high first pass metabolism appear to be the most susceptible to large increases in AUC (> 3-fold) when co-administered with Kaletra. Thus, co-administration of Kaletra with drugs highly dependent on CYP3A for clearance and for which elevated plasma concentrations are associated with serious and/or life-threatening events is contraindicated. Co-administration with other CYP3A substrates may require a dose adjustment or additional monitoring). Products include:

Uniphyl 2817

Theophylline Calcium Salicylate (Kaletra is an inhibitor of CYP3A and may increase plasma concentrations of agents that are primarily metabolized by CYP3A. Agents that are extensively metabolized by CYP3A and have high first pass metabolism appear to be the most susceptible to large increases in AUC (> 3-fold) when co-administered with Kaletra. Thus, co-administration of Kaletra with drugs highly dependent on CYP3A for clearance and for which elevated plasma concentrations are associated with serious and/or life-threatening events is contraindicated. Co-administration with other CYP3A substrates may require a dose adjustment or additional monitoring).

No products indexed under this heading.

Theophylline Sodium Glycinate (Kaletra is an inhibitor of CYP3A and may increase plasma concentrations of agents that are primarily metabolized by CYP3A. Agents that are extensively metabolized by CYP3A and have high first pass metabolism appear to be the most susceptible to large increases in AUC (> 3-fold) when co-administered with Kaletra. Thus, co-administration of Kaletra with drugs highly dependent on CYP3A for clearance and for which elevated plasma concentrations are associated with serious and/or life-threatening events is contraindicated. Co-administration with other CYP3A substrates may require a dose adjustment or additional monitoring).

No products indexed under this heading.

Thioridazine Hydrochloride (Cases of QT interval prolongation and torsade de pointes have been reported although causality of Kaletra could not be established. Avoid use in patients with congenital long QT syndrome, those with hypokalemia, and with other drugs that prolong the QT interval). Products include:

Thioridazine Hydrochloride 2384

Thiothixene (Cases of QT interval prolongation and torsade de pointes have been reported although causality of Kaletra could not be established. Avoid use in patients with congenital long QT syndrome, those with hypokalemia, and with other drugs that prolong the QT interval). Products include:

Thiothixene 2386

Tiagabine Hydrochloride (Kaletra is an inhibitor of CYP3A and may increase plasma concentrations of agents that are primarily metabolized by CYP3A. Agents that are extensively metabolized by CYP3A and have high first pass metabolism appear to be the most susceptible to large increases in AUC (> 3-fold) when co-administered with Kaletra. Thus, co-administration of Kaletra with drugs highly dependent on CYP3A for clearance and for which elevated plasma concentrations are associated with serious and/or life-threatening events is contraindicated. Co-administration with other CYP3A substrates may require a dose adjustment or additional monitoring). Products include:

Gabitril 972

Timolol Hemihydrate (PR interval prolongation may occur in some patients. Cases of second and third degree heart block have been reported. Caution must be used in patients with pre-existing conduction system disease, ischemic heart disease, cardiomyopathy, underlying structural heart disease or when administering with other drugs that may prolong the PR interval including β-adrenergic blockers). Products include:

Betimol 3490

Timolol Maleate (PR interval prolongation may occur in some patients. Cases of second and third degree heart block have been reported. Caution must be used in patients with pre-existing conduction system disease, ischemic heart disease, cardiomyopathy, underlying structural heart disease or when administering with other drugs that may prolong the PR interval including β-adrenergic blockers). Products include:

Combigan 601

Dorzolamide Hydrochloride/Timolol Maleate Ophthalmic Solution .... ⊙ 243

Timoptic in Ocudose .... ⊙ 231

Tipranavir (Co-administration may result in a decrease in lopinavir AUC and C_{min}. Kaletra should not be administered with tipranavir (500 mg twice-daily) or co-administered with ritonavir (200 mg twice-daily)).

No products indexed under this heading.

Tocainide Hydrochloride (Cases of QT interval prolongation and torsade de pointes have been reported although causality of Kaletra could not be established. Avoid use in patients with congenital long QT syndrome, those with hypokalemia, and with other drugs that prolong the QT interval).

No products indexed under this heading.

Tolazamide (New onset diabetes mellitus, exacerbation of pre-existing diabetes mellitus, and hyperglycemia have been reported during post-marketing surveillance in HIV-1 infected patients receiving protease inhibitor therapy. Some patients required either initiation or dose adjustments of oral hypoglycemic agents for treatment of these events).

No products indexed under this heading.

Tolbutamide (New onset diabetes mellitus, exacerbation of pre-existing diabetes mellitus, and hyperglycemia have been reported during post-marketing surveillance in HIV-1 infected patients receiving protease inhibitor therapy. Some patients required either initiation or dose adjustments of oral hypoglycemic agents for treatment of these events).

No products indexed under this heading.

Tolterodine Tartrate (Kaletra is an inhibitor of CYP3A and may increase plasma concentrations of agents that are primarily metabolized by CYP3A. Agents that are extensively metabolized by CYP3A and have high first pass metabolism appear to be the most susceptible to large increases in AUC (> 3-fold) when co-administered with Kaletra. Thus, co-administration of Kaletra with drugs highly dependent on CYP3A for clearance and for which elevated plasma concentrations are associated with serious and/or life-threatening events is contraindicated. Co-administration with other CYP3A substrates may require a dose adjustment or additional monitoring).

No products indexed under this heading.

Tranylcypromine Sulfate (Cases of QT interval prolongation and torsade de pointes have been reported although causality of Kaletra could not be established. Avoid use in patients with congenital long QT syndrome, those with hypokalemia, and with other drugs that prolong the QT interval). Products include:

Parnate 1584

Trazodone Hydrochloride (Concomitant use of trazodone and Kaletra may increase concentrations of trazodone. Adverse events of nausea, dizziness, hypotension and syncope have been observed following co-administration of trazodone and ritonavir. If trazodone is used with a CYP3A4 inhibitor, such as ritonavir, the combination should be used with caution and a lower dose of trazodone should be considered).

No products indexed under this heading.

Triazolam (Kaletra is an inhibitor of CYP3A and may increase plasma concentrations of agents that are primarily metabolized by CYP3A, such as triazolam. Concurrent administration of kaletra and triazolam may result to prolonged or increased sedation or respiratory depression).

No products indexed under this heading.

Trifluoperazine Hydrochloride (Cases of QT interval prolongation and torsade de pointes have been reported although causality of Kaletra could not be established. Avoid use in patients with congenital long QT syndrome, those with hypokalemia, and with other drugs that prolong the QT interval).

No products indexed under this heading.

Trimipramine Maleate (Cases of QT interval prolongation and torsade de pointes have been reported although causality of Kaletra could not be established. Avoid use in patients with congenital long QT syndrome, those with hypokalemia, and with other drugs that prolong the QT interval).

No products indexed under this heading.

Troglitazone (New onset diabetes mellitus, exacerbation of pre-existing diabetes mellitus, and hyperglycemia have been reported during post-marketing surveillance in HIV-1 infected patients receiving protease inhibitor therapy. Some patients required either initiation or dose adjustments of oral hypoglycemic agents for treatment of these events).

No products indexed under this heading.

Troleandomycin (Although not noted with concurrent ketoconazole, co-administration of Kaletra and other drugs that inhibit CYP3A may increase lopinavir plasma concentrations).

No products indexed under this heading.

Vardenafil Hydrochloride (Particular caution should be used when prescribing vardenafil in patients receiving Kaletra. Co-administration of Kaletra with these drugs is expected to substantially increase their concentrations and may result in an increase in associated adverse reactions including hypotension, syncope, visual changes and prolonged erection. It is recommended not to exceed the following dose of 2.5 mg every 72 hours). Products include:

Levitra 3157

Venlafaxine Hydrochloride (Kaletra is an inhibitor of CYP3A and may increase plasma concentrations of agents that are primarily metabolized by CYP3A. Agents that are extensively metabolized by CYP3A and have high first pass metabolism appear to be the most susceptible to large increases in AUC (> 3-fold) when co-administered with Kaletra. Thus, co-administration of Kaletra with drugs highly dependent on CYP3A for clearance and for which elevated plasma concentrations are associated with serious and/or life-threatening events is contraindicated. Co-administration with other CYP3A substrates may require a dose adjustment or additional monitoring). Products include:

Effexor XR 3504

Venlafaxine Hydrochloride Tablets ... 2388

Verapamil Hydrochloride (PR interval prolongation may occur in some patients. Cases of second and third degree heart block have been reported. Caution must be used in patients with pre-existing conduction system disease, ischemic heart disease, cardiomyopathy, underlying structural heart disease or when administering with other drugs that may prolong the PR interval including calcium channel blockers). Products include:

Tarka 534

Vinblastine Sulfate (Concentrations of vinblastine may be increased when co-administered with Kaletra resulting in the potential for increased adverse events usually associated with these anticancer agents).

No products indexed under this heading.

Vincristine Sulfate (Concentrations of vincristine may be increased when co-administered with Kaletra resulting in the potential for increased adverse events usually associated with these anticancer agents).

No products indexed under this heading.

Voriconazole (Co-administration of voriconazole with Kaletra has not been studied. However, a study has been shown that administration of voriconazole with ritonavir 100 mg every 12

(⊙ Described in PDR® for Ophthalmic Medicines)

hours decreased voriconazole steady-state AUC by an average of 39%; therefore, co-administration of Kaletra and voriconazole may result in decreased voriconazole concentrations and the potential for decreased voriconazole effectiveness and should be avoided, unless an assessment of the benefit/risk to the patient justifies the use of voriconazole).
No products indexed under this heading.

Warfarin Sodium (Concentrations of warfarin may be affected. It is recommended that INR (international normalized ratio) be monitored).
No products indexed under this heading.

Zafirlukast (Although not noted with concurrent ketoconazole, co-administration of Kaletra and other drugs that inhibit CYP3A may increase lopinavir plasma concentrations). Products include:
Accolate **3612**

Zidovudine (Kaletra induces glucuronidation; therefore, Kaletra has the potential to reduce zidovudine plasma concentrations; the clinical significance is unknown). Products include:
Combivir **1404**
Retrovir **1634**
Retrovir IV **1640**
Trizivir **1688**

Zileuton (Although not noted with concurrent ketoconazole, co-administration of Kaletra and other drugs that inhibit CYP3A may increase lopinavir plasma concentrations).
No products indexed under this heading.

Ziprasidone Hydrochloride (Cases of QT interval prolongation and torsade de pointes have been reported although causality of Kaletra could not be established. Avoid use in patients with congenital long QT syndrome, those with hypokalemia, and with other drugs that prolong the QT interval). Products include:
Geodon **2723**

Food Interactions

Food, unspecified (Relative to fasting, administration of Kaletra tablets with a moderate fat meal (500 - 682 Kcal, 23 to 25% calories from fat) increased lopinavir AUC and C_{max} by 26.9% and 17.6%, respectively. Relative to fasting, administration of KALETRA tablets with a high fat meal (872 Kcal, 56% from fat) increased lopinavir AUC by 18.9% but not C_{max}. Therefore, KALETRA tablets may be taken with or without food).

Grapefruit (Although not noted with concurrent ketoconazole, co-administration of Kaletra and other drugs that inhibit CYP3A may increase lopinavir plasma concentrations).

Grapefruit Juice (Although not noted with concurrent ketoconazole, co-administration of Kaletra and other drugs that inhibit CYP3A may increase lopinavir plasma concentrations).

Meal, unspecified (Relative to fasting, administration of Kaletra tablets with a moderate fat meal (500 - 682 Kcal, 23 to 25% calories from fat) increased lopinavir AUC and C_{max} by 26.9% and 17.6%, respectively. Relative to fasting, administration of Kaletra tablets with a high fat meal (872 Kcal, 56% from fat) increased lopinavir AUC by 18.9% but not C_{max}. Therefore, Kaletra tablets may be taken with or without food).

KAPIDEX DELAYED RELEASE CAPSULES

(Dexlansoprazole) **3362**
May interact with absorption of drugs where gastric ph is an important determinant in their bioavailability, ampicillins, iron salts, and certain other agents. Compounds in these categories include:

Ampicillin (It is theoretically possible that dexlansoprazole may interfere with the absorption of other drugs where gastric pH is an important determinant of oral bioavailability (eg, ampicillin esters)).
No products indexed under this heading.

Ampicillin Sodium (It is theoretically possible that dexlansoprazole may interfere with the absorption of other drugs where gastric pH is an important determinant of oral bioavailability (eg, ampicillin esters)).
No products indexed under this heading.

Ampicillin Trihydrate (It is theoretically possible that dexlansoprazole may interfere with the absorption of other drugs where gastric pH is an important determinant of oral bioavailability (eg, ampicillin esters)).
No products indexed under this heading.

Atazanavir (Dexlansoprazole causes inhibition of gastric acid secretion. Dexlansoprazole is likely to substantially decrease the systemic concentrations of the HIV protease inhibitor atazanavir, which is dependent upon the presence of gastric acid for absorption, and may result in a loss of therapeutic effect of atazanavir and the development of HIV resistance. Therefore, dexlansoprazole should not be co-administered with atazanavir).
No products indexed under this heading.

Atazanavir Sulfate (Dexlansoprazole causes inhibition of gastric acid secretion. Dexlansoprazole is likely to substantially decrease the systemic concentrations of the HIV protease inhibitor atazanavir, which is dependent upon the presence of gastric acid for absorption, and may result in a loss of therapeutic effect of atazanavir and the development of HIV resistance. Therefore, dexlansoprazole should not be co-administered with atazanavir).
No products indexed under this heading.

Bacampicillin Hydrochloride (It is theoretically possible that dexlansoprazole may interfere with the absorption of other drugs where gastric pH is an important determinant of oral bioavailability (eg, ampicillin esters)).
No products indexed under this heading.

Digoxin (It is theoretically possible that dexlansoprazole may interfere with the absorption of other drugs where gastric pH is an important determinant of oral bioavailability (eg, digoxin)). Products include:
Lanoxin Injection **1546**
Lanoxin Injection Pediatric **1549**
Lanoxin Tablets **1553**

Ferrous Fumarate (It is theoretically possible that dexlansoprazole may interfere with the absorption of other drugs where gastric pH is an important determinant of oral bioavailability (eg, iron salts)). Products include:
PreNexa **3473**

Ferrous Gluconate (It is theoretically possible that dexlansoprazole may interfere with the absorption of other drugs where gastric pH is an important determinant of oral bioavailability (eg, iron salts)). Products include:
CitraNatal Assure **2332**
CitraNatal Rx **2332**

Ferrous Sulfate (It is theoretically possible that dexlansoprazole may interfere with the absorption of other drugs where gastric pH is an important determinant of oral bioavailability (eg, iron salts)).
No products indexed under this heading.

Iron (It is theoretically possible that dexlansoprazole may interfere with the absorption of other drugs where gastric pH is an important determinant of oral bioavailability (eg, iron salts)).
No products indexed under this heading.

Iron, Peptonized (It is theoretically possible that dexlansoprazole may interfere with the absorption of other drugs where gastric pH is an important determinant of oral bioavailability (eg, iron salts)).
No products indexed under this heading.

Iron Cacodylate (It is theoretically possible that dexlansoprazole may interfere with the absorption of other drugs where gastric pH is an important determinant of oral bioavailability (eg, iron salts)).
No products indexed under this heading.

Iron Carbonyl (It is theoretically possible that dexlansoprazole may interfere with the absorption of other drugs where gastric pH is an important determinant of oral bioavailability (eg, iron salts)). Products include:
CitraNatal 90 DHA Capsules **2332**
CitraNatal Assure **2332**
CitraNatal Harmony **2332**
CitraNatal Rx **2332**
Ferralet **2333**

Iron Dextran (It is theoretically possible that dexlansoprazole may interfere with the absorption of other drugs where gastric pH is an important determinant of oral bioavailability (eg, iron salts)).
No products indexed under this heading.

Iron Polysaccharide Complex (It is theoretically possible that dexlansoprazole may interfere with the absorption of other drugs where gastric pH is an important determinant of oral bioavailability (eg, iron salts)).
No products indexed under this heading.

Iron Sucrose (It is theoretically possible that dexlansoprazole may interfere with the absorption of other drugs where gastric pH is an important determinant of oral bioavailability (eg, iron salts)).
No products indexed under this heading.

Iron Supplements (It is theoretically possible that dexlansoprazole may interfere with the absorption of other drugs where gastric pH is an important determinant of oral bioavailability (eg, iron salts)).
No products indexed under this heading.

Ketoconazole (It is theoretically possible that dexlansoprazole may interfere with the absorption of other drugs where gastric pH is an important determinant of oral bioavailability (eg, ketoconazole)). Products include:
Extina **3319**
Xolegel **3337**

Polysaccharide Iron Complex (It is theoretically possible that dexlansoprazole may interfere with the absorption of other drugs where gastric pH is an important determinant of oral bioavailability (eg, iron salts)). Products include:
Nu-Iron 150 .... **2321**

Tacrolimus (Concomitant administration of dexlansoprazole and tacrolimus may increase whole blood levels of tacrolimus, especially in transplant patients who are intermediate or poor metabolizers of CYP2C19). Products include:
Prograf Capsules **677**
Prograf Injection **677**
Protopic **685**

Warfarin Sodium (Co-administration of dexlansoprazole 90 mg and warfarin 25 mg did not affect the pharmacokinetics of warfarin or INR. However, there have been reports of increased INR and prothrombin time in patients receiving PPIs and warfarin concomitantly. Increases in INR and prothrombin time may lead to abnormal bleeding and even death. Patients treated with dexlansoprazole and warfarin concomitantly may need to be monitored for increases in INR and prothrombin time).
No products indexed under this heading.

Food Interactions

Food, unspecified (In food-effect studies in healthy subjects receiving dexlansoprazole under various fed conditions compared to fasting, increases in C_{max} ranged from 12% to 55%, increases in AUC ranged from 9% to 37%, and T_{max} varied (ranging from a decrease of 0.7 hours to an increase of 3 hours). No significant differences in mean intragastric pH were observed between fasted and various fed conditions. However, the percentage of time intragastric pH exceeded 4 over the 24-hour dosing interval decreased slightly when dexlansoprazole was administered after a meal (57%) relative to fasting (64%), primarily due to a decreased response in intragastric pH during the first 4 hours after dosing. Because of this, while dexlansoprazole can be taken without regard to food, some patients may benefit from administering the dose prior to a meal if post-meal symptoms do not resolve under post-fed conditions).

Meal, unspecified (In food-effect studies in healthy subjects receiving dexlansoprazole under various fed conditions compared to fasting, increases in C_{max} ranged from 12% to 55%, increases in AUC ranged from 9% to 37%, and T_{max} varied (ranging from a decrease of 0.7 hours to an increase of 3 hours). No significant differences in mean intragastric pH were observed between fasted and various fed conditions. However, the percentage of time intragastric pH exceeded 4 over the 24-hour dosing interval decreased slightly when dexlansoprazole was administered after a meal (57%) relative to fasting (64%), primarily due to a decreased response in intragastric pH during the first 4 hours after dosing. Because of this, while dexlansoprazole can be taken without regard to food, some patients may benefit from administering the dose prior to a meal if post-meal symptoms do not resolve under post-fed conditions).

KEPIVANCE

(Palifermin) **875**
May interact with antineoplastics, low molecular weight heparins, and certain other agents. Compounds in these categories include:

Altretamine (Palifermin should not be administered within 24 hours before, during infusion of, or within 24 hours after administration of myelotoxic chemotherapy. In a clinical trial, administration of palifermin whitin 24 hours of chemotherapy resulted in increased severity and duration of oral mucositis). Products include:
Hexalen **1066**

Anastrozole (Palifermin should not be administered within 24 hours before, during infusion of, or within 24 hours after administration of myelotoxic chemotherapy. In a clinical trial, administration of palifermin whitin 24 hours of chemotherapy resulted in increased severity and duration of oral mucositis).
No products indexed under this heading.

Asparaginase (Palifermin should not be administered within 24 hours before, during infusion of, or within 24 hours after administration of myelotoxic chemotherapy. In a clinical trial, administration of palifermin whitin 24 hours of chemotherapy resulted in increased severity and duration of oral mucositis). Products include:
Elspar **2005, 2122**

Kepivance Interactions Index 934

Bicalutamide (Palifermin should not be administered within 24 hours before, during infusion of, or within 24 hours after administration of myelotoxic chemotherapy. In a clinical trial, administration of palifermin whitin 24 hours of chemotherapy resulted in increased severity and duration of oral mucositis).
No products indexed under this heading.

Bleomycin Sulfate (Palifermin should not be administered within 24 hours before, during infusion of, or within 24 hours after administration of myelotoxic chemotherapy. In a clinical trial, administration of palifermin whitin 24 hours of chemotherapy resulted in increased severity and duration of oral mucositis).
No products indexed under this heading.

Busulfan (Palifermin should not be administered within 24 hours before, during infusion of, or within 24 hours after administration of myelotoxic chemotherapy. In a clinical trial, administration of palifermin whitin 24 hours of chemotherapy resulted in increased severity and duration of oral mucositis). Products include:
Myleran 1581

Carboplatin (Palifermin should not be administered within 24 hours before, during infusion of, or within 24 hours after administration of myelotoxic chemotherapy. In a clinical trial, administration of palifermin whitin 24 hours of chemotherapy resulted in increased severity and duration of oral mucositis).
No products indexed under this heading.

Carmustine (BCNU) (Palifermin should not be administered within 24 hours before, during infusion of, or within 24 hours after administration of myelotoxic chemotherapy. In a clinical trial, administration of palifermin whitin 24 hours of chemotherapy resulted in increased severity and duration of oral mucositis).
No products indexed under this heading.

Chlorambucil (Palifermin should not be administered within 24 hours before, during infusion of, or within 24 hours after administration of myelotoxic chemotherapy. In a clinical trial, administration of palifermin whitin 24 hours of chemotherapy resulted in increased severity and duration of oral mucositis). Products include:
Leukeran 1557

Cisplatin (Palifermin should not be administered within 24 hours before, during infusion of, or within 24 hours after administration of myelotoxic chemotherapy. In a clinical trial, administration of palifermin whitin 24 hours of chemotherapy resulted in increased severity and duration of oral mucositis).
No products indexed under this heading.

Cyclophosphamide (Palifermin should not be administered within 24 hours before, during infusion of, or within 24 hours after administration of myelotoxic chemotherapy. In a clinical trial, administration of palifermin whitin 24 hours of chemotherapy resulted in increased severity and duration of oral mucositis).
No products indexed under this heading.

Dacarbazine (Palifermin should not be administered within 24 hours before, during infusion of, or within 24 hours after administration of myelotoxic chemotherapy. In a clinical trial, administration of palifermin whitin 24 hours of chemotherapy resulted in increased severity and duration of oral mucositis).
No products indexed under this heading.

Dalteparin Sodium (*In vitro* and *in vivo* data suggests that palifermin interacts with unfractioned as well as low molecular weight heparins. Heparin co-administration resulted in a 5-fold increase in palifermin systemic exposure. Thus, heparin should be used with care in patients who are concomitantly administered palifermin. If heparin is used to maintain an IV line, saline should be used to rinse the line prior to and after palifermin administration). Products include:
Fragmin 1058

Daunorubicin Citrate (Palifermin should not be administered within 24 hours before, during infusion of, or within 24 hours after administration of myelotoxic chemotherapy. In a clinical trial, administration of palifermin whitin 24 hours of chemotherapy resulted in increased severity and duration of oral mucositis).
No products indexed under this heading.

Daunorubicin Hydrochloride (Palifermin should not be administered within 24 hours before, during infusion of, or within 24 hours after administration of myelotoxic chemotherapy. In a clinical trial, administration of palifermin whitin 24 hours of chemotherapy resulted in increased severity and duration of oral mucositis).
No products indexed under this heading.

Denileukin Diftitox (Palifermin should not be administered within 24 hours before, during infusion of, or within 24 hours after administration of myelotoxic chemotherapy. In a clinical trial, administration of palifermin whitin 24 hours of chemotherapy resulted in increased severity and duration of oral mucositis). Products include:
Ontak 1068

Docetaxel (Palifermin should not be administered within 24 hours before, during infusion of, or within 24 hours after administration of myelotoxic chemotherapy. In a clinical trial, administration of palifermin whitin 24 hours of chemotherapy resulted in increased severity and duration of oral mucositis). Products include:
Taxotere 3035

Doxorubicin Hydrochloride (Palifermin should not be administered within 24 hours before, during infusion of, or within 24 hours after administration of myelotoxic chemotherapy. In a clinical trial, administration of palifermin whitin 24 hours of chemotherapy resulted in increased severity and duration of oral mucositis).
No products indexed under this heading.

Enoxaparin Sodium (*In vitro* and *in vivo* data suggests that palifermin interacts with unfractioned as well as low molecular weight heparins. Heparin co-administration resulted in a 5-fold increase in palifermin systemic exposure. Thus, heparin should be used with care in patients who are concomitantly administered palifermin. If heparin is used to maintain an IV line, saline should be used to rinse the line prior to and after palifermin administration). Products include:
Lovenox 3005

Epirubicin Hydrochloride (Palifermin should not be administered within 24 hours before, during infusion of, or within 24 hours after administration of myelotoxic chemotherapy. In a clinical trial, administration of palifermin whitin 24 hours of chemotherapy resulted in increased severity and duration of oral mucositis).
No products indexed under this heading.

Estramustine Phosphate Sodium (Palifermin should not be administered within 24 hours before, during infusion of, or within 24 hours after administration of myelotoxic chemotherapy. In a clinical trial, administration of palifermin whitin 24 hours of chemotherapy resulted in increased severity and duration of oral mucositis).
No products indexed under this heading.

Etoposide (Palifermin should not be administered within 24 hours before, during infusion of, or within 24 hours after administration of myelotoxic chemotherapy. In a clinical trial, administration of palifermin whitin 24 hours of chemotherapy resulted in increased severity and duration of oral mucositis).
No products indexed under this heading.

Exemestane (Palifermin should not be administered within 24 hours before, during infusion of, or within 24 hours after administration of myelotoxic chemotherapy. In a clinical trial, administration of palifermin whitin 24 hours of chemotherapy resulted in increased severity and duration of oral mucositis). Products include:
Aromasin 2758

Floxuridine (Palifermin should not be administered within 24 hours before, during infusion of, or within 24 hours after administration of myelotoxic chemotherapy. In a clinical trial, administration of palifermin whitin 24 hours of chemotherapy resulted in increased severity and duration of oral mucositis).
No products indexed under this heading.

Fluorouracil (Palifermin should not be administered within 24 hours before, during infusion of, or within 24 hours after administration of myelotoxic chemotherapy. In a clinical trial, administration of palifermin whitin 24 hours of chemotherapy resulted in increased severity and duration of oral mucositis). Products include:
Carac 2966

Flutamide (Palifermin should not be administered within 24 hours before, during infusion of, or within 24 hours after administration of myelotoxic chemotherapy. In a clinical trial, administration of palifermin whitin 24 hours of chemotherapy resulted in increased severity and duration of oral mucositis).
No products indexed under this heading.

Gemcitabine Hydrochloride (Palifermin should not be administered within 24 hours before, during infusion of, or within 24 hours after administration of myelotoxic chemotherapy. In a clinical trial, administration of palifermin whitin 24 hours of chemotherapy resulted in increased severity and duration of oral mucositis). Products include:
Gemzar 1900

Heparin (*In vitro* and *in vivo* data suggests that palifermin interacts with unfractioned as well as low molecular weight heparins. Heparin co-administration resulted in a 5-fold increase in palifermin systemic exposure. Thus, heparin should be used with care in patients who are concomitantly administered palifermin. If heparin is used to maintain an IV line, saline should be used to rinse the line prior to and after palifermin administration).
No products indexed under this heading.

Heparin Calcium (*In vitro* and *in vivo* data suggests that palifermin interacts with unfractioned as well as low molecular weight heparins. Heparin co-administration resulted in a 5-fold increase in palifermin systemic exposure. Thus, heparin should be used with care in patients who are concomitantly administered palifermin. If heparin is used to maintain an IV line, saline should be used to rinse the line prior to and after palifermin administration).
No products indexed under this heading.

Heparin Sodium (*In vitro* and *in vivo* data suggests that palifermin interacts with unfractioned as well as low molecular weight heparins. Heparin co-administration resulted in a 5-fold increase in palifermin systemic exposure. Thus, heparin should be used with care in patients who are concomitantly administered palifermin. If heparin is used to maintain an IV line, saline should be used to rinse the line prior to and after palifermin administration).
No products indexed under this heading.

Hydroxyurea (Palifermin should not be administered within 24 hours before, during infusion of, or within 24 hours after administration of myelotoxic chemotherapy. In a clinical trial, administration of palifermin whitin 24 hours of chemotherapy resulted in increased severity and duration of oral mucositis).
No products indexed under this heading.

Idarubicin Hydrochloride (Palifermin should not be administered within 24 hours before, during infusion of, or within 24 hours after administration of myelotoxic chemotherapy. In a clinical trial, administration of palifermin whitin 24 hours of chemotherapy resulted in increased severity and duration of oral mucositis).
No products indexed under this heading.

Ifosfamide (Palifermin should not be administered within 24 hours before, during infusion of, or within 24 hours after administration of myelotoxic chemotherapy. In a clinical trial, administration of palifermin whitin 24 hours of chemotherapy resulted in increased severity and duration of oral mucositis).
No products indexed under this heading.

Interferon alfa-2a, Recombinant (Palifermin should not be administered within 24 hours before, during infusion of, or within 24 hours after administration of myelotoxic chemotherapy. In a clinical trial, administration of palifermin whitin 24 hours of chemotherapy resulted in increased severity and duration of oral mucositis).
No products indexed under this heading.

Interferon alfa-2b, Recombinant (Palifermin should not be administered within 24 hours before, during infusion of, or within 24 hours after administration of myelotoxic chemotherapy. In a clinical trial, administration of palifermin whitin 24 hours of chemotherapy resulted in increased severity and duration of oral mucositis). Products include:
Intron A 3140

Irinotecan Hydrochloride (Palifermin should not be administered within 24 hours before, during infusion of, or within 24 hours after administration of myelotoxic chemotherapy. In a clinical trial, administration of palifermin whitin 24 hours of chemotherapy resulted in increased severity and duration of oral mucositis).
No products indexed under this heading.

Levamisole Hydrochloride (Palifermin should not be administered within 24 hours before, during infusion of, or within 24 hours after administration of myelotoxic chemotherapy. In a clinical trial, administration of palifermin whitin 24 hours of chemotherapy resulted in increased severity and duration of oral mucositis).
No products indexed under this heading.

Lomustine (CCNU) (Palifermin should not be administered within 24 hours before, during infusion of, or within 24 hours after administration of myelotoxic chemotherapy. In a clinical trial, administration of palifermin whitin 24 hours of chemotherapy resulted in increased severity and duration of oral mucositis).
No products indexed under this heading.

Mechlorethamine Hydrochloride (Palifermin should not be administered within 24 hours before, during infusion of, or within 24 hours after administration of myelotoxic chemotherapy. In a clinical trial, administration of palifermin whitin 24 hours of chemotherapy resulted in increased severity and duration of oral mucositis). Products include:
Mustargen 2010

KEPPRA XR EXTENDED-RELEASE TABLETS
(Levetiracetam) 3434

Fat (Intake of a high fat, high calorie breakfast before the administration of extended-release levetiracetam tablets resulted in a higher peak concentration, and longer median time to peak. The median time to peak (T_{max}) was 2 hours longer in the fed state).
No products indexed under this heading.

Probenecid (Probenecid, a renal tubular secretion blocking agent, administered at a dose of 500 mg four times a day, did not change the pharmacokinetics of levetiracetam 1000 mg twice daily. C^{ss}_{max} of the metabolite, ucb L057, was approximately doubled in the presence of probenecid while the fraction of drug excreted unchanged in the urine remained the same. Renal clearance of ucb L057 in the presence of probenecid decreased 60%, probably related to competitive inhibition of tubular secretion of ucb L057).
No products indexed under this heading.

Food Interactions

Food, unspecified (Intake of a high fat, high calorie breakfast before the administration of extended-release levetiracetam tablets resulted in a higher peak concentration, and longer median time to peak. The median time to peak (T_{max}) was 2 hours longer in the fed state).

Meal, unspecified (Intake of a high fat, high calorie breakfast before the administration of extended-release levetiracetam tablets resulted in a higher peak concentration, and longer median time to peak. The median time to peak (T_{max}) was 2 hours longer in the fed state).

KETEK TABLETS
(Telithromycin) 2991

May interact with benzodiazepine that are metabolized by CYP3A4, class 1A antiarrhythmics, class III antiarrhythmics, cytochrome p450 3a4 inducers (selected), cytochrome p450 3a4 substrates (selected), drugs which undergo biotransformation by cytochrome p-450 mixed function oxidase, ergot-containing drugs, HMG-CoA reductase inhibitors, oral anticoagulants, phenytoin, quinidine, theophyllines, and certain other agents. Compounds in these categories include:

Acarbose (Elevated levels of drugs metabolized by the CYP450 system may be observed when co-administered with telithromycin; therefore, increases or prolongation of the therapeutic and/or adverse effects of the concomitant drug may be observed).
No products indexed under this heading.

Alatrofloxacin Mesylate (Elevated levels of drugs metabolized by the CYP450 system may be observed when co-administered with telithromycin; therefore, increases or prolongation of the therapeutic and/or adverse effects of the concomitant drug may be observed).
No products indexed under this heading.

Alfentanil Hydrochloride (Co-administration of telithromycin with a drug primarily metabolized by the CYP 3A4 enzyme system may result in increased plasma concentrations of the drug co-administered with telithromycin that could increase or prolong both the therapeutic and adverse effects).
No products indexed under this heading.

Allium sativum (Concomitant administration of CYP 3A4 inducers is likely to result in subtherapeutic levels of telithromycin and loss of effect).
No products indexed under this heading.

Alprazolam (Concomitant administration of telithromycin with midazolam increased the AUC of midazolam; therefore, precaution should be used with other benzodiazepines metabolized by CYP 3A4 and that undergo a high first-pass effect (eg, triazolam)).
No products indexed under this heading.

Aminoglutethimide (Concomitant administration of CYP 3A4 inducers is likely to result in subtherapeutic levels of telithromycin and loss of effect).
No products indexed under this heading.

Aminophylline (Elevated levels of drugs metabolized by the CYP450 system may be observed when co-administered with telithromycin; therefore, increases or prolongation of the therapeutic and/or adverse effects of the concomitant drug may be observed).
No products indexed under this heading.

Amiodarone Hydrochloride (Telithromycin should be avoided in patients with congenital prolongation of

Ketek Interactions Index 936

the QT_c interval, and in patients with ongoing proarrhythmic conditions, such as uncorrected hypokalemia or hypomagnesemia, clinically significant bradycardia, and in patients receiving Class IA (eg, quinidine and procainamide) or Class III (eg, dofetilide) antiarrhythmic agents).
No products indexed under this heading.

Amitriptyline Hydrochloride (Co-administration of telithromycin with a drug primarily metabolized by the CYP 3A4 enzyme system may result in increased plasma concentrations of the drug co-administered with telithromycin that could increase or prolong both the therapeutic and adverse effects).
No products indexed under this heading.

Amlodipine Besylate (Co-administration of telithromycin with a drug primarily metabolized by the CYP 3A4 enzyme system may result in increased plasma concentrations of the drug co-administered with telithromycin that could increase or prolong both the therapeutic and adverse effects). Products include:
Azor ... **1010**
Exforge ... **2443**
Exforge HCT ... **2449**

Amoxapine (Elevated levels of drugs metabolized by the CYP450 system may be observed when co-administered with telithromycin; therefore, increases or prolongation of the therapeutic and/or adverse effects of the concomitant drug may be observed).
No products indexed under this heading.

Amphetamine Aspartate (Elevated levels of drugs metabolized by the CYP450 system may be observed when co-administered with telithromycin; therefore, increases or prolongation of the therapeutic and/or adverse effects of the concomitant drug may be observed).
No products indexed under this heading.

Amphetamine Aspartate Monohydrate (Elevated levels of drugs metabolized by the CYP450 system may be observed when co-administered with telithromycin; therefore, increases or prolongation of the therapeutic and/or adverse effects of the concomitant drug may be observed).
No products indexed under this heading.

Amphetamine Sulfate (Elevated levels of drugs metabolized by the CYP450 system may be observed when co-administered with telithromycin; therefore, increases or prolongation of the therapeutic and/or adverse effects of the concomitant drug may be observed).
No products indexed under this heading.

Anagrelide Hydrochloride (Elevated levels of drugs metabolized by the CYP450 system may be observed when co-administered with telithromycin; therefore, increases or prolongation of the therapeutic and/or adverse effects of the concomitant drug may be observed).
No products indexed under this heading.

Anisindione (Spontaneous post-marketing reports suggest that administration of telithromycin and oral anticoagulants concomitantly may potentiate the effects of the oral anticoagulants. Consideration should be given to monitoring prothrombin times/INR while patients are receiving telithromycin and oral anticoagulants simultaneously).
No products indexed under this heading.

Aprepitant (Co-administration of telithromycin with a drug primarily metabolized by the CYP 3A4 enzyme system may result in increased plasma concentrations of the drug co-administered with telithromycin that could increase or prolong both the therapeutic and adverse effects). Products include:
Emend ... **2124**

Astemizole (Co-administration of telithromycin with a drug primarily metabolized by the CYP 3A4 enzyme system may result in increased plasma concentrations of the drug co-administered with telithromycin that could increase or prolong both the therapeutic and adverse effects).
No products indexed under this heading.

Atomoxetine Hydrochloride (Elevated levels of drugs metabolized by the CYP450 system may be observed when co-administered with telithromycin; therefore, increases or prolongation of the therapeutic and/or adverse effects of the concomitant drug may be observed). Products include:
Strattera ... **1957**

Atorvastatin Calcium (High levels of HMG-CoA reductase inhibitors increase the risk of myopathy. Use of simvastatin, lovastatin, or atorvastatin concomitantly with telithromycin should be avoided. If telithromycin is prescribed, therapy with simvastatin, lovastatin, or atorvastatin should be suspended during the course of treatment. Patients concomitantly treated with statins should be carefully monitored for signs and symptoms of myopathy and rhabdomyolysis). Products include:
Lipitor ... **2703**

Belladonna Ergotamine (Co-administration of telithromycin with a drug primarily metabolized by the CYP 3A4 enzyme system may result in increased plasma concentrations of the drug co-administered with telithromycin that could increase or prolong both the therapeutic and adverse effects).
No products indexed under this heading.

Benzphetamine Hydrochloride (Elevated levels of drugs metabolized by the CYP450 system may be observed when co-administered with telithromycin; therefore, increases or prolongation of the therapeutic and/or adverse effects of the concomitant drug may be observed).
No products indexed under this heading.

Betamethasone (Concomitant administration of CYP 3A4 inducers is likely to result in subtherapeutic levels of telithromycin and loss of effect).
No products indexed under this heading.

Betamethasone Acetate (Concomitant administration of CYP 3A4 inducers is likely to result in subtherapeutic levels of telithromycin and loss of effect).
No products indexed under this heading.

Betamethasone Benzoate (Concomitant administration of CYP 3A4 inducers is likely to result in subtherapeutic levels of telithromycin and loss of effect).
No products indexed under this heading.

Betamethasone Dipropionate (Concomitant administration of CYP 3A4 inducers is likely to result in subtherapeutic levels of telithromycin and loss of effect). Products include:
Diprolene Lotion 0.05% ... **3108**
Diprolene Ointment 0.05% ... **3109**
Diprolene AF Cream 0.05% ... **3107**
Lotrisone ... **3163**

Betamethasone Sodium Phosphate (Concomitant administration of CYP 3A4 inducers is likely to result in subtherapeutic levels of telithromycin and loss of effect).
No products indexed under this heading.

Betamethasone Valerate (Concomitant administration of CYP 3A4 inducers is likely to result in subtherapeutic levels of telithromycin and loss of effect). Products include:
Luxiq ... **3321**

Bisoprolol Fumarate (Elevated levels of drugs metabolized by the CYP450 system may be observed when co-administered with telithromycin; therefore, increases or prolongation of the therapeutic and/or adverse effects of the concomitant drug may be observed).
No products indexed under this heading.

Bosentan (Concomitant administration of CYP 3A4 inducers is likely to result in subtherapeutic levels of telithromycin and loss of effect). Products include:
Tracleer ... **573**

Bretylium Tosylate (Telithromycin should be avoided in patients with congenital prolongation of the QT_c interval, and in patients with ongoing proarrhythmic conditions, such as uncorrected hypokalemia or hypomagnesemia, clinically significant bradycardia, and in patients receiving Class IA (eg, quinidine and procainamide) or Class III (eg, dofetilide) antiarrhythmic agents).
No products indexed under this heading.

Bromocriptine Mesylate (Elevated levels of drugs metabolized by the CYP450 system may be observed when co-administered with telithromycin; therefore, increases or prolongation of the therapeutic and/or adverse effects of the concomitant drug may be observed).
No products indexed under this heading.

Buspirone Hydrochloride (Co-administration of telithromycin with a drug primarily metabolized by the CYP 3A4 enzyme system may result in increased plasma concentrations of the drug co-administered with telithromycin that could increase or prolong both the therapeutic and adverse effects).
No products indexed under this heading.

Busulfan (Co-administration of telithromycin with a drug primarily metabolized by the CYP 3A4 enzyme system may result in increased plasma concentrations of the drug co-administered with telithromycin that could increase or prolong both the therapeutic and adverse effects). Products include:
Myleran ... **1581**

Caffeine (Elevated levels of drugs metabolized by the CYP450 system may be observed when co-administered with telithromycin; therefore, increases or prolongation of the therapeutic and/or adverse effects of the concomitant drug may be observed).
No products indexed under this heading.

Caffeine Anhydrous (Elevated levels of drugs metabolized by the CYP450 system may be observed when co-administered with telithromycin; therefore, increases or prolongation of the therapeutic and/or adverse effects of the concomitant drug may be observed).
No products indexed under this heading.

Caffeine Citrate (Elevated levels of drugs metabolized by the CYP450 system may be observed when co-administered with telithromycin; therefore, increases or prolongation of the therapeutic and/or adverse effects of the concomitant drug may be observed).
No products indexed under this heading.

Caffeine-containing medications (Elevated levels of drugs metabolized by the CYP450 system may be observed when co-administered with telithromycin; therefore, increases or prolongation of the therapeutic and/or adverse effects of the concomitant drug may be observed).
No products indexed under this heading.

Caffeine Sodium Benzoate (Elevated levels of drugs metabolized by the CYP450 system may be observed when co-administered with telithromycin; therefore, increases or prolongation of the therapeutic and/or adverse effects of the concomitant drug may be observed).
No products indexed under this heading.

Candesartan Cilexetil (Elevated levels of drugs metabolized by the CYP450 system may be observed when co-administered with telithromycin; therefore, increases or prolongation of the therapeutic and/or adverse effects of the concomitant drug may be observed). Products include:
Atacand ... **697**
Atacand HCT ... **700**

Captopril (Elevated levels of drugs metabolized by the CYP450 system may be observed when co-administered with telithromycin; therefore, increases or prolongation of the therapeutic and/or adverse effects of the concomitant drug may be observed). Products include:
Captopril ... **2341**

Carbamazepine (Concomitant administration of other CYP 3A4 inducers, such as phenytoin, carbamazepine, or phenobarbital, is likely to result in subtherapeutic levels of telithromycin and loss of effect). Products include:
Carbatrol ... **3280**
Equetro ... **3477**

Carisoprodol (Elevated levels of drugs metabolized by the CYP450 system may be observed when co-administered with telithromycin; therefore, increases or prolongation of the therapeutic and/or adverse effects of the concomitant drug may be observed).
No products indexed under this heading.

Carvedilol (Elevated levels of drugs metabolized by the CYP450 system may be observed when co-administered with telithromycin; therefore, increases or prolongation of the therapeutic and/or adverse effects of the concomitant drug may be observed). Products include:
Coreg ... **1409**

Celecoxib (Elevated levels of drugs metabolized by the CYP450 system may be observed when co-administered with telithromycin; therefore, increases or prolongation of the therapeutic and/or adverse effects of the concomitant drug may be observed). Products include:
Celebrex ... **3272**

Cerivastatin Sodium (High levels of HMG-CoA reductase inhibitors increase the risk of myopathy. Use of simvastatin, lovastatin, or atorvastatin concomitantly with telithromycin should be avoided. If telithromycin is prescribed, therapy with simvastatin, lovastatin, or atorvastatin should be suspended during the course of treatment. Patients concomitantly treated with statins should be carefully monitored for signs and symptoms of myopathy and rhabdomyolysis).
No products indexed under this heading.

Cevimeline Hydrochloride (Elevated levels of drugs metabolized by the CYP450 system may be observed when co-administered with telithromycin; therefore, increases or prolongation of the therapeutic and/or adverse effects of the concomitant drug may be observed). Products include:
Evoxac ... **1027**

(⊙ Described in PDR® for Ophthalmic Medicines)

Chlordiazepoxide (Elevated levels of drugs metabolized by the CYP450 system may be observed when co-administered with telithromycin; therefore, increases or prolongation of the therapeutic and/or adverse effects of the concomitant drug may be observed).
No products indexed under this heading.

Chlordiazepoxide Hydrochloride (Elevated levels of drugs metabolized by the CYP450 system may be observed when co-administered with telithromycin; therefore, increases or prolongation of the therapeutic and/or adverse effects of the concomitant drug may be observed).
No products indexed under this heading.

Chlorpheniramine (Co-administration of telithromycin with a drug primarily metabolized by the CYP 3A4 enzyme system may result in increased plasma concentrations of the drug co-administered with telithromycin that could increase or prolong both the therapeutic and adverse effects).
No products indexed under this heading.

Chlorpheniramine Maleate (Co-administration of telithromycin with a drug primarily metabolized by the CYP 3A4 enzyme system may result in increased plasma concentrations of the drug co-administered with telithromycin that could increase or prolong both the therapeutic and adverse effects).
No products indexed under this heading.

Chlorpheniramine Polistirex (Co-administration of telithromycin with a drug primarily metabolized by the CYP 3A4 enzyme system may result in increased plasma concentrations of the drug co-administered with telithromycin that could increase or prolong both the therapeutic and adverse effects). Products include:
Tussionex 3443

Chlorpheniramine Tannate (Co-administration of telithromycin with a drug primarily metabolized by the CYP 3A4 enzyme system may result in increased plasma concentrations of the drug co-administered with telithromycin that could increase or prolong both the therapeutic and adverse effects).
No products indexed under this heading.

Chlorpromazine (Elevated levels of drugs metabolized by the CYP450 system may be observed when co-administered with telithromycin; therefore, increases or prolongation of the therapeutic and/or adverse effects of the concomitant drug may be observed).
No products indexed under this heading.

Chlorpromazine Hydrochloride (Elevated levels of drugs metabolized by the CYP450 system may be observed when co-administered with telithromycin; therefore, increases or prolongation of the therapeutic and/or adverse effects of the concomitant drug may be observed).
No products indexed under this heading.

Chlorpropamide (Elevated levels of drugs metabolized by the CYP450 system may be observed when co-administered with telithromycin; therefore, increases or prolongation of the therapeutic and/or adverse effects of the concomitant drug may be observed).
No products indexed under this heading.

Cilostazol (Elevated levels of drugs metabolized by the CYP450 system may be observed when co-administered with telithromycin; therefore, increases or prolongation of the therapeutic and/or adverse effects of the concomitant drug may be observed).
No products indexed under this heading.

Cimetidine Hydrochloride (Elevated levels of drugs metabolized by the CYP450 system may be observed when co-administered with telithromycin; therefore, increases or prolongation of the therapeutic and/or adverse effects of the concomitant drug may be observed).
No products indexed under this heading.

Ciprofloxacin (Concomitant administration of CYP 3A4 inducers is likely to result in subtherapeutic levels of telithromycin and loss of effect). Products include:
Cipro I.V. 3082
Cipro 3073
Cipro XR 3091
Ciprodex 583

Ciprofloxacin Hydrochloride (Concomitant administration of CYP 3A4 inducers is likely to result in subtherapeutic levels of telithromycin and loss of effect). Products include:
Cipro 3073

Cisapride (Co-administration of telithromycin with cisapride is contraindicated. Steady-state peak plasma concentrations of cisapride (an agent with the potential to increase QT interval) were increased by 95% when co-administered with repeated doses of telithromycin, resulting in significant increases in QT_c).
No products indexed under this heading.

Cisplatin (Concomitant administration of CYP 3A4 inducers is likely to result in subtherapeutic levels of telithromycin and loss of effect).
No products indexed under this heading.

Citalopram Hydrobromide (Elevated levels of drugs metabolized by the CYP450 system may be observed when co-administered with telithromycin; therefore, increases or prolongation of the therapeutic and/or adverse effects of the concomitant drug may be observed). Products include:
Celexa 1153

Clarithromycin (Co-administration of telithromycin with a drug primarily metabolized by the CYP 3A4 enzyme system may result in increased plasma concentrations of the drug co-administered with telithromycin that could increase or prolong both the therapeutic and adverse effects). Products include:
Biaxin/Biaxin XL 412

Clomipramine Hydrochloride (Elevated levels of drugs metabolized by the CYP450 system may be observed when co-administered with telithromycin; therefore, increases or prolongation of the therapeutic and/or adverse effects of the concomitant drug may be observed).
No products indexed under this heading.

Clopidogrel Bisulfate (Elevated levels of drugs metabolized by the CYP450 system may be observed when co-administered with telithromycin; therefore, increases or prolongation of the therapeutic and/or adverse effects of the concomitant drug may be observed). Products include:
Plavix 3027

Clopidogrel Hydrogen Sulfate (Elevated levels of drugs metabolized by the CYP450 system may be observed when co-administered with telithromycin; therefore, increases or prolongation of the therapeutic and/or adverse effects of the concomitant drug may be observed).
No products indexed under this heading.

Clozapine (Elevated levels of drugs metabolized by the CYP450 system may be observed when co-administered with telithromycin; therefore, increases or prolongation of the therapeutic and/or adverse effects of the concomitant drug may be observed).
No products indexed under this heading.

Codeine Phosphate (Elevated levels of drugs metabolized by the CYP450 system may be observed when co-administered with telithromycin; therefore, increases or prolongation of the therapeutic and/or adverse effects of the concomitant drug may be observed). Products include:
Tylenol with Codeine 2691

Codeine Sulfate (Elevated levels of drugs metabolized by the CYP450 system may be observed when co-administered with telithromycin; therefore, increases or prolongation of the therapeutic and/or adverse effects of the concomitant drug may be observed).
No products indexed under this heading.

Cortisone Acetate (Concomitant administration of CYP 3A4 inducers is likely to result in subtherapeutic levels of telithromycin and loss of effect).
No products indexed under this heading.

Cyclobenzaprine (Elevated levels of drugs metabolized by the CYP450 system may be observed when co-administered with telithromycin; therefore, increases or prolongation of the therapeutic and/or adverse effects of the concomitant drug may be observed).
No products indexed under this heading.

Cyclobenzaprine Hydrochloride (Elevated levels of drugs metabolized by the CYP450 system may be observed when co-administered with telithromycin; therefore, increases or prolongation of the therapeutic and/or adverse effects of the concomitant drug may be observed). Products include:
Amrix 964

Cyclophosphamide (Elevated levels of drugs metabolized by the CYP450 system may be observed when co-administered with telithromycin; therefore, increases or prolongation of the therapeutic and/or adverse effects of the concomitant drug may be observed).
No products indexed under this heading.

Cyclosporine (Drugs metabolized by the cytochrome P450 system, such as carbamazepine, cyclosporine, tacrolimus, sirolimus, hexobarbital, and phenytoin; elevation of serum levels of these drugs may be observed when co-administered with telithromycin. As a result, increases or prolongation of the therapeutic and/or adverse effects of the concomitant drug may be observed). Products include:
Gengraf 440
Neoral Oral Solution 2496
Neoral Capsules 2496
Restasis 605

Desipramine Hydrochloride (Elevated levels of drugs metabolized by the CYP450 system may be observed when co-administered with telithromycin; therefore, increases or prolongation of the therapeutic and/or adverse effects of the concomitant drug may be observed).
No products indexed under this heading.

Desogestrel (Co-administration of telithromycin with a drug primarily metabolized by the CYP 3A4 enzyme system may result in increased plasma concentrations of the drug co-administered with telithromycin that could increase or prolong both the therapeutic and adverse effects).
No products indexed under this heading.

Dexamethasone (Concomitant administration of CYP 3A4 inducers is likely to result in subtherapeutic levels of telithromycin and loss of effect). Products include:
Ciprodex 583
Ozurdex .... ⊙223
Tobramycin and Dexamethasone
Ophthalmic Suspension .... ⊙251

Dexamethasone Acetate (Concomitant administration of CYP 3A4 inducers is likely to result in subtherapeutic levels of telithromycin and loss of effect).
No products indexed under this heading.

Dexamethasone Phosphate (Concomitant administration of CYP 3A4 inducers is likely to result in subtherapeutic levels of telithromycin and loss of effect).
No products indexed under this heading.

Dexamethasone Sodium (Concomitant administration of CYP 3A4 inducers is likely to result in subtherapeutic levels of telithromycin and loss of effect).
No products indexed under this heading.

Dexamethasone Sodium Phosphate (Concomitant administration of CYP 3A4 inducers is likely to result in subtherapeutic levels of telithromycin and loss of effect).
No products indexed under this heading.

Dexamethasone Sodium Phosphate Injection (Concomitant administration of CYP 3A4 inducers is likely to result in subtherapeutic levels of telithromycin and loss of effect).
No products indexed under this heading.

Dexfenfluramine Hydrochloride (Elevated levels of drugs metabolized by the CYP450 system may be observed when co-administered with telithromycin; therefore, increases or prolongation of the therapeutic and/or adverse effects of the concomitant drug may be observed).
No products indexed under this heading.

Dextromethorphan (Elevated levels of drugs metabolized by the CYP450 system may be observed when co-administered with telithromycin; therefore, increases or prolongation of the therapeutic and/or adverse effects of the concomitant drug may be observed).
No products indexed under this heading.

Dextromethorphan Hydrobromide (Elevated levels of drugs metabolized by the CYP450 system may be observed when co-administered with telithromycin; therefore, increases or prolongation of the therapeutic and/or adverse effects of the concomitant drug may be observed).
No products indexed under this heading.

Dextromethorphan Polistirex (Elevated levels of drugs metabolized by the CYP450 system may be observed when co-administered with telithromycin; therefore, increases or prolongation of the therapeutic and/or adverse effects of the concomitant drug may be observed).
No products indexed under this heading.

Diazepam (Concomitant administration of telithromycin with midazolam increased the AUC of midazolam; therefore, precaution should be used with other benzodiazepines metabolized by CYP 3A4 and that undergo a high first-pass effect (eg, triazolam)). Products include:
Valium Tablets 2880

Diclofenac Potassium (Elevated levels of drugs metabolized by the CYP450 system may be observed when co-administered with telithromycin; therefore, increases or prolongation of the therapeutic and/or adverse effects of the concomitant drug may be observed).
No products indexed under this heading.

Diclofenac Sodium (Elevated levels of drugs metabolized by the CYP450 system may be observed when co-administered with telithromycin; therefore, increases or prolongation of the therapeutic and/or adverse effects of the concomitant drug may be observed).
No products indexed under this heading.

Dicumarol (Spontaneous post-marketing reports suggest that administration of telithromycin and oral anticoagulants concomitantly may potentiate the effects of the oral anticoagulants. Consideration should be given to monitoring prothrombin times/INR while patients are receiving telithromycin and oral anticoagulants simultaneously).
No products indexed under this heading.

Digoxin (The plasma peak and trough levels of digoxin were increased by 73% and 21%, respectively, in healthy volunteers when co-administered with telithromycin. However, trough plasma concentrations of digoxin (when equilibrium between plasma and tissue concentrations has been achieved) ranged from 0.74 to 2.17 ng/mL. There were no significant changes in ECG parameters and no signs of digoxin toxicity. Monitoring of digoxin side effects or serum levels should be considered during concomitant administration of digoxin and telithromycin). Products include:
Lanoxin Injection 1546
Lanoxin Injection Pediatric 1549
Lanoxin Tablets 1553

Dihydroergotamine Mesylate (Co-administration is not recommended because acute ergot toxicity characterized by severe peripheral vasospasm and dyesthesia have been reported with macrolide antibiotics).
No products indexed under this heading.

Diltiazem Hydrochloride (Co-administration of telithromycin with a drug primarily metabolized by the CYP 3A4 enzyme system may result in increased plasma concentrations of the drug co-administered with telithromycin that could increase or prolong both the therapeutic and adverse effects). Products include:
Cardizem LA 423

Diltiazem Maleate (Co-administration of telithromycin with a drug primarily metabolized by the CYP 3A4 enzyme system may result in increased plasma concentrations of the drug co-administered with telithromycin that could increase or prolong both the therapeutic and adverse effects).
No products indexed under this heading.

Disopyramide (Telithromycin should be avoided in patients with congenital prolongation of the QT_c interval, and in patients with ongoing proarrhythmic conditions, such as uncorrected hypokalemia or hypomagnesemia, clinically significant bradycardia, and in patients receiving Class IA (eg, quinidine and procainamide) or Class III (eg, dofetilide) antiarrhythmic agents).
No products indexed under this heading.

Disopyramide Phosphate (Telithromycin should be avoided in patients with congenital prolongation of the QT_c interval, and in patients with ongoing proarrhythmic conditions, such as uncorrected hypokalemia or hypomagnesemia, clinically significant bradycardia, and in patients receiving Class IA (eg, quinidine and procainamide) or Class III (eg, dofetilide) antiarrhythmic agents).
No products indexed under this heading.

Disulfiram (Co-administration of telithromycin with a drug primarily metabolized by the CYP 3A4 enzyme system may result in increased plasma concentrations of the drug co-administered with telithromycin that could increase or prolong both the therapeutic and adverse effects).
No products indexed under this heading.

Divalproex Sodium (Elevated levels of drugs metabolized by the CYP450 system may be observed when co-administered with telithromycin; therefore, increases or prolongation of the therapeutic and/or adverse effects of the concomitant drug may be observed). Products include:
Depakote ER 426

Docetaxel (Elevated levels of drugs metabolized by the CYP450 system may be observed when co-administered with telithromycin; therefore, increases or prolongation of the therapeutic and/or adverse effects of the concomitant drug may be observed). Products include:
Taxotere 3035

Dolasetron Mesylate (Elevated levels of drugs metabolized by the CYP450 system may be observed when co-administered with telithromycin; therefore, increases or prolongation of the therapeutic and/or adverse effects of the concomitant drug may be observed). Products include:
Anzemet Injection 2931
Anzemet Tablets 2934

Donepezil Hydrochloride (Elevated levels of drugs metabolized by the CYP450 system may be observed when co-administered with telithromycin; therefore, increases or prolongation of the therapeutic and/or adverse effects of the concomitant drug may be observed). Products include:
Aricept 1045
Aricept ODT 1045

Doxepin Hydrochloride (Elevated levels of drugs metabolized by the CYP450 system may be observed when co-administered with telithromycin; therefore, increases or prolongation of the therapeutic and/or adverse effects of the concomitant drug may be observed).
No products indexed under this heading.

Doxorubicin Hydrochloride (Co-administration of telithromycin with a drug primarily metabolized by the CYP 3A4 enzyme system may result in increased plasma concentrations of the drug co-administered with telithromycin that could increase or prolong both the therapeutic and adverse effects).
No products indexed under this heading.

Dronabinol (Co-administration of telithromycin with a drug primarily metabolized by the CYP 3A4 enzyme system may result in increased plasma concentrations of the drug co-administered with telithromycin that could increase or prolong both the therapeutic and adverse effects).
No products indexed under this heading.

Drugs that Undergo Biotransformation by Cytochrome P-450 Mixed Function Oxidase (Elevated levels of drugs metabolized by the CYP450 system may be observed when co-administered with telithromycin; therefore, increases or prolongation of the therapeutic and/or adverse effects of the concomitant drug may be observed).
No products indexed under this heading.

Dyphylline (Elevated levels of drugs metabolized by the CYP450 system may be observed when co-administered with telithromycin; therefore, increases or prolongation of the therapeutic and/or adverse effects of the concomitant drug may be observed).
No products indexed under this heading.

Efavirenz (Concomitant administration of CYP 3A4 inducers is likely to result in subtherapeutic levels of telithromycin and loss of effect). Products include:
Atripla 906

Encainide Hydrochloride (Elevated levels of drugs metabolized by the CYP450 system may be observed when co-administered with telithromycin; therefore, increases or prolongation of the therapeutic and/or adverse effects of the concomitant drug may be observed).
No products indexed under this heading.

Enoxacin (Elevated levels of drugs metabolized by the CYP450 system may be observed when co-administered with telithromycin; therefore, increases or prolongation of the therapeutic and/or adverse effects of the concomitant drug may be observed).
No products indexed under this heading.

Eprosartan Mesylate (Elevated levels of drugs metabolized by the CYP450 system may be observed when co-administered with telithromycin; therefore, increases or prolongation of the therapeutic and/or adverse effects of the concomitant drug may be observed). Products include:
Teveten 538
Teveten HCT 541

Ergonovine Maleate (Co-administration is not recommended because acute ergot toxicity characterized by severe peripheral vasospasm and dyesthesia have been reported with macrolide antibiotics).
No products indexed under this heading.

Ergotamine Tartrate (Co-administration is not recommended because acute ergot toxicity characterized by severe peripheral vasospasm and dyesthesia have been reported with macrolide antibiotics).
No products indexed under this heading.

Erythromycin (Co-administration of telithromycin with a drug primarily metabolized by the CYP 3A4 enzyme system may result in increased plasma concentrations of the drug co-administered with telithromycin that could increase or prolong both the therapeutic and adverse effects).
No products indexed under this heading.

Erythromycin Estolate (Co-administration of telithromycin with a drug primarily metabolized by the CYP 3A4 enzyme system may result in increased plasma concentrations of the drug co-administered with telithromycin that could increase or prolong both the therapeutic and adverse effects).
No products indexed under this heading.

Erythromycin Ethylsuccinate (Co-administration of telithromycin with a drug primarily metabolized by the CYP 3A4 enzyme system may result in increased plasma concentrations of the drug co-administered with telithromycin that could increase or prolong both the therapeutic and adverse effects). Products include:
E.E.S. 437
EryPed 435

Erythromycin Gluceptate (Co-administration of telithromycin with a drug primarily metabolized by the CYP 3A4 enzyme system may result in increased plasma concentrations of the drug co-administered with telithromycin that could increase or prolong both the therapeutic and adverse effects).
No products indexed under this heading.

Erythromycin Lactobionate (Co-administration of telithromycin with a drug primarily metabolized by the CYP 3A4 enzyme system may result in increased plasma concentrations of the drug co-administered with telithromycin that could increase or prolong both the therapeutic and adverse effects).
No products indexed under this heading.

Erythromycin Stearate (Co-administration of telithromycin with a drug primarily metabolized by the CYP 3A4 enzyme system may result in increased plasma concentrations of the drug co-administered with telithromycin that could increase or prolong both the therapeutic and adverse effects).
No products indexed under this heading.

Esomeprazole Magnesium (Elevated levels of drugs metabolized by the CYP450 system may be observed when co-administered with telithromycin; therefore, increases or prolongation of the therapeutic and/or adverse effects of the concomitant drug may be observed). Products include:
Nexium Capsules 704
Nexium Oral Suspension 704

Esomeprazole Sodium (Elevated levels of drugs metabolized by the CYP450 system may be observed when co-administered with telithromycin; therefore, increases or prolongation of the therapeutic and/or adverse effects of the concomitant drug may be observed). Products include:
Nexium I.V. 712

Estradiol (Co-administration of telithromycin with a drug primarily metabolized by the CYP 3A4 enzyme system may result in increased plasma concentrations of the drug co-administered with telithromycin that could increase or prolong both the therapeutic and adverse effects). Products include:
Activella 2561
Angeliq 831
Climara 841
Climara Pro 847
Divigel 3467
Estrasorb 1777
Vagifem 2589

Estradiol Benzoate (Co-administration of telithromycin with a drug primarily metabolized by the CYP 3A4 enzyme system may result in increased plasma concentrations of the drug co-administered with telithromycin that could increase or prolong both the therapeutic and adverse effects).
No products indexed under this heading.

Estradiol Cypionate (Co-administration of telithromycin with a drug primarily metabolized by the CYP 3A4 enzyme system may result in increased plasma concentrations of the drug co-administered with telithromycin that could increase or prolong both the therapeutic and adverse effects).
No products indexed under this heading.

Estradiol Valerate (Co-administration of telithromycin with a drug primarily metabolized by the CYP 3A4 enzyme system may result in increased plasma concentrations of the drug co-administered with telithromycin that could increase or prolong both the therapeutic and adverse effects).
No products indexed under this heading.

Estrogen (Elevated levels of drugs metabolized by the CYP450 system may be observed when co-administered with telithromycin; therefore, increases or prolongation of the therapeutic and/or adverse effects of the concomitant drug may be observed).
No products indexed under this heading.

Estrogens, Conjugated (Elevated levels of drugs metabolized by the CYP450 system may be observed when co-administered with telithromycin; therefore, increases or prolongation of

the therapeutic and/or adverse effects of the concomitant drug may be observed). Products include:

Estrogens, Conjugated, Synthetic A (Elevated levels of drugs metabolized by the CYP450 system may be observed when co-administered with telithromycin; therefore, increases or prolongation of the therapeutic and/or adverse effects of the concomitant drug may be observed).
No products indexed under this heading.

Estrogens, Esterified (Elevated levels of drugs metabolized by the CYP450 system may be observed when co-administered with telithromycin; therefore, increases or prolongation of the therapeutic and/or adverse effects of the concomitant drug may be observed).
No products indexed under this heading.

Ethinyl Estradiol (Co-administration of telithromycin with a drug primarily metabolized by the CYP 3A4 enzyme system may result in increased plasma concentrations of the drug co-administered with telithromycin that could increase or prolong both the therapeutic and adverse effects). Products include:

Ethosuximide (Co-administration of telithromycin with a drug primarily metabolized by the CYP 3A4 enzyme system may result in increased plasma concentrations of the drug co-administered with telithromycin that could increase or prolong both the therapeutic and adverse effects).
No products indexed under this heading.

Ethotoin (Elevated levels of drugs metabolized by the CYP450 system may be observed when co-administered with telithromycin; therefore, increases or prolongation of the therapeutic and/or adverse effects of the concomitant drug may be observed).
No products indexed under this heading.

Ethynodiol Diacetate (Co-administration of telithromycin with a drug primarily metabolized by the CYP 3A4 enzyme system may result in increased plasma concentrations of the drug co-administered with telithromycin that could increase or prolong both the therapeutic and adverse effects).
No products indexed under this heading.

Etodolac (Elevated levels of drugs metabolized by the CYP450 system may be observed when co-administered with telithromycin; therefore, increases or prolongation of the therapeutic and/or adverse effects of the concomitant drug may be observed).
No products indexed under this heading.

Etoposide (Co-administration of telithromycin with a drug primarily metabolized by the CYP 3A4 enzyme system may result in increased plasma concentrations of the drug co-administered with telithromycin that could increase or prolong both the therapeutic and adverse effects).
No products indexed under this heading.

Etoposide Phosphate (Co-administration of telithromycin with a drug primarily metabolized by the CYP 3A4 enzyme system may result in increased plasma concentrations of the drug co-administered with telithromycin that could increase or prolong both the therapeutic and adverse effects).
No products indexed under this heading.

Felbamate (Concomitant administration of CYP 3A4 inducers is likely to result in subtherapeutic levels of telithromycin and loss of effect).
No products indexed under this heading.

Felodipine (Co-administration of telithromycin with a drug primarily metabolized by the CYP 3A4 enzyme system may result in increased plasma concentrations of the drug co-administered with telithromycin that could increase or prolong both the therapeutic and adverse effects).
No products indexed under this heading.

Fenoprofen Calcium (Elevated levels of drugs metabolized by the CYP450 system may be observed when co-administered with telithromycin; therefore, increases or prolongation of the therapeutic and/or adverse effects of the concomitant drug may be observed).
No products indexed under this heading.

Fentanyl (Co-administration of telithromycin with a drug primarily metabolized by the CYP 3A4 enzyme system may result in increased plasma concentrations of the drug co-administered with telithromycin that could increase or prolong both the therapeutic and adverse effects). Products include:

Fentanyl Citrate (Co-administration of telithromycin with a drug primarily metabolized by the CYP 3A4 enzyme system may result in increased plasma concentrations of the drug co-administered with telithromycin that could increase or prolong both the therapeutic and adverse effects). Products include:

Flecainide Acetate (Elevated levels of drugs metabolized by the CYP450 system may be observed when co-administered with telithromycin; therefore, increases or prolongation of the therapeutic and/or adverse effects of the concomitant drug may be observed).
No products indexed under this heading.

Fludrocortisone Acetate (Concomitant administration of CYP 3A4 inducers is likely to result in subtherapeutic levels of telithromycin and loss of effect).
No products indexed under this heading.

Fluoxetine (Elevated levels of drugs metabolized by the CYP450 system may be observed when co-administered with telithromycin; therefore, increases or prolongation of the therapeutic and/or adverse effects of the concomitant drug may be observed).
No products indexed under this heading.

Fluoxetine Hydrochloride (Elevated levels of drugs metabolized by the CYP450 system may be observed when co-administered with telithromycin; therefore, increases or prolongation of the therapeutic and/or adverse effects of the concomitant drug may be observed). Products include:

Fluphenazine Decanoate (Elevated levels of drugs metabolized by the CYP450 system may be observed when co-administered with telithromycin; therefore, increases or prolongation of the therapeutic and/or adverse effects of the concomitant drug may be observed).
No products indexed under this heading.

Fluphenazine Enanthate (Elevated levels of drugs metabolized by the CYP450 system may be observed when co-administered with telithromycin; therefore, increases or prolongation of the therapeutic and/or adverse effects of the concomitant drug may be observed).
No products indexed under this heading.

Fluphenazine Hydrochloride (Elevated levels of drugs metabolized by the CYP450 system may be observed when co-administered with telithromycin; therefore, increases or prolongation of the therapeutic and/or adverse effects of the concomitant drug may be observed).
No products indexed under this heading.

Flurbiprofen (Elevated levels of drugs metabolized by the CYP450 system may be observed when co-administered with telithromycin; therefore, increases or prolongation of the therapeutic and/or adverse effects of the concomitant drug may be observed).
No products indexed under this heading.

Flurbiprofen Sodium (Elevated levels of drugs metabolized by the CYP450 system may be observed when co-administered with telithromycin; therefore, increases or prolongation of the therapeutic and/or adverse effects of the concomitant drug may be observed).
No products indexed under this heading.

Flutamide (Elevated levels of drugs metabolized by the CYP450 system may be observed when co-administered with telithromycin; therefore, increases or prolongation of the therapeutic and/or adverse effects of the concomitant drug may be observed).
No products indexed under this heading.

Fluticasone Propionate (Elevated levels of drugs metabolized by the CYP450 system may be observed when co-administered with telithromycin; therefore, increases or prolongation of the therapeutic and/or adverse effects of the concomitant drug may be observed). Products include:

Fluvastatin Sodium (High levels of HMG-CoA reductase inhibitors increase the risk of myopathy. Use of simvastatin, lovastatin, or atorvastatin concomitantly with telithromycin should be avoided. If telithromycin is prescribed, therapy with simvastatin, lovastatin, or atorvastatin should be suspended during the course of treatment. Patients concomitantly treated with statins should be carefully monitored for signs and symptoms of myopathy and rhabdomyolysis).
No products indexed under this heading.

Fluvoxamine Maleate (Elevated levels of drugs metabolized by the CYP450 system may be observed when co-administered with telithromycin; therefore, increases or prolongation of the therapeutic and/or adverse effects of the concomitant drug may be observed).
No products indexed under this heading.

Formoterol Fumarate (Elevated levels of drugs metabolized by the CYP450 system may be observed when co-administered with telithromycin; therefore, increases or prolongation of the therapeutic and/or adverse effects of the concomitant drug may be observed). Products include:

Fosphenytoin (Concomitant administration of other CYP 3A4 inducers, such as phenytoin, carbamazepine, or phenobarbital, is likely to result in subtherapeutic levels of telithromycin and loss of effect).
No products indexed under this heading.

Fosphenytoin Sodium (Concomitant administration of other CYP 3A4 inducers, such as phenytoin, carbamazepine, or phenobarbital, is likely to result in subtherapeutic levels of telithromycin and loss of effect).
No products indexed under this heading.

Gabapentin (Elevated levels of drugs metabolized by the CYP450 system may be observed when co-administered with telithromycin; therefore, increases or prolongation of the therapeutic and/or adverse effects of the concomitant drug may be observed).
No products indexed under this heading.

Galantamine Hydrobromide (Elevated levels of drugs metabolized by the CYP450 system may be observed when co-administered with telithromycin; therefore, increases or prolongation of the therapeutic and/or adverse effects of the concomitant drug may be observed).
No products indexed under this heading.

Garlic Extract (Concomitant administration of CYP 3A4 inducers is likely to result in subtherapeutic levels of telithromycin and loss of effect).
No products indexed under this heading.

Garlic Oil (Concomitant administration of CYP 3A4 inducers is likely to result in subtherapeutic levels of telithromycin and loss of effect).
No products indexed under this heading.

Glimepiride (Elevated levels of drugs metabolized by the CYP450 system may be observed when co-administered with telithromycin; therefore, increases or prolongation of the therapeutic and/or adverse effects of the concomitant drug may be observed). Products include:

Glipizide (Elevated levels of drugs metabolized by the CYP450 system may be observed when co-administered with telithromycin; therefore, increases or prolongation of the therapeutic and/or adverse effects of the concomitant drug may be observed).
No products indexed under this heading.

Glyburide (Elevated levels of drugs metabolized by the CYP450 system may be observed when co-administered with telithromycin; therefore, increases or prolongation of the therapeutic and/or adverse effects of the concomitant drug may be observed).
No products indexed under this heading.

Grepafloxacin Hydrochloride (Elevated levels of drugs metabolized by the CYP450 system may be observed when co-administered with telithromycin; therefore, increases or prolongation of the therapeutic and/or adverse effects of the concomitant drug may be observed).
No products indexed under this heading.

IMPORTANT NOTE: Always consult each drug listing in the patient's regimen for possible interactions.

Haloperidol (Co-administration of telithromycin with a drug primarily metabolized by the CYP 3A4 enzyme system may result in increased plasma concentrations of the drug co-administered with telithromycin that could increase or prolong both the therapeutic and adverse effects).
    No products indexed under this heading.

Haloperidol Decanoate (Co-administration of telithromycin with a drug primarily metabolized by the CYP 3A4 enzyme system may result in increased plasma concentrations of the drug co-administered with telithromycin that could increase or prolong both the therapeutic and adverse effects).
    No products indexed under this heading.

Haloperidol Lactate (Co-administration of telithromycin with a drug primarily metabolized by the CYP 3A4 enzyme system may result in increased plasma concentrations of the drug co-administered with telithromycin that could increase or prolong both the therapeutic and adverse effects).
    No products indexed under this heading.

Hexobarbital (Drugs metabolized by the cytochrome P450 system, such as carbamazepine, cyclosporine, tacrolimus, sirolimus, hexobarbital, and phenytoin; elevation of serum levels of these drugs may be observed when co-administered with telithromycin. As a result, increases or prolongation of the therapeutic and/or adverse effects of the concomitant drug may be observed).
    No products indexed under this heading.

Hydrocodone Bitartrate (Elevated levels of drugs metabolized by the CYP450 system may be observed when co-administered with telithromycin; therefore, increases or prolongation of the therapeutic and/or adverse effects of the concomitant drug may be observed). Products include:

Hydrocortisone (Concomitant administration of CYP 3A4 inducers is likely to result in subtherapeutic levels of telithromycin and loss of effect).
    No products indexed under this heading.

Hydrocortisone (Alcohol) (Concomitant administration of CYP 3A4 inducers is likely to result in subtherapeutic levels of telithromycin and loss of effect).
    No products indexed under this heading.

Hydrocortisone Acetate (Concomitant administration of CYP 3A4 inducers is likely to result in subtherapeutic levels of telithromycin and loss of effect).
    No products indexed under this heading.

Hydrocortisone Butyrate (Concomitant administration of CYP 3A4 inducers is likely to result in subtherapeutic levels of telithromycin and loss of effect).
    No products indexed under this heading.

Hydrocortisone Cypionate (Concomitant administration of CYP 3A4 inducers is likely to result in subtherapeutic levels of telithromycin and loss of effect).
    No products indexed under this heading.

Hydrocortisone Hemisuccinate (Concomitant administration of CYP 3A4 inducers is likely to result in subtherapeutic levels of telithromycin and loss of effect).
    No products indexed under this heading.

Hydrocortisone Probutate (Concomitant administration of CYP 3A4 inducers is likely to result in subtherapeutic levels of telithromycin and loss of effect).
    No products indexed under this heading.

Hydrocortisone Sodium Phosphate (Concomitant administration of CYP 3A4 inducers is likely to result in subtherapeutic levels of telithromycin and loss of effect).
    No products indexed under this heading.

Hydrocortisone Sodium Succinate (Concomitant administration of CYP 3A4 inducers is likely to result in subtherapeutic levels of telithromycin and loss of effect).
    No products indexed under this heading.

Hydrocortisone Valerate (Concomitant administration of CYP 3A4 inducers is likely to result in subtherapeutic levels of telithromycin and loss of effect).
    No products indexed under this heading.

Hypericum (Concomitant administration of CYP 3A4 inducers is likely to result in subtherapeutic levels of telithromycin and loss of effect).
    No products indexed under this heading.

Hypericum Perforatum (Concomitant administration of CYP 3A4 inducers is likely to result in subtherapeutic levels of telithromycin and loss of effect). Products include:

Ibuprofen (Elevated levels of drugs metabolized by the CYP450 system may be observed when co-administered with telithromycin; therefore, increases or prolongation of the therapeutic and/or adverse effects of the concomitant drug may be observed). Products include:

Imipramine Hydrochloride (Elevated levels of drugs metabolized by the CYP450 system may be observed when co-administered with telithromycin; therefore, increases or prolongation of the therapeutic and/or adverse effects of the concomitant drug may be observed).
    No products indexed under this heading.

Imipramine Pamoate (Elevated levels of drugs metabolized by the CYP450 system may be observed when co-administered with telithromycin; therefore, increases or prolongation of the therapeutic and/or adverse effects of the concomitant drug may be observed).
    No products indexed under this heading.

Indinavir Sulfate (Co-administration of telithromycin with a drug primarily metabolized by the CYP 3A4 enzyme system may result in increased plasma concentrations of the drug co-administered with telithromycin that could increase or prolong both the therapeutic and adverse effects). Products include:

Indomethacin (Elevated levels of drugs metabolized by the CYP450 system may be observed when co-administered with telithromycin; therefore, increases or prolongation of the therapeutic and/or adverse effects of the concomitant drug may be observed). Products include:

Indomethacin Sodium Trihydrate (Elevated levels of drugs metabolized by the CYP450 system may be observed when co-administered with telithromycin; therefore, increases or prolongation of the therapeutic and/or adverse effects of the concomitant drug may be observed). Products include:

Indoramin Hydrochloride (Elevated levels of drugs metabolized by the CYP450 system may be observed when co-administered with telithromycin; therefore, increases or prolongation of the therapeutic and/or adverse effects of the concomitant drug may be observed).
    No products indexed under this heading.

Irbesartan (Elevated levels of drugs metabolized by the CYP450 system may be observed when co-administered with telithromycin; therefore, increases or prolongation of the therapeutic and/or adverse effects of the concomitant drug may be observed). Products include:

Isotretinoin (Elevated levels of drugs metabolized by the CYP450 system may be observed when co-administered with telithromycin; therefore, increases or prolongation of the therapeutic and/or adverse effects of the concomitant drug may be observed). Products include:

Isradipine (Co-administration of telithromycin with a drug primarily metabolized by the CYP 3A4 enzyme system may result in increased plasma concentrations of the drug co-administered with telithromycin that could increase or prolong both the therapeutic and adverse effects). Products include:

Itraconazole (A multiple-dose interaction study with itraconazole showed that C_{max} of telithromycin was increased by 22% and AUC by 54%).
    No products indexed under this heading.

Ixabepilone (Co-administration of telithromycin with a drug primarily metabolized by the CYP 3A4 enzyme system may result in increased plasma concentrations of the drug co-administered with telithromycin that could increase or prolong both the therapeutic and adverse effects).
    No products indexed under this heading.

Ketoconazole (A multiple-dose interaction study with ketoconazole showed that C_{max} of telithromycin was increased by 51% and AUC by 95%). Products include:

Ketoprofen (Elevated levels of drugs metabolized by the CYP450 system may be observed when co-administered with telithromycin; therefore, increases or prolongation of the therapeutic and/or adverse effects of the concomitant drug may be observed).
    No products indexed under this heading.

Ketorolac Tromethamine (Elevated levels of drugs metabolized by the CYP450 system may be observed when co-administered with telithromycin; therefore, increases or prolongation of the therapeutic and/or adverse effects of the concomitant drug may be observed). Products include:

Labetalol Hydrochloride (Elevated levels of drugs metabolized by the CYP450 system may be observed when co-administered with telithromycin; therefore, increases or prolongation of the therapeutic and/or adverse effects of the concomitant drug may be observed).
    No products indexed under this heading.

Lamotrigine (Elevated levels of drugs metabolized by the CYP450 system may be observed when co-administered with telithromycin; therefore, increases or prolongation of the therapeutic and/

or adverse effects of the concomitant drug may be observed). Products include:

Lansoprazole (Elevated levels of drugs metabolized by the CYP450 system may be observed when co-administered with telithromycin; therefore, increases or prolongation of the therapeutic and/or adverse effects of the concomitant drug may be observed).
    No products indexed under this heading.

Levetiracetam (Elevated levels of drugs metabolized by the CYP450 system may be observed when co-administered with telithromycin; therefore, increases or prolongation of the therapeutic and/or adverse effects of the concomitant drug may be observed). Products include:

Levobupivacaine Hydrochloride (Elevated levels of drugs metabolized by the CYP450 system may be observed when co-administered with telithromycin; therefore, increases or prolongation of the therapeutic and/or adverse effects of the concomitant drug may be observed).
    No products indexed under this heading.

Levonorgestrel (When oral contraceptives containing ethinyl estradiol and levonorgestrel were co-administered with telithromycin, the steady-state AUC of ethinyl estradiol did not change and the steady-state AUC of levonorgestrel was increased by 50%. The pharmacokinetic/pharmacodynamic study showed that telithromycin did not interfere with the antiovulatory effect of oral contraceptives containing ethinyl estradiol and levonorgestrel). Products include:

Lidocaine (Co-administration of telithromycin with a drug primarily metabolized by the CYP 3A4 enzyme system may result in increased plasma concentrations of the drug co-administered with telithromycin that could increase or prolong both the therapeutic and adverse effects). Products include:

Lidocaine Base (Elevated levels of drugs metabolized by the CYP450 system may be observed when co-administered with telithromycin; therefore, increases or prolongation of the therapeutic and/or adverse effects of the concomitant drug may be observed).
    No products indexed under this heading.

Lidocaine Hydrochloride (Co-administration of telithromycin with a drug primarily metabolized by the CYP 3A4 enzyme system may result in increased plasma concentrations of the drug co-administered with telithromycin that could increase or prolong both the therapeutic and adverse effects).
    No products indexed under this heading.

Lomefloxacin Hydrochloride (Elevated levels of drugs metabolized by the CYP450 system may be observed when co-administered with telithromycin; therefore, increases or prolongation of the therapeutic and/or adverse effects of the concomitant drug may be observed).
    No products indexed under this heading.

Losartan Potassium (Elevated levels of drugs metabolized by the CYP450 system may be observed when co-

administered with telithromycin; therefore, increases or prolongation of the therapeutic and/or adverse effects of the concomitant drug may be observed). Products include:

Cozaar 2106
Hyzaar 2162
Hyzaar 100-12.5 2162

Lovastatin (High levels of HMG-CoA reductase inhibitors increase the risk of myopathy. Use of simvastatin, lovastatin, or atorvastatin concomitantly with telithromycin should be avoided. If telithromycin is prescribed, therapy with simvastatin, lovastatin, or atorvastatin should be suspended during the course of treatment. Patients concomitantly treated with statins should be carefully monitored for signs and symptoms of myopathy and rhabdomyolysis).
Products include:

Advicor 402
Mevacor 2212

Maprotiline Hydrochloride (Elevated levels of drugs metabolized by the CYP450 system may be observed when co-administered with telithromycin; therefore, increases or prolongation of the therapeutic and/or adverse effects of the concomitant drug may be observed).
No products indexed under this heading.

Meclofenamate Sodium (Elevated levels of drugs metabolized by the CYP450 system may be observed when co-administered with telithromycin; therefore, increases or prolongation of the therapeutic and/or adverse effects of the concomitant drug may be observed).
No products indexed under this heading.

Mefenamic Acid (Elevated levels of drugs metabolized by the CYP450 system may be observed when co-administered with telithromycin; therefore, increases or prolongation of the therapeutic and/or adverse effects of the concomitant drug may be observed).
No products indexed under this heading.

Meloxicam (Elevated levels of drugs metabolized by the CYP450 system may be observed when co-administered with telithromycin; therefore, increases or prolongation of the therapeutic and/or adverse effects of the concomitant drug may be observed).
No products indexed under this heading.

Meperidine Hydrochloride (Elevated levels of drugs metabolized by the CYP450 system may be observed when co-administered with telithromycin; therefore, increases or prolongation of the therapeutic and/or adverse effects of the concomitant drug may be observed).
No products indexed under this heading.

Mephenytoin (Concomitant administration of CYP 3A4 inducers is likely to result in subtherapeutic levels of telithromycin and loss of effect).
No products indexed under this heading.

Mephobarbital (Elevated levels of drugs metabolized by the CYP450 system may be observed when co-administered with telithromycin; therefore, increases or prolongation of the therapeutic and/or adverse effects of the concomitant drug may be observed).
No products indexed under this heading.

Meprobamate (Elevated levels of drugs metabolized by the CYP450 system may be observed when co-administered with telithromycin; therefore, increases or prolongation of the therapeutic and/or adverse effects of the concomitant drug may be observed).
No products indexed under this heading.

Mestranol (Co-administration of telithromycin with a drug primarily metabolized by the CYP 3A4 enzyme system may result in increased plasma concentrations of the drug co-administered with telithromycin that could increase or prolong both the therapeutic and adverse effects).
No products indexed under this heading.

Metformin Hydrochloride (Elevated levels of drugs metabolized by the CYP450 system may be observed when co-administered with telithromycin; therefore, increases or prolongation of the therapeutic and/or adverse effects of the concomitant drug may be observed). Products include:

ActoPlus 3338
Avandamet 1345
Janumet 2188

Methadone Hydrochloride (Co-administration of telithromycin with a drug primarily metabolized by the CYP 3A4 enzyme system may result in increased plasma concentrations of the drug co-administered with telithromycin that could increase or prolong both the therapeutic and adverse effects).
No products indexed under this heading.

Methamphetamine Hydrochloride (Elevated levels of drugs metabolized by the CYP450 system may be observed when co-administered with telithromycin; therefore, increases or prolongation of the therapeutic and/or adverse effects of the concomitant drug may be observed).
No products indexed under this heading.

Methsuximide (Concomitant administration of CYP 3A4 inducers is likely to result in subtherapeutic levels of telithromycin and loss of effect).
No products indexed under this heading.

Methylergonovine Maleate (Co-administration is not recommended because acute ergot toxicity characterized by severe peripheral vasospasm and dyesthesia have been reported with macrolide antibiotics).
No products indexed under this heading.

Methylprednisolone (Concomitant administration of CYP 3A4 inducers is likely to result in subtherapeutic levels of telithromycin and loss of effect).
No products indexed under this heading.

Methylprednisolone Acetate (Concomitant administration of CYP 3A4 inducers is likely to result in subtherapeutic levels of telithromycin and loss of effect).
No products indexed under this heading.

Methylprednisolone Sodium Succinate (Concomitant administration of CYP 3A4 inducers is likely to result in subtherapeutic levels of telithromycin and loss of effect).
No products indexed under this heading.

Methysergide Maleate (Co-administration is not recommended because acute ergot toxicity characterized by severe peripheral vasospasm and dyesthesia have been reported with macrolide antibiotics).
No products indexed under this heading.

Metoprolol Succinate (In patients treated with metoprolol for heart failure, the increased exposure to metoprolol, a CYP 2D6 substrate, may be of clinical importance. Therefore, co-administration of telithromycin and metoprolol in patients with heart failure should be considered with caution).
Products include:

Toprol XL 732

Metoprolol Tartrate (In patients treated with metoprolol for heart failure, the increased exposure to metoprolol, a CYP 2D6 substrate, may be of clinical importance. Therefore, co-administration of telithromycin and metoprolol in patients with heart failure should be considered with caution).
No products indexed under this heading.

Mexiletine Hydrochloride (Elevated levels of drugs metabolized by the CYP450 system may be observed when co-administered with telithromycin; therefore, increases or prolongation of the therapeutic and/or adverse effects of the concomitant drug may be observed).
No products indexed under this heading.

Midazolam Hydrochloride (Concomitant administration of telithromycin with intravenous or oral midazolam resulted in 2- and 6-fold increases, respectively, in the AUC of midazolam due to inhibition of CYP 3A4-dependent metabolism of midazolam. Patients should be monitored with concomitant administration of midazolam and dosage adjustment of midazolam should be considered if necessary).
No products indexed under this heading.

Miglitol (Elevated levels of drugs metabolized by the CYP450 system may be observed when co-administered with telithromycin; therefore, increases or prolongation of the therapeutic and/or adverse effects of the concomitant drug may be observed).
No products indexed under this heading.

Mirtazapine (Elevated levels of drugs metabolized by the CYP450 system may be observed when co-administered with telithromycin; therefore, increases or prolongation of the therapeutic and/or adverse effects of the concomitant drug may be observed). Products include:

Remeron Tablets 3214
RemeronSolTab Tablets 3219

Modafinil (Concomitant administration of CYP 3A4 inducers is likely to result in subtherapeutic levels of telithromycin and loss of effect). Products include:

Provigil 983

Montelukast Sodium (Elevated levels of drugs metabolized by the CYP450 system may be observed when co-administered with telithromycin; therefore, increases or prolongation of the therapeutic and/or adverse effects of the concomitant drug may be observed). Products include:

Singulair 2270

Moricizine Hydrochloride (Telithromycin should be avoided in patients with congenital prolongation of the QT_c interval, and in patients with ongoing proarrhythmic conditions, such as uncorrected hypokalemia or hypomagnesemia, clinically significant bradycardia, and in patients receiving Class IA (eg, quinidine and procainamide) or Class III (eg, dofetilide) antiarrhythmic agents).
No products indexed under this heading.

Morphine Sulfate (Elevated levels of drugs metabolized by the CYP450 system may be observed when co-administered with telithromycin; therefore, increases or prolongation of the therapeutic and/or adverse effects of the concomitant drug may be observed). Products include:

Avinza 1822
Embeda 1831
MS Contin 2803

Moxifloxacin Hydrochloride (Elevated levels of drugs metabolized by the CYP450 system may be observed when co-administered with telithromycin; therefore, increases or prolongation of

the therapeutic and/or adverse effects of the concomitant drug may be observed). Products include:

Avelox 3064
Vigamox 589

Nabumetone (Elevated levels of drugs metabolized by the CYP450 system may be observed when co-administered with telithromycin; therefore, increases or prolongation of the therapeutic and/or adverse effects of the concomitant drug may be observed).
No products indexed under this heading.

Nafcillin Sodium (Concomitant administration of CYP 3A4 inducers is likely to result in subtherapeutic levels of telithromycin and loss of effect).
No products indexed under this heading.

Naproxen (Elevated levels of drugs metabolized by the CYP450 system may be observed when co-administered with telithromycin; therefore, increases or prolongation of the therapeutic and/or adverse effects of the concomitant drug may be observed). Products include:

EC-Naprosyn 2850
Naprosyn 2850
Anaprox/Naprosyn 2850

Naproxen Sodium (Elevated levels of drugs metabolized by the CYP450 system may be observed when co-administered with telithromycin; therefore, increases or prolongation of the therapeutic and/or adverse effects of the concomitant drug may be observed). Products include:

Anaprox 2850
Anaprox DS 2850
Treximet 1681

Nateglinide (Elevated levels of drugs metabolized by the CYP450 system may be observed when co-administered with telithromycin; therefore, increases or prolongation of the therapeutic and/or adverse effects of the concomitant drug may be observed).
No products indexed under this heading.

Nefazodone Hydrochloride (Co-administration of telithromycin with a drug primarily metabolized by the CYP 3A4 enzyme system may result in increased plasma concentrations of the drug co-administered with telithromycin that could increase or prolong both the therapeutic and adverse effects).
No products indexed under this heading.

Nelfinavir Mesylate (Co-administration of telithromycin with a drug primarily metabolized by the CYP 3A4 enzyme system may result in increased plasma concentrations of the drug co-administered with telithromycin that could increase or prolong both the therapeutic and adverse effects).
No products indexed under this heading.

Nevirapine (Concomitant administration of CYP 3A4 inducers is likely to result in subtherapeutic levels of telithromycin and loss of effect).
Products include:

Viramune Oral Suspension 897
Viramune Tablets 897

Nicardipine (Co-administration of telithromycin with a drug primarily metabolized by the CYP 3A4 enzyme system may result in increased plasma concentrations of the drug co-administered with telithromycin that could increase or prolong both the therapeutic and adverse effects).
No products indexed under this heading.

Nicardipine Hydrochloride (Co-administration of telithromycin with a drug primarily metabolized by the CYP 3A4 enzyme system may result in increased plasma concentrations of the drug co-administered with telithromycin that could increase or prolong both the therapeutic and adverse effects).
No products indexed under this heading.

IMPORTANT NOTE: Always consult each drug listing in the patient's regimen for possible interactions.

Ketek Interactions Index 942

Nicotine Polacrilex (Elevated levels of drugs metabolized by the CYP450 system may be observed when co-administered with telithromycin; therefore, increases or prolongation of the therapeutic and/or adverse effects of the concomitant drug may be observed).
No products indexed under this heading.

Nicotine Salicylate (Elevated levels of drugs metabolized by the CYP450 system may be observed when co-administered with telithromycin; therefore, increases or prolongation of the therapeutic and/or adverse effects of the concomitant drug may be observed).
No products indexed under this heading.

Nicotine Sulfate (Elevated levels of drugs metabolized by the CYP450 system may be observed when co-administered with telithromycin; therefore, increases or prolongation of the therapeutic and/or adverse effects of the concomitant drug may be observed).
No products indexed under this heading.

Nifedipine (Co-administration of telithromycin with a drug primarily metabolized by the CYP 3A4 enzyme system may result in increased plasma concentrations of the drug co-administered with telithromycin that could increase or prolong both the therapeutic and adverse effects).
No products indexed under this heading.

Nilutamide (Elevated levels of drugs metabolized by the CYP450 system may be observed when co-administered with telithromycin; therefore, increases or prolongation of the therapeutic and/or adverse effects of the concomitant drug may be observed).
No products indexed under this heading.

Nimodipine (Co-administration of telithromycin with a drug primarily metabolized by the CYP 3A4 enzyme system may result in increased plasma concentrations of the drug co-administered with telithromycin that could increase or prolong both the therapeutic and adverse effects).
No products indexed under this heading.

Nisoldipine (Co-administration of telithromycin with a drug primarily metabolized by the CYP 3A4 enzyme system may result in increased plasma concentrations of the drug co-administered with telithromycin that could increase or prolong both the therapeutic and adverse effects).
No products indexed under this heading.

Nitrendipine (Co-administration of telithromycin with a drug primarily metabolized by the CYP 3A4 enzyme system may result in increased plasma concentrations of the drug co-administered with telithromycin that could increase or prolong both the therapeutic and adverse effects).
No products indexed under this heading.

Norethindrone (Co-administration of telithromycin with a drug primarily metabolized by the CYP 3A4 enzyme system may result in increased plasma concentrations of the drug co-administered with telithromycin that could increase or prolong both the therapeutic and adverse effects). Products include:
Ortho Micronor 2660

Norethindrone Acetate (Co-administration of telithromycin with a drug primarily metabolized by the CYP 3A4 enzyme system may result in increased plasma concentrations of the drug co-administered with telithromycin that could increase or prolong both the therapeutic and adverse effects). Products include:
Activella 2561

Norfloxacin (Elevated levels of drugs metabolized by the CYP450 system may be observed when co-administered with telithromycin; therefore, increases or prolongation of the therapeutic and/or adverse effects of the concomitant drug may be observed). Products include:
Noroxin 2220

Norgestrel (Co-administration of telithromycin with a drug primarily metabolized by the CYP 3A4 enzyme system may result in increased plasma concentrations of the drug co-administered with telithromycin that could increase or prolong both the therapeutic and adverse effects).
No products indexed under this heading.

Nortriptyline Hydrochloride (Elevated levels of drugs metabolized by the CYP450 system may be observed when co-administered with telithromycin; therefore, increases or prolongation of the therapeutic and/or adverse effects of the concomitant drug may be observed).
No products indexed under this heading.

Ofloxacin (Elevated levels of drugs metabolized by the CYP450 system may be observed when co-administered with telithromycin; therefore, increases or prolongation of the therapeutic and/or adverse effects of the concomitant drug may be observed).
No products indexed under this heading.

Olanzapine (Elevated levels of drugs metabolized by the CYP450 system may be observed when co-administered with telithromycin; therefore, increases or prolongation of the therapeutic and/or adverse effects of the concomitant drug may be observed). Products include:
Symbyax 1965
Zyprexa 1984
Zyprexa IntraMuscular 1984
Zyprexa ZYDIS 1984

Omeprazole (Elevated levels of drugs metabolized by the CYP450 system may be observed when co-administered with telithromycin; therefore, increases or prolongation of the therapeutic and/or adverse effects of the concomitant drug may be observed).
No products indexed under this heading.

Omeprazole Magnesium (Elevated levels of drugs metabolized by the CYP450 system may be observed when co-administered with telithromycin; therefore, increases or prolongation of the therapeutic and/or adverse effects of the concomitant drug may be observed).
No products indexed under this heading.

Ondansetron (Co-administration of telithromycin with a drug primarily metabolized by the CYP 3A4 enzyme system may result in increased plasma concentrations of the drug co-administered with telithromycin that could increase or prolong both the therapeutic and adverse effects).
No products indexed under this heading.

Ondansetron Hydrochloride (Co-administration of telithromycin with a drug primarily metabolized by the CYP 3A4 enzyme system may result in increased plasma concentrations of the drug co-administered with telithromycin that could increase or prolong both the therapeutic and adverse effects). Products include:
Zofran Injection 1750
Zofran 1756
Zofran ODT 1756

Oxaprozin (Elevated levels of drugs metabolized by the CYP450 system may be observed when co-administered with telithromycin; therefore, increases or prolongation of the therapeutic and/or adverse effects of the concomitant drug may be observed).
No products indexed under this heading.

Oxcarbazepine (Concomitant administration of CYP 3A4 inducers is likely to result in subtherapeutic levels of telithromycin and loss of effect).
No products indexed under this heading.

Oxycodone Hydrochloride (Elevated levels of drugs metabolized by the CYP450 system may be observed when co-administered with telithromycin; therefore, increases or prolongation of the therapeutic and/or adverse effects of the concomitant drug may be observed). Products include:
OxyContin 2807
Percocet 1121
Percodan 1124

Paclitaxel (Co-administration of telithromycin with a drug primarily metabolized by the CYP 3A4 enzyme system may result in increased plasma concentrations of the drug co-administered with telithromycin that could increase or prolong both the therapeutic and adverse effects).
No products indexed under this heading.

Pantoprazole Sodium (Elevated levels of drugs metabolized by the CYP450 system may be observed when co-administered with telithromycin; therefore, increases or prolongation of the therapeutic and/or adverse effects of the concomitant drug may be observed). Products include:
Protonix Tablets 3571
Protonix 3575

Paramethadione (Elevated levels of drugs metabolized by the CYP450 system may be observed when co-administered with telithromycin; therefore, increases or prolongation of the therapeutic and/or adverse effects of the concomitant drug may be observed).
No products indexed under this heading.

Paroxetine Hydrochloride (Elevated levels of drugs metabolized by the CYP450 system may be observed when co-administered with telithromycin; therefore, increases or prolongation of the therapeutic and/or adverse effects of the concomitant drug may be observed). Products include:
Paroxetine CR 2361
Paroxetine ER 2371
Paxil 1586
Paxil CR 1596

Pentamidine Isethionate (Elevated levels of drugs metabolized by the CYP450 system may be observed when co-administered with telithromycin; therefore, increases or prolongation of the therapeutic and/or adverse effects of the concomitant drug may be observed).
No products indexed under this heading.

Phenacemide (Elevated levels of drugs metabolized by the CYP450 system may be observed when co-administered with telithromycin; therefore, increases or prolongation of the therapeutic and/or adverse effects of the concomitant drug may be observed).
No products indexed under this heading.

Phenobarbital (Concomitant administration of other CYP 3A4 inducers, such as phenytoin, carbamazepine, or phenobarbital, is likely to result in subtherapeutic levels of telithromycin and loss of effect). Products include:
Donnatal 2711

Phenobarbital Sodium (Concomitant administration of other CYP 3A4 inducers, such as phenytoin, carbamazepine, or phenobarbital, is likely to result in subtherapeutic levels of telithromycin and loss of effect).
No products indexed under this heading.

Phensuximide (Elevated levels of drugs metabolized by the CYP450 system may be observed when co-administered with telithromycin; therefore, increases or prolongation of the therapeutic and/or adverse effects of the concomitant drug may be observed).
No products indexed under this heading.

Phenylbutazone (Elevated levels of drugs metabolized by the CYP450 system may be observed when co-administered with telithromycin; therefore, increases or prolongation of the therapeutic and/or adverse effects of the concomitant drug may be observed).
No products indexed under this heading.

Phenytoin (Concomitant administration of other CYP 3A4 inducers, such as phenytoin, carbamazepine, or phenobarbital, is likely to result in subtherapeutic levels of telithromycin and loss of effect).
No products indexed under this heading.

Phenytoin Sodium (Concomitant administration of other CYP 3A4 inducers, such as phenytoin, carbamazepine, or phenobarbital, is likely to result in subtherapeutic levels of telithromycin and loss of effect). Products include:
Phenytek Capsules 2380

Pimozide (The use of telithromycin is contraindicated with pimozide. Although there are no studies looking at the interaction between telithromycin and pimozide, there is a potential risk of increased pimozide plasma levels by inhibition of CYP 3A4 pathways by telithromycin as with macrolides).
No products indexed under this heading.

Pindolol (Elevated levels of drugs metabolized by the CYP450 system may be observed when co-administered with telithromycin; therefore, increases or prolongation of the therapeutic and/or adverse effects of the concomitant drug may be observed).
No products indexed under this heading.

Pioglitazone Hydrochloride (Elevated levels of drugs metabolized by the CYP450 system may be observed when co-administered with telithromycin; therefore, increases or prolongation of the therapeutic and/or adverse effects of the concomitant drug may be observed). Products include:
ActoPlus 3338
Actos 3345
Duetact 3354

Piroxicam (Elevated levels of drugs metabolized by the CYP450 system may be observed when co-administered with telithromycin; therefore, increases or prolongation of the therapeutic and/or adverse effects of the concomitant drug may be observed).
No products indexed under this heading.

Polyestradiol Phosphate (Co-administration of telithromycin with a drug primarily metabolized by the CYP 3A4 enzyme system may result in increased plasma concentrations of the drug co-administered with telithromycin that could increase or prolong both the therapeutic and adverse effects).
No products indexed under this heading.

Pravastatin Sodium (Although pravastatin is not metabolized by CYPs, hepatic cell OATP1 transporters play an important role in its elimination from the body. *In vitro* OATP1 transporter inhibition has been demonstrated for macrolides and telithromycin. Telithromycin

slightly inhibits the *in vitro* transporter uptake of pravastatin. The *in vivo* relevance of this *in vitro* finding has not been established for telithromycin).

No products indexed under this heading.

Prednisolone (Concomitant administration of CYP 3A4 inducers is likely to result in subtherapeutic levels of telithromycin and loss of effect).

No products indexed under this heading.

Prednisolone Acetate (Concomitant administration of CYP 3A4 inducers is likely to result in subtherapeutic levels of telithromycin and loss of effect). Products include:

Blephamide	⊙212, ⊙214
Pred Forte	⊙225
Pred Mild	⊙230
Pred-G	⊙226, 227

Prednisolone Sodium Phosphate (Concomitant administration of CYP 3A4 inducers is likely to result in subtherapeutic levels of telithromycin and loss of effect).

No products indexed under this heading.

Prednisolone Tebutate (Concomitant administration of CYP 3A4 inducers is likely to result in subtherapeutic levels of telithromycin and loss of effect).

No products indexed under this heading.

Prednisone (Concomitant administration of CYP 3A4 inducers is likely to result in subtherapeutic levels of telithromycin and loss of effect).

No products indexed under this heading.

Prednisone sodium phosphate (Concomitant administration of CYP 3A4 inducers is likely to result in subtherapeutic levels of telithromycin and loss of effect).

No products indexed under this heading.

Primidone (Concomitant administration of CYP 3A4 inducers is likely to result in subtherapeutic levels of telithromycin and loss of effect).

No products indexed under this heading.

Procainamide (Telithromycin should be avoided in patients with congenital prolongation of the QT$_c$ interval, and in patients with ongoing proarrhythmic conditions, such as uncorrected hypokalemia or hypomagnesemia, clinically significant bradycardia, and in patients receiving Class IA (eg, quinidine and procainamide) or Class III (eg, dofetilide) antiarrhythmic agents).

No products indexed under this heading.

Progesterone (Elevated levels of drugs metabolized by the CYP450 system may be observed when co-administered with telithromycin; therefore, increases or prolongation of the therapeutic and/or adverse effects of the concomitant drug may be observed). Products include:

Crinone 4%	996
Crinone 8%	996
Prometrium	3307

Proguanil Hydrochloride (Elevated levels of drugs metabolized by the CYP450 system may be observed when co-administered with telithromycin; therefore, increases or prolongation of the therapeutic and/or adverse effects of the concomitant drug may be observed). Products include:

Malarone Pediatric Tablets	1572
Malarone	1572

Propafenone Hydrochloride (Elevated levels of drugs metabolized by the CYP450 system may be observed when co-administered with telithromycin; therefore, increases or prolongation of the therapeutic and/or adverse effects of the concomitant drug may be observed). Products include:

Rythmol	1648
Rythmol SR	1652

Propoxyphene Hydrochloride (Elevated levels of drugs metabolized by the CYP450 system may be observed when co-administered with telithromycin; therefore, increases or prolongation of the therapeutic and/or adverse effects of the concomitant drug may be observed).

No products indexed under this heading.

Propoxyphene Napsylate (Elevated levels of drugs metabolized by the CYP450 system may be observed when co-administered with telithromycin; therefore, increases or prolongation of the therapeutic and/or adverse effects of the concomitant drug may be observed).

No products indexed under this heading.

Propranolol Hydrochloride (Elevated levels of drugs metabolized by the CYP450 system may be observed when co-administered with telithromycin; therefore, increases or prolongation of the therapeutic and/or adverse effects of the concomitant drug may be observed). Products include:

InnoPran XL	1517

Protriptyline Hydrochloride (Elevated levels of drugs metabolized by the CYP450 system may be observed when co-administered with telithromycin; therefore, increases or prolongation of the therapeutic and/or adverse effects of the concomitant drug may be observed).

No products indexed under this heading.

Quetiapine Fumarate (Elevated levels of drugs metabolized by the CYP450 system may be observed when co-administered with telithromycin; therefore, increases or prolongation of the therapeutic and/or adverse effects of the concomitant drug may be observed). Products include:

Seroquel	750
Seroquel XR	759

Quinidine (Telithromycin should be avoided in patients with congenital prolongation of the QT$_c$ interval, and in patients with ongoing proarrhythmic conditions, such as uncorrected hypokalemia or hypomagnesemia, clinically significant bradycardia, and in patients receiving Class IA (eg, quinidine and procainamide) or Class III (eg, dofetilide) antiarrhythmic agents).

No products indexed under this heading.

Quinidine Gluconate (Telithromycin should be avoided in patients with congenital prolongation of the QT$_c$ interval, and in patients with ongoing proarrhythmic conditions, such as uncorrected hypokalemia or hypomagnesemia, clinically significant bradycardia, and in patients receiving Class IA (eg, quinidine and procainamide) or Class III (eg, dofetilide) antiarrhythmic agents).

No products indexed under this heading.

Quinidine Hydrochloride (Telithromycin should be avoided in patients with congenital prolongation of the QT$_c$ interval, and in patients with ongoing proarrhythmic conditions, such as uncorrected hypokalemia or hypomagnesemia, clinically significant bradycardia, and in patients receiving Class IA (eg, quinidine and procainamide) or Class III (eg, dofetilide) antiarrhythmic agents).

No products indexed under this heading.

Quinidine Polygalacturonate (Telithromycin should be avoided in patients with congenital prolongation of the QT$_c$ interval, and in patients with ongoing proarrhythmic conditions, such as uncorrected hypokalemia or hypomagnesemia, clinically significant bradycardia, and in patients receiving Class IA (eg, quinidine and procainamide) or Class III (eg, dofetilide) antiarrhythmic agents).

No products indexed under this heading.

Quinidine Sulfate (Telithromycin should be avoided in patients with congenital prolongation of the QT$_c$ interval, and in patients with ongoing proarrhythmic conditions, such as uncorrected hypokalemia or hypomagnesemia, clinically significant bradycardia, and in patients receiving Class IA (eg, quinidine and procainamide) or Class III (eg, dofetilide) antiarrhythmic agents).

No products indexed under this heading.

Quinine (Elevated levels of drugs metabolized by the CYP450 system may be observed when co-administered with telithromycin; therefore, increases or prolongation of the therapeutic and/or adverse effects of the concomitant drug may be observed). Products include:

Hyland's Leg Cramps PM with Quinine	3315

Quinine Sulfate (Elevated levels of drugs metabolized by the CYP450 system may be observed when co-administered with telithromycin; therefore, increases or prolongation of the therapeutic and/or adverse effects of the concomitant drug may be observed).

No products indexed under this heading.

Rabeprazole Sodium (Elevated levels of drugs metabolized by the CYP450 system may be observed when co-administered with telithromycin; therefore, increases or prolongation of the therapeutic and/or adverse effects of the concomitant drug may be observed). Products include:

Aciphex	1035

Repaglinide (Elevated levels of drugs metabolized by the CYP450 system may be observed when co-administered with telithromycin; therefore, increases or prolongation of the therapeutic and/or adverse effects of the concomitant drug may be observed).

No products indexed under this heading.

Rifabutin (Co-administration of telithromycin with a drug primarily metabolized by the CYP 3A4 enzyme system may result in increased plasma concentrations of the drug co-administered with telithromycin that could increase or prolong both the therapeutic and adverse effects).

No products indexed under this heading.

Rifampicin (Concomitant administration of CYP 3A4 inducers is likely to result in subtherapeutic levels of telithromycin and loss of effect).

No products indexed under this heading.

Rifampin (During concomitant administration of rifampin and telithromycin in repeated doses, C$_{max}$ and AUC of telithromycin were decreased by 79%, and 86%, respectively. Concomitant treatment of telithromycin with rifampin, a CYP 3A4 inducer, should be avoided).

No products indexed under this heading.

Rifapentine (Concomitant administration of CYP 3A4 inducers is likely to result in subtherapeutic levels of telithromycin and loss of effect).

No products indexed under this heading.

Riluzole (Elevated levels of drugs metabolized by the CYP450 system may be observed when co-administered with telithromycin; therefore, increases or prolongation of the therapeutic and/or adverse effects of the concomitant drug may be observed). Products include:

Rilutek	3032

Risperidone (Elevated levels of drugs metabolized by the CYP450 system may be observed when co-administered with telithromycin; therefore, increases or prolongation of the therapeutic and/or adverse effects of the concomitant drug may be observed). Products include:

Risperdal Consta	2682

Ritonavir (Co-administration of telithromycin with a drug primarily metabolized by the CYP 3A4 enzyme system may result in increased plasma concentrations of the drug co-administered with telithromycin that could increase or prolong both the therapeutic and adverse effects). Products include:

Kaletra	458
Norvir	509

Rofecoxib (Elevated levels of drugs metabolized by the CYP450 system may be observed when co-administered with telithromycin; therefore, increases or prolongation of the therapeutic and/or adverse effects of the concomitant drug may be observed).

No products indexed under this heading.

Ropinirole Hydrochloride (Elevated levels of drugs metabolized by the CYP450 system may be observed when co-administered with telithromycin; therefore, increases or prolongation of the therapeutic and/or adverse effects of the concomitant drug may be observed). Products include:

Requip	1620
Requip XL	1628

Ropivacaine Hydrochloride (Elevated levels of drugs metabolized by the CYP450 system may be observed when co-administered with telithromycin; therefore, increases or prolongation of the therapeutic and/or adverse effects of the concomitant drug may be observed).

No products indexed under this heading.

Rosiglitazone (Elevated levels of drugs metabolized by the CYP450 system may be observed when co-administered with telithromycin; therefore, increases or prolongation of the therapeutic and/or adverse effects of the concomitant drug may be observed).

No products indexed under this heading.

Rosiglitazone Maleate (Elevated levels of drugs metabolized by the CYP450 system may be observed when co-administered with telithromycin; therefore, increases or prolongation of the therapeutic and/or adverse effects of the concomitant drug may be observed). Products include:

Avandamet	1345
Avandaryl	1356
Avandia	1366

Rosiglitazone/Metformin (Elevated levels of drugs metabolized by the CYP450 system may be observed when co-administered with telithromycin; therefore, increases or prolongation of the therapeutic and/or adverse effects of the concomitant drug may be observed).

No products indexed under this heading.

Rosuvastatin Calcium (High levels of HMG-CoA reductase inhibitors increase the risk of myopathy. Use of simvastatin, lovastatin, or atorvastatin concomitantly with telithromycin should be avoided. If telithromycin is prescribed, therapy with simvastatin, lovastatin, or atorvastatin should be suspended during the course of treatment. Patients concomitantly treated with statins should be carefully monitored for signs and symptoms of myopathy and rhabdomyolysis). Products include:

Crestor	736

Saquinavir (Co-administration of telithromycin with a drug primarily metabolized by the CYP 3A4 enzyme system may result in increased plasma concentrations of the drug co-administered with telithromycin that could increase or prolong both the therapeutic and adverse effects).

No products indexed under this heading.

IMPORTANT NOTE: Always consult each drug listing in the patient's regimen for possible interactions.

Saquinavir Mesylate (Co-administration of telithromycin with a drug primarily metabolized by the CYP 3A4 enzyme system may result in increased plasma concentrations of the drug co-administered with telithromycin that could increase or prolong both the therapeutic and adverse effects).
No products indexed under this heading.

Sertraline Hydrochloride (Co-administration of telithromycin with a drug primarily metabolized by the CYP 3A4 enzyme system may result in increased plasma concentrations of the drug co-administered with telithromycin that could increase or prolong both the therapeutic and adverse effects).
No products indexed under this heading.

Sildenafil Citrate (Co-administration of telithromycin with a drug primarily metabolized by the CYP 3A4 enzyme system may result in increased plasma concentrations of the drug co-administered with telithromycin that could increase or prolong both the therapeutic and adverse effects).
No products indexed under this heading.

Simvastatin (High levels of HMG-CoA reductase inhibitors increase the risk of myopathy. Use of simvastatin, lovastatin, or atorvastatin concomitantly with telithromycin should be avoided. If telithromycin is prescribed, therapy with simvastatin, lovastatin, or atorvastatin should be suspended during the course of treatment. Patients concomitantly treated with statins should be carefully monitored for signs and symptoms of myopathy and rhabdomyolysis). Products include:

Simcor	524
Vytorin 10/10	2303, 3240
Vytorin 10/20	2303, 3240
Vytorin 10/40	2303, 3240
Vytorin 10/80	2303, 3240
Zocor	2289

Sirolimus (Drugs metabolized by the cytochrome P450 system, such as carbamazepine, cyclosporine, tacrolimus, sirolimus, hexobarbital, and phenytoin; elevation of serum levels of these drugs may be observed when co-administered with telithromycin. As a result, increases or prolongation of the therapeutic and/or adverse effects of the concomitant drug may be observed). Products include:

Rapamune	3579

Sotalol Hydrochloride (Telithromycin has been shown to decrease the C_{max} and AUC of sotalol by 34% and 20%, respectively, due to decreased absorption).
No products indexed under this heading.

Sulfamethoxazole (Elevated levels of drugs metabolized by the CYP450 system may be observed when co-administered with telithromycin; therefore, increases or prolongation of the therapeutic and/or adverse effects of the concomitant drug may be observed).
No products indexed under this heading.

Sulfinpyrazone (Concomitant administration of CYP 3A4 inducers is likely to result in subtherapeutic levels of telithromycin and loss of effect).
No products indexed under this heading.

Sulindac (Elevated levels of drugs metabolized by the CYP450 system may be observed when co-administered with telithromycin; therefore, increases or prolongation of the therapeutic and/or adverse effects of the concomitant drug may be observed). Products include:

Clinoril	2098

Suprofen (Elevated levels of drugs metabolized by the CYP450 system may be observed when co-administered with telithromycin; therefore, increases or prolongation of the therapeutic and/or adverse effects of the concomitant drug may be observed).
No products indexed under this heading.

Tacrine Hydrochloride (Elevated levels of drugs metabolized by the CYP450 system may be observed when co-administered with telithromycin; therefore, increases or prolongation of the therapeutic and/or adverse effects of the concomitant drug may be observed).
No products indexed under this heading.

Tacrolimus (Drugs metabolized by the cytochrome P450 system, such as carbamazepine, cyclosporine, tacrolimus, sirolimus, hexobarbital, and phenytoin; elevation of serum levels of these drugs may be observed when co-administered with telithromycin. As a result, increases or prolongation of the therapeutic and/or adverse effects of the concomitant drug may be observed). Products include:

Prograf Capsules	677
Prograf Injection	677
Protopic	685

Tadalafil (Co-administration of telithromycin with a drug primarily metabolized by the CYP 3A4 enzyme system may result in increased plasma concentrations of the drug co-administered with telithromycin that could increase or prolong both the therapeutic and adverse effects). Products include:

Adcirca	3461
Cialis	1861

Tamoxifen Citrate (Co-administration of telithromycin with a drug primarily metabolized by the CYP 3A4 enzyme system may result in increased plasma concentrations of the drug co-administered with telithromycin that could increase or prolong both the therapeutic and adverse effects).
No products indexed under this heading.

Telmisartan (Elevated levels of drugs metabolized by the CYP450 system may be observed when co-administered with telithromycin; therefore, increases or prolongation of the therapeutic and/or adverse effects of the concomitant drug may be observed). Products include:

Micardis	887
Micardis HCT	889

Teniposide (Elevated levels of drugs metabolized by the CYP450 system may be observed when co-administered with telithromycin; therefore, increases or prolongation of the therapeutic and/or adverse effects of the concomitant drug may be observed).
No products indexed under this heading.

Terfenadine (Co-administration of telithromycin with a drug primarily metabolized by the CYP 3A4 enzyme system may result in increased plasma concentrations of the drug co-administered with telithromycin that could increase or prolong both the therapeutic and adverse effects).
No products indexed under this heading.

Testosterone (Elevated levels of drugs metabolized by the CYP450 system may be observed when co-administered with telithromycin; therefore, increases or prolongation of the therapeutic and/or adverse effects of the concomitant drug may be observed). Products include:

AndroGel	3456

Testosterone Cypionate (Elevated levels of drugs metabolized by the CYP450 system may be observed when co-administered with telithromycin; therefore, increases or prolongation of the therapeutic and/or adverse effects of the concomitant drug may be observed).
No products indexed under this heading.

Testosterone Enanthate (Elevated levels of drugs metabolized by the CYP450 system may be observed when co-administered with telithromycin; therefore, increases or prolongation of the therapeutic and/or adverse effects of the concomitant drug may be observed). Products include:

Delatestryl	1102

Testosterone Propionate (Elevated levels of drugs metabolized by the CYP450 system may be observed when co-administered with telithromycin; therefore, increases or prolongation of the therapeutic and/or adverse effects of the concomitant drug may be observed).
No products indexed under this heading.

Theophyllinate (Concomitant administration of CYP 3A4 inducers is likely to result in subtherapeutic levels of telithromycin and loss of effect).
No products indexed under this heading.

Theophylline (When theophylline was co-administered with repeated doses of telithromycin, there was an increase of approximately 16% and 17% on the steady-state C_{max} and AUC of theophylline. Co-administration of theophylline may worsen gastrointestinal side effects, such as nausea and vomiting, especially in female patients. It is recommended that telithromycin should be taken with theophylline 1 hour apart to decrease the likelihood of gastrointestinal side effects).
No products indexed under this heading.

Theophylline Anhydrous (When theophylline was co-administered with repeated doses of telithromycin, there was an increase of approximately 16% and 17% on the steady-state C_{max} and AUC of theophylline. Co-administration of theophylline may worsen gastrointestinal side effects, such as nausea and vomiting, especially in female patients. It is recommended that telithromycin should be taken with theophylline 1 hour apart to decrease the likelihood of gastrointestinal side effects). Products include:

Uniphyl	2817

Theophylline Calcium Salicylate (When theophylline was co-administered with repeated doses of telithromycin, there was an increase of approximately 16% and 17% on the steady-state C_{max} and AUC of theophylline. Co-administration of theophylline may worsen gastrointestinal side effects, such as nausea and vomiting, especially in female patients. It is recommended that telithromycin should be taken with theophylline 1 hour apart to decrease the likelihood of gastrointestinal side effects).
No products indexed under this heading.

Theophylline Dihydroxypropyl (Glyceryl) (When theophylline was co-administered with repeated doses of telithromycin, there was an increase of approximately 16% and 17% on the steady-state C_{max} and AUC of theophylline. Co-administration of theophylline may worsen gastrointestinal side effects, such as nausea and vomiting, especially in female patients. It is recommended that telithromycin should be taken with theophylline 1 hour apart to decrease the likelihood of gastrointestinal side effects).
No products indexed under this heading.

Theophylline Ethylenediamine (When theophylline was co-administered with repeated doses of telithromycin, there was an increase of approximately 16% and 17% on the steady-state C_{max} and AUC of theophylline. Co-administration of theophylline may worsen gastrointestinal side effects, such as nausea and vomiting, especially in female patients. It is recommended that telithromycin should be taken with theophylline 1 hour apart to decrease the likelihood of gastrointestinal side effects).
No products indexed under this heading.

Theophylline Sodium Glycinate (When theophylline was co-administered with repeated doses of telithromycin, there was an increase of approximately 16% and 17% on the steady-state C_{max} and AUC of theophylline. Co-administration of theophylline may worsen gastrointestinal side effects, such as nausea and vomiting, especially in female patients. It is recommended that telithromycin should be taken with theophylline 1 hour apart to decrease the likelihood of gastrointestinal side effects).
No products indexed under this heading.

Thioridazine (Elevated levels of drugs metabolized by the CYP450 system may be observed when co-administered with telithromycin; therefore, increases or prolongation of the therapeutic and/or adverse effects of the concomitant drug may be observed).
No products indexed under this heading.

Thioridazine Hydrochloride (Elevated levels of drugs metabolized by the CYP450 system may be observed when co-administered with telithromycin; therefore, increases or prolongation of the therapeutic and/or adverse effects of the concomitant drug may be observed). Products include:

Thioridazine Hydrochloride	2384

Tiagabine Hydrochloride (Co-administration of telithromycin with a drug primarily metabolized by the CYP 3A4 enzyme system may result in increased plasma concentrations of the drug co-administered with telithromycin that could increase or prolong both the therapeutic and adverse effects). Products include:

Gabitril	972

Timolol Maleate (Elevated levels of drugs metabolized by the CYP450 system may be observed when co-administered with telithromycin; therefore, increases or prolongation of the therapeutic and/or adverse effects of the concomitant drug may be observed). Products include:

Combigan	601
Dorzolamide Hydrochloride/Timolol Maleate Ophthalmic Solution	⊙243
Timoptic in Ocudose	⊙231

Tolazamide (Elevated levels of drugs metabolized by the CYP450 system may be observed when co-administered with telithromycin; therefore, increases or prolongation of the therapeutic and/or adverse effects of the concomitant drug may be observed).
No products indexed under this heading.

Tolbutamide (Elevated levels of drugs metabolized by the CYP450 system may be observed when co-administered with telithromycin; therefore, increases or prolongation of the therapeutic and/or adverse effects of the concomitant drug may be observed).
No products indexed under this heading.

Tolbutamide Sodium (Elevated levels of drugs metabolized by the CYP450 system may be observed when co-administered with telithromycin; therefore, increases or prolongation of the therapeutic and/or adverse effects of the concomitant drug may be observed).
No products indexed under this heading.

Tolmetin Sodium (Elevated levels of drugs metabolized by the CYP450 system may be observed when co-administered with telithromycin; therefore, increases or prolongation of the therapeutic and/or adverse effects of the concomitant drug may be observed).
No products indexed under this heading.

Tolterodine Tartrate (Co-administration of telithromycin with a drug primarily metabolized by the CYP 3A4 enzyme system may result in increased plasma concentrations of the drug co-administered with telithromycin that could increase or prolong both the therapeutic and adverse effects).
No products indexed under this heading.

Topiramate (Elevated levels of drugs metabolized by the CYP450 system may be observed when co-administered with telithromycin; therefore, increases or prolongation of the therapeutic and/or adverse effects of the concomitant drug may be observed).
No products indexed under this heading.

Torsemide (Elevated levels of drugs metabolized by the CYP450 system may be observed when co-administered with telithromycin; therefore, increases or prolongation of the therapeutic and/or adverse effects of the concomitant drug may be observed).
No products indexed under this heading.

Tramadol Hydrochloride (Elevated levels of drugs metabolized by the CYP450 system may be observed when co-administered with telithromycin; therefore, increases or prolongation of the therapeutic and/or adverse effects of the concomitant drug may be observed). Products include:

Trazodone Hydrochloride (Co-administration of telithromycin with a drug primarily metabolized by the CYP 3A4 enzyme system may result in increased plasma concentrations of the drug co-administered with telithromycin that could increase or prolong both the therapeutic and adverse effects).
No products indexed under this heading.

Tretinoin (Elevated levels of drugs metabolized by the CYP450 system may be observed when co-administered with telithromycin; therefore, increases or prolongation of the therapeutic and/or adverse effects of the concomitant drug may be observed).
No products indexed under this heading.

Triamcinolone (Concomitant administration of CYP 3A4 inducers is likely to result in subtherapeutic levels of telithromycin and loss of effect).
No products indexed under this heading.

Triamcinolone Acetonide (Concomitant administration of CYP 3A4 inducers is likely to result in subtherapeutic levels of telithromycin and loss of effect). Products include:

Triamcinolone Diacetate (Concomitant administration of CYP 3A4 inducers is likely to result in subtherapeutic levels of telithromycin and loss of effect).
No products indexed under this heading.

Triamcinolone Hexacetonide (Concomitant administration of CYP 3A4 inducers is likely to result in subtherapeutic levels of telithromycin and loss of effect).
No products indexed under this heading.

Triazolam (Concomitant administration of telithromycin with midazolam increased the AUC of midazolam; therefore, precaution should be used with other benzodiazepines metabolized by CYP 3A4 and that undergo a high first-pass effect (eg, triazolam)).
No products indexed under this heading.

Trimethadione (Elevated levels of drugs metabolized by the CYP450 system may be observed when co-administered with telithromycin; therefore, increases or prolongation of the therapeutic and/or adverse effects of the concomitant drug may be observed).
No products indexed under this heading.

Trimethaphan Camsylate (Elevated levels of drugs metabolized by the CYP450 system may be observed when co-administered with telithromycin; therefore, increases or prolongation of the therapeutic and/or adverse effects of the concomitant drug may be observed).
No products indexed under this heading.

Trimipramine Maleate (Elevated levels of drugs metabolized by the CYP450 system may be observed when co-administered with telithromycin; therefore, increases or prolongation of the therapeutic and/or adverse effects of the concomitant drug may be observed).
No products indexed under this heading.

Troglitazone (Concomitant administration of CYP 3A4 inducers is likely to result in subtherapeutic levels of telithromycin and loss of effect).
No products indexed under this heading.

Trovafloxacin Mesylate (Elevated levels of drugs metabolized by the CYP450 system may be observed when co-administered with telithromycin; therefore, increases or prolongation of the therapeutic and/or adverse effects of the concomitant drug may be observed).
No products indexed under this heading.

Valdecoxib (Elevated levels of drugs metabolized by the CYP450 system may be observed when co-administered with telithromycin; therefore, increases or prolongation of the therapeutic and/or adverse effects of the concomitant drug may be observed).
No products indexed under this heading.

Valproate Sodium (Elevated levels of drugs metabolized by the CYP450 system may be observed when co-administered with telithromycin; therefore, increases or prolongation of the therapeutic and/or adverse effects of the concomitant drug may be observed).
No products indexed under this heading.

Valproic Acid (Elevated levels of drugs metabolized by the CYP450 system may be observed when co-administered with telithromycin; therefore, increases or prolongation of the therapeutic and/or adverse effects of the concomitant drug may be observed).
No products indexed under this heading.

Valsartan (Elevated levels of drugs metabolized by the CYP450 system may be observed when co-administered with telithromycin; therefore, increases or prolongation of the therapeutic and/or adverse effects of the concomitant drug may be observed). Products include:

Vardenafil Hydrochloride (Co-administration of telithromycin with a drug primarily metabolized by the CYP 3A4 enzyme system may result in increased plasma concentrations of the drug co-administered with telithromycin that could increase or prolong both the therapeutic and adverse effects). Products include:

Venlafaxine Hydrochloride (Elevated levels of drugs metabolized by the CYP450 system may be observed when co-administered with telithromycin; therefore, increases or prolongation of the therapeutic and/or adverse effects of the concomitant drug may be observed). Products include:

Verapamil Hydrochloride (Co-administration of telithromycin with a drug primarily metabolized by the CYP 3A4 enzyme system may result in increased plasma concentrations of the drug co-administered with telithromycin that could increase or prolong both the therapeutic and adverse effects). Products include:

Vinblastine Sulfate (Co-administration of telithromycin with a drug primarily metabolized by the CYP 3A4 enzyme system may result in increased plasma concentrations of the drug co-administered with telithromycin that could increase or prolong both the therapeutic and adverse effects).
No products indexed under this heading.

Vincristine Sulfate (Co-administration of telithromycin with a drug primarily metabolized by the CYP 3A4 enzyme system may result in increased plasma concentrations of the drug co-administered with telithromycin that could increase or prolong both the therapeutic and adverse effects).
No products indexed under this heading.

Vitamin A (Elevated levels of drugs metabolized by the CYP450 system may be observed when co-administered with telithromycin; therefore, increases or prolongation of the therapeutic and/or adverse effects of the concomitant drug may be observed). Products include:

Vitamin A Acetate (Elevated levels of drugs metabolized by the CYP450 system may be observed when co-administered with telithromycin; therefore, increases or prolongation of the therapeutic and/or adverse effects of the concomitant drug may be observed).
No products indexed under this heading.

Voriconazole (Elevated levels of drugs metabolized by the CYP450 system may be observed when co-administered with telithromycin; therefore, increases or prolongation of the therapeutic and/or adverse effects of the concomitant drug may be observed).
No products indexed under this heading.

Warfarin Sodium (Spontaneous post-marketing reports suggest that administration of telithromycin and oral anticoagulants concomitantly may potentiate the effects of the oral anticoagulants. Consideration should be given to monitoring prothrombin times/INR while patients are receiving telithromycin and oral anticoagulants simultaneously).
No products indexed under this heading.

Zafirlukast (Elevated levels of drugs metabolized by the CYP450 system may be observed when co-administered with telithromycin; therefore, increases or prolongation of the therapeutic and/or adverse effects of the concomitant drug may be observed). Products include:

Zileuton (Elevated levels of drugs metabolized by the CYP450 system may be observed when co-administered with telithromycin; therefore, increases or prolongation of the therapeutic and/or adverse effects of the concomitant drug may be observed).
No products indexed under this heading.

Zolmitriptan (Elevated levels of drugs metabolized by the CYP450 system may be observed when co-administered with telithromycin; therefore, increases or prolongation of the therapeutic and/or adverse effects of the concomitant drug may be observed). Products include:

Zonisamide (Elevated levels of drugs metabolized by the CYP450 system may be observed when co-administered with telithromycin; therefore, increases or prolongation of the therapeutic and/or adverse effects of the concomitant drug may be observed). Products include:

Zopiclone (Elevated levels of drugs metabolized by the CYP450 system may be observed when co-administered with telithromycin; therefore, increases or prolongation of the therapeutic and/or adverse effects of the concomitant drug may be observed).
No products indexed under this heading.

Food Interactions

Beverages, caffeine-containing (Elevated levels of drugs metabolized by the CYP450 system may be observed when co-administered with telithromycin; therefore, increases or prolongation of the therapeutic and/or adverse effects of the concomitant drug may be observed).

Food, caffeine-containing (Elevated levels of drugs metabolized by the CYP450 system may be observed when co-administered with telithromycin; therefore, increases or prolongation of the therapeutic and/or adverse effects of the concomitant drug may be observed).

KINERET INJECTION

May interact with immunosuppressive agents, TNF antagonists, vaccines, live, and certain other agents. Compounds in these categories include:

Adalimumab (A higher rate of serious infections has been observed in patients treated with concurrent anakinra and etanercept therapy than in patients treated with etanercept alone. Two percent of patients treated concurrently with anakinra and etanercept developed neutropenia (ANC < 1x10^9/L). Use of anakinra in combination with TNF blocking agents is not recommended). Products include:

Azathioprine (Infections have been noted in all organ systems and have been reported in patients receiving anakinra alone or in combination with immunosuppressive agents).
No products indexed under this heading.

Basiliximab (Infections have been noted in all organ systems and have been reported in patients receiving anakinra alone or in combination with immunosuppressive agents). Products include:

Simulect 2524

BCG Vaccine (No data is available on either the effects of live vaccination or the secondary transmission of infection by live vaccines in patients receiving anakinra. Therefore, live vaccines should not be given concurrently with anakinra).
No products indexed under this heading.

Cyclosporine (Infections have been noted in all organ systems and have been reported in patients receiving anakinra alone or in combination with immunosuppressive agents). Products include:

Etanercept (In a 24 week study of concurrent anakinra and etanercept therapy, the rate of serious infections in the combination arm (7%) was higher than with etanercept alone (0%). The combination of anakinra and etanercept did not result in higher ACR response rates compared to etanercept alone. Two percent of patients treated concurrently with anakinra and etanercept developed neutropenia (ANC $< 1 \times 10^9$/L). Use of anakinra in combination with TNF blocking agents is not recommended). Products include:

Infliximab (A higher rate of serious infections has been observed in patients treated with concurrent anakinra and etanercept therapy than in patients treated with etanercept alone. Two percent of patients treated concurrently with anakinra and etanercept developed neutropenia (ANC $< 1 \times 10^9$/L). Use of anakinra in combination with TNF blocking agents is not recommended). Products include:

Influenza Vaccine, Live Attenuated (No data is available on either the effects of live vaccination or the secondary transmission of infection by live vaccines in patients receiving anakinra. Therefore, live vaccines should not be given concurrently with anakinra).
No products indexed under this heading.

Influenza Virus Vaccine Live, Intranasal (No data is available on either the effects of live vaccination or the secondary transmission of infection by live vaccines in patients receiving anakinra. Therefore, live vaccines should not be given concurrently with anakinra). Products include:

Measles, Mumps, Rubella and Varicella Virus Vaccine Live (No data is available on either the effects of live vaccination or the secondary transmission of infection by live vaccines in patients receiving anakinra. Therefore, live vaccines should not be given concurrently with anakinra). Products include:

Measles, Mumps & Rubella Virus Vaccine, Live (No data is available on either the effects of live vaccination or the secondary transmission of infection by live vaccines in patients receiving anakinra. Therefore, live vaccines should not be given concurrently with anakinra). Products include:

Measles & Rubella Virus Vaccine Live (No data is available on either the effects of live vaccination or the secondary transmission of infection by live vaccines in patients receiving anakinra. Therefore, live vaccines should not be given concurrently with anakinra).
No products indexed under this heading.

Measles Virus Vaccine Live (No data is available on either the effects of live vaccination or the secondary transmission of infection by live vaccines in patients receiving anakinra. Therefore, live vaccines should not be given concurrently with anakinra). Products include:

Mumps Virus Vaccine, Live (No data is available on either the effects of live vaccination or the secondary transmission of infection by live vaccines in patients receiving anakinra. Therefore, live vaccines should not be given concurrently with anakinra). Products include:

Muromonab-CD3 (Infections have been noted in all organ systems and have been reported in patients receiving anakinra alone or in combination with immunosuppressive agents). Products include:

Mycophenolate Mofetil (Infections have been noted in all organ systems and have been reported in patients receiving anakinra alone or in combination with immunosuppressive agents).
No products indexed under this heading.

Poliovirus Vaccine, Live, Oral, Trivalent, Types 1,2,3 (Sabin) (No data is available on either the effects of live vaccination or the secondary transmission of infection by live vaccines in patients receiving anakinra. Therefore, live vaccines should not be given concurrently with anakinra).
No products indexed under this heading.

Rapamycin (Infections have been noted in all organ systems and have been reported in patients receiving anakinra alone or in combination with immunosuppressive agents).
No products indexed under this heading.

Rotavirus Vaccine, Live, Oral, Tetravalent (No data is available on either the effects of live vaccination or the secondary transmission of infection by live vaccines in patients receiving anakinra. Therefore, live vaccines should not be given concurrently with anakinra).
No products indexed under this heading.

Rubella & Mumps Virus Vaccine Live (No data is available on either the effects of live vaccination or the secondary transmission of infection by live vaccines in patients receiving anakinra. Therefore, live vaccines should not be given concurrently with anakinra).
No products indexed under this heading.

Rubella Virus Vaccine Live (No data is available on either the effects of live vaccination or the secondary transmission of infection by live vaccines in patients receiving anakinra. Therefore, live vaccines should not be given concurrently with anakinra). Products include:

Sirolimus (Infections have been noted in all organ systems and have been reported in patients receiving anakinra alone or in combination with immunosuppressive agents). Products include:

Smallpox Vaccine (No data is available on either the effects of live vaccination or the secondary transmission of infection by live vaccines in patients receiving anakinra. Therefore, live vaccines should not be given concurrently with anakinra).
No products indexed under this heading.

Tacrolimus (Infections have been noted in all organ systems and have been reported in patients receiving anakinra alone or in combination with immunosuppressive agents). Products include:

Prograf Capsules 677
Prograf Injection 677
Protopic 685

Typhoid Vaccine (No data is available on either the effects of live vaccination or the secondary transmission of infection by live vaccines in patients receiving anakinra. Therefore, live vaccines should not be given concurrently with anakinra).
No products indexed under this heading.

Varicella Virus Vaccine, Live (No data is available on either the effects of live vaccination or the secondary transmission of infection by live vaccines in patients receiving anakinra. Therefore, live vaccines should not be given concurrently with anakinra). Products include:

Yellow Fever Vaccine (No data is available on either the effects of live vaccination or the secondary transmission of infection by live vaccines in patients receiving anakinra. Therefore, live vaccines should not be given concurrently with anakinra).
No products indexed under this heading.

Zoster Vaccine Live (No data is available on either the effects of live vaccination or the secondary transmission of infection by live vaccines in patients receiving anakinra. Therefore, live vaccines should not be given concurrently with anakinra). Products include:

KINRIX INJECTION VACCINE

(Diptheria and Tetanus Toxoids and Acellular Pertussis Adsorbed and Inactivated Poliovirus Vaccine) 1519
May interact with alkylating agents, antimetabolites, corticosteroids, cytotoxic drugs, immunosuppressive agents, and certain other agents. Compounds in these categories include:

Alclometasone Dipropionate (Immunosuppressive therapies, including corticosteroids (used in greater than physiologic doses), may reduce the immune response to vaccines).
No products indexed under this heading.

Azathioprine (Immunosuppressive therapies, including irradiation, antimetabolites, alkylating agents, cytotoxic drugs, and corticosteroids (used in greater than physiologic doses), may reduce the immune response to vaccines).
No products indexed under this heading.

Basiliximab (Immunosuppressive therapies, including irradiation, antimetabolites, alkylating agents, cytotoxic drugs, and corticosteroids (used in greater than physiologic doses), may reduce the immune response to vaccines). Products include:

Beclomethasone Dipropionate (Immunosuppressive therapies, including corticosteroids (used in greater than physiologic doses), may reduce the immune response to vaccines). Products include:

Beclomethasone Dipropionate Monohydrate (Immunosuppressive therapies, including corticosteroids (used in greater than physiologic doses), may reduce the immune response to vaccines). Products include:

Betamethasone (Immunosuppressive therapies, including corticosteroids (used in greater than physiologic doses), may reduce the immune response to vaccines).
No products indexed under this heading.

Betamethasone Acetate (Immunosuppressive therapies, including corticosteroids (used in greater than physiologic doses), may reduce the immune response to vaccines).
No products indexed under this heading.

Betamethasone Benzoate (Immunosuppressive therapies, including corticosteroids (used in greater than physiologic doses), may reduce the immune response to vaccines).
No products indexed under this heading.

Betamethasone Dipropionate (Immunosuppressive therapies, including corticosteroids (used in greater than physiologic doses), may reduce the immune response to vaccines). Products include:

Betamethasone Sodium Phosphate (Immunosuppressive therapies, including corticosteroids (used in greater than physiologic doses), may reduce the immune response to vaccines).
No products indexed under this heading.

Betamethasone Valerate (Immunosuppressive therapies, including corticosteroids (used in greater than physiologic doses), may reduce the immune response to vaccines). Products include:

Bleomycin Sulfate (Immunosuppressive therapies, including cytotoxic drugs, may reduce the immune response to vaccines).
No products indexed under this heading.

Budesonide (Immunosuppressive therapies, including corticosteroids (used in greater than physiologic doses), may reduce the immune response to vaccines). Products include:

Busulfan (Immunosuppressive therapies, including alkylating agents, may reduce the immune response to vaccines). Products include:

Capecitabine (Immunosuppressive therapies, including antimetabolites, may reduce the immune response to vaccines). Products include:

Carmustine (BCNU) (Immunosuppressive therapies, including alkylating agents, may reduce the immune response to vaccines).
No products indexed under this heading.

Chlorambucil (Immunosuppressive therapies, including alkylating agents, may reduce the immune response to vaccines). Products include:

Ciclesonide (Immunosuppressive therapies, including corticosteroids (used in greater than physiologic doses), may reduce the immune response to vaccines).
No products indexed under this heading.

Cladribine (Immunosuppressive therapies, including antimetabolites, may reduce the immune response to vaccines). Products include:

Cortisone Acetate (Immunosuppressive therapies, including corticosteroids (used in greater than physiologic doses), may reduce the immune response to vaccines).
No products indexed under this heading.

Cyclophosphamide (Immunosuppressive therapies, including alkylating agents, may reduce the immune response to vaccines).
No products indexed under this heading.

(⊙ Described in PDR® for Ophthalmic Medicines)

IMPORTANT NOTE: Always consult each drug listing in the patient's regimen for possible interactions.

Procarbazine Hydrochloride
(Immunosuppressive therapies, including cytotoxic drugs, may reduce the immune response to vaccines).
No products indexed under this heading.

Radiation (Immunosuppressive therapies, including irradiation, may reduce the immune response to vaccines).
No products indexed under this heading.

Rapamycin (Immunosuppressive therapies, including irradiation, antimetabolites, alkylating agents, cytotoxic drugs, and corticosteroids (used in greater than physiologic doses), may reduce the immune response to vaccines).
No products indexed under this heading.

Sirolimus (Immunosuppressive therapies, including irradiation, antimetabolites, alkylating agents, cytotoxic drugs, and corticosteroids (used in greater than physiologic doses), may reduce the immune response to vaccines).
Products include:
Rapamune 3579

Tacrolimus (Immunosuppressive therapies, including irradiation, antimetabolites, alkylating agents, cytotoxic drugs, and corticosteroids (used in greater than physiologic doses), may reduce the immune response to vaccines).
Products include:
Prograf Capsules 677
Prograf Injection 677
Protopic 685

Tamoxifen Citrate (Immunosuppressive therapies, including cytotoxic drugs, may reduce the immune response to vaccines).
No products indexed under this heading.

Thioguanine (Immunosuppressive therapies, including antimetabolites, may reduce the immune response to vaccines). Products include:
Tabloid 1664

Thiotepa (Immunosuppressive therapies, including alkylating agents, may reduce the immune response to vaccines).
No products indexed under this heading.

Triamcinolone (Immunosuppressive therapies, including corticosteroids (used in greater than physiologic doses), may reduce the immune response to vaccines).
No products indexed under this heading.

Triamcinolone Acetonide (Immunosuppressive therapies, including corticosteroids (used in greater than physiologic doses), may reduce the immune response to vaccines). Products include:
Azmacort 408
Nasacort AQ 3019

Triamcinolone Diacetate (Immunosuppressive therapies, including corticosteroids (used in greater than physiologic doses), may reduce the immune response to vaccines).
No products indexed under this heading.

Triamcinolone Hexacetonide (Immunosuppressive therapies, including corticosteroids (used in greater than physiologic doses), may reduce the immune response to vaccines).
No products indexed under this heading.

Vinblastine Sulfate (Immunosuppressive therapies, including cytotoxic drugs, may reduce the immune response to vaccines).
No products indexed under this heading.

Vincristine Sulfate (Immunosuppressive therapies, including cytotoxic drugs, may reduce the immune response to vaccines).
No products indexed under this heading.

Vinorelbine Tartrate (Immunosuppressive therapies, including cytotoxic drugs, may reduce the immune response to vaccines).
No products indexed under this heading.

KLONOPIN TABLETS

(Clonazepam) 2855
May interact with alcohols, anti-anxiety agents, anticonvulsants, antifungals, barbiturates, butyrophenones, central nervous system depressants, cytochrome p450 3a inhibitors (selected), cytochrome p450 inducers (selected), hypnotics and sedatives, monoamine oxidase inhibitors, narcotic analgesics, phenothiazines, phenytoin, tricyclic antidepressants, and certain other agents. Compounds in these categories include:

Alfentanil Hydrochloride (The CNS-depressant action of the benzodiazepine class of drugs may be potentiated by alcohol, narcotics, barbiturates, nonbarbiturate hypnotics, antianxiety agents, phenothiazines, thioxanthene and butyrophenone classes of antipsychotic agents, monoamine oxidase inhibitors and tricyclic antidepressants, and by other anticonvulsant drugs).
No products indexed under this heading.

Allium cepa (Cytochrome P-450 inducers, such as phenytoin, carbamazepine and phenobarbital induce clonazepam metabolism, causing an approximately 30% decrease in plasma clonazepam levels). Products include:
Hyland's Cold 'N Cough 3314
Mederma 2319
Mederma for Kids 2319

Allium sativum (Cytochrome P-450 inducers, such as phenytoin, carbamazepine and phenobarbital induce clonazepam metabolism, causing an approximately 30% decrease in plasma clonazepam levels).
No products indexed under this heading.

Allium schoenoprasum (Cytochrome P-450 inducers, such as phenytoin, carbamazepine and phenobarbital induce clonazepam metabolism, causing an approximately 30% decrease in plasma clonazepam levels).
No products indexed under this heading.

Allium ursinum (Cytochrome P-450 inducers, such as phenytoin, carbamazepine and phenobarbital induce clonazepam metabolism, causing an approximately 30% decrease in plasma clonazepam levels).
No products indexed under this heading.

Alprazolam (The CNS-depressant action of the benzodiazepine class of drugs may be potentiated by alcohol, narcotics, barbiturates, nonbarbiturate hypnotics, antianxiety agents, the phenothiazines, thioxanthene and butyrophenone classes of antipsychotic agents, monoamine oxidase inhibitors and tricyclic antidepressants, and by other anticonvulsant drugs).
No products indexed under this heading.

Aminoglutethimide (Cytochrome P-450 inducers, such as phenytoin, carbamazepine and phenobarbital induce clonazepam metabolism, causing an approximately 30% decrease in plasma clonazepam levels).
No products indexed under this heading.

Amiodarone Hydrochloride (Although clinical studies have not been performed, based on the involvement of the cytochrome P-450 3A family in clonazepam metabolism, inhibitors of this enzyme system, notably oral antifungal agents, should be used cautiously in patients receiving clonazepam).
No products indexed under this heading.

Amitriptyline Hydrochloride (The CNS-depressant action of the benzodiazepine class of drugs may be potentiated by alcohol, narcotics, barbiturates, nonbarbiturate hypnotics, antianxiety agents, the phenothiazines, thioxanthene and butyrophenone classes of antipsychotic agents, monoamine oxidase inhibitors and tricyclic antidepressants, and by other anticonvulsant drugs).
No products indexed under this heading.

Amobarbital (The CNS-depressant action of the benzodiazepine class of drugs may be potentiated by alcohol, narcotics, barbiturates, nonbarbiturate hypnotics, antianxiety agents, phenothiazines, thioxanthene and butyrophenone classes of antipsychotic agents, monoamine oxidase inhibitors and tricyclic antidepressants, and by other anticonvulsant drugs).
No products indexed under this heading.

Amobarbital Sodium (The CNS-depressant action of the benzodiazepine class of drugs may be potentiated by alcohol, narcotics, barbiturates, nonbarbiturate hypnotics, antianxiety agents, phenothiazines, thioxanthene and butyrophenone classes of antipsychotic agents, monoamine oxidase inhibitors and tricyclic antidepressants, and by other anticonvulsant drugs).
No products indexed under this heading.

Amoxapine (The CNS-depressant action of the benzodiazepine class of drugs may be potentiated by alcohol, narcotics, barbiturates, nonbarbiturate hypnotics, antianxiety agents, the phenothiazines, thioxanthene and butyrophenone classes of antipsychotic agents, monoamine oxidase inhibitors and tricyclic antidepressants, and by other anticonvulsant drugs).
No products indexed under this heading.

Amphotericin B (Although clinical studies have not been performed, based on the involvement of the cytochrome P-450 3A family in clonazepam metabolism, inhibitors of this enzyme system, notably oral antifungal agents, should be used cautiously in patients receiving clonazepam).
No products indexed under this heading.

Amphotericin B, liposomal (Although clinical studies have not been performed, based on the involvement of the cytochrome P-450 3A family in clonazepam metabolism, inhibitors of this enzyme system, notably oral antifungal agents, should be used cautiously in patients receiving clonazepam).
Products include:
AmBisome 659

Amphotericin B Cholesteryl Sulfate (Although clinical studies have not been performed, based on the involvement of the cytochrome P-450 3A family in clonazepam metabolism, inhibitors of this enzyme system, notably oral antifungal agents, should be used cautiously in patients receiving clonazepam).
No products indexed under this heading.

Amphotericin B Lipid Complex (Although clinical studies have not been performed, based on the involvement of the cytochrome P-450 3A family in clonazepam metabolism, inhibitors of this enzyme system, notably oral antifungal agents, should be used cautiously in patients receiving clonazepam).
No products indexed under this heading.

Amprenavir (Although clinical studies have not been performed, based on the involvement of the cytochrome P-450 3A family in clonazepam metabolism, inhibitors of this enzyme system, notably oral antifungal agents, should be used cautiously in patients receiving clonazepam).
No products indexed under this heading.

Anidulafungin (Although clinical studies have not been performed, based on the involvement of the cytochrome P-450 3A family in clonazepam metabolism, inhibitors of this enzyme system, notably oral antifungal agents, should be used cautiously in patients receiving clonazepam).
No products indexed under this heading.

Apomorphine (The CNS-depressant action of the benzodiazepine class of drugs may be potentiated by alcohol, narcotics, barbiturates, nonbarbiturate hypnotics, antianxiety agents, phenothiazines, thioxanthene and butyrophenone classes of antipsychotic agents, monoamine oxidase inhibitors and tricyclic antidepressants, and by other anticonvulsant drugs).
No products indexed under this heading.

Apomorphine Hydrochloride (The CNS-depressant action of the benzodiazepine class of drugs may be potentiated by alcohol, narcotics, barbiturates, nonbarbiturate hypnotics, antianxiety agents, phenothiazines, thioxanthene and butyrophenone classes of antipsychotic agents, monoamine oxidase inhibitors and tricyclic antidepressants, and by other anticonvulsant drugs).
No products indexed under this heading.

Aprepitant (Although clinical studies have not been performed, based on the involvement of the cytochrome P-450 3A family in clonazepam metabolism, inhibitors of this enzyme system, notably oral antifungal agents, should be used cautiously in patients receiving clonazepam). Products include:
Emend 2124

Aprobarbital (The CNS-depressant action of the benzodiazepine class of drugs may be potentiated by alcohol, narcotics, barbiturates, nonbarbiturate hypnotics, antianxiety agents, phenothiazines, thioxanthene and butyrophenone classes of antipsychotic agents, monoamine oxidase inhibitors and tricyclic antidepressants, and by other anticonvulsant drugs).
No products indexed under this heading.

Betamethasone (Cytochrome P-450 inducers, such as phenytoin, carbamazepine and phenobarbital induce clonazepam metabolism, causing an approximately 30% decrease in plasma clonazepam levels).
No products indexed under this heading.

Betamethasone Acetate (Cytochrome P-450 inducers, such as phenytoin, carbamazepine and phenobarbital induce clonazepam metabolism, causing an approximately 30% decrease in plasma clonazepam levels).
No products indexed under this heading.

Betamethasone Benzoate (Cytochrome P-450 inducers, such as phenytoin, carbamazepine and phenobarbital induce clonazepam metabolism, causing an approximately 30% decrease in plasma clonazepam levels).
No products indexed under this heading.

Betamethasone Dipropionate (Cytochrome P-450 inducers, such as phenytoin, carbamazepine and phenobarbital induce clonazepam metabolism, causing an approximately 30% decrease in plasma clonazepam levels). Products include:
Diprolene Lotion 0.05% 3108
Diprolene Ointment 0.05% 3109
Diprolene AF Cream 0.05% 3107
Lotrisone 3163

Betamethasone Sodium Phosphate (Cytochrome P-450 inducers, such as phenytoin, carbamazepine and phenobarbital induce clonazepam metabolism, causing an approximately 30% decrease in plasma clonazepam levels).
No products indexed under this heading.

(⊙ Described in PDR® for Ophthalmic Medicines)

949 Interactions Index Klonopin

Betamethasone Valerate (Cytochrome P-450 inducers, such as phenytoin, carbamazepine and phenobarbital induce clonazepam metabolism, causing an approximately 30% decrease in plasma clonazepam levels). Products include:
Luxiq 3321

Bosentan (Cytochrome P-450 inducers, such as phenytoin, carbamazepine and phenobarbital induce clonazepam metabolism, causing an approximately 30% decrease in plasma clonazepam levels). Products include:
Tracleer 573

Buprenorphine Hydrochloride (The CNS-depressant action of the benzodiazepine class of drugs may be potentiated by alcohol, narcotics, barbiturates, nonbarbiturate hypnotics, antianxiety agents, phenothiazines, thioxanthene and butyrophenone classes of antipsychotic agents, monoamine oxidase inhibitors and tricyclic antidepressants, and by other anticonvulsant drugs).
No products indexed under this heading.

Buspirone Hydrochloride (The CNS-depressant action of the benzodiazepine class of drugs may be potentiated by alcohol, narcotics, barbiturates, nonbarbiturate hypnotics, antianxiety agents, the phenothiazines, thioxanthene and butyrophenone classes of antipsychotic agents, monoamine oxidase inhibitors and tricyclic antidepressants, and by other anticonvulsant drugs).
No products indexed under this heading.

Butabarbital (The CNS-depressant action of the benzodiazepine class of drugs may be potentiated by alcohol, narcotics, barbiturates, nonbarbiturate hypnotics, antianxiety agents, phenothiazines, thioxanthene and butyrophenone classes of antipsychotic agents, monoamine oxidase inhibitors and tricyclic antidepressants, and by other anticonvulsant drugs).
No products indexed under this heading.

Butabarbital Sodium (The CNS-depressant action of the benzodiazepine class of drugs may be potentiated by alcohol, narcotics, barbiturates, nonbarbiturate hypnotics, antianxiety agents, phenothiazines, thioxanthene and butyrophenone classes of antipsychotic agents, monoamine oxidase inhibitors and tricyclic antidepressants, and by other anticonvulsant drugs).
No products indexed under this heading.

Butalbital (The CNS-depressant action of the benzodiazepine class of drugs may be potentiated by alcohol, narcotics, barbiturates, nonbarbiturate hypnotics, antianxiety agents, phenothiazines, thioxanthene and butyrophenone classes of antipsychotic agents, monoamine oxidase inhibitors and tricyclic antidepressants, and by other anticonvulsant drugs).
No products indexed under this heading.

Butoconazole Nitrate (Although clinical studies have not been performed, based on the involvement of the cytochrome P-450 3A family in clonazepam metabolism, inhibitors of this enzyme system, notably oral antifungal agents, should be used cautiously in patients receiving clonazepam).
No products indexed under this heading.

Carbamazepine (Induces clonazepam metabolism causing an approximately 30% decrease in plasma clonazepam levels). Products include:
Carbatrol 3280
Equetro 3477

Caspofungin acetate (Although clinical studies have not been performed, based on the involvement of the cytochrome P-450 3A family in clonazepam metabolism, inhibitors of this enzyme system, notably oral antifungal agents, should be used cautiously in patients receiving clonazepam). Products include:
Cancidas 2088

Chloral Hydrate (The CNS-depressant action of the benzodiazepine class of drugs may be potentiated by alcohol, narcotics, barbiturates, nonbarbiturate hypnotics, antianxiety agents, the phenothiazines, thioxanthene and butyrophenone classes of antipsychotic agents, monoamine oxidase inhibitors and tricyclic antidepressants, and by other anticonvulsant drugs).
No products indexed under this heading.

Chlordiazepoxide (Since clonazepam produces CNS depression, patients receiving this drug should be warned about the concomitant use of alcohol or other CNS-depressant drugs during clonazepam therapy).
No products indexed under this heading.

Chlordiazepoxide Hydrochloride (Since clonazepam produces CNS depression, patients receiving this drug should be warned about the concomitant use of alcohol or other CNS-depressant drugs during clonazepam therapy).
No products indexed under this heading.

Chlorpromazine (The CNS-depressant action of the benzodiazepine class of drugs may be potentiated by alcohol, narcotics, barbiturates, nonbarbiturate hypnotics, antianxiety agents, the phenothiazines, thioxanthene and butyrophenone classes of antipsychotic agents, monoamine oxidase inhibitors and tricyclic antidepressants, and by other anticonvulsant drugs).
No products indexed under this heading.

Chlorpromazine Hydrochloride (The CNS-depressant action of the benzodiazepine class of drugs may be potentiated by alcohol, narcotics, barbiturates, nonbarbiturate hypnotics, antianxiety agents, the phenothiazines, thioxanthene and butyrophenone classes of antipsychotic agents, monoamine oxidase inhibitors and tricyclic antidepressants, and by other anticonvulsant drugs).
No products indexed under this heading.

Chlorprothixene (Since clonazepam produces CNS depression, patients receiving this drug should be warned about the concomitant use of alcohol or other CNS-depressant drugs during clonazepam therapy).
No products indexed under this heading.

Chlorprothixene Hydrochloride (Since clonazepam produces CNS depression, patients receiving this drug should be warned about the concomitant use of alcohol or other CNS-depressant drugs during clonazepam therapy).
No products indexed under this heading.

Chlorprothixene Lactate (Since clonazepam produces CNS depression, patients receiving this drug should be warned about the concomitant use of alcohol or other CNS-depressant drugs during clonazepam therapy).
No products indexed under this heading.

Cimetidine (Although clinical studies have not been performed, based on the involvement of the cytochrome P-450 3A family in clonazepam metabolism, inhibitors of this enzyme system, notably oral antifungal agents, should be used cautiously in patients receiving clonazepam).
No products indexed under this heading.

Cimetidine Hydrochloride (Although clinical studies have not been performed, based on the involvement of the cytochrome P-450 3A family in clonazepam metabolism, inhibitors of this enzyme system, notably oral antifungal agents, should be used cautiously in patients receiving clonazepam).
No products indexed under this heading.

Ciprofloxacin (Although clinical studies have not been performed, based on the involvement of the cytochrome P-450 3A family in clonazepam metabolism, inhibitors of this enzyme system, notably oral antifungal agents, should be used cautiously in patients receiving clonazepam). Products include:
Cipro I.V. 3082
Cipro 3073
Cipro XR 3091
Ciprodex 583

Ciprofloxacin Hydrochloride (Although clinical studies have not been performed, based on the involvement of the cytochrome P-450 3A family in clonazepam metabolism, inhibitors of this enzyme system, notably oral antifungal agents, should be used cautiously in patients receiving clonazepam). Products include:
Cipro 3073

Cisplatin (Cytochrome P-450 inducers, such as phenytoin, carbamazepine and phenobarbital induce clonazepam metabolism, causing an approximately 30% decrease in plasma clonazepam levels).
No products indexed under this heading.

Citalopram Hydrobromide (Cytochrome P-450 inducers, such as phenytoin, carbamazepine and phenobarbital induce clonazepam metabolism, causing an approximately 30% decrease in plasma clonazepam levels). Products include:
Celexa 1153

Clarithromycin (Although clinical studies have not been performed, based on the involvement of the cytochrome P-450 3A family in clonazepam metabolism, inhibitors of this enzyme system, notably oral antifungal agents, should be used cautiously in patients receiving clonazepam). Products include:
Biaxin/Biaxin XL 412

Clomipramine Hydrochloride (The CNS-depressant action of the benzodiazepine class of drugs may be potentiated by alcohol, narcotics, barbiturates, nonbarbiturate hypnotics, antianxiety agents, the phenothiazines, thioxanthene and butyrophenone classes of antipsychotic agents, monoamine oxidase inhibitors and tricyclic antidepressants, and by other anticonvulsant drugs).
No products indexed under this heading.

Clorazepate Dipotassium (The CNS-depressant action of the benzodiazepine class of drugs may be potentiated by alcohol, narcotics, barbiturates, nonbarbiturate hypnotics, antianxiety agents, the phenothiazines, thioxanthene and butyrophenone classes of antipsychotic agents, monoamine oxidase inhibitors and tricyclic antidepressants, and by other anticonvulsant drugs).
No products indexed under this heading.

Clotrimazole (Although clinical studies have not been performed, based on the involvement of the cytochrome P-450 3A family in clonazepam metabolism, inhibitors of this enzyme system, notably oral antifungal agents, should be used cautiously in patients receiving clonazepam). Products include:
Lotrisone 3163

Clotrimazole, Topical (Although clinical studies have not been performed, based on the involvement of the cytochrome P-450 3A family in clonazepam metabolism, inhibitors of this enzyme system, notably oral antifungal agents, should be used cautiously in patients receiving clonazepam).
No products indexed under this heading.

Clozapine (Since clonazepam produces CNS depression, patients receiving this drug should be warned about the concomitant use of alcohol or other CNS-depressant drugs during clonazepam therapy).
No products indexed under this heading.

Codeine Phosphate (The CNS-depressant action of the benzodiazepine class of drugs may be potentiated by alcohol, narcotics, barbiturates, nonbarbiturate hypnotics, antianxiety agents, phenothiazines, thioxanthene and butyrophenone classes of antipsychotic agents, monoamine oxidase inhibitors and tricyclic antidepressants, and by other anticonvulsant drugs). Products include:
Tylenol with Codeine 2691

Codeine Sulfate (The CNS-depressant action of the benzodiazepine class of drugs may be potentiated by alcohol, narcotics, barbiturates, nonbarbiturate hypnotics, antianxiety agents, phenothiazines, thioxanthene and butyrophenone classes of antipsychotic agents, monoamine oxidase inhibitors and tricyclic antidepressants, and by other anticonvulsant drugs).
No products indexed under this heading.

Cortisone Acetate (Cytochrome P-450 inducers, such as phenytoin, carbamazepine and phenobarbital induce clonazepam metabolism, causing an approximately 30% decrease in plasma clonazepam levels).
No products indexed under this heading.

Cyclosporine (Although clinical studies have not been performed, based on the involvement of the cytochrome P-450 3A family in clonazepam metabolism, inhibitors of this enzyme system, notably oral antifungal agents, should be used cautiously in patients receiving clonazepam). Products include:
Gengraf 440
Neoral Oral Solution 2496
Neoral Capsules 2496
Restasis 605

Delavirdine Mesylate (Although clinical studies have not been performed, based on the involvement of the cytochrome P-450 3A family in clonazepam metabolism, inhibitors of this enzyme system, notably oral antifungal agents, should be used cautiously in patients receiving clonazepam).
No products indexed under this heading.

Desflurane (Since clonazepam produces CNS depression, patients receiving this drug should be warned about the concomitant use of alcohol or other CNS-depressant drugs during clonazepam therapy).
No products indexed under this heading.

Desipramine Hydrochloride (The CNS-depressant action of the benzodiazepine class of drugs may be potentiated by alcohol, narcotics, barbiturates, nonbarbiturate hypnotics, antianxiety agents, the phenothiazines, thioxanthene and butyrophenone classes of antipsychotic agents, monoamine oxidase inhibitors and tricyclic antidepressants, and by other anticonvulsant drugs).
No products indexed under this heading.

Dexamethasone (Cytochrome P-450 inducers, such as phenytoin, carbamazepine and phenobarbital induce clonazepam metabolism, causing an approximately 30% decrease in plasma clonazepam levels). Products include:

IMPORTANT NOTE: Always consult each drug listing in the patient's regimen for possible interactions.

Klonopin | Interactions Index | 950

Ciprodex 583
Ozurdex .... ⊙223
Tobramycin and Dexamethasone Ophthalmic Suspension .... ⊙251

Dexamethasone Acetate (Cytochrome P-450 inducers, such as phenytoin, carbamazepine and phenobarbital induce clonazepam metabolism, causing an approximately 30% decrease in plasma clonazepam levels).
No products indexed under this heading.

Dexamethasone Phosphate (Cytochrome P-450 inducers, such as phenytoin, carbamazepine and phenobarbital induce clonazepam metabolism, causing an approximately 30% decrease in plasma clonazepam levels).
No products indexed under this heading.

Dexamethasone Sodium (Cytochrome P-450 inducers, such as phenytoin, carbamazepine and phenobarbital induce clonazepam metabolism, causing an approximately 30% decrease in plasma clonazepam levels).
No products indexed under this heading.

Dexamethasone Sodium Phosphate (Cytochrome P-450 inducers, such as phenytoin, carbamazepine and phenobarbital induce clonazepam metabolism, causing an approximately 30% decrease in plasma clonazepam levels).
No products indexed under this heading.

Dexamethasone Sodium Phosphate Injection (Cytochrome P-450 inducers, such as phenytoin, carbamazepine and phenobarbital induce clonazepam metabolism, causing an approximately 30% decrease in plasma clonazepam levels).
No products indexed under this heading.

Dezocine (The CNS-depressant action of the benzodiazepine class of drugs may be potentiated by alcohol, narcotics, barbiturates, nonbarbiturate hypnotics, antianxiety agents, phenothiazines, thioxanthene and butyrophenone classes of antipsychotic agents, monoamine oxidase inhibitors and tricyclic antidepressants, and by other anticonvulsant drugs).
No products indexed under this heading.

Diazepam (Since clonazepam produces CNS depression, patients receiving this drug should be warned about the concomitant use of alcohol or other CNS-depressant drugs during clonazepam therapy). Products include:
Valium Tablets 2880

Dihydrocodeine Bitartrate (The CNS-depressant action of the benzodiazepine class of drugs may be potentiated by alcohol, narcotics, barbiturates, nonbarbiturate hypnotics, antianxiety agents, phenothiazines, thioxanthene and butyrophenone classes of antipsychotic agents, monoamine oxidase inhibitors and tricyclic antidepressants, and by other anticonvulsant drugs).
No products indexed under this heading.

Dihydrocodeinone Bitartrate (The CNS-depressant action of the benzodiazepine class of drugs may be potentiated by alcohol, narcotics, barbiturates, nonbarbiturate hypnotics, antianxiety agents, phenothiazines, thioxanthene and butyrophenone classes of antipsychotic agents, monoamine oxidase inhibitors and tricyclic antidepressants, and by other anticonvulsant drugs).
No products indexed under this heading.

Diltiazem Hydrochloride (Although clinical studies have not been performed, based on the involvement of the cytochrome P-450 3A family in clonazepam metabolism, inhibitors of this enzyme system, notably oral antifungal agents, should be used cautiously in patients receiving clonazepam). Products include:
Cardizem LA 423

Diltiazem Maleate (Although clinical studies have not been performed, based on the involvement of the cytochrome P-450 3A family in clonazepam metabolism, inhibitors of this enzyme system, notably oral antifungal agents, should be used cautiously in patients receiving clonazepam).
No products indexed under this heading.

Divalproex Sodium (The CNS-depressant action of the benzodiazepine class of drugs may be potentiated by alcohol, narcotics, barbiturates, nonbarbiturate hypnotics, antianxiety agents, the phenothiazines, thioxanthene and butyrophenone classes of antipsychotic agents, monoamine oxidase inhibitors and tricyclic antidepressants, and by other anticonvulsant drugs). Products include:
Depakote ER 426

Doxepin Hydrochloride (The CNS-depressant action of the benzodiazepine class of drugs may be potentiated by alcohol, narcotics, barbiturates, nonbarbiturate hypnotics, antianxiety agents, the phenothiazines, thioxanthene and butyrophenone classes of antipsychotic agents, monoamine oxidase inhibitors and tricyclic antidepressants, and by other anticonvulsant drugs).
No products indexed under this heading.

Doxorubicin Hydrochloride (Cytochrome P-450 inducers, such as phenytoin, carbamazepine and phenobarbital induce clonazepam metabolism, causing an approximately 30% decrease in plasma clonazepam levels).
No products indexed under this heading.

Droperidol (Since clonazepam produces CNS depression, patients receiving this drug should be warned about the concomitant use of alcohol or other CNS-depressant drugs during clonazepam therapy).
No products indexed under this heading.

Duloxetine Hydrochloride (The CNS-depressant action of the benzodiazepine class of drugs may be potentiated by alcohol, narcotics, barbiturates, nonbarbiturate hypnotics, antianxiety agents, the phenothiazines, thioxanthene and butyrophenone classes of antipsychotic agents, monoamine oxidase inhibitors and tricyclic antidepressants, and by other anticonvulsant drugs). Products include:
Cymbalta 1871

Econazole Nitrate (Although clinical studies have not been performed, based on the involvement of the cytochrome P-450 3A family in clonazepam metabolism, inhibitors of this enzyme system, notably oral antifungal agents, should be used cautiously in patients receiving clonazepam).
No products indexed under this heading.

Efavirenz (Although clinical studies have not been performed, based on the involvement of the cytochrome P-450 3A family in clonazepam metabolism, inhibitors of this enzyme system, notably oral antifungal agents, should be used cautiously in patients receiving clonazepam). Products include:
Atripla 906

Enflurane (Since clonazepam produces CNS depression, patients receiving this drug should be warned about the concomitant use of alcohol or other CNS-depressant drugs during clonazepam therapy).
No products indexed under this heading.

Erythromycin (Although clinical studies have not been performed, based on the involvement of the cytochrome P-450 3A family in clonazepam metabolism, inhibitors of this enzyme system, notably oral antifungal agents, should be used cautiously in patients receiving clonazepam).
No products indexed under this heading.

Erythromycin, Topical (Cytochrome P-450 inducers, such as phenytoin, carbamazepine and phenobarbital induce clonazepam metabolism, causing an approximately 30% decrease in plasma clonazepam levels).
No products indexed under this heading.

Erythromycin Estolate (Cytochrome P-450 inducers, such as phenytoin, carbamazepine and phenobarbital induce clonazepam metabolism, causing an approximately 30% decrease in plasma clonazepam levels).
No products indexed under this heading.

Erythromycin Ethylsuccinate (Cytochrome P-450 inducers, such as phenytoin, carbamazepine and phenobarbital induce clonazepam metabolism, causing an approximately 30% decrease in plasma clonazepam levels). Products include:
E.E.S. 437
EryPed 435

Erythromycin Gluceptate (Cytochrome P-450 inducers, such as phenytoin, carbamazepine and phenobarbital induce clonazepam metabolism, causing an approximately 30% decrease in plasma clonazepam levels).
No products indexed under this heading.

Erythromycin Lactobionate (Cytochrome P-450 inducers, such as phenytoin, carbamazepine and phenobarbital induce clonazepam metabolism, causing an approximately 30% decrease in plasma clonazepam levels).
No products indexed under this heading.

Erythromycin Stearate (Cytochrome P-450 inducers, such as phenytoin, carbamazepine and phenobarbital induce clonazepam metabolism, causing an approximately 30% decrease in plasma clonazepam levels).
No products indexed under this heading.

Escitalopram Oxalate (The CNS-depressant action of the benzodiazepine class of drugs may be potentiated by alcohol, narcotics, barbiturates, nonbarbiturate hypnotics, antianxiety agents, the phenothiazines, thioxanthene and butyrophenone classes of antipsychotic agents, monoamine oxidase inhibitors and tricyclic antidepressants, and by other anticonvulsant drugs). Products include:
Lexapro Oral Suspension 1160
Lexapro Tablets 1160

Esomeprazole Magnesium (Cytochrome P-450 inducers, such as phenytoin, carbamazepine and phenobarbital induce clonazepam metabolism, causing an approximately 30% decrease in plasma clonazepam levels). Products include:
Nexium Capsules 704
Nexium Oral Suspension 704

Esomeprazole Sodium (Cytochrome P-450 inducers, such as phenytoin, carbamazepine and phenobarbital induce clonazepam metabolism, causing an approximately 30% decrease in plasma clonazepam levels). Products include:
Nexium I.V. 712

Estazolam (The CNS-depressant action of the benzodiazepine class of drugs may be potentiated by alcohol, narcotics, barbiturates, nonbarbiturate hypnotics, antianxiety agents, the phenothiazines, thioxanthene and butyrophenone classes of antipsychotic agents, monoamine oxidase inhibitors and tricyclic antidepressants, and by other anticonvulsant drugs).
No products indexed under this heading.

Ethanol (The CNS-depressant action of the benzodiazepine class of drugs may be potentiated by alcohol. Patients should be advised to avoid alcohol while taking clonazepam).
No products indexed under this heading.

Ethchlorvynol (The CNS-depressant action of the benzodiazepine class of drugs may be potentiated by alcohol, narcotics, barbiturates, nonbarbiturate hypnotics, antianxiety agents, the phenothiazines, thioxanthene and butyrophenone classes of antipsychotic agents, monoamine oxidase inhibitors and tricyclic antidepressants, and by other anticonvulsant drugs).
No products indexed under this heading.

Ethinamate (The CNS-depressant action of the benzodiazepine class of drugs may be potentiated by alcohol, narcotics, barbiturates, nonbarbiturate hypnotics, antianxiety agents, the phenothiazines, thioxanthene and butyrophenone classes of antipsychotic agents, monoamine oxidase inhibitors and tricyclic antidepressants, and by other anticonvulsant drugs).
No products indexed under this heading.

Ethosuximide (The CNS-depressant action of the benzodiazepine class of drugs may be potentiated by alcohol, narcotics, barbiturates, nonbarbiturate hypnotics, antianxiety agents, the phenothiazines, thioxanthene and butyrophenone classes of antipsychotic agents, monoamine oxidase inhibitors and tricyclic antidepressants, and by other anticonvulsant drugs).
No products indexed under this heading.

Ethotoin (The CNS-depressant action of the benzodiazepine class of drugs may be potentiated by alcohol, narcotics, barbiturates, nonbarbiturate hypnotics, antianxiety agents, the phenothiazines, thioxanthene and butyrophenone classes of antipsychotic agents, monoamine oxidase inhibitors and tricyclic antidepressants, and by other anticonvulsant drugs).
No products indexed under this heading.

Ethyl Alcohol (The CNS-depressant action of the benzodiazepine class of drugs may be potentiated by alcohol. Patients should be advised to avoid alcohol while taking clonazepam).
No products indexed under this heading.

Felbamate (The CNS-depressant action of the benzodiazepine class of drugs may be potentiated by alcohol, narcotics, barbiturates, nonbarbiturate hypnotics, antianxiety agents, the phenothiazines, thioxanthene and butyrophenone classes of antipsychotic agents, monoamine oxidase inhibitors and tricyclic antidepressants, and by other anticonvulsant drugs).
No products indexed under this heading.

Fentanyl (The CNS-depressant action of the benzodiazepine class of drugs may be potentiated by alcohol, narcotics, barbiturates, nonbarbiturate hypnotics, antianxiety agents, phenothiazines, thioxanthene and butyrophenone classes of antipsychotic agents, monoamine oxidase inhibitors and tricyclic antidepressants, and by other anticonvulsant drugs). Products include:
Duragesic 2604
Fentanyl Transdermal System 2346
Onsolis 2054

(⊙ Described in PDR® for Ophthalmic Medicines)

951 Interactions Index Klonopin

Fentanyl Citrate (The CNS-depressant action of the benzodiazepine class of drugs may be potentiated by alcohol, narcotics, barbiturates, nonbarbiturate hypnotics, antianxiety agents, phenothiazines, thioxanthene and butyrophenone classes of antipsychotic agents, monoamine oxidase inhibitors and tricyclic antidepressants, and by other anticonvulsant drugs).
Products include:
Fentora 966

Fluconazole (Although clinical studies have not been performed, based on the involvement of the cytochrome P-450 3A family in clonazepam metabolism, inhibitors of this enzyme system, notably oral antifungal agents, should be used cautiously in patients receiving clonazepam).
No products indexed under this heading.

Flucytosine (Although clinical studies have not been performed, based on the involvement of the cytochrome P-450 3A family in clonazepam metabolism, inhibitors of this enzyme system, notably oral antifungal agents, should be used cautiously in patients receiving clonazepam).
No products indexed under this heading.

Fludrocortisone Acetate (Cytochrome P-450 inducers, such as phenytoin, carbamazepine and phenobarbital induce clonazepam metabolism, causing an approximately 30% decrease in plasma clonazepam levels).
No products indexed under this heading.

Fluoxetine (Although clinical studies have not been performed, based on the involvement of the cytochrome P-450 3A family in clonazepam metabolism, inhibitors of this enzyme system, notably oral antifungal agents, should be used cautiously in patients receiving clonazepam).
No products indexed under this heading.

Fluoxetine Hydrochloride (Although clinical studies have not been performed, based on the involvement of the cytochrome P-450 3A family in clonazepam metabolism, inhibitors of this enzyme system, notably oral antifungal agents, should be used cautiously in patients receiving clonazepam).
Products include:
Prozac Weekly 1941
Prozac Pulvules 1941
Symbyax 1965

Fluphenazine Decanoate (The CNS-depressant action of the benzodiazepine class of drugs may be potentiated by alcohol, narcotics, barbiturates, nonbarbiturate hypnotics, antianxiety agents, the phenothiazines, thioxanthene and butyrophenone classes of antipsychotic agents, monoamine oxidase inhibitors and tricyclic antidepressants, and by other anticonvulsant drugs).
No products indexed under this heading.

Fluphenazine Enanthate (The CNS-depressant action of the benzodiazepine class of drugs may be potentiated by alcohol, narcotics, barbiturates, nonbarbiturate hypnotics, antianxiety agents, the phenothiazines, thioxanthene and butyrophenone classes of antipsychotic agents, monoamine oxidase inhibitors and tricyclic antidepressants, and by other anticonvulsant drugs).
No products indexed under this heading.

Fluphenazine Hydrochloride (The CNS-depressant action of the benzodiazepine class of drugs may be potentiated by alcohol, narcotics, barbiturates, nonbarbiturate hypnotics, antianxiety agents, the phenothiazines, thioxanthene and butyrophenone classes of antipsychotic agents, monoamine oxidase inhibitors and tricyclic antidepressants, and by other anticonvulsant drugs).
No products indexed under this heading.

Flurazepam Hydrochloride (The CNS-depressant action of the benzodiazepine class of drugs may be potentiated by alcohol, narcotics, barbiturates, nonbarbiturate hypnotics, antianxiety agents, the phenothiazines, thioxanthene and butyrophenone classes of antipsychotic agents, monoamine oxidase inhibitors and tricyclic antidepressants, and by other anticonvulsant drugs).
No products indexed under this heading.

Fluvoxamine (The CNS-depressant action of the benzodiazepine class of drugs may be potentiated by alcohol, narcotics, barbiturates, nonbarbiturate hypnotics, antianxiety agents, the phenothiazines, thioxanthene and butyrophenone classes of antipsychotic agents, monoamine oxidase inhibitors and tricyclic antidepressants, and by other anticonvulsant drugs).
No products indexed under this heading.

Fluvoxamine Maleate (The CNS-depressant action of the benzodiazepine class of drugs may be potentiated by alcohol, narcotics, barbiturates, nonbarbiturate hypnotics, antianxiety agents, the phenothiazines, thioxanthene and butyrophenone classes of antipsychotic agents, monoamine oxidase inhibitors and tricyclic antidepressants, and by other anticonvulsant drugs).
No products indexed under this heading.

Fosphenytoin (Cytochrome P-450 inducers, such as phenytoin, carbamazepine and phenobarbital, induce clonazepam metabolism, causing an approximately 30% decrease in plasma clonazepam levels).
No products indexed under this heading.

Fosphenytoin Sodium (Cytochrome P-450 inducers, such as phenytoin, carbamazepine and phenobarbital, induce clonazepam metabolism, causing an approximately 30% decrease in plasma clonazepam levels).
No products indexed under this heading.

Gabapentin (The CNS-depressant action of the benzodiazepine class of drugs may be potentiated by alcohol, narcotics, barbiturates, nonbarbiturate hypnotics, antianxiety agents, the phenothiazines, thioxanthene and butyrophenone classes of antipsychotic agents, monoamine oxidase inhibitors and tricyclic antidepressants, and by other anticonvulsant drugs).
No products indexed under this heading.

Garlic Extract (Cytochrome P-450 inducers, such as phenytoin, carbamazepine and phenobarbital induce clonazepam metabolism, causing an approximately 30% decrease in plasma clonazepam levels).
No products indexed under this heading.

Garlic Oil (Cytochrome P-450 inducers, such as phenytoin, carbamazepine and phenobarbital induce clonazepam metabolism, causing an approximately 30% decrease in plasma clonazepam levels).
No products indexed under this heading.

Glutethimide (The CNS-depressant action of the benzodiazepine class of drugs may be potentiated by alcohol, narcotics, barbiturates, nonbarbiturate hypnotics, antianxiety agents, the phenothiazines, thioxanthene and butyrophenone classes of antipsychotic agents, monoamine oxidase inhibitors and tricyclic antidepressants, and by other anticonvulsant drugs).
No products indexed under this heading.

Griseofulvin (Although clinical studies have not been performed, based on the involvement of the cytochrome P-450 3A family in clonazepam metabolism, inhibitors of this enzyme system, notably oral antifungal agents, should be used cautiously in patients receiving clonazepam).
No products indexed under this heading.

Halazepam (Since clonazepam produces CNS depression, patients receiving this drug should be warned about the concomitant use of alcohol or other CNS-depressant drugs during clonazepam therapy).
No products indexed under this heading.

Haloperidol (The CNS-depressant action of the benzodiazepine class of drugs may be potentiated by alcohol, narcotics, barbiturates, nonbarbiturate hypnotics, antianxiety agents, the phenothiazines, thioxanthene and butyrophenone classes of antipsychotic agents, monoamine oxidase inhibitors and tricyclic antidepressants, and by other anticonvulsant drugs).
No products indexed under this heading.

Haloperidol Decanoate (The CNS-depressant action of the benzodiazepine class of drugs may be potentiated by alcohol, narcotics, barbiturates, nonbarbiturate hypnotics, antianxiety agents, the phenothiazines, thioxanthene and butyrophenone classes of antipsychotic agents, monoamine oxidase inhibitors and tricyclic antidepressants, and by other anticonvulsant drugs).
No products indexed under this heading.

Haloperidol Lactate (Since clonazepam produces CNS depression, patients receiving this drug should be warned about the concomitant use of alcohol or other CNS-depressant drugs during clonazepam therapy).
No products indexed under this heading.

Hexobarbital (The CNS-depressant action of the benzodiazepine class of drugs may be potentiated by alcohol, narcotics, barbiturates, nonbarbiturate hypnotics, antianxiety agents, phenothiazines, thioxanthene and butyrophenone classes of antipsychotic agents, monoamine oxidase inhibitors and tricyclic antidepressants, and by other anticonvulsant drugs).
No products indexed under this heading.

Hydrocodone Bitartrate (The CNS-depressant action of the benzodiazepine class of drugs may be potentiated by alcohol, narcotics, barbiturates, nonbarbiturate hypnotics, antianxiety agents, phenothiazines, thioxanthene and butyrophenone classes of antipsychotic agents, monoamine oxidase inhibitors and tricyclic antidepressants, and by other anticonvulsant drugs).
Products include:
Vicodin 560
Vicodin ES 561
Vicodin HP 563
Vicoprofen 564
Zydone 1138

Hydrocodone Polistirex (The CNS-depressant action of the benzodiazepine class of drugs may be potentiated by alcohol, narcotics, barbiturates, nonbarbiturate hypnotics, antianxiety agents, phenothiazines, thioxanthene and butyrophenone classes of antipsychotic agents, monoamine oxidase inhibitors and tricyclic antidepressants, and by other anticonvulsant drugs).
Products include:
Tussionex 3443

Hydrocortisone (Cytochrome P-450 inducers, such as phenytoin, carbamazepine and phenobarbital induce clonazepam metabolism, causing an approximately 30% decrease in plasma clonazepam levels).
No products indexed under this heading.

Hydrocortisone (Alcohol) (Cytochrome P-450 inducers, such as phenytoin, carbamazepine and phenobarbital induce clonazepam metabolism, causing an approximately 30% decrease in plasma clonazepam levels).
No products indexed under this heading.

Hydrocortisone Acetate (Cytochrome P-450 inducers, such as phenytoin, carbamazepine and phenobarbital induce clonazepam metabolism, causing an approximately 30% decrease in plasma clonazepam levels).
No products indexed under this heading.

Hydrocortisone Butyrate (Cytochrome P-450 inducers, such as phenytoin, carbamazepine and phenobarbital induce clonazepam metabolism, causing an approximately 30% decrease in plasma clonazepam levels).
No products indexed under this heading.

Hydrocortisone Cypionate (Cytochrome P-450 inducers, such as phenytoin, carbamazepine and phenobarbital induce clonazepam metabolism, causing an approximately 30% decrease in plasma clonazepam levels).
No products indexed under this heading.

Hydrocortisone Hemisuccinate (Cytochrome P-450 inducers, such as phenytoin, carbamazepine and phenobarbital induce clonazepam metabolism, causing an approximately 30% decrease in plasma clonazepam levels).
No products indexed under this heading.

Hydrocortisone Probutate (Cytochrome P-450 inducers, such as phenytoin, carbamazepine and phenobarbital induce clonazepam metabolism, causing an approximately 30% decrease in plasma clonazepam levels).
No products indexed under this heading.

Hydrocortisone Sodium Phosphate (Cytochrome P-450 inducers, such as phenytoin, carbamazepine and phenobarbital induce clonazepam metabolism, causing an approximately 30% decrease in plasma clonazepam levels).
No products indexed under this heading.

Hydrocortisone Sodium Succinate (Cytochrome P-450 inducers, such as phenytoin, carbamazepine and phenobarbital induce clonazepam metabolism, causing an approximately 30% decrease in plasma clonazepam levels).
No products indexed under this heading.

Hydrocortisone Valerate (Cytochrome P-450 inducers, such as phenytoin, carbamazepine and phenobarbital induce clonazepam metabolism, causing an approximately 30% decrease in plasma clonazepam levels).
No products indexed under this heading.

Hydromorphone (The CNS-depressant action of the benzodiazepine class of drugs may be potentiated by alcohol, narcotics, barbiturates, nonbarbiturate hypnotics, antianxiety agents, phenothiazines, thioxanthene and butyrophenone classes of antipsychotic agents, monoamine oxidase inhibitors and tricyclic antidepressants, and by other anticonvulsant drugs).
No products indexed under this heading.

Hydromorphone Hydrochloride (The CNS-depressant action of the ben-

953 **Interactions Index** **Klonopin**

Maprotiline Hydrochloride (The CNS-depressant action of the benzodiazepine class of drugs may be potentiated by alcohol, narcotics, barbiturates, nonbarbiturate hypnotics, antianxiety agents, the phenothiazines, thioxanthene and butyrophenone classes of antipsychotic agents, monoamine oxidase inhibitors and tricyclic antidepressants, and by other anticonvulsant drugs).
No products indexed under this heading.

Meperidine Hydrochloride (The CNS-depressant action of the benzodiazepine class of drugs may be potentiated by alcohol, narcotics, barbiturates, nonbarbiturate hypnotics, antianxiety agents, phenothiazines, thioxanthene and butyrophenone classes of antipsychotic agents, monoamine oxidase inhibitors and tricyclic antidepressants, and by other anticonvulsant drugs).
No products indexed under this heading.

Mephenytoin (The CNS-depressant action of the benzodiazepine class of drugs may be potentiated by alcohol, narcotics, barbiturates, nonbarbiturate hypnotics, antianxiety agents, the phenothiazines, thioxanthene and butyrophenone classes of antipsychotic agents, monoamine oxidase inhibitors and tricyclic antidepressants, and by other anticonvulsant drugs).
No products indexed under this heading.

Mephobarbital (The CNS-depressant action of the benzodiazepine class of drugs may be potentiated by alcohol, narcotics, barbiturates, nonbarbiturate hypnotics, antianxiety agents, phenothiazines, thioxanthene and butyrophenone classes of antipsychotic agents, monoamine oxidase inhibitors and tricyclic antidepressants, and by other anticonvulsant drugs).
No products indexed under this heading.

Meprobamate (Since clonazepam produces CNS depression, patients receiving this drug should be warned about the concomitant use of alcohol or other CNS-depressant drugs during clonazepam therapy).
No products indexed under this heading.

Mesoridazine Besylate (The CNS-depressant action of the benzodiazepine class of drugs may be potentiated by alcohol, narcotics, barbiturates, nonbarbiturate hypnotics, antianxiety agents, the phenothiazines, thioxanthene and butyrophenone classes of antipsychotic agents, monoamine oxidase inhibitors and tricyclic antidepressants, and by other anticonvulsant drugs).
No products indexed under this heading.

Methadone Hydrochloride (The CNS-depressant action of the benzodiazepine class of drugs may be potentiated by alcohol, narcotics, barbiturates, nonbarbiturate hypnotics, antianxiety agents, phenothiazines, thioxanthene and butyrophenone classes of antipsychotic agents, monoamine oxidase inhibitors and tricyclic antidepressants, and by other anticonvulsant drugs).
No products indexed under this heading.

Methohexital Sodium (Since clonazepam produces CNS depression, patients receiving this drug should be warned about the concomitant use of alcohol or other CNS-depressant drugs during clonazepam therapy).
No products indexed under this heading.

Methotrimeprazine (The CNS-depressant action of the benzodiazepine class of drugs may be potentiated by alcohol, narcotics, barbiturates, nonbarbiturate hypnotics, antianxiety agents, the phenothiazines, thioxanthene and butyrophenone classes of antipsychotic agents, monoamine oxidase inhibitors and tricyclic antidepressants, and by other anticonvulsant drugs).
No products indexed under this heading.

Methoxyflurane (Since clonazepam produces CNS depression, patients receiving this drug should be warned about the concomitant use of alcohol or other CNS-depressant drugs during clonazepam therapy).
No products indexed under this heading.

Methsuximide (The CNS-depressant action of the benzodiazepine class of drugs may be potentiated by alcohol, narcotics, barbiturates, nonbarbiturate hypnotics, antianxiety agents, the phenothiazines, thioxanthene and butyrophenone classes of antipsychotic agents, monoamine oxidase inhibitors and tricyclic antidepressants, and by other anticonvulsant drugs).
No products indexed under this heading.

Methylprednisolone (Cytochrome P-450 inducers, such as phenytoin, carbamazepine and phenobarbital induce clonazepam metabolism, causing an approximately 30% decrease in plasma clonazepam levels).
No products indexed under this heading.

Methylprednisolone Acetate (Cytochrome P-450 inducers, such as phenytoin, carbamazepine and phenobarbital induce clonazepam metabolism, causing an approximately 30% decrease in plasma clonazepam levels).
No products indexed under this heading.

Methylprednisolone Sodium Succinate (Cytochrome P-450 inducers, such as phenytoin, carbamazepine and phenobarbital induce clonazepam metabolism, causing an approximately 30% decrease in plasma clonazepam levels).
No products indexed under this heading.

Metronidazole (Although clinical studies have not been performed, based on the involvement of the cytochrome P-450 3A family in clonazepam metabolism, inhibitors of this enzyme system, notably oral antifungal agents, should be used cautiously in patients receiving clonazepam). Products include:
Pylera 793

Metronidazole Benzoate (Although clinical studies have not been performed, based on the involvement of the cytochrome P-450 3A family in clonazepam metabolism, inhibitors of this enzyme system, notably oral antifungal agents, should be used cautiously in patients receiving clonazepam).
No products indexed under this heading.

Metronidazole Hydrochloride (Although clinical studies have not been performed, based on the involvement of the cytochrome P-450 3A family in clonazepam metabolism, inhibitors of this enzyme system, notably oral antifungal agents, should be used cautiously in patients receiving clonazepam).
No products indexed under this heading.

Micafungin Sodium (Although clinical studies have not been performed, based on the involvement of the cytochrome P-450 3A family in clonazepam metabolism, inhibitors of this enzyme system, notably oral antifungal agents, should be used cautiously in patients receiving clonazepam). Products include:
Mycamine 670

Miconazole (Although clinical studies have not been performed, based on the involvement of the cytochrome P-450 3A family in clonazepam metabolism, inhibitors of this enzyme system, notably oral antifungal agents, should be used cautiously in patients receiving clonazepam).
No products indexed under this heading.

Midazolam Hydrochloride (The CNS-depressant action of the benzodiazepine class of drugs may be potentiated by alcohol, narcotics, barbiturates, nonbarbiturate hypnotics, antianxiety agents, the phenothiazines, thioxanthene and butyrophenone classes of antipsychotic agents, monoamine oxidase inhibitors and tricyclic antidepressants, and by other anticonvulsant drugs).
No products indexed under this heading.

Moclobemide (The CNS-depressant action of the benzodiazepine class of drugs may be potentiated by alcohol, narcotics, barbiturates, nonbarbiturate hypnotics, antianxiety agents, the phenothiazines, thioxanthene and butyrophenone classes of antipsychotic agents, monoamine oxidase inhibitors and tricyclic antidepressants, and by other anticonvulsant drugs).
No products indexed under this heading.

Modafinil (Cytochrome P-450 inducers, such as phenytoin, carbamazepine and phenobarbital induce clonazepam metabolism, causing an approximately 30% decrease in plasma clonazepam levels). Products include:
Provigil 983

Molindone Hydrochloride (Since clonazepam produces CNS depression, patients receiving this drug should be warned about the concomitant use of alcohol or other CNS-depressant drugs during clonazepam therapy). Products include:
Moban 1108

Morphine Sulfate (The CNS-depressant action of the benzodiazepine class of drugs may be potentiated by alcohol, narcotics, barbiturates, nonbarbiturate hypnotics, antianxiety agents, phenothiazines, thioxanthene and butyrophenone classes of antipsychotic agents, monoamine oxidase inhibitors and tricyclic antidepressants, and by other anticonvulsant drugs). Products include:
Avinza 1822
Embeda 1831
MS Contin 2803

Morphine Sulfate, Liposomal (The CNS-depressant action of the benzodiazepine class of drugs may be potentiated by alcohol, narcotics, barbiturates, nonbarbiturate hypnotics, antianxiety agents, phenothiazines, thioxanthene and butyrophenone classes of antipsychotic agents, monoamine oxidase inhibitors and tricyclic antidepressants, and by other anticonvulsant drugs).
No products indexed under this heading.

Nafcillin Sodium (Cytochrome P-450 inducers, such as phenytoin, carbamazepine and phenobarbital induce clonazepam metabolism, causing an approximately 30% decrease in plasma clonazepam levels).
No products indexed under this heading.

Nefazodone Hydrochloride (Although clinical studies have not been performed, based on the involvement of the cytochrome P-450 3A family in clonazepam metabolism, inhibitors of this enzyme system, notably oral antifungal agents, should be used cautiously in patients receiving clonazepam).
No products indexed under this heading.

Nelfinavir Mesylate (Although clinical studies have not been performed, based on the involvement of the cytochrome P-450 3A family in clonazepam metabolism, inhibitors of this enzyme system, notably oral antifungal agents, should be used cautiously in patients receiving clonazepam).
No products indexed under this heading.

Nevirapine (Cytochrome P-450 inducers, such as phenytoin, carbamazepine and phenobarbital induce clonazepam metabolism, causing an approximately 30% decrease in plasma clonazepam levels). Products include:
Viramune Oral Suspension 897
Viramune Tablets 897

Nicotine (Cytochrome P-450 inducers, such as phenytoin, carbamazepine and phenobarbital induce clonazepam metabolism, causing an approximately 30% decrease in plasma clonazepam levels).
No products indexed under this heading.

Nicotine Polacrilex (Cytochrome P-450 inducers, such as phenytoin, carbamazepine and phenobarbital induce clonazepam metabolism, causing an approximately 30% decrease in plasma clonazepam levels).
No products indexed under this heading.

Nicotine Salicylate (Cytochrome P-450 inducers, such as phenytoin, carbamazepine and phenobarbital induce clonazepam metabolism, causing an approximately 30% decrease in plasma clonazepam levels).
No products indexed under this heading.

Nicotine Sulfate (Cytochrome P-450 inducers, such as phenytoin, carbamazepine and phenobarbital induce clonazepam metabolism, causing an approximately 30% decrease in plasma clonazepam levels).
No products indexed under this heading.

Nifedipine (Although clinical studies have not been performed, based on the involvement of the cytochrome P-450 3A family in clonazepam metabolism, inhibitors of this enzyme system, notably oral antifungal agents, should be used cautiously in patients receiving clonazepam).
No products indexed under this heading.

Norethindrone (Cytochrome P-450 inducers, such as phenytoin, carbamazepine and phenobarbital induce clonazepam metabolism, causing an approximately 30% decrease in plasma clonazepam levels). Products include:
Ortho Micronor 2660

Norethindrone Acetate (Cytochrome P-450 inducers, such as phenytoin, carbamazepine and phenobarbital induce clonazepam metabolism, causing an approximately 30% decrease in plasma clonazepam levels). Products include:
Activella 2561

Norfloxacin (Although clinical studies have not been performed, based on the involvement of the cytochrome P-450 3A family in clonazepam metabolism, inhibitors of this enzyme system, notably oral antifungal agents, should be used cautiously in patients receiving clonazepam). Products include:
Noroxin 2220

Nortriptyline Hydrochloride (The CNS-depressant action of the benzodiazepine class of drugs may be potentiated by alcohol, narcotics, barbiturates, nonbarbiturate hypnotics, antianxiety agents, the phenothiazines, thioxanthene and butyrophenone classes of antipsychotic agents, monoamine oxidase inhibitors and tricyclic antidepressants, and by other anticonvulsant drugs).
No products indexed under this heading.

Olanzapine (Since clonazepam produces CNS depression, patients receiv-

ing this drug should be warned about the concomitant use of alcohol or other CNS-depressant drugs during clonazepam therapy). Products include:

Omeprazole (Cytochrome P-450 inducers, such as phenytoin, carbamazepine and phenobarbital induce clonazepam metabolism, causing an approximately 30% decrease in plasma clonazepam levels).
No products indexed under this heading.

Omeprazole Magnesium (Cytochrome P-450 inducers, such as phenytoin, carbamazepine and phenobarbital induce clonazepam metabolism, causing an approximately 30% decrease in plasma clonazepam levels).
No products indexed under this heading.

Oxazepam (Since clonazepam produces CNS depression, patients receiving this drug should be warned about the concomitant use of alcohol or other CNS-depressant drugs during clonazepam therapy).
No products indexed under this heading.

Oxcarbazepine (The CNS-depressant action of the benzodiazepine class of drugs may be potentiated by alcohol, narcotics, barbiturates, nonbarbiturate hypnotics, antianxiety agents, the phenothiazines, thioxanthene and butyrophenone classes of antipsychotic agents, monoamine oxidase inhibitors and tricyclic antidepressants, and by other anticonvulsant drugs).
No products indexed under this heading.

Oxiconazole Nitrate (Although clinical studies have not been performed, based on the involvement of the cytochrome P-450 3A family in clonazepam metabolism, inhibitors of this enzyme system, notably oral antifungal agents, should be used cautiously in patients receiving clonazepam).
No products indexed under this heading.

Oxycodone Hydrochloride (The CNS-depressant action of the benzodiazepine class of drugs may be potentiated by alcohol, narcotics, barbiturates, nonbarbiturate hypnotics, antianxiety agents, phenothiazines, thioxanthene and butyrophenone classes of antipsychotic agents, monoamine oxidase inhibitors and tricyclic antidepressants, and by other anticonvulsant drugs). Products include:

Oxycodone Terephthalate (The CNS-depressant action of the benzodiazepine class of drugs may be potentiated by alcohol, narcotics, barbiturates, nonbarbiturate hypnotics, antianxiety agents, phenothiazines, thioxanthene and butyrophenone classes of antipsychotic agents, monoamine oxidase inhibitors and tricyclic antidepressants, and by other anticonvulsant drugs).
No products indexed under this heading.

Oxymorphone Hydrochloride (The CNS-depressant action of the benzodiazepine class of drugs may be potentiated by alcohol, narcotics, barbiturates, nonbarbiturate hypnotics, antianxiety agents, phenothiazines, thioxanthene and butyrophenone classes of antipsychotic agents, monoamine oxidase inhibitors and tricyclic antidepressants, and by other anticonvulsant drugs). Products include:

Paramethadione (The CNS-depressant action of the benzodiazepine class of drugs may be potentiated by alcohol, narcotics, barbiturates, nonbarbiturate hypnotics, antianxiety agents, the phenothiazines, thioxanthene and butyrophenone classes of antipsychotic agents, monoamine oxidase inhibitors and tricyclic antidepressants, and by other anticonvulsant drugs).
No products indexed under this heading.

Pargyline Hydrochloride (The CNS-depressant action of the benzodiazepine class of drugs may be potentiated by alcohol, narcotics, barbiturates, nonbarbiturate hypnotics, antianxiety agents, the phenothiazines, thioxanthene and butyrophenone classes of antipsychotic agents, monoamine oxidase inhibitors and tricyclic antidepressants, and by other anticonvulsant drugs).
No products indexed under this heading.

Paroxetine (The CNS-depressant action of the benzodiazepine class of drugs may be potentiated by alcohol, narcotics, barbiturates, nonbarbiturate hypnotics, antianxiety agents, the phenothiazines, thioxanthene and butyrophenone classes of antipsychotic agents, monoamine oxidase inhibitors and tricyclic antidepressants, and by other anticonvulsant drugs).
No products indexed under this heading.

Paroxetine Hydrochloride (The CNS-depressant action of the benzodiazepine class of drugs may be potentiated by alcohol, narcotics, barbiturates, nonbarbiturate hypnotics, antianxiety agents, the phenothiazines, thioxanthene and butyrophenone classes of antipsychotic agents, monoamine oxidase inhibitors and tricyclic antidepressants, and by other anticonvulsant drugs). Products include:

Paroxetine Mesylate (The CNS-depressant action of the benzodiazepine class of drugs may be potentiated by alcohol, narcotics, barbiturates, nonbarbiturate hypnotics, antianxiety agents, the phenothiazines, thioxanthene and butyrophenone classes of antipsychotic agents, monoamine oxidase inhibitors and tricyclic antidepressants, and by other anticonvulsant drugs).
No products indexed under this heading.

Pentobarbital (The CNS-depressant action of the benzodiazepine class of drugs may be potentiated by alcohol, narcotics, barbiturates, nonbarbiturate hypnotics, antianxiety agents, phenothiazines, thioxanthene and butyrophenone classes of antipsychotic agents, monoamine oxidase inhibitors and tricyclic antidepressants, and by other anticonvulsant drugs).
No products indexed under this heading.

Pentobarbital Sodium (The CNS-depressant action of the benzodiazepine class of drugs may be potentiated by alcohol, narcotics, barbiturates, nonbarbiturate hypnotics, antianxiety agents, phenothiazines, thioxanthene and butyrophenone classes of antipsychotic agents, monoamine oxidase inhibitors and tricyclic antidepressants, and by other anticonvulsant drugs). Products include:

Perphenazine (The CNS-depressant action of the benzodiazepine class of drugs may be potentiated by alcohol, narcotics, barbiturates, nonbarbiturate hypnotics, antianxiety agents, the phenothiazines, thioxanthene and butyrophenone classes of antipsychotic agents, monoamine oxidase inhibitors and tricyclic antidepressants, and by other anticonvulsant drugs).
No products indexed under this heading.

Phenacemide (The CNS-depressant action of the benzodiazepine class of drugs may be potentiated by alcohol, narcotics, barbiturates, nonbarbiturate hypnotics, antianxiety agents, the phenothiazines, thioxanthene and butyrophenone classes of antipsychotic agents, monoamine oxidase inhibitors and tricyclic antidepressants, and by other anticonvulsant drugs).
No products indexed under this heading.

Phenelzine Sulfate (The CNS-depressant action of the benzodiazepine class of drugs may be potentiated by alcohol, narcotics, barbiturates, nonbarbiturate hypnotics, antianxiety agents, the phenothiazines, thioxanthene and butyrophenone classes of antipsychotic agents, monoamine oxidase inhibitors and tricyclic antidepressants, and by other anticonvulsant drugs).
No products indexed under this heading.

Phenobarbital (Induces clonazepam metabolism, causing an approximately 30% decrease in plasma clonazepam levels; CNS depressant action may be potentiated). Products include:

Phenobarbital Sodium (Induces clonazepam metabolism, causing an approximately 30% decrease in plasma clonazepam levels; CNS depressant action may be potentiated).
No products indexed under this heading.

Phenothiazine Derivatives (The CNS-depressant action of the benzodiazepine class of drugs may be potentiated by alcohol, narcotics, barbiturates, nonbarbiturate hypnotics, antianxiety agents, the phenothiazines, thioxanthene and butyrophenone classes of antipsychotic agents, monoamine oxidase inhibitors and tricyclic antidepressants, and by other anticonvulsant drugs).
No products indexed under this heading.

Phenothiazines (The CNS-depressant action of the benzodiazepine class of drugs may be potentiated by alcohol, narcotics, barbiturates, nonbarbiturate hypnotics, antianxiety agents, the phenothiazines, thioxanthene and butyrophenone classes of antipsychotic agents, monoamine oxidase inhibitors and tricyclic antidepressants, and by other anticonvulsant drugs).
No products indexed under this heading.

Phensuximide (The CNS-depressant action of the benzodiazepine class of drugs may be potentiated by alcohol, narcotics, barbiturates, nonbarbiturate hypnotics, antianxiety agents, the phenothiazines, thioxanthene and butyrophenone classes of antipsychotic agents, monoamine oxidase inhibitors and tricyclic antidepressants, and by other anticonvulsant drugs).
No products indexed under this heading.

Phenytoin (Cytochrome P-450 inducers, such as phenytoin, carbamazepine and phenobarbital, induce clonazepam metabolism, causing an approximately 30% decrease in plasma clonazepam levels).
No products indexed under this heading.

Phenytoin Sodium (Cytochrome P-450 inducers, such as phenytoin, carbamazepine and phenobarbital, induce

clonazepam metabolism, causing an approximately 30% decrease in plasma clonazepam levels). Products include:

Posaconazole (Although clinical studies have not been performed, based on the involvement of the cytochrome P-450 3A family in clonazepam metabolism, inhibitors of this enzyme system, notably oral antifungal agents, should be used cautiously in patients receiving clonazepam). Products include:

Prazepam (Since clonazepam produces CNS depression, patients receiving this drug should be warned about the concomitant use of alcohol or other CNS-depressant drugs during clonazepam therapy).
No products indexed under this heading.

Prednisolone (Cytochrome P-450 inducers, such as phenytoin, carbamazepine and phenobarbital induce clonazepam metabolism, causing an approximately 30% decrease in plasma clonazepam levels).
No products indexed under this heading.

Prednisolone Acetate (Cytochrome P-450 inducers, such as phenytoin, carbamazepine and phenobarbital induce clonazepam metabolism, causing an approximately 30% decrease in plasma clonazepam levels). Products include:

Prednisolone Sodium Phosphate (Cytochrome P-450 inducers, such as phenytoin, carbamazepine and phenobarbital induce clonazepam metabolism, causing an approximately 30% decrease in plasma clonazepam levels).
No products indexed under this heading.

Prednisolone Tebutate (Cytochrome P-450 inducers, such as phenytoin, carbamazepine and phenobarbital induce clonazepam metabolism, causing an approximately 30% decrease in plasma clonazepam levels).
No products indexed under this heading.

Prednisone (Cytochrome P-450 inducers, such as phenytoin, carbamazepine and phenobarbital induce clonazepam metabolism, causing an approximately 30% decrease in plasma clonazepam levels).
No products indexed under this heading.

Prednisone sodium phosphate (Cytochrome P-450 inducers, such as phenytoin, carbamazepine and phenobarbital induce clonazepam metabolism, causing an approximately 30% decrease in plasma clonazepam levels).
No products indexed under this heading.

Primidone (The CNS-depressant action of the benzodiazepine class of drugs may be potentiated by alcohol, narcotics, barbiturates, nonbarbiturate hypnotics, antianxiety agents, the phenothiazines, thioxanthene and butyrophenone classes of antipsychotic agents, monoamine oxidase inhibitors and tricyclic antidepressants, and by other anticonvulsant drugs).
No products indexed under this heading.

Procarbazine Hydrochloride (The CNS-depressant action of the benzodiazepine class of drugs may be potentiated by alcohol, narcotics, barbiturates, nonbarbiturate hypnotics, antianxiety agents, the phenothiazines, thioxanthene and butyrophenone classes of antipsychotic agents, monoamine oxidase inhibitors and tricyclic antidepressants, and by other anticonvulsant drugs).
No products indexed under this heading.

955 Interactions Index Klonopin

Prochlorperazine (The CNS-depressant action of the benzodiazepine class of drugs may be potentiated by alcohol, narcotics, barbiturates, nonbarbiturate hypnotics, antianxiety agents, the phenothiazines, thioxanthene and butyrophenone classes of antipsychotic agents, monoamine oxidase inhibitors and tricyclic antidepressants, and by other anticonvulsant drugs).
No products indexed under this heading.

Prochlorperazine Edisylate (The CNS-depressant action of the benzodiazepine class of drugs may be potentiated by alcohol, narcotics, barbiturates, nonbarbiturate hypnotics, antianxiety agents, the phenothiazines, thioxanthene and butyrophenone classes of antipsychotic agents, monoamine oxidase inhibitors and tricyclic antidepressants, and by other anticonvulsant drugs).
No products indexed under this heading.

Prochlorperazine Maleate (The CNS-depressant action of the benzodiazepine class of drugs may be potentiated by alcohol, narcotics, barbiturates, nonbarbiturate hypnotics, antianxiety agents, the phenothiazines, thioxanthene and butyrophenone classes of antipsychotic agents, monoamine oxidase inhibitors and tricyclic antidepressants, and by other anticonvulsant drugs).
No products indexed under this heading.

Promethazine (The CNS-depressant action of the benzodiazepine class of drugs may be potentiated by alcohol, narcotics, barbiturates, nonbarbiturate hypnotics, antianxiety agents, the phenothiazines, thioxanthene and butyrophenone classes of antipsychotic agents, monoamine oxidase inhibitors and tricyclic antidepressants, and by other anticonvulsant drugs).
No products indexed under this heading.

Promethazine Hydrochloride (The CNS-depressant action of the benzodiazepine class of drugs may be potentiated by alcohol, narcotics, barbiturates, nonbarbiturate hypnotics, antianxiety agents, the phenothiazines, thioxanthene and butyrophenone classes of antipsychotic agents, monoamine oxidase inhibitors and tricyclic antidepressants, and by other anticonvulsant drugs).
No products indexed under this heading.

Propofol (The CNS-depressant action of the benzodiazepine class of drugs may be potentiated by alcohol, narcotics, barbiturates, nonbarbiturate hypnotics, antianxiety agents, the phenothiazines, thioxanthene and butyrophenone classes of antipsychotic agents, monoamine oxidase inhibitors and tricyclic antidepressants, and by other anticonvulsant drugs).
No products indexed under this heading.

Propoxyphene Hydrochloride (The CNS-depressant action of the benzodiazepine class of drugs may be potentiated by alcohol, narcotics, barbiturates, nonbarbiturate hypnotics, antianxiety agents, phenothiazines, thioxanthene and butyrophenone classes of antipsychotic agents, monoamine oxidase inhibitors and tricyclic antidepressants, and by other anticonvulsant drugs).
No products indexed under this heading.

Propoxyphene Napsylate (The CNS-depressant action of the benzodiazepine class of drugs may be potentiated by alcohol, narcotics, barbiturates, nonbarbiturate hypnotics, antianxiety agents, phenothiazines, thioxanthene and butyrophenone classes of antipsychotic agents, monoamine oxidase inhibitors and tricyclic antidepressants, and by other anticonvulsant drugs).
No products indexed under this heading.

Protriptyline Hydrochloride (The CNS-depressant action of the benzodiazepine class of drugs may be potentiated by alcohol, narcotics, barbiturates, nonbarbiturate hypnotics, antianxiety agents, the phenothiazines, thioxanthene and butyrophenone classes of antipsychotic agents, monoamine oxidase inhibitors and tricyclic antidepressants, and by other anticonvulsant drugs).
No products indexed under this heading.

Quazepam (The CNS-depressant action of the benzodiazepine class of drugs may be potentiated by alcohol, narcotics, barbiturates, nonbarbiturate hypnotics, antianxiety agents, the phenothiazines, thioxanthene and butyrophenone classes of antipsychotic agents, monoamine oxidase inhibitors and tricyclic antidepressants, and by other anticonvulsant drugs).
No products indexed under this heading.

Quetiapine Fumarate (Since clonazepam produces CNS depression, patients receiving this drug should be warned about the concomitant use of alcohol or other CNS-depressant drugs during clonazepam therapy). Products include:
Seroquel 750
Seroquel XR 759

Quinine (Although clinical studies have not been performed, based on the involvement of the cytochrome P-450 3A family in clonazepam metabolism, inhibitors of this enzyme system, notably oral antifungal agents, should be used cautiously in patients receiving clonazepam). Products include:
Hyland's Leg Cramps PM with Quinine 3315

Quinine Sulfate (Although clinical studies have not been performed, based on the involvement of the cytochrome P-450 3A family in clonazepam metabolism, inhibitors of this enzyme system, notably oral antifungal agents, should be used cautiously in patients receiving clonazepam).
No products indexed under this heading.

Ramelteon (The CNS-depressant action of the benzodiazepine class of drugs may be potentiated by alcohol, narcotics, barbiturates, nonbarbiturate hypnotics, antianxiety agents, the phenothiazines, thioxanthene and butyrophenone classes of antipsychotic agents, monoamine oxidase inhibitors and tricyclic antidepressants, and by other anticonvulsant drugs). Products include:
Rozerem 3366

Rasagiline Mesylate (The CNS-depressant action of the benzodiazepine class of drugs may be potentiated by alcohol, narcotics, barbiturates, nonbarbiturate hypnotics, antianxiety agents, the phenothiazines, thioxanthene and butyrophenone classes of antipsychotic agents, monoamine oxidase inhibitors and tricyclic antidepressants, and by other anticonvulsant drugs). Products include:
Azilect 3383

Remifentanil Hydrochloride (The CNS-depressant action of the benzodiazepine class of drugs may be potentiated by alcohol, narcotics, barbiturates, nonbarbiturate hypnotics, antianxiety agents, phenothiazines, thioxanthene and butyrophenone classes of antipsychotic agents, monoamine oxidase inhibitors and tricyclic antidepressants, and by other anticonvulsant drugs).
No products indexed under this heading.

Rifabutin (Cytochrome P-450 inducers, such as phenytoin, carbamazepine and phenobarbital induce clonazepam metabolism, causing an approximately 30% decrease in plasma clonazepam levels).
No products indexed under this heading.

Rifampicin (Cytochrome P-450 inducers, such as phenytoin, carbamazepine and phenobarbital induce clonazepam metabolism, causing an approximately 30% decrease in plasma clonazepam levels).
No products indexed under this heading.

Rifampin (Cytochrome P-450 inducers, such as phenytoin, carbamazepine and phenobarbital induce clonazepam metabolism, causing an approximately 30% decrease in plasma clonazepam levels).
No products indexed under this heading.

Rifapentine (Cytochrome P-450 inducers, such as phenytoin, carbamazepine and phenobarbital induce clonazepam metabolism, causing an approximately 30% decrease in plasma clonazepam levels).
No products indexed under this heading.

Risperidone (Since clonazepam produces CNS depression, patients receiving this drug should be warned about the concomitant use of alcohol or other CNS-depressant drugs during clonazepam therapy). Products include:
Risperdal Consta 2682

Ritonavir (Although clinical studies have not been performed, based on the involvement of the cytochrome P-450 3A family in clonazepam metabolism, inhibitors of this enzyme system, notably oral antifungal agents, should be used cautiously in patients receiving clonazepam). Products include:
Kaletra 458
Norvir 509

Rufinamide (The CNS-depressant action of the benzodiazepine class of drugs may be potentiated by alcohol, narcotics, barbiturates, nonbarbiturate hypnotics, antianxiety agents, the phenothiazines, thioxanthene and butyrophenone classes of antipsychotic agents, monoamine oxidase inhibitors and tricyclic antidepressants, and by other anticonvulsant drugs). Products include:
Banzel 1050

Saquinavir (Although clinical studies have not been performed, based on the involvement of the cytochrome P-450 3A family in clonazepam metabolism, inhibitors of this enzyme system, notably oral antifungal agents, should be used cautiously in patients receiving clonazepam).
No products indexed under this heading.

Saquinavir Mesylate (Although clinical studies have not been performed, based on the involvement of the cytochrome P-450 3A family in clonazepam metabolism, inhibitors of this enzyme system, notably oral antifungal agents, should be used cautiously in patients receiving clonazepam).
No products indexed under this heading.

Secobarbital Sodium (The CNS-depressant action of the benzodiazepine class of drugs may be potentiated by alcohol, narcotics, barbiturates, nonbarbiturate hypnotics, antianxiety agents, phenothiazines, thioxanthene and butyrophenone classes of antipsychotic agents, monoamine oxidase inhibitors and tricyclic antidepressants, and by other anticonvulsant drugs).
No products indexed under this heading.

Selegiline (The CNS-depressant action of the benzodiazepine class of drugs may be potentiated by alcohol, narcotics, barbiturates, nonbarbiturate hypnotics, antianxiety agents, the phenothiazines, thioxanthene and butyrophenone classes of antipsychotic agents, monoamine oxidase inhibitors and tricyclic antidepressants, and by other anticonvulsant drugs). Products include:
Emsam 3623

Selegiline Hydrochloride (The CNS-depressant action of the benzodiazepine class of drugs may be potentiated by alcohol, narcotics, barbiturates, nonbarbiturate hypnotics, antianxiety agents, the phenothiazines, thioxanthene and butyrophenone classes of antipsychotic agents, monoamine oxidase inhibitors and tricyclic antidepressants, and by other anticonvulsant drugs). Products include:
Eldepryl 3312

Sertaconazole Nitrate (Although clinical studies have not been performed, based on the involvement of the cytochrome P-450 3A family in clonazepam metabolism, inhibitors of this enzyme system, notably oral antifungal agents, should be used cautiously in patients receiving clonazepam).
No products indexed under this heading.

Sertraline Hydrochloride (The CNS-depressant action of the benzodiazepine class of drugs may be potentiated by alcohol, narcotics, barbiturates, nonbarbiturate hypnotics, antianxiety agents, the phenothiazines, thioxanthene and butyrophenone classes of antipsychotic agents, monoamine oxidase inhibitors and tricyclic antidepressants, and by other anticonvulsant drugs).
No products indexed under this heading.

Sevoflurane (Since clonazepam produces CNS depression, patients receiving this drug should be warned about the concomitant use of alcohol or other CNS-depressant drugs during clonazepam therapy). Products include:
Ultane 554

Sodium Butabarbital (The CNS-depressant action of the benzodiazepine class of drugs may be potentiated by alcohol, narcotics, barbiturates, nonbarbiturate hypnotics, antianxiety agents, phenothiazines, thioxanthene and butyrophenone classes of antipsychotic agents, monoamine oxidase inhibitors and tricyclic antidepressants, and by other anticonvulsant drugs).
No products indexed under this heading.

Sodium Oxybate (Since clonazepam produces CNS depression, patients receiving this drug should be warned about the concomitant use of alcohol or other CNS-depressant drugs during clonazepam therapy).
No products indexed under this heading.

Sodium Pentobarbital (The CNS-depressant action of the benzodiazepine class of drugs may be potentiated by alcohol, narcotics, barbiturates, nonbarbiturate hypnotics, antianxiety agents, phenothiazines, thioxanthene and butyrophenone classes of antipsychotic agents, monoamine oxidase inhibitors and tricyclic antidepressants, and by other anticonvulsant drugs).
No products indexed under this heading.

Sufentanil Citrate (The CNS-depressant action of the benzodiazepine class of drugs may be potentiated by alcohol, narcotics, barbiturates, nonbarbiturate hypnotics, antianxiety agents, phenothiazines, thioxanthene and butyrophenone classes of antipsychotic agents, monoamine oxidase inhibitors and tricyclic antidepressants, and by other anticonvulsant drugs).
No products indexed under this heading.

Sulfinpyrazone (Cytochrome P-450 inducers, such as phenytoin, carbamazepine and phenobarbital induce clonazepam metabolism, causing an approximately 30% decrease in plasma clonazepam levels).
No products indexed under this heading.

IMPORTANT NOTE: Always consult each drug listing in the patient's regimen for possible interactions.

Klonopin Interactions Index 956

Talbutal (Since clonazepam produces CNS depression, patients receiving this drug should be warned about the concomitant use of alcohol or other CNS-depressant drugs during clonazepam therapy).
No products indexed under this heading.

Temazepam (The CNS-depressant action of the benzodiazepine class of drugs may be potentiated by alcohol, narcotics, barbiturates, nonbarbiturate hypnotics, antianxiety agents, the phenothiazines, thioxanthene and butyrophenone classes of antipsychotic agents, monoamine oxidase inhibitors and tricyclic antidepressants, and by other anticonvulsant drugs).
No products indexed under this heading.

Terbinafine Hydrochloride (Although clinical studies have not been performed, based on the involvement of the cytochrome P-450 3A family in clonazepam metabolism, inhibitors of this enzyme system, notably oral antifungal agents, should be used cautiously in patients receiving clonazepam).
No products indexed under this heading.

Terconazole (Although clinical studies have not been performed, based on the involvement of the cytochrome P-450 3A family in clonazepam metabolism, inhibitors of this enzyme system, notably oral antifungal agents, should be used cautiously in patients receiving clonazepam).
No products indexed under this heading.

Theophyllinate (Cytochrome P-450 inducers, such as phenytoin, carbamazepine and phenobarbital induce clonazepam metabolism, causing an approximately 30% decrease in plasma clonazepam levels).
No products indexed under this heading.

Theophylline (Cytochrome P-450 inducers, such as phenytoin, carbamazepine and phenobarbital induce clonazepam metabolism, causing an approximately 30% decrease in plasma clonazepam levels).
No products indexed under this heading.

Theophylline Anhydrous (Cytochrome P-450 inducers, such as phenytoin, carbamazepine and phenobarbital induce clonazepam metabolism, causing an approximately 30% decrease in plasma clonazepam levels). Products include:
Uniphyl 2817

Theophylline Calcium Salicylate (Cytochrome P-450 inducers, such as phenytoin, carbamazepine and phenobarbital induce clonazepam metabolism, causing an approximately 30% decrease in plasma clonazepam levels).
No products indexed under this heading.

Theophylline Dihydroxypropyl (Glyceryl) (Cytochrome P-450 inducers, such as phenytoin, carbamazepine and phenobarbital induce clonazepam metabolism, causing an approximately 30% decrease in plasma clonazepam levels).
No products indexed under this heading.

Theophylline Ethylenediamine (Cytochrome P-450 inducers, such as phenytoin, carbamazepine and phenobarbital induce clonazepam metabolism, causing an approximately 30% decrease in plasma clonazepam levels).
No products indexed under this heading.

Theophylline Sodium Glycinate (Cytochrome P-450 inducers, such as phenytoin, carbamazepine and phenobarbital induce clonazepam metabolism, causing an approximately 30% decrease in plasma clonazepam levels).
No products indexed under this heading.

Thiamylal Sodium (The CNS-depressant action of the benzodiazepine class of drugs may be potentiated by alcohol, narcotics, barbiturates, nonbarbiturate hypnotics, antianxiety agents, phenothiazines, thioxanthene and butyrophenone classes of antipsychotic agents, monoamine oxidase inhibitors and tricyclic antidepressants, and by other anticonvulsant drugs).
No products indexed under this heading.

Thioridazine (The CNS-depressant action of the benzodiazepine class of drugs may be potentiated by alcohol, narcotics, barbiturates, nonbarbiturate hypnotics, antianxiety agents, the phenothiazines, thioxanthene and butyrophenone classes of antipsychotic agents, monoamine oxidase inhibitors and tricyclic antidepressants, and by other anticonvulsant drugs).
No products indexed under this heading.

Thioridazine Hydrochloride (The CNS-depressant action of the benzodiazepine class of drugs may be potentiated by alcohol, narcotics, barbiturates, nonbarbiturate hypnotics, antianxiety agents, the phenothiazines, thioxanthene and butyrophenone classes of antipsychotic agents, monoamine oxidase inhibitors and tricyclic antidepressants, and by other anticonvulsant drugs). Products include:
Thioridazine Hydrochloride 2384

Thiothixene (Since clonazepam produces CNS depression, patients receiving this drug should be warned about the concomitant use of alcohol or other CNS-depressant drugs during clonazepam therapy). Products include:
Thiothixene 2386

Thiothixene Hydrochloride (Since clonazepam produces CNS depression, patients receiving this drug should be warned about the concomitant use of alcohol or other CNS-depressant drugs during clonazepam therapy).
No products indexed under this heading.

Thioxanthene Derivatives (The CNS-depressant action of the benzodiazepine class of drugs may be potentiated by alcohol, narcotics, barbiturates, nonbarbiturate hypnotics, antianxiety agents, the phenothiazines, thioxanthene and butyrophenone classes of antipsychotic agents, monoamine oxidase inhibitors and tricyclic antidepressants, and by other anticonvulsant drugs).
No products indexed under this heading.

Tiagabine Hydrochloride (The CNS-depressant action of the benzodiazepine class of drugs may be potentiated by alcohol, narcotics, barbiturates, nonbarbiturate hypnotics, antianxiety agents, the phenothiazines, thioxanthene and butyrophenone classes of antipsychotic agents, monoamine oxidase inhibitors and tricyclic antidepressants, and by other anticonvulsant drugs). Products include:
Gabitril 972

Tobacco (Cytochrome P-450 inducers, such as phenytoin, carbamazepine and phenobarbital induce clonazepam metabolism, causing an approximately 30% decrease in plasma clonazepam levels).
No products indexed under this heading.

Topiramate (The CNS-depressant action of the benzodiazepine class of drugs may be potentiated by alcohol, narcotics, barbiturates, nonbarbiturate hypnotics, antianxiety agents, the phenothiazines, thioxanthene and butyrophenone classes of antipsychotic agents, monoamine oxidase inhibitors and tricyclic antidepressants, and by other anticonvulsant drugs).
No products indexed under this heading.

Tranylcypromine Sulfate (The CNS-depressant action of the benzodiazepine class of drugs may be potentiated by alcohol, narcotics, barbiturates, nonbarbiturate hypnotics, antianxiety agents, the phenothiazines, thioxanthene and butyrophenone classes of antipsychotic agents, monoamine oxidase inhibitors and tricyclic antidepressants, and by other anticonvulsant drugs). Products include:
Parnate 1584

Triamcinolone (Cytochrome P-450 inducers, such as phenytoin, carbamazepine and phenobarbital induce clonazepam metabolism, causing an approximately 30% decrease in plasma clonazepam levels).
No products indexed under this heading.

Triamcinolone Acetonide (Cytochrome P-450 inducers, such as phenytoin, carbamazepine and phenobarbital induce clonazepam metabolism, causing an approximately 30% decrease in plasma clonazepam levels). Products include:
Azmacort 408
Nasacort AQ 3019

Triamcinolone Diacetate (Cytochrome P-450 inducers, such as phenytoin, carbamazepine and phenobarbital induce clonazepam metabolism, causing an approximately 30% decrease in plasma clonazepam levels).
No products indexed under this heading.

Triamcinolone Hexacetonide (Cytochrome P-450 inducers, such as phenytoin, carbamazepine and phenobarbital induce clonazepam metabolism, causing an approximately 30% decrease in plasma clonazepam levels).
No products indexed under this heading.

Triazolam (The CNS-depressant action of the benzodiazepine class of drugs may be potentiated by alcohol, narcotics, barbiturates, nonbarbiturate hypnotics, antianxiety agents, the phenothiazines, thioxanthene and butyrophenone classes of antipsychotic agents, monoamine oxidase inhibitors and tricyclic antidepressants, and by other anticonvulsant drugs).
No products indexed under this heading.

Trifluoperazine Hydrochloride (The CNS-depressant action of the benzodiazepine class of drugs may be potentiated by alcohol, narcotics, barbiturates, nonbarbiturate hypnotics, antianxiety agents, the phenothiazines, thioxanthene and butyrophenone classes of antipsychotic agents, monoamine oxidase inhibitors and tricyclic antidepressants, and by other anticonvulsant drugs).
No products indexed under this heading.

Trimethadione (The CNS-depressant action of the benzodiazepine class of drugs may be potentiated by alcohol, narcotics, barbiturates, nonbarbiturate hypnotics, antianxiety agents, the phenothiazines, thioxanthene and butyrophenone classes of antipsychotic agents, monoamine oxidase inhibitors and tricyclic antidepressants, and by other anticonvulsant drugs).
No products indexed under this heading.

Trimipramine Maleate (The CNS-depressant action of the benzodiazepine class of drugs may be potentiated by alcohol, narcotics, barbiturates, nonbarbiturate hypnotics, antianxiety agents, the phenothiazines, thioxanthene and butyrophenone classes of antipsychotic agents, monoamine oxidase inhibitors and tricyclic antidepressants, and by other anticonvulsant drugs).
No products indexed under this heading.

Troglitazone (Cytochrome P-450 inducers, such as phenytoin, carbamazepine and phenobarbital induce clonazepam metabolism, causing an approximately 30% decrease in plasma clonazepam levels).
No products indexed under this heading.

Troleandomycin (Although clinical studies have not been performed, based on the involvement of the cytochrome P-450 3A family in clonazepam metabolism, inhibitors of this enzyme system, notably oral antifungal agents, should be used cautiously in patients receiving clonazepam).
No products indexed under this heading.

Valproate Sodium (The CNS-depressant action of the benzodiazepine class of drugs may be potentiated by alcohol, narcotics, barbiturates, nonbarbiturate hypnotics, antianxiety agents, the phenothiazines, thioxanthene and butyrophenone classes of antipsychotic agents, monoamine oxidase inhibitors and tricyclic antidepressants, and by other anticonvulsant drugs).
No products indexed under this heading.

Valproic Acid (The CNS-depressant action of the benzodiazepine class of drugs may be potentiated by alcohol, narcotics, barbiturates, nonbarbiturate hypnotics, antianxiety agents, the phenothiazines, thioxanthene and butyrophenone classes of antipsychotic agents, monoamine oxidase inhibitors and tricyclic antidepressants, and by other anticonvulsant drugs).
No products indexed under this heading.

Venlafaxine Hydrochloride (The CNS-depressant action of the benzodiazepine class of drugs may be potentiated by alcohol, narcotics, barbiturates, nonbarbiturate hypnotics, antianxiety agents, the phenothiazines, thioxanthene and butyrophenone classes of antipsychotic agents, monoamine oxidase inhibitors and tricyclic antidepressants, and by other anticonvulsant drugs). Products include:
Effexor XR 3504
Venlafaxine Hydrochloride Tablets ... 2388

Verapamil Hydrochloride (Although clinical studies have not been performed, based on the involvement of the cytochrome P-450 3A family in clonazepam metabolism, inhibitors of this enzyme system, notably oral antifungal agents, should be used cautiously in patients receiving clonazepam). Products include:
Tarka 534

Voriconazole (Although clinical studies have not been performed, based on the involvement of the cytochrome P-450 3A family in clonazepam metabolism, inhibitors of this enzyme system, notably oral antifungal agents, should be used cautiously in patients receiving clonazepam).
No products indexed under this heading.

Zafirlukast (Although clinical studies have not been performed, based on the involvement of the cytochrome P-450 3A family in clonazepam metabolism, inhibitors of this enzyme system, notably oral antifungal agents, should be used cautiously in patients receiving clonazepam). Products include:
Accolate 3612

Zaleplon (The CNS-depressant action of the benzodiazepine class of drugs may be potentiated by alcohol, narcotics, barbiturates, nonbarbiturate hypnotics, antianxiety agents, the phenothiazines, thioxanthene and butyrophenone classes of antipsychotic agents, monoamine oxidase inhibitors and tricyclic antidepressants, and by other anticonvulsant drugs).
No products indexed under this heading.

Zileuton (Although clinical studies have not been performed, based on the involvement of the cytochrome P-450 3A family in clonazepam metabolism, inhibitors of this enzyme system, notably oral antifungal agents, should be used cautiously in patients receiving clonazepam).
No products indexed under this heading.

Ziprasidone Hydrochloride (Since clonazepam produces CNS depression, patients receiving this drug should be warned about the concomitant use of alcohol or other CNS-depressant drugs during clonazepam therapy). Products include:
Geodon 2723

Zolpidem Tartrate (The CNS-depressant action of the benzodiazepine class of drugs may be potentiated by alcohol, narcotics, barbiturates, nonbarbiturate hypnotics, antianxiety agents, the phenothiazines, thioxanthene and butyrophenone classes of antipsychotic agents, monoamine oxidase inhibitors and tricyclic antidepressants, and by other anticonvulsant drugs). Products include:
Ambien 2920
Ambien CR 2925

Zonisamide (The CNS-depressant action of the benzodiazepine class of drugs may be potentiated by alcohol, narcotics, barbiturates, nonbarbiturate hypnotics, antianxiety agents, the phenothiazines, thioxanthene and butyrophenone classes of antipsychotic agents, monoamine oxidase inhibitors and tricyclic antidepressants, and by other anticonvulsant drugs). Products include:
Zonegran 1081

Food Interactions

Alcohol (The CNS-depressant action of the benzodiazepine class of drugs may be potentiated by alcohol. Patients should be advised to avoid alcohol while taking clonazepam).

Beer, reduced-alcohol (The CNS-depressant action of the benzodiazepine class of drugs may be potentiated by alcohol. Patients should be advised to avoid alcohol while taking clonazepam).

Beer, unspecified (The CNS-depressant action of the benzodiazepine class of drugs may be potentiated by alcohol. Patients should be advised to avoid alcohol while taking clonazepam).

Broccoli (Cytochrome P-450 inducers, such as phenytoin, carbamazepine and phenobarbital induce clonazepam metabolism, causing an approximately 30% decrease in plasma clonazepam levels).

Brussel Sprouts (Cytochrome P-450 inducers, such as phenytoin, carbamazepine and phenobarbital induce clonazepam metabolism, causing an approximately 30% decrease in plasma clonazepam levels).

Charbroiled Food (Cytochrome P-450 inducers, such as phenytoin, carbamazepine and phenobarbital induce clonazepam metabolism, causing an approximately 30% decrease in plasma clonazepam levels).

Grapefruit (Although clinical studies have not been performed, based on the involvement of the cytochrome P-450 3A family in clonazepam metabolism, inhibitors of this enzyme system, notably oral antifungal agents, should be used cautiously in patients receiving clonazepam).

Grapefruit Juice (Although clinical studies have not been performed, based on the involvement of the cytochrome P-450 3A family in clonazepam metabo-

---

lism, inhibitors of this enzyme system, notably oral antifungal agents, should be used cautiously in patients receiving clonazepam).

Wine, Chianti (The CNS-depressant action of the benzodiazepine class of drugs may be potentiated by alcohol. Patients should be advised to avoid alcohol while taking clonazepam).

Wine, Red (The CNS-depressant action of the benzodiazepine class of drugs may be potentiated by alcohol. Patients should be advised to avoid alcohol while taking clonazepam).

Wine, unspecified (The CNS-depressant action of the benzodiazepine class of drugs may be potentiated by alcohol. Patients should be advised to avoid alcohol while taking clonazepam).

Wine products (The CNS-depressant action of the benzodiazepine class of drugs may be potentiated by alcohol. Patients should be advised to avoid alcohol while taking clonazepam).

KLONOPIN WAFERS
(Clonazepam) 2855
See Klonopin Tablets

K-PHOS ORIGINAL (SODIUM FREE) TABLETS
(Potassium Acid Phosphate) 874
May interact with antacids, potassium preparations, potassium sparing diuretics, salicylates, and certain other agents. Compounds in these categories include:

Aluminum Carbonate (May bind phosphate and prevent its absorption).
No products indexed under this heading.

Aluminum Hydroxide (May bind phosphate and prevent its absorption).
No products indexed under this heading.

Amiloride Hydrochloride (Hyperkalemia).
No products indexed under this heading.

Aspirin (Increased serum salicylate levels; possible toxicity). Products include:
Aggrenox 880
Bayer Aspirin 829
Percodan 1124
St. Joseph Aspirin 2045

Aspirin, Enteric Coated (Increased serum salicylate levels; possible toxicity).
No products indexed under this heading.

Aspirin Buffered (Increased serum salicylate levels; possible toxicity).
No products indexed under this heading.

Calcium Carbonate (May bind phosphate and prevent its absorption). Products include:
Chelated Mineral 3476
Pepcid Complete 1822
Extra Strength Rolaids Softchews Vanilla Creme 2045

Choline Magnesium Trisalicylate (Increased serum salicylate levels; possible toxicity).
No products indexed under this heading.

Diflunisal (Increased serum salicylate levels; possible toxicity).
No products indexed under this heading.

Magaldrate (May bind phosphate and prevent its absorption).
No products indexed under this heading.

Magnesium Carbonate (May bind phosphate and prevent its absorption).
No products indexed under this heading.

Magnesium Hydroxide (May bind phosphate and prevent its absorption). Products include:
Fleet Pedia-Lax Chewable Tablets 1144
Pepcid Complete 1822

Magnesium Oxide (May bind phosphate and prevent its absorption).
Products include:
Beelith 873

Magnesium Salicylate (Increased serum salicylate levels; possible toxicity).
No products indexed under this heading.

Magnesium Trisilicate (May bind phosphate and prevent its absorption).
No products indexed under this heading.

Potassium Bicarbonate (Potential for hyperkalemia).
No products indexed under this heading.

Potassium Chloride (Potential for hyperkalemia). Products include:
MoviPrep Oral Solution 2905

Potassium Citrate (Potential for hyperkalemia). Products include:
Urocit-K 2333

Potassium Gluconate (Potential for hyperkalemia).
No products indexed under this heading.

Potassium Phosphate (Potential for hyperkalemia). Products include:
K-Phos Neutral 873

Salsalate (Increased serum salicylate levels; possible toxicity).
No products indexed under this heading.

Sodium Bicarbonate (May bind phosphate and prevent its absorption).
No products indexed under this heading.

Spironolactone (Hyperkalemia).
No products indexed under this heading.

Triamterene (Hyperkalemia). Products include:
Dyazide 1429
Dyrenium 3495

K-PHOS NEUTRAL TABLETS
(Potassium Phosphate, Sodium Phosphate) 873
May interact with antacids containing aluminum, calcium and magnesium, calcium preparations, potassium preparations, potassium sparing diuretics, and certain other agents. Compounds in these categories include:

ACTH (Concurrent use with corticotropin may result in hypernatremia).
No products indexed under this heading.

Aluminum Carbonate (Co-administration with antacids may bind the phosphate and prevent its absorption).
No products indexed under this heading.

Aluminum Hydroxide (Co-administration with antacids may bind the phosphate and prevent its absorption).
No products indexed under this heading.

Amiloride Hydrochloride (Concurrent use with potassium-sparing diuretics may cause hyperkalemia).
No products indexed under this heading.

Calcium Carbonate (Co-administration with antacids may bind the phosphate and prevent its absorption). Products include:
Chelated Mineral 3476
Pepcid Complete 1822
Extra Strength Rolaids Softchews Vanilla Creme 2045

Calcium Carbonate (Concurrent use with calcium-containing preparations may antagonize the effects of phosphates in the treatment of hypercalcemia). Products include:
Chelated Mineral 3476
Pepcid Complete 1822
Extra Strength Rolaids Softchews Vanilla Creme 2045

Calcium Chloride (Concurrent use with calcium-containing preparations may antagonize the effects of phosphates in the treatment of hypercalcemia).
No products indexed under this heading.

Calcium Citrate (Concurrent use with calcium-containing preparations may antagonize the effects of phosphates in the treatment of hypercalcemia). Products include:
Active Calcium 3476
Chelated Mineral 3476
CitraNatal 90 DHA Capsules 2332
CitraNatal Assure 2332
CitraNatal Harmony 2332
CitraNatal Rx 2332

Calcium Glubionate (Concurrent use with calcium-containing preparations may antagonize the effects of phosphates in the treatment of hypercalcemia).
No products indexed under this heading.

Deserpidine (Concurrent use with antihypertensives, such as rauwolfia alkaloids, may result in hypernatremia).
No products indexed under this heading.

Diazoxide (Concurrent use with antihypertensives, such as diazoxide, may result in hypernatremia). Products include:
Proglycem 1179
Proglycem Suspension 1179

Fludrocortisone Acetate (Concurrent use with mineralocorticoids may result in hypernatremia).
No products indexed under this heading.

Guanethidine Monosulfate (Concurrent use with antihypertensives, such as guanethidine, may result in hypernatremia).
No products indexed under this heading.

Hydralazine Hydrochloride (Concurrent use with antihypertensives, such as hydralazine, may result in hypernatremia).
No products indexed under this heading.

Magaldrate (Co-administration with antacids may bind the phosphate and prevent its absorption).
No products indexed under this heading.

Magnesium Carbonate (Co-administration with antacids may bind the phosphate and prevent its absorption).
No products indexed under this heading.

Magnesium Hydroxide (Co-administration with antacids may bind the phosphate and prevent its absorption). Products include:
Fleet Pedia-Lax Chewable Tablets 1144
Pepcid Complete 1822

Magnesium Oxide (Co-administration with antacids may bind the phosphate and prevent its absorption). Products include:
Beelith 873

Magnesium Trisilicate (Co-administration with antacids may bind the phosphate and prevent its absorption).
No products indexed under this heading.

Methyldopa (Concurrent use with antihypertensives, such as methyldopa, may result in hypernatremia).
No products indexed under this heading.

Potassium Acid Phosphate (Concurrent use with potassium-containing medications may cause hyperkalemia). Products include:
K-Phos Original 874

Potassium Bicarbonate (Concurrent use with potassium-containing medications may cause hyperkalemia).
No products indexed under this heading.

Potassium Chloride (Concurrent use with potassium-containing medications may cause hyperkalemia). Products include:

IMPORTANT NOTE: Always consult each drug listing in the patient's regimen for possible interactions.

Potassium Citrate (Concurrent use with potassium-containing medications may cause hyperkalemia). Products include:

Potassium Gluconate (Concurrent use with potassium-containing medications may cause hyperkalemia).
No products indexed under this heading.

Rauwolfia Serpentina (Concurrent use with antihypertensives, such as rauwolfia alkaloids, may result in hypernatremia).
No products indexed under this heading.

Rescinnamine (Concurrent use with antihypertensives, such as rauwolfia alkaloids, may result in hypernatremia).
No products indexed under this heading.

Reserpine (Concurrent use with antihypertensives, such as rauwolfia alkaloids, may result in hypernatremia).
No products indexed under this heading.

Spironolactone (Concurrent use with potassium-sparing diuretics may cause hyperkalemia).
No products indexed under this heading.

Triamterene (Concurrent use with potassium-sparing diuretics may cause hyperkalemia). Products include:

Vitamin D (Concurrent use with vitamin D may antagonize the effects of phosphates in the treatment of hypercalcemia). Products include:

KRISTALOSE FOR ORAL SOLUTION

May interact with nonabsorbable antacids. Compounds in these categories include:

Aluminum Carbonate (Results of preliminary studies suggests that nonabsorbable antacids given concurrently with lactulose may inhibit the desired lactulose-induced drop in colonic pH).
No products indexed under this heading.

Aluminum Hydroxide (Results of preliminary studies suggests that nonabsorbable antacids given concurrently with lactulose may inhibit the desired lactulose-induced drop in colonic pH).
No products indexed under this heading.

Calcium Carbonate (Results of preliminary studies suggests that nonabsorbable antacids given concurrently with lactulose may inhibit the desired lactulose-induced drop in colonic pH). Products include:

Magnesium Carbonate (Results of preliminary studies suggests that nonabsorbable antacids given concurrently with lactulose may inhibit the desired lactulose-induced drop in colonic pH).
No products indexed under this heading.

Magnesium Hydroxide (Results of preliminary studies suggests that nonabsorbable antacids given concurrently with lactulose may inhibit the desired lactulose-induced drop in colonic pH). Products include:

LACRISERT STERILE OPHTHALMIC INSERT

None cited in PDR database.

LAMICTAL CHEWABLE DISPERSIBLE TABLETS

See Lamictal Tablets

LAMICTAL ODT ORALLY DISINTEGRATING TABLETS

See Lamictal Tablets

LAMICTAL TABLETS

May interact with dihydrofolate reductase inhibitors, drugs affecting hepatic drug metabolizing enzyme systems, estrogens, oral contraceptives, phenytoin, valproate, and certain other agents. Compounds in these categories include:

Carbamazepine (Concomitant use with carbamazepine may decrease lamotrigine concentrations by approximately 40%. Concomitant use may also increase increase CBZ epoxide levels (the active metabolite of carbamazepine). Lamotrigine has no appreciable effect on steady-state carbamazepine plasma concentrations. There is limited clinical data suggesting there is a higher incidence of dizziness, diplopia, ataxia, and blurred vision in patients receiving carbamazepine with lamotrigine than in patients receiving other AEDs with lamotrigine). Products include:

Chlorotrianisene (Some estrogen-containing oral contraceptives have been shown to decrease serum concentrations of lamotrigine. Dosage adjustments will be necessary in most patients who start or stop estrogen-containing oral contraceptives while taking lamotrigine. During the week of inactive hormone preparation ("pill-free" week) of oral contraceptive therapy, plasma levels are expected to rise, as much as doubling by the end of the week. Adverse events consistent with elevated levels of lamotrigine, such as dizziness, ataxia and diplopia, could occur. In addition, a decrease in levonorgestrel concentrations by 19% was seen when an oral contraceptive containing 150 mcg of levonorgestrel was concomitantly used with lamotrigine).
No products indexed under this heading.

Cimetidine (Since lamotrigine is metabolized predominately by glucuronic acid conjugation, drugs that are known to induce or inhibit glucuronidation may affect the apparent clearance of lamotrigine and doses of lamotrigine may require adjustment based on clinical response).
No products indexed under this heading.

Cimetidine Hydrochloride (Since lamotrigine is metabolized predominately by glucuronic acid conjugation, drugs that are known to induce or inhibit glucuronidation may affect the apparent clearance of lamotrigine and doses of lamotrigine may require adjustment based on clinical response).
No products indexed under this heading.

Desogestrel (Some estrogen-containing oral contraceptives have been shown to decrease serum concentrations of lamotrigine. Dosage adjustments will be necessary in most patients who start or stop estrogen-containing oral contraceptives while taking lamotrigine. During the week of inactive hormone preparation ("pill-free" week) of oral contraceptive therapy, plasma levels are expected to rise, as much as doubling by the end of the week. Adverse events consistent with elevated levels of lamotrigine, such as dizziness, ataxia and diplopia, could occur. In addition, a decrease in levonorgestrel concentrations by 19% was seen when an oral contraceptive containing 150 mcg of levonorgestrel was concomitantly used with lamotrigine).
No products indexed under this heading.

Dienestrol (Some estrogen-containing oral contraceptives have been shown to decrease serum concentrations of lamotrigine. Dosage adjustments will be necessary in most patients who start or stop estrogen-containing oral contraceptives while taking lamotrigine. During the week of inactive hormone preparation ("pill-free" week) of oral contraceptive therapy, plasma levels are expected to rise, as much as doubling by the end of the week. Adverse events consistent with elevated levels of lamotrigine, such as dizziness, ataxia and diplopia, could occur. In addition, a decrease in levonorgestrel concentrations by 19% was seen when an oral contraceptive containing 150 mcg of levonorgestrel was concomitantly used with lamotrigine).
No products indexed under this heading.

Diethylstilbestrol (Some estrogen-containing oral contraceptives have been shown to decrease serum concentrations of lamotrigine. Dosage adjustments will be necessary in most patients who start or stop estrogen-containing oral contraceptives while taking lamotrigine. During the week of inactive hormone preparation ("pill-free" week) of oral contraceptive therapy, plasma levels are expected to rise, as much as doubling by the end of the week. Adverse events consistent with elevated levels of lamotrigine, such as dizziness, ataxia and diplopia, could occur. In addition, a decrease in levonorgestrel concentrations by 19% was seen when an oral contraceptive containing 150 mcg of levonorgestrel was concomitantly used with lamotrigine).
No products indexed under this heading.

Divalproex Sodium (Concomitant use of lamotrigine with valproate may increase lamotrigine concentrations slightly more than 2-fold. In addition, when lamotrigine was administered to healthy volunteers receiving valproate, the trough steady-state valproate plasma concentrations decreased by an average of 25% over a 3-week period, and then stabilized. However, adding lamotrigine to the existing therapy did not cause a change in valproate plasma concentrations in either adult or pediatric patients in controlled clinical trials. Also, co-administration with valproate may increase the risk of rash). Products include:

Drugs, unspecified (Since lamotrigine is metabolized predominately by glucuronic acid conjugation, drugs that are known to induce or inhibit glucuronidation may affect the apparent clearance of lamotrigine and doses of lamotrigine may require adjustment based on clinical response).
No products indexed under this heading.

Erythromycin (Since lamotrigine is metabolized predominately by glucuronic acid conjugation, drugs that are known to induce or inhibit glucuronidation may affect the apparent clearance of lamotrigine and doses of lamotrigine may require adjustment based on clinical response).
No products indexed under this heading.

Erythromycin Estolate (Since lamotrigine is metabolized predominately by glucuronic acid conjugation, drugs that are known to induce or inhibit glucuronidation may affect the apparent clearance of lamotrigine and doses of lamotrigine may require adjustment based on clinical response).
No products indexed under this heading.

Erythromycin Ethylsuccinate (Since lamotrigine is metabolized predominately by glucuronic acid conjugation, drugs that are known to induce or inhibit glucuronidation may affect the apparent clearance of lamotrigine and doses of lamotrigine may require adjustment based on clinical response). Products include:

Erythromycin Gluceptate (Since lamotrigine is metabolized predominately by glucuronic acid conjugation, drugs that are known to induce or inhibit glucuronidation may affect the apparent clearance of lamotrigine and doses of lamotrigine may require adjustment based on clinical response).
No products indexed under this heading.

Erythromycin Lactobionate (Since lamotrigine is metabolized predominately by glucuronic acid conjugation, drugs that are known to induce or inhibit glucuronidation may affect the apparent clearance of lamotrigine and doses of lamotrigine may require adjustment based on clinical response).
No products indexed under this heading.

Erythromycin Stearate (Since lamotrigine is metabolized predominately by glucuronic acid conjugation, drugs that are known to induce or inhibit glucuronidation may affect the apparent clearance of lamotrigine and doses of lamotrigine may require adjustment based on clinical response).
No products indexed under this heading.

Estradiol (Some estrogen-containing oral contraceptives have been shown to decrease serum concentrations of lamotrigine. Dosage adjustments will be necessary in most patients who start or stop estrogen-containing oral contraceptives while taking lamotrigine. During the week of inactive hormone preparation ("pill-free" week) of oral contraceptive therapy, plasma levels are expected to rise, as much as doubling by the end of the week. Adverse events consistent with elevated levels of lamotrigine, such as dizziness, ataxia and diplopia, could occur. In addition, a decrease in levonorgestrel concentrations by 19% was seen when an oral contraceptive containing 150 mcg of levonorgestrel was concomitantly used with lamotrigine). Products include:

Estrogens, Conjugated (Some estrogen-containing oral contraceptives have been shown to decrease serum concentrations of lamotrigine. Dosage adjustments will be necessary in most patients who start or stop estrogen-containing oral contraceptives while taking lamotrigine. During the week of inactive hormone preparation ("pill-free" week) of oral contraceptive therapy, plasma levels are expected to rise, as much as doubling by the end of the week. Adverse events consistent with elevated levels of lamotrigine, such as dizziness, ataxia and diplopia, could occur. In addition, a decrease in levonorgestrel concentrations by 19% was seen when an oral contraceptive

containing 150 mcg of levonorgestrel was concomitantly used with lamotrigine). Products include:

Estrogens, Esterified (Some estrogen-containing oral contraceptives have been shown to decrease serum concentrations of lamotrigine. Dosage adjustments will be necessary in most patients who start or stop estrogen-containing oral contraceptives while taking lamotrigine. During the week of inactive hormone preparation ("pill-free" week) of oral contraceptive therapy, plasma levels are expected to rise, as much as doubling by the end of the week. Adverse events consistent with elevated levels of lamotrigine, such as dizziness, ataxia and diplopia, could occur. In addition, a decrease in levonorgestrel concentrations by 19% was seen when an oral contraceptive containing 150 mcg of levonorgestrel was concomitantly used with lamotrigine).
No products indexed under this heading.

Estropipate (Some estrogen-containing oral contraceptives have been shown to decrease serum concentrations of lamotrigine. Dosage adjustments will be necessary in most patients who start or stop estrogen-containing oral contraceptives while taking lamotrigine. During the week of inactive hormone preparation ("pill-free" week) of oral contraceptive therapy, plasma levels are expected to rise, as much as doubling by the end of the week. Adverse events consistent with elevated levels of lamotrigine, such as dizziness, ataxia and diplopia, could occur. In addition, a decrease in levonorgestrel concentrations by 19% was seen when an oral contraceptive containing 150 mcg of levonorgestrel was concomitantly used with lamotrigine).
No products indexed under this heading.

Ethinyl Estradiol (Some estrogen-containing oral contraceptives have been shown to decrease serum concentrations of lamotrigine. Dosage adjustments will be necessary in most patients who start or stop estrogen-containing oral contraceptives while taking lamotrigine. During the week of inactive hormone preparation ("pill-free" week) of oral contraceptive therapy, plasma levels are expected to rise, as much as doubling by the end of the week. Adverse events consistent with elevated levels of lamotrigine, such as dizziness, ataxia and diplopia, could occur. In addition, a decrease in levonorgestrel concentrations by 19% was seen when an oral contraceptive containing 150 mcg of levonorgestrel was concomitantly used with lamotrigine). Products include:

Ethynodiol Diacetate (Some estrogen-containing oral contraceptives have been shown to decrease serum concentrations of lamotrigine. Dosage adjustments will be necessary in most patients who start or stop estrogen-containing oral contraceptives while taking lamotrigine. During the week of inactive hormone preparation ("pill-free" week) of oral contraceptive therapy, plasma levels are expected to rise, as much as doubling by the end of the

week. Adverse events consistent with elevated levels of lamotrigine, such as dizziness, ataxia and diplopia, could occur. In addition, a decrease in levonorgestrel concentrations by 19% was seen when an oral contraceptive containing 150 mcg of levonorgestrel was concomitantly used with lamotrigine).
No products indexed under this heading.

Fosphenytoin (Concomitant use of phenytoin with lamotrigine may decrease lamotrigine steady-state concentrations by approximately 40%).
No products indexed under this heading.

Fosphenytoin Sodium (Concomitant use of phenytoin with lamotrigine may decrease lamotrigine steady-state concentrations by approximately 40%).
No products indexed under this heading.

Levonorgestrel (A decrease in levonorgestrel concentrations by 19% was seen when an oral contraceptive containing 150 mcg of levonorgestrel was concomitantly used with lamotrigine). Products include:

Mestranol (Some estrogen-containing oral contraceptives have been shown to decrease serum concentrations of lamotrigine. Dosage adjustments will be necessary in most patients who start or stop estrogen-containing oral contraceptives while taking lamotrigine. During the week of inactive hormone preparation ("pill-free" week) of oral contraceptive therapy, plasma levels are expected to rise, as much as doubling by the end of the week. Adverse events consistent with elevated levels of lamotrigine, such as dizziness, ataxia and diplopia, could occur. In addition, a decrease in levonorgestrel concentrations by 19% was seen when an oral contraceptive containing 150 mcg of levonorgestrel was concomitantly used with lamotrigine).
No products indexed under this heading.

Methotrexate Sodium (Lamotrigine is a weak inhibitor of dihydrofolate reductase; use caution when prescribing other medications that inhibit folate metabolism).
No products indexed under this heading.

Norethindrone (Some estrogen-containing oral contraceptives have been shown to decrease serum concentrations of lamotrigine. Dosage adjustments will be necessary in most patients who start or stop estrogen-containing oral contraceptives while taking lamotrigine. During the week of inactive hormone preparation ("pill-free" week) of oral contraceptive therapy, plasma levels are expected to rise, as much as doubling by the end of the week. Adverse events consistent with elevated levels of lamotrigine, such as dizziness, ataxia and diplopia, could occur. In addition, a decrease in levonorgestrel concentrations by 19% was seen when an oral contraceptive containing 150 mcg of levonorgestrel was concomitantly used with lamotrigine). Products include:

Norethynodrel (Some estrogen-containing oral contraceptives have been shown to decrease serum concentrations of lamotrigine. Dosage adjustments will be necessary in most patients who start or stop estrogen-containing oral contraceptives while taking lamotrigine. During the week of inactive hormone preparation ("pill-free" week) of oral contraceptive therapy, plasma levels are expected to rise, as

much as doubling by the end of the week. Adverse events consistent with elevated levels of lamotrigine, such as dizziness, ataxia and diplopia, could occur. In addition, a decrease in levonorgestrel concentrations by 19% was seen when an oral contraceptive containing 150 mcg of levonorgestrel was concomitantly used with lamotrigine).
No products indexed under this heading.

Norgestimate (Some estrogen-containing oral contraceptives have been shown to decrease serum concentrations of lamotrigine. Dosage adjustments will be necessary in most patients who start or stop estrogen-containing oral contraceptives while taking lamotrigine. During the week of inactive hormone preparation ("pill-free" week) of oral contraceptive therapy, plasma levels are expected to rise, as much as doubling by the end of the week. Adverse events consistent with elevated levels of lamotrigine, such as dizziness, ataxia and diplopia, could occur. In addition, a decrease in levonorgestrel concentrations by 19% was seen when an oral contraceptive containing 150 mcg of levonorgestrel was concomitantly used with lamotrigine). Products include:

Norgestrel (Some estrogen-containing oral contraceptives have been shown to decrease serum concentrations of lamotrigine. Dosage adjustments will be necessary in most patients who start or stop estrogen-containing oral contraceptives while taking lamotrigine. During the week of inactive hormone preparation ("pill-free" week) of oral contraceptive therapy, plasma levels are expected to rise, as much as doubling by the end of the week. Adverse events consistent with elevated levels of lamotrigine, such as dizziness, ataxia and diplopia, could occur. In addition, a decrease in levonorgestrel concentrations by 19% was seen when an oral contraceptive containing 150 mcg of levonorgestrel was concomitantly used with lamotrigine).
No products indexed under this heading.

Olanzapine (The AUC and C_{max} of lamotrigine was reduced on average by 24% and 20%, respectively, following the addition of olanzapine to lamotrigine in healthy male volunteers compared to healthy male volunteers receiving lamotrigine alone. This reduction in lamotrigine plasma concentration is not expected to be clinically relevant). Products include:

Oxcarbazepine (Limited clinical data suggests a higher incidence of headache, dizziness, nausea, and somnolence with co-administration of lamotrigine and oxcarbazepine compared to lamotrigine alone or oxcarbazepine alone).
No products indexed under this heading.

Phenobarbital (Concomitant use of lamotrigine with phenobarbital may decrease lamotrigine steady-state concentrations by approximately 40%). Products include:

Phenobarbital Sodium (Concomitant use of lamotrigine with phenobarbital may decrease lamotrigine steady-state concentrations by approximately 40%).
No products indexed under this heading.

Phenytoin (Concomitant use of phenytoin with lamotrigine may decrease lamotrigine steady-state concentrations by approximately 40%).
No products indexed under this heading.

Phenytoin Sodium (Concomitant use of phenytoin with lamotrigine may decrease lamotrigine steady-state concentrations by approximately 40%). Products include:

Polyestradiol Phosphate (Some estrogen-containing oral contraceptives have been shown to decrease serum concentrations of lamotrigine. Dosage adjustments will be necessary in most patients who start or stop estrogen-containing oral contraceptives while taking lamotrigine. During the week of inactive hormone preparation ("pill-free" week) of oral contraceptive therapy, plasma levels are expected to rise, as much as doubling by the end of the week. Adverse events consistent with elevated levels of lamotrigine, such as dizziness, ataxia and diplopia, could occur. In addition, a decrease in levonorgestrel concentrations by 19% was seen when an oral contraceptive containing 150 mcg of levonorgestrel was concomitantly used with lamotrigine).
No products indexed under this heading.

Primidone (Concomitant use of lamotrigine with primidone may decrease lamotrigine steady-state concentrations by approximately 40%).
No products indexed under this heading.

Quinestrol (Some estrogen-containing oral contraceptives have been shown to decrease serum concentrations of lamotrigine. Dosage adjustments will be necessary in most patients who start or stop estrogen-containing oral contraceptives while taking lamotrigine. During the week of inactive hormone preparation ("pill-free" week) of oral contraceptive therapy, plasma levels are expected to rise, as much as doubling by the end of the week. Adverse events consistent with elevated levels of lamotrigine, such as dizziness, ataxia and diplopia, could occur. In addition, a decrease in levonorgestrel concentrations by 19% was seen when an oral contraceptive containing 150 mcg of levonorgestrel was concomitantly used with lamotrigine).
No products indexed under this heading.

Rifampin (Concomitant use of lamotrigine with rifampin may decrease lamotrigine concentrations. The AUC of lamotrigine may be decreased by approximately 40% when co-administered with rifampin).
No products indexed under this heading.

Theophyllinate (Since lamotrigine is metabolized predominately by glucuronic acid conjugation, drugs that are known to induce or inhibit glucuronidation may affect the apparent clearance of lamotrigine and doses of lamotrigine may require adjustment based on clinical response).
No products indexed under this heading.

Theophylline (Since lamotrigine is metabolized predominately by glucuronic acid conjugation, drugs that are known to induce or inhibit glucuronidation may affect the apparent clearance of lamotrigine and doses of lamotrigine may require adjustment based on clinical response).
No products indexed under this heading.

Theophylline Anhydrous (Since lamotrigine is metabolized predominately by glucuronic acid conjugation, drugs that are known to induce or inhibit glucuronidation may affect the apparent clearance of lamotrigine and doses of lamotrigine may require adjustment based on clinical response). Products include:

IMPORTANT NOTE: Always consult each drug listing in the patient's regimen for possible interactions.

Lamictal Interactions Index 960

Theophylline Calcium Salicylate (Since lamotrigine is metabolized predominately by glucuronic acid conjugation, drugs that are known to induce or inhibit glucuronidation may affect the apparent clearance of lamotrigine and doses of lamotrigine may require adjustment based on clinical response).
No products indexed under this heading.

Theophylline Dihydroxypropyl (Glyceryl) (Since lamotrigine is metabolized predominately by glucuronic acid conjugation, drugs that are known to induce or inhibit glucuronidation may affect the apparent clearance of lamotrigine and doses of lamotrigine may require adjustment based on clinical response).
No products indexed under this heading.

Theophylline Ethylenediamine (Since lamotrigine is metabolized predominately by glucuronic acid conjugation, drugs that are known to induce or inhibit glucuronidation may affect the apparent clearance of lamotrigine and doses of lamotrigine may require adjustment based on clinical response).
No products indexed under this heading.

Theophylline Sodium Glycinate (Since lamotrigine is metabolized predominately by glucuronic acid conjugation, drugs that are known to induce or inhibit glucuronidation may affect the apparent clearance of lamotrigine and doses of lamotrigine may require adjustment based on clinical response).
No products indexed under this heading.

Topiramate (Topiramate resulted in no change in plasma concentrations of lamotrigine. Administration of lamotrigine resulted in a 15% increase in topiramate concentrations).
No products indexed under this heading.

Trimethoprim (Lamotrigine is a weak inhibitor of dihydrofolate reductase; use caution when prescribing other medications that inhibit folate metabolism).
No products indexed under this heading.

Trimetrexate Glucuronate (Lamotrigine is a weak inhibitor of dihydrofolate reductase; use caution when prescribing other medications that inhibit folate metabolism).
No products indexed under this heading.

Valproate Sodium (Concomitant use of lamotrigine with valproate may increase lamotrigine concentrations slightly more than 2-fold. In addition, when lamotrigine was administered to healthy volunteers receiving valproate, the trough steady-state valproate plasma concentrations decreased by an average of 25% over a 3-week period, and then stabilized. However, adding lamotrigine to the existing therapy did not cause a change in valproate plasma concentrations in either adult or pediatric patients in controlled clinical trials. Also, co-administration with valproate may increase the risk of rash).
No products indexed under this heading.

Valproic Acid (Concomitant use of lamotrigine with valproate may increase lamotrigine concentrations slightly more than 2-fold. In addition, when lamotrigine was administered to healthy volunteers receiving valproate, the trough steady-state valproate plasma concentrations decreased by an average of 25% over a 3-week period, and then stabilized. However, adding lamotrigine to the existing therapy did not cause a change in valproate plasma concentrations in either adult or pediatric patients in controlled clinical trials. Also, co-administration with valproate may increase the risk of rash).
No products indexed under this heading.

LAMICTAL XR EXTENDED-RELEASE TABLETS
(Lamotrigine) 1536
See Lamictal Tablets

LANOXIN INJECTION
(Digoxin) 1546
See Lanoxin Tablets

LANOXIN INJECTION PEDIATRIC
(Digoxin) 1549
See Lanoxin Tablets

LANOXIN TABLETS
(Digoxin) 1553
May interact with amphotericins, antacids, antineoplastics, beta-blockers, calcium channel blockers, calcium preparations, corticosteroids, diuretics, erythromycin, inhibitors of renal tubular secretion or resorption, macrolide antibiotics, nephrotoxic agents, potassium-depleting diuretics, quinidine, sympathomimetics, tetracyclines, thyroid preparations, and certain other agents. Compounds in these categories include:

Abacavir Sulfate (Caution should be exercised when combining digoxin with any drug that may cause a significant deterioration in renal function, since a decline in glomerular filtration or tubular secretion may impair the excretion of digoxin). Products include:
Epzicom 1448
Trizivir 1688
Ziagen 1740

Acebutolol Hydrochloride (Both digitalis glycosides and β-blockers slow atrioventricular conduction and decrease heart rate. Concomitant use can increase the risk of bradycardia).
No products indexed under this heading.

Acyclovir (Caution should be exercised when combining digoxin with any drug that may cause a significant deterioration in renal function, since a decline in glomerular filtration or tubular secretion may impair the excretion of digoxin). Products include:
Zovirax 1760

Acyclovir Sodium (Caution should be exercised when combining digoxin with any drug that may cause a significant deterioration in renal function, since a decline in glomerular filtration or tubular secretion may impair the excretion of digoxin).
No products indexed under this heading.

Alatrofloxacin Mesylate (Caution should be exercised when combining digoxin with any drug that may cause a significant deterioration in renal function, since a decline in glomerular filtration or tubular secretion may impair the excretion of digoxin).
No products indexed under this heading.

Albuterol (Concomitant use of digoxin and sympathomimetics increases the risk of cardiac arrhythmias).
No products indexed under this heading.

Albuterol Sulfate (Concomitant use of digoxin and sympathomimetics increases the risk of cardiac arrhythmias). Products include:
ProAir HFA 3393
Proventil HFA 3204
Ventolin HFA 1708

Alclometasone Dipropionate (In patients with hypokalemia or hypomagnesemia, toxicity may occur despite serum digoxin concentrations below 2.0 ng/mL, because potassium or magnesium depletion sensitizes the myocardium to digoxin. Therefore, it is desirable to maintain normal serum potassium and magnesium concentrations in patients being treated with digoxin. Deficiencies of these electrolytes may result from concomitant use with corticosteroids).
No products indexed under this heading.

Aldesleukin (Caution should be exercised when combining digoxin with any drug that may cause a significant deterioration in renal function, since a decline in glomerular filtration or tubular secretion may impair the excretion of digoxin). Products include:
Proleukin 2504

Alprazolam (Alprazolam may raise the serum digoxin concentration due to a reduction in clearance and/or in volume of distribution of the drug, with the implication that digitalis intoxication may result).
No products indexed under this heading.

Altretamine (Certain anticancer drugs may interfere with intestinal digoxin absorption, resulting in unexpectedly low serum concentrations). Products include:
Hexalen 1066

Aluminum Carbonate (In patients with hypokalemia or hypomagnesemia, toxicity may occur despite serum digoxin concentrations below 2.0 ng/mL, because potassium or magnesium depletion sensitizes the myocardium to digoxin. Therefore, it is desirable to maintain normal serum potassium and magnesium concentrations in patients being treated with digoxin. Deficiencies of these electrolytes may result from concomitant use with antacids. In addition, antacids may interfere with intestinal digoxin absorption, resulting in unexpectedly low serum concentrations).
No products indexed under this heading.

Aluminum Hydroxide (In patients with hypokalemia or hypomagnesemia, toxicity may occur despite serum digoxin concentrations below 2.0 ng/mL, because potassium or magnesium depletion sensitizes the myocardium to digoxin. Therefore, it is desirable to maintain normal serum potassium and magnesium concentrations in patients being treated with digoxin. Deficiencies of these electrolytes may result from concomitant use with antacids. In addition, antacids may interfere with intestinal digoxin absorption, resulting in unexpectedly low serum concentrations).
No products indexed under this heading.

Amikacin Sulfate (Caution should be exercised when combining digoxin with any drug that may cause a significant deterioration in renal function, since a decline in glomerular filtration or tubular secretion may impair the excretion of digoxin).
No products indexed under this heading.

Amiloride Hydrochloride (In patients with hypokalemia or hypomagnesemia, toxicity may occur despite serum digoxin concentrations below 2.0 ng/mL, because potassium or magnesium depletion sensitizes the myocardium to digoxin. Therefore, it is desirable to maintain normal serum potassium and magnesium concentrations in patients being treated with digoxin. Deficiencies of these electrolytes may result from concomitant use with diuretics).
No products indexed under this heading.

Amiodarone Hydrochloride (Amiodarone may raise the serum digoxin concentration due to a reduction in clearance and/or in volume of distribution of the drug, with the implication that digitalis intoxication may result).
No products indexed under this heading.

Amlodipine Besylate (Although calcium channel blockers and digoxin may be useful in combination to control atrial fibrillation, their additive effects on AV node conduction can result in advanced or complete heart block). Products include:
Azor 1010
Exforge 2443
Exforge HCT 2449

Amoxicillin (Caution should be exercised when combining digoxin with any drug that may cause a significant deterioration in renal function, since a decline in glomerular filtration or tubular secretion may impair the excretion of digoxin). Products include:
Amoxil Capsules 1311
Amoxil Chewable Tablets 1311
Amoxil 1311
Amoxil Powder 1311
Augmentin 1331
Augmentin Tablets 1335
Augmentin ES-600 1338
Augmentin XR 1342
Moxatag 2321

Amoxicillin Trihydrate (Caution should be exercised when combining digoxin with any drug that may cause a significant deterioration in renal function, since a decline in glomerular filtration or tubular secretion may impair the excretion of digoxin).
No products indexed under this heading.

Amphotericin B (In patients with hypokalemia or hypomagnesemia, toxicity may occur despite serum digoxin concentrations below 2.0 ng/mL, because potassium or magnesium depletion sensitizes the myocardium to digoxin. Therefore, it is desirable to maintain normal serum potassium and magnesium concentrations in patients being treated with digoxin. Deficiencies of these electrolytes may result from concomitant use with amphotercin B).
No products indexed under this heading.

Amphotericin B, liposomal (In patients with hypokalemia or hypomagnesemia, toxicity may occur despite serum digoxin concentrations below 2.0 ng/mL, because potassium or magnesium depletion sensitizes the myocardium to digoxin. Therefore, it is desirable to maintain normal serum potassium and magnesium concentrations in patients being treated with digoxin. Deficiencies of these electrolytes may result from concomitant use with amphotercin B). Products include:
AmBisome 659

Amphotericin B Cholesteryl Sulfate (In patients with hypokalemia or hypomagnesemia, toxicity may occur despite serum digoxin concentrations below 2.0 ng/mL, because potassium or magnesium depletion sensitizes the myocardium to digoxin. Therefore, it is desirable to maintain normal serum potassium and magnesium concentrations in patients being treated with digoxin. Deficiencies of these electrolytes may result from concomitant use with amphotercin B).
No products indexed under this heading.

Amphotericin B Lipid Complex (In patients with hypokalemia or hypomagnesemia, toxicity may occur despite serum digoxin concentrations below 2.0 ng/mL, because potassium or magnesium depletion sensitizes the myocardium to digoxin. Therefore, it is desirable to maintain normal serum potassium and magnesium concentrations in patients being treated with digoxin. Deficiencies of these electrolytes may result from concomitant use with amphotercin B).
No products indexed under this heading.

Ampicillin (Caution should be exercised when combining digoxin with any drug that may cause a significant deterioration in renal function, since a decline in glomerular filtration or tubular secretion may impair the excretion of digoxin).
No products indexed under this heading.

IMPORTANT NOTE: Always consult each drug listing in the patient's regimen for possible interactions.

Lanoxin Interactions Index 962

CitraNatal 90 DHA Capsules 2332
CitraNatal Assure 2332
CitraNatal Harmony 2332
CitraNatal Rx 2332

Calcium Glubionate (Calcium, particularly if administered rapidly by the intravenous route, may produce serious arrhythmias in digitalized patients).
No products indexed under this heading.

Captopril (Caution should be exercised when combining digoxin with any drug that may cause a significant deterioration in renal function, since a decline in glomerular filtration or tubular secretion may impair the excretion of digoxin). Products include:
Captopril 2341

Carbenicillin Disodium (Caution should be exercised when combining digoxin with any drug that may cause a significant deterioration in renal function, since a decline in glomerular filtration or tubular secretion may impair the excretion of digoxin).
No products indexed under this heading.

Carbenicillin Indanyl Sodium (Caution should be exercised when combining digoxin with any drug that may cause a significant deterioration in renal function, since a decline in glomerular filtration or tubular secretion may impair the excretion of digoxin).
No products indexed under this heading.

Carboplatin (Certain anticancer drugs may interfere with intestinal digoxin absorption, resulting in unexpectedly low serum concentrations).
No products indexed under this heading.

Carmustine (BCNU) (Certain anticancer drugs may interfere with intestinal digoxin absorption, resulting in unexpectedly low serum concentrations).
No products indexed under this heading.

Carteolol Hydrochloride (Both digitalis glycosides and β-blockers slow atrioventricular conduction and decrease heart rate. Concomitant use can increase the risk of bradycardia).
No products indexed under this heading.

Carvedilol (Both digitalis glycosides and β-blockers slow atrioventricular conduction and decrease heart rate. Concomitant use can increase the risk of bradycardia. Digoxin concentrations are increased by about 15% when digoxin and carvedilol are administered concomitantly. Therefore, increased monitoring of digoxin is recommended when initiating, adjusting, or discontinuing carvedilol). Products include:
Coreg 1409

Carvedilol Phosphate (Both digitalis glycosides and β-blockers slow atrioventricular conduction and decrease heart rate. Concomitant use can increase the risk of bradycardia. Digoxin concentrations are increased by about 15% when digoxin and carvedilol are administered concomitantly. Therefore, increased monitoring of digoxin is recommended when initiating, adjusting, or discontinuing carvedilol). Products include:
Coreg CR 1416

Cefaclor (Caution should be exercised when combining digoxin with any drug that may cause a significant deterioration in renal function, since a decline in glomerular filtration or tubular secretion may impair the excretion of digoxin).
No products indexed under this heading.

Cefadroxil (Caution should be exercised when combining digoxin with any drug that may cause a significant deterioration in renal function, since a decline in glomerular filtration or tubular secretion may impair the excretion of digoxin).
No products indexed under this heading.

Cefamandole Nafate (Caution should be exercised when combining digoxin with any drug that may cause a significant deterioration in renal function, since a decline in glomerular filtration or tubular secretion may impair the excretion of digoxin).
No products indexed under this heading.

Cefazolin Sodium (Caution should be exercised when combining digoxin with any drug that may cause a significant deterioration in renal function, since a decline in glomerular filtration or tubular secretion may impair the excretion of digoxin).
No products indexed under this heading.

Cefdinir (Caution should be exercised when combining digoxin with any drug that may cause a significant deterioration in renal function, since a decline in glomerular filtration or tubular secretion may impair the excretion of digoxin). Products include:
Omnicef Capsules 518
Omnicef Oral Suspension 518

Cefepime Hydrochloride (Caution should be exercised when combining digoxin with any drug that may cause a significant deterioration in renal function, since a decline in glomerular filtration or tubular secretion may impair the excretion of digoxin).
No products indexed under this heading.

Cefixime (Caution should be exercised when combining digoxin with any drug that may cause a significant deterioration in renal function, since a decline in glomerular filtration or tubular secretion may impair the excretion of digoxin). Products include:
Suprax for Oral Suspension 2038
Suprax Tablets 2038

Cefmetazole Sodium (Caution should be exercised when combining digoxin with any drug that may cause a significant deterioration in renal function, since a decline in glomerular filtration or tubular secretion may impair the excretion of digoxin).
No products indexed under this heading.

Cefonicid Sodium (Caution should be exercised when combining digoxin with any drug that may cause a significant deterioration in renal function, since a decline in glomerular filtration or tubular secretion may impair the excretion of digoxin).
No products indexed under this heading.

Cefoperazone Sodium (Caution should be exercised when combining digoxin with any drug that may cause a significant deterioration in renal function, since a decline in glomerular filtration or tubular secretion may impair the excretion of digoxin).
No products indexed under this heading.

Ceforanide (Caution should be exercised when combining digoxin with any drug that may cause a significant deterioration in renal function, since a decline in glomerular filtration or tubular secretion may impair the excretion of digoxin).
No products indexed under this heading.

Cefotaxime Sodium (Caution should be exercised when combining digoxin with any drug that may cause a significant deterioration in renal function, since a decline in glomerular filtration or tubular secretion may impair the excretion of digoxin).
No products indexed under this heading.

Cefotetan (Caution should be exercised when combining digoxin with any drug that may cause a significant deterioration in renal function, since a decline in glomerular filtration or tubular secretion may impair the excretion of digoxin).
No products indexed under this heading.

Cefoxitin Sodium (Caution should be exercised when combining digoxin with any drug that may cause a significant deterioration in renal function, since a decline in glomerular filtration or tubular secretion may impair the excretion of digoxin).
No products indexed under this heading.

Cefpodoxime Proxetil (Caution should be exercised when combining digoxin with any drug that may cause a significant deterioration in renal function, since a decline in glomerular filtration or tubular secretion may impair the excretion of digoxin).
No products indexed under this heading.

Cefprozil (Caution should be exercised when combining digoxin with any drug that may cause a significant deterioration in renal function, since a decline in glomerular filtration or tubular secretion may impair the excretion of digoxin).
No products indexed under this heading.

Ceftazidime (Caution should be exercised when combining digoxin with any drug that may cause a significant deterioration in renal function, since a decline in glomerular filtration or tubular secretion may impair the excretion of digoxin). Products include:
Fortaz 1481

Ceftizoxime Sodium (Caution should be exercised when combining digoxin with any drug that may cause a significant deterioration in renal function, since a decline in glomerular filtration or tubular secretion may impair the excretion of digoxin).
No products indexed under this heading.

Ceftriaxone Sodium (Caution should be exercised when combining digoxin with any drug that may cause a significant deterioration in renal function, since a decline in glomerular filtration or tubular secretion may impair the excretion of digoxin). Products include:
Rocephin 2859

Cefuroxime Axetil (Caution should be exercised when combining digoxin with any drug that may cause a significant deterioration in renal function, since a decline in glomerular filtration or tubular secretion may impair the excretion of digoxin). Products include:
Ceftin 1399

Cefuroxime Sodium (Caution should be exercised when combining digoxin with any drug that may cause a significant deterioration in renal function, since a decline in glomerular filtration or tubular secretion may impair the excretion of digoxin).
No products indexed under this heading.

Celecoxib (Caution should be exercised when combining digoxin with any drug that may cause a significant deterioration in renal function, since a decline in glomerular filtration or tubular secretion may impair the excretion of digoxin). Products include:
Celebrex 3272

Cephalexin (Caution should be exercised when combining digoxin with any drug that may cause a significant deterioration in renal function, since a decline in glomerular filtration or tubular secretion may impair the excretion of digoxin).
No products indexed under this heading.

Cephalothin Sodium (Caution should be exercised when combining digoxin with any drug that may cause a significant deterioration in renal function, since a decline in glomerular filtration or tubular secretion may impair the excretion of digoxin).
No products indexed under this heading.

Cephapirin Sodium (Caution should be exercised when combining digoxin with any drug that may cause a significant deterioration in renal function, since a decline in glomerular filtration or tubular secretion may impair the excretion of digoxin).
No products indexed under this heading.

Cephradine (Caution should be exercised when combining digoxin with any drug that may cause a significant deterioration in renal function, since a decline in glomerular filtration or tubular secretion may impair the excretion of digoxin).
No products indexed under this heading.

Cerivastatin Sodium (Caution should be exercised when combining digoxin with any drug that may cause a significant deterioration in renal function, since a decline in glomerular filtration or tubular secretion may impair the excretion of digoxin).
No products indexed under this heading.

Chlorambucil (Certain anticancer drugs may interfere with intestinal digoxin absorption, resulting in unexpectedly low serum concentrations). Products include:
Leukeran 1557

Chlorothiazide (In patients with hypokalemia or hypomagnesemia, toxicity may occur despite serum digoxin concentrations below 2.0 ng/mL, because potassium or magnesium depletion sensitizes the myocardium to digoxin. Therefore, it is desirable to maintain normal serum potassium and magnesium concentrations in patients being treated with digoxin. Deficiencies of these electrolytes may result from concomitant use with diuretics. Potassium-depleting diuretics are a major contributing factor to digitalis toxicity).
No products indexed under this heading.

Chlorothiazide Sodium (In patients with hypokalemia or hypomagnesemia, toxicity may occur despite serum digoxin concentrations below 2.0 ng/mL, because potassium or magnesium depletion sensitizes the myocardium to digoxin. Therefore, it is desirable to maintain normal serum potassium and magnesium concentrations in patients being treated with digoxin. Deficiencies of these electrolytes may result from concomitant use with diuretics. Potassium-depleting diuretics are a major contributing factor to digitalis toxicity). Products include:
Diuril Intravenous 2009

Chlorpropamide (Caution should be exercised when combining digoxin with any drug that may cause a significant deterioration in renal function, since a decline in glomerular filtration or tubular secretion may impair the excretion of digoxin).
No products indexed under this heading.

Chlorthalidone (In patients with hypokalemia or hypomagnesemia, toxicity may occur despite serum digoxin concentrations below 2.0 ng/mL, because potassium or magnesium depletion sensitizes the myocardium to digoxin. Therefore, it is desirable to maintain normal serum potassium and magnesium concentrations in patients being treated with digoxin. Deficiencies of these electrolytes may result from concomitant use with diuretics). Products include:
Clorpres 2344

Cholestyramine (Cholestyramine may interfere with intestinal digoxin absorption, resulting in unexpectedly low serum concentrations).
No products indexed under this heading.

Ciclesonide (In patients with hypokalemia or hypomagnesemia, toxicity may occur despite serum digoxin concentrations below 2.0 ng/mL, because potas-

sium or magnesium depletion sensitizes the myocardium to digoxin. Therefore, it is desirable to maintain normal serum potassium and magnesium concentrations in patients being treated with digoxin. Deficiencies of these electrolytes may result from concomitant use with corticosteroids).
No products indexed under this heading.

Cidofovir (Caution should be exercised when combining digoxin with any drug that may cause a significant deterioration in renal function, since a decline in glomerular filtration or tubular secretion may impair the excretion of digoxin).
No products indexed under this heading.

Cilastatin Sodium (Caution should be exercised when combining digoxin with any drug that may cause a significant deterioration in renal function, since a decline in glomerular filtration or tubular secretion may impair the excretion of digoxin). Products include:
Primaxin I.M. 2232
Primaxin I.V. 2235

Cimetidine (Caution should be exercised when combining digoxin with any drug that may cause a significant deterioration in renal function, since a decline in glomerular filtration or tubular secretion may impair the excretion of digoxin).
No products indexed under this heading.

Cimetidine Hydrochloride (Caution should be exercised when combining digoxin with any drug that may cause a significant deterioration in renal function, since a decline in glomerular filtration or tubular secretion may impair the excretion of digoxin).
No products indexed under this heading.

Cisplatin (Certain anticancer drugs may interfere with intestinal digoxin absorption, resulting in unexpectedly low serum concentrations).
No products indexed under this heading.

Cladribine (Caution should be exercised when combining digoxin with any drug that may cause a significant deterioration in renal function, since a decline in glomerular filtration or tubular secretion may impair the excretion of digoxin). Products include:
Leustatin 946

Clarithromycin (Clarithromycin may increase digoxin absorption in patients who inactivate digoxin by bacterial metabolism in the lower intestine, so that digitalis intoxication may result). Products include:
Biaxin/Biaxin XL 412

Clozapine (Caution should be exercised when combining digoxin with any drug that may cause a significant deterioration in renal function, since a decline in glomerular filtration or tubular secretion may impair the excretion of digoxin).
No products indexed under this heading.

Colistimethate Sodium (Caution should be exercised when combining digoxin with any drug that may cause a significant deterioration in renal function, since a decline in glomerular filtration or tubular secretion may impair the excretion of digoxin).
No products indexed under this heading.

Colistin Sulfate (Caution should be exercised when combining digoxin with any drug that may cause a significant deterioration in renal function, since a decline in glomerular filtration or tubular secretion may impair the excretion of digoxin).
No products indexed under this heading.

Cortisone Acetate (In patients with hypokalemia or hypomagnesemia, toxicity may occur despite serum digoxin concentrations below 2.0 ng/mL, because potassium or magnesium depletion sensitizes the myocardium to digoxin. Therefore, it is desirable to maintain normal serum potassium and magnesium concentrations in patients being treated with digoxin. Deficiencies of these electrolytes may result from concomitant use with corticosteroids).
No products indexed under this heading.

Cyclophosphamide (Certain anticancer drugs may interfere with intestinal digoxin absorption, resulting in unexpectedly low serum concentrations).
No products indexed under this heading.

Cyclosporine (Caution should be exercised when combining digoxin with any drug that may cause a significant deterioration in renal function, since a decline in glomerular filtration or tubular secretion may impair the excretion of digoxin). Products include:
Gengraf 440
Neoral Oral Solution 2496
Neoral Capsules 2496
Restasis 605

Cytarabine (Caution should be exercised when combining digoxin with any drug that may cause a significant deterioration in renal function, since a decline in glomerular filtration or tubular secretion may impair the excretion of digoxin).
No products indexed under this heading.

Cytarabine Liposome (Caution should be exercised when combining digoxin with any drug that may cause a significant deterioration in renal function, since a decline in glomerular filtration or tubular secretion may impair the excretion of digoxin).
No products indexed under this heading.

Dacarbazine (Certain anticancer drugs may interfere with intestinal digoxin absorption, resulting in unexpectedly low serum concentrations).
No products indexed under this heading.

Daunorubicin Citrate (Certain anticancer drugs may interfere with intestinal digoxin absorption, resulting in unexpectedly low serum concentrations).
No products indexed under this heading.

Daunorubicin Hydrochloride (Certain anticancer drugs may interfere with intestinal digoxin absorption, resulting in unexpectedly low serum concentrations).
No products indexed under this heading.

Delavirdine Mesylate (Caution should be exercised when combining digoxin with any drug that may cause a significant deterioration in renal function, since a decline in glomerular filtration or tubular secretion may impair the excretion of digoxin).
No products indexed under this heading.

Demeclocycline Hydrochloride (Tetracycline may increase digoxin absorption in patients who inactivate digoxin by bacterial metabolism in the lower intestine, so that digitalis intoxication may result).
No products indexed under this heading.

Denileukin Diftitox (Certain anticancer drugs may interfere with intestinal digoxin absorption, resulting in unexpectedly low serum concentrations). Products include:
Ontak 1068

Desoximetasone (In patients with hypokalemia or hypomagnesemia, toxicity may occur despite serum digoxin concentrations below 2.0 ng/mL, because potassium or magnesium depletion sensitizes the myocardium to digoxin. Therefore, it is desirable to maintain normal serum potassium and magnesium concentrations in patients being treated with digoxin. Deficiencies of these electrolytes may result from concomitant use with corticosteroids).
No products indexed under this heading.

Dexamethasone (In patients with hypokalemia or hypomagnesemia, toxicity may occur despite serum digoxin concentrations below 2.0 ng/mL, because potassium or magnesium depletion sensitizes the myocardium to digoxin. Therefore, it is desirable to maintain normal serum potassium and magnesium concentrations in patients being treated with digoxin. Deficiencies of these electrolytes may result from concomitant use with corticosteroids).
Products include:
Ciprodex 583
Ozurdex .... ⊙223
Tobramycin and Dexamethasone Ophthalmic Suspension .... ⊙251

Dexamethasone Acetate (In patients with hypokalemia or hypomagnesemia, toxicity may occur despite serum digoxin concentrations below 2.0 ng/mL, because potassium or magnesium depletion sensitizes the myocardium to digoxin. Therefore, it is desirable to maintain normal serum potassium and magnesium concentrations in patients being treated with digoxin. Deficiencies of these electrolytes may result from concomitant use with corticosteroids).
No products indexed under this heading.

Dexamethasone Phosphate (In patients with hypokalemia or hypomagnesemia, toxicity may occur despite serum digoxin concentrations below 2.0 ng/mL, because potassium or magnesium depletion sensitizes the myocardium to digoxin. Therefore, it is desirable to maintain normal serum potassium and magnesium concentrations in patients being treated with digoxin. Deficiencies of these electrolytes may result from concomitant use with corticosteroids).
No products indexed under this heading.

Dexamethasone Sodium (In patients with hypokalemia or hypomagnesemia, toxicity may occur despite serum digoxin concentrations below 2.0 ng/mL, because potassium or magnesium depletion sensitizes the myocardium to digoxin. Therefore, it is desirable to maintain normal serum potassium and magnesium concentrations in patients being treated with digoxin. Deficiencies of these electrolytes may result from concomitant use with corticosteroids).
No products indexed under this heading.

Dexamethasone Sodium Phosphate (In patients with hypokalemia or hypomagnesemia, toxicity may occur despite serum digoxin concentrations below 2.0 ng/mL, because potassium or magnesium depletion sensitizes the myocardium to digoxin. Therefore, it is desirable to maintain normal serum potassium and magnesium concentrations in patients being treated with digoxin. Deficiencies of these electrolytes may result from concomitant use with corticosteroids).
No products indexed under this heading.

Dexamethasone Sodium Phosphate Injection (In patients with hypokalemia or hypomagnesemia, toxicity may occur despite serum digoxin concentrations below 2.0 ng/mL, because potassium or magnesium depletion sensitizes the myocardium to digoxin. Therefore, it is desirable to maintain normal serum potassium and magnesium concentrations in patients being treated with digoxin. Deficiencies of these electrolytes may result from concomitant use with corticosteroids).
No products indexed under this heading.

Diatrizoate Meglumine (Caution should be exercised when combining digoxin with any drug that may cause a significant deterioration in renal function, since a decline in glomerular filtration or tubular secretion may impair the excretion of digoxin).
No products indexed under this heading.

Diatrizoate Sodium (Caution should be exercised when combining digoxin with any drug that may cause a significant deterioration in renal function, since a decline in glomerular filtration or tubular secretion may impair the excretion of digoxin).
No products indexed under this heading.

Diclofenac Potassium (Caution should be exercised when combining digoxin with any drug that may cause a significant deterioration in renal function, since a decline in glomerular filtration or tubular secretion may impair the excretion of digoxin).
No products indexed under this heading.

Diclofenac Sodium (Caution should be exercised when combining digoxin with any drug that may cause a significant deterioration in renal function, since a decline in glomerular filtration or tubular secretion may impair the excretion of digoxin).
No products indexed under this heading.

Dicloxacillin Sodium (Caution should be exercised when combining digoxin with any drug that may cause a significant deterioration in renal function, since a decline in glomerular filtration or tubular secretion may impair the excretion of digoxin).
No products indexed under this heading.

Didanosine (Caution should be exercised when combining digoxin with any drug that may cause a significant deterioration in renal function, since a decline in glomerular filtration or tubular secretion may impair the excretion of digoxin).
No products indexed under this heading.

Diflorasone Diacetate (In patients with hypokalemia or hypomagnesemia, toxicity may occur despite serum digoxin concentrations below 2.0 ng/mL, because potassium or magnesium depletion sensitizes the myocardium to digoxin. Therefore, it is desirable to maintain normal serum potassium and magnesium concentrations in patients being treated with digoxin. Deficiencies of these electrolytes may result from concomitant use with corticosteroids).
No products indexed under this heading.

Diltiazem Hydrochloride (Although calcium channel blockers and digoxin may be useful in combination to control atrial fibrillation, their additive effects on AV node conduction can result in advanced or complete heart block). Products include:
Cardizem LA 423

Diphenoxylate (Diphenoxylate, by decreasing gut motility, may increase digoxin absorption).
No products indexed under this heading.

Diphenoxylate Hydrochloride (Diphenoxylate, by decreasing gut motility, may increase digoxin absorption).
No products indexed under this heading.

Dirithromycin (Erythromycin and clarithromycin (and possibly other macrolide antibiotics) may increase digoxin absorption in patients who inactivate digoxin by bacterial metabolism in the lower intestine, so that digitalis intoxication may result).
No products indexed under this heading.

Dobutamine Hydrochloride (Concomitant use of digoxin and sympathomimetics increases the risk of cardiac arrhythmias).
No products indexed under this heading.

Docetaxel (Certain anticancer drugs may interfere with intestinal digoxin absorption, resulting in unexpectedly low serum concentrations). Products include:
Taxotere 3035

Dopamine Hydrochloride (Concomitant use of digoxin and sympathomimetics increases the risk of cardiac arrhythmias).

No products indexed under this heading.

Doxorubicin Hydrochloride (Certain anticancer drugs may interfere with intestinal digoxin absorption, resulting in unexpectedly low serum concentrations).

No products indexed under this heading.

Doxycycline (Tetracycline may increase digoxin absorption in patients who inactivate digoxin by bacterial metabolism in the lower intestine, so that digitalis intoxication may result).

No products indexed under this heading.

Doxycycline Calcium (Tetracycline may increase digoxin absorption in patients who inactivate digoxin by bacterial metabolism in the lower intestine, so that digitalis intoxication may result).

No products indexed under this heading.

Doxycycline Hyclate (Tetracycline may increase digoxin absorption in patients who inactivate digoxin by bacterial metabolism in the lower intestine, so that digitalis intoxication may result).

No products indexed under this heading.

Doxycycline Monohydrate (Tetracycline may increase digoxin absorption in patients who inactivate digoxin by bacterial metabolism in the lower intestine, so that digitalis intoxication may result).

No products indexed under this heading.

Efavirenz (Caution should be exercised when combining digoxin with any drug that may cause a significant deterioration in renal function, since a decline in glomerular filtration or tubular secretion may impair the excretion of digoxin). Products include:

Atripla 906

Emtricitabine (Caution should be exercised when combining digoxin with any drug that may cause a significant deterioration in renal function, since a decline in glomerular filtration or tubular secretion may impair the excretion of digoxin). Products include:

Atripla 906
Emtriva 1238
Emtriva Oral Solution 1238
Truvada 1258

Enalapril Maleate (Caution should be exercised when combining digoxin with any drug that may cause a significant deterioration in renal function, since a decline in glomerular filtration or tubular secretion may impair the excretion of digoxin).

No products indexed under this heading.

Enalaprilat (Caution should be exercised when combining digoxin with any drug that may cause a significant deterioration in renal function, since a decline in glomerular filtration or tubular secretion may impair the excretion of digoxin).

No products indexed under this heading.

Enfuvirtide (Caution should be exercised when combining digoxin with any drug that may cause a significant deterioration in renal function, since a decline in glomerular filtration or tubular secretion may impair the excretion of digoxin).

No products indexed under this heading.

Ephedrine Hydrochloride (Concomitant use of digoxin and sympathomimetics increases the risk of cardiac arrhythmias).

No products indexed under this heading.

Ephedrine Sulfate (Concomitant use of digoxin and sympathomimetics increases the risk of cardiac arrhythmias).

No products indexed under this heading.

Ephedrine Tannate (Concomitant use of digoxin and sympathomimetics increases the risk of cardiac arrhythmias).

No products indexed under this heading.

Epinephrine (Concomitant use of digoxin and sympathomimetics increases the risk of cardiac arrhythmias). Products include:

EpiPen 3631
Twinject 3268

Epinephrine Bitartrate (Concomitant use of digoxin and sympathomimetics increases the risk of cardiac arrhythmias).

No products indexed under this heading.

Epinephrine Hydrochloride (Concomitant use of digoxin and sympathomimetics increases the risk of cardiac arrhythmias).

No products indexed under this heading.

Epirubicin Hydrochloride (Certain anticancer drugs may interfere with intestinal digoxin absorption, resulting in unexpectedly low serum concentrations).

No products indexed under this heading.

Erythromycin (Erythromycin may increase digoxin absorption in patients who inactivate digoxin by bacterial metabolism in the lower intestine, so that digitalis intoxication may result).

No products indexed under this heading.

Erythromycin, Topical (Erythromycin may increase digoxin absorption in patients who inactivate digoxin by bacterial metabolism in the lower intestine, so that digitalis intoxication may result).

No products indexed under this heading.

Erythromycin Estolate (Erythromycin may increase digoxin absorption in patients who inactivate digoxin by bacterial metabolism in the lower intestine, so that digitalis intoxication may result).

No products indexed under this heading.

Erythromycin Ethylsuccinate (Erythromycin may increase digoxin absorption in patients who inactivate digoxin by bacterial metabolism in the lower intestine, so that digitalis intoxication may result). Products include:

E.E.S. 437
EryPed 435

Erythromycin Gluceptate (Erythromycin may increase digoxin absorption in patients who inactivate digoxin by bacterial metabolism in the lower intestine, so that digitalis intoxication may result).

No products indexed under this heading.

Erythromycin Lactobionate (Erythromycin may increase digoxin absorption in patients who inactivate digoxin by bacterial metabolism in the lower intestine, so that digitalis intoxication may result).

No products indexed under this heading.

Erythromycin Stearate (Erythromycin may increase digoxin absorption in patients who inactivate digoxin by bacterial metabolism in the lower intestine, so that digitalis intoxication may result).

No products indexed under this heading.

Esmolol Hydrochloride (Both digitalis glycosides and β-blockers slow atrioventricular conduction and decrease heart rate. Concomitant use can increase the risk of bradycardia).

No products indexed under this heading.

Estramustine Phosphate Sodium (Certain anticancer drugs may interfere with intestinal digoxin absorption, resulting in unexpectedly low serum concentrations).

No products indexed under this heading.

Ethacrynic Acid (In patients with hypokalemia or hypomagnesemia, toxicity may occur despite serum digoxin concentrations below 2.0 ng/mL, because potassium or magnesium depletion sensitizes the myocardium to digoxin. Therefore, it is desirable to maintain normal serum potassium and magnesium concentrations in patients being treated with digoxin. Deficiencies of these electrolytes may result from concomitant use with diuretics. Potassium-depleting diuretics are a major contributing factor to digitalis toxicity).

No products indexed under this heading.

Ethiodized Oil (Caution should be exercised when combining digoxin with any drug that may cause a significant deterioration in renal function, since a decline in glomerular filtration or tubular secretion may impair the excretion of digoxin).

No products indexed under this heading.

Etodolac (Caution should be exercised when combining digoxin with any drug that may cause a significant deterioration in renal function, since a decline in glomerular filtration or tubular secretion may impair the excretion of digoxin).

No products indexed under this heading.

Etoposide (Certain anticancer drugs may interfere with intestinal digoxin absorption, resulting in unexpectedly low serum concentrations).

No products indexed under this heading.

Exemestane (Certain anticancer drugs may interfere with intestinal digoxin absorption, resulting in unexpectedly low serum concentrations). Products include:

Aromasin 2758

Felodipine (Although calcium channel blockers and digoxin may be useful in combination to control atrial fibrillation, their additive effects on AV node conduction can result in advanced or complete heart block).

No products indexed under this heading.

Fenoprofen Calcium (Caution should be exercised when combining digoxin with any drug that may cause a significant deterioration in renal function, since a decline in glomerular filtration or tubular secretion may impair the excretion of digoxin).

No products indexed under this heading.

Filgrastim (Caution should be exercised when combining digoxin with any drug that may cause a significant deterioration in renal function, since a decline in glomerular filtration or tubular secretion may impair the excretion of digoxin). Products include:

Neupogen 631

Floxuridine (Certain anticancer drugs may interfere with intestinal digoxin absorption, resulting in unexpectedly low serum concentrations).

No products indexed under this heading.

Fludrocortisone Acetate (In patients with hypokalemia or hypomagnesemia, toxicity may occur despite serum digoxin concentrations below 2.0 ng/mL, because potassium or magnesium depletion sensitizes the myocardium to digoxin. Therefore, it is desirable to maintain normal serum potassium and magnesium concentrations in patients being treated with digoxin. Deficiencies of these electrolytes may result from concomitant use with corticosteroids).

No products indexed under this heading.

Flumethasone Pivalate (In patients with hypokalemia or hypomagnesemia, toxicity may occur despite serum digoxin concentrations below 2.0 ng/mL, because potassium or magnesium depletion sensitizes the myocardium to digoxin. Therefore, it is desirable to maintain normal serum potassium and magnesium concentrations in patients being treated with digoxin. Deficiencies of these electrolytes may result from concomitant use with corticosteroids).

No products indexed under this heading.

Flunisolide Hemihydrate (In patients with hypokalemia or hypomagnesemia, toxicity may occur despite serum digoxin concentrations below 2.0 ng/mL, because potassium or magnesium depletion sensitizes the myocardium to digoxin. Therefore, it is desirable to maintain normal serum potassium and magnesium concentrations in patients being treated with digoxin. Deficiencies of these electrolytes may result from concomitant use with corticosteroids).

No products indexed under this heading.

Fluorouracil (Certain anticancer drugs may interfere with intestinal digoxin absorption, resulting in unexpectedly low serum concentrations). Products include:

Carac 2966

Flurbiprofen (Caution should be exercised when combining digoxin with any drug that may cause a significant deterioration in renal function, since a decline in glomerular filtration or tubular secretion may impair the excretion of digoxin).

No products indexed under this heading.

Flutamide (Certain anticancer drugs may interfere with intestinal digoxin absorption, resulting in unexpectedly low serum concentrations).

No products indexed under this heading.

Fluticasone Furoate (In patients with hypokalemia or hypomagnesemia, toxicity may occur despite serum digoxin concentrations below 2.0 ng/mL, because potassium or magnesium depletion sensitizes the myocardium to digoxin. Therefore, it is desirable to maintain normal serum potassium and magnesium concentrations in patients being treated with digoxin. Deficiencies of these electrolytes may result from concomitant use with corticosteroids). Products include:

Veramyst 1713

Fluticasone Propionate (In patients with hypokalemia or hypomagnesemia, toxicity may occur despite serum digoxin concentrations below 2.0 ng/mL, because potassium or magnesium depletion sensitizes the myocardium to digoxin. Therefore, it is desirable to maintain normal serum potassium and magnesium concentrations in patients being treated with digoxin. Deficiencies of these electrolytes may result from concomitant use with corticosteroids). Products include:

Advair 100/50 1275
Advair 250/50 1275
Advair 500/50 1275
Advair HFA 45/21 1288
Advair HFA 115/21 1288
Advair HFA 230/21 1288
Flonase 1459
Flovent Diskus 1463
Flovent HFA 1470

Fluvastatin Sodium (Caution should be exercised when combining digoxin with any drug that may cause a significant deterioration in renal function, since a decline in glomerular filtration or tubular secretion may impair the excretion of digoxin).

No products indexed under this heading.

Foscarnet Sodium (Caution should be exercised when combining digoxin with any drug that may cause a significant deterioration in renal function, since a decline in glomerular filtration or tubular secretion may impair the excretion of digoxin).

No products indexed under this heading.

Fosinopril Sodium (Caution should be exercised when combining digoxin with any drug that may cause a significant deterioration in renal function, since a decline in glomerular filtration or tubular secretion may impair the excretion of digoxin).

No products indexed under this heading.

Furosemide (In patients with hypokalemia or hypomagnesemia, toxicity may occur despite serum digoxin concentrations below 2.0 ng/mL, because potassium or magnesium depletion sensitizes the myocardium to digoxin. Therefore, it is desirable to maintain normal serum potassium and magnesium concentrations in patients being treated with digoxin. Deficiencies of these electrolytes may result from concomitant use with diuretics. Potassium-depleting diuretics are a major contributing factor to digitalis toxicity). Products include:
Furosemide 2354

Gadopentetate Dimeglumine (Caution should be exercised when combining digoxin with any drug that may cause a significant deterioration in renal function, since a decline in glomerular filtration or tubular secretion may impair the excretion of digoxin).
No products indexed under this heading.

Gemcitabine Hydrochloride (Certain anticancer drugs may interfere with intestinal digoxin absorption, resulting in unexpectedly low serum concentrations). Products include:
Gemzar 1900

Gentamicin (Caution should be exercised when combining digoxin with any drug that may cause a significant deterioration in renal function, since a decline in glomerular filtration or tubular secretion may impair the excretion of digoxin).
No products indexed under this heading.

Gentamicin Sulfate (Caution should be exercised when combining digoxin with any drug that may cause a significant deterioration in renal function, since a decline in glomerular filtration or tubular secretion may impair the excretion of digoxin). Products include:
Pred-G .... ⊙ 226, ⊙ 227

Glipizide (Caution should be exercised when combining digoxin with any drug that may cause a significant deterioration in renal function, since a decline in glomerular filtration or tubular secretion may impair the excretion of digoxin).
No products indexed under this heading.

Globulin, Immune (Human) (Caution should be exercised when combining digoxin with any drug that may cause a significant deterioration in renal function, since a decline in glomerular filtration or tubular secretion may impair the excretion of digoxin). Products include:

Glyburide (Caution should be exercised when combining digoxin with any drug that may cause a significant deterioration in renal function, since a decline in glomerular filtration or tubular secretion may impair the excretion of digoxin).
No products indexed under this heading.

Gold Therapy (Caution should be exercised when combining digoxin with any drug that may cause a significant deterioration in renal function, since a decline in glomerular filtration or tubular secretion may impair the excretion of digoxin).
No products indexed under this heading.

HMG-CoA Reductase Inhibitors (Caution should be exercised when combining digoxin with any drug that may cause a significant deterioration in renal function, since a decline in glomerular filtration or tubular secretion may impair the excretion of digoxin).
No products indexed under this heading.

Hydrochlorothiazide (In patients with hypokalemia or hypomagnesemia, toxicity may occur despite serum digoxin concentrations below 2.0 ng/mL, because potassium or magnesium depletion sensitizes the myocardium to digoxin. Therefore, it is desirable to maintain normal serum potassium and

magnesium concentrations in patients being treated with digoxin. Deficiencies of these electrolytes may result from concomitant use with diuretics. Potassium-depleting diuretics are a major contributing factor to digitalis toxicity). Products include:

Atacand HCT	700
Avalide	2956
Benicar HCT	1017
Diovan HCT	2419
Dyazide	1429
Exforge HCT	2449
Hyzaar	2162
Hyzaar 100-12.5	2162
Micardis HCT	889
Prinzide	2246
Tekturna HCT	2541
Teveten HCT	541

Hydrocortisone (In patients with hypokalemia or hypomagnesemia, toxicity may occur despite serum digoxin concentrations below 2.0 ng/mL, because potassium or magnesium depletion sensitizes the myocardium to digoxin. Therefore, it is desirable to maintain normal serum potassium and magnesium concentrations in patients being treated with digoxin. Deficiencies of these electrolytes may result from concomitant use with corticosteroids).
No products indexed under this heading.

Hydrocortisone (Alcohol) (In patients with hypokalemia or hypomagnesemia, toxicity may occur despite serum digoxin concentrations below 2.0 ng/mL, because potassium or magnesium depletion sensitizes the myocardium to digoxin. Therefore, it is desirable to maintain normal serum potassium and magnesium concentrations in patients being treated with digoxin. Deficiencies of these electrolytes may result from concomitant use with corticosteroids).
No products indexed under this heading.

Hydrocortisone Acetate (In patients with hypokalemia or hypomagnesemia, toxicity may occur despite serum digoxin concentrations below 2.0 ng/mL, because potassium or magnesium depletion sensitizes the myocardium to digoxin. Therefore, it is desirable to maintain normal serum potassium and magnesium concentrations in patients being treated with digoxin. Deficiencies of these electrolytes may result from concomitant use with corticosteroids).
No products indexed under this heading.

Hydrocortisone Butyrate (In patients with hypokalemia or hypomagnesemia, toxicity may occur despite serum digoxin concentrations below 2.0 ng/mL, because potassium or magnesium depletion sensitizes the myocardium to digoxin. Therefore, it is desirable to maintain normal serum potassium and magnesium concentrations in patients being treated with digoxin. Deficiencies of these electrolytes may result from concomitant use with corticosteroids).
No products indexed under this heading.

Hydrocortisone Cypionate (In patients with hypokalemia or hypomagnesemia, toxicity may occur despite serum digoxin concentrations below 2.0 ng/mL, because potassium or magnesium depletion sensitizes the myocardium to digoxin. Therefore, it is desirable to maintain normal serum potassium and magnesium concentrations in patients being treated with digoxin. Deficiencies of these electrolytes may result from concomitant use with corticosteroids).
No products indexed under this heading.

Hydrocortisone Hemisuccinate (In patients with hypokalemia or hypomagnesemia, toxicity may occur despite serum digoxin concentrations below 2.0 ng/mL, because potassium or magnesium depletion sensitizes the myocar-

dium to digoxin. Therefore, it is desirable to maintain normal serum potassium and magnesium concentrations in patients being treated with digoxin. Deficiencies of these electrolytes may result from concomitant use with corticosteroids).
No products indexed under this heading.

Hydrocortisone Probutate (In patients with hypokalemia or hypomagnesemia, toxicity may occur despite serum digoxin concentrations below 2.0 ng/mL, because potassium or magnesium depletion sensitizes the myocardium to digoxin. Therefore, it is desirable to maintain normal serum potassium and magnesium concentrations in patients being treated with digoxin. Deficiencies of these electrolytes may result from concomitant use with corticosteroids).
No products indexed under this heading.

Hydrocortisone Sodium Phosphate (In patients with hypokalemia or hypomagnesemia, toxicity may occur despite serum digoxin concentrations below 2.0 ng/mL, because potassium or magnesium depletion sensitizes the myocardium to digoxin. Therefore, it is desirable to maintain normal serum potassium and magnesium concentrations in patients being treated with digoxin. Deficiencies of these electrolytes may result from concomitant use with corticosteroids).
No products indexed under this heading.

Hydrocortisone Sodium Succinate (In patients with hypokalemia or hypomagnesemia, toxicity may occur despite serum digoxin concentrations below 2.0 ng/mL, because potassium or magnesium depletion sensitizes the myocardium to digoxin. Therefore, it is desirable to maintain normal serum potassium and magnesium concentrations in patients being treated with digoxin. Deficiencies of these electrolytes may result from concomitant use with corticosteroids).
No products indexed under this heading.

Hydrocortisone Valerate (In patients with hypokalemia or hypomagnesemia, toxicity may occur despite serum digoxin concentrations below 2.0 ng/mL, because potassium or magnesium depletion sensitizes the myocardium to digoxin. Therefore, it is desirable to maintain normal serum potassium and magnesium concentrations in patients being treated with digoxin. Deficiencies of these electrolytes may result from concomitant use with corticosteroids).
No products indexed under this heading.

Hydroflumethiazide (In patients with hypokalemia or hypomagnesemia, toxicity may occur despite serum digoxin concentrations below 2.0 ng/mL, because potassium or magnesium depletion sensitizes the myocardium to digoxin. Therefore, it is desirable to maintain normal serum potassium and magnesium concentrations in patients being treated with digoxin. Deficiencies of these electrolytes may result from concomitant use with diuretics. Potassium-depleting diuretics are a major contributing factor to digitalis toxicity).
No products indexed under this heading.

Hydroxyurea (Certain anticancer drugs may interfere with intestinal digoxin absorption, resulting in unexpectedly low serum concentrations).
No products indexed under this heading.

Ibuprofen (Caution should be exercised when combining digoxin with any drug that may cause a significant deterioration in renal function, since a decline in glomerular filtration or tubular secretion may impair the excretion of digoxin). Products include:
Motrin IB 2043

Children's Motrin	2044
Children's Motrin Non-Staining Dye-Free	2044
Infants' Motrin	2044
Infants' Motrin Dye-Free	2044
Junior Strength Motrin	2044
Vicoprofen	564

Idarubicin Hydrochloride (Certain anticancer drugs may interfere with intestinal digoxin absorption, resulting in unexpectedly low serum concentrations).
No products indexed under this heading.

Ifosfamide (Certain anticancer drugs may interfere with intestinal digoxin absorption, resulting in unexpectedly low serum concentrations).
No products indexed under this heading.

Imipenem (Caution should be exercised when combining digoxin with any drug that may cause a significant deterioration in renal function, since a decline in glomerular filtration or tubular secretion may impair the excretion of digoxin). Products include:
Primaxin I.M. 2232
Primaxin I.V. 2235

Immune Globulin Intravenous (Human) (Caution should be exercised when combining digoxin with any drug that may cause a significant deterioration in renal function, since a decline in glomerular filtration or tubular secretion may impair the excretion of digoxin). Products include:
Flebogamma 5% DIF 1794
Gammagard 812, 815
Gamunex 3374

Indapamide (In patients with hypokalemia or hypomagnesemia, toxicity may occur despite serum digoxin concentrations below 2.0 ng/mL, because potassium or magnesium depletion sensitizes the myocardium to digoxin. Therefore, it is desirable to maintain normal serum potassium and magnesium concentrations in patients being treated with digoxin. Deficiencies of these electrolytes may result from concomitant use with diuretics). Products include:
Indapamide 2356

Indinavir Sulfate (Caution should be exercised when combining digoxin with any drug that may cause a significant deterioration in renal function, since a decline in glomerular filtration or tubular secretion may impair the excretion of digoxin). Products include:
Crixivan 2113

Indomethacin (Indomethacin may raise the serum digoxin concentration due to a reduction in clearance and/or in volume of distribution of the drug, with the implication that digitalis intoxication may result). Products include:
Indocin 2167

Indomethacin Sodium Trihydrate (Indomethacin may raise the serum digoxin concentration due to a reduction in clearance and/or in volume of distribution of the drug, with the implication that digitalis intoxication may result). Products include:
Indocin I.V. 2007

Interferon alfa-2a, Recombinant (Certain anticancer drugs may interfere with intestinal digoxin absorption, resulting in unexpectedly low serum concentrations).
No products indexed under this heading.

Interferon alfa-2b, Recombinant (Certain anticancer drugs may interfere with intestinal digoxin absorption, resulting in unexpectedly low serum concentrations). Products include:
Intron A 3140

Interferon Beta-1b (Caution should be exercised when combining digoxin with any drug that may cause a significant deterioration in renal function,

---

IMPORTANT NOTE: Always consult each drug listing in the patient's regimen for possible interactions.

Lanoxin Interactions Index 966

since a decline in glomerular filtration or tubular secretion may impair the excretion of digoxin). Products include:
Betaseron 836
Extavia 2459

Interleuken-2 (Caution should be exercised when combining digoxin with any drug that may cause a significant deterioration in renal function, since a decline in glomerular filtration or tubular secretion may impair the excretion of digoxin).
No products indexed under this heading.

Iodamide Meglumine (Caution should be exercised when combining digoxin with any drug that may cause a significant deterioration in renal function, since a decline in glomerular filtration or tubular secretion may impair the excretion of digoxin).
No products indexed under this heading.

Iohexol (Caution should be exercised when combining digoxin with any drug that may cause a significant deterioration in renal function, since a decline in glomerular filtration or tubular secretion may impair the excretion of digoxin).
No products indexed under this heading.

Iopamidol (Caution should be exercised when combining digoxin with any drug that may cause a significant deterioration in renal function, since a decline in glomerular filtration or tubular secretion may impair the excretion of digoxin).
No products indexed under this heading.

Iopanoic Acid (Caution should be exercised when combining digoxin with any drug that may cause a significant deterioration in renal function, since a decline in glomerular filtration or tubular secretion may impair the excretion of digoxin).
No products indexed under this heading.

Iothalamate Meglumine (Caution should be exercised when combining digoxin with any drug that may cause a significant deterioration in renal function, since a decline in glomerular filtration or tubular secretion may impair the excretion of digoxin).
No products indexed under this heading.

Ioxaglate Meglumine (Caution should be exercised when combining digoxin with any drug that may cause a significant deterioration in renal function, since a decline in glomerular filtration or tubular secretion may impair the excretion of digoxin).
No products indexed under this heading.

Ioxaglate Sodium (Caution should be exercised when combining digoxin with any drug that may cause a significant deterioration in renal function, since a decline in glomerular filtration or tubular secretion may impair the excretion of digoxin).
No products indexed under this heading.

Irinotecan Hydrochloride (Certain anticancer drugs may interfere with intestinal digoxin absorption, resulting in unexpectedly low serum concentrations).
No products indexed under this heading.

Isoproterenol Hydrochloride (Concomitant use of digoxin and sympathomimetics increases the risk of cardiac arrhythmias).
No products indexed under this heading.

Isoproterenol Sulfate (Concomitant use of digoxin and sympathomimetics increases the risk of cardiac arrhythmias).
No products indexed under this heading.

Isradipine (Although calcium channel blockers and digoxin may be useful in combination to control atrial fibrillation, their additive effects on AV node conduction can result in advanced or complete heart block). Products include:
DynaCirc CR 1432

Itraconazole (Itraconazole may raise the serum digoxin concentration due to a reduction in clearance and/or in volume of distribution of the drug, with the implication that digitalis intoxication may result).
No products indexed under this heading.

Kanamycin Sulfate (Caution should be exercised when combining digoxin with any drug that may cause a significant deterioration in renal function, since a decline in glomerular filtration or tubular secretion may impair the excretion of digoxin).
No products indexed under this heading.

Kaolin (Kaolin-pectin may interfere with intestinal digoxin absorption, resulting in unexpectedly low serum concentrations).
No products indexed under this heading.

Ketoprofen (Caution should be exercised when combining digoxin with any drug that may cause a significant deterioration in renal function, since a decline in glomerular filtration or tubular secretion may impair the excretion of digoxin).
No products indexed under this heading.

Ketorolac Tromethamine (Caution should be exercised when combining digoxin with any drug that may cause a significant deterioration in renal function, since a decline in glomerular filtration or tubular secretion may impair the excretion of digoxin). Products include:
Acuvail .... ⊙ 209

Labetalol Hydrochloride (Both digitalis glycosides and β-blockers slow atrioventricular conduction and decrease heart rate. Concomitant use can increase the risk of bradycardia).
No products indexed under this heading.

Lamium album (Caution should be exercised when combining digoxin with any drug that may cause a significant deterioration in renal function, since a decline in glomerular filtration or tubular secretion may impair the excretion of digoxin).
No products indexed under this heading.

Levalbuterol Hydrochloride (Concomitant use of digoxin and sympathomimetics increases the risk of cardiac arrhythmias).
No products indexed under this heading.

Levamisole Hydrochloride (Certain anticancer drugs may interfere with intestinal digoxin absorption, resulting in unexpectedly low serum concentrations).
No products indexed under this heading.

Levobunolol Hydrochloride (Both digitalis glycosides and β-blockers slow atrioventricular conduction and decrease heart rate. Concomitant use can increase the risk of bradycardia).
No products indexed under this heading.

Levothyroxine Sodium (Thyroid administration to a digitalized, hypothyroid patient may increase the dose requirement of digoxin). Products include:
Levoxyl Tablets 1843
Synthroid 529

Liothyronine Sodium (Thyroid administration to a digitalized, hypothyroid patient may increase the dose requirement of digoxin). Products include:
Cytomel 1830

Liotrix (Thyroid administration to a digitalized, hypothyroid patient may increase the dose requirement of digoxin).
No products indexed under this heading.

Lisinopril (Caution should be exercised when combining digoxin with any drug that may cause a significant deterioration in renal function, since a decline in glomerular filtration or tubular secretion may impair the excretion of digoxin). Products include:
Prinivil 2241
Prinzide 2246

Lithium (Caution should be exercised when combining digoxin with any drug that may cause a significant deterioration in renal function, since a decline in glomerular filtration or tubular secretion may impair the excretion of digoxin).
No products indexed under this heading.

Lithium Carbonate (Caution should be exercised when combining digoxin with any drug that may cause a significant deterioration in renal function, since a decline in glomerular filtration or tubular secretion may impair the excretion of digoxin).
No products indexed under this heading.

Lithium Citrate (Caution should be exercised when combining digoxin with any drug that may cause a significant deterioration in renal function, since a decline in glomerular filtration or tubular secretion may impair the excretion of digoxin).
No products indexed under this heading.

Lomustine (CCNU) (Certain anticancer drugs may interfere with intestinal digoxin absorption, resulting in unexpectedly low serum concentrations).
No products indexed under this heading.

Lopinavir (Caution should be exercised when combining digoxin with any drug that may cause a significant deterioration in renal function, since a decline in glomerular filtration or tubular secretion may impair the excretion of digoxin). Products include:
Kaletra 458

Loracarbef (Caution should be exercised when combining digoxin with any drug that may cause a significant deterioration in renal function, since a decline in glomerular filtration or tubular secretion may impair the excretion of digoxin).
No products indexed under this heading.

Lovastatin (Caution should be exercised when combining digoxin with any drug that may cause a significant deterioration in renal function, since a decline in glomerular filtration or tubular secretion may impair the excretion of digoxin). Products include:
Advicor 402
Mevacor 2212

Magaldrate (In patients with hypokalemia or hypomagnesemia, toxicity may occur despite serum digoxin concentrations below 2.0 ng/mL, because potassium or magnesium depletion sensitizes the myocardium to digoxin. Therefore, it is desirable to maintain normal serum potassium and magnesium concentrations in patients being treated with digoxin. Deficiencies of these electrolytes may result from concomitant use with antacids. In addition, antacids may interfere with intestinal digoxin absorption, resulting in unexpectedly low serum concentrations).
No products indexed under this heading.

Magnesium Carbonate (In patients with hypokalemia or hypomagnesemia, toxicity may occur despite serum digoxin concentrations below 2.0 ng/mL, because potassium or magnesium depletion sensitizes the myocardium to digoxin. Therefore, it is desirable to maintain normal serum potassium and magnesium concentrations in patients being treated with digoxin. Deficiencies of these electrolytes may result from concomitant use with antacids. In addition, antacids may interfere with intestinal digoxin absorption, resulting in unexpectedly low serum concentrations).
No products indexed under this heading.

Magnesium Hydroxide (In patients with hypokalemia or hypomagnesemia, toxicity may occur despite serum digoxin concentrations below 2.0 ng/mL, because potassium or magnesium depletion sensitizes the myocardium to digoxin. Therefore, it is desirable to maintain normal serum potassium and magnesium concentrations in patients being treated with digoxin. Deficiencies of these electrolytes may result from concomitant use with antacids. In addition, antacids may interfere with intestinal digoxin absorption, resulting in unexpectedly low serum concentrations). Products include:
Fleet Pedia-Lax Chewable Tablets 1144
Pepcid Complete 1822

Magnesium Oxide (In patients with hypokalemia or hypomagnesemia, toxicity may occur despite serum digoxin concentrations below 2.0 ng/mL, because potassium or magnesium depletion sensitizes the myocardium to digoxin. Therefore, it is desirable to maintain normal serum potassium and magnesium concentrations in patients being treated with digoxin. Deficiencies of these electrolytes may result from concomitant use with antacids. In addition, antacids may interfere with intestinal digoxin absorption, resulting in unexpectedly low serum concentrations). Products include:
Beelith 873

Magnesium Trisilicate (In patients with hypokalemia or hypomagnesemia, toxicity may occur despite serum digoxin concentrations below 2.0 ng/mL, because potassium or magnesium depletion sensitizes the myocardium to digoxin. Therefore, it is desirable to maintain normal serum potassium and magnesium concentrations in patients being treated with digoxin. Deficiencies of these electrolytes may result from concomitant use with antacids. In addition, antacids may interfere with intestinal digoxin absorption, resulting in unexpectedly low serum concentrations).
No products indexed under this heading.

Mechlorethamine Hydrochloride (Certain anticancer drugs may interfere with intestinal digoxin absorption, resulting in unexpectedly low serum concentrations). Products include:
Mustargen 2010

Meclofenamate Sodium (Caution should be exercised when combining digoxin with any drug that may cause a significant deterioration in renal function, since a decline in glomerular filtration or tubular secretion may impair the excretion of digoxin).
No products indexed under this heading.

Mefenamic Acid (Caution should be exercised when combining digoxin with any drug that may cause a significant deterioration in renal function, since a decline in glomerular filtration or tubular secretion may impair the excretion of digoxin).
No products indexed under this heading.

Megestrol Acetate (Certain anticancer drugs may interfere with intestinal digoxin absorption, resulting in unexpectedly low serum concentrations). Products include:
Megace ES 2698

Meloxicam (Caution should be exercised when combining digoxin with any drug that may cause a significant deterioration in renal function, since a decline in glomerular filtration or tubular secretion may impair the excretion of digoxin).
No products indexed under this heading.

Melphalan (Certain anticancer drugs may interfere with intestinal digoxin absorption, resulting in unexpectedly low serum concentrations). Products include:
Alkeran 1302

Melphalan Hydrochloride (Caution should be exercised when combining digoxin with any drug that may cause a significant deterioration in renal function, since a decline in glomerular filtration or tubular secretion may impair the excretion of digoxin). Products include:
Alkeran for Injection 1300

Mercaptopurine (Certain anticancer drugs may interfere with intestinal digoxin absorption, resulting in unexpectedly low serum concentrations).
No products indexed under this heading.

Mesalamine (Caution should be exercised when combining digoxin with any drug that may cause a significant deterioration in renal function, since a decline in glomerular filtration or tubular secretion may impair the excretion of digoxin). Products include:
Apriso 2899
Asacol 2786
Asacol HD 2787
Canasa 782
Lialda 3295
Pentasa 3297

Metaproterenol Sulfate (Concomitant use of digoxin and sympathomimetics increases the risk of cardiac arrhythmias).
No products indexed under this heading.

Metaraminol Bitartrate (Concomitant use of digoxin and sympathomimetics increases the risk of cardiac arrhythmias).
No products indexed under this heading.

Methacycline Hydrochloride (Tetracycline may increase digoxin absorption in patients who inactivate digoxin by bacterial metabolism in the lower intestine, so that digitalis intoxication may result).
No products indexed under this heading.

Methimazole (Caution should be exercised when combining digoxin with any drug that may cause a significant deterioration in renal function, since a decline in glomerular filtration or tubular secretion may impair the excretion of digoxin).
No products indexed under this heading.

Methotrexate (Certain anticancer drugs may interfere with intestinal digoxin absorption, resulting in unexpectedly low serum concentrations).
No products indexed under this heading.

Methotrexate Sodium (Certain anticancer drugs may interfere with intestinal digoxin absorption, resulting in unexpectedly low serum concentrations).
No products indexed under this heading.

Methoxamine Hydrochloride (Concomitant use of digoxin and sympathomimetics increases the risk of cardiac arrhythmias).
No products indexed under this heading.

Methyclothiazide (In patients with hypokalemia or hypomagnesemia, toxicity may occur despite serum digoxin concentrations below 2.0 ng/mL, because potassium or magnesium depletion sensitizes the myocardium to digoxin. Therefore, it is desirable to maintain normal serum potassium and magnesium concentrations in patients being treated with digoxin. Deficiencies of these electrolytes may result from concomitant use with diuretics. Potassium-depleting diuretics are a major contributing factor to digitalis toxicity).
No products indexed under this heading.

Methylprednisolone (In patients with hypokalemia or hypomagnesemia, toxicity may occur despite serum digoxin concentrations below 2.0 ng/mL, because potassium or magnesium depletion sensitizes the myocardium to digoxin. Therefore, it is desirable to maintain normal serum potassium and magnesium concentrations in patients being treated with digoxin. Deficiencies of these electrolytes may result from concomitant use with corticosteroids).
No products indexed under this heading.

Methylprednisolone Acetate (In patients with hypokalemia or hypomagnesemia, toxicity may occur despite serum digoxin concentrations below 2.0 ng/mL, because potassium or magnesium depletion sensitizes the myocardium to digoxin. Therefore, it is desirable to maintain normal serum potassium and magnesium concentrations in patients being treated with digoxin. Deficiencies of these electrolytes may result from concomitant use with corticosteroids).
No products indexed under this heading.

Methylprednisolone Sodium Succinate (In patients with hypokalemia or hypomagnesemia, toxicity may occur despite serum digoxin concentrations below 2.0 ng/mL, because potassium or magnesium depletion sensitizes the myocardium to digoxin. Therefore, it is desirable to maintain normal serum potassium and magnesium concentrations in patients being treated with digoxin. Deficiencies of these electrolytes may result from concomitant use with corticosteroids).
No products indexed under this heading.

Metipranolol Hydrochloride (Both digitalis glycosides and β-blockers slow atrioventricular conduction and decrease heart rate. Concomitant use can increase the risk of bradycardia).
No products indexed under this heading.

Metoclopramide Hydrochloride (Metoclopramide may interfere with intestinal digoxin absorption, resulting in unexpectedly low serum concentrations). Products include:
Metozolv ODT 2901

Metolazone (In patients with hypokalemia or hypomagnesemia, toxicity may occur despite serum digoxin concentrations below 2.0 ng/mL, because potassium or magnesium depletion sensitizes the myocardium to digoxin. Therefore, it is desirable to maintain normal serum potassium and magnesium concentrations in patients being treated with digoxin. Deficiencies of these electrolytes may result from concomitant use with diuretics).
No products indexed under this heading.

Metoprolol Succinate (Both digitalis glycosides and β-blockers slow atrioventricular conduction and decrease heart rate. Concomitant use can increase the risk of bradycardia). Products include:
Toprol XL 732

Metoprolol Tartrate (Both digitalis glycosides and β-blockers slow atrioventricular conduction and decrease heart rate. Concomitant use can increase the risk of bradycardia).
No products indexed under this heading.

Mezlocillin Sodium (Caution should be exercised when combining digoxin with any drug that may cause a significant deterioration in renal function, since a decline in glomerular filtration or tubular secretion may impair the excretion of digoxin).
No products indexed under this heading.

Mibefradil Dihydrochloride (Although calcium channel blockers and digoxin may be useful in combination to control atrial fibrillation, their additive effects on AV node conduction can result in advanced or complete heart block).
No products indexed under this heading.

Minocycline Hydrochloride (Tetracycline may increase digoxin absorption in patients who inactivate digoxin by bacterial metabolism in the lower intestine, so that digitalis intoxication may result). Products include:
Solodyn 2073

Mitomycin (Mitomycin-C) (Certain anticancer drugs may interfere with intestinal digoxin absorption, resulting in unexpectedly low serum concentrations).
No products indexed under this heading.

Mitotane (Certain anticancer drugs may interfere with intestinal digoxin absorption, resulting in unexpectedly low serum concentrations).
No products indexed under this heading.

Mitoxantrone Hydrochloride (Certain anticancer drugs may interfere with intestinal digoxin absorption, resulting in unexpectedly low serum concentrations). Products include:
Novantrone 1088

Moexipril Hydrochloride (Caution should be exercised when combining digoxin with any drug that may cause a significant deterioration in renal function, since a decline in glomerular filtration or tubular secretion may impair the excretion of digoxin).
No products indexed under this heading.

Mometasone Furoate (In patients with hypokalemia or hypomagnesemia, toxicity may occur despite serum digoxin concentrations below 2.0 ng/mL, because potassium or magnesium depletion sensitizes the myocardium to digoxin. Therefore, it is desirable to maintain normal serum potassium and magnesium concentrations in patients being treated with digoxin. Deficiencies of these electrolytes may result from concomitant use with corticosteroids). Products include:
Asmanex 3058
Elocon Cream 3111
Elocon Lotion 3112
Elocon Ointment 3114

Mometasone Furoate Monohydrate (In patients with hypokalemia or hypomagnesemia, toxicity may occur despite serum digoxin concentrations below 2.0 ng/mL, because potassium or magnesium depletion sensitizes the myocardium to digoxin. Therefore, it is desirable to maintain normal serum potassium and magnesium concentrations in patients being treated with digoxin. Deficiencies of these electrolytes may result from concomitant use with corticosteroids). Products include:
Nasonex 3166

Muromonab-CD3 (Caution should be exercised when combining digoxin with any drug that may cause a significant deterioration in renal function, since a decline in glomerular filtration or tubular secretion may impair the excretion of digoxin). Products include:
Orthoclone OKT3 949

Nabumetone (Caution should be exercised when combining digoxin with any drug that may cause a significant deterioration in renal function, since a decline in glomerular filtration or tubular secretion may impair the excretion of digoxin).
No products indexed under this heading.

Nadolol (Both digitalis glycosides and β-blockers slow atrioventricular conduction and decrease heart rate. Concomitant use can increase the risk of bradycardia). Products include:
Nadolol 2359

Nafcillin Sodium (Caution should be exercised when combining digoxin with any drug that may cause a significant deterioration in renal function, since a decline in glomerular filtration or tubular secretion may impair the excretion of digoxin).
No products indexed under this heading.

Naproxen (Caution should be exercised when combining digoxin with any drug that may cause a significant deterioration in renal function, since a decline in glomerular filtration or tubular secretion may impair the excretion of digoxin). Products include:
EC-Naprosyn 2850
Naprosyn 2850
Anaprox/Naprosyn 2850

Naproxen Sodium (Caution should be exercised when combining digoxin with any drug that may cause a significant deterioration in renal function, since a decline in glomerular filtration or tubular secretion may impair the excretion of digoxin). Products include:
Anaprox 2850
Anaprox DS 2850
Treximet 1681

Nebivolol (Both digitalis glycosides and β-blockers slow atrioventricular conduction and decrease heart rate. Concomitant use can increase the risk of bradycardia). Products include:
Bystolic 1147

Nelfinavir Mesylate (Caution should be exercised when combining digoxin with any drug that may cause a significant deterioration in renal function, since a decline in glomerular filtration or tubular secretion may impair the excretion of digoxin).
No products indexed under this heading.

Neomycin (Neomycin may interfere with intestinal digoxin absorption, resulting in unexpectedly low serum concentrations).
No products indexed under this heading.

Neomycin, oral (Neomycin may interfere with intestinal digoxin absorption, resulting in unexpectedly low serum concentrations).
No products indexed under this heading.

Neomycin Sulfate (Neomycin may interfere with intestinal digoxin absorption, resulting in unexpectedly low serum concentrations).
No products indexed under this heading.

Nevirapine (Caution should be exercised when combining digoxin with any drug that may cause a significant deterioration in renal function, since a decline in glomerular filtration or tubular secretion may impair the excretion of digoxin). Products include:
Viramune Oral Suspension 897
Viramune Tablets 897

Nicardipine (Although calcium channel blockers and digoxin may be useful in combination to control atrial fibrillation, their additive effects on AV node conduction can result in advanced or complete heart block).
No products indexed under this heading.

Nicardipine Hydrochloride (Although calcium channel blockers and digoxin may be useful in combination to control atrial fibrillation, their additive effects on AV node conduction can result in advanced or complete heart block).
No products indexed under this heading.

Nifedipine (Although calcium channel blockers and digoxin may be useful in combination to control atrial fibrillation, their additive effects on AV node conduction can result in advanced or complete heart block).
No products indexed under this heading.

Nimodipine (Although calcium channel blockers and digoxin may be useful in combination to control atrial fibrillation, their additive effects on AV node conduction can result in advanced or complete heart block).
No products indexed under this heading.

Nisoldipine (Although calcium channel blockers and digoxin may be useful in combination to control atrial fibrillation, their additive effects on AV node conduction can result in advanced or complete heart block).
No products indexed under this heading.

IMPORTANT NOTE: Always consult each drug listing in the patient's regimen for possible interactions.

Norepinephrine Bitartrate (Concomitant use of digoxin and sympathomimetics increases the risk of cardiac arrhythmias).
No products indexed under this heading.

Norfloxacin (Caution should be exercised when combining digoxin with any drug that may cause a significant deterioration in renal function, since a decline in glomerular filtration or tubular secretion may impair the excretion of digoxin). Products include:
Noroxin 2220

Olsalazine Sodium (Caution should be exercised when combining digoxin with any drug that may cause a significant deterioration in renal function, since a decline in glomerular filtration or tubular secretion may impair the excretion of digoxin).
No products indexed under this heading.

Omeprazole (Caution should be exercised when combining digoxin with any drug that may cause a significant deterioration in renal function, since a decline in glomerular filtration or tubular secretion may impair the excretion of digoxin).
No products indexed under this heading.

Oxaliplatin (Certain anticancer drugs may interfere with intestinal digoxin absorption, resulting in unexpectedly low serum concentrations). Products include:
Eloxatin 2975

Oxaprozin (Caution should be exercised when combining digoxin with any drug that may cause a significant deterioration in renal function, since a decline in glomerular filtration or tubular secretion may impair the excretion of digoxin).
No products indexed under this heading.

Oxytetracycline (Tetracycline may increase digoxin absorption in patients who inactivate digoxin by bacterial metabolism in the lower intestine, so that digitalis intoxication may result).
No products indexed under this heading.

Oxytetracycline Hydrochloride (Tetracycline may increase digoxin absorption in patients who inactivate digoxin by bacterial metabolism in the lower intestine, so that digitalis intoxication may result).
No products indexed under this heading.

Paclitaxel (Certain anticancer drugs may interfere with intestinal digoxin absorption, resulting in unexpectedly low serum concentrations).
No products indexed under this heading.

Pamidronate Disodium (Caution should be exercised when combining digoxin with any drug that may cause a significant deterioration in renal function, since a decline in glomerular filtration or tubular secretion may impair the excretion of digoxin).
No products indexed under this heading.

Paroxetine Hydrochloride (Caution should be exercised when combining digoxin with any drug that may cause a significant deterioration in renal function, since a decline in glomerular filtration or tubular secretion may impair the excretion of digoxin). Products include:
Paroxetine CR 2361
Paroxetine ER 2371
Paxil 1586
Paxil CR 1596

Pectin (Kaolin-pectin may interfere with intestinal digoxin absorption, resulting in unexpectedly low serum concentrations).
No products indexed under this heading.

Penbutolol Sulfate (Both digitalis glycosides and β-blockers slow atrioventricular conduction and decrease heart rate. Concomitant use can increase the risk of bradycardia).
No products indexed under this heading.

Penicillamine (Co-administration has resulted in inconsistent reports regarding the effects of penicillamine on serum digoxin concentration).
No products indexed under this heading.

Penicillin G Benzathine (Caution should be exercised when combining digoxin with any drug that may cause a significant deterioration in renal function, since a decline in glomerular filtration or tubular secretion may impair the excretion of digoxin). Products include:
Bicillin C-R Injectable Suspension 1826
Bicillin L-A 1828

Penicillin G Potassium (Caution should be exercised when combining digoxin with any drug that may cause a significant deterioration in renal function, since a decline in glomerular filtration or tubular secretion may impair the excretion of digoxin).
No products indexed under this heading.

Penicillin G Procaine (Caution should be exercised when combining digoxin with any drug that may cause a significant deterioration in renal function, since a decline in glomerular filtration or tubular secretion may impair the excretion of digoxin). Products include:
Bicillin C-R Injectable Suspension 1826
Bicillin L-A 1828

Penicillin G Sodium (Caution should be exercised when combining digoxin with any drug that may cause a significant deterioration in renal function, since a decline in glomerular filtration or tubular secretion may impair the excretion of digoxin).
No products indexed under this heading.

Penicillin V Potassium (Caution should be exercised when combining digoxin with any drug that may cause a significant deterioration in renal function, since a decline in glomerular filtration or tubular secretion may impair the excretion of digoxin).
No products indexed under this heading.

Pentamidine Isethionate (Caution should be exercised when combining digoxin with any drug that may cause a significant deterioration in renal function, since a decline in glomerular filtration or tubular secretion may impair the excretion of digoxin).
No products indexed under this heading.

Perindopril Erbumine (Caution should be exercised when combining digoxin with any drug that may cause a significant deterioration in renal function, since a decline in glomerular filtration or tubular secretion may impair the excretion of digoxin).
No products indexed under this heading.

Phenylbutazone (Caution should be exercised when combining digoxin with any drug that may cause a significant deterioration in renal function, since a decline in glomerular filtration or tubular secretion may impair the excretion of digoxin).
No products indexed under this heading.

Phenylephrine Bitartrate (Concomitant use of digoxin and sympathomimetics increases the risk of cardiac arrhythmias).
No products indexed under this heading.

Phenylephrine Hydrochloride (Concomitant use of digoxin and sympathomimetics increases the risk of cardiac arrhythmias). Products include:
Sudafed PE Nasal Decongestant 2048
Children's Sudafed PE Nasal
Decongestant 2047

Phenylephrine Tannate (Concomitant use of digoxin and sympathomimetics increases the risk of cardiac arrhythmias).
No products indexed under this heading.

Phenylpropanolamine Hydrochloride (Concomitant use of digoxin and sympathomimetics increases the risk of cardiac arrhythmias).
No products indexed under this heading.

Pindolol (Both digitalis glycosides and β-blockers slow atrioventricular conduction and decrease heart rate. Concomitant use can increase the risk of bradycardia).
No products indexed under this heading.

Pirbuterol Acetate (Concomitant use of digoxin and sympathomimetics increases the risk of cardiac arrhythmias). Products include:
Maxair Autohaler 1782

Piroxicam (Caution should be exercised when combining digoxin with any drug that may cause a significant deterioration in renal function, since a decline in glomerular filtration or tubular secretion may impair the excretion of digoxin).
No products indexed under this heading.

Plicamycin (Caution should be exercised when combining digoxin with any drug that may cause a significant deterioration in renal function, since a decline in glomerular filtration or tubular secretion may impair the excretion of digoxin).
No products indexed under this heading.

Polymyxin (Caution should be exercised when combining digoxin with any drug that may cause a significant deterioration in renal function, since a decline in glomerular filtration or tubular secretion may impair the excretion of digoxin).
No products indexed under this heading.

Polymyxin B Sulfate (Caution should be exercised when combining digoxin with any drug that may cause a significant deterioration in renal function, since a decline in glomerular filtration or tubular secretion may impair the excretion of digoxin).
No products indexed under this heading.

Polythiazide (In patients with hypokalemia or hypomagnesemia, toxicity may occur despite serum digoxin concentrations below 2.0 ng/mL, because potassium or magnesium depletion sensitizes the myocardium to digoxin. Therefore, it is desirable to maintain normal serum potassium and magnesium concentrations in patients being treated with digoxin. Deficiencies of these electrolytes may result from concomitant use with diuretics. Potassium-depleting diuretics are a major contributing factor to digitalis toxicity).
No products indexed under this heading.

Pravastatin Sodium (Caution should be exercised when combining digoxin with any drug that may cause a significant deterioration in renal function, since a decline in glomerular filtration or tubular secretion may impair the excretion of digoxin).
No products indexed under this heading.

Prednisolone (In patients with hypokalemia or hypomagnesemia, toxicity may occur despite serum digoxin concentrations below 2.0 ng/mL, because potassium or magnesium depletion sensitizes the myocardium to digoxin. Therefore, it is desirable to maintain normal serum potassium and magnesium concentrations in patients being treated with digoxin. Deficiencies of these electrolytes may result from concomitant use with corticosteroids).
No products indexed under this heading.

Prednisolone Acetate (In patients with hypokalemia or hypomagnesemia, toxicity may occur despite serum digoxin concentrations below 2.0 ng/mL, because potassium or magnesium depletion sensitizes the myocardium to digoxin. Therefore, it is desirable to

maintain normal serum potassium and magnesium concentrations in patients being treated with digoxin. Deficiencies of these electrolytes may result from concomitant use with corticosteroids). Products include:
Blephamide .... ⊙**212**, ⊙**214**
Pred Forte .... ⊙**225**
Pred Mild .... ⊙**230**
Pred-G .... ⊙**226**, ⊙**227**

Prednisolone Sodium Phosphate (In patients with hypokalemia or hypomagnesemia, toxicity may occur despite serum digoxin concentrations below 2.0 ng/mL, because potassium or magnesium depletion sensitizes the myocardium to digoxin. Therefore, it is desirable to maintain normal serum potassium and magnesium concentrations in patients being treated with digoxin. Deficiencies of these electrolytes may result from concomitant use with corticosteroids).
No products indexed under this heading.

Prednisolone Tebutate (In patients with hypokalemia or hypomagnesemia, toxicity may occur despite serum digoxin concentrations below 2.0 ng/mL, because potassium or magnesium depletion sensitizes the myocardium to digoxin. Therefore, it is desirable to maintain normal serum potassium and magnesium concentrations in patients being treated with digoxin. Deficiencies of these electrolytes may result from concomitant use with corticosteroids).
No products indexed under this heading.

Prednisone (In patients with hypokalemia or hypomagnesemia, toxicity may occur despite serum digoxin concentrations below 2.0 ng/mL, because potassium or magnesium depletion sensitizes the myocardium to digoxin. Therefore, it is desirable to maintain normal serum potassium and magnesium concentrations in patients being treated with digoxin. Deficiencies of these electrolytes may result from concomitant use with corticosteroids).
No products indexed under this heading.

Prednisone sodium phosphate (In patients with hypokalemia or hypomagnesemia, toxicity may occur despite serum digoxin concentrations below 2.0 ng/mL, because potassium or magnesium depletion sensitizes the myocardium to digoxin. Therefore, it is desirable to maintain normal serum potassium and magnesium concentrations in patients being treated with digoxin. Deficiencies of these electrolytes may result from concomitant use with corticosteroids).
No products indexed under this heading.

Probenecid (Caution should be exercised when combining digoxin with any drug that may cause a significant deterioration in renal function, since a decline in glomerular filtration or tubular secretion may impair the excretion of digoxin).
No products indexed under this heading.

Procarbazine Hydrochloride (Certain anticancer drugs may interfere with intestinal digoxin absorption, resulting in unexpectedly low serum concentrations).
No products indexed under this heading.

Propafenone Hydrochloride (Propafenone may raise the serum digoxin concentration due to a reduction in clearance and/or in volume of distribution of the drug, with the implication that digitalis intoxication may result). Products include:
Rythmol 1648
Rythmol SR 1652

Propantheline Bromide (Propantheline by decreasing gut motility may increase digoxin absorption).
No products indexed under this heading.

Propranolol Hydrochloride (Both digitalis glycosides and β-blockers slow atrioventricular conduction and decrease heart rate. Concomitant use can increase the risk of bradycardia). Products include:
InnoPran XL 1517

Pseudoephedrine Hydrochloride (Concomitant use of digoxin and sympathomimetics increases the risk of cardiac arrhythmias). Products include:
Allegra-D 2915
Allegra-D 24 2918
Sudafed 12 Hour Nasal Decongestant Non-Drowsy 2048
Sudafed 24 Hour 2048
Sudafed Nasal Decongestant 2047
Children's Sudafed Nasal Decongestant Liquid 2047
Zyrtec-D Allergy & Congestion 2054

Pseudoephedrine Sulfate (Concomitant use of digoxin and sympathomimetics increases the risk of cardiac arrhythmias). Products include:
Clarinex-D 12-Hour 3101
Clarinex-D 3104

Quinapril Hydrochloride (Caution should be exercised when combining digoxin with any drug that may cause a significant deterioration in renal function, since a decline in glomerular filtration or tubular secretion may impair the excretion of digoxin).
No products indexed under this heading.

Quinidine (Quinidine may raise the serum digoxin concentration due to a reduction in clearance and/or in volume of distribution of the drug, with the implication that digitalis intoxication may result).
No products indexed under this heading.

Quinidine Gluconate (Quinidine may raise the serum digoxin concentration due to a reduction in clearance and/or in volume of distribution of the drug, with the implication that digitalis intoxication may result).
No products indexed under this heading.

Quinidine Hydrochloride (Quinidine may raise the serum digoxin concentration due to a reduction in clearance and/or in volume of distribution of the drug, with the implication that digitalis intoxication may result).
No products indexed under this heading.

Quinidine Polygalacturonate (Quinidine may raise the serum digoxin concentration due to a reduction in clearance and/or in volume of distribution of the drug, with the implication that digitalis intoxication may result).
No products indexed under this heading.

Quinidine Sulfate (Quinidine may raise the serum digoxin concentration due to a reduction in clearance and/or in volume of distribution of the drug, with the implication that digitalis intoxication may result).
No products indexed under this heading.

Quinine (Co-administration has resulted in inconsistent reports regarding the effects of quinine on serum digoxin concentrations). Products include:
Hyland's Leg Cramps PM with Quinine 3315

Quinine Sulfate (Co-administration has resulted in inconsistent reports regarding the effects of quinine on serum digoxin concentrations).
No products indexed under this heading.

Rabeprazole Sodium (Caution should be exercised when combining digoxin with any drug that may cause a significant deterioration in renal function, since a decline in glomerular filtration or tubular secretion may impair the excretion of digoxin). Products include:
Aciphex 1035

Ramipril (Caution should be exercised when combining digoxin with any drug that may cause a significant deterioration in renal function, since a decline in glomerular filtration or tubular secretion may impair the excretion of digoxin).
No products indexed under this heading.

Rifampin (Rifampin may decrease serum digoxin concentration, especially in patients with renal dysfunction, by increasing the non-renal clearance of digoxin).
No products indexed under this heading.

Riluzole (Caution should be exercised when combining digoxin with any drug that may cause a significant deterioration in renal function, since a decline in glomerular filtration or tubular secretion may impair the excretion of digoxin). Products include:
Rilutek 3032

Ritonavir (Caution should be exercised when combining digoxin with any drug that may cause a significant deterioration in renal function, since a decline in glomerular filtration or tubular secretion may impair the excretion of digoxin). Products include:
Kaletra 458
Norvir 509

Rofecoxib (Caution should be exercised when combining digoxin with any drug that may cause a significant deterioration in renal function, since a decline in glomerular filtration or tubular secretion may impair the excretion of digoxin).
No products indexed under this heading.

Salmeterol Xinafoate (Concomitant use of digoxin and sympathomimetics increases the risk of cardiac arrhythmias). Products include:
Advair 100/50 1275
Advair 250/50 1275
Advair 500/50 1275
Advair HFA 45/21 1288
Advair HFA 115/21 1288
Advair HFA 230/21 1288
Serevent Diskus 1656

Saquinavir (Caution should be exercised when combining digoxin with any drug that may cause a significant deterioration in renal function, since a decline in glomerular filtration or tubular secretion may impair the excretion of digoxin).
No products indexed under this heading.

Sibutramine Hydrochloride Monohydrate (Caution should be exercised when combining digoxin with any drug that may cause a significant deterioration in renal function, since a decline in glomerular filtration or tubular secretion may impair the excretion of digoxin). Products include:
Meridia 492

Simvastatin (Caution should be exercised when combining digoxin with any drug that may cause a significant deterioration in renal function, since a decline in glomerular filtration or tubular secretion may impair the excretion of digoxin). Products include:
Simcor 524
Vytorin 10/10 .... 2303, 3240
Vytorin 10/20 .... 2303, 3240
Vytorin 10/40 .... 2303, 3240
Vytorin 10/80 .... 2303, 3240
Zocor 2289

Sodium Bicarbonate (In patients with hypokalemia or hypomagnesemia, toxicity may occur despite serum digoxin concentrations below 2.0 ng/mL, because potassium or magnesium depletion sensitizes the myocardium to digoxin. Therefore, it is desirable to maintain normal serum potassium and magnesium concentrations in patients being treated with digoxin. Deficiencies of these electrolytes may result from concomitant use with antacids. In addition, antacids may interfere with intestinal digoxin absorption, resulting in unexpectedly low serum concentrations).
No products indexed under this heading.

Sotalol Hydrochloride (Both digitalis glycosides and β-blockers slow atrioventricular conduction and decrease heart rate. Concomitant use can increase the risk of bradycardia).
No products indexed under this heading.

Spirapril Hydrochloride (Caution should be exercised when combining digoxin with any drug that may cause a significant deterioration in renal function, since a decline in glomerular filtration or tubular secretion may impair the excretion of digoxin).
No products indexed under this heading.

Spironolactone (Spironolactone may raise the serum digoxin concentration due to a reduction in clearance and/or in volume of distribution of the drug, with the implication that digitalis intoxication may result).
No products indexed under this heading.

Stavudine (Caution should be exercised when combining digoxin with any drug that may cause a significant deterioration in renal function, since a decline in glomerular filtration or tubular secretion may impair the excretion of digoxin).
No products indexed under this heading.

Streptomycin Sulfate (Caution should be exercised when combining digoxin with any drug that may cause a significant deterioration in renal function, since a decline in glomerular filtration or tubular secretion may impair the excretion of digoxin).
No products indexed under this heading.

Streptozocin (Certain anticancer drugs may interfere with intestinal digoxin absorption, resulting in unexpectedly low serum concentrations).
No products indexed under this heading.

Succinylcholine Chloride (May cause a sudden extrusion of potassium from muscle cells, and may thereby cause arrhythmias in digitalized patients).
No products indexed under this heading.

Sulfacytine (Caution should be exercised when combining digoxin with any drug that may cause a significant deterioration in renal function, since a decline in glomerular filtration or tubular secretion may impair the excretion of digoxin).
No products indexed under this heading.

Sulfamethizole (Caution should be exercised when combining digoxin with any drug that may cause a significant deterioration in renal function, since a decline in glomerular filtration or tubular secretion may impair the excretion of digoxin).
No products indexed under this heading.

Sulfamethoxazole (Caution should be exercised when combining digoxin with any drug that may cause a significant deterioration in renal function, since a decline in glomerular filtration or tubular secretion may impair the excretion of digoxin).
No products indexed under this heading.

Sulfasalazine (Sulfasalazine may interfere with intestinal digoxin absorption, resulting in unexpectedly low serum concentrations).
No products indexed under this heading.

Sulfinpyrazone (Caution should be exercised when combining digoxin with any drug that may cause a significant deterioration in renal function, since a decline in glomerular filtration or tubular secretion may impair the excretion of digoxin).
No products indexed under this heading.

Sulfisoxazole Acetyl (Caution should be exercised when combining digoxin with any drug that may cause a significant deterioration in renal function, since a decline in glomerular filtration or tubular secretion may impair the excretion of digoxin).
No products indexed under this heading.

Sulfisoxazole Diolamine (Caution should be exercised when combining digoxin with any drug that may cause a significant deterioration in renal function, since a decline in glomerular filtration or tubular secretion may impair the excretion of digoxin).
No products indexed under this heading.

Sulindac (Caution should be exercised when combining digoxin with any drug that may cause a significant deterioration in renal function, since a decline in glomerular filtration or tubular secretion may impair the excretion of digoxin). Products include:
Clinoril 2098

Tacrolimus (Caution should be exercised when combining digoxin with any drug that may cause a significant deterioration in renal function, since a decline in glomerular filtration or tubular secretion may impair the excretion of digoxin). Products include:
Prograf Capsules 677
Prograf Injection 677
Protopic 685

Tamoxifen Citrate (Certain anticancer drugs may interfere with intestinal digoxin absorption, resulting in unexpectedly low serum concentrations).
No products indexed under this heading.

Teniposide (Certain anticancer drugs may interfere with intestinal digoxin absorption, resulting in unexpectedly low serum concentrations).
No products indexed under this heading.

Tenofovir Disoproxil Fumarate (Caution should be exercised when combining digoxin with any drug that may cause a significant deterioration in renal function, since a decline in glomerular filtration or tubular secretion may impair the excretion of digoxin). Products include:
Atripla 906
Truvada 1258
Viread 1266

Terbutaline Sulfate (Concomitant use of digoxin and sympathomimetics increases the risk of cardiac arrhythmias).
No products indexed under this heading.

Tetracycline Hydrochloride (Tetracycline may increase digoxin absorption in patients who inactivate digoxin by bacterial metabolism in the lower intestine, so that digitalis intoxication may result). Products include:
Pylera 793

Tetracycline Phosphate Complex (Tetracycline may increase digoxin absorption in patients who inactivate digoxin by bacterial metabolism in the lower intestine, so that digitalis intoxication may result).
No products indexed under this heading.

Thioguanine (Certain anticancer drugs may interfere with intestinal digoxin absorption, resulting in unexpectedly low serum concentrations). Products include:
Tabloid 1664

Thiotepa (Certain anticancer drugs may interfere with intestinal digoxin absorption, resulting in unexpectedly low serum concentrations).
No products indexed under this heading.

Thyroglobulin (Thyroid administration to a digitalized, hypothyroid patient may increase the dose requirement of digoxin).
No products indexed under this heading.

IMPORTANT NOTE: Always consult each drug listing in the patient's regimen for possible interactions.

Thyroid (Thyroid administration to a digitalized, hypothyroid patient may increase the dose requirement of digoxin). Products include:
Naturethroid 2830

Thyroxine (Thyroid administration to a digitalized, hypothyroid patient may increase the dose requirement of digoxin).
No products indexed under this heading.

Thyroxine Sodium (Thyroid administration to a digitalized, hypothyroid patient may increase the dose requirement of digoxin).
No products indexed under this heading.

Ticarcillin Disodium (Caution should be exercised when combining digoxin with any drug that may cause a significant deterioration in renal function, since a decline in glomerular filtration or tubular secretion may impair the excretion of digoxin). Products include:
Timentin ADD-Vantage 1670
Timentin Galaxy 1674
Timentin 1666
Timentin Pharmacy 1678

Timolol Hemihydrate (Both digitalis glycosides and β-blockers slow atrioventricular conduction and decrease heart rate. Concomitant use can increase the risk of bradycardia). Products include:
Betimol 3490

Timolol Maleate (Both digitalis glycosides and β-blockers slow atrioventricular conduction and decrease heart rate. Concomitant use can increase the risk of bradycardia). Products include:
Combigan 601
Dorzolamide
Hydrochloride/Timolol Maleate
Ophthalmic Solution .... ⊙243
Timoptic in Ocudose .... ⊙231

Tobramycin (Caution should be exercised when combining digoxin with any drug that may cause a significant deterioration in renal function, since a decline in glomerular filtration or tubular secretion may impair the excretion of digoxin). Products include:
Tobi Nebulizer 2546
Tobramycin and Dexamethasone
Ophthalmic Suspension .... ⊙251
Zylet .... ⊙252

Tobramycin Sulfate (Caution should be exercised when combining digoxin with any drug that may cause a significant deterioration in renal function, since a decline in glomerular filtration or tubular secretion may impair the excretion of digoxin).
No products indexed under this heading.

Tolazamide (Caution should be exercised when combining digoxin with any drug that may cause a significant deterioration in renal function, since a decline in glomerular filtration or tubular secretion may impair the excretion of digoxin).
No products indexed under this heading.

Tolbutamide (Caution should be exercised when combining digoxin with any drug that may cause a significant deterioration in renal function, since a decline in glomerular filtration or tubular secretion may impair the excretion of digoxin).
No products indexed under this heading.

Tolmetin Sodium (Caution should be exercised when combining digoxin with any drug that may cause a significant deterioration in renal function, since a decline in glomerular filtration or tubular secretion may impair the excretion of digoxin).
No products indexed under this heading.

Topotecan Hydrochloride (Certain anticancer drugs may interfere with intestinal digoxin absorption, resulting in unexpectedly low serum concentrations). Products include:

Hycamtin 1491
Hycamtin Capsules 1488

Toremifene Citrate (Certain anticancer drugs may interfere with intestinal digoxin absorption, resulting in unexpectedly low serum concentrations).
No products indexed under this heading.

Torsemide (In patients with hypokalemia or hypomagnesemia, toxicity may occur despite serum digoxin concentrations below 2.0 ng/mL, because potassium or magnesium depletion sensitizes the myocardium to digoxin. Therefore, it is desirable to maintain normal serum potassium and magnesium concentrations in patients being treated with digoxin. Deficiencies of these electrolytes may result from concomitant use with diuretics. Potassium-depleting diuretics are a major contributing factor to digitalis toxicity).
No products indexed under this heading.

Trandolapril (Caution should be exercised when combining digoxin with any drug that may cause a significant deterioration in renal function, since a decline in glomerular filtration or tubular secretion may impair the excretion of digoxin). Products include:
Mavik 489
Tarka 534

Triamcinolone (In patients with hypokalemia or hypomagnesemia, toxicity may occur despite serum digoxin concentrations below 2.0 ng/mL, because potassium or magnesium depletion sensitizes the myocardium to digoxin. Therefore, it is desirable to maintain normal serum potassium and magnesium concentrations in patients being treated with digoxin. Deficiencies of these electrolytes may result from concomitant use with corticosteroids).
No products indexed under this heading.

Triamcinolone Acetonide (In patients with hypokalemia or hypomagnesemia, toxicity may occur despite serum digoxin concentrations below 2.0 ng/mL, because potassium or magnesium depletion sensitizes the myocardium to digoxin. Therefore, it is desirable to maintain normal serum potassium and magnesium concentrations in patients being treated with digoxin. Deficiencies of these electrolytes may result from concomitant use with corticosteroids). Products include:
Azmacort 408
Nasacort AQ 3019

Triamcinolone Diacetate (In patients with hypokalemia or hypomagnesemia, toxicity may occur despite serum digoxin concentrations below 2.0 ng/mL, because potassium or magnesium depletion sensitizes the myocardium to digoxin. Therefore, it is desirable to maintain normal serum potassium and magnesium concentrations in patients being treated with digoxin. Deficiencies of these electrolytes may result from concomitant use with corticosteroids).
No products indexed under this heading.

Triamcinolone Hexacetonide (In patients with hypokalemia or hypomagnesemia, toxicity may occur despite serum digoxin concentrations below 2.0 ng/mL, because potassium or magnesium depletion sensitizes the myocardium to digoxin. Therefore, it is desirable to maintain normal serum potassium and magnesium concentrations in patients being treated with digoxin. Deficiencies of these electrolytes may result from concomitant use with corticosteroids).
No products indexed under this heading.

Triamterene (In patients with hypokalemia or hypomagnesemia, toxicity may occur despite serum digoxin concentrations below 2.0 ng/mL, because potassium or magnesium depletion sensitizes

the myocardium to digoxin. Therefore, it is desirable to maintain normal serum potassium and magnesium concentrations in patients being treated with digoxin. Deficiencies of these electrolytes may result from concomitant use with diuretics). Products include:
Dyazide 1429
Dyrenium 3495

Trimethadione (Caution should be exercised when combining digoxin with any drug that may cause a significant deterioration in renal function, since a decline in glomerular filtration or tubular secretion may impair the excretion of digoxin).
No products indexed under this heading.

Troleandomycin (Erythromycin and clarithromycin (and possibly other macrolide antibiotics) may increase digoxin absorption in patients who inactivate digoxin by bacterial metabolism in the lower intestine, so that digitalis intoxication may result).
No products indexed under this heading.

Trovafloxacin Mesylate (Caution should be exercised when combining digoxin with any drug that may cause a significant deterioration in renal function, since a decline in glomerular filtration or tubular secretion may impair the excretion of digoxin).
No products indexed under this heading.

Tyropanoate Sodium (Caution should be exercised when combining digoxin with any drug that may cause a significant deterioration in renal function, since a decline in glomerular filtration or tubular secretion may impair the excretion of digoxin).
No products indexed under this heading.

Valacyclovir Hydrochloride (Caution should be exercised when combining digoxin with any drug that may cause a significant deterioration in renal function, since a decline in glomerular filtration or tubular secretion may impair the excretion of digoxin). Products include:
Valtrex 1702

Valdecoxib (Caution should be exercised when combining digoxin with any drug that may cause a significant deterioration in renal function, since a decline in glomerular filtration or tubular secretion may impair the excretion of digoxin).
No products indexed under this heading.

Valrubicin (Certain anticancer drugs may interfere with intestinal digoxin absorption, resulting in unexpectedly low serum concentrations). Products include:
Valstar 1131

Vancomycin Hydrochloride (Caution should be exercised when combining digoxin with any drug that may cause a significant deterioration in renal function, since a decline in glomerular filtration or tubular secretion may impair the excretion of digoxin).
No products indexed under this heading.

Verapamil Hydrochloride (Verapamil may raise the serum digoxin concentration due to a reduction in clearance and/or in volume of distribution of the drug, with the implication that digitalis intoxication may result). Products include:
Tarka 534

Vincristine Sulfate (Certain anticancer drugs may interfere with intestinal digoxin absorption, resulting in unexpectedly low serum concentrations).
No products indexed under this heading.

Vinorelbine Tartrate (Certain anticancer drugs may interfere with intestinal digoxin absorption, resulting in unexpectedly low serum concentrations).
No products indexed under this heading.

Voriconazole (Caution should be exercised when combining digoxin with any drug that may cause a significant deterioration in renal function, since a decline in glomerular filtration or tubular secretion may impair the excretion of digoxin).
No products indexed under this heading.

Zalcitabine (Caution should be exercised when combining digoxin with any drug that may cause a significant deterioration in renal function, since a decline in glomerular filtration or tubular secretion may impair the excretion of digoxin).
No products indexed under this heading.

Zidovudine (Caution should be exercised when combining digoxin with any drug that may cause a significant deterioration in renal function, since a decline in glomerular filtration or tubular secretion may impair the excretion of digoxin). Products include:
Combivir 1404
Retrovir 1634
Retrovir IV 1640
Trizivir 1688

Zoledronic Acid (Caution should be exercised when combining digoxin with any drug that may cause a significant deterioration in renal function, since a decline in glomerular filtration or tubular secretion may impair the excretion of digoxin). Products include:
Reclast 2509
Zometa 2554

Food Interactions

Food, unspecified (When digoxin tablets are taken after meals, the rate of absorption is slowed, but the total amount of digoxin absorbed is usually unchanged. When taken with meals high in bran fiber, however, the amount absorbed from an oral dose may be reduced).

Meal, high in bran fiber (When digoxin tablets are taken after meals, the rate of absorption is slowed, but the total amount of digoxin absorbed is usually unchanged. When taken with meals high in bran fiber, however, the amount absorbed from an oral dose may be reduced).

Meal, unspecified (When digoxin tablets are taken after meals, the rate of absorption is slowed, but the total amount of digoxin absorbed is usually unchanged. When taken with meals high in bran fiber, however, the amount absorbed from an oral dose may be reduced).

LANTUS INJECTION

(Insulin Glargine) 2996
May interact with ACE inhibitors, alcohols, beta-blockers, corticosteroids, diuretics, fibrates, lithium preparations, monoamine oxidase inhibitors, oral contraceptives, oral hypoglycemic agents, phenothiazines, protease inhibitors, salicylates, sympathomimetics, thyroid preparations, and certain other agents. Compounds in these categories include:

Acarbose (May increase the blood-glucose-lowering effect and susceptibility to hypoglycemia).
No products indexed under this heading.

Acebutolol Hydrochloride (Beta-blockers may either potentiate or weaken the blood-glucose-lowering effect of insulin; signs of hypoglycemia may be reduced or absent with co-administration).
No products indexed under this heading.

Albuterol (Sympathomimetic agents may reduce the blood-glucose-lowering effect of insulin).
No products indexed under this heading.

Albuterol Sulfate (Sympathomimetic agents may reduce the blood-glucose-lowering effect of insulin). Products include:
- ProAir HFA 3393
- Proventil HFA 3204
- Ventolin HFA 1708

Alclometasone Dipropionate (Co-administration with corticosteroids may reduce the blood-glucose-lowering effect of insulin).
No products indexed under this heading.

Amiloride Hydrochloride (Diuretics may reduce the blood-glucose-lowering effect of insulin).
No products indexed under this heading.

Amprenavir (May reduce the blood-glucose lowering effect of insulin).
No products indexed under this heading.

Aspirin (May increase the blood-glucose-lowering effect and susceptibility to hypoglycemia). Products include:
- Aggrenox 880
- Bayer Aspirin 829
- Percodan 1124
- St. Joseph Aspirin 2045

Aspirin, Enteric Coated (May increase the blood-glucose-lowering effect and susceptibility to hypoglycemia).
No products indexed under this heading.

Aspirin Buffered (May increase the blood-glucose-lowering effect and susceptibility to hypoglycemia).
No products indexed under this heading.

Atazanavir (May reduce the blood-glucose lowering effect of insulin).
No products indexed under this heading.

Atazanavir Sulfate (May reduce the blood-glucose lowering effect of insulin).
No products indexed under this heading.

Atenolol (Beta-blockers may either potentiate or weaken the blood-glucose-lowering effect of insulin; signs of hypoglycemia may be reduced or absent with co-administration).
No products indexed under this heading.

Beclomethasone Dipropionate (Co-administration with corticosteroids may reduce the blood-glucose-lowering effect of insulin). Products include:
- Qvar 3398

Beclomethasone Dipropionate Monohydrate (Co-administration with corticosteroids may reduce the blood-glucose-lowering effect of insulin). Products include:
- Beconase AQ 1386

Benazepril Hydrochloride (May increase the blood-glucose-lowering effect and susceptibility to hypoglycemia).
No products indexed under this heading.

Bendroflumethiazide (Diuretics may reduce the blood-glucose-lowering effect of insulin).
No products indexed under this heading.

Betamethasone (Co-administration with corticosteroids may reduce the blood-glucose-lowering effect of insulin).
No products indexed under this heading.

Betamethasone Acetate (Co-administration with corticosteroids may reduce the blood-glucose-lowering effect of insulin).
No products indexed under this heading.

Betamethasone Benzoate (Co-administration with corticosteroids may reduce the blood-glucose-lowering effect of insulin).
No products indexed under this heading.

Betamethasone Dipropionate (Co-administration with corticosteroids may reduce the blood-glucose-lowering effect of insulin). Products include:
- Diprolene Lotion 0.05% 3108
- Diprolene Ointment 0.05% 3109
- Diprolene AF Cream 0.05% 3107
- Lotrisone 3163

Betamethasone Sodium Phosphate (Co-administration with corticosteroids may reduce the blood-glucose-lowering effect of insulin).
No products indexed under this heading.

Betamethasone Valerate (Co-administration with corticosteroids may reduce the blood-glucose-lowering effect of insulin). Products include:
- Luxíq 3321

Betaxolol Hydrochloride (Beta-blockers may either potentiate or weaken the blood-glucose-lowering effect of insulin; signs of hypoglycemia may be reduced or absent with co-administration).
No products indexed under this heading.

Bisoprolol Fumarate (Beta-blockers may either potentiate or weaken the blood-glucose-lowering effect of insulin; signs of hypoglycemia may be reduced or absent with co-administration).
No products indexed under this heading.

Budesonide (Co-administration with corticosteroids may reduce the blood-glucose-lowering effect of insulin). Products include:
- Pulmicort Flexhaler 714
- Symbicort 80/4.5 720
- Symbicort 160/4.5 720

Bumetanide (Diuretics may reduce the blood-glucose-lowering effect of insulin).
No products indexed under this heading.

Captopril (May increase the blood-glucose-lowering effect and susceptibility to hypoglycemia). Products include:
- Captopril 2341

Carteolol Hydrochloride (Beta-blockers may either potentiate or weaken the blood-glucose-lowering effect of insulin; signs of hypoglycemia may be reduced or absent with co-administration).
No products indexed under this heading.

Carvedilol (Beta-blockers may either potentiate or weaken the blood-glucose-lowering effect of insulin; signs of hypoglycemia may be reduced or absent with co-administration). Products include:
- Coreg 1409

Carvedilol Phosphate (Beta-blockers may either potentiate or weaken the blood-glucose-lowering effect of insulin; signs of hypoglycemia may be reduced or absent with co-administration). Products include:
- Coreg CR 1416

Chlorothiazide (Diuretics may reduce the blood-glucose-lowering effect of insulin).
No products indexed under this heading.

Chlorothiazide Sodium (Diuretics may reduce the blood-glucose-lowering effect of insulin). Products include:
- Diuril Intravenous 2009

Chlorpromazine (Phenothiazine derivatives may reduce the blood-glucose-lowering effect of insulin).
No products indexed under this heading.

Chlorpromazine Hydrochloride (Phenothiazine derivatives may reduce the blood-glucose-lowering effect of insulin).
No products indexed under this heading.

Chlorpropamide (May increase the blood-glucose-lowering effect and susceptibility to hypoglycemia).
No products indexed under this heading.

Chlorthalidone (Diuretics may reduce the blood-glucose-lowering effect of insulin). Products include:
- Clorpres 2344

Choline Magnesium Trisalicylate (May increase the blood-glucose-lowering effect and susceptibility to hypoglycemia).
No products indexed under this heading.

Ciclesonide (Co-administration with corticosteroids may reduce the blood-glucose-lowering effect of insulin).
No products indexed under this heading.

Clofibrate (May increase the blood-glucose-lowering effect and susceptibility to hypoglycemia).
No products indexed under this heading.

Clonidine (Signs of hypoglycemia may be reduced or absent with co-administration). Products include:
- Catapres-TTS 884

Clonidine Hydrochloride (Signs of hypoglycemia may be reduced or absent with co-administration). Products include:
- Clorpres 2344

Cortisone Acetate (Co-administration with corticosteroids may reduce the blood-glucose-lowering effect of insulin).
No products indexed under this heading.

Danazol (May reduce the blood-glucose-lowering effect of insulin).
No products indexed under this heading.

Darunavir (May reduce the blood-glucose lowering effect of insulin).
No products indexed under this heading.

Desogestrel (Oral contraceptives may reduce the blood-glucose-lowering effect of insulin).
No products indexed under this heading.

Desoximetasone (Co-administration with corticosteroids may reduce the blood-glucose-lowering effect of insulin).
No products indexed under this heading.

Dexamethasone (Co-administration with corticosteroids may reduce the blood-glucose-lowering effect of insulin). Products include:
- Ciprodex 583
- Ozurdex .... ⊙ 223
- Tobramycin and Dexamethasone Ophthalmic Suspension .... ⊙ 251

Dexamethasone Acetate (Co-administration with corticosteroids may reduce the blood-glucose-lowering effect of insulin).
No products indexed under this heading.

Dexamethasone Phosphate (Co-administration with corticosteroids may reduce the blood-glucose-lowering effect of insulin).
No products indexed under this heading.

Dexamethasone Sodium (Co-administration with corticosteroids may reduce the blood-glucose-lowering effect of insulin).
No products indexed under this heading.

Dexamethasone Sodium Phosphate (Co-administration with corticosteroids may reduce the blood-glucose-lowering effect of insulin).
No products indexed under this heading.

Dexamethasone Sodium Phosphate Injection (Co-administration with corticosteroids may reduce the blood-glucose-lowering effect of insulin).
No products indexed under this heading.

Diflorasone Diacetate (Co-administration with corticosteroids may reduce the blood-glucose-lowering effect of insulin).
No products indexed under this heading.

Diflunisal (May increase the blood-glucose-lowering effect and susceptibility to hypoglycemia).
No products indexed under this heading.

Disopyramide Phosphate (May increase the blood-glucose-lowering effect and susceptibility to hypoglycemia).
No products indexed under this heading.

Dobutamine Hydrochloride (Sympathomimetic agents may reduce the blood-glucose-lowering effect of insulin).
No products indexed under this heading.

Dopamine Hydrochloride (Sympathomimetic agents may reduce the blood-glucose-lowering effect of insulin).
No products indexed under this heading.

Enalapril Maleate (May increase the blood-glucose-lowering effect and susceptibility to hypoglycemia).
No products indexed under this heading.

Enalaprilat (May increase the blood-glucose-lowering effect and susceptibility to hypoglycemia).
No products indexed under this heading.

Ephedrine Hydrochloride (Sympathomimetic agents may reduce the blood-glucose-lowering effect of insulin).
No products indexed under this heading.

Ephedrine Sulfate (Sympathomimetic agents may reduce the blood-glucose-lowering effect of insulin).
No products indexed under this heading.

Ephedrine Tannate (Sympathomimetic agents may reduce the blood-glucose-lowering effect of insulin).
No products indexed under this heading.

Epinephrine (Sympathomimetic agents may reduce the blood-glucose-lowering effect of insulin). Products include:
- EpiPen 3631
- Twinject 3268

Epinephrine Bitartrate (Sympathomimetic agents may reduce the blood-glucose-lowering effect of insulin).
No products indexed under this heading.

Epinephrine Hydrochloride (Sympathomimetic agents may reduce the blood-glucose-lowering effect of insulin).
No products indexed under this heading.

Esmolol Hydrochloride (Beta-blockers may either potentiate or weaken the blood-glucose-lowering effect of insulin; signs of hypoglycemia may be reduced or absent with co-administration).
No products indexed under this heading.

Ethacrynic Acid (Diuretics may reduce the blood-glucose-lowering effect of insulin).
No products indexed under this heading.

Ethanol (May either potentiate or weaken the blood-glucose-lowering effect of insulin).
No products indexed under this heading.

Ethinyl Estradiol (Oral contraceptives may reduce the blood-glucose-lowering effect of insulin). Products include:
- LoSeasonique 3407
- Lybrel 3514
- NuvaRing 3181
- Ortho Evra 2648
- Ortho-Cyclen/Ortho Tri-Cyclen 2663
- Ortho Tri-Cyclen Lo Tablets 2673
- Seasonique 3418
- Yaz 864

Ethyl Alcohol (May either potentiate or weaken the blood-glucose-lowering effect of insulin).
No products indexed under this heading.

Ethynodiol Diacetate (Oral contraceptives may reduce the blood-glucose-lowering effect of insulin).
No products indexed under this heading.

Fenofibrate (May increase the blood-glucose-lowering effect and susceptibility to hypoglycemia). Products include:
- Fenoglide 3263
- Tricor 544
- Trilipix 548

Fludrocortisone Acetate (Co-administration with corticosteroids may reduce the blood-glucose-lowering effect of insulin).
No products indexed under this heading.

IMPORTANT NOTE: Always consult each drug listing in the patient's regimen for possible interactions.

(⊙ Described in PDR® for Ophthalmic Medicines)

973 **Interactions Index** **Lantus**

Nebivolol (Beta-blockers may either potentiate or weaken the blood-glucose-lowering effect of insulin; signs of hypoglycemia may be reduced or absent with co-administration). Products include:
Bystolic 1147

Nelfinavir Mesylate (May reduce the blood-glucose lowering effect of insulin).
No products indexed under this heading.

Norepinephrine Bitartrate (Sympathomimetic agents may reduce the blood-glucose-lowering effect of insulin).
No products indexed under this heading.

Norethindrone (Oral contraceptives may reduce the blood-glucose-lowering effect of insulin). Products include:
Ortho Micronor 2660

Norethynodrel (Oral contraceptives may reduce the blood-glucose-lowering effect of insulin).
No products indexed under this heading.

Norgestimate (Oral contraceptives may reduce the blood-glucose-lowering effect of insulin). Products include:
Ortho-Cyclen/Ortho Tri-Cyclen 2663
Ortho Tri-Cyclen Lo Tablets 2673

Norgestrel (Oral contraceptives may reduce the blood-glucose-lowering effect of insulin).
No products indexed under this heading.

Octreotide Acetate (May increase the blood-glucose-lowering effect and susceptibility to hypoglycemia).
Products include:
Sandostatin 2517
Sandostatin LAR 2519

Pargyline Hydrochloride (May increase the blood-glucose-lowering effect and susceptibility to hypoglycemia).
No products indexed under this heading.

Penbutolol Sulfate (Beta-blockers may either potentiate or weaken the blood-glucose-lowering effect of insulin; signs of hypoglycemia may be reduced or absent with co-administration).
No products indexed under this heading.

Pentamidine Isethionate (May cause hypoglycemia, which may sometimes be followed by hyperglycemia).
No products indexed under this heading.

Perindopril Erbumine (May increase the blood-glucose-lowering effect and susceptibility to hypoglycemia).
No products indexed under this heading.

Perphenazine (Phenothiazine derivatives may reduce the blood-glucose-lowering effect of insulin).
No products indexed under this heading.

Phenelzine Sulfate (May increase the blood-glucose-lowering effect and susceptibility to hypoglycemia).
No products indexed under this heading.

Phenothiazine Derivatives (Phenothiazine derivatives may reduce the blood-glucose-lowering effect of insulin).
No products indexed under this heading.

Phenothiazines (Phenothiazine derivatives may reduce the blood-glucose-lowering effect of insulin).
No products indexed under this heading.

Phenylephrine Bitartrate (Sympathomimetic agents may reduce the blood-glucose-lowering effect of insulin).
No products indexed under this heading.

Phenylephrine Hydrochloride (Sympathomimetic agents may reduce the blood-glucose-lowering effect of insulin). Products include:
Sudafed PE Nasal Decongestant 2048
Children's Sudafed PE Nasal Decongestant 2047

Phenylephrine Tannate (Sympathomimetic agents may reduce the blood-glucose-lowering effect of insulin).
No products indexed under this heading.

Phenylpropanolamine Hydrochloride (Sympathomimetic agents may reduce the blood-glucose-lowering effect of insulin).
No products indexed under this heading.

Pindolol (Beta-blockers may either potentiate or weaken the blood-glucose-lowering effect of insulin; signs of hypoglycemia may be reduced or absent with co-administration).
No products indexed under this heading.

Pioglitazone Hydrochloride (May increase the blood-glucose-lowering effect and susceptibility to hypoglycemia). Products include:
ActoPlus 3338
Actos 3345
Duetact 3354

Pirbuterol Acetate (Sympathomimetic agents may reduce the blood-glucose-lowering effect of insulin).
Products include:
Maxair Autohaler 1782

Polythiazide (Diuretics may reduce the blood-glucose-lowering effect of insulin).
No products indexed under this heading.

Prednisolone (Co-administration with corticosteroids may reduce the blood-glucose-lowering effect of insulin).
No products indexed under this heading.

Prednisolone Acetate (Co-administration with corticosteroids may reduce the blood-glucose-lowering effect of insulin). Products include:
Blephamide .... ⊙212, ⊙214
Pred Forte .... ⊙225
Pred Mild .... ⊙230
Pred-G .... ⊙226, ⊙227

Prednisolone Sodium Phosphate (Co-administration with corticosteroids may reduce the blood-glucose-lowering effect of insulin).
No products indexed under this heading.

Prednisolone Tebutate (Co-administration with corticosteroids may reduce the blood-glucose-lowering effect of insulin).
No products indexed under this heading.

Prednisone (Co-administration with corticosteroids may reduce the blood-glucose-lowering effect of insulin).
No products indexed under this heading.

Prednisone sodium phosphate (Co-administration with corticosteroids may reduce the blood-glucose-lowering effect of insulin).
No products indexed under this heading.

Procarbazine Hydrochloride (May increase the blood-glucose-lowering effect and susceptibility to hypoglycemia).
No products indexed under this heading.

Prochlorperazine (Phenothiazine derivatives may reduce the blood-glucose-lowering effect of insulin).
No products indexed under this heading.

Prochlorperazine Edisylate (Phenothiazine derivatives may reduce the blood-glucose-lowering effect of insulin).
No products indexed under this heading.

Prochlorperazine Maleate (Phenothiazine derivatives may reduce the blood-glucose-lowering effect of insulin).
No products indexed under this heading.

Promethazine (Phenothiazine derivatives may reduce the blood-glucose-lowering effect of insulin).
No products indexed under this heading.

Promethazine Hydrochloride (Phenothiazine derivatives may reduce the blood-glucose-lowering effect of insulin).
No products indexed under this heading.

Propoxyphene Hydrochloride (May increase the blood-glucose-lowering effect and susceptibility to hypoglycemia).
No products indexed under this heading.

Propoxyphene Napsylate (May increase the blood-glucose-lowering effect and susceptibility to hypoglycemia).
No products indexed under this heading.

Propranolol Hydrochloride (Beta-blockers may either potentiate or weaken the blood-glucose-lowering effect of insulin; signs of hypoglycemia may be reduced or absent with co-administration). Products include:
InnoPran XL 1517

Pseudoephedrine Hydrochloride (Sympathomimetic agents may reduce the blood-glucose-lowering effect of insulin). Products include:
Allegra-D 2915
Allegra-D 24 2918
Sudafed 12 Hour Nasal Decongestant Non-Drowsy 2048
Sudafed 24 Hour 2048
Sudafed Nasal Decongestant 2047
Children's Sudafed Nasal Decongestant Liquid 2047
Zyrtec-D Allergy & Congestion 2054

Pseudoephedrine Sulfate (Sympathomimetic agents may reduce the blood-glucose-lowering effect of insulin).
Products include:
Clarinex-D 12-Hour 3101
Clarinex-D 3104

Quinapril Hydrochloride (May increase the blood-glucose-lowering effect and susceptibility to hypoglycemia).
No products indexed under this heading.

Ramipril (May increase the blood-glucose-lowering effect and susceptibility to hypoglycemia).
No products indexed under this heading.

Rasagiline Mesylate (May increase the blood-glucose-lowering effect and susceptibility to hypoglycemia).
Products include:
Azilect 3383

Repaglinide (May increase the blood-glucose-lowering effect and susceptibility to hypoglycemia).
No products indexed under this heading.

Reserpine (Signs of hypoglycemia may be reduced or absent with co-administration).
No products indexed under this heading.

Ritonavir (May reduce the blood-glucose lowering effect of insulin).
Products include:
Kaletra 458
Norvir 509

Rosiglitazone Maleate (May increase the blood-glucose-lowering effect and susceptibility to hypoglycemia). Products include:
Avandamet 1345
Avandaryl 1356
Avandia 1366

Salmeterol Xinafoate (Sympathomimetic agents may reduce the blood-glucose-lowering effect of insulin).
Products include:
Advair 100/50 1275
Advair 250/50 1275
Advair 500/50 1275
Advair HFA 45/21 1288
Advair HFA 115/21 1288
Advair HFA 230/21 1288
Serevent Diskus 1656

Salsalate (May increase the blood-glucose-lowering effect and susceptibility to hypoglycemia).
No products indexed under this heading.

Saquinavir (May reduce the blood-glucose lowering effect of insulin).
No products indexed under this heading.

Saquinavir Mesylate (May reduce the blood-glucose lowering effect of insulin).
No products indexed under this heading.

Selegiline (May increase the blood-glucose-lowering effect and susceptibility to hypoglycemia). Products include:
Emsam 3623

Selegiline Hydrochloride (May increase the blood-glucose-lowering effect and susceptibility to hypoglycemia). Products include:
Eldepryl 3312

Sitagliptin Phosphate (May increase the blood-glucose-lowering effect and susceptibility to hypoglycemia).
Products include:
Janumet 2188
Januvia 2196

Somatropin (May reduce the blood-glucose-lowering effect of insulin).
Products include:
Nutropin 1204
Nutropin AQ 1209
Nutropin AQ NuSpin 1209
Nutropin AQ Pen 1209
Nutropin AQ Pen Cartridge 1209

Sotalol Hydrochloride (Beta-blockers may either potentiate or weaken the blood-glucose-lowering effect of insulin; signs of hypoglycemia may be reduced or absent with co-administration).
No products indexed under this heading.

Spirapril Hydrochloride (May increase the blood-glucose-lowering effect and susceptibility to hypoglycemia).
No products indexed under this heading.

Spironolactone (Diuretics may reduce the blood-glucose-lowering effect of insulin).
No products indexed under this heading.

Sulfamethoxazole (Co-administration with sulfonamide antibiotics may increase the blood-glucose-lowering effect and susceptibility to hypoglycemia).
No products indexed under this heading.

Sulfisoxazole Acetyl (Co-administration with sulfonamide antibiotics may increase the blood-glucose-lowering effect and susceptibility to hypoglycemia).
No products indexed under this heading.

Terbutaline Sulfate (Sympathomimetic agents may reduce the blood-glucose-lowering effect of insulin).
No products indexed under this heading.

Thioridazine (Phenothiazine derivatives may reduce the blood-glucose-lowering effect of insulin).
No products indexed under this heading.

Thioridazine Hydrochloride (Phenothiazine derivatives may reduce the blood-glucose-lowering effect of insulin).
Products include:
Thioridazine Hydrochloride 2384

Thyroglobulin (May reduce the blood-glucose-lowering effect of insulin).
No products indexed under this heading.

Thyroid (May reduce the blood-glucose-lowering effect of insulin).
Products include:
Naturethroid 2830

Thyroxine (May reduce the blood-glucose-lowering effect of insulin).
No products indexed under this heading.

Thyroxine Sodium (May reduce the blood-glucose-lowering effect of insulin).
No products indexed under this heading.

Timolol Hemihydrate (Beta-blockers may either potentiate or weaken the blood-glucose-lowering effect of insulin; signs of hypoglycemia may be reduced or absent with co-administration).
Products include:
Betimol 3490

Timolol Maleate (Beta-blockers may either potentiate or weaken the blood-glucose-lowering effect of insulin; signs of hypoglycemia may be reduced or absent with co-administration). Products include:
Combigan 601

IMPORTANT NOTE: Always consult each drug listing in the patient's regimen for possible interactions.

Lantus
Interactions Index
974

Dorzolamide Hydrochloride/Timolol Maleate Ophthalmic Solution ⊙243
Timoptic in Ocudose ⊙231

Tipranavir (May reduce the blood-glucose lowering effect of insulin).
No products indexed under this heading.

Tolazamide (May increase the blood-glucose-lowering effect and susceptibility to hypoglycemia).
No products indexed under this heading.

Tolbutamide (May increase the blood-glucose-lowering effect and susceptibility to hypoglycemia).
No products indexed under this heading.

Torsemide (Diuretics may reduce the blood-glucose-lowering effect of insulin).
No products indexed under this heading.

Trandolapril (May increase the blood-glucose-lowering effect and susceptibility to hypoglycemia). Products include:
Mavik 489
Tarka 534

Tranylcypromine Sulfate (May increase the blood-glucose-lowering effect and susceptibility to hypoglycemia). Products include:
Parnate 1584

Triamcinolone (Co-administration with corticosteroids may reduce the blood-glucose-lowering effect of insulin).
No products indexed under this heading.

Triamcinolone Acetonide (Co-administration with corticosteroids may reduce the blood-glucose-lowering effect of insulin). Products include:
Azmacort 408
Nasacort AQ 3019

Triamcinolone Diacetate (Co-administration with corticosteroids may reduce the blood-glucose-lowering effect of insulin).
No products indexed under this heading.

Triamcinolone Hexacetonide (Co-administration with corticosteroids may reduce the blood-glucose-lowering effect of insulin).
No products indexed under this heading.

Triamterene (Diuretics may reduce the blood-glucose-lowering effect of insulin). Products include:
Dyazide 1429
Dyrenium 3495

Trifluoperazine Hydrochloride (Phenothiazine derivatives may reduce the blood-glucose-lowering effect of insulin).
No products indexed under this heading.

Troglitazone (May increase the blood-glucose-lowering effect and susceptibility to hypoglycemia).
No products indexed under this heading.

Food Interactions

Alcohol (May either potentiate or weaken the blood-glucose-lowering effect of insulin).

Beer, reduced-alcohol (May either potentiate or weaken the blood-glucose-lowering effect of insulin).

Beer, unspecified (May either potentiate or weaken the blood-glucose-lowering effect of insulin).

Wine, Chianti (May either potentiate or weaken the blood-glucose-lowering effect of insulin).

Wine, Red (May either potentiate or weaken the blood-glucose-lowering effect of insulin).

Wine, unspecified (May either potentiate or weaken the blood-glucose-lowering effect of insulin).

Wine products (May either potentiate or weaken the blood-glucose-lowering effect of insulin).

LETAIRIS TABLETS

(Ambrisentan) 1250

May interact with cytochrome p450 2c19 inhibitors (selected), cytochrome p450 3a inhibitors (selected), cytochrome p450 3a4 inhibitors (selected), cytochrome p450 inducers (selected), P-glycoprotein inducers, P-glycoprotein inhibitors, UDP-glucuronosyltransferase (UGT) inducers (selected), and certain other agents. Compounds in these categories include:

Acetazolamide (Based on *in vitro* data, interactions with strong inhibitors of P-glycoprotein (P-gp), the Organic Anion Transport Protein (OATP), CYP3A4, CYP2C19, and uridine 5' diphosphate glucuronosyltransferases (UGTs) are possible).
No products indexed under this heading.

Acetazolamide Sodium (Based on *in vitro* data, interactions with strong inhibitors of P-glycoprotein (P-gp), the Organic Anion Transport Protein (OATP), CYP3A4, CYP2C19, and uridine 5' diphosphate glucuronosyltransferases (UGTs) are possible).
No products indexed under this heading.

Allium cepa (Use caution when ambrisentan is co-administered with inducers of CYPs). Products include:
Hyland's Cold 'N Cough 3314
Mederma 2319
Mederma for Kids 2319

Allium sativum (Use caution when ambrisentan is co-administered with inducers of CYPs).
No products indexed under this heading.

Allium schoenoprasum (Use caution when ambrisentan is co-administered with inducers of CYPs).
No products indexed under this heading.

Allium ursinum (Use caution when ambrisentan is co-administered with inducers of CYPs).
No products indexed under this heading.

Aminoglutethimide (Use caution when ambrisentan is co-administered with inducers of CYPs).
No products indexed under this heading.

Amiodarone Hydrochloride (Use caution when ambrisentan is co-administered with strong CYP3A-inhibitors).
No products indexed under this heading.

Amlodipine Besylate (Based on *in vitro* data, interactions with strong inhibitors of P-glycoprotein (P-gp), the Organic Anion Transport Protein (OATP), CYP3A4, CYP2C19, and uridine 5' diphosphate glucuronosyltransferases (UGTs) are possible). Products include:
Azor 1010
Exforge 2443
Exforge HCT 2449

Amprenavir (Use caution when ambrisentan is co-administered with strong CYP3A-inhibitors).
No products indexed under this heading.

Anastrozole (Based on *in vitro* data, interactions with strong inhibitors of P-glycoprotein (P-gp), the Organic Anion Transport Protein (OATP), CYP3A4, CYP2C19, and uridine 5' diphosphate glucuronosyltransferases (UGTs) are possible).
No products indexed under this heading.

Aprepitant (Use caution when ambrisentan is co-administered with strong CYP3A-inhibitors). Products include:
Emend 2124

Atazanavir (Based on *in vitro* data, interactions with strong inhibitors of P-glycoprotein (P-gp), the Organic Anion Transport Protein (OATP), CYP3A4, CYP2C19, and uridine 5' diphosphate glucuronosyltransferases (UGTs) are possible).
No products indexed under this heading.

Atazanavir Sulfate (Based on *in vitro* data, interactions with strong inhibitors of P-glycoprotein (P-gp), the Organic Anion Transport Protein (OATP), CYP3A4, CYP2C19, and uridine 5' diphosphate glucuronosyltransferases (UGTs) are possible).
No products indexed under this heading.

Atenolol (Based on *in vitro* data, interactions with strong inhibitors of P-glycoprotein (P-gp), the Organic Anion Transport Protein (OATP), CYP3A4, CYP2C19, and uridine 5' diphosphate glucuronosyltransferases (UGTs) are possible).
No products indexed under this heading.

Atorvastatin Calcium (Based on *in vitro* data, interactions with strong inhibitors of P-glycoprotein (P-gp), the Organic Anion Transport Protein (OATP), CYP3A4, CYP2C19, and uridine 5' diphosphate glucuronosyltransferases (UGTs) are possible). Products include:
Lipitor 2703

Azithromycin Dihydrate (Based on *in vitro* data, interactions with strong inhibitors of P-glycoprotein (P-gp), the Organic Anion Transport Protein (OATP), CYP3A4, CYP2C19, and uridine 5' diphosphate glucuronosyltransferases (UGTs) are possible).
No products indexed under this heading.

Betamethasone (Use caution when ambrisentan is co-administered with inducers of CYPs).
No products indexed under this heading.

Betamethasone Acetate (Use caution when ambrisentan is co-administered with inducers of CYPs).
No products indexed under this heading.

Betamethasone Benzoate (Use caution when ambrisentan is co-administered with inducers of CYPs).
No products indexed under this heading.

Betamethasone Dipropionate (Use caution when ambrisentan is co-administered with inducers of CYPs). Products include:
Diprolene Lotion 0.05% 3108
Diprolene Ointment 0.05% 3109
Diprolene AF Cream 0.05% 3107
Lotrisone 3163

Betamethasone Sodium Phosphate (Use caution when ambrisentan is co-administered with inducers of CYPs).
No products indexed under this heading.

Betamethasone Valerate (Use caution when ambrisentan is co-administered with inducers of CYPs). Products include:
Luxíq 3321

Bosentan (Use caution when ambrisentan is co-administered with inducers of CYPs). Products include:
Tracleer 573

Carbamazepine (Use caution when ambrisentan is co-administered with inducers of CYPs). Products include:
Carbatrol 3280
Equetro 3477

Carvedilol (Based on *in vitro* data, interactions with strong inhibitors of P-glycoprotein (P-gp), the Organic Anion Transport Protein (OATP), CYP3A4, CYP2C19, and uridine 5' diphosphate glucuronosyltransferases (UGTs) are possible). Products include:
Coreg 1409

Carvedilol Phosphate (Based on *in vitro* data, interactions with strong inhibitors of P-glycoprotein (P-gp), the Organic Anion Transport Protein (OATP), CYP3A4, CYP2C19, and uridine 5' diphosphate glucuronosyltransferases (UGTs) are possible). Products include:
Coreg CR 1416

Chlorpromazine (Use caution when ambrisentan is co-administered with inducers of P-gp).
No products indexed under this heading.

Chlorpromazine Hydrochloride (Use caution when ambrisentan is co-administered with inducers of P-gp).
No products indexed under this heading.

Cimetidine (Use caution when ambrisentan is co-administered with strong CYP3A-inhibitors).
No products indexed under this heading.

Cimetidine Hydrochloride (Use caution when ambrisentan is co-administered with strong CYP3A-inhibitors).
No products indexed under this heading.

Ciprofloxacin (Use caution when ambrisentan is co-administered with strong CYP3A-inhibitors). Products include:
Cipro I.V. 3082
Cipro 3073
Cipro XR 3091
Ciprodex 583

Ciprofloxacin Hydrochloride (Use caution when ambrisentan is co-administered with strong CYP3A-inhibitors). Products include:
Cipro 3073

Cisplatin (Use caution when ambrisentan is co-administered with inducers of CYPs).
No products indexed under this heading.

Citalopram Hydrobromide (Use caution when ambrisentan is co-administered with strong CYP219-inhibitors). Products include:
Celexa 1153

Clarithromycin (Use caution when ambrisentan is co-administered with strong CYP3A-inhibitors). Products include:
Biaxin/Biaxin XL 412

Clotrimazole (Use caution when ambrisentan is co-administered with inducers of P-gp). Products include:
Lotrisone 3163

Clotrimazole, Topical (Use caution when ambrisentan is co-administered with inducers of P-gp).
No products indexed under this heading.

Conivaptan Hydrochloride (Based on *in vitro* data, interactions with strong inhibitors of P-glycoprotein (P-gp), the Organic Anion Transport Protein (OATP), CYP3A4, CYP2C19, and uridine 5' diphosphate glucuronosyltransferases (UGTs) are possible). Products include:
Vaprisol 689

Cortisone Acetate (Use caution when ambrisentan is co-administered with inducers of CYPs).
No products indexed under this heading.

Cyclosporine (Cyclosporine is a strong inhibitor of P-glycoprotein (P-gp), Organic Anion transport Protein (OATP), and CYP3A4. *In vitro* data indicate ambrisentan is a substrate of P-gp, OATP and CYP3A. Therefore, use caution when ambrisentan is co-administered with cyclosporine A, because cyclosporine A may cause increased exposure to ambrisentan). Products include:
Gengraf 440
Neoral Oral Solution 2496
Neoral Capsules 2496
Restasis 605

Dalfopristin (Based on *in vitro* data, interactions with strong inhibitors of P-glycoprotein (P-gp), the Organic Anion Transport Protein (OATP), CYP3A4, CYP2C19, and uridine 5' diphosphate glucuronosyltransferases (UGTs) are possible).
No products indexed under this heading.

IMPORTANT NOTE: Always consult each drug listing in the patient's regimen for possible interactions.

(⊙ Described in PDR® for Ophthalmic Medicines)

IMPORTANT NOTE: Always consult each drug listing in the patient's regimen for possible interactions.

(⊙ Described in PDR® for Ophthalmic Medicines)

Aluminum Carbonate (Levaquin Injection should not be co-administered with any solution containing multivalent cations, such as magnesium, through the same intravenous line).
No products indexed under this heading.

Aluminum Chlorhydroxide (Levaquin Injection should not be co-administered with any solution containing multivalent cations, such as magnesium, through the same intravenous line).
No products indexed under this heading.

Aluminum Chloride (Levaquin Injection should not be co-administered with any solution containing multivalent cations, such as magnesium, through the same intravenous line).
No products indexed under this heading.

Aluminum Chlorohydrate (Levaquin Injection should not be co-administered with any solution containing multivalent cations, such as magnesium, through the same intravenous line).
No products indexed under this heading.

Aluminum Glycinate (Levaquin Injection should not be co-administered with any solution containing multivalent cations, such as magnesium, through the same intravenous line).
No products indexed under this heading.

Aluminum Hydroxide (Levaquin Injection should not be co-administered with any solution containing multivalent cations, such as magnesium, through the same intravenous line).
No products indexed under this heading.

Aluminum Hydroxide Preparations (Levaquin Injection should not be co-administered with any solution containing multivalent cations, such as magnesium, through the same intravenous line).
No products indexed under this heading.

Aluminum Sulfate (Levaquin Injection should not be co-administered with any solution containing multivalent cations, such as magnesium, through the same intravenous line).
No products indexed under this heading.

Amiodarone Hydrochloride (Levofloxacin should be avoided in patients with known prolongation of the QT interval, patients with uncorrected hypokalemia, and patients receiving Class III (eg, amiodarone) antiarrhythmic agents. Elderly patients may be more susceptible to drug-associated effects on the QT interval).
No products indexed under this heading.

Amitriptyline Hydrochloride (Prolongation of the QT interval and isolated cases of torsade de pointes have been reported due to levofloxacin. Levofloxacin should be avoided with other drugs that prolong the QT interval. Levofloxacin should be avoided in patients with known prolongation of the QT interval, patients with uncorrected hypokalemia, and patients receiving Class IA (quinidine, procainamide), or Class III (amiodarone, sotalol) antiarrhythmic agents. Elderly patients may be more susceptible to drug-associated effects on the QT interval).
No products indexed under this heading.

Amoxapine (Prolongation of the QT interval and isolated cases of torsade de pointes have been reported due to levofloxacin. Levofloxacin should be avoided with other drugs that prolong the QT interval. Levofloxacin should be avoided in patients with known prolongation of the QT interval, patients with uncorrected hypokalemia, and patients receiving Class IA (quinidine, procainamide), or Class III (amiodarone, sotalol) antiarrhythmic agents. Elderly patients may be more susceptible to drug-associated effects on the QT interval).
No products indexed under this heading.

Astemizole (Prolongation of the QT interval and isolated cases of torsade de pointes have been reported due to levofloxacin. Levofloxacin should be avoided with other drugs that prolong the QT interval. Levofloxacin should be avoided in patients with known prolongation of the QT interval, patients with uncorrected hypokalemia, and patients receiving Class IA (quinidine, procainamide), or Class III (amiodarone, sotalol) antiarrhythmic agents. Elderly patients may be more susceptible to drug-associated effects on the QT interval).
No products indexed under this heading.

Beclomethasone Dipropionate (Fluoroquinolones, including levofloxacin, are associated with an increased risk of tendinitis and tendon rupture in all ages. This risk is further increased in patients taking corticosteroid drugs). Products include:
Qvar 3398

Beclomethasone Dipropionate Monohydrate (Fluoroquinolones, including levofloxacin, are associated with an increased risk of tendinitis and tendon rupture in all ages. This risk is further increased in patients taking corticosteroid drugs). Products include:
Beconase AQ 1386

Betamethasone (Fluoroquinolones, including levofloxacin, are associated with an increased risk of tendinitis and tendon rupture in all ages. This risk is further increased in patients taking corticosteroid drugs).
No products indexed under this heading.

Betamethasone Acetate (Fluoroquinolones, including levofloxacin, are associated with an increased risk of tendinitis and tendon rupture in all ages. This risk is further increased in patients taking corticosteroid drugs).
No products indexed under this heading.

Betamethasone Benzoate (Fluoroquinolones, including levofloxacin, are associated with an increased risk of tendinitis and tendon rupture in all ages. This risk is further increased in patients taking corticosteroid drugs).
No products indexed under this heading.

Betamethasone Dipropionate (Fluoroquinolones, including levofloxacin, are associated with an increased risk of tendinitis and tendon rupture in all ages. This risk is further increased in patients taking corticosteroid drugs). Products include:
Diprolene Lotion 0.05% 3108
Diprolene Ointment 0.05% 3109
Diprolene AF Cream 0.05% 3107
Lotrisone 3163

Betamethasone Sodium Phosphate (Fluoroquinolones, including levofloxacin, are associated with an increased risk of tendinitis and tendon rupture in all ages. This risk is further increased in patients taking corticosteroid drugs).
No products indexed under this heading.

Betamethasone Valerate (Fluoroquinolones, including levofloxacin, are associated with an increased risk of tendinitis and tendon rupture in all ages. This risk is further increased in patients taking corticosteroid drugs). Products include:
Luxíq 3321

Bretylium Tosylate (Levofloxacin should be avoided in patients with known prolongation of the QT interval, patients with uncorrected hypokalemia, and patients receiving Class III (amiodarone, sotalol) antiarrhythmic agents. Elderly patients may be more susceptible to drug-associated effects on the QT interval).
No products indexed under this heading.

Budesonide (Fluoroquinolones, including levofloxacin, are associated with an increased risk of tendinitis and tendon rupture in all ages. This risk is further increased in patients taking corticosteroid drugs). Products include:
Pulmicort Flexhaler 714
Symbicort 80/4.5 720
Symbicort 160/4.5 720

Buspirone Hydrochloride (Prolongation of the QT interval and isolated cases of torsade de pointes have been reported due to levofloxacin. Levofloxacin should be avoided with other drugs that prolong the QT interval. Levofloxacin should be avoided in patients with known prolongation of the QT interval, patients with uncorrected hypokalemia, and patients receiving Class IA (quinidine, procainamide), or Class III (amiodarone, sotalol) antiarrhythmic agents. Elderly patients may be more susceptible to drug-associated effects on the QT interval).
No products indexed under this heading.

Calcium (Levaquin Injection should not be co-administered with any solution containing multivalent cations, such as magnesium, through the same intravenous line). Products include:
BoneMate Plus 3454
Cardio Basics 3455
Chelated Mineral 3476
CitraNatal 90 DHA Capsules 2332
CitraNatal Harmony 2332

Calcium (Oyster Shell) (Levaquin Injection should not be co-administered with any solution containing multivalent cations, such as magnesium, through the same intravenous line).
No products indexed under this heading.

Calcium Acetate (Levaquin Injection should not be co-administered with any solution containing multivalent cations, such as magnesium, through the same intravenous line).
No products indexed under this heading.

Calcium Ascorbate (Levaquin Injection should not be co-administered with any solution containing multivalent cations, such as magnesium, through the same intravenous line). Products include:
Bio-C 3454
Procosa II 3476
Proflavanol 90 3476

Calcium Carbaspirin (Levaquin Injection should not be co-administered with any solution containing multivalent cations, such as magnesium, through the same intravenous line).
No products indexed under this heading.

Calcium Carbonate (Levaquin Injection should not be co-administered with any solution containing multivalent cations, such as magnesium, through the same intravenous line). Products include:
Chelated Mineral 3476
Pepcid Complete 1822
Extra Strength Rolaids Softchews
Vanilla Creme 2045

Calcium Carbonate, Precipitated (Levaquin Injection should not be co-administered with any solution containing multivalent cations, such as magnesium, through the same intravenous line).
No products indexed under this heading.

Calcium Caseinate (Levaquin Injection should not be co-administered with any solution containing multivalent cations, such as magnesium, through the same intravenous line).
No products indexed under this heading.

Calcium Chloride (Levaquin Injection should not be co-administered with any solution containing multivalent cations, such as magnesium, through the same intravenous line).
No products indexed under this heading.

Calcium Citrate (Levaquin Injection should not be co-administered with any solution containing multivalent cations, such as magnesium, through the same intravenous line). Products include:
Active Calcium 3476
Chelated Mineral 3476
CitraNatal 90 DHA Capsules 2332
CitraNatal Assure 2332
CitraNatal Harmony 2332
CitraNatal Rx 2332

Calcium Disodium Edetate (Levaquin Injection should not be co-administered with any solution containing multivalent cations, such as magnesium, through the same intravenous line).
No products indexed under this heading.

Calcium Glubionate (Levaquin Injection should not be co-administered with any solution containing multivalent cations, such as magnesium, through the same intravenous line).
No products indexed under this heading.

Calcium Gluconate (Levaquin Injection should not be co-administered with any solution containing multivalent cations, such as magnesium, through the same intravenous line).
No products indexed under this heading.

Calcium Glycerophosphate (Levaquin Injection should not be co-administered with any solution containing multivalent cations, such as magnesium, through the same intravenous line).
No products indexed under this heading.

Calcium Iodide (Levaquin Injection should not be co-administered with any solution containing multivalent cations, such as magnesium, through the same intravenous line).
No products indexed under this heading.

Calcium Lactate (Levaquin Injection should not be co-administered with any solution containing multivalent cations, such as magnesium, through the same intravenous line).
No products indexed under this heading.

Calcium Levulinate (Levaquin Injection should not be co-administered with any solution containing multivalent cations, such as magnesium, through the same intravenous line).
No products indexed under this heading.

Calcium Pantothenate (Levaquin Injection should not be co-administered with any solution containing multivalent cations, such as magnesium, through the same intravenous line). Products include:
Cardio Basics 3455

Calcium Phosphate (Levaquin Injection should not be co-administered with any solution containing multivalent cations, such as magnesium, through the same intravenous line).
No products indexed under this heading.

Calcium Phosphate, Dibasic (Levaquin Injection should not be co-administered with any solution containing multivalent cations, such as magnesium, through the same intravenous line).
No products indexed under this heading.

Calcium Phosphate, Tribasic (Levaquin Injection should not be co-administered with any solution containing multivalent cations, such as magnesium, through the same intravenous line).
No products indexed under this heading.

Calcium Phosphorus Preparations (Levaquin Injection should not be co-administered with any solution containing multivalent cations, such as magnesium, through the same intravenous line).
No products indexed under this heading.

IMPORTANT NOTE: Always consult each drug listing in the patient's regimen for possible interactions.

Calcium Polycarbophil (Levaquin Injection should not be co-administered with any solution containing multivalent cations, such as magnesium, through the same intravenous line).
No products indexed under this heading.

Calcium Salts (Levaquin Injection should not be co-administered with any solution containing multivalent cations, such as magnesium, through the same intravenous line).
No products indexed under this heading.

Calcium Sodium Alginate Fiber (Levaquin Injection should not be co-administered with any solution containing multivalent cations, such as magnesium, through the same intravenous line).
No products indexed under this heading.

Calcium Undecylenate (Levaquin Injection should not be co-administered with any solution containing multivalent cations, such as magnesium, through the same intravenous line).
No products indexed under this heading.

Celecoxib (Concomitant administration of a non-steroidal anti-inflammatory drug with a fluoroquinolone, including levofloxacin, may increase the risk of CNS stimulation and convulsive seizures). Products include:
Celebrex 3272

Chlordiazepoxide (Prolongation of the QT interval and isolated cases of torsade de pointes have been reported due to levofloxacin. Levofloxacin should be avoided with other drugs that prolong the QT interval. Levofloxacin should be avoided in patients with known prolongation of the QT interval, patients with uncorrected hypokalemia, and patients receiving Class IA (quinidine, procainamide), or Class III (amiodarone, sotalol) antiarrhythmic agents. Elderly patients may be more susceptible to drug-associated effects on the QT interval).
No products indexed under this heading.

Chlordiazepoxide Hydrochloride (Prolongation of the QT interval and isolated cases of torsade de pointes have been reported due to levofloxacin. Levofloxacin should be avoided with other drugs that prolong the QT interval. Levofloxacin should be avoided in patients with known prolongation of the QT interval, patients with uncorrected hypokalemia, and patients receiving Class IA (quinidine, procainamide), or Class III (amiodarone, sotalol) antiarrhythmic agents. Elderly patients may be more susceptible to drug-associated effects on the QT interval).
No products indexed under this heading.

Chlorpromazine (Prolongation of the QT interval and isolated cases of torsade de pointes have been reported due to levofloxacin. Levofloxacin should be avoided with other drugs that prolong the QT interval. Levofloxacin should be avoided in patients with known prolongation of the QT interval, patients with uncorrected hypokalemia, and patients receiving Class IA (quinidine, procainamide), or Class III (amiodarone, sotalol) antiarrhythmic agents. Elderly patients may be more susceptible to drug-associated effects on the QT interval).
No products indexed under this heading.

Chlorpromazine Hydrochloride (Prolongation of the QT interval and isolated cases of torsade de pointes have been reported due to levofloxacin. Levofloxacin should be avoided with other drugs that prolong the QT interval. Levofloxacin should be avoided in patients with known prolongation of the QT interval, patients with uncorrected hypokalemia, and patients receiving Class IA (quinidine, procainamide), or Class III (amiodarone, sotalol) antiar-

rhythmic agents. Elderly patients may be more susceptible to drug-associated effects on the QT interval).
No products indexed under this heading.

Chlorpropamide (Disturbances of blood glucose, including symptomatic hyper- and hypoglycemia, have been reported with levofloxacin, usually in diabetic patients receiving concomitant treatment with an oral hypoglycemic agent (eg, glyburide). In these patients, careful monitoring of blood glucose is recommended. If a hypoglycemic reaction occurs in a patient being treated with levofloxacin, levofloxacin should be discontinued and appropriate therapy should be initiated immediately).
No products indexed under this heading.

Chlorprothixene (Prolongation of the QT interval and isolated cases of torsade de pointes have been reported due to levofloxacin. Levofloxacin should be avoided with other drugs that prolong the QT interval. Levofloxacin should be avoided in patients with known prolongation of the QT interval, patients with uncorrected hypokalemia, and patients receiving Class IA (quinidine, procainamide), or Class III (amiodarone, sotalol) antiarrhythmic agents. Elderly patients may be more susceptible to drug-associated effects on the QT interval).
No products indexed under this heading.

Chlorprothixene Hydrochloride (Prolongation of the QT interval and isolated cases of torsade de pointes have been reported due to levofloxacin. Levofloxacin should be avoided with other drugs that prolong the QT interval. Levofloxacin should be avoided in patients with known prolongation of the QT interval, patients with uncorrected hypokalemia, and patients receiving Class IA (quinidine, procainamide), or Class III (amiodarone, sotalol) antiarrhythmic agents. Elderly patients may be more susceptible to drug-associated effects on the QT interval).
No products indexed under this heading.

Ciclesonide (Fluoroquinolones, including levofloxacin, are associated with an increased risk of tendinitis and tendon rupture in all ages. This risk is further increased in patients taking corticosteroid drugs).
No products indexed under this heading.

Cimetidine (The AUC and $t_{1/2}$ of levofloxacin were higher while CL/F and CL_R were lower during concomitant treatment of levofloxacin with cimetidine compared to levofloxacin alone).
No products indexed under this heading.

Cimetidine Hydrochloride (The AUC and $t_{1/2}$ of levofloxacin were higher while CL/F and CL_R were lower during concomitant treatment of levofloxacin with cimetidine compared to levofloxacin alone).
No products indexed under this heading.

Clomipramine Hydrochloride (Prolongation of the QT interval and isolated cases of torsade de pointes have been reported due to levofloxacin. Levofloxacin should be avoided with other drugs that prolong the QT interval. Levofloxacin should be avoided in patients with known prolongation of the QT interval, patients with uncorrected hypokalemia, and patients receiving Class IA (quinidine, procainamide), or Class III (amiodarone, sotalol) antiarrhythmic agents. Elderly patients may be more susceptible to drug-associated effects on the QT interval).
No products indexed under this heading.

Clorazepate Dipotassium (Prolongation of the QT interval and isolated cases of torsade de pointes have been reported due to levofloxacin. Levofloxacin should be avoided with other drugs that prolong the QT interval. Levofloxa-

cin should be avoided in patients with known prolongation of the QT interval, patients with uncorrected hypokalemia, and patients receiving Class IA (quinidine, procainamide), or Class III (amiodarone, sotalol) antiarrhythmic agents. Elderly patients may be more susceptible to drug-associated effects on the QT interval).
No products indexed under this heading.

Clozapine (Prolongation of the QT interval and isolated cases of torsade de pointes have been reported due to levofloxacin. Levofloxacin should be avoided with other drugs that prolong the QT interval. Levofloxacin should be avoided in patients with known prolongation of the QT interval, patients with uncorrected hypokalemia, and patients receiving Class IA (quinidine, procainamide), or Class III (amiodarone, sotalol) antiarrhythmic agents. Elderly patients may be more susceptible to drug-associated effects on the QT interval).
No products indexed under this heading.

Cortisone Acetate (Fluoroquinolones, including levofloxacin, are associated with an increased risk of tendinitis and tendon rupture in all ages. This risk is further increased in patients taking corticosteroid drugs).
No products indexed under this heading.

Cyclosporine (Elevated serum levels of cyclosporine have been reported in the patient population when co-administered with some other fluoroquinolones. Levofloxacin C_{max} and k_e were slightly lower while T_{max} and $t_{1/2}$ were slightly longer in the presence of cyclosporine than those observed in other studies without concomitant medication). Products include:
Gengraf 440
Neoral Oral Solution 2496
Neoral Capsules 2496
Restasis 605

Desipramine Hydrochloride (Prolongation of the QT interval and isolated cases of torsade de pointes have been reported due to levofloxacin. Levofloxacin should be avoided with other drugs that prolong the QT interval. Levofloxacin should be avoided in patients with known prolongation of the QT interval, patients with uncorrected hypokalemia, and patients receiving Class IA (quinidine, procainamide), or Class III (amiodarone, sotalol) antiarrhythmic agents. Elderly patients may be more susceptible to drug-associated effects on the QT interval).
No products indexed under this heading.

Desoximetasone (Fluoroquinolones, including levofloxacin, are associated with an increased risk of tendinitis and tendon rupture in all ages. This risk is further increased in patients taking corticosteroid drugs).
No products indexed under this heading.

Dexamethasone (Fluoroquinolones, including levofloxacin, are associated with an increased risk of tendinitis and tendon rupture in all ages. This risk is further increased in patients taking corticosteroid drugs). Products include:
Ciprodex 583
Ozurdex .... ⊙ 223
Tobramycin and Dexamethasone
Ophthalmic Suspension .... ⊙ 251

Dexamethasone Acetate (Fluoroquinolones, including levofloxacin, are associated with an increased risk of tendinitis and tendon rupture in all ages. This risk is further increased in patients taking corticosteroid drugs).
No products indexed under this heading.

Dexamethasone Phosphate (Fluoroquinolones, including levofloxacin, are associated with an increased risk of tendinitis and tendon rupture in all ages. This risk is further increased in patients taking corticosteroid drugs).
No products indexed under this heading.

Dexamethasone Sodium (Fluoroquinolones, including levofloxacin, are associated with an increased risk of tendinitis and tendon rupture in all ages. This risk is further increased in patients taking corticosteroid drugs).
No products indexed under this heading.

Dexamethasone Sodium Phosphate (Fluoroquinolones, including levofloxacin, are associated with an increased risk of tendinitis and tendon rupture in all ages. This risk is further increased in patients taking corticosteroid drugs).
No products indexed under this heading.

Dexamethasone Sodium Phosphate Injection (Fluoroquinolones, including levofloxacin, are associated with an increased risk of tendinitis and tendon rupture in all ages. This risk is further increased in patients taking corticosteroid drugs).
No products indexed under this heading.

Diazepam (Prolongation of the QT interval and isolated cases of torsade de pointes have been reported due to levofloxacin. Levofloxacin should be avoided with other drugs that prolong the QT interval. Levofloxacin should be avoided in patients with known prolongation of the QT interval, patients with uncorrected hypokalemia, and patients receiving Class IA (quinidine, procainamide), or Class III (amiodarone, sotalol) antiarrhythmic agents. Elderly patients may be more susceptible to drug-associated effects on the QT interval).
Products include:
Valium Tablets 2880

Diclofenac Epolamine (Concomitant administration of a non-steroidal anti-inflammatory drug with a fluoroquinolone, including levofloxacin, may increase the risk of CNS stimulation and convulsive seizures). Products include:
Flector 1839

Diclofenac Potassium (Concomitant administration of a non-steroidal anti-inflammatory drug with a fluoroquinolone, including levofloxacin, may increase the risk of CNS stimulation and convulsive seizures).
No products indexed under this heading.

Diclofenac Sodium (Concomitant administration of a non-steroidal anti-inflammatory drug with a fluoroquinolone, including levofloxacin, may increase the risk of CNS stimulation and convulsive seizures).
No products indexed under this heading.

Diflorasone Diacetate (Fluoroquinolones, including levofloxacin, are associated with an increased risk of tendinitis and tendon rupture in all ages. This risk is further increased in patients taking corticosteroid drugs).
No products indexed under this heading.

Disopyramide (Levofloxacin should be avoided in patients with known prolongation of the QT interval, patients with uncorrected hypokalemia, and patients receiving Class IA (quinidine, procainamide) antiarrhythmic agents. Elderly patients may be more susceptible to drug-associated effects on the QT interval).
No products indexed under this heading.

(⊙ Described in PDR® for Ophthalmic Medicines)

Disopyramide Phosphate (Levofloxacin should be avoided in patients with known prolongation of the QT interval, patients with uncorrected hypokalemia, and patients receiving Class IA (quinidine, procainamide) antiarrhythmic agents. Elderly patients may be more susceptible to drug-associated effects on the QT interval.

No products indexed under this heading.

Dofetilide (Prolongation of the QT interval and isolated cases of torsade de pointes have been reported due to levofloxacin. Levofloxacin should be avoided with other drugs that prolong the QT interval. Levofloxacin should be avoided in patients with known prolongation of the QT interval, patients with uncorrected hypokalemia, and patients receiving Class IA (quinidine, procainamide), or Class III (amiodarone, sotalol) antiarrhythmic agents. Elderly patients may be more susceptible to drug-associated effects on the QT interval).

No products indexed under this heading.

Doxepin Hydrochloride (Prolongation of the QT interval and isolated cases of torsade de pointes have been reported due to levofloxacin. Levofloxacin should be avoided with other drugs that prolong the QT interval. Levofloxacin should be avoided in patients with known prolongation of the QT interval, patients with uncorrected hypokalemia, and patients receiving Class IA (quinidine, procainamide), or Class III (amiodarone, sotalol) antiarrhythmic agents. Elderly patients may be more susceptible to drug-associated effects on the QT interval).

No products indexed under this heading.

Droperidol (Prolongation of the QT interval and isolated cases of torsade de pointes have been reported due to levofloxacin. Levofloxacin should be avoided with other drugs that prolong the QT interval. Levofloxacin should be avoided in patients with known prolongation of the QT interval, patients with uncorrected hypokalemia, and patients receiving Class IA (quinidine, procainamide), or Class III (amiodarone, sotalol) antiarrhythmic agents. Elderly patients may be more susceptible to drug-associated effects on the QT interval).

No products indexed under this heading.

Erythromycin (Prolongation of the QT interval and isolated cases of torsade de pointes have been reported due to levofloxacin. Levofloxacin should be avoided with other drugs that prolong the QT interval. Levofloxacin should be avoided in patients with known prolongation of the QT interval, patients with uncorrected hypokalemia, and patients receiving Class IA (quinidine, procainamide), or Class III (amiodarone, sotalol) antiarrhythmic agents. Elderly patients may be more susceptible to drug-associated effects on the QT interval).

No products indexed under this heading.

Erythromycin Estolate (Prolongation of the QT interval and isolated cases of torsade de pointes have been reported due to levofloxacin. Levofloxacin should be avoided with other drugs that prolong the QT interval. Levofloxacin should be avoided in patients with known prolongation of the QT interval, patients with uncorrected hypokalemia, and patients receiving Class IA (quinidine, procainamide), or Class III (amiodarone, sotalol) antiarrhythmic agents. Elderly patients may be more susceptible to drug-associated effects on the QT interval).

No products indexed under this heading.

Erythromycin Ethylsuccinate (Prolongation of the QT interval and isolated cases of torsade de pointes have been reported due to levofloxacin. Levofloxacin should be avoided with other drugs that prolong the QT interval. Levofloxa-

cin should be avoided in patients with known prolongation of the QT interval, patients with uncorrected hypokalemia, and patients receiving Class IA (quinidine, procainamide), or Class III (amiodarone, sotalol) antiarrhythmic agents. Elderly patients may be more susceptible to drug-associated effects on the QT interval). Products include:

Erythromycin Gluceptate (Prolongation of the QT interval and isolated cases of torsade de pointes have been reported due to levofloxacin. Levofloxacin should be avoided with other drugs that prolong the QT interval. Levofloxacin should be avoided in patients with known prolongation of the QT interval, patients with uncorrected hypokalemia, and patients receiving Class IA (quinidine, procainamide), or Class III (amiodarone, sotalol) antiarrhythmic agents. Elderly patients may be more susceptible to drug-associated effects on the QT interval).

No products indexed under this heading.

Erythromycin Lactobionate (Prolongation of the QT interval and isolated cases of torsade de pointes have been reported due to levofloxacin. Levofloxacin should be avoided with other drugs that prolong the QT interval. Levofloxacin should be avoided in patients with known prolongation of the QT interval, patients with uncorrected hypokalemia, and patients receiving Class IA (quinidine, procainamide), or Class III (amiodarone, sotalol) antiarrhythmic agents. Elderly patients may be more susceptible to drug-associated effects on the QT interval).

No products indexed under this heading.

Erythromycin Stearate (Prolongation of the QT interval and isolated cases of torsade de pointes have been reported due to levofloxacin. Levofloxacin should be avoided with other drugs that prolong the QT interval. Levofloxacin should be avoided in patients with known prolongation of the QT interval, patients with uncorrected hypokalemia, and patients receiving Class IA (quinidine, procainamide), or Class III (amiodarone, sotalol) antiarrhythmic agents. Elderly patients may be more susceptible to drug-associated effects on the QT interval).

No products indexed under this heading.

Etodolac (Concomitant administration of a non-steroidal anti-inflammatory drug with a fluoroquinolone, including levofloxacin, may increase the risk of CNS stimulation and convulsive seizures).

No products indexed under this heading.

Fenoprofen Calcium (Concomitant administration of a non-steroidal anti-inflammatory drug with a fluoroquinolone, including levofloxacin, may increase the risk of CNS stimulation and convulsive seizures).

No products indexed under this heading.

Ferrous Fumarate (Levaquin Injection should not be co-administered with any solution containing multivalent cations, such as magnesium, through the same intravenous line). Products include:

Ferrous Gluconate (Levaquin Injection should not be co-administered with any solution containing multivalent cations, such as magnesium, through the same intravenous line). Products include:

Ferrous Sulfate (Levaquin Injection should not be co-administered with any solution containing multivalent cations, such as magnesium, through the same intravenous line).

No products indexed under this heading.

Flecainide Acetate (Prolongation of the QT interval and isolated cases of torsade de pointes have been reported due to levofloxacin. Levofloxacin should be avoided with other drugs that prolong the QT interval. Levofloxacin should be avoided in patients with known prolongation of the QT interval, patients with uncorrected hypokalemia, and patients receiving Class IA (quinidine, procainamide), or Class III (amiodarone, sotalol) antiarrhythmic agents. Elderly patients may be more susceptible to drug-associated effects on the QT interval).

No products indexed under this heading.

Fludrocortisone Acetate (Fluoroquinolones, including levofloxacin, are associated with an increased risk of tendinitis and tendon rupture in all ages. This risk is further increased in patients taking corticosteroid drugs).

No products indexed under this heading.

Flumethasone Pivalate (Fluoroquinolones, including levofloxacin, are associated with an increased risk of tendinitis and tendon rupture in all ages. This risk is further increased in patients taking corticosteroid drugs).

No products indexed under this heading.

Flunisolide Hemihydrate (Fluoroquinolones, including levofloxacin, are associated with an increased risk of tendinitis and tendon rupture in all ages. This risk is further increased in patients taking corticosteroid drugs).

No products indexed under this heading.

Fluphenazine Decanoate (Prolongation of the QT interval and isolated cases of torsade de pointes have been reported due to levofloxacin. Levofloxacin should be avoided with other drugs that prolong the QT interval. Levofloxacin should be avoided in patients with known prolongation of the QT interval, patients with uncorrected hypokalemia, and patients receiving Class IA (quinidine, procainamide), or Class III (amiodarone, sotalol) antiarrhythmic agents. Elderly patients may be more susceptible to drug-associated effects on the QT interval).

No products indexed under this heading.

Fluphenazine Enanthate (Prolongation of the QT interval and isolated cases of torsade de pointes have been reported due to levofloxacin. Levofloxacin should be avoided with other drugs that prolong the QT interval. Levofloxacin should be avoided in patients with known prolongation of the QT interval, patients with uncorrected hypokalemia, and patients receiving Class IA (quinidine, procainamide), or Class III (amiodarone, sotalol) antiarrhythmic agents. Elderly patients may be more susceptible to drug-associated effects on the QT interval).

No products indexed under this heading.

Fluphenazine Hydrochloride (Prolongation of the QT interval and isolated cases of torsade de pointes have been reported due to levofloxacin. Levofloxacin should be avoided with other drugs that prolong the QT interval. Levofloxacin should be avoided in patients with known prolongation of the QT interval, patients with uncorrected hypokalemia, and patients receiving Class IA (quinidine, procainamide), or Class III (amiodarone, sotalol) antiarrhythmic agents. Elderly patients may be more susceptible to drug-associated effects on the QT interval).

No products indexed under this heading.

Flurbiprofen (Concomitant administration of a non-steroidal anti-inflammatory drug with a fluoroquinolone, including levofloxacin, may increase the risk of CNS stimulation and convulsive seizures).

No products indexed under this heading.

Fluticasone Furoate (Fluoroquinolones, including levofloxacin, are associated with an increased risk of tendinitis and tendon rupture in all ages. This risk is further increased in patients taking corticosteroid drugs). Products include:

Fluticasone Propionate (Fluoroquinolones, including levofloxacin, are associated with an increased risk of tendinitis and tendon rupture in all ages. This risk is further increased in patients taking corticosteroid drugs). Products include:

Glibenclamide (Disturbances of blood glucose, including symptomatic hyper- and hypoglycemia, have been reported with levofloxacin, usually in diabetic patients receiving concomitant treatment with an oral hypoglycemic agent (eg, glyburide). In these patients, careful monitoring of blood glucose is recommended. If a hypoglycemic reaction occurs in a patient being treated with levofloxacin, levofloxacin, should be discontinued and appropriate therapy should be initiated immediately).

No products indexed under this heading.

Glimepiride (Disturbances of blood glucose, including symptomatic hyper- and hypoglycemia, have been reported with levofloxacin, usually in diabetic patients receiving concomitant treatment with an oral hypoglycemic agent (eg, glyburide). In these patients, careful monitoring of blood glucose is recommended. If a hypoglycemic reaction occurs in a patient being treated with levofloxacin, levofloxacin, should be discontinued and appropriate therapy should be initiated immediately). Products include:

Glipizide (Disturbances of blood glucose, including symptomatic hyper- and hypoglycemia, have been reported with levofloxacin, usually in diabetic patients receiving concomitant treatment with an oral hypoglycemic agent (eg, glyburide). In these patients, careful monitoring of blood glucose is recommended. If a hypoglycemic reaction occurs in a patient being treated with levofloxacin, levofloxacin, should be discontinued and appropriate therapy should be initiated immediately).

No products indexed under this heading.

Glyburide (Disturbances of blood glucose, including symptomatic hyper- and hypoglycemia, have been reported with levofloxacin, usually in diabetic patients receiving concomitant treatment with an oral hypoglycemic agent (eg, glyburide). In these patients, careful monitoring of blood glucose is recommended. If a hypoglycemic reaction occurs in a patient being treated with levofloxacin, levofloxacin, should be discontinued and appropriate therapy should be initiated immediately).

No products indexed under this heading.

Haloperidol (Prolongation of the QT interval and isolated cases of torsade de pointes have been reported due to levofloxacin. Levofloxacin should be avoided with other drugs that prolong

IMPORTANT NOTE: Always consult each drug listing in the patient's regimen for possible interactions.

the QT interval. Levofloxacin should be avoided in patients with known prolongation of the QT interval, patients with uncorrected hypokalemia, and patients receiving Class IA (quinidine, procainamide), or Class III (amiodarone, sotalol) antiarrhythmic agents. Elderly patients may be more susceptible to drug-associated effects on the QT interval).

No products indexed under this heading.

Haloperidol Decanoate (Prolongation of the QT interval and isolated cases of torsade de pointes have been reported due to levofloxacin. Levofloxacin should be avoided with other drugs that prolong the QT interval. Levofloxacin should be avoided in patients with known prolongation of the QT interval, patients with uncorrected hypokalemia, and patients receiving Class IA (quinidine, procainamide), or Class III (amiodarone, sotalol) antiarrhythmic agents. Elderly patients may be more susceptible to drug-associated effects on the QT interval).

No products indexed under this heading.

Haloperidol Lactate (Prolongation of the QT interval and isolated cases of torsade de pointes have been reported due to levofloxacin. Levofloxacin should be avoided with other drugs that prolong the QT interval. Levofloxacin should be avoided in patients with known prolongation of the QT interval, patients with uncorrected hypokalemia, and patients receiving Class IA (quinidine, procainamide), or Class III (amiodarone, sotalol) antiarrhythmic agents. Elderly patients may be more susceptible to drug-associated effects on the QT interval).

No products indexed under this heading.

Hydrocortisone (Fluoroquinolones, including levofloxacin, are associated with an increased risk of tendinitis and tendon rupture in all ages. This risk is further increased in patients taking corticosteroid drugs).

No products indexed under this heading.

Hydrocortisone (Alcohol) (Fluoroquinolones, including levofloxacin, are associated with an increased risk of tendinitis and tendon rupture in all ages. This risk is further increased in patients taking corticosteroid drugs).

No products indexed under this heading.

Hydrocortisone Acetate (Fluoroquinolones, including levofloxacin, are associated with an increased risk of tendinitis and tendon rupture in all ages. This risk is further increased in patients taking corticosteroid drugs).

No products indexed under this heading.

Hydrocortisone Butyrate (Fluoroquinolones, including levofloxacin, are associated with an increased risk of tendinitis and tendon rupture in all ages. This risk is further increased in patients taking corticosteroid drugs).

No products indexed under this heading.

Hydrocortisone Cypionate (Fluoroquinolones, including levofloxacin, are associated with an increased risk of tendinitis and tendon rupture in all ages. This risk is further increased in patients taking corticosteroid drugs).

No products indexed under this heading.

Hydrocortisone Hemisuccinate (Fluoroquinolones, including levofloxacin, are associated with an increased risk of tendinitis and tendon rupture in all ages. This risk is further increased in patients taking corticosteroid drugs).

No products indexed under this heading.

Hydrocortisone Probutate (Fluoroquinolones, including levofloxacin, are associated with an increased risk of tendinitis and tendon rupture in all ages. This risk is further increased in patients taking corticosteroid drugs).

No products indexed under this heading.

Hydrocortisone Sodium Phosphate (Fluoroquinolones, including levofloxacin, are associated with an increased risk of tendinitis and tendon rupture in all ages. This risk is further increased in patients taking corticosteroid drugs).

No products indexed under this heading.

Hydrocortisone Sodium Succinate (Fluoroquinolones, including levofloxacin, are associated with an increased risk of tendinitis and tendon rupture in all ages. This risk is further increased in patients taking corticosteroid drugs).

No products indexed under this heading.

Hydrocortisone Valerate (Fluoroquinolones, including levofloxacin, are associated with an increased risk of tendinitis and tendon rupture in all ages. This risk is further increased in patients taking corticosteroid drugs).

No products indexed under this heading.

Hydroxyzine Hydrochloride (Prolongation of the QT interval and isolated cases of torsade de pointes have been reported due to levofloxacin. Levofloxacin should be avoided with other drugs that prolong the QT interval. Levofloxacin should be avoided in patients with known prolongation of the QT interval, patients with uncorrected hypokalemia, and patients receiving Class IA (quinidine, procainamide), or Class III (amiodarone, sotalol) antiarrhythmic agents. Elderly patients may be more susceptible to drug-associated effects on the QT interval).

No products indexed under this heading.

Ibuprofen (Concomitant administration of a non-steroidal anti-inflammatory drug with a fluoroquinolone, including levofloxacin, may increase the risk of CNS stimulation and convulsive seizures). Products include:

Imipramine Hydrochloride (Prolongation of the QT interval and isolated cases of torsade de pointes have been reported due to levofloxacin. Levofloxacin should be avoided with other drugs that prolong the QT interval. Levofloxacin should be avoided in patients with known prolongation of the QT interval, patients with uncorrected hypokalemia, and patients receiving Class IA (quinidine, procainamide), or Class III (amiodarone, sotalol) antiarrhythmic agents. Elderly patients may be more susceptible to drug-associated effects on the QT interval).

No products indexed under this heading.

Imipramine Pamoate (Prolongation of the QT interval and isolated cases of torsade de pointes have been reported due to levofloxacin. Levofloxacin should be avoided with other drugs that prolong the QT interval. Levofloxacin should be avoided in patients with known prolongation of the QT interval, patients with uncorrected hypokalemia, and patients receiving Class IA (quinidine, procainamide), or Class III (amiodarone, sotalol) antiarrhythmic agents. Elderly patients may be more susceptible to drug-associated effects on the QT interval).

No products indexed under this heading.

Indomethacin (Concomitant administration of a non-steroidal anti-inflammatory drug with a fluoroquinolone, including levofloxacin, may increase the risk of CNS stimulation and convulsive seizures). Products include:

Indomethacin Sodium Trihydrate (Concomitant administration of a non-steroidal anti-inflammatory drug with a fluoroquinolone, including levofloxacin, may increase the risk of CNS stimulation and convulsive seizures). Products include:

Insulin (Disturbances of blood glucose, including symptomatic hyper- and hypoglycemia, have been reported with levofloxacin, usually in diabetic patients receiving concomitant treatment with insulin. In these patients, careful monitoring of blood glucose is recommended. If a hypoglycemic reaction occurs in a patient being treated with levofloxacin, levofloxacin, should be discontinued and appropriate therapy should be initiated immediately).

No products indexed under this heading.

Insulin, Human, Zinc Suspension (Disturbances of blood glucose, including symptomatic hyper- and hypoglycemia, have been reported with levofloxacin, usually in diabetic patients receiving concomitant treatment with insulin. In these patients, careful monitoring of blood glucose is recommended. If a hypoglycemic reaction occurs in a patient being treated with levofloxacin, levofloxacin, should be discontinued and appropriate therapy should be initiated immediately).

No products indexed under this heading.

Insulin, Human (rDNA origin) (Disturbances of blood glucose, including symptomatic hyper- and hypoglycemia, have been reported with levofloxacin, usually in diabetic patients receiving concomitant treatment with insulin. In these patients, careful monitoring of blood glucose is recommended. If a hypoglycemic reaction occurs in a patient being treated with levofloxacin, levofloxacin, should be discontinued and appropriate therapy should be initiated immediately). Products include:

Insulin, Human NPH (Disturbances of blood glucose, including symptomatic hyper- and hypoglycemia, have been reported with levofloxacin, usually in diabetic patients receiving concomitant treatment with insulin. In these patients, careful monitoring of blood glucose is recommended. If a hypoglycemic reaction occurs in a patient being treated with levofloxacin, levofloxacin, should be discontinued and appropriate therapy should be initiated immediately). Products include:

Insulin, Human Regular (Disturbances of blood glucose, including symptomatic hyper- and hypoglycemia, have been reported with levofloxacin, usually in diabetic patients receiving concomitant treatment with insulin. In these patients, careful monitoring of blood glucose is recommended. If a hypoglycemic reaction occurs in a patient being treated with levofloxacin, levofloxacin, should be discontinued and appropriate therapy should be initiated immediately). Products include:

Insulin, Human Regular and Human NPH Mixture (Disturbances of blood glucose, including symptomatic hyper- and hypoglycemia, have been reported with levofloxacin, usually in diabetic patients receiving concomitant treatment with insulin. In these patients, careful monitoring of blood glucose is recommended. If a hypoglycemic reaction occurs in a patient being treated with levofloxacin, levofloxacin, should be discontinued and appropriate therapy should be initiated immediately). Products include:

Insulin, NPH (Disturbances of blood glucose, including symptomatic hyper- and hypoglycemia, have been reported with levofloxacin, usually in diabetic patients receiving concomitant treatment with insulin. In these patients, careful monitoring of blood glucose is recommended. If a hypoglycemic reaction occurs in a patient being treated with levofloxacin, levofloxacin, should be discontinued and appropriate therapy should be initiated immediately).

No products indexed under this heading.

Insulin, Regular (Disturbances of blood glucose, including symptomatic hyper- and hypoglycemia, have been reported with levofloxacin, usually in diabetic patients receiving concomitant treatment with insulin. In these patients, careful monitoring of blood glucose is recommended. If a hypoglycemic reaction occurs in a patient being treated with levofloxacin, levofloxacin, should be discontinued and appropriate therapy should be initiated immediately).

No products indexed under this heading.

Insulin, Regular and NPH mixture (Disturbances of blood glucose, including symptomatic hyper- and hypoglycemia, have been reported with levofloxacin, usually in diabetic patients receiving concomitant treatment with insulin. In these patients, careful monitoring of blood glucose is recommended. If a hypoglycemic reaction occurs in a patient being treated with levofloxacin, levofloxacin, should be discontinued and appropriate therapy should be initiated immediately).

No products indexed under this heading.

Insulin, Zinc Crystals (Disturbances of blood glucose, including symptomatic hyper- and hypoglycemia, have been reported with levofloxacin, usually in diabetic patients receiving concomitant treatment with insulin. In these patients, careful monitoring of blood glucose is recommended. If a hypoglycemic reaction occurs in a patient being treated with levofloxacin, levofloxacin, should be discontinued and appropriate therapy should be initiated immediately).

No products indexed under this heading.

Insulin, Zinc Suspension (Disturbances of blood glucose, including symptomatic hyper- and hypoglycemia, have been reported with levofloxacin, usually in diabetic patients receiving concomitant treatment with insulin. In these patients, careful monitoring of blood glucose is recommended. If a hypoglycemic reaction occurs in a patient being treated with levofloxacin, levofloxacin, should be discontinued and appropriate therapy should be initiated immediately).

No products indexed under this heading.

Insulin Aspart (Disturbances of blood glucose, including symptomatic hyper- and hypoglycemia, have been reported with levofloxacin, usually in diabetic patients receiving concomitant treatment with insulin. In these patients, careful monitoring of blood glucose is recommended. If a hypoglycemic reaction occurs in a patient being treated with levofloxacin, levofloxacin, should be discontinued and appropriate therapy should be initiated immediately).

No products indexed under this heading.

Insulin Aspart, Human (Disturbances of blood glucose, including symptomatic hyper- and hypoglycemia, have been reported with levofloxacin, usually in diabetic patients receiving concomitant treatment with insulin. In these patients, careful monitoring of blood glucose is recommended. If a hypoglycemic reaction occurs in a patient being treated with levofloxacin, levofloxacin, should

(⊙ Described in PDR® for Ophthalmic Medicines)

be discontinued and appropriate therapy should be initiated immediately).
Products include:

Insulin Aspart, Human Regular
(Disturbances of blood glucose, including symptomatic hyper- and hypoglycemia, have been reported with levofloxacin, usually in diabetic patients receiving concomitant treatment with insulin. In these patients, careful monitoring of blood glucose is recommended. If a hypoglycemic reaction occurs in a patient being treated with levofloxacin, levofloxacin, should be discontinued and appropriate therapy should be initiated immediately). Products include:

Insulin Aspart Protamine, Human
(Disturbances of blood glucose, including symptomatic hyper- and hypoglycemia, have been reported with levofloxacin, usually in diabetic patients receiving concomitant treatment with insulin. In these patients, careful monitoring of blood glucose is recommended. If a hypoglycemic reaction occurs in a patient being treated with levofloxacin, levofloxacin, should be discontinued and appropriate therapy should be initiated immediately). Products include:

Insulin Detemir (rDNA Origin) (Disturbances of blood glucose, including symptomatic hyper- and hypoglycemia, have been reported with levofloxacin, usually in diabetic patients receiving concomitant treatment with insulin. In these patients, careful monitoring of blood glucose is recommended. If a hypoglycemic reaction occurs in a patient being treated with levofloxacin, levofloxacin, should be discontinued and appropriate therapy should be initiated immediately). Products include:

Insulin Glargine (Disturbances of blood glucose, including symptomatic hyper- and hypoglycemia, have been reported with levofloxacin, usually in diabetic patients receiving concomitant treatment with insulin. In these patients, careful monitoring of blood glucose is recommended. If a hypoglycemic reaction occurs in a patient being treated with levofloxacin, levofloxacin, should be discontinued and appropriate therapy should be initiated immediately). Products include:

Insulin Glulisine (Disturbances of blood glucose, including symptomatic hyper- and hypoglycemia, have been reported with levofloxacin, usually in diabetic patients receiving concomitant treatment with insulin. In these patients, careful monitoring of blood glucose is recommended. If a hypoglycemic reaction occurs in a patient being treated with levofloxacin, levofloxacin, should be discontinued and appropriate therapy should be initiated immediately). Products include:

Insulin Lispro, Human (Disturbances of blood glucose, including symptomatic hyper- and hypoglycemia, have been reported with levofloxacin, usually in diabetic patients receiving concomitant treatment with insulin. In these patients, careful monitoring of blood glucose is recommended. If a hypoglycemic reaction occurs in a patient being treated with levofloxacin, levofloxacin, should be discontinued and appropriate therapy should be initiated immediately). Products include:

Insulin Lispro Protamine, Human
(Disturbances of blood glucose, includ-

ing symptomatic hyper- and hypoglycemia, have been reported with levofloxacin, usually in diabetic patients receiving concomitant treatment with insulin. In these patients, careful monitoring of blood glucose is recommended. If a hypoglycemic reaction occurs in a patient being treated with levofloxacin, levofloxacin, should be discontinued and appropriate therapy should be initiated immediately). Products include:

Iron (Levaquin Injection should not be co-administered with any solution containing multivalent cations, such as magnesium, through the same intravenous line).
No products indexed under this heading.

Iron, Peptonized (Levaquin Injection should not be co-administered with any solution containing multivalent cations, such as magnesium, through the same intravenous line).
No products indexed under this heading.

Iron & Ammonium Citrate (Levaquin Injection should not be co-administered with any solution containing multivalent cations, such as magnesium, through the same intravenous line).
No products indexed under this heading.

Iron Cacodylate (Levaquin Injection should not be co-administered with any solution containing multivalent cations, such as magnesium, through the same intravenous line).
No products indexed under this heading.

Iron Carbonyl (Levaquin Injection should not be co-administered with any solution containing multivalent cations, such as magnesium, through the same intravenous line). Products include:

Iron Supplements (Levaquin Injection should not be co-administered with any solution containing multivalent cations, such as magnesium, through the same intravenous line).
No products indexed under this heading.

Isocarboxazid (Prolongation of the QT interval and isolated cases of torsade de pointes have been reported due to levofloxacin. Levofloxacin should be avoided with other drugs that prolong the QT interval. Levofloxacin should be avoided in patients with known prolongation of the QT interval, patients with uncorrected hypokalemia, and patients receiving Class IA (quinidine, procainamide), or Class III (amiodarone, sotalol) antiarrhythmic agents. Elderly patients may be more susceptible to drug-associated effects on the QT interval). Products include:

Ketoprofen (Concomitant administration of a non-steroidal anti-inflammatory drug with a fluoroquinolone, including levofloxacin, may increase the risk of CNS stimulation and convulsive seizures).
No products indexed under this heading.

Ketorolac Tromethamine (Concomitant administration of a non-steroidal anti-inflammatory drug with a fluoroquinolone, including levofloxacin, may increase the risk of CNS stimulation and convulsive seizures). Products include:

Lidocaine (Prolongation of the QT interval and isolated cases of torsade de pointes have been reported due to levofloxacin. Levofloxacin should be avoided with other drugs that prolong the QT interval. Levofloxacin should be avoided in patients with known prolongation of the QT interval, patients with

uncorrected hypokalemia, and patients receiving Class IA (quinidine, procainamide), or Class III (amiodarone, sotalol) antiarrhythmic agents. Elderly patients may be more susceptible to drug-associated effects on the QT interval).
Products include:

Lidocaine Hydrochloride (Prolongation of the QT interval and isolated cases of torsade de pointes have been reported due to levofloxacin. Levofloxacin should be avoided with other drugs that prolong the QT interval. Levofloxacin should be avoided in patients with known prolongation of the QT interval, patients with uncorrected hypokalemia, and patients receiving Class IA (quinidine, procainamide), or Class III (amiodarone, sotalol) antiarrhythmic agents. Elderly patients may be more susceptible to drug-associated effects on the QT interval).
No products indexed under this heading.

Lithium Carbonate (Prolongation of the QT interval and isolated cases of torsade de pointes have been reported due to levofloxacin. Levofloxacin should be avoided with other drugs that prolong the QT interval. Levofloxacin should be avoided in patients with known prolongation of the QT interval, patients with uncorrected hypokalemia, and patients receiving Class IA (quinidine, procainamide), or Class III (amiodarone, sotalol) antiarrhythmic agents. Elderly patients may be more susceptible to drug-associated effects on the QT interval).
No products indexed under this heading.

Lithium Citrate (Prolongation of the QT interval and isolated cases of torsade de pointes have been reported due to levofloxacin. Levofloxacin should be avoided with other drugs that prolong the QT interval. Levofloxacin should be avoided in patients with known prolongation of the QT interval, patients with uncorrected hypokalemia, and patients receiving Class IA (quinidine, procainamide), or Class III (amiodarone, sotalol) antiarrhythmic agents. Elderly patients may be more susceptible to drug-associated effects on the QT interval).
No products indexed under this heading.

Lorazepam (Prolongation of the QT interval and isolated cases of torsade de pointes have been reported due to levofloxacin. Levofloxacin should be avoided with other drugs that prolong the QT interval. Levofloxacin should be avoided in patients with known prolongation of the QT interval, patients with uncorrected hypokalemia, and patients receiving Class IA (quinidine, procainamide), or Class III (amiodarone, sotalol) antiarrhythmic agents. Elderly patients may be more susceptible to drug-associated effects on the QT interval).
No products indexed under this heading.

Loxapine Hydrochloride (Prolongation of the QT interval and isolated cases of torsade de pointes have been reported due to levofloxacin. Levofloxacin should be avoided with other drugs that prolong the QT interval. Levofloxacin should be avoided in patients with known prolongation of the QT interval, patients with uncorrected hypokalemia, and patients receiving Class IA (quinidine, procainamide), or Class III (amiodarone, sotalol) antiarrhythmic agents. Elderly patients may be more susceptible to drug-associated effects on the QT interval).
No products indexed under this heading.

Loxapine Succinate (Prolongation of the QT interval and isolated cases of torsade de pointes have been reported due to levofloxacin. Levofloxacin should be avoided with other drugs that prolong the QT interval. Levofloxacin

should be avoided in patients with known prolongation of the QT interval, patients with uncorrected hypokalemia, and patients receiving Class IA (quinidine, procainamide), or Class III (amiodarone, sotalol) antiarrhythmic agents. Elderly patients may be more susceptible to drug-associated effects on the QT interval).
No products indexed under this heading.

Magnesium (Levaquin Injection should not be co-administered with any solution containing multivalent cations, such as magnesium, through the same intravenous line). Products include:

Magnesium Aluminum Silicate (Levaquin Injection should not be co-administered with any solution containing multivalent cations, such as magnesium, through the same intravenous line).
No products indexed under this heading.

Magnesium Carbonate (Levaquin Injection should not be co-administered with any solution containing multivalent cations, such as magnesium, through the same intravenous line).
No products indexed under this heading.

Magnesium Chloride (Levaquin Injection should not be co-administered with any solution containing multivalent cations, such as magnesium, through the same intravenous line).
No products indexed under this heading.

Magnesium Citrate (Levaquin Injection should not be co-administered with any solution containing multivalent cations, such as magnesium, through the same intravenous line). Products include:

Magnesium Gluconate (Levaquin Injection should not be co-administered with any solution containing multivalent cations, such as magnesium, through the same intravenous line).
No products indexed under this heading.

Magnesium Hydroxide (Levaquin Injection should not be co-administered with any solution containing multivalent cations, such as magnesium, through the same intravenous line). Products include:

Magnesium Lactate (Levaquin Injection should not be co-administered with any solution containing multivalent cations, such as magnesium, through the same intravenous line).
No products indexed under this heading.

Magnesium Oxide (Levaquin Injection should not be co-administered with any solution containing multivalent cations, such as magnesium, through the same intravenous line). Products include:

Magnesium Salicylate (Levaquin Injection should not be co-administered with any solution containing multivalent cations, such as magnesium, through the same intravenous line).
No products indexed under this heading.

Magnesium Salicylate Tetrahydrate (Levaquin Injection should not be co-administered with any solution containing multivalent cations, such as magnesium, through the same intravenous line).
No products indexed under this heading.

Magnesium Salts (Levaquin Injection should not be co-administered with any solution containing multivalent cations, such as magnesium, through the same intravenous line).
No products indexed under this heading.

Magnesium Sulfate (Levaquin Injection should not be co-administered with any solution containing multivalent cations, such as magnesium, through the same intravenous line).

No products indexed under this heading.

Magnesium Trisilicate (Levaquin Injection should not be co-administered with any solution containing multivalent cations, such as magnesium, through the same intravenous line).

No products indexed under this heading.

Maprotiline Hydrochloride (Prolongation of the QT interval and isolated cases of torsade de pointes have been reported due to levofloxacin. Levofloxacin should be avoided with other drugs that prolong the QT interval. Levofloxacin should be avoided in patients with known prolongation of the QT interval, patients with uncorrected hypokalemia, and patients receiving Class IA (quinidine, procainamide), or Class III (amiodarone, sotalol) antiarrhythmic agents. Elderly patients may be more susceptible to drug-associated effects on the QT interval).

No products indexed under this heading.

Meclofenamate Sodium (Concomitant administration of a non-steroidal anti-inflammatory drug with a fluoroquinolone, including levofloxacin, may increase the risk of CNS stimulation and convulsive seizures).

No products indexed under this heading.

Mefenamic Acid (Concomitant administration of a non-steroidal anti-inflammatory drug with a fluoroquinolone, including levofloxacin, may increase the risk of CNS stimulation and convulsive seizures).

No products indexed under this heading.

Meloxicam (Concomitant administration of a non-steroidal anti-inflammatory drug with a fluoroquinolone, including levofloxacin, may increase the risk of CNS stimulation and convulsive seizures).

No products indexed under this heading.

Meprobamate (Prolongation of the QT interval and isolated cases of torsade de pointes have been reported due to levofloxacin. Levofloxacin should be avoided with other drugs that prolong the QT interval. Levofloxacin should be avoided in patients with known prolongation of the QT interval, patients with uncorrected hypokalemia, and patients receiving Class IA (quinidine, procainamide), or Class III (amiodarone, sotalol) antiarrhythmic agents. Elderly patients may be more susceptible to drug-associated effects on the QT interval).

No products indexed under this heading.

Mesoridazine Besylate (Prolongation of the QT interval and isolated cases of torsade de pointes have been reported due to levofloxacin. Levofloxacin should be avoided with other drugs that prolong the QT interval. Levofloxacin should be avoided in patients with known prolongation of the QT interval, patients with uncorrected hypokalemia, and patients receiving Class IA (quinidine, procainamide), or Class III (amiodarone, sotalol) antiarrhythmic agents. Elderly patients may be more susceptible to drug-associated effects on the QT interval).

No products indexed under this heading.

Metformin Hydrochloride (Disturbances of blood glucose, including symptomatic hyper- and hypoglycemia, have been reported with levofloxacin, usually in diabetic patients receiving concomitant treatment with an oral hypoglycemic agent (eg, glyburide). In these patients, careful monitoring of blood glucose is recommended. If a hypoglycemic reaction occurs in a patient being treated with levofloxacin, levofloxacin,

should be discontinued and appropriate therapy should be initiated immediately). Products include:

Methylprednisolone (Fluoroquinolones, including levofloxacin, are associated with an increased risk of tendinitis and tendon rupture in all ages. This risk is further increased in patients taking corticosteroid drugs).

No products indexed under this heading.

Methylprednisolone Acetate (Fluoroquinolones, including levofloxacin, are associated with an increased risk of tendinitis and tendon rupture in all ages. This risk is further increased in patients taking corticosteroid drugs).

No products indexed under this heading.

Methylprednisolone Sodium Succinate (Fluoroquinolones, including levofloxacin, are associated with an increased risk of tendinitis and tendon rupture in all ages. This risk is further increased in patients taking corticosteroid drugs).

No products indexed under this heading.

Mexiletine Hydrochloride (Prolongation of the QT interval and isolated cases of torsade de pointes have been reported due to levofloxacin. Levofloxacin should be avoided with other drugs that prolong the QT interval. Levofloxacin should be avoided in patients with known prolongation of the QT interval, patients with uncorrected hypokalemia, and patients receiving Class IA (quinidine, procainamide), or Class III (amiodarone, sotalol) antiarrhythmic agents. Elderly patients may be more susceptible to drug-associated effects on the QT interval).

No products indexed under this heading.

Midazolam Hydrochloride (Prolongation of the QT interval and isolated cases of torsade de pointes have been reported due to levofloxacin. Levofloxacin should be avoided with other drugs that prolong the QT interval. Levofloxacin should be avoided in patients with known prolongation of the QT interval, patients with uncorrected hypokalemia, and patients receiving Class IA (quinidine, procainamide), or Class III (amiodarone, sotalol) antiarrhythmic agents. Elderly patients may be more susceptible to drug-associated effects on the QT interval).

No products indexed under this heading.

Miglitol (Disturbances of blood glucose, including symptomatic hyper- and hypoglycemia, have been reported with levofloxacin, usually in diabetic patients receiving concomitant treatment with an oral hypoglycemic agent (eg, glyburide). In these patients, careful monitoring of blood glucose is recommended. If a hypoglycemic reaction occurs in a patient being treated with levofloxacin, levofloxacin, should be discontinued and appropriate therapy should be initiated immediately).

No products indexed under this heading.

Molindone Hydrochloride (Prolongation of the QT interval and isolated cases of torsade de pointes have been reported due to levofloxacin. Levofloxacin should be avoided with other drugs that prolong the QT interval. Levofloxacin should be avoided in patients with known prolongation of the QT interval, patients with uncorrected hypokalemia, and patients receiving Class IA (quinidine, procainamide), or Class III (amiodarone, sotalol) antiarrhythmic agents. Elderly patients may be more susceptible to drug-associated effects on the QT interval). Products include:

Mometasone Furoate (Fluoroquinolones, including levofloxacin, are associat-

ed with an increased risk of tendinitis and tendon rupture in all ages. This risk is further increased in patients taking corticosteroid drugs). Products include:

Mometasone Furoate Monohydrate (Fluoroquinolones, including levofloxacin, are associated with an increased risk of tendinitis and tendon rupture in all ages. This risk is further increased in patients taking corticosteroid drugs). Products include:

Moricizine Hydrochloride (Levofloxacin should be avoided in patients with known prolongation of the QT interval, patients with uncorrected hypokalemia, and patients receiving Class IA (quinidine, procainamide) antiarrhythmic agents. Elderly patients may be more susceptible to drug-associated effects on the QT interval).

No products indexed under this heading.

Nabumetone (Concomitant administration of a non-steroidal anti-inflammatory drug with a fluoroquinolone, including levofloxacin, may increase the risk of CNS stimulation and convulsive seizures).

No products indexed under this heading.

Naproxen (Concomitant administration of a non-steroidal anti-inflammatory drug with a fluoroquinolone, including levofloxacin, may increase the risk of CNS stimulation and convulsive seizures). Products include:

Naproxen Sodium (Concomitant administration of a non-steroidal anti-inflammatory drug with a fluoroquinolone, including levofloxacin, may increase the risk of CNS stimulation and convulsive seizures). Products include:

Nateglinide (Disturbances of blood glucose, including symptomatic hyper- and hypoglycemia, have been reported with levofloxacin, usually in diabetic patients receiving concomitant treatment with an oral hypoglycemic agent (eg, glyburide). In these patients, careful monitoring of blood glucose is recommended. If a hypoglycemic reaction occurs in a patient being treated with levofloxacin, levofloxacin, should be discontinued and appropriate therapy should be initiated immediately).

No products indexed under this heading.

Nortriptyline Hydrochloride (Prolongation of the QT interval and isolated cases of torsade de pointes have been reported due to levofloxacin. Levofloxacin should be avoided with other drugs that prolong the QT interval. Levofloxacin should be avoided in patients with known prolongation of the QT interval, patients with uncorrected hypokalemia, and patients receiving Class IA (quinidine, procainamide), or Class III (amiodarone, sotalol) antiarrhythmic agents. Elderly patients may be more susceptible to drug-associated effects on the QT interval).

No products indexed under this heading.

Olanzapine (Prolongation of the QT interval and isolated cases of torsade de pointes have been reported due to levofloxacin. Levofloxacin should be avoided with other drugs that prolong the QT interval. Levofloxacin should be avoided in patients with known prolongation of the QT interval, patients with uncorrected hypokalemia, and patients receiving Class IA (quinidine, procainamide), or Class III (amiodarone, sotalol)

antiarrhythmic agents. Elderly patients may be more susceptible to drug-associated effects on the QT interval). Products include:

Oxaprozin (Concomitant administration of a non-steroidal anti-inflammatory drug with a fluoroquinolone, including levofloxacin, may increase the risk of CNS stimulation and convulsive seizures).

No products indexed under this heading.

Oxazepam (Prolongation of the QT interval and isolated cases of torsade de pointes have been reported due to levofloxacin. Levofloxacin should be avoided with other drugs that prolong the QT interval. Levofloxacin should be avoided in patients with known prolongation of the QT interval, patients with uncorrected hypokalemia, and patients receiving Class IA (quinidine, procainamide), or Class III (amiodarone, sotalol) antiarrhythmic agents. Elderly patients may be more susceptible to drug-associated effects on the QT interval).

No products indexed under this heading.

Perphenazine (Prolongation of the QT interval and isolated cases of torsade de pointes have been reported due to levofloxacin. Levofloxacin should be avoided with other drugs that prolong the QT interval. Levofloxacin should be avoided in patients with known prolongation of the QT interval, patients with uncorrected hypokalemia, and patients receiving Class IA (quinidine, procainamide), or Class III (amiodarone, sotalol) antiarrhythmic agents. Elderly patients may be more susceptible to drug-associated effects on the QT interval).

No products indexed under this heading.

Phenelzine Sulfate (Prolongation of the QT interval and isolated cases of torsade de pointes have been reported due to levofloxacin. Levofloxacin should be avoided with other drugs that prolong the QT interval. Levofloxacin should be avoided in patients with known prolongation of the QT interval, patients with uncorrected hypokalemia, and patients receiving Class IA (quinidine, procainamide), or Class III (amiodarone, sotalol) antiarrhythmic agents. Elderly patients may be more susceptible to drug-associated effects on the QT interval).

No products indexed under this heading.

Phenylbutazone (Concomitant administration of a non-steroidal anti-inflammatory drug with a fluoroquinolone, including levofloxacin, may increase the risk of CNS stimulation and convulsive seizures).

No products indexed under this heading.

Pioglitazone Hydrochloride (Disturbances of blood glucose, including symptomatic hyper- and hypoglycemia, have been reported with levofloxacin, usually in diabetic patients receiving concomitant treatment with an oral hypoglycemic agent (eg, glyburide). In these patients, careful monitoring of blood glucose is recommended. If a hypoglycemic reaction occurs in a patient being treated with levofloxacin, levofloxacin, should be discontinued and appropriate therapy should be initiated immediately). Products include:

Piroxicam (Concomitant administration of a non-steroidal anti-inflammatory drug with a fluoroquinolone, including levofloxacin, may increase the risk of CNS stimulation and convulsive seizures).

No products indexed under this heading.

Prazepam (Prolongation of the QT interval and isolated cases of torsade de pointes have been reported due to levofloxacin. Levofloxacin should be avoided with other drugs that prolong the QT interval. Levofloxacin should be avoided in patients with known prolongation of the QT interval, patients with uncorrected hypokalemia, and patients receiving Class IA (quinidine, procainamide), or Class III (amiodarone, sotalol) antiarrhythmic agents. Elderly patients may be more susceptible to drug-associated effects on the QT interval).
No products indexed under this heading.

Prednisolone (Fluoroquinolones, including levofloxacin, are associated with an increased risk of tendinitis and tendon rupture in all ages. This risk is further increased in patients taking corticosteroid drugs).
No products indexed under this heading.

Prednisolone Acetate (Fluoroquinolones, including levofloxacin, are associated with an increased risk of tendinitis and tendon rupture in all ages. This risk is further increased in patients taking corticosteroid drugs). Products include:
Blephamide ....⊙**212**, ⊙**214**
Pred Forte .... ⊙**225**
Pred Mild .... ⊙**230**
Pred-G .... ⊙**226**, ⊙**227**

Prednisolone Sodium Phosphate (Fluoroquinolones, including levofloxacin, are associated with an increased risk of tendinitis and tendon rupture in all ages. This risk is further increased in patients taking corticosteroid drugs).
No products indexed under this heading.

Prednisolone Tebutate (Fluoroquinolones, including levofloxacin, are associated with an increased risk of tendinitis and tendon rupture in all ages. This risk is further increased in patients taking corticosteroid drugs).
No products indexed under this heading.

Prednisone (Fluoroquinolones, including levofloxacin, are associated with an increased risk of tendinitis and tendon rupture in all ages. This risk is further increased in patients taking corticosteroid drugs).
No products indexed under this heading.

Prednisone sodium phosphate (Fluoroquinolones, including levofloxacin, are associated with an increased risk of tendinitis and tendon rupture in all ages. This risk is further increased in patients taking corticosteroid drugs).
No products indexed under this heading.

Probenecid (The AUC and $t_{1/2}$ of levofloxacin were higher while CL/F and CL$_R$ were lower during concomitant treatment of levofloxacin with probenecid compared to levofloxacin alone).
No products indexed under this heading.

Procainamide (Levofloxacin should be avoided in patients with known prolongation of the QT interval, patients with uncorrected hypokalemia, and patients receiving Class IA (eg, procainamide) antiarrhythmic agents. Elderly patients may be more susceptible to drug-associated effects on the QT interval).
No products indexed under this heading.

Procainamide Hydrochloride (Levofloxacin should be avoided in patients with known prolongation of the QT interval, patients with uncorrected hypokalemia, and patients receiving Class IA (eg, procainamide) antiarrhythmic agents. Elderly patients may be more susceptible to drug-associated effects on the QT interval).
No products indexed under this heading.

Prochlorperazine (Prolongation of the QT interval and isolated cases of torsade de pointes have been reported due to levofloxacin. Levofloxacin should be avoided with other drugs that pro-

long the QT interval. Levofloxacin should be avoided in patients with known prolongation of the QT interval, patients with uncorrected hypokalemia, and patients receiving Class IA (quinidine, procainamide), or Class III (amiodarone, sotalol) antiarrhythmic agents. Elderly patients may be more susceptible to drug-associated effects on the QT interval).
No products indexed under this heading.

Promethazine Hydrochloride (Prolongation of the QT interval and isolated cases of torsade de pointes have been reported due to levofloxacin. Levofloxacin should be avoided with other drugs that prolong the QT interval. Levofloxacin should be avoided in patients with known prolongation of the QT interval, patients with uncorrected hypokalemia, and patients receiving Class IA (quinidine, procainamide), or Class III (amiodarone, sotalol) antiarrhythmic agents. Elderly patients may be more susceptible to drug-associated effects on the QT interval).
No products indexed under this heading.

Propafenone Hydrochloride (Prolongation of the QT interval and isolated cases of torsade de pointes have been reported due to levofloxacin. Levofloxacin should be avoided with other drugs that prolong the QT interval. Levofloxacin should be avoided in patients with known prolongation of the QT interval, patients with uncorrected hypokalemia, and patients receiving Class IA (quinidine, procainamide), or Class III (amiodarone, sotalol) antiarrhythmic agents. Elderly patients may be more susceptible to drug-associated effects on the QT interval). Products include:
Rythmol 1648
Rythmol SR 1652

Protriptyline Hydrochloride (Prolongation of the QT interval and isolated cases of torsade de pointes have been reported due to levofloxacin. Levofloxacin should be avoided with other drugs that prolong the QT interval. Levofloxacin should be avoided in patients with known prolongation of the QT interval, patients with uncorrected hypokalemia, and patients receiving Class IA (quinidine, procainamide), or Class III (amiodarone, sotalol) antiarrhythmic agents. Elderly patients may be more susceptible to drug-associated effects on the QT interval).
No products indexed under this heading.

Quetiapine Fumarate (Prolongation of the QT interval and isolated cases of torsade de pointes have been reported due to levofloxacin. Levofloxacin should be avoided with other drugs that prolong the QT interval. Levofloxacin should be avoided in patients with known prolongation of the QT interval, patients with uncorrected hypokalemia, and patients receiving Class IA (quinidine, procainamide), or Class III (amiodarone, sotalol) antiarrhythmic agents. Elderly patients may be more susceptible to drug-associated effects on the QT interval). Products include:
Seroquel 750
Seroquel XR 759

Quinidine (Levofloxacin should be avoided in patients with known prolongation of the QT interval, patients with uncorrected hypokalemia, and patients receiving Class IA (eg, quinidine) antiarrhythmic agents. Elderly patients may be more susceptible to drug-associated effects on the QT interval).
No products indexed under this heading.

Quinidine Gluconate (Levofloxacin should be avoided in patients with known prolongation of the QT interval, patients with uncorrected hypokalemia, and patients receiving Class IA (eg, quinidine) antiarrhythmic agents. Elderly patients may be more susceptible to drug-associated effects on the QT interval).
No products indexed under this heading.

Quinidine Hydrochloride (Levofloxacin should be avoided in patients with known prolongation of the QT interval, patients with uncorrected hypokalemia, and patients receiving Class IA (eg, quinidine) antiarrhythmic agents. Elderly patients may be more susceptible to drug-associated effects on the QT interval).
No products indexed under this heading.

Quinidine Polygalacturonate (Levofloxacin should be avoided in patients with known prolongation of the QT interval, patients with uncorrected hypokalemia, and patients receiving Class IA (eg, quinidine) antiarrhythmic agents. Elderly patients may be more susceptible to drug-associated effects on the QT interval).
No products indexed under this heading.

Quinidine Sulfate (Levofloxacin should be avoided in patients with known prolongation of the QT interval, patients with uncorrected hypokalemia, and patients receiving Class IA (eg, quinidine) antiarrhythmic agents. Elderly patients may be more susceptible to drug-associated effects on the QT interval).
No products indexed under this heading.

Repaglinide (Disturbances of blood glucose, including symptomatic hyper- and hypoglycemia, have been reported with levofloxacin, usually in diabetic patients receiving concomitant treatment with an oral hypoglycemic agent (eg, glyburide). In these patients, careful monitoring of blood glucose is recommended. If a hypoglycemic reaction occurs in a patient being treated with levofloxacin, levofloxacin, should be discontinued and appropriate therapy should be initiated immediately).
No products indexed under this heading.

Risperidone (Prolongation of the QT interval and isolated cases of torsade de pointes have been reported due to levofloxacin. Levofloxacin should be avoided with other drugs that prolong the QT interval. Levofloxacin should be avoided in patients with known prolongation of the QT interval, patients with uncorrected hypokalemia, and patients receiving Class IA (quinidine, procainamide), or Class III (amiodarone, sotalol) antiarrhythmic agents. Elderly patients may be more susceptible to drug-associated effects on the QT interval). Products include:
Risperdal Consta 2682

Rofecoxib (Concomitant administration of a non-steroidal anti-inflammatory drug with a fluoroquinolone, including levofloxacin, may increase the risk of CNS stimulation and convulsive seizures).
No products indexed under this heading.

Rosiglitazone Maleate (Disturbances of blood glucose, including symptomatic hyper- and hypoglycemia, have been reported with levofloxacin, usually in diabetic patients receiving concomitant treatment with an oral hypoglycemic agent (eg, glyburide). In these patients, careful monitoring of blood glucose is recommended. If a hypoglycemic reaction occurs in a patient being treated with levofloxacin, levofloxacin, should be discontinued and appropriate therapy should be initiated immediately). Products include:
Avandamet 1345

Avandaryl 1356
Avandia 1366

Selenium (Levaquin Injection should not be co-administered with any solution containing multivalent cations, such as magnesium, through the same intravenous line). Products include:
Cardio Basics 3455
Chelated Mineral 3476

Selenium Sulfide (Levaquin Injection should not be co-administered with any solution containing multivalent cations, such as magnesium, through the same intravenous line).
No products indexed under this heading.

Sitagliptin Phosphate (Disturbances of blood glucose, including symptomatic hyper- and hypoglycemia, have been reported with levofloxacin, usually in diabetic patients receiving concomitant treatment with an oral hypoglycemic agent (eg, glyburide. In these patients, careful monitoring of blood glucose is recommended. If a hypoglycemic reaction occurs in a patient being treated with levofloxacin, levofloxacin, should be discontinued and appropriate therapy should be initiated immediately). Products include:
Janumet 2188
Januvia 2196

Sotalol Hydrochloride (Levofloxacin should be avoided in patients with known prolongation of the QT interval, patients with uncorrected hypokalemia, and patients receiving Class III (eg, sotalol) antiarrhythmic agents. Elderly patients may be more susceptible to drug-associated effects on the QT interval).
No products indexed under this heading.

Sulindac (Concomitant administration of a non-steroidal anti-inflammatory drug with a fluoroquinolone, including levofloxacin, may increase the risk of CNS stimulation and convulsive seizures). Products include:
Clinoril 2098

Theophylline (Concomitant administration of other fluoroquinolones with theophylline has resulted in prolonged elimination half-life, elevated serum theophylline levels, and a subsequent increase in the risk of theophylline-related adverse reactions in the patient population. Therefore, theophylline levels should be closely monitored and appropriate dosage adjustments made when levofloxacin is co-administered. Adverse reactions, including seizures, may occur with or without an elevation in serum theophylline levels).
No products indexed under this heading.

Theophylline Anhydrous (Concomitant administration of other fluoroquinolones with theophylline has resulted in prolonged elimination half-life, elevated serum theophylline levels, and a subsequent increase in the risk of theophylline-related adverse reactions in the patient population. Therefore, theophylline levels should be closely monitored and appropriate dosage adjustments made when levofloxacin is co-administered. Adverse reactions, including seizures, may occur with or without an elevation in serum theophylline levels). Products include:
Uniphyl 2817

Theophylline Calcium Salicylate (Concomitant administration of other fluoroquinolones with theophylline has resulted in prolonged elimination half-life, elevated serum theophylline levels, and a subsequent increase in the risk of theophylline-related adverse reactions in the patient population. Therefore, theophylline levels should be closely monitored and appropriate dosage adjustments made when levofloxacin is co-administered. Adverse reactions,

IMPORTANT NOTE: Always consult each drug listing in the patient's regimen for possible interactions.

including seizures, may occur with or without an elevation in serum theophylline levels).

No products indexed under this heading.

Theophylline Dihydroxypropyl (Glyceryl) (Concomitant administration of other fluoroquinolones with theophylline has resulted in prolonged elimination half-life, elevated serum theophylline levels, and a subsequent increase in the risk of theophylline-related adverse reactions in the patient population. Therefore, theophylline levels should be closely monitored and appropriate dosage adjustments made when levofloxacin is co-administered. Adverse reactions, including seizures, may occur with or without an elevation in serum theophylline levels).

No products indexed under this heading.

Theophylline Ethylenediamine (Concomitant administration of other fluoroquinolones with theophylline has resulted in prolonged elimination half-life, elevated serum theophylline levels, and a subsequent increase in the risk of theophylline-related adverse reactions in the patient population. Therefore, theophylline levels should be closely monitored and appropriate dosage adjustments made when levofloxacin is co-administered. Adverse reactions, including seizures, may occur with or without an elevation in serum theophylline levels).

No products indexed under this heading.

Theophylline Sodium Glycinate (Concomitant administration of other fluoroquinolones with theophylline has resulted in prolonged elimination half-life, elevated serum theophylline levels, and a subsequent increase in the risk of theophylline-related adverse reactions in the patient population. Therefore, theophylline levels should be closely monitored and appropriate dosage adjustments made when levofloxacin is co-administered. Adverse reactions, including seizures, may occur with or without an elevation in serum theophylline levels).

No products indexed under this heading.

Thioridazine Hydrochloride (Prolongation of the QT interval and isolated cases of torsade de pointes have been reported due to levofloxacin. Levofloxacin should be avoided with other drugs that prolong the QT interval. Levofloxacin should be avoided in patients with known prolongation of the QT interval, patients with uncorrected hypokalemia, and patients receiving Class IA (quinidine, procainamide), or Class III (amiodarone, sotalol) antiarrhythmic agents. Elderly patients may be more susceptible to drug-associated effects on the QT interval). Products include:
Thioridazine Hydrochloride 2384

Thiothixene (Prolongation of the QT interval and isolated cases of torsade de pointes have been reported due to levofloxacin. Levofloxacin should be avoided with other drugs that prolong the QT interval. Levofloxacin should be avoided in patients with known prolongation of the QT interval, patients with uncorrected hypokalemia, and patients receiving Class IA (quinidine, procainamide), or Class III (amiodarone, sotalol) antiarrhythmic agents. Elderly patients may be more susceptible to drug-associated effects on the QT interval). Products include:
Thiothixene 2386

Tocainide Hydrochloride (Prolongation of the QT interval and isolated cases of torsade de pointes have been reported due to levofloxacin. Levofloxacin should be avoided with other drugs that prolong the QT interval. Levofloxacin should be avoided in patients with known prolongation of the QT interval, patients with uncorrected hypokalemia,

and patients receiving Class IA (quinidine, procainamide), or Class III (amiodarone, sotalol) antiarrhythmic agents. Elderly patients may be more susceptible to drug-associated effects on the QT interval).

No products indexed under this heading.

Tolazamide (Disturbances of blood glucose, including symptomatic hyper- and hypoglycemia, have been reported with levofloxacin, usually in diabetic patients receiving concomitant treatment with an oral hypoglycemic agent (eg, glyburide). In these patients, careful monitoring of blood glucose is recommended. If a hypoglycemic reaction occurs in a patient being treated with levofloxacin, levofloxacin, should be discontinued and appropriate therapy should be initiated immediately).

No products indexed under this heading.

Tolbutamide (Disturbances of blood glucose, including symptomatic hyper- and hypoglycemia, have been reported with levofloxacin, usually in diabetic patients receiving concomitant treatment with an oral hypoglycemic agent (eg, glyburide). In these patients, careful monitoring of blood glucose is recommended. If a hypoglycemic reaction occurs in a patient being treated with levofloxacin, levofloxacin, should be discontinued and appropriate therapy should be initiated immediately).

No products indexed under this heading.

Tolmetin Sodium (Concomitant administration of a non-steroidal anti-inflammatory drug with a fluoroquinolone, including levofloxacin, may increase the risk of CNS stimulation and convulsive seizures).

No products indexed under this heading.

Tranylcypromine Sulfate (Prolongation of the QT interval and isolated cases of torsade de pointes have been reported due to levofloxacin. Levofloxacin should be avoided with other drugs that prolong the QT interval. Levofloxacin should be avoided in patients with known prolongation of the QT interval, patients with uncorrected hypokalemia, and patients receiving Class IA (quinidine, procainamide), or Class III (amiodarone, sotalol) antiarrhythmic agents. Elderly patients may be more susceptible to drug-associated effects on the QT interval). Products include:
Parnate 1584

Triamcinolone (Fluoroquinolones, including levofloxacin, are associated with an increased risk of tendinitis and tendon rupture in all ages. This risk is further increased in patients taking corticosteroid drugs).

No products indexed under this heading.

Triamcinolone Acetonide (Fluoroquinolones, including levofloxacin, are associated with an increased risk of tendinitis and tendon rupture in all ages. This risk is further increased in patients taking corticosteroid drugs). Products include:
Azmacort 408
Nasacort AQ 3019

Triamcinolone Diacetate (Fluoroquinolones, including levofloxacin, are associated with an increased risk of tendinitis and tendon rupture in all ages. This risk is further increased in patients taking corticosteroid drugs).

No products indexed under this heading.

Triamcinolone Hexacetonide (Fluoroquinolones, including levofloxacin, are associated with an increased risk of tendinitis and tendon rupture in all ages. This risk is further increased in patients taking corticosteroid drugs).

No products indexed under this heading.

Trifluoperazine Hydrochloride (Prolongation of the QT interval and isolated cases of torsade de pointes have been reported due to levofloxacin. Levofloxa-

cin should be avoided with other drugs that prolong the QT interval. Levofloxacin should be avoided in patients with known prolongation of the QT interval, patients with uncorrected hypokalemia, and patients receiving Class IA (quinidine, procainamide), or Class III (amiodarone, sotalol) antiarrhythmic agents. Elderly patients may be more susceptible to drug-associated effects on the QT interval).

No products indexed under this heading.

Trimipramine Maleate (Prolongation of the QT interval and isolated cases of torsade de pointes have been reported due to levofloxacin. Levofloxacin should be avoided with other drugs that prolong the QT interval. Levofloxacin should be avoided in patients with known prolongation of the QT interval, patients with uncorrected hypokalemia, and patients receiving Class IA (quinidine, procainamide), or Class III (amiodarone, sotalol) antiarrhythmic agents. Elderly patients may be more susceptible to drug-associated effects on the QT interval).

No products indexed under this heading.

Troglitazone (Disturbances of blood glucose, including symptomatic hyper- and hypoglycemia, have been reported with levofloxacin, usually in diabetic patients receiving concomitant treatment with an oral hypoglycemic agent (eg, glyburide). In these patients, careful monitoring of blood glucose is recommended. If a hypoglycemic reaction occurs in a patient being treated with levofloxacin, levofloxacin, should be discontinued and appropriate therapy should be initiated immediately).

No products indexed under this heading.

Ultraviolet radiation (Patients should be advised that photosensitivity/phototoxicity has been reported in patients receiving fluoroquinolone antibiotics. Patients should minimize or avoid exposure to natural or artificial sunlight (tanning beds or UVA/B treatment) while taking fluoroquinolones).

No products indexed under this heading.

Valdecoxib (Concomitant administration of a non-steroidal anti-inflammatory drug with a fluoroquinolone, including levofloxacin, may increase the risk of CNS stimulation and convulsive seizures).

No products indexed under this heading.

Warfarin Sodium (There have been reports during the postmarketing experience in patients that levofloxacin enhances the effects of warfarin. Elevations of the prothrombin time in the setting of concurrent warfarin and levofloxacin use have been associated with episodes of bleeding. Prothrombin time, International Normalized Ratio (INR), or other suitable anticoagulation tests should be closely monitored if levofloxacin is administered concomitantly with warfarin. Patients should also be monitored for evidence of bleeding).

No products indexed under this heading.

Zinc (Levaquin Injection should not be co-administered with any solution containing multivalent cations, such as magnesium, through the same intravenous line). Products include:
BoneMate Plus 3454
Cardio Basics 3455
Chelated Mineral 3476
CitraNatal 90 DHA Capsules 2332
CitraNatal Assure 2332
Heplive 607
Visutein 3456

Zinc Acetate (Levaquin Injection should not be co-administered with any solution containing multivalent cations, such as magnesium, through the same intravenous line).

No products indexed under this heading.

Zinc Bisglycinate (Levaquin Injection should not be co-administered with any solution containing multivalent cations, such as magnesium, through the same intravenous line).

No products indexed under this heading.

Zinc Chloride (Levaquin Injection should not be co-administered with any solution containing multivalent cations, such as magnesium, through the same intravenous line).

No products indexed under this heading.

Zinc Citrate (Levaquin Injection should not be co-administered with any solution containing multivalent cations, such as magnesium, through the same intravenous line). Products include:
Chelated Mineral 3476

Zinc-Containing Multivitamins (Levaquin Injection should not be co-administered with any solution containing multivalent cations, such as magnesium, through the same intravenous line).

No products indexed under this heading.

Zinc Gluconate (Levaquin Injection should not be co-administered with any solution containing multivalent cations, such as magnesium, through the same intravenous line).

No products indexed under this heading.

Zinc Oxide (Levaquin Injection should not be co-administered with any solution containing multivalent cations, such as magnesium, through the same intravenous line). Products include:
Bausch & Lomb Ocuvite Adult 50+ .... ⊙ 238
CitraNatal Rx 2332
Vusion Ointment 3335

Zinc Phenosulfonate (Levaquin Injection should not be co-administered with any solution containing multivalent cations, such as magnesium, through the same intravenous line).

No products indexed under this heading.

Zinc Sulfate (Levaquin Injection should not be co-administered with any solution containing multivalent cations, such as magnesium, through the same intravenous line). Products include:
Heplive 607
Zinc-220 606

Ziprasidone Hydrochloride (Prolongation of the QT interval and isolated cases of torsade de pointes have been reported due to levofloxacin. Levofloxacin should be avoided with other drugs that prolong the QT interval. Levofloxacin should be avoided in patients with known prolongation of the QT interval, patients with uncorrected hypokalemia, and patients receiving Class IA (quinidine, procainamide), or Class III (amiodarone, sotalol) antiarrhythmic agents. Elderly patients may be more susceptible to drug-associated effects on the QT interval). Products include:
Geodon 2723

Food Interactions
Iron Amino Acid Chelate (Levaquin Injection should not be co-administered with any solution containing multivalent cations, such as magnesium, through the same intravenous line).

LEVAQUIN ORAL SOLUTION
(Levofloxacin) 2629
May interact with antacids containing aluminum, calcium and magnesium, cations, class 1A antiarrhythmics, class III antiarrhythmics, corticosteroids, drugs that prolong the QT interval, insulin, iron containing oral preparations, non-steroidal anti-inflammatory agents, oral hypoglycemic agents, quinidine, theophyllines, and certain other agents. Compounds in these categories include:

Acarbose (Disturbances of blood glucose, including symptomatic hyper- and

hypoglycemia, have been reported with levofloxacin, usually in diabetic patients receiving concomitant treatment with an oral hypoglycemic agent (eg, glyburide). In these patients, careful monitoring of blood glucose is recommended. If a hypoglycemic reaction occurs in a patient being treated with levofloxacin, levofloxacin, should be discontinued and appropriate therapy should be initiated immediately).

No products indexed under this heading.

Alclometasone Dipropionate (Fluoroquinolones, including levofloxacin, are associated with an increased risk of tendinitis and tendon rupture in all ages. This risk is further increased in patients taking corticosteroid drugs).

No products indexed under this heading.

Alprazolam (Prolongation of the QT interval and isolated cases of torsade de pointes have been reported due to levofloxacin. Levofloxacin should be avoided with other drugs that prolong the QT interval. Levofloxacin should be avoided in patients with known prolongation of the QT interval, patients with uncorrected hypokalemia, and patients receiving Class IA (quinidine, procainamide), or Class III (amiodarone, sotalol) antiarrhythmic agents. Elderly patients may be more susceptible to drug-associated effects on the QT interval).

No products indexed under this heading.

Aluminum Acetate (Concurrent administration of levofloxacin tablets/oral solution with metal cations such as iron may interfere with the gastrointestinal absorption of levofloxacin, resulting in systemic levels considerably lower than desired. These agents should be taken at least two hours before or two hours after levofloxacin administration).

No products indexed under this heading.

Aluminum Carbonate (Concurrent administration of levofloxacin tablets/oral solution with antacids containing magnesium, or aluminum may interfere with the gastrointestinal absorption of levofloxacin, resulting in systemic levels considerably lower than desired. These agents should be taken at least two hours before or two hours after levofloxacin administration).

No products indexed under this heading.

Aluminum Chlorhydroxide (Concurrent administration of levofloxacin tablets/oral solution with metal cations such as iron may interfere with the gastrointestinal absorption of levofloxacin, resulting in systemic levels considerably lower than desired. These agents should be taken at least two hours before or two hours after levofloxacin administration).

No products indexed under this heading.

Aluminum Chloride (Concurrent administration of levofloxacin tablets/oral solution with metal cations such as iron may interfere with the gastrointestinal absorption of levofloxacin, resulting in systemic levels considerably lower than desired. These agents should be taken at least two hours before or two hours after levofloxacin administration).

No products indexed under this heading.

Aluminum Chlorohydrate (Concurrent administration of levofloxacin tablets/oral solution with metal cations such as iron may interfere with the gastrointestinal absorption of levofloxacin, resulting in systemic levels considerably lower than desired. These agents should be taken at least two hours before or two hours after levofloxacin administration).

No products indexed under this heading.

Aluminum Glycinate (Concurrent administration of levofloxacin tablets/oral solution with metal cations such as iron may interfere with the gastrointestinal absorption of levofloxacin, resulting in systemic levels considerably lower than desired. These agents should be taken at least two hours before or two hours after levofloxacin administration).

No products indexed under this heading.

Aluminum Hydroxide (Concurrent administration of levofloxacin tablets/oral solution with antacids containing magnesium, or aluminum may interfere with the gastrointestinal absorption of levofloxacin, resulting in systemic levels considerably lower than desired. These agents should be taken at least two hours before or two hours after levofloxacin administration).

No products indexed under this heading.

Aluminum Hydroxide Preparations (Concurrent administration of levofloxacin tablets/oral solution with metal cations such as iron may interfere with the gastrointestinal absorption of levofloxacin, resulting in systemic levels considerably lower than desired. These agents should be taken at least two hours before or two hours after levofloxacin administration).

No products indexed under this heading.

Aluminum Sulfate (Concurrent administration of levofloxacin tablets/oral solution with metal cations such as iron may interfere with the gastrointestinal absorption of levofloxacin, resulting in systemic levels considerably lower than desired. These agents should be taken at least two hours before or two hours after levofloxacin administration).

No products indexed under this heading.

Amiodarone Hydrochloride (Levofloxacin should be avoided in patients with known prolongation of the QT interval, patients with uncorrected hypokalemia, and patients receiving Class III (eg, amiodarone) antiarrhythmic agents. Elderly patients may be more susceptible to drug-associated effects on the QT interval).

No products indexed under this heading.

Amitriptyline Hydrochloride (Prolongation of the QT interval and isolated cases of torsade de pointes have been reported due to levofloxacin. Levofloxacin should be avoided with other drugs that prolong the QT interval. Levofloxacin should be avoided in patients with known prolongation of the QT interval, patients with uncorrected hypokalemia, and patients receiving Class IA (quinidine, procainamide), or Class III (amiodarone, sotalol) antiarrhythmic agents. Elderly patients may be more susceptible to drug-associated effects on the QT interval).

No products indexed under this heading.

Amoxapine (Prolongation of the QT interval and isolated cases of torsade de pointes have been reported due to levofloxacin. Levofloxacin should be avoided with other drugs that prolong the QT interval. Levofloxacin should be avoided in patients with known prolongation of the QT interval, patients with uncorrected hypokalemia, and patients receiving Class IA (quinidine, procainamide), or Class III (amiodarone, sotalol) antiarrhythmic agents. Elderly patients may be more susceptible to drug-associated effects on the QT interval).

No products indexed under this heading.

Astemizole (Prolongation of the QT interval and isolated cases of torsade de pointes have been reported due to levofloxacin. Levofloxacin should be avoided with other drugs that prolong the QT interval. Levofloxacin should be avoided in patients with known prolongation of the QT interval, patients with uncorrected hypokalemia, and patients

receiving Class IA (quinidine, procainamide), or Class III (amiodarone, sotalol) antiarrhythmic agents. Elderly patients may be more susceptible to drug-associated effects on the QT interval).

No products indexed under this heading.

Beclomethasone Dipropionate (Fluoroquinolones, including levofloxacin, are associated with an increased risk of tendinitis and tendon rupture in all ages. This risk is further increased in patients taking corticosteroid drugs). Products include:

Qvar 3398

Beclomethasone Dipropionate Monohydrate (Fluoroquinolones, including levofloxacin, are associated with an increased risk of tendinitis and tendon rupture in all ages. This risk is further increased in patients taking corticosteroid drugs). Products include:

Beconase AQ 1386

Betamethasone (Fluoroquinolones, including levofloxacin, are associated with an increased risk of tendinitis and tendon rupture in all ages. This risk is further increased in patients taking corticosteroid drugs).

No products indexed under this heading.

Betamethasone Acetate (Fluoroquinolones, including levofloxacin, are associated with an increased risk of tendinitis and tendon rupture in all ages. This risk is further increased in patients taking corticosteroid drugs).

No products indexed under this heading.

Betamethasone Benzoate (Fluoroquinolones, including levofloxacin, are associated with an increased risk of tendinitis and tendon rupture in all ages. This risk is further increased in patients taking corticosteroid drugs).

No products indexed under this heading.

Betamethasone Dipropionate (Fluoroquinolones, including levofloxacin, are associated with an increased risk of tendinitis and tendon rupture in all ages. This risk is further increased in patients taking corticosteroid drugs). Products include:

Diprolene Lotion 0.05% 3108
Diprolene Ointment 0.05% 3109
Diprolene AF Cream 0.05% 3107
Lotrisone 3163

Betamethasone Sodium Phosphate (Fluoroquinolones, including levofloxacin, are associated with an increased risk of tendinitis and tendon rupture in all ages. This risk is further increased in patients taking corticosteroid drugs).

No products indexed under this heading.

Betamethasone Valerate (Fluoroquinolones, including levofloxacin, are associated with an increased risk of tendinitis and tendon rupture in all ages. This risk is further increased in patients taking corticosteroid drugs). Products include:

Luxiq 3321

Bretylium Tosylate (Levofloxacin should be avoided in patients with known prolongation of the QT interval, patients with uncorrected hypokalemia, and patients receiving Class III (amiodarone, sotalol) antiarrhythmic agents. Elderly patients may be more susceptible to drug-associated effects on the QT interval).

No products indexed under this heading.

Budesonide (Fluoroquinolones, including levofloxacin, are associated with an increased risk of tendinitis and tendon rupture in all ages. This risk is further increased in patients taking corticosteroid drugs). Products include:

Pulmicort Flexhaler 714
Symbicort 80/4.5 720
Symbicort 160/4.5 720

Buspirone Hydrochloride (Prolongation of the QT interval and isolated

cases of torsade de pointes have been reported due to levofloxacin. Levofloxacin should be avoided with other drugs that prolong the QT interval. Levofloxacin should be avoided in patients with known prolongation of the QT interval, patients with uncorrected hypokalemia, and patients receiving Class IA (quinidine, procainamide), or Class III (amiodarone, sotalol) antiarrhythmic agents. Elderly patients may be more susceptible to drug-associated effects on the QT interval).

No products indexed under this heading.

Calcium (Concurrent administration of levofloxacin tablets/oral solution with metal cations such as iron may interfere with the gastrointestinal absorption of levofloxacin, resulting in systemic levels considerably lower than desired. These agents should be taken at least two hours before or two hours after levofloxacin administration). Products include:

BoneMate Plus 3454
Cardio Basics 3455
Chelated Mineral 3476
CitraNatal 90 DHA Capsules 2332
CitraNatal Harmony 2332

Calcium (Oyster Shell) (Concurrent administration of levofloxacin tablets/oral solution with metal cations such as iron may interfere with the gastrointestinal absorption of levofloxacin, resulting in systemic levels considerably lower than desired. These agents should be taken at least two hours before or two hours after levofloxacin administration).

No products indexed under this heading.

Calcium Acetate (Concurrent administration of levofloxacin tablets/oral solution with metal cations such as iron may interfere with the gastrointestinal absorption of levofloxacin, resulting in systemic levels considerably lower than desired. These agents should be taken at least two hours before or two hours after levofloxacin administration).

No products indexed under this heading.

Calcium Ascorbate (Concurrent administration of levofloxacin tablets/oral solution with metal cations such as iron may interfere with the gastrointestinal absorption of levofloxacin, resulting in systemic levels considerably lower than desired. These agents should be taken at least two hours before or two hours after levofloxacin administration). Products include:

Bio-C 3454
Procosa II 3476
Proflavanol 90 3476

Calcium Carbaspirin (Concurrent administration of levofloxacin tablets/oral solution with metal cations such as iron may interfere with the gastrointestinal absorption of levofloxacin, resulting in systemic levels considerably lower than desired. These agents should be taken at least two hours before or two hours after levofloxacin administration).

No products indexed under this heading.

Calcium Carbonate (Concurrent administration of levofloxacin tablets/oral solution with antacids containing magnesium, or aluminum may interfere with the gastrointestinal absorption of levofloxacin, resulting in systemic levels considerably lower than desired. These agents should be taken at least two hours before or two hours after levofloxacin administration). Products include:

Chelated Mineral 3476
Pepcid Complete 1822
Extra Strength Rolaids Softchews
Vanilla Creme 2045

IMPORTANT NOTE: Always consult each drug listing in the patient's regimen for possible interactions.

Calcium Carbonate, Precipitated (Concurrent administration of levofloxacin tablets/oral solution with metal cations such as iron may interfere with the gastrointestinal absorption of levofloxacin, resulting in systemic levels considerably lower than desired. These agents should be taken at least two hours before or two hours after levofloxacin administration).
No products indexed under this heading.

Calcium Caseinate (Concurrent administration of levofloxacin tablets/oral solution with metal cations such as iron may interfere with the gastrointestinal absorption of levofloxacin, resulting in systemic levels considerably lower than desired. These agents should be taken at least two hours before or two hours after levofloxacin administration).
No products indexed under this heading.

Calcium Chloride (Concurrent administration of levofloxacin tablets/oral solution with metal cations such as iron may interfere with the gastrointestinal absorption of levofloxacin, resulting in systemic levels considerably lower than desired. These agents should be taken at least two hours before or two hours after levofloxacin administration).
No products indexed under this heading.

Calcium Citrate (Concurrent administration of levofloxacin tablets/oral solution with metal cations such as iron may interfere with the gastrointestinal absorption of levofloxacin, resulting in systemic levels considerably lower than desired. These agents should be taken at least two hours before or two hours after levofloxacin administration).
Products include:
Active Calcium 3476
Chelated Mineral 3476
CitraNatal 90 DHA Capsules 2332
CitraNatal Assure 2332
CitraNatal Harmony 2332
CitraNatal Rx 2332

Calcium Disodium Edetate (Concurrent administration of levofloxacin tablets/oral solution with metal cations such as iron may interfere with the gastrointestinal absorption of levofloxacin, resulting in systemic levels considerably lower than desired. These agents should be taken at least two hours before or two hours after levofloxacin administration).
No products indexed under this heading.

Calcium Glubionate (Concurrent administration of levofloxacin tablets/oral solution with metal cations such as iron may interfere with the gastrointestinal absorption of levofloxacin, resulting in systemic levels considerably lower than desired. These agents should be taken at least two hours before or two hours after levofloxacin administration).
No products indexed under this heading.

Calcium Gluconate (Concurrent administration of levofloxacin tablets/oral solution with metal cations such as iron may interfere with the gastrointestinal absorption of levofloxacin, resulting in systemic levels considerably lower than desired. These agents should be taken at least two hours before or two hours after levofloxacin administration).
No products indexed under this heading.

Calcium Glycerophosphate (Concurrent administration of levofloxacin tablets/oral solution with metal cations such as iron may interfere with the gastrointestinal absorption of levofloxacin, resulting in systemic levels considerably lower than desired. These agents should be taken at least two hours before or two hours after levofloxacin administration).
No products indexed under this heading.

Calcium Iodide (Concurrent administration of levofloxacin tablets/oral solution with metal cations such as iron may interfere with the gastrointestinal absorption of levofloxacin, resulting in systemic levels considerably lower than desired. These agents should be taken at least two hours before or two hours after levofloxacin administration).
No products indexed under this heading.

Calcium Lactate (Concurrent administration of levofloxacin tablets/oral solution with metal cations such as iron may interfere with the gastrointestinal absorption of levofloxacin, resulting in systemic levels considerably lower than desired. These agents should be taken at least two hours before or two hours after levofloxacin administration).
No products indexed under this heading.

Calcium Levulinate (Concurrent administration of levofloxacin tablets/oral solution with metal cations such as iron may interfere with the gastrointestinal absorption of levofloxacin, resulting in systemic levels considerably lower than desired. These agents should be taken at least two hours before or two hours after levofloxacin administration).
No products indexed under this heading.

Calcium Pantothenate (Concurrent administration of levofloxacin tablets/oral solution with metal cations such as iron may interfere with the gastrointestinal absorption of levofloxacin, resulting in systemic levels considerably lower than desired. These agents should be taken at least two hours before or two hours after levofloxacin administration).
Products include:
Cardio Basics 3455

Calcium Phosphate (Concurrent administration of levofloxacin tablets/oral solution with metal cations such as iron may interfere with the gastrointestinal absorption of levofloxacin, resulting in systemic levels considerably lower than desired. These agents should be taken at least two hours before or two hours after levofloxacin administration).
No products indexed under this heading.

Calcium Phosphate, Dibasic (Concurrent administration of levofloxacin tablets/oral solution with metal cations such as iron may interfere with the gastrointestinal absorption of levofloxacin, resulting in systemic levels considerably lower than desired. These agents should be taken at least two hours before or two hours after levofloxacin administration).
No products indexed under this heading.

Calcium Phosphate, Tribasic (Concurrent administration of levofloxacin tablets/oral solution with metal cations such as iron may interfere with the gastrointestinal absorption of levofloxacin, resulting in systemic levels considerably lower than desired. These agents should be taken at least two hours before or two hours after levofloxacin administration).
No products indexed under this heading.

Calcium Phosphorus Preparations (Concurrent administration of levofloxacin tablets/oral solution with metal cations such as iron may interfere with the gastrointestinal absorption of levofloxacin, resulting in systemic levels considerably lower than desired. These agents should be taken at least two hours before or two hours after levofloxacin administration).
No products indexed under this heading.

Calcium Polycarbophil (Concurrent administration of levofloxacin tablets/oral solution with metal cations such as iron may interfere with the gastrointestinal absorption of levofloxacin, resulting in systemic levels considerably lower than desired. These agents should be taken at least two hours before or two hours after levofloxacin administration).
No products indexed under this heading.

Calcium Salts (Concurrent administration of levofloxacin tablets/oral solution with metal cations such as iron may interfere with the gastrointestinal absorption of levofloxacin, resulting in systemic levels considerably lower than desired. These agents should be taken at least two hours before or two hours after levofloxacin administration).
No products indexed under this heading.

Calcium Sodium Alginate Fiber (Concurrent administration of levofloxacin tablets/oral solution with metal cations such as iron may interfere with the gastrointestinal absorption of levofloxacin, resulting in systemic levels considerably lower than desired. These agents should be taken at least two hours before or two hours after levofloxacin administration).
No products indexed under this heading.

Calcium Undecylenate (Concurrent administration of levofloxacin tablets/oral solution with metal cations such as iron may interfere with the gastrointestinal absorption of levofloxacin, resulting in systemic levels considerably lower than desired. These agents should be taken at least two hours before or two hours after levofloxacin administration).
No products indexed under this heading.

Celecoxib (Concomitant administration of a non-steroidal anti-inflammatory drug with a fluoroquinolone, including levofloxacin, may increase the risk of CNS stimulation and convulsive seizures). Products include:
Celebrex 3272

Chlordiazepoxide (Prolongation of the QT interval and isolated cases of torsade de pointes have been reported due to levofloxacin. Levofloxacin should be avoided with other drugs that prolong the QT interval. Levofloxacin should be avoided in patients with known prolongation of the QT interval, patients with uncorrected hypokalemia, and patients receiving Class IA (quinidine, procainamide), or Class III (amiodarone, sotalol) antiarrhythmic agents. Elderly patients may be more susceptible to drug-associated effects on the QT interval).
No products indexed under this heading.

Chlordiazepoxide Hydrochloride (Prolongation of the QT interval and isolated cases of torsade de pointes have been reported due to levofloxacin. Levofloxacin should be avoided with other drugs that prolong the QT interval. Levofloxacin should be avoided in patients with known prolongation of the QT interval, patients with uncorrected hypokalemia, and patients receiving Class IA (quinidine, procainamide), or Class III (amiodarone, sotalol) antiarrhythmic agents. Elderly patients may be more susceptible to drug-associated effects on the QT interval).
No products indexed under this heading.

Chlorpromazine (Prolongation of the QT interval and isolated cases of torsade de pointes have been reported due to levofloxacin. Levofloxacin should be avoided with other drugs that prolong the QT interval. Levofloxacin should be avoided in patients with known prolongation of the QT interval, patients with uncorrected hypokalemia, and patients receiving Class IA (quinidine, procainamide), or Class III (amiodarone, sotalol) antiarrhythmic agents. Elderly patients may be more susceptible to drug-associated effects on the QT interval).
No products indexed under this heading.

Chlorpromazine Hydrochloride (Prolongation of the QT interval and isolated cases of torsade de pointes have been reported due to levofloxacin. Levofloxacin should be avoided with other drugs that prolong the QT interval. Levofloxacin should be avoided in patients with known prolongation of the QT interval, patients with uncorrected hypokalemia, and patients receiving Class IA (quinidine, procainamide), or Class III (amiodarone, sotalol) antiarrhythmic agents. Elderly patients may be more susceptible to drug-associated effects on the QT interval).
No products indexed under this heading.

Chlorpropamide (Disturbances of blood glucose, including symptomatic hyper- and hypoglycemia, have been reported with levofloxacin, usually in diabetic patients receiving concomitant treatment with an oral hypoglycemic agent (eg, glyburide). In these patients, careful monitoring of blood glucose is recommended. If a hypoglycemic reaction occurs in a patient being treated with levofloxacin, levofloxacin, should be discontinued and appropriate therapy should be initiated immediately).
No products indexed under this heading.

Chlorprothixene (Prolongation of the QT interval and isolated cases of torsade de pointes have been reported due to levofloxacin. Levofloxacin should be avoided with other drugs that prolong the QT interval. Levofloxacin should be avoided in patients with known prolongation of the QT interval, patients with uncorrected hypokalemia, and patients receiving Class IA (quinidine, procainamide), or Class III (amiodarone, sotalol) antiarrhythmic agents. Elderly patients may be more susceptible to drug-associated effects on the QT interval).
No products indexed under this heading.

Chlorprothixene Hydrochloride (Prolongation of the QT interval and isolated cases of torsade de pointes have been reported due to levofloxacin. Levofloxacin should be avoided with other drugs that prolong the QT interval. Levofloxacin should be avoided in patients with known prolongation of the QT interval, patients with uncorrected hypokalemia, and patients receiving Class IA (quinidine, procainamide), or Class III (amiodarone, sotalol) antiarrhythmic agents. Elderly patients may be more susceptible to drug-associated effects on the QT interval).
No products indexed under this heading.

Ciclesonide (Fluoroquinolones, including levofloxacin, are associated with an increased risk of tendinitis and tendon rupture in all ages. This risk is further increased in patients taking corticosteroid drugs).
No products indexed under this heading.

Cimetidine (The AUC and $t_{1/2}$ of levofloxacin were higher while CL/F and CL_R were lower during concomitant treatment of levofloxacin with cimetidine compared to levofloxacin alone).
No products indexed under this heading.

Cimetidine Hydrochloride (The AUC and $t_{1/2}$ of levofloxacin were higher while CL/F and CL_R were lower during concomitant treatment of levofloxacin with cimetidine compared to levofloxacin alone).
No products indexed under this heading.

Clomipramine Hydrochloride (Prolongation of the QT interval and isolated cases of torsade de pointes have been reported due to levofloxacin. Levofloxacin should be avoided with other drugs that prolong the QT interval. Levofloxa-

cin should be avoided in patients with known prolongation of the QT interval, patients with uncorrected hypokalemia, and patients receiving Class IA (quinidine, procainamide), or Class III (amiodarone, sotalol) antiarrhythmic agents. Elderly patients may be more susceptible to drug-associated effects on the QT interval).

No products indexed under this heading.

Clorazepate Dipotassium (Prolongation of the QT interval and isolated cases of torsade de pointes have been reported due to levofloxacin. Levofloxacin should be avoided with other drugs that prolong the QT interval. Levofloxacin should be avoided in patients with known prolongation of the QT interval, patients with uncorrected hypokalemia, and patients receiving Class IA (quinidine, procainamide), or Class III (amiodarone, sotalol) antiarrhythmic agents. Elderly patients may be more susceptible to drug-associated effects on the QT interval).

No products indexed under this heading.

Clozapine (Prolongation of the QT interval and isolated cases of torsade de pointes have been reported due to levofloxacin. Levofloxacin should be avoided with other drugs that prolong the QT interval. Levofloxacin should be avoided in patients with known prolongation of the QT interval, patients with uncorrected hypokalemia, and patients receiving Class IA (quinidine, procainamide), or Class III (amiodarone, sotalol) antiarrhythmic agents. Elderly patients may be more susceptible to drug-associated effects on the QT interval).

No products indexed under this heading.

Cortisone Acetate (Fluoroquinolones, including levofloxacin, are associated with an increased risk of tendinitis and tendon rupture in all ages. This risk is further increased in patients taking corticosteroid drugs).

No products indexed under this heading.

Cyclosporine (Elevated serum levels of cyclosporine have been reported in the patient population when co-administered with some other fluoroquinolones. Levofloxacin C_{max} and k_e were slightly lower while T_{max} and $t_{1/2}$ were slightly longer in the presence of cyclosporine than those observed in other studies without concomitant medication). Products include:

Desipramine Hydrochloride (Prolongation of the QT interval and isolated cases of torsade de pointes have been reported due to levofloxacin. Levofloxacin should be avoided with other drugs that prolong the QT interval. Levofloxacin should be avoided in patients with known prolongation of the QT interval, patients with uncorrected hypokalemia, and patients receiving Class IA (quinidine, procainamide), or Class III (amiodarone, sotalol) antiarrhythmic agents. Elderly patients may be more susceptible to drug-associated effects on the QT interval).

No products indexed under this heading.

Desoximetasone (Fluoroquinolones, including levofloxacin, are associated with an increased risk of tendinitis and tendon rupture in all ages. This risk is further increased in patients taking corticosteroid drugs).

No products indexed under this heading.

Dexamethasone (Fluoroquinolones, including levofloxacin, are associated with an increased risk of tendinitis and tendon rupture in all ages. This risk is further increased in patients taking corticosteroid drugs). Products include:

Dexamethasone Acetate (Fluoroquinolones, including levofloxacin, are associated with an increased risk of tendinitis and tendon rupture in all ages. This risk is further increased in patients taking corticosteroid drugs).

No products indexed under this heading.

Dexamethasone Phosphate (Fluoroquinolones, including levofloxacin, are associated with an increased risk of tendinitis and tendon rupture in all ages. This risk is further increased in patients taking corticosteroid drugs).

No products indexed under this heading.

Dexamethasone Sodium (Fluoroquinolones, including levofloxacin, are associated with an increased risk of tendinitis and tendon rupture in all ages. This risk is further increased in patients taking corticosteroid drugs).

No products indexed under this heading.

Dexamethasone Sodium Phosphate (Fluoroquinolones, including levofloxacin, are associated with an increased risk of tendinitis and tendon rupture in all ages. This risk is further increased in patients taking corticosteroid drugs).

No products indexed under this heading.

Dexamethasone Sodium Phosphate Injection (Fluoroquinolones, including levofloxacin, are associated with an increased risk of tendinitis and tendon rupture in all ages. This risk is further increased in patients taking corticosteroid drugs).

No products indexed under this heading.

Diazepam (Prolongation of the QT interval and isolated cases of torsade de pointes have been reported due to levofloxacin. Levofloxacin should be avoided with other drugs that prolong the QT interval. Levofloxacin should be avoided in patients with known prolongation of the QT interval, patients with uncorrected hypokalemia, and patients receiving Class IA (quinidine, procainamide), or Class III (amiodarone, sotalol) antiarrhythmic agents. Elderly patients may be more susceptible to drug-associated effects on the QT interval). Products include:

Diclofenac Epolamine (Concomitant administration of a non-steroidal anti-inflammatory drug with a fluoroquinolone, including levofloxacin, may increase the risk of CNS stimulation and convulsive seizures). Products include:

Diclofenac Potassium (Concomitant administration of a non-steroidal anti-inflammatory drug with a fluoroquinolone, including levofloxacin, may increase the risk of CNS stimulation and convulsive seizures).

No products indexed under this heading.

Diclofenac Sodium (Concomitant administration of a non-steroidal anti-inflammatory drug with a fluoroquinolone, including levofloxacin, may increase the risk of CNS stimulation and convulsive seizures).

No products indexed under this heading.

Didanosine (Didanosine may substantially interfere with the gastrointestinal absorption of levofloxacin tablets/oral solution, resulting in systemic levels considerably lower than desired. Didanosine should be taken at least two hours before or two hours after levofloxacin administration).

No products indexed under this heading.

Diflorasone Diacetate (Fluoroquinolones, including levofloxacin, are associated with an increased risk of tendinitis and tendon rupture in all ages. This risk is further increased in patients taking corticosteroid drugs).

No products indexed under this heading.

Disopyramide (Levofloxacin should be avoided in patients with known prolongation of the QT interval, patients with uncorrected hypokalemia, and patients receiving Class IA (quinidine, procainamide) antiarrhythmic agents. Elderly patients may be more susceptible to drug-associated effects on the QT interval).

No products indexed under this heading.

Disopyramide Phosphate (Levofloxacin should be avoided in patients with known prolongation of the QT interval, patients with uncorrected hypokalemia, and patients receiving Class IA (quinidine, procainamide) antiarrhythmic agents. Elderly patients may be more susceptible to drug-associated effects on the QT interval).

No products indexed under this heading.

Dofetilide (Prolongation of the QT interval and isolated cases of torsade de pointes have been reported due to levofloxacin. Levofloxacin should be avoided with other drugs that prolong the QT interval. Levofloxacin should be avoided in patients with known prolongation of the QT interval, patients with uncorrected hypokalemia, and patients receiving Class IA (quinidine, procainamide), or Class III (amiodarone, sotalol) antiarrhythmic agents. Elderly patients may be more susceptible to drug-associated effects on the QT interval).

No products indexed under this heading.

Doxepin Hydrochloride (Prolongation of the QT interval and isolated cases of torsade de pointes have been reported due to levofloxacin. Levofloxacin should be avoided with other drugs that prolong the QT interval. Levofloxacin should be avoided in patients with known prolongation of the QT interval, patients with uncorrected hypokalemia, and patients receiving Class IA (quinidine, procainamide), or Class III (amiodarone, sotalol) antiarrhythmic agents. Elderly patients may be more susceptible to drug-associated effects on the QT interval).

No products indexed under this heading.

Droperidol (Prolongation of the QT interval and isolated cases of torsade de pointes have been reported due to levofloxacin. Levofloxacin should be avoided with other drugs that prolong the QT interval. Levofloxacin should be avoided in patients with known prolongation of the QT interval, patients with uncorrected hypokalemia, and patients receiving Class IA (quinidine, procainamide), or Class III (amiodarone, sotalol) antiarrhythmic agents. Elderly patients may be more susceptible to drug-associated effects on the QT interval).

No products indexed under this heading.

Erythromycin (Prolongation of the QT interval and isolated cases of torsade de pointes have been reported due to levofloxacin. Levofloxacin should be avoided with other drugs that prolong the QT interval. Levofloxacin should be avoided in patients with known prolongation of the QT interval, patients with uncorrected hypokalemia, and patients receiving Class IA (quinidine, procainamide), or Class III (amiodarone, sotalol) antiarrhythmic agents. Elderly patients may be more susceptible to drug-associated effects on the QT interval).

No products indexed under this heading.

Erythromycin Estolate (Prolongation of the QT interval and isolated cases of torsade de pointes have been reported due to levofloxacin. Levofloxacin should

be avoided with other drugs that prolong the QT interval. Levofloxacin should be avoided in patients with known prolongation of the QT interval, patients with uncorrected hypokalemia, and patients receiving Class IA (quinidine, procainamide), or Class III (amiodarone, sotalol) antiarrhythmic agents. Elderly patients may be more susceptible to drug-associated effects on the QT interval).

No products indexed under this heading.

Erythromycin Ethylsuccinate (Prolongation of the QT interval and isolated cases of torsade de pointes have been reported due to levofloxacin. Levofloxacin should be avoided with other drugs that prolong the QT interval. Levofloxacin should be avoided in patients with known prolongation of the QT interval, patients with uncorrected hypokalemia, and patients receiving Class IA (quinidine, procainamide), or Class III (amiodarone, sotalol) antiarrhythmic agents. Elderly patients may be more susceptible to drug-associated effects on the QT interval). Products include:

Erythromycin Gluceptate (Prolongation of the QT interval and isolated cases of torsade de pointes have been reported due to levofloxacin. Levofloxacin should be avoided with other drugs that prolong the QT interval. Levofloxacin should be avoided in patients with known prolongation of the QT interval, patients with uncorrected hypokalemia, and patients receiving Class IA (quinidine, procainamide), or Class III (amiodarone, sotalol) antiarrhythmic agents. Elderly patients may be more susceptible to drug-associated effects on the QT interval).

No products indexed under this heading.

Erythromycin Lactobionate (Prolongation of the QT interval and isolated cases of torsade de pointes have been reported due to levofloxacin. Levofloxacin should be avoided with other drugs that prolong the QT interval. Levofloxacin should be avoided in patients with known prolongation of the QT interval, patients with uncorrected hypokalemia, and patients receiving Class IA (quinidine, procainamide), or Class III (amiodarone, sotalol) antiarrhythmic agents. Elderly patients may be more susceptible to drug-associated effects on the QT interval).

No products indexed under this heading.

Erythromycin Stearate (Prolongation of the QT interval and isolated cases of torsade de pointes have been reported due to levofloxacin. Levofloxacin should be avoided with other drugs that prolong the QT interval. Levofloxacin should be avoided in patients with known prolongation of the QT interval, patients with uncorrected hypokalemia, and patients receiving Class IA (quinidine, procainamide), or Class III (amiodarone, sotalol) antiarrhythmic agents. Elderly patients may be more susceptible to drug-associated effects on the QT interval).

No products indexed under this heading.

Etodolac (Concomitant administration of a non-steroidal anti-inflammatory drug with a fluoroquinolone, including levofloxacin, may increase the risk of CNS stimulation and convulsive seizures).

No products indexed under this heading.

Fenoprofen Calcium (Concomitant administration of a non-steroidal anti-inflammatory drug with a fluoroquinolone, including levofloxacin, may increase the risk of CNS stimulation and convulsive seizures).

No products indexed under this heading.

Ferrous Fumarate (Concurrent administration of levofloxacin tablets/

oral solution with metal cations such as iron may interfere with the gastrointestinal absorption of levofloxacin, resulting in systemic levels considerably lower than desired. These agents should be taken at least two hours before or two hours after levofloxacin administration). Products include:
PreNexa 3473

Ferrous Gluconate (Concurrent administration of levofloxacin tablets/oral solution with metal cations such as iron may interfere with the gastrointestinal absorption of levofloxacin, resulting in systemic levels considerably lower than desired. These agents should be taken at least two hours before or two hours after levofloxacin administration). Products include:
CitraNatal Assure 2332
CitraNatal Rx 2332

Ferrous Sulfate (Concurrent administration of levofloxacin tablets/oral solution with metal cations such as iron may interfere with the gastrointestinal absorption of levofloxacin, resulting in systemic levels considerably lower than desired. These agents should be taken at least two hours before or two hours after levofloxacin administration).
No products indexed under this heading.

Flecainide Acetate (Prolongation of the QT interval and isolated cases of torsade de pointes have been reported due to levofloxacin. Levofloxacin should be avoided with other drugs that prolong the QT interval. Levofloxacin should be avoided in patients with known prolongation of the QT interval, patients with uncorrected hypokalemia, and patients receiving Class IA (quinidine, procainamide), or Class III (amiodarone, sotalol) antiarrhythmic agents. Elderly patients may be more susceptible to drug-associated effects on the QT interval).
No products indexed under this heading.

Fludrocortisone Acetate (Fluoroquinolones, including levofloxacin, are associated with an increased risk of tendinitis and tendon rupture in all ages. This risk is further increased in patients taking corticosteroid drugs).
No products indexed under this heading.

Flumethasone Pivalate (Fluoroquinolones, including levofloxacin, are associated with an increased risk of tendinitis and tendon rupture in all ages. This risk is further increased in patients taking corticosteroid drugs).
No products indexed under this heading.

Flunisolide Hemihydrate (Fluoroquinolones, including levofloxacin, are associated with an increased risk of tendinitis and tendon rupture in all ages. This risk is further increased in patients taking corticosteroid drugs).
No products indexed under this heading.

Fluphenazine Decanoate (Prolongation of the QT interval and isolated cases of torsade de pointes have been reported due to levofloxacin. Levofloxacin should be avoided with other drugs that prolong the QT interval. Levofloxacin should be avoided in patients with known prolongation of the QT interval, patients with uncorrected hypokalemia, and patients receiving Class IA (quinidine, procainamide), or Class III (amiodarone, sotalol) antiarrhythmic agents. Elderly patients may be more susceptible to drug-associated effects on the QT interval).
No products indexed under this heading.

Fluphenazine Enanthate (Prolongation of the QT interval and isolated cases of torsade de pointes have been reported due to levofloxacin. Levofloxacin should be avoided with other drugs that prolong the QT interval. Levofloxacin should be avoided in patients with known prolongation of the QT interval, patients with uncorrected hypokalemia, and patients receiving Class IA (quinidine, procainamide), or Class III (amiodarone, sotalol) antiarrhythmic agents. Elderly patients may be more susceptible to drug-associated effects on the QT interval).
No products indexed under this heading.

Fluphenazine Hydrochloride (Prolongation of the QT interval and isolated cases of torsade de pointes have been reported due to levofloxacin. Levofloxacin should be avoided with other drugs that prolong the QT interval. Levofloxacin should be avoided in patients with known prolongation of the QT interval, patients with uncorrected hypokalemia, and patients receiving Class IA (quinidine, procainamide), or Class III (amiodarone, sotalol) antiarrhythmic agents. Elderly patients may be more susceptible to drug-associated effects on the QT interval).
No products indexed under this heading.

Flurbiprofen (Concomitant administration of a non-steroidal anti-inflammatory drug with a fluoroquinolone, including levofloxacin, may increase the risk of CNS stimulation and convulsive seizures).
No products indexed under this heading.

Fluticasone Furoate (Fluoroquinolones, including levofloxacin, are associated with an increased risk of tendinitis and tendon rupture in all ages. This risk is further increased in patients taking corticosteroid drugs). Products include:
Veramyst 1713

Fluticasone Propionate (Fluoroquinolones, including levofloxacin, are associated with an increased risk of tendinitis and tendon rupture in all ages. This risk is further increased in patients taking corticosteroid drugs). Products include:
Advair 100/50 1275
Advair 250/50 1275
Advair 500/50 1275
Advair HFA 45/21 1288
Advair HFA 115/21 1288
Advair HFA 230/21 1288
Flonase 1459
Flovent Diskus 1463
Flovent HFA 1470

Glibenclamide (Disturbances of blood glucose, including symptomatic hyper- and hypoglycemia, have been reported with levofloxacin, usually in diabetic patients receiving concomitant treatment with an oral hypoglycemic agent (eg, glyburide). In these patients, careful monitoring of blood glucose is recommended. If a hypoglycemic reaction occurs in a patient being treated with levofloxacin, levofloxacin, should be discontinued and appropriate therapy should be initiated immediately).
No products indexed under this heading.

Glimepiride (Disturbances of blood glucose, including symptomatic hyper- and hypoglycemia, have been reported with levofloxacin, usually in diabetic patients receiving concomitant treatment with an oral hypoglycemic agent (eg, glyburide). In these patients, careful monitoring of blood glucose is recommended. If a hypoglycemic reaction occurs in a patient being treated with levofloxacin, levofloxacin, should be discontinued and appropriate therapy should be initiated immediately). Products include:
Avandaryl 1356
Duetact 3354

Glipizide (Disturbances of blood glucose, including symptomatic hyper- and hypoglycemia, have been reported with levofloxacin, usually in diabetic patients receiving concomitant treatment with an oral hypoglycemic agent (eg, glyburide). In these patients, careful monitoring of blood glucose is recommended. If a hypoglycemic reaction occurs in a patient being treated with levofloxacin, levofloxacin, should be discontinued and appropriate therapy should be initiated immediately).
No products indexed under this heading.

Glyburide (Disturbances of blood glucose, including symptomatic hyper- and hypoglycemia, have been reported with levofloxacin, usually in diabetic patients receiving concomitant treatment with an oral hypoglycemic agent (eg, glyburide). In these patients, careful monitoring of blood glucose is recommended. If a hypoglycemic reaction occurs in a patient being treated with levofloxacin, levofloxacin, should be discontinued and appropriate therapy should be initiated immediately).
No products indexed under this heading.

Haloperidol (Prolongation of the QT interval and isolated cases of torsade de pointes have been reported due to levofloxacin. Levofloxacin should be avoided with other drugs that prolong the QT interval. Levofloxacin should be avoided in patients with known prolongation of the QT interval, patients with uncorrected hypokalemia, and patients receiving Class IA (quinidine, procainamide), or Class III (amiodarone, sotalol) antiarrhythmic agents. Elderly patients may be more susceptible to drug-associated effects on the QT interval).
No products indexed under this heading.

Haloperidol Decanoate (Prolongation of the QT interval and isolated cases of torsade de pointes have been reported due to levofloxacin. Levofloxacin should be avoided with other drugs that prolong the QT interval. Levofloxacin should be avoided in patients with known prolongation of the QT interval, patients with uncorrected hypokalemia, and patients receiving Class IA (quinidine, procainamide), or Class III (amiodarone, sotalol) antiarrhythmic agents. Elderly patients may be more susceptible to drug-associated effects on the QT interval).
No products indexed under this heading.

Haloperidol Lactate (Prolongation of the QT interval and isolated cases of torsade de pointes have been reported due to levofloxacin. Levofloxacin should be avoided with other drugs that prolong the QT interval. Levofloxacin should be avoided in patients with known prolongation of the QT interval, patients with uncorrected hypokalemia, and patients receiving Class IA (quinidine, procainamide), or Class III (amiodarone, sotalol) antiarrhythmic agents. Elderly patients may be more susceptible to drug-associated effects on the QT interval).
No products indexed under this heading.

Hydrocortisone (Fluoroquinolones, including levofloxacin, are associated with an increased risk of tendinitis and tendon rupture in all ages. This risk is further increased in patients taking corticosteroid drugs).
No products indexed under this heading.

Hydrocortisone (Alcohol) (Fluoroquinolones, including levofloxacin, are associated with an increased risk of tendinitis and tendon rupture in all ages. This risk is further increased in patients taking corticosteroid drugs).
No products indexed under this heading.

Hydrocortisone Acetate (Fluoroquinolones, including levofloxacin, are associated with an increased risk of tendinitis and tendon rupture in all ages. This risk is further increased in patients taking corticosteroid drugs).
No products indexed under this heading.

Hydrocortisone Butyrate (Fluoroquinolones, including levofloxacin, are associated with an increased risk of tendinitis and tendon rupture in all ages. This risk is further increased in patients taking corticosteroid drugs).
No products indexed under this heading.

Hydrocortisone Cypionate (Fluoroquinolones, including levofloxacin, are associated with an increased risk of tendinitis and tendon rupture in all ages. This risk is further increased in patients taking corticosteroid drugs).
No products indexed under this heading.

Hydrocortisone Hemisuccinate (Fluoroquinolones, including levofloxacin, are associated with an increased risk of tendinitis and tendon rupture in all ages. This risk is further increased in patients taking corticosteroid drugs).
No products indexed under this heading.

Hydrocortisone Probutate (Fluoroquinolones, including levofloxacin, are associated with an increased risk of tendinitis and tendon rupture in all ages. This risk is further increased in patients taking corticosteroid drugs).
No products indexed under this heading.

Hydrocortisone Sodium Phosphate (Fluoroquinolones, including levofloxacin, are associated with an increased risk of tendinitis and tendon rupture in all ages. This risk is further increased in patients taking corticosteroid drugs).
No products indexed under this heading.

Hydrocortisone Sodium Succinate (Fluoroquinolones, including levofloxacin, are associated with an increased risk of tendinitis and tendon rupture in all ages. This risk is further increased in patients taking corticosteroid drugs).
No products indexed under this heading.

Hydrocortisone Valerate (Fluoroquinolones, including levofloxacin, are associated with an increased risk of tendinitis and tendon rupture in all ages. This risk is further increased in patients taking corticosteroid drugs).
No products indexed under this heading.

Hydroxyzine Hydrochloride (Prolongation of the QT interval and isolated cases of torsade de pointes have been reported due to levofloxacin. Levofloxacin should be avoided with other drugs that prolong the QT interval. Levofloxacin should be avoided in patients with known prolongation of the QT interval, patients with uncorrected hypokalemia, and patients receiving Class IA (quinidine, procainamide), or Class III (amiodarone, sotalol) antiarrhythmic agents. Elderly patients may be more susceptible to drug-associated effects on the QT interval).
No products indexed under this heading.

Ibuprofen (Concomitant administration of a non-steroidal anti-inflammatory drug with a fluoroquinolone, including levofloxacin, may increase the risk of CNS stimulation and convulsive seizures). Products include:
Motrin IB 2043
Children's Motrin 2044
Children's Motrin Non-Staining Dye-Free 2044
Infants' Motrin 2044
Infants' Motrin Dye-Free 2044
Junior Strength Motrin 2044
Vicoprofen 564

Imipramine Hydrochloride (Prolongation of the QT interval and isolated cases of torsade de pointes have been reported due to levofloxacin. Levofloxacin should be avoided with other drugs that prolong the QT interval. Levofloxacin should be avoided in patients with known prolongation of the QT interval, patients with uncorrected hypokalemia, and patients receiving Class IA (quinidine, procainamide), or Class III (amio-

991 **Interactions Index** **Levaquin Oral Solution**

darone, sotalol) antiarrhythmic agents. Elderly patients may be more susceptible to drug-associated effects on the QT interval).
No products indexed under this heading.

Imipramine Pamoate (Prolongation of the QT interval and isolated cases of torsade de pointes have been reported due to levofloxacin. Levofloxacin should be avoided with other drugs that prolong the QT interval. Levofloxacin should be avoided in patients with known prolongation of the QT interval, patients with uncorrected hypokalemia, and patients receiving Class IA (quinidine, procainamide), or Class III (amiodarone, sotalol) antiarrhythmic agents. Elderly patients may be more susceptible to drug-associated effects on the QT interval).
No products indexed under this heading.

Indomethacin (Concomitant administration of a non-steroidal anti-inflammatory drug with a fluoroquinolone, including levofloxacin, may increase the risk of CNS stimulation and convulsive seizures). Products include:
Indocin **2167**

Indomethacin Sodium Trihydrate (Concomitant administration of a non-steroidal anti-inflammatory drug with a fluoroquinolone, including levofloxacin, may increase the risk of CNS stimulation and convulsive seizures). Products include:
Indocin I.V. **2007**

Insulin (Disturbances of blood glucose, including symptomatic hyper- and hypoglycemia, have been reported with levofloxacin, usually in diabetic patients receiving concomitant treatment with insulin. In these patients, careful monitoring of blood glucose is recommended. If a hypoglycemic reaction occurs in a patient being treated with levofloxacin, levofloxacin, should be discontinued and appropriate therapy should be initiated immediately).
No products indexed under this heading.

Insulin, Human, Zinc Suspension (Disturbances of blood glucose, including symptomatic hyper- and hypoglycemia, have been reported with levofloxacin, usually in diabetic patients receiving concomitant treatment with insulin. In these patients, careful monitoring of blood glucose is recommended. If a hypoglycemic reaction occurs in a patient being treated with levofloxacin, levofloxacin, should be discontinued and appropriate therapy should be initiated immediately).
No products indexed under this heading.

Insulin, Human (rDNA origin) (Disturbances of blood glucose, including symptomatic hyper- and hypoglycemia, have been reported with levofloxacin, usually in diabetic patients receiving concomitant treatment with insulin. In these patients, careful monitoring of blood glucose is recommended. If a hypoglycemic reaction occurs in a patient being treated with levofloxacin, levofloxacin, should be discontinued and appropriate therapy should be initiated immediately). Products include:
Exubera **2717**

Insulin, Human NPH (Disturbances of blood glucose, including symptomatic hyper- and hypoglycemia, have been reported with levofloxacin, usually in diabetic patients receiving concomitant treatment with insulin. In these patients, careful monitoring of blood glucose is recommended. If a hypoglycemic reaction occurs in a patient being treated with levofloxacin, levofloxacin, should be discontinued and appropriate therapy should be initiated immediately).
Products include:
Humulin N Vial **1934**

Insulin, Human Regular (Disturbances of blood glucose, including symptomatic hyper- and hypoglycemia, have been reported with levofloxacin, usually in diabetic patients receiving concomitant treatment with insulin. In these patients, careful monitoring of blood glucose is recommended. If a hypoglycemic reaction occurs in a patient being treated with levofloxacin, levofloxacin, should be discontinued and appropriate therapy should be initiated immediately). Products include:
Humulin R **1937**
Humulin R (U-500) **1939**

Insulin, Human Regular and Human NPH Mixture (Disturbances of blood glucose, including symptomatic hyper- and hypoglycemia, have been reported with levofloxacin, usually in diabetic patients receiving concomitant treatment with insulin. In these patients, careful monitoring of blood glucose is recommended. If a hypoglycemic reaction occurs in a patient being treated with levofloxacin, levofloxacin, should be discontinued and appropriate therapy should be initiated immediately).
Products include:
Humulin 50/50 .... **1930**
Humulin 70/30 Vial **1931**

Insulin, NPH (Disturbances of blood glucose, including symptomatic hyper- and hypoglycemia, have been reported with levofloxacin, usually in diabetic patients receiving concomitant treatment with insulin. In these patients, careful monitoring of blood glucose is recommended. If a hypoglycemic reaction occurs in a patient being treated with levofloxacin, levofloxacin, should be discontinued and appropriate therapy should be initiated immediately).
No products indexed under this heading.

Insulin, Regular (Disturbances of blood glucose, including symptomatic hyper- and hypoglycemia, have been reported with levofloxacin, usually in diabetic patients receiving concomitant treatment with insulin. In these patients, careful monitoring of blood glucose is recommended. If a hypoglycemic reaction occurs in a patient being treated with levofloxacin, levofloxacin, should be discontinued and appropriate therapy should be initiated immediately).
No products indexed under this heading.

Insulin, Regular and NPH mixture (Disturbances of blood glucose, including symptomatic hyper- and hypoglycemia, have been reported with levofloxacin, usually in diabetic patients receiving concomitant treatment with insulin. In these patients, careful monitoring of blood glucose is recommended. If a hypoglycemic reaction occurs in a patient being treated with levofloxacin, levofloxacin, should be discontinued and appropriate therapy should be initiated immediately).
No products indexed under this heading.

Insulin, Zinc Crystals (Disturbances of blood glucose, including symptomatic hyper- and hypoglycemia, have been reported with levofloxacin, usually in diabetic patients receiving concomitant treatment with insulin. In these patients, careful monitoring of blood glucose is recommended. If a hypoglycemic reaction occurs in a patient being treated with levofloxacin, levofloxacin, should be discontinued and appropriate therapy should be initiated immediately).
No products indexed under this heading.

Insulin, Zinc Suspension (Disturbances of blood glucose, including symptomatic hyper- and hypoglycemia, have been reported with levofloxacin, usually in diabetic patients receiving concomitant treatment with insulin. In these patients, careful monitoring of blood glucose is recommended. If a hypoglycemic reaction occurs in a patient being treated with levofloxacin, levofloxacin, should be discontinued and appropriate therapy should be initiated immediately).
No products indexed under this heading.

Insulin Aspart (Disturbances of blood glucose, including symptomatic hyper- and hypoglycemia, have been reported with levofloxacin, usually in diabetic patients receiving concomitant treatment with insulin. In these patients, careful monitoring of blood glucose is recommended. If a hypoglycemic reaction occurs in a patient being treated with levofloxacin, levofloxacin, should be discontinued and appropriate therapy should be initiated immediately).
No products indexed under this heading.

Insulin Aspart, Human (Disturbances of blood glucose, including symptomatic hyper- and hypoglycemia, have been reported with levofloxacin, usually in diabetic patients receiving concomitant treatment with insulin. In these patients, careful monitoring of blood glucose is recommended. If a hypoglycemic reaction occurs in a patient being treated with levofloxacin, levofloxacin, should be discontinued and appropriate therapy should be initiated immediately).
Products include:
NovoLog Mix 70/30 .... **2581**

Insulin Aspart, Human Regular (Disturbances of blood glucose, including symptomatic hyper- and hypoglycemia, have been reported with levofloxacin, usually in diabetic patients receiving concomitant treatment with insulin. In these patients, careful monitoring of blood glucose is recommended. If a hypoglycemic reaction occurs in a patient being treated with levofloxacin, levofloxacin, should be discontinued and appropriate therapy should be initiated immediately). Products include:
NovoLog **2575**

Insulin Aspart Protamine, Human (Disturbances of blood glucose, including symptomatic hyper- and hypoglycemia, have been reported with levofloxacin, usually in diabetic patients receiving concomitant treatment with insulin. In these patients, careful monitoring of blood glucose is recommended. If a hypoglycemic reaction occurs in a patient being treated with levofloxacin, levofloxacin, should be discontinued and appropriate therapy should be initiated immediately). Products include:
NovoLog Mix 70/30 .... **2581**

Insulin Detemir (rDNA Origin) (Disturbances of blood glucose, including symptomatic hyper- and hypoglycemia, have been reported with levofloxacin, usually in diabetic patients receiving concomitant treatment with insulin. In these patients, careful monitoring of blood glucose is recommended. If a hypoglycemic reaction occurs in a patient being treated with levofloxacin, levofloxacin, should be discontinued and appropriate therapy should be initiated immediately). Products include:
Levemir **2566**

Insulin Glargine (Disturbances of blood glucose, including symptomatic hyper- and hypoglycemia, have been reported with levofloxacin, usually in diabetic patients receiving concomitant treatment with insulin. In these patients, careful monitoring of blood glucose is recommended. If a hypoglycemic reaction occurs in a patient being treated with levofloxacin, levofloxacin, should be discontinued and appropriate therapy should be initiated immediately).
Products include:
Lantus **2996**

Insulin Glulisine (Disturbances of blood glucose, including symptomatic hyper- and hypoglycemia, have been reported with levofloxacin, usually in diabetic patients receiving concomitant treatment with insulin. In these patients, careful monitoring of blood glucose is recommended. If a hypoglycemic reaction occurs in a patient being treated with levofloxacin, levofloxacin, should be discontinued and appropriate therapy should be initiated immediately).
Products include:
Apidra **2937**
Apidra SoloStar **2937**

Insulin Lispro, Human (Disturbances of blood glucose, including symptomatic hyper- and hypoglycemia, have been reported with levofloxacin, usually in diabetic patients receiving concomitant treatment with insulin. In these patients, careful monitoring of blood glucose is recommended. If a hypoglycemic reaction occurs in a patient being treated with levofloxacin, levofloxacin, should be discontinued and appropriate therapy should be initiated immediately).
Products include:
Humalog **1910**
Humalog Mix **1914**
Humalog Mix75/25 .... **1917**

Insulin Lispro Protamine, Human (Disturbances of blood glucose, including symptomatic hyper- and hypoglycemia, have been reported with levofloxacin, usually in diabetic patients receiving concomitant treatment with insulin. In these patients, careful monitoring of blood glucose is recommended. If a hypoglycemic reaction occurs in a patient being treated with levofloxacin, levofloxacin, should be discontinued and appropriate therapy should be initiated immediately). Products include:
Humalog Mix **1914**
Humalog Mix75/25 .... **1917**

Iron (Concurrent administration of levofloxacin tablets/oral solution with metal cations such as iron may interfere with the gastrointestinal absorption of levofloxacin, resulting in systemic levels considerably lower than desired. These agents should be taken at least two hours before or two hours after levofloxacin administration).
No products indexed under this heading.

Iron, Peptonized (Concurrent administration of levofloxacin tablets/oral solution with metal cations such as iron may interfere with the gastrointestinal absorption of levofloxacin, resulting in systemic levels considerably lower than desired. These agents should be taken at least two hours before or two hours after levofloxacin administration).
No products indexed under this heading.

Iron & Ammonium Citrate (Concurrent administration of levofloxacin tablets/oral solution with metal cations such as iron may interfere with the gastrointestinal absorption of levofloxacin, resulting in systemic levels considerably lower than desired. These agents should be taken at least two hours before or two hours after levofloxacin administration).
No products indexed under this heading.

Iron Cacodylate (Concurrent administration of levofloxacin tablets/oral solution with metal cations such as iron may interfere with the gastrointestinal absorption of levofloxacin, resulting in systemic levels considerably lower than desired. These agents should be taken at least two hours before or two hours after levofloxacin administration).
No products indexed under this heading.

Iron Carbonyl (Concurrent administration of levofloxacin tablets/oral solution with metal cations such as iron may interfere with the gastrointestinal absorption of levofloxacin, resulting in systemic levels considerably lower than desired. These agents should be taken at least two hours before or two hours after levofloxacin administration).
Products include:

IMPORTANT NOTE: Always consult each drug listing in the patient's regimen for possible interactions.

Levaquin Oral Solution — Interactions Index — 992

CitraNatal 90 DHA Capsules 2332
CitraNatal Assure 2332
CitraNatal Harmony 2332
CitraNatal Rx 2332
Ferralet 2333

Iron Supplements (Concurrent administration of levofloxacin tablets/oral solution with metal cations such as iron may interfere with the gastrointestinal absorption of levofloxacin, resulting in systemic levels considerably lower than desired. These agents should be taken at least two hours before or two hours after levofloxacin administration).
No products indexed under this heading.

Isocarboxazid (Prolongation of the QT interval and isolated cases of torsade de pointes have been reported due to levofloxacin. Levofloxacin should be avoided with other drugs that prolong the QT interval. Levofloxacin should be avoided in patients with known prolongation of the QT interval, patients with uncorrected hypokalemia, and patients receiving Class IA (quinidine, procainamide), or Class III (amiodarone, sotalol) antiarrhythmic agents. Elderly patients may be more susceptible to drug-associated effects on the QT interval). Products include:
Marplan 3481

Ketoprofen (Concomitant administration of a non-steroidal anti-inflammatory drug with a fluoroquinolone, including levofloxacin, may increase the risk of CNS stimulation and convulsive seizures).
No products indexed under this heading.

Ketorolac Tromethamine (Concomitant administration of a non-steroidal anti-inflammatory drug with a fluoroquinolone, including levofloxacin, may increase the risk of CNS stimulation and convulsive seizures). Products include:
Acuvail .... ⊙209

Lidocaine (Prolongation of the QT interval and isolated cases of torsade de pointes have been reported due to levofloxacin. Levofloxacin should be avoided with other drugs that prolong the QT interval. Levofloxacin should be avoided in patients with known prolongation of the QT interval, patients with uncorrected hypokalemia, and patients receiving Class IA (quinidine, procainamide), or Class III (amiodarone, sotalol) antiarrhythmic agents. Elderly patients may be more susceptible to drug-associated effects on the QT interval). Products include:
Lidoderm 1107

Lidocaine Hydrochloride (Prolongation of the QT interval and isolated cases of torsade de pointes have been reported due to levofloxacin. Levofloxacin should be avoided with other drugs that prolong the QT interval. Levofloxacin should be avoided in patients with known prolongation of the QT interval, patients with uncorrected hypokalemia, and patients receiving Class IA (quinidine, procainamide), or Class III (amiodarone, sotalol) antiarrhythmic agents. Elderly patients may be more susceptible to drug-associated effects on the QT interval).
No products indexed under this heading.

Lithium Carbonate (Prolongation of the QT interval and isolated cases of torsade de pointes have been reported due to levofloxacin. Levofloxacin should be avoided with other drugs that prolong the QT interval. Levofloxacin should be avoided in patients with known prolongation of the QT interval, patients with uncorrected hypokalemia, and patients receiving Class IA (quinidine, procainamide), or Class III (amiodarone, sotalol) antiarrhythmic agents. Elderly patients may be more susceptible to drug-associated effects on the QT interval).
No products indexed under this heading.

Lithium Citrate (Prolongation of the QT interval and isolated cases of torsade de pointes have been reported due to levofloxacin. Levofloxacin should be avoided with other drugs that prolong the QT interval. Levofloxacin should be avoided in patients with known prolongation of the QT interval, patients with uncorrected hypokalemia, and patients receiving Class IA (quinidine, procainamide), or Class III (amiodarone, sotalol) antiarrhythmic agents. Elderly patients may be more susceptible to drug-associated effects on the QT interval).
No products indexed under this heading.

Lorazepam (Prolongation of the QT interval and isolated cases of torsade de pointes have been reported due to levofloxacin. Levofloxacin should be avoided with other drugs that prolong the QT interval. Levofloxacin should be avoided in patients with known prolongation of the QT interval, patients with uncorrected hypokalemia, and patients receiving Class IA (quinidine, procainamide), or Class III (amiodarone, sotalol) antiarrhythmic agents. Elderly patients may be more susceptible to drug-associated effects on the QT interval).
No products indexed under this heading.

Loxapine Hydrochloride (Prolongation of the QT interval and isolated cases of torsade de pointes have been reported due to levofloxacin. Levofloxacin should be avoided with other drugs that prolong the QT interval. Levofloxacin should be avoided in patients with known prolongation of the QT interval, patients with uncorrected hypokalemia, and patients receiving Class IA (quinidine, procainamide), or Class III (amiodarone, sotalol) antiarrhythmic agents. Elderly patients may be more susceptible to drug-associated effects on the QT interval).
No products indexed under this heading.

Loxapine Succinate (Prolongation of the QT interval and isolated cases of torsade de pointes have been reported due to levofloxacin. Levofloxacin should be avoided with other drugs that prolong the QT interval. Levofloxacin should be avoided in patients with known prolongation of the QT interval, patients with uncorrected hypokalemia, and patients receiving Class IA (quinidine, procainamide), or Class III (amiodarone, sotalol) antiarrhythmic agents. Elderly patients may be more susceptible to drug-associated effects on the QT interval).
No products indexed under this heading.

Magaldrate (Concurrent administration of levofloxacin tablets/oral solution with antacids containing magnesium, or aluminum may interfere with the gastrointestinal absorption of levofloxacin, resulting in systemic levels considerably lower than desired. These agents should be taken at least two hours before or two hours after levofloxacin administration).
No products indexed under this heading.

Magnesium (Concurrent administration of levofloxacin tablets/oral solution with metal cations such as iron may interfere with the gastrointestinal absorption of levofloxacin, resulting in systemic levels considerably lower than desired. These agents should be taken at least two hours before or two hours after levofloxacin administration). Products include:
BoneMate Plus 3454
Cardio Basics 3455
Chelated Mineral 3476

Magnesium Aluminum Silicate (Concurrent administration of levofloxacin tablets/oral solution with metal cations such as iron may interfere with the gastrointestinal absorption of levofloxacin, resulting in systemic levels considerably lower than desired. These agents should be taken at least two hours before or two hours after levofloxacin administration).
No products indexed under this heading.

Magnesium Carbonate (Concurrent administration of levofloxacin tablets/oral solution with antacids containing magnesium, or aluminum may interfere with the gastrointestinal absorption of levofloxacin, resulting in systemic levels considerably lower than desired. These agents should be taken at least two hours before or two hours after levofloxacin administration).
No products indexed under this heading.

Magnesium Chloride (Concurrent administration of levofloxacin tablets/oral solution with metal cations such as iron may interfere with the gastrointestinal absorption of levofloxacin, resulting in systemic levels considerably lower than desired. These agents should be taken at least two hours before or two hours after levofloxacin administration).
No products indexed under this heading.

Magnesium Citrate (Concurrent administration of levofloxacin tablets/oral solution with metal cations such as iron may interfere with the gastrointestinal absorption of levofloxacin, resulting in systemic levels considerably lower than desired. These agents should be taken at least two hours before or two hours after levofloxacin administration). Products include:
Chelated Mineral 3476

Magnesium Gluconate (Concurrent administration of levofloxacin tablets/oral solution with metal cations such as iron may interfere with the gastrointestinal absorption of levofloxacin, resulting in systemic levels considerably lower than desired. These agents should be taken at least two hours before or two hours after levofloxacin administration).
No products indexed under this heading.

Magnesium Hydroxide (Concurrent administration of levofloxacin tablets/oral solution with antacids containing magnesium, or aluminum may interfere with the gastrointestinal absorption of levofloxacin, resulting in systemic levels considerably lower than desired. These agents should be taken at least two hours before or two hours after levofloxacin administration). Products include:
Fleet Pedia-Lax Chewable Tablets 1144
Pepcid Complete 1822

Magnesium Lactate (Concurrent administration of levofloxacin tablets/oral solution with metal cations such as iron may interfere with the gastrointestinal absorption of levofloxacin, resulting in systemic levels considerably lower than desired. These agents should be taken at least two hours before or two hours after levofloxacin administration).
No products indexed under this heading.

Magnesium Oxide (Concurrent administration of levofloxacin tablets/oral solution with antacids containing magnesium, or aluminum may interfere with the gastrointestinal absorption of levofloxacin, resulting in systemic levels considerably lower than desired. These agents should be taken at least two hours before or two hours after levofloxacin administration). Products include:
Beelith 873

Magnesium Salicylate (Concurrent administration of levofloxacin tablets/oral solution with metal cations such as iron may interfere with the gastrointestinal absorption of levofloxacin, resulting in systemic levels considerably lower than desired. These agents should be taken at least two hours before or two hours after levofloxacin administration).
No products indexed under this heading.

Magnesium Salicylate Tetrahydrate (Concurrent administration of levofloxacin tablets/oral solution with metal cations such as iron may interfere with the gastrointestinal absorption of levofloxacin, resulting in systemic levels considerably lower than desired. These agents should be taken at least two hours before or two hours after levofloxacin administration).
No products indexed under this heading.

Magnesium Salts (Concurrent administration of levofloxacin tablets/oral solution with metal cations such as iron may interfere with the gastrointestinal absorption of levofloxacin, resulting in systemic levels considerably lower than desired. These agents should be taken at least two hours before or two hours after levofloxacin administration).
No products indexed under this heading.

Magnesium Sulfate (Concurrent administration of levofloxacin tablets/oral solution with metal cations such as iron may interfere with the gastrointestinal absorption of levofloxacin, resulting in systemic levels considerably lower than desired. These agents should be taken at least two hours before or two hours after levofloxacin administration).
No products indexed under this heading.

Magnesium Trisilicate (Concurrent administration of levofloxacin tablets/oral solution with antacids containing magnesium, or aluminum may interfere with the gastrointestinal absorption of levofloxacin, resulting in systemic levels considerably lower than desired. These agents should be taken at least two hours before or two hours after levofloxacin administration).
No products indexed under this heading.

Maprotiline Hydrochloride (Prolongation of the QT interval and isolated cases of torsade de pointes have been reported due to levofloxacin. Levofloxacin should be avoided with other drugs that prolong the QT interval. Levofloxacin should be avoided in patients with known prolongation of the QT interval, patients with uncorrected hypokalemia, and patients receiving Class IA (quinidine, procainamide), or Class III (amiodarone, sotalol) antiarrhythmic agents. Elderly patients may be more susceptible to drug-associated effects on the QT interval).
No products indexed under this heading.

Meclofenamate Sodium (Concomitant administration of a non-steroidal anti-inflammatory drug with a fluoroquinolone, including levofloxacin, may increase the risk of CNS stimulation and convulsive seizures).
No products indexed under this heading.

Mefenamic Acid (Concomitant administration of a non-steroidal anti-inflammatory drug with a fluoroquinolone, including levofloxacin, may increase the risk of CNS stimulation and convulsive seizures).
No products indexed under this heading.

Meloxicam (Concomitant administration of a non-steroidal anti-inflammatory drug with a fluoroquinolone, including levofloxacin, may increase the risk of CNS stimulation and convulsive seizures).
No products indexed under this heading.

Meprobamate (Prolongation of the QT interval and isolated cases of tor-

sade de pointes have been reported due to levofloxacin. Levofloxacin should be avoided with other drugs that prolong the QT interval. Levofloxacin should be avoided in patients with known prolongation of the QT interval, patients with uncorrected hypokalemia, and patients receiving Class IA (quinidine, procainamide), or Class III (amiodarone, sotalol) antiarrhythmic agents. Elderly patients may be more susceptible to drug-associated effects on the QT interval).

No products indexed under this heading.

Mesoridazine Besylate (Prolongation of the QT interval and isolated cases of torsade de pointes have been reported due to levofloxacin. Levofloxacin should be avoided with other drugs that prolong the QT interval. Levofloxacin should be avoided in patients with known prolongation of the QT interval, patients with uncorrected hypokalemia, and patients receiving Class IA (quinidine, procainamide), or Class III (amiodarone, sotalol) antiarrhythmic agents. Elderly patients may be more susceptible to drug-associated effects on the QT interval).

No products indexed under this heading.

Metformin Hydrochloride (Disturbances of blood glucose, including symptomatic hyper- and hypoglycemia, have been reported with levofloxacin, usually in diabetic patients receiving concomitant treatment with an oral hypoglycemic agent (eg, glyburide). In these patients, careful monitoring of blood glucose is recommended. If a hypoglycemic reaction occurs in a patient being treated with levofloxacin, levofloxacin, should be discontinued and appropriate therapy should be initiated immediately). Products include:

ActoPlus 3338
Avandamet 1345
Janumet 2188

Methylprednisolone (Fluoroquinolones, including levofloxacin, are associated with an increased risk of tendinitis and tendon rupture in all ages. This risk is further increased in patients taking corticosteroid drugs).

No products indexed under this heading.

Methylprednisolone Acetate (Fluoroquinolones, including levofloxacin, are associated with an increased risk of tendinitis and tendon rupture in all ages. This risk is further increased in patients taking corticosteroid drugs).

No products indexed under this heading.

Methylprednisolone Sodium Succinate (Fluoroquinolones, including levofloxacin, are associated with an increased risk of tendinitis and tendon rupture in all ages. This risk is further increased in patients taking corticosteroid drugs).

No products indexed under this heading.

Mexiletine Hydrochloride (Prolongation of the QT interval and isolated cases of torsade de pointes have been reported due to levofloxacin. Levofloxacin should be avoided with other drugs that prolong the QT interval. Levofloxacin should be avoided in patients with known prolongation of the QT interval, patients with uncorrected hypokalemia, and patients receiving Class IA (quinidine, procainamide), or Class III (amiodarone, sotalol) antiarrhythmic agents. Elderly patients may be more susceptible to drug-associated effects on the QT interval).

No products indexed under this heading.

Midazolam Hydrochloride (Prolongation of the QT interval and isolated cases of torsade de pointes have been reported due to levofloxacin. Levofloxacin should be avoided with other drugs that prolong the QT interval. Levofloxacin should be avoided in patients with

known prolongation of the QT interval, patients with uncorrected hypokalemia, and patients receiving Class IA (quinidine, procainamide), or Class III (amiodarone, sotalol) antiarrhythmic agents. Elderly patients may be more susceptible to drug-associated effects on the QT interval).

No products indexed under this heading.

Miglitol (Disturbances of blood glucose, including symptomatic hyper- and hypoglycemia, have been reported with levofloxacin, usually in diabetic patients receiving concomitant treatment with an oral hypoglycemic agent (eg, glyburide). In these patients, careful monitoring of blood glucose is recommended. If a hypoglycemic reaction occurs in a patient being treated with levofloxacin, levofloxacin, should be discontinued and appropriate therapy should be initiated immediately).

No products indexed under this heading.

Molindone Hydrochloride (Prolongation of the QT interval and isolated cases of torsade de pointes have been reported due to levofloxacin. Levofloxacin should be avoided with other drugs that prolong the QT interval. Levofloxacin should be avoided in patients with known prolongation of the QT interval, patients with uncorrected hypokalemia, and patients receiving Class IA (quinidine, procainamide), or Class III (amiodarone, sotalol) antiarrhythmic agents. Elderly patients may be more susceptible to drug-associated effects on the QT interval). Products include:

Moban 1108

Mometasone Furoate (Fluoroquinolones, including levofloxacin, are associated with an increased risk of tendinitis and tendon rupture in all ages. This risk is further increased in patients taking corticosteroid drugs). Products include:

Asmanex 3058
Elocon Cream 3111
Elocon Lotion 3112
Elocon Ointment 3114

Mometasone Furoate Monohydrate (Fluoroquinolones, including levofloxacin, are associated with an increased risk of tendinitis and tendon rupture in all ages. This risk is further increased in patients taking corticosteroid drugs). Products include:

Nasonex 3166

Moricizine Hydrochloride (Levofloxacin should be avoided in patients with known prolongation of the QT interval, patients with uncorrected hypokalemia, and patients receiving Class IA (quinidine, procainamide) antiarrhythmic agents. Elderly patients may be more susceptible to drug-associated effects on the QT interval).

No products indexed under this heading.

Nabumetone (Concomitant administration of a non-steroidal anti-inflammatory drug with a fluoroquinolone, including levofloxacin, may increase the risk of CNS stimulation and convulsive seizures).

No products indexed under this heading.

Naproxen (Concomitant administration of a non-steroidal anti-inflammatory drug with a fluoroquinolone, including levofloxacin, may increase the risk of CNS stimulation and convulsive seizures). Products include:

EC-Naprosyn 2850
Naprosyn 2850
Anaprox/Naprosyn 2850

Naproxen Sodium (Concomitant administration of a non-steroidal anti-inflammatory drug with a fluoroquinolone, including levofloxacin, may increase the risk of CNS stimulation and convulsive seizures). Products include:

Anaprox 2850
Anaprox DS 2850
Treximet 1681

Nateglinide (Disturbances of blood glucose, including symptomatic hyper- and hypoglycemia, have been reported with levofloxacin, usually in diabetic patients receiving concomitant treatment with an oral hypoglycemic agent (eg, glyburide). In these patients, careful monitoring of blood glucose is recommended. If a hypoglycemic reaction occurs in a patient being treated with levofloxacin, levofloxacin, should be discontinued and appropriate therapy should be initiated immediately).

No products indexed under this heading.

Nortriptyline Hydrochloride (Prolongation of the QT interval and isolated cases of torsade de pointes have been reported due to levofloxacin. Levofloxacin should be avoided with other drugs that prolong the QT interval. Levofloxacin should be avoided in patients with known prolongation of the QT interval, patients with uncorrected hypokalemia, and patients receiving Class IA (quinidine, procainamide), or Class III (amiodarone, sotalol) antiarrhythmic agents. Elderly patients may be more susceptible to drug-associated effects on the QT interval).

No products indexed under this heading.

Olanzapine (Prolongation of the QT interval and isolated cases of torsade de pointes have been reported due to levofloxacin. Levofloxacin should be avoided with other drugs that prolong the QT interval. Levofloxacin should be avoided in patients with known prolongation of the QT interval, patients with uncorrected hypokalemia, and patients receiving Class IA (quinidine, procainamide), or Class III (amiodarone, sotalol) antiarrhythmic agents. Elderly patients may be more susceptible to drug-associated effects on the QT interval). Products include:

Symbyax 1965
Zyprexa 1984
Zyprexa IntraMuscular 1984
Zyprexa ZYDIS 1984

Oxaprozin (Concomitant administration of a non-steroidal anti-inflammatory drug with a fluoroquinolone, including levofloxacin, may increase the risk of CNS stimulation and convulsive seizures).

No products indexed under this heading.

Oxazepam (Prolongation of the QT interval and isolated cases of torsade de pointes have been reported due to levofloxacin. Levofloxacin should be avoided with other drugs that prolong the QT interval. Levofloxacin should be avoided in patients with known prolongation of the QT interval, patients with uncorrected hypokalemia, and patients receiving Class IA (quinidine, procainamide), or Class III (amiodarone, sotalol) antiarrhythmic agents. Elderly patients may be more susceptible to drug-associated effects on the QT interval).

No products indexed under this heading.

Perphenazine (Prolongation of the QT interval and isolated cases of torsade de pointes have been reported due to levofloxacin. Levofloxacin should be avoided with other drugs that prolong the QT interval. Levofloxacin should be avoided in patients with known prolongation of the QT interval, patients with uncorrected hypokalemia, and patients receiving Class IA (quinidine, procainamide), or Class III (amiodarone, sotalol) antiarrhythmic agents. Elderly patients may be more susceptible to drug-associated effects on the QT interval).

No products indexed under this heading.

Phenelzine Sulfate (Prolongation of the QT interval and isolated cases of torsade de pointes have been reported due to levofloxacin. Levofloxacin should be avoided with other drugs that prolong the QT interval. Levofloxacin should be avoided in patients with

known prolongation of the QT interval, patients with uncorrected hypokalemia, and patients receiving Class IA (quinidine, procainamide), or Class III (amiodarone, sotalol) antiarrhythmic agents. Elderly patients may be more susceptible to drug-associated effects on the QT interval).

No products indexed under this heading.

Phenylbutazone (Concomitant administration of a non-steroidal anti-inflammatory drug with a fluoroquinolone, including levofloxacin, may increase the risk of CNS stimulation and convulsive seizures).

No products indexed under this heading.

Pioglitazone Hydrochloride (Disturbances of blood glucose, including symptomatic hyper- and hypoglycemia, have been reported with levofloxacin, usually in diabetic patients receiving concomitant treatment with an oral hypoglycemic agent (eg, glyburide). In these patients, careful monitoring of blood glucose is recommended. If a hypoglycemic reaction occurs in a patient being treated with levofloxacin, levofloxacin, should be discontinued and appropriate therapy should be initiated immediately). Products include:

ActoPlus 3338
Actos 3345
Duetact 3354

Piroxicam (Concomitant administration of a non-steroidal anti-inflammatory drug with a fluoroquinolone, including levofloxacin, may increase the risk of CNS stimulation and convulsive seizures).

No products indexed under this heading.

Polysaccharide Iron Complex (Concurrent administration of levofloxacin tablets/oral solution with metal cations such as iron may interfere with the gastrointestinal absorption of levofloxacin, resulting in systemic levels considerably lower than desired. These agents should be taken at least two hours before or two hours after levofloxacin administration). Products include:

Nu-Iron 150 2321

Prazepam (Prolongation of the QT interval and isolated cases of torsade de pointes have been reported due to levofloxacin. Levofloxacin should be avoided with other drugs that prolong the QT interval. Levofloxacin should be avoided in patients with known prolongation of the QT interval, patients with uncorrected hypokalemia, and patients receiving Class IA (quinidine, procainamide), or Class III (amiodarone, sotalol) antiarrhythmic agents. Elderly patients may be more susceptible to drug-associated effects on the QT interval).

No products indexed under this heading.

Prednisolone (Fluoroquinolones, including levofloxacin, are associated with an increased risk of tendinitis and tendon rupture in all ages. This risk is further increased in patients taking corticosteroid drugs).

No products indexed under this heading.

Prednisolone Acetate (Fluoroquinolones, including levofloxacin, are associated with an increased risk of tendinitis and tendon rupture in all ages. This risk is further increased in patients taking corticosteroid drugs). Products include:

Blephamide .... ⊙212, ⊙214
Pred Forte .... ⊙225
Pred Mild .... ⊙230
Pred-G .... ⊙226, ⊙227

Prednisolone Sodium Phosphate (Fluoroquinolones, including levofloxacin, are associated with an increased risk of tendinitis and tendon rupture in all ages. This risk is further increased in patients taking corticosteroid drugs).

No products indexed under this heading.

IMPORTANT NOTE: Always consult each drug listing in the patient's regimen for possible interactions.

Levaquin Oral Solution Interactions Index 994

Prednisolone Tebutate (Fluoroquinolones, including levofloxacin, are associated with an increased risk of tendinitis and tendon rupture in all ages. This risk is further increased in patients taking corticosteroid drugs).
No products indexed under this heading.

Prednisone (Fluoroquinolones, including levofloxacin, are associated with an increased risk of tendinitis and tendon rupture in all ages. This risk is further increased in patients taking corticosteroid drugs).
No products indexed under this heading.

Prednisone sodium phosphate (Fluoroquinolones, including levofloxacin, are associated with an increased risk of tendinitis and tendon rupture in all ages. This risk is further increased in patients taking corticosteroid drugs).
No products indexed under this heading.

Probenecid (The AUC and $t_{1/2}$ of levofloxacin were higher while CL/F and CL_R were lower during concomitant treatment of levofloxacin with probenecid compared to levofloxacin alone).
No products indexed under this heading.

Procainamide (Levofloxacin should be avoided in patients with known prolongation of the QT interval, patients with uncorrected hypokalemia, and patients receiving Class IA (eg, procainamide) antiarrhythmic agents. Elderly patients may be more susceptible to drug-associated effects on the QT interval).
No products indexed under this heading.

Procainamide Hydrochloride (Levofloxacin should be avoided in patients with known prolongation of the QT interval, patients with uncorrected hypokalemia, and patients receiving Class IA (eg, procainamide) antiarrhythmic agents. Elderly patients may be more susceptible to drug-associated effects on the QT interval).
No products indexed under this heading.

Prochlorperazine (Prolongation of the QT interval and isolated cases of torsade de pointes have been reported due to levofloxacin. Levofloxacin should be avoided with other drugs that prolong the QT interval. Levofloxacin should be avoided in patients with known prolongation of the QT interval, patients with uncorrected hypokalemia, and patients receiving Class IA (quinidine, procainamide), or Class III (amiodarone, sotalol) antiarrhythmic agents. Elderly patients may be more susceptible to drug-associated effects on the QT interval).
No products indexed under this heading.

Promethazine Hydrochloride (Prolongation of the QT interval and isolated cases of torsade de pointes have been reported due to levofloxacin. Levofloxacin should be avoided with other drugs that prolong the QT interval. Levofloxacin should be avoided in patients with known prolongation of the QT interval, patients with uncorrected hypokalemia, and patients receiving Class IA (quinidine, procainamide), or Class III (amiodarone, sotalol) antiarrhythmic agents. Elderly patients may be more susceptible to drug-associated effects on the QT interval).
No products indexed under this heading.

Propafenone Hydrochloride (Prolongation of the QT interval and isolated cases of torsade de pointes have been reported due to levofloxacin. Levofloxacin should be avoided with other drugs that prolong the QT interval. Levofloxacin should be avoided in patients with known prolongation of the QT interval, patients with uncorrected hypokalemia, and patients receiving Class IA (quinidine, procainamide), or Class III (amiodarone, sotalol) antiarrhythmic agents. Elderly patients may be more susceptible to drug-associated effects on the QT interval). Products include:
Rythmol 1648
Rythmol SR 1652

Protriptyline Hydrochloride (Prolongation of the QT interval and isolated cases of torsade de pointes have been reported due to levofloxacin. Levofloxacin should be avoided with other drugs that prolong the QT interval. Levofloxacin should be avoided in patients with known prolongation of the QT interval, patients with uncorrected hypokalemia, and patients receiving Class IA (quinidine, procainamide), or Class III (amiodarone, sotalol) antiarrhythmic agents. Elderly patients may be more susceptible to drug-associated effects on the QT interval).
No products indexed under this heading.

Quetiapine Fumarate (Prolongation of the QT interval and isolated cases of torsade de pointes have been reported due to levofloxacin. Levofloxacin should be avoided with other drugs that prolong the QT interval. Levofloxacin should be avoided in patients with known prolongation of the QT interval, patients with uncorrected hypokalemia, and patients receiving Class IA (quinidine, procainamide), or Class III (amiodarone, sotalol) antiarrhythmic agents. Elderly patients may be more susceptible to drug-associated effects on the QT interval). Products include:
Seroquel 750
Seroquel XR 759

Quinidine (Levofloxacin should be avoided in patients with known prolongation of the QT interval, patients with uncorrected hypokalemia, and patients receiving Class IA (eg, quinidine) antiarrhythmic agents. Elderly patients may be more susceptible to drug-associated effects on the QT interval).
No products indexed under this heading.

Quinidine Gluconate (Levofloxacin should be avoided in patients with known prolongation of the QT interval, patients with uncorrected hypokalemia, and patients receiving Class IA (eg, quinidine) antiarrhythmic agents. Elderly patients may be more susceptible to drug-associated effects on the QT interval).
No products indexed under this heading.

Quinidine Hydrochloride (Levofloxacin should be avoided in patients with known prolongation of the QT interval, patients with uncorrected hypokalemia, and patients receiving Class IA (eg, quinidine) antiarrhythmic agents. Elderly patients may be more susceptible to drug-associated effects on the QT interval).
No products indexed under this heading.

Quinidine Polygalacturonate (Levofloxacin should be avoided in patients with known prolongation of the QT interval, patients with uncorrected hypokalemia, and patients receiving Class IA (eg, quinidine) antiarrhythmic agents. Elderly patients may be more susceptible to drug-associated effects on the QT interval).
No products indexed under this heading.

Quinidine Sulfate (Levofloxacin should be avoided in patients with known prolongation of the QT interval, patients with uncorrected hypokalemia, and patients receiving Class IA (eg, quinidine) antiarrhythmic agents. Elderly patients may be more susceptible to drug-associated effects on the QT interval).
No products indexed under this heading.

Repaglinide (Disturbances of blood glucose, including symptomatic hyper- and hypoglycemia, have been reported with levofloxacin, usually in diabetic patients receiving concomitant treatment with an oral hypoglycemic agent (eg, glyburide). In these patients, careful monitoring of blood glucose is recommended. If a hypoglycemic reaction occurs in a patient being treated with levofloxacin, levofloxacin, should be discontinued and appropriate therapy should be initiated immediately).
No products indexed under this heading.

Risperidone (Prolongation of the QT interval and isolated cases of torsade de pointes have been reported due to levofloxacin. Levofloxacin should be avoided with other drugs that prolong the QT interval. Levofloxacin should be avoided in patients with known prolongation of the QT interval, patients with uncorrected hypokalemia, and patients receiving Class IA (quinidine, procainamide), or Class III (amiodarone, sotalol) antiarrhythmic agents. Elderly patients may be more susceptible to drug-associated effects on the QT interval). Products include:
Risperdal Consta 2682

Rofecoxib (Concomitant administration of a non-steroidal anti-inflammatory drug with a fluoroquinolone, including levofloxacin, may increase the risk of CNS stimulation and convulsive seizures).
No products indexed under this heading.

Rosiglitazone Maleate (Disturbances of blood glucose, including symptomatic hyper- and hypoglycemia, have been reported with levofloxacin, usually in diabetic patients receiving concomitant treatment with an oral hypoglycemic agent (eg, glyburide). In these patients, careful monitoring of blood glucose is recommended. If a hypoglycemic reaction occurs in a patient being treated with levofloxacin, levofloxacin, should be discontinued and appropriate therapy should be initiated immediately). Products include:
Avandamet 1345
Avandaryl 1356
Avandia 1366

Selenium (Concurrent administration of levofloxacin tablets/oral solution with metal cations such as iron may interfere with the gastrointestinal absorption of levofloxacin, resulting in systemic levels considerably lower than desired. These agents should be taken at least two hours before or two hours after levofloxacin administration). Products include:
Cardio Basics 3455
Chelated Mineral 3476

Selenium Sulfide (Concurrent administration of levofloxacin tablets/oral solution with metal cations such as iron may interfere with the gastrointestinal absorption of levofloxacin, resulting in systemic levels considerably lower than desired. These agents should be taken at least two hours before or two hours after levofloxacin administration).
No products indexed under this heading.

Sitagliptin Phosphate (Disturbances of blood glucose, including symptomatic hyper- and hypoglycemia, have been reported with levofloxacin, usually in diabetic patients receiving concomitant treatment with an oral hypoglycemic agent (eg, glyburide). In these patients, careful monitoring of blood glucose is recommended. If a hypoglycemic reaction occurs in a patient being treated with levofloxacin, levofloxacin, should be discontinued and appropriate therapy should be initiated immediately). Products include:
Janumet 2188
Januvia 2196

Sotalol Hydrochloride (Levofloxacin should be avoided in patients with known prolongation of the QT interval, patients with uncorrected hypokalemia, and patients receiving Class III (eg, sotalol) antiarrhythmic agents. Elderly patients may be more susceptible to drug-associated effects on the QT interval).
No products indexed under this heading.

Sucralfate (Concurrent administration of levofloxacin tablets/oral solution with sucralfate may interfere with the gastrointestinal absorption of levofloxacin, resulting in systemic levels considerably lower than desired. Sucralfate should be taken at least two hours before or two hours after levofloxacin administration). Products include:
Carafate Suspension 784
Carafate Tablets 785

Sulindac (Concomitant administration of a non-steroidal anti-inflammatory drug with a fluoroquinolone, including levofloxacin, may increase the risk of CNS stimulation and convulsive seizures). Products include:
Clinoril 2098

Theophylline (Concomitant administration of other fluoroquinolones with theophylline has resulted in prolonged elimination half-life, elevated serum theophylline levels, and a subsequent increase in the risk of theophylline-related adverse reactions in the patient population. Therefore, theophylline levels should be closely monitored and appropriate dosage adjustments made when levofloxacin is co-administered. Adverse reactions, including seizures, may occur with or without an elevation in serum theophylline levels).
No products indexed under this heading.

Theophylline Anhydrous (Concomitant administration of other fluoroquinolones with theophylline has resulted in prolonged elimination half-life, elevated serum theophylline levels, and a subsequent increase in the risk of theophylline-related adverse reactions in the patient population. Therefore, theophylline levels should be closely monitored and appropriate dosage adjustments made when levofloxacin is co-administered. Adverse reactions, including seizures, may occur with or without an elevation in serum theophylline levels). Products include:
Uniphyl 2817

Theophylline Calcium Salicylate (Concomitant administration of other fluoroquinolones with theophylline has resulted in prolonged elimination half-life, elevated serum theophylline levels, and a subsequent increase in the risk of theophylline-related adverse reactions in the patient population. Therefore, theophylline levels should be closely monitored and appropriate dosage adjustments made when levofloxacin is co-administered. Adverse reactions, including seizures, may occur with or without an elevation in serum theophylline levels).
No products indexed under this heading.

Theophylline Dihydroxypropyl (Glyceryl) (Concomitant administration of other fluoroquinolones with theophylline has resulted in prolonged elimination half-life, elevated serum theophylline levels, and a subsequent increase in the risk of theophylline-related adverse reactions in the patient population. Therefore, theophylline levels should be closely monitored and appropriate dosage adjustments made when levofloxacin is co-administered. Adverse reactions, including seizures, may occur with or without an elevation in serum theophylline levels).
No products indexed under this heading.

Theophylline Ethylenediamine (Concomitant administration of other

fluoroquinolones with theophylline has resulted in prolonged elimination half-life, elevated serum theophylline levels, and a subsequent increase in the risk of theophylline-related adverse reactions in the patient population. Therefore, theophylline levels should be closely monitored and appropriate dosage adjustments made when levofloxacin is co-administered. Adverse reactions, including seizures, may occur with or without an elevation in serum theophylline levels.

No products indexed under this heading.

Theophylline Sodium Glycinate (Concomitant administration of other fluoroquinolones with theophylline has resulted in prolonged elimination half-life, elevated serum theophylline levels, and a subsequent increase in the risk of theophylline-related adverse reactions in the patient population. Therefore, theophylline levels should be closely monitored and appropriate dosage adjustments made when levofloxacin is co-administered. Adverse reactions, including seizures, may occur with or without an elevation in serum theophylline levels.

No products indexed under this heading.

Thioridazine Hydrochloride (Prolongation of the QT interval and isolated cases of torsade de pointes have been reported due to levofloxacin. Levofloxacin should be avoided with other drugs that prolong the QT interval. Levofloxacin should be avoided in patients with known prolongation of the QT interval, patients with uncorrected hypokalemia, and patients receiving Class IA (quinidine, procainamide), or Class III (amiodarone, sotalol) antiarrhythmic agents. Elderly patients may be more susceptible to drug-associated effects on the QT interval). Products include:
Thioridazine Hydrochloride 2384

Thiothixene (Prolongation of the QT interval and isolated cases of torsade de pointes have been reported due to levofloxacin. Levofloxacin should be avoided with other drugs that prolong the QT interval. Levofloxacin should be avoided in patients with known prolongation of the QT interval, patients with uncorrected hypokalemia, and patients receiving Class IA (quinidine, procainamide), or Class III (amiodarone, sotalol) antiarrhythmic agents. Elderly patients may be more susceptible to drug-associated effects on the QT interval). Products include:
Thiothixene 2386

Tocainide Hydrochloride (Prolongation of the QT interval and isolated cases of torsade de pointes have been reported due to levofloxacin. Levofloxacin should be avoided with other drugs that prolong the QT interval. Levofloxacin should be avoided in patients with known prolongation of the QT interval, patients with uncorrected hypokalemia, and patients receiving Class IA (quinidine, procainamide), or Class III (amiodarone, sotalol) antiarrhythmic agents. Elderly patients may be more susceptible to drug-associated effects on the QT interval).

No products indexed under this heading.

Tolazamide (Disturbances of blood glucose, including symptomatic hyper- and hypoglycemia, have been reported with levofloxacin, usually in diabetic patients receiving concomitant treatment with an oral hypoglycemic agent (eg, glyburide). In these patients, careful monitoring of blood glucose is recommended. If a hypoglycemic reaction occurs in a patient being treated with levofloxacin, levofloxacin, should be discontinued and appropriate therapy should be initiated immediately).

No products indexed under this heading.

Tolbutamide (Disturbances of blood glucose, including symptomatic hyper- and hypoglycemia, have been reported with levofloxacin, usually in diabetic patients receiving concomitant treatment with an oral hypoglycemic agent (eg, glyburide). In these patients, careful monitoring of blood glucose is recommended. If a hypoglycemic reaction occurs in a patient being treated with levofloxacin, levofloxacin, should be discontinued and appropriate therapy should be initiated immediately).

No products indexed under this heading.

Tolmetin Sodium (Concomitant administration of a non-steroidal anti-inflammatory drug with a fluoroquinolone, including levofloxacin, may increase the risk of CNS stimulation and convulsive seizures).

No products indexed under this heading.

Tranylcypromine Sulfate (Prolongation of the QT interval and isolated cases of torsade de pointes have been reported due to levofloxacin. Levofloxacin should be avoided with other drugs that prolong the QT interval. Levofloxacin should be avoided in patients with known prolongation of the QT interval, patients with uncorrected hypokalemia, and patients receiving Class IA (quinidine, procainamide), or Class III (amiodarone, sotalol) antiarrhythmic agents. Elderly patients may be more susceptible to drug-associated effects on the QT interval). Products include:
Parnate 1584

Triamcinolone (Fluoroquinolones, including levofloxacin, are associated with an increased risk of tendinitis and tendon rupture in all ages. This risk is further increased in patients taking corticosteroid drugs).

No products indexed under this heading.

Triamcinolone Acetonide (Fluoroquinolones, including levofloxacin, are associated with an increased risk of tendinitis and tendon rupture in all ages. This risk is further increased in patients taking corticosteroid drugs). Products include:
Azmacort 408
Nasacort AQ 3019

Triamcinolone Diacetate (Fluoroquinolones, including levofloxacin, are associated with an increased risk of tendinitis and tendon rupture in all ages. This risk is further increased in patients taking corticosteroid drugs).

No products indexed under this heading.

Triamcinolone Hexacetonide (Fluoroquinolones, including levofloxacin, are associated with an increased risk of tendinitis and tendon rupture in all ages. This risk is further increased in patients taking corticosteroid drugs).

No products indexed under this heading.

Trifluoperazine Hydrochloride (Prolongation of the QT interval and isolated cases of torsade de pointes have been reported due to levofloxacin. Levofloxacin should be avoided with other drugs that prolong the QT interval. Levofloxacin should be avoided in patients with known prolongation of the QT interval, patients with uncorrected hypokalemia, and patients receiving Class IA (quinidine, procainamide), or Class III (amiodarone, sotalol) antiarrhythmic agents. Elderly patients may be more susceptible to drug-associated effects on the QT interval).

No products indexed under this heading.

Trimipramine Maleate (Prolongation of the QT interval and isolated cases of torsade de pointes have been reported due to levofloxacin. Levofloxacin should be avoided with other drugs that prolong the QT interval. Levofloxacin should be avoided in patients with known prolongation of the QT interval, patients with uncorrected hypokalemia,

and patients receiving Class IA (quinidine, procainamide), or Class III (amiodarone, sotalol) antiarrhythmic agents. Elderly patients may be more susceptible to drug-associated effects on the QT interval).

No products indexed under this heading.

Troglitazone (Disturbances of blood glucose, including symptomatic hyper- and hypoglycemia, have been reported with levofloxacin, usually in diabetic patients receiving concomitant treatment with an oral hypoglycemic agent (eg, glyburide). In these patients, careful monitoring of blood glucose is recommended. If a hypoglycemic reaction occurs in a patient being treated with levofloxacin, levofloxacin, should be discontinued and appropriate therapy should be initiated immediately).

No products indexed under this heading.

Ultraviolet radiation (Patients should be advised that photosensitivity/phototoxicity has been reported in patients receiving fluoroquinolone antibiotics. Patients should minimize or avoid exposure to natural or artificial sunlight (tanning beds or UVA/B treatment) while taking fluoroquinolones).

No products indexed under this heading.

Valdecoxib (Concomitant administration of a non-steroidal anti-inflammatory drug with a fluoroquinolone, including levofloxacin, may increase the risk of CNS stimulation and convulsive seizures).

No products indexed under this heading.

Warfarin Sodium (There have been reports during the postmarketing experience in patients that levofloxacin enhances the effects of warfarin. Elevations of the prothrombin time in the setting of concurrent warfarin and levofloxacin use have been associated with episodes of bleeding. Prothrombin time, International Normalized Ratio (INR), or other suitable anticoagulation tests should be closely monitored if levofloxacin is administered concomitantly with warfarin. Patients should also be monitored for evidence of bleeding).

No products indexed under this heading.

Zinc (Concurrent administration of levofloxacin tablets/oral solution with metal cations such as iron may interfere with the gastrointestinal absorption of levofloxacin, resulting in systemic levels considerably lower than desired. These agents should be taken at least two hours before or two hours after levofloxacin administration). Products include:
BoneMate Plus 3454
Cardio Basics 3455
Chelated Mineral 3476
CitraNatal 90 DHA Capsules 2332
CitraNatal Assure 2332
Heplive 607
Visutein 3456

Zinc Acetate (Concurrent administration of levofloxacin tablets/oral solution with metal cations such as iron may interfere with the gastrointestinal absorption of levofloxacin, resulting in systemic levels considerably lower than desired. These agents should be taken at least two hours before or two hours after levofloxacin administration).

No products indexed under this heading.

Zinc Bisglycinate (Concurrent administration of levofloxacin tablets/oral solution with metal cations such as iron may interfere with the gastrointestinal absorption of levofloxacin, resulting in systemic levels considerably lower than desired. These agents should be taken at least two hours before or two hours after levofloxacin administration).

No products indexed under this heading.

Zinc Chloride (Concurrent administration of levofloxacin tablets/oral solution with metal cations such as iron may interfere with the gastrointestinal absorption of levofloxacin, resulting in systemic levels considerably lower than desired. These agents should be taken at least two hours before or two hours after levofloxacin administration).

No products indexed under this heading.

Zinc Citrate (Concurrent administration of levofloxacin tablets/oral solution with metal cations such as iron may interfere with the gastrointestinal absorption of levofloxacin, resulting in systemic levels considerably lower than desired. These agents should be taken at least two hours before or two hours after levofloxacin administration). Products include:
Chelated Mineral 3476

Zinc-Containing Multivitamins (Concurrent administration of levofloxacin tablets/oral solution and multivitamin preparations with zinc may interfere with the gastrointestinal absorption of levofloxacin, resulting in systemic levels considerably lower than desired. These agents should be taken at least two hours before or two hours after oral levofloxacin administration).

No products indexed under this heading.

Zinc Gluconate (Concurrent administration of levofloxacin tablets/oral solution with metal cations such as iron may interfere with the gastrointestinal absorption of levofloxacin, resulting in systemic levels considerably lower than desired. These agents should be taken at least two hours before or two hours after levofloxacin administration).

No products indexed under this heading.

Zinc Oxide (Concurrent administration of levofloxacin tablets/oral solution with metal cations such as iron may interfere with the gastrointestinal absorption of levofloxacin, resulting in systemic levels considerably lower than desired. These agents should be taken at least two hours before or two hours after levofloxacin administration). Products include:
Bausch & Lomb Ocuvite Adult
50+ .... ☉ 238
CitraNatal Rx 2332
Vusion Ointment 3335

Zinc Phenosulfonate (Concurrent administration of levofloxacin tablets/oral solution with metal cations such as iron may interfere with the gastrointestinal absorption of levofloxacin, resulting in systemic levels considerably lower than desired. These agents should be taken at least two hours before or two hours after levofloxacin administration).

No products indexed under this heading.

Zinc Sulfate (Concurrent administration of levofloxacin tablets/oral solution with metal cations such as iron may interfere with the gastrointestinal absorption of levofloxacin, resulting in systemic levels considerably lower than desired. These agents should be taken at least two hours before or two hours after levofloxacin administration). Products include:
Heplive 607
Zinc-220 606

Ziprasidone Hydrochloride (Prolongation of the QT interval and isolated cases of torsade de pointes have been reported due to levofloxacin. Levofloxacin should be avoided with other drugs that prolong the QT interval. Levofloxacin should be avoided in patients with known prolongation of the QT interval, patients with uncorrected hypokalemia, and patients receiving Class IA (quinidine, procainamide), or Class III (amiodarone, sotalol) antiarrhythmic agents.

IMPORTANT NOTE: Always consult each drug listing in the patient's regimen for possible interactions.

Elderly patients may be more suscepti-ble to drug-associated effects on the QT interval). Products include:

Food Interactions

Food, unspecified (Oral administration of a 500 mg dose of levofloxacin with food prolongs the time to peak concen-tration by approximately 1 hour and decreases the peak concentration by approximately 25% (following oral solu-tion administration). It is recommended that levofloxacin oral solution be taken 1 hour before, or 2 hours after eating).

Iron Amino Acid Chelate (Concurrent administration of levofloxacin tablets/oral solution with metal cations such as iron may interfere with the gastrointesti-nal absorption of levofloxacin, resulting in systemic levels considerably lower than desired. These agents should be taken at least two hours before or two hours after levofloxacin administration).

Meal, unspecified (Oral administration of a 500 mg dose of levofloxacin with food prolongs the time to peak concen-tration by approximately 1 hour and decreases the peak concentration by approximately 25% (following oral solu-tion administration). It is recommended that levofloxacin oral solution be taken 1 hour before, or 2 hours after eating).

LEVAQUIN TABLETS

May interact with antacids containing aluminum, calcium and magnesium, cations, class IA antiarrhythmics, class III antiarrhythmics, corticosteroids, drugs that prolong the QT interval, insu-lin, iron containing oral preparations, non-steroidal anti-inflammatory agents, oral hypoglycemic agents, quinidine, theophyllines, and certain other agents. Compounds in these categories in-clude:

Acarbose (Disturbances of blood glu-cose, including symptomatic hyper- and hypoglycemia, have been reported with levofloxacin, usually in diabetic patients receiving concomitant treatment with an oral hypoglycemic agent (eg, gly-buride). In these patients, careful moni-toring of blood glucose is recom-mended. If a hypoglycemic reaction occurs in a patient being treated with levofloxacin, levofloxacin, should be discontinued and appropriate therapy should be initiated immediately).

No products indexed under this heading.

Alclometasone Dipropionate (Fluo-roquinolones, including levofloxacin, are associated with an increased risk of tendinitis and tendon rupture in all ages. This risk is further increased in patients taking corticosteroid drugs).

No products indexed under this heading.

Alprazolam (Prolongation of the QT interval and isolated cases of torsade de pointes have been reported due to levofloxacin. Levofloxacin should be avoided with other drugs that prolong the QT interval. Levofloxacin should be avoided in patients with known prolon-gation of the QT interval, patients with uncorrected hypokalemia, and patients receiving Class IA (quinidine, procaina-mide), or Class III (amiodarone, sotalol) antiarrhythmic agents. Elderly patients may be more susceptible to drug-associated effects on the QT interval).

No products indexed under this heading.

Aluminum Acetate (Concurrent administration of levofloxacin tablets/oral solution with metal cations such as iron may interfere with the gastrointesti-nal absorption of levofloxacin, resulting in systemic levels considerably lower than desired. These agents should be taken at least two hours before or two hours after levofloxacin administration).

No products indexed under this heading.

Aluminum Carbonate (Concurrent administration of levofloxacin tablets/oral solution with antacids containing magnesium, or aluminum may interfere with the gastrointestinal absorption of levofloxacin, resulting in systemic levels considerably lower than desired. These agents should be taken at least two hours before or two hours after levof-loxacin administration).

No products indexed under this heading.

Aluminum Chlorhydroxide (Concur-rent administration of levofloxacin tablets/oral solution with metal cations such as iron may interfere with the gas-trointestinal absorption of levofloxacin, resulting in systemic levels considerably lower than desired. These agents should be taken at least two hours before or two hours after levofloxacin administration).

No products indexed under this heading.

Aluminum Chloride (Concurrent administration of levofloxacin tablets/oral solution with metal cations such as iron may interfere with the gastrointesti-nal absorption of levofloxacin, resulting in systemic levels considerably lower than desired. These agents should be taken at least two hours before or two hours after levofloxacin administration).

No products indexed under this heading.

Aluminum Chlorohydrate (Concur-rent administration of levofloxacin tablets/oral solution with metal cations such as iron may interfere with the gas-trointestinal absorption of levofloxacin, resulting in systemic levels considerably lower than desired. These agents should be taken at least two hours before or two hours after levofloxacin administration).

No products indexed under this heading.

Aluminum Glycinate (Concurrent administration of levofloxacin tablets/oral solution with metal cations such as iron may interfere with the gastrointesti-nal absorption of levofloxacin, resulting in systemic levels considerably lower than desired. These agents should be taken at least two hours before or two hours after levofloxacin administration).

No products indexed under this heading.

Aluminum Hydroxide (Concurrent administration of levofloxacin tablets/oral solution with antacids containing magnesium, or aluminum may interfere with the gastrointestinal absorption of levofloxacin, resulting in systemic levels considerably lower than desired. These agents should be taken at least two hours before or two hours after levof-loxacin administration).

No products indexed under this heading.

Aluminum Hydroxide Prepara-tions (Concurrent administration of levofloxacin tablets/oral solution with metal cations such as iron may interfere with the gastrointestinal absorption of levofloxacin, resulting in systemic levels considerably lower than desired. These agents should be taken at least two hours before or two hours after levof-loxacin administration).

No products indexed under this heading.

Aluminum Sulfate (Concurrent administration of levofloxacin tablets/oral solution with metal cations such as iron may interfere with the gastrointesti-nal absorption of levofloxacin, resulting in systemic levels considerably lower than desired. These agents should be taken at least two hours before or two hours after levofloxacin administration).

No products indexed under this heading.

Amiodarone Hydrochloride (Levof-loxacin should be avoided in patients with known prolongation of the QT inter-val, patients with uncorrected hypoka-lemia, and patients receiving Class III (eg, amiodarone) antiarrhythmic agents. Elderly patients may be more suscepti-ble to drug-associated effects on the QT interval).

No products indexed under this heading.

Amitriptyline Hydrochloride (Pro-longation of the QT interval and isolated cases of torsade de pointes have been reported due to levofloxacin. Levofloxa-cin should be avoided with other drugs that prolong the QT interval. Levofloxa-cin should be avoided in patients with known prolongation of the QT interval, patients with uncorrected hypokalemia, and patients receiving Class IA (quini-dine, procainamide), or Class III (amio-darone, sotalol) antiarrhythmic agents. Elderly patients may be more suscepti-ble to drug-associated effects on the QT interval).

No products indexed under this heading.

Amoxapine (Prolongation of the QT interval and isolated cases of torsade de pointes have been reported due to levofloxacin. Levofloxacin should be avoided with other drugs that prolong the QT interval. Levofloxacin should be avoided in patients with known prolon-gation of the QT interval, patients with uncorrected hypokalemia, and patients receiving Class IA (quinidine, procaina-mide), or Class III (amiodarone, sotalol) antiarrhythmic agents. Elderly patients may be more susceptible to drug-associated effects on the QT interval).

No products indexed under this heading.

Astemizole (Prolongation of the QT interval and isolated cases of torsade de pointes have been reported due to levofloxacin. Levofloxacin should be avoided with other drugs that prolong the QT interval. Levofloxacin should be avoided in patients with known prolon-gation of the QT interval, patients with uncorrected hypokalemia, and patients receiving Class IA (quinidine, procaina-mide), or Class III (amiodarone, sotalol) antiarrhythmic agents. Elderly patients may be more susceptible to drug-associated effects on the QT interval).

No products indexed under this heading.

Beclomethasone Dipropionate (Fluoroquinolones, including levofloxa-cin, are associated with an increased risk of tendinitis and tendon rupture in all ages. This risk is further increased in patients taking corticosteroid drugs). Products include:

Beclomethasone Dipropionate Monohydrate (Fluoroquinolones, including levofloxacin, are associated with an increased risk of tendinitis and tendon rupture in all ages. This risk is further increased in patients taking cor-ticosteroid drugs). Products include:

Betamethasone (Fluoroquinolones, including levofloxacin, are associated with an increased risk of tendinitis and tendon rupture in all ages. This risk is further increased in patients taking cor-ticosteroid drugs).

No products indexed under this heading.

Betamethasone Acetate (Fluoroqui-nolones, including levofloxacin, are associated with an increased risk of tendinitis and tendon rupture in all ages. This risk is further increased in patients taking corticosteroid drugs).

No products indexed under this heading.

Betamethasone Benzoate (Fluoro-quinolones, including levofloxacin, are associated with an increased risk of tendinitis and tendon rupture in all ages. This risk is further increased in patients taking corticosteroid drugs).

No products indexed under this heading.

Betamethasone Dipropionate (Fluo-roquinolones, including levofloxacin, are associated with an increased risk of tendinitis and tendon rupture in all ages. This risk is further increased in patients taking corticosteroid drugs). Products include:

Betamethasone Sodium Phos-phate (Fluoroquinolones, including levofloxacin, are associated with an increased risk of tendinitis and tendon rupture in all ages. This risk is further increased in patients taking corticoster-oid drugs).

No products indexed under this heading.

Betamethasone Valerate (Fluoroqui-nolones, including levofloxacin, are associated with an increased risk of tendinitis and tendon rupture in all ages. This risk is further increased in patients taking corticosteroid drugs). Products include:

Bretylium Tosylate (Levofloxacin should be avoided in patients with known prolongation of the QT interval, patients with uncorrected hypokalemia, and patients receiving Class III (amio-darone, sotalol) antiarrhythmic agents. Elderly patients may be more suscepti-ble to drug-associated effects on the QT interval).

No products indexed under this heading.

Budesonide (Fluoroquinolones, includ-ing levofloxacin, are associated with an increased risk of tendinitis and tendon rupture in all ages. This risk is further increased in patients taking corticoster-oid drugs). Products include:

Buspirone Hydrochloride (Prolonga-tion of the QT interval and isolated cases of torsade de pointes have been reported due to levofloxacin. Levofloxa-cin should be avoided with other drugs that prolong the QT interval. Levofloxa-cin should be avoided in patients with known prolongation of the QT interval, patients with uncorrected hypokalemia, and patients receiving Class IA (quini-dine, procainamide), or Class III (amio-darone, sotalol) antiarrhythmic agents. Elderly patients may be more suscepti-ble to drug-associated effects on the QT interval).

No products indexed under this heading.

Calcium (Concurrent administration of levofloxacin tablets/oral solution with metal cations such as iron may interfere with the gastrointestinal absorption of levofloxacin, resulting in systemic levels considerably lower than desired. These agents should be taken at least two hours before or two hours after levof-loxacin administration). Products include:

Calcium (Oyster Shell) (Concurrent administration of levofloxacin tablets/oral solution with metal cations such as iron may interfere with the gastrointestinal absorption of levofloxacin, resulting in systemic levels considerably lower than desired. These agents should be taken at least two hours before or two hours after levofloxacin administration).
No products indexed under this heading.

Calcium Acetate (Concurrent administration of levofloxacin tablets/oral solution with metal cations such as iron may interfere with the gastrointestinal absorption of levofloxacin, resulting in systemic levels considerably lower than desired. These agents should be taken at least two hours before or two hours after levofloxacin administration).
No products indexed under this heading.

Calcium Ascorbate (Concurrent administration of levofloxacin tablets/oral solution with metal cations such as iron may interfere with the gastrointestinal absorption of levofloxacin, resulting in systemic levels considerably lower than desired. These agents should be taken at least two hours before or two hours after levofloxacin administration).
Products include:

Calcium Carbaspirin (Concurrent administration of levofloxacin tablets/oral solution with metal cations such as iron may interfere with the gastrointestinal absorption of levofloxacin, resulting in systemic levels considerably lower than desired. These agents should be taken at least two hours before or two hours after levofloxacin administration).
No products indexed under this heading.

Calcium Carbonate (Concurrent administration of levofloxacin tablets/oral solution with antacids containing magnesium, or aluminum may interfere with the gastrointestinal absorption of levofloxacin, resulting in systemic levels considerably lower than desired. These agents should be taken at least two hours before or two hours after levofloxacin administration). Products include:

Calcium Carbonate, Precipitated (Concurrent administration of levofloxacin tablets/oral solution with metal cations such as iron may interfere with the gastrointestinal absorption of levofloxacin, resulting in systemic levels considerably lower than desired. These agents should be taken at least two hours before or two hours after levofloxacin administration).
No products indexed under this heading.

Calcium Caseinate (Concurrent administration of levofloxacin tablets/oral solution with metal cations such as iron may interfere with the gastrointestinal absorption of levofloxacin, resulting in systemic levels considerably lower than desired. These agents should be taken at least two hours before or two hours after levofloxacin administration).
No products indexed under this heading.

Calcium Chloride (Concurrent administration of levofloxacin tablets/oral solution with metal cations such as iron may interfere with the gastrointestinal absorption of levofloxacin, resulting in systemic levels considerably lower than desired. These agents should be taken at least two hours before or two hours after levofloxacin administration).
No products indexed under this heading.

Calcium Citrate (Concurrent administration of levofloxacin tablets/oral solution with metal cations such as iron may

interfere with the gastrointestinal absorption of levofloxacin, resulting in systemic levels considerably lower than desired. These agents should be taken at least two hours before or two hours after levofloxacin administration). Products include:

Calcium Disodium Edetate (Concurrent administration of levofloxacin tablets/oral solution with metal cations such as iron may interfere with the gastrointestinal absorption of levofloxacin, resulting in systemic levels considerably lower than desired. These agents should be taken at least two hours before or two hours after levofloxacin administration).
No products indexed under this heading.

Calcium Glubionate (Concurrent administration of levofloxacin tablets/oral solution with metal cations such as iron may interfere with the gastrointestinal absorption of levofloxacin, resulting in systemic levels considerably lower than desired. These agents should be taken at least two hours before or two hours after levofloxacin administration).
No products indexed under this heading.

Calcium Gluconate (Concurrent administration of levofloxacin tablets/oral solution with metal cations such as iron may interfere with the gastrointestinal absorption of levofloxacin, resulting in systemic levels considerably lower than desired. These agents should be taken at least two hours before or two hours after levofloxacin administration).
No products indexed under this heading.

Calcium Glycerophosphate (Concurrent administration of levofloxacin tablets/oral solution with metal cations such as iron may interfere with the gastrointestinal absorption of levofloxacin, resulting in systemic levels considerably lower than desired. These agents should be taken at least two hours before or two hours after levofloxacin administration).
No products indexed under this heading.

Calcium Iodide (Concurrent administration of levofloxacin tablets/oral solution with metal cations such as iron may interfere with the gastrointestinal absorption of levofloxacin, resulting in systemic levels considerably lower than desired. These agents should be taken at least two hours before or two hours after levofloxacin administration).
No products indexed under this heading.

Calcium Lactate (Concurrent administration of levofloxacin tablets/oral solution with metal cations such as iron may interfere with the gastrointestinal absorption of levofloxacin, resulting in systemic levels considerably lower than desired. These agents should be taken at least two hours before or two hours after levofloxacin administration).
No products indexed under this heading.

Calcium Levulinate (Concurrent administration of levofloxacin tablets/oral solution with metal cations such as iron may interfere with the gastrointestinal absorption of levofloxacin, resulting in systemic levels considerably lower than desired. These agents should be taken at least two hours before or two hours after levofloxacin administration).
No products indexed under this heading.

Calcium Pantothenate (Concurrent administration of levofloxacin tablets/oral solution with metal cations such as iron may interfere with the gastrointestinal absorption of levofloxacin, resulting in systemic levels considerably lower than desired. These agents should be

taken at least two hours before or two hours after levofloxacin administration). Products include:

Calcium Phosphate (Concurrent administration of levofloxacin tablets/oral solution with metal cations such as iron may interfere with the gastrointestinal absorption of levofloxacin, resulting in systemic levels considerably lower than desired. These agents should be taken at least two hours before or two hours after levofloxacin administration).
No products indexed under this heading.

Calcium Phosphate, Dibasic (Concurrent administration of levofloxacin tablets/oral solution with metal cations such as iron may interfere with the gastrointestinal absorption of levofloxacin, resulting in systemic levels considerably lower than desired. These agents should be taken at least two hours before or two hours after levofloxacin administration).
No products indexed under this heading.

Calcium Phosphate, Tribasic (Concurrent administration of levofloxacin tablets/oral solution with metal cations such as iron may interfere with the gastrointestinal absorption of levofloxacin, resulting in systemic levels considerably lower than desired. These agents should be taken at least two hours before or two hours after levofloxacin administration).
No products indexed under this heading.

Calcium Phosphorus Preparations (Concurrent administration of levofloxacin tablets/oral solution with metal cations such as iron may interfere with the gastrointestinal absorption of levofloxacin, resulting in systemic levels considerably lower than desired. These agents should be taken at least two hours before or two hours after levofloxacin administration).
No products indexed under this heading.

Calcium Polycarbophil (Concurrent administration of levofloxacin tablets/oral solution with metal cations such as iron may interfere with the gastrointestinal absorption of levofloxacin, resulting in systemic levels considerably lower than desired. These agents should be taken at least two hours before or two hours after levofloxacin administration).
No products indexed under this heading.

Calcium Salts (Concurrent administration of levofloxacin tablets/oral solution with metal cations such as iron may interfere with the gastrointestinal absorption of levofloxacin, resulting in systemic levels considerably lower than desired. These agents should be taken at least two hours before or two hours after levofloxacin administration).
No products indexed under this heading.

Calcium Sodium Alginate Fiber (Concurrent administration of levofloxacin tablets/oral solution with metal cations such as iron may interfere with the gastrointestinal absorption of levofloxacin, resulting in systemic levels considerably lower than desired. These agents should be taken at least two hours before or two hours after levofloxacin administration).
No products indexed under this heading.

Calcium Undecylenate (Concurrent administration of levofloxacin tablets/oral solution with metal cations such as iron may interfere with the gastrointestinal absorption of levofloxacin, resulting in systemic levels considerably lower than desired. These agents should be taken at least two hours before or two hours after levofloxacin administration).
No products indexed under this heading.

Celecoxib (Concomitant administration of a non-steroidal anti-inflammatory drug with a fluoroquinolone, including

levofloxacin, may increase the risk of CNS stimulation and convulsive seizures). Products include:

Chlordiazepoxide (Prolongation of the QT interval and isolated cases of torsade de pointes have been reported due to levofloxacin. Levofloxacin should be avoided with other drugs that prolong the QT interval. Levofloxacin should be avoided in patients with known prolongation of the QT interval, patients with uncorrected hypokalemia, and patients receiving Class IA (quinidine, procainamide), or Class III (amiodarone, sotalol) antiarrhythmic agents. Elderly patients may be more susceptible to drug-associated effects on the QT interval).
No products indexed under this heading.

Chlordiazepoxide Hydrochloride (Prolongation of the QT interval and isolated cases of torsade de pointes have been reported due to levofloxacin. Levofloxacin should be avoided with other drugs that prolong the QT interval. Levofloxacin should be avoided in patients with known prolongation of the QT interval, patients with uncorrected hypokalemia, and patients receiving Class IA (quinidine, procainamide), or Class III (amiodarone, sotalol) antiarrhythmic agents. Elderly patients may be more susceptible to drug-associated effects on the QT interval).
No products indexed under this heading.

Chlorpromazine (Prolongation of the QT interval and isolated cases of torsade de pointes have been reported due to levofloxacin. Levofloxacin should be avoided with other drugs that prolong the QT interval. Levofloxacin should be avoided in patients with known prolongation of the QT interval, patients with uncorrected hypokalemia, and patients receiving Class IA (quinidine, procainamide), or Class III (amiodarone, sotalol) antiarrhythmic agents. Elderly patients may be more susceptible to drug-associated effects on the QT interval).
No products indexed under this heading.

Chlorpromazine Hydrochloride (Prolongation of the QT interval and isolated cases of torsade de pointes have been reported due to levofloxacin. Levofloxacin should be avoided with other drugs that prolong the QT interval. Levofloxacin should be avoided in patients with known prolongation of the QT interval, patients with uncorrected hypokalemia, and patients receiving Class IA (quinidine, procainamide), or Class III (amiodarone, sotalol) antiarrhythmic agents. Elderly patients may be more susceptible to drug-associated effects on the QT interval).
No products indexed under this heading.

Chlorpropamide (Disturbances of blood glucose, including symptomatic hyper- and hypoglycemia, have been reported with levofloxacin, usually in diabetic patients receiving concomitant treatment with an oral hypoglycemic agent (eg, glyburide). In these patients, careful monitoring of blood glucose is recommended. If a hypoglycemic reaction occurs in a patient being treated with levofloxacin, levofloxacin, should be discontinued and appropriate therapy should be initiated immediately).
No products indexed under this heading.

Chlorprothixene (Prolongation of the QT interval and isolated cases of torsade de pointes have been reported due to levofloxacin. Levofloxacin should be avoided with other drugs that prolong the QT interval. Levofloxacin should be avoided in patients with known prolongation of the QT interval, patients with uncorrected hypokalemia, and patients receiving Class IA (quinidine, procainamide), or Class III (amio-

darone, sotalol) antiarrhythmic agents. Elderly patients may be more susceptible to drug-associated effects on the QT interval).
No products indexed under this heading.

Chlorprothixene Hydrochloride (Prolongation of the QT interval and isolated cases of torsade de pointes have been reported due to levofloxacin. Levofloxacin should be avoided with other drugs that prolong the QT interval. Levofloxacin should be avoided in patients with known prolongation of the QT interval, patients with uncorrected hypokalemia, and patients receiving Class IA (quinidine, procainamide), or Class III (amiodarone, sotalol) antiarrhythmic agents. Elderly patients may be more susceptible to drug-associated effects on the QT interval).
No products indexed under this heading.

Ciclesonide (Fluoroquinolones, including levofloxacin, are associated with an increased risk of tendinitis and tendon rupture in all ages. This risk is further increased in patients taking corticosteroid drugs).
No products indexed under this heading.

Cimetidine (The AUC and $t_{1/2}$ of levofloxacin were higher while CL/F and CL_R were lower during concomitant treatment of levofloxacin with cimetidine compared to levofloxacin alone).
No products indexed under this heading.

Cimetidine Hydrochloride (The AUC and $t_{1/2}$ of levofloxacin were higher while CL/F and CL_R were lower during concomitant treatment of levofloxacin with cimetidine compared to levofloxacin alone).
No products indexed under this heading.

Clomipramine Hydrochloride (Prolongation of the QT interval and isolated cases of torsade de pointes have been reported due to levofloxacin. Levofloxacin should be avoided with other drugs that prolong the QT interval. Levofloxacin should be avoided in patients with known prolongation of the QT interval, patients with uncorrected hypokalemia, and patients receiving Class IA (quinidine, procainamide), or Class III (amiodarone, sotalol) antiarrhythmic agents. Elderly patients may be more susceptible to drug-associated effects on the QT interval).
No products indexed under this heading.

Clorazepate Dipotassium (Prolongation of the QT interval and isolated cases of torsade de pointes have been reported due to levofloxacin. Levofloxacin should be avoided with other drugs that prolong the QT interval. Levofloxacin should be avoided in patients with known prolongation of the QT interval, patients with uncorrected hypokalemia, and patients receiving Class IA (quinidine, procainamide), or Class III (amiodarone, sotalol) antiarrhythmic agents. Elderly patients may be more susceptible to drug-associated effects on the QT interval).
No products indexed under this heading.

Clozapine (Prolongation of the QT interval and isolated cases of torsade de pointes have been reported due to levofloxacin. Levofloxacin should be avoided with other drugs that prolong the QT interval. Levofloxacin should be avoided in patients with known prolongation of the QT interval, patients with uncorrected hypokalemia, and patients receiving Class IA (quinidine, procainamide), or Class III (amiodarone, sotalol) antiarrhythmic agents. Elderly patients may be more susceptible to drug-associated effects on the QT interval).
No products indexed under this heading.

Cortisone Acetate (Fluoroquinolones, including levofloxacin, are associated with an increased risk of tendinitis and tendon rupture in all ages. This risk is further increased in patients taking corticosteroid drugs).
No products indexed under this heading.

Cyclosporine (Elevated serum levels of cyclosporine have been reported in the patient population when coadministered with some other fluoroquinolones. Levofloxacin C_{max} and k_e were slightly lower while T_{max} and $t_{1/2}$ were slightly longer in the presence of cyclosporine than those observed in other studies without concomitant medication). Products include:
Gengraf 440
Neoral Oral Solution 2496
Neoral Capsules 2496
Restasis 605

Desipramine Hydrochloride (Prolongation of the QT interval and isolated cases of torsade de pointes have been reported due to levofloxacin. Levofloxacin should be avoided with other drugs that prolong the QT interval. Levofloxacin should be avoided in patients with known prolongation of the QT interval, patients with uncorrected hypokalemia, and patients receiving Class IA (quinidine, procainamide), or Class III (amiodarone, sotalol) antiarrhythmic agents. Elderly patients may be more susceptible to drug-associated effects on the QT interval).
No products indexed under this heading.

Desoximetasone (Fluoroquinolones, including levofloxacin, are associated with an increased risk of tendinitis and tendon rupture in all ages. This risk is further increased in patients taking corticosteroid drugs).
No products indexed under this heading.

Dexamethasone (Fluoroquinolones, including levofloxacin, are associated with an increased risk of tendinitis and tendon rupture in all ages. This risk is further increased in patients taking corticosteroid drugs). Products include:
Ciprodex 583
Ozurdex .... ⊙ 223
Tobramycin and Dexamethasone Ophthalmic Suspension .... ⊙ 251

Dexamethasone Acetate (Fluoroquinolones, including levofloxacin, are associated with an increased risk of tendinitis and tendon rupture in all ages. This risk is further increased in patients taking corticosteroid drugs).
No products indexed under this heading.

Dexamethasone Phosphate (Fluoroquinolones, including levofloxacin, are associated with an increased risk of tendinitis and tendon rupture in all ages. This risk is further increased in patients taking corticosteroid drugs).
No products indexed under this heading.

Dexamethasone Sodium (Fluoroquinolones, including levofloxacin, are associated with an increased risk of tendinitis and tendon rupture in all ages. This risk is further increased in patients taking corticosteroid drugs).
No products indexed under this heading.

Dexamethasone Sodium Phosphate (Fluoroquinolones, including levofloxacin, are associated with an increased risk of tendinitis and tendon rupture in all ages. This risk is further increased in patients taking corticosteroid drugs).
No products indexed under this heading.

Dexamethasone Sodium Phosphate Injection (Fluoroquinolones, including levofloxacin, are associated with an increased risk of tendinitis and tendon rupture in all ages. This risk is further increased in patients taking corticosteroid drugs).
No products indexed under this heading.

Diazepam (Prolongation of the QT interval and isolated cases of torsade de pointes have been reported due to levofloxacin. Levofloxacin should be avoided with other drugs that prolong the QT interval. Levofloxacin should be avoided in patients with known prolongation of the QT interval, patients with uncorrected hypokalemia, and patients receiving Class IA (quinidine, procainamide), or Class III (amiodarone, sotalol) antiarrhythmic agents. Elderly patients may be more susceptible to drug-associated effects on the QT interval). Products include:
Valium Tablets 2880

Diclofenac Epolamine (Concomitant administration of a non-steroidal anti-inflammatory drug with a fluoroquinolone, including levofloxacin, may increase the risk of CNS stimulation and convulsive seizures). Products include:
Flector 1839

Diclofenac Potassium (Concomitant administration of a non-steroidal anti-inflammatory drug with a fluoroquinolone, including levofloxacin, may increase the risk of CNS stimulation and convulsive seizures).
No products indexed under this heading.

Diclofenac Sodium (Concomitant administration of a non-steroidal anti-inflammatory drug with a fluoroquinolone, including levofloxacin, may increase the risk of CNS stimulation and convulsive seizures).
No products indexed under this heading.

Didanosine (Didanosine may substantially interfere with the gastrointestinal absorption of levofloxacin tablets/oral solution, resulting in systemic levels considerably lower than desired. Didanosine should be taken at least two hours before or two hours after levofloxacin administration).
No products indexed under this heading.

Diflorasone Diacetate (Fluoroquinolones, including levofloxacin, are associated with an increased risk of tendinitis and tendon rupture in all ages. This risk is further increased in patients taking corticosteroid drugs).
No products indexed under this heading.

Disopyramide (Levofloxacin should be avoided in patients with known prolongation of the QT interval, patients with uncorrected hypokalemia, and patients receiving Class IA (quinidine, procainamide) antiarrhythmic agents. Elderly patients may be more susceptible to drug-associated effects on the QT interval).
No products indexed under this heading.

Disopyramide Phosphate (Levofloxacin should be avoided in patients with known prolongation of the QT interval, patients with uncorrected hypokalemia, and patients receiving Class IA (quinidine, procainamide) antiarrhythmic agents. Elderly patients may be more susceptible to drug-associated effects on the QT interval).
No products indexed under this heading.

Dofetilide (Prolongation of the QT interval and isolated cases of torsade de pointes have been reported due to levofloxacin. Levofloxacin should be avoided with other drugs that prolong the QT interval. Levofloxacin should be avoided in patients with known prolongation of the QT interval, patients with uncorrected hypokalemia, and patients receiving Class IA (quinidine, procainamide), or Class III (amiodarone, sotalol) antiarrhythmic agents. Elderly patients may be more susceptible to drug-associated effects on the QT interval).
No products indexed under this heading.

Doxepin Hydrochloride (Prolongation of the QT interval and isolated cases of torsade de pointes have been reported due to levofloxacin. Levofloxacin should be avoided with other drugs that prolong the QT interval. Levofloxacin should be avoided in patients with known prolongation of the QT interval, patients with uncorrected hypokalemia, and patients receiving Class IA (quinidine, procainamide), or Class III (amiodarone, sotalol) antiarrhythmic agents. Elderly patients may be more susceptible to drug-associated effects on the QT interval).
No products indexed under this heading.

Droperidol (Prolongation of the QT interval and isolated cases of torsade de pointes have been reported due to levofloxacin. Levofloxacin should be avoided with other drugs that prolong the QT interval. Levofloxacin should be avoided in patients with known prolongation of the QT interval, patients with uncorrected hypokalemia, and patients receiving Class IA (quinidine, procainamide), or Class III (amiodarone, sotalol) antiarrhythmic agents. Elderly patients may be more susceptible to drug-associated effects on the QT interval).
No products indexed under this heading.

Erythromycin (Prolongation of the QT interval and isolated cases of torsade de pointes have been reported due to levofloxacin. Levofloxacin should be avoided with other drugs that prolong the QT interval. Levofloxacin should be avoided in patients with known prolongation of the QT interval, patients with uncorrected hypokalemia, and patients receiving Class IA (quinidine, procainamide), or Class III (amiodarone, sotalol) antiarrhythmic agents. Elderly patients may be more susceptible to drug-associated effects on the QT interval).
No products indexed under this heading.

Erythromycin Estolate (Prolongation of the QT interval and isolated cases of torsade de pointes have been reported due to levofloxacin. Levofloxacin should be avoided with other drugs that prolong the QT interval. Levofloxacin should be avoided in patients with known prolongation of the QT interval, patients with uncorrected hypokalemia, and patients receiving Class IA (quinidine, procainamide), or Class III (amiodarone, sotalol) antiarrhythmic agents. Elderly patients may be more susceptible to drug-associated effects on the QT interval).
No products indexed under this heading.

Erythromycin Ethylsuccinate (Prolongation of the QT interval and isolated cases of torsade de pointes have been reported due to levofloxacin. Levofloxacin should be avoided with other drugs that prolong the QT interval. Levofloxacin should be avoided in patients with known prolongation of the QT interval, patients with uncorrected hypokalemia, and patients receiving Class IA (quinidine, procainamide), or Class III (amiodarone, sotalol) antiarrhythmic agents. Elderly patients may be more susceptible to drug-associated effects on the QT interval). Products include:
E.E.S. 437
EryPed 435

Erythromycin Gluceptate (Prolongation of the QT interval and isolated cases of torsade de pointes have been reported due to levofloxacin. Levofloxacin should be avoided with other drugs that prolong the QT interval. Levofloxacin should be avoided in patients with known prolongation of the QT interval, patients with uncorrected hypokalemia, and patients receiving Class IA (quinidine, procainamide), or Class III (amiodarone, sotalol) antiarrhythmic agents. Elderly patients may be more susceptible to drug-associated effects on the QT interval).
No products indexed under this heading.

999 Interactions Index Levaquin Tablets

Erythromycin Lactobionate (Prolongation of the QT interval and isolated cases of torsade de pointes have been reported due to levofloxacin. Levofloxacin should be avoided with other drugs that prolong the QT interval. Levofloxacin should be avoided in patients with known prolongation of the QT interval, patients with uncorrected hypokalemia, and patients receiving Class IA (quinidine, procainamide), or Class III (amiodarone, sotalol) antiarrhythmic agents. Elderly patients may be more susceptible to drug-associated effects on the QT interval).
No products indexed under this heading.

Erythromycin Stearate (Prolongation of the QT interval and isolated cases of torsade de pointes have been reported due to levofloxacin. Levofloxacin should be avoided with other drugs that prolong the QT interval. Levofloxacin should be avoided in patients with known prolongation of the QT interval, patients with uncorrected hypokalemia, and patients receiving Class IA (quinidine, procainamide), or Class III (amiodarone, sotalol) antiarrhythmic agents. Elderly patients may be more susceptible to drug-associated effects on the QT interval).
No products indexed under this heading.

Etodolac (Concomitant administration of a non-steroidal anti-inflammatory drug with a fluoroquinolone, including levofloxacin, may increase the risk of CNS stimulation and convulsive seizures).
No products indexed under this heading.

Fenoprofen Calcium (Concomitant administration of a non-steroidal anti-inflammatory drug with a fluoroquinolone, including levofloxacin, may increase the risk of CNS stimulation and convulsive seizures).
No products indexed under this heading.

Ferrous Fumarate (Concurrent administration of levofloxacin tablets/oral solution with metal cations such as iron may interfere with the gastrointestinal absorption of levofloxacin, resulting in systemic levels considerably lower than desired. These agents should be taken at least two hours before or two hours after levofloxacin administration). Products include:
PreNexa **3473**

Ferrous Gluconate (Concurrent administration of levofloxacin tablets/oral solution with metal cations such as iron may interfere with the gastrointestinal absorption of levofloxacin, resulting in systemic levels considerably lower than desired. These agents should be taken at least two hours before or two hours after levofloxacin administration). Products include:
CitraNatal Assure **2332**
CitraNatal Rx **2332**

Ferrous Sulfate (Concurrent administration of levofloxacin tablets/oral solution with metal cations such as iron may interfere with the gastrointestinal absorption of levofloxacin, resulting in systemic levels considerably lower than desired. These agents should be taken at least two hours before or two hours after levofloxacin administration).
No products indexed under this heading.

Flecainide Acetate (Prolongation of the QT interval and isolated cases of torsade de pointes have been reported due to levofloxacin. Levofloxacin should be avoided with other drugs that prolong the QT interval. Levofloxacin should be avoided in patients with known prolongation of the QT interval, patients with uncorrected hypokalemia, and patients receiving Class IA (quinidine, procainamide), or Class III (amiodarone, sotalol) antiarrhythmic agents. Elderly patients may be more susceptible to drug-associated effects on the QT interval).
No products indexed under this heading.

Fludrocortisone Acetate (Fluoroquinolones, including levofloxacin, are associated with an increased risk of tendinitis and tendon rupture in all ages. This risk is further increased in patients taking corticosteroid drugs).
No products indexed under this heading.

Flumethasone Pivalate (Fluoroquinolones, including levofloxacin, are associated with an increased risk of tendinitis and tendon rupture in all ages. This risk is further increased in patients taking corticosteroid drugs).
No products indexed under this heading.

Flunisolide Hemihydrate (Fluoroquinolones, including levofloxacin, are associated with an increased risk of tendinitis and tendon rupture in all ages. This risk is further increased in patients taking corticosteroid drugs).
No products indexed under this heading.

Fluphenazine Decanoate (Prolongation of the QT interval and isolated cases of torsade de pointes have been reported due to levofloxacin. Levofloxacin should be avoided with other drugs that prolong the QT interval. Levofloxacin should be avoided in patients with known prolongation of the QT interval, patients with uncorrected hypokalemia, and patients receiving Class IA (quinidine, procainamide), or Class III (amiodarone, sotalol) antiarrhythmic agents. Elderly patients may be more susceptible to drug-associated effects on the QT interval).
No products indexed under this heading.

Fluphenazine Enanthate (Prolongation of the QT interval and isolated cases of torsade de pointes have been reported due to levofloxacin. Levofloxacin should be avoided with other drugs that prolong the QT interval. Levofloxacin should be avoided in patients with known prolongation of the QT interval, patients with uncorrected hypokalemia, and patients receiving Class IA (quinidine, procainamide), or Class III (amiodarone, sotalol) antiarrhythmic agents. Elderly patients may be more susceptible to drug-associated effects on the QT interval).
No products indexed under this heading.

Fluphenazine Hydrochloride (Prolongation of the QT interval and isolated cases of torsade de pointes have been reported due to levofloxacin. Levofloxacin should be avoided with other drugs that prolong the QT interval. Levofloxacin should be avoided in patients with known prolongation of the QT interval, patients with uncorrected hypokalemia, and patients receiving Class IA (quinidine, procainamide), or Class III (amiodarone, sotalol) antiarrhythmic agents. Elderly patients may be more susceptible to drug-associated effects on the QT interval).
No products indexed under this heading.

Flurbiprofen (Concomitant administration of a non-steroidal anti-inflammatory drug with a fluoroquinolone, including levofloxacin, may increase the risk of CNS stimulation and convulsive seizures).
No products indexed under this heading.

Fluticasone Furoate (Fluoroquinolones, including levofloxacin, are associated with an increased risk of tendinitis and tendon rupture in all ages. This risk is further increased in patients taking corticosteroid drugs). Products include:
Veramyst **1713**

Fluticasone Propionate (Fluoroquinolones, including levofloxacin, are associated with an increased risk of tendinitis and tendon rupture in all ages. This risk is further increased in patients taking corticosteroid drugs). Products include:
Advair 100/50 .... **1275**
Advair 250/50 .... **1275**
Advair 500/50 .... **1275**
Advair HFA 45/21 .... **1288**
Advair HFA 115/21 .... **1288**
Advair HFA 230/21 .... **1288**
Flonase **1459**
Flovent Diskus **1463**
Flovent HFA **1470**

Glibenclamide (Disturbances of blood glucose, including symptomatic hyper- and hypoglycemia, have been reported with levofloxacin, usually in diabetic patients receiving concomitant treatment with an oral hypoglycemic agent (eg, glyburide). In these patients, careful monitoring of blood glucose is recommended. If a hypoglycemic reaction occurs in a patient being treated with levofloxacin, levofloxacin, should be discontinued and appropriate therapy should be initiated immediately).
No products indexed under this heading.

Glimepiride (Disturbances of blood glucose, including symptomatic hyper- and hypoglycemia, have been reported with levofloxacin, usually in diabetic patients receiving concomitant treatment with an oral hypoglycemic agent (eg, glyburide). In these patients, careful monitoring of blood glucose is recommended. If a hypoglycemic reaction occurs in a patient being treated with levofloxacin, levofloxacin, should be discontinued and appropriate therapy should be initiated immediately). Products include:
Avandaryl **1356**
Duetact **3354**

Glipizide (Disturbances of blood glucose, including symptomatic hyper- and hypoglycemia, have been reported with levofloxacin, usually in diabetic patients receiving concomitant treatment with an oral hypoglycemic agent (eg, glyburide). In these patients, careful monitoring of blood glucose is recommended. If a hypoglycemic reaction occurs in a patient being treated with levofloxacin, levofloxacin, should be discontinued and appropriate therapy should be initiated immediately).
No products indexed under this heading.

Glyburide (Disturbances of blood glucose, including symptomatic hyper- and hypoglycemia, have been reported with levofloxacin, usually in diabetic patients receiving concomitant treatment with an oral hypoglycemic agent (eg, glyburide). In these patients, careful monitoring of blood glucose is recommended. If a hypoglycemic reaction occurs in a patient being treated with levofloxacin, levofloxacin, should be discontinued and appropriate therapy should be initiated immediately).
No products indexed under this heading.

Haloperidol (Prolongation of the QT interval and isolated cases of torsade de pointes have been reported due to levofloxacin. Levofloxacin should be avoided with other drugs that prolong the QT interval. Levofloxacin should be avoided in patients with known prolongation of the QT interval, patients with uncorrected hypokalemia, and patients receiving Class IA (quinidine, procainamide), or Class III (amiodarone, sotalol) antiarrhythmic agents. Elderly patients may be more susceptible to drug-associated effects on the QT interval).
No products indexed under this heading.

Haloperidol Decanoate (Prolongation of the QT interval and isolated cases of torsade de pointes have been reported due to levofloxacin. Levofloxacin should be avoided with other drugs that prolong the QT interval. Levofloxacin should be avoided in patients with known prolongation of the QT interval, patients with uncorrected hypokalemia, and patients receiving Class IA (quinidine, procainamide), or Class III (amiodarone, sotalol) antiarrhythmic agents. Elderly patients may be more susceptible to drug-associated effects on the QT interval).
No products indexed under this heading.

Haloperidol Lactate (Prolongation of the QT interval and isolated cases of torsade de pointes have been reported due to levofloxacin. Levofloxacin should be avoided with other drugs that prolong the QT interval. Levofloxacin should be avoided in patients with known prolongation of the QT interval, patients with uncorrected hypokalemia, and patients receiving Class IA (quinidine, procainamide), or Class III (amiodarone, sotalol) antiarrhythmic agents. Elderly patients may be more susceptible to drug-associated effects on the QT interval).
No products indexed under this heading.

Hydrocortisone (Fluoroquinolones, including levofloxacin, are associated with an increased risk of tendinitis and tendon rupture in all ages. This risk is further increased in patients taking corticosteroid drugs).
No products indexed under this heading.

Hydrocortisone (Alcohol) (Fluoroquinolones, including levofloxacin, are associated with an increased risk of tendinitis and tendon rupture in all ages. This risk is further increased in patients taking corticosteroid drugs).
No products indexed under this heading.

Hydrocortisone Acetate (Fluoroquinolones, including levofloxacin, are associated with an increased risk of tendinitis and tendon rupture in all ages. This risk is further increased in patients taking corticosteroid drugs).
No products indexed under this heading.

Hydrocortisone Butyrate (Fluoroquinolones, including levofloxacin, are associated with an increased risk of tendinitis and tendon rupture in all ages. This risk is further increased in patients taking corticosteroid drugs).
No products indexed under this heading.

Hydrocortisone Cypionate (Fluoroquinolones, including levofloxacin, are associated with an increased risk of tendinitis and tendon rupture in all ages. This risk is further increased in patients taking corticosteroid drugs).
No products indexed under this heading.

Hydrocortisone Hemisuccinate (Fluoroquinolones, including levofloxacin, are associated with an increased risk of tendinitis and tendon rupture in all ages. This risk is further increased in patients taking corticosteroid drugs).
No products indexed under this heading.

Hydrocortisone Probutate (Fluoroquinolones, including levofloxacin, are associated with an increased risk of tendinitis and tendon rupture in all ages. This risk is further increased in patients taking corticosteroid drugs).
No products indexed under this heading.

Hydrocortisone Sodium Phosphate (Fluoroquinolones, including levofloxacin, are associated with an increased risk of tendinitis and tendon rupture in all ages. This risk is further increased in patients taking corticosteroid drugs).
No products indexed under this heading.

Hydrocortisone Sodium Succinate (Fluoroquinolones, including levofloxacin, are associated with an increased risk of tendinitis and tendon rupture in all ages. This risk is further increased in patients taking corticosteroid drugs).
No products indexed under this heading.

IMPORTANT NOTE: Always consult each drug listing in the patient's regimen for possible interactions.

Hydrocortisone Valerate (Fluoroquinolones, including levofloxacin, are associated with an increased risk of tendinitis and tendon rupture in all ages. This risk is further increased in patients taking corticosteroid drugs).
No products indexed under this heading.

Hydroxyzine Hydrochloride (Prolongation of the QT interval and isolated cases of torsade de pointes have been reported due to levofloxacin. Levofloxacin should be avoided with other drugs that prolong the QT interval. Levofloxacin should be avoided in patients with known prolongation of the QT interval, patients with uncorrected hypokalemia, and patients receiving Class IA (quinidine, procainamide), or Class III (amiodarone, sotalol) antiarrhythmic agents. Elderly patients may be more susceptible to drug-associated effects on the QT interval).
No products indexed under this heading.

Ibuprofen (Concomitant administration of a non-steroidal anti-inflammatory drug with a fluoroquinolone, including levofloxacin, may increase the risk of CNS stimulation and convulsive seizures). Products include:

Imipramine Hydrochloride (Prolongation of the QT interval and isolated cases of torsade de pointes have been reported due to levofloxacin. Levofloxacin should be avoided with other drugs that prolong the QT interval. Levofloxacin should be avoided in patients with known prolongation of the QT interval, patients with uncorrected hypokalemia, and patients receiving Class IA (quinidine, procainamide), or Class III (amiodarone, sotalol) antiarrhythmic agents. Elderly patients may be more susceptible to drug-associated effects on the QT interval).
No products indexed under this heading.

Imipramine Pamoate (Prolongation of the QT interval and isolated cases of torsade de pointes have been reported due to levofloxacin. Levofloxacin should be avoided with other drugs that prolong the QT interval. Levofloxacin should be avoided in patients with known prolongation of the QT interval, patients with uncorrected hypokalemia, and patients receiving Class IA (quinidine, procainamide), or Class III (amiodarone, sotalol) antiarrhythmic agents. Elderly patients may be more susceptible to drug-associated effects on the QT interval).
No products indexed under this heading.

Indomethacin (Concomitant administration of a non-steroidal anti-inflammatory drug with a fluoroquinolone, including levofloxacin, may increase the risk of CNS stimulation and convulsive seizures). Products include:

Indomethacin Sodium Trihydrate (Concomitant administration of a non-steroidal anti-inflammatory drug with a fluoroquinolone, including levofloxacin, may increase the risk of CNS stimulation and convulsive seizures). Products include:

Insulin (Disturbances of blood glucose, including symptomatic hyper- and hypoglycemia, have been reported with levofloxacin, usually in diabetic patients receiving concomitant treatment with insulin. In these patients, careful monitoring of blood glucose is recommended. If a hypoglycemic reaction occurs in a patient being treated with levofloxacin, levofloxacin, should be discontinued and appropriate therapy should be initiated immediately).
No products indexed under this heading.

Insulin, Human, Zinc Suspension (Disturbances of blood glucose, including symptomatic hyper- and hypoglycemia, have been reported with levofloxacin, usually in diabetic patients receiving concomitant treatment with insulin. In these patients, careful monitoring of blood glucose is recommended. If a hypoglycemic reaction occurs in a patient being treated with levofloxacin, levofloxacin, should be discontinued and appropriate therapy should be initiated immediately).
No products indexed under this heading.

Insulin, Human (rDNA origin) (Disturbances of blood glucose, including symptomatic hyper- and hypoglycemia, have been reported with levofloxacin, usually in diabetic patients receiving concomitant treatment with insulin. In these patients, careful monitoring of blood glucose is recommended. If a hypoglycemic reaction occurs in a patient being treated with levofloxacin, levofloxacin, should be discontinued and appropriate therapy should be initiated immediately). Products include:

Insulin, Human NPH (Disturbances of blood glucose, including symptomatic hyper- and hypoglycemia, have been reported with levofloxacin, usually in diabetic patients receiving concomitant treatment with insulin. In these patients, careful monitoring of blood glucose is recommended. If a hypoglycemic reaction occurs in a patient being treated with levofloxacin, levofloxacin, should be discontinued and appropriate therapy should be initiated immediately). Products include:

Insulin, Human Regular (Disturbances of blood glucose, including symptomatic hyper- and hypoglycemia, have been reported with levofloxacin, usually in diabetic patients receiving concomitant treatment with insulin. In these patients, careful monitoring of blood glucose is recommended. If a hypoglycemic reaction occurs in a patient being treated with levofloxacin, levofloxacin, should be discontinued and appropriate therapy should be initiated immediately). Products include:

Insulin, Human Regular and Human NPH Mixture (Disturbances of blood glucose, including symptomatic hyper- and hypoglycemia, have been reported with levofloxacin, usually in diabetic patients receiving concomitant treatment with insulin. In these patients, careful monitoring of blood glucose is recommended. If a hypoglycemic reaction occurs in a patient being treated with levofloxacin, levofloxacin, should be discontinued and appropriate therapy should be initiated immediately). Products include:

Insulin, NPH (Disturbances of blood glucose, including symptomatic hyper- and hypoglycemia, have been reported with levofloxacin, usually in diabetic patients receiving concomitant treatment with insulin. In these patients, careful monitoring of blood glucose is recommended. If a hypoglycemic reaction occurs in a patient being treated with levofloxacin, levofloxacin, should be discontinued and appropriate therapy should be initiated immediately).
No products indexed under this heading.

Insulin, Regular (Disturbances of blood glucose, including symptomatic hyper- and hypoglycemia, have been reported with levofloxacin, usually in diabetic patients receiving concomitant treatment with insulin. In these patients, careful monitoring of blood glucose is recommended. If a hypoglycemic reaction occurs in a patient being treated with levofloxacin, levofloxacin, should be discontinued and appropriate therapy should be initiated immediately).
No products indexed under this heading.

Insulin, Regular and NPH mixture (Disturbances of blood glucose, including symptomatic hyper- and hypoglycemia, have been reported with levofloxacin, usually in diabetic patients receiving concomitant treatment with insulin. In these patients, careful monitoring of blood glucose is recommended. If a hypoglycemic reaction occurs in a patient being treated with levofloxacin, levofloxacin, should be discontinued and appropriate therapy should be initiated immediately).
No products indexed under this heading.

Insulin, Zinc Crystals (Disturbances of blood glucose, including symptomatic hyper- and hypoglycemia, have been reported with levofloxacin, usually in diabetic patients receiving concomitant treatment with insulin. In these patients, careful monitoring of blood glucose is recommended. If a hypoglycemic reaction occurs in a patient being treated with levofloxacin, levofloxacin, should be discontinued and appropriate therapy should be initiated immediately).
No products indexed under this heading.

Insulin, Zinc Suspension (Disturbances of blood glucose, including symptomatic hyper- and hypoglycemia, have been reported with levofloxacin, usually in diabetic patients receiving concomitant treatment with insulin. In these patients, careful monitoring of blood glucose is recommended. If a hypoglycemic reaction occurs in a patient being treated with levofloxacin, levofloxacin, should be discontinued and appropriate therapy should be initiated immediately).
No products indexed under this heading.

Insulin Aspart (Disturbances of blood glucose, including symptomatic hyper- and hypoglycemia, have been reported with levofloxacin, usually in diabetic patients receiving concomitant treatment with insulin. In these patients, careful monitoring of blood glucose is recommended. If a hypoglycemic reaction occurs in a patient being treated with levofloxacin, levofloxacin, should be discontinued and appropriate therapy should be initiated immediately).
No products indexed under this heading.

Insulin Aspart, Human (Disturbances of blood glucose, including symptomatic hyper- and hypoglycemia, have been reported with levofloxacin, usually in diabetic patients receiving concomitant treatment with insulin. In these patients, careful monitoring of blood glucose is recommended. If a hypoglycemic reaction occurs in a patient being treated with levofloxacin, levofloxacin, should be discontinued and appropriate therapy should be initiated immediately). Products include:

Insulin Aspart, Human Regular (Disturbances of blood glucose, including symptomatic hyper- and hypoglycemia, have been reported with levofloxacin, usually in diabetic patients receiving concomitant treatment with insulin. In these patients, careful monitoring of blood glucose is recommended. If a hypoglycemic reaction occurs in a patient being treated with levofloxacin, levofloxacin, should be discontinued and appropriate therapy should be initiated immediately). Products include:

Insulin Aspart Protamine, Human (Disturbances of blood glucose, including symptomatic hyper- and hypoglycemia, have been reported with levofloxacin, usually in diabetic patients receiving concomitant treatment with insulin. In these patients, careful monitoring of blood glucose is recommended. If a hypoglycemic reaction occurs in a patient being treated with levofloxacin, levofloxacin, should be discontinued and appropriate therapy should be initiated immediately). Products include:

Insulin Detemir (rDNA Origin) (Disturbances of blood glucose, including symptomatic hyper- and hypoglycemia, have been reported with levofloxacin, usually in diabetic patients receiving concomitant treatment with insulin. In these patients, careful monitoring of blood glucose is recommended. If a hypoglycemic reaction occurs in a patient being treated with levofloxacin, levofloxacin, should be discontinued and appropriate therapy should be initiated immediately). Products include:

Insulin Glargine (Disturbances of blood glucose, including symptomatic hyper- and hypoglycemia, have been reported with levofloxacin, usually in diabetic patients receiving concomitant treatment with insulin. In these patients, careful monitoring of blood glucose is recommended. If a hypoglycemic reaction occurs in a patient being treated with levofloxacin, levofloxacin, should be discontinued and appropriate therapy should be initiated immediately). Products include:

Insulin Glulisine (Disturbances of blood glucose, including symptomatic hyper- and hypoglycemia, have been reported with levofloxacin, usually in diabetic patients receiving concomitant treatment with insulin. In these patients, careful monitoring of blood glucose is recommended. If a hypoglycemic reaction occurs in a patient being treated with levofloxacin, levofloxacin, should be discontinued and appropriate therapy should be initiated immediately). Products include:

Insulin Lispro, Human (Disturbances of blood glucose, including symptomatic hyper- and hypoglycemia, have been reported with levofloxacin, usually in diabetic patients receiving concomitant treatment with insulin. In these patients, careful monitoring of blood glucose is recommended. If a hypoglycemic reaction occurs in a patient being treated with levofloxacin, levofloxacin, should be discontinued and appropriate therapy should be initiated immediately). Products include:

Insulin Lispro Protamine, Human (Disturbances of blood glucose, including symptomatic hyper- and hypoglycemia, have been reported with levofloxacin, usually in diabetic patients receiving concomitant treatment with insulin. In these patients, careful monitoring of blood glucose is recommended. If a hypoglycemic reaction occurs in a patient being treated with levofloxacin, levofloxacin, should be discontinued and appropriate therapy should be initiated immediately). Products include:

(⊙ Described in PDR® for Ophthalmic Medicines)

1001 Interactions Index Levaquin Tablets

Iron (Concurrent administration of levofloxacin tablets/oral solution with metal cations such as iron may interfere with the gastrointestinal absorption of levofloxacin, resulting in systemic levels considerably lower than desired. These agents should be taken at least two hours before or two hours after levofloxacin administration).
No products indexed under this heading.

Iron, Peptonized (Concurrent administration of levofloxacin tablets/oral solution with metal cations such as iron may interfere with the gastrointestinal absorption of levofloxacin, resulting in systemic levels considerably lower than desired. These agents should be taken at least two hours before or two hours after levofloxacin administration).
No products indexed under this heading.

Iron & Ammonium Citrate (Concurrent administration of levofloxacin tablets/oral solution with metal cations such as iron may interfere with the gastrointestinal absorption of levofloxacin, resulting in systemic levels considerably lower than desired. These agents should be taken at least two hours before or two hours after levofloxacin administration).
No products indexed under this heading.

Iron Cacodylate (Concurrent administration of levofloxacin tablets/oral solution with metal cations such as iron may interfere with the gastrointestinal absorption of levofloxacin, resulting in systemic levels considerably lower than desired. These agents should be taken at least two hours before or two hours after levofloxacin administration).
No products indexed under this heading.

Iron Carbonyl (Concurrent administration of levofloxacin tablets/oral solution with metal cations such as iron may interfere with the gastrointestinal absorption of levofloxacin, resulting in systemic levels considerably lower than desired. These agents should be taken at least two hours before or two hours after levofloxacin administration).
Products include:
CitraNatal 90 DHA Capsules 2332
CitraNatal Assure 2332
CitraNatal Harmony 2332
CitraNatal Rx 2332
Ferralet 2333

Iron Supplements (Concurrent administration of levofloxacin tablets/oral solution with metal cations such as iron may interfere with the gastrointestinal absorption of levofloxacin, resulting in systemic levels considerably lower than desired. These agents should be taken at least two hours before or two hours after levofloxacin administration).
No products indexed under this heading.

Isocarboxazid (Prolongation of the QT interval and isolated cases of torsade de pointes have been reported due to levofloxacin. Levofloxacin should be avoided with other drugs that prolong the QT interval. Levofloxacin should be avoided in patients with known prolongation of the QT interval, patients with uncorrected hypokalemia, and patients receiving Class IA (quinidine, procainamide), or Class III (amiodarone, sotalol) antiarrhythmic agents. Elderly patients may be more susceptible to drug-associated effects on the QT interval). Products include:
Marplan 3481

Ketoprofen (Concomitant administration of a non-steroidal anti-inflammatory drug with a fluoroquinolone, including levofloxacin, may increase the risk of CNS stimulation and convulsive seizures).
No products indexed under this heading.

Ketorolac Tromethamine (Concomitant administration of a non-steroidal anti-inflammatory drug with a fluoroquinolone, including levofloxacin, may increase the risk of CNS stimulation and convulsive seizures). Products include:
Acuvail .... ⊙ 209

Lidocaine (Prolongation of the QT interval and isolated cases of torsade de pointes have been reported due to levofloxacin. Levofloxacin should be avoided with other drugs that prolong the QT interval. Levofloxacin should be avoided in patients with known prolongation of the QT interval, patients with uncorrected hypokalemia, and patients receiving Class IA (quinidine, procainamide), or Class III (amiodarone, sotalol) antiarrhythmic agents. Elderly patients may be more susceptible to drug-associated effects on the QT interval).
Products include:
Lidoderm 1107

Lidocaine Hydrochloride (Prolongation of the QT interval and isolated cases of torsade de pointes have been reported due to levofloxacin. Levofloxacin should be avoided with other drugs that prolong the QT interval. Levofloxacin should be avoided in patients with known prolongation of the QT interval, patients with uncorrected hypokalemia, and patients receiving Class IA (quinidine, procainamide), or Class III (amiodarone, sotalol) antiarrhythmic agents. Elderly patients may be more susceptible to drug-associated effects on the QT interval).
No products indexed under this heading.

Lithium Carbonate (Prolongation of the QT interval and isolated cases of torsade de pointes have been reported due to levofloxacin. Levofloxacin should be avoided with other drugs that prolong the QT interval. Levofloxacin should be avoided in patients with known prolongation of the QT interval, patients with uncorrected hypokalemia, and patients receiving Class IA (quinidine, procainamide), or Class III (amiodarone, sotalol) antiarrhythmic agents. Elderly patients may be more susceptible to drug-associated effects on the QT interval).
No products indexed under this heading.

Lithium Citrate (Prolongation of the QT interval and isolated cases of torsade de pointes have been reported due to levofloxacin. Levofloxacin should be avoided with other drugs that prolong the QT interval. Levofloxacin should be avoided in patients with known prolongation of the QT interval, patients with uncorrected hypokalemia, and patients receiving Class IA (quinidine, procainamide), or Class III (amiodarone, sotalol) antiarrhythmic agents. Elderly patients may be more susceptible to drug-associated effects on the QT interval).
No products indexed under this heading.

Lorazepam (Prolongation of the QT interval and isolated cases of torsade de pointes have been reported due to levofloxacin. Levofloxacin should be avoided with other drugs that prolong the QT interval. Levofloxacin should be avoided in patients with known prolongation of the QT interval, patients with uncorrected hypokalemia, and patients receiving Class IA (quinidine, procainamide), or Class III (amiodarone, sotalol) antiarrhythmic agents. Elderly patients may be more susceptible to drug-associated effects on the QT interval).
No products indexed under this heading.

Loxapine Hydrochloride (Prolongation of the QT interval and isolated cases of torsade de pointes have been reported due to levofloxacin. Levofloxacin should be avoided with other drugs that prolong the QT interval. Levofloxacin should be avoided in patients with known prolongation of the QT interval, patients with uncorrected hypokalemia, and patients receiving Class IA (quinidine, procainamide), or Class III (amiodarone, sotalol) antiarrhythmic agents. Elderly patients may be more susceptible to drug-associated effects on the QT interval).
No products indexed under this heading.

Loxapine Succinate (Prolongation of the QT interval and isolated cases of torsade de pointes have been reported due to levofloxacin. Levofloxacin should be avoided with other drugs that prolong the QT interval. Levofloxacin should be avoided in patients with known prolongation of the QT interval, patients with uncorrected hypokalemia, and patients receiving Class IA (quinidine, procainamide), or Class III (amiodarone, sotalol) antiarrhythmic agents. Elderly patients may be more susceptible to drug-associated effects on the QT interval).
No products indexed under this heading.

Magaldrate (Concurrent administration of levofloxacin tablets/oral solution with antacids containing magnesium, or aluminum may interfere with the gastrointestinal absorption of levofloxacin, resulting in systemic levels considerably lower than desired. These agents should be taken at least two hours before or two hours after levofloxacin administration).
No products indexed under this heading.

Magnesium (Concurrent administration of levofloxacin tablets/oral solution with metal cations such as iron may interfere with the gastrointestinal absorption of levofloxacin, resulting in systemic levels considerably lower than desired. These agents should be taken at least two hours before or two hours after levofloxacin administration).
Products include:
BoneMate Plus 3454
Cardio Basics 3455
Chelated Mineral 3476

Magnesium Aluminum Silicate (Concurrent administration of levofloxacin tablets/oral solution with metal cations such as iron may interfere with the gastrointestinal absorption of levofloxacin, resulting in systemic levels considerably lower than desired. These agents should be taken at least two hours before or two hours after levofloxacin administration).
No products indexed under this heading.

Magnesium Carbonate (Concurrent administration of levofloxacin tablets/oral solution with antacids containing magnesium, or aluminum may interfere with the gastrointestinal absorption of levofloxacin, resulting in systemic levels considerably lower than desired. These agents should be taken at least two hours before or two hours after levofloxacin administration).
No products indexed under this heading.

Magnesium Chloride (Concurrent administration of levofloxacin tablets/oral solution with metal cations such as iron may interfere with the gastrointestinal absorption of levofloxacin, resulting in systemic levels considerably lower than desired. These agents should be taken at least two hours before or two hours after levofloxacin administration).
No products indexed under this heading.

Magnesium Citrate (Concurrent administration of levofloxacin tablets/oral solution with metal cations such as iron may interfere with the gastrointestinal absorption of levofloxacin, resulting in systemic levels considerably lower than desired. These agents should be taken at least two hours before or two hours after levofloxacin administration).
Products include:
Chelated Mineral 3476

Magnesium Gluconate (Concurrent administration of levofloxacin tablets/oral solution with metal cations such as iron may interfere with the gastrointestinal absorption of levofloxacin, resulting in systemic levels considerably lower than desired. These agents should be taken at least two hours before or two hours after levofloxacin administration).
No products indexed under this heading.

Magnesium Hydroxide (Concurrent administration of levofloxacin tablets/oral solution with antacids containing magnesium, or aluminum may interfere with the gastrointestinal absorption of levofloxacin, resulting in systemic levels considerably lower than desired. These agents should be taken at least two hours before or two hours after levofloxacin administration). Products include:
Fleet Pedia-Lax Chewable Tablets 1144
Pepcid Complete 1822

Magnesium Lactate (Concurrent administration of levofloxacin tablets/oral solution with metal cations such as iron may interfere with the gastrointestinal absorption of levofloxacin, resulting in systemic levels considerably lower than desired. These agents should be taken at least two hours before or two hours after levofloxacin administration).
No products indexed under this heading.

Magnesium Oxide (Concurrent administration of levofloxacin tablets/oral solution with antacids containing magnesium, or aluminum may interfere with the gastrointestinal absorption of levofloxacin, resulting in systemic levels considerably lower than desired. These agents should be taken at least two hours before or two hours after levofloxacin administration). Products include:
Beelith 873

Magnesium Salicylate (Concurrent administration of levofloxacin tablets/oral solution with metal cations such as iron may interfere with the gastrointestinal absorption of levofloxacin, resulting in systemic levels considerably lower than desired. These agents should be taken at least two hours before or two hours after levofloxacin administration).
No products indexed under this heading.

Magnesium Salicylate Tetrahydrate (Concurrent administration of levofloxacin tablets/oral solution with metal cations such as iron may interfere with the gastrointestinal absorption of levofloxacin, resulting in systemic levels considerably lower than desired. These agents should be taken at least two hours before or two hours after levofloxacin administration).
No products indexed under this heading.

Magnesium Salts (Concurrent administration of levofloxacin tablets/oral solution with metal cations such as iron may interfere with the gastrointestinal absorption of levofloxacin, resulting in systemic levels considerably lower than desired. These agents should be taken at least two hours before or two hours after levofloxacin administration).
No products indexed under this heading.

Magnesium Sulfate (Concurrent administration of levofloxacin tablets/oral solution with metal cations such as iron may interfere with the gastrointestinal absorption of levofloxacin, resulting in systemic levels considerably lower than desired. These agents should be taken at least two hours before or two hours after levofloxacin administration).
No products indexed under this heading.

IMPORTANT NOTE: Always consult each drug listing in the patient's regimen for possible interactions.

Magnesium Trisilicate (Concurrent administration of levofloxacin tablets/oral solution with antacids containing magnesium, or aluminum may interfere with the gastrointestinal absorption of levofloxacin, resulting in systemic levels considerably lower than desired. These agents should be taken at least two hours before or two hours after levofloxacin administration).

No products indexed under this heading.

Maprotiline Hydrochloride (Prolongation of the QT interval and isolated cases of torsade de pointes have been reported due to levofloxacin. Levofloxacin should be avoided with other drugs that prolong the QT interval. Levofloxacin should be avoided in patients with known prolongation of the QT interval, patients with uncorrected hypokalemia, and patients receiving Class IA (quinidine, procainamide), or Class III (amiodarone, sotalol) antiarrhythmic agents. Elderly patients may be more susceptible to drug-associated effects on the QT interval).

No products indexed under this heading.

Meclofenamate Sodium (Concomitant administration of a non-steroidal anti-inflammatory drug with a fluoroquinolone, including levofloxacin, may increase the risk of CNS stimulation and convulsive seizures).

No products indexed under this heading.

Mefenamic Acid (Concomitant administration of a non-steroidal anti-inflammatory drug with a fluoroquinolone, including levofloxacin, may increase the risk of CNS stimulation and convulsive seizures).

No products indexed under this heading.

Meloxicam (Concomitant administration of a non-steroidal anti-inflammatory drug with a fluoroquinolone, including levofloxacin, may increase the risk of CNS stimulation and convulsive seizures).

No products indexed under this heading.

Meprobamate (Prolongation of the QT interval and isolated cases of torsade de pointes have been reported due to levofloxacin. Levofloxacin should be avoided with other drugs that prolong the QT interval. Levofloxacin should be avoided in patients with known prolongation of the QT interval, patients with uncorrected hypokalemia, and patients receiving Class IA (quinidine, procainamide), or Class III (amiodarone, sotalol) antiarrhythmic agents. Elderly patients may be more susceptible to drug-associated effects on the QT interval).

No products indexed under this heading.

Mesoridazine Besylate (Prolongation of the QT interval and isolated cases of torsade de pointes have been reported due to levofloxacin. Levofloxacin should be avoided with other drugs that prolong the QT interval. Levofloxacin should be avoided in patients with known prolongation of the QT interval, patients with uncorrected hypokalemia, and patients receiving Class IA (quinidine, procainamide), or Class III (amiodarone, sotalol) antiarrhythmic agents. Elderly patients may be more susceptible to drug-associated effects on the QT interval).

No products indexed under this heading.

Metformin Hydrochloride (Disturbances of blood glucose, including symptomatic hyper- and hypoglycemia, have been reported with levofloxacin, usually in diabetic patients receiving concomitant treatment with an oral hypoglycemic agent (eg, glyburide). In these patients, careful monitoring of blood glucose is recommended. If a hypoglycemic reaction occurs in a patient being treated with levofloxacin, levofloxacin,

should be discontinued and appropriate therapy should be initiated immediately). Products include:

Methylprednisolone (Fluoroquinolones, including levofloxacin, are associated with an increased risk of tendinitis and tendon rupture in all ages. This risk is further increased in patients taking corticosteroid drugs).

No products indexed under this heading.

Methylprednisolone Acetate (Fluoroquinolones, including levofloxacin, are associated with an increased risk of tendinitis and tendon rupture in all ages. This risk is further increased in patients taking corticosteroid drugs).

No products indexed under this heading.

Methylprednisolone Sodium Succinate (Fluoroquinolones, including levofloxacin, are associated with an increased risk of tendinitis and tendon rupture in all ages. This risk is further increased in patients taking corticosteroid drugs).

No products indexed under this heading.

Mexiletine Hydrochloride (Prolongation of the QT interval and isolated cases of torsade de pointes have been reported due to levofloxacin. Levofloxacin should be avoided with other drugs that prolong the QT interval. Levofloxacin should be avoided in patients with known prolongation of the QT interval, patients with uncorrected hypokalemia, and patients receiving Class IA (quinidine, procainamide), or Class III (amiodarone, sotalol) antiarrhythmic agents. Elderly patients may be more susceptible to drug-associated effects on the QT interval).

No products indexed under this heading.

Midazolam Hydrochloride (Prolongation of the QT interval and isolated cases of torsade de pointes have been reported due to levofloxacin. Levofloxacin should be avoided with other drugs that prolong the QT interval. Levofloxacin should be avoided in patients with known prolongation of the QT interval, patients with uncorrected hypokalemia, and patients receiving Class IA (quinidine, procainamide), or Class III (amiodarone, sotalol) antiarrhythmic agents. Elderly patients may be more susceptible to drug-associated effects on the QT interval).

No products indexed under this heading.

Miglitol (Disturbances of blood glucose, including symptomatic hyper- and hypoglycemia, have been reported with levofloxacin, usually in diabetic patients receiving concomitant treatment with an oral hypoglycemic agent (eg, glyburide). In these patients, careful monitoring of blood glucose is recommended. If a hypoglycemic reaction occurs in a patient being treated with levofloxacin, levofloxacin, should be discontinued and appropriate therapy should be initiated immediately).

No products indexed under this heading.

Molindone Hydrochloride (Prolongation of the QT interval and isolated cases of torsade de pointes have been reported due to levofloxacin. Levofloxacin should be avoided with other drugs that prolong the QT interval. Levofloxacin should be avoided in patients with known prolongation of the QT interval, patients with uncorrected hypokalemia, and patients receiving Class IA (quinidine, procainamide), or Class III (amiodarone, sotalol) antiarrhythmic agents. Elderly patients may be more susceptible to drug-associated effects on the QT interval). Products include:

Mometasone Furoate (Fluoroquinolones, including levofloxacin, are associated with an increased risk of tendinitis and tendon rupture in all ages. This risk is further increased in patients taking corticosteroid drugs). Products include:

Mometasone Furoate Monohydrate (Fluoroquinolones, including levofloxacin, are associated with an increased risk of tendinitis and tendon rupture in all ages. This risk is further increased in patients taking corticosteroid drugs). Products include:

Moricizine Hydrochloride (Levofloxacin should be avoided in patients with known prolongation of the QT interval, patients with uncorrected hypokalemia, and patients receiving Class IA (quinidine, procainamide) antiarrhythmic agents. Elderly patients may be more susceptible to drug-associated effects on the QT interval).

No products indexed under this heading.

Nabumetone (Concomitant administration of a non-steroidal anti-inflammatory drug with a fluoroquinolone, including levofloxacin, may increase the risk of CNS stimulation and convulsive seizures).

No products indexed under this heading.

Naproxen (Concomitant administration of a non-steroidal anti-inflammatory drug with a fluoroquinolone, including levofloxacin, may increase the risk of CNS stimulation and convulsive seizures). Products include:

Naproxen Sodium (Concomitant administration of a non-steroidal anti-inflammatory drug with a fluoroquinolone, including levofloxacin, may increase the risk of CNS stimulation and convulsive seizures). Products include:

Nateglinide (Disturbances of blood glucose, including symptomatic hyper- and hypoglycemia, have been reported with levofloxacin, usually in diabetic patients receiving concomitant treatment with an oral hypoglycemic agent (eg, glyburide). In these patients, careful monitoring of blood glucose is recommended. If a hypoglycemic reaction occurs in a patient being treated with levofloxacin, levofloxacin, should be discontinued and appropriate therapy should be initiated immediately).

No products indexed under this heading.

Nortriptyline Hydrochloride (Prolongation of the QT interval and isolated cases of torsade de pointes have been reported due to levofloxacin. Levofloxacin should be avoided with other drugs that prolong the QT interval. Levofloxacin should be avoided in patients with known prolongation of the QT interval, patients with uncorrected hypokalemia, and patients receiving Class IA (quinidine, procainamide), or Class III (amiodarone, sotalol) antiarrhythmic agents. Elderly patients may be more susceptible to drug-associated effects on the QT interval).

No products indexed under this heading.

Olanzapine (Prolongation of the QT interval and isolated cases of torsade de pointes have been reported due to levofloxacin. Levofloxacin should be avoided with other drugs that prolong the QT interval. Levofloxacin should be avoided in patients with known prolongation of the QT interval, patients with uncorrected hypokalemia, and patients receiving Class IA (quinidine, procainamide), or Class III (amiodarone, sotalol)

antiarrhythmic agents. Elderly patients may be more susceptible to drug-associated effects on the QT interval). Products include:

Oxaprozin (Concomitant administration of a non-steroidal anti-inflammatory drug with a fluoroquinolone, including levofloxacin, may increase the risk of CNS stimulation and convulsive seizures).

No products indexed under this heading.

Oxazepam (Prolongation of the QT interval and isolated cases of torsade de pointes have been reported due to levofloxacin. Levofloxacin should be avoided with other drugs that prolong the QT interval. Levofloxacin should be avoided in patients with known prolongation of the QT interval, patients with uncorrected hypokalemia, and patients receiving Class IA (quinidine, procainamide), or Class III (amiodarone, sotalol) antiarrhythmic agents. Elderly patients may be more susceptible to drug-associated effects on the QT interval).

No products indexed under this heading.

Perphenazine (Prolongation of the QT interval and isolated cases of torsade de pointes have been reported due to levofloxacin. Levofloxacin should be avoided with other drugs that prolong the QT interval. Levofloxacin should be avoided in patients with known prolongation of the QT interval, patients with uncorrected hypokalemia, and patients receiving Class IA (quinidine, procainamide), or Class III (amiodarone, sotalol) antiarrhythmic agents. Elderly patients may be more susceptible to drug-associated effects on the QT interval).

No products indexed under this heading.

Phenelzine Sulfate (Prolongation of the QT interval and isolated cases of torsade de pointes have been reported due to levofloxacin. Levofloxacin should be avoided with other drugs that prolong the QT interval. Levofloxacin should be avoided in patients with known prolongation of the QT interval, patients with uncorrected hypokalemia, and patients receiving Class IA (quinidine, procainamide), or Class III (amiodarone, sotalol) antiarrhythmic agents. Elderly patients may be more susceptible to drug-associated effects on the QT interval).

No products indexed under this heading.

Phenylbutazone (Concomitant administration of a non-steroidal anti-inflammatory drug with a fluoroquinolone, including levofloxacin, may increase the risk of CNS stimulation and convulsive seizures).

No products indexed under this heading.

Pioglitazone Hydrochloride (Disturbances of blood glucose, including symptomatic hyper- and hypoglycemia, have been reported with levofloxacin, usually in diabetic patients receiving concomitant treatment with an oral hypoglycemic agent (eg, glyburide). In these patients, careful monitoring of blood glucose is recommended. If a hypoglycemic reaction occurs in a patient being treated with levofloxacin, levofloxacin, should be discontinued and appropriate therapy should be initiated immediately). Products include:

Piroxicam (Concomitant administration of a non-steroidal anti-inflammatory drug with a fluoroquinolone, including levofloxacin, may increase the risk of CNS stimulation and convulsive seizures).

No products indexed under this heading.

(⊙ Described in PDR® for Ophthalmic Medicines)

Polysaccharide Iron Complex (Concurrent administration of levofloxacin tablets/oral solution with metal cations such as iron may interfere with the gastrointestinal absorption of levofloxacin, resulting in systemic levels considerably lower than desired. These agents should be taken at least two hours before or two hours after levofloxacin administration). Products include:

Prazepam (Prolongation of the QT interval and isolated cases of torsade de pointes have been reported due to levofloxacin. Levofloxacin should be avoided with other drugs that prolong the QT interval. Levofloxacin should be avoided in patients with known prolongation of the QT interval, patients with uncorrected hypokalemia, and patients receiving Class IA (quinidine, procainamide), or Class III (amiodarone, sotalol) antiarrhythmic agents. Elderly patients may be more susceptible to drug-associated effects on the QT interval).
No products indexed under this heading.

Prednisolone (Fluoroquinolones, including levofloxacin, are associated with an increased risk of tendinitis and tendon rupture in all ages. This risk is further increased in patients taking corticosteroid drugs).
No products indexed under this heading.

Prednisolone Acetate (Fluoroquinolones, including levofloxacin, are associated with an increased risk of tendinitis and tendon rupture in all ages. This risk is further increased in patients taking corticosteroid drugs). Products include:

Prednisolone Sodium Phosphate (Fluoroquinolones, including levofloxacin, are associated with an increased risk of tendinitis and tendon rupture in all ages. This risk is further increased in patients taking corticosteroid drugs).
No products indexed under this heading.

Prednisolone Tebutate (Fluoroquinolones, including levofloxacin, are associated with an increased risk of tendinitis and tendon rupture in all ages. This risk is further increased in patients taking corticosteroid drugs).
No products indexed under this heading.

Prednisone (Fluoroquinolones, including levofloxacin, are associated with an increased risk of tendinitis and tendon rupture in all ages. This risk is further increased in patients taking corticosteroid drugs).
No products indexed under this heading.

Prednisone sodium phosphate (Fluoroquinolones, including levofloxacin, are associated with an increased risk of tendinitis and tendon rupture in all ages. This risk is further increased in patients taking corticosteroid drugs).
No products indexed under this heading.

Probenecid (The AUC and $t_{1/2}$ of levofloxacin were higher while CL/F and CL_R were lower during concomitant treatment of levofloxacin with probenecid compared to levofloxacin alone).
No products indexed under this heading.

Procainamide (Levofloxacin should be avoided in patients with known prolongation of the QT interval, patients with uncorrected hypokalemia, and patients receiving Class IA (eg, procainamide) antiarrhythmic agents. Elderly patients may be more susceptible to drug-associated effects on the QT interval).
No products indexed under this heading.

Procainamide Hydrochloride (Levofloxacin should be avoided in patients with known prolongation of the QT interval, patients with uncorrected hypokalemia, and patients receiving Class IA (eg, procainamide) antiarrhythmic agents. Elderly patients may be more susceptible to drug-associated effects on the QT interval).
No products indexed under this heading.

Prochlorperazine (Prolongation of the QT interval and isolated cases of torsade de pointes have been reported due to levofloxacin. Levofloxacin should be avoided with other drugs that prolong the QT interval. Levofloxacin should be avoided in patients with known prolongation of the QT interval, patients with uncorrected hypokalemia, and patients receiving Class IA (quinidine, procainamide), or Class III (amiodarone, sotalol) antiarrhythmic agents. Elderly patients may be more susceptible to drug-associated effects on the QT interval).
No products indexed under this heading.

Promethazine Hydrochloride (Prolongation of the QT interval and isolated cases of torsade de pointes have been reported due to levofloxacin. Levofloxacin should be avoided with other drugs that prolong the QT interval. Levofloxacin should be avoided in patients with known prolongation of the QT interval, patients with uncorrected hypokalemia, and patients receiving Class IA (quinidine, procainamide), or Class III (amiodarone, sotalol) antiarrhythmic agents. Elderly patients may be more susceptible to drug-associated effects on the QT interval).
No products indexed under this heading.

Propafenone Hydrochloride (Prolongation of the QT interval and isolated cases of torsade de pointes have been reported due to levofloxacin. Levofloxacin should be avoided with other drugs that prolong the QT interval. Levofloxacin should be avoided in patients with known prolongation of the QT interval, patients with uncorrected hypokalemia, and patients receiving Class IA (quinidine, procainamide), or Class III (amiodarone, sotalol) antiarrhythmic agents. Elderly patients may be more susceptible to drug-associated effects on the QT interval). Products include:

Protriptyline Hydrochloride (Prolongation of the QT interval and isolated cases of torsade de pointes have been reported due to levofloxacin. Levofloxacin should be avoided with other drugs that prolong the QT interval. Levofloxacin should be avoided in patients with known prolongation of the QT interval, patients with uncorrected hypokalemia, and patients receiving Class IA (quinidine, procainamide), or Class III (amiodarone, sotalol) antiarrhythmic agents. Elderly patients may be more susceptible to drug-associated effects on the QT interval).
No products indexed under this heading.

Quetiapine Fumarate (Prolongation of the QT interval and isolated cases of torsade de pointes have been reported due to levofloxacin. Levofloxacin should be avoided with other drugs that prolong the QT interval. Levofloxacin should be avoided in patients with known prolongation of the QT interval, patients with uncorrected hypokalemia, and patients receiving Class IA (quinidine, procainamide), or Class III (amiodarone, sotalol) antiarrhythmic agents. Elderly patients may be more susceptible to drug-associated effects on the QT interval). Products include:

Quinidine (Levofloxacin should be avoided in patients with known prolongation of the QT interval, patients with uncorrected hypokalemia, and patients receiving Class IA (eg, quinidine) antiarrhythmic agents. Elderly patients may be more susceptible to drug-associated effects on the QT interval).
No products indexed under this heading.

Quinidine Gluconate (Levofloxacin should be avoided in patients with known prolongation of the QT interval, patients with uncorrected hypokalemia, and patients receiving Class IA (eg, quinidine) antiarrhythmic agents. Elderly patients may be more susceptible to drug-associated effects on the QT interval).
No products indexed under this heading.

Quinidine Hydrochloride (Levofloxacin should be avoided in patients with known prolongation of the QT interval, patients with uncorrected hypokalemia, and patients receiving Class IA (eg, quinidine) antiarrhythmic agents. Elderly patients may be more susceptible to drug-associated effects on the QT interval).
No products indexed under this heading.

Quinidine Polygalacturonate (Levofloxacin should be avoided in patients with known prolongation of the QT interval, patients with uncorrected hypokalemia, and patients receiving Class IA (eg, quinidine) antiarrhythmic agents. Elderly patients may be more susceptible to drug-associated effects on the QT interval).
No products indexed under this heading.

Quinidine Sulfate (Levofloxacin should be avoided in patients with known prolongation of the QT interval, patients with uncorrected hypokalemia, and patients receiving Class IA (eg, quinidine) antiarrhythmic agents. Elderly patients may be more susceptible to drug-associated effects on the QT interval).
No products indexed under this heading.

Repaglinide (Disturbances of blood glucose, including symptomatic hyper- and hypoglycemia, have been reported with levofloxacin, usually in diabetic patients receiving concomitant treatment with an oral hypoglycemic agent (eg, glyburide). In these patients, careful monitoring of blood glucose is recommended. If a hypoglycemic reaction occurs in a patient being treated with levofloxacin, levofloxacin, should be discontinued and appropriate therapy should be initiated immediately).
No products indexed under this heading.

Risperidone (Prolongation of the QT interval and isolated cases of torsade de pointes have been reported due to levofloxacin. Levofloxacin should be avoided with other drugs that prolong the QT interval. Levofloxacin should be avoided in patients with known prolongation of the QT interval, patients with uncorrected hypokalemia, and patients receiving Class IA (quinidine, procainamide), or Class III (amiodarone, sotalol) antiarrhythmic agents. Elderly patients may be more susceptible to drug-associated effects on the QT interval). Products include:

Rofecoxib (Concomitant administration of a non-steroidal anti-inflammatory drug with a fluoroquinolone, including levofloxacin, may increase the risk of CNS stimulation and convulsive seizures).
No products indexed under this heading.

Rosiglitazone Maleate (Disturbances of blood glucose, including symptomatic hyper- and hypoglycemia, have been reported with levofloxacin, usually in diabetic patients receiving concomitant treatment with an oral hypoglyce-

mic agent (eg, glyburide). In these patients, careful monitoring of blood glucose is recommended. If a hypoglycemic reaction occurs in a patient being treated with levofloxacin, levofloxacin, should be discontinued and appropriate therapy should be initiated immediately). Products include:

Selenium (Concurrent administration of levofloxacin tablets/oral solution with metal cations such as iron may interfere with the gastrointestinal absorption of levofloxacin, resulting in systemic levels considerably lower than desired. These agents should be taken at least two hours before or two hours after levofloxacin administration). Products include:

Selenium Sulfide (Concurrent administration of levofloxacin tablets/oral solution with metal cations such as iron may interfere with the gastrointestinal absorption of levofloxacin, resulting in systemic levels considerably lower than desired. These agents should be taken at least two hours before or two hours after levofloxacin administration).
No products indexed under this heading.

Sitagliptin Phosphate (Disturbances of blood glucose, including symptomatic hyper- and hypoglycemia, have been reported with levofloxacin, usually in diabetic patients receiving concomitant treatment with an oral hypoglycemic agent (eg, glyburide). In these patients, careful monitoring of blood glucose is recommended. If a hypoglycemic reaction occurs in a patient being treated with levofloxacin, levofloxacin, should be discontinued and appropriate therapy should be initiated immediately). Products include:

Sotalol Hydrochloride (Levofloxacin should be avoided in patients with known prolongation of the QT interval, patients with uncorrected hypokalemia, and patients receiving Class III (eg, sotalol) antiarrhythmic agents. Elderly patients may be more susceptible to drug-associated effects on the QT interval).
No products indexed under this heading.

Sucralfate (Concurrent administration of levofloxacin tablets/oral solution with sucralfate may interfere with the gastrointestinal absorption of levofloxacin, resulting in systemic levels considerably lower than desired. Sucralfate should be taken at least two hours before or two hours after levofloxacin administration). Products include:

Sulindac (Concomitant administration of a non-steroidal anti-inflammatory drug with a fluoroquinolone, including levofloxacin, may increase the risk of CNS stimulation and convulsive seizures). Products include:

Theophylline (Concomitant administration of other fluoroquinolones with theophylline has resulted in prolonged elimination half-life, elevated serum theophylline levels, and a subsequent increase in the risk of theophylline-related adverse reactions in the patient population. Therefore, theophylline levels should be closely monitored and appropriate dosage adjustments made when levofloxacin is co-administered. Adverse reactions, including seizures, may occur with or without an elevation in serum theophylline levels).
No products indexed under this heading.

IMPORTANT NOTE: Always consult each drug listing in the patient's regimen for possible interactions.

Theophylline Anhydrous (Concomitant administration of other fluoroquinolones with theophylline has resulted in prolonged elimination half-life, elevated serum theophylline levels, and a subsequent increase in the risk of theophylline-related adverse reactions in the patient population. Therefore, theophylline levels should be closely monitored and appropriate dosage adjustments made when levofloxacin is co-administered. Adverse reactions, including seizures, may occur with or without an elevation in serum theophylline levels). Products include:

Theophylline Calcium Salicylate (Concomitant administration of other fluoroquinolones with theophylline has resulted in prolonged elimination half-life, elevated serum theophylline levels, and a subsequent increase in the risk of theophylline-related adverse reactions in the patient population. Therefore, theophylline levels should be closely monitored and appropriate dosage adjustments made when levofloxacin is co-administered. Adverse reactions, including seizures, may occur with or without an elevation in serum theophylline levels).
No products indexed under this heading.

Theophylline Dihydroxypropyl (Glyceryl) (Concomitant administration of other fluoroquinolones with theophylline has resulted in prolonged elimination half-life, elevated serum theophylline levels, and a subsequent increase in the risk of theophylline-related adverse reactions in the patient population. Therefore, theophylline levels should be closely monitored and appropriate dosage adjustments made when levofloxacin is co-administered. Adverse reactions, including seizures, may occur with or without an elevation in serum theophylline levels).
No products indexed under this heading.

Theophylline Ethylenediamine (Concomitant administration of other fluoroquinolones with theophylline has resulted in prolonged elimination half-life, elevated serum theophylline levels, and a subsequent increase in the risk of theophylline-related adverse reactions in the patient population. Therefore, theophylline levels should be closely monitored and appropriate dosage adjustments made when levofloxacin is co-administered. Adverse reactions, including seizures, may occur with or without an elevation in serum theophylline levels).
No products indexed under this heading.

Theophylline Sodium Glycinate (Concomitant administration of other fluoroquinolones with theophylline has resulted in prolonged elimination half-life, elevated serum theophylline levels, and a subsequent increase in the risk of theophylline-related adverse reactions in the patient population. Therefore, theophylline levels should be closely monitored and appropriate dosage adjustments made when levofloxacin is co-administered. Adverse reactions, including seizures, may occur with or without an elevation in serum theophylline levels).
No products indexed under this heading.

Thioridazine Hydrochloride (Prolongation of the QT interval and isolated cases of torsade de pointes have been reported due to levofloxacin. Levofloxacin should be avoided with other drugs that prolong the QT interval. Levofloxacin should be avoided in patients with known prolongation of the QT interval, patients with uncorrected hypokalemia, and patients receiving Class IA (quinidine, procainamide), or Class III (amiodarone, sotalol) antiarrhythmic agents.

Elderly patients may be more susceptible to drug-associated effects on the QT interval). Products include:

Thiothixene (Prolongation of the QT interval and isolated cases of torsade de pointes have been reported due to levofloxacin. Levofloxacin should be avoided with other drugs that prolong the QT interval. Levofloxacin should be avoided in patients with known prolongation of the QT interval, patients with uncorrected hypokalemia, and patients receiving Class IA (quinidine, procainamide), or Class III (amiodarone, sotalol) antiarrhythmic agents. Elderly patients may be more susceptible to drug-associated effects on the QT interval). Products include:

Tocainide Hydrochloride (Prolongation of the QT interval and isolated cases of torsade de pointes have been reported due to levofloxacin. Levofloxacin should be avoided with other drugs that prolong the QT interval. Levofloxacin should be avoided in patients with known prolongation of the QT interval, patients with uncorrected hypokalemia, and patients receiving Class IA (quinidine, procainamide), or Class III (amiodarone, sotalol) antiarrhythmic agents. Elderly patients may be more susceptible to drug-associated effects on the QT interval).
No products indexed under this heading.

Tolazamide (Disturbances of blood glucose, including symptomatic hyper- and hypoglycemia, have been reported with levofloxacin, usually in diabetic patients receiving concomitant treatment with an oral hypoglycemic agent (eg, glyburide). In these patients, careful monitoring of blood glucose is recommended. If a hypoglycemic reaction occurs in a patient being treated with levofloxacin, levofloxacin, should be discontinued and appropriate therapy should be initiated immediately).
No products indexed under this heading.

Tolbutamide (Disturbances of blood glucose, including symptomatic hyper- and hypoglycemia, have been reported with levofloxacin, usually in diabetic patients receiving concomitant treatment with an oral hypoglycemic agent (eg, glyburide). In these patients, careful monitoring of blood glucose is recommended. If a hypoglycemic reaction occurs in a patient being treated with levofloxacin, levofloxacin, should be discontinued and appropriate therapy should be initiated immediately).
No products indexed under this heading.

Tolmetin Sodium (Concomitant administration of a non-steroidal anti-inflammatory drug with a fluoroquinolone, including levofloxacin, may increase the risk of CNS stimulation and convulsive seizures).
No products indexed under this heading.

Tranylcypromine Sulfate (Prolongation of the QT interval and isolated cases of torsade de pointes have been reported due to levofloxacin. Levofloxacin should be avoided with other drugs that prolong the QT interval. Levofloxacin should be avoided in patients with known prolongation of the QT interval, patients with uncorrected hypokalemia, and patients receiving Class IA (quinidine, procainamide), or Class III (amiodarone, sotalol) antiarrhythmic agents. Elderly patients may be more susceptible to drug-associated effects on the QT interval). Products include:

Triamcinolone (Fluoroquinolones, including levofloxacin, are associated with an increased risk of tendinitis and tendon rupture in all ages. This risk is further increased in patients taking corticosteroid drugs).
No products indexed under this heading.

Triamcinolone Acetonide (Fluoroquinolones, including levofloxacin, are associated with an increased risk of tendinitis and tendon rupture in all ages. This risk is further increased in patients taking corticosteroid drugs). Products include:

Triamcinolone Diacetate (Fluoroquinolones, including levofloxacin, are associated with an increased risk of tendinitis and tendon rupture in all ages. This risk is further increased in patients taking corticosteroid drugs).
No products indexed under this heading.

Triamcinolone Hexacetonide (Fluoroquinolones, including levofloxacin, are associated with an increased risk of tendinitis and tendon rupture in all ages. This risk is further increased in patients taking corticosteroid drugs).
No products indexed under this heading.

Trifluoperazine Hydrochloride (Prolongation of the QT interval and isolated cases of torsade de pointes have been reported due to levofloxacin. Levofloxacin should be avoided with other drugs that prolong the QT interval. Levofloxacin should be avoided in patients with known prolongation of the QT interval, patients with uncorrected hypokalemia, and patients receiving Class IA (quinidine, procainamide), or Class III (amiodarone, sotalol) antiarrhythmic agents. Elderly patients may be more susceptible to drug-associated effects on the QT interval).
No products indexed under this heading.

Trimipramine Maleate (Prolongation of the QT interval and isolated cases of torsade de pointes have been reported due to levofloxacin. Levofloxacin should be avoided with other drugs that prolong the QT interval. Levofloxacin should be avoided in patients with known prolongation of the QT interval, patients with uncorrected hypokalemia, and patients receiving Class IA (quinidine, procainamide), or Class III (amiodarone, sotalol) antiarrhythmic agents. Elderly patients may be more susceptible to drug-associated effects on the QT interval).
No products indexed under this heading.

Troglitazone (Disturbances of blood glucose, including symptomatic hyper- and hypoglycemia, have been reported with levofloxacin, usually in diabetic patients receiving concomitant treatment with an oral hypoglycemic agent (eg, glyburide). In these patients, careful monitoring of blood glucose is recommended. If a hypoglycemic reaction occurs in a patient being treated with levofloxacin, levofloxacin, should be discontinued and appropriate therapy should be initiated immediately).
No products indexed under this heading.

Ultraviolet radiation (Patients should be advised that photosensitivity/phototoxicity has been reported in patients receiving fluoroquinolone antibiotics. Patients should minimize or avoid exposure to natural or artificial sunlight (tanning beds or UVA/B treatment) while taking fluoroquinolones).
No products indexed under this heading.

Valdecoxib (Concomitant administration of a non-steroidal anti-inflammatory drug with a fluoroquinolone, including levofloxacin, may increase the risk of CNS stimulation and convulsive seizures).
No products indexed under this heading.

Warfarin Sodium (There have been reports during the postmarketing experience in patients that levofloxacin enhances the effects of warfarin. Elevations of the prothrombin time in the setting of concurrent warfarin and levofloxacin use have been associated with episodes of bleeding. Prothrombin time, International Normalized Ratio (INR), or other suitable anticoagulation tests should be closely monitored if levofloxacin is administered concomitantly with warfarin. Patients should also be monitored for evidence of bleeding).
No products indexed under this heading.

Zinc (Concurrent administration of levofloxacin tablets/oral solution with metal cations such as iron may interfere with the gastrointestinal absorption of levofloxacin, resulting in systemic levels considerably lower than desired. These agents should be taken at least two hours before or two hours after levofloxacin administration). Products include:

Zinc Acetate (Concurrent administration of levofloxacin tablets/oral solution with metal cations such as iron may interfere with the gastrointestinal absorption of levofloxacin, resulting in systemic levels considerably lower than desired. These agents should be taken at least two hours before or two hours after levofloxacin administration).
No products indexed under this heading.

Zinc Bisglycinate (Concurrent administration of levofloxacin tablets/oral solution with metal cations such as iron may interfere with the gastrointestinal absorption of levofloxacin, resulting in systemic levels considerably lower than desired. These agents should be taken at least two hours before or two hours after levofloxacin administration).
No products indexed under this heading.

Zinc Chloride (Concurrent administration of levofloxacin tablets/oral solution with metal cations such as iron may interfere with the gastrointestinal absorption of levofloxacin, resulting in systemic levels considerably lower than desired. These agents should be taken at least two hours before or two hours after levofloxacin administration).
No products indexed under this heading.

Zinc Citrate (Concurrent administration of levofloxacin tablets/oral solution with metal cations such as iron may interfere with the gastrointestinal absorption of levofloxacin, resulting in systemic levels considerably lower than desired. These agents should be taken at least two hours before or two hours after levofloxacin administration). Products include:

Zinc-Containing Multivitamins (Concurrent administration of levofloxacin tablets/oral solution and multivitamin preparations with zinc may interfere with the gastrointestinal absorption of levofloxacin, resulting in systemic levels considerably lower than desired. These agents should be taken at least two hours before or two hours after oral levofloxacin administration).
No products indexed under this heading.

Zinc Gluconate (Concurrent administration of levofloxacin tablets/oral solution with metal cations such as iron may interfere with the gastrointestinal absorption of levofloxacin, resulting in systemic levels considerably lower than desired. These agents should be taken at least two hours before or two hours after levofloxacin administration).
No products indexed under this heading.

Zinc Oxide (Concurrent administration of levofloxacin tablets/oral solution with metal cations such as iron may interfere with the gastrointestinal absorption of levofloxacin, resulting in systemic levels considerably lower than desired. These agents should be taken at least two hours before or two hours after levofloxacin administration). Products include:
Bausch & Lomb Ocuvite Adult 50+ .... ⊙238
CitraNatal Rx 2332
Vusion Ointment 3335

Zinc Phenosulfonate (Concurrent administration of levofloxacin tablets/oral solution with metal cations such as iron may interfere with the gastrointestinal absorption of levofloxacin, resulting in systemic levels considerably lower than desired. These agents should be taken at least two hours before or two hours after levofloxacin administration).
No products indexed under this heading.

Zinc Sulfate (Concurrent administration of levofloxacin tablets/oral solution with metal cations such as iron may interfere with the gastrointestinal absorption of levofloxacin, resulting in systemic levels considerably lower than desired. These agents should be taken at least two hours before or two hours after levofloxacin administration). Products include:
Heplive 607
Zinc-220 606

Ziprasidone Hydrochloride (Prolongation of the QT interval and isolated cases of torsade de pointes have been reported due to levofloxacin. Levofloxacin should be avoided with other drugs that prolong the QT interval. Levofloxacin should be avoided in patients with known prolongation of the QT interval, patients with uncorrected hypokalemia, and patients receiving Class IA (quinidine, procainamide), or Class III (amiodarone, sotalol) antiarrhythmic agents. Elderly patients may be more susceptible to drug-associated effects on the QT interval). Products include:
Geodon 2723

Food Interactions

Food, unspecified (Oral administration of a 500 mg dose of levofloxacin with food prolongs the time to peak concentration by approximately 1 hour and decreases the peak concentration by approximately 14% (following tablet administration). Therefore, levofloxacin can be administered without regard to food).

Iron Amino Acid Chelate (Concurrent administration of levofloxacin tablets/oral solution with metal cations such as iron may interfere with the gastrointestinal absorption of levofloxacin, resulting in systemic levels considerably lower than desired. These agents should be taken at least two hours before or two hours after levofloxacin administration).

Meal, unspecified (Oral administration of a 500 mg dose of levofloxacin with food prolongs the time to peak concentration by approximately 1 hour and decreases the peak concentration by approximately 14% (following tablet administration). Therefore, levofloxacin can be administered without regard to food).

LEVAQUIN IN 5% DEXTROSE INJECTION

(Levofloxacin) 2629
See Levaquin Injection

LEVEMIR INJECTION

(Insulin Detemir (rDNA Origin)) 2566
May interact with ACE inhibitors, alcohols, beta-blockers, corticosteroids, diuretics, estrogens, fibrates, lithium preparations, monoamine oxidase inhibitors, oral hypoglycemic agents, phenothiazines, progestins, salicylates, sulfonamides, sympathomimetics, thyroid preparations, and certain other agents. Compounds in these categories include:

Acarbose (Co-administration may reduce the blood-glucose-lowering effect of insulin and susceptibility to hypoglycemia).
No products indexed under this heading.

Acebutolol Hydrochloride (Co-administration may either potentiate or weaken the blood-glucose-lowering effect of insulin. Signs of hypoglycemia may be reduced or absent).
No products indexed under this heading.

Albuterol (Co-administration may reduce the blood-glucose-lowering effect of insulin).
No products indexed under this heading.

Albuterol Sulfate (Co-administration may reduce the blood-glucose-lowering effect of insulin). Products include:
ProAir HFA 3393
Proventil HFA 3204
Ventolin HFA 1708

Alclometasone Dipropionate (Co-administration may reduce the blood-glucose-lowering effect of insulin).
No products indexed under this heading.

Amiloride Hydrochloride (Co-administration may reduce the blood-glucose-lowering effect of insulin).
No products indexed under this heading.

Aspirin (Co-administration may reduce the blood-glucose-lowering effect of insulin and susceptibility to hypoglycemia). Products include:
Aggrenox 880
Bayer Aspirin 829
Percodan 1124
St. Joseph Aspirin 2045

Aspirin, Enteric Coated (Co-administration may reduce the blood-glucose-lowering effect of insulin and susceptibility to hypoglycemia).
No products indexed under this heading.

Aspirin Buffered (Co-administration may reduce the blood-glucose-lowering effect of insulin and susceptibility to hypoglycemia).
No products indexed under this heading.

Atenolol (Co-administration may either potentiate or weaken the blood-glucose-lowering effect of insulin. Signs of hypoglycemia may be reduced or absent).
No products indexed under this heading.

Beclomethasone Dipropionate (Co-administration may reduce the blood-glucose-lowering effect of insulin). Products include:
Qvar 3398

Beclomethasone Dipropionate Monohydrate (Co-administration may reduce the blood-glucose-lowering effect of insulin). Products include:
Beconase AQ 1386

Benazepril Hydrochloride (Co-administration may reduce the blood-glucose-lowering effect of insulin and susceptibility to hypoglycemia).
No products indexed under this heading.

Bendroflumethiazide (Co-administration may reduce the blood-glucose-lowering effect of insulin).
No products indexed under this heading.

Betamethasone (Co-administration may reduce the blood-glucose-lowering effect of insulin).
No products indexed under this heading.

Betamethasone Acetate (Co-administration may reduce the blood-glucose-lowering effect of insulin).
No products indexed under this heading.

Betamethasone Benzoate (Co-administration may reduce the blood-glucose-lowering effect of insulin).
No products indexed under this heading.

Betamethasone Dipropionate (Co-administration may reduce the blood-glucose-lowering effect of insulin). Products include:
Diprolene Lotion 0.05% 3108
Diprolene Ointment 0.05% 3109
Diprolene AF Cream 0.05% 3107
Lotrisone 3163

Betamethasone Sodium Phosphate (Co-administration may reduce the blood-glucose-lowering effect of insulin).
No products indexed under this heading.

Betamethasone Valerate (Co-administration may reduce the blood-glucose-lowering effect of insulin). Products include:
Luxíq 3321

Betaxolol Hydrochloride (Co-administration may either potentiate or weaken the blood-glucose-lowering effect of insulin. Signs of hypoglycemia may be reduced or absent).
No products indexed under this heading.

Bisoprolol Fumarate (Co-administration may either potentiate or weaken the blood-glucose-lowering effect of insulin. Signs of hypoglycemia may be reduced or absent).
No products indexed under this heading.

Budesonide (Co-administration may reduce the blood-glucose-lowering effect of insulin). Products include:
Pulmicort Flexhaler 714
Symbicort 80/4.5 720
Symbicort 160/4.5 720

Bumetanide (Co-administration may reduce the blood-glucose-lowering effect of insulin).
No products indexed under this heading.

Captopril (Co-administration may reduce the blood-glucose-lowering effect of insulin and susceptibility to hypoglycemia). Products include:
Captopril 2341

Carteolol Hydrochloride (Co-administration may either potentiate or weaken the blood-glucose-lowering effect of insulin. Signs of hypoglycemia may be reduced or absent).
No products indexed under this heading.

Carvedilol (Co-administration may either potentiate or weaken the blood-glucose-lowering effect of insulin. Signs of hypoglycemia may be reduced or absent). Products include:
Coreg 1409

Carvedilol Phosphate (Co-administration may either potentiate or weaken the blood-glucose-lowering effect of insulin. Signs of hypoglycemia may be reduced or absent). Products include:
Coreg CR 1416

Chlorothiazide (Co-administration may reduce the blood-glucose-lowering effect of insulin).
No products indexed under this heading.

Chlorothiazide Sodium (Co-administration may reduce the blood-glucose-lowering effect of insulin). Products include:
Diuril Intravenous 2009

Chlorotrianisene (Co-administration may reduce the blood-glucose-lowering effect of insulin).
No products indexed under this heading.

Chlorpromazine (Co-administration may reduce the blood-glucose-lowering effect of insulin).
No products indexed under this heading.

Chlorpromazine Hydrochloride (Co-administration may reduce the blood-glucose-lowering effect of insulin).
No products indexed under this heading.

Chlorpropamide (Co-administration may reduce the blood-glucose-lowering effect of insulin and susceptibility to hypoglycemia).
No products indexed under this heading.

Chlorthalidone (Co-administration may reduce the blood-glucose-lowering effect of insulin). Products include:
Clorpres 2344

Choline Magnesium Trisalicylate (Co-administration may reduce the blood-glucose-lowering effect of insulin and susceptibility to hypoglycemia).
No products indexed under this heading.

Ciclesonide (Co-administration may reduce the blood-glucose-lowering effect of insulin).
No products indexed under this heading.

Clofibrate (Co-administration may reduce the blood-glucose-lowering effect of insulin and susceptibility to hypoglycemia).
No products indexed under this heading.

Clonidine (Co-administration may either potentiate or weaken the blood-glucose lowering effect of insulin. Signs of hypoglycemia may be reduced or absent). Products include:
Catapres-TTS 884

Cortisone Acetate (Co-administration may reduce the blood-glucose-lowering effect of insulin).
No products indexed under this heading.

Danazol (Co-administration may reduce the blood-glucose-lowering effect of insulin).
No products indexed under this heading.

Desogestrel (Co-administration may reduce the blood-glucose-lowering effect of insulin).
No products indexed under this heading.

Desoximetasone (Co-administration may reduce the blood-glucose-lowering effect of insulin).
No products indexed under this heading.

Dexamethasone (Co-administration may reduce the blood-glucose-lowering effect of insulin). Products include:
Ciprodex 583
Ozurdex .... ⊙223
Tobramycin and Dexamethasone Ophthalmic Suspension .... ⊙251

Dexamethasone Acetate (Co-administration may reduce the blood-glucose-lowering effect of insulin).
No products indexed under this heading.

Dexamethasone Phosphate (Co-administration may reduce the blood-glucose-lowering effect of insulin).
No products indexed under this heading.

Dexamethasone Sodium (Co-administration may reduce the blood-glucose-lowering effect of insulin).
No products indexed under this heading.

Dexamethasone Sodium Phosphate (Co-administration may reduce the blood-glucose-lowering effect of insulin).
No products indexed under this heading.

Dexamethasone Sodium Phosphate Injection (Co-administration may reduce the blood-glucose-lowering effect of insulin).
No products indexed under this heading.

Dienestrol (Co-administration may reduce the blood-glucose-lowering effect of insulin).
No products indexed under this heading.

Diethylstilbestrol (Co-administration may reduce the blood-glucose-lowering effect of insulin).
No products indexed under this heading.

Diflorasone Diacetate (Co-administration may reduce the blood-glucose-lowering effect of insulin).
No products indexed under this heading.

Diflunisal (Co-administration may reduce the blood-glucose-lowering effect of insulin and susceptibility to hypoglycemia).
No products indexed under this heading.

Disopyramide (Co-administration may reduce the blood-glucose-lowering effect of insulin and susceptibility to hypoglycemia).
No products indexed under this heading.

Dobutamine Hydrochloride (Co-administration may reduce the blood-glucose-lowering effect of insulin).
No products indexed under this heading.

Dopamine Hydrochloride (Co-administration may reduce the blood-glucose-lowering effect of insulin).
No products indexed under this heading.

Enalapril Maleate (Co-administration may reduce the blood-glucose-lowering effect of insulin and susceptibility to hypoglycemia).
No products indexed under this heading.

Enalaprilat (Co-administration may reduce the blood-glucose-lowering effect of insulin and susceptibility to hypoglycemia).
No products indexed under this heading.

Ephedrine Hydrochloride (Co-administration may reduce the blood-glucose-lowering effect of insulin).
No products indexed under this heading.

Ephedrine Sulfate (Co-administration may reduce the blood-glucose-lowering effect of insulin).
No products indexed under this heading.

Ephedrine Tannate (Co-administration may reduce the blood-glucose-lowering effect of insulin).
No products indexed under this heading.

Epinephrine (Co-administration may reduce the blood-glucose-lowering effect of insulin). Products include:
EpiPen 3631
Twinject 3268

Epinephrine Bitartrate (Co-administration may reduce the blood-glucose-lowering effect of insulin).
No products indexed under this heading.

Epinephrine Hydrochloride (Co-administration may reduce the blood-glucose-lowering effect of insulin).
No products indexed under this heading.

Esmolol Hydrochloride (Co-administration may either potentiate or weaken the blood-glucose-lowering effect of insulin. Signs of hypoglycemia may be reduced or absent).
No products indexed under this heading.

Estradiol (Co-administration may reduce the blood-glucose-lowering effect of insulin). Products include:
Activella 2561
Angeliq 831
Climara 841
Climara Pro 847
Divigel 3467
Estrasorb 1777
Vagifem 2589

Estrogens, Conjugated (Co-administration may reduce the blood-glucose-lowering effect of insulin).
Products include:
Premarin Intravenous 3528
Premarin Tablets 3533
Premarin Vaginal Cream 3540
Premphase 3549
Prempro 3549

Estrogens, Esterified (Co-administration may reduce the blood-glucose-lowering effect of insulin).
No products indexed under this heading.

Estropipate (Co-administration may reduce the blood-glucose-lowering effect of insulin).
No products indexed under this heading.

Ethacrynic Acid (Co-administration may reduce the blood-glucose-lowering effect of insulin).
No products indexed under this heading.

Ethanol (Co-administration may either potentiate or weaken the blood-glucose lowering effect of insulin).
No products indexed under this heading.

Ethinyl Estradiol (Co-administration may reduce the blood-glucose-lowering effect of insulin). Products include:
LoSeasonique 3407
Lybrel 3514
NuvaRing 3181
Ortho Evra 2648
Ortho-Cyclen/Ortho Tri-Cyclen 2663
Ortho Tri-Cyclen Lo Tablets 2673
Seasonique 3418
Yaz 864

Ethyl Alcohol (Co-administration may either potentiate or weaken the blood-glucose lowering effect of insulin).
No products indexed under this heading.

Fenofibrate (Co-administration may reduce the blood-glucose-lowering effect of insulin and susceptibility to hypoglycemia). Products include:
Fenoglide 3263
Tricor 544
Trilipix 548

Fludrocortisone Acetate (Co-administration may reduce the blood-glucose-lowering effect of insulin).
No products indexed under this heading.

Flumethasone Pivalate (Co-administration may reduce the blood-glucose-lowering effect of insulin).
No products indexed under this heading.

Flunisolide Hemihydrate (Co-administration may reduce the blood-glucose-lowering effect of insulin).
No products indexed under this heading.

Fluoxetine (Co-administration may reduce the blood-glucose-lowering effect of insulin and susceptibility to hypoglycemia).
No products indexed under this heading.

Fluphenazine Decanoate (Co-administration may reduce the blood-glucose-lowering effect of insulin).
No products indexed under this heading.

Fluphenazine Enanthate (Co-administration may reduce the blood-glucose-lowering effect of insulin).
No products indexed under this heading.

Fluphenazine Hydrochloride (Co-administration may reduce the blood-glucose-lowering effect of insulin).
No products indexed under this heading.

Fluticasone Furoate (Co-administration may reduce the blood-glucose-lowering effect of insulin).
Products include:
Veramyst 1713

Fluticasone Propionate (Co-administration may reduce the blood-glucose-lowering effect of insulin).
Products include:
Advair 100/50 1275
Advair 250/50 1275
Advair 500/50 1275
Advair HFA 45/21 1288
Advair HFA 115/21 1288
Advair HFA 230/21 1288
Flonase 1459
Flovent Diskus 1463
Flovent HFA 1470

Fosinopril Sodium (Co-administration may reduce the blood-glucose-lowering effect of insulin and susceptibility to hypoglycemia).
No products indexed under this heading.

Furosemide (Co-administration may reduce the blood-glucose-lowering effect of insulin). Products include:
Furosemide 2354

Gemfibrozil (Co-administration may reduce the blood-glucose-lowering effect of insulin and susceptibility to hypoglycemia).
No products indexed under this heading.

Glibenclamide (Co-administration may reduce the blood-glucose-lowering effect of insulin and susceptibility to hypoglycemia).
No products indexed under this heading.

Glimepiride (Co-administration may reduce the blood-glucose-lowering effect of insulin and susceptibility to hypoglycemia). Products include:
Avandaryl 1356
Duetact 3354

Glipizide (Co-administration may reduce the blood-glucose-lowering effect of insulin and susceptibility to hypoglycemia).
No products indexed under this heading.

Glyburide (Co-administration may reduce the blood-glucose-lowering effect of insulin and susceptibility to hypoglycemia).
No products indexed under this heading.

Guanethidine (Signs of hypoglycemia may be reduced or absent).
No products indexed under this heading.

Hydrochlorothiazide (Co-administration may reduce the blood-glucose-lowering effect of insulin).
Products include:
Atacand HCT 700
Avalide 2956
Benicar HCT 1017
Diovan HCT 2419
Dyazide 1429
Exforge HCT 2449
Hyzaar 2162
Hyzaar 100-12.5 2162
Micardis HCT 889
Prinzide 2246
Tekturna HCT 2541
Teveten HCT 541

Hydrocortisone (Co-administration may reduce the blood-glucose-lowering effect of insulin).
No products indexed under this heading.

Hydrocortisone (Alcohol) (Co-administration may reduce the blood-glucose-lowering effect of insulin).
No products indexed under this heading.

Hydrocortisone Acetate (Co-administration may reduce the blood-glucose-lowering effect of insulin).
No products indexed under this heading.

Hydrocortisone Butyrate (Co-administration may reduce the blood-glucose-lowering effect of insulin).
No products indexed under this heading.

Hydrocortisone Cypionate (Co-administration may reduce the blood-glucose-lowering effect of insulin).
No products indexed under this heading.

Hydrocortisone Hemisuccinate (Co-administration may reduce the blood-glucose-lowering effect of insulin).
No products indexed under this heading.

Hydrocortisone Probutate (Co-administration may reduce the blood-glucose-lowering effect of insulin).
No products indexed under this heading.

Hydrocortisone Sodium Phosphate (Co-administration may reduce the blood-glucose-lowering effect of insulin).
No products indexed under this heading.

Hydrocortisone Sodium Succinate (Co-administration may reduce the blood-glucose-lowering effect of insulin).
No products indexed under this heading.

Hydrocortisone Valerate (Co-administration may reduce the blood-glucose-lowering effect of insulin).
No products indexed under this heading.

Hydroflumethiazide (Co-administration may reduce the blood-glucose-lowering effect of insulin).
No products indexed under this heading.

Indapamide (Co-administration may reduce the blood-glucose-lowering effect of insulin). Products include:
Indapamide 2356

Isocarboxazid (Co-administration may reduce the blood-glucose-lowering effect of insulin and susceptibility to hypoglycemia). Products include:
Marplan 3481

Isoniazid (Co-administration may reduce the blood-glucose-lowering effect of insulin).
No products indexed under this heading.

Isoproterenol Hydrochloride (Co-administration may reduce the blood-glucose-lowering effect of insulin).
No products indexed under this heading.

Isoproterenol Sulfate (Co-administration may reduce the blood-glucose-lowering effect of insulin).
No products indexed under this heading.

Labetalol Hydrochloride (Co-administration may either potentiate or weaken the blood-glucose-lowering effect of insulin. Signs of hypoglycemia may be reduced or absent).
No products indexed under this heading.

Levalbuterol Hydrochloride (Co-administration may reduce the blood-glucose-lowering effect of insulin).
No products indexed under this heading.

Levobunolol Hydrochloride (Co-administration may either potentiate or weaken the blood-glucose-lowering effect of insulin. Signs of hypoglycemia may be reduced or absent).
No products indexed under this heading.

Levothyroxine Sodium (Co-administration may reduce the blood-glucose-lowering effect of insulin).
Products include:
Levoxyl Tablets 1843
Synthroid 529

Liothyronine Sodium (Co-administration may reduce the blood-glucose-lowering effect of insulin).
Products include:
Cytomel 1830

Liotrix (Co-administration may reduce the blood-glucose-lowering effect of insulin).
No products indexed under this heading.

Lisinopril (Co-administration may reduce the blood-glucose-lowering effect of insulin and susceptibility to hypoglycemia). Products include:
Prinivil 2241
Prinzide 2246

Lithium (Co-administration may either potentiate or weaken the blood-glucose-lowering effect of insulin).
No products indexed under this heading.

Lithium Carbonate (Co-administration may either potentiate or weaken the blood-glucose-lowering effect of insulin).
No products indexed under this heading.

Lithium Citrate (Co-administration may either potentiate or weaken the blood-glucose-lowering effect of insulin).
No products indexed under this heading.

Magnesium Salicylate (Co-administration may reduce the blood-glucose-lowering effect of insulin and susceptibility to hypoglycemia).
No products indexed under this heading.

Medroxyprogesterone Acetate (Co-administration may reduce the blood-glucose-lowering effect of insulin). Products include:
- Premphase 3549
- Prempro 3549

Megestrol Acetate (Co-administration may reduce the blood-glucose-lowering effect of insulin). Products include:
- Megace ES 2698

Mesoridazine Besylate (Co-administration may reduce the blood-glucose-lowering effect of insulin).
No products indexed under this heading.

Metaproterenol Sulfate (Co-administration may reduce the blood-glucose-lowering effect of insulin).
No products indexed under this heading.

Metaraminol Bitartrate (Co-administration may reduce the blood-glucose-lowering effect of insulin).
No products indexed under this heading.

Metformin Hydrochloride (Co-administration may reduce the blood-glucose-lowering effect of insulin and susceptibility to hypoglycemia).
Products include:
- ActoPlus 3338
- Avandamet 1345
- Janumet 2188

Methotrimeprazine (Co-administration may reduce the blood-glucose-lowering effect of insulin).
No products indexed under this heading.

Methoxamine Hydrochloride (Co-administration may reduce the blood-glucose-lowering effect of insulin).
No products indexed under this heading.

Methyclothiazide (Co-administration may reduce the blood-glucose-lowering effect of insulin).
No products indexed under this heading.

Methylprednisolone (Co-administration may reduce the blood-glucose-lowering effect of insulin).
No products indexed under this heading.

Methylprednisolone Acetate (Co-administration may reduce the blood-glucose-lowering effect of insulin).
No products indexed under this heading.

Methylprednisolone Sodium Succinate (Co-administration may reduce the blood-glucose-lowering effect of insulin).
No products indexed under this heading.

Metipranolol Hydrochloride (Co-administration may either potentiate or weaken the blood-glucose-lowering effect of insulin. Signs of hypoglycemia may be reduced or absent).
No products indexed under this heading.

Metolazone (Co-administration may reduce the blood-glucose-lowering effect of insulin).
No products indexed under this heading.

Metoprolol Succinate (Co-administration may either potentiate or weaken the blood-glucose-lowering effect of insulin. Signs of hypoglycemia may be reduced or absent). Products include:
- Toprol XL 732

Metoprolol Tartrate (Co-administration may either potentiate or weaken the blood-glucose-lowering effect of insulin. Signs of hypoglycemia may be reduced or absent).
No products indexed under this heading.

Miglitol (Co-administration may reduce the blood-glucose-lowering effect of insulin and susceptibility to hypoglycemia).
No products indexed under this heading.

Moclobemide (Co-administration may reduce the blood-glucose-lowering effect of insulin and susceptibility to hypoglycemia).
No products indexed under this heading.

Moexipril Hydrochloride (Co-administration may reduce the blood-glucose-lowering effect of insulin and susceptibility to hypoglycemia).
No products indexed under this heading.

Mometasone Furoate (Co-administration may reduce the blood-glucose-lowering effect of insulin).
Products include:
- Asmanex 3058
- Elocon Cream 3111
- Elocon Lotion 3112
- Elocon Ointment 3114

Mometasone Furoate Monohydrate (Co-administration may reduce the blood-glucose-lowering effect of insulin). Products include:
- Nasonex 3166

Nadolol (Co-administration may either potentiate or weaken the blood-glucose-lowering effect of insulin. Signs of hypoglycemia may be reduced or absent).
Products include:
- Nadolol 2359

Nateglinide (Co-administration may reduce the blood-glucose-lowering effect of insulin and susceptibility to hypoglycemia).
No products indexed under this heading.

Nebivolol (Co-administration may either potentiate or weaken the blood-glucose-lowering effect of insulin. Signs of hypoglycemia may be reduced or absent). Products include:
- Bystolic 1147

Norepinephrine Bitartrate (Co-administration may reduce the blood-glucose-lowering effect of insulin).
No products indexed under this heading.

Norethindrone (Co-administration may reduce the blood-glucose-lowering effect of insulin). Products include:
- Ortho Micronor 2660

Norethindrone Acetate (Co-administration may reduce the blood-glucose-lowering effect of insulin).
Products include:
- Activella 2561

Norgestimate (Co-administration may reduce the blood-glucose-lowering effect of insulin). Products include:
- Ortho-Cyclen/Ortho Tri-Cyclen 2663
- Ortho Tri-Cyclen Lo Tablets 2673

Octreotide Acetate (Co-administration may increase the blood-glucose-lowering effect of insulin and susceptibility to hypoglycemia).
Products include:
- Sandostatin 2517
- Sandostatin LAR 2519

Pargyline Hydrochloride (Co-administration may reduce the blood-glucose-lowering effect of insulin and susceptibility to hypoglycemia).
No products indexed under this heading.

Penbutolol Sulfate (Co-administration may either potentiate or weaken the blood-glucose-lowering effect of insulin. Signs of hypoglycemia may be reduced or absent).
No products indexed under this heading.

Pentamidine Isethionate (Co-administration may cause hypoglycemia, which may sometimes be followed by hyperglycemia).
No products indexed under this heading.

Perindopril Erbumine (Co-administration may reduce the blood-glucose-lowering effect of insulin and susceptibility to hypoglycemia).
No products indexed under this heading.

Perphenazine (Co-administration may reduce the blood-glucose-lowering effect of insulin).
No products indexed under this heading.

Phenelzine Sulfate (Co-administration may reduce the blood-glucose-lowering effect of insulin and susceptibility to hypoglycemia).
No products indexed under this heading.

Phenothiazine Derivatives (Co-administration may reduce the blood-glucose-lowering effect of insulin).
No products indexed under this heading.

Phenothiazines (Co-administration may reduce the blood-glucose-lowering effect of insulin).
No products indexed under this heading.

Phenylephrine Bitartrate (Co-administration may reduce the blood-glucose-lowering effect of insulin).
No products indexed under this heading.

Phenylephrine Hydrochloride (Co-administration may reduce the blood-glucose-lowering effect of insulin).
Products include:
- Sudafed PE Nasal Decongestant 2048
- Children's Sudafed PE Nasal Decongestant 2047

Phenylephrine Tannate (Co-administration may reduce the blood-glucose-lowering effect of insulin).
No products indexed under this heading.

Phenylpropanolamine Hydrochloride (Co-administration may reduce the blood-glucose-lowering effect of insulin).
No products indexed under this heading.

Pindolol (Co-administration may either potentiate or weaken the blood-glucose-lowering effect of insulin. Signs of hypoglycemia may be reduced or absent).
No products indexed under this heading.

Pioglitazone Hydrochloride (Co-administration may reduce the blood-glucose-lowering effect of insulin and susceptibility to hypoglycemia).
Products include:
- ActoPlus 3338
- Actos 3345
- Duetact 3354

Pirbuterol Acetate (Co-administration may reduce the blood-glucose-lowering effect of insulin). Products include:
- Maxair Autohaler 1782

Polyestradiol Phosphate (Co-administration may reduce the blood-glucose-lowering effect of insulin).
No products indexed under this heading.

Polythiazide (Co-administration may reduce the blood-glucose-lowering effect of insulin).
No products indexed under this heading.

Prednisolone (Co-administration may reduce the blood-glucose-lowering effect of insulin).
No products indexed under this heading.

Prednisolone Acetate (Co-administration may reduce the blood-glucose-lowering effect of insulin).
Products include:
- Blephamide .... ⊙212, ⊙214
- Pred Forte .... ⊙225
- Pred Mild .... ⊙230
- Pred-G .... ⊙226, ⊙227

Prednisolone Sodium Phosphate (Co-administration may reduce the blood-glucose-lowering effect of insulin).
No products indexed under this heading.

Prednisolone Tebutate (Co-administration may reduce the blood-glucose-lowering effect of insulin).
No products indexed under this heading.

Prednisone (Co-administration may reduce the blood-glucose-lowering effect of insulin).
No products indexed under this heading.

Prednisone sodium phosphate (Co-administration may reduce the blood-glucose-lowering effect of insulin).
No products indexed under this heading.

Procarbazine Hydrochloride (Co-administration may reduce the blood-glucose-lowering effect of insulin and susceptibility to hypoglycemia).
No products indexed under this heading.

Prochlorperazine (Co-administration may reduce the blood-glucose-lowering effect of insulin).
No products indexed under this heading.

Prochlorperazine Edisylate (Co-administration may reduce the blood-glucose-lowering effect of insulin).
No products indexed under this heading.

Prochlorperazine Maleate (Co-administration may reduce the blood-glucose-lowering effect of insulin).
No products indexed under this heading.

Promethazine (Co-administration may reduce the blood-glucose-lowering effect of insulin).
No products indexed under this heading.

Promethazine Hydrochloride (Co-administration may reduce the blood-glucose-lowering effect of insulin).
No products indexed under this heading.

Propoxyphene Hydrochloride (Co-administration may increase the blood-glucose-lowering effect of insulin and susceptibility to hypoglycemia).
No products indexed under this heading.

Propoxyphene Napsylate (Co-administration may increase the blood-glucose-lowering effect of insulin and susceptibility to hypoglycemia).
No products indexed under this heading.

Propranolol Hydrochloride (Co-administration may either potentiate or weaken the blood-glucose-lowering effect of insulin. Signs of hypoglycemia may be reduced or absent). Products include:
- InnoPran XL 1517

Pseudoephedrine Hydrochloride (Co-administration may reduce the blood-glucose-lowering effect of insulin).
Products include:
- Allegra-D 2915
- Allegra-D 24 2918
- Sudafed 12 Hour Nasal Decongestant Non-Drowsy 2048
- Sudafed 24 Hour 2048
- Sudafed Nasal Decongestant 2047
- Children's Sudafed Nasal Decongestant Liquid 2047
- Zyrtec-D Allergy & Congestion 2054

Pseudoephedrine Sulfate (Co-administration may reduce the blood-glucose-lowering effect of insulin).
Products include:
- Clarinex-D 12-Hour 3101
- Clarinex-D 3104

Quinapril Hydrochloride (Co-administration may reduce the blood-glucose-lowering effect of insulin and susceptibility to hypoglycemia).
No products indexed under this heading.

Quinestrol (Co-administration may reduce the blood-glucose-lowering effect of insulin).
No products indexed under this heading.

Ramipril (Co-administration may reduce the blood-glucose-lowering effect of insulin and susceptibility to hypoglycemia).
No products indexed under this heading.

Rasagiline Mesylate (Co-administration may reduce the blood-glucose-lowering effect of insulin and susceptibility to hypoglycemia).
Products include:
- Azilect 3383

Repaglinide (Co-administration may reduce the blood-glucose-lowering effect of insulin and susceptibility to hypoglycemia).
No products indexed under this heading.

Reserpine (Signs of hypoglycemia may be reduced or absent).
No products indexed under this heading.

Rosiglitazone Maleate (Co-administration may reduce the blood-glucose-lowering effect of insulin and susceptibility to hypoglycemia).
Products include:
- Avandamet 1345
- Avandaryl 1356
- Avandia 1366

IMPORTANT NOTE: Always consult each drug listing in the patient's regimen for possible interactions.

Salmeterol Xinafoate (Co-administration may reduce the blood-glucose-lowering effect of insulin). Products include:

Salsalate (Co-administration may reduce the blood-glucose-lowering effect of insulin and susceptibility to hypoglycemia).
No products indexed under this heading.

Selegiline (Co-administration may reduce the blood-glucose-lowering effect of insulin and susceptibility to hypoglycemia). Products include:

Selegiline Hydrochloride (Co-administration may reduce the blood-glucose-lowering effect of insulin and susceptibility to hypoglycemia). Products include:

Sitagliptin Phosphate (Co-administration may reduce the blood-glucose-lowering effect of insulin and susceptibility to hypoglycemia). Products include:

Somatropin (Co-administration may reduce the blood-glucose-lowering effect of insulin). Products include:

Sotalol Hydrochloride (Co-administration may either potentiate or weaken the blood-glucose-lowering effect of insulin. Signs of hypoglycemia may be reduced or absent).
No products indexed under this heading.

Spirapril Hydrochloride (Co-administration may reduce the blood-glucose-lowering effect of insulin and susceptibility to hypoglycemia).
No products indexed under this heading.

Spironolactone (Co-administration may reduce the blood-glucose-lowering effect of insulin).
No products indexed under this heading.

Sulfacytine (Co-administration may reduce the blood-glucose-lowering effect of insulin and susceptibility to hypoglycemia).
No products indexed under this heading.

Sulfamethizole (Co-administration may reduce the blood-glucose-lowering effect of insulin and susceptibility to hypoglycemia).
No products indexed under this heading.

Sulfamethoxazole (Co-administration may reduce the blood-glucose-lowering effect of insulin and susceptibility to hypoglycemia).
No products indexed under this heading.

Sulfasalazine (Co-administration may reduce the blood-glucose-lowering effect of insulin and susceptibility to hypoglycemia).
No products indexed under this heading.

Sulfinpyrazone (Co-administration may reduce the blood-glucose-lowering effect of insulin and susceptibility to hypoglycemia).
No products indexed under this heading.

Sulfisoxazole Acetyl (Co-administration may reduce the blood-glucose-lowering effect of insulin and susceptibility to hypoglycemia).
No products indexed under this heading.

Sulfisoxazole Diolamine (Co-administration may reduce the blood-glucose-lowering effect of insulin and susceptibility to hypoglycemia).
No products indexed under this heading.

Terbutaline Sulfate (Co-administration may reduce the blood-glucose-lowering effect of insulin).
No products indexed under this heading.

Thioridazine (Co-administration may reduce the blood-glucose-lowering effect of insulin).
No products indexed under this heading.

Thioridazine Hydrochloride (Co-administration may reduce the blood-glucose-lowering effect of insulin). Products include:

Thyroglobulin (Co-administration may reduce the blood-glucose-lowering effect of insulin).
No products indexed under this heading.

Thyroid (Co-administration may reduce the blood-glucose-lowering effect of insulin). Products include:

Thyroxine (Co-administration may reduce the blood-glucose-lowering effect of insulin).
No products indexed under this heading.

Thyroxine Sodium (Co-administration may either reduce the blood-glucose-lowering effect of insulin).
No products indexed under this heading.

Timolol Hemihydrate (Co-administration may either potentiate or weaken the blood-glucose-lowering effect of insulin. Signs of hypoglycemia may be reduced or absent). Products include:

Timolol Maleate (Co-administration may either potentiate or weaken the blood-glucose-lowering effect of insulin. Signs of hypoglycemia may be reduced or absent). Products include:

Tolazamide (Co-administration may reduce the blood-glucose-lowering effect of insulin and susceptibility to hypoglycemia).
No products indexed under this heading.

Tolbutamide (Co-administration may reduce the blood-glucose-lowering effect of insulin and susceptibility to hypoglycemia).
No products indexed under this heading.

Torsemide (Co-administration may reduce the blood-glucose-lowering effect of insulin).
No products indexed under this heading.

Trandolapril (Co-administration may reduce the blood-glucose-lowering effect of insulin and susceptibility to hypoglycemia). Products include:

Tranylcypromine Sulfate (Co-administration may reduce the blood-glucose-lowering effect of insulin and susceptibility to hypoglycemia). Products include:

Triamcinolone (Co-administration may reduce the blood-glucose-lowering effect of insulin).
No products indexed under this heading.

Triamcinolone Acetonide (Co-administration may reduce the blood-glucose-lowering effect of insulin). Products include:

Triamcinolone Diacetate (Co-administration may reduce the blood-glucose-lowering effect of insulin).
No products indexed under this heading.

Triamcinolone Hexacetonide (Co-administration may reduce the blood-glucose-lowering effect of insulin).
No products indexed under this heading.

Triamterene (Co-administration may reduce the blood-glucose-lowering effect of insulin). Products include:

Trifluoperazine Hydrochloride (Co-administration may reduce the blood-glucose-lowering effect of insulin).
No products indexed under this heading.

Troglitazone (Co-administration may reduce the blood-glucose-lowering effect of insulin and susceptibility to hypoglycemia).
No products indexed under this heading.

Food Interactions

Alcohol (Co-administration may either potentiate or weaken the blood-glucose lowering effect of insulin).

Beer, reduced-alcohol (Co-administration may either potentiate or weaken the blood-glucose lowering effect of insulin).

Beer, unspecified (Co-administration may either potentiate or weaken the blood-glucose lowering effect of insulin).

Wine, Chianti (Co-administration may either potentiate or weaken the blood-glucose lowering effect of insulin).

Wine, Red (Co-administration may either potentiate or weaken the blood-glucose lowering effect of insulin).

Wine, unspecified (Co-administration may either potentiate or weaken the blood-glucose lowering effect of insulin).

Wine products (Co-administration may either potentiate or weaken the blood-glucose lowering effect of insulin).

LEVITRA TABLETS

(Vardenafil Hydrochloride) 3157
May interact with alpha adrenergic blockers, class 1A antiarrhythmics, class III antiarrhythmics, cytochrome p450 2c9 inhibitors (selected), cytochrome p450 3a4 inhibitors (selected), cytochrome p450 3a4 inhibitors, potent (selected), drugs that prolong the QT interval, erythromycin, nitrates and nitrites, protease inhibitors, quinidine, and certain other agents. Compounds in these categories include:

Acetazolamide (Studies in human liver microsomes showed that vardenafil is metabolized primarily by cytochrome P450 (CYP) isoforms 3A4/5, and to a lesser degree, by CYP2C9. Therefore, inhibitors of CYP3A4 are expected to reduce vardenafil clearance).
No products indexed under this heading.

Acetazolamide Sodium (Studies in human liver microsomes showed that vardenafil is metabolized primarily by cytochrome P450 (CYP) isoforms 3A4/5, and to a lesser degree, by CYP2C9. Therefore, inhibitors of CYP3A4 are expected to reduce vardenafil clearance).
No products indexed under this heading.

Alfuzosin Hydrochloride (Caution is advised when phosphodiesterase type 5 (PDE5) inhibitors are co-administered with α-blockers. PDE5 inhibitors, including vardenafil, and α-adrenergic blocking agents are both vasodilators with blood pressure lowering effects. When vasodilators are used in combination, an additive effect on blood pressure may be anticipated. In some patients, concomitant use of these two drug classes can lower blood pressure signifi-

cantly, leading to symptomatic hypotension (eg, fainting). Concomitant treatment with vardenafil and α-blockers should be initiated only if the patient is stable on his α-blocker therapy. Vardenafil should be initiated at the lowest recommended starting dose). Products include:

Alprazolam (In a study of the effect of vardenafil on QT interval in 59 healthy males, therapeutic (10 mg) and supratherapeutic (80 mg) doses of vardenafil and the active control moxifloxacin (400 mg) produced similar increases in QTc interval. A postmarketing study evaluating the effect of combining vardenafil with another drug of comparable QT effect showed an additive QT effect when compared with either drug alone. These observations should be considered in clinical decisions when prescribing vardenafil to patients taking medications known to prolong the QT interval).
No products indexed under this heading.

Amiodarone Hydrochloride (Patients taking Class III antiarrhythmic medications should avoid using vardenafil).
No products indexed under this heading.

Amitriptyline Hydrochloride (In a study of the effect of vardenafil on QT interval in 59 healthy males, therapeutic (10 mg) and supratherapeutic (80 mg) doses of vardenafil and the active control moxifloxacin (400 mg) produced similar increases in QTc interval. A postmarketing study evaluating the effect of combining vardenafil with another drug of comparable QT effect showed an additive QT effect when compared with either drug alone. These observations should be considered in clinical decisions when prescribing vardenafil to patients taking medications known to prolong the QT interval).
No products indexed under this heading.

Amoxapine (In a study of the effect of vardenafil on QT interval in 59 healthy males, therapeutic (10 mg) and supratherapeutic (80 mg) doses of vardenafil and the active control moxifloxacin (400 mg) produced similar increases in QTc interval. A postmarketing study evaluating the effect of combining vardenafil with another drug of comparable QT effect showed an additive QT effect when compared with either drug alone. These observations should be considered in clinical decisions when prescribing vardenafil to patients taking medications known to prolong the QT interval).
No products indexed under this heading.

Amprenavir (Long-term safety information is not available on the concomitant administration of vardenafil with HIV protease inhibitors).
No products indexed under this heading.

Amyl Nitrite (Administration of vardenafil with nitrates (either regularly and/or intermittently) and nitric oxide donors is contraindicated. Consistent with the effects of PDE5 inhibition on the nitric oxide/cyclic guanosine monophosphate pathway, PDE5 inhibitors may potentiate the hypotensive effects of nitrates. A suitable time interval following vardenafil dosing for the safe administration of nitrates or nitric oxide donors has not been determined).
No products indexed under this heading.

Anastrozole (Studies in human liver microsomes showed that vardenafil is metabolized primarily by cytochrome P450 (CYP) isoforms 3A4/5, and to a lesser degree, by CYP2C9. Therefore, inhibitors of CYP3A4 are expected to reduce vardenafil clearance).
No products indexed under this heading.

Apraclonidine Hydrochloride (Caution is advised when phosphodiesterase type 5 (PDE5) inhibitors are co-

1009 **Interactions Index** **Levitra**

administered with α-blockers. PDE5 inhibitors, including vardenafil, and α-adrenergic blocking agents are both vasodilators with blood pressure lowering effects. When vasodilators are used in combination, an additive effect on blood pressure may be anticipated. In some patients, concomitant use of these two drug classes can lower blood pressure significantly, leading to symptomatic hypotension (eg, fainting). Concomitant treatment with vardenafil and α-blockers should be initiated only if the patient is stable on his α-blocker therapy. Vardenafil should be initiated at the lowest recommended starting dose).
No products indexed under this heading.

Aprepitant (Studies in human liver microsomes showed that vardenafil is metabolized primarily by cytochrome P450 (CYP) isoforms 3A4/5, and to a lesser degree, by CYP2C9. Therefore, inhibitors of CYP3A4 are expected to reduce vardenafil clearance). Products include:
Emend **2124**

Astemizole (In a study of the effect of vardenafil on QT interval in 59 healthy males, therapeutic (10 mg) and supratherapeutic (80 mg) doses of vardenafil and the active control moxifloxacin (400 mg) produced similar increases in QTc interval. A postmarketing study evaluating the effect of combining vardenafil with another drug of comparable QT effect showed an additive QT effect when compared with either drug alone. These observations should be considered in clinical decisions when prescribing vardenafil to patients taking medications known to prolong the QT interval).
No products indexed under this heading.

Atazanavir (Patients taking atazanavir, a potent CYP3A4 inhibitor, should not exceed a dose of vardenafil 2.5 mg once daily).
No products indexed under this heading.

Atazanavir Sulfate (Patients taking atazanavir, a potent CYP3A4 inhibitor, should not exceed a dose of vardenafil 2.5 mg once daily).
No products indexed under this heading.

Bendroflumethiazide (Studies in human liver microsomes showed that vardenafil is metabolized primarily by cytochrome P450 (CYP) isoforms 3A4/5, and to a lesser degree, by CYP2C9. Therefore, inhibitors of CYP2C9 are expected to reduce vardenafil clearance).
No products indexed under this heading.

Bretylium Tosylate (Patients taking Class III antiarrhythmic medications should avoid using vardenafil).
No products indexed under this heading.

Buspirone Hydrochloride (In a study of the effect of vardenafil on QT interval in 59 healthy males, therapeutic (10 mg) and supratherapeutic (80 mg) doses of vardenafil and the active control moxifloxacin (400 mg) produced similar increases in QTc interval. A postmarketing study evaluating the effect of combining vardenafil with another drug of comparable QT effect showed an additive QT effect when compared with either drug alone. These observations should be considered in clinical decisions when prescribing vardenafil to patients taking medications known to prolong the QT interval).
No products indexed under this heading.

Chloramphenicol (Studies in human liver microsomes showed that vardenafil is metabolized primarily by cytochrome P450 (CYP) isoforms 3A4/5, and to a lesser degree, by CYP2C9. Therefore, inhibitors of CYP2C9 are expected to reduce vardenafil clearance).
No products indexed under this heading.

Chloramphenicol Palmitate (Studies in human liver microsomes showed that vardenafil is metabolized primarily by cytochrome P450 (CYP) isoforms 3A4/5, and to a lesser degree, by CYP2C9. Therefore, inhibitors of CYP2C9 are expected to reduce vardenafil clearance).
No products indexed under this heading.

Chloramphenicol Sodium Succinate (Studies in human liver microsomes showed that vardenafil is metabolized primarily by cytochrome P450 (CYP) isoforms 3A4/5, and to a lesser degree, by CYP2C9. Therefore, inhibitors of CYP2C9 are expected to reduce vardenafil clearance).
No products indexed under this heading.

Chlordiazepoxide (In a study of the effect of vardenafil on QT interval in 59 healthy males, therapeutic (10 mg) and supratherapeutic (80 mg) doses of vardenafil and the active control moxifloxacin (400 mg) produced similar increases in QTc interval. A postmarketing study evaluating the effect of combining vardenafil with another drug of comparable QT effect showed an additive QT effect when compared with either drug alone. These observations should be considered in clinical decisions when prescribing vardenafil to patients taking medications known to prolong the QT interval).
No products indexed under this heading.

Chlordiazepoxide Hydrochloride (In a study of the effect of vardenafil on QT interval in 59 healthy males, therapeutic (10 mg) and supratherapeutic (80 mg) doses of vardenafil and the active control moxifloxacin (400 mg) produced similar increases in QTc interval. A postmarketing study evaluating the effect of combining vardenafil with another drug of comparable QT effect showed an additive QT effect when compared with either drug alone. These observations should be considered in clinical decisions when prescribing vardenafil to patients taking medications known to prolong the QT interval).
No products indexed under this heading.

Chlorothiazide (Studies in human liver microsomes showed that vardenafil is metabolized primarily by cytochrome P450 (CYP) isoforms 3A4/5, and to a lesser degree, by CYP2C9. Therefore, inhibitors of CYP2C9 are expected to reduce vardenafil clearance).
No products indexed under this heading.

Chlorothiazide Sodium (Studies in human liver microsomes showed that vardenafil is metabolized primarily by cytochrome P450 (CYP) isoforms 3A4/5, and to a lesser degree, by CYP2C9. Therefore, inhibitors of CYP2C9 are expected to reduce vardenafil clearance). Products include:
Diuril Intravenous **2009**

Chlorpromazine (In a study of the effect of vardenafil on QT interval in 59 healthy males, therapeutic (10 mg) and supratherapeutic (80 mg) doses of vardenafil and the active control moxifloxacin (400 mg) produced similar increases in QTc interval. A postmarketing study evaluating the effect of combining vardenafil with another drug of comparable QT effect showed an additive QT effect when compared with either drug alone. These observations should be considered in clinical decisions when prescribing vardenafil to patients taking medications known to prolong the QT interval).
No products indexed under this heading.

Chlorpromazine Hydrochloride (In a study of the effect of vardenafil on QT interval in 59 healthy males, therapeutic (10 mg) and supratherapeutic (80 mg) doses of vardenafil and the active control moxifloxacin (400 mg) produced similar increases in QTc interval. A postmarketing study evaluating the effect of combining vardenafil with another drug of comparable QT effect showed an additive QT effect when compared with either drug alone. These observations should be considered in clinical decisions when prescribing vardenafil to patients taking medications known to prolong the QT interval).
No products indexed under this heading.

Chlorpropamide (Studies in human liver microsomes showed that vardenafil is metabolized primarily by cytochrome P450 (CYP) isoforms 3A4/5, and to a lesser degree, by CYP2C9. Therefore, inhibitors of CYP2C9 are expected to reduce vardenafil clearance).
No products indexed under this heading.

Chlorprothixene (In a study of the effect of vardenafil on QT interval in 59 healthy males, therapeutic (10 mg) and supratherapeutic (80 mg) doses of vardenafil and the active control moxifloxacin (400 mg) produced similar increases in QTc interval. A postmarketing study evaluating the effect of combining vardenafil with another drug of comparable QT effect showed an additive QT effect when compared with either drug alone. These observations should be considered in clinical decisions when prescribing vardenafil to patients taking medications known to prolong the QT interval).
No products indexed under this heading.

Chlorprothixene Hydrochloride (In a study of the effect of vardenafil on QT interval in 59 healthy males, therapeutic (10 mg) and supratherapeutic (80 mg) doses of vardenafil and the active control moxifloxacin (400 mg) produced similar increases in QTc interval. A postmarketing study evaluating the effect of combining vardenafil with another drug of comparable QT effect showed an additive QT effect when compared with either drug alone. These observations should be considered in clinical decisions when prescribing vardenafil to patients taking medications known to prolong the QT interval).
No products indexed under this heading.

Cimetidine (Studies in human liver microsomes showed that vardenafil is metabolized primarily by cytochrome P450 (CYP) isoforms 3A4/5, and to a lesser degree, by CYP2C9. Therefore, inhibitors of CYP3A4 are expected to reduce vardenafil clearance).
No products indexed under this heading.

Cimetidine Hydrochloride (Studies in human liver microsomes showed that vardenafil is metabolized primarily by cytochrome P450 (CYP) isoforms 3A4/5, and to a lesser degree, by CYP2C9. Therefore, inhibitors of CYP3A4 are expected to reduce vardenafil clearance).
No products indexed under this heading.

Ciprofloxacin (Studies in human liver microsomes showed that vardenafil is metabolized primarily by cytochrome P450 (CYP) isoforms 3A4/5, and to a lesser degree, by CYP2C9. Therefore, inhibitors of CYP3A4 are expected to reduce vardenafil clearance). Products include:
Cipro I.V. **3082**
Cipro **3073**
Cipro XR **3091**
Ciprodex **583**

Clarithromycin (Patients taking clarithromycin, a potent CYP3A4 inhibitor, should not exceed a dose of vardenafil 2.5 mg once daily). Products include:
Biaxin/Biaxin XL **412**

Clomipramine Hydrochloride (In a study of the effect of vardenafil on QT interval in 59 healthy males, therapeutic (10 mg) and supratherapeutic (80 mg) doses of vardenafil and the active control moxifloxacin (400 mg) produced similar increases in QTc interval. A postmarketing study evaluating the effect of combining vardenafil with another drug of comparable QT effect showed an additive QT effect when compared with either drug alone. These observations should be considered in clinical decisions when prescribing vardenafil to patients taking medications known to prolong the QT interval).
No products indexed under this heading.

Clonidine (Caution is advised when phosphodiesterase type 5 (PDE5) inhibitors are co-administered with α-blockers. PDE5 inhibitors, including vardenafil, and α-adrenergic blocking agents are both vasodilators with blood pressure lowering effects. When vasodilators are used in combination, an additive effect on blood pressure may be anticipated. In some patients, concomitant use of these two drug classes can lower blood pressure significantly, leading to symptomatic hypotension (eg, fainting). Concomitant treatment with vardenafil and α-blockers should be initiated only if the patient is stable on his α-blocker therapy. Vardenafil should be initiated at the lowest recommended starting dose). Products include:
Catapres-TTS **884**

Clonidine Hydrochloride (Caution is advised when phosphodiesterase type 5 (PDE5) inhibitors are co-administered with α-blockers. PDE5 inhibitors, including vardenafil, and α-adrenergic blocking agents are both vasodilators with blood pressure lowering effects. When vasodilators are used in combination, an additive effect on blood pressure may be anticipated. In some patients, concomitant use of these two drug classes can lower blood pressure significantly, leading to symptomatic hypotension (eg, fainting). Concomitant treatment with vardenafil and α-blockers should be initiated only if the patient is stable on his α-blocker therapy. Vardenafil should be initiated at the lowest recommended starting dose). Products include:
Clorpres **2344**

Clopidogrel Bisulfate (Studies in human liver microsomes showed that vardenafil is metabolized primarily by cytochrome P450 (CYP) isoforms 3A4/5, and to a lesser degree, by CYP2C9. Therefore, inhibitors of CYP2C9 are expected to reduce vardenafil clearance). Products include:
Plavix **3027**

Clopidogrel Hydrogen Sulfate (Studies in human liver microsomes showed that vardenafil is metabolized primarily by cytochrome P450 (CYP) isoforms 3A4/5, and to a lesser degree, by CYP2C9. Therefore, inhibitors of CYP2C9 are expected to reduce vardenafil clearance).
No products indexed under this heading.

Clorazepate Dipotassium (In a study of the effect of vardenafil on QT interval in 59 healthy males, therapeutic (10 mg) and supratherapeutic (80 mg) doses of vardenafil and the active control moxifloxacin (400 mg) produced similar increases in QTc interval. A postmarketing study evaluating the effect of combining vardenafil with another drug of comparable QT effect showed an additive QT effect when compared with either drug alone. These observations should be considered in clinical decisions when prescribing vardenafil to patients taking medications known to prolong the QT interval).
No products indexed under this heading.

Clotrimazole (Studies in human liver microsomes showed that vardenafil is metabolized primarily by cytochrome

P450 (CYP) isoforms 3A4/5, and to a lesser degree, by CYP2C9. Therefore, inhibitors of CYP3A4 are expected to reduce vardenafil clearance). Products include:

Lotrisone 3163

Clozapine (In a study of the effect of vardenafil on QT interval in 59 healthy males, therapeutic (10 mg) and supratherapeutic (80 mg) doses of vardenafil and the active control moxifloxacin (400 mg) produced similar increases in QTc interval. A postmarketing study evaluating the effect of combining vardenafil with another drug of comparable QT effect showed an additive QT effect when compared with either drug alone. These observations should be considered in clinical decisions when prescribing vardenafil to patients taking medications known to prolong the QT interval).

No products indexed under this heading.

Conivaptan Hydrochloride (Studies in human liver microsomes showed that vardenafil is metabolized primarily by cytochrome P450 (CYP) isoforms 3A4/5, and to a lesser degree, by CYP2C9. Therefore, inhibitors of CYP3A4 are expected to reduce vardenafil clearance). Products include:

Vaprisol 689

Cyclosporine (Studies in human liver microsomes showed that vardenafil is metabolized primarily by cytochrome P450 (CYP) isoforms 3A4/5, and to a lesser degree, by CYP2C9. Therefore, inhibitors of CYP3A4 are expected to reduce vardenafil clearance). Products include:

Gengraf 440
Neoral Oral Solution 2496
Neoral Capsules 2496
Restasis 605

Dalfopristin (Studies in human liver microsomes showed that vardenafil is metabolized primarily by cytochrome P450 (CYP) isoforms 3A4/5, and to a lesser degree, by CYP2C9. Therefore, inhibitors of CYP3A4 are expected to reduce vardenafil clearance).

No products indexed under this heading.

Danazol (Studies in human liver microsomes showed that vardenafil is metabolized primarily by cytochrome P450 (CYP) isoforms 3A4/5, and to a lesser degree, by CYP2C9. Therefore, inhibitors of CYP3A4 are expected to reduce vardenafil clearance).

No products indexed under this heading.

Darunavir (Long-term safety information is not available on the concomitant administration of vardenafil with HIV protease inhibitors).

No products indexed under this heading.

Dasatinib (Studies in human liver microsomes showed that vardenafil is metabolized primarily by cytochrome P450 (CYP) isoforms 3A4/5, and to a lesser degree, by CYP2C9. Therefore, inhibitors of CYP3A4 are expected to reduce vardenafil clearance).

No products indexed under this heading.

Delavirdine Mesylate (Studies in human liver microsomes showed that vardenafil is metabolized primarily by cytochrome P450 (CYP) isoforms 3A4/5, and to a lesser degree, by CYP2C9. Therefore, inhibitors of CYP3A4 are expected to reduce vardenafil clearance. Patients taking potent CYP3A4 inhibitors should not exceed a dose of vardenafil 2.5 mg once daily).

No products indexed under this heading.

Delavirine (Studies in human liver microsomes showed that vardenafil is metabolized primarily by cytochrome P450 (CYP) isoforms 3A4/5, and to a lesser degree, by CYP2C9. Therefore, inhibitors of CYP3A4 are expected to reduce vardenafil clearance. Patients taking potent CYP3A4 inhibitors should not exceed a dose of vardenafil 2.5 mg once daily).

No products indexed under this heading.

Desipramine Hydrochloride (In a study of the effect of vardenafil on QT interval in 59 healthy males, therapeutic (10 mg) and supratherapeutic (80 mg) doses of vardenafil and the active control moxifloxacin (400 mg) produced similar increases in QTc interval. A postmarketing study evaluating the effect of combining vardenafil with another drug of comparable QT effect showed an additive QT effect when compared with either drug alone. These observations should be considered in clinical decisions when prescribing vardenafil to patients taking medications known to prolong the QT interval).

No products indexed under this heading.

Desloratadine (Studies in human liver microsomes showed that vardenafil is metabolized primarily by cytochrome P450 (CYP) isoforms 3A4/5, and to a lesser degree, by CYP2C9. Therefore, inhibitors of CYP3A4 are expected to reduce vardenafil clearance). Products include:

Clarinex Syrup 3098
Clarinex 3098
Clarinex Reditabs 3098
Clarinex-D 12-Hour 3101
Clarinex-D 3104

Diazepam (In a study of the effect of vardenafil on QT interval in 59 healthy males, therapeutic (10 mg) and supratherapeutic (80 mg) doses of vardenafil and the active control moxifloxacin (400 mg) produced similar increases in QTc interval. A postmarketing study evaluating the effect of combining vardenafil with another drug of comparable QT effect showed an additive QT effect when compared with either drug alone. These observations should be considered in clinical decisions when prescribing vardenafil to patients taking medications known to prolong the QT interval). Products include:

Valium Tablets 2880

Diclofenac Epolamine (Studies in human liver microsomes showed that vardenafil is metabolized primarily by cytochrome P450 (CYP) isoforms 3A4/5, and to a lesser degree, by CYP2C9. Therefore, inhibitors of CYP2C9 are expected to reduce vardenafil clearance). Products include:

Flector 1839

Diclofenac Potassium (Studies in human liver microsomes showed that vardenafil is metabolized primarily by cytochrome P450 (CYP) isoforms 3A4/5, and to a lesser degree, by CYP2C9. Therefore, inhibitors of CYP2C9 are expected to reduce vardenafil clearance).

No products indexed under this heading.

Diclofenac Sodium (Studies in human liver microsomes showed that vardenafil is metabolized primarily by cytochrome P450 (CYP) isoforms 3A4/5, and to a lesser degree, by CYP2C9. Therefore, inhibitors of CYP2C9 are expected to reduce vardenafil clearance).

No products indexed under this heading.

Diltiazem Hydrochloride (Studies in human liver microsomes showed that vardenafil is metabolized primarily by cytochrome P450 (CYP) isoforms 3A4/5, and to a lesser degree, by CYP2C9. Therefore, inhibitors of CYP3A4 are expected to reduce vardenafil clearance). Products include:

Cardizem LA 423

Diltiazem Maleate (Studies in human liver microsomes showed that vardenafil is metabolized primarily by cytochrome P450 (CYP) isoforms 3A4/5, and to a lesser degree, by CYP2C9. Therefore, inhibitors of CYP3A4 are expected to reduce vardenafil clearance).

No products indexed under this heading.

Disopyramide (Patients taking Class 1A antiarrhythmic medications should avoid using vardenafil).

No products indexed under this heading.

Disopyramide Phosphate (Patients taking Class 1A antiarrhythmic medications should avoid using vardenafil).

No products indexed under this heading.

Disulfiram (Studies in human liver microsomes showed that vardenafil is metabolized primarily by cytochrome P450 (CYP) isoforms 3A4/5, and to a lesser degree, by CYP2C9. Therefore, inhibitors of CYP2C9 are expected to reduce vardenafil clearance).

No products indexed under this heading.

Dofetilide (In a study of the effect of vardenafil on QT interval in 59 healthy males, therapeutic (10 mg) and supratherapeutic (80 mg) doses of vardenafil and the active control moxifloxacin (400 mg) produced similar increases in QTc interval. A postmarketing study evaluating the effect of combining vardenafil with another drug of comparable QT effect showed an additive QT effect when compared with either drug alone. These observations should be considered in clinical decisions when prescribing vardenafil to patients taking medications known to prolong the QT interval).

No products indexed under this heading.

Doxazosin Mesylate (Caution is advised when phosphodiesterase type 5 (PDE5) inhibitors are co-administered with α-blockers. PDE5 inhibitors, including vardenafil, and α-adrenergic blocking agents are both vasodilators with blood pressure lowering effects. When vasodilators are used in combination, an additive effect on blood pressure may be anticipated. In some patients, concomitant use of these two drug classes can lower blood pressure significantly, leading to symptomatic hypotension (eg, fainting). Concomitant treatment with vardenafil and α-blockers should be initiated only if the patient is stable on his α-blocker therapy. Vardenafil should be initiated at the lowest recommended starting dose).

No products indexed under this heading.

Doxepin Hydrochloride (In a study of the effect of vardenafil on QT interval in 59 healthy males, therapeutic (10 mg) and supratherapeutic (80 mg) doses of vardenafil and the active control moxifloxacin (400 mg) produced similar increases in QTc interval. A postmarketing study evaluating the effect of combining vardenafil with another drug of comparable QT effect showed an additive QT effect when compared with either drug alone. These observations should be considered in clinical decisions when prescribing vardenafil to patients taking medications known to prolong the QT interval).

No products indexed under this heading.

Droperidol (In a study of the effect of vardenafil on QT interval in 59 healthy males, therapeutic (10 mg) and supratherapeutic (80 mg) doses of vardenafil and the active control moxifloxacin (400 mg) produced similar increases in QTc interval. A postmarketing study evaluating the effect of combining vardenafil with another drug of comparable QT effect showed an additive QT effect when compared with either drug alone. These observations should be considered in clinical decisions when prescribing vardenafil to patients taking medications known to prolong the QT interval).

No products indexed under this heading.

Efavirenz (Studies in human liver microsomes showed that vardenafil is metabolized primarily by cytochrome P450 (CYP) isoforms 3A4/5, and to a lesser degree, by CYP2C9. Therefore, inhibitors of CYP3A4 are expected to reduce vardenafil clearance). Products include:

Atripla 906

Erythrityl Tetranitrate (Administration of vardenafil with nitrates (either regularly and/or intermittently) and nitric oxide donors is contraindicated. Consistent with the effects of PDE5 inhibition on the nitric oxide/cyclic guanosine monophosphate pathway, PDE5 inhibitors may potentiate the hypotensive effects of nitrates. A suitable time interval following vardenafil dosing for the safe administration of nitrates or nitric oxide donors has not been determined).

No products indexed under this heading.

Erythromycin (In a study of the effect of vardenafil on QT interval in 59 healthy males, therapeutic (10 mg) and supratherapeutic (80 mg) doses of vardenafil and the active control moxifloxacin (400 mg) produced similar increases in QTc interval. A postmarketing study evaluating the effect of combining vardenafil with another drug of comparable QT effect showed an additive QT effect when compared with either drug alone. These observations should be considered in clinical decisions when prescribing vardenafil to patients taking medications known to prolong the QT interval).

No products indexed under this heading.

Erythromycin, Topical (Erythromycin (500 mg t.i.d.) produced a 4-fold increase in vardenafil AUC and a 3-fold increase in C_{max} when co-administered with vardenafil 5 mg in healthy volunteers. It is recommended not to exceed a single 5 mg dose of vardenafil in a 24 hour period when used in combination with erythromycin).

No products indexed under this heading.

Erythromycin Estolate (In a study of the effect of vardenafil on QT interval in 59 healthy males, therapeutic (10 mg) and supratherapeutic (80 mg) doses of vardenafil and the active control moxifloxacin (400 mg) produced similar increases in QTc interval. A postmarketing study evaluating the effect of combining vardenafil with another drug of comparable QT effect showed an additive QT effect when compared with either drug alone. These observations should be considered in clinical decisions when prescribing vardenafil to patients taking medications known to prolong the QT interval).

No products indexed under this heading.

Erythromycin Ethylsuccinate (In a study of the effect of vardenafil on QT interval in 59 healthy males, therapeutic (10 mg) and supratherapeutic (80 mg) doses of vardenafil and the active control moxifloxacin (400 mg) produced similar increases in QTc interval. A postmarketing study evaluating the effect of combining vardenafil with another drug of comparable QT effect showed an additive QT effect when compared with either drug alone. These observations should be considered in clinical decisions when prescribing vardenafil to patients taking medications known to prolong the QT interval). Products include:

E.E.S. 437
EryPed 435

Erythromycin Gluceptate (In a study of the effect of vardenafil on QT interval in 59 healthy males, therapeutic (10 mg) and supratherapeutic (80 mg)

1011 Interactions Index Levitra

doses of vardenafil and the active control moxifloxacin (400 mg) produced similar increases in QTc interval. A postmarketing study evaluating the effect of combining vardenafil with another drug of comparable QT effect showed an additive QT effect when compared with either drug alone. These observations should be considered in clinical decisions when prescribing vardenafil to patients taking medications known to prolong the QT interval).
No products indexed under this heading.

Erythromycin Lactobionate (In a study of the effect of vardenafil on QT interval in 59 healthy males, therapeutic (10 mg) and supratherapeutic (80 mg) doses of vardenafil and the active control moxifloxacin (400 mg) produced similar increases in QTc interval. A postmarketing study evaluating the effect of combining vardenafil with another drug of comparable QT effect showed an additive QT effect when compared with either drug alone. These observations should be considered in clinical decisions when prescribing vardenafil to patients taking medications known to prolong the QT interval).
No products indexed under this heading.

Erythromycin Stearate (In a study of the effect of vardenafil on QT interval in 59 healthy males, therapeutic (10 mg) and supratherapeutic (80 mg) doses of vardenafil and the active control moxifloxacin (400 mg) produced similar increases in QTc interval. A postmarketing study evaluating the effect of combining vardenafil with another drug of comparable QT effect showed an additive QT effect when compared with either drug alone. These observations should be considered in clinical decisions when prescribing vardenafil to patients taking medications known to prolong the QT interval).
No products indexed under this heading.

Esomeprazole Magnesium (Studies in human liver microsomes showed that vardenafil is metabolized primarily by cytochrome P450 (CYP) isoforms 3A4/5, and to a lesser degree, by CYP2C9. Therefore, inhibitors of CYP3A4 are expected to reduce vardenafil clearance). Products include:
Nexium Capsules 704
Nexium Oral Suspension 704

Esomeprazole Sodium (Studies in human liver microsomes showed that vardenafil is metabolized primarily by cytochrome P450 (CYP) isoforms 3A4/5, and to a lesser degree, by CYP2C9. Therefore, inhibitors of CYP3A4 are expected to reduce vardenafil clearance). Products include:
Nexium I.V. 712

Fat (Two food-effect studies were conducted which showed that high-fat meals caused a reduction in C_{max} by 18%-50%).
No products indexed under this heading.

Fenofibrate (Studies in human liver microsomes showed that vardenafil is metabolized primarily by cytochrome P450 (CYP) isoforms 3A4/5, and to a lesser degree, by CYP2C9. Therefore, inhibitors of CYP2C9 are expected to reduce vardenafil clearance). Products include:
Fenoglide 3263
Tricor 544
Trilipix 548

Flecainide Acetate (In a study of the effect of vardenafil on QT interval in 59 healthy males, therapeutic (10 mg) and supratherapeutic (80 mg) doses of vardenafil and the active control moxifloxacin (400 mg) produced similar increases in QTc interval. A postmarketing study evaluating the effect of combining vardenafil with another drug of comparable QT effect showed an additive QT effect when compared with either drug alone. These observations should be considered in clinical decisions when prescribing vardenafil to patients taking medications known to prolong the QT interval).
No products indexed under this heading.

Fluconazole (Studies in human liver microsomes showed that vardenafil is metabolized primarily by cytochrome P450 (CYP) isoforms 3A4/5, and to a lesser degree, by CYP2C9. Therefore, inhibitors of CYP3A4 are expected to reduce vardenafil clearance).
No products indexed under this heading.

Fluorouracil (Studies in human liver microsomes showed that vardenafil is metabolized primarily by cytochrome P450 (CYP) isoforms 3A4/5, and to a lesser degree, by CYP2C9. Therefore, inhibitors of CYP2C9 are expected to reduce vardenafil clearance). Products include:
Carac 2966

Fluoxetine (Studies in human liver microsomes showed that vardenafil is metabolized primarily by cytochrome P450 (CYP) isoforms 3A4/5, and to a lesser degree, by CYP2C9. Therefore, inhibitors of CYP3A4 are expected to reduce vardenafil clearance).
No products indexed under this heading.

Fluoxetine Hydrochloride (Studies in human liver microsomes showed that vardenafil is metabolized primarily by cytochrome P450 (CYP) isoforms 3A4/5, and to a lesser degree, by CYP2C9. Therefore, inhibitors of CYP3A4 are expected to reduce vardenafil clearance). Products include:
Prozac Weekly 1941
Prozac Pulvules 1941
Symbyax 1965

Fluphenazine Decanoate (In a study of the effect of vardenafil on QT interval in 59 healthy males, therapeutic (10 mg) and supratherapeutic (80 mg) doses of vardenafil and the active control moxifloxacin (400 mg) produced similar increases in QTc interval. A postmarketing study evaluating the effect of combining vardenafil with another drug of comparable QT effect showed an additive QT effect when compared with either drug alone. These observations should be considered in clinical decisions when prescribing vardenafil to patients taking medications known to prolong the QT interval).
No products indexed under this heading.

Fluphenazine Enanthate (In a study of the effect of vardenafil on QT interval in 59 healthy males, therapeutic (10 mg) and supratherapeutic (80 mg) doses of vardenafil and the active control moxifloxacin (400 mg) produced similar increases in QTc interval. A postmarketing study evaluating the effect of combining vardenafil with another drug of comparable QT effect showed an additive QT effect when compared with either drug alone. These observations should be considered in clinical decisions when prescribing vardenafil to patients taking medications known to prolong the QT interval).
No products indexed under this heading.

Fluphenazine Hydrochloride (In a study of the effect of vardenafil on QT interval in 59 healthy males, therapeutic (10 mg) and supratherapeutic (80 mg) doses of vardenafil and the active control moxifloxacin (400 mg) produced similar increases in QTc interval. A postmarketing study evaluating the effect of combining vardenafil with another drug of comparable QT effect showed an additive QT effect when compared with either drug alone. These observations should be considered in clinical decisions when prescribing vardenafil to patients taking medications known to prolong the QT interval).
No products indexed under this heading.

Flurbiprofen (Studies in human liver microsomes showed that vardenafil is metabolized primarily by cytochrome P450 (CYP) isoforms 3A4/5, and to a lesser degree, by CYP2C9. Therefore, inhibitors of CYP2C9 are expected to reduce vardenafil clearance).
No products indexed under this heading.

Flurbiprofen Sodium (Studies in human liver microsomes showed that vardenafil is metabolized primarily by cytochrome P450 (CYP) isoforms 3A4/5, and to a lesser degree, by CYP2C9. Therefore, inhibitors of CYP2C9 are expected to reduce vardenafil clearance).
No products indexed under this heading.

Fluvastatin Sodium (Studies in human liver microsomes showed that vardenafil is metabolized primarily by cytochrome P450 (CYP) isoforms 3A4/5, and to a lesser degree, by CYP2C9. Therefore, inhibitors of CYP2C9 are expected to reduce vardenafil clearance).
No products indexed under this heading.

Fluvoxamine Maleate (Studies in human liver microsomes showed that vardenafil is metabolized primarily by cytochrome P450 (CYP) isoforms 3A4/5, and to a lesser degree, by CYP2C9. Therefore, inhibitors of CYP3A4 are expected to reduce vardenafil clearance).
No products indexed under this heading.

Fosamprenavir Calcium (Long-term safety information is not available on the concomitant administration of vardenafil with HIV protease inhibitors). Products include:
Lexiva Oral Suspension 1558
Lexiva 1558

Gemfibrozil (Studies in human liver microsomes showed that vardenafil is metabolized primarily by cytochrome P450 (CYP) isoforms 3A4/5, and to a lesser degree, by CYP2C9. Therefore, inhibitors of CYP2C9 are expected to reduce vardenafil clearance).
No products indexed under this heading.

Glipizide (Studies in human liver microsomes showed that vardenafil is metabolized primarily by cytochrome P450 (CYP) isoforms 3A4/5, and to a lesser degree, by CYP2C9. Therefore, inhibitors of CYP2C9 are expected to reduce vardenafil clearance).
No products indexed under this heading.

Glyburide (Studies in human liver microsomes showed that vardenafil is metabolized primarily by cytochrome P450 (CYP) isoforms 3A4/5, and to a lesser degree, by CYP2C9. Therefore, inhibitors of CYP2C9 are expected to reduce vardenafil clearance).
No products indexed under this heading.

Glyceryl Trinitrate (Administration of vardenafil with nitrates (either regularly and/or intermittently) and nitric oxide donors is contraindicated. Consistent with the effects of PDE5 inhibition on the nitric oxide/cyclic guanosine monophosphate pathway, PDE5 inhibitors may potentiate the hypotensive effects of nitrates. A suitable time interval following vardenafil dosing for the safe administration of nitrates or nitric oxide donors has not been determined).
No products indexed under this heading.

Haloperidol (In a study of the effect of vardenafil on QT interval in 59 healthy males, therapeutic (10 mg) and supratherapeutic (80 mg) doses of vardenafil and the active control moxifloxacin (400 mg) produced similar increases in QTc interval. A postmarketing study evaluating the effect of combining vardenafil with another drug of comparable QT effect showed an additive QT effect when compared with either drug alone. These observations should be considered in clinical decisions when prescribing vardenafil to patients taking medications known to prolong the QT interval).
No products indexed under this heading.

Haloperidol Decanoate (In a study of the effect of vardenafil on QT interval in 59 healthy males, therapeutic (10 mg) and supratherapeutic (80 mg) doses of vardenafil and the active control moxifloxacin (400 mg) produced similar increases in QTc interval. A postmarketing study evaluating the effect of combining vardenafil with another drug of comparable QT effect showed an additive QT effect when compared with either drug alone. These observations should be considered in clinical decisions when prescribing vardenafil to patients taking medications known to prolong the QT interval).
No products indexed under this heading.

Haloperidol Lactate (In a study of the effect of vardenafil on QT interval in 59 healthy males, therapeutic (10 mg) and supratherapeutic (80 mg) doses of vardenafil and the active control moxifloxacin (400 mg) produced similar increases in QTc interval. A postmarketing study evaluating the effect of combining vardenafil with another drug of comparable QT effect showed an additive QT effect when compared with either drug alone. These observations should be considered in clinical decisions when prescribing vardenafil to patients taking medications known to prolong the QT interval).
No products indexed under this heading.

Hydrochlorothiazide (Studies in human liver microsomes showed that vardenafil is metabolized primarily by cytochrome P450 (CYP) isoforms 3A4/5, and to a lesser degree, by CYP2C9. Therefore, inhibitors of CYP2C9 are expected to reduce vardenafil clearance). Products include:
Atacand HCT 700
Avalide 2956
Benicar HCT 1017
Diovan HCT 2419
Dyazide 1429
Exforge HCT 2449
Hyzaar 2162
Hyzaar 100-12.5 2162
Micardis HCT 889
Prinzide 2246
Tekturna HCT 2541
Teveten HCT 541

Hydrochlorothiazide Hydrochloride (Studies in human liver microsomes showed that vardenafil is metabolized primarily by cytochrome P450 (CYP) isoforms 3A4/5, and to a lesser degree, by CYP2C9. Therefore, inhibitors of CYP2C9 are expected to reduce vardenafil clearance).
No products indexed under this heading.

Hydroflumethiazide (Studies in human liver microsomes showed that vardenafil is metabolized primarily by cytochrome P450 (CYP) isoforms 3A4/5, and to a lesser degree, by CYP2C9. Therefore, inhibitors of CYP2C9 are expected to reduce vardenafil clearance).
No products indexed under this heading.

Hydroxyzine Hydrochloride (In a study of the effect of vardenafil on QT interval in 59 healthy males, therapeutic (10 mg) and supratherapeutic (80 mg) doses of vardenafil and the active control moxifloxacin (400 mg) produced similar increases in QTc interval. A postmarketing study evaluating the effect of combining vardenafil with another drug of comparable QT effect showed an additive QT effect when compared with either drug alone. These observations should be considered in clinical deci-

IMPORTANT NOTE: Always consult each drug listing in the patient's regimen for possible interactions.

sions when prescribing vardenafil to patients taking medications known to prolong the QT interval).
No products indexed under this heading.

Imatinib Mesylate (Studies in human liver microsomes showed that vardenafil is metabolized primarily by cytochrome P450 (CYP) isoforms 3A4/5, and to a lesser degree, by CYP2C9. Therefore, inhibitors of CYP3A4 are expected to reduce vardenafil clearance). Products include:
Gleevec 2477

Imipramine Hydrochloride (In a study of the effect of vardenafil on QT interval in 59 healthy males, therapeutic (10 mg) and supratherapeutic (80 mg) doses of vardenafil and the active control moxifloxacin (400 mg) produced similar increases in QTc interval. A postmarketing study evaluating the effect of combining vardenafil with another drug of comparable QT effect showed an additive QT effect when compared with either drug alone. These observations should be considered in clinical decisions when prescribing vardenafil to patients taking medications known to prolong the QT interval).
No products indexed under this heading.

Imipramine Pamoate (In a study of the effect of vardenafil on QT interval in 59 healthy males, therapeutic (10 mg) and supratherapeutic (80 mg) doses of vardenafil and the active control moxifloxacin (400 mg) produced similar increases in QTc interval. A postmarketing study evaluating the effect of combining vardenafil with another drug of comparable QT effect showed an additive QT effect when compared with either drug alone. These observations should be considered in clinical decisions when prescribing vardenafil to patients taking medications known to prolong the QT interval).
No products indexed under this heading.

Indinavir Sulfate (Indinavir (800 mg t.i.d.) co-administered with vardenafil 10 mg resulted in a 16-fold increase in vardenafil AUC a 7-fold increase in vardenafil C_{max} and a 2-fold increase in vardenafil half-life. It is recommended not to exceed a single 2.5 mg vardenafil dose in a 24 hour period when used in combination with indinavir. Long-term safety information is not available on the concomitant administration of vardenafil with HIV protease inhibitors). Products include:
Crixivan 2113

Isocarboxazid (In a study of the effect of vardenafil on QT interval in 59 healthy males, therapeutic (10 mg) and supratherapeutic (80 mg) doses of vardenafil and the active control moxifloxacin (400 mg) produced similar increases in QTc interval. A postmarketing study evaluating the effect of combining vardenafil with another drug of comparable QT effect showed an additive QT effect when compared with either drug alone. These observations should be considered in clinical decisions when prescribing vardenafil to patients taking medications known to prolong the QT interval). Products include:
Marplan 3481

Isoniazid (Studies in human liver microsomes showed that vardenafil is metabolized primarily by cytochrome P450 (CYP) isoforms 3A4/5, and to a lesser degree, by CYP2C9. Therefore, inhibitors of CYP3A4 are expected to reduce vardenafil clearance).
No products indexed under this heading.

Isosorbide Dinitrate (Administration of vardenafil with nitrates (either regularly and/or intermittently) and nitric oxide donors is contraindicated. Consistent with the effects of PDE5 inhibition on the nitric oxide/cyclic guanosine monophosphate pathway, PDE5 inhibitors may potentiate the hypotensive effects of nitrates. A suitable time interval following vardenafil dosing for the safe administration of nitrates or nitric oxide donors has not been determined).
No products indexed under this heading.

Isosorbide Mononitrate (Administration of vardenafil with nitrates (either regularly and/or intermittently) and nitric oxide donors is contraindicated. Consistent with the effects of PDE5 inhibition on the nitric oxide/cyclic guanosine monophosphate pathway, PDE5 inhibitors may potentiate the hypotensive effects of nitrates. A suitable time interval following vardenafil dosing for the safe administration of nitrates or nitric oxide donors has not been determined).
No products indexed under this heading.

Itraconazole (Patients taking itraconazole 400 mg daily should not exceed a dose of vardenafil 2.5 mg once daily. For patients taking itraconazole 200 mg daily, a single dose of 5 mg of vardenafil should not be exceeded in a 24 hour period).
No products indexed under this heading.

Ketoconazole (Ketoconazole (200 mg once daily), produced a 10-fold increase in vardenafil AUC and a 4-fold increase in C_{max} when co-administered with vardenafil (5 mg) in healthy volunteers. A 5 mg vardenafil dose should not be exceeded when used in combination with 200 mg once daily ketoconazole. Since higher doses of ketoconazole (400 mg daily) may result in higher increases in C_{max} and AUC, a single 2.5 mg dose of vardenafil should not be exceeded in a 24 hour period when used in combination with ketoconazole 400 mg daily). Products include:
Extina 3319
Xolegel 3337

Ketoprofen (Studies in human liver microsomes showed that vardenafil is metabolized primarily by cytochrome P450 (CYP) isoforms 3A4/5, and to a lesser degree, by CYP2C9. Therefore, inhibitors of CYP2C9 are expected to reduce vardenafil clearance).
No products indexed under this heading.

Lapatinib (Studies in human liver microsomes showed that vardenafil is metabolized primarily by cytochrome P450 (CYP) isoforms 3A4/5, and to a lesser degree, by CYP2C9. Therefore, inhibitors of CYP3A4 are expected to reduce vardenafil clearance). Products include:
Tykerb 1698

Leflunomide (Studies in human liver microsomes showed that vardenafil is metabolized primarily by cytochrome P450 (CYP) isoforms 3A4/5, and to a lesser degree, by CYP2C9. Therefore, inhibitors of CYP2C9 are expected to reduce vardenafil clearance).
No products indexed under this heading.

Lidocaine (In a study of the effect of vardenafil on QT interval in 59 healthy males, therapeutic (10 mg) and supratherapeutic (80 mg) doses of vardenafil and the active control moxifloxacin (400 mg) produced similar increases in QTc interval. A postmarketing study evaluating the effect of combining vardenafil with another drug of comparable QT effect showed an additive QT effect when compared with either drug alone. These observations should be considered in clinical decisions when prescribing vardenafil to patients taking medications known to prolong the QT interval). Products include:
Lidoderm 1107

Lidocaine Hydrochloride (In a study of the effect of vardenafil on QT interval in 59 healthy males, therapeutic (10 mg) and supratherapeutic (80 mg) doses of vardenafil and the active control moxifloxacin (400 mg) produced similar increases in QTc interval. A postmarketing study evaluating the effect of combining vardenafil with another drug of comparable QT effect showed an additive QT effect when compared with either drug alone. These observations should be considered in clinical decisions when prescribing vardenafil to patients taking medications known to prolong the QT interval).
No products indexed under this heading.

Lithium Carbonate (In a study of the effect of vardenafil on QT interval in 59 healthy males, therapeutic (10 mg) and supratherapeutic (80 mg) doses of vardenafil and the active control moxifloxacin (400 mg) produced similar increases in QTc interval. A postmarketing study evaluating the effect of combining vardenafil with another drug of comparable QT effect showed an additive QT effect when compared with either drug alone. These observations should be considered in clinical decisions when prescribing vardenafil to patients taking medications known to prolong the QT interval).
No products indexed under this heading.

Lithium Citrate (In a study of the effect of vardenafil on QT interval in 59 healthy males, therapeutic (10 mg) and supratherapeutic (80 mg) doses of vardenafil and the active control moxifloxacin (400 mg) produced similar increases in QTc interval. A postmarketing study evaluating the effect of combining vardenafil with another drug of comparable QT effect showed an additive QT effect when compared with either drug alone. These observations should be considered in clinical decisions when prescribing vardenafil to patients taking medications known to prolong the QT interval).
No products indexed under this heading.

Lopinavir (Long-term safety information is not available on the concomitant administration of vardenafil with HIV protease inhibitors). Products include:
Kaletra 458

Loratadine (Studies in human liver microsomes showed that vardenafil is metabolized primarily by cytochrome P450 (CYP) isoforms 3A4/5, and to a lesser degree, by CYP2C9. Therefore, inhibitors of CYP3A4 are expected to reduce vardenafil clearance).
No products indexed under this heading.

Lorazepam (In a study of the effect of vardenafil on QT interval in 59 healthy males, therapeutic (10 mg) and supratherapeutic (80 mg) doses of vardenafil and the active control moxifloxacin (400 mg) produced similar increases in QTc interval. A postmarketing study evaluating the effect of combining vardenafil with another drug of comparable QT effect showed an additive QT effect when compared with either drug alone. These observations should be considered in clinical decisions when prescribing vardenafil to patients taking medications known to prolong the QT interval).
No products indexed under this heading.

Lovastatin (Studies in human liver microsomes showed that vardenafil is metabolized primarily by cytochrome P450 (CYP) isoforms 3A4/5, and to a lesser degree, by CYP2C9. Therefore, inhibitors of CYP2C9 are expected to reduce vardenafil clearance). Products include:
Advicor 402
Mevacor 2212

Loxapine Hydrochloride (In a study of the effect of vardenafil on QT interval in 59 healthy males, therapeutic (10 mg) and supratherapeutic (80 mg) doses of vardenafil and the active control moxifloxacin (400 mg) produced similar increases in QTc interval. A postmarketing study evaluating the effect of combining vardenafil with another drug of comparable QT effect showed an additive QT effect when compared with either drug alone. These observations should be considered in clinical decisions when prescribing vardenafil to patients taking medications known to prolong the QT interval).
No products indexed under this heading.

Loxapine Succinate (In a study of the effect of vardenafil on QT interval in 59 healthy males, therapeutic (10 mg) and supratherapeutic (80 mg) doses of vardenafil and the active control moxifloxacin (400 mg) produced similar increases in QTc interval. A postmarketing study evaluating the effect of combining vardenafil with another drug of comparable QT effect showed an additive QT effect when compared with either drug alone. These observations should be considered in clinical decisions when prescribing vardenafil to patients taking medications known to prolong the QT interval).
No products indexed under this heading.

Maprotiline Hydrochloride (In a study of the effect of vardenafil on QT interval in 59 healthy males, therapeutic (10 mg) and supratherapeutic (80 mg) doses of vardenafil and the active control moxifloxacin (400 mg) produced similar increases in QTc interval. A postmarketing study evaluating the effect of combining vardenafil with another drug of comparable QT effect showed an additive QT effect when compared with either drug alone. These observations should be considered in clinical decisions when prescribing vardenafil to patients taking medications known to prolong the QT interval).
No products indexed under this heading.

Meprobamate (In a study of the effect of vardenafil on QT interval in 59 healthy males, therapeutic (10 mg) and supratherapeutic (80 mg) doses of vardenafil and the active control moxifloxacin (400 mg) produced similar increases in QTc interval. A postmarketing study evaluating the effect of combining vardenafil with another drug of comparable QT effect showed an additive QT effect when compared with either drug alone. These observations should be considered in clinical decisions when prescribing vardenafil to patients taking medications known to prolong the QT interval).
No products indexed under this heading.

Mesoridazine Besylate (In a study of the effect of vardenafil on QT interval in 59 healthy males, therapeutic (10 mg) and supratherapeutic (80 mg) doses of vardenafil and the active control moxifloxacin (400 mg) produced similar increases in QTc interval. A postmarketing study evaluating the effect of combining vardenafil with another drug of comparable QT effect showed an additive QT effect when compared with either drug alone. These observations should be considered in clinical decisions when prescribing vardenafil to patients taking medications known to prolong the QT interval).
No products indexed under this heading.

Methyclothiazide (Studies in human liver microsomes showed that vardenafil is metabolized primarily by cytochrome P450 (CYP) isoforms 3A4/5, and to a lesser degree, by CYP2C9. Therefore, inhibitors of CYP2C9 are expected to reduce vardenafil clearance).
No products indexed under this heading.

Metronidazole (Studies in human liver microsomes showed that vardenafil is metabolized primarily by cytochrome P450 (CYP) isoforms 3A4/5, and to a

lesser degree, by CYP2C9. Therefore, inhibitors of CYP3A4 are expected to reduce vardenafil clearance). Products include:

Pylera **793**

Metronidazole Benzoate (Studies in human liver microsomes showed that vardenafil is metabolized primarily by cytochrome P450 (CYP) isoforms 3A4/5, and to a lesser degree, by CYP2C9. Therefore, inhibitors of CYP3A4 are expected to reduce vardenafil clearance).

No products indexed under this heading.

Metronidazole Hydrochloride (Studies in human liver microsomes showed that vardenafil is metabolized primarily by cytochrome P450 (CYP) isoforms 3A4/5, and to a lesser degree, by CYP2C9. Therefore, inhibitors of CYP3A4 are expected to reduce vardenafil clearance).

No products indexed under this heading.

Metronidazole Sodium (Studies in human liver microsomes showed that vardenafil is metabolized primarily by cytochrome P450 (CYP) isoforms 3A4/5, and to a lesser degree, by CYP2C9. Therefore, inhibitors of CYP3A4 are expected to reduce vardenafil clearance).

No products indexed under this heading.

Mexiletine Hydrochloride (In a study of the effect of vardenafil on QT interval in 59 healthy males, therapeutic (10 mg) and supratherapeutic (80 mg) doses of vardenafil and the active control moxifloxacin (400 mg) produced similar increases in QTc interval. A postmarketing study evaluating the effect of combining vardenafil with another drug of comparable QT effect showed an additive QT effect when compared with either drug alone. These observations should be considered in clinical decisions when prescribing vardenafil to patients taking medications known to prolong the QT interval).

No products indexed under this heading.

Miconazole (Studies in human liver microsomes showed that vardenafil is metabolized primarily by cytochrome P450 (CYP) isoforms 3A4/5, and to a lesser degree, by CYP2C9. Therefore, inhibitors of CYP3A4 are expected to reduce vardenafil clearance).

No products indexed under this heading.

Miconazole Nitrate (Studies in human liver microsomes showed that vardenafil is metabolized primarily by cytochrome P450 (CYP) isoforms 3A4/5, and to a lesser degree, by CYP2C9. Therefore, inhibitors of CYP3A4 are expected to reduce vardenafil clearance). Products include:

Vusion Ointment **3335**

Midazolam Hydrochloride (In a study of the effect of vardenafil on QT interval in 59 healthy males, therapeutic (10 mg) and supratherapeutic (80 mg) doses of vardenafil and the active control moxifloxacin (400 mg) produced similar increases in QTc interval. A postmarketing study evaluating the effect of combining vardenafil with another drug of comparable QT effect showed an additive QT effect when compared with either drug alone. These observations should be considered in clinical decisions when prescribing vardenafil to patients taking medications known to prolong the QT interval).

No products indexed under this heading.

Mifepristone (Studies in human liver microsomes showed that vardenafil is metabolized primarily by cytochrome P450 (CYP) isoforms 3A4/5, and to a lesser degree, by CYP2C9. Therefore, inhibitors of CYP3A4 are expected to reduce vardenafil clearance).

No products indexed under this heading.

Modafinil (Studies in human liver microsomes showed that vardenafil is metabolized primarily by cytochrome P450 (CYP) isoforms 3A4/5, and to a lesser degree, by CYP2C9. Therefore, inhibitors of CYP2C9 are expected to reduce vardenafil clearance). Products include:

Provigil **983**

Molindone Hydrochloride (In a study of the effect of vardenafil on QT interval in 59 healthy males, therapeutic (10 mg) and supratherapeutic (80 mg) doses of vardenafil and the active control moxifloxacin (400 mg) produced similar increases in QTc interval. A postmarketing study evaluating the effect of combining vardenafil with another drug of comparable QT effect showed an additive QT effect when compared with either drug alone. These observations should be considered in clinical decisions when prescribing vardenafil to patients taking medications known to prolong the QT interval). Products include:

Moban **1108**

Moricizine Hydrochloride (Patients taking Class 1A antiarrhythmic medications should avoid using vardenafil).

No products indexed under this heading.

Nefazodone Hydrochloride (Studies in human liver microsomes showed that vardenafil is metabolized primarily by cytochrome P450 (CYP) isoforms 3A4/5, and to a lesser degree, by CYP2C9. Therefore, inhibitors of CYP3A4 are expected to reduce vardenafil clearance. Patients taking potent CYP3A4 inhibitors should not exceed a dose of vardenafil 2.5 mg once daily).

No products indexed under this heading.

Nelfinavir Mesylate (Long-term safety information is not available on the concomitant administration of vardenafil with HIV protease inhibitors).

No products indexed under this heading.

Nevirapine (Studies in human liver microsomes showed that vardenafil is metabolized primarily by cytochrome P450 (CYP) isoforms 3A4/5, and to a lesser degree, by CYP2C9. Therefore, inhibitors of CYP3A4 are expected to reduce vardenafil clearance). Products include:

Viramune Oral Suspension **897**
Viramune Tablets **897**

Niacin (Studies in human liver microsomes showed that vardenafil is metabolized primarily by cytochrome P450 (CYP) isoforms 3A4/5, and to a lesser degree, by CYP2C9. Therefore, inhibitors of CYP3A4 are expected to reduce vardenafil clearance). Products include:

Advicor **402**
Cardio Basics **3455**
Niaspan **497**
Simcor **524**

Niacinamide (Studies in human liver microsomes showed that vardenafil is metabolized primarily by cytochrome P450 (CYP) isoforms 3A4/5, and to a lesser degree, by CYP2C9. Therefore, inhibitors of CYP3A4 are expected to reduce vardenafil clearance). Products include:

CitraNatal 90 DHA Capsules **2332**
CitraNatal Assure **2332**
CitraNatal Rx **2332**
Heplive **607**

Niacinamide Hydroiodide (Studies in human liver microsomes showed that vardenafil is metabolized primarily by cytochrome P450 (CYP) isoforms 3A4/5, and to a lesser degree, by CYP2C9. Therefore, inhibitors of CYP3A4 are expected to reduce vardenafil clearance).

No products indexed under this heading.

Nicotinamide (Studies in human liver microsomes showed that vardenafil is metabolized primarily by cytochrome P450 (CYP) isoforms 3A4/5, and to a lesser degree, by CYP2C9. Therefore, inhibitors of CYP3A4 are expected to reduce vardenafil clearance).

No products indexed under this heading.

Nifedipine (In patients whose hypertension was controlled with nifedipine, vardenafil 20 mg produced mean additional supine systolic/diastolic blood pressure reductions of 6/5 mmHg compared to placebo).

No products indexed under this heading.

Nitrate & Nitrite Preparations (Administration of vardenafil with nitrates (either regularly and/or intermittently) and nitric oxide donors is contraindicated. Consistent with the effects of PDE5 inhibition on the nitric oxide/ cyclic guanosine monophosphate pathway, PDE5 inhibitors may potentiate the hypotensive effects of nitrates. A suitable time interval following vardenafil dosing for the safe administration of nitrates or nitric oxide donors has not been determined).

No products indexed under this heading.

Nitrates, organic (Administration of vardenafil with nitrates (either regularly and/or intermittently) and nitric oxide donors is contraindicated. Consistent with the effects of PDE5 inhibition on the nitric oxide/cyclic guanosine monophosphate pathway, PDE5 inhibitors may potentiate the hypotensive effects of nitrates. A suitable time interval following vardenafil dosing for the safe administration of nitrates or nitric oxide donors has not been determined).

No products indexed under this heading.

Nitrates and Nitrites (Administration of vardenafil with nitrates (either regularly and/or intermittently) and nitric oxide donors is contraindicated. Consistent with the effects of PDE5 inhibition on the nitric oxide/cyclic guanosine monophosphate pathway, PDE5 inhibitors may potentiate the hypotensive effects of nitrates. A suitable time interval following vardenafil dosing for the safe administration of nitrates or nitric oxide donors has not been determined).

No products indexed under this heading.

Nitroglycerin (Administration of vardenafil with nitrates (either regularly and/ or intermittently) and nitric oxide donors is contraindicated. Consistent with the effects of PDE5 inhibition on the nitric oxide/cyclic guanosine monophosphate pathway, PDE5 inhibitors may potentiate the hypotensive effects of nitrates. A suitable time interval following vardenafil dosing for the safe administration of nitrates or nitric oxide donors has not been determined). Products include:

Nitro-Dur **3170**
Nitrolingual **3266**

Nitroglycerin, long-acting formulations (Administration of vardenafil with nitrates (either regularly and/or intermittently) and nitric oxide donors is contraindicated. Consistent with the effects of PDE5 inhibition on the nitric oxide/cyclic guanosine monophosphate pathway, PDE5 inhibitors may potentiate the hypotensive effects of nitrates. A suitable time interval following vardenafil dosing for the safe administration of nitrates or nitric oxide donors has not been determined).

No products indexed under this heading.

Nitroglycerin Intravenous (Administration of vardenafil with nitrates (either regularly and/or intermittently) and nitric oxide donors is contraindicated. Consistent with the effects of PDE5 inhibition on the nitric oxide/cyclic guanosine monophosphate pathway, PDE5 inhibitors may potentiate the hypotensive effects of nitrates. A suitable time

interval following vardenafil dosing for the safe administration of nitrates or nitric oxide donors has not been determined).

No products indexed under this heading.

Norfloxacin (Studies in human liver microsomes showed that vardenafil is metabolized primarily by cytochrome P450 (CYP) isoforms 3A4/5, and to a lesser degree, by CYP2C9. Therefore, inhibitors of CYP3A4 are expected to reduce vardenafil clearance). Products include:

Noroxin **2220**

Nortriptyline Hydrochloride (In a study of the effect of vardenafil on QT interval in 59 healthy males, therapeutic (10 mg) and supratherapeutic (80 mg) doses of vardenafil and the active control moxifloxacin (400 mg) produced similar increases in QTc interval. A postmarketing study evaluating the effect of combining vardenafil with another drug of comparable QT effect showed an additive QT effect when compared with either drug alone. These observations should be considered in clinical decisions when prescribing vardenafil to patients taking medications known to prolong the QT interval).

No products indexed under this heading.

Olanzapine (In a study of the effect of vardenafil on QT interval in 59 healthy males, therapeutic (10 mg) and supratherapeutic (80 mg) doses of vardenafil and the active control moxifloxacin (400 mg) produced similar increases in QTc interval. A postmarketing study evaluating the effect of combining vardenafil with another drug of comparable QT effect showed an additive QT effect when compared with either drug alone. These observations should be considered in clinical decisions when prescribing vardenafil to patients taking medications known to prolong the QT interval). Products include:

Symbyax **1965**
Zyprexa **1984**
Zyprexa IntraMuscular **1984**
Zyprexa ZYDIS **1984**

Omeprazole (Studies in human liver microsomes showed that vardenafil is metabolized primarily by cytochrome P450 (CYP) isoforms 3A4/5, and to a lesser degree, by CYP2C9. Therefore, inhibitors of CYP3A4 are expected to reduce vardenafil clearance).

No products indexed under this heading.

Oxazepam (In a study of the effect of vardenafil on QT interval in 59 healthy males, therapeutic (10 mg) and supratherapeutic (80 mg) doses of vardenafil and the active control moxifloxacin (400 mg) produced similar increases in QTc interval. A postmarketing study evaluating the effect of combining vardenafil with another drug of comparable QT effect showed an additive QT effect when compared with either drug alone. These observations should be considered in clinical decisions when prescribing vardenafil to patients taking medications known to prolong the QT interval).

No products indexed under this heading.

Oxiconazole Nitrate (Studies in human liver microsomes showed that vardenafil is metabolized primarily by cytochrome P450 (CYP) isoforms 3A4/5, and to a lesser degree, by CYP2C9. Therefore, inhibitors of CYP2C9 are expected to reduce vardenafil clearance).

No products indexed under this heading.

Paroxetine Hydrochloride (Studies in human liver microsomes showed that vardenafil is metabolized primarily by cytochrome P450 (CYP) isoforms 3A4/5, and to a lesser degree, by CYP2C9. Therefore, inhibitors of CYP3A4 are expected to reduce vardenafil clearance). Products include:

Paroxetine CR ... 2361
Paroxetine ER ... 2371
Paxil ... 1586
Paxil CR ... 1596

Pentaerythritol Tetranitrate (Administration of vardenafil with nitrates (either regularly and/or intermittently) and nitric oxide donors is contraindicated. Consistent with the effects of PDE5 inhibition on the nitric oxide/cyclic guanosine monophosphate pathway, PDE5 inhibitors may potentiate the hypotensive effects of nitrates. A suitable time interval following vardenafil dosing for the safe administration of nitrates or nitric oxide donors has not been determined).
No products indexed under this heading.

Perphenazine (In a study of the effect of vardenafil on QT interval in 59 healthy males, therapeutic (10 mg) and supratherapeutic (80 mg) doses of vardenafil and the active control moxifloxacin (400 mg) produced similar increases in QTc interval. A postmarketing study evaluating the effect of combining vardenafil with another drug of comparable QT effect showed an additive QT effect when compared with either drug alone. These observations should be considered in clinical decisions when prescribing vardenafil to patients taking medications known to prolong the QT interval).
No products indexed under this heading.

Phenelzine Sulfate (In a study of the effect of vardenafil on QT interval in 59 healthy males, therapeutic (10 mg) and supratherapeutic (80 mg) doses of vardenafil and the active control moxifloxacin (400 mg) produced similar increases in QTc interval. A postmarketing study evaluating the effect of combining vardenafil with another drug of comparable QT effect showed an additive QT effect when compared with either drug alone. These observations should be considered in clinical decisions when prescribing vardenafil to patients taking medications known to prolong the QT interval).
No products indexed under this heading.

Phenylbutazone (Studies in human liver microsomes showed that vardenafil is metabolized primarily by cytochrome P450 (CYP) isoforms 3A4/5, and to a lesser degree, by CYP2C9. Therefore, inhibitors of CYP2C9 are expected to reduce vardenafil clearance).
No products indexed under this heading.

Polythiazide (Studies in human liver microsomes showed that vardenafil is metabolized primarily by cytochrome P450 (CYP) isoforms 3A4/5, and to a lesser degree, by CYP2C9. Therefore, inhibitors of CYP2C9 are expected to reduce vardenafil clearance).
No products indexed under this heading.

Posaconazole (Studies in human liver microsomes showed that vardenafil is metabolized primarily by cytochrome P450 (CYP) isoforms 3A4/5, and to a lesser degree, by CYP2C9. Therefore, inhibitors of CYP3A4 are expected to reduce vardenafil clearance). Products include:
Noxafil ... 3172

Prazepam (In a study of the effect of vardenafil on QT interval in 59 healthy males, therapeutic (10 mg) and supratherapeutic (80 mg) doses of vardenafil and the active control moxifloxacin (400 mg) produced similar increases in QTc interval. A postmarketing study evaluating the effect of combining vardenafil with another drug of comparable QT effect showed an additive QT effect when compared with either drug alone. These observations should be considered in clinical decisions when prescribing vardenafil to patients taking medications known to prolong the QT interval).
No products indexed under this heading.

Prazosin Hydrochloride (Caution is advised when phosphodiesterase type 5 (PDE5) inhibitors are co-administered with α-blockers. PDE5 inhibitors, including vardenafil, and α-adrenergic blocking agents are both vasodilators with blood pressure lowering effects. When vasodilators are used in combination, an additive effect on blood pressure may be anticipated. In some patients, concomitant use of these two drug classes can lower blood pressure significantly, leading to symptomatic hypotension (eg, fainting). Concomitant treatment with vardenafil and α-blockers should be initiated only if the patient is stable on his α-blocker therapy. Vardenafil should be initiated at the lowest recommended starting dose).
No products indexed under this heading.

Procainamide (Patients taking Class 1A antiarrhythmic medications should avoid using vardenafil).
No products indexed under this heading.

Procainamide Hydrochloride (In a study of the effect of vardenafil on QT interval in 59 healthy males, therapeutic (10 mg) and supratherapeutic (80 mg) doses of vardenafil and the active control moxifloxacin (400 mg) produced similar increases in QTc interval. A postmarketing study evaluating the effect of combining vardenafil with another drug of comparable QT effect showed an additive QT effect when compared with either drug alone. These observations should be considered in clinical decisions when prescribing vardenafil to patients taking medications known to prolong the QT interval).
No products indexed under this heading.

Prochlorperazine (In a study of the effect of vardenafil on QT interval in 59 healthy males, therapeutic (10 mg) and supratherapeutic (80 mg) doses of vardenafil and the active control moxifloxacin (400 mg) produced similar increases in QTc interval. A postmarketing study evaluating the effect of combining vardenafil with another drug of comparable QT effect showed an additive QT effect when compared with either drug alone. These observations should be considered in clinical decisions when prescribing vardenafil to patients taking medications known to prolong the QT interval).
No products indexed under this heading.

Promethazine Hydrochloride (In a study of the effect of vardenafil on QT interval in 59 healthy males, therapeutic (10 mg) and supratherapeutic (80 mg) doses of vardenafil and the active control moxifloxacin (400 mg) produced similar increases in QTc interval. A postmarketing study evaluating the effect of combining vardenafil with another drug of comparable QT effect showed an additive QT effect when compared with either drug alone. These observations should be considered in clinical decisions when prescribing vardenafil to patients taking medications known to prolong the QT interval).
No products indexed under this heading.

Propafenone Hydrochloride (In a study of the effect of vardenafil on QT interval in 59 healthy males, therapeutic (10 mg) and supratherapeutic (80 mg) doses of vardenafil and the active control moxifloxacin (400 mg) produced similar increases in QTc interval. A postmarketing study evaluating the effect of combining vardenafil with another drug of comparable QT effect showed an additive QT effect when compared with either drug alone. These observations should be considered in clinical decisions when prescribing vardenafil to patients taking medications known to prolong the QT interval). Products include:
Rythmol ... 1648
Rythmol SR ... 1652

Propoxyphene Hydrochloride (Studies in human liver microsomes showed that vardenafil is metabolized primarily by cytochrome P450 (CYP) isoforms 3A4/5, and to a lesser degree, by CYP2C9. Therefore, inhibitors of CYP3A4 are expected to reduce vardenafil clearance).
No products indexed under this heading.

Propoxyphene Napsylate (Studies in human liver microsomes showed that vardenafil is metabolized primarily by cytochrome P450 (CYP) isoforms 3A4/5, and to a lesser degree, by CYP2C9. Therefore, inhibitors of CYP3A4 are expected to reduce vardenafil clearance).
No products indexed under this heading.

Protriptyline Hydrochloride (In a study of the effect of vardenafil on QT interval in 59 healthy males, therapeutic (10 mg) and supratherapeutic (80 mg) doses of vardenafil and the active control moxifloxacin (400 mg) produced similar increases in QTc interval. A postmarketing study evaluating the effect of combining vardenafil with another drug of comparable QT effect showed an additive QT effect when compared with either drug alone. These observations should be considered in clinical decisions when prescribing vardenafil to patients taking medications known to prolong the QT interval).
No products indexed under this heading.

Quetiapine Fumarate (In a study of the effect of vardenafil on QT interval in 59 healthy males, therapeutic (10 mg) and supratherapeutic (80 mg) doses of vardenafil and the active control moxifloxacin (400 mg) produced similar increases in QTc interval. A postmarketing study evaluating the effect of combining vardenafil with another drug of comparable QT effect showed an additive QT effect when compared with either drug alone. These observations should be considered in clinical decisions when prescribing vardenafil to patients taking medications known to prolong the QT interval). Products include:
Seroquel ... 750
Seroquel XR ... 759

Quinidine (Patients taking Class 1A antiarrhythmic medications should avoid using vardenafil).
No products indexed under this heading.

Quinidine Gluconate (Patients taking Class 1A antiarrhythmic medications should avoid using vardenafil).
No products indexed under this heading.

Quinidine Hydrochloride (Patients taking Class 1A antiarrhythmic medications should avoid using vardenafil).
No products indexed under this heading.

Quinidine Polygalacturonate (Patients taking Class 1A antiarrhythmic medications should avoid using vardenafil).
No products indexed under this heading.

Quinidine Sulfate (Patients taking Class 1A antiarrhythmic medications should avoid using vardenafil).
No products indexed under this heading.

Quinine (Studies in human liver microsomes showed that vardenafil is metabolized primarily by cytochrome P450 (CYP) isoforms 3A4/5, and to a lesser degree, by CYP2C9. Therefore, inhibitors of CYP3A4 are expected to reduce vardenafil clearance). Products include:
Hyland's Leg Cramps PM with Quinine ... 3315

Quinine Sulfate (Studies in human liver microsomes showed that vardenafil is metabolized primarily by cytochrome P450 (CYP) isoforms 3A4/5, and to a lesser degree, by CYP2C9. Therefore, inhibitors of CYP3A4 are expected to reduce vardenafil clearance).
No products indexed under this heading.

Quinupristin (Studies in human liver microsomes showed that vardenafil is metabolized primarily by cytochrome P450 (CYP) isoforms 3A4/5, and to a lesser degree, by CYP2C9. Therefore, inhibitors of CYP3A4 are expected to reduce vardenafil clearance).
No products indexed under this heading.

Ranitidine Bismuth Citrate (Studies in human liver microsomes showed that vardenafil is metabolized primarily by cytochrome P450 (CYP) isoforms 3A4/5, and to a lesser degree, by CYP2C9. Therefore, inhibitors of CYP3A4 are expected to reduce vardenafil clearance).
No products indexed under this heading.

Ranitidine Hydrochloride (Studies in human liver microsomes showed that vardenafil is metabolized primarily by cytochrome P450 (CYP) isoforms 3A4/5, and to a lesser degree, by CYP2C9. Therefore, inhibitors of CYP3A4 are expected to reduce vardenafil clearance). Products include:
Zantac ... 1737
Zantac Injection ... 1732
Zantac Pharmacy ... 1735

Risperidone (In a study of the effect of vardenafil on QT interval in 59 healthy males, therapeutic (10 mg) and supratherapeutic (80 mg) doses of vardenafil and the active control moxifloxacin (400 mg) produced similar increases in QTc interval. A postmarketing study evaluating the effect of combining vardenafil with another drug of comparable QT effect showed an additive QT effect when compared with either drug alone. These observations should be considered in clinical decisions when prescribing vardenafil to patients taking medications known to prolong the QT interval). Products include:
Risperdal Consta ... 2682

Ritonavir (Ritonavir (600 mg b.i.d.) co-administered with vardenafil 5 mg resulted in a 49-fold increase in vardenafil AUC and a 13-fold increase in vardenafil C_{max}. The interaction is a consequence of blocking hepatic metabolism of vardenafil by ritonavir, a highly potent CYP3A4 inhibitor, which also inhibits CYP2C9. Ritonavir significantly prolonged the half-life of vardenafil to 26 hours. Consequently, it is recommended not to exceed a single 2.5 mg vardenafil dose in a 72 hour period when used in combination with ritonavir. Long-term safety information is not available on the concomitant administration of vardenafil with HIV protease inhibitors). Products include:
Kaletra ... 458
Norvir ... 509

Saquinavir (Patients taking saquinavir, a potent CYP3A4 inhibitor, should not exceed a dose of vardenafil 2.5 mg once daily).
No products indexed under this heading.

Saquinavir Mesylate (Patients taking saquinavir, a potent CYP3A4 inhibitor, should not exceed a dose of vardenafil 2.5 mg once daily).
No products indexed under this heading.

Sertraline Hydrochloride (Studies in human liver microsomes showed that vardenafil is metabolized primarily by cytochrome P450 (CYP) isoforms 3A4/5, and to a lesser degree, by CYP2C9. Therefore, inhibitors of CYP3A4 are expected to reduce vardenafil clearance).
No products indexed under this heading.

1015 Interactions Index Levitra

Sildenafil Citrate (Studies in human liver microsomes showed that vardenafil is metabolized primarily by cytochrome P450 (CYP) isoforms 3A4/5, and to a lesser degree, by CYP2C9. Therefore, inhibitors of CYP3A4 are expected to reduce vardenafil clearance).
No products indexed under this heading.

Sotalol Hydrochloride (Patients taking Class III antiarrhythmic medications should avoid using vardenafil).
No products indexed under this heading.

Sulfacytine (Studies in human liver microsomes showed that vardenafil is metabolized primarily by cytochrome P450 (CYP) isoforms 3A4/5, and to a lesser degree, by CYP2C9. Therefore, inhibitors of CYP2C9 are expected to reduce vardenafil clearance).
No products indexed under this heading.

Sulfamethizole (Studies in human liver microsomes showed that vardenafil is metabolized primarily by cytochrome P450 (CYP) isoforms 3A4/5, and to a lesser degree, by CYP2C9. Therefore, inhibitors of CYP2C9 are expected to reduce vardenafil clearance).
No products indexed under this heading.

Sulfamethoxazole (Studies in human liver microsomes showed that vardenafil is metabolized primarily by cytochrome P450 (CYP) isoforms 3A4/5, and to a lesser degree, by CYP2C9. Therefore, inhibitors of CYP2C9 are expected to reduce vardenafil clearance).
No products indexed under this heading.

Sulfasalazine (Studies in human liver microsomes showed that vardenafil is metabolized primarily by cytochrome P450 (CYP) isoforms 3A4/5, and to a lesser degree, by CYP2C9. Therefore, inhibitors of CYP2C9 are expected to reduce vardenafil clearance).
No products indexed under this heading.

Sulfinpyrazone (Studies in human liver microsomes showed that vardenafil is metabolized primarily by cytochrome P450 (CYP) isoforms 3A4/5, and to a lesser degree, by CYP2C9. Therefore, inhibitors of CYP2C9 are expected to reduce vardenafil clearance).
No products indexed under this heading.

Sulfisoxazole Acetyl (Studies in human liver microsomes showed that vardenafil is metabolized primarily by cytochrome P450 (CYP) isoforms 3A4/5, and to a lesser degree, by CYP2C9. Therefore, inhibitors of CYP2C9 are expected to reduce vardenafil clearance).
No products indexed under this heading.

Sulfisoxazole Diolamine (Studies in human liver microsomes showed that vardenafil is metabolized primarily by cytochrome P450 (CYP) isoforms 3A4/5, and to a lesser degree, by CYP2C9. Therefore, inhibitors of CYP2C9 are expected to reduce vardenafil clearance).
No products indexed under this heading.

Tamsulosin Hydrochloride (Caution is advised when phosphodiesterase type 5 (PDE5) inhibitors are co-administered with α-blockers. PDE5 inhibitors, including vardenafil, and α-adrenergic blocking agents are both vasodilators with blood pressure lowering effects. When vasodilators are used in combination, an additive effect on blood pressure may be anticipated. In some patients, concomitant use of these two drug classes can lower blood pressure significantly, leading to symptomatic hypotension (eg, fainting). Concomitant treatment with vardenafil and α-blockers should be initiated only if the patient is stable on his α-blocker therapy. Vardenafil should be initiated at the lowest recommended starting dose).
No products indexed under this heading.

Telithromycin (Studies in human liver microsomes showed that vardenafil is metabolized primarily by cytochrome P450 (CYP) isoforms 3A4/5, and to a lesser degree, by CYP2C9. Therefore, inhibitors of CYP3A4 are expected to reduce vardenafil clearance. Patients taking potent CYP3A4 inhibitors should not exceed a dose of vardenafil 2.5 mg once daily). Products include:
Ketek 2991

Terazosin Hydrochloride (Caution is advised when phosphodiesterase type 5 (PDE5) inhibitors are co-administered with α-blockers. PDE5 inhibitors, including vardenafil, and α-adrenergic blocking agents are both vasodilators with blood pressure lowering effects. When vasodilators are used in combination, an additive effect on blood pressure may be anticipated. In some patients, concomitant use of these two drug classes can lower blood pressure significantly, leading to symptomatic hypotension (eg, fainting). Concomitant treatment with vardenafil and α-blockers should be initiated only if the patient is stable on his α-blocker therapy. Vardenafil should be initiated at the lowest recommended starting dose).
No products indexed under this heading.

Terconazole (Studies in human liver microsomes showed that vardenafil is metabolized primarily by cytochrome P450 (CYP) isoforms 3A4/5, and to a lesser degree, by CYP2C9. Therefore, inhibitors of CYP2C9 are expected to reduce vardenafil clearance).
No products indexed under this heading.

Thioridazine Hydrochloride (In a study of the effect of vardenafil on QT interval in 59 healthy males, therapeutic (10 mg) and supratherapeutic (80 mg) doses of vardenafil and the active control moxifloxacin (400 mg) produced similar increases in QTc interval. A postmarketing study evaluating the effect of combining vardenafil with another drug of comparable QT effect showed an additive QT effect when compared with either drug alone. These observations should be considered in clinical decisions when prescribing vardenafil to patients taking medications known to prolong the QT interval). Products include:
Thioridazine Hydrochloride 2384

Thiothixene (In a study of the effect of vardenafil on QT interval in 59 healthy males, therapeutic (10 mg) and supratherapeutic (80 mg) doses of vardenafil and the active control moxifloxacin (400 mg) produced similar increases in QTc interval. A postmarketing study evaluating the effect of combining vardenafil with another drug of comparable QT effect showed an additive QT effect when compared with either drug alone. These observations should be considered in clinical decisions when prescribing vardenafil to patients taking medications known to prolong the QT interval). Products include:
Thiothixene 2386

Ticlopidine Hydrochloride (Studies in human liver microsomes showed that vardenafil is metabolized primarily by cytochrome P450 (CYP) isoforms 3A4/5, and to a lesser degree, by CYP2C9. Therefore, inhibitors of CYP2C9 are expected to reduce vardenafil clearance).
No products indexed under this heading.

Tipranavir (Long-term safety information is not available on the concomitant administration of vardenafil with HIV protease inhibitors).
No products indexed under this heading.

Tocainide Hydrochloride (In a study of the effect of vardenafil on QT interval in 59 healthy males, therapeutic (10 mg) and supratherapeutic (80 mg) doses of vardenafil and the active control moxifloxacin (400 mg) produced similar increases in QTc interval. A postmarketing study evaluating the effect of combining vardenafil with another drug of comparable QT effect showed an additive QT effect when compared with either drug alone. These observations should be considered in clinical decisions when prescribing vardenafil to patients taking medications known to prolong the QT interval).
No products indexed under this heading.

Tolazamide (Studies in human liver microsomes showed that vardenafil is metabolized primarily by cytochrome P450 (CYP) isoforms 3A4/5, and to a lesser degree, by CYP2C9. Therefore, inhibitors of CYP2C9 are expected to reduce vardenafil clearance).
No products indexed under this heading.

Tolbutamide (Studies in human liver microsomes showed that vardenafil is metabolized primarily by cytochrome P450 (CYP) isoforms 3A4/5, and to a lesser degree, by CYP2C9. Therefore, inhibitors of CYP2C9 are expected to reduce vardenafil clearance).
No products indexed under this heading.

Tolbutamide Sodium (Studies in human liver microsomes showed that vardenafil is metabolized primarily by cytochrome P450 (CYP) isoforms 3A4/5, and to a lesser degree, by CYP2C9. Therefore, inhibitors of CYP2C9 are expected to reduce vardenafil clearance).
No products indexed under this heading.

Tranylcypromine Sulfate (In a study of the effect of vardenafil on QT interval in 59 healthy males, therapeutic (10 mg) and supratherapeutic (80 mg) doses of vardenafil and the active control moxifloxacin (400 mg) produced similar increases in QTc interval. A postmarketing study evaluating the effect of combining vardenafil with another drug of comparable QT effect showed an additive QT effect when compared with either drug alone. These observations should be considered in clinical decisions when prescribing vardenafil to patients taking medications known to prolong the QT interval). Products include:
Parnate 1584

Trifluoperazine Hydrochloride (In a study of the effect of vardenafil on QT interval in 59 healthy males, therapeutic (10 mg) and supratherapeutic (80 mg) doses of vardenafil and the active control moxifloxacin (400 mg) produced similar increases in QTc interval. A postmarketing study evaluating the effect of combining vardenafil with another drug of comparable QT effect showed an additive QT effect when compared with either drug alone. These observations should be considered in clinical decisions when prescribing vardenafil to patients taking medications known to prolong the QT interval).
No products indexed under this heading.

Trimipramine Maleate (In a study of the effect of vardenafil on QT interval in 59 healthy males, therapeutic (10 mg) and supratherapeutic (80 mg) doses of vardenafil and the active control moxifloxacin (400 mg) produced similar increases in QTc interval. A postmarketing study evaluating the effect of combining vardenafil with another drug of comparable QT effect showed an additive QT effect when compared with either drug alone. These observations should be considered in clinical decisions when prescribing vardenafil to patients taking medications known to prolong the QT interval).
No products indexed under this heading.

Troglitazone (Studies in human liver microsomes showed that vardenafil is metabolized primarily by cytochrome P450 (CYP) isoforms 3A4/5, and to a lesser degree, by CYP2C9. Therefore, inhibitors of CYP3A4 are expected to reduce vardenafil clearance).
No products indexed under this heading.

Troleandomycin (Studies in human liver microsomes showed that vardenafil is metabolized primarily by cytochrome P450 (CYP) isoforms 3A4/5, and to a lesser degree, by CYP2C9. Therefore, inhibitors of CYP3A4 are expected to reduce vardenafil clearance. Patients taking potent CYP3A4 inhibitors should not exceed a dose of vardenafil 2.5 mg once daily).
No products indexed under this heading.

Valproate Sodium (Studies in human liver microsomes showed that vardenafil is metabolized primarily by cytochrome P450 (CYP) isoforms 3A4/5, and to a lesser degree, by CYP2C9. Therefore, inhibitors of CYP3A4 are expected to reduce vardenafil clearance).
No products indexed under this heading.

Verapamil Hydrochloride (Studies in human liver microsomes showed that vardenafil is metabolized primarily by cytochrome P450 (CYP) isoforms 3A4/5, and to a lesser degree, by CYP2C9. Therefore, inhibitors of CYP3A4 are expected to reduce vardenafil clearance). Products include:
Tarka 534

Voriconazole (Studies in human liver microsomes showed that vardenafil is metabolized primarily by cytochrome P450 (CYP) isoforms 3A4/5, and to a lesser degree, by CYP2C9. Therefore, inhibitors of CYP3A4 are expected to reduce vardenafil clearance. Patients taking potent CYP3A4 inhibitors should not exceed a dose of vardenafil 2.5 mg once daily).
No products indexed under this heading.

Zafirlukast (Studies in human liver microsomes showed that vardenafil is metabolized primarily by cytochrome P450 (CYP) isoforms 3A4/5, and to a lesser degree, by CYP2C9. Therefore, inhibitors of CYP3A4 are expected to reduce vardenafil clearance). Products include:
Accolate 3612

Zileuton (Studies in human liver microsomes showed that vardenafil is metabolized primarily by cytochrome P450 (CYP) isoforms 3A4/5, and to a lesser degree, by CYP2C9. Therefore, inhibitors of CYP3A4 are expected to reduce vardenafil clearance).
No products indexed under this heading.

Ziprasidone Hydrochloride (In a study of the effect of vardenafil on QT interval in 59 healthy males, therapeutic (10 mg) and supratherapeutic (80 mg) doses of vardenafil and the active control moxifloxacin (400 mg) produced similar increases in QTc interval. A postmarketing study evaluating the effect of combining vardenafil with another drug of comparable QT effect showed an additive QT effect when compared with either drug alone. These observations should be considered in clinical decisions when prescribing vardenafil to patients taking medications known to prolong the QT interval). Products include:
Geodon 2723

IMPORTANT NOTE: Always consult each drug listing in the patient's regimen for possible interactions.

Food Interactions

Food, unspecified (Two food-effect studies were conducted which showed that high-fat meals caused a reduction in C_{max} by 18%-50%).

Grapefruit (Although specific interactions have not been studied, other CYP3A4 inhibitors, including grapefruit juice, would likely increase vardenafil exposure).

Grapefruit Juice (Although specific interactions have not been studied, other CYP3A4 inhibitors, including grapefruit juice, would likely increase vardenafil exposure).

Meal, unspecified (Two food-effect studies were conducted which showed that high-fat meals caused a reduction in C_{max} by 18%-50%).

LEVOXYL TABLETS

(Levothyroxine Sodium) 1843

May interact with androgens, antacids containing aluminum, calcium and magnesium, beta-blockers, cardiac glycosides, dopamine agonists, estrogens, glucocorticoids, hydantoin anticonvulsants, insulin, lithium preparations, oral anticoagulants, oral hypoglycemic agents, phenytoin, radiographic iodinated contrast media, salicylates, sympathomimetics, thiazides, tricyclic antidepressants, xanthines. Compounds in these categories include:

Acarbose (Addition of levothyroxine to antidiabetic therapy may result in increased antidiabetic agent requirements).
No products indexed under this heading.

Acebutolol Hydrochloride (Co-administration with beta-blockers may decrease T4 5'-deiodinase activity; action of beta-blocker may be impaired when the hypothyroid patient is converted to euthyroid).
No products indexed under this heading.

Albuterol (Co-administration of sympathomimetic agents may increase the effects of sympathomimetics or thyroid hormone; thyroid hormones may increase risk of coronary insufficiency when sympathomimetic agents are administered to patients with coronary disease).
No products indexed under this heading.

Albuterol Sulfate (Co-administration of sympathomimetic agents may increase the effects of sympathomimetics or thyroid hormone; thyroid hormones may increase risk of coronary insufficiency when sympathomimetic agents are administered to patients with coronary disease). Products include:
ProAir HFA 3393
Proventil HFA 3204
Ventolin HFA 1708

Aldesleukin (Co-administration has been associated with transient painless thyroiditis in 20% of patients). Products include:
Proleukin 2504

Aluminum Carbonate (Co-administration with antacids may reduce the efficacy of levothyroxine by binding and delaying or preventing absorption, potentially resulting in hypothyroidism; administer levothyroxine at least 4 hours apart from these agents).
No products indexed under this heading.

Aluminum Hydroxide (Co-administration with antacids may reduce the efficacy of levothyroxine by binding and delaying or preventing absorption, potentially resulting in hypothyroidism; administer levothyroxine at least 4 hours apart from these agents).
No products indexed under this heading.

Aminoglutethimide (May decrease thyroid hormone secretion, which may result in hypothyroidism).
No products indexed under this heading.

Aminophylline (Decreased theophylline clearance may occur in hypothyroid patients; clearance returns to normal when euthyroid state is achieved).
No products indexed under this heading.

p-Aminosalicylic Acid (Co-administration has been associated with thyroid hormone and/or TSH level alterations by various mechanisms).
No products indexed under this heading.

Amiodarone Hydrochloride (May decrease thyroid hormone secretion, which may result in hypothyroidism; amiodarone is slowly excreted, producing more prolonged hypothyroidism; amiodarone may induce hyperthyroidism by causing thyroiditis).
No products indexed under this heading.

Amitriptyline Hydrochloride (Co-administration may increase the therapeutic and toxic effects of both drugs possibly due to increased receptor sensitivity to catecholamines; toxic effects may include increased risk of arrhythmias and CNS stimulation; onset of tricyclics may be accelerated).
No products indexed under this heading.

Amoxapine (Co-administration may increase the therapeutic and toxic effects of both drugs possibly due to increased receptor sensitivity to catecholamines; toxic effects may include increased risk of arrhythmias and CNS stimulation; onset of tricyclics may be accelerated).
No products indexed under this heading.

Anisindione (Thyroid hormones appear to increase the catabolism of vitamin K-dependent clotting factors, thereby increasing the anticoagulant activity of oral anticoagulants).
No products indexed under this heading.

Asparaginase (Co-administration may result in decreased serum TBG concentration). Products include:
Elspar 2005, 2122

Aspirin (Co-administration with salicylates at greater than 2 gm inhibit binding of T4 and T3 to TBG and transthyrelin; an initial increase in serum FT4 is followed by return of FT4 to normal levels with sustained therapeutic salicylate concentrations, although total T4 levels may decrease by as much as 30%). Products include:
Aggrenox 880
Bayer Aspirin 829
Percodan 1124
St. Joseph Aspirin 2045

Aspirin, Enteric Coated (Co-administration with salicylates at greater than 2 gm inhibit binding of T4 and T3 to TBG and transthyrelin; an initial increase in serum FT4 is followed by return of FT4 to normal levels with sustained therapeutic salicylate concentrations, although total T4 levels may decrease by as much as 30%).
No products indexed under this heading.

Aspirin Buffered (Co-administration with salicylates at greater than 2 gm inhibit binding of T4 and T3 to TBG and transthyrelin; an initial increase in serum FT4 is followed by return of FT4 to normal levels with sustained therapeutic salicylate concentrations, although total T4 levels may decrease by as much as 30%).
No products indexed under this heading.

Atenolol (Co-administration with beta-blockers may decrease T4 5'-deiodinase activity; action of beta-blocker may be impaired when the hypothyroid patient is converted to euthyroid).
No products indexed under this heading.

Bendroflumethiazide (Co-administration has been associated with thyroid hormone and/or TSH level alterations by various mechanisms).
No products indexed under this heading.

Betamethasone Acetate (Co-administration with glucocorticoids may result in a transient reduction in TSH secretion; the reduction is not sustained, therefore, hypothyroidism does not occur; glucocorticoids may decrease serum TBG concentration).
No products indexed under this heading.

Betamethasone Sodium Phosphate (Co-administration with glucocorticoids may result in a transient reduction in TSH secretion; the reduction is not sustained, therefore, hypothyroidism does not occur; glucocorticoids may decrease serum TBG concentration).
No products indexed under this heading.

Betaxolol Hydrochloride (Co-administration with beta-blockers may decrease T4 5'-deiodinase activity; action of beta-blocker may be impaired when the hypothyroid patient is converted to euthyroid).
No products indexed under this heading.

Bisoprolol Fumarate (Co-administration with beta-blockers may decrease T4 5'-deiodinase activity; action of beta-blocker may be impaired when the hypothyroid patient is converted to euthyroid).
No products indexed under this heading.

Bromocriptine Mesylate (Co-administration with dopamine agonists may result in a transient reduction in TSH secretion; the reduction is not sustained, therefore, hypothyroidism does not occur).
No products indexed under this heading.

Budesonide (Co-administration with glucocorticoids may result in a transient reduction in TSH secretion; the reduction is not sustained, therefore, hypothyroidism does not occur; glucocorticoids may decrease serum TBG concentration). Products include:
Pulmicort Flexhaler 714
Symbicort 80/4.5 720
Symbicort 160/4.5 720

Calcium Carbonate (Co-administration with calcium carbonate may form insoluble chelate with levothyroxine, which may result in hypothyroidism; administer levothyroxine at least 4 hours apart from these agents). Products include:
Chelated Mineral 3476
Pepcid Complete 1822
Extra Strength Rolaids Softchews Vanilla Creme 2045

Carbamazepine (Co-administration may increase hepatic metabolism, which may result in hypothyroidism, resulting in increased levothyroxine requirements; carbamazepine reduces serum protein binding of levothyroxine, and total- and free-T4 may be reduced by 20% to 40%, but most patients have normal serum TSH levels and are clinically euthyroid). Products include:
Carbatrol 3280
Equetro 3477

Carteolol Hydrochloride (Co-administration with beta-blockers may decrease T4 5'-deiodinase activity; action of beta-blocker may be impaired when the hypothyroid patient is converted to euthyroid).
No products indexed under this heading.

Carvedilol (Co-administration with beta-blockers may decrease T4 5'-deiodinase activity; action of beta-blocker may be impaired when the hypothyroid patient is converted to euthyroid). Products include:
Coreg 1409

Carvedilol Phosphate (Co-administration with beta-blockers may decrease T4 5'-deiodinase activity; action of beta-blocker may be impaired when the hypothyroid patient is converted to euthyroid). Products include:
Coreg CR 1416

Chloral Hydrate (Co-administration has been associated with thyroid hormone and/or TSH level alterations by various mechanisms).
No products indexed under this heading.

Chlorothiazide (Co-administration has been associated with thyroid hormone and/or TSH level alterations by various mechanisms).
No products indexed under this heading.

Chlorothiazide Sodium (Co-administration has been associated with thyroid hormone and/or TSH level alterations by various mechanisms). Products include:
Diuril Intravenous 2009

Chlorotrianisene (Co-administration with oral estrogens may result in increased serum TBG concentrations).
No products indexed under this heading.

Chlorpropamide (Addition of levothyroxine to antidiabetic therapy may result in increased antidiabetic agent requirements).
No products indexed under this heading.

Cholestyramine (Co-administration may result in decreased T4 absorption, which may result in hypothyroidism; administer levothyroxine at least 4 hours apart from these agents).
No products indexed under this heading.

Choline Magnesium Trisalicylate (Co-administration with salicylates at greater than 2 gm inhibit binding of T4 and T3 to TBG and transthyrelin; an initial increase in serum FT4 is followed by return of FT4 to normal levels with sustained therapeutic salicylate concentrations, although total T4 levels may decrease by as much as 30%).
No products indexed under this heading.

Clofibrate (Co-administration may result in increased serum TBG concentrations).
No products indexed under this heading.

Clomipramine Hydrochloride (Co-administration may increase the therapeutic and toxic effects of both drugs possibly due to increased receptor sensitivity to catecholamines; toxic effects may include increased risk of arrhythmias and CNS stimulation; onset of tricyclics may be accelerated).
No products indexed under this heading.

Colestipol Hydrochloride (Co-administration may result in decreased T4 absorption, which may result in hypothyroidism; administer levothyroxine at least 4 hours apart from these agents).
No products indexed under this heading.

Cortisone Acetate (Co-administration with glucocorticoids may result in a transient reduction in TSH secretion; the reduction is not sustained, therefore, hypothyroidism does not occur; glucocorticoids may decrease serum TBG concentration).
No products indexed under this heading.

Desipramine Hydrochloride (Co-administration may increase the therapeutic and toxic effects of both drugs possibly due to increased receptor sensitivity to catecholamines; toxic effects may include increased risk of arrhythmias and CNS stimulation; onset of tricyclics may be accelerated).
No products indexed under this heading.

Deslanoside (Co-administration may result in reduced serum digitalis glycosides in hyperthyroidism or when the hypothyroid patient is converted to euthyroid state; therapeutic effect of digitalis glycoside may be reduced).
No products indexed under this heading.

Dexamethasone (Co-administration with glucocorticoids may result in a transient reduction in TSH secretion;

the reduction is not sustained, therefore, hypothyroidism does not occur; glucocorticoids may decrease serum TBG concentration). Products include:

Dexamethasone Acetate (Co-administration with glucocorticoids may result in a transient reduction in TSH secretion; the reduction is not sustained, therefore, hypothyroidism does not occur; glucocorticoids may decrease serum TBG concentration).
No products indexed under this heading.

Dexamethasone Sodium Phosphate (Co-administration with glucocorticoids may result in a transient reduction in TSH secretion; the reduction is not sustained, therefore, hypothyroidism does not occur; glucocorticoids may decrease serum TBG concentration).
No products indexed under this heading.

Diatrizoate Meglumine (May decrease thyroid hormone secretion, which may result in hypothyrodism; the fetus, elderly, and euthyroid patients with underlying thyroid disease are among those individuals who are susceptible to iodine-induced hypothyroidism; oral cholecytographic agents slowly excreted, producing more prolonged hypothyroidism; iodide drugs that contain pharmacologic amounts of iodide may cause hypothyroidism in euthyroid patients with Grave's disease previously treated with thyroid autonomy; hyperthyroidism may develop over several weeks and may persist for several months after therapy discontinuation).
No products indexed under this heading.

Diatrizoate Sodium (May decrease thyroid hormone secretion, which may result in hypothyrodism; the fetus, elderly, and euthyroid patients with underlying thyroid disease are among those individuals who are susceptible to iodine-induced hypothyroidism; oral cholecytographic agents slowly excreted, producing more prolonged hypothyroidism; iodide drugs that contain pharmacologic amounts of iodide may cause hypothyroidism in euthyroid patients with Grave's disease previously treated with thyroid autonomy; hyperthyroidism may develop over several weeks and may persist for several months after therapy discontinuation).
No products indexed under this heading.

Diazepam (Co-administration has been associated with thyroid hormone and/or TSH level alterations by various mechanisms). Products include:

Dicumarol (Thyroid hormones appear to increase the catabolism of vitamin K-dependent clotting factors, thereby increasing the anticoagulant activity of oral anticoagulants).
No products indexed under this heading.

Dienestrol (Co-administration with oral estrogens may result in increased serum TBG concentrations).
No products indexed under this heading.

Diethylstilbestrol (Co-administration with oral estrogens may result in increased serum TBG concentrations).
No products indexed under this heading.

Diflunisal (Co-administration with salicylates at greater than 2 gm inhibit binding of T4 and T3 to TBG and transthyrelin; an initial increase in serum FT4 is followed by return of FT4 to normal levels with sustained therapeutic salicylate concentrations, although total T4 levels may decrease by as much as 30%).
No products indexed under this heading.

Digitalis Glycoside Preparations (Co-administration may result in reduced serum digitalis glycosides in hyperthyroidism or when the hypothyroid patient is converted to euthyroid state; therapeutic effect of digitalis glycoside may be reduced).
No products indexed under this heading.

Digitalis Lanata (Co-administration may result in reduced serum digitalis glycosides in hyperthyroidism or when the hypothyroid patient is converted to euthyroid state; therapeutic effect of digitalis glycoside may be reduced).
No products indexed under this heading.

Digitalis Purpurea (Co-administration may result in reduced serum digitalis glycosides in hyperthyroidism or when the hypothyroid patient is converted to euthyroid state; therapeutic effect of digitalis glycoside may be reduced).
No products indexed under this heading.

Digitoxin (Co-administration may result in reduced serum digitalis glycosides in hyperthyroidism or when the hypothyroid patient is converted to euthyroid state; therapeutic effect of digitalis glycoside may be reduced).
No products indexed under this heading.

Digoxin (Co-administration may result in reduced serum digitalis glycosides in hyperthyroidism or when the hypothyroid patient is converted to euthyroid state; therapeutic effect of digitalis glycoside may be reduced). Products include:

Dobutamine Hydrochloride (Co-administration of sympathomimetic agents may increase the effects of sympathomimetics or thyroid hormone; thyroid hormones may increase risk of coronary insufficiency when sympathomimetic agents are administered to patients with coronary disease).
No products indexed under this heading.

Dopamine Hydrochloride (Co-administration with dopamine may result in a transient reduction in TSH secretion; the reduction is not sustained, therefore, hypothyroidism does not occur).
No products indexed under this heading.

Doxepin Hydrochloride (Co-administration may increase the therapeutic and toxic effects of both drugs possibly due to increased receptor sensitivity to catecholamines; toxic effects may include increased risk of arrhythmias and CNS stimulation; onset of tricyclics may be accelerated).
No products indexed under this heading.

Dyphylline (Decreased theophylline clearance may occur in hypothyroid patients; clearance returns to normal when euthyroid state is achieved).
No products indexed under this heading.

Ephedrine Hydrochloride (Co-administration of sympathomimetic agents may increase the effects of sympathomimetics or thyroid hormone; thyroid hormones may increase risk of coronary insufficiency when sympathomimetic agents are administered to patients with coronary disease).
No products indexed under this heading.

Ephedrine Sulfate (Co-administration of sympathomimetic agents may increase the effects of sympathomimetics or thyroid hormone; thyroid hormones may increase risk of coronary insufficiency when sympathomimetic agents are administered to patients with coronary disease).
No products indexed under this heading.

Ephedrine Tannate (Co-administration of sympathomimetic agents may increase the effects of sympathomimetics or thyroid hormone; thyroid hormones may increase risk of coronary insufficiency when sympathomimetic agents are administered to patients with coronary disease).
No products indexed under this heading.

Epinephrine (Co-administration of sympathomimetic agents may increase the effects of sympathomimetics or thyroid hormone; thyroid hormones may increase risk of coronary insufficiency when sympathomimetic agents are administered to patients with coronary disease). Products include:

Epinephrine Bitartrate (Co-administration of sympathomimetic agents may increase the effects of sympathomimetics or thyroid hormone; thyroid hormones may increase risk of coronary insufficiency when sympathomimetic agents are administered to patients with coronary disease).
No products indexed under this heading.

Epinephrine Hydrochloride (Co-administration of sympathomimetic agents may increase the effects of sympathomimetics or thyroid hormone; thyroid hormones may increase risk of coronary insufficiency when sympathomimetic agents are administered to patients with coronary disease).
No products indexed under this heading.

Esmolol Hydrochloride (Co-administration with beta-blockers may decrease T4 5'-deiodinase activity; action of beta-blocker may be impaired when the hypothyroid patient is converted to euthyroid).
No products indexed under this heading.

Estradiol (Co-administration with oral estrogens may result in increased serum TBG concentrations). Products include:

Estrogens, Conjugated (Co-administration with oral estrogens may result in increased serum TBG concentrations). Products include:

Estrogens, Esterified (Co-administration with oral estrogens may result in increased serum TBG concentrations).
No products indexed under this heading.

Estropipate (Co-administration with oral estrogens may result in increased serum TBG concentrations).
No products indexed under this heading.

Ethinyl Estradiol (Co-administration with estrogen containing oral contraceptives may result in increased serum TBG concentrations). Products include:

Ethiodized Oil (May decrease thyroid hormone secretion, which may result in hypothyrodism; the fetus, elderly, and

euthyroid patients with underlying thyroid disease are among those individuals who are susceptible to iodine-induced hypothyroidism; oral cholecytographic agents slowly excreted, producing more prolonged hypothyroidism; iodide drugs that contain pharmacologic amounts of iodide may cause hypothyroidism in euthyroid patients with Grave's disease previously treated with thyroid autonomy; hyperthyroidism may develop over several weeks and may persist for several months after therapy discontinuation).
No products indexed under this heading.

Ethionamide (Co-administration has been associated with thyroid hormone and/or TSH level alterations by various mechanisms).
No products indexed under this heading.

Ethotoin (Hydantoins may cause protein-binding site displacement; co-administration results in an initial transient increase in FT4; continued administration results in a decrease in serum T4 and normal FT4 and TSH concentrations and, therefore, patients are clinically euthyroid).
No products indexed under this heading.

Ferrous Sulfate (Co-administration may result in decreased T4 absorption, which may result in hypothyroidism; ferrous sulfate may form a ferricthyroxine complex; administer levothyroxine at least 4 hours apart from these agents).
No products indexed under this heading.

Fiber Supplement (Concurrent use of dietary fiber may bind and decrease the absorption of levothyroxine sodium from GI tract). Products include:

Fludrocortisone Acetate (Co-administration with glucocorticoids may result in a transient reduction in TSH secretion; the reduction is not sustained, therefore, hypothyroidism does not occur; glucocorticoids may decrease serum TBG concentration).
No products indexed under this heading.

Fluorouracil (Co-administration with 5-FU may result in increased serum TBG concentrations). Products include:

Fluoxymesterone (Co-administration with androgens/anabolic steroids may result in decreased serum TBG concentration).
No products indexed under this heading.

Fosphenytoin (Hydantoins may cause protein-binding site displacement; co-administration results in an initial transient increase in FT4; co-administration may increase hepatic metabolism, which may result in hypothyroidism, resulting in increased levothyroxine requirements; phenytoin reduces serum protein binding of levothyroxine, and total- and free-T4 may be reduced by 20% to 40%, but most patients have normal serum TSH levels and are clinically euthyroid).
No products indexed under this heading.

Fosphenytoin Sodium (Hydantoins may cause protein-binding site displacement; co-administration results in an initial transient increase in FT4; co-administration may increase hepatic metabolism, which may result in hypothyroidism, resulting in increased levothyroxine requirements; phenytoin reduces serum protein binding of levothyroxine, and total- and free-T4 may be reduced by 20% to 40%, but most patients have normal serum TSH levels and are clinically euthyroid).
No products indexed under this heading.

Furosemide (May cause protein-binding site displacement at greater than 80 mg IV; co-administration results

in an initial transient increase in FT4; continued administration results in a decrease in serum T4 and normal FT4 and TSH concentrations and, therefore, patients are clinically euthyroid). Products include:

Gadopentetate Dimeglumine (May decrease thyroid hormone secretion, which may result in hypothyrodism; the fetus, elderly, and euthyroid patients with underlying thyroid disease are among those individuals who are susceptible to iodine-induced hypothyroidism; oral cholecytographic agents slowly excreted, producing more prolonged hypothyroidism; iodide drugs that contain pharmacologic amounts of iodide may cause hypothyroidism in euthyroid patients with Grave's disease previously treated with thyroid autonomy; hyperthyroidism may develop over several weeks and may persist for several months after therapy discontinuation).
No products indexed under this heading.

Glibenclamide (Addition of levothyroxine to antidiabetic therapy may result in increased antidiabetic agent requirements).
No products indexed under this heading.

Glimepiride (Addition of levothyroxine to antidiabetic therapy may result in increased antidiabetic agent requirements). Products include:

Glipizide (Addition of levothyroxine to antidiabetic therapy may result in increased antidiabetic agent requirements).
No products indexed under this heading.

Glyburide (Addition of levothyroxine to antidiabetic therapy may result in increased antidiabetic agent requirements).
No products indexed under this heading.

Heparin Sodium (May cause protein-binding site displacement; co-administration results in an initial transient increase in FT4; continued administration results in a decrease in serum T4 and normal FT4 and TSH concentrations and, therefore, patients are clinically euthyroid).
No products indexed under this heading.

Heroin (Co-administration may result in increased serum TBG concentrations).
No products indexed under this heading.

Hydrochlorothiazide (Co-administration has been associated with thyroid hormone and/or TSH level alterations by various mechanisms). Products include:

Hydrocortisone (Co-administration with glucocorticoids may result in a transient reduction in TSH secretion; the reduction is not sustained, therefore, hypothyroidism does not occur; glucocorticoids may decrease serum TBG concentration).
No products indexed under this heading.

Hydrocortisone Acetate (Co-administration with glucocorticoids may result in a transient reduction in TSH secretion; the reduction is not sustained, therefore, hypothyroidism does not occur; glucocorticoids may decrease serum TBG concentration).
No products indexed under this heading.

Hydrocortisone Sodium Phosphate (Co-administration with glucocorticoids may result in a transient reduction in TSH secretion; the reduction is not sustained, therefore, hypothyroidism does not occur; glucocorticoids may decrease serum TBG concentration).
No products indexed under this heading.

Hydrocortisone Sodium Succinate (Co-administration with glucocorticoids may result in a transient reduction in TSH secretion; the reduction is not sustained, therefore, hypothyroidism does not occur; glucocorticoids may decrease serum TBG concentration).
No products indexed under this heading.

Hydroflumethiazide (Co-administration has been associated with thyroid hormone and/or TSH level alterations by various mechanisms).
No products indexed under this heading.

Imipramine Hydrochloride (Co-administration may increase the therapeutic and toxic effects of both drugs possibly due to increased receptor sensitivity to catecholamines; toxic effects may include increased risk of arrhythmias and CNS stimulation; onset of tricyclics may be accelerated).
No products indexed under this heading.

Imipramine Pamoate (Co-administration may increase the therapeutic and toxic effects of both drugs possibly due to increased receptor sensitivity to catecholamines; toxic effects may include increased risk of arrhythmias and CNS stimulation; onset of tricyclics may be accelerated).
No products indexed under this heading.

Infant Formula (Concurrent use of soybean flour may bind and decrease the absorption of levothyroxine sodium from GI tract).
No products indexed under this heading.

Insulin (Addition of levothyroxine to insulin therapy may result in increased insulin requirements).
No products indexed under this heading.

Insulin, Human, Zinc Suspension (Addition of levothyroxine to insulin therapy may result in increased insulin requirements).
No products indexed under this heading.

Insulin, Human (rDNA origin) (Addition of levothyroxine to insulin therapy may result in increased insulin requirements). Products include:

Insulin, Human NPH (Addition of levothyroxine to insulin therapy may result in increased insulin requirements). Products include:

Insulin, Human Regular (Addition of levothyroxine to insulin therapy may result in increased insulin requirements). Products include:

Insulin, Human Regular and Human NPH Mixture (Addition of levothyroxine to insulin therapy may result in increased insulin requirements). Products include:

Insulin, NPH (Addition of levothyroxine to insulin therapy may result in increased insulin requirements).
No products indexed under this heading.

Insulin, Regular (Addition of levothyroxine to insulin therapy may result in increased insulin requirements).
No products indexed under this heading.

Insulin, Regular and NPH mixture (Addition of levothyroxine to insulin therapy may result in increased insulin requirements).
No products indexed under this heading.

Insulin, Zinc Crystals (Addition of levothyroxine to insulin therapy may result in increased insulin requirements).
No products indexed under this heading.

Insulin, Zinc Suspension (Addition of levothyroxine to insulin therapy may result in increased insulin requirements).
No products indexed under this heading.

Insulin Aspart (Addition of levothyroxine to insulin therapy may result in increased insulin requirements).
No products indexed under this heading.

Insulin Aspart, Human (Addition of levothyroxine to insulin therapy may result in increased insulin requirements). Products include:

Insulin Aspart, Human Regular (Addition of levothyroxine to insulin therapy may result in increased insulin requirements). Products include:

Insulin Aspart Protamine, Human (Addition of levothyroxine to insulin therapy may result in increased insulin requirements). Products include:

Insulin Detemir (rDNA Origin) (Addition of levothyroxine to insulin therapy may result in increased insulin requirements). Products include:

Insulin Glargine (Addition of levothyroxine to insulin therapy may result in increased insulin requirements). Products include:

Insulin Glulisine (Addition of levothyroxine to insulin therapy may result in increased insulin requirements). Products include:

Insulin Lispro, Human (Addition of levothyroxine to insulin therapy may result in increased insulin requirements). Products include:

Insulin Lispro Protamine, Human (Addition of levothyroxine to insulin therapy may result in increased insulin requirements). Products include:

Interferon alfa-2a, Recombinant (Co-administration with interferon alpha has been associated with the development of antithyroid microsomal antibodies in 20% of patients and some have transient hypothyroidism, hyperthyroidism, or both; patients who have antithyroid antibodies before treatment are at higher risk for thyroid dysfunction).
No products indexed under this heading.

Interferon alfa-2b, Recombinant (Co-administration with interferon alpha has been associated with the development of antithyroid microsomal antibodies in 20% of patients and some have transient hypothyroidism, hyperthyroidism, or both; patients who have antithyroid antibodies before treatment are at higher risk for thyroid dysfunction). Products include:

Interferon alfa-N3 (Human Leukocyte Derived) (Co-administration with interferon alpha has been associated with the development of antithyroid microsomal antibodies in 20% of patients and some have transient hypothyroidism, hyperthyroidism, or both; patients who have antithyroid antibodies before treatment are at higher risk for thyroid dysfunction). Products include:

Iodamide Meglumine (May decrease thyroid hormone secretion, which may result in hypothyrodism; the fetus,

elderly, and euthyroid patients with underlying thyroid disease are among those individuals who are susceptible to iodine-induced hypothyroidism; oral cholecytographic agents slowly excreted, producing more prolonged hypothyroidism; iodide drugs that contain pharmacologic amounts of iodide may cause hypothyroidism in euthyroid patients with Grave's disease previously treated with thyroid autonomy; hyperthyroidism may develop over several weeks and may persist for several months after therapy discontinuation).
No products indexed under this heading.

Iohexol (May decrease thyroid hormone secretion, which may result in hypothyrodism; the fetus, elderly, and euthyroid patients with underlying thyroid disease are among those individuals who are susceptible to iodine-induced hypothyroidism; oral cholecytographic agents slowly excreted, producing more prolonged hypothyroidism; iodide drugs that contain pharmacologic amounts of iodide may cause hypothyroidism in euthyroid patients with Grave's disease previously treated with thyroid autonomy; hyperthyroidism may develop over several weeks and may persist for several months after therapy discontinuation).
No products indexed under this heading.

Iopamidol (May decrease thyroid hormone secretion, which may result in hypothyrodism; the fetus, elderly, and euthyroid patients with underlying thyroid disease are among those individuals who are susceptible to iodine-induced hypothyroidism; oral cholecytographic agents slowly excreted, producing more prolonged hypothyroidism; iodide drugs that contain pharmacologic amounts of iodide may cause hypothyroidism in euthyroid patients with Grave's disease previously treated with thyroid autonomy; hyperthyroidism may develop over several weeks and may persist for several months after therapy discontinuation).
No products indexed under this heading.

Iopanoic Acid (May decrease thyroid hormone secretion, which may result in hypothyrodism; the fetus, elderly, and euthyroid patients with underlying thyroid disease are among those individuals who are susceptible to iodine-induced hypothyroidism; oral cholecytographic agents slowly excreted, producing more prolonged hypothyroidism; iodide drugs that contain pharmacologic amounts of iodide may cause hypothyroidism in euthyroid patients with Grave's disease previously treated with thyroid autonomy; hyperthyroidism may develop over several weeks and may persist for several months after therapy discontinuation).
No products indexed under this heading.

Iothalamate Meglumine (May decrease thyroid hormone secretion, which may result in hypothyrodism; the fetus, elderly, and euthyroid patients with underlying thyroid disease are among those individuals who are susceptible to iodine-induced hypothyroidism; oral cholecytographic agents slowly excreted, producing more prolonged hypothyroidism; iodide drugs that contain pharmacologic amounts of iodide may cause hypothyroidism in euthyroid patients with Grave's disease previously treated with thyroid autonomy; hyperthyroidism may develop over several weeks and may persist for several months after therapy discontinuation).
No products indexed under this heading.

Ioxaglate Meglumine (May decrease thyroid hormone secretion, which may result in hypothyrodism; the fetus, elderly, and euthyroid patients with underlying thyroid disease are among those individuals who are susceptible to

iodine-induced hypothyroidism; oral cholecystographic agents slowly excreted, producing more prolonged hypothyroidism; iodide drugs that contain pharmacologic amounts of iodide may cause hypothyroidism in euthyroid patients with Grave's disease previously treated with thyroid autonomy; hyperthyroidism may develop over several weeks and may persist for several months after therapy discontinuation).
No products indexed under this heading.

Ioxaglate Sodium (May decrease thyroid hormone secretion, which may result in hypothyrodism; the fetus, elderly, and euthyroid patients with underlying thyroid disease are among those individuals who are susceptible to iodine-induced hypothyroidism; oral cholecytographic agents slowly excreted, producing more prolonged hypothyroidism; iodide drugs that contain pharmacologic amounts of iodide may cause hypothyroidism in euthyroid patients with Grave's disease previously treated with thyroid autonomy; hyperthyroidism may develop over several weeks and may persist for several months after therapy discontinuation).
No products indexed under this heading.

Isoproterenol Hydrochloride (Co-administration of sympathomimetic agents may increase the effects of sympathomimetics or thyroid hormone; thyroid hormones may increase risk of coronary insufficiency when sympathomimetic agents are administered to patients with coronary disease).
No products indexed under this heading.

Isoproterenol Sulfate (Co-administration of sympathomimetic agents may increase the effects of sympathomimetics or thyroid hormone; thyroid hormones may increase risk of coronary insufficiency when sympathomimetic agents are administered to patients with coronary disease).
No products indexed under this heading.

Ketamine Hydrochloride (Co-administration may produce marked hypertension and tachycardia).
No products indexed under this heading.

Labetalol Hydrochloride (Co-administration with beta-blockers may decrease T4 5'-deiodinase activity; action of beta-blocker may be impaired when the hypothyroid patient is converted to euthyroid).
No products indexed under this heading.

Levalbuterol Hydrochloride (Co-administration of sympathomimetic agents may increase the effects of sympathomimetics or thyroid hormone; thyroid hormones may increase risk of coronary insufficiency when sympathomimetic agents are administered to patients with coronary disease).
No products indexed under this heading.

Levobunolol Hydrochloride (Co-administration with beta-blockers may decrease T4 5'-deiodinase activity; action of beta-blocker may be impaired when the hypothyroid patient is converted to euthyroid).
No products indexed under this heading.

Levodopa (Co-administration with dopamine agonists may result in a transient reduction in TSH secretion; the reduction is not sustained, therefore, hypothyroidism does not occur). Products include:

Lithium (May decrease thyroid hormone secretion, which may result in hypothyrodism; long-term lithium therapy can result in goiter in up to 50% of patients, and either subclinical or overt hypothyroidism, each in up to 20% of patients).
No products indexed under this heading.

Lithium Carbonate (May decrease thyroid hormone secretion, which may result in hypothyrodism; long-term lithium therapy can result in goiter in up to 50% of patients, and either subclinical or overt hypothyroidism, each in up to 20% of patients).
No products indexed under this heading.

Lithium Citrate (May decrease thyroid hormone secretion, which may result in hypothyrodism; long-term lithium therapy can result in goiter in up to 50% of patients, and either subclinical or overt hypothyroidism, each in up to 20% of patients).
No products indexed under this heading.

Lovastatin (Co-administration has been associated with thyroid hormone and/or TSH level alterations by various mechanisms). Products include:

Magaldrate (Co-administration with antacids may reduce the efficacy of levothyroxine by binding and delaying or preventing absorption, potentially resulting in hypothyroidism; administer levothyroxine at least 4 hours apart from these agents).
No products indexed under this heading.

Magnesium Carbonate (Co-administration with antacids may reduce the efficacy of levothyroxine by binding and delaying or preventing absorption, potentially resulting in hypothyroidism; administer levothyroxine at least 4 hours apart from these agents).
No products indexed under this heading.

Magnesium Hydroxide (Co-administration with antacids may reduce the efficacy of levothyroxine by binding and delaying or preventing absorption, potentially resulting in hypothyroidism; administer levothyroxine at least 4 hours apart from these agents). Products include:

Magnesium Oxide (Co-administration with antacids may reduce the efficacy of levothyroxine by binding and delaying or preventing absorption, potentially resulting in hypothyroidism; administer levothyroxine at least 4 hours apart from these agents). Products include:

Magnesium Salicylate (Co-administration with salicylates at greater than 2 gm inhibit binding of T4 and T3 to TBG and transthyrelin; an initial increase in serum FT4 is followed by return of FT4 to normal levels with sustained therapeutic salicylate concentrations, although total T4 levels may decrease by as much as 30%).
No products indexed under this heading.

Magnesium Trisilicate (Co-administration with antacids may reduce the efficacy of levothyroxine by binding and delaying or preventing absorption, potentially resulting in hypothyroidism; administer levothyroxine at least 4 hours apart from these agents).
No products indexed under this heading.

Maprotiline Hydrochloride (Co-administration may increase the therapeutic and toxic effects of both drugs possibly due to increased receptor sensitivity to catecholamines; toxic effects may include increased risk of arrhythmias and CNS stimulation; onset of tricyclics may be accelerated).
No products indexed under this heading.

Meclofenamate Sodium (Co-administration with fenamate NSAID may result in decreased serum TBG concentration).
No products indexed under this heading.

Mefenamic Acid (Co-administration with fenamate NSAID may result in decreased serum TBG concentration).
No products indexed under this heading.

Mephenytoin (Hydantoins may cause protein-binding site displacement; co-administration results in an initial transient increase in FT4; continued administration results in a decrease in serum T4 and normal FT4 and TSH concentrations and, therefore, patients are clinically euthyroid).
No products indexed under this heading.

Mercaptopurine (Co-administration has been associated with thyroid hormone and/or TSH level alterations by various mechanisms).
No products indexed under this heading.

Mestranol (Co-administration with estrogen containing oral contraceptives may result in increased serum TBG concentrations).
No products indexed under this heading.

Metaproterenol Sulfate (Co-administration of sympathomimetic agents may increase the effects of sympathomimetics or thyroid hormone; thyroid hormones may increase risk of coronary insufficiency when sympathomimetic agents are administered to patients with coronary disease).
No products indexed under this heading.

Metaraminol Bitartrate (Co-administration of sympathomimetic agents may increase the effects of sympathomimetics or thyroid hormone; thyroid hormones may increase risk of coronary insufficiency when sympathomimetic agents are administered to patients with coronary disease).
No products indexed under this heading.

Metformin Hydrochloride (Addition of levothyroxine to antidiabetic therapy may result in increased antidiabetic agent requirements). Products include:

Methadone Hydrochloride (Co-administration may result in increased serum TBG concentrations).
No products indexed under this heading.

Methimazole (May decrease thyroid hormone secretion, which may result in hypothyrodism).
No products indexed under this heading.

Methoxamine Hydrochloride (Co-administration of sympathomimetic agents may increase the effects of sympathomimetics or thyroid hormone; thyroid hormones may increase risk of coronary insufficiency when sympathomimetic agents are administered to patients with coronary disease).
No products indexed under this heading.

Methyclothiazide (Co-administration has been associated with thyroid hormone and/or TSH level alterations by various mechanisms).
No products indexed under this heading.

Methylprednisolone Acetate (Co-administration with glucocorticoids may result in a transient reduction in TSH secretion; the reduction is not sustained, therefore, hypothyroidism does not occur; glucocorticoids may decrease serum TBG concentration).
No products indexed under this heading.

Methylprednisolone Sodium Succinate (Co-administration with glucocorticoids may result in a transient reduction in TSH secretion; the reduction is not sustained, therefore, hypothyroidism does not occur; glucocorticoids may decrease serum TBG concentration).
No products indexed under this heading.

Methyltestosterone (Co-administration with androgens/anabolic steroids may result in decreased serum TBG concentration).
No products indexed under this heading.

Metipranolol Hydrochloride (Co-administration with beta-blockers may decrease T4 5'-deiodinase activity; action of beta-blocker may be impaired when the hypothyroid patient is converted to euthyroid).
No products indexed under this heading.

Metoclopramide Hydrochloride (Co-administration has been associated with thyroid hormone and/or TSH level alterations by various mechanisms). Products include:

Metoprolol Succinate (Co-administration with beta-blockers may decrease T4 5'-deiodinase activity; action of beta-blocker may be impaired when the hypothyroid patient is converted to euthyroid). Products include:

Metoprolol Tartrate (Co-administration with beta-blockers may decrease T4 5'-deiodinase activity; action of beta-blocker may be impaired when the hypothyroid patient is converted to euthyroid).
No products indexed under this heading.

Miglitol (Addition of levothyroxine to antidiabetic therapy may result in increased antidiabetic agent requirements).
No products indexed under this heading.

Mitotane (Co-administration may result in increased serum TBG concentrations).
No products indexed under this heading.

Nadolol (Co-administration with beta-blockers may decrease T4 5'-deiodinase activity; action of beta-blocker may be impaired when the hypothyroid patient is converted to euthyroid). Products include:

Nateglinide (Addition of levothyroxine to antidiabetic therapy may result in increased antidiabetic agent requirements).
No products indexed under this heading.

Nebivolol (Co-administration with beta-blockers may decrease T4 5'-deiodinase activity; action of beta-blocker may be impaired when the hypothyroid patient is converted to euthyroid). Products include:

Niacin (Co-administration with slow-release nicotinic acid may result in decreased serum TBG concentration). Products include:

Norepinephrine Bitartrate (Co-administration of sympathomimetic agents may increase the effects of sympathomimetics or thyroid hormone; thyroid hormones may increase risk of coronary insufficiency when sympathomimetic agents are administered to patients with coronary disease).
No products indexed under this heading.

IMPORTANT NOTE: Always consult each drug listing in the patient's regimen for possible interactions.

Sodium Polystyrene Sulfonate (Co-administration may result in decreased T4 absorption, which may result in hypothyroidism; administer levothyroxine at least 4 hours apart from these agents).
No products indexed under this heading.

Somatrem (Excessive use of thyroid hormone with growth hormones may accelerate epiphyseal closure; however, untreated hypothyroidism may interfere with growth response to growth hormone).
No products indexed under this heading.

Somatropin (Excessive use of thyroid hormone with growth hormones may accelerate epiphyseal closure; however, untreated hypothyroidism may interfere with growth response to growth hormone). Products include:
Nutropin **1204**
Nutropin AQ **1209**
Nutropin AQ NuSpin **1209**
Nutropin AQ Pen **1209**
Nutropin AQ Pen Cartridge **1209**

Sotalol Hydrochloride (Co-administration with beta-blockers may decrease T4 5'-deiodinase activity; action of beta-blocker may be impaired when the hypothyroid patient is converted to euthyroid).
No products indexed under this heading.

Soybean Preparations (Concurrent use of soybean flour may bind and decrease the absorption of levothyroxine sodium from GI tract).
No products indexed under this heading.

Stanozolol (Co-administration with androgens/anabolic steroids may result in decreased serum TBG concentration).
No products indexed under this heading.

Sucralfate (Co-administration may result in decreased T4 absorption, which may result in hypothyroidism; administer levothyroxine at least 4 hours apart from these agents). Products include:
Carafate Suspension **784**
Carafate Tablets **785**

Sulfamethoxazole (May decrease thyroid hormone secretion, which may result in hypothyrodism).
No products indexed under this heading.

Sulfisoxazole Acetyl (May decrease thyroid hormone secretion, which may result in hypothyrodism).
No products indexed under this heading.

Tamoxifen Citrate (Co-administration may result in increased serum TBG concentrations).
No products indexed under this heading.

Terbutaline Sulfate (Co-administration of sympathomimetic agents may increase the effects of sympathomimetics or thyroid hormone; thyroid hormones may increase risk of coronary insufficiency when sympathomimetic agents are administered to patients with coronary disease).
No products indexed under this heading.

Theophylline (Decreased theophylline clearance may occur in hypothyroid patients; clearance returns to normal when euthyroid state is achieved).
No products indexed under this heading.

Theophylline Anhydrous (Decreased theophylline clearance may occur in hypothyroid patients; clearance returns to normal when euthyroid state is achieved). Products include:
Uniphyl **2817**

Theophylline Calcium Salicylate (Decreased theophylline clearance may occur in hypothyroid patients; clearance returns to normal when euthyroid state is achieved).
No products indexed under this heading.

Theophylline Dihydroxypropyl (Glyceryl) (Decreased theophylline clearance may occur in hypothyroid patients; clearance returns to normal when euthyroid state is achieved).
No products indexed under this heading.

Theophylline Ethylenediamine (Decreased theophylline clearance may occur in hypothyroid patients; clearance returns to normal when euthyroid state is achieved).
No products indexed under this heading.

Theophylline Sodium Glycinate (Decreased theophylline clearance may occur in hypothyroid patients; clearance returns to normal when euthyroid state is achieved).
No products indexed under this heading.

Timolol Hemihydrate (Co-administration with beta-blockers may decrease T4 5'-deiodinase activity; action of beta-blocker may be impaired when the hypothyroid patient is converted to euthyroid). Products include:
Betimol **3490**

Timolol Maleate (Co-administration with beta-blockers may decrease T4 5'-deiodinase activity; action of beta-blocker may be impaired when the hypothyroid patient is converted to euthyroid). Products include:
Combigan **601**
Dorzolamide Hydrochloride/Timolol Maleate Ophthalmic Solution .... ⊙ **243**
Timoptic in Ocudose .... ⊙ **231**

Tolazamide (Addition of levothyroxine to antidiabetic therapy may result in increased antidiabetic agent requirements).
No products indexed under this heading.

Tolbutamide (May decrease thyroid hormone secretion, which may result in hypothyrodism).
No products indexed under this heading.

Triamcinolone (Co-administration with glucocorticoids may result in a transient reduction in TSH secretion; the reduction is not sustained, therefore, hypothyroidism does not occur; glucocorticoids may decrease serum TBG concentration).
No products indexed under this heading.

Triamcinolone Acetonide (Co-administration with glucocorticoids may result in a transient reduction in TSH secretion; the reduction is not sustained, therefore, hypothyroidism does not occur; glucocorticoids may decrease serum TBG concentration). Products include:
Azmacort **408**
Nasacort AQ **3019**

Triamcinolone Diacetate (Co-administration with glucocorticoids may result in a transient reduction in TSH secretion; the reduction is not sustained, therefore, hypothyroidism does not occur; glucocorticoids may decrease serum TBG concentration).
No products indexed under this heading.

Triamcinolone Hexacetonide (Co-administration with glucocorticoids may result in a transient reduction in TSH secretion; the reduction is not sustained, therefore, hypothyroidism does not occur; glucocorticoids may decrease serum TBG concentration).
No products indexed under this heading.

Trimipramine Maleate (Co-administration may increase the therapeutic and toxic effects of both drugs possibly due to increased receptor sensitivity to catecholamines; toxic effects may include increased risk of arrhythmias and CNS stimulation; onset of tricyclics may be accelerated).
No products indexed under this heading.

Troglitazone (Addition of levothyroxine to antidiabetic therapy may result in increased antidiabetic agent requirements).
No products indexed under this heading.

Tyropanoate Sodium (May decrease thyroid hormone secretion, which may result in hypothyroidism; the fetus, elderly, and euthyroid patients with underlying thyroid disease are among those individuals who are susceptible to iodine-induced hypothyroidism; oral cholecytographic agents slowly excreted, producing more prolonged hypothyroidism; iodide drugs that contain pharmacologic amounts of iodide may cause hypothyroidism in euthyroid patients with Grave's disease previously treated with thyroid autonomy; hyperthyroidism may develop over several weeks and may persist for several months after therapy discontinuation).
No products indexed under this heading.

Warfarin Sodium (Thyroid hormones appear to increase the catabolism of vitamin K-dependent clotting factors, thereby increasing the anticoagulant activity of oral anticoagulants).
No products indexed under this heading.

Food Interactions

Cotton seed meal (Concurrent use of cotton seed meal may bind and decrease the absorption of levothyroxine sodium from GI tract).

Dietary Fiber (Concurrent use of dietary fiber may bind and decrease the absorption of levothyroxine sodium from GI tract).

Soybean Formula, Children's (Concurrent use of soybean flour may bind and decrease the absorption of levothyroxine sodium from GI tract).

Walnuts (Concurrent use of walnuts may bind and decrease the absorption of levothyroxine sodium from GI tract).

LEXAPRO ORAL SUSPENSION

(Escitalopram Oxalate) **1160**
See Lexapro Tablets

LEXAPRO TABLETS

(Escitalopram Oxalate) **1160**
May interact with alcohols, anticoagulants, antipsychotic agents, aspirin-acetylsalicylic acid, central nervous system depressants, central nervous system stimulants, cytochrome p450 2c19 inhibitors (selected), cytochrome p450 2d6 substrates (selected), cytochrome p450 3a4 inhibitors (selected), diuretics, dopamine antagonists, lithium preparations, monoamine oxidase inhibitors, non-steroidal anti-inflammatory agents, serotonin and norepinephrine reuptake inhibitors, serotoninergic agents, triptans, and certain other agents. Compounds in these categories include:

Acetazolamide (*In vitro* studies indicated that CYP3A4 and -2C19 are the primary enzymes involved in the metabolism of escitalopram. However, co-administration of escitalopram (20 mg) and ritonavir (600 mg), a potent inhibitor of CYP3A4, did not significantly affect the pharmacokinetics of escitalopram oxalate. Because escitalopram oxalate is metabolized by multiple enzyme systems, inhibition of a single enzyme may not appreciably decrease escitalopram clearance).
No products indexed under this heading.

Acetazolamide Sodium (*In vitro* studies indicated that CYP3A4 and -2C19 are the primary enzymes involved in the metabolism of escitalopram. However, co-administration of escitalopram (20 mg) and ritonavir (600 mg), a potent inhibitor of CYP3A4, did not significantly affect the pharmacokinetics of escitalopram oxalate. Because escitalopram oxalate is metabolized by multiple enzyme systems, inhibition of a single enzyme may not appreciably decrease escitalopram clearance).
No products indexed under this heading.

Alfentanil Hydrochloride (Given the primary CNS effects of escitalopram, caution should be used when it is taken in combination of other centrally acting drugs).
No products indexed under this heading.

Almotriptan Malate (There have been rare post-marketing reports of serotonin syndrome with use of a SSRI and a triptan. If concomitant treatment of escitalopram with a triptan is clinically warranted, careful observation of the patient is advised, particularly during treatment initiation and dose increases). Products include:
Axert **2593**

Alprazolam (Given the primary CNS effects of escitalopram, caution should be used when it is taken in combination of other centrally acting drugs).
No products indexed under this heading.

Amiloride Hydrochloride (Hyponatremia may occur as a result of treatment with escitalopram. Patients taking diuretics may be at greater risk. Discontinuation of escitalopram should be considered in patients with symptomatic hyponatremia and appropriate medical intervention should be instituted).
No products indexed under this heading.

Amiodarone Hydrochloride (*In vitro* studies indicated that CYP3A4 and -2C19 are the primary enzymes involved in the metabolism of escitalopram. However, co-administration of escitalopram (20 mg) and ritonavir (600 mg), a potent inhibitor of CYP3A4, did not significantly affect the pharmacokinetics of escitalopram oxalate. Because escitalopram oxalate is metabolized by multiple enzyme systems, inhibition of a single enzyme may not appreciably decrease escitalopram clearance).
No products indexed under this heading.

Amitriptyline Hydrochloride (*In vitro* studies did not reveal an inhibitory effect of escitalopram on CYP2D6. In addition, steady state levels of racemic citalopram were not significantly different in poor metabolizers and extensive CYP2D6 metabolizers after multi-dose administration of citalopram, suggesting that co-administration, with escitalopram, of a drug that inhibits CYP2D6, is unlikely to have clinically significant effects on escitalopram metabolism. However, there are limited *in vivo* data suggesting a modest CYP2D6 inhibitory effect for escitalopram, ie co-administration of escitalopram (20 mg/day for 21 days) with the tricyclic antidepressant desipramine (single dose of 50 mg), a substrate for CYP2D6 resulted in a 40% increase in C_{max} and a 100% increase in AUC of desipramine. The clinical significance of this finding is unknown. Nevertheless, caution is indicated in the co-administration of escitalopram and drugs metabolized by CYP2D6).
No products indexed under this heading.

Amobarbital (Given the primary CNS effects of escitalopram, caution should be used when it is taken in combination of other centrally acting drugs).
No products indexed under this heading.

Amobarbital Sodium (Given the primary CNS effects of escitalopram, caution should be used when it is taken in combination of other centrally acting drugs).
No products indexed under this heading.

Lexapro Interactions Index 1022

Amphetamine Aspartate (Given the primary CNS effects of escitalopram, caution should be used when it is taken in combination of other centrally acting drugs).
No products indexed under this heading.

Amphetamine Aspartate Monohydrate (Given the primary CNS effects of escitalopram, caution should be used when it is taken in combination of other centrally acting drugs).
No products indexed under this heading.

Amphetamine Resins (Given the primary CNS effects of escitalopram, caution should be used when it is taken in combination of other centrally acting drugs).
No products indexed under this heading.

Amphetamine Sulfate (Given the primary CNS effects of escitalopram, caution should be used when it is taken in combination of other centrally acting drugs).
No products indexed under this heading.

Amprenavir (*In vitro* studies indicated that CYP3A4 and -2C19 are the primary enzymes involved in the metabolism of escitalopram. However, co-administration of escitalopram (20 mg) and ritonavir (600 mg), a potent inhibitor of CYP3A4, did not significantly affect the pharmacokinetics of escitalopram oxalate. Because escitalopram oxalate is metabolized by multiple enzyme systems, inhibition of a single enzyme may not appreciably decrease escitalopram clearance).
No products indexed under this heading.

Anastrozole (*In vitro* studies indicated that CYP3A4 and -2C19 are the primary enzymes involved in the metabolism of escitalopram. However, co-administration of escitalopram (20 mg) and ritonavir (600 mg), a potent inhibitor of CYP3A4, did not significantly affect the pharmacokinetics of escitalopram oxalate. Because escitalopram oxalate is metabolized by multiple enzyme systems, inhibition of a single enzyme may not appreciably decrease escitalopram clearance).
No products indexed under this heading.

Anisindione (Escitalopram may increase the risk of bleeding events. Concomitant use of anticoagulants may add to this risk. Case reports and epidemiological studies of the case-control and cohort design have demonstrated an association between use of drugs that interfere with serotonin reuptake and the occurrence of gastrointestinal bleeding. Patients should be cautioned about the risk of bleeding associated with the concomitant use of escitalopram and anticoagulants).
No products indexed under this heading.

Aprepitant (*In vitro* studies indicated that CYP3A4 and -2C19 are the primary enzymes involved in the metabolism of escitalopram. However, co-administration of escitalopram (20 mg) and ritonavir (600 mg), a potent inhibitor of CYP3A4, did not significantly affect the pharmacokinetics of escitalopram oxalate. Because escitalopram oxalate is metabolized by multiple enzyme systems, inhibition of a single enzyme may not appreciably decrease escitalopram clearance). Products include:
Emend 2124

Aprobarbital (Given the primary CNS effects of escitalopram, caution should be used when it is taken in combination of other centrally acting drugs).
No products indexed under this heading.

Ardeparin Sodium (Escitalopram may increase the risk of bleeding events. Concomitant use of anticoagulants may add to this risk. Case reports and epidemiological studies of the case-control and cohort design have demonstrated an association between use of drugs that interfere with serotonin reuptake and the occurrence of gastrointestinal bleeding. Patients should be cautioned about the risk of bleeding associated with the concomitant use of escitalopram and anticoagulants).
No products indexed under this heading.

Aripiprazole (The development of a potentially life-threatening serotonin syndrome or Neuroleptic Malignant Syndrome (NMS)-like reactions have been reported with SNRIs and SSRIs alone, including escitalopram treatment, but particularly with concomitant use of serotonergic drugs (including triptans) with drugs which impair metabolism of serotonin (including MAOIs), or with antipsychotics or other dopamine antagonists. Patients should be monitored for the emergence of serotonin syndrome or NMS-like signs and symptoms. Treatment with escitalopram and any concomitant serotonergic or antidopaminergic agents, including antipsychotics, should be discontinued immediately if the above events occur and supportive symptomatic treatment should be initiated).
No products indexed under this heading.

Aspirin (Escitalopram may increase the risk of bleeding events. Concomitant use of aspirin may add to this risk. Case reports and epidemiological studies of the case-control and cohort design have demonstrated an association between use of drugs that interfere with serotonin reuptake and the occurrence of gastrointestinal bleeding. Patients should be cautioned about the risk of bleeding associated with the concomitant use of escitalopram and aspirin). Products include:
Aggrenox 880
Bayer Aspirin 829
Percodan 1124
St. Joseph Aspirin 2045

Aspirin, Enteric Coated (Escitalopram may increase the risk of bleeding events. Concomitant use of aspirin may add to this risk. Case reports and epidemiological studies of the case-control and cohort design have demonstrated an association between use of drugs that interfere with serotonin reuptake and the occurrence of gastrointestinal bleeding. Patients should be cautioned about the risk of bleeding associated with the concomitant use of escitalopram and aspirin).
No products indexed under this heading.

Aspirin Buffered (Escitalopram may increase the risk of bleeding events. Concomitant use of aspirin may add to this risk. Case reports and epidemiological studies of the case-control and cohort design have demonstrated an association between use of drugs that interfere with serotonin reuptake and the occurrence of gastrointestinal bleeding. Patients should be cautioned about the risk of bleeding associated with the concomitant use of escitalopram and aspirin).
No products indexed under this heading.

Atazanavir (*In vitro* studies indicated that CYP3A4 and -2C19 are the primary enzymes involved in the metabolism of escitalopram. However, co-administration of escitalopram (20 mg) and ritonavir (600 mg), a potent inhibitor of CYP3A4, did not significantly affect the pharmacokinetics of escitalopram oxalate. Because escitalopram oxalate is metabolized by multiple enzyme systems, inhibition of a single enzyme may not appreciably decrease escitalopram clearance).
No products indexed under this heading.

Atazanavir Sulfate (*In vitro* studies indicated that CYP3A4 and -2C19 are the primary enzymes involved in the metabolism of escitalopram. However, co-administration of escitalopram (20 mg) and ritonavir (600 mg), a potent inhibitor of CYP3A4, did not significantly affect the pharmacokinetics of escitalopram oxalate. Because escitalopram oxalate is metabolized by multiple enzyme systems, inhibition of a single enzyme may not appreciably decrease escitalopram clearance).
No products indexed under this heading.

Atomoxetine Hydrochloride (*In vitro* studies did not reveal an inhibitory effect of escitalopram on CYP2D6. In addition, steady state levels of racemic citalopram were not significantly different in poor metabolizers and extensive CYP2D6 metabolizers after multi-dose administration of citalopram, suggesting that co-administration, with escitalopram, of a drug that inhibits CYP2D6, is unlikely to have clinically significant effects on escitalopram metabolism. However, there are limited *in vivo* data suggesting a modest CYP2D6 inhibitory effect for escitalopram, ie co-administration of escitalopram (20 mg/day for 21 days) with the tricyclic antidepressant desipramine (single dose of 50 mg), a substrate for CYP2D6 resulted in a 40% increase in C_{max} and a 100% increase in AUC of desipramine. The clinical significance of this finding is unknown. Nevertheless, caution is indicated in the co-administration of escitalopram and drugs metabolized by CYP2D6). Products include:
Strattera 1957

Bendroflumethiazide (Hyponatremia may occur as a result of treatment with escitalopram. Patients taking diuretics may be at greater risk. Discontinuation of escitalopram should be considered in patients with symptomatic hyponatremia and appropriate medical intervention should be instituted).
No products indexed under this heading.

Bisoprolol Fumarate (*In vitro* studies did not reveal an inhibitory effect of escitalopram on CYP2D6. In addition, steady state levels of racemic citalopram were not significantly different in poor metabolizers and extensive CYP2D6 metabolizers after multi-dose administration of citalopram, suggesting that co-administration, with escitalopram, of a drug that inhibits CYP2D6, is unlikely to have clinically significant effects on escitalopram metabolism. However, there are limited *in vivo* data suggesting a modest CYP2D6 inhibitory effect for escitalopram, ie co-administration of escitalopram (20 mg/day for 21 days) with the tricyclic antidepressant desipramine (single dose of 50 mg), a substrate for CYP2D6 resulted in a 40% increase in C_{max} and a 100% increase in AUC of desipramine. The clinical significance of this finding is unknown. Nevertheless, caution is indicated in the co-administration of escitalopram and drugs metabolized by CYP2D6).
No products indexed under this heading.

Bumetanide (Hyponatremia may occur as a result of treatment with escitalopram. Patients taking diuretics may be at greater risk. Discontinuation of escitalopram should be considered in patients with symptomatic hyponatremia and appropriate medical intervention should be instituted).
No products indexed under this heading.

Buprenorphine Hydrochloride (Given the primary CNS effects of escitalopram, caution should be used when it is taken in combination of other centrally acting drugs).
No products indexed under this heading.

Buspirone Hydrochloride (Given the primary CNS effects of escitalopram, caution should be used when it is taken in combination of other centrally acting drugs).
No products indexed under this heading.

Butabarbital (Given the primary CNS effects of escitalopram, caution should be used when it is taken in combination of other centrally acting drugs).
No products indexed under this heading.

Butabarbital Sodium (Given the primary CNS effects of escitalopram, caution should be used when it is taken in combination of other centrally acting drugs).
No products indexed under this heading.

Butalbital (Given the primary CNS effects of escitalopram, caution should be used when it is taken in combination of other centrally acting drugs).
No products indexed under this heading.

Captopril (*In vitro* studies did not reveal an inhibitory effect of escitalopram on CYP2D6. In addition, steady state levels of racemic citalopram were not significantly different in poor metabolizers and extensive CYP2D6 metabolizers after multi-dose administration of citalopram, suggesting that co-administration, with escitalopram, of a drug that inhibits CYP2D6, is unlikely to have clinically significant effects on escitalopram metabolism. However, there are limited *in vivo* data suggesting a modest CYP2D6 inhibitory effect for escitalopram, ie co-administration of escitalopram (20 mg/day for 21 days) with the tricyclic antidepressant desipramine (single dose of 50 mg), a substrate for CYP2D6 resulted in a 40% increase in C_{max} and a 100% increase in AUC of desipramine. The clinical significance of this finding is unknown. Nevertheless, caution is indicated in the co-administration of escitalopram and drugs metabolized by CYP2D6). Products include:
Captopril 2341

Carbamazepine (Combined administration of racemic citalopram (40 mg/day for 14 days) and carbamazepine (titrated to 400 mg/day for 35 days) did not significantly affect the pharmacokinetics of carbamazepine, a CYP3A4 substrate. Although trough citalopram plasma levels were unaffected, given the enzyme inducing properties of carbamazepine, the possibility that carbamazepine might increase the clearance of escitalopram should be considered if the two drugs are co-administered). Products include:
Carbatrol 3280
Equetro 3477

Carvedilol (*In vitro* studies did not reveal an inhibitory effect of escitalopram on CYP2D6. In addition, steady state levels of racemic citalopram were not significantly different in poor metabolizers and extensive CYP2D6 metabolizers after multi-dose administration of citalopram, suggesting that co-administration, with escitalopram, of a drug that inhibits CYP2D6, is unlikely to have clinically significant effects on escitalopram metabolism. However, there are limited *in vivo* data suggesting a modest CYP2D6 inhibitory effect for escitalopram, ie co-administration of escitalopram (20 mg/day for 21 days) with the tricyclic antidepressant desipramine (single dose of 50 mg), a substrate for CYP2D6 resulted in a 40% increase in C_{max} and a 100% increase in AUC of desipramine. The clinical significance of this finding is unknown. Nevertheless, caution is indicated in the co-administration of escitalopram and drugs metabolized by CYP2D6). Products include:
Coreg 1409

Celecoxib (Epidemiological studies of the case-control and cohort design that have demonstrated an association between use of psychotropic drugs that interfere with serotonin reuptake and the occurrence of upper gastrointestinal bleeding have also shown that concurrent use of an NSAID may potentiate the risk of bleeding; use caution when administering). Products include:

Celebrex 3272

Cevimeline Hydrochloride (*In vitro* studies did not reveal an inhibitory effect of escitalopram on CYP2D6. In addition, steady state levels of racemic citalopram were not significantly different in poor metabolizers and extensive CYP2D6 metabolizers after multi-dose administration of citalopram, suggesting that co-administration, with escitalopram, of a drug that inhibits CYP2D6, is unlikely to have clinically significant effects on escitalopram metabolism. However, there are limited *in vivo* data suggesting a modest CYP2D6 inhibitory effect for escitalopram, ie co-administration of escitalopram (20 mg/day for 21 days) with the tricyclic antidepressant desipramine (single dose of 50 mg), a substrate for CYP2D6 resulted in a 40% increase in C_{max} and a 100% increase in AUC of desipramine. The clinical significance of this finding is unknown. Nevertheless, caution is indicated in the co-administration of escitalopram and drugs metabolized by CYP2D6). Products include:

Evoxac 1027

Chlordiazepoxide (Given the primary CNS effects of escitalopram, caution should be used when it is taken in combination of other centrally acting drugs).
No products indexed under this heading.

Chlordiazepoxide Hydrochloride (Given the primary CNS effects of escitalopram, caution should be used when it is taken in combination of other centrally acting drugs).
No products indexed under this heading.

Chlorothiazide (Hyponatremia may occur as a result of treatment with escitalopram. Patients taking diuretics may be at greater risk. Discontinuation of escitalopram should be considered in patients with symptomatic hyponatremia and appropriate medical intervention should be instituted).
No products indexed under this heading.

Chlorothiazide Sodium (Hyponatremia may occur as a result of treatment with escitalopram. Patients taking diuretics may be at greater risk. Discontinuation of escitalopram should be considered in patients with symptomatic hyponatremia and appropriate medical intervention should be instituted). Products include:

Diuril Intravenous 2009

Chlorpromazine (The development of a potentially life-threatening serotonin syndrome or Neuroleptic Malignant Syndrome (NMS)-like reactions have been reported with SNRIs and SSRIs alone, including escitalopram treatment, but particularly with concomitant use of serotonergic drugs (including triptans) with drugs which impair metabolism of serotonin (including MAOIs), or with antipsychotics or other dopamine antagonists. Patients should be monitored for the emergence of serotonin syndrome or NMS-like signs and symptoms. Treatment with escitalopram and any concomitant serotonergic or antidopaminergic agents, including antipsychotics, should be discontinued immediately if the above events occur and supportive symptomatic treatment should be initiated).
No products indexed under this heading.

Chlorpromazine Hydrochloride (The development of a potentially life-threatening serotonin syndrome or Neu-

roleptic Malignant Syndrome (NMS)-like reactions have been reported with SNRIs and SSRIs alone, including escitalopram treatment, but particularly with concomitant use of serotonergic drugs (including triptans) with drugs which impair metabolism of serotonin (including MAOIs), or with antipsychotics or other dopamine antagonists. Patients should be monitored for the emergence of serotonin syndrome or NMS-like signs and symptoms. Treatment with escitalopram and any concomitant serotonergic or antidopaminergic agents, including antipsychotics, should be discontinued immediately if the above events occur and supportive symptomatic treatment should be initiated).
No products indexed under this heading.

Chlorpropamide (*In vitro* studies did not reveal an inhibitory effect of escitalopram on CYP2D6. In addition, steady state levels of racemic citalopram were not significantly different in poor metabolizers and extensive CYP2D6 metabolizers after multi-dose administration of citalopram, suggesting that co-administration, with escitalopram, of a drug that inhibits CYP2D6, is unlikely to have clinically significant effects on escitalopram metabolism. However, there are limited *in vivo* data suggesting a modest CYP2D6 inhibitory effect for escitalopram, ie co-administration of escitalopram (20 mg/day for 21 days) with the tricyclic antidepressant desipramine (single dose of 50 mg), a substrate for CYP2D6 resulted in a 40% increase in C_{max} and a 100% increase in AUC of desipramine. The clinical significance of this finding is unknown. Nevertheless, caution is indicated in the co-administration of escitalopram and drugs metabolized by CYP2D6).
No products indexed under this heading.

Chlorprothixene (The development of a potentially life-threatening serotonin syndrome or Neuroleptic Malignant Syndrome (NMS)-like reactions have been reported with SNRIs and SSRIs alone, including escitalopram treatment, but particularly with concomitant use of serotonergic drugs (including triptans) with drugs which impair metabolism of serotonin (including MAOIs), or with antipsychotics or other dopamine antagonists. Patients should be monitored for the emergence of serotonin syndrome or NMS-like signs and symptoms. Treatment with escitalopram and any concomitant serotonergic or antidopaminergic agents, including antipsychotics, should be discontinued immediately if the above events occur and supportive symptomatic treatment should be initiated).
No products indexed under this heading.

Chlorprothixene Hydrochloride (The development of a potentially life-threatening serotonin syndrome or Neuroleptic Malignant Syndrome (NMS)-like reactions have been reported with SNRIs and SSRIs alone, including escitalopram treatment, but particularly with concomitant use of serotonergic drugs (including triptans) with drugs which impair metabolism of serotonin (including MAOIs), or with antipsychotics or other dopamine antagonists. Patients should be monitored for the emergence of serotonin syndrome or NMS-like signs and symptoms. Treatment with escitalopram and any concomitant serotonergic or antidopaminergic agents, including antipsychotics, should be discontinued immediately if the above events occur and supportive symptomatic treatment should be initiated).
No products indexed under this heading.

Chlorprothixene Lactate (The development of a potentially life-threatening serotonin syndrome or Neuroleptic Malignant Syndrome (NMS)-like reac-

tions have been reported with SNRIs and SSRIs alone, including escitalopram treatment, but particularly with concomitant use of serotonergic drugs (including triptans) with drugs which impair metabolism of serotonin (including MAOIs), or with antipsychotics or other dopamine antagonists. Patients should be monitored for the emergence of serotonin syndrome or NMS-like signs and symptoms. Treatment with escitalopram and any concomitant serotonergic or antidopaminergic agents, including antipsychotics, should be discontinued immediately if the above events occur and supportive symptomatic treatment should be initiated).
No products indexed under this heading.

Chlorthalidone (Hyponatremia may occur as a result of treatment with escitalopram. Patients taking diuretics may be at greater risk. Discontinuation of escitalopram should be considered in patients with symptomatic hyponatremia and appropriate medical intervention should be instituted). Products include:

Clorpres 2344

Cimetidine (In subjects who received 21 days of 40mg/day racemic citalopram, combined administration of 400 mg/day cimetidine for 8 days resulted in an increase in citalopram AUC and C_{max} of 43% and 39%, respectively. The clinical significance of these findings is unknown).
No products indexed under this heading.

Cimetidine Hydrochloride (In subjects who received 21 days of 40mg/day racemic citalopram, combined administration of 400 mg/day cimetidine for 8 days resulted in an increase in citalopram AUC and C_{max} of 43% and 39%, respectively. The clinical significance of these findings is unknown).
No products indexed under this heading.

Ciprofloxacin (*In vitro* studies indicated that CYP3A4 and -2C19 are the primary enzymes involved in the metabolism of escitalopram. However, co-administration of escitalopram (20 mg) and ritonavir (600 mg), a potent inhibitor of CYP3A4, did not significantly affect the pharmacokinetics of escitalopram oxalate. Because escitalopram oxalate is metabolized by multiple enzyme systems, inhibition of a single enzyme may not appreciably decrease escitalopram clearance). Products include:

Cipro I.V. 3082
Cipro 3073
Cipro XR 3091
Ciprodex 583

Citalopram Hydrobromide (The development of a potentially life-threatening serotonin syndrome or Neuroleptic Malignant Syndrome (NMS)-like reactions have been reported with SNRIs and SSRIs alone, including escitalopram treatment, but particularly with concomitant use of serotonergic drugs (including triptans) with drugs which impair metabolism of serotonin (including MAOIs), or with antipsychotics or other dopamine antagonists. Patients should be monitored for the emergence of serotonin syndrome or NMS-like signs and symptoms. Treatment with escitalopram and any concomitant serotonergic or antidopaminergic agents, including antipsychotics, should be discontinued immediately if the above events occur and supportive symptomatic treatment should be initiated). Products include:

Celexa 1153

Clarithromycin (*In vitro* studies indicated that CYP3A4 and -2C19 are the primary enzymes involved in the metabolism of escitalopram. However, co-administration of escitalopram (20 mg) and ritonavir (600 mg), a potent inhibi-

tor of CYP3A4, did not significantly affect the pharmacokinetics of escitalopram oxalate. Because escitalopram oxalate is metabolized by multiple enzyme systems, inhibition of a single enzyme may not appreciably decrease escitalopram clearance). Products include:

Biaxin/Biaxin XL 412

Clomipramine Hydrochloride (*In vitro* studies did not reveal an inhibitory effect of escitalopram on CYP2D6. In addition, steady state levels of racemic citalopram were not significantly different in poor metabolizers and extensive CYP2D6 metabolizers after multi-dose administration of citalopram, suggesting that co-administration, with escitalopram, of a drug that inhibits CYP2D6, is unlikely to have clinically significant effects on escitalopram metabolism. However, there are limited *in vivo* data suggesting a modest CYP2D6 inhibitory effect for escitalopram, ie co-administration of escitalopram (20 mg/day for 21 days) with the tricyclic antidepressant desipramine (single dose of 50 mg), a substrate for CYP2D6 resulted in a 40% increase in C_{max} and a 100% increase in AUC of desipramine. The clinical significance of this finding is unknown. Nevertheless, caution is indicated in the co-administration of escitalopram and drugs metabolized by CYP2D6).
No products indexed under this heading.

Clonazepam (Given the primary CNS effects of escitalopram, caution should be used when it is taken in combination of other centrally acting drugs). Products include:

Klonopin 2855

Clorazepate Dipotassium (Given the primary CNS effects of escitalopram, caution should be used when it is taken in combination of other centrally acting drugs).
No products indexed under this heading.

Clotrimazole (*In vitro* studies indicated that CYP3A4 and -2C19 are the primary enzymes involved in the metabolism of escitalopram. However, co-administration of escitalopram (20 mg) and ritonavir (600 mg), a potent inhibitor of CYP3A4, did not significantly affect the pharmacokinetics of escitalopram oxalate. Because escitalopram oxalate is metabolized by multiple enzyme systems, inhibition of a single enzyme may not appreciably decrease escitalopram clearance). Products include:

Lotrisone 3163

Clozapine (The development of a potentially life-threatening serotonin syndrome or Neuroleptic Malignant Syndrome (NMS)-like reactions have been reported with SNRIs and SSRIs alone, including escitalopram treatment, but particularly with concomitant use of serotonergic drugs (including triptans) with drugs which impair metabolism of serotonin (including MAOIs), or with antipsychotics or other dopamine antagonists. Patients should be monitored for the emergence of serotonin syndrome or NMS-like signs and symptoms. Treatment with escitalopram and any concomitant serotonergic or antidopaminergic agents, including antipsychotics, should be discontinued immediately if the above events occur and supportive symptomatic treatment should be initiated).
No products indexed under this heading.

Codeine Phosphate (Given the primary CNS effects of escitalopram, caution should be used when it is taken in combination of other centrally acting drugs). Products include:

Tylenol with Codeine 2691

IMPORTANT NOTE: Always consult each drug listing in the patient's regimen for possible interactions.

Codeine Sulfate (Given the primary CNS effects of escitalopram, caution should be used when it is taken in combination of other centrally acting drugs).
No products indexed under this heading.

Conivaptan Hydrochloride (*In vitro* studies indicated that CYP3A4 and -2C19 are the primary enzymes involved in the metabolism of escitalopram. However, co-administration of escitalopram (20 mg) and ritonavir (600 mg), a potent inhibitor of CYP3A4, did not significantly affect the pharmacokinetics of escitalopram oxalate. Because escitalopram oxalate is metabolized by multiple enzyme systems, inhibition of a single enzyme may not appreciably decrease escitalopram clearance). Products include:
Vaprisol 689

Cyclobenzaprine Hydrochloride (*In vitro* studies did not reveal an inhibitory effect of escitalopram on CYP2D6. In addition, steady state levels of racemic citalopram were not significantly different in poor metabolizers and extensive CYP2D6 metabolizers after multi-dose administration of citalopram, suggesting that co-administration, with escitalopram, of a drug that inhibits CYP2D6, is unlikely to have clinically significant effects on escitalopram metabolism. However, there are limited *in vivo* data suggesting a modest CYP2D6 inhibitory effect for escitalopram, ie co-administration of escitalopram (20 mg/day for 21 days) with the tricyclic antidepressant desipramine (single dose of 50 mg), a substrate for CYP2D6 resulted in a 40% increase in C_{max} and a 100% increase in AUC of desipramine. The clinical significance of this finding is unknown. Nevertheless, caution is indicated in the co-administration of escitalopram and drugs metabolized by CYP2D6). Products include:
Amrix 964

Cyclosporine (*In vitro* studies indicated that CYP3A4 and -2C19 are the primary enzymes involved in the metabolism of escitalopram. However, co-administration of escitalopram (20 mg) and ritonavir (600 mg), a potent inhibitor of CYP3A4, did not significantly affect the pharmacokinetics of escitalopram oxalate. Because escitalopram oxalate is metabolized by multiple enzyme systems, inhibition of a single enzyme may not appreciably decrease escitalopram clearance). Products include:
Gengraf 440
Neoral Oral Solution 2496
Neoral Capsules 2496
Restasis 605

Dalfopristin (*In vitro* studies indicated that CYP3A4 and -2C19 are the primary enzymes involved in the metabolism of escitalopram. However, co-administration of escitalopram (20 mg) and ritonavir (600 mg), a potent inhibitor of CYP3A4, did not significantly affect the pharmacokinetics of escitalopram oxalate. Because escitalopram oxalate is metabolized by multiple enzyme systems, inhibition of a single enzyme may not appreciably decrease escitalopram clearance).
No products indexed under this heading.

Dalteparin Sodium (Escitalopram may increase the risk of bleeding events. Concomitant use of anticoagulants may add to this risk. Case reports and epidemiological studies of the case-control and cohort design have demonstrated an association between use of drugs that interfere with serotonin reuptake and the occurrence of gastrointestinal bleeding. Patients should be cautioned about the risk of bleeding associated with the concomitant use of escitalopram and anticoagulants). Products include:
Fragmin 1058

Danaparoid Sodium (Escitalopram may increase the risk of bleeding events. Concomitant use of anticoagulants may add to this risk. Case reports and epidemiological studies of the case-control and cohort design have demonstrated an association between use of drugs that interfere with serotonin reuptake and the occurrence of gastrointestinal bleeding. Patients should be cautioned about the risk of bleeding associated with the concomitant use of escitalopram and anticoagulants).
No products indexed under this heading.

Danazol (*In vitro* studies indicated that CYP3A4 and -2C19 are the primary enzymes involved in the metabolism of escitalopram. However, co-administration of escitalopram (20 mg) and ritonavir (600 mg), a potent inhibitor of CYP3A4, did not significantly affect the pharmacokinetics of escitalopram oxalate. Because escitalopram oxalate is metabolized by multiple enzyme systems, inhibition of a single enzyme may not appreciably decrease escitalopram clearance).
No products indexed under this heading.

Darunavir (*In vitro* studies indicated that CYP3A4 and -2C19 are the primary enzymes involved in the metabolism of escitalopram. However, co-administration of escitalopram (20 mg) and ritonavir (600 mg), a potent inhibitor of CYP3A4, did not significantly affect the pharmacokinetics of escitalopram oxalate. Because escitalopram oxalate is metabolized by multiple enzyme systems, inhibition of a single enzyme may not appreciably decrease escitalopram clearance).
No products indexed under this heading.

Dasatinib (*In vitro* studies indicated that CYP3A4 and -2C19 are the primary enzymes involved in the metabolism of escitalopram. However, co-administration of escitalopram (20 mg) and ritonavir (600 mg), a potent inhibitor of CYP3A4, did not significantly affect the pharmacokinetics of escitalopram oxalate. Because escitalopram oxalate is metabolized by multiple enzyme systems, inhibition of a single enzyme may not appreciably decrease escitalopram clearance).
No products indexed under this heading.

Debrisoquine (*In vitro* studies did not reveal an inhibitory effect of escitalopram on CYP2D6. In addition, steady state levels of racemic citalopram were not significantly different in poor metabolizers and extensive CYP2D6 metabolizers after multi-dose administration of citalopram, suggesting that co-administration, with escitalopram, of a drug that inhibits CYP2D6, is unlikely to have clinically significant effects on escitalopram metabolism. However, there are limited *in vivo* data suggesting a modest CYP2D6 inhibitory effect for escitalopram, ie co-administration of escitalopram (20 mg/day for 21 days) with the tricyclic antidepressant desipramine (single dose of 50 mg), a substrate for CYP2D6 resulted in a 40% increase in C_{max} and a 100% increase in AUC of desipramine. The clinical significance of this finding is unknown. Nevertheless, caution is indicated in the co-administration of escitalopram and drugs metabolized by CYP2D6).
No products indexed under this heading.

Delavirdine Mesylate (*In vitro* studies indicated that CYP3A4 and -2C19 are the primary enzymes involved in the metabolism of escitalopram. However, co-administration of escitalopram (20 mg) and ritonavir (600 mg), a potent inhibitor of CYP3A4, did not significantly affect the pharmacokinetics of escitalopram oxalate. Because escitalopram oxalate is metabolized by multiple enzyme systems, inhibition of a single enzyme may not appreciably decrease escitalopram clearance).
No products indexed under this heading.

Delavirine (*In vitro* studies indicated that CYP3A4 and -2C19 are the primary enzymes involved in the metabolism of escitalopram. However, co-administration of escitalopram (20 mg) and ritonavir (600 mg), a potent inhibitor of CYP3A4, did not significantly affect the pharmacokinetics of escitalopram oxalate. Because escitalopram oxalate is metabolized by multiple enzyme systems, inhibition of a single enzyme may not appreciably decrease escitalopram clearance).
No products indexed under this heading.

Desflurane (Given the primary CNS effects of escitalopram, caution should be used when it is taken in combination of other centrally acting drugs).
No products indexed under this heading.

Desipramine Hydrochloride (*In vitro* studies did not reveal an inhibitory effect of escitalopram on CYP2D6. In addition, steady state levels of racemic citalopram were not significantly different in poor metabolizers and extensive CYP2D6 metabolizers after multi-dose administration of citalopram, suggesting that co-administration, with escitalopram, of a drug that inhibits CYP2D6, is unlikely to have clinically significant effects on escitalopram metabolism. However, there are limited *in vivo* data suggesting a modest CYP2D6 inhibitory effect for escitalopram, ie co-administration of escitalopram (20 mg/day for 21 days) with the tricyclic antidepressant desipramine (single dose of 50 mg), a substrate for CYP2D6 resulted in a 40% increase in C_{max} and a 100% increase in AUC of desipramine. The clinical significance of this finding is unknown. Nevertheless, caution is indicated in the co-administration of escitalopram and drugs metabolized by CYP2D6).
No products indexed under this heading.

Desloratadine (*In vitro* studies indicated that CYP3A4 and -2C19 are the primary enzymes involved in the metabolism of escitalopram. However, co-administration of escitalopram (20 mg) and ritonavir (600 mg), a potent inhibitor of CYP3A4, did not significantly affect the pharmacokinetics of escitalopram oxalate. Because escitalopram oxalate is metabolized by multiple enzyme systems, inhibition of a single enzyme may not appreciably decrease escitalopram clearance). Products include:
Clarinex Syrup 3098
Clarinex 3098
Clarinex Reditabs 3098
Clarinex-D 12-Hour 3101
Clarinex-D 3104

Desogestrel (*In vitro* studies indicated that CYP3A4 and -2C19 are the primary enzymes involved in the metabolism of escitalopram. However, co-administration of escitalopram (20 mg) and ritonavir (600 mg), a potent inhibitor of CYP3A4, did not significantly affect the pharmacokinetics of escitalopram oxalate. Because escitalopram oxalate is metabolized by multiple enzyme systems, inhibition of a single enzyme may not appreciably decrease escitalopram clearance).
No products indexed under this heading.

Desvenlafaxine Succinate (The development of a potentially life threatening serotonin syndrome or Neuroleptic Malignant syndrome-like reactions have been reported with SSRIs alone, including escitalopram, but particularly with concomitant use of serotonergic drugs. Serotonin syndrome, in its most severe form, can resemble neuroleptic malignant syndrome. The concomitant use of escitalopram with SNRIs is not recommended). Products include:
Pristiq 3564

Dexfenfluramine Hydrochloride (*In vitro* studies did not reveal an inhibitory effect of escitalopram on CYP2D6. In addition, steady state levels of racemic citalopram were not significantly different in poor metabolizers and extensive CYP2D6 metabolizers after multi-dose administration of citalopram, suggesting that co-administration, with escitalopram, of a drug that inhibits CYP2D6, is unlikely to have clinically significant effects on escitalopram metabolism. However, there are limited *in vivo* data suggesting a modest CYP2D6 inhibitory effect for escitalopram, ie co-administration of escitalopram (20 mg/day for 21 days) with the tricyclic antidepressant desipramine (single dose of 50 mg), a substrate for CYP2D6 resulted in a 40% increase in C_{max} and a 100% increase in AUC of desipramine. The clinical significance of this finding is unknown. Nevertheless, caution is indicated in the co-administration of escitalopram and drugs metabolized by CYP2D6).
No products indexed under this heading.

Dexmethylphenidate Hydrochloride (Given the primary CNS effects of escitalopram, caution should be used when it is taken in combination of other centrally acting drugs). Products include:
Focalin XR 2472

Dextroamphetamine (Given the primary CNS effects of escitalopram, caution should be used when it is taken in combination of other centrally acting drugs).
No products indexed under this heading.

Dextroamphetamine Saccharate (Given the primary CNS effects of escitalopram, caution should be used when it is taken in combination of other centrally acting drugs).
No products indexed under this heading.

Dextroamphetamine Sulfate (Given the primary CNS effects of escitalopram, caution should be used when it is taken in combination of other centrally acting drugs). Products include:
Dexedrine 1425

Dextromethorphan Hydrobromide (*In vitro* studies did not reveal an inhibitory effect of escitalopram on CYP2D6. In addition, steady state levels of racemic citalopram were not significantly different in poor metabolizers and extensive CYP2D6 metabolizers after multi-dose administration of citalopram, suggesting that co-administration, with escitalopram, of a drug that inhibits CYP2D6, is unlikely to have clinically significant effects on escitalopram metabolism. However, there are limited *in vivo* data suggesting a modest CYP2D6 inhibitory effect for escitalopram, ie co-administration of escitalopram (20 mg/day for 21 days) with the tricyclic antidepressant desipramine (single dose of 50 mg), a substrate for CYP2D6 resulted in a 40% increase in C_{max} and a 100% increase in AUC of desipramine. The clinical significance of this finding is unknown. Nevertheless, caution is indicated in the co-administration of escitalopram and drugs metabolized by CYP2D6).
No products indexed under this heading.

Dextromethorphan Polistirex (*In vitro* studies did not reveal an inhibitory effect of escitalopram on CYP2D6. In addition, steady state levels of racemic citalopram were not significantly different in poor metabolizers and extensive CYP2D6 metabolizers after multi-dose administration of citalopram, suggesting that co-administration, with escitalopram, of a drug that inhibits CYP2D6, is

1025 Interactions Index Lexapro

unlikely to have clinically significant effects on escitalopram metabolism. However, there are limited *in vivo* data suggesting a modest CYP2D6 inhibitory effect for escitalopram, ie co-administration of escitalopram (20 mg/day for 21 days) with the tricyclic antidepressant desipramine (single dose of 50 mg), a substrate for CYP2D6 resulted in a 40% increase in C_{max} and a 100% increase in AUC of desipramine. The clinical significance of this finding is unknown. Nevertheless, caution is indicated in the co-administration of escitalopram and drugs metabolized by CYP2D6).
No products indexed under this heading.

Dezocine (Given the primary CNS effects of escitalopram, caution should be used when it is taken in combination of other centrally acting drugs).
No products indexed under this heading.

Diazepam (Given the primary CNS effects of escitalopram, caution should be used when it is taken in combination of other centrally acting drugs). Products include:
Valium Tablets 2880

Diclofenac Epolamine (Epidemiological studies of the case-control and cohort design that have demonstrated an association between use of psychotropic drugs that interfere with serotonin reuptake and the occurrence of upper gastrointestinal bleeding have also shown that concurrent use of an NSAID may potentiate the risk of bleeding; use caution when administering). Products include:
Flector 1839

Diclofenac Potassium (Epidemiological studies of the case-control and cohort design that have demonstrated an association between use of psychotropic drugs that interfere with serotonin reuptake and the occurrence of upper gastrointestinal bleeding have also shown that concurrent use of an NSAID may potentiate the risk of bleeding; use caution when administering).
No products indexed under this heading.

Diclofenac Sodium (Epidemiological studies of the case-control and cohort design that have demonstrated an association between use of psychotropic drugs that interfere with serotonin reuptake and the occurrence of upper gastrointestinal bleeding have also shown that concurrent use of an NSAID may potentiate the risk of bleeding; use caution when administering).
No products indexed under this heading.

Dicumarol (Escitalopram may increase the risk of bleeding events. Concomitant use of anticoagulants may add to this risk. Case reports and epidemiological studies of the case-control and cohort design have demonstrated an association between use of drugs that interfere with serotonin reuptake and the occurrence of gastrointestinal bleeding. Patients should be cautioned about the risk of bleeding associated with the concomitant use of escitalopram and anticoagulants).
No products indexed under this heading.

Diltiazem Hydrochloride (*In vitro* studies indicated that CYP3A4 and -2C19 are the primary enzymes involved in the metabolism of escitalopram. However, co-administration of escitalopram (20 mg) and ritonavir (600 mg), a potent inhibitor of CYP3A4, did not significantly affect the pharmacokinetics of escitalopram oxalate. Because escitalopram oxalate is metabolized by multiple enzyme systems, inhibition of a single enzyme may not appreciably decrease escitalopram clearance). Products include:
Cardizem LA 423

Diltiazem Maleate (*In vitro* studies indicated that CYP3A4 and -2C19 are the primary enzymes involved in the metabolism of escitalopram. However, co-administration of escitalopram (20 mg) and ritonavir (600 mg), a potent inhibitor of CYP3A4, did not significantly affect the pharmacokinetics of escitalopram oxalate. Because escitalopram oxalate is metabolized by multiple enzyme systems, inhibition of a single enzyme may not appreciably decrease escitalopram clearance).
No products indexed under this heading.

Dolasetron Mesylate (*In vitro* studies did not reveal an inhibitory effect of escitalopram on CYP2D6. In addition, steady state levels of racemic citalopram were not significantly different in poor metabolizers and extensive CYP2D6 metabolizers after multi-dose administration of citalopram, suggesting that co-administration, with escitalopram, of a drug that inhibits CYP2D6, is unlikely to have clinically significant effects on escitalopram metabolism. However, there are limited *in vivo* data suggesting a modest CYP2D6 inhibitory effect for escitalopram, ie co-administration of escitalopram (20 mg/day for 21 days) with the tricyclic antidepressant desipramine (single dose of 50 mg), a substrate for CYP2D6 resulted in a 40% increase in C_{max} and a 100% increase in AUC of desipramine. The clinical significance of this finding is unknown. Nevertheless, caution is indicated in the co-administration of escitalopram and drugs metabolized by CYP2D6). Products include:
Anzemet Injection 2931
Anzemet Tablets 2934

Donepezil Hydrochloride (*In vitro* studies did not reveal an inhibitory effect of escitalopram on CYP2D6. In addition, steady state levels of racemic citalopram were not significantly different in poor metabolizers and extensive CYP2D6 metabolizers after multi-dose administration of citalopram, suggesting that co-administration, with escitalopram, of a drug that inhibits CYP2D6, is unlikely to have clinically significant effects on escitalopram metabolism. However, there are limited *in vivo* data suggesting a modest CYP2D6 inhibitory effect for escitalopram, ie co-administration of escitalopram (20 mg/day for 21 days) with the tricyclic antidepressant desipramine (single dose of 50 mg), a substrate for CYP2D6 resulted in a 40% increase in C_{max} and a 100% increase in AUC of desipramine. The clinical significance of this finding is unknown. Nevertheless, caution is indicated in the co-administration of escitalopram and drugs metabolized by CYP2D6). Products include:
Aricept 1045
Aricept ODT 1045

Doxepin Hydrochloride (*In vitro* studies did not reveal an inhibitory effect of escitalopram on CYP2D6. In addition, steady state levels of racemic citalopram were not significantly different in poor metabolizers and extensive CYP2D6 metabolizers after multi-dose administration of citalopram, suggesting that co-administration, with escitalopram, of a drug that inhibits CYP2D6, is unlikely to have clinically significant effects on escitalopram metabolism. However, there are limited *in vivo* data suggesting a modest CYP2D6 inhibitory effect for escitalopram, ie co-administration of escitalopram (20 mg/day for 21 days) with the tricyclic antidepressant desipramine (single dose of 50 mg), a substrate for CYP2D6 resulted in a 40% increase in C_{max} and a 100% increase in AUC of desipramine. The clinical significance of this finding is unknown. Nevertheless, caution is indicated in the co-administration of escitalopram and drugs metabolized by CYP2D6).
No products indexed under this heading.

Droperidol (Given the primary CNS effects of escitalopram, caution should be used when it is taken in combination of other centrally acting drugs).
No products indexed under this heading.

Duloxetine Hydrochloride (The development of a potentially life threatening serotonin syndrome or Neuroleptic Malignant syndrome-like reactions have been reported with SSRIs alone, including escitalopram, but particularly with concomitant use of serotonergic drugs. Serotonin syndrome, in its most severe form, can resemble neuroleptic malignant syndrome. The concomitant use of escitalopram with SNRIs is not recommended). Products include:
Cymbalta 1871

Efavirenz (*In vitro* studies indicated that CYP3A4 and -2C19 are the primary enzymes involved in the metabolism of escitalopram. However, co-administration of escitalopram (20 mg) and ritonavir (600 mg), a potent inhibitor of CYP3A4, did not significantly affect the pharmacokinetics of escitalopram oxalate. Because escitalopram oxalate is metabolized by multiple enzyme systems, inhibition of a single enzyme may not appreciably decrease escitalopram clearance). Products include:
Atripla 906

Eletriptan Hydrobromide (There have been rare post-marketing reports of serotonin syndrome with use of a SSRI and a triptan. If concomitant treatment of escitalopram with a triptan is clinically warranted, careful observation of the patient is advised, particularly during treatment initiation and dose increases).
No products indexed under this heading.

Encainide Hydrochloride (*In vitro* studies did not reveal an inhibitory effect of escitalopram on CYP2D6. In addition, steady state levels of racemic citalopram were not significantly different in poor metabolizers and extensive CYP2D6 metabolizers after multi-dose administration of citalopram, suggesting that co-administration, with escitalopram, of a drug that inhibits CYP2D6, is unlikely to have clinically significant effects on escitalopram metabolism. However, there are limited *in vivo* data suggesting a modest CYP2D6 inhibitory effect for escitalopram, ie co-administration of escitalopram (20 mg/day for 21 days) with the tricyclic antidepressant desipramine (single dose of 50 mg), a substrate for CYP2D6 resulted in a 40% increase in C_{max} and a 100% increase in AUC of desipramine. The clinical significance of this finding is unknown. Nevertheless, caution is indicated in the co-administration of escitalopram and drugs metabolized by CYP2D6).
No products indexed under this heading.

Enflurane (Given the primary CNS effects of escitalopram, caution should be used when it is taken in combination of other centrally acting drugs).
No products indexed under this heading.

Enoxaparin Sodium (Escitalopram may increase the risk of bleeding events. Concomitant use of anticoagulants may add to this risk. Case reports and epidemiological studies of the case-control and cohort design have demonstrated an association between use of drugs that interfere with serotonin reuptake and the occurrence of gastrointestinal bleeding. Patients should be cautioned about the risk of bleeding associated with the concomitant use of escitalopram and anticoagulants). Products include:
Lovenox 3005

Erythromycin (*In vitro* studies indicated that CYP3A4 and -2C19 are the primary enzymes involved in the metabolism of escitalopram. However, co-administration of escitalopram (20 mg) and ritonavir (600 mg), a potent inhibitor of CYP3A4, did not significantly affect the pharmacokinetics of escitalopram oxalate. Because escitalopram oxalate is metabolized by multiple enzyme systems, inhibition of a single enzyme may not appreciably decrease escitalopram clearance).
No products indexed under this heading.

Erythromycin Estolate (*In vitro* studies indicated that CYP3A4 and -2C19 are the primary enzymes involved in the metabolism of escitalopram. However, co-administration of escitalopram (20 mg) and ritonavir (600 mg), a potent inhibitor of CYP3A4, did not significantly affect the pharmacokinetics of escitalopram oxalate. Because escitalopram oxalate is metabolized by multiple enzyme systems, inhibition of a single enzyme may not appreciably decrease escitalopram clearance).
No products indexed under this heading.

Erythromycin Ethylsuccinate (*In vitro* studies indicated that CYP3A4 and -2C19 are the primary enzymes involved in the metabolism of escitalopram. However, co-administration of escitalopram (20 mg) and ritonavir (600 mg), a potent inhibitor of CYP3A4, did not significantly affect the pharmacokinetics of escitalopram oxalate. Because escitalopram oxalate is metabolized by multiple enzyme systems, inhibition of a single enzyme may not appreciably decrease escitalopram clearance). Products include:
E.E.S. 437
EryPed 435

Erythromycin Gluceptate (*In vitro* studies indicated that CYP3A4 and -2C19 are the primary enzymes involved in the metabolism of escitalopram. However, co-administration of escitalopram (20 mg) and ritonavir (600 mg), a potent inhibitor of CYP3A4, did not significantly affect the pharmacokinetics of escitalopram oxalate. Because escitalopram oxalate is metabolized by multiple enzyme systems, inhibition of a single enzyme may not appreciably decrease escitalopram clearance).
No products indexed under this heading.

Erythromycin Lactobionate (*In vitro* studies indicated that CYP3A4 and -2C19 are the primary enzymes involved in the metabolism of escitalopram. However, co-administration of escitalopram (20 mg) and ritonavir (600 mg), a potent inhibitor of CYP3A4, did not significantly affect the pharmacokinetics of escitalopram oxalate. Because escitalopram oxalate is metabolized by multiple enzyme systems, inhibition of a single enzyme may not appreciably decrease escitalopram clearance).
No products indexed under this heading.

Erythromycin Stearate (*In vitro* studies indicated that CYP3A4 and -2C19 are the primary enzymes involved in the metabolism of escitalopram. However, co-administration of escitalopram (20 mg) and ritonavir (600 mg), a potent inhibitor of CYP3A4, did not significantly affect the pharmacokinetics of escitalopram oxalate. Because escitalopram oxalate is metabolized by multiple enzyme systems, inhibition of a single enzyme may not appreciably decrease escitalopram clearance).
No products indexed under this heading.

Esomeprazole Magnesium (*In vitro* studies indicated that CYP3A4 and -2C19 are the primary enzymes involved in the metabolism of escitalo-

IMPORTANT NOTE: Always consult each drug listing in the patient's regimen for possible interactions.

pram. However, co-administration of escitalopram (20 mg) and ritonavir (600 mg), a potent inhibitor of CYP3A4, did not significantly affect the pharmacokinetics of escitalopram oxalate. Because escitalopram oxalate is metabolized by multiple enzyme systems, inhibition of a single enzyme may not appreciably decrease escitalopram clearance). Products include:

Nexium Capsules 704
Nexium Oral Suspension 704

Esomeprazole Sodium (*In vitro* studies indicated that CYP3A4 and -2C19 are the primary enzymes involved in the metabolism of escitalopram. However, co-administration of escitalopram (20 mg) and ritonavir (600 mg), a potent inhibitor of CYP3A4, did not significantly affect the pharmacokinetics of escitalopram oxalate. Because escitalopram oxalate is metabolized by multiple enzyme systems, inhibition of a single enzyme may not appreciably decrease escitalopram clearance). Products include:

Nexium I.V. 712

Estazolam (Given the primary CNS effects of escitalopram, caution should be used when it is taken in combination of other centrally acting drugs).
No products indexed under this heading.

Ethacrynic Acid (Hyponatremia may occur as a result of treatment with escitalopram. Patients taking diuretics may be at greater risk. Discontinuation of escitalopram should be considered in patients with symptomatic hyponatremia and appropriate medical intervention should be instituted).
No products indexed under this heading.

Ethanol (Although escitalopram did not potentiate the cognitive and motor effects of alcohol in a clinical trial, as with other psychotropic medications, the use of alcohol by patients taking escitalopram is not recommended).
No products indexed under this heading.

Ethchlorvynol (Given the primary CNS effects of escitalopram, caution should be used when it is taken in combination of other centrally acting drugs).
No products indexed under this heading.

Ethinamate (Given the primary CNS effects of escitalopram, caution should be used when it is taken in combination of other centrally acting drugs).
No products indexed under this heading.

Ethinyl Estradiol (*In vitro* studies indicated that CYP3A4 and -2C19 are the primary enzymes involved in the metabolism of escitalopram. However, co-administration of escitalopram (20 mg) and ritonavir (600 mg), a potent inhibitor of CYP3A4, did not significantly affect the pharmacokinetics of escitalopram oxalate. Because escitalopram oxalate is metabolized by multiple enzyme systems, inhibition of a single enzyme may not appreciably decrease escitalopram clearance). Products include:

LoSeasonique 3407
Lybrel 3514
NuvaRing 3181
Ortho Evra 2648
Ortho-Cyclen/Ortho Tri-Cyclen 2663
Ortho Tri-Cyclen Lo Tablets 2673
Seasonique 3418
Yaz 864

Ethyl Alcohol (Although escitalopram did not potentiate the cognitive and motor effects of alcohol in a clinical trial, as with other psychotropic medications, the use of alcohol by patients taking escitalopram is not recommended).
No products indexed under this heading.

Ethynodiol Diacetate (*In vitro* studies indicated that CYP3A4 and -2C19 are the primary enzymes involved in the metabolism of escitalopram. However, co-administration of escitalopram (20 mg) and ritonavir (600 mg), a potent inhibitor of CYP3A4, did not significantly affect the pharmacokinetics of escitalopram oxalate. Because escitalopram oxalate is metabolized by multiple enzyme systems, inhibition of a single enzyme may not appreciably decrease escitalopram clearance).
No products indexed under this heading.

Etodolac (Epidemiological studies of the case-control and cohort design that have demonstrated an association between use of psychotropic drugs that interfere with serotonin reuptake and the occurrence of upper gastrointestinal bleeding have also shown that concurrent use of an NSAID may potentiate the risk of bleeding; use caution when administering).
No products indexed under this heading.

Felbamate (*In vitro* studies indicated that CYP3A4 and -2C19 are the primary enzymes involved in the metabolism of escitalopram. However, co-administration of escitalopram (20 mg) and ritonavir (600 mg), a potent inhibitor of CYP3A4, did not significantly affect the pharmacokinetics of escitalopram oxalate. Because escitalopram oxalate is metabolized by multiple enzyme systems, inhibition of a single enzyme may not appreciably decrease escitalopram clearance).
No products indexed under this heading.

Fenoprofen Calcium (Epidemiological studies of the case-control and cohort design that have demonstrated an association between use of psychotropic drugs that interfere with serotonin reuptake and the occurrence of upper gastrointestinal bleeding have also shown that concurrent use of an NSAID may potentiate the risk of bleeding; use caution when administering).
No products indexed under this heading.

Fentanyl (Given the primary CNS effects of escitalopram, caution should be used when it is taken in combination of other centrally acting drugs). Products include:

Duragesic 2604
Fentanyl Transdermal System 2346
Onsolis 2054

Fentanyl Citrate (Given the primary CNS effects of escitalopram, caution should be used when it is taken in combination of other centrally acting drugs). Products include:

Fentora 966

Flecainide Acetate (*In vitro* studies did not reveal an inhibitory effect of escitalopram on CYP2D6. In addition, steady state levels of racemic citalopram were not significantly different in poor metabolizers and extensive CYP2D6 metabolizers after multi-dose administration of citalopram, suggesting that co-administration, with escitalopram, of a drug that inhibits CYP2D6, is unlikely to have clinically significant effects on escitalopram metabolism. However, there are limited *in vivo* data suggesting a modest CYP2D6 inhibitory effect for escitalopram, ie co-administration of escitalopram (20 mg/day for 21 days) with the tricyclic antidepressant desipramine (single dose of 50 mg), a substrate for CYP2D6 resulted in a 40% increase in C_{max} and a 100% increase in AUC of desipramine. The clinical significance of this finding is unknown. Nevertheless, caution is indicated in the co-administration of escitalopram and drugs metabolized by CYP2D6).
No products indexed under this heading.

Fluconazole (*In vitro* studies indicated that CYP3A4 and -2C19 are the primary enzymes involved in the metabolism of escitalopram. However, co-administration of escitalopram (20 mg) and ritonavir (600 mg), a potent inhibitor of CYP3A4, did not significantly affect the pharmacokinetics of escitalopram oxalate. Because escitalopram oxalate is metabolized by multiple enzyme systems, inhibition of a single enzyme may not appreciably decrease escitalopram clearance).
No products indexed under this heading.

Fluoxetine (*In vitro* studies did not reveal an inhibitory effect of escitalopram on CYP2D6. In addition, steady state levels of racemic citalopram were not significantly different in poor metabolizers and extensive CYP2D6 metabolizers after multi-dose administration of citalopram, suggesting that co-administration, with escitalopram, of a drug that inhibits CYP2D6, is unlikely to have clinically significant effects on escitalopram metabolism. However, there are limited *in vivo* data suggesting a modest CYP2D6 inhibitory effect for escitalopram, ie co-administration of escitalopram (20 mg/day for 21 days) with the tricyclic antidepressant desipramine (single dose of 50 mg), a substrate for CYP2D6 resulted in a 40% increase in C_{max} and a 100% increase in AUC of desipramine. The clinical significance of this finding is unknown. Nevertheless, caution is indicated in the co-administration of escitalopram and drugs metabolized by CYP2D6).
No products indexed under this heading.

Fluoxetine Hydrochloride (The development of a potentially life-threatening serotonin syndrome or Neuroleptic Malignant Syndrome (NMS)-like reactions have been reported with SNRIs and SSRIs alone, including escitalopram treatment, but particularly with concomitant use of serotonergic drugs (including triptans) with drugs which impair metabolism of serotonin (including MAOIs), or with antipsychotics or other dopamine antagonists. Patients should be monitored for the emergence of serotonin syndrome or NMS-like signs and symptoms. Treatment with escitalopram and any concomitant serotonergic or antidopaminergic agents, including antipsychotics, should be discontinued immediately if the above events occur and supportive symptomatic treatment should be initiated). Products include:

Prozac Weekly 1941
Prozac Pulvules 1941
Symbyax 1965

Fluphenazine Decanoate (The development of a potentially life-threatening serotonin syndrome or Neuroleptic Malignant Syndrome (NMS)-like reactions have been reported with SNRIs and SSRIs alone, including escitalopram treatment, but particularly with concomitant use of serotonergic drugs (including triptans) with drugs which impair metabolism of serotonin (including MAOIs), or with antipsychotics or other dopamine antagonists. Patients should be monitored for the emergence of serotonin syndrome or NMS-like signs and symptoms. Treatment with escitalopram and any concomitant serotonergic or antidopaminergic agents, including antipsychotics, should be discontinued immediately if the above events occur and supportive symptomatic treatment should be initiated).
No products indexed under this heading.

Fluphenazine Enanthate (The development of a potentially life-threatening serotonin syndrome or Neuroleptic Malignant Syndrome (NMS)-like reactions have been reported with SNRIs and SSRIs alone, including escitalopram treatment, but particularly with concomitant use of serotonergic drugs (including triptans) with drugs which impair metabolism of serotonin (including MAOIs), or with antipsychotics or other dopamine antagonists. Patients should be monitored for the emergence of serotonin syndrome or NMS-like signs and symptoms. Treatment with escitalopram and any concomitant serotonergic or antidopaminergic agents, including antipsychotics, should be discontinued immediately if the above events occur and supportive symptomatic treatment should be initiated).
No products indexed under this heading.

Fluphenazine Hydrochloride (The development of a potentially life-threatening serotonin syndrome or Neuroleptic Malignant Syndrome (NMS)-like reactions have been reported with SNRIs and SSRIs alone, including escitalopram treatment, but particularly with concomitant use of serotonergic drugs (including triptans) with drugs which impair metabolism of serotonin (including MAOIs), or with antipsychotics or other dopamine antagonists. Patients should be monitored for the emergence of serotonin syndrome or NMS-like signs and symptoms. Treatment with escitalopram and any concomitant serotonergic or antidopaminergic agents, including antipsychotics, should be discontinued immediately if the above events occur and supportive symptomatic treatment should be initiated).
No products indexed under this heading.

Flurazepam Hydrochloride (Given the primary CNS effects of escitalopram, caution should be used when it is taken in combination of other centrally acting drugs).
No products indexed under this heading.

Flurbiprofen (Epidemiological studies of the case-control and cohort design that have demonstrated an association between use of psychotropic drugs that interfere with serotonin reuptake and the occurrence of upper gastrointestinal bleeding have also shown that concurrent use of an NSAID may potentiate the risk of bleeding; use caution when administering).
No products indexed under this heading.

Fluvastatin Sodium (*In vitro* studies indicated that CYP3A4 and -2C19 are the primary enzymes involved in the metabolism of escitalopram. However, co-administration of escitalopram (20 mg) and ritonavir (600 mg), a potent inhibitor of CYP3A4, did not significantly affect the pharmacokinetics of escitalopram oxalate. Because escitalopram oxalate is metabolized by multiple enzyme systems, inhibition of a single enzyme may not appreciably decrease escitalopram clearance).
No products indexed under this heading.

Fluvoxamine (*In vitro* studies indicated that CYP3A4 and -2C19 are the primary enzymes involved in the metabolism of escitalopram. However, co-administration of escitalopram (20 mg) and ritonavir (600 mg), a potent inhibitor of CYP3A4, did not significantly affect the pharmacokinetics of escitalopram oxalate. Because escitalopram oxalate is metabolized by multiple enzyme systems, inhibition of a single enzyme may not appreciably decrease escitalopram clearance).
No products indexed under this heading.

Fluvoxamine Maleate (The development of a potentially life-threatening serotonin syndrome or Neuroleptic Malignant Syndrome (NMS)-like reactions have been reported with SNRIs and SSRIs alone, including escitalopram treatment, but particularly with concomitant use of serotonergic drugs (including triptans) with drugs which impair metabolism of serotonin (including MAOIs), or with antipsychotics or other dopamine antagonists. Patients should be monitored for the emergence of serotonin syndrome or NMS-like signs and symptoms. Treatment with escitalo-

1027 Interactions Index Lexapro

pram and any concomitant serotonergic or antidopaminergic agents, including antipsychotics, should be discontinued immediately if the above events occur and supportive symptomatic treatment should be initiated).
No products indexed under this heading.

Fondaparinux Sodium (Escitalopram may increase the risk of bleeding events. Concomitant use of anticoagulants may add to this risk. Case reports and epidemiological studies of the case-control and cohort design have demonstrated an association between use of drugs that interfere with serotonin reuptake and the occurrence of gastrointestinal bleeding. Patients should be cautioned about the risk of bleeding associated with the concomitant use of escitalopram and anticoagulants). Products include:
Arixtra 1320

Formoterol Fumarate (*In vitro* studies did not reveal an inhibitory effect of escitalopram on CYP2D6. In addition, steady state levels of racemic citalopram were not significantly different in poor metabolizers and extensive CYP2D6 metabolizers after multi-dose administration of citalopram, suggesting that co-administration, with escitalopram, of a drug that inhibits CYP2D6, is unlikely to have clinically significant effects on escitalopram metabolism. However, there are limited *in vivo* data suggesting a modest CYP2D6 inhibitory effect for escitalopram, ie co-administration of escitalopram (20 mg/day for 21 days) with the tricyclic antidepressant desipramine (single dose of 50 mg), a substrate for CYP2D6 resulted in a 40% increase in C_{max} and a 100% increase in AUC of desipramine. The clinical significance of this finding is unknown. Nevertheless, caution is indicated in the co-administration of escitalopram and drugs metabolized by CYP2D6). Products include:
Foradil 3121
Perforomist 3634

Fosamprenavir Calcium (*In vitro* studies indicated that CYP3A4 and -2C19 are the primary enzymes involved in the metabolism of escitalopram. However, co-administration of escitalopram (20 mg) and ritonavir (600 mg), a potent inhibitor of CYP3A4, did not significantly affect the pharmacokinetics of escitalopram oxalate. Because escitalopram oxalate is metabolized by multiple enzyme systems, inhibition of a single enzyme may not appreciably decrease escitalopram clearance). Products include:
Lexiva Oral Suspension 1558
Lexiva 1558

Frovatriptan Succinate (There have been rare post-marketing reports of serotonin syndrome with use of a SSRI and a triptan. If concomitant treatment of escitalopram with a triptan is clinically warranted, careful observation of the patient is advised, particularly during treatment initiation and dose increases). Products include:
Frova 1103

Furosemide (Hyponatremia may occur as a result of treatment with escitalopram. Patients taking diuretics may be at greater risk. Discontinuation of escitalopram should be considered in patients with symptomatic hyponatremia and appropriate medical intervention should be instituted). Products include:
Furosemide 2354

Galantamine Hydrobromide (*In vitro* studies did not reveal an inhibitory effect of escitalopram on CYP2D6. In addition, steady state levels of racemic citalopram were not significantly different in poor metabolizers and extensive CYP2D6 metabolizers after multi-dose administration of citalopram, suggesting that co-administration, with escitalopram, of a drug that inhibits CYP2D6, is unlikely to have clinically significant effects on escitalopram metabolism. However, there are limited *in vivo* data suggesting a modest CYP2D6 inhibitory effect for escitalopram, ie co-administration of escitalopram (20 mg/day for 21 days) with the tricyclic antidepressant desipramine (single dose of 50 mg), a substrate for CYP2D6 resulted in a 40% increase in C_{max} and a 100% increase in AUC of desipramine. The clinical significance of this finding is unknown. Nevertheless, caution is indicated in the co-administration of escitalopram and drugs metabolized by CYP2D6).
No products indexed under this heading.

Glutethimide (Given the primary CNS effects of escitalopram, caution should be used when it is taken in combination of other centrally acting drugs).
No products indexed under this heading.

Halazepam (Given the primary CNS effects of escitalopram, caution should be used when it is taken in combination of other centrally acting drugs).
No products indexed under this heading.

Haloperidol (The development of a potentially life-threatening serotonin syndrome or Neuroleptic Malignant Syndrome (NMS)-like reactions have been reported with SNRIs and SSRIs alone, including escitalopram treatment, but particularly with concomitant use of serotonergic drugs (including triptans) with drugs which impair metabolism of serotonin (including MAOIs), or with antipsychotics or other dopamine antagonists. Patients should be monitored for the emergence of serotonin syndrome or NMS-like signs and symptoms. Treatment with escitalopram and any concomitant serotonergic or antidopaminergic agents, including antipsychotics, should be discontinued immediately if the above events occur and supportive symptomatic treatment should be initiated).
No products indexed under this heading.

Haloperidol Decanoate (The development of a potentially life-threatening serotonin syndrome or Neuroleptic Malignant Syndrome (NMS)-like reactions have been reported with SNRIs and SSRIs alone, including escitalopram treatment, but particularly with concomitant use of serotonergic drugs (including triptans) with drugs which impair metabolism of serotonin (including MAOIs), or with antipsychotics or other dopamine antagonists. Patients should be monitored for the emergence of serotonin syndrome or NMS-like signs and symptoms. Treatment with escitalopram and any concomitant serotonergic or antidopaminergic agents, including antipsychotics, should be discontinued immediately if the above events occur and supportive symptomatic treatment should be initiated).
No products indexed under this heading.

Haloperidol Lactate (The development of a potentially life-threatening serotonin syndrome or Neuroleptic Malignant Syndrome (NMS)-like reactions have been reported with SNRIs and SSRIs alone, including escitalopram treatment, but particularly with concomitant use of serotonergic drugs (including triptans) with drugs which impair metabolism of serotonin (including MAOIs), or with antipsychotics or other dopamine antagonists. Patients should be monitored for the emergence of serotonin syndrome or NMS-like signs and symptoms. Treatment with escitalopram and any concomitant serotonergic or antidopaminergic agents, including antipsychotics, should be discontinued immediately if the above events occur and supportive symptomatic treatment should be initiated).
No products indexed under this heading.

Heparin Calcium (Escitalopram may increase the risk of bleeding events. Concomitant use of anticoagulants may add to this risk. Case reports and epidemiological studies of the case-control and cohort design have demonstrated an association between use of drugs that interfere with serotonin reuptake and the occurrence of gastrointestinal bleeding. Patients should be cautioned about the risk of bleeding associated with the concomitant use of escitalopram and anticoagulants).
No products indexed under this heading.

Heparin Sodium (Escitalopram may increase the risk of bleeding events. Concomitant use of anticoagulants may add to this risk. Case reports and epidemiological studies of the case-control and cohort design have demonstrated an association between use of drugs that interfere with serotonin reuptake and the occurrence of gastrointestinal bleeding. Patients should be cautioned about the risk of bleeding associated with the concomitant use of escitalopram and anticoagulants).
No products indexed under this heading.

Hexobarbital (Given the primary CNS effects of escitalopram, caution should be used when it is taken in combination of other centrally acting drugs).
No products indexed under this heading.

Hydrochlorothiazide (Hyponatremia may occur as a result of treatment with escitalopram. Patients taking diuretics may be at greater risk. Discontinuation of escitalopram should be considered in patients with symptomatic hyponatremia and appropriate medical intervention should be instituted). Products include:
Atacand HCT 700
Avalide 2956
Benicar HCT 1017
Diovan HCT 2419
Dyazide 1429
Exforge HCT 2449
Hyzaar 2162
Hyzaar 100-12.5 2162
Micardis HCT 889
Prinzide 2246
Tekturna HCT 2541
Teveten HCT 541

Hydrocodone Bitartrate (Given the primary CNS effects of escitalopram, caution should be used when it is taken in combination of other centrally acting drugs). Products include:
Vicodin 560
Vicodin ES 561
Vicodin HP 563
Vicoprofen 564
Zydone 1138

Hydrocodone Polistirex (Given the primary CNS effects of escitalopram, caution should be used when it is taken in combination of other centrally acting drugs). Products include:
Tussionex 3443

Hydroflumethiazide (Hyponatremia may occur as a result of treatment with escitalopram. Patients taking diuretics may be at greater risk. Discontinuation of escitalopram should be considered in patients with symptomatic hyponatremia and appropriate medical intervention should be instituted).
No products indexed under this heading.

Hydromorphone (Given the primary CNS effects of escitalopram, caution should be used when it is taken in combination of other centrally acting drugs).
No products indexed under this heading.

Hydromorphone Hydrochloride (Given the primary CNS effects of escitalopram, caution should be used when it is taken in combination of other centrally acting drugs). Products include:
Dilaudid Injection 2800
Dilaudid Oral 2797
Dilaudid Tablets 2797
Dilaudid-HP 2800

Hydroxyamphetamine Hydrobromide (Given the primary CNS effects of escitalopram, caution should be used when it is taken in combination of other centrally acting drugs).
No products indexed under this heading.

Hydroxyzine Hydrochloride (Given the primary CNS effects of escitalopram, caution should be used when it is taken in combination of other centrally acting drugs).
No products indexed under this heading.

Hypericum (Based on the mechanism of action of escitalopram and the potential for serotonin syndrome, caution is advised when escitalopram is co-administered with other drugs that may effect the serotonergic neurotransmitter systems such as St. John's Wort).
No products indexed under this heading.

Ibuprofen (Epidemiological studies of the case-control and cohort design that have demonstrated an association between use of psychotropic drugs that interfere with serotonin reuptake and the occurrence of upper gastrointestinal bleeding have also shown that concurrent use of an NSAID may potentiate the risk of bleeding; use caution when administering). Products include:
Motrin IB 2043
Children's Motrin 2044
Children's Motrin Non-Staining Dye-Free 2044
Infants' Motrin 2044
Infants' Motrin Dye-Free 2044
Junior Strength Motrin 2044
Vicoprofen 564

Imatinib Mesylate (*In vitro* studies indicated that CYP3A4 and -2C19 are the primary enzymes involved in the metabolism of escitalopram. However, co-administration of escitalopram (20 mg) and ritonavir (600 mg), a potent inhibitor of CYP3A4, did not significantly affect the pharmacokinetics of escitalopram oxalate. Because escitalopram oxalate is metabolized by multiple enzyme systems, inhibition of a single enzyme may not appreciably decrease escitalopram clearance). Products include:
Gleevec 2477

Imipramine Hydrochloride (*In vitro* studies did not reveal an inhibitory effect of escitalopram on CYP2D6. In addition, steady state levels of racemic citalopram were not significantly different in poor metabolizers and extensive CYP2D6 metabolizers after multi-dose administration of citalopram, suggesting that co-administration, with escitalopram, of a drug that inhibits CYP2D6, is unlikely to have clinically significant effects on escitalopram metabolism. However, there are limited *in vivo* data suggesting a modest CYP2D6 inhibitory effect for escitalopram, ie co-administration of escitalopram (20 mg/day for 21 days) with the tricyclic antidepressant desipramine (single dose of 50 mg), a substrate for CYP2D6 resulted in a 40% increase in C_{max} and a 100% increase in AUC of desipramine. The clinical significance of this finding is unknown. Nevertheless, caution is indicated in the co-administration of escitalopram and drugs metabolized by CYP2D6).
No products indexed under this heading.

Imipramine Pamoate (*In vitro* studies did not reveal an inhibitory effect of escitalopram on CYP2D6. In addition, steady state levels of racemic citalopram were not significantly different in poor metabolizers and extensive

IMPORTANT NOTE: Always consult each drug listing in the patient's regimen for possible interactions.

Lexapro Interactions Index 1028

CYP2D6 metabolizers after multi-dose administration of citalopram, suggesting that co-administration, with escitalopram, of a drug that inhibits CYP2D6, is unlikely to have clinically significant effects on escitalopram metabolism. However, there are limited *in vivo* data suggesting a modest CYP2D6 inhibitory effect for escitalopram, ie co-administration of escitalopram (20 mg/day for 21 days) with the tricyclic antidepressant desipramine (single dose of 50 mg), a substrate for CYP2D6 resulted in a 40% increase in C_{max} and a 100% increase in AUC of desipramine. The clinical significance of this finding is unknown. Nevertheless, caution is indicated in the co-administration of escitalopram and drugs metabolized by CYP2D6).
No products indexed under this heading.

Indapamide (Hyponatremia may occur as a result of treatment with escitalopram. Patients taking diuretics may be at greater risk. Discontinuation of escitalopram should be considered in patients with symptomatic hyponatremia and appropriate medical intervention should be instituted). Products include:
Indapamide 2356

Indinavir Sulfate (*In vitro* studies indicated that CYP3A4 and -2C19 are the primary enzymes involved in the metabolism of escitalopram. However, co-administration of escitalopram (20 mg) and ritonavir (600 mg), a potent inhibitor of CYP3A4, did not significantly affect the pharmacokinetics of escitalopram oxalate. Because escitalopram oxalate is metabolized by multiple enzyme systems, inhibition of a single enzyme may not appreciably decrease escitalopram clearance). Products include:
Crixivan 2113

Indomethacin (Epidemiological studies of the case-control and cohort design that have demonstrated an association between use of psychotropic drugs that interfere with serotonin reuptake and the occurrence of upper gastrointestinal bleeding have also shown that concurrent use of an NSAID may potentiate the risk of bleeding; use caution when administering). Products include:
Indocin 2167

Indomethacin Sodium Trihydrate (Epidemiological studies of the case-control and cohort design that have demonstrated an association between use of psychotropic drugs that interfere with serotonin reuptake and the occurrence of upper gastrointestinal bleeding have also shown that concurrent use of an NSAID may potentiate the risk of bleeding; use caution when administering). Products include:
Indocin I.V. 2007

Indoramin Hydrochloride (*In vitro* studies did not reveal an inhibitory effect of escitalopram on CYP2D6. In addition, steady state levels of racemic citalopram were not significantly different in poor metabolizers and extensive CYP2D6 metabolizers after multi-dose administration of citalopram, suggesting that co-administration, with escitalopram, of a drug that inhibits CYP2D6, is unlikely to have clinically significant effects on escitalopram metabolism. However, there are limited *in vivo* data suggesting a modest CYP2D6 inhibitory effect for escitalopram, ie co-administration of escitalopram (20 mg/day for 21 days) with the tricyclic antidepressant desipramine (single dose of 50 mg), a substrate for CYP2D6 resulted in a 40% increase in C_{max} and a 100% increase in AUC of desipramine. The clinical significance of this finding is unknown. Nevertheless, caution is indicated in the co-administration of escitalopram and drugs metabolized by CYP2D6).
No products indexed under this heading.

Isocarboxazid (Concomitant use of MAO inhibitors and escitalopram is contraindicated. In patients receiving SSRIs in combination with a MAO inhibitor, there have been reports of serious, sometimes fatal reactions including hyperthermia, rigidity, myoclonus, and autonomic instability. These reactions have also been reported in patients who have recently discontinued SSRI treatment and have been started on an MAO inhibitor. Some cases presented with features resembling neuroleptic malignant syndrome. Furthermore, additional data suggests that the combined use of SSRIs and MAO inhibitors may act synergistically to elevate blood pressure and evoke behavioral excitation. Therefore, it is recommended that escitalopram should not be used in combination with an MAO inhibitor, or within 14 days of discontinuing treatment with an MAO inhibitor. Similarily, at least 14 days should be allowed after stopping escitalopram before starting an MAO inhibitor). Products include:
Marplan 3481

Isoflurane (Given the primary CNS effects of escitalopram, caution should be used when it is taken in combination of other centrally acting drugs).
No products indexed under this heading.

Isoniazid (*In vitro* studies indicated that CYP3A4 and -2C19 are the primary enzymes involved in the metabolism of escitalopram. However, co-administration of escitalopram (20 mg) and ritonavir (600 mg), a potent inhibitor of CYP3A4, did not significantly affect the pharmacokinetics of escitalopram oxalate. Because escitalopram oxalate is metabolized by multiple enzyme systems, inhibition of a single enzyme may not appreciably decrease escitalopram clearance).
No products indexed under this heading.

Itraconazole (*In vitro* studies indicated that CYP3A4 and -2C19 are the primary enzymes involved in the metabolism of escitalopram. However, co-administration of escitalopram (20 mg) and ritonavir (600 mg), a potent inhibitor of CYP3A4, did not significantly affect the pharmacokinetics of escitalopram oxalate. Because escitalopram oxalate is metabolized by multiple enzyme systems, inhibition of a single enzyme may not appreciably decrease escitalopram clearance).
No products indexed under this heading.

Ketamine Hydrochloride (Given the primary CNS effects of escitalopram, caution should be used when it is taken in combination of other centrally acting drugs).
No products indexed under this heading.

Ketoconazole (Combined administration of racemic citalopram (40 mg) and ketoconazole (200 mg), a potent CYP3A4 inhibitor, decreased the C_{max} and AUC of ketoconazole by 21% and 10%, respectively, and did not significantly affect the pharmacokinetics of citalopram). Products include:
Extina 3319
Xolegel 3337

Ketoprofen (Epidemiological studies of the case-control and cohort design that have demonstrated an association between use of psychotropic drugs that interfere with serotonin reuptake and the occurrence of upper gastrointestinal bleeding have also shown that concurrent use of an NSAID may potentiate the risk of bleeding; use caution when administering).
No products indexed under this heading.

Ketorolac Tromethamine (Epidemiological studies of the case-control and cohort design that have demonstrated an association between use of psychotropic drugs that interfere with serotonin reuptake and the occurrence of upper gastrointestinal bleeding have also shown that concurrent use of an NSAID may potentiate the risk of bleeding; use caution when administering). Products include:
Acuvail .... ⊙ 209

Labetalol Hydrochloride (*In vitro* studies did not reveal an inhibitory effect of escitalopram on CYP2D6. In addition, steady state levels of racemic citalopram were not significantly different in poor metabolizers and extensive CYP2D6 metabolizers after multi-dose administration of citalopram, suggesting that co-administration, with escitalopram, of a drug that inhibits CYP2D6, is unlikely to have clinically significant effects on escitalopram metabolism. However, there are limited *in vivo* data suggesting a modest CYP2D6 inhibitory effect for escitalopram, ie co-administration of escitalopram (20 mg/day for 21 days) with the tricyclic antidepressant desipramine (single dose of 50 mg), a substrate for CYP2D6 resulted in a 40% increase in C_{max} and a 100% increase in AUC of desipramine. The clinical significance of this finding is unknown. Nevertheless, caution is indicated in the co-administration of escitalopram and drugs metabolized by CYP2D6).
No products indexed under this heading.

Lansoprazole (*In vitro* studies indicated that CYP3A4 and -2C19 are the primary enzymes involved in the metabolism of escitalopram. However, co-administration of escitalopram (20 mg) and ritonavir (600 mg), a potent inhibitor of CYP3A4, did not significantly affect the pharmacokinetics of escitalopram oxalate. Because escitalopram oxalate is metabolized by multiple enzyme systems, inhibition of a single enzyme may not appreciably decrease escitalopram clearance).
No products indexed under this heading.

Lapatinib (*In vitro* studies indicated that CYP3A4 and -2C19 are the primary enzymes involved in the metabolism of escitalopram. However, co-administration of escitalopram (20 mg) and ritonavir (600 mg), a potent inhibitor of CYP3A4, did not significantly affect the pharmacokinetics of escitalopram oxalate. Because escitalopram oxalate is metabolized by multiple enzyme systems, inhibition of a single enzyme may not appreciably decrease escitalopram clearance). Products include:
Tykerb 1698

Letrozole (*In vitro* studies indicated that CYP3A4 and -2C19 are the primary enzymes involved in the metabolism of escitalopram. However, co-administration of escitalopram (20 mg) and ritonavir (600 mg), a potent inhibitor of CYP3A4, did not significantly affect the pharmacokinetics of escitalopram oxalate. Because escitalopram oxalate is metabolized by multiple enzyme systems, inhibition of a single enzyme may not appreciably decrease escitalopram clearance). Products include:
Femara 2466

Levomethadyl Acetate Hydrochloride (Given the primary CNS effects of escitalopram, caution should be used when it is taken in combination of other centrally acting drugs).
No products indexed under this heading.

Levonorgestrel (*In vitro* studies indicated that CYP3A4 and -2C19 are the primary enzymes involved in the metabolism of escitalopram. However, co-administration of escitalopram (20 mg) and ritonavir (600 mg), a potent inhibitor of CYP3A4, did not significantly affect the pharmacokinetics of escitalopram oxalate. Because escitalopram oxalate is metabolized by multiple enzyme systems, inhibition of a single enzyme may not appreciably decrease escitalopram clearance). Products include:
Climara Pro 847
LoSeasonique 3407
Lybrel 3514
Mirena 854
Plan B 3416
Seasonique 3418

Levorphanol Tartrate (Given the primary CNS effects of escitalopram, caution should be used when it is taken in combination of other centrally acting drugs).
No products indexed under this heading.

Lidocaine (*In vitro* studies did not reveal an inhibitory effect of escitalopram on CYP2D6. In addition, steady state levels of racemic citalopram were not significantly different in poor metabolizers and extensive CYP2D6 metabolizers after multi-dose administration of citalopram, suggesting that co-administration, with escitalopram, of a drug that inhibits CYP2D6, is unlikely to have clinically significant effects on escitalopram metabolism. However, there are limited *in vivo* data suggesting a modest CYP2D6 inhibitory effect for escitalopram, ie co-administration of escitalopram (20 mg/day for 21 days) with the tricyclic antidepressant desipramine (single dose of 50 mg), a substrate for CYP2D6 resulted in a 40% increase in C_{max} and a 100% increase in AUC of desipramine. The clinical significance of this finding is unknown. Nevertheless, caution is indicated in the co-administration of escitalopram and drugs metabolized by CYP2D6). Products include:
Lidoderm 1107

Lidocaine Hydrochloride (*In vitro* studies did not reveal an inhibitory effect of escitalopram on CYP2D6. In addition, steady state levels of racemic citalopram were not significantly different in poor metabolizers and extensive CYP2D6 metabolizers after multi-dose administration of citalopram, suggesting that co-administration, with escitalopram, of a drug that inhibits CYP2D6, is unlikely to have clinically significant effects on escitalopram metabolism. However, there are limited *in vivo* data suggesting a modest CYP2D6 inhibitory effect for escitalopram, ie co-administration of escitalopram (20 mg/day for 21 days) with the tricyclic antidepressant desipramine (single dose of 50 mg), a substrate for CYP2D6 resulted in a 40% increase in C_{max} and a 100% increase in AUC of desipramine. The clinical significance of this finding is unknown. Nevertheless, caution is indicated in the co-administration of escitalopram and drugs metabolized by CYP2D6).
No products indexed under this heading.

Linezolid (Based on the mechanism of action of escitalopram and the potential for serotonin syndrome, caution is advised when escitalopram is co-administered with other drugs that may effect the serotonergic neurotransmitter system such as linezolid). Products include:
Zyvox 2769

Lisdexamfetamine Dimesylate (Given the primary CNS effects of escitalopram, caution should be used when it is taken in combination of other centrally acting drugs). Products include:
Vyvanse 3298

Lithium (The development of a potentially life-threatening serotonin syn-

drome or Neuroleptic Malignant Syndrome (NMS)-like reactions have been reported with SNRIs and SSRIs alone, including escitalopram treatment, but particularly with concomitant use of serotonergic drugs (including triptans) with drugs which impair metabolism of serotonin (including MAOIs), or with antipsychotics or other dopamine antagonists. Patients should be monitored for the emergence of serotonin syndrome or NMS-like signs and symptoms. Treatment with escitalopram and any concomitant serotonergic or antidopaminergic agents, including antipsychotics, should be discontinued immediately if the above events occur and supportive symptomatic treatment should be initiated.
No products indexed under this heading.

Lithium Carbonate (The development of a potentially life-threatening serotonin syndrome or Neuroleptic Malignant Syndrome (NMS)-like reactions have been reported with SNRIs and SSRIs alone, including escitalopram treatment, but particularly with concomitant use of serotonergic drugs (including triptans) with drugs which impair metabolism of serotonin (including MAOIs), or with antipsychotics or other dopamine antagonists. Patients should be monitored for the emergence of serotonin syndrome or NMS-like signs and symptoms. Treatment with escitalopram and any concomitant serotonergic or antidopaminergic agents, including antipsychotics, should be discontinued immediately if the above events occur and supportive symptomatic treatment should be initiated).
No products indexed under this heading.

Lithium Citrate (The development of a potentially life-threatening serotonin syndrome or Neuroleptic Malignant Syndrome (NMS)-like reactions have been reported with SNRIs and SSRIs alone, including escitalopram treatment, but particularly with concomitant use of serotonergic drugs (including triptans) with drugs which impair metabolism of serotonin (including MAOIs), or with antipsychotics or other dopamine antagonists. Patients should be monitored for the emergence of serotonin syndrome or NMS-like signs and symptoms. Treatment with escitalopram and any concomitant serotonergic or antidopaminergic agents, including antipsychotics, should be discontinued immediately if the above events occur and supportive symptomatic treatment should be initiated).
No products indexed under this heading.

Lopinavir (In vitro studies indicated that CYP3A4 and -2C19 are the primary enzymes involved in the metabolism of escitalopram. However, co-administration of escitalopram (20 mg) and ritonavir (600 mg), a potent inhibitor of CYP3A4, did not significantly affect the pharmacokinetics of escitalopram oxalate. Because escitalopram oxalate is metabolized by multiple enzyme systems, inhibition of a single enzyme may not appreciably decrease escitalopram clearance). Products include:
Kaletra 458

Loratadine (In vitro studies indicated that CYP3A4 and -2C19 are the primary enzymes involved in the metabolism of escitalopram. However, co-administration of escitalopram (20 mg) and ritonavir (600 mg), a potent inhibitor of CYP3A4, did not significantly affect the pharmacokinetics of escitalopram oxalate. Because escitalopram oxalate is metabolized by multiple enzyme systems, inhibition of a single enzyme may not appreciably decrease escitalopram clearance).
No products indexed under this heading.

Lorazepam (Given the primary CNS effects of escitalopram, caution should be used when it is taken in combination of other centrally acting drugs).
No products indexed under this heading.

Low Molecular Weight Heparins (Escitalopram may increase the risk of bleeding events. Concomitant use of anticoagulants may add to this risk. Case reports and epidemiological studies of the case-control and cohort design have demonstrated an association between use of drugs that interfere with serotonin reuptake and the occurrence of gastrointestinal bleeding. Patients should be cautioned about the risk of bleeding associated with the concomitant use of escitalopram and anticoagulants).
No products indexed under this heading.

Loxapine Hydrochloride (The development of a potentially life-threatening serotonin syndrome or Neuroleptic Malignant Syndrome (NMS)-like reactions have been reported with SNRIs and SSRIs alone, including escitalopram treatment, but particularly with concomitant use of serotonergic drugs (including triptans) with drugs which impair metabolism of serotonin (including MAOIs), or with antipsychotics or other dopamine antagonists. Patients should be monitored for the emergence of serotonin syndrome or NMS-like signs and symptoms. Treatment with escitalopram and any concomitant serotonergic or antidopaminergic agents, including antipsychotics, should be discontinued immediately if the above events occur and supportive symptomatic treatment should be initiated).
No products indexed under this heading.

Loxapine Succinate (The development of a potentially life-threatening serotonin syndrome or Neuroleptic Malignant Syndrome (NMS)-like reactions have been reported with SNRIs and SSRIs alone, including escitalopram treatment, but particularly with concomitant use of serotonergic drugs (including triptans) with drugs which impair metabolism of serotonin (including MAOIs), or with antipsychotics or other dopamine antagonists. Patients should be monitored for the emergence of serotonin syndrome or NMS-like signs and symptoms. Treatment with escitalopram and any concomitant serotonergic or antidopaminergic agents, including antipsychotics, should be discontinued immediately if the above events occur and supportive symptomatic treatment should be initiated).
No products indexed under this heading.

Maprotiline Hydrochloride (In vitro studies did not reveal an inhibitory effect of escitalopram on CYP2D6. In addition, steady state levels of racemic citalopram were not significantly different in poor metabolizers and extensive CYP2D6 metabolizers after multi-dose administration of citalopram, suggesting that co-administration, with escitalopram, of a drug that inhibits CYP2D6, is unlikely to have clinically significant effects on escitalopram metabolism. However, there are limited in vivo data suggesting a modest CYP2D6 inhibitory effect for escitalopram, ie co-administration of escitalopram (20 mg/day for 21 days) with the tricyclic antidepressant desipramine (single dose of 50 mg), a substrate for CYP2D6 resulted in a 40% increase in C_{max} and a 100% increase in AUC of desipramine. The clinical significance of this finding is unknown. Nevertheless, caution is indicated in the co-administration of escitalopram and drugs metabolized by CYP2D6).
No products indexed under this heading.

Meclofenamate Sodium (Epidemiological studies of the case-control and cohort design that have demonstrated an association between use of psychotropic drugs that interfere with serotonin reuptake and the occurrence of upper gastrointestinal bleeding have also shown that concurrent use of an NSAID may potentiate the risk of bleeding; use caution when administering).
No products indexed under this heading.

Mefenamic Acid (Epidemiological studies of the case-control and cohort design that have demonstrated an association between use of psychotropic drugs that interfere with serotonin reuptake and the occurrence of upper gastrointestinal bleeding have also shown that concurrent use of an NSAID may potentiate the risk of bleeding; use caution when administering).
No products indexed under this heading.

Meloxicam (Epidemiological studies of the case-control and cohort design that have demonstrated an association between use of psychotropic drugs that interfere with serotonin reuptake and the occurrence of upper gastrointestinal bleeding have also shown that concurrent use of an NSAID may potentiate the risk of bleeding; use caution when administering).
No products indexed under this heading.

Meperidine Hydrochloride (Given the primary CNS effects of escitalopram, caution should be used when it is taken in combination of other centrally acting drugs).
No products indexed under this heading.

Mephobarbital (Given the primary CNS effects of escitalopram, caution should be used when it is taken in combination of other centrally acting drugs).
No products indexed under this heading.

Meprobamate (Given the primary CNS effects of escitalopram, caution should be used when it is taken in combination of other centrally acting drugs).
No products indexed under this heading.

Mesoridazine Besylate (The development of a potentially life-threatening serotonin syndrome or Neuroleptic Malignant Syndrome (NMS)-like reactions have been reported with SNRIs and SSRIs alone, including escitalopram treatment, but particularly with concomitant use of serotonergic drugs (including triptans) with drugs which impair metabolism of serotonin (including MAOIs), or with antipsychotics or other dopamine antagonists. Patients should be monitored for the emergence of serotonin syndrome or NMS-like signs and symptoms. Treatment with escitalopram and any concomitant serotonergic or antidopaminergic agents, including antipsychotics, should be discontinued immediately if the above events occur and supportive symptomatic treatment should be initiated).
No products indexed under this heading.

Mestranol (In vitro studies indicated that CYP3A4 and -2C19 are the primary enzymes involved in the metabolism of escitalopram. However, co-administration of escitalopram (20 mg) and ritonavir (600 mg), a potent inhibitor of CYP3A4, did not significantly affect the pharmacokinetics of escitalopram oxalate. Because escitalopram oxalate is metabolized by multiple enzyme systems, inhibition of a single enzyme may not appreciably decrease escitalopram clearance).
No products indexed under this heading.

Methadone Hydrochloride (Given the primary CNS effects of escitalopram, caution should be used when it is taken in combination of other centrally acting drugs).
No products indexed under this heading.

Methamphetamine Hydrochloride (Given the primary CNS effects of escitalopram, caution should be used when it is taken in combination of other centrally acting drugs).
No products indexed under this heading.

Methohexital Sodium (Given the primary CNS effects of escitalopram, caution should be used when it is taken in combination of other centrally acting drugs).
No products indexed under this heading.

Methotrimeprazine (The development of a potentially life-threatening serotonin syndrome or Neuroleptic Malignant Syndrome (NMS)-like reactions have been reported with SNRIs and SSRIs alone, including escitalopram treatment, but particularly with concomitant use of serotonergic drugs (including triptans) with drugs which impair metabolism of serotonin (including MAOIs), or with antipsychotics or other dopamine antagonists. Patients should be monitored for the emergence of serotonin syndrome or NMS-like signs and symptoms. Treatment with escitalopram and any concomitant serotonergic or antidopaminergic agents, including antipsychotics, should be discontinued immediately if the above events occur and supportive symptomatic treatment should be initiated).
No products indexed under this heading.

Methoxyflurane (Given the primary CNS effects of escitalopram, caution should be used when it is taken in combination of other centrally acting drugs).
No products indexed under this heading.

Methoxyphenamine (In vitro studies did not reveal an inhibitory effect of escitalopram on CYP2D6. In addition, steady state levels of racemic citalopram were not significantly different in poor metabolizers and extensive CYP2D6 metabolizers after multi-dose administration of citalopram, suggesting that co-administration, with escitalopram, of a drug that inhibits CYP2D6, is unlikely to have clinically significant effects on escitalopram metabolism. However, there are limited in vivo data suggesting a modest CYP2D6 inhibitory effect for escitalopram, ie co-administration of escitalopram (20 mg/day for 21 days) with the tricyclic antidepressant desipramine (single dose of 50 mg), a substrate for CYP2D6 resulted in a 40% increase in C_{max} and a 100% increase in AUC of desipramine. The clinical significance of this finding is unknown. Nevertheless, caution is indicated in the co-administration of escitalopram and drugs metabolized by CYP2D6).
No products indexed under this heading.

Methyclothiazide (Hyponatremia may occur as a result of treatment with escitalopram. Patients taking diuretics may be at greater risk. Discontinuation of escitalopram should be considered in patients with symptomatic hyponatremia and appropriate medical intervention should be instituted).
No products indexed under this heading.

Methylphenidate (Given the primary CNS effects of escitalopram, caution should be used when it is taken in combination of other centrally acting drugs). Products include:
Daytrana 3283

Methylphenidate Hydrochloride (Given the primary CNS effects of escitalopram, caution should be used when it is taken in combination of other centrally acting drugs). Products include:
Concerta 2598
Metadate CD 3439

Metoclopramide Hydrochloride (The development of a potentially life-threatening serotonin syndrome or Neuroleptic Malignant Syndrome (NMS)-like

IMPORTANT NOTE: Always consult each drug listing in the patient's regimen for possible interactions.

Lexapro Interactions Index 1030

reactions have been reported with SNRIs and SSRIs alone, including escitalopram treatment, but particularly with concomitant use of serotonergic drugs (including triptans) with drugs which impair metabolism of serotonin (including MAOIs), or with antipsychotics or other dopamine antagonists. Patients should be monitored for the emergence of serotonin syndrome or NMS-like signs and symptoms. Treatment with escitalopram and any concomitant serotonergic or antidopaminergic agents, including antipsychotics, should be discontinued immediately if the above events occur and supportive symptomatic treatment should be initiated). Products include:

Metozolv ODT ... 2901

Metolazone (Hyponatremia may occur as a result of treatment with escitalopram. Patients taking diuretics may be at greater risk. Discontinuation of escitalopram should be considered in patients with symptomatic hyponatremia and appropriate medical intervention should be instituted).

No products indexed under this heading.

Metoprolol Succinate (Administration of 20 mg/day escitalopram for 21 days in healthy volunteers resulted in a 50% increase in C_{max} and 82% increase in AUC of the beta-adrenergic blocker metoprolol (given in a single dose of 100 mg). Increased metoprolol plasma levels have been associated with decreased cardioselectivity. Co-administration of escitalopram and metoprolol had no clinically significant effects on blood pressure or heart rate). Products include:

Toprol XL ... 732

Metoprolol Tartrate (Administration of 20 mg/day escitalopram for 21 days in healthy volunteers resulted in a 50% increase in C_{max} and 82% increase in AUC of the beta-adrenergic blocker metoprolol (given in a single dose of 100 mg). Increased metoprolol plasma levels have been associated with decreased cardioselectivity. Co-administration of escitalopram and metoprolol had no clinically significant effects on blood pressure or heart rate).

No products indexed under this heading.

Metronidazole (*In vitro* studies indicated that CYP3A4 and -2C19 are the primary enzymes involved in the metabolism of escitalopram. However, co-administration of escitalopram (20 mg) and ritonavir (600 mg), a potent inhibitor of CYP3A4, did not significantly affect the pharmacokinetics of escitalopram oxalate. Because escitalopram oxalate is metabolized by multiple enzyme systems, inhibition of a single enzyme may not appreciably decrease escitalopram clearance). Products include:

Pylera ... 793

Metronidazole Benzoate (*In vitro* studies indicated that CYP3A4 and -2C19 are the primary enzymes involved in the metabolism of escitalopram. However, co-administration of escitalopram (20 mg) and ritonavir (600 mg), a potent inhibitor of CYP3A4, did not significantly affect the pharmacokinetics of escitalopram oxalate. Because escitalopram oxalate is metabolized by multiple enzyme systems, inhibition of a single enzyme may not appreciably decrease escitalopram clearance).

No products indexed under this heading.

Metronidazole Hydrochloride (*In vitro* studies indicated that CYP3A4 and -2C19 are the primary enzymes involved in the metabolism of escitalopram. However, co-administration of escitalopram (20 mg) and ritonavir (600 mg), a potent inhibitor of CYP3A4, did not significantly affect the pharmacokinetics of escitalopram oxalate. Because escitalopram oxalate is metabolized by multiple enzyme systems, inhibition of a single enzyme may not appreciably decrease escitalopram clearance).

No products indexed under this heading.

Metronidazole Sodium (*In vitro* studies indicated that CYP3A4 and -2C19 are the primary enzymes involved in the metabolism of escitalopram. However, co-administration of escitalopram (20 mg) and ritonavir (600 mg), a potent inhibitor of CYP3A4, did not significantly affect the pharmacokinetics of escitalopram oxalate. Because escitalopram oxalate is metabolized by multiple enzyme systems, inhibition of a single enzyme may not appreciably decrease escitalopram clearance).

No products indexed under this heading.

Mexiletine Hydrochloride (*In vitro* studies did not reveal an inhibitory effect of escitalopram on CYP2D6. In addition, steady state levels of racemic citalopram were not significantly different in poor metabolizers and extensive CYP2D6 metabolizers after multi-dose administration of citalopram, suggesting that co-administration, with escitalopram, of a drug that inhibits CYP2D6, is unlikely to have clinically significant effects on escitalopram metabolism. However, there are limited *in vivo* data suggesting a modest CYP2D6 inhibitory effect for escitalopram, ie co-administration of escitalopram (20 mg/day for 21 days) with the tricyclic antidepressant desipramine (single dose of 50 mg), a substrate for CYP2D6 resulted in a 40% increase in C_{max} and a 100% increase in AUC of desipramine. The clinical significance of this finding is unknown. Nevertheless, caution is indicated in the co-administration of escitalopram and drugs metabolized by CYP2D6).

No products indexed under this heading.

Miconazole (*In vitro* studies indicated that CYP3A4 and -2C19 are the primary enzymes involved in the metabolism of escitalopram. However, co-administration of escitalopram (20 mg) and ritonavir (600 mg), a potent inhibitor of CYP3A4, did not significantly affect the pharmacokinetics of escitalopram oxalate. Because escitalopram oxalate is metabolized by multiple enzyme systems, inhibition of a single enzyme may not appreciably decrease escitalopram clearance).

No products indexed under this heading.

Miconazole Nitrate (*In vitro* studies indicated that CYP3A4 and -2C19 are the primary enzymes involved in the metabolism of escitalopram. However, co-administration of escitalopram (20 mg) and ritonavir (600 mg), a potent inhibitor of CYP3A4, did not significantly affect the pharmacokinetics of escitalopram oxalate. Because escitalopram oxalate is metabolized by multiple enzyme systems, inhibition of a single enzyme may not appreciably decrease escitalopram clearance). Products include:

Vusion Ointment ... 3335

Midazolam Hydrochloride (Given the primary CNS effects of escitalopram, caution should be used when it is taken in combination of other centrally acting drugs).

No products indexed under this heading.

Mifepristone (*In vitro* studies indicated that CYP3A4 and -2C19 are the primary enzymes involved in the metabolism of escitalopram. However, co-administration of escitalopram (20 mg) and ritonavir (600 mg), a potent inhibitor of CYP3A4, did not significantly affect the pharmacokinetics of escitalopram oxalate. Because escitalopram oxalate is metabolized by multiple enzyme systems, inhibition of a single enzyme may not appreciably decrease escitalopram clearance).

No products indexed under this heading.

Mirtazapine (*In vitro* studies did not reveal an inhibitory effect of escitalopram on CYP2D6. In addition, steady state levels of racemic citalopram were not significantly different in poor metabolizers and extensive CYP2D6 metabolizers after multi-dose administration of citalopram, suggesting that co-administration, with escitalopram, of a drug that inhibits CYP2D6, is unlikely to have clinically significant effects on escitalopram metabolism. However, there are limited *in vivo* data suggesting a modest CYP2D6 inhibitory effect for escitalopram, ie co-administration of escitalopram (20 mg/day for 21 days) with the tricyclic antidepressant desipramine (single dose of 50 mg), a substrate for CYP2D6 resulted in a 40% increase in C_{max} and a 100% increase in AUC of desipramine. The clinical significance of this finding is unknown. Nevertheless, caution is indicated in the co-administration of escitalopram and drugs metabolized by CYP2D6). Products include:

Remeron Tablets ... 3214
RemeronSolTab Tablets ... 3219

Moclobemide (Concomitant use of MAO inhibitors and escitalopram is contraindicated. In patients receiving SSRIs in combination with a MAO inhibitor, there have been reports of serious, sometimes fatal reactions including hyperthermia, rigidity, myoclonus, and autonomic instability. These reactions have also been reported in patients who have recently discontinued SSRI treatment and have been started on an MAO inhibitor. Some cases presented with features resembling neuroleptic malignant syndrome. Furthermore, additional data suggests that the combined use of SSRIs and MAO inhibitors may act synergistically to elevate blood pressure and evoke behavioral excitation. Therefore, it is recommended that escitalopram should not be used in combination with an MAO inhibitor, or within 14 days of discontinuing treatment with an MAO inhibitor. Similarly, at least 14 days should be allowed after stopping escitalopram before starting an MAO inhibitor).

No products indexed under this heading.

Modafinil (*In vitro* studies indicated that CYP3A4 and -2C19 are the primary enzymes involved in the metabolism of escitalopram. However, co-administration of escitalopram (20 mg) and ritonavir (600 mg), a potent inhibitor of CYP3A4, did not significantly affect the pharmacokinetics of escitalopram oxalate. Because escitalopram oxalate is metabolized by multiple enzyme systems, inhibition of a single enzyme may not appreciably decrease escitalopram clearance). Products include:

Provigil ... 983

Molindone Hydrochloride (The development of a potentially life-threatening serotonin syndrome or Neuroleptic Malignant Syndrome (NMS)-like reactions have been reported with SNRIs and SSRIs alone, including escitalopram treatment, but particularly with concomitant use of serotonergic drugs (including triptans) with drugs which impair metabolism of serotonin (including MAOIs), or with antipsychotics or other dopamine antagonists. Patients should be monitored for the emergence of serotonin syndrome or NMS-like signs and symptoms. Treatment with escitalopram and any concomitant serotonergic or antidopaminergic agents, including antipsychotics, should be discontinued immediately if the above events occur and supportive symptomatic treatment should be initiated). Products include:

Moban ... 1108

Morphine Sulfate (Given the primary CNS effects of escitalopram, caution should be used when it is taken in combination of other centrally acting drugs). Products include:

Avinza ... 1822
Embeda ... 1831
MS Contin ... 2803

Morphine Sulfate, Liposomal (Given the primary CNS effects of escitalopram, caution should be used when it is taken in combination of other centrally acting drugs).

No products indexed under this heading.

Nabumetone (Epidemiological studies of the case-control and cohort design that have demonstrated an association between use of psychotropic drugs that interfere with serotonin reuptake and the occurrence of upper gastrointestinal bleeding have also shown that concurrent use of an NSAID may potentiate the risk of bleeding; use caution when administering).

No products indexed under this heading.

Naproxen (Epidemiological studies of the case-control and cohort design that have demonstrated an association between use of psychotropic drugs that interfere with serotonin reuptake and the occurrence of upper gastrointestinal bleeding have also shown that concurrent use of an NSAID may potentiate the risk of bleeding; use caution when administering). Products include:

EC-Naprosyn ... 2850
Naprosyn ... 2850
Anaprox/Naprosyn ... 2850

Naproxen Sodium (Epidemiological studies of the case-control and cohort design that have demonstrated an association between use of psychotropic drugs that interfere with serotonin reuptake and the occurrence of upper gastrointestinal bleeding have also shown that concurrent use of an NSAID may potentiate the risk of bleeding; use caution when administering). Products include:

Anaprox ... 2850
Anaprox DS ... 2850
Treximet ... 1681

Naratriptan Hydrochloride (There have been rare post-marketing reports of serotonin syndrome with use of a SSRI and a triptan. If concomitant treatment of escitalopram with a triptan is clinically warranted, careful observation of the patient is advised, particularly during treatment initiation and dose increases). Products include:

Amerge ... 1306

Nefazodone Hydrochloride (The development of a potentially life threatening serotonin syndrome or Neuroleptic Malignant syndrome-like reactions have been reported with SSRIs alone, including escitalopram, but particularly with concomitant use of serotonergic drugs. Serotonin syndrome, in its most severe form, can resemble neuroleptic malignant syndrome. The concomitant use of escitalopram with SNRIs is not recommended).

No products indexed under this heading.

Nelfinavir Mesylate (*In vitro* studies did not reveal an inhibitory effect of escitalopram on CYP2D6. In addition, steady state levels of racemic citalopram were not significantly different in poor metabolizers and extensive CYP2D6 metabolizers after multi-dose administration of citalopram, suggesting that co-administration, with escitalopram, of a drug that inhibits CYP2D6, is unlikely to have clinically significant effects on escitalopram metabolism.

However, there are limited *in vivo* data suggesting a modest CYP2D6 inhibitory effect for escitalopram, ie co-administration of escitalopram (20 mg/day for 21 days) with the tricyclic antidepressant desipramine (single dose of 50 mg), a substrate for CYP2D6 resulted in a 40% increase in C_{max} and a 100% increase in AUC of desipramine. The clinical significance of this finding is unknown. Nevertheless, caution is indicated in the co-administration of escitalopram and drugs metabolized by CYP2D6).

No products indexed under this heading.

Nevirapine (*In vitro* studies indicated that CYP3A4 and -2C19 are the primary enzymes involved in the metabolism of escitalopram. However, co-administration of escitalopram (20 mg) and ritonavir (600 mg), a potent inhibitor of CYP3A4, did not significantly affect the pharmacokinetics of escitalopram oxalate. Because escitalopram oxalate is metabolized by multiple enzyme systems, inhibition of a single enzyme may not appreciably decrease escitalopram clearance). Products include:

Viramune Oral Suspension 897
Viramune Tablets 897

Niacin (*In vitro* studies indicated that CYP3A4 and -2C19 are the primary enzymes involved in the metabolism of escitalopram. However, co-administration of escitalopram (20 mg) and ritonavir (600 mg), a potent inhibitor of CYP3A4, did not significantly affect the pharmacokinetics of escitalopram oxalate. Because escitalopram oxalate is metabolized by multiple enzyme systems, inhibition of a single enzyme may not appreciably decrease escitalopram clearance). Products include:

Advicor 402
Cardio Basics 3455
Niaspan 497
Simcor 524

Niacinamide (*In vitro* studies indicated that CYP3A4 and -2C19 are the primary enzymes involved in the metabolism of escitalopram. However, co-administration of escitalopram (20 mg) and ritonavir (600 mg), a potent inhibitor of CYP3A4, did not significantly affect the pharmacokinetics of escitalopram oxalate. Because escitalopram oxalate is metabolized by multiple enzyme systems, inhibition of a single enzyme may not appreciably decrease escitalopram clearance). Products include:

CitraNatal 90 DHA Capsules 2332
CitraNatal Assure 2332
CitraNatal Rx 2332
Heplive 607

Niacinamide Hydroiodide (*In vitro* studies indicated that CYP3A4 and -2C19 are the primary enzymes involved in the metabolism of escitalopram. However, co-administration of escitalopram (20 mg) and ritonavir (600 mg), a potent inhibitor of CYP3A4, did not significantly affect the pharmacokinetics of escitalopram oxalate. Because escitalopram oxalate is metabolized by multiple enzyme systems, inhibition of a single enzyme may not appreciably decrease escitalopram clearance).

No products indexed under this heading.

Nicotinamide (*In vitro* studies indicated that CYP3A4 and -2C19 are the primary enzymes involved in the metabolism of escitalopram. However, co-administration of escitalopram (20 mg) and ritonavir (600 mg), a potent inhibitor of CYP3A4, did not significantly affect the pharmacokinetics of escitalopram oxalate. Because escitalopram oxalate is metabolized by multiple

enzyme systems, inhibition of a single enzyme may not appreciably decrease escitalopram clearance).

No products indexed under this heading.

Nifedipine (*In vitro* studies indicated that CYP3A4 and -2C19 are the primary enzymes involved in the metabolism of escitalopram. However, co-administration of escitalopram (20 mg) and ritonavir (600 mg), a potent inhibitor of CYP3A4, did not significantly affect the pharmacokinetics of escitalopram oxalate. Because escitalopram oxalate is metabolized by multiple enzyme systems, inhibition of a single enzyme may not appreciably decrease escitalopram clearance).

No products indexed under this heading.

Norethindrone (*In vitro* studies indicated that CYP3A4 and -2C19 are the primary enzymes involved in the metabolism of escitalopram. However, co-administration of escitalopram (20 mg) and ritonavir (600 mg), a potent inhibitor of CYP3A4, did not significantly affect the pharmacokinetics of escitalopram oxalate. Because escitalopram oxalate is metabolized by multiple enzyme systems, inhibition of a single enzyme may not appreciably decrease escitalopram clearance). Products include:

Ortho Micronor 2660

Norethynodrel (*In vitro* studies indicated that CYP3A4 and -2C19 are the primary enzymes involved in the metabolism of escitalopram. However, co-administration of escitalopram (20 mg) and ritonavir (600 mg), a potent inhibitor of CYP3A4, did not significantly affect the pharmacokinetics of escitalopram oxalate. Because escitalopram oxalate is metabolized by multiple enzyme systems, inhibition of a single enzyme may not appreciably decrease escitalopram clearance).

No products indexed under this heading.

Norfloxacin (*In vitro* studies indicated that CYP3A4 and -2C19 are the primary enzymes involved in the metabolism of escitalopram. However, co-administration of escitalopram (20 mg) and ritonavir (600 mg), a potent inhibitor of CYP3A4, did not significantly affect the pharmacokinetics of escitalopram oxalate. Because escitalopram oxalate is metabolized by multiple enzyme systems, inhibition of a single enzyme may not appreciably decrease escitalopram clearance). Products include:

Noroxin 2220

Norgestimate (*In vitro* studies indicated that CYP3A4 and -2C19 are the primary enzymes involved in the metabolism of escitalopram. However, co-administration of escitalopram (20 mg) and ritonavir (600 mg), a potent inhibitor of CYP3A4, did not significantly affect the pharmacokinetics of escitalopram oxalate. Because escitalopram oxalate is metabolized by multiple enzyme systems, inhibition of a single enzyme may not appreciably decrease escitalopram clearance). Products include:

Ortho-Cyclen/Ortho Tri-Cyclen 2663
Ortho Tri-Cyclen Lo Tablets 2673

Norgestrel (*In vitro* studies indicated that CYP3A4 and -2C19 are the primary enzymes involved in the metabolism of escitalopram. However, co-administration of escitalopram (20 mg) and ritonavir (600 mg), a potent inhibitor of CYP3A4, did not significantly affect the pharmacokinetics of escitalopram oxalate. Because escitalopram oxalate is metabolized by multiple enzyme systems, inhibition of a single enzyme may not appreciably decrease escitalopram clearance).

No products indexed under this heading.

Nortriptyline Hydrochloride (*In vitro* studies did not reveal an inhibitory effect of escitalopram on CYP2D6. In addition, steady state levels of racemic citalopram were not significantly different in poor metabolizers and extensive CYP2D6 metabolizers after multi-dose administration of citalopram, suggesting that co-administration, with escitalopram, of a drug that inhibits CYP2D6, is unlikely to have clinically significant effects on escitalopram metabolism. However, there are limited *in vivo* data suggesting a modest CYP2D6 inhibitory effect for escitalopram, ie co-administration of escitalopram (20 mg/day for 21 days) with the tricyclic antidepressant desipramine (single dose of 50 mg), a substrate for CYP2D6 resulted in a 40% increase in C_{max} and a 100% increase in AUC of desipramine. The clinical significance of this finding is unknown. Nevertheless, caution is indicated in the co-administration of escitalopram and drugs metabolized by CYP2D6).

No products indexed under this heading.

Olanzapine (The development of a potentially life-threatening serotonin syndrome or Neuroleptic Malignant Syndrome (NMS)-like reactions have been reported with SNRIs and SSRIs alone, including escitalopram treatment, but particularly with concomitant use of serotonergic drugs (including triptans) with drugs which impair metabolism of serotonin (including MAOIs), or with antipsychotics or other dopamine antagonists. Patients should be monitored for the emergence of serotonin syndrome or NMS-like signs and symptoms. Treatment with escitalopram and any concomitant serotonergic or anti-dopaminergic agents, including antipsychotics, should be discontinued immediately if the above events occur and supportive symptomatic treatment should be initiated). Products include:

Symbyax 1965
Zyprexa 1984
Zyprexa IntraMuscular 1984
Zyprexa ZYDIS 1984

Omeprazole (*In vitro* studies did not reveal an inhibitory effect of escitalopram on CYP2D6. In addition, steady state levels of racemic citalopram were not significantly different in poor metabolizers and extensive CYP2D6 metabolizers after multi-dose administration of citalopram, suggesting that co-administration, with escitalopram, of a drug that inhibits CYP2D6, is unlikely to have clinically significant effects on escitalopram metabolism. However, there are limited *in vivo* data suggesting a modest CYP2D6 inhibitory effect for escitalopram, ie co-administration of escitalopram (20 mg/day for 21 days) with the tricyclic antidepressant desipramine (single dose of 50 mg), a substrate for CYP2D6 resulted in a 40% increase in C_{max} and a 100% increase in AUC of desipramine. The clinical significance of this finding is unknown. Nevertheless, caution is indicated in the co-administration of escitalopram and drugs metabolized by CYP2D6).

No products indexed under this heading.

Ondansetron (*In vitro* studies did not reveal an inhibitory effect of escitalopram on CYP2D6. In addition, steady state levels of racemic citalopram were not significantly different in poor metabolizers and extensive CYP2D6 metabolizers after multi-dose administration of citalopram, suggesting that co-administration, with escitalopram, of a drug that inhibits CYP2D6, is unlikely to have clinically significant effects on escitalopram metabolism. However, there are limited *in vivo* data suggesting a modest CYP2D6 inhibitory effect for escitalopram, ie co-administration of escitalopram (20 mg/day for 21 days)

with the tricyclic antidepressant desipramine (single dose of 50 mg), a substrate for CYP2D6 resulted in a 40% increase in C_{max} and a 100% increase in AUC of desipramine. The clinical significance of this finding is unknown. Nevertheless, caution is indicated in the co-administration of escitalopram and drugs metabolized by CYP2D6).

No products indexed under this heading.

Ondansetron Hydrochloride (*In vitro* studies did not reveal an inhibitory effect of escitalopram on CYP2D6. In addition, steady state levels of racemic citalopram were not significantly different in poor metabolizers and extensive CYP2D6 metabolizers after multi-dose administration of citalopram, suggesting that co-administration, with escitalopram, of a drug that inhibits CYP2D6, is unlikely to have clinically significant effects on escitalopram metabolism. However, there are limited *in vivo* data suggesting a modest CYP2D6 inhibitory effect for escitalopram, ie co-administration of escitalopram (20 mg/day for 21 days) with the tricyclic antidepressant desipramine (single dose of 50 mg), a substrate for CYP2D6 resulted in a 40% increase in C_{max} and a 100% increase in AUC of desipramine. The clinical significance of this finding is unknown. Nevertheless, caution is indicated in the co-administration of escitalopram and drugs metabolized by CYP2D6). Products include:

Zofran Injection 1750
Zofran 1756
Zofran ODT 1756

Oxaprozin (Epidemiological studies of the case-control and cohort design that have demonstrated an association between use of psychotropic drugs that interfere with serotonin reuptake and the occurrence of upper gastrointestinal bleeding have also shown that concurrent use of an NSAID may potentiate the risk of bleeding; use caution when administering).

No products indexed under this heading.

Oxazepam (Given the primary CNS effects of escitalopram, caution should be used when it is taken in combination of other centrally acting drugs).

No products indexed under this heading.

Oxcarbazepine (*In vitro* studies indicated that CYP3A4 and -2C19 are the primary enzymes involved in the metabolism of escitalopram. However, co-administration of escitalopram (20 mg) and ritonavir (600 mg), a potent inhibitor of CYP3A4, did not significantly affect the pharmacokinetics of escitalopram oxalate. Because escitalopram oxalate is metabolized by multiple enzyme systems, inhibition of a single enzyme may not appreciably decrease escitalopram clearance).

No products indexed under this heading.

Oxycodone Hydrochloride (Given the primary CNS effects of escitalopram, caution should be used when it is taken in combination of other centrally acting drugs). Products include:

OxyContin 2807
Percocet 1121
Percodan 1124

Oxycodone Terephthalate (Given the primary CNS effects of escitalopram, caution should be used when it is taken in combination of other centrally acting drugs).

No products indexed under this heading.

Oxymorphone Hydrochloride (Given the primary CNS effects of escitalopram, caution should be used when it is taken in combination of other centrally acting drugs). Products include:

Opana 1110
Opana ER 1114

Paclitaxel (*In vitro* studies did not reveal an inhibitory effect of escitalo-

Lexapro
Interactions Index
1032

pram on CYP2D6. In addition, steady state levels of racemic citalopram were not significantly different in poor metabolizers and extensive CYP2D6 metabolizers after multi-dose administration of citalopram, suggesting that co-administration, with escitalopram, of a drug that inhibits CYP2D6, is unlikely to have clinically significant effects on escitalopram metabolism. However, there are limited *in vivo* data suggesting a modest CYP2D6 inhibitory effect for escitalopram, ie co-administration of escitalopram (20 mg/day for 21 days) with the tricyclic antidepressant desipramine (single dose of 50 mg), a substrate for CYP2D6 resulted in a 40% increase in C_{max} and a 100% increase in AUC of desipramine. The clinical significance of this finding is unknown. Nevertheless, caution is indicated in the co-administration of escitalopram and drugs metabolized by CYP2D6).
No products indexed under this heading.

Paliperidone (The development of a potentially life-threatening serotonin syndrome or Neuroleptic Malignant Syndrome (NMS)-like reactions have been reported with SNRIs and SSRIs alone, including escitalopram treatment, but particularly with concomitant use of serotonergic drugs (including triptans) with drugs which impair metabolism of serotonin (including MAOIs), or with antipsychotics or other dopamine antagonists. Patients should be monitored for the emergence of serotonin syndrome or NMS-like signs and symptoms. Treatment with escitalopram and any concomitant serotonergic or antidopaminergic agents, including antipsychotics, should be discontinued immediately if the above events occur and supportive symptomatic treatment should be initiated). Products include:
Invega 2613
Invega Sustenna 2621

Pargyline Hydrochloride (Concomitant use of MAO inhibitors and escitalopram is contraindicated. In patients receiving SSRIs in combination with a MAO inhibitor, there have been reports of serious, sometimes fatal reactions including hyperthermia, rigidity, myoclonus, and autonomic instability. These reactions have also been reported in patients who have recently discontinued SSRI treatment and have been started on an MAO inhibitor. Some cases presented with features resembling neuroleptic malignant syndrome. Furthermore, additional data suggests that the combined use of SSRIs and MAO inhibitors may act synergistically to elevate blood pressure and evoke behavioral excitation. Therefore, it is recommended that escitalopram should not be used in combination with an MAO inhibitor, or within 14 days of discontinuing treatment with an MAO inhibitor. Similarly, at least 14 days should be allowed after stopping escitalopram before starting an MAO inhibitor).
No products indexed under this heading.

Paroxetine Hydrochloride (The development of a potentially life-threatening serotonin syndrome or Neuroleptic Malignant Syndrome (NMS)-like reactions have been reported with SNRIs and SSRIs alone, including escitalopram treatment, but particularly with concomitant use of serotonergic drugs (including triptans) with drugs which impair metabolism of serotonin (including MAOIs), or with antipsychotics or other dopamine antagonists. Patients should be monitored for the emergence of serotonin syndrome or NMS-like signs and symptoms. Treatment with escitalopram and any concomitant serotonergic or antidopaminergic agents, including antipsychotics, should be discontinued immediately if the above events occur and supportive symptomatic treatment should be initiated). Products include:
Paroxetine CR 2361
Paroxetine ER 2371
Paxil 1586
Paxil CR 1596

Pemoline (Given the primary CNS effects of escitalopram, caution should be used when it is taken in combination of other centrally acting drugs).
No products indexed under this heading.

Pentobarbital (Given the primary CNS effects of escitalopram, caution should be used when it is taken in combination of other centrally acting drugs).
No products indexed under this heading.

Pentobarbital Sodium (Given the primary CNS effects of escitalopram, caution should be used when it is taken in combination of other centrally acting drugs). Products include:
Nembutal 2012

Perphenazine (The development of a potentially life-threatening serotonin syndrome or Neuroleptic Malignant Syndrome (NMS)-like reactions have been reported with SNRIs and SSRIs alone, including escitalopram treatment, but particularly with concomitant use of serotonergic drugs (including triptans) with drugs which impair metabolism of serotonin (including MAOIs), or with antipsychotics or other dopamine antagonists. Patients should be monitored for the emergence of serotonin syndrome or NMS-like signs and symptoms. Treatment with escitalopram and any concomitant serotonergic or antidopaminergic agents, including antipsychotics, should be discontinued immediately if the above events occur and supportive symptomatic treatment should be initiated).
No products indexed under this heading.

Phenelzine Sulfate (Concomitant use of MAO inhibitors and escitalopram is contraindicated. In patients receiving SSRIs in combination with a MAO inhibitor, there have been reports of serious, sometimes fatal reactions including hyperthermia, rigidity, myoclonus, and autonomic instability. These reactions have also been reported in patients who have recently discontinued SSRI treatment and have been started on an MAO inhibitor. Some cases presented with features resembling neuroleptic malignant syndrome. Furthermore, additional data suggests that the combined use of SSRIs and MAO inhibitors may act synergistically to elevate blood pressure and evoke behavioral excitation. Therefore, it is recommended that escitalopram should not be used in combination with an MAO inhibitor, or within 14 days of discontinuing treatment with an MAO inhibitor. Similarly, at least 14 days should be allowed after stopping escitalopram before starting an MAO inhibitor).
No products indexed under this heading.

Phenobarbital (Given the primary CNS effects of escitalopram, caution should be used when it is taken in combination of other centrally acting drugs). Products include:
Donnatal 2711

Phenobarbital Sodium (Given the primary CNS effects of escitalopram, caution should be used when it is taken in combination of other centrally acting drugs).
No products indexed under this heading.

Phenylbutazone (Epidemiological studies of the case-control and cohort design that have demonstrated an association between use of psychotropic drugs that interfere with serotonin reuptake and the occurrence of upper gastrointestinal bleeding have also shown that concurrent use of an NSAID may potentiate the risk of bleeding; use caution when administering).
No products indexed under this heading.

Pimozide (Concomitant use of escitalopram in patients taking pimozide is contraindicated. In a controlled study, a single dose of pimozide 2 mg co-administered with racemic citalopram 40 mg given once daily for 11 days was associated with a mean increase in QTc values of approximately 10 msec compared to pimozide given alone. Racemic citalopram did not alter the mean AUC or C_{max} of pimozide. The mechanism of this pharmacodynamic interaction is not known).
No products indexed under this heading.

Pindolol (*In vitro* studies did not reveal an inhibitory effect of escitalopram on CYP2D6. In addition, steady state levels of racemic citalopram were not significantly different in poor metabolizers and extensive CYP2D6 metabolizers after multi-dose administration of citalopram, suggesting that co-administration, with escitalopram, of a drug that inhibits CYP2D6, is unlikely to have clinically significant effects on escitalopram metabolism. However, there are limited *in vivo* data suggesting a modest CYP2D6 inhibitory effect for escitalopram, ie co-administration of escitalopram (20 mg/day for 21 days) with the tricyclic antidepressant desipramine (single dose of 50 mg), a substrate for CYP2D6 resulted in a 40% increase in C_{max} and a 100% increase in AUC of desipramine. The clinical significance of this finding is unknown. Nevertheless, caution is indicated in the co-administration of escitalopram and drugs metabolized by CYP2D6).
No products indexed under this heading.

Piroxicam (Epidemiological studies of the case-control and cohort design that have demonstrated an association between use of psychotropic drugs that interfere with serotonin reuptake and the occurrence of upper gastrointestinal bleeding have also shown that concurrent use of an NSAID may potentiate the risk of bleeding; use caution when administering).
No products indexed under this heading.

Polythiazide (Hyponatremia may occur as a result of treatment with escitalopram. Patients taking diuretics may be at greater risk. Discontinuation of escitalopram should be considered in patients with symptomatic hyponatremia and appropriate medical intervention should be instituted).
No products indexed under this heading.

Posaconazole (*In vitro* studies indicated that CYP3A4 and -2C19 are the primary enzymes involved in the metabolism of escitalopram. However, co-administration of escitalopram (20 mg) and ritonavir (600 mg), a potent inhibitor of CYP3A4, did not significantly affect the pharmacokinetics of escitalopram oxalate. Because escitalopram oxalate is metabolized by multiple enzyme systems, inhibition of a single enzyme may not appreciably decrease escitalopram clearance). Products include:
Noxafil 3172

Prazepam (Given the primary CNS effects of escitalopram, caution should be used when it is taken in combination of other centrally acting drugs).
No products indexed under this heading.

Procarbazine Hydrochloride (Concomitant use of MAO inhibitors and escitalopram is contraindicated. In patients receiving SSRIs in combination with a MAO inhibitor, there have been reports of serious, sometimes fatal reactions including hyperthermia, rigidity, myoclonus, and autonomic instability. These reactions have also been reported in patients who have recently discontinued SSRI treatment and have been started on an MAO inhibitor. Some cases presented with features resembling neuroleptic malignant syndrome. Furthermore, additional data suggests that the combined use of SSRIs and MAO inhibitors may act synergistically to elevate blood pressure and evoke behavioral excitation. Therefore, it is recommended that escitalopram should not be used in combination with an MAO inhibitor, or within 14 days of discontinuing treatment with an MAO inhibitor. Similarly, at least 14 days should be allowed after stopping escitalopram before starting an MAO inhibitor).
No products indexed under this heading.

Prochlorperazine (The development of a potentially life-threatening serotonin syndrome or Neuroleptic Malignant Syndrome (NMS)-like reactions have been reported with SNRIs and SSRIs alone, including escitalopram treatment, but particularly with concomitant use of serotonergic drugs (including triptans) with drugs which impair metabolism of serotonin (including MAOIs), or with antipsychotics or other dopamine antagonists. Patients should be monitored for the emergence of serotonin syndrome or NMS-like signs and symptoms. Treatment with escitalopram and any concomitant serotonergic or antidopaminergic agents, including antipsychotics, should be discontinued immediately if the above events occur and supportive symptomatic treatment should be initiated).
No products indexed under this heading.

Prochlorperazine Edisylate (Given the primary CNS effects of escitalopram, caution should be used when it is taken in combination of other centrally acting drugs).
No products indexed under this heading.

Prochlorperazine Maleate (Given the primary CNS effects of escitalopram, caution should be used when it is taken in combination of other centrally acting drugs).
No products indexed under this heading.

Promethazine (The development of a potentially life-threatening serotonin syndrome or Neuroleptic Malignant Syndrome (NMS)-like reactions have been reported with SNRIs and SSRIs alone, including escitalopram treatment, but particularly with concomitant use of serotonergic drugs (including triptans) with drugs which impair metabolism of serotonin (including MAOIs), or with antipsychotics or other dopamine antagonists. Patients should be monitored for the emergence of serotonin syndrome or NMS-like signs and symptoms. Treatment with escitalopram and any concomitant serotonergic or antidopaminergic agents, including antipsychotics, should be discontinued immediately if the above events occur and supportive symptomatic treatment should be initiated).
No products indexed under this heading.

Promethazine Hydrochloride (The development of a potentially life-threatening serotonin syndrome or Neuroleptic Malignant Syndrome (NMS)-like reactions have been reported with SNRIs and SSRIs alone, including escitalopram treatment, but particularly with concomitant use of serotonergic drugs (including triptans) with drugs which impair metabolism of serotonin (includ-

1033 **Interactions Index** **Lexapro**

ing MAOIs), or with antipsychotics or other dopamine antagonists. Patients should be monitored for the emergence of serotonin syndrome or NMS-like signs and symptoms. Treatment with escitalopram and any concomitant serotonergic or antidopaminergic agents, including antipsychotics, should be discontinued immediately if the above events occur and supportive symptomatic treatment should be initiated).
No products indexed under this heading.

Propafenone Hydrochloride (*In vitro* studies did not reveal an inhibitory effect of escitalopram on CYP2D6. In addition, steady state levels of racemic citalopram were not significantly different in poor metabolizers and extensive CYP2D6 metabolizers after multi-dose administration of citalopram, suggesting that co-administration, with escitalopram, of a drug that inhibits CYP2D6, is unlikely to have clinically significant effects on escitalopram metabolism. However, there are limited *in vivo* data suggesting a modest CYP2D6 inhibitory effect for escitalopram, ie co-administration of escitalopram (20 mg/day for 21 days) with the tricyclic antidepressant desipramine (single dose of 50 mg), a substrate for CYP2D6 resulted in a 40% increase in C_{max} and a 100% increase in AUC of desipramine. The clinical significance of this finding is unknown. Nevertheless, caution is indicated in the co-administration of escitalopram and drugs metabolized by CYP2D6). Products include:
Rythmol 1648
Rythmol SR 1652

Propofol (Given the primary CNS effects of escitalopram, caution should be used when it is taken in combination of other centrally acting drugs).
No products indexed under this heading.

Propoxyphene Hydrochloride (Given the primary CNS effects of escitalopram, caution should be used when it is taken in combination of other centrally acting drugs).
No products indexed under this heading.

Propoxyphene Napsylate (Given the primary CNS effects of escitalopram, caution should be used when it is taken in combination of other centrally acting drugs).
No products indexed under this heading.

Propranolol Hydrochloride (*In vitro* studies did not reveal an inhibitory effect of escitalopram on CYP2D6. In addition, steady state levels of racemic citalopram were not significantly different in poor metabolizers and extensive CYP2D6 metabolizers after multi-dose administration of citalopram, suggesting that co-administration, with escitalopram, of a drug that inhibits CYP2D6, is unlikely to have clinically significant effects on escitalopram metabolism. However, there are limited *in vivo* data suggesting a modest CYP2D6 inhibitory effect for escitalopram, ie co-administration of escitalopram (20 mg/day for 21 days) with the tricyclic antidepressant desipramine (single dose of 50 mg), a substrate for CYP2D6 resulted in a 40% increase in C_{max} and a 100% increase in AUC of desipramine. The clinical significance of this finding is unknown. Nevertheless, caution is indicated in the co-administration of escitalopram and drugs metabolized by CYP2D6). Products include:
InnoPran XL 1517

Quazepam (Given the primary CNS effects of escitalopram, caution should be used when it is taken in combination of other centrally acting drugs).
No products indexed under this heading.

Quetiapine Fumarate (The development of a potentially life-threatening serotonin syndrome or Neuroleptic Malignant Syndrome (NMS)-like reactions have been reported with SNRIs and SSRIs alone, including escitalopram treatment, but particularly with concomitant use of serotonergic drugs (including triptans) with drugs which impair metabolism of serotonin (including MAOIs), or with antipsychotics or other dopamine antagonists. Patients should be monitored for the emergence of serotonin syndrome or NMS-like signs and symptoms. Treatment with escitalopram and any concomitant serotonergic or antidopaminergic agents, including antipsychotics, should be discontinued immediately if the above events occur and supportive symptomatic treatment should be initiated). Products include:
Seroquel 750
Seroquel XR 759

Quinidine (*In vitro* studies indicated that CYP3A4 and -2C19 are the primary enzymes involved in the metabolism of escitalopram. However, co-administration of escitalopram (20 mg) and ritonavir (600 mg), a potent inhibitor of CYP3A4, did not significantly affect the pharmacokinetics of escitalopram oxalate. Because escitalopram oxalate is metabolized by multiple enzyme systems, inhibition of a single enzyme may not appreciably decrease escitalopram clearance).
No products indexed under this heading.

Quinidine Gluconate (*In vitro* studies did not reveal an inhibitory effect of escitalopram on CYP2D6. In addition, steady state levels of racemic citalopram were not significantly different in poor metabolizers and extensive CYP2D6 metabolizers after multi-dose administration of citalopram, suggesting that co-administration, with escitalopram, of a drug that inhibits CYP2D6, is unlikely to have clinically significant effects on escitalopram metabolism. However, there are limited *in vivo* data suggesting a modest CYP2D6 inhibitory effect for escitalopram, ie co-administration of escitalopram (20 mg/day for 21 days) with the tricyclic antidepressant desipramine (single dose of 50 mg), a substrate for CYP2D6 resulted in a 40% increase in C_{max} and a 100% increase in AUC of desipramine. The clinical significance of this finding is unknown. Nevertheless, caution is indicated in the co-administration of escitalopram and drugs metabolized by CYP2D6).
No products indexed under this heading.

Quinidine Hydrochloride (*In vitro* studies did not reveal an inhibitory effect of escitalopram on CYP2D6. In addition, steady state levels of racemic citalopram were not significantly different in poor metabolizers and extensive CYP2D6 metabolizers after multi-dose administration of citalopram, suggesting that co-administration, with escitalopram, of a drug that inhibits CYP2D6, is unlikely to have clinically significant effects on escitalopram metabolism. However, there are limited *in vivo* data suggesting a modest CYP2D6 inhibitory effect for escitalopram, ie co-administration of escitalopram (20 mg/day for 21 days) with the tricyclic antidepressant desipramine (single dose of 50 mg), a substrate for CYP2D6 resulted in a 40% increase in C_{max} and a 100% increase in AUC of desipramine. The clinical significance of this finding is unknown. Nevertheless, caution is indicated in the co-administration of escitalopram and drugs metabolized by CYP2D6).
No products indexed under this heading.

Quinidine Polygalacturonate (*In vitro* studies did not reveal an inhibitory effect of escitalopram on CYP2D6. In addition, steady state levels of racemic citalopram were not significantly different in poor metabolizers and extensive CYP2D6 metabolizers after multi-dose administration of citalopram, suggesting that co-administration, with escitalopram, of a drug that inhibits CYP2D6, is unlikely to have clinically significant effects on escitalopram metabolism. However, there are limited *in vivo* data suggesting a modest CYP2D6 inhibitory effect for escitalopram, ie co-administration of escitalopram (20 mg/day for 21 days) with the tricyclic antidepressant desipramine (single dose of 50 mg), a substrate for CYP2D6 resulted in a 40% increase in C_{max} and a 100% increase in AUC of desipramine. The clinical significance of this finding is unknown. Nevertheless, caution is indicated in the co-administration of escitalopram and drugs metabolized by CYP2D6).
No products indexed under this heading.

Quinidine Sulfate (*In vitro* studies did not reveal an inhibitory effect of escitalopram on CYP2D6. In addition, steady state levels of racemic citalopram were not significantly different in poor metabolizers and extensive CYP2D6 metabolizers after multi-dose administration of citalopram, suggesting that co-administration, with escitalopram, of a drug that inhibits CYP2D6, is unlikely to have clinically significant effects on escitalopram metabolism. However, there are limited *in vivo* data suggesting a modest CYP2D6 inhibitory effect for escitalopram, ie co-administration of escitalopram (20 mg/day for 21 days) with the tricyclic antidepressant desipramine (single dose of 50 mg), a substrate for CYP2D6 resulted in a 40% increase in C_{max} and a 100% increase in AUC of desipramine. The clinical significance of this finding is unknown. Nevertheless, caution is indicated in the co-administration of escitalopram and drugs metabolized by CYP2D6).
No products indexed under this heading.

Quinine (*In vitro* studies indicated that CYP3A4 and -2C19 are the primary enzymes involved in the metabolism of escitalopram. However, co-administration of escitalopram (20 mg) and ritonavir (600 mg), a potent inhibitor of CYP3A4, did not significantly affect the pharmacokinetics of escitalopram oxalate. Because escitalopram oxalate is metabolized by multiple enzyme systems, inhibition of a single enzyme may not appreciably decrease escitalopram clearance). Products include:
Hyland's Leg Cramps PM with Quinine 3315

Quinine Sulfate (*In vitro* studies indicated that CYP3A4 and -2C19 are the primary enzymes involved in the metabolism of escitalopram. However, co-administration of escitalopram (20 mg) and ritonavir (600 mg), a potent inhibitor of CYP3A4, did not significantly affect the pharmacokinetics of escitalopram oxalate. Because escitalopram oxalate is metabolized by multiple enzyme systems, inhibition of a single enzyme may not appreciably decrease escitalopram clearance).
No products indexed under this heading.

Quinupristin (*In vitro* studies indicated that CYP3A4 and -2C19 are the primary enzymes involved in the metabolism of escitalopram. However, co-administration of escitalopram (20 mg) and ritonavir (600 mg), a potent inhibitor of CYP3A4, did not significantly affect the pharmacokinetics of escitalopram oxalate. Because escitalopram oxalate is metabolized by multiple enzyme systems, inhibition of a single enzyme may not appreciably decrease escitalopram clearance).
No products indexed under this heading.

Ranitidine Bismuth Citrate (*In vitro* studies indicated that CYP3A4 and -2C19 are the primary enzymes involved in the metabolism of escitalopram. However, co-administration of escitalopram (20 mg) and ritonavir (600 mg), a potent inhibitor of CYP3A4, did not significantly affect the pharmacokinetics of escitalopram oxalate. Because escitalopram oxalate is metabolized by multiple enzyme systems, inhibition of a single enzyme may not appreciably decrease escitalopram clearance).
No products indexed under this heading.

Ranitidine Hydrochloride (*In vitro* studies indicated that CYP3A4 and -2C19 are the primary enzymes involved in the metabolism of escitalopram. However, co-administration of escitalopram (20 mg) and ritonavir (600 mg), a potent inhibitor of CYP3A4, did not significantly affect the pharmacokinetics of escitalopram oxalate. Because escitalopram oxalate is metabolized by multiple enzyme systems, inhibition of a single enzyme may not appreciably decrease escitalopram clearance). Products include:
Zantac 1737
Zantac Injection 1732
Zantac Pharmacy 1735

Rasagiline Mesylate (Concomitant use of MAO inhibitors and escitalopram is contraindicated. In patients receiving SSRIs in combination with a MAO inhibitor, there have been reports of serious, sometimes fatal reactions including hyperthermia, rigidity, myoclonus, and autonomic instability. These reactions have also been reported in patients who have recently discontinued SSRI treatment and have been started on an MAO inhibitor. Some cases presented with features resembling neuroleptic malignant syndrome. Furthermore, additional data suggests that the combined use of SSRIs and MAO inhibitors may act synergistically to elevate blood pressure and evoke behavioral excitation. Therefore, it is recommended that escitalopram should not be used in combination with an MAO inhibitor, or within 14 days of discontinuing treatment with an MAO inhibitor. Similarly, at least 14 days should be allowed after stopping escitalopram before starting an MAO inhibitor). Products include:
Azilect 3383

Remifentanil Hydrochloride (Given the primary CNS effects of escitalopram, caution should be used when it is taken in combination of other centrally acting drugs).
No products indexed under this heading.

Risperidone (The development of a potentially life-threatening serotonin syndrome or Neuroleptic Malignant Syndrome (NMS)-like reactions have been reported with SNRIs and SSRIs alone, including escitalopram treatment, but particularly with concomitant use of serotonergic drugs (including triptans) with drugs which impair metabolism of serotonin (including MAOIs), or with antipsychotics or other dopamine antagonists. Patients should be monitored for the emergence of serotonin syndrome or NMS-like signs and symptoms. Treatment with escitalopram and any concomitant serotonergic or antidopaminergic agents, including antipsychotics, should be discontinued immediately if the above events occur and supportive symptomatic treatment should be initiated). Products include:
Risperdal Consta 2682

Ritonavir (*In vitro* studies did not reveal an inhibitory effect of escitalopram on CYP2D6. In addition, steady state levels of racemic citalopram were not significantly different in poor metabolizers and extensive CYP2D6

IMPORTANT NOTE: Always consult each drug listing in the patient's regimen for possible interactions.

Lexapro Interactions Index 1034

metabolizers after multi-dose administration of citalopram, suggesting that co-administration, with escitalopram, of a drug that inhibits CYP2D6, is unlikely to have clinically significant effects on escitalopram metabolism. However, there are limited *in vivo* data suggesting a modest CYP2D6 inhibitory effect for escitalopram, ie co-administration of escitalopram (20 mg/day for 21 days) with the tricyclic antidepressant desipramine (single dose of 50 mg), a substrate for CYP2D6 resulted in a 40% increase in C_{max} and a 100% increase in AUC of desipramine. The clinical significance of this finding is unknown. Nevertheless, caution is indicated in the co-administration of escitalopram and drugs metabolized by CYP2D6). Products include:
Kaletra 458
Norvir 509

Rizatriptan Benzoate (There have been rare post-marketing reports of serotonin syndrome with use of a SSRI and a triptan. If concomitant treatment of escitalopram with a triptan is clinically warranted, careful observation of the patient is advised, particularly during treatment initiation and dose increases). Products include:
Maxalt 2206
Maxalt-MLT 2206

Rofecoxib (Epidemiological studies of the case-control and cohort design that have demonstrated an association between use of psychotropic drugs that interfere with serotonin reuptake and the occurrence of upper gastrointestinal bleeding have also shown that concurrent use of an NSAID may potentiate the risk of bleeding; use caution when administering).
No products indexed under this heading.

Saquinavir (*In vitro* studies indicated that CYP3A4 and -2C19 are the primary enzymes involved in the metabolism of escitalopram. However, co-administration of escitalopram (20 mg) and ritonavir (600 mg), a potent inhibitor of CYP3A4, did not significantly affect the pharmacokinetics of escitalopram oxalate. Because escitalopram oxalate is metabolized by multiple enzyme systems, inhibition of a single enzyme may not appreciably decrease escitalopram clearance).
No products indexed under this heading.

Saquinavir Mesylate (*In vitro* studies indicated that CYP3A4 and -2C19 are the primary enzymes involved in the metabolism of escitalopram. However, co-administration of escitalopram (20 mg) and ritonavir (600 mg), a potent inhibitor of CYP3A4, did not significantly affect the pharmacokinetics of escitalopram oxalate. Because escitalopram oxalate is metabolized by multiple enzyme systems, inhibition of a single enzyme may not appreciably decrease escitalopram clearance).
No products indexed under this heading.

Secobarbital Sodium (Given the primary CNS effects of escitalopram, caution should be used when it is taken in combination of other centrally acting drugs).
No products indexed under this heading.

Selegiline (Concomitant use of MAO inhibitors and escitalopram is contraindicated. In patients receiving SSRIs in combination with a MAO inhibitor, there have been reports of serious, sometimes fatal reactions including hyperthermia, rigidity, myoclonus, and autonomic instability. These reactions have also been reported in patients who have recently discontinued SSRI treatment and have been started on an MAO inhibitor. Some cases presented with features resembling neuroleptic malignant syndrome. Furthermore, additional data suggests that the combined use of SSRIs and MAO inhibitors may act synergistically to elevate blood pressure and evoke behavioral excitation. Therefore, it is recommended that escitalopram should not be used in combination with an MAO inhibitor, or within 14 days of discontinuing treatment with an MAO inhibitor. Similarly, at least 14 days should be allowed after stopping escitalopram before starting an MAO inhibitor). Products include:
Emsam 3623

Selegiline Hydrochloride (Concomitant use of MAO inhibitors and escitalopram is contraindicated. In patients receiving SSRIs in combination with a MAO inhibitor, there have been reports of serious, sometimes fatal reactions including hyperthermia, rigidity, myoclonus, and autonomic instability. These reactions have also been reported in patients who have recently discontinued SSRI treatment and have been started on an MAO inhibitor. Some cases presented with features resembling neuroleptic malignant syndrome. Furthermore, additional data suggests that the combined use of SSRIs and MAO inhibitors may act synergistically to elevate blood pressure and evoke behavioral excitation. Therefore, it is recommended that escitalopram should not be used in combination with an MAO inhibitor, or within 14 days of discontinuing treatment with an MAO inhibitor. Similarly, at least 14 days should be allowed after stopping escitalopram before starting an MAO inhibitor). Products include:
Eldepryl 3312

Sertraline Hydrochloride (The development of a potentially life-threatening serotonin syndrome or Neuroleptic Malignant Syndrome (NMS)-like reactions have been reported with SNRIs and SSRIs alone, including escitalopram treatment, but particularly with concomitant use of serotonergic drugs (including triptans) with drugs which impair metabolism of serotonin (including MAOIs), or with antipsychotics or other dopamine antagonists. Patients should be monitored for the emergence of serotonin syndrome or NMS-like signs and symptoms. Treatment with escitalopram and any concomitant serotonergic or antidopaminergic agents, including antipsychotics, should be discontinued immediately if the above events occur and supportive symptomatic treatment should be initiated).
No products indexed under this heading.

Sevoflurane (Given the primary CNS effects of escitalopram, caution should be used when it is taken in combination of other centrally acting drugs). Products include:
Ultane 554

Sildenafil Citrate (*In vitro* studies indicated that CYP3A4 and -2C19 are the primary enzymes involved in the metabolism of escitalopram. However, co-administration of escitalopram (20 mg) and ritonavir (600 mg), a potent inhibitor of CYP3A4, did not significantly affect the pharmacokinetics of escitalopram oxalate. Because escitalopram oxalate is metabolized by multiple enzyme systems, inhibition of a single enzyme may not appreciably decrease escitalopram clearance).
No products indexed under this heading.

Sodium Butabarbital (Given the primary CNS effects of escitalopram, caution should be used when it is taken in combination of other centrally acting drugs).
No products indexed under this heading.

Sodium Oxybate (Given the primary CNS effects of escitalopram, caution should be used when it is taken in combination of other centrally acting drugs).
No products indexed under this heading.

Sodium Pentobarbital (Given the primary CNS effects of escitalopram, caution should be used when it is taken in combination of other centrally acting drugs).
No products indexed under this heading.

Spironolactone (Hyponatremia may occur as a result of treatment with escitalopram. Patients taking diuretics may be at greater risk. Discontinuation of escitalopram should be considered in patients with symptomatic hyponatremia and appropriate medical intervention should be instituted).
No products indexed under this heading.

Sufentanil Citrate (Given the primary CNS effects of escitalopram, caution should be used when it is taken in combination of other centrally acting drugs).
No products indexed under this heading.

Sulfaphenazole (*In vitro* studies indicated that CYP3A4 and -2C19 are the primary enzymes involved in the metabolism of escitalopram. However, co-administration of escitalopram (20 mg) and ritonavir (600 mg), a potent inhibitor of CYP3A4, did not significantly affect the pharmacokinetics of escitalopram oxalate. Because escitalopram oxalate is metabolized by multiple enzyme systems, inhibition of a single enzyme may not appreciably decrease escitalopram clearance).
No products indexed under this heading.

Sulindac (Epidemiological studies of the case-control and cohort design that have demonstrated an association between use of psychotropic drugs that interfere with serotonin reuptake and the occurrence of upper gastrointestinal bleeding have also shown that concurrent use of an NSAID may potentiate the risk of bleeding; use caution when administering). Products include:
Clinoril 2098

Sumatriptan (There have been rare post-maketing reports describing patients with weakness, hyperreflexia, and incoordination following the use of an SSRI and sumatriptan. If concomitant treatment with sumatriptan and escitalopram is clinically warranted, appropriate observation of the patient is advised). Products include:
Imitrex Nasal 1503

Sumatriptan Succinate (There have been rare post-maketing reports describing patients with weakness, hyperreflexia, and incoordination following the use of an SSRI and sumatriptan. If concomitant treatment with sumatriptan and escitalopram is clinically warranted, appropriate observation of the patient is advised). Products include:
Imitrex 1497
Imitrex Tablets 1508
Treximet 1681

Talbutal (Given the primary CNS effects of escitalopram, caution should be used when it is taken in combination of other centrally acting drugs).
No products indexed under this heading.

Tamoxifen Citrate (*In vitro* studies did not reveal an inhibitory effect of escitalopram on CYP2D6. In addition, steady state levels of racemic citalopram were not significantly different in poor metabolizers and extensive CYP2D6 metabolizers after multi-dose administration of citalopram, suggesting that co-administration, with escitalopram, of a drug that inhibits CYP2D6, is unlikely to have clinically significant effects on escitalopram metabolism. However, there are limited *in vivo* data suggesting a modest CYP2D6 inhibitory effect for escitalopram, ie co-administration of escitalopram (20 mg/day for 21 days) with the tricyclic antidepressant desipramine (single dose of 50 mg), a substrate for CYP2D6 resulted in a 40% increase in C_{max} and a 100% increase in AUC of desipramine. The clinical significance of this finding is unknown. Nevertheless, caution is indicated in the co-administration of escitalopram and drugs metabolized by CYP2D6).
No products indexed under this heading.

Telithromycin (*In vitro* studies indicated that CYP3A4 and -2C19 are the primary enzymes involved in the metabolism of escitalopram. However, co-administration of escitalopram (20 mg) and ritonavir (600 mg), a potent inhibitor of CYP3A4, did not significantly affect the pharmacokinetics of escitalopram oxalate. Because escitalopram oxalate is metabolized by multiple enzyme systems, inhibition of a single enzyme may not appreciably decrease escitalopram clearance). Products include:
Ketek 2991

Telmisartan (*In vitro* studies indicated that CYP3A4 and -2C19 are the primary enzymes involved in the metabolism of escitalopram. However, co-administration of escitalopram (20 mg) and ritonavir (600 mg), a potent inhibitor of CYP3A4, did not significantly affect the pharmacokinetics of escitalopram oxalate. Because escitalopram oxalate is metabolized by multiple enzyme systems, inhibition of a single enzyme may not appreciably decrease escitalopram clearance). Products include:
Micardis 887
Micardis HCT 889

Temazepam (Given the primary CNS effects of escitalopram, caution should be used when it is taken in combination of other centrally acting drugs).
No products indexed under this heading.

Teniposide (*In vitro* studies did not reveal an inhibitory effect of escitalopram on CYP2D6. In addition, steady state levels of racemic citalopram were not significantly different in poor metabolizers and extensive CYP2D6 metabolizers after multi-dose administration of citalopram, suggesting that co-administration, with escitalopram, of a drug that inhibits CYP2D6, is unlikely to have clinically significant effects on escitalopram metabolism. However, there are limited *in vivo* data suggesting a modest CYP2D6 inhibitory effect for escitalopram, ie co-administration of escitalopram (20 mg/day for 21 days) with the tricyclic antidepressant desipramine (single dose of 50 mg), a substrate for CYP2D6 resulted in a 40% increase in C_{max} and a 100% increase in AUC of desipramine. The clinical significance of this finding is unknown. Nevertheless, caution is indicated in the co-administration of escitalopram and drugs metabolized by CYP2D6).
No products indexed under this heading.

Testosterone (*In vitro* studies did not reveal an inhibitory effect of escitalopram on CYP2D6. In addition, steady state levels of racemic citalopram were not significantly different in poor metabolizers and extensive CYP2D6 metabolizers after multi-dose administration of citalopram, suggesting that co-administration, with escitalopram, of a drug that inhibits CYP2D6, is unlikely to have clinically significant effects on escitalopram metabolism. However, there are limited *in vivo* data suggesting a modest CYP2D6 inhibitory effect for escitalopram, ie co-administration of escitalopram (20 mg/day for 21 days) with the tricyclic antidepressant desipramine (single dose of 50 mg), a substrate for CYP2D6 resulted in a 40% increase in C_{max} and a 100% increase in AUC of desipramine. The clinical significance of this finding is unknown. Nevertheless, caution is indicated in the

(⊙ Described in PDR® for Ophthalmic Medicines)

co-administration of escitalopram and drugs metabolized by CYP2D6).
Products include:

Testosterone Cypionate (*In vitro* studies did not reveal an inhibitory effect of escitalopram on CYP2D6. In addition, steady state levels of racemic citalopram were not significantly different in poor metabolizers and extensive CYP2D6 metabolizers after multi-dose administration of citalopram, suggesting that co-administration, with escitalopram, of a drug that inhibits CYP2D6, is unlikely to have clinically significant effects on escitalopram metabolism. However, there are limited *in vivo* data suggesting a modest CYP2D6 inhibitory effect for escitalopram, ie co-administration of escitalopram (20 mg/day for 21 days) with the tricyclic antidepressant desipramine (single dose of 50 mg), a substrate for CYP2D6 resulted in a 40% increase in C_{max} and a 100% increase in AUC of desipramine. The clinical significance of this finding is unknown. Nevertheless, caution is indicated in the co-administration of escitalopram and drugs metabolized by CYP2D6).
No products indexed under this heading.

Testosterone Enanthate (*In vitro* studies did not reveal an inhibitory effect of escitalopram on CYP2D6. In addition, steady state levels of racemic citalopram were not significantly different in poor metabolizers and extensive CYP2D6 metabolizers after multi-dose administration of citalopram, suggesting that co-administration, with escitalopram, of a drug that inhibits CYP2D6, is unlikely to have clinically significant effects on escitalopram metabolism. However, there are limited *in vivo* data suggesting a modest CYP2D6 inhibitory effect for escitalopram, ie co-administration of escitalopram (20 mg/day for 21 days) with the tricyclic antidepressant desipramine (single dose of 50 mg), a substrate for CYP2D6 resulted in a 40% increase in C_{max} and a 100% increase in AUC of desipramine. The clinical significance of this finding is unknown. Nevertheless, caution is indicated in the co-administration of escitalopram and drugs metabolized by CYP2D6). Products include:

Testosterone Propionate (*In vitro* studies did not reveal an inhibitory effect of escitalopram on CYP2D6. In addition, steady state levels of racemic citalopram were not significantly different in poor metabolizers and extensive CYP2D6 metabolizers after multi-dose administration of citalopram, suggesting that co-administration, with escitalopram, of a drug that inhibits CYP2D6, is unlikely to have clinically significant effects on escitalopram metabolism. However, there are limited *in vivo* data suggesting a modest CYP2D6 inhibitory effect for escitalopram, ie co-administration of escitalopram (20 mg/day for 21 days) with the tricyclic antidepressant desipramine (single dose of 50 mg), a substrate for CYP2D6 resulted in a 40% increase in C_{max} and a 100% increase in AUC of desipramine. The clinical significance of this finding is unknown. Nevertheless, caution is indicated in the co-administration of escitalopram and drugs metabolized by CYP2D6).
No products indexed under this heading.

Thiamylal Sodium (Given the primary CNS effects of escitalopram, caution should be used when it is taken in combination of other centrally acting drugs).
No products indexed under this heading.

Thioridazine (Given the primary CNS effects of escitalopram, caution should be used when it is taken in combination of other centrally acting drugs).
No products indexed under this heading.

Thioridazine Hydrochloride (The development of a potentially life-threatening serotonin syndrome or Neuroleptic Malignant Syndrome (NMS)-like reactions have been reported with SNRIs and SSRIs alone, including escitalopram treatment, but particularly with concomitant use of serotonergic drugs (including triptans) with drugs which impair metabolism of serotonin (including MAOIs), or with antipsychotics or other dopamine antagonists. Patients should be monitored for the emergence of serotonin syndrome or NMS-like signs and symptoms. Treatment with escitalopram and any concomitant serotonergic or antidopaminergic agents, including antipsychotics, should be discontinued immediately if the above events occur and supportive symptomatic treatment should be initiated).
Products include:

Thiothixene (The development of a potentially life-threatening serotonin syndrome or Neuroleptic Malignant Syndrome (NMS)-like reactions have been reported with SNRIs and SSRIs alone, including escitalopram treatment, but particularly with concomitant use of serotonergic drugs (including triptans) with drugs which impair metabolism of serotonin (including MAOIs), or with antipsychotics or other dopamine antagonists. Patients should be monitored for the emergence of serotonin syndrome or NMS-like signs and symptoms. Treatment with escitalopram and any concomitant serotonergic or antidopaminergic agents, including antipsychotics, should be discontinued immediately if the above events occur and supportive symptomatic treatment should be initiated). Products include:

Thiothixene Hydrochloride (Given the primary CNS effects of escitalopram, caution should be used when it is taken in combination of other centrally acting drugs).
No products indexed under this heading.

Ticlopidine Hydrochloride (*In vitro* studies indicated that CYP3A4 and -2C19 are the primary enzymes involved in the metabolism of escitalopram. However, co-administration of escitalopram (20 mg) and ritonavir (600 mg), a potent inhibitor of CYP3A4, did not significantly affect the pharmacokinetics of escitalopram oxalate. Because escitalopram oxalate is metabolized by multiple enzyme systems, inhibition of a single enzyme may not appreciably decrease escitalopram clearance).
No products indexed under this heading.

Timolol Maleate (*In vitro* studies did not reveal an inhibitory effect of escitalopram on CYP2D6. In addition, steady state levels of racemic citalopram were not significantly different in poor metabolizers and extensive CYP2D6 metabolizers after multi-dose administration of citalopram, suggesting that co-administration, with escitalopram, of a drug that inhibits CYP2D6, is unlikely to have clinically significant effects on escitalopram metabolism. However, there are limited *in vivo* data suggesting a modest CYP2D6 inhibitory effect for escitalopram, ie co-administration of escitalopram (20 mg/day for 21 days) with the tricyclic antidepressant desipramine (single dose of 50 mg), a substrate for CYP2D6 resulted in a 40% increase in C_{max} and a 100% increase in AUC of desipramine. The clinical significance of this finding is unknown.

Nevertheless, caution is indicated in the co-administration of escitalopram and drugs metabolized by CYP2D6).
Products include:

Tinzaparin Sodium (Escitalopram may increase the risk of bleeding events. Concomitant use of anticoagulants may add to this risk. Case reports and epidemiological studies of the case-control and cohort design have demonstrated an association between use of drugs that interfere with serotonin reuptake and the occurrence of gastrointestinal bleeding. Patients should be cautioned about the risk of bleeding associated with the concomitant use of escitalopram and anticoagulants).
No products indexed under this heading.

Tolbutamide (*In vitro* studies indicated that CYP3A4 and -2C19 are the primary enzymes involved in the metabolism of escitalopram. However, co-administration of escitalopram (20 mg) and ritonavir (600 mg), a potent inhibitor of CYP3A4, did not significantly affect the pharmacokinetics of escitalopram oxalate. Because escitalopram oxalate is metabolized by multiple enzyme systems, inhibition of a single enzyme may not appreciably decrease escitalopram clearance).
No products indexed under this heading.

Tolbutamide Sodium (*In vitro* studies indicated that CYP3A4 and -2C19 are the primary enzymes involved in the metabolism of escitalopram. However, co-administration of escitalopram (20 mg) and ritonavir (600 mg), a potent inhibitor of CYP3A4, did not significantly affect the pharmacokinetics of escitalopram oxalate. Because escitalopram oxalate is metabolized by multiple enzyme systems, inhibition of a single enzyme may not appreciably decrease escitalopram clearance).
No products indexed under this heading.

Tolmetin Sodium (Epidemiological studies of the case-control and cohort design that have demonstrated an association between use of psychotropic drugs that interfere with serotonin reuptake and the occurrence of upper gastrointestinal bleeding have also shown that concurrent use of an NSAID may potentiate the risk of bleeding; use caution when administering).
No products indexed under this heading.

Tolterodine Tartrate (*In vitro* studies did not reveal an inhibitory effect of escitalopram on CYP2D6. In addition, steady state levels of racemic citalopram were not significantly different in poor metabolizers and extensive CYP2D6 metabolizers after multi-dose administration of citalopram, suggesting that co-administration, with escitalopram, of a drug that inhibits CYP2D6, is unlikely to have clinically significant effects on escitalopram metabolism. However, there are limited *in vivo* data suggesting a modest CYP2D6 inhibitory effect for escitalopram, ie co-administration of escitalopram (20 mg/day for 21 days) with the tricyclic antidepressant desipramine (single dose of 50 mg), a substrate for CYP2D6 resulted in a 40% increase in C_{max} and a 100% increase in AUC of desipramine. The clinical significance of this finding is unknown. Nevertheless, caution is indicated in the co-administration of escitalopram and drugs metabolized by CYP2D6).
No products indexed under this heading.

Topiramate (*In vitro* studies indicated that CYP3A4 and -2C19 are the primary enzymes involved in the metabolism of escitalopram. However, co-

administration of escitalopram (20 mg) and ritonavir (600 mg), a potent inhibitor of CYP3A4, did not significantly affect the pharmacokinetics of escitalopram oxalate. Because escitalopram oxalate is metabolized by multiple enzyme systems, inhibition of a single enzyme may not appreciably decrease escitalopram clearance).
No products indexed under this heading.

Torsemide (Hyponatremia may occur as a result of treatment with escitalopram. Patients taking diuretics may be at greater risk. Discontinuation of escitalopram should be considered in patients with symptomatic hyponatremia and appropriate medical intervention should be instituted).
No products indexed under this heading.

Tramadol Hydrochloride (Based on the mechanism of action of escitalopram and the potential for serotonin syndrome, caution is advised when escitalopram is co-administered with other drugs that may affect the serotonergic neurotransmitter systems, such as tramadol). Products include:

Tranylcypromine Sulfate (Concomitant use of MAO inhibitors and escitalopram is contraindicated. In patients receiving SSRIs in combination with a MAO inhibitor, there have been reports of serious, sometimes fatal reactions including hyperthermia, rigidity, myoclonus, and autonomic instability. These reactions have also been reported in patients who have recently discontinued SSRI treatment and have been started on an MAO inhibitor. Some cases presented with features resembling neuroleptic malignant syndrome. Furthermore, additional data suggests that the combined use of SSRIs and MAO inhibitors may act synergistically to elevate blood pressure and evoke behavioral excitation. Therefore, it is recommended that escitalopram should not be used in combination with an MAO inhibitor, or within 14 days of discontinuing treatment with an MAO inhibitor. Similarly, at least 14 days should be allowed after stopping escitalopram before starting an MAO inhibitor). Products include:

Trazodone Hydrochloride (*In vitro* studies did not reveal an inhibitory effect of escitalopram on CYP2D6. In addition, steady state levels of racemic citalopram were not significantly different in poor metabolizers and extensive CYP2D6 metabolizers after multi-dose administration of citalopram, suggesting that co-administration, with escitalopram, of a drug that inhibits CYP2D6, is unlikely to have clinically significant effects on escitalopram metabolism. However, there are limited *in vivo* data suggesting a modest CYP2D6 inhibitory effect for escitalopram, ie co-administration of escitalopram (20 mg/day for 21 days) with the tricyclic antidepressant desipramine (single dose of 50 mg), a substrate for CYP2D6 resulted in a 40% increase in C_{max} and a 100% increase in AUC of desipramine. The clinical significance of this finding is unknown. Nevertheless, caution is indicated in the co-administration of escitalopram and drugs metabolized by CYP2D6).
No products indexed under this heading.

Triamterene (Hyponatremia may occur as a result of treatment with escitalopram. Patients taking diuretics may be at greater risk. Discontinuation of escitalopram should be considered in patients with symptomatic hyponatremia and appropriate medical intervention should be instituted). Products include:

Triazolam (Given the primary CNS effects of escitalopram, caution should be used when it is taken in combination of other centrally acting drugs).

No products indexed under this heading.

Trifluoperazine Hydrochloride (The development of a potentially life-threatening serotonin syndrome or Neuroleptic Malignant Syndrome (NMS)-like reactions have been reported with SNRIs and SSRIs alone, including escitalopram treatment, but particularly with concomitant use of serotonergic drugs (including triptans) with drugs which impair metabolism of serotonin (including MAOIs), or with antipsychotics or other dopamine antagonists. Patients should be monitored for the emergence of serotonin syndrome or NMS-like signs and symptoms. Treatment with escitalopram and any concomitant serotonergic or antidopaminergic agents, including antipsychotics, should be discontinued immediately if the above events occur and supportive symptomatic treatment should be initiated).

No products indexed under this heading.

Trimipramine Maleate (In vitro studies did not reveal an inhibitory effect of escitalopram on CYP2D6. In addition, steady state levels of racemic citalopram were not significantly different in poor metabolizers and extensive CYP2D6 metabolizers after multi-dose administration of citalopram, suggesting that co-administration, with escitalopram, of a drug that inhibits CYP2D6, is unlikely to have clinically significant effects on escitalopram metabolism. However, there are limited in vivo data suggesting a modest CYP2D6 inhibitory effect for escitalopram, ie co-administration of escitalopram (20 mg/day for 21 days) with the tricyclic antidepressant desipramine (single dose of 50 mg), a substrate for CYP2D6 resulted in a 40% increase in C_{max} and a 100% increase in AUC of desipramine. The clinical significance of this finding is unknown. Nevertheless, caution is indicated in the co-administration of escitalopram and drugs metabolized by CYP2D6).

No products indexed under this heading.

Troglitazone (In vitro studies indicated that CYP3A4 and -2C19 are the primary enzymes involved in the metabolism of escitalopram. However, co-administration of escitalopram (20 mg) and ritonavir (600 mg), a potent inhibitor of CYP3A4, did not significantly affect the pharmacokinetics of escitalopram oxalate. Because escitalopram oxalate is metabolized by multiple enzyme systems, inhibition of a single enzyme may not appreciably decrease escitalopram clearance).

No products indexed under this heading.

Troleandomycin (In vitro studies indicated that CYP3A4 and -2C19 are the primary enzymes involved in the metabolism of escitalopram. However, co-administration of escitalopram (20 mg) and ritonavir (600 mg), a potent inhibitor of CYP3A4, did not significantly affect the pharmacokinetics of escitalopram oxalate. Because escitalopram oxalate is metabolized by multiple enzyme systems, inhibition of a single enzyme may not appreciably decrease escitalopram clearance).

No products indexed under this heading.

Tryptophan (The concomitant use of escitalopram with serotonin precursors, such as tryptophan, is not recommended).

No products indexed under this heading.

Valdecoxib (Epidemiological studies of the case-control and cohort design that have demonstrated an association between use of psychotropic drugs that interfere with serotonin reuptake and the occurrence of upper gastrointestinal bleeding have also shown that concurrent use of an NSAID may potentiate the risk of bleeding; use caution when administering).

No products indexed under this heading.

Valproate Sodium (In vitro studies indicated that CYP3A4 and -2C19 are the primary enzymes involved in the metabolism of escitalopram. However, co-administration of escitalopram (20 mg) and ritonavir (600 mg), a potent inhibitor of CYP3A4, did not significantly affect the pharmacokinetics of escitalopram oxalate. Because escitalopram oxalate is metabolized by multiple enzyme systems, inhibition of a single enzyme may not appreciably decrease escitalopram clearance).

No products indexed under this heading.

Vardenafil Hydrochloride (In vitro studies indicated that CYP3A4 and -2C19 are the primary enzymes involved in the metabolism of escitalopram. However, co-administration of escitalopram (20 mg) and ritonavir (600 mg), a potent inhibitor of CYP3A4, did not significantly affect the pharmacokinetics of escitalopram oxalate. Because escitalopram oxalate is metabolized by multiple enzyme systems, inhibition of a single enzyme may not appreciably decrease escitalopram clearance). Products include:

Venlafaxine Hydrochloride (The development of a potentially life threatening serotonin syndrome or Neuroleptic Malignant syndrome-like reactions have been reported with SSRIs alone, including escitalopram, but particularly with concomitant use of serotonergic drugs. Serotonin syndrome, in its most severe form, can resemble neuroleptic malignant syndrome. The concomitant use of escitalopram with SNRIs is not recommended). Products include:

Verapamil Hydrochloride (In vitro studies indicated that CYP3A4 and -2C19 are the primary enzymes involved in the metabolism of escitalopram. However, co-administration of escitalopram (20 mg) and ritonavir (600 mg), a potent inhibitor of CYP3A4, did not significantly affect the pharmacokinetics of escitalopram oxalate. Because escitalopram oxalate is metabolized by multiple enzyme systems, inhibition of a single enzyme may not appreciably decrease escitalopram clearance). Products include:

Vinblastine Sulfate (In vitro studies did not reveal an inhibitory effect of escitalopram on CYP2D6. In addition, steady state levels of racemic citalopram were not significantly different in poor metabolizers and extensive CYP2D6 metabolizers after multi-dose administration of citalopram, suggesting that co-administration, with escitalopram, of a drug that inhibits CYP2D6, is unlikely to have clinically significant effects on escitalopram metabolism. However, there are limited in vivo data suggesting a modest CYP2D6 inhibitory effect for escitalopram, ie co-administration of escitalopram (20 mg/day for 21 days) with the tricyclic antidepressant desipramine (single dose of 50 mg), a substrate for CYP2D6 resulted in a 40% increase in C_{max} and a 100% increase in AUC of desipramine. The clinical significance of this finding is unknown. Nevertheless, caution is indi-

cated in the co-administration of escitalopram and drugs metabolized by CYP2D6).

No products indexed under this heading.

Voriconazole (In vitro studies indicated that CYP3A4 and -2C19 are the primary enzymes involved in the metabolism of escitalopram. However, co-administration of escitalopram (20 mg) and ritonavir (600 mg), a potent inhibitor of CYP3A4, did not significantly affect the pharmacokinetics of escitalopram oxalate. Because escitalopram oxalate is metabolized by multiple enzyme systems, inhibition of a single enzyme may not appreciably decrease escitalopram clearance).

No products indexed under this heading.

Warfarin Sodium (Altered anticoagulant effects, including increased bleeding, have been reported when SSRIs are co-administered with warfarin. Patients receiving warfarin therapy should be carefully monitored when escitalopram is initiated or discontinued).

No products indexed under this heading.

Zafirlukast (In vitro studies indicated that CYP3A4 and -2C19 are the primary enzymes involved in the metabolism of escitalopram. However, co-administration of escitalopram (20 mg) and ritonavir (600 mg), a potent inhibitor of CYP3A4, did not significantly affect the pharmacokinetics of escitalopram oxalate. Because escitalopram oxalate is metabolized by multiple enzyme systems, inhibition of a single enzyme may not appreciably decrease escitalopram clearance). Products include:

Zaleplon (Given the primary CNS effects of escitalopram, caution should be used when it is taken in combination of other centrally acting drugs).

No products indexed under this heading.

Zileuton (In vitro studies indicated that CYP3A4 and -2C19 are the primary enzymes involved in the metabolism of escitalopram. However, co-administration of escitalopram (20 mg) and ritonavir (600 mg), a potent inhibitor of CYP3A4, did not significantly affect the pharmacokinetics of escitalopram oxalate. Because escitalopram oxalate is metabolized by multiple enzyme systems, inhibition of a single enzyme may not appreciably decrease escitalopram clearance).

No products indexed under this heading.

Ziprasidone Hydrochloride (The development of a potentially life-threatening serotonin syndrome or Neuroleptic Malignant Syndrome (NMS)-like reactions have been reported with SNRIs and SSRIs alone, including escitalopram treatment, but particularly with concomitant use of serotonergic drugs (including triptans) with drugs which impair metabolism of serotonin (including MAOIs), or with antipsychotics or other dopamine antagonists. Patients should be monitored for the emergence of serotonin syndrome or NMS-like signs and symptoms. Treatment with escitalopram and any concomitant serotonergic or antidopaminergic agents, including antipsychotics, should be discontinued immediately if the above events occur and supportive symptomatic treatment should be initiated). Products include:

Zolmitriptan (There have been rare post-marketing reports of serotonin syndrome with use of a SSRI and a triptan. If concomitant treatment of escitalopram with a triptan is clinically warranted, careful observation of the patient is advised, particularly during treatment initiation and dose increases). Products include:

Zolpidem Tartrate (Given the primary CNS effects of escitalopram, caution should be used when it is taken in combination of other centrally acting drugs). Products include:

Zonisamide (In vitro studies did not reveal an inhibitory effect of escitalopram on CYP2D6. In addition, steady state levels of racemic citalopram were not significantly different in poor metabolizers and extensive CYP2D6 metabolizers after multi-dose administration of citalopram, suggesting that co-administration, with escitalopram, of a drug that inhibits CYP2D6, is unlikely to have clinically significant effects on escitalopram metabolism. However, there are limited in vivo data suggesting a modest CYP2D6 inhibitory effect for escitalopram, ie co-administration of escitalopram (20 mg/day for 21 days) with the tricyclic antidepressant desipramine (single dose of 50 mg), a substrate for CYP2D6 resulted in a 40% increase in C_{max} and a 100% increase in AUC of desipramine. The clinical significance of this finding is unknown. Nevertheless, caution is indicated in the co-administration of escitalopram and drugs metabolized by CYP2D6). Products include:

Food Interactions

Alcohol (Although escitalopram did not potentiate the cognitive and motor effects of alcohol in a clinical trial, as with other psychotropic medications, the use of alcohol by patients taking escitalopram is not recommended).

Beer, reduced-alcohol (Although escitalopram did not potentiate the cognitive and motor effects of alcohol in a clinical trial, as with other psychotropic medications, the use of alcohol by patients taking escitalopram is not recommended).

Beer, unspecified (Although escitalopram did not potentiate the cognitive and motor effects of alcohol in a clinical trial, as with other psychotropic medications, the use of alcohol by patients taking escitalopram is not recommended).

Grapefruit (In vitro studies indicated that CYP3A4 and -2C19 are the primary enzymes involved in the metabolism of escitalopram. However, co-administration of escitalopram (20 mg) and ritonavir (600 mg), a potent inhibitor of CYP3A4, did not significantly affect the pharmacokinetics of escitalopram oxalate. Because escitalopram oxalate is metabolized by multiple enzyme systems, inhibition of a single enzyme may not appreciably decrease escitalopram clearance).

Grapefruit Juice (In vitro studies indicated that CYP3A4 and -2C19 are the primary enzymes involved in the metabolism of escitalopram. However, co-administration of escitalopram (20 mg) and ritonavir (600 mg), a potent inhibitor of CYP3A4, did not significantly affect the pharmacokinetics of escitalopram oxalate. Because escitalopram oxalate is metabolized by multiple enzyme systems, inhibition of a single enzyme may not appreciably decrease escitalopram clearance).

Wine, Chianti (Although escitalopram did not potentiate the cognitive and motor effects of alcohol in a clinical trial, as with other psychotropic medications, the use of alcohol by patients taking escitalopram is not recommended).

Wine, Red (Although escitalopram did not potentiate the cognitive and motor effects of alcohol in a clinical trial, as with other psychotropic medications, the use of alcohol by patients taking escitalopram is not recommended).

Wine, unspecified (Although escitalopram did not potentiate the cognitive and motor effects of alcohol in a clinical trial, as with other psychotropic medications, the use of alcohol by patients taking escitalopram is not recommended).

Wine products (Although escitalopram did not potentiate the cognitive and motor effects of alcohol in a clinical trial, as with other psychotropic medications, the use of alcohol by patients taking escitalopram is not recommended).

LEXISCAN INJECTION

(Regadenoson) 668
May interact with caffeines, theophyllines, xanthines, and certain other agents. Compounds in these categories include:

Aminophylline (Aminophylline (100 mg, administered by slow IV injection over 60 seconds) injected 1 minute after 0.4 mg regadenoson in subjects undergoing cardiac catheterization, was shown to shorten the duration of the coronary blood flow response to regadenosn as measured by pulsed-wave Doppler ultrasonography).
No products indexed under this heading.

Caffeine (Methylxanthines (eg, caffeine) are non-specific adenosine receptor antagonists and may interfere with the vasodilation activity of regadenoson. Patients should avoid consumption of any products containing methylxanthines as well as any drugs containing theophylline for at least 12 hours before regadenoson administration).
No products indexed under this heading.

Caffeine Anhydrous (Methylxanthines (eg, caffeine) are non-specific adenosine receptor antagonists and may interfere with the vasodilation activity of regadenoson. Patients should avoid consumption of any products containing methylxanthines as well as any drugs containing theophylline for at least 12 hours before regadenoson administration).
No products indexed under this heading.

Caffeine Citrate (Methylxanthines (eg, caffeine) are non-specific adenosine receptor antagonists and may interfere with the vasodilation activity of regadenoson. Patients should avoid consumption of any products containing methylxanthines as well as any drugs containing theophylline for at least 12 hours before regadenoson administration).
No products indexed under this heading.

Caffeine-containing medications (Methylxanthines (eg, caffeine) are non-specific adenosine receptor antagonists and may interfere with the vasodilation activity of regadenoson. Patients should avoid consumption of any products containing methylxanthines as well as any drugs containing theophylline for at least 12 hours before regadenoson administration).
No products indexed under this heading.

Caffeine Sodium Benzoate (Methylxanthines (eg, caffeine) are non-specific adenosine receptor antagonists and may interfere with the vasodilation activity of regadenoson. Patients should avoid consumption of any products containing methylxanthines as well as any drugs containing theophylline for at least 12 hours before regadenoson administration).
No products indexed under this heading.

Dipyridamole (Dipyridamole may change the effects of regadenoson.

When possible, withhold dipyridamole for at least two days prior to regadenoson administration). Products include:
Aggrenox 880

Dyphylline (Methylxanthines (eg, caffeine and theophylline) are non-specific adenosine receptor antagonists and may interfere with the vasodilation activity of regadenoson. Patients should avoid consumption of any products containing methylxanthines as well as any drugs containing theophylline for at least 12 hours before regadenoson administration).
No products indexed under this heading.

Theophylline (Methylxanthines (eg, theophylline) are non-specific adenosine receptor antagonists and may interfere with the vasodilation activity of regadenoson. Patients should avoid consumption of any products containing methylxanthines as well as any drugs containing theophylline for at least 12 hour before regadenoson administration).
No products indexed under this heading.

Theophylline Anhydrous (Methylxanthines (eg, theophylline) are non-specific adenosine receptor antagonists and may interfere with the vasodilation activity of regadenoson. Patients should avoid consumption of any products containing methylxanthines as well as any drugs containing theophylline for at least 12 hour before regadenoson administration). Products include:
Uniphyl 2817

Theophylline Calcium Salicylate (Methylxanthines (eg, theophylline) are non-specific adenosine receptor antagonists and may interfere with the vasodilation activity of regadenoson. Patients should avoid consumption of any products containing methylxanthines as well as any drugs containing theophylline for at least 12 hour before regadenoson administration).
No products indexed under this heading.

Theophylline Dihydroxypropyl (Glyceryl) (Methylxanthines (eg, theophylline) are non-specific adenosine receptor antagonists and may interfere with the vasodilation activity of regadenoson. Patients should avoid consumption of any products containing methylxanthines as well as any drugs containing theophylline for at least 12 hour before regadenoson administration).
No products indexed under this heading.

Theophylline Ethylenediamine (Methylxanthines (eg, theophylline) are non-specific adenosine receptor antagonists and may interfere with the vasodilation activity of regadenoson. Patients should avoid consumption of any products containing methylxanthines as well as any drugs containing theophylline for at least 12 hour before regadenoson administration).
No products indexed under this heading.

Theophylline Sodium Glycinate (Methylxanthines (eg, theophylline) are non-specific adenosine receptor antagonists and may interfere with the vasodilation activity of regadenoson. Patients should avoid consumption of any products containing methylxanthines as well as any drugs containing theophylline for at least 12 hour before regadenoson administration).
No products indexed under this heading.

Food Interactions

Beverages, caffeine-containing (Methylxanthines (eg, caffeine) are non-specific adenosine receptor antagonists and may interfere with the vasodilation activity of regadenoson. Patients should avoid consumption of any products containing methylxanthines as well as any drugs containing theophylline for at least

12 hours before regadenoson administration).

Food, caffeine-containing (Methylxanthines (eg, caffeine) are non-specific adenosine receptor antagonists and may interfere with the vasodilation activity of regadenoson. Patients should avoid consumption of any products containing methylxanthines as well as any drugs containing theophylline for at least 12 hours before regadenoson administration).

LEXIVA ORAL SUSPENSION

(Fosamprenavir Calcium) 1558
See Lexiva Tablets

LEXIVA TABLETS

(Fosamprenavir Calcium) 1558
May interact with antiarrhythmics, benzodiazepines, calcium channel blockers, cytochrome p450 3a4 inducers (selected), cytochrome p450 3a4 inhibitors (selected), cytochrome p450 3a4 substrates (selected), dexamethasones, ergot-containing drugs, histamine H2-receptor antagonists, immunosuppressive agents, insulin, oral contraceptives, oral hypoglycemic agents, PDE5 inhibitors, phenytoin, proton pump inhibitor, quinidine, tricyclic antidepressants, and certain other agents. Compounds in these categories include:

Acarbose (New onset diabetes mellitus, exacerbation of pre-existing diabetes mellitus, and hyperglycemia have been reported during post-marketing surveillance in HIV-infected patients receiving protease inhibitor therapy. Some patients required either initiation or dose adjustments of insulin or oral hypoglycemic agents for treatment of these events).
No products indexed under this heading.

Acebutolol Hydrochloride (Caution must be used when fosamprenavir calcium is administered concomitantly with antiarrhythmics (eg, amiodarone, bepridil, lidocaine (systemic), quinidine). Co-administration of fosamprenavir calcium with antiarrhythmics may lead to increased levels of antiarrhythmics. Increased exposure may be associated with life-threatening reactions such as cardiac arrhythmias. Therapeutic concentration monitoring is recommended, if available, for antiarrhythmics when co-administered with fosamprenavir).
No products indexed under this heading.

Acetazolamide (Amprenavir is metabolized by CYP3A4. Co-administration of fosamprenavir calcium and drugs that inhibit CYP3A4 may increase amprenavir concentrations and increase the incidence of adverse effects).
No products indexed under this heading.

Acetazolamide Sodium (Amprenavir is metabolized by CYP3A4. Co-administration of fosamprenavir calcium and drugs that inhibit CYP3A4 may increase amprenavir concentrations and increase the incidence of adverse effects).
No products indexed under this heading.

Adenosine (Caution must be used when fosamprenavir calcium is administered concomitantly with antiarrhythmics (eg, amiodarone, bepridil, lidocaine (systemic), quinidine). Co-administration of fosamprenavir calcium with antiarrhythmics may lead to increased levels of antiarrhythmics. Increased exposure may be associated with life-threatening reactions such as cardiac arrhythmias. Therapeutic concentration monitoring is recommended, if available, for antiarrhythmics when co-administered with fosamprenavir). Products include:
Adenocard 656

Adenoscan 657

Alfentanil Hydrochloride (Co-administration with drugs that are highly dependent on CYP3A4 for clearance and for which elevated plasma concentrations are associated with serious and/or life-threatening events are contraindicated).
No products indexed under this heading.

Allium sativum (Amprenavir is metabolized by CYP3A4. Co-administration of fosamprenavir calcium and drugs that induce CYP3A4 may decrease amprenavir concentrations and reduce its therapeutic effect).
No products indexed under this heading.

Alprazolam (Co-administration of alprazolam with fosamprenavir calcium may lead to increased concentrations of alprazolam. A decrease in the alprazolam dose may be needed).
No products indexed under this heading.

Aluminum Hydroxide (Co-administration of the antacid MAALOX TC, a 30 ml single dose and fosamprenavir calcium, a 1,400 mg single dose, may lead to a decrease in fosamprenavir C_{max} by 35%, a decrease in fosamprenavir AUC by 18% and increase in fosamprenavir C_{min} by 14%).
No products indexed under this heading.

Aminoglutethimide (Amprenavir is metabolized by CYP3A4. Co-administration of fosamprenavir calcium and drugs that induce CYP3A4 may decrease amprenavir concentrations and reduce its therapeutic effect).
No products indexed under this heading.

Amiodarone Hydrochloride (Caution must be used when fosamprenavir calcium is administered concomitantly with amiodarone. Co-administration of fosamprenavir calcium with amiodarone may lead to increased levels of amiodarone. Increased exposure may be associated with life-threatening reactions such as cardiac arrhythmias. Therapeutic concentration monitoring is recommended, if available, for amiodarone when co-administered with fosamprenavir).
No products indexed under this heading.

Amitriptyline Hydrochloride (Co-administration of tricyclic antidepressants (eg, amitriptyline, imipramine) with fosamprenavir calcium may lead to increased concentrations of the tricyclics. Therapeutic concentration monitoring is recommended for tricyclic antidepressants).
No products indexed under this heading.

Amlodipine Besylate (Co-administration of fosamprenavir calcium with the calcium channel blocker amlodipine may increase levels of amlodipine. Caution is warranted and clinical monitoring is recommended). Products include:
Azor 1010
Exforge 2443
Exforge HCT 2449

Amoxapine (Co-administration of tricyclic antidepressants (eg, amitriptyline, imipramine) with fosamprenavir calcium may lead to increased concentrations of the tricyclics. Therapeutic concentration monitoring is recommended for tricyclic antidepressants).
No products indexed under this heading.

Amprenavir (Amprenavir is metabolized by CYP3A4. Co-administration of fosamprenavir calcium and drugs that inhibit CYP3A4 may increase amprenavir concentrations and increase the incidence of adverse effects).
No products indexed under this heading.

IMPORTANT NOTE: Always consult each drug listing in the patient's regimen for possible interactions.

Lexiva Interactions Index 1038

Anastrozole (Amprenavir is metabolized by CYP3A4. Co-administration of fosamprenavir calcium and drugs that inhibit CYP3A4 may increase amprenavir concentrations and increase the incidence of adverse effects).
No products indexed under this heading.

Aprepitant (Co-administration with drugs that are highly dependent on CYP3A4 for clearance and for which elevated plasma concentrations are associated with serious and/or life-threatening events are contraindicated). Products include:
Emend 2124

Astemizole (Co-administration with drugs that are highly dependent on CYP3A4 for clearance and for which elevated plasma concentrations are associated with serious and/or life-threatening events are contraindicated).
No products indexed under this heading.

Atazanavir (Co-administration of fosamprenavir/ritonavir combination with atazanavir may lead to decreased levels of atazanavir).
No products indexed under this heading.

Atazanavir Sulfate (Co-administration of fosamprenavir/ritonavir combination with atazanavir may lead to decreased levels of atazanavir).
No products indexed under this heading.

Atorvastatin Calcium (Co-administration of fosamprenavir calcium with atorvastatin may lead to increased atorvastatin levels. The lowest possible dose of atorvastatin must be used with careful monitoring, or other HMG-CoA reductase inhibitors such as fluvastatin or pravastatin must be considered). Products include:
Lipitor 2703

Azathioprine (Co-administration of fosamprenavir calcium with immunosuppressants (eg, cyclosporine, tacrolimus, rapamycin) may lead to increased levels of immunosuppressants. Therapeutic concentration monitoring is recommended for immunosuppressant agents when co-administered with fosamprenavir).
No products indexed under this heading.

Basiliximab (Co-administration of fosamprenavir calcium with immunosuppressants (eg, cyclosporine, tacrolimus, rapamycin) may lead to increased levels of immunosuppressants. Therapeutic concentration monitoring is recommended for immunosuppressant agents when co-administered with fosamprenavir). Products include:
Simulect 2524

Belladonna Ergotamine (Co-administration with drugs that are highly dependent on CYP3A4 for clearance and for which elevated plasma concentrations are associated with serious and/or life-threatening events are contraindicated).
No products indexed under this heading.

Bepridil Hydrochloride (Caution must be used when fosamprenavir calcium is administered concomitantly with bepridil. Co-administration of fosamprenavir calcium with bepridil may lead to increased levels of bepridil. Increased exposure may be associated with life-threatening reactions such as cardiac arrhythmias. Therapeutic concentration monitoring is recommended, if available, for bepridil when co-administered with fosamprenavir).
No products indexed under this heading.

Betamethasone (Amprenavir is metabolized by CYP3A4. Co-administration of fosamprenavir calcium and drugs that induce CYP3A4 may decrease amprenavir concentrations and reduce its therapeutic effect).
No products indexed under this heading.

Betamethasone Acetate (Amprenavir is metabolized by CYP3A4. Co-administration of fosamprenavir calcium and drugs that induce CYP3A4 may decrease amprenavir concentrations and reduce its therapeutic effect).
No products indexed under this heading.

Betamethasone Benzoate (Amprenavir is metabolized by CYP3A4. Co-administration of fosamprenavir calcium and drugs that induce CYP3A4 may decrease amprenavir concentrations and reduce its therapeutic effect).
No products indexed under this heading.

Betamethasone Dipropionate (Amprenavir is metabolized by CYP3A4. Co-administration of fosamprenavir calcium and drugs that induce CYP3A4 may decrease amprenavir concentrations and reduce its therapeutic effect). Products include:
Diprolene Lotion 0.05% 3108
Diprolene Ointment 0.05% 3109
Diprolene AF Cream 0.05% 3107
Lotrisone 3163

Betamethasone Sodium Phosphate (Amprenavir is metabolized by CYP3A4. Co-administration of fosamprenavir calcium and drugs that induce CYP3A4 may decrease amprenavir concentrations and reduce its therapeutic effect).
No products indexed under this heading.

Betamethasone Valerate (Amprenavir is metabolized by CYP3A4. Co-administration of fosamprenavir calcium and drugs that induce CYP3A4 may decrease amprenavir concentrations and reduce its therapeutic effect). Products include:
Luxiq 3321

Bosentan (Amprenavir is metabolized by CYP3A4. Co-administration of fosamprenavir calcium and drugs that induce CYP3A4 may decrease amprenavir concentrations and reduce its therapeutic effect). Products include:
Tracleer 573

Bretylium Tosylate (Caution must be used when fosamprenavir calcium is administered concomitantly with antiarrhythmics (eg, amiodarone, bepridil, lidocaine (systemic), quinidine). Co-administration of fosamprenavir calcium with antiarrhythmics may lead to increased levels of antiarrhythmics. Increased exposure may be associated with life-threatening reactions such as cardiac arrhythmias. Therapeutic concentration monitoring is recommended, if available, for antiarrhythmics when co-administered with fosamprenavir).
No products indexed under this heading.

Buspirone Hydrochloride (Co-administration with drugs that are highly dependent on CYP3A4 for clearance and for which elevated plasma concentrations are associated with serious and/or life-threatening events are contraindicated).
No products indexed under this heading.

Busulfan (Co-administration with drugs that are highly dependent on CYP3A4 for clearance and for which elevated plasma concentrations are associated with serious and/or life-threatening events are contraindicated). Products include:
Myleran 1581

Carbamazepine (Co-administration of carbamazepine with fosamprenavir calcium may lead to decreased amprenavir levels. Caution must be used when fosamprenavir and anticonvulsants such as carbamazepine are administered concomitantly. Fosamprenavir may be less effective due to decreased plasma concentrations in patients taking these agents concomitantly). Products include:
Carbatrol 3280
Equetro 3477

Cerivastatin Sodium (Co-administration with drugs that are highly dependent on CYP3A4 for clearance and for which elevated plasma concentrations are associated with serious and/or life-threatening events are contraindicated).
No products indexed under this heading.

Chlordiazepoxide (Co-administration of benzodiazepines (eg, alprazolam, clorazepate, diazepam, flurazepam) with fosamprenavir calcium may lead to increased concentrations of the benzodiazepines. A decrease in benzodiazepine dose may be needed).
No products indexed under this heading.

Chlordiazepoxide Hydrochloride (Co-administration of benzodiazepines (eg, alprazolam, clorazepate, diazepam, flurazepam) with fosamprenavir calcium may lead to increased concentrations of the benzodiazepines. A decrease in benzodiazepine dose may be needed).
No products indexed under this heading.

Chlorpheniramine (Co-administration with drugs that are highly dependent on CYP3A4 for clearance and for which elevated plasma concentrations are associated with serious and/or life-threatening events are contraindicated).
No products indexed under this heading.

Chlorpheniramine Maleate (Co-administration with drugs that are highly dependent on CYP3A4 for clearance and for which elevated plasma concentrations are associated with serious and/or life-threatening events are contraindicated).
No products indexed under this heading.

Chlorpheniramine Polistirex (Co-administration with drugs that are highly dependent on CYP3A4 for clearance and for which elevated plasma concentrations are associated with serious and/or life-threatening events are contraindicated). Products include:
Tussionex 3443

Chlorpheniramine Tannate (Co-administration with drugs that are highly dependent on CYP3A4 for clearance and for which elevated plasma concentrations are associated with serious and/or life-threatening events are contraindicated).
No products indexed under this heading.

Chlorpropamide (New onset diabetes mellitus, exacerbation of pre-existing diabetes mellitus, and hyperglycemia have been reported during post-marketing surveillance in HIV-infected patients receiving protease inhibitor therapy. Some patients required either initiation or dose adjustments of insulin or oral hypoglycemic agents for treatment of these events).
No products indexed under this heading.

Cimetidine (Co-administration of fosamprenavir and the histamine H_2-receptor antagonist cimetidine may lead to decreased levels of amprenavir. Caution must be used during co-administration because fosamprenavir may be less effective due to decreased amprenavir plasma concentrations in patients taking cimetidine concomitantly).
No products indexed under this heading.

Cimetidine Hydrochloride (Co-administration of fosamprenavir and the histamine H_2-receptor antagonist cimetidine may lead to decreased levels of amprenavir. Caution must be used during co-administration because fosamprenavir may be less effective due to decreased amprenavir plasma concentrations in patients taking cimetidine concomitantly).
No products indexed under this heading.

Ciprofloxacin (Amprenavir is metabolized by CYP3A4. Co-administration of fosamprenavir calcium and drugs that inhibit CYP3A4 may increase amprenavir concentrations and increase the incidence of adverse effects). Products include:
Cipro I.V. 3082
Cipro 3073
Cipro XR 3091
Ciprodex 583

Ciprofloxacin Hydrochloride (Amprenavir is metabolized by CYP3A4. Co-administration of fosamprenavir calcium and drugs that induce CYP3A4 may decrease amprenavir concentrations and reduce its therapeutic effect). Products include:
Cipro 3073

Cisapride (Co-administration of fosamprenavir calcium with cisapride is contraindicated due to the potential for serious and/or life-threatening reactions such as cardiac arrhythmias).
No products indexed under this heading.

Cisplatin (Amprenavir is metabolized by CYP3A4. Co-administration of fosamprenavir calcium and drugs that induce CYP3A4 may decrease amprenavir concentrations and reduce its therapeutic effect).
No products indexed under this heading.

Clarithromycin (Co-administration with drugs that are highly dependent on CYP3A4 for clearance and for which elevated plasma concentrations are associated with serious and/or life-threatening events are contraindicated). Products include:
Biaxin/Biaxin XL 412

Clomipramine Hydrochloride (Co-administration of tricyclic antidepressants (eg, amitriptyline, imipramine) with fosamprenavir calcium may lead to increased concentrations of the tricyclics. Therapeutic concentration monitoring is recommended for tricyclic antidepressants).
No products indexed under this heading.

Clorazepate Dipotassium (Co-administration of clorazepate with fosamprenavir calcium may lead to increased concentrations of clorazepate. A decrease in the clorazepate dose may be needed).
No products indexed under this heading.

Clotrimazole (Amprenavir is metabolized by CYP3A4. Co-administration of fosamprenavir calcium and drugs that inhibit CYP3A4 may increase amprenavir concentrations and increase the incidence of adverse effects). Products include:
Lotrisone 3163

Conivaptan Hydrochloride (Amprenavir is metabolized by CYP3A4. Co-administration of fosamprenavir calcium and drugs that inhibit CYP3A4 may increase amprenavir concentrations and increase the incidence of adverse effects). Products include:
Vaprisol 689

Cortisone Acetate (Amprenavir is metabolized by CYP3A4. Co-administration of fosamprenavir calcium and drugs that induce CYP3A4 may decrease amprenavir concentrations and reduce its therapeutic effect).
No products indexed under this heading.

Cyclosporine (Co-administration of fosamprenavir calcium with the immunosuppressant cyclosporine may lead to increased levels of cyclosporine. Therapeutic concentration monitoring is recommended for cyclosporine when co-administered with fosamprenavir). Products include:
Gengraf 440
Neoral Oral Solution 2496
Neoral Capsules 2496
Restasis 605

1039 **Interactions Index** **Lexiva**

Dalfopristin (Amprenavir is metabolized by CYP3A4. Co-administration of fosamprenavir calcium and drugs that inhibit CYP3A4 may increase amprenavir concentrations and increase the incidence of adverse effects).
No products indexed under this heading.

Danazol (Amprenavir is metabolized by CYP3A4. Co-administration of fosamprenavir calcium and drugs that inhibit CYP3A4 may increase amprenavir concentrations and increase the incidence of adverse effects).
No products indexed under this heading.

Darunavir (Amprenavir is metabolized by CYP3A4. Co-administration of fosamprenavir calcium and drugs that inhibit CYP3A4 may increase amprenavir concentrations and increase the incidence of adverse effects).
No products indexed under this heading.

Dasatinib (Amprenavir is metabolized by CYP3A4. Co-administration of fosamprenavir calcium and drugs that inhibit CYP3A4 may increase amprenavir concentrations and increase the incidence of adverse effects).
No products indexed under this heading.

Delavirdine Mesylate (Co-administration of fosamprenavir calcium with delavirdine is contraindicated because it may lead to loss of virologic response and possible resistance to delavirdine).
No products indexed under this heading.

Delavirine (Amprenavir is metabolized by CYP3A4. Co-administration of fosamprenavir calcium and drugs that inhibit CYP3A4 may increase amprenavir concentrations and increase the incidence of adverse effects).
No products indexed under this heading.

Desipramine Hydrochloride (Co-administration of tricyclic antidepressants (eg, amitriptyline, imipramine) with fosamprenavir calcium may lead to increased concentrations of the tricyclics. Therapeutic concentration monitoring is recommended for tricyclic antidepressants).
No products indexed under this heading.

Desloratadine (Amprenavir is metabolized by CYP3A4. Co-administration of fosamprenavir calcium and drugs that inhibit CYP3A4 may increase amprenavir concentrations and increase the incidence of adverse effects). Products include:
Clarinex Syrup **3098**
Clarinex **3098**
Clarinex Reditabs **3098**
Clarinex-D 12-Hour **3101**
Clarinex-D **3104**

Desogestrel (Co-administration of fosamprenavir calcium with oral contraceptives containing the combination ethinyl estradiol/norethindrone may lead to decreased levels of amprenavir and ethinyl estradiol. Co-administration of fosamprenavir calcium/ ritonavir with oral contraceptives containing ethinyl estradiol/ norethindrone may lead to decreased levels of ethinyl estradiol. Alternative methods of non-hormonal contraception are recommended. May lead to loss of virologic response. There may be an increased risk of transaminase elevations. No data are available on the use of fosamprenavir/ritonavir with other hormonal therapies, such as hormone replacement therapy (HRT) for postmenopausal women).
No products indexed under this heading.

Dexamethasone (Caution must be used when fosamprenavir and corticosteroids such as dexamethasone are administered concomitantly. Co-administration of dexamethasone with fosamprenavir calcium may decrease amprenavir levels. Fosamprenavir calcium may be less effective due to decreased amprenavir plasma concentrations in patients taking these agents concomitantly). Products include:
Ciprodex **583**
Ozurdex .... ⊙**223**
Tobramycin and Dexamethasone Ophthalmic Suspension .... ⊙**251**

Dexamethasone Acetate (Caution must be used when fosamprenavir and corticosteroids such as dexamethasone are administered concomitantly. Co-administration of dexamethasone with fosamprenavir calcium may decrease amprenavir levels. Fosamprenavir calcium may be less effective due to decreased amprenavir plasma concentrations in patients taking these agents concomitantly).
No products indexed under this heading.

Dexamethasone Phosphate (Caution must be used when fosamprenavir and corticosteroids such as dexamethasone are administered concomitantly. Co-administration of dexamethasone with fosamprenavir calcium may decrease amprenavir levels. Fosamprenavir calcium may be less effective due to decreased amprenavir plasma concentrations in patients taking these agents concomitantly).
No products indexed under this heading.

Dexamethasone Sodium (Caution must be used when fosamprenavir and corticosteroids such as dexamethasone are administered concomitantly. Co-administration of dexamethasone with fosamprenavir calcium may decrease amprenavir levels. Fosamprenavir calcium may be less effective due to decreased amprenavir plasma concentrations in patients taking these agents concomitantly).
No products indexed under this heading.

Dexamethasone Sodium Phosphate (Caution must be used when fosamprenavir and corticosteroids such as dexamethasone are administered concomitantly. Co-administration of dexamethasone with fosamprenavir calcium may decrease amprenavir levels. Fosamprenavir calcium may be less effective due to decreased amprenavir plasma concentrations in patients taking these agents concomitantly).
No products indexed under this heading.

Dexamethasone Sodium Phosphate Injection (Caution must be used when fosamprenavir and corticosteroids such as dexamethasone are administered concomitantly. Co-administration of dexamethasone with fosamprenavir calcium may decrease amprenavir levels. Fosamprenavir calcium may be less effective due to decreased amprenavir plasma concentrations in patients taking these agents concomitantly).
No products indexed under this heading.

Dexlansoprazole (Proton pump inhibitors (eg, esomeprazole, lansoprazole, omeprazole, pantoprazole, rabeprazole) can be administered at the same time as a dose of fosamprenavir calcium with no change in plasma amprenavir concentrations). Products include:
Kapidex **3362**

Diazepam (Co-administration of diazepam with fosamprenavir calcium may lead to increased concentrations of diazepam. A decrease in the diazepam dose may be needed). Products include:
Valium Tablets **2880**

Dihydroergotamine Mesylate (Co-administration of fosamprenavir calcium with ergot derivatives such as dihydroergotamine is contraindicated due to potential for serious and/or life-threatening reactions such as acute ergot toxicity characterized by peripheral vasospasm and ischemia of the extremities and other tissues).
No products indexed under this heading.

Diltiazem Hydrochloride (Co-administration of fosamprenavir calcium with the calcium channel blocker diltiazem may increase levels of diltiazem. Caution is warranted and clinical monitoring is recommended). Products include:
Cardizem LA **423**

Diltiazem Maleate (Co-administration of fosamprenavir calcium with the calcium channel blocker diltiazem may increase levels of diltiazem. Caution is warranted and clinical monitoring is recommended).
No products indexed under this heading.

Disopyramide (Co-administration with drugs that are highly dependent on CYP3A4 for clearance and for which elevated plasma concentrations are associated with serious and/or life-threatening events are contraindicated).
No products indexed under this heading.

Disopyramide Phosphate (Caution must be used when fosamprenavir calcium is administered concomitantly with antiarrhythmics (eg, amiodarone, bepridil, lidocaine (systemic), quinidine). Co-administration of fosamprenavir calcium with antiarrhythmics may lead to increased levels of antiarrhythmics. Increased exposure may be associated with life-threatening reactions such as cardiac arrhythmias. Therapeutic concentration monitoring is recommended, if available, for antiarrhythmics when co-administered with fosamprenavir).
No products indexed under this heading.

Disulfiram (Co-administration with drugs that are highly dependent on CYP3A4 for clearance and for which elevated plasma concentrations are associated with serious and/or life-threatening events are contraindicated).
No products indexed under this heading.

Dofetilide (Caution must be used when fosamprenavir calcium is administered concomitantly with antiarrhythmics (eg, amiodarone, bepridil, lidocaine (systemic), quinidine). Co-administration of fosamprenavir calcium with antiarrhythmics may lead to increased levels of antiarrhythmics. Increased exposure may be associated with life-threatening reactions such as cardiac arrhythmias. Therapeutic concentration monitoring is recommended, if available, for antiarrhythmics when co-administered with fosamprenavir).
No products indexed under this heading.

Doxepin Hydrochloride (Co-administration of tricyclic antidepressants (eg, amitriptyline, imipramine) with fosamprenavir calcium may lead to increased concentrations of the tricyclics. Therapeutic concentration monitoring is recommended for tricyclic antidepressants).
No products indexed under this heading.

Doxorubicin Hydrochloride (Co-administration with drugs that are highly dependent on CYP3A4 for clearance and for which elevated plasma concentrations are associated with serious and/or life-threatening events are contraindicated).
No products indexed under this heading.

Dronabinol (Co-administration with drugs that are highly dependent on CYP3A4 for clearance and for which elevated plasma concentrations are associated with serious and/or life-threatening events are contraindicated).
No products indexed under this heading.

Efavirenz (Co-administration of fosamprenavir calcium with efavirenz may lead to decreased amprenavir levels. Appropriate doses of the combinations with respect to safety and efficacy have not been established. An additional 100 mg/day (300 mg total) of ritonavir is recommended when efavirenz is administered with fosamprenavir/ ritonavir once daily. No change in the ritonavir dose is required when efavirenz is administered with fosamprenavir plus ritonavir twice daily). Products include:
Atripla **906**

Ergonovine Maleate (Co-administration of fosamprenavir calcium with ergot derivatives such as ergonovine is contraindicated due to potential for serious and/or life-threatening reactions such as acute ergot toxicity characterized by peripheral vasospasm and ischemia of the extremities and other tissues).
No products indexed under this heading.

Ergotamine Tartrate (Co-administration of fosamprenavir calcium with ergot derivatives such as ergotamine is contraindicated due to potential for serious and/or life-threatening reactions such as acute ergot toxicity characterized by peripheral vasospasm and ischemia of the extremities and other tissues).
No products indexed under this heading.

Erythromycin (Co-administration with drugs that are highly dependent on CYP3A4 for clearance and for which elevated plasma concentrations are associated with serious and/or life-threatening events are contraindicated).
No products indexed under this heading.

Erythromycin Estolate (Co-administration with drugs that are highly dependent on CYP3A4 for clearance and for which elevated plasma concentrations are associated with serious and/or life-threatening events are contraindicated).
No products indexed under this heading.

Erythromycin Ethylsuccinate (Co-administration with drugs that are highly dependent on CYP3A4 for clearance and for which elevated plasma concentrations are associated with serious and/or life-threatening events are contraindicated). Products include:
E.E.S. **437**
EryPed **435**

Erythromycin Gluceptate (Co-administration with drugs that are highly dependent on CYP3A4 for clearance and for which elevated plasma concentrations are associated with serious and/or life-threatening events are contraindicated).
No products indexed under this heading.

Erythromycin Lactobionate (Co-administration with drugs that are highly dependent on CYP3A4 for clearance and for which elevated plasma concentrations are associated with serious and/or life-threatening events are contraindicated).
No products indexed under this heading.

Erythromycin Stearate (Co-administration with drugs that are highly dependent on CYP3A4 for clearance and for which elevated plasma concentrations are associated with serious and/or life-threatening events are contraindicated).
No products indexed under this heading.

Esomeprazole Magnesium (Concurrent administration of esomeprazole

IMPORTANT NOTE: Always consult each drug listing in the patient's regimen for possible interactions.

with fosamprenavir calcium may lead to increased levels of esomeprazole. Proton pump inhibitors (eg, esomeprazole) can be administered at the same time as a dose of fosamprenavir calcium with no change in plasma amprenavir concentrations). Products include:

Esomeprazole Sodium (Concurrent administration of esomeprazole with fosamprenavir calcium may lead to increased levels of esomeprazole. Proton pump inhibitors (eg, esomeprazole) can be administered at the same time as a dose of fosamprenavir calcium with no change in plasma amprenavir concentrations). Products include:

Estazolam (Co-administration of benzodiazepines (eg, alprazolam, clorazepate, diazepam, flurazepam) with fosamprenavir calcium may lead to increased concentrations of the benzodiazepines. A decrease in benzodiazepine dose may be needed).
No products indexed under this heading.

Estradiol (Co-administration with drugs that are highly dependent on CYP3A4 for clearance and for which elevated plasma concentrations are associated with serious and/or life-threatening events are contraindicated). Products include:

Estradiol Benzoate (Co-administration with drugs that are highly dependent on CYP3A4 for clearance and for which elevated plasma concentrations are associated with serious and/or life-threatening events are contraindicated).
No products indexed under this heading.

Estradiol Cypionate (Co-administration with drugs that are highly dependent on CYP3A4 for clearance and for which elevated plasma concentrations are associated with serious and/or life-threatening events are contraindicated).
No products indexed under this heading.

Estradiol Valerate (Co-administration with drugs that are highly dependent on CYP3A4 for clearance and for which elevated plasma concentrations are associated with serious and/or life-threatening events are contraindicated).
No products indexed under this heading.

Ethinyl Estradiol (Co-administration of fosamprenavir calcium with oral contraceptives containing the combination ethinyl estradiol/norethindrone may lead to decreased levels of amprenavir and ethinyl estradiol. Co-administration of fosamprenavir calcium/ ritonavir with oral contraceptives containing ethinyl estradiol/ norethindrone may lead to decreased levels of ethinyl estradiol. Alternative methods of non-hormonal contraception are recommended. May lead to loss of virologic response. There may be an increased risk of transaminase elevations. No data are available on the use of fosamprenavir/ritonavir with other hormonal therapies, such as hormone replacement therapy (HRT) for postmenopausal women). Products include:

Ethosuximide (Co-administration with drugs that are highly dependent on CYP3A4 for clearance and for which elevated plasma concentrations are associated with serious and/or life-threatening events are contraindicated).
No products indexed under this heading.

Ethynodiol Diacetate (Co-administration of fosamprenavir calcium with oral contraceptives containing the combination ethinyl estradiol/ norethindrone may lead to decreased levels of amprenavir and ethinyl estradiol. Co-administration of fosamprenavir calcium/ ritonavir with oral contraceptives containing ethinyl estradiol/ norethindrone may lead to decreased levels of ethinyl estradiol. Alternative methods of non-hormonal contraception are recommended. May lead to loss of virologic response. There may be an increased risk of transaminase elevations. No data are available on the use of fosamprenavir/ritonavir with other hormonal therapies, such as hormone replacement therapy (HRT) for postmenopausal women).
No products indexed under this heading.

Etoposide (Co-administration with drugs that are highly dependent on CYP3A4 for clearance and for which elevated plasma concentrations are associated with serious and/or life-threatening events are contraindicated).
No products indexed under this heading.

Etoposide Phosphate (Co-administration with drugs that are highly dependent on CYP3A4 for clearance and for which elevated plasma concentrations are associated with serious and/or life-threatening events are contraindicated).
No products indexed under this heading.

Famotidine (Co-administration of fosamprenavir and the histamine H2-receptor antagonist famotidine may lead to decreased levels of amprenavir. Caution must be used during co-administration because fosamprenavir may be less effective due to decreased amprenavir plasma concentrations in patients taking famotidine concomitantly). Products include:

Felbamate (Amprenavir is metabolized by CYP3A4. Co-administration of fosamprenavir calcium and drugs that induce CYP3A4 may decrease amprenavir concentrations and reduce its therapeutic effect).
No products indexed under this heading.

Felodipine (Co-administration of fosamprenavir calcium with the calcium channel blocker felodipine may increase levels of felodipine. Caution is warranted and clinical monitoring is recommended).
No products indexed under this heading.

Fentanyl (Co-administration with drugs that are highly dependent on CYP3A4 for clearance and for which elevated plasma concentrations are associated with serious and/or life-threatening events are contraindicated). Products include:

Fentanyl Citrate (Co-administration with drugs that are highly dependent on CYP3A4 for clearance and for which elevated plasma concentrations are associated with serious and/or life-threatening events are contraindicated). Products include:

Flecainide Acetate (If fosamprenavir is co-administered with ritonavir, concomitant use of the antiarrhythmic agent flecainide is contraindicated due to the potential for serious and/or life-threatening reactions such as cardiac arrhythmias secondary to increases in plasma concentrations of flecainide).
No products indexed under this heading.

Fluconazole (Amprenavir is metabolized by CYP3A4. Co-administration of fosamprenavir calcium and drugs that inhibit CYP3A4 may increase amprenavir concentrations and increase the incidence of adverse effects).
No products indexed under this heading.

Fludrocortisone Acetate (Amprenavir is metabolized by CYP3A4. Co-administration of fosamprenavir calcium and drugs that induce CYP3A4 may decrease amprenavir concentrations and reduce its therapeutic effect).
No products indexed under this heading.

Fluoxetine (Amprenavir is metabolized by CYP3A4. Co-administration of fosamprenavir calcium and drugs that inhibit CYP3A4 may increase amprenavir concentrations and increase the incidence of adverse effects).
No products indexed under this heading.

Fluoxetine Hydrochloride (Amprenavir is metabolized by CYP3A4. Co-administration of fosamprenavir calcium and drugs that inhibit CYP3A4 may increase amprenavir concentrations and increase the incidence of adverse effects). Products include:

Flurazepam Hydrochloride (Co-administration of flurazepam with fosamprenavir calcium may lead to increased concentrations of flurazepam. A decrease in the flurazepam dose may be needed).
No products indexed under this heading.

Fluticasone Furoate (Co-administration of fosamprenavir calcium (with or without ritonavir) with fluticasone may lead to increased fluticasone levels. Caution must be used and alternatives to fluticasone should be considered, particularly for long term use. Concomitant use may result in significantly reduced serum cortisol concentrations. Systemic effects including Cushing's syndrome and adrenal suppression have been reported during postmarketing use in patients receiving ritonavir and inhaled or intranasally administered fluticasone. Co-administration of fluticasone and fosamprenavir / ritonavir is not recommended unless the potential benefit to the patient outweighs the risk of systemic corticosteroid side effects). Products include:

Fluticasone Propionate (Co-administration of fosamprenavir calcium (with or without ritonavir) with fluticasone may lead to increased fluticasone levels. Caution must be used and alternatives to fluticasone should be considered, particularly for long term use. Concomitant use may result in significantly reduced serum cortisol concentrations. Systemic effects including Cushing's syndrome and adrenal suppression have been reported during postmarketing use in patients receiving ritonavir and inhaled or intranasally administered fluticasone. Co-administration of fluticasone and fosamprenavir / ritonavir is not recommended unless the potential benefit to the patient outweighs the risk of systemic corticosteroid side effects). Products include:

Fluvoxamine Maleate (Amprenavir is metabolized by CYP3A4. Co-administration of fosamprenavir calcium and drugs that inhibit CYP3A4 may increase amprenavir concentrations and increase the incidence of adverse effects).
No products indexed under this heading.

Fosphenytoin (Caution must be used when fosamprenavir is co-administered with phenytoin. Co-administration of fosamprenavir with phenytoin may decrease amprenavir levels. Fosamprenavir may be less effective due to decreased amprenavir concentrations when taken concomitantly with phenytoin. When phenytoin is co-administered with fosamprenavir/ritonavir, an increase in amprenavir levels and a decrease in phenytoin levels may occur. Plasma phenytoin levels concentrations should be monitored and phenytoin dose should be increased as appropriate. No change in fosamprenavir/ ritonavir dose is recommended).
No products indexed under this heading.

Fosphenytoin Sodium (Caution must be used when fosamprenavir is co-administered with phenytoin. Co-administration of fosamprenavir with phenytoin may decrease amprenavir levels. Fosamprenavir may be less effective due to decreased amprenavir concentrations when taken concomitantly with phenytoin. When phenytoin is co-administered with fosamprenavir/ ritonavir, an increase in amprenavir levels and a decrease in phenytoin levels may occur. Plasma phenytoin levels concentrations should be monitored and phenytoin dose should be increased as appropriate. No change in fosamprenavir/ritonavir dose is recommended).
No products indexed under this heading.

Garlic Extract (Amprenavir is metabolized by CYP3A4. Co-administration of fosamprenavir calcium and drugs that induce CYP3A4 may decrease amprenavir concentrations and reduce its therapeutic effect).
No products indexed under this heading.

Garlic Oil (Amprenavir is metabolized by CYP3A4. Co-administration of fosamprenavir calcium and drugs that induce CYP3A4 may decrease amprenavir concentrations and reduce its therapeutic effect).
No products indexed under this heading.

Glibenclamide (New onset diabetes mellitus, exacerbation of pre-existing diabetes mellitus, and hyperglycemia have been reported during postmarketing surveillance in HIV-infected patients receiving protease inhibitor therapy. Some patients required either initiation or dose adjustments of insulin or oral hypoglycemic agents for treatment of these events).
No products indexed under this heading.

Glimepiride (New onset diabetes mellitus, exacerbation of pre-existing diabetes mellitus, and hyperglycemia have been reported during post-marketing surveillance in HIV-infected patients receiving protease inhibitor therapy. Some patients required either initiation or dose adjustments of insulin or oral hypoglycemic agents for treatment of these events). Products include:

1041 Interactions Index Lexiva

Glipizide (New onset diabetes mellitus, exacerbation of pre-existing diabetes mellitus, and hyperglycemia have been reported during post-marketing surveillance in HIV-infected patients receiving protease inhibitor therapy. Some patients required either initiation or dose adjustments of insulin or oral hypoglycemic agents for treatment of these events).
No products indexed under this heading.

Glyburide (New onset diabetes mellitus, exacerbation of pre-existing diabetes mellitus, and hyperglycemia have been reported during post-marketing surveillance in HIV-infected patients receiving protease inhibitor therapy. Some patients required either initiation or dose adjustments of insulin or oral hypoglycemic agents for treatment of these events).
No products indexed under this heading.

Halazepam (Co-administration of benzodiazepines (eg, alprazolam, clorazepate, diazepam, flurazepam) with fosamprenavir calcium may lead to increased concentrations of the benzodiazepines. A decrease in benzodiazepine dose may be needed).
No products indexed under this heading.

Haloperidol (Co-administration with drugs that are highly dependent on CYP3A4 for clearance and for which elevated plasma concentrations are associated with serious and/or life-threatening events are contraindicated).
No products indexed under this heading.

Haloperidol Decanoate (Co-administration with drugs that are highly dependent on CYP3A4 for clearance and for which elevated plasma concentrations are associated with serious and/or life-threatening events are contraindicated).
No products indexed under this heading.

Haloperidol Lactate (Co-administration with drugs that are highly dependent on CYP3A4 for clearance and for which elevated plasma concentrations are associated with serious and/or life-threatening events are contraindicated).
No products indexed under this heading.

Hydrocortisone (Amprenavir is metabolized by CYP3A4. Co-administration of fosamprenavir calcium and drugs that induce CYP3A4 may decrease amprenavir concentrations and reduce its therapeutic effect).
No products indexed under this heading.

Hydrocortisone (Alcohol) (Amprenavir is metabolized by CYP3A4. Co-administration of fosamprenavir calcium and drugs that induce CYP3A4 may decrease amprenavir concentrations and reduce its therapeutic effect).
No products indexed under this heading.

Hydrocortisone Acetate (Amprenavir is metabolized by CYP3A4. Co-administration of fosamprenavir calcium and drugs that induce CYP3A4 may decrease amprenavir concentrations and reduce its therapeutic effect).
No products indexed under this heading.

Hydrocortisone Butyrate (Amprenavir is metabolized by CYP3A4. Co-administration of fosamprenavir calcium and drugs that induce CYP3A4 may decrease amprenavir concentrations and reduce its therapeutic effect).
No products indexed under this heading.

Hydrocortisone Cypionate (Amprenavir is metabolized by CYP3A4. Co-administration of fosamprenavir calcium and drugs that induce CYP3A4 may decrease amprenavir concentrations and reduce its therapeutic effect).
No products indexed under this heading.

Hydrocortisone Hemisuccinate (Amprenavir is metabolized by CYP3A4. Co-administration of fosamprenavir calcium and drugs that induce CYP3A4 may decrease amprenavir concentrations and reduce its therapeutic effect).
No products indexed under this heading.

Hydrocortisone Probutate (Amprenavir is metabolized by CYP3A4. Co-administration of fosamprenavir calcium and drugs that induce CYP3A4 may decrease amprenavir concentrations and reduce its therapeutic effect).
No products indexed under this heading.

Hydrocortisone Sodium Phosphate (Amprenavir is metabolized by CYP3A4. Co-administration of fosamprenavir calcium and drugs that induce CYP3A4 may decrease amprenavir concentrations and reduce its therapeutic effect).
No products indexed under this heading.

Hydrocortisone Sodium Succinate (Amprenavir is metabolized by CYP3A4. Co-administration of fosamprenavir calcium and drugs that induce CYP3A4 may decrease amprenavir concentrations and reduce its therapeutic effect).
No products indexed under this heading.

Hydrocortisone Valerate (Amprenavir is metabolized by CYP3A4. Co-administration of fosamprenavir calcium and drugs that induce CYP3A4 may decrease amprenavir concentrations and reduce its therapeutic effect).
No products indexed under this heading.

Hypericum (Amprenavir is metabolized by CYP3A4. Co-administration of fosamprenavir calcium and drugs that induce CYP3A4 may decrease amprenavir concentrations and reduce its therapeutic effect).
No products indexed under this heading.

Hypericum Perforatum (Co-administration of fosamprenavir calcium with hypericum perforatum is contraindicated because it may lead to loss of virologic response and possible resistance to fosamprenavir or other protease inhibitors). Products include:
Traumeel 1800

Imatinib Mesylate (Amprenavir is metabolized by CYP3A4. Co-administration of fosamprenavir calcium and drugs that inhibit CYP3A4 may increase amprenavir concentrations and increase the incidence of adverse effects). Products include:
Gleevec 2477

Imipramine Hydrochloride (Co-administration of tricyclic antidepressants (eg, amitriptyline, imipramine) with fosamprenavir calcium may lead to increased concentrations of the tricyclics. Therapeutic concentration monitoring is recommended for tricyclic antidepressants).
No products indexed under this heading.

Imipramine Pamoate (Co-administration of tricyclic antidepressants (eg, amitriptyline, imipramine) with fosamprenavir calcium may lead to increased concentrations of the tricyclics. Therapeutic concentration monitoring is recommended for tricyclic antidepressants).
No products indexed under this heading.

Indinavir Sulfate (Co-administration of fosamprenavir calcium with indinavir may lead to increased amprenavir levels. The effect on indinavir is not well established). Products include:
Crixivan 2113

Insulin (New onset diabetes mellitus, exacerbation of pre-existing diabetes mellitus, and hyperglycemia have been reported during post-marketing surveillance in HIV-infected patients receiving protease inhibitor therapy. Some patients required either initiation or dose adjustments of insulin or oral hypoglycemic agents for treatment of these events).
No products indexed under this heading.

Insulin, Human, Zinc Suspension (New onset diabetes mellitus, exacerbation of pre-existing diabetes mellitus, and hyperglycemia have been reported during post-marketing surveillance in HIV-infected patients receiving protease inhibitor therapy. Some patients required either initiation or dose adjustments of insulin or oral hypoglycemic agents for treatment of these events).
No products indexed under this heading.

Insulin, Human (rDNA origin) (New onset diabetes mellitus, exacerbation of pre-existing diabetes mellitus, and hyperglycemia have been reported during post-marketing surveillance in HIV-infected patients receiving protease inhibitor therapy. Some patients required either initiation or dose adjustments of insulin or oral hypoglycemic agents for treatment of these events). Products include:
Exubera 2717

Insulin, Human NPH (New onset diabetes mellitus, exacerbation of pre-existing diabetes mellitus, and hyperglycemia have been reported during post-marketing surveillance in HIV-infected patients receiving protease inhibitor therapy. Some patients required either initiation or dose adjustments of insulin or oral hypoglycemic agents for treatment of these events). Products include:
Humulin N Vial 1934

Insulin, Human Regular (New onset diabetes mellitus, exacerbation of pre-existing diabetes mellitus, and hyperglycemia have been reported during post-marketing surveillance in HIV-infected patients receiving protease inhibitor therapy. Some patients required either initiation or dose adjustments of insulin or oral hypoglycemic agents for treatment of these events). Products include:
Humulin R 1937
Humulin R (U-500) 1939

Insulin, Human Regular and Human NPH Mixture (New onset diabetes mellitus, exacerbation of pre-existing diabetes mellitus, and hyperglycemia have been reported during post-marketing surveillance in HIV-infected patients receiving protease inhibitor therapy. Some patients required either initiation or dose adjustments of insulin or oral hypoglycemic agents for treatment of these events). Products include:
Humulin 50/50 1930
Humulin 70/30 Vial 1931

Insulin, NPH (New onset diabetes mellitus, exacerbation of pre-existing diabetes mellitus, and hyperglycemia have been reported during post-marketing surveillance in HIV-infected patients receiving protease inhibitor therapy. Some patients required either initiation or dose adjustments of insulin or oral hypoglycemic agents for treatment of these events).
No products indexed under this heading.

Insulin, Regular (New onset diabetes mellitus, exacerbation of pre-existing diabetes mellitus, and hyperglycemia have been reported during post-marketing surveillance in HIV-infected patients receiving protease inhibitor therapy. Some patients required either initiation or dose adjustments of insulin or oral hypoglycemic agents for treatment of these events).
No products indexed under this heading.

Insulin, Regular and NPH mixture (New onset diabetes mellitus, exacerbation of pre-existing diabetes mellitus, and hyperglycemia have been reported during post-marketing surveillance in HIV-infected patients receiving protease inhibitor therapy. Some patients required either initiation or dose adjustments of insulin or oral hypoglycemic agents for treatment of these events).
No products indexed under this heading.

Insulin, Zinc Crystals (New onset diabetes mellitus, exacerbation of pre-existing diabetes mellitus, and hyperglycemia have been reported during post-marketing surveillance in HIV-infected patients receiving protease inhibitor therapy. Some patients required either initiation or dose adjustments of insulin or oral hypoglycemic agents for treatment of these events).
No products indexed under this heading.

Insulin, Zinc Suspension (New onset diabetes mellitus, exacerbation of pre-existing diabetes mellitus, and hyperglycemia have been reported during post-marketing surveillance in HIV-infected patients receiving protease inhibitor therapy. Some patients required either initiation or dose adjustments of insulin or oral hypoglycemic agents for treatment of these events).
No products indexed under this heading.

Insulin Aspart (New onset diabetes mellitus, exacerbation of pre-existing diabetes mellitus, and hyperglycemia have been reported during post-marketing surveillance in HIV-infected patients receiving protease inhibitor therapy. Some patients required either initiation or dose adjustments of insulin or oral hypoglycemic agents for treatment of these events).
No products indexed under this heading.

Insulin Aspart, Human (New onset diabetes mellitus, exacerbation of pre-existing diabetes mellitus, and hyperglycemia have been reported during post-marketing surveillance in HIV-infected patients receiving protease inhibitor therapy. Some patients required either initiation or dose adjustments of insulin or oral hypoglycemic agents for treatment of these events). Products include:
NovoLog Mix 70/30 2581

Insulin Aspart, Human Regular (New onset diabetes mellitus, exacerbation of pre-existing diabetes mellitus, and hyperglycemia have been reported during post-marketing surveillance in HIV-infected patients receiving protease inhibitor therapy. Some patients required either initiation or dose adjustments of insulin or oral hypoglycemic agents for treatment of these events). Products include:
NovoLog 2575

Insulin Aspart Protamine, Human (New onset diabetes mellitus, exacerbation of pre-existing diabetes mellitus, and hyperglycemia have been reported during post-marketing surveillance in HIV-infected patients receiving protease inhibitor therapy. Some patients required either initiation or dose adjustments of insulin or oral hypoglycemic agents for treatment of these events). Products include:
NovoLog Mix 70/30 2581

IMPORTANT NOTE: Always consult each drug listing in the patient's regimen for possible interactions.

Lexiva Interactions Index 1042

Insulin Detemir (rDNA Origin) (New onset diabetes mellitus, exacerbation of pre-existing diabetes mellitus, and hyperglycemia have been reported during post-marketing surveillance in HIV-infected patients receiving protease inhibitor therapy. Some patients required either initiation or dose adjustments of insulin or oral hypoglycemic agents for treatment of these events). Products include:
Levemir 2566

Insulin Glargine (New onset diabetes mellitus, exacerbation of pre-existing diabetes mellitus, and hyperglycemia have been reported during post-marketing surveillance in HIV-infected patients receiving protease inhibitor therapy. Some patients required either initiation or dose adjustments of insulin or oral hypoglycemic agents for treatment of these events). Products include:
Lantus 2996

Insulin Glulisine (New onset diabetes mellitus, exacerbation of pre-existing diabetes mellitus, and hyperglycemia have been reported during post-marketing surveillance in HIV-infected patients receiving protease inhibitor therapy. Some patients required either initiation or dose adjustments of insulin or oral hypoglycemic agents for treatment of these events). Products include:
Apidra 2937
Apidra SoloStar 2937

Insulin Lispro, Human (New onset diabetes mellitus, exacerbation of pre-existing diabetes mellitus, and hyperglycemia have been reported during post-marketing surveillance in HIV-infected patients receiving protease inhibitor therapy. Some patients required either initiation or dose adjustments of insulin or oral hypoglycemic agents for treatment of these events). Products include:
Humalog 1910
Humalog Mix 1914
Humalog Mix75/25 1917

Insulin Lispro Protamine, Human (New onset diabetes mellitus, exacerbation of pre-existing diabetes mellitus, and hyperglycemia have been reported during post-marketing surveillance in HIV-infected patients receiving protease inhibitor therapy. Some patients required either initiation or dose adjustments of insulin or oral hypoglycemic agents for treatment of these events). Products include:
Humalog Mix 1914
Humalog Mix75/25 1917

Isoniazid (Amprenavir is metabolized by CYP3A4. Co-administration of fosamprenavir calcium and drugs that inhibit CYP3A4 may increase amprenavir concentrations and increase the incidence of adverse effects).
No products indexed under this heading.

Isradipine (Co-administration of fosamprenavir calcium with the calcium channel blocker isradipine may increase levels of isradipine. Caution is warranted and clinical monitoring is recommended). Products include:
DynaCirc CR 1432

Itraconazole (Co-administration of fosamprenavir calcium with itraconazole may increase itraconazole levels. Increased monitoring for adverse events is recommended during concomitant use. When co-administered with fosamprenavir alone, a dose reduction of itraconazole may be needed for patients receiving more than 400 mg of itraconazole per day. If the patient is receiving the fosamprenavir/ritonavir combination, co-administration of high doses of itraconazole (>200 mg/day) is not recommended).
No products indexed under this heading.

Ixabepilone (Co-administration with drugs that are highly dependent on CYP3A4 for clearance and for which elevated plasma concentrations are associated with serious and/or life-threatening events are contraindicated).
No products indexed under this heading.

Ketoconazole (Co-administration of fosamprenavir calcium with ketoconazole may increase ketoconazole levels. Increased monitoring for adverse events is recommended during concomitant use. When co-administered with fosamprenavir alone, a dose reduction of ketoconazole may be needed for patients receiving more than 400 mg of ketoconazole per day. If the patient is receiving the fosamprenavir/ritonavir combination, co-administration of high doses of ketoconazole (>200 mg/day) is not recommended). Products include:
Extina 3319
Xolegel 3337

Lansoprazole (Proton pump inhibitors (eg, esomeprazole, lansoprazole, omeprazole, pantoprazole, rabeprazole) can be administered at the same time as a dose of fosamprenavir calcium with no change in plasma amprenavir concentrations).
No products indexed under this heading.

Lapatinib (Amprenavir is metabolized by CYP3A4. Co-administration of fosamprenavir calcium and drugs that inhibit CYP3A4 may increase amprenavir concentrations and increase the incidence of adverse effects). Products include:
Tykerb 1698

Levonorgestrel (Co-administration of fosamprenavir calcium with oral contraceptives containing the combination ethinyl estradiol/norethindrone may lead to decreased levels of amprenavir and ethinyl estradiol. Co-administration of fosamprenavir calcium/ ritonavir with oral contraceptives containing ethinyl estradiol/ norethindrone may lead to decreased levels of ethinyl estradiol. Alternative methods of non-hormonal contraception are recommended. May lead to loss of virologic response. There may be an increased risk of transaminase elevations. No data are available on the use of fosamprenavir/ritonavir with other hormonal therapies, such as hormone replacement therapy (HRT) for postmenopausal women). Products include:
Climara Pro 847
LoSeasonique 3407
Lybrel 3514
Mirena 854
Plan B 3416
Seasonique 3418

Lidocaine (Caution must be used when fosamprenavir calcium is administered concomitantly with lidocaine (systemic). Co-administration of fosamprenavir calcium with lidocaine (systemic) may lead to increased levels of lidocaine (systemic). Increased exposure may be associated with life-threatening reactions such as cardiac arrhythmias. Therapeutic concentration monitoring, if available, is recommended for lidocaine (systemic) when co-administered with fosamprenavir). Products include:
Lidoderm 1107

Lidocaine Base (Caution must be used when fosamprenavir calcium is administered concomitantly with lidocaine (systemic). Co-administration of fosamprenavir calcium with lidocaine (systemic) may lead to increased levels of lidocaine (systemic). Increased exposure may be associated with life-threatening reactions such as cardiac arrhythmias. Therapeutic concentration monitoring, if available, is recommended for lidocaine (systemic) when co-administered with fosamprenavir).
No products indexed under this heading.

Lidocaine Hydrochloride (Caution must be used when fosamprenavir calcium is administered concomitantly with lidocaine (systemic). Co-administration of fosamprenavir calcium with lidocaine (systemic) may lead to increased levels of lidocaine (systemic). Increased exposure may be associated with life-threatening reactions such as cardiac arrhythmias. Therapeutic concentration monitoring, if available, is recommended for lidocaine (systemic) when co-administered with fosamprenavir).
No products indexed under this heading.

Lopinavir (Co-administration of lopinavir/ritonavir combination with fosamprenavir may lead to decreased levels of amprenavir and lopinavir. An increased rate of adverse events has also been observed with co-administration of these medications). Products include:
Kaletra 458

Loratadine (Amprenavir is metabolized by CYP3A4. Co-administration of fosamprenavir calcium and drugs that inhibit CYP3A4 may increase amprenavir concentrations and increase the incidence of adverse effects).
No products indexed under this heading.

Lorazepam (Co-administration of benzodiazepines (eg, alprazolam, clorazepate, diazepam, flurazepam) with fosamprenavir calcium may lead to increased concentrations of the benzodiazepines. A decrease in benzodiazepine dose may be needed).
No products indexed under this heading.

Lovastatin (Co-administration of fosamprenavir calcium with lovastatin is contraindicated due to the potential for serious reactions such as the risk of myopathy including rhabdomyolysis). Products include:
Advicor 402
Mevacor 2212

Magnesium Hydroxide (Co-administration of the antacid MAALOX TC, a 30 ml single dose and fosamprenavir calcium, a 1,400 mg single dose, may lead to a decrease in fosamprenavir C_{max} by 35%, a decrease in fosamprenavir AUC by 18% and increase in fosamprenavir C_{min} by 14%). Products include:
Fleet Pedia-Lax Chewable Tablets 1144
Pepcid Complete 1822

Maprotiline Hydrochloride (Co-administration of tricyclic antidepressants (eg, amitriptyline, imipramine) with fosamprenavir calcium may lead to increased concentrations of the tricyclics. Therapeutic concentration monitoring is recommended for tricyclic antidepressants).
No products indexed under this heading.

Mephenytoin (Amprenavir is metabolized by CYP3A4. Co-administration of fosamprenavir calcium and drugs that induce CYP3A4 may decrease amprenavir concentrations and reduce its therapeutic effect).
No products indexed under this heading.

Mestranol (Co-administration of fosamprenavir calcium with oral contraceptives containing the combination ethinyl estradiol/norethindrone may lead to decreased levels of amprenavir and ethinyl estradiol. Co-administration of fosamprenavir calcium/ ritonavir with oral contraceptives containing ethinyl estradiol/ norethindrone may lead to decreased levels of ethinyl estradiol. Alternative methods of non-hormonal contraception are recommended. May lead to loss of virologic response. There may be an increased risk of transaminase elevations. No data are available on the use of fosamprenavir/ritonavir with other hormonal therapies, such as hormone replacement therapy (HRT) for postmenopausal women).
No products indexed under this heading.

Metformin Hydrochloride (New onset diabetes mellitus, exacerbation of pre-existing diabetes mellitus, and hyperglycemia have been reported during post-marketing surveillance in HIV-infected patients receiving protease inhibitor therapy. Some patients required either initiation or dose adjustments of insulin or oral hypoglycemic agents for treatment of these events). Products include:
ActoPlus 3338
Avandamet 1345
Janumet 2188

Methadone Hydrochloride (Co-administration of fosamprenavir calcium with methadone may lead to decreased levels of methadone. Data suggest that the interaction is not clinically relevant; however, patients should be monitored for opiate withdrawal symptoms).
No products indexed under this heading.

Methsuximide (Amprenavir is metabolized by CYP3A4. Co-administration of fosamprenavir calcium and drugs that induce CYP3A4 may decrease amprenavir concentrations and reduce its therapeutic effect).
No products indexed under this heading.

Methylergonovine Maleate (Co-administration of fosamprenavir calcium with ergot derivatives, such as methylergonovine, is contraindicated due to potential for serious and/or life-threatening reactions such as acute ergot toxicity characterized by peripheral vasospasm and ischemia of the extremities and other tissues).
No products indexed under this heading.

Methylprednisolone (Amprenavir is metabolized by CYP3A4. Co-administration of fosamprenavir calcium and drugs that induce CYP3A4 may decrease amprenavir concentrations and reduce its therapeutic effect).
No products indexed under this heading.

Methylprednisolone Acetate (Amprenavir is metabolized by CYP3A4. Co-administration of fosamprenavir calcium and drugs that induce CYP3A4 may decrease amprenavir concentrations and reduce its therapeutic effect).
No products indexed under this heading.

Methylprednisolone Sodium Succinate (Amprenavir is metabolized by CYP3A4. Co-administration of fosamprenavir calcium and drugs that induce CYP3A4 may decrease amprenavir concentrations and reduce its therapeutic effect).
No products indexed under this heading.

Methysergide Maleate (Co-administration of fosamprenavir calcium with ergot derivatives such as dihydroergotamine, ergonovine, ergotamine, methylergonovine is contraindicated due to potential for serious and/or life-threatening reactions such as acute ergot toxicity characterized by peripheral vasospasm and ischemia of the extremities and other tissues).
No products indexed under this heading.

Metronidazole (Amprenavir is metabolized by CYP3A4. Co-administration of fosamprenavir calcium and drugs that inhibit CYP3A4 may increase amprenavir concentrations and increase the incidence of adverse effects). Products include:
Pylera 793

1043 Interactions Index Lexiva

Metronidazole Benzoate (Amprenavir is metabolized by CYP3A4. Co-administration of fosamprenavir calcium and drugs that inhibit CYP3A4 may increase amprenavir concentrations and increase the incidence of adverse effects).
No products indexed under this heading.

Metronidazole Hydrochloride (Amprenavir is metabolized by CYP3A4. Co-administration of fosamprenavir calcium and drugs that inhibit CYP3A4 may increase amprenavir concentrations and increase the incidence of adverse effects).
No products indexed under this heading.

Metronidazole Sodium (Amprenavir is metabolized by CYP3A4. Co-administration of fosamprenavir calcium and drugs that inhibit CYP3A4 may increase amprenavir concentrations and increase the incidence of adverse effects).
No products indexed under this heading.

Mexiletine Hydrochloride (Caution must be used when fosamprenavir calcium is administered concomitantly with antiarrhythmics (eg, amiodarone, bepridil, lidocaine (systemic), quinidine). Co-administration of fosamprenavir calcium with antiarrhythmics may lead to increased levels of antiarrhythmics. Increased exposure may be associated with life-threatening reactions such as cardiac arrhythmias. Therapeutic concentration monitoring is recommended, if available, for antiarrhythmics when co-administered with fosamprenavir).
No products indexed under this heading.

Mibefradil Dihydrochloride (Co-administration of fosamprenavir calcium with calcium channel blockers (eg, diltiazem, felodipine, nifedepine, nicardepine, nimodipine, verapamil, amlodipine, nisoldipine, isradipine) may increase levels of calcium channel blockers. Caution is warranted and clinical monitoring is recommended).
No products indexed under this heading.

Miconazole (Amprenavir is metabolized by CYP3A4. Co-administration of fosamprenavir calcium and drugs that inhibit CYP3A4 may increase amprenavir concentrations and increase the incidence of adverse effects).
No products indexed under this heading.

Miconazole Nitrate (Amprenavir is metabolized by CYP3A4. Co-administration of fosamprenavir calcium and drugs that inhibit CYP3A4 may increase amprenavir concentrations and increase the incidence of adverse effects). Products include:
Vusion Ointment **3335**

Midazolam Hydrochloride (Co-administration of fosamprenavir calcium with midazolam is contraindicated due to potential for serious and/or life-threatening reactions such as prolonged or increased sedation or respiratory depression).
No products indexed under this heading.

Mifepristone (Amprenavir is metabolized by CYP3A4. Co-administration of fosamprenavir calcium and drugs that inhibit CYP3A4 may increase amprenavir concentrations and increase the incidence of adverse effects).
No products indexed under this heading.

Miglitol (New onset diabetes mellitus, exacerbation of pre-existing diabetes mellitus, and hyperglycemia have been reported during post-marketing surveillance in HIV-infected patients receiving protease inhibitor therapy. Some patients required either initiation or dose adjustments of insulin or oral hypoglycemic agents for treatment of these events).
No products indexed under this heading.

Modafinil (Amprenavir is metabolized by CYP3A4. Co-administration of fosamprenavir calcium and drugs that induce CYP3A4 may decrease amprenavir concentrations and reduce its therapeutic effect). Products include:
Provigil **983**

Moricizine Hydrochloride (Caution must be used when fosamprenavir calcium is administered concomitantly with antiarrhythmics (eg, amiodarone, bepridil, lidocaine (systemic), quinidine). Co-administration of fosamprenavir calcium with antiarrhythmics may lead to increased levels of antiarrhythmics. Increased exposure may be associated with life-threatening reactions such as cardiac arrhythmias. Therapeutic concentration monitoring is recommended, if available, for antiarrhythmics when co-administered with fosamprenavir).
No products indexed under this heading.

Muromonab-CD3 (Co-administration of fosamprenavir calcium with immunosuppressants (eg, cyclosporine, tacrolimus, rapamycin) may lead to increased levels of immunosuppressants. Therapeutic concentration monitoring is recommended for immunosuppressant agents when co-administered with fosamprenavir). Products include:
Orthoclone OKT3 .... **949**

Mycophenolate Mofetil (Co-administration of fosamprenavir calcium with immunosuppressants (eg, cyclosporine, tacrolimus, rapamycin) may lead to increased levels of immunosuppressants. Therapeutic concentration monitoring is recommended for immunosuppressant agents when co-administered with fosamprenavir).
No products indexed under this heading.

Nafcillin Sodium (Amprenavir is metabolized by CYP3A4. Co-administration of fosamprenavir calcium and drugs that induce CYP3A4 may decrease amprenavir concentrations and reduce its therapeutic effect).
No products indexed under this heading.

Nateglinide (New onset diabetes mellitus, exacerbation of pre-existing diabetes mellitus, and hyperglycemia have been reported during post-marketing surveillance in HIV-infected patients receiving protease inhibitor therapy. Some patients required either initiation or dose adjustments of insulin or oral hypoglycemic agents for treatment of these events).
No products indexed under this heading.

Nefazodone Hydrochloride (Co-administration with drugs that are highly dependent on CYP3A4 for clearance and for which elevated plasma concentrations are associated with serious and/or life-threatening events are contraindicated).
No products indexed under this heading.

Nelfinavir Mesylate (Co-administration of fosamprenavir calcium with nelfinavir may lead to increased amprenavir levels. The effect on nelfinavir is not well established).
No products indexed under this heading.

Nevirapine (Co-administration of fosamprenavir calcium with nevirapine may lead to decreased amprenavir levels and increased nevirapine levels. Co-administration of nevirapine and fosamprenavir calcium without ritonavir is not recommended). Products include:
Viramune Oral Suspension **897**
Viramune Tablets **897**

Niacin (Amprenavir is metabolized by CYP3A4. Co-administration of fosamprenavir calcium and drugs that inhibit CYP3A4 may increase amprenavir concentrations and increase the incidence of adverse effects). Products include:
Advicor **402**
Cardio Basics **3455**
Niaspan **497**
Simcor **524**

Niacinamide (Amprenavir is metabolized by CYP3A4. Co-administration of fosamprenavir calcium and drugs that inhibit CYP3A4 may increase amprenavir concentrations and increase the incidence of adverse effects). Products include:
CitraNatal 90 DHA Capsules **2332**
CitraNatal Assure **2332**
CitraNatal Rx **2332**
Heplive **607**

Niacinamide Hydroiodide (Amprenavir is metabolized by CYP3A4. Co-administration of fosamprenavir calcium and drugs that inhibit CYP3A4 may increase amprenavir concentrations and increase the incidence of adverse effects).
No products indexed under this heading.

Nicardipine (Co-administration of fosamprenavir calcium with the calcium channel blocker nicardipine may increase levels of nicardipine. Caution is warranted and clinical monitoring is recommended).
No products indexed under this heading.

Nicardipine Hydrochloride (Co-administration of fosamprenavir calcium with the calcium channel blocker nicardipine may increase levels of nicardipine. Caution is warranted and clinical monitoring is recommended).
No products indexed under this heading.

Nicotinamide (Amprenavir is metabolized by CYP3A4. Co-administration of fosamprenavir calcium and drugs that inhibit CYP3A4 may increase amprenavir concentrations and increase the incidence of adverse effects).
No products indexed under this heading.

Nifedipine (Co-administration of fosamprenavir calcium with the calcium channel blocker nifedepine may increase levels of nifedipine. Caution is warranted and clinical monitoring is recommended).
No products indexed under this heading.

Nimodipine (Co-administration of fosamprenavir calcium with the calcium channel blocker nimodipine may increase levels of nimodipine. Caution is warranted and clinical monitoring is recommended).
No products indexed under this heading.

Nisoldipine (Co-administration of fosamprenavir calcium with the calcium channel blocker nisoldipine may increase levels of nisoldipine. Caution is warranted and clinical monitoring is recommended).
No products indexed under this heading.

Nitrendipine (Co-administration with drugs that are highly dependent on CYP3A4 for clearance and for which elevated plasma concentrations are associated with serious and/or life-threatening events are contraindicated).
No products indexed under this heading.

Nizatidine (Co-administration of fosamprenavir and the histamine H_2-receptor antagonist nizatidine may lead to decreased levels of amprenavir. Caution must be used during co-administration because fosamprenavir may be less effective due to decreased amprenavir plasma concentrations in patients taking nizatidine concomitantly). Products include:
Axid **1381**

Norethindrone (Co-administration of fosamprenavir calcium with oral contraceptives containing the combination ethinyl estradiol/norethindrone may lead to decreased levels of amprenavir and ethinyl estradiol. Co-administration of fosamprenavir calcium/ ritonavir with oral contraceptives containing ethinyl estradiol/ norethindrone may lead to decreased levels of ethinyl estradiol. Alternative methods of non-hormonal contraception are recommended. May lead to loss of virologic response. There may be an increased risk of transaminase elevations. No data are available on the use of fosamprenavir/ritonavir with other hormonal therapies, such as hormone replacement therapy (HRT) for postmenopausal women). Products include:
Ortho Micronor **2660**

Norethindrone Acetate (Co-administration of fosamprenavir calcium with oral contraceptives containing the combination ethinyl estradiol/ norethindrone may lead to decreased levels of amprenavir and ethinyl estradiol. Co-administration of fosamprenavir calcium/ ritonavir with oral contraceptives containing ethinyl estradiol/ norethindrone may lead to decreased levels of ethinyl estradiol. Alternative methods of non-hormonal contraception are recommended. May lead to loss of virologic response. There may be an increased risk of transaminase elevations. No data are available on the use of fosamprenavir/ritonavir with other hormonal therapies, such as hormone replacement therapy (HRT) for postmenopausal women). Products include:
Activella **2561**

Norethynodrel (Co-administration of fosamprenavir calcium with oral contraceptives containing the combination ethinyl estradiol/norethindrone may lead to decreased levels of amprenavir and ethinyl estradiol. Co-administration of fosamprenavir calcium/ ritonavir with oral contraceptives containing ethinyl estradiol/ norethindrone may lead to decreased levels of ethinyl estradiol. Alternative methods of non-hormonal contraception are recommended. May lead to loss of virologic response. There may be an increased risk of transaminase elevations. No data are available on the use of fosamprenavir/ritonavir with other hormonal therapies, such as hormone replacement therapy (HRT) for postmenopausal women).
No products indexed under this heading.

Norfloxacin (Amprenavir is metabolized by CYP3A4. Co-administration of fosamprenavir calcium and drugs that inhibit CYP3A4 may increase amprenavir concentrations and increase the incidence of adverse effects). Products include:
Noroxin **2220**

Norgestimate (Co-administration of fosamprenavir calcium with oral contraceptives containing the combination ethinyl estradiol/norethindrone may lead to decreased levels of amprenavir and ethinyl estradiol. Co-administration of fosamprenavir calcium/ ritonavir with oral contraceptives containing ethinyl estradiol/ norethindrone may lead to decreased levels of ethinyl estradiol. Alternative methods of non-hormonal contraception are recommended. May lead to loss of virologic response. There may be an increased risk of transaminase elevations. No data are available on the use of fosamprenavir/ritonavir with other hormonal therapies, such as hormone replacement therapy (HRT) for postmenopausal women). Products include:
Ortho-Cyclen/Ortho Tri-Cyclen **2663**
Ortho Tri-Cyclen Lo Tablets **2673**

Norgestrel (Co-administration of fosamprenavir calcium with oral contraceptives containing the combination ethinyl estradiol/norethindrone may lead to decreased levels of amprenavir and ethinyl estradiol. Co-administration of fosamprenavir calcium/ ritonavir with oral contraceptives containing ethinyl estradiol/ norethindrone may lead to decreased levels of ethinyl estradiol. Alternative methods of non-hormonal

IMPORTANT NOTE: Always consult each drug listing in the patient's regimen for possible interactions.

contraception are recommended. May lead to loss of virologic response. There may be an increased risk of transaminase elevations. No data are available on the use of fosamprenavir/ritonavir with other hormonal therapies, such as hormone replacement therapy (HRT) for postmenopausal women).
No products indexed under this heading.

Nortriptyline Hydrochloride (Co-administration of tricyclic antidepressants (eg, amitriptyline, imipramine) with fosamprenavir calcium may lead to increased concentrations of the tricyclics. Therapeutic concentration monitoring is recommended for tricyclic antidepressants).
No products indexed under this heading.

Omeprazole (Proton pump inhibitors (eg, esomeprazole, lansoprazole, omeprazole, pantoprazole, rabeprazole) can be administered at the same time as a dose of fosamprenavir calcium with no change in plasma amprenavir concentrations).
No products indexed under this heading.

Omeprazole Magnesium (Proton pump inhibitors (eg, esomeprazole, lansoprazole, omeprazole, pantoprazole, rabeprazole) can be administered at the same time as a dose of fosamprenavir calcium with no change in plasma amprenavir concentrations).
No products indexed under this heading.

Ondansetron (Co-administration with drugs that are highly dependent on CYP3A4 for clearance and for which elevated plasma concentrations are associated with serious and/or life-threatening events are contraindicated).
No products indexed under this heading.

Ondansetron Hydrochloride (Co-administration with drugs that are highly dependent on CYP3A4 for clearance and for which elevated plasma concentrations are associated with serious and/or life-threatening events are contraindicated). Products include:
Zofran Injection **1750**
Zofran **1756**
Zofran ODT **1756**

Oxazepam (Co-administration of benzodiazepines (eg, alprazolam, clorazepate, diazepam, flurazepam) with fosamprenavir calcium may lead to increased concentrations of the benzodiazepines. A decrease in benzodiazepine dose may be needed).
No products indexed under this heading.

Oxcarbazepine (Amprenavir is metabolized by CYP3A4. Co-administration of fosamprenavir calcium and drugs that induce CYP3A4 may decrease amprenavir concentrations and reduce its therapeutic effect).
No products indexed under this heading.

Paclitaxel (Co-administration with drugs that are highly dependent on CYP3A4 for clearance and for which elevated plasma concentrations are associated with serious and/or life-threatening events are contraindicated).
No products indexed under this heading.

Pantoprazole Sodium (Proton pump inhibitors (eg, esomeprazole, lansoprazole, omeprazole, pantoprazole, rabeprazole) can be administered at the same time as a dose of fosamprenavir calcium with no change in plasma amprenavir concentrations). Products include:
Protonix Tablets **3571**
Protonix **3575**

Paroxetine (Co-administration of paroxetine with fosamprenavir calcium/ritonavir may significantly decrease plasma levels of paroxetine. Any paroxetine dose adjustment should be guided by clinical effect (tolerability and efficacy)).
No products indexed under this heading.

Paroxetine Hydrochloride (Co-administration of paroxetine with fosamprenavir calcium/ritonavir may significantly decrease plasma levels of paroxetine. Any paroxetine dose adjustment should be guided by clinical effect (tolerability and efficacy)). Products include:
Paroxetine CR **2361**
Paroxetine ER **2371**
Paxil **1586**
Paxil CR **1596**

Paroxetine Mesylate (Co-administration of paroxetine with fosamprenavir calcium/ritonavir may significantly decrease plasma levels of paroxetine. Any paroxetine dose adjustment should be guided by clinical effect (tolerability and efficacy)).
No products indexed under this heading.

Phenobarbital (Caution must be used when fosamprenavir and anticonvulsants such as phenobarbital are administered concomitantly. Co-administration of phenobarbital with fosamprenavir calcium may lead to decreased amprenavir levels. Fosamprenavir may be less effective due to decreased plasma concentrations in patients taking these agents concomitantly). Products include:
Donnatal **2711**

Phenobarbital Sodium (Caution must be used when fosamprenavir and anticonvulsants such as phenobarbital are administered concomitantly. Co-administration of phenobarbital with fosamprenavir calcium may lead to decreased amprenavir levels. Fosamprenavir may be less effective due to decreased plasma concentrations in patients taking these agents concomitantly).
No products indexed under this heading.

Phenytoin (Caution must be used when fosamprenavir is co-administered with phenytoin. Co-administration of fosamprenavir with phenytoin may decrease amprenavir levels. Fosamprenavir may be less effective due to decreased amprenavir concentrations when taken concomitantly with phenytoin. When phenytoin is co-administered with fosamprenavir/ritonavir, an increase in amprenavir levels and a decrease in phenytoin levels may occur. Plasma phenytoin levels concentrations should be monitored and phenytoin dose should be increased as appropriate. No change in fosamprenavir/ritonavir dose is recommended).
No products indexed under this heading.

Phenytoin Sodium (Caution must be used when fosamprenavir is co-administered with phenytoin. Co-administration of fosamprenavir with phenytoin may decrease amprenavir levels. Fosamprenavir may be less effective due to decreased amprenavir concentrations when taken concomitantly with phenytoin. When phenytoin is co-administered with fosamprenavir/ritonavir, an increase in amprenavir levels and a decrease in phenytoin levels may occur. Plasma phenytoin levels concentrations should be monitored and phenytoin dose should be increased as appropriate. No change in fosamprenavir/ritonavir dose is recommended). Products include:
Phenytek Capsules **2380**

Pimozide (Co-administration of fosamprenavir with pimozide is contraindicated due to potential for serious and/or life-threatening reactions such as cardiac arrhythmias).
No products indexed under this heading.

Pioglitazone Hydrochloride (New onset diabetes mellitus, exacerbation of pre-existing diabetes mellitus, and hyperglycemia have been reported during post-marketing surveillance in HIV-infected patients receiving protease inhibitor therapy. Some patients required either initiation or dose adjustments of insulin or oral hypoglycemic agents for treatment of these events). Products include:
ActoPlus **3338**
Actos **3345**
Duetact **3354**

Polyestradiol Phosphate (Co-administration with drugs that are highly dependent on CYP3A4 for clearance and for which elevated plasma concentrations are associated with serious and/or life-threatening events are contraindicated).
No products indexed under this heading.

Posaconazole (Amprenavir is metabolized by CYP3A4. Co-administration of fosamprenavir calcium and drugs that inhibit CYP3A4 may increase amprenavir concentrations and increase the incidence of adverse effects). Products include:
Noxafil **3172**

Prazepam (Co-administration of benzodiazepines (eg, alprazolam, clorazepate, diazepam, flurazepam) with fosamprenavir calcium may lead to increased concentrations of the benzodiazepines. A decrease in benzodiazepine dose may be needed).
No products indexed under this heading.

Prednisolone (Amprenavir is metabolized by CYP3A4. Co-administration of fosamprenavir calcium and drugs that induce CYP3A4 may decrease amprenavir concentrations and reduce its therapeutic effect).
No products indexed under this heading.

Prednisolone Acetate (Amprenavir is metabolized by CYP3A4. Co-administration of fosamprenavir calcium and drugs that induce CYP3A4 may decrease amprenavir concentrations and reduce its therapeutic effect). Products include:
Blephamide .... ⊙**212**, ⊙**214**
Pred Forte .... ⊙**225**
Pred Mild .... ⊙**230**
Pred-G .... ⊙**226**, ⊙**227**

Prednisolone Sodium Phosphate (Amprenavir is metabolized by CYP3A4. Co-administration of fosamprenavir calcium and drugs that induce CYP3A4 may decrease amprenavir concentrations and reduce its therapeutic effect).
No products indexed under this heading.

Prednisolone Tebutate (Amprenavir is metabolized by CYP3A4. Co-administration of fosamprenavir calcium and drugs that induce CYP3A4 may decrease amprenavir concentrations and reduce its therapeutic effect).
No products indexed under this heading.

Prednisone (Amprenavir is metabolized by CYP3A4. Co-administration of fosamprenavir calcium and drugs that induce CYP3A4 may decrease amprenavir concentrations and reduce its therapeutic effect).
No products indexed under this heading.

Prednisone sodium phosphate (Amprenavir is metabolized by CYP3A4. Co-administration of fosamprenavir calcium and drugs that induce CYP3A4 may decrease amprenavir concentrations and reduce its therapeutic effect).
No products indexed under this heading.

Primidone (Amprenavir is metabolized by CYP3A4. Co-administration of fosamprenavir calcium and drugs that induce CYP3A4 may decrease amprenavir concentrations and reduce its therapeutic effect).
No products indexed under this heading.

Procainamide Hydrochloride (Caution must be used when fosamprenavir calcium is administered concomitantly with antiarrhythmics (eg, amiodarone, bepridil, lidocaine (systemic), quinidine). Co-administration of fosamprenavir calcium with antiarrhythmics may lead to increased levels of antiarrhythmics. Increased exposure may be associated with life-threatening reactions such as cardiac arrhythmias. Therapeutic concentration monitoring is recommended, if available, for antiarrhythmics when co-administered with fosamprenavir).
No products indexed under this heading.

Propafenone Hydrochloride (If fosamprenavir is co-administered with ritonavir, concomitant use of the antiarrhythmic agent propafenone is contraindicated due to the potential for serious and/or life-threatening reactions such as cardiac arrhythmias secondary to increases in plasma concentrations of propafenone). Products include:
Rythmol **1648**
Rythmol SR **1652**

Propoxyphene Hydrochloride (Amprenavir is metabolized by CYP3A4. Co-administration of fosamprenavir calcium and drugs that inhibit CYP3A4 may increase amprenavir concentrations and increase the incidence of adverse effects).
No products indexed under this heading.

Propoxyphene Napsylate (Amprenavir is metabolized by CYP3A4. Co-administration of fosamprenavir calcium and drugs that inhibit CYP3A4 may increase amprenavir concentrations and increase the incidence of adverse effects).
No products indexed under this heading.

Propranolol Hydrochloride (Caution must be used when fosamprenavir calcium is administered concomitantly with antiarrhythmics (eg, amiodarone, bepridil, lidocaine (systemic), quinidine). Co-administration of fosamprenavir calcium with antiarrhythmics may lead to increased levels of antiarrhythmics. Increased exposure may be associated with life-threatening reactions such as cardiac arrhythmias. Therapeutic concentration monitoring is recommended, if available, for antiarrhythmics when co-administered with fosamprenavir). Products include:
InnoPran XL **1517**

Protriptyline Hydrochloride (Co-administration of tricyclic antidepressants (eg, amitriptyline, imipramine) with fosamprenavir calcium may lead to increased concentrations of the tricyclics. Therapeutic concentration monitoring is recommended for tricyclic antidepressants).
No products indexed under this heading.

Quazepam (Co-administration of benzodiazepines (eg, alprazolam, clorazepate, diazepam, flurazepam) with fosamprenavir calcium may lead to increased concentrations of the benzodiazepines. A decrease in benzodiazepine dose may be needed).
No products indexed under this heading.

Quinidine (Caution must be used when fosamprenavir calcium is administered concomitantly with quinidine. Co-administration of fosamprenavir calcium with quinidine may lead to increased levels of quinidine. Increased exposure may be associated with life-threatening reactions such as cardiac arrhythmias. Therapeutic concentration monitoring is recommended for quinidine, if available, when co-administered with fosamprenavir).
No products indexed under this heading.

Quinidine Gluconate (Caution must be used when fosamprenavir calcium is administered concomitantly with quinidine. Co-administration of fosamprenavir calcium with quinidine may lead to increased levels of quinidine. Increased exposure may be associated with life-threatening reactions such as cardiac arrhythmias. Therapeutic con-

centration monitoring is recommended for quinidine, if available, when co-administered with fosamprenavir).
No products indexed under this heading.

Quinidine Hydrochloride (Caution must be used when fosamprenavir calcium is administered concomitantly with quinidine. Co-administration of fosamprenavir calcium with quinidine may lead to increased levels of quinidine. Increased exposure may be associated with life-threatening reactions such as cardiac arrhythmias. Therapeutic concentration monitoring is recommended for quinidine, if available, when co-administered with fosamprenavir).
No products indexed under this heading.

Quinidine Polygalacturonate (Caution must be used when fosamprenavir calcium is administered concomitantly with quinidine. Co-administration of fosamprenavir calcium with quinidine may lead to increased levels of quinidine. Increased exposure may be associated with life-threatening reactions such as cardiac arrhythmias. Therapeutic concentration monitoring is recommended for quinidine, if available, when co-administered with fosamprenavir).
No products indexed under this heading.

Quinidine Sulfate (Caution must be used when fosamprenavir calcium is administered concomitantly with quinidine. Co-administration of fosamprenavir calcium with quinidine may lead to increased levels of quinidine. Increased exposure may be associated with life-threatening reactions such as cardiac arrhythmias. Therapeutic concentration monitoring is recommended for quinidine, if available, when co-administered with fosamprenavir).
No products indexed under this heading.

Quinine (Amprenavir is metabolized by CYP3A4. Co-administration of fosamprenavir calcium and drugs that inhibit CYP3A4 may increase amprenavir concentrations and increase the incidence of adverse effects). Products include:
Hyland's Leg Cramps PM with Quinine **3315**

Quinine Sulfate (Amprenavir is metabolized by CYP3A4. Co-administration of fosamprenavir calcium and drugs that inhibit CYP3A4 may increase amprenavir concentrations and increase the incidence of adverse effects).
No products indexed under this heading.

Quinupristin (Amprenavir is metabolized by CYP3A4. Co-administration of fosamprenavir calcium and drugs that inhibit CYP3A4 may increase amprenavir concentrations and increase the incidence of adverse effects).
No products indexed under this heading.

Rabeprazole Sodium (Proton pump inhibitors (eg, esomeprazole, lansoprazole, omeprazole, pantoprazole, rabeprazole) can be administered at the same time as a dose of fosamprenavir calcium with no change in plasma amprenavir concentrations). Products include:
Aciphex **1035**

Ranitidine Bismuth Citrate (Co-administration of fosamprenavir and the histamine H_2-receptor antagonist ranitidine may lead to decreased levels of amprenavir. Caution must be used during co-administration because fosamprenavir may be less effective due to decreased amprenavir plasma concentrations in patients taking ranitidine concomitantly).
No products indexed under this heading.

Ranitidine Hydrochloride (Co-administration of fosamprenavir and the histamine H_2-receptor antagonist ranitidine may lead to decreased levels of amprenavir. Caution must be used during co-administration because fosamprenavir may be less effective due to decreased amprenavir plasma concentrations in patients taking ranitidine concomitantly). Products include:
Zantac **1737**
Zantac Injection **1732**
Zantac Pharmacy **1735**

Rapamycin (Co-administration of fosamprenavir calcium with the immunosuppressant rapamycin may lead to increased levels of rapamycin. Therapeutic concentration monitoring is recommended for rapamycin when co-administered with fosamprenavir).
No products indexed under this heading.

Repaglinide (New onset diabetes mellitus, exacerbation of pre-existing diabetes mellitus, and hyperglycemia have been reported during post-marketing surveillance in HIV-infected patients receiving protease inhibitor therapy. Some patients required either initiation or dose adjustments of insulin or oral hypoglycemic agents for treatment of these events).
No products indexed under this heading.

Rifabutin (Co-administration of fosamprenavir calcium with rifabutin may cause increased levels of rifabutin and its metabolite. A complete blood count should be performed weekly and as clinically indicated in order to monitor for neutropenia in patients receiving concurrent administration. In patients receiving fosamprenavir alone, a dosage reduction of rifabutin by at least half the recommended dose is required. In patients receiving fosamprenavir/ritonavir combination, dosage reduction of rifabutin by at least 75% of the usual dose of 300 mg/day is recommended (maximum dose of 150 mg every other day or three times weekly)).
No products indexed under this heading.

Rifampicin (Amprenavir is metabolized by CYP3A4. Co-administration of fosamprenavir calcium and drugs that induce CYP3A4 may decrease amprenavir concentrations and reduce its therapeutic effect).
No products indexed under this heading.

Rifampin (Co-administration of fosamprenavir calcium with rifampin is contraindicated because it may lead to loss of virologic response and possible resistance to fosamprenavir or other protease inhibitors).
No products indexed under this heading.

Rifapentine (Amprenavir is metabolized by CYP3A4. Co-administration of fosamprenavir calcium and drugs that induce CYP3A4 may decrease amprenavir concentrations and reduce its therapeutic effect).
No products indexed under this heading.

Ritonavir (Co-administration of lopinavir/ritonavir and fosamprenavir may lead to decreased levels of amprenavir and lopinavir (when given in combination with ritonavir). An increased rate of adverse events has also been observed with co-administration of these medications. Higher than approved dose combinations of fosamprenavir calcium and ritonavir are not recommended due to an increased risk of transaminase elevations). Products include:
Kaletra **458**
Norvir **509**

Rosiglitazone Maleate (New onset diabetes mellitus, exacerbation of pre-existing diabetes mellitus, and hyperglycemia have been reported during post-marketing surveillance in HIV-infected patients receiving protease inhibitor therapy. Some patients required either initiation or dose adjustments of insulin or oral hypoglycemic agents for treatment of these events). Products include:
Avandamet **1345**
Avandaryl **1356**
Avandia **1366**

Rosuvastatin Calcium (Co-administration of fosamprenavir calcium with rosuvastatin may lead to increased rosuvastatin levels. Use the lowest possible dose of rosuvastatin with careful monitoring, or consider other HMG-CoA reductase inhibitors such as fluvastatin or pravastatin). Products include:
Crestor **736**

Saquinavir (Co-administration of fosamprenavir calcium with saquinavir may lead to decreased levels of amprenavir. The effect on saquinavir is not well established).
No products indexed under this heading.

Saquinavir Mesylate (Co-administration of fosamprenavir calcium with saquinavir may lead to decreased levels of amprenavir. The effect on saquinavir is not well established).
No products indexed under this heading.

Sertraline Hydrochloride (Co-administration with drugs that are highly dependent on CYP3A4 for clearance and for which elevated plasma concentrations are associated with serious and/or life-threatening events are contraindicated).
No products indexed under this heading.

Sildenafil Citrate (Co-administration of fosamprenavir calcium with sildenafil may lead to increased levels of sildenafil. Concomitant use may result in an increase in PDE5 inhibitor-associated adverse events, including hypotension, visual changes, and priapism. When co-administered with fosamprenavir alone or in combination with ritonavir, sildenafil dosage should be 25 mg every 48 hours).
No products indexed under this heading.

Simvastatin (Co-administration of fosamprenavir calcium with simvastatin is contraindicated due to the potential for serious reactions such as risk of myopathy including rhabdomyolysis).
Products include:
Simcor **524**
Vytorin 10/10 .... **2303, 3240**
Vytorin 10/20 .... **2303, 3240**
Vytorin 10/40 .... **2303, 3240**
Vytorin 10/80 .... **2303, 3240**
Zocor **2289**

Sirolimus (Co-administration of fosamprenavir calcium with immunosuppressants (eg, cyclosporine, tacrolimus, rapamycin) may lead to increased levels of immunosuppressants. Therapeutic concentration monitoring is recommended for immunosuppressant agents when co-administered with fosamprenavir). Products include:
Rapamune **3579**

Sitagliptin Phosphate (New onset diabetes mellitus, exacerbation of pre-existing diabetes mellitus, and hyperglycemia have been reported during post-marketing surveillance in HIV-infected patients receiving protease inhibitor therapy. Some patients required either initiation or dose adjustments of insulin or oral hypoglycemic agents for treatment of these events). Products include:
Janumet **2188**
Januvia **2196**

Sotalol Hydrochloride (Caution must be used when fosamprenavir calcium is administered concomitantly with antiarrhythmics (eg, amiodarone, bepridil, lidocaine (systemic), quinidine). Co-administration of fosamprenavir calcium with antiarrhythmics may lead to increased levels of antiarrhythmics. Increased exposure may be associated with life-threatening reactions such as cardiac arrhythmias. Therapeutic concentration monitoring is recommended, if available, for antiarrhythmics when co-administered with fosamprenavir).
No products indexed under this heading.

Sulfinpyrazone (Amprenavir is metabolized by CYP3A4. Co-administration of fosamprenavir calcium and drugs that induce CYP3A4 may decrease amprenavir concentrations and reduce its therapeutic effect).
No products indexed under this heading.

Tacrolimus (Co-administration of fosamprenavir calcium with the immunosuppressant tacrolimus may lead to increased levels of tacrolimus. Therapeutic concentration monitoring is recommended for tacrolimus when co-administered with fosamprenavir).
Products include:
Prograf Capsules **677**
Prograf Injection **677**
Protopic **685**

Tadalafil (Co-administration of fosamprenavir calcium with tadalafil may lead to increased levels of tadalafil. Concomitant use may result in an increase in PDE5 inhibitor-associated adverse events, including hypotension, visual changes, and priapism. When co-administered with fosamprenavir alone or in combination with ritonavir, tadalafil dosage should be no more than 10 mg every 72 hours). Products include:
Adcirca **3461**
Cialis **1861**

Tamoxifen Citrate (Co-administration with drugs that are highly dependent on CYP3A4 for clearance and for which elevated plasma concentrations are associated with serious and/or life-threatening events are contraindicated).
No products indexed under this heading.

Telithromycin (Amprenavir is metabolized by CYP3A4. Co-administration of fosamprenavir calcium and drugs that inhibit CYP3A4 may increase amprenavir concentrations and increase the incidence of adverse effects).
Products include:
Ketek **2991**

Temazepam (Co-administration of benzodiazepines (eg, alprazolam, clorazepate, diazepam, flurazepam) with fosamprenavir calcium may lead to increased concentrations of the benzodiazepines. A decrease in benzodiazepine dose may be needed).
No products indexed under this heading.

Terfenadine (Co-administration with drugs that are highly dependent on CYP3A4 for clearance and for which elevated plasma concentrations are associated with serious and/or life-threatening events are contraindicated).
No products indexed under this heading.

Theophyllinate (Amprenavir is metabolized by CYP3A4. Co-administration of fosamprenavir calcium and drugs that induce CYP3A4 may decrease amprenavir concentrations and reduce its therapeutic effect).
No products indexed under this heading.

Theophylline (Co-administration with drugs that are highly dependent on CYP3A4 for clearance and for which elevated plasma concentrations are associated with serious and/or life-threatening events are contraindicated).
No products indexed under this heading.

Theophylline Anhydrous (Co-administration with drugs that are highly dependent on CYP3A4 for clearance and for which elevated plasma concentrations are associated with serious and/or life-threatening events are contraindicated). Products include:
Uniphyl **2817**

Theophylline Calcium Salicylate (Co-administration with drugs that are highly dependent on CYP3A4 for clearance and for which elevated plasma concentrations are associated with serious and/or life-threatening events are contraindicated).
No products indexed under this heading.

Theophylline Dihydroxypropyl (Glyceryl) (Co-administration with drugs that are highly dependent on CYP3A4 for clearance and for which elevated plasma concentrations are associated with serious and/or life-threatening events are contraindicated).
No products indexed under this heading.

Theophylline Ethylenediamine (Co-administration with drugs that are highly dependent on CYP3A4 for clearance and for which elevated plasma concentrations are associated with serious and/or life-threatening events are contraindicated).
No products indexed under this heading.

Theophylline Sodium Glycinate (Co-administration with drugs that are highly dependent on CYP3A4 for clearance and for which elevated plasma concentrations are associated with serious and/or life-threatening events are contraindicated).
No products indexed under this heading.

Tiagabine Hydrochloride (Co-administration with drugs that are highly dependent on CYP3A4 for clearance and for which elevated plasma concentrations are associated with serious and/or life-threatening events are contraindicated). Products include:
Gabitril 972

Tocainide Hydrochloride (Caution must be used when fosamprenavir calcium is administered concomitantly with antiarrhythmics (eg, amiodarone, bepridil, lidocaine (systemic), quinidine). Co-administration of fosamprenavir calcium with antiarrhythmics may lead to increased levels of antiarrhythmics. Increased exposure may be associated with life-threatening reactions such as cardiac arrhythmias. Therapeutic concentration monitoring is recommended, if available, for antiarrhythmics when co-administered with fosamprenavir).
No products indexed under this heading.

Tolazamide (New onset diabetes mellitus, exacerbation of pre-existing diabetes mellitus, and hyperglycemia have been reported during post-marketing surveillance in HIV-infected patients receiving protease inhibitor therapy. Some patients required either initiation or dose adjustments of insulin or oral hypoglycemic agents for treatment of these events).
No products indexed under this heading.

Tolbutamide (New onset diabetes mellitus, exacerbation of pre-existing diabetes mellitus, and hyperglycemia have been reported during post-marketing surveillance in HIV-infected patients receiving protease inhibitor therapy. Some patients required either initiation or dose adjustments of insulin or oral hypoglycemic agents for treatment of these events).
No products indexed under this heading.

Tolterodine Tartrate (Co-administration with drugs that are highly dependent on CYP3A4 for clearance and for which elevated plasma concentrations are associated with serious and/or life-threatening events are contraindicated).
No products indexed under this heading.

Trazodone Hydrochloride (Concomitant use of trazodone and fosamprenavir calcium with or without ritonavir may increase plasma concentrations of trazodone. Adverse events of nausea, dizziness, hypotension, and syncope have been observed following co-administration of trazodone and ritonavir. If trazodone is used with a CYP3A4 inhibitor such as fosamprenavir calcium, the combination should be used with caution and a lower dose of trazodone should be considered).
No products indexed under this heading.

Triamcinolone (Amprenavir is metabolized by CYP3A4. Co-administration of fosamprenavir calcium and drugs that induce CYP3A4 may decrease amprenavir concentrations and reduce its therapeutic effect).
No products indexed under this heading.

Triamcinolone Acetonide (Amprenavir is metabolized by CYP3A4. Co-administration of fosamprenavir calcium and drugs that induce CYP3A4 may decrease amprenavir concentrations and reduce its therapeutic effect). Products include:
Azmacort 408
Nasacort AQ 3019

Triamcinolone Diacetate (Amprenavir is metabolized by CYP3A4. Co-administration of fosamprenavir calcium and drugs that induce CYP3A4 may decrease amprenavir concentrations and reduce its therapeutic effect).
No products indexed under this heading.

Triamcinolone Hexacetonide (Amprenavir is metabolized by CYP3A4. Co-administration of fosamprenavir calcium and drugs that induce CYP3A4 may decrease amprenavir concentrations and reduce its therapeutic effect).
No products indexed under this heading.

Triazolam (Co-administration of fosamprenavir calcium with triazolam is contraindicated due to potential for serious and/or life-threatening reactions such as prolonged or increased sedation or respiratory depression).
No products indexed under this heading.

Trimipramine Maleate (Co-administration of tricyclic antidepressants (eg, amitriptyline, imipramine) with fosamprenavir calcium may lead to increased concentrations of the tricyclics. Therapeutic concentration monitoring is recommended for tricyclic antidepressants).
No products indexed under this heading.

Troglitazone (New onset diabetes mellitus, exacerbation of pre-existing diabetes mellitus, and hyperglycemia have been reported during post-marketing surveillance in HIV-infected patients receiving protease inhibitor therapy. Some patients required either initiation or dose adjustments of insulin or oral hypoglycemic agents for treatment of these events).
No products indexed under this heading.

Troleandomycin (Amprenavir is metabolized by CYP3A4. Co-administration of fosamprenavir calcium and drugs that inhibit CYP3A4 may increase amprenavir concentrations and increase the incidence of adverse effects).
No products indexed under this heading.

Valproate Sodium (Amprenavir is metabolized by CYP3A4. Co-administration of fosamprenavir calcium and drugs that inhibit CYP3A4 may increase amprenavir concentrations and increase the incidence of adverse effects).
No products indexed under this heading.

Vardenafil Hydrochloride (Co-administration of fosamprenavir calcium with vardenafil may lead to increased levels of vardenafil. Concomitant use may result in an increase in PDE5 inhibitor-associated adverse events, including hypotension, visual changes, and priapism. When co-administered with fosamprenavir alone, vardenafil dosage should be no more than 2.5 mg every 24 hours. If co-administered with fosamprenavir/ritonavir combination, the vardenafil dosage should be no more than 2.5 mg every 72 hours). Products include:
Levitra 3157

Verapamil Hydrochloride (Co-administration of fosamprenavir calcium

with the calcium channel blocker verapamil may increase levels of verapamil. Caution is warranted and clinical monitoring is recommended). Products include:
Tarka 534

Vinblastine Sulfate (Co-administration with drugs that are highly dependent on CYP3A4 for clearance and for which elevated plasma concentrations are associated with serious and/or life-threatening events are contraindicated).
No products indexed under this heading.

Vincristine Sulfate (Co-administration with drugs that are highly dependent on CYP3A4 for clearance and for which elevated plasma concentrations are associated with serious and/or life-threatening events are contraindicated).
No products indexed under this heading.

Voriconazole (Amprenavir is metabolized by CYP3A4. Co-administration of fosamprenavir calcium and drugs that inhibit CYP3A4 may increase amprenavir concentrations and increase the incidence of adverse effects).
No products indexed under this heading.

Warfarin Sodium (Concentrations of warfarin may be affected when co-administered with fosamprenavir. It is recommended that INR (International Normalized Ratio) be monitored).
No products indexed under this heading.

Zafirlukast (Amprenavir is metabolized by CYP3A4. Co-administration of fosamprenavir calcium and drugs that inhibit CYP3A4 may increase amprenavir concentrations and increase the incidence of adverse effects). Products include:
Accolate 3612

Zileuton (Amprenavir is metabolized by CYP3A4. Co-administration of fosamprenavir calcium and drugs that inhibit CYP3A4 may increase amprenavir concentrations and increase the incidence of adverse effects).
No products indexed under this heading.

Food Interactions

Grapefruit (Amprenavir is metabolized by CYP3A4. Co-administration of fosamprenavir calcium and drugs that inhibit CYP3A4 may increase amprenavir concentrations and increase the incidence of adverse effects).

Grapefruit Juice (Amprenavir is metabolized by CYP3A4. Co-administration of fosamprenavir calcium and drugs that inhibit CYP3A4 may increase amprenavir concentrations and increase the incidence of adverse effects).

LIALDA TABLETS

(Mesalamine) 3295
May interact with nephrotoxic agents, non-steroidal anti-inflammatory agents, and certain other agents. Compounds in these categories include:

Abacavir Sulfate (The concurrent use of mesalamine with known nephrotoxic agents, may increase the risk of renal reactions). Products include:
Epzicom 1448
Trizivir 1688
Ziagen 1740

Acyclovir (The concurrent use of mesalamine with known nephrotoxic agents, may increase the risk of renal reactions). Products include:
Zovirax 1760

Acyclovir Sodium (The concurrent use of mesalamine with known nephrotoxic agents, may increase the risk of renal reactions).
No products indexed under this heading.

Alatrofloxacin Mesylate (The concurrent use of mesalamine with known nephrotoxic agents, may increase the risk of renal reactions).
No products indexed under this heading.

Aldesleukin (The concurrent use of mesalamine with known nephrotoxic agents, may increase the risk of renal reactions). Products include:
Proleukin 2504

Amikacin Sulfate (The concurrent use of mesalamine with known nephrotoxic agents, may increase the risk of renal reactions).
No products indexed under this heading.

Amoxicillin (The concurrent use of mesalamine with known nephrotoxic agents, may increase the risk of renal reactions). Products include:
Amoxil Capsules 1311
Amoxil Chewable Tablets 1311
Amoxil 1311
Amoxil Powder 1311
Augmentin 1331
Augmentin Tablets 1335
Augmentin ES-600 1338
Augmentin XR 1342
Moxatag 2321

Amoxicillin Trihydrate (The concurrent use of mesalamine with known nephrotoxic agents, may increase the risk of renal reactions).
No products indexed under this heading.

Amphotericin B (The concurrent use of mesalamine with known nephrotoxic agents, may increase the risk of renal reactions).
No products indexed under this heading.

Amphotericin B, liposomal (The concurrent use of mesalamine with known nephrotoxic agents, may increase the risk of renal reactions). Products include:
AmBisome 659

Amphotericin B Cholesteryl Sulfate (The concurrent use of mesalamine with known nephrotoxic agents, may increase the risk of renal reactions).
No products indexed under this heading.

Amphotericin B Lipid Complex (The concurrent use of mesalamine with known nephrotoxic agents, may increase the risk of renal reactions).
No products indexed under this heading.

Ampicillin (The concurrent use of mesalamine with known nephrotoxic agents, may increase the risk of renal reactions).
No products indexed under this heading.

Ampicillin Sodium (The concurrent use of mesalamine with known nephrotoxic agents, may increase the risk of renal reactions).
No products indexed under this heading.

Ampicillin Trihydrate (The concurrent use of mesalamine with known nephrotoxic agents, may increase the risk of renal reactions).
No products indexed under this heading.

Amprenavir (The concurrent use of mesalamine with known nephrotoxic agents, may increase the risk of renal reactions).
No products indexed under this heading.

Aspirin (The concurrent use of mesalamine with known nephrotoxic agents, may increase the risk of renal reactions). Products include:
Aggrenox 880
Bayer Aspirin 829
Percodan 1124
St. Joseph Aspirin 2045

Atazanavir (The concurrent use of mesalamine with known nephrotoxic agents, may increase the risk of renal reactions).
No products indexed under this heading.

Atorvastatin Calcium (The concurrent use of mesalamine with known

IMPORTANT NOTE: Always consult each drug listing in the patient's regimen for possible interactions.

(⊙ Described in PDR® for Ophthalmic Medicines)

1049 Interactions Index Lialda

Methyclothiazide (The concurrent use of mesalamine with known nephrotoxic agents, may increase the risk of renal reactions).
No products indexed under this heading.

Mezlocillin Sodium (The concurrent use of mesalamine with known nephrotoxic agents, may increase the risk of renal reactions).
No products indexed under this heading.

Minocycline Hydrochloride (The concurrent use of mesalamine with known nephrotoxic agents, may increase the risk of renal reactions). Products include:
Solodyn ... 2073

Mitomycin (Mitomycin-C) (The concurrent use of mesalamine with known nephrotoxic agents, may increase the risk of renal reactions).
No products indexed under this heading.

Moexipril Hydrochloride (The concurrent use of mesalamine with known nephrotoxic agents, may increase the risk of renal reactions).
No products indexed under this heading.

Muromonab-CD3 (The concurrent use of mesalamine with known nephrotoxic agents, may increase the risk of renal reactions). Products include:
Orthoclone OKT3 ... 949

Nabumetone (The concurrent use of mesalamine with known nephrotoxic agents, including non-steroidal anti-inflammatory drugs (NSAIDs) may increase the risk of renal reactions).
No products indexed under this heading.

Nafcillin Sodium (The concurrent use of mesalamine with known nephrotoxic agents, may increase the risk of renal reactions).
No products indexed under this heading.

Naproxen (The concurrent use of mesalamine with known nephrotoxic agents, including non-steroidal anti-inflammatory drugs (NSAIDs) may increase the risk of renal reactions). Products include:
EC-Naprosyn ... 2850
Naprosyn ... 2850
Anaprox/Naprosyn ... 2850

Naproxen Sodium (The concurrent use of mesalamine with known nephrotoxic agents, including non-steroidal anti-inflammatory drugs (NSAIDs) may increase the risk of renal reactions). Products include:
Anaprox ... 2850
Anaprox DS ... 2850
Treximet ... 1681

Nelfinavir Mesylate (The concurrent use of mesalamine with known nephrotoxic agents, may increase the risk of renal reactions).
No products indexed under this heading.

Neomycin (The concurrent use of mesalamine with known nephrotoxic agents, may increase the risk of renal reactions).
No products indexed under this heading.

Neomycin, oral (The concurrent use of mesalamine with known nephrotoxic agents, may increase the risk of renal reactions).
No products indexed under this heading.

Neomycin Sulfate (The concurrent use of mesalamine with known nephrotoxic agents, may increase the risk of renal reactions).
No products indexed under this heading.

Nevirapine (The concurrent use of mesalamine with known nephrotoxic agents, may increase the risk of renal reactions). Products include:
Viramune Oral Suspension ... 897
Viramune Tablets ... 897

Norfloxacin (The concurrent use of mesalamine with known nephrotoxic agents, may increase the risk of renal reactions). Products include:
Noroxin ... 2220

Olsalazine Sodium (The concurrent use of mesalamine with known nephrotoxic agents, may increase the risk of renal reactions).
No products indexed under this heading.

Omeprazole (The concurrent use of mesalamine with known nephrotoxic agents, may increase the risk of renal reactions).
No products indexed under this heading.

Oxaprozin (The concurrent use of mesalamine with known nephrotoxic agents, including non-steroidal anti-inflammatory drugs (NSAIDs) may increase the risk of renal reactions).
No products indexed under this heading.

Pamidronate Disodium (The concurrent use of mesalamine with known nephrotoxic agents, may increase the risk of renal reactions).
No products indexed under this heading.

Paroxetine Hydrochloride (The concurrent use of mesalamine with known nephrotoxic agents, may increase the risk of renal reactions). Products include:
Paroxetine CR ... 2361
Paroxetine ER ... 2371
Paxil ... 1586
Paxil CR ... 1596

Penicillamine (The concurrent use of mesalamine with known nephrotoxic agents, may increase the risk of renal reactions).
No products indexed under this heading.

Penicillin G Benzathine (The concurrent use of mesalamine with known nephrotoxic agents, may increase the risk of renal reactions). Products include:
Bicillin C-R Injectable Suspension ... 1826
Bicillin L-A ... 1828

Penicillin G Potassium (The concurrent use of mesalamine with known nephrotoxic agents, may increase the risk of renal reactions).
No products indexed under this heading.

Penicillin G Procaine (The concurrent use of mesalamine with known nephrotoxic agents, may increase the risk of renal reactions). Products include:
Bicillin C-R Injectable Suspension ... 1826
Bicillin L-A ... 1828

Penicillin G Sodium (The concurrent use of mesalamine with known nephrotoxic agents, may increase the risk of renal reactions).
No products indexed under this heading.

Penicillin V Potassium (The concurrent use of mesalamine with known nephrotoxic agents, may increase the risk of renal reactions).
No products indexed under this heading.

Pentamidine Isethionate (The concurrent use of mesalamine with known nephrotoxic agents, may increase the risk of renal reactions).
No products indexed under this heading.

Perindopril Erbumine (The concurrent use of mesalamine with known nephrotoxic agents, may increase the risk of renal reactions).
No products indexed under this heading.

Phenylbutazone (The concurrent use of mesalamine with known nephrotoxic agents, including non-steroidal anti-inflammatory drugs (NSAIDs) may increase the risk of renal reactions).
No products indexed under this heading.

Piroxicam (The concurrent use of mesalamine with known nephrotoxic agents, including non-steroidal anti-inflammatory drugs (NSAIDs) may increase the risk of renal reactions).
No products indexed under this heading.

Plicamycin (The concurrent use of mesalamine with known nephrotoxic agents, may increase the risk of renal reactions).
No products indexed under this heading.

Polymyxin (The concurrent use of mesalamine with known nephrotoxic agents, may increase the risk of renal reactions).
No products indexed under this heading.

Polymyxin B Sulfate (The concurrent use of mesalamine with known nephrotoxic agents, may increase the risk of renal reactions).
No products indexed under this heading.

Polythiazide (The concurrent use of mesalamine with known nephrotoxic agents, may increase the risk of renal reactions).
No products indexed under this heading.

Pravastatin Sodium (The concurrent use of mesalamine with known nephrotoxic agents, may increase the risk of renal reactions).
No products indexed under this heading.

Quinapril Hydrochloride (The concurrent use of mesalamine with known nephrotoxic agents, may increase the risk of renal reactions).
No products indexed under this heading.

Rabeprazole Sodium (The concurrent use of mesalamine with known nephrotoxic agents, may increase the risk of renal reactions). Products include:
Aciphex ... 1035

Ramipril (The concurrent use of mesalamine with known nephrotoxic agents, may increase the risk of renal reactions).
No products indexed under this heading.

Rifampin (The concurrent use of mesalamine with known nephrotoxic agents, may increase the risk of renal reactions).
No products indexed under this heading.

Riluzole (The concurrent use of mesalamine with known nephrotoxic agents, may increase the risk of renal reactions). Products include:
Rilutek ... 3032

Ritonavir (The concurrent use of mesalamine with known nephrotoxic agents, may increase the risk of renal reactions). Products include:
Kaletra ... 458
Norvir ... 509

Rofecoxib (The concurrent use of mesalamine with known nephrotoxic agents, including non-steroidal anti-inflammatory drugs (NSAIDs) may increase the risk of renal reactions).
No products indexed under this heading.

Saquinavir (The concurrent use of mesalamine with known nephrotoxic agents, may increase the risk of renal reactions).
No products indexed under this heading.

Sibutramine Hydrochloride Monohydrate (The concurrent use of mesalamine with known nephrotoxic agents, may increase the risk of renal reactions). Products include:
Meridia ... 492

Simvastatin (The concurrent use of mesalamine with known nephrotoxic agents, may increase the risk of renal reactions). Products include:
Simcor ... 524
Vytorin 10/10 ... 2303, 3240
Vytorin 10/20 ... 2303, 3240
Vytorin 10/40 ... 2303, 3240
Vytorin 10/80 ... 2303, 3240
Zocor ... 2289

Spirapril Hydrochloride (The concurrent use of mesalamine with known nephrotoxic agents, may increase the risk of renal reactions).
No products indexed under this heading.

Stavudine (The concurrent use of mesalamine with known nephrotoxic agents, may increase the risk of renal reactions).
No products indexed under this heading.

Streptomycin Sulfate (The concurrent use of mesalamine with known nephrotoxic agents, may increase the risk of renal reactions).
No products indexed under this heading.

Streptozocin (The concurrent use of mesalamine with known nephrotoxic agents, may increase the risk of renal reactions).
No products indexed under this heading.

Sulfacytine (The concurrent use of mesalamine with known nephrotoxic agents, may increase the risk of renal reactions).
No products indexed under this heading.

Sulfamethizole (The concurrent use of mesalamine with known nephrotoxic agents, may increase the risk of renal reactions).
No products indexed under this heading.

Sulfamethoxazole (The concurrent use of mesalamine with known nephrotoxic agents, may increase the risk of renal reactions).
No products indexed under this heading.

Sulfasalazine (The concurrent use of mesalamine with known nephrotoxic agents, may increase the risk of renal reactions).
No products indexed under this heading.

Sulfinpyrazone (The concurrent use of mesalamine with known nephrotoxic agents, may increase the risk of renal reactions).
No products indexed under this heading.

Sulfisoxazole Acetyl (The concurrent use of mesalamine with known nephrotoxic agents, may increase the risk of renal reactions).
No products indexed under this heading.

Sulfisoxazole Diolamine (The concurrent use of mesalamine with known nephrotoxic agents, may increase the risk of renal reactions).
No products indexed under this heading.

Sulindac (The concurrent use of mesalamine with known nephrotoxic agents, including non-steroidal anti-inflammatory drugs (NSAIDs) may increase the risk of renal reactions). Products include:
Clinoril ... 2098

Tacrolimus (The concurrent use of mesalamine with known nephrotoxic agents, may increase the risk of renal reactions). Products include:
Prograf Capsules ... 677
Prograf Injection ... 677
Protopic ... 685

Tenofovir Disoproxil Fumarate (The concurrent use of mesalamine with known nephrotoxic agents, may increase the risk of renal reactions). Products include:
Atripla ... 906
Truvada ... 1258
Viread ... 1266

Thioguanine (The concurrent use of mesalamine with known nephrotoxic agents, may increase the risk of renal reactions). Products include:
Tabloid ... 1664

Ticarcillin Disodium (The concurrent use of mesalamine with known nephrotoxic agents, may increase the risk of renal reactions). Products include:
Timentin ADD-Vantage ... 1670
Timentin Galaxy ... 1674
Timentin ... 1666
Timentin Pharmacy ... 1678

Tobramycin (The concurrent use of mesalamine with known nephrotoxic agents, may increase the risk of renal reactions). Products include:

IMPORTANT NOTE: Always consult each drug listing in the patient's regimen for possible interactions.

Tobi Nebulizer 2546
Tobramycin and Dexamethasone
   Ophthalmic Suspension............... ⊙251
Zylet .... ⊙252

Tobramycin Sulfate (The concurrent use of mesalamine with known nephrotoxic agents, may increase the risk of renal reactions).
   No products indexed under this heading.

Tolazamide (The concurrent use of mesalamine with known nephrotoxic agents, may increase the risk of renal reactions).
   No products indexed under this heading.

Tolbutamide (The concurrent use of mesalamine with known nephrotoxic agents, may increase the risk of renal reactions).
   No products indexed under this heading.

Tolmetin Sodium (The concurrent use of mesalamine with known nephrotoxic agents, including non-steroidal anti-inflammatory drugs (NSAIDs) may increase the risk of renal reactions).
   No products indexed under this heading.

Trandolapril (The concurrent use of mesalamine with known nephrotoxic agents, may increase the risk of renal reactions). Products include:
   Mavik 489
   Tarka 534

Triamterene (The concurrent use of mesalamine with known nephrotoxic agents, may increase the risk of renal reactions). Products include:
   Dyazide 1429
   Dyrenium 3495

Trimethadione (The concurrent use of mesalamine with known nephrotoxic agents, may increase the risk of renal reactions).
   No products indexed under this heading.

Trovafloxacin Mesylate (The concurrent use of mesalamine with known nephrotoxic agents, may increase the risk of renal reactions).
   No products indexed under this heading.

Tyropanoate Sodium (The concurrent use of mesalamine with known nephrotoxic agents, may increase the risk of renal reactions).
   No products indexed under this heading.

Valacyclovir Hydrochloride (The concurrent use of mesalamine with known nephrotoxic agents, may increase the risk of renal reactions). Products include:
   Valtrex 1702

Valdecoxib (The concurrent use of mesalamine with known nephrotoxic agents, including non-steroidal anti-inflammatory drugs (NSAIDs) may increase the risk of renal reactions).
   No products indexed under this heading.

Vancomycin Hydrochloride (The concurrent use of mesalamine with known nephrotoxic agents, may increase the risk of renal reactions).
   No products indexed under this heading.

Voriconazole (The concurrent use of mesalamine with known nephrotoxic agents, may increase the risk of renal reactions).
   No products indexed under this heading.

Zalcitabine (The concurrent use of mesalamine with known nephrotoxic agents, may increase the risk of renal reactions).
   No products indexed under this heading.

Zidovudine (The concurrent use of mesalamine with known nephrotoxic agents, may increase the risk of renal reactions). Products include:
   Combivir 1404
   Retrovir 1634
   Retrovir IV 1640
   Trizivir 1688

Zoledronic Acid (The concurrent use of mesalamine with known nephrotoxic agents, may increase the risk of renal reactions). Products include:
   Reclast 2509
   Zometa 2554

LIDODERM PATCH

(Lidocaine) 1107
May interact with class 1A antiarrhythmics, local anesthetics, and certain other agents. Compounds in these categories include:

Articaine Hydrochloride (When used concomitantly with other products containing local anesthetic agents, the amount absorbed from all formulations must be considered).
   No products indexed under this heading.

Bupivacaine Hydrochloride (When used concomitantly with other products containing local anesthetic agents, the amount absorbed from all formulations must be considered).
   No products indexed under this heading.

Chloroprocaine Hydrochloride (When used concomitantly with other products containing local anesthetic agents, the amount absorbed from all formulations must be considered).
   No products indexed under this heading.

Cocaine Hydrochloride (When used concomitantly with other products containing local anesthetic agents, the amount absorbed from all formulations must be considered).
   No products indexed under this heading.

Disopyramide (Should be used with caution in patients receiving Class I antiarrhythmic drugs since the toxic effects are additive and potentially synergistic).
   No products indexed under this heading.

Disopyramide Phosphate (Should be used with caution in patients receiving Class I antiarrhythmic drugs since the toxic effects are additive and potentially synergistic).
   No products indexed under this heading.

Etidocaine Hydrochloride (When used concomitantly with other products containing local anesthetic agents, the amount absorbed from all formulations must be considered).
   No products indexed under this heading.

Levobupivacaine Hydrochloride (When used concomitantly with other products containing local anesthetic agents, the amount absorbed from all formulations must be considered).
   No products indexed under this heading.

Lidocaine Hydrochloride (When used concomitantly with other products containing local anesthetic agents, the amount absorbed from all formulations must be considered).
   No products indexed under this heading.

Mepivacaine Hydrochloride (When used concomitantly with other products containing local anesthetic agents, the amount absorbed from all formulations must be considered).
   No products indexed under this heading.

Mexiletine Hydrochloride (Co-administration in patients receiving Class-1 antiarrhythmic drugs, such as mexiletine, may result in additive toxic effects).
   No products indexed under this heading.

Moricizine Hydrochloride (Should be used with caution in patients receiving Class I antiarrhythmic drugs since the toxic effects are additive and potentially synergistic).
   No products indexed under this heading.

Procainamide (Should be used with caution in patients receiving Class I antiarrhythmic drugs since the toxic effects are additive and potentially synergistic).
   No products indexed under this heading.

Procaine Hydrochloride (When used concomitantly with other products containing local anesthetic agents, the amount absorbed from all formulations must be considered).
   No products indexed under this heading.

Quinidine (Should be used with caution in patients receiving Class I antiarrhythmic drugs since the toxic effects are additive and potentially synergistic).
   No products indexed under this heading.

Quinidine Gluconate (Should be used with caution in patients receiving Class I antiarrhythmic drugs since the toxic effects are additive and potentially synergistic).
   No products indexed under this heading.

Quinidine Hydrochloride (Should be used with caution in patients receiving Class I antiarrhythmic drugs since the toxic effects are additive and potentially synergistic).
   No products indexed under this heading.

Quinidine Polygalacturonate (Should be used with caution in patients receiving Class I antiarrhythmic drugs since the toxic effects are additive and potentially synergistic).
   No products indexed under this heading.

Quinidine Sulfate (Should be used with caution in patients receiving Class I antiarrhythmic drugs since the toxic effects are additive and potentially synergistic).
   No products indexed under this heading.

Tetracaine Hydrochloride (When used concomitantly with other products containing local anesthetic agents, the amount absorbed from all formulations must be considered).
   No products indexed under this heading.

Tocainide Hydrochloride (Co-administration in patients receiving Class-1 antiarrhythmic drugs, such as tocainide, may result in additive toxic effects).
   No products indexed under this heading.

LIFEPAK CAPSULES

(Vitamins with Minerals) 2778
None cited in PDR database.

LIPITOR TABLETS

(Atorvastatin Calcium) 2703
May interact with azole antifungals, cytochrome p450 3a4 inducers (selected), cytochrome p450 3a4 inhibitors (selected), cytochrome p450 3a4 inhibitors, potent (selected), erythromycin, fibrates, immunosuppressive agents, oral contraceptives, protease inhibitors, and certain other agents. Compounds in these categories include:

Acetazolamide (Atorvastatin is metabolized by cytochrome P450 3A4. Concomitant administration of atorvastatin with strong inhibitors of cytochrome P450 3A4 can lead to increases in plasma concentrations of atorvastatin. The extent of interaction and potentiation of effects depends on the variability of effect on cytochrome P450 3A4. The concomitant use of higher doses of atorvastatin with certain drugs such as strong CYP3A4 inhibitors increases the risk of myopathy/rhabdomyolysis).
   No products indexed under this heading.

Acetazolamide Sodium (Atorvastatin is metabolized by cytochrome P450 3A4. Concomitant administration of atorvastatin with strong inhibitors of cytochrome P450 3A4 can lead to increases in plasma concentrations of atorvastatin. The extent of interaction and potentiation of effects depends on the variability of effect on cytochrome P450 3A4. The concomitant use of higher doses of atorvastatin with cer-

tain drugs such as strong CYP3A4 inhibitors increases the risk of myopathy/rhabdomyolysis).
   No products indexed under this heading.

Allium sativum (Concomitant administration of atorvastatin with inducers of cytochrome P450 3A4 can lead to variable reductions in plasma concentrations of atorvastatin).
   No products indexed under this heading.

Aluminum Hydroxide (Co-administration with aluminum hydroxide resulted in a 33% decrease in the AUC and 34% decrease in the C_{max} of atorvastatin).
   No products indexed under this heading.

Aminoglutethimide (Concomitant administration of atorvastatin with inducers of cytochrome P450 3A4 can lead to variable reductions in plasma concentrations of atorvastatin).
   No products indexed under this heading.

Amiodarone Hydrochloride (Atorvastatin is metabolized by cytochrome P450 3A4. Concomitant administration of atorvastatin with strong inhibitors of cytochrome P450 3A4 can lead to increases in plasma concentrations of atorvastatin. The extent of interaction and potentiation of effects depends on the variability of effect on cytochrome P450 3A4. The concomitant use of higher doses of atorvastatin with certain drugs such as strong CYP3A4 inhibitors increases the risk of myopathy/rhabdomyolysis).
   No products indexed under this heading.

Amlodipine Besylate (Co-administration with amlodipine resulted in a 15% increase in AUC and 12% decrease in C_{max} of atorvastatin). Products include:
   Azor 1010
   Exforge 2443
   Exforge HCT 2449

Amprenavir (Atorvastatin AUC was significantly increased with concomitant administration of atorvastatin 40 mg with ritonavir plus saquinavir (400 mg twice daily) or atorvastatin 20 mg with lopinavir plus ritonavir (400 mg + 100 mg twice daily) compared to that of atorvastatin alone. The concomitant use of higher doses of atorvastatin with certain drugs such as strong CYP3A4 inhibitors (eg, HIV protease inhibitors) increases the risk of myopathy/rhabdomyolysis. Caution should be used when exceeding>20 mg atorvastatin daily; the lowest dose necessary should be used).
   No products indexed under this heading.

Anastrozole (Atorvastatin is metabolized by cytochrome P450 3A4. Concomitant administration of atorvastatin with strong inhibitors of cytochrome P450 3A4 can lead to increases in plasma concentrations of atorvastatin. The extent of interaction and potentiation of effects depends on the variability of effect on cytochrome P450 3A4. The concomitant use of higher doses of atorvastatin with certain drugs such as strong CYP3A4 inhibitors increases the risk of myopathy/rhabdomyolysis).
   No products indexed under this heading.

Antipyrine (Co-administration with antipyrine resulted in a 3% increase in the AUC and 11% decrease in the C_{max} of antipyrine).
   No products indexed under this heading.

Aprepitant (Atorvastatin is metabolized by cytochrome P450 3A4. Concomitant administration of atorvastatin with strong inhibitors of cytochrome P450 3A4 can lead to increases in plasma concentrations of atorvastatin. The extent of interaction and potentiation of effects depends on the variability of effect on cytochrome P450 3A4. The concomitant use of higher doses of atorvastatin with certain drugs such as

1051 Interactions Index Lipitor

strong CYP3A4 inhibitors increases the risk of myopathy/rhabdomyolysis). Products include:

Emend 2124

Atazanavir (Atorvastatin AUC was significantly increased with concomitant administration of atorvastatin 40 mg with ritonavir plus saquinavir (400 mg twice daily) or atorvastatin 20 mg with lopinavir plus ritonavir (400 mg + 100 mg twice daily) compared to that of atorvastatin alone. The concomitant use of higher doses of atorvastatin with certain drugs such as strong CYP3A4 inhibitors (eg, HIV protease inhibitors) increases the risk of myopathy/rhabdomyolysis. Caution should be used when exceeding>20 mg atorvastatin daily; the lowest dose necessary should be used).

No products indexed under this heading.

Atazanavir Sulfate (Atorvastatin AUC was significantly increased with concomitant administration of atorvastatin 40 mg with ritonavir plus saquinavir (400 mg twice daily) or atorvastatin 20 mg with lopinavir plus ritonavir (400 mg + 100 mg twice daily) compared to that of atorvastatin alone. The concomitant use of higher doses of atorvastatin with certain drugs such as strong CYP3A4 inhibitors (eg, HIV protease inhibitors) increases the risk of myopathy/rhabdomyolysis. Caution should be used when exceeding>20 mg atorvastatin daily; the lowest dose necessary should be used).

No products indexed under this heading.

Azathioprine (Physicians considering combined therapy with atorvastatin and immunosuppressive drugs should carefully weigh the potential benefits and risks and should carefully monitor patients for any signs or symptoms of muscle pain, tenderness, or weakness, particularly during the initial months of therapy and during any periods of upward dosage titration of either drug. Lower starting and maintenance doses of atorvastatin should be considered when taken concomitantly with immunosuppressive drugs. Periodic creatine phosphokinase (CPK) determinations may be considered in such situations).

No products indexed under this heading.

Basiliximab (Physicians considering combined therapy with atorvastatin and immunosuppressive drugs should carefully weigh the potential benefits and risks and should carefully monitor patients for any signs or symptoms of muscle pain, tenderness, or weakness, particularly during the initial months of therapy and during any periods of upward dosage titration of either drug. Lower starting and maintenance doses of atorvastatin should be considered when taken concomitantly with immunosuppressive drugs. Periodic creatine phosphokinase (CPK) determinations may be considered in such situations). Products include:

Simulect 2524

Betamethasone (Concomitant administration of atorvastatin with inducers of cytochrome P450 3A4 can lead to variable reductions in plasma concentrations of atorvastatin).

No products indexed under this heading.

Betamethasone Acetate (Concomitant administration of atorvastatin with inducers of cytochrome P450 3A4 can lead to variable reductions in plasma concentrations of atorvastatin).

No products indexed under this heading.

Betamethasone Benzoate (Concomitant administration of atorvastatin with inducers of cytochrome P450 3A4 can lead to variable reductions in plasma concentrations of atorvastatin).

No products indexed under this heading.

Betamethasone Dipropionate (Concomitant administration of atorvastatin with inducers of cytochrome P450 3A4 can lead to variable reductions in plasma concentrations of atorvastatin). Products include:

Diprolene Lotion 0.05% 3108

Diprolene Ointment 0.05% 3109

Diprolene AF Cream 0.05% 3107

Lotrisone 3163

Betamethasone Sodium Phosphate (Concomitant administration of atorvastatin with inducers of cytochrome P450 3A4 can lead to variable reductions in plasma concentrations of atorvastatin).

No products indexed under this heading.

Betamethasone Valerate (Concomitant administration of atorvastatin with inducers of cytochrome P450 3A4 can lead to variable reductions in plasma concentrations of atorvastatin). Products include:

Luxiq 3321

Bosentan (Concomitant administration of atorvastatin with inducers of cytochrome P450 3A4 can lead to variable reductions in plasma concentrations of atorvastatin). Products include:

Tracleer 573

Butoconazole Nitrate (The risk of myopathy during treatment with drugs in this class is increased with concurrent administration of azole antifungals. Physicians considering combined therapy with atorvastatin and azole antifungals should carefully weigh the potential benefits and risks and should carefully monitor patients for any signs or symptoms of muscle pain, tenderness, or weakness, particularly during the initial months of therapy and during any periods of upward dosage titration of either drug. Lower starting and maintenance doses of atorvastatin should be considered when taken concomitantly with azole antifungals. Periodic creatine phosphokinase (CPK) determinations may be considered in such situations).

No products indexed under this heading.

Carbamazepine (Concomitant administration of atorvastatin with inducers of cytochrome P450 3A4 can lead to variable reductions in plasma concentrations of atorvastatin). Products include:

Carbatrol 3280

Equetro 3477

Cimetidine (HMG-CoA reductase inhibitors interfere with cholesterol synthesis and theoretically might blunt adrenal and/or gonadal steroid production. Clinical studies have shown that atorvastatin does not reduce basal plasma cortisol concentration or impair adrenal reserve. Caution should be exercised if an HMG-CoA reductase inhibitor is administered concomitantly with drugs that may decrease levels or activity of endogenous steroid hormones, such as cimetidine).

No products indexed under this heading.

Cimetidine Hydrochloride (HMG-CoA reductase inhibitors interfere with cholesterol synthesis and theoretically might blunt adrenal and/or gonadal steroid production. Clinical studies have shown that atorvastatin does not reduce basal plasma cortisol concentration or impair adrenal reserve. Caution should be exercised if an HMG-CoA reductase inhibitor is administered concomitantly with drugs that may decrease levels or activity of endogenous steroid hormones, such as cimetidine).

No products indexed under this heading.

Ciprofloxacin (Atorvastatin is metabolized by cytochrome P450 3A4. Concomitant administration of atorvastatin with strong inhibitors of cytochrome P450 3A4 can lead to increases in plasma concentrations of atorvastatin. The extent of interaction and potentiation of effects depends on the variability of effect on cytochrome P450 3A4. The concomitant use of higher doses of atorvastatin with certain drugs such as strong CYP3A4 inhibitors increases the risk of myopathy/rhabdomyolysis). Products include:

Cipro I.V. 3082

Cipro 3073

Cipro XR 3091

Ciprodex 583

Ciprofloxacin Hydrochloride (Concomitant administration of atorvastatin with inducers of cytochrome P450 3A4 can lead to variable reductions in plasma concentrations of atorvastatin). Products include:

Cipro 3073

Cisplatin (Concomitant administration of atorvastatin with inducers of cytochrome P450 3A4 can lead to variable reductions in plasma concentrations of atorvastatin).

No products indexed under this heading.

Clarithromycin (Atorvastatin AUC was significantly increased with concomitant administration of atorvastatin 80 mg with clarithromycin (500 mg twice daily) compared to that of atorvastatin alone. The concomitant use of higher doses of atorvastatin with certain drugs such as strong CYP3A4 inhibitors (eg, clarithromycin) increases the risk of myopathy/rhabdomyolysis. Physicians considering combined therapy with atorvastatin and clarithromycin, should carefully weigh the benefits and risks and should carefully monitor patients for any signs or symptoms of muscle pain, tenderness, weakness, particularly during initial months of therapy and during any periods of upward dosage titration of either drug. Periodic creatine phosphokinase (CPK) determinations may be considered in such situations. Caution when exceeding atorvastatin doses> 20 mg daily; the lowest dose necessary should be used). Products include:

Biaxin/Biaxin XL 412

Clofibrate (The risk of myopathy during treatment with drugs in this class is increased with concurrent fibric acid derivatives. Physicians considering combined therapy with atorvastatin and fibric acid derivatives should carefully weigh the potential benefits and risks and should carefully monitor patients for any signs or symptoms of muscle pain, tenderness, or weakness, particularly during the initial months of therapy and during any periods of upward dosage titration of either drug. Lower starting and maintenance doses of atorvastatin should be considered when taken concomitantly with fibrates. Periodic creatine phosphokinase (CPK) determinations may be considered in such situations).

No products indexed under this heading.

Clotrimazole (The risk of myopathy during treatment with drugs in this class is increased with concurrent administration of azole antifungals. Physicians considering combined therapy with atorvastatin and azole antifungals should carefully weigh the potential benefits and risks and should carefully monitor patients for any signs or symptoms of muscle pain, tenderness, or weakness, particularly during the initial months of therapy and during any periods of upward dosage titration of either drug. Lower starting and maintenance doses of atorvastatin should be considered when taken concomitantly with azole antifungals. Periodic creatine phosphokinase (CPK) determinations may be considered in such situations). Products include:

Lotrisone 3163

Colestipol (Co-administration with colestipol resulted in a 26% decrease in the C_{max} of atorvastatin).

No products indexed under this heading.

Colestipol Hydrochloride (Co-administration with colestipol resulted in a 26% decrease in the C_{max} of atorvastatin).

No products indexed under this heading.

Conivaptan Hydrochloride (Atorvastatin is metabolized by cytochrome P450 3A4. Concomitant administration of atorvastatin with strong inhibitors of cytochrome P450 3A4 can lead to increases in plasma concentrations of atorvastatin. The extent of interaction and potentiation of effects depends on the variability of effect on cytochrome P450 3A4. The concomitant use of higher doses of atorvastatin with certain drugs such as strong CYP3A4 inhibitors increases the risk of myopathy/rhabdomyolysis). Products include:

Vaprisol 689

Cortisone Acetate (Concomitant administration of atorvastatin with inducers of cytochrome P450 3A4 can lead to variable reductions in plasma concentrations of atorvastatin).

No products indexed under this heading.

Cyclosporine (Atorvastatin and atorvastatin-metabolites are substrates of the OATP1B1 transporter. Inhibitors of the OATP1B1 (eg, cyclosporine) can increase the bioavailability of atorvastatin. Atorvastatin AUC was significantly increased with concomitant administration of atorvastatin 10 mg and cyclosporine 5.2 mg/kg/day compared to that of atorvastatin alone. The risk of myopathy during treatment with drugs in this class is increased with concurrent administration of cyclosporine. In cases where co-administration of atorvastatin with cyclosporine is necessary, the dose of atorvastatin should not exceed 10 mg). Products include:

Gengraf 440

Neoral Oral Solution 2496

Neoral Capsules 2496

Restasis 605

Dalfopristin (Atorvastatin is metabolized by cytochrome P450 3A4. Concomitant administration of atorvastatin with strong inhibitors of cytochrome P450 3A4 can lead to increases in plasma concentrations of atorvastatin. The extent of interaction and potentiation of effects depends on the variability of effect on cytochrome P450 3A4. The concomitant use of higher doses of atorvastatin with certain drugs such as strong CYP3A4 inhibitors increases the risk of myopathy/rhabdomyolysis).

No products indexed under this heading.

Danazol (Atorvastatin is metabolized by cytochrome P450 3A4. Concomitant administration of atorvastatin with strong inhibitors of cytochrome P450 3A4 can lead to increases in plasma concentrations of atorvastatin. The extent of interaction and potentiation of effects depends on the variability of effect on cytochrome P450 3A4. The concomitant use of higher doses of atorvastatin with certain drugs such as strong CYP3A4 inhibitors increases the risk of myopathy/rhabdomyolysis).

No products indexed under this heading.

Darunavir (Atorvastatin AUC was significantly increased with concomitant administration of atorvastatin 40 mg with ritonavir plus saquinavir (400 mg twice daily) or atorvastatin 20 mg with lopinavir plus ritonavir (400 mg + 100 mg twice daily) compared to that of atorvastatin alone. The concomitant use of higher doses of atorvastatin with certain drugs such as strong CYP3A4 inhibitors (eg, HIV protease inhibitors) increases the risk of myopathy/rhabdomyolysis. Caution should be

IMPORTANT NOTE: Always consult each drug listing in the patient's regimen for possible interactions.

Lipitor Interactions Index 1052

used when exceeding>20 mg atorvastatin daily; the lowest dose necessary should be used).
No products indexed under this heading.

Dasatinib (Atorvastatin is metabolized by cytochrome P450 3A4. Concomitant administration of atorvastatin with strong inhibitors of cytochrome P450 3A4 can lead to increases in plasma concentrations of atorvastatin. The extent of interaction and potentiation of effects depends on the variability of effect on cytochrome P450 3A4. The concomitant use of higher doses of atorvastatin with certain drugs such as strong CYP3A4 inhibitors increases the risk of myopathy/rhabdomyolysis).
No products indexed under this heading.

Delavirdine Mesylate (Atorvastatin is metabolized by cytochrome P450 3A4. Concomitant administration of atorvastatin with strong inhibitors of cytochrome P450 3A4 can lead to increases in plasma concentrations of atorvastatin. The extent of interaction and potentiation of effects depends on the variability of effect on cytochrome P450 3A4. The concomitant use of higher doses of atorvastatin with certain drugs such as strong CYP3A4 inhibitors increases the risk of myopathy/rhabdomyolysis).
No products indexed under this heading.

Delavirine (Atorvastatin is metabolized by cytochrome P450 3A4. Concomitant administration of atorvastatin with strong inhibitors of cytochrome P450 3A4 can lead to increases in plasma concentrations of atorvastatin. The extent of interaction and potentiation of effects depends on the variability of effect on cytochrome P450 3A4. The concomitant use of higher doses of atorvastatin with certain drugs such as strong CYP3A4 inhibitors increases the risk of myopathy/rhabdomyolysis).
No products indexed under this heading.

Desloratadine (Atorvastatin is metabolized by cytochrome P450 3A4. Concomitant administration of atorvastatin with strong inhibitors of cytochrome P450 3A4 can lead to increases in plasma concentrations of atorvastatin. The extent of interaction and potentiation of effects depends on the variability of effect on cytochrome P450 3A4. The concomitant use of higher doses of atorvastatin with certain drugs such as strong CYP3A4 inhibitors increases the risk of myopathy/rhabdomyolysis). Products include:
Clarinex Syrup 3098
Clarinex 3098
Clarinex Reditabs 3098
Clarinex-D 12-Hour 3101
Clarinex-D 3104

Desogestrel (Co-administration of atorvastatin and oral contraceptive increased AUC values for norethindrone and ethinyl estradiol. These increases should be considered when selecting an oral contraceptive for a woman taking atorvastatin).
No products indexed under this heading.

Dexamethasone (Concomitant administration of atorvastatin with inducers of cytochrome P450 3A4 can lead to variable reductions in plasma concentrations of atorvastatin). Products include:
Ciprodex 583
Ozurdex .... ⊙ 223
Tobramycin and Dexamethasone Ophthalmic Suspension .... ⊙ 251

Dexamethasone Acetate (Concomitant administration of atorvastatin with inducers of cytochrome P450 3A4 can lead to variable reductions in plasma concentrations of atorvastatin).
No products indexed under this heading.

Dexamethasone Phosphate (Concomitant administration of atorvastatin with inducers of cytochrome P450 3A4 can lead to variable reductions in plasma concentrations of atorvastatin).
No products indexed under this heading.

Dexamethasone Sodium (Concomitant administration of atorvastatin with inducers of cytochrome P450 3A4 can lead to variable reductions in plasma concentrations of atorvastatin).
No products indexed under this heading.

Dexamethasone Sodium Phosphate (Concomitant administration of atorvastatin with inducers of cytochrome P450 3A4 can lead to variable reductions in plasma concentrations of atorvastatin).
No products indexed under this heading.

Dexamethasone Sodium Phosphate Injection (Concomitant administration of atorvastatin with inducers of cytochrome P450 3A4 can lead to variable reductions in plasma concentrations of atorvastatin).
No products indexed under this heading.

Digoxin (When multiple doses of atorvastatin and digoxin were co-administered, steady state plasma digoxin concentrations increased by approximately 20%. Patients taking digoxin should be monitored appropriately). Products include:
Lanoxin Injection 1546
Lanoxin Injection Pediatric 1549
Lanoxin Tablets 1553

Diltiazem Hydrochloride (Co-administration with diltiazem resulted in a 51% increase in AUC of atorvastatin). Products include:
Cardizem LA 423

Diltiazem Maleate (Co-administration with diltiazem resulted in a 51% increase in AUC of atorvastatin).
No products indexed under this heading.

Doxorubicin Hydrochloride (Concomitant administration of atorvastatin with inducers of cytochrome P450 3A4 can lead to variable reductions in plasma concentrations of atorvastatin).
No products indexed under this heading.

Econazole Nitrate (The risk of myopathy during treatment with drugs in this class is increased with concurrent administration of azole antifungals. Physicians considering combined therapy with atorvastatin and azole antifungals should carefully weigh the potential benefits and risks and should carefully monitor patients for any signs or symptoms of muscle pain, tenderness, or weakness, particularly during the initial months of therapy and during any periods of upward dosage titration of either drug. Lower starting and maintenance doses of atorvastatin should be considered when taken concomitantly with azole antifungals. Periodic creatine phosphokinase (CPK) determinations may be considered in such situations).
No products indexed under this heading.

Efavirenz (Concomitant administration of atorvastatin with inducers of cytochrome P450 3A4 (eg, efavirenz) can lead to variable reductions in plasma concentrations of atorvastatin). Products include:
Atripla 906

Erythromycin (The risk of myopathy during treatment with drugs in this class is increased with concurrent erythromycin. Physicians considering combined therapy with atorvastatin and erythromycin should carefully weigh the potential benefits and risks and should carefully monitor patients for any signs or symptoms of muscle pain, tenderness, or weakness, particularly during the initial months of therapy and during any periods of upward dosage titration of either drug. Lower starting and maintenance doses of atorvastatin should be considered when taken concomitantly with erythromycin. Periodic creatine phosphokinase (CPK) determinations may be considered in such situations).
No products indexed under this heading.

Erythromycin, Topical (The risk of myopathy during treatment with drugs in this class is increased with concurrent erythromycin. Physicians considering combined therapy with atorvastatin and erythromycin should carefully weigh the potential benefits and risks and should carefully monitor patients for any signs or symptoms of muscle pain, tenderness, or weakness, particularly during the initial months of therapy and during any periods of upward dosage titration of either drug. Lower starting and maintenance doses of atorvastatin should be considered when taken concomitantly with erythromycin. Periodic creatine phosphokinase (CPK) determinations may be considered in such situations).
No products indexed under this heading.

Erythromycin Estolate (The risk of myopathy during treatment with drugs in this class is increased with concurrent erythromycin. Physicians considering combined therapy with atorvastatin and erythromycin should carefully weigh the potential benefits and risks and should carefully monitor patients for any signs or symptoms of muscle pain, tenderness, or weakness, particularly during the initial months of therapy and during any periods of upward dosage titration of either drug. Lower starting and maintenance doses of atorvastatin should be considered when taken concomitantly with erythromycin. Periodic creatine phosphokinase (CPK) determinations may be considered in such situations).
No products indexed under this heading.

Erythromycin Ethylsuccinate (The risk of myopathy during treatment with drugs in this class is increased with concurrent erythromycin. Physicians considering combined therapy with atorvastatin and erythromycin should carefully weigh the potential benefits and risks and should carefully monitor patients for any signs or symptoms of muscle pain, tenderness, or weakness, particularly during the initial months of therapy and during any periods of upward dosage titration of either drug. Lower starting and maintenance doses of atorvastatin should be considered when taken concomitantly with erythromycin. Periodic creatine phosphokinase (CPK) determinations may be considered in such situations). Products include:
E.E.S. 437
EryPed 435

Erythromycin Gluceptate (The risk of myopathy during treatment with drugs in this class is increased with concurrent erythromycin. Physicians considering combined therapy with atorvastatin and erythromycin should carefully weigh the potential benefits and risks and should carefully monitor patients for any signs or symptoms of muscle pain, tenderness, or weakness, particularly during the initial months of therapy and during any periods of upward dosage titration of either drug. Lower starting and maintenance doses of atorvastatin should be considered when taken concomitantly with erythromycin. Periodic creatine phosphokinase (CPK) determinations may be considered in such situations).
No products indexed under this heading.

Erythromycin Lactobionate (The risk of myopathy during treatment with drugs in this class is increased with concurrent erythromycin. Physicians considering combined therapy with atorvastatin and erythromycin should carefully weigh the potential benefits and risks and should carefully monitor patients for any signs or symptoms of muscle pain, tenderness, or weakness, particularly during the initial months of therapy and during any periods of upward dosage titration of either drug. Lower starting and maintenance doses of atorvastatin should be considered when taken concomitantly with erythromycin. Periodic creatine phosphokinase (CPK) determinations may be considered in such situations).
No products indexed under this heading.

Erythromycin Stearate (The risk of myopathy during treatment with drugs in this class is increased with concurrent erythromycin. Physicians considering combined therapy with atorvastatin and erythromycin should carefully weigh the potential benefits and risks and should carefully monitor patients for any signs or symptoms of muscle pain, tenderness, or weakness, particularly during the initial months of therapy and during any periods of upward dosage titration of either drug. Lower starting and maintenance doses of atorvastatin should be considered when taken concomitantly with erythromycin. Periodic creatine phosphokinase (CPK) determinations may be considered in such situations).
No products indexed under this heading.

Esomeprazole Magnesium (Atorvastatin is metabolized by cytochrome P450 3A4. Concomitant administration of atorvastatin with strong inhibitors of cytochrome P450 3A4 can lead to increases in plasma concentrations of atorvastatin. The extent of interaction and potentiation of effects depends on the variability of effect on cytochrome P450 3A4. The concomitant use of higher doses of atorvastatin with certain drugs such as strong CYP3A4 inhibitors increases the risk of myopathy/rhabdomyolysis). Products include:
Nexium Capsules 704
Nexium Oral Suspension 704

Esomeprazole Sodium (Atorvastatin is metabolized by cytochrome P450 3A4. Concomitant administration of atorvastatin with strong inhibitors of cytochrome P450 3A4 can lead to increases in plasma concentrations of atorvastatin. The extent of interaction and potentiation of effects depends on the variability of effect on cytochrome P450 3A4. The concomitant use of higher doses of atorvastatin with certain drugs such as strong CYP3A4 inhibitors increases the risk of myopathy/rhabdomyolysis). Products include:
Nexium I.V. 712

Ethinyl Estradiol (Co-administration of atorvastatin and oral contraceptive increased AUC values for norethindrone and ethinyl estradiol. These increases should be considered when selecting an oral contraceptive for a woman taking atorvastatin). Products include:
LoSeasonique 3407
Lybrel 3514
NuvaRing 3181
Ortho Evra 2648
Ortho-Cyclen/Ortho Tri-Cyclen 2663
Ortho Tri-Cyclen Lo Tablets 2673
Seasonique 3418
Yaz 864

Ethosuximide (Concomitant administration of atorvastatin with inducers of cytochrome P450 3A4 can lead to variable reductions in plasma concentrations of atorvastatin).
No products indexed under this heading.

1053 Interactions Index Lipitor

Ethynodiol Diacetate (Co-administration of atorvastatin and oral contraceptive increased AUC values for norethindrone and ethinyl estradiol. These increases should be considered when selecting an oral contraceptive for a woman taking atorvastatin).
No products indexed under this heading.

Felbamate (Concomitant administration of atorvastatin with inducers of cytochrome P450 3A4 can lead to variable reductions in plasma concentrations of atorvastatin).
No products indexed under this heading.

Fenofibrate (Co-administration with fenofibrate resulted in a 3% increase in the AUC and 2% increase in the C_{max} of atorvastatin. The risk of myopathy during treatment with drugs in this class is increased with concurrent fibric acid derivatives. Physicians considering combined therapy with atorvastatin and fibric acid derivatives should carefully weigh the potential benefits and risks and should carefully monitor patients for any signs or symptoms of muscle pain, tenderness, or weakness, particularly during the initial months of therapy and during any periods of upward dosage titration of either drug. Lower starting and maintenance doses of atorvastatin should be considered when taken concomitantly with fibrates. Periodic creatine phosphokinase (CPK) determinations may be considered in such situations). Products include:
Fenoglide ... 3263
Tricor ... 544
Trilipix ... 548

Fluconazole (The risk of myopathy during treatment with drugs in this class is increased with concurrent administration of azole antifungals. Physicians considering combined therapy with atorvastatin and azole antifungals should carefully weigh the potential benefits and risks and should carefully monitor patients for any signs or symptoms of muscle pain, tenderness, or weakness, particularly during the initial months of therapy and during any periods of upward dosage titration of either drug. Lower starting and maintenance doses of atorvastatin should be considered when taken concomitantly with azole antifungals. Periodic creatine phosphokinase (CPK) determinations may be considered in such situations).
No products indexed under this heading.

Fludrocortisone Acetate (Concomitant administration of atorvastatin with inducers of cytochrome P450 3A4 can lead to variable reductions in plasma concentrations of atorvastatin).
No products indexed under this heading.

Fluoxetine (Atorvastatin is metabolized by cytochrome P450 3A4. Concomitant administration of atorvastatin with strong inhibitors of cytochrome P450 3A4 can lead to increases in plasma concentrations of atorvastatin. The extent of interaction and potentiation of effects depends on the variability of effect on cytochrome P450 3A4. The concomitant use of higher doses of atorvastatin with certain drugs such as strong CYP3A4 inhibitors increases the risk of myopathy/rhabdomyolysis).
No products indexed under this heading.

Fluoxetine Hydrochloride (Atorvastatin is metabolized by cytochrome P450 3A4. Concomitant administration of atorvastatin with strong inhibitors of cytochrome P450 3A4 can lead to increases in plasma concentrations of atorvastatin. The extent of interaction and potentiation of effects depends on the variability of effect on cytochrome P450 3A4. The concomitant use of higher doses of atorvastatin with certain drugs such as strong CYP3A4 inhibitors increases the risk of myopathy/rhabdomyolysis). Products include:
Prozac Weekly ... 1941
Prozac Pulvules ... 1941
Symbyax ... 1965

Fluvoxamine Maleate (Atorvastatin is metabolized by cytochrome P450 3A4. Concomitant administration of atorvastatin with strong inhibitors of cytochrome P450 3A4 can lead to increases in plasma concentrations of atorvastatin. The extent of interaction and potentiation of effects depends on the variability of effect on cytochrome P450 3A4. The concomitant use of higher doses of atorvastatin with certain drugs such as strong CYP3A4 inhibitors increases the risk of myopathy/rhabdomyolysis).
No products indexed under this heading.

Fosamprenavir Calcium (Atorvastatin AUC was significantly increased with concomitant administration of atorvastatin 40 mg with ritonavir plus saquinavir (400 mg twice daily) or atorvastatin 20 mg with lopinavir plus ritonavir (400 mg + 100 mg twice daily) compared to that of atorvastatin alone. The concomitant use of higher doses of atorvastatin with certain drugs such as strong CYP3A4 inhibitors (eg, HIV protease inhibitors) increases the risk of myopathy/rhabdomyolysis. Caution should be used when exceeding>20 mg atorvastatin daily; the lowest dose necessary should be used). Products include:
Lexiva Oral Suspension ... 1558
Lexiva ... 1558

Fosphenytoin Sodium (Concomitant administration of atorvastatin with inducers of cytochrome P450 3A4 can lead to variable reductions in plasma concentrations of atorvastatin).
No products indexed under this heading.

Garlic Extract (Concomitant administration of atorvastatin with inducers of cytochrome P450 3A4 can lead to variable reductions in plasma concentrations of atorvastatin).
No products indexed under this heading.

Garlic Oil (Concomitant administration of atorvastatin with inducers of cytochrome P450 3A4 can lead to variable reductions in plasma concentrations of atorvastatin).
No products indexed under this heading.

Gemfibrozil (Co-administration with gemfibrozil resulted in a 33% increase in the AUC and <1% decrease in the C_{max} of atorvastatin. The risk of myopathy during treatment with drugs in this class is increased with concurrent fibric acid derivatives. Physicians considering combined therapy with atorvastatin and fibric acid derivatives should carefully weigh the potential benefits and risks and should carefully monitor patients for any signs or symptoms of muscle pain, tenderness, or weakness, particularly during the initial months of therapy and during any periods of upward dosage titration of either drug. Lower starting and maintenance doses of atorvastatin should be considered when taken concomitantly with fibrates. Periodic creatine phosphokinase (CPK) determinations may be considered in such situations).
No products indexed under this heading.

Hydrocortisone (Concomitant administration of atorvastatin with inducers of cytochrome P450 3A4 can lead to variable reductions in plasma concentrations of atorvastatin).
No products indexed under this heading.

Hydrocortisone (Alcohol) (Concomitant administration of atorvastatin with inducers of cytochrome P450 3A4 can lead to variable reductions in plasma concentrations of atorvastatin).
No products indexed under this heading.

Hydrocortisone Acetate (Concomitant administration of atorvastatin with inducers of cytochrome P450 3A4 can lead to variable reductions in plasma concentrations of atorvastatin).
No products indexed under this heading.

Hydrocortisone Butyrate (Concomitant administration of atorvastatin with inducers of cytochrome P450 3A4 can lead to variable reductions in plasma concentrations of atorvastatin).
No products indexed under this heading.

Hydrocortisone Cypionate (Concomitant administration of atorvastatin with inducers of cytochrome P450 3A4 can lead to variable reductions in plasma concentrations of atorvastatin).
No products indexed under this heading.

Hydrocortisone Hemisuccinate (Concomitant administration of atorvastatin with inducers of cytochrome P450 3A4 can lead to variable reductions in plasma concentrations of atorvastatin).
No products indexed under this heading.

Hydrocortisone Probutate (Concomitant administration of atorvastatin with inducers of cytochrome P450 3A4 can lead to variable reductions in plasma concentrations of atorvastatin).
No products indexed under this heading.

Hydrocortisone Sodium Phosphate (Concomitant administration of atorvastatin with inducers of cytochrome P450 3A4 can lead to variable reductions in plasma concentrations of atorvastatin).
No products indexed under this heading.

Hydrocortisone Sodium Succinate (Concomitant administration of atorvastatin with inducers of cytochrome P450 3A4 can lead to variable reductions in plasma concentrations of atorvastatin).
No products indexed under this heading.

Hydrocortisone Valerate (Concomitant administration of atorvastatin with inducers of cytochrome P450 3A4 can lead to variable reductions in plasma concentrations of atorvastatin).
No products indexed under this heading.

Hypericum (Concomitant administration of atorvastatin with inducers of cytochrome P450 3A4 can lead to variable reductions in plasma concentrations of atorvastatin).
No products indexed under this heading.

Hypericum Perforatum (Concomitant administration of atorvastatin with inducers of cytochrome P450 3A4 can lead to variable reductions in plasma concentrations of atorvastatin).
Products include:
Traumeel ... 1800

Imatinib Mesylate (Atorvastatin is metabolized by cytochrome P450 3A4. Concomitant administration of atorvastatin with strong inhibitors of cytochrome P450 3A4 can lead to increases in plasma concentrations of atorvastatin. The extent of interaction and potentiation of effects depends on the variability of effect on cytochrome P450 3A4. The concomitant use of higher doses of atorvastatin with certain drugs such as strong CYP3A4 inhibitors increases the risk of myopathy/rhabdomyolysis). Products include:
Gleevec ... 2477

Indinavir Sulfate (Atorvastatin AUC was significantly increased with concomitant administration of atorvastatin 40 mg with ritonavir plus saquinavir (400 mg twice daily) or atorvastatin 20 mg with lopinavir plus ritonavir (400 mg + 100 mg twice daily) compared to that of atorvastatin alone. The concomitant use of higher doses of atorvastatin with certain drugs such as strong CYP3A4 inhibitors (eg, HIV protease inhibitors) increases the risk of myopathy/rhabdomyolysis. Caution should be used when exceeding>20 mg atorvastatin daily; the lowest dose necessary should be used). Products include:
Crixivan ... 2113

Isoniazid (Atorvastatin is metabolized by cytochrome P450 3A4. Concomitant administration of atorvastatin with strong inhibitors of cytochrome P450 3A4 can lead to increases in plasma concentrations of atorvastatin. The extent of interaction and potentiation of effects depends on the variability of effect on cytochrome P450 3A4. The concomitant use of higher doses of atorvastatin with certain drugs such as strong CYP3A4 inhibitors increases the risk of myopathy/rhabdomyolysis).
No products indexed under this heading.

Itraconazole (Atorvastatin AUC was significantly increased with concomitant administration of atorvastatin 40 mg and itraconazole 200 mg. Therefore, in patients taking itraconazole, caution should be used when the atorvastatin dose exceeds 20 mg; the lowest dose necessary should be used. The risk of myopathy during treatment with statins is increased with concurrent administration with strong CYP 3A4 inhibitors (eg, itraconazole). Periodic creatine phosphokinase (CPK) determinations may be considered in such situations).
No products indexed under this heading.

Ketoconazole (The risk of myopathy during treatment with drugs in this class is increased with concurrent administration of azole antifungals. Physicians considering combined therapy with atorvastatin and azole antifungals should carefully weigh the potential benefits and risks and should carefully monitor patients for any signs or symptoms of muscle pain, tenderness, or weakness, particularly during the initial months of therapy and during any periods of upward dosage titration of either drug. Lower starting and maintenance doses of atorvastatin should be considered when taken concomitantly with azole antifungals. Periodic creatine phosphokinase (CPK) determinations may be considered in such situations. In addition, caution should be exercised if a statin is administered concomitantly with drugs that may decrease the levels or activity of endogenous steroid hormones, such as ketoconazole).
Products include:
Extina ... 3319
Xolegel ... 3337

Lapatinib (Atorvastatin is metabolized by cytochrome P450 3A4. Concomitant administration of atorvastatin with strong inhibitors of cytochrome P450 3A4 can lead to increases in plasma concentrations of atorvastatin. The extent of interaction and potentiation of effects depends on the variability of effect on cytochrome P450 3A4. The concomitant use of higher doses of atorvastatin with certain drugs such as strong CYP3A4 inhibitors increases the risk of myopathy/rhabdomyolysis).
Products include:
Tykerb ... 1698

Levonorgestrel (Co-administration of atorvastatin and oral contraceptive increased AUC values for norethindrone and ethinyl estradiol. These increases should be considered when selecting an oral contraceptive for a woman taking atorvastatin). Products include:
Climara Pro ... 847
LoSeasonique ... 3407
Lybrel ... 3514
Mirena ... 854

IMPORTANT NOTE: Always consult each drug listing in the patient's regimen for possible interactions.

Lipitor Interactions Index 1054

Plan B 3416
Seasonique 3418

Lopinavir (Atorvastatin AUC was significantly increased with concomitant administration of atorvastatin 20 mg with lopinavir plus ritonavir (400 mg + 100 mg bid) compared to that of atorvastatin alone. Therefore, in patients taking HIV protease inhibitors, caution should be used when the atorvastatin dose exceeds 20 mg. The risk of myopathy during treatment with atorvastatin is increased with concurrent administration of combination of lopinavir plus ritonavir. Physicians considering combined therapy with atorvastatin and a combination of lopinavir plus ritonavir, should carefully weigh the potential benefits and risks, and should carefully monitor for any signs or symptoms of muscle pain, tenderness, or weakness, particuarly during initial months of therapy and during any periods of upward dosage titration of either drug. Periodic CPK determinations may be considered in such situations). Products include:
Kaletra 458

Loratadine (Atorvastatin is metabolized by cytochrome P450 3A4. Concomitant administration of atorvastatin with strong inhibitors of cytochrome P450 3A4 can lead to increases in plasma concentrations of atorvastatin. The extent of interaction and potentiation of effects depends on the variability of effect on cytochrome P450 3A4. The concomitant use of higher doses of atorvastatin with certain drugs such as strong CYP3A4 inhibitors increases the risk of myopathy/rhabdomyolysis).
No products indexed under this heading.

Magnesium Hydroxide (Co-administration with magnesium hydroxide resulted in a 33% decrease in the AUC and 34% decrease in the C_{max} of atorvastatin). Products include:
Fleet Pedia-Lax Chewable Tablets 1144
Pepcid Complete 1822

Mephenytoin (Concomitant administration of atorvastatin with inducers of cytochrome P450 3A4 can lead to variable reductions in plasma concentrations of atorvastatin).
No products indexed under this heading.

Mestranol (Co-administration of atorvastatin and oral contraceptive increased AUC values for norethindrone and ethinyl estradiol. These increases should be considered when selecting an oral contraceptive for a woman taking atorvastatin).
No products indexed under this heading.

Methsuximide (Concomitant administration of atorvastatin with inducers of cytochrome P450 3A4 can lead to variable reductions in plasma concentrations of atorvastatin).
No products indexed under this heading.

Methylprednisolone (Concomitant administration of atorvastatin with inducers of cytochrome P450 3A4 can lead to variable reductions in plasma concentrations of atorvastatin).
No products indexed under this heading.

Methylprednisolone Acetate (Concomitant administration of atorvastatin with inducers of cytochrome P450 3A4 can lead to variable reductions in plasma concentrations of atorvastatin).
No products indexed under this heading.

Methylprednisolone Sodium Succinate (Concomitant administration of atorvastatin with inducers of cytochrome P450 3A4 can lead to variable reductions in plasma concentrations of atorvastatin).
No products indexed under this heading.

Metronidazole (Atorvastatin is metabolized by cytochrome P450 3A4. Concomitant administration of atorvastatin with strong inhibitors of cytochrome P450 3A4 can lead to increases in plasma concentrations of atorvastatin. The extent of interaction and potentiation of effects depends on the variability of effect on cytochrome P450 3A4. The concomitant use of higher doses of atorvastatin with certain drugs such as strong CYP3A4 inhibitors increases the risk of myopathy/rhabdomyolysis). Products include:
Pylera 793

Metronidazole Benzoate (Atorvastatin is metabolized by cytochrome P450 3A4. Concomitant administration of atorvastatin with strong inhibitors of cytochrome P450 3A4 can lead to increases in plasma concentrations of atorvastatin. The extent of interaction and potentiation of effects depends on the variability of effect on cytochrome P450 3A4. The concomitant use of higher doses of atorvastatin with certain drugs such as strong CYP3A4 inhibitors increases the risk of myopathy/rhabdomyolysis).
No products indexed under this heading.

Metronidazole Hydrochloride (Atorvastatin is metabolized by cytochrome P450 3A4. Concomitant administration of atorvastatin with strong inhibitors of cytochrome P450 3A4 can lead to increases in plasma concentrations of atorvastatin. The extent of interaction and potentiation of effects depends on the variability of effect on cytochrome P450 3A4. The concomitant use of higher doses of atorvastatin with certain drugs such as strong CYP3A4 inhibitors increases the risk of myopathy/rhabdomyolysis).
No products indexed under this heading.

Metronidazole Sodium (Atorvastatin is metabolized by cytochrome P450 3A4. Concomitant administration of atorvastatin with strong inhibitors of cytochrome P450 3A4 can lead to increases in plasma concentrations of atorvastatin. The extent of interaction and potentiation of effects depends on the variability of effect on cytochrome P450 3A4. The concomitant use of higher doses of atorvastatin with certain drugs such as strong CYP3A4 inhibitors increases the risk of myopathy/rhabdomyolysis).
No products indexed under this heading.

Miconazole (The risk of myopathy during treatment with drugs in this class is increased with concurrent administration of azole antifungals. Physicians considering combined therapy with atorvastatin and azole antifungals should carefully weigh the potential benefits and risks and should carefully monitor patients for any signs or symptoms of muscle pain, tenderness, or weakness, particularly during the initial months of therapy and during any periods of upward dosage titration of either drug. Lower starting and maintenance doses of atorvastatin should be considered when taken concomitantly with azole antifungals. Periodic creatine phosphokinase (CPK) determinations may be considered in such situations).
No products indexed under this heading.

Miconazole Nitrate (Atorvastatin is metabolized by cytochrome P450 3A4. Concomitant administration of atorvastatin with strong inhibitors of cytochrome P450 3A4 can lead to increases in plasma concentrations of atorvastatin. The extent of interaction and potentiation of effects depends on the variability of effect on cytochrome P450 3A4. The concomitant use of higher doses of atorvastatin with certain drugs such as strong CYP3A4 inhibitors increases the risk of myopathy/rhabdomyolysis). Products include:
Vusion Ointment 3335

Mifepristone (Atorvastatin is metabolized by cytochrome P450 3A4. Concomitant administration of atorvastatin with strong inhibitors of cytochrome P450 3A4 can lead to increases in plasma concentrations of atorvastatin. The extent of interaction and potentiation of effects depends on the variability of effect on cytochrome P450 3A4. The concomitant use of higher doses of atorvastatin with certain drugs such as strong CYP3A4 inhibitors increases the risk of myopathy/rhabdomyolysis).
No products indexed under this heading.

Modafinil (Concomitant administration of atorvastatin with inducers of cytochrome P450 3A4 can lead to variable reductions in plasma concentrations of atorvastatin). Products include:
Provigil 983

Muromonab-CD3 (Physicians considering combined therapy with atorvastatin and immunosuppressive drugs should carefully weigh the potential benefits and risks and should carefully monitor patients for any signs or symptoms of muscle pain, tenderness, or weakness, particularly during the initial months of therapy and during any periods of upward dosage titration of either drug. Lower starting and maintenance doses of atorvastatin should be considered when taken concomitantly with immunosuppressive drugs. Periodic creatine phosphokinase (CPK) determinations may be considered in such situations). Products include:
Orthoclone OKT3 949

Mycophenolate Mofetil (Physicians considering combined therapy with atorvastatin and immunosuppressive drugs should carefully weigh the potential benefits and risks and should carefully monitor patients for any signs or symptoms of muscle pain, tenderness, or weakness, particularly during the initial months of therapy and during any periods of upward dosage titration of either drug. Lower starting and maintenance doses of atorvastatin should be considered when taken concomitantly with immunosuppressive drugs. Periodic creatine phosphokinase (CPK) determinations may be considered in such situations).
No products indexed under this heading.

Nafcillin Sodium (Concomitant administration of atorvastatin with inducers of cytochrome P450 3A4 can lead to variable reductions in plasma concentrations of atorvastatin).
No products indexed under this heading.

Nefazodone Hydrochloride (Atorvastatin is metabolized by cytochrome P450 3A4. Concomitant administration of atorvastatin with strong inhibitors of cytochrome P450 3A4 can lead to increases in plasma concentrations of atorvastatin. The extent of interaction and potentiation of effects depends on the variability of effect on cytochrome P450 3A4. The concomitant use of higher doses of atorvastatin with certain drugs such as strong CYP3A4 inhibitors increases the risk of myopathy/rhabdomyolysis).
No products indexed under this heading.

Nelfinavir Mesylate (Atorvastatin AUC was significantly increased with concomitant administration of atorvastatin 40 mg with ritonavir plus saquinavir (400 mg twice daily) or atorvastatin 20 mg with lopinavir plus ritonavir (400 mg + 100 mg twice daily) compared to that of atorvastatin alone. The concomitant use of higher doses of atorvastatin with certain drugs such as strong CYP3A4 inhibitors (eg, HIV protease inhibitors) increases the risk of myopathy/rhabdomyolysis. Caution should be used when exceeding>20 mg atorvastatin daily; the lowest dose necessary should be used).
No products indexed under this heading.

Nevirapine (Atorvastatin is metabolized by cytochrome P450 3A4. Concomitant administration of atorvastatin with strong inhibitors of cytochrome P450 3A4 can lead to increases in plasma concentrations of atorvastatin. The extent of interaction and potentiation of effects depends on the variability of effect on cytochrome P450 3A4. The concomitant use of higher doses of atorvastatin with certain drugs such as strong CYP3A4 inhibitors increases the risk of myopathy/rhabdomyolysis). Products include:
Viramune Oral Suspension 897
Viramune Tablets 897

Niacin (The risk of myopathy during treatment with atorvastatin is increased with concurrent administration of niacin. Physicians considering combined therapy with atorvastatin and lipid-modifying doses of niacin should carefully weigh the potential benefits and risks, and should carefully monitor patients for any signs or symptoms of muscle pain, tenderness, or weakness, particularly during the initial months of therapy and during any periods of upward dosage titration of either drug. Lower starting and maintenance doses of atorvastatin should be considered when taken concomitantly with lipid modifying doses of niacin. Periodic CPK determinations may be considered in such situations). Products include:
Advicor 402
Cardio Basics 3455
Niaspan 497
Simcor 524

Niacinamide (The risk of myopathy during treatment with atorvastatin is increased with concurrent administration of niacin. Physicians considering combined therapy with atorvastatin and lipid-modifying doses of niacin should carefully weigh the potential benefits and risks, and should carefully monitor patients for any signs or symptoms of muscle pain, tenderness, or weakness, particularly during the initial months of therapy and during any periods of upward dosage titration of either drug. Lower starting and maintenance doses of atorvastatin should be considered when taken concomitantly with lipid modifying doses of niacin. Periodic CPK determinations may be considered in such situations). Products include:
CitraNatal 90 DHA Capsules 2332
CitraNatal Assure 2332
CitraNatal Rx 2332
Heplive 607

Niacinamide Hydroiodide (The risk of myopathy during treatment with atorvastatin is increased with concurrent administration of niacin. Physicians considering combined therapy with atorvastatin and lipid-modifying doses of niacin should carefully weigh the potential benefits and risks, and should carefully monitor patients for any signs or symptoms of muscle pain, tenderness, or weakness, particularly during the initial months of therapy and during any periods of upward dosage titration of either drug. Lower starting and maintenance doses of atorvastatin should be considered when taken concomitantly with lipid modifying doses of niacin. Periodic CPK determinations may be considered in such situations).
No products indexed under this heading.

Nicotinamide (Atorvastatin is metabolized by cytochrome P450 3A4. Concomitant administration of atorvastatin with strong inhibitors of cytochrome P450 3A4 can lead to increases in plasma concentrations of atorvastatin. The extent of interaction and potentiation of

effects depends on the variability of effect on cytochrome P450 3A4. The concomitant use of higher doses of atorvastatin with certain drugs such as strong CYP3A4 inhibitors increases the risk of myopathy/rhabdomyolysis).

No products indexed under this heading.

Nifedipine (Atorvastatin is metabolized by cytochrome P450 3A4. Concomitant administration of atorvastatin with strong inhibitors of cytochrome P450 3A4 can lead to increases in plasma concentrations of atorvastatin. The extent of interaction and potentiation of effects depends on the variability of effect on cytochrome P450 3A4. The concomitant use of higher doses of atorvastatin with certain drugs such as strong CYP3A4 inhibitors increases the risk of myopathy/rhabdomyolysis).

No products indexed under this heading.

Norethindrone (Co-administration of atorvastatin and oral contraceptive increased AUC values for norethindrone and ethinyl estradiol. These increases should be considered when selecting an oral contraceptive for a woman taking atorvastatin). Products include:

Ortho Micronor 2660

Norethynodrel (Co-administration of atorvastatin and oral contraceptive increased AUC values for norethindrone and ethinyl estradiol. These increases should be considered when selecting an oral contraceptive for a woman taking atorvastatin).

No products indexed under this heading.

Norfloxacin (Atorvastatin is metabolized by cytochrome P450 3A4. Concomitant administration of atorvastatin with strong inhibitors of cytochrome P450 3A4 can lead to increases in plasma concentrations of atorvastatin. The extent of interaction and potentiation of effects depends on the variability of effect on cytochrome P450 3A4. The concomitant use of higher doses of atorvastatin with certain drugs such as strong CYP3A4 inhibitors increases the risk of myopathy/rhabdomyolysis). Products include:

Noroxin 2220

Norgestimate (Co-administration of atorvastatin and oral contraceptive increased AUC values for norethindrone and ethinyl estradiol. These increases should be considered when selecting an oral contraceptive for a woman taking atorvastatin). Products include:

Ortho-Cyclen/Ortho Tri-Cyclen 2663
Ortho Tri-Cyclen Lo Tablets 2673

Norgestrel (Co-administration of atorvastatin and oral contraceptive increased AUC values for norethindrone and ethinyl estradiol. These increases should be considered when selecting an oral contraceptive for a woman taking atorvastatin).

No products indexed under this heading.

Omeprazole (Atorvastatin is metabolized by cytochrome P450 3A4. Concomitant administration of atorvastatin with strong inhibitors of cytochrome P450 3A4 can lead to increases in plasma concentrations of atorvastatin. The extent of interaction and potentiation of effects depends on the variability of effect on cytochrome P450 3A4. The concomitant use of higher doses of atorvastatin with certain drugs such as strong CYP3A4 inhibitors increases the risk of myopathy/rhabdomyolysis).

No products indexed under this heading.

Oxcarbazepine (Concomitant administration of atorvastatin with inducers of cytochrome P450 3A4 can lead to variable reductions in plasma concentrations of atorvastatin).

No products indexed under this heading.

Oxiconazole Nitrate (The risk of myopathy during treatment with drugs in this class is increased with concur-

rent administration of azole antifungals. Physicians considering combined therapy with atorvastatin and azole antifungals should carefully weigh the potential benefits and risks and should carefully monitor patients for any signs or symptoms of muscle pain, tenderness, or weakness, particularly during the initial months of therapy and during any periods of upward dosage titration of either drug. Lower starting and maintenance doses of atorvastatin should be considered when taken concomitantly with azole antifungals. Periodic creatine phosphokinase (CPK) determinations may be considered in such situations).

No products indexed under this heading.

Paroxetine Hydrochloride (Atorvastatin is metabolized by cytochrome P450 3A4. Concomitant administration of atorvastatin with strong inhibitors of cytochrome P450 3A4 can lead to increases in plasma concentrations of atorvastatin. The extent of interaction and potentiation of effects depends on the variability of effect on cytochrome P450 3A4. The concomitant use of higher doses of atorvastatin with certain drugs such as strong CYP3A4 inhibitors increases the risk of myopathy/rhabdomyolysis). Products include:

Paroxetine CR 2361
Paroxetine ER 2371
Paxil 1586
Paxil CR 1596

Phenobarbital (Concomitant administration of atorvastatin with inducers of cytochrome P450 3A4 can lead to variable reductions in plasma concentrations of atorvastatin). Products include:

Donnatal 2711

Phenobarbital Sodium (Concomitant administration of atorvastatin with inducers of cytochrome P450 3A4 can lead to variable reductions in plasma concentrations of atorvastatin).

No products indexed under this heading.

Phenytoin (Concomitant administration of atorvastatin with inducers of cytochrome P450 3A4 can lead to variable reductions in plasma concentrations of atorvastatin).

No products indexed under this heading.

Phenytoin Sodium (Concomitant administration of atorvastatin with inducers of cytochrome P450 3A4 can lead to variable reductions in plasma concentrations of atorvastatin). Products include:

Phenytek Capsules 2380

Posaconazole (The risk of myopathy during treatment with drugs in this class is increased with concurrent administration of azole antifungals. Physicians considering combined therapy with atorvastatin and azole antifungals should carefully weigh the potential benefits and risks and should carefully monitor patients for any signs or symptoms of muscle pain, tenderness, or weakness, particularly during the initial months of therapy and during any periods of upward dosage titration of either drug. Lower starting and maintenance doses of atorvastatin should be considered when taken concomitantly with azole antifungals. Periodic creatine phosphokinase (CPK) determinations may be considered in such situations). Products include:

Noxafil 3172

Prednisolone (Concomitant administration of atorvastatin with inducers of cytochrome P450 3A4 can lead to variable reductions in plasma concentrations of atorvastatin).

No products indexed under this heading.

Prednisolone Acetate (Concomitant administration of atorvastatin with inducers of cytochrome P450 3A4 can

lead to variable reductions in plasma concentrations of atorvastatin). Products include:

Blephamide .... ⊙212, ⊙214
Pred Forte .... ⊙225
Pred Mild .... ⊙230
Pred-G .... ⊙226, ⊙227

Prednisolone Sodium Phosphate (Concomitant administration of atorvastatin with inducers of cytochrome P450 3A4 can lead to variable reductions in plasma concentrations of atorvastatin).

No products indexed under this heading.

Prednisolone Tebutate (Concomitant administration of atorvastatin with inducers of cytochrome P450 3A4 can lead to variable reductions in plasma concentrations of atorvastatin).

No products indexed under this heading.

Prednisone (Concomitant administration of atorvastatin with inducers of cytochrome P450 3A4 can lead to variable reductions in plasma concentrations of atorvastatin).

No products indexed under this heading.

Prednisone sodium phosphate (Concomitant administration of atorvastatin with inducers of cytochrome P450 3A4 can lead to variable reductions in plasma concentrations of atorvastatin).

No products indexed under this heading.

Primidone (Concomitant administration of atorvastatin with inducers of cytochrome P450 3A4 can lead to variable reductions in plasma concentrations of atorvastatin).

No products indexed under this heading.

Propoxyphene Hydrochloride (Atorvastatin is metabolized by cytochrome P450 3A4. Concomitant administration of atorvastatin with strong inhibitors of cytochrome P450 3A4 can lead to increases in plasma concentrations of atorvastatin. The extent of interaction and potentiation of effects depends on the variability of effect on cytochrome P450 3A4. The concomitant use of higher doses of atorvastatin with certain drugs such as strong CYP3A4 inhibitors increases the risk of myopathy/rhabdomyolysis).

No products indexed under this heading.

Propoxyphene Napsylate (Atorvastatin is metabolized by cytochrome P450 3A4. Concomitant administration of atorvastatin with strong inhibitors of cytochrome P450 3A4 can lead to increases in plasma concentrations of atorvastatin. The extent of interaction and potentiation of effects depends on the variability of effect on cytochrome P450 3A4. The concomitant use of higher doses of atorvastatin with certain drugs such as strong CYP3A4 inhibitors increases the risk of myopathy/rhabdomyolysis).

No products indexed under this heading.

Quinidine (Atorvastatin is metabolized by cytochrome P450 3A4. Concomitant administration of atorvastatin with strong inhibitors of cytochrome P450 3A4 can lead to increases in plasma concentrations of atorvastatin. The extent of interaction and potentiation of effects depends on the variability of effect on cytochrome P450 3A4. The concomitant use of higher doses of atorvastatin with certain drugs such as strong CYP3A4 inhibitors increases the risk of myopathy/rhabdomyolysis).

No products indexed under this heading.

Quinidine Hydrochloride (Atorvastatin is metabolized by cytochrome P450 3A4. Concomitant administration of atorvastatin with strong inhibitors of cytochrome P450 3A4 can lead to increases in plasma concentrations of atorvastatin. The extent of interaction and potentiation of effects depends on the variability of effect on cytochrome P450 3A4. The concomitant use of

higher doses of atorvastatin with certain drugs such as strong CYP3A4 inhibitors increases the risk of myopathy/rhabdomyolysis).

No products indexed under this heading.

Quinidine Polygalacturonate (Atorvastatin is metabolized by cytochrome P450 3A4. Concomitant administration of atorvastatin with strong inhibitors of cytochrome P450 3A4 can lead to increases in plasma concentrations of atorvastatin. The extent of interaction and potentiation of effects depends on the variability of effect on cytochrome P450 3A4. The concomitant use of higher doses of atorvastatin with certain drugs such as strong CYP3A4 inhibitors increases the risk of myopathy/rhabdomyolysis).

No products indexed under this heading.

Quinidine Sulfate (Atorvastatin is metabolized by cytochrome P450 3A4. Concomitant administration of atorvastatin with strong inhibitors of cytochrome P450 3A4 can lead to increases in plasma concentrations of atorvastatin. The extent of interaction and potentiation of effects depends on the variability of effect on cytochrome P450 3A4. The concomitant use of higher doses of atorvastatin with certain drugs such as strong CYP3A4 inhibitors increases the risk of myopathy/rhabdomyolysis).

No products indexed under this heading.

Quinine (Atorvastatin is metabolized by cytochrome P450 3A4. Concomitant administration of atorvastatin with strong inhibitors of cytochrome P450 3A4 can lead to increases in plasma concentrations of atorvastatin. The extent of interaction and potentiation of effects depends on the variability of effect on cytochrome P450 3A4. The concomitant use of higher doses of atorvastatin with certain drugs such as strong CYP3A4 inhibitors increases the risk of myopathy/rhabdomyolysis). Products include:

Hyland's Leg Cramps PM with
   Quinine 3315

Quinine Sulfate (Atorvastatin is metabolized by cytochrome P450 3A4. Concomitant administration of atorvastatin with strong inhibitors of cytochrome P450 3A4 can lead to increases in plasma concentrations of atorvastatin. The extent of interaction and potentiation of effects depends on the variability of effect on cytochrome P450 3A4. The concomitant use of higher doses of atorvastatin with certain drugs such as strong CYP3A4 inhibitors increases the risk of myopathy/rhabdomyolysis).

No products indexed under this heading.

Quinupristin (Atorvastatin is metabolized by cytochrome P450 3A4. Concomitant administration of atorvastatin with strong inhibitors of cytochrome P450 3A4 can lead to increases in plasma concentrations of atorvastatin. The extent of interaction and potentiation of effects depends on the variability of effect on cytochrome P450 3A4. The concomitant use of higher doses of atorvastatin with certain drugs such as strong CYP3A4 inhibitors increases the risk of myopathy/rhabdomyolysis).

No products indexed under this heading.

Ranitidine Bismuth Citrate (Atorvastatin is metabolized by cytochrome P450 3A4. Concomitant administration of atorvastatin with strong inhibitors of cytochrome P450 3A4 can lead to increases in plasma concentrations of atorvastatin. The extent of interaction and potentiation of effects depends on the variability of effect on cytochrome P450 3A4. The concomitant use of higher doses of atorvastatin with cer-

---

IMPORTANT NOTE: Always consult each drug listing in the patient's regimen for possible interactions.

Lipitor Interactions Index 1056

tain drugs such as strong CYP3A4 inhibitors increases the risk of myopathy/rhabdomyolysis).
No products indexed under this heading.

Ranitidine Hydrochloride (Atorvastatin is metabolized by cytochrome P450 3A4. Concomitant administration of atorvastatin with strong inhibitors of cytochrome P450 3A4 can lead to increases in plasma concentrations of atorvastatin. The extent of interaction and potentiation of effects depends on the variability of effect on cytochrome P450 3A4. The concomitant use of higher doses of atorvastatin with certain drugs such as strong CYP3A4 inhibitors increases the risk of myopathy/rhabdomyolysis). Products include:
Zantac 1737
Zantac Injection 1732
Zantac Pharmacy 1735

Rapamycin (Physicians considering combined therapy with atorvastatin and immunosuppressive drugs should carefully weigh the potential benefits and risks and should carefully monitor patients for any signs or symptoms of muscle pain, tenderness, or weakness, particularly during the initial months of therapy and during any periods of upward dosage titration of either drug. Lower starting and maintenance doses of atorvastatin should be considered when taken concomitantly with immunosuppressive drugs. Periodic creatine phosphokinase (CPK) determinations may be considered in such situations).
No products indexed under this heading.

Rifabutin (Concomitant administration of atorvastatin with inducers of cytochrome P450 3A4 can lead to variable reductions in plasma concentrations of atorvastatin).
No products indexed under this heading.

Rifampicin (Concomitant administration of atorvastatin with inducers of cytochrome P450 3A4 can lead to variable reductions in plasma concentrations of atorvastatin).
No products indexed under this heading.

Rifampin (Concomitant administration of atorvastatin with inducers of cytochrome P450 3A4 (eg, rifampin) can lead to variable reductions in plasma concentrations of atorvastatin. Due to the dual interaction mechanism of rifampin, simultaneous co-administration of atorvastatin with rifampin is recommended, as delayed administration of atorvastatin after administration of rifampin has been associated with a significant reduction in atorvastatin plasma concentrations).
No products indexed under this heading.

Rifapentine (Concomitant administration of atorvastatin with inducers of cytochrome P450 3A4 can lead to variable reductions in plasma concentrations of atorvastatin).
No products indexed under this heading.

Ritonavir (Atorvastatin AUC was significantly increased with concomitant administration of atorvastatin 40 mg with ritonavir plus saquinavir (400 mg bid) or atorvastatin 20 mg with lopinavir plus ritonavir (400 mg + 100 mg bid) compared to that of atorvastatin alone. Therefore, in patients taking HIV protease inhibitors, caution should be used when the atorvastatin dose exceeds 20 mg. The risk of myopathy during treatment with atorvastatin is increased with concurrent administration of combination of ritonavir plus saquinavir or lopinavir plus ritonavir. Physicians considering combined therapy with atorvastatin and a combination of ritonavir plus saquinavir or lopinavir plus ritonavir, should carefully weigh the potential benefits and risks, and should carefully monitor for any signs or symptoms of muscle pain, tenderness, or weakness, particularly during initial months of therapy and during any periods of upward dosage titration of either drug. Periodic CPK determinations may be considered in such situations). Products include:
Kaletra 458
Norvir 509

Saquinavir (Atorvastatin AUC was significantly increased with concomitant administration of atorvastatin 40 mg with ritonavir plus saquinavir (400 mg bid) compared to that of atorvastatin alone. Therefore, in patients taking HIV protease inhibitors, caution should be used when the atorvastatin dose exceeds 20 mg. The risk of myopathy during treatment with atorvastatin is increased with concurrent administration of combination of ritonavir plus saquinavir. Physicians considering combined therapy with atorvastatin and a combination of ritonavir plus saquinavir, should carefully weigh the potential benefits and risks, and should carefully monitor for any signs or symptoms of muscle pain, tenderness, or weakness, particularly during initial months of therapy and during any periods of upward dosage titration of either drug. Periodic CPK determinations may be considered in such situations).
No products indexed under this heading.

Saquinavir Mesylate (Atorvastatin AUC was significantly increased with concomitant administration of atorvastatin 40 mg with ritonavir plus saquinavir (400 mg bid) compared to that of atorvastatin alone. Therefore, in patients taking HIV protease inhibitors, caution should be used when the atorvastatin dose exceeds 20 mg. The risk of myopathy during treatment with atorvastatin is increased with concurrent administration of combination of ritonavir plus saquinavir. Physicians considering combined therapy with atorvastatin and a combination of ritonavir plus saquinavir, should carefully weigh the potential benefits and risks, and should carefully monitor for any signs or symptoms of muscle pain, tenderness, or weakness, particularly during initial months of therapy and during any periods of upward dosage titration of either drug. Periodic CPK determinations may be considered in such situations).
No products indexed under this heading.

Sertaconazole Nitrate (The risk of myopathy during treatment with drugs in this class is increased with concurrent administration of azole antifungals. Physicians considering combined therapy with atorvastatin and azole antifungals should carefully weigh the potential benefits and risks and should carefully monitor patients for any signs or symptoms of muscle pain, tenderness, or weakness, particularly during the initial months of therapy and during any periods of upward dosage titration of either drug. Lower starting and maintenance doses of atorvastatin should be considered when taken concomitantly with azole antifungals. Periodic creatine phosphokinase (CPK) determinations may be considered in such situations).
No products indexed under this heading.

Sertraline Hydrochloride (Atorvastatin is metabolized by cytochrome P450 3A4. Concomitant administration of atorvastatin with strong inhibitors of cytochrome P450 3A4 can lead to increases in plasma concentrations of atorvastatin. The extent of interaction and potentiation of effects depends on the variability of effect on cytochrome P450 3A4. The concomitant use of higher doses of atorvastatin with certain drugs such as strong CYP3A4 inhibitors increases the risk of myopathy/rhabdomyolysis).
No products indexed under this heading.

Sildenafil Citrate (Atorvastatin is metabolized by cytochrome P450 3A4. Concomitant administration of atorvastatin with strong inhibitors of cytochrome P450 3A4 can lead to increases in plasma concentrations of atorvastatin. The extent of interaction and potentiation of effects depends on the variability of effect on cytochrome P450 3A4. The concomitant use of higher doses of atorvastatin with certain drugs such as strong CYP3A4 inhibitors increases the risk of myopathy/rhabdomyolysis).
No products indexed under this heading.

Sirolimus (Physicians considering combined therapy with atorvastatin and immunosuppressive drugs should carefully weigh the potential benefits and risks and should carefully monitor patients for any signs or symptoms of muscle pain, tenderness, or weakness, particularly during the initial months of therapy and during any periods of upward dosage titration of either drug. Lower starting and maintenance doses of atorvastatin should be considered when taken concomitantly with immunosuppressive drugs. Periodic creatine phosphokinase (CPK) determinations may be considered in such situations). Products include:
Rapamune 3579

Spironolactone (HMG-CoA reductase inhibitors interfere with cholesterol synthesis and theoretically might blunt adrenal and/or gonadal steroid production. Clinical studies have shown that atorvastatin does not reduce basal plasma cortisol concentration or impair adrenal reserve. Caution should be exercised if an HMG-CoA reductase inhibitor is administered concomitantly with drugs that may decrease levels or activity of endogenous steroid hormones, such as spironolactone).
No products indexed under this heading.

Sulfinpyrazone (Concomitant administration of atorvastatin with inducers of cytochrome P450 3A4 can lead to variable reductions in plasma concentrations of atorvastatin).
No products indexed under this heading.

Tacrolimus (Physicians considering combined therapy with atorvastatin and immunosuppressive drugs should carefully weigh the potential benefits and risks and should carefully monitor patients for any signs or symptoms of muscle pain, tenderness, or weakness, particularly during the initial months of therapy and during any periods of upward dosage titration of either drug. Lower starting and maintenance doses of atorvastatin should be considered when taken concomitantly with immunosuppressive drugs. Periodic creatine phosphokinase (CPK) determinations may be considered in such situations). Products include:
Prograf Capsules 677
Prograf Injection 677
Protopic 685

Telithromycin (Atorvastatin is metabolized by cytochrome P450 3A4. Concomitant administration of atorvastatin with strong inhibitors of cytochrome P450 3A4 can lead to increases in plasma concentrations of atorvastatin. The extent of interaction and potentiation of effects depends on the variability of effect on cytochrome P450 3A4. The concomitant use of higher doses of atorvastatin with certain drugs such as strong CYP3A4 inhibitors increases the risk of myopathy/rhabdomyolysis). Products include:
Ketek 2991

Terconazole (The risk of myopathy during treatment with drugs in this class is increased with concurrent administration of azole antifungals. Physicians considering combined therapy with atorvastatin and azole antifungals should carefully weigh the potential benefits and risks and should carefully monitor patients for any signs or symptoms of muscle pain, tenderness, or weakness, particularly during the initial months of therapy and during any periods of upward dosage titration of either drug. Lower starting and maintenance doses of atorvastatin should be considered when taken concomitantly with azole antifungals. Periodic creatine phosphokinase (CPK) determinations may be considered in such situations).
No products indexed under this heading.

Theophyllinate (Concomitant administration of atorvastatin with inducers of cytochrome P450 3A4 can lead to variable reductions in plasma concentrations of atorvastatin).
No products indexed under this heading.

Theophylline (Concomitant administration of atorvastatin with inducers of cytochrome P450 3A4 can lead to variable reductions in plasma concentrations of atorvastatin).
No products indexed under this heading.

Theophylline Anhydrous (Concomitant administration of atorvastatin with inducers of cytochrome P450 3A4 can lead to variable reductions in plasma concentrations of atorvastatin). Products include:
Uniphyl 2817

Theophylline Calcium Salicylate (Concomitant administration of atorvastatin with inducers of cytochrome P450 3A4 can lead to variable reductions in plasma concentrations of atorvastatin).
No products indexed under this heading.

Theophylline Dihydroxypropyl (Glyceryl) (Concomitant administration of atorvastatin with inducers of cytochrome P450 3A4 can lead to variable reductions in plasma concentrations of atorvastatin).
No products indexed under this heading.

Theophylline Ethylenediamine (Concomitant administration of atorvastatin with inducers of cytochrome P450 3A4 can lead to variable reductions in plasma concentrations of atorvastatin).
No products indexed under this heading.

Theophylline Sodium Glycinate (Concomitant administration of atorvastatin with inducers of cytochrome P450 3A4 can lead to variable reductions in plasma concentrations of atorvastatin).
No products indexed under this heading.

Tipranavir (Atorvastatin AUC was significantly increased with concomitant administration of atorvastatin 40 mg with ritonavir plus saquinavir (400 mg twice daily) or atorvastatin 20 mg with lopinavir plus ritonavir (400 mg + 100 mg twice daily) compared to that of atorvastatin alone. The concomitant use of higher doses of atorvastatin with certain drugs such as strong CYP3A4 inhibitors (eg, HIV protease inhibitors) increases the risk of myopathy/rhabdomyolysis. Caution should be used when exceeding>20 mg atorvastatin daily; the lowest dose necessary should be used).
No products indexed under this heading.

Triamcinolone (Concomitant administration of atorvastatin with inducers of cytochrome P450 3A4 can lead to variable reductions in plasma concentrations of atorvastatin).
No products indexed under this heading.

Triamcinolone Acetonide (Concomitant administration of atorvastatin with inducers of cytochrome P450 3A4 can lead to variable reductions in plasma concentrations of atorvastatin). Products include:
Azmacort 408
Nasacort AQ 3019

Triamcinolone Diacetate (Concomitant administration of atorvastatin with inducers of cytochrome P450 3A4 can lead to variable reductions in plasma concentrations of atorvastatin).
No products indexed under this heading.

Triamcinolone Hexacetonide (Concomitant administration of atorvastatin with inducers of cytochrome P450 3A4 can lead to variable reductions in plasma concentrations of atorvastatin).
No products indexed under this heading.

Troglitazone (Atorvastatin is metabolized by cytochrome P450 3A4. Concomitant administration of atorvastatin with strong inhibitors of cytochrome P450 3A4 can lead to increases in plasma concentrations of atorvastatin. The extent of interaction and potentiation of effects depends on the variability of effect on cytochrome P450 3A4. The concomitant use of higher doses of atorvastatin with certain drugs such as strong CYP3A4 inhibitors increases the risk of myopathy/rhabdomyolysis).
No products indexed under this heading.

Troleandomycin (Atorvastatin is metabolized by cytochrome P450 3A4. Concomitant administration of atorvastatin with strong inhibitors of cytochrome P450 3A4 can lead to increases in plasma concentrations of atorvastatin. The extent of interaction and potentiation of effects depends on the variability of effect on cytochrome P450 3A4. The concomitant use of higher doses of atorvastatin with certain drugs such as strong CYP3A4 inhibitors increases the risk of myopathy/rhabdomyolysis).
No products indexed under this heading.

Valproate Sodium (Atorvastatin is metabolized by cytochrome P450 3A4. Concomitant administration of atorvastatin with strong inhibitors of cytochrome P450 3A4 can lead to increases in plasma concentrations of atorvastatin. The extent of interaction and potentiation of effects depends on the variability of effect on cytochrome P450 3A4. The concomitant use of higher doses of atorvastatin with certain drugs such as strong CYP3A4 inhibitors increases the risk of myopathy/rhabdomyolysis).
No products indexed under this heading.

Vardenafil Hydrochloride (Atorvastatin is metabolized by cytochrome P450 3A4. Concomitant administration of atorvastatin with strong inhibitors of cytochrome P450 3A4 can lead to increases in plasma concentrations of atorvastatin. The extent of interaction and potentiation of effects depends on the variability of effect on cytochrome P450 3A4. The concomitant use of higher doses of atorvastatin with certain drugs such as strong CYP3A4 inhibitors increases the risk of myopathy/rhabdomyolysis). Products include:

Verapamil Hydrochloride (Atorvastatin is metabolized by cytochrome P450 3A4. Concomitant administration of atorvastatin with strong inhibitors of cytochrome P450 3A4 can lead to increases in plasma concentrations of atorvastatin. The extent of interaction and potentiation of effects depends on the variability of effect on cytochrome P450 3A4. The concomitant use of higher doses of atorvastatin with certain drugs such as strong CYP3A4 inhibitors increases the risk of myopathy/rhabdomyolysis). Products include:

Voriconazole (The risk of myopathy during treatment with drugs in this class is increased with concurrent administration of azole antifungals. Physicians considering combined therapy with atorvastatin and azole antifungals should carefully weigh the potential benefits and risks and should carefully monitor patients for any signs or symptoms of muscle pain, tenderness, or weakness, particularly during the initial months of therapy and during any periods of upward dosage titration of either drug. Lower starting and maintenance doses of atorvastatin should be considered when taken concomitantly with azole antifungals. Periodic creatine phosphokinase (CPK) determinations may be considered in such situations).
No products indexed under this heading.

Zafirlukast (Atorvastatin is metabolized by cytochrome P450 3A4. Concomitant administration of atorvastatin with strong inhibitors of cytochrome P450 3A4 can lead to increases in plasma concentrations of atorvastatin. The extent of interaction and potentiation of effects depends on the variability of effect on cytochrome P450 3A4. The concomitant use of higher doses of atorvastatin with certain drugs such as strong CYP3A4 inhibitors increases the risk of myopathy/rhabdomyolysis). Products include:

Zileuton (Atorvastatin is metabolized by cytochrome P450 3A4. Concomitant administration of atorvastatin with strong inhibitors of cytochrome P450 3A4 can lead to increases in plasma concentrations of atorvastatin. The extent of interaction and potentiation of effects depends on the variability of effect on cytochrome P450 3A4. The concomitant use of higher doses of atorvastatin with certain drugs such as strong CYP3A4 inhibitors increases the risk of myopathy/rhabdomyolysis).
No products indexed under this heading.

Food Interactions

Grapefruit (Grapefruit juice contains one or more components that inhibit CYP 3A4 and can increase plasma concentrations of atorvastatin, especially with excessive grapefruit juice consumption (>1.2 liters per day)).

Grapefruit Juice (Grapefruit juice contains one or more components that inhibit CYP 3A4 and can increase plasma concentrations of atorvastatin, especially with excessive grapefruit juice consumption (>1.2 liters per day)).

LOSEASONIQUE TABLETS

May interact with antibiotics, barbiturates, cytochrome p450 3a4 inducers (selected), cytochrome p450 3a4 inhibitors (selected), phenytoin, protease inhibitors, thyroid preparations, and certain other agents. Compounds in these categories include:

Acetaminophen (Acetaminophen may increase plasma ethinyl estradiol levels, possibly by inhibition of conjugation). Products include:

Acetaminophen-containing products (Acetaminophen may increase plasma ethinyl estradiol levels, possibly by inhibition of conjugation).
No products indexed under this heading.

Acetazolamide (CYP3A4 inhibitors may increase plasma hormone levels).
No products indexed under this heading.

Acetazolamide Sodium (CYP3A4 inhibitors may increase plasma hormone levels).
No products indexed under this heading.

Alatrofloxacin Mesylate (There have been reports of pregnancy while taking hormonal contraceptives and antibiotics, but clinical pharmacokinetic studies have not shown consistent effects of antibiotics on plasma concentrations of synthetic steroids).
No products indexed under this heading.

Allium sativum (If a woman on hormonal contraceptives takes a drug or herbal product that induces enzymes, including CYP3A4, that metabolize contraceptive hormones, counsel her to use additional contraception or a different method of contraception. Drugs or herbal products that induce such enzymes may decrease the plasma concentrations of contraceptive hormones, and may decrease the effectiveness of hormonal contraceptives or increase breakthrough bleeding).
No products indexed under this heading.

Amikacin Sulfate (There have been reports of pregnancy while taking hormonal contraceptives and antibiotics, but clinical pharmacokinetic studies have not shown consistent effects of antibiotics on plasma concentrations of synthetic steroids).
No products indexed under this heading.

Aminoglutethimide (If a woman on hormonal contraceptives takes a drug or herbal product that induces enzymes, including CYP3A4, that metabolize contraceptive hormones, counsel her to use additional contraception or a different method of contraception. Drugs or herbal products that induce such enzymes may decrease the plasma concentrations of contraceptive hormones, and may decrease the effectiveness of hormonal contraceptives or increase breakthrough bleeding).
No products indexed under this heading.

Amiodarone Hydrochloride (CYP3A4 inhibitors may increase plasma hormone levels).
No products indexed under this heading.

Amobarbital (Barbiturates may decrease the plasma concentrations of contraceptive hormones, and may decrease the effectiveness of hormonal contraceptives or increase breakthrough bleeding).
No products indexed under this heading.

Amobarbital Sodium (Barbiturates may decrease the plasma concentrations of contraceptive hormones, and may decrease the effectiveness of hormonal contraceptives or increase breakthrough bleeding).
No products indexed under this heading.

Amoxicillin (There have been reports of pregnancy while taking hormonal contraceptives and antibiotics, but clinical pharmacokinetic studies have not shown consistent effects of antibiotics on plasma concentrations of synthetic steroids). Products include:

Amoxicillin Trihydrate (There have been reports of pregnancy while taking hormonal contraceptives and antibiotics, but clinical pharmacokinetic studies have not shown consistent effects of antibiotics on plasma concentrations of synthetic steroids).
No products indexed under this heading.

Ampicillin (There have been reports of pregnancy while taking hormonal contraceptives and antibiotics, but clinical pharmacokinetic studies have not shown consistent effects of antibiotics on plasma concentrations of synthetic steroids).
No products indexed under this heading.

Ampicillin Sodium (There have been reports of pregnancy while taking hormonal contraceptives and antibiotics, but clinical pharmacokinetic studies have not shown consistent effects of antibiotics on plasma concentrations of synthetic steroids).
No products indexed under this heading.

Ampicillin Trihydrate (There have been reports of pregnancy while taking hormonal contraceptives and antibiotics, but clinical pharmacokinetic studies have not shown consistent effects of antibiotics on plasma concentrations of synthetic steroids).
No products indexed under this heading.

Amprenavir (Significant changes (increase or decrease) in the plasma levels of the estrogen and progestin have been noted in some cases of co-administration of HIV protease inhibitors).
No products indexed under this heading.

Anastrozole (CYP3A4 inhibitors may increase plasma hormone levels).
No products indexed under this heading.

Antibiotics, non-penicillin, unspecified (There have been reports of pregnancy while taking hormonal contraceptives and antibiotics, but clinical pharmacokinetic studies have not shown consistent effects of antibiotics on plasma concentrations of synthetic steroids).
No products indexed under this heading.

Aprepitant (If a woman on hormonal contraceptives takes a drug or herbal product that induces enzymes, including CYP3A4, that metabolize contraceptive hormones, counsel her to use additional contraception or a different method of contraception. Drugs or herbal products that induce such enzymes may decrease the plasma concentrations of contraceptive hormones, and may decrease the effectiveness of hormonal contraceptives or increase breakthrough bleeding). Products include:

Aprobarbital (Barbiturates may decrease the plasma concentrations of contraceptive hormones, and may decrease the effectiveness of hormonal contraceptives or increase breakthrough bleeding).
No products indexed under this heading.

Ascorbic Acid (Ascorbic acid may increase plasma ethinyl estradiol levels, possibly by inhibition of conjugation).
No products indexed under this heading.

Atazanavir (Significant changes (increase or decrease) in the plasma levels of the estrogen and progestin have been noted in some cases of co-administration of HIV protease inhibitors).
No products indexed under this heading.

Atazanavir Sulfate (Significant changes (increase or decrease) in the plasma levels of the estrogen and progestin have been noted in some cases of co-administration of HIV protease inhibitors).
No products indexed under this heading.

Atorvastatin Calcium (Co-administration of atorvastatin and certain combination oral contraceptives containing ethinyl estradiol increase AUC values for ethinyl estradiol by approximately 20%). Products include:
Lipitor 2703

Azithromycin Dihydrate (There have been reports of pregnancy while taking hormonal contraceptives and antibiotics, but clinical pharmacokinetic studies have not shown consistent effects of antibiotics on plasma concentrations of synthetic steroids).
No products indexed under this heading.

Azlocillin Sodium (There have been reports of pregnancy while taking hormonal contraceptives and antibiotics, but clinical pharmacokinetic studies have not shown consistent effects of antibiotics on plasma concentrations of synthetic steroids).
No products indexed under this heading.

Aztreonam (There have been reports of pregnancy while taking hormonal contraceptives and antibiotics, but clinical pharmacokinetic studies have not shown consistent effects of antibiotics on plasma concentrations of synthetic steroids).
No products indexed under this heading.

Bacampicillin Hydrochloride (There have been reports of pregnancy while taking hormonal contraceptives and antibiotics, but clinical pharmacokinetic studies have not shown consistent effects of antibiotics on plasma concentrations of synthetic steroids).
No products indexed under this heading.

Betamethasone (If a woman on hormonal contraceptives takes a drug or herbal product that induces enzymes, including CYP3A4, that metabolize contraceptive hormones, counsel her to use additional contraception or a different method of contraception. Drugs or herbal products that induce such enzymes may decrease the plasma concentrations of contraceptive hormones, and may decrease the effectiveness of hormonal contraceptives or increase breakthrough bleeding).
No products indexed under this heading.

Betamethasone Acetate (If a woman on hormonal contraceptives takes a drug or herbal product that induces enzymes, including CYP3A4, that metabolize contraceptive hormones, counsel her to use additional contraception or a different method of contraception. Drugs or herbal products that induce such enzymes may decrease the plasma concentrations of contraceptive hormones, and may decrease the effectiveness of hormonal contraceptives or increase breakthrough bleeding).
No products indexed under this heading.

Betamethasone Benzoate (If a woman on hormonal contraceptives takes a drug or herbal product that induces enzymes, including CYP3A4, that metabolize contraceptive hormones, counsel her to use additional contraception or a different method of contraception. Drugs or herbal products that induce such enzymes may decrease the plasma concentrations of contraceptive hormones, and may decrease the effectiveness of hormonal contraceptives or increase breakthrough bleeding).
No products indexed under this heading.

Betamethasone Dipropionate (If a woman on hormonal contraceptives

takes a drug or herbal product that induces enzymes, including CYP3A4, that metabolize contraceptive hormones, counsel her to use additional contraception or a different method of contraception. Drugs or herbal products that induce such enzymes may decrease the plasma concentrations of contraceptive hormones, and may decrease the effectiveness of hormonal contraceptives or increase breakthrough bleeding). Products include:
Diprolene Lotion 0.05% 3108
Diprolene Ointment 0.05% 3109
Diprolene AF Cream 0.05% 3107
Lotrisone 3163

Betamethasone Sodium Phosphate (If a woman on hormonal contraceptives takes a drug or herbal product that induces enzymes, including CYP3A4, that metabolize contraceptive hormones, counsel her to use additional contraception or a different method of contraception. Drugs or herbal products that induce such enzymes may decrease the plasma concentrations of contraceptive hormones, and may decrease the effectiveness of hormonal contraceptives or increase breakthrough bleeding).
No products indexed under this heading.

Betamethasone Valerate (If a woman on hormonal contraceptives takes a drug or herbal product that induces enzymes, including CYP3A4, that metabolize contraceptive hormones, counsel her to use additional contraception or a different method of contraception. Drugs or herbal products that induce such enzymes may decrease the plasma concentrations of contraceptive hormones, and may decrease the effectiveness of hormonal contraceptives or increase breakthrough bleeding). Products include:
Luxíq 3321

Bosentan (Bosentan may decrease the plasma concentrations of contraceptive hormones, and may decrease the effectiveness of hormonal contraceptives or increase breakthrough bleeding). Products include:
Tracleer 573

Butabarbital (Barbiturates may decrease the plasma concentrations of contraceptive hormones, and may decrease the effectiveness of hormonal contraceptives or increase breakthrough bleeding).
No products indexed under this heading.

Butabarbital Sodium (Barbiturates may decrease the plasma concentrations of contraceptive hormones, and may decrease the effectiveness of hormonal contraceptives or increase breakthrough bleeding).
No products indexed under this heading.

Butalbital (Barbiturates may decrease the plasma concentrations of contraceptive hormones, and may decrease the effectiveness of hormonal contraceptives or increase breakthrough bleeding).
No products indexed under this heading.

Carbamazepine (Carbamazepine may decrease the plasma concentrations of contraceptive hormones, and may decrease the effectiveness of hormonal contraceptives or increase breakthrough bleeding). Products include:
Carbatrol 3280
Equetro 3477

Carbenicillin Disodium (There have been reports of pregnancy while taking hormonal contraceptives and antibiotics, but clinical pharmacokinetic studies have not shown consistent effects of antibiotics on plasma concentrations of synthetic steroids).
No products indexed under this heading.

Carbenicillin Indanyl Sodium (There have been reports of pregnancy while taking hormonal contraceptives and antibiotics, but clinical pharmacokinetic studies have not shown consistent effects of antibiotics on plasma concentrations of synthetic steroids).
No products indexed under this heading.

Cefaclor (There have been reports of pregnancy while taking hormonal contraceptives and antibiotics, but clinical pharmacokinetic studies have not shown consistent effects of antibiotics on plasma concentrations of synthetic steroids).
No products indexed under this heading.

Cefadroxil (There have been reports of pregnancy while taking hormonal contraceptives and antibiotics, but clinical pharmacokinetic studies have not shown consistent effects of antibiotics on plasma concentrations of synthetic steroids).
No products indexed under this heading.

Cefamandole Nafate (There have been reports of pregnancy while taking hormonal contraceptives and antibiotics, but clinical pharmacokinetic studies have not shown consistent effects of antibiotics on plasma concentrations of synthetic steroids).
No products indexed under this heading.

Cefazolin Sodium (There have been reports of pregnancy while taking hormonal contraceptives and antibiotics, but clinical pharmacokinetic studies have not shown consistent effects of antibiotics on plasma concentrations of synthetic steroids).
No products indexed under this heading.

Cefixime (There have been reports of pregnancy while taking hormonal contraceptives and antibiotics, but clinical pharmacokinetic studies have not shown consistent effects of antibiotics on plasma concentrations of synthetic steroids). Products include:
Suprax for Oral Suspension 2038
Suprax Tablets 2038

Cefmetazole Sodium (There have been reports of pregnancy while taking hormonal contraceptives and antibiotics, but clinical pharmacokinetic studies have not shown consistent effects of antibiotics on plasma concentrations of synthetic steroids).
No products indexed under this heading.

Cefonicid Sodium (There have been reports of pregnancy while taking hormonal contraceptives and antibiotics, but clinical pharmacokinetic studies have not shown consistent effects of antibiotics on plasma concentrations of synthetic steroids).
No products indexed under this heading.

Cefoperazone Sodium (There have been reports of pregnancy while taking hormonal contraceptives and antibiotics, but clinical pharmacokinetic studies have not shown consistent effects of antibiotics on plasma concentrations of synthetic steroids).
No products indexed under this heading.

Ceforanide (There have been reports of pregnancy while taking hormonal contraceptives and antibiotics, but clinical pharmacokinetic studies have not shown consistent effects of antibiotics on plasma concentrations of synthetic steroids).
No products indexed under this heading.

Cefotaxime Sodium (There have been reports of pregnancy while taking hormonal contraceptives and antibiotics, but clinical pharmacokinetic studies have not shown consistent effects of antibiotics on plasma concentrations of synthetic steroids).
No products indexed under this heading.

Cefotetan (There have been reports of pregnancy while taking hormonal contraceptives and antibiotics, but clinical pharmacokinetic studies have not shown consistent effects of antibiotics on plasma concentrations of synthetic steroids).
No products indexed under this heading.

Cefoxitin Sodium (There have been reports of pregnancy while taking hormonal contraceptives and antibiotics, but clinical pharmacokinetic studies have not shown consistent effects of antibiotics on plasma concentrations of synthetic steroids).
No products indexed under this heading.

Cefpodoxime Proxetil (There have been reports of pregnancy while taking hormonal contraceptives and antibiotics, but clinical pharmacokinetic studies have not shown consistent effects of antibiotics on plasma concentrations of synthetic steroids).
No products indexed under this heading.

Cefprozil (There have been reports of pregnancy while taking hormonal contraceptives and antibiotics, but clinical pharmacokinetic studies have not shown consistent effects of antibiotics on plasma concentrations of synthetic steroids).
No products indexed under this heading.

Ceftazidime (There have been reports of pregnancy while taking hormonal contraceptives and antibiotics, but clinical pharmacokinetic studies have not shown consistent effects of antibiotics on plasma concentrations of synthetic steroids). Products include:
Fortaz 1481

Ceftizoxime Sodium (There have been reports of pregnancy while taking hormonal contraceptives and antibiotics, but clinical pharmacokinetic studies have not shown consistent effects of antibiotics on plasma concentrations of synthetic steroids).
No products indexed under this heading.

Ceftriaxone Sodium (There have been reports of pregnancy while taking hormonal contraceptives and antibiotics, but clinical pharmacokinetic studies have not shown consistent effects of antibiotics on plasma concentrations of synthetic steroids). Products include:
Rocephin 2859

Cefuroxime Axetil (There have been reports of pregnancy while taking hormonal contraceptives and antibiotics, but clinical pharmacokinetic studies have not shown consistent effects of antibiotics on plasma concentrations of synthetic steroids). Products include:
Ceftin 1399

Cefuroxime Sodium (There have been reports of pregnancy while taking hormonal contraceptives and antibiotics, but clinical pharmacokinetic studies have not shown consistent effects of antibiotics on plasma concentrations of synthetic steroids).
No products indexed under this heading.

Cephalexin (There have been reports of pregnancy while taking hormonal contraceptives and antibiotics, but clinical pharmacokinetic studies have not shown consistent effects of antibiotics on plasma concentrations of synthetic steroids).
No products indexed under this heading.

Cephalothin Sodium (There have been reports of pregnancy while taking hormonal contraceptives and antibiotics, but clinical pharmacokinetic studies have not shown consistent effects of antibiotics on plasma concentrations of synthetic steroids).
No products indexed under this heading.

Cephapirin Sodium (There have been reports of pregnancy while taking hormonal contraceptives and antibiotics, but clinical pharmacokinetic studies have not shown consistent effects of antibiotics on plasma concentrations of synthetic steroids).
No products indexed under this heading.

Cephradine (There have been reports of pregnancy while taking hormonal contraceptives and antibiotics, but clinical pharmacokinetic studies have not shown consistent effects of antibiotics on plasma concentrations of synthetic steroids).
No products indexed under this heading.

Chloramphenicol (There have been reports of pregnancy while taking hormonal contraceptives and antibiotics, but clinical pharmacokinetic studies have not shown consistent effects of antibiotics on plasma concentrations of synthetic steroids).
No products indexed under this heading.

Chloramphenicol Palmitate (There have been reports of pregnancy while taking hormonal contraceptives and antibiotics, but clinical pharmacokinetic studies have not shown consistent effects of antibiotics on plasma concentrations of synthetic steroids).
No products indexed under this heading.

Chloramphenicol Sodium Succinate (There have been reports of pregnancy while taking hormonal contraceptives and antibiotics, but clinical pharmacokinetic studies have not shown consistent effects of antibiotics on plasma concentrations of synthetic steroids).
No products indexed under this heading.

Cilastatin Sodium (There have been reports of pregnancy while taking hormonal contraceptives and antibiotics, but clinical pharmacokinetic studies have not shown consistent effects of antibiotics on plasma concentrations of synthetic steroids). Products include:
Primaxin I.M. **2232**
Primaxin I.V. **2235**

Cimetidine (CYP3A4 inhibitors may increase plasma hormone levels).
No products indexed under this heading.

Cimetidine Hydrochloride (CYP3A4 inhibitors may increase plasma hormone levels).
No products indexed under this heading.

Ciprofloxacin (There have been reports of pregnancy while taking hormonal contraceptives and antibiotics, but clinical pharmacokinetic studies have not shown consistent effects of antibiotics on plasma concentrations of synthetic steroids). Products include:
Cipro I.V. **3082**
Cipro **3073**
Cipro XR **3091**
Ciprodex **583**

Ciprofloxacin Hydrochloride (There have been reports of pregnancy while taking hormonal contraceptives and antibiotics, but clinical pharmacokinetic studies have not shown consistent effects of antibiotics on plasma concentrations of synthetic steroids). Products include:
Cipro **3073**

Cisplatin (If a woman on hormonal contraceptives takes a drug or herbal product that induces enzymes, including CYP3A4, that metabolize contraceptive hormones, counsel her to use additional contraception or a different method of contraception. Drugs or herbal products that induce such enzymes may decrease the plasma concentrations of contraceptive hormones, and may decrease the effectiveness of hormonal contraceptives or increase breakthrough bleeding).
No products indexed under this heading.

Clarithromycin (There have been reports of pregnancy while taking hormonal contraceptives and antibiotics, but clinical pharmacokinetic studies have not shown consistent effects of antibiotics on plasma concentrations of synthetic steroids). Products include:
Biaxin/Biaxin XL **412**

Clotrimazole (There have been reports of pregnancy while taking hormonal contraceptives and antibiotics, but clinical pharmacokinetic studies have not shown consistent effects of antibiotics on plasma concentrations of synthetic steroids). Products include:
Lotrisone **3163**

Cloxacillin (There have been reports of pregnancy while taking hormonal contraceptives and antibiotics, but clinical pharmacokinetic studies have not shown consistent effects of antibiotics on plasma concentrations of synthetic steroids).
No products indexed under this heading.

Cloxacillin Sodium (There have been reports of pregnancy while taking hormonal contraceptives and antibiotics, but clinical pharmacokinetic studies have not shown consistent effects of antibiotics on plasma concentrations of synthetic steroids).
No products indexed under this heading.

Cloxacillin Sodium Monohydrate (There have been reports of pregnancy while taking hormonal contraceptives and antibiotics, but clinical pharmacokinetic studies have not shown consistent effects of antibiotics on plasma concentrations of synthetic steroids).
No products indexed under this heading.

Conivaptan Hydrochloride (CYP3A4 inhibitors may increase plasma hormone levels). Products include:
Vaprisol **689**

Cortisone Acetate (If a woman on hormonal contraceptives takes a drug or herbal product that induces enzymes, including CYP3A4, that metabolize contraceptive hormones, counsel her to use additional contraception or a different method of contraception. Drugs or herbal products that induce such enzymes may decrease the plasma concentrations of contraceptive hormones, and may decrease the effectiveness of hormonal contraceptives or increase breakthrough bleeding).
No products indexed under this heading.

Cyclosporine (CYP3A4 inhibitors may increase plasma hormone levels). Products include:
Gengraf **440**
Neoral Oral Solution **2496**
Neoral Capsules **2496**
Restasis **605**

Dalfopristin (CYP3A4 inhibitors may increase plasma hormone levels).
No products indexed under this heading.

Danazol (CYP3A4 inhibitors may increase plasma hormone levels).
No products indexed under this heading.

Darunavir (Significant changes (increase or decrease) in the plasma levels of the estrogen and progestin have been noted in some cases of co-administration of HIV protease inhibitors).
No products indexed under this heading.

Dasatinib (CYP3A4 inhibitors may increase plasma hormone levels).
No products indexed under this heading.

Daunorubicin Hydrochloride (There have been reports of pregnancy while taking hormonal contraceptives and antibiotics, but clinical pharmacokinetic studies have not shown consistent effects of antibiotics on plasma concentrations of synthetic steroids).
No products indexed under this heading.

Delavirdine Mesylate (CYP3A4 inhibitors may increase plasma hormone levels).
No products indexed under this heading.

Delavirine (CYP3A4 inhibitors may increase plasma hormone levels).
No products indexed under this heading.

Demeclocycline Hydrochloride (There have been reports of pregnancy while taking hormonal contraceptives and antibiotics, but clinical pharmacokinetic studies have not shown consistent effects of antibiotics on plasma concentrations of synthetic steroids).
No products indexed under this heading.

Desloratadine (CYP3A4 inhibitors may increase plasma hormone levels). Products include:
Clarinex Syrup **3098**
Clarinex **3098**
Clarinex Reditabs **3098**
Clarinex-D 12-Hour **3101**
Clarinex-D **3104**

Dexamethasone (If a woman on hormonal contraceptives takes a drug or herbal product that induces enzymes, including CYP3A4, that metabolize contraceptive hormones, counsel her to use additional contraception or a different method of contraception. Drugs or herbal products that induce such enzymes may decrease the plasma concentrations of contraceptive hormones, and may decrease the effectiveness of hormonal contraceptives or increase breakthrough bleeding). Products include:
Ciprodex **583**
Ozurdex .... ⊙ **223**
Tobramycin and Dexamethasone Ophthalmic Suspension .... ⊙ **251**

Dexamethasone Acetate (If a woman on hormonal contraceptives takes a drug or herbal product that induces enzymes, including CYP3A4, that metabolize contraceptive hormones, counsel her to use additional contraception or a different method of contraception. Drugs or herbal products that induce such enzymes may decrease the plasma concentrations of contraceptive hormones, and may decrease the effectiveness of hormonal contraceptives or increase breakthrough bleeding).
No products indexed under this heading.

Dexamethasone Phosphate (If a woman on hormonal contraceptives takes a drug or herbal product that induces enzymes, including CYP3A4, that metabolize contraceptive hormones, counsel her to use additional contraception or a different method of contraception. Drugs or herbal products that induce such enzymes may decrease the plasma concentrations of contraceptive hormones, and may decrease the effectiveness of hormonal contraceptives or increase breakthrough bleeding).
No products indexed under this heading.

Dexamethasone Sodium (If a woman on hormonal contraceptives takes a drug or herbal product that induces enzymes, including CYP3A4, that metabolize contraceptive hormones, counsel her to use additional contraception or a different method of contraception. Drugs or herbal products that induce such enzymes may decrease the plasma concentrations of contraceptive hormones, and may decrease the effectiveness of hormonal contraceptives or increase breakthrough bleeding).
No products indexed under this heading.

Dexamethasone Sodium Phosphate (If a woman on hormonal contraceptives takes a drug or herbal product that induces enzymes, including CYP3A4, that metabolize contraceptive hormones, counsel her to use additional contraception or a different method of contraception. Drugs or herbal products that induce such enzymes may decrease the plasma concentrations of contraceptive hormones, and may decrease the effectiveness of hormonal contraceptives or increase breakthrough bleeding).
No products indexed under this heading.

Dexamethasone Sodium Phosphate Injection (If a woman on hormonal contraceptives takes a drug or herbal product that induces enzymes, including CYP3A4, that metabolize contraceptive hormones, counsel her to use additional contraception or a different method of contraception. Drugs or herbal products that induce such enzymes may decrease the plasma concentrations of contraceptive hormones, and may decrease the effectiveness of hormonal contraceptives or increase breakthrough bleeding).
No products indexed under this heading.

Dicloxacillin (There have been reports of pregnancy while taking hormonal contraceptives and antibiotics, but clinical pharmacokinetic studies have not shown consistent effects of antibiotics on plasma concentrations of synthetic steroids).
No products indexed under this heading.

Dicloxacillin Sodium (There have been reports of pregnancy while taking hormonal contraceptives and antibiotics, but clinical pharmacokinetic studies have not shown consistent effects of antibiotics on plasma concentrations of synthetic steroids).
No products indexed under this heading.

Diltiazem Hydrochloride (CYP3A4 inhibitors may increase plasma hormone levels). Products include:
Cardizem LA **423**

Diltiazem Maleate (CYP3A4 inhibitors may increase plasma hormone levels).
No products indexed under this heading.

Dirithromycin (There have been reports of pregnancy while taking hormonal contraceptives and antibiotics, but clinical pharmacokinetic studies have not shown consistent effects of antibiotics on plasma concentrations of synthetic steroids).
No products indexed under this heading.

Disodium Carbenicillin (There have been reports of pregnancy while taking hormonal contraceptives and antibiotics, but clinical pharmacokinetic studies have not shown consistent effects of antibiotics on plasma concentrations of synthetic steroids).
No products indexed under this heading.

Doxorubicin Hydrochloride (If a woman on hormonal contraceptives takes a drug or herbal product that induces enzymes, including CYP3A4, that metabolize contraceptive hormones, counsel her to use additional contraception or a different method of contraception. Drugs or herbal products that induce such enzymes may decrease the plasma concentrations of contraceptive hormones, and may decrease the effectiveness of hormonal contraceptives or increase breakthrough bleeding).
No products indexed under this heading.

Doxycycline Calcium (There have been reports of pregnancy while taking hormonal contraceptives and antibiotics, but clinical pharmacokinetic studies have not shown consistent effects of antibiotics on plasma concentrations of synthetic steroids).
No products indexed under this heading.

IMPORTANT NOTE: Always consult each drug listing in the patient's regimen for possible interactions.

Doxycycline Hyclate (There have been reports of pregnancy while taking hormonal contraceptives and antibiotics, but clinical pharmacokinetic studies have not shown consistent effects of antibiotics on plasma concentrations of synthetic steroids).
No products indexed under this heading.

Doxycycline Monohydrate (There have been reports of pregnancy while taking hormonal contraceptives and antibiotics, but clinical pharmacokinetic studies have not shown consistent effects of antibiotics on plasma concentrations of synthetic steroids).
No products indexed under this heading.

Efavirenz (If a woman on hormonal contraceptives takes a drug or herbal product that induces enzymes, including CYP3A4, that metabolize contraceptive hormones, counsel her to use additional contraception or a different method of contraception. Drugs or herbal products that induce such enzymes may decrease the plasma concentrations of contraceptive hormones, and may decrease the effectiveness of hormonal contraceptives or increase breakthrough bleeding). Products include:
Atripla 906

Enoxacin (There have been reports of pregnancy while taking hormonal contraceptives and antibiotics, but clinical pharmacokinetic studies have not shown consistent effects of antibiotics on plasma concentrations of synthetic steroids).
No products indexed under this heading.

Epirubicin Hydrochloride (There have been reports of pregnancy while taking hormonal contraceptives and antibiotics, but clinical pharmacokinetic studies have not shown consistent effects of antibiotics on plasma concentrations of synthetic steroids).
No products indexed under this heading.

Erythromycin (There have been reports of pregnancy while taking hormonal contraceptives and antibiotics, but clinical pharmacokinetic studies have not shown consistent effects of antibiotics on plasma concentrations of synthetic steroids).
No products indexed under this heading.

Erythromycin, Topical (There have been reports of pregnancy while taking hormonal contraceptives and antibiotics, but clinical pharmacokinetic studies have not shown consistent effects of antibiotics on plasma concentrations of synthetic steroids).
No products indexed under this heading.

Erythromycin Estolate (There have been reports of pregnancy while taking hormonal contraceptives and antibiotics, but clinical pharmacokinetic studies have not shown consistent effects of antibiotics on plasma concentrations of synthetic steroids).
No products indexed under this heading.

Erythromycin Ethylsuccinate (There have been reports of pregnancy while taking hormonal contraceptives and antibiotics, but clinical pharmacokinetic studies have not shown consistent effects of antibiotics on plasma concentrations of synthetic steroids). Products include:
E.E.S. 437
EryPed 435

Erythromycin Gluceptate (There have been reports of pregnancy while taking hormonal contraceptives and antibiotics, but clinical pharmacokinetic studies have not shown consistent effects of antibiotics on plasma concentrations of synthetic steroids).
No products indexed under this heading.

Erythromycin Lactobionate (There have been reports of pregnancy while taking hormonal contraceptives and antibiotics, but clinical pharmacokinetic studies have not shown consistent effects of antibiotics on plasma concentrations of synthetic steroids).
No products indexed under this heading.

Erythromycin Stearate (There have been reports of pregnancy while taking hormonal contraceptives and antibiotics, but clinical pharmacokinetic studies have not shown consistent effects of antibiotics on plasma concentrations of synthetic steroids).
No products indexed under this heading.

Esomeprazole Magnesium (CYP3A4 inhibitors may increase plasma hormone levels). Products include:
Nexium Capsules 704
Nexium Oral Suspension 704

Esomeprazole Sodium (CYP3A4 inhibitors may increase plasma hormone levels). Products include:
Nexium I.V. 712

Ethosuximide (If a woman on hormonal contraceptives takes a drug or herbal product that induces enzymes, including CYP3A4, that metabolize contraceptive hormones, counsel her to use additional contraception or a different method of contraception. Drugs or herbal products that induce such enzymes may decrease the plasma concentrations of contraceptive hormones, and may decrease the effectiveness of hormonal contraceptives or increase breakthrough bleeding).
No products indexed under this heading.

Felbamate (Felbamate may decrease the plasma concentrations of contraceptive hormones, and may decrease the effectiveness of hormonal contraceptives or increase breakthrough bleeding).
No products indexed under this heading.

Fluconazole (CYP3A4 inhibitors may increase plasma hormone levels).
No products indexed under this heading.

Fludrocortisone Acetate (If a woman on hormonal contraceptives takes a drug or herbal product that induces enzymes, including CYP3A4, that metabolize contraceptive hormones, counsel her to use additional contraception or a different method of contraception. Drugs or herbal products that induce such enzymes may decrease the plasma concentrations of contraceptive hormones, and may decrease the effectiveness of hormonal contraceptives or increase breakthrough bleeding).
No products indexed under this heading.

Fluoxetine (CYP3A4 inhibitors may increase plasma hormone levels).
No products indexed under this heading.

Fluoxetine Hydrochloride (CYP3A4 inhibitors may increase plasma hormone levels). Products include:
Prozac Weekly 1941
Prozac Pulvules 1941
Symbyax 1965

Fluvoxamine Maleate (CYP3A4 inhibitors may increase plasma hormone levels).
No products indexed under this heading.

Fosamprenavir Calcium (Significant changes (increase or decrease) in the plasma levels of the estrogen and progestin have been noted in some cases of co-administration of HIV protease inhibitors). Products include:
Lexiva Oral Suspension 1558
Lexiva 1558

Fosphenytoin (Phenytoin may decrease the plasma concentrations of contraceptive hormones, and may decrease the effectiveness of hormonal contraceptives or increase breakthrough bleeding).
No products indexed under this heading.

Fosphenytoin Sodium (Phenytoin may decrease the plasma concentrations of contraceptive hormones, and may decrease the effectiveness of hormonal contraceptives or increase breakthrough bleeding).
No products indexed under this heading.

Garlic Extract (If a woman on hormonal contraceptives takes a drug or herbal product that induces enzymes, including CYP3A4, that metabolize contraceptive hormones, counsel her to use additional contraception or a different method of contraception. Drugs or herbal products that induce such enzymes may decrease the plasma concentrations of contraceptive hormones, and may decrease the effectiveness of hormonal contraceptives or increase breakthrough bleeding).
No products indexed under this heading.

Garlic Oil (If a woman on hormonal contraceptives takes a drug or herbal product that induces enzymes, including CYP3A4, that metabolize contraceptive hormones, counsel her to use additional contraception or a different method of contraception. Drugs or herbal products that induce such enzymes may decrease the plasma concentrations of contraceptive hormones, and may decrease the effectiveness of hormonal contraceptives or increase breakthrough bleeding).
No products indexed under this heading.

Gatifloxacin (There have been reports of pregnancy while taking hormonal contraceptives and antibiotics, but clinical pharmacokinetic studies have not shown consistent effects of antibiotics on plasma concentrations of synthetic steroids).
No products indexed under this heading.

Gemifloxacin Mesylate (There have been reports of pregnancy while taking hormonal contraceptives and antibiotics, but clinical pharmacokinetic studies have not shown consistent effects of antibiotics on plasma concentrations of synthetic steroids).
No products indexed under this heading.

Gentamicin Sulfate (There have been reports of pregnancy while taking hormonal contraceptives and antibiotics, but clinical pharmacokinetic studies have not shown consistent effects of antibiotics on plasma concentrations of synthetic steroids). Products include:
Pred-G .... ⊙226, ⊙227

Grepafloxacin Hydrochloride (There have been reports of pregnancy while taking hormonal contraceptives and antibiotics, but clinical pharmacokinetic studies have not shown consistent effects of antibiotics on plasma concentrations of synthetic steroids).
No products indexed under this heading.

Griseofulvin (Griseofulvin may decrease the plasma concentrations of contraceptive hormones, and may decrease the effectiveness of hormonal contraceptives or increase breakthrough bleeding).
No products indexed under this heading.

Hexobarbital (Barbiturates may decrease the plasma concentrations of contraceptive hormones, and may decrease the effectiveness of hormonal contraceptives or increase breakthrough bleeding).
No products indexed under this heading.

Hydrocortisone (If a woman on hormonal contraceptives takes a drug or herbal product that induces enzymes, including CYP3A4, that metabolize contraceptive hormones, counsel her to use additional contraception or a different method of contraception. Drugs or herbal products that induce such enzymes may decrease the plasma concentrations of contraceptive hormones, and may decrease the effectiveness of hormonal contraceptives or increase breakthrough bleeding).
No products indexed under this heading.

Hydrocortisone (Alcohol) (If a woman on hormonal contraceptives takes a drug or herbal product that induces enzymes, including CYP3A4, that metabolize contraceptive hormones, counsel her to use additional contraception or a different method of contraception. Drugs or herbal products that induce such enzymes may decrease the plasma concentrations of contraceptive hormones, and may decrease the effectiveness of hormonal contraceptives or increase breakthrough bleeding).
No products indexed under this heading.

Hydrocortisone Acetate (If a woman on hormonal contraceptives takes a drug or herbal product that induces enzymes, including CYP3A4, that metabolize contraceptive hormones, counsel her to use additional contraception or a different method of contraception. Drugs or herbal products that induce such enzymes may decrease the plasma concentrations of contraceptive hormones, and may decrease the effectiveness of hormonal contraceptives or increase breakthrough bleeding).
No products indexed under this heading.

Hydrocortisone Butyrate (If a woman on hormonal contraceptives takes a drug or herbal product that induces enzymes, including CYP3A4, that metabolize contraceptive hormones, counsel her to use additional contraception or a different method of contraception. Drugs or herbal products that induce such enzymes may decrease the plasma concentrations of contraceptive hormones, and may decrease the effectiveness of hormonal contraceptives or increase breakthrough bleeding).
No products indexed under this heading.

Hydrocortisone Cypionate (If a woman on hormonal contraceptives takes a drug or herbal product that induces enzymes, including CYP3A4, that metabolize contraceptive hormones, counsel her to use additional contraception or a different method of contraception. Drugs or herbal products that induce such enzymes may decrease the plasma concentrations of contraceptive hormones, and may decrease the effectiveness of hormonal contraceptives or increase breakthrough bleeding).
No products indexed under this heading.

Hydrocortisone Hemisuccinate (If a woman on hormonal contraceptives takes a drug or herbal product that induces enzymes, including CYP3A4, that metabolize contraceptive hormones, counsel her to use additional contraception or a different method of contraception. Drugs or herbal products that induce such enzymes may decrease the plasma concentrations of contraceptive hormones, and may decrease the effectiveness of hormonal contraceptives or increase breakthrough bleeding).
No products indexed under this heading.

Hydrocortisone Probutate (If a woman on hormonal contraceptives takes a drug or herbal product that induces enzymes, including CYP3A4, that metabolize contraceptive hormones, counsel her to use additional contraception or a different method of contraception. Drugs or herbal products that induce such enzymes may decrease the plasma concentrations of

Nefazodone Hydrochloride
(CYP3A4 inhibitors may increase plasma hormone levels).
   No products indexed under this heading.

Nelfinavir Mesylate (Significant changes (increase or decrease) in the plasma levels of the estrogen and progestin have been noted in some cases of co-administration of HIV protease inhibitors).
   No products indexed under this heading.

Nevirapine (If a woman on hormonal contraceptives takes a drug or herbal product that induces enzymes, including CYP3A4, that metabolize contraceptive hormones, counsel her to use additional contraception or a different method of contraception. Drugs or herbal products that induce such enzymes may decrease the plasma concentrations of contraceptive hormones, and may decrease the effectiveness of hormonal contraceptives or increase breakthrough bleeding). Products include:
   Viramune Oral Suspension 897
   Viramune Tablets 897

Niacin (CYP3A4 inhibitors may increase plasma hormone levels). Products include:
   Advicor 402
   Cardio Basics 3455
   Niaspan 497
   Simcor 524

Niacinamide (CYP3A4 inhibitors may increase plasma hormone levels). Products include:
   CitraNatal 90 DHA Capsules 2332
   CitraNatal Assure 2332
   CitraNatal Rx 2332
   Heplive 607

Niacinamide Hydroiodide (CYP3A4 inhibitors may increase plasma hormone levels).
   No products indexed under this heading.

Nicotinamide (CYP3A4 inhibitors may increase plasma hormone levels).
   No products indexed under this heading.

Nifedipine (CYP3A4 inhibitors may increase plasma hormone levels).
   No products indexed under this heading.

Norfloxacin (There have been reports of pregnancy while taking hormonal contraceptives and antibiotics, but clinical pharmacokinetic studies have not shown consistent effects of antibiotics on plasma concentrations of synthetic steroids). Products include:
   Noroxin 2220

Ofloxacin (There have been reports of pregnancy while taking hormonal contraceptives and antibiotics, but clinical pharmacokinetic studies have not shown consistent effects of antibiotics on plasma concentrations of synthetic steroids).
   No products indexed under this heading.

Omeprazole (CYP3A4 inhibitors may increase plasma hormone levels).
   No products indexed under this heading.

Oxacillin (There have been reports of pregnancy while taking hormonal contraceptives and antibiotics, but clinical pharmacokinetic studies have not shown consistent effects of antibiotics on plasma concentrations of synthetic steroids).
   No products indexed under this heading.

Oxacillin Sodium (There have been reports of pregnancy while taking hormonal contraceptives and antibiotics, but clinical pharmacokinetic studies have not shown consistent effects of antibiotics on plasma concentrations of synthetic steroids).
   No products indexed under this heading.

Oxcarbazepine (Oxcarbazepine may decrease the plasma concentrations of contraceptive hormones, and may decrease the effectiveness of hormonal contraceptives or increase breakthrough bleeding).
   No products indexed under this heading.

Oxytetracycline Hydrochloride
(There have been reports of pregnancy while taking hormonal contraceptives and antibiotics, but clinical pharmacokinetic studies have not shown consistent effects of antibiotics on plasma concentrations of synthetic steroids).
   No products indexed under this heading.

Paroxetine Hydrochloride (CYP3A4 inhibitors may increase plasma hormone levels). Products include:
   Paroxetine CR 2361
   Paroxetine ER 2371
   Paxil 1586
   Paxil CR 1596

Penicillin, Potassium Phenoxymethyl (There have been reports of pregnancy while taking hormonal contraceptives and antibiotics, but clinical pharmacokinetic studies have not shown consistent effects of antibiotics on plasma concentrations of synthetic steroids).
   No products indexed under this heading.

Penicillin G Benzathine (There have been reports of pregnancy while taking hormonal contraceptives and antibiotics, but clinical pharmacokinetic studies have not shown consistent effects of antibiotics on plasma concentrations of synthetic steroids). Products include:
   Bicillin C-R Injectable Suspension 1826
   Bicillin L-A 1828

Penicillin G Dibenzylethyenediamine (There have been reports of pregnancy while taking hormonal contraceptives and antibiotics, but clinical pharmacokinetic studies have not shown consistent effects of antibiotics on plasma concentrations of synthetic steroids).
   No products indexed under this heading.

Penicillin G Potassium (There have been reports of pregnancy while taking hormonal contraceptives and antibiotics, but clinical pharmacokinetic studies have not shown consistent effects of antibiotics on plasma concentrations of synthetic steroids).
   No products indexed under this heading.

Penicillin G Procaine (There have been reports of pregnancy while taking hormonal contraceptives and antibiotics, but clinical pharmacokinetic studies have not shown consistent effects of antibiotics on plasma concentrations of synthetic steroids). Products include:
   Bicillin C-R Injectable Suspension 1826
   Bicillin L-A 1828

Penicillin G Sodium (There have been reports of pregnancy while taking hormonal contraceptives and antibiotics, but clinical pharmacokinetic studies have not shown consistent effects of antibiotics on plasma concentrations of synthetic steroids).
   No products indexed under this heading.

Penicillin V (There have been reports of pregnancy while taking hormonal contraceptives and antibiotics, but clinical pharmacokinetic studies have not shown consistent effects of antibiotics on plasma concentrations of synthetic steroids).
   No products indexed under this heading.

Penicillin V Potassium (There have been reports of pregnancy while taking hormonal contraceptives and antibiotics, but clinical pharmacokinetic studies have not shown consistent effects of antibiotics on plasma concentrations of synthetic steroids).
   No products indexed under this heading.

Penicillins (There have been reports of pregnancy while taking hormonal contraceptives and antibiotics, but clinical pharmacokinetic studies have not shown consistent effects of antibiotics on plasma concentrations of synthetic steroids).
   No products indexed under this heading.

Pentobarbital (Barbiturates may decrease the plasma concentrations of contraceptive hormones, and may decrease the effectiveness of hormonal contraceptives or increase breakthrough bleeding).
   No products indexed under this heading.

Pentobarbital Sodium (Barbiturates may decrease the plasma concentrations of contraceptive hormones, and may decrease the effectiveness of hormonal contraceptives or increase breakthrough bleeding). Products include:
   Nembutal 2012

Phenobarbital (Barbiturates may decrease the plasma concentrations of contraceptive hormones, and may decrease the effectiveness of hormonal contraceptives or increase breakthrough bleeding). Products include:
   Donnatal 2711

Phenobarbital Sodium (Barbiturates may decrease the plasma concentrations of contraceptive hormones, and may decrease the effectiveness of hormonal contraceptives or increase breakthrough bleeding).
   No products indexed under this heading.

Phenytoin (Phenytoin may decrease the plasma concentrations of contraceptive hormones, and may decrease the effectiveness of hormonal contraceptives or increase breakthrough bleeding).
   No products indexed under this heading.

Phenytoin Sodium (Phenytoin may decrease the plasma concentrations of contraceptive hormones, and may decrease the effectiveness of hormonal contraceptives or increase breakthrough bleeding). Products include:
   Phenytek Capsules 2380

Piperacillin Sodium (There have been reports of pregnancy while taking hormonal contraceptives and antibiotics, but clinical pharmacokinetic studies have not shown consistent effects of antibiotics on plasma concentrations of synthetic steroids). Products include:
   Zosyn 3607

Posaconazole (CYP3A4 inhibitors may increase plasma hormone levels). Products include:
   Noxafil 3172

Prednisolone (If a woman on hormonal contraceptives takes a drug or herbal product that induces enzymes, including CYP3A4, that metabolize contraceptive hormones, counsel her to use additional contraception or a different method of contraception. Drugs or herbal products that induce such enzymes may decrease the plasma concentrations of contraceptive hormones, and may decrease the effectiveness of hormonal contraceptives or increase breakthrough bleeding).
   No products indexed under this heading.

Prednisolone Acetate (If a woman on hormonal contraceptives takes a drug or herbal product that induces enzymes, including CYP3A4, that metabolize contraceptive hormones, counsel her to use additional contraception or a different method of contraception. Drugs or herbal products that induce such enzymes may decrease the plasma concentrations of contraceptive hormones, and may decrease the effectiveness of hormonal contraceptives or increase breakthrough bleeding). Products include:
   Blephamide .... ⊙212, ⊙214

   Pred Forte .... ⊙225
   Pred Mild .... ⊙230
   Pred-G .... ⊙226, ⊙227

Prednisolone Sodium Phosphate
(If a woman on hormonal contraceptives takes a drug or herbal product that induces enzymes, including CYP3A4, that metabolize contraceptive hormones, counsel her to use additional contraception or a different method of contraception. Drugs or herbal products that induce such enzymes may decrease the plasma concentrations of contraceptive hormones, and may decrease the effectiveness of hormonal contraceptives or increase breakthrough bleeding).
   No products indexed under this heading.

Prednisolone Tebutate (If a woman on hormonal contraceptives takes a drug or herbal product that induces enzymes, including CYP3A4, that metabolize contraceptive hormones, counsel her to use additional contraception or a different method of contraception. Drugs or herbal products that induce such enzymes may decrease the plasma concentrations of contraceptive hormones, and may decrease the effectiveness of hormonal contraceptives or increase breakthrough bleeding).
   No products indexed under this heading.

Prednisone (If a woman on hormonal contraceptives takes a drug or herbal product that induces enzymes, including CYP3A4, that metabolize contraceptive hormones, counsel her to use additional contraception or a different method of contraception. Drugs or herbal products that induce such enzymes may decrease the plasma concentrations of contraceptive hormones, and may decrease the effectiveness of hormonal contraceptives or increase breakthrough bleeding).
   No products indexed under this heading.

Prednisone sodium phosphate (If a woman on hormonal contraceptives takes a drug or herbal product that induces enzymes, including CYP3A4, that metabolize contraceptive hormones, counsel her to use additional contraception or a different method of contraception. Drugs or herbal products that induce such enzymes may decrease the plasma concentrations of contraceptive hormones, and may decrease the effectiveness of hormonal contraceptives or increase breakthrough bleeding).
   No products indexed under this heading.

Primidone (If a woman on hormonal contraceptives takes a drug or herbal product that induces enzymes, including CYP3A4, that metabolize contraceptive hormones, counsel her to use additional contraception or a different method of contraception. Drugs or herbal products that induce such enzymes may decrease the plasma concentrations of contraceptive hormones, and may decrease the effectiveness of hormonal contraceptives or increase breakthrough bleeding).
   No products indexed under this heading.

Propoxyphene Hydrochloride
(CYP3A4 inhibitors may increase plasma hormone levels).
   No products indexed under this heading.

Propoxyphene Napsylate (CYP3A4 inhibitors may increase plasma hormone levels).
   No products indexed under this heading.

Quinidine (CYP3A4 inhibitors may increase plasma hormone levels).
   No products indexed under this heading.

Quinidine Hydrochloride (CYP3A4 inhibitors may increase plasma hormone levels).
   No products indexed under this heading.

IMPORTANT NOTE: Always consult each drug listing in the patient's regimen for possible interactions.

Tipranavir (Significant changes (increase or decrease) in the plasma levels of the estrogen and progestin have been noted in some cases of co-administration of HIV protease inhibitors).
No products indexed under this heading.

Tobacco (Cigarette smoking increases the risk of serious cardiovascular events from combination oral contraceptives (COC) use).
No products indexed under this heading.

Tobramycin (There have been reports of pregnancy while taking hormonal contraceptives and antibiotics, but clinical pharmacokinetic studies have not shown consistent effects of antibiotics on plasma concentrations of synthetic steroids). Products include:
Tobi Nebulizer 2546
Tobramycin and Dexamethasone Ophthalmic Suspension............... ⊙251
Zylet .... ⊙252

Tobramycin Sulfate (There have been reports of pregnancy while taking hormonal contraceptives and antibiotics, but clinical pharmacokinetic studies have not shown consistent effects of antibiotics on plasma concentrations of synthetic steroids).
No products indexed under this heading.

Topiramate (Topiramate may decrease the plasma concentrations of contraceptive hormones, and may decrease the effectiveness of hormonal contraceptives or increase breakthrough bleeding).
No products indexed under this heading.

Triamcinolone (If a woman on hormonal contraceptives takes a drug or herbal product that induces enzymes, including CYP3A4, that metabolize contraceptive hormones, counsel her to use additional contraception or a different method of contraception. Drugs or herbal products that induce such enzymes may decrease the plasma concentrations of contraceptive hormones, and may decrease the effectiveness of hormonal contraceptives or increase breakthrough bleeding).
No products indexed under this heading.

Triamcinolone Acetonide (If a woman on hormonal contraceptives takes a drug or herbal product that induces enzymes, including CYP3A4, that metabolize contraceptive hormones, counsel her to use additional contraception or a different method of contraception. Drugs or herbal products that induce such enzymes may decrease the plasma concentrations of contraceptive hormones, and may decrease the effectiveness of hormonal contraceptives or increase breakthrough bleeding). Products include:
Azmacort 408
Nasacort AQ 3019

Triamcinolone Diacetate (If a woman on hormonal contraceptives takes a drug or herbal product that induces enzymes, including CYP3A4, that metabolize contraceptive hormones, counsel her to use additional contraception or a different method of contraception. Drugs or herbal products that induce such enzymes may decrease the plasma concentrations of contraceptive hormones, and may decrease the effectiveness of hormonal contraceptives or increase breakthrough bleeding).
No products indexed under this heading.

Triamcinolone Hexacetonide (If a woman on hormonal contraceptives takes a drug or herbal product that induces enzymes, including CYP3A4, that metabolize contraceptive hormones, counsel her to use additional contraception or a different method of contraception. Drugs or herbal products that induce such enzymes may decrease the plasma concentrations of

contraceptive hormones, and may decrease the effectiveness of hormonal contraceptives or increase breakthrough bleeding).
No products indexed under this heading.

Troglitazone (If a woman on hormonal contraceptives takes a drug or herbal product that induces enzymes, including CYP3A4, that metabolize contraceptive hormones, counsel her to use additional contraception or a different method of contraception. Drugs or herbal products that induce such enzymes may decrease the plasma concentrations of contraceptive hormones, and may decrease the effectiveness of hormonal contraceptives or increase breakthrough bleeding).
No products indexed under this heading.

Troleandomycin (There have been reports of pregnancy while taking hormonal contraceptives and antibiotics, but clinical pharmacokinetic studies have not shown consistent effects of antibiotics on plasma concentrations of synthetic steroids).
No products indexed under this heading.

Trovafloxacin Mesylate (There have been reports of pregnancy while taking hormonal contraceptives and antibiotics, but clinical pharmacokinetic studies have not shown consistent effects of antibiotics on plasma concentrations of synthetic steroids).
No products indexed under this heading.

Valproate Sodium (CYP3A4 inhibitors may increase plasma hormone levels).
No products indexed under this heading.

Vardenafil Hydrochloride (CYP3A4 inhibitors may increase plasma hormone levels). Products include:
Levitra 3157

Verapamil Hydrochloride (CYP3A4 inhibitors may increase plasma hormone levels). Products include:
Tarka 534

Vitamin C (Ascorbic acid may increase plasma ethinyl estradiol levels, possibly by inhibition of conjugation). Products include:
Bausch & Lomb Ocuvite Adult 50+ .... ⊙238
Bio-C 3454
BoneMate Plus 3454
Cardio Basics 3455
CitraNatal 90 DHA Capsules 2332
CitraNatal Assure 2332
CitraNatal Rx 2332
Ferralet 2333
Heplive 607
Meili Clear 607
MoviPrep Oral Solution 2905
PreNexa 3473
Proflavanol 90 3476

Voriconazole (CYP3A4 inhibitors may increase plasma hormone levels).
No products indexed under this heading.

Zafirlukast (CYP3A4 inhibitors may increase plasma hormone levels). Products include:
Accolate 3612

Zileuton (CYP3A4 inhibitors may increase plasma hormone levels).
No products indexed under this heading.

Food Interactions

Grapefruit (CYP3A4 inhibitors may increase plasma hormone levels).

Grapefruit Juice (CYP3A4 inhibitors may increase plasma hormone levels).

LOTEMAX OPHTHALMIC SUSPENSION 0.5%
(Loteprednol Etabonate) .... ⊙247
None cited in PDR database.

LOTRISONE CREAM
(Betamethasone Dipropionate, Clotrimazole) 3163
None cited in PDR database.

LOTRISONE LOTION
(Betamethasone Dipropionate, Clotrimazole) 3163
None cited in PDR database.

LOVAZA CAPSULES
(Omega-3-Acid Ethyl Esters) 1569
May interact with anticoagulants, aspirin-acetylsalicylic acid, beta-blockers, estrogens, non-steroidal anti-inflammatory agents, thiazides, and certain other agents. Compounds in these categories include:

Acebutolol Hydrochloride (Medications known to exacerbate hypertriglyceridemia (eg, β-blockers) should be discontinued or changed if possible prior considering triglyceride lowering therapy).
No products indexed under this heading.

Anisindione (Possible prolongation of bleeding time with concomitant anticoagulants administration. Patients receiving treatment with both omega-3-acids and anticoagulants should be monitored periodically).
No products indexed under this heading.

Anticoagulant drugs, unspecified (Possible prolongation of bleeding time with concomitant anticoagulants administration. Patients receiving treatment with both omega-3-acids and anticoagulants should be monitored periodically).
No products indexed under this heading.

Ardeparin Sodium (Possible prolongation of bleeding time with concomitant anticoagulants administration. Patients receiving treatment with both omega-3-acids and anticoagulants should be monitored periodically).
No products indexed under this heading.

Aspirin (Possible prolongation of bleeding time with concomitant anticoagulants administration. Patients receiving treatment with both omega-3-acids and drugs affecting coagulation (eg, aspirin) should be monitored periodically). Products include:
Aggrenox 880
Bayer Aspirin 829
Percodan 1124
St. Joseph Aspirin 2045

Aspirin, Enteric Coated (Possible prolongation of bleeding time with concomitant anticoagulants administration. Patients receiving treatment with both omega-3-acids and drugs affecting coagulation (eg, aspirin) should be monitored periodically).
No products indexed under this heading.

Aspirin Buffered (Possible prolongation of bleeding time with concomitant anticoagulants administration. Patients receiving treatment with both omega-3-acids and drugs affecting coagulation (eg, aspirin) should be monitored periodically).
No products indexed under this heading.

Atenolol (Medications known to exacerbate hypertriglyceridemia (eg, β-blockers) should be discontinued or changed if possible prior considering triglyceride lowering therapy).
No products indexed under this heading.

Bendroflumethiazide (Medications known to exacerbate hypertriglyceridemia (eg, thiazides) should be discontinued or changed if possible before considering triglyceride lowering therapy).
No products indexed under this heading.

Betaxolol Hydrochloride (Medications known to exacerbate hypertriglyceridemia (eg, β-blockers) should be discontinued or changed if possible prior considering triglyceride lowering therapy).
No products indexed under this heading.

Bisoprolol Fumarate (Medications known to exacerbate hypertriglyceridemia (eg, β-blockers) should be discontinued or changed if possible prior considering triglyceride lowering therapy).
No products indexed under this heading.

Carteolol Hydrochloride (Medications known to exacerbate hypertriglyceridemia (eg, β-blockers) should be discontinued or changed if possible prior considering triglyceride lowering therapy).
No products indexed under this heading.

Carvedilol (Medications known to exacerbate hypertriglyceridemia (eg, β-blockers) should be discontinued or changed if possible prior considering triglyceride lowering therapy). Products include:
Coreg 1409

Carvedilol Phosphate (Medications known to exacerbate hypertriglyceridemia (eg, β-blockers) should be discontinued or changed if possible prior considering triglyceride lowering therapy). Products include:
Coreg CR 1416

Celecoxib (Possible prolongation of bleeding time with concomitant anticoagulants administration. Patients receiving treatment with both omega-3-acids and drugs affecting coagulation (eg, NSAIDs) should be monitored periodically). Products include:
Celebrex 3272

Chlorothiazide (Medications known to exacerbate hypertriglyceridemia (eg, thiazides) should be discontinued or changed if possible before considering triglyceride lowering therapy).
No products indexed under this heading.

Chlorothiazide Sodium (Medications known to exacerbate hypertriglyceridemia (eg, thiazides) should be discontinued or changed if possible before considering triglyceride lowering therapy). Products include:
Diuril Intravenous 2009

Chlorotrianisene (Medications known to exacerbate hypertriglyceridemia (eg, estrogens) should be discontinued or changed if possible before considering triglyceride lowering therapy).
No products indexed under this heading.

Coumarin Derivatives (Possible prolongation of bleeding time with concomitant anticoagulants administration. Patients receiving treatment with both omega-3-acids and anticoagulants (eg, coumarin) should be monitored periodically).
No products indexed under this heading.

Dalteparin Sodium (Possible prolongation of bleeding time with concomitant anticoagulants administration. Patients receiving treatment with both omega-3-acids and anticoagulants should be monitored periodically). Products include:
Fragmin 1058

Danaparoid Sodium (Possible prolongation of bleeding time with concomitant anticoagulants administration. Patients receiving treatment with both omega-3-acids and anticoagulants should be monitored periodically).
No products indexed under this heading.

Diclofenac Epolamine (Possible prolongation of bleeding time with concomitant anticoagulants administration. Patients receiving treatment with both omega-3-acids and drugs affecting coagulation (eg, NSAIDs) should be monitored periodically). Products include:
Flector 1839

IMPORTANT NOTE: Always consult each drug listing in the patient's regimen for possible interactions.

Piroxicam (Possible prolongation of bleeding time with concomitant anticoagulants administration. Patients receiving treatment with both omega-3-acids and drugs affecting coagulation (eg, NSAIDs) should be monitored periodically).

No products indexed under this heading.

Polyestradiol Phosphate (Medications known to exacerbate hypertriglyceridemia (eg, estrogens) should be discontinued or changed if possible before considering triglyceride lowering therapy).

No products indexed under this heading.

Polythiazide (Medications known to exacerbate hypertriglyceridemia (eg, thiazides) should be discontinued or changed if possible before considering triglyceride lowering therapy).

No products indexed under this heading.

Propranolol Hydrochloride (Medications known to exacerbate hypertriglyceridemia (eg, β-blockers) should be discontinued or changed if possible prior considering triglyceride lowering therapy). Products include:
InnoPran XL 1517

Quinestrol (Medications known to exacerbate hypertriglyceridemia (eg, estrogens) should be discontinued or changed if possible before considering triglyceride lowering therapy).

No products indexed under this heading.

Rofecoxib (Possible prolongation of bleeding time with concomitant anticoagulants administration. Patients receiving treatment with both omega-3-acids and drugs affecting coagulation (eg, NSAIDs) should be monitored periodically).

No products indexed under this heading.

Sotalol Hydrochloride (Medications known to exacerbate hypertriglyceridemia (eg, β-blockers) should be discontinued or changed if possible prior considering triglyceride lowering therapy).

No products indexed under this heading.

Sulindac (Possible prolongation of bleeding time with concomitant anticoagulants administration. Patients receiving treatment with both omega-3-acids and drugs affecting coagulation (eg, NSAIDs) should be monitored periodically). Products include:
Clinoril 2098

Timolol Hemihydrate (Medications known to exacerbate hypertriglyceridemia (eg, β-blockers) should be discontinued or changed if possible prior considering triglyceride lowering therapy). Products include:
Betimol 3490

Timolol Maleate (Medications known to exacerbate hypertriglyceridemia (eg, β-blockers) should be discontinued or changed if possible prior considering triglyceride lowering therapy). Products include:
Combigan 601
Dorzolamide
Hydrochloride/Timolol Maleate
Ophthalmic Solution .... ⊙243
Timoptic in Ocudose ....⊙231

Tinzaparin Sodium (Possible prolongation of bleeding time with concomitant anticoagulants administration. Patients receiving treatment with both omega-3-acids and anticoagulants should be monitored periodically).

No products indexed under this heading.

Tolmetin Sodium (Possible prolongation of bleeding time with concomitant anticoagulants administration. Patients receiving treatment with both omega-3-acids and drugs affecting coagulation (eg, NSAIDs) should be monitored periodically).

No products indexed under this heading.

Valdecoxib (Possible prolongation of bleeding time with concomitant anticoagulants administration. Patients receiving treatment with both omega-3-acids and drugs affecting coagulation (eg, NSAIDs) should be monitored periodically).

No products indexed under this heading.

Warfarin Sodium (Possible prolongation of bleeding time with concomitant anticoagulants administration. Patients receiving treatment with both omega-3-acids and anticoagulants (eg, warfarin) should be monitored periodically).

No products indexed under this heading.

LOVENOX INJECTION

(Enoxaparin Sodium) 3005
May interact with anticoagulants, aspirin-acetylsalicylic acid, non-steroidal anti-inflammatory agents, platelet inhibitors, potassium sparing diuretics, salicylates, spinal and peridural anesthetics, and certain other agents. Compounds in these categories include:

Abciximab (Whenever possible, agents which may enhance the risk of hemorrhage should be discontinued prior to initiation of enoxaparin therapy. These agents include medications such as: anticoagulants, platelet inhibitors including acetylsalicylic acid, salicylates, NSAIDs (including ketorolac tromethamine), dipyridamole, or sulfinpyrazone. If co-administration is essential, conduct close clinical and laboratory monitoring). Products include:
ReoPro 1952

Amiloride Hydrochloride (Cases of hyperkalemia have been reported. Most of these reports occurred in patients who also had conditions that tend toward the development of hyperkalemia (eg, renal dysfunction, concomitant potassium-sparing drugs, administration of potassium, hematoma in body tissues)).

No products indexed under this heading.

Anisindione (Whenever possible, agents which may enhance the risk of hemorrhage should be discontinued prior to initiation of enoxaparin therapy. These agents include medications such as: anticoagulants, platelet inhibitors including acetylsalicylic acid, salicylates, NSAIDs (including ketorolac tromethamine), dipyridamole, or sulfinpyrazone. If co-administration is essential, conduct close clinical and laboratory monitoring).

No products indexed under this heading.

Ardeparin Sodium (Whenever possible, agents which may enhance the risk of hemorrhage should be discontinued prior to initiation of enoxaparin therapy. These agents include medications such as: anticoagulants, platelet inhibitors including acetylsalicylic acid, salicylates, NSAIDs (including ketorolac tromethamine), dipyridamole, or sulfinpyrazone. If co-administration is essential, conduct close clinical and laboratory monitoring).

No products indexed under this heading.

Aspirin (The use of aspirin and other NSAIDs may enhance the risk of hemorrhage. Their use should be discontinued prior to enoxaparin therapy whenever possible; if co-administration is essential, the patient's clinical and laboratory status should be closely monitored). Products include:
Aggrenox 880
Bayer Aspirin 829
Percodan 1124
St. Joseph Aspirin 2045

Aspirin, Enteric Coated (Whenever possible, agents which may enhance the risk of hemorrhage should be discontinued prior to initiation of enoxaparin therapy. These agents include

medications such as: anticoagulants, platelet inhibitors including acetylsalicylic acid, salicylates, NSAIDs (including ketorolac tromethamine), dipyridamole, or sulfinpyrazone. If co-administration is essential, conduct close clinical and laboratory monitoring).

No products indexed under this heading.

Aspirin Buffered (Whenever possible, agents which may enhance the risk of hemorrhage should be discontinued prior to initiation of enoxaparin therapy. These agents include medications such as: anticoagulants, platelet inhibitors including acetylsalicylic acid, salicylates, NSAIDs (including ketorolac tromethamine), dipyridamole, or sulfinpyrazone. If co-administration is essential, conduct close clinical and laboratory monitoring).

No products indexed under this heading.

Azlocillin Sodium (Whenever possible, agents which may enhance the risk of hemorrhage should be discontinued prior to initiation of enoxaparin therapy. These agents include medications such as: anticoagulants, platelet inhibitors including acetylsalicylic acid, salicylates, NSAIDs (including ketorolac tromethamine), dipyridamole, or sulfinpyrazone. If co-administration is essential, conduct close clinical and laboratory monitoring).

No products indexed under this heading.

Bupivacaine Hydrochloride (There have been reports of epidural or spinal hematoma formation with concurrent use of enoxaparin and spinal/epidural anesthesia or spinal puncture).

No products indexed under this heading.

Carbenicillin Indanyl Sodium (Whenever possible, agents which may enhance the risk of hemorrhage should be discontinued prior to initiation of enoxaparin therapy. These agents include medications such as: anticoagulants, platelet inhibitors including acetylsalicylic acid, salicylates, NSAIDs (including ketorolac tromethamine), dipyridamole, or sulfinpyrazone. If co-administration is essential, conduct close clinical and laboratory monitoring).

No products indexed under this heading.

Celecoxib (Whenever possible, agents which may enhance the risk of hemorrhage should be discontinued prior to initiation of enoxaparin therapy. These agents include medications such as: anticoagulants, platelet inhibitors including acetylsalicylic acid, salicylates, NSAIDs (including ketorolac tromethamine), dipyridamole, or sulfinpyrazone. If co-administration is essential, conduct close clinical and laboratory monitoring). Products include:
Celebrex 3272

Choline Magnesium Trisalicylate (Whenever possible, agents which may enhance the risk of hemorrhage should be discontinued prior to initiation of enoxaparin therapy. These agents include medications such as: anticoagulants, platelet inhibitors including acetylsalicylic acid, salicylates, NSAIDs (including ketorolac tromethamine), dipyridamole, or sulfinpyrazone. If co-administration is essential, conduct close clinical and laboratory monitoring).

No products indexed under this heading.

Clopidogrel Bisulfate (Whenever possible, agents which may enhance the risk of hemorrhage should be discontinued prior to initiation of enoxaparin therapy. These agents include medications such as: anticoagulants, platelet inhibitors including acetylsalicylic acid, salicylates, NSAIDs (including ketorolac tromethamine), dipyridamole, or sulfinpyrazone. If co-administration is

essential, conduct close clinical and laboratory monitoring). Products include:
Plavix 3027

Dalteparin Sodium (Whenever possible, agents which may enhance the risk of hemorrhage should be discontinued prior to initiation of enoxaparin therapy. These agents include medications such as: anticoagulants, platelet inhibitors including acetylsalicylic acid, salicylates, NSAIDs (including ketorolac tromethamine), dipyridamole, or sulfinpyrazone. If co-administration is essential, conduct close clinical and laboratory monitoring). Products include:
Fragmin 1058

Danaparoid Sodium (Whenever possible, agents which may enhance the risk of hemorrhage should be discontinued prior to initiation of enoxaparin therapy. These agents include medications such as: anticoagulants, platelet inhibitors including acetylsalicylic acid, salicylates, NSAIDs (including ketorolac tromethamine), dipyridamole, or sulfinpyrazone. If co-administration is essential, conduct close clinical and laboratory monitoring).

No products indexed under this heading.

Dextran (Whenever possible, agents which may enhance the risk of hemorrhage should be discontinued prior to initiation of enoxaparin therapy. These agents include medications such as: anticoagulants, platelet inhibitors including acetylsalicylic acid, salicylates, NSAIDs (including ketorolac tromethamine), dipyridamole, or sulfinpyrazone. If co-administration is essential, conduct close clinical and laboratory monitoring).

No products indexed under this heading.

Dextran 40 (Whenever possible, agents which may enhance the risk of hemorrhage should be discontinued prior to initiation of enoxaparin therapy. These agents include medications such as: anticoagulants, platelet inhibitors including acetylsalicylic acid, salicylates, NSAIDs (including ketorolac tromethamine), dipyridamole, or sulfinpyrazone. If co-administration is essential, conduct close clinical and laboratory monitoring).

No products indexed under this heading.

Dextran 70 (Whenever possible, agents which may enhance the risk of hemorrhage should be discontinued prior to initiation of enoxaparin therapy. These agents include medications such as: anticoagulants, platelet inhibitors including acetylsalicylic acid, salicylates, NSAIDs (including ketorolac tromethamine), dipyridamole, or sulfinpyrazone. If co-administration is essential, conduct close clinical and laboratory monitoring).

No products indexed under this heading.

Dextran I (Whenever possible, agents which may enhance the risk of hemorrhage should be discontinued prior to initiation of enoxaparin therapy. These agents include medications such as: anticoagulants, platelet inhibitors including acetylsalicylic acid, salicylates, NSAIDs (including ketorolac tromethamine), dipyridamole, or sulfinpyrazone. If co-administration is essential, conduct close clinical and laboratory monitoring).

No products indexed under this heading.

Dextrans (Low Molecular Weight) (Whenever possible, agents which may enhance the risk of hemorrhage should be discontinued prior to initiation of enoxaparin therapy. These agents include medications such as: anticoagulants, platelet inhibitors including acetylsalicylic acid, salicylates, NSAIDs (including ketorolac tromethamine), dipyridamole, or sulfinpyrazone. If co-

1067 **Interactions Index** **Lovenox**

administration is essential, conduct close clinical and laboratory monitoring).
No products indexed under this heading.

Diclofenac Epolamine (Whenever possible, agents which may enhance the risk of hemorrhage should be discontinued prior to initiation of enoxaparin therapy. These agents include medications such as: anticoagulants, platelet inhibitors including acetylsalicylic acid, salicylates, NSAIDs (including ketorolac tromethamine), dipyridamole, or sulfinpyrazone. If co-administration is essential, conduct close clinical and laboratory monitoring). Products include:
Flector 1839

Diclofenac Potassium (Whenever possible, agents which may enhance the risk of hemorrhage should be discontinued prior to initiation of enoxaparin therapy. These agents include medications such as: anticoagulants, platelet inhibitors including acetylsalicylic acid, salicylates, NSAIDs (including ketorolac tromethamine), dipyridamole, or sulfinpyrazone. If co-administration is essential, conduct close clinical and laboratory monitoring).
No products indexed under this heading.

Diclofenac Sodium (Whenever possible, agents which may enhance the risk of hemorrhage should be discontinued prior to initiation of enoxaparin therapy. These agents include medications such as: anticoagulants, platelet inhibitors including acetylsalicylic acid, salicylates, NSAIDs (including ketorolac tromethamine), dipyridamole, or sulfinpyrazone. If co-administration is essential, conduct close clinical and laboratory monitoring).
No products indexed under this heading.

Dicumarol (Whenever possible, agents which may enhance the risk of hemorrhage should be discontinued prior to initiation of enoxaparin therapy. These agents include medications such as: anticoagulants, platelet inhibitors including acetylsalicylic acid, salicylates, NSAIDs (including ketorolac tromethamine), dipyridamole, or sulfinpyrazone. If co-administration is essential, conduct close clinical and laboratory monitoring).
No products indexed under this heading.

Diflunisal (Whenever possible, agents which may enhance the risk of hemorrhage should be discontinued prior to initiation of enoxaparin therapy. These agents include medications such as: anticoagulants, platelet inhibitors including acetylsalicylic acid, salicylates, NSAIDs (including ketorolac tromethamine), dipyridamole, or sulfinpyrazone. If co-administration is essential, conduct close clinical and laboratory monitoring).
No products indexed under this heading.

Dipyridamole (Whenever possible, agents which may enhance the risk of hemorrhage should be discontinued prior to initiation of enoxaparin therapy. These agents include medications such as: anticoagulants, platelet inhibitors including acetylsalicylic acid, salicylates, NSAIDs (including ketorolac tromethamine), dipyridamole, or sulfinpyrazone. If co-administration is essential, conduct close clinical and laboratory monitoring). Products include:
Aggrenox 880

Eptifibatide (Whenever possible, agents which may enhance the risk of hemorrhage should be discontinued prior to initiation of enoxaparin therapy. These agents include medications such as: anticoagulants, platelet inhibitors including acetylsalicylic acid, salicylates, NSAIDs (including ketorolac tromethamine), dipyridamole, or sulfinpyrazone. If co-administration is essential, conduct close clinical and laboratory monitoring). Products include:
Integrilin 3135

Etidocaine Hydrochloride (There have been reports of epidural or spinal hematoma formation with concurrent use of enoxaparin and spinal/epidural anesthesia or spinal puncture).
No products indexed under this heading.

Etodolac (Whenever possible, agents which may enhance the risk of hemorrhage should be discontinued prior to initiation of enoxaparin therapy. These agents include medications such as: anticoagulants, platelet inhibitors including acetylsalicylic acid, salicylates, NSAIDs (including ketorolac tromethamine), dipyridamole, or sulfinpyrazone. If co-administration is essential, conduct close clinical and laboratory monitoring).
No products indexed under this heading.

Fenoprofen Calcium (Whenever possible, agents which may enhance the risk of hemorrhage should be discontinued prior to initiation of enoxaparin therapy. These agents include medications such as: anticoagulants, platelet inhibitors including acetylsalicylic acid, salicylates, NSAIDs (including ketorolac tromethamine), dipyridamole, or sulfinpyrazone. If co-administration is essential, conduct close clinical and laboratory monitoring).
No products indexed under this heading.

Flurbiprofen (Whenever possible, agents which may enhance the risk of hemorrhage should be discontinued prior to initiation of enoxaparin therapy. These agents include medications such as: anticoagulants, platelet inhibitors including acetylsalicylic acid, salicylates, NSAIDs (including ketorolac tromethamine), dipyridamole, or sulfinpyrazone. If co-administration is essential, conduct close clinical and laboratory monitoring).
No products indexed under this heading.

Fondaparinux Sodium (Whenever possible, agents which may enhance the risk of hemorrhage should be discontinued prior to initiation of enoxaparin therapy. These agents include medications such as: anticoagulants, platelet inhibitors including acetylsalicylic acid, salicylates, NSAIDs (including ketorolac tromethamine), dipyridamole, or sulfinpyrazone. If co-administration is essential, conduct close clinical and laboratory monitoring). Products include:
Arixtra 1320

Heparin Calcium (Whenever possible, agents which may enhance the risk of hemorrhage should be discontinued prior to initiation of enoxaparin therapy. These agents include medications such as: anticoagulants, platelet inhibitors including acetylsalicylic acid, salicylates, NSAIDs (including ketorolac tromethamine), dipyridamole, or sulfinpyrazone. If co-administration is essential, conduct close clinical and laboratory monitoring).
No products indexed under this heading.

Heparin Sodium (Whenever possible, agents which may enhance the risk of hemorrhage should be discontinued prior to initiation of enoxaparin therapy. These agents include medications such as: anticoagulants, platelet inhibitors including acetylsalicylic acid, salicylates, NSAIDs (including ketorolac tromethamine), dipyridamole, or sulfinpyrazone. If co-administration is essential, conduct close clinical and laboratory monitoring).
No products indexed under this heading.

Hydroxychloroquine Sulfate (Whenever possible, agents which may enhance the risk of hemorrhage should be discontinued prior to initiation of enoxaparin therapy. These agents include medications such as: anticoagulants, platelet inhibitors including acetylsalicylic acid, salicylates, NSAIDs (including ketorolac tromethamine), dipyridamole, or sulfinpyrazone. If co-administration is essential, conduct close clinical and laboratory monitoring).
No products indexed under this heading.

Ibuprofen (Whenever possible, agents which may enhance the risk of hemorrhage should be discontinued prior to initiation of enoxaparin therapy. These agents include medications such as: anticoagulants, platelet inhibitors including acetylsalicylic acid, salicylates, NSAIDs (including ketorolac tromethamine), dipyridamole, or sulfinpyrazone. If co-administration is essential, conduct close clinical and laboratory monitoring). Products include:
Motrin IB 2043
Children's Motrin 2044
Children's Motrin Non-Staining Dye-Free 2044
Infants' Motrin 2044
Infants' Motrin Dye-Free 2044
Junior Strength Motrin 2044
Vicoprofen 564

Indomethacin (Whenever possible, agents which may enhance the risk of hemorrhage should be discontinued prior to initiation of enoxaparin therapy. These agents include medications such as: anticoagulants, platelet inhibitors including acetylsalicylic acid, salicylates, NSAIDs (including ketorolac tromethamine), dipyridamole, or sulfinpyrazone. If co-administration is essential, conduct close clinical and laboratory monitoring). Products include:
Indocin 2167

Indomethacin Sodium Trihydrate (Whenever possible, agents which may enhance the risk of hemorrhage should be discontinued prior to initiation of enoxaparin therapy. These agents include medications such as: anticoagulants, platelet inhibitors including acetylsalicylic acid, salicylates, NSAIDs (including ketorolac tromethamine), dipyridamole, or sulfinpyrazone. If co-administration is essential, conduct close clinical and laboratory monitoring). Products include:
Indocin I.V. 2007

Ketoprofen (Whenever possible, agents which may enhance the risk of hemorrhage should be discontinued prior to initiation of enoxaparin therapy. These agents include medications such as: anticoagulants, platelet inhibitors including acetylsalicylic acid, salicylates, NSAIDs (including ketorolac tromethamine), dipyridamole, or sulfinpyrazone. If co-administration is essential, conduct close clinical and laboratory monitoring).
No products indexed under this heading.

Ketorolac Tromethamine (Whenever possible, agents which may enhance the risk of hemorrhage should be discontinued prior to initiation of enoxaparin therapy. These agents include medications such as: anticoagulants, platelet inhibitors including acetylsalicylic acid, salicylates, NSAIDs (including ketorolac tromethamine), dipyridamole, or sulfinpyrazone. If co-administration is essential, conduct close clinical and laboratory monitoring). Products include:
Acuvail .... ⊙ 209

Lidocaine Hydrochloride (There have been reports of epidural or spinal hematoma formation with concurrent use of enoxaparin and spinal/epidural anesthesia or spinal puncture).
No products indexed under this heading.

Low Molecular Weight Heparins (Whenever possible, agents which may enhance the risk of hemorrhage should be discontinued prior to initiation of enoxaparin therapy. These agents include medications such as: anticoagulants, platelet inhibitors including acetylsalicylic acid, salicylates, NSAIDs (including ketorolac tromethamine), dipyridamole, or sulfinpyrazone. If co-administration is essential, conduct close clinical and laboratory monitoring).
No products indexed under this heading.

Magnesium Salicylate (Whenever possible, agents which may enhance the risk of hemorrhage should be discontinued prior to initiation of enoxaparin therapy. These agents include medications such as: anticoagulants, platelet inhibitors including acetylsalicylic acid, salicylates, NSAIDs (including ketorolac tromethamine), dipyridamole, or sulfinpyrazone. If co-administration is essential, conduct close clinical and laboratory monitoring).
No products indexed under this heading.

Meclofenamate Sodium (Whenever possible, agents which may enhance the risk of hemorrhage should be discontinued prior to initiation of enoxaparin therapy. These agents include medications such as: anticoagulants, platelet inhibitors including acetylsalicylic acid, salicylates, NSAIDs (including ketorolac tromethamine), dipyridamole, or sulfinpyrazone. If co-administration is essential, conduct close clinical and laboratory monitoring).
No products indexed under this heading.

Mefenamic Acid (Whenever possible, agents which may enhance the risk of hemorrhage should be discontinued prior to initiation of enoxaparin therapy. These agents include medications such as: anticoagulants, platelet inhibitors including acetylsalicylic acid, salicylates, NSAIDs (including ketorolac tromethamine), dipyridamole, or sulfinpyrazone. If co-administration is essential, conduct close clinical and laboratory monitoring).
No products indexed under this heading.

Meloxicam (Whenever possible, agents which may enhance the risk of hemorrhage should be discontinued prior to initiation of enoxaparin therapy. These agents include medications such as: anticoagulants, platelet inhibitors including acetylsalicylic acid, salicylates, NSAIDs (including ketorolac tromethamine), dipyridamole, or sulfinpyrazone. If co-administration is essential, conduct close clinical and laboratory monitoring).
No products indexed under this heading.

Mepivacaine Hydrochloride (There have been reports of epidural or spinal hematoma formation with concurrent use of enoxaparin and spinal/epidural anesthesia or spinal puncture).
No products indexed under this heading.

Mezlocillin Sodium (Whenever possible, agents which may enhance the risk of hemorrhage should be discontinued prior to initiation of enoxaparin therapy. These agents include medications such as: anticoagulants, platelet inhibitors including acetylsalicylic acid, salicylates, NSAIDs (including ketorolac tromethamine), dipyridamole, or sulfinpyrazone. If co-administration is essential, conduct close clinical and laboratory monitoring).
No products indexed under this heading.

Nabumetone (Whenever possible, agents which may enhance the risk of hemorrhage should be discontinued prior to initiation of enoxaparin therapy. These agents include medications such as: anticoagulants, platelet inhibitors including acetylsalicylic acid, salicylates, NSAIDs (including ketorolac tromethamine), dipyridamole, or sulfin-

IMPORTANT NOTE: Always consult each drug listing in the patient's regimen for possible interactions.

Lovenox Interactions Index 1068

pyrazone. If co-administration is essential, conduct close clinical and laboratory monitoring).
No products indexed under this heading.

Nafcillin Sodium (Whenever possible, agents which may enhance the risk of hemorrhage should be discontinued prior to initiation of enoxaparin therapy. These agents include medications such as: anticoagulants, platelet inhibitors including acetylsalicylic acid, salicylates, NSAIDs (including ketorolac tromethamine), dipyridamole, or sulfinpyrazone. If co-administration is essential, conduct close clinical and laboratory monitoring).
No products indexed under this heading.

Naproxen (Whenever possible, agents which may enhance the risk of hemorrhage should be discontinued prior to initiation of enoxaparin therapy. These agents include medications such as: anticoagulants, platelet inhibitors including acetylsalicylic acid, salicylates, NSAIDs (including ketorolac tromethamine), dipyridamole, or sulfinpyrazone. If co-administration is essential, conduct close clinical and laboratory monitoring). Products include:
EC-Naprosyn 2850
Naprosyn 2850
Anaprox/Naprosyn 2850

Naproxen Sodium (Whenever possible, agents which may enhance the risk of hemorrhage should be discontinued prior to initiation of enoxaparin therapy. These agents include medications such as: anticoagulants, platelet inhibitors including acetylsalicylic acid, salicylates, NSAIDs (including ketorolac tromethamine), dipyridamole, or sulfinpyrazone. If co-administration is essential, conduct close clinical and laboratory monitoring). Products include:
Anaprox 2850
Anaprox DS 2850
Treximet 1681

Oxaprozin (Whenever possible, agents which may enhance the risk of hemorrhage should be discontinued prior to initiation of enoxaparin therapy. These agents include medications such as: anticoagulants, platelet inhibitors including acetylsalicylic acid, salicylates, NSAIDs (including ketorolac tromethamine), dipyridamole, or sulfinpyrazone. If co-administration is essential, conduct close clinical and laboratory monitoring).
No products indexed under this heading.

Penicillin G Benzathine (Whenever possible, agents which may enhance the risk of hemorrhage should be discontinued prior to initiation of enoxaparin therapy. These agents include medications such as: anticoagulants, platelet inhibitors including acetylsalicylic acid, salicylates, NSAIDs (including ketorolac tromethamine), dipyridamole, or sulfinpyrazone. If co-administration is essential, conduct close clinical and laboratory monitoring). Products include:
Bicillin C-R Injectable Suspension 1826
Bicillin L-A 1828

Penicillin G Procaine (Whenever possible, agents which may enhance the risk of hemorrhage should be discontinued prior to initiation of enoxaparin therapy. These agents include medications such as: anticoagulants, platelet inhibitors including acetylsalicylic acid, salicylates, NSAIDs (including ketorolac tromethamine), dipyridamole, or sulfinpyrazone. If co-administration is essential, conduct close clinical and laboratory monitoring). Products include:
Bicillin C-R Injectable Suspension 1826
Bicillin L-A 1828

Phenylbutazone (Whenever possible, agents which may enhance the risk of hemorrhage should be discontinued prior to initiation of enoxaparin therapy. These agents include medications such as: anticoagulants, platelet inhibitors including acetylsalicylic acid, salicylates, NSAIDs (including ketorolac tromethamine), dipyridamole, or sulfinpyrazone. If co-administration is essential, conduct close clinical and laboratory monitoring).
No products indexed under this heading.

Piroxicam (Whenever possible, agents which may enhance the risk of hemorrhage should be discontinued prior to initiation of enoxaparin therapy. These agents include medications such as: anticoagulants, platelet inhibitors including acetylsalicylic acid, salicylates, NSAIDs (including ketorolac tromethamine), dipyridamole, or sulfinpyrazone. If co-administration is essential, conduct close clinical and laboratory monitoring).
No products indexed under this heading.

Procaine Hydrochloride (There have been reports of epidural or spinal hematoma formation with concurrent use of enoxaparin and spinal/epidural anesthesia or spinal puncture).
No products indexed under this heading.

Rofecoxib (Whenever possible, agents which may enhance the risk of hemorrhage should be discontinued prior to initiation of enoxaparin therapy. These agents include medications such as: anticoagulants, platelet inhibitors including acetylsalicylic acid, salicylates, NSAIDs (including ketorolac tromethamine), dipyridamole, or sulfinpyrazone. If co-administration is essential, conduct close clinical and laboratory monitoring).
No products indexed under this heading.

Salsalate (Whenever possible, agents which may enhance the risk of hemorrhage should be discontinued prior to initiation of enoxaparin therapy. These agents include medications such as: anticoagulants, platelet inhibitors including acetylsalicylic acid, salicylates, NSAIDs (including ketorolac tromethamine), dipyridamole, or sulfinpyrazone. If co-administration is essential, conduct close clinical and laboratory monitoring).
No products indexed under this heading.

Spironolactone (Cases of hyperkalemia have been reported. Most of these reports occurred in patients who also had conditions that tend toward the development of hyperkalemia (eg, renal dysfunction, concomitant potassium-sparing drugs, administration of potassium, hematoma in body tissues)).
No products indexed under this heading.

Sulfinpyrazone (Whenever possible, agents which may enhance the risk of hemorrhage should be discontinued prior to initiation of enoxaparin therapy. These agents include medications such as: anticoagulants, platelet inhibitors including acetylsalicylic acid, salicylates, NSAIDs (including ketorolac tromethamine), dipyridamole, or sulfinpyrazone. If co-administration is essential, conduct close clinical and laboratory monitoring).
No products indexed under this heading.

Sulindac (Whenever possible, agents which may enhance the risk of hemorrhage should be discontinued prior to initiation of enoxaparin therapy. These agents include medications such as: anticoagulants, platelet inhibitors including acetylsalicylic acid, salicylates, NSAIDs (including ketorolac tromethamine), dipyridamole, or sulfinpyrazone. If co-administration is essential, conduct close clinical and laboratory monitoring). Products include:
Clinoril 2098

Tetracaine Hydrochloride (There have been reports of epidural or spinal hematoma formation with concurrent use of enoxaparin and spinal/epidural anesthesia or spinal puncture).
No products indexed under this heading.

Ticarcillin Disodium (Whenever possible, agents which may enhance the risk of hemorrhage should be discontinued prior to initiation of enoxaparin therapy. These agents include medications such as: anticoagulants, platelet inhibitors including acetylsalicylic acid, salicylates, NSAIDs (including ketorolac tromethamine), dipyridamole, or sulfinpyrazone. If co-administration is essential, conduct close clinical and laboratory monitoring). Products include:
Timentin ADD-Vantage 1670
Timentin Galaxy 1674
Timentin 1666
Timentin Pharmacy 1678

Ticlopidine Hydrochloride (Whenever possible, agents which may enhance the risk of hemorrhage should be discontinued prior to initiation of enoxaparin therapy. These agents include medications such as: anticoagulants, platelet inhibitors including acetylsalicylic acid, salicylates, NSAIDs (including ketorolac tromethamine), dipyridamole, or sulfinpyrazone. If co-administration is essential, conduct close clinical and laboratory monitoring).
No products indexed under this heading.

Tinzaparin Sodium (Whenever possible, agents which may enhance the risk of hemorrhage should be discontinued prior to initiation of enoxaparin therapy. These agents include medications such as: anticoagulants, platelet inhibitors including acetylsalicylic acid, salicylates, NSAIDs (including ketorolac tromethamine), dipyridamole, or sulfinpyrazone. If co-administration is essential, conduct close clinical and laboratory monitoring).
No products indexed under this heading.

Tirofiban Hydrochloride (Whenever possible, agents which may enhance the risk of hemorrhage should be discontinued prior to initiation of enoxaparin therapy. These agents include medications such as: anticoagulants, platelet inhibitors including acetylsalicylic acid, salicylates, NSAIDs (including ketorolac tromethamine), dipyridamole, or sulfinpyrazone. If co-administration is essential, conduct close clinical and laboratory monitoring).
No products indexed under this heading.

Tolmetin Sodium (Whenever possible, agents which may enhance the risk of hemorrhage should be discontinued prior to initiation of enoxaparin therapy. These agents include medications such as: anticoagulants, platelet inhibitors including acetylsalicylic acid, salicylates, NSAIDs (including ketorolac tromethamine), dipyridamole, or sulfinpyrazone. If co-administration is essential, conduct close clinical and laboratory monitoring).
No products indexed under this heading.

Triamterene (Cases of hyperkalemia have been reported. Most of these reports occurred in patients who also had conditions that tend toward the development of hyperkalemia (eg, renal dysfunction, concomitant potassium-sparing drugs, administration of potassium, hematoma in body tissues)). Products include:
Dyazide 1429
Dyrenium 3495

Valdecoxib (Whenever possible, agents which may enhance the risk of hemorrhage should be discontinued prior to initiation of enoxaparin therapy. These agents include medications such as: anticoagulants, platelet inhibitors including acetylsalicylic acid, salicylates, NSAIDs (including ketorolac tromethamine), dipyridamole, or sulfinpyrazone. If co-administration is essential, conduct close clinical and laboratory monitoring).
No products indexed under this heading.

Warfarin Sodium (Whenever possible, agents which may enhance the risk of hemorrhage should be discontinued prior to initiation of enoxaparin therapy. These agents include medications such as: anticoagulants, platelet inhibitors including acetylsalicylic acid, salicylates, NSAIDs (including ketorolac tromethamine), dipyridamole, or sulfinpyrazone. If co-administration is essential, conduct close clinical and laboratory monitoring).
No products indexed under this heading.

LUCENTIS INJECTION

(Ranibizumab) 1201

Verteporfin (11% of patients developed serious intraocular inflammation when ranibizumab was used concomitantly with verteporfin). Products include:
Visudyne 2549

LUMIGAN OPHTHALMIC SOLUTION

(Bimatoprost) 604
None cited in PDR database.

LUPRON DEPOT 3.75 MG

(Leuprolide Acetate) 472
May interact with alcohols, anticonvulsants, corticosteroids, and certain other agents. Compounds in these categories include:

Alclometasone Dipropionate (In patients with major risk factors for decreased bone mineral content such as chronic use of drugs that can reduce bone mass (eg, corticosteroids), leuprolide acetate depot may pose an additional risk. In these patients, the risks and benefits must be weighed carefully before therapy with leuprolide acetate depot alone is instituted, and concomitant treatment with norethindrone acetate 5 mg daily should be considered. Retreatment with gonadotropin-releasing hormone analogs, including leuprolide acetate, is not advisable in patients with major risk factors for loss of bone mineral content).
No products indexed under this heading.

Beclomethasone Dipropionate (In patients with major risk factors for decreased bone mineral content such as chronic use of drugs that can reduce bone mass (eg, corticosteroids), leuprolide acetate depot may pose an additional risk. In these patients, the risks and benefits must be weighed carefully before therapy with leuprolide acetate depot alone is instituted, and concomitant treatment with norethindrone acetate 5 mg daily should be considered. Retreatment with gonadotropin-releasing hormone analogs, including leuprolide acetate, is not advisable in patients with major risk factors for loss of bone mineral content). Products include:
Qvar 3398

Beclomethasone Dipropionate Monohydrate (In patients with major risk factors for decreased bone mineral content such as chronic use of drugs that can reduce bone mass (eg, corticosteroids), leuprolide acetate depot may pose an additional risk. In these patients, the risks and benefits must be weighed carefully before therapy with leuprolide acetate depot alone is instituted, and concomitant treatment with norethindrone acetate 5 mg daily should be considered. Retreatment with gonadotropin-releasing hormone analogs, including leuprolide acetate, is not

(⊙ Described in PDR® for Ophthalmic Medicines)

advisable in patients with major risk factors for loss of bone mineral content). Products include:

Beconase AQ 1386

Betamethasone (In patients with major risk factors for decreased bone mineral content such as chronic use of drugs that can reduce bone mass (eg, corticosteroids), leuprolide acetate depot may pose an additional risk. In these patients, the risks and benefits must be weighed carefully before therapy with leuprolide acetate depot alone is instituted, and concomitant treatment with norethindrone acetate 5 mg daily should be considered. Retreatment with gonadotropin-releasing hormone analogs, including leuprolide acetate, is not advisable in patients with major risk factors for loss of bone mineral content).

No products indexed under this heading.

Betamethasone Acetate (In patients with major risk factors for decreased bone mineral content such as chronic use of drugs that can reduce bone mass (eg, corticosteroids), leuprolide acetate depot may pose an additional risk. In these patients, the risks and benefits must be weighed carefully before therapy with leuprolide acetate depot alone is instituted, and concomitant treatment with norethindrone acetate 5 mg daily should be considered. Retreatment with gonadotropin-releasing hormone analogs, including leuprolide acetate, is not advisable in patients with major risk factors for loss of bone mineral content).

No products indexed under this heading.

Betamethasone Benzoate (In patients with major risk factors for decreased bone mineral content such as chronic use of drugs that can reduce bone mass (eg, corticosteroids), leuprolide acetate depot may pose an additional risk. In these patients, the risks and benefits must be weighed carefully before therapy with leuprolide acetate depot alone is instituted, and concomitant treatment with norethindrone acetate 5 mg daily should be considered. Retreatment with gonadotropin-releasing hormone analogs, including leuprolide acetate, is not advisable in patients with major risk factors for loss of bone mineral content).

No products indexed under this heading.

Betamethasone Dipropionate (In patients with major risk factors for decreased bone mineral content such as chronic use of drugs that can reduce bone mass (eg, corticosteroids), leuprolide acetate depot may pose an additional risk. In these patients, the risks and benefits must be weighed carefully before therapy with leuprolide acetate depot alone is instituted, and concomitant treatment with norethindrone acetate 5 mg daily should be considered. Retreatment with gonadotropin-releasing hormone analogs, including leuprolide acetate, is not advisable in patients with major risk factors for loss of bone mineral content). Products include:

Diprolene Lotion 0.05% 3108
Diprolene Ointment 0.05% 3109
Diprolene AF Cream 0.05% 3107
Lotrisone 3163

Betamethasone Sodium Phosphate (In patients with major risk factors for decreased bone mineral content such as chronic use of drugs that can reduce bone mass (eg, corticosteroids), leuprolide acetate depot may pose an additional risk. In these patients, the risks and benefits must be weighed carefully before therapy with leuprolide acetate depot alone is instituted, and concomitant treatment with norethindrone acetate 5 mg daily should be considered. Retreatment with gonadotropin-releasing hormone analogs, including leuprolide acetate, is not advisable in patients with major risk factors for loss of bone mineral content).

No products indexed under this heading.

Betamethasone Valerate (In patients with major risk factors for decreased bone mineral content such as chronic use of drugs that can reduce bone mass (eg, corticosteroids), leuprolide acetate depot may pose an additional risk. In these patients, the risks and benefits must be weighed carefully before therapy with leuprolide acetate depot alone is instituted, and concomitant treatment with norethindrone acetate 5 mg daily should be considered. Retreatment with gonadotropin-releasing hormone analogs, including leuprolide acetate, is not advisable in patients with major risk factors for loss of bone mineral content). Products include:

Luxíq 3321

Budesonide (In patients with major risk factors for decreased bone mineral content such as chronic use of drugs that can reduce bone mass (eg, corticosteroids), leuprolide acetate depot may pose an additional risk. In these patients, the risks and benefits must be weighed carefully before therapy with leuprolide acetate depot alone is instituted, and concomitant treatment with norethindrone acetate 5 mg daily should be considered. Retreatment with gonadotropin-releasing hormone analogs, including leuprolide acetate, is not advisable in patients with major risk factors for loss of bone mineral content). Products include:

Pulmicort Flexhaler 714
Symbicort 80/4.5 720
Symbicort 160/4.5 720

Carbamazepine (In patients with major risk factors for decreased bone mineral content such as chronic use of drugs that can reduce bone mass (eg, anticonvulsants), leuprolide acetate depot therapy may pose an additional risk. In these patients, the risks and benefits must be weighed carefully before therapy with leuprolide acetate depot alone is instituted, and concomitant treatment with norethindrone acetate 5 mg daily should be considered. Retreatment with gonadotropin-releasing hormone analogs, including leuprolide acetate, is not advisable in patients with major risk factors for loss of bone mineral content). Products include:

Carbatrol 3280
Equetro 3477

Ciclesonide (In patients with major risk factors for decreased bone mineral content such as chronic use of drugs that can reduce bone mass (eg, corticosteroids), leuprolide acetate depot may pose an additional risk. In these patients, the risks and benefits must be weighed carefully before therapy with leuprolide acetate depot alone is instituted, and concomitant treatment with norethindrone acetate 5 mg daily should be considered. Retreatment with gonadotropin-releasing hormone analogs, including leuprolide acetate, is not advisable in patients with major risk factors for loss of bone mineral content).

No products indexed under this heading.

Cortisone Acetate (In patients with major risk factors for decreased bone mineral content such as chronic use of drugs that can reduce bone mass (eg, corticosteroids), leuprolide acetate depot may pose an additional risk. In these patients, the risks and benefits must be weighed carefully before therapy with leuprolide acetate depot alone is instituted, and concomitant treatment with norethindrone acetate 5 mg daily should be considered. Retreatment with gonadotropin-releasing hormone analogs, including leuprolide acetate, is not advisable in patients with major risk factors for loss of bone mineral content).

No products indexed under this heading.

Desoximetasone (In patients with major risk factors for decreased bone mineral content such as chronic use of drugs that can reduce bone mass (eg, corticosteroids), leuprolide acetate depot may pose an additional risk. In these patients, the risks and benefits must be weighed carefully before therapy with leuprolide acetate depot alone is instituted, and concomitant treatment with norethindrone acetate 5 mg daily should be considered. Retreatment with gonadotropin-releasing hormone analogs, including leuprolide acetate, is not advisable in patients with major risk factors for loss of bone mineral content).

No products indexed under this heading.

Dexamethasone (In patients with major risk factors for decreased bone mineral content such as chronic use of drugs that can reduce bone mass (eg, corticosteroids), leuprolide acetate depot may pose an additional risk. In these patients, the risks and benefits must be weighed carefully before therapy with leuprolide acetate depot alone is instituted, and concomitant treatment with norethindrone acetate 5 mg daily should be considered. Retreatment with gonadotropin-releasing hormone analogs, including leuprolide acetate, is not advisable in patients with major risk factors for loss of bone mineral content). Products include:

Ciprodex 583
Ozurdex .... ⊙223
Tobramycin and Dexamethasone Ophthalmic Suspension .... ⊙251

Dexamethasone Acetate (In patients with major risk factors for decreased bone mineral content such as chronic use of drugs that can reduce bone mass (eg, corticosteroids), leuprolide acetate depot may pose an additional risk. In these patients, the risks and benefits must be weighed carefully before therapy with leuprolide acetate depot alone is instituted, and concomitant treatment with norethindrone acetate 5 mg daily should be considered. Retreatment with gonadotropin-releasing hormone analogs, including leuprolide acetate, is not advisable in patients with major risk factors for loss of bone mineral content).

No products indexed under this heading.

Dexamethasone Phosphate (In patients with major risk factors for decreased bone mineral content such as chronic use of drugs that can reduce bone mass (eg, corticosteroids), leuprolide acetate depot may pose an additional risk. In these patients, the risks and benefits must be weighed carefully before therapy with leuprolide acetate depot alone is instituted, and concomitant treatment with norethindrone acetate 5 mg daily should be considered. Retreatment with gonadotropin-releasing hormone analogs, including leuprolide acetate, is not advisable in patients with major risk factors for loss of bone mineral content).

No products indexed under this heading.

Dexamethasone Sodium (In patients with major risk factors for decreased bone mineral content such as chronic use of drugs that can reduce bone mass (eg, corticosteroids), leuprolide acetate depot may pose an additional risk. In these patients, the risks and benefits must be weighed carefully before therapy with leuprolide acetate depot alone is instituted, and concomitant treatment with norethindrone acetate 5 mg daily should be considered. Retreatment with gonadotropin-releasing hormone analogs, including leuprolide acetate, is not advisable in patients with major risk factors for loss of bone mineral content).

No products indexed under this heading.

Dexamethasone Sodium Phosphate (In patients with major risk factors for decreased bone mineral content such as chronic use of drugs that can reduce bone mass (eg, corticosteroids), leuprolide acetate depot may pose an additional risk. In these patients, the risks and benefits must be weighed carefully before therapy with leuprolide acetate depot alone is instituted, and concomitant treatment with norethindrone acetate 5 mg daily should be considered. Retreatment with gonadotropin-releasing hormone analogs, including leuprolide acetate, is not advisable in patients with major risk factors for loss of bone mineral content).

No products indexed under this heading.

Dexamethasone Sodium Phosphate Injection (In patients with major risk factors for decreased bone mineral content such as chronic use of drugs that can reduce bone mass (eg, corticosteroids), leuprolide acetate depot may pose an additional risk. In these patients, the risks and benefits must be weighed carefully before therapy with leuprolide acetate depot alone is instituted, and concomitant treatment with norethindrone acetate 5 mg daily should be considered. Retreatment with gonadotropin-releasing hormone analogs, including leuprolide acetate, is not advisable in patients with major risk factors for loss of bone mineral content).

No products indexed under this heading.

Diflorasone Diacetate (In patients with major risk factors for decreased bone mineral content such as chronic use of drugs that can reduce bone mass (eg, corticosteroids), leuprolide acetate depot may pose an additional risk. In these patients, the risks and benefits must be weighed carefully before therapy with leuprolide acetate depot alone is instituted, and concomitant treatment with norethindrone acetate 5 mg daily should be considered. Retreatment with gonadotropin-releasing hormone analogs, including leuprolide acetate, is not advisable in patients with major risk factors for loss of bone mineral content).

No products indexed under this heading.

Divalproex Sodium (In patients with major risk factors for decreased bone mineral content such as chronic use of drugs that can reduce bone mass (eg, anticonvulsants), leuprolide acetate depot therapy may pose an additional risk. In these patients, the risks and benefits must be weighed carefully before therapy with leuprolide acetate depot alone is instituted, and concomitant treatment with norethindrone acetate 5 mg daily should be considered. Retreatment with gonadotropin-releasing hormone analogs, including leuprolide acetate, is not advisable in patients with major risk factors for loss of bone mineral content). Products include:

Depakote ER 426

Ethanol (In patients with major risk factors for decreased bone mineral content such as chronic alcohol use, leuprolide acetate depot may pose an additional risk. In these patients, the risks and benefits must be weighed carefully before therapy with leuprolide acetate depot alone is instituted, and concomitant treatment with norethindrone acetate 5 mg daily should be con-

sidered. Retreatment with gonadotropin-releasing hormone analogs, including leuprolide acetate, is not advisable in patients with major risk factors for loss of bone mineral content).
No products indexed under this heading.

Ethosuximide (In patients with major risk factors for decreased bone mineral content such as chronic use of drugs that can reduce bone mass (eg, anticonvulsants), leuprolide acetate depot therapy may pose an additional risk. In these patients, the risks and benefits must be weighed carefully before therapy with leuprolide acetate depot alone is instituted, and concomitant treatment with norethindrone acetate 5 mg daily should be considered. Retreatment with gonadotropin-releasing hormone analogs, including leuprolide acetate, is not advisable in patients with major risk factors for loss of bone mineral content).
No products indexed under this heading.

Ethotoin (In patients with major risk factors for decreased bone mineral content such as chronic use of drugs that can reduce bone mass (eg, anticonvulsants), leuprolide acetate depot therapy may pose an additional risk. In these patients, the risks and benefits must be weighed carefully before therapy with leuprolide acetate depot alone is instituted, and concomitant treatment with norethindrone acetate 5 mg daily should be considered. Retreatment with gonadotropin-releasing hormone analogs, including leuprolide acetate, is not advisable in patients with major risk factors for loss of bone mineral content).
No products indexed under this heading.

Ethyl Alcohol (In patients with major risk factors for decreased bone mineral content such as chronic alcohol use, leuprolide acetate depot may pose an additional risk. In these patients, the risks and benefits must be weighed carefully before therapy with leuprolide acetate depot alone is instituted, and concomitant treatment with norethindrone acetate 5 mg daily should be considered. Retreatment with gonadotropin-releasing hormone analogs, including leuprolide acetate, is not advisable in patients with major risk factors for loss of bone mineral content).
No products indexed under this heading.

Felbamate (In patients with major risk factors for decreased bone mineral content such as chronic use of drugs that can reduce bone mass (eg, anticonvulsants), leuprolide acetate depot therapy may pose an additional risk. In these patients, the risks and benefits must be weighed carefully before therapy with leuprolide acetate depot alone is instituted, and concomitant treatment with norethindrone acetate 5 mg daily should be considered. Retreatment with gonadotropin-releasing hormone analogs, including leuprolide acetate, is not advisable in patients with major risk factors for loss of bone mineral content).
No products indexed under this heading.

Fludrocortisone Acetate (In patients with major risk factors for decreased bone mineral content such as chronic use of drugs that can reduce bone mass (eg, corticosteroids), leuprolide acetate depot may pose an additional risk. In these patients, the risks and benefits must be weighed carefully before therapy with leuprolide acetate depot alone is instituted, and concomitant treatment with norethindrone acetate 5 mg daily should be considered. Retreatment with gonadotropin-releasing hormone analogs, including leuprolide acetate, is not advisable in patients with major risk factors for loss of bone mineral content).
No products indexed under this heading.

Flumethasone Pivalate (In patients with major risk factors for decreased bone mineral content such as chronic use of drugs that can reduce bone mass (eg, corticosteroids), leuprolide acetate depot may pose an additional risk. In these patients, the risks and benefits must be weighed carefully before therapy with leuprolide acetate depot alone is instituted, and concomitant treatment with norethindrone acetate 5 mg daily should be considered. Retreatment with gonadotropin-releasing hormone analogs, including leuprolide acetate, is not advisable in patients with major risk factors for loss of bone mineral content).
No products indexed under this heading.

Flunisolide Hemihydrate (In patients with major risk factors for decreased bone mineral content such as chronic use of drugs that can reduce bone mass (eg, corticosteroids), leuprolide acetate depot may pose an additional risk. In these patients, the risks and benefits must be weighed carefully before therapy with leuprolide acetate depot alone is instituted, and concomitant treatment with norethindrone acetate 5 mg daily should be considered. Retreatment with gonadotropin-releasing hormone analogs, including leuprolide acetate, is not advisable in patients with major risk factors for loss of bone mineral content).
No products indexed under this heading.

Fluticasone Furoate (In patients with major risk factors for decreased bone mineral content such as chronic use of drugs that can reduce bone mass (eg, corticosteroids), leuprolide acetate depot may pose an additional risk. In these patients, the risks and benefits must be weighed carefully before therapy with leuprolide acetate depot alone is instituted, and concomitant treatment with norethindrone acetate 5 mg daily should be considered. Retreatment with gonadotropin-releasing hormone analogs, including leuprolide acetate, is not advisable in patients with major risk factors for loss of bone mineral content). Products include:
Veramyst 1713

Fluticasone Propionate (In patients with major risk factors for decreased bone mineral content such as chronic use of drugs that can reduce bone mass (eg, corticosteroids), leuprolide acetate depot may pose an additional risk. In these patients, the risks and benefits must be weighed carefully before therapy with leuprolide acetate depot alone is instituted, and concomitant treatment with norethindrone acetate 5 mg daily should be considered. Retreatment with gonadotropin-releasing hormone analogs, including leuprolide acetate, is not advisable in patients with major risk factors for loss of bone mineral content). Products include:
Advair 100/50 1275
Advair 250/50 1275
Advair 500/50 1275
Advair HFA 45/21 1288
Advair HFA 115/21 1288
Advair HFA 230/21 1288
Flonase 1459
Flovent Diskus 1463
Flovent HFA 1470

Fosphenytoin (In patients with major risk factors for decreased bone mineral content such as chronic use of drugs that can reduce bone mass (eg, anticonvulsants), leuprolide acetate depot therapy may pose an additional risk. In these patients, the risks and benefits must be weighed carefully before therapy with leuprolide acetate depot alone is instituted, and concomitant treatment with norethindrone acetate 5 mg daily should be considered. Retreatment with gonadotropin-releasing hormone analogs, including leuprolide acetate, is not advisable in patients with major risk factors for loss of bone mineral content).
No products indexed under this heading.

Fosphenytoin Sodium (In patients with major risk factors for decreased bone mineral content such as chronic use of drugs that can reduce bone mass (eg, anticonvulsants), leuprolide acetate depot therapy may pose an additional risk. In these patients, the risks and benefits must be weighed carefully before therapy with leuprolide acetate depot alone is instituted, and concomitant treatment with norethindrone acetate 5 mg daily should be considered. Retreatment with gonadotropin-releasing hormone analogs, including leuprolide acetate, is not advisable in patients with major risk factors for loss of bone mineral content).
No products indexed under this heading.

Gabapentin (In patients with major risk factors for decreased bone mineral content such as chronic use of drugs that can reduce bone mass (eg, anticonvulsants), leuprolide acetate depot therapy may pose an additional risk. In these patients, the risks and benefits must be weighed carefully before therapy with leuprolide acetate depot alone is instituted, and concomitant treatment with norethindrone acetate 5 mg daily should be considered. Retreatment with gonadotropin-releasing hormone analogs, including leuprolide acetate, is not advisable in patients with major risk factors for loss of bone mineral content).
No products indexed under this heading.

Hydrocortisone (In patients with major risk factors for decreased bone mineral content such as chronic use of drugs that can reduce bone mass (eg, corticosteroids), leuprolide acetate depot may pose an additional risk. In these patients, the risks and benefits must be weighed carefully before therapy with leuprolide acetate depot alone is instituted, and concomitant treatment with norethindrone acetate 5 mg daily should be considered. Retreatment with gonadotropin-releasing hormone analogs, including leuprolide acetate, is not advisable in patients with major risk factors for loss of bone mineral content).
No products indexed under this heading.

Hydrocortisone (Alcohol) (In patients with major risk factors for decreased bone mineral content such as chronic use of drugs that can reduce bone mass (eg, corticosteroids), leuprolide acetate depot may pose an additional risk. In these patients, the risks and benefits must be weighed carefully before therapy with leuprolide acetate depot alone is instituted, and concomitant treatment with norethindrone acetate 5 mg daily should be considered. Retreatment with gonadotropin-releasing hormone analogs, including leuprolide acetate, is not advisable in patients with major risk factors for loss of bone mineral content).
No products indexed under this heading.

Hydrocortisone Acetate (In patients with major risk factors for decreased bone mineral content such as chronic use of drugs that can reduce bone mass (eg, corticosteroids), leuprolide acetate depot may pose an additional risk. In these patients, the risks and benefits must be weighed carefully before therapy with leuprolide acetate depot alone is instituted, and concomitant treatment with norethindrone acetate 5 mg daily should be considered. Retreatment with gonadotropin-releasing hormone analogs, including leuprolide acetate, is not advisable in patients with major risk factors for loss of bone mineral content).
No products indexed under this heading.

Hydrocortisone Butyrate (In patients with major risk factors for decreased bone mineral content such as chronic use of drugs that can reduce bone mass (eg, corticosteroids), leuprolide acetate depot may pose an additional risk. In these patients, the risks and benefits must be weighed carefully before therapy with leuprolide acetate depot alone is instituted, and concomitant treatment with norethindrone acetate 5 mg daily should be considered. Retreatment with gonadotropin-releasing hormone analogs, including leuprolide acetate, is not advisable in patients with major risk factors for loss of bone mineral content).
No products indexed under this heading.

Hydrocortisone Cypionate (In patients with major risk factors for decreased bone mineral content such as chronic use of drugs that can reduce bone mass (eg, corticosteroids), leuprolide acetate depot may pose an additional risk. In these patients, the risks and benefits must be weighed carefully before therapy with leuprolide acetate depot alone is instituted, and concomitant treatment with norethindrone acetate 5 mg daily should be considered. Retreatment with gonadotropin-releasing hormone analogs, including leuprolide acetate, is not advisable in patients with major risk factors for loss of bone mineral content).
No products indexed under this heading.

Hydrocortisone Hemisuccinate (In patients with major risk factors for decreased bone mineral content such as chronic use of drugs that can reduce bone mass (eg, corticosteroids), leuprolide acetate depot may pose an additional risk. In these patients, the risks and benefits must be weighed carefully before therapy with leuprolide acetate depot alone is instituted, and concomitant treatment with norethindrone acetate 5 mg daily should be considered. Retreatment with gonadotropin-releasing hormone analogs, including leuprolide acetate, is not advisable in patients with major risk factors for loss of bone mineral content).
No products indexed under this heading.

Hydrocortisone Probutate (In patients with major risk factors for decreased bone mineral content such as chronic use of drugs that can reduce bone mass (eg, corticosteroids), leuprolide acetate depot may pose an additional risk. In these patients, the risks and benefits must be weighed carefully before therapy with leuprolide acetate depot alone is instituted, and concomitant treatment with norethindrone acetate 5 mg daily should be considered. Retreatment with gonadotropin-releasing hormone analogs, including leuprolide acetate, is not advisable in patients with major risk factors for loss of bone mineral content).
No products indexed under this heading.

Hydrocortisone Sodium Phosphate (In patients with major risk factors for decreased bone mineral content such as chronic use of drugs that can reduce bone mass (eg, corticosteroids), leuprolide acetate depot may pose an additional risk. In these patients, the risks and benefits must be weighed carefully before therapy with leuprolide acetate depot alone is instituted, and concomitant treatment with norethindrone acetate 5 mg daily should be considered. Retreatment with gonadotropin-releasing hormone ana-

logs, including leuprolide acetate, is not advisable in patients with major risk factors for loss of bone mineral content).
No products indexed under this heading.

Hydrocortisone Sodium Succinate (In patients with major risk factors for decreased bone mineral content such as chronic use of drugs that can reduce bone mass (eg, corticosteroids), leuprolide acetate depot may pose an additional risk. In these patients, the risks and benefits must be weighed carefully before therapy with leuprolide acetate depot alone is instituted, and concomitant treatment with norethindrone acetate 5 mg daily should be considered. Retreatment with gonadotropin-releasing hormone analogs, including leuprolide acetate, is not advisable in patients with major risk factors for loss of bone mineral content).
No products indexed under this heading.

Hydrocortisone Valerate (In patients with major risk factors for decreased bone mineral content such as chronic use of drugs that can reduce bone mass (eg, corticosteroids), leuprolide acetate depot may pose an additional risk. In these patients, the risks and benefits must be weighed carefully before therapy with leuprolide acetate depot alone is instituted, and concomitant treatment with norethindrone acetate 5 mg daily should be considered. Retreatment with gonadotropin-releasing hormone analogs, including leuprolide acetate, is not advisable in patients with major risk factors for loss of bone mineral content).
No products indexed under this heading.

Lamotrigine (In patients with major risk factors for decreased bone mineral content such as chronic use of drugs that can reduce bone mass (eg, anticonvulsants), leuprolide acetate depot therapy may pose an additional risk. In these patients, the risks and benefits must be weighed carefully before therapy with leuprolide acetate depot alone is instituted, and concomitant treatment with norethindrone acetate 5 mg daily should be considered. Retreatment with gonadotropin-releasing hormone analogs, including leuprolide acetate, is not advisable in patients with major risk factors for loss of bone mineral content). Products include:
Lamictal **1522**
Lamictal ODT **1522**
Lamictal XR **1536**

Levetiracetam (In patients with major risk factors for decreased bone mineral content such as chronic use of drugs that can reduce bone mass (eg, anticonvulsants), leuprolide acetate depot therapy may pose an additional risk. In these patients, the risks and benefits must be weighed carefully before therapy with leuprolide acetate depot alone is instituted, and concomitant treatment with norethindrone acetate 5 mg daily should be considered. Retreatment with gonadotropin-releasing hormone analogs, including leuprolide acetate, is not advisable in patients with major risk factors for loss of bone mineral content). Products include:
Keppra XR **3434**

Mephenytoin (In patients with major risk factors for decreased bone mineral content such as chronic use of drugs that can reduce bone mass (eg, anticonvulsants), leuprolide acetate depot therapy may pose an additional risk. In these patients, the risks and benefits must be weighed carefully before therapy with leuprolide acetate depot alone is instituted, and concomitant treatment with norethindrone acetate 5 mg daily should be considered. Retreatment with gonadotropin-releasing hormone analogs, including leuprolide acetate, is not advisable in patients with major risk factors for loss of bone mineral content).
No products indexed under this heading.

Methsuximide (In patients with major risk factors for decreased bone mineral content such as chronic use of drugs that can reduce bone mass (eg, anticonvulsants), leuprolide acetate depot therapy may pose an additional risk. In these patients, the risks and benefits must be weighed carefully before therapy with leuprolide acetate depot alone is instituted, and concomitant treatment with norethindrone acetate 5 mg daily should be considered. Retreatment with gonadotropin-releasing hormone analogs, including leuprolide acetate, is not advisable in patients with major risk factors for loss of bone mineral content).
No products indexed under this heading.

Methylprednisolone (In patients with major risk factors for decreased bone mineral content such as chronic use of drugs that can reduce bone mass (eg, corticosteroids), leuprolide acetate depot may pose an additional risk. In these patients, the risks and benefits must be weighed carefully before therapy with leuprolide acetate depot alone is instituted, and concomitant treatment with norethindrone acetate 5 mg daily should be considered. Retreatment with gonadotropin-releasing hormone analogs, including leuprolide acetate, is not advisable in patients with major risk factors for loss of bone mineral content).
No products indexed under this heading.

Methylprednisolone Acetate (In patients with major risk factors for decreased bone mineral content such as chronic use of drugs that can reduce bone mass (eg, corticosteroids), leuprolide acetate depot may pose an additional risk. In these patients, the risks and benefits must be weighed carefully before therapy with leuprolide acetate depot alone is instituted, and concomitant treatment with norethindrone acetate 5 mg daily should be considered. Retreatment with gonadotropin-releasing hormone analogs, including leuprolide acetate, is not advisable in patients with major risk factors for loss of bone mineral content).
No products indexed under this heading.

Methylprednisolone Sodium Succinate (In patients with major risk factors for decreased bone mineral content such as chronic use of drugs that can reduce bone mass (eg, corticosteroids), leuprolide acetate depot may pose an additional risk. In these patients, the risks and benefits must be weighed carefully before therapy with leuprolide acetate depot alone is instituted, and concomitant treatment with norethindrone acetate 5 mg daily should be considered. Retreatment with gonadotropin-releasing hormone analogs, including leuprolide acetate, is not advisable in patients with major risk factors for loss of bone mineral content).
No products indexed under this heading.

Mometasone Furoate (In patients with major risk factors for decreased bone mineral content such as chronic use of drugs that can reduce bone mass (eg, corticosteroids), leuprolide acetate depot may pose an additional risk. In these patients, the risks and benefits must be weighed carefully before therapy with leuprolide acetate depot alone is instituted, and concomitant treatment with norethindrone acetate 5 mg daily should be considered. Retreatment with gonadotropin-releasing hormone analogs, including leuprolide acetate, is not advisable in patients with major risk factors for loss of bone mineral content). Products include:
Asmanex **3058**
Elocon Cream **3111**
Elocon Lotion **3112**
Elocon Ointment **3114**

Mometasone Furoate Monohydrate (In patients with major risk factors for decreased bone mineral content such as chronic use of drugs that can reduce bone mass (eg, corticosteroids), leuprolide acetate depot may pose an additional risk. In these patients, the risks and benefits must be weighed carefully before therapy with leuprolide acetate depot alone is instituted, and concomitant treatment with norethindrone acetate 5 mg daily should be considered. Retreatment with gonadotropin-releasing hormone analogs, including leuprolide acetate, is not advisable in patients with major risk factors for loss of bone mineral content). Products include:
Nasonex **3166**

Oxcarbazepine (In patients with major risk factors for decreased bone mineral content such as chronic use of drugs that can reduce bone mass (eg, anticonvulsants), leuprolide acetate depot therapy may pose an additional risk. In these patients, the risks and benefits must be weighed carefully before therapy with leuprolide acetate depot alone is instituted, and concomitant treatment with norethindrone acetate 5 mg daily should be considered. Retreatment with gonadotropin-releasing hormone analogs, including leuprolide acetate, is not advisable in patients with major risk factors for loss of bone mineral content).
No products indexed under this heading.

Paramethadione (In patients with major risk factors for decreased bone mineral content such as chronic use of drugs that can reduce bone mass (eg, anticonvulsants), leuprolide acetate depot therapy may pose an additional risk. In these patients, the risks and benefits must be weighed carefully before therapy with leuprolide acetate depot alone is instituted, and concomitant treatment with norethindrone acetate 5 mg daily should be considered. Retreatment with gonadotropin-releasing hormone analogs, including leuprolide acetate, is not advisable in patients with major risk factors for loss of bone mineral content).
No products indexed under this heading.

Phenacemide (In patients with major risk factors for decreased bone mineral content such as chronic use of drugs that can reduce bone mass (eg, anticonvulsants), leuprolide acetate depot therapy may pose an additional risk. In these patients, the risks and benefits must be weighed carefully before therapy with leuprolide acetate depot alone is instituted, and concomitant treatment with norethindrone acetate 5 mg daily should be considered. Retreatment with gonadotropin-releasing hormone analogs, including leuprolide acetate, is not advisable in patients with major risk factors for loss of bone mineral content).
No products indexed under this heading.

Phenobarbital (In patients with major risk factors for decreased bone mineral content such as chronic use of drugs that can reduce bone mass (eg, anticonvulsants), leuprolide acetate depot therapy may pose an additional risk. In these patients, the risks and benefits must be weighed carefully before therapy with leuprolide acetate depot alone is instituted, and concomitant treatment with norethindrone acetate 5 mg daily should be considered. Retreatment with gonadotropin-releasing hormone analogs, including leuprolide acetate, is not advisable in patients with major risk factors for loss of bone mineral content). Products include:
Donnatal **2711**

Phenobarbital Sodium (In patients with major risk factors for decreased bone mineral content such as chronic use of drugs that can reduce bone mass (eg, anticonvulsants), leuprolide acetate depot therapy may pose an additional risk. In these patients, the risks and benefits must be weighed carefully before therapy with leuprolide acetate depot alone is instituted, and concomitant treatment with norethindrone acetate 5 mg daily should be considered. Retreatment with gonadotropin-releasing hormone analogs, including leuprolide acetate, is not advisable in patients with major risk factors for loss of bone mineral content).
No products indexed under this heading.

Phensuximide (In patients with major risk factors for decreased bone mineral content such as chronic use of drugs that can reduce bone mass (eg, anticonvulsants), leuprolide acetate depot therapy may pose an additional risk. In these patients, the risks and benefits must be weighed carefully before therapy with leuprolide acetate depot alone is instituted, and concomitant treatment with norethindrone acetate 5 mg daily should be considered. Retreatment with gonadotropin-releasing hormone analogs, including leuprolide acetate, is not advisable in patients with major risk factors for loss of bone mineral content).
No products indexed under this heading.

Phenytoin (In patients with major risk factors for decreased bone mineral content such as chronic use of drugs that can reduce bone mass (eg, anticonvulsants), leuprolide acetate depot therapy may pose an additional risk. In these patients, the risks and benefits must be weighed carefully before therapy with leuprolide acetate depot alone is instituted, and concomitant treatment with norethindrone acetate 5 mg daily should be considered. Retreatment with gonadotropin-releasing hormone analogs, including leuprolide acetate, is not advisable in patients with major risk factors for loss of bone mineral content).
No products indexed under this heading.

Phenytoin Sodium (In patients with major risk factors for decreased bone mineral content such as chronic use of drugs that can reduce bone mass (eg, anticonvulsants), leuprolide acetate depot therapy may pose an additional risk. In these patients, the risks and benefits must be weighed carefully before therapy with leuprolide acetate depot alone is instituted, and concomitant treatment with norethindrone acetate 5 mg daily should be considered. Retreatment with gonadotropin-releasing hormone analogs, including leuprolide acetate, is not advisable in patients with major risk factors for loss of bone mineral content). Products include:
Phenytek Capsules **2380**

Prednisolone (In patients with major risk factors for decreased bone mineral content such as chronic use of drugs that can reduce bone mass (eg, corticosteroids), leuprolide acetate depot may pose an additional risk. In these patients, the risks and benefits must be weighed carefully before therapy with leuprolide acetate depot alone is instituted, and concomitant treatment with norethindrone acetate 5 mg daily should be considered. Retreatment with gonadotropin-releasing hormone analogs, including leuprolide acetate, is not

IMPORTANT NOTE: Always consult each drug listing in the patient's regimen for possible interactions.

advisable in patients with major risk factors for loss of bone mineral content).

No products indexed under this heading.

Prednisolone Acetate (In patients with major risk factors for decreased bone mineral content such as chronic use of drugs that can reduce bone mass (eg, corticosteroids), leuprolide acetate depot may pose an additional risk. In these patients, the risks and benefits must be weighed carefully before therapy with leuprolide acetate depot alone is instituted, and concomitant treatment with norethindrone acetate 5 mg daily should be considered. Retreatment with gonadotropin-releasing hormone analogs, including leuprolide acetate, is not advisable in patients with major risk factors for loss of bone mineral content). Products include:

Blephamide .... ⊙212, ⊙214
Pred Forte ....⊙225
Pred Mild ....⊙230
Pred-G ....⊙226, ⊙227

Prednisolone Sodium Phosphate (In patients with major risk factors for decreased bone mineral content such as chronic use of drugs that can reduce bone mass (eg, corticosteroids), leuprolide acetate depot may pose an additional risk. In these patients, the risks and benefits must be weighed carefully before therapy with leuprolide acetate depot alone is instituted, and concomitant treatment with norethindrone acetate 5 mg daily should be considered. Retreatment with gonadotropin-releasing hormone analogs, including leuprolide acetate, is not advisable in patients with major risk factors for loss of bone mineral content).

No products indexed under this heading.

Prednisolone Tebutate (In patients with major risk factors for decreased bone mineral content such as chronic use of drugs that can reduce bone mass (eg, corticosteroids), leuprolide acetate depot may pose an additional risk. In these patients, the risks and benefits must be weighed carefully before therapy with leuprolide acetate depot alone is instituted, and concomitant treatment with norethindrone acetate 5 mg daily should be considered. Retreatment with gonadotropin-releasing hormone analogs, including leuprolide acetate, is not advisable in patients with major risk factors for loss of bone mineral content).

No products indexed under this heading.

Prednisone (In patients with major risk factors for decreased bone mineral content such as chronic use of drugs that can reduce bone mass (eg, corticosteroids), leuprolide acetate depot may pose an additional risk. In these patients, the risks and benefits must be weighed carefully before therapy with leuprolide acetate depot alone is instituted, and concomitant treatment with norethindrone acetate 5 mg daily should be considered. Retreatment with gonadotropin-releasing hormone analogs, including leuprolide acetate, is not advisable in patients with major risk factors for loss of bone mineral content).

No products indexed under this heading.

Prednisone sodium phosphate (In patients with major risk factors for decreased bone mineral content such as chronic use of drugs that can reduce bone mass (eg, corticosteroids), leuprolide acetate depot may pose an additional risk. In these patients, the risks and benefits must be weighed carefully before therapy with leuprolide acetate depot alone is instituted, and concomitant treatment with norethindrone acetate 5 mg daily should be considered. Retreatment with gonadotropin-

releasing hormone analogs, including leuprolide acetate, is not advisable in patients with major risk factors for loss of bone mineral content).

No products indexed under this heading.

Primidone (In patients with major risk factors for decreased bone mineral content such as chronic use of drugs that can reduce bone mass (eg, anticonvulsants), leuprolide acetate depot therapy may pose an additional risk. In these patients, the risks and benefits must be weighed carefully before therapy with leuprolide acetate depot alone is instituted, and concomitant treatment with norethindrone acetate 5 mg daily should be considered. Retreatment with gonadotropin-releasing hormone analogs, including leuprolide acetate, is not advisable in patients with major risk factors for loss of bone mineral content).

No products indexed under this heading.

Rufinamide (In patients with major risk factors for decreased bone mineral content such as chronic use of drugs that can reduce bone mass (eg, anticonvulsants), leuprolide acetate depot therapy may pose an additional risk. In these patients, the risks and benefits must be weighed carefully before therapy with leuprolide acetate depot alone is instituted, and concomitant treatment with norethindrone acetate 5 mg daily should be considered. Retreatment with gonadotropin-releasing hormone analogs, including leuprolide acetate, is not advisable in patients with major risk factors for loss of bone mineral content). Products include:

Banzel 1050

Tiagabine Hydrochloride (In patients with major risk factors for decreased bone mineral content such as chronic use of drugs that can reduce bone mass (eg, anticonvulsants), leuprolide acetate depot therapy may pose an additional risk. In these patients, the risks and benefits must be weighed carefully before therapy with leuprolide acetate depot alone is instituted, and concomitant treatment with norethindrone acetate 5 mg daily should be considered. Retreatment with gonadotropin-releasing hormone analogs, including leuprolide acetate, is not advisable in patients with major risk factors for loss of bone mineral content). Products include:

Gabitril 972

Tobacco (In patients with major risk factors for decreased bone mineral content such as chronic tobacco use, leuprolide acetate depot may pose an additional risk. In these patients, the risks and benefits must be weighed carefully before therapy with leuprolide acetate depot alone is instituted, and concomitant treatment with norethindrone acetate 5 mg daily should be considered. Retreatment with gonadotropin-releasing hormone analogs, including leuprolide acetate, is not advisable in patients with major risk factors for loss of bone mineral content).

No products indexed under this heading.

Topiramate (In patients with major risk factors for decreased bone mineral content such as chronic use of drugs that can reduce bone mass (eg, anticonvulsants), leuprolide acetate depot therapy may pose an additional risk. In these patients, the risks and benefits must be weighed carefully before therapy with leuprolide acetate depot alone is instituted, and concomitant treatment with norethindrone acetate 5 mg daily should be considered. Retreatment with gonadotropin-releasing hormone analogs, including leuprolide acetate, is not

advisable in patients with major risk factors for loss of bone mineral content).

No products indexed under this heading.

Triamcinolone (In patients with major risk factors for decreased bone mineral content such as chronic use of drugs that can reduce bone mass (eg, corticosteroids), leuprolide acetate depot may pose an additional risk. In these patients, the risks and benefits must be weighed carefully before therapy with leuprolide acetate depot alone is instituted, and concomitant treatment with norethindrone acetate 5 mg daily should be considered. Retreatment with gonadotropin-releasing hormone analogs, including leuprolide acetate, is not advisable in patients with major risk factors for loss of bone mineral content).

No products indexed under this heading.

Triamcinolone Acetonide (In patients with major risk factors for decreased bone mineral content such as chronic use of drugs that can reduce bone mass (eg, corticosteroids), leuprolide acetate depot may pose an additional risk. In these patients, the risks and benefits must be weighed carefully before therapy with leuprolide acetate depot alone is instituted, and concomitant treatment with norethindrone acetate 5 mg daily should be considered. Retreatment with gonadotropin-releasing hormone analogs, including leuprolide acetate, is not advisable in patients with major risk factors for loss of bone mineral content). Products include:

Azmacort 408
Nasacort AQ 3019

Triamcinolone Diacetate (In patients with major risk factors for decreased bone mineral content such as chronic use of drugs that can reduce bone mass (eg, corticosteroids), leuprolide acetate depot may pose an additional risk. In these patients, the risks and benefits must be weighed carefully before therapy with leuprolide acetate depot alone is instituted, and concomitant treatment with norethindrone acetate 5 mg daily should be considered. Retreatment with gonadotropin-releasing hormone analogs, including leuprolide acetate, is not advisable in patients with major risk factors for loss of bone mineral content).

No products indexed under this heading.

Triamcinolone Hexacetonide (In patients with major risk factors for decreased bone mineral content such as chronic use of drugs that can reduce bone mass (eg, corticosteroids), leuprolide acetate depot may pose an additional risk. In these patients, the risks and benefits must be weighed carefully before therapy with leuprolide acetate depot alone is instituted, and concomitant treatment with norethindrone acetate 5 mg daily should be considered. Retreatment with gonadotropin-releasing hormone analogs, including leuprolide acetate, is not advisable in patients with major risk factors for loss of bone mineral content).

No products indexed under this heading.

Trimethadione (In patients with major risk factors for decreased bone mineral content such as chronic use of drugs that can reduce bone mass (eg, anticonvulsants), leuprolide acetate depot therapy may pose an additional risk. In these patients, the risks and benefits must be weighed carefully before therapy with leuprolide acetate depot alone is instituted, and concomitant treatment with norethindrone acetate 5 mg daily should be considered. Retreatment with gonadotropin-releasing hormone analogs, including leuprolide acetate, is not

advisable in patients with major risk factors for loss of bone mineral content).

No products indexed under this heading.

Valproate Sodium (In patients with major risk factors for decreased bone mineral content such as chronic use of drugs that can reduce bone mass (eg, anticonvulsants), leuprolide acetate depot therapy may pose an additional risk. In these patients, the risks and benefits must be weighed carefully before therapy with leuprolide acetate depot alone is instituted, and concomitant treatment with norethindrone acetate 5 mg daily should be considered. Retreatment with gonadotropin-releasing hormone analogs, including leuprolide acetate, is not advisable in patients with major risk factors for loss of bone mineral content).

No products indexed under this heading.

Valproic Acid (In patients with major risk factors for decreased bone mineral content such as chronic use of drugs that can reduce bone mass (eg, anticonvulsants), leuprolide acetate depot therapy may pose an additional risk. In these patients, the risks and benefits must be weighed carefully before therapy with leuprolide acetate depot alone is instituted, and concomitant treatment with norethindrone acetate 5 mg daily should be considered. Retreatment with gonadotropin-releasing hormone analogs, including leuprolide acetate, is not advisable in patients with major risk factors for loss of bone mineral content).

No products indexed under this heading.

Zonisamide (In patients with major risk factors for decreased bone mineral content such as chronic use of drugs that can reduce bone mass (eg, anticonvulsants), leuprolide acetate depot therapy may pose an additional risk. In these patients, the risks and benefits must be weighed carefully before therapy with leuprolide acetate depot alone is instituted, and concomitant treatment with norethindrone acetate 5 mg daily should be considered. Retreatment with gonadotropin-releasing hormone analogs, including leuprolide acetate, is not advisable in patients with major risk factors for loss of bone mineral content). Products include:

Zonegran 1081

Food Interactions

Alcohol (In patients with major risk factors for decreased bone mineral content such as chronic alcohol use, leuprolide acetate depot may pose an additional risk. In these patients, the risks and benefits must be weighed carefully before therapy with leuprolide acetate depot alone is instituted, and concomitant treatment with norethindrone acetate 5 mg daily should be considered. Retreatment with gonadotropin-releasing hormone analogs, including leuprolide acetate, is not advisable in patients with major risk factors for loss of bone mineral content).

Beer, reduced-alcohol (In patients with major risk factors for decreased bone mineral content such as chronic alcohol use, leuprolide acetate depot may pose an additional risk. In these patients, the risks and benefits must be weighed carefully before therapy with leuprolide acetate depot alone is instituted, and concomitant treatment with norethindrone acetate 5 mg daily should be considered. Retreatment with gonadotropin-releasing hormone analogs, including leuprolide acetate, is not advisable in patients with major risk factors for loss of bone mineral content).

1073 Interactions Index Lybrel

Beer, unspecified (In patients with major risk factors for decreased bone mineral content such as chronic alcohol use, leuprolide acetate depot may pose an additional risk. In these patients, the risks and benefits must be weighed carefully before therapy with leuprolide acetate depot alone is instituted, and concomitant treatment with norethindrone acetate 5 mg daily should be considered. Retreatment with gonadotropin-releasing hormone analogs, including leuprolide acetate, is not advisable in patients with major risk factors for loss of bone mineral content).

Wine, Chianti (In patients with major risk factors for decreased bone mineral content such as chronic alcohol use, leuprolide acetate depot may pose an additional risk. In these patients, the risks and benefits must be weighed carefully before therapy with leuprolide acetate depot alone is instituted, and concomitant treatment with norethindrone acetate 5 mg daily should be considered. Retreatment with gonadotropin-releasing hormone analogs, including leuprolide acetate, is not advisable in patients with major risk factors for loss of bone mineral content).

Wine, Red (In patients with major risk factors for decreased bone mineral content such as chronic alcohol use, leuprolide acetate depot may pose an additional risk. In these patients, the risks and benefits must be weighed carefully before therapy with leuprolide acetate depot alone is instituted, and concomitant treatment with norethindrone acetate 5 mg daily should be considered. Retreatment with gonadotropin-releasing hormone analogs, including leuprolide acetate, is not advisable in patients with major risk factors for loss of bone mineral content).

Wine, unspecified (In patients with major risk factors for decreased bone mineral content such as chronic alcohol use, leuprolide acetate depot may pose an additional risk. In these patients, the risks and benefits must be weighed carefully before therapy with leuprolide acetate depot alone is instituted, and concomitant treatment with norethindrone acetate 5 mg daily should be considered. Retreatment with gonadotropin-releasing hormone analogs, including leuprolide acetate, is not advisable in patients with major risk factors for loss of bone mineral content).

Wine products (In patients with major risk factors for decreased bone mineral content such as chronic alcohol use, leuprolide acetate depot may pose an additional risk. In these patients, the risks and benefits must be weighed carefully before therapy with leuprolide acetate depot alone is instituted, and concomitant treatment with norethindrone acetate 5 mg daily should be considered. Retreatment with gonadotropin-releasing hormone analogs, including leuprolide acetate, is not advisable in patients with major risk factors for loss of bone mineral content).

LUPRON DEPOT 7.5 MG

(Leuprolide Acetate) 476
None cited in PDR database.

LUPRON DEPOT--3 MONTH 11.25 MG

(Leuprolide Acetate) 478
See Lupron Depot 3.75 mg

LUPRON DEPOT-- 3 MONTH 22.5 MG

(Leuprolide Acetate) 483
None cited in PDR database.

LUPRON DEPOT-- 4 MONTH 30 MG

(Leuprolide Acetate) 484
None cited in PDR database.

LUPRON DEPOT-PED 7.5 MG, 11.25 MG AND 15 MG

(Leuprolide Acetate) 487
None cited in PDR database.

LUXÍQ FOAM

(Betamethasone Valerate) 3321
None cited in PDR database.

LYBREL TABLETS

(Ethinyl Estradiol, Levonorgestrel) 3514
May interact with antibiotics, anticonvulsants, aspirin and acetaminophen containing products, barbiturates, corticosteroids, cytochrome p450 3a4 inducers (selected), cytochrome p450 3a4 inhibitors (selected), drugs affecting gastrointestinal motility, drugs which undergo biotransformation by cytochrome p-450 mixed function oxidase, penicillins, protease inhibitors, tetracyclines, theophyllines, and certain other agents. Compounds in these categories include:

Acarbose (Contraceptive effectiveness may be reduced when hormonal contraceptives are co-administered with antibiotics, anticonvulsants, and other drugs that increase the metabolism of contraceptive steroids. This could result in unintended pregnancy or unscheduled bleeding. In such cases a nonhormonal back-up method of birth control should be considered).
No products indexed under this heading.

Acetaminophen (Contraceptive effectiveness may be reduced when hormonal contraceptives are co-administered with antibiotics, anticonvulsants, and other drugs that increase the metabolism of contraceptive steroids. This could result in unintended pregnancy or unscheduled bleeding. In such cases a nonhormonal back-up method of birth control should be considered). Products include:
Percocet 1121
Tylenol 2049
Tylenol 8 Hour 2049
Extra Strength Tylenol Caplets, Cool Caplets, and EZ Tabs 2049
Extra Strength Tylenol Adult Rapid Blast Liquid 2049
Extra Strength Tylenol Rapid Release 2049
Tylenol with Codeine 2691
Tylenol Arthritis Pain Extended Release Geltabs/Caplets 2049
Children's Tylenol Suspension Liquid 2048
Chlidren's Tylenol Meltaways 2048
Tylenol, Infants' Drops 2048
Junior Tylenol 2048
Vicodin 560
Vicodin ES 561
Vicodin HP 563
Zydone 1138

Acetazolamide (CYP 3A4 inhibitors such as indinavir, itraconazole, ketoconazole, fluconazole, and troleandomycin may increase plasma hormone levels).
No products indexed under this heading.

Acetazolamide Sodium (CYP 3A4 inhibitors such as indinavir, itraconazole, ketoconazole, fluconazole, and troleandomycin may increase plasma hormone levels).
No products indexed under this heading.

Alatrofloxacin Mesylate (Contraceptive effectiveness may be reduced when hormonal contraceptives are co-administered with antibiotics, anticonvulsants, and other drugs that increase the metabolism of contraceptive steroids. This could result in unintended pregnancy or unscheduled bleeding. In such cases a nonhormonal back-up method of birth control should be considered).
No products indexed under this heading.

Albuterol (Enterohepatic recirculation of estrogens may also be decreased by substances that reduce gut transit time).
No products indexed under this heading.

Albuterol Sulfate (Enterohepatic recirculation of estrogens may also be decreased by substances that reduce gut transit time). Products include:
ProAir HFA 3393
Proventil HFA 3204
Ventolin HFA 1708

Alclometasone Dipropionate (Increased plasma concentrations of cyclosporine, prednisolone and other corticosteroids, have been reported with concomitant administration of oral contraceptives).
No products indexed under this heading.

Alfentanil Hydrochloride (Contraceptive effectiveness may be reduced when hormonal contraceptives are co-administered with antibiotics, anticonvulsants, and other drugs that increase the metabolism of contraceptive steroids. This could result in unintended pregnancy or unscheduled bleeding. In such cases a nonhormonal back-up method of birth control should be considered).
No products indexed under this heading.

Allium sativum (Contraceptive effectiveness may be reduced when hormonal contraceptives are co-administered with antibiotics, anticonvulsants, and other drugs that increase the metabolism of contraceptive steroids. This could result in unintended pregnancy or unscheduled bleeding. In such cases a nonhormonal back-up method of birth control should be considered).
No products indexed under this heading.

Alprazolam (Contraceptive effectiveness may be reduced when hormonal contraceptives are co-administered with antibiotics, anticonvulsants, and other drugs that increase the metabolism of contraceptive steroids. This could result in unintended pregnancy or unscheduled bleeding. In such cases a nonhormonal back-up method of birth control should be considered).
No products indexed under this heading.

Amikacin Sulfate (Contraceptive effectiveness may be reduced when hormonal contraceptives are co-administered with antibiotics, anticonvulsants, and other drugs that increase the metabolism of contraceptive steroids. This could result in unintended pregnancy or unscheduled bleeding. In such cases a nonhormonal back-up method of birth control should be considered).
No products indexed under this heading.

Aminoglutethimide (Contraceptive effectiveness may be reduced when hormonal contraceptives are co-administered with antibiotics, anticonvulsants, and other drugs that increase the metabolism of contraceptive steroids. This could result in unintended pregnancy or unscheduled bleeding. In such cases a nonhormonal back-up method of birth control should be considered).
No products indexed under this heading.

Aminophylline (Contraceptive effectiveness may be reduced when hormonal contraceptives are co-administered with antibiotics, anticonvulsants, and other drugs that increase the metabolism of contraceptive steroids. This could result in unintended pregnancy or unscheduled bleeding. In such cases a nonhormonal back-up method of birth control should be considered).
No products indexed under this heading.

Amiodarone Hydrochloride (Contraceptive effectiveness may be reduced when hormonal contraceptives are co-administered with antibiotics, anticonvulsants, and other drugs that increase the metabolism of contraceptive steroids. This could result in unintended pregnancy or unscheduled bleeding. In such cases a nonhormonal back-up method of birth control should be considered).
No products indexed under this heading.

Amitriptyline Hydrochloride (Contraceptive effectiveness may be reduced when hormonal contraceptives are co-administered with antibiotics, anticonvulsants, and other drugs that increase the metabolism of contraceptive steroids. This could result in unintended pregnancy or unscheduled bleeding. In such cases a nonhormonal back-up method of birth control should be considered).
No products indexed under this heading.

Amlodipine Besylate (Contraceptive effectiveness may be reduced when hormonal contraceptives are co-administered with antibiotics, anticonvulsants, and other drugs that increase the metabolism of contraceptive steroids. This could result in unintended pregnancy or unscheduled bleeding. In such cases a nonhormonal back-up method of birth control should be considered). Products include:
Azor 1010
Exforge 2443
Exforge HCT 2449

Amobarbital (Contraceptive effectiveness may be reduced when hormonal contraceptives are co-administered with antibiotics, anticonvulsants, and other drugs that increase the metabolism of contraceptive steroids. This could result in unintended pregnancy or unscheduled bleeding. In such cases a nonhormonal back-up method of birth control should be considered).
No products indexed under this heading.

Amobarbital Sodium (Contraceptive effectiveness may be reduced when hormonal contraceptives are co-administered with antibiotics, anticonvulsants, and other drugs that increase the metabolism of contraceptive steroids. This could result in unintended pregnancy or unscheduled bleeding. In such cases a nonhormonal back-up method of birth control should be considered).
No products indexed under this heading.

Amoxapine (Contraceptive effectiveness may be reduced when hormonal contraceptives are co-administered with antibiotics, anticonvulsants, and other drugs that increase the metabolism of contraceptive steroids. This could result in unintended pregnancy or unscheduled bleeding. In such cases a nonhormonal back-up method of birth control should be considered).
No products indexed under this heading.

Amoxicillin (Contraceptive effectiveness may be reduced when hormonal contraceptives are co-administered with antibiotics, anticonvulsants, and other drugs that increase the metabolism of contraceptive steroids. This could result in unintended pregnancy or unscheduled bleeding. In such cases a nonhor-

monal back-up method of birth control should be considered). Products include:

Amoxicillin Trihydrate (Contraceptive effectiveness may be reduced when hormonal contraceptives are co-administered with antibiotics, anticonvulsants, and other drugs that increase the metabolism of contraceptive steroids. This could result in unintended pregnancy or unscheduled bleeding. In such cases a nonhormonal back-up method of birth control should be considered).

No products indexed under this heading.

Amphetamine Aspartate (Contraceptive effectiveness may be reduced when hormonal contraceptives are co-administered with antibiotics, anticonvulsants, and other drugs that increase the metabolism of contraceptive steroids. This could result in unintended pregnancy or unscheduled bleeding. In such cases a nonhormonal back-up method of birth control should be considered).

No products indexed under this heading.

Amphetamine Aspartate Monohydrate (Contraceptive effectiveness may be reduced when hormonal contraceptives are co-administered with antibiotics, anticonvulsants, and other drugs that increase the metabolism of contraceptive steroids. This could result in unintended pregnancy or unscheduled bleeding. In such cases a nonhormonal back-up method of birth control should be considered).

No products indexed under this heading.

Amphetamine Sulfate (Contraceptive effectiveness may be reduced when hormonal contraceptives are co-administered with antibiotics, anticonvulsants, and other drugs that increase the metabolism of contraceptive steroids. This could result in unintended pregnancy or unscheduled bleeding. In such cases a nonhormonal back-up method of birth control should be considered).

No products indexed under this heading.

Ampicillin (Contraceptive effectiveness may be reduced when hormonal contraceptives are co-administered with antibiotics, anticonvulsants, and other drugs that increase the metabolism of contraceptive steroids. This could result in unintended pregnancy or unscheduled bleeding. In such cases a nonhormonal back-up method of birth control should be considered).

No products indexed under this heading.

Ampicillin Sodium (Contraceptive effectiveness may be reduced when hormonal contraceptives are co-administered with antibiotics, anticonvulsants, and other drugs that increase the metabolism of contraceptive steroids. This could result in unintended pregnancy or unscheduled bleeding. In such cases a nonhormonal back-up method of birth control should be considered).

No products indexed under this heading.

Ampicillin Trihydrate (Contraceptive effectiveness may be reduced when hormonal contraceptives are co-administered with antibiotics, anticonvulsants, and other drugs that increase the metabolism of contraceptive steroids. This could result in unintended pregnancy or unscheduled bleeding. In such cases a nonhormonal back-up method of birth control should be considered).

No products indexed under this heading.

Amprenavir (Several of the anti-HIV protease inhibitors have been studied with co-administration of oral combination hormonal contraceptives; significant changes (increase and decrease) in the plasma levels of the estrogen and progestin have been noted in some cases. The safety and efficacy of oral contraceptive products may be affected with co-administration of anti-HIV protease inhibitors. Health care professionals should refer to the label of the individual anti-HIV protease inhibitors for further drug-drug interaction information).

No products indexed under this heading.

Anagrelide Hydrochloride (Contraceptive effectiveness may be reduced when hormonal contraceptives are co-administered with antibiotics, anticonvulsants, and other drugs that increase the metabolism of contraceptive steroids. This could result in unintended pregnancy or unscheduled bleeding. In such cases a nonhormonal back-up method of birth control should be considered).

No products indexed under this heading.

Anastrozole (CYP 3A4 inhibitors such as indinavir, itraconazole, ketoconazole, fluconazole, and troleandomycin may increase plasma hormone levels).

No products indexed under this heading.

Antibiotics, non-penicillin, unspecified (Contraceptive effectiveness may be reduced when hormonal contraceptives are co-administered with antibiotics, anticonvulsants, and other drugs that increase the metabolism of contraceptive steroids. This could result in unintended pregnancy or unscheduled bleeding. In such cases a nonhormonal back-up method of birth control should be considered).

No products indexed under this heading.

Apomorphine (Enterohepatic recirculation of estrogens may also be decreased by substances that reduce gut transit time).

No products indexed under this heading.

Apomorphine Hydrochloride (Enterohepatic recirculation of estrogens may also be decreased by substances that reduce gut transit time).

No products indexed under this heading.

Aprepitant (Contraceptive effectiveness may be reduced when hormonal contraceptives are co-administered with antibiotics, anticonvulsants, and other drugs that increase the metabolism of contraceptive steroids. This could result in unintended pregnancy or unscheduled bleeding. In such cases a nonhormonal back-up method of birth control should be considered). Products include:

Aprobarbital (Contraceptive effectiveness may be reduced when hormonal contraceptives are co-administered with antibiotics, anticonvulsants, and other drugs that increase the metabolism of contraceptive steroids. This could result in unintended pregnancy or unscheduled bleeding. In such cases a nonhormonal back-up method of birth control should be considered).

No products indexed under this heading.

Aspirin (Acetaminophen increases the bioavailability of ethinyl estradiol since these drugs act as competitive inhibitors for sulfation of ethinyl estradiol in the gastrointestinal wall, a known pathway of elimination for ethinyl estradiol. Decreased plasma concentrations of acetaminophen due to induction of conjugation (particularly glucuronidation) have been noted when this drug is administered with oral contraceptives). Products include:

Astemizole (Contraceptive effectiveness may be reduced when hormonal contraceptives are co-administered with antibiotics, anticonvulsants, and other drugs that increase the metabolism of contraceptive steroids. This could result in unintended pregnancy or unscheduled bleeding. In such cases a nonhormonal back-up method of birth control should be considered).

No products indexed under this heading.

Atazanavir (Several of the anti-HIV protease inhibitors have been studied with co-administration of oral combination hormonal contraceptives; significant changes (increase and decrease) in the plasma levels of the estrogen and progestin have been noted in some cases. The safety and efficacy of oral contraceptive products may be affected with co-administration of anti-HIV protease inhibitors. Health care professionals should refer to the label of the individual anti-HIV protease inhibitors for further drug-drug interaction information).

No products indexed under this heading.

Atazanavir Sulfate (Several of the anti-HIV protease inhibitors have been studied with co-administration of oral combination hormonal contraceptives; significant changes (increase and decrease) in the plasma levels of the estrogen and progestin have been noted in some cases. The safety and efficacy of oral contraceptive products may be affected with co-administration of anti-HIV protease inhibitors. Health care professionals should refer to the label of the individual anti-HIV protease inhibitors for further drug-drug interaction information).

No products indexed under this heading.

Atomoxetine Hydrochloride (Contraceptive effectiveness may be reduced when hormonal contraceptives are co-administered with antibiotics, anticonvulsants, and other drugs that increase the metabolism of contraceptive steroids. This could result in unintended pregnancy or unscheduled bleeding. In such cases a nonhormonal back-up method of birth control should be considered). Products include:

Atorvastatin Calcium (Co-administration of atorvastatin increases AUC values for ethinyl estradiol by approximately 20%). Products include:

Atropine Sulfate (Enterohepatic recirculation of estrogens may also be decreased by substances that reduce gut transit time). Products include:

Azatadine Maleate (Enterohepatic recirculation of estrogens may also be decreased by substances that reduce gut transit time).

No products indexed under this heading.

Azithromycin Dihydrate (Contraceptive effectiveness may be reduced when hormonal contraceptives are co-administered with antibiotics, anticonvulsants, and other drugs that increase the metabolism of contraceptive steroids. This could result in unintended pregnancy or unscheduled bleeding. In such cases a nonhormonal back-up method of birth control should be considered).

No products indexed under this heading.

Azlocillin Sodium (Contraceptive effectiveness may be reduced when hormonal contraceptives are co-administered with antibiotics, anticonvulsants, and other drugs that increase the metabolism of contraceptive steroids. This could result in unintended pregnancy or unscheduled bleeding. In such cases a nonhormonal back-up method of birth control should be considered).

No products indexed under this heading.

Aztreonam (Contraceptive effectiveness may be reduced when hormonal contraceptives are co-administered with antibiotics, anticonvulsants, and other drugs that increase the metabolism of contraceptive steroids. This could result in unintended pregnancy or unscheduled bleeding. In such cases a nonhormonal back-up method of birth control should be considered).

No products indexed under this heading.

Bacampicillin Hydrochloride (Contraceptive effectiveness may be reduced when hormonal contraceptives are co-administered with antibiotics, anticonvulsants, and other drugs that increase the metabolism of contraceptive steroids. This could result in unintended pregnancy or unscheduled bleeding. In such cases a nonhormonal back-up method of birth control should be considered).

No products indexed under this heading.

Beclomethasone Dipropionate (Increased plasma concentrations of cyclosporine, prednisolone and other corticosteroids, have been reported with concomitant administration of oral contraceptives). Products include:

Beclomethasone Dipropionate Monohydrate (Increased plasma concentrations of cyclosporine, prednisolone and other corticosteroids, have been reported with concomitant administration of oral contraceptives). Products include:

Belladonna Alkaloids (Enterohepatic recirculation of estrogens may also be decreased by substances that reduce gut transit time). Products include:

Belladonna Ergotamine (Contraceptive effectiveness may be reduced when hormonal contraceptives are co-administered with antibiotics, anticonvulsants, and other drugs that increase the metabolism of contraceptive steroids. This could result in unintended pregnancy or unscheduled bleeding. In such cases a nonhormonal back-up method of birth control should be considered).

No products indexed under this heading.

Benzphetamine Hydrochloride (Contraceptive effectiveness may be reduced when hormonal contraceptives are co-administered with antibiotics, anticonvulsants, and other drugs that increase the metabolism of contraceptive steroids. This could result in unintended pregnancy or unscheduled bleeding. In such cases a nonhormonal back-up method of birth control should be considered).

No products indexed under this heading.

1075 Interactions Index Lybrel

Benztropine Mesylate (Enterohepatic recirculation of estrogens may also be decreased by substances that reduce gut transit time).
No products indexed under this heading.

Bepridil Hydrochloride (Enterohepatic recirculation of estrogens may also be decreased by substances that reduce gut transit time).
No products indexed under this heading.

Betamethasone (Contraceptive effectiveness may be reduced when hormonal contraceptives are co-administered with antibiotics, anticonvulsants, and other drugs that increase the metabolism of contraceptive steroids. This could result in unintended pregnancy or unscheduled bleeding. In such cases a nonhormonal back-up method of birth control should be considered).
No products indexed under this heading.

Betamethasone Acetate (Contraceptive effectiveness may be reduced when hormonal contraceptives are co-administered with antibiotics, anticonvulsants, and other drugs that increase the metabolism of contraceptive steroids. This could result in unintended pregnancy or unscheduled bleeding. In such cases a nonhormonal back-up method of birth control should be considered).
No products indexed under this heading.

Betamethasone Benzoate (Contraceptive effectiveness may be reduced when hormonal contraceptives are co-administered with antibiotics, anticonvulsants, and other drugs that increase the metabolism of contraceptive steroids. This could result in unintended pregnancy or unscheduled bleeding. In such cases a nonhormonal back-up method of birth control should be considered).
No products indexed under this heading.

Betamethasone Dipropionate (Contraceptive effectiveness may be reduced when hormonal contraceptives are co-administered with antibiotics, anticonvulsants, and other drugs that increase the metabolism of contraceptive steroids. This could result in unintended pregnancy or unscheduled bleeding. In such cases a nonhormonal back-up method of birth control should be considered). Products include:
Diprolene Lotion 0.05% **3108**
Diprolene Ointment 0.05% **3109**
Diprolene AF Cream 0.05% **3107**
Lotrisone **3163**

Betamethasone Sodium Phosphate (Contraceptive effectiveness may be reduced when hormonal contraceptives are co-administered with antibiotics, anticonvulsants, and other drugs that increase the metabolism of contraceptive steroids. This could result in unintended pregnancy or unscheduled bleeding. In such cases a nonhormonal back-up method of birth control should be considered).
No products indexed under this heading.

Betamethasone Valerate (Contraceptive effectiveness may be reduced when hormonal contraceptives are co-administered with antibiotics, anticonvulsants, and other drugs that increase the metabolism of contraceptive steroids. This could result in unintended pregnancy or unscheduled bleeding. In such cases a nonhormonal back-up method of birth control should be considered). Products include:
Luxíq **3321**

Bethanechol Chloride (Enterohepatic recirculation of estrogens may also be decreased by substances that reduce gut transit time).
No products indexed under this heading.

Biperiden Hydrochloride (Enterohepatic recirculation of estrogens may also be decreased by substances that reduce gut transit time).
No products indexed under this heading.

Bisoprolol Fumarate (Contraceptive effectiveness may be reduced when hormonal contraceptives are co-administered with antibiotics, anticonvulsants, and other drugs that increase the metabolism of contraceptive steroids. This could result in unintended pregnancy or unscheduled bleeding. In such cases a nonhormonal back-up method of birth control should be considered).
No products indexed under this heading.

Bitolterol Mesylate (Enterohepatic recirculation of estrogens may also be decreased by substances that reduce gut transit time).
No products indexed under this heading.

Bosentan (Contraceptive effectiveness may be reduced when hormonal contraceptives are co-administered with antibiotics, anticonvulsants, and other drugs that increase the metabolism of contraceptive steroids. This could result in unintended pregnancy or unscheduled bleeding. In such cases a nonhormonal back-up method of birth control should be considered). Products include:
Tracleer **573**

Bromocriptine Mesylate (Contraceptive effectiveness may be reduced when hormonal contraceptives are co-administered with antibiotics, anticonvulsants, and other drugs that increase the metabolism of contraceptive steroids. This could result in unintended pregnancy or unscheduled bleeding. In such cases a nonhormonal back-up method of birth control should be considered).
No products indexed under this heading.

Bromodiphenhydramine Hydrochloride (Enterohepatic recirculation of estrogens may also be decreased by substances that reduce gut transit time).
No products indexed under this heading.

Brompheniramine Maleate (Enterohepatic recirculation of estrogens may also be decreased by substances that reduce gut transit time).
No products indexed under this heading.

Budesonide (Increased plasma concentrations of cyclosporine, prednisolone and other corticosteroids, have been reported with concomitant administration of oral contraceptives).
Products include:
Pulmicort Flexhaler **714**
Symbicort 80/4.5 .... **720**
Symbicort 160/4.5 .... **720**

Buprenorphine Hydrochloride (Enterohepatic recirculation of estrogens may also be decreased by substances that reduce gut transit time).
No products indexed under this heading.

Buspirone Hydrochloride (Contraceptive effectiveness may be reduced when hormonal contraceptives are co-administered with antibiotics, anticonvulsants, and other drugs that increase the metabolism of contraceptive steroids. This could result in unintended pregnancy or unscheduled bleeding. In such cases a nonhormonal back-up method of birth control should be considered).
No products indexed under this heading.

Busulfan (Contraceptive effectiveness may be reduced when hormonal contraceptives are co-administered with antibiotics, anticonvulsants, and other drugs that increase the metabolism of contraceptive steroids. This could result in unintended pregnancy or unscheduled bleeding. In such cases a nonhormonal back-up method of birth control should be considered). Products include:
Myleran **1581**

Butabarbital (Contraceptive effectiveness may be reduced when hormonal contraceptives are co-administered with antibiotics, anticonvulsants, and other drugs that increase the metabolism of contraceptive steroids. This could result in unintended pregnancy or unscheduled bleeding. In such cases a nonhormonal back-up method of birth control should be considered).
No products indexed under this heading.

Butabarbital Sodium (Contraceptive effectiveness may be reduced when hormonal contraceptives are co-administered with antibiotics, anticonvulsants, and other drugs that increase the metabolism of contraceptive steroids. This could result in unintended pregnancy or unscheduled bleeding. In such cases a nonhormonal back-up method of birth control should be considered).
No products indexed under this heading.

Butalbital (Contraceptive effectiveness may be reduced when hormonal contraceptives are co-administered with antibiotics, anticonvulsants, and other drugs that increase the metabolism of contraceptive steroids. This could result in unintended pregnancy or unscheduled bleeding. In such cases a nonhormonal back-up method of birth control should be considered).
No products indexed under this heading.

Caffeine (Contraceptive effectiveness may be reduced when hormonal contraceptives are co-administered with antibiotics, anticonvulsants, and other drugs that increase the metabolism of contraceptive steroids. This could result in unintended pregnancy or unscheduled bleeding. In such cases a nonhormonal back-up method of birth control should be considered).
No products indexed under this heading.

Caffeine Anhydrous (Contraceptive effectiveness may be reduced when hormonal contraceptives are co-administered with antibiotics, anticonvulsants, and other drugs that increase the metabolism of contraceptive steroids. This could result in unintended pregnancy or unscheduled bleeding. In such cases a nonhormonal back-up method of birth control should be considered).
No products indexed under this heading.

Caffeine Citrate (Contraceptive effectiveness may be reduced when hormonal contraceptives are co-administered with antibiotics, anticonvulsants, and other drugs that increase the metabolism of contraceptive steroids. This could result in unintended pregnancy or unscheduled bleeding. In such cases a nonhormonal back-up method of birth control should be considered).
No products indexed under this heading.

Caffeine-containing medications (Contraceptive effectiveness may be reduced when hormonal contraceptives are co-administered with antibiotics, anticonvulsants, and other drugs that increase the metabolism of contraceptive steroids. This could result in unintended pregnancy or unscheduled bleeding. In such cases a nonhormonal back-up method of birth control should be considered).
No products indexed under this heading.

Caffeine Sodium Benzoate (Contraceptive effectiveness may be reduced when hormonal contraceptives are co-administered with antibiotics, anticonvulsants, and other drugs that increase the metabolism of contraceptive steroids. This could result in unintended pregnancy or unscheduled bleeding. In such cases a nonhormonal back-up method of birth control should be considered).
No products indexed under this heading.

Candesartan Cilexetil (Contraceptive effectiveness may be reduced when hormonal contraceptives are co-administered with antibiotics, anticonvulsants, and other drugs that increase the metabolism of contraceptive steroids. This could result in unintended pregnancy or unscheduled bleeding. In such cases a nonhormonal back-up method of birth control should be considered). Products include:
Atacand **697**
Atacand HCT **700**

Captopril (Contraceptive effectiveness may be reduced when hormonal contraceptives are co-administered with antibiotics, anticonvulsants, and other drugs that increase the metabolism of contraceptive steroids. This could result in unintended pregnancy or unscheduled bleeding. In such cases a nonhormonal back-up method of birth control should be considered). Products include:
Captopril **2341**

Carbamazepine (Contraceptive effectiveness may be reduced when hormonal contraceptives are co-administered with antibiotics, anticonvulsants, and other drugs that increase the metabolism of contraceptive steroids. This could result in unintended pregnancy or unscheduled bleeding. In such cases a nonhormonal back-up method of birth control should be considered). Products include:
Carbatrol **3280**
Equetro **3477**

Carbenicillin Disodium (Contraceptive effectiveness may be reduced when hormonal contraceptives are co-administered with antibiotics, anticonvulsants, and other drugs that increase the metabolism of contraceptive steroids. This could result in unintended pregnancy or unscheduled bleeding. In such cases a nonhormonal back-up method of birth control should be considered).
No products indexed under this heading.

Carbenicillin Indanyl Sodium (Contraceptive effectiveness may be reduced when hormonal contraceptives are co-administered with antibiotics, anticonvulsants, and other drugs that increase the metabolism of contraceptive steroids. This could result in unintended pregnancy or unscheduled bleeding. In such cases a nonhormonal back-up method of birth control should be considered).
No products indexed under this heading.

Carisoprodol (Contraceptive effectiveness may be reduced when hormonal contraceptives are co-administered with antibiotics, anticonvulsants, and other drugs that increase the metabolism of contraceptive steroids. This could result in unintended pregnancy or unscheduled bleeding. In such cases a nonhormonal back-up method of birth control should be considered).
No products indexed under this heading.

Carvedilol (Contraceptive effectiveness may be reduced when hormonal contraceptives are co-administered with antibiotics, anticonvulsants, and other drugs that increase the metabolism of contraceptive steroids. This could result in unintended pregnancy or unscheduled bleeding. In such cases a nonhor-

IMPORTANT NOTE: Always consult each drug listing in the patient's regimen for possible interactions.

monal back-up method of birth control should be considered). Products include:

Cefaclor (Contraceptive effectiveness may be reduced when hormonal contraceptives are co-administered with antibiotics, anticonvulsants, and other drugs that increase the metabolism of contraceptive steroids. This could result in unintended pregnancy or unscheduled bleeding. In such cases a nonhormonal back-up method of birth control should be considered).
No products indexed under this heading.

Cefadroxil (Contraceptive effectiveness may be reduced when hormonal contraceptives are co-administered with antibiotics, anticonvulsants, and other drugs that increase the metabolism of contraceptive steroids. This could result in unintended pregnancy or unscheduled bleeding. In such cases a nonhormonal back-up method of birth control should be considered).
No products indexed under this heading.

Cefamandole Nafate (Contraceptive effectiveness may be reduced when hormonal contraceptives are co-administered with antibiotics, anticonvulsants, and other drugs that increase the metabolism of contraceptive steroids. This could result in unintended pregnancy or unscheduled bleeding. In such cases a nonhormonal back-up method of birth control should be considered).
No products indexed under this heading.

Cefazolin Sodium (Contraceptive effectiveness may be reduced when hormonal contraceptives are co-administered with antibiotics, anticonvulsants, and other drugs that increase the metabolism of contraceptive steroids. This could result in unintended pregnancy or unscheduled bleeding. In such cases a nonhormonal back-up method of birth control should be considered).
No products indexed under this heading.

Cefixime (Contraceptive effectiveness may be reduced when hormonal contraceptives are co-administered with antibiotics, anticonvulsants, and other drugs that increase the metabolism of contraceptive steroids. This could result in unintended pregnancy or unscheduled bleeding. In such cases a nonhormonal back-up method of birth control should be considered). Products include:

Cefmetazole Sodium (Contraceptive effectiveness may be reduced when hormonal contraceptives are co-administered with antibiotics, anticonvulsants, and other drugs that increase the metabolism of contraceptive steroids. This could result in unintended pregnancy or unscheduled bleeding. In such cases a nonhormonal back-up method of birth control should be considered).
No products indexed under this heading.

Cefonicid Sodium (Contraceptive effectiveness may be reduced when hormonal contraceptives are co-administered with antibiotics, anticonvulsants, and other drugs that increase the metabolism of contraceptive steroids. This could result in unintended pregnancy or unscheduled bleeding. In such cases a nonhormonal back-up method of birth control should be considered).
No products indexed under this heading.

Cefoperazone Sodium (Contraceptive effectiveness may be reduced when hormonal contraceptives are co-administered with antibiotics, anticonvulsants, and other drugs that increase the metabolism of contraceptive steroids. This could result in unintended pregnancy or unscheduled bleeding. In such cases a nonhormonal back-up method of birth control should be considered).
No products indexed under this heading.

Ceforanide (Contraceptive effectiveness may be reduced when hormonal contraceptives are co-administered with antibiotics, anticonvulsants, and other drugs that increase the metabolism of contraceptive steroids. This could result in unintended pregnancy or unscheduled bleeding. In such cases a nonhormonal back-up method of birth control should be considered).
No products indexed under this heading.

Cefotaxime Sodium (Contraceptive effectiveness may be reduced when hormonal contraceptives are co-administered with antibiotics, anticonvulsants, and other drugs that increase the metabolism of contraceptive steroids. This could result in unintended pregnancy or unscheduled bleeding. In such cases a nonhormonal back-up method of birth control should be considered).
No products indexed under this heading.

Cefotetan (Contraceptive effectiveness may be reduced when hormonal contraceptives are co-administered with antibiotics, anticonvulsants, and other drugs that increase the metabolism of contraceptive steroids. This could result in unintended pregnancy or unscheduled bleeding. In such cases a nonhormonal back-up method of birth control should be considered).
No products indexed under this heading.

Cefoxitin Sodium (Contraceptive effectiveness may be reduced when hormonal contraceptives are co-administered with antibiotics, anticonvulsants, and other drugs that increase the metabolism of contraceptive steroids. This could result in unintended pregnancy or unscheduled bleeding. In such cases a nonhormonal back-up method of birth control should be considered).
No products indexed under this heading.

Cefpodoxime Proxetil (Contraceptive effectiveness may be reduced when hormonal contraceptives are co-administered with antibiotics, anticonvulsants, and other drugs that increase the metabolism of contraceptive steroids. This could result in unintended pregnancy or unscheduled bleeding. In such cases a nonhormonal back-up method of birth control should be considered).
No products indexed under this heading.

Cefprozil (Contraceptive effectiveness may be reduced when hormonal contraceptives are co-administered with antibiotics, anticonvulsants, and other drugs that increase the metabolism of contraceptive steroids. This could result in unintended pregnancy or unscheduled bleeding. In such cases a nonhormonal back-up method of birth control should be considered).
No products indexed under this heading.

Ceftazidime (Contraceptive effectiveness may be reduced when hormonal contraceptives are co-administered with antibiotics, anticonvulsants, and other drugs that increase the metabolism of contraceptive steroids. This could result in unintended pregnancy or unscheduled bleeding. In such cases a nonhormonal back-up method of birth control should be considered). Products include:

Ceftizoxime Sodium (Contraceptive effectiveness may be reduced when hormonal contraceptives are co-administered with antibiotics, anticonvulsants, and other drugs that increase the metabolism of contraceptive steroids. This could result in unintended pregnancy or unscheduled bleeding. In such cases a nonhormonal back-up method of birth control should be considered).
No products indexed under this heading.

Ceftriaxone Sodium (Contraceptive effectiveness may be reduced when hormonal contraceptives are co-administered with antibiotics, anticonvulsants, and other drugs that increase the metabolism of contraceptive steroids. This could result in unintended pregnancy or unscheduled bleeding. In such cases a nonhormonal back-up method of birth control should be considered). Products include:

Cefuroxime Axetil (Contraceptive effectiveness may be reduced when hormonal contraceptives are co-administered with antibiotics, anticonvulsants, and other drugs that increase the metabolism of contraceptive steroids. This could result in unintended pregnancy or unscheduled bleeding. In such cases a nonhormonal back-up method of birth control should be considered). Products include:

Cefuroxime Sodium (Contraceptive effectiveness may be reduced when hormonal contraceptives are co-administered with antibiotics, anticonvulsants, and other drugs that increase the metabolism of contraceptive steroids. This could result in unintended pregnancy or unscheduled bleeding. In such cases a nonhormonal back-up method of birth control should be considered).
No products indexed under this heading.

Celecoxib (Contraceptive effectiveness may be reduced when hormonal contraceptives are co-administered with antibiotics, anticonvulsants, and other drugs that increase the metabolism of contraceptive steroids. This could result in unintended pregnancy or unscheduled bleeding. In such cases a nonhormonal back-up method of birth control should be considered). Products include:

Cephalexin (Contraceptive effectiveness may be reduced when hormonal contraceptives are co-administered with antibiotics, anticonvulsants, and other drugs that increase the metabolism of contraceptive steroids. This could result in unintended pregnancy or unscheduled bleeding. In such cases a nonhormonal back-up method of birth control should be considered).
No products indexed under this heading.

Cephalothin Sodium (Contraceptive effectiveness may be reduced when hormonal contraceptives are co-administered with antibiotics, anticonvulsants, and other drugs that increase the metabolism of contraceptive steroids. This could result in unintended pregnancy or unscheduled bleeding. In such cases a nonhormonal back-up method of birth control should be considered).
No products indexed under this heading.

Cephapirin Sodium (Contraceptive effectiveness may be reduced when hormonal contraceptives are co-administered with antibiotics, anticonvulsants, and other drugs that increase the metabolism of contraceptive steroids. This could result in unintended pregnancy or unscheduled bleeding. In such cases a nonhormonal back-up method of birth control should be considered).
No products indexed under this heading.

Cephradine (Contraceptive effectiveness may be reduced when hormonal contraceptives are co-administered with antibiotics, anticonvulsants, and other drugs that increase the metabolism of contraceptive steroids. This could result in unintended pregnancy or unscheduled bleeding. In such cases a nonhormonal back-up method of birth control should be considered).
No products indexed under this heading.

Cerivastatin Sodium (Contraceptive effectiveness may be reduced when hormonal contraceptives are co-administered with antibiotics, anticonvulsants, and other drugs that increase the metabolism of contraceptive steroids. This could result in unintended pregnancy or unscheduled bleeding. In such cases a nonhormonal back-up method of birth control should be considered).
No products indexed under this heading.

Cevimeline Hydrochloride (Contraceptive effectiveness may be reduced when hormonal contraceptives are co-administered with antibiotics, anticonvulsants, and other drugs that increase the metabolism of contraceptive steroids. This could result in unintended pregnancy or unscheduled bleeding. In such cases a nonhormonal back-up method of birth control should be considered). Products include:

Chloramphenicol (Contraceptive effectiveness may be reduced when hormonal contraceptives are co-administered with antibiotics, anticonvulsants, and other drugs that increase the metabolism of contraceptive steroids. This could result in unintended pregnancy or unscheduled bleeding. In such cases a nonhormonal back-up method of birth control should be considered).
No products indexed under this heading.

Chloramphenicol Palmitate (Contraceptive effectiveness may be reduced when hormonal contraceptives are co-administered with antibiotics, anticonvulsants, and other drugs that increase the metabolism of contraceptive steroids. This could result in unintended pregnancy or unscheduled bleeding. In such cases a nonhormonal back-up method of birth control should be considered).
No products indexed under this heading.

Chloramphenicol Sodium Succinate (Contraceptive effectiveness may be reduced when hormonal contraceptives are co-administered with antibiotics, anticonvulsants, and other drugs that increase the metabolism of contraceptive steroids. This could result in unintended pregnancy or unscheduled bleeding. In such cases a nonhormonal back-up method of birth control should be considered).
No products indexed under this heading.

(⊙ Described in PDR® for Ophthalmic Medicines)

IMPORTANT NOTE: Always consult each drug listing in the patient's regimen for possible interactions.

Lybrel Interactions Index 1078

Codeine Sulfate (Contraceptive effectiveness may be reduced when hormonal contraceptives are co-administered with antibiotics, anticonvulsants, and other drugs that increase the metabolism of contraceptive steroids. This could result in unintended pregnancy or unscheduled bleeding. In such cases a nonhormonal back-up method of birth control should be considered).
No products indexed under this heading.

Conivaptan Hydrochloride (CYP 3A4 inhibitors such as indinavir, itraconazole, ketoconazole, fluconazole, and troleandomycin may increase plasma hormone levels). Products include:
Vaprisol 689

Cortisone Acetate (Contraceptive effectiveness may be reduced when hormonal contraceptives are co-administered with antibiotics, anticonvulsants, and other drugs that increase the metabolism of contraceptive steroids. This could result in unintended pregnancy or unscheduled bleeding. In such cases a nonhormonal back-up method of birth control should be considered).
No products indexed under this heading.

Cyclobenzaprine (Contraceptive effectiveness may be reduced when hormonal contraceptives are co-administered with antibiotics, anticonvulsants, and other drugs that increase the metabolism of contraceptive steroids. This could result in unintended pregnancy or unscheduled bleeding. In such cases a nonhormonal back-up method of birth control should be considered).
No products indexed under this heading.

Cyclobenzaprine Hydrochloride (Contraceptive effectiveness may be reduced when hormonal contraceptives are co-administered with antibiotics, anticonvulsants, and other drugs that increase the metabolism of contraceptive steroids. This could result in unintended pregnancy or unscheduled bleeding. In such cases a nonhormonal back-up method of birth control should be considered). Products include:
Amrix 964

Cyclophosphamide (Contraceptive effectiveness may be reduced when hormonal contraceptives are co-administered with antibiotics, anticonvulsants, and other drugs that increase the metabolism of contraceptive steroids. This could result in unintended pregnancy or unscheduled bleeding. In such cases a nonhormonal back-up method of birth control should be considered).
No products indexed under this heading.

Cyclosporine (Contraceptive effectiveness may be reduced when hormonal contraceptives are co-administered with antibiotics, anticonvulsants, and other drugs that increase the metabolism of contraceptive steroids. This could result in unintended pregnancy or unscheduled bleeding. In such cases a nonhormonal back-up method of birth control should be considered). Products include:
Gengraf 440
Neoral Oral Solution 2496
Neoral Capsules 2496
Restasis 605

Cyproheptadine Hydrochloride (Enterohepatic recirculation of estrogens may also be decreased by substances that reduce gut transit time).
No products indexed under this heading.

Dalfopristin (CYP 3A4 inhibitors such as indinavir, itraconazole, ketoconazole, fluconazole, and troleandomycin may increase plasma hormone levels).
No products indexed under this heading.

Danazol (CYP 3A4 inhibitors such as indinavir, itraconazole, ketoconazole, fluconazole, and troleandomycin may increase plasma hormone levels).
No products indexed under this heading.

Darunavir (Several of the anti-HIV protease inhibitors have been studied with co-administration of oral combination hormonal contraceptives; significant changes (increase and decrease) in the plasma levels of the estrogen and progestin have been noted in some cases. The safety and efficacy of oral contraceptive products may be affected with co-administration of anti-HIV protease inhibitors. Health care professionals should refer to the label of the individual anti-HIV protease inhibitors for further drug-drug interaction information).
No products indexed under this heading.

Dasatinib (CYP 3A4 inhibitors such as indinavir, itraconazole, ketoconazole, fluconazole, and troleandomycin may increase plasma hormone levels).
No products indexed under this heading.

Daunorubicin Hydrochloride (Contraceptive effectiveness may be reduced when hormonal contraceptives are co-administered with antibiotics, anticonvulsants, and other drugs that increase the metabolism of contraceptive steroids. This could result in unintended pregnancy or unscheduled bleeding. In such cases a nonhormonal back-up method of birth control should be considered).
No products indexed under this heading.

Delavirdine Mesylate (CYP 3A4 inhibitors such as indinavir, itraconazole, ketoconazole, fluconazole, and troleandomycin may increase plasma hormone levels).
No products indexed under this heading.

Delavirine (CYP 3A4 inhibitors such as indinavir, itraconazole, ketoconazole, fluconazole, and troleandomycin may increase plasma hormone levels).
No products indexed under this heading.

Demeclocycline Hydrochloride (Contraceptive effectiveness may be reduced when hormonal contraceptives are co-administered with antibiotics, anticonvulsants, and other drugs that increase the metabolism of contraceptive steroids. This could result in unintended pregnancy or unscheduled bleeding. In such cases a nonhormonal back-up method of birth control should be considered).
No products indexed under this heading.

Desipramine Hydrochloride (Contraceptive effectiveness may be reduced when hormonal contraceptives are co-administered with antibiotics, anticonvulsants, and other drugs that increase the metabolism of contraceptive steroids. This could result in unintended pregnancy or unscheduled bleeding. In such cases a nonhormonal back-up method of birth control should be considered).
No products indexed under this heading.

Desloratadine (CYP 3A4 inhibitors such as indinavir, itraconazole, ketoconazole, fluconazole, and troleandomycin may increase plasma hormone levels). Products include:
Clarinex Syrup 3098
Clarinex 3098
Clarinex Reditabs 3098
Clarinex-D 12-Hour 3101
Clarinex-D 3104

Desogestrel (Contraceptive effectiveness may be reduced when hormonal contraceptives are co-administered with antibiotics, anticonvulsants, and other drugs that increase the metabolism of contraceptive steroids. This could result in unintended pregnancy or unscheduled bleeding. In such cases a nonhormonal back-up method of birth control should be considered).
No products indexed under this heading.

Desoximetasone (Increased plasma concentrations of cyclosporine, prednisolone and other corticosteroids, have been reported with concomitant administration of oral contraceptives).
No products indexed under this heading.

Dexamethasone (Contraceptive effectiveness may be reduced when hormonal contraceptives are co-administered with antibiotics, anticonvulsants, and other drugs that increase the metabolism of contraceptive steroids. This could result in unintended pregnancy or unscheduled bleeding. In such cases a nonhormonal back-up method of birth control should be considered). Products include:
Ciprodex 583
Ozurdex .... ⊙ 223
Tobramycin and Dexamethasone Ophthalmic Suspension .... ⊙ 251

Dexamethasone Acetate (Contraceptive effectiveness may be reduced when hormonal contraceptives are co-administered with antibiotics, anticonvulsants, and other drugs that increase the metabolism of contraceptive steroids. This could result in unintended pregnancy or unscheduled bleeding. In such cases a nonhormonal back-up method of birth control should be considered).
No products indexed under this heading.

Dexamethasone Phosphate (Contraceptive effectiveness may be reduced when hormonal contraceptives are co-administered with antibiotics, anticonvulsants, and other drugs that increase the metabolism of contraceptive steroids. This could result in unintended pregnancy or unscheduled bleeding. In such cases a nonhormonal back-up method of birth control should be considered).
No products indexed under this heading.

Dexamethasone Sodium (Contraceptive effectiveness may be reduced when hormonal contraceptives are co-administered with antibiotics, anticonvulsants, and other drugs that increase the metabolism of contraceptive steroids. This could result in unintended pregnancy or unscheduled bleeding. In such cases a nonhormonal back-up method of birth control should be considered).
No products indexed under this heading.

Dexamethasone Sodium Phosphate (Contraceptive effectiveness may be reduced when hormonal contraceptives are co-administered with antibiotics, anticonvulsants, and other drugs that increase the metabolism of contraceptive steroids. This could result in unintended pregnancy or unscheduled bleeding. In such cases a nonhormonal back-up method of birth control should be considered).
No products indexed under this heading.

Dexamethasone Sodium Phosphate Injection (Contraceptive effectiveness may be reduced when hormonal contraceptives are co-administered with antibiotics, anticonvulsants, and other drugs that increase the metabolism of contraceptive steroids. This could result in unintended pregnancy or unscheduled bleeding. In such cases a nonhormonal back-up method of birth control should be considered).
No products indexed under this heading.

Dexchlorpheniramine Maleate (Enterohepatic recirculation of estrogens may also be decreased by substances that reduce gut transit time).
No products indexed under this heading.

Dexfenfluramine Hydrochloride (Contraceptive effectiveness may be reduced when hormonal contraceptives are co-administered with antibiotics, anticonvulsants, and other drugs that increase the metabolism of contraceptive steroids. This could result in unintended pregnancy or unscheduled bleeding. In such cases a nonhormonal back-up method of birth control should be considered).
No products indexed under this heading.

Dextromethorphan (Contraceptive effectiveness may be reduced when hormonal contraceptives are co-administered with antibiotics, anticonvulsants, and other drugs that increase the metabolism of contraceptive steroids. This could result in unintended pregnancy or unscheduled bleeding. In such cases a nonhormonal back-up method of birth control should be considered).
No products indexed under this heading.

Dextromethorphan Hydrobromide (Contraceptive effectiveness may be reduced when hormonal contraceptives are co-administered with antibiotics, anticonvulsants, and other drugs that increase the metabolism of contraceptive steroids. This could result in unintended pregnancy or unscheduled bleeding. In such cases a nonhormonal back-up method of birth control should be considered).
No products indexed under this heading.

Dextromethorphan Polistirex (Contraceptive effectiveness may be reduced when hormonal contraceptives are co-administered with antibiotics, anticonvulsants, and other drugs that increase the metabolism of contraceptive steroids. This could result in unintended pregnancy or unscheduled bleeding. In such cases a nonhormonal back-up method of birth control should be considered).
No products indexed under this heading.

Dezocine (Enterohepatic recirculation of estrogens may also be decreased by substances that reduce gut transit time).
No products indexed under this heading.

Diazepam (Contraceptive effectiveness may be reduced when hormonal contraceptives are co-administered with antibiotics, anticonvulsants, and other drugs that increase the metabolism of contraceptive steroids. This could result in unintended pregnancy or unscheduled bleeding. In such cases a nonhormonal back-up method of birth control should be considered). Products include:
Valium Tablets 2880

Diclofenac Potassium (Contraceptive effectiveness may be reduced when hormonal contraceptives are co-administered with antibiotics, anticonvulsants, and other drugs that increase the metabolism of contraceptive steroids. This could result in unintended pregnancy or unscheduled bleeding. In such cases a nonhormonal back-up method of birth control should be considered).
No products indexed under this heading.

(⊙ Described in PDR® for Ophthalmic Medicines)

1079 Interactions Index Lybrel

Diclofenac Sodium (Contraceptive effectiveness may be reduced when hormonal contraceptives are co-administered with antibiotics, anticonvulsants, and other drugs that increase the metabolism of contraceptive steroids. This could result in unintended pregnancy or unscheduled bleeding. In such cases a nonhormonal back-up method of birth control should be considered).
No products indexed under this heading.

Dicloxacillin (Contraceptive effectiveness may be reduced when hormonal contraceptives are co-administered with antibiotics, anticonvulsants, and other drugs that increase the metabolism of contraceptive steroids. This could result in unintended pregnancy or unscheduled bleeding. In such cases a nonhormonal back-up method of birth control should be considered).
No products indexed under this heading.

Dicloxacillin Sodium (Contraceptive effectiveness may be reduced when hormonal contraceptives are co-administered with antibiotics, anticonvulsants, and other drugs that increase the metabolism of contraceptive steroids. This could result in unintended pregnancy or unscheduled bleeding. In such cases a nonhormonal back-up method of birth control should be considered).
No products indexed under this heading.

Dicyclomine Hydrochloride (Enterohepatic recirculation of estrogens may also be decreased by substances that reduce gut transit time). Products include:
Bentyl Capsules 780
Bentyl Injection 780
Bentyl Syrup 780
Bentyl Tablets 780

Diflorasone Diacetate (Increased plasma concentrations of cyclosporine, prednisolone and other corticosteroids, have been reported with concomitant administration of oral contraceptives).
No products indexed under this heading.

Dihydrocodeine Bitartrate (Enterohepatic recirculation of estrogens may also be decreased by substances that reduce gut transit time).
No products indexed under this heading.

Dihydroergotamine Mesylate (Contraceptive effectiveness may be reduced when hormonal contraceptives are co-administered with antibiotics, anticonvulsants, and other drugs that increase the metabolism of contraceptive steroids. This could result in unintended pregnancy or unscheduled bleeding. In such cases a nonhormonal back-up method of birth control should be considered).
No products indexed under this heading.

Diltiazem Hydrochloride (Contraceptive effectiveness may be reduced when hormonal contraceptives are co-administered with antibiotics, anticonvulsants, and other drugs that increase the metabolism of contraceptive steroids. This could result in unintended pregnancy or unscheduled bleeding. In such cases a nonhormonal back-up method of birth control should be considered). Products include:
Cardizem LA 423

Diltiazem Maleate (Contraceptive effectiveness may be reduced when hormonal contraceptives are co-administered with antibiotics, anticonvulsants, and other drugs that increase the metabolism of contraceptive steroids. This could result in unintended pregnancy or unscheduled bleeding. In such cases a nonhormonal back-up method of birth control should be considered).
No products indexed under this heading.

Diphenhydramine Hydrochloride (Enterohepatic recirculation of estrogens may also be decreased by substances that reduce gut transit time). Products include:
Benadryl Allergy Ultratab 2042
Children's Benadryl Allergy Liquid 2042

Diphenoxylate (Enterohepatic recirculation of estrogens may also be decreased by substances that reduce gut transit time).
No products indexed under this heading.

Diphenoxylate Hydrochloride (Enterohepatic recirculation of estrogens may also be decreased by substances that reduce gut transit time).
No products indexed under this heading.

Diphenylpyraline Hydrochloride (Enterohepatic recirculation of estrogens may also be decreased by substances that reduce gut transit time).
No products indexed under this heading.

Dirithromycin (Contraceptive effectiveness may be reduced when hormonal contraceptives are co-administered with antibiotics, anticonvulsants, and other drugs that increase the metabolism of contraceptive steroids. This could result in unintended pregnancy or unscheduled bleeding. In such cases a nonhormonal back-up method of birth control should be considered).
No products indexed under this heading.

Disodium Carbenicillin (Contraceptive effectiveness may be reduced when hormonal contraceptives are co-administered with antibiotics, anticonvulsants, and other drugs that increase the metabolism of contraceptive steroids. This could result in unintended pregnancy or unscheduled bleeding. In such cases a nonhormonal back-up method of birth control should be considered).
No products indexed under this heading.

Disopyramide (Contraceptive effectiveness may be reduced when hormonal contraceptives are co-administered with antibiotics, anticonvulsants, and other drugs that increase the metabolism of contraceptive steroids. This could result in unintended pregnancy or unscheduled bleeding. In such cases a nonhormonal back-up method of birth control should be considered).
No products indexed under this heading.

Disopyramide Phosphate (Contraceptive effectiveness may be reduced when hormonal contraceptives are co-administered with antibiotics, anticonvulsants, and other drugs that increase the metabolism of contraceptive steroids. This could result in unintended pregnancy or unscheduled bleeding. In such cases a nonhormonal back-up method of birth control should be considered).
No products indexed under this heading.

Disulfiram (Contraceptive effectiveness may be reduced when hormonal contraceptives are co-administered with antibiotics, anticonvulsants, and other drugs that increase the metabolism of contraceptive steroids. This could result in unintended pregnancy or unscheduled bleeding. In such cases a nonhormonal back-up method of birth control should be considered).
No products indexed under this heading.

Divalproex Sodium (Contraceptive effectiveness may be reduced when hormonal contraceptives are co-administered with antibiotics, anticonvulsants, and other drugs that increase the metabolism of contraceptive steroids. This could result in unintended pregnancy or unscheduled bleeding. In such cases a nonhormonal back-up method of birth control should be considered). Products include:
Depakote ER 426

Dobutamine (Enterohepatic recirculation of estrogens may also be decreased by substances that reduce gut transit time).
No products indexed under this heading.

Dobutamine Hydrochloride (Enterohepatic recirculation of estrogens may also be decreased by substances that reduce gut transit time).
No products indexed under this heading.

Docetaxel (Contraceptive effectiveness may be reduced when hormonal contraceptives are co-administered with antibiotics, anticonvulsants, and other drugs that increase the metabolism of contraceptive steroids. This could result in unintended pregnancy or unscheduled bleeding. In such cases a nonhormonal back-up method of birth control should be considered). Products include:
Taxotere 3035

Dolasetron Mesylate (Contraceptive effectiveness may be reduced when hormonal contraceptives are co-administered with antibiotics, anticonvulsants, and other drugs that increase the metabolism of contraceptive steroids. This could result in unintended pregnancy or unscheduled bleeding. In such cases a nonhormonal back-up method of birth control should be considered). Products include:
Anzemet Injection 2931
Anzemet Tablets 2934

Domperidone (Enterohepatic recirculation of estrogens may also be decreased by substances that reduce gut transit time).
No products indexed under this heading.

Donepezil Hydrochloride (Contraceptive effectiveness may be reduced when hormonal contraceptives are co-administered with antibiotics, anticonvulsants, and other drugs that increase the metabolism of contraceptive steroids. This could result in unintended pregnancy or unscheduled bleeding. In such cases a nonhormonal back-up method of birth control should be considered). Products include:
Aricept 1045
Aricept ODT 1045

Dopamine Hydrochloride (Enterohepatic recirculation of estrogens may also be decreased by substances that reduce gut transit time).
No products indexed under this heading.

Doxepin Hydrochloride (Contraceptive effectiveness may be reduced when hormonal contraceptives are co-administered with antibiotics, anticonvulsants, and other drugs that increase the metabolism of contraceptive steroids. This could result in unintended pregnancy or unscheduled bleeding. In such cases a nonhormonal back-up method of birth control should be considered).
No products indexed under this heading.

Doxorubicin Hydrochloride (Contraceptive effectiveness may be reduced when hormonal contraceptives are co-administered with antibiotics, anticonvulsants, and other drugs that increase the metabolism of contraceptive steroids. This could result in unintended pregnancy or unscheduled bleeding. In such cases a nonhormonal back-up method of birth control should be considered).
No products indexed under this heading.

Doxycycline (Several cases of contraceptive failure and unscheduled bleeding have been reported in the literature with concomitant administration of antibiotics such as ampicillin and other penicillins, and tetracyclines. However, clinical pharmacology studies investigating drug interactions between combined oral contraceptives and these antibiotics have reported inconsistent results).
No products indexed under this heading.

Doxycycline Calcium (Contraceptive effectiveness may be reduced when hormonal contraceptives are co-administered with antibiotics, anticonvulsants, and other drugs that increase the metabolism of contraceptive steroids. This could result in unintended pregnancy or unscheduled bleeding. In such cases a nonhormonal back-up method of birth control should be considered).
No products indexed under this heading.

Doxycycline Hyclate (Contraceptive effectiveness may be reduced when hormonal contraceptives are co-administered with antibiotics, anticonvulsants, and other drugs that increase the metabolism of contraceptive steroids. This could result in unintended pregnancy or unscheduled bleeding. In such cases a nonhormonal back-up method of birth control should be considered).
No products indexed under this heading.

Doxycycline Monohydrate (Contraceptive effectiveness may be reduced when hormonal contraceptives are co-administered with antibiotics, anticonvulsants, and other drugs that increase the metabolism of contraceptive steroids. This could result in unintended pregnancy or unscheduled bleeding. In such cases a nonhormonal back-up method of birth control should be considered).
No products indexed under this heading.

Dronabinol (Contraceptive effectiveness may be reduced when hormonal contraceptives are co-administered with antibiotics, anticonvulsants, and other drugs that increase the metabolism of contraceptive steroids. This could result in unintended pregnancy or unscheduled bleeding. In such cases a nonhormonal back-up method of birth control should be considered).
No products indexed under this heading.

Drugs that Undergo Biotransformation by Cytochrome P-450 Mixed Function Oxidase (Contraceptive effectiveness may be reduced when hormonal contraceptives are co-administered with antibiotics, anticonvulsants, and other drugs that increase the metabolism of contraceptive steroids. This could result in unintended pregnancy or unscheduled bleeding. In such cases a nonhormonal back-up method of birth control should be considered).
No products indexed under this heading.

Dyphylline (Contraceptive effectiveness may be reduced when hormonal contraceptives are co-administered with antibiotics, anticonvulsants, and other drugs that increase the metabolism of contraceptive steroids. This could result in unintended pregnancy or unscheduled bleeding. In such cases a nonhormonal back-up method of birth control should be considered).
No products indexed under this heading.

Edrophonium Chloride (Enterohepatic recirculation of estrogens may also be decreased by substances that reduce gut transit time).
No products indexed under this heading.

Efavirenz (Contraceptive effectiveness may be reduced when hormonal contra-

IMPORTANT NOTE: Always consult each drug listing in the patient's regimen for possible interactions.

ceptives are co-administered with antibiotics, anticonvulsants, and other drugs that increase the metabolism of contraceptive steroids. This could result in unintended pregnancy or unscheduled bleeding. In such cases a nonhormonal back-up method of birth control should be considered). Products include:
Atripla 906

Encainide Hydrochloride (Contraceptive effectiveness may be reduced when hormonal contraceptives are co-administered with antibiotics, anticonvulsants, and other drugs that increase the metabolism of contraceptive steroids. This could result in unintended pregnancy or unscheduled bleeding. In such cases a nonhormonal back-up method of birth control should be considered).
No products indexed under this heading.

Enoxacin (Contraceptive effectiveness may be reduced when hormonal contraceptives are co-administered with antibiotics, anticonvulsants, and other drugs that increase the metabolism of contraceptive steroids. This could result in unintended pregnancy or unscheduled bleeding. In such cases a nonhormonal back-up method of birth control should be considered).
No products indexed under this heading.

Ephedrine Hydrochloride (Enterohepatic recirculation of estrogens may also be decreased by substances that reduce gut transit time).
No products indexed under this heading.

Ephedrine Sulfate (Enterohepatic recirculation of estrogens may also be decreased by substances that reduce gut transit time).
No products indexed under this heading.

Ephedrine Tannate (Enterohepatic recirculation of estrogens may also be decreased by substances that reduce gut transit time).
No products indexed under this heading.

Epinephrine (Enterohepatic recirculation of estrogens may also be decreased by substances that reduce gut transit time). Products include:
EpiPen 3631
Twinject 3268

Epinephrine Hydrochloride (Enterohepatic recirculation of estrogens may also be decreased by substances that reduce gut transit time).
No products indexed under this heading.

Epirubicin Hydrochloride (Contraceptive effectiveness may be reduced when hormonal contraceptives are co-administered with antibiotics, anticonvulsants, and other drugs that increase the metabolism of contraceptive steroids. This could result in unintended pregnancy or unscheduled bleeding. In such cases a nonhormonal back-up method of birth control should be considered).
No products indexed under this heading.

Eprosartan Mesylate (Contraceptive effectiveness may be reduced when hormonal contraceptives are co-administered with antibiotics, anticonvulsants, and other drugs that increase the metabolism of contraceptive steroids. This could result in unintended pregnancy or unscheduled bleeding. In such cases a nonhormonal back-up method of birth control should be considered). Products include:
Teveten 538
Teveten HCT 541

Ergotamine Tartrate (Contraceptive effectiveness may be reduced when hormonal contraceptives are co-administered with antibiotics, anticonvulsants, and other drugs that increase the metabolism of contraceptive steroids. This could result in unintended pregnancy or unscheduled bleeding. In such cases a nonhormonal back-up method of birth control should be considered).
No products indexed under this heading.

Erythromycin (Contraceptive effectiveness may be reduced when hormonal contraceptives are co-administered with antibiotics, anticonvulsants, and other drugs that increase the metabolism of contraceptive steroids. This could result in unintended pregnancy or unscheduled bleeding. In such cases a nonhormonal back-up method of birth control should be considered).
No products indexed under this heading.

Erythromycin, Topical (Contraceptive effectiveness may be reduced when hormonal contraceptives are co-administered with antibiotics, anticonvulsants, and other drugs that increase the metabolism of contraceptive steroids. This could result in unintended pregnancy or unscheduled bleeding. In such cases a nonhormonal back-up method of birth control should be considered).
No products indexed under this heading.

Erythromycin Estolate (Contraceptive effectiveness may be reduced when hormonal contraceptives are co-administered with antibiotics, anticonvulsants, and other drugs that increase the metabolism of contraceptive steroids. This could result in unintended pregnancy or unscheduled bleeding. In such cases a nonhormonal back-up method of birth control should be considered).
No products indexed under this heading.

Erythromycin Ethylsuccinate (Contraceptive effectiveness may be reduced when hormonal contraceptives are co-administered with antibiotics, anticonvulsants, and other drugs that increase the metabolism of contraceptive steroids. This could result in unintended pregnancy or unscheduled bleeding. In such cases a nonhormonal back-up method of birth control should be considered). Products include:
E.E.S. 437
EryPed 435

Erythromycin Gluceptate (Contraceptive effectiveness may be reduced when hormonal contraceptives are co-administered with antibiotics, anticonvulsants, and other drugs that increase the metabolism of contraceptive steroids. This could result in unintended pregnancy or unscheduled bleeding. In such cases a nonhormonal back-up method of birth control should be considered).
No products indexed under this heading.

Erythromycin Lactobionate (Contraceptive effectiveness may be reduced when hormonal contraceptives are co-administered with antibiotics, anticonvulsants, and other drugs that increase the metabolism of contraceptive steroids. This could result in unintended pregnancy or unscheduled bleeding. In such cases a nonhormonal back-up method of birth control should be considered).
No products indexed under this heading.

Erythromycin Stearate (Contraceptive effectiveness may be reduced when hormonal contraceptives are co-administered with antibiotics, anticonvulsants, and other drugs that increase the metabolism of contraceptive steroids. This could result in unintended pregnancy or unscheduled bleeding. In such cases a nonhormonal back-up method of birth control should be considered).
No products indexed under this heading.

Esomeprazole Magnesium (Contraceptive effectiveness may be reduced when hormonal contraceptives are co-administered with antibiotics, anticonvulsants, and other drugs that increase the metabolism of contraceptive steroids. This could result in unintended pregnancy or unscheduled bleeding. In such cases a nonhormonal back-up method of birth control should be considered). Products include:
Nexium Capsules 704
Nexium Oral Suspension 704

Esomeprazole Sodium (Contraceptive effectiveness may be reduced when hormonal contraceptives are co-administered with antibiotics, anticonvulsants, and other drugs that increase the metabolism of contraceptive steroids. This could result in unintended pregnancy or unscheduled bleeding. In such cases a nonhormonal back-up method of birth control should be considered). Products include:
Nexium I.V. 712

Estradiol (Contraceptive effectiveness may be reduced when hormonal contraceptives are co-administered with antibiotics, anticonvulsants, and other drugs that increase the metabolism of contraceptive steroids. This could result in unintended pregnancy or unscheduled bleeding. In such cases a nonhormonal back-up method of birth control should be considered). Products include:
Activella 2561
Angeliq 831
Climara 841
Climara Pro 847
Divigel 3467
Estrasorb 1777
Vagifem 2589

Estradiol Benzoate (Contraceptive effectiveness may be reduced when hormonal contraceptives are co-administered with antibiotics, anticonvulsants, and other drugs that increase the metabolism of contraceptive steroids. This could result in unintended pregnancy or unscheduled bleeding. In such cases a nonhormonal back-up method of birth control should be considered).
No products indexed under this heading.

Estradiol Cypionate (Contraceptive effectiveness may be reduced when hormonal contraceptives are co-administered with antibiotics, anticonvulsants, and other drugs that increase the metabolism of contraceptive steroids. This could result in unintended pregnancy or unscheduled bleeding. In such cases a nonhormonal back-up method of birth control should be considered).
No products indexed under this heading.

Estradiol Valerate (Contraceptive effectiveness may be reduced when hormonal contraceptives are co-administered with antibiotics, anticonvulsants, and other drugs that increase the metabolism of contraceptive steroids. This could result in unintended pregnancy or unscheduled bleeding. In such cases a nonhormonal back-up method of birth control should be considered).
No products indexed under this heading.

Estrogen (Contraceptive effectiveness may be reduced when hormonal contraceptives are co-administered with antibiotics, anticonvulsants, and other drugs that increase the metabolism of contraceptive steroids. This could result in unintended pregnancy or unscheduled bleeding. In such cases a nonhormonal back-up method of birth control should be considered).
No products indexed under this heading.

Estrogens, Conjugated (Contraceptive effectiveness may be reduced when hormonal contraceptives are co-administered with antibiotics, anticonvulsants, and other drugs that increase the metabolism of contraceptive steroids. This could result in unintended pregnancy or unscheduled bleeding. In such cases a nonhormonal back-up method of birth control should be considered). Products include:
Premarin Intravenous 3528
Premarin Tablets 3533
Premarin Vaginal Cream 3540
Premphase 3549
Prempro 3549

Estrogens, Conjugated, Synthetic A (Contraceptive effectiveness may be reduced when hormonal contraceptives are co-administered with antibiotics, anticonvulsants, and other drugs that increase the metabolism of contraceptive steroids. This could result in unintended pregnancy or unscheduled bleeding. In such cases a nonhormonal back-up method of birth control should be considered).
No products indexed under this heading.

Estrogens, Esterified (Contraceptive effectiveness may be reduced when hormonal contraceptives are co-administered with antibiotics, anticonvulsants, and other drugs that increase the metabolism of contraceptive steroids. This could result in unintended pregnancy or unscheduled bleeding. In such cases a nonhormonal back-up method of birth control should be considered).
No products indexed under this heading.

Ethosuximide (Contraceptive effectiveness may be reduced when hormonal contraceptives are co-administered with antibiotics, anticonvulsants, and other drugs that increase the metabolism of contraceptive steroids. This could result in unintended pregnancy or unscheduled bleeding. In such cases a nonhormonal back-up method of birth control should be considered).
No products indexed under this heading.

Ethotoin (Contraceptive effectiveness may be reduced when hormonal contraceptives are co-administered with antibiotics, anticonvulsants, and other drugs that increase the metabolism of contraceptive steroids. This could result in unintended pregnancy or unscheduled bleeding. In such cases a nonhormonal back-up method of birth control should be considered).
No products indexed under this heading.

Ethynodiol Diacetate (Contraceptive effectiveness may be reduced when hormonal contraceptives are co-administered with antibiotics, anticonvulsants, and other drugs that increase the metabolism of contraceptive steroids. This could result in unintended pregnancy or unscheduled bleeding. In such cases a nonhormonal back-up method of birth control should be considered).
No products indexed under this heading.

(⊙ Described in PDR® for Ophthalmic Medicines)

1081 Interactions Index Lybrel

Etodolac (Contraceptive effectiveness may be reduced when hormonal contraceptives are co-administered with antibiotics, anticonvulsants, and other drugs that increase the metabolism of contraceptive steroids. This could result in unintended pregnancy or unscheduled bleeding. In such cases a nonhormonal back-up method of birth control should be considered).
No products indexed under this heading.

Etoposide (Contraceptive effectiveness may be reduced when hormonal contraceptives are co-administered with antibiotics, anticonvulsants, and other drugs that increase the metabolism of contraceptive steroids. This could result in unintended pregnancy or unscheduled bleeding. In such cases a nonhormonal back-up method of birth control should be considered).
No products indexed under this heading.

Etoposide Phosphate (Contraceptive effectiveness may be reduced when hormonal contraceptives are co-administered with antibiotics, anticonvulsants, and other drugs that increase the metabolism of contraceptive steroids. This could result in unintended pregnancy or unscheduled bleeding. In such cases a nonhormonal back-up method of birth control should be considered).
No products indexed under this heading.

Felbamate (Contraceptive effectiveness may be reduced when hormonal contraceptives are co-administered with antibiotics, anticonvulsants, and other drugs that increase the metabolism of contraceptive steroids. This could result in unintended pregnancy or unscheduled bleeding. In such cases a nonhormonal back-up method of birth control should be considered).
No products indexed under this heading.

Felodipine (Contraceptive effectiveness may be reduced when hormonal contraceptives are co-administered with antibiotics, anticonvulsants, and other drugs that increase the metabolism of contraceptive steroids. This could result in unintended pregnancy or unscheduled bleeding. In such cases a nonhormonal back-up method of birth control should be considered).
No products indexed under this heading.

Fenoprofen Calcium (Contraceptive effectiveness may be reduced when hormonal contraceptives are co-administered with antibiotics, anticonvulsants, and other drugs that increase the metabolism of contraceptive steroids. This could result in unintended pregnancy or unscheduled bleeding. In such cases a nonhormonal back-up method of birth control should be considered).
No products indexed under this heading.

Fentanyl (Contraceptive effectiveness may be reduced when hormonal contraceptives are co-administered with antibiotics, anticonvulsants, and other drugs that increase the metabolism of contraceptive steroids. This could result in unintended pregnancy or unscheduled bleeding. In such cases a nonhormonal back-up method of birth control should be considered). Products include:
Duragesic 2604
Fentanyl Transdermal System 2346
Onsolis 2054

Fentanyl Citrate (Contraceptive effectiveness may be reduced when hormonal contraceptives are co-administered with antibiotics, anticonvulsants, and other drugs that increase the metabolism of contraceptive steroids. This could result in unintended pregnancy or unscheduled bleeding. In such cases a nonhormonal back-up method of birth control should be considered). Products include:
Fentora 966

Flecainide Acetate (Contraceptive effectiveness may be reduced when hormonal contraceptives are co-administered with antibiotics, anticonvulsants, and other drugs that increase the metabolism of contraceptive steroids. This could result in unintended pregnancy or unscheduled bleeding. In such cases a nonhormonal back-up method of birth control should be considered).
No products indexed under this heading.

Fluconazole (CYP 3A4 inhibitors such as indinavir, itraconazole, ketoconazole, fluconazole, and troleandomycin may increase plasma hormone levels).
No products indexed under this heading.

Fludrocortisone Acetate (Contraceptive effectiveness may be reduced when hormonal contraceptives are co-administered with antibiotics, anticonvulsants, and other drugs that increase the metabolism of contraceptive steroids. This could result in unintended pregnancy or unscheduled bleeding. In such cases a nonhormonal back-up method of birth control should be considered).
No products indexed under this heading.

Flumethasone Pivalate (Increased plasma concentrations of cyclosporine, prednisolone and other corticosteroids, have been reported with concomitant administration of oral contraceptives).
No products indexed under this heading.

Flunisolide Hemihydrate (Increased plasma concentrations of cyclosporine, prednisolone and other corticosteroids, have been reported with concomitant administration of oral contraceptives).
No products indexed under this heading.

Fluoxetine (Contraceptive effectiveness may be reduced when hormonal contraceptives are co-administered with antibiotics, anticonvulsants, and other drugs that increase the metabolism of contraceptive steroids. This could result in unintended pregnancy or unscheduled bleeding. In such cases a nonhormonal back-up method of birth control should be considered).
No products indexed under this heading.

Fluoxetine Hydrochloride (Contraceptive effectiveness may be reduced when hormonal contraceptives are co-administered with antibiotics, anticonvulsants, and other drugs that increase the metabolism of contraceptive steroids. This could result in unintended pregnancy or unscheduled bleeding. In such cases a nonhormonal back-up method of birth control should be considered). Products include:
Prozac Weekly 1941
Prozac Pulvules 1941
Symbyax 1965

Fluphenazine Decanoate (Contraceptive effectiveness may be reduced when hormonal contraceptives are co-administered with antibiotics, anticonvulsants, and other drugs that increase the metabolism of contraceptive steroids. This could result in unintended pregnancy or unscheduled bleeding. In such cases a nonhormonal back-up method of birth control should be considered).
No products indexed under this heading.

Fluphenazine Enanthate (Contraceptive effectiveness may be reduced when hormonal contraceptives are co-administered with antibiotics, anticonvulsants, and other drugs that increase the metabolism of contraceptive steroids. This could result in unintended pregnancy or unscheduled bleeding. In such cases a nonhormonal back-up method of birth control should be considered).
No products indexed under this heading.

Fluphenazine Hydrochloride (Contraceptive effectiveness may be reduced when hormonal contraceptives are co-administered with antibiotics, anticonvulsants, and other drugs that increase the metabolism of contraceptive steroids. This could result in unintended pregnancy or unscheduled bleeding. In such cases a nonhormonal back-up method of birth control should be considered).
No products indexed under this heading.

Flurbiprofen (Contraceptive effectiveness may be reduced when hormonal contraceptives are co-administered with antibiotics, anticonvulsants, and other drugs that increase the metabolism of contraceptive steroids. This could result in unintended pregnancy or unscheduled bleeding. In such cases a nonhormonal back-up method of birth control should be considered).
No products indexed under this heading.

Flurbiprofen Sodium (Contraceptive effectiveness may be reduced when hormonal contraceptives are co-administered with antibiotics, anticonvulsants, and other drugs that increase the metabolism of contraceptive steroids. This could result in unintended pregnancy or unscheduled bleeding. In such cases a nonhormonal back-up method of birth control should be considered).
No products indexed under this heading.

Flutamide (Contraceptive effectiveness may be reduced when hormonal contraceptives are co-administered with antibiotics, anticonvulsants, and other drugs that increase the metabolism of contraceptive steroids. This could result in unintended pregnancy or unscheduled bleeding. In such cases a nonhormonal back-up method of birth control should be considered).
No products indexed under this heading.

Fluticasone Furoate (Increased plasma concentrations of cyclosporine, prednisolone and other corticosteroids, have been reported with concomitant administration of oral contraceptives). Products include:
Veramyst 1713

Fluticasone Propionate (Contraceptive effectiveness may be reduced when hormonal contraceptives are co-administered with antibiotics, anticonvulsants, and other drugs that increase the metabolism of contraceptive steroids. This could result in unintended pregnancy or unscheduled bleeding. In such cases a nonhormonal back-up method of birth control should be considered). Products include:
Advair 100/50 1275
Advair 250/50 1275
Advair 500/50 1275
Advair HFA 45/21 1288
Advair HFA 115/21 1288
Advair HFA 230/21 1288
Flonase 1459
Flovent Diskus 1463
Flovent HFA 1470

Fluvastatin Sodium (Contraceptive effectiveness may be reduced when hormonal contraceptives are co-administered with antibiotics, anticonvulsants, and other drugs that increase the metabolism of contraceptive steroids. This could result in unintended pregnancy or unscheduled bleeding. In such cases a nonhormonal back-up method of birth control should be considered).
No products indexed under this heading.

Fluvoxamine Maleate (Contraceptive effectiveness may be reduced when hormonal contraceptives are co-administered with antibiotics, anticonvulsants, and other drugs that increase the metabolism of contraceptive steroids. This could result in unintended pregnancy or unscheduled bleeding. In such cases a nonhormonal back-up method of birth control should be considered).
No products indexed under this heading.

Formoterol Fumarate (Contraceptive effectiveness may be reduced when hormonal contraceptives are co-administered with antibiotics, anticonvulsants, and other drugs that increase the metabolism of contraceptive steroids. This could result in unintended pregnancy or unscheduled bleeding. In such cases a nonhormonal back-up method of birth control should be considered). Products include:
Foradil 3121
Perforomist 3634

Fosamprenavir Calcium (Several of the anti-HIV protease inhibitors have been studied with co-administration of oral combination hormonal contraceptives; significant changes (increase and decrease) in the plasma levels of the estrogen and progestin have been noted in some cases. The safety and efficacy of oral contraceptive products may be affected with co-administration of anti-HIV protease inhibitors. Health care professionals should refer to the label of the individual anti-HIV protease inhibitors for further drug-drug interaction information). Products include:
Lexiva Oral Suspension 1558
Lexiva 1558

Fosphenytoin (Contraceptive effectiveness may be reduced when hormonal contraceptives are co-administered with antibiotics, anticonvulsants, and other drugs that increase the metabolism of contraceptive steroids. This could result in unintended pregnancy or unscheduled bleeding. In such cases a nonhormonal back-up method of birth control should be considered).
No products indexed under this heading.

Fosphenytoin Sodium (Contraceptive effectiveness may be reduced when hormonal contraceptives are co-administered with antibiotics, anticonvulsants, and other drugs that increase the metabolism of contraceptive steroids. This could result in unintended pregnancy or unscheduled bleeding. In such cases a nonhormonal back-up method of birth control should be considered).
No products indexed under this heading.

Gabapentin (Contraceptive effectiveness may be reduced when hormonal contraceptives are co-administered with antibiotics, anticonvulsants, and other drugs that increase the metabolism of contraceptive steroids. This could result in unintended pregnancy or unscheduled bleeding. In such cases a nonhormonal back-up method of birth control should be considered).
No products indexed under this heading.

Galantamine Hydrobromide (Contraceptive effectiveness may be reduced when hormonal contraceptives are co-administered with antibiotics, anticonvulsants, and other drugs that increase the metabolism of contraceptive steroids. This could result in unintended pregnancy or unscheduled bleeding. In such cases a nonhormonal back-up method of birth control should be considered).
No products indexed under this heading.

IMPORTANT NOTE: Always consult each drug listing in the patient's regimen for possible interactions.

Garlic Extract (Contraceptive effectiveness may be reduced when hormonal contraceptives are co-administered with antibiotics, anticonvulsants, and other drugs that increase the metabolism of contraceptive steroids. This could result in unintended pregnancy or unscheduled bleeding. In such cases a nonhormonal back-up method of birth control should be considered).
No products indexed under this heading.

Garlic Oil (Contraceptive effectiveness may be reduced when hormonal contraceptives are co-administered with antibiotics, anticonvulsants, and other drugs that increase the metabolism of contraceptive steroids. This could result in unintended pregnancy or unscheduled bleeding. In such cases a nonhormonal back-up method of birth control should be considered).
No products indexed under this heading.

Gatifloxacin (Contraceptive effectiveness may be reduced when hormonal contraceptives are co-administered with antibiotics, anticonvulsants, and other drugs that increase the metabolism of contraceptive steroids. This could result in unintended pregnancy or unscheduled bleeding. In such cases a nonhormonal back-up method of birth control should be considered).
No products indexed under this heading.

Gemifloxacin Mesylate (Contraceptive effectiveness may be reduced when hormonal contraceptives are co-administered with antibiotics, anticonvulsants, and other drugs that increase the metabolism of contraceptive steroids. This could result in unintended pregnancy or unscheduled bleeding. In such cases a nonhormonal back-up method of birth control should be considered).
No products indexed under this heading.

Gentamicin Sulfate (Contraceptive effectiveness may be reduced when hormonal contraceptives are co-administered with antibiotics, anticonvulsants, and other drugs that increase the metabolism of contraceptive steroids. This could result in unintended pregnancy or unscheduled bleeding. In such cases a nonhormonal back-up method of birth control should be considered). Products include:
Pred-G .... ⊙ **226**, ⊙ **227**

Glimepiride (Contraceptive effectiveness may be reduced when hormonal contraceptives are co-administered with antibiotics, anticonvulsants, and other drugs that increase the metabolism of contraceptive steroids. This could result in unintended pregnancy or unscheduled bleeding. In such cases a nonhormonal back-up method of birth control should be considered). Products include:
Avandaryl **1356**
Duetact **3354**

Glipizide (Contraceptive effectiveness may be reduced when hormonal contraceptives are co-administered with antibiotics, anticonvulsants, and other drugs that increase the metabolism of contraceptive steroids. This could result in unintended pregnancy or unscheduled bleeding. In such cases a nonhormonal back-up method of birth control should be considered).
No products indexed under this heading.

Glyburide (Contraceptive effectiveness may be reduced when hormonal contraceptives are co-administered with antibiotics, anticonvulsants, and other drugs that increase the metabolism of contraceptive steroids. This could result in unintended pregnancy or unscheduled bleeding. In such cases a nonhormonal back-up method of birth control should be considered).
No products indexed under this heading.

Glycopyrrolate (Enterohepatic recirculation of estrogens may also be decreased by substances that reduce gut transit time).
No products indexed under this heading.

Grepafloxacin Hydrochloride (Contraceptive effectiveness may be reduced when hormonal contraceptives are co-administered with antibiotics, anticonvulsants, and other drugs that increase the metabolism of contraceptive steroids. This could result in unintended pregnancy or unscheduled bleeding. In such cases a nonhormonal back-up method of birth control should be considered).
No products indexed under this heading.

Griseofulvin (Contraceptive effectiveness may be reduced when hormonal contraceptives are co-administered with antibiotics, anticonvulsants, and other drugs that increase the metabolism of contraceptive steroids. This could result in unintended pregnancy or unscheduled bleeding. In such cases a nonhormonal back-up method of birth control should be considered).
No products indexed under this heading.

Haloperidol (Contraceptive effectiveness may be reduced when hormonal contraceptives are co-administered with antibiotics, anticonvulsants, and other drugs that increase the metabolism of contraceptive steroids. This could result in unintended pregnancy or unscheduled bleeding. In such cases a nonhormonal back-up method of birth control should be considered).
No products indexed under this heading.

Haloperidol Decanoate (Contraceptive effectiveness may be reduced when hormonal contraceptives are co-administered with antibiotics, anticonvulsants, and other drugs that increase the metabolism of contraceptive steroids. This could result in unintended pregnancy or unscheduled bleeding. In such cases a nonhormonal back-up method of birth control should be considered).
No products indexed under this heading.

Haloperidol Lactate (Contraceptive effectiveness may be reduced when hormonal contraceptives are co-administered with antibiotics, anticonvulsants, and other drugs that increase the metabolism of contraceptive steroids. This could result in unintended pregnancy or unscheduled bleeding. In such cases a nonhormonal back-up method of birth control should be considered).
No products indexed under this heading.

Hexobarbital (Contraceptive effectiveness may be reduced when hormonal contraceptives are co-administered with antibiotics, anticonvulsants, and other drugs that increase the metabolism of contraceptive steroids. This could result in unintended pregnancy or unscheduled bleeding. In such cases a nonhormonal back-up method of birth control should be considered).
No products indexed under this heading.

Hydrocodone Bitartrate (Contraceptive effectiveness may be reduced when hormonal contraceptives are co-administered with antibiotics, anticonvulsants, and other drugs that increase the metabolism of contraceptive steroids. This could result in unintended pregnancy or unscheduled bleeding. In such cases a nonhormonal back-up method of birth control should be considered). Products include:
Vicodin **560**
Vicodin ES **561**
Vicodin HP **563**
Vicoprofen **564**
Zydone **1138**

Hydrocodone Polistirex (Enterohepatic recirculation of estrogens may also be decreased by substances that reduce gut transit time). Products include:
Tussionex **3443**

Hydrocortisone (Contraceptive effectiveness may be reduced when hormonal contraceptives are co-administered with antibiotics, anticonvulsants, and other drugs that increase the metabolism of contraceptive steroids. This could result in unintended pregnancy or unscheduled bleeding. In such cases a nonhormonal back-up method of birth control should be considered).
No products indexed under this heading.

Hydrocortisone (Alcohol) (Contraceptive effectiveness may be reduced when hormonal contraceptives are co-administered with antibiotics, anticonvulsants, and other drugs that increase the metabolism of contraceptive steroids. This could result in unintended pregnancy or unscheduled bleeding. In such cases a nonhormonal back-up method of birth control should be considered).
No products indexed under this heading.

Hydrocortisone Acetate (Contraceptive effectiveness may be reduced when hormonal contraceptives are co-administered with antibiotics, anticonvulsants, and other drugs that increase the metabolism of contraceptive steroids. This could result in unintended pregnancy or unscheduled bleeding. In such cases a nonhormonal back-up method of birth control should be considered).
No products indexed under this heading.

Hydrocortisone Butyrate (Contraceptive effectiveness may be reduced when hormonal contraceptives are co-administered with antibiotics, anticonvulsants, and other drugs that increase the metabolism of contraceptive steroids. This could result in unintended pregnancy or unscheduled bleeding. In such cases a nonhormonal back-up method of birth control should be considered).
No products indexed under this heading.

Hydrocortisone Cypionate (Contraceptive effectiveness may be reduced when hormonal contraceptives are co-administered with antibiotics, anticonvulsants, and other drugs that increase the metabolism of contraceptive steroids. This could result in unintended pregnancy or unscheduled bleeding. In such cases a nonhormonal back-up method of birth control should be considered).
No products indexed under this heading.

Hydrocortisone Hemisuccinate (Contraceptive effectiveness may be reduced when hormonal contraceptives are co-administered with antibiotics, anticonvulsants, and other drugs that increase the metabolism of contraceptive steroids. This could result in unintended pregnancy or unscheduled bleeding. In such cases a nonhormonal back-up method of birth control should be considered).
No products indexed under this heading.

Hydrocortisone Probutate (Contraceptive effectiveness may be reduced when hormonal contraceptives are co-administered with antibiotics, anticonvulsants, and other drugs that increase the metabolism of contraceptive steroids. This could result in unintended pregnancy or unscheduled bleeding. In such cases a nonhormonal back-up method of birth control should be considered).
No products indexed under this heading.

Hydrocortisone Sodium Phosphate (Contraceptive effectiveness may be reduced when hormonal contraceptives are co-administered with antibiotics, anticonvulsants, and other drugs that increase the metabolism of contraceptive steroids. This could result in unintended pregnancy or unscheduled bleeding. In such cases a nonhormonal back-up method of birth control should be considered).
No products indexed under this heading.

Hydrocortisone Sodium Succinate (Contraceptive effectiveness may be reduced when hormonal contraceptives are co-administered with antibiotics, anticonvulsants, and other drugs that increase the metabolism of contraceptive steroids. This could result in unintended pregnancy or unscheduled bleeding. In such cases a nonhormonal back-up method of birth control should be considered).
No products indexed under this heading.

Hydrocortisone Valerate (Contraceptive effectiveness may be reduced when hormonal contraceptives are co-administered with antibiotics, anticonvulsants, and other drugs that increase the metabolism of contraceptive steroids. This could result in unintended pregnancy or unscheduled bleeding. In such cases a nonhormonal back-up method of birth control should be considered).
No products indexed under this heading.

Hydromorphone (Enterohepatic recirculation of estrogens may also be decreased by substances that reduce gut transit time).
No products indexed under this heading.

Hydromorphone Hydrochloride (Enterohepatic recirculation of estrogens may also be decreased by substances that reduce gut transit time). Products include:
Dilaudid Injection **2800**
Dilaudid Oral **2797**
Dilaudid Tablets **2797**
Dilaudid-HP **2800**

Hyoscyamine (Enterohepatic recirculation of estrogens may also be decreased by substances that reduce gut transit time).
No products indexed under this heading.

Hyoscyamine Sulfate (Enterohepatic recirculation of estrogens may also be decreased by substances that reduce gut transit time). Products include:
Donnatal **2711**

Hypericum (Contraceptive effectiveness may be reduced when hormonal contraceptives are co-administered with antibiotics, anticonvulsants, and other drugs that increase the metabolism of contraceptive steroids. This could result in unintended pregnancy or unscheduled bleeding. In such cases a nonhormonal back-up method of birth control should be considered).
No products indexed under this heading.

Hypericum Perforatum (Contraceptive effectiveness may be reduced when hormonal contraceptives are co-administered with antibiotics, anticonvulsants, and other drugs that increase the metabolism of contraceptive steroids. This could result in unintended pregnancy or unscheduled bleeding. In such cases a nonhormonal back-up method of birth control should be considered). Products include:
Traumeel **1800**

Ibuprofen (Contraceptive effectiveness may be reduced when hormonal contraceptives are co-administered with antibiotics, anticonvulsants, and other drugs that increase the metabolism of contraceptive steroids. This could result in unintended pregnancy or unscheduled bleeding. In such cases a nonhor-

monal back-up method of birth control should be considered). Products include:

Idarubicin Hydrochloride (Contraceptive effectiveness may be reduced when hormonal contraceptives are co-administered with antibiotics, anticonvulsants, and other drugs that increase the metabolism of contraceptive steroids. This could result in unintended pregnancy or unscheduled bleeding. In such cases a nonhormonal back-up method of birth control should be considered).

No products indexed under this heading.

Imatinib Mesylate (CYP 3A4 inhibitors such as indinavir, itraconazole, ketoconazole, fluconazole, and troleandomycin may increase plasma hormone levels). Products include:

Imipenem (Contraceptive effectiveness may be reduced when hormonal contraceptives are co-administered with antibiotics, anticonvulsants, and other drugs that increase the metabolism of contraceptive steroids. This could result in unintended pregnancy or unscheduled bleeding. In such cases a nonhormonal back-up method of birth control should be considered). Products include:

Imipramine Hydrochloride (Contraceptive effectiveness may be reduced when hormonal contraceptives are co-administered with antibiotics, anticonvulsants, and other drugs that increase the metabolism of contraceptive steroids. This could result in unintended pregnancy or unscheduled bleeding. In such cases a nonhormonal back-up method of birth control should be considered).

No products indexed under this heading.

Imipramine Pamoate (Contraceptive effectiveness may be reduced when hormonal contraceptives are co-administered with antibiotics, anticonvulsants, and other drugs that increase the metabolism of contraceptive steroids. This could result in unintended pregnancy or unscheduled bleeding. In such cases a nonhormonal back-up method of birth control should be considered).

No products indexed under this heading.

Indinavir Sulfate (Contraceptive effectiveness may be reduced when hormonal contraceptives are co-administered with antibiotics, anticonvulsants, and other drugs that increase the metabolism of contraceptive steroids. This could result in unintended pregnancy or unscheduled bleeding. In such cases a nonhormonal back-up method of birth control should be considered). Products include:

Indomethacin (Contraceptive effectiveness may be reduced when hormonal contraceptives are co-administered with antibiotics, anticonvulsants, and other drugs that increase the metabolism of contraceptive steroids. This could result in unintended pregnancy or unscheduled bleeding. In such cases a nonhormonal back-up method of birth control should be considered). Products include:

Indomethacin Sodium Trihydrate (Contraceptive effectiveness may be reduced when hormonal contraceptives are co-administered with antibiotics, anticonvulsants, and other drugs that increase the metabolism of contraceptive steroids. This could result in unintended pregnancy or unscheduled bleeding. In such cases a nonhormonal back-up method of birth control should be considered). Products include:

Indoramin Hydrochloride (Contraceptive effectiveness may be reduced when hormonal contraceptives are co-administered with antibiotics, anticonvulsants, and other drugs that increase the metabolism of contraceptive steroids. This could result in unintended pregnancy or unscheduled bleeding. In such cases a nonhormonal back-up method of birth control should be considered).

No products indexed under this heading.

Ipratropium Bromide (Enterohepatic recirculation of estrogens may also be decreased by substances that reduce gut transit time).

No products indexed under this heading.

Irbesartan (Contraceptive effectiveness may be reduced when hormonal contraceptives are co-administered with antibiotics, anticonvulsants, and other drugs that increase the metabolism of contraceptive steroids. This could result in unintended pregnancy or unscheduled bleeding. In such cases a nonhormonal back-up method of birth control should be considered). Products include:

Isoetharine (Enterohepatic recirculation of estrogens may also be decreased by substances that reduce gut transit time).

No products indexed under this heading.

Isoniazid (CYP 3A4 inhibitors such as indinavir, itraconazole, ketoconazole, fluconazole, and troleandomycin may increase plasma hormone levels).

No products indexed under this heading.

Isoproterenol Hydrochloride (Enterohepatic recirculation of estrogens may also be decreased by substances that reduce gut transit time).

No products indexed under this heading.

Isoproterenol Sulfate (Enterohepatic recirculation of estrogens may also be decreased by substances that reduce gut transit time).

No products indexed under this heading.

Isotretinoin (Contraceptive effectiveness may be reduced when hormonal contraceptives are co-administered with antibiotics, anticonvulsants, and other drugs that increase the metabolism of contraceptive steroids. This could result in unintended pregnancy or unscheduled bleeding. In such cases a nonhormonal back-up method of birth control should be considered). Products include:

Isradipine (Contraceptive effectiveness may be reduced when hormonal contraceptives are co-administered with antibiotics, anticonvulsants, and other drugs that increase the metabolism of contraceptive steroids. This could result in unintended pregnancy or unscheduled bleeding. In such cases a nonhormonal back-up method of birth control should be considered). Products include:

Itraconazole (Contraceptive effectiveness may be reduced when hormonal contraceptives are co-administered with antibiotics, anticonvulsants, and other drugs that increase the metabolism of contraceptive steroids. This could result in unintended pregnancy or unscheduled bleeding. In such cases a nonhormonal back-up method of birth control should be considered).

No products indexed under this heading.

Ixabepilone (Contraceptive effectiveness may be reduced when hormonal contraceptives are co-administered with antibiotics, anticonvulsants, and other drugs that increase the metabolism of contraceptive steroids. This could result in unintended pregnancy or unscheduled bleeding. In such cases a nonhormonal back-up method of birth control should be considered).

No products indexed under this heading.

Kanamycin Sulfate (Contraceptive effectiveness may be reduced when hormonal contraceptives are co-administered with antibiotics, anticonvulsants, and other drugs that increase the metabolism of contraceptive steroids. This could result in unintended pregnancy or unscheduled bleeding. In such cases a nonhormonal back-up method of birth control should be considered).

No products indexed under this heading.

Ketoconazole (Contraceptive effectiveness may be reduced when hormonal contraceptives are co-administered with antibiotics, anticonvulsants, and other drugs that increase the metabolism of contraceptive steroids. This could result in unintended pregnancy or unscheduled bleeding. In such cases a nonhormonal back-up method of birth control should be considered). Products include:

Ketoprofen (Contraceptive effectiveness may be reduced when hormonal contraceptives are co-administered with antibiotics, anticonvulsants, and other drugs that increase the metabolism of contraceptive steroids. This could result in unintended pregnancy or unscheduled bleeding. In such cases a nonhormonal back-up method of birth control should be considered).

No products indexed under this heading.

Ketorolac Tromethamine (Contraceptive effectiveness may be reduced when hormonal contraceptives are co-administered with antibiotics, anticonvulsants, and other drugs that increase the metabolism of contraceptive steroids. This could result in unintended pregnancy or unscheduled bleeding. In such cases a nonhormonal back-up method of birth control should be considered). Products include:

Labetalol Hydrochloride (Contraceptive effectiveness may be reduced when hormonal contraceptives are co-administered with antibiotics, anticonvulsants, and other drugs that increase the metabolism of contraceptive steroids. This could result in unintended pregnancy or unscheduled bleeding. In such cases a nonhormonal back-up method of birth control should be considered).

No products indexed under this heading.

Lamotrigine (Decreased plasma concentrations of lamotrigine due to induction of conjugation (particularly glucuronidation), have been noted when this drug is administered with oral contraceptives). Products include:

Lansoprazole (Contraceptive effectiveness may be reduced when hormonal contraceptives are co-administered with antibiotics, anticonvulsants, and other drugs that increase the metabolism of contraceptive steroids. This could result in unintended pregnancy or unscheduled bleeding. In such cases a nonhormonal back-up method of birth control should be considered).

No products indexed under this heading.

Lapatinib (CYP 3A4 inhibitors such as indinavir, itraconazole, ketoconazole, fluconazole, and troleandomycin may increase plasma hormone levels). Products include:

Levalbuterol Hydrochloride (Enterohepatic recirculation of estrogens may also be decreased by substances that reduce gut transit time).

No products indexed under this heading.

Levetiracetam (Contraceptive effectiveness may be reduced when hormonal contraceptives are co-administered with antibiotics, anticonvulsants, and other drugs that increase the metabolism of contraceptive steroids. This could result in unintended pregnancy or unscheduled bleeding. In such cases a nonhormonal back-up method of birth control should be considered). Products include:

Levobupivacaine Hydrochloride (Contraceptive effectiveness may be reduced when hormonal contraceptives are co-administered with antibiotics, anticonvulsants, and other drugs that increase the metabolism of contraceptive steroids. This could result in unintended pregnancy or unscheduled bleeding. In such cases a nonhormonal back-up method of birth control should be considered).

No products indexed under this heading.

Levofloxacin (Contraceptive effectiveness may be reduced when hormonal contraceptives are co-administered with antibiotics, anticonvulsants, and other drugs that increase the metabolism of contraceptive steroids. This could result in unintended pregnancy or unscheduled bleeding. In such cases a nonhormonal back-up method of birth control should be considered). Products include:

Levorphanol Tartrate (Enterohepatic recirculation of estrogens may also be decreased by substances that reduce gut transit time).

No products indexed under this heading.

Lidocaine (Contraceptive effectiveness may be reduced when hormonal contraceptives are co-administered with antibiotics, anticonvulsants, and other drugs that increase the metabolism of contraceptive steroids. This could result in unintended pregnancy or unscheduled bleeding. In such cases a nonhormonal back-up method of birth control should be considered). Products include:

Lidocaine Base (Contraceptive effectiveness may be reduced when hormonal contraceptives are co-administered with antibiotics, anticonvulsants, and other drugs that increase the metabolism of contraceptive steroids. This could result in unintended pregnancy or unscheduled bleeding. In such cases a nonhormonal back-up method of birth control should be considered).

No products indexed under this heading.

Lidocaine Hydrochloride (Contraceptive effectiveness may be reduced when hormonal contraceptives are co-administered with antibiotics, anticonvulsants, and other drugs that increase the metabolism of contraceptive steroids. This could result in unintended pregnancy or unscheduled bleeding. In such cases a nonhormonal back-up method of birth control should be considered).
No products indexed under this heading.

Lomefloxacin Hydrochloride (Contraceptive effectiveness may be reduced when hormonal contraceptives are co-administered with antibiotics, anticonvulsants, and other drugs that increase the metabolism of contraceptive steroids. This could result in unintended pregnancy or unscheduled bleeding. In such cases a nonhormonal back-up method of birth control should be considered).
No products indexed under this heading.

Lopinavir (Several of the anti-HIV protease inhibitors have been studied with co-administration of oral combination hormonal contraceptives; significant changes (increase and decrease) in the plasma levels of the estrogen and progestin have been noted in some cases. The safety and efficacy of oral contraceptive products may be affected with co-administration of anti-HIV protease inhibitors. Health care professionals should refer to the label of the individual anti-HIV protease inhibitors for further drug-drug interaction information). Products include:
Kaletra 458

Loracarbef (Contraceptive effectiveness may be reduced when hormonal contraceptives are co-administered with antibiotics, anticonvulsants, and other drugs that increase the metabolism of contraceptive steroids. This could result in unintended pregnancy or unscheduled bleeding. In such cases a nonhormonal back-up method of birth control should be considered).
No products indexed under this heading.

Loratadine (CYP 3A4 inhibitors such as indinavir, itraconazole, ketoconazole, fluconazole, and troleandomycin may increase plasma hormone levels).
No products indexed under this heading.

Losartan Potassium (Contraceptive effectiveness may be reduced when hormonal contraceptives are co-administered with antibiotics, anticonvulsants, and other drugs that increase the metabolism of contraceptive steroids. This could result in unintended pregnancy or unscheduled bleeding. In such cases a nonhormonal back-up method of birth control should be considered). Products include:
Cozaar 2106
Hyzaar 2162
Hyzaar 100-12.5 2162

Lovastatin (Contraceptive effectiveness may be reduced when hormonal contraceptives are co-administered with antibiotics, anticonvulsants, and other drugs that increase the metabolism of contraceptive steroids. This could result in unintended pregnancy or unscheduled bleeding. In such cases a nonhormonal back-up method of birth control should be considered). Products include:
Advicor 402
Mevacor 2212

Maprotiline Hydrochloride (Contraceptive effectiveness may be reduced when hormonal contraceptives are co-administered with antibiotics, anticonvulsants, and other drugs that increase the metabolism of contraceptive steroids. This could result in unintended pregnancy or unscheduled bleeding. In such cases a nonhormonal back-up method of birth control should be considered).
No products indexed under this heading.

Meclofenamate Sodium (Contraceptive effectiveness may be reduced when hormonal contraceptives are co-administered with antibiotics, anticonvulsants, and other drugs that increase the metabolism of contraceptive steroids. This could result in unintended pregnancy or unscheduled bleeding. In such cases a nonhormonal back-up method of birth control should be considered).
No products indexed under this heading.

Mefenamic Acid (Contraceptive effectiveness may be reduced when hormonal contraceptives are co-administered with antibiotics, anticonvulsants, and other drugs that increase the metabolism of contraceptive steroids. This could result in unintended pregnancy or unscheduled bleeding. In such cases a nonhormonal back-up method of birth control should be considered).
No products indexed under this heading.

Meloxicam (Contraceptive effectiveness may be reduced when hormonal contraceptives are co-administered with antibiotics, anticonvulsants, and other drugs that increase the metabolism of contraceptive steroids. This could result in unintended pregnancy or unscheduled bleeding. In such cases a nonhormonal back-up method of birth control should be considered).
No products indexed under this heading.

Mepenzolate Bromide (Enterohepatic recirculation of estrogens may also be decreased by substances that reduce gut transit time).
No products indexed under this heading.

Meperidine Hydrochloride (Contraceptive effectiveness may be reduced when hormonal contraceptives are co-administered with antibiotics, anticonvulsants, and other drugs that increase the metabolism of contraceptive steroids. This could result in unintended pregnancy or unscheduled bleeding. In such cases a nonhormonal back-up method of birth control should be considered).
No products indexed under this heading.

Mephenytoin (Contraceptive effectiveness may be reduced when hormonal contraceptives are co-administered with antibiotics, anticonvulsants, and other drugs that increase the metabolism of contraceptive steroids. This could result in unintended pregnancy or unscheduled bleeding. In such cases a nonhormonal back-up method of birth control should be considered).
No products indexed under this heading.

Mephobarbital (Contraceptive effectiveness may be reduced when hormonal contraceptives are co-administered with antibiotics, anticonvulsants, and other drugs that increase the metabolism of contraceptive steroids. This could result in unintended pregnancy or unscheduled bleeding. In such cases a nonhormonal back-up method of birth control should be considered).
No products indexed under this heading.

Meprobamate (Contraceptive effectiveness may be reduced when hormonal contraceptives are co-administered with antibiotics, anticonvulsants, and other drugs that increase the metabolism of contraceptive steroids. This could result in unintended pregnancy or unscheduled bleeding. In such cases a nonhormonal back-up method of birth control should be considered).
No products indexed under this heading.

Mestranol (Contraceptive effectiveness may be reduced when hormonal contraceptives are co-administered with antibiotics, anticonvulsants, and other drugs that increase the metabolism of contraceptive steroids. This could result in unintended pregnancy or unscheduled bleeding. In such cases a nonhormonal back-up method of birth control should be considered).
No products indexed under this heading.

Metaproterenol Sulfate (Enterohepatic recirculation of estrogens may also be decreased by substances that reduce gut transit time).
No products indexed under this heading.

Metformin Hydrochloride (Contraceptive effectiveness may be reduced when hormonal contraceptives are co-administered with antibiotics, anticonvulsants, and other drugs that increase the metabolism of contraceptive steroids. This could result in unintended pregnancy or unscheduled bleeding. In such cases a nonhormonal back-up method of birth control should be considered). Products include:
ActoPlus 3338
Avandamet 1345
Janumet 2188

Methacycline Hydrochloride (Contraceptive effectiveness may be reduced when hormonal contraceptives are co-administered with antibiotics, anticonvulsants, and other drugs that increase the metabolism of contraceptive steroids. This could result in unintended pregnancy or unscheduled bleeding. In such cases a nonhormonal back-up method of birth control should be considered).
No products indexed under this heading.

Methadone Hydrochloride (Contraceptive effectiveness may be reduced when hormonal contraceptives are co-administered with antibiotics, anticonvulsants, and other drugs that increase the metabolism of contraceptive steroids. This could result in unintended pregnancy or unscheduled bleeding. In such cases a nonhormonal back-up method of birth control should be considered).
No products indexed under this heading.

Methamphetamine Hydrochloride (Contraceptive effectiveness may be reduced when hormonal contraceptives are co-administered with antibiotics, anticonvulsants, and other drugs that increase the metabolism of contraceptive steroids. This could result in unintended pregnancy or unscheduled bleeding. In such cases a nonhormonal back-up method of birth control should be considered).
No products indexed under this heading.

Methdilazine Hydrochloride (Enterohepatic recirculation of estrogens may also be decreased by substances that reduce gut transit time).
No products indexed under this heading.

Methicillin Sodium (Contraceptive effectiveness may be reduced when hormonal contraceptives are co-administered with antibiotics, anticonvulsants, and other drugs that increase the metabolism of contraceptive steroids. This could result in unintended pregnancy or unscheduled bleeding. In such cases a nonhormonal back-up method of birth control should be considered).
No products indexed under this heading.

Methsuximide (Contraceptive effectiveness may be reduced when hormonal contraceptives are co-administered with antibiotics, anticonvulsants, and other drugs that increase the metabolism of contraceptive steroids. This could result in unintended pregnancy or unscheduled bleeding. In such cases a nonhormonal back-up method of birth control should be considered).
No products indexed under this heading.

Methylprednisolone (Contraceptive effectiveness may be reduced when hormonal contraceptives are co-administered with antibiotics, anticonvulsants, and other drugs that increase the metabolism of contraceptive steroids. This could result in unintended pregnancy or unscheduled bleeding. In such cases a nonhormonal back-up method of birth control should be considered).
No products indexed under this heading.

Methylprednisolone Acetate (Contraceptive effectiveness may be reduced when hormonal contraceptives are co-administered with antibiotics, anticonvulsants, and other drugs that increase the metabolism of contraceptive steroids. This could result in unintended pregnancy or unscheduled bleeding. In such cases a nonhormonal back-up method of birth control should be considered).
No products indexed under this heading.

Methylprednisolone Sodium Succinate (Contraceptive effectiveness may be reduced when hormonal contraceptives are co-administered with antibiotics, anticonvulsants, and other drugs that increase the metabolism of contraceptive steroids. This could result in unintended pregnancy or unscheduled bleeding. In such cases a nonhormonal back-up method of birth control should be considered).
No products indexed under this heading.

Metoclopramide Hydrochloride (Enterohepatic recirculation of estrogens may also be decreased by substances that reduce gut transit time). Products include:
Metozolv ODT 2901

Metoprolol Succinate (Contraceptive effectiveness may be reduced when hormonal contraceptives are co-administered with antibiotics, anticonvulsants, and other drugs that increase the metabolism of contraceptive steroids. This could result in unintended pregnancy or unscheduled bleeding. In such cases a nonhormonal back-up method of birth control should be considered). Products include:
Toprol XL 732

Metoprolol Tartrate (Contraceptive effectiveness may be reduced when hormonal contraceptives are co-administered with antibiotics, anticonvulsants, and other drugs that increase the metabolism of contraceptive steroids. This could result in unintended pregnancy or unscheduled bleeding. In such cases a nonhormonal back-up method of birth control should be considered).
No products indexed under this heading.

Metronidazole (CYP 3A4 inhibitors such as indinavir, itraconazole, keto-

1085 **Interactions Index** **Lybrel**

conazole, fluconazole, and troleandomycin may increase plasma hormone levels). Products include:
Pylera 793

Metronidazole Benzoate (CYP 3A4 inhibitors such as indinavir, itraconazole, ketoconazole, fluconazole, and troleandomycin may increase plasma hormone levels).
No products indexed under this heading.

Metronidazole Hydrochloride (CYP 3A4 inhibitors such as indinavir, itraconazole, ketoconazole, fluconazole, and troleandomycin may increase plasma hormone levels).
No products indexed under this heading.

Metronidazole Sodium (CYP 3A4 inhibitors such as indinavir, itraconazole, ketoconazole, fluconazole, and troleandomycin may increase plasma hormone levels).
No products indexed under this heading.

Mexiletine Hydrochloride (Contraceptive effectiveness may be reduced when hormonal contraceptives are co-administered with antibiotics, anticonvulsants, and other drugs that increase the metabolism of contraceptive steroids. This could result in unintended pregnancy or unscheduled bleeding. In such cases a nonhormonal back-up method of birth control should be considered).
No products indexed under this heading.

Mezlocillin Sodium (Contraceptive effectiveness may be reduced when hormonal contraceptives are co-administered with antibiotics, anticonvulsants, and other drugs that increase the metabolism of contraceptive steroids. This could result in unintended pregnancy or unscheduled bleeding. In such cases a nonhormonal back-up method of birth control should be considered).
No products indexed under this heading.

Mibefradil Dihydrochloride (Enterohepatic recirculation of estrogens may also be decreased by substances that reduce gut transit time).
No products indexed under this heading.

Miconazole (CYP 3A4 inhibitors such as indinavir, itraconazole, ketoconazole, fluconazole, and troleandomycin may increase plasma hormone levels).
No products indexed under this heading.

Miconazole Nitrate (CYP 3A4 inhibitors such as indinavir, itraconazole, ketoconazole, fluconazole, and troleandomycin may increase plasma hormone levels). Products include:
Vusion Ointment 3335

Midazolam Hydrochloride (Contraceptive effectiveness may be reduced when hormonal contraceptives are co-administered with antibiotics, anticonvulsants, and other drugs that increase the metabolism of contraceptive steroids. This could result in unintended pregnancy or unscheduled bleeding. In such cases a nonhormonal back-up method of birth control should be considered).
No products indexed under this heading.

Mifepristone (CYP 3A4 inhibitors such as indinavir, itraconazole, ketoconazole, fluconazole, and troleandomycin may increase plasma hormone levels).
No products indexed under this heading.

Miglitol (Contraceptive effectiveness may be reduced when hormonal contraceptives are co-administered with antibiotics, anticonvulsants, and other drugs that increase the metabolism of contraceptive steroids. This could result in unintended pregnancy or unscheduled bleeding. In such cases a nonhormonal back-up method of birth control should be considered).
No products indexed under this heading.

Minocycline Hydrochloride (Contraceptive effectiveness may be reduced when hormonal contraceptives are co-administered with antibiotics, anticonvulsants, and other drugs that increase the metabolism of contraceptive steroids. This could result in unintended pregnancy or unscheduled bleeding. In such cases a nonhormonal back-up method of birth control should be considered). Products include:
Solodyn 2073

Mirtazapine (Contraceptive effectiveness may be reduced when hormonal contraceptives are co-administered with antibiotics, anticonvulsants, and other drugs that increase the metabolism of contraceptive steroids. This could result in unintended pregnancy or unscheduled bleeding. In such cases a nonhormonal back-up method of birth control should be considered). Products include:
Remeron Tablets 3214
RemeronSolTab Tablets 3219

Modafinil (Contraceptive effectiveness may be reduced when hormonal contraceptives are co-administered with antibiotics, anticonvulsants, and other drugs that increase the metabolism of contraceptive steroids. This could result in unintended pregnancy or unscheduled bleeding. In such cases a nonhormonal back-up method of birth control should be considered). Products include:
Provigil 983

Mometasone Furoate (Increased plasma concentrations of cyclosporine, prednisolone and other corticosteroids, have been reported with concomitant administration of oral contraceptives). Products include:
Asmanex 3058
Elocon Cream 3111
Elocon Lotion 3112
Elocon Ointment 3114

Mometasone Furoate Monohydrate (Increased plasma concentrations of cyclosporine, prednisolone and other corticosteroids, have been reported with concomitant administration of oral contraceptives). Products include:
Nasonex 3166

Montelukast Sodium (Contraceptive effectiveness may be reduced when hormonal contraceptives are co-administered with antibiotics, anticonvulsants, and other drugs that increase the metabolism of contraceptive steroids. This could result in unintended pregnancy or unscheduled bleeding. In such cases a nonhormonal back-up method of birth control should be considered). Products include:
Singulair 2270

Morphine Sulfate (Increased clearance of morphine, due to induction of conjugation (particularly glucuronidation), have been noted when this drug is administered with oral contraceptives). Products include:
Avinza 1822
Embeda 1831
MS Contin 2803

Morphine Sulfate, Liposomal (Increased clearance of morphine, due to induction of conjugation (particularly glucuronidation), have been noted when this drug is administered with oral contraceptives).
No products indexed under this heading.

Moxifloxacin Hydrochloride (Contraceptive effectiveness may be reduced when hormonal contraceptives are co-administered with antibiotics, anticonvulsants, and other drugs that increase the metabolism of contraceptive steroids. This could result in unintended pregnancy or unscheduled bleeding. In such cases a nonhormonal back-up method of birth control should be considered). Products include:
Avelox 3064
Vigamox 589

Nabumetone (Contraceptive effectiveness may be reduced when hormonal contraceptives are co-administered with antibiotics, anticonvulsants, and other drugs that increase the metabolism of contraceptive steroids. This could result in unintended pregnancy or unscheduled bleeding. In such cases a nonhormonal back-up method of birth control should be considered).
No products indexed under this heading.

Nafcillin Sodium (Contraceptive effectiveness may be reduced when hormonal contraceptives are co-administered with antibiotics, anticonvulsants, and other drugs that increase the metabolism of contraceptive steroids. This could result in unintended pregnancy or unscheduled bleeding. In such cases a nonhormonal back-up method of birth control should be considered).
No products indexed under this heading.

Naproxen (Contraceptive effectiveness may be reduced when hormonal contraceptives are co-administered with antibiotics, anticonvulsants, and other drugs that increase the metabolism of contraceptive steroids. This could result in unintended pregnancy or unscheduled bleeding. In such cases a nonhormonal back-up method of birth control should be considered). Products include:
EC-Naprosyn 2850
Naprosyn 2850
Anaprox/Naprosyn 2850

Naproxen Sodium (Contraceptive effectiveness may be reduced when hormonal contraceptives are co-administered with antibiotics, anticonvulsants, and other drugs that increase the metabolism of contraceptive steroids. This could result in unintended pregnancy or unscheduled bleeding. In such cases a nonhormonal back-up method of birth control should be considered). Products include:
Anaprox 2850
Anaprox DS 2850
Treximet 1681

Nateglinide (Contraceptive effectiveness may be reduced when hormonal contraceptives are co-administered with antibiotics, anticonvulsants, and other drugs that increase the metabolism of contraceptive steroids. This could result in unintended pregnancy or unscheduled bleeding. In such cases a nonhormonal back-up method of birth control should be considered).
No products indexed under this heading.

Nefazodone Hydrochloride (Contraceptive effectiveness may be reduced when hormonal contraceptives are co-administered with antibiotics, anticonvulsants, and other drugs that increase the metabolism of contraceptive steroids. This could result in unintended pregnancy or unscheduled bleeding. In such cases a nonhormonal back-up method of birth control should be considered).
No products indexed under this heading.

Nelfinavir Mesylate (Contraceptive effectiveness may be reduced when hormonal contraceptives are co-administered with antibiotics, anticonvulsants, and other drugs that increase the metabolism of contraceptive steroids. This could result in unintended pregnancy or unscheduled bleeding. In such cases a nonhormonal back-up method of birth control should be considered).
No products indexed under this heading.

Neostigmine Bromide (Enterohepatic recirculation of estrogens may also be decreased by substances that reduce gut transit time).
No products indexed under this heading.

Neostigmine Methylsulfate (Enterohepatic recirculation of estrogens may also be decreased by substances that reduce gut transit time).
No products indexed under this heading.

Nevirapine (Contraceptive effectiveness may be reduced when hormonal contraceptives are co-administered with antibiotics, anticonvulsants, and other drugs that increase the metabolism of contraceptive steroids. This could result in unintended pregnancy or unscheduled bleeding. In such cases a nonhormonal back-up method of birth control should be considered). Products include:
Viramune Oral Suspension 897
Viramune Tablets 897

Niacin (CYP 3A4 inhibitors such as indinavir, itraconazole, ketoconazole, fluconazole, and troleandomycin may increase plasma hormone levels). Products include:
Advicor 402
Cardio Basics 3455
Niaspan 497
Simcor 524

Niacinamide (CYP 3A4 inhibitors such as indinavir, itraconazole, ketoconazole, fluconazole, and troleandomycin may increase plasma hormone levels). Products include:
CitraNatal 90 DHA Capsules 2332
CitraNatal Assure 2332
CitraNatal Rx 2332
Heplive 607

Niacinamide Hydroiodide (CYP 3A4 inhibitors such as indinavir, itraconazole, ketoconazole, fluconazole, and troleandomycin may increase plasma hormone levels).
No products indexed under this heading.

Nicardipine (Contraceptive effectiveness may be reduced when hormonal contraceptives are co-administered with antibiotics, anticonvulsants, and other drugs that increase the metabolism of contraceptive steroids. This could result in unintended pregnancy or unscheduled bleeding. In such cases a nonhormonal back-up method of birth control should be considered).
No products indexed under this heading.

Nicardipine Hydrochloride (Contraceptive effectiveness may be reduced when hormonal contraceptives are co-administered with antibiotics, anticonvulsants, and other drugs that increase the metabolism of contraceptive steroids. This could result in unintended pregnancy or unscheduled bleeding. In such cases a nonhormonal back-up method of birth control should be considered).
No products indexed under this heading.

Nicotinamide (CYP 3A4 inhibitors such as indinavir, itraconazole, ketoconazole, fluconazole, and troleandomycin may increase plasma hormone levels).
No products indexed under this heading.

Nicotine Polacrilex (Contraceptive effectiveness may be reduced when hormonal contraceptives are co-administered with antibiotics, anticonvulsants, and other drugs that increase the metabolism of contraceptive steroids. This could result in unintended pregnancy or unscheduled bleeding. In such cases a nonhormonal back-up method of birth control should be considered).
No products indexed under this heading.

IMPORTANT NOTE: Always consult each drug listing in the patient's regimen for possible interactions.

Lybrel Interactions Index 1086

Nicotine Salicylate (Contraceptive effectiveness may be reduced when hormonal contraceptives are co-administered with antibiotics, anticonvulsants, and other drugs that increase the metabolism of contraceptive steroids. This could result in unintended pregnancy or unscheduled bleeding. In such cases a nonhormonal back-up method of birth control should be considered).
No products indexed under this heading.

Nicotine Sulfate (Contraceptive effectiveness may be reduced when hormonal contraceptives are co-administered with antibiotics, anticonvulsants, and other drugs that increase the metabolism of contraceptive steroids. This could result in unintended pregnancy or unscheduled bleeding. In such cases a nonhormonal back-up method of birth control should be considered).
No products indexed under this heading.

Nifedipine (Contraceptive effectiveness may be reduced when hormonal contraceptives are co-administered with antibiotics, anticonvulsants, and other drugs that increase the metabolism of contraceptive steroids. This could result in unintended pregnancy or unscheduled bleeding. In such cases a nonhormonal back-up method of birth control should be considered).
No products indexed under this heading.

Nilutamide (Contraceptive effectiveness may be reduced when hormonal contraceptives are co-administered with antibiotics, anticonvulsants, and other drugs that increase the metabolism of contraceptive steroids. This could result in unintended pregnancy or unscheduled bleeding. In such cases a nonhormonal back-up method of birth control should be considered).
No products indexed under this heading.

Nimodipine (Contraceptive effectiveness may be reduced when hormonal contraceptives are co-administered with antibiotics, anticonvulsants, and other drugs that increase the metabolism of contraceptive steroids. This could result in unintended pregnancy or unscheduled bleeding. In such cases a nonhormonal back-up method of birth control should be considered).
No products indexed under this heading.

Nisoldipine (Contraceptive effectiveness may be reduced when hormonal contraceptives are co-administered with antibiotics, anticonvulsants, and other drugs that increase the metabolism of contraceptive steroids. This could result in unintended pregnancy or unscheduled bleeding. In such cases a nonhormonal back-up method of birth control should be considered).
No products indexed under this heading.

Nitrendipine (Contraceptive effectiveness may be reduced when hormonal contraceptives are co-administered with antibiotics, anticonvulsants, and other drugs that increase the metabolism of contraceptive steroids. This could result in unintended pregnancy or unscheduled bleeding. In such cases a nonhormonal back-up method of birth control should be considered).
No products indexed under this heading.

Norethindrone (Contraceptive effectiveness may be reduced when hormonal contraceptives are co-administered with antibiotics, anticonvulsants, and other drugs that increase the metabolism of contraceptive steroids. This could result in unintended pregnancy or unscheduled bleeding. In such cases a nonhormonal back-up method of birth control should be considered). Products include:
Ortho Micronor **2660**

Norethindrone Acetate (Contraceptive effectiveness may be reduced when hormonal contraceptives are co-administered with antibiotics, anticonvulsants, and other drugs that increase the metabolism of contraceptive steroids. This could result in unintended pregnancy or unscheduled bleeding. In such cases a nonhormonal back-up method of birth control should be considered). Products include:
Activella **2561**

Norfloxacin (Contraceptive effectiveness may be reduced when hormonal contraceptives are co-administered with antibiotics, anticonvulsants, and other drugs that increase the metabolism of contraceptive steroids. This could result in unintended pregnancy or unscheduled bleeding. In such cases a nonhormonal back-up method of birth control should be considered). Products include:
Noroxin **2220**

Norgestrel (Contraceptive effectiveness may be reduced when hormonal contraceptives are co-administered with antibiotics, anticonvulsants, and other drugs that increase the metabolism of contraceptive steroids. This could result in unintended pregnancy or unscheduled bleeding. In such cases a nonhormonal back-up method of birth control should be considered).
No products indexed under this heading.

Nortriptyline Hydrochloride (Contraceptive effectiveness may be reduced when hormonal contraceptives are co-administered with antibiotics, anticonvulsants, and other drugs that increase the metabolism of contraceptive steroids. This could result in unintended pregnancy or unscheduled bleeding. In such cases a nonhormonal back-up method of birth control should be considered).
No products indexed under this heading.

Octreotide Acetate (Enterohepatic recirculation of estrogens may also be decreased by substances that reduce gut transit time). Products include:
Sandostatin **2517**
Sandostatin LAR **2519**

Ofloxacin (Contraceptive effectiveness may be reduced when hormonal contraceptives are co-administered with antibiotics, anticonvulsants, and other drugs that increase the metabolism of contraceptive steroids. This could result in unintended pregnancy or unscheduled bleeding. In such cases a nonhormonal back-up method of birth control should be considered).
No products indexed under this heading.

Olanzapine (Contraceptive effectiveness may be reduced when hormonal contraceptives are co-administered with antibiotics, anticonvulsants, and other drugs that increase the metabolism of contraceptive steroids. This could result in unintended pregnancy or unscheduled bleeding. In such cases a nonhormonal back-up method of birth control should be considered). Products include:
Symbyax **1965**
Zyprexa **1984**
Zyprexa IntraMuscular **1984**
Zyprexa ZYDIS **1984**

Omeprazole (Contraceptive effectiveness may be reduced when hormonal contraceptives are co-administered with antibiotics, anticonvulsants, and other drugs that increase the metabolism of contraceptive steroids. This could result in unintended pregnancy or unscheduled bleeding. In such cases a nonhormonal back-up method of birth control should be considered).
No products indexed under this heading.

Omeprazole Magnesium (Contraceptive effectiveness may be reduced when hormonal contraceptives are co-administered with antibiotics, anticonvulsants, and other drugs that increase the metabolism of contraceptive steroids. This could result in unintended pregnancy or unscheduled bleeding. In such cases a nonhormonal back-up method of birth control should be considered).
No products indexed under this heading.

Ondansetron (Contraceptive effectiveness may be reduced when hormonal contraceptives are co-administered with antibiotics, anticonvulsants, and other drugs that increase the metabolism of contraceptive steroids. This could result in unintended pregnancy or unscheduled bleeding. In such cases a nonhormonal back-up method of birth control should be considered).
No products indexed under this heading.

Ondansetron Hydrochloride (Contraceptive effectiveness may be reduced when hormonal contraceptives are co-administered with antibiotics, anticonvulsants, and other drugs that increase the metabolism of contraceptive steroids. This could result in unintended pregnancy or unscheduled bleeding. In such cases a nonhormonal back-up method of birth control should be considered). Products include:
Zofran Injection **1750**
Zofran **1756**
Zofran ODT **1756**

Oxacillin (Contraceptive effectiveness may be reduced when hormonal contraceptives are co-administered with antibiotics, anticonvulsants, and other drugs that increase the metabolism of contraceptive steroids. This could result in unintended pregnancy or unscheduled bleeding. In such cases a nonhormonal back-up method of birth control should be considered).
No products indexed under this heading.

Oxacillin Sodium (Contraceptive effectiveness may be reduced when hormonal contraceptives are co-administered with antibiotics, anticonvulsants, and other drugs that increase the metabolism of contraceptive steroids. This could result in unintended pregnancy or unscheduled bleeding. In such cases a nonhormonal back-up method of birth control should be considered).
No products indexed under this heading.

Oxaprozin (Contraceptive effectiveness may be reduced when hormonal contraceptives are co-administered with antibiotics, anticonvulsants, and other drugs that increase the metabolism of contraceptive steroids. This could result in unintended pregnancy or unscheduled bleeding. In such cases a nonhormonal back-up method of birth control should be considered).
No products indexed under this heading.

Oxcarbazepine (Contraceptive effectiveness may be reduced when hormonal contraceptives are co-administered with antibiotics, anticonvulsants, and other drugs that increase the metabolism of contraceptive steroids. This could result in unintended pregnancy or unscheduled bleeding. In such cases a nonhormonal back-up method of birth control should be considered).
No products indexed under this heading.

Oxybutynin Chloride (Enterohepatic recirculation of estrogens may also be decreased by substances that reduce gut transit time).
No products indexed under this heading.

Oxycodone Hydrochloride (Contraceptive effectiveness may be reduced when hormonal contraceptives are co-administered with antibiotics, anticonvulsants, and other drugs that increase the metabolism of contraceptive steroids. This could result in unintended pregnancy or unscheduled bleeding. In such cases a nonhormonal back-up method of birth control should be considered). Products include:
OxyContin **2807**
Percocet **1121**
Percodan **1124**

Oxycodone Terephthalate (Enterohepatic recirculation of estrogens may also be decreased by substances that reduce gut transit time).
No products indexed under this heading.

Oxymorphone Hydrochloride (Enterohepatic recirculation of estrogens may also be decreased by substances that reduce gut transit time). Products include:
Opana **1110**
Opana ER **1114**

Oxyphenonium Bromide (Enterohepatic recirculation of estrogens may also be decreased by substances that reduce gut transit time).
No products indexed under this heading.

Oxytetracycline (Several cases of contraceptive failure and unscheduled bleeding have been reported in the literature with concomitant administration of antibiotics such as ampicillin and other penicillins, and tetracyclines. However, clinical pharmacology studies investigating drug interactions between combined oral contraceptives and these antibiotics have reported inconsistent results).
No products indexed under this heading.

Oxytetracycline Hydrochloride (Contraceptive effectiveness may be reduced when hormonal contraceptives are co-administered with antibiotics, anticonvulsants, and other drugs that increase the metabolism of contraceptive steroids. This could result in unintended pregnancy or unscheduled bleeding. In such cases a nonhormonal back-up method of birth control should be considered).
No products indexed under this heading.

Paclitaxel (Contraceptive effectiveness may be reduced when hormonal contraceptives are co-administered with antibiotics, anticonvulsants, and other drugs that increase the metabolism of contraceptive steroids. This could result in unintended pregnancy or unscheduled bleeding. In such cases a nonhormonal back-up method of birth control should be considered).
No products indexed under this heading.

Pantoprazole Sodium (Contraceptive effectiveness may be reduced when hormonal contraceptives are co-administered with antibiotics, anticonvulsants, and other drugs that increase the metabolism of contraceptive steroids. This could result in unintended pregnancy or unscheduled bleeding. In such cases a nonhormonal back-up method of birth control should be considered). Products include:
Protonix Tablets **3571**
Protonix **3575**

Paramethadione (Contraceptive effectiveness may be reduced when hormonal contraceptives are co-administered with antibiotics, anticonvulsants, and other drugs that increase the metabolism of contraceptive steroids. This could result in unintended pregnancy or unscheduled bleeding. In such cases a nonhormonal back-up method of birth control should be considered).
No products indexed under this heading.

Paroxetine Hydrochloride (Contraceptive effectiveness may be reduced when hormonal contraceptives are co-administered with antibiotics, anticonvulsants, and other drugs that increase the metabolism of contraceptive ste-

roids. This could result in unintended pregnancy or unscheduled bleeding. In such cases a nonhormonal back-up method of birth control should be considered). Products include:

Penicillin, Potassium Phenoxymethyl (Contraceptive effectiveness may be reduced when hormonal contraceptives are co-administered with antibiotics, anticonvulsants, and other drugs that increase the metabolism of contraceptive steroids. This could result in unintended pregnancy or unscheduled bleeding. In such cases a nonhormonal back-up method of birth control should be considered).

No products indexed under this heading.

Penicillin G Benzathine (Contraceptive effectiveness may be reduced when hormonal contraceptives are co-administered with antibiotics, anticonvulsants, and other drugs that increase the metabolism of contraceptive steroids. This could result in unintended pregnancy or unscheduled bleeding. In such cases a nonhormonal back-up method of birth control should be considered). Products include:

Penicillin G Dibenzylethyenediamine (Contraceptive effectiveness may be reduced when hormonal contraceptives are co-administered with antibiotics, anticonvulsants, and other drugs that increase the metabolism of contraceptive steroids. This could result in unintended pregnancy or unscheduled bleeding. In such cases a nonhormonal back-up method of birth control should be considered).

No products indexed under this heading.

Penicillin G Potassium (Contraceptive effectiveness may be reduced when hormonal contraceptives are co-administered with antibiotics, anticonvulsants, and other drugs that increase the metabolism of contraceptive steroids. This could result in unintended pregnancy or unscheduled bleeding. In such cases a nonhormonal back-up method of birth control should be considered).

No products indexed under this heading.

Penicillin G Procaine (Contraceptive effectiveness may be reduced when hormonal contraceptives are co-administered with antibiotics, anticonvulsants, and other drugs that increase the metabolism of contraceptive steroids. This could result in unintended pregnancy or unscheduled bleeding. In such cases a nonhormonal back-up method of birth control should be considered). Products include:

Penicillin G Sodium (Contraceptive effectiveness may be reduced when hormonal contraceptives are co-administered with antibiotics, anticonvulsants, and other drugs that increase the metabolism of contraceptive steroids. This could result in unintended pregnancy or unscheduled bleeding. In such cases a nonhormonal back-up method of birth control should be considered).

No products indexed under this heading.

Penicillin V (Contraceptive effectiveness may be reduced when hormonal contraceptives are co-administered with antibiotics, anticonvulsants, and other drugs that increase the metabolism of contraceptive steroids. This could result in unintended pregnancy or unscheduled bleeding. In such cases a nonhormonal back-up method of birth control should be considered).

No products indexed under this heading.

Penicillin V Potassium (Contraceptive effectiveness may be reduced when hormonal contraceptives are co-administered with antibiotics, anticonvulsants, and other drugs that increase the metabolism of contraceptive steroids. This could result in unintended pregnancy or unscheduled bleeding. In such cases a nonhormonal back-up method of birth control should be considered).

No products indexed under this heading.

Penicillins (Contraceptive effectiveness may be reduced when hormonal contraceptives are co-administered with antibiotics, anticonvulsants, and other drugs that increase the metabolism of contraceptive steroids. This could result in unintended pregnancy or unscheduled bleeding. In such cases a nonhormonal back-up method of birth control should be considered).

No products indexed under this heading.

Pentamidine Isethionate (Contraceptive effectiveness may be reduced when hormonal contraceptives are co-administered with antibiotics, anticonvulsants, and other drugs that increase the metabolism of contraceptive steroids. This could result in unintended pregnancy or unscheduled bleeding. In such cases a nonhormonal back-up method of birth control should be considered).

No products indexed under this heading.

Pentobarbital (Contraceptive effectiveness may be reduced when hormonal contraceptives are co-administered with antibiotics, anticonvulsants, and other drugs that increase the metabolism of contraceptive steroids. This could result in unintended pregnancy or unscheduled bleeding. In such cases a nonhormonal back-up method of birth control should be considered).

No products indexed under this heading.

Pentobarbital Sodium (Contraceptive effectiveness may be reduced when hormonal contraceptives are co-administered with antibiotics, anticonvulsants, and other drugs that increase the metabolism of contraceptive steroids. This could result in unintended pregnancy or unscheduled bleeding. In such cases a nonhormonal back-up method of birth control should be considered). Products include:

Pergolide Mesylate (Enterohepatic recirculation of estrogens may also be decreased by substances that reduce gut transit time).

No products indexed under this heading.

Phenacemide (Contraceptive effectiveness may be reduced when hormonal contraceptives are co-administered with antibiotics, anticonvulsants, and other drugs that increase the metabolism of contraceptive steroids. This could result in unintended pregnancy or unscheduled bleeding. In such cases a nonhormonal back-up method of birth control should be considered).

No products indexed under this heading.

Phenobarbital (Contraceptive effectiveness may be reduced when hormonal contraceptives are co-administered with antibiotics, anticonvulsants, and other drugs that increase the metabolism of contraceptive steroids. This

could result in unintended pregnancy or unscheduled bleeding. In such cases a nonhormonal back-up method of birth control should be considered). Products include:

Phenobarbital Sodium (Contraceptive effectiveness may be reduced when hormonal contraceptives are co-administered with antibiotics, anticonvulsants, and other drugs that increase the metabolism of contraceptive steroids. This could result in unintended pregnancy or unscheduled bleeding. In such cases a nonhormonal back-up method of birth control should be considered).

No products indexed under this heading.

Phensuximide (Contraceptive effectiveness may be reduced when hormonal contraceptives are co-administered with antibiotics, anticonvulsants, and other drugs that increase the metabolism of contraceptive steroids. This could result in unintended pregnancy or unscheduled bleeding. In such cases a nonhormonal back-up method of birth control should be considered).

No products indexed under this heading.

Phenylbutazone (Contraceptive effectiveness may be reduced when hormonal contraceptives are co-administered with antibiotics, anticonvulsants, and other drugs that increase the metabolism of contraceptive steroids. This could result in unintended pregnancy or unscheduled bleeding. In such cases a nonhormonal back-up method of birth control should be considered).

No products indexed under this heading.

Phenytoin (Contraceptive effectiveness may be reduced when hormonal contraceptives are co-administered with antibiotics, anticonvulsants, and other drugs that increase the metabolism of contraceptive steroids. This could result in unintended pregnancy or unscheduled bleeding. In such cases a nonhormonal back-up method of birth control should be considered).

No products indexed under this heading.

Phenytoin Sodium (Contraceptive effectiveness may be reduced when hormonal contraceptives are co-administered with antibiotics, anticonvulsants, and other drugs that increase the metabolism of contraceptive steroids. This could result in unintended pregnancy or unscheduled bleeding. In such cases a nonhormonal back-up method of birth control should be considered). Products include:

Pimozide (Contraceptive effectiveness may be reduced when hormonal contraceptives are co-administered with antibiotics, and other drugs that increase the metabolism of contraceptive steroids. This could result in unintended pregnancy or unscheduled bleeding. In such cases a nonhormonal back-up method of birth control should be considered).

No products indexed under this heading.

Pindolol (Contraceptive effectiveness may be reduced when hormonal contraceptives are co-administered with antibiotics, and other drugs that increase the metabolism of contraceptive steroids. This could result in unintended pregnancy or unscheduled bleeding. In such cases a nonhormonal back-up method of birth control should be considered).

No products indexed under this heading.

Pioglitazone Hydrochloride (Contraceptive effectiveness may be reduced when hormonal contraceptives are co-administered with antibiotics, anticonvulsants, and other drugs that increase the metabolism of contracep-

tive steroids. This could result in unintended pregnancy or unscheduled bleeding. In such cases a nonhormonal back-up method of birth control should be considered). Products include:

Piperacillin Sodium (Contraceptive effectiveness may be reduced when hormonal contraceptives are co-administered with antibiotics, anticonvulsants, and other drugs that increase the metabolism of contraceptive steroids. This could result in unintended pregnancy or unscheduled bleeding. In such cases a nonhormonal back-up method of birth control should be considered). Products include:

Pirbuterol Acetate (Enterohepatic recirculation of estrogens may also be decreased by substances that reduce gut transit time). Products include:

Piroxicam (Contraceptive effectiveness may be reduced when hormonal contraceptives are co-administered with antibiotics, anticonvulsants, and other drugs that increase the metabolism of contraceptive steroids. This could result in unintended pregnancy or unscheduled bleeding. In such cases a nonhormonal back-up method of birth control should be considered).

No products indexed under this heading.

Polyestradiol Phosphate (Contraceptive effectiveness may be reduced when hormonal contraceptives are co-administered with antibiotics, anticonvulsants, and other drugs that increase the metabolism of contraceptive steroids. This could result in unintended pregnancy or unscheduled bleeding. In such cases a nonhormonal back-up method of birth control should be considered).

No products indexed under this heading.

Posaconazole (CYP 3A4 inhibitors such as indinavir, itraconazole, ketoconazole, fluconazole, and troleandomycin may increase plasma hormone levels). Products include:

Pramipexole Dihydrochloride (Enterohepatic recirculation of estrogens may also be decreased by substances that reduce gut transit time).

No products indexed under this heading.

Prednisolone (Contraceptive effectiveness may be reduced when hormonal contraceptives are co-administered with antibiotics, anticonvulsants, and other drugs that increase the metabolism of contraceptive steroids. This could result in unintended pregnancy or unscheduled bleeding. In such cases a nonhormonal back-up method of birth control should be considered).

No products indexed under this heading.

Prednisolone Acetate (Contraceptive effectiveness may be reduced when hormonal contraceptives are co-administered with antibiotics, anticonvulsants, and other drugs that increase the metabolism of contraceptive steroids. This could result in unintended pregnancy or unscheduled bleeding. In such cases a nonhormonal back-up method of birth control should be considered). Products include:

IMPORTANT NOTE: Always consult each drug listing in the patient's regimen for possible interactions.

1089 Interactions Index Lybrel

Riluzole (Contraceptive effectiveness may be reduced when hormonal contraceptives are co-administered with antibiotics, anticonvulsants, and other drugs that increase the metabolism of contraceptive steroids. This could result in unintended pregnancy or unscheduled bleeding. In such cases a nonhormonal back-up method of birth control should be considered). Products include:
Rilutek 3032

Risperidone (Contraceptive effectiveness may be reduced when hormonal contraceptives are co-administered with antibiotics, anticonvulsants, and other drugs that increase the metabolism of contraceptive steroids. This could result in unintended pregnancy or unscheduled bleeding. In such cases a nonhormonal back-up method of birth control should be considered). Products include:
Risperdal Consta 2682

Ritonavir (Contraceptive effectiveness may be reduced when hormonal contraceptives are co-administered with antibiotics, anticonvulsants, and other drugs that increase the metabolism of contraceptive steroids. This could result in unintended pregnancy or unscheduled bleeding. In such cases a nonhormonal back-up method of birth control should be considered). Products include:
Kaletra 458
Norvir 509

Rivastigmine Tartrate (Enterohepatic recirculation of estrogens may also be decreased by substances that reduce gut transit time). Products include:
Exelon 2432
Exelon Oral 2432
Exelon Patch 2437

Rofecoxib (Contraceptive effectiveness may be reduced when hormonal contraceptives are co-administered with antibiotics, anticonvulsants, and other drugs that increase the metabolism of contraceptive steroids. This could result in unintended pregnancy or unscheduled bleeding. In such cases a nonhormonal back-up method of birth control should be considered).
No products indexed under this heading.

Ropinirole Hydrochloride (Contraceptive effectiveness may be reduced when hormonal contraceptives are co-administered with antibiotics, anticonvulsants, and other drugs that increase the metabolism of contraceptive steroids. This could result in unintended pregnancy or unscheduled bleeding. In such cases a nonhormonal back-up method of birth control should be considered). Products include:
Requip 1620
Requip XL 1628

Ropivacaine Hydrochloride (Contraceptive effectiveness may be reduced when hormonal contraceptives are co-administered with antibiotics, anticonvulsants, and other drugs that increase the metabolism of contraceptive steroids. This could result in unintended pregnancy or unscheduled bleeding. In such cases a nonhormonal back-up method of birth control should be considered).
No products indexed under this heading.

Rosiglitazone (Contraceptive effectiveness may be reduced when hormonal contraceptives are co-administered with antibiotics, anticonvulsants, and other drugs that increase the metabolism of contraceptive steroids. This could result in unintended pregnancy or unscheduled bleeding. In such cases a nonhormonal back-up method of birth control should be considered).
No products indexed under this heading.

Rosiglitazone Maleate (Contraceptive effectiveness may be reduced when hormonal contraceptives are co-administered with antibiotics, anticonvulsants, and other drugs that increase the metabolism of contraceptive steroids. This could result in unintended pregnancy or unscheduled bleeding. In such cases a nonhormonal back-up method of birth control should be considered). Products include:
Avandamet 1345
Avandaryl 1356
Avandia 1366

Rosiglitazone/Metformin (Contraceptive effectiveness may be reduced when hormonal contraceptives are co-administered with antibiotics, anticonvulsants, and other drugs that increase the metabolism of contraceptive steroids. This could result in unintended pregnancy or unscheduled bleeding. In such cases a nonhormonal back-up method of birth control should be considered).
No products indexed under this heading.

Rufinamide (Contraceptive effectiveness may be reduced when hormonal contraceptives are co-administered with antibiotics, anticonvulsants, and other drugs that increase the metabolism of contraceptive steroids. This could result in unintended pregnancy or unscheduled bleeding. In such cases a nonhormonal back-up method of birth control should be considered). Products include:
Banzel 1050

Salicylic Acid (Increased clearance of salicylic adid, due to induction of conjugation (particularly glucuronidation), have been noted when this drug is administered with oral contraceptives).
No products indexed under this heading.

Salmeterol Xinafoate (Enterohepatic recirculation of estrogens may also be decreased by substances that reduce gut transit time). Products include:
Advair 100/50 1275
Advair 250/50 1275
Advair 500/50 1275
Advair HFA 45/21 1288
Advair HFA 115/21 1288
Advair HFA 230/21 1288
Serevent Diskus 1656

Saquinavir (Contraceptive effectiveness may be reduced when hormonal contraceptives are co-administered with antibiotics, anticonvulsants, and other drugs that increase the metabolism of contraceptive steroids. This could result in unintended pregnancy or unscheduled bleeding. In such cases a nonhormonal back-up method of birth control should be considered).
No products indexed under this heading.

Saquinavir Mesylate (Contraceptive effectiveness may be reduced when hormonal contraceptives are co-administered with antibiotics, anticonvulsants, and other drugs that increase the metabolism of contraceptive steroids. This could result in unintended pregnancy or unscheduled bleeding. In such cases a nonhormonal back-up method of birth control should be considered).
No products indexed under this heading.

Scopolamine (Enterohepatic recirculation of estrogens may also be decreased by substances that reduce gut transit time). Products include:
Transderm Scōp 2397

Scopolamine Hydrobromide (Enterohepatic recirculation of estrogens may also be decreased by substances that reduce gut transit time). Products include:
Donnatal 2711

Secobarbital Sodium (Contraceptive effectiveness may be reduced when hormonal contraceptives are co-administered with antibiotics, anticonvulsants, and other drugs that increase the metabolism of contraceptive steroids. This could result in unintended pregnancy or unscheduled bleeding. In such cases a nonhormonal back-up method of birth control should be considered).
No products indexed under this heading.

Sertraline Hydrochloride (Contraceptive effectiveness may be reduced when hormonal contraceptives are co-administered with antibiotics, anticonvulsants, and other drugs that increase the metabolism of contraceptive steroids. This could result in unintended pregnancy or unscheduled bleeding. In such cases a nonhormonal back-up method of birth control should be considered).
No products indexed under this heading.

Sildenafil Citrate (Contraceptive effectiveness may be reduced when hormonal contraceptives are co-administered with antibiotics, anticonvulsants, and other drugs that increase the metabolism of contraceptive steroids. This could result in unintended pregnancy or unscheduled bleeding. In such cases a nonhormonal back-up method of birth control should be considered).
No products indexed under this heading.

Simvastatin (Contraceptive effectiveness may be reduced when hormonal contraceptives are co-administered with antibiotics, anticonvulsants, and other drugs that increase the metabolism of contraceptive steroids. This could result in unintended pregnancy or unscheduled bleeding. In such cases a nonhormonal back-up method of birth control should be considered). Products include:
Simcor 524
Vytorin 10/10 .... 2303, 3240
Vytorin 10/20 .... 2303, 3240
Vytorin 10/40 .... 2303, 3240
Vytorin 10/80 .... 2303, 3240
Zocor 2289

Sirolimus (Contraceptive effectiveness may be reduced when hormonal contraceptives are co-administered with antibiotics, anticonvulsants, and other drugs that increase the metabolism of contraceptive steroids. This could result in unintended pregnancy or unscheduled bleeding. In such cases a nonhormonal back-up method of birth control should be considered). Products include:
Rapamune 3579

Sodium Butabarbital (Contraceptive effectiveness may be reduced when hormonal contraceptives are co-administered with antibiotics, anticonvulsants, and other drugs that increase the metabolism of contraceptive steroids. This could result in unintended pregnancy or unscheduled bleeding. In such cases a nonhormonal back-up method of birth control should be considered).
No products indexed under this heading.

Sodium Cloxacillin Monohydrate (Contraceptive effectiveness may be reduced when hormonal contraceptives are co-administered with antibiotics, anticonvulsants, and other drugs that increase the metabolism of contraceptive steroids. This could result in unintended pregnancy or unscheduled bleeding. In such cases a nonhormonal back-up method of birth control should be considered).
No products indexed under this heading.

Sodium Pentobarbital (Contraceptive effectiveness may be reduced when hormonal contraceptives are co-administered with antibiotics, anticonvulsants, and other drugs that increase the metabolism of contraceptive steroids. This could result in unintended pregnancy or unscheduled bleeding. In such cases a nonhormonal back-up method of birth control should be considered).
No products indexed under this heading.

Sparfloxacin (Contraceptive effectiveness may be reduced when hormonal contraceptives are co-administered with antibiotics, anticonvulsants, and other drugs that increase the metabolism of contraceptive steroids. This could result in unintended pregnancy or unscheduled bleeding. In such cases a nonhormonal back-up method of birth control should be considered).
No products indexed under this heading.

Streptomycin Sulfate (Contraceptive effectiveness may be reduced when hormonal contraceptives are co-administered with antibiotics, anticonvulsants, and other drugs that increase the metabolism of contraceptive steroids. This could result in unintended pregnancy or unscheduled bleeding. In such cases a nonhormonal back-up method of birth control should be considered).
No products indexed under this heading.

Sucralfate (Enterohepatic recirculation of estrogens may also be decreased by substances that reduce gut transit time). Products include:
Carafate Suspension 784
Carafate Tablets 785

Sufentanil Citrate (Enterohepatic recirculation of estrogens may also be decreased by substances that reduce gut transit time).
No products indexed under this heading.

Sulfamethizole (Contraceptive effectiveness may be reduced when hormonal contraceptives are co-administered with antibiotics, anticonvulsants, and other drugs that increase the metabolism of contraceptive steroids. This could result in unintended pregnancy or unscheduled bleeding. In such cases a nonhormonal back-up method of birth control should be considered).
No products indexed under this heading.

Sulfamethoxazole (Contraceptive effectiveness may be reduced when hormonal contraceptives are co-administered with antibiotics, anticonvulsants, and other drugs that increase the metabolism of contraceptive steroids. This could result in unintended pregnancy or unscheduled bleeding. In such cases a nonhormonal back-up method of birth control should be considered).
No products indexed under this heading.

Sulfinpyrazone (Contraceptive effectiveness may be reduced when hormonal contraceptives are co-administered with antibiotics, anticonvulsants, and other drugs that increase the metabolism of contraceptive steroids. This could result in unintended pregnancy or unscheduled bleeding. In such cases a nonhormonal back-up method of birth control should be considered).
No products indexed under this heading.

Sulfisoxazole Acetyl (Contraceptive effectiveness may be reduced when hormonal contraceptives are co-administered with antibiotics, anticonvulsants, and other drugs that increase the metabolism of contraceptive steroids. This could result in unintended pregnancy or unscheduled bleeding. In such cases a nonhormonal back-up method of birth control should be considered).
No products indexed under this heading.

IMPORTANT NOTE: Always consult each drug listing in the patient's regimen for possible interactions.

Sulfisoxazole Diolamine (Contraceptive effectiveness may be reduced when hormonal contraceptives are co-administered with antibiotics, anticonvulsants, and other drugs that increase the metabolism of contraceptive steroids. This could result in unintended pregnancy or unscheduled bleeding. In such cases a nonhormonal back-up method of birth control should be considered).

No products indexed under this heading.

Sulindac (Contraceptive effectiveness may be reduced when hormonal contraceptives are co-administered with antibiotics, anticonvulsants, and other drugs that increase the metabolism of contraceptive steroids. This could result in unintended pregnancy or unscheduled bleeding. In such cases a nonhormonal back-up method of birth control should be considered). Products include:

Clinoril 2098

Suprofen (Contraceptive effectiveness may be reduced when hormonal contraceptives are co-administered with antibiotics, anticonvulsants, and other drugs that increase the metabolism of contraceptive steroids. This could result in unintended pregnancy or unscheduled bleeding. In such cases a nonhormonal back-up method of birth control should be considered).

No products indexed under this heading.

Tacrine Hydrochloride (Contraceptive effectiveness may be reduced when hormonal contraceptives are co-administered with antibiotics, anticonvulsants, and other drugs that increase the metabolism of contraceptive steroids. This could result in unintended pregnancy or unscheduled bleeding. In such cases a nonhormonal back-up method of birth control should be considered).

No products indexed under this heading.

Tacrolimus (Contraceptive effectiveness may be reduced when hormonal contraceptives are co-administered with antibiotics, anticonvulsants, and other drugs that increase the metabolism of contraceptive steroids. This could result in unintended pregnancy or unscheduled bleeding. In such cases a nonhormonal back-up method of birth control should be considered). Products include:

Prograf Capsules 677
Prograf Injection 677
Protopic 685

Tadalafil (Contraceptive effectiveness may be reduced when hormonal contraceptives are co-administered with antibiotics, anticonvulsants, and other drugs that increase the metabolism of contraceptive steroids. This could result in unintended pregnancy or unscheduled bleeding. In such cases a nonhormonal back-up method of birth control should be considered). Products include:

Adcirca 3461
Cialis 1861

Tamoxifen Citrate (Contraceptive effectiveness may be reduced when hormonal contraceptives are co-administered with antibiotics, anticonvulsants, and other drugs that increase the metabolism of contraceptive steroids. This could result in unintended pregnancy or unscheduled bleeding. In such cases a nonhormonal back-up method of birth control should be considered).

No products indexed under this heading.

Telithromycin (CYP 3A4 inhibitors such as indinavir, itraconazole, ketoconazole, fluconazole, and troleandomycin may increase plasma hormone levels). Products include:

Ketek 2991

Telmisartan (Contraceptive effectiveness may be reduced when hormonal

contraceptives are co-administered with antibiotics, anticonvulsants, and other drugs that increase the metabolism of contraceptive steroids. This could result in unintended pregnancy or unscheduled bleeding. In such cases a nonhormonal back-up method of birth control should be considered). Products include:

Micardis 887
Micardis HCT 889

Temazepam (Increased clearance of temazepam, due to induction of conjugation (particularly glucuronidation), have been noted when this drug is administered with oral contraceptives).

No products indexed under this heading.

Teniposide (Contraceptive effectiveness may be reduced when hormonal contraceptives are co-administered with antibiotics, anticonvulsants, and other drugs that increase the metabolism of contraceptive steroids. This could result in unintended pregnancy or unscheduled bleeding. In such cases a nonhormonal back-up method of birth control should be considered).

No products indexed under this heading.

Terbutaline Sulfate (Enterohepatic recirculation of estrogens may also be decreased by substances that reduce gut transit time).

No products indexed under this heading.

Terfenadine (Contraceptive effectiveness may be reduced when hormonal contraceptives are co-administered with antibiotics, anticonvulsants, and other drugs that increase the metabolism of contraceptive steroids. This could result in unintended pregnancy or unscheduled bleeding. In such cases a nonhormonal back-up method of birth control should be considered).

No products indexed under this heading.

Testosterone (Contraceptive effectiveness may be reduced when hormonal contraceptives are co-administered with antibiotics, anticonvulsants, and other drugs that increase the metabolism of contraceptive steroids. This could result in unintended pregnancy or unscheduled bleeding. In such cases a nonhormonal back-up method of birth control should be considered). Products include:

AndroGel 3456

Testosterone Cypionate (Contraceptive effectiveness may be reduced when hormonal contraceptives are co-administered with antibiotics, anticonvulsants, and other drugs that increase the metabolism of contraceptive steroids. This could result in unintended pregnancy or unscheduled bleeding. In such cases a nonhormonal back-up method of birth control should be considered).

No products indexed under this heading.

Testosterone Enanthate (Contraceptive effectiveness may be reduced when hormonal contraceptives are co-administered with antibiotics, anticonvulsants, and other drugs that increase the metabolism of contraceptive steroids. This could result in unintended pregnancy or unscheduled bleeding. In such cases a nonhormonal back-up method of birth control should be considered). Products include:

Delatestryl 1102

Testosterone Propionate (Contraceptive effectiveness may be reduced when hormonal contraceptives are co-administered with antibiotics, anticonvulsants, and other drugs that increase the metabolism of contraceptive steroids. This could result in unintended pregnancy or unscheduled bleeding. In such cases a nonhormonal back-up method of birth control should be considered).

No products indexed under this heading.

Tetracycline Hydrochloride (Contraceptive effectiveness may be reduced when hormonal contraceptives are co-administered with antibiotics, anticonvulsants, and other drugs that increase the metabolism of contraceptive steroids. This could result in unintended pregnancy or unscheduled bleeding. In such cases a nonhormonal back-up method of birth control should be considered). Products include:

Pylera 793

Tetracycline Phosphate Complex (Several cases of contraceptive failure and unscheduled bleeding have been reported in the literature with concomitant administration of antibiotics such as ampicillin and other penicillins, and tetracyclines. However, clinical pharmacology studies investigating drug interactions between combined oral contraceptives and these antibiotics have reported inconsistent results).

No products indexed under this heading.

Theophyllinate (Contraceptive effectiveness may be reduced when hormonal contraceptives are co-administered with antibiotics, anticonvulsants, and other drugs that increase the metabolism of contraceptive steroids. This could result in unintended pregnancy or unscheduled bleeding. In such cases a nonhormonal back-up method of birth control should be considered).

No products indexed under this heading.

Theophylline (Contraceptive effectiveness may be reduced when hormonal contraceptives are co-administered with antibiotics, anticonvulsants, and other drugs that increase the metabolism of contraceptive steroids. This could result in unintended pregnancy or unscheduled bleeding. In such cases a nonhormonal back-up method of birth control should be considered).

No products indexed under this heading.

Theophylline Anhydrous (Contraceptive effectiveness may be reduced when hormonal contraceptives are co-administered with antibiotics, anticonvulsants, and other drugs that increase the metabolism of contraceptive steroids. This could result in unintended pregnancy or unscheduled bleeding. In such cases a nonhormonal back-up method of birth control should be considered). Products include:

Uniphyl 2817

Theophylline Calcium Salicylate (Contraceptive effectiveness may be reduced when hormonal contraceptives are co-administered with antibiotics, anticonvulsants, and other drugs that increase the metabolism of contraceptive steroids. This could result in unintended pregnancy or unscheduled bleeding. In such cases a nonhormonal back-up method of birth control should be considered).

No products indexed under this heading.

Theophylline Dihydroxypropyl (Glyceryl) (Contraceptive effectiveness may be reduced when hormonal contraceptives are co-administered with antibiotics, anticonvulsants, and other drugs that increase the metabolism of contraceptive steroids. This could result in unintended pregnancy or unscheduled bleeding. In such cases a nonhormonal back-up method of birth control should be considered).

No products indexed under this heading.

Theophylline Ethylenediamine (Contraceptive effectiveness may be reduced when hormonal contraceptives are co-administered with antibiotics, anticonvulsants, and other drugs that increase the metabolism of contraceptive steroids. This could result in unintended pregnancy or unscheduled bleeding. In such cases a nonhormonal back-up method of birth control should be considered).

No products indexed under this heading.

Theophylline Sodium Glycinate (Contraceptive effectiveness may be reduced when hormonal contraceptives are co-administered with antibiotics, anticonvulsants, and other drugs that increase the metabolism of contraceptive steroids. This could result in unintended pregnancy or unscheduled bleeding. In such cases a nonhormonal back-up method of birth control should be considered).

No products indexed under this heading.

Thiamylal Sodium (Contraceptive effectiveness may be reduced when hormonal contraceptives are co-administered with antibiotics, anticonvulsants, and other drugs that increase the metabolism of contraceptive steroids. This could result in unintended pregnancy or unscheduled bleeding. In such cases a nonhormonal back-up method of birth control should be considered).

No products indexed under this heading.

Thioridazine (Contraceptive effectiveness may be reduced when hormonal contraceptives are co-administered with antibiotics, anticonvulsants, and other drugs that increase the metabolism of contraceptive steroids. This could result in unintended pregnancy or unscheduled bleeding. In such cases a nonhormonal back-up method of birth control should be considered).

No products indexed under this heading.

Thioridazine Hydrochloride (Contraceptive effectiveness may be reduced when hormonal contraceptives are co-administered with antibiotics, anticonvulsants, and other drugs that increase the metabolism of contraceptive steroids. This could result in unintended pregnancy or unscheduled bleeding. In such cases a nonhormonal back-up method of birth control should be considered). Products include:

Thioridazine Hydrochloride 2384

Tiagabine Hydrochloride (Contraceptive effectiveness may be reduced when hormonal contraceptives are co-administered with antibiotics, anticonvulsants, and other drugs that increase the metabolism of contraceptive steroids. This could result in unintended pregnancy or unscheduled bleeding. In such cases a nonhormonal back-up method of birth control should be considered). Products include:

Gabitril 972

Ticarcillin Disodium (Contraceptive effectiveness may be reduced when hormonal contraceptives are co-administered with antibiotics, anticonvulsants, and other drugs that increase the metabolism of contraceptive steroids. This could result in unintended pregnancy or unscheduled bleeding. In such cases a nonhormonal back-up method of birth control should be considered). Products include:

Timentin ADD-Vantage 1670
Timentin Galaxy 1674
Timentin 1666
Timentin Pharmacy 1678

Timolol Maleate (Contraceptive effectiveness may be reduced when hormonal contraceptives are co-administered with antibiotics, anticonvulsants, and other drugs that increase the metabolism of contraceptive ste-

roids. This could result in unintended pregnancy or unscheduled bleeding. In such cases a nonhormonal back-up method of birth control should be considered). Products include:

Combigan 601
Dorzolamide Hydrochloride/Timolol Maleate Ophthalmic Solution .... ⊙243
Timoptic in Ocudose .... ⊙231

Tipranavir (Several of the anti-HIV protease inhibitors have been studied with co-administration of oral combination hormonal contraceptives; significant changes (increase and decrease) in the plasma levels of the estrogen and progestin have been noted in some cases. The safety and efficacy of oral contraceptive products may be affected with co-administration of anti-HIV protease inhibitors. Health care professionals should refer to the label of the individual anti-HIV protease inhibitors for further drug-drug interaction information).
No products indexed under this heading.

Tobramycin (Contraceptive effectiveness may be reduced when hormonal contraceptives are co-administered with antibiotics, anticonvulsants, and other drugs that increase the metabolism of contraceptive steroids. This could result in unintended pregnancy or unscheduled bleeding. In such cases a nonhormonal back-up method of birth control should be considered). Products include:

Tobi Nebulizer 2546
Tobramycin and Dexamethasone Ophthalmic Suspension .... ⊙251
Zylet .... ⊙252

Tobramycin Sulfate (Contraceptive effectiveness may be reduced when hormonal contraceptives are co-administered with antibiotics, anticonvulsants, and other drugs that increase the metabolism of contraceptive steroids. This could result in unintended pregnancy or unscheduled bleeding. In such cases a nonhormonal back-up method of birth control should be considered).
No products indexed under this heading.

Tolazamide (Contraceptive effectiveness may be reduced when hormonal contraceptives are co-administered with antibiotics, anticonvulsants, and other drugs that increase the metabolism of contraceptive steroids. This could result in unintended pregnancy or unscheduled bleeding. In such cases a nonhormonal back-up method of birth control should be considered).
No products indexed under this heading.

Tolbutamide (Contraceptive effectiveness may be reduced when hormonal contraceptives are co-administered with antibiotics, anticonvulsants, and other drugs that increase the metabolism of contraceptive steroids. This could result in unintended pregnancy or unscheduled bleeding. In such cases a nonhormonal back-up method of birth control should be considered).
No products indexed under this heading.

Tolbutamide Sodium (Contraceptive effectiveness may be reduced when hormonal contraceptives are co-administered with antibiotics, anticonvulsants, and other drugs that increase the metabolism of contraceptive steroids. This could result in unintended pregnancy or unscheduled bleeding. In such cases a nonhormonal back-up method of birth control should be considered).
No products indexed under this heading.

Tolmetin Sodium (Contraceptive effectiveness may be reduced when hormonal contraceptives are co-administered with antibiotics, anticonvulsants, and other drugs that increase the metabolism of contraceptive steroids. This could result in unintended pregnancy or unscheduled bleeding. In such cases a nonhormonal back-up method of birth control should be considered).
No products indexed under this heading.

Tolterodine Tartrate (Contraceptive effectiveness may be reduced when hormonal contraceptives are co-administered with antibiotics, anticonvulsants, and other drugs that increase the metabolism of contraceptive steroids. This could result in unintended pregnancy or unscheduled bleeding. In such cases a nonhormonal back-up method of birth control should be considered).
No products indexed under this heading.

Topiramate (Contraceptive effectiveness may be reduced when hormonal contraceptives are co-administered with antibiotics, anticonvulsants, and other drugs that increase the metabolism of contraceptive steroids. This could result in unintended pregnancy or unscheduled bleeding. In such cases a nonhormonal back-up method of birth control should be considered).
No products indexed under this heading.

Torsemide (Contraceptive effectiveness may be reduced when hormonal contraceptives are co-administered with antibiotics, anticonvulsants, and other drugs that increase the metabolism of contraceptive steroids. This could result in unintended pregnancy or unscheduled bleeding. In such cases a nonhormonal back-up method of birth control should be considered).
No products indexed under this heading.

Tramadol Hydrochloride (Contraceptive effectiveness may be reduced when hormonal contraceptives are co-administered with antibiotics, anticonvulsants, and other drugs that increase the metabolism of contraceptive steroids. This could result in unintended pregnancy or unscheduled bleeding. In such cases a nonhormonal back-up method of birth control should be considered). Products include:

Ryzolt 2813
Ultram ER 2693

Trazodone Hydrochloride (Contraceptive effectiveness may be reduced when hormonal contraceptives are co-administered with antibiotics, anticonvulsants, and other drugs that increase the metabolism of contraceptive steroids. This could result in unintended pregnancy or unscheduled bleeding. In such cases a nonhormonal back-up method of birth control should be considered).
No products indexed under this heading.

Tretinoin (Contraceptive effectiveness may be reduced when hormonal contraceptives are co-administered with antibiotics, anticonvulsants, and other drugs that increase the metabolism of contraceptive steroids. This could result in unintended pregnancy or unscheduled bleeding. In such cases a nonhormonal back-up method of birth control should be considered).
No products indexed under this heading.

Triamcinolone (Contraceptive effectiveness may be reduced when hormonal contraceptives are co-administered with antibiotics, anticonvulsants, and other drugs that increase the metabolism of contraceptive steroids. This could result in unintended pregnancy or unscheduled bleeding. In such cases a nonhormonal back-up method of birth control should be considered).
No products indexed under this heading.

Triamcinolone Acetonide (Contraceptive effectiveness may be reduced when hormonal contraceptives are co-administered with antibiotics, anticonvulsants, and other drugs that increase the metabolism of contraceptive steroids. This could result in unintended pregnancy or unscheduled bleeding. In such cases a nonhormonal back-up method of birth control should be considered). Products include:

Azmacort 408
Nasacort AQ 3019

Triamcinolone Diacetate (Contraceptive effectiveness may be reduced when hormonal contraceptives are co-administered with antibiotics, anticonvulsants, and other drugs that increase the metabolism of contraceptive steroids. This could result in unintended pregnancy or unscheduled bleeding. In such cases a nonhormonal back-up method of birth control should be considered).
No products indexed under this heading.

Triamcinolone Hexacetonide (Contraceptive effectiveness may be reduced when hormonal contraceptives are co-administered with antibiotics, anticonvulsants, and other drugs that increase the metabolism of contraceptive steroids. This could result in unintended pregnancy or unscheduled bleeding. In such cases a nonhormonal back-up method of birth control should be considered).
No products indexed under this heading.

Triazolam (Contraceptive effectiveness may be reduced when hormonal contraceptives are co-administered with antibiotics, anticonvulsants, and other drugs that increase the metabolism of contraceptive steroids. This could result in unintended pregnancy or unscheduled bleeding. In such cases a nonhormonal back-up method of birth control should be considered).
No products indexed under this heading.

Tridihexethyl Chloride (Enterohepatic recirculation of estrogens may also be decreased by substances that reduce gut transit time).
No products indexed under this heading.

Trihexyphenidyl Hydrochloride (Enterohepatic recirculation of estrogens may also be decreased by substances that reduce gut transit time).
No products indexed under this heading.

Trimeprazine Tartrate (Enterohepatic recirculation of estrogens may also be decreased by substances that reduce gut transit time).
No products indexed under this heading.

Trimethadione (Contraceptive effectiveness may be reduced when hormonal contraceptives are co-administered with antibiotics, anticonvulsants, and other drugs that increase the metabolism of contraceptive steroids. This could result in unintended pregnancy or unscheduled bleeding. In such cases a nonhormonal back-up method of birth control should be considered).
No products indexed under this heading.

Trimethaphan Camsylate (Contraceptive effectiveness may be reduced when hormonal contraceptives are co-administered with antibiotics, anticonvulsants, and other drugs that increase the metabolism of contraceptive steroids. This could result in unintended pregnancy or unscheduled bleeding. In such cases a nonhormonal back-up method of birth control should be considered).
No products indexed under this heading.

Trimipramine Maleate (Contraceptive effectiveness may be reduced when hormonal contraceptives are co-administered with antibiotics, anticonvulsants, and other drugs that increase the metabolism of contraceptive steroids. This could result in unintended pregnancy or unscheduled bleeding. In such cases a nonhormonal back-up method of birth control should be considered).
No products indexed under this heading.

Tripelennamine Hydrochloride (Enterohepatic recirculation of estrogens may also be decreased by substances that reduce gut transit time).
No products indexed under this heading.

Triprolidine Hydrochloride (Enterohepatic recirculation of estrogens may also be decreased by substances that reduce gut transit time).
No products indexed under this heading.

Troglitazone (Contraceptive effectiveness may be reduced when hormonal contraceptives are co-administered with antibiotics, anticonvulsants, and other drugs that increase the metabolism of contraceptive steroids. This could result in unintended pregnancy or unscheduled bleeding. In such cases a nonhormonal back-up method of birth control should be considered).
No products indexed under this heading.

Troleandomycin (Troleandomycin may also increase the risk of intrahepatic cholestasis during co-administration with combination oral contraceptives. May also increase plasma hormone levels).
No products indexed under this heading.

Trovafloxacin Mesylate (Contraceptive effectiveness may be reduced when hormonal contraceptives are co-administered with antibiotics, anticonvulsants, and other drugs that increase the metabolism of contraceptive steroids. This could result in unintended pregnancy or unscheduled bleeding. In such cases a nonhormonal back-up method of birth control should be considered).
No products indexed under this heading.

Valdecoxib (Contraceptive effectiveness may be reduced when hormonal contraceptives are co-administered with antibiotics, anticonvulsants, and other drugs that increase the metabolism of contraceptive steroids. This could result in unintended pregnancy or unscheduled bleeding. In such cases a nonhormonal back-up method of birth control should be considered).
No products indexed under this heading.

Valproate Sodium (Contraceptive effectiveness may be reduced when hormonal contraceptives are co-administered with antibiotics, anticonvulsants, and other drugs that increase the metabolism of contraceptive steroids. This could result in unintended pregnancy or unscheduled bleeding. In such cases a nonhormonal back-up method of birth control should be considered).
No products indexed under this heading.

Valproic Acid (Contraceptive effectiveness may be reduced when hormonal contraceptives are co-administered with antibiotics, anticonvulsants, and other drugs that increase the metabolism of contraceptive steroids. This could result in unintended pregnancy or unscheduled bleeding. In such cases a nonhormonal back-up method of birth control should be considered).
No products indexed under this heading.

Valsartan (Contraceptive effectiveness may be reduced when hormonal contraceptives are co-administered with antibiotics, anticonvulsants, and other drugs that increase the metabolism of

Food Interactions

Beverages, caffeine-containing (Contraceptive effectiveness may be reduced when hormonal contraceptives are co-administered with antibiotics, anticonvulsants, and other drugs that increase the metabolism of contraceptive steroids. This could result in unintended pregnancy or unscheduled bleeding. In such cases a nonhormonal back-up method of birth control should be considered).

Food, caffeine-containing (Contraceptive effectiveness may be reduced when hormonal contraceptives are co-administered with antibiotics, anticonvulsants, and other drugs that increase the metabolism of contraceptive steroids. This could result in unintended pregnancy or unscheduled bleeding. In such cases a nonhormonal back-up method of birth control should be considered).

Grapefruit (CYP 3A4 inhibitors such as indinavir, itraconazole, ketoconazole, fluconazole, and troleandomycin may increase plasma hormone levels).

Grapefruit Juice (CYP 3A4 inhibitors such as indinavir, itraconazole, ketoconazole, fluconazole, and troleandomycin may increase plasma hormone levels).

LYRICA CAPSULES

May interact with ACE inhibitors, alcohols, benzodiazepines, central nervous system depressants, narcotic analgesics, and certain other agents. Compounds in these categories include:

Alfentanil Hydrochloride (Patients who require concomitant treatment with central nervous system depressants such as opiates or benzodiazepines should be informed that they may experience additive CNS side effects, such as somnolence).
No products indexed under this heading.

Alprazolam (Patients who require concomitant treatment with central nervous system depressants such as opiates or benzodiazepines should be informed that they may experience additive CNS side effects, such as somnolence).
No products indexed under this heading.

Amobarbital (Patients who require concomitant treatment with central nervous system depressants such as opiates or benzodiazepines should be informed that they may experience additive CNS side effects, such as somnolence).
No products indexed under this heading.

Amobarbital Sodium (Patients who require concomitant treatment with central nervous system depressants such as opiates or benzodiazepines should be informed that they may experience additive CNS side effects, such as somnolence).
No products indexed under this heading.

Apomorphine (Patients who require concomitant treatment with central nervous system depressants such as opiates or benzodiazepines should be informed that they may experience additive CNS side effects, such as somnolence).
No products indexed under this heading.

Apomorphine Hydrochloride (Patients who require concomitant treatment with central nervous system depressants such as opiates or benzodiazepines should be informed that they may experience additive CNS side effects, such as somnolence).
No products indexed under this heading.

Aprobarbital (Patients who require concomitant treatment with central nervous system depressants such as opiates or benzodiazepines should be informed that they may experience additive CNS side effects, such as somnolence).
No products indexed under this heading.

Benazepril Hydrochloride (Patients who are taking other drugs associated with angioedema (eg, angiotensin converting enzyme inhibitors [ACE inhibitors]) may be at increased risk of developing angioedema).
No products indexed under this heading.

Buprenorphine Hydrochloride (Patients who require concomitant treatment with central nervous system depressants such as opiates or benzodiazepines should be informed that they may experience additive CNS side effects, such as somnolence).
No products indexed under this heading.

Buspirone Hydrochloride (Patients who require concomitant treatment with central nervous system depressants such as opiates or benzodiazepines should be informed that they may experience additive CNS side effects, such as somnolence).
No products indexed under this heading.

Butabarbital (Patients who require concomitant treatment with central nervous system depressants such as opiates or benzodiazepines should be informed that they may experience additive CNS side effects, such as somnolence).
No products indexed under this heading.

Butabarbital Sodium (Patients who require concomitant treatment with central nervous system depressants such as opiates or benzodiazepines should be informed that they may experience additive CNS side effects, such as somnolence).
No products indexed under this heading.

Butalbital (Patients who require concomitant treatment with central nervous system depressants such as opiates or benzodiazepines should be informed that they may experience additive CNS side effects, such as somnolence).
No products indexed under this heading.

Captopril (Patients who are taking other drugs associated with angioedema (eg, angiotensin converting enzyme inhibitors [ACE inhibitors]) may be at increased risk of developing angioedema). Products include:

1093 Interactions Index Lyrica

Chlordiazepoxide (Patients who require concomitant treatment with central nervous system depressants such as opiates or benzodiazepines should be informed that they may experience additive CNS side effects, such as somnolence).
No products indexed under this heading.

Chlordiazepoxide Hydrochloride (Patients who require concomitant treatment with central nervous system depressants such as opiates or benzodiazepines should be informed that they may experience additive CNS side effects, such as somnolence).
No products indexed under this heading.

Chlorpromazine (Patients who require concomitant treatment with central nervous system depressants such as opiates or benzodiazepines should be informed that they may experience additive CNS side effects, such as somnolence).
No products indexed under this heading.

Chlorpromazine Hydrochloride (Patients who require concomitant treatment with central nervous system depressants such as opiates or benzodiazepines should be informed that they may experience additive CNS side effects, such as somnolence).
No products indexed under this heading.

Chlorprothixene (Patients who require concomitant treatment with central nervous system depressants such as opiates or benzodiazepines should be informed that they may experience additive CNS side effects, such as somnolence).
No products indexed under this heading.

Chlorprothixene Hydrochloride (Patients who require concomitant treatment with central nervous system depressants such as opiates or benzodiazepines should be informed that they may experience additive CNS side effects, such as somnolence).
No products indexed under this heading.

Chlorprothixene Lactate (Patients who require concomitant treatment with central nervous system depressants such as opiates or benzodiazepines should be informed that they may experience additive CNS side effects, such as somnolence).
No products indexed under this heading.

Clonazepam (Patients who require concomitant treatment with central nervous system depressants such as opiates or benzodiazepines should be informed that they may experience additive CNS side effects, such as somnolence). Products include:
Klonopin 2855

Clorazepate Dipotassium (Patients who require concomitant treatment with central nervous system depressants such as opiates or benzodiazepines should be informed that they may experience additive CNS side effects, such as somnolence).
No products indexed under this heading.

Clozapine (Patients who require concomitant treatment with central nervous system depressants such as opiates or benzodiazepines should be informed that they may experience additive CNS side effects, such as somnolence).
No products indexed under this heading.

Codeine Phosphate (Patients who require concomitant treatment with central nervous system depressants such as opiates or benzodiazepines should be informed that they may experience additive CNS side effects, such as somnolence). Products include:
Tylenol with Codeine 2691

Codeine Sulfate (Patients who require concomitant treatment with central nervous system depressants such as opiates or benzodiazepines should be informed that they may experience additive CNS side effects, such as somnolence).
No products indexed under this heading.

Desflurane (Patients who require concomitant treatment with central nervous system depressants such as opiates or benzodiazepines should be informed that they may experience additive CNS side effects, such as somnolence).
No products indexed under this heading.

Dezocine (Patients who require concomitant treatment with central nervous system depressants such as opiates or benzodiazepines should be informed that they may experience additive CNS side effects, such as somnolence).
No products indexed under this heading.

Diazepam (Patients who require concomitant treatment with central nervous system depressants such as opiates or benzodiazepines should be informed that they may experience additive CNS side effects, such as somnolence). Products include:
Valium Tablets 2880

Dihydrocodeine Bitartrate (Patients who require concomitant treatment with central nervous system depressants such as opiates or benzodiazepines should be informed that they may experience additive CNS side effects, such as somnolence).
No products indexed under this heading.

Dihydrocodeinone Bitartrate (Patients who require concomitant treatment with central nervous system depressants such as opiates or benzodiazepines should be informed that they may experience additive CNS side effects, such as somnolence).
No products indexed under this heading.

Droperidol (Patients who require concomitant treatment with central nervous system depressants such as opiates or benzodiazepines should be informed that they may experience additive CNS side effects, such as somnolence).
No products indexed under this heading.

Enalapril Maleate (Patients who are taking other drugs associated with angioedema (eg, angiotensin converting enzyme inhibitors [ACE inhibitors]) may be at increased risk of developing angioedema).
No products indexed under this heading.

Enalaprilat (Patients who are taking other drugs associated with angioedema (eg, angiotensin converting enzyme inhibitors [ACE inhibitors]) may be at increased risk of developing angioedema).
No products indexed under this heading.

Enflurane (Patients who require concomitant treatment with central nervous system depressants such as opiates or benzodiazepines should be informed that they may experience additive CNS side effects, such as somnolence).
No products indexed under this heading.

Estazolam (Patients who require concomitant treatment with central nervous system depressants such as opiates or benzodiazepines should be informed that they may experience additive CNS side effects, such as somnolence).
No products indexed under this heading.

Ethanol (Multiple oral doses of pregabalin were co-administered with oxycodone, lorazepam, or ethanol. Although no pharmacokinetic interactions were seen, additive effects on cognitive and gross motor functioning were seen when pregabalin was co-administered with these drugs).
No products indexed under this heading.

Ethchlorvynol (Patients who require concomitant treatment with central nervous system depressants such as opiates or benzodiazepines should be informed that they may experience additive CNS side effects, such as somnolence).
No products indexed under this heading.

Ethinamate (Patients who require concomitant treatment with central nervous system depressants such as opiates or benzodiazepines should be informed that they may experience additive CNS side effects, such as somnolence).
No products indexed under this heading.

Ethyl Alcohol (Patients who are taking other drugs associated with angioedema (eg, angiotensin converting enzyme inhibitors [ACE inhibitors]) may be at increased risk of developing angioedema).
No products indexed under this heading.

Fentanyl (Patients who require concomitant treatment with central nervous system depressants such as opiates or benzodiazepines should be informed that they may experience additive CNS side effects, such as somnolence). Products include:
Duragesic 2604
Fentanyl Transdermal System 2346
Onsolis 2054

Fentanyl Citrate (Patients who require concomitant treatment with central nervous system depressants such as opiates or benzodiazepines should be informed that they may experience additive CNS side effects, such as somnolence). Products include:
Fentora 966

Fluphenazine Decanoate (Patients who require concomitant treatment with central nervous system depressants such as opiates or benzodiazepines should be informed that they may experience additive CNS side effects, such as somnolence).
No products indexed under this heading.

Fluphenazine Enanthate (Patients who require concomitant treatment with central nervous system depressants such as opiates or benzodiazepines should be informed that they may experience additive CNS side effects, such as somnolence).
No products indexed under this heading.

Fluphenazine Hydrochloride (Patients who require concomitant treatment with central nervous system depressants such as opiates or benzodiazepines should be informed that they may experience additive CNS side effects, such as somnolence).
No products indexed under this heading.

Flurazepam Hydrochloride (Patients who require concomitant treatment with central nervous system depressants such as opiates or benzodiazepines should be informed that they may experience additive CNS side effects, such as somnolence).
No products indexed under this heading.

Fosinopril Sodium (Patients who are taking other drugs associated with angioedema (eg, angiotensin converting enzyme inhibitors [ACE inhibitors]) may be at increased risk of developing angioedema).
No products indexed under this heading.

Glutethimide (Patients who require concomitant treatment with central nervous system depressants such as opiates or benzodiazepines should be informed that they may experience additive CNS side effects, such as somnolence).
No products indexed under this heading.

Halazepam (Patients who require concomitant treatment with central nervous system depressants such as opiates or benzodiazepines should be informed that they may experience additive CNS side effects, such as somnolence).
No products indexed under this heading.

Haloperidol (Patients who require concomitant treatment with central nervous system depressants such as opiates or benzodiazepines should be informed that they may experience additive CNS side effects, such as somnolence).
No products indexed under this heading.

Haloperidol Decanoate (Patients who require concomitant treatment with central nervous system depressants such as opiates or benzodiazepines should be informed that they may experience additive CNS side effects, such as somnolence).
No products indexed under this heading.

Haloperidol Lactate (Patients who require concomitant treatment with central nervous system depressants such as opiates or benzodiazepines should be informed that they may experience additive CNS side effects, such as somnolence).
No products indexed under this heading.

Hexobarbital (Patients who require concomitant treatment with central nervous system depressants such as opiates or benzodiazepines should be informed that they may experience additive CNS side effects, such as somnolence).
No products indexed under this heading.

Hydrocodone Bitartrate (Patients who require concomitant treatment with central nervous system depressants such as opiates or benzodiazepines should be informed that they may experience additive CNS side effects, such as somnolence). Products include:
Vicodin 560
Vicodin ES 561
Vicodin HP 563
Vicoprofen 564
Zydone 1138

Hydrocodone Polistirex (Patients who require concomitant treatment with central nervous system depressants such as opiates or benzodiazepines should be informed that they may experience additive CNS side effects, such as somnolence). Products include:
Tussionex 3443

Hydromorphone (Patients who require concomitant treatment with central nervous system depressants such as opiates or benzodiazepines should be informed that they may experience additive CNS side effects, such as somnolence).
No products indexed under this heading.

Hydromorphone Hydrochloride (Patients who require concomitant treatment with central nervous system depressants such as opiates or benzodiazepines should be informed that they may experience additive CNS side effects, such as somnolence). Products include:
Dilaudid Injection 2800
Dilaudid Oral 2797
Dilaudid Tablets 2797
Dilaudid-HP 2800

Hydroxyzine Hydrochloride (Patients who require concomitant treatment with central nervous system depressants such as opiates or benzodiazepines should be informed that they may experience additive CNS side effects, such as somnolence).
No products indexed under this heading.

Lyrica | Interactions Index | 1094

Isoflurane (Patients who require concomitant treatment with central nervous system depressants such as opiates or benzodiazepines should be informed that they may experience additive CNS side effects, such as somnolence).
No products indexed under this heading.

Ketamine Hydrochloride (Patients who require concomitant treatment with central nervous system depressants such as opiates or benzodiazepines should be informed that they may experience additive CNS side effects, such as somnolence).
No products indexed under this heading.

Levomethadyl Acetate Hydrochloride (Patients who require concomitant treatment with central nervous system depressants such as opiates or benzodiazepines should be informed that they may experience additive CNS side effects, such as somnolence).
No products indexed under this heading.

Levorphanol Tartrate (Patients who require concomitant treatment with central nervous system depressants such as opiates or benzodiazepines should be informed that they may experience additive CNS side effects, such as somnolence).
No products indexed under this heading.

Lisinopril (Patients who are taking other drugs associated with angioedema (eg, angiotensin converting enzyme inhibitors [ACE inhibitors]) may be at increased risk of developing angioedema). Products include:
Prinivil ... 2241
Prinzide ... 2246

Lorazepam (Multiple oral doses of pregabalin were co-administered with oxycodone, lorazepam, or ethanol. Although no pharmacokinetic interactions were seen, additive effects on cognitive and gross motor functioning were seen when pregabalin was co-administered with these drugs).
No products indexed under this heading.

Loxapine Hydrochloride (Patients who require concomitant treatment with central nervous system depressants such as opiates or benzodiazepines should be informed that they may experience additive CNS side effects, such as somnolence).
No products indexed under this heading.

Loxapine Succinate (Patients who require concomitant treatment with central nervous system depressants such as opiates or benzodiazepines should be informed that they may experience additive CNS side effects, such as somnolence).
No products indexed under this heading.

Meperidine Hydrochloride (Patients who require concomitant treatment with central nervous system depressants such as opiates or benzodiazepines should be informed that they may experience additive CNS side effects, such as somnolence).
No products indexed under this heading.

Mephobarbital (Patients who require concomitant treatment with central nervous system depressants such as opiates or benzodiazepines should be informed that they may experience additive CNS side effects, such as somnolence).
No products indexed under this heading.

Meprobamate (Patients who require concomitant treatment with central nervous system depressants such as opiates or benzodiazepines should be informed that they may experience additive CNS side effects, such as somnolence).
No products indexed under this heading.

Mesoridazine Besylate (Patients who require concomitant treatment with central nervous system depressants such as opiates or benzodiazepines should be informed that they may experience additive CNS side effects, such as somnolence).
No products indexed under this heading.

Methadone Hydrochloride (Patients who require concomitant treatment with central nervous system depressants such as opiates or benzodiazepines should be informed that they may experience additive CNS side effects, such as somnolence).
No products indexed under this heading.

Methohexital Sodium (Patients who require concomitant treatment with central nervous system depressants such as opiates or benzodiazepines should be informed that they may experience additive CNS side effects, such as somnolence).
No products indexed under this heading.

Methotrimeprazine (Patients who require concomitant treatment with central nervous system depressants such as opiates or benzodiazepines should be informed that they may experience additive CNS side effects, such as somnolence).
No products indexed under this heading.

Methoxyflurane (Patients who require concomitant treatment with central nervous system depressants such as opiates or benzodiazepines should be informed that they may experience additive CNS side effects, such as somnolence).
No products indexed under this heading.

Midazolam Hydrochloride (Patients who require concomitant treatment with central nervous system depressants such as opiates or benzodiazepines should be informed that they may experience additive CNS side effects, such as somnolence).
No products indexed under this heading.

Moexipril Hydrochloride (Patients who are taking other drugs associated with angioedema (eg, angiotensin converting enzyme inhibitors [ACE inhibitors]) may be at increased risk of developing angioedema).
No products indexed under this heading.

Molindone Hydrochloride (Patients who require concomitant treatment with central nervous system depressants such as opiates or benzodiazepines should be informed that they may experience additive CNS side effects, such as somnolence). Products include:
Moban ... 1108

Morphine Sulfate (Patients who require concomitant treatment with central nervous system depressants such as opiates or benzodiazepines should be informed that they may experience additive CNS side effects, such as somnolence). Products include:
Avinza ... 1822
Embeda ... 1831
MS Contin ... 2803

Morphine Sulfate, Liposomal (Patients who require concomitant treatment with central nervous system depressants such as opiates or benzodiazepines should be informed that they may experience additive CNS side effects, such as somnolence).
No products indexed under this heading.

Olanzapine (Patients who require concomitant treatment with central nervous system depressants such as opiates or benzodiazepines should be informed that they may experience additive CNS side effects, such as somnolence). Products include:
Symbyax ... 1965
Zyprexa ... 1984
Zyprexa IntraMuscular ... 1984
Zyprexa ZYDIS ... 1984

Oxazepam (Patients who require concomitant treatment with central nervous system depressants such as opiates or benzodiazepines should be informed that they may experience additive CNS side effects, such as somnolence).
No products indexed under this heading.

Oxycodone Hydrochloride (Multiple oral doses of pregabalin were co-administered with oxycodone, lorazepam, or ethanol. Although no pharmacokinetic interactions were seen, additive effects on cognitive and gross motor functioning were seen when pregabalin was co-administered with these drugs). Products include:
OxyContin ... 2807
Percocet ... 1121
Percodan ... 1124

Oxycodone Terephthalate (Multiple oral doses of pregabalin were co-administered with oxycodone, lorazepam, or ethanol. Although no pharmacokinetic interactions were seen, additive effects on cognitive and gross motor functioning were seen when pregabalin was co-administered with these drugs).
No products indexed under this heading.

Oxymorphone Hydrochloride (Patients who require concomitant treatment with central nervous system depressants such as opiates or benzodiazepines should be informed that they may experience additive CNS side effects, such as somnolence). Products include:
Opana ... 1110
Opana ER ... 1114

Pentobarbital (Patients who require concomitant treatment with central nervous system depressants such as opiates or benzodiazepines should be informed that they may experience additive CNS side effects, such as somnolence).
No products indexed under this heading.

Pentobarbital Sodium (Patients who require concomitant treatment with central nervous system depressants such as opiates or benzodiazepines should be informed that they may experience additive CNS side effects, such as somnolence). Products include:
Nembutal ... 2012

Perindopril Erbumine (Patients who are taking other drugs associated with angioedema (eg, angiotensin converting enzyme inhibitors [ACE inhibitors]) may be at increased risk of developing angioedema).
No products indexed under this heading.

Perphenazine (Patients who require concomitant treatment with central nervous system depressants such as opiates or benzodiazepines should be informed that they may experience additive CNS side effects, such as somnolence).
No products indexed under this heading.

Phenobarbital (Patients who require concomitant treatment with central nervous system depressants such as opiates or benzodiazepines should be informed that they may experience additive CNS side effects, such as somnolence). Products include:
Donnatal ... 2711

Phenobarbital Sodium (Patients who require concomitant treatment with central nervous system depressants such as opiates or benzodiazepines should be informed that they may experience additive CNS side effects, such as somnolence).
No products indexed under this heading.

Pioglitazone Hydrochloride (Concomitant treatment with pregabalin and thiazolidinedione antididabetic agents may lead to an additive effect on edema and weight gain). Products include:
ActoPlus ... 3338
Actos ... 3345
Duetact ... 3354

Prazepam (Patients who require concomitant treatment with central nervous system depressants such as opiates or benzodiazepines should be informed that they may experience additive CNS side effects, such as somnolence).
No products indexed under this heading.

Prochlorperazine (Patients who require concomitant treatment with central nervous system depressants such as opiates or benzodiazepines should be informed that they may experience additive CNS side effects, such as somnolence).
No products indexed under this heading.

Prochlorperazine Edisylate (Patients who require concomitant treatment with central nervous system depressants such as opiates or benzodiazepines should be informed that they may experience additive CNS side effects, such as somnolence).
No products indexed under this heading.

Prochlorperazine Maleate (Patients who require concomitant treatment with central nervous system depressants such as opiates or benzodiazepines should be informed that they may experience additive CNS side effects, such as somnolence).
No products indexed under this heading.

Promethazine (Patients who require concomitant treatment with central nervous system depressants such as opiates or benzodiazepines should be informed that they may experience additive CNS side effects, such as somnolence).
No products indexed under this heading.

Promethazine Hydrochloride (Patients who require concomitant treatment with central nervous system depressants such as opiates or benzodiazepines should be informed that they may experience additive CNS side effects, such as somnolence).
No products indexed under this heading.

Propofol (Patients who require concomitant treatment with central nervous system depressants such as opiates or benzodiazepines should be informed that they may experience additive CNS side effects, such as somnolence).
No products indexed under this heading.

Propoxyphene Hydrochloride (Patients who require concomitant treatment with central nervous system depressants such as opiates or benzodiazepines should be informed that they may experience additive CNS side effects, such as somnolence).
No products indexed under this heading.

Propoxyphene Napsylate (Patients who require concomitant treatment with central nervous system depressants such as opiates or benzodiazepines should be informed that they may experience additive CNS side effects, such as somnolence).
No products indexed under this heading.

Quazepam (Patients who require concomitant treatment with central nervous system depressants such as opiates or benzodiazepines should be informed that they may experience additive CNS side effects, such as somnolence).
No products indexed under this heading.

Quetiapine Fumarate (Patients who require concomitant treatment with central nervous system depressants such as opiates or benzodiazepines should be informed that they may experience additive CNS side effects, such as somnolence). Products include:
Seroquel ... 750
Seroquel XR ... 759

Quinapril Hydrochloride (Patients who are taking other drugs associated with angioedema (eg, angiotensin converting enzyme inhibitors [ACE inhibitors]) may be at increased risk of developing angioedema).
No products indexed under this heading.

Ramipril (Patients who are taking other drugs associated with angioedema (eg, angiotensin converting enzyme inhibitors [ACE inhibitors]) may be at increased risk of developing angioedema).
No products indexed under this heading.

Remifentanil Hydrochloride (Patients who require concomitant treatment with central nervous system depressants such as opiates or benzodiazepines should be informed that they may experience additive CNS side effects, such as somnolence).
No products indexed under this heading.

Risperidone (Patients who require concomitant treatment with central nervous system depressants such as opiates or benzodiazepines should be informed that they may experience additive CNS side effects, such as somnolence). Products include:
Risperdal Consta 2682

Rosiglitazone (Concomitant treatment with pregabalin and thiazolidinedione antididabetic agents may lead to an additive effect on edema and weight gain).
No products indexed under this heading.

Rosiglitazone Maleate (Concomitant treatment with pregabalin and thiazolidinedione antididabetic agents may lead to an additive effect on edema and weight gain). Products include:
Avandamet 1345
Avandaryl 1356
Avandia 1366

Rosiglitazone/Metformin (Concomitant treatment with pregabalin and thiazolidinedione antididabetic agents may lead to an additive effect on edema and weight gain).
No products indexed under this heading.

Secobarbital Sodium (Patients who require concomitant treatment with central nervous system depressants such as opiates or benzodiazepines should be informed that they may experience additive CNS side effects, such as somnolence).
No products indexed under this heading.

Sevoflurane (Patients who require concomitant treatment with central nervous system depressants such as opiates or benzodiazepines should be informed that they may experience additive CNS side effects, such as somnolence). Products include:
Ultane 554

Sodium Butabarbital (Patients who require concomitant treatment with central nervous system depressants such as opiates or benzodiazepines should be informed that they may experience additive CNS side effects, such as somnolence).
No products indexed under this heading.

Sodium Oxybate (Patients who require concomitant treatment with central nervous system depressants such as opiates or benzodiazepines should be informed that they may experience additive CNS side effects, such as somnolence).
No products indexed under this heading.

Sodium Pentobarbital (Patients who require concomitant treatment with central nervous system depressants such as opiates or benzodiazepines should be informed that they may experience additive CNS side effects, such as somnolence).
No products indexed under this heading.

Spirapril Hydrochloride (Patients who are taking other drugs associated with angioedema (eg, angiotensin converting enzyme inhibitors [ACE inhibitors]) may be at increased risk of developing angioedema).
No products indexed under this heading.

Sufentanil Citrate (Patients who require concomitant treatment with central nervous system depressants such as opiates or benzodiazepines should be informed that they may experience additive CNS side effects, such as somnolence).
No products indexed under this heading.

Talbutal (Patients who require concomitant treatment with central nervous system depressants such as opiates or benzodiazepines should be informed that they may experience additive CNS side effects, such as somnolence).
No products indexed under this heading.

Temazepam (Patients who require concomitant treatment with central nervous system depressants such as opiates or benzodiazepines should be informed that they may experience additive CNS side effects, such as somnolence).
No products indexed under this heading.

Thiamylal Sodium (Patients who require concomitant treatment with central nervous system depressants such as opiates or benzodiazepines should be informed that they may experience additive CNS side effects, such as somnolence).
No products indexed under this heading.

Thioridazine (Patients who require concomitant treatment with central nervous system depressants such as opiates or benzodiazepines should be informed that they may experience additive CNS side effects, such as somnolence).
No products indexed under this heading.

Thioridazine Hydrochloride (Patients who require concomitant treatment with central nervous system depressants such as opiates or benzodiazepines should be informed that they may experience additive CNS side effects, such as somnolence). Products include:
Thioridazine Hydrochloride 2384

Thiothixene (Patients who require concomitant treatment with central nervous system depressants such as opiates or benzodiazepines should be informed that they may experience additive CNS side effects, such as somnolence). Products include:
Thiothixene 2386

Thiothixene Hydrochloride (Patients who require concomitant treatment with central nervous system depressants such as opiates or benzodiazepines should be informed that they may experience additive CNS side effects, such as somnolence).
No products indexed under this heading.

Trandolapril (Patients who are taking other drugs associated with angioedema (eg, angiotensin converting enzyme inhibitors [ACE inhibitors]) may be at increased risk of developing angioedema). Products include:
Mavik 489
Tarka 534

Triazolam (Patients who require concomitant treatment with central nervous system depressants such as opiates or benzodiazepines should be informed that they may experience additive CNS side effects, such as somnolence).
No products indexed under this heading.

Trifluoperazine Hydrochloride (Patients who require concomitant treatment with central nervous system depressants such as opiates or benzodiazepines should be informed that they may experience additive CNS side effects, such as somnolence).
No products indexed under this heading.

Zaleplon (Patients who require concomitant treatment with central nervous system depressants such as opiates or benzodiazepines should be informed that they may experience additive CNS side effects, such as somnolence).
No products indexed under this heading.

Ziprasidone Hydrochloride (Patients who require concomitant treatment with central nervous system depressants such as opiates or benzodiazepines should be informed that they may experience additive CNS side effects, such as somnolence). Products include:
Geodon 2723

Zolpidem Tartrate (Patients who require concomitant treatment with central nervous system depressants such as opiates or benzodiazepines should be informed that they may experience additive CNS side effects, such as somnolence). Products include:
Ambien 2920
Ambien CR 2925

Food Interactions

Alcohol (Patients who are taking other drugs associated with angioedema (eg, angiotensin converting enzyme inhibitors [ACE inhibitors]) may be at increased risk of developing angioedema).

Beer, reduced-alcohol (Patients who are taking other drugs associated with angioedema (eg, angiotensin converting enzyme inhibitors [ACE inhibitors]) may be at increased risk of developing angioedema).

Beer, unspecified (Patients who are taking other drugs associated with angioedema (eg, angiotensin converting enzyme inhibitors [ACE inhibitors]) may be at increased risk of developing angioedema).

Wine, Chianti (Patients who are taking other drugs associated with angioedema (eg, angiotensin converting enzyme inhibitors [ACE inhibitors]) may be at increased risk of developing angioedema).

Wine, Red (Patients who are taking other drugs associated with angioedema (eg, angiotensin converting enzyme inhibitors [ACE inhibitors]) may be at increased risk of developing angioedema).

Wine, unspecified (Patients who are taking other drugs associated with angioedema (eg, angiotensin converting enzyme inhibitors [ACE inhibitors]) may be at increased risk of developing angioedema).

Wine products (Patients who are taking other drugs associated with angioedema (eg, angiotensin converting enzyme inhibitors [ACE inhibitors]) may be at increased risk of developing angioedema).

MALARONE PEDIATRIC TABLETS

(Atovaquone, Proguanil Hydrochloride) 1572
See Malarone Tablets

MALARONE TABLETS

(Atovaquone, Proguanil Hydrochloride) 1572
May interact with oral anticoagulants, tetracyclines, and certain other agents. Compounds in these categories include:

Anisindione (Proguanil may potentiate the anticoagulant effect of warfarin and other coumarin-based anticoagulants. Caution is advised when initiating or withdrawing malaria prophylaxis or treatment in patients on continuous treatment with coumarin-based anticoagulants; suitable coagulation tests should be closely monitored).
No products indexed under this heading.

Demeclocycline Hydrochloride (Co-administration with tetracyclines has been associated with approximately a 40% reduction in plasma concentrations of atovaquone).
No products indexed under this heading.

Dicumarol (Proguanil may potentiate the anticoagulant effect of warfarin and other coumarin-based anticoagulants. Caution is advised when initiating or withdrawing malaria prophylaxis or treatment in patients on continuous treatment with coumarin-based anticoagulants; suitable coagulation tests should be closely monitored).
No products indexed under this heading.

Doxycycline (Co-administration with tetracyclines has been associated with approximately a 40% reduction in plasma concentrations of atovaquone).
No products indexed under this heading.

Doxycycline Calcium (Co-administration with tetracyclines has been associated with approximately a 40% reduction in plasma concentrations of atovaquone).
No products indexed under this heading.

Doxycycline Hyclate (Co-administration with tetracyclines has been associated with approximately a 40% reduction in plasma concentrations of atovaquone).
No products indexed under this heading.

Doxycycline Monohydrate (Co-administration with tetracyclines has been associated with approximately a 40% reduction in plasma concentrations of atovaquone).
No products indexed under this heading.

Indinavir Sulfate (Concomitant administration of atovaquone (750 mg BID with food for 14 days) and indinavir (800 mg TID without food for 14 days) resulted in a decrease in the C_{trough} of indinavir (23% decrease [90% CI 8%, 35%]). Caution should be exercised when prescribing atovaquone with indinavir due to the decrease in trough levels of indinavir). Products include:
Crixivan 2113

Methacycline Hydrochloride (Co-administration with tetracyclines has been associated with approximately a 40% reduction in plasma concentrations of atovaquone).
No products indexed under this heading.

Metoclopramide Hydrochloride (May reduce the bioavailability of atovaquone and should be used only if other antiemetics are not available). Products include:
Metozolv ODT 2901

Minocycline Hydrochloride (Co-administration with tetracyclines has been associated with approximately a 40% reduction in plasma concentrations of atovaquone). Products include:
Solodyn 2073

Oxytetracycline (Co-administration with tetracyclines has been associated with approximately a 40% reduction in plasma concentrations of atovaquone).
No products indexed under this heading.

Oxytetracycline Hydrochloride (Co-administration with tetracyclines has been associated with approximately a 40% reduction in plasma concentrations of atovaquone).
No products indexed under this heading.

IMPORTANT NOTE: Always consult each drug listing in the patient's regimen for possible interactions.

Malarone Interactions Index 1096

Rifabutin (Co-administration of rifabutin is known to reduce atovaquone levels by approximately 34%; concomitant therapy is not recommended).
No products indexed under this heading.

Rifampin (Co-administration of rifampin is known to reduce atovaquone levels by approximately 50%; concomitant therapy is not recommended).
No products indexed under this heading.

Tetracycline Hydrochloride (Co-administration with tetracyclines has been associated with approximately a 40% reduction in plasma concentrations of atovaquone). Products include:
Pylera 793

Tetracycline Phosphate Complex (Co-administration with tetracyclines has been associated with approximately a 40% reduction in plasma concentrations of atovaquone).
No products indexed under this heading.

Warfarin Sodium (Proguanil may potentiate the anticoagulant effect of warfarin and other coumarin-based anticoagulants. Caution is advised when initiating or withdrawing malaria prophylaxis or treatment in patients on continuous treatment with coumarin-based anticoagulants; suitable coagulation tests should be closely monitored).
No products indexed under this heading.

Food Interactions

Food, unspecified (Dietary fat intake with atovaquone increases the rate and extent of absorption; Malarone should be taken with food or milky drink).

MARINEOMEGA SOFTGEL CAPSULES

(Fatty Acids, Vitamin E) 2778
None cited in PDR database.

MARPLAN TABLETS

(Isocarboxazid) 3481
May interact with alcohols, amphetamines, anesthetics, antihistamines, antihypertensives, central nervous system depressants, dibenzazepines, diuretics, hypnotics and sedatives, monoamine oxidase inhibitors, narcotic analgesics, selective serotonin reuptake inhibitors, sympathomimetics, and certain other agents. Compounds in these categories include:

Acebutolol Hydrochloride (Isocarboxazid should not be used in combination with anti-hypertensive agents, including thiazide diuretics. A marked potentiating effect on these drugs has been reported, resulting in hypotension).
No products indexed under this heading.

Acrivastine (Isocarboxazid should not be administered in combination with antihistamines).
No products indexed under this heading.

Albuterol (Isocarboxazid should not be administered in combination with sympathomimetics, including amphetamines, or with over-the-counter drugs such as cold, hay fever, or weight-reducing preparations that contain vasoconstrictors).
No products indexed under this heading.

Albuterol Sulfate (Isocarboxazid should not be administered in combination with sympathomimetics, including amphetamines, or with over-the-counter drugs such as cold, hay fever, or weight-reducing preparations that contain vasoconstrictors). Products include:
ProAir HFA 3393
Proventil HFA 3204
Ventolin HFA 1708

Alfentanil Hydrochloride (Isocarboxazid should not be administered in combination with some central nervous system depressants including narcotic analgesics).
No products indexed under this heading.

Aliskiren (Isocarboxazid should not be used in combination with anti-hypertensive agents, including thiazide diuretics. A marked potentiating effect on these drugs has been reported, resulting in hypotension). Products include:
Tekturna 2538
Tekturna HCT 2541
Valturna 3637

Alprazolam (Isocarboxazid should not be administered in combination with central nervous system depressants).
No products indexed under this heading.

Amiloride Hydrochloride (Isocarboxazid should not be used in combination with anti-hypertensive agents, including thiazide diuretics. A marked potentiating effect on these drugs has been reported, resulting in hypotension).
No products indexed under this heading.

Amitriptyline Hydrochloride (Isocarboxazid should not be administered in combination with dibenzazepines. In patients being transferred to isocarboxazid from dibenzazepine-related entities, a medication-free interval of at least 1 week should be allowed, after which isocarboxazid therapy should be started using half the normal starting dosage for at least the first week of therapy. Similarly, at least 1 week should elapse between the discontinuation of isocarboxazid and initiation of other dibenzazepine-related entities, or the re-administration of isocarboxazid).
No products indexed under this heading.

Amlodipine Besylate (Isocarboxazid should not be used in combination with anti-hypertensive agents, including thiazide diuretics. A marked potentiating effect on these drugs has been reported, resulting in hypotension). Products include:
Azor 1010
Exforge 2443
Exforge HCT 2449

Amobarbital (Isocarboxazid should not be administered in combination with central nervous system depressants).
No products indexed under this heading.

Amobarbital Sodium (Isocarboxazid should not be administered in combination with central nervous system depressants).
No products indexed under this heading.

Amoxapine (Isocarboxazid should not be administered in combination with dibenzazepines. In patients being transferred to isocarboxazid from dibenzazepine-related entities, a medication-free interval of at least 1 week should be allowed, after which isocarboxazid therapy should be started using half the normal starting dosage for at least the first week of therapy. Similarly, at least 1 week should elapse between the discontinuation of isocarboxazid and initiation of other dibenzazepine-related entities, or the re-administration of isocarboxazid).
No products indexed under this heading.

Amphetamine Resins (Isocarboxazid should not be administered in combination with sympathomimetics including amphetamines).
No products indexed under this heading.

Amphetamine Sulfate (Isocarboxazid should not be administered in combination with sympathomimetics including amphetamines).
No products indexed under this heading.

Apomorphine (Isocarboxazid should not be administered in combination with some central nervous system depressants including narcotic analgesics).
No products indexed under this heading.

Apomorphine Hydrochloride (Isocarboxazid should not be administered in combination with some central nervous system depressants including narcotic analgesics).
No products indexed under this heading.

Aprobarbital (Isocarboxazid should not be administered in combination with central nervous system depressants).
No products indexed under this heading.

Articaine Hydrochloride (Isocarboxazid should not be administered in combination with anesthetic drugs. Patients taking isocarboxazid should not undergo elective surgery requiring general anesthesia. Also, they should not be given cocaine or local anesthesia containing sympathomimetic vasoconstrictors. The possible combined hypotensive effects of isocarboxazid and spinal anesthesia should be kept in mind. Isocarboxazid should be discontinued at least 10 days before elective surgery).
No products indexed under this heading.

Astemizole (Isocarboxazid should not be administered in combination with antihistamines).
No products indexed under this heading.

Atenolol (Isocarboxazid should not be used in combination with anti-hypertensive agents, including thiazide diuretics. A marked potentiating effect on these drugs has been reported, resulting in hypotension).
No products indexed under this heading.

Azatadine Maleate (Isocarboxazid should not be administered in combination with antihistamines).
No products indexed under this heading.

Benazepril Hydrochloride (Isocarboxazid should not be used in combination with anti-hypertensive agents, including thiazide diuretics. A marked potentiating effect on these drugs has been reported, resulting in hypotension).
No products indexed under this heading.

Bendroflumethiazide (Isocarboxazid should not be used in combination with anti-hypertensive agents, including thiazide diuretics. A marked potentiating effect on these drugs has been reported, resulting in hypotension).
No products indexed under this heading.

Benzocaine (Isocarboxazid should not be administered in combination with anesthetic drugs. Patients taking isocarboxazid should not undergo elective surgery requiring general anesthesia. Also, they should not be given cocaine or local anesthesia containing sympathomimetic vasoconstrictors. The possible combined hypotensive effects of isocarboxazid and spinal anesthesia should be kept in mind. Isocarboxazid should be discontinued at least 10 days before elective surgery).
No products indexed under this heading.

Betaxolol Hydrochloride (Isocarboxazid should not be used in combination with anti-hypertensive agents, including thiazide diuretics. A marked potentiating effect on these drugs has been reported, resulting in hypotension).
No products indexed under this heading.

Bisoprolol Fumarate (Isocarboxazid should not be used in combination with anti-hypertensive agents, including thiazide diuretics. A marked potentiating effect on these drugs has been reported, resulting in hypotension).
No products indexed under this heading.

Bromodiphenhydramine Hydrochloride (Isocarboxazid should not be administered in combination with antihistamines).
No products indexed under this heading.

Brompheniramine Maleate (Isocarboxazid should not be administered in combination with antihistamines).
No products indexed under this heading.

Bumetanide (Isocarboxazid should not be used in combination with anti-hypertensive agents, including thiazide diuretics. A marked potentiating effect on these drugs has been reported, resulting in hypotension).
No products indexed under this heading.

Bupivacaine Hydrochloride (Isocarboxazid should not be administered in combination with anesthetic drugs. Patients taking isocarboxazid should not undergo elective surgery requiring general anesthesia. Also, they should not be given cocaine or local anesthesia containing sympathomimetic vasoconstrictors. The possible combined hypotensive effects of isocarboxazid and spinal anesthesia should be kept in mind. Isocarboxazid should be discontinued at least 10 days before elective surgery).
No products indexed under this heading.

Buprenorphine Hydrochloride (Isocarboxazid should not be administered in combination with some central nervous system depressants including narcotic analgesics).
No products indexed under this heading.

Bupropion Hydrochloride (Isocarboxazid should not be administered in combination with bupropion hydrochloride. The concurrent administration of a MAOI and bupropion hydrochloride is contraindicated. At least 14 days should elapse between discontinuation of an MAOI and initiationof treatment with bupropion hydrochloride). Products include:
Aplenzin 2948
Wellbutrin 1719
Wellbutrin SR 1725
Zyban 1762

Buspirone Hydrochloride (Isocarboxazid should not be administered in combination with buspirone hydrochloride. At least 10 days should elapse between the discontinuation of isocarboxazid and the institution of buspirone hydrochloride).
No products indexed under this heading.

Butabarbital (Isocarboxazid should not be administered in combination with hypnotics and sedatives).
No products indexed under this heading.

Butabarbital Sodium (Isocarboxazid should not be administered in combination with hypnotics and sedatives).
No products indexed under this heading.

Butalbital (Isocarboxazid should not be administered in combination with hypnotics and sedatives).
No products indexed under this heading.

Caffeine (Isocarboxazid should not be administered in combination with excessive quantities of caffeine).
No products indexed under this heading.

Candesartan Cilexetil (Isocarboxazid should not be used in combination with anti-hypertensive agents, including thiazide diuretics. A marked potentiating effect on these drugs has been reported, resulting in hypotension). Products include:
Atacand 697
Atacand HCT 700

Captopril (Isocarboxazid should not be used in combination with anti-hypertensive agents, including thiazide diuretics. A marked potentiating effect

1097 Interactions Index Marplan

on these drugs has been reported, resulting in hypotension). Products include:
Captopril 2341

Carbamazepine (Isocarboxazid should not be administered in combination with dibenzazepines. In patients being transferred to isocarboxazid from dibenzazepine-related entities, a medication-free interval of at least 1 week should be allowed, after which isocarboxazid therapy should be started using half the normal starting dosage for at least the first week of therapy. Similarly, at least 1 week should elapse between the discontinuation of isocarboxazid and initiation of other dibenzazepine-related entities, or the re-administration of isocarboxazid). Products include:
Carbatrol 3280
Equetro 3477

Carteolol Hydrochloride (Isocarboxazid should not be used in combination with anti-hypertensive agents, including thiazide diuretics. A marked potentiating effect on these drugs has been reported, resulting in hypotension).
No products indexed under this heading.

Carvedilol (Isocarboxazid should not be used in combination with anti-hypertensive agents, including thiazide diuretics. A marked potentiating effect on these drugs has been reported, resulting in hypotension). Products include:
Coreg 1409

Carvedilol Phosphate (Isocarboxazid should not be used in combination with anti-hypertensive agents, including thiazide diuretics. A marked potentiating effect on these drugs has been reported, resulting in hypotension). Products include:
Coreg CR 1416

Cetirizine Hydrochloride (Isocarboxazid should not be administered in combination with antihistamines). Products include:
Zyrtec Allergy 2052
Children's Zyrtec Allergy Syrup 2053
Children's Zyrtec Allergy 2053
Children's Zyrtec Hives Relief 2053
Zyrtec-D Allergy & Congestion 2054

Chloral Hydrate (Isocarboxazid should not be administered in combination with hypnotics and sedatives).
No products indexed under this heading.

Chlordiazepoxide (Isocarboxazid should not be administered in combination with central nervous system depressants).
No products indexed under this heading.

Chlordiazepoxide Hydrochloride (Isocarboxazid should not be administered in combination with central nervous system depressants).
No products indexed under this heading.

Chloroprocaine Hydrochloride (Isocarboxazid should not be administered in combination with anesthetic drugs. Patients taking isocarboxazid should not undergo elective surgery requiring general anesthesia. Also, they should not be given cocaine or local anesthesia containing sympathomimetic vasoconstrictors. The possible combined hypotensive effects of isocarboxazid and spinal anesthesia should be kept in mind. Isocarboxazid should be discontinued at least 10 days before elective surgery).
No products indexed under this heading.

Chlorothiazide (Isocarboxazid should not be used in combination with anti-hypertensive agents, including thiazide diuretics. A marked potentiating effect on these drugs has been reported, resulting in hypotension).
No products indexed under this heading.

Chlorothiazide Sodium (Isocarboxazid should not be used in combination with anti-hypertensive agents, including thiazide diuretics. A marked potentiating effect on these drugs has been reported, resulting in hypotension). Products include:
Diuril Intravenous 2009

Chlorpheniramine Maleate (Isocarboxazid should not be administered in combination with antihistamines).
No products indexed under this heading.

Chlorpheniramine Polistirex (Isocarboxazid should not be administered in combination with antihistamines). Products include:
Tussionex 3443

Chlorpheniramine Tannate (Isocarboxazid should not be administered in combination with antihistamines).
No products indexed under this heading.

Chlorpromazine (Isocarboxazid should not be administered in combination with central nervous system depressants).
No products indexed under this heading.

Chlorpromazine Hydrochloride (Isocarboxazid should not be administered in combination with central nervous system depressants).
No products indexed under this heading.

Chlorprothixene (Isocarboxazid should not be administered in combination with central nervous system depressants).
No products indexed under this heading.

Chlorprothixene Hydrochloride (Isocarboxazid should not be administered in combination with central nervous system depressants).
No products indexed under this heading.

Chlorprothixene Lactate (Isocarboxazid should not be administered in combination with central nervous system depressants).
No products indexed under this heading.

Chlorthalidone (Isocarboxazid should not be used in combination with anti-hypertensive agents, including thiazide diuretics. A marked potentiating effect on these drugs has been reported, resulting in hypotension). Products include:
Clorpres 2344

Citalopram Hydrobromide (Isocarboxazid should not be administered in combination with any selective serotonin reuptake inhibitors. At least 2 weeks should be allowed after stopping sertraline or paroxetine before starting isocarboxazid. In addition, there should be an interval of at least 10 days between discontinuation of isocarboxazid and initiation of SSRIs). Products include:
Celexa 1153

Clemastine Fumarate (Isocarboxazid should not be administered in combination with antihistamines).
No products indexed under this heading.

Clomipramine Hydrochloride (Isocarboxazid should not be administered in combination with dibenzazepines. In patients being transferred to isocarboxazid from dibenzazepine-related entities, a medication-free interval of at least 1 week should be allowed, after which isocarboxazid therapy should be started using half the normal starting dosage for at least the first week of therapy. Similarly, at least 1 week should elapse between the discontinuation of isocarboxazid and initiation of other dibenzazepine-related entities, or the re-administration of isocarboxazid).
No products indexed under this heading.

Clonazepam (Isocarboxazid should not be administered in combination with central nervous system depressants). Products include:
Klonopin 2855

Clonidine (Isocarboxazid should not be used in combination with anti-hypertensive agents, including thiazide diuretics. A marked potentiating effect on these drugs has been reported, resulting in hypotension). Products include:
Catapres-TTS 884

Clonidine Hydrochloride (Isocarboxazid should not be used in combination with anti-hypertensive agents, including thiazide diuretics. A marked potentiating effect on these drugs has been reported, resulting in hypotension). Products include:
Clorpres 2344

Clorazepate Dipotassium (Isocarboxazid should not be administered in combination with central nervous system depressants).
No products indexed under this heading.

Clozapine (Isocarboxazid should not be administered in combination with dibenzazepines. In patients being transferred to isocarboxazid from dibenzazepine-related entities, a medication-free interval of at least 1 week should be allowed, after which isocarboxazid therapy should be started using half the normal starting dosage for at least the first week of therapy. Similarly, at least 1 week should elapse between the discontinuation of isocarboxazid and initiation of other dibenzazepine-related entities, or the re-administration of isocarboxazid).
No products indexed under this heading.

Cocaine Hydrochloride (Isocarboxazid should not be administered in combination with anesthetic drugs. Patients taking isocarboxazid should not undergo elective surgery requiring general anesthesia. Also, they should not be given cocaine or local anesthesia containing sympathomimetic vasoconstrictors. The possible combined hypotensive effects of isocarboxazid and spinal anesthesia should be kept in mind. Isocarboxazid should be discontinued at least 10 days before elective surgery).
No products indexed under this heading.

Codeine Phosphate (Isocarboxazid should not be administered in combination with some central nervous system depressants including narcotic analgesics). Products include:
Tylenol with Codeine 2691

Codeine Sulfate (Isocarboxazid should not be administered in combination with some central nervous system depressants including narcotic analgesics).
No products indexed under this heading.

Cyclobenzaprine Hydrochloride (Isocarboxazid should not be administered in combination with dibenzazepines. In patients being transferred to isocarboxazid from dibenzazepine-related entities, a medication-free interval of at least 1 week should be allowed, after which isocarboxazid therapy should be started using half the normal starting dosage for at least the first week of therapy. Similarly, at least 1 week should elapse between the discontinuation of isocarboxazid and initiation of other dibenzazepine-related entities, or the re-administration of isocarboxazid). Products include:
Amrix 964

Cyproheptadine Hydrochloride (Isocarboxazid should not be administered in combination with antihistamines).
No products indexed under this heading.

Deserpidine (Isocarboxazid should not be used in combination with anti-hypertensive agents, including thiazide diuretics. A marked potentiating effect on these drugs has been reported, resulting in hypotension).
No products indexed under this heading.

Desflurane (Isocarboxazid should not be administered in combination with central nervous system depressants).
No products indexed under this heading.

Desipramine Hydrochloride (Isocarboxazid should not be administered in combination with dibenzazepines. In patients being transferred to isocarboxazid from dibenzazepine-related entities, a medication-free interval of at least 1 week should be allowed, after which isocarboxazid therapy should be started using half the normal starting dosage for at least the first week of therapy. Similarly, at least 1 week should elapse between the discontinuation of isocarboxazid and initiation of other dibenzazepine-related entities, or the re-administration of isocarboxazid).
No products indexed under this heading.

Dexchlorpheniramine Maleate (Isocarboxazid should not be administered in combination with antihistamines).
No products indexed under this heading.

Dextroamphetamine Sulfate (Isocarboxazid should not be administered in combination with sympathomimetics including amphetamines). Products include:
Dexedrine 1425

Dextromethorphan (Isocarboxazid should not be administered in combination with dextromethorphan. The combination of MAO inhibitors and dextromethorphan has been reported to cause brief episodes of psychosis or bizarre behavior).
No products indexed under this heading.

Dezocine (Isocarboxazid should not be administered in combination with some central nervous system depressants including narcotic analgesics).
No products indexed under this heading.

Diazepam (Isocarboxazid should not be administered in combination with central nervous system depressants). Products include:
Valium Tablets 2880

Diazoxide (Isocarboxazid should not be used in combination with anti-hypertensive agents, including thiazide diuretics. A marked potentiating effect on these drugs has been reported, resulting in hypotension). Products include:
Proglycem 1179
Proglycem Suspension 1179

Dibucaine (Isocarboxazid should not be administered in combination with anesthetic drugs. Patients taking isocarboxazid should not undergo elective surgery requiring general anesthesia. Also, they should not be given cocaine or local anesthesia containing sympathomimetic vasoconstrictors. The possible combined hypotensive effects of isocarboxazid and spinal anesthesia should be kept in mind. Isocarboxazid should be discontinued at least 10 days before elective surgery).
No products indexed under this heading.

Dibucaine Hydrochloride (Isocarboxazid should not be administered in combination with anesthetic drugs. Patients taking isocarboxazid should not undergo elective surgery requiring general anesthesia. Also, they should not be given cocaine or local anesthesia containing sympathomimetic vasoconstrictors. The possible combined hypotensive effects of isocarboxazid and spinal anesthesia should be kept in mind. Isocarboxazid should be discontinued at least 10 days before elective surgery).
No products indexed under this heading.

IMPORTANT NOTE: Always consult each drug listing in the patient's regimen for possible interactions.

Marplan Interactions Index 1098

Dihydrocodeine Bitartrate (Isocarboxazid should not be administered in combination with some central nervous system depressants including narcotic analgesics).
No products indexed under this heading.

Dihydrocodeinone Bitartrate (Isocarboxazid should not be administered in combination with some central nervous system depressants including narcotic analgesics).
No products indexed under this heading.

Diltiazem Hydrochloride (Isocarboxazid should not be used in combination with anti-hypertensive agents, including thiazide diuretics. A marked potentiating effect on these drugs has been reported, resulting in hypotension). Products include:
Cardizem LA 423

Diltiazem Maleate (Isocarboxazid should not be used in combination with anti-hypertensive agents, including thiazide diuretics. A marked potentiating effect on these drugs has been reported, resulting in hypotension).
No products indexed under this heading.

Diphenhydramine Hydrochloride (Isocarboxazid should not be administered in combination with antihistamines). Products include:
Benadryl Allergy Ultratab 2042
Children's Benadryl Allergy Liquid 2042

Diphenylpyraline Hydrochloride (Isocarboxazid should not be administered in combination with antihistamines).
No products indexed under this heading.

Dobutamine Hydrochloride (Isocarboxazid should not be administered in combination with sympathomimetics, including amphetamines, or with over-the-counter drugs such as cold, hay fever, or weight-reducing preparations that contain vasoconstrictors).
No products indexed under this heading.

Dopamine Hydrochloride (Isocarboxazid should not be administered in combination with sympathomimetics, including amphetamines, or with over-the-counter drugs such as cold, hay fever, or weight-reducing preparations that contain vasoconstrictors).
No products indexed under this heading.

Doxazosin Mesylate (Isocarboxazid should not be used in combination with anti-hypertensive agents, including thiazide diuretics. A marked potentiating effect on these drugs has been reported, resulting in hypotension).
No products indexed under this heading.

Doxepin Hydrochloride (Isocarboxazid should not be administered in combination with dibenzazepines. In patients being transferred to isocarboxazid from dibenzazepine-related entities, a medication-free interval of at least 1 week should be allowed, after which isocarboxazid therapy should be started using half the normal starting dosage for at least the first week of therapy. Similarly, at least 1 week should elapse between the discontinuation of isocarboxazid and initiation of other dibenzazepine-related entities, or the re-administration of isocarboxazid).
No products indexed under this heading.

Droperidol (Isocarboxazid should not be administered in combination with central nervous system depressants).
No products indexed under this heading.

Enalapril Maleate (Isocarboxazid should not be used in combination with anti-hypertensive agents, including thiazide diuretics. A marked potentiating effect on these drugs has been reported, resulting in hypotension).
No products indexed under this heading.

Enalaprilat (Isocarboxazid should not be used in combination with anti-hypertensive agents, including thiazide diuretics. A marked potentiating effect on these drugs has been reported, resulting in hypotension).
No products indexed under this heading.

Enflurane (Isocarboxazid should not be administered in combination with anesthetic drugs. Patients taking isocarboxazid should not undergo elective surgery requiring general anesthesia. Also, they should not be given cocaine or local anesthesia containing sympathomimetic vasoconstrictors. The possible combined hypotensive effects of isocarboxazid and spinal anesthesia should be kept in mind. Isocarboxazid should be discontinued at least 10 days before elective surgery).
No products indexed under this heading.

Ephedrine Hydrochloride (Isocarboxazid should not be administered in combination with sympathomimetics, including amphetamines, or with over-the-counter drugs such as cold, hay fever, or weight-reducing preparations that contain vasoconstrictors).
No products indexed under this heading.

Ephedrine Sulfate (Isocarboxazid should not be administered in combination with sympathomimetics, including amphetamines, or with over-the-counter drugs such as cold, hay fever, or weight-reducing preparations that contain vasoconstrictors).
No products indexed under this heading.

Ephedrine Tannate (Isocarboxazid should not be administered in combination with sympathomimetics, including amphetamines, or with over-the-counter drugs such as cold, hay fever, or weight-reducing preparations that contain vasoconstrictors).
No products indexed under this heading.

Epinephrine (Isocarboxazid should not be administered in combination with sympathomimetics, including amphetamines, or with over-the-counter drugs such as cold, hay fever, or weight-reducing preparations that contain vasoconstrictors). Products include:
EpiPen 3631
Twinject 3268

Epinephrine Bitartrate (Isocarboxazid should not be administered in combination with sympathomimetics, including amphetamines, or with over-the-counter drugs such as cold, hay fever, or weight-reducing preparations that contain vasoconstrictors).
No products indexed under this heading.

Epinephrine Hydrochloride (Isocarboxazid should not be administered in combination with sympathomimetics, including amphetamines, or with over-the-counter drugs such as cold, hay fever, or weight-reducing preparations that contain vasoconstrictors).
No products indexed under this heading.

Eprosartan Mesylate (Isocarboxazid should not be used in combination with anti-hypertensive agents, including thiazide diuretics. A marked potentiating effect on these drugs has been reported, resulting in hypotension). Products include:
Teveten 538
Teveten HCT 541

Escitalopram Oxalate (Isocarboxazid should not be administered in combination with any selective serotonin reuptake inhibitors. At least 2 weeks should be allowed after stopping sertraline or paroxetine before starting isocarboxazid. In addition, there should be an interval of at least 10 days between discontinuation of isocarboxazid and initiation of SSRIs). Products include:
Lexapro Oral Suspension 1160
Lexapro Tablets 1160

Esmolol Hydrochloride (Isocarboxazid should not be used in combination with anti-hypertensive agents, including thiazide diuretics. A marked potentiating effect on these drugs has been reported, resulting in hypotension).
No products indexed under this heading.

Estazolam (Isocarboxazid should not be administered in combination with hypnotics and sedatives).
No products indexed under this heading.

Ethacrynic Acid (Isocarboxazid should not be used in combination with anti-hypertensive agents, including thiazide diuretics. A marked potentiating effect on these drugs has been reported, resulting in hypotension).
No products indexed under this heading.

Ethanol (Isocarboxazid should not be administered in combination with central nervous system depressants).
No products indexed under this heading.

Ethchlorvynol (Isocarboxazid should not be administered in combination with hypnotics and sedatives).
No products indexed under this heading.

Ethinamate (Isocarboxazid should not be administered in combination with hypnotics and sedatives).
No products indexed under this heading.

Ethyl Alcohol (Isocarboxazid should not be administered in combination with central nervous system depressants).
No products indexed under this heading.

Etidocaine Hydrochloride (Isocarboxazid should not be administered in combination with anesthetic drugs. Patients taking isocarboxazid should not undergo elective surgery requiring general anesthesia. Also, they should not be given cocaine or local anesthesia containing sympathomimetic vasoconstrictors. The possible combined hypotensive effects of isocarboxazid and spinal anesthesia should be kept in mind. Isocarboxazid should be discontinued at least 10 days before elective surgery).
No products indexed under this heading.

Felodipine (Isocarboxazid should not be used in combination with anti-hypertensive agents, including thiazide diuretics. A marked potentiating effect on these drugs has been reported, resulting in hypotension).
No products indexed under this heading.

Fentanyl (Isocarboxazid should not be administered in combination with some central nervous system depressants including narcotic analgesics). Products include:
Duragesic 2604
Fentanyl Transdermal System 2346
Onsolis 2054

Fentanyl Citrate (Isocarboxazid should not be administered in combination with some central nervous system depressants including narcotic analgesics). Products include:
Fentora 966

Fexofenadine Hydrochloride (Isocarboxazid should not be administered in combination with antihistamines). Products include:
Allegra ODT 2911
Allegra Oral Solution 2911
Allegra 2911
Allegra-D 2915
Allegra-D 24 2918

Fluoxetine (Isocarboxazid should not be administered in combination with any SSRI. There have been reports of serious, sometimes fatal, reactions in patients receiving fluoxetine in combination with a MAOI, and in patients who have recently discontinued fluoxetine and are then started on a MAOI. Fluoxetine and other SSRIs should not be used in combination with isocarboxazid, or within 14 days of discontinuing therapy with isocarboxazid. As fluoxetine and its major metabolite have very long elimination half-lives, at least 5 weeks should be allowed after stopping fluoxetine before starting isocarboxazid).
No products indexed under this heading.

Fluoxetine Hydrochloride (Isocarboxazid should not be administered in combination with any selective serotonin reuptake inhibitors. At least 2 weeks should be allowed after stopping sertraline or paroxetine before starting isocarboxazid. In addition, there should be an interval of at least 10 days between discontinuation of isocarboxazid and initiation of SSRIs). Products include:
Prozac Weekly 1941
Prozac Pulvules 1941
Symbyax 1965

Fluphenazine Decanoate (Isocarboxazid should not be administered in combination with central nervous system depressants).
No products indexed under this heading.

Fluphenazine Enanthate (Isocarboxazid should not be administered in combination with central nervous system depressants).
No products indexed under this heading.

Fluphenazine Hydrochloride (Isocarboxazid should not be administered in combination with central nervous system depressants).
No products indexed under this heading.

Flurazepam Hydrochloride (Isocarboxazid should not be administered in combination with hypnotics and sedatives).
No products indexed under this heading.

Fluvoxamine (Isocarboxazid should not be administered in combination with any selective serotonin reuptake inhibitors. At least 2 weeks should be allowed after stopping sertraline or paroxetine before starting isocarboxazid. In addition, there should be an interval of at least 10 days between discontinuation of isocarboxazid and initiation of SSRIs).
No products indexed under this heading.

Fluvoxamine Maleate (Isocarboxazid should not be administered in combination with any selective serotonin reuptake inhibitors. At least 2 weeks should be allowed after stopping sertraline or paroxetine before starting isocarboxazid. In addition, there should be an interval of at least 10 days between discontinuation of isocarboxazid and initiation of SSRIs).
No products indexed under this heading.

Fosinopril Sodium (Isocarboxazid should not be used in combination with anti-hypertensive agents, including thiazide diuretics. A marked potentiating effect on these drugs has been reported, resulting in hypotension).
No products indexed under this heading.

Furosemide (Isocarboxazid should not be used in combination with anti-hypertensive agents, including thiazide diuretics. A marked potentiating effect on these drugs has been reported, resulting in hypotension). Products include:
Furosemide 2354

Glutethimide (Isocarboxazid should not be administered in combination with hypnotics and sedatives).
No products indexed under this heading.

Guanabenz Acetate (Isocarboxazid should not be used in combination with anti-hypertensive agents, including thiazide diuretics. A marked potentiating effect on these drugs has been reported, resulting in hypotension).
No products indexed under this heading.

Guanethidine (Isocarboxazid should not be used in combination with anti-hypertensive agents, including thiazide diuretics. A marked potentiating effect on these drugs has been reported, resulting in hypotension).
No products indexed under this heading.

Guanethidine Monosulfate (Isocarboxazid should not be used in combination with anti-hypertensive agents, including thiazide diuretics. A marked potentiating effect on these drugs has been reported, resulting in hypotension).
No products indexed under this heading.

Guanethidine Sulfate (Isocarboxazid should not be used in combination with anti-hypertensive agents, including thiazide diuretics. A marked potentiating effect on these drugs has been reported, resulting in hypotension).
No products indexed under this heading.

Halazepam (Isocarboxazid should not be administered in combination with central nervous system depressants).
No products indexed under this heading.

Haloperidol (Isocarboxazid should not be administered in combination with central nervous system depressants).
No products indexed under this heading.

Haloperidol Decanoate (Isocarboxazid should not be administered in combination with central nervous system depressants).
No products indexed under this heading.

Haloperidol Lactate (Isocarboxazid should not be administered in combination with central nervous system depressants).
No products indexed under this heading.

Halothane (Isocarboxazid should not be administered in combination with anesthetic drugs. Patients taking isocarboxazid should not undergo elective surgery requiring general anesthesia. Also, they should not be given cocaine or local anesthesia containing sympathomimetic vasoconstrictors. The possible combined hypotensive effects of isocarboxazid and spinal anesthesia should be kept in mind. Isocarboxazid should be discontinued at least 10 days before elective surgery).
No products indexed under this heading.

Hexobarbital (Isocarboxazid should not be administered in combination with central nervous system depressants).
No products indexed under this heading.

Hydralazine Hydrochloride (Isocarboxazid should not be used in combination with anti-hypertensive agents, including thiazide diuretics. A marked potentiating effect on these drugs has been reported, resulting in hypotension).
No products indexed under this heading.

Hydrochlorothiazide (Isocarboxazid should not be used in combination with anti-hypertensive agents, including thiazide diuretics. A marked potentiating effect on these drugs has been reported, resulting in hypotension). Products include:
- Atacand HCT **700**
- Avalide **2956**
- Benicar HCT **1017**
- Diovan HCT **2419**
- Dyazide **1429**
- Exforge HCT **2449**
- Hyzaar **2162**
- Hyzaar 100-12.5 .... **2162**
- Micardis HCT **889**
- Prinzide **2246**
- Tekturna HCT **2541**
- Teveten HCT **541**

Hydrocodone Bitartrate (Isocarboxazid should not be administered in combination with some central nervous system depressants including narcotic analgesics). Products include:
- Vicodin **560**
- Vicodin ES **561**
- Vicodin HP **563**
- Vicoprofen **564**
- Zydone **1138**

Hydrocodone Polistirex (Isocarboxazid should not be administered in combination with some central nervous system depressants including narcotic analgesics). Products include:
- Tussionex **3443**

Hydroflumethiazide (Isocarboxazid should not be used in combination with anti-hypertensive agents, including thiazide diuretics. A marked potentiating effect on these drugs has been reported, resulting in hypotension).
No products indexed under this heading.

Hydromorphone (Isocarboxazid should not be administered in combination with some central nervous system depressants including narcotic analgesics).
No products indexed under this heading.

Hydromorphone Hydrochloride (Isocarboxazid should not be administered in combination with some central nervous system depressants including narcotic analgesics). Products include:
- Dilaudid Injection **2800**
- Dilaudid Oral **2797**
- Dilaudid Tablets **2797**
- Dilaudid-HP **2800**

Hydroxyzine Hydrochloride (Isocarboxazid should not be administered in combination with central nervous system depressants).
No products indexed under this heading.

Imipramine Hydrochloride (Isocarboxazid should not be administered in combination with dibenzazepines. In patients being transferred to isocarboxazid from dibenzazepine-related entities, a medication-free interval of at least 1 week should be allowed, after which isocarboxazid therapy should be started using half the normal starting dosage for at least the first week of therapy. Similarly, at least 1 week should elapse between the discontinuation of isocarboxazid and initiation of other dibenzazepine-related entities, or the re-administration of isocarboxazid).
No products indexed under this heading.

Imipramine Pamoate (Isocarboxazid should not be administered in combination with dibenzazepines. In patients being transferred to isocarboxazid from dibenzazepine-related entities, a medication-free interval of at least 1 week should be allowed, after which isocarboxazid therapy should be started using half the normal starting dosage for at least the first week of therapy. Similarly, at least 1 week should elapse between the discontinuation of isocarboxazid and initiation of other dibenzazepine-related entities, or the re-administration of isocarboxazid).
No products indexed under this heading.

Indapamide (Isocarboxazid should not be used in combination with anti-hypertensive agents, including thiazide diuretics. A marked potentiating effect on these drugs has been reported, resulting in hypotension). Products include:
- Indapamide **2356**

Irbesartan (Isocarboxazid should not be used in combination with anti-hypertensive agents, including thiazide diuretics. A marked potentiating effect on these drugs has been reported, resulting in hypotension). Products include:
- Avalide **2956**
- Avapro **2962**

Isoflurane (Isocarboxazid should not be administered in combination with anesthetic drugs. Patients taking isocarboxazid should not undergo elective surgery requiring general anesthesia. Also, they should not be given cocaine or local anesthesia containing sympathomimetic vasoconstrictors. The possible combined hypotensive effects of isocarboxazid and spinal anesthesia should be kept in mind. Isocarboxazid should be discontinued at least 10 days before elective surgery).
No products indexed under this heading.

Isoproterenol Hydrochloride (Isocarboxazid should not be administered in combination with sympathomimetics, including amphetamines, or with over-the-counter drugs such as cold, hay fever, or weight-reducing preparations that contain vasoconstrictors).
No products indexed under this heading.

Isoproterenol Sulfate (Isocarboxazid should not be administered in combination with sympathomimetics, including amphetamines, or with over-the-counter drugs such as cold, hay fever, or weight-reducing preparations that contain vasoconstrictors).
No products indexed under this heading.

Isradipine (Isocarboxazid should not be used in combination with anti-hypertensive agents, including thiazide diuretics. A marked potentiating effect on these drugs has been reported, resulting in hypotension). Products include:
- DynaCirc CR **1432**

Ketamine Hydrochloride (Isocarboxazid should not be administered in combination with anesthetic drugs. Patients taking isocarboxazid should not undergo elective surgery requiring general anesthesia. Also, they should not be given cocaine or local anesthesia containing sympathomimetic vasoconstrictors. The possible combined hypotensive effects of isocarboxazid and spinal anesthesia should be kept in mind. Isocarboxazid should be discontinued at least 10 days before elective surgery).
No products indexed under this heading.

Labetalol Hydrochloride (Isocarboxazid should not be used in combination with anti-hypertensive agents, including thiazide diuretics. A marked potentiating effect on these drugs has been reported, resulting in hypotension).
No products indexed under this heading.

Levalbuterol Hydrochloride (Isocarboxazid should not be administered in combination with sympathomimetics, including amphetamines, or with over-the-counter drugs such as cold, hay fever, or weight-reducing preparations that contain vasoconstrictors).
No products indexed under this heading.

Levobupivacaine Hydrochloride (Isocarboxazid should not be administered in combination with anesthetic drugs. Patients taking isocarboxazid should not undergo elective surgery requiring general anesthesia. Also, they should not be given cocaine or local anesthesia containing sympathomimetic vasoconstrictors. The possible combined hypotensive effects of isocarboxazid and spinal anesthesia should be kept in mind. Isocarboxazid should be discontinued at least 10 days before elective surgery).
No products indexed under this heading.

Levomethadyl Acetate Hydrochloride (Isocarboxazid should not be administered in combination with central nervous system depressants).
No products indexed under this heading.

Levorphanol Tartrate (Isocarboxazid should not be administered in combination with some central nervous system depressants including narcotic analgesics).
No products indexed under this heading.

Lidocaine (Isocarboxazid should not be administered in combination with anesthetic drugs. Patients taking isocarboxazid should not undergo elective surgery requiring general anesthesia. Also, they should not be given cocaine or local anesthesia containing sympathomimetic vasoconstrictors. The possible combined hypotensive effects of isocarboxazid and spinal anesthesia should be kept in mind. Isocarboxazid should be discontinued at least 10 days before elective surgery). Products include:
- Lidoderm **1107**

Lidocaine Base (Isocarboxazid should not be administered in combination with anesthetic drugs. Patients taking isocarboxazid should not undergo elective surgery requiring general anesthesia. Also, they should not be given cocaine or local anesthesia containing sympathomimetic vasoconstrictors. The possible combined hypotensive effects of isocarboxazid and spinal anesthesia should be kept in mind. Isocarboxazid should be discontinued at least 10 days before elective surgery).
No products indexed under this heading.

Lidocaine Hydrochloride (Isocarboxazid should not be administered in combination with anesthetic drugs. Patients taking isocarboxazid should not undergo elective surgery requiring general anesthesia. Also, they should not be given cocaine or local anesthesia containing sympathomimetic vasoconstrictors. The possible combined hypotensive effects of isocarboxazid and spinal anesthesia should be kept in mind. Isocarboxazid should be discontinued at least 10 days before elective surgery).
No products indexed under this heading.

Lisinopril (Isocarboxazid should not be used in combination with anti-hypertensive agents, including thiazide diuretics. A marked potentiating effect on these drugs has been reported, resulting in hypotension). Products include:
- Prinivil **2241**
- Prinzide **2246**

Loratadine (Isocarboxazid should not be administered in combination with antihistamines).
No products indexed under this heading.

Lorazepam (Isocarboxazid should not be administered in combination with hypnotics and sedatives).
No products indexed under this heading.

Losartan Potassium (Isocarboxazid should not be used in combination with anti-hypertensive agents, including thiazide diuretics. A marked potentiating effect on these drugs has been reported, resulting in hypotension). Products include:
- Cozaar **2106**
- Hyzaar **2162**
- Hyzaar 100-12.5 .... **2162**

Loxapine Hydrochloride (Isocarboxazid should not be administered in combination with central nervous system depressants).
No products indexed under this heading.

Loxapine Succinate (Isocarboxazid should not be administered in combination with central nervous system depressants).
No products indexed under this heading.

Maprotiline Hydrochloride (Isocarboxazid should not be administered in combination with dibenzazepines. In patients being transferred to isocarboxazid from dibenzazepine-related entities, a medication-free interval of at least 1 week should be allowed, after which isocarboxazid therapy should be started using half the normal starting dosage for at least the first week of therapy. Similarly, at least 1 week should elapse between the discontinuation of isocarboxazid and initiation of

Marplan Interactions Index 1100

other dibenzazepine-related entities, or the re-administration of isocarboxazid).
No products indexed under this heading.

Mecamylamine Hydrochloride (Isocarboxazid should not be used in combination with anti-hypertensive agents, including thiazide diuretics. A marked potentiating effect on these drugs has been reported, resulting in hypotension).
No products indexed under this heading.

Meperidine Hydrochloride (Meperidine should not be used concomitantly with MAOI or within 2 or 3 weeks following MAO therapy. Serious reactions have been precipitated with concomitant use).
No products indexed under this heading.

Mephobarbital (Isocarboxazid should not be administered in combination with central nervous system depressants).
No products indexed under this heading.

Mepivacaine Hydrochloride (Isocarboxazid should not be administered in combination with anesthetic drugs. Patients taking isocarboxazid should not undergo elective surgery requiring general anesthesia. Also, they should not be given cocaine or local anesthesia containing sympathomimetic vasoconstrictors. The possible combined hypotensive effects of isocarboxazid and spinal anesthesia should be kept in mind. Isocarboxazid should be discontinued at least 10 days before elective surgery).
No products indexed under this heading.

Meprobamate (Isocarboxazid should not be administered in combination with central nervous system depressants).
No products indexed under this heading.

Mesoridazine Besylate (Isocarboxazid should not be administered in combination with central nervous system depressants).
No products indexed under this heading.

Metaproterenol Sulfate (Isocarboxazid should not be administered in combination with sympathomimetics, including amphetamines, or with over-the-counter drugs such as cold, hay fever, or weight-reducing preparations that contain vasoconstrictors).
No products indexed under this heading.

Metaraminol Bitartrate (Isocarboxazid should not be administered in combination with sympathomimetics, including amphetamines, or with over-the-counter drugs such as cold, hay fever, or weight-reducing preparations that contain vasoconstrictors).
No products indexed under this heading.

Methadone Hydrochloride (Isocarboxazid should not be administered in combination with some central nervous system depressants including narcotic analgesics).
No products indexed under this heading.

Methamphetamine Hydrochloride (Isocarboxazid should not be administered in combination with sympathomimetics including amphetamines).
No products indexed under this heading.

Methdilazine Hydrochloride (Isocarboxazid should not be administered in combination with antihistamines).
No products indexed under this heading.

Methohexital Sodium (Isocarboxazid should not be administered in combination with anesthetic drugs. Patients taking isocarboxazid should not undergo elective surgery requiring general anesthesia. Also, they should not be given cocaine or local anesthesia containing sympathomimetic vasoconstrictors. The possible combined hypotensive effects of isocarboxazid and spinal anesthesia should be kept in mind. Isocarboxazid should be discontinued at least 10 days before elective surgery).
No products indexed under this heading.

Methotrimeprazine (Isocarboxazid should not be administered in combination with central nervous system depressants).
No products indexed under this heading.

Methoxamine Hydrochloride (Isocarboxazid should not be administered in combination with sympathomimetics, including amphetamines, or with over-the-counter drugs such as cold, hay fever, or weight-reducing preparations that contain vasoconstrictors).
No products indexed under this heading.

Methoxyflurane (Isocarboxazid should not be administered in combination with central nervous system depressants).
No products indexed under this heading.

Methyclothiazide (Isocarboxazid should not be used in combination with anti-hypertensive agents, including thiazide diuretics. A marked potentiating effect on these drugs has been reported, resulting in hypotension).
No products indexed under this heading.

Methyldopa (Isocarboxazid should not be used in combination with anti-hypertensive agents, including thiazide diuretics. A marked potentiating effect on these drugs has been reported, resulting in hypotension).
No products indexed under this heading.

Methyldopate Hydrochloride (Isocarboxazid should not be used in combination with anti-hypertensive agents, including thiazide diuretics. A marked potentiating effect on these drugs has been reported, resulting in hypotension).
No products indexed under this heading.

Metolazone (Isocarboxazid should not be used in combination with anti-hypertensive agents, including thiazide diuretics. A marked potentiating effect on these drugs has been reported, resulting in hypotension).
No products indexed under this heading.

Metoprolol Succinate (Isocarboxazid should not be used in combination with anti-hypertensive agents, including thiazide diuretics. A marked potentiating effect on these drugs has been reported, resulting in hypotension). Products include:
Toprol XL **732**

Metoprolol Tartrate (Isocarboxazid should not be used in combination with anti-hypertensive agents, including thiazide diuretics. A marked potentiating effect on these drugs has been reported, resulting in hypotension).
No products indexed under this heading.

Metyrosine (Isocarboxazid should not be used in combination with anti-hypertensive agents, including thiazide diuretics. A marked potentiating effect on these drugs has been reported, resulting in hypotension).
No products indexed under this heading.

Mibefradil Dihydrochloride (Isocarboxazid should not be used in combination with anti-hypertensive agents, including thiazide diuretics. A marked potentiating effect on these drugs has been reported, resulting in hypotension).
No products indexed under this heading.

Midazolam Hydrochloride (Isocarboxazid should not be administered in combination with anesthetic drugs. Patients taking isocarboxazid should not undergo elective surgery requiring general anesthesia. Also, they should not be given cocaine or local anesthesia containing sympathomimetic vasoconstrictors. The possible combined hypotensive effects of isocarboxazid and spinal anesthesia should be kept in mind. Isocarboxazid should be discontinued at least 10 days before elective surgery).
No products indexed under this heading.

Minoxidil (Isocarboxazid should not be used in combination with anti-hypertensive agents, including thiazide diuretics. A marked potentiating effect on these drugs has been reported, resulting in hypotension).
No products indexed under this heading.

Moclobemide (Isocarboxazid should not be administered in combination with monoamine oxidase inhibitors. In patients being transferred to isocarboxazid from other MAOI, a medication-free interval of at least 1 week should be allowed, after which isocarboxazid therapy should be started using half the normal starting dosage for at least the first week of therapy. Similarly, at least 1 week should elapse between the discontinuation of isocarboxazid and initiation of another MAOI, or the re-administration of isocarboxazid).
No products indexed under this heading.

Moexipril Hydrochloride (Isocarboxazid should not be used in combination with anti-hypertensive agents, including thiazide diuretics. A marked potentiating effect on these drugs has been reported, resulting in hypotension).
No products indexed under this heading.

Molindone Hydrochloride (Isocarboxazid should not be administered in combination with central nervous system depressants). Products include:
Moban **1108**

Morphine Sulfate (Isocarboxazid should not be administered in combination with some central nervous system depressants including narcotic analgesics). Products include:
Avinza **1822**
Embeda **1831**
MS Contin **2803**

Morphine Sulfate, Liposomal (Isocarboxazid should not be administered in combination with some central nervous system depressants including narcotic analgesics).
No products indexed under this heading.

Nadolol (Isocarboxazid should not be used in combination with anti-hypertensive agents, including thiazide diuretics. A marked potentiating effect on these drugs has been reported, resulting in hypotension). Products include:
Nadolol **2359**

Nebivolol (Isocarboxazid should not be used in combination with anti-hypertensive agents, including thiazide diuretics. A marked potentiating effect on these drugs has been reported, resulting in hypotension). Products include:
Bystolic **1147**

Nicardipine Hydrochloride (Isocarboxazid should not be used in combination with anti-hypertensive agents, including thiazide diuretics. A marked potentiating effect on these drugs has been reported, resulting in hypotension).
No products indexed under this heading.

Nifedipine (Isocarboxazid should not be used in combination with anti-hypertensive agents, including thiazide diuretics. A marked potentiating effect on these drugs has been reported, resulting in hypotension).
No products indexed under this heading.

Nisoldipine (Isocarboxazid should not be used in combination with anti-hypertensive agents, including thiazide diuretics. A marked potentiating effect on these drugs has been reported, resulting in hypotension).
No products indexed under this heading.

Nitroglycerin (Isocarboxazid should not be used in combination with anti-hypertensive agents, including thiazide diuretics. A marked potentiating effect on these drugs has been reported, resulting in hypotension). Products include:
Nitro-Dur **3170**
Nitrolingual **3266**

Norepinephrine Bitartrate (Isocarboxazid should not be administered in combination with sympathomimetics, including amphetamines, or with over-the-counter drugs such as cold, hay fever, or weight-reducing preparations that contain vasoconstrictors).
No products indexed under this heading.

Nortriptyline Hydrochloride (Isocarboxazid should not be administered in combination with dibenzazepines. In patients being transferred to isocarboxazid from dibenzazepine-related entities, a medication-free interval of at least 1 week should be allowed, after which isocarboxazid therapy should be started using half the normal starting dosage for at least the first week of therapy. Similarly, at least 1 week should elapse between the discontinuation of isocarboxazid and initiation of other dibenzazepine-related entities, or the re-administration of isocarboxazid).
No products indexed under this heading.

Olanzapine (Isocarboxazid should not be administered in combination with central nervous system depressants). Products include:
Symbyax **1965**
Zyprexa **1984**
Zyprexa IntraMuscular **1984**
Zyprexa ZYDIS **1984**

Oxazepam (Isocarboxazid should not be administered in combination with central nervous system depressants).
No products indexed under this heading.

Oxycodone Hydrochloride (Isocarboxazid should not be administered in combination with some central nervous system depressants including narcotic analgesics). Products include:
OxyContin **2807**
Percocet **1121**
Percodan **1124**

Oxycodone Terephthalate (Isocarboxazid should not be administered in combination with some central nervous system depressants including narcotic analgesics).
No products indexed under this heading.

Oxymorphone Hydrochloride (Isocarboxazid should not be administered in combination with some central nervous system depressants including narcotic analgesics). Products include:
Opana **1110**
Opana ER **1114**

Pargyline Hydrochloride (Isocarboxazid should not be administered in combination with monoamine oxidase inhibitors. In patients being transferred to isocarboxazid from other MAOI, a medication-free interval of at least 1 week should be allowed, after which isocarboxazid therapy should be started using half the normal starting dosage for at least the first week of therapy. Similarly, at least 1 week should elapse between the discontinuation of isocarboxazid and initiation of another MAOI, or the re-administration of isocarboxazid).
No products indexed under this heading.

Paroxetine (Isocarboxazid should not be administered in combination with any selective serotonin reuptake inhibitors. At least 2 weeks should be allowed after stopping sertraline or paroxetine before starting isocarboxazid. In addition, there should be an interval of at least 10 days between discontinuation of isocarboxazid and initiation of SSRIs).
No products indexed under this heading.

(⊙ Described in PDR® for Ophthalmic Medicines)

Paroxetine Hydrochloride (Isocarboxazid should not be administered in combination with any selective serotonin reuptake inhibitors. At least 2 weeks should be allowed after stopping paroxetine before starting isocarboxazid. In addition, there should be an interval of at least 10 days between discontinuation of isocarboxazid and initiation of SSRIs). Products include:

Paroxetine CR **2361**
Paroxetine ER **2371**
Paxil **1586**
Paxil CR **1596**

Paroxetine Mesylate (Isocarboxazid should not be administered in combination with any selective serotonin reuptake inhibitors. At least 2 weeks should be allowed after stopping sertraline or paroxetine before starting isocarboxazid. In addition, there should be an interval of at least 10 days between discontinuation of isocarboxazid and initiation of SSRIs).
No products indexed under this heading.

Penbutolol Sulfate (Isocarboxazid should not be used in combination with anti-hypertensive agents, including thiazide diuretics. A marked potentiating effect on these drugs has been reported, resulting in hypotension).
No products indexed under this heading.

Pentobarbital (Isocarboxazid should not be administered in combination with central nervous system depressants).
No products indexed under this heading.

Pentobarbital Sodium (Isocarboxazid should not be administered in combination with central nervous system depressants). Products include:

Nembutal **2012**

Perindopril Erbumine (Isocarboxazid should not be used in combination with anti-hypertensive agents, including thiazide diuretics. A marked potentiating effect on these drugs has been reported, resulting in hypotension).
No products indexed under this heading.

Perphenazine (Isocarboxazid should not be administered in combination with central nervous system depressants).
No products indexed under this heading.

Phenelzine Sulfate (Isocarboxazid should not be administered in combination with monoamine oxidase inhibitors. In patients being transferred to isocarboxazid from other MAOI, a medication-free interval of at least 1 week should be allowed, after which isocarboxazid therapy should be started using half the normal starting dosage for at least the first week of therapy. Similarly, at least 1 week should elapse between the discontinuation of isocarboxazid and initiation of another MAOI, or the re-administration of isocarboxazid).
No products indexed under this heading.

Phenobarbital (Isocarboxazid should not be administered in combination with central nervous system depressants). Products include:

Donnatal **2711**

Phenobarbital Sodium (Isocarboxazid should not be administered in combination with central nervous system depressants).
No products indexed under this heading.

Phenoxybenzamine Hydrochloride (Isocarboxazid should not be used in combination with anti-hypertensive agents, including thiazide diuretics. A marked potentiating effect on these drugs has been reported, resulting in hypotension). Products include:

Dibenzyline **3495**

Phentolamine Mesylate (Isocarboxazid should not be used in combination with anti-hypertensive agents, including thiazide diuretics. A marked potentiating effect on these drugs has been reported, resulting in hypotension).
No products indexed under this heading.

Phenylephrine Bitartrate (Isocarboxazid should not be administered in combination with sympathomimetics, including amphetamines, or with over-the-counter drugs such as cold, hay fever, or weight-reducing preparations that contain vasoconstrictors).
No products indexed under this heading.

Phenylephrine Hydrochloride (Isocarboxazid should not be administered in combination with sympathomimetics, including amphetamines, or with over-the-counter drugs such as cold, hay fever, or weight-reducing preparations that contain vasoconstrictors). Products include:

Sudafed PE Nasal Decongestant **2048**
Children's Sudafed PE Nasal Decongestant **2047**

Phenylephrine Tannate (Isocarboxazid should not be administered in combination with sympathomimetics, including amphetamines, or with over-the-counter drugs such as cold, hay fever, or weight-reducing preparations that contain vasoconstrictors).
No products indexed under this heading.

Phenylpropanolamine Hydrochloride (Isocarboxazid should not be administered in combination with sympathomimetics, including amphetamines, or with over-the-counter drugs such as cold, hay fever, or weight-reducing preparations that contain vasoconstrictors).
No products indexed under this heading.

Pindolol (Isocarboxazid should not be used in combination with anti-hypertensive agents, including thiazide diuretics. A marked potentiating effect on these drugs has been reported, resulting in hypotension).
No products indexed under this heading.

Pirbuterol Acetate (Isocarboxazid should not be administered in combination with sympathomimetics, including amphetamines, or with over-the-counter drugs such as cold, hay fever, or weight-reducing preparations that contain vasoconstrictors). Products include:

Maxair Autohaler **1782**

Polythiazide (Isocarboxazid should not be used in combination with anti-hypertensive agents, including thiazide diuretics. A marked potentiating effect on these drugs has been reported, resulting in hypotension).
No products indexed under this heading.

Prazepam (Isocarboxazid should not be administered in combination with central nervous system depressants).
No products indexed under this heading.

Prazosin Hydrochloride (Isocarboxazid should not be used in combination with anti-hypertensive agents, including thiazide diuretics. A marked potentiating effect on these drugs has been reported, resulting in hypotension).
No products indexed under this heading.

Prilocaine (Isocarboxazid should not be administered in combination with anesthetic drugs. Patients taking isocarboxazid should not undergo elective surgery requiring general anesthesia. Also, they should not be given cocaine or local anesthesia containing sympathomimetic vasoconstrictors. The possible combined hypotensive effects of isocarboxazid and spinal anesthesia should be kept in mind. Isocarboxazid should be discontinued at least 10 days before elective surgery).
No products indexed under this heading.

Prilocaine Hydrochloride (Isocarboxazid should not be administered in combination with anesthetic drugs. Patients taking isocarboxazid should not undergo elective surgery requiring general anesthesia. Also, they should not be given cocaine or local anesthesia containing sympathomimetic vasoconstrictors. The possible combined hypotensive effects of isocarboxazid and spinal anesthesia should be kept in mind. Isocarboxazid should be discontinued at least 10 days before elective surgery).
No products indexed under this heading.

Procaine (Isocarboxazid should not be administered in combination with anesthetic drugs. Patients taking isocarboxazid should not undergo elective surgery requiring general anesthesia. Also, they should not be given cocaine or local anesthesia containing sympathomimetic vasoconstrictors. The possible combined hypotensive effects of isocarboxazid and spinal anesthesia should be kept in mind. Isocarboxazid should be discontinued at least 10 days before elective surgery).
No products indexed under this heading.

Procaine Hydrochloride (Isocarboxazid should not be administered in combination with anesthetic drugs. Patients taking isocarboxazid should not undergo elective surgery requiring general anesthesia. Also, they should not be given cocaine or local anesthesia containing sympathomimetic vasoconstrictors. The possible combined hypotensive effects of isocarboxazid and spinal anesthesia should be kept in mind. Isocarboxazid should be discontinued at least 10 days before elective surgery).
No products indexed under this heading.

Procarbazine Hydrochloride (Isocarboxazid should not be administered in combination with monoamine oxidase inhibitors. In patients being transferred to isocarboxazid from other MAOI, a medication-free interval of at least 1 week should be allowed, after which isocarboxazid therapy should be started using half the normal starting dosage for at least the first week of therapy. Similarly, at least 1 week should elapse between the discontinuation of isocarboxazid and initiation of another MAOI, or the re-administration of isocarboxazid).
No products indexed under this heading.

Prochlorperazine (Isocarboxazid should not be administered in combination with central nervous system depressants).
No products indexed under this heading.

Prochlorperazine Edisylate (Isocarboxazid should not be administered in combination with central nervous system depressants).
No products indexed under this heading.

Prochlorperazine Maleate (Isocarboxazid should not be administered in combination with central nervous system depressants).
No products indexed under this heading.

Promethazine (Isocarboxazid should not be administered in combination with central nervous system depressants).
No products indexed under this heading.

Promethazine Hydrochloride (Isocarboxazid should not be administered in combination with antihistamines).
No products indexed under this heading.

Proparacaine Hydrochloride (Isocarboxazid should not be administered in combination with anesthetic drugs. Patients taking isocarboxazid should not undergo elective surgery requiring general anesthesia. Also, they should not be given cocaine or local anesthesia containing sympathomimetic vasoconstrictors. The possible combined hypotensive effects of isocarboxazid and spinal anesthesia should be kept in mind. Isocarboxazid should be discontinued at least 10 days before elective surgery).
No products indexed under this heading.

Propofol (Isocarboxazid should not be administered in combination with anesthetic drugs. Patients taking isocarboxazid should not undergo elective surgery requiring general anesthesia. Also, they should not be given cocaine or local anesthesia containing sympathomimetic vasoconstrictors. The possible combined hypotensive effects of isocarboxazid and spinal anesthesia should be kept in mind. Isocarboxazid should be discontinued at least 10 days before elective surgery).
No products indexed under this heading.

Propoxyphene Hydrochloride (Isocarboxazid should not be administered in combination with some central nervous system depressants including narcotic analgesics).
No products indexed under this heading.

Propoxyphene Napsylate (Isocarboxazid should not be administered in combination with some central nervous system depressants including narcotic analgesics).
No products indexed under this heading.

Propranolol Hydrochloride (Isocarboxazid should not be used in combination with anti-hypertensive agents, including thiazide diuretics. A marked potentiating effect on these drugs has been reported, resulting in hypotension). Products include:

InnoPran XL **1517**

Protriptyline Hydrochloride (Isocarboxazid should not be administered in combination with dibenzazepines. In patients being transferred to isocarboxazid from dibenzazepine-related entities, a medication-free interval of at least 1 week should be allowed, after which isocarboxazid therapy should be started using half the normal starting dosage for at least the first week of therapy. Similarly, at least 1 week should elapse between the discontinuation of isocarboxazid and initiation of other dibenzazepine-related entities, or the re-administration of isocarboxazid).
No products indexed under this heading.

Pseudoephedrine Hydrochloride (Isocarboxazid should not be administered in combination with sympathomimetics, including amphetamines, or with over-the-counter drugs such as cold, hay fever, or weight-reducing preparations that contain vasoconstrictors). Products include:

Allegra-D **2915**
Allegra-D 24 .... **2918**
Sudafed 12 Hour Nasal Decongestant Non-Drowsy **2048**
Sudafed 24 Hour **2048**
Sudafed Nasal Decongestant **2047**
Children's Sudafed Nasal Decongestant Liquid **2047**
Zyrtec-D Allergy & Congestion **2054**

Pseudoephedrine Sulfate (Isocarboxazid should not be administered in combination with sympathomimetics, including amphetamines, or with over-the-counter drugs such as cold, hay fever, or weight-reducing preparations that contain vasoconstrictors). Products include:

Clarinex-D 12-Hour **3101**
Clarinex-D **3104**

Pyrilamine Maleate (Isocarboxazid should not be administered in combination with antihistamines).
No products indexed under this heading.

Pyrilamine Tannate (Isocarboxazid should not be administered in combination with antihistamines).
No products indexed under this heading.

IMPORTANT NOTE: Always consult each drug listing in the patient's regimen for possible interactions.

Marplan Interactions Index 1102

Quazepam (Isocarboxazid should not be administered in combination with hypnotics and sedatives).
No products indexed under this heading.

Quetiapine Fumarate (Isocarboxazid should not be administered in combination with central nervous system depressants). Products include:
Seroquel **750**
Seroquel XR **759**

Quinapril Hydrochloride (Isocarboxazid should not be used in combination with anti-hypertensive agents, including thiazide diuretics. A marked potentiating effect on these drugs has been reported, resulting in hypotension).
No products indexed under this heading.

Ramelteon (Isocarboxazid should not be administered in combination with hypnotics and sedatives). Products include:
Rozerem **3366**

Ramipril (Isocarboxazid should not be used in combination with anti-hypertensive agents, including thiazide diuretics. A marked potentiating effect on these drugs has been reported, resulting in hypotension).
No products indexed under this heading.

Rasagiline Mesylate (Isocarboxazid should not be administered in combination with monoamine oxidase inhibitors. In patients being transferred to isocarboxazid from other MAOI, a medication-free interval of at least 1 week should be allowed, after which isocarboxazid therapy should be started using half the normal starting dosage for at least the first week of therapy. Similarly, at least 1 week should elapse between the discontinuation of isocarboxazid and initiation of another MAOI, or the re-administration of isocarboxazid). Products include:
Azilect **3383**

Rauwolfia Serpentina (Isocarboxazid should not be used in combination with anti-hypertensive agents, including thiazide diuretics. A marked potentiating effect on these drugs has been reported, resulting in hypotension).
No products indexed under this heading.

Remifentanil Hydrochloride (Isocarboxazid should not be administered in combination with some central nervous system depressants including narcotic analgesics).
No products indexed under this heading.

Rescinnamine (Isocarboxazid should not be used in combination with anti-hypertensive agents, including thiazide diuretics. A marked potentiating effect on these drugs has been reported, resulting in hypotension).
No products indexed under this heading.

Reserpine (Isocarboxazid should not be used in combination with anti-hypertensive agents, including thiazide diuretics. A marked potentiating effect on these drugs has been reported, resulting in hypotension).
No products indexed under this heading.

Risperidone (Isocarboxazid should not be administered in combination with central nervous system depressants). Products include:
Risperdal Consta **2682**

Ropivacaine Hydrochloride (Isocarboxazid should not be administered in combination with anesthetic drugs. Patients taking isocarboxazid should not undergo elective surgery requiring general anesthesia. Also, they should not be given cocaine or local anesthesia containing sympathomimetic vasoconstrictors. The possible combined hypotensive effects of isocarboxazid and spinal anesthesia should be kept in mind. Isocarboxazid should be discontinued at least 10 days before elective surgery).
No products indexed under this heading.

Salmeterol Xinafoate (Isocarboxazid should not be administered in combination with sympathomimetics, including amphetamines, or with over-the-counter drugs such as cold, hay fever, or weight-reducing preparations that contain vasoconstrictors). Products include:
Advair 100/50 .... **1275**
Advair 250/50 .... **1275**
Advair 500/50 .... **1275**
Advair HFA 45/21 .... **1288**
Advair HFA 115/21 .... **1288**
Advair HFA 230/21 .... **1288**
Serevent Diskus **1656**

Secobarbital Sodium (Isocarboxazid should not be administered in combination with hypnotics and sedatives).
No products indexed under this heading.

Selegiline (Isocarboxazid should not be administered in combination with monoamine oxidase inhibitors. In patients being transferred to isocarboxazid from other MAOI, a medication-free interval of at least 1 week should be allowed, after which isocarboxazid therapy should be started using half the normal starting dosage for at least the first week of therapy. Similarly, at least 1 week should elapse between the discontinuation of isocarboxazid and initiation of another MAOI, or the re-administration of isocarboxazid). Products include:
Emsam **3623**

Selegiline Hydrochloride (Isocarboxazid should not be administered in combination with monoamine oxidase inhibitors. In patients being transferred to isocarboxazid from other MAOI, a medication-free interval of at least 1 week should be allowed, after which isocarboxazid therapy should be started using half the normal starting dosage for at least the first week of therapy. Similarly, at least 1 week should elapse between the discontinuation of isocarboxazid and initiation of another MAOI, or the re-administration of isocarboxazid). Products include:
Eldepryl **3312**

Sertraline Hydrochloride (Isocarboxazid should not be administered in combination with any selective serotonin reuptake inhibitors. At least 2 weeks should be allowed after stopping sertraline before starting isocarboxazid. In addition, there should be an interval of at least 10 days between discontinuation of isocarboxazid and initiation of SSRIs).
No products indexed under this heading.

Sevoflurane (Isocarboxazid should not be administered in combination with central nervous system depressants). Products include:
Ultane **554**

Sodium Butabarbital (Isocarboxazid should not be administered in combination with hypnotics and sedatives).
No products indexed under this heading.

Sodium Nitroprusside (Isocarboxazid should not be used in combination with anti-hypertensive agents, including thiazide diuretics. A marked potentiating effect on these drugs has been reported, resulting in hypotension).
No products indexed under this heading.

Sodium Oxybate (Isocarboxazid should not be administered in combination with central nervous system depressants).
No products indexed under this heading.

Sodium Pentobarbital (Isocarboxazid should not be administered in combination with central nervous system depressants).
No products indexed under this heading.

Sotalol Hydrochloride (Isocarboxazid should not be used in combination with anti-hypertensive agents, including thiazide diuretics. A marked potentiating effect on these drugs has been reported, resulting in hypotension).
No products indexed under this heading.

Spirapril Hydrochloride (Isocarboxazid should not be used in combination with anti-hypertensive agents, including thiazide diuretics. A marked potentiating effect on these drugs has been reported, resulting in hypotension).
No products indexed under this heading.

Spironolactone (Isocarboxazid should not be used in combination with anti-hypertensive agents, including thiazide diuretics. A marked potentiating effect on these drugs has been reported, resulting in hypotension).
No products indexed under this heading.

Sufentanil Citrate (Isocarboxazid should not be administered in combination with some central nervous system depressants including narcotic analgesics).
No products indexed under this heading.

Talbutal (Isocarboxazid should not be administered in combination with central nervous system depressants).
No products indexed under this heading.

Telmisartan (Isocarboxazid should not be used in combination with anti-hypertensive agents, including thiazide diuretics. A marked potentiating effect on these drugs has been reported, resulting in hypotension). Products include:
Micardis **887**
Micardis HCT **889**

Temazepam (Isocarboxazid should not be administered in combination with hypnotics and sedatives).
No products indexed under this heading.

Terazosin Hydrochloride (Isocarboxazid should not be used in combination with anti-hypertensive agents, including thiazide diuretics. A marked potentiating effect on these drugs has been reported, resulting in hypotension).
No products indexed under this heading.

Terbutaline Sulfate (Isocarboxazid should not be administered in combination with sympathomimetics, including amphetamines, or with over-the-counter drugs such as cold, hay fever, or weight-reducing preparations that contain vasoconstrictors).
No products indexed under this heading.

Terfenadine (Isocarboxazid should not be administered in combination with antihistamines).
No products indexed under this heading.

Tetracaine (Isocarboxazid should not be administered in combination with anesthetic drugs. Patients taking isocarboxazid should not undergo elective surgery requiring general anesthesia. Also, they should not be given cocaine or local anesthesia containing sympathomimetic vasoconstrictors. The possible combined hypotensive effects of isocarboxazid and spinal anesthesia should be kept in mind. Isocarboxazid should be discontinued at least 10 days before elective surgery).
No products indexed under this heading.

Tetracaine Hydrochloride (Isocarboxazid should not be administered in combination with anesthetic drugs. Patients taking isocarboxazid should not undergo elective surgery requiring general anesthesia. Also, they should not be given cocaine or local anesthesia containing sympathomimetic vasoconstrictors. The possible combined hypotensive effects of isocarboxazid and spinal anesthesia should be kept in mind. Isocarboxazid should be discontinued at least 10 days before elective surgery).
No products indexed under this heading.

Thiamylal Sodium (Isocarboxazid should not be administered in combination with anesthetic drugs. Patients taking isocarboxazid should not undergo elective surgery requiring general anesthesia. Also, they should not be given cocaine or local anesthesia containing sympathomimetic vasoconstrictors. The possible combined hypotensive effects of isocarboxazid and spinal anesthesia should be kept in mind. Isocarboxazid should be discontinued at least 10 days before elective surgery).
No products indexed under this heading.

Thioridazine (Isocarboxazid should not be administered in combination with central nervous system depressants).
No products indexed under this heading.

Thioridazine Hydrochloride (Isocarboxazid should not be administered in combination with central nervous system depressants). Products include:
Thioridazine Hydrochloride **2384**

Thiothixene (Isocarboxazid should not be administered in combination with central nervous system depressants). Products include:
Thiothixene **2386**

Thiothixene Hydrochloride (Isocarboxazid should not be administered in combination with central nervous system depressants).
No products indexed under this heading.

Timolol Maleate (Isocarboxazid should not be used in combination with anti-hypertensive agents, including thiazide diuretics. A marked potentiating effect on these drugs has been reported, resulting in hypotension). Products include:
Combigan **601**
Dorzolamide Hydrochloride/Timolol Maleate Ophthalmic Solution .... ⊙**243**
Timoptic in Ocudose .... ⊙**231**

Torsemide (Isocarboxazid should not be used in combination with anti-hypertensive agents, including thiazide diuretics. A marked potentiating effect on these drugs has been reported, resulting in hypotension).
No products indexed under this heading.

Trandolapril (Isocarboxazid should not be used in combination with anti-hypertensive agents, including thiazide diuretics. A marked potentiating effect on these drugs has been reported, resulting in hypotension). Products include:
Mavik **489**
Tarka **534**

Tranylcypromine Sulfate (Isocarboxazid should not be administered in combination with monoamine oxidase inhibitors. In patients being transferred to isocarboxazid from other MAOI, a medication-free interval of at least 1 week should be allowed, after which isocarboxazid therapy should be started using half the normal starting dosage for at least the first week of therapy. Similarly, at least 1 week should elapse between the discontinuation of isocarboxazid and initiation of another MAOI, or the re-administration of isocarboxazid). Products include:
Parnate **1584**

Triamterene (Isocarboxazid should not be used in combination with anti-hypertensive agents, including thiazide diuretics. A marked potentiating effect on these drugs has been reported, resulting in hypotension). Products include:
Dyazide **1429**
Dyrenium **3495**

(⊙ Described in PDR® for Ophthalmic Medicines)

Triazolam (Isocarboxazid should not be administered in combination with hypnotics and sedatives).

No products indexed under this heading.

Trifluoperazine Hydrochloride (Isocarboxazid should not be administered in combination with central nervous system depressants).

No products indexed under this heading.

Trimeprazine Tartrate (Isocarboxazid should not be administered in combination with antihistamines).

No products indexed under this heading.

Trimethaphan Camsylate (Isocarboxazid should not be used in combination with anti-hypertensive agents, including thiazide diuretics. A marked potentiating effect on these drugs has been reported, resulting in hypotension).

No products indexed under this heading.

Trimipramine Maleate (Isocarboxazid should not be administered in combination with dibenzazepines. In patients being transferred to isocarboxazid from dibenzazepine-related entities, a medication-free interval of at least 1 week should be allowed, after which isocarboxazid therapy should be started using half the normal starting dosage for at least the first week of therapy. Similarly, at least 1 week should elapse between the discontinuation of isocarboxazid and initiation of other dibenzazepine-related entities, or the re-administration of isocarboxazid).

No products indexed under this heading.

Tripelennamine Hydrochloride (Isocarboxazid should not be administered in combination with antihistamines).

No products indexed under this heading.

Triprolidine Hydrochloride (Isocarboxazid should not be administered in combination with antihistamines).

No products indexed under this heading.

Valsartan (Isocarboxazid should not be used in combination with anti-hypertensive agents, including thiazide diuretics. A marked potentiating effect on these drugs has been reported, resulting in hypotension). Products include:

Verapamil Hydrochloride (Isocarboxazid should not be used in combination with anti-hypertensive agents, including thiazide diuretics. A marked potentiating effect on these drugs has been reported, resulting in hypotension). Products include:

Zaleplon (Isocarboxazid should not be administered in combination with hypnotics and sedatives).

No products indexed under this heading.

Ziprasidone Hydrochloride (Isocarboxazid should not be administered in combination with central nervous system depressants). Products include:

Zolpidem Tartrate (Isocarboxazid should not be administered in combination with hypnotics and sedatives). Products include:

Food Interactions

Alcohol (Isocarboxazid should not be administered in combination with central nervous system depressants).

Beer, reduced-alcohol (Isocarboxazid should not be administered in combination with some central nervous systems depressants including alcohol).

Beer, unspecified (Isocarboxazid should not be administered in combination with some central nervous systems depressants including alcohol).

Food high in tyramine (Isocarboxazid should not be administered in combination with cheese or other foods with a high tyramine content. Hypertensive crises have sometimes occurred during isocarboxazid therapy after ingestion of foods with a high tyramine content. In general, patients should avoid protein foods in which aging or protein breakdown is used to increase flavor. In particular, patients should be instructed not to take foods such as cheese, sour cream, Chianti wine, sherry, beer (including non-alcoholic beer), liqueurs, pickled herring, anchovies, caviar, liver, canned figs, raisins, bananas or avocados, chocolate, soy sauce, sauerkraut, the pods of broad beans (fava beans), yeast extracts, yogurt, meat extracts, meat prepared with tenderizers, or dry sausage).

Wine, Chianti (Isocarboxazid should not be administered in combination with some central nervous systems depressants including alcohol).

Wine, Red (Isocarboxazid should not be administered in combination with some central nervous systems depressants including alcohol).

Wine, unspecified (Isocarboxazid should not be administered in combination with some central nervous systems depressants including alcohol).

Wine products (Isocarboxazid should not be administered in combination with some central nervous systems depressants including alcohol).

MAVIK TABLETS

May interact with diuretics, lithium preparations, potassium preparations, potassium sparing diuretics, and certain other agents. Compounds in these categories include:

Amiloride Hydrochloride (Co-administration increases the risk of hyperkalemia; patients on diuretics, especially those on recently instituted diuretic therapy, may experience an excessive reduction in blood pressure after initiation of therapy with trandolapril).

No products indexed under this heading.

Bendroflumethiazide (Patients on diuretics, especially those on recently instituted diuretic therapy, may experience an excessive reduction in blood pressure after initiation of therapy with trandolapril).

No products indexed under this heading.

Bumetanide (Patients on diuretics, especially those on recently instituted diuretic therapy, may experience an excessive reduction in blood pressure after initiation of therapy with trandolapril).

No products indexed under this heading.

Chlorothiazide (Patients on diuretics, especially those on recently instituted diuretic therapy, may experience an excessive reduction in blood pressure after initiation of therapy with trandolapril).

No products indexed under this heading.

Chlorothiazide Sodium (Patients on diuretics, especially those on recently instituted diuretic therapy, may experience an excessive reduction in blood pressure after initiation of therapy with trandolapril). Products include:

Chlorthalidone (Patients on diuretics, especially those on recently instituted diuretic therapy, may experience an

excessive reduction in blood pressure after initiation of therapy with trandolapril). Products include:

Cimetidine (Co-administration has led to an increase of about 44% in C_{max} for trandolapril with no effect on ACE inhibition).

No products indexed under this heading.

Cimetidine Hydrochloride (Co-administration has led to an increase of about 44% in C_{max} for trandolapril with no effect on ACE inhibition).

No products indexed under this heading.

Ethacrynic Acid (Patients on diuretics, especially those on recently instituted diuretic therapy, may experience an excessive reduction in blood pressure after initiation of therapy with trandolapril).

No products indexed under this heading.

Furosemide (Co-administration has led to an increase of about 25% in the renal clearance of trandolapril with no effect on ACE inhibition; patients on diuretics, especially those on recently instituted diuretic therapy, may experience an excessive reduction in blood pressure after initiation of therapy with trandolapril). Products include:

Hydrochlorothiazide (Patients on diuretics, especially those on recently instituted diuretic therapy, may experience an excessive reduction in blood pressure after initiation of therapy with trandolapril). Products include:

Hydroflumethiazide (Patients on diuretics, especially those on recently instituted diuretic therapy, may experience an excessive reduction in blood pressure after initiation of therapy with trandolapril).

No products indexed under this heading.

Indapamide (Patients on diuretics, especially those on recently instituted diuretic therapy, may experience an excessive reduction in blood pressure after initiation of therapy with trandolapril). Products include:

Lithium (Co-administration of ACE inhibitors and lithium has resulted in increased serum lithium levels and symptoms of lithium toxicity).

No products indexed under this heading.

Lithium Carbonate (Co-administration of ACE inhibitors and lithium has resulted in increased serum lithium levels and symptoms of lithium toxicity).

No products indexed under this heading.

Lithium Citrate (Co-administration of ACE inhibitors and lithium has resulted in increased serum lithium levels and symptoms of lithium toxicity).

No products indexed under this heading.

Methyclothiazide (Patients on diuretics, especially those on recently instituted diuretic therapy, may experience an excessive reduction in blood pressure after initiation of therapy with trandolapril).

No products indexed under this heading.

Metolazone (Patients on diuretics, especially those on recently instituted diuretic therapy, may experience an excessive reduction in blood pressure after initiation of therapy with trandolapril).

No products indexed under this heading.

Polythiazide (Patients on diuretics, especially those on recently instituted diuretic therapy, may experience an excessive reduction in blood pressure after initiation of therapy with trandolapril).

No products indexed under this heading.

Potassium Acid Phosphate (Co-administration increases the risk of hyperkalemia). Products include:

Potassium Bicarbonate (Co-administration increases the risk of hyperkalemia).

No products indexed under this heading.

Potassium Chloride (Co-administration increases the risk of hyperkalemia). Products include:

Potassium Citrate (Co-administration increases the risk of hyperkalemia). Products include:

Potassium Gluconate (Co-administration increases the risk of hyperkalemia).

No products indexed under this heading.

Potassium Phosphate (Co-administration increases the risk of hyperkalemia). Products include:

Spironolactone (Co-administration increases the risk of hyperkalemia; patients on diuretics, especially those on recently instituted diuretic therapy, may experience an excessive reduction in blood pressure after initiation of therapy with trandolapril).

No products indexed under this heading.

Torsemide (Patients on diuretics, especially those on recently instituted diuretic therapy, may experience an excessive reduction in blood pressure after initiation of therapy with trandolapril).

No products indexed under this heading.

Triamterene (Co-administration increases the risk of hyperkalemia; patients on diuretics, especially those on recently instituted diuretic therapy, may experience an excessive reduction in blood pressure after initiation of therapy with trandolapril). Products include:

Food Interactions

Food, unspecified (Slows absorption of trandolapril but does not affect AUC or C_{max}).

MAXAIR AUTOHALER

May interact with beta-blockers, monoamine oxidase inhibitors, potassium-depleting diuretics, sympathomimetic aerosol bronchodilators, tricyclic antidepressants. Compounds in these categories include:

Acebutolol Hydrochloride (Co-administration with beta adrenergic receptor blocking agents blocks the pulmonary effect of pirbuterol and may produce severe bronchospasm in asthmatic patients).

No products indexed under this heading.

Albuterol (Potential for additive effects).

No products indexed under this heading.

IMPORTANT NOTE: Always consult each drug listing in the patient's regimen for possible interactions.

Maxair | Interactions Index | 1104

Amitriptyline Hydrochloride (Concurrent and/or sequential use with tricyclic antidepressants can result in the potentiation of pirbuterol's action on the vascular system).
No products indexed under this heading.

Amoxapine (Concurrent and/or sequential use with tricyclic antidepressants can result in the potentiation of pirbuterol's action on the vascular system).
No products indexed under this heading.

Atenolol (Co-administration with beta adrenergic receptor blocking agents blocks the pulmonary effect of pirbuterol and may produce severe bronchospasm in asthmatic patients).
No products indexed under this heading.

Bendroflumethiazide (The ECG changes and/or hypokalemia that may result from administration of non-potassium sparing diuretics can be acutely worsened by beta-agonists; clinical significance is not known).
No products indexed under this heading.

Betaxolol Hydrochloride (Co-administration with beta adrenergic receptor blocking agents blocks the pulmonary effect of pirbuterol and may produce severe bronchospasm in asthmatic patients).
No products indexed under this heading.

Bisoprolol Fumarate (Co-administration with beta adrenergic receptor blocking agents blocks the pulmonary effect of pirbuterol and may produce severe bronchospasm in asthmatic patients).
No products indexed under this heading.

Bitolterol Mesylate (Potential for additive effects).
No products indexed under this heading.

Bumetanide (The ECG changes and/or hypokalemia that may result from administration of non-potassium sparing diuretics can be acutely worsened by beta-agonists; clinical significance is not known).
No products indexed under this heading.

Carteolol Hydrochloride (Co-administration with beta adrenergic receptor blocking agents blocks the pulmonary effect of pirbuterol and may produce severe bronchospasm in asthmatic patients).
No products indexed under this heading.

Carvedilol (Co-administration with beta adrenergic receptor blocking agents blocks the pulmonary effect of pirbuterol and may produce severe bronchospasm in asthmatic patients). Products include:
Coreg 1409

Carvedilol Phosphate (Co-administration with beta adrenergic receptor blocking agents blocks the pulmonary effect of pirbuterol and may produce severe bronchospasm in asthmatic patients). Products include:
Coreg CR 1416

Chlorothiazide (The ECG changes and/or hypokalemia that may result from administration of non-potassium sparing diuretics can be acutely worsened by beta-agonists; clinical significance is not known).
No products indexed under this heading.

Chlorothiazide Sodium (The ECG changes and/or hypokalemia that may result from administration of non-potassium sparing diuretics can be acutely worsened by beta-agonists; clinical significance is not known). Products include:
Diuril Intravenous 2009

Clomipramine Hydrochloride (Concurrent and/or sequential use with tricyclic antidepressants can result in the potentiation of pirbuterol's action on the vascular system).
No products indexed under this heading.

Desipramine Hydrochloride (Concurrent and/or sequential use with tricyclic antidepressants can result in the potentiation of pirbuterol's action on the vascular system).
No products indexed under this heading.

Doxepin Hydrochloride (Concurrent and/or sequential use with tricyclic antidepressants can result in the potentiation of pirbuterol's action on the vascular system).
No products indexed under this heading.

Esmolol Hydrochloride (Co-administration with beta adrenergic receptor blocking agents blocks the pulmonary effect of pirbuterol and may produce severe bronchospasm in asthmatic patients).
No products indexed under this heading.

Ethacrynic Acid (The ECG changes and/or hypokalemia that may result from administration of non-potassium sparing diuretics can be acutely worsened by beta-agonists; clinical significance is not known).
No products indexed under this heading.

Furosemide (The ECG changes and/or hypokalemia that may result from administration of non-potassium sparing diuretics can be acutely worsened by beta-agonists; clinical significance is not known). Products include:
Furosemide 2354

Hydrochlorothiazide (The ECG changes and/or hypokalemia that may result from administration of non-potassium sparing diuretics can be acutely worsened by beta-agonists; clinical significance is not known). Products include:
Atacand HCT 700
Avalide 2956
Benicar HCT 1017
Diovan HCT 2419
Dyazide 1429
Exforge HCT 2449
Hyzaar 2162
Hyzaar 100-12.5 2162
Micardis HCT 889
Prinzide 2246
Tekturna HCT 2541
Teveten HCT 541

Hydroflumethiazide (The ECG changes and/or hypokalemia that may result from administration of non-potassium sparing diuretics can be acutely worsened by beta-agonists; clinical significance is not known).
No products indexed under this heading.

Imipramine Hydrochloride (Concurrent and/or sequential use with tricyclic antidepressants can result in the potentiation of pirbuterol's action on the vascular system).
No products indexed under this heading.

Imipramine Pamoate (Concurrent and/or sequential use with tricyclic antidepressants can result in the potentiation of pirbuterol's action on the vascular system).
No products indexed under this heading.

Isocarboxazid (Concurrent and/or sequential use with MAO inhibitors can result in the potentiation of pirbuterol's action on the vascular system). Products include:
Marplan 3481

Isoetharine (Potential for additive effects).
No products indexed under this heading.

Isoproterenol Hydrochloride (Potential for additive effects).
No products indexed under this heading.

Labetalol Hydrochloride (Co-administration with beta adrenergic receptor blocking agents blocks the pulmonary effect of pirbuterol and may produce severe bronchospasm in asthmatic patients).
No products indexed under this heading.

Levalbuterol Hydrochloride (Potential for additive effects).
No products indexed under this heading.

Levobunolol Hydrochloride (Co-administration with beta adrenergic receptor blocking agents blocks the pulmonary effect of pirbuterol and may produce severe bronchospasm in asthmatic patients).
No products indexed under this heading.

Maprotiline Hydrochloride (Concurrent and/or sequential use with tricyclic antidepressants can result in the potentiation of pirbuterol's action on the vascular system).
No products indexed under this heading.

Metaproterenol Sulfate (Potential for additive effects).
No products indexed under this heading.

Methyclothiazide (The ECG changes and/or hypokalemia that may result from administration of non-potassium sparing diuretics can be acutely worsened by beta-agonists; clinical significance is not known).
No products indexed under this heading.

Metipranolol Hydrochloride (Co-administration with beta adrenergic receptor blocking agents blocks the pulmonary effect of pirbuterol and may produce severe bronchospasm in asthmatic patients).
No products indexed under this heading.

Metoprolol Succinate (Co-administration with beta adrenergic receptor blocking agents blocks the pulmonary effect of pirbuterol and may produce severe bronchospasm in asthmatic patients). Products include:
Toprol XL 732

Metoprolol Tartrate (Co-administration with beta adrenergic receptor blocking agents blocks the pulmonary effect of pirbuterol and may produce severe bronchospasm in asthmatic patients).
No products indexed under this heading.

Moclobemide (Concurrent and/or sequential use with MAO inhibitors can result in the potentiation of pirbuterol's action on the vascular system).
No products indexed under this heading.

Nadolol (Co-administration with beta adrenergic receptor blocking agents blocks the pulmonary effect of pirbuterol and may produce severe bronchospasm in asthmatic patients). Products include:
Nadolol 2359

Nebivolol (Co-administration with beta adrenergic receptor blocking agents blocks the pulmonary effect of pirbuterol and may produce severe bronchospasm in asthmatic patients). Products include:
Bystolic 1147

Nortriptyline Hydrochloride (Concurrent and/or sequential use with tricyclic antidepressants can result in the potentiation of pirbuterol's action on the vascular system).
No products indexed under this heading.

Pargyline Hydrochloride (Concurrent and/or sequential use with MAO inhibitors can result in the potentiation of pirbuterol's action on the vascular system).
No products indexed under this heading.

Penbutolol Sulfate (Co-administration with beta adrenergic receptor blocking agents blocks the pulmonary effect of pirbuterol and may produce severe bronchospasm in asthmatic patients).
No products indexed under this heading.

Phenelzine Sulfate (Concurrent and/or sequential use with MAO inhibitors can result in the potentiation of pirbuterol's action on the vascular system).
No products indexed under this heading.

Pindolol (Co-administration with beta adrenergic receptor blocking agents blocks the pulmonary effect of pirbuterol and may produce severe bronchospasm in asthmatic patients).
No products indexed under this heading.

Polythiazide (The ECG changes and/or hypokalemia that may result from administration of non-potassium sparing diuretics can be acutely worsened by beta-agonists; clinical significance is not known).
No products indexed under this heading.

Procarbazine Hydrochloride (Concurrent and/or sequential use with MAO inhibitors can result in the potentiation of pirbuterol's action on the vascular system).
No products indexed under this heading.

Propranolol Hydrochloride (Co-administration with beta adrenergic receptor blocking agents blocks the pulmonary effect of pirbuterol and may produce severe bronchospasm in asthmatic patients). Products include:
InnoPran XL 1517

Protriptyline Hydrochloride (Concurrent and/or sequential use with tricyclic antidepressants can result in the potentiation of pirbuterol's action on the vascular system).
No products indexed under this heading.

Rasagiline Mesylate (Concurrent and/or sequential use with MAO inhibitors can result in the potentiation of pirbuterol's action on the vascular system). Products include:
Azilect 3383

Salmeterol Xinafoate (Potential for additive effects). Products include:
Advair 100/50 1275
Advair 250/50 1275
Advair 500/50 1275
Advair HFA 45/21 1288
Advair HFA 115/21 1288
Advair HFA 230/21 1288
Serevent Diskus 1656

Selegiline (Concurrent and/or sequential use with MAO inhibitors can result in the potentiation of pirbuterol's action on the vascular system). Products include:
Emsam 3623

Selegiline Hydrochloride (Concurrent and/or sequential use with MAO inhibitors can result in the potentiation of pirbuterol's action on the vascular system). Products include:
Eldepryl 3312

Sotalol Hydrochloride (Co-administration with beta adrenergic receptor blocking agents blocks the pulmonary effect of pirbuterol and may produce severe bronchospasm in asthmatic patients).
No products indexed under this heading.

Terbutaline Sulfate (Potential for additive effects).
No products indexed under this heading.

Timolol Hemihydrate (Co-administration with beta adrenergic receptor blocking agents blocks the pulmonary effect of pirbuterol and may produce severe bronchospasm in asthmatic patients). Products include:
Betimol 3490

Timolol Maleate (Co-administration with beta adrenergic receptor blocking agents blocks the pulmonary effect of pirbuterol and may produce severe bronchospasm in asthmatic patients). Products include:
Combigan 601
Dorzolamide Hydrochloride/Timolol Maleate Ophthalmic Solution .... ⊙243
Timoptic in Ocudose .... ⊙231

(⊙ Described in PDR® for Ophthalmic Medicines)

Torsemide (The ECG changes and/or hypokalemia that may result from administration of non-potassium sparing diuretics can be acutely worsened by beta-agonists; clinical significance is not known).

No products indexed under this heading.

Tranylcypromine Sulfate (Concurrent and/or sequential use with MAO inhibitors can result in the potentiation of pirbuterol's action on the vascular system). Products include:
Parnate 1584

Trimipramine Maleate (Concurrent and/or sequential use with tricyclic antidepressants can result in the potentiation of pirbuterol's action on the vascular system).

No products indexed under this heading.

MAXALT TABLETS
(Rizatriptan Benzoate) 2206
May interact with 5HT1-receptor agonists, ergot-containing drugs, monoamine oxidase inhibitors, selective serotonin reuptake inhibitors, serotonin and norepinephrine reuptake inhibitors, and certain other agents. Compounds in these categories include:

Almotriptan Malate (Co-administration with other 5-HT1 agonists within 24 hours of each other is contraindicated because the vasospastic effects may be additive). Products include:
Axert 2593

Citalopram Hydrobromide (Co-administration of 5-HT1 agonists with selective serotonin reuptake inhibitors (SSRIs) has resulted, rarely, in hyperreflexia, weakness, and incoordination. The development of a potentially life-threatening serotonin syndrome may occur with triptans, including rizatriptan benzoate treatment, particularly during combined use with SSRIs. If concomitant treatment with rizatriptan benzoate and an SSRI (eg, fluoxetine, paroxetine, sertraline, fluvoxamine, citalopram escitalopram) is clinically warranted, careful observation of patient is advised, particularly during treatment initiation and dose increases). Products include:
Celexa 1153

Desipramine Hydrochloride (Cases of life-threatening serotonin syndrome have been reported during combined use of serotonin-norepinephrine reuptake inhibitors).

No products indexed under this heading.

Desvenlafaxine Succinate (The development of a potentially life-threatening serotonin syndrome may occur with triptans, including rizatriptan benzoate treatment, particularly during combined use with serotonin norepinephrine reuptake inhibitors (SNRI). If concomitant treatment with rizatriptan benzoate and an SNRI (eg, venlafaxine, duloxetine) is clinically warranted, careful observation of patient is advised, particularly during treatment initiation and dose increases). Products include:
Pristiq 3564

Dihydroergotamine Mesylate (Ergot-containing drugs have been reported to cause prolonged vasospastic reactions; because there is a theoretical basis that these effects may be additive, use of ergot-type agents and rizatriptan within 24 hours is contraindicated).

No products indexed under this heading.

Duloxetine Hydrochloride (The development of a potentially life-threatening serotonin syndrome may occur with triptans, including rizatriptan benzoate treatment, particularly during combined use with serotonin norepinephrine reuptake inhibitors (SNRI). If concomitant treatment with rizatriptan benzoate and an SNRI (eg, venlafaxine, duloxetine) is clinically warranted, careful observation of patient is advised, particularly during treatment initiation and dose increases). Products include:
Cymbalta 1871

Eletriptan Hydrobromide (Co-administration with other 5-HT1 agonists within 24 hours of each other is contraindicated because the vasospastic effects may be additive).

No products indexed under this heading.

Ergonovine Maleate (Ergot-containing drugs have been reported to cause prolonged vasospastic reactions; because there is a theoretical basis that these effects may be additive, use of ergot-type agents and rizatriptan within 24 hours is contraindicated).

No products indexed under this heading.

Ergotamine Tartrate (Ergot-containing drugs have been reported to cause prolonged vasospastic reactions; because there is a theoretical basis that these effects may be additive, use of ergot-type agents and rizatriptan within 24 hours is contraindicated).

No products indexed under this heading.

Escitalopram Oxalate (Co-administration of 5-HT1 agonists with selective serotonin reuptake inhibitors (SSRIs) has resulted, rarely, in hyperreflexia, weakness, and incoordination. The development of a potentially life-threatening serotonin syndrome may occur with triptans, including rizatriptan benzoate treatment, particularly during combined use with SSRIs. If concomitant treatment with rizatriptan benzoate and an SSRI (eg, fluoxetine, paroxetine, sertraline, fluvoxamine, citalopram escitalopram) is clinically warranted, careful observation of patient is advised, particularly during treatment initiation and dose increases). Products include:
Lexapro Oral Suspension 1160
Lexapro Tablets 1160

Fluoxetine (Co-administration of 5-HT1 agonists with selective serotonin reuptake inhibitors (SSRIs) has resulted, rarely, in hyperreflexia, weakness, and incoordination. The development of a potentially life-threatening serotonin syndrome may occur with triptans, including rizatriptan benzoate treatment, particularly during combined use with SSRIs. If concomitant treatment with rizatriptan benzoate and an SSRI (eg, fluoxetine, paroxetine, sertraline, fluvoxamine, citalopram escitalopram) is clinically warranted, careful observation of patient is advised, particularly during treatment initiation and dose increases).

No products indexed under this heading.

Fluoxetine Hydrochloride (Co-administration of 5-HT1 agonists with selective serotonin reuptake inhibitors (SSRIs) has resulted, rarely, in hyperreflexia, weakness, and incoordination. The development of a potentially life-threatening serotonin syndrome may occur with triptans, including rizatriptan benzoate treatment, particularly during combined use with SSRIs. If concomitant treatment with rizatriptan benzoate and an SSRI (eg, fluoxetine, paroxetine, sertraline, fluvoxamine, citalopram escitalopram) is clinically warranted, careful observation of patient is advised, particularly during treatment initiation and dose increases). Products include:
Prozac Weekly 1941
Prozac Pulvules 1941
Symbyax 1965

Fluvoxamine (Co-administration of 5-HT1 agonists with selective serotonin reuptake inhibitors (SSRIs) has resulted, rarely, in hyperreflexia, weakness, and incoordination. The development of a potentially life-threatening serotonin syndrome may occur with triptans, including rizatriptan benzoate treat-

ment, particularly during combined use with SSRIs. If concomitant treatment with rizatriptan benzoate and an SSRI (eg, fluoxetine, paroxetine, sertraline, fluvoxamine, citalopram escitalopram) is clinically warranted, careful observation of patient is advised, particularly during treatment initiation and dose increases).

No products indexed under this heading.

Fluvoxamine Maleate (Co-administration of 5-HT1 agonists with selective serotonin reuptake inhibitors (SSRIs) has resulted, rarely, in hyperreflexia, weakness, and incoordination. The development of a potentially life-threatening serotonin syndrome may occur with triptans, including rizatriptan benzoate treatment, particularly during combined use with SSRIs. If concomitant treatment with rizatriptan benzoate and an SSRI (eg, fluoxetine, paroxetine, sertraline, fluvoxamine, citalopram escitalopram) is clinically warranted, careful observation of patient is advised, particularly during treatment initiation and dose increases).

No products indexed under this heading.

Frovatriptan Succinate (Co-administration with other 5-HT1 agonists within 24 hours of each other is contraindicated because the vasospastic effects may be additive). Products include:
Frova 1103

Isocarboxazid (Plasma concentrations of rizatriptan may be increased by MAO inhibitors; concurrent and/or sequential use is contraindicated). Products include:
Marplan 3481

Methylergonovine Maleate (Ergot-containing drugs have been reported to cause prolonged vasospastic reactions; because there is a theoretical basis that these effects may be additive, use of ergot-type agents and rizatriptan within 24 hours is contraindicated).

No products indexed under this heading.

Methysergide Maleate (Ergot-containing drugs have been reported to cause prolonged vasospastic reactions; because there is a theoretical basis that these effects may be additive, use of ergot-type agents and rizatriptan within 24 hours is contraindicated).

No products indexed under this heading.

Moclobemide (Concomitant therapy with the selective, reversible MAO-A inhibitor, moclobemide, has resulted in increased systemic exposure of rizatriptan and its metabolite; concurrent and/or sequential use is contraindicated).

No products indexed under this heading.

Naratriptan Hydrochloride (Co-administration with other 5-HT1 agonists within 24 hours of each other is contraindicated because the vasospastic effects may be additive). Products include:
Amerge 1306

Nefazodone Hydrochloride (Cases of life-threatening serotonin syndrome have been reported during combined use of serotonin-norepinephrine reuptake inhibitors).

No products indexed under this heading.

Pargyline Hydrochloride (Plasma concentrations of rizatriptan may be increased by MAO inhibitors; concurrent and/or sequential use is contraindicated).

No products indexed under this heading.

Paroxetine (Co-administration of 5-HT1 agonists with selective serotonin reuptake inhibitors (SSRIs) has resulted, rarely, in hyperreflexia, weakness, and incoordination. The development of a potentially life-threatening serotonin syndrome may occur with triptans, including rizatriptan benzoate treatment, particularly during combined use

with SSRIs. If concomitant treatment with rizatriptan benzoate and an SSRI (eg, fluoxetine, paroxetine, sertraline, fluvoxamine, citalopram escitalopram) is clinically warranted, careful observation of patient is advised, particularly during treatment initiation and dose increases).

No products indexed under this heading.

Paroxetine Hydrochloride (Co-administration of 5-HT1 agonists with selective serotonin reuptake inhibitors (SSRIs) has resulted, rarely, in hyperreflexia, weakness, and incoordination; no pharmacokinetic interaction was observed with a single dose study). Products include:
Paroxetine CR 2361
Paroxetine ER 2371
Paxil 1586
Paxil CR 1596

Paroxetine Mesylate (Co-administration of 5-HT1 agonists with selective serotonin reuptake inhibitors (SSRIs) has resulted, rarely, in hyperreflexia, weakness, and incoordination. The development of a potentially life-threatening serotonin syndrome may occur with triptans, including rizatriptan benzoate treatment, particularly during combined use with SSRIs. If concomitant treatment with rizatriptan benzoate and an SSRI (eg, fluoxetine, paroxetine, sertraline, fluvoxamine, citalopram escitalopram) is clinically warranted, careful observation of patient is advised, particularly during treatment initiation and dose increases).

No products indexed under this heading.

Phenelzine Sulfate (Plasma concentrations of rizatriptan may be increased by MAO inhibitors; concurrent and/or sequential use is contraindicated).

No products indexed under this heading.

Procarbazine Hydrochloride (Plasma concentrations of rizatriptan may be increased by MAO inhibitors; concurrent and/or sequential use is contraindicated).

No products indexed under this heading.

Propranolol Hydrochloride (Co-administration has resulted in an increase in mean plasma AUC for rizatriptan by 70%). Products include:
InnoPran XL 1517

Rasagiline Mesylate (Plasma concentrations of rizatriptan may be increased by MAO inhibitors; concurrent and/or sequential use is contraindicated). Products include:
Azilect 3383

Selegiline (Plasma concentrations of rizatriptan may be increased by MAO inhibitors; concurrent and/or sequential use is contraindicated). Products include:
Emsam 3623

Selegiline Hydrochloride (Plasma concentrations of rizatriptan may be increased by MAO inhibitors; concurrent and/or sequential use is contraindicated). Products include:
Eldepryl 3312

Sertraline Hydrochloride (Co-administration of 5-HT1 agonists with selective serotonin reuptake inhibitors (SSRIs) has resulted, rarely, in hyperreflexia, weakness, and incoordination. The development of a potentially life-threatening serotonin syndrome may occur with triptans, including rizatriptan benzoate treatment, particularly during combined use with SSRIs. If concomitant treatment with rizatriptan benzoate and an SSRI (eg, fluoxetine, paroxetine, sertraline, fluvoxamine, citalopram escitalopram) is clinically warranted, careful observation of patient is advised, particularly during treatment initiation and dose increases).

No products indexed under this heading.

Maxalt Interactions Index 1106

Sumatriptan (Co-administration with other 5-HT1 agonists within 24 hours of each other is contraindicated because the vasospastic effects may be additive). Products include:
Imitrex Nasal ... 1503

Sumatriptan Succinate (Co-administration with other 5-HT1 agonists within 24 hours of each other is contraindicated because the vasospastic effects may be additive). Products include:
Imitrex ... 1497
Imitrex Tablets ... 1508
Treximet ... 1681

Tranylcypromine Sulfate (Plasma concentrations of rizatriptan may be increased by MAO inhibitors; concurrent and/or sequential use is contraindicated). Products include:
Parnate ... 1584

Venlafaxine Hydrochloride (The development of a potentially life-threatening serotonin syndrome may occur with triptans, including rizatriptan benzoate treatment, particularly during combined use with serotonin norepinephrine reuptake inhibitors (SNRI). If concomitant treatment with rizatriptan benzoate and an SNRI (eg, venlafaxine, duloxetine) is clinically warranted, careful observation of patient is advised, particularly during treatment initiation and dose increases). Products include:
Effexor XR ... 3504
Venlafaxine Hydrochloride Tablets ... 2388

Zolmitriptan (Co-administration with other 5-HT1 agonists within 24 hours of each other is contraindicated because the vasospastic effects may be additive). Products include:
Zomig Tablets ... 773
Zomig Nasal Spray ... 768
Zomig-ZMT Tablets ... 773

Food Interactions

Food, unspecified (Delays the time to reach peak concentration by an hour; no significant effect on the bioavailability).

MAXALT-MLT ORALLY DISINTEGRATING TABLETS

(Rizatriptan Benzoate) ... 2206
See Maxalt Tablets

MED OMEGA FISH OIL 2800

(Docosahexaenoic Acid (DHA), Eicosapentaenoic Acid (EPA), Omega-3 Acids) ... 918
None cited in PDR database.

MEDERMA TOPICAL GEL

(Allantoin, Allium cepa) ... 2319
None cited in PDR database.

MEDERMA CREAM PLUS SPF 30

(Avobenzone, Octocrylene, Oxybenzone) ... 2319
None cited in PDR database.

MEDERMA FOR KIDS TOPICAL GEL

(Allantoin, Allium cepa) ... 2319
None cited in PDR database.

MEDIZYM TABLETS

(Ananas comosus, Bromelains, Carica papaya, Chymotrypsin, Pancreatin, Papain, Trypsin) ... 2041
None cited in PDR database.

MEGA ANTIOXIDANT TABLETS

(Dietary Supplement, Vitamins, Multiple) ... 3476
None cited in PDR database.

MEGACE ES ORAL SUSPENSION

(Megestrol Acetate) ... 2698
May interact with insulin, and certain other agents. Compounds in these categories include:

Indinavir Sulfate (A pharmacokinetic study demonstrated that co-administration of megestrol acetate and indinavir results in a significant decrease in the pharmacokinetic parameters (approximately 36% for C_{max} and approximately 28% for AUC) of indinavir. Administration of a higher dose of indinavir should be considered when co-administering with megestrol acetate). Products include:
Crixivan ... 2113

Insulin (Exacerbation of pre-existing diabetes with increased insulin requirements has been reported in association with concomitant use of megestrol acetate).
No products indexed under this heading.

Insulin, Human, Zinc Suspension (Exacerbation of pre-existing diabetes with increased insulin requirements has been reported in association with concomitant use of megestrol acetate).
No products indexed under this heading.

Insulin, Human (rDNA origin) (Exacerbation of pre-existing diabetes with increased insulin requirements has been reported in association with concomitant use of megestrol acetate). Products include:
Exubera ... 2717

Insulin, Human NPH (Exacerbation of pre-existing diabetes with increased insulin requirements has been reported in association with concomitant use of megestrol acetate). Products include:
Humulin N Vial ... 1934

Insulin, Human Regular (Exacerbation of pre-existing diabetes with increased insulin requirements has been reported in association with concomitant use of megestrol acetate). Products include:
Humulin R ... 1937
Humulin R (U-500) ... 1939

Insulin, Human Regular and Human NPH Mixture (Exacerbation of pre-existing diabetes with increased insulin requirements has been reported in association with concomitant use of megestrol acetate). Products include:
Humulin 50/50 ... 1930
Humulin 70/30 Vial ... 1931

Insulin, NPH (Exacerbation of pre-existing diabetes with increased insulin requirements has been reported in association with concomitant use of megestrol acetate).
No products indexed under this heading.

Insulin, Regular (Exacerbation of pre-existing diabetes with increased insulin requirements has been reported in association with concomitant use of megestrol acetate).
No products indexed under this heading.

Insulin, Regular and NPH mixture (Exacerbation of pre-existing diabetes with increased insulin requirements has been reported in association with concomitant use of megestrol acetate).
No products indexed under this heading.

Insulin, Zinc Crystals (Exacerbation of pre-existing diabetes with increased insulin requirements has been reported in association with concomitant use of megestrol acetate).
No products indexed under this heading.

Insulin, Zinc Suspension (Exacerbation of pre-existing diabetes with increased insulin requirements has been reported in association with concomitant use of megestrol acetate).
No products indexed under this heading.

Insulin Aspart (Exacerbation of pre-existing diabetes with increased insulin requirements has been reported in association with concomitant use of megestrol acetate).
No products indexed under this heading.

Insulin Aspart, Human (Exacerbation of pre-existing diabetes with increased insulin requirements has been reported in association with concomitant use of megestrol acetate). Products include:
NovoLog Mix 70/30 ... 2581

Insulin Aspart, Human Regular (Exacerbation of pre-existing diabetes with increased insulin requirements has been reported in association with concomitant use of megestrol acetate). Products include:
NovoLog ... 2575

Insulin Aspart Protamine, Human (Exacerbation of pre-existing diabetes with increased insulin requirements has been reported in association with concomitant use of megestrol acetate). Products include:
NovoLog Mix 70/30 ... 2581

Insulin Detemir (rDNA Origin) (Exacerbation of pre-existing diabetes with increased insulin requirements has been reported in association with concomitant use of megestrol acetate). Products include:
Levemir ... 2566

Insulin Glargine (Exacerbation of pre-existing diabetes with increased insulin requirements has been reported in association with concomitant use of megestrol acetate). Products include:
Lantus ... 2996

Insulin Glulisine (Exacerbation of pre-existing diabetes with increased insulin requirements has been reported in association with concomitant use of megestrol acetate). Products include:
Apidra ... 2937
Apidra SoloStar ... 2937

Insulin Lispro, Human (Exacerbation of pre-existing diabetes with increased insulin requirements has been reported in association with concomitant use of megestrol acetate). Products include:
Humalog ... 1910
Humalog Mix ... 1914
Humalog Mix75/25 ... 1917

Insulin Lispro Protamine, Human (Exacerbation of pre-existing diabetes with increased insulin requirements has been reported in association with concomitant use of megestrol acetate). Products include:
Humalog Mix ... 1914
Humalog Mix75/25 ... 1917

MEILI CLEAR SOFT CAPSULES

(Beta-Carotene, Bilberry, Euphrasia officinalis, Folic Acid, Herbals, Multiple, Lutein, Lycium barbarum, Vitamin C, Zeaxanthin) ... 607
None cited in PDR database.

MEILI SOFT CAPSULES

(Avocado Oil, Bee Pollen, Collagen, Herbals, Multiple, Laminaria hyperborea, Liver, Desiccated, Ribes nigrum, Spirulina) ... 607
None cited in PDR database.

MENTAX CREAM

(Butenafine Hydrochloride) ... 2358
None cited in PDR database.

MEPRON SUSPENSION

(Atovaquone) ... 1576
May interact with highly protein bound drugs (selected), and certain other agents. Compounds in these categories include:

Amiodarone Hydrochloride (Atovaquone is highly bound to plasma protein (greater than 99.9%); caution is advised when co-administered with other highly protein bound drugs with narrow therapeutic indices).
No products indexed under this heading.

Amitriptyline Hydrochloride (Atovaquone is highly bound to plasma protein (greater than 99.9%); caution is advised when co-administered with other highly protein bound drugs with narrow therapeutic indices).
No products indexed under this heading.

Cefonicid Sodium (Atovaquone is highly bound to plasma protein (greater than 99.9%); caution is advised when co-administered with other highly protein bound drugs with narrow therapeutic indices).
No products indexed under this heading.

Celecoxib (Atovaquone is highly bound to plasma protein (greater than 99.9%); caution is advised when co-administered with other highly protein bound drugs with narrow therapeutic indices). Products include:
Celebrex ... 3272

Chlordiazepoxide (Atovaquone is highly bound to plasma protein (greater than 99.9%); caution is advised when co-administered with other highly protein bound drugs with narrow therapeutic indices).
No products indexed under this heading.

Chlordiazepoxide Hydrochloride (Atovaquone is highly bound to plasma protein (greater than 99.9%); caution is advised when co-administered with other highly protein bound drugs with narrow therapeutic indices).
No products indexed under this heading.

Chlorpromazine (Atovaquone is highly bound to plasma protein (greater than 99.9%); caution is advised when co-administered with other highly protein bound drugs with narrow therapeutic indices).
No products indexed under this heading.

Chlorpromazine Hydrochloride (Atovaquone is highly bound to plasma protein (greater than 99.9%); caution is advised when co-administered with other highly protein bound drugs with narrow therapeutic indices).
No products indexed under this heading.

Clomipramine Hydrochloride (Atovaquone is highly bound to plasma protein (greater than 99.9%); caution is advised when co-administered with other highly protein bound drugs with narrow therapeutic indices).
No products indexed under this heading.

Clozapine (Atovaquone is highly bound to plasma protein (greater than 99.9%); caution is advised when co-administered with other highly protein bound drugs with narrow therapeutic indices).
No products indexed under this heading.

Cyclosporine (Atovaquone is highly bound to plasma protein (greater than 99.9%); caution is advised when co-administered with other highly protein bound drugs with narrow therapeutic indices). Products include:
Gengraf ... 440
Neoral Oral Solution ... 2496
Neoral Capsules ... 2496
Restasis ... 605

Diazepam (Atovaquone is highly bound to plasma protein (greater than 99.9%); caution is advised when co-administered with other highly protein bound drugs with narrow therapeutic indices). Products include:
Valium Tablets ... 2880

(⊙ Described in PDR® for Ophthalmic Medicines)

Diclofenac Potassium (Atovaquone is highly bound to plasma protein (greater than 99.9%); caution is advised when co-administered with other highly protein bound drugs with narrow therapeutic indices).
No products indexed under this heading.

Diclofenac Sodium (Atovaquone is highly bound to plasma protein (greater than 99.9%); caution is advised when co-administered with other highly protein bound drugs with narrow therapeutic indices).
No products indexed under this heading.

Digitalis Glycoside Preparations (Atovaquone is highly bound to plasma protein (greater than 99.9%); caution is advised when co-administered with other highly protein bound drugs with narrow therapeutic indices).
No products indexed under this heading.

Digitalis Lanata (Atovaquone is highly bound to plasma protein (greater than 99.9%); caution is advised when co-administered with other highly protein bound drugs with narrow therapeutic indices).
No products indexed under this heading.

Digitalis Purpurea (Atovaquone is highly bound to plasma protein (greater than 99.9%); caution is advised when co-administered with other highly protein bound drugs with narrow therapeutic indices).
No products indexed under this heading.

Dipyridamole (Atovaquone is highly bound to plasma protein (greater than 99.9%); caution is advised when co-administered with other highly protein bound drugs with narrow therapeutic indices). Products include:

Fenoprofen Calcium (Atovaquone is highly bound to plasma protein (greater than 99.9%); caution is advised when co-administered with other highly protein bound drugs with narrow therapeutic indices).
No products indexed under this heading.

Flurazepam Hydrochloride (Atovaquone is highly bound to plasma protein (greater than 99.9%); caution is advised when co-administered with other highly protein bound drugs with narrow therapeutic indices).
No products indexed under this heading.

Flurbiprofen (Atovaquone is highly bound to plasma protein (greater than 99.9%); caution is advised when co-administered with other highly protein bound drugs with narrow therapeutic indices).
No products indexed under this heading.

Glipizide (Atovaquone is highly bound to plasma protein (greater than 99.9%); caution is advised when co-administered with other highly protein bound drugs with narrow therapeutic indices).
No products indexed under this heading.

Ibuprofen (Atovaquone is highly bound to plasma protein (greater than 99.9%); caution is advised when co-administered with other highly protein bound drugs with narrow therapeutic indices). Products include:

Imipramine Hydrochloride (Atovaquone is highly bound to plasma protein (greater than 99.9%); caution is advised when co-administered with other highly protein bound drugs with narrow therapeutic indices).
No products indexed under this heading.

Imipramine Pamoate (Atovaquone is highly bound to plasma protein (greater than 99.9%); caution is advised when co-administered with other highly protein bound drugs with narrow therapeutic indices).
No products indexed under this heading.

Indomethacin (Atovaquone is highly bound to plasma protein (greater than 99.9%); caution is advised when co-administered with other highly protein bound drugs with narrow therapeutic indices). Products include:

Indomethacin Sodium Trihydrate (Atovaquone is highly bound to plasma protein (greater than 99.9%); caution is advised when co-administered with other highly protein bound drugs with narrow therapeutic indices). Products include:

Ketoprofen (Atovaquone is highly bound to plasma protein (greater than 99.9%); caution is advised when co-administered with other highly protein bound drugs with narrow therapeutic indices).
No products indexed under this heading.

Ketorolac Tromethamine (Atovaquone is highly bound to plasma protein (greater than 99.9%); caution is advised when co-administered with other highly protein bound drugs with narrow therapeutic indices). Products include:

Meclofenamate Sodium (Atovaquone is highly bound to plasma protein (greater than 99.9%); caution is advised when co-administered with other highly protein bound drugs with narrow therapeutic indices).
No products indexed under this heading.

Mefenamic Acid (Atovaquone is highly bound to plasma protein (greater than 99.9%); caution is advised when co-administered with other highly protein bound drugs with narrow therapeutic indices).
No products indexed under this heading.

Midazolam Hydrochloride (Atovaquone is highly bound to plasma protein (greater than 99.9%); caution is advised when co-administered with other highly protein bound drugs with narrow therapeutic indices).
No products indexed under this heading.

Naproxen (Atovaquone is highly bound to plasma protein (greater than 99.9%); caution is advised when co-administered with other highly protein bound drugs with narrow therapeutic indices). Products include:

Naproxen Sodium (Atovaquone is highly bound to plasma protein (greater than 99.9%); caution is advised when co-administered with other highly protein bound drugs with narrow therapeutic indices). Products include:

Nortriptyline Hydrochloride (Atovaquone is highly bound to plasma protein (greater than 99.9%); caution is advised when co-administered with other highly protein bound drugs with narrow therapeutic indices).
No products indexed under this heading.

Oxaprozin (Atovaquone is highly bound to plasma protein (greater than 99.9%); caution is advised when co-administered with other highly protein bound drugs with narrow therapeutic indices).
No products indexed under this heading.

Oxazepam (Atovaquone is highly bound to plasma protein (greater than 99.9%); caution is advised when co-administered with other highly protein bound drugs with narrow therapeutic indices).
No products indexed under this heading.

Phenylbutazone (Atovaquone is highly bound to plasma protein (greater than 99.9%); caution is advised when co-administered with other highly protein bound drugs with narrow therapeutic indices).
No products indexed under this heading.

Piroxicam (Atovaquone is highly bound to plasma protein (greater than 99.9%); caution is advised when co-administered with other highly protein bound drugs with narrow therapeutic indices).
No products indexed under this heading.

Propranolol Hydrochloride (Atovaquone is highly bound to plasma protein (greater than 99.9%); caution is advised when co-administered with other highly protein bound drugs with narrow therapeutic indices). Products include:

Rifabutin (Due to structural similarity to rifampin, rifabutin may decrease average steady-state plasma atovaquone concentration).
No products indexed under this heading.

Rifampin (Co-administration with oral rifampin in HIV-infected individuals may result in a 52% +/- 13% decrease in the average steady-state plasma atovaquone concentration and a 37% +/- 42% increase in the average steady-state plasma rifampin concentration).
No products indexed under this heading.

Sulfamethoxazole (Co-administration with TMP-SMX may result in slight decrease in average steady-state concentrations of TMP-SMX; this effect is minor and would not expect to produce clinically significant events).
No products indexed under this heading.

Sulindac (Atovaquone is highly bound to plasma protein (greater than 99.9%); caution is advised when co-administered with other highly protein bound drugs with narrow therapeutic indices). Products include:

Temazepam (Atovaquone is highly bound to plasma protein (greater than 99.9%); caution is advised when co-administered with other highly protein bound drugs with narrow therapeutic indices).
No products indexed under this heading.

Tolbutamide (Atovaquone is highly bound to plasma protein (greater than 99.9%); caution is advised when co-administered with other highly protein bound drugs with narrow therapeutic indices).
No products indexed under this heading.

Tolmetin Sodium (Atovaquone is highly bound to plasma protein (greater than 99.9%); caution is advised when co-administered with other highly protein bound drugs with narrow therapeutic indices).
No products indexed under this heading.

Trimethoprim (Co-administration with TMP-SMX may result in slight decrease in average steady-state concentrations of TMP-SMX; this effect is minor and would not expect to produce clinically significant events).
No products indexed under this heading.

Trimipramine Maleate (Atovaquone is highly bound to plasma protein (greater than 99.9%); caution is advised when co-administered with other highly protein bound drugs with narrow therapeutic indices).
No products indexed under this heading.

Warfarin Sodium (Atovaquone is highly bound to plasma protein (greater than 99.9%); caution is advised when co-administered with other highly protein bound drugs with narrow therapeutic indices).
No products indexed under this heading.

Zidovudine (Atovaquone tablets have shown to decrease zidovudine apparent oral clearance leading to an increase in plasma zidovudine AUC; this effect is minor and would not expect to produce clinically significant events). Products include:

Food Interactions

Food, unspecified (Food enhances absorption by approximately two-fold).

MERIDIA CAPSULES

May interact with alcohols, antidepressant drugs, antipsychotic agents, centrally-acting drugs, dopamine antagonists, ephedrine, erythromycin, lithium preparations, mixed agonist/antagonist opioid analgesics, monoamine oxidase inhibitors, nasal decongestants, selective serotonin reuptake inhibitors, serotoninergic agents, sympathomimetics, triptans, and certain other agents. Compounds in these categories include:

Albuterol (Concomitant use of sibutramine and other agents that may raise blood pressure or heart rate have not been evaluated. These include certain decongestants, cough, cold, and allergy medications that contain agents, such as ephedrine, or pseudoephedrine. Caution should be used when prescribing sibutramine to patients who use these medications).
No products indexed under this heading.

Albuterol Sulfate (Concomitant use of sibutramine and other agents that may raise blood pressure or heart rate have not been evaluated. These include certain decongestants, cough, cold, and allergy medications that contain agents, such as ephedrine, or pseudoephedrine. Caution should be used when prescribing sibutramine to patients who use these medications). Products include:

Alfentanil Hydrochloride (The use of sibutramine in combination with other CNS-active drugs, particularly serotonergic agents, has not been systematically evaluated. Consequently, caution is advised if the concomitant administration of sibutramine with other centrally-acting drugs is indicated. Sibutramine is contraindicated in patients taking other centrally acting weight loss drugs).
No products indexed under this heading.

Almotriptan Malate (The development of a potentially life-threatening serotonin syndrome, or Neuroleptic Malignant Syndrome (NMS)-like reactions, has been reported with SNRIs and SSRIs alone, including sibutramine treatment, but particularly with concomitant use of serotonergic drugs (including triptans)). Products include:

IMPORTANT NOTE: Always consult each drug listing in the patient's regimen for possible interactions.

Meridia Interactions Index 1108

Alprazolam (The use of sibutramine in combination with other CNS-active drugs, particularly serotonergic agents, has not been systematically evaluated. Consequently, caution is advised if the concomitant administration of sibutramine with other centrally-acting drugs is indicated. Sibutramine is contraindicated in patients taking other centrally acting weight loss drugs).
No products indexed under this heading.

Amitriptyline Hydrochloride (Patients should be advised to inform their physicians if they are taking, or plan to take, any prescription or over-the-counter drugs, especially antidepressants, since there is a potential for interactions).
No products indexed under this heading.

Amoxapine (Patients should be advised to inform their physicians if they are taking, or plan to take, any prescription or over-the-counter drugs, especially antidepressants, since there is a potential for interactions).
No products indexed under this heading.

Amphetamine Aspartate (The use of sibutramine in combination with other CNS-active drugs, particularly serotonergic agents, has not been systematically evaluated. Consequently, caution is advised if the concomitant administration of sibutramine with other centrally-acting drugs is indicated. Sibutramine is contraindicated in patients taking other centrally acting weight loss drugs).
No products indexed under this heading.

Amphetamine Aspartate Monohydrate (The use of sibutramine in combination with other CNS-active drugs, particularly serotonergic agents, has not been systematically evaluated. Consequently, caution is advised if the concomitant administration of sibutramine with other centrally-acting drugs is indicated. Sibutramine is contraindicated in patients taking other centrally acting weight loss drugs).
No products indexed under this heading.

Amphetamine Resins (The use of sibutramine in combination with other CNS-active drugs, particularly serotonergic agents, has not been systematically evaluated. Consequently, caution is advised if the concomitant administration of sibutramine with other centrally-acting drugs is indicated. Sibutramine is contraindicated in patients taking other centrally acting weight loss drugs).
No products indexed under this heading.

Amphetamine Sulfate (The use of sibutramine in combination with other CNS-active drugs, particularly serotonergic agents, has not been systematically evaluated. Consequently, caution is advised if the concomitant administration of sibutramine with other centrally-acting drugs is indicated. Sibutramine is contraindicated in patients taking other centrally acting weight loss drugs).
No products indexed under this heading.

Aprobarbital (The use of sibutramine in combination with other CNS-active drugs, particularly serotonergic agents, has not been systematically evaluated. Consequently, caution is advised if the concomitant administration of sibutramine with other centrally-acting drugs is indicated. Sibutramine is contraindicated in patients taking other centrally acting weight loss drugs).
No products indexed under this heading.

Aripiprazole (The development of a potentially life-threatening serotonin syndrome, or Neuroleptic Malignant Syndrome (NMS)-like reactions, has been reported with SNRIs and SSRIs alone, including sibutramine treatment, but particularly with concomitant use with antipsychotics).
No products indexed under this heading.

Buprenorphine Hydrochloride (The rare, but serious, constellation of symptoms termed "serotonin syndrome" has also been reported with the concomitant use of selective serotonin reuptake inhibitors and certain opioids, such as dextromethorphan, meperidine, pentazocine and fentanyl, lithium, or tryptophan).
No products indexed under this heading.

Bupropion Hydrochloride (Patients should be advised to inform their physicians if they are taking, or plan to take, any prescription or over-the-counter drugs, especially antidepressants, since there is a potential for interactions). Products include:
Aplenzin 2948
Wellbutrin 1719
Wellbutrin SR 1725
Zyban 1762

Buspirone Hydrochloride (The use of sibutramine in combination with other CNS-active drugs, particularly serotonergic agents, has not been systematically evaluated. Consequently, caution is advised if the concomitant administration of sibutramine with other centrally-acting drugs is indicated. Sibutramine is contraindicated in patients taking other centrally acting weight loss drugs).
No products indexed under this heading.

Butabarbital (The use of sibutramine in combination with other CNS-active drugs, particularly serotonergic agents, has not been systematically evaluated. Consequently, caution is advised if the concomitant administration of sibutramine with other centrally-acting drugs is indicated. Sibutramine is contraindicated in patients taking other centrally acting weight loss drugs).
No products indexed under this heading.

Butalbital (The use of sibutramine in combination with other CNS-active drugs, particularly serotonergic agents, has not been systematically evaluated. Consequently, caution is advised if the concomitant administration of sibutramine with other centrally-acting drugs is indicated. Sibutramine is contraindicated in patients taking other centrally acting weight loss drugs).
No products indexed under this heading.

Butorphanol Tartrate (The rare, but serious, constellation of symptoms termed "serotonin syndrome" has also been reported with the concomitant use of selective serotonin reuptake inhibitors and certain opioids, such as dextromethorphan, meperidine, pentazocine and fentanyl, lithium, or tryptophan).
No products indexed under this heading.

Chlordiazepoxide (The use of sibutramine in combination with other CNS-active drugs, particularly serotonergic agents, has not been systematically evaluated. Consequently, caution is advised if the concomitant administration of sibutramine with other centrally-acting drugs is indicated. Sibutramine is contraindicated in patients taking other centrally acting weight loss drugs).
No products indexed under this heading.

Chlordiazepoxide Hydrochloride (The use of sibutramine in combination with other CNS-active drugs, particularly serotonergic agents, has not been systematically evaluated. Consequently, caution is advised if the concomitant administration of sibutramine with other centrally-acting drugs is indicated. Sibutramine is contraindicated in patients taking other centrally acting weight loss drugs).
No products indexed under this heading.

Chlorpromazine (The development of a potentially life-threatening serotonin syndrome, or Neuroleptic Malignant Syndrome (NMS)-like reactions, has been reported with SNRIs and SSRIs alone, including sibutramine treatment, but particularly with concomitant use with antipsychotics).
No products indexed under this heading.

Chlorpromazine Hydrochloride (The development of a potentially life-threatening serotonin syndrome, or Neuroleptic Malignant Syndrome (NMS)-like reactions, has been reported with SNRIs and SSRIs alone, including sibutramine treatment, but particularly with concomitant use with antipsychotics).
No products indexed under this heading.

Chlorprothixene (The development of a potentially life-threatening serotonin syndrome, or Neuroleptic Malignant Syndrome (NMS)-like reactions, has been reported with SNRIs and SSRIs alone, including sibutramine treatment, but particularly with concomitant use with antipsychotics).
No products indexed under this heading.

Chlorprothixene Hydrochloride (The development of a potentially life-threatening serotonin syndrome, or Neuroleptic Malignant Syndrome (NMS)-like reactions, has been reported with SNRIs and SSRIs alone, including sibutramine treatment, but particularly with concomitant use with antipsychotics).
No products indexed under this heading.

Chlorprothixene Lactate (The development of a potentially life-threatening serotonin syndrome, or Neuroleptic Malignant Syndrome (NMS)-like reactions, has been reported with SNRIs and SSRIs alone, including sibutramine treatment, but particularly with concomitant use with antipsychotics).
No products indexed under this heading.

Cimetidine (Concomitant administration of cimetidine 400 mg twice daily and sibutramine 15 mg once daily for 7 days in 12 volunteers resulted in small increases in combined (M_1 and M_2) plasma C_{max} (3.4%) and AUC (7.3%)).
No products indexed under this heading.

Cimetidine Hydrochloride (Concomitant administration of cimetidine 400 mg twice daily and sibutramine 15 mg once daily for 7 days in 12 volunteers resulted in small increases in combined (M_1 and M_2) plasma C_{max} (3.4%) and AUC (7.3%)).
No products indexed under this heading.

Citalopram Hydrobromide (The development of a potentially life-threatening serotonin syndrome, or Neuroleptic Malignant Syndrome (NMS)-like reactions, has been reported with SNRIs and SSRIs alone, including sibutramine treatment, but particularly with concomitant use of serotonergic drugs (including triptans)). Products include:
Celexa 1153

Clorazepate Dipotassium (The use of sibutramine in combination with other CNS-active drugs, particularly serotonergic agents, has not been systematically evaluated. Consequently, caution is advised if the concomitant administration of sibutramine with other centrally-acting drugs is indicated. Sibutramine is contraindicated in patients taking other centrally acting weight loss drugs).
No products indexed under this heading.

Clozapine (The development of a potentially life-threatening serotonin syndrome, or Neuroleptic Malignant Syndrome (NMS)-like reactions, has been reported with SNRIs and SSRIs alone, including sibutramine treatment, but particularly with concomitant use with antipsychotics).
No products indexed under this heading.

Codeine Phosphate (The use of sibutramine in combination with other CNS-active drugs, particularly serotonergic agents, has not been systematically evaluated. Consequently, caution is advised if the concomitant administration of sibutramine with other centrally-acting drugs is indicated. Sibutramine is contraindicated in patients taking other centrally acting weight loss drugs). Products include:
Tylenol with Codeine 2691

Codeine Sulfate (The use of sibutramine in combination with other CNS-active drugs, particularly serotonergic agents, has not been systematically evaluated. Consequently, caution is advised if the concomitant administration of sibutramine with other centrally-acting drugs is indicated. Sibutramine is contraindicated in patients taking other centrally acting weight loss drugs).
No products indexed under this heading.

Desflurane (The use of sibutramine in combination with other CNS-active drugs, particularly serotonergic agents, has not been systematically evaluated. Consequently, caution is advised if the concomitant administration of sibutramine with other centrally-acting drugs is indicated. Sibutramine is contraindicated in patients taking other centrally acting weight loss drugs).
No products indexed under this heading.

Desipramine Hydrochloride (Patients should be advised to inform their physicians if they are taking, or plan to take, any prescription or over-the-counter drugs, especially antidepressants, since there is a potential for interactions).
No products indexed under this heading.

Desoxyephedrine (Patients should be advised to inform their physicians if they are taking, or plan to take, any prescription or over-the-counter drugs, especially decongestants, since there is a potential for interactions).
No products indexed under this heading.

Dexmethylphenidate Hydrochloride (The use of sibutramine in combination with other CNS-active drugs, particularly serotonergic agents, has not been systematically evaluated. Consequently, caution is advised if the concomitant administration of sibutramine with other centrally-acting drugs is indicated. Sibutramine is contraindicated in patients taking other centrally acting weight loss drugs). Products include:
Focalin XR 2472

Dextroamphetamine (The use of sibutramine in combination with other CNS-active drugs, particularly serotonergic agents, has not been systematically evaluated. Consequently, caution is advised if the concomitant administration of sibutramine with other centrally-acting drugs is indicated. Sibutramine is contraindicated in patients taking other centrally acting weight loss drugs).
No products indexed under this heading.

Dextroamphetamine Saccharate (The use of sibutramine in combination with other CNS-active drugs, particularly serotonergic agents, has not been systematically evaluated. Consequently, caution is advised if the concomitant administration of sibutramine with other centrally-acting drugs is indicated.

1109 **Interactions Index** **Meridia**

Sibutramine is contraindicated in patients taking other centrally acting weight loss drugs).
No products indexed under this heading.

Dextroamphetamine Sulfate (The use of sibutramine in combination with other CNS-active drugs, particularly serotonergic agents, has not been systematically evaluated. Consequently, caution is advised if the concomitant administration of sibutramine with other centrally-acting drugs is indicated. Sibutramine is contraindicated in patients taking other centrally acting weight loss drugs). Products include:
Dexedrine **1425**

Dextromethorphan Hydrobromide (The rare, but serious, constellation of symptoms termed "serotonin syndrome" has also been reported with the concomitant use of selective serotonin reuptake inhibitors and certain opioids, such as dextromethorphan).
No products indexed under this heading.

Dextromethorphan Polistirex (The rare, but serious, constellation of symptoms termed "serotonin syndrome" has also been reported with the concomitant use of selective serotonin reuptake inhibitors and certain opioids, such as dextromethorphan).
No products indexed under this heading.

Dezocine (The use of sibutramine in combination with other CNS-active drugs, particularly serotonergic agents, has not been systematically evaluated. Consequently, caution is advised if the concomitant administration of sibutramine with other centrally-acting drugs is indicated. Sibutramine is contraindicated in patients taking other centrally acting weight loss drugs).
No products indexed under this heading.

Diazepam (The use of sibutramine in combination with other CNS-active drugs, particularly serotonergic agents, has not been systematically evaluated. Consequently, caution is advised if the concomitant administration of sibutramine with other centrally-acting drugs is indicated. Sibutramine is contraindicated in patients taking other centrally acting weight loss drugs). Products include:
Valium Tablets **2880**

Dihydroergotamine Mesylate (The rare, but serious, constellation of symptoms termed "serotonin syndrome" has also been reported with the concomitant use of selective serotonin reuptake inhibitors and agents for migraine therapy, such as dihydroergotamine).
No products indexed under this heading.

Dobutamine Hydrochloride (Concomitant use of sibutramine and other agents that may raise blood pressure or heart rate have not been evaluated. These include certain decongestants, cough, cold, and allergy medications that contain agents, such as ephedrine, or pseudoephedrine. Caution should be used when prescribing sibutramine to patients who use these medications).
No products indexed under this heading.

Dopamine Hydrochloride (Concomitant use of sibutramine and other agents that may raise blood pressure or heart rate have not been evaluated. These include certain decongestants, cough, cold, and allergy medications that contain agents, such as ephedrine, or pseudoephedrine. Caution should be used when prescribing sibutramine to patients who use these medications).
No products indexed under this heading.

Doxepin Hydrochloride (Patients should be advised to inform their physicians if they are taking, or plan to take, any prescription or over-the-counter drugs, especially antidepressants, since there is a potential for interactions).
No products indexed under this heading.

Droperidol (The use of sibutramine in combination with other CNS-active drugs, particularly serotonergic agents, has not been systematically evaluated. Consequently, caution is advised if the concomitant administration of sibutramine with other centrally-acting drugs is indicated. Sibutramine is contraindicated in patients taking other centrally acting weight loss drugs).
No products indexed under this heading.

Drugs, unspecified (Patients should be advised to inform their physicians if they are taking, or plan to take, any prescription or over-the-counter drugs, especially weight-reducing agents, decongestants, antidepressants, cough suppressants, lithium, dihydroergotamine, sumatriptan, or tryptophan, since there is a potential for interactions).
No products indexed under this heading.

Eletriptan Hydrobromide (The development of a potentially life-threatening serotonin syndrome, or Neuroleptic Malignant Syndrome (NMS)-like reactions, has been reported with SNRIs and SSRIs alone, including sibutramine treatment, but particularly with concomitant use of serotonergic drugs (including triptans)).
No products indexed under this heading.

Enflurane (The use of sibutramine in combination with other CNS-active drugs, particularly serotonergic agents, has not been systematically evaluated. Consequently, caution is advised if the concomitant administration of sibutramine with other centrally-acting drugs is indicated. Sibutramine is contraindicated in patients taking other centrally acting weight loss drugs).
No products indexed under this heading.

Ephedrine Hydrochloride (Caution should be used when prescribing sibutramine to patients who use allergy medications, such as ephedrine).
No products indexed under this heading.

Ephedrine Sulfate (Patients should be advised to inform their physicians if they are taking, or plan to take, any prescription or over-the-counter drugs, especially decongestants, since there is a potential for interactions).
No products indexed under this heading.

Ephedrine Tannate (Caution should be used when prescribing sibutramine to patients who use allergy medications, such as ephedrine).
No products indexed under this heading.

Epinephrine (Concomitant use of sibutramine and other agents that may raise blood pressure or heart rate have not been evaluated. These include certain decongestants, cough, cold, and allergy medications that contain agents, such as ephedrine, or pseudoephedrine. Caution should be used when prescribing sibutramine to patients who use these medications). Products include:
EpiPen **3631**
Twinject **3268**

Epinephrine Bitartrate (Concomitant use of sibutramine and other agents that may raise blood pressure or heart rate have not been evaluated. These include certain decongestants, cough, cold, and allergy medications that contain agents, such as ephedrine, or pseudoephedrine. Caution should be used when prescribing sibutramine to patients who use these medications).
No products indexed under this heading.

Epinephrine Hydrochloride (Patients should be advised to inform their physicians if they are taking, or plan to take, any prescription or over-the-counter drugs, especially decongestants, since there is a potential for interactions).
No products indexed under this heading.

Erythromycin (Concomitant administration of sibutramine with erythromycin resulted in small increases in the AUC (less than 14%) for M_1 and M_2. A small reduction in C_{max} for M_1 (11%) and a slight increase in C_{max} for M_2(10%) were observed).
No products indexed under this heading.

Erythromycin, Topical (Concomitant administration of sibutramine with erythromycin resulted in small increases in the AUC (less than 14%) for M_1 and M_2. A small reduction in C_{max} for M_1 (11%) and a slight increase in C_{max} for M_2(10%) were observed).
No products indexed under this heading.

Erythromycin Estolate (Concomitant administration of sibutramine with erythromycin resulted in small increases in the AUC (less than 14%) for M_1 and M_2. A small reduction in C_{max} for M_1 (11%) and a slight increase in C_{max} for M_2(10%) were observed).
No products indexed under this heading.

Erythromycin Ethylsuccinate (Concomitant administration of sibutramine with erythromycin resulted in small increases in the AUC (less than 14%) for M_1 and M_2. A small reduction in C_{max} for M_1 (11%) and a slight increase in C_{max} for M_2(10%) were observed). Products include:
E.E.S. **437**
EryPed **435**

Erythromycin Gluceptate (Concomitant administration of sibutramine with erythromycin resulted in small increases in the AUC (less than 14%) for M_1 and M_2. A small reduction in C_{max} for M_1 (11%) and a slight increase in C_{max} for M_2(10%) were observed).
No products indexed under this heading.

Erythromycin Lactobionate (Concomitant administration of sibutramine with erythromycin resulted in small increases in the AUC (less than 14%) for M_1 and M_2. A small reduction in C_{max} for M_1 (11%) and a slight increase in C_{max} for M_2(10%) were observed).
No products indexed under this heading.

Erythromycin Stearate (Concomitant administration of sibutramine with erythromycin resulted in small increases in the AUC (less than 14%) for M_1 and M_2. A small reduction in C_{max} for M_1 (11%) and a slight increase in C_{max} for M_2(10%) were observed).
No products indexed under this heading.

Escitalopram Oxalate (The development of a potentially life-threatening serotonin syndrome, or Neuroleptic Malignant Syndrome (NMS)-like reactions, has been reported with SNRIs and SSRIs alone, including sibutramine treatment, but particularly with concomitant use of serotonergic drugs (including triptans)). Products include:
Lexapro Oral Suspension **1160**
Lexapro Tablets **1160**

Estazolam (The use of sibutramine in combination with other CNS-active drugs, particularly serotonergic agents, has not been systematically evaluated. Consequently, caution is advised if the concomitant administration of sibutramine with other centrally-acting drugs is indicated. Sibutramine is contraindicated in patients taking other centrally acting weight loss drugs).
No products indexed under this heading.

Ethanol (In a double-blind, placebo-controlled, crossover study in 19 volunteers, administration of a single dose of ethanol (0.5 mL/kg) together with 20 mg of sibutramine resulted in no psychomotor interactions of clinical significance between alcohol and sibutramine. However, the concomitant use of sibutramine and excess alcohol is not recommended).
No products indexed under this heading.

Ethchlorvynol (The use of sibutramine in combination with other CNS-active drugs, particularly serotonergic agents, has not been systematically evaluated. Consequently, caution is advised if the concomitant administration of sibutramine with other centrally-acting drugs is indicated. Sibutramine is contraindicated in patients taking other centrally acting weight loss drugs).
No products indexed under this heading.

Ethinamate (The use of sibutramine in combination with other CNS-active drugs, particularly serotonergic agents, has not been systematically evaluated. Consequently, caution is advised if the concomitant administration of sibutramine with other centrally-acting drugs is indicated. Sibutramine is contraindicated in patients taking other centrally acting weight loss drugs).
No products indexed under this heading.

Ethyl Alcohol (In a double-blind, placebo-controlled, crossover study in 19 volunteers, administration of a single dose of ethanol (0.5 mL/kg) together with 20 mg of sibutramine resulted in no psychomotor interactions of clinical significance between alcohol and sibutramine. However, the concomitant use of sibutramine and excess alcohol is not recommended).
No products indexed under this heading.

Fentanyl (The rare, but serious, constellation of symptoms termed "serotonin syndrome" has also been reported with the concomitant use of selective serotonin reuptake inhibitors and certain opioids, such as fentanyl). Products include:
Duragesic **2604**
Fentanyl Transdermal System **2346**
Onsolis **2054**

Fentanyl Citrate (The rare, but serious, constellation of symptoms termed "serotonin syndrome" has also been reported with the concomitant use of selective serotonin reuptake inhibitors and certain opioids, such as fentanyl). Products include:
Fentora **966**

Fluoxetine (The rare, but serious, constellation of symptoms termed "serotonin syndrome" has also been reported with the concomitant use of selective serotonin reuptake inhibitors and agents for migraine therapy, such as sumatriptan succinate and dihydroergotamine, certain opioids, such as dextromethorphan, meperidine, pentazocine and fentanyl, lithium, or tryptophan. Serotonin syndrome has also been reported with the concomitant use of two serotonin reuptake inhibitors. The syndrome requires immediate medical attention and may include one or more of the following symptoms: excitement, hypomania, restlessness, loss of consciousness, confusion, disorientation, anxiety, agitation, motor weakness, myoclonus, tremor, hemiballismus, hyperreflexia, ataxia, dysarthria, incoordination, hyperthermia, shivering, pupillary dilation, diaphoresis, emesis, and tachycardia).
No products indexed under this heading.

Fluoxetine Hydrochloride (The development of a potentially life-threatening serotonin syndrome, or Neuroleptic Malignant Syndrome (NMS)-like reactions, has been reported with SNRIs and SSRIs alone, including sibutramine treatment, but particularly with concomitant use of serotonergic drugs (including triptans)). Products include:
Prozac Weekly **1941**
Prozac Pulvules **1941**
Symbyax **1965**

IMPORTANT NOTE: Always consult each drug listing in the patient's regimen for possible interactions.

Fluphenazine Decanoate (The development of a potentially life-threatening serotonin syndrome, or Neuroleptic Malignant Syndrome (NMS)-like reactions, has been reported with SNRIs and SSRIs alone, including sibutramine treatment, but particularly with concomitant use with antipsychotics).

No products indexed under this heading.

Fluphenazine Enanthate (The development of a potentially life-threatening serotonin syndrome, or Neuroleptic Malignant Syndrome (NMS)-like reactions, has been reported with SNRIs and SSRIs alone, including sibutramine treatment, but particularly with concomitant use with antipsychotics).

No products indexed under this heading.

Fluphenazine Hydrochloride (The development of a potentially life-threatening serotonin syndrome, or Neuroleptic Malignant Syndrome (NMS)-like reactions, has been reported with SNRIs and SSRIs alone, including sibutramine treatment, but particularly with concomitant use with antipsychotics).

No products indexed under this heading.

Flurazepam Hydrochloride (The use of sibutramine in combination with other CNS-active drugs, particularly serotonergic agents, has not been systematically evaluated. Consequently, caution is advised if the concomitant administration of sibutramine with other centrally-acting drugs is indicated. Sibutramine is contraindicated in patients taking other centrally acting weight loss drugs).

No products indexed under this heading.

Fluvoxamine (Patients should be advised to inform their physicians if they are taking, or plan to take, any prescription or over-the-counter drugs, especially antidepressants, since there is a potential for interactions).

No products indexed under this heading.

Fluvoxamine Maleate (The development of a potentially life-threatening serotonin syndrome, or Neuroleptic Malignant Syndrome (NMS)-like reactions, has been reported with SNRIs and SSRIs alone, including sibutramine treatment, but particularly with concomitant use of serotonergic drugs (including triptans)).

No products indexed under this heading.

Frovatriptan Succinate (The development of a potentially life-threatening serotonin syndrome, or Neuroleptic Malignant Syndrome (NMS)-like reactions, has been reported with SNRIs and SSRIs alone, including sibutramine treatment, but particularly with concomitant use of serotonergic drugs (including triptans)). Products include:

Frova 1103

Glutethimide (The use of sibutramine in combination with other CNS-active drugs, particularly serotonergic agents, has not been systematically evaluated. Consequently, caution is advised if the concomitant administration of sibutramine with other centrally-acting drugs is indicated. Sibutramine is contraindicated in patients taking other centrally acting weight loss drugs).

No products indexed under this heading.

Haloperidol (The development of a potentially life-threatening serotonin syndrome, or Neuroleptic Malignant Syndrome (NMS)-like reactions, has been reported with SNRIs and SSRIs alone, including sibutramine treatment, but particularly with concomitant use with antipsychotics).

No products indexed under this heading.

Haloperidol Decanoate (The development of a potentially life-threatening serotonin syndrome, or Neuroleptic Malignant Syndrome (NMS)-like reactions, has been reported with SNRIs and SSRIs alone, including sibutramine treatment, but particularly with concomitant use with antipsychotics).

No products indexed under this heading.

Haloperidol Lactate (The development of a potentially life-threatening serotonin syndrome, or Neuroleptic Malignant Syndrome (NMS)-like reactions, has been reported with SNRIs and SSRIs alone, including sibutramine treatment, but particularly with concomitant use with antipsychotics).

No products indexed under this heading.

Hydrocodone Bitartrate (The use of sibutramine in combination with other CNS-active drugs, particularly serotonergic agents, has not been systematically evaluated. Consequently, caution is advised if the concomitant administration of sibutramine with other centrally-acting drugs is indicated. Sibutramine is contraindicated in patients taking other centrally acting weight loss drugs). Products include:

Vicodin	560
Vicodin ES	561
Vicodin HP	563
Vicoprofen	564
Zydone	1138

Hydrocodone Polistirex (The use of sibutramine in combination with other CNS-active drugs, particularly serotonergic agents, has not been systematically evaluated. Consequently, caution is advised if the concomitant administration of sibutramine with other centrally-acting drugs is indicated. Sibutramine is contraindicated in patients taking other centrally acting weight loss drugs). Products include:

Tussionex 3443

Hydromorphone Hydrochloride (The use of sibutramine in combination with other CNS-active drugs, particularly serotonergic agents, has not been systematically evaluated. Consequently, caution is advised if the concomitant administration of sibutramine with other centrally-acting drugs is indicated. Sibutramine is contraindicated in patients taking other centrally acting weight loss drugs). Products include:

Dilaudid Injection	2800
Dilaudid Oral	2797
Dilaudid Tablets	2797
Dilaudid-HP	2800

Hydroxyamphetamine Hydrobromide (The use of sibutramine in combination with other CNS-active drugs, particularly serotonergic agents, has not been systematically evaluated. Consequently, caution is advised if the concomitant administration of sibutramine with other centrally-acting drugs is indicated. Sibutramine is contraindicated in patients taking other centrally acting weight loss drugs).

No products indexed under this heading.

Hydroxyzine Hydrochloride (The use of sibutramine in combination with other CNS-active drugs, particularly serotonergic agents, has not been systematically evaluated. Consequently, caution is advised if the concomitant administration of sibutramine with other centrally-acting drugs is indicated. Sibutramine is contraindicated in patients taking other centrally acting weight loss drugs).

No products indexed under this heading.

Imipramine Hydrochloride (Patients should be advised to inform their physicians if they are taking, or plan to take, any prescription or over-the-counter drugs, especially antidepressants, since there is a potential for interactions).

No products indexed under this heading.

Imipramine Pamoate (Patients should be advised to inform their physicians if they are taking, or plan to take, any prescription or over-the-counter drugs, especially antidepressants, since there is a potential for interactions).

No products indexed under this heading.

Isocarboxazid (Sibutramine is contraindicated in patients receiving monoamine oxidase inhibitors (MAOIs). In patients receiving MAOIs (eg, phenelzine, selegiline) in combination with serotonergic agents (eg, fluoxetine, fluvoxamine, paroxetine, sertraline, venlafaxine), there have been reports of serious, sometimes fatal, reactions ("serotonin syndrome"). Because sibutramine inhibits serotonin reuptake, sibutramine should not be used concomitantly with a MAOI). Products include:

Marplan 3481

Isoflurane (The use of sibutramine in combination with other CNS-active drugs, particularly serotonergic agents, has not been systematically evaluated. Consequently, caution is advised if the concomitant administration of sibutramine with other centrally-acting drugs is indicated. Sibutramine is contraindicated in patients taking other centrally acting weight loss drugs).

No products indexed under this heading.

Isoproterenol Hydrochloride (Concomitant use of sibutramine and other agents that may raise blood pressure or heart rate have not been evaluated. These include certain decongestants, cough, cold, and allergy medications that contain agents, such as ephedrine, or pseudoephedrine. Caution should be used when prescribing sibutramine to patients who use these medications).

No products indexed under this heading.

Isoproterenol Sulfate (Concomitant use of sibutramine and other agents that may raise blood pressure or heart rate have not been evaluated. These include certain decongestants, cough, cold, and allergy medications that contain agents, such as ephedrine, or pseudoephedrine. Caution should be used when prescribing sibutramine to patients who use these medications).

No products indexed under this heading.

Ketamine Hydrochloride (The use of sibutramine in combination with other CNS-active drugs, particularly serotonergic agents, has not been systematically evaluated. Consequently, caution is advised if the concomitant administration of sibutramine with other centrally-acting drugs is indicated. Sibutramine is contraindicated in patients taking other centrally acting weight loss drugs).

No products indexed under this heading.

Ketoconazole (Concomitant administration of 200 mg doses of ketoconazole twice daily and 20 mg sibutramine once daily for 7 days in 12 uncomplicated obese subjects resulted in moderate increases in AUC and C_{max} of 58% and 36% for M_1 and of 20% and 19% for M_2, respectively). Products include:

| Extina .... | 3319 |
| Xolegel .... | 3337 |

Levalbuterol Hydrochloride (Concomitant use of sibutramine and other agents that may raise blood pressure or heart rate have not been evaluated. These include certain decongestants, cough, cold, and allergy medications that contain agents, such as ephedrine, or pseudoephedrine. Caution should be used when prescribing sibutramine to patients who use these medications).

No products indexed under this heading.

Levomethadyl Acetate Hydrochloride (The use of sibutramine in combination with other CNS-active drugs, particularly serotonergic agents, has not

been systematically evaluated. Consequently, caution is advised if the concomitant administration of sibutramine with other centrally-acting drugs is indicated. Sibutramine is contraindicated in patients taking other centrally acting weight loss drugs).

No products indexed under this heading.

Levorphanol Tartrate (The use of sibutramine in combination with other CNS-active drugs, particularly serotonergic agents, has not been systematically evaluated. Consequently, caution is advised if the concomitant administration of sibutramine with other centrally-acting drugs is indicated. Sibutramine is contraindicated in patients taking other centrally acting weight loss drugs).

No products indexed under this heading.

Lisdexamfetamine Dimesylate (The use of sibutramine in combination with other CNS-active drugs, particularly serotonergic agents, has not been systematically evaluated. Consequently, caution is advised if the concomitant administration of sibutramine with other centrally-acting drugs is indicated. Sibutramine is contraindicated in patients taking other centrally acting weight loss drugs). Products include:

Vyvanse 3298

Lithium (The rare, but serious, constellation of symptoms termed "serotonin syndrome" has also been reported with the concomitant use of lithium).

No products indexed under this heading.

Lithium Carbonate (The rare, but serious, constellation of symptoms termed "serotonin syndrome" has also been reported with the concomitant use of lithium).

No products indexed under this heading.

Lithium Citrate (The rare, but serious, constellation of symptoms termed "serotonin syndrome" has also been reported with the concomitant use of lithium).

No products indexed under this heading.

Lorazepam (The use of sibutramine in combination with other CNS-active drugs, particularly serotonergic agents, has not been systematically evaluated. Consequently, caution is advised if the concomitant administration of sibutramine with other centrally-acting drugs is indicated. Sibutramine is contraindicated in patients taking other centrally acting weight loss drugs).

No products indexed under this heading.

Loxapine Hydrochloride (The development of a potentially life-threatening serotonin syndrome, or Neuroleptic Malignant Syndrome (NMS)-like reactions, has been reported with SNRIs and SSRIs alone, including sibutramine treatment, but particularly with concomitant use with antipsychotics).

No products indexed under this heading.

Loxapine Succinate (The development of a potentially life-threatening serotonin syndrome, or Neuroleptic Malignant Syndrome (NMS)-like reactions, has been reported with SNRIs and SSRIs alone, including sibutramine treatment, but particularly with concomitant use with antipsychotics).

No products indexed under this heading.

Maprotiline Hydrochloride (Patients should be advised to inform their physicians if they are taking, or plan to take, any prescription or over-the-counter drugs, especially antidepressants, since there is a potential for interactions).

No products indexed under this heading.

Meperidine Hydrochloride (The rare, but serious, constellation of symptoms termed "serotonin syndrome" has also been reported with the concomitant use of selective serotonin reuptake inhibitors and certain opioids, such as meperidine).
No products indexed under this heading.

Mephobarbital (The use of sibutramine in combination with other CNS-active drugs, particularly serotonergic agents, has not been systematically evaluated. Consequently, caution is advised if the concomitant administration of sibutramine with other centrally-acting drugs is indicated. Sibutramine is contraindicated in patients taking other centrally acting weight loss drugs).
No products indexed under this heading.

Meprobamate (The use of sibutramine in combination with other CNS-active drugs, particularly serotonergic agents, has not been systematically evaluated. Consequently, caution is advised if the concomitant administration of sibutramine with other centrally-acting drugs is indicated. Sibutramine is contraindicated in patients taking other centrally acting weight loss drugs).
No products indexed under this heading.

Mesoridazine Besylate (The development of a potentially life-threatening serotonin syndrome, or Neuroleptic Malignant Syndrome (NMS)-like reactions, has been reported with SNRIs and SSRIs alone, including sibutramine treatment, but particularly with concomitant use with antipsychotics).
No products indexed under this heading.

Metaproterenol Sulfate (Concomitant use of sibutramine and other agents that may raise blood pressure or heart rate have not been evaluated. These include certain decongestants, cough, cold, and allergy medications that contain agents, such as ephedrine, or pseudoephedrine. Caution should be used when prescribing sibutramine to patients who use these medications).
No products indexed under this heading.

Metaraminol Bitartrate (Concomitant use of sibutramine and other agents that may raise blood pressure or heart rate have not been evaluated. These include certain decongestants, cough, cold, and allergy medications that contain agents, such as ephedrine, or pseudoephedrine. Caution should be used when prescribing sibutramine to patients who use these medications).
No products indexed under this heading.

Methadone Hydrochloride (The use of sibutramine in combination with other CNS-active drugs, particularly serotonergic agents, has not been systematically evaluated. Consequently, caution is advised if the concomitant administration of sibutramine with other centrally-acting drugs is indicated. Sibutramine is contraindicated in patients taking other centrally acting weight loss drugs).
No products indexed under this heading.

Methamphetamine Hydrochloride (The use of sibutramine in combination with other CNS-active drugs, particularly serotonergic agents, has not been systematically evaluated. Consequently, caution is advised if the concomitant administration of sibutramine with other centrally-acting drugs is indicated. Sibutramine is contraindicated in patients taking other centrally acting weight loss drugs).
No products indexed under this heading.

Methohexital Sodium (The use of sibutramine in combination with other CNS-active drugs, particularly serotonergic agents, has not been systematically evaluated. Consequently, caution is advised if the concomitant administration of sibutramine with other centrally-acting drugs is indicated. Sibutramine is contraindicated in patients taking other centrally acting weight loss drugs).
No products indexed under this heading.

Methotrimeprazine (The development of a potentially life-threatening serotonin syndrome, or Neuroleptic Malignant Syndrome (NMS)-like reactions, has been reported with SNRIs and SSRIs alone, including sibutramine treatment, but particularly with concomitant use with antipsychotics).
No products indexed under this heading.

Methoxamine Hydrochloride (Concomitant use of sibutramine and other agents that may raise blood pressure or heart rate have not been evaluated. These include certain decongestants, cough, cold, and allergy medications that contain agents, such as ephedrine, or pseudoephedrine. Caution should be used when prescribing sibutramine to patients who use these medications).
No products indexed under this heading.

Methoxyflurane (The use of sibutramine in combination with other CNS-active drugs, particularly serotonergic agents, has not been systematically evaluated. Consequently, caution is advised if the concomitant administration of sibutramine with other centrally-acting drugs is indicated. Sibutramine is contraindicated in patients taking other centrally acting weight loss drugs).
No products indexed under this heading.

Methylphenidate (The use of sibutramine in combination with other CNS-active drugs, particularly serotonergic agents, has not been systematically evaluated. Consequently, caution is advised if the concomitant administration of sibutramine with other centrally-acting drugs is indicated. Sibutramine is contraindicated in patients taking other centrally acting weight loss drugs). Products include:
Daytrana **3283**

Methylphenidate Hydrochloride (The use of sibutramine in combination with other CNS-active drugs, particularly serotonergic agents, has not been systematically evaluated. Consequently, caution is advised if the concomitant administration of sibutramine with other centrally-acting drugs is indicated. Sibutramine is contraindicated in patients taking other centrally acting weight loss drugs). Products include:
Concerta **2598**
Metadate CD **3439**

Metoclopramide Hydrochloride (The development of a potentially life-threatening serotonin syndrome, or Neuroleptic Malignant Syndrome (NMS)-like reactions, has been reported with SNRIs and SSRIs alone, including sibutramine treatment, but particularly with concomitant use with dopamine antagonists). Products include:
Metozolv ODT **2901**

Midazolam Hydrochloride (The use of sibutramine in combination with other CNS-active drugs, particularly serotonergic agents, has not been systematically evaluated. Consequently, caution is advised if the concomitant administration of sibutramine with other centrally-acting drugs is indicated. Sibutramine is contraindicated in patients taking other centrally acting weight loss drugs).
No products indexed under this heading.

Mirtazapine (Patients should be advised to inform their physicians if they are taking, or plan to take, any prescription or over-the-counter drugs, especially antidepressants, since there is a potential for interactions). Products include:
Remeron Tablets **3214**
RemeronSolTab Tablets **3219**

Moclobemide (Sibutramine is contraindicated in patients receiving monoamine oxidase inhibitors (MAOIs). In patients receiving MAOIs (eg, phenelzine, selegiline) in combination with serotonergic agents (eg, fluoxetine, fluvoxamine, paroxetine, sertraline, venlafaxine), there have been reports of serious, sometimes fatal, reactions ("serotonin syndrome"). Because sibutramine inhibits serotonin reuptake, sibutramine should not be used concomitantly with a MAOI).
No products indexed under this heading.

Molindone Hydrochloride (The development of a potentially life-threatening serotonin syndrome, or Neuroleptic Malignant Syndrome (NMS)-like reactions, has been reported with SNRIs and SSRIs alone, including sibutramine treatment, but particularly with concomitant use with antipsychotics). Products include:
Moban **1108**

Morphine Sulfate (The use of sibutramine in combination with other CNS-active drugs, particularly serotonergic agents, has not been systematically evaluated. Consequently, caution is advised if the concomitant administration of sibutramine with other centrally-acting drugs is indicated. Sibutramine is contraindicated in patients taking other centrally acting weight loss drugs). Products include:
Avinza **1822**
Embeda **1831**
MS Contin **2803**

Nalbuphine Hydrochloride (The rare, but serious, constellation of symptoms termed "serotonin syndrome" has also been reported with the concomitant use of selective serotonin reuptake inhibitors and certain opioids, such as dextromethorphan, meperidine, pentazocine and fentanyl, lithium, or tryptophan).
No products indexed under this heading.

Naphazoline Hydrochloride (Patients should be advised to inform their physicians if they are taking, or plan to take, any prescription or over-the-counter drugs, especially decongestants, since there is a potential for interactions). Products include:
Visine-A .... ⊙ **257**

Naratriptan Hydrochloride (The development of a potentially life-threatening serotonin syndrome, or Neuroleptic Malignant Syndrome (NMS)-like reactions, has been reported with SNRIs and SSRIs alone, including sibutramine treatment, but particularly with concomitant use of serotonergic drugs (including triptans)). Products include:
Amerge **1306**

Nefazodone Hydrochloride (Patients should be advised to inform their physicians if they are taking, or plan to take, any prescription or over-the-counter drugs, especially antidepressants, since there is a potential for interactions).
No products indexed under this heading.

Norepinephrine Bitartrate (Concomitant use of sibutramine and other agents that may raise blood pressure or heart rate have not been evaluated. These include certain decongestants, cough, cold, and allergy medications that contain agents, such as ephedrine, or pseudoephedrine. Caution should be used when prescribing sibutramine to patients who use these medications).
No products indexed under this heading.

Nortriptyline Hydrochloride (Patients should be advised to inform their physicians if they are taking, or plan to take, any prescription or over-the-counter drugs, especially antidepressants, since there is a potential for interactions).
No products indexed under this heading.

Olanzapine (Steady-state pharmacokinetics of sibutramine and metabolites M_1 and M_2 were evaluated in 24 healthy volunteers after the co-administration of sibutramine 15 mg once daily with olanzapine 5 mg twice daily for 3 days and 10 mg once daily thereafter for 7 days. Olanzapine slightly increased M_1 C_{max} (19%), and moderately increased sibutramine C_{max} (47%) and AUC (63%)). Products include:
Symbyax **1965**
Zyprexa **1984**
Zyprexa IntraMuscular **1984**
Zyprexa ZYDIS **1984**

Oxazepam (The use of sibutramine in combination with other CNS-active drugs, particularly serotonergic agents, has not been systematically evaluated. Consequently, caution is advised if the concomitant administration of sibutramine with other centrally-acting drugs is indicated. Sibutramine is contraindicated in patients taking other centrally acting weight loss drugs).
No products indexed under this heading.

Oxycodone Hydrochloride (The use of sibutramine in combination with other CNS-active drugs, particularly serotonergic agents, has not been systematically evaluated. Consequently, caution is advised if the concomitant administration of sibutramine with other centrally-acting drugs is indicated. Sibutramine is contraindicated in patients taking other centrally acting weight loss drugs). Products include:
OxyContin **2807**
Percocet **1121**
Percodan **1124**

Paliperidone (The development of a potentially life-threatening serotonin syndrome, or Neuroleptic Malignant Syndrome (NMS)-like reactions, has been reported with SNRIs and SSRIs alone, including sibutramine treatment, but particularly with concomitant use with antipsychotics). Products include:
Invega **2613**
Invega Sustenna **2621**

Pargyline Hydrochloride (Sibutramine is contraindicated in patients receiving monoamine oxidase inhibitors (MAOIs). In patients receiving MAOIs (eg, phenelzine, selegiline) in combination with serotonergic agents (eg, fluoxetine, fluvoxamine, paroxetine, sertraline, venlafaxine), there have been reports of serious, sometimes fatal, reactions ("serotonin syndrome"). Because sibutramine inhibits serotonin reuptake, sibutramine should not be used concomitantly with a MAOI).
No products indexed under this heading.

Paroxetine (Patients should be advised to inform their physicians if they are taking, or plan to take, any prescription or over-the-counter drugs, especially antidepressants, since there is a potential for interactions).
No products indexed under this heading.

Paroxetine Hydrochloride (The development of a potentially life-threatening serotonin syndrome, or Neuroleptic Malignant Syndrome (NMS)-like reactions, has been reported with SNRIs and SSRIs alone, including sibutramine treatment, but particularly with concomitant use of serotonergic drugs (including triptans)). Products include:
Paroxetine CR **2361**
Paroxetine ER **2371**
Paxil **1586**

Paxil CR 1596

Paroxetine Mesylate (Patients should be advised to inform their physicians if they are taking, or plan to take, any prescription or over-the-counter drugs, especially antidepressants, since there is a potential for interactions).
No products indexed under this heading.

Pemoline (The use of sibutramine in combination with other CNS-active drugs, particularly serotonergic agents, has not been systematically evaluated. Consequently, caution is advised if the concomitant administration of sibutramine with other centrally-acting drugs is indicated. Sibutramine is contraindicated in patients taking other centrally acting weight loss drugs).
No products indexed under this heading.

Pentazocine Hydrochloride (The rare, but serious, constellation of symptoms termed "serotonin syndrome" has also been reported with the concomitant use of selective serotonin reuptake inhibitors and certain opioids, such as pentazocine).
No products indexed under this heading.

Pentazocine Lactate (The rare, but serious, constellation of symptoms termed "serotonin syndrome" has also been reported with the concomitant use of selective serotonin reuptake inhibitors and certain opioids, such as pentazocine).
No products indexed under this heading.

Pentobarbital Sodium (The use of sibutramine in combination with other CNS-active drugs, particularly serotonergic agents, has not been systematically evaluated. Consequently, caution is advised if the concomitant administration of sibutramine with other centrally-acting drugs is indicated. Sibutramine is contraindicated in patients taking other centrally acting weight loss drugs). Products include:
Nembutal 2012

Perphenazine (The development of a potentially life-threatening serotonin syndrome, or Neuroleptic Malignant Syndrome (NMS)-like reactions, has been reported with SNRIs and SSRIs alone, including sibutramine treatment, but particularly with concomitant use with antipsychotics).
No products indexed under this heading.

Phenelzine Sulfate (Sibutramine is contraindicated in patients receiving monoamine oxidase inhibitors (MAOIs). In patients receiving MAOIs (eg, phenelzine, selegiline) in combination with serotonergic agents (eg, fluoxetine, fluvoxamine, paroxetine, sertraline, venlafaxine), there have been reports of serious, sometimes fatal, reactions ("serotonin syndrome"). Because sibutramine inhibits serotonin reuptake, sibutramine should not be used concomitantly with a MAOI).
No products indexed under this heading.

Phenobarbital (The use of sibutramine in combination with other CNS-active drugs, particularly serotonergic agents, has not been systematically evaluated. Consequently, caution is advised if the concomitant administration of sibutramine with other centrally-acting drugs is indicated. Sibutramine is contraindicated in patients taking other centrally acting weight loss drugs). Products include:
Donnatal 2711

Phenobarbital Sodium (The use of sibutramine in combination with other CNS-active drugs, particularly serotonergic agents, has not been systematically evaluated. Consequently, caution is advised if the concomitant administration of sibutramine with other centrally-acting drugs is indicated. Sibutramine is contraindicated in patients taking other centrally acting weight loss drugs).
No products indexed under this heading.

Phenylephrine Bitartrate (Concomitant use of sibutramine and other agents that may raise blood pressure or heart rate have not been evaluated. These include certain decongestants, cough, cold, and allergy medications that contain agents, such as ephedrine, or pseudoephedrine. Caution should be used when prescribing sibutramine to patients who use these medications).
No products indexed under this heading.

Phenylephrine Hydrochloride (Patients should be advised to inform their physicians if they are taking, or plan to take, any prescription or over-the-counter drugs, especially decongestants, since there is a potential for interactions). Products include:
Sudafed PE Nasal Decongestant 2048
Children's Sudafed PE Nasal Decongestant 2047

Phenylephrine Tannate (Concomitant use of sibutramine and other agents that may raise blood pressure or heart rate have not been evaluated. These include certain decongestants, cough, cold, and allergy medications that contain agents, such as ephedrine, or pseudoephedrine. Caution should be used when prescribing sibutramine to patients who use these medications).
No products indexed under this heading.

Phenylpropanolamine Hydrochloride (Concomitant use of sibutramine and other agents that may raise blood pressure or heart rate have not been evaluated. These include certain decongestants, cough, cold, and allergy medications that contain agents, such as ephedrine, or pseudoephedrine. Caution should be used when prescribing sibutramine to patients who use these medications).
No products indexed under this heading.

Pimozide (The development of a potentially life-threatening serotonin syndrome, or Neuroleptic Malignant Syndrome (NMS)-like reactions, has been reported with SNRIs and SSRIs alone, including sibutramine treatment, but particularly with concomitant use with antipsychotics).
No products indexed under this heading.

Pirbuterol Acetate (Concomitant use of sibutramine and other agents that may raise blood pressure or heart rate have not been evaluated. These include certain decongestants, cough, cold, and allergy medications that contain agents, such as ephedrine, or pseudoephedrine. Caution should be used when prescribing sibutramine to patients who use these medications). Products include:
Maxair Autohaler 1782

Prazepam (The use of sibutramine in combination with other CNS-active drugs, particularly serotonergic agents, has not been systematically evaluated. Consequently, caution is advised if the concomitant administration of sibutramine with other centrally-acting drugs is indicated. Sibutramine is contraindicated in patients taking other centrally acting weight loss drugs).
No products indexed under this heading.

Procarbazine Hydrochloride (Sibutramine is contraindicated in patients receiving monoamine oxidase inhibitors (MAOIs). In patients receiving MAOIs (eg, phenelzine, selegiline) in combination with serotonergic agents (eg, fluoxetine, fluvoxamine, paroxetine, sertraline, venlafaxine), there have been reports of serious, sometimes fatal, reactions ("serotonin syndrome"). Because sibutramine inhibits serotonin reuptake, sibutramine should not be used concomitantly with a MAOI).
No products indexed under this heading.

Prochlorperazine (The development of a potentially life-threatening serotonin syndrome, or Neuroleptic Malignant Syndrome (NMS)-like reactions, has been reported with SNRIs and SSRIs alone, including sibutramine treatment, but particularly with concomitant use with antipsychotics).
No products indexed under this heading.

Promethazine (The development of a potentially life-threatening serotonin syndrome, or Neuroleptic Malignant Syndrome (NMS)-like reactions, has been reported with SNRIs and SSRIs alone, including sibutramine treatment, but particularly with concomitant use with dopamine antagonists).
No products indexed under this heading.

Promethazine Hydrochloride (The development of a potentially life-threatening serotonin syndrome, or Neuroleptic Malignant Syndrome (NMS)-like reactions, has been reported with SNRIs and SSRIs alone, including sibutramine treatment, but particularly with concomitant use with dopamine antagonists).
No products indexed under this heading.

Propofol (The use of sibutramine in combination with other CNS-active drugs, particularly serotonergic agents, has not been systematically evaluated. Consequently, caution is advised if the concomitant administration of sibutramine with other centrally-acting drugs is indicated. Sibutramine is contraindicated in patients taking other centrally acting weight loss drugs).
No products indexed under this heading.

Propoxyphene Hydrochloride (The use of sibutramine in combination with other CNS-active drugs, particularly serotonergic agents, has not been systematically evaluated. Consequently, caution is advised if the concomitant administration of sibutramine with other centrally-acting drugs is indicated. Sibutramine is contraindicated in patients taking other centrally acting weight loss drugs).
No products indexed under this heading.

Propoxyphene Napsylate (The use of sibutramine in combination with other CNS-active drugs, particularly serotonergic agents, has not been systematically evaluated. Consequently, caution is advised if the concomitant administration of sibutramine with other centrally-acting drugs is indicated. Sibutramine is contraindicated in patients taking other centrally acting weight loss drugs).
No products indexed under this heading.

Propylhexedrine (Patients should be advised to inform their physicians if they are taking, or plan to take, any prescription or over-the-counter drugs, especially decongestants, since there is a potential for interactions).
No products indexed under this heading.

Protriptyline Hydrochloride (Patients should be advised to inform their physicians if they are taking, or plan to take, any prescription or over-the-counter drugs, especially antidepressants, since there is a potential for interactions).
No products indexed under this heading.

Pseudoephedrine (Caution should be used when prescribing sibutramine to patients who use allergy medications that contain agents, such as pseudoephedrine).
No products indexed under this heading.

Pseudoephedrine Hydrochloride (Caution should be used when prescribing sibutramine to patients who use allergy medications that contain agents, such as pseudoephedrine). Products include:
Allegra-D 2915
Allegra-D 24 2918
Sudafed 12 Hour Nasal Decongestant Non-Drowsy 2048
Sudafed 24 Hour 2048
Sudafed Nasal Decongestant 2047
Children's Sudafed Nasal Decongestant Liquid..................... 2047
Zyrtec-D Allergy & Congestion 2054

Pseudoephedrine Preparations (Caution should be used when prescribing sibutramine to patients who use allergy medications that contain agents, such as pseudoephedrine).
No products indexed under this heading.

Pseudoephedrine Sulfate (Sibutramine substantially raises blood in some patients and concomitant use of sibutramine and drugs that raise blood pressure and/or heart rate, such as decongestants, requires caution). Products include:
Clarinex-D 12-Hour 3101
Clarinex-D 3104

Pseudoephedrine Tannate (Caution should be used when prescribing sibutramine to patients who use allergy medications that contain agents, such as pseudoephedrine).
No products indexed under this heading.

Quazepam (The use of sibutramine in combination with other CNS-active drugs, particularly serotonergic agents, has not been systematically evaluated. Consequently, caution is advised if the concomitant administration of sibutramine with other centrally-acting drugs is indicated. Sibutramine is contraindicated in patients taking other centrally acting weight loss drugs).
No products indexed under this heading.

Quetiapine Fumarate (The development of a potentially life-threatening serotonin syndrome, or Neuroleptic Malignant Syndrome (NMS)-like reactions, has been reported with SNRIs and SSRIs alone, including sibutramine treatment, but particularly with concomitant use with antipsychotics). Products include:
Seroquel 750
Seroquel XR 759

Rasagiline Mesylate (Sibutramine is contraindicated in patients receiving monoamine oxidase inhibitors (MAOIs). In patients receiving MAOIs (eg, phenelzine, selegiline) in combination with serotonergic agents (eg, fluoxetine, fluvoxamine, paroxetine, sertraline, venlafaxine), there have been reports of serious, sometimes fatal, reactions ("serotonin syndrome"). Because sibutramine inhibits serotonin reuptake, sibutramine should not be used concomitantly with a MAOI). Products include:
Azilect 3383

Remifentanil Hydrochloride (The use of sibutramine in combination with other CNS-active drugs, particularly serotonergic agents, has not been systematically evaluated. Consequently, caution is advised if the concomitant administration of sibutramine with other centrally-acting drugs is indicated. Sibutramine is contraindicated in patients taking other centrally acting weight loss drugs).
No products indexed under this heading.

Risperidone (The development of a potentially life-threatening serotonin syndrome, or Neuroleptic Malignant Syndrome (NMS)-like reactions, has been reported with SNRIs and SSRIs alone, including sibutramine treatment, but particularly with concomitant use with antipsychotics). Products include:
Risperdal Consta **2682**

Rizatriptan Benzoate (The development of a potentially life-threatening serotonin syndrome, or Neuroleptic Malignant Syndrome (NMS)-like reactions, has been reported with SNRIs and SSRIs alone, including sibutramine treatment, but particularly with concomitant use of serotonergic drugs (including triptans). Products include:
Maxalt **2206**
Maxalt-MLT **2206**

Salmeterol Xinafoate (Concomitant use of sibutramine and other agents that may raise blood pressure or heart rate have not been evaluated. These include certain decongestants, cough, cold, and allergy medications that contain agents, such as ephedrine, or pseudoephedrine. Caution should be used when prescribing sibutramine to patients who use these medications). Products include:
Advair 100/50 .... **1275**
Advair 250/50 .... **1275**
Advair 500/50 .... **1275**
Advair HFA 45/21 .... **1288**
Advair HFA 115/21 .... **1288**
Advair HFA 230/21 .... **1288**
Serevent Diskus **1656**

Secobarbital Sodium (The use of sibutramine in combination with other CNS-active drugs, particularly serotonergic agents, has not been systematically evaluated. Consequently, caution is advised if the concomitant administration of sibutramine with other centrally-acting drugs is indicated. Sibutramine is contraindicated in patients taking other centrally acting weight loss drugs).
No products indexed under this heading.

Selegiline (Sibutramine is contraindicated in patients receiving monoamine oxidase inhibitors (MAOIs). In patients receiving MAOIs (eg, phenelzine, selegiline) in combination with serotonergic agents (eg, fluoxetine, fluvoxamine, paroxetine, sertraline, venlafaxine), there have been reports of serious, sometimes fatal, reactions ("serotonin syndrome"). Because sibutramine inhibits serotonin reuptake, sibutramine should not be used concomitantly with a MAOI). Products include:
Emsam **3623**

Selegiline Hydrochloride (Sibutramine is contraindicated in patients receiving monoamine oxidase inhibitors (MAOIs). In patients receiving MAOIs (eg, phenelzine, selegiline) in combination with serotonergic agents (eg, fluoxetine, fluvoxamine, paroxetine, sertraline, venlafaxine), there have been reports of serious, sometimes fatal, reactions ("serotonin syndrome"). Because sibutramine inhibits serotonin reuptake, sibutramine should not be used concomitantly with a MAOI). Products include:
Eldepryl **3312**

Sertraline Hydrochloride (The development of a potentially life-threatening serotonin syndrome, or Neuroleptic Malignant Syndrome (NMS)-like reactions, has been reported with SNRIs and SSRIs alone, including sibutramine treatment, but particularly with concomitant use of serotonergic drugs (including triptans)).
No products indexed under this heading.

Sevoflurane (The use of sibutramine in combination with other CNS-active drugs, particularly serotonergic agents, has not been systematically evaluated.

Consequently, caution is advised if the concomitant administration of sibutramine with other centrally-acting drugs is indicated. Sibutramine is contraindicated in patients taking other centrally acting weight loss drugs). Products include:
Ultane **554**

Simvastatin (Steady-state pharmacokinetics of sibutramine and metabolites M_1 and M_2 were evaluated in 27 healthy volunteers after the administration of simvastatin 20 mg once daily in the evening and sibutramine 15 mg once daily in the morning for 7 days. The C_{max} (16%) and AUC (12%) of M_1 were slightly decreased. Simvastatin slightly decreased sibutramine C_{max} (14%) and AUC (21%). Sibutramine increased the AUC (7%) of the pharmacologically active moiety, simvastatin acid and reduced the C_{max} (25%) and AUC (15%) of inactive simvastatin). Products include:
Simcor **524**
Vytorin 10/10 .... **2303, 3240**
Vytorin 10/20 .... **2303, 3240**
Vytorin 10/40 .... **2303, 3240**
Vytorin 10/80 .... **2303, 3240**
Zocor **2289**

Sodium Oxybate (The use of sibutramine in combination with other CNS-active drugs, particularly serotonergic agents, has not been systematically evaluated. Consequently, caution is advised if the concomitant administration of sibutramine with other centrally-acting drugs is indicated. Sibutramine is contraindicated in patients taking other centrally acting weight loss drugs).
No products indexed under this heading.

Sufentanil Citrate (The use of sibutramine in combination with other CNS-active drugs, particularly serotonergic agents, has not been systematically evaluated. Consequently, caution is advised if the concomitant administration of sibutramine with other centrally-acting drugs is indicated. Sibutramine is contraindicated in patients taking other centrally acting weight loss drugs).
No products indexed under this heading.

Sumatriptan (The development of a potentially life-threatening serotonin syndrome, or Neuroleptic Malignant Syndrome (NMS)-like reactions, has been reported with SNRIs and SSRIs alone, including sibutramine treatment, but particularly with concomitant use of serotonergic drugs (including triptans)). Products include:
Imitrex Nasal **1503**

Sumatriptan Succinate (The rare, but serious, constellation of symptoms termed "serotonin syndrome" has also been reported with the concomitant use of selective serotonin reuptake inhibitors and agents for migraine therapy, such as sumatriptan succinate). Products include:
Imitrex **1497**
Imitrex Tablets **1508**
Treximet **1681**

Temazepam (The use of sibutramine in combination with other CNS-active drugs, particularly serotonergic agents, has not been systematically evaluated. Consequently, caution is advised if the concomitant administration of sibutramine with other centrally-acting drugs is indicated. Sibutramine is contraindicated in patients taking other centrally acting weight loss drugs).
No products indexed under this heading.

Terbutaline Sulfate (Concomitant use of sibutramine and other agents that may raise blood pressure or heart rate have not been evaluated. These include certain decongestants, cough, cold, and allergy medications that contain agents, such as ephedrine, or pseudoephedrine. Caution should be used when prescribing sibutramine to patients who use these medications).
No products indexed under this heading.

Tetrahydrozoline Hydrochloride (Patients should be advised to inform their physicians if they are taking, or plan to take, any prescription or over-the-counter drugs, especially decongestants, since there is a potential for interactions).
No products indexed under this heading.

Thiamylal Sodium (The use of sibutramine in combination with other CNS-active drugs, particularly serotonergic agents, has not been systematically evaluated. Consequently, caution is advised if the concomitant administration of sibutramine with other centrally-acting drugs is indicated. Sibutramine is contraindicated in patients taking other centrally acting weight loss drugs).
No products indexed under this heading.

Thioridazine Hydrochloride (The development of a potentially life-threatening serotonin syndrome, or Neuroleptic Malignant Syndrome (NMS)-like reactions, has been reported with SNRIs and SSRIs alone, including sibutramine treatment, but particularly with concomitant use with antipsychotics). Products include:
Thioridazine Hydrochloride **2384**

Thiothixene (The development of a potentially life-threatening serotonin syndrome, or Neuroleptic Malignant Syndrome (NMS)-like reactions, has been reported with SNRIs and SSRIs alone, including sibutramine treatment, but particularly with concomitant use with antipsychotics). Products include:
Thiothixene **2386**

Tranylcypromine Sulfate (Sibutramine is contraindicated in patients receiving monoamine oxidase inhibitors (MAOIs). In patients receiving MAOIs (eg, phenelzine, selegiline) in combination with serotonergic agents (eg, fluoxetine, fluvoxamine, paroxetine, sertraline, venlafaxine), there have been reports of serious, sometimes fatal, reactions ("serotonin syndrome"). Because sibutramine inhibits serotonin reuptake, sibutramine should not be used concomitantly with a MAOI). Products include:
Parnate **1584**

Trazodone Hydrochloride (Patients should be advised to inform their physicians if they are taking, or plan to take, any prescription or over-the-counter drugs, especially antidepressants, since there is a potential for interactions).
No products indexed under this heading.

Triazolam (The use of sibutramine in combination with other CNS-active drugs, particularly serotonergic agents, has not been systematically evaluated. Consequently, caution is advised if the concomitant administration of sibutramine with other centrally-acting drugs is indicated. Sibutramine is contraindicated in patients taking other centrally acting weight loss drugs).
No products indexed under this heading.

Trifluoperazine Hydrochloride (The development of a potentially life-threatening serotonin syndrome, or Neuroleptic Malignant Syndrome (NMS)-like reactions, has been reported with SNRIs and SSRIs alone, including sibutramine treatment, but particularly with concomitant use with antipsychotics).
No products indexed under this heading.

Trimipramine Maleate (Patients should be advised to inform their physicians if they are taking, or plan to take, any prescription or over-the-counter drugs, especially antidepressants, since there is a potential for interactions).
No products indexed under this heading.

Tryptophan (The rare, but serious, constellation of symptoms termed "serotonin syndrome" has also been reported with the concomitant use of selective serotonin reuptake inhibitors and certain opioids, such as tryptophan).
No products indexed under this heading.

L-Tryptophan (Sibutramine inhibits serotonin reuptake and combination of SSRIs and tryptophan has resulted in serious, sometimes fatal, reactions, serotonin syndrome).
No products indexed under this heading.

Venlafaxine Hydrochloride (The development of a potentially life-threatening serotonin syndrome, or Neuroleptic Malignant Syndrome (NMS)-like reactions, has been reported with SNRIs and SSRIs alone, including sibutramine treatment, but particularly with concomitant use of serotonergic drugs (including triptans)). Products include:
Effexor XR **3504**
Venlafaxine Hydrochloride Tablets ... **2388**

Xylometazoline Hydrochloride (Patients should be advised to inform their physicians if they are taking, or plan to take, any prescription or over-the-counter drugs, especially decongestants, since there is a potential for interactions).
No products indexed under this heading.

Zaleplon (The use of sibutramine in combination with other CNS-active drugs, particularly serotonergic agents, has not been systematically evaluated. Consequently, caution is advised if the concomitant administration of sibutramine with other centrally-acting drugs is indicated. Sibutramine is contraindicated in patients taking other centrally acting weight loss drugs).
No products indexed under this heading.

Ziprasidone Hydrochloride (The development of a potentially life-threatening serotonin syndrome, or Neuroleptic Malignant Syndrome (NMS)-like reactions, has been reported with SNRIs and SSRIs alone, including sibutramine treatment, but particularly with concomitant use with antipsychotics). Products include:
Geodon **2723**

Zolmitriptan (The development of a potentially life-threatening serotonin syndrome, or Neuroleptic Malignant Syndrome (NMS)-like reactions, has been reported with SNRIs and SSRIs alone, including sibutramine treatment, but particularly with concomitant use of serotonergic drugs (including triptans)). Products include:
Zomig Tablets **773**
Zomig Nasal Spray **768**
Zomig-ZMT Tablets **773**

Zolpidem Tartrate (The use of sibutramine in combination with other CNS-active drugs, particularly serotonergic agents, has not been systematically evaluated. Consequently, caution is advised if the concomitant administration of sibutramine with other centrally-acting drugs is indicated.

IMPORTANT NOTE: Always consult each drug listing in the patient's regimen for possible interactions.

Sibutramine is contraindicated in patients taking other centrally acting weight loss drugs). Products include:
Ambien 2920
Ambien CR 2925

Food Interactions

Alcohol (In a double-blind, placebo-controlled, crossover study in 19 volunteers, administration of a single dose of ethanol (0.5 mL/kg) together with 20 mg of sibutramine resulted in no psychomotor interactions of clinical significance between alcohol and sibutramine. However, the concomitant use of sibutramine and excess alcohol is not recommended).

Beer, reduced-alcohol (In a double-blind, placebo-controlled, crossover study in 19 volunteers, administration of a single dose of ethanol (0.5 mL/kg) together with 20 mg of sibutramine resulted in no psychomotor interactions of clinical significance between alcohol and sibutramine. However, the concomitant use of sibutramine and excess alcohol is not recommended).

Beer, unspecified (In a double-blind, placebo-controlled, crossover study in 19 volunteers, administration of a single dose of ethanol (0.5 mL/kg) together with 20 mg of sibutramine resulted in no psychomotor interactions of clinical significance between alcohol and sibutramine. However, the concomitant use of sibutramine and excess alcohol is not recommended).

Food, unspecified (Administration of a single 20 mg dose of sibutramine with a standard breakfast resulted in reduced peak M_1 and M_2 concentrations (by 27% and 32%, respectively) and delayed the time to peak by approximately three hours. However, the AUCs of M_1 and M_2 were not significantly altered).

Meal, unspecified (Administration of a single 20 mg dose of sibutramine with a standard breakfast resulted in reduced peak M_1 and M_2 concentrations (by 27% and 32%, respectively) and delayed the time to peak by approximately three hours. However, the AUCs of M_1 and M_2 were not significantly altered).

Wine, Chianti (In a double-blind, placebo-controlled, crossover study in 19 volunteers, administration of a single dose of ethanol (0.5 mL/kg) together with 20 mg of sibutramine resulted in no psychomotor interactions of clinical significance between alcohol and sibutramine. However, the concomitant use of sibutramine and excess alcohol is not recommended).

Wine, Red (In a double-blind, placebo-controlled, crossover study in 19 volunteers, administration of a single dose of ethanol (0.5 mL/kg) together with 20 mg of sibutramine resulted in no psychomotor interactions of clinical significance between alcohol and sibutramine. However, the concomitant use of sibutramine and excess alcohol is not recommended).

Wine, unspecified (In a double-blind, placebo-controlled, crossover study in 19 volunteers, administration of a single dose of ethanol (0.5 mL/kg) together with 20 mg of sibutramine resulted in no psychomotor interactions of clinical significance between alcohol and sibutramine. However, the concomitant use of sibutramine and excess alcohol is not recommended).

Wine products (In a double-blind, placebo-controlled, crossover study in 19 volunteers, administration of a single dose of ethanol (0.5 mL/kg) together with 20 mg of sibutramine resulted in no psychomotor interactions of clinical significance between alcohol and sibutramine. However, the concomitant use of sibutramine and excess alcohol is not recommended).

MERREM I.V.

(Meropenem) 745
May interact with valproate, and certain other agents. Compounds in these categories include:

Divalproex Sodium (A clinically significant reduction in serum valproic acid concentrations has been reported in patients receiving carbapenem antibiotics and may result in loss of seizure control. Although the mechanism of this interaction is not fully understood, data from *in vivo* and animal studies suggest that carbapenem antibiotics may inhibit valproic acid glucuronide hydrolysis. Serum valproic acid concentrations should be monitored frequently after initiating carbapenem therapy. Alternative antibacterial or anticonvulsant therapy should be considered if serum valproic acid concentrations drop below the therapeutic range or a seizure occurs). Products include:
Depakote ER 426

Probenecid (Competes with meropenem for active tubular secretion and, thus, inhibits the renal excretion of meropenem. Statistically significant increases in the elimination half-life and the extent of systemic exposure have been reported; co-administration is not recommended).
No products indexed under this heading.

Valproate Sodium (A clinically significant reduction in serum valproic acid concentrations has been reported in patients receiving carbapenem antibiotics and may result in loss of seizure control. Although the mechanism of this interaction is not fully understood, data from *in vivo* and animal studies suggest that carbapenem antibiotics may inhibit valproic acid glucuronide hydrolysis. Serum valproic acid concentrations should be monitored frequently after initiating carbapenem therapy. Alternative antibacterial or anticonvulsant therapy should be considered if serum valproic acid concentrations drop below the therapeutic range or a seizure occurs).
No products indexed under this heading.

Valproic Acid (A clinically significant reduction in serum valproic acid concentrations has been reported in patients receiving carbapenem antibiotics and may result in loss of seizure control. Although the mechanism of this interaction is not fully understood, data from *in vivo* and animal studies suggest that carbapenem antibiotics may inhibit valproic acid glucuronide hydrolysis. Serum valproic acid concentrations should be monitored frequently after initiating carbapenem therapy. Alternative antibacterial or anticonvulsant therapy should be considered if serum valproic acid concentrations drop below the therapeutic range or a seizure occurs).
No products indexed under this heading.

MERUVAX II

(Rubella Virus Vaccine Live) 2210
May interact with immunosuppressive agents. Compounds in these categories include:

Azathioprine (Concurrent immunosuppressive therapy is contraindicated).
No products indexed under this heading.

Basiliximab (Concurrent immunosuppressive therapy is contraindicated). Products include:
Simulect 2524

Cyclosporine (Concurrent immunosuppressive therapy is contraindicated). Products include:
Gengraf 440
Neoral Oral Solution 2496
Neoral Capsules 2496
Restasis 605

Muromonab-CD3 (Concurrent immunosuppressive therapy is contraindicated). Products include:
Orthoclone OKT3 949

Mycophenolate Mofetil (Concurrent immunosuppressive therapy is contraindicated).
No products indexed under this heading.

Rapamycin (Concurrent immunosuppressive therapy is contraindicated).
No products indexed under this heading.

Sirolimus (Concurrent immunosuppressive therapy is contraindicated). Products include:
Rapamune 3579

Tacrolimus (Concurrent immunosuppressive therapy is contraindicated). Products include:
Prograf Capsules 677
Prograf Injection 677
Protopic 685

METADATE CD CAPSULES

(Methylphenidate Hydrochloride) 3439
May interact with halogenated hydrocarbon anesthetics, monoamine oxidase inhibitors, oral anticoagulants, phenytoin, selective serotonin reuptake inhibitors, tricyclic antidepressants, urinary acidifying agents, urinary alkalinizing agents, vasopressors, and certain other agents. Compounds in these categories include:

Amitriptyline Hydrochloride (Methylphenidate may inhibit the metabolism of tricyclic antidepressants; downward dosage adjustment of tricyclic antidepressants may be required).
No products indexed under this heading.

Ammonium Chloride (Clearance of methylphenidate might be affected by urinary pH, increasing with the use of acidifying agents. This should be considered when methylphenidate is given in combination with agents that alter urinary pH).
No products indexed under this heading.

Amoxapine (Methylphenidate may inhibit the metabolism of tricyclic antidepressants; downward dosage adjustment of tricyclic antidepressants may be required).
No products indexed under this heading.

Anisindione (Methylphenidate may inhibit the metabolism of coumarin anticoagulants; downward dosage adjustment of anticoagulants may be required).
No products indexed under this heading.

Citalopram Hydrobromide (Methylphenidate may inhibit the metabolism of selective serotonin reuptake inhibitors; downward dosage adjustment of SSRI may be required). Products include:
Celexa 1153

Clomipramine Hydrochloride (Methylphenidate may inhibit the metabolism of tricyclic antidepressants; downward dosage adjustment of tricyclic antidepressants may be required).
No products indexed under this heading.

Clonidine (Co-administration has resulted in serious adverse events, although no causality for the combination has been established). Products include:
Catapres-TTS 884

Clonidine Hydrochloride (Co-administration has resulted in serious adverse events, although no causality for the combination has been established). Products include:
Clorpres 2344

Desflurane (There is a risk of sudden blood pressure increase during surgery. If surgery is planned, methylphenidate should not be taken the day of the surgery).
No products indexed under this heading.

Desipramine Hydrochloride (Methylphenidate may inhibit the metabolism of tricyclic antidepressants; downward dosage adjustment of tricyclic antidepressants may be required).
No products indexed under this heading.

Dibasic Sodium Phosphate (Clearance of methylphenidate might be affected by urinary pH, increasing with the use of acidifying agents. This should be considered when methylphenidate is given in combination with agents that alter urinary pH). Products include:
Fleet Prep Kit 3 1145

Dicumarol (Methylphenidate may inhibit the metabolism of coumarin anticoagulants; downward dosage adjustment of anticoagulants may be required).
No products indexed under this heading.

Dipotassium Phosphate (Clearance of methylphenidate might be affected by urinary pH, increasing with the use of acidifying agents. This should be considered when methylphenidate is given in combination with agents that alter urinary pH).
No products indexed under this heading.

Disodium Phosphate (Clearance of methylphenidate might be affected by urinary pH, increasing with the use of acidifying agents. This should be considered when methylphenidate is given in combination with agents that alter urinary pH).
No products indexed under this heading.

Dobutamine (Methylphenidate causes rise in blood pressure; co-administration with other pressor agents should be undertaken with caution).
No products indexed under this heading.

Dobutamine Hydrochloride (Methylphenidate causes rise in blood pressure; co-administration with other pressor agents should be undertaken with caution).
No products indexed under this heading.

Dopamine Hydrochloride (Methylphenidate causes rise in blood pressure; co-administration with other pressor agents should be undertaken with caution).
No products indexed under this heading.

Doxepin Hydrochloride (Methylphenidate may inhibit the metabolism of tricyclic antidepressants; downward dosage adjustment of tricyclic antidepressants may be required).
No products indexed under this heading.

Enflurane (There is a risk of sudden blood pressure increase during surgery. If surgery is planned, methylphenidate should not be taken the day of the surgery).
No products indexed under this heading.

Ephedrine Sulfate (Methylphenidate causes rise in blood pressure; co-administration with other pressor agents should be undertaken with caution).
No products indexed under this heading.

Epinephrine Bitartrate (Methylphenidate causes rise in blood pressure; co-administration with other pressor agents should be undertaken with caution).
No products indexed under this heading.

Epinephrine Hydrochloride (Methylphenidate causes rise in blood pressure; co-administration with other pressor agents should be undertaken with caution).
No products indexed under this heading.

Escitalopram Oxalate (Methylphenidate may inhibit the metabolism of

selective serotonin reuptake inhibitors; downward dosage adjustment of SSRI may be required). Products include:

Fluoxetine (Methylphenidate may inhibit the metabolism of selective serotonin reuptake inhibitors; downward dosage adjustment of SSRI may be required).
No products indexed under this heading.

Fluoxetine Hydrochloride (Methylphenidate may inhibit the metabolism of selective serotonin reuptake inhibitors; downward dosage adjustment of SSRI may be required). Products include:

Fluvoxamine (Methylphenidate may inhibit the metabolism of selective serotonin reuptake inhibitors; downward dosage adjustment of SSRI may be required).
No products indexed under this heading.

Fluvoxamine Maleate (Methylphenidate may inhibit the metabolism of selective serotonin reuptake inhibitors; downward dosage adjustment of SSRI may be required).
No products indexed under this heading.

Fosphenytoin (Methylphenidate may inhibit the metabolism of anticonvulsants, such as phenytoin; additionally methylphenidate may lower the convulsive threshold in patients with prior history of seizures).
No products indexed under this heading.

Fosphenytoin Sodium (Methylphenidate may inhibit the metabolism of anticonvulsants, such as phenytoin; additionally methylphenidate may lower the convulsive threshold in patients with prior history of seizures).
No products indexed under this heading.

Halothane (There is a risk of sudden blood pressure increase during surgery. If surgery is planned, methylphenidate should not be taken the day of the surgery).
No products indexed under this heading.

Imipramine Hydrochloride (Methylphenidate may inhibit the metabolism of tricyclic antidepressants; downward dosage adjustment of tricyclic antidepressants may be required).
No products indexed under this heading.

Imipramine Pamoate (Methylphenidate may inhibit the metabolism of tricyclic antidepressants; downward dosage adjustment of tricyclic antidepressants may be required).
No products indexed under this heading.

Isocarboxazid (Co-administration is contraindicated during treatment with monoamine oxidase inhibitors, and also within a minimum of 14 days following discontinuation of a monoamine oxidase inhibitor (hypertensive crises may result)). Products include:

Isoflurane (There is a risk of sudden blood pressure increase during surgery. If surgery is planned, methylphenidate should not be taken the day of the surgery).
No products indexed under this heading.

Isoproterenol Hydrochloride (Methylphenidate causes rise in blood pressure; co-administration with other pressor agents should be undertaken with caution).
No products indexed under this heading.

Isoproterenol Sulfate (Methylphenidate causes rise in blood pressure; co-administration with other pressor agents should be undertaken with caution).
No products indexed under this heading.

Maprotiline Hydrochloride (Methylphenidate may inhibit the metabolism of tricyclic antidepressants; downward dosage adjustment of tricyclic antidepressants may be required).
No products indexed under this heading.

Mephentermine Sulfate (Methylphenidate causes rise in blood pressure; co-administration with other pressor agents should be undertaken with caution).
No products indexed under this heading.

Metaraminol Bitartrate (Methylphenidate causes rise in blood pressure; co-administration with other pressor agents should be undertaken with caution).
No products indexed under this heading.

Methoxamine Hydrochloride (Methylphenidate causes rise in blood pressure; co-administration with other pressor agents should be undertaken with caution).
No products indexed under this heading.

Methoxyflurane (There is a risk of sudden blood pressure increase during surgery. If surgery is planned, methylphenidate should not be taken the day of the surgery).
No products indexed under this heading.

Moclobemide (Co-administration is contraindicated during treatment with monoamine oxidase inhibitors, and also within a minimum of 14 days following discontinuation of a monoamine oxidase inhibitor (hypertensive crises may result)).
No products indexed under this heading.

Monobasic Potassium Phosphate (Clearance of methylphenidate might be affected by urinary pH, increasing with the use of acidifying agents. This should be considered when methylphenidate is given in combination with agents that alter urinary pH).
No products indexed under this heading.

Monobasic Sodium Phosphate (Clearance of methylphenidate might be affected by urinary pH, increasing with the use of acidifying agents. This should be considered when methylphenidate is given in combination with agents that alter urinary pH). Products include:

Norepinephrine Bitartrate (Methylphenidate causes rise in blood pressure; co-administration with other pressor agents should be undertaken with caution).
No products indexed under this heading.

Nortriptyline Hydrochloride (Methylphenidate may inhibit the metabolism of tricyclic antidepressants; downward dosage adjustment of tricyclic antidepressants may be required).
No products indexed under this heading.

Pargyline Hydrochloride (Co-administration is contraindicated during treatment with monoamine oxidase inhibitors, and also within a minimum of 14 days following discontinuation of a monoamine oxidase inhibitor (hypertensive crises may result)).
No products indexed under this heading.

Paroxetine (Methylphenidate may inhibit the metabolism of selective serotonin reuptake inhibitors; downward dosage adjustment of SSRI may be required).
No products indexed under this heading.

Paroxetine Hydrochloride (Methylphenidate may inhibit the metabolism of selective serotonin reuptake inhibitors; downward dosage adjustment of SSRI may be required). Products include:

Paroxetine Mesylate (Methylphenidate may inhibit the metabolism of selective serotonin reuptake inhibitors; downward dosage adjustment of SSRI may be required).
No products indexed under this heading.

Phenelzine Sulfate (Co-administration is contraindicated during treatment with monoamine oxidase inhibitors, and also within a minimum of 14 days following discontinuation of a monoamine oxidase inhibitor (hypertensive crises may result)).
No products indexed under this heading.

Phenobarbital (Methylphenidate may inhibit the metabolism of anticonvulsants, such as phenobarbital; additionally methylphenidate may lower the convulsive threshold in patients with prior history of seizures). Products include:

Phenylbutazone (Human pharmacologic studies have shown the methylphenidate may inhibit the metabolism of phenylbutazone. Downward dose adjustment of these drugs may be required when given concomitantly with methylphenidate).
No products indexed under this heading.

Phenylephrine Hydrochloride (Methylphenidate causes rise in blood pressure; co-administration with other pressor agents should be undertaken with caution). Products include:

Phenytoin (Methylphenidate may inhibit the metabolism of anticonvulsants, such as phenytoin; additionally methylphenidate may lower the convulsive threshold in patients with prior history of seizures).
No products indexed under this heading.

Phenytoin Sodium (Methylphenidate may inhibit the metabolism of anticonvulsants, such as phenytoin; additionally methylphenidate may lower the convulsive threshold in patients with prior history of seizures). Products include:

Potassium Acid Phosphate (Clearance of methylphenidate might be affected by urinary pH, increasing with the use of acidifying agents. This should be considered when methylphenidate is given in combination with agents that alter urinary pH). Products include:

Potassium Citrate (Clearance of methylphenidate might be affected by urinary pH, decreasing with the use of alkalizing agents. This should be considered when methylphenidate is given in combination with agents that alter urinary pH). Products include:

Primidone (Methylphenidate may inhibit the metabolism of anticonvulsants, such as primidone; additionally methylphenidate may lower the convulsive threshold in patients with prior history of seizures).
No products indexed under this heading.

Procarbazine Hydrochloride (Co-administration is contraindicated during treatment with monoamine oxidase inhibitors, and also within a minimum of 14 days following discontinuation of a monoamine oxidase inhibitor (hypertensive crises may result)).
No products indexed under this heading.

Protriptyline Hydrochloride (Methylphenidate may inhibit the metabolism of tricyclic antidepressants; downward dosage adjustment of tricyclic antidepressants may be required).
No products indexed under this heading.

Rasagiline Mesylate (Co-administration is contraindicated during treatment with monoamine oxidase

inhibitors, and also within a minimum of 14 days following discontinuation of a monoamine oxidase inhibitor (hypertensive crises may result)). Products include:

Selegiline (Co-administration is contraindicated during treatment with monoamine oxidase inhibitors, and also within a minimum of 14 days following discontinuation of a monoamine oxidase inhibitor (hypertensive crises may result)). Products include:

Selegiline Hydrochloride (Co-administration is contraindicated during treatment with monoamine oxidase inhibitors, and also within a minimum of 14 days following discontinuation of a monoamine oxidase inhibitor (hypertensive crises may result)). Products include:

Sertraline Hydrochloride (Methylphenidate may inhibit the metabolism of selective serotonin reuptake inhibitors; downward dosage adjustment of SSRI may be required).
No products indexed under this heading.

Sevoflurane (There is a risk of sudden blood pressure increase during surgery. If surgery is planned, methylphenidate should not be taken the day of the surgery). Products include:

Sodium Acid Phosphate (Clearance of methylphenidate might be affected by urinary pH, increasing with the use of acidifying agents. This should be considered when methylphenidate is given in combination with agents that alter urinary pH). Products include:

Sodium Bicarbonate (Clearance of methylphenidate might be affected by urinary pH, decreasing with the use of alkalizing agents. This should be considered when methylphenidate is given in combination with agents that alter urinary pH).
No products indexed under this heading.

Sodium Citrate (Clearance of methylphenidate might be affected by urinary pH, decreasing with the use of alkalizing agents. This should be considered when methylphenidate is given in combination with agents that alter urinary pH).
No products indexed under this heading.

Sodium Phosphate (Clearance of methylphenidate might be affected by urinary pH, increasing with the use of acidifying agents. This should be considered when methylphenidate is given in combination with agents that alter urinary pH). Products include:

Tranylcypromine Sulfate (Co-administration is contraindicated during treatment with monoamine oxidase inhibitors, and also within a minimum of 14 days following discontinuation of a monoamine oxidase inhibitor (hypertensive crises may result)). Products include:

Trimipramine Maleate (Methylphenidate may inhibit the metabolism of tricyclic antidepressants; downward dosage adjustment of tricyclic antidepressants may be required).
No products indexed under this heading.

Venlafaxine Hydrochloride (Co-administration in a patient on methylphenidate for 18 months has resulted in neuroleptic malignant syndrome within 45 minutes of ingesting his first dose of venlafaxine). Products include:

IMPORTANT NOTE: Always consult each drug listing in the patient's regimen for possible interactions.

Vitamin C (Clearance of methylphenidate might be affected by urinary pH, increasing with the use of acidifying agents. This should be considered when methylphenidate is given in combination with agents that alter urinary pH).
Products include:

Warfarin Sodium (Methylphenidate may inhibit the metabolism of coumarin anticoagulants; downward dosage adjustment of anticoagulants may be required).
No products indexed under this heading.

METOZOLV ODT ORALLY DISINTEGRATING TABLETS

(Metoclopramide Hydrochloride) 2901
May interact with alcohols, anticholinergics, anticonvulsants, antidepressant drugs, antipsychotic agents, hepatotoxic drugs, hypnotics and sedatives, insulin, monoamine oxidase inhibitors, narcotic analgesics, tetracyclines, tranquilizers, and certain other agents. Compounds in these categories include:

Acetaminophen (Absorption of drugs from the stomach may be diminished by metoclopramide (eg, digoxin), whereas the rate and/or extent of absorption of drugs from the small bowel may be increased (eg, acetaminophen, tetracycline, levodopa, ethanol, cyclosporine)).
Products include:

Alfentanil Hydrochloride (The effects of metoclopramide on gastrointestinal motility are antagonized by anticholinergic drugs and narcotic analgesics. Additive sedative effects can occur when metoclopramide is given with alcohol, sedatives, hypnotics, narcotics, or tranquilizers).
No products indexed under this heading.

Alprazolam (Additive sedative effects can occur when metoclopramide is given with alcohol, sedatives, hypnotics, narcotics, or tranquilizers).
No products indexed under this heading.

Amiodarone Hydrochloride (Rarely, cases of hepatotoxicity characterized by such findings as jaundice and altered liver function tests, when metoclopramide was administered with other drugs with known hepatotoxic potential).
No products indexed under this heading.

Amitriptyline Hydrochloride (Co-administration of metoclopramide with drugs likely to cause extrapyramidal reactions is contraindicated. Concomitant use of metoclopramide should be avoided in patients taking antidepressants, antipsychotics, and/or neuroleptics that have been associated with extrapyramidal reactions such as tardive dyskinesia or Neuroleptic Malignant Syndrome (NMS) that have occurred in association with metoclopramide).
No products indexed under this heading.

Amoxapine (Co-administration of metoclopramide with drugs likely to cause extrapyramidal reactions is contraindicated. Concomitant use of metoclopramide should be avoided in patients taking antidepressants, antipsychotics, and/or neuroleptics that have been associated with extrapyramidal reactions such as tardive dyskinesia or Neuroleptic Malignant Syndrome (NMS) that have occurred in association with metoclopramide).
No products indexed under this heading.

Amoxicillin (Rarely, cases of hepatotoxicity characterized by such findings as jaundice and altered liver function tests, when metoclopramide was administered with other drugs with known hepatotoxic potential). Products include:

Amoxicillin Trihydrate (Rarely, cases of hepatotoxicity characterized by such findings as jaundice and altered liver function tests, when metoclopramide was administered with other drugs with known hepatotoxic potential).
No products indexed under this heading.

Ampicillin (Rarely, cases of hepatotoxicity characterized by such findings as jaundice and altered liver function tests, when metoclopramide was administered with other drugs with known hepatotoxic potential).
No products indexed under this heading.

Ampicillin Sodium (Rarely, cases of hepatotoxicity characterized by such findings as jaundice and altered liver function tests, when metoclopramide was administered with other drugs with known hepatotoxic potential).
No products indexed under this heading.

Ampicillin Trihydrate (Rarely, cases of hepatotoxicity characterized by such findings as jaundice and altered liver function tests, when metoclopramide was administered with other drugs with known hepatotoxic potential).
No products indexed under this heading.

Amprenavir (Rarely, cases of hepatotoxicity characterized by such findings as jaundice and altered liver function tests, when metoclopramide was administered with other drugs with known hepatotoxic potential).
No products indexed under this heading.

Apomorphine (The effects of metoclopramide on gastrointestinal motility are antagonized by anticholinergic drugs and narcotic analgesics. Additive sedative effects can occur when metoclopramide is given with alcohol, sedatives, hypnotics, narcotics, or tranquilizers).
No products indexed under this heading.

Apomorphine Hydrochloride (The effects of metoclopramide on gastrointestinal motility are antagonized by anticholinergic drugs and narcotic analgesics. Additive sedative effects can occur when metoclopramide is given with alcohol, sedatives, hypnotics, narcotics, or tranquilizers).
No products indexed under this heading.

Aripiprazole (Co-administration of metoclopramide with drugs likely to cause extrapyramidal reactions is contraindicated. Concomitant use of metoclopramide should be avoided in patients taking antidepressants, antipsychotics, and/or neuroleptics that have been associated with extrapyramidal reactions such as tardive dyskinesia or Neuroleptic Malignant Syndrome (NMS) that have occurred in association with metoclopramide).
No products indexed under this heading.

Atazanavir (Rarely, cases of hepatotoxicity characterized by such findings as jaundice and altered liver function tests, when metoclopramide was administered with other drugs with known hepatotoxic potential).
No products indexed under this heading.

Atazanavir Sulfate (Rarely, cases of hepatotoxicity characterized by such findings as jaundice and altered liver function tests, when metoclopramide was administered with other drugs with known hepatotoxic potential).
No products indexed under this heading.

Atorvastatin Calcium (Rarely, cases of hepatotoxicity characterized by such findings as jaundice and altered liver function tests, when metoclopramide was administered with other drugs with known hepatotoxic potential). Products include:

Atropine Sulfate (The effects of metoclopramide on gastrointestinal motility are antagonized by anticholinergic drugs and narcotic analgesics). Products include:

Azathioprine (Rarely, cases of hepatotoxicity characterized by such findings as jaundice and altered liver function tests, when metoclopramide was administered with other drugs with known hepatotoxic potential).
No products indexed under this heading.

Azathioprine Sodium (Rarely, cases of hepatotoxicity characterized by such findings as jaundice and altered liver function tests, when metoclopramide was administered with other drugs with known hepatotoxic potential).
No products indexed under this heading.

Azlocillin Sodium (Rarely, cases of hepatotoxicity characterized by such findings as jaundice and altered liver function tests, when metoclopramide was administered with other drugs with known hepatotoxic potential).
No products indexed under this heading.

Bacampicillin Hydrochloride (Rarely, cases of hepatotoxicity characterized by such findings as jaundice and altered liver function tests, when metoclopramide was administered with other drugs with known hepatotoxic potential).
No products indexed under this heading.

Belladonna Alkaloids (The effects of metoclopramide on gastrointestinal motility are antagonized by anticholinergic drugs and narcotic analgesics). Products include:

Bendroflumethiazide (Rarely, cases of hepatotoxicity characterized by such findings as jaundice and altered liver function tests, when metoclopramide was administered with other drugs with known hepatotoxic potential).
No products indexed under this heading.

Benztropine Mesylate (The effects of metoclopramide on gastrointestinal motility are antagonized by anticholinergic drugs and narcotic analgesics).
No products indexed under this heading.

Biperiden Hydrochloride (The effects of metoclopramide on gastrointestinal motility are antagonized by anticholinergic drugs and narcotic analgesics).
No products indexed under this heading.

Buprenorphine Hydrochloride (The effects of metoclopramide on gastrointestinal motility are antagonized by anticholinergic drugs and narcotic analgesics. Additive sedative effects can occur when metoclopramide is given with alcohol, sedatives, hypnotics, narcotics, or tranquilizers).
No products indexed under this heading.

Bupropion (Rarely, cases of hepatotoxicity characterized by such findings as jaundice and altered liver function tests, when metoclopramide was administered with other drugs with known hepatotoxic potential).
No products indexed under this heading.

Bupropion Hydrochloride (Co-administration of metoclopramide with drugs likely to cause extrapyramidal reactions is contraindicated. Concomitant use of metoclopramide should be avoided in patients taking antidepressants, antipsychotics, and/or neuroleptics that have been associated with extrapyramidal reactions such as tardive dyskinesia or Neuroleptic Malignant Syndrome (NMS) that have occurred in association with metoclopramide). Products include:

Buspirone Hydrochloride (Additive sedative effects can occur when metoclopramide is given with alcohol, sedatives, hypnotics, narcotics, or tranquilizers).
No products indexed under this heading.

Butabarbital (Additive sedative effects can occur when metoclopramide is given with alcohol, sedatives, hypnotics, narcotics, or tranquilizers).
No products indexed under this heading.

Butabarbital Sodium (Additive sedative effects can occur when metoclopramide is given with alcohol, sedatives, hypnotics, narcotics, or tranquilizers).
No products indexed under this heading.

Butalbital (Additive sedative effects can occur when metoclopramide is given with alcohol, sedatives, hypnotics, narcotics, or tranquilizers).
No products indexed under this heading.

Carbamazepine (Co-administration of metoclopramide with drugs likely to cause extrapyramidal reactions is contraindicated. Concomitant use of metoclopramide should be avoided in patients taking antidepressants, antipsychotics, and/or neuroleptics that have been associated with extrapyramidal reactions such as tardive dyskinesia or Neuroleptic Malignant Syndrome (NMS) that have occurred in association with metoclopramide). Products include:

(⊙ Described in PDR® for Ophthalmic Medicines)

Carbenicillin Disodium (Rarely, cases of hepatotoxicity characterized by such findings as jaundice and altered liver function tests, when metoclopramide was administered with other drugs with known hepatotoxic potential).
No products indexed under this heading.

Carbenicillin Indanyl Sodium (Rarely, cases of hepatotoxicity characterized by such findings as jaundice and altered liver function tests, when metoclopramide was administered with other drugs with known hepatotoxic potential).
No products indexed under this heading.

Celecoxib (Rarely, cases of hepatotoxicity characterized by such findings as jaundice and altered liver function tests, when metoclopramide was administered with other drugs with known hepatotoxic potential). Products include:
Celebrex 3272

Cerivastatin Sodium (Rarely, cases of hepatotoxicity characterized by such findings as jaundice and altered liver function tests, when metoclopramide was administered with other drugs with known hepatotoxic potential).
No products indexed under this heading.

Chloral Hydrate (Additive sedative effects can occur when metoclopramide is given with alcohol, sedatives, hypnotics, narcotics, or tranquilizers).
No products indexed under this heading.

Chlordiazepoxide (Additive sedative effects can occur when metoclopramide is given with alcohol, sedatives, hypnotics, narcotics, or tranquilizers).
No products indexed under this heading.

Chlordiazepoxide Hydrochloride (Additive sedative effects can occur when metoclopramide is given with alcohol, sedatives, hypnotics, narcotics, or tranquilizers).
No products indexed under this heading.

Chlorothiazide (Rarely, cases of hepatotoxicity characterized by such findings as jaundice and altered liver function tests, when metoclopramide was administered with other drugs with known hepatotoxic potential).
No products indexed under this heading.

Chlorothiazide Sodium (Rarely, cases of hepatotoxicity characterized by such findings as jaundice and altered liver function tests, when metoclopramide was administered with other drugs with known hepatotoxic potential). Products include:
Diuril Intravenous 2009

Chlorpromazine (Co-administration of metoclopramide with drugs likely to cause extrapyramidal reactions is contraindicated. Concomitant use of metoclopramide should be avoided in patients taking antidepressants, antipsychotics, and/or neuroleptics that have been associated with extrapyramidal reactions such as tardive dyskinesia or Neuroleptic Malignant Syndrome (NMS) that have occurred in association with metoclopramide).
No products indexed under this heading.

Chlorpromazine Hydrochloride (Co-administration of metoclopramide with drugs likely to cause extrapyramidal reactions is contraindicated. Concomitant use of metoclopramide should be avoided in patients taking antidepressants, antipsychotics, and/or neuroleptics that have been associated with extrapyramidal reactions such as tardive dyskinesia or Neuroleptic Malignant Syndrome (NMS) that have occurred in association with metoclopramide).
No products indexed under this heading.

Chlorpropamide (Rarely, cases of hepatotoxicity characterized by such findings as jaundice and altered liver function tests, when metoclopramide was administered with other drugs with known hepatotoxic potential).
No products indexed under this heading.

Chlorprothixene (Co-administration of metoclopramide with drugs likely to cause extrapyramidal reactions is contraindicated. Concomitant use of metoclopramide should be avoided in patients taking antidepressants, antipsychotics, and/or neuroleptics that have been associated with extrapyramidal reactions such as tardive dyskinesia or Neuroleptic Malignant Syndrome (NMS) that have occurred in association with metoclopramide).
No products indexed under this heading.

Chlorprothixene Hydrochloride (Co-administration of metoclopramide with drugs likely to cause extrapyramidal reactions is contraindicated. Concomitant use of metoclopramide should be avoided in patients taking antidepressants, antipsychotics, and/or neuroleptics that have been associated with extrapyramidal reactions such as tardive dyskinesia or Neuroleptic Malignant Syndrome (NMS) that have occurred in association with metoclopramide).
No products indexed under this heading.

Chlorprothixene Lactate (Co-administration of metoclopramide with drugs likely to cause extrapyramidal reactions is contraindicated. Concomitant use of metoclopramide should be avoided in patients taking antidepressants, antipsychotics, and/or neuroleptics that have been associated with extrapyramidal reactions such as tardive dyskinesia or Neuroleptic Malignant Syndrome (NMS) that have occurred in association with metoclopramide).
No products indexed under this heading.

Citalopram Hydrobromide (Co-administration of metoclopramide with drugs likely to cause extrapyramidal reactions is contraindicated. Concomitant use of metoclopramide should be avoided in patients taking antidepressants, antipsychotics, and/or neuroleptics that have been associated with extrapyramidal reactions such as tardive dyskinesia or Neuroleptic Malignant Syndrome (NMS) that have occurred in association with metoclopramide). Products include:
Celexa 1153

Clidinium Bromide (The effects of metoclopramide on gastrointestinal motility are antagonized by anticholinergic drugs and narcotic analgesics).
No products indexed under this heading.

Clomipramine Hydrochloride (Rarely, cases of hepatotoxicity characterized by such findings as jaundice and altered liver function tests, when metoclopramide was administered with other drugs with known hepatotoxic potential).
No products indexed under this heading.

Clorazepate Dipotassium (Additive sedative effects can occur when metoclopramide is given with alcohol, sedatives, hypnotics, narcotics, or tranquilizers).
No products indexed under this heading.

Cloxacillin (Rarely, cases of hepatotoxicity characterized by such findings as jaundice and altered liver function tests, when metoclopramide was administered with other drugs with known hepatotoxic potential).
No products indexed under this heading.

Cloxacillin Sodium (Rarely, cases of hepatotoxicity characterized by such findings as jaundice and altered liver function tests, when metoclopramide was administered with other drugs with known hepatotoxic potential).
No products indexed under this heading.

Cloxacillin Sodium Monohydrate (Rarely, cases of hepatotoxicity characterized by such findings as jaundice and altered liver function tests, when metoclopramide was administered with other drugs with known hepatotoxic potential).
No products indexed under this heading.

Clozapine (Co-administration of metoclopramide with drugs likely to cause extrapyramidal reactions is contraindicated. Concomitant use of metoclopramide should be avoided in patients taking antidepressants, antipsychotics, and/or neuroleptics that have been associated with extrapyramidal reactions such as tardive dyskinesia or Neuroleptic Malignant Syndrome (NMS) that have occurred in association with metoclopramide).
No products indexed under this heading.

Codeine Phosphate (The effects of metoclopramide on gastrointestinal motility are antagonized by anticholinergic drugs and narcotic analgesics. Additive sedative effects can occur when metoclopramide is given with alcohol, sedatives, hypnotics, narcotics, or tranquilizers). Products include:
Tylenol with Codeine 2691

Codeine Sulfate (The effects of metoclopramide on gastrointestinal motility are antagonized by anticholinergic drugs and narcotic analgesics. Additive sedative effects can occur when metoclopramide is given with alcohol, sedatives, hypnotics, narcotics, or tranquilizers).
No products indexed under this heading.

Cyclosporine (Absorption of drugs from the stomach may be diminished by metoclopramide (eg, digoxin), whereas the rate and/or extent of absorption of drugs from the small bowel may be increased (eg, acetaminophen, tetracycline, levodopa, ethanol, cyclosporine)). Products include:
Gengraf 440
Neoral Oral Solution 2496
Neoral Capsules 2496
Restasis 605

Darunavir (Rarely, cases of hepatotoxicity characterized by such findings as jaundice and altered liver function tests, when metoclopramide was administered with other drugs with known hepatotoxic potential).
No products indexed under this heading.

Demeclocycline Hydrochloride (Absorption of drugs from the stomach may be diminished by metoclopramide (eg, digoxin), whereas the rate and/or extent of absorption of drugs from the small bowel may be increased (eg, acetaminophen, tetracycline, levodopa, ethanol, cyclosporine)).
No products indexed under this heading.

Desipramine Hydrochloride (Co-administration of metoclopramide with drugs likely to cause extrapyramidal reactions is contraindicated. Concomitant use of metoclopramide should be avoided in patients taking antidepressants, antipsychotics, and/or neuroleptics that have been associated with extrapyramidal reactions such as tardive dyskinesia or Neuroleptic Malignant Syndrome (NMS) that have occurred in association with metoclopramide).
No products indexed under this heading.

Dezocine (The effects of metoclopramide on gastrointestinal motility are antagonized by anticholinergic drugs and narcotic analgesics. Additive sedative effects can occur when metoclopramide is given with alcohol, sedatives, hypnotics, narcotics, or tranquilizers).
No products indexed under this heading.

Diazepam (Additive sedative effects can occur when metoclopramide is given with alcohol, sedatives, hypnotics, narcotics, or tranquilizers). Products include:
Valium Tablets 2880

Diclofenac Epolamine (Rarely, cases of hepatotoxicity characterized by such findings as jaundice and altered liver function tests, when metoclopramide was administered with other drugs with known hepatotoxic potential). Products include:
Flector 1839

Diclofenac Potassium (Rarely, cases of hepatotoxicity characterized by such findings as jaundice and altered liver function tests, when metoclopramide was administered with other drugs with known hepatotoxic potential).
No products indexed under this heading.

Diclofenac Sodium (Rarely, cases of hepatotoxicity characterized by such findings as jaundice and altered liver function tests, when metoclopramide was administered with other drugs with known hepatotoxic potential).
No products indexed under this heading.

Dicloxacillin (Rarely, cases of hepatotoxicity characterized by such findings as jaundice and altered liver function tests, when metoclopramide was administered with other drugs with known hepatotoxic potential).
No products indexed under this heading.

Dicloxacillin Sodium (Rarely, cases of hepatotoxicity characterized by such findings as jaundice and altered liver function tests, when metoclopramide was administered with other drugs with known hepatotoxic potential).
No products indexed under this heading.

Dicyclomine Hydrochloride (The effects of metoclopramide on gastrointestinal motility are antagonized by anticholinergic drugs and narcotic analgesics). Products include:
Bentyl Capsules 780
Bentyl Injection 780
Bentyl Syrup 780
Bentyl Tablets 780

Digoxin (Absorption of drugs from the stomach may be diminished by metoclopramide (eg, digoxin), whereas the rate and/or extent of absorption of drugs from the small bowel may be increased (eg, acetaminophen, tetracycline, levodopa, ethanol, cyclosporine)). Products include:
Lanoxin Injection 1546
Lanoxin Injection Pediatric 1549
Lanoxin Tablets 1553

Dihydrocodeine Bitartrate (The effects of metoclopramide on gastrointestinal motility are antagonized by anticholinergic drugs and narcotic analgesics. Additive sedative effects can occur when metoclopramide is given with alcohol, sedatives, hypnotics, narcotics, or tranquilizers).
No products indexed under this heading.

Dihydrocodeinone Bitartrate (The effects of metoclopramide on gastrointestinal motility are antagonized by anticholinergic drugs and narcotic analgesics. Additive sedative effects can occur when metoclopramide is given with alcohol, sedatives, hypnotics, narcotics, or tranquilizers).
No products indexed under this heading.

IMPORTANT NOTE: Always consult each drug listing in the patient's regimen for possible interactions.

Disodium Carbenicillin (Rarely, cases of hepatotoxicity characterized by such findings as jaundice and altered liver function tests, when metoclopramide was administered with other drugs with known hepatotoxic potential).
No products indexed under this heading.

Divalproex Sodium (Co-administration of metoclopramide with drugs likely to cause extrapyramidal reactions is contraindicated. Concomitant use of metoclopramide should be avoided in patients taking antidepressants, antipsychotics, and/or neuroleptics that have been associated with extrapyramidal reactions such as tardive dyskinesia or Neuroleptic Malignant Syndrome (NMS) that have occurred in association with metoclopramide). Products include:
Depakote ER 426

Doxepin Hydrochloride (Co-administration of metoclopramide with drugs likely to cause extrapyramidal reactions is contraindicated. Concomitant use of metoclopramide should be avoided in patients taking antidepressants, antipsychotics, and/or neuroleptics that have been associated with extrapyramidal reactions such as tardive dyskinesia or Neuroleptic Malignant Syndrome (NMS) that have occurred in association with metoclopramide).
No products indexed under this heading.

Doxycycline (Absorption of drugs from the stomach may be diminished by metoclopramide (eg, digoxin), whereas the rate and/or extent of absorption of drugs from the small bowel may be increased (eg, acetaminophen, tetracycline, levodopa, ethanol, cyclosporine)).
No products indexed under this heading.

Doxycycline Calcium (Absorption of drugs from the stomach may be diminished by metoclopramide (eg, digoxin), whereas the rate and/or extent of absorption of drugs from the small bowel may be increased (eg, acetaminophen, tetracycline, levodopa, ethanol, cyclosporine)).
No products indexed under this heading.

Doxycycline Hyclate (Absorption of drugs from the stomach may be diminished by metoclopramide (eg, digoxin), whereas the rate and/or extent of absorption of drugs from the small bowel may be increased (eg, acetaminophen, tetracycline, levodopa, ethanol, cyclosporine)).
No products indexed under this heading.

Doxycycline Monohydrate (Absorption of drugs from the stomach may be diminished by metoclopramide (eg, digoxin), whereas the rate and/or extent of absorption of drugs from the small bowel may be increased (eg, acetaminophen, tetracycline, levodopa, ethanol, cyclosporine)).
No products indexed under this heading.

Droperidol (Additive sedative effects can occur when metoclopramide is given with alcohol, sedatives, hypnotics, narcotics, or tranquilizers).
No products indexed under this heading.

Duloxetine Hydrochloride (Rarely, cases of hepatotoxicity characterized by such findings as jaundice and altered liver function tests, when metoclopramide was administered with other drugs with known hepatotoxic potential). Products include:
Cymbalta 1871

Erythromycin (Rarely, cases of hepatotoxicity characterized by such findings as jaundice and altered liver function tests, when metoclopramide was administered with other drugs with known hepatotoxic potential).
No products indexed under this heading.

Erythromycin, Topical (Rarely, cases of hepatotoxicity characterized by such findings as jaundice and altered liver function tests, when metoclopramide was administered with other drugs with known hepatotoxic potential).
No products indexed under this heading.

Erythromycin Estolate (Rarely, cases of hepatotoxicity characterized by such findings as jaundice and altered liver function tests, when metoclopramide was administered with other drugs with known hepatotoxic potential).
No products indexed under this heading.

Erythromycin Ethylsuccinate (Rarely, cases of hepatotoxicity characterized by such findings as jaundice and altered liver function tests, when metoclopramide was administered with other drugs with known hepatotoxic potential). Products include:
E.E.S. 437
EryPed 435

Erythromycin Gluceptate (Rarely, cases of hepatotoxicity characterized by such findings as jaundice and altered liver function tests, when metoclopramide was administered with other drugs with known hepatotoxic potential).
No products indexed under this heading.

Erythromycin Lactobionate (Rarely, cases of hepatotoxicity characterized by such findings as jaundice and altered liver function tests, when metoclopramide was administered with other drugs with known hepatotoxic potential).
No products indexed under this heading.

Erythromycin Stearate (Rarely, cases of hepatotoxicity characterized by such findings as jaundice and altered liver function tests, when metoclopramide was administered with other drugs with known hepatotoxic potential).
No products indexed under this heading.

Escitalopram Oxalate (Co-administration of metoclopramide with drugs likely to cause extrapyramidal reactions is contraindicated. Concomitant use of metoclopramide should be avoided in patients taking antidepressants, antipsychotics, and/or neuroleptics that have been associated with extrapyramidal reactions such as tardive dyskinesia or Neuroleptic Malignant Syndrome (NMS) that have occurred in association with metoclopramide). Products include:
Lexapro Oral Suspension 1160
Lexapro Tablets 1160

Estazolam (Additive sedative effects can occur when metoclopramide is given with alcohol, sedatives, hypnotics, narcotics, or tranquilizers).
No products indexed under this heading.

Ethanol (Absorption of drugs from the stomach may be diminished by metoclopramide (eg, digoxin), whereas the rate and/or extent of absorption of drugs from the small bowel may be increased (eg, acetaminophen, tetracycline, levodopa, ethanol, cyclosporine)).
No products indexed under this heading.

Ethchlorvynol (Additive sedative effects can occur when metoclopramide is given with alcohol, sedatives, hypnotics, narcotics, or tranquilizers).
No products indexed under this heading.

Ethinamate (Additive sedative effects can occur when metoclopramide is given with alcohol, sedatives, hypnotics, narcotics, or tranquilizers).
No products indexed under this heading.

Ethosuximide (Co-administration of metoclopramide with drugs likely to cause extrapyramidal reactions is contraindicated. Concomitant use of metoclopramide should be avoided in patients taking antidepressants, antipsychotics, and/or neuroleptics that have been associated with extrapyramidal reactions such as tardive dyskinesia

or Neuroleptic Malignant Syndrome (NMS) that have occurred in association with metoclopramide).
No products indexed under this heading.

Ethotoin (Co-administration of metoclopramide with drugs likely to cause extrapyramidal reactions is contraindicated. Concomitant use of metoclopramide should be avoided in patients taking antidepressants, antipsychotics, and/or neuroleptics that have been associated with extrapyramidal reactions such as tardive dyskinesia or Neuroleptic Malignant Syndrome (NMS) that have occurred in association with metoclopramide).
No products indexed under this heading.

Ethyl Alcohol (Additive sedative effects can occur when metoclopramide is given with alcohol, sedatives, hypnotics, narcotics, or tranquilizers).
No products indexed under this heading.

Etodolac (Rarely, cases of hepatotoxicity characterized by such findings as jaundice and altered liver function tests, when metoclopramide was administered with other drugs with known hepatotoxic potential).
No products indexed under this heading.

Fat (In a food-effect study with 28 subjects, metoclopramide taken immediately after a high-fat meal had a 17% lower peak blood level than when taken after an overnight fast. The time to peak blood levels increased from about 1.75 hours under fasted conditions to 3 hours when taken immediately after a high-fat meal. The extent of metoclopramide absorbed (area under the curve) was comparable whether metoclopramide was administered with or without food. The clinical effect of the decrease in peak plasma level if metoclopramide is inadvertently taken with food is unknown).
No products indexed under this heading.

Felbamate (Co-administration of metoclopramide with drugs likely to cause extrapyramidal reactions is contraindicated. Concomitant use of metoclopramide should be avoided in patients taking antidepressants, antipsychotics, and/or neuroleptics that have been associated with extrapyramidal reactions such as tardive dyskinesia or Neuroleptic Malignant Syndrome (NMS) that have occurred in association with metoclopramide).
No products indexed under this heading.

Fenofibrate (Rarely, cases of hepatotoxicity characterized by such findings as jaundice and altered liver function tests, when metoclopramide was administered with other drugs with known hepatotoxic potential). Products include:
Fenoglide 3263
Tricor 544
Trilipix 548

Fenoprofen Calcium (Rarely, cases of hepatotoxicity characterized by such findings as jaundice and altered liver function tests, when metoclopramide was administered with other drugs with known hepatotoxic potential).
No products indexed under this heading.

Fentanyl (The effects of metoclopramide on gastrointestinal motility are antagonized by anticholinergic drugs and narcotic analgesics. Additive sedative effects can occur when metoclopramide is given with alcohol, sedatives, hypnotics, narcotics, or tranquilizers). Products include:
Duragesic 2604
Fentanyl Transdermal System 2346
Onsolis 2054

Fentanyl Citrate (The effects of metoclopramide on gastrointestinal motility are antagonized by anticholinergic drugs and narcotic analgesics.

Additive sedative effects can occur when metoclopramide is given with alcohol, sedatives, hypnotics, narcotics, or tranquilizers). Products include:
Fentora 966

Fluconazole (Rarely, cases of hepatotoxicity characterized by such findings as jaundice and altered liver function tests, when metoclopramide was administered with other drugs with known hepatotoxic potential).
No products indexed under this heading.

Fluoxetine Hydrochloride (Co-administration of metoclopramide with drugs likely to cause extrapyramidal reactions is contraindicated. Concomitant use of metoclopramide should be avoided in patients taking antidepressants, antipsychotics, and/or neuroleptics that have been associated with extrapyramidal reactions such as tardive dyskinesia or Neuroleptic Malignant Syndrome (NMS) that have occurred in association with metoclopramide). Products include:
Prozac Weekly 1941
Prozac Pulvules 1941
Symbyax 1965

Fluphenazine Decanoate (Co-administration of metoclopramide with drugs likely to cause extrapyramidal reactions is contraindicated. Concomitant use of metoclopramide should be avoided in patients taking antidepressants, antipsychotics, and/or neuroleptics that have been associated with extrapyramidal reactions such as tardive dyskinesia or Neuroleptic Malignant Syndrome (NMS) that have occurred in association with metoclopramide).
No products indexed under this heading.

Fluphenazine Enanthate (Co-administration of metoclopramide with drugs likely to cause extrapyramidal reactions is contraindicated. Concomitant use of metoclopramide should be avoided in patients taking antidepressants, antipsychotics, and/or neuroleptics that have been associated with extrapyramidal reactions such as tardive dyskinesia or Neuroleptic Malignant Syndrome (NMS) that have occurred in association with metoclopramide).
No products indexed under this heading.

Fluphenazine Hydrochloride (Co-administration of metoclopramide with drugs likely to cause extrapyramidal reactions is contraindicated. Concomitant use of metoclopramide should be avoided in patients taking antidepressants, antipsychotics, and/or neuroleptics that have been associated with extrapyramidal reactions such as tardive dyskinesia or Neuroleptic Malignant Syndrome (NMS) that have occurred in association with metoclopramide).
No products indexed under this heading.

Flurazepam Hydrochloride (Additive sedative effects can occur when metoclopramide is given with alcohol, sedatives, hypnotics, narcotics, or tranquilizers).
No products indexed under this heading.

Flurbiprofen (Rarely, cases of hepatotoxicity characterized by such findings as jaundice and altered liver function tests, when metoclopramide was administered with other drugs with known hepatotoxic potential).
No products indexed under this heading.

Flurbiprofen Sodium (Rarely, cases of hepatotoxicity characterized by such findings as jaundice and altered liver function tests, when metoclopramide was administered with other drugs with known hepatotoxic potential).
No products indexed under this heading.

Fluvastatin Sodium (Rarely, cases of hepatotoxicity characterized by such findings as jaundice and altered liver function tests, when metoclopramide was administered with other drugs with known hepatotoxic potential).
No products indexed under this heading.

Fluvoxamine (Co-administration of metoclopramide with drugs likely to cause extrapyramidal reactions is contraindicated. Concomitant use of metoclopramide should be avoided in patients taking antidepressants, antipsychotics, and/or neuroleptics that have been associated with extrapyramidal reactions such as tardive dyskinesia or Neuroleptic Malignant Syndrome (NMS) that have occurred in association with metoclopramide).
No products indexed under this heading.

Fluvoxamine Maleate (Co-administration of metoclopramide with drugs likely to cause extrapyramidal reactions is contraindicated. Concomitant use of metoclopramide should be avoided in patients taking antidepressants, antipsychotics, and/or neuroleptics that have been associated with extrapyramidal reactions such as tardive dyskinesia or Neuroleptic Malignant Syndrome (NMS) that have occurred in association with metoclopramide).
No products indexed under this heading.

Fosamprenavir Calcium (Rarely, cases of hepatotoxicity characterized by such findings as jaundice and altered liver function tests, when metoclopramide was administered with other drugs with known hepatotoxic potential). Products include:
Lexiva Oral Suspension 1558
Lexiva 1558

Fosphenytoin (Co-administration of metoclopramide with drugs likely to cause extrapyramidal reactions is contraindicated. Concomitant use of metoclopramide should be avoided in patients taking antidepressants, antipsychotics, and/or neuroleptics that have been associated with extrapyramidal reactions such as tardive dyskinesia or Neuroleptic Malignant Syndrome (NMS) that have occurred in association with metoclopramide).
No products indexed under this heading.

Fosphenytoin Sodium (Co-administration of metoclopramide with drugs likely to cause extrapyramidal reactions is contraindicated. Concomitant use of metoclopramide should be avoided in patients taking antidepressants, antipsychotics, and/or neuroleptics that have been associated with extrapyramidal reactions such as tardive dyskinesia or Neuroleptic Malignant Syndrome (NMS) that have occurred in association with metoclopramide).
No products indexed under this heading.

Gabapentin (Co-administration of metoclopramide with drugs likely to cause extrapyramidal reactions is contraindicated. Concomitant use of metoclopramide should be avoided in patients taking antidepressants, antipsychotics, and/or neuroleptics that have been associated with extrapyramidal reactions such as tardive dyskinesia or Neuroleptic Malignant Syndrome (NMS) that have occurred in association with metoclopramide).
No products indexed under this heading.

Gemfibrozil (Rarely, cases of hepatotoxicity characterized by such findings as jaundice and altered liver function tests, when metoclopramide was administered with other drugs with known hepatotoxic potential).
No products indexed under this heading.

Glimepiride (Rarely, cases of hepatotoxicity characterized by such findings as jaundice and altered liver function tests, when metoclopramide was

administered with other drugs with known hepatotoxic potential). Products include:
Avandaryl 1356
Duetact 3354

Glipizide (Rarely, cases of hepatotoxicity characterized by such findings as jaundice and altered liver function tests, when metoclopramide was administered with other drugs with known hepatotoxic potential).
No products indexed under this heading.

Glutethimide (Additive sedative effects can occur when metoclopramide is given with alcohol, sedatives, hypnotics, narcotics, or tranquilizers).
No products indexed under this heading.

Glyburide (Rarely, cases of hepatotoxicity characterized by such findings as jaundice and altered liver function tests, when metoclopramide was administered with other drugs with known hepatotoxic potential).
No products indexed under this heading.

Glycopyrrolate (The effects of metoclopramide on gastrointestinal motility are antagonized by anticholinergic drugs and narcotic analgesics).
No products indexed under this heading.

Griseofulvin (Rarely, cases of hepatotoxicity characterized by such findings as jaundice and altered liver function tests, when metoclopramide was administered with other drugs with known hepatotoxic potential).
No products indexed under this heading.

Haloperidol (Co-administration of metoclopramide with drugs likely to cause extrapyramidal reactions is contraindicated. Concomitant use of metoclopramide should be avoided in patients taking antidepressants, antipsychotics, and/or neuroleptics that have been associated with extrapyramidal reactions such as tardive dyskinesia or Neuroleptic Malignant Syndrome (NMS) that have occurred in association with metoclopramide).
No products indexed under this heading.

Haloperidol Decanoate (Co-administration of metoclopramide with drugs likely to cause extrapyramidal reactions is contraindicated. Concomitant use of metoclopramide should be avoided in patients taking antidepressants, antipsychotics, and/or neuroleptics that have been associated with extrapyramidal reactions such as tardive dyskinesia or Neuroleptic Malignant Syndrome (NMS) that have occurred in association with metoclopramide).
No products indexed under this heading.

Haloperidol Lactate (Co-administration of metoclopramide with drugs likely to cause extrapyramidal reactions is contraindicated. Concomitant use of metoclopramide should be avoided in patients taking antidepressants, antipsychotics, and/or neuroleptics that have been associated with extrapyramidal reactions such as tardive dyskinesia or Neuroleptic Malignant Syndrome (NMS) that have occurred in association with metoclopramide).
No products indexed under this heading.

Halothane (Rarely, cases of hepatotoxicity characterized by such findings as jaundice and altered liver function tests, when metoclopramide was administered with other drugs with known hepatotoxic potential).
No products indexed under this heading.

Heparin (Rarely, cases of hepatotoxicity characterized by such findings as jaundice and altered liver function tests, when metoclopramide was administered with other drugs with known hepatotoxic potential).
No products indexed under this heading.

Heparin Calcium (Rarely, cases of hepatotoxicity characterized by such findings as jaundice and altered liver function tests, when metoclopramide was administered with other drugs with known hepatotoxic potential).
No products indexed under this heading.

Heparin Sodium (Rarely, cases of hepatotoxicity characterized by such findings as jaundice and altered liver function tests, when metoclopramide was administered with other drugs with known hepatotoxic potential).
No products indexed under this heading.

Hydralazine (Rarely, cases of hepatotoxicity characterized by such findings as jaundice and altered liver function tests, when metoclopramide was administered with other drugs with known hepatotoxic potential).
No products indexed under this heading.

Hydralazine Hydrochloride (Rarely, cases of hepatotoxicity characterized by such findings as jaundice and altered liver function tests, when metoclopramide was administered with other drugs with known hepatotoxic potential).
No products indexed under this heading.

Hydrochlorothiazide (Rarely, cases of hepatotoxicity characterized by such findings as jaundice and altered liver function tests, when metoclopramide was administered with other drugs with known hepatotoxic potential). Products include:
Atacand HCT 700
Avalide 2956
Benicar HCT 1017
Diovan HCT 2419
Dyazide 1429
Exforge HCT 2449
Hyzaar 2162
Hyzaar 100-12.5 2162
Micardis HCT 889
Prinzide 2246
Tekturna HCT 2541
Teveten HCT 541

Hydrochlorothiazide Hydrochloride (Rarely, cases of hepatotoxicity characterized by such findings as jaundice and altered liver function tests, when metoclopramide was administered with other drugs with known hepatotoxic potential).
No products indexed under this heading.

Hydrocodone Bitartrate (The effects of metoclopramide on gastrointestinal motility are antagonized by anticholinergic drugs and narcotic analgesics. Additive sedative effects can occur when metoclopramide is given with alcohol, sedatives, hypnotics, narcotics, or tranquilizers). Products include:
Vicodin 560
Vicodin ES 561
Vicodin HP 563
Vicoprofen 564
Zydone 1138

Hydrocodone Polistirex (The effects of metoclopramide on gastrointestinal motility are antagonized by anticholinergic drugs and narcotic analgesics. Additive sedative effects can occur when metoclopramide is given with alcohol, sedatives, hypnotics, narcotics, or tranquilizers). Products include:
Tussionex 3443

Hydroflumethiazide (Rarely, cases of hepatotoxicity characterized by such findings as jaundice and altered liver function tests, when metoclopramide was administered with other drugs with known hepatotoxic potential).
No products indexed under this heading.

Hydromorphone (The effects of metoclopramide on gastrointestinal motility are antagonized by anticholinergic drugs and narcotic analgesics. Additive sedative effects can occur when metoclopramide is given with alcohol, sedatives, hypnotics, narcotics, or tranquilizers).
No products indexed under this heading.

Hydromorphone Hydrochloride (The effects of metoclopramide on gastrointestinal motility are antagonized by anticholinergic drugs and narcotic analgesics. Additive sedative effects can occur when metoclopramide is given with alcohol, sedatives, hypnotics, narcotics, or tranquilizers). Products include:
Dilaudid Injection 2800
Dilaudid Oral 2797
Dilaudid Tablets 2797
Dilaudid-HP 2800

Hydroxyzine Hydrochloride (Additive sedative effects can occur when metoclopramide is given with alcohol, sedatives, hypnotics, narcotics, or tranquilizers).
No products indexed under this heading.

Hyoscyamine (The effects of metoclopramide on gastrointestinal motility are antagonized by anticholinergic drugs and narcotic analgesics).
No products indexed under this heading.

Hyoscyamine Sulfate (The effects of metoclopramide on gastrointestinal motility are antagonized by anticholinergic drugs and narcotic analgesics). Products include:
Donnatal 2711

Ibuprofen (Rarely, cases of hepatotoxicity characterized by such findings as jaundice and altered liver function tests, when metoclopramide was administered with other drugs with known hepatotoxic potential). Products include:
Motrin IB 2043
Children's Motrin 2044
Children's Motrin Non-Staining
Dye-Free 2044
Infants' Motrin 2044
Infants' Motrin Dye-Free 2044
Junior Strength Motrin 2044
Vicoprofen 564

Imatinib Mesylate (Rarely, cases of hepatotoxicity characterized by such findings as jaundice and altered liver function tests, when metoclopramide was administered with other drugs with known hepatotoxic potential). Products include:
Gleevec 2477

Imipramine Hydrochloride (Co-administration of metoclopramide with drugs likely to cause extrapyramidal reactions is contraindicated. Concomitant use of metoclopramide should be avoided in patients taking antidepressants, antipsychotics, and/or neuroleptics that have been associated with extrapyramidal reactions such as tardive dyskinesia or Neuroleptic Malignant Syndrome (NMS) that have occurred in association with metoclopramide).
No products indexed under this heading.

Imipramine Pamoate (Co-administration of metoclopramide with drugs likely to cause extrapyramidal reactions is contraindicated. Concomitant use of metoclopramide should be avoided in patients taking antidepressants, antipsychotics, and/or neuroleptics that have been associated with extrapyramidal reactions such as tardive dyskinesia or Neuroleptic Malignant Syndrome (NMS) that have occurred in association with metoclopramide).
No products indexed under this heading.

Indinavir Sulfate (Rarely, cases of hepatotoxicity characterized by such findings as jaundice and altered liver function tests, when metoclopramide

was administered with other drugs with known hepatotoxic potential). Products include:
Crixivan 2113

Indomethacin (Rarely, cases of hepatotoxicity characterized by such findings as jaundice and altered liver function tests, when metoclopramide was administered with other drugs with known hepatotoxic potential). Products include:
Indocin 2167

Indomethacin Sodium Trihydrate (Rarely, cases of hepatotoxicity characterized by such findings as jaundice and altered liver function tests, when metoclopramide was administered with other drugs with known hepatotoxic potential). Products include:
Indocin I.V. 2007

Insulin (Because the action of metoclopramide will hasten the movement of food to the intestines and therefore the rate of absorption, insulin dosage or timing of dosage may require adjustment. Increasing movement of food to the intestines may lead to absorption of less glucose from a meal, hence less glucose in the circulation for a particular dose of administered insulin to act upon, resulting in hypoglycemia).
No products indexed under this heading.

Insulin, Human, Zinc Suspension (Because the action of metoclopramide will hasten the movement of food to the intestines and therefore the rate of absorption, insulin dosage or timing of dosage may require adjustment. Increasing movement of food to the intestines may lead to absorption of less glucose from a meal, hence less glucose in the circulation for a particular dose of administered insulin to act upon, resulting in hypoglycemia).
No products indexed under this heading.

Insulin, Human (rDNA origin) (Because the action of metoclopramide will hasten the movement of food to the intestines and therefore the rate of absorption, insulin dosage or timing of dosage may require adjustment. Increasing movement of food to the intestines may lead to absorption of less glucose from a meal, hence less glucose in the circulation for a particular dose of administered insulin to act upon, resulting in hypoglycemia). Products include:
Exubera 2717

Insulin, Human NPH (Because the action of metoclopramide will hasten the movement of food to the intestines and therefore the rate of absorption, insulin dosage or timing of dosage may require adjustment. Increasing movement of food to the intestines may lead to absorption of less glucose from a meal, hence less glucose in the circulation for a particular dose of administered insulin to act upon, resulting in hypoglycemia). Products include:
Humulin N Vial 1934

Insulin, Human Regular (Because the action of metoclopramide will hasten the movement of food to the intestines and therefore the rate of absorption, insulin dosage or timing of dosage may require adjustment. Increasing movement of food to the intestines may lead to absorption of less glucose from a meal, hence less glucose in the circulation for a particular dose of administered insulin to act upon, resulting in hypoglycemia). Products include:
Humulin R 1937
Humulin R (U-500) 1939

Insulin, Human Regular and Human NPH Mixture (Because the action of metoclopramide will hasten the movement of food to the intestines and therefore the rate of absorption, insulin dosage or timing of dosage may require adjustment. Increasing movement of food to the intestines may lead to absorption of less glucose from a meal, hence less glucose in the circulation for a particular dose of administered insulin to act upon, resulting in hypoglycemia). Products include:
Humulin 50/50 1930
Humulin 70/30 Vial 1931

Insulin, NPH (Because the action of metoclopramide will hasten the movement of food to the intestines and therefore the rate of absorption, insulin dosage or timing of dosage may require adjustment. Increasing movement of food to the intestines may lead to absorption of less glucose from a meal, hence less glucose in the circulation for a particular dose of administered insulin to act upon, resulting in hypoglycemia).
No products indexed under this heading.

Insulin, Regular (Because the action of metoclopramide will hasten the movement of food to the intestines and therefore the rate of absorption, insulin dosage or timing of dosage may require adjustment. Increasing movement of food to the intestines may lead to absorption of less glucose from a meal, hence less glucose in the circulation for a particular dose of administered insulin to act upon, resulting in hypoglycemia).
No products indexed under this heading.

Insulin, Regular and NPH mixture (Because the action of metoclopramide will hasten the movement of food to the intestines and therefore the rate of absorption, insulin dosage or timing of dosage may require adjustment. Increasing movement of food to the intestines may lead to absorption of less glucose from a meal, hence less glucose in the circulation for a particular dose of administered insulin to act upon, resulting in hypoglycemia).
No products indexed under this heading.

Insulin, Zinc Crystals (Because the action of metoclopramide will hasten the movement of food to the intestines and therefore the rate of absorption, insulin dosage or timing of dosage may require adjustment. Increasing movement of food to the intestines may lead to absorption of less glucose from a meal, hence less glucose in the circulation for a particular dose of administered insulin to act upon, resulting in hypoglycemia).
No products indexed under this heading.

Insulin, Zinc Suspension (Because the action of metoclopramide will hasten the movement of food to the intestines and therefore the rate of absorption, insulin dosage or timing of dosage may require adjustment. Increasing movement of food to the intestines may lead to absorption of less glucose from a meal, hence less glucose in the circulation for a particular dose of administered insulin to act upon, resulting in hypoglycemia).
No products indexed under this heading.

Insulin Aspart (Because the action of metoclopramide will hasten the movement of food to the intestines and therefore the rate of absorption, insulin dosage or timing of dosage may require adjustment. Increasing movement of food to the intestines may lead to absorption of less glucose from a meal, hence less glucose in the circulation for a particular dose of administered insulin to act upon, resulting in hypoglycemia).
No products indexed under this heading.

Insulin Aspart, Human (Because the action of metoclopramide will hasten the movement of food to the intestines and therefore the rate of absorption, insulin dosage or timing of dosage may require adjustment. Increasing movement of food to the intestines may lead to absorption of less glucose from a meal, hence less glucose in the circulation for a particular dose of administered insulin to act upon, resulting in hypoglycemia). Products include:
NovoLog Mix 70/30 2581

Insulin Aspart, Human Regular (Because the action of metoclopramide will hasten the movement of food to the intestines and therefore the rate of absorption, insulin dosage or timing of dosage may require adjustment. Increasing movement of food to the intestines may lead to absorption of less glucose from a meal, hence less glucose in the circulation for a particular dose of administered insulin to act upon, resulting in hypoglycemia). Products include:
NovoLog 2575

Insulin Aspart Protamine, Human (Because the action of metoclopramide will hasten the movement of food to the intestines and therefore the rate of absorption, insulin dosage or timing of dosage may require adjustment. Increasing movement of food to the intestines may lead to absorption of less glucose from a meal, hence less glucose in the circulation for a particular dose of administered insulin to act upon, resulting in hypoglycemia). Products include:
NovoLog Mix 70/30 2581

Insulin Detemir (rDNA Origin) (Because the action of metoclopramide will hasten the movement of food to the intestines and therefore the rate of absorption, insulin dosage or timing of dosage may require adjustment. Increasing movement of food to the intestines may lead to absorption of less glucose from a meal, hence less glucose in the circulation for a particular dose of administered insulin to act upon, resulting in hypoglycemia). Products include:
Levemir 2566

Insulin Glargine (Because the action of metoclopramide will hasten the movement of food to the intestines and therefore the rate of absorption, insulin dosage or timing of dosage may require adjustment. Increasing movement of food to the intestines may lead to absorption of less glucose from a meal, hence less glucose in the circulation for a particular dose of administered insulin to act upon, resulting in hypoglycemia). Products include:
Lantus 2996

Insulin Glulisine (Because the action of metoclopramide will hasten the movement of food to the intestines and therefore the rate of absorption, insulin dosage or timing of dosage may require adjustment. Increasing movement of food to the intestines may lead to absorption of less glucose from a meal, hence less glucose in the circulation for a particular dose of administered insulin to act upon, resulting in hypoglycemia). Products include:
Apidra 2937
Apidra SoloStar 2937

Insulin Lispro, Human (Because the action of metoclopramide will hasten the movement of food to the intestines and therefore the rate of absorption, insulin dosage or timing of dosage may require adjustment. Increasing movement of food to the intestines may lead to absorption of less glucose from a meal, hence less glucose in the circulation for a particular dose of administered insulin to act upon, resulting in hypoglycemia). Products include:
Humalog 1910
Humalog Mix 1914
Humalog Mix75/25 1917

Insulin Lispro Protamine, Human (Because the action of metoclopramide will hasten the movement of food to the intestines and therefore the rate of absorption, insulin dosage or timing of dosage may require adjustment. Increasing movement of food to the intestines may lead to absorption of less glucose from a meal, hence less glucose in the circulation for a particular dose of administered insulin to act upon, resulting in hypoglycemia). Products include:
Humalog Mix 1914
Humalog Mix75/25 1917

Interferon Beta-1a (Rarely, cases of hepatotoxicity characterized by such findings as jaundice and altered liver function tests, when metoclopramide was administered with other drugs with known hepatotoxic potential). Products include:
Rebif 1096

Ipratropium Bromide (The effects of metoclopramide on gastrointestinal motility are antagonized by anticholinergic drugs and narcotic analgesics).
No products indexed under this heading.

Isocarboxazid (Co-administration of metoclopramide with drugs likely to cause extrapyramidal reactions is contraindicated. Concomitant use of metoclopramide should be avoided in patients taking antidepressants, antipsychotics, and/or neuroleptics that have been associated with extrapyramidal reactions such as tardive dyskinesia or Neuroleptic Malignant Syndrome (NMS) that have occurred in association with metoclopramide). Products include:
Marplan 3481

Isoniazid (Rarely, cases of hepatotoxicity characterized by such findings as jaundice and altered liver function tests, when metoclopramide was administered with other drugs with known hepatotoxic potential).
No products indexed under this heading.

Isotretinoin (Rarely, cases of hepatotoxicity characterized by such findings as jaundice and altered liver function tests, when metoclopramide was administered with other drugs with known hepatotoxic potential). Products include:
Accutane 2832

Itraconazole (Rarely, cases of hepatotoxicity characterized by such findings as jaundice and altered liver function tests, when metoclopramide was administered with other drugs with known hepatotoxic potential).
No products indexed under this heading.

Ketoconazole (Rarely, cases of hepatotoxicity characterized by such findings as jaundice and altered liver function tests, when metoclopramide was administered with other drugs with known hepatotoxic potential). Products include:
Extina 3319
Xolegel 3337

Ketoprofen (Rarely, cases of hepatotoxicity characterized by such findings as jaundice and altered liver function tests, when metoclopramide was administered with other drugs with known hepatotoxic potential).
No products indexed under this heading.

Ketorolac Tromethamine (Rarely, cases of hepatotoxicity characterized by such findings as jaundice and altered liver function tests, when metoclopramide was administered with other drugs with known hepatotoxic potential). Products include:
Acuvail .... ⊙ 209

Labetalol Hydrochloride (Rarely, cases of hepatotoxicity characterized by such findings as jaundice and altered liver function tests, when metoclopramide was administered with other drugs with known hepatotoxic potential).
No products indexed under this heading.

1121 Interactions Index Metozolv ODT

Lamotrigine (Co-administration of metoclopramide with drugs likely to cause extrapyramidal reactions is contraindicated. Concomitant use of metoclopramide should be avoided in patients taking antidepressants, antipsychotics, and/or neuroleptics that have been associated with extrapyramidal reactions such as tardive dyskinesia or Neuroleptic Malignant Syndrome (NMS) that have occurred in association with metoclopramide). Products include:
- Lamictal 1522
- Lamictal ODT 1522
- Lamictal XR 1536

Leflunomide (Rarely, cases of hepatotoxicity characterized by such findings as jaundice and altered liver function tests, when metoclopramide was administered with other drugs with known hepatotoxic potential).
No products indexed under this heading.

Levetiracetam (Co-administration of metoclopramide with drugs likely to cause extrapyramidal reactions is contraindicated. Concomitant use of metoclopramide should be avoided in patients taking antidepressants, antipsychotics, and/or neuroleptics that have been associated with extrapyramidal reactions such as tardive dyskinesia or Neuroleptic Malignant Syndrome (NMS) that have occurred in association with metoclopramide). Products include:
- Keppra XR 3434

Levodopa (Absorption of drugs from the stomach may be diminished by metoclopramide (eg, digoxin), whereas the rate and/or extent of absorption of drugs from the small bowel may be increased (eg, acetaminophen, tetracycline, levodopa, ethanol, cyclosporine)). Products include:
- Stalevo 2526

Levorphanol Tartrate (The effects of metoclopramide on gastrointestinal motility are antagonized by anticholinergic drugs and narcotic analgesics. Additive sedative effects can occur when metoclopramide is given with alcohol, sedatives, hypnotics, narcotics, or tranquilizers).
No products indexed under this heading.

Lithium (Co-administration of metoclopramide with drugs likely to cause extrapyramidal reactions is contraindicated. Concomitant use of metoclopramide should be avoided in patients taking antidepressants, antipsychotics, and/or neuroleptics that have been associated with extrapyramidal reactions such as tardive dyskinesia or Neuroleptic Malignant Syndrome (NMS) that have occurred in association with metoclopramide).
No products indexed under this heading.

Lithium Carbonate (Co-administration of metoclopramide with drugs likely to cause extrapyramidal reactions is contraindicated. Concomitant use of metoclopramide should be avoided in patients taking antidepressants, antipsychotics, and/or neuroleptics that have been associated with extrapyramidal reactions such as tardive dyskinesia or Neuroleptic Malignant Syndrome (NMS) that have occurred in association with metoclopramide).
No products indexed under this heading.

Lithium Citrate (Co-administration of metoclopramide with drugs likely to cause extrapyramidal reactions is contraindicated. Concomitant use of metoclopramide should be avoided in patients taking antidepressants, antipsychotics, and/or neuroleptics that have been associated with extrapyramidal reactions such as tardive dyskinesia or Neuroleptic Malignant Syndrome (NMS) that have occurred in association with metoclopramide).
No products indexed under this heading.

Lopinavir (Rarely, cases of hepatotoxicity characterized by such findings as jaundice and altered liver function tests, when metoclopramide was administered with other drugs with known hepatotoxic potential). Products include:
- Kaletra 458

Lorazepam (Additive sedative effects can occur when metoclopramide is given with alcohol, sedatives, hypnotics, narcotics, or tranquilizers).
No products indexed under this heading.

Lovastatin (Rarely, cases of hepatotoxicity characterized by such findings as jaundice and altered liver function tests, when metoclopramide was administered with other drugs with known hepatotoxic potential). Products include:
- Advicor 402
- Mevacor 2212

Loxapine Hydrochloride (Co-administration of metoclopramide with drugs likely to cause extrapyramidal reactions is contraindicated. Concomitant use of metoclopramide should be avoided in patients taking antidepressants, antipsychotics, and/or neuroleptics that have been associated with extrapyramidal reactions such as tardive dyskinesia or Neuroleptic Malignant Syndrome (NMS) that have occurred in association with metoclopramide).
No products indexed under this heading.

Loxapine Succinate (Co-administration of metoclopramide with drugs likely to cause extrapyramidal reactions is contraindicated. Concomitant use of metoclopramide should be avoided in patients taking antidepressants, antipsychotics, and/or neuroleptics that have been associated with extrapyramidal reactions such as tardive dyskinesia or Neuroleptic Malignant Syndrome (NMS) that have occurred in association with metoclopramide).
No products indexed under this heading.

Maprotiline Hydrochloride (Co-administration of metoclopramide with drugs likely to cause extrapyramidal reactions is contraindicated. Concomitant use of metoclopramide should be avoided in patients taking antidepressants, antipsychotics, and/or neuroleptics that have been associated with extrapyramidal reactions such as tardive dyskinesia or Neuroleptic Malignant Syndrome (NMS) that have occurred in association with metoclopramide).
No products indexed under this heading.

Maraviroc (Rarely, cases of hepatotoxicity characterized by such findings as jaundice and altered liver function tests, when metoclopramide was administered with other drugs with known hepatotoxic potential). Products include:
- Selzentry 2740

Meclofenamate Sodium (Rarely, cases of hepatotoxicity characterized by such findings as jaundice and altered liver function tests, when metoclopramide was administered with other drugs with known hepatotoxic potential).
No products indexed under this heading.

Mefenamic Acid (Rarely, cases of hepatotoxicity characterized by such findings as jaundice and altered liver function tests, when metoclopramide was administered with other drugs with known hepatotoxic potential).
No products indexed under this heading.

Meloxicam (Rarely, cases of hepatotoxicity characterized by such findings as jaundice and altered liver function tests, when metoclopramide was administered with other drugs with known hepatotoxic potential).
No products indexed under this heading.

Mepenzolate Bromide (The effects of metoclopramide on gastrointestinal motility are antagonized by anticholinergic drugs and narcotic analgesics).
No products indexed under this heading.

Meperidine Hydrochloride (The effects of metoclopramide on gastrointestinal motility are antagonized by anticholinergic drugs and narcotic analgesics. Additive sedative effects can occur when metoclopramide is given with alcohol, sedatives, hypnotics, narcotics, or tranquilizers).
No products indexed under this heading.

Mephenytoin (Co-administration of metoclopramide with drugs likely to cause extrapyramidal reactions is contraindicated. Concomitant use of metoclopramide should be avoided in patients taking antidepressants, antipsychotics, and/or neuroleptics that have been associated with extrapyramidal reactions such as tardive dyskinesia or Neuroleptic Malignant Syndrome (NMS) that have occurred in association with metoclopramide).
No products indexed under this heading.

Meprobamate (Additive sedative effects can occur when metoclopramide is given with alcohol, sedatives, hypnotics, narcotics, or tranquilizers).
No products indexed under this heading.

Mesoridazine Besylate (Co-administration of metoclopramide with drugs likely to cause extrapyramidal reactions is contraindicated. Concomitant use of metoclopramide should be avoided in patients taking antidepressants, antipsychotics, and/or neuroleptics that have been associated with extrapyramidal reactions such as tardive dyskinesia or Neuroleptic Malignant Syndrome (NMS) that have occurred in association with metoclopramide).
No products indexed under this heading.

Methacycline Hydrochloride (Absorption of drugs from the stomach may be diminished by metoclopramide (eg, digoxin), whereas the rate and/or extent of absorption of drugs from the small bowel may be increased (eg, acetaminophen, tetracycline, levodopa, ethanol, cyclosporine)).
No products indexed under this heading.

Methadone Hydrochloride (The effects of metoclopramide on gastrointestinal motility are antagonized by anticholinergic drugs and narcotic analgesics. Additive sedative effects can occur when metoclopramide is given with alcohol, sedatives, hypnotics, narcotics, or tranquilizers).
No products indexed under this heading.

Methicillin Sodium (Rarely, cases of hepatotoxicity characterized by such findings as jaundice and altered liver function tests, when metoclopramide was administered with other drugs with known hepatotoxic potential).
No products indexed under this heading.

Methimazole (Rarely, cases of hepatotoxicity characterized by such findings as jaundice and altered liver function tests, when metoclopramide was administered with other drugs with known hepatotoxic potential).
No products indexed under this heading.

Methotrexate (Rarely, cases of hepatotoxicity characterized by such findings as jaundice and altered liver function tests, when metoclopramide was administered with other drugs with known hepatotoxic potential).
No products indexed under this heading.

Methotrexate Sodium (Rarely, cases of hepatotoxicity characterized by such findings as jaundice and altered liver function tests, when metoclopramide was administered with other drugs with known hepatotoxic potential).
No products indexed under this heading.

Methotrimeprazine (Co-administration of metoclopramide with drugs likely to cause extrapyramidal reactions is contraindicated. Concomitant use of metoclopramide should be avoided in patients taking antidepressants, antipsychotics, and/or neuroleptics that have been associated with extrapyramidal reactions such as tardive dyskinesia or Neuroleptic Malignant Syndrome (NMS) that have occurred in association with metoclopramide).
No products indexed under this heading.

Methsuximide (Co-administration of metoclopramide with drugs likely to cause extrapyramidal reactions is contraindicated. Concomitant use of metoclopramide should be avoided in patients taking antidepressants, antipsychotics, and/or neuroleptics that have been associated with extrapyramidal reactions such as tardive dyskinesia or Neuroleptic Malignant Syndrome (NMS) that have occurred in association with metoclopramide).
No products indexed under this heading.

Methyclothiazide (Rarely, cases of hepatotoxicity characterized by such findings as jaundice and altered liver function tests, when metoclopramide was administered with other drugs with known hepatotoxic potential).
No products indexed under this heading.

Mezlocillin Sodium (Rarely, cases of hepatotoxicity characterized by such findings as jaundice and altered liver function tests, when metoclopramide was administered with other drugs with known hepatotoxic potential).
No products indexed under this heading.

Midazolam Hydrochloride (Additive sedative effects can occur when metoclopramide is given with alcohol, sedatives, hypnotics, narcotics, or tranquilizers).
No products indexed under this heading.

Minocycline Hydrochloride (Absorption of drugs from the stomach may be diminished by metoclopramide (eg, digoxin), whereas the rate and/or extent of absorption of drugs from the small bowel may be increased (eg, acetaminophen, tetracycline, levodopa, ethanol, cyclosporine)). Products include:
- Solodyn 2073

Mirtazapine (Co-administration of metoclopramide with drugs likely to cause extrapyramidal reactions is contraindicated. Concomitant use of metoclopramide should be avoided in patients taking antidepressants, antipsychotics, and/or neuroleptics that have been associated with extrapyramidal reactions such as tardive dyskinesia or Neuroleptic Malignant Syndrome (NMS) that have occurred in association with metoclopramide). Products include:
- Remeron Tablets 3214
- RemeronSolTab Tablets 3219

Moclobemide (Metoclopramide has been shown to release catecholamines in patients with essential hypertension suggests that it should be used cautiously, if at all, in patients taking monoamine oxidase (MAO) inhibitors).
No products indexed under this heading.

Molindone Hydrochloride (Co-administration of metoclopramide with drugs likely to cause extrapyramidal reactions is contraindicated. Concomitant use of metoclopramide should be avoided in patients taking antidepressants, antipsychotics, and/or neuroleptics that have been associated with

IMPORTANT NOTE: Always consult each drug listing in the patient's regimen for possible interactions.

extrapyramidal reactions such as tardive dyskinesia or Neuroleptic Malignant Syndrome (NMS) that have occurred in association with metoclopramide). Products include:

Morphine Sulfate (The effects of metoclopramide on gastrointestinal motility are antagonized by anticholinergic drugs and narcotic analgesics. Additive sedative effects can occur when metoclopramide is given with alcohol, sedatives, hypnotics, narcotics, or tranquilizers). Products include:

Morphine Sulfate, Liposomal (The effects of metoclopramide on gastrointestinal motility are antagonized by anticholinergic drugs and narcotic analgesics. Additive sedative effects can occur when metoclopramide is given with alcohol, sedatives, hypnotics, narcotics, or tranquilizers).
No products indexed under this heading.

Nabumetone (Rarely, cases of hepatotoxicity characterized by such findings as jaundice and altered liver function tests, when metoclopramide was administered with other drugs with known hepatotoxic potential).
No products indexed under this heading.

Nafcillin Sodium (Rarely, cases of hepatotoxicity characterized by such findings as jaundice and altered liver function tests, when metoclopramide was administered with other drugs with known hepatotoxic potential).
No products indexed under this heading.

Naproxen (Rarely, cases of hepatotoxicity characterized by such findings as jaundice and altered liver function tests, when metoclopramide was administered with other drugs with known hepatotoxic potential). Products include:

Naproxen Sodium (Rarely, cases of hepatotoxicity characterized by such findings as jaundice and altered liver function tests, when metoclopramide was administered with other drugs with known hepatotoxic potential). Products include:

Nefazodone Hydrochloride (Co-administration of metoclopramide with drugs likely to cause extrapyramidal reactions is contraindicated. Concomitant use of metoclopramide should be avoided in patients taking antidepressants, antipsychotics, and/or neuroleptics that have been associated with extrapyramidal reactions such as tardive dyskinesia or Neuroleptic Malignant Syndrome (NMS) that have occurred in association with metoclopramide).
No products indexed under this heading.

Nelfinavir Mesylate (Rarely, cases of hepatotoxicity characterized by such findings as jaundice and altered liver function tests, when metoclopramide was administered with other drugs with known hepatotoxic potential).
No products indexed under this heading.

Nevirapine (Rarely, cases of hepatotoxicity characterized by such findings as jaundice and altered liver function tests, when metoclopramide was administered with other drugs with known hepatotoxic potential). Products include:

Niacin (Rarely, cases of hepatotoxicity characterized by such findings as jaundice and altered liver function tests,

when metoclopramide was administered with other drugs with known hepatotoxic potential). Products include:

Niacinamide (Rarely, cases of hepatotoxicity characterized by such findings as jaundice and altered liver function tests, when metoclopramide was administered with other drugs with known hepatotoxic potential). Products include:

Niacinamide Hydroiodide (Rarely, cases of hepatotoxicity characterized by such findings as jaundice and altered liver function tests, when metoclopramide was administered with other drugs with known hepatotoxic potential).
No products indexed under this heading.

Nicotinic Acid (Rarely, cases of hepatotoxicity characterized by such findings as jaundice and altered liver function tests, when metoclopramide was administered with other drugs with known hepatotoxic potential).
No products indexed under this heading.

Nitrofurantoin (Rarely, cases of hepatotoxicity characterized by such findings as jaundice and altered liver function tests, when metoclopramide was administered with other drugs with known hepatotoxic potential).
No products indexed under this heading.

Nitrofurantoin Macrocrystals (Rarely, cases of hepatotoxicity characterized by such findings as jaundice and altered liver function tests, when metoclopramide was administered with other drugs with known hepatotoxic potential).
No products indexed under this heading.

Nitrofurantoin Monohydrate (Rarely, cases of hepatotoxicity characterized by such findings as jaundice and altered liver function tests, when metoclopramide was administered with other drugs with known hepatotoxic potential).
No products indexed under this heading.

Nitrofurantoin Sodium (Rarely, cases of hepatotoxicity characterized by such findings as jaundice and altered liver function tests, when metoclopramide was administered with other drugs with known hepatotoxic potential).
No products indexed under this heading.

Nortriptyline Hydrochloride (Co-administration of metoclopramide with drugs likely to cause extrapyramidal reactions is contraindicated. Concomitant use of metoclopramide should be avoided in patients taking antidepressants, antipsychotics, and/or neuroleptics that have been associated with extrapyramidal reactions such as tardive dyskinesia or Neuroleptic Malignant Syndrome (NMS) that have occurred in association with metoclopramide).
No products indexed under this heading.

Olanzapine (Co-administration of metoclopramide with drugs likely to cause extrapyramidal reactions is contraindicated. Concomitant use of metoclopramide should be avoided in patients taking antidepressants, antipsychotics, and/or neuroleptics that have been associated with extrapyramidal reactions such as tardive dyskinesia or Neuroleptic Malignant Syndrome (NMS) that have occurred in association with metoclopramide). Products include:

Oxacillin (Rarely, cases of hepatotoxicity characterized by such findings as jaundice and altered liver function tests, when metoclopramide was administered with other drugs with known hepatotoxic potential).
No products indexed under this heading.

Oxacillin Sodium (Rarely, cases of hepatotoxicity characterized by such findings as jaundice and altered liver function tests, when metoclopramide was administered with other drugs with known hepatotoxic potential).
No products indexed under this heading.

Oxaprozin (Rarely, cases of hepatotoxicity characterized by such findings as jaundice and altered liver function tests, when metoclopramide was administered with other drugs with known hepatotoxic potential).
No products indexed under this heading.

Oxazepam (Additive sedative effects can occur when metoclopramide is given with alcohol, sedatives, hypnotics, narcotics, or tranquilizers).
No products indexed under this heading.

Oxcarbazepine (Co-administration of metoclopramide with drugs likely to cause extrapyramidal reactions is contraindicated. Concomitant use of metoclopramide should be avoided in patients taking antidepressants, antipsychotics, and/or neuroleptics that have been associated with extrapyramidal reactions such as tardive dyskinesia or Neuroleptic Malignant Syndrome (NMS) that have occurred in association with metoclopramide).
No products indexed under this heading.

Oxybutynin Chloride (The effects of metoclopramide on gastrointestinal motility are antagonized by anticholinergic drugs and narcotic analgesics).
No products indexed under this heading.

Oxycodone Hydrochloride (The effects of metoclopramide on gastrointestinal motility are antagonized by anticholinergic drugs and narcotic analgesics. Additive sedative effects can occur when metoclopramide is given with alcohol, sedatives, hypnotics, narcotics, or tranquilizers). Products include:

Oxycodone Terephthalate (The effects of metoclopramide on gastrointestinal motility are antagonized by anticholinergic drugs and narcotic analgesics. Additive sedative effects can occur when metoclopramide is given with alcohol, sedatives, hypnotics, narcotics, or tranquilizers).
No products indexed under this heading.

Oxymetholone (Rarely, cases of hepatotoxicity characterized by such findings as jaundice and altered liver function tests, when metoclopramide was administered with other drugs with known hepatotoxic potential).
No products indexed under this heading.

Oxymorphone Hydrochloride (The effects of metoclopramide on gastrointestinal motility are antagonized by anticholinergic drugs and narcotic analgesics. Additive sedative effects can occur when metoclopramide is given with alcohol, sedatives, hypnotics, narcotics, or tranquilizers). Products include:

Oxytetracycline (Absorption of drugs from the stomach may be diminished by metoclopramide (eg, digoxin), whereas the rate and/or extent of absorption of drugs from the small bowel may be increased (eg, acetaminophen, tetracycline, levodopa, ethanol, cyclosporine)).
No products indexed under this heading.

Oxytetracycline Hydrochloride (Absorption of drugs from the stomach may be diminished by metoclopramide (eg, digoxin), whereas the rate and/or extent of absorption of drugs from the small bowel may be increased (eg, acetaminophen, tetracycline, levodopa, ethanol, cyclosporine)).
No products indexed under this heading.

Paliperidone (Co-administration of metoclopramide with drugs likely to cause extrapyramidal reactions is contraindicated. Concomitant use of metoclopramide should be avoided in patients taking antidepressants, antipsychotics, and/or neuroleptics that have been associated with extrapyramidal reactions such as tardive dyskinesia or Neuroleptic Malignant Syndrome (NMS) that have occurred in association with metoclopramide). Products include:

Paramethadione (Co-administration of metoclopramide with drugs likely to cause extrapyramidal reactions is contraindicated. Concomitant use of metoclopramide should be avoided in patients taking antidepressants, antipsychotics, and/or neuroleptics that have been associated with extrapyramidal reactions such as tardive dyskinesia or Neuroleptic Malignant Syndrome (NMS) that have occurred in association with metoclopramide).
No products indexed under this heading.

Pargyline Hydrochloride (Metoclopramide has been shown to release catecholamines in patients with essential hypertension suggests that it should be used cautiously, if at all, in patients taking monoamine oxidase (MAO) inhibitors).
No products indexed under this heading.

Paroxetine (Co-administration of metoclopramide with drugs likely to cause extrapyramidal reactions is contraindicated. Concomitant use of metoclopramide should be avoided in patients taking antidepressants, antipsychotics, and/or neuroleptics that have been associated with extrapyramidal reactions such as tardive dyskinesia or Neuroleptic Malignant Syndrome (NMS) that have occurred in association with metoclopramide).
No products indexed under this heading.

Paroxetine Hydrochloride (Co-administration of metoclopramide with drugs likely to cause extrapyramidal reactions is contraindicated. Concomitant use of metoclopramide should be avoided in patients taking antidepressants, antipsychotics, and/or neuroleptics that have been associated with extrapyramidal reactions such as tardive dyskinesia or Neuroleptic Malignant Syndrome (NMS) that have occurred in association with metoclopramide). Products include:

Paroxetine Mesylate (Co-administration of metoclopramide with drugs likely to cause extrapyramidal reactions is contraindicated. Concomitant use of metoclopramide should be avoided in patients taking antidepressants, antipsychotics, and/or neuroleptics that have been associated with extrapyramidal reactions such as tar-

dive dyskinesia or Neuroleptic Malignant Syndrome (NMS) that have occurred in association with metoclopramide).
No products indexed under this heading.

Penicillin, Potassium Phenoxymethyl (Rarely, cases of hepatotoxicity characterized by such findings as jaundice and altered liver function tests, when metoclopramide was administered with other drugs with known hepatotoxic potential).
No products indexed under this heading.

Penicillin G Benzathine (Rarely, cases of hepatotoxicity characterized by such findings as jaundice and altered liver function tests, when metoclopramide was administered with other drugs with known hepatotoxic potential).
Products include:
Bicillin C-R Injectable Suspension 1826
Bicillin L-A 1828

Penicillin G Dibenzylethyenediamine (Rarely, cases of hepatotoxicity characterized by such findings as jaundice and altered liver function tests, when metoclopramide was administered with other drugs with known hepatotoxic potential).
No products indexed under this heading.

Penicillin G Potassium (Rarely, cases of hepatotoxicity characterized by such findings as jaundice and altered liver function tests, when metoclopramide was administered with other drugs with known hepatotoxic potential).
No products indexed under this heading.

Penicillin G Procaine (Rarely, cases of hepatotoxicity characterized by such findings as jaundice and altered liver function tests, when metoclopramide was administered with other drugs with known hepatotoxic potential). Products include:
Bicillin C-R Injectable Suspension 1826
Bicillin L-A 1828

Penicillin G Sodium (Rarely, cases of hepatotoxicity characterized by such findings as jaundice and altered liver function tests, when metoclopramide was administered with other drugs with known hepatotoxic potential).
No products indexed under this heading.

Penicillin V (Rarely, cases of hepatotoxicity characterized by such findings as jaundice and altered liver function tests, when metoclopramide was administered with other drugs with known hepatotoxic potential).
No products indexed under this heading.

Penicillin V Potassium (Rarely, cases of hepatotoxicity characterized by such findings as jaundice and altered liver function tests, when metoclopramide was administered with other drugs with known hepatotoxic potential).
No products indexed under this heading.

Penicillins (Rarely, cases of hepatotoxicity characterized by such findings as jaundice and altered liver function tests, when metoclopramide was administered with other drugs with known hepatotoxic potential).
No products indexed under this heading.

Perphenazine (Co-administration of metoclopramide with drugs likely to cause extrapyramidal reactions is contraindicated. Concomitant use of metoclopramide should be avoided in patients taking antidepressants, antipsychotics, and/or neuroleptics that have been associated with extrapyramidal reactions such as tardive dyskinesia or Neuroleptic Malignant Syndrome (NMS) that have occurred in association with metoclopramide).
No products indexed under this heading.

Phenacemide (Co-administration of metoclopramide with drugs likely to cause extrapyramidal reactions is contraindicated. Concomitant use of metoclopramide should be avoided in patients taking antidepressants, antipsychotics, and/or neuroleptics that have been associated with extrapyramidal reactions such as tardive dyskinesia or Neuroleptic Malignant Syndrome (NMS) that have occurred in association with metoclopramide).
No products indexed under this heading.

Phenelzine Sulfate (Co-administration of metoclopramide with drugs likely to cause extrapyramidal reactions is contraindicated. Concomitant use of metoclopramide should be avoided in patients taking antidepressants, antipsychotics, and/or neuroleptics that have been associated with extrapyramidal reactions such as tardive dyskinesia or Neuroleptic Malignant Syndrome (NMS) that have occurred in association with metoclopramide).
No products indexed under this heading.

Phenobarbital (Co-administration of metoclopramide with drugs likely to cause extrapyramidal reactions is contraindicated. Concomitant use of metoclopramide should be avoided in patients taking antidepressants, antipsychotics, and/or neuroleptics that have been associated with extrapyramidal reactions such as tardive dyskinesia or Neuroleptic Malignant Syndrome (NMS) that have occurred in association with metoclopramide). Products include:
Donnatal 2711

Phenobarbital Sodium (Co-administration of metoclopramide with drugs likely to cause extrapyramidal reactions is contraindicated. Concomitant use of metoclopramide should be avoided in patients taking antidepressants, antipsychotics, and/or neuroleptics that have been associated with extrapyramidal reactions such as tardive dyskinesia or Neuroleptic Malignant Syndrome (NMS) that have occurred in association with metoclopramide).
No products indexed under this heading.

Phensuximide (Co-administration of metoclopramide with drugs likely to cause extrapyramidal reactions is contraindicated. Concomitant use of metoclopramide should be avoided in patients taking antidepressants, antipsychotics, and/or neuroleptics that have been associated with extrapyramidal reactions such as tardive dyskinesia or Neuroleptic Malignant Syndrome (NMS) that have occurred in association with metoclopramide).
No products indexed under this heading.

Phenylbutazone (Rarely, cases of hepatotoxicity characterized by such findings as jaundice and altered liver function tests, when metoclopramide was administered with other drugs with known hepatotoxic potential).
No products indexed under this heading.

Phenytoin (Co-administration of metoclopramide with drugs likely to cause extrapyramidal reactions is contraindicated. Concomitant use of metoclopramide should be avoided in patients taking antidepressants, antipsychotics, and/or neuroleptics that have been associated with extrapyramidal reactions such as tardive dyskinesia or Neuroleptic Malignant Syndrome (NMS) that have occurred in association with metoclopramide).
No products indexed under this heading.

Phenytoin Sodium (Co-administration of metoclopramide with drugs likely to cause extrapyramidal reactions is contraindicated. Concomitant use of metoclopramide should be avoided in patients taking antidepressants, antipsychotics, and/or neuroleptics that have been associated with extrapyramidal reactions such as tardive dyskinesia or Neuroleptic Malignant Syndrome (NMS) that have occurred in association with metoclopramide). Products include:
Phenytek Capsules 2380

Pimozide (Co-administration of metoclopramide with drugs likely to cause extrapyramidal reactions is contraindicated. Concomitant use of metoclopramide should be avoided in patients taking antidepressants, antipsychotics, and/or neuroleptics that have been associated with extrapyramidal reactions such as tardive dyskinesia or Neuroleptic Malignant Syndrome (NMS) that have occurred in association with metoclopramide).
No products indexed under this heading.

Pioglitazone Hydrochloride (Rarely, cases of hepatotoxicity characterized by such findings as jaundice and altered liver function tests, when metoclopramide was administered with other drugs with known hepatotoxic potential).
Products include:
ActoPlus 3338
Actos 3345
Duetact 3354

Piperacillin Sodium (Rarely, cases of hepatotoxicity characterized by such findings as jaundice and altered liver function tests, when metoclopramide was administered with other drugs with known hepatotoxic potential). Products include:
Zosyn 3607

Piroxicam (Rarely, cases of hepatotoxicity characterized by such findings as jaundice and altered liver function tests, when metoclopramide was administered with other drugs with known hepatotoxic potential).
No products indexed under this heading.

Polythiazide (Rarely, cases of hepatotoxicity characterized by such findings as jaundice and altered liver function tests, when metoclopramide was administered with other drugs with known hepatotoxic potential).
No products indexed under this heading.

Pravastatin Sodium (Rarely, cases of hepatotoxicity characterized by such findings as jaundice and altered liver function tests, when metoclopramide was administered with other drugs with known hepatotoxic potential).
No products indexed under this heading.

Prazepam (Additive sedative effects can occur when metoclopramide is given with alcohol, sedatives, hypnotics, narcotics, or tranquilizers).
No products indexed under this heading.

Primidone (Co-administration of metoclopramide with drugs likely to cause extrapyramidal reactions is contraindicated. Concomitant use of metoclopramide should be avoided in patients taking antidepressants, antipsychotics, and/or neuroleptics that have been associated with extrapyramidal reactions such as tardive dyskinesia or Neuroleptic Malignant Syndrome (NMS) that have occurred in association with metoclopramide).
No products indexed under this heading.

Procainamide (Rarely, cases of hepatotoxicity characterized by such findings as jaundice and altered liver function tests, when metoclopramide was administered with other drugs with known hepatotoxic potential).
No products indexed under this heading.

Procainamide Hydrochloride (Rarely, cases of hepatotoxicity characterized by such findings as jaundice and altered liver function tests, when metoclopramide was administered with other drugs with known hepatotoxic potential).
No products indexed under this heading.

Procarbazine Hydrochloride (Metoclopramide has been shown to release catecholamines in patients with essential hypertension suggests that it should be used cautiously, if at all, in patients taking monoamine oxidase (MAO) inhibitors).
No products indexed under this heading.

Prochlorperazine (Co-administration of metoclopramide with drugs likely to cause extrapyramidal reactions is contraindicated. Concomitant use of metoclopramide should be avoided in patients taking antidepressants, antipsychotics, and/or neuroleptics that have been associated with extrapyramidal reactions such as tardive dyskinesia or Neuroleptic Malignant Syndrome (NMS) that have occurred in association with metoclopramide).
No products indexed under this heading.

Procyclidine Hydrochloride (The effects of metoclopramide on gastrointestinal motility are antagonized by anticholinergic drugs and narcotic analgesics).
No products indexed under this heading.

Promethazine Hydrochloride (Additive sedative effects can occur when metoclopramide is given with alcohol, sedatives, hypnotics, narcotics, or tranquilizers).
No products indexed under this heading.

Propantheline Bromide (The effects of metoclopramide on gastrointestinal motility are antagonized by anticholinergic drugs and narcotic analgesics).
No products indexed under this heading.

Propofol (Additive sedative effects can occur when metoclopramide is given with alcohol, sedatives, hypnotics, narcotics, or tranquilizers).
No products indexed under this heading.

Propoxyphene Hydrochloride (The effects of metoclopramide on gastrointestinal motility are antagonized by anticholinergic drugs and narcotic analgesics. Additive sedative effects can occur when metoclopramide is given with alcohol, sedatives, hypnotics, narcotics, or tranquilizers).
No products indexed under this heading.

Propoxyphene Napsylate (The effects of metoclopramide on gastrointestinal motility are antagonized by anticholinergic drugs and narcotic analgesics. Additive sedative effects can occur when metoclopramide is given with alcohol, sedatives, hypnotics, narcotics, or tranquilizers).
No products indexed under this heading.

Propylthiouracil (Rarely, cases of hepatotoxicity characterized by such findings as jaundice and altered liver function tests, when metoclopramide was administered with other drugs with known hepatotoxic potential).
No products indexed under this heading.

Protriptyline Hydrochloride (Co-administration of metoclopramide with drugs likely to cause extrapyramidal reactions is contraindicated. Concomitant use of metoclopramide should be avoided in patients taking antidepressants, antipsychotics, and/or neuroleptics that have been associated with extrapyramidal reactions such as tardive dyskinesia or Neuroleptic Malignant Syndrome (NMS) that have occurred in association with metoclopramide).
No products indexed under this heading.

Quazepam (Additive sedative effects can occur when metoclopramide is given with alcohol, sedatives, hypnotics, narcotics, or tranquilizers).
No products indexed under this heading.

Quetiapine Fumarate (Co-administration of metoclopramide with drugs likely to cause extrapyramidal reactions is contraindicated. Concomi-

tant use of metoclopramide should be avoided in patients taking antidepressants, antipsychotics, and/or neuroleptics that have been associated with extrapyramidal reactions such as tardive dyskinesia or Neuroleptic Malignant Syndrome (NMS) that have occurred in association with metoclopramide). Products include:

Seroquel 750
Seroquel XR 759

Ramelteon (Additive sedative effects can occur when metoclopramide is given with alcohol, sedatives, hypnotics, narcotics, or tranquilizers). Products include:

Rozerem 3366

Rasagiline Mesylate (Metoclopramide has been shown to release catecholamines in patients with essential hypertension suggests that it should be used cautiously, if at all, in patients taking monoamine oxidase (MAO) inhibitors). Products include:

Azilect 3383

Remifentanil Hydrochloride (The effects of metoclopramide on gastrointestinal motility are antagonized by anticholinergic drugs and narcotic analgesics. Additive sedative effects can occur when metoclopramide is given with alcohol, sedatives, hypnotics, narcotics, or tranquilizers).

No products indexed under this heading.

Rifampin (Rarely, cases of hepatotoxicity characterized by such findings as jaundice and altered liver function tests, when metoclopramide was administered with other drugs with known hepatotoxic potential).

No products indexed under this heading.

Risperidone (Co-administration of metoclopramide with drugs likely to cause extrapyramidal reactions is contraindicated. Concomitant use of metoclopramide should be avoided in patients taking antidepressants, antipsychotics, and/or neuroleptics that have been associated with extrapyramidal reactions such as tardive dyskinesia or Neuroleptic Malignant Syndrome (NMS) that have occurred in association with metoclopramide). Products include:

Risperdal Consta 2682

Ritonavir (Rarely, cases of hepatotoxicity characterized by such findings as jaundice and altered liver function tests, when metoclopramide was administered with other drugs with known hepatotoxic potential). Products include:

Kaletra 458
Norvir 509

Rofecoxib (Rarely, cases of hepatotoxicity characterized by such findings as jaundice and altered liver function tests, when metoclopramide was administered with other drugs with known hepatotoxic potential).

No products indexed under this heading.

Rosuvastatin Calcium (Rarely, cases of hepatotoxicity characterized by such findings as jaundice and altered liver function tests, when metoclopramide was administered with other drugs with known hepatotoxic potential). Products include:

Crestor 736

Rufinamide (Co-administration of metoclopramide with drugs likely to cause extrapyramidal reactions is contraindicated. Concomitant use of metoclopramide should be avoided in patients taking antidepressants, antipsychotics, and/or neuroleptics that have been associated with extrapyramidal reactions such as tardive dyskinesia or Neuroleptic Malignant Syndrome (NMS) that have occurred in association with metoclopramide). Products include:

Banzel 1050

Saquinavir (Rarely, cases of hepatotoxicity characterized by such findings as jaundice and altered liver function tests, when metoclopramide was administered with other drugs with known hepatotoxic potential).

No products indexed under this heading.

Saquinavir Mesylate (Rarely, cases of hepatotoxicity characterized by such findings as jaundice and altered liver function tests, when metoclopramide was administered with other drugs with known hepatotoxic potential).

No products indexed under this heading.

Scopolamine (The effects of metoclopramide on gastrointestinal motility are antagonized by anticholinergic drugs and narcotic analgesics). Products include:

Transderm Scōp 2397

Scopolamine Hydrobromide (The effects of metoclopramide on gastrointestinal motility are antagonized by anticholinergic drugs and narcotic analgesics). Products include:

Donnatal 2711

Secobarbital Sodium (Additive sedative effects can occur when metoclopramide is given with alcohol, sedatives, hypnotics, narcotics, or tranquilizers).

No products indexed under this heading.

Selegiline (Co-administration of metoclopramide with drugs likely to cause extrapyramidal reactions is contraindicated. Concomitant use of metoclopramide should be avoided in patients taking antidepressants, antipsychotics, and/or neuroleptics that have been associated with extrapyramidal reactions such as tardive dyskinesia or Neuroleptic Malignant Syndrome (NMS) that have occurred in association with metoclopramide). Products include:

Emsam 3623

Selegiline Hydrochloride (Co-administration of metoclopramide with drugs likely to cause extrapyramidal reactions is contraindicated. Concomitant use of metoclopramide should be avoided in patients taking antidepressants, antipsychotics, and/or neuroleptics that have been associated with extrapyramidal reactions such as tardive dyskinesia or Neuroleptic Malignant Syndrome (NMS) that have occurred in association with metoclopramide). Products include:

Eldepryl 3312

Sertraline Hydrochloride (Co-administration of metoclopramide with drugs likely to cause extrapyramidal reactions is contraindicated. Concomitant use of metoclopramide should be avoided in patients taking antidepressants, antipsychotics, and/or neuroleptics that have been associated with extrapyramidal reactions such as tardive dyskinesia or Neuroleptic Malignant Syndrome (NMS) that have occurred in association with metoclopramide).

No products indexed under this heading.

Simvastatin (Rarely, cases of hepatotoxicity characterized by such findings as jaundice and altered liver function tests, when metoclopramide was administered with other drugs with known hepatotoxic potential). Products include:

Simcor 524
Vytorin 10/10 .... 2303, 3240
Vytorin 10/20 .... 2303, 3240
Vytorin 10/40 .... 2303, 3240
Vytorin 10/80 .... 2303, 3240
Zocor 2289

Sodium Butabarbital (Additive sedative effects can occur when metoclopramide is given with alcohol, sedatives, hypnotics, narcotics, or tranquilizers).

No products indexed under this heading.

Sodium Cloxacillin Monohydrate (Rarely, cases of hepatotoxicity characterized by such findings as jaundice and altered liver function tests, when metoclopramide was administered with other drugs with known hepatotoxic potential).

No products indexed under this heading.

Statins (Rarely, cases of hepatotoxicity characterized by such findings as jaundice and altered liver function tests, when metoclopramide was administered with other drugs with known hepatotoxic potential).

No products indexed under this heading.

Sufentanil Citrate (The effects of metoclopramide on gastrointestinal motility are antagonized by anticholinergic drugs and narcotic analgesics. Additive sedative effects can occur when metoclopramide is given with alcohol, sedatives, hypnotics, narcotics, or tranquilizers).

No products indexed under this heading.

Sulfacytine (Rarely, cases of hepatotoxicity characterized by such findings as jaundice and altered liver function tests, when metoclopramide was administered with other drugs with known hepatotoxic potential).

No products indexed under this heading.

Sulfamethizole (Rarely, cases of hepatotoxicity characterized by such findings as jaundice and altered liver function tests, when metoclopramide was administered with other drugs with known hepatotoxic potential).

No products indexed under this heading.

Sulfamethoxazole (Rarely, cases of hepatotoxicity characterized by such findings as jaundice and altered liver function tests, when metoclopramide was administered with other drugs with known hepatotoxic potential).

No products indexed under this heading.

Sulfasalazine (Rarely, cases of hepatotoxicity characterized by such findings as jaundice and altered liver function tests, when metoclopramide was administered with other drugs with known hepatotoxic potential).

No products indexed under this heading.

Sulfinpyrazone (Rarely, cases of hepatotoxicity characterized by such findings as jaundice and altered liver function tests, when metoclopramide was administered with other drugs with known hepatotoxic potential).

No products indexed under this heading.

Sulfisoxazole Acetyl (Rarely, cases of hepatotoxicity characterized by such findings as jaundice and altered liver function tests, when metoclopramide was administered with other drugs with known hepatotoxic potential).

No products indexed under this heading.

Sulfisoxazole Diolamine (Rarely, cases of hepatotoxicity characterized by such findings as jaundice and altered liver function tests, when metoclopramide was administered with other drugs with known hepatotoxic potential).

No products indexed under this heading.

Sulindac (Rarely, cases of hepatotoxicity characterized by such findings as jaundice and altered liver function tests, when metoclopramide was administered with other drugs with known hepatotoxic potential). Products include:

Clinoril 2098

Tacrine Hydrochloride (Rarely, cases of hepatotoxicity characterized by such findings as jaundice and altered liver function tests, when metoclopramide was administered with other drugs with known hepatotoxic potential).

No products indexed under this heading.

Tamoxifen Citrate (Rarely, cases of hepatotoxicity characterized by such findings as jaundice and altered liver function tests, when metoclopramide was administered with other drugs with known hepatotoxic potential).

No products indexed under this heading.

Telithromycin (Rarely, cases of hepatotoxicity characterized by such findings as jaundice and altered liver function tests, when metoclopramide was administered with other drugs with known hepatotoxic potential). Products include:

Ketek 2991

Temazepam (Additive sedative effects can occur when metoclopramide is given with alcohol, sedatives, hypnotics, narcotics, or tranquilizers).

No products indexed under this heading.

Tetracycline Hydrochloride (Absorption of drugs from the stomach may be diminished by metoclopramide (eg, digoxin), whereas the rate and/or extent of absorption of drugs from the small bowel may be increased (eg, acetaminophen, tetracycline, levodopa, ethanol, cyclosporine)). Products include:

Pylera 793

Tetracycline Phosphate Complex (Absorption of drugs from the stomach may be diminished by metoclopramide (eg, digoxin), whereas the rate and/or extent of absorption of drugs from the small bowel may be increased (eg, acetaminophen, tetracycline, levodopa, ethanol, cyclosporine)).

No products indexed under this heading.

Thiazide Diuretics (Rarely, cases of hepatotoxicity characterized by such findings as jaundice and altered liver function tests, when metoclopramide was administered with other drugs with known hepatotoxic potential).

No products indexed under this heading.

Thiazides (Rarely, cases of hepatotoxicity characterized by such findings as jaundice and altered liver function tests, when metoclopramide was administered with other drugs with known hepatotoxic potential).

No products indexed under this heading.

Thioridazine Hydrochloride (Co-administration of metoclopramide with drugs likely to cause extrapyramidal reactions is contraindicated. Concomitant use of metoclopramide should be avoided in patients taking antidepressants, antipsychotics, and/or neuroleptics that have been associated with extrapyramidal reactions such as tardive dyskinesia or Neuroleptic Malignant Syndrome (NMS) that have occurred in association with metoclopramide). Products include:

Thioridazine Hydrochloride 2384

Thiothixene (Co-administration of metoclopramide with drugs likely to cause extrapyramidal reactions is contraindicated. Concomitant use of metoclopramide should be avoided in patients taking antidepressants, antipsychotics, and/or neuroleptics that have been associated with extrapyramidal reactions such as tardive dyskinesia or Neuroleptic Malignant Syndrome (NMS) that have occurred in association with metoclopramide). Products include:

Thiothixene 2386

Tiagabine Hydrochloride (Co-administration of metoclopramide with drugs likely to cause extrapyramidal reactions is contraindicated. Concomitant use of metoclopramide should be avoided in patients taking antidepressants, antipsychotics, and/or neuroleptics that have been associated with extrapyramidal reactions such as tardive dyskinesia or Neuroleptic Malignant

Syndrome (NMS) that have occurred in association with metoclopramide). Products include:
Gabitril 972

Ticarcillin Disodium (Rarely, cases of hepatotoxicity characterized by such findings as jaundice and altered liver function tests, when metoclopramide was administered with other drugs with known hepatotoxic potential). Products include:
Timentin ADD-Vantage 1670
Timentin Galaxy 1674
Timentin 1666
Timentin Pharmacy 1678

Tipranavir (Rarely, cases of hepatotoxicity characterized by such findings as jaundice and altered liver function tests, when metoclopramide was administered with other drugs with known hepatotoxic potential).
No products indexed under this heading.

Tolazamide (Rarely, cases of hepatotoxicity characterized by such findings as jaundice and altered liver function tests, when metoclopramide was administered with other drugs with known hepatotoxic potential).
No products indexed under this heading.

Tolbutamide (Rarely, cases of hepatotoxicity characterized by such findings as jaundice and altered liver function tests, when metoclopramide was administered with other drugs with known hepatotoxic potential).
No products indexed under this heading.

Tolbutamide Sodium (Rarely, cases of hepatotoxicity characterized by such findings as jaundice and altered liver function tests, when metoclopramide was administered with other drugs with known hepatotoxic potential).
No products indexed under this heading.

Tolmetin Sodium (Rarely, cases of hepatotoxicity characterized by such findings as jaundice and altered liver function tests, when metoclopramide was administered with other drugs with known hepatotoxic potential).
No products indexed under this heading.

Tolterodine Tartrate (The effects of metoclopramide on gastrointestinal motility are antagonized by anticholinergic drugs and narcotic analgesics).
No products indexed under this heading.

Topiramate (Co-administration of metoclopramide with drugs likely to cause extrapyramidal reactions is contraindicated. Concomitant use of metoclopramide should be avoided in patients taking antidepressants, antipsychotics, and/or neuroleptics that have been associated with extrapyramidal reactions such as tardive dyskinesia or Neuroleptic Malignant Syndrome (NMS) that have occurred in association with metoclopramide).
No products indexed under this heading.

Tranylcypromine Sulfate (Co-administration of metoclopramide with drugs likely to cause extrapyramidal reactions is contraindicated. Concomitant use of metoclopramide should be avoided in patients taking antidepressants, antipsychotics, and/or neuroleptics that have been associated with extrapyramidal reactions such as tardive dyskinesia or Neuroleptic Malignant Syndrome (NMS) that have occurred in association with metoclopramide). Products include:
Parnate 1584

Trazodone Hydrochloride (Co-administration of metoclopramide with drugs likely to cause extrapyramidal reactions is contraindicated. Concomitant use of metoclopramide should be avoided in patients taking antidepressants, antipsychotics, and/or neuroleptics that have been associated with extrapyramidal reactions such as tardive dyskinesia or Neuroleptic Malignant Syndrome (NMS) that have occurred in association with metoclopramide).
No products indexed under this heading.

Triazolam (Additive sedative effects can occur when metoclopramide is given with alcohol, sedatives, hypnotics, narcotics, or tranquilizers).
No products indexed under this heading.

Tridihexethyl Chloride (The effects of metoclopramide on gastrointestinal motility are antagonized by anticholinergic drugs and narcotic analgesics).
No products indexed under this heading.

Trifluoperazine Hydrochloride (Co-administration of metoclopramide with drugs likely to cause extrapyramidal reactions is contraindicated. Concomitant use of metoclopramide should be avoided in patients taking antidepressants, antipsychotics, and/or neuroleptics that have been associated with extrapyramidal reactions such as tardive dyskinesia or Neuroleptic Malignant Syndrome (NMS) that have occurred in association with metoclopramide).
No products indexed under this heading.

Trihexyphenidyl Hydrochloride (The effects of metoclopramide on gastrointestinal motility are antagonized by anticholinergic drugs and narcotic analgesics).
No products indexed under this heading.

Trimethadione (Co-administration of metoclopramide with drugs likely to cause extrapyramidal reactions is contraindicated. Concomitant use of metoclopramide should be avoided in patients taking antidepressants, antipsychotics, and/or neuroleptics that have been associated with extrapyramidal reactions such as tardive dyskinesia or Neuroleptic Malignant Syndrome (NMS) that have occurred in association with metoclopramide).
No products indexed under this heading.

Trimethoprim (Rarely, cases of hepatotoxicity characterized by such findings as jaundice and altered liver function tests, when metoclopramide was administered with other drugs with known hepatotoxic potential).
No products indexed under this heading.

Trimethoprim Hydrochloride (Rarely, cases of hepatotoxicity characterized by such findings as jaundice and altered liver function tests, when metoclopramide was administered with other drugs with known hepatotoxic potential).
No products indexed under this heading.

Trimethoprim Sulfate (Rarely, cases of hepatotoxicity characterized by such findings as jaundice and altered liver function tests, when metoclopramide was administered with other drugs with known hepatotoxic potential).
No products indexed under this heading.

Trimipramine Maleate (Co-administration of metoclopramide with drugs likely to cause extrapyramidal reactions is contraindicated. Concomitant use of metoclopramide should be avoided in patients taking antidepressants, antipsychotics, and/or neuroleptics that have been associated with extrapyramidal reactions such as tardive dyskinesia or Neuroleptic Malignant Syndrome (NMS) that have occurred in association with metoclopramide).
No products indexed under this heading.

Valdecoxib (Rarely, cases of hepatotoxicity characterized by such findings as jaundice and altered liver function tests, when metoclopramide was administered with other drugs with known hepatotoxic potential).
No products indexed under this heading.

Valproate Sodium (Co-administration of metoclopramide with drugs likely to cause extrapyramidal reactions is contraindicated. Concomitant use of metoclopramide should be avoided in patients taking antidepressants, antipsychotics, and/or neuroleptics that have been associated with extrapyramidal reactions such as tardive dyskinesia or Neuroleptic Malignant Syndrome (NMS) that have occurred in association with metoclopramide).
No products indexed under this heading.

Valproic Acid (Co-administration of metoclopramide with drugs likely to cause extrapyramidal reactions is contraindicated. Concomitant use of metoclopramide should be avoided in patients taking antidepressants, antipsychotics, and/or neuroleptics that have been associated with extrapyramidal reactions such as tardive dyskinesia or Neuroleptic Malignant Syndrome (NMS) that have occurred in association with metoclopramide).
No products indexed under this heading.

Venlafaxine Hydrochloride (Co-administration of metoclopramide with drugs likely to cause extrapyramidal reactions is contraindicated. Concomitant use of metoclopramide should be avoided in patients taking antidepressants, antipsychotics, and/or neuroleptics that have been associated with extrapyramidal reactions such as tardive dyskinesia or Neuroleptic Malignant Syndrome (NMS) that have occurred in association with metoclopramide). Products include:
Effexor XR 3504
Venlafaxine Hydrochloride Tablets ... 2388

Voriconazole (Rarely, cases of hepatotoxicity characterized by such findings as jaundice and altered liver function tests, when metoclopramide was administered with other drugs with known hepatotoxic potential).
No products indexed under this heading.

Zaleplon (Additive sedative effects can occur when metoclopramide is given with alcohol, sedatives, hypnotics, narcotics, or tranquilizers).
No products indexed under this heading.

Ziprasidone Hydrochloride (Co-administration of metoclopramide with drugs likely to cause extrapyramidal reactions is contraindicated. Concomitant use of metoclopramide should be avoided in patients taking antidepressants, antipsychotics, and/or neuroleptics that have been associated with extrapyramidal reactions such as tardive dyskinesia or Neuroleptic Malignant Syndrome (NMS) that have occurred in association with metoclopramide). Products include:
Geodon 2723

Zolpidem Tartrate (Additive sedative effects can occur when metoclopramide is given with alcohol, sedatives, hypnotics, narcotics, or tranquilizers). Products include:
Ambien 2920
Ambien CR 2925

Zonisamide (Co-administration of metoclopramide with drugs likely to cause extrapyramidal reactions is contraindicated. Concomitant use of metoclopramide should be avoided in patients taking antidepressants, antipsychotics, and/or neuroleptics that have been associated with extrapyramidal reactions such as tardive dyskinesia or Neuroleptic Malignant Syndrome (NMS) that have occurred in association with metoclopramide). Products include:
Zonegran 1081

Food Interactions

Alcohol (Additive sedative effects can occur when metoclopramide is given with alcohol, sedatives, hypnotics, narcotics, or tranquilizers).

Beer, reduced-alcohol (Additive sedative effects can occur when metoclopramide is given with alcohol, sedatives, hypnotics, narcotics, or tranquilizers).

Beer, unspecified (Additive sedative effects can occur when metoclopramide is given with alcohol, sedatives, hypnotics, narcotics, or tranquilizers).

Food, unspecified (In a food-effect study with 28 subjects, metoclopramide taken immediately after a high-fat meal had a 17% lower peak blood level than when taken after an overnight fast. The time to peak blood levels increased from about 1.75 hours under fasted conditions to 3 hours when taken immediately after a high-fat meal. The extent of metoclopramide absorbed (area under the curve) was comparable whether metoclopramide was administered with or without food. The clinical effect of the decrease in peak plasma level if metoclopramide is inadvertently taken with food is unknown).

Meal, unspecified (In a food-effect study with 28 subjects, metoclopramide taken immediately after a high-fat meal had a 17% lower peak blood level than when taken after an overnight fast. The time to peak blood levels increased from about 1.75 hours under fasted conditions to 3 hours when taken immediately after a high-fat meal. The extent of metoclopramide absorbed (area under the curve) was comparable whether metoclopramide was administered with or without food. The clinical effect of the decrease in peak plasma level if metoclopramide is inadvertently taken with food is unknown).

Wine, Chianti (Additive sedative effects can occur when metoclopramide is given with alcohol, sedatives, hypnotics, narcotics, or tranquilizers).

Wine, Red (Additive sedative effects can occur when metoclopramide is given with alcohol, sedatives, hypnotics, narcotics, or tranquilizers).

Wine, unspecified (Additive sedative effects can occur when metoclopramide is given with alcohol, sedatives, hypnotics, narcotics, or tranquilizers).

Wine products (Additive sedative effects can occur when metoclopramide is given with alcohol, sedatives, hypnotics, narcotics, or tranquilizers).

MEVACOR TABLETS

(Lovastatin) 2212
May interact with alcohols, azole antifungals, cytochrome p450 3a4 inhibitors (selected), erythromycin, fibrates, oral anticoagulants, protease inhibitors, and certain other agents. Compounds in these categories include:

Acetazolamide (The risk of myopathy/rhabdomyolysis is increased by concomitant use of lovastatin with potent inhibitors of CYP3A4, particularly with higher doses of lovastatin; concomitant use should be avoided unless the benefits of combined therapy outweigh the increased risk).
No products indexed under this heading.

Acetazolamide Sodium (The risk of myopathy/rhabdomyolysis is increased by concomitant use of lovastatin with potent inhibitors of CYP3A4, particularly with higher doses of lovastatin; concomitant use should be avoided unless the benefits of combined therapy outweigh the increased risk).
No products indexed under this heading.

IMPORTANT NOTE: Always consult each drug listing in the patient's regimen for possible interactions.

Amiodarone Hydrochloride (The combined use of lovastatin at doses higher than 40 mg daily with amiodarone should be avoided unless the clinical benefit is likely to outweigh the increased risk of myopathy).
No products indexed under this heading.

Amprenavir (The risk of myopathy/ rhabdomyolysis is increased by concomitant use of lovastatin with potent inhibitors of CYP3A4, particularly with higher doses of lovastatin; concomitant use should be avoided unless the benefits of combined therapy outweigh the increased risk).
No products indexed under this heading.

Anastrozole (The risk of myopathy/ rhabdomyolysis is increased by concomitant use of lovastatin with potent inhibitors of CYP3A4, particularly with higher doses of lovastatin; concomitant use should be avoided unless the benefits of combined therapy outweigh the increased risk).
No products indexed under this heading.

Anisindione (Co-administration has resulted in bleeding and/or increased prothrombin time in few patients).
No products indexed under this heading.

Aprepitant (The risk of myopathy/ rhabdomyolysis is increased by concomitant use of lovastatin with potent inhibitors of CYP3A4, particularly with higher doses of lovastatin; concomitant use should be avoided unless the benefits of combined therapy outweigh the increased risk). Products include:
Emend 2124

Atazanavir (The risk of myopathy/ rhabdomyolysis is increased by concomitant use of lovastatin with potent inhibitors of CYP3A4, particularly with higher doses of lovastatin; concomitant use should be avoided unless the benefits of combined therapy outweigh the increased risk).
No products indexed under this heading.

Atazanavir Sulfate (The risk of myopathy/rhabdomyolysis is increased by concomitant use of lovastatin with potent inhibitors of CYP3A4, particularly with higher doses of lovastatin; concomitant use should be avoided unless the benefits of combined therapy outweigh the increased risk).
No products indexed under this heading.

Butoconazole Nitrate (The risk of myopathy appears to be increased by high levels of HMG-CoA reductase inhibitory activity in plasma; lovastatin is metabolized by CYP3A4 isoenzyme, certain agents, such as azole antifungals, share this metabolic pathway and can raise the plasma levels of lovastatin and may increase the risk of myopathy).
No products indexed under this heading.

Cimetidine (The risk of myopathy/ rhabdomyolysis is increased by concomitant use of lovastatin with potent inhibitors of CYP3A4, particularly with higher doses of lovastatin; concomitant use should be avoided unless the benefits of combined therapy outweigh the increased risk).
No products indexed under this heading.

Cimetidine Hydrochloride (The risk of myopathy/rhabdomyolysis is increased by concomitant use of lovastatin with potent inhibitors of CYP3A4, particularly with higher doses of lovastatin; concomitant use should be avoided unless the benefits of combined therapy outweigh the increased risk).
No products indexed under this heading.

Ciprofloxacin (The risk of myopathy/ rhabdomyolysis is increased by concomitant use of lovastatin with potent inhibitors of CYP3A4, particularly with higher doses of lovastatin; concomitant

use should be avoided unless the benefits of combined therapy outweigh the increased risk). Products include:
Cipro I.V. 3082
Cipro 3073
Cipro XR 3091
Ciprodex 583

Clarithromycin (The risk of myopathy appears to be increased by high levels of HMG-CoA reductase inhibitory activity in plasma; lovastatin is metabolized by CYP3A4 isoenzyme, certain agents, such as macrolide antibiotics clarithromycin, share this metabolic pathway and can raise the plasma levels of lovastatin and may increase the risk of myopathy). Products include:
Biaxin/Biaxin XL 412

Clofibrate (The incidence and severity of myopathy are increased by co-administration of HMG-CoA reductase inhibitors with drugs that cause myopathy when given alone, such as fibrates; combined use should be avoided; if used concurrently, the dose of lovastatin should generally not exceed 20 mg).
No products indexed under this heading.

Clotrimazole (The risk of myopathy appears to be increased by high levels of HMG-CoA reductase inhibitory activity in plasma; lovastatin is metabolized by CYP3A4 isoenzyme, certain agents, such as azole antifungals, share this metabolic pathway and can raise the plasma levels of lovastatin and may increase the risk of myopathy). Products include:
Lotrisone 3163

Conivaptan Hydrochloride (The risk of myopathy/rhabdomyolysis is increased by concomitant use of lovastatin with potent inhibitors of CYP3A4, particularly with higher doses of lovastatin; concomitant use should be avoided unless the benefits of combined therapy outweigh the increased risk). Products include:
Vaprisol 689

Cyclosporine (The risk of myopathy appears to be increased by high levels of HMG-CoA reductase inhibitory activity in plasma; lovastatin is metabolized by CYP3A4 isoenzyme, certain agents, such as cyclosporine, share this metabolic pathway and can raise the plasma levels of lovastatin and may increase the risk of myopathy; the dose of lovastatin should generally not exceed 20 mg if used concomitantly). Products include:
Gengraf 440
Neoral Oral Solution 2496
Neoral Capsules 2496
Restasis 605

Dalfopristin (The risk of myopathy/ rhabdomyolysis is increased by concomitant use of lovastatin with potent inhibitors of CYP3A4, particularly with higher doses of lovastatin; concomitant use should be avoided unless the benefits of combined therapy outweigh the increased risk).
No products indexed under this heading.

Danazol (The risk of rhabdomyolysis/ myopathy is increased by concomitant administration of danazol, particularly with higher doses of lovastatin. The dose of lovastatin should not exceed 20 mg daily in patients receiving concomitant medication with danazol).
No products indexed under this heading.

Darunavir (The risk of myopathy/ rhabdomyolysis is increased by concomitant use of lovastatin with potent inhibitors of CYP3A4, particularly with higher doses of lovastatin; concomitant use should be avoided unless the benefits of combined therapy outweigh the increased risk).
No products indexed under this heading.

Dasatinib (The risk of myopathy/ rhabdomyolysis is increased by concomitant use of lovastatin with potent inhibitors of CYP3A4, particularly with higher doses of lovastatin; concomitant use should be avoided unless the benefits of combined therapy outweigh the increased risk).
No products indexed under this heading.

Delavirdine Mesylate (The risk of myopathy/rhabdomyolysis is increased by concomitant use of lovastatin with potent inhibitors of CYP3A4, particularly with higher doses of lovastatin; concomitant use should be avoided unless the benefits of combined therapy outweigh the increased risk).
No products indexed under this heading.

Delavirine (The risk of myopathy/ rhabdomyolysis is increased by concomitant use of lovastatin with potent inhibitors of CYP3A4, particularly with higher doses of lovastatin; concomitant use should be avoided unless the benefits of combined therapy outweigh the increased risk).
No products indexed under this heading.

Desloratadine (The risk of myopathy/ rhabdomyolysis is increased by concomitant use of lovastatin with potent inhibitors of CYP3A4, particularly with higher doses of lovastatin; concomitant use should be avoided unless the benefits of combined therapy outweigh the increased risk). Products include:
Clarinex Syrup 3098
Clarinex 3098
Clarinex Reditabs 3098
Clarinex-D 12-Hour 3101
Clarinex-D 3104

Dicumarol (Co-administration has resulted in bleeding and/or increased prothrombin time in few patients).
No products indexed under this heading.

Diltiazem Hydrochloride (The risk of myopathy/rhabdomyolysis is increased by concomitant use of lovastatin with potent inhibitors of CYP3A4, particularly with higher doses of lovastatin; concomitant use should be avoided unless the benefits of combined therapy outweigh the increased risk). Products include:
Cardizem LA 423

Diltiazem Maleate (The risk of myopathy/rhabdomyolysis is increased by concomitant use of lovastatin with potent inhibitors of CYP3A4, particularly with higher doses of lovastatin; concomitant use should be avoided unless the benefits of combined therapy outweigh the increased risk).
No products indexed under this heading.

Econazole Nitrate (The risk of myopathy appears to be increased by high levels of HMG-CoA reductase inhibitory activity in plasma; lovastatin is metabolized by CYP3A4 isoenzyme, certain agents, such as azole antifungals, share this metabolic pathway and can raise the plasma levels of lovastatin and may increase the risk of myopathy).
No products indexed under this heading.

Efavirenz (The risk of myopathy/ rhabdomyolysis is increased by concomitant use of lovastatin with potent inhibitors of CYP3A4, particularly with higher doses of lovastatin; concomitant use should be avoided unless the benefits of combined therapy outweigh the increased risk). Products include:
Atripla 906

Erythromycin (The risk of myopathy/ rhabdomyolysis is increased by concomitant use of lovastatin with potent inhibitors of CYP3A4, particularly with higher doses of lovastatin; concomitant use should be avoided unless the benefits of combined therapy outweigh the increased risk).
No products indexed under this heading.

Erythromycin, Topical (The risk of myopathy appears to be increased by high levels of HMG-CoA reductase inhibitory activity in plasma; lovastatin is metabolized by CYP3A4 isoenzyme, certain agents, such as macrolide antibiotics erythromycin, share this metabolic pathway and can raise the plasma levels of lovastatin and may increase the risk of myopathy).
No products indexed under this heading.

Erythromycin Estolate (The risk of myopathy/rhabdomyolysis is increased by concomitant use of lovastatin with potent inhibitors of CYP3A4, particularly with higher doses of lovastatin; concomitant use should be avoided unless the benefits of combined therapy outweigh the increased risk).
No products indexed under this heading.

Erythromycin Ethylsuccinate (The risk of myopathy/rhabdomyolysis is increased by concomitant use of lovastatin with potent inhibitors of CYP3A4, particularly with higher doses of lovastatin; concomitant use should be avoided unless the benefits of combined therapy outweigh the increased risk). Products include:
E.E.S. 437
EryPed 435

Erythromycin Gluceptate (The risk of myopathy/rhabdomyolysis is increased by concomitant use of lovastatin with potent inhibitors of CYP3A4, particularly with higher doses of lovastatin; concomitant use should be avoided unless the benefits of combined therapy outweigh the increased risk).
No products indexed under this heading.

Erythromycin Lactobionate (The risk of myopathy/rhabdomyolysis is increased by concomitant use of lovastatin with potent inhibitors of CYP3A4, particularly with higher doses of lovastatin; concomitant use should be avoided unless the benefits of combined therapy outweigh the increased risk).
No products indexed under this heading.

Erythromycin Stearate (The risk of myopathy/rhabdomyolysis is increased by concomitant use of lovastatin with potent inhibitors of CYP3A4, particularly with higher doses of lovastatin; concomitant use should be avoided unless the benefits of combined therapy outweigh the increased risk).
No products indexed under this heading.

Esomeprazole Magnesium (The risk of myopathy/rhabdomyolysis is increased by concomitant use of lovastatin with potent inhibitors of CYP3A4, particularly with higher doses of lovastatin; concomitant use should be avoided unless the benefits of combined therapy outweigh the increased risk). Products include:
Nexium Capsules 704
Nexium Oral Suspension 704

Esomeprazole Sodium (The risk of myopathy/rhabdomyolysis is increased by concomitant use of lovastatin with potent inhibitors of CYP3A4, particularly with higher doses of lovastatin; concomitant use should be avoided unless the benefits of combined therapy outweigh the increased risk). Products include:
Nexium I.V. 712

Ethanol (Lovastatin should be used with caution in patients who have consumed substantial quantity of alcohol and have a past history of liver disease; active liver disease and unexplained elevation in transaminase are contraindications to the use of lovastatin).
No products indexed under this heading.

Ethyl Alcohol (Lovastatin should be used with caution in patients who have consumed substantial quantity of alcohol and have a past history of liver disease; active liver disease and unexplained elevation in transaminase are contraindications to the use of lovastatin).

No products indexed under this heading.

Fenofibrate (The incidence and severity of myopathy are increased by co-administration of HMG-CoA reductase inhibitors with drugs that cause myopathy when given alone, such as fibrates; combined use should be avoided; if used concurrently, the dose of lovastatin should generally not exceed 20 mg). Products include:

Fluconazole (The risk of myopathy appears to be increased by high levels of HMG-CoA reductase inhibitory activity in plasma; lovastatin is metabolized by CYP3A4 isoenzyme, certain agents, such as azole antifungals, share this metabolic pathway and can raise the plasma levels of lovastatin and may increase the risk of myopathy).

No products indexed under this heading.

Fluoxetine (The risk of myopathy/rhabdomyolysis is increased by concomitant use of lovastatin with potent inhibitors of CYP3A4, particularly with higher doses of lovastatin; concomitant use should be avoided unless the benefits of combined therapy outweigh the increased risk).

No products indexed under this heading.

Fluoxetine Hydrochloride (The risk of myopathy/rhabdomyolysis is increased by concomitant use of lovastatin with potent inhibitors of CYP3A4, particularly with higher doses of lovastatin; concomitant use should be avoided unless the benefits of combined therapy outweigh the increased risk). Products include:

Fluvoxamine Maleate (The risk of myopathy/rhabdomyolysis is increased by concomitant use of lovastatin with potent inhibitors of CYP3A4, particularly with higher doses of lovastatin; concomitant use should be avoided unless the benefits of combined therapy outweigh the increased risk).

No products indexed under this heading.

Fosamprenavir Calcium (The risk of myopathy/rhabdomyolysis is increased by concomitant use of lovastatin with potent inhibitors of CYP3A4, particularly with higher doses of lovastatin; concomitant use should be avoided unless the benefits of combined therapy outweigh the increased risk). Products include:

Gemfibrozil (The incidence and severity of myopathy are increased by co-administration of HMG-CoA reductase inhibitors with drugs that cause myopathy when given alone, such as fibrates; combined use should be avoided; if used concurrently, the dose of lovastatin should generally not exceed 20 mg).

No products indexed under this heading.

Imatinib Mesylate (The risk of myopathy/rhabdomyolysis is increased by concomitant use of lovastatin with potent inhibitors of CYP3A4, particularly with higher doses of lovastatin; concomitant use should be avoided unless the benefits of combined therapy outweigh the increased risk). Products include:

Indinavir Sulfate (The risk of myopathy/rhabdomyolysis is increased by concomitant use of lovastatin with potent inhibitors of CYP3A4, particularly with higher doses of lovastatin; concomitant use should be avoided unless the benefits of combined therapy outweigh the increased risk). Products include:

Isoniazid (The risk of myopathy/rhabdomyolysis is increased by concomitant use of lovastatin with potent inhibitors of CYP3A4, particularly with higher doses of lovastatin; concomitant use should be avoided unless the benefits of combined therapy outweigh the increased risk).

No products indexed under this heading.

Itraconazole (The risk of myopathy appears to be increased by high levels of HMG-CoA reductase inhibitory activity in plasma; lovastatin is metabolized by CYP3A4 isoenzyme, certain agents, such as itraconazole, share this metabolic pathway and can raise the plasma levels of lovastatin and may increase the risk of myopathy).

No products indexed under this heading.

Ketoconazole (The risk of myopathy appears to be increased by high levels of HMG-CoA reductase inhibitory activity in plasma; lovastatin is metabolized by CYP3A4 isoenzyme, certain agents, such as ketoconazole, share this metabolic pathway and can raise the plasma levels of lovastatin and may increase the risk of myopathy). Products include:

Lapatinib (The risk of myopathy/rhabdomyolysis is increased by concomitant use of lovastatin with potent inhibitors of CYP3A4, particularly with higher doses of lovastatin; concomitant use should be avoided unless the benefits of combined therapy outweigh the increased risk). Products include:

Lopinavir (The risk of myopathy/rhabdomyolysis is increased by concomitant use of lovastatin with potent inhibitors of CYP3A4, particularly with higher doses of lovastatin; concomitant use should be avoided unless the benefits of combined therapy outweigh the increased risk). Products include:

Loratadine (The risk of myopathy/rhabdomyolysis is increased by concomitant use of lovastatin with potent inhibitors of CYP3A4, particularly with higher doses of lovastatin; concomitant use should be avoided unless the benefits of combined therapy outweigh the increased risk).

No products indexed under this heading.

Metronidazole (The risk of myopathy/rhabdomyolysis is increased by concomitant use of lovastatin with potent inhibitors of CYP3A4, particularly with higher doses of lovastatin; concomitant use should be avoided unless the benefits of combined therapy outweigh the increased risk). Products include:

Metronidazole Benzoate (The risk of myopathy/rhabdomyolysis is increased by concomitant use of lovastatin with potent inhibitors of CYP3A4, particularly with higher doses of lovastatin; concomitant use should be avoided unless the benefits of combined therapy outweigh the increased risk).

No products indexed under this heading.

Metronidazole Hydrochloride (The risk of myopathy/rhabdomyolysis is increased by concomitant use of lovastatin with potent inhibitors of CYP3A4, particularly with higher doses of lovastatin; concomitant use should be avoided unless the benefits of combined therapy outweigh the increased risk).

No products indexed under this heading.

Metronidazole Sodium (The risk of myopathy/rhabdomyolysis is increased by concomitant use of lovastatin with potent inhibitors of CYP3A4, particularly with higher doses of lovastatin; concomitant use should be avoided unless the benefits of combined therapy outweigh the increased risk).

No products indexed under this heading.

Miconazole (The risk of myopathy appears to be increased by high levels of HMG-CoA reductase inhibitory activity in plasma; lovastatin is metabolized by CYP3A4 isoenzyme, certain agents, such as azole antifungals, share this metabolic pathway and can raise the plasma levels of lovastatin and may increase the risk of myopathy).

No products indexed under this heading.

Miconazole Nitrate (The risk of myopathy/rhabdomyolysis is increased by concomitant use of lovastatin with potent inhibitors of CYP3A4, particularly with higher doses of lovastatin; concomitant use should be avoided unless the benefits of combined therapy outweigh the increased risk). Products include:

Mifepristone (The risk of myopathy/rhabdomyolysis is increased by concomitant use of lovastatin with potent inhibitors of CYP3A4, particularly with higher doses of lovastatin; concomitant use should be avoided unless the benefits of combined therapy outweigh the increased risk).

No products indexed under this heading.

Nefazodone Hydrochloride (The risk of myopathy appears to be increased by high levels of HMG-CoA reductase inhibitory activity in plasma; lovastatin is metabolized by CYP3A4 isoenzyme, certain agents, such as antidepressant nefazodone, share this metabolic pathway and can raise the plasma levels of lovastatin and may increase the risk of myopathy).

No products indexed under this heading.

Nelfinavir Mesylate (The risk of myopathy/rhabdomyolysis is increased by concomitant use of lovastatin with potent inhibitors of CYP3A4, particularly with higher doses of lovastatin; concomitant use should be avoided unless the benefits of combined therapy outweigh the increased risk).

No products indexed under this heading.

Nevirapine (The risk of myopathy/rhabdomyolysis is increased by concomitant use of lovastatin with potent inhibitors of CYP3A4, particularly with higher doses of lovastatin; concomitant use should be avoided unless the benefits of combined therapy outweigh the increased risk). Products include:

Niacin (The incidence and severity of myopathy are increased by co-administration of HMG-CoA reductase inhibitors with drugs that cause myopathy when given alone, such as lipid-lowering doses of niacin; combined use should be avoided; if used concurrently, the dose of lovastatin should generally not exceed 20 mg). Products include:

Niacinamide (The risk of myopathy/rhabdomyolysis is increased by concomitant use of lovastatin with potent inhibitors of CYP3A4, particularly with higher doses of lovastatin; concomitant use should be avoided unless the benefits of combined therapy outweigh the increased risk). Products include:

Niacinamide Hydroiodide (The risk of myopathy/rhabdomyolysis is increased by concomitant use of lovastatin with potent inhibitors of CYP3A4, particularly with higher doses of lovastatin; concomitant use should be avoided unless the benefits of combined therapy outweigh the increased risk).

No products indexed under this heading.

Nicotinamide (The risk of myopathy/rhabdomyolysis is increased by concomitant use of lovastatin with potent inhibitors of CYP3A4, particularly with higher doses of lovastatin; concomitant use should be avoided unless the benefits of combined therapy outweigh the increased risk).

No products indexed under this heading.

Nifedipine (The risk of myopathy/rhabdomyolysis is increased by concomitant use of lovastatin with potent inhibitors of CYP3A4, particularly with higher doses of lovastatin; concomitant use should be avoided unless the benefits of combined therapy outweigh the increased risk).

No products indexed under this heading.

Norfloxacin (The risk of myopathy/rhabdomyolysis is increased by concomitant use of lovastatin with potent inhibitors of CYP3A4, particularly with higher doses of lovastatin; concomitant use should be avoided unless the benefits of combined therapy outweigh the increased risk). Products include:

Omeprazole (The risk of myopathy/rhabdomyolysis is increased by concomitant use of lovastatin with potent inhibitors of CYP3A4, particularly with higher doses of lovastatin; concomitant use should be avoided unless the benefits of combined therapy outweigh the increased risk).

No products indexed under this heading.

Oxiconazole Nitrate (The risk of myopathy appears to be increased by high levels of HMG-CoA reductase inhibitory activity in plasma; lovastatin is metabolized by CYP3A4 isoenzyme, certain agents, such as azole antifungals, share this metabolic pathway and can raise the plasma levels of lovastatin and may increase the risk of myopathy).

No products indexed under this heading.

Paroxetine Hydrochloride (The risk of myopathy/rhabdomyolysis is increased by concomitant use of lovastatin with potent inhibitors of CYP3A4, particularly with higher doses of lovastatin; concomitant use should be avoided unless the benefits of combined therapy outweigh the increased risk). Products include:

Posaconazole (The risk of myopathy appears to be increased by high levels of HMG-CoA reductase inhibitory activity in plasma; lovastatin is metabolized by CYP3A4 isoenzyme, certain agents, such as azole antifungals, share this metabolic pathway and can raise the plasma levels of lovastatin and may increase the risk of myopathy). Products include:

IMPORTANT NOTE: Always consult each drug listing in the patient's regimen for possible interactions.

Propoxyphene Hydrochloride (The risk of myopathy/rhabdomyolysis is increased by concomitant use of lovastatin with potent inhibitors of CYP3A4, particularly with higher doses of lovastatin; concomitant use should be avoided unless the benefits of combined therapy outweigh the increased risk).
No products indexed under this heading.

Propoxyphene Napsylate (The risk of myopathy/rhabdomyolysis is increased by concomitant use of lovastatin with potent inhibitors of CYP3A4, particularly with higher doses of lovastatin; concomitant use should be avoided unless the benefits of combined therapy outweigh the increased risk).
No products indexed under this heading.

Quinidine (The risk of myopathy/rhabdomyolysis is increased by concomitant use of lovastatin with potent inhibitors of CYP3A4, particularly with higher doses of lovastatin; concomitant use should be avoided unless the benefits of combined therapy outweigh the increased risk).
No products indexed under this heading.

Quinidine Hydrochloride (The risk of myopathy/rhabdomyolysis is increased by concomitant use of lovastatin with potent inhibitors of CYP3A4, particularly with higher doses of lovastatin; concomitant use should be avoided unless the benefits of combined therapy outweigh the increased risk).
No products indexed under this heading.

Quinidine Polygalacturonate (The risk of myopathy/rhabdomyolysis is increased by concomitant use of lovastatin with potent inhibitors of CYP3A4, particularly with higher doses of lovastatin; concomitant use should be avoided unless the benefits of combined therapy outweigh the increased risk).
No products indexed under this heading.

Quinidine Sulfate (The risk of myopathy/rhabdomyolysis is increased by concomitant use of lovastatin with potent inhibitors of CYP3A4, particularly with higher doses of lovastatin; concomitant use should be avoided unless the benefits of combined therapy outweigh the increased risk).
No products indexed under this heading.

Quinine (The risk of myopathy/rhabdomyolysis is increased by concomitant use of lovastatin with potent inhibitors of CYP3A4, particularly with higher doses of lovastatin; concomitant use should be avoided unless the benefits of combined therapy outweigh the increased risk). Products include:
Hyland's Leg Cramps PM with Quinine 3315

Quinine Sulfate (The risk of myopathy/rhabdomyolysis is increased by concomitant use of lovastatin with potent inhibitors of CYP3A4, particularly with higher doses of lovastatin; concomitant use should be avoided unless the benefits of combined therapy outweigh the increased risk).
No products indexed under this heading.

Quinupristin (The risk of myopathy/rhabdomyolysis is increased by concomitant use of lovastatin with potent inhibitors of CYP3A4, particularly with higher doses of lovastatin; concomitant use should be avoided unless the benefits of combined therapy outweigh the increased risk).
No products indexed under this heading.

Ranitidine Bismuth Citrate (The risk of myopathy/rhabdomyolysis is increased by concomitant use of lovastatin with potent inhibitors of CYP3A4, particularly with higher doses of lovastatin; concomitant use should be avoided unless the benefits of combined therapy outweigh the increased risk).
No products indexed under this heading.

Ranitidine Hydrochloride (The risk of myopathy/rhabdomyolysis is increased by concomitant use of lovastatin with potent inhibitors of CYP3A4, particularly with higher doses of lovastatin; concomitant use should be avoided unless the benefits of combined therapy outweigh the increased risk). Products include:
Zantac 1737
Zantac Injection 1732
Zantac Pharmacy 1735

Ritonavir (The risk of myopathy/rhabdomyolysis is increased by concomitant use of lovastatin with potent inhibitors of CYP3A4, particularly with higher doses of lovastatin; concomitant use should be avoided unless the benefits of combined therapy outweigh the increased risk). Products include:
Kaletra 458
Norvir 509

Saquinavir (The risk of myopathy/rhabdomyolysis is increased by concomitant use of lovastatin with potent inhibitors of CYP3A4, particularly with higher doses of lovastatin; concomitant use should be avoided unless the benefits of combined therapy outweigh the increased risk).
No products indexed under this heading.

Saquinavir Mesylate (The risk of myopathy/rhabdomyolysis is increased by concomitant use of lovastatin with potent inhibitors of CYP3A4, particularly with higher doses of lovastatin; concomitant use should be avoided unless the benefits of combined therapy outweigh the increased risk).
No products indexed under this heading.

Sertaconazole Nitrate (The risk of myopathy appears to be increased by high levels of HMG-CoA reductase inhibitory activity in plasma; lovastatin is metabolized by CYP3A4 isoenzyme, certain agents, such as azole antifungals, share this metabolic pathway and can raise the plasma levels of lovastatin and may increase the risk of myopathy).
No products indexed under this heading.

Sertraline Hydrochloride (The risk of myopathy/rhabdomyolysis is increased by concomitant use of lovastatin with potent inhibitors of CYP3A4, particularly with higher doses of lovastatin; concomitant use should be avoided unless the benefits of combined therapy outweigh the increased risk).
No products indexed under this heading.

Sildenafil Citrate (The risk of myopathy/rhabdomyolysis is increased by concomitant use of lovastatin with potent inhibitors of CYP3A4, particularly with higher doses of lovastatin; concomitant use should be avoided unless the benefits of combined therapy outweigh the increased risk).
No products indexed under this heading.

Telithromycin (The risk of myopathy appears to be increased by high levels of HMG-CoA reductase inhibitory activity in plasma; lovastatin is metabolized by CYP3A4 isoenzyme, certain agents, such as macrolide antibiotics telithromycin, share this metabolic pathway and can raise the plasma levels of lovastatin and may increase the risk of myopathy). Products include:
Ketek 2991

Terconazole (The risk of myopathy appears to be increased by high levels of HMG-CoA reductase inhibitory activity in plasma; lovastatin is metabolized by CYP3A4 isoenzyme, certain agents, such as azole antifungals, share this metabolic pathway and can raise the plasma levels of lovastatin and may increase the risk of myopathy).
No products indexed under this heading.

Tipranavir (The risk of myopathy/rhabdomyolysis is increased by concomitant use of lovastatin with potent inhibitors of CYP3A4, particularly with higher doses of lovastatin; concomitant use should be avoided unless the benefits of combined therapy outweigh the increased risk).
No products indexed under this heading.

Troglitazone (The risk of myopathy/rhabdomyolysis is increased by concomitant use of lovastatin with potent inhibitors of CYP3A4, particularly with higher doses of lovastatin; concomitant use should be avoided unless the benefits of combined therapy outweigh the increased risk).
No products indexed under this heading.

Troleandomycin (The risk of myopathy/rhabdomyolysis is increased by concomitant use of lovastatin with potent inhibitors of CYP3A4, particularly with higher doses of lovastatin; concomitant use should be avoided unless the benefits of combined therapy outweigh the increased risk).
No products indexed under this heading.

Valproate Sodium (The risk of myopathy/rhabdomyolysis is increased by concomitant use of lovastatin with potent inhibitors of CYP3A4, particularly with higher doses of lovastatin; concomitant use should be avoided unless the benefits of combined therapy outweigh the increased risk).
No products indexed under this heading.

Vardenafil Hydrochloride (The risk of myopathy/rhabdomyolysis is increased by concomitant use of lovastatin with potent inhibitors of CYP3A4, particularly with higher doses of lovastatin; concomitant use should be avoided unless the benefits of combined therapy outweigh the increased risk). Products include:
Levitra 3157

Verapamil Hydrochloride (The combined use of lovastatin at doses higher than 40 mg daily with verapamil should be avoided unless the clinical benefit is likely to outweigh the increased risk of myopathy). Products include:
Tarka 534

Voriconazole (The risk of myopathy appears to be increased by high levels of HMG-CoA reductase inhibitory activity in plasma; lovastatin is metabolized by CYP3A4 isoenzyme, certain agents, such as azole antifungals, share this metabolic pathway and can raise the plasma levels of lovastatin and may increase the risk of myopathy).
No products indexed under this heading.

Warfarin Sodium (Co-administration has resulted in bleeding and/or increased prothrombin time in few patients).
No products indexed under this heading.

Zafirlukast (The risk of myopathy/rhabdomyolysis is increased by concomitant use of lovastatin with potent inhibitors of CYP3A4, particularly with higher doses of lovastatin; concomitant use should be avoided unless the benefits of combined therapy outweigh the increased risk). Products include:
Accolate 3612

Zileuton (The risk of myopathy/rhabdomyolysis is increased by concomitant use of lovastatin with potent inhibitors of CYP3A4, particularly with higher doses of lovastatin; concomitant use should be avoided unless the benefits of combined therapy outweigh the increased risk).
No products indexed under this heading.

Food Interactions

Alcohol (Lovastatin should be used with caution in patients who have consumed substantial quantity of alcohol and have a past history of liver disease; active liver disease and unexplained elevation in transaminase are contraindications to the use of lovastatin).

Beer, reduced-alcohol (Lovastatin should be used with caution in patients who have consumed substantial quantity of alcohol and have a past history of liver disease; active liver disease and unexplained elevation in transaminase are contraindications to the use of lovastatin).

Beer, unspecified (Lovastatin should be used with caution in patients who have consumed substantial quantity of alcohol and have a past history of liver disease; active liver disease and unexplained elevation in transaminase are contraindications to the use of lovastatin).

Grapefruit (The risk of myopathy/rhabdomyolysis is increased by concomitant use of lovastatin with potent inhibitors of CYP3A4, particularly with higher doses of lovastatin; concomitant use should be avoided unless the benefits of combined therapy outweigh the increased risk).

Grapefruit Juice (The risk of myopathy/rhabdomyolysis is increased by concomitant use of lovastatin with potent inhibitors of CYP3A4, particularly with higher doses of lovastatin; concomitant use should be avoided unless the benefits of combined therapy outweigh the increased risk).

Meal, unspecified (When lovastatin was given under fasting conditions, plasma concentrations of total inhibitors were on average about two-thirds those found when lovastatin was administered immediately after a standard meal).

Wine, Chianti (Lovastatin should be used with caution in patients who have consumed substantial quantity of alcohol and have a past history of liver disease; active liver disease and unexplained elevation in transaminase are contraindications to the use of lovastatin).

Wine, Red (Lovastatin should be used with caution in patients who have consumed substantial quantity of alcohol and have a past history of liver disease; active liver disease and unexplained elevation in transaminase are contraindications to the use of lovastatin).

Wine, unspecified (Lovastatin should be used with caution in patients who have consumed substantial quantity of alcohol and have a past history of liver disease; active liver disease and unexplained elevation in transaminase are contraindications to the use of lovastatin).

Wine products (Lovastatin should be used with caution in patients who have consumed substantial quantity of alcohol and have a past history of liver disease; active liver disease and unexplained elevation in transaminase are contraindications to the use of lovastatin).

MICARDIS TABLETS

(Telmisartan) 887

1129 Interactions Index Micardis

May interact with ACE inhibitors, cytochrome p450 2c19 substrates (selected), and certain other agents. Compounds in these categories include:

Amitriptyline Hydrochloride (Telmisartan is not metabolized by the cytochrome P450 system and had no effects *in vitro* on cytochrome P450 enzymes, except for some inhibition of CYP2C19).
No products indexed under this heading.

Amoxapine (Telmisartan is not metabolized by the cytochrome P450 system and had no effects *in vitro* on cytochrome P450 enzymes, except for some inhibition of CYP2C19).
No products indexed under this heading.

Benazepril Hydrochloride (As a consequence of inhibiting the renin-angiotensin-aldosterone system, changes in renal function (including acute renal failure) have been reported. Dual blockade of the renin-angiotensin aldosterone system (eg, by adding an ACE-inhibitor to an angiotensin II receptor antagonist) should be used with caution and should include close monitoring of renal function).
No products indexed under this heading.

Captopril (As a consequence of inhibiting the renin-angiotensin-aldosterone system, changes in renal function (including acute renal failure) have been reported. Dual blockade of the renin-angiotensin aldosterone system (eg, by adding an ACE-inhibitor to an angiotensin II receptor antagonist) should be used with caution and should include close monitoring of renal function).
Products include:
Captopril **2341**

Carisoprodol (Telmisartan is not metabolized by the cytochrome P450 system and had no effects *in vitro* on cytochrome P450 enzymes, except for some inhibition of CYP2C19).
No products indexed under this heading.

Cilostazol (Telmisartan is not metabolized by the cytochrome P450 system and had no effects *in vitro* on cytochrome P450 enzymes, except for some inhibition of CYP2C19).
No products indexed under this heading.

Citalopram Hydrobromide (Telmisartan is not metabolized by the cytochrome P450 system and had no effects *in vitro* on cytochrome P450 enzymes, except for some inhibition of CYP2C19). Products include:
Celexa **1153**

Clomipramine Hydrochloride (Telmisartan is not metabolized by the cytochrome P450 system and had no effects *in vitro* on cytochrome P450 enzymes, except for some inhibition of CYP2C19).
No products indexed under this heading.

Cyclophosphamide (Telmisartan is not metabolized by the cytochrome P450 system and had no effects *in vitro* on cytochrome P450 enzymes, except for some inhibition of CYP2C19).
No products indexed under this heading.

Desipramine Hydrochloride (Telmisartan is not metabolized by the cytochrome P450 system and had no effects *in vitro* on cytochrome P450 enzymes, except for some inhibition of CYP2C19).
No products indexed under this heading.

Dextromethorphan (Telmisartan is not metabolized by the cytochrome P450 system and had no effects *in vitro* on cytochrome P450 enzymes, except for some inhibition of CYP2C19).
No products indexed under this heading.

Dextromethorphan Hydrobromide (Telmisartan is not metabolized by the cytochrome P450 system and had no effects *in vitro* on cytochrome P450 enzymes, except for some inhibition of CYP2C19).
No products indexed under this heading.

Diazepam (Telmisartan is not metabolized by the cytochrome P450 system and had no effects *in vitro* on cytochrome P450 enzymes, except for some inhibition of CYP2C19). Products include:
Valium Tablets **2880**

Digoxin (When telmisartan was co-administered with digoxin, median increases in digoxin peak plasma concentration (49%) and in trough concentration (20%) were observed. It is, therefore, recommended that digoxin levels be monitored when initiating, adjusting, and discontinuing telmisartan to avoid possible over- or under-digitalization).
Products include:
Lanoxin Injection **1546**
Lanoxin Injection Pediatric **1549**
Lanoxin Tablets **1553**

Divalproex Sodium (Telmisartan is not metabolized by the cytochrome P450 system and had no effects *in vitro* on cytochrome P450 enzymes, except for some inhibition of CYP2C19).
Products include:
Depakote ER **426**

Doxepin Hydrochloride (Telmisartan is not metabolized by the cytochrome P450 system and had no effects *in vitro* on cytochrome P450 enzymes, except for some inhibition of CYP2C19).
No products indexed under this heading.

Enalapril Maleate (As a consequence of inhibiting the renin-angiotensin-aldosterone system, changes in renal function (including acute renal failure) have been reported. Dual blockade of the renin-angiotensin aldosterone system (eg, by adding an ACE-inhibitor to an angiotensin II receptor antagonist) should be used with caution and should include close monitoring of renal function).
No products indexed under this heading.

Enalaprilat (As a consequence of inhibiting the renin-angiotensin-aldosterone system, changes in renal function (including acute renal failure) have been reported. Dual blockade of the renin-angiotensin aldosterone system (eg, by adding an ACE-inhibitor to an angiotensin II receptor antagonist) should be used with caution and should include close monitoring of renal function).
No products indexed under this heading.

Esomeprazole Magnesium (Telmisartan is not metabolized by the cytochrome P450 system and had no effects *in vitro* on cytochrome P450 enzymes, except for some inhibition of CYP2C19). Products include:
Nexium Capsules **704**
Nexium Oral Suspension **704**

Esomeprazole Sodium (Telmisartan is not metabolized by the cytochrome P450 system and had no effects *in vitro* on cytochrome P450 enzymes, except for some inhibition of CYP2C19).
Products include:
Nexium I.V. **712**

Ethosuximide (Telmisartan is not metabolized by the cytochrome P450 system and had no effects *in vitro* on cytochrome P450 enzymes, except for some inhibition of CYP2C19).
No products indexed under this heading.

Ethotoin (Telmisartan is not metabolized by the cytochrome P450 system and had no effects *in vitro* on cytochrome P450 enzymes, except for some inhibition of CYP2C19).
No products indexed under this heading.

Felbamate (Telmisartan is not metabolized by the cytochrome P450 system and had no effects *in vitro* on cytochrome P450 enzymes, except for some inhibition of CYP2C19).
No products indexed under this heading.

Formoterol Fumarate (Telmisartan is not metabolized by the cytochrome P450 system and had no effects *in vitro* on cytochrome P450 enzymes, except for some inhibition of CYP2C19).
Products include:
Foradil **3121**
Perforomist **3634**

Fosinopril Sodium (As a consequence of inhibiting the renin-angiotensin-aldosterone system, changes in renal function (including acute renal failure) have been reported. Dual blockade of the renin-angiotensin aldosterone system (eg, by adding an ACE-inhibitor to an angiotensin II receptor antagonist) should be used with caution and should include close monitoring of renal function).
No products indexed under this heading.

Fosphenytoin (Telmisartan is not metabolized by the cytochrome P450 system and had no effects *in vitro* on cytochrome P450 enzymes, except for some inhibition of CYP2C19).
No products indexed under this heading.

Fosphenytoin Sodium (Telmisartan is not metabolized by the cytochrome P450 system and had no effects *in vitro* on cytochrome P450 enzymes, except for some inhibition of CYP2C19).
No products indexed under this heading.

Gabapentin (Telmisartan is not metabolized by the cytochrome P450 system and had no effects *in vitro* on cytochrome P450 enzymes, except for some inhibition of CYP2C19).
No products indexed under this heading.

Imipramine Hydrochloride (Telmisartan is not metabolized by the cytochrome P450 system and had no effects *in vitro* on cytochrome P450 enzymes, except for some inhibition of CYP2C19).
No products indexed under this heading.

Imipramine Pamoate (Telmisartan is not metabolized by the cytochrome P450 system and had no effects *in vitro* on cytochrome P450 enzymes, except for some inhibition of CYP2C19).
No products indexed under this heading.

Indomethacin (Telmisartan is not metabolized by the cytochrome P450 system and had no effects *in vitro* on cytochrome P450 enzymes, except for some inhibition of CYP2C19). Products include:
Indocin **2167**

Indomethacin Sodium Trihydrate (Telmisartan is not metabolized by the cytochrome P450 system and had no effects *in vitro* on cytochrome P450 enzymes, except for some inhibition of CYP2C19). Products include:
Indocin I.V. **2007**

Lamotrigine (Telmisartan is not metabolized by the cytochrome P450 system and had no effects *in vitro* on cytochrome P450 enzymes, except for some inhibition of CYP2C19). Products include:
Lamictal **1522**
Lamictal ODT **1522**
Lamictal XR **1536**

Lansoprazole (Telmisartan is not metabolized by the cytochrome P450 system and had no effects *in vitro* on cytochrome P450 enzymes, except for some inhibition of CYP2C19).
No products indexed under this heading.

Levetiracetam (Telmisartan is not metabolized by the cytochrome P450 system and had no effects *in vitro* on cytochrome P450 enzymes, except for some inhibition of CYP2C19). Products include:
Keppra XR **3434**

Lisinopril (As a consequence of inhibiting the renin-angiotensin-aldosterone system, changes in renal function (including acute renal failure) have been reported. Dual blockade of the renin-angiotensin aldosterone system (eg, by adding an ACE-inhibitor to an angiotensin II receptor antagonist) should be used with caution and should include close monitoring of renal function).
Products include:
Prinivil **2241**
Prinzide **2246**

Maprotiline Hydrochloride (Telmisartan is not metabolized by the cytochrome P450 system and had no effects *in vitro* on cytochrome P450 enzymes, except for some inhibition of CYP2C19).
No products indexed under this heading.

Mephenytoin (Telmisartan is not metabolized by the cytochrome P450 system and had no effects *in vitro* on cytochrome P450 enzymes, except for some inhibition of CYP2C19).
No products indexed under this heading.

Mephobarbital (Telmisartan is not metabolized by the cytochrome P450 system and had no effects *in vitro* on cytochrome P450 enzymes, except for some inhibition of CYP2C19).
No products indexed under this heading.

Meprobamate (Telmisartan is not metabolized by the cytochrome P450 system and had no effects *in vitro* on cytochrome P450 enzymes, except for some inhibition of CYP2C19).
No products indexed under this heading.

Methsuximide (Telmisartan is not metabolized by the cytochrome P450 system and had no effects *in vitro* on cytochrome P450 enzymes, except for some inhibition of CYP2C19).
No products indexed under this heading.

Midazolam Hydrochloride (Telmisartan is not metabolized by the cytochrome P450 system and had no effects *in vitro* on cytochrome P450 enzymes, except for some inhibition of CYP2C19).
No products indexed under this heading.

Moexipril Hydrochloride (As a consequence of inhibiting the renin-angiotensin-aldosterone system, changes in renal function (including acute renal failure) have been reported. Dual blockade of the renin-angiotensin aldosterone system (eg, by adding an ACE-inhibitor to an angiotensin II receptor antagonist) should be used with caution and should include close monitoring of renal function).
No products indexed under this heading.

Nelfinavir Mesylate (Telmisartan is not metabolized by the cytochrome P450 system and had no effects *in vitro* on cytochrome P450 enzymes, except for some inhibition of CYP2C19).
No products indexed under this heading.

Nilutamide (Telmisartan is not metabolized by the cytochrome P450 system and had no effects *in vitro* on cytochrome P450 enzymes, except for some inhibition of CYP2C19).
No products indexed under this heading.

Nortriptyline Hydrochloride (Telmisartan is not metabolized by the cytochrome P450 system and had no effects *in vitro* on cytochrome P450 enzymes, except for some inhibition of CYP2C19).
No products indexed under this heading.

IMPORTANT NOTE: Always consult each drug listing in the patient's regimen for possible interactions.

Omeprazole (Telmisartan is not metabolized by the cytochrome P450 system and had no effects *in vitro* on cytochrome P450 enzymes, except for some inhibition of CYP2C19).
No products indexed under this heading.

Omeprazole Magnesium (Telmisartan is not metabolized by the cytochrome P450 system and had no effects *in vitro* on cytochrome P450 enzymes, except for some inhibition of CYP2C19).
No products indexed under this heading.

Oxcarbazepine (Telmisartan is not metabolized by the cytochrome P450 system and had no effects *in vitro* on cytochrome P450 enzymes, except for some inhibition of CYP2C19).
No products indexed under this heading.

Pantoprazole Sodium (Telmisartan is not metabolized by the cytochrome P450 system and had no effects *in vitro* on cytochrome P450 enzymes, except for some inhibition of CYP2C19). Products include:
Protonix Tablets 3571
Protonix 3575

Paramethadione (Telmisartan is not metabolized by the cytochrome P450 system and had no effects *in vitro* on cytochrome P450 enzymes, except for some inhibition of CYP2C19).
No products indexed under this heading.

Pentamidine Isethionate (Telmisartan is not metabolized by the cytochrome P450 system and had no effects *in vitro* on cytochrome P450 enzymes, except for some inhibition of CYP2C19).
No products indexed under this heading.

Perindopril Erbumine (As a consequence of inhibiting the renin-angiotensin-aldosterone system, changes in renal function (including acute renal failure) have been reported. Dual blockade of the renin-angiotensin aldosterone system (eg, by adding an ACE-inhibitor to an angiotensin II receptor antagonist) should be used with caution and should include close monitoring of renal function).
No products indexed under this heading.

Phenacemide (Telmisartan is not metabolized by the cytochrome P450 system and had no effects *in vitro* on cytochrome P450 enzymes, except for some inhibition of CYP2C19).
No products indexed under this heading.

Phenobarbital (Telmisartan is not metabolized by the cytochrome P450 system and had no effects *in vitro* on cytochrome P450 enzymes, except for some inhibition of CYP2C19). Products include:
Donnatal 2711

Phenobarbital Sodium (Telmisartan is not metabolized by the cytochrome P450 system and had no effects *in vitro* on cytochrome P450 enzymes, except for some inhibition of CYP2C19).
No products indexed under this heading.

Phensuximide (Telmisartan is not metabolized by the cytochrome P450 system and had no effects *in vitro* on cytochrome P450 enzymes, except for some inhibition of CYP2C19).
No products indexed under this heading.

Phenytoin (Telmisartan is not metabolized by the cytochrome P450 system and had no effects *in vitro* on cytochrome P450 enzymes, except for some inhibition of CYP2C19).
No products indexed under this heading.

Phenytoin Sodium (Telmisartan is not metabolized by the cytochrome P450 system and had no effects *in vitro* on cytochrome P450 enzymes, except for some inhibition of CYP2C19). Products include:
Phenytek Capsules 2380

Primidone (Telmisartan is not metabolized by the cytochrome P450 system and had no effects *in vitro* on cytochrome P450 enzymes, except for some inhibition of CYP2C19).
No products indexed under this heading.

Progesterone (Telmisartan is not metabolized by the cytochrome P450 system and had no effects *in vitro* on cytochrome P450 enzymes, except for some inhibition of CYP2C19). Products include:
Crinone 4% 996
Crinone 8% 996
Prometrium 3307

Proguanil Hydrochloride (Telmisartan is not metabolized by the cytochrome P450 system and had no effects *in vitro* on cytochrome P450 enzymes, except for some inhibition of CYP2C19). Products include:
Malarone Pediatric Tablets 1572
Malarone 1572

Propranolol Hydrochloride (Telmisartan is not metabolized by the cytochrome P450 system and had no effects *in vitro* on cytochrome P450 enzymes, except for some inhibition of CYP2C19). Products include:
InnoPran XL 1517

Protriptyline Hydrochloride (Telmisartan is not metabolized by the cytochrome P450 system and had no effects *in vitro* on cytochrome P450 enzymes, except for some inhibition of CYP2C19).
No products indexed under this heading.

Quinapril Hydrochloride (As a consequence of inhibiting the renin-angiotensin-aldosterone system, changes in renal function (including acute renal failure) have been reported. Dual blockade of the renin-angiotensin aldosterone system (eg, by adding an ACE-inhibitor to an angiotensin II receptor antagonist) should be used with caution and should include close monitoring of renal function).
No products indexed under this heading.

Rabeprazole Sodium (Telmisartan is not metabolized by the cytochrome P450 system and had no effects *in vitro* on cytochrome P450 enzymes, except for some inhibition of CYP2C19). Products include:
Aciphex 1035

Ramipril (As a consequence of inhibiting the renin-angiotensin-aldosterone system, changes in renal function (including acute renal failure) have been reported. Dual blockade of the renin-angiotensin aldosterone system (eg, by adding an ACE-inhibitor to an angiotensin II receptor antagonist) should be used with caution and should include close monitoring of renal function).
No products indexed under this heading.

Sertraline Hydrochloride (Telmisartan is not metabolized by the cytochrome P450 system and had no effects *in vitro* on cytochrome P450 enzymes, except for some inhibition of CYP2C19).
No products indexed under this heading.

Spirapril Hydrochloride (As a consequence of inhibiting the renin-angiotensin-aldosterone system, changes in renal function (including acute renal failure) have been reported. Dual blockade of the renin-angiotensin aldosterone system (eg, by adding an ACE-inhibitor to an angiotensin II receptor antagonist) should be used with caution and should include close monitoring of renal function).
No products indexed under this heading.

Teniposide (Telmisartan is not metabolized by the cytochrome P450 system and had no effects *in vitro* on cytochrome P450 enzymes, except for some inhibition of CYP2C19).
No products indexed under this heading.

Thioridazine (Telmisartan is not metabolized by the cytochrome P450 system and had no effects *in vitro* on cytochrome P450 enzymes, except for some inhibition of CYP2C19).
No products indexed under this heading.

Thioridazine Hydrochloride (Telmisartan is not metabolized by the cytochrome P450 system and had no effects *in vitro* on cytochrome P450 enzymes, except for some inhibition of CYP2C19). Products include:
Thioridazine Hydrochloride 2384

Tiagabine Hydrochloride (Telmisartan is not metabolized by the cytochrome P450 system and had no effects *in vitro* on cytochrome P450 enzymes, except for some inhibition of CYP2C19). Products include:
Gabitril 972

Tolbutamide (Telmisartan is not metabolized by the cytochrome P450 system and had no effects *in vitro* on cytochrome P450 enzymes, except for some inhibition of CYP2C19).
No products indexed under this heading.

Tolbutamide Sodium (Telmisartan is not metabolized by the cytochrome P450 system and had no effects *in vitro* on cytochrome P450 enzymes, except for some inhibition of CYP2C19).
No products indexed under this heading.

Topiramate (Telmisartan is not metabolized by the cytochrome P450 system and had no effects *in vitro* on cytochrome P450 enzymes, except for some inhibition of CYP2C19).
No products indexed under this heading.

Trandolapril (As a consequence of inhibiting the renin-angiotensin-aldosterone system, changes in renal function (including acute renal failure) have been reported. Dual blockade of the renin-angiotensin aldosterone system (eg, by adding an ACE-inhibitor to an angiotensin II receptor antagonist) should be used with caution and should include close monitoring of renal function). Products include:
Mavik 489
Tarka 534

Trimethadione (Telmisartan is not metabolized by the cytochrome P450 system and had no effects *in vitro* on cytochrome P450 enzymes, except for some inhibition of CYP2C19).
No products indexed under this heading.

Trimipramine Maleate (Telmisartan is not metabolized by the cytochrome P450 system and had no effects *in vitro* on cytochrome P450 enzymes, except for some inhibition of CYP2C19).
No products indexed under this heading.

Valproate Sodium (Telmisartan is not metabolized by the cytochrome P450 system and had no effects *in vitro* on cytochrome P450 enzymes, except for some inhibition of CYP2C19).
No products indexed under this heading.

Valproic Acid (Telmisartan is not metabolized by the cytochrome P450 system and had no effects *in vitro* on cytochrome P450 enzymes, except for some inhibition of CYP2C19).
No products indexed under this heading.

Voriconazole (Telmisartan is not metabolized by the cytochrome P450 system and had no effects *in vitro* on cytochrome P450 enzymes, except for some inhibition of CYP2C19).
No products indexed under this heading.

Warfarin Sodium (Telmisartan administered for 10 days slightly decreased the mean warfarin trough plasma concentration; this decrease did not result in a change in International Normalized Ratio (INR).
No products indexed under this heading.

Zonisamide (Telmisartan is not metabolized by the cytochrome P450 system

and had no effects *in vitro* on cytochrome P450 enzymes, except for some inhibition of CYP2C19). Products include:
Zonegran 1081

Food Interactions

Food, unspecified (Food slightly reduces the bioavailability of telmisartan, with a reduction in the area under the plasma concentration-time curve (AUC) of about 6% with the 40 mg tablet and about 20% after a 160 mg dose. The absolute bioavailability of telmisartan is dose dependent. At 40 and 160 mg the bioavailability was 42% and 58%, respectively).

Meal, unspecified (Food slightly reduces the bioavailability of telmisartan, with a reduction in the area under the plasma concentration-time curve (AUC) of about 6% with the 40 mg tablet and about 20% after a 160 mg dose. The absolute bioavailability of telmisartan is dose dependent. At 40 and 160 mg the bioavailability was 42% and 58%, respectively).

MICARDIS HCT TABLETS

(Hydrochlorothiazide, Telmisartan) **889**
May interact with ACE inhibitors, alcohols, antihypertensives, barbiturates, cardiac glycosides, corticosteroids, cytochrome p450 2c19 substrates (selected), insulin, lithium preparations, narcotic analgesics, non-steroidal anti-inflammatory agents, nondepolarizing neuromuscular blocking agents, oral hypoglycemic agents, potassium preparations, vasopressors, and certain other agents. Compounds in these categories include:

Acarbose (Concurrent administration of hydrochlorothiazides with oral hypoglycemic agents in diabetic patients may require dosage adjustments of oral hypoglycemic agents).
No products indexed under this heading.

Acebutolol Hydrochloride (Thiazides may add to or potentiate the action of other antihypertensive drugs; this may be enhanced in the post-sympathectomy patient. Hypotension, including orthostatic hypotension, may also be aggravated by antihypertensive drugs).
No products indexed under this heading.

ACTH (ACTH, when administered concurrently with thiazide diuretics, intensifies electrolyte depletion, particularly hypokalemia).
No products indexed under this heading.

Alclometasone Dipropionate (Corticosteroids, when administered concurrently with thiazide diuretics, intensify electrolyte depletion, particularly hypokalemia).
No products indexed under this heading.

Alfentanil Hydrochloride (Potentiation of orthostatic hypotension may occur with concurrent administration of narcotics).
No products indexed under this heading.

Aliskiren (Thiazides may add to or potentiate the action of other antihypertensive drugs; this may be enhanced in the post-sympathectomy patient. Hypotension, including orthostatic hypotension, may also be aggravated by antihypertensive drugs). Products include:
Tekturna 2538
Tekturna HCT 2541
Valturna 3637

Amitriptyline Hydrochloride (Telmisartan is not metabolized by the cytochrome P450 system and had no effects *in vitro* on cytochrome P450 enzymes, except for some inhibition of CYP2C19).
No products indexed under this heading.

Amlodipine Besylate (Thiazides may add to or potentiate the action of other

antihypertensive drugs; this may be enhanced in the post-sympathectomy patient. Hypotension, including orthostatic hypotension, may also be aggravated by antihypertensive drugs). Products include:

Azor **1010**
Exforge **2443**
Exforge HCT **2449**

Amobarbital (Potentiation of orthostatic hypotension may occur with concurrent administration of barbiturates).
No products indexed under this heading.

Amobarbital Sodium (Potentiation of orthostatic hypotension may occur with concurrent administration of barbiturates).
No products indexed under this heading.

Amoxapine (Telmisartan is not metabolized by the cytochrome P450 system and had no effects *in vitro* on cytochrome P450 enzymes, except for some inhibition of CYP2C19).
No products indexed under this heading.

Apomorphine (Potentiation of orthostatic hypotension may occur with concurrent administration of narcotics).
No products indexed under this heading.

Apomorphine Hydrochloride (Potentiation of orthostatic hypotension may occur with concurrent administration of narcotics).
No products indexed under this heading.

Aprobarbital (Potentiation of orthostatic hypotension may occur with concurrent administration of barbiturates).
No products indexed under this heading.

Atenolol (Thiazides may add to or potentiate the action of other antihypertensive drugs; this may be enhanced in the post-sympathectomy patient. Hypotension, including orthostatic hypotension, may also be aggravated by antihypertensive drugs).
No products indexed under this heading.

Atracurium Besylate (Concurrent administration of non-depolarizing skeletal muscle relaxants (eg, tubocurarine) with hydrochlorothiazide may cause possible increased responsiveness to the muscle relaxant).
No products indexed under this heading.

Beclomethasone Dipropionate (Corticosteroids, when administered concurrently with thiazide diuretics, intensify electrolyte depletion, particularly hypokalemia). Products include:

Qvar **3398**

Beclomethasone Dipropionate Monohydrate (Corticosteroids, when administered concurrently with thiazide diuretics, intensify electrolyte depletion, particularly hypokalemia). Products include:

Beconase AQ **1386**

Benazepril Hydrochloride (As a consequence of inhibiting the renin-angiotensin-aldosterone system, changes in renal function (including acute renal failure) have been reported. Dual blockade of the renin-angiotensin-aldosterone system (eg, by adding an ACE-inhibitor to an angiotensin II receptor antagonist) should be used with caution and should include close monitoring of renal function).
No products indexed under this heading.

Bendroflumethiazide (Thiazides may add to or potentiate the action of other antihypertensive drugs; this may be enhanced in the post-sympathectomy patient. Hypotension, including orthostatic hypotension, may also be aggravated by antihypertensive drugs).
No products indexed under this heading.

Betamethasone (Corticosteroids, when administered concurrently with thiazide diuretics, intensify electrolyte depletion, particularly hypokalemia).
No products indexed under this heading.

Betamethasone Acetate (Corticosteroids, when administered concurrently with thiazide diuretics, intensify electrolyte depletion, particularly hypokalemia).
No products indexed under this heading.

Betamethasone Benzoate (Corticosteroids, when administered concurrently with thiazide diuretics, intensify electrolyte depletion, particularly hypokalemia).
No products indexed under this heading.

Betamethasone Dipropionate (Corticosteroids, when administered concurrently with thiazide diuretics, intensify electrolyte depletion, particularly hypokalemia). Products include:

Diprolene Lotion 0.05% **3108**
Diprolene Ointment 0.05% **3109**
Diprolene AF Cream 0.05% **3107**
Lotrisone **3163**

Betamethasone Sodium Phosphate (Corticosteroids, when administered concurrently with thiazide diuretics, intensify electrolyte depletion, particularly hypokalemia).
No products indexed under this heading.

Betamethasone Valerate (Corticosteroids, when administered concurrently with thiazide diuretics, intensify electrolyte depletion, particularly hypokalemia). Products include:

Luxíq **3321**

Betaxolol Hydrochloride (Thiazides may add to or potentiate the action of other antihypertensive drugs; this may be enhanced in the post-sympathectomy patient. Hypotension, including orthostatic hypotension, may also be aggravated by antihypertensive drugs).
No products indexed under this heading.

Bisoprolol Fumarate (Thiazides may add to or potentiate the action of other antihypertensive drugs; this may be enhanced in the post-sympathectomy patient. Hypotension, including orthostatic hypotension, may also be aggravated by antihypertensive drugs).
No products indexed under this heading.

Budesonide (Corticosteroids, when administered concurrently with thiazide diuretics, intensify electrolyte depletion, particularly hypokalemia). Products include:

Pulmicort Flexhaler **714**
Symbicort 80/4.5 .... **720**
Symbicort 160/4.5 .... **720**

Buprenorphine Hydrochloride (Potentiation of orthostatic hypotension may occur with concurrent administration of narcotics).
No products indexed under this heading.

Butabarbital (Potentiation of orthostatic hypotension may occur with concurrent administration of barbiturates).
No products indexed under this heading.

Butabarbital Sodium (Potentiation of orthostatic hypotension may occur with concurrent administration of barbiturates).
No products indexed under this heading.

Butalbital (Potentiation of orthostatic hypotension may occur with concurrent administration of barbiturates).
No products indexed under this heading.

Candesartan Cilexetil (Thiazides may add to or potentiate the action of other antihypertensive drugs; this may be enhanced in the post-sympathectomy patient. Hypotension, including orthostatic hypotension, may also be aggravated by antihypertensive drugs). Products include:

Atacand **697**
Atacand HCT **700**

Captopril (As a consequence of inhibiting the renin-angiotensin-aldosterone system, changes in renal function (including acute renal failure) have been reported. Dual blockade of the renin-angiotensin-aldosterone system (eg, by adding an ACE-inhibitor to an angiotensin II receptor antagonist) should be used with caution and should include close monitoring of renal function). Products include:

Captopril **2341**

Carisoprodol (Telmisartan is not metabolized by the cytochrome P450 system and had no effects *in vitro* on cytochrome P450 enzymes, except for some inhibition of CYP2C19).
No products indexed under this heading.

Carteolol Hydrochloride (Thiazides may add to or potentiate the action of other antihypertensive drugs; this may be enhanced in the post-sympathectomy patient. Hypotension, including orthostatic hypotension, may also be aggravated by antihypertensive drugs).
No products indexed under this heading.

Carvedilol (Thiazides may add to or potentiate the action of other antihypertensive drugs; this may be enhanced in the post-sympathectomy patient. Hypotension, including orthostatic hypotension, may also be aggravated by antihypertensive drugs). Products include:

Coreg **1409**

Carvedilol Phosphate (Thiazides may add to or potentiate the action of other antihypertensive drugs; this may be enhanced in the post-sympathectomy patient. Hypotension, including orthostatic hypotension, may also be aggravated by antihypertensive drugs). Products include:

Coreg CR **1416**

Celecoxib (In some patients, the administration of a non-steroidal anti-inflammatory agent can reduce the diuretic, natriuretic, and antihypertensive effects of loop, potassium-sparing and thiazide diuretics. Therefore, when hydrochlorothiazide and non-steroidal anti-inflammatory agents are used concomitantly, the patient should be observed closely to determine if the desired effect of the diuretic is obtained). Products include:

Celebrex **3272**

Chlorothiazide (Thiazides may add to or potentiate the action of other antihypertensive drugs; this may be enhanced in the post-sympathectomy patient. Hypotension, including orthostatic hypotension, may also be aggravated by antihypertensive drugs).
No products indexed under this heading.

Chlorothiazide Sodium (Thiazides may add to or potentiate the action of other antihypertensive drugs; this may be enhanced in the post-sympathectomy patient. Hypotension, including orthostatic hypotension, may also be aggravated by antihypertensive drugs). Products include:

Diuril Intravenous **2009**

Chlorpropamide (Concurrent administration of hydrochlorothiazides with oral hypoglycemic agents in diabetic patients may require dosage adjustments of oral hypoglycemic agents).
No products indexed under this heading.

Chlorthalidone (Thiazides may add to or potentiate the action of other antihypertensive drugs; this may be enhanced in the post-sympathectomy patient. Hypotension, including orthostatic hypotension, may also be aggravated by antihypertensive drugs). Products include:

Clorpres **2344**

Cholestyramine (Absorption of hydrochlorothiazide is impaired in the presence of anionic exchange resins. Single dose of cholestyramine bind the hydrochlorothiazide and reduce its absorption from the gastrointestinal tract by up to 85%).
No products indexed under this heading.

Ciclesonide (Corticosteroids, when administered concurrently with thiazide diuretics, intensify electrolyte depletion, particularly hypokalemia).
No products indexed under this heading.

Cilostazol (Telmisartan is not metabolized by the cytochrome P450 system and had no effects *in vitro* on cytochrome P450 enzymes, except for some inhibition of CYP2C19).
No products indexed under this heading.

Cisatracurium Besylate (Concurrent administration of non-depolarizing skeletal muscle relaxants (eg, tubocurarine) with hydrochlorothiazide may cause possible increased responsiveness to the muscle relaxant). Products include:

Nimbex **503**

Citalopram Hydrobromide (Telmisartan is not metabolized by the cytochrome P450 system and had no effects *in vitro* on cytochrome P450 enzymes, except for some inhibition of CYP2C19). Products include:

Celexa **1153**

Clomipramine Hydrochloride (Telmisartan is not metabolized by the cytochrome P450 system and had no effects *in vitro* on cytochrome P450 enzymes, except for some inhibition of CYP2C19).
No products indexed under this heading.

Clonidine (Thiazides may add to or potentiate the action of other antihypertensive drugs; this may be enhanced in the post-sympathectomy patient. Hypotension, including orthostatic hypotension, may also be aggravated by antihypertensive drugs). Products include:

Catapres-TTS **884**

Clonidine Hydrochloride (Thiazides may add to or potentiate the action of other antihypertensive drugs; this may be enhanced in the post-sympathectomy patient. Hypotension, including orthostatic hypotension, may also be aggravated by antihypertensive drugs). Products include:

Clorpres **2344**

Codeine Phosphate (Potentiation of orthostatic hypotension may occur with concurrent administration of narcotics). Products include:

Tylenol with Codeine **2691**

Codeine Sulfate (Potentiation of orthostatic hypotension may occur with concurrent administration of narcotics).
No products indexed under this heading.

Colestipol (Absorption of hydrochlorothiazide is impaired in the presence of anionic exchange resins. Single dose of colestipol resins bind the hydrochlorothiazide and reduce its absorption from the gastrointestinal tract by up to 43%).
No products indexed under this heading.

Colestipol Hydrochloride (Absorption of hydrochlorothiazide is impaired in the presence of anionic exchange resins. Single dose of colestipol resins bind the hydrochlorothiazide and reduce its absorption from the gastrointestinal tract by up to 43%).
No products indexed under this heading.

Cortisone Acetate (Corticosteroids, when administered concurrently with thiazide diuretics, intensify electrolyte depletion, particularly hypokalemia).
No products indexed under this heading.

IMPORTANT NOTE: Always consult each drug listing in the patient's regimen for possible interactions.

Cyclophosphamide (Telmisartan is not metabolized by the cytochrome P450 system and had no effects in vitro on cytochrome P450 enzymes, except for some inhibition of CYP2C19).
   No products indexed under this heading.

Deserpidine (Thiazides may add to or potentiate the action of other antihypertensive drugs; this may be enhanced in the post-sympathectomy patient. Hypotension, including orthostatic hypotension, may also be aggravated by antihypertensive drugs).
   No products indexed under this heading.

Desipramine Hydrochloride (Telmisartan is not metabolized by the cytochrome P450 system and had no effects in vitro on cytochrome P450 enzymes, except for some inhibition of CYP2C19).
   No products indexed under this heading.

Deslanoside (Hypokalemia may cause cardiac arrhythmia and may also sensitize or exaggerate the response of the heart to the toxic effects of digitalis (eg, increased ventricular irritability)).
   No products indexed under this heading.

Desoximetasone (Corticosteroids, when administered concurrently with thiazide diuretics, intensify electrolyte depletion, particularly hypokalemia).
   No products indexed under this heading.

Dexamethasone (Corticosteroids, when administered concurrently with thiazide diuretics, intensify electrolyte depletion, particularly hypokalemia).
Products include:

Ciprodex	583
Ozurdex	⊙223
Tobramycin and Dexamethasone Ophthalmic Suspension	⊙251

Dexamethasone Acetate (Corticosteroids, when administered concurrently with thiazide diuretics, intensify electrolyte depletion, particularly hypokalemia).
   No products indexed under this heading.

Dexamethasone Phosphate (Corticosteroids, when administered concurrently with thiazide diuretics, intensify electrolyte depletion, particularly hypokalemia).
   No products indexed under this heading.

Dexamethasone Sodium (Corticosteroids, when administered concurrently with thiazide diuretics, intensify electrolyte depletion, particularly hypokalemia).
   No products indexed under this heading.

Dexamethasone Sodium Phosphate (Corticosteroids, when administered concurrently with thiazide diuretics, intensify electrolyte depletion, particularly hypokalemia).
   No products indexed under this heading.

Dexamethasone Sodium Phosphate Injection (Corticosteroids, when administered concurrently with thiazide diuretics, intensify electrolyte depletion, particularly hypokalemia).
   No products indexed under this heading.

Dextromethorphan (Telmisartan is not metabolized by the cytochrome P450 system and had no effects in vitro on cytochrome P450 enzymes, except for some inhibition of CYP2C19).
   No products indexed under this heading.

Dextromethorphan Hydrobromide (Telmisartan is not metabolized by the cytochrome P450 system and had no effects in vitro on cytochrome P450 enzymes, except for some inhibition of CYP2C19).
   No products indexed under this heading.

Dezocine (Potentiation of orthostatic hypotension may occur with concurrent administration of narcotics).
   No products indexed under this heading.

Diazepam (Telmisartan is not metabolized by the cytochrome P450 system and had no effects in vitro on cytochrome P450 enzymes, except for some inhibition of CYP2C19). Products include:

Valium Tablets	2880

Diazoxide (Thiazides may add to or potentiate the action of other antihypertensive drugs; this may be enhanced in the post-sympathectomy patient. Hypotension, including orthostatic hypotension, may also be aggravated by antihypertensive drugs). Products include:

Proglycem	1179
Proglycem Suspension	1179

Diclofenac Epolamine (In some patients, the administration of a non-steroidal anti-inflammatory agent can reduce the diuretic, natriuretic, and antihypertensive effects of loop, potassium-sparing and thiazide diuretics. Therefore, when hydrochlorothiazide and non-steroidal anti-inflammatory agents are used concomitantly, the patient should be observed closely to determine if the desired effect of the diuretic is obtained). Products include:

Flector	1839

Diclofenac Potassium (In some patients, the administration of a non-steroidal anti-inflammatory agent can reduce the diuretic, natriuretic, and antihypertensive effects of loop, potassium-sparing and thiazide diuretics. Therefore, when hydrochlorothiazide and non-steroidal anti-inflammatory agents are used concomitantly, the patient should be observed closely to determine if the desired effect of the diuretic is obtained).
   No products indexed under this heading.

Diclofenac Sodium (In some patients, the administration of a non-steroidal anti-inflammatory agent can reduce the diuretic, natriuretic, and antihypertensive effects of loop, potassium-sparing and thiazide diuretics. Therefore, when hydrochlorothiazide and non-steroidal anti-inflammatory agents are used concomitantly, the patient should be observed closely to determine if the desired effect of the diuretic is obtained).
   No products indexed under this heading.

Diflorasone Diacetate (Corticosteroids, when administered concurrently with thiazide diuretics, intensify electrolyte depletion, particularly hypokalemia).
   No products indexed under this heading.

Digitalis Glycoside Preparations (Hypokalemia may cause cardiac arrhythmia and may also sensitize or exaggerate the response of the heart to the toxic effects of digitalis (eg, increased ventricular irritability)).
   No products indexed under this heading.

Digitalis Lanata (Hypokalemia may cause cardiac arrhythmia and may also sensitize or exaggerate the response of the heart to the toxic effects of digitalis (eg, increased ventricular irritability)).
   No products indexed under this heading.

Digitalis Purpurea (Hypokalemia may cause cardiac arrhythmia and may also sensitize or exaggerate the response of the heart to the toxic effects of digitalis (eg, increased ventricular irritability)).
   No products indexed under this heading.

Digitoxin (Hypokalemia may cause cardiac arrhythmia and may also sensitize or exaggerate the response of the heart to the toxic effects of digitalis (eg, increased ventricular irritability)).
   No products indexed under this heading.

Digoxin (When telmisartan was co-administered with digoxin, median increases in digoxin peak plasma concentration (49%) and in trough concentration (20%) were observed. It is, therefore, recommended that digoxin levels be monitored when initiating, adjusting, and discontinuing telmisartan to avoid possible over- or under-digitalization). Products include:

Lanoxin Injection	1546
Lanoxin Injection Pediatric	1549
Lanoxin Tablets	1553

Dihydrocodeine Bitartrate (Potentiation of orthostatic hypotension may occur with concurrent administration of narcotics).
   No products indexed under this heading.

Dihydrocodeinone Bitartrate (Potentiation of orthostatic hypotension may occur with concurrent administration of narcotics).
   No products indexed under this heading.

Diltiazem Hydrochloride (Thiazides may add to or potentiate the action of other antihypertensive drugs; this may be enhanced in the post-sympathectomy patient. Hypotension, including orthostatic hypotension, may also be aggravated by antihypertensive drugs). Products include:

Cardizem LA	423

Diltiazem Maleate (Thiazides may add to or potentiate the action of other antihypertensive drugs; this may be enhanced in the post-sympathectomy patient. Hypotension, including orthostatic hypotension, may also be aggravated by antihypertensive drugs).
   No products indexed under this heading.

Divalproex Sodium (Telmisartan is not metabolized by the cytochrome P450 system and had no effects in vitro on cytochrome P450 enzymes, except for some inhibition of CYP2C19). Products include:

Depakote ER	426

Dobutamine (Concurrent administration of pressor amines with hydrochlorothiazides may cause possible decreased response to pressor amines but not sufficient to preclude their use).
   No products indexed under this heading.

Dobutamine Hydrochloride (Concurrent administration of pressor amines with hydrochlorothiazides may cause possible decreased response to pressor amines but not sufficient to preclude their use).
   No products indexed under this heading.

Dopamine Hydrochloride (Concurrent administration of pressor amines with hydrochlorothiazides may cause possible decreased response to pressor amines but not sufficient to preclude their use).
   No products indexed under this heading.

Doxacurium Chloride (Concurrent administration of non-depolarizing skeletal muscle relaxants (eg, tubocurarine) with hydrochlorothiazide may cause possible increased responsiveness to the muscle relaxant).
   No products indexed under this heading.

Doxazosin Mesylate (Thiazides may add to or potentiate the action of other antihypertensive drugs; this may be enhanced in the post-sympathectomy patient. Hypotension, including orthostatic hypotension, may also be aggravated by antihypertensive drugs).
   No products indexed under this heading.

Doxepin Hydrochloride (Telmisartan is not metabolized by the cytochrome P450 system and had no effects in vitro on cytochrome P450 enzymes, except for some inhibition of CYP2C19).
   No products indexed under this heading.

d-Tubocurarine (Concurrent administration of non-depolarizing skeletal muscle relaxants (eg, tubocurarine) with hydrochlorothiazide may cause possible increased responsiveness to the muscle relaxant).
   No products indexed under this heading.

Enalapril Maleate (As a consequence of inhibiting the renin-angiotensin-aldosterone system, changes in renal function (including acute renal failure) have been reported. Dual blockade of the renin-angiotensin-aldosterone system (eg, by adding an ACE-inhibitor to an angiotensin II receptor antagonist) should be used with caution and should include close monitoring of renal function).
   No products indexed under this heading.

Enalaprilat (As a consequence of inhibiting the renin-angiotensin-aldosterone system, changes in renal function (including acute renal failure) have been reported. Dual blockade of the renin-angiotensin-aldosterone system (eg, by adding an ACE-inhibitor to an angiotensin II receptor antagonist) should be used with caution and should include close monitoring of renal function).
   No products indexed under this heading.

Ephedrine Sulfate (Concurrent administration of pressor amines with hydrochlorothiazides may cause possible decreased response to pressor amines but not sufficient to preclude their use).
   No products indexed under this heading.

Epinephrine Bitartrate (Concurrent administration of pressor amines with hydrochlorothiazides may cause possible decreased response to pressor amines but not sufficient to preclude their use).
   No products indexed under this heading.

Epinephrine Hydrochloride (Concurrent administration of pressor amines with hydrochlorothiazides may cause possible decreased response to pressor amines but not sufficient to preclude their use).
   No products indexed under this heading.

Eprosartan Mesylate (Thiazides may add to or potentiate the action of other antihypertensive drugs; this may be enhanced in the post-sympathectomy patient. Hypotension, including orthostatic hypotension, may also be aggravated by antihypertensive drugs). Products include:

Teveten	538
Teveten HCT	541

Esmolol Hydrochloride (Thiazides may add to or potentiate the action of other antihypertensive drugs; this may be enhanced in the post-sympathectomy patient. Hypotension, including orthostatic hypotension, may also be aggravated by antihypertensive drugs).
   No products indexed under this heading.

Esomeprazole Magnesium (Telmisartan is not metabolized by the cytochrome P450 system and had no effects in vitro on cytochrome P450 enzymes, except for some inhibition of CYP2C19). Products include:

Nexium Capsules	704
Nexium Oral Suspension	704

Esomeprazole Sodium (Telmisartan is not metabolized by the cytochrome P450 system and had no effects in vitro on cytochrome P450 enzymes, except for some inhibition of CYP2C19). Products include:

Nexium I.V.	712

Ethanol (Potentiation of orthostatic hypotension may occur with alcohol, barbiturates, or narcotics when administered concurrently with thiazide diuretics).
   No products indexed under this heading.

Ethosuximide (Telmisartan is not metabolized by the cytochrome P450 system and had no effects in vitro on cytochrome P450 enzymes, except for some inhibition of CYP2C19).
   No products indexed under this heading.

1133 Interactions Index Micardis HCT

Ethotoin (Telmisartan is not metabolized by the cytochrome P450 system and had no effects *in vitro* on cytochrome P450 enzymes, except for some inhibition of CYP2C19).
No products indexed under this heading.

Ethyl Alcohol (Potentiation of orthostatic hypotension may occur with alcohol, barbiturates, or narcotics when administered concurrently with thiazide diuretics).
No products indexed under this heading.

Etodolac (In some patients, the administration of a non-steroidal anti-inflammatory agent can reduce the diuretic, natriuretic, and antihypertensive effects of loop, potassium-sparing and thiazide diuretics. Therefore, when hydrochlorothiazide and non-steroidal anti-inflammatory agents are used concomitantly, the patient should be observed closely to determine if the desired effect of the diuretic is obtained).
No products indexed under this heading.

Felbamate (Telmisartan is not metabolized by the cytochrome P450 system and had no effects *in vitro* on cytochrome P450 enzymes, except for some inhibition of CYP2C19).
No products indexed under this heading.

Felodipine (Thiazides may add to or potentiate the action of other antihypertensive drugs; this may be enhanced in the post-sympathectomy patient. Hypotension, including orthostatic hypotension, may also be aggravated by antihypertensive drugs).
No products indexed under this heading.

Fenoprofen Calcium (In some patients, the administration of a non-steroidal anti-inflammatory agent can reduce the diuretic, natriuretic, and antihypertensive effects of loop, potassium-sparing and thiazide diuretics. Therefore, when hydrochlorothiazide and non-steroidal anti-inflammatory agents are used concomitantly, the patient should be observed closely to determine if the desired effect of the diuretic is obtained).
No products indexed under this heading.

Fentanyl (Potentiation of orthostatic hypotension may occur with concurrent administration of narcotics). Products include:
Duragesic 2604
Fentanyl Transdermal System 2346
Onsolis 2054

Fentanyl Citrate (Potentiation of orthostatic hypotension may occur with concurrent administration of narcotics). Products include:
Fentora 966

Fludrocortisone Acetate (Corticosteroids, when administered concurrently with thiazide diuretics, intensify electrolyte depletion, particularly hypokalemia).
No products indexed under this heading.

Flumethasone Pivalate (Corticosteroids, when administered concurrently with thiazide diuretics, intensify electrolyte depletion, particularly hypokalemia).
No products indexed under this heading.

Flunisolide Hemihydrate (Corticosteroids, when administered concurrently with thiazide diuretics, intensify electrolyte depletion, particularly hypokalemia).
No products indexed under this heading.

Flurbiprofen (In some patients, the administration of a non-steroidal anti-inflammatory agent can reduce the diuretic, natriuretic, and antihypertensive effects of loop, potassium-sparing and thiazide diuretics. Therefore, when hydrochlorothiazide and non-steroidal anti-inflammatory agents are used concomitantly, the patient should be observed closely to determine if the desired effect of the diuretic is obtained).
No products indexed under this heading.

Fluticasone Furoate (Corticosteroids, when administered concurrently with thiazide diuretics, intensify electrolyte depletion, particularly hypokalemia). Products include:
Veramyst 1713

Fluticasone Propionate (Corticosteroids, when administered concurrently with thiazide diuretics, intensify electrolyte depletion, particularly hypokalemia). Products include:
Advair 100/50 1275
Advair 250/50 1275
Advair 500/50 1275
Advair HFA 45/21 1288
Advair HFA 115/21 1288
Advair HFA 230/21 1288
Flonase 1459
Flovent Diskus 1463
Flovent HFA 1470

Formoterol Fumarate (Telmisartan is not metabolized by the cytochrome P450 system and had no effects *in vitro* on cytochrome P450 enzymes, except for some inhibition of CYP2C19). Products include:
Foradil 3121
Perforomist 3634

Fosinopril Sodium (As a consequence of inhibiting the renin-angiotensin-aldosterone system, changes in renal function (including acute renal failure) have been reported. Dual blockade of the renin-angiotensin-aldosterone system (eg, by adding an ACE-inhibitor to an angiotensin II receptor antagonist) should be used with caution and should include close monitoring of renal function).
No products indexed under this heading.

Fosphenytoin (Telmisartan is not metabolized by the cytochrome P450 system and had no effects *in vitro* on cytochrome P450 enzymes, except for some inhibition of CYP2C19).
No products indexed under this heading.

Fosphenytoin Sodium (Telmisartan is not metabolized by the cytochrome P450 system and had no effects *in vitro* on cytochrome P450 enzymes, except for some inhibition of CYP2C19).
No products indexed under this heading.

Furosemide (Thiazides may add to or potentiate the action of other antihypertensive drugs; this may be enhanced in the post-sympathectomy patient. Hypotension, including orthostatic hypotension, may also be aggravated by antihypertensive drugs). Products include:
Furosemide 2354

Gabapentin (Telmisartan is not metabolized by the cytochrome P450 system and had no effects *in vitro* on cytochrome P450 enzymes, except for some inhibition of CYP2C19).
No products indexed under this heading.

Gallamine (Concurrent administration of non-depolarizing skeletal muscle relaxants (eg, tubocurarine) with hydrochlorothiazide may cause possible increased responsiveness to the muscle relaxant).
No products indexed under this heading.

Gallamine Triethiodide (Concurrent administration of non-depolarizing skeletal muscle relaxants (eg, tubocurarine) with hydrochlorothiazide may cause possible increased responsiveness to the muscle relaxant).
No products indexed under this heading.

Glibenclamide (Concurrent administration of hydrochlorothiazides with oral hypoglycemic agents in diabetic patients may require dosage adjustments of oral hypoglycemic agents).
No products indexed under this heading.

Glimepiride (Concurrent administration of hydrochlorothiazides with oral hypoglycemic agents in diabetic patients may require dosage adjustments of oral hypoglycemic agents). Products include:
Avandaryl 1356
Duetact 3354

Glipizide (Concurrent administration of hydrochlorothiazides with oral hypoglycemic agents in diabetic patients may require dosage adjustments of oral hypoglycemic agents).
No products indexed under this heading.

Glyburide (Concurrent administration of hydrochlorothiazides with oral hypoglycemic agents in diabetic patients may require dosage adjustments of oral hypoglycemic agents).
No products indexed under this heading.

Guanabenz Acetate (Thiazides may add to or potentiate the action of other antihypertensive drugs; this may be enhanced in the post-sympathectomy patient. Hypotension, including orthostatic hypotension, may also be aggravated by antihypertensive drugs).
No products indexed under this heading.

Guanethidine (Thiazides may add to or potentiate the action of other antihypertensive drugs; this may be enhanced in the post-sympathectomy patient. Hypotension, including orthostatic hypotension, may also be aggravated by antihypertensive drugs).
No products indexed under this heading.

Guanethidine Monosulfate (Thiazides may add to or potentiate the action of other antihypertensive drugs; this may be enhanced in the post-sympathectomy patient. Hypotension, including orthostatic hypotension, may also be aggravated by antihypertensive drugs).
No products indexed under this heading.

Guanethidine Sulfate (Thiazides may add to or potentiate the action of other antihypertensive drugs; this may be enhanced in the post-sympathectomy patient. Hypotension, including orthostatic hypotension, may also be aggravated by antihypertensive drugs).
No products indexed under this heading.

Hexobarbital (Potentiation of orthostatic hypotension may occur with concurrent administration of barbiturates).
No products indexed under this heading.

Hydralazine Hydrochloride (Thiazides may add to or potentiate the action of other antihypertensive drugs; this may be enhanced in the post-sympathectomy patient. Hypotension, including orthostatic hypotension, may also be aggravated by antihypertensive drugs).
No products indexed under this heading.

Hydrocodone Bitartrate (Potentiation of orthostatic hypotension may occur with concurrent administration of narcotics). Products include:
Vicodin 560
Vicodin ES 561
Vicodin HP 563
Vicoprofen 564
Zydone 1138

Hydrocodone Polistirex (Potentiation of orthostatic hypotension may occur with concurrent administration of narcotics). Products include:
Tussionex 3443

Hydrocortisone (Corticosteroids, when administered concurrently with thiazide diuretics, intensify electrolyte depletion, particularly hypokalemia).
No products indexed under this heading.

Hydrocortisone (Alcohol) (Corticosteroids, when administered concurrently with thiazide diuretics, intensify electrolyte depletion, particularly hypokalemia).
No products indexed under this heading.

Hydrocortisone Acetate (Corticosteroids, when administered concurrently with thiazide diuretics, intensify electrolyte depletion, particularly hypokalemia).
No products indexed under this heading.

Hydrocortisone Butyrate (Corticosteroids, when administered concurrently with thiazide diuretics, intensify electrolyte depletion, particularly hypokalemia).
No products indexed under this heading.

Hydrocortisone Cypionate (Corticosteroids, when administered concurrently with thiazide diuretics, intensify electrolyte depletion, particularly hypokalemia).
No products indexed under this heading.

Hydrocortisone Hemisuccinate (Corticosteroids, when administered concurrently with thiazide diuretics, intensify electrolyte depletion, particularly hypokalemia).
No products indexed under this heading.

Hydrocortisone Probutate (Corticosteroids, when administered concurrently with thiazide diuretics, intensify electrolyte depletion, particularly hypokalemia).
No products indexed under this heading.

Hydrocortisone Sodium Phosphate (Corticosteroids, when administered concurrently with thiazide diuretics, intensify electrolyte depletion, particularly hypokalemia).
No products indexed under this heading.

Hydrocortisone Sodium Succinate (Corticosteroids, when administered concurrently with thiazide diuretics, intensify electrolyte depletion, particularly hypokalemia).
No products indexed under this heading.

Hydrocortisone Valerate (Corticosteroids, when administered concurrently with thiazide diuretics, intensify electrolyte depletion, particularly hypokalemia).
No products indexed under this heading.

Hydroflumethiazide (Thiazides may add to or potentiate the action of other antihypertensive drugs; this may be enhanced in the post-sympathectomy patient. Hypotension, including orthostatic hypotension, may also be aggravated by antihypertensive drugs).
No products indexed under this heading.

Hydromorphone (Potentiation of orthostatic hypotension may occur with concurrent administration of narcotics).
No products indexed under this heading.

Hydromorphone Hydrochloride (Potentiation of orthostatic hypotension may occur with concurrent administration of narcotics). Products include:
Dilaudid Injection 2800
Dilaudid Oral 2797
Dilaudid Tablets 2797
Dilaudid-HP 2800

Ibuprofen (In some patients, the administration of a non-steroidal anti-inflammatory agent can reduce the diuretic, natriuretic, and antihypertensive effects of loop, potassium-sparing and thiazide diuretics. Therefore, when hydrochlorothiazide and non-steroidal anti-inflammatory agents are used concomitantly, the patient should be observed closely to determine if the desired effect of the diuretic is obtained). Products include:
Motrin IB 2043
Children's Motrin 2044
Children's Motrin Non-Staining Dye-Free 2044
Infants' Motrin 2044
Infants' Motrin Dye-Free 2044
Junior Strength Motrin 2044
Vicoprofen 564

IMPORTANT NOTE: Always consult each drug listing in the patient's regimen for possible interactions.

Imipramine Hydrochloride (Telmisartan is not metabolized by the cytochrome P450 system and had no effects *in vitro* on cytochrome P450 enzymes, except for some inhibition of CYP2C19).
No products indexed under this heading.

Imipramine Pamoate (Telmisartan is not metabolized by the cytochrome P450 system and had no effects *in vitro* on cytochrome P450 enzymes, except for some inhibition of CYP2C19).
No products indexed under this heading.

Indapamide (Thiazides may add to or potentiate the action of other antihypertensive drugs; this may be enhanced in the post-sympathectomy patient. Hypotension, including orthostatic hypotension, may also be aggravated by antihypertensive drugs). Products include:
Indapamide 2356

Indomethacin (In some patients, the administration of a non-steroidal anti-inflammatory agent can reduce the diuretic, natriuretic, and antihypertensive effects of loop, potassium-sparing and thiazide diuretics. Therefore, when hydrochlorothiazide and non-steroidal anti-inflammatory agents are used concomitantly, the patient should be observed closely to determine if the desired effect of the diuretic is obtained). Products include:
Indocin 2167

Indomethacin Sodium Trihydrate (In some patients, the administration of a non-steroidal anti-inflammatory agent can reduce the diuretic, natriuretic, and antihypertensive effects of loop, potassium-sparing and thiazide diuretics. Therefore, when hydrochlorothiazide and non-steroidal anti-inflammatory agents are used concomitantly, the patient should be observed closely to determine if the desired effect of the diuretic is obtained). Products include:
Indocin I.V. 2007

Insulin (Concurrent administration of hydrochlorothiazides with insulin in diabetic patients may require dosage adjustments of insulin).
No products indexed under this heading.

Insulin, Human, Zinc Suspension (Concurrent administration of hydrochlorothiazides with insulin in diabetic patients may require dosage adjustments of insulin).
No products indexed under this heading.

Insulin, Human (rDNA origin) (Concurrent administration of hydrochlorothiazides with insulin in diabetic patients may require dosage adjustments of insulin). Products include:
Exubera 2717

Insulin, Human NPH (Concurrent administration of hydrochlorothiazides with insulin in diabetic patients may require dosage adjustments of insulin). Products include:
Humulin N Vial 1934

Insulin, Human Regular (Concurrent administration of hydrochlorothiazides with insulin in diabetic patients may require dosage adjustments of insulin). Products include:
Humulin R 1937
Humulin R (U-500) 1939

Insulin, Human Regular and Human NPH Mixture (Concurrent administration of hydrochlorothiazides with insulin in diabetic patients may require dosage adjustments of insulin). Products include:
Humulin 50/50 1930
Humulin 70/30 Vial 1931

Insulin, NPH (Concurrent administration of hydrochlorothiazides with insulin in diabetic patients may require dosage adjustments of insulin).
No products indexed under this heading.

Insulin, Regular (Concurrent administration of hydrochlorothiazides with insulin in diabetic patients may require dosage adjustments of insulin).
No products indexed under this heading.

Insulin, Regular and NPH mixture (Concurrent administration of hydrochlorothiazides with insulin in diabetic patients may require dosage adjustments of insulin).
No products indexed under this heading.

Insulin, Zinc Crystals (Concurrent administration of hydrochlorothiazides with insulin in diabetic patients may require dosage adjustments of insulin).
No products indexed under this heading.

Insulin, Zinc Suspension (Concurrent administration of hydrochlorothiazides with insulin in diabetic patients may require dosage adjustments of insulin).
No products indexed under this heading.

Insulin Aspart (Concurrent administration of hydrochlorothiazides with insulin in diabetic patients may require dosage adjustments of insulin).
No products indexed under this heading.

Insulin Aspart, Human (Concurrent administration of hydrochlorothiazides with insulin in diabetic patients may require dosage adjustments of insulin). Products include:
NovoLog Mix 70/30 2581

Insulin Aspart, Human Regular (Concurrent administration of hydrochlorothiazides with insulin in diabetic patients may require dosage adjustments of insulin). Products include:
NovoLog 2575

Insulin Aspart Protamine, Human (Concurrent administration of hydrochlorothiazides with insulin in diabetic patients may require dosage adjustments of insulin). Products include:
NovoLog Mix 70/30 2581

Insulin Detemir (rDNA Origin) (Concurrent administration of hydrochlorothiazides with insulin in diabetic patients may require dosage adjustments of insulin). Products include:
Levemir 2566

Insulin Glargine (Concurrent administration of hydrochlorothiazides with insulin in diabetic patients may require dosage adjustments of insulin). Products include:
Lantus 2996

Insulin Glulisine (Concurrent administration of hydrochlorothiazides with insulin in diabetic patients may require dosage adjustments of insulin). Products include:
Apidra 2937
Apidra SoloStar 2937

Insulin Lispro, Human (Concurrent administration of hydrochlorothiazides with insulin in diabetic patients may require dosage adjustments of insulin). Products include:
Humalog 1910
Humalog Mix 1914
Humalog Mix75/25 1917

Insulin Lispro Protamine, Human (Concurrent administration of hydrochlorothiazides with insulin in diabetic patients may require dosage adjustments of insulin). Products include:
Humalog Mix 1914
Humalog Mix75/25 1917

Irbesartan (Thiazides may add to or potentiate the action of other antihypertensive drugs; this may be enhanced in the post-sympathectomy patient. Hypotension, including orthostatic hypotension, may also be aggravated by antihypertensive drugs). Products include:
Avalide 2956
Avapro 2962

Isoproterenol Hydrochloride (Concurrent administration of pressor amines with hydrochlorothiazides may cause possible decreased response to pressor amines but not sufficient to preclude their use).
No products indexed under this heading.

Isoproterenol Sulfate (Concurrent administration of pressor amines with hydrochlorothiazides may cause possible decreased response to pressor amines but not sufficient to preclude their use).
No products indexed under this heading.

Isradipine (Thiazides may add to or potentiate the action of other antihypertensive drugs; this may be enhanced in the post-sympathectomy patient. Hypotension, including orthostatic hypotension, may also be aggravated by antihypertensive drugs). Products include:
DynaCirc CR 1432

Ketoprofen (In some patients, the administration of a non-steroidal anti-inflammatory agent can reduce the diuretic, natriuretic, and antihypertensive effects of loop, potassium-sparing and thiazide diuretics. Therefore, when hydrochlorothiazide and non-steroidal anti-inflammatory agents are used concomitantly, the patient should be observed closely to determine if the desired effect of the diuretic is obtained).
No products indexed under this heading.

Ketorolac Tromethamine (In some patients, the administration of a non-steroidal anti-inflammatory agent can reduce the diuretic, natriuretic, and antihypertensive effects of loop, potassium-sparing and thiazide diuretics. Therefore, when hydrochlorothiazide and non-steroidal anti-inflammatory agents are used concomitantly, the patient should be observed closely to determine if the desired effect of the diuretic is obtained). Products include:
Acuvail .... ⊙ 209

Labetalol Hydrochloride (Thiazides may add to or potentiate the action of other antihypertensive drugs; this may be enhanced in the post-sympathectomy patient. Hypotension, including orthostatic hypotension, may also be aggravated by antihypertensive drugs).
No products indexed under this heading.

Lamotrigine (Telmisartan is not metabolized by the cytochrome P450 system and had no effects *in vitro* on cytochrome P450 enzymes, except for some inhibition of CYP2C19). Products include:
Lamictal 1522
Lamictal ODT 1522
Lamictal XR 1536

Lansoprazole (Telmisartan is not metabolized by the cytochrome P450 system and had no effects *in vitro* on cytochrome P450 enzymes, except for some inhibition of CYP2C19).
No products indexed under this heading.

Levetiracetam (Telmisartan is not metabolized by the cytochrome P450 system and had no effects *in vitro* on cytochrome P450 enzymes, except for some inhibition of CYP2C19). Products include:
Keppra XR 3434

Levorphanol Tartrate (Potentiation of orthostatic hypotension may occur with concurrent administration of narcotics).
No products indexed under this heading.

Lisinopril (As a consequence of inhibiting the renin-angiotensin-aldosterone system, changes in renal function (including acute renal failure) have been reported. Dual blockade of the renin-angiotensin-aldosterone system (eg, by adding an ACE-inhibitor to an angiotensin II receptor antagonist) should be used with caution and should include close monitoring of renal function). Products include:
Prinivil 2241
Prinzide 2246

Lithium (Lithium generally should not be given with diuretics. Diuretic agents reduce the renal clearance of lithium and add a high risk of lithium toxicity).
No products indexed under this heading.

Lithium Carbonate (Lithium generally should not be given with diuretics. Diuretic agents reduce the renal clearance of lithium and add a high risk of lithium toxicity).
No products indexed under this heading.

Lithium Citrate (Lithium generally should not be given with diuretics. Diuretic agents reduce the renal clearance of lithium and add a high risk of lithium toxicity).
No products indexed under this heading.

Losartan Potassium (Thiazides may add to or potentiate the action of other antihypertensive drugs; this may be enhanced in the post-sympathectomy patient. Hypotension, including orthostatic hypotension, may also be aggravated by antihypertensive drugs). Products include:
Cozaar 2106
Hyzaar 2162
Hyzaar 100-12.5 2162

Maprotiline Hydrochloride (Telmisartan is not metabolized by the cytochrome P450 system and had no effects *in vitro* on cytochrome P450 enzymes, except for some inhibition of CYP2C19).
No products indexed under this heading.

Mecamylamine Hydrochloride (Thiazides may add to or potentiate the action of other antihypertensive drugs; this may be enhanced in the post-sympathectomy patient. Hypotension, including orthostatic hypotension, may also be aggravated by antihypertensive drugs).
No products indexed under this heading.

Meclofenamate Sodium (In some patients, the administration of a non-steroidal anti-inflammatory agent can reduce the diuretic, natriuretic, and antihypertensive effects of loop, potassium-sparing and thiazide diuretics. Therefore, when hydrochlorothiazide and non-steroidal anti-inflammatory agents are used concomitantly, the patient should be observed closely to determine if the desired effect of the diuretic is obtained).
No products indexed under this heading.

Mefenamic Acid (In some patients, the administration of a non-steroidal anti-inflammatory agent can reduce the diuretic, natriuretic, and antihypertensive effects of loop, potassium-sparing and thiazide diuretics. Therefore, when hydrochlorothiazide and non-steroidal anti-inflammatory agents are used concomitantly, the patient should be observed closely to determine if the desired effect of the diuretic is obtained).
No products indexed under this heading.

Meloxicam (In some patients, the administration of a non-steroidal anti-inflammatory agent can reduce the diuretic, natriuretic, and antihypertensive effects of loop, potassium-sparing and thiazide diuretics. Therefore, when hydrochlorothiazide and non-steroidal anti-inflammatory agents are used concomitantly, the patient should be observed closely to determine if the desired effect of the diuretic is obtained).
No products indexed under this heading.

(⊙ Described in PDR® for Ophthalmic Medicines)

1135 Interactions Index Micardis HCT

Meperidine Hydrochloride (Potentiation of orthostatic hypotension may occur with concurrent administration of narcotics).
No products indexed under this heading.

Mephentermine Sulfate (Concurrent administration of pressor amines with hydrochlorothiazides may cause possible decreased response to pressor amines but not sufficient to preclude their use).
No products indexed under this heading.

Mephenytoin (Telmisartan is not metabolized by the cytochrome P450 system and had no effects *in vitro* on cytochrome P450 enzymes, except for some inhibition of CYP2C19).
No products indexed under this heading.

Mephobarbital (Potentiation of orthostatic hypotension may occur with concurrent administration of barbiturates).
No products indexed under this heading.

Meprobamate (Telmisartan is not metabolized by the cytochrome P450 system and had no effects *in vitro* on cytochrome P450 enzymes, except for some inhibition of CYP2C19).
No products indexed under this heading.

Metaraminol Bitartrate (Concurrent administration of pressor amines with hydrochlorothiazides may cause possible decreased response to pressor amines but not sufficient to preclude their use).
No products indexed under this heading.

Metformin Hydrochloride (Concurrent administration of hydrochlorothiazides with oral hypoglycemic agents in diabetic patients may require dosage adjustments of oral hypoglycemic agents). Products include:
ActoPlus 3338
Avandamet 1345
Janumet 2188

Methadone Hydrochloride (Potentiation of orthostatic hypotension may occur with concurrent administration of narcotics).
No products indexed under this heading.

Methoxamine Hydrochloride (Concurrent administration of pressor amines with hydrochlorothiazides may cause possible decreased response to pressor amines but not sufficient to preclude their use).
No products indexed under this heading.

Methsuximide (Telmisartan is not metabolized by the cytochrome P450 system and had no effects *in vitro* on cytochrome P450 enzymes, except for some inhibition of CYP2C19).
No products indexed under this heading.

Methyclothiazide (Thiazides may add to or potentiate the action of other antihypertensive drugs; this may be enhanced in the post-sympathectomy patient. Hypotension, including orthostatic hypotension, may also be aggravated by antihypertensive drugs).
No products indexed under this heading.

Methyldopa (Thiazides may add to or potentiate the action of other antihypertensive drugs; this may be enhanced in the post-sympathectomy patient. Hypotension, including orthostatic hypotension, may also be aggravated by antihypertensive drugs).
No products indexed under this heading.

Methyldopate Hydrochloride (Thiazides may add to or potentiate the action of other antihypertensive drugs; this may be enhanced in the post-sympathectomy patient. Hypotension, including orthostatic hypotension, may also be aggravated by antihypertensive drugs).
No products indexed under this heading.

Methylprednisolone (Corticosteroids, when administered concurrently with thiazide diuretics, intensify electrolyte depletion, particularly hypokalemia).
No products indexed under this heading.

Methylprednisolone Acetate (Corticosteroids, when administered concurrently with thiazide diuretics, intensify electrolyte depletion, particularly hypokalemia).
No products indexed under this heading.

Methylprednisolone Sodium Succinate (Corticosteroids, when administered concurrently with thiazide diuretics, intensify electrolyte depletion, particularly hypokalemia).
No products indexed under this heading.

Metocurine Iodide (Concurrent administration of non-depolarizing skeletal muscle relaxants (eg, tubocurarine) with hydrochlorothiazide may cause possible increased responsiveness to the muscle relaxant).
No products indexed under this heading.

Metolazone (Thiazides may add to or potentiate the action of other antihypertensive drugs; this may be enhanced in the post-sympathectomy patient. Hypotension, including orthostatic hypotension, may also be aggravated by antihypertensive drugs).
No products indexed under this heading.

Metoprolol Succinate (Thiazides may add to or potentiate the action of other antihypertensive drugs; this may be enhanced in the post-sympathectomy patient. Hypotension, including orthostatic hypotension, may also be aggravated by antihypertensive drugs). Products include:
Toprol XL 732

Metoprolol Tartrate (Thiazides may add to or potentiate the action of other antihypertensive drugs; this may be enhanced in the post-sympathectomy patient. Hypotension, including orthostatic hypotension, may also be aggravated by antihypertensive drugs).
No products indexed under this heading.

Metyrosine (Thiazides may add to or potentiate the action of other antihypertensive drugs; this may be enhanced in the post-sympathectomy patient. Hypotension, including orthostatic hypotension, may also be aggravated by antihypertensive drugs).
No products indexed under this heading.

Mibefradil Dihydrochloride (Thiazides may add to or potentiate the action of other antihypertensive drugs; this may be enhanced in the post-sympathectomy patient. Hypotension, including orthostatic hypotension, may also be aggravated by antihypertensive drugs).
No products indexed under this heading.

Midazolam Hydrochloride (Telmisartan is not metabolized by the cytochrome P450 system and had no effects *in vitro* on cytochrome P450 enzymes, except for some inhibition of CYP2C19).
No products indexed under this heading.

Miglitol (Concurrent administration of hydrochlorothiazides with oral hypoglycemic agents in diabetic patients may require dosage adjustments of oral hypoglycemic agents).
No products indexed under this heading.

Minoxidil (Thiazides may add to or potentiate the action of other antihypertensive drugs; this may be enhanced in the post-sympathectomy patient. Hypotension, including orthostatic hypotension, may also be aggravated by antihypertensive drugs).
No products indexed under this heading.

Mivacurium Chloride (Concurrent administration of non-depolarizing skeletal muscle relaxants (eg, tubocurarine) with hydrochlorothiazide may cause possible increased responsiveness to the muscle relaxant).
No products indexed under this heading.

Moexipril Hydrochloride (As a consequence of inhibiting the renin-angiotensin-aldosterone system, changes in renal function (including acute renal failure) have been reported. Dual blockade of the renin-angiotensin-aldosterone system (eg, by adding an ACE-inhibitor to an angiotensin II receptor antagonist) should be used with caution and should include close monitoring of renal function).
No products indexed under this heading.

Mometasone Furoate (Corticosteroids, when administered concurrently with thiazide diuretics, intensify electrolyte depletion, particularly hypokalemia). Products include:
Asmanex 3058
Elocon Cream 3111
Elocon Lotion 3112
Elocon Ointment 3114

Mometasone Furoate Monohydrate (Corticosteroids, when administered concurrently with thiazide diuretics, intensify electrolyte depletion, particularly hypokalemia). Products include:
Nasonex 3166

Morphine Sulfate (Potentiation of orthostatic hypotension may occur with concurrent administration of narcotics). Products include:
Avinza 1822
Embeda 1831
MS Contin 2803

Morphine Sulfate, Liposomal (Potentiation of orthostatic hypotension may occur with concurrent administration of narcotics).
No products indexed under this heading.

Nabumetone (In some patients, the administration of a non-steroidal anti-inflammatory agent can reduce the diuretic, natriuretic, and antihypertensive effects of loop, potassium-sparing and thiazide diuretics. Therefore, when hydrochlorothiazide and non-steroidal anti-inflammatory agents are used concomitantly, the patient should be observed closely to determine if the desired effect of the diuretic is obtained).
No products indexed under this heading.

Nadolol (Thiazides may add to or potentiate the action of other antihypertensive drugs; this may be enhanced in the post-sympathectomy patient. Hypotension, including orthostatic hypotension, may also be aggravated by antihypertensive drugs). Products include:
Nadolol 2359

Naproxen (In some patients, the administration of a non-steroidal anti-inflammatory agent can reduce the diuretic, natriuretic, and antihypertensive effects of loop, potassium-sparing and thiazide diuretics. Therefore, when hydrochlorothiazide and non-steroidal anti-inflammatory agents are used concomitantly, the patient should be observed closely to determine if the desired effect of the diuretic is obtained). Products include:
EC-Naprosyn 2850
Naprosyn 2850
Anaprox/Naprosyn 2850

Naproxen Sodium (In some patients, the administration of a non-steroidal anti-inflammatory agent can reduce the diuretic, natriuretic, and antihypertensive effects of loop, potassium-sparing and thiazide diuretics. Therefore, when hydrochlorothiazide and non-steroidal anti-inflammatory agents are used concomitantly, the patient should be observed closely to determine if the desired effect of the diuretic is obtained). Products include:
Anaprox 2850
Anaprox DS 2850
Treximet 1681

Nateglinide (Concurrent administration of hydrochlorothiazides with oral hypoglycemic agents in diabetic patients may require dosage adjustments of oral hypoglycemic agents).
No products indexed under this heading.

Nebivolol (Thiazides may add to or potentiate the action of other antihypertensive drugs; this may be enhanced in the post-sympathectomy patient. Hypotension, including orthostatic hypotension, may also be aggravated by antihypertensive drugs). Products include:
Bystolic 1147

Nelfinavir Mesylate (Telmisartan is not metabolized by the cytochrome P450 system and had no effects *in vitro* on cytochrome P450 enzymes, except for some inhibition of CYP2C19).
No products indexed under this heading.

Nicardipine Hydrochloride (Thiazides may add to or potentiate the action of other antihypertensive drugs; this may be enhanced in the post-sympathectomy patient. Hypotension, including orthostatic hypotension, may also be aggravated by antihypertensive drugs).
No products indexed under this heading.

Nifedipine (Thiazides may add to or potentiate the action of other antihypertensive drugs; this may be enhanced in the post-sympathectomy patient. Hypotension, including orthostatic hypotension, may also be aggravated by antihypertensive drugs).
No products indexed under this heading.

Nilutamide (Telmisartan is not metabolized by the cytochrome P450 system and had no effects *in vitro* on cytochrome P450 enzymes, except for some inhibition of CYP2C19).
No products indexed under this heading.

Nisoldipine (Thiazides may add to or potentiate the action of other antihypertensive drugs; this may be enhanced in the post-sympathectomy patient. Hypotension, including orthostatic hypotension, may also be aggravated by antihypertensive drugs).
No products indexed under this heading.

Nitroglycerin (Thiazides may add to or potentiate the action of other antihypertensive drugs; this may be enhanced in the post-sympathectomy patient. Hypotension, including orthostatic hypotension, may also be aggravated by antihypertensive drugs). Products include:
Nitro-Dur 3170
Nitrolingual 3266

Norepinephrine Bitartrate (Possible decreased response to pressor amines).
No products indexed under this heading.

Nortriptyline Hydrochloride (Telmisartan is not metabolized by the cytochrome P450 system and had no effects *in vitro* on cytochrome P450 enzymes, except for some inhibition of CYP2C19).
No products indexed under this heading.

Omeprazole (Telmisartan is not metabolized by the cytochrome P450 system and had no effects *in vitro* on cytochrome P450 enzymes, except for some inhibition of CYP2C19).
No products indexed under this heading.

Omeprazole Magnesium (Telmisartan is not metabolized by the cytochrome P450 system and had no effects *in vitro* on cytochrome P450 enzymes, except for some inhibition of CYP2C19).
No products indexed under this heading.

IMPORTANT NOTE: Always consult each drug listing in the patient's regimen for possible interactions.

Oxaprozin (In some patients, the administration of a non-steroidal anti-inflammatory agent can reduce the diuretic, natriuretic, and antihypertensive effects of loop, potassium-sparing and thiazide diuretics. Therefore, when hydrochlorothiazide and non-steroidal anti-inflammatory agents are used concomitantly, the patient should be observed closely to determine if the desired effect of the diuretic is obtained).
No products indexed under this heading.

Oxcarbazepine (Telmisartan is not metabolized by the cytochrome P450 system and had no effects *in vitro* on cytochrome P450 enzymes, except for some inhibition of CYP2C19).
No products indexed under this heading.

Oxycodone Hydrochloride (Potentiation of orthostatic hypotension may occur with concurrent administration of narcotics). Products include:
OxyContin 2807
Percocet 1121
Percodan 1124

Oxycodone Terephthalate (Potentiation of orthostatic hypotension may occur with concurrent administration of narcotics).
No products indexed under this heading.

Oxymorphone Hydrochloride (Potentiation of orthostatic hypotension may occur with concurrent administration of narcotics). Products include:
Opana 1110
Opana ER 1114

Pancuronium Bromide (Concurrent administration of non-depolarizing skeletal muscle relaxants (eg, tubocurarine) with hydrochlorothiazide may cause possible increased responsiveness to the muscle relaxant).
No products indexed under this heading.

Pantoprazole Sodium (Telmisartan is not metabolized by the cytochrome P450 system and had no effects *in vitro* on cytochrome P450 enzymes, except for some inhibition of CYP2C19). Products include:
Protonix Tablets 3571
Protonix 3575

Paramethadione (Telmisartan is not metabolized by the cytochrome P450 system and had no effects *in vitro* on cytochrome P450 enzymes, except for some inhibition of CYP2C19).
No products indexed under this heading.

Penbutolol Sulfate (Thiazides may add to or potentiate the action of other antihypertensive drugs; this may be enhanced in the post-sympathectomy patient. Hypotension, including orthostatic hypotension, may also be aggravated by antihypertensive drugs).
No products indexed under this heading.

Pentamidine Isethionate (Telmisartan is not metabolized by the cytochrome P450 system and had no effects *in vitro* on cytochrome P450 enzymes, except for some inhibition of CYP2C19).
No products indexed under this heading.

Pentobarbital (Potentiation of orthostatic hypotension may occur with concurrent administration of barbiturates).
No products indexed under this heading.

Pentobarbital Sodium (Potentiation of orthostatic hypotension may occur with concurrent administration of barbiturates). Products include:
Nembutal 2012

Perindopril Erbumine (As a consequence of inhibiting the renin-angiotensin-aldosterone system, changes in renal function (including acute renal failure) have been reported. Dual blockade of the renin-angiotensin-aldosterone system (eg, by adding an ACE-inhibitor to an angiotensin II receptor antagonist) should be used with caution and should include close monitoring of renal function).
No products indexed under this heading.

Phenacemide (Telmisartan is not metabolized by the cytochrome P450 system and had no effects *in vitro* on cytochrome P450 enzymes, except for some inhibition of CYP2C19).
No products indexed under this heading.

Phenobarbital (Potentiation of orthostatic hypotension may occur with concurrent administration of barbiturates). Products include:
Donnatal 2711

Phenobarbital Sodium (Potentiation of orthostatic hypotension may occur with concurrent administration of barbiturates).
No products indexed under this heading.

Phenoxybenzamine Hydrochloride (Thiazides may add to or potentiate the action of other antihypertensive drugs; this may be enhanced in the post-sympathectomy patient. Hypotension, including orthostatic hypotension, may also be aggravated by antihypertensive drugs). Products include:
Dibenzyline 3495

Phensuximide (Telmisartan is not metabolized by the cytochrome P450 system and had no effects *in vitro* on cytochrome P450 enzymes, except for some inhibition of CYP2C19).
No products indexed under this heading.

Phentolamine Mesylate (Thiazides may add to or potentiate the action of other antihypertensive drugs; this may be enhanced in the post-sympathectomy patient. Hypotension, including orthostatic hypotension, may also be aggravated by antihypertensive drugs).
No products indexed under this heading.

Phenylbutazone (In some patients, the administration of a non-steroidal anti-inflammatory agent can reduce the diuretic, natriuretic, and antihypertensive effects of loop, potassium-sparing and thiazide diuretics. Therefore, when hydrochlorothiazide and non-steroidal anti-inflammatory agents are used concomitantly, the patient should be observed closely to determine if the desired effect of the diuretic is obtained).
No products indexed under this heading.

Phenylephrine Hydrochloride (Concurrent administration of pressor amines with hydrochlorothiazides may cause possible decreased response to pressor amines but not sufficient to preclude their use). Products include:
Sudafed PE Nasal Decongestant 2048
Children's Sudafed PE Nasal
Decongestant 2047

Phenytoin (Telmisartan is not metabolized by the cytochrome P450 system and had no effects *in vitro* on cytochrome P450 enzymes, except for some inhibition of CYP2C19).
No products indexed under this heading.

Phenytoin Sodium (Telmisartan is not metabolized by the cytochrome P450 system and had no effects *in vitro* on cytochrome P450 enzymes, except for some inhibition of CYP2C19). Products include:
Phenytek Capsules 2380

Pindolol (Thiazides may add to or potentiate the action of other antihypertensive drugs; this may be enhanced in the post-sympathectomy patient. Hypotension, including orthostatic hypotension, may also be aggravated by antihypertensive drugs).
No products indexed under this heading.

Pioglitazone Hydrochloride (Concurrent administration of hydrochlorothiazides with oral hypoglycemic agents in diabetic patients may require dosage adjustments of oral hypoglycemic agents). Products include:
ActoPlus 3338
Actos 3345
Duetact 3354

Pipecuronium Bromide (Concurrent administration of non-depolarizing skeletal muscle relaxants (eg, tubocurarine) with hydrochlorothiazide may cause possible increased responsiveness to the muscle relaxant).
No products indexed under this heading.

Piroxicam (In some patients, the administration of a non-steroidal anti-inflammatory agent can reduce the diuretic, natriuretic, and antihypertensive effects of loop, potassium-sparing and thiazide diuretics. Therefore, when hydrochlorothiazide and non-steroidal anti-inflammatory agents are used concomitantly, the patient should be observed closely to determine if the desired effect of the diuretic is obtained).
No products indexed under this heading.

Polythiazide (Thiazides may add to or potentiate the action of other antihypertensive drugs; this may be enhanced in the post-sympathectomy patient. Hypotension, including orthostatic hypotension, may also be aggravated by antihypertensive drugs).
No products indexed under this heading.

Potassium Acid Phosphate (Concurrent use of potassium supplements or salt substitute is not recommended). Products include:
K-Phos Original 874

Potassium Bicarbonate (Concurrent use of potassium supplements or salt substitute is not recommended).
No products indexed under this heading.

Potassium Chloride (Concurrent use of potassium supplements or salt substitute is not recommended). Products include:
MoviPrep Oral Solution 2905

Potassium Citrate (Concurrent use of potassium supplements or salt substitute is not recommended). Products include:
Urocit-K 2333

Potassium Gluconate (Concurrent use of potassium supplements or salt substitute is not recommended).
No products indexed under this heading.

Potassium Phosphate (Concurrent use of potassium supplements or salt substitute is not recommended). Products include:
K-Phos Neutral 873

Prazosin Hydrochloride (Thiazides may add to or potentiate the action of other antihypertensive drugs; this may be enhanced in the post-sympathectomy patient. Hypotension, including orthostatic hypotension, may also be aggravated by antihypertensive drugs).
No products indexed under this heading.

Prednisolone (Corticosteroids, when administered concurrently with thiazide diuretics, intensify electrolyte depletion, particularly hypokalemia).
No products indexed under this heading.

Prednisolone Acetate (Corticosteroids, when administered concurrently

with thiazide diuretics, intensify electrolyte depletion, particularly hypokalemia). Products include:
Blephamide .... ⊙212, ⊙214
Pred Forte .... ⊙225
Pred Mild .... ⊙230
Pred-G .... ⊙226, ⊙227

Prednisolone Sodium Phosphate (Corticosteroids, when administered concurrently with thiazide diuretics, intensify electrolyte depletion, particularly hypokalemia).
No products indexed under this heading.

Prednisolone Tebutate (Corticosteroids, when administered concurrently with thiazide diuretics, intensify electrolyte depletion, particularly hypokalemia).
No products indexed under this heading.

Prednisone (Corticosteroids, when administered concurrently with thiazide diuretics, intensify electrolyte depletion, particularly hypokalemia).
No products indexed under this heading.

Prednisone sodium phosphate (Corticosteroids, when administered concurrently with thiazide diuretics, intensify electrolyte depletion, particularly hypokalemia).
No products indexed under this heading.

Pressor Amines (Pressor amines, (eg, norepinephrine) when administered concurrently with thiazide diuretics, may possibly decrease response to pressor amines but not sufficient to preclude their use).
No products indexed under this heading.

Primidone (Telmisartan is not metabolized by the cytochrome P450 system and had no effects *in vitro* on cytochrome P450 enzymes, except for some inhibition of CYP2C19).
No products indexed under this heading.

Progesterone (Telmisartan is not metabolized by the cytochrome P450 system and had no effects *in vitro* on cytochrome P450 enzymes, except for some inhibition of CYP2C19). Products include:
Crinone 4% 996
Crinone 8% 996
Prometrium 3307

Proguanil Hydrochloride (Telmisartan is not metabolized by the cytochrome P450 system and had no effects *in vitro* on cytochrome P450 enzymes, except for some inhibition of CYP2C19). Products include:
Malarone Pediatric Tablets 1572
Malarone 1572

Propoxyphene Hydrochloride (Potentiation of orthostatic hypotension may occur with concurrent administration of narcotics).
No products indexed under this heading.

Propoxyphene Napsylate (Potentiation of orthostatic hypotension may occur with concurrent administration of narcotics).
No products indexed under this heading.

Propranolol Hydrochloride (Thiazides may add to or potentiate the action of other antihypertensive drugs; this may be enhanced in the post-sympathectomy patient. Hypotension, including orthostatic hypotension, may also be aggravated by antihypertensive drugs). Products include:
InnoPran XL 1517

Protriptyline Hydrochloride (Telmisartan is not metabolized by the cytochrome P450 system and had no effects *in vitro* on cytochrome P450 enzymes, except for some inhibition of CYP2C19).
No products indexed under this heading.

Quinapril Hydrochloride (As a consequence of inhibiting the renin-angiotensin-aldosterone system, changes in renal function (including acute renal failure) have been reported. Dual

1137 Interactions Index Micardis HCT

blockade of the renin-angiotensin-aldosterone system (eg, by adding an ACE-inhibitor to an angiotensin II receptor antagonist) should be used with caution and should include close monitoring of renal function).
No products indexed under this heading.

Rabeprazole Sodium (Telmisartan is not metabolized by the cytochrome P450 system and had no effects *in vitro* on cytochrome P450 enzymes, except for some inhibition of CYP2C19). Products include:
Aciphex 1035

Ramipril (As a consequence of inhibiting the renin-angiotensin-aldosterone system, changes in renal function (including acute renal failure) have been reported. Dual blockade of the renin-angiotensin-aldosterone system (eg, by adding an ACE-inhibitor to an angiotensin II receptor antagonist) should be used with caution and should include close monitoring of renal function).
No products indexed under this heading.

Rapacuronium Bromide (Concurrent administration of non-depolarizing skeletal muscle relaxants (eg, tubocurarine) with hydrochlorothiazide may cause possible increased responsiveness to the muscle relaxant).
No products indexed under this heading.

Rauwolfia Serpentina (Thiazides may add to or potentiate the action of other antihypertensive drugs; this may be enhanced in the post-sympathectomy patient. Hypotension, including orthostatic hypotension, may also be aggravated by antihypertensive drugs).
No products indexed under this heading.

Remifentanil Hydrochloride (Potentiation of orthostatic hypotension may occur with concurrent administration of narcotics).
No products indexed under this heading.

Repaglinide (Concurrent administration of hydrochlorothiazides with oral hypoglycemic agents in diabetic patients may require dosage adjustments of oral hypoglycemic agents).
No products indexed under this heading.

Rescinnamine (Thiazides may add to or potentiate the action of other antihypertensive drugs; this may be enhanced in the post-sympathectomy patient. Hypotension, including orthostatic hypotension, may also be aggravated by antihypertensive drugs).
No products indexed under this heading.

Reserpine (Thiazides may add to or potentiate the action of other antihypertensive drugs; this may be enhanced in the post-sympathectomy patient. Hypotension, including orthostatic hypotension, may also be aggravated by antihypertensive drugs).
No products indexed under this heading.

Rocuronium Bromide (Concurrent administration of non-depolarizing skeletal muscle relaxants (eg, tubocurarine) with hydrochlorothiazide may cause possible increased responsiveness to the muscle relaxant). Products include:
Zemuron 3249

Rofecoxib (In some patients, the administration of a non-steroidal anti-inflammatory agent can reduce the diuretic, natriuretic, and antihypertensive effects of loop, potassium-sparing and thiazide diuretics. Therefore, when hydrochlorothiazide and non-steroidal anti-inflammatory agents are used concomitantly, the patient should be observed closely to determine if the desired effect of the diuretic is obtained).
No products indexed under this heading.

Rosiglitazone Maleate (Concurrent administration of hydrochlorothiazides with oral hypoglycemic agents in diabetic patients may require dosage adjustments of oral hypoglycemic agents). Products include:
Avandamet 1345
Avandaryl 1356
Avandia 1366

Secobarbital Sodium (Potentiation of orthostatic hypotension may occur with concurrent administration of barbiturates).
No products indexed under this heading.

Sertraline Hydrochloride (Telmisartan is not metabolized by the cytochrome P450 system and had no effects *in vitro* on cytochrome P450 enzymes, except for some inhibition of CYP2C19).
No products indexed under this heading.

Sitagliptin Phosphate (Concurrent administration of hydrochlorothiazides with oral hypoglycemic agents in diabetic patients may require dosage adjustments of oral hypoglycemic agents). Products include:
Janumet 2188
Januvia 2196

Sodium Butabarbital (Potentiation of orthostatic hypotension may occur with concurrent administration of barbiturates).
No products indexed under this heading.

Sodium Nitroprusside (Thiazides may add to or potentiate the action of other antihypertensive drugs; this may be enhanced in the post-sympathectomy patient. Hypotension, including orthostatic hypotension, may also be aggravated by antihypertensive drugs).
No products indexed under this heading.

Sodium Pentobarbital (Potentiation of orthostatic hypotension may occur with concurrent administration of barbiturates).
No products indexed under this heading.

Sotalol Hydrochloride (Thiazides may add to or potentiate the action of other antihypertensive drugs; this may be enhanced in the post-sympathectomy patient. Hypotension, including orthostatic hypotension, may also be aggravated by antihypertensive drugs).
No products indexed under this heading.

Spirapril Hydrochloride (As a consequence of inhibiting the renin-angiotensin-aldosterone system, changes in renal function (including acute renal failure) have been reported. Dual blockade of the renin-angiotensin-aldosterone system (eg, by adding an ACE-inhibitor to an angiotensin II receptor antagonist) should be used with caution and should include close monitoring of renal function).
No products indexed under this heading.

Sufentanil Citrate (Potentiation of orthostatic hypotension may occur with concurrent administration of narcotics).
No products indexed under this heading.

Sulindac (In some patients, the administration of a non-steroidal anti-inflammatory agent can reduce the diuretic, natriuretic, and antihypertensive effects of loop, potassium-sparing and thiazide diuretics. Therefore, when hydrochlorothiazide and non-steroidal anti-inflammatory agents are used concomitantly, the patient should be observed closely to determine if the desired effect of the diuretic is obtained). Products include:
Clinoril 2098

Teniposide (Telmisartan is not metabolized by the cytochrome P450 system and had no effects *in vitro* on cytochrome P450 enzymes, except for some inhibition of CYP2C19).
No products indexed under this heading.

Terazosin Hydrochloride (Thiazides may add to or potentiate the action of other antihypertensive drugs; this may be enhanced in the post-sympathectomy patient. Hypotension, including orthostatic hypotension, may also be aggravated by antihypertensive drugs).
No products indexed under this heading.

Thiamylal Sodium (Potentiation of orthostatic hypotension may occur with concurrent administration of barbiturates).
No products indexed under this heading.

Thioridazine (Telmisartan is not metabolized by the cytochrome P450 system and had no effects *in vitro* on cytochrome P450 enzymes, except for some inhibition of CYP2C19).
No products indexed under this heading.

Thioridazine Hydrochloride (Telmisartan is not metabolized by the cytochrome P450 system and had no effects *in vitro* on cytochrome P450 enzymes, except for some inhibition of CYP2C19). Products include:
Thioridazine Hydrochloride 2384

Tiagabine Hydrochloride (Telmisartan is not metabolized by the cytochrome P450 system and had no effects *in vitro* on cytochrome P450 enzymes, except for some inhibition of CYP2C19). Products include:
Gabitril 972

Timolol Maleate (Thiazides may add to or potentiate the action of other antihypertensive drugs; this may be enhanced in the post-sympathectomy patient. Hypotension, including orthostatic hypotension, may also be aggravated by antihypertensive drugs). Products include:
Combigan 601
Dorzolamide Hydrochloride/Timolol Maleate Ophthalmic Solution .... ⊙ 243
Timoptic in Ocudose .... ⊙ 231

Tolazamide (Concurrent administration of hydrochlorothiazides with oral hypoglycemic agents in diabetic patients may require dosage adjustments of oral hypoglycemic agents).
No products indexed under this heading.

Tolbutamide (Concurrent administration of hydrochlorothiazides with oral hypoglycemic agents in diabetic patients may require dosage adjustments of oral hypoglycemic agents).
No products indexed under this heading.

Tolbutamide Sodium (Telmisartan is not metabolized by the cytochrome P450 system and had no effects *in vitro* on cytochrome P450 enzymes, except for some inhibition of CYP2C19).
No products indexed under this heading.

Tolmetin Sodium (In some patients, the administration of a non-steroidal anti-inflammatory agent can reduce the diuretic, natriuretic, and antihypertensive effects of loop, potassium-sparing and thiazide diuretics. Therefore, when hydrochlorothiazide and non-steroidal anti-inflammatory agents are used concomitantly, the patient should be observed closely to determine if the desired effect of the diuretic is obtained).
No products indexed under this heading.

Topiramate (Telmisartan is not metabolized by the cytochrome P450 system and had no effects *in vitro* on cytochrome P450 enzymes, except for some inhibition of CYP2C19).
No products indexed under this heading.

Torsemide (Thiazides may add to or potentiate the action of other antihypertensive drugs; this may be enhanced in the post-sympathectomy patient. Hypotension, including orthostatic hypotension, may also be aggravated by antihypertensive drugs).
No products indexed under this heading.

Trandolapril (As a consequence of inhibiting the renin-angiotensin-aldosterone system, changes in renal function (including acute renal failure) have been reported. Dual blockade of the renin-angiotensin-aldosterone system (eg, by adding an ACE-inhibitor to an angiotensin II receptor antagonist) should be used with caution and should include close monitoring of renal function). Products include:
Mavik 489
Tarka 534

Triamcinolone (Corticosteroids, when administered concurrently with thiazide diuretics, intensify electrolyte depletion, particularly hypokalemia).
No products indexed under this heading.

Triamcinolone Acetonide (Corticosteroids, when administered concurrently with thiazide diuretics, intensify electrolyte depletion, particularly hypokalemia). Products include:
Azmacort 408
Nasacort AQ 3019

Triamcinolone Diacetate (Corticosteroids, when administered concurrently with thiazide diuretics, intensify electrolyte depletion, particularly hypokalemia).
No products indexed under this heading.

Triamcinolone Hexacetonide (Corticosteroids, when administered concurrently with thiazide diuretics, intensify electrolyte depletion, particularly hypokalemia).
No products indexed under this heading.

Trimethadione (Telmisartan is not metabolized by the cytochrome P450 system and had no effects *in vitro* on cytochrome P450 enzymes, except for some inhibition of CYP2C19).
No products indexed under this heading.

Trimethaphan Camsylate (Thiazides may add to or potentiate the action of other antihypertensive drugs; this may be enhanced in the post-sympathectomy patient. Hypotension, including orthostatic hypotension, may also be aggravated by antihypertensive drugs).
No products indexed under this heading.

Trimipramine Maleate (Telmisartan is not metabolized by the cytochrome P450 system and had no effects *in vitro* on cytochrome P450 enzymes, except for some inhibition of CYP2C19).
No products indexed under this heading.

Troglitazone (Concurrent administration of hydrochlorothiazides with oral hypoglycemic agents in diabetic patients may require dosage adjustments of oral hypoglycemic agents).
No products indexed under this heading.

Tubocurarine Chloride (Concurrent administration of non-depolarizing skeletal muscle relaxants (eg, tubocurarine) with hydrochlorothiazide may cause possible increased responsiveness to the muscle relaxant).
No products indexed under this heading.

Valdecoxib (In some patients, the administration of a non-steroidal anti-inflammatory agent can reduce the diuretic, natriuretic, and antihypertensive effects of loop, potassium-sparing and thiazide diuretics. Therefore, when hydrochlorothiazide and non-steroidal anti-inflammatory agents are used concomitantly, the patient should be observed closely to determine if the desired effect of the diuretic is obtained).
No products indexed under this heading.

Valproate Sodium (Telmisartan is not metabolized by the cytochrome P450 system and had no effects *in vitro* on cytochrome P450 enzymes, except for some inhibition of CYP2C19).
No products indexed under this heading.

IMPORTANT NOTE: Always consult each drug listing in the patient's regimen for possible interactions.

Valproic Acid (Telmisartan is not metabolized by the cytochrome P450 system and had no effects in vitro on cytochrome P450 enzymes, except for some inhibition of CYP2C19).

No products indexed under this heading.

Valsartan (Thiazides may add to or potentiate the action of other antihypertensive drugs; this may be enhanced in the post-sympathectomy patient. Hypotension, including orthostatic hypotension, may also be aggravated by antihypertensive drugs). Products include:

Vecuronium Bromide (Concurrent administration of non-depolarizing skeletal muscle relaxants (eg, tubocurarine) with hydrochlorothiazide may cause possible increased responsiveness to the muscle relaxant).

No products indexed under this heading.

Verapamil Hydrochloride (Thiazides may add to or potentiate the action of other antihypertensive drugs; this may be enhanced in the post-sympathectomy patient. Hypotension, including orthostatic hypotension, may also be aggravated by antihypertensive drugs). Products include:

Voriconazole (Telmisartan is not metabolized by the cytochrome P450 system and had no effects in vitro on cytochrome P450 enzymes, except for some inhibition of CYP2C19).

No products indexed under this heading.

Warfarin Sodium (Telmisartan administered for 10 days slightly decreased the mean warfarin trough plasma concentration; this decrease did not result in a change in International Normalized Ratio (INR)).

No products indexed under this heading.

Zonisamide (Telmisartan is not metabolized by the cytochrome P450 system and had no effects in vitro on cytochrome P450 enzymes, except for some inhibition of CYP2C19). Products include:

Food Interactions

Alcohol (Potentiation of orthostatic hypotension may occur with alcohol, barbiturates, or narcotics when administered concurrently with thiazide diuretics).

Beer, reduced-alcohol (Potentiation of orthostatic hypotension may occur with alcohol, barbiturates, or narcotics when administered concurrently with thiazide diuretics).

Beer, unspecified (Potentiation of orthostatic hypotension may occur with alcohol, barbiturates, or narcotics when administered concurrently with thiazide diuretics).

Food, unspecified (Food slightly reduces the bioavailability of telmisartan, with a reduction in the area under the plasma concentration-time curve (AUC) of about 6% with the 40 mg tablet and about 20% after a 160 mg dose. The absolute bioavailability of telmisartan is dose dependent. At 40 mg and 160 mg the bioavailability was 42% and 58%, respectively).

Meal, unspecified (Food slightly reduces the bioavailability of telmisartan, with a reduction in the area under the plasma concentration-time curve (AUC) of about 6% with the 40 mg tablet and about 20% after a 160 mg dose. The absolute bioavailability of telmisartan is dose dependent. At 40 mg and 160 mg the bioavailability was 42% and 58%, respectively).

Wine, Chianti (Potentiation of orthostatic hypotension may occur with alcohol, barbiturates, or narcotics when administered concurrently with thiazide diuretics).

Wine, Red (Potentiation of orthostatic hypotension may occur with alcohol, barbiturates, or narcotics when administered concurrently with thiazide diuretics).

Wine, unspecified (Potentiation of orthostatic hypotension may occur with alcohol, barbiturates, or narcotics when administered concurrently with thiazide diuretics).

Wine products (Potentiation of orthostatic hypotension may occur with alcohol, barbiturates, or narcotics when administered concurrently with thiazide diuretics).

MIMYX CREAM

None cited in PDR database.

MIRENA INTRAUTERINE SYSTEM

May interact with anticoagulants, corticosteroids, cytochrome p450 inducers (selected), hepatic microsomal enzyme inducers, insulin. Compounds in these categories include:

Alclometasone Dipropionate (Patients requiring chronic corticosteroid therapy should be monitored with special care for infection).

No products indexed under this heading.

Allium cepa (The metabolism of progestogens may be increased by concomitant use of substances known to induce drug-metabolizing liver enzymes, specifically cytochrome P450 enzymes). Products include:

Allium sativum (The metabolism of progestogens may be increased by concomitant use of substances known to induce drug-metabolizing liver enzymes, specifically cytochrome P450 enzymes).

No products indexed under this heading.

Allium schoenoprasum (The metabolism of progestogens may be increased by concomitant use of substances known to induce drug-metabolizing liver enzymes, specifically cytochrome P450 enzymes).

No products indexed under this heading.

Allium ursinum (The metabolism of progestogens may be increased by concomitant use of substances known to induce drug-metabolizing liver enzymes, specifically cytochrome P450 enzymes).

No products indexed under this heading.

Aminoglutethimide (The metabolism of progestogens may be increased by concomitant use of substances known to induce drug-metabolizing liver enzymes, specifically cytochrome P450 enzymes).

No products indexed under this heading.

Anisindione (Levonorgestrel releasing intrauterine system should be used with caution in patients who are receiving anticoagulants).

No products indexed under this heading.

Aprepitant (The metabolism of progestogens may be increased by concomitant use of substances known to induce drug-metabolizing liver enzymes, specifically cytochrome P450 enzymes). Products include:

Ardeparin Sodium (Levonorgestrel releasing intrauterine system should be used with caution in patients who are receiving anticoagulants).

No products indexed under this heading.

Beclomethasone Dipropionate (Patients requiring chronic corticosteroid therapy should be monitored with special care for infection). Products include:

Beclomethasone Dipropionate Monohydrate (Patients requiring chronic corticosteroid therapy should be monitored with special care for infection). Products include:

Betamethasone (Patients requiring chronic corticosteroid therapy should be monitored with special care for infection).

No products indexed under this heading.

Betamethasone Acetate (Patients requiring chronic corticosteroid therapy should be monitored with special care for infection).

No products indexed under this heading.

Betamethasone Benzoate (Patients requiring chronic corticosteroid therapy should be monitored with special care for infection).

No products indexed under this heading.

Betamethasone Dipropionate (Patients requiring chronic corticosteroid therapy should be monitored with special care for infection). Products include:

Betamethasone Sodium Phosphate (Patients requiring chronic corticosteroid therapy should be monitored with special care for infection).

No products indexed under this heading.

Betamethasone Valerate (Patients requiring chronic corticosteroid therapy should be monitored with special care for infection). Products include:

Bosentan (The metabolism of progestogens may be increased by concomitant use of substances known to induce drug-metabolizing liver enzymes, specifically cytochrome P450 enzymes). Products include:

Budesonide (Patients requiring chronic corticosteroid therapy should be monitored with special care for infection). Products include:

Carbamazepine (The metabolism of progestogens may be increased by concomitant use of substances known to induce drug-metabolizing liver enzymes, specifically cytochrome P450 enzymes). Products include:

Chlorpropamide (The metabolism of progestogens may be increased by concomitant use of substances known to induce drug-metabolizing liver enzymes, specifically cytochrome P450 enzymes).

No products indexed under this heading.

Ciclesonide (Patients requiring chronic corticosteroid therapy should be monitored with special care for infection).

No products indexed under this heading.

Ciprofloxacin (The metabolism of progestogens may be increased by concomitant use of substances known to induce drug-metabolizing liver enzymes, specifically cytochrome P450 enzymes). Products include:

Ciprofloxacin Hydrochloride (The metabolism of progestogens may be increased by concomitant use of substances known to induce drug-metabolizing liver enzymes, specifically cytochrome P450 enzymes). Products include:

Cisplatin (The metabolism of progestogens may be increased by concomitant use of substances known to induce drug-metabolizing liver enzymes, specifically cytochrome P450 enzymes).

No products indexed under this heading.

Citalopram Hydrobromide (The metabolism of progestogens may be increased by concomitant use of substances known to induce drug-metabolizing liver enzymes, specifically cytochrome P450 enzymes). Products include:

Cortisone Acetate (Patients requiring chronic corticosteroid therapy should be monitored with special care for infection).

No products indexed under this heading.

Dalteparin Sodium (Levonorgestrel releasing intrauterine system should be used with caution in patients who are receiving anticoagulants). Products include:

Danaparoid Sodium (Levonorgestrel releasing intrauterine system should be used with caution in patients who are receiving anticoagulants).

No products indexed under this heading.

Desoximetasone (Patients requiring chronic corticosteroid therapy should be monitored with special care for infection).

No products indexed under this heading.

Dexamethasone (Patients requiring chronic corticosteroid therapy should be monitored with special care for infection). Products include:

Dexamethasone Acetate (Patients requiring chronic corticosteroid therapy should be monitored with special care for infection).

No products indexed under this heading.

Dexamethasone Phosphate (Patients requiring chronic corticosteroid therapy should be monitored with special care for infection).

No products indexed under this heading.

Dexamethasone Sodium (Patients requiring chronic corticosteroid therapy should be monitored with special care for infection).

No products indexed under this heading.

Dexamethasone Sodium Phosphate (Patients requiring chronic corticosteroid therapy should be monitored with special care for infection).

No products indexed under this heading.

Dexamethasone Sodium Phosphate Injection (Patients requiring chronic corticosteroid therapy should be monitored with special care for infection).

No products indexed under this heading.

Dicumarol (Levonorgestrel releasing intrauterine system should be used with caution in patients who are receiving anticoagulants).

No products indexed under this heading.

Diflorasone Diacetate (Patients requiring chronic corticosteroid therapy should be monitored with special care for infection).
   No products indexed under this heading.

Diltiazem Hydrochloride (The metabolism of progestogens may be increased by concomitant use of substances known to induce drug-metabolizing liver enzymes, specifically cytochrome P450 enzymes). Products include:

Diltiazem Maleate (The metabolism of progestogens may be increased by concomitant use of substances known to induce drug-metabolizing liver enzymes, specifically cytochrome P450 enzymes).
   No products indexed under this heading.

Doxorubicin Hydrochloride (The metabolism of progestogens may be increased by concomitant use of substances known to induce drug-metabolizing liver enzymes, specifically cytochrome P450 enzymes).
   No products indexed under this heading.

Efavirenz (The metabolism of progestogens may be increased by concomitant use of substances known to induce drug-metabolizing liver enzymes, specifically cytochrome P450 enzymes). Products include:

Enoxaparin Sodium (Levonorgestrel releasing intrauterine system should be used with caution in patients who are receiving anticoagulants). Products include:

Erythromycin (The metabolism of progestogens may be increased by concomitant use of substances known to induce drug-metabolizing liver enzymes, specifically cytochrome P450 enzymes).
   No products indexed under this heading.

Erythromycin, Topical (The metabolism of progestogens may be increased by concomitant use of substances known to induce drug-metabolizing liver enzymes, specifically cytochrome P450 enzymes).
   No products indexed under this heading.

Erythromycin Estolate (The metabolism of progestogens may be increased by concomitant use of substances known to induce drug-metabolizing liver enzymes, specifically cytochrome P450 enzymes).
   No products indexed under this heading.

Erythromycin Ethylsuccinate (The metabolism of progestogens may be increased by concomitant use of substances known to induce drug-metabolizing liver enzymes, specifically cytochrome P450 enzymes). Products include:

Erythromycin Gluceptate (The metabolism of progestogens may be increased by concomitant use of substances known to induce drug-metabolizing liver enzymes, specifically cytochrome P450 enzymes).
   No products indexed under this heading.

Erythromycin Lactobionate (The metabolism of progestogens may be increased by concomitant use of substances known to induce drug-metabolizing liver enzymes, specifically cytochrome P450 enzymes).
   No products indexed under this heading.

Erythromycin Stearate (The metabolism of progestogens may be increased by concomitant use of substances known to induce drug-metabolizing liver enzymes, specifically cytochrome P450 enzymes).
   No products indexed under this heading.

Escitalopram Oxalate (The metabolism of progestogens may be increased by concomitant use of substances known to induce drug-metabolizing liver enzymes, specifically cytochrome P450 enzymes). Products include:

Esomeprazole Magnesium (The metabolism of progestogens may be increased by concomitant use of substances known to induce drug-metabolizing liver enzymes, specifically cytochrome P450 enzymes). Products include:

Esomeprazole Sodium (The metabolism of progestogens may be increased by concomitant use of substances known to induce drug-metabolizing liver enzymes, specifically cytochrome P450 enzymes). Products include:

Ethanol (The metabolism of progestogens may be increased by concomitant use of substances known to induce drug-metabolizing liver enzymes, specifically cytochrome P450 enzymes).
   No products indexed under this heading.

Ethosuximide (The metabolism of progestogens may be increased by concomitant use of substances known to induce drug-metabolizing liver enzymes, specifically cytochrome P450 enzymes).
   No products indexed under this heading.

Ethyl Alcohol (The metabolism of progestogens may be increased by concomitant use of substances known to induce drug-metabolizing liver enzymes, specifically cytochrome P450 enzymes).
   No products indexed under this heading.

Felbamate (The metabolism of progestogens may be increased by concomitant use of substances known to induce drug-metabolizing liver enzymes, specifically cytochrome P450 enzymes).
   No products indexed under this heading.

Fludrocortisone Acetate (Patients requiring chronic corticosteroid therapy should be monitored with special care for infection).
   No products indexed under this heading.

Flumethasone Pivalate (Patients requiring chronic corticosteroid therapy should be monitored with special care for infection).
   No products indexed under this heading.

Flunisolide Hemihydrate (Patients requiring chronic corticosteroid therapy should be monitored with special care for infection).
   No products indexed under this heading.

Fluticasone Furoate (Patients requiring chronic corticosteroid therapy should be monitored with special care for infection). Products include:

Fluticasone Propionate (Patients requiring chronic corticosteroid therapy should be monitored with special care for infection). Products include:

Fluvoxamine (The metabolism of progestogens may be increased by concomitant use of substances known to induce drug-metabolizing liver enzymes, specifically cytochrome P450 enzymes).
   No products indexed under this heading.

Fluvoxamine Maleate (The metabolism of progestogens may be increased by concomitant use of substances known to induce drug-metabolizing liver enzymes, specifically cytochrome P450 enzymes).
   No products indexed under this heading.

Fondaparinux Sodium (Levonorgestrel releasing intrauterine system should be used with caution in patients who are receiving anticoagulants). Products include:

Fosphenytoin (The metabolism of progestogens may be increased by concomitant use of substances known to induce drug-metabolizing liver enzymes, specifically cytochrome P450 enzymes).
   No products indexed under this heading.

Fosphenytoin Sodium (The metabolism of progestogens may be increased by concomitant use of substances known to induce drug-metabolizing liver enzymes, specifically cytochrome P450 enzymes).
   No products indexed under this heading.

Garlic Extract (The metabolism of progestogens may be increased by concomitant use of substances known to induce drug-metabolizing liver enzymes, specifically cytochrome P450 enzymes).
   No products indexed under this heading.

Garlic Oil (The metabolism of progestogens may be increased by concomitant use of substances known to induce drug-metabolizing liver enzymes, specifically cytochrome P450 enzymes).
   No products indexed under this heading.

Glipizide (The metabolism of progestogens may be increased by concomitant use of substances known to induce drug-metabolizing liver enzymes, specifically cytochrome P450 enzymes).
   No products indexed under this heading.

Glyburide (The metabolism of progestogens may be increased by concomitant use of substances known to induce drug-metabolizing liver enzymes, specifically cytochrome P450 enzymes).
   No products indexed under this heading.

Heparin Calcium (Levonorgestrel releasing intrauterine system should be used with caution in patients who are receiving anticoagulants).
   No products indexed under this heading.

Heparin Sodium (Levonorgestrel releasing intrauterine system should be used with caution in patients who are receiving anticoagulants).
   No products indexed under this heading.

Hepatic Enzyme-Inducing Agents (The metabolism of progestogens may be increased by concomitant use of substances known to induce drug-metabolizing liver enzymes, specifically cytochrome P450 enzymes).
   No products indexed under this heading.

Hydrocortisone (Patients requiring chronic corticosteroid therapy should be monitored with special care for infection).
   No products indexed under this heading.

Hydrocortisone (Alcohol) (Patients requiring chronic corticosteroid therapy should be monitored with special care for infection).
   No products indexed under this heading.

Hydrocortisone Acetate (Patients requiring chronic corticosteroid therapy should be monitored with special care for infection).
   No products indexed under this heading.

Hydrocortisone Butyrate (Patients requiring chronic corticosteroid therapy should be monitored with special care for infection).
   No products indexed under this heading.

Hydrocortisone Cypionate (Patients requiring chronic corticosteroid therapy should be monitored with special care for infection).
   No products indexed under this heading.

Hydrocortisone Hemisuccinate (Patients requiring chronic corticosteroid therapy should be monitored with special care for infection).
   No products indexed under this heading.

Hydrocortisone Probutate (Patients requiring chronic corticosteroid therapy should be monitored with special care for infection).
   No products indexed under this heading.

Hydrocortisone Sodium Phosphate (Patients requiring chronic corticosteroid therapy should be monitored with special care for infection).
   No products indexed under this heading.

Hydrocortisone Sodium Succinate (Patients requiring chronic corticosteroid therapy should be monitored with special care for infection).
   No products indexed under this heading.

Hydrocortisone Valerate (Patients requiring chronic corticosteroid therapy should be monitored with special care for infection).
   No products indexed under this heading.

Hypericum (The metabolism of progestogens may be increased by concomitant use of substances known to induce drug-metabolizing liver enzymes, specifically cytochrome P450 enzymes).
   No products indexed under this heading.

Hypericum Perforatum (The metabolism of progestogens may be increased by concomitant use of substances known to induce drug-metabolizing liver enzymes, specifically cytochrome P450 enzymes). Products include:

Insulin (Patients receiving insulin for diabetes should be monitored with special care for infection).
   No products indexed under this heading.

Insulin, Human, Zinc Suspension (Patients receiving insulin for diabetes should be monitored with special care for infection).
   No products indexed under this heading.

Insulin, Human (rDNA origin) (Patients receiving insulin for diabetes should be monitored with special care for infection). Products include:

Insulin, Human NPH (Patients receiving insulin for diabetes should be monitored with special care for infection). Products include:

Insulin, Human Regular (Patients receiving insulin for diabetes should be monitored with special care for infection). Products include:

Insulin, Human Regular and Human NPH Mixture (Patients receiving insulin for diabetes should be monitored with special care for infection). Products include:

IMPORTANT NOTE: Always consult each drug listing in the patient's regimen for possible interactions.

Insulin, NPH (Patients receiving insulin for diabetes should be monitored with special care for infection).
No products indexed under this heading.

Insulin, Regular (Patients receiving insulin for diabetes should be monitored with special care for infection).
No products indexed under this heading.

Insulin, Regular and NPH mixture (Patients receiving insulin for diabetes should be monitored with special care for infection).
No products indexed under this heading.

Insulin, Zinc Crystals (Patients receiving insulin for diabetes should be monitored with special care for infection).
No products indexed under this heading.

Insulin, Zinc Suspension (Patients receiving insulin for diabetes should be monitored with special care for infection).
No products indexed under this heading.

Insulin Aspart (Patients receiving insulin for diabetes should be monitored with special care for infection).
No products indexed under this heading.

Insulin Aspart, Human (Patients receiving insulin for diabetes should be monitored with special care for infection). Products include:
NovoLog Mix 70/30 2581

Insulin Aspart, Human Regular (Patients receiving insulin for diabetes should be monitored with special care for infection). Products include:
NovoLog 2575

Insulin Aspart Protamine, Human (Patients receiving insulin for diabetes should be monitored with special care for infection). Products include:
NovoLog Mix 70/30 2581

Insulin Detemir (rDNA Origin) (Patients receiving insulin for diabetes should be monitored with special care for infection). Products include:
Levemir 2566

Insulin Glargine (Patients receiving insulin for diabetes should be monitored with special care for infection). Products include:
Lantus 2996

Insulin Glulisine (Patients receiving insulin for diabetes should be monitored with special care for infection). Products include:
Apidra 2937
Apidra SoloStar 2937

Insulin Lispro, Human (Patients receiving insulin for diabetes should be monitored with special care for infection). Products include:
Humalog 1910
Humalog Mix 1914
Humalog Mix 75/25 1917

Insulin Lispro Protamine, Human (Patients receiving insulin for diabetes should be monitored with special care for infection). Products include:
Humalog Mix 1914
Humalog Mix 75/25 1917

Lansoprazole (The metabolism of progestogens may be increased by concomitant use of substances known to induce drug-metabolizing liver enzymes, specifically cytochrome P450 enzymes).
No products indexed under this heading.

Low Molecular Weight Heparins (Levonorgestrel releasing intrauterine system should be used with caution in patients who are receiving anticoagulants).
No products indexed under this heading.

Mephenytoin (The metabolism of progestogens may be increased by concomitant use of substances known to induce drug-metabolizing liver enzymes, specifically cytochrome P450 enzymes).
No products indexed under this heading.

Methsuximide (The metabolism of progestogens may be increased by concomitant use of substances known to induce drug-metabolizing liver enzymes, specifically cytochrome P450 enzymes).
No products indexed under this heading.

Methylprednisolone (Patients requiring chronic corticosteroid therapy should be monitored with special care for infection).
No products indexed under this heading.

Methylprednisolone Acetate (Patients requiring chronic corticosteroid therapy should be monitored with special care for infection).
No products indexed under this heading.

Methylprednisolone Sodium Succinate (Patients requiring chronic corticosteroid therapy should be monitored with special care for infection).
No products indexed under this heading.

Modafinil (The metabolism of progestogens may be increased by concomitant use of substances known to induce drug-metabolizing liver enzymes, specifically cytochrome P450 enzymes). Products include:
Provigil 983

Mometasone Furoate (Patients requiring chronic corticosteroid therapy should be monitored with special care for infection). Products include:
Asmanex 3058
Elocon Cream 3111
Elocon Lotion 3112
Elocon Ointment 3114

Mometasone Furoate Monohydrate (Patients requiring chronic corticosteroid therapy should be monitored with special care for infection). Products include:
Nasonex 3166

Nafcillin Sodium (The metabolism of progestogens may be increased by concomitant use of substances known to induce drug-metabolizing liver enzymes, specifically cytochrome P450 enzymes).
No products indexed under this heading.

Nevirapine (The metabolism of progestogens may be increased by concomitant use of substances known to induce drug-metabolizing liver enzymes, specifically cytochrome P450 enzymes). Products include:
Viramune Oral Suspension 897
Viramune Tablets 897

Nicotine (The metabolism of progestogens may be increased by concomitant use of substances known to induce drug-metabolizing liver enzymes, specifically cytochrome P450 enzymes).
No products indexed under this heading.

Nicotine Polacrilex (The metabolism of progestogens may be increased by concomitant use of substances known to induce drug-metabolizing liver enzymes, specifically cytochrome P450 enzymes).
No products indexed under this heading.

Nicotine Salicylate (The metabolism of progestogens may be increased by concomitant use of substances known to induce drug-metabolizing liver enzymes, specifically cytochrome P450 enzymes).
No products indexed under this heading.

Nicotine Sulfate (The metabolism of progestogens may be increased by concomitant use of substances known to induce drug-metabolizing liver enzymes, specifically cytochrome P450 enzymes).
No products indexed under this heading.

Norethindrone (The metabolism of progestogens may be increased by concomitant use of substances known to induce drug-metabolizing liver enzymes, specifically cytochrome P450 enzymes). Products include:
Ortho Micronor 2660

Norethindrone Acetate (The metabolism of progestogens may be increased by concomitant use of substances known to induce drug-metabolizing liver enzymes, specifically cytochrome P450 enzymes). Products include:
Activella 2561

Omeprazole (The metabolism of progestogens may be increased by concomitant use of substances known to induce drug-metabolizing liver enzymes, specifically cytochrome P450 enzymes).
No products indexed under this heading.

Omeprazole Magnesium (The metabolism of progestogens may be increased by concomitant use of substances known to induce drug-metabolizing liver enzymes, specifically cytochrome P450 enzymes).
No products indexed under this heading.

Oxcarbazepine (The metabolism of progestogens may be increased by concomitant use of substances known to induce drug-metabolizing liver enzymes, specifically cytochrome P450 enzymes).
No products indexed under this heading.

Phenobarbital (The metabolism of progestogens may be increased by concomitant use of substances known to induce drug-metabolizing liver enzymes, specifically cytochrome P450 enzymes). Products include:
Donnatal 2711

Phenobarbital Sodium (The metabolism of progestogens may be increased by concomitant use of substances known to induce drug-metabolizing liver enzymes, specifically cytochrome P450 enzymes).
No products indexed under this heading.

Phenylbutazone (The metabolism of progestogens may be increased by concomitant use of substances known to induce drug-metabolizing liver enzymes, specifically cytochrome P450 enzymes).
No products indexed under this heading.

Phenytoin (The metabolism of progestogens may be increased by concomitant use of substances known to induce drug-metabolizing liver enzymes, specifically cytochrome P450 enzymes).
No products indexed under this heading.

Phenytoin Sodium (The metabolism of progestogens may be increased by concomitant use of substances known to induce drug-metabolizing liver enzymes, specifically cytochrome P450 enzymes). Products include:
Phenytek Capsules 2380

Prednisolone (Patients requiring chronic corticosteroid therapy should be monitored with special care for infection).
No products indexed under this heading.

Prednisolone Acetate (Patients requiring chronic corticosteroid therapy should be monitored with special care for infection). Products include:
Blephamide .... ⊙212, ⊙214
Pred Forte .... ⊙225
Pred Mild .... ⊙230

Pred-G .... ⊙226, ⊙227

Prednisolone Sodium Phosphate (Patients requiring chronic corticosteroid therapy should be monitored with special care for infection).
No products indexed under this heading.

Prednisolone Tebutate (Patients requiring chronic corticosteroid therapy should be monitored with special care for infection).
No products indexed under this heading.

Prednisone (Patients requiring chronic corticosteroid therapy should be monitored with special care for infection).
No products indexed under this heading.

Prednisone sodium phosphate (Patients requiring chronic corticosteroid therapy should be monitored with special care for infection).
No products indexed under this heading.

Primidone (The metabolism of progestogens may be increased by concomitant use of substances known to induce drug-metabolizing liver enzymes, specifically cytochrome P450 enzymes).
No products indexed under this heading.

Rifabutin (The metabolism of progestogens may be increased by concomitant use of substances known to induce drug-metabolizing liver enzymes, specifically cytochrome P450 enzymes).
No products indexed under this heading.

Rifampicin (The metabolism of progestogens may be increased by concomitant use of substances known to induce drug-metabolizing liver enzymes, specifically cytochrome P450 enzymes).
No products indexed under this heading.

Rifampin (The metabolism of progestogens may be increased by concomitant use of substances known to induce drug-metabolizing liver enzymes, specifically cytochrome P450 enzymes).
No products indexed under this heading.

Rifapentine (The metabolism of progestogens may be increased by concomitant use of substances known to induce drug-metabolizing liver enzymes, specifically cytochrome P450 enzymes).
No products indexed under this heading.

Ritonavir (The metabolism of progestogens may be increased by concomitant use of substances known to induce drug-metabolizing liver enzymes, specifically cytochrome P450 enzymes). Products include:
Kaletra 458
Norvir 509

Secobarbital Sodium (The metabolism of progestogens may be increased by concomitant use of substances known to induce drug-metabolizing liver enzymes, specifically cytochrome P450 enzymes).
No products indexed under this heading.

Sulfinpyrazone (The metabolism of progestogens may be increased by concomitant use of substances known to induce drug-metabolizing liver enzymes, specifically cytochrome P450 enzymes).
No products indexed under this heading.

Theophyllinate (The metabolism of progestogens may be increased by concomitant use of substances known to induce drug-metabolizing liver enzymes, specifically cytochrome P450 enzymes).
No products indexed under this heading.

1141 Interactions Index Moban

Theophylline (The metabolism of progestogens may be increased by concomitant use of substances known to induce drug-metabolizing liver enzymes, specifically cytochrome P450 enzymes).
No products indexed under this heading.

Theophylline Anhydrous (The metabolism of progestogens may be increased by concomitant use of substances known to induce drug-metabolizing liver enzymes, specifically cytochrome P450 enzymes). Products include:
Uniphyl ... 2817

Theophylline Calcium Salicylate (The metabolism of progestogens may be increased by concomitant use of substances known to induce drug-metabolizing liver enzymes, specifically cytochrome P450 enzymes).
No products indexed under this heading.

Theophylline Dihydroxypropyl (Glyceryl) (The metabolism of progestogens may be increased by concomitant use of substances known to induce drug-metabolizing liver enzymes, specifically cytochrome P450 enzymes).
No products indexed under this heading.

Theophylline Ethylenediamine (The metabolism of progestogens may be increased by concomitant use of substances known to induce drug-metabolizing liver enzymes, specifically cytochrome P450 enzymes).
No products indexed under this heading.

Theophylline Sodium Glycinate (The metabolism of progestogens may be increased by concomitant use of substances known to induce drug-metabolizing liver enzymes, specifically cytochrome P450 enzymes).
No products indexed under this heading.

Tinzaparin Sodium (Levonorgestrel releasing intrauterine system should be used with caution in patients who are receiving anticoagulants).
No products indexed under this heading.

Tobacco (The metabolism of progestogens may be increased by concomitant use of substances known to induce drug-metabolizing liver enzymes, specifically cytochrome P450 enzymes).
No products indexed under this heading.

Tolazamide (The metabolism of progestogens may be increased by concomitant use of substances known to induce drug-metabolizing liver enzymes, specifically cytochrome P450 enzymes).
No products indexed under this heading.

Tolbutamide (The metabolism of progestogens may be increased by concomitant use of substances known to induce drug-metabolizing liver enzymes, specifically cytochrome P450 enzymes).
No products indexed under this heading.

Triamcinolone (Patients requiring chronic corticosteroid therapy should be monitored with special care for infection).
No products indexed under this heading.

Triamcinolone Acetonide (Patients requiring chronic corticosteroid therapy should be monitored with special care for infection). Products include:
Azmacort ... 408
Nasacort AQ ... 3019

Triamcinolone Diacetate (Patients requiring chronic corticosteroid therapy should be monitored with special care for infection).
No products indexed under this heading.

Triamcinolone Hexacetonide (Patients requiring chronic corticosteroid therapy should be monitored with special care for infection).
No products indexed under this heading.

Troglitazone (The metabolism of progestogens may be increased by concomitant use of substances known to induce drug-metabolizing liver enzymes, specifically cytochrome P450 enzymes).
No products indexed under this heading.

Warfarin Sodium (Levonorgestrel releasing intrauterine system should be used with caution in patients who are receiving anticoagulants).
No products indexed under this heading.

Food Interactions

Broccoli (The metabolism of progestogens may be increased by concomitant use of substances known to induce drug-metabolizing liver enzymes, specifically cytochrome P450 enzymes).

Brussel Sprouts (The metabolism of progestogens may be increased by concomitant use of substances known to induce drug-metabolizing liver enzymes, specifically cytochrome P450 enzymes).

Charbroiled Food (The metabolism of progestogens may be increased by concomitant use of substances known to induce drug-metabolizing liver enzymes, specifically cytochrome P450 enzymes).

M-M-R II
(Measles, Mumps & Rubella Virus Vaccine, Live) ... 2203
May interact with immunosuppressive agents. Compounds in these categories include:

Azathioprine (Concurrent administration with immunosuppressant is contraindicated).
No products indexed under this heading.

Basiliximab (Concurrent administration with immunosuppressant is contraindicated). Products include:
Simulect ... 2524

Cyclosporine (Concurrent administration with immunosuppressant is contraindicated). Products include:
Gengraf ... 440
Neoral Oral Solution ... 2496
Neoral Capsules ... 2496
Restasis ... 605

Muromonab-CD3 (Concurrent administration with immunosuppressant is contraindicated). Products include:
Orthoclone OKT3 ... 949

Mycophenolate Mofetil (Concurrent administration with immunosuppressant is contraindicated).
No products indexed under this heading.

Rapamycin (Concurrent administration with immunosuppressant is contraindicated).
No products indexed under this heading.

Sirolimus (Concurrent administration with immunosuppressant is contraindicated). Products include:
Rapamune ... 3579

Tacrolimus (Concurrent administration with immunosuppressant is contraindicated). Products include:
Prograf Capsules ... 677
Prograf Injection ... 677
Protopic ... 685

MOBAN TABLETS
(Molindone Hydrochloride) ... 1108
May interact with alcohols, barbiturates, narcotic analgesics, phenytoin, tetracyclines. Compounds in these categories include:

Alfentanil Hydrochloride (Concomitant use of molindone with narcotics is contraindicated).
No products indexed under this heading.

Amobarbital (Concomitant use of molindone with barbiturates is contraindicated).
No products indexed under this heading.

Amobarbital Sodium (Concomitant use of molindone with barbiturates is contraindicated).
No products indexed under this heading.

Apomorphine (Concomitant use of molindone with narcotics is contraindicated).
No products indexed under this heading.

Apomorphine Hydrochloride (Concomitant use of molindone with narcotics is contraindicated).
No products indexed under this heading.

Aprobarbital (Concomitant use of molindone with barbiturates is contraindicated).
No products indexed under this heading.

Buprenorphine Hydrochloride (Concomitant use of molindone with narcotics is contraindicated).
No products indexed under this heading.

Butabarbital (Concomitant use of molindone with barbiturates is contraindicated).
No products indexed under this heading.

Butabarbital Sodium (Concomitant use of molindone with barbiturates is contraindicated).
No products indexed under this heading.

Butalbital (Concomitant use of molindone with barbiturates is contraindicated).
No products indexed under this heading.

Codeine Phosphate (Concomitant use of molindone with narcotics is contraindicated). Products include:
Tylenol with Codeine ... 2691

Codeine Sulfate (Concomitant use of molindone with narcotics is contraindicated).
No products indexed under this heading.

Demeclocycline Hydrochloride (Molindone contains calcium sulfate as an excipient and that calcium ions may interfere with the absorption of preparations containingphenytoin sodium and tetracyclines).
No products indexed under this heading.

Dezocine (Concomitant use of molindone with narcotics is contraindicated).
No products indexed under this heading.

Dihydrocodeine Bitartrate (Concomitant use of molindone with narcotics is contraindicated).
No products indexed under this heading.

Dihydrocodeinone Bitartrate (Concomitant use of molindone with narcotics is contraindicated).
No products indexed under this heading.

Doxycycline (Molindone contains calcium sulfate as an excipient and that calcium ions may interfere with the absorption of preparations containing-phenytoin sodium and tetracyclines).
No products indexed under this heading.

Doxycycline Calcium (Molindone contains calcium sulfate as an excipient and that calcium ions may interfere with the absorption of preparations containingphenytoin sodium and tetracyclines).
No products indexed under this heading.

Doxycycline Hyclate (Molindone contains calcium sulfate as an excipient and that calcium ions may interfere with the absorption of preparations containingphenytoin sodium and tetracyclines).
No products indexed under this heading.

Doxycycline Monohydrate (Molindone contains calcium sulfate as an excipient and that calcium ions may interfere with the absorption of preparations containingphenytoin sodium and tetracyclines).
No products indexed under this heading.

Ethanol (Concomitant use of molindone with alcohol is contraindicated).
No products indexed under this heading.

Ethyl Alcohol (Concomitant use of molindone with alcohol is contraindicated).
No products indexed under this heading.

Fentanyl (Concomitant use of molindone with narcotics is contraindicated). Products include:
Duragesic ... 2604
Fentanyl Transdermal System ... 2346
Onsolis ... 2054

Fentanyl Citrate (Concomitant use of molindone with narcotics is contraindicated). Products include:
Fentora ... 966

Fosphenytoin (Molindone contains calcium sulfate as an excipient and that calcium ions may interfere with the absorption of preparations contaning phenytoin sodium).
No products indexed under this heading.

Fosphenytoin Sodium (Molindone contains calcium sulfate as an excipient and that calcium ions may interfere with the absorption of preparations contaning phenytoin sodium).
No products indexed under this heading.

Hexobarbital (Concomitant use of molindone with barbiturates is contraindicated).
No products indexed under this heading.

Hydrocodone Bitartrate (Concomitant use of molindone with narcotics is contraindicated). Products include:
Vicodin ... 560
Vicodin ES ... 561
Vicodin HP ... 563
Vicoprofen ... 564
Zydone ... 1138

Hydrocodone Polistirex (Concomitant use of molindone with narcotics is contraindicated). Products include:
Tussionex ... 3443

Hydromorphone (Concomitant use of molindone with narcotics is contraindicated).
No products indexed under this heading.

Hydromorphone Hydrochloride (Concomitant use of molindone with narcotics is contraindicated). Products include:
Dilaudid Injection ... 2800
Dilaudid Oral ... 2797
Dilaudid Tablets ... 2797
Dilaudid-HP ... 2800

Levorphanol Tartrate (Concomitant use of molindone with narcotics is contraindicated).
No products indexed under this heading.

Meperidine Hydrochloride (Concomitant use of molindone with narcotics is contraindicated).
No products indexed under this heading.

Mephobarbital (Concomitant use of molindone with barbiturates is contraindicated).
No products indexed under this heading.

Methacycline Hydrochloride (Molindone contains calcium sulfate as an excipient and that calcium ions may interfere with the absorption of preparations containingphenytoin sodium and tetracyclines).
No products indexed under this heading.

Methadone Hydrochloride (Concomitant use of molindone with narcotics is contraindicated).
No products indexed under this heading.

Minocycline Hydrochloride (Molindone contains calcium sulfate as an excipient and that calcium ions may interfere with the absorption of preparations containingphenytoin sodium and tetracyclines). Products include:
Solodyn ... 2073

Morphine Sulfate (Concomitant use of molindone with narcotics is contraindicated). Products include:
Avinza ... 1822
Embeda ... 1831

IMPORTANT NOTE: Always consult each drug listing in the patient's regimen for possible interactions.

Food Interactions

Alcohol (Concomitant use of molindone with alcohol is contraindicated).

Beer, reduced-alcohol (Concomitant use of molindone with alcohol is contraindicated).

Beer, unspecified (Concomitant use of molindone with alcohol is contraindicated).

Wine, Chianti (Concomitant use of molindone with alcohol is contraindicated).

Wine, Red (Concomitant use of molindone with alcohol is contraindicated).

Wine, unspecified (Concomitant use of molindone with alcohol is contraindicated).

Wine products (Concomitant use of molindone with alcohol is contraindicated).

MOTRIN IB TABLETS AND CAPLETS

(Ibuprofen) 2043
May interact with anticoagulants, aspirin-acetylsalicylic acid, corticosteroids, non-steroidal anti-inflammatory agents, and certain other agents. Compounds in these categories include:

1143 **Interactions Index** **Children's Motrin**

Heparin Calcium (Increased risk of stomach bleeding if co-administered with anticoagulants).
No products indexed under this heading.

Heparin Sodium (Increased risk of stomach bleeding if co-administered with anticoagulants).
No products indexed under this heading.

Hydrocortisone (Increased risk of stomach bleeding if co-administered with steroidal drugs).
No products indexed under this heading.

Hydrocortisone (Alcohol) (Increased risk of stomach bleeding if co-administered with steroidal drugs).
No products indexed under this heading.

Hydrocortisone Acetate (Increased risk of stomach bleeding if co-administered with steroidal drugs).
No products indexed under this heading.

Hydrocortisone Butyrate (Increased risk of stomach bleeding if co-administered with steroidal drugs).
No products indexed under this heading.

Hydrocortisone Cypionate (Increased risk of stomach bleeding if co-administered with steroidal drugs).
No products indexed under this heading.

Hydrocortisone Hemisuccinate (Increased risk of stomach bleeding if co-administered with steroidal drugs).
No products indexed under this heading.

Hydrocortisone Probutate (Increased risk of stomach bleeding if co-administered with steroidal drugs).
No products indexed under this heading.

Hydrocortisone Sodium Phosphate (Increased risk of stomach bleeding if co-administered with steroidal drugs).
No products indexed under this heading.

Hydrocortisone Sodium Succinate (Increased risk of stomach bleeding if co-administered with steroidal drugs).
No products indexed under this heading.

Hydrocortisone Valerate (Increased risk of stomach bleeding if co-administered with steroidal drugs).
No products indexed under this heading.

Indomethacin (Increased risk of stomach bleeding if co-administered with non-steroidal anti-inflammatory drugs). Products include:
Indocin 2167

Indomethacin Sodium Trihydrate (Increased risk of stomach bleeding if co-administered with non-steroidal anti-inflammatory drugs). Products include:
Indocin I.V. 2007

Ketoprofen (Increased risk of stomach bleeding if co-administered with non-steroidal anti-inflammatory drugs).
No products indexed under this heading.

Ketorolac Tromethamine (Increased risk of stomach bleeding if co-administered with non-steroidal anti-inflammatory drugs). Products include:
Acuvail .... ⊙209

Low Molecular Weight Heparins (Increased risk of stomach bleeding if co-administered with anticoagulants).
No products indexed under this heading.

Meclofenamate Sodium (Increased risk of stomach bleeding if co-administered with non-steroidal anti-inflammatory drugs).
No products indexed under this heading.

Mefenamic Acid (Increased risk of stomach bleeding if co-administered with non-steroidal anti-inflammatory drugs).
No products indexed under this heading.

Meloxicam (Increased risk of stomach bleeding if co-administered with non-steroidal anti-inflammatory drugs).
No products indexed under this heading.

Methylprednisolone (Increased risk of stomach bleeding if co-administered with steroidal drugs).
No products indexed under this heading.

Methylprednisolone Acetate (Increased risk of stomach bleeding if co-administered with steroidal drugs).
No products indexed under this heading.

Methylprednisolone Sodium Succinate (Increased risk of stomach bleeding if co-administered with steroidal drugs).
No products indexed under this heading.

Mometasone Furoate (Increased risk of stomach bleeding if co-administered with steroidal drugs). Products include:
Asmanex 3058
Elocon Cream 3111
Elocon Lotion 3112
Elocon Ointment 3114

Mometasone Furoate Monohydrate (Increased risk of stomach bleeding if co-administered with steroidal drugs). Products include:
Nasonex 3166

Nabumetone (Increased risk of stomach bleeding if co-administered with non-steroidal anti-inflammatory drugs).
No products indexed under this heading.

Naproxen (Increased risk of stomach bleeding if co-administered with non-steroidal anti-inflammatory drugs). Products include:
EC-Naprosyn 2850
Naprosyn 2850
Anaprox/Naprosyn 2850

Naproxen Sodium (Increased risk of stomach bleeding if co-administered with non-steroidal anti-inflammatory drugs). Products include:
Anaprox 2850
Anaprox DS 2850
Treximet 1681

Oxaprozin (Increased risk of stomach bleeding if co-administered with non-steroidal anti-inflammatory drugs).
No products indexed under this heading.

Phenylbutazone (Increased risk of stomach bleeding if co-administered with non-steroidal anti-inflammatory drugs).
No products indexed under this heading.

Piroxicam (Increased risk of stomach bleeding if co-administered with non-steroidal anti-inflammatory drugs).
No products indexed under this heading.

Prednisolone (Increased risk of stomach bleeding if co-administered with steroidal drugs).
No products indexed under this heading.

Prednisolone Acetate (Increased risk of stomach bleeding if co-administered with steroidal drugs). Products include:
Blephamide .... ⊙212, ⊙214
Pred Forte .... ⊙225
Pred Mild .... ⊙230
Pred-G .... ⊙226, ⊙227

Prednisolone Sodium Phosphate (Increased risk of stomach bleeding if co-administered with steroidal drugs).
No products indexed under this heading.

Prednisolone Tebutate (Increased risk of stomach bleeding if co-administered with steroidal drugs).
No products indexed under this heading.

Prednisone (Increased risk of stomach bleeding if co-administered with steroidal drugs).
No products indexed under this heading.

Prednisone sodium phosphate (Increased risk of stomach bleeding if co-administered with steroidal drugs).
No products indexed under this heading.

Rofecoxib (Increased risk of stomach bleeding if co-administered with non-steroidal anti-inflammatory drugs).
No products indexed under this heading.

Sulindac (Increased risk of stomach bleeding if co-administered with non-steroidal anti-inflammatory drugs). Products include:
Clinoril 2098

Tinzaparin Sodium (Increased risk of stomach bleeding if co-administered with anticoagulants).
No products indexed under this heading.

Tolmetin Sodium (Increased risk of stomach bleeding if co-administered with non-steroidal anti-inflammatory drugs).
No products indexed under this heading.

Triamcinolone (Increased risk of stomach bleeding if co-administered with steroidal drugs).
No products indexed under this heading.

Triamcinolone Acetonide (Increased risk of stomach bleeding if co-administered with steroidal drugs). Products include:
Azmacort 408
Nasacort AQ 3019

Triamcinolone Diacetate (Increased risk of stomach bleeding if co-administered with steroidal drugs).
No products indexed under this heading.

Triamcinolone Hexacetonide (Increased risk of stomach bleeding if co-administered with steroidal drugs).
No products indexed under this heading.

Valdecoxib (Increased risk of stomach bleeding if co-administered with non-steroidal anti-inflammatory drugs).
No products indexed under this heading.

Warfarin Sodium (Increased risk of stomach bleeding if co-administered with anticoagulants).
No products indexed under this heading.

CHILDREN'S MOTRIN DOSING CHART 2043

CHILDREN'S MOTRIN ORAL SUSPENSION

(Ibuprofen) 2044
May interact with anticoagulants, aspirin-acetylsalicylic acid, corticosteroids, diuretics, non-steroidal anti-inflammatory agents, and certain other agents. Compounds in these categories include:

Alclometasone Dipropionate (Ibuprofen is a non-steroidal anti-inflammatory drug (NSAID), which may cause stomach bleeding. The chance of this is higher if the patient (child) is taking a steroid drug).
No products indexed under this heading.

Amiloride Hydrochloride (Consult a doctor before use if taking a diuretic).
No products indexed under this heading.

Anisindione (Ibuprofen is a non-steroidal anti-inflammatory drug (NSAID), which may cause stomach bleeding. The chance of this is higher if the patient (child) is taking a blood thinning (anticoagulant) drug).
No products indexed under this heading.

Ardeparin Sodium (Ibuprofen is a non-steroidal anti-inflammatory drug (NSAID), which may cause stomach bleeding. The chance of this is higher if the patient (child) is taking a blood thinning (anticoagulant) drug).
No products indexed under this heading.

Aspirin (Ibuprofen is a non-steroidal anti-inflammatory drug (NSAID), which may cause stomach bleeding. The chance of this is higher if the patient (child) is taking other drugs containing an NSAID (eg, aspirin, ibuprofen, naproxen, or others)). Products include:
Aggrenox 880
Bayer Aspirin 829
Percodan 1124
St. Joseph Aspirin 2045

Aspirin, Enteric Coated (Ibuprofen is a non-steroidal anti-inflammatory drug (NSAID), which may cause stomach bleeding. The chance of this is higher if the patient (child) is taking other drugs containing an NSAID (eg, aspirin, ibuprofen, naproxen, or others)).
No products indexed under this heading.

Aspirin Buffered (Ibuprofen is a non-steroidal anti-inflammatory drug (NSAID), which may cause stomach bleeding. The chance of this is higher if the patient (child) is taking other drugs containing an NSAID (eg, aspirin, ibuprofen, naproxen, or others)).
No products indexed under this heading.

Beclomethasone Dipropionate (Ibuprofen is a non-steroidal anti-inflammatory drug (NSAID), which may cause stomach bleeding. The chance of this is higher if the patient (child) is taking a steroid drug). Products include:
Qvar 3398

Beclomethasone Dipropionate Monohydrate (Ibuprofen is a non-steroidal anti-inflammatory drug (NSAID), which may cause stomach bleeding. The chance of this is higher if the patient (child) is taking a steroid drug). Products include:
Beconase AQ 1386

Bendroflumethiazide (Consult a doctor before use if taking a diuretic).
No products indexed under this heading.

Betamethasone (Ibuprofen is a non-steroidal anti-inflammatory drug (NSAID), which may cause stomach bleeding. The chance of this is higher if the patient (child) is taking a steroid drug).
No products indexed under this heading.

Betamethasone Acetate (Ibuprofen is a non-steroidal anti-inflammatory drug (NSAID), which may cause stomach bleeding. The chance of this is higher if the patient (child) is taking a steroid drug).
No products indexed under this heading.

Betamethasone Benzoate (Ibuprofen is a non-steroidal anti-inflammatory drug (NSAID), which may cause stomach bleeding. The chance of this is higher if the patient (child) is taking a steroid drug).
No products indexed under this heading.

Betamethasone Dipropionate (Ibuprofen is a non-steroidal anti-inflammatory drug (NSAID), which may cause stomach bleeding. The chance of this is higher if the patient (child) is taking a steroid drug). Products include:
Diprolene Lotion 0.05% 3108
Diprolene Ointment 0.05% 3109
Diprolene AF Cream 0.05% 3107
Lotrisone 3163

Betamethasone Sodium Phosphate (Ibuprofen is a non-steroidal anti-inflammatory drug (NSAID), which may cause stomach bleeding. The chance of this is higher if the patient (child) is taking a steroid drug).
No products indexed under this heading.

Betamethasone Valerate (Ibuprofen is a non-steroidal anti-inflammatory drug (NSAID), which may cause stomach bleeding. The chance of this is higher if the patient (child) is taking a steroid drug). Products include:
Luxíq 3321

Budesonide (Ibuprofen is a non-steroidal anti-inflammatory drug (NSAID), which may cause stomach bleeding. The chance of this is higher if the patient (child) is taking a steroid drug). Products include:
Pulmicort Flexhaler 714
Symbicort 80/4.5 720
Symbicort 160/4.5 720

Bumetanide (Consult a doctor before use if taking a diuretic).
No products indexed under this heading.

IMPORTANT NOTE: Always consult each drug listing in the patient's regimen for possible interactions.

Celecoxib (Ibuprofen is a non-steroidal anti-inflammatory drug (NSAID), which may cause stomach bleeding. The chance of this is higher if the patient (child) is taking other drugs containing an NSAID (eg, aspirin, ibuprofen, naproxen, or others)). Products include:

Chlorothiazide (Consult a doctor before use if taking a diuretic).
No products indexed under this heading.

Chlorothiazide Sodium (Consult a doctor before use if taking a diuretic). Products include:

Chlorthalidone (Consult a doctor before use if taking a diuretic). Products include:

Ciclesonide (Ibuprofen is a non-steroidal anti-inflammatory drug (NSAID), which may cause stomach bleeding. The chance of this is higher if the patient (child) is taking a steroid drug).
No products indexed under this heading.

Cortisone Acetate (Ibuprofen is a non-steroidal anti-inflammatory drug (NSAID), which may cause stomach bleeding. The chance of this is higher if the patient (child) is taking a steroid drug).
No products indexed under this heading.

Dalteparin Sodium (Ibuprofen is a non-steroidal anti-inflammatory drug (NSAID), which may cause stomach bleeding. The chance of this is higher if the patient (child) is taking a blood thinning (anticoagulant) drug). Products include:

Danaparoid Sodium (Ibuprofen is a non-steroidal anti-inflammatory drug (NSAID), which may cause stomach bleeding. The chance of this is higher if the patient (child) is taking a blood thinning (anticoagulant) drug).
No products indexed under this heading.

Desoximetasone (Ibuprofen is a non-steroidal anti-inflammatory drug (NSAID), which may cause stomach bleeding. The chance of this is higher if the patient (child) is taking a steroid drug).
No products indexed under this heading.

Dexamethasone (Ibuprofen is a non-steroidal anti-inflammatory drug (NSAID), which may cause stomach bleeding. The chance of this is higher if the patient (child) is taking a steroid drug). Products include:

Dexamethasone Acetate (Ibuprofen is a non-steroidal anti-inflammatory drug (NSAID), which may cause stomach bleeding. The chance of this is higher if the patient (child) is taking a steroid drug).
No products indexed under this heading.

Dexamethasone Phosphate (Ibuprofen is a non-steroidal anti-inflammatory drug (NSAID), which may cause stomach bleeding. The chance of this is higher if the patient (child) is taking a steroid drug).
No products indexed under this heading.

Dexamethasone Sodium (Ibuprofen is a non-steroidal anti-inflammatory drug (NSAID), which may cause stomach bleeding. The chance of this is higher if the patient (child) is taking a steroid drug).
No products indexed under this heading.

Dexamethasone Sodium Phosphate (Ibuprofen is a non-steroidal anti-inflammatory drug (NSAID), which may cause stomach bleeding. The chance of this is higher if the patient (child) is taking a steroid drug).
No products indexed under this heading.

Dexamethasone Sodium Phosphate Injection (Ibuprofen is a non-steroidal anti-inflammatory drug (NSAID), which may cause stomach bleeding. The chance of this is higher if the patient (child) is taking a steroid drug).
No products indexed under this heading.

Diclofenac Epolamine (Ibuprofen is a non-steroidal anti-inflammatory drug (NSAID), which may cause stomach bleeding. The chance of this is higher if the patient (child) is taking other drugs containing an NSAID (eg, aspirin, ibuprofen, naproxen, or others)). Products include:

Diclofenac Potassium (Ibuprofen is a non-steroidal anti-inflammatory drug (NSAID), which may cause stomach bleeding. The chance of this is higher if the patient (child) is taking other drugs containing an NSAID (eg, aspirin, ibuprofen, naproxen, or others)).
No products indexed under this heading.

Diclofenac Sodium (Ibuprofen is a non-steroidal anti-inflammatory drug (NSAID), which may cause stomach bleeding. The chance of this is higher if the patient (child) is taking other drugs containing an NSAID (eg, aspirin, ibuprofen, naproxen, or others)).
No products indexed under this heading.

Dicumarol (Ibuprofen is a non-steroidal anti-inflammatory drug (NSAID), which may cause stomach bleeding. The chance of this is higher if the patient (child) is taking a blood thinning (anticoagulant) drug).
No products indexed under this heading.

Diflorasone Diacetate (Ibuprofen is a non-steroidal anti-inflammatory drug (NSAID), which may cause stomach bleeding. The chance of this is higher if the patient (child) is taking a steroid drug).
No products indexed under this heading.

Enoxaparin Sodium (Ibuprofen is a non-steroidal anti-inflammatory drug (NSAID), which may cause stomach bleeding. The chance of this is higher if the patient (child) is taking a blood thinning (anticoagulant) drug). Products include:

Ethacrynic Acid (Consult a doctor before use if taking a diuretic).
No products indexed under this heading.

Etodolac (Ibuprofen is a non-steroidal anti-inflammatory drug (NSAID), which may cause stomach bleeding. The chance of this is higher if the patient (child) is taking other drugs containing an NSAID (eg, aspirin, ibuprofen, naproxen, or others)).
No products indexed under this heading.

Fenoprofen Calcium (Ibuprofen is a non-steroidal anti-inflammatory drug (NSAID), which may cause stomach bleeding. The chance of this is higher if the patient (child) is taking other drugs containing an NSAID (eg, aspirin, ibuprofen, naproxen, or others)).
No products indexed under this heading.

Fludrocortisone Acetate (Ibuprofen is a non-steroidal anti-inflammatory drug (NSAID), which may cause stomach bleeding. The chance of this is higher if the patient (child) is taking a steroid drug).
No products indexed under this heading.

Flumethasone Pivalate (Ibuprofen is a non-steroidal anti-inflammatory drug (NSAID), which may cause stomach bleeding. The chance of this is higher if the patient (child) is taking a steroid drug).
No products indexed under this heading.

Flunisolide Hemihydrate (Ibuprofen is a non-steroidal anti-inflammatory drug (NSAID), which may cause stomach bleeding. The chance of this is higher if the patient (child) is taking a steroid drug).
No products indexed under this heading.

Flurbiprofen (Ibuprofen is a non-steroidal anti-inflammatory drug (NSAID), which may cause stomach bleeding. The chance of this is higher if the patient (child) is taking other drugs containing an NSAID (eg, aspirin, ibuprofen, naproxen, or others)).
No products indexed under this heading.

Fluticasone Furoate (Ibuprofen is a non-steroidal anti-inflammatory drug (NSAID), which may cause stomach bleeding. The chance of this is higher if the patient (child) is taking a steroid drug). Products include:

Fluticasone Propionate (Ibuprofen is a non-steroidal anti-inflammatory drug (NSAID), which may cause stomach bleeding. The chance of this is higher if the patient (child) is taking a steroid drug). Products include:

Fondaparinux Sodium (Ibuprofen is a non-steroidal anti-inflammatory drug (NSAID), which may cause stomach bleeding. The chance of this is higher if the patient (child) is taking a blood thinning (anticoagulant) drug). Products include:

Furosemide (Consult a doctor before use if taking a diuretic). Products include:

Heparin Calcium (Ibuprofen is a non-steroidal anti-inflammatory drug (NSAID), which may cause stomach bleeding. The chance of this is higher if the patient (child) is taking a blood thinning (anticoagulant) drug).
No products indexed under this heading.

Heparin Sodium (Ibuprofen is a non-steroidal anti-inflammatory drug (NSAID), which may cause stomach bleeding. The chance of this is higher if the patient (child) is taking a blood thinning (anticoagulant) drug).
No products indexed under this heading.

Hydrochlorothiazide (Consult a doctor before use if taking a diuretic). Products include:

Hydrocortisone (Ibuprofen is a non-steroidal anti-inflammatory drug (NSAID), which may cause stomach bleeding. The chance of this is higher if the patient (child) is taking a steroid drug).
No products indexed under this heading.

Hydrocortisone (Alcohol) (Ibuprofen is a non-steroidal anti-inflammatory drug (NSAID), which may cause stomach bleeding. The chance of this is higher if the patient (child) is taking a steroid drug).
No products indexed under this heading.

Hydrocortisone Acetate (Ibuprofen is a non-steroidal anti-inflammatory drug (NSAID), which may cause stomach bleeding. The chance of this is higher if the patient (child) is taking a steroid drug).
No products indexed under this heading.

Hydrocortisone Butyrate (Ibuprofen is a non-steroidal anti-inflammatory drug (NSAID), which may cause stomach bleeding. The chance of this is higher if the patient (child) is taking a steroid drug).
No products indexed under this heading.

Hydrocortisone Cypionate (Ibuprofen is a non-steroidal anti-inflammatory drug (NSAID), which may cause stomach bleeding. The chance of this is higher if the patient (child) is taking a steroid drug).
No products indexed under this heading.

Hydrocortisone Hemisuccinate (Ibuprofen is a non-steroidal anti-inflammatory drug (NSAID), which may cause stomach bleeding. The chance of this is higher if the patient (child) is taking a steroid drug).
No products indexed under this heading.

Hydrocortisone Probutate (Ibuprofen is a non-steroidal anti-inflammatory drug (NSAID), which may cause stomach bleeding. The chance of this is higher if the patient (child) is taking a steroid drug).
No products indexed under this heading.

Hydrocortisone Sodium Phosphate (Ibuprofen is a non-steroidal anti-inflammatory drug (NSAID), which may cause stomach bleeding. The chance of this is higher if the patient (child) is taking a steroid drug).
No products indexed under this heading.

Hydrocortisone Sodium Succinate (Ibuprofen is a non-steroidal anti-inflammatory drug (NSAID), which may cause stomach bleeding. The chance of this is higher if the patient (child) is taking a steroid drug).
No products indexed under this heading.

Hydrocortisone Valerate (Ibuprofen is a non-steroidal anti-inflammatory drug (NSAID), which may cause stomach bleeding. The chance of this is higher if the patient (child) is taking a steroid drug).
No products indexed under this heading.

Hydroflumethiazide (Consult a doctor before use if taking a diuretic).
No products indexed under this heading.

Ibuprofen Lysine (Ibuprofen is a non-steroidal anti-inflammatory drug (NSAID), which may cause stomach bleeding. The chance of this is higher if the patient (child) is taking other drugs containing an NSAID (eg, aspirin, ibuprofen, naproxen, or others)). Products include:

Indapamide (Consult a doctor before use if taking a diuretic). Products include:

Indomethacin (Ibuprofen is a non-steroidal anti-inflammatory drug (NSAID), which may cause stomach bleeding. The chance of this is higher if

the patient (child) is taking other drugs containing an NSAID (eg, aspirin, ibuprofen, naproxen, or others)). Products include:

Indomethacin Sodium Trihydrate (Ibuprofen is a non-steroidal anti-inflammatory drug (NSAID), which may cause stomach bleeding. The chance of this is higher if the patient (child) is taking other drugs containing an NSAID (eg, aspirin, ibuprofen, naproxen, or others)). Products include:

Ketoprofen (Ibuprofen is a non-steroidal anti-inflammatory drug (NSAID), which may cause stomach bleeding. The chance of this is higher if the patient (child) is taking other drugs containing an NSAID (eg, aspirin, ibuprofen, naproxen, or others)).
No products indexed under this heading.

Ketorolac Tromethamine (Ibuprofen is a non-steroidal anti-inflammatory drug (NSAID), which may cause stomach bleeding. The chance of this is higher if the patient (child) is taking other drugs containing an NSAID (eg, aspirin, ibuprofen, naproxen, or others)). Products include:

Low Molecular Weight Heparins (Ibuprofen is a non-steroidal anti-inflammatory drug (NSAID), which may cause stomach bleeding. The chance of this is higher if the patient (child) is taking a blood thinning (anticoagulant) drug).
No products indexed under this heading.

Meclofenamate Sodium (Ibuprofen is a non-steroidal anti-inflammatory drug (NSAID), which may cause stomach bleeding. The chance of this is higher if the patient (child) is taking other drugs containing an NSAID (eg, aspirin, ibuprofen, naproxen, or others)).
No products indexed under this heading.

Mefenamic Acid (Ibuprofen is a non-steroidal anti-inflammatory drug (NSAID), which may cause stomach bleeding. The chance of this is higher if the patient (child) is taking other drugs containing an NSAID (eg, aspirin, ibuprofen, naproxen, or others)).
No products indexed under this heading.

Meloxicam (Ibuprofen is a non-steroidal anti-inflammatory drug (NSAID), which may cause stomach bleeding. The chance of this is higher if the patient (child) is taking other drugs containing an NSAID (eg, aspirin, ibuprofen, naproxen, or others)).
No products indexed under this heading.

Methyclothiazide (Consult a doctor before use if taking a diuretic).
No products indexed under this heading.

Methylprednisolone (Ibuprofen is a non-steroidal anti-inflammatory drug (NSAID), which may cause stomach bleeding. The chance of this is higher if the patient (child) is taking a steroid drug).
No products indexed under this heading.

Methylprednisolone Acetate (Ibuprofen is a non-steroidal anti-inflammatory drug (NSAID), which may cause stomach bleeding. The chance of this is higher if the patient (child) is taking a steroid drug).
No products indexed under this heading.

Methylprednisolone Sodium Succinate (Ibuprofen is a non-steroidal anti-inflammatory drug (NSAID), which may cause stomach bleeding. The chance of this is higher if the patient (child) is taking a steroid drug).
No products indexed under this heading.

Metolazone (Consult a doctor before use if taking a diuretic).
No products indexed under this heading.

Mometasone Furoate (Ibuprofen is a non-steroidal anti-inflammatory drug

(NSAID), which may cause stomach bleeding. The chance of this is higher if the patient (child) is taking a steroid drug). Products include:

Mometasone Furoate Monohydrate (Ibuprofen is a non-steroidal anti-inflammatory drug (NSAID), which may cause stomach bleeding. The chance of this is higher if the patient (child) is taking a steroid drug). Products include:

Nabumetone (Ibuprofen is a non-steroidal anti-inflammatory drug (NSAID), which may cause stomach bleeding. The chance of this is higher if the patient (child) is taking other drugs containing an NSAID (eg, aspirin, ibuprofen, naproxen, or others)).
No products indexed under this heading.

Naproxen (Ibuprofen is a non-steroidal anti-inflammatory drug (NSAID), which may cause stomach bleeding. The chance of this is higher if the patient (child) is taking other drugs containing an NSAID (eg, aspirin, ibuprofen, naproxen, or others)). Products include:

Naproxen Sodium (Ibuprofen is a non-steroidal anti-inflammatory drug (NSAID), which may cause stomach bleeding. The chance of this is higher if the patient (child) is taking other drugs containing an NSAID (eg, aspirin, ibuprofen, naproxen, or others)). Products include:

Oxaprozin (Ibuprofen is a non-steroidal anti-inflammatory drug (NSAID), which may cause stomach bleeding. The chance of this is higher if the patient (child) is taking other drugs containing an NSAID (eg, aspirin, ibuprofen, naproxen, or others)).
No products indexed under this heading.

Phenylbutazone (Ibuprofen is a non-steroidal anti-inflammatory drug (NSAID), which may cause stomach bleeding. The chance of this is higher if the patient (child) is taking other drugs containing an NSAID (eg, aspirin, ibuprofen, naproxen, or others)).
No products indexed under this heading.

Piroxicam (Ibuprofen is a non-steroidal anti-inflammatory drug (NSAID), which may cause stomach bleeding. The chance of this is higher if the patient (child) is taking other drugs containing an NSAID (eg, aspirin, ibuprofen, naproxen, or others)).
No products indexed under this heading.

Polythiazide (Consult a doctor before use if taking a diuretic).
No products indexed under this heading.

Prednisolone (Ibuprofen is a non-steroidal anti-inflammatory drug (NSAID), which may cause stomach bleeding. The chance of this is higher if the patient (child) is taking a steroid drug).
No products indexed under this heading.

Prednisolone Acetate (Ibuprofen is a non-steroidal anti-inflammatory drug (NSAID), which may cause stomach bleeding. The chance of this is higher if the patient (child) is taking a steroid drug). Products include:

Prednisolone Sodium Phosphate (Ibuprofen is a non-steroidal anti-inflammatory drug (NSAID), which may cause stomach bleeding. The chance of this is higher if the patient (child) is taking a steroid drug).
No products indexed under this heading.

Prednisolone Tebutate (Ibuprofen is a non-steroidal anti-inflammatory drug (NSAID), which may cause stomach bleeding. The chance of this is higher if the patient (child) is taking a steroid drug).
No products indexed under this heading.

Prednisone (Ibuprofen is a non-steroidal anti-inflammatory drug (NSAID), which may cause stomach bleeding. The chance of this is higher if the patient (child) is taking a steroid drug).
No products indexed under this heading.

Prednisone sodium phosphate (Ibuprofen is a non-steroidal anti-inflammatory drug (NSAID), which may cause stomach bleeding. The chance of this is higher if the patient (child) is taking a steroid drug).
No products indexed under this heading.

Rofecoxib (Ibuprofen is a non-steroidal anti-inflammatory drug (NSAID), which may cause stomach bleeding. The chance of this is higher if the patient (child) is taking other drugs containing an NSAID (eg, aspirin, ibuprofen, naproxen, or others)).
No products indexed under this heading.

Spironolactone (Consult a doctor before use if taking a diuretic).
No products indexed under this heading.

Steroids, unspecified (Ibuprofen is a non-steroidal anti-inflammatory drug (NSAID), which may cause stomach bleeding. The chance of this is higher if the patient (child) is taking a steroid drug).
No products indexed under this heading.

Sulindac (Ibuprofen is a non-steroidal anti-inflammatory drug (NSAID), which may cause stomach bleeding. The chance of this is higher if the patient (child) is taking other drugs containing an NSAID (eg, aspirin, ibuprofen, naproxen, or others)). Products include:

Tinzaparin Sodium (Ibuprofen is a non-steroidal anti-inflammatory drug (NSAID), which may cause stomach bleeding. The chance of this is higher if the patient (child) is taking a blood thinning (anticoagulant) drug).
No products indexed under this heading.

Tolmetin Sodium (Ibuprofen is a non-steroidal anti-inflammatory drug (NSAID), which may cause stomach bleeding. The chance of this is higher if the patient (child) is taking other drugs containing an NSAID (eg, aspirin, ibuprofen, naproxen, or others)).
No products indexed under this heading.

Torsemide (Consult a doctor before use if taking a diuretic).
No products indexed under this heading.

Triamcinolone (Ibuprofen is a non-steroidal anti-inflammatory drug (NSAID), which may cause stomach bleeding. The chance of this is higher if the patient (child) is taking a steroid drug).
No products indexed under this heading.

Triamcinolone Acetonide (Ibuprofen is a non-steroidal anti-inflammatory drug (NSAID), which may cause stomach bleeding. The chance of this is higher if the patient (child) is taking a steroid drug). Products include:

Triamcinolone Diacetate (Ibuprofen is a non-steroidal anti-inflammatory drug (NSAID), which may cause stomach bleeding. The chance of this is higher if the patient (child) is taking a steroid drug).
No products indexed under this heading.

Triamcinolone Hexacetonide (Ibuprofen is a non-steroidal anti-inflammatory drug (NSAID), which may cause stomach bleeding. The chance of this is higher if the patient (child) is taking a steroid drug).
No products indexed under this heading.

Triamterene (Consult a doctor before use if taking a diuretic). Products include:

Valdecoxib (Ibuprofen is a non-steroidal anti-inflammatory drug (NSAID), which may cause stomach bleeding. The chance of this is higher if the patient (child) is taking other drugs containing an NSAID (eg, aspirin, ibuprofen, naproxen, or others)).
No products indexed under this heading.

Warfarin Sodium (Ibuprofen is a non-steroidal anti-inflammatory drug (NSAID), which may cause stomach bleeding. The chance of this is higher if the patient (child) is taking a blood thinning (anticoagulant) drug).
No products indexed under this heading.

CHILDREN'S MOTRIN NON-STAINING DYE-FREE ORAL SUSPENSION

See Children's Motrin Oral Suspension

INFANTS' MOTRIN CONCENTRATED DROPS

See Children's Motrin Oral Suspension

INFANTS' MOTRIN NON-STAINING DYE-FREE CONCENTRATED DROPS

See Children's Motrin Oral Suspension

JUNIOR STRENGTH MOTRIN CAPLETS AND CHEWABLE TABLETS

See Children's Motrin Oral Suspension

MOVIPREP ORAL SOLUTION

Oral Medications, unspecified (Oral medication administered within 1 hour of the start of administration of MoviPrep may be flushed from the gastrointestinal tract and the medication may not be absorbed).
No products indexed under this heading.

MOXATAG TABLETS

May interact with chloramphenicol, macrolide antibiotics, oral contraceptives, sulfonamides, tetracyclines, and certain other agents. Compounds in these categories include:

Azithromycin Dihydrate (Macrolides may interfere with the bactericidal effects of penicillin. This has been demonstrated *in vitro*; however, the clinical significance of this interaction is not well documented).
No products indexed under this heading.

Moxatag Interactions Index 1146

Bendroflumethiazide (Sulfonamides may interfere with the bactericidal effects of penicillin. This has been demonstrated *in vitro*; however, the clinical significance of this interaction is not well documented).
No products indexed under this heading.

Chloramphenicol (Chloramphenicol may interfere with the bactericidal effects of penicillin. This has been demonstrated *in vitro*; however, the clinical significance of this interaction is not well documented).
No products indexed under this heading.

Chloramphenicol Palmitate (Chloramphenicol may interfere with the bactericidal effects of penicillin. This has been demonstrated *in vitro*; however, the clinical significance of this interaction is not well documented).
No products indexed under this heading.

Chloramphenicol Sodium Succinate (Chloramphenicol may interfere with the bactericidal effects of penicillin. This has been demonstrated *in vitro*; however, the clinical significance of this interaction is not well documented).
No products indexed under this heading.

Chlorothiazide (Sulfonamides may interfere with the bactericidal effects of penicillin. This has been demonstrated *in vitro*; however, the clinical significance of this interaction is not well documented).
No products indexed under this heading.

Chlorothiazide Sodium (Sulfonamides may interfere with the bactericidal effects of penicillin. This has been demonstrated *in vitro*; however, the clinical significance of this interaction is not well documented). Products include:
Diuril Intravenous **2009**

Chlorpropamide (Sulfonamides may interfere with the bactericidal effects of penicillin. This has been demonstrated *in vitro*; however, the clinical significance of this interaction is not well documented).
No products indexed under this heading.

Clarithromycin (Macrolides may interfere with the bactericidal effects of penicillin. This has been demonstrated *in vitro*; however, the clinical significance of this interaction is not well documented). Products include:
Biaxin/Biaxin XL **412**

Demeclocycline Hydrochloride (Tetracyclines may interfere with the bactericidal effects of penicillin. This has been demonstrated *in vitro*; however, the clinical significance of this interaction is not well documented).
No products indexed under this heading.

Desogestrel (Amoxicillin may affect the gut flora, leading to lower estrogen reabsorption and potentially resulting in reduced efficacy of combined oral estrogen/progesterone contraceptives).
No products indexed under this heading.

Dirithromycin (Macrolides may interfere with the bactericidal effects of penicillin. This has been demonstrated *in vitro*; however, the clinical significance of this interaction is not well documented).
No products indexed under this heading.

Doxycycline (Tetracyclines may interfere with the bactericidal effects of penicillin. This has been demonstrated *in vitro*; however, the clinical significance of this interaction is not well documented).
No products indexed under this heading.

Doxycycline Calcium (Tetracyclines may interfere with the bactericidal effects of penicillin. This has been demonstrated *in vitro*; however, the clinical significance of this interaction is not well documented).
No products indexed under this heading.

Doxycycline Hyclate (Tetracyclines may interfere with the bactericidal effects of penicillin. This has been demonstrated *in vitro*; however, the clinical significance of this interaction is not well documented).
No products indexed under this heading.

Doxycycline Monohydrate (Tetracyclines may interfere with the bactericidal effects of penicillin. This has been demonstrated *in vitro*; however, the clinical significance of this interaction is not well documented).
No products indexed under this heading.

Erythromycin (Macrolides may interfere with the bactericidal effects of penicillin. This has been demonstrated *in vitro*; however, the clinical significance of this interaction is not well documented).
No products indexed under this heading.

Erythromycin Estolate (Macrolides may interfere with the bactericidal effects of penicillin. This has been demonstrated *in vitro*; however, the clinical significance of this interaction is not well documented).
No products indexed under this heading.

Erythromycin Ethylsuccinate (Macrolides may interfere with the bactericidal effects of penicillin. This has been demonstrated *in vitro*; however, the clinical significance of this interaction is not well documented). Products include:
E.E.S. **437**
EryPed **435**

Erythromycin Gluceptate (Macrolides may interfere with the bactericidal effects of penicillin. This has been demonstrated *in vitro*; however, the clinical significance of this interaction is not well documented).
No products indexed under this heading.

Erythromycin Stearate (Macrolides may interfere with the bactericidal effects of penicillin. This has been demonstrated *in vitro*; however, the clinical significance of this interaction is not well documented).
No products indexed under this heading.

Ethinyl Estradiol (Amoxicillin may affect the gut flora, leading to lower estrogen reabsorption and potentially resulting in reduced efficacy of combined oral estrogen/progesterone contraceptives). Products include:
LoSeasonique **3407**
Lybrel **3514**
NuvaRing **3181**
Ortho Evra **2648**
Ortho-Cyclen/Ortho Tri-Cyclen **2663**
Ortho Tri-Cyclen Lo Tablets **2673**
Seasonique **3418**
Yaz **864**

Ethynodiol Diacetate (Amoxicillin may affect the gut flora, leading to lower estrogen reabsorption and potentially resulting in reduced efficacy of combined oral estrogen/progesterone contraceptives).
No products indexed under this heading.

Glipizide (Sulfonamides may interfere with the bactericidal effects of penicillin. This has been demonstrated *in vitro*; however, the clinical significance of this interaction is not well documented).
No products indexed under this heading.

Glyburide (Sulfonamides may interfere with the bactericidal effects of penicillin. This has been demonstrated *in vitro*; however, the clinical significance of this interaction is not well documented).
No products indexed under this heading.

Hydrochlorothiazide (Sulfonamides may interfere with the bactericidal effects of penicillin. This has been demonstrated *in vitro*; however, the clinical significance of this interaction is not well documented). Products include:
Atacand HCT **700**
Avalide **2956**
Benicar HCT **1017**
Diovan HCT **2419**
Dyazide **1429**
Exforge HCT **2449**
Hyzaar **2162**
Hyzaar 100-12.5 .... **2162**
Micardis HCT **889**
Prinzide **2246**
Tekturna HCT **2541**
Teveten HCT **541**

Hydroflumethiazide (Sulfonamides may interfere with the bactericidal effects of penicillin. This has been demonstrated *in vitro*; however, the clinical significance of this interaction is not well documented).
No products indexed under this heading.

Lansoprazole (In a study of healthy adult subjects, amoxicillin AUC was similar whereas C_{max} increased approximately 35% following the administration of lansoprazole with amoxicillin extended release tablets given with food).
No products indexed under this heading.

Levonorgestrel (Amoxicillin may affect the gut flora, leading to lower estrogen reabsorption and potentially resulting in reduced efficacy of combined oral estrogen/progesterone contraceptives). Products include:
Climara Pro **847**
LoSeasonique **3407**
Lybrel **3514**
Mirena **854**
Plan B **3416**
Seasonique **3418**

Mestranol (Amoxicillin may affect the gut flora, leading to lower estrogen reabsorption and potentially resulting in reduced efficacy of combined oral estrogen/progesterone contraceptives).
No products indexed under this heading.

Methacycline Hydrochloride (Tetracyclines may interfere with the bactericidal effects of penicillin. This has been demonstrated *in vitro*; however, the clinical significance of this interaction is not well documented).
No products indexed under this heading.

Methyclothiazide (Sulfonamides may interfere with the bactericidal effects of penicillin. This has been demonstrated *in vitro*; however, the clinical significance of this interaction is not well documented).
No products indexed under this heading.

Minocycline Hydrochloride (Tetracyclines may interfere with the bactericidal effects of penicillin. This has been demonstrated *in vitro*; however, the clinical significance of this interaction is not well documented). Products include:
Solodyn **2073**

Norethindrone (Amoxicillin may affect the gut flora, leading to lower estrogen reabsorption and potentially resulting in reduced efficacy of combined oral estrogen/progesterone contraceptives). Products include:
Ortho Micronor **2660**

Norethynodrel (Amoxicillin may affect the gut flora, leading to lower estrogen reabsorption and potentially resulting in reduced efficacy of combined oral estrogen/progesterone contraceptives).
No products indexed under this heading.

Norgestimate (Amoxicillin may affect the gut flora, leading to lower estrogen reabsorption and potentially resulting in reduced efficacy of combined oral estrogen/progesterone contraceptives). Products include:
Ortho-Cyclen/Ortho Tri-Cyclen **2663**
Ortho Tri-Cyclen Lo Tablets **2673**

Norgestrel (Amoxicillin may affect the gut flora, leading to lower estrogen reabsorption and potentially resulting in reduced efficacy of combined oral estrogen/progesterone contraceptives).
No products indexed under this heading.

Oxytetracycline (Tetracyclines may interfere with the bactericidal effects of penicillin. This has been demonstrated *in vitro*; however, the clinical significance of this interaction is not well documented).
No products indexed under this heading.

Oxytetracycline Hydrochloride (Tetracyclines may interfere with the bactericidal effects of penicillin. This has been demonstrated *in vitro*; however, the clinical significance of this interaction is not well documented).
No products indexed under this heading.

Polythiazide (Sulfonamides may interfere with the bactericidal effects of penicillin. This has been demonstrated *in vitro*; however, the clinical significance of this interaction is not well documented).
No products indexed under this heading.

Probenecid (Probenecid decreases the renal tubular secretion of amoxicillin. Concurrent use of amoxicillin extended release tablets and probenecid may result in increased and prolonged blood levels of amoxicillin. The clinical relevance of this finding has not been evaluated).
No products indexed under this heading.

Sulfacytine (Sulfonamides may interfere with the bactericidal effects of penicillin. This has been demonstrated *in vitro*; however, the clinical significance of this interaction is not well documented).
No products indexed under this heading.

Sulfamethizole (Sulfonamides may interfere with the bactericidal effects of penicillin. This has been demonstrated *in vitro*; however, the clinical significance of this interaction is not well documented).
No products indexed under this heading.

Sulfamethoxazole (Sulfonamides may interfere with the bactericidal effects of penicillin. This has been demonstrated *in vitro*; however, the clinical significance of this interaction is not well documented).
No products indexed under this heading.

Sulfasalazine (Sulfonamides may interfere with the bactericidal effects of penicillin. This has been demonstrated *in vitro*; however, the clinical significance of this interaction is not well documented).
No products indexed under this heading.

Sulfinpyrazone (Sulfonamides may interfere with the bactericidal effects of penicillin. This has been demonstrated *in vitro*; however, the clinical significance of this interaction is not well documented).
No products indexed under this heading.

Sulfisoxazole Acetyl (Sulfonamides may interfere with the bactericidal effects of penicillin. This has been demonstrated *in vitro*; however, the clinical significance of this interaction is not well documented).
No products indexed under this heading.

Sulfisoxazole Diolamine (Sulfonamides may interfere with the bactericidal effects of penicillin. This has been demonstrated *in vitro*; however, the clinical significance of this interaction is not well documented).
No products indexed under this heading.

Tetracycline Hydrochloride (Tetracyclines may interfere with the bactericidal effects of penicillin. This has been demonstrated *in vitro*; however, the

clinical significance of this interaction is not well documented). Products include:
Pylera 793

Tetracycline Phosphate Complex (Tetracyclines may interfere with the bactericidal effects of penicillin. This has been demonstrated *in vitro*; however, the clinical significance of this interaction is not well documented).
No products indexed under this heading.

Tolazamide (Sulfonamides may interfere with the bactericidal effects of penicillin. This has been demonstrated *in vitro*; however, the clinical significance of this interaction is not well documented).
No products indexed under this heading.

Tolbutamide (Sulfonamides may interfere with the bactericidal effects of penicillin. This has been demonstrated *in vitro*; however, the clinical significance of this interaction is not well documented).
No products indexed under this heading.

Troleandomycin (Macrolides may interfere with the bactericidal effects of penicillin. This has been demonstrated *in vitro*; however, the clinical significance of this interaction is not well documented).
No products indexed under this heading.

MS CONTIN TABLETS
(Morphine Sulfate) 2803
May interact with alcohols, central nervous system depressants, general anesthetics, hypnotics and sedatives, mixed agonist/antagonist opioid analgesics, neuromuscular blocking agents, phenothiazines, tranquilizers. Compounds in these categories include:

Alfentanil Hydrochloride (Profound sedation, coma, severe hypotension, respiratory depression).
No products indexed under this heading.

Alprazolam (Profound sedation, coma, severe hypotension, respiratory depression).
No products indexed under this heading.

Amobarbital (Profound sedation, coma, severe hypotension, respiratory depression).
No products indexed under this heading.

Amobarbital Sodium (Profound sedation, coma, severe hypotension, respiratory depression).
No products indexed under this heading.

Aprobarbital (Profound sedation, coma, severe hypotension, respiratory depression).
No products indexed under this heading.

Atracurium Besylate (Increased respiratory depression).
No products indexed under this heading.

Buprenorphine Hydrochloride (Mixed agonist/antagonist analgesics may reduce the analgesic effect or may precipitate withdrawal symptoms).
No products indexed under this heading.

Buspirone Hydrochloride (Profound sedation, coma, severe hypotension, respiratory depression).
No products indexed under this heading.

Butabarbital (Profound sedation, coma, severe hypotension, respiratory depression).
No products indexed under this heading.

Butabarbital Sodium (Profound sedation, coma, severe hypotension, respiratory depression).
No products indexed under this heading.

Butalbital (Profound sedation, coma, severe hypotension, respiratory depression).
No products indexed under this heading.

Butorphanol Tartrate (Mixed agonist/antagonist analgesics may reduce the analgesic effect or may precipitate withdrawal symptoms).
No products indexed under this heading.

Chloral Hydrate (Profound sedation, coma, severe hypotension, respiratory depression).
No products indexed under this heading.

Chlordiazepoxide (Profound sedation, coma, severe hypotension, respiratory depression).
No products indexed under this heading.

Chlordiazepoxide Hydrochloride (Profound sedation, coma, severe hypotension, respiratory depression).
No products indexed under this heading.

Chlorpromazine (Profound sedation, coma, severe hypotension, respiratory depression).
No products indexed under this heading.

Chlorpromazine Hydrochloride (Profound sedation, coma, severe hypotension, respiratory depression).
No products indexed under this heading.

Chlorprothixene (Profound sedation, coma, severe hypotension, respiratory depression).
No products indexed under this heading.

Chlorprothixene Hydrochloride (Profound sedation, coma, severe hypotension, respiratory depression).
No products indexed under this heading.

Chlorprothixene Lactate (Profound sedation, coma, severe hypotension, respiratory depression).
No products indexed under this heading.

Cisatracurium Besylate (Increased respiratory depression). Products include:
Nimbex 503

Clonazepam (Profound sedation, coma, severe hypotension, respiratory depression). Products include:
Klonopin 2855

Clorazepate Dipotassium (Profound sedation, coma, severe hypotension, respiratory depression).
No products indexed under this heading.

Clozapine (Profound sedation, coma, severe hypotension, respiratory depression).
No products indexed under this heading.

Codeine Phosphate (Profound sedation, coma, severe hypotension, respiratory depression). Products include:
Tylenol with Codeine 2691

Codeine Sulfate (Profound sedation, coma, severe hypotension, respiratory depression).
No products indexed under this heading.

Decamethonium (Increased respiratory depression).
No products indexed under this heading.

Desflurane (Profound sedation, coma, severe hypotension, respiratory depression).
No products indexed under this heading.

Dezocine (Profound sedation, coma, severe hypotension, respiratory depression).
No products indexed under this heading.

Diazepam (Profound sedation, coma, severe hypotension, respiratory depression). Products include:
Valium Tablets 2880

Doxacurium Chloride (Increased respiratory depression).
No products indexed under this heading.

Droperidol (Profound sedation, coma, severe hypotension, respiratory depression).
No products indexed under this heading.

d-Tubocurarine (Increased respiratory depression).
No products indexed under this heading.

Enflurane (Profound sedation, coma, severe hypotension, respiratory depression).
No products indexed under this heading.

Estazolam (Profound sedation, coma, severe hypotension, respiratory depression).
No products indexed under this heading.

Ethanol (Profound sedation, coma, severe hypotension, respiratory depression).
No products indexed under this heading.

Ethchlorvynol (Profound sedation, coma, severe hypotension, respiratory depression).
No products indexed under this heading.

Ethinamate (Profound sedation, coma, severe hypotension, respiratory depression).
No products indexed under this heading.

Ethyl Alcohol (Profound sedation, coma, severe hypotension, respiratory depression).
No products indexed under this heading.

Fentanyl (Profound sedation, coma, severe hypotension, respiratory depression). Products include:
Duragesic 2604
Fentanyl Transdermal System 2346
Onsolis 2054

Fentanyl Citrate (Profound sedation, coma, severe hypotension, respiratory depression). Products include:
Fentora 966

Fluphenazine Decanoate (Profound sedation, coma, severe hypotension, respiratory depression).
No products indexed under this heading.

Fluphenazine Enanthate (Profound sedation, coma, severe hypotension, respiratory depression).
No products indexed under this heading.

Fluphenazine Hydrochloride (Profound sedation, coma, severe hypotension, respiratory depression).
No products indexed under this heading.

Flurazepam Hydrochloride (Profound sedation, coma, severe hypotension, respiratory depression).
No products indexed under this heading.

Gallamine (Increased respiratory depression).
No products indexed under this heading.

Gallamine Triethiodide (Increased respiratory depression).
No products indexed under this heading.

Glutethimide (Profound sedation, coma, severe hypotension, respiratory depression).
No products indexed under this heading.

Halazepam (Profound sedation, coma, severe hypotension, respiratory depression).
No products indexed under this heading.

Haloperidol (Profound sedation, coma, severe hypotension, respiratory depression).
No products indexed under this heading.

Haloperidol Decanoate (Profound sedation, coma, severe hypotension, respiratory depression).
No products indexed under this heading.

Haloperidol Lactate (Profound sedation, coma, severe hypotension, respiratory depression).
No products indexed under this heading.

Halothane (Profound sedation, coma, severe hypotension, respiratory depression).
No products indexed under this heading.

Hexobarbital (Profound sedation, coma, severe hypotension, respiratory depression).
No products indexed under this heading.

Hydrocodone Bitartrate (Profound sedation, coma, severe hypotension, respiratory depression). Products include:

Vicodin 560
Vicodin ES 561
Vicodin HP 563
Vicoprofen 564
Zydone 1138

Hydrocodone Polistirex (Profound sedation, coma, severe hypotension, respiratory depression). Products include:
Tussionex 3443

Hydromorphone (Profound sedation, coma, severe hypotension, respiratory depression).
No products indexed under this heading.

Hydromorphone Hydrochloride (Profound sedation, coma, severe hypotension, respiratory depression). Products include:
Dilaudid Injection 2800
Dilaudid Oral 2797
Dilaudid Tablets 2797
Dilaudid-HP 2800

Hydroxyzine Hydrochloride (Profound sedation, coma, severe hypotension, respiratory depression).
No products indexed under this heading.

Isoflurane (Profound sedation, coma, severe hypotension, respiratory depression).
No products indexed under this heading.

Ketamine Hydrochloride (Profound sedation, coma, severe hypotension, respiratory depression).
No products indexed under this heading.

Levomethadyl Acetate Hydrochloride (Profound sedation, coma, severe hypotension, respiratory depression).
No products indexed under this heading.

Levorphanol Tartrate (Profound sedation, coma, severe hypotension, respiratory depression).
No products indexed under this heading.

Lorazepam (Profound sedation, coma, severe hypotension, respiratory depression).
No products indexed under this heading.

Loxapine Hydrochloride (Profound sedation, coma, severe hypotension, respiratory depression).
No products indexed under this heading.

Loxapine Succinate (Profound sedation, coma, severe hypotension, respiratory depression).
No products indexed under this heading.

Meperidine Hydrochloride (Profound sedation, coma, severe hypotension, respiratory depression).
No products indexed under this heading.

Mephobarbital (Profound sedation, coma, severe hypotension, respiratory depression).
No products indexed under this heading.

Meprobamate (Profound sedation, coma, severe hypotension, respiratory depression).
No products indexed under this heading.

Mesoridazine Besylate (Profound sedation, coma, severe hypotension, respiratory depression).
No products indexed under this heading.

Methadone Hydrochloride (Profound sedation, coma, severe hypotension, respiratory depression).
No products indexed under this heading.

Methohexital Sodium (Profound sedation, coma, severe hypotension, respiratory depression).
No products indexed under this heading.

Methotrimeprazine (Profound sedation, coma, severe hypotension, respiratory depression).
No products indexed under this heading.

Methoxyflurane (Profound sedation, coma, severe hypotension, respiratory depression).
No products indexed under this heading.

IMPORTANT NOTE: Always consult each drug listing in the patient's regimen for possible interactions.

MS Interactions Index 1148

Metocurine Iodide (Increased respiratory depression).
No products indexed under this heading.

Midazolam Hydrochloride (Profound sedation, coma, severe hypotension, respiratory depression).
No products indexed under this heading.

Mivacurium Chloride (Increased respiratory depression).
No products indexed under this heading.

Molindone Hydrochloride (Profound sedation, coma, severe hypotension, respiratory depression). Products include:
Moban 1108

Morphine Sulfate, Liposomal (Profound sedation, coma, severe hypotension, respiratory depression).
No products indexed under this heading.

Nalbuphine Hydrochloride (Mixed agonist/antagonist analgesics may reduce the analgesic effect or may precipitate withdrawal symptoms).
No products indexed under this heading.

Nitrous Oxide (Profound sedation, coma, severe hypotension, respiratory depression).
No products indexed under this heading.

Olanzapine (Profound sedation, coma, severe hypotension, respiratory depression). Products include:
Symbyax 1965
Zyprexa 1984
Zyprexa IntraMuscular 1984
Zyprexa ZYDIS 1984

Oxazepam (Profound sedation, coma, severe hypotension, respiratory depression).
No products indexed under this heading.

Oxycodone Hydrochloride (Profound sedation, coma, severe hypotension, respiratory depression). Products include:
OxyContin 2807
Percocet 1121
Percodan 1124

Oxycodone Terephthalate (Profound sedation, coma, severe hypotension, respiratory depression).
No products indexed under this heading.

Oxymorphone Hydrochloride (Profound sedation, coma, severe hypotension, respiratory depression). Products include:
Opana 1110
Opana ER 1114

Pancuronium Bromide (Increased respiratory depression).
No products indexed under this heading.

Pentazocine Hydrochloride (Mixed agonist/antagonist analgesics may reduce the analgesic effect or may precipitate withdrawal symptoms).
No products indexed under this heading.

Pentazocine Lactate (Mixed agonist/antagonist analgesics may reduce the analgesic effect or may precipitate withdrawal symptoms).
No products indexed under this heading.

Pentobarbital (Profound sedation, coma, severe hypotension, respiratory depression).
No products indexed under this heading.

Pentobarbital Sodium (Profound sedation, coma, severe hypotension, respiratory depression). Products include:
Nembutal 2012

Perphenazine (Profound sedation, coma, severe hypotension, respiratory depression).
No products indexed under this heading.

Phenobarbital (Profound sedation, coma, severe hypotension, respiratory depression). Products include:
Donnatal 2711

Phenobarbital Sodium (Profound sedation, coma, severe hypotension, respiratory depression).
No products indexed under this heading.

Phenothiazine Derivatives (Profound sedation, coma, severe hypotension, respiratory depression).
No products indexed under this heading.

Phenothiazines (Profound sedation, coma, severe hypotension, respiratory depression).
No products indexed under this heading.

Prazepam (Profound sedation, coma, severe hypotension, respiratory depression).
No products indexed under this heading.

Prochlorperazine (Profound sedation, coma, severe hypotension, respiratory depression).
No products indexed under this heading.

Prochlorperazine Edisylate (Profound sedation, coma, severe hypotension, respiratory depression).
No products indexed under this heading.

Prochlorperazine Maleate (Profound sedation, coma, severe hypotension, respiratory depression).
No products indexed under this heading.

Promethazine (Profound sedation, coma, severe hypotension, respiratory depression).
No products indexed under this heading.

Promethazine Hydrochloride (Profound sedation, coma, severe hypotension, respiratory depression).
No products indexed under this heading.

Propofol (Profound sedation, coma, severe hypotension, respiratory depression).
No products indexed under this heading.

Propoxyphene Hydrochloride (Profound sedation, coma, severe hypotension, respiratory depression).
No products indexed under this heading.

Propoxyphene Napsylate (Profound sedation, coma, severe hypotension, respiratory depression).
No products indexed under this heading.

Quazepam (Profound sedation, coma, severe hypotension, respiratory depression).
No products indexed under this heading.

Quetiapine Fumarate (Profound sedation, coma, severe hypotension, respiratory depression). Products include:
Seroquel 750
Seroquel XR 759

Ramelteon (Profound sedation, coma, severe hypotension, respiratory depression). Products include:
Rozerem 3366

Rapacuronium Bromide (Increased respiratory depression).
No products indexed under this heading.

Remifentanil Hydrochloride (Profound sedation, coma, severe hypotension, respiratory depression).
No products indexed under this heading.

Risperidone (Profound sedation, coma, severe hypotension, respiratory depression). Products include:
Risperdal Consta 2682

Rocuronium Bromide (Increased respiratory depression). Products include:
Zemuron 3249

Secobarbital Sodium (Profound sedation, coma, severe hypotension, respiratory depression).
No products indexed under this heading.

Sevoflurane (Profound sedation, coma, severe hypotension, respiratory depression). Products include:
Ultane 554

Sodium Butabarbital (Profound sedation, coma, severe hypotension, respiratory depression).
No products indexed under this heading.

Sodium Oxybate (Profound sedation, coma, severe hypotension, respiratory depression).
No products indexed under this heading.

Sodium Pentobarbital (Profound sedation, coma, severe hypotension, respiratory depression).
No products indexed under this heading.

Succinylcholine Chloride (Increased respiratory depression).
No products indexed under this heading.

Sufentanil Citrate (Profound sedation, coma, severe hypotension, respiratory depression).
No products indexed under this heading.

Talbutal (Profound sedation, coma, severe hypotension, respiratory depression).
No products indexed under this heading.

Temazepam (Profound sedation, coma, severe hypotension, respiratory depression).
No products indexed under this heading.

Thiamylal Sodium (Profound sedation, coma, severe hypotension, respiratory depression).
No products indexed under this heading.

Thioridazine (Profound sedation, coma, severe hypotension, respiratory depression).
No products indexed under this heading.

Thioridazine Hydrochloride (Profound sedation, coma, severe hypotension, respiratory depression). Products include:
Thioridazine Hydrochloride 2384

Thiothixene (Profound sedation, coma, severe hypotension, respiratory depression). Products include:
Thiothixene 2386

Thiothixene Hydrochloride (Profound sedation, coma, severe hypotension, respiratory depression).
No products indexed under this heading.

Triazolam (Profound sedation, coma, severe hypotension, respiratory depression).
No products indexed under this heading.

Trifluoperazine Hydrochloride (Profound sedation, coma, severe hypotension, respiratory depression).
No products indexed under this heading.

Tubocurarine Chloride (Increased respiratory depression).
No products indexed under this heading.

Vecuronium Bromide (Increased respiratory depression).
No products indexed under this heading.

Zaleplon (Profound sedation, coma, severe hypotension, respiratory depression).
No products indexed under this heading.

Ziprasidone Hydrochloride (Profound sedation, coma, severe hypotension, respiratory depression). Products include:
Geodon 2723

Zolpidem Tartrate (Profound sedation, coma, severe hypotension, respiratory depression). Products include:
Ambien 2920
Ambien CR 2925

Food Interactions

Alcohol (Profound sedation, coma, severe hypotension, respiratory depression).

Beer, reduced-alcohol (Respiratory depression, hypotension and profound sedation or coma may result).

Beer, unspecified (Respiratory depression, hypotension and profound sedation or coma may result).

Wine, Chianti (Respiratory depression, hypotension and profound sedation or coma may result).

Wine, Red (Respiratory depression, hypotension and profound sedation or coma may result).

Wine, unspecified (Respiratory depression, hypotension and profound sedation or coma may result).

Wine products (Respiratory depression, hypotension and profound sedation or coma may result).

MULTAQ TABLETS

(Dronedarone) 3015

May interact with antipsychotic agents, beta-blockers, calcium channel blockers, class I antiarrhythmics, class III antiarrhythmics, cytochrome p450 2d6 substrates (selected), cytochrome p450 3a inducers (selected), cytochrome p450 3a inhibitors (selected), cytochrome p450 3a substrates (selected), drugs that prolong the QT interval, macrolide antibiotics, P-glycoprotein substrates (selected), phenothiazines, phenytoin, selective serotonin reuptake inhibitors, tricyclic antidepressants, and certain other agents. Compounds in these categories include:

Acebutolol Hydrochloride (Co-administration of dronedarone with other CYP 2D6 substrates, including other beta-blockers, may have increased exposure. In clinical trials, bradycardia was more frequently observed when dronedarone was given in combination with β-blockers. Give low dose of β-blockers initially, and increase only after ECG verification of good tolerability).
No products indexed under this heading.

Alfentanil Hydrochloride (Dronedarone is metabolized primarily by CYP 3A and is a moderate inhibitor of CYP 3A and CYP 2D6. Dronedarone's blood levels can therefore be affected by inhibitors and inducers of CYP 3A, and dronedarone can interact with drugs that are substrates of CYP 3A and CYP 2D6. Co-administration of dronedarone with CYP 3A substrates may increase plasma concentrations of tacrolimus, sirolimus, and other CYP 3A substrates with a narrow therapeutic range when given orally. Monitor plasma concentrations and adjust dosage appropriately).
No products indexed under this heading.

Allium sativum (Dronedarone is metabolized primarily by CYP 3A and is a moderate inhibitor of CYP 3A and CYP 2D6. Dronedarone's blood levels can therefore be affected by inhibitors and inducers of CYP 3A, and dronedarone can interact with drugs that are substrates of CYP 3A and CYP 2D6. Avoid other CYP 3A inducers such as phenobarbital, carbamazepine, phenytoin, and St John's wort with dronedarone because they decrease its exposure significantly).
No products indexed under this heading.

Alprazolam (Concomitant use of drugs or herbal products that prolong the QT interval might increase the risk of Torsade de Pointes, such as phenothiazine anti-psychotics, tricyclic antidepressants, certain oral macrolide antibiotics, and Class I and III antiarrhythmics. Co-administration of drugs prolonging the QT interval (such as certain phenothiazines, tricyclic antidepressants, certain macrolide antibiotics, and Class I and III antiarrhythmics) is contraindicated because of the potential risk of Torsade de Pointes-type ventricular tachycardia).
No products indexed under this heading.

Ambrisentan (Dronedarone has no significant potential to inhibit CYP 1A2, CYP 2C9, CYP 2C19, CYP 2C8 and CYP 2B6. It has the potential to inhibit

1149 **Interactions Index** **Multaq**

P-glycoprotein (P-gP) transport. Dronedarone increased digoxin exposure by 2.5-fold by inhibiting the P-gP transporter. Other P-gP substrates are expected to have increased exposure when co-administered with dronedarone).
Products include:
Letairis Tablets 1250

Aminophylline (Dronedarone is metabolized primarily by CYP 3A and is a moderate inhibitor of CYP 3A and CYP 2D6. Dronedarone's blood levels can therefore be affected by inhibitors and inducers of CYP 3A, and dronedarone can interact with drugs that are substrates of CYP 3A and CYP 2D6. Co-administration of dronedarone with CYP 3A substrates may increase plasma concentrations of tacrolimus, sirolimus, and other CYP 3A substrates with a narrow therapeutic range when given orally. Monitor plasma concentrations and adjust dosage appropriately).
No products indexed under this heading.

Amiodarone Hydrochloride (Concomitant use of drugs or herbal products that prolong the QT interval might increase the risk of Torsade de Pointes, such as phenothiazine anti-psychotics, tricyclic antidepressants, certain oral macrolide antibiotics, and Class I and III antiarrhythmics. Co-administration of drugs prolonging the QT interval (such as certain phenothiazines, tricyclic antidepressants, certain macrolide antibiotics, and Class I and III antiarrhythmics) is contraindicated because of the potential risk of Torsade de Pointes-type ventricular tachycardia).
No products indexed under this heading.

Amitriptyline Hydrochloride (Concomitant use of drugs or herbal products that prolong the QT interval might increase the risk of Torsade de Pointes, such as phenothiazine anti-psychotics, tricyclic antidepressants, certain oral macrolide antibiotics, and Class I and III antiarrhythmics. Co-administration of drugs prolonging the QT interval (such as certain phenothiazines, tricyclic antidepressants, certain macrolide antibiotics, and Class I and III antiarrhythmics) is contraindicated because of the potential risk of Torsade de Pointes-type ventricular tachycardia).
No products indexed under this heading.

Amlodipine Besylate (Co-administration of dronedarone with calcium channel blockers may increase calcium channel blocker (verapamil, diltiazem or nifedipine) exposure by 1.4- to 1.5-fold. Calcium channel blockers with depressant effects on the sinus and AV nodes could potentiate dronedarone's effects on conduction. Give low doses of calcium channel blockers initially and increase only after ECG verification of good tolerability). Products include:
Azor 1010
Exforge 2443
Exforge HCT 2449

Amoxapine (Concomitant use of drugs or herbal products that prolong the QT interval might increase the risk of Torsade de Pointes, such as phenothiazine anti-psychotics, tricyclic antidepressants, certain oral macrolide antibiotics, and Class I and III antiarrhythmics. Co-administration of drugs prolonging the QT interval (such as certain phenothiazines, tricyclic antidepressants, certain macrolide antibiotics, and Class I and III antiarrhythmics) is contraindicated because of the potential risk of Torsade de Pointes-type ventricular tachycardia).
No products indexed under this heading.

Amphetamine Aspartate (Dronedarone is metabolized primarily by CYP 3A and is a moderate inhibitor of CYP 3A and CYP 2D6. Dronedarone's blood levels can therefore be affected by inhibitors and inducers of CYP 3A, and dronedarone can interact with drugs that are substrates of CYP 3A and CYP 2D6. Other CYP 2D6 substrates, including other β-blockers, tricyclic antidepressants, and selective serotonin reuptake inhibitors (SSRIs) may have increased exposure upon co-administration with dronedarone).
No products indexed under this heading.

Amphetamine Aspartate Monohydrate (Dronedarone is metabolized primarily by CYP 3A and is a moderate inhibitor of CYP 3A and CYP 2D6. Dronedarone's blood levels can therefore be affected by inhibitors and inducers of CYP 3A, and dronedarone can interact with drugs that are substrates of CYP 3A and CYP 2D6. Other CYP 2D6 substrates, including other β-blockers, tricyclic antidepressants, and selective serotonin reuptake inhibitors (SSRIs) may have increased exposure upon co-administration with dronedarone).
No products indexed under this heading.

Amphetamine Sulfate (Dronedarone is metabolized primarily by CYP 3A and is a moderate inhibitor of CYP 3A and CYP 2D6. Dronedarone's blood levels can therefore be affected by inhibitors and inducers of CYP 3A, and dronedarone can interact with drugs that are substrates of CYP 3A and CYP 2D6. Other CYP 2D6 substrates, including other β-blockers, tricyclic antidepressants, and selective serotonin reuptake inhibitors (SSRIs) may have increased exposure upon co-administration with dronedarone).
No products indexed under this heading.

Amprenavir (Dronedarone is metabolized primarily by CYP 3A and is a moderate inhibitor of CYP 3A and CYP 2D6. Dronedarone's blood levels can therefore be affected by inhibitors and inducers of CYP 3A, and dronedarone can interact with drugs that are substrates of CYP 3A and CYP 2D6. Concomitant use of other potent CYP 3A inhibitors such as itraconazole, voriconazole, ritonavir, clarithromycin, and nefazodone is contraindicated).
No products indexed under this heading.

Aprepitant (Dronedarone is metabolized primarily by CYP 3A and is a moderate inhibitor of CYP 3A and CYP 2D6. Dronedarone's blood levels can therefore be affected by inhibitors and inducers of CYP 3A, and dronedarone can interact with drugs that are substrates of CYP 3A and CYP 2D6. Concomitant use of other potent CYP 3A inhibitors such as itraconazole, voriconazole, ritonavir, clarithromycin, and nefazodone is contraindicated). Products include:
Emend 2124

Aripiprazole (Concomitant use of drugs or herbal products that prolong the QT interval and might increase the risk of Torsade de Pointes, such as phenothiazine anti-psychotics, tricyclic antidepressants, certain oral macrolide antibiotics, and Class I and III antiarrhythmics is contraindicated).
No products indexed under this heading.

Astemizole (Concomitant use of drugs or herbal products that prolong the QT interval might increase the risk of Torsade de Pointes, such as phenothiazine anti-psychotics, tricyclic antidepressants, certain oral macrolide antibiotics, and Class I and III antiarrhythmics. Co-administration of drugs prolonging the QT interval (such as certain phenothiazines, tricyclic antidepressants, certain macrolide antibiotics, and Class I and III antiarrhythmics) is contraindicated because of the potential risk of Torsade de Pointes-type ventricular tachycardia).
No products indexed under this heading.

Atenolol (Co-administration of dronedarone with other CYP 2D6 substrates, including other beta-blockers, may have increased exposure. In clinical trials, bradycardia was more frequently observed when dronedarone was given in combination with β-blockers. Give low dose of β-blockers initially, and increase only after ECG verification of good tolerability).
No products indexed under this heading.

Atomoxetine Hydrochloride (Dronedarone is metabolized primarily by CYP 3A and is a moderate inhibitor of CYP 3A and CYP 2D6. Dronedarone's blood levels can therefore be affected by inhibitors and inducers of CYP 3A, and dronedarone can interact with drugs that are substrates of CYP 3A and CYP 2D6. Other CYP 2D6 substrates, including other β-blockers, tricyclic antidepressants, and selective serotonin reuptake inhibitors (SSRIs) may have increased exposure upon co-administration with dronedarone).
Products include:
Strattera 1957

Atorvastatin Calcium (Dronedarone has no significant potential to inhibit CYP 1A2, CYP 2C9, CYP 2C19, CYP 2C8 and CYP 2B6. It has the potential to inhibit P-glycoprotein (P-gP) transport. Dronedarone increased digoxin exposure by 2.5-fold by inhibiting the P-gP transporter. Other P-gP substrates are expected to have increased exposure when co-administered with dronedarone). Products include:
Lipitor 2703

Azithromycin Dihydrate (Co-administration of drugs prolonging the QT interval (such as certain phenothiazines, tricyclic antidepressants, certain macrolide antibiotics, and Class I and III antiarrhythmics) is contraindicated because of the potential risk of Torsade de Pointes-type ventricular tachycardia).
No products indexed under this heading.

Bepridil Hydrochloride (Co-administration of dronedarone with calcium channel blockers may increase calcium channel blocker (verapamil, diltiazem or nifedipine) exposure by 1.4- to 1.5-fold. Calcium channel blockers with depressant effects on the sinus and AV nodes could potentiate dronedarone's effects on conduction. Give low doses of calcium channel blockers initially and increase only after ECG verification of good tolerability).
No products indexed under this heading.

Betaxolol Hydrochloride (Co-administration of dronedarone with other CYP 2D6 substrates, including other beta-blockers, may have increased exposure. In clinical trials, bradycardia was more frequently observed when dronedarone was given in combination with β-blockers. Give low dose of β-blockers initially, and increase only after ECG verification of good tolerability).
No products indexed under this heading.

Bisoprolol Fumarate (Co-administration of dronedarone with other CYP 2D6 substrates, including other beta-blockers, may have increased exposure. In clinical trials, bradycardia was more frequently observed when dronedarone was given in combination with β-blockers. Give low dose of β-blockers initially, and increase only after ECG verification of good tolerability).
No products indexed under this heading.

Bretylium Tosylate (Concomitant use of drugs or herbal products that prolong the QT interval might increase the risk of Torsade de Pointes, such as phenothiazine anti-psychotics, tricyclic antidepressants, certain oral macrolide antibiotics, and Class I and III antiarrhythmics. Co-administration of drugs prolonging the QT interval (such as certain phenothiazines, tricyclic antidepressants, certain macrolide antibiotics, and Class I and III antiarrhythmics) is contraindicated because of the potential risk of Torsade de Pointes-type ventricular tachycardia).
No products indexed under this heading.

Bromocriptine Mesylate (Dronedarone is metabolized primarily by CYP 3A and is a moderate inhibitor of CYP 3A and CYP 2D6. Dronedarone's blood levels can therefore be affected by inhibitors and inducers of CYP 3A, and dronedarone can interact with drugs that are substrates of CYP 3A and CYP 2D6. Co-administration of dronedarone with CYP 3A substrates may increase plasma concentrations of tacrolimus, sirolimus, and other CYP 3A substrates with a narrow therapeutic range when given orally. Monitor plasma concentrations and adjust dosage appropriately).
No products indexed under this heading.

Buspirone Hydrochloride (Concomitant use of drugs or herbal products that prolong the QT interval might increase the risk of Torsade de Pointes, such as phenothiazine anti-psychotics, tricyclic antidepressants, certain oral macrolide antibiotics, and Class I and III antiarrhythmics. Co-administration of drugs prolonging the QT interval (such as certain phenothiazines, tricyclic antidepressants, certain macrolide antibiotics, and Class I and III antiarrhythmics) is contraindicated because of the potential risk of Torsade de Pointes-type ventricular tachycardia).
No products indexed under this heading.

Busulfan (Dronedarone is metabolized primarily by CYP 3A and is a moderate inhibitor of CYP 3A and CYP 2D6. Dronedarone's blood levels can therefore be affected by inhibitors and inducers of CYP 3A, and dronedarone can interact with drugs that are substrates of CYP 3A and CYP 2D6. Co-administration of dronedarone with CYP 3A substrates may increase plasma concentrations of tacrolimus, sirolimus, and other CYP 3A substrates with a narrow therapeutic range when given orally. Monitor plasma concentrations and adjust dosage appropriately).
Products include:
Myleran 1581

Captopril (Dronedarone is metabolized primarily by CYP 3A and is a moderate inhibitor of CYP 3A and CYP 2D6. Dronedarone's blood levels can therefore be affected by inhibitors and inducers of CYP 3A, and dronedarone can interact with drugs that are substrates of CYP 3A and CYP 2D6. Other CYP 2D6 substrates, including other β-blockers, tricyclic antidepressants, and selective serotonin reuptake inhibitors (SSRIs) may have increased exposure upon co-administration with dronedarone). Products include:
Captopril 2341

Carbamazepine (Dronedarone is metabolized primarily by CYP 3A and is a moderate inhibitor of CYP 3A and CYP 2D6. Dronedarone's blood levels can therefore be affected by inhibitors and inducers of CYP 3A, and dronedarone can interact with drugs that are substrates of CYP 3A and CYP 2D6. Avoid other CYP 3A inducers such as phenobarbital, carbamazepine, phenytoin, and St John's wort with dronedarone because they decrease its exposure significantly). Products include:
Carbatrol 3280
Equetro 3477

IMPORTANT NOTE: Always consult each drug listing in the patient's regimen for possible interactions.

Multaq Interactions Index 1150

Carteolol Hydrochloride (Co-administration of dronedarone with other CYP 2D6 substrates, including other beta-blockers, may have increased exposure. In clinical trials, bradycardia was more frequently observed when dronedarone was given in combination with β-blockers. Give low dose of β-blockers initially, and increase only after ECG verification of good tolerability).
No products indexed under this heading.

Carvedilol (Co-administration of dronedarone with other CYP 2D6 substrates, including other beta-blockers, may have increased exposure. In clinical trials, bradycardia was more frequently observed when dronedarone was given in combination with β-blockers. Give low dose of β-blockers initially, and increase only after ECG verification of good tolerability). Products include:
Coreg **1409**

Carvedilol Phosphate (Co-administration of dronedarone with other CYP 2D6 substrates, including other beta-blockers, may have increased exposure. In clinical trials, bradycardia was more frequently observed when dronedarone was given in combination with β-blockers. Give low dose of β-blockers initially, and increase only after ECG verification of good tolerability). Products include:
Coreg CR **1416**

Cerivastatin Sodium (Dronedarone is metabolized primarily by CYP 3A and is a moderate inhibitor of CYP 3A and CYP 2D6. Dronedarone's blood levels can therefore be affected by inhibitors and inducers of CYP 3A, and dronedarone can interact with drugs that are substrates of CYP 3A and CYP 2D6. Co-administration of dronedarone with CYP 3A substrates may increase plasma concentrations of tacrolimus, sirolimus, and other CYP 3A substrates with a narrow therapeutic range when given orally. Monitor plasma concentrations and adjust dosage appropriately).
No products indexed under this heading.

Cevimeline Hydrochloride (Dronedarone is metabolized primarily by CYP 3A and is a moderate inhibitor of CYP 3A and CYP 2D6. Dronedarone's blood levels can therefore be affected by inhibitors and inducers of CYP 3A, and dronedarone can interact with drugs that are substrates of CYP 3A and CYP 2D6. Other CYP 2D6 substrates, including other β-blockers, tricyclic antidepressants, and selective serotonin reuptake inhibitors (SSRIs) may have increased exposure upon co-administration with dronedarone). Products include:
Evoxac **1027**

Chlordiazepoxide (Concomitant use of drugs or herbal products that prolong the QT interval might increase the risk of Torsade de Pointes, such as phenothiazine anti-psychotics, tricyclic antidepressants, certain oral macrolide antibiotics, and Class I and III antiarrhythmics. Co-administration of drugs prolonging the QT interval (such as certain phenothiazines, tricyclic antidepressants, certain macrolide antibiotics, and Class I and III antiarrhythmics) is contraindicated because of the potential risk of Torsade de Pointes-type ventricular tachycardia).
No products indexed under this heading.

Chlordiazepoxide Hydrochloride (Concomitant use of drugs or herbal products that prolong the QT interval might increase the risk of Torsade de Pointes, such as phenothiazine anti-psychotics, tricyclic antidepressants, certain oral macrolide antibiotics, and Class I and III antiarrhythmics. Co-administration of drugs prolonging the QT interval (such as certain phenothiazines, tricyclic antidepressants, certain macrolide antibiotics, and Class I and III antiarrhythmics) is contraindicated because of the potential risk of Torsade de Pointes-type ventricular tachycardia).
No products indexed under this heading.

Chlorpheniramine (Dronedarone is metabolized primarily by CYP 3A and is a moderate inhibitor of CYP 3A and CYP 2D6. Dronedarone's blood levels can therefore be affected by inhibitors and inducers of CYP 3A, and dronedarone can interact with drugs that are substrates of CYP 3A and CYP 2D6. Co-administration of dronedarone with CYP 3A substrates may increase plasma concentrations of tacrolimus, sirolimus, and other CYP 3A substrates with a narrow therapeutic range when given orally. Monitor plasma concentrations and adjust dosage appropriately).
No products indexed under this heading.

Chlorpheniramine Maleate (Dronedarone is metabolized primarily by CYP 3A and is a moderate inhibitor of CYP 3A and CYP 2D6. Dronedarone's blood levels can therefore be affected by inhibitors and inducers of CYP 3A, and dronedarone can interact with drugs that are substrates of CYP 3A and CYP 2D6. Co-administration of dronedarone with CYP 3A substrates may increase plasma concentrations of tacrolimus, sirolimus, and other CYP 3A substrates with a narrow therapeutic range when given orally. Monitor plasma concentrations and adjust dosage appropriately).
No products indexed under this heading.

Chlorpheniramine Polistirex (Dronedarone is metabolized primarily by CYP 3A and is a moderate inhibitor of CYP 3A and CYP 2D6. Dronedarone's blood levels can therefore be affected by inhibitors and inducers of CYP 3A, and dronedarone can interact with drugs that are substrates of CYP 3A and CYP 2D6. Co-administration of dronedarone with CYP 3A substrates may increase plasma concentrations of tacrolimus, sirolimus, and other CYP 3A substrates with a narrow therapeutic range when given orally. Monitor plasma concentrations and adjust dosage appropriately). Products include:
Tussionex **3443**

Chlorpheniramine Tannate (Dronedarone is metabolized primarily by CYP 3A and is a moderate inhibitor of CYP 3A and CYP 2D6. Dronedarone's blood levels can therefore be affected by inhibitors and inducers of CYP 3A, and dronedarone can interact with drugs that are substrates of CYP 3A and CYP 2D6. Co-administration of dronedarone with CYP 3A substrates may increase plasma concentrations of tacrolimus, sirolimus, and other CYP 3A substrates with a narrow therapeutic range when given orally. Monitor plasma concentrations and adjust dosage appropriately).
No products indexed under this heading.

Chlorpromazine (Co-administration of drugs prolonging the QT interval (such as certain phenothiazines, tricyclic antidepressants, certain macrolide antibiotics, and Class I and III antiarrhythmics) is contraindicated because of the potential risk of Torsade de Pointes-type ventricular tachycardia).
No products indexed under this heading.

Chlorpromazine Hydrochloride (Co-administration of drugs prolonging the QT interval (such as certain phenothiazines, tricyclic antidepressants, certain macrolide antibiotics, and Class I and III antiarrhythmics) is contraindicated because of the potential risk of Torsade de Pointes-type ventricular tachycardia).
No products indexed under this heading.

Chlorpropamide (Dronedarone is metabolized primarily by CYP 3A and is a moderate inhibitor of CYP 3A and CYP 2D6. Dronedarone's blood levels can therefore be affected by inhibitors and inducers of CYP 3A, and dronedarone can interact with drugs that are substrates of CYP 3A and CYP 2D6. Other CYP 2D6 substrates, including other β-blockers, tricyclic antidepressants, and selective serotonin reuptake inhibitors (SSRIs) may have increased exposure upon co-administration with dronedarone).
No products indexed under this heading.

Chlorprothixene (Concomitant use of drugs or herbal products that prolong the QT interval might increase the risk of Torsade de Pointes, such as phenothiazine anti-psychotics, tricyclic antidepressants, certain oral macrolide antibiotics, and Class I and III antiarrhythmics. Co-administration of drugs prolonging the QT interval (such as certain phenothiazines, tricyclic antidepressants, certain macrolide antibiotics, and Class I and III antiarrhythmics) is contraindicated because of the potential risk of Torsade de Pointes-type ventricular tachycardia).
No products indexed under this heading.

Chlorprothixene Hydrochloride (Concomitant use of drugs or herbal products that prolong the QT interval might increase the risk of Torsade de Pointes, such as phenothiazine anti-psychotics, tricyclic antidepressants, certain oral macrolide antibiotics, and Class I and III antiarrhythmics. Co-administration of drugs prolonging the QT interval (such as certain phenothiazines, tricyclic antidepressants, certain macrolide antibiotics, and Class I and III antiarrhythmics) is contraindicated because of the potential risk of Torsade de Pointes-type ventricular tachycardia).
No products indexed under this heading.

Chlorprothixene Lactate (Concomitant use of drugs or herbal products that prolong the QT interval and might increase the risk of Torsade de Pointes, such as phenothiazine anti-psychotics, tricyclic antidepressants, certain oral macrolide antibiotics, and Class I and III antiarrhythmics is contraindicated).
No products indexed under this heading.

Cilostazol (Dronedarone is metabolized primarily by CYP 3A and is a moderate inhibitor of CYP 3A and CYP 2D6. Dronedarone's blood levels can therefore be affected by inhibitors and inducers of CYP 3A, and dronedarone can interact with drugs that are substrates of CYP 3A and CYP 2D6. Co-administration of dronedarone with CYP 3A substrates may increase plasma concentrations of tacrolimus, sirolimus, and other CYP 3A substrates with a narrow therapeutic range when given orally. Monitor plasma concentrations and adjust dosage appropriately).
No products indexed under this heading.

Cimetidine (Dronedarone is metabolized primarily by CYP 3A and is a moderate inhibitor of CYP 3A and CYP 2D6. Dronedarone's blood levels can therefore be affected by inhibitors and inducers of CYP 3A, and dronedarone can interact with drugs that are substrates of CYP 3A and CYP 2D6. Concomitant use of other potent CYP 3A inhibitors such as itraconazole, voriconazole, ritonavir, clarithromycin, and nefazodone is contraindicated).
No products indexed under this heading.

Cimetidine Hydrochloride (Dronedarone is metabolized primarily by CYP 3A and is a moderate inhibitor of CYP 3A and CYP 2D6. Dronedarone's blood levels can therefore be affected by inhibitors and inducers of CYP 3A, and dronedarone can interact with drugs that are substrates of CYP 3A and CYP 2D6. Concomitant use of other potent CYP 3A inhibitors such as itraconazole, voriconazole, ritonavir, clarithromycin, and nefazodone is contraindicated).
No products indexed under this heading.

Ciprofloxacin (Dronedarone is metabolized primarily by CYP 3A and is a moderate inhibitor of CYP 3A and CYP 2D6. Dronedarone's blood levels can therefore be affected by inhibitors and inducers of CYP 3A, and dronedarone can interact with drugs that are substrates of CYP 3A and CYP 2D6. Concomitant use of other potent CYP 3A inhibitors such as itraconazole, voriconazole, ritonavir, clarithromycin, and nefazodone is contraindicated).
Products include:
Cipro I.V. **3082**
Cipro **3073**
Cipro XR **3091**
Ciprodex **583**

Ciprofloxacin Hydrochloride (Dronedarone is metabolized primarily by CYP 3A and is a moderate inhibitor of CYP 3A and CYP 2D6. Dronedarone's blood levels can therefore be affected by inhibitors and inducers of CYP 3A, and dronedarone can interact with drugs that are substrates of CYP 3A and CYP 2D6. Concomitant use of other potent CYP 3A inhibitors such as itraconazole, voriconazole, ritonavir, clarithromycin, and nefazodone is contraindicated). Products include:
Cipro **3073**

Cisapride (Dronedarone is metabolized primarily by CYP 3A and is a moderate inhibitor of CYP 3A and CYP 2D6. Dronedarone's blood levels can therefore be affected by inhibitors and inducers of CYP 3A, and dronedarone can interact with drugs that are substrates of CYP 3A and CYP 2D6. Co-administration of dronedarone with CYP 3A substrates may increase plasma concentrations of tacrolimus, sirolimus, and other CYP 3A substrates with a narrow therapeutic range when given orally. Monitor plasma concentrations and adjust dosage appropriately).
No products indexed under this heading.

Citalopram Hydrobromide (Other CYP 2D6 substrates, including serotonin reuptake inhibitors (SSRIs), may have increased exposure upon co-administration with dronedarone).
Products include:
Celexa **1153**

Clarithromycin (Concomitant use of other potent CYP 3A inhibitors such as itraconazole, voriconazole, ritonavir, clarithromycin, and nefazodone is contraindicated). Products include:
Biaxin/Biaxin XL **412**

Clomipramine Hydrochloride (Concomitant use of drugs or herbal products that prolong the QT interval might increase the risk of Torsade de Pointes, such as phenothiazine anti-psychotics, tricyclic antidepressants, certain oral macrolide antibiotics, and Class I and III antiarrhythmics. Co-administration of drugs prolonging the QT interval (such as certain phenothiazines, tricyclic antidepressants, certain macrolide antibiotics, and Class I and III antiarrhythmics) is contraindicated because of the potential risk of Torsade de Pointes-type ventricular tachycardia).
No products indexed under this heading.

Clorazepate Dipotassium (Concomitant use of drugs or herbal products that prolong the QT interval might increase the risk of Torsade de Pointes, such as phenothiazine anti-psychotics, tricyclic antidepressants, certain oral macrolide antibiotics, and Class I and III antiarrhythmics. Co-administration of drugs prolonging the QT interval (such as certain phenothiazines, tricyclic antidepressants, certain macrolide antibiotics, and Class I and III antiarrhythmics)

is contraindicated because of the potential risk of Torsade de Pointes-type ventricular tachycardia).
No products indexed under this heading.

Clozapine (Concomitant use of drugs or herbal products that prolong the QT interval might increase the risk of Torsade de Pointes, such as phenothiazine anti-psychotics, tricyclic antidepressants, certain oral macrolide antibiotics, and Class I and III antiarrhythmics. Co-administration of drugs prolonging the QT interval (such as certain phenothiazines, tricyclic antidepressants, certain macrolide antibiotics, and Class I and III antiarrhythmics) is contraindicated because of the potential risk of Torsade de Pointes-type ventricular tachycardia).
No products indexed under this heading.

Codeine Phosphate (Dronedarone is metabolized primarily by CYP 3A and is a moderate inhibitor of CYP 3A and CYP 2D6. Dronedarone's blood levels can therefore be affected by inhibitors and inducers of CYP 3A, and dronedarone can interact with drugs that are substrates of CYP 3A and CYP 2D6. Other CYP 2D6 substrates, including other β-blockers, tricyclic antidepressants, and selective serotonin reuptake inhibitors (SSRIs) may have increased exposure upon co-administration with dronedarone). Products include:
Tylenol with Codeine 2691

Codeine Sulfate (Dronedarone is metabolized primarily by CYP 3A and is a moderate inhibitor of CYP 3A and CYP 2D6. Dronedarone's blood levels can therefore be affected by inhibitors and inducers of CYP 3A, and dronedarone can interact with drugs that are substrates of CYP 3A and CYP 2D6. Other CYP 2D6 substrates, including other β-blockers, tricyclic antidepressants, and selective serotonin reuptake inhibitors (SSRIs) may have increased exposure upon co-administration with dronedarone).
No products indexed under this heading.

Cyclobenzaprine Hydrochloride (Dronedarone is metabolized primarily by CYP 3A and is a moderate inhibitor of CYP 3A and CYP 2D6. Dronedarone's blood levels can therefore be affected by inhibitors and inducers of CYP 3A, and dronedarone can interact with drugs that are substrates of CYP 3A and CYP 2D6. Other CYP 2D6 substrates, including other β-blockers, tricyclic antidepressants, and selective serotonin reuptake inhibitors (SSRIs) may have increased exposure upon co-administration with dronedarone).
Products include:
Amrix 964

Cyclosporine (Dronedarone is metabolized primarily by CYP 3A and is a moderate inhibitor of CYP 3A and CYP 2D6. Dronedarone's blood levels can therefore be affected by inhibitors and inducers of CYP 3A, and dronedarone can interact with drugs that are substrates of CYP 3A and CYP 2D6. Concomitant use of other potent CYP 3A inhibitors such as itraconazole, voriconazole, ritonavir, clarithromycin, and nefazodone is contraindicated).
Products include:
Gengraf 440
Neoral Oral Solution 2496
Neoral Capsules 2496
Restasis 605

Debrisoquine (Dronedarone is metabolized primarily by CYP 3A and is a moderate inhibitor of CYP 3A and CYP 2D6. Dronedarone's blood levels can therefore be affected by inhibitors and inducers of CYP 3A, and dronedarone can interact with drugs that are substrates of CYP 3A and CYP 2D6. Other CYP 2D6 substrates, including other β-blockers, tricyclic antidepressants, and selective serotonin reuptake inhibitors (SSRIs) may have increased exposure upon co-administration with dronedarone).
No products indexed under this heading.

Delavirdine Mesylate (Dronedarone is metabolized primarily by CYP 3A and is a moderate inhibitor of CYP 3A and CYP 2D6. Dronedarone's blood levels can therefore be affected by inhibitors and inducers of CYP 3A, and dronedarone can interact with drugs that are substrates of CYP 3A and CYP 2D6. Concomitant use of other potent CYP 3A inhibitors such as itraconazole, voriconazole, ritonavir, clarithromycin, and nefazodone is contraindicated).
No products indexed under this heading.

Desipramine Hydrochloride (Concomitant use of drugs or herbal products that prolong the QT interval might increase the risk of Torsade de Pointes, such as phenothiazine anti-psychotics, tricyclic antidepressants, certain oral macrolide antibiotics, and Class I and III antiarrhythmics. Co-administration of drugs prolonging the QT interval (such as certain phenothiazines, tricyclic antidepressants, certain macrolide antibiotics, and Class I and III antiarrhythmics) is contraindicated because of the potential risk of Torsade de Pointes-type ventricular tachycardia).
No products indexed under this heading.

Desogestrel (Dronedarone is metabolized primarily by CYP 3A and is a moderate inhibitor of CYP 3A and CYP 2D6. Dronedarone's blood levels can therefore be affected by inhibitors and inducers of CYP 3A, and dronedarone can interact with drugs that are substrates of CYP 3A and CYP 2D6. Co-administration of dronedarone with CYP 3A substrates may increase plasma concentrations of tacrolimus, sirolimus, and other CYP 3A substrates with a narrow therapeutic range when given orally. Monitor plasma concentrations and adjust dosage appropriately).
No products indexed under this heading.

Dexamethasone (Dronedarone has no significant potential to inhibit CYP 1A2, CYP 2C9, CYP 2C19, CYP 2C8 and CYP 2B6. It has the potential to inhibit P-glycoprotein (P-gP) transport. Dronedarone increased digoxin exposure by 2.5-fold by inhibiting the P-gP transporter. Other P-gP substrates are expected to have increased exposure when co-administered with dronedarone). Products include:
Ciprodex 583
Ozurdex ....⊙223
Tobramycin and Dexamethasone Ophthalmic Suspension ....⊙251

Dexamethasone Acetate (Dronedarone has no significant potential to inhibit CYP 1A2, CYP 2C9, CYP 2C19, CYP 2C8 and CYP 2B6. It has the potential to inhibit P-glycoprotein (P-gP) transport. Dronedarone increased digoxin exposure by 2.5-fold by inhibiting the P-gP transporter. Other P-gP substrates are expected to have increased exposure when co-administered with dronedarone).
No products indexed under this heading.

Dexamethasone Phosphate (Dronedarone has no significant potential to inhibit CYP 1A2, CYP 2C9, CYP 2C19, CYP 2C8 and CYP 2B6. It has the potential to inhibit P-glycoprotein (P-gP) transport. Dronedarone increased digoxin exposure by 2.5-fold by inhibiting the P-gP transporter. Other P-gP substrates are expected to have increased exposure when co-administered with dronedarone).
No products indexed under this heading.

Dexamethasone Sodium (Dronedarone has no significant potential to inhibit CYP 1A2, CYP 2C9, CYP 2C19, CYP 2C8 and CYP 2B6. It has the potential to inhibit P-glycoprotein (P-gP) transport. Dronedarone increased digoxin exposure by 2.5-fold by inhibiting the P-gP transporter. Other P-gP substrates are expected to have increased exposure when co-administered with dronedarone).
No products indexed under this heading.

Dexamethasone Sodium Phosphate (Dronedarone has no significant potential to inhibit CYP 1A2, CYP 2C9, CYP 2C19, CYP 2C8 and CYP 2B6. It has the potential to inhibit P-glycoprotein (P-gP) transport. Dronedarone increased digoxin exposure by 2.5-fold by inhibiting the P-gP transporter. Other P-gP substrates are expected to have increased exposure when co-administered with dronedarone).
No products indexed under this heading.

Dexamethasone Sodium Phosphate Injection (Dronedarone has no significant potential to inhibit CYP 1A2, CYP 2C9, CYP 2C19, CYP 2C8 and CYP 2B6. It has the potential to inhibit P-glycoprotein (P-gP) transport. Dronedarone increased digoxin exposure by 2.5-fold by inhibiting the P-gP transporter. Other P-gP substrates are expected to have increased exposure when co-administered with dronedarone).
No products indexed under this heading.

Dexfenfluramine Hydrochloride (Dronedarone is metabolized primarily by CYP 3A and is a moderate inhibitor of CYP 3A and CYP 2D6. Dronedarone's blood levels can therefore be affected by inhibitors and inducers of CYP 3A, and dronedarone can interact with drugs that are substrates of CYP 3A and CYP 2D6. Other CYP 2D6 substrates, including other β-blockers, tricyclic antidepressants, and selective serotonin reuptake inhibitors (SSRIs) may have increased exposure upon co-administration with dronedarone).
No products indexed under this heading.

Dextromethorphan Hydrobromide (Dronedarone is metabolized primarily by CYP 3A and is a moderate inhibitor of CYP 3A and CYP 2D6. Dronedarone's blood levels can therefore be affected by inhibitors and inducers of CYP 3A, and dronedarone can interact with drugs that are substrates of CYP 3A and CYP 2D6. Other CYP 2D6 substrates, including other β-blockers, tricyclic antidepressants, and selective serotonin reuptake inhibitors (SSRIs) may have increased exposure upon co-administration with dronedarone).
No products indexed under this heading.

Dextromethorphan Polistirex (Dronedarone is metabolized primarily by CYP 3A and is a moderate inhibitor of CYP 3A and CYP 2D6. Dronedarone's blood levels can therefore be affected by inhibitors and inducers of CYP 3A, and dronedarone can interact with drugs that are substrates of CYP 3A and CYP 2D6. Other CYP 2D6 substrates, including other β-blockers, tricyclic antidepressants, and selective serotonin reuptake inhibitors (SSRIs) may have increased exposure upon co-administration with dronedarone).
No products indexed under this heading.

Diazepam (Concomitant use of drugs or herbal products that prolong the QT interval might increase the risk of Torsade de Pointes, such as phenothiazine anti-psychotics, tricyclic antidepressants, certain oral macrolide antibiotics, and Class I and III antiarrhythmics. Co-administration of drugs prolonging the QT interval (such as certain phenothiazines, tricyclic antidepressants, certain macrolide antibiotics, and Class I and III antiarrhythmics) is contraindicated because of the potential risk of Torsade de Pointes-type ventricular tachycardia). Products include:
Valium Tablets 2880

Digoxin (Digoxin can potentiate the electrophysiologic effects of dronedarone (such as decreased AV-node conduction). In clinical trials, increased levels of digoxin were observed when dronedarone was co-administered with digoxin. Gastrointestinal disorders were also increased. Because of the pharmacokinetic interaction and possible pharmacodynamic interaction, reconsider the need for digoxin therapy. If digoxin treatment is continued, halve the dose of digoxin, monitor serum levels closely, and observe for toxicity. Dronedarone increased digoxin exposure by 2.5-fold by inhibiting the P-gP transporter). Products include:
Lanoxin Injection 1546
Lanoxin Injection Pediatric 1549
Lanoxin Tablets 1553

Digoxin Immune Fab (Ovine) (Dronedarone has no significant potential to inhibit CYP 1A2, CYP 2C9, CYP 2C19, CYP 2C8 and CYP 2B6. It has the potential to inhibit P-glycoprotein (P-gP) transport. Dronedarone increased digoxin exposure by 2.5-fold by inhibiting the P-gP transporter. Other P-gP substrates are expected to have increased exposure when co-administered with dronedarone).
Products include:
Digibind 1427

Dihydroergotamine Mesylate (Dronedarone is metabolized primarily by CYP 3A and is a moderate inhibitor of CYP 3A and CYP 2D6. Dronedarone's blood levels can therefore be affected by inhibitors and inducers of CYP 3A, and dronedarone can interact with drugs that are substrates of CYP 3A and CYP 2D6. Co-administration of dronedarone with CYP 3A substrates may increase plasma concentrations of tacrolimus, sirolimus, and other CYP 3A substrates with a narrow therapeutic range when given orally. Monitor plasma concentrations and adjust dosage appropriately).
No products indexed under this heading.

Diltiazem Hydrochloride (Co-administration of dronedarone with a moderate CYP 3A inhibitor such as diltiazem may increase dronedarone exposure by approximately 1.4- to 1.7-fold).
Products include:
Cardizem LA 423

Diltiazem Maleate (Co-administration of dronedarone with a moderate CYP 3A inhibitor such as diltiazem may increase dronedarone exposure by approximately 1.4- to 1.7-fold).
No products indexed under this heading.

Dirithromycin (Co-administration of drugs prolonging the QT interval (such as certain phenothiazines, tricyclic antidepressants, certain macrolide antibiotics, and Class I and III antiarrhythmics) is contraindicated because of the potential risk of Torsade de Pointes-type ventricular tachycardia).
No products indexed under this heading.

Disopyramide (Concomitant use of drugs or herbal products that prolong the QT interval might increase the risk of Torsade de Pointes, such as phenothiazine anti-psychotics, tricyclic antidepressants, certain oral macrolide antibiotics, and Class I and III antiarrhythmics. Co-administration of drugs prolonging the QT interval (such as certain phenothiazines, tricyclic antidepressants, certain macrolide antibiotics, and Class I and III antiarrhythmics) is contraindicated because of the potential risk of Torsade de Pointes-type ventricular tachycardia).
No products indexed under this heading.

IMPORTANT NOTE: Always consult each drug listing in the patient's regimen for possible interactions.

Multaq Interactions Index 1152

Disopyramide Phosphate (Concomitant use of drugs or herbal products that prolong the QT interval might increase the risk of Torsade de Pointes, such as phenothiazine anti-psychotics, tricyclic antidepressants, certain oral macrolide antibiotics, and Class I and III antiarrhythmics. Co-administration of drugs prolonging the QT interval (such as certain phenothiazines, tricyclic antidepressants, certain macrolide antibiotics, and Class I and III antiarrhythmics) is contraindicated because of the potential risk of Torsade de Pointes-type ventricular tachycardia).
No products indexed under this heading.

Dofetilide (Concomitant use of drugs or herbal products that prolong the QT interval might increase the risk of Torsade de Pointes, such as phenothiazine anti-psychotics, tricyclic antidepressants, certain oral macrolide antibiotics, and Class I and III antiarrhythmics. Co-administration of drugs prolonging the QT interval (such as certain phenothiazines, tricyclic antidepressants, certain macrolide antibiotics, and Class I and III antiarrhythmics) is contraindicated because of the potential risk of Torsade de Pointes-type ventricular tachycardia).
No products indexed under this heading.

Dolasetron Mesylate (Dronedarone is metabolized primarily by CYP 3A and is a moderate inhibitor of CYP 3A and CYP 2D6. Dronedarone's blood levels can therefore be affected by inhibitors and inducers of CYP 3A, and dronedarone can interact with drugs that are substrates of CYP 3A and CYP 2D6. Other CYP 2D6 substrates, including other β-blockers, tricyclic antidepressants, and selective serotonin reuptake inhibitors (SSRIs) may have increased exposure upon co-administration with dronedarone). Products include:
Anzemet Injection 2931
Anzemet Tablets 2934

Domperidone (Dronedarone has no significant potential to inhibit CYP 1A2, CYP 2C9, CYP 2C19, CYP 2C8 and CYP 2B6. It has the potential to inhibit P-glycoprotein (P-gP) transport. Dronedarone increased digoxin exposure by 2.5-fold by inhibiting the P-gP transporter. Other P-gP substrates are expected to have increased exposure when co-administered with dronedarone).
No products indexed under this heading.

Donepezil Hydrochloride (Dronedarone is metabolized primarily by CYP 3A and is a moderate inhibitor of CYP 3A and CYP 2D6. Dronedarone's blood levels can therefore be affected by inhibitors and inducers of CYP 3A, and dronedarone can interact with drugs that are substrates of CYP 3A and CYP 2D6. Other CYP 2D6 substrates, including other β-blockers, tricyclic antidepressants, and selective serotonin reuptake inhibitors (SSRIs) may have increased exposure upon co-administration with dronedarone). Products include:
Aricept 1045
Aricept ODT 1045

Doxepin Hydrochloride (Concomitant use of drugs or herbal products that prolong the QT interval might increase the risk of Torsade de Pointes, such as phenothiazine anti-psychotics, tricyclic antidepressants, certain oral macrolide antibiotics, and Class I and III antiarrhythmics. Co-administration of drugs prolonging the QT interval (such as certain phenothiazines, tricyclic antidepressants, certain macrolide antibiotics, and Class I and III antiarrhythmics) is contraindicated because of the potential risk of Torsade de Pointes-type ventricular tachycardia).
No products indexed under this heading.

Doxorubicin Hydrochloride (Dronedarone has no significant potential to inhibit CYP 1A2, CYP 2C9, CYP 2C19, CYP 2C8 and CYP 2B6. It has the potential to inhibit P-glycoprotein (P-gP) transport. Dronedarone increased digoxin exposure by 2.5-fold by inhibiting the P-gP transporter. Other P-gP substrates are expected to have increased exposure when co-administered with dronedarone).
No products indexed under this heading.

Doxorubicin Hydrochloride Liposome (Dronedarone has no significant potential to inhibit CYP 1A2, CYP 2C9, CYP 2C19, CYP 2C8 and CYP 2B6. It has the potential to inhibit P-glycoprotein (P-gP) transport. Dronedarone increased digoxin exposure by 2.5-fold by inhibiting the P-gP transporter. Other P-gP substrates are expected to have increased exposure when co-administered with dronedarone). Products include:
Doxil 939

Dronabinol (Dronedarone is metabolized primarily by CYP 3A and is a moderate inhibitor of CYP 3A and CYP 2D6. Dronedarone's blood levels can therefore be affected by inhibitors and inducers of CYP 3A, and dronedarone can interact with drugs that are substrates of CYP 3A and CYP 2D6. Co-administration of dronedarone with CYP 3A substrates may increase plasma concentrations of tacrolimus, sirolimus, and other CYP 3A substrates with a narrow therapeutic range when given orally. Monitor plasma concentrations and adjust dosage appropriately).
No products indexed under this heading.

Droperidol (Concomitant use of drugs or herbal products that prolong the QT interval might increase the risk of Torsade de Pointes, such as phenothiazine anti-psychotics, tricyclic antidepressants, certain oral macrolide antibiotics, and Class I and III antiarrhythmics. Co-administration of drugs prolonging the QT interval (such as certain phenothiazines, tricyclic antidepressants, certain macrolide antibiotics, and Class I and III antiarrhythmics) is contraindicated because of the potential risk of Torsade de Pointes-type ventricular tachycardia).
No products indexed under this heading.

Dyphylline (Dronedarone is metabolized primarily by CYP 3A and is a moderate inhibitor of CYP 3A and CYP 2D6. Dronedarone's blood levels can therefore be affected by inhibitors and inducers of CYP 3A, and dronedarone can interact with drugs that are substrates of CYP 3A and CYP 2D6. Co-administration of dronedarone with CYP 3A substrates may increase plasma concentrations of tacrolimus, sirolimus, and other CYP 3A substrates with a narrow therapeutic range when given orally. Monitor plasma concentrations and adjust dosage appropriately).
No products indexed under this heading.

Efavirenz (Dronedarone is metabolized primarily by CYP 3A and is a moderate inhibitor of CYP 3A and CYP 2D6. Dronedarone's blood levels can therefore be affected by inhibitors and inducers of CYP 3A, and dronedarone can interact with drugs that are substrates of CYP 3A and CYP 2D6. Concomitant use of other potent CYP 3A inhibitors such as itraconazole, voriconazole, ritonavir, clarithromycin, and nefazodone is contraindicated). Products include:
Atripla 906

Encainide Hydrochloride (Dronedarone is metabolized primarily by CYP 3A and is a moderate inhibitor of CYP 3A and CYP 2D6. Dronedarone's blood levels can therefore be affected by inhibitors and inducers of CYP 3A, and dronedarone can interact with drugs that are substrates of CYP 3A and CYP 2D6. Other CYP 2D6 substrates, including other β-blockers, tricyclic antidepressants, and selective serotonin reuptake inhibitors (SSRIs) may have increased exposure upon co-administration with dronedarone).
No products indexed under this heading.

Ergotamine Tartrate (Dronedarone is metabolized primarily by CYP 3A and is a moderate inhibitor of CYP 3A and CYP 2D6. Dronedarone's blood levels can therefore be affected by inhibitors and inducers of CYP 3A, and dronedarone can interact with drugs that are substrates of CYP 3A and CYP 2D6. Co-administration of dronedarone with CYP 3A substrates may increase plasma concentrations of tacrolimus, sirolimus, and other CYP 3A substrates with a narrow therapeutic range when given orally. Monitor plasma concentrations and adjust dosage appropriately).
No products indexed under this heading.

Erythromycin (Concomitant use of drugs or herbal products that prolong the QT interval might increase the risk of Torsade de Pointes, such as phenothiazine anti-psychotics, tricyclic antidepressants, certain oral macrolide antibiotics, and Class I and III antiarrhythmics. Co-administration of drugs prolonging the QT interval (such as certain phenothiazines, tricyclic antidepressants, certain macrolide antibiotics, and Class I and III antiarrhythmics) is contraindicated because of the potential risk of Torsade de Pointes-type ventricular tachycardia).
No products indexed under this heading.

Erythromycin, Topical (Dronedarone has no significant potential to inhibit CYP 1A2, CYP 2C9, CYP 2C19, CYP 2C8 and CYP 2B6. It has the potential to inhibit P-glycoprotein (P-gP) transport. Dronedarone increased digoxin exposure by 2.5-fold by inhibiting the P-gP transporter. Other P-gP substrates are expected to have increased exposure when co-administered with dronedarone).
No products indexed under this heading.

Erythromycin Estolate (Concomitant use of drugs or herbal products that prolong the QT interval might increase the risk of Torsade de Pointes, such as phenothiazine anti-psychotics, tricyclic antidepressants, certain oral macrolide antibiotics, and Class I and III antiarrhythmics. Co-administration of drugs prolonging the QT interval (such as certain phenothiazines, tricyclic antidepressants, certain macrolide antibiotics, and Class I and III antiarrhythmics) is contraindicated because of the potential risk of Torsade de Pointes-type ventricular tachycardia).
No products indexed under this heading.

Erythromycin Ethylsuccinate (Concomitant use of drugs or herbal products that prolong the QT interval might increase the risk of Torsade de Pointes, such as phenothiazine anti-psychotics, tricyclic antidepressants, certain oral macrolide antibiotics, and Class I and III antiarrhythmics. Co-administration of drugs prolonging the QT interval (such as certain phenothiazines, tricyclic antidepressants, certain macrolide antibiotics, and Class I and III antiarrhythmics) is contraindicated because of the potential risk of Torsade de Pointes-type ventricular tachycardia). Products include:
E.E.S. 437
EryPed 435

Erythromycin Gluceptate (Concomitant use of drugs or herbal products that prolong the QT interval might increase the risk of Torsade de Pointes, such as phenothiazine anti-psychotics, tricyclic antidepressants, certain oral macrolide antibiotics, and Class I and III antiarrhythmics. Co-administration of drugs prolonging the QT interval (such as certain phenothiazines, tricyclic antidepressants, certain macrolide antibiotics, and Class I and III antiarrhythmics) is contraindicated because of the potential risk of Torsade de Pointes-type ventricular tachycardia).
No products indexed under this heading.

Erythromycin Lactobionate (Concomitant use of drugs or herbal products that prolong the QT interval might increase the risk of Torsade de Pointes, such as phenothiazine anti-psychotics, tricyclic antidepressants, certain oral macrolide antibiotics, and Class I and III antiarrhythmics. Co-administration of drugs prolonging the QT interval (such as certain phenothiazines, tricyclic antidepressants, certain macrolide antibiotics, and Class I and III antiarrhythmics) is contraindicated because of the potential risk of Torsade de Pointes-type ventricular tachycardia).
No products indexed under this heading.

Erythromycin Stearate (Concomitant use of drugs or herbal products that prolong the QT interval might increase the risk of Torsade de Pointes, such as phenothiazine anti-psychotics, tricyclic antidepressants, certain oral macrolide antibiotics, and Class I and III antiarrhythmics. Co-administration of drugs prolonging the QT interval (such as certain phenothiazines, tricyclic antidepressants, certain macrolide antibiotics, and Class I and III antiarrhythmics) is contraindicated because of the potential risk of Torsade de Pointes-type ventricular tachycardia).
No products indexed under this heading.

Escitalopram Oxalate (Other CYP 2D6 substrates, including serotonin reuptake inhibitors (SSRIs), may have increased exposure upon co-administration with dronedarone). Products include:
Lexapro Oral Suspension 1160
Lexapro Tablets 1160

Esmolol Hydrochloride (Co-administration of dronedarone with other CYP 2D6 substrates, including other beta-blockers, may have increased exposure. In clinical trials, bradycardia was more frequently observed when dronedarone was given in combination with β-blockers. Give low dose of β-blockers initially, and increase only after ECG verification of good tolerability).
No products indexed under this heading.

Estrogen (Dronedarone is metabolized primarily by CYP 3A and is a moderate inhibitor of CYP 3A and CYP 2D6. Dronedarone's blood levels can therefore be affected by inhibitors and inducers of CYP 3A, and dronedarone can interact with drugs that are substrates of CYP 3A and CYP 2D6. Co-administration of dronedarone with CYP 3A substrates may increase plasma concentrations of tacrolimus, sirolimus, and other CYP 3A substrates with a narrow therapeutic range when given orally. Monitor plasma concentrations and adjust dosage appropriately).
No products indexed under this heading.

Estrogens, Conjugated (Dronedarone is metabolized primarily by CYP 3A and is a moderate inhibitor of CYP 3A and CYP 2D6. Dronedarone's blood levels can therefore be affected by inhibitors and inducers of CYP 3A, and dronedarone can interact with drugs that are substrates of CYP 3A and CYP 2D6. Co-administration of dronedarone with CYP 3A substrates may increase plasma concentrations of tacrolimus, sirolimus, and other CYP 3A substrates with a narrow therapeutic range when given orally. Monitor plasma concentrations and adjust dosage appropriately). Products include:

1153 Interactions Index Multaq

Premarin Intravenous 3528
Premarin Tablets 3533
Premarin Vaginal Cream 3540
Premphase 3549
Prempro 3549

Estrogens, Conjugated, Synthetic A (Dronedarone is metabolized primarily by CYP 3A and is a moderate inhibitor of CYP 3A and CYP 2D6. Dronedarone's blood levels can therefore be affected by inhibitors and inducers of CYP 3A, and dronedarone can interact with drugs that are substrates of CYP 3A and CYP 2D6. Co-administration of dronedarone with CYP 3A substrates may increase plasma concentrations of tacrolimus, sirolimus, and other CYP 3A substrates with a narrow therapeutic range when given orally. Monitor plasma concentrations and adjust dosage appropriately).
No products indexed under this heading.

Estrogens, Esterified (Dronedarone is metabolized primarily by CYP 3A and is a moderate inhibitor of CYP 3A and CYP 2D6. Dronedarone's blood levels can therefore be affected by inhibitors and inducers of CYP 3A, and dronedarone can interact with drugs that are substrates of CYP 3A and CYP 2D6. Co-administration of dronedarone with CYP 3A substrates may increase plasma concentrations of tacrolimus, sirolimus, and other CYP 3A substrates with a narrow therapeutic range when given orally. Monitor plasma concentrations and adjust dosage appropriately).
No products indexed under this heading.

Ethinyl Estradiol (Dronedarone is metabolized primarily by CYP 3A and is a moderate inhibitor of CYP 3A and CYP 2D6. Dronedarone's blood levels can therefore be affected by inhibitors and inducers of CYP 3A, and dronedarone can interact with drugs that are substrates of CYP 3A and CYP 2D6. Co-administration of dronedarone with CYP 3A substrates may increase plasma concentrations of tacrolimus, sirolimus, and other CYP 3A substrates with a narrow therapeutic range when given orally. Monitor plasma concentrations and adjust dosage appropriately).
Products include:
LoSeasonique 3407
Lybrel 3514
NuvaRing 3181
Ortho Evra 2648
Ortho-Cyclen/Ortho Tri-Cyclen 2663
Ortho Tri-Cyclen Lo Tablets 2673
Seasonique 3418
Yaz 864

Ethosuximide (Dronedarone is metabolized primarily by CYP 3A and is a moderate inhibitor of CYP 3A and CYP 2D6. Dronedarone's blood levels can therefore be affected by inhibitors and inducers of CYP 3A, and dronedarone can interact with drugs that are substrates of CYP 3A and CYP 2D6. Avoid other CYP 3A inducers such as phenobarbital, carbamazepine, phenytoin, and St John's wort with dronedarone because they decrease its exposure significantly).
No products indexed under this heading.

Ethynodiol Diacetate (Dronedarone is metabolized primarily by CYP 3A and is a moderate inhibitor of CYP 3A and CYP 2D6. Dronedarone's blood levels can therefore be affected by inhibitors and inducers of CYP 3A, and dronedarone can interact with drugs that are substrates of CYP 3A and CYP 2D6. Co-administration of dronedarone with CYP 3A substrates may increase plasma concentrations of tacrolimus, sirolimus, and other CYP 3A substrates with a narrow therapeutic range when given orally. Monitor plasma concentrations and adjust dosage appropriately).
No products indexed under this heading.

Etoposide (Dronedarone has no significant potential to inhibit CYP 1A2, CYP 2C9, CYP 2C19, CYP 2C8 and CYP 2B6. It has the potential to inhibit P-glycoprotein (P-gP) transport. Dronedarone increased digoxin exposure by 2.5-fold by inhibiting the P-gP transporter. Other P-gP substrates are expected to have increased exposure when co-administered with dronedarone).
No products indexed under this heading.

Etoposide Phosphate (Dronedarone has no significant potential to inhibit CYP 1A2, CYP 2C9, CYP 2C19, CYP 2C8 and CYP 2B6. It has the potential to inhibit P-glycoprotein (P-gP) transport. Dronedarone increased digoxin exposure by 2.5-fold by inhibiting the P-gP transporter. Other P-gP substrates are expected to have increased exposure when co-administered with dronedarone).
No products indexed under this heading.

Felodipine (Co-administration of dronedarone with calcium channel blockers may increase calcium channel blocker (verapamil, diltiazem or nifedipine) exposure by 1.4- to 1.5-fold. Calcium channel blockers with depressant effects on the sinus and AV nodes could potentiate dronedarone's effects on conduction. Give low doses of calcium channel blockers initially and increase only after ECG verification of good tolerability).
No products indexed under this heading.

Fentanyl (Dronedarone is metabolized primarily by CYP 3A and is a moderate inhibitor of CYP 3A and CYP 2D6. Dronedarone's blood levels can therefore be affected by inhibitors and inducers of CYP 3A, and dronedarone can interact with drugs that are substrates of CYP 3A and CYP 2D6. Co-administration of dronedarone with CYP 3A substrates may increase plasma concentrations of tacrolimus, sirolimus, and other CYP 3A substrates with a narrow therapeutic range when given orally. Monitor plasma concentrations and adjust dosage appropriately).
Products include:
Duragesic 2604
Fentanyl Transdermal System 2346
Onsolis 2054

Fentanyl Citrate (Dronedarone is metabolized primarily by CYP 3A and is a moderate inhibitor of CYP 3A and CYP 2D6. Dronedarone's blood levels can therefore be affected by inhibitors and inducers of CYP 3A, and dronedarone can interact with drugs that are substrates of CYP 3A and CYP 2D6. Co-administration of dronedarone with CYP 3A substrates may increase plasma concentrations of tacrolimus, sirolimus, and other CYP 3A substrates with a narrow therapeutic range when given orally. Monitor plasma concentrations and adjust dosage appropriately).
Products include:
Fentora 966

Fexofenadine Hydrochloride (Dronedarone has no significant potential to inhibit CYP 1A2, CYP 2C9, CYP 2C19, CYP 2C8 and CYP 2B6. It has the potential to inhibit P-glycoprotein (P-gP) transport. Dronedarone increased digoxin exposure by 2.5-fold by inhibiting the P-gP transporter. Other P-gP substrates are expected to have increased exposure when co-administered with dronedarone).
Products include:
Allegra ODT 2911
Allegra Oral Solution 2911
Allegra 2911
Allegra-D 2915
Allegra-D 24 2918

Flecainide Acetate (Concomitant use of drugs or herbal products that prolong the QT interval might increase the risk of Torsade de Pointes, such as phenothiazine anti-psychotics, tricyclic antidepressants, certain oral macrolide antibiotics, and Class I and III antiarrhythmics. Co-administration of drugs prolonging the QT interval (such as certain phenothiazines, tricyclic antidepressants, certain macrolide antibiotics, and Class I and III antiarrhythmics) is contraindicated because of the potential risk of Torsade de Pointes-type ventricular tachycardia).
No products indexed under this heading.

Fluconazole (Dronedarone is metabolized primarily by CYP 3A and is a moderate inhibitor of CYP 3A and CYP 2D6. Dronedarone's blood levels can therefore be affected by inhibitors and inducers of CYP 3A, and dronedarone can interact with drugs that are substrates of CYP 3A and CYP 2D6. Concomitant use of other potent CYP 3A inhibitors such as itraconazole, voriconazole, ritonavir, clarithromycin, and nefazodone is contraindicated).
No products indexed under this heading.

Fluoxetine (Dronedarone is metabolized primarily by CYP 3A and is a moderate inhibitor of CYP 3A and CYP 2D6. Dronedarone's blood levels can therefore be affected by inhibitors and inducers of CYP 3A, and dronedarone can interact with drugs that are substrates of CYP 3A and CYP 2D6. Concomitant use of other potent CYP 3A inhibitors such as itraconazole, voriconazole, ritonavir, clarithromycin, and nefazodone is contraindicated).
No products indexed under this heading.

Fluoxetine Hydrochloride (Dronedarone is metabolized primarily by CYP 3A and is a moderate inhibitor of CYP 3A and CYP 2D6. Dronedarone's blood levels can therefore be affected by inhibitors and inducers of CYP 3A, and dronedarone can interact with drugs that are substrates of CYP 3A and CYP 2D6. Concomitant use of other potent CYP 3A inhibitors such as itraconazole, voriconazole, ritonavir, clarithromycin, and nefazodone is contraindicated).
Products include:
Prozac Weekly 1941
Prozac Pulvules 1941
Symbyax 1965

Fluphenazine Decanoate (Co-administration of drugs prolonging the QT interval (such as certain phenothiazines, tricyclic antidepressants, certain macrolide antibiotics, and Class I and III antiarrhythmics) is contraindicated because of the potential risk of Torsade de Pointes-type ventricular tachycardia).
No products indexed under this heading.

Fluphenazine Enanthate (Co-administration of drugs prolonging the QT interval (such as certain phenothiazines, tricyclic antidepressants, certain macrolide antibiotics, and Class I and III antiarrhythmics) is contraindicated because of the potential risk of Torsade de Pointes-type ventricular tachycardia).
No products indexed under this heading.

Fluphenazine Hydrochloride (Co-administration of drugs prolonging the QT interval (such as certain phenothiazines, tricyclic antidepressants, certain macrolide antibiotics, and Class I and III antiarrhythmics) is contraindicated because of the potential risk of Torsade de Pointes-type ventricular tachycardia).
No products indexed under this heading.

Fluvoxamine (Other CYP 2D6 substrates, including serotonin reuptake inhibitors (SSRIs), may have increased exposure upon co-administration with dronedarone).
No products indexed under this heading.

Fluvoxamine Maleate (Dronedarone is metabolized primarily by CYP 3A and is a moderate inhibitor of CYP 3A and CYP 2D6. Dronedarone's blood levels can therefore be affected by inhibitors and inducers of CYP 3A, and dronedarone can interact with drugs that are substrates of CYP 3A and CYP 2D6. Concomitant use of other potent CYP 3A inhibitors such as itraconazole, voriconazole, ritonavir, clarithromycin, and nefazodone is contraindicated).
No products indexed under this heading.

Formoterol Fumarate (Dronedarone is metabolized primarily by CYP 3A and is a moderate inhibitor of CYP 3A and CYP 2D6. Dronedarone's blood levels can therefore be affected by inhibitors and inducers of CYP 3A, and dronedarone can interact with drugs that are substrates of CYP 3A and CYP 2D6. Other CYP 2D6 substrates, including other β-blockers, tricyclic antidepressants, and selective serotonin reuptake inhibitors (SSRIs) may have increased exposure upon co-administration with dronedarone). Products include:
Foradil 3121
Perforomist 3634

Fosamprenavir Calcium (Dronedarone has no significant potential to inhibit CYP 1A2, CYP 2C9, CYP 2C19, CYP 2C8 and CYP 2B6. It has the potential to inhibit P-glycoprotein (P-gP) transport. Dronedarone increased digoxin exposure by 2.5-fold by inhibiting the P-gP transporter. Other P-gP substrates are expected to have increased exposure when co-administered with dronedarone). Products include:
Lexiva Oral Suspension 1558
Lexiva 1558

Fosphenytoin (Co-administration of dronedarone with CYP 3A inducers such as phenytoin should be avoided because phenytoin may decrease dronedarone exposure significantly).
No products indexed under this heading.

Fosphenytoin Sodium (Co-administration of dronedarone with CYP 3A inducers such as phenytoin should be avoided because phenytoin may decrease dronedarone exposure significantly).
No products indexed under this heading.

Galantamine Hydrobromide (Dronedarone is metabolized primarily by CYP 3A and is a moderate inhibitor of CYP 3A and CYP 2D6. Dronedarone's blood levels can therefore be affected by inhibitors and inducers of CYP 3A, and dronedarone can interact with drugs that are substrates of CYP 3A and CYP 2D6. Other CYP 2D6 substrates, including other β-blockers, tricyclic antidepressants, and selective serotonin reuptake inhibitors (SSRIs) may have increased exposure upon co-administration with dronedarone).
No products indexed under this heading.

Glyburide (Dronedarone is metabolized primarily by CYP 3A and is a moderate inhibitor of CYP 3A and CYP 2D6. Dronedarone's blood levels can therefore be affected by inhibitors and inducers of CYP 3A, and dronedarone can interact with drugs that are substrates of CYP 3A and CYP 2D6. Co-administration of dronedarone with CYP 3A substrates may increase plasma concentrations of tacrolimus, sirolimus, and other CYP 3A substrates with a narrow therapeutic range when given orally. Monitor plasma concentrations and adjust dosage appropriately).
No products indexed under this heading.

Haloperidol (Concomitant use of drugs or herbal products that prolong the QT interval might increase the risk of Torsade de Pointes, such as phenothiazine anti-psychotics, tricyclic antidepressants, certain oral macrolide antibiotics, and Class I and III antiarrhythmics. Co-administration of drugs prolonging the QT interval (such as certain phenothiazines, tricyclic antidepressants, certain macrolide antibiot-

ics, and Class I and III antiarrhythmics) is contraindicated because of the potential risk of Torsade de Pointes-type ventricular tachycardia).
No products indexed under this heading.

Haloperidol Decanoate (Concomitant use of drugs or herbal products that prolong the QT interval might increase the risk of Torsade de Pointes, such as phenothiazine anti-psychotics, tricyclic antidepressants, certain oral macrolide antibiotics, and Class I and III antiarrhythmics. Co-administration of drugs prolonging the QT interval (such as certain phenothiazines, tricyclic antidepressants, certain macrolide antibiotics, and Class I and III antiarrhythmics) is contraindicated because of the potential risk of Torsade de Pointes-type ventricular tachycardia).
No products indexed under this heading.

Haloperidol Lactate (Concomitant use of drugs or herbal products that prolong the QT interval might increase the risk of Torsade de Pointes, such as phenothiazine anti-psychotics, tricyclic antidepressants, certain oral macrolide antibiotics, and Class I and III antiarrhythmics. Co-administration of drugs prolonging the QT interval (such as certain phenothiazines, tricyclic antidepressants, certain macrolide antibiotics, and Class I and III antiarrhythmics) is contraindicated because of the potential risk of Torsade de Pointes-type ventricular tachycardia).
No products indexed under this heading.

Herbal Medicines, unspecified (Concomitant use of drugs or herbal products that prolong the QT interval and might increase the risk of Torsade de Pointes, such as phenothiazine antipsychotics, tricyclic antidepressants, certain oral macrolide antibiotics, and Class I and III antiarrhythmics is contraindicated).
No products indexed under this heading.

Hydrocodone Bitartrate (Dronedarone is metabolized primarily by CYP 3A and is a moderate inhibitor of CYP 3A and CYP 2D6. Dronedarone's blood levels can therefore be affected by inhibitors and inducers of CYP 3A, and dronedarone can interact with drugs that are substrates of CYP 3A and CYP 2D6. Other CYP 2D6 substrates, including other β-blockers, tricyclic antidepressants, and selective serotonin reuptake inhibitors (SSRIs) may have increased exposure upon co-administration with dronedarone).
Products include:
Vicodin 560
Vicodin ES 561
Vicodin HP 563
Vicoprofen 564
Zydone 1138

Hydrocortisone (Dronedarone has no significant potential to inhibit CYP 1A2, CYP 2C9, CYP 2C19, CYP 2C8 and CYP 2B6. It has the potential to inhibit P-glycoprotein (P-gP) transport. Dronedarone increased digoxin exposure by 2.5-fold by inhibiting the P-gP transporter. Other P-gP substrates are expected to have increased exposure when co-administered with dronedarone).
No products indexed under this heading.

Hydrocortisone (Alcohol) (Dronedarone has no significant potential to inhibit CYP 1A2, CYP 2C9, CYP 2C19, CYP 2C8 and CYP 2B6. It has the potential to inhibit P-glycoprotein (P-gP) transport. Dronedarone increased digoxin exposure by 2.5-fold by inhibiting the P-gP transporter. Other P-gP substrates are expected to have increased exposure when co-administered with dronedarone).
No products indexed under this heading.

Hydrocortisone Acetate (Dronedarone has no significant potential to inhibit CYP 1A2, CYP 2C9, CYP 2C19, CYP 2C8 and CYP 2B6. It has the potential to inhibit P-glycoprotein (P-gP) transport. Dronedarone increased digoxin exposure by 2.5-fold by inhibiting the P-gP transporter. Other P-gP substrates are expected to have increased exposure when co-administered with dronedarone).
No products indexed under this heading.

Hydrocortisone Butyrate (Dronedarone has no significant potential to inhibit CYP 1A2, CYP 2C9, CYP 2C19, CYP 2C8 and CYP 2B6. It has the potential to inhibit P-glycoprotein (P-gP) transport. Dronedarone increased digoxin exposure by 2.5-fold by inhibiting the P-gP transporter. Other P-gP substrates are expected to have increased exposure when co-administered with dronedarone).
No products indexed under this heading.

Hydrocortisone Cypionate (Dronedarone has no significant potential to inhibit CYP 1A2, CYP 2C9, CYP 2C19, CYP 2C8 and CYP 2B6. It has the potential to inhibit P-glycoprotein (P-gP) transport. Dronedarone increased digoxin exposure by 2.5-fold by inhibiting the P-gP transporter. Other P-gP substrates are expected to have increased exposure when co-administered with dronedarone).
No products indexed under this heading.

Hydrocortisone Hemisuccinate (Dronedarone has no significant potential to inhibit CYP 1A2, CYP 2C9, CYP 2C19, CYP 2C8 and CYP 2B6. It has the potential to inhibit P-glycoprotein (P-gP) transport. Dronedarone increased digoxin exposure by 2.5-fold by inhibiting the P-gP transporter. Other P-gP substrates are expected to have increased exposure when co-administered with dronedarone).
No products indexed under this heading.

Hydrocortisone Probutate (Dronedarone has no significant potential to inhibit CYP 1A2, CYP 2C9, CYP 2C19, CYP 2C8 and CYP 2B6. It has the potential to inhibit P-glycoprotein (P-gP) transport. Dronedarone increased digoxin exposure by 2.5-fold by inhibiting the P-gP transporter. Other P-gP substrates are expected to have increased exposure when co-administered with dronedarone).
No products indexed under this heading.

Hydrocortisone Sodium Phosphate (Dronedarone has no significant potential to inhibit CYP 1A2, CYP 2C9, CYP 2C19, CYP 2C8 and CYP 2B6. It has the potential to inhibit P-glycoprotein (P-gP) transport. Dronedarone increased digoxin exposure by 2.5-fold by inhibiting the P-gP transporter. Other P-gP substrates are expected to have increased exposure when co-administered with dronedarone).
No products indexed under this heading.

Hydrocortisone Sodium Succinate (Dronedarone has no significant potential to inhibit CYP 1A2, CYP 2C9, CYP 2C19, CYP 2C8 and CYP 2B6. It has the potential to inhibit P-glycoprotein (P-gP) transport. Dronedarone increased digoxin exposure by 2.5-fold by inhibiting the P-gP transporter. Other P-gP substrates are expected to have increased exposure when co-administered with dronedarone).
No products indexed under this heading.

Hydrocortisone Valerate (Dronedarone has no significant potential to inhibit CYP 1A2, CYP 2C9, CYP 2C19, CYP 2C8 and CYP 2B6. It has the potential to inhibit P-glycoprotein (P-gP) transport. Dronedarone increased digoxin exposure by 2.5-fold by inhibiting the P-gP transporter. Other P-gP substrates are expected to have increased exposure when co-administered with dronedarone).
No products indexed under this heading.

Hydroxyzine Hydrochloride (Concomitant use of drugs or herbal products that prolong the QT interval might increase the risk of Torsade de Pointes, such as phenothiazine anti-psychotics, tricyclic antidepressants, certain oral macrolide antibiotics, and Class I and III antiarrhythmics. Co-administration of drugs prolonging the QT interval (such as certain phenothiazines, tricyclic antidepressants, certain macrolide antibiotics, and Class I and III antiarrhythmics) is contraindicated because of the potential risk of Torsade de Pointes-type ventricular tachycardia).
No products indexed under this heading.

Hypericum Perforatum (Co-administration of dronedarone with CYP 3A inducers such as St. John's Wort should be avoided because phenytoin may decrease dronedarone exposure significantly). Products include:
Traumeel 1800

Imipramine Hydrochloride (Concomitant use of drugs or herbal products that prolong the QT interval might increase the risk of Torsade de Pointes, such as phenothiazine anti-psychotics, tricyclic antidepressants, certain oral macrolide antibiotics, and Class I and III antiarrhythmics. Co-administration of drugs prolonging the QT interval (such as certain phenothiazines, tricyclic antidepressants, certain macrolide antibiotics, and Class I and III antiarrhythmics) is contraindicated because of the potential risk of Torsade de Pointes-type ventricular tachycardia).
No products indexed under this heading.

Imipramine Pamoate (Concomitant use of drugs or herbal products that prolong the QT interval might increase the risk of Torsade de Pointes, such as phenothiazine anti-psychotics, tricyclic antidepressants, certain oral macrolide antibiotics, and Class I and III antiarrhythmics. Co-administration of drugs prolonging the QT interval (such as certain phenothiazines, tricyclic antidepressants, certain macrolide antibiotics, and Class I and III antiarrhythmics) is contraindicated because of the potential risk of Torsade de Pointes-type ventricular tachycardia).
No products indexed under this heading.

Indinavir Sulfate (Dronedarone is metabolized primarily by CYP 3A and is a moderate inhibitor of CYP 3A and CYP 2D6. Dronedarone's blood levels can therefore be affected by inhibitors and inducers of CYP 3A, and dronedarone can interact with drugs that are substrates of CYP 3A and CYP 2D6. Concomitant use of other potent CYP 3A inhibitors such as itraconazole, voriconazole, ritonavir, clarithromycin, and nefazodone is contraindicated).
Products include:
Crixivan 2113

Indoramin Hydrochloride (Dronedarone is metabolized primarily by CYP 3A and is a moderate inhibitor of CYP 3A and CYP 2D6. Dronedarone's blood levels can therefore be affected by inhibitors and inducers of CYP 3A, and dronedarone can interact with drugs that are substrates of CYP 3A and CYP 2D6. Other CYP 2D6 substrates, including other β-blockers, tricyclic antidepressants, and selective serotonin reuptake inhibitors (SSRIs) may have increased exposure upon co-administration with dronedarone).
No products indexed under this heading.

Isocarboxazid (Concomitant use of drugs or herbal products that prolong the QT interval might increase the risk of Torsade de Pointes, such as phenothiazine anti-psychotics, tricyclic antidepressants, certain oral macrolide antibiotics, and Class I and III antiarrhythmics. Co-administration of drugs prolonging the QT interval (such as certain phenothiazines, tricyclic antidepressants, certain macrolide antibiotics, and Class I and III antiarrhythmics) is contraindicated because of the potential risk of Torsade de Pointes-type ventricular tachycardia). Products include:
Marplan 3481

Isoniazid (Dronedarone is metabolized primarily by CYP 3A and is a moderate inhibitor of CYP 3A and CYP 2D6. Dronedarone's blood levels can therefore be affected by inhibitors and inducers of CYP 3A, and dronedarone can interact with drugs that are substrates of CYP 3A and CYP 2D6. Concomitant use of other potent CYP 3A inhibitors such as itraconazole, voriconazole, ritonavir, clarithromycin, and nefazodone is contraindicated).
No products indexed under this heading.

Isradipine (Co-administration of dronedarone with calcium channel blockers may increase calcium channel blocker (verapamil, diltiazem or nifedipine) exposure by 1.4- to 1.5-fold. Calcium channel blockers with depressant effects on the sinus and AV nodes could potentiate dronedarone's effects on conduction. Give low doses of calcium channel blockers initially and increase only after ECG verification of good tolerability).
Products include:
DynaCirc CR 1432

Itraconazole (Concomitant use of strong CYP 3A inhibitors, such as ketoconazole, itraconazole, voriconazole, cyclosporine, telithromycin, clarithromycin, nefazodone, and ritonavir is contraindicated).
No products indexed under this heading.

Ivermectin (Dronedarone has no significant potential to inhibit CYP 1A2, CYP 2C9, CYP 2C19, CYP 2C8 and CYP 2B6. It has the potential to inhibit P-glycoprotein (P-gP) transport. Dronedarone increased digoxin exposure by 2.5-fold by inhibiting the P-gP transporter. Other P-gP substrates are expected to have increased exposure when co-administered with dronedarone).
Products include:
Stromectol 2277

Ketoconazole (Concomitant use of ketoconazole as well as other potent CYP 3A inhibitors such as itraconazole, voriconazole, ritonavir, clarithromycin, and nefazodone is contraindicated. Repeated doses of ketoconazole, a strong CYP 3A inhibitor, resulted in a 17-fold increase in dronedarone exposure and a 9-fold increase in C_{max}).
Products include:
Extina 3319
Xolegel 3337

Labetalol Hydrochloride (Co-administration of dronedarone with other CYP 2D6 substrates, including other beta-blockers, may have increased exposure. In clinical trials, bradycardia was more frequently observed when dronedarone was given in combination with β-blockers. Give low dose of β-blockers initially, and increase only after ECG verification of good tolerability).
No products indexed under this heading.

Lapatinib (Dronedarone has no significant potential to inhibit CYP 1A2, CYP 2C9, CYP 2C19, CYP 2C8 and CYP

1155 Interactions Index Multaq

2B6. It has the potential to inhibit P-glycoprotein (P-gP) transport. Dronedarone increased digoxin exposure by 2.5-fold by inhibiting the P-gP transporter. Other P-gP substrates are expected to have increased exposure when co-administered with dronedarone).
Products include:
Tykerb 1698

Levobunolol Hydrochloride (Co-administration of dronedarone with other CYP 2D6 substrates, including other beta-blockers, may have increased exposure. In clinical trials, bradycardia was more frequently observed when dronedarone was given in combination with β-blockers. Give low dose of β-blockers initially, and increase only after ECG verification of good tolerability).
No products indexed under this heading.

Levonorgestrel (Dronedarone is metabolized primarily by CYP 3A and is a moderate inhibitor of CYP 3A and CYP 2D6. Dronedarone's blood levels can therefore be affected by inhibitors and inducers of CYP 3A, and dronedarone can interact with drugs that are substrates of CYP 3A and CYP 2D6. Co-administration of dronedarone with CYP 3A substrates may increase plasma concentrations of tacrolimus, sirolimus, and other CYP 3A substrates with a narrow therapeutic range when given orally. Monitor plasma concentrations and adjust dosage appropriately).
Products include:
Climara Pro 847
LoSeasonique 3407
Lybrel 3514
Mirena 854
Plan B 3416
Seasonique 3418

Lidocaine (Concomitant use of drugs or herbal products that prolong the QT interval might increase the risk of Torsade de Pointes, such as phenothiazine anti-psychotics, tricyclic antidepressants, certain oral macrolide antibiotics, and Class I and III antiarrhythmics. Co-administration of drugs prolonging the QT interval (such as certain phenothiazines, tricyclic antidepressants, certain macrolide antibiotics, and Class I and III antiarrhythmics) is contraindicated because of the potential risk of Torsade de Pointes-type ventricular tachycardia).
Products include:
Lidoderm 1107

Lidocaine Hydrochloride (Concomitant use of drugs or herbal products that prolong the QT interval might increase the risk of Torsade de Pointes, such as phenothiazine anti-psychotics, tricyclic antidepressants, certain oral macrolide antibiotics, and Class I and III antiarrhythmics. Co-administration of drugs prolonging the QT interval (such as certain phenothiazines, tricyclic antidepressants, certain macrolide antibiotics, and Class I and III antiarrhythmics) is contraindicated because of the potential risk of Torsade de Pointes-type ventricular tachycardia).
No products indexed under this heading.

Lithium (Concomitant use of drugs or herbal products that prolong the QT interval and might increase the risk of Torsade de Pointes, such as phenothiazine anti-psychotics, tricyclic antidepressants, certain oral macrolide antibiotics, and Class I and III antiarrhythmics is contraindicated).
No products indexed under this heading.

Lithium Carbonate (Concomitant use of drugs or herbal products that prolong the QT interval might increase the risk of Torsade de Pointes, such as phenothiazine anti-psychotics, tricyclic antidepressants, certain oral macrolide antibiotics, and Class I and III antiarrhythmics. Co-administration of drugs prolonging the QT interval (such as certain phenothiazines, tricyclic antidepressants, certain macrolide antibiotics, and Class I and III antiarrhythmics) is contraindicated because of the potential risk of Torsade de Pointes-type ventricular tachycardia).
No products indexed under this heading.

Lithium Citrate (Concomitant use of drugs or herbal products that prolong the QT interval might increase the risk of Torsade de Pointes, such as phenothiazine anti-psychotics, tricyclic antidepressants, certain oral macrolide antibiotics, and Class I and III antiarrhythmics. Co-administration of drugs prolonging the QT interval (such as certain phenothiazines, tricyclic antidepressants, certain macrolide antibiotics, and Class I and III antiarrhythmics) is contraindicated because of the potential risk of Torsade de Pointes-type ventricular tachycardia).
No products indexed under this heading.

Loperamide Hydrochloride (Dronedarone has no significant potential to inhibit CYP 1A2, CYP 2C9, CYP 2C19, CYP 2C8 and CYP 2B6. It has the potential to inhibit P-glycoprotein (P-gP) transport. Dronedarone increased digoxin exposure by 2.5-fold by inhibiting the P-gP transporter. Other P-gP substrates are expected to have increased exposure when co-administered with dronedarone).
Products include:
Imodium A-D 2042
Imodium Multi-Symptom Relief 2043

Lopinavir (Dronedarone is metabolized primarily by CYP 3A and is a moderate inhibitor of CYP 3A and CYP 2D6. Dronedarone's blood levels can therefore be affected by inhibitors and inducers of CYP 3A, and dronedarone can interact with drugs that are substrates of CYP 3A and CYP 2D6. Concomitant use of other potent CYP 3A inhibitors such as itraconazole, voriconazole, ritonavir, clarithromycin, and nefazodone is contraindicated). Products include:
Kaletra 458

Lorazepam (Concomitant use of drugs or herbal products that prolong the QT interval might increase the risk of Torsade de Pointes, such as phenothiazine anti-psychotics, tricyclic antidepressants, certain oral macrolide antibiotics, and Class I and III antiarrhythmics. Co-administration of drugs prolonging the QT interval (such as certain phenothiazines, tricyclic antidepressants, certain macrolide antibiotics, and Class I and III antiarrhythmics) is contraindicated because of the potential risk of Torsade de Pointes-type ventricular tachycardia).
No products indexed under this heading.

Lovastatin (Dronedarone has no significant potential to inhibit CYP 1A2, CYP 2C9, CYP 2C19, CYP 2C8 and CYP 2B6. It has the potential to inhibit P-glycoprotein (P-gP) transport. Dronedarone increased digoxin exposure by 2.5-fold by inhibiting the P-gP transporter. Other P-gP substrates are expected to have increased exposure when co-administered with dronedarone).
Products include:
Advicor 402
Mevacor 2212

Loxapine Hydrochloride (Concomitant use of drugs or herbal products that prolong the QT interval might increase the risk of Torsade de Pointes, such as phenothiazine anti-psychotics, tricyclic antidepressants, certain oral macrolide antibiotics, and Class I and III antiarrhythmics. Co-administration of drugs prolonging the QT interval (such as certain phenothiazines, tricyclic antidepressants, certain macrolide antibiotics, and Class I and III antiarrhythmics) is contraindicated because of the potential risk of Torsade de Pointes-type ventricular tachycardia).
No products indexed under this heading.

Loxapine Succinate (Concomitant use of drugs or herbal products that prolong the QT interval might increase the risk of Torsade de Pointes, such as phenothiazine anti-psychotics, tricyclic antidepressants, certain oral macrolide antibiotics, and Class I and III antiarrhythmics. Co-administration of drugs prolonging the QT interval (such as certain phenothiazines, tricyclic antidepressants, certain macrolide antibiotics, and Class I and III antiarrhythmics) is contraindicated because of the potential risk of Torsade de Pointes-type ventricular tachycardia).
No products indexed under this heading.

Maprotiline Hydrochloride (Concomitant use of drugs or herbal products that prolong the QT interval might increase the risk of Torsade de Pointes, such as phenothiazine anti-psychotics, tricyclic antidepressants, certain oral macrolide antibiotics, and Class I and III antiarrhythmics. Co-administration of drugs prolonging the QT interval (such as certain phenothiazines, tricyclic antidepressants, certain macrolide antibiotics, and Class I and III antiarrhythmics) is contraindicated because of the potential risk of Torsade de Pointes-type ventricular tachycardia).
No products indexed under this heading.

Maraviroc (Dronedarone has no significant potential to inhibit CYP 1A2, CYP 2C9, CYP 2C19, CYP 2C8 and CYP 2B6. It has the potential to inhibit P-glycoprotein (P-gP) transport. Dronedarone increased digoxin exposure by 2.5-fold by inhibiting the P-gP transporter. Other P-gP substrates are expected to have increased exposure when co-administered with dronedarone).
Products include:
Selzentry 2740

Meperidine Hydrochloride (Dronedarone is metabolized primarily by CYP 3A and is a moderate inhibitor of CYP 3A and CYP 2D6. Dronedarone's blood levels can therefore be affected by inhibitors and inducers of CYP 3A, and dronedarone can interact with drugs that are substrates of CYP 3A and CYP 2D6. Other CYP 2D6 substrates, including other β-blockers, tricyclic antidepressants, and selective serotonin reuptake inhibitors (SSRIs) may have increased exposure upon co-administration with dronedarone).
No products indexed under this heading.

Meprobamate (Concomitant use of drugs or herbal products that prolong the QT interval might increase the risk of Torsade de Pointes, such as phenothiazine anti-psychotics, tricyclic antidepressants, certain oral macrolide antibiotics, and Class I and III antiarrhythmics. Co-administration of drugs prolonging the QT interval (such as certain phenothiazines, tricyclic antidepressants, certain macrolide antibiotics, and Class I and III antiarrhythmics) is contraindicated because of the potential risk of Torsade de Pointes-type ventricular tachycardia).
No products indexed under this heading.

Mesoridazine Besylate (Co-administration of drugs prolonging the QT interval (such as certain phenothiazines, tricyclic antidepressants, certain macrolide antibiotics, and Class I and III antiarrhythmics) is contraindicated because of the potential risk of Torsade de Pointes-type ventricular tachycardia).
No products indexed under this heading.

Mestranol (Dronedarone is metabolized primarily by CYP 3A and is a moderate inhibitor of CYP 3A and CYP 2D6. Dronedarone's blood levels can therefore be affected by inhibitors and inducers of CYP 3A, and dronedarone can interact with drugs that are substrates of CYP 3A and CYP 2D6. Co-administration of dronedarone with CYP 3A substrates may increase plasma concentrations of tacrolimus, sirolimus, and other CYP 3A substrates with a narrow therapeutic range when given orally. Monitor plasma concentrations and adjust dosage appropriately).
No products indexed under this heading.

Methadone Hydrochloride (Dronedarone is metabolized primarily by CYP 3A and is a moderate inhibitor of CYP 3A and CYP 2D6. Dronedarone's blood levels can therefore be affected by inhibitors and inducers of CYP 3A, and dronedarone can interact with drugs that are substrates of CYP 3A and CYP 2D6. Co-administration of dronedarone with CYP 3A substrates may increase plasma concentrations of tacrolimus, sirolimus, and other CYP 3A substrates with a narrow therapeutic range when given orally. Monitor plasma concentrations and adjust dosage appropriately).
No products indexed under this heading.

Methamphetamine Hydrochloride (Dronedarone is metabolized primarily by CYP 3A and is a moderate inhibitor of CYP 3A and CYP 2D6. Dronedarone's blood levels can therefore be affected by inhibitors and inducers of CYP 3A, and dronedarone can interact with drugs that are substrates of CYP 3A and CYP 2D6. Other CYP 2D6 substrates, including other β-blockers, tricyclic antidepressants, and selective serotonin reuptake inhibitors (SSRIs) may have increased exposure upon co-administration with dronedarone).
No products indexed under this heading.

Methotrimeprazine (Co-administration of drugs prolonging the QT interval (such as certain phenothiazines, tricyclic antidepressants, certain macrolide antibiotics, and Class I and III antiarrhythmics) is contraindicated because of the potential risk of Torsade de Pointes-type ventricular tachycardia).
No products indexed under this heading.

Methoxyphenamine (Dronedarone is metabolized primarily by CYP 3A and is a moderate inhibitor of CYP 3A and CYP 2D6. Dronedarone's blood levels can therefore be affected by inhibitors and inducers of CYP 3A, and dronedarone can interact with drugs that are substrates of CYP 3A and CYP 2D6. Other CYP 2D6 substrates, including other β-blockers, tricyclic antidepressants, and selective serotonin reuptake inhibitors (SSRIs) may have increased exposure upon co-administration with dronedarone).
No products indexed under this heading.

Methylprednisolone (Dronedarone is metabolized primarily by CYP 3A and is a moderate inhibitor of CYP 3A and CYP 2D6. Dronedarone's blood levels can therefore be affected by inhibitors and inducers of CYP 3A, and dronedarone can interact with drugs that are substrates of CYP 3A and CYP 2D6. Co-administration of dronedarone with CYP 3A substrates may increase plasma concentrations of tacrolimus, sirolimus, and other CYP 3A substrates with a narrow therapeutic range when given orally. Monitor plasma concentrations and adjust dosage appropriately).
No products indexed under this heading.

Methylprednisolone Acetate (Dronedarone is metabolized primarily by CYP 3A and is a moderate inhibitor of CYP 3A and CYP 2D6. Dronedarone's blood levels can therefore be affected by inhibitors and inducers of CYP 3A, and dronedarone can interact with drugs that are substrates of CYP 3A and CYP 2D6. Co-administration of dronedarone with CYP 3A substrates

Multaq **Interactions Index** **1156**

may increase plasma concentrations of tacrolimus, sirolimus, and other CYP 3A substrates with a narrow therapeutic range when given orally. Monitor plasma concentrations and adjust dosage appropriately).
No products indexed under this heading.

Methylprednisolone Sodium Succinate (Dronedarone is metabolized primarily by CYP 3A and is a moderate inhibitor of CYP 3A and CYP 2D6. Dronedarone's blood levels can therefore be affected by inhibitors and inducers of CYP 3A, and dronedarone can interact with drugs that are substrates of CYP 3A and CYP 2D6. Co-administration of dronedarone with CYP 3A substrates may increase plasma concentrations of tacrolimus, sirolimus, and other CYP 3A substrates with a narrow therapeutic range when given orally. Monitor plasma concentrations and adjust dosage appropriately).
No products indexed under this heading.

Metipranolol Hydrochloride (Co-administration of dronedarone with other CYP 2D6 substrates, including other beta-blockers, may have increased exposure. In clinical trials, bradycardia was more frequently observed when dronedarone was given in combination with β-blockers. Give low dose of β-blockers initially, and increase only after ECG verification of good tolerability).
No products indexed under this heading.

Metoprolol Succinate (Co-administration of dronedarone with metroprolol may increase metoprolol exposure by 1.6-fold following multiple dose administration). Products include:
Toprol XL 732

Metoprolol Tartrate (Co-administration of dronedarone with metroprolol may increase metoprolol exposure by 1.6-fold following multiple dose administration).
No products indexed under this heading.

Metronidazole (Dronedarone is metabolized primarily by CYP 3A and is a moderate inhibitor of CYP 3A and CYP 2D6. Dronedarone's blood levels can therefore be affected by inhibitors and inducers of CYP 3A, and dronedarone can interact with drugs that are substrates of CYP 3A and CYP 2D6. Concomitant use of other potent CYP 3A inhibitors such as itraconazole, voriconazole, ritonavir, clarithromycin, and nefazodone is contraindicated). Products include:
Pylera 793

Metronidazole Benzoate (Dronedarone is metabolized primarily by CYP 3A and is a moderate inhibitor of CYP 3A and CYP 2D6. Dronedarone's blood levels can therefore be affected by inhibitors and inducers of CYP 3A, and dronedarone can interact with drugs that are substrates of CYP 3A and CYP 2D6. Concomitant use of other potent CYP 3A inhibitors such as itraconazole, voriconazole, ritonavir, clarithromycin, and nefazodone is contraindicated).
No products indexed under this heading.

Metronidazole Hydrochloride (Dronedarone is metabolized primarily by CYP 3A and is a moderate inhibitor of CYP 3A and CYP 2D6. Dronedarone's blood levels can therefore be affected by inhibitors and inducers of CYP 3A, and dronedarone can interact with drugs that are substrates of CYP 3A and CYP 2D6. Concomitant use of other potent CYP 3A inhibitors such as itraconazole, voriconazole, ritonavir, clarithromycin, and nefazodone is contraindicated).
No products indexed under this heading.

Mexiletine Hydrochloride (Concomitant use of drugs or herbal products that prolong the QT interval might increase the risk of Torsade de Pointes, such as phenothiazine anti-psychotics, tricyclic antidepressants, certain oral macrolide antibiotics, and Class I and III antiarrhythmics. Co-administration of drugs prolonging the QT interval (such as certain phenothiazines, tricyclic antidepressants, certain macrolide antibiotics, and Class I and III antiarrhythmics) is contraindicated because of the potential risk of Torsade de Pointes-type ventricular tachycardia).
No products indexed under this heading.

Mibefradil Dihydrochloride (Co-administration of dronedarone with calcium channel blockers may increase calcium channel blocker (verapamil, diltiazem or nifedipine) exposure by 1.4- to 1.5-fold. Calcium channel blockers with depressant effects on the sinus and AV nodes could potentiate dronedarone's effects on conduction. Give low doses of calcium channel blockers initially and increase only after ECG verification of good tolerability).
No products indexed under this heading.

Miconazole (Dronedarone is metabolized primarily by CYP 3A and is a moderate inhibitor of CYP 3A and CYP 2D6. Dronedarone's blood levels can therefore be affected by inhibitors and inducers of CYP 3A, and dronedarone can interact with drugs that are substrates of CYP 3A and CYP 2D6. Concomitant use of other potent CYP 3A inhibitors such as itraconazole, voriconazole, ritonavir, clarithromycin, and nefazodone is contraindicated).
No products indexed under this heading.

Midazolam Hydrochloride (Concomitant use of drugs or herbal products that prolong the QT interval might increase the risk of Torsade de Pointes, such as phenothiazine anti-psychotics, tricyclic antidepressants, certain oral macrolide antibiotics, and Class I and III antiarrhythmics. Co-administration of drugs prolonging the QT interval (such as certain phenothiazines, tricyclic antidepressants, certain macrolide antibiotics, and Class I and III antiarrhythmics) is contraindicated because of the potential risk of Torsade de Pointes-type ventricular tachycardia).
No products indexed under this heading.

Mirtazapine (Dronedarone is metabolized primarily by CYP 3A and is a moderate inhibitor of CYP 3A and CYP 2D6. Dronedarone's blood levels can therefore be affected by inhibitors and inducers of CYP 3A, and dronedarone can interact with drugs that are substrates of CYP 3A and CYP 2D6. Other CYP 2D6 substrates, including other β-blockers, tricyclic antidepressants, and selective serotonin reuptake inhibitors (SSRIs) may have increased exposure upon co-administration with dronedarone). Products include:
Remeron Tablets 3214
RemeronSolTab Tablets 3219

Modafinil (Dronedarone is metabolized primarily by CYP 3A and is a moderate inhibitor of CYP 3A and CYP 2D6. Dronedarone's blood levels can therefore be affected by inhibitors and inducers of CYP 3A, and dronedarone can interact with drugs that are substrates of CYP 3A and CYP 2D6. Avoid other CYP 3A inducers such as phenobarbital, carbamazepine, phenytoin, and St John's wort with dronedarone because they decrease its exposure significantly). Products include:
Provigil 983

Molindone Hydrochloride (Concomitant use of drugs or herbal products that prolong the QT interval might increase the risk of Torsade de Pointes, such as phenothiazine anti-psychotics, tricyclic antidepressants, certain oral macrolide antibiotics, and Class I and III antiarrhythmics. Co-administration of drugs prolonging the QT interval (such as certain phenothiazines, tricyclic antidepressants, certain macrolide antibiotics, and Class I and III antiarrhythmics) is contraindicated because of the potential risk of Torsade de Pointes-type ventricular tachycardia). Products include:
Moban 1108

Moricizine Hydrochloride (Co-administration of drugs prolonging the QT interval (such as certain phenothiazines, tricyclic antidepressants, certain macrolide antibiotics, and Class I and III antiarrhythmics) is contraindicated because of the potential risk of Torsade de Pointes-type ventricular tachycardia).
No products indexed under this heading.

Morphine Sulfate (Dronedarone is metabolized primarily by CYP 3A and is a moderate inhibitor of CYP 3A and CYP 2D6. Dronedarone's blood levels can therefore be affected by inhibitors and inducers of CYP 3A, and dronedarone can interact with drugs that are substrates of CYP 3A and CYP 2D6. Other CYP 2D6 substrates, including other β-blockers, tricyclic antidepressants, and selective serotonin reuptake inhibitors (SSRIs) may have increased exposure upon co-administration with dronedarone). Products include:
Avinza 1822
Embeda 1831
MS Contin 2803

Nadolol (Co-administration of dronedarone with other CYP 2D6 substrates, including other beta-blockers, may have increased exposure. In clinical trials, bradycardia was more frequently observed when dronedarone was given in combination with β-blockers. Give low dose of β-blockers initially, and increase only after ECG verification of good tolerability). Products include:
Nadolol 2359

Nebivolol (Co-administration of dronedarone with other CYP 2D6 substrates, including other beta-blockers, may have increased exposure. In clinical trials, bradycardia was more frequently observed when dronedarone was given in combination with β-blockers. Give low dose of β-blockers initially, and increase only after ECG verification of good tolerability). Products include:
Bystolic 1147

Nefazodone Hydrochloride (Concomitant use of other potent CYP 3A inhibitors such as itraconazole, voriconazole, ritonavir, clarithromycin, and nefazodone is contraindicated).
No products indexed under this heading.

Nelfinavir Mesylate (Dronedarone is metabolized primarily by CYP 3A and is a moderate inhibitor of CYP 3A and CYP 2D6. Dronedarone's blood levels can therefore be affected by inhibitors and inducers of CYP 3A, and dronedarone can interact with drugs that are substrates of CYP 3A and CYP 2D6. Concomitant use of other potent CYP 3A inhibitors such as itraconazole, voriconazole, ritonavir, clarithromycin, and nefazodone is contraindicated).
No products indexed under this heading.

Nevirapine (Dronedarone is metabolized primarily by CYP 3A and is a moderate inhibitor of CYP 3A and CYP 2D6. Dronedarone's blood levels can therefore be affected by inhibitors and inducers of CYP 3A, and dronedarone can interact with drugs that are substrates of CYP 3A and CYP 2D6. Avoid other CYP 3A inducers such as phenobarbital, carbamazepine, phenytoin, and St John's wort with dronedarone because they decrease its exposure significantly). Products include:
Viramune Oral Suspension 897
Viramune Tablets 897

Nicardipine (Co-administration of dronedarone with calcium channel blockers may increase calcium channel blocker (verapamil, diltiazem or nifedipine) exposure by 1.4- to 1.5-fold. Calcium channel blockers with depressant effects on the sinus and AV nodes could potentiate dronedarone's effects on conduction. Give low doses of calcium channel blockers initially and increase only after ECG verification of good tolerability).
No products indexed under this heading.

Nicardipine Hydrochloride (Co-administration of dronedarone with calcium channel blockers may increase calcium channel blocker (verapamil, diltiazem or nifedipine) exposure by 1.4- to 1.5-fold. Calcium channel blockers with depressant effects on the sinus and AV nodes could potentiate dronedarone's effects on conduction. Give low doses of calcium channel blockers initially and increase only after ECG verification of good tolerability).
No products indexed under this heading.

Nifedipine (Dronedarone is metabolized primarily by CYP 3A and is a moderate inhibitor of CYP 3A and CYP 2D6. Dronedarone's blood levels can therefore be affected by inhibitors and inducers of CYP 3A, and dronedarone can interact with drugs that are substrates of CYP 3A and CYP 2D6. Concomitant use of other potent CYP 3A inhibitors such as itraconazole, voriconazole, ritonavir, clarithromycin, and nefazodone is contraindicated).
No products indexed under this heading.

Nimodipine (Co-administration of dronedarone with calcium channel blockers may increase calcium channel blocker (verapamil, diltiazem or nifedipine) exposure by 1.4- to 1.5-fold. Calcium channel blockers with depressant effects on the sinus and AV nodes could potentiate dronedarone's effects on conduction. Give low doses of calcium channel blockers initially and increase only after ECG verification of good tolerability).
No products indexed under this heading.

Nisoldipine (Co-administration of dronedarone with calcium channel blockers may increase calcium channel blocker (verapamil, diltiazem or nifedipine) exposure by 1.4- to 1.5-fold. Calcium channel blockers with depressant effects on the sinus and AV nodes could potentiate dronedarone's effects on conduction. Give low doses of calcium channel blockers initially and increase only after ECG verification of good tolerability).
No products indexed under this heading.

Norethindrone (Dronedarone is metabolized primarily by CYP 3A and is a moderate inhibitor of CYP 3A and CYP 2D6. Dronedarone's blood levels can therefore be affected by inhibitors and inducers of CYP 3A, and dronedarone can interact with drugs that are substrates of CYP 3A and CYP 2D6. Co-administration of dronedarone with CYP 3A substrates may increase plasma concentrations of tacrolimus, sirolimus, and other CYP 3A substrates with a narrow therapeutic range when given orally. Monitor plasma concentrations and adjust dosage appropriately). Products include:
Ortho Micronor 2660

Norfloxacin (Dronedarone is metabolized primarily by CYP 3A and is a moderate inhibitor of CYP 3A and CYP 2D6. Dronedarone's blood levels can therefore be affected by inhibitors and inducers of CYP 3A, and dronedarone can interact with drugs that are substrates of CYP 3A and CYP 2D6. Concomitant use of other potent CYP 3A inhibitors such as itraconazole, voriconazole, ritonavir, clarithromycin, and nefazodone is contraindicated). Products include:

IMPORTANT NOTE: Always consult each drug listing in the patient's regimen for possible interactions.

Multaq Interactions Index 1158

Prochlorperazine (Co-administration of drugs prolonging the QT interval (such as certain phenothiazines, tricyclic antidepressants, certain macrolide antibiotics, and Class I and III antiarrhythmics) is contraindicated because of the potential risk of Torsade de Pointes-type ventricular tachycardia).
No products indexed under this heading.

Prochlorperazine Edisylate (Co-administration of drugs prolonging the QT interval (such as certain phenothiazines, tricyclic antidepressants, certain macrolide antibiotics, and Class I and III antiarrhythmics) is contraindicated because of the potential risk of Torsade de Pointes-type ventricular tachycardia).
No products indexed under this heading.

Prochlorperazine Maleate (Co-administration of drugs prolonging the QT interval (such as certain phenothiazines, tricyclic antidepressants, certain macrolide antibiotics, and Class I and III antiarrhythmics) is contraindicated because of the potential risk of Torsade de Pointes-type ventricular tachycardia).
No products indexed under this heading.

Promethazine (Co-administration of drugs prolonging the QT interval (such as certain phenothiazines, tricyclic antidepressants, certain macrolide antibiotics, and Class I and III antiarrhythmics) is contraindicated because of the potential risk of Torsade de Pointes-type ventricular tachycardia).
No products indexed under this heading.

Promethazine Hydrochloride (Co-administration of drugs prolonging the QT interval (such as certain phenothiazines, tricyclic antidepressants, certain macrolide antibiotics, and Class I and III antiarrhythmics) is contraindicated because of the potential risk of Torsade de Pointes-type ventricular tachycardia).
No products indexed under this heading.

Propafenone Hydrochloride (Concomitant use of drugs or herbal products that prolong the QT interval might increase the risk of Torsade de Pointes, such as phenothiazine anti-psychotics, tricyclic antidepressants, certain oral macrolide antibiotics, and Class I and III antiarrhythmics. Co-administration of drugs prolonging the QT interval (such as certain phenothiazines, tricyclic antidepressants, certain macrolide antibiotics, and Class I and III antiarrhythmics) is contraindicated because of the potential risk of Torsade de Pointes-type ventricular tachycardia). Products include:
Rythmol 1648
Rythmol SR 1652

Propoxyphene Hydrochloride (Dronedarone is metabolized primarily by CYP 3A and is a moderate inhibitor of CYP 3A and CYP 2D6. Dronedarone's blood levels can therefore be affected by inhibitors and inducers of CYP 3A, and dronedarone can interact with drugs that are substrates of CYP 3A and CYP 2D6. Other CYP 2D6 substrates, including other β-blockers, tricyclic antidepressants, and selective serotonin reuptake inhibitors (SSRIs) may have increased exposure upon co-administration with dronedarone).
No products indexed under this heading.

Propoxyphene Napsylate (Dronedarone is metabolized primarily by CYP 3A and is a moderate inhibitor of CYP 3A and CYP 2D6. Dronedarone's blood levels can therefore be affected by inhibitors and inducers of CYP 3A, and dronedarone can interact with drugs that are substrates of CYP 3A and CYP 2D6. Other CYP 2D6 substrates, including other β-blockers, tricyclic antidepressants, and selective serotonin reuptake inhibitors (SSRIs) may have increased exposure upon co-administration with dronedarone).
No products indexed under this heading.

Propranolol (Co-administration of dronedarone with propranolol may increase propranolol exposure by approximately 1.3-fold following single dose administration).
No products indexed under this heading.

Propranolol Hydrochloride (Co-administration of dronedarone with propranolol may increase propranolol exposure by approximately 1.3-fold following single dose administration). Products include:
InnoPran XL 1517

Protriptyline Hydrochloride (Concomitant use of drugs or herbal products that prolong the QT interval might increase the risk of Torsade de Pointes, such as phenothiazine anti-psychotics, tricyclic antidepressants, certain oral macrolide antibiotics, and Class I and III antiarrhythmics. Co-administration of drugs prolonging the QT interval (such as certain phenothiazines, tricyclic antidepressants, certain macrolide antibiotics, and Class I and III antiarrhythmics) is contraindicated because of the potential risk of Torsade de Pointes-type ventricular tachycardia).
No products indexed under this heading.

Quetiapine Fumarate (Concomitant use of drugs or herbal products that prolong the QT interval might increase the risk of Torsade de Pointes, such as phenothiazine anti-psychotics, tricyclic antidepressants, certain oral macrolide antibiotics, and Class I and III antiarrhythmics. Co-administration of drugs prolonging the QT interval (such as certain phenothiazines, tricyclic antidepressants, certain macrolide antibiotics, and Class I and III antiarrhythmics) is contraindicated because of the potential risk of Torsade de Pointes-type ventricular tachycardia). Products include:
Seroquel 750
Seroquel XR 759

Quinidine (Concomitant use of drugs or herbal products that prolong the QT interval might increase the risk of Torsade de Pointes, such as phenothiazine anti-psychotics, tricyclic antidepressants, certain oral macrolide antibiotics, and Class I and III antiarrhythmics. Co-administration of drugs prolonging the QT interval (such as certain phenothiazines, tricyclic antidepressants, certain macrolide antibiotics, and Class I and III antiarrhythmics) is contraindicated because of the potential risk of Torsade de Pointes-type ventricular tachycardia).
No products indexed under this heading.

Quinidine Gluconate (Concomitant use of drugs or herbal products that prolong the QT interval might increase the risk of Torsade de Pointes, such as phenothiazine anti-psychotics, tricyclic antidepressants, certain oral macrolide antibiotics, and Class I and III antiarrhythmics. Co-administration of drugs prolonging the QT interval (such as certain phenothiazines, tricyclic antidepressants, certain macrolide antibiotics, and Class I and III antiarrhythmics) is contraindicated because of the potential risk of Torsade de Pointes-type ventricular tachycardia).
No products indexed under this heading.

Quinidine Hydrochloride (Concomitant use of drugs or herbal products that prolong the QT interval might increase the risk of Torsade de Pointes, such as phenothiazine anti-psychotics, tricyclic antidepressants, certain oral macrolide antibiotics, and Class I and III antiarrhythmics. Co-administration of drugs prolonging the QT interval (such as certain phenothiazines, tricyclic antidepressants, certain macrolide antibiotics, and Class I and III antiarrhythmics) is contraindicated because of the potential risk of Torsade de Pointes-type ventricular tachycardia).
No products indexed under this heading.

Quinidine Polygalacturonate (Concomitant use of drugs or herbal products that prolong the QT interval might increase the risk of Torsade de Pointes, such as phenothiazine anti-psychotics, tricyclic antidepressants, certain oral macrolide antibiotics, and Class I and III antiarrhythmics. Co-administration of drugs prolonging the QT interval (such as certain phenothiazines, tricyclic antidepressants, certain macrolide antibiotics, and Class I and III antiarrhythmics) is contraindicated because of the potential risk of Torsade de Pointes-type ventricular tachycardia).
No products indexed under this heading.

Quinidine Sulfate (Concomitant use of drugs or herbal products that prolong the QT interval might increase the risk of Torsade de Pointes, such as phenothiazine anti-psychotics, tricyclic antidepressants, certain oral macrolide antibiotics, and Class I and III antiarrhythmics. Co-administration of drugs prolonging the QT interval (such as certain phenothiazines, tricyclic antidepressants, certain macrolide antibiotics, and Class I and III antiarrhythmics) is contraindicated because of the potential risk of Torsade de Pointes-type ventricular tachycardia).
No products indexed under this heading.

Quinine (Dronedarone is metabolized primarily by CYP 3A and is a moderate inhibitor of CYP 3A and CYP 2D6. Dronedarone's blood levels can therefore be affected by inhibitors and inducers of CYP 3A, and dronedarone can interact with drugs that are substrates of CYP 3A and CYP 2D6. Concomitant use of other potent CYP 3A inhibitors such as itraconazole, voriconazole, ritonavir, clarithromycin, and nefazodone is contraindicated). Products include:
Hyland's Leg Cramps PM with Quinine 3315

Quinine Sulfate (Dronedarone is metabolized primarily by CYP 3A and is a moderate inhibitor of CYP 3A and CYP 2D6. Dronedarone's blood levels can therefore be affected by inhibitors and inducers of CYP 3A, and dronedarone can interact with drugs that are substrates of CYP 3A and CYP 2D6. Concomitant use of other potent CYP 3A inhibitors such as itraconazole, voriconazole, ritonavir, clarithromycin, and nefazodone is contraindicated).
No products indexed under this heading.

Ranolazine (Dronedarone has no significant potential to inhibit CYP 1A2, CYP 2C9, CYP 2C19, CYP 2C8 and CYP 2B6. It has the potential to inhibit P-glycoprotein (P-gP) transport. Dronedarone increased digoxin exposure by 2.5-fold by inhibiting the P-gP transporter. Other P-gP substrates are expected to have increased exposure when co-administered with dronedarone). Products include:
Ranexa 1255

Rifabutin (Dronedarone is metabolized primarily by CYP 3A and is a moderate inhibitor of CYP 3A and CYP 2D6. Dronedarone's blood levels can therefore be affected by inhibitors and inducers of CYP 3A, and dronedarone can interact with drugs that are substrates of CYP 3A and CYP 2D6. Avoid other CYP 3A inducers such as phenobarbital, carbamazepine, phenytoin, and St John's wort with dronedarone because they decrease its exposure significantly).
No products indexed under this heading.

Rifampicin (Dronedarone is metabolized primarily by CYP 3A and is a moderate inhibitor of CYP 3A and CYP 2D6. Dronedarone's blood levels can therefore be affected by inhibitors and inducers of CYP 3A, and dronedarone can interact with drugs that are substrates of CYP 3A and CYP 2D6. Avoid other CYP 3A inducers such as phenobarbital, carbamazepine, phenytoin, and St John's wort with dronedarone because they decrease its exposure significantly).
No products indexed under this heading.

Rifampin (Rifampin decreased dronedarone exposure by 80%. Avoid rifampin with dronedarone because it may decrease its exposure significantly).
No products indexed under this heading.

Rifapentine (Dronedarone is metabolized primarily by CYP 3A and is a moderate inhibitor of CYP 3A and CYP 2D6. Dronedarone's blood levels can therefore be affected by inhibitors and inducers of CYP 3A, and dronedarone can interact with drugs that are substrates of CYP 3A and CYP 2D6. Avoid other CYP 3A inducers such as phenobarbital, carbamazepine, phenytoin, and St John's wort with dronedarone because they decrease its exposure significantly).
No products indexed under this heading.

Risperidone (Concomitant use of drugs or herbal products that prolong the QT interval might increase the risk of Torsade de Pointes, such as phenothiazine anti-psychotics, tricyclic antidepressants, certain oral macrolide antibiotics, and Class I and III antiarrhythmics. Co-administration of drugs prolonging the QT interval (such as certain phenothiazines, tricyclic antidepressants, certain macrolide antibiotics, and Class I and III antiarrhythmics) is contraindicated because of the potential risk of Torsade de Pointes-type ventricular tachycardia). Products include:
Risperdal Consta 2682

Ritonavir (Dronedarone is metabolized primarily by CYP 3A and is a moderate inhibitor of CYP 3A and CYP 2D6. Dronedarone's blood levels can therefore be affected by inhibitors and inducers of CYP 3A, and dronedarone can interact with drugs that are substrates of CYP 3A and CYP 2D6. Concomitant use of other potent CYP 3A inhibitors such as itraconazole, voriconazole, ritonavir, clarithromycin, and nefazodone is contraindicated). Products include:
Kaletra 458
Norvir 509

Saquinavir (Dronedarone is metabolized primarily by CYP 3A and is a moderate inhibitor of CYP 3A and CYP 2D6. Dronedarone's blood levels can therefore be affected by inhibitors and inducers of CYP 3A, and dronedarone can interact with drugs that are substrates of CYP 3A and CYP 2D6. Concomitant use of other potent CYP 3A inhibitors such as itraconazole, voriconazole, ritonavir, clarithromycin, and nefazodone is contraindicated).
No products indexed under this heading.

Saquinavir Mesylate (Dronedarone is metabolized primarily by CYP 3A and is a moderate inhibitor of CYP 3A and CYP 2D6. Dronedarone's blood levels can therefore be affected by inhibitors and inducers of CYP 3A, and dronedarone can interact with drugs that are substrates of CYP 3A and CYP 2D6. Concomitant use of other potent CYP 3A inhibitors such as itraconazole, voriconazole, ritonavir, clarithromycin, and nefazodone is contraindicated).
No products indexed under this heading.

Sertraline Hydrochloride (Dronedarone is metabolized primarily by CYP 3A and is a moderate inhibitor of CYP 3A and CYP 2D6. Dronedarone's blood levels can therefore be affected by inhibitors and inducers of CYP 3A, and dronedarone can interact with drugs that are substrates of CYP 3A and CYP 2D6. Concomitant use of other potent

1159 **Interactions Index** **Multaq**

CYP 3A inhibitors such as itraconazole, voriconazole, ritonavir, clarithromycin, and nefazodone is contraindicated).
No products indexed under this heading.

Sildenafil Citrate (Dronedarone is metabolized primarily by CYP 3A and is a moderate inhibitor of CYP 3A and CYP 2D6. Dronedarone's blood levels can therefore be affected by inhibitors and inducers of CYP 3A, and dronedarone can interact with drugs that are substrates of CYP 3A and CYP 2D6. Co-administration of dronedarone with CYP 3A substrates may increase plasma concentrations of tacrolimus, sirolimus, and other CYP 3A substrates with a narrow therapeutic range when given orally. Monitor plasma concentrations and adjust dosage appropriately).
No products indexed under this heading.

Simvastatin (Co-administration of dronedarone with simvastatin may increase simvastatin/simvastatin acid exposure by 4- and 2-fold, respectively). Products include:
Simcor 524
Vytorin 10/10 .... 2303, 3240
Vytorin 10/20 .... 2303, 3240
Vytorin 10/40 .... 2303, 3240
Vytorin 10/80 .... 2303, 3240
Zocor 2289

Sirolimus (Co-administration of dronedarone with sirolimus may increase plasma concentrations of sirolimus with a narrow therapeutic range when given orally. Monitor plasma concentrations and adjust dosage appropriately). Products include:
Rapamune 3579

Sitagliptin Phosphate (Dronedarone has no significant potential to inhibit CYP 1A2, CYP 2C9, CYP 2C19, CYP 2C8 and CYP 2B6. It has the potential to inhibit P-glycoprotein (P-gP) transport. Dronedarone increased digoxin exposure by 2.5-fold by inhibiting the P-gP transporter. Other P-gP substrates are expected to have increased exposure when co-administered with dronedarone). Products include:
Janumet 2188
Januvia 2196

Sotalol Hydrochloride (Co-administration of drugs prolonging the QT interval (such as certain phenothiazines, tricyclic antidepressants, certain macrolide antibiotics, and Class I and III antiarrhythmics) is contraindicated because of the potential risk of Torsade de Pointes-type ventricular tachycardia).
No products indexed under this heading.

Tacrolimus (Co-administration of dronedarone with tacrolimus may increase plasma concentrations of tacrolimus with a narrow therapeutic range when given orally. Monitor plasma concentrations and adjust dosage appropriately). Products include:
Prograf Capsules 677
Prograf Injection 677
Protopic 685

Tamoxifen Citrate (Dronedarone is metabolized primarily by CYP 3A and is a moderate inhibitor of CYP 3A and CYP 2D6. Dronedarone's blood levels can therefore be affected by inhibitors and inducers of CYP 3A, and dronedarone can interact with drugs that are substrates of CYP 3A and CYP 2D6. Co-administration of dronedarone with CYP 3A substrates may increase plasma concentrations of tacrolimus, sirolimus, and other CYP 3A substrates with a narrow therapeutic range when given orally. Monitor plasma concentrations and adjust dosage appropriately).
No products indexed under this heading.

Telithromycin (Concomitant use of strong CYP 3A inhibitors, such as ketoconazole, itraconazole, voriconazole, cyclosporine, telithromycin, clarithromycin, nefazodone, and ritonavir is contraindicated). Products include:
Ketek 2991

Temsirolimus (Dronedarone has no significant potential to inhibit CYP 1A2, CYP 2C9, CYP 2C19, CYP 2C8 and CYP 2B6. It has the potential to inhibit P-glycoprotein (P-gP) transport. Dronedarone increased digoxin exposure by 2.5-fold by inhibiting the P-gP transporter. Other P-gP substrates are expected to have increased exposure when co-administered with dronedarone). Products include:
Torisel 3592

Teniposide (Dronedarone is metabolized primarily by CYP 3A and is a moderate inhibitor of CYP 3A and CYP 2D6. Dronedarone's blood levels can therefore be affected by inhibitors and inducers of CYP 3A, and dronedarone can interact with drugs that are substrates of CYP 3A and CYP 2D6. Other CYP 2D6 substrates, including other β-blockers, tricyclic antidepressants, and selective serotonin reuptake inhibitors (SSRIs) may have increased exposure upon co-administration with dronedarone).
No products indexed under this heading.

Terfenadine (Dronedarone is metabolized primarily by CYP 3A and is a moderate inhibitor of CYP 3A and CYP 2D6. Dronedarone's blood levels can therefore be affected by inhibitors and inducers of CYP 3A, and dronedarone can interact with drugs that are substrates of CYP 3A and CYP 2D6. Co-administration of dronedarone with CYP 3A substrates may increase plasma concentrations of tacrolimus, sirolimus, and other CYP 3A substrates with a narrow therapeutic range when given orally. Monitor plasma concentrations and adjust dosage appropriately).
No products indexed under this heading.

Testosterone (Dronedarone is metabolized primarily by CYP 3A and is a moderate inhibitor of CYP 3A and CYP 2D6. Dronedarone's blood levels can therefore be affected by inhibitors and inducers of CYP 3A, and dronedarone can interact with drugs that are substrates of CYP 3A and CYP 2D6. Co-administration of dronedarone with CYP 3A substrates may increase plasma concentrations of tacrolimus, sirolimus, and other CYP 3A substrates with a narrow therapeutic range when given orally. Monitor plasma concentrations and adjust dosage appropriately). Products include:
AndroGel 3456

Testosterone Cypionate (Dronedarone is metabolized primarily by CYP 3A and is a moderate inhibitor of CYP 3A and CYP 2D6. Dronedarone's blood levels can therefore be affected by inhibitors and inducers of CYP 3A, and dronedarone can interact with drugs that are substrates of CYP 3A and CYP 2D6. Co-administration of dronedarone with CYP 3A substrates may increase plasma concentrations of tacrolimus, sirolimus, and other CYP 3A substrates with a narrow therapeutic range when given orally. Monitor plasma concentrations and adjust dosage appropriately).
No products indexed under this heading.

Testosterone Enanthate (Dronedarone is metabolized primarily by CYP 3A and is a moderate inhibitor of CYP 3A and CYP 2D6. Dronedarone's blood levels can therefore be affected by inhibitors and inducers of CYP 3A, and dronedarone can interact with drugs that are substrates of CYP 3A and CYP 2D6. Co-administration of dronedarone with CYP 3A substrates may increase plasma concentrations of tacrolimus, sirolimus, and other CYP 3A substrates with a narrow therapeutic range when given orally. Monitor plasma concentrations and adjust dosage appropriately). Products include:
Delatestryl 1102

Testosterone Propionate (Dronedarone is metabolized primarily by CYP 3A and is a moderate inhibitor of CYP 3A and CYP 2D6. Dronedarone's blood levels can therefore be affected by inhibitors and inducers of CYP 3A, and dronedarone can interact with drugs that are substrates of CYP 3A and CYP 2D6. Co-administration of dronedarone with CYP 3A substrates may increase plasma concentrations of tacrolimus, sirolimus, and other CYP 3A substrates with a narrow therapeutic range when given orally. Monitor plasma concentrations and adjust dosage appropriately).
No products indexed under this heading.

Theophylline (Dronedarone is metabolized primarily by CYP 3A and is a moderate inhibitor of CYP 3A and CYP 2D6. Dronedarone's blood levels can therefore be affected by inhibitors and inducers of CYP 3A, and dronedarone can interact with drugs that are substrates of CYP 3A and CYP 2D6. Co-administration of dronedarone with CYP 3A substrates may increase plasma concentrations of tacrolimus, sirolimus, and other CYP 3A substrates with a narrow therapeutic range when given orally. Monitor plasma concentrations and adjust dosage appropriately).
No products indexed under this heading.

Theophylline Anhydrous (Dronedarone is metabolized primarily by CYP 3A and is a moderate inhibitor of CYP 3A and CYP 2D6. Dronedarone's blood levels can therefore be affected by inhibitors and inducers of CYP 3A, and dronedarone can interact with drugs that are substrates of CYP 3A and CYP 2D6. Co-administration of dronedarone with CYP 3A substrates may increase plasma concentrations of tacrolimus, sirolimus, and other CYP 3A substrates with a narrow therapeutic range when given orally. Monitor plasma concentrations and adjust dosage appropriately). Products include:
Uniphyl 2817

Theophylline Calcium Salicylate (Dronedarone is metabolized primarily by CYP 3A and is a moderate inhibitor of CYP 3A and CYP 2D6. Dronedarone's blood levels can therefore be affected by inhibitors and inducers of CYP 3A, and dronedarone can interact with drugs that are substrates of CYP 3A and CYP 2D6. Co-administration of dronedarone with CYP 3A substrates may increase plasma concentrations of tacrolimus, sirolimus, and other CYP 3A substrates with a narrow therapeutic range when given orally. Monitor plasma concentrations and adjust dosage appropriately).
No products indexed under this heading.

Theophylline Sodium Glycinate (Dronedarone is metabolized primarily by CYP 3A and is a moderate inhibitor of CYP 3A and CYP 2D6. Dronedarone's blood levels can therefore be affected by inhibitors and inducers of CYP 3A, and dronedarone can interact with drugs that are substrates of CYP 3A and CYP 2D6. Co-administration of dronedarone with CYP 3A substrates may increase plasma concentrations of tacrolimus, sirolimus, and other CYP 3A substrates with a narrow therapeutic range when given orally. Monitor plasma concentrations and adjust dosage appropriately).
No products indexed under this heading.

Thioridazine (Co-administration of drugs prolonging the QT interval (such as certain phenothiazines, tricyclic antidepressants, certain macrolide antibiotics, and Class I and III antiarrhythmics) is contraindicated because of the potential risk of Torsade de Pointes-type ventricular tachycardia).
No products indexed under this heading.

Thioridazine Hydrochloride (Co-administration of drugs prolonging the QT interval (such as certain phenothiazines, tricyclic antidepressants, certain macrolide antibiotics, and Class I and III antiarrhythmics) is contraindicated because of the potential risk of Torsade de Pointes-type ventricular tachycardia). Products include:
Thioridazine Hydrochloride 2384

Thiothixene (Concomitant use of drugs or herbal products that prolong the QT interval might increase the risk of Torsade de Pointes, such as phenothiazine anti-psychotics, tricyclic antidepressants, certain oral macrolide antibiotics, and Class I and III antiarrhythmics. Co-administration of drugs prolonging the QT interval (such as certain phenothiazines, tricyclic antidepressants, certain macrolide antibiotics, and Class I and III antiarrhythmics) is contraindicated because of the potential risk of Torsade de Pointes-type ventricular tachycardia). Products include:
Thiothixene 2386

Tiagabine Hydrochloride (Dronedarone is metabolized primarily by CYP 3A and is a moderate inhibitor of CYP 3A and CYP 2D6. Dronedarone's blood levels can therefore be affected by inhibitors and inducers of CYP 3A, and dronedarone can interact with drugs that are substrates of CYP 3A and CYP 2D6. Co-administration of dronedarone with CYP 3A substrates may increase plasma concentrations of tacrolimus, sirolimus, and other CYP 3A substrates with a narrow therapeutic range when given orally. Monitor plasma concentrations and adjust dosage appropriately). Products include:
Gabitril 972

Timolol Hemihydrate (Co-administration of dronedarone with other CYP 2D6 substrates, including other beta-blockers, may have increased exposure. In clinical trials, bradycardia was more frequently observed when dronedarone was given in combination with β-blockers. Give low dose of β-blockers initially, and increase only after ECG verification of good tolerability). Products include:
Betimol 3490

Timolol Maleate (Co-administration of dronedarone with other CYP 2D6 substrates, including other beta-blockers, may have increased exposure. In clinical trials, bradycardia was more frequently observed when dronedarone was given in combination with β-blockers. Give low dose of β-blockers initially, and increase only after ECG verification of good tolerability). Products include:
Combigan 601
Dorzolamide Hydrochloride/Timolol Maleate Ophthalmic Solution .... ⊙243
Timoptic in Ocudose .... ⊙231

Tipranavir (Dronedarone has no significant potential to inhibit CYP 1A2, CYP 2C9, CYP 2C19, CYP 2C8 and CYP 2B6. It has the potential to inhibit P-glycoprotein (P-gP) transport. Dronedarone increased digoxin exposure by 2.5-fold by inhibiting the P-gP transporter. Other P-gP substrates are expected to have increased exposure when co-administered with dronedarone).
No products indexed under this heading.

Tocainide Hydrochloride (Concomitant use of drugs or herbal products that prolong the QT interval might

increase the risk of Torsade de Pointes, such as phenothiazine anti-psychotics, tricyclic antidepressants, certain oral macrolide antibiotics, and Class I and III antiarrhythmics. Co-administration of drugs prolonging the QT interval (such as certain phenothiazines, tricyclic antidepressants, certain macrolide antibiotics, and Class I and III antiarrhythmics) is contraindicated because of the potential risk of Torsade de Pointes-type ventricular tachycardia).
No products indexed under this heading.

Tolterodine Tartrate (Dronedarone is metabolized primarily by CYP 3A and is a moderate inhibitor of CYP 3A and CYP 2D6. Dronedarone's blood levels can therefore be affected by inhibitors and inducers of CYP 3A, and dronedarone can interact with drugs that are substrates of CYP 3A and CYP 2D6. Co-administration of dronedarone with CYP 3A substrates may increase plasma concentrations of tacrolimus, sirolimus, and other CYP 3A substrates with a narrow therapeutic range when given orally. Monitor plasma concentrations and adjust dosage appropriately).
No products indexed under this heading.

Tramadol Hydrochloride (Dronedarone is metabolized primarily by CYP 3A and is a moderate inhibitor of CYP 3A and CYP 2D6. Dronedarone's blood levels can therefore be affected by inhibitors and inducers of CYP 3A, and dronedarone can interact with drugs that are substrates of CYP 3A and CYP 2D6. Other CYP 2D6 substrates, including other β-blockers, tricyclic antidepressants, and selective serotonin reuptake inhibitors (SSRIs) may have increased exposure upon co-administration with dronedarone). Products include:
Ryzolt 2813
Ultram ER 2693

Tranylcypromine Sulfate (Concomitant use of drugs or herbal products that prolong the QT interval might increase the risk of Torsade de Pointes, such as phenothiazine anti-psychotics, tricyclic antidepressants, certain oral macrolide antibiotics, and Class I and III antiarrhythmics. Co-administration of drugs prolonging the QT interval (such as certain phenothiazines, tricyclic antidepressants, certain macrolide antibiotics, and Class I and III antiarrhythmics) is contraindicated because of the potential risk of Torsade de Pointes-type ventricular tachycardia). Products include:
Parnate 1584

Trazodone Hydrochloride (Dronedarone is metabolized primarily by CYP 3A and is a moderate inhibitor of CYP 3A and CYP 2D6. Dronedarone's blood levels can therefore be affected by inhibitors and inducers of CYP 3A, and dronedarone can interact with drugs that are substrates of CYP 3A and CYP 2D6. Co-administration of dronedarone with CYP 3A substrates may increase plasma concentrations of tacrolimus, sirolimus, and other CYP 3A substrates with a narrow therapeutic range when given orally. Monitor plasma concentrations and adjust dosage appropriately).
No products indexed under this heading.

Triazolam (Dronedarone is metabolized primarily by CYP 3A and is a moderate inhibitor of CYP 3A and CYP 2D6. Dronedarone's blood levels can therefore be affected by inhibitors and inducers of CYP 3A, and dronedarone can interact with drugs that are substrates of CYP 3A and CYP 2D6. Co-administration of dronedarone with CYP 3A substrates may increase plasma concentrations of tacrolimus, sirolimus, and other CYP 3A substrates with a narrow therapeutic range when given orally. Monitor plasma concentrations and adjust dosage appropriately).
No products indexed under this heading.

Trifluoperazine Hydrochloride (Co-administration of drugs prolonging the QT interval (such as certain phenothiazines, tricyclic antidepressants, certain macrolide antibiotics, and Class I and III antiarrhythmics) is contraindicated because of the potential risk of Torsade de Pointes-type ventricular tachycardia).
No products indexed under this heading.

Trimipramine Maleate (Concomitant use of drugs or herbal products that prolong the QT interval might increase the risk of Torsade de Pointes, such as phenothiazine anti-psychotics, tricyclic antidepressants, certain oral macrolide antibiotics, and Class I and III antiarrhythmics. Co-administration of drugs prolonging the QT interval (such as certain phenothiazines, tricyclic antidepressants, certain macrolide antibiotics, and Class I and III antiarrhythmics) is contraindicated because of the potential risk of Torsade de Pointes-type ventricular tachycardia).
No products indexed under this heading.

Troleandomycin (Dronedarone is metabolized primarily by CYP 3A and is a moderate inhibitor of CYP 3A and CYP 2D6. Dronedarone's blood levels can therefore be affected by inhibitors and inducers of CYP 3A, and dronedarone can interact with drugs that are substrates of CYP 3A and CYP 2D6. Concomitant use of other potent CYP 3A inhibitors such as itraconazole, voriconazole, ritonavir, clarithromycin, and nefazodone is contraindicated).
No products indexed under this heading.

Venlafaxine Hydrochloride (Dronedarone is metabolized primarily by CYP 3A and is a moderate inhibitor of CYP 3A and CYP 2D6. Dronedarone's blood levels can therefore be affected by inhibitors and inducers of CYP 3A, and dronedarone can interact with drugs that are substrates of CYP 3A and CYP 2D6. Concomitant use of other potent CYP 3A inhibitors such as itraconazole, voriconazole, ritonavir, clarithromycin, and nefazodone is contraindicated). Products include:
Effexor XR 3504
Venlafaxine Hydrochloride Tablets ... 2388

Verapamil Hydrochloride (Co-administration of dronedarone with a moderate CYP 3A inhibitor such as verapamil may increase dronedarone exposure by approximately 1.4- to 1.7-fold). Products include:
Tarka 534

Vinblastine Sulfate (Dronedarone has no significant potential to inhibit CYP 1A2, CYP 2C9, CYP 2C19, CYP 2C8 and CYP 2B6. It has the potential to inhibit P-glycoprotein (P-gP) transport. Dronedarone increased digoxin exposure by 2.5-fold by inhibiting the P-gP transporter. Other P-gP substrates are expected to have increased exposure when co-administered with dronedarone).
No products indexed under this heading.

Vincristine Sulfate (Dronedarone has no significant potential to inhibit CYP 1A2, CYP 2C9, CYP 2C19, CYP 2C8 and CYP 2B6. It has the potential to inhibit P-glycoprotein (P-gP) transport. Dronedarone increased digoxin exposure by 2.5-fold by inhibiting the P-gP transporter. Other P-gP substrates are expected to have increased exposure when co-administered with dronedarone).
No products indexed under this heading.

Voriconazole (Concomitant use of strong CYP 3A inhibitors, such as ketoconazole, itraconazole, voriconazole, cyclosporine, telithromycin, clarithromycin, nefazodone, and ritonavir is contraindicated).
No products indexed under this heading.

Warfarin Sodium (Dronedarone is metabolized primarily by CYP 3A and is a moderate inhibitor of CYP 3A and CYP 2D6. Dronedarone's blood levels can therefore be affected by inhibitors and inducers of CYP 3A, and dronedarone can interact with drugs that are substrates of CYP 3A and CYP 2D6. Co-administration of dronedarone with CYP 3A substrates may increase plasma concentrations of tacrolimus, sirolimus, and other CYP 3A substrates with a narrow therapeutic range when given orally. Monitor plasma concentrations and adjust dosage appropriately).
No products indexed under this heading.

Zafirlukast (Dronedarone is metabolized primarily by CYP 3A and is a moderate inhibitor of CYP 3A and CYP 2D6. Dronedarone's blood levels can therefore be affected by inhibitors and inducers of CYP 3A, and dronedarone can interact with drugs that are substrates of CYP 3A and CYP 2D6. Concomitant use of other potent CYP 3A inhibitors such as itraconazole, voriconazole, ritonavir, clarithromycin, and nefazodone is contraindicated). Products include:
Accolate 3612

Zileuton (Dronedarone is metabolized primarily by CYP 3A and is a moderate inhibitor of CYP 3A and CYP 2D6. Dronedarone's blood levels can therefore be affected by inhibitors and inducers of CYP 3A, and dronedarone can interact with drugs that are substrates of CYP 3A and CYP 2D6. Concomitant use of other potent CYP 3A inhibitors such as itraconazole, voriconazole, ritonavir, clarithromycin, and nefazodone is contraindicated).
No products indexed under this heading.

Ziprasidone Hydrochloride (Concomitant use of drugs or herbal products that prolong the QT interval might increase the risk of Torsade de Pointes, such as phenothiazine anti-psychotics, tricyclic antidepressants, certain oral macrolide antibiotics, and Class I and III antiarrhythmics. Co-administration of drugs prolonging the QT interval (such as certain phenothiazines, tricyclic antidepressants, certain macrolide antibiotics, and Class I and III antiarrhythmics) is contraindicated because of the potential risk of Torsade de Pointes-type ventricular tachycardia). Products include:
Geodon 2723

Zonisamide (Dronedarone is metabolized primarily by CYP 3A and is a moderate inhibitor of CYP 3A and CYP 2D6. Dronedarone's blood levels can therefore be affected by inhibitors and inducers of CYP 3A, and dronedarone can interact with drugs that are substrates of CYP 3A and CYP 2D6. Other CYP 2D6 substrates, including other β-blockers, tricyclic antidepressants, and selective serotonin reuptake inhibitors (SSRIs) may have increased exposure upon co-administration with dronedarone). Products include:
Zonegran 1081

Food Interactions

Grapefruit (Dronedarone is metabolized primarily by CYP 3A and is a moderate inhibitor of CYP 3A and CYP 2D6. Dronedarone's blood levels can therefore be affected by inhibitors and inducers of CYP 3A, and dronedarone can interact with drugs that are substrates of CYP 3A and CYP 2D6. Concomitant use of other potent CYP 3A inhibitors such as itraconazole, voriconazole, ritonavir, clarithromycin, and nefazodone is contraindicated).

Grapefruit Juice (Grapefruit juice, a moderate inhibitor of CYP 3A, resulted in a 3-fold increase in dronedarone exposure and a 2.5-fold increase in C_{max}. Therefore, patients should avoid grapefruit juice beverages while taking dronedarone).

MUMPSVAX

(Mumps Virus Vaccine, Live) 2218
May interact with immunosuppressive agents. Compounds in these categories include:

Azathioprine (Concurrent immunosuppressive therapy is contraindicated).
No products indexed under this heading.

Basiliximab (Concurrent immunosuppressive therapy is contraindicated). Products include:
Simulect 2524

Cyclosporine (Concurrent immunosuppressive therapy is contraindicated). Products include:
Gengraf 440
Neoral Oral Solution 2496
Neoral Capsules 2496
Restasis 605

Muromonab-CD3 (Concurrent immunosuppressive therapy is contraindicated). Products include:
Orthoclone OKT3 949

Mycophenolate Mofetil (Concurrent immunosuppressive therapy is contraindicated).
No products indexed under this heading.

Rapamycin (Concurrent immunosuppressive therapy is contraindicated).
No products indexed under this heading.

Sirolimus (Concurrent immunosuppressive therapy is contraindicated). Products include:
Rapamune 3579

Tacrolimus (Concurrent immunosuppressive therapy is contraindicated). Products include:
Prograf Capsules 677
Prograf Injection 677
Protopic 685

MURO 128 OPHTHALMIC OINTMENT

(Sodium Chloride) .... ⊙249
None cited in PDR database.

MURO 128 OPHTHALMIC SOLUTION 2% AND 5%

(Sodium Chloride) .... ⊙249
None cited in PDR database.

MUSTARGEN FOR INJECTION

(Mechlorethamine Hydrochloride) 2010
May interact with antineoplastics, and certain other agents. Compounds in these categories include:

Altretamine (Precautions must be observed with the use of mechlorethamine and chemotheraphy in alternating courses. Hematopoiesis may be further compromised, and leukopenia, thrombocytopenia and anemia may become more severe in patients who have been previously treated with chemotherapeutic agents). Products include:
Hexalen 1066

Anastrozole (Precautions must be observed with the use of mechlorethamine and chemotheraphy in alternating courses. Hematopoiesis may be further compromised, and leukopenia, thrombocytopenia and anemia may become more severe in patients who have been previously treated with chemotherapeutic agents).
No products indexed under this heading.

Asparaginase (Precautions must be observed with the use of mechloretha-

---

IMPORTANT NOTE: Always consult each drug listing in the patient's regimen for possible interactions.

Mitomycin (Mitomycin-C) (Precautions must be observed with the use of mechlorethamine and chemotheraphy in alternating courses. Hematopoiesis may be further compromised, and leukopenia, thrombocytopenia and anemia may become more severe in patients who have been previously treated with chemotherapeutic agents).
No products indexed under this heading.

Mitotane (Precautions must be observed with the use of mechlorethamine and chemotheraphy in alternating courses. Hematopoiesis may be further compromised, and leukopenia, thrombocytopenia and anemia may become more severe in patients who have been previously treated with chemotherapeutic agents).
No products indexed under this heading.

Mitoxantrone Hydrochloride (Precautions must be observed with the use of mechlorethamine and chemotheraphy in alternating courses. Hematopoiesis may be further compromised, and leukopenia, thrombocytopenia and anemia may become more severe in patients who have been previously treated with chemotherapeutic agents). Products include:
Novantrone 1088

Oxaliplatin (Precautions must be observed with the use of mechlorethamine and chemotheraphy in alternating courses. Hematopoiesis may be further compromised, and leukopenia, thrombocytopenia and anemia may become more severe in patients who have been previously treated with chemotherapeutic agents). Products include:
Eloxatin 2975

Paclitaxel (Precautions must be observed with the use of mechlorethamine and chemotheraphy in alternating courses. Hematopoiesis may be further compromised, and leukopenia, thrombocytopenia and anemia may become more severe in patients who have been previously treated with chemotherapeutic agents).
No products indexed under this heading.

Procarbazine Hydrochloride (Precautions must be observed with the use of mechlorethamine and chemotheraphy in alternating courses. Hematopoiesis may be further compromised, and leukopenia, thrombocytopenia and anemia may become more severe in patients who have been previously treated with chemotherapeutic agents).
No products indexed under this heading.

Radiation (Precautions must be observed with the use of mechlorethamine and x-ray therapy in alternating courses. Irradiation of such areas as sternum, ribs, and vertebrae shortly after a course of nitrogen mustard may lead to hematologic complications).
No products indexed under this heading.

Streptozocin (Precautions must be observed with the use of mechlorethamine and chemotheraphy in alternating courses. Hematopoiesis may be further compromised, and leukopenia, thrombocytopenia and anemia may become more severe in patients who have been previously treated with chemotherapeutic agents).
No products indexed under this heading.

Tamoxifen Citrate (Precautions must be observed with the use of mechlorethamine and chemotheraphy in alternating courses. Hematopoiesis may be further compromised, and leukopenia, thrombocytopenia and anemia may become more severe in patients who have been previously treated with chemotherapeutic agents).
No products indexed under this heading.

Teniposide (Precautions must be observed with the use of mechlorethamine and chemotheraphy in alternating courses. Hematopoiesis may be further compromised, and leukopenia, thrombocytopenia and anemia may become more severe in patients who have been previously treated with chemotherapeutic agents).
No products indexed under this heading.

Thioguanine (Precautions must be observed with the use of mechlorethamine and chemotheraphy in alternating courses. Hematopoiesis may be further compromised, and leukopenia, thrombocytopenia and anemia may become more severe in patients who have been previously treated with chemotherapeutic agents). Products include:
Tabloid 1664

Thiotepa (Precautions must be observed with the use of mechlorethamine and chemotheraphy in alternating courses. Hematopoiesis may be further compromised, and leukopenia, thrombocytopenia and anemia may become more severe in patients who have been previously treated with chemotherapeutic agents).
No products indexed under this heading.

Topotecan Hydrochloride (Precautions must be observed with the use of mechlorethamine and chemotheraphy in alternating courses. Hematopoiesis may be further compromised, and leukopenia, thrombocytopenia and anemia may become more severe in patients who have been previously treated with chemotherapeutic agents). Products include:
Hycamtin 1491
Hycamtin Capsules 1488

Toremifene Citrate (Precautions must be observed with the use of mechlorethamine and chemotheraphy in alternating courses. Hematopoiesis may be further compromised, and leukopenia, thrombocytopenia and anemia may become more severe in patients who have been previously treated with chemotherapeutic agents).
No products indexed under this heading.

Valrubicin (Precautions must be observed with the use of mechlorethamine and chemotheraphy in alternating courses. Hematopoiesis may be further compromised, and leukopenia, thrombocytopenia and anemia may become more severe in patients who have been previously treated with chemotherapeutic agents). Products include:
Valstar 1131

Vincristine Sulfate (Precautions must be observed with the use of mechlorethamine and chemotheraphy in alternating courses. Hematopoiesis may be further compromised, and leukopenia, thrombocytopenia and anemia may become more severe in patients who have been previously treated with chemotherapeutic agents).
No products indexed under this heading.

Vinorelbine Tartrate (Precautions must be observed with the use of mechlorethamine and chemotheraphy in alternating courses. Hematopoiesis may be further compromised, and leukopenia, thrombocytopenia and anemia may become more severe in patients who have been previously treated with chemotherapeutic agents).
No products indexed under this heading.

MYCAMINE FOR INJECTION

(Micafungin Sodium) 670

Itraconazole (When used concomitantly, itraconazole AUC and C_{max} were increased by 22% and 11%, respectively. Patients receiving itraconazole in combination with micafungin sodium should be monitored for itraconazole toxicity and itraconazole dosage should be reduced if necessary).
No products indexed under this heading.

Nifedipine (Nifedipine AUC and C_{max} were increased by 18% and 42%, respectively, in the presence of steady state micafungin sodium compared with nifedipine alone. Patients receiving nifedipine in combination with micafungin sodium should be monitored for nifedipine toxicity and nifedipine dosage should be reduced if necessary).
No products indexed under this heading.

Sirolimus (Sirolimus AUC was increased by 21% with no effect on C_{max} in the presence of steady-state micafungin sodium compared with sirolimus alone. Patients receiving sirolimus in combination with micafungin sodium should be monitored for sirolimus toxicity and sirolimus dosage should be reduced if necessary). Products include:
Rapamune 3579

MYFORTIC TABLETS

(Mycophenolic Acid) 2491
May interact with antacids, bacteriostatic antibiotics, bile acid sequestering agents, immunosuppressive agents, oral contraceptives, vaccines, live, and certain other agents. Compounds in these categories include:

Acyclovir (May be taken with mycophenolic acid; however, during the period of treatment, physicians should monitor blood cell counts. Both acyclovir and MPAG concentrations are increased in the presence of renal impairment; their co-existence may compete for tubular secretion and further increase in the concentrations of the two). Products include:
Zovirax 1760

Acyclovir Sodium (May be taken with mycophenolic acid; however, during the period of treatment, physicians should monitor blood cell counts. Both acyclovir and MPAG concentrations are increased in the presence of renal impairment; their co-existence may compete for tubular secretion and further increase in the concentrations of the two).
No products indexed under this heading.

Aluminum Carbonate (Absorption of a single dose of mycophenolic acid was decreased when administered to 12 stable renal transplant patients also taking magnesium-aluminum-containing antacids (30 mL): the mean C_{max} and $AUC_{(0-t)}$ values for MPA were 25% and 37% lower, respectively, than when mycophenolic acid was administered alone under fasting conditions. It is recommended that mycophenolic acid and antacids not be administered simultaneously).
No products indexed under this heading.

Aluminum Hydroxide (Absorption of a single dose of mycophenolic acid was decreased when administered to 12 stable renal transplant patients also taking magnesium-aluminum-containing antacids (30 mL): the mean C_{max} and $AUC_{(0-t)}$ values for MPA were 25% and 37% lower, respectively, than when mycophenolic acid was administered alone under fasting conditions. It is recommended that mycophenolic acid and antacids not be administered simultaneously).
No products indexed under this heading.

Azathioprine (Given that azathioprine inhibits purine metabolism, it is recommended that mycophenolic acid not be administered concomitantly with azathioprine).
No products indexed under this heading.

Azathioprine Sodium (Given that azathioprine inhibits purine metabolism, it is recommended that mycophenolic acid not be administered concomitantly with azathioprine).
No products indexed under this heading.

Basiliximab (Cases of pure red cell aplasia (PRCA) have been reported in patients treated with mycophenolate mofetil (MMF) in combination with other immunosuppressive agents). Products include:
Simulect 2524

BCG Vaccine (During treatment with mycophenolic acid, the use of live attenuated vaccines should be avoided and patients should be advised that vaccinations may be less effective. Influenza vaccination may be of value).
No products indexed under this heading.

Calcium Carbonate (Absorption of a single dose of mycophenolic acid was decreased when administered to 12 stable renal transplant patients also taking magnesium-aluminum-containing antacids (30 mL): the mean C_{max} and $AUC_{(0-t)}$ values for MPA were 25% and 37% lower, respectively, than when mycophenolic acid was administered alone under fasting conditions. It is recommended that mycophenolic acid and antacids not be administered simultaneously). Products include:
Chelated Mineral 3476
Pepcid Complete 1822
Extra Strength Rolaids Softchews
Vanilla Creme 2045

Charcoal, Activated (Do not administer mycophenolic acid with agents that may interfere with enterohepatic recirculation, or drugs that may bind bile acids, for example oral activated charcoal, because of the potential to reduce the efficacy of mycophenolic acid).
No products indexed under this heading.

Chloramphenicol (Drugs that alter the gastrointestinal flora may interact with mycophenolic acid by disrupting enterohepatic recirculation. Interference of MPAG hydrolysis may lead to less mycophenolic acid available for absorption).
No products indexed under this heading.

Chloramphenicol Palmitate (Drugs that alter the gastrointestinal flora may interact with mycophenolic acid by disrupting enterohepatic recirculation. Interference of MPAG hydrolysis may lead to less mycophenolic acid available for absorption).
No products indexed under this heading.

Chloramphenicol Sodium Succinate (Drugs that alter the gastrointestinal flora may interact with mycophenolic acid by disrupting enterohepatic recirculation. Interference of MPAG hydrolysis may lead to less mycophenolic acid available for absorption).
No products indexed under this heading.

Cholestyramine (Do not administer mycophenolic acid with cholestyramine or other agents that may interfere with enterohepatic recirculation or drugs that may bind bile acids because of the potential to reduce the efficacy of mycophenolic acid).
No products indexed under this heading.

Colesevelam Hydrochloride (Do not administer mycophenolic acid with agents that may interfere with enterohepatic recirculation or drugs that may bind bile acids because of the potential to reduce the efficacy of mycophenolic acid). Products include:
Welchol 1029

IMPORTANT NOTE: Always consult each drug listing in the patient's regimen for possible interactions.

Norgestrel (It is recommended that oral contraceptives are co-administered with mycophenolic acid with caution, and additional birth control methods be considered).
No products indexed under this heading.

Oxytetracycline Hydrochloride (Drugs that alter the gastrointestinal flora may interact with mycophenolic acid by disrupting enterohepatic recirculation. Interference of MPAG hydrolysis may lead to less mycophenolic acid available for absorption).
No products indexed under this heading.

Poliovirus Vaccine, Live, Oral, Trivalent, Types 1,2,3 (Sabin) (During treatment with mycophenolic acid, the use of live attenuated vaccines should be avoided and patients should be advised that vaccinations may be less effective. Influenza vaccination may be of value).
No products indexed under this heading.

Rapamycin (Cases of pure red cell aplasia (PRCA) have been reported in patients treated with mycophenolate mofetil (MMF) in combination with other immunosuppressive agents).
No products indexed under this heading.

Rotavirus Vaccine, Live, Oral, Tetravalent (During treatment with mycophenolic acid, the use of live attenuated vaccines should be avoided and patients should be advised that vaccinations may be less effective. Influenza vaccination may be of value).
No products indexed under this heading.

Rubella & Mumps Virus Vaccine Live (During treatment with mycophenolic acid, the use of live attenuated vaccines should be avoided and patients should be advised that vaccinations may be less effective. Influenza vaccination may be of value).
No products indexed under this heading.

Rubella Virus Vaccine Live (During treatment with mycophenolic acid, the use of live attenuated vaccines should be avoided and patients should be advised that vaccinations may be less effective. Influenza vaccination may be of value). Products include:
Meruvax II 2210

Sirolimus (Cases of pure red cell aplasia (PRCA) have been reported in patients treated with mycophenolate mofetil (MMF) in combination with other immunosuppressive agents). Products include:
Rapamune 3579

Smallpox Vaccine (During treatment with mycophenolic acid, the use of live attenuated vaccines should be avoided and patients should be advised that vaccinations may be less effective. Influenza vaccination may be of value).
No products indexed under this heading.

Sodium Bicarbonate (Absorption of a single dose of mycophenolic acid was decreased when administered to 12 stable renal transplant patients also taking magnesium-aluminum-containing antacids (30 mL): the mean C_{max} and $AUC_{(0-t)}$ values for MPA were 25% and 37% lower, respectively, than when mycophenolic acid was administered alone under fasting conditions. It is recommended that mycophenolic acid and antacids not be administered simultaneously).
No products indexed under this heading.

Sulfamethizole (Drugs that alter the gastrointestinal flora may interact with mycophenolic acid by disrupting enterohepatic recirculation. Interference of MPAG hydrolysis may lead to less mycophenolic acid available for absorption).
No products indexed under this heading.

Sulfamethoxazole (Drugs that alter the gastrointestinal flora may interact with mycophenolic acid by disrupting enterohepatic recirculation. Interference of MPAG hydrolysis may lead to less mycophenolic acid available for absorption).
No products indexed under this heading.

Sulfisoxazole Acetyl (Drugs that alter the gastrointestinal flora may interact with mycophenolic acid by disrupting enterohepatic recirculation. Interference of MPAG hydrolysis may lead to less mycophenolic acid available for absorption).
No products indexed under this heading.

Tacrolimus (Cases of pure red cell aplasia (PRCA) have been reported in patients treated with mycophenolate mofetil (MMF) in combination with other immunosuppressive agents). Products include:
Prograf Capsules 677
Prograf Injection 677
Protopic 685

Tetracycline Hydrochloride (Drugs that alter the gastrointestinal flora may interact with mycophenolic acid by disrupting enterohepatic recirculation. Interference of MPAG hydrolysis may lead to less mycophenolic acid available for absorption). Products include:
Pylera 793

Typhoid Vaccine (During treatment with mycophenolic acid, the use of live attenuated vaccines should be avoided and patients should be advised that vaccinations may be less effective. Influenza vaccination may be of value).
No products indexed under this heading.

Varicella Virus Vaccine, Live (During treatment with mycophenolic acid, the use of live attenuated vaccines should be avoided and patients should be advised that vaccinations may be less effective. Influenza vaccination may be of value). Products include:
Varivax 2285

Yellow Fever Vaccine (During treatment with mycophenolic acid, the use of live attenuated vaccines should be avoided and patients should be advised that vaccinations may be less effective. Influenza vaccination may be of value).
No products indexed under this heading.

Zoster Vaccine Live (During treatment with mycophenolic acid, the use of live attenuated vaccines should be avoided and patients should be advised that vaccinations may be less effective. Influenza vaccination may be of value). Products include:
Zostavax 2299

Food Interactions

Food, unspecified (Co-administration of mycophenolic acid with a high fat meal decreased C_{max} by 33%, a 3.5-hour delay in the T_{lag} (range, -6 to 18 hours), and 5.0-hour delay in the T_{max} (range, -9 to 20 hours) of MPA. To avoid the variability in MPA absorption between doses, mycophenolic acid should be taken on an empty stomach).

Meal, unspecified (Co-administration of mycophenolic acid with a high fat meal decreased C_{max} by 33%, a 3.5-hour delay in the T_{lag} (range, -6 to 18 hours), and 5.0-hour delay in the T_{max} (range, -9 to 20 hours) of MPA. To avoid the variability in MPA absorption between doses, mycophenolic acid should be taken on an empty stomach).

MYLERAN TABLETS

(Busulfan) 1581
May interact with agents associated with myelosuppression, antineoplastics, cytotoxic drugs, and certain other agents. Compounds in these categories include:

Altretamine (Potential for rare life-threatening hepatic veno-occlusive disease). Products include:
Hexalen 1066

Anastrozole (Potential for rare life-threatening hepatic veno-occlusive disease).
No products indexed under this heading.

Asparaginase (Potential for rare life-threatening hepatic veno-occlusive disease). Products include:
Elspar 2005, 2122

Bicalutamide (Potential for rare life-threatening hepatic veno-occlusive disease).
No products indexed under this heading.

Bleomycin Sulfate (Busulfan-induced pulmonary toxicity may be additive to the effects produced by other cytotoxic agents).
No products indexed under this heading.

Bone Marrow Depressants, unspecified (Additive myelosuppression).
No products indexed under this heading.

Carboplatin (Potential for rare life-threatening hepatic veno-occlusive disease).
No products indexed under this heading.

Carmustine (BCNU) (Potential for rare life-threatening hepatic veno-occlusive disease).
No products indexed under this heading.

Chlorambucil (Potential for rare life-threatening hepatic veno-occlusive disease). Products include:
Leukeran 1557

Chloramphenicol (Busulfan may cause additive myelosuppression when used with other myelosuppressive drugs).
No products indexed under this heading.

Chloramphenicol Palmitate (Busulfan may cause additive myelosuppression when used with other myelosuppressive drugs).
No products indexed under this heading.

Chloramphenicol Sodium Succinate (Busulfan may cause additive myelosuppression when used with other myelosuppressive drugs).
No products indexed under this heading.

Cisplatin (Potential for rare life-threatening hepatic veno-occlusive disease).
No products indexed under this heading.

Cladribine (Busulfan may cause additive myelosuppression when used with other myelosuppressive drugs). Products include:
Leustatin 946

Cyclophosphamide (Potential for rare life-threatening hepatic veno-occlusive disease; potential for cardiac temponade; co-administration may result in reduced busulfan clearance).
No products indexed under this heading.

Dacarbazine (Potential for rare life-threatening hepatic veno-occlusive disease).
No products indexed under this heading.

Daunorubicin Citrate (Potential for rare life-threatening hepatic veno-occlusive disease).
No products indexed under this heading.

Daunorubicin Citrate Liposome (Busulfan may cause additive myelosuppression when used with other myelosuppressive drugs).
No products indexed under this heading.

Daunorubicin Hydrochloride (Busulfan-induced pulmonary toxicity may be additive to the effects produced by other cytotoxic agents).
No products indexed under this heading.

Denileukin Diftitox (Potential for rare life-threatening hepatic veno-occlusive disease). Products include:
Ontak 1068

Dexrazoxane (Busulfan may cause additive myelosuppression when used with other myelosuppressive drugs).
No products indexed under this heading.

Docetaxel (Potential for rare life-threatening hepatic veno-occlusive disease). Products include:
Taxotere 3035

Doxorubicin Hydrochloride (Busulfan-induced pulmonary toxicity may be additive to the effects produced by other cytotoxic agents).
No products indexed under this heading.

Doxorubicin Hydrochloride Liposome (Busulfan may cause additive myelosuppression when used with other myelosuppressive drugs). Products include:
Doxil 939

Epirubicin Hydrochloride (Busulfan-induced pulmonary toxicity may be additive to the effects produced by other cytotoxic agents).
No products indexed under this heading.

Estramustine Phosphate Sodium (Potential for rare life-threatening hepatic veno-occlusive disease).
No products indexed under this heading.

Etoposide (Potential for rare life-threatening hepatic veno-occlusive disease).
No products indexed under this heading.

Exemestane (Potential for rare life-threatening hepatic veno-occlusive disease). Products include:
Aromasin 2758

Floxuridine (Potential for rare life-threatening hepatic veno-occlusive disease).
No products indexed under this heading.

Fludarabine Phosphate (Busulfan may cause additive myelosuppression when used with other myelosuppressive drugs). Products include:
Oforta 3023

Fluorouracil (Busulfan-induced pulmonary toxicity may be additive to the effects produced by other cytotoxic agents). Products include:
Carac 2966

Flutamide (Potential for rare life-threatening hepatic veno-occlusive disease).
No products indexed under this heading.

Gemcitabine Hydrochloride (Potential for rare life-threatening hepatic veno-occlusive disease). Products include:
Gemzar 1900

Gemtuzumab Ozogamicin (Busulfan may cause additive myelosuppression when used with other myelosuppressive drugs). Products include:
Mylotarg 3524

Hydroxyurea (Busulfan-induced pulmonary toxicity may be additive to the effects produced by other cytotoxic agents).
No products indexed under this heading.

Idarubicin Hydrochloride (Potential for rare life-threatening hepatic veno-occlusive disease).
No products indexed under this heading.

Ifosfamide (Potential for rare life-threatening hepatic veno-occlusive disease).
No products indexed under this heading.

Interferon alfa-2a, Recombinant (Potential for rare life-threatening hepatic veno-occlusive disease).
No products indexed under this heading.

Interferon alfa-2b, Recombinant (Potential for rare life-threatening hepatic veno-occlusive disease). Products include:
Intron A 3140

IMPORTANT NOTE: Always consult each drug listing in the patient's regimen for possible interactions.

Chlordiazepoxide Hydrochloride (Potential for drug-drug interaction with drugs affected by CYP450 enzymes).
No products indexed under this heading.

Chlorpheniramine (Potential for drug-drug interaction with drugs affected by CYP450 enzymes).
No products indexed under this heading.

Chlorpheniramine Maleate (Potential for drug-drug interaction with drugs affected by CYP450 enzymes).
No products indexed under this heading.

Chlorpheniramine Polistirex (Potential for drug-drug interaction with drugs affected by CYP450 enzymes). Products include:

Chlorpheniramine Tannate (Potential for drug-drug interaction with drugs affected by CYP450 enzymes).
No products indexed under this heading.

Chlorpromazine (Potential for drug-drug interaction with drugs affected by CYP450 enzymes).
No products indexed under this heading.

Chlorpromazine Hydrochloride (Potential for drug-drug interaction with drugs affected by CYP450 enzymes).
No products indexed under this heading.

Chlorpropamide (Potential for drug-drug interaction with drugs affected by CYP450 enzymes).
No products indexed under this heading.

Cilostazol (Potential for drug-drug interaction with drugs affected by CYP450 enzymes).
No products indexed under this heading.

Cimetidine Hydrochloride (Potential for drug-drug interaction with drugs affected by CYP450 enzymes).
No products indexed under this heading.

Ciprofloxacin (Potential for drug-drug interaction with drugs affected by CYP450 enzymes). Products include:

Ciprofloxacin Hydrochloride (Potential for drug-drug interaction with drugs affected by CYP450 enzymes). Products include:

Cisapride (Potential for drug-drug interaction with drugs affected by CYP450 enzymes).
No products indexed under this heading.

Citalopram Hydrobromide (Potential for drug-drug interaction with drugs affected by CYP450 enzymes). Products include:

Clarithromycin (Potential for drug-drug interaction with drugs affected by CYP450 enzymes). Products include:

Clomipramine Hydrochloride (Potential for drug-drug interaction with drugs affected by CYP450 enzymes).
No products indexed under this heading.

Clopidogrel Bisulfate (Potential for drug-drug interaction with drugs affected by CYP450 enzymes). Products include:

Clopidogrel Hydrogen Sulfate (Potential for drug-drug interaction with drugs affected by CYP450 enzymes).
No products indexed under this heading.

Clozapine (Potential for drug-drug interaction with drugs affected by CYP450 enzymes).
No products indexed under this heading.

Codeine Phosphate (Potential for drug-drug interaction with drugs affected by CYP450 enzymes). Products include:

Codeine Sulfate (Potential for drug-drug interaction with drugs affected by CYP450 enzymes).
No products indexed under this heading.

Cyclobenzaprine (Potential for drug-drug interaction with drugs affected by CYP450 enzymes).
No products indexed under this heading.

Cyclobenzaprine Hydrochloride (Potential for drug-drug interaction with drugs affected by CYP450 enzymes). Products include:

Cyclophosphamide (Potential for drug-drug interaction with drugs affected by CYP450 enzymes).
No products indexed under this heading.

Cyclosporine (Potential for drug-drug interaction with drugs affected by CYP450 enzymes). Products include:

Desipramine Hydrochloride (Potential for drug-drug interaction with drugs affected by CYP450 enzymes).
No products indexed under this heading.

Desogestrel (Potential for drug-drug interaction with drugs affected by CYP450 enzymes).
No products indexed under this heading.

Dexamethasone (Potential for drug-drug interaction with drugs affected by CYP450 enzymes). Products include:

Dexamethasone Acetate (Potential for drug-drug interaction with drugs affected by CYP450 enzymes).
No products indexed under this heading.

Dexamethasone Phosphate (Potential for drug-drug interaction with drugs affected by CYP450 enzymes).
No products indexed under this heading.

Dexamethasone Sodium (Potential for drug-drug interaction with drugs affected by CYP450 enzymes).
No products indexed under this heading.

Dexamethasone Sodium Phosphate (Potential for drug-drug interaction with drugs affected by CYP450 enzymes).
No products indexed under this heading.

Dexfenfluramine Hydrochloride (Potential for drug-drug interaction with drugs affected by CYP450 enzymes).
No products indexed under this heading.

Dextromethorphan (Potential for drug-drug interaction with drugs affected by CYP450 enzymes).
No products indexed under this heading.

Dextromethorphan Hydrobromide (Potential for drug-drug interaction with drugs affected by CYP450 enzymes).
No products indexed under this heading.

Dextromethorphan Polistirex (Potential for drug-drug interaction with drugs affected by CYP450 enzymes).
No products indexed under this heading.

Diazepam (Potential for drug-drug interaction with drugs affected by CYP450 enzymes). Products include:

Diclofenac Potassium (Potential for drug-drug interaction with drugs affected by CYP450 enzymes).
No products indexed under this heading.

Diclofenac Sodium (Potential for drug-drug interaction with drugs affected by CYP450 enzymes).
No products indexed under this heading.

Dihydroergotamine Mesylate (Potential for drug-drug interaction with drugs affected by CYP450 enzymes).
No products indexed under this heading.

Diltiazem Hydrochloride (Potential for drug-drug interaction with drugs affected by CYP450 enzymes). Products include:

Diltiazem Maleate (Potential for drug-drug interaction with drugs affected by CYP450 enzymes).
No products indexed under this heading.

Disopyramide (Potential for drug-drug interaction with drugs affected by CYP450 enzymes).
No products indexed under this heading.

Disopyramide Phosphate (Potential for drug-drug interaction with drugs affected by CYP450 enzymes).
No products indexed under this heading.

Disulfiram (Potential for drug-drug interaction with drugs affected by CYP450 enzymes).
No products indexed under this heading.

Divalproex Sodium (Potential for drug-drug interaction with drugs affected by CYP450 enzymes). Products include:

Docetaxel (Potential for drug-drug interaction with drugs affected by CYP450 enzymes). Products include:

Dolasetron Mesylate (Potential for drug-drug interaction with drugs affected by CYP450 enzymes). Products include:

Donepezil Hydrochloride (Potential for drug-drug interaction with drugs affected by CYP450 enzymes). Products include:

Doxepin Hydrochloride (Potential for drug-drug interaction with drugs affected by CYP450 enzymes).
No products indexed under this heading.

Doxorubicin Hydrochloride (Potential for drug-drug interaction with drugs affected by CYP450 enzymes).
No products indexed under this heading.

Dronabinol (Potential for drug-drug interaction with drugs affected by CYP450 enzymes).
No products indexed under this heading.

Drugs that Undergo Biotransformation by Cytochrome P-450 Mixed Function Oxidase (Potential for drug-drug interaction with drugs affected by CYP450 enzymes).
No products indexed under this heading.

Dyphylline (Potential for drug-drug interaction with drugs affected by CYP450 enzymes).
No products indexed under this heading.

Encainide Hydrochloride (Potential for drug-drug interaction with drugs affected by CYP450 enzymes).
No products indexed under this heading.

Enoxacin (Potential for drug-drug interaction with drugs affected by CYP450 enzymes).
No products indexed under this heading.

Eprosartan Mesylate (Potential for drug-drug interaction with drugs affected by CYP450 enzymes). Products include:

Ergotamine Tartrate (Potential for drug-drug interaction with drugs affected by CYP450 enzymes).
No products indexed under this heading.

Erythromycin (Potential for drug-drug interaction with drugs affected by CYP450 enzymes).
No products indexed under this heading.

Erythromycin Estolate (Potential for drug-drug interaction with drugs affected by CYP450 enzymes).
No products indexed under this heading.

Erythromycin Ethylsuccinate (Potential for drug-drug interaction with drugs affected by CYP450 enzymes). Products include:

Erythromycin Gluceptate (Potential for drug-drug interaction with drugs affected by CYP450 enzymes).
No products indexed under this heading.

Erythromycin Lactobionate (Potential for drug-drug interaction with drugs affected by CYP450 enzymes).
No products indexed under this heading.

Erythromycin Stearate (Potential for drug-drug interaction with drugs affected by CYP450 enzymes).
No products indexed under this heading.

Esomeprazole Magnesium (Potential for drug-drug interaction with drugs affected by CYP450 enzymes). Products include:

Esomeprazole Sodium (Potential for drug-drug interaction with drugs affected by CYP450 enzymes). Products include:

Estradiol (Potential for drug-drug interaction with drugs affected by CYP450 enzymes). Products include:

Estradiol Benzoate (Potential for drug-drug interaction with drugs affected by CYP450 enzymes).
No products indexed under this heading.

Estradiol Cypionate (Potential for drug-drug interaction with drugs affected by CYP450 enzymes).
No products indexed under this heading.

Estradiol Valerate (Potential for drug-drug interaction with drugs affected by CYP450 enzymes).
No products indexed under this heading.

Estrogen (Potential for drug-drug interaction with drugs affected by CYP450 enzymes).
No products indexed under this heading.

Estrogens, Conjugated (Potential for drug-drug interaction with drugs affected by CYP450 enzymes). Products include:

Estrogens, Conjugated, Synthetic A (Potential for drug-drug interaction with drugs affected by CYP450 enzymes).
No products indexed under this heading.

Estrogens, Esterified (Potential for drug-drug interaction with drugs affected by CYP450 enzymes).
No products indexed under this heading.

Ethinyl Estradiol (Potential for drug-drug interaction with drugs affected by CYP450 enzymes). Products include:

IMPORTANT NOTE: Always consult each drug listing in the patient's regimen for possible interactions.

Food Interactions

Beverages, caffeine-containing (Potential for drug-drug interaction with drugs affected by CYP450 enzymes).

Food, caffeine-containing (Potential for drug-drug interaction with drugs affected by CYP450 enzymes).

NADOLOL TABLETS

May interact with general anesthetics, insulin, oral hypoglycemic agents, and certain other agents. Compounds in these categories include:

Acarbose (Beta-adrenergic blockade may prevent the appearance of premonitory signs and symptoms, such as tachycardia and blood pressure changes, of acute hypoglycemia; beta-blockade also reduces the release of insulin in response to hyperglycemia; adjust dosage of oral antidiabetic drugs).
No products indexed under this heading.

IMPORTANT NOTE: Always consult each drug listing in the patient's regimen for possible interactions.

Nadolol Interactions Index 1170

Chlorpropamide (Beta-adrenergic blockade may prevent the appearance of premonitory signs and symptoms, such as tachycardia and blood pressure changes, of acute hypoglycemia; beta-blockade also reduces the release of insulin in response to hyperglycemia; adjust dosage of oral antidiabetic drugs).
No products indexed under this heading.

Desflurane (Co-administration may result in exaggeration of the hypotension induced by general anesthetics).
No products indexed under this heading.

Enflurane (Co-administration may result in exaggeration of the hypotension induced by general anesthetics).
No products indexed under this heading.

Epinephrine (Patients with a history of severe anaphylactic reaction to variety of allergens may be more reactive to repeated challenge; potential for unresponsiveness to the usual dose of epinephrine). Products include:
EpiPen 3631
Twinject 3268

Epinephrine Hydrochloride (Patients with a history of severe anaphylactic reaction to variety of allergens may be more reactive to repeated challenge; potential for unresponsiveness to the usual dose of epinephrine).
No products indexed under this heading.

Glibenclamide (Beta-adrenergic blockade may prevent the appearance of premonitory signs and symptoms, such as tachycardia and blood pressure changes, of acute hypoglycemia; beta-blockade also reduces the release of insulin in response to hyperglycemia; adjust dosage of oral antidiabetic drugs).
No products indexed under this heading.

Glimepiride (Beta-adrenergic blockade may prevent the appearance of premonitory signs and symptoms, such as tachycardia and blood pressure changes, of acute hypoglycemia; beta-blockade also reduces the release of insulin in response to hyperglycemia; adjust dosage of oral antidiabetic drugs). Products include:
Avandaryl 1356
Duetact 3354

Glipizide (Beta-adrenergic blockade may prevent the appearance of premonitory signs and symptoms, such as tachycardia and blood pressure changes, of acute hypoglycemia; beta-blockade also reduces the release of insulin in response to hyperglycemia; adjust dosage of oral antidiabetic drugs).
No products indexed under this heading.

Glyburide (Beta-adrenergic blockade may prevent the appearance of premonitory signs and symptoms, such as tachycardia and blood pressure changes, of acute hypoglycemia; beta-blockade also reduces the release of insulin in response to hyperglycemia; adjust dosage of oral antidiabetic drugs).
No products indexed under this heading.

Halothane (Co-administration may result in exaggeration of the hypotension induced by general anesthetics).
No products indexed under this heading.

Insulin (Beta-adrenergic blockade may prevent the appearance of premonitory signs and symptoms, such as tachycardia and blood pressure changes, of acute hypoglycemia; beta-blockade also reduces the release of insulin in response to hyperglycemia; adjust dosage of insulin).
No products indexed under this heading.

Insulin, Human, Zinc Suspension (Beta-adrenergic blockade may prevent the appearance of premonitory signs and symptoms, such as tachycardia and blood pressure changes, of acute hypoglycemia; beta-blockade also reduces the release of insulin in response to hyperglycemia; adjust dosage of insulin).
No products indexed under this heading.

Insulin, Human (rDNA origin) (Beta-adrenergic blockade may prevent the appearance of premonitory signs and symptoms, such as tachycardia and blood pressure changes, of acute hypoglycemia; beta-blockade also reduces the release of insulin in response to hyperglycemia; adjust dosage of insulin). Products include:
Exubera 2717

Insulin, Human NPH (Beta-adrenergic blockade may prevent the appearance of premonitory signs and symptoms, such as tachycardia and blood pressure changes, of acute hypoglycemia; beta-blockade also reduces the release of insulin in response to hyperglycemia; adjust dosage of insulin). Products include:
Humulin N Vial 1934

Insulin, Human Regular (Beta-adrenergic blockade may prevent the appearance of premonitory signs and symptoms, such as tachycardia and blood pressure changes, of acute hypoglycemia; beta-blockade also reduces the release of insulin in response to hyperglycemia; adjust dosage of insulin). Products include:
Humulin R 1937
Humulin R (U-500) 1939

Insulin, Human Regular and Human NPH Mixture (Beta-adrenergic blockade may prevent the appearance of premonitory signs and symptoms, such as tachycardia and blood pressure changes, of acute hypoglycemia; beta-blockade also reduces the release of insulin in response to hyperglycemia; adjust dosage of insulin). Products include:
Humulin 50/50 1930
Humulin 70/30 Vial 1931

Insulin, NPH (Beta-adrenergic blockade may prevent the appearance of premonitory signs and symptoms, such as tachycardia and blood pressure changes, of acute hypoglycemia; beta-blockade also reduces the release of insulin in response to hyperglycemia; adjust dosage of insulin).
No products indexed under this heading.

Insulin, Regular (Beta-adrenergic blockade may prevent the appearance of premonitory signs and symptoms, such as tachycardia and blood pressure changes, of acute hypoglycemia; beta-blockade also reduces the release of insulin in response to hyperglycemia; adjust dosage of insulin).
No products indexed under this heading.

Insulin, Regular and NPH mixture (Beta-adrenergic blockade may prevent the appearance of premonitory signs and symptoms, such as tachycardia and blood pressure changes, of acute hypoglycemia; beta-blockade also reduces the release of insulin in response to hyperglycemia; adjust dosage of insulin).
No products indexed under this heading.

Insulin, Zinc Crystals (Beta-adrenergic blockade may prevent the appearance of premonitory signs and symptoms, such as tachycardia and blood pressure changes, of acute hypoglycemia; beta-blockade also reduces the release of insulin in response to hyperglycemia; adjust dosage of insulin).
No products indexed under this heading.

Insulin, Zinc Suspension (Beta-adrenergic blockade may prevent the appearance of premonitory signs and symptoms, such as tachycardia and blood pressure changes, of acute hypoglycemia; beta-blockade also reduces the release of insulin in response to hyperglycemia; adjust dosage of insulin).
No products indexed under this heading.

Insulin Aspart (Beta-adrenergic blockade may prevent the appearance of premonitory signs and symptoms, such as tachycardia and blood pressure changes, of acute hypoglycemia; beta-blockade also reduces the release of insulin in response to hyperglycemia; adjust dosage of insulin).
No products indexed under this heading.

Insulin Aspart, Human (Beta-adrenergic blockade may prevent the appearance of premonitory signs and symptoms, such as tachycardia and blood pressure changes, of acute hypoglycemia; beta-blockade also reduces the release of insulin in response to hyperglycemia; adjust dosage of insulin). Products include:
NovoLog Mix 70/30 2581

Insulin Aspart, Human Regular (Beta-adrenergic blockade may prevent the appearance of premonitory signs and symptoms, such as tachycardia and blood pressure changes, of acute hypoglycemia; beta-blockade also reduces the release of insulin in response to hyperglycemia; adjust dosage of insulin). Products include:
NovoLog 2575

Insulin Aspart Protamine, Human (Beta-adrenergic blockade may prevent the appearance of premonitory signs and symptoms, such as tachycardia and blood pressure changes, of acute hypoglycemia; beta-blockade also reduces the release of insulin in response to hyperglycemia; adjust dosage of insulin). Products include:
NovoLog Mix 70/30 2581

Insulin Detemir (rDNA Origin) (Beta-adrenergic blockade may prevent the appearance of premonitory signs and symptoms, such as tachycardia and blood pressure changes, of acute hypoglycemia; beta-blockade also reduces the release of insulin in response to hyperglycemia; adjust dosage of insulin). Products include:
Levemir 2566

Insulin Glargine (Beta-adrenergic blockade may prevent the appearance of premonitory signs and symptoms, such as tachycardia and blood pressure changes, of acute hypoglycemia; beta-blockade also reduces the release of insulin in response to hyperglycemia; adjust dosage of insulin). Products include:
Lantus 2996

Insulin Glulisine (Beta-adrenergic blockade may prevent the appearance of premonitory signs and symptoms, such as tachycardia and blood pressure changes, of acute hypoglycemia; beta-blockade also reduces the release of insulin in response to hyperglycemia; adjust dosage of insulin). Products include:
Apidra 2937
Apidra SoloStar 2937

Insulin Lispro, Human (Beta-adrenergic blockade may prevent the appearance of premonitory signs and symptoms, such as tachycardia and blood pressure changes, of acute hypoglycemia; beta-blockade also reduces the release of insulin in response to hyperglycemia; adjust dosage of insulin). Products include:
Humalog 1910
Humalog Mix 1914
Humalog Mix75/25 1917

Insulin Lispro Protamine, Human (Beta-adrenergic blockade may prevent the appearance of premonitory signs and symptoms, such as tachycardia and blood pressure changes, of acute hypoglycemia; beta-blockade also reduces the release of insulin in response to hyperglycemia; adjust dosage of insulin). Products include:
Humalog Mix 1914
Humalog Mix75/25 1917

Isoflurane (Co-administration may result in exaggeration of the hypotension induced by general anesthetics).
No products indexed under this heading.

Ketamine Hydrochloride (Co-administration may result in exaggeration of the hypotension induced by general anesthetics).
No products indexed under this heading.

Metformin Hydrochloride (Beta-adrenergic blockade may prevent the appearance of premonitory signs and symptoms, such as tachycardia and blood pressure changes, of acute hypoglycemia; beta-blockade also reduces the release of insulin in response to hyperglycemia; adjust dosage of oral antidiabetic drugs). Products include:
ActoPlus 3338
Avandamet 1345
Janumet 2188

Methohexital Sodium (Co-administration may result in exaggeration of the hypotension induced by general anesthetics).
No products indexed under this heading.

Methoxyflurane (Co-administration may result in exaggeration of the hypotension induced by general anesthetics).
No products indexed under this heading.

Miglitol (Beta-adrenergic blockade may prevent the appearance of premonitory signs and symptoms, such as tachycardia and blood pressure changes, of acute hypoglycemia; beta-blockade also reduces the release of insulin in response to hyperglycemia; adjust dosage of oral antidiabetic drugs).
No products indexed under this heading.

Nateglinide (Beta-adrenergic blockade may prevent the appearance of premonitory signs and symptoms, such as tachycardia and blood pressure changes, of acute hypoglycemia; beta-blockade also reduces the release of insulin in response to hyperglycemia; adjust dosage of oral antidiabetic drugs).
No products indexed under this heading.

Nitrous Oxide (Co-administration may result in exaggeration of the hypotension induced by general anesthetics).
No products indexed under this heading.

Pioglitazone Hydrochloride (Beta-adrenergic blockade may prevent the appearance of premonitory signs and symptoms, such as tachycardia and blood pressure changes, of acute hypoglycemia; beta-blockade also reduces the release of insulin in response to hyperglycemia; adjust dosage of oral antidiabetic drugs). Products include:
ActoPlus 3338
Actos 3345
Duetact 3354

Propofol (Co-administration may result in exaggeration of the hypotension induced by general anesthetics).
No products indexed under this heading.

(⊙ Described in PDR® for Ophthalmic Medicines)

Repaglinide (Beta-adrenergic blockade may prevent the appearance of premonitory signs and symptoms, such as tachycardia and blood pressure changes, of acute hypoglycemia; beta-blockade also reduces the release of insulin in response to hyperglycemia; adjust dosage of oral antidiabetic drugs).
No products indexed under this heading.

Reserpine (Potential for additive effects resulting in hypotension and/or excessive bradycardia (vertigo, syncope, postural hypotension)).
No products indexed under this heading.

Rosiglitazone Maleate (Beta-adrenergic blockade may prevent the appearance of premonitory signs and symptoms, such as tachycardia and blood pressure changes, of acute hypoglycemia; beta-blockade also reduces the release of insulin in response to hyperglycemia; adjust dosage of oral antidiabetic drugs). Products include:

Sevoflurane (Co-administration may result in exaggeration of the hypotension induced by general anesthetics). Products include:

Sitagliptin Phosphate (Beta-adrenergic blockade may prevent the appearance of premonitory signs and symptoms, such as tachycardia and blood pressure changes, of acute hypoglycemia; beta-blockade also reduces the release of insulin in response to hyperglycemia; adjust dosage of oral antidiabetic drugs). Products include:

Tolazamide (Beta-adrenergic blockade may prevent the appearance of premonitory signs and symptoms, such as tachycardia and blood pressure changes, of acute hypoglycemia; beta-blockade also reduces the release of insulin in response to hyperglycemia; adjust dosage of oral antidiabetic drugs).
No products indexed under this heading.

Tolbutamide (Beta-adrenergic blockade may prevent the appearance of premonitory signs and symptoms, such as tachycardia and blood pressure changes, of acute hypoglycemia; beta-blockade also reduces the release of insulin in response to hyperglycemia; adjust dosage of oral antidiabetic drugs).
No products indexed under this heading.

Troglitazone (Beta-adrenergic blockade may prevent the appearance of premonitory signs and symptoms, such as tachycardia and blood pressure changes, of acute hypoglycemia; beta-blockade also reduces the release of insulin in response to hyperglycemia; adjust dosage of oral antidiabetic drugs).
No products indexed under this heading.

NAFTIN CREAM
(Naftifine Hydrochloride) 2320
None cited in PDR database.

NAFTIN GEL
(Naftifine Hydrochloride) 2320
None cited in PDR database.

NAMENDA ORAL SOLUTION
(Memantine Hydrochloride) 1168
See Namenda Tablets

NAMENDA TABLETS
(Memantine Hydrochloride) 1168
May interact with carbonic anhydrase inhibitors, quinidine, urinary alkalinizing agents, and certain other agents. Compounds in these categories include:

Acetazolamide (Alterations of urine pH towards the alkaline condition by drugs that make the urine alkaline (eg, carbonic anhydrase inhibitors) may lead to an accumulation of memantine with a possible increase in adverse effects; use with caution).
No products indexed under this heading.

Amantadine Hydrochloride (The combined use of memantine with other NMDA antagonists, like amantadine, has not been systemically evaluated and such use should be approached with caution).
No products indexed under this heading.

Cimetidine (Co-administration with drugs that use the same renal cationic system, including cimetidine, could potentially result in altered plasma levels of both drugs).
No products indexed under this heading.

Cimetidine Hydrochloride (Co-administration with drugs that use the same renal cationic system, including cimetidine, could potentially result in altered plasma levels of both drugs).
No products indexed under this heading.

Dextromethorphan (The combined use of memantine with other NMDA antagonists, like dextromethorphan, has not been systemically evaluated and such use should be approached with caution).
No products indexed under this heading.

Dextromethorphan Hydrobromide (The combined use of memantine with other NMDA antagonists, like dextromethorphan, has not been systemically evaluated and such use should be approached with caution).
No products indexed under this heading.

Dextromethorphan Polistirex (The combined use of memantine with other NMDA antagonists, like dextromethorphan, has not been systemically evaluated and such use should be approached with caution).
No products indexed under this heading.

Dextromethorphan Tannate (The combined use of memantine with other NMDA antagonists, like dextromethorphan, has not been systemically evaluated and such use should be approached with caution).
No products indexed under this heading.

Dichlorphenamide (Alterations of urine pH towards the alkaline condition by drugs that make the urine alkaline (eg, carbonic anhydrase inhibitors) may lead to an accumulation of memantine with a possible increase in adverse effects; use with caution).
No products indexed under this heading.

Dorzolamide Hydrochloride (Alterations of urine pH towards the alkaline condition by drugs that make the urine alkaline (eg, carbonic anhydrase inhibitors) may lead to an accumulation of memantine with a possible increase in adverse effects; use with caution). Products include:

Hydrochlorothiazide (Co-administration with drugs that use the same renal cationic system, including hydrochlorothiazide, could potentially result in altered plasma levels of both drugs. The co-administration of memantine and hydrochlorothiazide/triamterene decreased the bioavailability of hydrochlorothiazide by 20%). Products include:

Hydrochlorothiazide Hydrochloride (Co-administration with drugs that use the same renal cationic system, including hydrochlorothiazide, could potentially result in altered plasma levels of both drugs. The co-administration of memantine and hydrochlorothiazide/triamterene decreased the bioavailability of hydrochlorothiazide by 20%).
No products indexed under this heading.

Ketamine (The combined use of memantine with other NMDA antagonists, like ketamine, has not been systemically evaluated and such use should be approached with caution).
No products indexed under this heading.

Ketamine Hydrochloride (The combined use of memantine with other NMDA antagonists, like ketamine, has not been systemically evaluated and such use should be approached with caution).
No products indexed under this heading.

Methazolamide (Alterations of urine pH towards the alkaline condition by drugs that make the urine alkaline (eg, carbonic anhydrase inhibitors) may lead to an accumulation of memantine with a possible increase in adverse effects; use with caution).
No products indexed under this heading.

Nicotine (Co-administration with drugs that use the same renal cationic system, including nicotine, could potentially result in altered plasma levels of both drugs).
No products indexed under this heading.

Nicotine Polacrilex (Co-administration with drugs that use the same renal cationic system, including nicotine, could potentially result in altered plasma levels of both drugs).
No products indexed under this heading.

Nicotine Salicylate (Co-administration with drugs that use the same renal cationic system, including nicotine, could potentially result in altered plasma levels of both drugs).
No products indexed under this heading.

Nicotine Sulfate (Co-administration with drugs that use the same renal cationic system, including nicotine, could potentially result in altered plasma levels of both drugs).
No products indexed under this heading.

Potassium Citrate (Alterations of urine pH towards the alkaline condition by drugs that make the urine alkaline may lead to an accumulation of memantine with a possible increase in adverse effects; use with caution). Products include:

Quinidine (Co-administration with drugs that use the same renal cationic system, including quinidine, could potentially result in altered plasma levels of both drugs).
No products indexed under this heading.

Quinidine Gluconate (Co-administration with drugs that use the same renal cationic system, including quinidine, could potentially result in altered plasma levels of both drugs).
No products indexed under this heading.

Quinidine Hydrochloride (Co-administration with drugs that use the same renal cationic system, including quinidine, could potentially result in altered plasma levels of both drugs).
No products indexed under this heading.

Quinidine Polygalacturonate (Co-administration with drugs that use the same renal cationic system, including quinidine, could result in altered plasma levels of both drugs).
No products indexed under this heading.

Quinidine Sulfate (Co-administration with drugs that use the same renal cationic system, including quinidine, could potentially result in altered plasma levels of both drugs).
No products indexed under this heading.

Ranitidine Bismuth Citrate (Co-administration with drugs that use the same renal cationic system, including ranitidine, could potentially result in altered plasma levels of both drugs).
No products indexed under this heading.

Ranitidine Hydrochloride (Co-administration with drugs that use the same renal cationic system, including ranitidine, could potentially result in altered plasma levels of both drugs). Products include:

Sodium Bicarbonate (Alterations of urine pH towards the alkaline condition by drugs that make the urine alkaline (eg, sodium bicarbonate) may lead to an accumulation of memantine with a possible increase in adverse effects; hence, use with caution).
No products indexed under this heading.

Sodium Citrate (Alterations of urine pH towards the alkaline condition by drugs that make the urine alkaline may lead to an accumulation of memantine with a possible increase in adverse effects; use with caution).
No products indexed under this heading.

Torsemide (Alterations of urine pH towards the alkaline condition by drugs that make the urine alkaline (eg, carbonic anhydrase inhibitors) may lead to an accumulation of memantine with a possible increase in adverse effects; use with caution).
No products indexed under this heading.

Triamterene (Co-administration with drugs that use the same renal cationic system, including triamterene, could potentially result in altered plasma levels of both drugs. However, co-administration of memantine and hydrochlorothiazide/triamterene did not affect the bioavailability of either memantine or triamterene). Products include:

NAPROSYN SUSPENSION
(Naproxen) 2850
See EC-Naprosyn Delayed-Release Tablets

NAPROSYN TABLETS
(Naproxen) 2850
See EC-Naprosyn Delayed-Release Tablets

NASACORT AQ NASAL SPRAY
(Triamcinolone Acetonide) 3019
None cited in PDR database.

NASCOBAL NASAL SPRAY
(Vitamin B12) 2700
May interact with agents associated with myelosuppression, alcohols, antibiotics, chloramphenicol, and certain other agents. Compounds in these categories include:

Alatrofloxacin Mesylate (Persons taking most antibiotics invalidate folic acid and vitamin B12 diagnostic blood assays).
No products indexed under this heading.

Altretamine (Blunted or impeded therapeutic response to vitamin B12 may

be due to such conditions as infection, uremia, drugs having bone marrow suppressant properties, and concurrent iron or folic acid deficiency). Products include:

Hexalen 1066

Amikacin Sulfate (Persons taking most antibiotics invalidate folic acid and vitamin B12 diagnostic blood assays).
No products indexed under this heading.

Amoxicillin (Persons taking most antibiotics invalidate folic acid and vitamin B12 diagnostic blood assays). Products include:

Amoxil Capsules 1311
Amoxil Chewable Tablets 1311
Amoxil 1311
Amoxil Powder 1311
Augmentin 1331
Augmentin Tablets 1335
Augmentin ES-600 1338
Augmentin XR 1342
Moxatag 2321

Amoxicillin Trihydrate (Persons taking most antibiotics invalidate folic acid and vitamin B12 diagnostic blood assays).
No products indexed under this heading.

Ampicillin (Persons taking most antibiotics invalidate folic acid and vitamin B12 diagnostic blood assays).
No products indexed under this heading.

Ampicillin Sodium (Persons taking most antibiotics invalidate folic acid and vitamin B12 diagnostic blood assays).
No products indexed under this heading.

Ampicillin Trihydrate (Persons taking most antibiotics invalidate folic acid and vitamin B12 diagnostic blood assays).
No products indexed under this heading.

Antibiotics, non-penicillin, unspecified (Persons taking most antibiotics invalidate folic acid and vitamin B12 diagnostic blood assays).
No products indexed under this heading.

Azithromycin Dihydrate (Persons taking most antibiotics invalidate folic acid and vitamin B12 diagnostic blood assays).
No products indexed under this heading.

Azlocillin Sodium (Persons taking most antibiotics invalidate folic acid and vitamin B12 diagnostic blood assays).
No products indexed under this heading.

Aztreonam (Persons taking most antibiotics invalidate folic acid and vitamin B12 diagnostic blood assays).
No products indexed under this heading.

Bacampicillin Hydrochloride (Persons taking most antibiotics invalidate folic acid and vitamin B12 diagnostic blood assays).
No products indexed under this heading.

Busulfan (Blunted or impeded therapeutic response to vitamin B12 may be due to such conditions as infection, uremia, drugs having bone marrow suppressant properties, and concurrent iron or folic acid deficiency). Products include:

Myleran 1581

Carbenicillin Disodium (Persons taking most antibiotics invalidate folic acid and vitamin B12 diagnostic blood assays).
No products indexed under this heading.

Carbenicillin Indanyl Sodium (Persons taking most antibiotics invalidate folic acid and vitamin B12 diagnostic blood assays).
No products indexed under this heading.

Cefaclor (Persons taking most antibiotics invalidate folic acid and vitamin B12 diagnostic blood assays).
No products indexed under this heading.

Cefadroxil (Persons taking most antibiotics invalidate folic acid and vitamin B12 diagnostic blood assays).
No products indexed under this heading.

Cefamandole Nafate (Persons taking most antibiotics invalidate folic acid and vitamin B12 diagnostic blood assays).
No products indexed under this heading.

Cefazolin Sodium (Persons taking most antibiotics invalidate folic acid and vitamin B12 diagnostic blood assays).
No products indexed under this heading.

Cefixime (Persons taking most antibiotics invalidate folic acid and vitamin B12 diagnostic blood assays). Products include:

Suprax for Oral Suspension 2038
Suprax Tablets 2038

Cefmetazole Sodium (Persons taking most antibiotics invalidate folic acid and vitamin B12 diagnostic blood assays).
No products indexed under this heading.

Cefonicid Sodium (Persons taking most antibiotics invalidate folic acid and vitamin B12 diagnostic blood assays).
No products indexed under this heading.

Cefoperazone Sodium (Persons taking most antibiotics invalidate folic acid and vitamin B12 diagnostic blood assays).
No products indexed under this heading.

Ceforanide (Persons taking most antibiotics invalidate folic acid and vitamin B12 diagnostic blood assays).
No products indexed under this heading.

Cefotaxime Sodium (Persons taking most antibiotics invalidate folic acid and vitamin B12 diagnostic blood assays).
No products indexed under this heading.

Cefotetan (Persons taking most antibiotics invalidate folic acid and vitamin B12 diagnostic blood assays).
No products indexed under this heading.

Cefoxitin Sodium (Persons taking most antibiotics invalidate folic acid and vitamin B12 diagnostic blood assays).
No products indexed under this heading.

Cefpodoxime Proxetil (Persons taking most antibiotics invalidate folic acid and vitamin B12 diagnostic blood assays).
No products indexed under this heading.

Cefprozil (Persons taking most antibiotics invalidate folic acid and vitamin B12 diagnostic blood assays).
No products indexed under this heading.

Ceftazidime (Persons taking most antibiotics invalidate folic acid and vitamin B12 diagnostic blood assays). Products include:

Fortaz 1481

Ceftizoxime Sodium (Persons taking most antibiotics invalidate folic acid and vitamin B12 diagnostic blood assays).
No products indexed under this heading.

Ceftriaxone Sodium (Persons taking most antibiotics invalidate folic acid and vitamin B12 diagnostic blood assays). Products include:

Rocephin 2859

Cefuroxime Axetil (Persons taking most antibiotics invalidate folic acid and vitamin B12 diagnostic blood assays). Products include:

Ceftin 1399

Cefuroxime Sodium (Persons taking most antibiotics invalidate folic acid and vitamin B12 diagnostic blood assays).
No products indexed under this heading.

Cephalexin (Persons taking most antibiotics invalidate folic acid and vitamin B12 diagnostic blood assays).
No products indexed under this heading.

Cephalothin Sodium (Persons taking most antibiotics invalidate folic acid and vitamin B12 diagnostic blood assays).
No products indexed under this heading.

Cephapirin Sodium (Persons taking most antibiotics invalidate folic acid and vitamin B12 diagnostic blood assays).
No products indexed under this heading.

Cephradine (Persons taking most antibiotics invalidate folic acid and vitamin B12 diagnostic blood assays).
No products indexed under this heading.

Chlorambucil (Blunted or impeded therapeutic response to vitamin B12 may be due to such conditions as infection, uremia, drugs having bone marrow suppressant properties, and concurrent iron or folic acid deficiency). Products include:

Leukeran 1557

Chloramphenicol (Blunted or impeded therapeutic response to vitamin B12 may be due to such conditions as infection, uremia, drugs having bone marrow suppressant properties such as chloramphenicol, and concurrent iron or folic acid deficiency).
No products indexed under this heading.

Chloramphenicol Palmitate (Blunted or impeded therapeutic response to vitamin B12 may be due to such conditions as infection, uremia, drugs having bone marrow suppressant properties such as chloramphenicol, and concurrent iron or folic acid deficiency).
No products indexed under this heading.

Chloramphenicol Sodium Succinate (Blunted or impeded therapeutic response to vitamin B12 may be due to such conditions as infection, uremia, drugs having bone marrow suppressant properties such as chloramphenicol, and concurrent iron or folic acid deficiency).
No products indexed under this heading.

Cilastatin Sodium (Persons taking most antibiotics invalidate folic acid and vitamin B12 diagnostic blood assays). Products include:

Primaxin I.M. 2232
Primaxin I.V. 2235

Ciprofloxacin (Persons taking most antibiotics invalidate folic acid and vitamin B12 diagnostic blood assays). Products include:

Cipro I.V. 3082
Cipro 3073
Cipro XR 3091
Ciprodex 583

Ciprofloxacin Hydrochloride (Persons taking most antibiotics invalidate folic acid and vitamin B12 diagnostic blood assays). Products include:

Cipro 3073

Cladribine (Blunted or impeded therapeutic response to vitamin B12 may be due to such conditions as infection, uremia, drugs having bone marrow suppressant properties, and concurrent iron or folic acid deficiency). Products include:

Leustatin 946

Clarithromycin (Persons taking most antibiotics invalidate folic acid and vitamin B12 diagnostic blood assays). Products include:

Biaxin/Biaxin XL 412

Clotrimazole (Persons taking most antibiotics invalidate folic acid and vitamin B12 diagnostic blood assays). Products include:

Lotrisone 3163

Cloxacillin (Persons taking most antibiotics invalidate folic acid and vitamin B12 diagnostic blood assays).
No products indexed under this heading.

Cloxacillin Sodium (Persons taking most antibiotics invalidate folic acid and vitamin B12 diagnostic blood assays).
No products indexed under this heading.

Cloxacillin Sodium Monohydrate (Persons taking most antibiotics invalidate folic acid and vitamin B12 diagnostic blood assays).
No products indexed under this heading.

Colchicine (Colchicine intake for longer than 2 weeks may produce malabsorption of vitamin B12).
No products indexed under this heading.

Daunorubicin Citrate Liposome (Blunted or impeded therapeutic response to vitamin B12 may be due to such conditions as infection, uremia, drugs having bone marrow suppressant properties, and concurrent iron or folic acid deficiency).
No products indexed under this heading.

Daunorubicin Hydrochloride (Blunted or impeded therapeutic response to vitamin B12 may be due to such conditions as infection, uremia, drugs having bone marrow suppressant properties, and concurrent iron or folic acid deficiency).
No products indexed under this heading.

Demeclocycline Hydrochloride (Persons taking most antibiotics invalidate folic acid and vitamin B12 diagnostic blood assays).
No products indexed under this heading.

Dexrazoxane (Blunted or impeded therapeutic response to vitamin B12 may be due to such conditions as infection, uremia, drugs having bone marrow suppressant properties, and concurrent iron or folic acid deficiency).
No products indexed under this heading.

Dicloxacillin (Persons taking most antibiotics invalidate folic acid and vitamin B12 diagnostic blood assays).
No products indexed under this heading.

Dicloxacillin Sodium (Persons taking most antibiotics invalidate folic acid and vitamin B12 diagnostic blood assays).
No products indexed under this heading.

Dirithromycin (Persons taking most antibiotics invalidate folic acid and vitamin B12 diagnostic blood assays).
No products indexed under this heading.

Disodium Carbenicillin (Persons taking most antibiotics invalidate folic acid and vitamin B12 diagnostic blood assays).
No products indexed under this heading.

Doxorubicin Hydrochloride (Blunted or impeded therapeutic response to vitamin B12 may be due to such conditions as infection, uremia, drugs having bone marrow suppressant properties, and concurrent iron or folic acid deficiency).
No products indexed under this heading.

Doxorubicin Hydrochloride Liposome (Blunted or impeded therapeutic response to vitamin B12 may be due to such conditions as infection, uremia, drugs having bone marrow suppressant properties, and concurrent iron or folic acid deficiency). Products include:

Doxil 939

Doxycycline Calcium (Persons taking most antibiotics invalidate folic acid and vitamin B12 diagnostic blood assays).
No products indexed under this heading.

Doxycycline Hyclate (Persons taking most antibiotics invalidate folic acid and vitamin B12 diagnostic blood assays).
No products indexed under this heading.

Doxycycline Monohydrate (Persons taking most antibiotics invalidate folic acid and vitamin B12 diagnostic blood assays).
No products indexed under this heading.

Enoxacin (Persons taking most antibiotics invalidate folic acid and vitamin B12 diagnostic blood assays).
No products indexed under this heading.

Epirubicin Hydrochloride (Persons taking most antibiotics invalidate folic acid and vitamin B12 diagnostic blood assays).
No products indexed under this heading.

Erythromycin (Persons taking most antibiotics invalidate folic acid and vitamin B12 diagnostic blood assays).
No products indexed under this heading.

Erythromycin, Topical (Persons taking most antibiotics invalidate folic acid and vitamin B12 diagnostic blood assays).
No products indexed under this heading.

Erythromycin Estolate (Persons taking most antibiotics invalidate folic acid and vitamin B12 diagnostic blood assays).
No products indexed under this heading.

Erythromycin Ethylsuccinate (Persons taking most antibiotics invalidate folic acid and vitamin B12 diagnostic blood assays). Products include:
E.E.S. 437
EryPed 435

Erythromycin Gluceptate (Persons taking most antibiotics invalidate folic acid and vitamin B12 diagnostic blood assays).
No products indexed under this heading.

Erythromycin Lactobionate (Persons taking most antibiotics invalidate folic acid and vitamin B12 diagnostic blood assays).
No products indexed under this heading.

Erythromycin Stearate (Persons taking most antibiotics invalidate folic acid and vitamin B12 diagnostic blood assays).
No products indexed under this heading.

Ethanol (Heavy alcohol intake for longer than 2 weeks may produce malabsorption of vitamin B12).
No products indexed under this heading.

Ethyl Alcohol (Heavy alcohol intake for longer than 2 weeks may produce malabsorption of vitamin B12).
No products indexed under this heading.

Fludarabine Phosphate (Blunted or impeded therapeutic response to vitamin B12 may be due to such conditions as infection, uremia, drugs having bone marrow suppressant properties, and concurrent iron or folic acid deficiency). Products include:
Oforta 3023

Gatifloxacin (Persons taking most antibiotics invalidate folic acid and vitamin B12 diagnostic blood assays).
No products indexed under this heading.

Gemcitabine Hydrochloride (Blunted or impeded therapeutic response to vitamin B12 may be due to such conditions as infection, uremia, drugs having bone marrow suppressant properties, and concurrent iron or folic acid deficiency). Products include:
Gemzar 1900

Gemifloxacin Mesylate (Persons taking most antibiotics invalidate folic acid and vitamin B12 diagnostic blood assays).
No products indexed under this heading.

Gemtuzumab Ozogamicin (Blunted or impeded therapeutic response to vitamin B12 may be due to such conditions as infection, uremia, drugs having bone marrow suppressant properties, and concurrent iron or folic acid deficiency). Products include:
Mylotarg 3524

Gentamicin Sulfate (Persons taking most antibiotics invalidate folic acid and vitamin B12 diagnostic blood assays). Products include:
Pred-G .... ⊙226, ⊙227

Grepafloxacin Hydrochloride (Persons taking most antibiotics invalidate folic acid and vitamin B12 diagnostic blood assays).
No products indexed under this heading.

Griseofulvin (Persons taking most antibiotics invalidate folic acid and vitamin B12 diagnostic blood assays).
No products indexed under this heading.

Idarubicin Hydrochloride (Blunted or impeded therapeutic response to vitamin B12 may be due to such conditions as infection, uremia, drugs having bone marrow suppressant properties, and concurrent iron or folic acid deficiency).
No products indexed under this heading.

Imipenem (Persons taking most antibiotics invalidate folic acid and vitamin B12 diagnostic blood assays). Products include:
Primaxin I.M. 2232
Primaxin I.V. 2235

Interferon alfa-2a, Recombinant (Blunted or impeded therapeutic response to vitamin B12 may be due to such conditions as infection, uremia, drugs having bone marrow suppressant properties, and concurrent iron or folic acid deficiency).
No products indexed under this heading.

Irinotecan Hydrochloride (Blunted or impeded therapeutic response to vitamin B12 may be due to such conditions as infection, uremia, drugs having bone marrow suppressant properties, and concurrent iron or folic acid deficiency).
No products indexed under this heading.

Kanamycin Sulfate (Persons taking most antibiotics invalidate folic acid and vitamin B12 diagnostic blood assays).
No products indexed under this heading.

Levofloxacin (Persons taking most antibiotics invalidate folic acid and vitamin B12 diagnostic blood assays). Products include:
Iquix 3492
Levaquin 2629
Levaquin in 5% Dextrose 2629
Quixin 3493

Lomefloxacin Hydrochloride (Persons taking most antibiotics invalidate folic acid and vitamin B12 diagnostic blood assays).
No products indexed under this heading.

Loracarbef (Persons taking most antibiotics invalidate folic acid and vitamin B12 diagnostic blood assays).
No products indexed under this heading.

Melphalan Hydrochloride (Blunted or impeded therapeutic response to vitamin B12 may be due to such conditions as infection, uremia, drugs having bone marrow suppressant properties, and concurrent iron or folic acid deficiency). Products include:
Alkeran for Injection 1300

Mercaptopurine (Blunted or impeded therapeutic response to vitamin B12 may be due to such conditions as infection, uremia, drugs having bone marrow suppressant properties, and concurrent iron or folic acid deficiency).
No products indexed under this heading.

Methacycline Hydrochloride (Persons taking most antibiotics invalidate folic acid and vitamin B12 diagnostic blood assays).
No products indexed under this heading.

Methicillin Sodium (Persons taking most antibiotics invalidate folic acid and vitamin B12 diagnostic blood assays).
No products indexed under this heading.

Methotrexate (Persons taking methotrexate invalidate folic acid and vitamin B12 diagnostic blood assays).
No products indexed under this heading.

Methotrexate Sodium (Persons taking methotrexate invalidate folic acid and vitamin B12 diagnostic blood assays).
No products indexed under this heading.

Mezlocillin Sodium (Persons taking most antibiotics invalidate folic acid and vitamin B12 diagnostic blood assays).
No products indexed under this heading.

Minocycline Hydrochloride (Persons taking most antibiotics invalidate folic acid and vitamin B12 diagnostic blood assays). Products include:
Solodyn 2073

Mitoxantrone Hydrochloride (Blunted or impeded therapeutic response to vitamin B12 may be due to such conditions as infection, uremia, drugs having bone marrow suppressant properties, and concurrent iron or folic acid deficiency). Products include:
Novantrone 1088

Moxifloxacin Hydrochloride (Persons taking most antibiotics invalidate folic acid and vitamin B12 diagnostic blood assays). Products include:
Avelox 3064
Vigamox 589

Nafcillin Sodium (Persons taking most antibiotics invalidate folic acid and vitamin B12 diagnostic blood assays).
No products indexed under this heading.

Norfloxacin (Persons taking most antibiotics invalidate folic acid and vitamin B12 diagnostic blood assays). Products include:
Noroxin 2220

Ofloxacin (Persons taking most antibiotics invalidate folic acid and vitamin B12 diagnostic blood assays).
No products indexed under this heading.

Oxacillin (Persons taking most antibiotics invalidate folic acid and vitamin B12 diagnostic blood assays).
No products indexed under this heading.

Oxacillin Sodium (Persons taking most antibiotics invalidate folic acid and vitamin B12 diagnostic blood assays).
No products indexed under this heading.

Oxytetracycline Hydrochloride (Persons taking most antibiotics invalidate folic acid and vitamin B12 diagnostic blood assays).
No products indexed under this heading.

Para-Aminosalicylic Acid (Para-aminosalicylic acid intake for longer than 2 weeks may produce malabsorption of vitamin B12).
No products indexed under this heading.

Penicillin, Potassium Phenoxymethyl (Persons taking most antibiotics invalidate folic acid and vitamin B12 diagnostic blood assays).
No products indexed under this heading.

Penicillin G Benzathine (Persons taking most antibiotics invalidate folic acid and vitamin B12 diagnostic blood assays). Products include:
Bicillin C-R Injectable Suspension 1826
Bicillin L-A 1828

Penicillin G Dibenzylethyenediamine (Persons taking most antibiotics invalidate folic acid and vitamin B12 diagnostic blood assays).
No products indexed under this heading.

Penicillin G Potassium (Persons taking most antibiotics invalidate folic acid and vitamin B12 diagnostic blood assays).
No products indexed under this heading.

Penicillin G Procaine (Persons taking most antibiotics invalidate folic acid and vitamin B12 diagnostic blood assays). Products include:
Bicillin C-R Injectable Suspension 1826
Bicillin L-A 1828

Penicillin G Sodium (Persons taking most antibiotics invalidate folic acid and vitamin B12 diagnostic blood assays).
No products indexed under this heading.

Penicillin V (Persons taking most antibiotics invalidate folic acid and vitamin B12 diagnostic blood assays).
No products indexed under this heading.

Penicillin V Potassium (Persons taking most antibiotics invalidate folic acid and vitamin B12 diagnostic blood assays).
No products indexed under this heading.

Penicillins (Persons taking most antibiotics invalidate folic acid and vitamin B12 diagnostic blood assays).
No products indexed under this heading.

Piperacillin Sodium (Persons taking most antibiotics invalidate folic acid and vitamin B12 diagnostic blood assays). Products include:
Zosyn 3607

Pyrimethamine (Persons taking pyrimethamine invalidate folic acid and vitamin B12 diagnostic blood assays). Products include:
Daraprim 1423

Sodium Cloxacillin Monohydrate (Persons taking most antibiotics invalidate folic acid and vitamin B12 diagnostic blood assays).
No products indexed under this heading.

Sparfloxacin (Persons taking most antibiotics invalidate folic acid and vitamin B12 diagnostic blood assays).
No products indexed under this heading.

Streptomycin Sulfate (Persons taking most antibiotics invalidate folic acid and vitamin B12 diagnostic blood assays).
No products indexed under this heading.

Sulfamethizole (Persons taking most antibiotics invalidate folic acid and vitamin B12 diagnostic blood assays).
No products indexed under this heading.

Sulfamethoxazole (Persons taking most antibiotics invalidate folic acid and vitamin B12 diagnostic blood assays).
No products indexed under this heading.

Sulfisoxazole Acetyl (Persons taking most antibiotics invalidate folic acid and vitamin B12 diagnostic blood assays).
No products indexed under this heading.

Sulfisoxazole Diolamine (Persons taking most antibiotics invalidate folic acid and vitamin B12 diagnostic blood assays).
No products indexed under this heading.

Temozolomide (Blunted or impeded therapeutic response to vitamin B12 may be due to such conditions as infection, uremia, drugs having bone marrow suppressant properties, and concurrent iron or folic acid deficiency). Products include:
Temodar 3230
Temodar Injection 3230

Tetracycline Hydrochloride (Persons taking most antibiotics invalidate folic acid and vitamin B12 diagnostic blood assays). Products include:
Pylera 793

Thioguanine (Blunted or impeded therapeutic response to vitamin B12 may be due to such conditions as infection, uremia, drugs having bone marrow suppressant properties, and concurrent iron or folic acid deficiency). Products include:
Tabloid 1664

Ticarcillin Disodium (Persons taking most antibiotics invalidate folic acid and vitamin B12 diagnostic blood assays). Products include:
Timentin ADD-Vantage 1670
Timentin Galaxy 1674
Timentin 1666
Timentin Pharmacy 1678

IMPORTANT NOTE: Always consult each drug listing in the patient's regimen for possible interactions.

Tobramycin (Persons taking most antibiotics invalidate folic acid and vitamin B12 diagnostic blood assays). Products include:

Tobramycin Sulfate (Persons taking most antibiotics invalidate folic acid and vitamin B12 diagnostic blood assays).
No products indexed under this heading.

Troleandomycin (Persons taking most antibiotics invalidate folic acid and vitamin B12 diagnostic blood assays).
No products indexed under this heading.

Trovafloxacin Mesylate (Persons taking most antibiotics invalidate folic acid and vitamin B12 diagnostic blood assays).
No products indexed under this heading.

Vinorelbine Tartrate (Blunted or impeded therapeutic response to vitamin B12 may be due to such conditions as infection, uremia, drugs having bone marrow suppressant properties, and concurrent iron or folic acid deficiency).
No products indexed under this heading.

Food Interactions

Alcohol (Heavy alcohol intake for longer than 2 weeks may produce malabsorption of vitamin B12).

Beer, reduced-alcohol (Heavy alcohol intake for longer than 2 weeks may produce malabsorption of vitamin B12).

Beer, unspecified (Heavy alcohol intake for longer than 2 weeks may produce malabsorption of vitamin B12).

Beverages, hot (Hot foods may cause nasal secretions and a resulting loss of medication; therefore, patients should be told to administer cyanocobalamin nasal spray at least one hour before or one hour after ingestion of hot foods or liquids).

Food, hot (Hot foods may cause nasal secretions and a resulting loss of medication; therefore, patients should be told to administer cyanocobalamin nasal spray at least one hour before or one hour after ingestion of hot foods or liquids).

Food, unspecified (A vegetarian diet which contains no animal products (including milk products or eggs) does not supply any vitamin B12. Therefore, patients following such a diet should be advised to take cyanocobalamin nasal spray weekly).

Wine, Chianti (Heavy alcohol intake for longer than 2 weeks may produce malabsorption of vitamin B12).

Wine, Red (Heavy alcohol intake for longer than 2 weeks may produce malabsorption of vitamin B12).

Wine, unspecified (Heavy alcohol intake for longer than 2 weeks may produce malabsorption of vitamin B12).

Wine products (Heavy alcohol intake for longer than 2 weeks may produce malabsorption of vitamin B12).

NASONEX NASAL SPRAY

None cited in PDR database.

NATURETHROID TABLETS

May interact with androgens, corticosteroids, estrogens, insulin, oral anticoagulants, oral contraceptives, oral hypoglycemic agents, salicylates, and certain other agents. Compounds in these categories include:

Acarbose (Initiating thyroid replacement therapy may cause increases in insulin or oral hypoglycemic requirements).
No products indexed under this heading.

Alclometasone Dipropionate (Corticosteroids are known to interfere with laboratory tests performed in patients on thryoid hormone therapy).
No products indexed under this heading.

Anisindione (Thryoid hormones appear to increase catabolism of vitamin K-dependent clotting factors. If oral anticoagulants are also being given, compensatory increases in clotting factor synthesis are impaired).
No products indexed under this heading.

Aspirin (Preparations containing salicylates are known to interfere with laboratory tests performed in patients on thyroid hormone therapy). Products include:

Aspirin, Enteric Coated (Preparations containing salicylates are known to interfere with laboratory tests performed in patients on thyroid hormone therapy).
No products indexed under this heading.

Aspirin Buffered (Preparations containing salicylates are known to interfere with laboratory tests performed in patients on thyroid hormone therapy).
No products indexed under this heading.

Beclomethasone Dipropionate (Corticosteroids are known to interfere with laboratory tests performed in patients on thryoid hormone therapy). Products include:

Beclomethasone Dipropionate Monohydrate (Corticosteroids are known to interfere with laboratory tests performed in patients on thryoid hormone therapy). Products include:

Betamethasone (Corticosteroids are known to interfere with laboratory tests performed in patients on thyroid hormone therapy).
No products indexed under this heading.

Betamethasone Acetate (Corticosteroids are known to interfere with laboratory tests performed in patients on thyroid hormone therapy).
No products indexed under this heading.

Betamethasone Benzoate (Corticosteroids are known to interfere with laboratory tests performed in patients on thryoid hormone therapy).
No products indexed under this heading.

Betamethasone Dipropionate (Corticosteroids are known to interfere with laboratory tests performed in patients on thryoid hormone therapy). Products include:

Betamethasone Sodium Phosphate (Corticosteroids are known to interfere with laboratory tests performed in patients on thryoid hormone therapy).
No products indexed under this heading.

Betamethasone Valerate (Corticosteroids are known to interfere with laboratory tests performed in patients on thyroid hormone therapy). Products include:

Budesonide (Corticosteroids are known to interfere with laboratory tests performed in patients on thyroid hormone therapy). Products include:

Chlorotrianisene (Patients without a functioning thyroid gland who are on thyroid replacemet therapy may need to increase their thyroid dose if estrogens are given. Estrogens are also known to interfere with laboratory tests performed in patients on thyroid hormone therapy).
No products indexed under this heading.

Chlorpropamide (Initiating thyroid replacement therapy may cause increases in insulin or oral hypoglycemic requirements).
No products indexed under this heading.

Cholestyramine (Cholestyramine binds both levothyroxine and liothyronine in the intestine, thus impairing absorption of these thyroid hormones. Four to five hours should elapse between administration of cholestyramine and thyroid hormones).
No products indexed under this heading.

Choline Magnesium Trisalicylate (Preparations containing salicylates are known to interfere with laboratory tests performed in patients on thyroid hormone therapy).
No products indexed under this heading.

Ciclesonide (Corticosteroids are known to interfere with laboratory tests performed in patients on thyroid hormone therapy).
No products indexed under this heading.

Colestipol (Colestipol binds both levothyroxine and liothyronine in the intestine, thus impairing absorption of these thyroid hormones. Four to five hours should elapse between administration of cholestyramine and thyroid hormones).
No products indexed under this heading.

Colestipol Hydrochloride (Colestipol binds both levothyroxine and liothyronine in the intestine, thus impairing absorption of these thyroid hormones. Four to five hours should elapse between administration of cholestyramine and thyroid hormones).
No products indexed under this heading.

Cortisone Acetate (Corticosteroids are known to interfere with laboratory tests performed in patients on thyroid hormone therapy).
No products indexed under this heading.

Desogestrel (Patients without a functioning thyroid gland who are on thyroid replacemet therapy may need to increase their thyroid dose if estrogens containing oral contraceptives are given. Estrogens containing oral contraceptives are also known to interfere with laboratory tests performed in patients on thyroid hormone therapy).
No products indexed under this heading.

Desoximetasone (Corticosteroids are known to interfere with laboratory tests performed in patients on thyroid hormone therapy).
No products indexed under this heading.

Dexamethasone (Corticosteroids are known to interfere with laboratory tests performed in patients on thyroid hormone therapy). Products include:

Dexamethasone Acetate (Corticosteroids are known to interfere with laboratory tests performed in patients on thyroid hormone therapy).
No products indexed under this heading.

Dexamethasone Phosphate (Corticosteroids are known to interfere with laboratory tests performed in patients on thyroid hormone therapy).
No products indexed under this heading.

Dexamethasone Sodium (Corticosteroids are known to interfere with laboratory tests performed in patients on thyroid hormone therapy).
No products indexed under this heading.

Dexamethasone Sodium Phosphate (Corticosteroids are known to interfere with laboratory tests performed in patients on thyroid hormone therapy).
No products indexed under this heading.

Dexamethasone Sodium Phosphate Injection (Corticosteroids are known to interfere with laboratory tests performed in patients on thryoid hormone therapy).
No products indexed under this heading.

Dicumarol (Thyroid hormones appear to increase catabolism of vitamin K-dependent clotting factors. If oral anticoagulants are also being given, compensatory increases in clotting factor synthesis are impaired).
No products indexed under this heading.

Dienestrol (Patients without a functioning thyroid gland who are on thyroid replacemet therapy may need to increase their thyroid dose if estrogens are given. Estrogens are also known to interfere with laboratory tests performed in patients on thyroid hormone therapy).
No products indexed under this heading.

Diethylstilbestrol (Patients without a functioning thyroid gland who are on thyroid replacemet therapy may need to increase their thyroid dose if estrogens are given. Estrogens are also known to interfere with laboratory tests performed in patients on thyroid hormone therapy).
No products indexed under this heading.

Diflorasone Diacetate (Corticosteroids are known to interfere with laboratory tests performed in patients on thryoid hormone therapy).
No products indexed under this heading.

Diflunisal (Preparations containing salicylates are known to interfere with laboratory tests performed in patients on thyroid hormone therapy).
No products indexed under this heading.

Estradiol (Patients without a functioning thyroid gland who are on thyroid replacemet therapy may need to increase their thyroid dose if estrogens are given. Estrogens are also known to interfere with laboratory tests performed in patients on thyroid hormone therapy). Products include:

Estrogens, Conjugated (Patients without a functioning thyroid gland who are on thyroid replacemet therapy may need to increase their thyroid dose if estrogens are given. Estrogens are also known to interfere with laboratory tests performed in patients on thyroid hormone therapy). Products include:

Estrogens, Esterified (Patients without a functioning thyroid gland who are on thyroid replacemet therapy may need to increase their thyroid dose if estrogens are given. Estrogens are also known to interfere with laboratory tests performed in patients on thyroid hormone therapy).
No products indexed under this heading.

(⊙ Described in PDR® for Ophthalmic Medicines)

Estropipate (Patients without a functioning thyroid gland who are on thyroid replacemet therapy may need to increase their thyroid dose if estrogens are given. Estrogens are also known to interfere with laboratory tests performed in patients on thyroid hormone therapy).
No products indexed under this heading.

Ethinyl Estradiol (Patients without a functioning thyroid gland who are on thyroid replacemet therapy may need to increase their thyroid dose if estrogens are given. Estrogens are also known to interfere with laboratory tests performed in patients on thyroid hormone therapy). Products include:

Ethynodiol Diacetate (Patients without a functioning thyroid gland who are on thyroid replacemet therapy may need to increase their thyroid dose if estrogens containing oral contraceptives are given. Estrogens containing oral contraceptives are also known to interfere with laboratory tests performed in patients on thyroid hormone therapy).
No products indexed under this heading.

Fludrocortisone Acetate (Corticosteroids are known to interfere with laboratory tests performed in patients on thryoid hormone therapy).
No products indexed under this heading.

Flumethasone Pivalate (Corticosteroids are known to interfere with laboratory tests performed in patients on thryoid hormone therapy).
No products indexed under this heading.

Flunisolide Hemihydrate (Corticosteroids are known to interfere with laboratory tests performed in patients on thryoid hormone therapy).
No products indexed under this heading.

Fluoxymesterone (Androgens are known to interfere with laboratory tests performed in patients on thryoid hormone therapy).
No products indexed under this heading.

Fluticasone Furoate (Corticosteroids are known to interfere with laboratory tests performed in patients on thryoid hormone therapy). Products include:

Fluticasone Propionate (Corticosteroids are known to interfere with laboratory tests performed in patients on thryoid hormone therapy). Products include:

Glibenclamide (Initiating thyroid replacement therapy may cause increases in insulin or oral hypoglycemic requirements).
No products indexed under this heading.

Glimepiride (Initiating thyroid replacement therapy may cause increases in insulin or oral hypoglycemic requirements). Products include:

Glipizide (Initiating thyroid replacement therapy may cause increases in insulin or oral hypoglycemic requirements).
No products indexed under this heading.

Glyburide (Initiating thyroid replacement therapy may cause increases in insulin or oral hypoglycemic requirements).
No products indexed under this heading.

Hydrocortisone (Corticosteroids are known to interfere with laboratory tests performed in patients on thyroid hormone therapy).
No products indexed under this heading.

Hydrocortisone (Alcohol) (Corticosteroids are known to interfere with laboratory tests performed in patients on thryoid hormone therapy).
No products indexed under this heading.

Hydrocortisone Acetate (Corticosteroids are known to interfere with laboratory tests performed in patients on thryoid hormone therapy).
No products indexed under this heading.

Hydrocortisone Butyrate (Corticosteroids are known to interfere with laboratory tests performed in patients on thryoid hormone therapy).
No products indexed under this heading.

Hydrocortisone Cypionate (Corticosteroids are known to interfere with laboratory tests performed in patients on thryoid hormone therapy).
No products indexed under this heading.

Hydrocortisone Hemisuccinate (Corticosteroids are known to interfere with laboratory tests performed in patients on thryoid hormone therapy).
No products indexed under this heading.

Hydrocortisone Probutate (Corticosteroids are known to interfere with laboratory tests performed in patients on thryoid hormone therapy).
No products indexed under this heading.

Hydrocortisone Sodium Phosphate (Corticosteroids are known to interfere with laboratory tests performed in patients on thryoid hormone therapy).
No products indexed under this heading.

Hydrocortisone Sodium Succinate (Corticosteroids are known to interfere with laboratory tests performed in patients on thryoid hormone therapy).
No products indexed under this heading.

Hydrocortisone Valerate (Corticosteroids are known to interfere with laboratory tests performed in patients on thryoid hormone therapy).
No products indexed under this heading.

Insulin (Initiating thyroid replacement therapy may cause increases in insulin or oral hypoglycemic requirements).
No products indexed under this heading.

Insulin, Human, Zinc Suspension (Initiating thyroid replacement therapy may cause increases in insulin or oral hypoglycemic requirements).
No products indexed under this heading.

Insulin, Human (rDNA origin) (Initiating thyroid replacement therapy may cause increases in insulin or oral hypoglycemic requirements). Products include:

Insulin, Human NPH (Initiating thyroid replacement therapy may cause increases in insulin or oral hypoglycemic requirements). Products include:

Insulin, Human Regular (Initiating thyroid replacement therapy may cause increases in insulin or oral hypoglycemic requirements). Products include:

Insulin, Human Regular and Human NPH Mixture (Initiating thyroid replacement therapy may cause increases in insulin or oral hypoglycemic requirements). Products include:

Insulin, NPH (Initiating thyroid replacement therapy may cause increases in insulin or oral hypoglycemic requirements).
No products indexed under this heading.

Insulin, Regular (Initiating thyroid replacement therapy may cause increases in insulin or oral hypoglycemic requirements).
No products indexed under this heading.

Insulin, Regular and NPH mixture (Initiating thyroid replacement therapy may cause increases in insulin or oral hypoglycemic requirements).
No products indexed under this heading.

Insulin, Zinc Crystals (Initiating thyroid replacement therapy may cause increases in insulin or oral hypoglycemic requirements).
No products indexed under this heading.

Insulin, Zinc Suspension (Initiating thyroid replacement therapy may cause increases in insulin or oral hypoglycemic requirements).
No products indexed under this heading.

Insulin Aspart (Initiating thyroid replacement therapy may cause increases in insulin or oral hypoglycemic requirements).
No products indexed under this heading.

Insulin Aspart, Human (Initiating thyroid replacement therapy may cause increases in insulin or oral hypoglycemic requirements). Products include:

Insulin Aspart, Human Regular (Initiating thyroid replacement therapy may cause increases in insulin or oral hypoglycemic requirements). Products include:

Insulin Aspart Protamine, Human (Initiating thyroid replacement therapy may cause increases in insulin or oral hypoglycemic requirements). Products include:

Insulin Detemir (rDNA Origin) (Initiating thyroid replacement therapy may cause increases in insulin or oral hypoglycemic requirements). Products include:

Insulin Glargine (Initiating thyroid replacement therapy may cause increases in insulin or oral hypoglycemic requirements). Products include:

Insulin Glulisine (Initiating thyroid replacement therapy may cause increases in insulin or oral hypoglycemic requirements). Products include:

Insulin Lispro, Human (Initiating thyroid replacement therapy may cause increases in insulin or oral hypoglycemic requirements). Products include:

Insulin Lispro Protamine, Human (Initiating thyroid replacement therapy may cause increases in insulin or oral hypoglycemic requirements). Products include:

Iodine Preparations (Iodine-containing preparations are known to interfere with laboratory tests performed in patients on thyroid hormone therapy).
No products indexed under this heading.

Levonorgestrel (Patients without a functioning thyroid gland who are on thyroid replacemet therapy may need to increase their thyroid dose if estrogens containing oral contraceptives are giv-

en. Estrogens containing oral contraceptives are also known to interfere with laboratory tests performed in patients on thyroid hormone therapy). Products include:

Magnesium Salicylate (Preparations containing salicylates are known to interfere with laboratory tests performed in patients on thyroid hormone therapy).
No products indexed under this heading.

Mestranol (Patients without a functioning thyroid gland who are on thyroid replacemet therapy may need to increase their thyroid dose if estrogens containing oral contraceptives are given. Estrogens containing oral contraceptives are also known to interfere with laboratory tests performed in patients on thyroid hormone therapy).
No products indexed under this heading.

Metformin Hydrochloride (Initiating thyroid replacement therapy may cause increases in insulin or oral hypoglycemic requirements). Products include:

Methylprednisolone (Corticosteroids are known to interfere with laboratory tests performed in patients on thryoid hormone therapy).
No products indexed under this heading.

Methylprednisolone Acetate (Corticosteroids are known to interfere with laboratory tests performed in patients on thryoid hormone therapy).
No products indexed under this heading.

Methylprednisolone Sodium Succinate (Corticosteroids are known to interfere with laboratory tests performed in patients on thyroid hormone therapy).
No products indexed under this heading.

Methyltestosterone (Androgens are known to interfere with laboratory tests performed in patients on thyroid hormone therapy).
No products indexed under this heading.

Miglitol (Initiating thyroid replacement therapy may cause increases in insulin or oral hypoglycemic requirements).
No products indexed under this heading.

Mometasone Furoate (Corticosteroids are known to interfere with laboratory tests performed in patients on thryoid hormone therapy). Products include:

Mometasone Furoate Monohydrate (Corticosteroids are known to interfere with laboratory tests performed in patients on thryoid hormone therapy). Products include:

Nateglinide (Initiating thyroid replacement therapy may cause increases in insulin or oral hypoglycemic requirements).
No products indexed under this heading.

Norethindrone (Patients without a functioning thyroid gland who are on thyroid replacemet therapy may need to increase their thyroid dose if estrogens containing oral contraceptives are given. Estrogens containing oral contraceptives are also known to interfere with laboratory tests performed in patients on thyroid hormone therapy). Products include:

IMPORTANT NOTE: Always consult each drug listing in the patient's regimen for possible interactions.

Norethynodrel (Patients without a functioning thyroid gland who are on thyroid replacemet therapy may need to increase their thyroid dose if estrogens containing oral contraceptives are given. Estrogens containing oral contraceptives are also known to interfere with laboratory tests performed in patients on thyroid hormone therapy).
No products indexed under this heading.

Norgestimate (Patients without a functioning thyroid gland who are on thyroid replacemet therapy may need to increase their thyroid dose if estrogens containing oral contraceptives are given. Estrogens containing oral contraceptives are also known to interfere with laboratory tests performed in patients on thyroid hormone therapy). Products include:
Ortho-Cyclen/Ortho Tri-Cyclen 2663
Ortho Tri-Cyclen Lo Tablets 2673

Norgestrel (Patients without a functioning thyroid gland who are on thyroid replacemet therapy may need to increase their thyroid dose if estrogens containing oral contraceptives are given. Estrogens containing oral contraceptives are also known to interfere with laboratory tests performed in patients on thyroid hormone therapy).
No products indexed under this heading.

Oxandrolone (Androgens are known to interfere with laboratory tests performed in patients on thryoid hormone therapy).
No products indexed under this heading.

Oxymetholone (Androgens are known to interfere with laboratory tests performed in patients on thryoid hormone therapy).
No products indexed under this heading.

Pioglitazone Hydrochloride (Initiating thyroid replacement therapy may cause increases in insulin or oral hypoglycemic requirements). Products include:
ActoPlus 3338
Actos 3345
Duetact 3354

Polyestradiol Phosphate (Patients without a functioning thyroid gland who are on thyroid replacemet therapy may need to increase their thyroid dose if estrogens are given. Estrogens are also known to interfere with laboratory tests performed in patients on thyroid hormone therapy).
No products indexed under this heading.

Prednisolone (Corticosteroids are known to interfere with laboratory tests performed in patients on thryoid hormone therapy).
No products indexed under this heading.

Prednisolone Acetate (Corticosteroids are known to interfere with laboratory tests performed in patients on thryoid hormone therapy). Products include:
Blephamide .... ⊙212, ⊙214
Pred Forte .... ⊙225
Pred Mild .... ⊙230
Pred-G .... ⊙226, ⊙227

Prednisolone Sodium Phosphate (Corticosteroids are known to interfere with laboratory tests performed in patients on thryoid hormone therapy).
No products indexed under this heading.

Prednisolone Tebutate (Corticosteroids are known to interfere with laboratory tests performed in patients on thryoid hormone therapy).
No products indexed under this heading.

Prednisone (Corticosteroids are known to interfere with laboratory tests performed in patients on thyroid hormone therapy).
No products indexed under this heading.

Prednisone sodium phosphate (Corticosteroids are known to interfere with laboratory tests performed in patients on thyroid hormone therapy).
No products indexed under this heading.

Quinestrol (Patients without a functioning thyroid gland who are on thyroid replacemet therapy may need to increase their thyroid dose if estrogens are given. Estrogens are also known to interfere with laboratory tests performed in patients on thyroid hormone therapy).
No products indexed under this heading.

Repaglinide (Initiating thyroid replacement therapy may cause increases in insulin or oral hypoglycemic requirements).
No products indexed under this heading.

Rosiglitazone Maleate (Initiating thyroid replacement therapy may cause increases in insulin or oral hypoglycemic requirements). Products include:
Avandamet 1345
Avandaryl 1356
Avandia 1366

Salsalate (Preparations containing salicylates are known to interfere with laboratory tests performed in patients on thyroid hormone therapy).
No products indexed under this heading.

Sitagliptin Phosphate (Initiating thyroid replacement therapy may cause increases in insulin or oral hypoglycemic requirements). Products include:
Janumet 2188
Januvia 2196

Stanozolol (Androgens are known to interfere with laboratory tests performed in patients on thryoid hormone therapy).
No products indexed under this heading.

Tolazamide (Initiating thyroid replacement therapy may cause increases in insulin or oral hypoglycemic requirements).
No products indexed under this heading.

Tolbutamide (Initiating thyroid replacement therapy may cause increases in insulin or oral hypoglycemic requirements).
No products indexed under this heading.

Triamcinolone (Corticosteroids are known to interfere with laboratory tests performed in patients on thyroid hormone therapy).
No products indexed under this heading.

Triamcinolone Acetonide (Corticosteroids are known to interfere with laboratory tests performed in patients on thryoid hormone therapy). Products include:
Azmacort 408
Nasacort AQ 3019

Triamcinolone Diacetate (Corticosteroids are known to interfere with laboratory tests performed in patients on thryoid hormone therapy).
No products indexed under this heading.

Triamcinolone Hexacetonide (Corticosteroids are known to interfere with laboratory tests performed in patients on thryoid hormone therapy).
No products indexed under this heading.

Troglitazone (Initiating thyroid replacement therapy may cause increases in insulin or oral hypoglycemic requirements).
No products indexed under this heading.

Warfarin Sodium (Thryoid hormones appear to increase catabolism of vitamin K-dependent clotting factors. If oral anticoagulants are also being given, compensatory increases in clotting factor synthesis are impaired).
No products indexed under this heading.

NEMBUTAL SODIUM SOLUTION
(Pentobarbital Sodium) 2012

May interact with alcohols, antihistamines, central nervous system depressants, corticosteroids, doxycycline, estrogens, hypnotics and sedatives, monoamine oxidase inhibitors, narcotic analgesics, oral anticoagulants, oral contraceptives, phenytoin, tranquilizers, valproate, and certain other agents. Compounds in these categories include:

Acrivastine (The concomitant use of other central nervous system depressants, including antihistamines, may produce additive depressant effects).
No products indexed under this heading.

Alclometasone Dipropionate (Barbiturates appear to enhance the metabolism of exogenous corticosteroids probably through the induction of hepatic microsomal enzymes. Patients stabilized on corticosteroid therapy may require dosage adjustments if barbiturates are added or withdrawn from their dosage regimen).
No products indexed under this heading.

Alfentanil Hydrochloride (Concurrent use of the barbiturates with other CNS depressants (eg, narcotics) may result in additional CNS depressant effects).
No products indexed under this heading.

Alprazolam (The concomitant use of other central nervous system depressants, including tranquilizers, may produce additive depressant effects).
No products indexed under this heading.

Amobarbital (The concomitant use of other central nervous system depressants, including other sedatives or hypnotics, antihistamines, tranquilizers, or alcohol, may produce additive depressant effects).
No products indexed under this heading.

Amobarbital Sodium (The concomitant use of other central nervous system depressants, including other sedatives or hypnotics, antihistamines, tranquilizers, or alcohol, may produce additive depressant effects).
No products indexed under this heading.

Anisindione (Barbiturates can induce hepatic microsomal enzymes resulting in increased metabolism and decreased anticoagulant response of oral anticoagulants (eg, warfarin, acenocoumarol, dicumarol, and phenprocoumon). Patients stabilized on anticoagulant therapy may require dosage adjustments if barbiturates are added or withdrawn from their dosage regimen).
No products indexed under this heading.

Apomorphine (Concurrent use of the barbiturates with other CNS depressants (eg, narcotics) may result in additional CNS depressant effects).
No products indexed under this heading.

Apomorphine Hydrochloride (Concurrent use of the barbiturates with other CNS depressants (eg, narcotics) may result in additional CNS depressant effects).
No products indexed under this heading.

Aprobarbital (The concomitant use of other central nervous system depressants, including other sedatives or hypnotics, antihistamines, tranquilizers, or alcohol, may produce additive depressant effects).
No products indexed under this heading.

Astemizole (The concomitant use of other central nervous system depressants, including antihistamines, may produce additive depressant effects).
No products indexed under this heading.

Azatadine Maleate (The concomitant use of other central nervous system depressants, including antihistamines, may produce additive depressant effects).
No products indexed under this heading.

Beclomethasone Dipropionate (Barbiturates appear to enhance the metabolism of exogenous corticosteroids probably through the induction of hepatic microsomal enzymes. Patients stabilized on corticosteroid therapy may require dosage adjustments if barbiturates are added or withdrawn from their dosage regimen). Products include:
Qvar 3398

Beclomethasone Dipropionate Monohydrate (Barbiturates appear to enhance the metabolism of exogenous corticosteroids probably through the induction of hepatic microsomal enzymes. Patients stabilized on corticosteroid therapy may require dosage adjustments if barbiturates are added or withdrawn from their dosage regimen). Products include:
Beconase AQ 1386

Betamethasone (Barbiturates appear to enhance the metabolism of exogenous corticosteroids probably through the induction of hepatic microsomal enzymes. Patients stabilized on corticosteroid therapy may require dosage adjustments if barbiturates are added or withdrawn from their dosage regimen).
No products indexed under this heading.

Betamethasone Acetate (Barbiturates appear to enhance the metabolism of exogenous corticosteroids probably through the induction of hepatic microsomal enzymes. Patients stabilized on corticosteroid therapy may require dosage adjustments if barbiturates are added or withdrawn from their dosage regimen).
No products indexed under this heading.

Betamethasone Benzoate (Barbiturates appear to enhance the metabolism of exogenous corticosteroids probably through the induction of hepatic microsomal enzymes. Patients stabilized on corticosteroid therapy may require dosage adjustments if barbiturates are added or withdrawn from their dosage regimen).
No products indexed under this heading.

Betamethasone Dipropionate (Barbiturates appear to enhance the metabolism of exogenous corticosteroids probably through the induction of hepatic microsomal enzymes. Patients stabilized on corticosteroid therapy may require dosage adjustments if barbiturates are added or withdrawn from their dosage regimen). Products include:
Diprolene Lotion 0.05% 3108
Diprolene Ointment 0.05% 3109
Diprolene AF Cream 0.05% 3107
Lotrisone 3163

Betamethasone Sodium Phosphate (Barbiturates appear to enhance the metabolism of exogenous corticosteroids probably through the induction of hepatic microsomal enzymes. Patients stabilized on corticosteroid therapy may require dosage adjustments if barbiturates are added or withdrawn from their dosage regimen).
No products indexed under this heading.

Betamethasone Valerate (Barbiturates appear to enhance the metabolism of exogenous corticosteroids probably through the induction of hepatic microsomal enzymes. Patients stabilized on corticosteroid therapy may require dosage adjustments if barbiturates are added or withdrawn from their dosage regimen). Products include:
Luxiq 3321

Bromodiphenhydramine Hydrochloride (The concomitant use of other central nervous system depressants, including antihistamines, may produce additive depressant effects).
No products indexed under this heading.

(⊙ Described in PDR® for Ophthalmic Medicines)

Brompheniramine Maleate (The concomitant use of other central nervous system depressants, including antihistamines, may produce additive depressant effects).
No products indexed under this heading.

Budesonide (Barbiturates appear to enhance the metabolism of exogenous corticosteroids probably through the induction of hepatic microsomal enzymes. Patients stabilized on corticosteroid therapy may require dosage adjustments if barbiturates are added or withdrawn from their dosage regimen). Products include:

Buprenorphine Hydrochloride (Concurrent use of the barbiturates with other CNS depressants (eg, narcotics) may result in additional CNS depressant effects).
No products indexed under this heading.

Buspirone Hydrochloride (The concomitant use of other central nervous system depressants, including tranquilizers, may produce additive depressant effects).
No products indexed under this heading.

Butabarbital (The concomitant use of other central nervous system depressants, including other sedatives or hypnotics, may produce additive depressant effects).
No products indexed under this heading.

Butabarbital Sodium (The concomitant use of other central nervous system depressants, including other sedatives or hypnotics, may produce additive depressant effects).
No products indexed under this heading.

Butalbital (The concomitant use of other central nervous system depressants, including other sedatives or hypnotics, may produce additive depressant effects).
No products indexed under this heading.

Cetirizine Hydrochloride (The concomitant use of other central nervous system depressants, including antihistamines, may produce additive depressant effects). Products include:

Chloral Hydrate (The concomitant use of other central nervous system depressants, including other sedatives or hypnotics, may produce additive depressant effects).
No products indexed under this heading.

Chlordiazepoxide (The concomitant use of other central nervous system depressants, including tranquilizers, may produce additive depressant effects).
No products indexed under this heading.

Chlordiazepoxide Hydrochloride (The concomitant use of other central nervous system depressants, including tranquilizers, may produce additive depressant effects).
No products indexed under this heading.

Chlorotrianisene (Pretreatment with or concurrent administration of phenobarbital may decrease the effect of estradiol by increasing its metabolism. An alternate contraceptive method might be suggested to women taking phenobarbital. The application of this data to other barbiturates appears valid).
No products indexed under this heading.

Chlorpheniramine Maleate (The concomitant use of other central nervous system depressants, including antihistamines, may produce additive depressant effects).
No products indexed under this heading.

Chlorpheniramine Polistirex (The concomitant use of other central nervous system depressants, including antihistamines, may produce additive depressant effects). Products include:

Chlorpheniramine Tannate (The concomitant use of other central nervous system depressants, including antihistamines, may produce additive depressant effects).
No products indexed under this heading.

Chlorpromazine (The concomitant use of other central nervous system depressants, including tranquilizers, may produce additive depressant effects).
No products indexed under this heading.

Chlorpromazine Hydrochloride (The concomitant use of other central nervous system depressants, including tranquilizers, may produce additive depressant effects).
No products indexed under this heading.

Chlorprothixene (The concomitant use of other central nervous system depressants, including tranquilizers, may produce additive depressant effects).
No products indexed under this heading.

Chlorprothixene Hydrochloride (The concomitant use of other central nervous system depressants, including tranquilizers, may produce additive depressant effects).
No products indexed under this heading.

Chlorprothixene Lactate (The concomitant use of other central nervous system depressants, including tranquilizers, may produce additive depressant effects).
No products indexed under this heading.

Ciclesonide (Barbiturates appear to enhance the metabolism of exogenous corticosteroids probably through the induction of hepatic microsomal enzymes. Patients stabilized on corticosteroid therapy may require dosage adjustments if barbiturates are added or withdrawn from their dosage regimen).
No products indexed under this heading.

Clemastine Fumarate (The concomitant use of other central nervous system depressants, including antihistamines, may produce additive depressant effects).
No products indexed under this heading.

Clonazepam (The concomitant use of other central nervous system depressants, including other sedatives or hypnotics, antihistamines, tranquilizers, or alcohol, may produce additive depressant effects). Products include:

Clorazepate Dipotassium (The concomitant use of other central nervous system depressants, including tranquilizers, may produce additive depressant effects).
No products indexed under this heading.

Clozapine (The concomitant use of other central nervous system depressants, including other sedatives or hypnotics, antihistamines, tranquilizers, or alcohol, may produce additive depressant effects).
No products indexed under this heading.

Codeine Phosphate (Concurrent use of the barbiturates with other CNS depressants (eg, narcotics) may result in additional CNS depressant effects).
Products include:

Codeine Sulfate (Concurrent use of the barbiturates with other CNS depressants (eg, narcotics) may result in additional CNS depressant effects).
No products indexed under this heading.

Cortisone Acetate (Barbiturates appear to enhance the metabolism of exogenous corticosteroids probably through the induction of hepatic microsomal enzymes. Patients stabilized on corticosteroid therapy may require dosage adjustments if barbiturates are added or withdrawn from their dosage regimen).
No products indexed under this heading.

Cyproheptadine Hydrochloride (The concomitant use of other central nervous system depressants, including antihistamines, may produce additive depressant effects).
No products indexed under this heading.

Desflurane (The concomitant use of other central nervous system depressants, including other sedatives or hypnotics, antihistamines, tranquilizers, or alcohol, may produce additive depressant effects).
No products indexed under this heading.

Desogestrel (Pretreatment with or concurrent administration of phenobarbital may decrease the effect of estradiol by increasing its metabolism. An alternate contraceptive method might be suggested to women taking phenobarbital. The application of this data to other barbiturates appears valid).
No products indexed under this heading.

Desoximetasone (Barbiturates appear to enhance the metabolism of exogenous corticosteroids probably through the induction of hepatic microsomal enzymes. Patients stabilized on corticosteroid therapy may require dosage adjustments if barbiturates are added or withdrawn from their dosage regimen).
No products indexed under this heading.

Dexamethasone (Barbiturates appear to enhance the metabolism of exogenous corticosteroids probably through the induction of hepatic microsomal enzymes. Patients stabilized on corticosteroid therapy may require dosage adjustments if barbiturates are added or withdrawn from their dosage regimen). Products include:

Dexamethasone Acetate (Barbiturates appear to enhance the metabolism of exogenous corticosteroids probably through the induction of hepatic microsomal enzymes. Patients stabilized on corticosteroid therapy may require dosage adjustments if barbiturates are added or withdrawn from their dosage regimen).
No products indexed under this heading.

Dexamethasone Phosphate (Barbiturates appear to enhance the metabolism of exogenous corticosteroids probably through the induction of hepatic microsomal enzymes. Patients stabilized on corticosteroid therapy may require dosage adjustments if barbiturates are added or withdrawn from their dosage regimen).
No products indexed under this heading.

Dexamethasone Sodium (Barbiturates appear to enhance the metabolism of exogenous corticosteroids probably through the induction of hepatic microsomal enzymes. Patients stabilized on corticosteroid therapy may require dosage adjustments if barbiturates are added or withdrawn from their dosage regimen).
No products indexed under this heading.

Dexamethasone Sodium Phosphate (Barbiturates appear to enhance the metabolism of exogenous corticosteroids probably through the induction of hepatic microsomal enzymes. Patients stabilized on corticosteroid therapy may require dosage adjustments if barbiturates are added or withdrawn from their dosage regimen).
No products indexed under this heading.

Dexamethasone Sodium Phosphate Injection (Barbiturates appear to enhance the metabolism of exogenous corticosteroids probably through the induction of hepatic microsomal enzymes. Patients stabilized on corticosteroid therapy may require dosage adjustments if barbiturates are added or withdrawn from their dosage regimen).
No products indexed under this heading.

Dexchlorpheniramine Maleate (The concomitant use of other central nervous system depressants, including antihistamines, may produce additive depressant effects).
No products indexed under this heading.

Dezocine (Concurrent use of the barbiturates with other CNS depressants (eg, narcotics) may result in additional CNS depressant effects).
No products indexed under this heading.

Diazepam (The concomitant use of other central nervous system depressants, including tranquilizers, may produce additive depressant effects).
Products include:

Dicumarol (Phenobarbital lowers the plasma levels of dicumarol (name previously used: bishydroxycoumarin) and causes a decrease in anticoagulant activity as measured by the prothrombin time. Barbiturates can induce hepatic microsomal enzymes, resulting in increased metabolism and decreased anticoagulant response of oral anticoagulants (eg, dicumarol). Patients stabilized on anticoagulant therapy may require dosage adjustments if barbiturates are added to or withdrawn from their dosage regimen).
No products indexed under this heading.

Dienestrol (Pretreatment with or concurrent administration of phenobarbital may decrease the effect of estradiol by increasing its metabolism. An alternate contraceptive method might be suggested to women taking phenobarbital. The application of this data to other barbiturates appears valid).
No products indexed under this heading.

Diethylstilbestrol (Pretreatment with or concurrent administration of phenobarbital may decrease the effect of estradiol by increasing its metabolism. An alternate contraceptive method might be suggested to women taking phenobarbital. The application of this data to other barbiturates appears valid).
No products indexed under this heading.

Diflorasone Diacetate (Barbiturates appear to enhance the metabolism of exogenous corticosteroids probably through the induction of hepatic microsomal enzymes. Patients stabilized on corticosteroid therapy may require dosage adjustments if barbiturates are added or withdrawn from their dosage regimen).
No products indexed under this heading.

Dihydrocodeine Bitartrate (Concurrent use of the barbiturates with other CNS depressants (eg, narcotics) may result in additional CNS depressant effects).
No products indexed under this heading.

IMPORTANT NOTE: Always consult each drug listing in the patient's regimen for possible interactions.

Dihydrocodeinone Bitartrate (Concurrent use of the barbiturates with other CNS depressants (eg, narcotics) may result in additional CNS depressant effects).

No products indexed under this heading.

Diphenhydramine Hydrochloride (The concomitant use of other central nervous system depressants, including antihistamines, may produce additive depressant effects). Products include:

Diphenylpyraline Hydrochloride (The concomitant use of other central nervous system depressants, including antihistamines, may produce additive depressant effects).

No products indexed under this heading.

Divalproex Sodium (Sodium valproate and valproic acid appear to decrease barbiturate metabolism; therefore, barbiturate blood levels should be monitored and appropriate dosage adjustments made as indicated). Products include:

Doxycycline Calcium (Phenobarbital has been shown to shorten the half-life of doxycycline for as long as 2 weeks after barbiturate therapy is discontinued).

No products indexed under this heading.

Doxycycline Hyclate (Phenobarbital has been shown to shorten the half-life of doxycycline for as long as 2 weeks after barbiturate therapy is discontinued).

No products indexed under this heading.

Doxycycline Monohydrate (Phenobarbital has been shown to shorten the half-life of doxycycline for as long as 2 weeks after barbiturate therapy is discontinued).

No products indexed under this heading.

Droperidol (The concomitant use of other central nervous system depressants, including tranquilizers, may produce additive depressant effects).

No products indexed under this heading.

Enflurane (The concomitant use of other central nervous system depressants, including other sedatives or hypnotics, antihistamines, tranquilizers, or alcohol, may produce additive depressant effects).

No products indexed under this heading.

Estazolam (The concomitant use of other central nervous system depressants, including other sedatives or hypnotics, may produce additive depressant effects).

No products indexed under this heading.

Estradiol (Pretreatment with or concurrent administration of phenobarbital may decrease the effect of estradiol by increasing its metabolism. An alternate contraceptive method might be suggested to women taking phenobarbital. The application of this data to other barbiturates appears valid). Products include:

Estrogens, Conjugated (Pretreatment with or concurrent administration of phenobarbital may decrease the effect of estradiol by increasing its metabolism. An alternate contraceptive method might be suggested to women taking phenobarbital. The application of this data to other barbiturates appears valid). Products include:

Estrogens, Esterified (Pretreatment with or concurrent administration of phenobarbital may decrease the effect of estradiol by increasing its metabolism. An alternate contraceptive method might be suggested to women taking phenobarbital. The application of this data to other barbiturates appears valid).

No products indexed under this heading.

Estropipate (Pretreatment with or concurrent administration of phenobarbital may decrease the effect of estradiol by increasing its metabolism. An alternate contraceptive method might be suggested to women taking phenobarbital. The application of this data to other barbiturates appears valid).

No products indexed under this heading.

Ethanol (Concurrent use of barbiturates with other CNS depressants (eg, alcohol) may result in additional CNS depressant effects. Alcohol should not be consumed while taking barbiturates).

No products indexed under this heading.

Ethchlorvynol (The concomitant use of other central nervous system depressants, including other sedatives or hypnotics, may produce additive depressant effects).

No products indexed under this heading.

Ethinamate (The concomitant use of other central nervous system depressants, including other sedatives or hypnotics, may produce additive depressant effects).

No products indexed under this heading.

Ethinyl Estradiol (Pretreatment with or concurrent administration of phenobarbital may decrease the effect of estradiol by increasing its metabolism. An alternate contraceptive method might be suggested to women taking phenobarbital. The application of this data to other barbiturates appears valid). Products include:

Ethyl Alcohol (Concurrent use of barbiturates with other CNS depressants (eg, alcohol) may result in additional CNS depressant effects. Alcohol should not be consumed while taking barbiturates).

No products indexed under this heading.

Ethynodiol Diacetate (Pretreatment with or concurrent administration of phenobarbital may decrease the effect of estradiol by increasing its metabolism. An alternate contraceptive method might be suggested to women taking phenobarbital. The application of this data to other barbiturates appears valid).

No products indexed under this heading.

Fentanyl (Concurrent use of the barbiturates with other CNS depressants (eg, narcotics) may result in additional CNS depressant effects). Products include:

Fentanyl Citrate (Concurrent use of the barbiturates with other CNS depressants (eg, narcotics) may result in additional CNS depressant effects). Products include:

Fexofenadine Hydrochloride (The concomitant use of other central ner-

vous system depressants, including antihistamines, may produce additive depressant effects). Products include:

Fludrocortisone Acetate (Barbiturates appear to enhance the metabolism of exogenous corticosteroids probably through the induction of hepatic microsomal enzymes. Patients stabilized on corticosteroid therapy may require dosage adjustments if barbiturates are added or withdrawn from their dosage regimen).

No products indexed under this heading.

Flumethasone Pivalate (Barbiturates appear to enhance the metabolism of exogenous corticosteroids probably through the induction of hepatic microsomal enzymes. Patients stabilized on corticosteroid therapy may require dosage adjustments if barbiturates are added or withdrawn from their dosage regimen).

No products indexed under this heading.

Flunisolide Hemihydrate (Barbiturates appear to enhance the metabolism of exogenous corticosteroids probably through the induction of hepatic microsomal enzymes. Patients stabilized on corticosteroid therapy may require dosage adjustments if barbiturates are added or withdrawn from their dosage regimen).

No products indexed under this heading.

Fluphenazine Decanoate (The concomitant use of other central nervous system depressants, including tranquilizers, may produce additive depressant effects).

No products indexed under this heading.

Fluphenazine Enanthate (The concomitant use of other central nervous system depressants, including tranquilizers, may produce additive depressant effects).

No products indexed under this heading.

Fluphenazine Hydrochloride (The concomitant use of other central nervous system depressants, including tranquilizers, may produce additive depressant effects).

No products indexed under this heading.

Flurazepam Hydrochloride (The concomitant use of other central nervous system depressants, including other sedatives or hypnotics, may produce additive depressant effects).

No products indexed under this heading.

Fluticasone Furoate (Barbiturates appear to enhance the metabolism of exogenous corticosteroids probably through the induction of hepatic microsomal enzymes. Patients stabilized on corticosteroid therapy may require dosage adjustments if barbiturates are added or withdrawn from their dosage regimen). Products include:

Fluticasone Propionate (Barbiturates appear to enhance the metabolism of exogenous corticosteroids probably through the induction of hepatic microsomal enzymes. Patients stabilized on corticosteroid therapy may require dosage adjustments if barbiturates are added or withdrawn from their dosage regimen). Products include:

Fosphenytoin (The effect of barbiturates on the metabolism of phenytoin appears to be variable. Some investigators report an accelerating effect, while others report no effect. Because the effect of barbiturates on the metabolism of phenytoin is not predictable, phenytoin and barbiturate blood levels should be monitored more frequently if these drugs are given concurrently).

No products indexed under this heading.

Fosphenytoin Sodium (The effect of barbiturates on the metabolism of phenytoin appears to be variable. Some investigators report an accelerating effect, while others report no effect. Because the effect of barbiturates on the metabolism of phenytoin is not predictable, phenytoin and barbiturate blood levels should be monitored more frequently if these drugs are given concurrently).

No products indexed under this heading.

Glutethimide (The concomitant use of other central nervous system depressants, including other sedatives or hypnotics, may produce additive depressant effects).

No products indexed under this heading.

Griseofulvin (Phenobarbital appears to interfere with the absorption of orally administered griseofulvin, thus decreasing its blood level. The effect of the resultant decreased blood levels of griseofulvin on therapeutic response has not been established. However, it would be preferable to avoid concomitant administration of these drugs).

No products indexed under this heading.

Halazepam (The concomitant use of other central nervous system depressants, including other sedatives or hypnotics, antihistamines, tranquilizers, or alcohol, may produce additive depressant effects).

No products indexed under this heading.

Haloperidol (The concomitant use of other central nervous system depressants, including tranquilizers, may produce additive depressant effects).

No products indexed under this heading.

Haloperidol Decanoate (The concomitant use of other central nervous system depressants, including tranquilizers, may produce additive depressant effects).

No products indexed under this heading.

Haloperidol Lactate (The concomitant use of other central nervous system depressants, including other sedatives or hypnotics, antihistamines, tranquilizers, or alcohol, may produce additive depressant effects).

No products indexed under this heading.

Hexobarbital (The concomitant use of other central nervous system depressants, including other sedatives or hypnotics, antihistamines, tranquilizers, or alcohol, may produce additive depressant effects).

No products indexed under this heading.

Hydrocodone Bitartrate (Concurrent use of the barbiturates with other CNS depressants (eg, narcotics) may result in additional CNS depressant effects). Products include:

Hydrocodone Polistirex (Concurrent use of the barbiturates with other CNS depressants (eg, narcotics) may result in additional CNS depressant effects). Products include:

Hydrocortisone (Barbiturates appear to enhance the metabolism of exogenous corticosteroids probably through the induction of hepatic microsomal enzymes. Patients stabilized on corticosteroid therapy may require dosage adjustments if barbiturates are added or withdrawn from their dosage regimen).
No products indexed under this heading.

Hydrocortisone (Alcohol) (Barbiturates appear to enhance the metabolism of exogenous corticosteroids probably through the induction of hepatic microsomal enzymes. Patients stabilized on corticosteroid therapy may require dosage adjustments if barbiturates are added or withdrawn from their dosage regimen).
No products indexed under this heading.

Hydrocortisone Acetate (Barbiturates appear to enhance the metabolism of exogenous corticosteroids probably through the induction of hepatic microsomal enzymes. Patients stabilized on corticosteroid therapy may require dosage adjustments if barbiturates are added or withdrawn from their dosage regimen).
No products indexed under this heading.

Hydrocortisone Butyrate (Barbiturates appear to enhance the metabolism of exogenous corticosteroids probably through the induction of hepatic microsomal enzymes. Patients stabilized on corticosteroid therapy may require dosage adjustments if barbiturates are added or withdrawn from their dosage regimen).
No products indexed under this heading.

Hydrocortisone Cypionate (Barbiturates appear to enhance the metabolism of exogenous corticosteroids probably through the induction of hepatic microsomal enzymes. Patients stabilized on corticosteroid therapy may require dosage adjustments if barbiturates are added or withdrawn from their dosage regimen).
No products indexed under this heading.

Hydrocortisone Hemisuccinate (Barbiturates appear to enhance the metabolism of exogenous corticosteroids probably through the induction of hepatic microsomal enzymes. Patients stabilized on corticosteroid therapy may require dosage adjustments if barbiturates are added or withdrawn from their dosage regimen).
No products indexed under this heading.

Hydrocortisone Probutate (Barbiturates appear to enhance the metabolism of exogenous corticosteroids probably through the induction of hepatic microsomal enzymes. Patients stabilized on corticosteroid therapy may require dosage adjustments if barbiturates are added or withdrawn from their dosage regimen).
No products indexed under this heading.

Hydrocortisone Sodium Phosphate (Barbiturates appear to enhance the metabolism of exogenous corticosteroids probably through the induction of hepatic microsomal enzymes. Patients stabilized on corticosteroid therapy may require dosage adjustments if barbiturates are added or withdrawn from their dosage regimen).
No products indexed under this heading.

Hydrocortisone Sodium Succinate (Barbiturates appear to enhance the metabolism of exogenous corticosteroids probably through the induction of hepatic microsomal enzymes. Patients stabilized on corticosteroid therapy may require dosage adjustments if barbiturates are added or withdrawn from their dosage regimen).
No products indexed under this heading.

Hydrocortisone Valerate (Barbiturates appear to enhance the metabolism of exogenous corticosteroids probably through the induction of hepatic microsomal enzymes. Patients stabilized on corticosteroid therapy may require dosage adjustments if barbiturates are added or withdrawn from their dosage regimen).
No products indexed under this heading.

Hydromorphone (Concurrent use of the barbiturates with other CNS depressants (eg, narcotics) may result in additional CNS depressant effects).
No products indexed under this heading.

Hydromorphone Hydrochloride (Concurrent use of the barbiturates with other CNS depressants (eg, narcotics) may result in additional CNS depressant effects). Products include:

Hydroxyzine Hydrochloride (The concomitant use of other central nervous system depressants, including tranquilizers, may produce additive depressant effects).
No products indexed under this heading.

Isocarboxazid (Co-administration with MAO inhibitors prolongs the effects of barbiturates probably because the metabolism of the barbiturate is inhibited). Products include:

Isoflurane (The concomitant use of other central nervous system depressants, including other sedatives or hypnotics, antihistamines, tranquilizers, or alcohol, may produce additive depressant effects).
No products indexed under this heading.

Ketamine Hydrochloride (The concomitant use of other central nervous system depressants, including other sedatives or hypnotics, antihistamines, tranquilizers, or alcohol, may produce additive depressant effects).
No products indexed under this heading.

Levomethadyl Acetate Hydrochloride (The concomitant use of other central nervous system depressants, including other sedatives or hypnotics, antihistamines, tranquilizers, or alcohol, may produce additive depressant effects).
No products indexed under this heading.

Levonorgestrel (Pretreatment with or concurrent administration of phenobarbital may decrease the effect of estradiol by increasing its metabolism. An alternate contraceptive method might be suggested to women taking phenobarbital. The application of this data to other barbiturates appears valid). Products include:

Levorphanol Tartrate (Concurrent use of the barbiturates with other CNS depressants (eg, narcotics) may result in additional CNS depressant effects).
No products indexed under this heading.

Loratadine (The concomitant use of other central nervous system depressants, including antihistamines, may produce additive depressant effects).
No products indexed under this heading.

Lorazepam (The concomitant use of other central nervous system depressants, including other sedatives or hypnotics, may produce additive depressant effects).
No products indexed under this heading.

Loxapine Hydrochloride (The concomitant use of other central nervous system depressants, including tranquilizers, may produce additive depressant effects).
No products indexed under this heading.

Loxapine Succinate (The concomitant use of other central nervous system depressants, including tranquilizers, may produce additive depressant effects).
No products indexed under this heading.

Meperidine Hydrochloride (Concurrent use of the barbiturates with other CNS depressants (eg, narcotics) may result in additional CNS depressant effects).
No products indexed under this heading.

Mephobarbital (The concomitant use of other central nervous system depressants, including other sedatives or hypnotics, antihistamines, tranquilizers, or alcohol, may produce additive depressant effects).
No products indexed under this heading.

Meprobamate (The concomitant use of other central nervous system depressants, including tranquilizers, may produce additive depressant effects).
No products indexed under this heading.

Mesoridazine Besylate (The concomitant use of other central nervous system depressants, including tranquilizers, may produce additive depressant effects).
No products indexed under this heading.

Mestranol (Pretreatment with or concurrent administration of phenobarbital may decrease the effect of estradiol by increasing its metabolism. An alternate contraceptive method might be suggested to women taking phenobarbital. The application of this data to other barbiturates appears valid).
No products indexed under this heading.

Methadone Hydrochloride (Concurrent use of the barbiturates with other CNS depressants (eg, narcotics) may result in additional CNS depressant effects).
No products indexed under this heading.

Methdilazine Hydrochloride (The concomitant use of other central nervous system depressants, including antihistamines, may produce additive depressant effects).
No products indexed under this heading.

Methohexital Sodium (The concomitant use of other central nervous system depressants, including other sedatives or hypnotics, antihistamines, tranquilizers, or alcohol, may produce additive depressant effects).
No products indexed under this heading.

Methotrimeprazine (The concomitant use of other central nervous system depressants, including other sedatives or hypnotics, antihistamines, tranquilizers, or alcohol, may produce additive depressant effects).
No products indexed under this heading.

Methoxyflurane (The concomitant use of other central nervous system depressants, including other sedatives or hypnotics, antihistamines, tranquilizers, or alcohol, may produce additive depressant effects).
No products indexed under this heading.

Methylprednisolone (Barbiturates appear to enhance the metabolism of exogenous corticosteroids probably through the induction of hepatic microsomal enzymes. Patients stabilized on corticosteroid therapy may require dosage adjustments if barbiturates are added or withdrawn from their dosage regimen).
No products indexed under this heading.

Methylprednisolone Acetate (Barbiturates appear to enhance the metabolism of exogenous corticosteroids probably through the induction of hepatic microsomal enzymes. Patients stabilized on corticosteroid therapy may require dosage adjustments if barbiturates are added or withdrawn from their dosage regimen).
No products indexed under this heading.

Methylprednisolone Sodium Succinate (Barbiturates appear to enhance the metabolism of exogenous corticosteroids probably through the induction of hepatic microsomal enzymes. Patients stabilized on corticosteroid therapy may require dosage adjustments if barbiturates are added or withdrawn from their dosage regimen).
No products indexed under this heading.

Midazolam Hydrochloride (The concomitant use of other central nervous system depressants, including other sedatives or hypnotics, may produce additive depressant effects).
No products indexed under this heading.

Moclobemide (Co-administration with MAO inhibitors prolongs the effects of barbiturates probably because the metabolism of the barbiturate is inhibited).
No products indexed under this heading.

Molindone Hydrochloride (The concomitant use of other central nervous system depressants, including tranquilizers, may produce additive depressant effects). Products include:

Mometasone Furoate (Barbiturates appear to enhance the metabolism of exogenous corticosteroids probably through the induction of hepatic microsomal enzymes. Patients stabilized on corticosteroid therapy may require dosage adjustments if barbiturates are added or withdrawn from their dosage regimen). Products include:

Mometasone Furoate Monohydrate (Barbiturates appear to enhance the metabolism of exogenous corticosteroids probably through the induction of hepatic microsomal enzymes. Patients stabilized on corticosteroid therapy may require dosage adjustments if barbiturates are added or withdrawn from their dosage regimen). Products include:

Morphine Sulfate (Concurrent use of the barbiturates with other CNS depressants (eg, narcotics) may result in additional CNS depressant effects). Products include:

Morphine Sulfate, Liposomal (Concurrent use of the barbiturates with other CNS depressants (eg, narcotics) may result in additional CNS depressant effects).
No products indexed under this heading.

Norethindrone (Pretreatment with or concurrent administration of phenobarbital may decrease the effect of estradiol by increasing its metabolism. An alternate contraceptive method might be suggested to women taking phenobarbital. The application of this data to other barbiturates appears valid). Products include:

IMPORTANT NOTE: Always consult each drug listing in the patient's regimen for possible interactions.

(⊙ Described in PDR® for Ophthalmic Medicines)

notics, antihistamines, tranquilizers, or alcohol, may produce additive depressant effects). Products include:

Ultane 554

Sodium Butabarbital (The concomitant use of other central nervous system depressants, including other sedatives or hypnotics, may produce additive depressant effects).

No products indexed under this heading.

Sodium Oxybate (The concomitant use of other central nervous system depressants, including other sedatives or hypnotics, antihistamines, tranquilizers, or alcohol, may produce additive depressant effects).

No products indexed under this heading.

Sodium Pentobarbital (The concomitant use of other central nervous system depressants, including other sedatives or hypnotics, antihistamines, tranquilizers, or alcohol, may produce additive depressant effects).

No products indexed under this heading.

Sufentanil Citrate (Concurrent use of the barbiturates with other CNS depressants (eg, narcotics) may result in additional CNS depressant effects).

No products indexed under this heading.

Talbutal (The concomitant use of other central nervous system depressants, including other sedatives or hypnotics, antihistamines, tranquilizers, or alcohol, may produce additive depressant effects).

No products indexed under this heading.

Temazepam (The concomitant use of other central nervous system depressants, including other sedatives or hypnotics, may produce additive depressant effects).

No products indexed under this heading.

Terfenadine (The concomitant use of other central nervous system depressants, including antihistamines, may produce additive depressant effects).

No products indexed under this heading.

Thiamylal Sodium (The concomitant use of other central nervous system depressants, including other sedatives or hypnotics, antihistamines, tranquilizers, or alcohol, may produce additive depressant effects).

No products indexed under this heading.

Thioridazine (The concomitant use of other central nervous system depressants, including other sedatives or hypnotics, antihistamines, tranquilizers, or alcohol, may produce additive depressant effects).

No products indexed under this heading.

Thioridazine Hydrochloride (The concomitant use of other central nervous system depressants, including tranquilizers, may produce additive depressant effects). Products include:

Thioridazine Hydrochloride 2384

Thiothixene (The concomitant use of other central nervous system depressants, including tranquilizers, may produce additive depressant effects). Products include:

Thiothixene 2386

Thiothixene Hydrochloride (The concomitant use of other central nervous system depressants, including other sedatives or hypnotics, antihistamines, tranquilizers, or alcohol, may produce additive depressant effects).

No products indexed under this heading.

Tranylcypromine Sulfate (Coadministration with MAO inhibitors prolongs the effects of barbiturates probably because the metabolism of the barbiturate is inhibited). Products include:

Parnate 1584

Triamcinolone (Barbiturates appear to enhance the metabolism of exogenous corticosteroids probably through the induction of hepatic microsomal enzymes. Patients stabilized on corticosteroid therapy may require dosage adjustments if barbiturates are added or withdrawn from their dosage regimen).

No products indexed under this heading.

Triamcinolone Acetonide (Barbiturates appear to enhance the metabolism of exogenous corticosteroids probably through the induction of hepatic microsomal enzymes. Patients stabilized on corticosteroid therapy may require dosage adjustments if barbiturates are added or withdrawn from their dosage regimen). Products include:

Azmacort 408

Nasacort AQ 3019

Triamcinolone Diacetate (Barbiturates appear to enhance the metabolism of exogenous corticosteroids probably through the induction of hepatic microsomal enzymes. Patients stabilized on corticosteroid therapy may require dosage adjustments if barbiturates are added or withdrawn from their dosage regimen).

No products indexed under this heading.

Triamcinolone Hexacetonide (Barbiturates appear to enhance the metabolism of exogenous corticosteroids probably through the induction of hepatic microsomal enzymes. Patients stabilized on corticosteroid therapy may require dosage adjustments if barbiturates are added or withdrawn from their dosage regimen).

No products indexed under this heading.

Triazolam (The concomitant use of other central nervous system depressants, including other sedatives or hypnotics, may produce additive depressant effects).

No products indexed under this heading.

Trifluoperazine Hydrochloride (The concomitant use of other central nervous system depressants, including tranquilizers, may produce additive depressant effects).

No products indexed under this heading.

Trimeprazine Tartrate (The concomitant use of other central nervous system depressants, including antihistamines, may produce additive depressant effects).

No products indexed under this heading.

Tripelennamine Hydrochloride (The concomitant use of other central nervous system depressants, including antihistamines, may produce additive depressant effects).

No products indexed under this heading.

Triprolidine Hydrochloride (The concomitant use of other central nervous system depressants, including antihistamines, may produce additive depressant effects).

No products indexed under this heading.

Valproate Sodium (Sodium valproate and valproic acid appear to decrease barbiturate metabolism; therefore, barbiturate blood levels should be monitored and appropriate dosage adjustments made as indicated).

No products indexed under this heading.

Valproic Acid (Sodium valproate and valproic acid appear to decrease barbiturate metabolism; therefore, barbiturate blood levels should be monitored and appropriate dosage adjustments made as indicated).

No products indexed under this heading.

Warfarin Sodium (Barbiturates can induce hepatic microsomal enzymes, resulting in increased metabolism and decreased anticoagulant response of oral anticoagulants (eg, warfarin). Patients stabilized on anticoagulant therapy may require dosage adjustments if barbiturates are added or withdrawn from their dosage regimen).

No products indexed under this heading.

Zaleplon (The concomitant use of other central nervous system depressants, including other sedatives or hypnotics, may produce additive depressant effects).

No products indexed under this heading.

Ziprasidone Hydrochloride (The concomitant use of other central nervous system depressants, including other sedatives or hypnotics, antihistamines, tranquilizers, or alcohol, may produce additive depressant effects). Products include:

Geodon 2723

Zolpidem Tartrate (The concomitant use of other central nervous system depressants, including other sedatives or hypnotics, may produce additive depressant effects). Products include:

Ambien 2920

Ambien CR 2925

Food Interactions

Alcohol (Concurrent use of barbiturates with other CNS depressants (eg, alcohol) may result in additional CNS depressant effects. Alcohol should not be consumed while taking barbiturates).

Beer, reduced-alcohol (Concurrent use of barbiturates with other CNS depressants (eg, alcohol) may result in additional CNS depressant effects. Alcohol should not be consumed while taking barbiturates).

Beer, unspecified (Concurrent use of barbiturates with other CNS depressants (eg, alcohol) may result in additional CNS depressant effects. Alcohol should not be consumed while taking barbiturates).

Wine, Chianti (Concurrent use of barbiturates with other CNS depressants (eg, alcohol) may result in additional CNS depressant effects. Alcohol should not be consumed while taking barbiturates).

Wine, Red (Concurrent use of barbiturates with other CNS depressants (eg, alcohol) may result in additional CNS depressant effects. Alcohol should not be consumed while taking barbiturates).

Wine, unspecified (Concurrent use of barbiturates with other CNS depressants (eg, alcohol) may result in additional CNS depressant effects. Alcohol should not be consumed while taking barbiturates).

Wine products (Concurrent use of barbiturates with other CNS depressants (eg, alcohol) may result in additional CNS depressant effects. Alcohol should not be consumed while taking barbiturates).

NEOPROFEN INJECTION

(Ibuprofen Lysine) 2015

None cited in PDR database.

NEORAL ORAL SOLUTION

(Cyclosporine) 2496

See Neoral Soft Gelatin Capsules

NEORAL SOFT GELATIN CAPSULES

(Cyclosporine) 2496

May interact with ACE inhibitors, angiotensin-II receptor antagonists, erythromycin, fibrates, HMG-CoA reductase inhibitors, non-steroidal anti-inflammatory agents, oral contraceptives, phenytoin, potassium preparations, potassium sparing diuretics, protease inhibitors, vaccines, live, and certain other agents. Compounds in these categories include:

Allopurinol (Increases cyclosporine concentrations).

No products indexed under this heading.

Amiloride Hydrochloride (Cyclosporine may cause hyperkalemia; concurrent use should be avoided).

No products indexed under this heading.

Amiodarone Hydrochloride (Increases cyclosporine concentrations).

No products indexed under this heading.

Amphotericin B (May potentiate renal dysfunction).

No products indexed under this heading.

Amprenavir (The HIV protease inhibitors are known to inhibit cytochrome P450IIIA and increase the concentration of drugs metabolized by this enzyme system; agents that inhibit this enzyme could decrease metabolism and increase cyclosporine concentrations; this interaction has not been studied; however, care should be exercised).

No products indexed under this heading.

Atazanavir (The HIV protease inhibitors are known to inhibit cytochrome P450IIIA and increase the concentration of drugs metabolized by this enzyme system; agents that inhibit this enzyme could decrease metabolism and increase cyclosporine concentrations; this interaction has not been studied; however, care should be exercised).

No products indexed under this heading.

Atazanavir Sulfate (The HIV protease inhibitors are known to inhibit cytochrome P450IIIA and increase the concentration of drugs metabolized by this enzyme system; agents that inhibit this enzyme could decrease metabolism and increase cyclosporine concentrations; this interaction has not been studied; however, care should be exercised).

No products indexed under this heading.

Atorvastatin Calcium (Coadministration may result in myotoxicity; atorvastatin dosage should be reduced according to label recommendations. Atorvastatin needs to be temporarily withheld or discontinued in patients with signs and symptoms of myopathy or those with risk factors predisposing to severe renal injury secondary to rhabdomyolysis). Products include:

Lipitor 2703

Azapropazon (May potentiate renal dysfunction).

No products indexed under this heading.

Azathioprine (May potentiate renal dysfunction).

No products indexed under this heading.

Azithromycin (Concomitant azithromycin may increase cyclosporine concentrations). Products include:

AzaSite 1806

BCG Vaccine (The use of live vaccines should be avoided).

No products indexed under this heading.

Benazepril Hydrochloride (Caution is required when cyclosporine is coadministered with potassium-sparing drugs, such as angiotensin-converting enzyme inhibitors).

No products indexed under this heading.

Bromocriptine Mesylate (Increases cyclosporine concentrations).

No products indexed under this heading.

Candesartan Cilexetil (Caution is required when cyclosporine is coadministered with potassium-sparing drugs, such as angiotensin II receptor antagonists). Products include:

IMPORTANT NOTE: Always consult each drug listing in the patient's regimen for possible interactions.

P450IIIA and increase the concentration of drugs metabolized by this enzyme system; agents that inhibit this enzyme could decrease metabolism and increase cyclosporine concentrations; this interaction has not been studied; however, care should be exercised. Products include:

Rofecoxib (Co-administration with NSAID's particularly in the setting of dehydration, may potentiate renal dysfunction).

No products indexed under this heading.

Rosuvastatin Calcium (Literature and post-marketing cases of myotoxicity, including muscle pain and weakness, myositis, and rhabdomyolysis, have been reported with concomitant administration of cyclosporine with lovastatin, simvastatin, atorvastatin, pravastatin, and rarely, fluvastatin. When concurrently administered with cyclosporine, the dosage of these statins should be reduced according to label recommendations. Statin therapy needs to be temporarily withheld or discontinued in patients with signs and symptoms of myopathy or those with risk factors predisposing to severe renal injury, including renal failure, secondary to rhabdomyolysis). Products include:

Rotavirus Vaccine, Live, Oral, Tetravalent (The use of live vaccines should be avoided).

No products indexed under this heading.

Rubella & Mumps Virus Vaccine Live (The use of live vaccines should be avoided).

No products indexed under this heading.

Rubella Virus Vaccine Live (The use of live vaccines should be avoided). Products include:

Saquinavir (The HIV protease inhibitors are known to inhibit cytochrome P450IIIA and increase the concentration of drugs metabolized by this enzyme system; agents that inhibit this enzyme could decrease metabolism and increase cyclosporine concentrations; this interaction has not been studied; however, care should be exercised).

No products indexed under this heading.

Saquinavir Mesylate (The HIV protease inhibitors are known to inhibit cytochrome P450IIIA and increase the concentration of drugs metabolized by this enzyme system; agents that inhibit this enzyme could decrease metabolism and increase cyclosporine concentrations; this interaction has not been studied; however, care should be exercised).

No products indexed under this heading.

Simvastatin (Co-administration may result in myotoxicity; simvastation dosage should be reduced according to label recommendations. Simvastatin needs to be temporarily withheld or discontinued in patients with signs and symptoms of myopathy or those with risk factors predisposing to severe renal injury secondary to rhabdomyolysis). Products include:

Sirolimus (Elevations in serum creatinine were observed in studies using sirolimus in combination with full-dose cyclosporine. The effect is often reversible with cyclosporine dose reduction. Simultaneous co-administration of cyclosproine significantly increases

blood levels of sirolimus. To minimize increases in sirolimus blood concentrations, it is recommended that sirolimus be given 4 hours after cyclosporine administration). Products include:

Smallpox Vaccine (The use of live vaccines should be avoided).

No products indexed under this heading.

Spirapril Hydrochloride (Caution is required when cyclosporine is co-administered with potassium-sparing drugs, such as angiotensin-converting enzyme inhibitors).

No products indexed under this heading.

Spironolactone (Cyclosporine may cause hyperkalemia; concurrent use should be avoided).

No products indexed under this heading.

Sulfamethoxazole (Co-administration with trimethoprim/sulfamethoxazole may potentiate renal dysfunction).

No products indexed under this heading.

Sulfinpyrazone (Concomitant sulfinpyrazone may decrease cyclosporine concentrations).

No products indexed under this heading.

Sulindac (Concomitant use is associated with additive decreases in renal function with possible potentiation of renal dysfunction). Products include:

Tacrolimus (May potentiate renal dysfunction). Products include:

Telmisartan (Caution is required when cyclosporine is co-administered with potassium-sparing drugs, such as angiotensin II receptor antagonists). Products include:

Terbinafine Hydrochloride (Concomitant terbinafine may decrease cyclosporine concentrations).

No products indexed under this heading.

Ticlopidine Hydrochloride (Decreases cyclosporine concentrations).

No products indexed under this heading.

Tipranavir (The HIV protease inhibitors are known to inhibit cytochrome P450IIIA and increase the concentration of drugs metabolized by this enzyme system; agents that inhibit this enzyme could decrease metabolism and increase cyclosporine concentrations; this interaction has not been studied; however, care should be exercised).

No products indexed under this heading.

Tobramycin (May potentiate renal dysfunction). Products include:

Tobramycin Sulfate (May potentiate renal dysfunction).

No products indexed under this heading.

Tolmetin Sodium (Co-administration with NSAID's particularly in the setting of dehydration, may potentiate renal dysfunction).

No products indexed under this heading.

Trandolapril (Caution is required when cyclosporine is co-administered with potassium-sparing drugs, such as angiotensin-converting enzyme inhibitors). Products include:

Triamterene (Cyclosporine may cause hyperkalemia; concurrent use should be avoided). Products include:

Trimethoprim (Co-administration with trimethoprim/sulfamethoxazole may potentiate renal dysfunction).

No products indexed under this heading.

Typhoid Vaccine (The use of live vaccines should be avoided).

No products indexed under this heading.

Vaccines (Live) (Vaccination may be less effective).

No products indexed under this heading.

Valdecoxib (Co-administration with NSAID's particularly in the setting of dehydration, may potentiate renal dysfunction).

No products indexed under this heading.

Valsartan (Caution is required when cyclosporine is co-administered with potassium-sparing drugs, such as angiotensin II receptor antagonists). Products include:

Vancomycin Hydrochloride (May potentiate renal dysfunction).

No products indexed under this heading.

Varicella Virus Vaccine, Live (The use of live vaccines should be avoided). Products include:

Verapamil Hydrochloride (Increases cyclosporine concentrations). Products include:

Yellow Fever Vaccine (The use of live vaccines should be avoided).

No products indexed under this heading.

Zoster Vaccine Live (The use of live vaccines should be avoided). Products include:

Food Interactions

Diet, high-lipid (A high-fat meal consumed within one-half hour before Neoral administration decreased the AUC by 13% and C_{max} by 33%).

Food, unspecified (Administration of food with Neoral decreases the AUC and C_{max}).

Grapefruit (Affects the metabolism of cyclosporine and should be avoided).

Grapefruit Juice (Affects the metabolism of cyclosporine and should be avoided).

NEURASTA

NEULASTA

May interact with cytotoxic drugs, drugs which potentiate the release of neutrophils, lithium preparations. Compounds in these categories include:

Bleomycin Sulfate (Neulasta should not be administered in the period between 14 days before and 24 hours after administration of cytotoxic chemotherapy because of the potential for an increase in sensitivity of rapidly dividing myeloid cells to cytotoxic chemotherapy).

No products indexed under this heading.

Cyclophosphamide (Neulasta should not be administered in the period between 14 days before and 24 hours after administration of cytotoxic chemotherapy because of the potential for an increase in sensitivity of rapidly dividing myeloid cells to cytotoxic chemotherapy).

No products indexed under this heading.

Daunorubicin Hydrochloride (Neulasta should not be administered in the period between 14 days before and 24 hours after administration of cytotoxic chemotherapy because of the potential for an increase in sensitivity of rapidly dividing myeloid cells to cytotoxic chemotherapy).

No products indexed under this heading.

Doxorubicin Hydrochloride (Neulasta should not be administered in the period between 14 days before and 24 hours after administration of cytotoxic chemotherapy because of the potential for an increase in sensitivity of rapidly dividing myeloid cells to cytotoxic chemotherapy).

No products indexed under this heading.

Epirubicin Hydrochloride (Neulasta should not be administered in the period between 14 days before and 24 hours after administration of cytotoxic chemotherapy because of the potential for an increase in sensitivity of rapidly dividing myeloid cells to cytotoxic chemotherapy).

No products indexed under this heading.

Fluorouracil (Neulasta should not be administered in the period between 14 days before and 24 hours after administration of cytotoxic chemotherapy because of the potential for an increase in sensitivity of rapidly dividing myeloid cells to cytotoxic chemotherapy). Products include:

Hydroxyurea (Neulasta should not be administered in the period between 14 days before and 24 hours after administration of cytotoxic chemotherapy because of the potential for an increase in sensitivity of rapidly dividing myeloid cells to cytotoxic chemotherapy).

No products indexed under this heading.

Lithium (Lithium may potentiate the release of neutrophils when co-administered with pegfilgrastim; monitor neutrophil counts more frequently).

No products indexed under this heading.

Lithium Carbonate (Lithium may potentiate the release of neutrophils when co-administered with pegfilgrastim; monitor neutrophil counts more frequently).

No products indexed under this heading.

Lithium Citrate (Lithium may potentiate the release of neutrophils when co-administered with pegfilgrastim; monitor neutrophil counts more frequently).

No products indexed under this heading.

Methotrexate Sodium (Neulasta should not be administered in the period between 14 days before and 24 hours after administration of cytotoxic chemotherapy because of the potential for an increase in sensitivity of rapidly dividing myeloid cells to cytotoxic chemotherapy).

No products indexed under this heading.

Mitotane (Neulasta should not be administered in the period between 14 days before and 24 hours after administration of cytotoxic chemotherapy because of the potential for an increase in sensitivity of rapidly dividing myeloid cells to cytotoxic chemotherapy).

No products indexed under this heading.

Mitoxantrone Hydrochloride (Neulasta should not be administered in the period between 14 days before and 24 hours after administration of cytotoxic chemotherapy because of the potential for an increase in sensitivity of rapidly dividing myeloid cells to cytotoxic chemotherapy). Products include:

Procarbazine Hydrochloride (Neulasta should not be administered in the period between 14 days before and 24 hours after administration of cytotoxic chemotherapy because of the potential for an increase in sensitivity of rapidly dividing myeloid cells to cytotoxic chemotherapy).
No products indexed under this heading.

Tamoxifen Citrate (Neulasta should not be administered in the period between 14 days before and 24 hours after administration of cytotoxic chemotherapy because of the potential for an increase in sensitivity of rapidly dividing myeloid cells to cytotoxic chemotherapy).
No products indexed under this heading.

Vinblastine Sulfate (Neulasta should not be administered in the period between 14 days before and 24 hours after administration of cytotoxic chemotherapy because of the potential for an increase in sensitivity of rapidly dividing myeloid cells to cytotoxic chemotherapy).
No products indexed under this heading.

Vincristine Sulfate (Neulasta should not be administered in the period between 14 days before and 24 hours after administration of cytotoxic chemotherapy because of the potential for an increase in sensitivity of rapidly dividing myeloid cells to cytotoxic chemotherapy).
No products indexed under this heading.

Vinorelbine Tartrate (Neulasta should not be administered in the period between 14 days before and 24 hours after administration of cytotoxic chemotherapy because of the potential for an increase in sensitivity of rapidly dividing myeloid cells to cytotoxic chemotherapy).
No products indexed under this heading.

NEUPOGEN FOR INJECTION

(Filgrastim) 631
May interact with drugs which potentiate the release of neutrophils. Compounds in these categories include:

Lithium Carbonate (Concurrent use should be undertaken with caution since lithium potentiates the release of neutrophils).
No products indexed under this heading.

Lithium Citrate (Concurrent use should be undertaken with caution since lithium potentiates the release of neutrophils).
No products indexed under this heading.

NEVANAC OPHTHALMIC SUSPENSION 0.1%

(Nepafenac) .... ⊙203
May interact with anticoagulants, corticosteroids. Compounds in these categories include:

Alclometasone Dipropionate (Concomitant use of topical NSAIDs and topical steroids may slow or delay healing).
No products indexed under this heading.

Anisindione (It is recommended that nepafenac ophthalmic suspension be used with caution in patients who are receiving other medications which may prolong bleeding time).
No products indexed under this heading.

Ardeparin Sodium (It is recommended that nepafenac ophthalmic suspension be used with caution in patients who are receiving other medications which may prolong bleeding time).
No products indexed under this heading.

Beclomethasone Dipropionate (Concomitant use of topical NSAIDs and topical steroids may slow or delay healing). Products include:

Qvar 3398

Beclomethasone Dipropionate Monohydrate (Concomitant use of topical NSAIDs and topical steroids may slow or delay healing). Products include:
Beconase AQ 1386

Betamethasone (Concomitant use of topical NSAIDs and topical steroids may slow or delay healing).
No products indexed under this heading.

Betamethasone Acetate (Concomitant use of topical NSAIDs and topical steroids may slow or delay healing).
No products indexed under this heading.

Betamethasone Benzoate (Concomitant use of topical NSAIDs and topical steroids may slow or delay healing).
No products indexed under this heading.

Betamethasone Dipropionate (Concomitant use of topical NSAIDs and topical steroids may slow or delay healing). Products include:
Diprolene Lotion 0.05% 3108
Diprolene Ointment 0.05% 3109
Diprolene AF Cream 0.05% 3107
Lotrisone 3163

Betamethasone Sodium Phosphate (Concomitant use of topical NSAIDs and topical steroids may slow or delay healing).
No products indexed under this heading.

Betamethasone Valerate (Concomitant use of topical NSAIDs and topical steroids may slow or delay healing). Products include:
Luxíq 3321

Budesonide (Concomitant use of topical NSAIDs and topical steroids may slow or delay healing). Products include:
Pulmicort Flexhaler 714
Symbicort 80/4.5 720
Symbicort 160/4.5 720

Ciclesonide (Concomitant use of topical NSAIDs and topical steroids may slow or delay healing).
No products indexed under this heading.

Cortisone Acetate (Concomitant use of topical NSAIDs and topical steroids may slow or delay healing).
No products indexed under this heading.

Dalteparin Sodium (It is recommended that nepafenac ophthalmic suspension be used with caution in patients who are receiving other medications which may prolong bleeding time). Products include:
Fragmin 1058

Danaparoid Sodium (It is recommended that nepafenac ophthalmic suspension be used with caution in patients who are receiving other medications which may prolong bleeding time).
No products indexed under this heading.

Desoximetasone (Concomitant use of topical NSAIDs and topical steroids may slow or delay healing).
No products indexed under this heading.

Dexamethasone (Concomitant use of topical NSAIDs and topical steroids may slow or delay healing). Products include:
Ciprodex 583
Ozurdex .... ⊙223
Tobramycin and Dexamethasone Ophthalmic Suspension .... ⊙251

Dexamethasone Acetate (Concomitant use of topical NSAIDs and topical steroids may slow or delay healing).
No products indexed under this heading.

Dexamethasone Phosphate (Concomitant use of topical NSAIDs and topical steroids may slow or delay healing).
No products indexed under this heading.

Dexamethasone Sodium (Concomitant use of topical NSAIDs and topical steroids may slow or delay healing).
No products indexed under this heading.

Dexamethasone Sodium Phosphate (Concomitant use of topical NSAIDs and topical steroids may slow or delay healing).
No products indexed under this heading.

Dexamethasone Sodium Phosphate Injection (Concomitant use of topical NSAIDs and topical steroids may slow or delay healing).
No products indexed under this heading.

Dicumarol (It is recommended that nepafenac ophthalmic suspension be used with caution in patients who are receiving other medications which may prolong bleeding time).
No products indexed under this heading.

Diflorasone Diacetate (Concomitant use of topical NSAIDs and topical steroids may slow or delay healing).
No products indexed under this heading.

Enoxaparin Sodium (It is recommended that nepafenac ophthalmic suspension be used with caution in patients who are receiving other medications which may prolong bleeding time). Products include:
Lovenox 3005

Fludrocortisone Acetate (Concomitant use of topical NSAIDs and topical steroids may slow or delay healing).
No products indexed under this heading.

Flumethasone Pivalate (Concomitant use of topical NSAIDs and topical steroids may slow or delay healing).
No products indexed under this heading.

Flunisolide Hemihydrate (Concomitant use of topical NSAIDs and topical steroids may slow or delay healing).
No products indexed under this heading.

Fluticasone Furoate (Concomitant use of topical NSAIDs and topical steroids may slow or delay healing). Products include:
Veramyst 1713

Fluticasone Propionate (Concomitant use of topical NSAIDs and topical steroids may slow or delay healing). Products include:
Advair 100/50 1275
Advair 250/50 1275
Advair 500/50 1275
Advair HFA 45/21 1288
Advair HFA 115/21 1288
Advair HFA 230/21 1288
Flonase 1459
Flovent Diskus 1463
Flovent HFA 1470

Fondaparinux Sodium (It is recommended that nepafenac ophthalmic suspension be used with caution in patients who are receiving other medications which may prolong bleeding time). Products include:
Arixtra 1320

Heparin Calcium (It is recommended that nepafenac ophthalmic suspension be used with caution in patients who are receiving other medications which may prolong bleeding time).
No products indexed under this heading.

Heparin Sodium (It is recommended that nepafenac ophthalmic suspension be used with caution in patients who are receiving other medications which may prolong bleeding time).
No products indexed under this heading.

Hydrocortisone (Concomitant use of topical NSAIDs and topical steroids may slow or delay healing).
No products indexed under this heading.

Hydrocortisone (Alcohol) (Concomitant use of topical NSAIDs and topical steroids may slow or delay healing).
No products indexed under this heading.

Hydrocortisone Acetate (Concomitant use of topical NSAIDs and topical steroids may slow or delay healing).
No products indexed under this heading.

Hydrocortisone Butyrate (Concomitant use of topical NSAIDs and topical steroids may slow or delay healing).
No products indexed under this heading.

Hydrocortisone Cypionate (Concomitant use of topical NSAIDs and topical steroids may slow or delay healing).
No products indexed under this heading.

Hydrocortisone Hemisuccinate (Concomitant use of topical NSAIDs and topical steroids may slow or delay healing).
No products indexed under this heading.

Hydrocortisone Probutate (Concomitant use of topical NSAIDs and topical steroids may slow or delay healing).
No products indexed under this heading.

Hydrocortisone Sodium Phosphate (Concomitant use of topical NSAIDs and topical steroids may slow or delay healing).
No products indexed under this heading.

Hydrocortisone Sodium Succinate (Concomitant use of topical NSAIDs and topical steroids may slow or delay healing).
No products indexed under this heading.

Hydrocortisone Valerate (Concomitant use of topical NSAIDs and topical steroids may slow or delay healing).
No products indexed under this heading.

Low Molecular Weight Heparins (It is recommended that nepafenac ophthalmic suspension be used with caution in patients who are receiving other medications which may prolong bleeding time).
No products indexed under this heading.

Methylprednisolone (Concomitant use of topical NSAIDs and topical steroids may slow or delay healing).
No products indexed under this heading.

Methylprednisolone Acetate (Concomitant use of topical NSAIDs and topical steroids may slow or delay healing).
No products indexed under this heading.

Methylprednisolone Sodium Succinate (Concomitant use of topical NSAIDs and topical steroids may slow or delay healing).
No products indexed under this heading.

Mometasone Furoate (Concomitant use of topical NSAIDs and topical steroids may slow or delay healing). Products include:
Asmanex 3058
Elocon Cream 3111
Elocon Lotion 3112
Elocon Ointment 3114

Mometasone Furoate Monohydrate (Concomitant use of topical NSAIDs and topical steroids may slow or delay healing). Products include:
Nasonex 3166

Prednisolone (Concomitant use of topical NSAIDs and topical steroids may slow or delay healing).
No products indexed under this heading.

Prednisolone Acetate (Concomitant use of topical NSAIDs and topical steroids may slow or delay healing). Products include:
Blephamide .... ⊙212, ⊙214
Pred Forte .... ⊙225
Pred Mild .... ⊙230
Pred-G .... ⊙226, ⊙227

Prednisolone Sodium Phosphate (Concomitant use of topical NSAIDs and topical steroids may slow or delay healing).
No products indexed under this heading.

Prednisolone Tebutate (Concomitant use of topical NSAIDs and topical steroids may slow or delay healing).
No products indexed under this heading.

Prednisone (Concomitant use of topical NSAIDs and topical steroids may slow or delay healing).
No products indexed under this heading.

IMPORTANT NOTE: Always consult each drug listing in the patient's regimen for possible interactions.

Prednisone sodium phosphate
(Concomitant use of topical NSAIDs and topical steroids may slow or delay healing).
No products indexed under this heading.

Tinzaparin Sodium (It is recommended that nepafenac ophthalmic suspension be used with caution in patients who are receiving other medications which may prolong bleeding time).
No products indexed under this heading.

Triamcinolone (Concomitant use of topical NSAIDs and topical steroids may slow or delay healing).
No products indexed under this heading.

Triamcinolone Acetonide (Concomitant use of topical NSAIDs and topical steroids may slow or delay healing).
Products include:

Triamcinolone Diacetate (Concomitant use of topical NSAIDs and topical steroids may slow or delay healing).
No products indexed under this heading.

Triamcinolone Hexacetonide (Concomitant use of topical NSAIDs and topical steroids may slow or delay healing).
No products indexed under this heading.

Warfarin Sodium (It is recommended that nepafenac ophthalmic suspension be used with caution in patients who are receiving other medications which may prolong bleeding time).
No products indexed under this heading.

NEXIUM DELAYED-RELEASE CAPSULES

(Esomeprazole Magnesium) 704
May interact with absorption of drugs where gastric ph is an important determinant in their bioavailability, antiretroviral agents, cytochrome p450 2c19 inhibitors (selected), cytochrome p450 2c19 substrates (selected), cytochrome p450 3a4 inhibitors (selected), iron containing oral preparations, iron salts, and certain other agents. Compounds in these categories include:

Abacavir Sulfate (Omeprazole, of which esomeprazole is an enantiomer, has been reported to interact with some antiretroviral drugs. The clinical importance and the mechanisms behind these interactions are not always known. Increased gastric pH during omeprazole treatment may change the absorption of the antiretroviral drug. Other possible interaction mechanisms are via CYP2C19). Products include:

Acetazolamide (Concomitant administration of esomeprazole and a combined inhibitor of CYP 2C19 and CYP 3A4, such as voriconazole, may result in more than doubling of the esomeprazole exposure. Dose adjustment of esomeprazole is not normally required. However, in patients with Zollinger-Ellison's Syndrome, who may require higher doses up to 240 mg/day, dose adjustment may be considered).
No products indexed under this heading.

Acetazolamide Sodium (Concomitant administration of esomeprazole and a combined inhibitor of CYP 2C19 and CYP 3A4, such as voriconazole, may result in more than doubling of the esomeprazole exposure. Dose adjustment of esomeprazole is not normally required. However, in patients with Zollinger-Ellison's Syndrome, who may require higher doses up to 240 mg/day, dose adjustment may be considered).
No products indexed under this heading.

Amiodarone Hydrochloride (Concomitant administration of esomeprazole and a combined inhibitor of CYP

2C19 and CYP 3A4, such as voriconazole, may result in more than doubling of the esomeprazole exposure. Dose adjustment of esomeprazole is not normally required. However, in patients with Zollinger-Ellison's Syndrome, who may require higher doses up to 240 mg/day, dose adjustment may be considered).
No products indexed under this heading.

Amitriptyline Hydrochloride (Esomeprazole may potentially interfere with CYP 2C19, the major esomeprazole metabolizing enzyme. Co-administration of esomeprazole 30 mg and diazepam, a CYP2C19 substrate, resulted in a 45% decrease in clearance of diazepam).
No products indexed under this heading.

Amoxapine (Esomeprazole may potentially interfere with CYP 2C19, the major esomeprazole metabolizing enzyme. Co-administration of esomeprazole 30 mg and diazepam, a CYP2C19 substrate, resulted in a 45% decrease in clearance of diazepam).
No products indexed under this heading.

Amoxicillin (Co-administration of esomeprazole, clarithromycin, and amoxicillin has resulted in increases in the plasma levels of esomeprazole and 14-hydroxyclarithromycin). Products include:

Amoxicillin Trihydrate (Co-administration of esomeprazole, clarithromycin, and amoxicillin has resulted in increases in the plasma levels of esomeprazole and 14-hydroxyclarithromycin).
No products indexed under this heading.

Amprenavir (Omeprazole, of which esomeprazole is an enantiomer, has been reported to interact with some antiretroviral drugs. The clinical importance and the mechanisms behind these interactions are not always known. Increased gastric pH during omeprazole treatment may change the absorption of the antiretroviral drug. Other possible interaction mechanisms are via CYP2C19).
No products indexed under this heading.

Anastrozole (Concomitant administration of esomeprazole and a combined inhibitor of CYP 2C19 and CYP 3A4, such as voriconazole, may result in more than doubling of the esomeprazole exposure. Dose adjustment of esomeprazole is not normally required. However, in patients with Zollinger-Ellison's Syndrome, who may require higher doses up to 240 mg/day, dose adjustment may be considered).
No products indexed under this heading.

Aprepitant (Concomitant administration of esomeprazole and a combined inhibitor of CYP 2C19 and CYP 3A4, such as voriconazole, may result in more than doubling of the esomeprazole exposure. Dose adjustment of esomeprazole is not normally required. However, in patients with Zollinger-Ellison's Syndrome, who may require higher doses up to 240 mg/day, dose adjustment may be considered).
Products include:

Atazanavir (Concomitant use of atazanavir with proton pump inhibitors is not recommended. Co-administration of atazanavir with proton pump inhibitors is expected to substantially decrease atazanavir plasma concentrations and

thereby reduce its therapeutic effect and lead to the development of drug resistance. Esomeprazole inhibits gastric acid secretion. Therefore, esomeprazole may interfere with the absorption of drugs where gastric pH is an important determinant of bioavailability (eg, atazanavir)).
No products indexed under this heading.

Atazanavir Sulfate (Concomitant use of atazanavir with proton pump inhibitors is not recommended. Co-administration of atazanavir with proton pump inhibitors is expected to substantially decrease atazanavir plasma concentrations and thereby reduce its therapeutic effect and lead to the development of drug resistance. Esomeprazole inhibits gastric acid secretion. Therefore, esomeprazole may interfere with the absorption of drugs where gastric pH is an important determinant of bioavailability (eg, atazanavir)).
No products indexed under this heading.

Bacampicillin Hydrochloride (Esomeprazole inhibits gastric acid secretion. Therefore, esomeprazole may interfere with the absorption of drugs where gastric pH is an important determinant of bioavailability (eg, ketoconazole, atazanavir, iron salts, and digoxin)).
No products indexed under this heading.

Carisoprodol (Esomeprazole may potentially interfere with CYP 2C19, the major esomeprazole metabolizing enzyme. Co-administration of esomeprazole 30 mg and diazepam, a CYP2C19 substrate, resulted in a 45% decrease in clearance of diazepam).
No products indexed under this heading.

Cilostazol (Esomeprazole may potentially interfere with CYP 2C19, the major esomeprazole metabolizing enzyme. Co-administration of esomeprazole 30 mg and diazepam, a CYP2C19 substrate, resulted in a 45% decrease in clearance of diazepam).
No products indexed under this heading.

Cimetidine (Concomitant administration of esomeprazole and a combined inhibitor of CYP 2C19 and CYP 3A4, such as voriconazole, may result in more than doubling of the esomeprazole exposure. Dose adjustment of esomeprazole is not normally required. However, in patients with Zollinger-Ellison's Syndrome, who may require higher doses up to 240 mg/day, dose adjustment may be considered).
No products indexed under this heading.

Cimetidine Hydrochloride (Concomitant administration of esomeprazole and a combined inhibitor of CYP 2C19 and CYP 3A4, such as voriconazole, may result in more than doubling of the esomeprazole exposure. Dose adjustment of esomeprazole is not normally required. However, in patients with Zollinger-Ellison's Syndrome, who may require higher doses up to 240 mg/day, dose adjustment may be considered).
No products indexed under this heading.

Ciprofloxacin (Concomitant administration of esomeprazole and a combined inhibitor of CYP 2C19 and CYP 3A4, such as voriconazole, may result in more than doubling of the esomeprazole exposure. Dose adjustment of esomeprazole is not normally required. However, in patients with Zollinger-Ellison's Syndrome, who may require higher doses up to 240 mg/day, dose adjustment may be considered).
Products include:

Citalopram Hydrobromide (Esomeprazole may potentially interfere with

CYP 2C19, the major esomeprazole metabolizing enzyme. Co-administration of esomeprazole 30 mg and diazepam, a CYP2C19 substrate, resulted in a 45% decrease in clearance of diazepam). Products include:

Clarithromycin (Co-administration of esomeprazole, clarithromycin, and amoxicillin has resulted in increases in the plasma levels of esomeprazole and 14-hydroxyclarithromycin). Products include:

Clomipramine Hydrochloride (Esomeprazole may potentially interfere with CYP 2C19, the major esomeprazole metabolizing enzyme. Co-administration of esomeprazole 30 mg and diazepam, a CYP2C19 substrate, resulted in a 45% decrease in clearance of diazepam).
No products indexed under this heading.

Clotrimazole (Concomitant administration of esomeprazole and a combined inhibitor of CYP 2C19 and CYP 3A4, such as voriconazole, may result in more than doubling of the esomeprazole exposure. Dose adjustment of esomeprazole is not normally required. However, in patients with Zollinger-Ellison's Syndrome, who may require higher doses up to 240 mg/day, dose adjustment may be considered). Products include:

Conivaptan Hydrochloride (Concomitant administration of esomeprazole and a combined inhibitor of CYP 2C19 and CYP 3A4, such as voriconazole, may result in more than doubling of the esomeprazole exposure. Dose adjustment of esomeprazole is not normally required. However, in patients with Zollinger-Ellison's Syndrome, who may require higher doses up to 240 mg/day, dose adjustment may be considered). Products include:

Cyclophosphamide (Esomeprazole may potentially interfere with CYP 2C19, the major esomeprazole metabolizing enzyme. Co-administration of esomeprazole 30 mg and diazepam, a CYP2C19 substrate, resulted in a 45% decrease in clearance of diazepam).
No products indexed under this heading.

Cyclosporine (Concomitant administration of esomeprazole and a combined inhibitor of CYP 2C19 and CYP 3A4, such as voriconazole, may result in more than doubling of the esomeprazole exposure. Dose adjustment of esomeprazole is not normally required. However, in patients with Zollinger-Ellison's Syndrome, who may require higher doses up to 240 mg/day, dose adjustment may be considered). Products include:

Dalfopristin (Concomitant administration of esomeprazole and a combined inhibitor of CYP 2C19 and CYP 3A4, such as voriconazole, may result in more than doubling of the esomeprazole exposure. Dose adjustment of esomeprazole is not normally required. However, in patients with Zollinger-Ellison's Syndrome, who may require higher doses up to 240 mg/day, dose adjustment may be considered).
No products indexed under this heading.

Danazol (Concomitant administration of esomeprazole and a combined inhibitor of CYP 2C19 and CYP 3A4, such as voriconazole, may result in more than doubling of the esomeprazole exposure. Dose adjustment of esomeprazole is not normally required. However, in patients with Zollinger-Ellison's Syndrome, who may require higher doses up to 240 mg/day, dose adjustment may be considered).
No products indexed under this heading.

Darunavir (Omeprazole, of which esomeprazole is an enantiomer, has been reported to interact with some antiretroviral drugs. The clinical importance and the mechanisms behind these interactions are not always known. Increased gastric pH during omeprazole treatment may change the absorption of the antiretroviral drug. Other possible interaction mechanisms are via CYP2C19).
No products indexed under this heading.

Dasatinib (Concomitant administration of esomeprazole and a combined inhibitor of CYP 2C19 and CYP 3A4, such as voriconazole, may result in more than doubling of the esomeprazole exposure. Dose adjustment of esomeprazole is not normally required. However, in patients with Zollinger-Ellison's Syndrome, who may require higher doses up to 240 mg/day, dose adjustment may be considered).
No products indexed under this heading.

Delavirdine Mesylate (Omeprazole, of which esomeprazole is an enantiomer, has been reported to interact with some antiretroviral drugs. The clinical importance and the mechanisms behind these interactions are not always known. Increased gastric pH during omeprazole treatment may change the absorption of the antiretroviral drug. Other possible interaction mechanisms are via CYP2C19).
No products indexed under this heading.

Delavirine (Concomitant administration of esomeprazole and a combined inhibitor of CYP 2C19 and CYP 3A4, such as voriconazole, may result in more than doubling of the esomeprazole exposure. Dose adjustment of esomeprazole is not normally required. However, in patients with Zollinger-Ellison's Syndrome, who may require higher doses up to 240 mg/day, dose adjustment may be considered).
No products indexed under this heading.

Desipramine Hydrochloride (Esomeprazole may potentially interfere with CYP 2C19, the major esomeprazole metabolizing enzyme. Co-administration of esomeprazole 30 mg and diazepam, a CYP2C19 substrate, resulted in a 45% decrease in clearance of diazepam).
No products indexed under this heading.

Desloratadine (Concomitant administration of esomeprazole and a combined inhibitor of CYP 2C19 and CYP 3A4, such as voriconazole, may result in more than doubling of the esomeprazole exposure. Dose adjustment of esomeprazole is not normally required. However, in patients with Zollinger-Ellison's Syndrome, who may require higher doses up to 240 mg/day, dose adjustment may be considered).
Products include:

Desogestrel (Concomitant administration of esomeprazole and a combined inhibitor of CYP 2C19 and CYP 3A4, such as voriconazole, may result in more than doubling of the esomeprazole exposure. Dose adjustment of

esomeprazole is not normally required. However, in patients with Zollinger-Ellison's Syndrome, who may require higher doses up to 240 mg/day, dose adjustment may be considered).
No products indexed under this heading.

Dextromethorphan (Esomeprazole may potentially interfere with CYP 2C19, the major esomeprazole metabolizing enzyme. Co-administration of esomeprazole 30 mg and diazepam, a CYP2C19 substrate, resulted in a 45% decrease in clearance of diazepam).
No products indexed under this heading.

Dextromethorphan Hydrobromide (Esomeprazole may potentially interfere with CYP 2C19, the major esomeprazole metabolizing enzyme. Co-administration of esomeprazole 30 mg and diazepam, a CYP2C19 substrate, resulted in a 45% decrease in clearance of diazepam).
No products indexed under this heading.

Diazepam (Esomeprazole may potentially interfere with CYP 2C19, the major esomeprazole metabolizing enzyme. Co-administration of esomeprazole 30 mg and diazepam, a CYP2C19 substrate, resulted in a 45% decrease in clearance of diazepam). Products include:

Didanosine (Omeprazole, of which esomeprazole is an enantiomer, has been reported to interact with some antiretroviral drugs. The clinical importance and the mechanisms behind these interactions are not always known. Increased gastric pH during omeprazole treatment may change the absorption of the antiretroviral drug. Other possible interaction mechanisms are via CYP2C19).
No products indexed under this heading.

Digoxin (Esomeprazole inhibits gastric acid secretion; therefore, esomeprazole may interfere with the absorption of drugs where gastric pH is an important determinant of bioavailability, such as digoxin). Products include:

Diltiazem Hydrochloride (Concomitant administration of esomeprazole and a combined inhibitor of CYP 2C19 and CYP 3A4, such as voriconazole, may result in more than doubling of the esomeprazole exposure. Dose adjustment of esomeprazole is not normally required. However, in patients with Zollinger-Ellison's Syndrome, who may require higher doses up to 240 mg/day, dose adjustment may be considered).
Products include:

Diltiazem Maleate (Concomitant administration of esomeprazole and a combined inhibitor of CYP 2C19 and CYP 3A4, such as voriconazole, may result in more than doubling of the esomeprazole exposure. Dose adjustment of esomeprazole is not normally required. However, in patients with Zollinger-Ellison's Syndrome, who may require higher doses up to 240 mg/day, dose adjustment may be considered).
No products indexed under this heading.

Divalproex Sodium (Esomeprazole may potentially interfere with CYP 2C19, the major esomeprazole metabolizing enzyme. Co-administration of esomeprazole 30 mg and diazepam, a CYP2C19 substrate, resulted in a 45% decrease in clearance of diazepam).
Products include:

Doxepin Hydrochloride (Esomeprazole may potentially interfere with CYP 2C19, the major esomeprazole metabolizing enzyme. Co-administration of esomeprazole 30 mg and diazepam, a CYP2C19 substrate, resulted in a 45% decrease in clearance of diazepam).
No products indexed under this heading.

Efavirenz (Omeprazole, of which esomeprazole is an enantiomer, has been reported to interact with some antiretroviral drugs. The clinical importance and the mechanisms behind these interactions are not always known. Increased gastric pH during omeprazole treatment may change the absorption of the antiretroviral drug. Other possible interaction mechanisms are via CYP2C19). Products include:

Emtricitabine (Omeprazole, of which esomeprazole is an enantiomer, has been reported to interact with some antiretroviral drugs. The clinical importance and the mechanisms behind these interactions are not always known. Increased gastric pH during omeprazole treatment may change the absorption of the antiretroviral drug. Other possible interaction mechanisms are via CYP2C19). Products include:

Enfuvirtide (Omeprazole, of which esomeprazole is an enantiomer, has been reported to interact with some antiretroviral drugs. The clinical importance and the mechanisms behind these interactions are not always known. Increased gastric pH during omeprazole treatment may change the absorption of the antiretroviral drug. Other possible interaction mechanisms are via CYP2C19).
No products indexed under this heading.

Erythromycin (Concomitant administration of esomeprazole and a combined inhibitor of CYP 2C19 and CYP 3A4, such as voriconazole, may result in more than doubling of the esomeprazole exposure. Dose adjustment of esomeprazole is not normally required. However, in patients with Zollinger-Ellison's Syndrome, who may require higher doses up to 240 mg/day, dose adjustment may be considered).
No products indexed under this heading.

Erythromycin Estolate (Concomitant administration of esomeprazole and a combined inhibitor of CYP 2C19 and CYP 3A4, such as voriconazole, may result in more than doubling of the esomeprazole exposure. Dose adjustment of esomeprazole is not normally required. However, in patients with Zollinger-Ellison's Syndrome, who may require higher doses up to 240 mg/day, dose adjustment may be considered).
No products indexed under this heading.

Erythromycin Ethylsuccinate (Concomitant administration of esomeprazole and a combined inhibitor of CYP 2C19 and CYP 3A4, such as voriconazole, may result in more than doubling of the esomeprazole exposure. Dose adjustment of esomeprazole is not normally required. However, in patients with Zollinger-Ellison's Syndrome, who may require higher doses up to 240 mg/day, dose adjustment may be considered). Products include:

Erythromycin Gluceptate (Concomitant administration of esomeprazole and a combined inhibitor of CYP 2C19 and CYP 3A4, such as voriconazole, may result in more than doubling of the esomeprazole exposure. Dose adjustment of esomeprazole is not normally

required. However, in patients with Zollinger-Ellison's Syndrome, who may require higher doses up to 240 mg/day, dose adjustment may be considered).
No products indexed under this heading.

Erythromycin Lactobionate (Concomitant administration of esomeprazole and a combined inhibitor of CYP 2C19 and CYP 3A4, such as voriconazole, may result in more than doubling of the esomeprazole exposure. Dose adjustment of esomeprazole is not normally required. However, in patients with Zollinger-Ellison's Syndrome, who may require higher doses up to 240 mg/day, dose adjustment may be considered).
No products indexed under this heading.

Erythromycin Stearate (Concomitant administration of esomeprazole and a combined inhibitor of CYP 2C19 and CYP 3A4, such as voriconazole, may result in more than doubling of the esomeprazole exposure. Dose adjustment of esomeprazole is not normally required. However, in patients with Zollinger-Ellison's Syndrome, who may require higher doses up to 240 mg/day, dose adjustment may be considered).
No products indexed under this heading.

Esomeprazole Sodium (Esomeprazole may potentially interfere with CYP 2C19, the major esomeprazole metabolizing enzyme. Co-administration of esomeprazole 30 mg and diazepam, a CYP2C19 substrate, resulted in a 45% decrease in clearance of diazepam). Products include:

Ethinyl Estradiol (Concomitant administration of esomeprazole and a combined inhibitor of CYP 2C19 and CYP 3A4, such as voriconazole, may result in more than doubling of the esomeprazole exposure. Dose adjustment of esomeprazole is not normally required. However, in patients with Zollinger-Ellison's Syndrome, who may require higher doses up to 240 mg/day, dose adjustment may be considered). Products include:

Ethosuximide (Esomeprazole may potentially interfere with CYP 2C19, the major esomeprazole metabolizing enzyme. Co-administration of esomeprazole 30 mg and diazepam, a CYP2C19 substrate, resulted in a 45% decrease in clearance of diazepam).
No products indexed under this heading.

Ethotoin (Esomeprazole may potentially interfere with CYP 2C19, the major esomeprazole metabolizing enzyme. Co-administration of esomeprazole 30 mg and diazepam, a CYP2C19 substrate, resulted in a 45% decrease in clearance of diazepam).
No products indexed under this heading.

Ethynodiol Diacetate (Concomitant administration of esomeprazole and a combined inhibitor of CYP 2C19 and CYP 3A4, such as voriconazole, may result in more than doubling of the esomeprazole exposure. Dose adjustment of esomeprazole is not normally required. However, in patients with Zollinger-Ellison's Syndrome, who may require higher doses up to 240 mg/day, dose adjustment may be considered).
No products indexed under this heading.

IMPORTANT NOTE: Always consult each drug listing in the patient's regimen for possible interactions.

Nexium Interactions Index 1188

Felbamate (Esomeprazole may potentially interfere with CYP 2C19, the major esomeprazole metabolizing enzyme. Co-administration of esomeprazole 30 mg and diazepam, a CYP2C19 substrate, resulted in a 45% decrease in clearance of diazepam).
No products indexed under this heading.

Ferrous Fumarate (Esomeprazole inhibits gastric acid secretion; therefore, esomeprazole may interfere with the absorption of drugs where gastric pH is an important determinant of bioavailability, such as oral iron salts). Products include:
PreNexa 3473

Ferrous Gluconate (Esomeprazole inhibits gastric acid secretion; therefore, esomeprazole may interfere with the absorption of drugs where gastric pH is an important determinant of bioavailability, such as oral iron salts). Products include:
CitraNatal Assure 2332
CitraNatal Rx 2332

Ferrous Sulfate (Esomeprazole inhibits gastric acid secretion; therefore, esomeprazole may interfere with the absorption of drugs where gastric pH is an important determinant of bioavailability, such as oral iron salts).
No products indexed under this heading.

Fluconazole (Concomitant administration of esomeprazole and a combined inhibitor of CYP 2C19 and CYP 3A4, such as voriconazole, may result in more than doubling of the esomeprazole exposure. Dose adjustment of esomeprazole is not normally required. However, in patients with Zollinger-Ellison's Syndrome, who may require higher doses up to 240 mg/day, dose adjustment may be considered).
No products indexed under this heading.

Fluoxetine (Concomitant administration of esomeprazole and a combined inhibitor of CYP 2C19 and CYP 3A4, such as voriconazole, may result in more than doubling of the esomeprazole exposure. Dose adjustment of esomeprazole is not normally required. However, in patients with Zollinger-Ellison's Syndrome, who may require higher doses up to 240 mg/day, dose adjustment may be considered).
No products indexed under this heading.

Fluoxetine Hydrochloride (Concomitant administration of esomeprazole and a combined inhibitor of CYP 2C19 and CYP 3A4, such as voriconazole, may result in more than doubling of the esomeprazole exposure. Dose adjustment of esomeprazole is not normally required. However, in patients with Zollinger-Ellison's Syndrome, who may require higher doses up to 240 mg/day, dose adjustment may be considered). Products include:
Prozac Weekly 1941
Prozac Pulvules 1941
Symbyax 1965

Fluvastatin Sodium (Concomitant administration of esomeprazole and a combined inhibitor of CYP 2C19 and CYP 3A4, such as voriconazole, may result in more than doubling of the esomeprazole exposure. Dose adjustment of esomeprazole is not normally required. However, in patients with Zollinger-Ellison's Syndrome, who may require higher doses up to 240 mg/day, dose adjustment may be considered).
No products indexed under this heading.

Fluvoxamine (Concomitant administration of esomeprazole and a combined inhibitor of CYP 2C19 and CYP 3A4, such as voriconazole, may result in more than doubling of the esomeprazole exposure. Dose adjustment of esomeprazole is not normally required. However, in patients with Zollinger-Ellison's Syndrome, who may require higher doses up to 240 mg/day, dose adjustment may be considered).
No products indexed under this heading.

Fluvoxamine Maleate (Concomitant administration of esomeprazole and a combined inhibitor of CYP 2C19 and CYP 3A4, such as voriconazole, may result in more than doubling of the esomeprazole exposure. Dose adjustment of esomeprazole is not normally required. However, in patients with Zollinger-Ellison's Syndrome, who may require higher doses up to 240 mg/day, dose adjustment may be considered).
No products indexed under this heading.

Formoterol Fumarate (Esomeprazole may potentially interfere with CYP 2C19, the major esomeprazole metabolizing enzyme. Co-administration of esomeprazole 30 mg and diazepam, a CYP2C19 substrate, resulted in a 45% decrease in clearance of diazepam). Products include:
Foradil 3121
Perforomist 3634

Fosamprenavir Calcium (Omeprazole, of which esomeprazole is an enantiomer, has been reported to interact with some antiretroviral drugs. The clinical importance and the mechanisms behind these interactions are not always known. Increased gastric pH during omeprazole treatment may change the absorption of the antiretroviral drug. Other possible interaction mechanisms are via CYP2C19). Products include:
Lexiva Oral Suspension 1558
Lexiva 1558

Fosphenytoin (Esomeprazole may potentially interfere with CYP 2C19, the major esomeprazole metabolizing enzyme. Co-administration of esomeprazole 30 mg and diazepam, a CYP2C19 substrate, resulted in a 45% decrease in clearance of diazepam).
No products indexed under this heading.

Fosphenytoin Sodium (Esomeprazole may potentially interfere with CYP 2C19, the major esomeprazole metabolizing enzyme. Co-administration of esomeprazole 30 mg and diazepam, a CYP2C19 substrate, resulted in a 45% decrease in clearance of diazepam).
No products indexed under this heading.

Gabapentin (Esomeprazole may potentially interfere with CYP 2C19, the major esomeprazole metabolizing enzyme. Co-administration of esomeprazole 30 mg and diazepam, a CYP2C19 substrate, resulted in a 45% decrease in clearance of diazepam).
No products indexed under this heading.

Imatinib Mesylate (Concomitant administration of esomeprazole and a combined inhibitor of CYP 2C19 and CYP 3A4, such as voriconazole, may result in more than doubling of the esomeprazole exposure. Dose adjustment of esomeprazole is not normally required. However, in patients with Zollinger-Ellison's Syndrome, who may require higher doses up to 240 mg/day, dose adjustment may be considered). Products include:
Gleevec 2477

Imipramine Hydrochloride (Esomeprazole may potentially interfere with CYP 2C19, the major esomeprazole metabolizing enzyme. Co-administration of esomeprazole 30 mg and diazepam, a CYP2C19 substrate, resulted in a 45% decrease in clearance of diazepam).
No products indexed under this heading.

Imipramine Pamoate (Esomeprazole may potentially interfere with CYP 2C19, the major esomeprazole metabolizing enzyme. Co-administration of esomeprazole 30 mg and diazepam, a CYP2C19 substrate, resulted in a 45% decrease in clearance of diazepam).
No products indexed under this heading.

Indinavir Sulfate (Omeprazole, of which esomeprazole is an enantiomer, has been reported to interact with some antiretroviral drugs. The clinical importance and the mechanisms behind these interactions are not always known. Increased gastric pH during omeprazole treatment may change the absorption of the antiretroviral drug. Other possible interaction mechanisms are via CYP2C19). Products include:
Crixivan 2113

Indomethacin (Esomeprazole may potentially interfere with CYP 2C19, the major esomeprazole metabolizing enzyme. Co-administration of esomeprazole 30 mg and diazepam, a CYP2C19 substrate, resulted in a 45% decrease in clearance of diazepam). Products include:
Indocin 2167

Indomethacin Sodium Trihydrate (Esomeprazole may potentially interfere with CYP 2C19, the major esomeprazole metabolizing enzyme. Co-administration of esomeprazole 30 mg and diazepam, a CYP2C19 substrate, resulted in a 45% decrease in clearance of diazepam). Products include:
Indocin I.V. 2007

Iron (Esomeprazole inhibits gastric acid secretion; therefore, esomeprazole may interfere with the absorption of drugs where gastric pH is an important determinant of bioavailability, such as oral iron salts).
No products indexed under this heading.

Iron, Peptonized (Esomeprazole inhibits gastric acid secretion; therefore, esomeprazole may interfere with the absorption of drugs where gastric pH is an important determinant of bioavailability, such as oral iron salts).
No products indexed under this heading.

Iron Cacodylate (Esomeprazole inhibits gastric acid secretion; therefore, esomeprazole may interfere with the absorption of drugs where gastric pH is an important determinant of bioavailability, such as oral iron salts).
No products indexed under this heading.

Iron Carbonyl (Esomeprazole inhibits gastric acid secretion; therefore, esomeprazole may interfere with the absorption of drugs where gastric pH is an important determinant of bioavailability, such as oral iron salts). Products include:
CitraNatal 90 DHA Capsules 2332
CitraNatal Assure 2332
CitraNatal Harmony 2332
CitraNatal Rx 2332
Ferralet 2333

Iron Dextran (Esomeprazole inhibits gastric acid secretion; therefore, esomeprazole may interfere with the absorption of drugs where gastric pH is an important determinant of bioavailability, such as oral iron salts).
No products indexed under this heading.

Iron Polysaccharide Complex (Esomeprazole inhibits gastric acid secretion; therefore, esomeprazole may interfere with the absorption of drugs where gastric pH is an important determinant of bioavailability, such as oral iron salts).
No products indexed under this heading.

Iron Sucrose (Esomeprazole inhibits gastric acid secretion; therefore, esomeprazole may interfere with the absorption of drugs where gastric pH is an important determinant of bioavailability, such as oral iron salts).
No products indexed under this heading.

Iron Supplements (Esomeprazole inhibits gastric acid secretion; therefore, esomeprazole may interfere with the absorption of drugs where gastric pH is an important determinant of bioavailability, such as oral iron salts).
No products indexed under this heading.

Isoniazid (Concomitant administration of esomeprazole and a combined inhibitor of CYP 2C19 and CYP 3A4, such as voriconazole, may result in more than doubling of the esomeprazole exposure. Dose adjustment of esomeprazole is not normally required. However, in patients with Zollinger-Ellison's Syndrome, who may require higher doses up to 240 mg/day, dose adjustment may be considered).
No products indexed under this heading.

Itraconazole (Concomitant administration of esomeprazole and a combined inhibitor of CYP 2C19 and CYP 3A4, such as voriconazole, may result in more than doubling of the esomeprazole exposure. Dose adjustment of esomeprazole is not normally required. However, in patients with Zollinger-Ellison's Syndrome, who may require higher doses up to 240 mg/day, dose adjustment may be considered).
No products indexed under this heading.

Ketoconazole (Esomeprazole inhibits gastric acid secretion; therefore, esomeprazole may interfere with the absorption of drugs where gastric pH is an important determinant of bioavailability, such as ketoconazole). Products include:
Extina 3319
Xolegel 3337

Lamium album (Omeprazole, of which esomeprazole is an enantiomer, has been reported to interact with some antiretroviral drugs. The clinical importance and the mechanisms behind these interactions are not always known. Increased gastric pH during omeprazole treatment may change the absorption of the antiretroviral drug. Other possible interaction mechanisms are via CYP2C19).
No products indexed under this heading.

Lamotrigine (Esomeprazole may potentially interfere with CYP 2C19, the major esomeprazole metabolizing enzyme. Co-administration of esomeprazole 30 mg and diazepam, a CYP2C19 substrate, resulted in a 45% decrease in clearance of diazepam). Products include:
Lamictal 1522
Lamictal ODT 1522
Lamictal XR 1536

Lansoprazole (Esomeprazole may potentially interfere with CYP 2C19, the major esomeprazole metabolizing enzyme. Co-administration of esomeprazole 30 mg and diazepam, a CYP2C19 substrate, resulted in a 45% decrease in clearance of diazepam).
No products indexed under this heading.

Lapatinib (Concomitant administration of esomeprazole and a combined inhibitor of CYP 2C19 and CYP 3A4, such as voriconazole, may result in more than doubling of the esomeprazole exposure. Dose adjustment of esomeprazole is not normally required. However, in patients with Zollinger-Ellison's Syndrome, who may require higher doses up to 240 mg/day, dose adjustment may be considered). Products include:
Tykerb 1698

Letrozole (Concomitant administration of esomeprazole and a combined inhibi-

tor of CYP 2C19 and CYP 3A4, such as voriconazole, may result in more than doubling of the esomeprazole exposure. Dose adjustment of esomeprazole is not normally required. However, in patients with Zollinger-Ellison's Syndrome, who may require higher doses up to 240 mg/day, dose adjustment may be considered). Products include:

Levetiracetam (Esomeprazole may potentially interfere with CYP 2C19, the major esomeprazole metabolizing enzyme. Co-administration of esomeprazole 30 mg and diazepam, a CYP2C19 substrate, resulted in a 45% decrease in clearance of diazepam). Products include:

Levonorgestrel (Concomitant administration of esomeprazole and a combined inhibitor of CYP 2C19 and CYP 3A4, such as voriconazole, may result in more than doubling of the esomeprazole exposure. Dose adjustment of esomeprazole is not normally required. However, in patients with Zollinger-Ellison's Syndrome, who may require higher doses up to 240 mg/day, dose adjustment may be considered). Products include:

Lopinavir (Omeprazole, of which esomeprazole is an enantiomer, has been reported to interact with some antiretroviral drugs. The clinical importance and the mechanisms behind these interactions are not always known. Increased gastric pH during omeprazole treatment may change the absorption of the antiretroviral drug. Other possible interaction mechanisms are via CYP2C19). Products include:

Loratadine (Concomitant administration of esomeprazole and a combined inhibitor of CYP 2C19 and CYP 3A4, such as voriconazole, may result in more than doubling of the esomeprazole exposure. Dose adjustment of esomeprazole is not normally required. However, in patients with Zollinger-Ellison's Syndrome, who may require higher doses up to 240 mg/day, dose adjustment may be considered).
No products indexed under this heading.

Maprotiline Hydrochloride (Esomeprazole may potentially interfere with CYP 2C19, the major esomeprazole metabolizing enzyme. Co-administration of esomeprazole 30 mg and diazepam, a CYP2C19 substrate, resulted in a 45% decrease in clearance of diazepam).
No products indexed under this heading.

Mephenytoin (Esomeprazole may potentially interfere with CYP 2C19, the major esomeprazole metabolizing enzyme. Co-administration of esomeprazole 30 mg and diazepam, a CYP2C19 substrate, resulted in a 45% decrease in clearance of diazepam).
No products indexed under this heading.

Mephobarbital (Esomeprazole may potentially interfere with CYP 2C19, the major esomeprazole metabolizing enzyme. Co-administration of esomeprazole 30 mg and diazepam, a CYP2C19 substrate, resulted in a 45% decrease in clearance of diazepam).
No products indexed under this heading.

Meprobamate (Esomeprazole may potentially interfere with CYP 2C19, the major esomeprazole metabolizing enzyme. Co-administration of esomeprazole 30 mg and diazepam, a CYP2C19 substrate, resulted in a 45% decrease in clearance of diazepam).
No products indexed under this heading.

Mestranol (Concomitant administration of esomeprazole and a combined inhibitor of CYP 2C19 and CYP 3A4, such as voriconazole, may result in more than doubling of the esomeprazole exposure. Dose adjustment of esomeprazole is not normally required. However, in patients with Zollinger-Ellison's Syndrome, who may require higher doses up to 240 mg/day, dose adjustment may be considered).
No products indexed under this heading.

Methsuximide (Esomeprazole may potentially interfere with CYP 2C19, the major esomeprazole metabolizing enzyme. Co-administration of esomeprazole 30 mg and diazepam, a CYP2C19 substrate, resulted in a 45% decrease in clearance of diazepam).
No products indexed under this heading.

Metronidazole (Concomitant administration of esomeprazole and a combined inhibitor of CYP 2C19 and CYP 3A4, such as voriconazole, may result in more than doubling of the esomeprazole exposure. Dose adjustment of esomeprazole is not normally required. However, in patients with Zollinger-Ellison's Syndrome, who may require higher doses up to 240 mg/day, dose adjustment may be considered). Products include:

Metronidazole Benzoate (Concomitant administration of esomeprazole and a combined inhibitor of CYP 2C19 and CYP 3A4, such as voriconazole, may result in more than doubling of the esomeprazole exposure. Dose adjustment of esomeprazole is not normally required. However, in patients with Zollinger-Ellison's Syndrome, who may require higher doses up to 240 mg/day, dose adjustment may be considered).
No products indexed under this heading.

Metronidazole Hydrochloride (Concomitant administration of esomeprazole and a combined inhibitor of CYP 2C19 and CYP 3A4, such as voriconazole, may result in more than doubling of the esomeprazole exposure. Dose adjustment of esomeprazole is not normally required. However, in patients with Zollinger-Ellison's Syndrome, who may require higher doses up to 240 mg/day, dose adjustment may be considered).
No products indexed under this heading.

Metronidazole Sodium (Concomitant administration of esomeprazole and a combined inhibitor of CYP 2C19 and CYP 3A4, such as voriconazole, may result in more than doubling of the esomeprazole exposure. Dose adjustment of esomeprazole is not normally required. However, in patients with Zollinger-Ellison's Syndrome, who may require higher doses up to 240 mg/day, dose adjustment may be considered).
No products indexed under this heading.

Miconazole (Concomitant administration of esomeprazole and a combined inhibitor of CYP 2C19 and CYP 3A4, such as voriconazole, may result in more than doubling of the esomeprazole exposure. Dose adjustment of esomeprazole is not normally required. However, in patients with Zollinger-Ellison's Syndrome, who may require higher doses up to 240 mg/day, dose adjustment may be considered).
No products indexed under this heading.

Miconazole Nitrate (Concomitant administration of esomeprazole and a

combined inhibitor of CYP 2C19 and CYP 3A4, such as voriconazole, may result in more than doubling of the esomeprazole exposure. Dose adjustment of esomeprazole is not normally required. However, in patients with Zollinger-Ellison's Syndrome, who may require higher doses up to 240 mg/day, dose adjustment may be considered). Products include:

Midazolam Hydrochloride (Esomeprazole may potentially interfere with CYP 2C19, the major esomeprazole metabolizing enzyme. Co-administration of esomeprazole 30 mg and diazepam, a CYP2C19 substrate, resulted in a 45% decrease in clearance of diazepam).
No products indexed under this heading.

Mifepristone (Concomitant administration of esomeprazole and a combined inhibitor of CYP 2C19 and CYP 3A4, such as voriconazole, may result in more than doubling of the esomeprazole exposure. Dose adjustment of esomeprazole is not normally required. However, in patients with Zollinger-Ellison's Syndrome, who may require higher doses up to 240 mg/day, dose adjustment may be considered).
No products indexed under this heading.

Modafinil (Concomitant administration of esomeprazole and a combined inhibitor of CYP 2C19 and CYP 3A4, such as voriconazole, may result in more than doubling of the esomeprazole exposure. Dose adjustment of esomeprazole is not normally required. However, in patients with Zollinger-Ellison's Syndrome, who may require higher doses up to 240 mg/day, dose adjustment may be considered). Products include:

Nefazodone Hydrochloride (Concomitant administration of esomeprazole and a combined inhibitor of CYP 2C19 and CYP 3A4, such as voriconazole, may result in more than doubling of the esomeprazole exposure. Dose adjustment of esomeprazole is not normally required. However, in patients with Zollinger-Ellison's Syndrome, who may require higher doses up to 240 mg/day, dose adjustment may be considered).
No products indexed under this heading.

Nelfinavir Mesylate (Concomitant use of nelfinavir with proton pump inhibitors is not recommended. Following multiple doses of nelfinavir (1250 mg, twice daily) and omeprazole (40 mg daily), AUC was decreased by 36% and 92%, C_{max} by 37% and 89% and C_{min} by 39% and 75% respectively for nelfinavir and M8).
No products indexed under this heading.

Nevirapine (Omeprazole, of which esomeprazole is an enantiomer, has been reported to interact with some antiretroviral drugs. The clinical importance and the mechanisms behind these interactions are not always known. Increased gastric pH during omeprazole treatment may change the absorption of the antiretroviral drug. Other possible interaction mechanisms are via CYP2C19). Products include:

Niacin (Concomitant administration of esomeprazole and a combined inhibitor of CYP 2C19 and CYP 3A4, such as voriconazole, may result in more than doubling of the esomeprazole exposure. Dose adjustment of esomeprazole is not normally required. However, in patients with Zollinger-Ellison's Syndrome, who may require higher doses up to 240 mg/day, dose adjustment may be considered). Products include:

Niacinamide (Concomitant administration of esomeprazole and a combined inhibitor of CYP 2C19 and CYP 3A4, such as voriconazole, may result in more than doubling of the esomeprazole exposure. Dose adjustment of esomeprazole is not normally required. However, in patients with Zollinger-Ellison's Syndrome, who may require higher doses up to 240 mg/day, dose adjustment may be considered). Products include:

Niacinamide Hydroiodide (Concomitant administration of esomeprazole and a combined inhibitor of CYP 2C19 and CYP 3A4, such as voriconazole, may result in more than doubling of the esomeprazole exposure. Dose adjustment of esomeprazole is not normally required. However, in patients with Zollinger-Ellison's Syndrome, who may require higher doses up to 240 mg/day, dose adjustment may be considered).
No products indexed under this heading.

Nicotinamide (Concomitant administration of esomeprazole and a combined inhibitor of CYP 2C19 and CYP 3A4, such as voriconazole, may result in more than doubling of the esomeprazole exposure. Dose adjustment of esomeprazole is not normally required. However, in patients with Zollinger-Ellison's Syndrome, who may require higher doses up to 240 mg/day, dose adjustment may be considered).
No products indexed under this heading.

Nifedipine (Concomitant administration of esomeprazole and a combined inhibitor of CYP 2C19 and CYP 3A4, such as voriconazole, may result in more than doubling of the esomeprazole exposure. Dose adjustment of esomeprazole is not normally required. However, in patients with Zollinger-Ellison's Syndrome, who may require higher doses up to 240 mg/day, dose adjustment may be considered).
No products indexed under this heading.

Nilutamide (Esomeprazole may potentially interfere with CYP 2C19, the major esomeprazole metabolizing enzyme. Co-administration of esomeprazole 30 mg and diazepam, a CYP2C19 substrate, resulted in a 45% decrease in clearance of diazepam).
No products indexed under this heading.

Norethindrone (Concomitant administration of esomeprazole and a combined inhibitor of CYP 2C19 and CYP 3A4, such as voriconazole, may result in more than doubling of the esomeprazole exposure. Dose adjustment of esomeprazole is not normally required. However, in patients with Zollinger-Ellison's Syndrome, who may require higher doses up to 240 mg/day, dose adjustment may be considered). Products include:

Norethynodrel (Concomitant administration of esomeprazole and a combined inhibitor of CYP 2C19 and CYP 3A4, such as voriconazole, may result in more than doubling of the esomeprazole exposure. Dose adjustment of esomeprazole is not normally required. However, in patients with Zollinger-Ellison's Syndrome, who may require higher doses up to 240 mg/day, dose adjustment may be considered).
No products indexed under this heading.

Norfloxacin (Concomitant administration of esomeprazole and a combined inhibitor of CYP 2C19 and CYP 3A4, such as voriconazole, may result in

more than doubling of the esomeprazole exposure. Dose adjustment of esomeprazole is not normally required. However, in patients with Zollinger-Ellison's Syndrome, who may require higher doses up to 240 mg/day, dose adjustment may be considered).
Products include:
Noroxin ... 2220

Norgestimate (Concomitant administration of esomeprazole and a combined inhibitor of CYP 2C19 and CYP 3A4, such as voriconazole, may result in more than doubling of the esomeprazole exposure. Dose adjustment of esomeprazole is not normally required. However, in patients with Zollinger-Ellison's Syndrome, who may require higher doses up to 240 mg/day, dose adjustment may be considered).
Products include:
Ortho-Cyclen/Ortho Tri-Cyclen ... 2663
Ortho Tri-Cyclen Lo Tablets ... 2673

Norgestrel (Concomitant administration of esomeprazole and a combined inhibitor of CYP 2C19 and CYP 3A4, such as voriconazole, may result in more than doubling of the esomeprazole exposure. Dose adjustment of esomeprazole is not normally required. However, in patients with Zollinger-Ellison's Syndrome, who may require higher doses up to 240 mg/day, dose adjustment may be considered).
No products indexed under this heading.

Nortriptyline Hydrochloride (Esomeprazole may potentially interfere with CYP 2C19, the major esomeprazole metabolizing enzyme. Co-administration of esomeprazole 30 mg and diazepam, a CYP2C19 substrate, resulted in a 45% decrease in clearance of diazepam).
No products indexed under this heading.

Omeprazole (Esomeprazole may potentially interfere with CYP 2C19, the major esomeprazole metabolizing enzyme. Co-administration of esomeprazole 30 mg and diazepam, a CYP2C19 substrate, resulted in a 45% decrease in clearance of diazepam).
No products indexed under this heading.

Omeprazole Magnesium (Esomeprazole may potentially interfere with CYP 2C19, the major esomeprazole metabolizing enzyme. Co-administration of esomeprazole 30 mg and diazepam, a CYP2C19 substrate, resulted in a 45% decrease in clearance of diazepam).
No products indexed under this heading.

Oxcarbazepine (Esomeprazole may potentially interfere with CYP 2C19, the major esomeprazole metabolizing enzyme. Co-administration of esomeprazole 30 mg and diazepam, a CYP2C19 substrate, resulted in a 45% decrease in clearance of diazepam).
No products indexed under this heading.

Pantoprazole Sodium (Esomeprazole may potentially interfere with CYP 2C19, the major esomeprazole metabolizing enzyme. Co-administration of esomeprazole 30 mg and diazepam, a CYP2C19 substrate, resulted in a 45% decrease in clearance of diazepam).
Products include:
Protonix Tablets ... 3571
Protonix ... 3575

Paramethadione (Esomeprazole may potentially interfere with CYP 2C19, the major esomeprazole metabolizing enzyme. Co-administration of esomeprazole 30 mg and diazepam, a CYP2C19 substrate, resulted in a 45% decrease in clearance of diazepam).
No products indexed under this heading.

Paroxetine Hydrochloride (Concomitant administration of esomeprazole and a combined inhibitor of CYP 2C19 and CYP 3A4, such as voriconazole, may result in more than doubling of the esomeprazole exposure. Dose adjustment of esomeprazole is not normally required. However, in patients with Zollinger-Ellison's Syndrome, who may require higher doses up to 240 mg/day, dose adjustment may be considered).
Products include:
Paroxetine CR ... 2361
Paroxetine ER ... 2371
Paxil ... 1586
Paxil CR ... 1596

Pentamidine Isethionate (Esomeprazole may potentially interfere with CYP 2C19, the major esomeprazole metabolizing enzyme. Co-administration of esomeprazole 30 mg and diazepam, a CYP2C19 substrate, resulted in a 45% decrease in clearance of diazepam).
No products indexed under this heading.

Phenacemide (Esomeprazole may potentially interfere with CYP 2C19, the major esomeprazole metabolizing enzyme. Co-administration of esomeprazole 30 mg and diazepam, a CYP2C19 substrate, resulted in a 45% decrease in clearance of diazepam).
No products indexed under this heading.

Phenobarbital (Esomeprazole may potentially interfere with CYP 2C19, the major esomeprazole metabolizing enzyme. Co-administration of esomeprazole 30 mg and diazepam, a CYP2C19 substrate, resulted in a 45% decrease in clearance of diazepam).
Products include:
Donnatal ... 2711

Phenobarbital Sodium (Esomeprazole may potentially interfere with CYP 2C19, the major esomeprazole metabolizing enzyme. Co-administration of esomeprazole 30 mg and diazepam, a CYP2C19 substrate, resulted in a 45% decrease in clearance of diazepam).
No products indexed under this heading.

Phensuximide (Esomeprazole may potentially interfere with CYP 2C19, the major esomeprazole metabolizing enzyme. Co-administration of esomeprazole 30 mg and diazepam, a CYP2C19 substrate, resulted in a 45% decrease in clearance of diazepam).
No products indexed under this heading.

Phenytoin (Esomeprazole may potentially interfere with CYP 2C19, the major esomeprazole metabolizing enzyme. Co-administration of esomeprazole 30 mg and diazepam, a CYP2C19 substrate, resulted in a 45% decrease in clearance of diazepam).
No products indexed under this heading.

Phenytoin Sodium (Esomeprazole may potentially interfere with CYP 2C19, the major esomeprazole metabolizing enzyme. Co-administration of esomeprazole 30 mg and diazepam, a CYP2C19 substrate, resulted in a 45% decrease in clearance of diazepam).
Products include:
Phenytek Capsules ... 2380

Polysaccharide Iron Complex (Esomeprazole inhibits gastric acid secretion; therefore, esomeprazole may interfere with the absorption of drugs where gastric pH is an important determinant of bioavailability, such as oral iron salts). Products include:
Nu-Iron 150 ... 2321

Posaconazole (Concomitant administration of esomeprazole and a combined inhibitor of CYP 2C19 and CYP 3A4, such as voriconazole, may result in more than doubling of the esomeprazole exposure. Dose adjustment of esomeprazole is not normally required. However, in patients with Zollinger-Ellison's Syndrome, who may require higher doses up to 240 mg/day, dose adjustment may be considered).
Products include:
Noxafil ... 3172

Primidone (Esomeprazole may potentially interfere with CYP 2C19, the major esomeprazole metabolizing enzyme. Co-administration of esomeprazole 30 mg and diazepam, a CYP2C19 substrate, resulted in a 45% decrease in clearance of diazepam).
No products indexed under this heading.

Progesterone (Esomeprazole may potentially interfere with CYP 2C19, the major esomeprazole metabolizing enzyme. Co-administration of esomeprazole 30 mg and diazepam, a CYP2C19 substrate, resulted in a 45% decrease in clearance of diazepam).
Products include:
Crinone 4% ... 996
Crinone 8% ... 996
Prometrium ... 3307

Proguanil Hydrochloride (Esomeprazole may potentially interfere with CYP 2C19, the major esomeprazole metabolizing enzyme. Co-administration of esomeprazole 30 mg and diazepam, a CYP2C19 substrate, resulted in a 45% decrease in clearance of diazepam). Products include:
Malarone Pediatric Tablets ... 1572
Malarone ... 1572

Propoxyphene Hydrochloride (Concomitant administration of esomeprazole and a combined inhibitor of CYP 2C19 and CYP 3A4, such as voriconazole, may result in more than doubling of the esomeprazole exposure. Dose adjustment of esomeprazole is not normally required. However, in patients with Zollinger-Ellison's Syndrome, who may require higher doses up to 240 mg/day, dose adjustment may be considered).
No products indexed under this heading.

Propoxyphene Napsylate (Concomitant administration of esomeprazole and a combined inhibitor of CYP 2C19 and CYP 3A4, such as voriconazole, may result in more than doubling of the esomeprazole exposure. Dose adjustment of esomeprazole is not normally required. However, in patients with Zollinger-Ellison's Syndrome, who may require higher doses up to 240 mg/day, dose adjustment may be considered).
No products indexed under this heading.

Propranolol Hydrochloride (Esomeprazole may potentially interfere with CYP 2C19, the major esomeprazole metabolizing enzyme. Co-administration of esomeprazole 30 mg and diazepam, a CYP2C19 substrate, resulted in a 45% decrease in clearance of diazepam). Products include:
InnoPran XL ... 1517

Protriptyline Hydrochloride (Esomeprazole may potentially interfere with CYP 2C19, the major esomeprazole metabolizing enzyme. Co-administration of esomeprazole 30 mg and diazepam, a CYP2C19 substrate, resulted in a 45% decrease in clearance of diazepam).
No products indexed under this heading.

Quinidine (Concomitant administration of esomeprazole and a combined inhibitor of CYP 2C19 and CYP 3A4, such as voriconazole, may result in more than doubling of the esomeprazole exposure. Dose adjustment of esomeprazole is not normally required. However, in patients with Zollinger-Ellison's Syndrome, who may require higher doses up to 240 mg/day, dose adjustment may be considered).
No products indexed under this heading.

Quinidine Gluconate (Concomitant administration of esomeprazole and a combined inhibitor of CYP 2C19 and CYP 3A4, such as voriconazole, may result in more than doubling of the esomeprazole exposure. Dose adjustment of esomeprazole is not normally required. However, in patients with Zollinger-Ellison's Syndrome, who may require higher doses up to 240 mg/day, dose adjustment may be considered).
No products indexed under this heading.

Quinidine Hydrochloride (Concomitant administration of esomeprazole and a combined inhibitor of CYP 2C19 and CYP 3A4, such as voriconazole, may result in more than doubling of the esomeprazole exposure. Dose adjustment of esomeprazole is not normally required. However, in patients with Zollinger-Ellison's Syndrome, who may require higher doses up to 240 mg/day, dose adjustment may be considered).
No products indexed under this heading.

Quinidine Polygalacturonate (Concomitant administration of esomeprazole and a combined inhibitor of CYP 2C19 and CYP 3A4, such as voriconazole, may result in more than doubling of the esomeprazole exposure. Dose adjustment of esomeprazole is not normally required. However, in patients with Zollinger-Ellison's Syndrome, who may require higher doses up to 240 mg/day, dose adjustment may be considered).
No products indexed under this heading.

Quinidine Sulfate (Concomitant administration of esomeprazole and a combined inhibitor of CYP 2C19 and CYP 3A4, such as voriconazole, may result in more than doubling of the esomeprazole exposure. Dose adjustment of esomeprazole is not normally required. However, in patients with Zollinger-Ellison's Syndrome, who may require higher doses up to 240 mg/day, dose adjustment may be considered).
No products indexed under this heading.

Quinine (Concomitant administration of esomeprazole and a combined inhibitor of CYP 2C19 and CYP 3A4, such as voriconazole, may result in more than doubling of the esomeprazole exposure. Dose adjustment of esomeprazole is not normally required. However, in patients with Zollinger-Ellison's Syndrome, who may require higher doses up to 240 mg/day, dose adjustment may be considered). Products include:
Hyland's Leg Cramps PM with Quinine ... 3315

Quinine Sulfate (Concomitant administration of esomeprazole and a combined inhibitor of CYP 2C19 and CYP 3A4, such as voriconazole, may result in more than doubling of the esomeprazole exposure. Dose adjustment of esomeprazole is not normally required. However, in patients with Zollinger-Ellison's Syndrome, who may require higher doses up to 240 mg/day, dose adjustment may be considered).
No products indexed under this heading.

Quinupristin (Concomitant administration of esomeprazole and a combined inhibitor of CYP 2C19 and CYP 3A4, such as voriconazole, may result in more than doubling of the esomeprazole exposure. Dose adjustment of esomeprazole is not normally required. However, in patients with Zollinger-Ellison's Syndrome, who may require higher doses up to 240 mg/day, dose adjustment may be considered).
No products indexed under this heading.

Rabeprazole Sodium (Esomeprazole may potentially interfere with CYP 2C19, the major esomeprazole metabolizing enzyme. Co-administration of esomeprazole 30 mg and diazepam, a CYP2C19 substrate, resulted in a 45% decrease in clearance of diazepam).
Products include:
Aciphex ... 1035

Ranitidine Bismuth Citrate (Concomitant administration of esomeprazole and a combined inhibitor of CYP 2C19 and CYP 3A4, such as voriconazole, may result in more than doubling

1191 Interactions Index Nexium

of the esomeprazole exposure. Dose adjustment of esomeprazole is not normally required. However, in patients with Zollinger-Ellison's Syndrome, who may require higher doses up to 240 mg/day, dose adjustment may be considered).
No products indexed under this heading.

Ranitidine Hydrochloride (Concomitant administration of esomeprazole and a combined inhibitor of CYP 2C19 and CYP 3A4, such as voriconazole, may result in more than doubling of the esomeprazole exposure. Dose adjustment of esomeprazole is not normally required. However, in patients with Zollinger-Ellison's Syndrome, who may require higher doses up to 240 mg/day, dose adjustment may be considered). Products include:
Zantac 1737
Zantac Injection 1732
Zantac Pharmacy 1735

Ritonavir (For antiretroviral drugs, such as saquinavir, elevated serum levels have been reported with an increase in AUC by 82%, in C_{max} by 75% and in C_{min} by 106% following multiple dosing of saquinavir/ritonavir (1000/100 mg) bid for 15 days with omeprazole 40 mg qd co-administered days 11 to 15. Therefore, clinical and laboratory monitoring for saquinavir toxicity is recommended during concurrent use with esomeprazole sodium. Dose reduction of saquinavir should be considered from the safety perspective for individual patients). Products include:
Kaletra 458
Norvir 509

Saquinavir (Co-administration of saquinavir with proton pump inhibitors is expected to increasesaquinavir concentrations, which may increase toxicity and require dose reduction. For antiretroviral drugs, such as saquinavir, elevated serum levels have been reported with an increase in AUC by 82%, in C_{max} by 75% and in C_{min} by 106% following multiple dosing of saquinavir/ritonavir (1000/100 mg) bid for 15 days with omeprazole 40 mg qd co-administered days 11 to 15. Therefore, clinical and laboratory monitoring for saquinavir toxicity is recommended during concurrent use with esomeprazole sodium. Dose reduction of saquinavir should be considered from the safety perspective for individual patients).
No products indexed under this heading.

Saquinavir Mesylate (Co-administration of saquinavir with proton pump inhibitors is expected to increasesaquinavir concentrations, which may increase toxicity and require dose reduction. For antiretroviral drugs, such as saquinavir, elevated serum levels have been reported with an increase in AUC by 82%, in C_{max} by 75% and in C_{min} by 106% following multiple dosing of saquinavir/ritonavir (1000/100 mg) bid for 15 days with omeprazole 40 mg qd co-administered days 11 to 15. Therefore, clinical and laboratory monitoring for saquinavir toxicity is recommended during concurrent use with esomeprazole sodium. Dose reduction of saquinavir should be considered from the safety perspective for individual patients).
No products indexed under this heading.

Sertraline Hydrochloride (Esomeprazole may potentially interfere with CYP 2C19, the major esomeprazole metabolizing enzyme. Co-administration of esomeprazole 30 mg and diazepam, a CYP2C19 substrate, resulted in a 45% decrease in clearance of diazepam).
No products indexed under this heading.

Sildenafil Citrate (Concomitant administration of esomeprazole and a combined inhibitor of CYP 2C19 and CYP 3A4, such as voriconazole, may result in more than doubling of the esomeprazole exposure. Dose adjustment of esomeprazole is not normally required. However, in patients with Zollinger-Ellison's Syndrome, who may require higher doses up to 240 mg/day, dose adjustment may be considered).
No products indexed under this heading.

Stavudine (Omeprazole, of which esomeprazole is an enantiomer, has been reported to interact with some antiretroviral drugs. The clinical importance and the mechanisms behind these interactions are not always known. Increased gastric pH during omeprazole treatment may change the absorption of the antiretroviral drug. Other possible interaction mechanisms are via CYP2C19).
No products indexed under this heading.

Sulfaphenazole (Concomitant administration of esomeprazole and a combined inhibitor of CYP 2C19 and CYP 3A4, such as voriconazole, may result in more than doubling of the esomeprazole exposure. Dose adjustment of esomeprazole is not normally required. However, in patients with Zollinger-Ellison's Syndrome, who may require higher doses up to 240 mg/day, dose adjustment may be considered).
No products indexed under this heading.

Telithromycin (Concomitant administration of esomeprazole and a combined inhibitor of CYP 2C19 and CYP 3A4, such as voriconazole, may result in more than doubling of the esomeprazole exposure. Dose adjustment of esomeprazole is not normally required. However, in patients with Zollinger-Ellison's Syndrome, who may require higher doses up to 240 mg/day, dose adjustment may be considered). Products include:
Ketek 2991

Telmisartan (Concomitant administration of esomeprazole and a combined inhibitor of CYP 2C19 and CYP 3A4, such as voriconazole, may result in more than doubling of the esomeprazole exposure. Dose adjustment of esomeprazole is not normally required. However, in patients with Zollinger-Ellison's Syndrome, who may require higher doses up to 240 mg/day, dose adjustment may be considered). Products include:
Micardis 887
Micardis HCT 889

Teniposide (Esomeprazole may potentially interfere with CYP 2C19, the major esomeprazole metabolizing enzyme. Co-administration of esomeprazole 30 mg and diazepam, a CYP2C19 substrate, resulted in a 45% decrease in clearance of diazepam).
No products indexed under this heading.

Tenofovir Disoproxil Fumarate (Omeprazole, of which esomeprazole is an enantiomer, has been reported to interact with some antiretroviral drugs. The clinical importance and the mechanisms behind these interactions are not always known. Increased gastric pH during omeprazole treatment may change the absorption of the antiretroviral drug. Other possible interaction mechanisms are via CYP2C19). Products include:
Atripla 906
Truvada 1258
Viread 1266

Thioridazine (Esomeprazole may potentially interfere with CYP 2C19, the major esomeprazole metabolizing enzyme. Co-administration of esomeprazole 30 mg and diazepam, a CYP2C19 substrate, resulted in a 45% decrease in clearance of diazepam).
No products indexed under this heading.

Thioridazine Hydrochloride (Esomeprazole may potentially interfere with CYP 2C19, the major esomeprazole metabolizing enzyme. Co-administration of esomeprazole 30 mg and diazepam, a CYP2C19 substrate, resulted in a 45% decrease in clearance of diazepam). Products include:
Thioridazine Hydrochloride 2384

Tiagabine Hydrochloride (Esomeprazole may potentially interfere with CYP 2C19, the major esomeprazole metabolizing enzyme. Co-administration of esomeprazole 30 mg and diazepam, a CYP2C19 substrate, resulted in a 45% decrease in clearance of diazepam). Products include:
Gabitril 972

Ticlopidine Hydrochloride (Concomitant administration of esomeprazole and a combined inhibitor of CYP 2C19 and CYP 3A4, such as voriconazole, may result in more than doubling of the esomeprazole exposure. Dose adjustment of esomeprazole is not normally required. However, in patients with Zollinger-Ellison's Syndrome, who may require higher doses up to 240 mg/day, dose adjustment may be considered).
No products indexed under this heading.

Tipranavir (Omeprazole, of which esomeprazole is an enantiomer, has been reported to interact with some antiretroviral drugs. The clinical importance and the mechanisms behind these interactions are not always known. Increased gastric pH during omeprazole treatment may change the absorption of the antiretroviral drug. Other possible interaction mechanisms are via CYP2C19).
No products indexed under this heading.

Tolbutamide (Esomeprazole may potentially interfere with CYP 2C19, the major esomeprazole metabolizing enzyme. Co-administration of esomeprazole 30 mg and diazepam, a CYP2C19 substrate, resulted in a 45% decrease in clearance of diazepam).
No products indexed under this heading.

Tolbutamide Sodium (Esomeprazole may potentially interfere with CYP 2C19, the major esomeprazole metabolizing enzyme. Co-administration of esomeprazole 30 mg and diazepam, a CYP2C19 substrate, resulted in a 45% decrease in clearance of diazepam).
No products indexed under this heading.

Topiramate (Esomeprazole may potentially interfere with CYP 2C19, the major esomeprazole metabolizing enzyme. Co-administration of esomeprazole 30 mg and diazepam, a CYP2C19 substrate, resulted in a 45% decrease in clearance of diazepam).
No products indexed under this heading.

Tranylcypromine Sulfate (Concomitant administration of esomeprazole and a combined inhibitor of CYP 2C19 and CYP 3A4, such as voriconazole, may result in more than doubling of the esomeprazole exposure. Dose adjustment of esomeprazole is not normally required. However, in patients with Zollinger-Ellison's Syndrome, who may require higher doses up to 240 mg/day, dose adjustment may be considered). Products include:
Parnate 1584

Trimethadione (Esomeprazole may potentially interfere with CYP 2C19, the major esomeprazole metabolizing enzyme. Co-administration of esomeprazole 30 mg and diazepam, a CYP2C19 substrate, resulted in a 45% decrease in clearance of diazepam).
No products indexed under this heading.

Trimipramine Maleate (Esomeprazole may potentially interfere with CYP 2C19, the major esomeprazole metabolizing enzyme. Co-administration of esomeprazole 30 mg and diazepam, a CYP2C19 substrate, resulted in a 45% decrease in clearance of diazepam).
No products indexed under this heading.

Troglitazone (Concomitant administration of esomeprazole and a combined inhibitor of CYP 2C19 and CYP 3A4, such as voriconazole, may result in more than doubling of the esomeprazole exposure. Dose adjustment of esomeprazole is not normally required. However, in patients with Zollinger-Ellison's Syndrome, who may require higher doses up to 240 mg/day, dose adjustment may be considered).
No products indexed under this heading.

Troleandomycin (Concomitant administration of esomeprazole and a combined inhibitor of CYP 2C19 and CYP 3A4, such as voriconazole, may result in more than doubling of the esomeprazole exposure. Dose adjustment of esomeprazole is not normally required. However, in patients with Zollinger-Ellison's Syndrome, who may require higher doses up to 240 mg/day, dose adjustment may be considered).
No products indexed under this heading.

Valproate Sodium (Esomeprazole may potentially interfere with CYP 2C19, the major esomeprazole metabolizing enzyme. Co-administration of esomeprazole 30 mg and diazepam, a CYP2C19 substrate, resulted in a 45% decrease in clearance of diazepam).
No products indexed under this heading.

Valproic Acid (Esomeprazole may potentially interfere with CYP 2C19, the major esomeprazole metabolizing enzyme. Co-administration of esomeprazole 30 mg and diazepam, a CYP2C19 substrate, resulted in a 45% decrease in clearance of diazepam).
No products indexed under this heading.

Vardenafil Hydrochloride (Concomitant administration of esomeprazole and a combined inhibitor of CYP 2C19 and CYP 3A4, such as voriconazole, may result in more than doubling of the esomeprazole exposure. Dose adjustment of esomeprazole is not normally required. However, in patients with Zollinger-Ellison's Syndrome, who may require higher doses up to 240 mg/day, dose adjustment may be considered). Products include:
Levitra 3157

Verapamil Hydrochloride (Concomitant administration of esomeprazole and a combined inhibitor of CYP 2C19 and CYP 3A4, such as voriconazole, may result in more than doubling of the esomeprazole exposure. Dose adjustment of esomeprazole is not normally required. However, in patients with Zollinger-Ellison's Syndrome, who may require higher doses up to 240 mg/day, dose adjustment may be considered). Products include:
Tarka 534

Voriconazole (Concomitant administration of esomeprazole and a combined inhibitor of CYP 2C19 and CYP 3A4, such as voriconazole, may result in more than doubling of the esomeprazole exposure. Dose adjustment of esomeprazole is not normally required. However, in patients with Zollinger-Ellison's Syndrome, who may require higher doses up to 240 mg/day, dose adjustment may be considered).
No products indexed under this heading.

IMPORTANT NOTE: Always consult each drug listing in the patient's regimen for possible interactions.

Warfarin Sodium (Changes in prothrombin measures have been reported among patients on concomitant warfarin and esomeprazole therapy. Increases in INR and prothrombin time may lead to abnormal bleeding and even death. Patients treated with proton pump inhibitors and warfarin concomitantly may need to be monitored for increases in INR and prothrombin time).
No products indexed under this heading.

Zafirlukast (Concomitant administration of esomeprazole and a combined inhibitor of CYP 2C19 and CYP 3A4, such as voriconazole, may result in more than doubling of the esomeprazole exposure. Dose adjustment of esomeprazole is not normally required. However, in patients with Zollinger-Ellison's Syndrome, who may require higher doses up to 240 mg/day, dose adjustment may be considered). Products include:
Accolate 3612

Zalcitabine (Omeprazole, of which esomeprazole is an enantiomer, has been reported to interact with some antiretroviral drugs. The clinical importance and the mechanisms behind these interactions are not always known. Increased gastric pH during omeprazole treatment may change the absorption of the antiretroviral drug. Other possible interaction mechanisms are via CYP2C19).
No products indexed under this heading.

Zidovudine (Omeprazole, of which esomeprazole is an enantiomer, has been reported to interact with some antiretroviral drugs. The clinical importance and the mechanisms behind these interactions are not always known. Increased gastric pH during omeprazole treatment may change the absorption of the antiretroviral drug. Other possible interaction mechanisms are via CYP2C19). Products include:
Combivir 1404
Retrovir 1634
Retrovir IV 1640
Trizivir 1688

Zileuton (Concomitant administration of esomeprazole and a combined inhibitor of CYP 2C19 and CYP 3A4, such as voriconazole, may result in more than doubling of the esomeprazole exposure. Dose adjustment of esomeprazole is not normally required. However, in patients with Zollinger-Ellison's Syndrome, who may require higher doses up to 240 mg/day, dose adjustment may be considered).
No products indexed under this heading.

Zonisamide (Esomeprazole may potentially interfere with CYP 2C19, the major esomeprazole metabolizing enzyme. Co-administration of esomeprazole 30 mg and diazepam, a CYP2C19 substrate, resulted in a 45% decrease in clearance of diazepam). Products include:
Zonegran 1081

Food Interactions

Food, unspecified (The AUC after administration of a single 40 mg dose of esomeprazole is decreased by 43%-53% after food intake compared to fasting conditions. Esomeprazole should be taken at least one hour before meals).

Grapefruit (Concomitant administration of esomeprazole and a combined inhibitor of CYP 2C19 and CYP 3A4, such as voriconazole, may result in more than doubling of the esomeprazole exposure. Dose adjustment of esomeprazole is not normally required. However, in patients with Zollinger-Ellison's Syndrome, who may require higher doses up to 240 mg/day, dose adjustment may be considered).

Grapefruit Juice (Concomitant administration of esomeprazole and a combined inhibitor of CYP 2C19 and CYP 3A4, such as voriconazole, may result in more than doubling of the esomeprazole exposure. Dose adjustment of esomeprazole is not normally required. However, in patients with Zollinger-Ellison's Syndrome, who may require higher doses up to 240 mg/day, dose adjustment may be considered).

Meal, unspecified (The AUC after administration of a single 40 mg dose of esomeprazole is decreased by 43%-53% after food intake compared to fasting conditions. Esomeprazole should be taken at least one hour before meals).

NEXIUM DELAYED-RELEASE ORAL SUSPENSION
(Esomeprazole Magnesium) 704
See Nexium Delayed-Release Capsules

NEXIUM I.V.
(Esomeprazole Sodium) 712
May interact with absorption of drugs where gastric ph is an important determinant in their bioavailability, antiretroviral agents, cytochrome p450 2c19 inhibitors (selected), cytochrome p450 2c19 substrates (selected), cytochrome p450 3a4 inhibitors (selected), iron containing oral preparations, iron salts, and certain other agents. Compounds in these categories include:

Abacavir Sulfate (Omeprazole has been reported to interact with some antiretroviral drugs. The clinical importance and the mechanisms behind these interactions are not always known. Increased gastric pH during omeprazole treatment may change the absorption of the antiretroviral drug. Other possible interaction mechanisms are via CYP2C19). Products include:
Epzicom 1448
Trizivir 1688
Ziagen 1740

Acetazolamide (Concomitant administration of esomeprazole and a combined inhibitor of CYP2C19 and CYP3A4, such as voriconazole, may result in more than doubling of the esomeprazole exposure. Dose adjustment of esomeprazole is not normally required for the recommended doses. However, in patients who may require higher doses, dose adjustment may be considered).
No products indexed under this heading.

Acetazolamide Sodium (Concomitant administration of esomeprazole and a combined inhibitor of CYP2C19 and CYP3A4, such as voriconazole, may result in more than doubling of the esomeprazole exposure. Dose adjustment of esomeprazole is not normally required for the recommended doses. However, in patients who may require higher doses, dose adjustment may be considered).
No products indexed under this heading.

Amiodarone Hydrochloride (Concomitant administration of esomeprazole and a combined inhibitor of CYP2C19 and CYP3A4, such as voriconazole, may result in more than doubling of the esomeprazole exposure. Dose adjustment of esomeprazole is not normally required for the recommended doses. However, in patients who may require higher doses, dose adjustment may be considered).
No products indexed under this heading.

Amitriptyline Hydrochloride (Esomeprazole may potentially interfere with CYP2C19, the major esomeprazole metabolizing enzyme. Co-administration of esomeprazole 30 mg and diazepam, a CYP2C19 substrate, resulted in a

45% decrease in clearance of diazepam. Increased plasma levels of diazepam were observed 12 hours after dosing and onwards. However, at that time, the plasma levels of diazepam were below the therapeutic interval, and thus this interaction is unlikely to be of clinical relevance).
No products indexed under this heading.

Amoxapine (Esomeprazole may potentially interfere with CYP2C19, the major esomeprazole metabolizing enzyme. Co-administration of esomeprazole 30 mg and diazepam, a CYP2C19 substrate, resulted in a 45% decrease in clearance of diazepam. Increased plasma levels of diazepam were observed 12 hours after dosing and onwards. However, at that time, the plasma levels of diazepam were below the therapeutic interval, and thus this interaction is unlikely to be of clinical relevance).
No products indexed under this heading.

Amprenavir (Omeprazole has been reported to interact with some antiretroviral drugs. The clinical importance and the mechanisms behind these interactions are not always known. Increased gastric pH during omeprazole treatment may change the absorption of the antiretroviral drug. Other possible interaction mechanisms are via CYP2C19).
No products indexed under this heading.

Anastrozole (Concomitant administration of esomeprazole and a combined inhibitor of CYP2C19 and CYP3A4, such as voriconazole, may result in more than doubling of the esomeprazole exposure. Dose adjustment of esomeprazole is not normally required for the recommended doses. However, in patients who may require higher doses, dose adjustment may be considered).
No products indexed under this heading.

Aprepitant (Concomitant administration of esomeprazole and a combined inhibitor of CYP2C19 and CYP3A4, such as voriconazole, may result in more than doubling of the esomeprazole exposure. Dose adjustment of esomeprazole is not normally required for the recommended doses. However, in patients who may require higher doses, dose adjustment may be considered). Products include:
Emend 2124

Atazanavir (Concomitant use of atazanavir with proton pump inhibitors is not recommended. Co-administration of atazanavir with proton pump inhibitors is expected to substantially decrease atazanavir plasma concentrations and thereby reduce its therapeutic effect. Following multiple doses of atazanavir (400 mg, qd) and omeprazole (40 mg, qd, 2 hr before atazanavir), AUC was decreased by 94%, C_{max} by 96%, and C_{min} by 95%).
No products indexed under this heading.

Atazanavir Sulfate (Concomitant use of atazanavir with proton pump inhibitors is not recommended. Co-administration of atazanavir with proton pump inhibitors is expected to substantially decrease atazanavir plasma concentrations and thereby reduce its therapeutic effect. Following multiple doses of atazanavir (400 mg, qd) and omeprazole (40 mg, qd, 2 hr before atazanavir), AUC was decreased by 94%, C_{max} by 96%, and C_{min} by 95%).
No products indexed under this heading.

Bacampicillin Hydrochloride (Esomeprazole inhibits gastric acid secretion. Therefore, esomeprazole may interfere with the absorption of drugs where gastric pH is an important determinant of bioavailability (eg, ketoconazole, iron salts and digoxin)).
No products indexed under this heading.

Carisoprodol (Esomeprazole may potentially interfere with CYP2C19, the major esomeprazole metabolizing enzyme. Co-administration of esomeprazole 30 mg and diazepam, a CYP2C19 substrate, resulted in a 45% decrease in clearance of diazepam. Increased plasma levels of diazepam were observed 12 hours after dosing and onwards. However, at that time, the plasma levels of diazepam were below the therapeutic interval, and thus this interaction is unlikely to be of clinical relevance).
No products indexed under this heading.

Cilostazol (Esomeprazole may potentially interfere with CYP2C19, the major esomeprazole metabolizing enzyme. Co-administration of esomeprazole 30 mg and diazepam, a CYP2C19 substrate, resulted in a 45% decrease in clearance of diazepam. Increased plasma levels of diazepam were observed 12 hours after dosing and onwards. However, at that time, the plasma levels of diazepam were below the therapeutic interval, and thus this interaction is unlikely to be of clinical relevance).
No products indexed under this heading.

Cimetidine (Concomitant administration of esomeprazole and a combined inhibitor of CYP2C19 and CYP3A4, such as voriconazole, may result in more than doubling of the esomeprazole exposure. Dose adjustment of esomeprazole is not normally required for the recommended doses. However, in patients who may require higher doses, dose adjustment may be considered).
No products indexed under this heading.

Cimetidine Hydrochloride (Concomitant administration of esomeprazole and a combined inhibitor of CYP2C19 and CYP3A4, such as voriconazole, may result in more than doubling of the esomeprazole exposure. Dose adjustment of esomeprazole is not normally required for the recommended doses. However, in patients who may require higher doses, dose adjustment may be considered).
No products indexed under this heading.

Ciprofloxacin (Concomitant administration of esomeprazole and a combined inhibitor of CYP2C19 and CYP3A4, such as voriconazole, may result in more than doubling of the esomeprazole exposure. Dose adjustment of esomeprazole is not normally required for the recommended doses. However, in patients who may require higher doses, dose adjustment may be considered). Products include:
Cipro I.V. 3082
Cipro 3073
Cipro XR 3091
Ciprodex 583

Citalopram Hydrobromide (Esomeprazole may potentially interfere with CYP2C19, the major esomeprazole metabolizing enzyme. Co-administration of esomeprazole 30 mg and diazepam, a CYP2C19 substrate, resulted in a 45% decrease in clearance of diazepam. Increased plasma levels of diazepam were observed 12 hours after dosing and onwards. However, at that time, the plasma levels of diazepam were below the therapeutic interval, and thus this interaction is unlikely to be of clinical relevance). Products include:
Celexa 1153

Clarithromycin (Concomitant administration of esomeprazole and a combined inhibitor of CYP2C19 and CYP3A4, such as voriconazole, may result in more than doubling of the esomeprazole exposure. Dose adjustment of esomeprazole is not normally required for the recommended doses.

However, in patients who may require higher doses, dose adjustment may be considered). Products include:

Clomipramine Hydrochloride (Esomeprazole may potentially interfere with CYP2C19, the major esomeprazole metabolizing enzyme. Co-administration of esomeprazole 30 mg and diazepam, a CYP2C19 substrate, resulted in a 45% decrease in clearance of diazepam. Increased plasma levels of diazepam were observed 12 hours after dosing and onwards. However, at that time, the plasma levels of diazepam were below the therapeutic interval, and thus this interaction is unlikely to be of clinical relevance).

No products indexed under this heading.

Clotrimazole (Concomitant administration of esomeprazole and a combined inhibitor of CYP2C19 and CYP3A4, such as voriconazole, may result in more than doubling of the esomeprazole exposure. Dose adjustment of esomeprazole is not normally required for the recommended doses. However, in patients who may require higher doses, dose adjustment may be considered). Products include:

Conivaptan Hydrochloride (Concomitant administration of esomeprazole and a combined inhibitor of CYP2C19 and CYP3A4, such as voriconazole, may result in more than doubling of the esomeprazole exposure. Dose adjustment of esomeprazole is not normally required for the recommended doses. However, in patients who may require higher doses, dose adjustment may be considered). Products include:

Cyclophosphamide (Esomeprazole may potentially interfere with CYP2C19, the major esomeprazole metabolizing enzyme. Co-administration of esomeprazole 30 mg and diazepam, a CYP2C19 substrate, resulted in a 45% decrease in clearance of diazepam. Increased plasma levels of diazepam were observed 12 hours after dosing and onwards. However, at that time, the plasma levels of diazepam were below the therapeutic interval, and thus this interaction is unlikely to be of clinical relevance).

No products indexed under this heading.

Cyclosporine (Concomitant administration of esomeprazole and a combined inhibitor of CYP2C19 and CYP3A4, such as voriconazole, may result in more than doubling of the esomeprazole exposure. Dose adjustment of esomeprazole is not normally required for the recommended doses. However, in patients who may require higher doses, dose adjustment may be considered). Products include:

Dalfopristin (Concomitant administration of esomeprazole and a combined inhibitor of CYP2C19 and CYP3A4, such as voriconazole, may result in more than doubling of the esomeprazole exposure. Dose adjustment of esomeprazole is not normally required for the recommended doses. However, in patients who may require higher doses, dose adjustment may be considered).

No products indexed under this heading.

Danazol (Concomitant administration of esomeprazole and a combined inhibitor of CYP2C19 and CYP3A4, such as voriconazole, may result in more than doubling of the esomeprazole exposure. Dose adjustment of esomeprazole is not normally required for the recommended doses. However, in patients who may require higher doses, dose adjustment may be considered).

No products indexed under this heading.

Darunavir (Omeprazole has been reported to interact with some antiretroviral drugs. The clinical importance and the mechanisms behind these interactions are not always known. Increased gastric pH during omeprazole treatment may change the absorption of the antiretroviral drug. Other possible interaction mechanisms are via CYP2C19).

No products indexed under this heading.

Dasatinib (Concomitant administration of esomeprazole and a combined inhibitor of CYP2C19 and CYP3A4, such as voriconazole, may result in more than doubling of the esomeprazole exposure. Dose adjustment of esomeprazole is not normally required for the recommended doses. However, in patients who may require higher doses, dose adjustment may be considered).

No products indexed under this heading.

Delavirdine Mesylate (Omeprazole has been reported to interact with some antiretroviral drugs. The clinical importance and the mechanisms behind these interactions are not always known. Increased gastric pH during omeprazole treatment may change the absorption of the antiretroviral drug. Other possible interaction mechanisms are via CYP2C19).

No products indexed under this heading.

Delavirine (Concomitant administration of esomeprazole and a combined inhibitor of CYP2C19 and CYP3A4, such as voriconazole, may result in more than doubling of the esomeprazole exposure. Dose adjustment of esomeprazole is not normally required for the recommended doses. However, in patients who may require higher doses, dose adjustment may be considered).

No products indexed under this heading.

Desipramine Hydrochloride (Esomeprazole may potentially interfere with CYP2C19, the major esomeprazole metabolizing enzyme. Co-administration of esomeprazole 30 mg and diazepam, a CYP2C19 substrate, resulted in a 45% decrease in clearance of diazepam. Increased plasma levels of diazepam were observed 12 hours after dosing and onwards. However, at that time, the plasma levels of diazepam were below the therapeutic interval, and thus this interaction is unlikely to be of clinical relevance).

No products indexed under this heading.

Desloratadine (Concomitant administration of esomeprazole and a combined inhibitor of CYP2C19 and CYP3A4, such as voriconazole, may result in more than doubling of the esomeprazole exposure. Dose adjustment of esomeprazole is not normally required for the recommended doses. However, in patients who may require higher doses, dose adjustment may be considered). Products include:

Desogestrel (Concomitant administration of esomeprazole and a combined inhibitor of CYP2C19 and CYP3A4, such as voriconazole, may result in more than doubling of the esomeprazole exposure. Dose adjustment of esomeprazole is not normally required for the recommended doses. However, in patients who may require higher doses, dose adjustment may be considered).

No products indexed under this heading.

Dextromethorphan (Esomeprazole may potentially interfere with CYP2C19, the major esomeprazole metabolizing enzyme. Co-administration of esomeprazole 30 mg and diazepam, a CYP2C19 substrate, resulted in a 45% decrease in clearance of diazepam. Increased plasma levels of diazepam were observed 12 hours after dosing and onwards. However, at that time, the plasma levels of diazepam were below the therapeutic interval, and thus this interaction is unlikely to be of clinical relevance).

No products indexed under this heading.

Dextromethorphan Hydrobromide (Esomeprazole may potentially interfere with CYP2C19, the major esomeprazole metabolizing enzyme. Co-administration of esomeprazole 30 mg and diazepam, a CYP2C19 substrate, resulted in a 45% decrease in clearance of diazepam. Increased plasma levels of diazepam were observed 12 hours after dosing and onwards. However, at that time, the plasma levels of diazepam were below the therapeutic interval, and thus this interaction is unlikely to be of clinical relevance).

No products indexed under this heading.

Diazepam (Esomeprazole may potentially interfere with CYP2C19, the major esomeprazole metabolizing enzyme. Co-administration of esomeprazole 30 mg and diazepam, a CYP2C19 substrate, resulted in a 45% decrease in clearance of diazepam. Increased plasma levels of diazepam were observed 12 hours after dosing and onwards. However, at that time, the plasma levels of diazepam were below the therapeutic interval, and thus this interaction is unlikely to be of clinical relevance). Products include:

Didanosine (Omeprazole has been reported to interact with some antiretroviral drugs. The clinical importance and the mechanisms behind these interactions are not always known. Increased gastric pH during omeprazole treatment may change the absorption of the antiretroviral drug. Other possible interaction mechanisms are via CYP2C19).

No products indexed under this heading.

Digoxin (Esomeprazole inhibits gastric acid secretion; therefore, esomeprazole may interfere with the absorption of drugs where gastric pH is an important determinant of bioavailability, such as digoxin). Products include:

Diltiazem Hydrochloride (Concomitant administration of esomeprazole and a combined inhibitor of CYP2C19 and CYP3A4, such as voriconazole, may result in more than doubling of the esomeprazole exposure. Dose adjustment of esomeprazole is not normally required for the recommended doses. However, in patients who may require higher doses, dose adjustment may be considered). Products include:

Diltiazem Maleate (Concomitant administration of esomeprazole and a combined inhibitor of CYP2C19 and CYP3A4, such as voriconazole, may result in more than doubling of the esomeprazole exposure. Dose adjustment of esomeprazole is not normally required for the recommended doses. However, in patients who may require higher doses, dose adjustment may be considered).

No products indexed under this heading.

Divalproex Sodium (Esomeprazole may potentially interfere with CYP2C19, the major esomeprazole metabolizing enzyme. Co-administration of esomeprazole 30 mg and diazepam, a CYP2C19 substrate, resulted in a 45% decrease in clearance of diazepam. Increased plasma levels of diazepam were observed 12 hours after dosing and onwards. However, at that time, the plasma levels of diazepam were below the therapeutic interval, and thus this interaction is unlikely to be of clinical relevance). Products include:

Doxepin Hydrochloride (Esomeprazole may potentially interfere with CYP2C19, the major esomeprazole metabolizing enzyme. Co-administration of esomeprazole 30 mg and diazepam, a CYP2C19 substrate, resulted in a 45% decrease in clearance of diazepam. Increased plasma levels of diazepam were observed 12 hours after dosing and onwards. However, at that time, the plasma levels of diazepam were below the therapeutic interval, and thus this interaction is unlikely to be of clinical relevance).

No products indexed under this heading.

Efavirenz (Omeprazole has been reported to interact with some antiretroviral drugs. The clinical importance and the mechanisms behind these interactions are not always known. Increased gastric pH during omeprazole treatment may change the absorption of the antiretroviral drug. Other possible interaction mechanisms are via CYP2C19). Products include:

Emtricitabine (Omeprazole has been reported to interact with some antiretroviral drugs. The clinical importance and the mechanisms behind these interactions are not always known. Increased gastric pH during omeprazole treatment may change the absorption of the antiretroviral drug. Other possible interaction mechanisms are via CYP2C19). Products include:

Enfuvirtide (Omeprazole has been reported to interact with some antiretroviral drugs. The clinical importance and the mechanisms behind these interactions are not always known. Increased gastric pH during omeprazole treatment may change the absorption of the antiretroviral drug. Other possible interaction mechanisms are via CYP2C19).

No products indexed under this heading.

Erythromycin (Concomitant administration of esomeprazole and a combined inhibitor of CYP2C19 and CYP3A4, such as voriconazole, may result in more than doubling of the esomeprazole exposure. Dose adjustment of esomeprazole is not normally required for the recommended doses. However, in patients who may require higher doses, dose adjustment may be considered).

No products indexed under this heading.

IMPORTANT NOTE: Always consult each drug listing in the patient's regimen for possible interactions.

Erythromycin Estolate (Concomitant administration of esomeprazole and a combined inhibitor of CYP2C19 and CYP3A4, such as voriconazole, may result in more than doubling of the esomeprazole exposure. Dose adjustment of esomeprazole is not normally required for the recommended doses. However, in patients who may require higher doses, dose adjustment may be considered).
No products indexed under this heading.

Erythromycin Ethylsuccinate (Concomitant administration of esomeprazole and a combined inhibitor of CYP2C19 and CYP3A4, such as voriconazole, may result in more than doubling of the esomeprazole exposure. Dose adjustment of esomeprazole is not normally required for the recommended doses. However, in patients who may require higher doses, dose adjustment may be considered). Products include:

Erythromycin Gluceptate (Concomitant administration of esomeprazole and a combined inhibitor of CYP2C19 and CYP3A4, such as voriconazole, may result in more than doubling of the esomeprazole exposure. Dose adjustment of esomeprazole is not normally required for the recommended doses. However, in patients who may require higher doses, dose adjustment may be considered).
No products indexed under this heading.

Erythromycin Lactobionate (Concomitant administration of esomeprazole and a combined inhibitor of CYP2C19 and CYP3A4, such as voriconazole, may result in more than doubling of the esomeprazole exposure. Dose adjustment of esomeprazole is not normally required for the recommended doses. However, in patients who may require higher doses, dose adjustment may be considered).
No products indexed under this heading.

Erythromycin Stearate (Concomitant administration of esomeprazole and a combined inhibitor of CYP2C19 and CYP3A4, such as voriconazole, may result in more than doubling of the esomeprazole exposure. Dose adjustment of esomeprazole is not normally required for the recommended doses. However, in patients who may require higher doses, dose adjustment may be considered).
No products indexed under this heading.

Esomeprazole Magnesium (Esomeprazole may potentially interfere with CYP2C19, the major esomeprazole metabolizing enzyme. Co-administration of esomeprazole 30 mg and diazepam, a CYP2C19 substrate, resulted in a 45% decrease in clearance of diazepam. Increased plasma levels of diazepam were observed 12 hours after dosing and onwards. However, at that time, the plasma levels of diazepam were below the therapeutic interval, and thus this interaction is unlikely to be of clinical relevance). Products include:

Ethinyl Estradiol (Concomitant administration of esomeprazole and a combined inhibitor of CYP2C19 and CYP3A4, such as voriconazole, may result in more than doubling of the esomeprazole exposure. Dose adjustment of esomeprazole is not normally required for the recommended doses. However, in patients who may require higher doses, dose adjustment may be considered). Products include:

Ethosuximide (Esomeprazole may potentially interfere with CYP2C19, the major esomeprazole metabolizing enzyme. Co-administration of esomeprazole 30 mg and diazepam, a CYP2C19 substrate, resulted in a 45% decrease in clearance of diazepam. Increased plasma levels of diazepam were observed 12 hours after dosing and onwards. However, at that time, the plasma levels of diazepam were below the therapeutic interval, and thus this interaction is unlikely to be of clinical relevance).
No products indexed under this heading.

Ethotoin (Esomeprazole may potentially interfere with CYP2C19, the major esomeprazole metabolizing enzyme. Co-administration of esomeprazole 30 mg and diazepam, a CYP2C19 substrate, resulted in a 45% decrease in clearance of diazepam. Increased plasma levels of diazepam were observed 12 hours after dosing and onwards. However, at that time, the plasma levels of diazepam were below the therapeutic interval, and thus this interaction is unlikely to be of clinical relevance).
No products indexed under this heading.

Ethynodiol Diacetate (Concomitant administration of esomeprazole and a combined inhibitor of CYP2C19 and CYP3A4, such as voriconazole, may result in more than doubling of the esomeprazole exposure. Dose adjustment of esomeprazole is not normally required for the recommended doses. However, in patients who may require higher doses, dose adjustment may be considered).
No products indexed under this heading.

Felbamate (Esomeprazole may potentially interfere with CYP2C19, the major esomeprazole metabolizing enzyme. Co-administration of esomeprazole 30 mg and diazepam, a CYP2C19 substrate, resulted in a 45% decrease in clearance of diazepam. Increased plasma levels of diazepam were observed 12 hours after dosing and onwards. However, at that time, the plasma levels of diazepam were below the therapeutic interval, and thus this interaction is unlikely to be of clinical relevance).
No products indexed under this heading.

Ferrous Fumarate (Esomeprazole inhibits gastric acid secretion; therefore, esomeprazole may interfere with the absorption of drugs where gastric pH is an important determinant of bioavailability, such as oral iron salts). Products include:

Ferrous Gluconate (Esomeprazole inhibits gastric acid secretion; therefore, esomeprazole may interfere with the absorption of drugs where gastric pH is an important determinant of bioavailability, such as oral iron salts). Products include:

Ferrous Sulfate (Esomeprazole inhibits gastric acid secretion; therefore, esomeprazole may interfere with the absorption of drugs where gastric pH is an important determinant of bioavailability, such as oral iron salts).
No products indexed under this heading.

Fluconazole (Concomitant administration of esomeprazole and a combined inhibitor of CYP2C19 and CYP3A4, such as voriconazole, may result in more than doubling of the esomeprazole exposure. Dose adjustment of esomeprazole is not normally required for the recommended doses. However, in patients who may require higher doses, dose adjustment may be considered).
No products indexed under this heading.

Fluoxetine (Concomitant administration of esomeprazole and a combined inhibitor of CYP2C19 and CYP3A4, such as voriconazole, may result in more than doubling of the esomeprazole exposure. Dose adjustment of esomeprazole is not normally required for the recommended doses. However, in patients who may require higher doses, dose adjustment may be considered).
No products indexed under this heading.

Fluoxetine Hydrochloride (Concomitant administration of esomeprazole and a combined inhibitor of CYP2C19 and CYP3A4, such as voriconazole, may result in more than doubling of the esomeprazole exposure. Dose adjustment of esomeprazole is not normally required for the recommended doses. However, in patients who may require higher doses, dose adjustment may be considered). Products include:

Fluvastatin Sodium (Concomitant administration of esomeprazole and a combined inhibitor of CYP2C19 and CYP3A4, such as voriconazole, may result in more than doubling of the esomeprazole exposure. Dose adjustment of esomeprazole is not normally required for the recommended doses. However, in patients who may require higher doses, dose adjustment may be considered).
No products indexed under this heading.

Fluvoxamine (Concomitant administration of esomeprazole and a combined inhibitor of CYP2C19 and CYP3A4, such as voriconazole, may result in more than doubling of the esomeprazole exposure. Dose adjustment of esomeprazole is not normally required for the recommended doses. However, in patients who may require higher doses, dose adjustment may be considered).
No products indexed under this heading.

Fluvoxamine Maleate (Concomitant administration of esomeprazole and a combined inhibitor of CYP2C19 and CYP3A4, such as voriconazole, may result in more than doubling of the esomeprazole exposure. Dose adjustment of esomeprazole is not normally required for the recommended doses. However, in patients who may require higher doses, dose adjustment may be considered).
No products indexed under this heading.

Formoterol Fumarate (Esomeprazole may potentially interfere with CYP2C19, the major esomeprazole metabolizing enzyme. Co-administration of esomeprazole 30 mg and diazepam, a CYP2C19 substrate, resulted in a 45% decrease in clearance of diazepam. Increased plasma levels of diazepam were observed 12 hours after dosing and onwards. However, at that time, the plasma levels of diazepam were below the therapeutic interval, and thus this interaction is unlikely to be of clinical relevance). Products include:

Fosamprenavir Calcium (Omeprazole has been reported to interact with some antiretroviral drugs. The clinical importance and the mechanisms behind these interactions are not always known. Increased gastric pH during omeprazole treatment may change the absorption of the antiretroviral drug. Other possible interaction mechanisms are via CYP2C19). Products include:

Fosphenytoin (Esomeprazole may potentially interfere with CYP2C19, the major esomeprazole metabolizing enzyme. Co-administration of esomeprazole 30 mg and diazepam, a CYP2C19 substrate, resulted in a 45% decrease in clearance of diazepam. Increased plasma levels of diazepam were observed 12 hours after dosing and onwards. However, at that time, the plasma levels of diazepam were below the therapeutic interval, and thus this interaction is unlikely to be of clinical relevance).
No products indexed under this heading.

Fosphenytoin Sodium (Esomeprazole may potentially interfere with CYP2C19, the major esomeprazole metabolizing enzyme. Co-administration of esomeprazole 30 mg and diazepam, a CYP2C19 substrate, resulted in a 45% decrease in clearance of diazepam. Increased plasma levels of diazepam were observed 12 hours after dosing and onwards. However, at that time, the plasma levels of diazepam were below the therapeutic interval, and thus this interaction is unlikely to be of clinical relevance).
No products indexed under this heading.

Gabapentin (Esomeprazole may potentially interfere with CYP2C19, the major esomeprazole metabolizing enzyme. Co-administration of esomeprazole 30 mg and diazepam, a CYP2C19 substrate, resulted in a 45% decrease in clearance of diazepam. Increased plasma levels of diazepam were observed 12 hours after dosing and onwards. However, at that time, the plasma levels of diazepam were below the therapeutic interval, and thus this interaction is unlikely to be of clinical relevance).
No products indexed under this heading.

Imatinib Mesylate (Concomitant administration of esomeprazole and a combined inhibitor of CYP2C19 and CYP3A4, such as voriconazole, may result in more than doubling of the esomeprazole exposure. Dose adjustment of esomeprazole is not normally required for the recommended doses. However, in patients who may require higher doses, dose adjustment may be considered). Products include:

Imipramine Hydrochloride (Esomeprazole may potentially interfere with CYP2C19, the major esomeprazole metabolizing enzyme. Co-administration of esomeprazole 30 mg and diazepam, a CYP2C19 substrate, resulted in a 45% decrease in clearance of diazepam. Increased plasma levels of diazepam were observed 12 hours after dosing and onwards. However, at that time, the plasma levels of diazepam were below the therapeutic interval, and thus this interaction is unlikely to be of clinical relevance).
No products indexed under this heading.

Imipramine Pamoate (Esomeprazole may potentially interfere with CYP2C19, the major esomeprazole metabolizing enzyme. Co-administration of esomeprazole 30 mg and diazepam, a CYP2C19 substrate, resulted in a 45% decrease in clearance of diazepam. Increased plasma levels of diazepam were observed 12 hours after dosing and onwards. However, at that time, the plasma levels of diazepam were

1195 Interactions Index Nexium I.V.

below the therapeutic interval, and thus this interaction is unlikely to be of clinical relevance).
No products indexed under this heading.

Indinavir Sulfate (Omeprazole has been reported to interact with some antiretroviral drugs. The clinical importance and the mechanisms behind these interactions are not always known. Increased gastric pH during omeprazole treatment may change the absorption of the antiretroviral drug. Other possible interaction mechanisms are via CYP2C19). Products include:
Crixivan 2113

Indomethacin (Esomeprazole may potentially interfere with CYP2C19, the major esomeprazole metabolizing enzyme. Co-administration of esomeprazole 30 mg and diazepam, a CYP2C19 substrate, resulted in a 45% decrease in clearance of diazepam. Increased plasma levels of diazepam were observed 12 hours after dosing and onwards. However, at that time, the plasma levels of diazepam were below the therapeutic interval, and thus this interaction is unlikely to be of clinical relevance). Products include:
Indocin 2167

Indomethacin Sodium Trihydrate (Esomeprazole may potentially interfere with CYP2C19, the major esomeprazole metabolizing enzyme. Co-administration of esomeprazole 30 mg and diazepam, a CYP2C19 substrate, resulted in a 45% decrease in clearance of diazepam. Increased plasma levels of diazepam were observed 12 hours after dosing and onwards. However, at that time, the plasma levels of diazepam were below the therapeutic interval, and thus this interaction is unlikely to be of clinical relevance). Products include:
Indocin I.V. 2007

Iron (Esomeprazole inhibits gastric acid secretion; therefore, esomeprazole may interfere with the absorption of drugs where gastric pH is an important determinant of bioavailability, such as oral iron salts).
No products indexed under this heading.

Iron, Peptonized (Esomeprazole inhibits gastric acid secretion; therefore, esomeprazole may interfere with the absorption of drugs where gastric pH is an important determinant of bioavailability, such as oral iron salts).
No products indexed under this heading.

Iron Cacodylate (Esomeprazole inhibits gastric acid secretion; therefore, esomeprazole may interfere with the absorption of drugs where gastric pH is an important determinant of bioavailability, such as oral iron salts).
No products indexed under this heading.

Iron Carbonyl (Esomeprazole inhibits gastric acid secretion; therefore, esomeprazole may interfere with the absorption of drugs where gastric pH is an important determinant of bioavailability, such as oral iron salts). Products include:
CitraNatal 90 DHA Capsules 2332
CitraNatal Assure 2332
CitraNatal Harmony 2332
CitraNatal Rx 2332
Ferralet 2333

Iron Dextran (Esomeprazole inhibits gastric acid secretion; therefore, esomeprazole may interfere with the absorption of drugs where gastric pH is an important determinant of bioavailability, such as oral iron salts).
No products indexed under this heading.

Iron Polysaccharide Complex (Esomeprazole inhibits gastric acid secretion; therefore, esomeprazole may interfere with the absorption of drugs where gastric pH is an important determinant of bioavailability, such as oral iron salts).
No products indexed under this heading.

Iron Sucrose (Esomeprazole inhibits gastric acid secretion; therefore, esomeprazole may interfere with the absorption of drugs where gastric pH is an important determinant of bioavailability, such as oral iron salts).
No products indexed under this heading.

Iron Supplements (Esomeprazole inhibits gastric acid secretion; therefore, esomeprazole may interfere with the absorption of drugs where gastric pH is an important determinant of bioavailability, such as oral iron salts).
No products indexed under this heading.

Isoniazid (Concomitant administration of esomeprazole and a combined inhibitor of CYP2C19 and CYP3A4, such as voriconazole, may result in more than doubling of the esomeprazole exposure. Dose adjustment of esomeprazole is not normally required for the recommended doses. However, in patients who may require higher doses, dose adjustment may be considered).
No products indexed under this heading.

Itraconazole (Concomitant administration of esomeprazole and a combined inhibitor of CYP2C19 and CYP3A4, such as voriconazole, may result in more than doubling of the esomeprazole exposure. Dose adjustment of esomeprazole is not normally required for the recommended doses. However, in patients who may require higher doses, dose adjustment may be considered).
No products indexed under this heading.

Ketoconazole (Esomeprazole inhibits gastric acid secretion; therefore, esomeprazole may interfere with the absorption of drugs where gastric pH is an important determinant of bioavailability, such as ketoconazole). Products include:
Extina 3319
Xolegel 3337

Lamium album (Omeprazole has been reported to interact with some antiretroviral drugs. The clinical importance and the mechanisms behind these interactions are not always known. Increased gastric pH during omeprazole treatment may change the absorption of the antiretroviral drug. Other possible interaction mechanisms are via CYP2C19).
No products indexed under this heading.

Lamotrigine (Esomeprazole may potentially interfere with CYP2C19, the major esomeprazole metabolizing enzyme. Co-administration of esomeprazole 30 mg and diazepam, a CYP2C19 substrate, resulted in a 45% decrease in clearance of diazepam. Increased plasma levels of diazepam were observed 12 hours after dosing and onwards. However, at that time, the plasma levels of diazepam were below the therapeutic interval, and thus this interaction is unlikely to be of clinical relevance). Products include:
Lamictal 1522
Lamictal ODT 1522
Lamictal XR 1536

Lansoprazole (Esomeprazole may potentially interfere with CYP2C19, the major esomeprazole metabolizing enzyme. Co-administration of esomeprazole 30 mg and diazepam, a CYP2C19 substrate, resulted in a 45% decrease in clearance of diazepam. Increased plasma levels of diazepam were observed 12 hours after dosing and onwards. However, at that time, the plasma levels of diazepam were below the therapeutic interval, and thus this interaction is unlikely to be of clinical relevance).
No products indexed under this heading.

Lapatinib (Concomitant administration of esomeprazole and a combined inhibitor of CYP2C19 and CYP3A4, such as voriconazole, may result in more than doubling of the esomeprazole exposure. Dose adjustment of esomeprazole is not normally required for the recommended doses. However, in patients who may require higher doses, dose adjustment may be considered). Products include:
Tykerb 1698

Letrozole (Concomitant administration of esomeprazole and a combined inhibitor of CYP2C19 and CYP3A4, such as voriconazole, may result in more than doubling of the esomeprazole exposure. Dose adjustment of esomeprazole is not normally required for the recommended doses. However, in patients who may require higher doses, dose adjustment may be considered). Products include:
Femara 2466

Levetiracetam (Esomeprazole may potentially interfere with CYP2C19, the major esomeprazole metabolizing enzyme. Co-administration of esomeprazole 30 mg and diazepam, a CYP2C19 substrate, resulted in a 45% decrease in clearance of diazepam. Increased plasma levels of diazepam were observed 12 hours after dosing and onwards. However, at that time, the plasma levels of diazepam were below the therapeutic interval, and thus this interaction is unlikely to be of clinical relevance). Products include:
Keppra XR 3434

Levonorgestrel (Concomitant administration of esomeprazole and a combined inhibitor of CYP2C19 and CYP3A4, such as voriconazole, may result in more than doubling of the esomeprazole exposure. Dose adjustment of esomeprazole is not normally required for the recommended doses. However, in patients who may require higher doses, dose adjustment may be considered). Products include:
Climara Pro 847
LoSeasonique 3407
Lybrel 3514
Mirena 854
Plan B 3416
Seasonique 3418

Lopinavir (Omeprazole has been reported to interact with some antiretroviral drugs. The clinical importance and the mechanisms behind these interactions are not always known. Increased gastric pH during omeprazole treatment may change the absorption of the antiretroviral drug. Other possible interaction mechanisms are via CYP2C19). Products include:
Kaletra 458

Loratadine (Concomitant administration of esomeprazole and a combined inhibitor of CYP2C19 and CYP3A4, such as voriconazole, may result in more than doubling of the esomeprazole exposure. Dose adjustment of esomeprazole is not normally required for the recommended doses. However, in patients who may require higher doses, dose adjustment may be considered).
No products indexed under this heading.

Maprotiline Hydrochloride (Esomeprazole may potentially interfere with CYP2C19, the major esomeprazole metabolizing enzyme. Co-administration of esomeprazole 30 mg and diazepam, a CYP2C19 substrate, resulted in a 45% decrease in clearance of diazepam. Increased plasma levels of diazepam were observed 12 hours after dosing and onwards. However, at that time, the plasma levels of diazepam were below the therapeutic interval, and thus this interaction is unlikely to be of clinical relevance).
No products indexed under this heading.

Mephenytoin (Esomeprazole may potentially interfere with CYP2C19, the major esomeprazole metabolizing enzyme. Co-administration of esomeprazole 30 mg and diazepam, a CYP2C19 substrate, resulted in a 45% decrease in clearance of diazepam. Increased plasma levels of diazepam were observed 12 hours after dosing and onwards. However, at that time, the plasma levels of diazepam were below the therapeutic interval, and thus this interaction is unlikely to be of clinical relevance).
No products indexed under this heading.

Mephobarbital (Esomeprazole may potentially interfere with CYP2C19, the major esomeprazole metabolizing enzyme. Co-administration of esomeprazole 30 mg and diazepam, a CYP2C19 substrate, resulted in a 45% decrease in clearance of diazepam. Increased plasma levels of diazepam were observed 12 hours after dosing and onwards. However, at that time, the plasma levels of diazepam were below the therapeutic interval, and thus this interaction is unlikely to be of clinical relevance).
No products indexed under this heading.

Meprobamate (Esomeprazole may potentially interfere with CYP2C19, the major esomeprazole metabolizing enzyme. Co-administration of esomeprazole 30 mg and diazepam, a CYP2C19 substrate, resulted in a 45% decrease in clearance of diazepam. Increased plasma levels of diazepam were observed 12 hours after dosing and onwards. However, at that time, the plasma levels of diazepam were below the therapeutic interval, and thus this interaction is unlikely to be of clinical relevance).
No products indexed under this heading.

Mestranol (Concomitant administration of esomeprazole and a combined inhibitor of CYP2C19 and CYP3A4, such as voriconazole, may result in more than doubling of the esomeprazole exposure. Dose adjustment of esomeprazole is not normally required for the recommended doses. However, in patients who may require higher doses, dose adjustment may be considered).
No products indexed under this heading.

Methsuximide (Esomeprazole may potentially interfere with CYP2C19, the major esomeprazole metabolizing enzyme. Co-administration of esomeprazole 30 mg and diazepam, a CYP2C19 substrate, resulted in a 45% decrease in clearance of diazepam. Increased plasma levels of diazepam were observed 12 hours after dosing and onwards. However, at that time, the plasma levels of diazepam were below the therapeutic interval, and thus this interaction is unlikely to be of clinical relevance).
No products indexed under this heading.

Metronidazole (Concomitant administration of esomeprazole and a combined inhibitor of CYP2C19 and CYP3A4, such as voriconazole, may result in more than doubling of the esomeprazole exposure. Dose adjustment of esomeprazole is not normally required for the recommended doses. However, in patients who may require higher doses, dose adjustment may be considered). Products include:
Pylera 793

IMPORTANT NOTE: Always consult each drug listing in the patient's regimen for possible interactions.

Metronidazole Benzoate (Concomitant administration of esomeprazole and a combined inhibitor of CYP2C19 and CYP3A4, such as voriconazole, may result in more than doubling of the esomeprazole exposure. Dose adjustment of esomeprazole is not normally required for the recommended doses. However, in patients who may require higher doses, dose adjustment may be considered).
No products indexed under this heading.

Metronidazole Hydrochloride (Concomitant administration of esomeprazole and a combined inhibitor of CYP2C19 and CYP3A4, such as voriconazole, may result in more than doubling of the esomeprazole exposure. Dose adjustment of esomeprazole is not normally required for the recommended doses. However, in patients who may require higher doses, dose adjustment may be considered).
No products indexed under this heading.

Metronidazole Sodium (Concomitant administration of esomeprazole and a combined inhibitor of CYP2C19 and CYP3A4, such as voriconazole, may result in more than doubling of the esomeprazole exposure. Dose adjustment of esomeprazole is not normally required for the recommended doses. However, in patients who may require higher doses, dose adjustment may be considered).
No products indexed under this heading.

Miconazole (Concomitant administration of esomeprazole and a combined inhibitor of CYP2C19 and CYP3A4, such as voriconazole, may result in more than doubling of the esomeprazole exposure. Dose adjustment of esomeprazole is not normally required for the recommended doses. However, in patients who may require higher doses, dose adjustment may be considered).
No products indexed under this heading.

Miconazole Nitrate (Concomitant administration of esomeprazole and a combined inhibitor of CYP2C19 and CYP3A4, such as voriconazole, may result in more than doubling of the esomeprazole exposure. Dose adjustment of esomeprazole is not normally required for the recommended doses. However, in patients who may require higher doses, dose adjustment may be considered). Products include:
Vusion Ointment 3335

Midazolam Hydrochloride (Esomeprazole may potentially interfere with CYP2C19, the major esomeprazole metabolizing enzyme. Co-administration of esomeprazole 30 mg and diazepam, a CYP2C19 substrate, resulted in a 45% decrease in clearance of diazepam. Increased plasma levels of diazepam were observed 12 hours after dosing and onwards. However, at that time, the plasma levels of diazepam were below the therapeutic interval, and thus this interaction is unlikely to be of clinical relevance).
No products indexed under this heading.

Mifepristone (Concomitant administration of esomeprazole and a combined inhibitor of CYP2C19 and CYP3A4, such as voriconazole, may result in more than doubling of the esomeprazole exposure. Dose adjustment of esomeprazole is not normally required for the recommended doses. However, in patients who may require higher doses, dose adjustment may be considered).
No products indexed under this heading.

Modafinil (Concomitant administration of esomeprazole and a combined inhibitor of CYP2C19 and CYP3A4, such as voriconazole, may result in more than doubling of the esomeprazole expo-

sure. Dose adjustment of esomeprazole is not normally required for the recommended doses. However, in patients who may require higher doses, dose adjustment may be considered).
Products include:
Provigil 983

Nefazodone Hydrochloride (Concomitant administration of esomeprazole and a combined inhibitor of CYP2C19 and CYP3A4, such as voriconazole, may result in more than doubling of the esomeprazole exposure. Dose adjustment of esomeprazole is not normally required for the recommended doses. However, in patients who may require higher doses, dose adjustment may be considered).
No products indexed under this heading.

Nelfinavir Mesylate (Concomitant use of nelfinavir with proton pump inhibitors is not recommended. Following multiple doses of nelfinavir (1250 mg, bid) and omeprazole (40 mg qd), AUC was decreased by 36% and 92%, C_{max} by 37% and 89% and C_{min} by 39% and 75% respectively for nelfinavir and M8).
No products indexed under this heading.

Nevirapine (Omeprazole has been reported to interact with some antiretroviral drugs. The clinical importance and the mechanisms behind these interactions are not always known. Increased gastric pH during omeprazole treatment may change the absorption of the antiretroviral drug. Other possible interaction mechanisms are via CYP2C19).
Products include:
Viramune Oral Suspension 897
Viramune Tablets 897

Niacin (Concomitant administration of esomeprazole and a combined inhibitor of CYP2C19 and CYP3A4, such as voriconazole, may result in more than doubling of the esomeprazole exposure. Dose adjustment of esomeprazole is not normally required for the recommended doses. However, in patients who may require higher doses, dose adjustment may be considered).
Products include:
Advicor 402
Cardio Basics 3455
Niaspan 497
Simcor 524

Niacinamide (Concomitant administration of esomeprazole and a combined inhibitor of CYP2C19 and CYP3A4, such as voriconazole, may result in more than doubling of the esomeprazole exposure. Dose adjustment of esomeprazole is not normally required for the recommended doses. However, in patients who may require higher doses, dose adjustment may be considered). Products include:
CitraNatal 90 DHA Capsules 2332
CitraNatal Assure 2332
CitraNatal Rx 2332
Heplive 607

Niacinamide Hydroiodide (Concomitant administration of esomeprazole and a combined inhibitor of CYP2C19 and CYP3A4, such as voriconazole, may result in more than doubling of the esomeprazole exposure. Dose adjustment of esomeprazole is not normally required for the recommended doses. However, in patients who may require higher doses, dose adjustment may be considered).
No products indexed under this heading.

Nicotinamide (Concomitant administration of esomeprazole and a combined inhibitor of CYP2C19 and CYP3A4, such as voriconazole, may result in more than doubling of the esomeprazole exposure. Dose adjustment of esomeprazole is not normally required for the recommended doses. However, in patients who may require higher doses, dose adjustment may be considered).
No products indexed under this heading.

Nifedipine (Concomitant administration of esomeprazole and a combined inhibitor of CYP2C19 and CYP3A4, such as voriconazole, may result in more than doubling of the esomeprazole exposure. Dose adjustment of esomeprazole is not normally required for the recommended doses. However, in patients who may require higher doses, dose adjustment may be considered).
No products indexed under this heading.

Nilutamide (Esomeprazole may potentially interfere with CYP2C19, the major esomeprazole metabolizing enzyme. Co-administration of esomeprazole 30 mg and diazepam, a CYP2C19 substrate, resulted in a 45% decrease in clearance of diazepam. Increased plasma levels of diazepam were observed 12 hours after dosing and onwards. However, at that time, the plasma levels of diazepam were below the therapeutic interval, and thus this interaction is unlikely to be of clinical relevance).
No products indexed under this heading.

Norethindrone (Concomitant administration of esomeprazole and a combined inhibitor of CYP2C19 and CYP3A4, such as voriconazole, may result in more than doubling of the esomeprazole exposure. Dose adjustment of esomeprazole is not normally required for the recommended doses. However, in patients who may require higher doses, dose adjustment may be considered). Products include:
Ortho Micronor 2660

Norethynodrel (Concomitant administration of esomeprazole and a combined inhibitor of CYP2C19 and CYP3A4, such as voriconazole, may result in more than doubling of the esomeprazole exposure. Dose adjustment of esomeprazole is not normally required for the recommended doses. However, in patients who may require higher doses, dose adjustment may be considered).
No products indexed under this heading.

Norfloxacin (Concomitant administration of esomeprazole and a combined inhibitor of CYP2C19 and CYP3A4, such as voriconazole, may result in more than doubling of the esomeprazole exposure. Dose adjustment of esomeprazole is not normally required for the recommended doses. However, in patients who may require higher doses, dose adjustment may be considered). Products include:
Noroxin 2220

Norgestimate (Concomitant administration of esomeprazole and a combined inhibitor of CYP2C19 and CYP3A4, such as voriconazole, may result in more than doubling of the esomeprazole exposure. Dose adjustment of esomeprazole is not normally required for the recommended doses. However, in patients who may require higher doses, dose adjustment may be considered). Products include:
Ortho-Cyclen/Ortho Tri-Cyclen 2663
Ortho Tri-Cyclen Lo Tablets 2673

Norgestrel (Concomitant administration of esomeprazole and a combined inhibitor of CYP2C19 and CYP3A4, such as voriconazole, may result in more than doubling of the esomeprazole exposure. Dose adjustment of esomeprazole is not normally required for the recommended doses. However, in patients who may require higher doses, dose adjustment may be considered).
No products indexed under this heading.

Nortriptyline Hydrochloride (Esomeprazole may potentially interfere with CYP2C19, the major esomeprazole metabolizing enzyme. Co-administration of esomeprazole 30 mg and diazepam, a CYP2C19 substrate, resulted in a 45% decrease in clearance of diazepam. Increased plasma levels of diazepam were observed 12 hours after dosing and onwards. However, at that time, the plasma levels of diazepam were below the therapeutic interval, and thus this interaction is unlikely to be of clinical relevance).
No products indexed under this heading.

Omeprazole (Esomeprazole may potentially interfere with CYP2C19, the major esomeprazole metabolizing enzyme. Co-administration of esomeprazole 30 mg and diazepam, a CYP2C19 substrate, resulted in a 45% decrease in clearance of diazepam. Increased plasma levels of diazepam were observed 12 hours after dosing and onwards. However, at that time, the plasma levels of diazepam were below the therapeutic interval, and thus this interaction is unlikely to be of clinical relevance).
No products indexed under this heading.

Omeprazole Magnesium (Esomeprazole may potentially interfere with CYP2C19, the major esomeprazole metabolizing enzyme. Co-administration of esomeprazole 30 mg and diazepam, a CYP2C19 substrate, resulted in a 45% decrease in clearance of diazepam. Increased plasma levels of diazepam were observed 12 hours after dosing and onwards. However, at that time, the plasma levels of diazepam were below the therapeutic interval, and thus this interaction is unlikely to be of clinical relevance).
No products indexed under this heading.

Oxcarbazepine (Esomeprazole may potentially interfere with CYP2C19, the major esomeprazole metabolizing enzyme. Co-administration of esomeprazole 30 mg and diazepam, a CYP2C19 substrate, resulted in a 45% decrease in clearance of diazepam. Increased plasma levels of diazepam were observed 12 hours after dosing and onwards. However, at that time, the plasma levels of diazepam were below the therapeutic interval, and thus this interaction is unlikely to be of clinical relevance).
No products indexed under this heading.

Pantoprazole Sodium (Esomeprazole may potentially interfere with CYP2C19, the major esomeprazole metabolizing enzyme. Co-administration of esomeprazole 30 mg and diazepam, a CYP2C19 substrate, resulted in a 45% decrease in clearance of diazepam. Increased plasma levels of diazepam were observed 12 hours after dosing and onwards. However, at that time, the plasma levels of diazepam were below the therapeutic interval, and thus this interaction is unlikely to be of clinical relevance). Products include:
Protonix Tablets 3571
Protonix 3575

Paramethadione (Esomeprazole may potentially interfere with CYP2C19, the major esomeprazole metabolizing enzyme. Co-administration of esome-

1197 Interactions Index Nexium I.V.

prazole 30 mg and diazepam, a CYP2C19 substrate, resulted in a 45% decrease in clearance of diazepam. Increased plasma levels of diazepam were observed 12 hours after dosing and onwards. However, at that time, the plasma levels of diazepam were below the therapeutic interval, and thus this interaction is unlikely to be of clinical relevance).
No products indexed under this heading.

Paroxetine Hydrochloride (Concomitant administration of esomeprazole and a combined inhibitor of CYP2C19 and CYP3A4, such as voriconazole, may result in more than doubling of the esomeprazole exposure. Dose adjustment of esomeprazole is not normally required for the recommended doses. However, in patients who may require higher doses, dose adjustment may be considered). Products include:
Paroxetine CR ... 2361
Paroxetine ER ... 2371
Paxil ... 1586
Paxil CR ... 1596

Pentamidine Isethionate (Esomeprazole may potentially interfere with CYP2C19, the major esomeprazole metabolizing enzyme. Co-administration of esomeprazole 30 mg and diazepam, a CYP2C19 substrate, resulted in a 45% decrease in clearance of diazepam. Increased plasma levels of diazepam were observed 12 hours after dosing and onwards. However, at that time, the plasma levels of diazepam were below the therapeutic interval, and thus this interaction is unlikely to be of clinical relevance).
No products indexed under this heading.

Phenacemide (Esomeprazole may potentially interfere with CYP2C19, the major esomeprazole metabolizing enzyme. Co-administration of esomeprazole 30 mg and diazepam, a CYP2C19 substrate, resulted in a 45% decrease in clearance of diazepam. Increased plasma levels of diazepam were observed 12 hours after dosing and onwards. However, at that time, the plasma levels of diazepam were below the therapeutic interval, and thus this interaction is unlikely to be of clinical relevance).
No products indexed under this heading.

Phenobarbital (Esomeprazole may potentially interfere with CYP2C19, the major esomeprazole metabolizing enzyme. Co-administration of esomeprazole 30 mg and diazepam, a CYP2C19 substrate, resulted in a 45% decrease in clearance of diazepam. Increased plasma levels of diazepam were observed 12 hours after dosing and onwards. However, at that time, the plasma levels of diazepam were below the therapeutic interval, and thus this interaction is unlikely to be of clinical relevance). Products include:
Donnatal ... 2711

Phenobarbital Sodium (Esomeprazole may potentially interfere with CYP2C19, the major esomeprazole metabolizing enzyme. Co-administration of esomeprazole 30 mg and diazepam, a CYP2C19 substrate, resulted in a 45% decrease in clearance of diazepam. Increased plasma levels of diazepam were observed 12 hours after dosing and onwards. However, at that time, the plasma levels of diazepam were below the therapeutic interval, and thus this interaction is unlikely to be of clinical relevance).
No products indexed under this heading.

Phensuximide (Esomeprazole may potentially interfere with CYP2C19, the major esomeprazole metabolizing enzyme. Co-administration of esomeprazole 30 mg and diazepam, a CYP2C19 substrate, resulted in a 45% decrease in clearance of diazepam. Increased plasma levels of diazepam were observed 12 hours after dosing and onwards. However, at that time, the plasma levels of diazepam were below the therapeutic interval, and thus this interaction is unlikely to be of clinical relevance).
No products indexed under this heading.

Phenytoin (Esomeprazole may potentially interfere with CYP2C19, the major esomeprazole metabolizing enzyme. Co-administration of esomeprazole 30 mg and diazepam, a CYP2C19 substrate, resulted in a 45% decrease in clearance of diazepam. Increased plasma levels of diazepam were observed 12 hours after dosing and onwards. However, at that time, the plasma levels of diazepam were below the therapeutic interval, and thus this interaction is unlikely to be of clinical relevance).
No products indexed under this heading.

Phenytoin Sodium (Esomeprazole may potentially interfere with CYP2C19, the major esomeprazole metabolizing enzyme. Co-administration of esomeprazole 30 mg and diazepam, a CYP2C19 substrate, resulted in a 45% decrease in clearance of diazepam. Increased plasma levels of diazepam were observed 12 hours after dosing and onwards. However, at that time, the plasma levels of diazepam were below the therapeutic interval, and thus this interaction is unlikely to be of clinical relevance). Products include:
Phenytek Capsules ... 2380

Polysaccharide Iron Complex (Esomeprazole inhibits gastric acid secretion; therefore, esomeprazole may interfere with the absorption of drugs where gastric pH is an important determinant of bioavailability, such as oral iron salts). Products include:
Nu-Iron 150 ... 2321

Posaconazole (Concomitant administration of esomeprazole and a combined inhibitor of CYP2C19 and CYP3A4, such as voriconazole, may result in more than doubling of the esomeprazole exposure. Dose adjustment of esomeprazole is not normally required for the recommended doses. However, in patients who may require higher doses, dose adjustment may be considered). Products include:
Noxafil ... 3172

Primidone (Esomeprazole may potentially interfere with CYP2C19, the major esomeprazole metabolizing enzyme. Co-administration of esomeprazole 30 mg and diazepam, a CYP2C19 substrate, resulted in a 45% decrease in clearance of diazepam. Increased plasma levels of diazepam were observed 12 hours after dosing and onwards. However, at that time, the plasma levels of diazepam were below the therapeutic interval, and thus this interaction is unlikely to be of clinical relevance).
No products indexed under this heading.

Progesterone (Esomeprazole may potentially interfere with CYP2C19, the major esomeprazole metabolizing enzyme. Co-administration of esomeprazole 30 mg and diazepam, a CYP2C19 substrate, resulted in a 45% decrease in clearance of diazepam. Increased plasma levels of diazepam were observed 12 hours after dosing and onwards. However, at that time, the plasma levels of diazepam were below the therapeutic interval, and thus this interaction is unlikely to be of clinical relevance). Products include:
Crinone 4% ... 996
Crinone 8% ... 996
Prometrium ... 3307

Proguanil Hydrochloride (Esomeprazole may potentially interfere with CYP2C19, the major esomeprazole metabolizing enzyme. Co-administration of esomeprazole 30 mg and diazepam, a CYP2C19 substrate, resulted in a 45% decrease in clearance of diazepam. Increased plasma levels of diazepam were observed 12 hours after dosing and onwards. However, at that time, the plasma levels of diazepam were below the therapeutic interval, and thus this interaction is unlikely to be of clinical relevance). Products include:
Malarone Pediatric Tablets ... 1572
Malarone ... 1572

Propoxyphene Hydrochloride (Concomitant administration of esomeprazole and a combined inhibitor of CYP2C19 and CYP3A4, such as voriconazole, may result in more than doubling of the esomeprazole exposure. Dose adjustment of esomeprazole is not normally required for the recommended doses. However, in patients who may require higher doses, dose adjustment may be considered).
No products indexed under this heading.

Propoxyphene Napsylate (Concomitant administration of esomeprazole and a combined inhibitor of CYP2C19 and CYP3A4, such as voriconazole, may result in more than doubling of the esomeprazole exposure. Dose adjustment of esomeprazole is not normally required for the recommended doses. However, in patients who may require higher doses, dose adjustment may be considered).
No products indexed under this heading.

Propranolol Hydrochloride (Esomeprazole may potentially interfere with CYP2C19, the major esomeprazole metabolizing enzyme. Co-administration of esomeprazole 30 mg and diazepam, a CYP2C19 substrate, resulted in a 45% decrease in clearance of diazepam. Increased plasma levels of diazepam were observed 12 hours after dosing and onwards. However, at that time, the plasma levels of diazepam were below the therapeutic interval, and thus this interaction is unlikely to be of clinical relevance). Products include:
InnoPran XL ... 1517

Protriptyline Hydrochloride (Esomeprazole may potentially interfere with CYP2C19, the major esomeprazole metabolizing enzyme. Co-administration of esomeprazole 30 mg and diazepam, a CYP2C19 substrate, resulted in a 45% decrease in clearance of diazepam. Increased plasma levels of diazepam were observed 12 hours after dosing and onwards. However, at that time, the plasma levels of diazepam were below the therapeutic interval, and thus this interaction is unlikely to be of clinical relevance).
No products indexed under this heading.

Quinidine (Concomitant administration of esomeprazole and a combined inhibitor of CYP2C19 and CYP3A4, such as voriconazole, may result in more than doubling of the esomeprazole exposure. Dose adjustment of esomeprazole is not normally required for the recommended doses. However, in patients who may require higher doses, dose adjustment may be considered).
No products indexed under this heading.

Quinidine Gluconate (Concomitant administration of esomeprazole and a combined inhibitor of CYP2C19 and CYP3A4, such as voriconazole, may result in more than doubling of the esomeprazole exposure. Dose adjustment of esomeprazole is not normally required for the recommended doses. However, in patients who may require higher doses, dose adjustment may be considered).
No products indexed under this heading.

Quinidine Hydrochloride (Concomitant administration of esomeprazole and a combined inhibitor of CYP2C19 and CYP3A4, such as voriconazole, may result in more than doubling of the esomeprazole exposure. Dose adjustment of esomeprazole is not normally required for the recommended doses. However, in patients who may require higher doses, dose adjustment may be considered).
No products indexed under this heading.

Quinidine Polygalacturonate (Concomitant administration of esomeprazole and a combined inhibitor of CYP2C19 and CYP3A4, such as voriconazole, may result in more than doubling of the esomeprazole exposure. Dose adjustment of esomeprazole is not normally required for the recommended doses. However, in patients who may require higher doses, dose adjustment may be considered).
No products indexed under this heading.

Quinidine Sulfate (Concomitant administration of esomeprazole and a combined inhibitor of CYP2C19 and CYP3A4, such as voriconazole, may result in more than doubling of the esomeprazole exposure. Dose adjustment of esomeprazole is not normally required for the recommended doses. However, in patients who may require higher doses, dose adjustment may be considered).
No products indexed under this heading.

Quinine (Concomitant administration of esomeprazole and a combined inhibitor of CYP2C19 and CYP3A4, such as voriconazole, may result in more than doubling of the esomeprazole exposure. Dose adjustment of esomeprazole is not normally required for the recommended doses. However, in patients who may require higher doses, dose adjustment may be considered). Products include:
Hyland's Leg Cramps PM with Quinine ... 3315

Quinine Sulfate (Concomitant administration of esomeprazole and a combined inhibitor of CYP2C19 and CYP3A4, such as voriconazole, may result in more than doubling of the esomeprazole exposure. Dose adjustment of esomeprazole is not normally required for the recommended doses. However, in patients who may require higher doses, dose adjustment may be considered).
No products indexed under this heading.

Quinupristin (Concomitant administration of esomeprazole and a combined inhibitor of CYP2C19 and CYP3A4, such as voriconazole, may result in more than doubling of the esomeprazole exposure. Dose adjustment of esomeprazole is not normally required for the recommended doses. However, in patients who may require higher doses, dose adjustment may be considered).
No products indexed under this heading.

Rabeprazole Sodium (Esomeprazole may potentially interfere with CYP2C19, the major esomeprazole metabolizing enzyme. Co-administration of esomeprazole 30 mg and diazepam, a CYP2C19 substrate, resulted in a 45% decrease in clearance of diazepam. Increased plasma levels of diazepam were observed 12 hours after dosing and onwards. However, at that time, the plasma levels of diazepam were below the therapeutic interval, and thus this interaction is unlikely to be of clinical relevance). Products include:
Aciphex ... 1035

IMPORTANT NOTE: Always consult each drug listing in the patient's regimen for possible interactions.

Ranitidine Bismuth Citrate (Concomitant administration of esomeprazole and a combined inhibitor of CYP2C19 and CYP3A4, such as voriconazole, may result in more than doubling of the esomeprazole exposure. Dose adjustment of esomeprazole is not normally required for the recommended doses. However, in patients who may require higher doses, dose adjustment may be considered).
No products indexed under this heading.

Ranitidine Hydrochloride (Concomitant administration of esomeprazole and a combined inhibitor of CYP2C19 and CYP3A4, such as voriconazole, may result in more than doubling of the esomeprazole exposure. Dose adjustment of esomeprazole is not normally required for the recommended doses. However, in patients who may require higher doses, dose adjustment may be considered). Products include:
Zantac **1737**
Zantac Injection **1732**
Zantac Pharmacy **1735**

Ritonavir (For antiretroviral drugs, such as saquinavir, elevated serum levels have been reported with an increase in AUC by 82%, in C_{max} by 75% and in C_{min} by 106% following multiple dosing of saquinavir/ritonavir (1000/100 mg) bid for 15 days with omeprazole 40 mg qd co-administered days 11 to 15. Therefore, clinical and laboratory monitoring for saquinavir toxicity is recommended during concurrent use with esomeprazole sodium. Dose reduction of saquinavir should be considered from the safety perspective for individual patients). Products include:
Kaletra **458**
Norvir **509**

Saquinavir (For antiretroviral drugs, such as saquinavir, elevated serum levels have been reported with an increase in AUC by 82%, in C_{max} by 75% and in C_{min} by 106% following multiple dosing of saquinavir/ritonavir (1000/100 mg) bid for 15 days with omeprazole 40 mg qd co-administered days 11 to 15. Therefore, clinical and laboratory monitoring for saquinavir toxicity is recommended during concurrent use with esomeprazole sodium. Dose reduction of saquinavir should be considered from the safety perspective for individual patients).
No products indexed under this heading.

Saquinavir Mesylate (For antiretroviral drugs, such as saquinavir, elevated serum levels have been reported with an increase in AUC by 82%, in C_{max} by 75% and in C_{min} by 106% following multiple dosing of saquinavir/ritonavir (1000/100 mg) bid for 15 days with omeprazole 40 mg qd co-administered days 11 to 15. Therefore, clinical and laboratory monitoring for saquinavir toxicity is recommended during concurrent use with esomeprazole sodium. Dose reduction of saquinavir should be considered from the safety perspective for individual patients).
No products indexed under this heading.

Sertraline Hydrochloride (Esomeprazole may potentially interfere with CYP2C19, the major esomeprazole metabolizing enzyme. Co-administration of esomeprazole 30 mg and diazepam, a CYP2C19 substrate, resulted in a 45% decrease in clearance of diazepam. Increased plasma levels of diazepam were observed 12 hours after dosing and onwards. However, at that time, the plasma levels of diazepam were below the therapeutic interval, and thus this interaction is unlikely to be of clinical relevance).
No products indexed under this heading.

Sildenafil Citrate (Concomitant administration of esomeprazole and a combined inhibitor of CYP2C19 and CYP3A4, such as voriconazole, may result in more than doubling of the esomeprazole exposure. Dose adjustment of esomeprazole is not normally required for the recommended doses. However, in patients who may require higher doses, dose adjustment may be considered).
No products indexed under this heading.

Stavudine (Omeprazole has been reported to interact with some antiretroviral drugs. The clinical importance and the mechanisms behind these interactions are not always known. Increased gastric pH during omeprazole treatment may change the absorption of the antiretroviral drug. Other possible interaction mechanisms are via CYP2C19).
No products indexed under this heading.

Sulfaphenazole (Concomitant administration of esomeprazole and a combined inhibitor of CYP2C19 and CYP3A4, such as voriconazole, may result in more than doubling of the esomeprazole exposure. Dose adjustment of esomeprazole is not normally required for the recommended doses. However, in patients who may require higher doses, dose adjustment may be considered).
No products indexed under this heading.

Telithromycin (Concomitant administration of esomeprazole and a combined inhibitor of CYP2C19 and CYP3A4, such as voriconazole, may result in more than doubling of the esomeprazole exposure. Dose adjustment of esomeprazole is not normally required for the recommended doses. However, in patients who may require higher doses, dose adjustment may be considered). Products include:
Ketek **2991**

Telmisartan (Concomitant administration of esomeprazole and a combined inhibitor of CYP2C19 and CYP3A4, such as voriconazole, may result in more than doubling of the esomeprazole exposure. Dose adjustment of esomeprazole is not normally required for the recommended doses. However, in patients who may require higher doses, dose adjustment may be considered). Products include:
Micardis **887**
Micardis HCT **889**

Teniposide (Esomeprazole may potentially interfere with CYP2C19, the major esomeprazole metabolizing enzyme. Co-administration of esomeprazole 30 mg and diazepam, a CYP2C19 substrate, resulted in a 45% decrease in clearance of diazepam. Increased plasma levels of diazepam were observed 12 hours after dosing and onwards. However, at that time, the plasma levels of diazepam were below the therapeutic interval, and thus this interaction is unlikely to be of clinical relevance).
No products indexed under this heading.

Tenofovir Disoproxil Fumarate (Omeprazole has been reported to interact with some antiretroviral drugs. The clinical importance and the mechanisms behind these interactions are not always known. Increased gastric pH during omeprazole treatment may change the absorption of the antiretroviral drug. Other possible interaction mechanisms are via CYP2C19). Products include:
Atripla **906**
Truvada **1258**
Viread **1266**

Thioridazine (Esomeprazole may potentially interfere with CYP2C19, the major esomeprazole metabolizing enzyme. Co-administration of esomeprazole 30 mg and diazepam, a CYP2C19 substrate, resulted in a 45% decrease in clearance of diazepam. Increased plasma levels of diazepam were observed 12 hours after dosing and onwards. However, at that time, the plasma levels of diazepam were below the therapeutic interval, and thus this interaction is unlikely to be of clinical relevance).
No products indexed under this heading.

Thioridazine Hydrochloride (Esomeprazole may potentially interfere with CYP2C19, the major esomeprazole metabolizing enzyme. Co-administration of esomeprazole 30 mg and diazepam, a CYP2C19 substrate, resulted in a 45% decrease in clearance of diazepam. Increased plasma levels of diazepam were observed 12 hours after dosing and onwards. However, at that time, the plasma levels of diazepam were below the therapeutic interval, and thus this interaction is unlikely to be of clinical relevance). Products include:
Thioridazine Hydrochloride **2384**

Tiagabine Hydrochloride (Esomeprazole may potentially interfere with CYP2C19, the major esomeprazole metabolizing enzyme. Co-administration of esomeprazole 30 mg and diazepam, a CYP2C19 substrate, resulted in a 45% decrease in clearance of diazepam. Increased plasma levels of diazepam were observed 12 hours after dosing and onwards. However, at that time, the plasma levels of diazepam were below the therapeutic interval, and thus this interaction is unlikely to be of clinical relevance). Products include:
Gabitril **972**

Ticlopidine Hydrochloride (Concomitant administration of esomeprazole and a combined inhibitor of CYP2C19 and CYP3A4, such as voriconazole, may result in more than doubling of the esomeprazole exposure. Dose adjustment of esomeprazole is not normally required for the recommended doses. However, in patients who may require higher doses, dose adjustment may be considered).
No products indexed under this heading.

Tipranavir (Omeprazole has been reported to interact with some antiretroviral drugs. The clinical importance and the mechanisms behind these interactions are not always known. Increased gastric pH during omeprazole treatment may change the absorption of the antiretroviral drug. Other possible interaction mechanisms are via CYP2C19).
No products indexed under this heading.

Tolbutamide (Esomeprazole may potentially interfere with CYP2C19, the major esomeprazole metabolizing enzyme. Co-administration of esomeprazole 30 mg and diazepam, a CYP2C19 substrate, resulted in a 45% decrease in clearance of diazepam. Increased plasma levels of diazepam were observed 12 hours after dosing and onwards. However, at that time, the plasma levels of diazepam were below the therapeutic interval, and thus this interaction is unlikely to be of clinical relevance).
No products indexed under this heading.

Tolbutamide Sodium (Esomeprazole may potentially interfere with CYP2C19, the major esomeprazole metabolizing enzyme. Co-administration of esomeprazole 30 mg and diazepam, a CYP2C19 substrate, resulted in a 45% decrease in clearance of diazepam. Increased plasma levels of diazepam were observed 12 hours after dosing and onwards. However, at that time, the plasma levels of diazepam were below the therapeutic interval, and thus this interaction is unlikely to be of clinical relevance).
No products indexed under this heading.

Topiramate (Esomeprazole may potentially interfere with CYP2C19, the major esomeprazole metabolizing enzyme. Co-administration of esomeprazole 30 mg and diazepam, a CYP2C19 substrate, resulted in a 45% decrease in clearance of diazepam. Increased plasma levels of diazepam were observed 12 hours after dosing and onwards. However, at that time, the plasma levels of diazepam were below the therapeutic interval, and thus this interaction is unlikely to be of clinical relevance).
No products indexed under this heading.

Tranylcypromine Sulfate (Concomitant administration of esomeprazole and a combined inhibitor of CYP2C19 and CYP3A4, such as voriconazole, may result in more than doubling of the esomeprazole exposure. Dose adjustment of esomeprazole is not normally required for the recommended doses. However, in patients who may require higher doses, dose adjustment may be considered). Products include:
Parnate **1584**

Trimethadione (Esomeprazole may potentially interfere with CYP2C19, the major esomeprazole metabolizing enzyme. Co-administration of esomeprazole 30 mg and diazepam, a CYP2C19 substrate, resulted in a 45% decrease in clearance of diazepam. Increased plasma levels of diazepam were observed 12 hours after dosing and onwards. However, at that time, the plasma levels of diazepam were below the therapeutic interval, and thus this interaction is unlikely to be of clinical relevance).
No products indexed under this heading.

Trimipramine Maleate (Esomeprazole may potentially interfere with CYP2C19, the major esomeprazole metabolizing enzyme. Co-administration of esomeprazole 30 mg and diazepam, a CYP2C19 substrate, resulted in a 45% decrease in clearance of diazepam. Increased plasma levels of diazepam were observed 12 hours after dosing and onwards. However, at that time, the plasma levels of diazepam were below the therapeutic interval, and thus this interaction is unlikely to be of clinical relevance).
No products indexed under this heading.

Troglitazone (Concomitant administration of esomeprazole and a combined inhibitor of CYP2C19 and CYP3A4, such as voriconazole, may result in more than doubling of the esomeprazole exposure. Dose adjustment of esomeprazole is not normally required for the recommended doses. However, in patients who may require higher doses, dose adjustment may be considered).
No products indexed under this heading.

Troleandomycin (Concomitant administration of esomeprazole and a combined inhibitor of CYP2C19 and CYP3A4, such as voriconazole, may result in more than doubling of the esomeprazole exposure. Dose adjustment of esomeprazole is not normally required for the recommended doses. However, in patients who may require higher doses, dose adjustment may be considered).
No products indexed under this heading.

Valproate Sodium (Esomeprazole may potentially interfere with CYP2C19, the major esomeprazole metabolizing enzyme. Co-administration of esomeprazole 30 mg and diazepam, a CYP2C19 substrate, resulted in a 45% decrease in clearance of diazepam. Increased plasma levels of diazepam were observed 12 hours after dosing and onwards. However, at that time, the plasma levels of diazepam were below

the therapeutic interval, and thus this interaction is unlikely to be of clinical relevance).
No products indexed under this heading.

Valproic Acid (Esomeprazole may potentially interfere with CYP2C19, the major esomeprazole metabolizing enzyme. Co-administration of esomeprazole 30 mg and diazepam, a CYP2C19 substrate, resulted in a 45% decrease in clearance of diazepam. Increased plasma levels of diazepam were observed 12 hours after dosing and onwards. However, at that time, the plasma levels of diazepam were below the therapeutic interval, and thus this interaction is unlikely to be of clinical relevance).
No products indexed under this heading.

Vardenafil Hydrochloride (Concomitant administration of esomeprazole and a combined inhibitor of CYP2C19 and CYP3A4, such as voriconazole, may result in more than doubling of the esomeprazole exposure. Dose adjustment of esomeprazole is not normally required for the recommended doses. However, in patients who may require higher doses, dose adjustment may be considered). Products include:
Levitra 3157

Verapamil Hydrochloride (Concomitant administration of esomeprazole and a combined inhibitor of CYP2C19 and CYP3A4, such as voriconazole, may result in more than doubling of the esomeprazole exposure. Dose adjustment of esomeprazole is not normally required for the recommended doses. However, in patients who may require higher doses, dose adjustment may be considered). Products include:
Tarka 534

Voriconazole (Concomitant administration of esomeprazole and a combined inhibitor of CYP2C19 and CYP3A4, such as voriconazole, may result in more than doubling of the esomeprazole exposure. Dose adjustment of esomeprazole is not normally required for the recommended doses. However, in patients who may require higher doses, dose adjustment may be considered).
No products indexed under this heading.

Warfarin Sodium (Changes in prothrombin measures have been reported among patients on concomitant warfarin and esomeprazole therapy. Increases in INR and prothrombin time may lead to abnormal bleeding and even death. Patients treated with proton pump inhibitors and warfarin concomitantly may need to be monitored for increases in INR and prothrombin time).
No products indexed under this heading.

Zafirlukast (Concomitant administration of esomeprazole and a combined inhibitor of CYP2C19 and CYP3A4, such as voriconazole, may result in more than doubling of the esomeprazole exposure. Dose adjustment of esomeprazole is not normally required for the recommended doses. However, in patients who may require higher doses, dose adjustment may be considered). Products include:
Accolate 3612

Zalcitabine (Omeprazole has been reported to interact with some antiretroviral drugs. The clinical importance and the mechanisms behind these interactions are not always known. Increased gastric pH during omeprazole treatment may change the absorption of the antiretroviral drug. Other possible interaction mechanisms are via CYP2C19).
No products indexed under this heading.

Zidovudine (Omeprazole has been reported to interact with some antiretroviral drugs. The clinical importance and the mechanisms behind these interactions are not always known. Increased gastric pH during omeprazole treatment may change the absorption of the antiretroviral drug. Other possible interaction mechanisms are via CYP2C19). Products include:
Combivir 1404
Retrovir 1634
Retrovir IV 1640
Trizivir 1688

Zileuton (Concomitant administration of esomeprazole and a combined inhibitor of CYP2C19 and CYP3A4, such as voriconazole, may result in more than doubling of the esomeprazole exposure. Dose adjustment of esomeprazole is not normally required for the recommended doses. However, in patients who may require higher doses, dose adjustment may be considered).
No products indexed under this heading.

Zonisamide (Esomeprazole may potentially interfere with CYP2C19, the major esomeprazole metabolizing enzyme. Co-administration of esomeprazole 30 mg and diazepam, a CYP2C19 substrate, resulted in a 45% decrease in clearance of diazepam. Increased plasma levels of diazepam were observed 12 hours after dosing and onwards. However, at that time, the plasma levels of diazepam were below the therapeutic interval, and thus this interaction is unlikely to be of clinical relevance). Products include:
Zonegran 1081

Food Interactions

Grapefruit (Concomitant administration of esomeprazole and a combined inhibitor of CYP2C19 and CYP3A4, such as voriconazole, may result in more than doubling of the esomeprazole exposure. Dose adjustment of esomeprazole is not normally required for the recommended doses. However, in patients who may require higher doses, dose adjustment may be considered).

Grapefruit Juice (Concomitant administration of esomeprazole and a combined inhibitor of CYP2C19 and CYP3A4, such as voriconazole, may result in more than doubling of the esomeprazole exposure. Dose adjustment of esomeprazole is not normally required for the recommended doses. However, in patients who may require higher doses, dose adjustment may be considered).

NIASPAN EXTENDED-RELEASE TABLETS

(Niacin) 497
May interact with alcohols, aspirin-acetylsalicylic acid, beta-blockers, bile acid sequestering agents, calcium channel blockers, ganglionic blocking agents, nitrates and nitrites, oral anticoagulants, vasopressors, and certain other agents. Compounds in these categories include:

Acebutolol Hydrochloride (Caution should also be used when niacin is used in patients with unstable angina or in the acute phase of an myocardial infarction, particularly when such patients are also receiving vasoactive drugs such as adrenergic blocking agents).
No products indexed under this heading.

Amlodipine Besylate (Caution should also be used when niacin is used in patients with unstable angina or in the acute phase of an myocardial infarction, particularly when such patients are also receiving vasoactive drugs such as calcium channel blockers). Products include:
Azor 1010
Exforge 2443
Exforge HCT 2449

Amyl Nitrite (Caution should also be used when niacin is used in patients with unstable angina or in the acute phase of an myocardial infarction, particularly when such patients are also receiving vasoactive drugs such as nitrates).
No products indexed under this heading.

Anisindione (Niacin has been associated with small but statistically significant dose-related reductions in platelet count (mean of -11% with 2000 mg). Caution should be observed when niacin is administered concomitantly with anticoagulants. Platelet counts should be monitored closely in such patients).
No products indexed under this heading.

Aspirin (Concomitant use of aspirin may decrease the metabolic clearance of nicotinic acid). Products include:
Aggrenox 880
Bayer Aspirin 829
Percodan 1124
St. Joseph Aspirin 2045

Aspirin, Enteric Coated (Concomitant use of aspirin may decrease the metabolic clearance of nicotinic acid).
No products indexed under this heading.

Aspirin Buffered (Concomitant use of aspirin may decrease the metabolic clearance of nicotinic acid).
No products indexed under this heading.

Atenolol (Caution should also be used when niacin is used in patients with unstable angina or in the acute phase of an myocardial infarction, particularly when such patients are also receiving vasoactive drugs such as adrenergic blocking agents).
No products indexed under this heading.

Bepridil Hydrochloride (Caution should also be used when niacin is used in patients with unstable angina or in the acute phase of an myocardial infarction, particularly when such patients are also receiving vasoactive drugs such as calcium channel blockers).
No products indexed under this heading.

Betaxolol Hydrochloride (Caution should also be used when niacin is used in patients with unstable angina or in the acute phase of an myocardial infarction, particularly when such patients are also receiving vasoactive drugs such as adrenergic blocking agents).
No products indexed under this heading.

Bisoprolol Fumarate (Caution should also be used when niacin is used in patients with unstable angina or in the acute phase of an myocardial infarction, particularly when such patients are also receiving vasoactive drugs such as adrenergic blocking agents).
No products indexed under this heading.

Carteolol Hydrochloride (Caution should also be used when niacin is used in patients with unstable angina or in the acute phase of an myocardial infarction, particularly when such patients are also receiving vasoactive drugs such as adrenergic blocking agents).
No products indexed under this heading.

Carvedilol (Caution should also be used when niacin is used in patients with unstable angina or in the acute phase of an myocardial infarction, particularly when such patients are also receiving vasoactive drugs such as adrenergic blocking agents). Products include:
Coreg 1409

Carvedilol Phosphate (Caution should also be used when niacin is used in patients with unstable angina or in the acute phase of an myocardial infarction, particularly when such patients are also receiving vasoactive drugs such as adrenergic blocking agents). Products include:
Coreg CR 1416

Cholestyramine (An *in vitro* study was carried out investigating the niacin-binding capacity of cholestyramine. About 98% of available niacin was bound to 10 to 30% cholestyramine. Therefore, 4 to 6 hours or as great an interval as possible, should elapse between the ingestion of bile acid-binding resins and the administration of niacin).
No products indexed under this heading.

Colesevelam Hydrochloride (An *in vitro* study results suggest that the bile acid-binding resins have high niacin binding capacity. Therefore, 4 to 6 hours or as great an interval as possible, should elapse between the ingestion of bile acid-binding resins and the administration of niacin). Products include:
Welchol 1029

Colestipol (An *in vitro* study was carried out investigating the niacin-binding capacity of colestipol. About 98% of available niacin was bound to colestipol. Therefore, 4 to 6 hours or as great an interval as possible, should elapse between the ingestion of bile acid-binding resins and the administration of niacin).
No products indexed under this heading.

Colestipol Hydrochloride (An *in vitro* study was carried out investigating the niacin-binding capacity of colestipol. About 98% of available niacin was bound to colestipol. Therefore, 4 to 6 hours or as great an interval as possible, should elapse between the ingestion of bile acid-binding resins and the administration of niacin).
No products indexed under this heading.

Dicumarol (Niacin has been associated with small but statistically significant dose-related reductions in platelet count (mean of -11% with 2000 mg). Caution should be observed when niacin is administered concomitantly with anticoagulants. Platelet counts should be monitored closely in such patients).
No products indexed under this heading.

Diltiazem Hydrochloride (Caution should also be used when niacin is used in patients with unstable angina or in the acute phase of an myocardial infarction, particularly when such patients are also receiving vasoactive drugs such as calcium channel blockers). Products include:
Cardizem LA 423

Dobutamine (Niacin may potentiate the effects of vasoactive drugs resulting in postural hypotension).
No products indexed under this heading.

Dobutamine Hydrochloride (Niacin may potentiate the effects of vasoactive drugs resulting in postural hypotension).
No products indexed under this heading.

Dopamine Hydrochloride (Niacin may potentiate the effects of vasoactive drugs resulting in postural hypotension).
No products indexed under this heading.

Ephedrine Sulfate (Niacin may potentiate the effects of vasoactive drugs resulting in postural hypotension).
No products indexed under this heading.

Epinephrine Bitartrate (Niacin may potentiate the effects of vasoactive drugs resulting in postural hypotension).
No products indexed under this heading.

Epinephrine Hydrochloride (Niacin may potentiate the effects of vasoactive drugs resulting in postural hypotension).
No products indexed under this heading.

Erythrityl Tetranitrate (Caution should also be used when niacin is used in patients with unstable angina or in the acute phase of an myocardial infarction, particularly when such patients are also receiving vasoactive drugs such as nitrates).
No products indexed under this heading.

IMPORTANT NOTE: Always consult each drug listing in the patient's regimen for possible interactions.

Esmolol Hydrochloride (Caution should also be used when niacin is used in patients with unstable angina or in the acute phase of an myocardial infarction, particularly when such patients are also receiving vasoactive drugs such as adrenergic blocking agents).
No products indexed under this heading.

Ethanol (Concomitant alcohol may increase the side effects of flushing and pruritus and should be avoided around the time of Niaspan ingestion).
No products indexed under this heading.

Ethyl Alcohol (Concomitant alcohol may increase the side effects of flushing and pruritus and should be avoided around the time of Niaspan ingestion).
No products indexed under this heading.

Felodipine (Caution should also be used when niacin is used in patients with unstable angina or in the acute phase of an myocardial infarction, particularly when such patients are also receiving vasoactive drugs such as calcium channel blockers).
No products indexed under this heading.

Glyceryl Trinitrate (Caution should also be used when niacin is used in patients with unstable angina or in the acute phase of an myocardial infarction, particularly when such patients are also receiving vasoactive drugs such as nitrates).
No products indexed under this heading.

Isoproterenol Hydrochloride (Niacin may potentiate the effects of vasoactive drugs resulting in postural hypotension).
No products indexed under this heading.

Isoproterenol Sulfate (Niacin may potentiate the effects of vasoactive drugs resulting in postural hypotension).
No products indexed under this heading.

Isosorbide Dinitrate (Caution should also be used when niacin is used in patients with unstable angina or in the acute phase of an myocardial infarction, particularly when such patients are also receiving vasoactive drugs such as nitrates).
No products indexed under this heading.

Isosorbide Mononitrate (Caution should also be used when niacin is used in patients with unstable angina or in the acute phase of an myocardial infarction, particularly when such patients are also receiving vasoactive drugs such as nitrates).
No products indexed under this heading.

Isradipine (Caution should also be used when niacin is used in patients with unstable angina or in the acute phase of an myocardial infarction, particularly when such patients are also receiving vasoactive drugs such as calcium channel blockers). Products include:
DynaCirc CR 1432

Labetalol Hydrochloride (Caution should also be used when niacin is used in patients with unstable angina or in the acute phase of an myocardial infarction, particularly when such patients are also receiving vasoactive drugs such as adrenergic blocking agents).
No products indexed under this heading.

Levobunolol Hydrochloride (Caution should also be used when niacin is used in patients with unstable angina or in the acute phase of an myocardial infarction, particularly when such patients are also receiving vasoactive drugs such as adrenergic blocking agents).
No products indexed under this heading.

Lovastatin (Caution should be used when prescribing niacin (1 gm/day) with statins as these drugs can increase risk of myopathy/rhabdomyolysis. Combination therapy with niacin and lovastatin should not exceed doses of 2000 mg niacin and 40 mg lovastatin daily. The risk for myopathy and rhabdomyolysis are increased when lovastatin are co-administered with niacin, particularly in elderly patients and patients with diabetes, renal failure, or uncontrolled hypothyroidism. When niacin 2000 mg and lovastatin 40 mg were co-administered, Niacin increased lovastatin C_{max} and AUC by 2% and 14%, respectively, and decreased lovastatin acid C_{max} and AUC by 22% and 2%, respectively. Lovastatin reduced niacin bioavailability by 2-3%). Products include:
Advicor 402
Mevacor 2212

Mecamylamine Hydrochloride (Niacin may potentiate the effects of ganglionic blocking agents resulting in postural hypotension).
No products indexed under this heading.

Mephentermine Sulfate (Niacin may potentiate the effects of vasoactive drugs resulting in postural hypotension).
No products indexed under this heading.

Metaraminol Bitartrate (Niacin may potentiate the effects of vasoactive drugs resulting in postural hypotension).
No products indexed under this heading.

Methoxamine Hydrochloride (Niacin may potentiate the effects of vasoactive drugs resulting in postural hypotension).
No products indexed under this heading.

Metipranolol Hydrochloride (Caution should also be used when niacin is used in patients with unstable angina or in the acute phase of an myocardial infarction, particularly when such patients are also receiving vasoactive drugs such as adrenergic blocking agents).
No products indexed under this heading.

Metoprolol Succinate (Caution should also be used when niacin is used in patients with unstable angina or in the acute phase of an myocardial infarction, particularly when such patients are also receiving vasoactive drugs such as adrenergic blocking agents). Products include:
Toprol XL 732

Metoprolol Tartrate (Caution should also be used when niacin is used in patients with unstable angina or in the acute phase of an myocardial infarction, particularly when such patients are also receiving vasoactive drugs such as adrenergic blocking agents).
No products indexed under this heading.

Mibefradil Dihydrochloride (Caution should also be used when niacin is used in patients with unstable angina or in the acute phase of an myocardial infarction, particularly when such patients are also receiving vasoactive drugs such as calcium channel blockers).
No products indexed under this heading.

Nadolol (Caution should also be used when niacin is used in patients with unstable angina or in the acute phase of an myocardial infarction, particularly when such patients are also receiving vasoactive drugs such as adrenergic blocking agents). Products include:
Nadolol 2359

Nebivolol (Caution should also be used when niacin is used in patients with unstable angina or in the acute phase of an myocardial infarction, particularly when such patients are also receiving vasoactive drugs such as adrenergic blocking agents). Products include:
Bystolic 1147

Nicardipine (Caution should also be used when niacin is used in patients with unstable angina or in the acute phase of an myocardial infarction, particularly when such patients are also receiving vasoactive drugs such as calcium channel blockers).
No products indexed under this heading.

Nicardipine Hydrochloride (Caution should also be used when niacin is used in patients with unstable angina or in the acute phase of an myocardial infarction, particularly when such patients are also receiving vasoactive drugs such as calcium channel blockers).
No products indexed under this heading.

Nicotinamide (Concomitant use of related compound such as nicotinamide may potentiate the adverse effects of niacin).
No products indexed under this heading.

Nifedipine (Caution should also be used when niacin is used in patients with unstable angina or in the acute phase of an myocardial infarction, particularly when such patients are also receiving vasoactive drugs such as calcium channel blockers).
No products indexed under this heading.

Nimodipine (Caution should also be used when niacin is used in patients with unstable angina or in the acute phase of an myocardial infarction, particularly when such patients are also receiving vasoactive drugs such as calcium channel blockers).
No products indexed under this heading.

Nisoldipine (Caution should also be used when niacin is used in patients with unstable angina or in the acute phase of an myocardial infarction, particularly when such patients are also receiving vasoactive drugs such as calcium channel blockers).
No products indexed under this heading.

Nitrate & Nitrite Preparations (Caution should also be used when niacin is used in patients with unstable angina or in the acute phase of an myocardial infarction, particularly when such patients are also receiving vasoactive drugs such as nitrates).
No products indexed under this heading.

Nitrates, organic (Caution should also be used when niacin is used in patients with unstable angina or in the acute phase of an myocardial infarction, particularly when such patients are also receiving vasoactive drugs such as nitrates).
No products indexed under this heading.

Nitrates and Nitrites (Caution should also be used when niacin is used in patients with unstable angina or in the acute phase of an myocardial infarction, particularly when such patients are also receiving vasoactive drugs such as nitrates).
No products indexed under this heading.

Nitroglycerin (Caution should also be used when niacin is used in patients with unstable angina or in the acute phase of an myocardial infarction, particularly when such patients are also receiving vasoactive drugs such as nitrates). Products include:
Nitro-Dur 3170
Nitrolingual 3266

Nitroglycerin, long-acting formulations (Caution should also be used when niacin is used in patients with unstable angina or in the acute phase of an myocardial infarction, particularly when such patients are also receiving vasoactive drugs such as nitrates).
No products indexed under this heading.

Nitroglycerin Intravenous (Caution should also be used when niacin is used in patients with unstable angina or in the acute phase of an myocardial infarction, particularly when such patients are also receiving vasoactive drugs such as nitrates).
No products indexed under this heading.

Norepinephrine Bitartrate (Niacin may potentiate the effects of vasoactive drugs resulting in postural hypotension).
No products indexed under this heading.

Nutritional Supplement (Concomitant use of nutritional supplements which contains large doses of niacin may potentiate the adverse effects of niacin).
No products indexed under this heading.

Penbutolol Sulfate (Caution should also be used when niacin is used in patients with unstable angina or in the acute phase of an myocardial infarction, particularly when such patients are also receiving vasoactive drugs such as adrenergic blocking agents).
No products indexed under this heading.

Pentaerythritol Tetranitrate (Caution should also be used when niacin is used in patients with unstable angina or in the acute phase of an myocardial infarction, particularly when such patients are also receiving vasoactive drugs such as nitrates).
No products indexed under this heading.

Phenylephrine Hydrochloride (Niacin may potentiate the effects of vasoactive drugs resulting in postural hypotension). Products include:
Sudafed PE Nasal Decongestant 2048
Children's Sudafed PE Nasal Decongestant 2047

Pindolol (Caution should also be used when niacin is used in patients with unstable angina or in the acute phase of an myocardial infarction, particularly when such patients are also receiving vasoactive drugs such as adrenergic blocking agents).
No products indexed under this heading.

Propranolol Hydrochloride (Caution should also be used when niacin is used in patients with unstable angina or in the acute phase of an myocardial infarction, particularly when such patients are also receiving vasoactive drugs such as adrenergic blocking agents). Products include:
InnoPran XL 1517

Simvastatin (Caution should be used when prescribing niacin (1 gm/day) with statins as these drugs can increase risk of myopathy/rhabdomyolysis. Combination therapy with niacin and simvastatin should not exceed doses of 2000 mg niacin and 40 mg simvastatin daily. The risk for myopathy and rhabdomyolysis are increased when simvastatin are co-administered with niacin, particularly in elderly patients and patients with diabetes, renal failure, or uncontrolled hypothyroidism. When niacin 2000 mg and simvastatin 40 mg were co-administered, Niacin increased simvastatin C_{max} and AUC by 1% and 9%, respectively, and simvastatin acid C_{max} and AUC by 2% and 18%, respectively. Simvastatin reduced niacin bioavailability by 2%). Products include:
Simcor 524
Vytorin 10/10 .... 2303, 3240
Vytorin 10/20 .... 2303, 3240
Vytorin 10/40 .... 2303, 3240
Vytorin 10/80 .... 2303, 3240
Zocor 2289

Sotalol Hydrochloride (Caution should also be used when niacin is used in patients with unstable angina or in the acute phase of an myocardial infarction, particularly when such patients are also receiving vasoactive drugs such as adrenergic blocking agents).
No products indexed under this heading.

Timolol Hemihydrate (Caution should also be used when niacin is used in patients with unstable angina or in the acute phase of an myocardial infarction, particularly when such patients are also receiving vasoactive drugs such as adrenergic blocking agents). Products include:

Timolol Maleate (Caution should also be used when niacin is used in patients with unstable angina or in the acute phase of an myocardial infarction, particularly when such patients are also receiving vasoactive drugs such as adrenergic blocking agents). Products include:

Trimethaphan Camsylate (Niacin may potentiate the effects of ganglionic blocking agents resulting in postural hypotension).
No products indexed under this heading.

Verapamil Hydrochloride (Caution should also be used when niacin is used in patients with unstable angina or in the acute phase of an myocardial infarction, particularly when such patients are also receiving vasoactive drugs such as calcium channel blockers). Products include:

Vitamins, Supplement (Concomitant use of vitamins which contains large doses of niacin may potentiate the adverse effects of niacin).
No products indexed under this heading.

Warfarin Sodium (Niacin has been associated with small but statistically significant dose-related reductions in platelet count (mean of -11% with 2000 mg). Caution should be observed when niacin is administered concomitantly with anticoagulants. Platelet counts should be monitored closely in such patients).
No products indexed under this heading.

Food Interactions

Alcohol (Concomitant alcohol may increase the side effects of flushing and pruritus and should be avoided around the time of Niaspan ingestion).

Beer, reduced-alcohol (Concomitant alcohol may increase the side effects of flushing and pruritis and should be avoided around the time of Niaspan ingestion).

Beer, unspecified (Concomitant alcohol may increase the side effects of flushing and pruritus and should be avoided around the time of Niaspan ingestion).

Drinks, hot, unspecified (Concomitant administration of hot drinks may increase the side effects of flushing and pruritus and should be avoided around the time of niacin ingestion).

Food, unspecified (Concomitant administration of spicy foods may increase the side effects of flushing and pruritus and should be avoided around the time of niacin ingestion).

Meal, unspecified (Concomitant administration of spicy foods may increase the side effects of flushing and pruritus and should be avoided around the time of niacin ingestion).

Wine, Chianti (Concomitant alcohol may increase the side effects of flushing and pruritus and should be avoided around the time of Niaspan ingestion).

Wine, Red (Concomitant alcohol may increase the side effects of flushing and pruritus and should be avoided around the time of Niaspan ingestion).

Wine, unspecified (Concomitant alcohol may increase the side effects of flushing and pruritus and should be avoided around the time of Niaspan ingestion).

Wine products (Concomitant alcohol may increase the side effects of flushing and pruritus and should be avoided around the time of Niaspan ingestion).

NIMBEX INJECTION
May interact with aminoglycosides, lithium preparations, local anesthetics, phenytoin, tetracyclines, and certain other agents. Compounds in these categories include:

Amikacin Sulfate (Enhances neuromuscular blocking action).
No products indexed under this heading.

Articaine Hydrochloride (Enhances neuromuscular blocking action).
No products indexed under this heading.

Bacitracin (Enhances neuromuscular blocking action).
No products indexed under this heading.

Bupivacaine Hydrochloride (Enhances neuromuscular blocking action).
No products indexed under this heading.

Carbamazepine (Chronic administration of carbamazepine may produce resistance to the neuromuscular blocking action; slightly shorter durations of neuromuscular block may be anticipated). Products include:

Chloroprocaine Hydrochloride (Enhances neuromuscular blocking action).
No products indexed under this heading.

Clindamycin Hydrochloride (Enhances neuromuscular blocking action).
No products indexed under this heading.

Clindamycin Palmitate Hydrochloride (Enhances neuromuscular blocking action).
No products indexed under this heading.

Clindamycin Phosphate (Enhances neuromuscular blocking action). Products include:

Cocaine Hydrochloride (Enhances neuromuscular blocking action).
No products indexed under this heading.

Colistimethate Sodium (Enhances neuromuscular blocking action).
No products indexed under this heading.

Colistin Sulfate (Enhances neuromuscular blocking action).
No products indexed under this heading.

Demeclocycline Hydrochloride (Enhances neuromuscular blocking action).
No products indexed under this heading.

Dihydrostreptomycin (Enhances neuromuscular blocking action).
No products indexed under this heading.

Doxycycline (Enhances neuromuscular blocking action).
No products indexed under this heading.

Doxycycline Calcium (Enhances neuromuscular blocking action).
No products indexed under this heading.

Doxycycline Hyclate (Enhances neuromuscular blocking action).
No products indexed under this heading.

Doxycycline Monohydrate (Enhances neuromuscular blocking action).
No products indexed under this heading.

Enflurane (Enflurane administered with nitrous oxide/oxygen may prolong the clinically effective duration of action of initial and maintenance doses of cisatracurium and decrease the required infusion rate of cisatracurium).
No products indexed under this heading.

Etidocaine Hydrochloride (Enhances neuromuscular blocking action).
No products indexed under this heading.

Fosphenytoin (Chronic administration of phenytoin may produce resistance to the neuromuscular blocking action; slightly shorter durations of neuromuscular block may be anticipated).
No products indexed under this heading.

Fosphenytoin Sodium (Chronic administration of phenytoin may produce resistance to the neuromuscular blocking action; slightly shorter durations of neuromuscular block may be anticipated).
No products indexed under this heading.

Gentamicin (Enhances neuromuscular blocking action).
No products indexed under this heading.

Gentamicin Sulfate (Enhances neuromuscular blocking action). Products include:

Isoflurane (Isoflurane administered with nitrous oxide/oxygen may prolong the clinically effective duration of action of initial and maintenance doses of cisatracurium and decrease the required infusion rate of cisatracurium).
No products indexed under this heading.

Kanamycin Sulfate (Enhances neuromuscular blocking action).
No products indexed under this heading.

Levobupivacaine Hydrochloride (Enhances neuromuscular blocking action).
No products indexed under this heading.

Lidocaine Hydrochloride (Enhances neuromuscular blocking action).
No products indexed under this heading.

Lincomycin Hydrochloride (Enhances neuromuscular blocking action).
No products indexed under this heading.

Lithium (Enhances neuromuscular blocking action).
No products indexed under this heading.

Lithium Carbonate (Enhances neuromuscular blocking action).
No products indexed under this heading.

Lithium Citrate (Enhances neuromuscular blocking action).
No products indexed under this heading.

Magnesium Salts (Enhances neuromuscular blocking action).
No products indexed under this heading.

Mepivacaine Hydrochloride (Enhances neuromuscular blocking action).
No products indexed under this heading.

Methacycline Hydrochloride (Enhances neuromuscular blocking action).
No products indexed under this heading.

Minocycline Hydrochloride (Enhances neuromuscular blocking action). Products include:

Neomycin (Enhances neuromuscular blocking action).
No products indexed under this heading.

Neomycin, oral (Enhances neuromuscular blocking action).
No products indexed under this heading.

Neomycin Sulfate (Enhances neuromuscular blocking action).
No products indexed under this heading.

Oxytetracycline (Enhances neuromuscular blocking action).
No products indexed under this heading.

Oxytetracycline Hydrochloride (Enhances neuromuscular blocking action).
No products indexed under this heading.

Phenytoin (Chronic administration of phenytoin may produce resistance to the neuromuscular blocking action; slightly shorter durations of neuromuscular block may be anticipated).
No products indexed under this heading.

Phenytoin Sodium (Chronic administration of phenytoin may produce resistance to the neuromuscular blocking action; slightly shorter durations of neuromuscular block may be anticipated). Products include:

Polymyxin Preparations (Enhances neuromuscular blocking action).
No products indexed under this heading.

Procainamide Hydrochloride (Enhances neuromuscular blocking action).
No products indexed under this heading.

Procaine Hydrochloride (Enhances neuromuscular blocking action).
No products indexed under this heading.

Quinidine Gluconate (Enhances neuromuscular blocking action).
No products indexed under this heading.

Quinidine Polygalacturonate (Enhances neuromuscular blocking action).
No products indexed under this heading.

Quinidine Sulfate (Enhances neuromuscular blocking action).
No products indexed under this heading.

Streptomycin Sulfate (Enhances neuromuscular blocking action).
No products indexed under this heading.

Tetracaine Hydrochloride (Enhances neuromuscular blocking action).
No products indexed under this heading.

Tetracycline Hydrochloride (Enhances neuromuscular blocking action). Products include:

Tetracycline Phosphate Complex (Enhances neuromuscular blocking action).
No products indexed under this heading.

Tobramycin (Enhances neuromuscular blocking action). Products include:

Tobramycin Sulfate (Enhances neuromuscular blocking action).
No products indexed under this heading.

NITRO-DUR TRANSDERMAL INFUSION SYSTEM
May interact with alcohols, calcium channel blockers, vasodilators, and certain other agents. Compounds in these categories include:

Amlodipine Besylate (Vasodilating effects of nitroglycerin may be additive with those of other vasodilators). Products include:

IMPORTANT NOTE: Always consult each drug listing in the patient's regimen for possible interactions.

Amyl Nitrite (Vasodilating effects of nitroglycerin may be additive with those of other vasodilators).
No products indexed under this heading.

Bepridil Hydrochloride (Vasodilating effects of nitroglycerin may be additive with those of other vasodilators).
No products indexed under this heading.

Diazoxide (Vasodilating effects of nitroglycerin may be additive with those of other vasodilators). Products include:
Proglycem 1179
Proglycem Suspension 1179

Diltiazem Hydrochloride (Vasodilating effects of nitroglycerin may be additive with those of other vasodilators). Products include:
Cardizem LA 423

Epoprostenol Sodium (Vasodilating effects of nitroglycerin may be additive with those of other vasodilators). Products include:
Flolan 1453

Ethanol (Enhances sensitivity to the hypotensive effects).
No products indexed under this heading.

Ethaverine Hydrochloride (Vasodilating effects of nitroglycerin may be additive with those of other vasodilators).
No products indexed under this heading.

Ethyl Alcohol (Enhances sensitivity to the hypotensive effects).
No products indexed under this heading.

Felodipine (Vasodilating effects of nitroglycerin may be additive with those of other vasodilators).
No products indexed under this heading.

Hydralazine Hydrochloride (Vasodilating effects of nitroglycerin may be additive with those of other vasodilators).
No products indexed under this heading.

Isosorbide Dinitrate (Vasodilating effects of nitroglycerin may be additive with those of other vasodilators).
No products indexed under this heading.

Isosorbide Mononitrate (Vasodilating effects of nitroglycerin may be additive with those of other vasodilators).
No products indexed under this heading.

Isoxsuprine Hydrochloride (Vasodilating effects of nitroglycerin may be additive with those of other vasodilators).
No products indexed under this heading.

Isradipine (Vasodilating effects of nitroglycerin may be additive with those of other vasodilators). Products include:
DynaCirc CR 1432

Mibefradil Dihydrochloride (Vasodilating effects of nitroglycerin may be additive with those of other vasodilators).
No products indexed under this heading.

Minoxidil (Vasodilating effects of nitroglycerin may be additive with those of other vasodilators).
No products indexed under this heading.

Nicardipine (Vasodilating effects of nitroglycerin may be additive with those of other vasodilators).
No products indexed under this heading.

Nicardipine Hydrochloride (Vasodilating effects of nitroglycerin may be additive with those of other vasodilators).
No products indexed under this heading.

Nifedipine (Vasodilating effects of nitroglycerin may be additive with those of other vasodilators).
No products indexed under this heading.

Nimodipine (Vasodilating effects of nitroglycerin may be additive with those of other vasodilators).
No products indexed under this heading.

Nisoldipine (Vasodilating effects of nitroglycerin may be additive with those of other vasodilators).
No products indexed under this heading.

Nitroglycerin, long-acting formulations (Vasodilating effects of nitroglycerin may be additive with those of other vasodilators).
No products indexed under this heading.

Nitroglycerin Intravenous (Vasodilating effects of nitroglycerin may be additive with those of other vasodilators).
No products indexed under this heading.

Papaverine (Vasodilating effects of nitroglycerin may be additive with those of other vasodilators).
No products indexed under this heading.

Papaverine Hydrochloride (Vasodilating effects of nitroglycerin may be additive with those of other vasodilators).
No products indexed under this heading.

Sildenafil Citrate (Amplification of the vasodilatory effects of the nitroglycerin patch by sildenafil can result in severe hypotension).
No products indexed under this heading.

Tolazoline Hydrochloride (Vasodilating effects of nitroglycerin may be additive with those of other vasodilators).
No products indexed under this heading.

Verapamil Hydrochloride (Vasodilating effects of nitroglycerin may be additive with those of other vasodilators). Products include:
Tarka 534

Food Interactions

Alcohol (Vasodilating effects of nitroglycerin may be additive with those of other vasodilators).

Beer, reduced-alcohol (Enhances sensitivity to the hypotensive effects).

Beer, unspecified (Enhances sensitivity to the hypotensive effects).

Wine, Chianti (Enhances sensitivity to the hypotensive effects).

Wine, Red (Enhances sensitivity to the hypotensive effects).

Wine, unspecified (Enhances sensitivity to the hypotensive effects).

Wine products (Enhances sensitivity to the hypotensive effects).

NITROLINGUAL PUMPSPRAY
(Nitroglycerin) 3266
May interact with alcohols, calcium channel blockers, diuretics, PDE5 inhibitors, vasodilators, vasopressors, and certain other agents. Compounds in these categories include:

Amiloride Hydrochloride (Severe hypotension, particularly with upright posture, may occur even with small doses of nitroglycerin. The drug, therefore, should be used with caution in subjects who may have volume depletion from diuretic therapy).
No products indexed under this heading.

Amlodipine Besylate (Marked symptomatic orthostatic hypotension reported when calcium channel blockers and oral controlled-release nitroglycerin were used in combination. Dose adjustments of either class of agents may be necessary). Products include:
Azor 1010
Exforge 2443
Exforge HCT 2449

Amyl Nitrite (Other agents that depend on vascular smooth muscle have decreased or increased effect depending upon the agent).
No products indexed under this heading.

Bendroflumethiazide (Severe hypotension, particularly with upright posture, may occur even with small doses of nitroglycerin. The drug, therefore, should be used with caution in subjects who may have volume depletion from diuretic therapy).
No products indexed under this heading.

Bepridil Hydrochloride (Marked symptomatic orthostatic hypotension reported when calcium channel blockers and oral controlled-release nitroglycerin were used in combination. Dose adjustments of either class of agents may be necessary).
No products indexed under this heading.

Bumetanide (Severe hypotension, particularly with upright posture, may occur even with small doses of nitroglycerin. The drug, therefore, should be used with caution in subjects who may have volume depletion from diuretic therapy).
No products indexed under this heading.

Chlorothiazide (Severe hypotension, particularly with upright posture, may occur even with small doses of nitroglycerin. The drug, therefore, should be used with caution in subjects who may have volume depletion from diuretic therapy).
No products indexed under this heading.

Chlorothiazide Sodium (Severe hypotension, particularly with upright posture, may occur even with small doses of nitroglycerin. The drug, therefore, should be used with caution in subjects who may have volume depletion from diuretic therapy). Products include:
Diuril Intravenous 2009

Chlorthalidone (Severe hypotension, particularly with upright posture, may occur even with small doses of nitroglycerin. The drug, therefore, should be used with caution in subjects who may have volume depletion from diuretic therapy). Products include:
Clorpres 2344

Diazoxide (Other agents that depend on vascular smooth muscle have decreased or increased effect depending upon the agent). Products include:
Proglycem 1179
Proglycem Suspension 1179

Diltiazem Hydrochloride (Marked symptomatic orthostatic hypotension reported when calcium channel blockers and oral controlled-release nitroglycerin were used in combination. Dose adjustments of either class of agents may be necessary). Products include:
Cardizem LA 423

Dobutamine (Other agents that depend on vascular smooth muscle have decreased or increased effect depending upon the agent).
No products indexed under this heading.

Dobutamine Hydrochloride (Other agents that depend on vascular smooth muscle have decreased or increased effect depending upon the agent).
No products indexed under this heading.

Dopamine Hydrochloride (Other agents that depend on vascular smooth muscle have decreased or increased effect depending upon the agent).
No products indexed under this heading.

Ephedrine Sulfate (Other agents that depend on vascular smooth muscle have decreased or increased effect depending upon the agent).
No products indexed under this heading.

Epinephrine Bitartrate (Other agents that depend on vascular smooth muscle have decreased or increased effect depending upon the agent).
No products indexed under this heading.

Epinephrine Hydrochloride (Other agents that depend on vascular smooth muscle have decreased or increased effect depending upon the agent).
No products indexed under this heading.

Epoprostenol Sodium (Other agents that depend on vascular smooth muscle have decreased or increased effect depending upon the agent). Products include:
Flolan 1453

Ethacrynic Acid (Severe hypotension, particularly with upright posture, may occur even with small doses of nitroglycerin. The drug, therefore, should be used with caution in subjects who may have volume depletion from diuretic therapy).
No products indexed under this heading.

Ethanol (Alcohol may enhance sensitivity to hypotensive effects of nitrates).
No products indexed under this heading.

Ethaverine Hydrochloride (Other agents that depend on vascular smooth muscle have decreased or increased effect depending upon the agent).
No products indexed under this heading.

Ethyl Alcohol (Alcohol may enhance sensitivity to hypotensive effects of nitrates).
No products indexed under this heading.

Felodipine (Marked symptomatic orthostatic hypotension reported when calcium channel blockers and oral controlled-release nitroglycerin were used in combination. Dose adjustments of either class of agents may be necessary).
No products indexed under this heading.

Furosemide (Severe hypotension, particularly with upright posture, may occur even with small doses of nitroglycerin. The drug, therefore, should be used with caution in subjects who may have volume depletion from diuretic therapy). Products include:
Furosemide 2354

Hydralazine Hydrochloride (Other agents that depend on vascular smooth muscle have decreased or increased effect depending upon the agent).
No products indexed under this heading.

Hydrochlorothiazide (Severe hypotension, particularly with upright posture, may occur even with small doses of nitroglycerin. The drug, therefore, should be used with caution in subjects who may have volume depletion from diuretic therapy). Products include:
Atacand HCT 700
Avalide 2956
Benicar HCT 1017
Diovan HCT 2419
Dyazide 1429
Exforge HCT 2449
Hyzaar 2162
Hyzaar 100-12.5 2162
Micardis HCT 889
Prinzide 2246
Tekturna HCT 2541
Teveten HCT 541

Hydroflumethiazide (Severe hypotension, particularly with upright posture, may occur even with small doses of nitroglycerin. The drug, therefore, should be used with caution in subjects who may have volume depletion from diuretic therapy).
No products indexed under this heading.

Indapamide (Severe hypotension, particularly with upright posture, may occur even with small doses of nitroglycerin. The drug, therefore, should be used with caution in subjects who may have volume depletion from diuretic therapy). Products include:
Indapamide 2356

Isoproterenol Hydrochloride (Other agents that depend on vascular smooth muscle have decreased or increased effect depending upon the agent).
No products indexed under this heading.

Isoproterenol Sulfate (Other agents that depend on vascular smooth muscle have decreased or increased effect depending upon the agent).
No products indexed under this heading.

Isosorbide Dinitrate (Other agents that depend on vascular smooth muscle have decreased or increased effect depending upon the agent).
No products indexed under this heading.

Isosorbide Mononitrate (Other agents that depend on vascular smooth muscle have decreased or increased effect depending upon the agent).
No products indexed under this heading.

Isoxsuprine Hydrochloride (Other agents that depend on vascular smooth muscle have decreased or increased effect depending upon the agent).
No products indexed under this heading.

Isradipine (Marked symptomatic orthostatic hypotension reported when calcium channel blockers and oral controlled-release nitroglycerin were used in combination. Dose adjustments of either class of agents may be necessary). Products include:
DynaCirc CR 1432

Mephentermine Sulfate (Other agents that depend on vascular smooth muscle have decreased or increased effect depending upon the agent).
No products indexed under this heading.

Metaraminol Bitartrate (Other agents that depend on vascular smooth muscle have decreased or increased effect depending upon the agent).
No products indexed under this heading.

Methoxamine Hydrochloride (Other agents that depend on vascular smooth muscle have decreased or increased effect depending upon the agent).
No products indexed under this heading.

Methyclothiazide (Severe hypotension, particularly with upright posture, may occur even with small doses of nitroglycerin. The drug, therefore, should be used with caution in subjects who may have volume depletion from diuretic therapy).
No products indexed under this heading.

Metolazone (Severe hypotension, particularly with upright posture, may occur even with small doses of nitroglycerin. The drug, therefore, should be used with caution in subjects who may have volume depletion from diuretic therapy).
No products indexed under this heading.

Mibefradil Dihydrochloride (Marked symptomatic orthostatic hypotension reported when calcium channel blockers and oral controlled-release nitroglycerin were used in combination. Dose adjustments of either class of agents may be necessary).
No products indexed under this heading.

Minoxidil (Other agents that depend on vascular smooth muscle have decreased or increased effect depending upon the agent).
No products indexed under this heading.

Nicardipine (Marked symptomatic orthostatic hypotension reported when calcium channel blockers and oral controlled-release nitroglycerin were used in combination. Dose adjustments of either class of agents may be necessary).
No products indexed under this heading.

Nicardipine Hydrochloride (Marked symptomatic orthostatic hypotension reported when calcium channel blockers and oral controlled-release nitroglycerin were used in combination. Dose adjustments of either class of agents may be necessary).
No products indexed under this heading.

Nifedipine (Marked symptomatic orthostatic hypotension reported when calcium channel blockers and oral controlled-release nitroglycerin were used in combination. Dose adjustments of either class of agents may be necessary).
No products indexed under this heading.

Nimodipine (Marked symptomatic orthostatic hypotension reported when calcium channel blockers and oral controlled-release nitroglycerin were used in combination. Dose adjustments of either class of agents may be necessary).
No products indexed under this heading.

Nisoldipine (Marked symptomatic orthostatic hypotension reported when calcium channel blockers and oral controlled-release nitroglycerin were used in combination. Dose adjustments of either class of agents may be necessary).
No products indexed under this heading.

Nitroglycerin, long-acting formulations (Other agents that depend on vascular smooth muscle have decreased or increased effect depending upon the agent).
No products indexed under this heading.

Nitroglycerin Intravenous (Other agents that depend on vascular smooth muscle have decreased or increased effect depending upon the agent).
No products indexed under this heading.

Norepinephrine Bitartrate (Other agents that depend on vascular smooth muscle have decreased or increased effect depending upon the agent).
No products indexed under this heading.

Papaverine (Other agents that depend on vascular smooth muscle have decreased or increased effect depending upon the agent).
No products indexed under this heading.

Papaverine Hydrochloride (Other agents that depend on vascular smooth muscle have decreased or increased effect depending upon the agent).
No products indexed under this heading.

Phenylephrine Hydrochloride (Other agents that depend on vascular smooth muscle have decreased or increased effect depending upon the agent). Products include:
Sudafed PE Nasal Decongestant 2048
Children's Sudafed PE Nasal
Decongestant 2047

Phosphodiesterase Inhibitors (Nitroglycerin lingual spray is contraindicated in patients taking certain drugs for erectile dysfunction (phosphodiesterase inhibitors), as their concomitant use can cause severe hypotension).
No products indexed under this heading.

Polythiazide (Severe hypotension, particularly with upright posture, may occur even with small doses of nitroglycerin. The drug, therefore, should be used with caution in subjects who may have volume depletion from diuretic therapy).
No products indexed under this heading.

Sildenafil Citrate (Nitroglycerin lingual spray is contraindicated in patients taking drugs for erectile dysfunction (phosphodiesterase inhibitors), as their concomitant use can cause severe hypotension).
No products indexed under this heading.

Spironolactone (Severe hypotension, particularly with upright posture, may occur even with small doses of nitroglycerin. The drug, therefore, should be used with caution in subjects who may have volume depletion from diuretic therapy).
No products indexed under this heading.

Tadalafil (Nitroglycerin lingual spray is contraindicated in patients taking drugs for erectile dysfunction (phosphodiesterase inhibitors), as their concomitant use can cause severe hypotension).
Products include:
Adcirca 3461
Cialis 1861

Tolazoline Hydrochloride (Other agents that depend on vascular smooth muscle have decreased or increased effect depending upon the agent).
No products indexed under this heading.

Torsemide (Severe hypotension, particularly with upright posture, may occur even with small doses of nitroglycerin. The drug, therefore, should be used with caution in subjects who may have volume depletion from diuretic therapy).
No products indexed under this heading.

Triamterene (Severe hypotension, particularly with upright posture, may occur even with small doses of nitroglycerin. The drug, therefore, should be used with caution in subjects who may have volume depletion from diuretic therapy). Products include:
Dyazide 1429
Dyrenium 3495

Vardenafil Hydrochloride (Nitroglycerin lingual spray is contraindicated in patients taking drugs for erectile dysfunction (phosphodiesterase inhibitors), as their concomitant use can cause severe hypotension). Products include:
Levitra 3157

Verapamil Hydrochloride (Marked symptomatic orthostatic hypotension reported when calcium channel blockers and oral controlled-release nitroglycerin were used in combination. Dose adjustments of either class of agents may be necessary). Products include:
Tarka 534

Food Interactions

Alcohol (Alcohol may enhance sensitivity to hypotensive effects of nitrates).

Beer, reduced-alcohol (Alcohol may enhance sensitivity to hypotensive effects of nitrates).

Beer, unspecified (Alcohol may enhance sensitivity to hypotensive effects of nitrates).

Wine, Chianti (Alcohol may enhance sensitivity to hypotensive effects of nitrates).

Wine, Red (Alcohol may enhance sensitivity to hypotensive effects of nitrates).

Wine, unspecified (Alcohol may enhance sensitivity to hypotensive effects of nitrates).

Wine products (Alcohol may enhance sensitivity to hypotensive effects of nitrates).

NORDITROPIN CARTRIDGES
(Somatropin (rDNA Origin)) 2569
May interact with anticonvulsants, corticosteroids, drugs which undergo biotransformation by cytochrome p-450 mixed function oxidase, estrogens, glucocorticoids, insulin, oral hypoglycemic agents, sex steroids, and certain other agents. Compounds in these categories include:

Acarbose (In patients with diabetes mellitus requiring drug therapy, the dose of insulin and/or oral agents may require adjustment when somatropin therapy is initiated).
No products indexed under this heading.

Acetaminophen (Limited published data indicate that somatropin treatment increases cytochrome P450 (CYP450)-mediated antipyrine clearance in man. These data suggest that somatropin administration may alter the clearance of compounds known to be metabolized by CYP450 liver enzymes (eg, corticosteroids, sex steroids, anticonvulsants, cyclosporine). Careful monitoring is advisable when somatropin is administered in combination with other drugs known to be metabolized by CYP450 liver enzymes). Products include:
Percocet 1121
Tylenol 2049
Tylenol 8 Hour 2049
Extra Strength Tylenol Caplets,
Cool Caplets, and EZ Tabs 2049
Extra Strength Tylenol Adult Rapid
Blast Liquid 2049
Extra Strength Tylenol Rapid
Release 2049
Tylenol with Codeine 2691
Tylenol Arthritis Pain Extended
Release Geltabs/Caplets 2049
Children's Tylenol Suspension
Liquid 2048
Children's Tylenol Meltaways 2048
Tylenol, Infants' Drops 2048
Junior Tylenol 2048
Vicodin 560
Vicodin ES 561
Vicodin HP 563
Zydone 1138

Alatrofloxacin Mesylate (Limited published data indicate that somatropin treatment increases cytochrome P450 (CYP450)-mediated antipyrine clearance in man. These data suggest that somatropin administration may alter the clearance of compounds known to be metabolized by CYP450 liver enzymes (eg, corticosteroids, sex steroids, anticonvulsants, cyclosporine). Careful monitoring is advisable when somatropin is administered in combination with other drugs known to be metabolized by CYP450 liver enzymes).
No products indexed under this heading.

Alclometasone Dipropionate (Somatropin inhibits 11β-hydroxysteroid dehydrogenase type 1 (11βHSD-1) in adipose/hepatic tissue and may significantly impact the metabolism of cortisol and cortisone. Patients treated with glucocorticoid replacement therapy for previously diagnosed hypoadrenalism may require an increase in their maintenance or stress doses; this may be especially true for patients treated with cortisone acetate and prednisone. In addition, excessive glucocorticoid therapy may attenuate the growth promoting effects of somatropin in children. Therefore, glucocorticoid replacement therapy should be carefully adjusted in children with concomitant GH and glucocorticoid deficiency to avoid both hypoadrenalism and an inhibitory effect on growth. Also, somatropin administration may alter the clearance of compounds known to be metabolized by CYP450 liver enzymes (eg, corticosteroids). Careful monitoring is advisable when somatropin is administered in combination with other drugs known to be metabolized by CYP450 liver enzymes).
No products indexed under this heading.

Alfentanil Hydrochloride (Limited published data indicate that somatropin treatment increases cytochrome P450 (CYP450)-mediated antipyrine clearance in man. These data suggest that somatropin administration may alter the clearance of compounds known to be metabolized by CYP450 liver enzymes (eg,

corticosteroids, sex steroids, anticonvulsants, cyclosporine). Careful monitoring is advisable when somatropin is administered in combination with other drugs known to be metabolized by CYP450 liver enzymes).

No products indexed under this heading.

Alprazolam (Limited published data indicate that somatropin treatment increases cytochrome P450 (CYP450)-mediated antipyrine clearance in man. These data suggest that somatropin administration may alter the clearance of compounds known to be metabolized by CYP450 liver enzymes (eg, corticosteroids, sex steroids, anticonvulsants, cyclosporine). Careful monitoring is advisable when somatropin is administered in combination with other drugs known to be metabolized by CYP450 liver enzymes).

No products indexed under this heading.

Aminophylline (Limited published data indicate that somatropin treatment increases cytochrome P450 (CYP450)-mediated antipyrine clearance in man. These data suggest that somatropin administration may alter the clearance of compounds known to be metabolized by CYP450 liver enzymes (eg, corticosteroids, sex steroids, anticonvulsants, cyclosporine). Careful monitoring is advisable when somatropin is administered in combination with other drugs known to be metabolized by CYP450 liver enzymes).

No products indexed under this heading.

Amiodarone Hydrochloride (Limited published data indicate that somatropin treatment increases cytochrome P450 (CYP450)-mediated antipyrine clearance in man. These data suggest that somatropin administration may alter the clearance of compounds known to be metabolized by CYP450 liver enzymes (eg, corticosteroids, sex steroids, anticonvulsants, cyclosporine). Careful monitoring is advisable when somatropin is administered in combination with other drugs known to be metabolized by CYP450 liver enzymes).

No products indexed under this heading.

Amitriptyline Hydrochloride (Limited published data indicate that somatropin treatment increases cytochrome P450 (CYP450)-mediated antipyrine clearance in man. These data suggest that somatropin administration may alter the clearance of compounds known to be metabolized by CYP450 liver enzymes (eg, corticosteroids, sex steroids, anticonvulsants, cyclosporine). Careful monitoring is advisable when somatropin is administered in combination with other drugs known to be metabolized by CYP450 liver enzymes).

No products indexed under this heading.

Amlodipine Besylate (Limited published data indicate that somatropin treatment increases cytochrome P450 (CYP450)-mediated antipyrine clearance in man. These data suggest that somatropin administration may alter the clearance of compounds known to be metabolized by CYP450 liver enzymes (eg, corticosteroids, sex steroids, anticonvulsants, cyclosporine). Careful monitoring is advisable when somatropin is administered in combination with other drugs known to be metabolized by CYP450 liver enzymes). Products include:

Azor 1010
Exforge 2443
Exforge HCT 2449

Amoxapine (Limited published data indicate that somatropin treatment increases cytochrome P450 (CYP450)-mediated antipyrine clearance in man. These data suggest that somatropin administration may alter the clearance of compounds known to be metabolized by CYP450 liver enzymes (eg, corticosteroids, sex steroids, anticonvulsants, cyclosporine). Careful monitoring is advisable when somatropin is administered in combination with other drugs known to be metabolized by CYP450 liver enzymes).

No products indexed under this heading.

Amphetamine Aspartate (Limited published data indicate that somatropin treatment increases cytochrome P450 (CYP450)-mediated antipyrine clearance in man. These data suggest that somatropin administration may alter the clearance of compounds known to be metabolized by CYP450 liver enzymes (eg, corticosteroids, sex steroids, anticonvulsants, cyclosporine). Careful monitoring is advisable when somatropin is administered in combination with other drugs known to be metabolized by CYP450 liver enzymes).

No products indexed under this heading.

Amphetamine Aspartate Monohydrate (Limited published data indicate that somatropin treatment increases cytochrome P450 (CYP450)-mediated antipyrine clearance in man. These data suggest that somatropin administration may alter the clearance of compounds known to be metabolized by CYP450 liver enzymes (eg, corticosteroids, sex steroids, anticonvulsants, cyclosporine). Careful monitoring is advisable when somatropin is administered in combination with other drugs known to be metabolized by CYP450 liver enzymes).

No products indexed under this heading.

Amphetamine Sulfate (Limited published data indicate that somatropin treatment increases cytochrome P450 (CYP450)-mediated antipyrine clearance in man. These data suggest that somatropin administration may alter the clearance of compounds known to be metabolized by CYP450 liver enzymes (eg, corticosteroids, sex steroids, anticonvulsants, cyclosporine). Careful monitoring is advisable when somatropin is administered in combination with other drugs known to be metabolized by CYP450 liver enzymes).

No products indexed under this heading.

Anagrelide Hydrochloride (Limited published data indicate that somatropin treatment increases cytochrome P450 (CYP450)-mediated antipyrine clearance in man. These data suggest that somatropin administration may alter the clearance of compounds known to be metabolized by CYP450 liver enzymes (eg, corticosteroids, sex steroids, anticonvulsants, cyclosporine). Careful monitoring is advisable when somatropin is administered in combination with other drugs known to be metabolized by CYP450 liver enzymes).

No products indexed under this heading.

Aprepitant (Limited published data indicate that somatropin treatment increases cytochrome P450 (CYP450)-mediated antipyrine clearance in man. These data suggest that somatropin administration may alter the clearance of compounds known to be metabolized by CYP450 liver enzymes (eg, corticosteroids, sex steroids, anticonvulsants, cyclosporine). Careful monitoring is advisable when somatropin is administered in combination with other drugs known to be metabolized by CYP450 liver enzymes). Products include:

Emend 2124

Astemizole (Limited published data indicate that somatropin treatment increases cytochrome P450 (CYP450)-mediated antipyrine clearance in man. These data suggest that somatropin administration may alter the clearance of compounds known to be metabolized by CYP450 liver enzymes (eg, corticosteroids, sex steroids, anticonvulsants, cyclosporine). Careful monitoring is advisable when somatropin is administered in combination with other drugs known to be metabolized by CYP450 liver enzymes).

No products indexed under this heading.

Atomoxetine Hydrochloride (Limited published data indicate that somatropin treatment increases cytochrome P450 (CYP450)-mediated antipyrine clearance in man. These data suggest that somatropin administration may alter the clearance of compounds known to be metabolized by CYP450 liver enzymes (eg, corticosteroids, sex steroids, anticonvulsants, cyclosporine). Careful monitoring is advisable when somatropin is administered in combination with other drugs known to be metabolized by CYP450 liver enzymes). Products include:

Strattera 1957

Atorvastatin Calcium (Limited published data indicate that somatropin treatment increases cytochrome P450 (CYP450)-mediated antipyrine clearance in man. These data suggest that somatropin administration may alter the clearance of compounds known to be metabolized by CYP450 liver enzymes (eg, corticosteroids, sex steroids, anticonvulsants, cyclosporine). Careful monitoring is advisable when somatropin is administered in combination with other drugs known to be metabolized by CYP450 liver enzymes). Products include:

Lipitor 2703

Beclomethasone Dipropionate (Somatropin inhibits 11β-hydroxysteroid dehydrogenase type 1 (11βHSD-1) in adipose/hepatic tissue and may significantly impact the metabolism of cortisol and cortisone. Patients treated with glucocorticoid replacement therapy for previously diagnosed hypoadrenalism may require an increase in their maintenance or stress doses; this may be especially true for patients treated with cortisone acetate and prednisone. In addition, excessive glucocorticoid therapy may attenuate the growth promoting effects of somatropin in children. Therefore, glucocorticoid replacement therapy should be carefully adjusted in children with concomitant GH and glucocorticoid deficiency to avoid both hypoadrenalism and an inhibitory effect on growth. Also, somatropin administration may alter the clearance of compounds known to be metabolized by CYP450 liver enzymes (eg, corticosteroids). Careful monitoring is advisable when somatropin is administered in combination with other drugs known to be metabolized by CYP450 liver enzymes). Products include:

Qvar 3398

Beclomethasone Dipropionate Monohydrate (Somatropin inhibits 11β-hydroxysteroid dehydrogenase type 1 (11βHSD-1) in adipose/hepatic tissue and may significantly impact the metabolism of cortisol and cortisone. Patients treated with glucocorticoid replacement therapy for previously diagnosed hypoadrenalism may require an increase in their maintenance or stress doses; this may be especially true for patients treated with cortisone acetate and prednisone. In addition, excessive glucocorticoid therapy may attenuate the growth promoting effects of somatropin in children. Therefore, glucocorticoid replacement therapy should be carefully adjusted in children with concomitant GH and glucocorticoid deficiency to avoid both hypoadrenalism and an inhibitory effect on growth. Also, somatropin administration may alter the clearance of compounds known to be metabolized by CYP450 liver enzymes (eg, corticosteroids). Careful monitoring is advisable when somatropin is administered in combination with other drugs known to be metabolized by CYP450 liver enzymes). Products include:

Beconase AQ 1386

Belladonna Ergotamine (Limited published data indicate that somatropin treatment increases cytochrome P450 (CYP450)-mediated antipyrine clearance in man. These data suggest that somatropin administration may alter the clearance of compounds known to be metabolized by CYP450 liver enzymes (eg, corticosteroids, sex steroids, anticonvulsants, cyclosporine). Careful monitoring is advisable when somatropin is administered in combination with other drugs known to be metabolized by CYP450 liver enzymes).

No products indexed under this heading.

Benzphetamine Hydrochloride (Limited published data indicate that somatropin treatment increases cytochrome P450 (CYP450)-mediated antipyrine clearance in man. These data suggest that somatropin administration may alter the clearance of compounds known to be metabolized by CYP450 liver enzymes (eg, corticosteroids, sex steroids, anticonvulsants, cyclosporine). Careful monitoring is advisable when somatropin is administered in combination with other drugs known to be metabolized by CYP450 liver enzymes).

No products indexed under this heading.

Betamethasone (Somatropin inhibits 11β-hydroxysteroid dehydrogenase type 1 (11βHSD-1) in adipose/hepatic tissue and may significantly impact the metabolism of cortisol and cortisone. Patients treated with glucocorticoid replacement therapy for previously diagnosed hypoadrenalism may require an increase in their maintenance or stress doses; this may be especially true for patients treated with cortisone acetate and prednisone. In addition, excessive glucocorticoid therapy may attenuate the growth promoting effects of somatropin in children. Therefore, glucocorticoid replacement therapy should be carefully adjusted in children with concomitant GH and glucocorticoid deficiency to avoid both hypoadrenalism and an inhibitory effect on growth. Also, somatropin administration may alter the clearance of compounds known to be metabolized by CYP450 liver enzymes (eg, corticosteroids). Careful monitoring is advisable when somatropin is administered in combination with other drugs known to be metabolized by CYP450 liver enzymes).

No products indexed under this heading.

Betamethasone Acetate (Somatropin inhibits 11β-hydroxysteroid dehydrogenase type 1 (11βHSD-1) in adipose/hepatic tissue and may significantly impact the metabolism of cortisol and cortisone. Patients treated with glucocorticoid replacement therapy for previously diagnosed hypoadrenalism may require an increase in their maintenance or stress doses; this may be especially true for patients treated with cortisone acetate and prednisone. In addition, excessive glucocorticoid therapy may attenuate the growth promoting effects of somatropin in children. Therefore, glucocorticoid replacement therapy should be carefully adjusted in children with concomitant GH and glucocorticoid deficiency to avoid both hypoadrenalism and an inhibitory effect on growth. Also, somatropin administration may alter the clearance of compounds known to be metabolized by CYP450 liver enzymes (eg, corticosteroids). Careful monitoring is advisable when somatropin is administered in combination with other drugs known to be metabolized by CYP450 liver enzymes).

No products indexed under this heading.

1205 Interactions Index Norditropin

Betamethasone Benzoate (Somatropin inhibits 11β-hydroxysteroid dehydrogenase type 1 (11βHSD-1) in adipose/hepatic tissue and may significantly impact the metabolism of cortisol and cortisone. Patients treated with glucocorticoid replacement therapy for previously diagnosed hypoadrenalism may require an increase in their maintenance or stress doses; this may be especially true for patients treated with cortisone acetate and prednisone. In addition, excessive glucocorticoid therapy may attenuate the growth promoting effects of somatropin in children. Therefore, glucocorticoid replacement therapy should be carefully adjusted in children with concomitant GH and glucocorticoid deficiency to avoid both hypoadrenalism and an inhibitory effect on growth. Also, somatropin administration may alter the clearance of compounds known to be metabolized by CYP450 liver enzymes (eg, corticosteroids). Careful monitoring is advisable when somatropin is administered in combination with other drugs known to be metabolized by CYP450 liver enzymes).
No products indexed under this heading.

Betamethasone Dipropionate (Somatropin inhibits 11β-hydroxysteroid dehydrogenase type 1 (11βHSD-1) in adipose/hepatic tissue and may significantly impact the metabolism of cortisol and cortisone. Patients treated with glucocorticoid replacement therapy for previously diagnosed hypoadrenalism may require an increase in their maintenance or stress doses; this may be especially true for patients treated with cortisone acetate and prednisone. In addition, excessive glucocorticoid therapy may attenuate the growth promoting effects of somatropin in children. Therefore, glucocorticoid replacement therapy should be carefully adjusted in children with concomitant GH and glucocorticoid deficiency to avoid both hypoadrenalism and an inhibitory effect on growth. Also, somatropin administration may alter the clearance of compounds known to be metabolized by CYP450 liver enzymes (eg, corticosteroids). Careful monitoring is advisable when somatropin is administered in combination with other drugs known to be metabolized by CYP450 liver enzymes). Products include:
Diprolene Lotion 0.05% 3108
Diprolene Ointment 0.05% 3109
Diprolene AF Cream 0.05% 3107
Lotrisone 3163

Betamethasone Sodium Phosphate (Somatropin inhibits 11β-hydroxysteroid dehydrogenase type 1 (11βHSD-1) in adipose/hepatic tissue and may significantly impact the metabolism of cortisol and cortisone. Patients treated with glucocorticoid replacement therapy for previously diagnosed hypoadrenalism may require an increase in their maintenance or stress doses; this may be especially true for patients treated with cortisone acetate and prednisone. In addition, excessive glucocorticoid therapy may attenuate the growth promoting effects of somatropin in children. Therefore, glucocorticoid replacement therapy should be carefully adjusted in children with concomitant GH and glucocorticoid deficiency to avoid both hypoadrenalism and an inhibitory effect on growth. Also, somatropin administration may alter the clearance of compounds known to be metabolized by CYP450 liver enzymes (eg, corticosteroids). Careful monitoring is advisable when somatropin is administered in combination with other drugs known to be metabolized by CYP450 liver enzymes).
No products indexed under this heading.

Betamethasone Valerate (Somatropin inhibits 11β-hydroxysteroid dehydrogenase type 1 (11βHSD-1) in adipose/hepatic tissue and may significantly impact the metabolism of cortisol and cortisone. Patients treated with glucocorticoid replacement therapy for previously diagnosed hypoadrenalism may require an increase in their maintenance or stress doses; this may be especially true for patients treated with cortisone acetate and prednisone. In addition, excessive glucocorticoid therapy may attenuate the growth promoting effects of somatropin in children. Therefore, glucocorticoid replacement therapy should be carefully adjusted in children with concomitant GH and glucocorticoid deficiency to avoid both hypoadrenalism and an inhibitory effect on growth. Also, somatropin administration may alter the clearance of compounds known to be metabolized by CYP450 liver enzymes (eg, corticosteroids). Careful monitoring is advisable when somatropin is administered in combination with other drugs known to be metabolized by CYP450 liver enzymes). Products include:
Luxíq 3321

Bisoprolol Fumarate (Limited published data indicate that somatropin treatment increases cytochrome P450 (CYP450)-mediated antipyrine clearance in man. These data suggest that somatropin administration may alter the clearance of compounds known to be metabolized by CYP450 liver enzymes (eg, corticosteroids, sex steroids, anticonvulsants, cyclosporine). Careful monitoring is advisable when somatropin is administered in combination with other drugs known to be metabolized by CYP450 liver enzymes).
No products indexed under this heading.

Bromocriptine Mesylate (Limited published data indicate that somatropin treatment increases cytochrome P450 (CYP450)-mediated antipyrine clearance in man. These data suggest that somatropin administration may alter the clearance of compounds known to be metabolized by CYP450 liver enzymes (eg, corticosteroids, sex steroids, anticonvulsants, cyclosporine). Careful monitoring is advisable when somatropin is administered in combination with other drugs known to be metabolized by CYP450 liver enzymes).
No products indexed under this heading.

Budesonide (Somatropin inhibits 11β-hydroxysteroid dehydrogenase type 1 (11βHSD-1) in adipose/hepatic tissue and may significantly impact the metabolism of cortisol and cortisone. Patients treated with glucocorticoid replacement therapy for previously diagnosed hypoadrenalism may require an increase in their maintenance or stress doses; this may be especially true for patients treated with cortisone acetate and prednisone. In addition, excessive glucocorticoid therapy may attenuate the growth promoting effects of somatropin in children. Therefore, glucocorticoid replacement therapy should be carefully adjusted in children with concomitant GH and glucocorticoid deficiency to avoid both hypoadrenalism and an inhibitory effect on growth. Also, somatropin administration may alter the clearance of compounds known to be metabolized by CYP450 liver enzymes (eg, corticosteroids). Careful monitoring is advisable when somatropin is administered in combination with other drugs known to be metabolized by CYP450 liver enzymes). Products include:
Pulmicort Flexhaler 714
Symbicort 80/4.5 720
Symbicort 160/4.5 720

Buspirone Hydrochloride (Limited published data indicate that somatropin treatment increases cytochrome P450 (CYP450)-mediated antipyrine clearance in man. These data suggest that somatropin administration may alter the clearance of compounds known to be metabolized by CYP450 liver enzymes (eg, corticosteroids, sex steroids, anticonvulsants, cyclosporine). Careful monitoring is advisable when somatropin is administered in combination with other drugs known to be metabolized by CYP450 liver enzymes).
No products indexed under this heading.

Busulfan (Limited published data indicate that somatropin treatment increases cytochrome P450 (CYP450)-mediated antipyrine clearance in man. These data suggest that somatropin administration may alter the clearance of compounds known to be metabolized by CYP450 liver enzymes (eg, corticosteroids, sex steroids, anticonvulsants, cyclosporine). Careful monitoring is advisable when somatropin is administered in combination with other drugs known to be metabolized by CYP450 liver enzymes). Products include:
Myleran 1581

Caffeine (Limited published data indicate that somatropin treatment increases cytochrome P450 (CYP450)-mediated antipyrine clearance in man. These data suggest that somatropin administration may alter the clearance of compounds known to be metabolized by CYP450 liver enzymes (eg, corticosteroids, sex steroids, anticonvulsants, cyclosporine). Careful monitoring is advisable when somatropin is administered in combination with other drugs known to be metabolized by CYP450 liver enzymes).
No products indexed under this heading.

Caffeine Anhydrous (Limited published data indicate that somatropin treatment increases cytochrome P450 (CYP450)-mediated antipyrine clearance in man. These data suggest that somatropin administration may alter the clearance of compounds known to be metabolized by CYP450 liver enzymes (eg, corticosteroids, sex steroids, anticonvulsants, cyclosporine). Careful monitoring is advisable when somatropin is administered in combination with other drugs known to be metabolized by CYP450 liver enzymes).
No products indexed under this heading.

Caffeine Citrate (Limited published data indicate that somatropin treatment increases cytochrome P450 (CYP450)-mediated antipyrine clearance in man. These data suggest that somatropin administration may alter the clearance of compounds known to be metabolized by CYP450 liver enzymes (eg, corticosteroids, sex steroids, anticonvulsants, cyclosporine). Careful monitoring is advisable when somatropin is administered in combination with other drugs known to be metabolized by CYP450 liver enzymes).
No products indexed under this heading.

Caffeine-containing medications (Limited published data indicate that somatropin treatment increases cytochrome P450 (CYP450)-mediated antipyrine clearance in man. These data suggest that somatropin administration may alter the clearance of compounds known to be metabolized by CYP450 liver enzymes (eg, corticosteroids, sex steroids, anticonvulsants, cyclosporine). Careful monitoring is advisable when somatropin is administered in combination with other drugs known to be metabolized by CYP450 liver enzymes).
No products indexed under this heading.

Caffeine Sodium Benzoate (Limited published data indicate that somatropin treatment increases cytochrome P450 (CYP450)-mediated antipyrine clearance in man. These data suggest that somatropin administration may alter the clearance of compounds known to be metabolized by CYP450 liver enzymes (eg, corticosteroids, sex steroids, anticonvulsants, cyclosporine). Careful monitoring is advisable when somatropin is administered in combination with other drugs known to be metabolized by CYP450 liver enzymes).
No products indexed under this heading.

Candesartan Cilexetil (Limited published data indicate that somatropin treatment increases cytochrome P450 (CYP450)-mediated antipyrine clearance in man. These data suggest that somatropin administration may alter the clearance of compounds known to be metabolized by CYP450 liver enzymes (eg, corticosteroids, sex steroids, anticonvulsants, cyclosporine). Careful monitoring is advisable when somatropin is administered in combination with other drugs known to be metabolized by CYP450 liver enzymes). Products include:
Atacand 697
Atacand HCT 700

Captopril (Limited published data indicate that somatropin treatment increases cytochrome P450 (CYP450)-mediated antipyrine clearance in man. These data suggest that somatropin administration may alter the clearance of compounds known to be metabolized by CYP450 liver enzymes (eg, corticosteroids, sex steroids, anticonvulsants, cyclosporine). Careful monitoring is advisable when somatropin is administered in combination with other drugs known to be metabolized by CYP450 liver enzymes). Products include:
Captopril 2341

Carbamazepine (Limited published data indicate that somatropin treatment increases cytochrome P450 (CYP450)-mediated antipyrine clearance in man. These data suggest that somatropin administration may alter the clearance of compounds known to be metabolized by CYP450 liver enzymes (eg, anticonvulsants). Careful monitoring is advisable when somatropin is administered in combination with other drugs known to be metabolized by CYP450 liver enzymes). Products include:
Carbatrol 3280
Equetro 3477

Carisoprodol (Limited published data indicate that somatropin treatment increases cytochrome P450 (CYP450)-mediated antipyrine clearance in man. These data suggest that somatropin administration may alter the clearance of compounds known to be metabolized by CYP450 liver enzymes (eg, corticosteroids, sex steroids, anticonvulsants, cyclosporine). Careful monitoring is advisable when somatropin is administered in combination with other drugs known to be metabolized by CYP450 liver enzymes).
No products indexed under this heading.

Carvedilol (Limited published data indicate that somatropin treatment increases cytochrome P450 (CYP450)-mediated antipyrine clearance in man. These data suggest that somatropin administration may alter the clearance of compounds known to be metabolized by CYP450 liver enzymes (eg, corticosteroids, sex steroids, anticonvulsants, cyclosporine). Careful monitoring is advisable when somatropin is administered in combination with other drugs known to be metabolized by CYP450 liver enzymes). Products include:
Coreg 1409

Celecoxib (Limited published data indicate that somatropin treatment increases cytochrome P450 (CYP450)-mediated antipyrine clearance in man. These data suggest that somat-

Norditropin Interactions Index 1206

ropin administration may alter the clearance of compounds known to be metabolized by CYP450 liver enzymes (eg, corticosteroids, sex steroids, anticonvulsants, cyclosporine). Careful monitoring is advisable when somatropin is administered in combination with other drugs known to be metabolized by CYP450 liver enzymes). Products include:

Celebrex 3272

Cerivastatin Sodium (Limited published data indicate that somatropin treatment increases cytochrome P450 (CYP450)-mediated antipyrine clearance in man. These data suggest that somatropin administration may alter the clearance of compounds known to be metabolized by CYP450 liver enzymes (eg, corticosteroids, sex steroids, anticonvulsants, cyclosporine). Careful monitoring is advisable when somatropin is administered in combination with other drugs known to be metabolized by CYP450 liver enzymes).

No products indexed under this heading.

Cevimeline Hydrochloride (Limited published data indicate that somatropin treatment increases cytochrome P450 (CYP450)-mediated antipyrine clearance in man. These data suggest that somatropin administration may alter the clearance of compounds known to be metabolized by CYP450 liver enzymes (eg, corticosteroids, sex steroids, anticonvulsants, cyclosporine). Careful monitoring is advisable when somatropin is administered in combination with other drugs known to be metabolized by CYP450 liver enzymes). Products include:

Evoxac 1027

Chlordiazepoxide (Limited published data indicate that somatropin treatment increases cytochrome P450 (CYP450)-mediated antipyrine clearance in man. These data suggest that somatropin administration may alter the clearance of compounds known to be metabolized by CYP450 liver enzymes (eg, corticosteroids, sex steroids, anticonvulsants, cyclosporine). Careful monitoring is advisable when somatropin is administered in combination with other drugs known to be metabolized by CYP450 liver enzymes).

No products indexed under this heading.

Chlordiazepoxide Hydrochloride (Limited published data indicate that somatropin treatment increases cytochrome P450 (CYP450)-mediated antipyrine clearance in man. These data suggest that somatropin administration may alter the clearance of compounds known to be metabolized by CYP450 liver enzymes (eg, corticosteroids, sex steroids, anticonvulsants, cyclosporine). Careful monitoring is advisable when somatropin is administered in combination with other drugs known to be metabolized by CYP450 liver enzymes).

No products indexed under this heading.

Chlorotrianisene (In adult women on oral estrogen replacement, a larger dose of somatropin may be required to achieve the defined treatment goal).

No products indexed under this heading.

Chlorpheniramine (Limited published data indicate that somatropin treatment increases cytochrome P450 (CYP450)-mediated antipyrine clearance in man. These data suggest that somatropin administration may alter the clearance of compounds known to be metabolized by CYP450 liver enzymes (eg, corticosteroids, sex steroids, anticonvulsants, cyclosporine). Careful monitoring is advisable when somatropin is administered in combination with other drugs known to be metabolized by CYP450 liver enzymes).

No products indexed under this heading.

Chlorpheniramine Maleate (Limited published data indicate that somatropin treatment increases cytochrome P450 (CYP450)-mediated antipyrine clearance in man. These data suggest that somatropin administration may alter the clearance of compounds known to be metabolized by CYP450 liver enzymes (eg, corticosteroids, sex steroids, anticonvulsants, cyclosporine). Careful monitoring is advisable when somatropin is administered in combination with other drugs known to be metabolized by CYP450 liver enzymes).

No products indexed under this heading.

Chlorpheniramine Polistirex (Limited published data indicate that somatropin treatment increases cytochrome P450 (CYP450)-mediated antipyrine clearance in man. These data suggest that somatropin administration may alter the clearance of compounds known to be metabolized by CYP450 liver enzymes (eg, corticosteroids, sex steroids, anticonvulsants, cyclosporine). Careful monitoring is advisable when somatropin is administered in combination with other drugs known to be metabolized by CYP450 liver enzymes). Products include:

Tussionex 3443

Chlorpheniramine Tannate (Limited published data indicate that somatropin treatment increases cytochrome P450 (CYP450)-mediated antipyrine clearance in man. These data suggest that somatropin administration may alter the clearance of compounds known to be metabolized by CYP450 liver enzymes (eg, corticosteroids, sex steroids, anticonvulsants, cyclosporine). Careful monitoring is advisable when somatropin is administered in combination with other drugs known to be metabolized by CYP450 liver enzymes).

No products indexed under this heading.

Chlorpromazine (Limited published data indicate that somatropin treatment increases cytochrome P450 (CYP450)-mediated antipyrine clearance in man. These data suggest that somatropin administration may alter the clearance of compounds known to be metabolized by CYP450 liver enzymes (eg, corticosteroids, sex steroids, anticonvulsants, cyclosporine). Careful monitoring is advisable when somatropin is administered in combination with other drugs known to be metabolized by CYP450 liver enzymes).

No products indexed under this heading.

Chlorpromazine Hydrochloride (Limited published data indicate that somatropin treatment increases cytochrome P450 (CYP450)-mediated antipyrine clearance in man. These data suggest that somatropin administration may alter the clearance of compounds known to be metabolized by CYP450 liver enzymes (eg, corticosteroids, sex steroids, anticonvulsants, cyclosporine). Careful monitoring is advisable when somatropin is administered in combination with other drugs known to be metabolized by CYP450 liver enzymes).

No products indexed under this heading.

Chlorpropamide (In patients with diabetes mellitus requiring drug therapy, the dose of insulin and/or oral agents may require adjustment when somatropin therapy is initiated).

No products indexed under this heading.

Ciclesonide (Somatropin inhibits 11β-hydroxysteroid dehydrogenase type 1 (11βHSD-1) in adipose/hepatic tissue and may significantly impact the metabolism of cortisol and cortisone. Patients treated with glucocorticoid replacement therapy for previously diagnosed hypoadrenalism may require an increase in their maintenance or stress doses; this may be especially true for patients treated with cortisone acetate and prednisone. In addition, excessive glucocorticoid therapy may attenuate the growth promoting effects of somatropin in children. Therefore, glucocorticoid replacement therapy should be carefully adjusted in children with concomitant GH and glucocorticoid deficiency to avoid both hypoadrenalism and an inhibitory effect on growth. Also, somatropin administration may alter the clearance of compounds known to be metabolized by CYP450 liver enzymes (eg, corticosteroids). Careful monitoring is advisable when somatropin is administered in combination with other drugs known to be metabolized by CYP450 liver enzymes).

No products indexed under this heading.

Cilostazol (Limited published data indicate that somatropin treatment increases cytochrome P450 (CYP450)-mediated antipyrine clearance in man. These data suggest that somatropin administration may alter the clearance of compounds known to be metabolized by CYP450 liver enzymes (eg, corticosteroids, sex steroids, anticonvulsants, cyclosporine). Careful monitoring is advisable when somatropin is administered in combination with other drugs known to be metabolized by CYP450 liver enzymes).

No products indexed under this heading.

Cimetidine Hydrochloride (Limited published data indicate that somatropin treatment increases cytochrome P450 (CYP450)-mediated antipyrine clearance in man. These data suggest that somatropin administration may alter the clearance of compounds known to be metabolized by CYP450 liver enzymes (eg, corticosteroids, sex steroids, anticonvulsants, cyclosporine). Careful monitoring is advisable when somatropin is administered in combination with other drugs known to be metabolized by CYP450 liver enzymes).

No products indexed under this heading.

Ciprofloxacin (Limited published data indicate that somatropin treatment increases cytochrome P450 (CYP450)-mediated antipyrine clearance in man. These data suggest that somatropin administration may alter the clearance of compounds known to be metabolized by CYP450 liver enzymes (eg, corticosteroids, sex steroids, anticonvulsants, cyclosporine). Careful monitoring is advisable when somatropin is administered in combination with other drugs known to be metabolized by CYP450 liver enzymes). Products include:

Cipro I.V. 3082
Cipro 3073
Cipro XR 3091
Ciprodex 583

Ciprofloxacin Hydrochloride (Limited published data indicate that somatropin treatment increases cytochrome P450 (CYP450)-mediated antipyrine clearance in man. These data suggest that somatropin administration may alter the clearance of compounds known to be metabolized by CYP450 liver enzymes (eg, corticosteroids, sex steroids, anticonvulsants, cyclosporine). Careful monitoring is advisable when somatropin is administered in combination with other drugs known to be metabolized by CYP450 liver enzymes). Products include:

Cipro 3073

Cisapride (Limited published data indicate that somatropin treatment increases cytochrome P450 (CYP450)-mediated antipyrine clearance in man. These data suggest that somatropin administration may alter the clearance of compounds known to be metabolized by CYP450 liver enzymes (eg, corticosteroids, sex steroids, anticonvulsants, cyclosporine). Careful monitoring is advisable when somatropin is administered in combination with other drugs known to be metabolized by CYP450 liver enzymes).

No products indexed under this heading.

Citalopram Hydrobromide (Limited published data indicate that somatropin treatment increases cytochrome P450 (CYP450)-mediated antipyrine clearance in man. These data suggest that somatropin administration may alter the clearance of compounds known to be metabolized by CYP450 liver enzymes (eg, corticosteroids, sex steroids, anticonvulsants, cyclosporine). Careful monitoring is advisable when somatropin is administered in combination with other drugs known to be metabolized by CYP450 liver enzymes). Products include:

Celexa 1153

Clarithromycin (Limited published data indicate that somatropin treatment increases cytochrome P450 (CYP450)-mediated antipyrine clearance in man. These data suggest that somatropin administration may alter the clearance of compounds known to be metabolized by CYP450 liver enzymes (eg, corticosteroids, sex steroids, anticonvulsants, cyclosporine). Careful monitoring is advisable when somatropin is administered in combination with other drugs known to be metabolized by CYP450 liver enzymes). Products include:

Biaxin/Biaxin XL 412

Clomipramine Hydrochloride (Limited published data indicate that somatropin treatment increases cytochrome P450 (CYP450)-mediated antipyrine clearance in man. These data suggest that somatropin administration may alter the clearance of compounds known to be metabolized by CYP450 liver enzymes (eg, corticosteroids, sex steroids, anticonvulsants, cyclosporine). Careful monitoring is advisable when somatropin is administered in combination with other drugs known to be metabolized by CYP450 liver enzymes).

No products indexed under this heading.

Clopidogrel Bisulfate (Limited published data indicate that somatropin treatment increases cytochrome P450 (CYP450)-mediated antipyrine clearance in man. These data suggest that somatropin administration may alter the clearance of compounds known to be metabolized by CYP450 liver enzymes (eg, corticosteroids, sex steroids, anticonvulsants, cyclosporine). Careful monitoring is advisable when somatropin is administered in combination with other drugs known to be metabolized by CYP450 liver enzymes). Products include:

Plavix 3027

Clopidogrel Hydrogen Sulfate (Limited published data indicate that somatropin treatment increases cytochrome P450 (CYP450)-mediated antipyrine clearance in man. These data suggest that somatropin administration may alter the clearance of compounds known to be metabolized by CYP450 liver enzymes (eg, corticosteroids, sex steroids, anticonvulsants, cyclosporine). Careful monitoring is advisable when somatropin is administered in combination with other drugs known to be metabolized by CYP450 liver enzymes).

No products indexed under this heading.

Clozapine (Limited published data indicate that somatropin treatment increases cytochrome P450 (CYP450)-mediated antipyrine clearance in man. These data suggest that somatropin administration may alter the clearance of compounds known to be metab-

olized by CYP450 liver enzymes (eg, corticosteroids, sex steroids, anticonvulsants, cyclosporine). Careful monitoring is advisable when somatropin is administered in combination with other drugs known to be metabolized by CYP450 liver enzymes).
No products indexed under this heading.

Codeine Phosphate (Limited published data indicate that somatropin treatment increases cytochrome P450 (CYP450)-mediated antipyrine clearance in man. These data suggest that somatropin administration may alter the clearance of compounds known to be metabolized by CYP450 liver enzymes (eg, corticosteroids, sex steroids, anticonvulsants, cyclosporine). Careful monitoring is advisable when somatropin is administered in combination with other drugs known to be metabolized by CYP450 liver enzymes). Products include:
Tylenol with Codeine **2691**

Codeine Sulfate (Limited published data indicate that somatropin treatment increases cytochrome P450 (CYP450)-mediated antipyrine clearance in man. These data suggest that somatropin administration may alter the clearance of compounds known to be metabolized by CYP450 liver enzymes (eg, corticosteroids, sex steroids, anticonvulsants, cyclosporine). Careful monitoring is advisable when somatropin is administered in combination with other drugs known to be metabolized by CYP450 liver enzymes).
No products indexed under this heading.

Cortisol (Somatropin inhibits 11β-hydroxysteroid dehydrogenase type 1 (11βHSD-1) in adipose/hepatic tissue and may significantly impact the metabolism of cortisol and cortisone. Patients treated with glucocorticoid replacement therapy for previously diagnosed hypoadrenalism may require an increase in their maintenance or stress doses; this may be especially true for patients treated with cortisone acetate and prednisone. In addition, excessive glucocorticoid therapy may attenuate the growth promoting effects of somatropin in children. Therefore, glucocorticoid replacement therapy should be carefully adjusted in children with concomitant GH and glucocorticoid deficiency to avoid both hypoadrenalism and an inhibitory effect on growth. Also, somatropin administration may alter the clearance of compounds known to be metabolized by CYP450 liver enzymes (eg, corticosteroids). Careful monitoring is advisable when somatropin is administered in combination with other drugs known to be metabolized by CYP450 liver enzymes).
No products indexed under this heading.

Cortisone Acetate (Somatropin inhibits 11β-hydroxysteroid dehydrogenase type 1 (11βHSD-1) in adipose/hepatic tissue and may significantly impact the metabolism of cortisol and cortisone. Patients treated with glucocorticoid replacement therapy for previously diagnosed hypoadrenalism may require an increase in their maintenance or stress doses; this may be especially true for patients treated with cortisone acetate and prednisone. In addition, excessive glucocorticoid therapy may attenuate the growth promoting effects of somatropin in children. Therefore, glucocorticoid replacement therapy should be carefully adjusted in children with concomitant GH and glucocorticoid deficiency to avoid both hypoadrenalism and an inhibitory effect on growth. Also, somatropin administration may alter the clearance of compounds known to be metabolized by CYP450 liver enzymes (eg, corticosteroids). Careful monitoring is advisable when somatropin is administered in combination with other drugs known to be metabolized by CYP450 liver enzymes).
No products indexed under this heading.

Cyclobenzaprine (Limited published data indicate that somatropin treatment increases cytochrome P450 (CYP450)-mediated antipyrine clearance in man. These data suggest that somatropin administration may alter the clearance of compounds known to be metabolized by CYP450 liver enzymes (eg, corticosteroids, sex steroids, anticonvulsants, cyclosporine). Careful monitoring is advisable when somatropin is administered in combination with other drugs known to be metabolized by CYP450 liver enzymes).
No products indexed under this heading.

Cyclobenzaprine Hydrochloride (Limited published data indicate that somatropin treatment increases cytochrome P450 (CYP450)-mediated antipyrine clearance in man. These data suggest that somatropin administration may alter the clearance of compounds known to be metabolized by CYP450 liver enzymes (eg, corticosteroids, sex steroids, anticonvulsants, cyclosporine). Careful monitoring is advisable when somatropin is administered in combination with other drugs known to be metabolized by CYP450 liver enzymes). Products include:
Amrix **964**

Cyclophosphamide (Limited published data indicate that somatropin treatment increases cytochrome P450 (CYP450)-mediated antipyrine clearance in man. These data suggest that somatropin administration may alter the clearance of compounds known to be metabolized by CYP450 liver enzymes (eg, corticosteroids, sex steroids, anticonvulsants, cyclosporine). Careful monitoring is advisable when somatropin is administered in combination with other drugs known to be metabolized by CYP450 liver enzymes).
No products indexed under this heading.

Cyclosporine (Limited published data indicate that somatropin treatment increases cytochrome P450 (CYP450)-mediated antipyrine clearance in man. These data suggest that somatropin administration may alter the clearance of compounds known to be metabolized by CYP450 liver enzymes (eg, cyclosporine). Careful monitoring is advisable when somatropin is administered in combination with other drugs known to be metabolized by CYP450 liver enzymes). Products include:
Gengraf **440**
Neoral Oral Solution **2496**
Neoral Capsules **2496**
Restasis **605**

Desipramine Hydrochloride (Limited published data indicate that somatropin treatment increases cytochrome P450 (CYP450)-mediated antipyrine clearance in man. These data suggest that somatropin administration may alter the clearance of compounds known to be metabolized by CYP450 liver enzymes (eg, corticosteroids, sex steroids, anticonvulsants, cyclosporine). Careful monitoring is advisable when somatropin is administered in combination with other drugs known to be metabolized by CYP450 liver enzymes).
No products indexed under this heading.

Desogestrel (Limited published data indicate that somatropin treatment increases cytochrome P450 (CYP450)-mediated antipyrine clearance in man. These data suggest that somatropin administration may alter the clearance of compounds known to be metabolized by CYP450 liver enzymes (eg, sex steroids). Careful monitoring is advisable when somatropin is administered in combination with other drugs known to be metabolized by CYP450 liver enzymes).
No products indexed under this heading.

Desoximetasone (Somatropin inhibits 11β-hydroxysteroid dehydrogenase type 1 (11βHSD-1) in adipose/hepatic tissue and may significantly impact the metabolism of cortisol and cortisone. Patients treated with glucocorticoid replacement therapy for previously diagnosed hypoadrenalism may require an increase in their maintenance or stress doses; this may be especially true for patients treated with cortisone acetate and prednisone. In addition, excessive glucocorticoid therapy may attenuate the growth promoting effects of somatropin in children. Therefore, glucocorticoid replacement therapy should be carefully adjusted in children with concomitant GH and glucocorticoid deficiency to avoid both hypoadrenalism and an inhibitory effect on growth. Also, somatropin administration may alter the clearance of compounds known to be metabolized by CYP450 liver enzymes (eg, corticosteroids). Careful monitoring is advisable when somatropin is administered in combination with other drugs known to be metabolized by CYP450 liver enzymes).
No products indexed under this heading.

Dexamethasone (Somatropin inhibits 11β-hydroxysteroid dehydrogenase type 1 (11βHSD-1) in adipose/hepatic tissue and may significantly impact the metabolism of cortisol and cortisone. Patients treated with glucocorticoid replacement therapy for previously diagnosed hypoadrenalism may require an increase in their maintenance or stress doses; this may be especially true for patients treated with cortisone acetate and prednisone. In addition, excessive glucocorticoid therapy may attenuate the growth promoting effects of somatropin in children. Therefore, glucocorticoid replacement therapy should be carefully adjusted in children with concomitant GH and glucocorticoid deficiency to avoid both hypoadrenalism and an inhibitory effect on growth. Also, somatropin administration may alter the clearance of compounds known to be metabolized by CYP450 liver enzymes (eg, corticosteroids). Careful monitoring is advisable when somatropin is administered in combination with other drugs known to be metabolized by CYP450 liver enzymes). Products include:
Ciprodex **583**
Ozurdex .... ⊙ **223**
Tobramycin and Dexamethasone Ophthalmic Suspension .... ⊙ **251**

Dexamethasone Acetate (Somatropin inhibits 11β-hydroxysteroid dehydrogenase type 1 (11βHSD-1) in adipose/hepatic tissue and may significantly impact the metabolism of cortisol and cortisone. Patients treated with glucocorticoid replacement therapy for previously diagnosed hypoadrenalism may require an increase in their maintenance or stress doses; this may be especially true for patients treated with cortisone acetate and prednisone. In addition, excessive glucocorticoid therapy may attenuate the growth promoting effects of somatropin in children. Therefore, glucocorticoid replacement therapy should be carefully adjusted in children with concomitant GH and glucocorticoid deficiency to avoid both hypoadrenalism and an inhibitory effect on growth. Also, somatropin administration may alter the clearance of compounds known to be metabolized by CYP450 liver enzymes (eg, corticosteroids). Careful monitoring is advisable when somatropin is administered in combination with other drugs known to be metabolized by CYP450 liver enzymes).
No products indexed under this heading.

Dexamethasone Phosphate (Somatropin inhibits 11β-hydroxysteroid dehydrogenase type 1 (11βHSD-1) in adipose/hepatic tissue and may significantly impact the metabolism of cortisol and cortisone. Patients treated with glucocorticoid replacement therapy for previously diagnosed hypoadrenalism may require an increase in their maintenance or stress doses; this may be especially true for patients treated with cortisone acetate and prednisone. In addition, excessive glucocorticoid therapy may attenuate the growth promoting effects of somatropin in children. Therefore, glucocorticoid replacement therapy should be carefully adjusted in children with concomitant GH and glucocorticoid deficiency to avoid both hypoadrenalism and an inhibitory effect on growth. Also, somatropin administration may alter the clearance of compounds known to be metabolized by CYP450 liver enzymes (eg, corticosteroids). Careful monitoring is advisable when somatropin is administered in combination with other drugs known to be metabolized by CYP450 liver enzymes).
No products indexed under this heading.

Dexamethasone Sodium (Somatropin inhibits 11β-hydroxysteroid dehydrogenase type 1 (11βHSD-1) in adipose/hepatic tissue and may significantly impact the metabolism of cortisol and cortisone. Patients treated with glucocorticoid replacement therapy for previously diagnosed hypoadrenalism may require an increase in their maintenance or stress doses; this may be especially true for patients treated with cortisone acetate and prednisone. In addition, excessive glucocorticoid therapy may attenuate the growth promoting effects of somatropin in children. Therefore, glucocorticoid replacement therapy should be carefully adjusted in children with concomitant GH and glucocorticoid deficiency to avoid both hypoadrenalism and an inhibitory effect on growth. Also, somatropin administration may alter the clearance of compounds known to be metabolized by CYP450 liver enzymes (eg, corticosteroids). Careful monitoring is advisable when somatropin is administered in combination with other drugs known to be metabolized by CYP450 liver enzymes).
No products indexed under this heading.

Dexamethasone Sodium Phosphate (Somatropin inhibits 11β-hydroxysteroid dehydrogenase type 1 (11βHSD-1) in adipose/hepatic tissue and may significantly impact the metabolism of cortisol and cortisone. Patients treated with glucocorticoid replacement therapy for previously diagnosed hypoadrenalism may require an increase in their maintenance or stress doses; this may be especially true for patients treated with cortisone acetate and prednisone. In addition, excessive glucocorticoid therapy may attenuate the growth promoting effects of somatropin in children. Therefore, glucocorticoid replacement therapy should be carefully adjusted in children with concomitant GH and glucocorticoid deficiency to avoid both hypoadrenalism and an inhibitory effect on growth. Also, somatropin administration may alter the clearance of compounds known to be metabolized by CYP450 liver enzymes (eg, corticosteroids). Careful monitoring is advisable when somatropin is administered in combination with other drugs known to be metabolized by CYP450 liver enzymes).
No products indexed under this heading.

Dexamethasone Sodium Phosphate Injection (Somatropin inhibits 11β-hydroxysteroid dehydrogenase type 1 (11βHSD-1) in adipose/hepatic tissue and may significantly impact the metabolism of cortisol and cortisone.

IMPORTANT NOTE: Always consult each drug listing in the patient's regimen for possible interactions.

Patients treated with glucocorticoid replacement therapy for previously diagnosed hypoadrenalism may require an increase in their maintenance or stress doses; this may be especially true for patients treated with cortisone acetate and prednisone. In addition, excessive glucocorticoid therapy may attenuate the growth promoting effects of somatropin in children. Therefore, glucocorticoid replacement therapy should be carefully adjusted in children with concomitant GH and glucocorticoid deficiency to avoid both hypoadrenalism and an inhibitory effect on growth. Also, somatropin administration may alter the clearance of compounds known to be metabolized by CYP450 liver enzymes (eg, corticosteroids). Careful monitoring is advisable when somatropin is administered in combination with other drugs known to be metabolized by CYP450 liver enzymes).

No products indexed under this heading.

Dexfenfluramine Hydrochloride (Limited published data indicate that somatropin treatment increases cytochrome P450 (CYP450)-mediated antipyrine clearance in man. These data suggest that somatropin administration may alter the clearance of compounds known to be metabolized by CYP450 liver enzymes (eg, corticosteroids, sex steroids, anticonvulsants, cyclosporine). Careful monitoring is advisable when somatropin is administered in combination with other drugs known to be metabolized by CYP450 liver enzymes).

No products indexed under this heading.

Dextromethorphan (Limited published data indicate that somatropin treatment increases cytochrome P450 (CYP450)-mediated antipyrine clearance in man. These data suggest that somatropin administration may alter the clearance of compounds known to be metabolized by CYP450 liver enzymes (eg, corticosteroids, sex steroids, anticonvulsants, cyclosporine). Careful monitoring is advisable when somatropin is administered in combination with other drugs known to be metabolized by CYP450 liver enzymes).

No products indexed under this heading.

Dextromethorphan Hydrobromide (Limited published data indicate that somatropin treatment increases cytochrome P450 (CYP450)-mediated antipyrine clearance in man. These data suggest that somatropin administration may alter the clearance of compounds known to be metabolized by CYP450 liver enzymes (eg, corticosteroids, sex steroids, anticonvulsants, cyclosporine). Careful monitoring is advisable when somatropin is administered in combination with other drugs known to be metabolized by CYP450 liver enzymes).

No products indexed under this heading.

Dextromethorphan Polistirex (Limited published data indicate that somatropin treatment increases cytochrome P450 (CYP450)-mediated antipyrine clearance in man. These data suggest that somatropin administration may alter the clearance of compounds known to be metabolized by CYP450 liver enzymes (eg, corticosteroids, sex steroids, anticonvulsants, cyclosporine). Careful monitoring is advisable when somatropin is administered in combination with other drugs known to be metabolized by CYP450 liver enzymes).

No products indexed under this heading.

Diazepam (Limited published data indicate that somatropin treatment increases cytochrome P450 (CYP450)-mediated antipyrine clearance in man. These data suggest that somatropin administration may alter the clear-

ance of compounds known to be metabolized by CYP450 liver enzymes (eg, corticosteroids, sex steroids, anticonvulsants, cyclosporine). Careful monitoring is advisable when somatropin is administered in combination with other drugs known to be metabolized by CYP450 liver enzymes). Products include:
Valium Tablets **2880**

Diclofenac Potassium (Limited published data indicate that somatropin treatment increases cytochrome P450 (CYP450)-mediated antipyrine clearance in man. These data suggest that somatropin administration may alter the clearance of compounds known to be metabolized by CYP450 liver enzymes (eg, corticosteroids, sex steroids, anticonvulsants, cyclosporine). Careful monitoring is advisable when somatropin is administered in combination with other drugs known to be metabolized by CYP450 liver enzymes).

No products indexed under this heading.

Diclofenac Sodium (Limited published data indicate that somatropin treatment increases cytochrome P450 (CYP450)-mediated antipyrine clearance in man. These data suggest that somatropin administration may alter the clearance of compounds known to be metabolized by CYP450 liver enzymes (eg, corticosteroids, sex steroids, anticonvulsants, cyclosporine). Careful monitoring is advisable when somatropin is administered in combination with other drugs known to be metabolized by CYP450 liver enzymes).

No products indexed under this heading.

Dienestrol (In adult women on oral estrogen replacement, a larger dose of somatropin may be required to achieve the defined treatment goal).

No products indexed under this heading.

Diethylstilbestrol (In adult women on oral estrogen replacement, a larger dose of somatropin may be required to achieve the defined treatment goal).

No products indexed under this heading.

Diflorasone Diacetate (Somatropin inhibits 11β-hydroxysteroid dehydrogenase type 1 (11βHSD-1) in adipose/hepatic tissue and may significantly impact the metabolism of cortisol and cortisone. Patients treated with glucocorticoid replacement therapy for previously diagnosed hypoadrenalism may require an increase in their maintenance or stress doses; this may be especially true for patients treated with cortisone acetate and prednisone. In addition, excessive glucocorticoid therapy may attenuate the growth promoting effects of somatropin in children. Therefore, glucocorticoid replacement therapy should be carefully adjusted in children with concomitant GH and glucocorticoid deficiency to avoid both hypoadrenalism and an inhibitory effect on growth. Also, somatropin administration may alter the clearance of compounds known to be metabolized by CYP450 liver enzymes (eg, corticosteroids). Careful monitoring is advisable when somatropin is administered in combination with other drugs known to be metabolized by CYP450 liver enzymes).

No products indexed under this heading.

Dihydroergotamine Mesylate (Limited published data indicate that somatropin treatment increases cytochrome P450 (CYP450)-mediated antipyrine clearance in man. These data suggest that somatropin administration may alter the clearance of compounds known to be metabolized by CYP450 liver enzymes (eg, corticosteroids, sex steroids, anticonvulsants, cyclosporine). Careful monitoring is advisable when somatropin is administered in

combination with other drugs known to be metabolized by CYP450 liver enzymes).

No products indexed under this heading.

Diltiazem Hydrochloride (Limited published data indicate that somatropin treatment increases cytochrome P450 (CYP450)-mediated antipyrine clearance in man. These data suggest that somatropin administration may alter the clearance of compounds known to be metabolized by CYP450 liver enzymes (eg, corticosteroids, sex steroids, anticonvulsants, cyclosporine). Careful monitoring is advisable when somatropin is administered in combination with other drugs known to be metabolized by CYP450 liver enzymes). Products include:
Cardizem LA **423**

Diltiazem Maleate (Limited published data indicate that somatropin treatment increases cytochrome P450 (CYP450)-mediated antipyrine clearance in man. These data suggest that somatropin administration may alter the clearance of compounds known to be metabolized by CYP450 liver enzymes (eg, corticosteroids, sex steroids, anticonvulsants, cyclosporine). Careful monitoring is advisable when somatropin is administered in combination with other drugs known to be metabolized by CYP450 liver enzymes).

No products indexed under this heading.

Disopyramide (Limited published data indicate that somatropin treatment increases cytochrome P450 (CYP450)-mediated antipyrine clearance in man. These data suggest that somatropin administration may alter the clearance of compounds known to be metabolized by CYP450 liver enzymes (eg, corticosteroids, sex steroids, anticonvulsants, cyclosporine). Careful monitoring is advisable when somatropin is administered in combination with other drugs known to be metabolized by CYP450 liver enzymes).

No products indexed under this heading.

Disopyramide Phosphate (Limited published data indicate that somatropin treatment increases cytochrome P450 (CYP450)-mediated antipyrine clearance in man. These data suggest that somatropin administration may alter the clearance of compounds known to be metabolized by CYP450 liver enzymes (eg, corticosteroids, sex steroids, anticonvulsants, cyclosporine). Careful monitoring is advisable when somatropin is administered in combination with other drugs known to be metabolized by CYP450 liver enzymes).

No products indexed under this heading.

Disulfiram (Limited published data indicate that somatropin treatment increases cytochrome P450 (CYP450)-mediated antipyrine clearance in man. These data suggest that somatropin administration may alter the clearance of compounds known to be metabolized by CYP450 liver enzymes (eg, corticosteroids, sex steroids, anticonvulsants, cyclosporine). Careful monitoring is advisable when somatropin is administered in combination with other drugs known to be metabolized by CYP450 liver enzymes).

No products indexed under this heading.

Divalproex Sodium (Limited published data indicate that somatropin treatment increases cytochrome P450 (CYP450)-mediated antipyrine clearance in man. These data suggest that somatropin administration may alter the clearance of compounds known to be metabolized by CYP450 liver enzymes (eg, anticonvulsants). Careful monitoring is advisable when somatropin is administered in combination with other drugs known to be metabolized by CYP450 liver enzymes). Products include:

Depakote ER **426**

Docetaxel (Limited published data indicate that somatropin treatment increases cytochrome P450 (CYP450)-mediated antipyrine clearance in man. These data suggest that somatropin administration may alter the clearance of compounds known to be metabolized by CYP450 liver enzymes (eg, corticosteroids, sex steroids, anticonvulsants, cyclosporine). Careful monitoring is advisable when somatropin is administered in combination with other drugs known to be metabolized by CYP450 liver enzymes). Products include:
Taxotere **3035**

Dolasetron Mesylate (Limited published data indicate that somatropin treatment increases cytochrome P450 (CYP450)-mediated antipyrine clearance in man. These data suggest that somatropin administration may alter the clearance of compounds known to be metabolized by CYP450 liver enzymes (eg, corticosteroids, sex steroids, anticonvulsants, cyclosporine). Careful monitoring is advisable when somatropin is administered in combination with other drugs known to be metabolized by CYP450 liver enzymes). Products include:
Anzemet Injection **2931**
Anzemet Tablets **2934**

Donepezil Hydrochloride (Limited published data indicate that somatropin treatment increases cytochrome P450 (CYP450)-mediated antipyrine clearance in man. These data suggest that somatropin administration may alter the clearance of compounds known to be metabolized by CYP450 liver enzymes (eg, corticosteroids, sex steroids, anticonvulsants, cyclosporine). Careful monitoring is advisable when somatropin is administered in combination with other drugs known to be metabolized by CYP450 liver enzymes). Products include:
Aricept **1045**
Aricept ODT **1045**

Doxepin Hydrochloride (Limited published data indicate that somatropin treatment increases cytochrome P450 (CYP450)-mediated antipyrine clearance in man. These data suggest that somatropin administration may alter the clearance of compounds known to be metabolized by CYP450 liver enzymes (eg, corticosteroids, sex steroids, anticonvulsants, cyclosporine). Careful monitoring is advisable when somatropin is administered in combination with other drugs known to be metabolized by CYP450 liver enzymes).

No products indexed under this heading.

Doxorubicin Hydrochloride (Limited published data indicate that somatropin treatment increases cytochrome P450 (CYP450)-mediated antipyrine clearance in man. These data suggest that somatropin administration may alter the clearance of compounds known to be metabolized by CYP450 liver enzymes (eg, corticosteroids, sex steroids, anticonvulsants, cyclosporine). Careful monitoring is advisable when somatropin is administered in combination with other drugs known to be metabolized by CYP450 liver enzymes).

No products indexed under this heading.

Dronabinol (Limited published data indicate that somatropin treatment increases cytochrome P450 (CYP450)-mediated antipyrine clearance in man. These data suggest that somatropin administration may alter the clearance of compounds known to be metabolized by CYP450 liver enzymes (eg, corticosteroids, sex steroids, anticonvulsants, cyclosporine). Careful monitoring is advisable when somatropin is

administered in combination with other drugs known to be metabolized by CYP450 liver enzymes).
No products indexed under this heading.

Drugs that Undergo Biotransformation by Cytochrome P-450 Mixed Function Oxidase (Limited published data indicate that somatropin treatment increases cytochrome P450 (CYP450)-mediated antipyrine clearance in man. These data suggest that somatropin administration may alter the clearance of compounds known to be metabolized by CYP450 liver enzymes (eg, corticosteroids, sex steroids, anticonvulsants, cyclosporine). Careful monitoring is advisable when somatropin is administered in combination with other drugs known to be metabolized by CYP450 liver enzymes).
No products indexed under this heading.

Dyphylline (Limited published data indicate that somatropin treatment increases cytochrome P450 (CYP450)-mediated antipyrine clearance in man. These data suggest that somatropin administration may alter the clearance of compounds known to be metabolized by CYP450 liver enzymes (eg, corticosteroids, sex steroids, anticonvulsants, cyclosporine). Careful monitoring is advisable when somatropin is administered in combination with other drugs known to be metabolized by CYP450 liver enzymes).
No products indexed under this heading.

Encainide Hydrochloride (Limited published data indicate that somatropin treatment increases cytochrome P450 (CYP450)-mediated antipyrine clearance in man. These data suggest that somatropin administration may alter the clearance of compounds known to be metabolized by CYP450 liver enzymes (eg, corticosteroids, sex steroids, anticonvulsants, cyclosporine). Careful monitoring is advisable when somatropin is administered in combination with other drugs known to be metabolized by CYP450 liver enzymes).
No products indexed under this heading.

Enoxacin (Limited published data indicate that somatropin treatment increases cytochrome P450 (CYP450)-mediated antipyrine clearance in man. These data suggest that somatropin administration may alter the clearance of compounds known to be metabolized by CYP450 liver enzymes (eg, corticosteroids, sex steroids, anticonvulsants, cyclosporine). Careful monitoring is advisable when somatropin is administered in combination with other drugs known to be metabolized by CYP450 liver enzymes).
No products indexed under this heading.

Eprosartan Mesylate (Limited published data indicate that somatropin treatment increases cytochrome P450 (CYP450)-mediated antipyrine clearance in man. These data suggest that somatropin administration may alter the clearance of compounds known to be metabolized by CYP450 liver enzymes (eg, corticosteroids, sex steroids, anticonvulsants, cyclosporine). Careful monitoring is advisable when somatropin is administered in combination with other drugs known to be metabolized by CYP450 liver enzymes). Products include:

Ergotamine Tartrate (Limited published data indicate that somatropin treatment increases cytochrome P450 (CYP450)-mediated antipyrine clearance in man. These data suggest that somatropin administration may alter the clearance of compounds known to be metabolized by CYP450 liver enzymes (eg, corticosteroids, sex steroids, anticonvulsants, cyclosporine). Careful monitoring is advisable when somatropin is administered in combination with other drugs known to be metabolized by CYP450 liver enzymes).
No products indexed under this heading.

Erythromycin (Limited published data indicate that somatropin treatment increases cytochrome P450 (CYP450)-mediated antipyrine clearance in man. These data suggest that somatropin administration may alter the clearance of compounds known to be metabolized by CYP450 liver enzymes (eg, corticosteroids, sex steroids, anticonvulsants, cyclosporine). Careful monitoring is advisable when somatropin is administered in combination with other drugs known to be metabolized by CYP450 liver enzymes).
No products indexed under this heading.

Erythromycin Estolate (Limited published data indicate that somatropin treatment increases cytochrome P450 (CYP450)-mediated antipyrine clearance in man. These data suggest that somatropin administration may alter the clearance of compounds known to be metabolized by CYP450 liver enzymes (eg, corticosteroids, sex steroids, anticonvulsants, cyclosporine). Careful monitoring is advisable when somatropin is administered in combination with other drugs known to be metabolized by CYP450 liver enzymes).
No products indexed under this heading.

Erythromycin Ethylsuccinate (Limited published data indicate that somatropin treatment increases cytochrome P450 (CYP450)-mediated antipyrine clearance in man. These data suggest that somatropin administration may alter the clearance of compounds known to be metabolized by CYP450 liver enzymes (eg, corticosteroids, sex steroids, anticonvulsants, cyclosporine). Careful monitoring is advisable when somatropin is administered in combination with other drugs known to be metabolized by CYP450 liver enzymes). Products include:

Erythromycin Gluceptate (Limited published data indicate that somatropin treatment increases cytochrome P450 (CYP450)-mediated antipyrine clearance in man. These data suggest that somatropin administration may alter the clearance of compounds known to be metabolized by CYP450 liver enzymes (eg, corticosteroids, sex steroids, anticonvulsants, cyclosporine). Careful monitoring is advisable when somatropin is administered in combination with other drugs known to be metabolized by CYP450 liver enzymes).
No products indexed under this heading.

Erythromycin Lactobionate (Limited published data indicate that somatropin treatment increases cytochrome P450 (CYP450)-mediated antipyrine clearance in man. These data suggest that somatropin administration may alter the clearance of compounds known to be metabolized by CYP450 liver enzymes (eg, corticosteroids, sex steroids, anticonvulsants, cyclosporine). Careful monitoring is advisable when somatropin is administered in combination with other drugs known to be metabolized by CYP450 liver enzymes).
No products indexed under this heading.

Erythromycin Stearate (Limited published data indicate that somatropin treatment increases cytochrome P450 (CYP450)-mediated antipyrine clearance in man. These data suggest that somatropin administration may alter the clearance of compounds known to be metabolized by CYP450 liver enzymes (eg, corticosteroids, sex steroids, anticonvulsants, cyclosporine). Careful monitoring is advisable when somatropin is administered in combination with other drugs known to be metabolized by CYP450 liver enzymes).
No products indexed under this heading.

Esomeprazole Magnesium (Limited published data indicate that somatropin treatment increases cytochrome P450 (CYP450)-mediated antipyrine clearance in man. These data suggest that somatropin administration may alter the clearance of compounds known to be metabolized by CYP450 liver enzymes (eg, corticosteroids, sex steroids, anticonvulsants, cyclosporine). Careful monitoring is advisable when somatropin is administered in combination with other drugs known to be metabolized by CYP450 liver enzymes). Products include:

Esomeprazole Sodium (Limited published data indicate that somatropin treatment increases cytochrome P450 (CYP450)-mediated antipyrine clearance in man. These data suggest that somatropin administration may alter the clearance of compounds known to be metabolized by CYP450 liver enzymes (eg, corticosteroids, sex steroids, anticonvulsants, cyclosporine). Careful monitoring is advisable when somatropin is administered in combination with other drugs known to be metabolized by CYP450 liver enzymes). Products include:

Estradiol (In adult women on oral estrogen replacement, a larger dose of somatropin may be required to achieve the defined treatment goal). Products include:

Estradiol Benzoate (Limited published data indicate that somatropin treatment increases cytochrome P450 (CYP450)-mediated antipyrine clearance in man. These data suggest that somatropin administration may alter the clearance of compounds known to be metabolized by CYP450 liver enzymes (eg, corticosteroids, sex steroids, anticonvulsants, cyclosporine). Careful monitoring is advisable when somatropin is administered in combination with other drugs known to be metabolized by CYP450 liver enzymes).
No products indexed under this heading.

Estradiol Cypionate (Limited published data indicate that somatropin treatment increases cytochrome P450 (CYP450)-mediated antipyrine clearance in man. These data suggest that somatropin administration may alter the clearance of compounds known to be metabolized by CYP450 liver enzymes (eg, corticosteroids, sex steroids, anticonvulsants, cyclosporine). Careful monitoring is advisable when somatropin is administered in combination with other drugs known to be metabolized by CYP450 liver enzymes).
No products indexed under this heading.

Estradiol Valerate (Limited published data indicate that somatropin treatment increases cytochrome P450 (CYP450)-mediated antipyrine clearance in man. These data suggest that somatropin administration may alter the clearance of compounds known to be metabolized by CYP450 liver enzymes (eg, corticosteroids, sex steroids, anticonvulsants, cyclosporine). Careful monitoring is advisable when somatropin is administered in combination with other drugs known to be metabolized by CYP450 liver enzymes).
No products indexed under this heading.

Estrogen (Limited published data indicate that somatropin treatment increases cytochrome P450 (CYP450)-mediated antipyrine clearance in man. These data suggest that somatropin administration may alter the clearance of compounds known to be metabolized by CYP450 liver enzymes (eg, corticosteroids, sex steroids, anticonvulsants, cyclosporine). Careful monitoring is advisable when somatropin is administered in combination with other drugs known to be metabolized by CYP450 liver enzymes).
No products indexed under this heading.

Estrogens, Conjugated (In adult women on oral estrogen replacement, a larger dose of somatropin may be required to achieve the defined treatment goal). Products include:

Estrogens, Conjugated, Synthetic A (Limited published data indicate that somatropin treatment increases cytochrome P450 (CYP450)-mediated antipyrine clearance in man. These data suggest that somatropin administration may alter the clearance of compounds known to be metabolized by CYP450 liver enzymes (eg, corticosteroids, sex steroids, anticonvulsants, cyclosporine). Careful monitoring is advisable when somatropin is administered in combination with other drugs known to be metabolized by CYP450 liver enzymes).
No products indexed under this heading.

Estrogens, Esterified (In adult women on oral estrogen replacement, a larger dose of somatropin may be required to achieve the defined treatment goal).
No products indexed under this heading.

Estropipate (In adult women on oral estrogen replacement, a larger dose of somatropin may be required to achieve the defined treatment goal).
No products indexed under this heading.

Ethinyl Estradiol (In adult women on oral estrogen replacement, a larger dose of somatropin may be required to achieve the defined treatment goal). Products include:

Ethosuximide (Limited published data indicate that somatropin treatment increases cytochrome P450 (CYP450)-mediated antipyrine clearance in man. These data suggest that somatropin administration may alter the clearance of compounds known to be metabolized by CYP450 liver enzymes (eg, anticonvulsants). Careful monitoring is advisable when somatropin is administered in combination with other drugs known to be metabolized by CYP450 liver enzymes).
No products indexed under this heading.

Ethotoin (Limited published data indicate that somatropin treatment increases cytochrome P450 (CYP450)-mediated antipyrine clearance in man. These data suggest that somatropin administration may alter the clearance of compounds known to be metabolized by CYP450 liver enzymes (eg, anticonvulsants). Careful monitoring is advisable when somatropin is adminis-

Norditropin Interactions Index 1210

tered in combination with other drugs known to be metabolized by CYP450 liver enzymes).
No products indexed under this heading.

Ethynodiol Diacetate (Limited published data indicate that somatropin treatment increases cytochrome P450 (CYP450)-mediated antipyrine clearance in man. These data suggest that somatropin administration may alter the clearance of compounds known to be metabolized by CYP450 liver enzymes (eg, sex steroids). Careful monitoring is advisable when somatropin is administered in combination with other drugs known to be metabolized by CYP450 liver enzymes).
No products indexed under this heading.

Etodolac (Limited published data indicate that somatropin treatment increases cytochrome P450 (CYP450)-mediated antipyrine clearance in man. These data suggest that somatropin administration may alter the clearance of compounds known to be metabolized by CYP450 liver enzymes (eg, corticosteroids, sex steroids, anticonvulsants, cyclosporine). Careful monitoring is advisable when somatropin is administered in combination with other drugs known to be metabolized by CYP450 liver enzymes).
No products indexed under this heading.

Etoposide (Limited published data indicate that somatropin treatment increases cytochrome P450 (CYP450)-mediated antipyrine clearance in man. These data suggest that somatropin administration may alter the clearance of compounds known to be metabolized by CYP450 liver enzymes (eg, corticosteroids, sex steroids, anticonvulsants, cyclosporine). Careful monitoring is advisable when somatropin is administered in combination with other drugs known to be metabolized by CYP450 liver enzymes).
No products indexed under this heading.

Etoposide Phosphate (Limited published data indicate that somatropin treatment increases cytochrome P450 (CYP450)-mediated antipyrine clearance in man. These data suggest that somatropin administration may alter the clearance of compounds known to be metabolized by CYP450 liver enzymes (eg, corticosteroids, sex steroids, anticonvulsants, cyclosporine). Careful monitoring is advisable when somatropin is administered in combination with other drugs known to be metabolized by CYP450 liver enzymes).
No products indexed under this heading.

Felbamate (Limited published data indicate that somatropin treatment increases cytochrome P450 (CYP450)-mediated antipyrine clearance in man. These data suggest that somatropin administration may alter the clearance of compounds known to be metabolized by CYP450 liver enzymes (eg, anticonvulsants). Careful monitoring is advisable when somatropin is administered in combination with other drugs known to be metabolized by CYP450 liver enzymes).
No products indexed under this heading.

Felodipine (Limited published data indicate that somatropin treatment increases cytochrome P450 (CYP450)-mediated antipyrine clearance in man. These data suggest that somatropin administration may alter the clearance of compounds known to be metabolized by CYP450 liver enzymes (eg, corticosteroids, sex steroids, anticonvulsants, cyclosporine). Careful monitoring is advisable when somatropin is administered in combination with other drugs known to be metabolized by CYP450 liver enzymes).
No products indexed under this heading.

Fenoprofen Calcium (Limited published data indicate that somatropin treatment increases cytochrome P450 (CYP450)-mediated antipyrine clearance in man. These data suggest that somatropin administration may alter the clearance of compounds known to be metabolized by CYP450 liver enzymes (eg, corticosteroids, sex steroids, anticonvulsants, cyclosporine). Careful monitoring is advisable when somatropin is administered in combination with other drugs known to be metabolized by CYP450 liver enzymes).
No products indexed under this heading.

Fentanyl (Limited published data indicate that somatropin treatment increases cytochrome P450 (CYP450)-mediated antipyrine clearance in man. These data suggest that somatropin administration may alter the clearance of compounds known to be metabolized by CYP450 liver enzymes (eg, corticosteroids, sex steroids, anticonvulsants, cyclosporine). Careful monitoring is advisable when somatropin is administered in combination with other drugs known to be metabolized by CYP450 liver enzymes). Products include:
Duragesic **2604**
Fentanyl Transdermal System **2346**
Onsolis **2054**

Fentanyl Citrate (Limited published data indicate that somatropin treatment increases cytochrome P450 (CYP450)-mediated antipyrine clearance in man. These data suggest that somatropin administration may alter the clearance of compounds known to be metabolized by CYP450 liver enzymes (eg, corticosteroids, sex steroids, anticonvulsants, cyclosporine). Careful monitoring is advisable when somatropin is administered in combination with other drugs known to be metabolized by CYP450 liver enzymes). Products include:
Fentora **966**

Flecainide Acetate (Limited published data indicate that somatropin treatment increases cytochrome P450 (CYP450)-mediated antipyrine clearance in man. These data suggest that somatropin administration may alter the clearance of compounds known to be metabolized by CYP450 liver enzymes (eg, corticosteroids, sex steroids, anticonvulsants, cyclosporine). Careful monitoring is advisable when somatropin is administered in combination with other drugs known to be metabolized by CYP450 liver enzymes).
No products indexed under this heading.

Fludrocortisone Acetate (Somatropin inhibits 11β-hydroxysteroid dehydrogenase type 1 (11βHSD-1) in adipose/hepatic tissue and may significantly impact the metabolism of cortisol and cortisone. Patients treated with glucocorticoid replacement therapy for previously diagnosed hypoadrenalism may require an increase in their maintenance or stress doses; this may be especially true for patients treated with cortisone acetate and prednisone. In addition, excessive glucocorticoid therapy may attenuate the growth promoting effects of somatropin in children. Therefore, glucocorticoid replacement therapy should be carefully adjusted in children with concomitant GH and glucocorticoid deficiency to avoid both hypoadrenalism and an inhibitory effect on growth. Also, somatropin administration may alter the clearance of compounds known to be metabolized by CYP450 liver enzymes (eg, corticosteroids). Careful monitoring is advisable when somatropin is administered in combination with other drugs known to be metabolized by CYP450 liver enzymes).
No products indexed under this heading.

Flumethasone Pivalate (Somatropin inhibits 11β-hydroxysteroid dehydrogenase type 1 (11βHSD-1) in adipose/hepatic tissue and may significantly impact the metabolism of cortisol and cortisone. Patients treated with glucocorticoid replacement therapy for previously diagnosed hypoadrenalism may require an increase in their maintenance or stress doses; this may be especially true for patients treated with cortisone acetate and prednisone. In addition, excessive glucocorticoid therapy may attenuate the growth promoting effects of somatropin in children. Therefore, glucocorticoid replacement therapy should be carefully adjusted in children with concomitant GH and glucocorticoid deficiency to avoid both hypoadrenalism and an inhibitory effect on growth. Also, somatropin administration may alter the clearance of compounds known to be metabolized by CYP450 liver enzymes (eg, corticosteroids). Careful monitoring is advisable when somatropin is administered in combination with other drugs known to be metabolized by CYP450 liver enzymes).
No products indexed under this heading.

Flunisolide Hemihydrate (Somatropin inhibits 11β-hydroxysteroid dehydrogenase type 1 (11βHSD-1) in adipose/hepatic tissue and may significantly impact the metabolism of cortisol and cortisone. Patients treated with glucocorticoid replacement therapy for previously diagnosed hypoadrenalism may require an increase in their maintenance or stress doses; this may be especially true for patients treated with cortisone acetate and prednisone. In addition, excessive glucocorticoid therapy may attenuate the growth promoting effects of somatropin in children. Therefore, glucocorticoid replacement therapy should be carefully adjusted in children with concomitant GH and glucocorticoid deficiency to avoid both hypoadrenalism and an inhibitory effect on growth. Also, somatropin administration may alter the clearance of compounds known to be metabolized by CYP450 liver enzymes (eg, corticosteroids). Careful monitoring is advisable when somatropin is administered in combination with other drugs known to be metabolized by CYP450 liver enzymes).
No products indexed under this heading.

Fluoxetine (Limited published data indicate that somatropin treatment increases cytochrome P450 (CYP450)-mediated antipyrine clearance in man. These data suggest that somatropin administration may alter the clearance of compounds known to be metabolized by CYP450 liver enzymes (eg, corticosteroids, sex steroids, anticonvulsants, cyclosporine). Careful monitoring is advisable when somatropin is administered in combination with other drugs known to be metabolized by CYP450 liver enzymes).
No products indexed under this heading.

Fluoxetine Hydrochloride (Limited published data indicate that somatropin treatment increases cytochrome P450 (CYP450)-mediated antipyrine clearance in man. These data suggest that somatropin administration may alter the clearance of compounds known to be metabolized by CYP450 liver enzymes (eg, corticosteroids, sex steroids, anticonvulsants, cyclosporine). Careful monitoring is advisable when somatropin is administered in combination with other drugs known to be metabolized by CYP450 liver enzymes). Products include:
Prozac Weekly **1941**
Prozac Pulvules **1941**
Symbyax **1965**

Fluoxymesterone (Limited published data indicate that somatropin treatment increases cytochrome P450 (CYP450)-mediated antipyrine clearance in man. These data suggest that somatropin administration may alter the clearance of compounds known to be metabolized by CYP450 liver enzymes (eg, sex steroids). Careful monitoring is advisable when somatropin is administered in combination with other drugs known to be metabolized by CYP450 liver enzymes).
No products indexed under this heading.

Fluphenazine Decanoate (Limited published data indicate that somatropin treatment increases cytochrome P450 (CYP450)-mediated antipyrine clearance in man. These data suggest that somatropin administration may alter the clearance of compounds known to be metabolized by CYP450 liver enzymes (eg, corticosteroids, sex steroids, anticonvulsants, cyclosporine). Careful monitoring is advisable when somatropin is administered in combination with other drugs known to be metabolized by CYP450 liver enzymes).
No products indexed under this heading.

Fluphenazine Enanthate (Limited published data indicate that somatropin treatment increases cytochrome P450 (CYP450)-mediated antipyrine clearance in man. These data suggest that somatropin administration may alter the clearance of compounds known to be metabolized by CYP450 liver enzymes (eg, corticosteroids, sex steroids, anticonvulsants, cyclosporine). Careful monitoring is advisable when somatropin is administered in combination with other drugs known to be metabolized by CYP450 liver enzymes).
No products indexed under this heading.

Fluphenazine Hydrochloride (Limited published data indicate that somatropin treatment increases cytochrome P450 (CYP450)-mediated antipyrine clearance in man. These data suggest that somatropin administration may alter the clearance of compounds known to be metabolized by CYP450 liver enzymes (eg, corticosteroids, sex steroids, anticonvulsants, cyclosporine). Careful monitoring is advisable when somatropin is administered in combination with other drugs known to be metabolized by CYP450 liver enzymes).
No products indexed under this heading.

Flurbiprofen (Limited published data indicate that somatropin treatment increases cytochrome P450 (CYP450)-mediated antipyrine clearance in man. These data suggest that somatropin administration may alter the clearance of compounds known to be metabolized by CYP450 liver enzymes (eg, corticosteroids, sex steroids, anticonvulsants, cyclosporine). Careful monitoring is advisable when somatropin is administered in combination with other drugs known to be metabolized by CYP450 liver enzymes).
No products indexed under this heading.

Flurbiprofen Sodium (Limited published data indicate that somatropin treatment increases cytochrome P450 (CYP450)-mediated antipyrine clearance in man. These data suggest that somatropin administration may alter the clearance of compounds known to be metabolized by CYP450 liver enzymes (eg, corticosteroids, sex steroids, anticonvulsants, cyclosporine). Careful monitoring is advisable when somatropin is administered in combination with other drugs known to be metabolized by CYP450 liver enzymes).
No products indexed under this heading.

Flutamide (Limited published data indicate that somatropin treatment increases cytochrome P450 (CYP450)-mediated antipyrine clearance in man. These data suggest that somat-

ropin administration may alter the clearance of compounds known to be metabolized by CYP450 liver enzymes (eg, corticosteroids, sex steroids, anticonvulsants, cyclosporine). Careful monitoring is advisable when somatropin is administered in combination with other drugs known to be metabolized by CYP450 liver enzymes).
No products indexed under this heading.

Fluticasone Furoate (Somatropin inhibits 11β-hydroxysteroid dehydrogenase type 1 (11βHSD-1) in adipose/hepatic tissue and may significantly impact the metabolism of cortisol and cortisone. Patients treated with glucocorticoid replacement therapy for previously diagnosed hypoadrenalism may require an increase in their maintenance or stress doses; this may be especially true for patients treated with cortisone acetate and prednisone. In addition, excessive glucocorticoid therapy may attenuate the growth promoting effects of somatropin in children. Therefore, glucocorticoid replacement therapy should be carefully adjusted in children with concomitant GH and glucocorticoid deficiency to avoid both hypoadrenalism and an inhibitory effect on growth. Also, somatropin administration may alter the clearance of compounds known to be metabolized by CYP450 liver enzymes (eg, corticosteroids). Careful monitoring is advisable when somatropin is administered in combination with other drugs known to be metabolized by CYP450 liver enzymes). Products include:
Veramyst **1713**

Fluticasone Propionate (Somatropin inhibits 11β-hydroxysteroid dehydrogenase type 1 (11βHSD-1) in adipose/hepatic tissue and may significantly impact the metabolism of cortisol and cortisone. Patients treated with glucocorticoid replacement therapy for previously diagnosed hypoadrenalism may require an increase in their maintenance or stress doses; this may be especially true for patients treated with cortisone acetate and prednisone. In addition, excessive glucocorticoid therapy may attenuate the growth promoting effects of somatropin in children. Therefore, glucocorticoid replacement therapy should be carefully adjusted in children with concomitant GH and glucocorticoid deficiency to avoid both hypoadrenalism and an inhibitory effect on growth. Also, somatropin administration may alter the clearance of compounds known to be metabolized by CYP450 liver enzymes (eg, corticosteroids). Careful monitoring is advisable when somatropin is administered in combination with other drugs known to be metabolized by CYP450 liver enzymes). Products include:
Advair 100/50 .... **1275**
Advair 250/50 .... **1275**
Advair 500/50 .... **1275**
Advair HFA 45/21 .... **1288**
Advair HFA 115/21 .... **1288**
Advair HFA 230/21 .... **1288**
Flonase **1459**
Flovent Diskus **1463**
Flovent HFA **1470**

Fluvastatin Sodium (Limited published data indicate that somatropin treatment increases cytochrome P450 (CYP450)-mediated antipyrine clearance in man. These data suggest that somatropin administration may alter the clearance of compounds known to be metabolized by CYP450 liver enzymes (eg, corticosteroids, sex steroids, anticonvulsants, cyclosporine). Careful monitoring is advisable when somatropin is administered in combination with other drugs known to be metabolized by CYP450 liver enzymes).
No products indexed under this heading.

Fluvoxamine Maleate (Limited published data indicate that somatropin treatment increases cytochrome P450 (CYP450)-mediated antipyrine clearance in man. These data suggest that somatropin administration may alter the clearance of compounds known to be metabolized by CYP450 liver enzymes (eg, corticosteroids, sex steroids, anticonvulsants, cyclosporine). Careful monitoring is advisable when somatropin is administered in combination with other drugs known to be metabolized by CYP450 liver enzymes).
No products indexed under this heading.

Formoterol Fumarate (Limited published data indicate that somatropin treatment increases cytochrome P450 (CYP450)-mediated antipyrine clearance in man. These data suggest that somatropin administration may alter the clearance of compounds known to be metabolized by CYP450 liver enzymes (eg, corticosteroids, sex steroids, anticonvulsants, cyclosporine). Careful monitoring is advisable when somatropin is administered in combination with other drugs known to be metabolized by CYP450 liver enzymes). Products include:
Foradil **3121**
Perforomist **3634**

Fosphenytoin (Limited published data indicate that somatropin treatment increases cytochrome P450 (CYP450)-mediated antipyrine clearance in man. These data suggest that somatropin administration may alter the clearance of compounds known to be metabolized by CYP450 liver enzymes (eg, anticonvulsants). Careful monitoring is advisable when somatropin is administered in combination with other drugs known to be metabolized by CYP450 liver enzymes).
No products indexed under this heading.

Fosphenytoin Sodium (Limited published data indicate that somatropin treatment increases cytochrome P450 (CYP450)-mediated antipyrine clearance in man. These data suggest that somatropin administration may alter the clearance of compounds known to be metabolized by CYP450 liver enzymes (eg, anticonvulsants). Careful monitoring is advisable when somatropin is administered in combination with other drugs known to be metabolized by CYP450 liver enzymes).
No products indexed under this heading.

Gabapentin (Limited published data indicate that somatropin treatment increases cytochrome P450 (CYP450)-mediated antipyrine clearance in man. These data suggest that somatropin administration may alter the clearance of compounds known to be metabolized by CYP450 liver enzymes (eg, anticonvulsants). Careful monitoring is advisable when somatropin is administered in combination with other drugs known to be metabolized by CYP450 liver enzymes).
No products indexed under this heading.

Galantamine Hydrobromide (Limited published data indicate that somatropin treatment increases cytochrome P450 (CYP450)-mediated antipyrine clearance in man. These data suggest that somatropin administration may alter the clearance of compounds known to be metabolized by CYP450 liver enzymes (eg, corticosteroids, sex steroids, anticonvulsants, cyclosporine). Careful monitoring is advisable when somatropin is administered in combination with other drugs known to be metabolized by CYP450 liver enzymes).
No products indexed under this heading.

Glibenclamide (In patients with diabetes mellitus requiring drug therapy, the dose of insulin and/or oral agents may require adjustment when somatropin therapy is initiated).
No products indexed under this heading.

Glimepiride (In patients with diabetes mellitus requiring drug therapy, the dose of insulin and/or oral agents may require adjustment when somatropin therapy is initiated). Products include:
Avandaryl **1356**
Duetact **3354**

Glipizide (In patients with diabetes mellitus requiring drug therapy, the dose of insulin and/or oral agents may require adjustment when somatropin therapy is initiated).
No products indexed under this heading.

Glyburide (In patients with diabetes mellitus requiring drug therapy, the dose of insulin and/or oral agents may require adjustment when somatropin therapy is initiated).
No products indexed under this heading.

Grepafloxacin Hydrochloride (Limited published data indicate that somatropin treatment increases cytochrome P450 (CYP450)-mediated antipyrine clearance in man. These data suggest that somatropin administration may alter the clearance of compounds known to be metabolized by CYP450 liver enzymes (eg, corticosteroids, sex steroids, anticonvulsants, cyclosporine). Careful monitoring is advisable when somatropin is administered in combination with other drugs known to be metabolized by CYP450 liver enzymes).
No products indexed under this heading.

Haloperidol (Limited published data indicate that somatropin treatment increases cytochrome P450 (CYP450)-mediated antipyrine clearance in man. These data suggest that somatropin administration may alter the clearance of compounds known to be metabolized by CYP450 liver enzymes (eg, corticosteroids, sex steroids, anticonvulsants, cyclosporine). Careful monitoring is advisable when somatropin is administered in combination with other drugs known to be metabolized by CYP450 liver enzymes).
No products indexed under this heading.

Haloperidol Decanoate (Limited published data indicate that somatropin treatment increases cytochrome P450 (CYP450)-mediated antipyrine clearance in man. These data suggest that somatropin administration may alter the clearance of compounds known to be metabolized by CYP450 liver enzymes (eg, corticosteroids, sex steroids, anticonvulsants, cyclosporine). Careful monitoring is advisable when somatropin is administered in combination with other drugs known to be metabolized by CYP450 liver enzymes).
No products indexed under this heading.

Haloperidol Lactate (Limited published data indicate that somatropin treatment increases cytochrome P450 (CYP450)-mediated antipyrine clearance in man. These data suggest that somatropin administration may alter the clearance of compounds known to be metabolized by CYP450 liver enzymes (eg, corticosteroids, sex steroids, anticonvulsants, cyclosporine). Careful monitoring is advisable when somatropin is administered in combination with other drugs known to be metabolized by CYP450 liver enzymes).
No products indexed under this heading.

Hexobarbital (Limited published data indicate that somatropin treatment increases cytochrome P450 (CYP450)-mediated antipyrine clearance in man. These data suggest that somatropin administration may alter the clearance of compounds known to be metabolized by CYP450 liver enzymes (eg, corticosteroids, sex steroids, anticonvulsants, cyclosporine). Careful monitoring is advisable when somatropin is administered in combination with other drugs known to be metabolized by CYP450 liver enzymes).
No products indexed under this heading.

Hydrocodone Bitartrate (Limited published data indicate that somatropin treatment increases cytochrome P450 (CYP450)-mediated antipyrine clearance in man. These data suggest that somatropin administration may alter the clearance of compounds known to be metabolized by CYP450 liver enzymes (eg, corticosteroids, sex steroids, anticonvulsants, cyclosporine). Careful monitoring is advisable when somatropin is administered in combination with other drugs known to be metabolized by CYP450 liver enzymes). Products include:
Vicodin **560**
Vicodin ES **561**
Vicodin HP **563**
Vicoprofen **564**
Zydone **1138**

Hydrocortisone (Somatropin inhibits 11β-hydroxysteroid dehydrogenase type 1 (11βHSD-1) in adipose/hepatic tissue and may significantly impact the metabolism of cortisol and cortisone. Patients treated with glucocorticoid replacement therapy for previously diagnosed hypoadrenalism may require an increase in their maintenance or stress doses; this may be especially true for patients treated with cortisone acetate and prednisone. In addition, excessive glucocorticoid therapy may attenuate the growth promoting effects of somatropin in children. Therefore, glucocorticoid replacement therapy should be carefully adjusted in children with concomitant GH and glucocorticoid deficiency to avoid both hypoadrenalism and an inhibitory effect on growth. Also, somatropin administration may alter the clearance of compounds known to be metabolized by CYP450 liver enzymes (eg, corticosteroids). Careful monitoring is advisable when somatropin is administered in combination with other drugs known to be metabolized by CYP450 liver enzymes).
No products indexed under this heading.

Hydrocortisone (Alcohol) (Somatropin inhibits 11β-hydroxysteroid dehydrogenase type 1 (11βHSD-1) in adipose/hepatic tissue and may significantly impact the metabolism of cortisol and cortisone. Patients treated with glucocorticoid replacement therapy for previously diagnosed hypoadrenalism may require an increase in their maintenance or stress doses; this may be especially true for patients treated with cortisone acetate and prednisone. In addition, excessive glucocorticoid therapy may attenuate the growth promoting effects of somatropin in children. Therefore, glucocorticoid replacement therapy should be carefully adjusted in children with concomitant GH and glucocorticoid deficiency to avoid both hypoadrenalism and an inhibitory effect on growth. Also, somatropin administration may alter the clearance of compounds known to be metabolized by CYP450 liver enzymes (eg, corticosteroids). Careful monitoring is advisable when somatropin is administered in combination with other drugs known to be metabolized by CYP450 liver enzymes).
No products indexed under this heading.

Hydrocortisone Acetate (Somatropin inhibits 11β-hydroxysteroid dehydrogenase type 1 (11βHSD-1) in adipose/hepatic tissue and may significantly impact the metabolism of cortisol and cortisone. Patients treated with gluco-

Norditropin Interactions Index 1212

corticoid replacement therapy for previously diagnosed hypoadrenalism may require an increase in their maintenance or stress doses; this may be especially true for patients treated with cortisone acetate and prednisone. In addition, excessive glucocorticoid therapy may attenuate the growth promoting effects of somatropin in children. Therefore, glucocorticoid replacement therapy should be carefully adjusted in children with concomitant GH and glucocorticoid deficiency to avoid both hypoadrenalism and an inhibitory effect on growth. Also, somatropin administration may alter the clearance of compounds known to be metabolized by CYP450 liver enzymes (eg, corticosteroids). Careful monitoring is advisable when somatropin is administered in combination with other drugs known to be metabolized by CYP450 liver enzymes).
No products indexed under this heading.

Hydrocortisone Butyrate (Somatropin inhibits 11β-hydroxysteroid dehydrogenase type 1 (11βHSD-1) in adipose/hepatic tissue and may significantly impact the metabolism of cortisol and cortisone. Patients treated with glucocorticoid replacement therapy for previously diagnosed hypoadrenalism may require an increase in their maintenance or stress doses; this may be especially true for patients treated with cortisone acetate and prednisone. In addition, excessive glucocorticoid therapy may attenuate the growth promoting effects of somatropin in children. Therefore, glucocorticoid replacement therapy should be carefully adjusted in children with concomitant GH and glucocorticoid deficiency to avoid both hypoadrenalism and an inhibitory effect on growth. Also, somatropin administration may alter the clearance of compounds known to be metabolized by CYP450 liver enzymes (eg, corticosteroids). Careful monitoring is advisable when somatropin is administered in combination with other drugs known to be metabolized by CYP450 liver enzymes).
No products indexed under this heading.

Hydrocortisone Cypionate (Somatropin inhibits 11β-hydroxysteroid dehydrogenase type 1 (11βHSD-1) in adipose/hepatic tissue and may significantly impact the metabolism of cortisol and cortisone. Patients treated with glucocorticoid replacement therapy for previously diagnosed hypoadrenalism may require an increase in their maintenance or stress doses; this may be especially true for patients treated with cortisone acetate and prednisone. In addition, excessive glucocorticoid therapy may attenuate the growth promoting effects of somatropin in children. Therefore, glucocorticoid replacement therapy should be carefully adjusted in children with concomitant GH and glucocorticoid deficiency to avoid both hypoadrenalism and an inhibitory effect on growth. Also, somatropin administration may alter the clearance of compounds known to be metabolized by CYP450 liver enzymes (eg, corticosteroids). Careful monitoring is advisable when somatropin is administered in combination with other drugs known to be metabolized by CYP450 liver enzymes).
No products indexed under this heading.

Hydrocortisone Hemisuccinate (Somatropin inhibits 11β-hydroxysteroid dehydrogenase type 1 (11βHSD-1) in adipose/hepatic tissue and may significantly impact the metabolism of cortisol and cortisone. Patients treated with glucocorticoid replacement therapy for previously diagnosed hypoadrenalism may require an increase in their maintenance or stress doses; this may be especially true for patients treated with cortisone acetate and prednisone. In addition, excessive glucocorticoid therapy may attenuate the growth promoting effects of somatropin in children. Therefore, glucocorticoid replacement therapy should be carefully adjusted in children with concomitant GH and glucocorticoid deficiency to avoid both hypoadrenalism and an inhibitory effect on growth. Also, somatropin administration may alter the clearance of compounds known to be metabolized by CYP450 liver enzymes (eg, corticosteroids). Careful monitoring is advisable when somatropin is administered in combination with other drugs known to be metabolized by CYP450 liver enzymes).
No products indexed under this heading.

Hydrocortisone Probutate (Somatropin inhibits 11β-hydroxysteroid dehydrogenase type 1 (11βHSD-1) in adipose/hepatic tissue and may significantly impact the metabolism of cortisol and cortisone. Patients treated with glucocorticoid replacement therapy for previously diagnosed hypoadrenalism may require an increase in their maintenance or stress doses; this may be especially true for patients treated with cortisone acetate and prednisone. In addition, excessive glucocorticoid therapy may attenuate the growth promoting effects of somatropin in children. Therefore, glucocorticoid replacement therapy should be carefully adjusted in children with concomitant GH and glucocorticoid deficiency to avoid both hypoadrenalism and an inhibitory effect on growth. Also, somatropin administration may alter the clearance of compounds known to be metabolized by CYP450 liver enzymes (eg, corticosteroids). Careful monitoring is advisable when somatropin is administered in combination with other drugs known to be metabolized by CYP450 liver enzymes).
No products indexed under this heading.

Hydrocortisone Sodium Phosphate (Somatropin inhibits 11β-hydroxysteroid dehydrogenase type 1 (11βHSD-1) in adipose/hepatic tissue and may significantly impact the metabolism of cortisol and cortisone. Patients treated with glucocorticoid replacement therapy for previously diagnosed hypoadrenalism may require an increase in their maintenance or stress doses; this may be especially true for patients treated with cortisone acetate and prednisone. In addition, excessive glucocorticoid therapy may attenuate the growth promoting effects of somatropin in children. Therefore, glucocorticoid replacement therapy should be carefully adjusted in children with concomitant GH and glucocorticoid deficiency to avoid both hypoadrenalism and an inhibitory effect on growth. Also, somatropin administration may alter the clearance of compounds known to be metabolized by CYP450 liver enzymes (eg, corticosteroids). Careful monitoring is advisable when somatropin is administered in combination with other drugs known to be metabolized by CYP450 liver enzymes).
No products indexed under this heading.

Hydrocortisone Sodium Succinate (Somatropin inhibits 11β-hydroxysteroid dehydrogenase type 1 (11βHSD-1) in adipose/hepatic tissue and may significantly impact the metabolism of cortisol and cortisone. Patients treated with glucocorticoid replacement therapy for previously diagnosed hypoadrenalism may require an increase in their maintenance or stress doses; this may be especially true for patients treated with cortisone acetate and prednisone. In addition, excessive glucocorticoid therapy may attenuate the growth promoting effects of somatropin in children. Therefore, glucocorticoid replacement therapy should be carefully adjusted in children with concomitant GH and glucocorticoid deficiency to avoid both hypoadrenalism and an inhibitory effect on growth. Also, somatropin administration may alter the clearance of compounds known to be metabolized by CYP450 liver enzymes (eg, corticosteroids). Careful monitoring is advisable when somatropin is administered in combination with other drugs known to be metabolized by CYP450 liver enzymes).
No products indexed under this heading.

Hydrocortisone Valerate (Somatropin inhibits 11β-hydroxysteroid dehydrogenase type 1 (11βHSD-1) in adipose/hepatic tissue and may significantly impact the metabolism of cortisol and cortisone. Patients treated with glucocorticoid replacement therapy for previously diagnosed hypoadrenalism may require an increase in their maintenance or stress doses; this may be especially true for patients treated with cortisone acetate and prednisone. In addition, excessive glucocorticoid therapy may attenuate the growth promoting effects of somatropin in children. Therefore, glucocorticoid replacement therapy should be carefully adjusted in children with concomitant GH and glucocorticoid deficiency to avoid both hypoadrenalism and an inhibitory effect on growth. Also, somatropin administration may alter the clearance of compounds known to be metabolized by CYP450 liver enzymes (eg, corticosteroids). Careful monitoring is advisable when somatropin is administered in combination with other drugs known to be metabolized by CYP450 liver enzymes).
No products indexed under this heading.

Ibuprofen (Limited published data indicate that somatropin treatment increases cytochrome P450 (CYP450)-mediated antipyrine clearance in man. These data suggest that somatropin administration may alter the clearance of compounds known to be metabolized by CYP450 liver enzymes (eg, corticosteroids, sex steroids, anticonvulsants, cyclosporine). Careful monitoring is advisable when somatropin is administered in combination with other drugs known to be metabolized by CYP450 liver enzymes). Products include:
Motrin IB 2043
Children's Motrin 2044
Children's Motrin Non-Staining Dye-Free 2044
Infants' Motrin 2044
Infants' Motrin Dye-Free 2044
Junior Strength Motrin 2044
Vicoprofen 564

Imipramine Hydrochloride (Limited published data indicate that somatropin treatment increases cytochrome P450 (CYP450)-mediated antipyrine clearance in man. These data suggest that somatropin administration may alter the clearance of compounds known to be metabolized by CYP450 liver enzymes (eg, corticosteroids, sex steroids, anticonvulsants, cyclosporine). Careful monitoring is advisable when somatropin is administered in combination with other drugs known to be metabolized by CYP450 liver enzymes).
No products indexed under this heading.

Imipramine Pamoate (Limited published data indicate that somatropin treatment increases cytochrome P450 (CYP450)-mediated antipyrine clearance in man. These data suggest that somatropin administration may alter the clearance of compounds known to be metabolized by CYP450 liver enzymes (eg, corticosteroids, sex steroids, anticonvulsants, cyclosporine). Careful monitoring is advisable when somatropin is administered in combination with other drugs known to be metabolized by CYP450 liver enzymes).
No products indexed under this heading.

Indinavir Sulfate (Limited published data indicate that somatropin treatment increases cytochrome P450 (CYP450)-mediated antipyrine clearance in man. These data suggest that somatropin administration may alter the clearance of compounds known to be metabolized by CYP450 liver enzymes (eg, corticosteroids, sex steroids, anticonvulsants, cyclosporine). Careful monitoring is advisable when somatropin is administered in combination with other drugs known to be metabolized by CYP450 liver enzymes). Products include:
Crixivan 2113

Indomethacin (Limited published data indicate that somatropin treatment increases cytochrome P450 (CYP450)-mediated antipyrine clearance in man. These data suggest that somatropin administration may alter the clearance of compounds known to be metabolized by CYP450 liver enzymes (eg, corticosteroids, sex steroids, anticonvulsants, cyclosporine). Careful monitoring is advisable when somatropin is administered in combination with other drugs known to be metabolized by CYP450 liver enzymes). Products include:
Indocin 2167

Indomethacin Sodium Trihydrate (Limited published data indicate that somatropin treatment increases cytochrome P450 (CYP450)-mediated antipyrine clearance in man. These data suggest that somatropin administration may alter the clearance of compounds known to be metabolized by CYP450 liver enzymes (eg, corticosteroids, sex steroids, anticonvulsants, cyclosporine). Careful monitoring is advisable when somatropin is administered in combination with other drugs known to be metabolized by CYP450 liver enzymes). Products include:
Indocin I.V. 2007

Indoramin Hydrochloride (Limited published data indicate that somatropin treatment increases cytochrome P450 (CYP450)-mediated antipyrine clearance in man. These data suggest that somatropin administration may alter the clearance of compounds known to be metabolized by CYP450 liver enzymes (eg, corticosteroids, sex steroids, anticonvulsants, cyclosporine). Careful monitoring is advisable when somatropin is administered in combination with other drugs known to be metabolized by CYP450 liver enzymes).
No products indexed under this heading.

Insulin (In patients with diabetes mellitus requiring drug therapy, the dose of insulin and/or oral agents may require adjustment when somatropin therapy is initiated).
No products indexed under this heading.

Insulin, Human, Zinc Suspension (In patients with diabetes mellitus requiring drug therapy, the dose of insulin and/or oral agents may require adjustment when somatropin therapy is initiated).
No products indexed under this heading.

Insulin, Human (rDNA origin) (In patients with diabetes mellitus requiring drug therapy, the dose of insulin and/or oral agents may require adjustment when somatropin therapy is initiated). Products include:
Exubera 2717

Insulin, Human NPH (In patients with diabetes mellitus requiring drug therapy, the dose of insulin and/or oral agents may require adjustment when somatropin therapy is initiated). Products include:
Humulin N Vial 1934

Insulin, Human Regular (In patients with diabetes mellitus requiring drug

IMPORTANT NOTE: Always consult each drug listing in the patient's regimen for possible interactions.

in man. These data suggest that somatropin administration may alter the clearance of compounds known to be metabolized by CYP450 liver enzymes (eg, corticosteroids, sex steroids, anticonvulsants, cyclosporine). Careful monitoring is advisable when somatropin is administered in combination with other drugs known to be metabolized by CYP450 liver enzymes).

No products indexed under this heading.

Lomefloxacin Hydrochloride (Limited published data indicate that somatropin treatment increases cytochrome P450 (CYP450)-mediated antipyrine clearance in man. These data suggest that somatropin administration may alter the clearance of compounds known to be metabolized by CYP450 liver enzymes (eg, corticosteroids, sex steroids, anticonvulsants, cyclosporine). Careful monitoring is advisable when somatropin is administered in combination with other drugs known to be metabolized by CYP450 liver enzymes).

No products indexed under this heading.

Losartan Potassium (Limited published data indicate that somatropin treatment increases cytochrome P450 (CYP450)-mediated antipyrine clearance in man. These data suggest that somatropin administration may alter the clearance of compounds known to be metabolized by CYP450 liver enzymes (eg, corticosteroids, sex steroids, anticonvulsants, cyclosporine). Careful monitoring is advisable when somatropin is administered in combination with other drugs known to be metabolized by CYP450 liver enzymes). Products include:

Cozaar **2106**
Hyzaar **2162**
Hyzaar 100-12.5 .... **2162**

Lovastatin (Limited published data indicate that somatropin treatment increases cytochrome P450 (CYP450)-mediated antipyrine clearance in man. These data suggest that somatropin administration may alter the clearance of compounds known to be metabolized by CYP450 liver enzymes (eg, corticosteroids, sex steroids, anticonvulsants, cyclosporine). Careful monitoring is advisable when somatropin is administered in combination with other drugs known to be metabolized by CYP450 liver enzymes). Products include:

Advicor **402**
Mevacor **2212**

Maprotiline Hydrochloride (Limited published data indicate that somatropin treatment increases cytochrome P450 (CYP450)-mediated antipyrine clearance in man. These data suggest that somatropin administration may alter the clearance of compounds known to be metabolized by CYP450 liver enzymes (eg, corticosteroids, sex steroids, anticonvulsants, cyclosporine). Careful monitoring is advisable when somatropin is administered in combination with other drugs known to be metabolized by CYP450 liver enzymes).

No products indexed under this heading.

Meclofenamate Sodium (Limited published data indicate that somatropin treatment increases cytochrome P450 (CYP450)-mediated antipyrine clearance in man. These data suggest that somatropin administration may alter the clearance of compounds known to be metabolized by CYP450 liver enzymes (eg, corticosteroids, sex steroids, anticonvulsants, cyclosporine). Careful monitoring is advisable when somatropin is administered in combination with other drugs known to be metabolized by CYP450 liver enzymes).

No products indexed under this heading.

Mefenamic Acid (Limited published data indicate that somatropin treatment increases cytochrome P450 (CYP450)-mediated antipyrine clearance in man. These data suggest that somatropin administration may alter the clearance of compounds known to be metabolized by CYP450 liver enzymes (eg, corticosteroids, sex steroids, anticonvulsants, cyclosporine). Careful monitoring is advisable when somatropin is administered in combination with other drugs known to be metabolized by CYP450 liver enzymes).

No products indexed under this heading.

Meloxicam (Limited published data indicate that somatropin treatment increases cytochrome P450 (CYP450)-mediated antipyrine clearance in man. These data suggest that somatropin administration may alter the clearance of compounds known to be metabolized by CYP450 liver enzymes (eg, corticosteroids, sex steroids, anticonvulsants, cyclosporine). Careful monitoring is advisable when somatropin is administered in combination with other drugs known to be metabolized by CYP450 liver enzymes).

No products indexed under this heading.

Meperidine Hydrochloride (Limited published data indicate that somatropin treatment increases cytochrome P450 (CYP450)-mediated antipyrine clearance in man. These data suggest that somatropin administration may alter the clearance of compounds known to be metabolized by CYP450 liver enzymes (eg, corticosteroids, sex steroids, anticonvulsants, cyclosporine). Careful monitoring is advisable when somatropin is administered in combination with other drugs known to be metabolized by CYP450 liver enzymes).

No products indexed under this heading.

Mephenytoin (Limited published data indicate that somatropin treatment increases cytochrome P450 (CYP450)-mediated antipyrine clearance in man. These data suggest that somatropin administration may alter the clearance of compounds known to be metabolized by CYP450 liver enzymes (eg, anticonvulsants). Careful monitoring is advisable when somatropin is administered in combination with other drugs known to be metabolized by CYP450 liver enzymes).

No products indexed under this heading.

Mephobarbital (Limited published data indicate that somatropin treatment increases cytochrome P450 (CYP450)-mediated antipyrine clearance in man. These data suggest that somatropin administration may alter the clearance of compounds known to be metabolized by CYP450 liver enzymes (eg, corticosteroids, sex steroids, anticonvulsants, cyclosporine). Careful monitoring is advisable when somatropin is administered in combination with other drugs known to be metabolized by CYP450 liver enzymes).

No products indexed under this heading.

Meprobamate (Limited published data indicate that somatropin treatment increases cytochrome P450 (CYP450)-mediated antipyrine clearance in man. These data suggest that somatropin administration may alter the clearance of compounds known to be metabolized by CYP450 liver enzymes (eg, corticosteroids, sex steroids, anticonvulsants, cyclosporine). Careful monitoring is advisable when somatropin is administered in combination with other drugs known to be metabolized by CYP450 liver enzymes).

No products indexed under this heading.

Mestranol (Limited published data indicate that somatropin treatment increases cytochrome P450 (CYP450)-mediated antipyrine clearance in man. These data suggest that somatropin administration may alter the clearance of compounds known to be metabolized by CYP450 liver enzymes (eg, sex steroids). Careful monitoring is advisable when somatropin is administered in combination with other drugs known to be metabolized by CYP450 liver enzymes).

No products indexed under this heading.

Metformin Hydrochloride (In patients with diabetes mellitus requiring drug therapy, the dose of insulin and/or oral agents may require adjustment when somatropin therapy is initiated). Products include:

ActoPlus **3338**
Avandamet **1345**
Janumet **2188**

Methadone Hydrochloride (Limited published data indicate that somatropin treatment increases cytochrome P450 (CYP450)-mediated antipyrine clearance in man. These data suggest that somatropin administration may alter the clearance of compounds known to be metabolized by CYP450 liver enzymes (eg, corticosteroids, sex steroids, anticonvulsants, cyclosporine). Careful monitoring is advisable when somatropin is administered in combination with other drugs known to be metabolized by CYP450 liver enzymes).

No products indexed under this heading.

Methamphetamine Hydrochloride (Limited published data indicate that somatropin treatment increases cytochrome P450 (CYP450)-mediated antipyrine clearance in man. These data suggest that somatropin administration may alter the clearance of compounds known to be metabolized by CYP450 liver enzymes (eg, corticosteroids, sex steroids, anticonvulsants, cyclosporine). Careful monitoring is advisable when somatropin is administered in combination with other drugs known to be metabolized by CYP450 liver enzymes).

No products indexed under this heading.

Methsuximide (Limited published data indicate that somatropin treatment increases cytochrome P450 (CYP450)-mediated antipyrine clearance in man. These data suggest that somatropin administration may alter the clearance of compounds known to be metabolized by CYP450 liver enzymes (eg, anticonvulsants). Careful monitoring is advisable when somatropin is administered in combination with other drugs known to be metabolized by CYP450 liver enzymes).

No products indexed under this heading.

Methylprednisolone (Somatropin inhibits 11β-hydroxysteroid dehydrogenase type 1 (11βHSD-1) in adipose/hepatic tissue and may significantly impact the metabolism of cortisol and cortisone. Patients treated with glucocorticoid replacement therapy for previously diagnosed hypoadrenalism may require an increase in their maintenance or stress doses; this may be especially true for patients treated with cortisone acetate and prednisone. In addition, excessive glucocorticoid therapy may attenuate the growth promoting effects of somatropin in children. Therefore, glucocorticoid replacement therapy should be carefully adjusted in children with concomitant GH and glucocorticoid deficiency to avoid both hypoadrenalism and an inhibitory effect on growth. Also, somatropin administration may alter the clearance of compounds known to be metabolized by CYP450 liver enzymes (eg, corticosteroids). Careful monitoring is advisable when somatropin is administered in combination with other drugs known to be metabolized by CYP450 liver enzymes).

No products indexed under this heading.

Methylprednisolone Acetate (Somatropin inhibits 11β-hydroxysteroid dehydrogenase type 1 (11βHSD-1) in adipose/hepatic tissue and may significantly impact the metabolism of cortisol and cortisone. Patients treated with glucocorticoid replacement therapy for previously diagnosed hypoadrenalism may require an increase in their maintenance or stress doses; this may be especially true for patients treated with cortisone acetate and prednisone. In addition, excessive glucocorticoid therapy may attenuate the growth promoting effects of somatropin in children. Therefore, glucocorticoid replacement therapy should be carefully adjusted in children with concomitant GH and glucocorticoid deficiency to avoid both hypoadrenalism and an inhibitory effect on growth. Also, somatropin administration may alter the clearance of compounds known to be metabolized by CYP450 liver enzymes (eg, corticosteroids). Careful monitoring is advisable when somatropin is administered in combination with other drugs known to be metabolized by CYP450 liver enzymes).

No products indexed under this heading.

Methylprednisolone Sodium Succinate (Somatropin inhibits 11β-hydroxysteroid dehydrogenase type 1 (11βHSD-1) in adipose/hepatic tissue and may significantly impact the metabolism of cortisol and cortisone. Patients treated with glucocorticoid replacement therapy for previously diagnosed hypoadrenalism may require an increase in their maintenance or stress doses; this may be especially true for patients treated with cortisone acetate and prednisone. In addition, excessive glucocorticoid therapy may attenuate the growth promoting effects of somatropin in children. Therefore, glucocorticoid replacement therapy should be carefully adjusted in children with concomitant GH and glucocorticoid deficiency to avoid both hypoadrenalism and an inhibitory effect on growth. Also, somatropin administration may alter the clearance of compounds known to be metabolized by CYP450 liver enzymes (eg, corticosteroids). Careful monitoring is advisable when somatropin is administered in combination with other drugs known to be metabolized by CYP450 liver enzymes).

No products indexed under this heading.

Methyltestosterone (Limited published data indicate that somatropin treatment increases cytochrome P450 (CYP450)-mediated antipyrine clearance in man. These data suggest that somatropin administration may alter the clearance of compounds known to be metabolized by CYP450 liver enzymes (eg, sex steroids). Careful monitoring is advisable when somatropin is administered in combination with other drugs known to be metabolized by CYP450 liver enzymes).

No products indexed under this heading.

Metoprolol Succinate (Limited published data indicate that somatropin treatment increases cytochrome P450 (CYP450)-mediated antipyrine clearance in man. These data suggest that somatropin administration may alter the clearance of compounds known to be metabolized by CYP450 liver enzymes (eg, corticosteroids, sex steroids, anticonvulsants, cyclosporine). Careful monitoring is advisable when somatropin is administered in combination with other drugs known to be metabolized by CYP450 liver enzymes). Products include:

Toprol XL **732**

Metoprolol Tartrate (Limited published data indicate that somatropin treatment increases cytochrome P450 (CYP450)-mediated antipyrine clearance

in man. These data suggest that somatropin administration may alter the clearance of compounds known to be metabolized by CYP450 liver enzymes (eg, corticosteroids, sex steroids, anticonvulsants, cyclosporine). Careful monitoring is advisable when somatropin is administered in combination with other drugs known to be metabolized by CYP450 liver enzymes).

No products indexed under this heading.

Mexiletine Hydrochloride (Limited published data indicate that somatropin treatment increases cytochrome P450 (CYP450)-mediated antipyrine clearance in man. These data suggest that somatropin administration may alter the clearance of compounds known to be metabolized by CYP450 liver enzymes (eg, corticosteroids, sex steroids, anticonvulsants, cyclosporine). Careful monitoring is advisable when somatropin is administered in combination with other drugs known to be metabolized by CYP450 liver enzymes.

No products indexed under this heading.

Midazolam Hydrochloride (Limited published data indicate that somatropin treatment increases cytochrome P450 (CYP450)-mediated antipyrine clearance in man. These data suggest that somatropin administration may alter the clearance of compounds known to be metabolized by CYP450 liver enzymes (eg, corticosteroids, sex steroids, anticonvulsants, cyclosporine). Careful monitoring is advisable when somatropin is administered in combination with other drugs known to be metabolized by CYP450 liver enzymes).

No products indexed under this heading.

Miglitol (In patients with diabetes mellitus requiring drug therapy, the dose of insulin and/or oral agents may require adjustment when somatropin therapy is initiated).

No products indexed under this heading.

Mirtazapine (Limited published data indicate that somatropin treatment increases cytochrome P450 (CYP450)-mediated antipyrine clearance in man. These data suggest that somatropin administration may alter the clearance of compounds known to be metabolized by CYP450 liver enzymes (eg, corticosteroids, sex steroids, anticonvulsants, cyclosporine). Careful monitoring is advisable when somatropin is administered in combination with other drugs known to be metabolized by CYP450 liver enzymes). Products include:

   Remeron Tablets 3214
   RemeronSolTab Tablets 3219

Mometasone Furoate (Somatropin inhibits 11β-hydroxysteroid dehydrogenase type 1 (11βHSD-1) in adipose/hepatic tissue and may significantly impact the metabolism of cortisol and cortisone. Patients treated with glucocorticoid replacement therapy for previously diagnosed hypoadrenalism may require an increase in their maintenance or stress doses; this may be especially true for patients treated with cortisone acetate and prednisone. In addition, excessive glucocorticoid therapy may attenuate the growth promoting effects of somatropin in children. Therefore, glucocorticoid replacement therapy should be carefully adjusted in children with concomitant GH and glucocorticoid deficiency to avoid both hypoadrenalism and an inhibitory effect on growth. Also, somatropin administration may alter the clearance of compounds known to be metabolized by CYP450 liver enzymes (eg, corticosteroids). Careful monitoring is advisable when somatropin is administered in combination with other drugs known to be metabolized by CYP450 liver enzymes). Products include:

   Asmanex 3058

Elocon Cream 3111
Elocon Lotion 3112
Elocon Ointment 3114

Mometasone Furoate Monohydrate (Somatropin inhibits 11β-hydroxysteroid dehydrogenase type 1 (11βHSD-1) in adipose/hepatic tissue and may significantly impact the metabolism of cortisol and cortisone. Patients treated with glucocorticoid replacement therapy for previously diagnosed hypoadrenalism may require an increase in their maintenance or stress doses; this may be especially true for patients treated with cortisone acetate and prednisone. In addition, excessive glucocorticoid therapy may attenuate the growth promoting effects of somatropin in children. Therefore, glucocorticoid replacement therapy should be carefully adjusted in children with concomitant GH and glucocorticoid deficiency to avoid both hypoadrenalism and an inhibitory effect on growth. Also, somatropin administration may alter the clearance of compounds known to be metabolized by CYP450 liver enzymes (eg, corticosteroids). Careful monitoring is advisable when somatropin is administered in combination with other drugs known to be metabolized by CYP450 liver enzymes). Products include:

   Nasonex 3166

Montelukast Sodium (Limited published data indicate that somatropin treatment increases cytochrome P450 (CYP450)-mediated antipyrine clearance in man. These data suggest that somatropin administration may alter the clearance of compounds known to be metabolized by CYP450 liver enzymes (eg, corticosteroids, sex steroids, anticonvulsants, cyclosporine). Careful monitoring is advisable when somatropin is administered in combination with other drugs known to be metabolized by CYP450 liver enzymes). Products include:

   Singulair 2270

Morphine Sulfate (Limited published data indicate that somatropin treatment increases cytochrome P450 (CYP450)-mediated antipyrine clearance in man. These data suggest that somatropin administration may alter the clearance of compounds known to be metabolized by CYP450 liver enzymes (eg, corticosteroids, sex steroids, anticonvulsants, cyclosporine). Careful monitoring is advisable when somatropin is administered in combination with other drugs known to be metabolized by CYP450 liver enzymes). Products include:

   Avinza 1822
   Embeda 1831
   MS Contin 2803

Moxifloxacin Hydrochloride (Limited published data indicate that somatropin treatment increases cytochrome P450 (CYP450)-mediated antipyrine clearance in man. These data suggest that somatropin administration may alter the clearance of compounds known to be metabolized by CYP450 liver enzymes (eg, corticosteroids, sex steroids, anticonvulsants, cyclosporine). Careful monitoring is advisable when somatropin is administered in combination with other drugs known to be metabolized by CYP450 liver enzymes). Products include:

   Avelox 3064
   Vigamox 589

Nabumetone (Limited published data indicate that somatropin treatment increases cytochrome P450 (CYP450)-mediated antipyrine clearance in man. These data suggest that somatropin administration may alter the clearance of compounds known to be metabolized by CYP450 liver enzymes (eg, corticosteroids, sex steroids, anticon-

vulsants, cyclosporine). Careful monitoring is advisable when somatropin is administered in combination with other drugs known to be metabolized by CYP450 liver enzymes).

No products indexed under this heading.

Nafcillin Sodium (Limited published data indicate that somatropin treatment increases cytochrome P450 (CYP450)-mediated antipyrine clearance in man. These data suggest that somatropin administration may alter the clearance of compounds known to be metabolized by CYP450 liver enzymes (eg, corticosteroids, sex steroids, anticonvulsants, cyclosporine). Careful monitoring is advisable when somatropin is administered in combination with other drugs known to be metabolized by CYP450 liver enzymes).

No products indexed under this heading.

Naproxen (Limited published data indicate that somatropin treatment increases cytochrome P450 (CYP450)-mediated antipyrine clearance in man. These data suggest that somatropin administration may alter the clearance of compounds known to be metabolized by CYP450 liver enzymes (eg, corticosteroids, sex steroids, anticonvulsants, cyclosporine). Careful monitoring is advisable when somatropin is administered in combination with other drugs known to be metabolized by CYP450 liver enzymes). Products include:

   EC-Naprosyn 2850
   Naprosyn 2850
   Anaprox/Naprosyn 2850

Naproxen Sodium (Limited published data indicate that somatropin treatment increases cytochrome P450 (CYP450)-mediated antipyrine clearance in man. These data suggest that somatropin administration may alter the clearance of compounds known to be metabolized by CYP450 liver enzymes (eg, corticosteroids, sex steroids, anticonvulsants, cyclosporine). Careful monitoring is advisable when somatropin is administered in combination with other drugs known to be metabolized by CYP450 liver enzymes). Products include:

   Anaprox 2850
   Anaprox DS 2850
   Treximet 1681

Nateglinide (In patients with diabetes mellitus requiring drug therapy, the dose of insulin and/or oral agents may require adjustment when somatropin therapy is initiated).

No products indexed under this heading.

Nefazodone Hydrochloride (Limited published data indicate that somatropin treatment increases cytochrome P450 (CYP450)-mediated antipyrine clearance in man. These data suggest that somatropin administration may alter the clearance of compounds known to be metabolized by CYP450 liver enzymes (eg, corticosteroids, sex steroids, anticonvulsants, cyclosporine). Careful monitoring is advisable when somatropin is administered in combination with other drugs known to be metabolized by CYP450 liver enzymes).

No products indexed under this heading.

Nelfinavir Mesylate (Limited published data indicate that somatropin treatment increases cytochrome P450 (CYP450)-mediated antipyrine clearance in man. These data suggest that somatropin administration may alter the clearance of compounds known to be metabolized by CYP450 liver enzymes (eg, corticosteroids, sex steroids, anticonvulsants, cyclosporine). Careful monitoring is advisable when somatropin is administered in combination with other drugs known to be metabolized by CYP450 liver enzymes).

No products indexed under this heading.

Nicardipine (Limited published data indicate that somatropin treatment increases cytochrome P450 (CYP450)-mediated antipyrine clearance in man. These data suggest that somatropin administration may alter the clearance of compounds known to be metabolized by CYP450 liver enzymes (eg, corticosteroids, sex steroids, anticonvulsants, cyclosporine). Careful monitoring is advisable when somatropin is administered in combination with other drugs known to be metabolized by CYP450 liver enzymes).

No products indexed under this heading.

Nicardipine Hydrochloride (Limited published data indicate that somatropin treatment increases cytochrome P450 (CYP450)-mediated antipyrine clearance in man. These data suggest that somatropin administration may alter the clearance of compounds known to be metabolized by CYP450 liver enzymes (eg, corticosteroids, sex steroids, anticonvulsants, cyclosporine). Careful monitoring is advisable when somatropin is administered in combination with other drugs known to be metabolized by CYP450 liver enzymes).

No products indexed under this heading.

Nicotine Polacrilex (Limited published data indicate that somatropin treatment increases cytochrome P450 (CYP450)-mediated antipyrine clearance in man. These data suggest that somatropin administration may alter the clearance of compounds known to be metabolized by CYP450 liver enzymes (eg, corticosteroids, sex steroids, anticonvulsants, cyclosporine). Careful monitoring is advisable when somatropin is administered in combination with other drugs known to be metabolized by CYP450 liver enzymes).

No products indexed under this heading.

Nicotine Salicylate (Limited published data indicate that somatropin treatment increases cytochrome P450 (CYP450)-mediated antipyrine clearance in man. These data suggest that somatropin administration may alter the clearance of compounds known to be metabolized by CYP450 liver enzymes (eg, corticosteroids, sex steroids, anticonvulsants, cyclosporine). Careful monitoring is advisable when somatropin is administered in combination with other drugs known to be metabolized by CYP450 liver enzymes).

No products indexed under this heading.

Nicotine Sulfate (Limited published data indicate that somatropin treatment increases cytochrome P450 (CYP450)-mediated antipyrine clearance in man. These data suggest that somatropin administration may alter the clearance of compounds known to be metabolized by CYP450 liver enzymes (eg, corticosteroids, sex steroids, anticonvulsants, cyclosporine). Careful monitoring is advisable when somatropin is administered in combination with other drugs known to be metabolized by CYP450 liver enzymes).

No products indexed under this heading.

Nifedipine (Limited published data indicate that somatropin treatment increases cytochrome P450 (CYP450)-mediated antipyrine clearance in man. These data suggest that somatropin administration may alter the clearance of compounds known to be metabolized by CYP450 liver enzymes (eg, corticosteroids, sex steroids, anticonvulsants, cyclosporine). Careful monitoring is advisable when somatropin is administered in combination with other drugs known to be metabolized by CYP450 liver enzymes).

No products indexed under this heading.

Nilutamide (Limited published data indicate that somatropin treatment increases cytochrome P450

IMPORTANT NOTE: Always consult each drug listing in the patient's regimen for possible interactions.

(CYP450)-mediated antipyrine clearance in man. These data suggest that somatropin administration may alter the clearance of compounds known to be metabolized by CYP450 liver enzymes (eg, corticosteroids, sex steroids, anticonvulsants, cyclosporine). Careful monitoring is advisable when somatropin is administered in combination with other drugs known to be metabolized by CYP450 liver enzymes).
No products indexed under this heading.

Nimodipine (Limited published data indicate that somatropin treatment increases cytochrome P450 (CYP450)-mediated antipyrine clearance in man. These data suggest that somatropin administration may alter the clearance of compounds known to be metabolized by CYP450 liver enzymes (eg, corticosteroids, sex steroids, anticonvulsants, cyclosporine). Careful monitoring is advisable when somatropin is administered in combination with other drugs known to be metabolized by CYP450 liver enzymes).
No products indexed under this heading.

Nisoldipine (Limited published data indicate that somatropin treatment increases cytochrome P450 (CYP450)-mediated antipyrine clearance in man. These data suggest that somatropin administration may alter the clearance of compounds known to be metabolized by CYP450 liver enzymes (eg, corticosteroids, sex steroids, anticonvulsants, cyclosporine). Careful monitoring is advisable when somatropin is administered in combination with other drugs known to be metabolized by CYP450 liver enzymes).
No products indexed under this heading.

Nitrendipine (Limited published data indicate that somatropin treatment increases cytochrome P450 (CYP450)-mediated antipyrine clearance in man. These data suggest that somatropin administration may alter the clearance of compounds known to be metabolized by CYP450 liver enzymes (eg, corticosteroids, sex steroids, anticonvulsants, cyclosporine). Careful monitoring is advisable when somatropin is administered in combination with other drugs known to be metabolized by CYP450 liver enzymes).
No products indexed under this heading.

Norethindrone (Limited published data indicate that somatropin treatment increases cytochrome P450 (CYP450)-mediated antipyrine clearance in man. These data suggest that somatropin administration may alter the clearance of compounds known to be metabolized by CYP450 liver enzymes (eg, sex steroids). Careful monitoring is advisable when somatropin is administered in combination with other drugs known to be metabolized by CYP450 liver enzymes). Products include:
Ortho Micronor **2660**

Norethindrone Acetate (Limited published data indicate that somatropin treatment increases cytochrome P450 (CYP450)-mediated antipyrine clearance in man. These data suggest that somatropin administration may alter the clearance of compounds known to be metabolized by CYP450 liver enzymes (eg, sex steroids). Careful monitoring is advisable when somatropin is administered in combination with other drugs known to be metabolized by CYP450 liver enzymes). Products include:
Activella **2561**

Norfloxacin (Limited published data indicate that somatropin treatment increases cytochrome P450 (CYP450)-mediated antipyrine clearance in man. These data suggest that somatropin administration may alter the clearance of compounds known to be metabolized by CYP450 liver enzymes (eg, corticosteroids, sex steroids, anticonvulsants, cyclosporine). Careful monitoring is advisable when somatropin is administered in combination with other drugs known to be metabolized by CYP450 liver enzymes). Products include:
Noroxin **2220**

Norgestimate (Limited published data indicate that somatropin treatment increases cytochrome P450 (CYP450)-mediated antipyrine clearance in man. These data suggest that somatropin administration may alter the clearance of compounds known to be metabolized by CYP450 liver enzymes (eg, sex steroids). Careful monitoring is advisable when somatropin is administered in combination with other drugs known to be metabolized by CYP450 liver enzymes). Products include:
Ortho-Cyclen/Ortho Tri-Cyclen **2663**
Ortho Tri-Cyclen Lo Tablets **2673**

Norgestrel (Limited published data indicate that somatropin treatment increases cytochrome P450 (CYP450)-mediated antipyrine clearance in man. These data suggest that somatropin administration may alter the clearance of compounds known to be metabolized by CYP450 liver enzymes (eg, corticosteroids, sex steroids, anticonvulsants, cyclosporine). Careful monitoring is advisable when somatropin is administered in combination with other drugs known to be metabolized by CYP450 liver enzymes).
No products indexed under this heading.

Nortriptyline Hydrochloride (Limited published data indicate that somatropin treatment increases cytochrome P450 (CYP450)-mediated antipyrine clearance in man. These data suggest that somatropin administration may alter the clearance of compounds known to be metabolized by CYP450 liver enzymes (eg, corticosteroids, sex steroids, anticonvulsants, cyclosporine). Careful monitoring is advisable when somatropin is administered in combination with other drugs known to be metabolized by CYP450 liver enzymes).
No products indexed under this heading.

Ofloxacin (Limited published data indicate that somatropin treatment increases cytochrome P450 (CYP450)-mediated antipyrine clearance in man. These data suggest that somatropin administration may alter the clearance of compounds known to be metabolized by CYP450 liver enzymes (eg, corticosteroids, sex steroids, anticonvulsants, cyclosporine). Careful monitoring is advisable when somatropin is administered in combination with other drugs known to be metabolized by CYP450 liver enzymes).
No products indexed under this heading.

Olanzapine (Limited published data indicate that somatropin treatment increases cytochrome P450 (CYP450)-mediated antipyrine clearance in man. These data suggest that somatropin administration may alter the clearance of compounds known to be metabolized by CYP450 liver enzymes (eg, corticosteroids, sex steroids, anticonvulsants, cyclosporine). Careful monitoring is advisable when somatropin is administered in combination with other drugs known to be metabolized by CYP450 liver enzymes). Products include:
Symbyax **1965**
Zyprexa **1984**
Zyprexa IntraMuscular **1984**
Zyprexa ZYDIS **1984**

Omeprazole (Limited published data indicate that somatropin treatment increases cytochrome P450 (CYP450)-mediated antipyrine clearance in man. These data suggest that somatropin administration may alter the clearance of compounds known to be metabolized by CYP450 liver enzymes (eg, corticosteroids, sex steroids, anticonvulsants, cyclosporine). Careful monitoring is advisable when somatropin is administered in combination with other drugs known to be metabolized by CYP450 liver enzymes).
No products indexed under this heading.

Omeprazole Magnesium (Limited published data indicate that somatropin treatment increases cytochrome P450 (CYP450)-mediated antipyrine clearance in man. These data suggest that somatropin administration may alter the clearance of compounds known to be metabolized by CYP450 liver enzymes (eg, corticosteroids, sex steroids, anticonvulsants, cyclosporine). Careful monitoring is advisable when somatropin is administered in combination with other drugs known to be metabolized by CYP450 liver enzymes).
No products indexed under this heading.

Ondansetron (Limited published data indicate that somatropin treatment increases cytochrome P450 (CYP450)-mediated antipyrine clearance in man. These data suggest that somatropin administration may alter the clearance of compounds known to be metabolized by CYP450 liver enzymes (eg, corticosteroids, sex steroids, anticonvulsants, cyclosporine). Careful monitoring is advisable when somatropin is administered in combination with other drugs known to be metabolized by CYP450 liver enzymes).
No products indexed under this heading.

Ondansetron Hydrochloride (Limited published data indicate that somatropin treatment increases cytochrome P450 (CYP450)-mediated antipyrine clearance in man. These data suggest that somatropin administration may alter the clearance of compounds known to be metabolized by CYP450 liver enzymes (eg, corticosteroids, sex steroids, anticonvulsants, cyclosporine). Careful monitoring is advisable when somatropin is administered in combination with other drugs known to be metabolized by CYP450 liver enzymes). Products include:
Zofran Injection **1750**
Zofran **1756**
Zofran ODT **1756**

Oxaprozin (Limited published data indicate that somatropin treatment increases cytochrome P450 (CYP450)-mediated antipyrine clearance in man. These data suggest that somatropin administration may alter the clearance of compounds known to be metabolized by CYP450 liver enzymes (eg, corticosteroids, sex steroids, anticonvulsants, cyclosporine). Careful monitoring is advisable when somatropin is administered in combination with other drugs known to be metabolized by CYP450 liver enzymes).
No products indexed under this heading.

Oxcarbazepine (Limited published data indicate that somatropin treatment increases cytochrome P450 (CYP450)-mediated antipyrine clearance in man. These data suggest that somatropin administration may alter the clearance of compounds known to be metabolized by CYP450 liver enzymes (eg, anticonvulsants). Careful monitoring is advisable when somatropin is administered in combination with other drugs known to be metabolized by CYP450 liver enzymes).
No products indexed under this heading.

Oxycodone Hydrochloride (Limited published data indicate that somatropin treatment increases cytochrome P450 (CYP450)-mediated antipyrine clearance in man. These data suggest that somatropin administration may alter the clearance of compounds known to be metabolized by CYP450 liver enzymes (eg, corticosteroids, sex steroids, anticonvulsants, cyclosporine). Careful monitoring is advisable when somatropin is administered in combination with other drugs known to be metabolized by CYP450 liver enzymes). Products include:
OxyContin **2807**
Percocet **1121**
Percodan **1124**

Paclitaxel (Limited published data indicate that somatropin treatment increases cytochrome P450 (CYP450)-mediated antipyrine clearance in man. These data suggest that somatropin administration may alter the clearance of compounds known to be metabolized by CYP450 liver enzymes (eg, corticosteroids, sex steroids, anticonvulsants, cyclosporine). Careful monitoring is advisable when somatropin is administered in combination with other drugs known to be metabolized by CYP450 liver enzymes).
No products indexed under this heading.

Pantoprazole Sodium (Limited published data indicate that somatropin treatment increases cytochrome P450 (CYP450)-mediated antipyrine clearance in man. These data suggest that somatropin administration may alter the clearance of compounds known to be metabolized by CYP450 liver enzymes (eg, corticosteroids, sex steroids, anticonvulsants, cyclosporine). Careful monitoring is advisable when somatropin is administered in combination with other drugs known to be metabolized by CYP450 liver enzymes). Products include:
Protonix Tablets **3571**
Protonix **3575**

Paramethadione (Limited published data indicate that somatropin treatment increases cytochrome P450 (CYP450)-mediated antipyrine clearance in man. These data suggest that somatropin administration may alter the clearance of compounds known to be metabolized by CYP450 liver enzymes (eg, anticonvulsants). Careful monitoring is advisable when somatropin is administered in combination with other drugs known to be metabolized by CYP450 liver enzymes).
No products indexed under this heading.

Paroxetine Hydrochloride (Limited published data indicate that somatropin treatment increases cytochrome P450 (CYP450)-mediated antipyrine clearance in man. These data suggest that somatropin administration may alter the clearance of compounds known to be metabolized by CYP450 liver enzymes (eg, corticosteroids, sex steroids, anticonvulsants, cyclosporine). Careful monitoring is advisable when somatropin is administered in combination with other drugs known to be metabolized by CYP450 liver enzymes). Products include:
Paroxetine CR **2361**
Paroxetine ER **2371**
Paxil **1586**
Paxil CR **1596**

Pentamidine Isethionate (Limited published data indicate that somatropin treatment increases cytochrome P450 (CYP450)-mediated antipyrine clearance in man. These data suggest that somatropin administration may alter the clearance of compounds known to be metabolized by CYP450 liver enzymes (eg, corticosteroids, sex steroids, anticonvulsants, cyclosporine). Careful monitoring is advisable when somatropin is administered in combination with other drugs known to be metabolized by CYP450 liver enzymes).
No products indexed under this heading.

Phenacemide (Limited published data indicate that somatropin treatment increases cytochrome P450 (CYP450)-mediated antipyrine clearance in man. These data suggest that somatropin administration may alter the clearance of compounds known to be metabolized by CYP450 liver enzymes (eg, anticonvulsants). Careful monitoring is advisable when somatropin is administered in combination with other drugs known to be metabolized by CYP450 liver enzymes).
No products indexed under this heading.

Phenobarbital (Limited published data indicate that somatropin treatment increases cytochrome P450 (CYP450)-mediated antipyrine clearance in man. These data suggest that somatropin administration may alter the clearance of compounds known to be metabolized by CYP450 liver enzymes (eg, anticonvulsants). Careful monitoring is advisable when somatropin is administered in combination with other drugs known to be metabolized by CYP450 liver enzymes). Products include:
Donnatal **2711**

Phenobarbital Sodium (Limited published data indicate that somatropin treatment increases cytochrome P450 (CYP450)-mediated antipyrine clearance in man. These data suggest that somatropin administration may alter the clearance of compounds known to be metabolized by CYP450 liver enzymes (eg, anticonvulsants). Careful monitoring is advisable when somatropin is administered in combination with other drugs known to be metabolized by CYP450 liver enzymes).
No products indexed under this heading.

Phensuximide (Limited published data indicate that somatropin treatment increases cytochrome P450 (CYP450)-mediated antipyrine clearance in man. These data suggest that somatropin administration may alter the clearance of compounds known to be metabolized by CYP450 liver enzymes (eg, anticonvulsants). Careful monitoring is advisable when somatropin is administered in combination with other drugs known to be metabolized by CYP450 liver enzymes).
No products indexed under this heading.

Phenylbutazone (Limited published data indicate that somatropin treatment increases cytochrome P450 (CYP450)-mediated antipyrine clearance in man. These data suggest that somatropin administration may alter the clearance of compounds known to be metabolized by CYP450 liver enzymes (eg, corticosteroids, sex steroids, anticonvulsants, cyclosporine). Careful monitoring is advisable when somatropin is administered in combination with other drugs known to be metabolized by CYP450 liver enzymes).
No products indexed under this heading.

Phenytoin (Limited published data indicate that somatropin treatment increases cytochrome P450 (CYP450)-mediated antipyrine clearance in man. These data suggest that somatropin administration may alter the clearance of compounds known to be metabolized by CYP450 liver enzymes (eg, anticonvulsants). Careful monitoring is advisable when somatropin is administered in combination with other drugs known to be metabolized by CYP450 liver enzymes).
No products indexed under this heading.

Phenytoin Sodium (Limited published data indicate that somatropin treatment increases cytochrome P450 (CYP450)-mediated antipyrine clearance in man. These data suggest that somatropin administration may alter the clearance of compounds known to be metabolized by CYP450 liver enzymes (eg, anticonvulsants). Careful monitoring is advisable when somatropin is administered in combination with other drugs known to be metabolized by CYP450 liver enzymes). Products include:
Phenytek Capsules **2380**

Pimozide (Limited published data indicate that somatropin treatment increases cytochrome P450 (CYP450)-mediated antipyrine clearance in man. These data suggest that somatropin administration may alter the clearance of compounds known to be metabolized by CYP450 liver enzymes (eg, corticosteroids, sex steroids, anticonvulsants, cyclosporine). Careful monitoring is advisable when somatropin is administered in combination with other drugs known to be metabolized by CYP450 liver enzymes).
No products indexed under this heading.

Pindolol (Limited published data indicate that somatropin treatment increases cytochrome P450 (CYP450)-mediated antipyrine clearance in man. These data suggest that somatropin administration may alter the clearance of compounds known to be metabolized by CYP450 liver enzymes (eg, corticosteroids, sex steroids, anticonvulsants, cyclosporine). Careful monitoring is advisable when somatropin is administered in combination with other drugs known to be metabolized by CYP450 liver enzymes).
No products indexed under this heading.

Pioglitazone Hydrochloride (In patients with diabetes mellitus requiring drug therapy, the dose of insulin and/or oral agents may require adjustment when somatropin therapy is initiated). Products include:
ActoPlus **3338**
Actos **3345**
Duetact **3354**

Piroxicam (Limited published data indicate that somatropin treatment increases cytochrome P450 (CYP450)-mediated antipyrine clearance in man. These data suggest that somatropin administration may alter the clearance of compounds known to be metabolized by CYP450 liver enzymes (eg, corticosteroids, sex steroids, anticonvulsants, cyclosporine). Careful monitoring is advisable when somatropin is administered in combination with other drugs known to be metabolized by CYP450 liver enzymes).
No products indexed under this heading.

Polyestradiol Phosphate (In adult women on oral estrogen replacement, a larger dose of somatropin may be required to achieve the defined treatment goal).
No products indexed under this heading.

Prednisolone (Somatropin inhibits 11β-hydroxysteroid dehydrogenase type 1 (11βHSD-1) in adipose/hepatic tissue and may significantly impact the metabolism of cortisol and cortisone. Patients treated with glucocorticoid replacement therapy for previously diagnosed hypoadrenalism may require an increase in their maintenance or stress doses; this may be especially true for patients treated with cortisone acetate and prednisone. In addition, excessive glucocorticoid therapy may attenuate the growth promoting effects of somatropin in children. Therefore, glucocorticoid replacement therapy should be carefully adjusted in children with concomitant GH and glucocorticoid deficiency to avoid both hypoadrenalism and an inhibitory effect on growth. Also, somatropin administration may alter the clearance of compounds known to be metabolized by CYP450 liver enzymes (eg, corticosteroids). Careful monitoring is advisable when somatropin is administered in combination with other drugs known to be metabolized by CYP450 liver enzymes).
No products indexed under this heading.

Prednisolone Acetate (Somatropin inhibits 11β-hydroxysteroid dehydrogenase type 1 (11βHSD-1) in adipose/hepatic tissue and may significantly impact the metabolism of cortisol and cortisone. Patients treated with glucocorticoid replacement therapy for previously diagnosed hypoadrenalism may require an increase in their maintenance or stress doses; this may be especially true for patients treated with cortisone acetate and prednisone. In addition, excessive glucocorticoid therapy may attenuate the growth promoting effects of somatropin in children. Therefore, glucocorticoid replacement therapy should be carefully adjusted in children with concomitant GH and glucocorticoid deficiency to avoid both hypoadrenalism and an inhibitory effect on growth. Also, somatropin administration may alter the clearance of compounds known to be metabolized by CYP450 liver enzymes (eg, corticosteroids). Careful monitoring is advisable when somatropin is administered in combination with other drugs known to be metabolized by CYP450 liver enzymes). Products include:
Blephamide .... ⊙**212**, ⊙**214**
Pred Forte .... ⊙**225**
Pred Mild .... ⊙**230**
Pred-G .... ⊙**226**, ⊙**227**

Prednisolone Sodium Phosphate (Somatropin inhibits 11β-hydroxysteroid dehydrogenase type 1 (11βHSD-1) in adipose/hepatic tissue and may significantly impact the metabolism of cortisol and cortisone. Patients treated with glucocorticoid replacement therapy for previously diagnosed hypoadrenalism may require an increase in their maintenance or stress doses; this may be especially true for patients treated with cortisone acetate and prednisone. In addition, excessive glucocorticoid therapy may attenuate the growth promoting effects of somatropin in children. Therefore, glucocorticoid replacement therapy should be carefully adjusted in children with concomitant GH and glucocorticoid deficiency to avoid both hypoadrenalism and an inhibitory effect on growth. Also, somatropin administration may alter the clearance of compounds known to be metabolized by CYP450 liver enzymes (eg, corticosteroids). Careful monitoring is advisable when somatropin is administered in combination with other drugs known to be metabolized by CYP450 liver enzymes).
No products indexed under this heading.

Prednisolone Tebutate (Somatropin inhibits 11β-hydroxysteroid dehydrogenase type 1 (11βHSD-1) in adipose/hepatic tissue and may significantly impact the metabolism of cortisol and cortisone. Patients treated with glucocorticoid replacement therapy for previously diagnosed hypoadrenalism may require an increase in their maintenance or stress doses; this may be especially true for patients treated with cortisone acetate and prednisone. In addition, excessive glucocorticoid therapy may attenuate the growth promoting effects of somatropin in children. Therefore, glucocorticoid replacement therapy should be carefully adjusted in children with concomitant GH and glucocorticoid deficiency to avoid both hypoadrenalism and an inhibitory effect on growth. Also, somatropin administration may alter the clearance of compounds known to be metabolized by CYP450 liver enzymes (eg, corticosteroids). Careful monitoring is advisable when somatropin is administered in combination with other drugs known to be metabolized by CYP450 liver enzymes).
No products indexed under this heading.

Prednisone (Somatropin inhibits 11β-hydroxysteroid dehydrogenase type 1 (11βHSD-1) in adipose/hepatic tissue and may significantly impact the metabolism of cortisol and cortisone. Patients treated with glucocorticoid replacement therapy for previously diagnosed hypoadrenalism may require an increase in their maintenance or stress doses; this may be especially true for patients treated with cortisone acetate and prednisone. In addition, excessive glucocorticoid therapy may attenuate the growth promoting effects of somatropin in children. Therefore, glucocorticoid replacement therapy should be carefully adjusted in children with concomitant GH and glucocorticoid deficiency to avoid both hypoadrenalism and an inhibitory effect on growth. Also, somatropin administration may alter the clearance of compounds known to be metabolized by CYP450 liver enzymes (eg, corticosteroids). Careful monitoring is advisable when somatropin is administered in combination with other drugs known to be metabolized by CYP450 liver enzymes).
No products indexed under this heading.

Prednisone sodium phosphate (Somatropin inhibits 11β-hydroxysteroid dehydrogenase type 1 (11βHSD-1) in adipose/hepatic tissue and may significantly impact the metabolism of cortisol and cortisone. Patients treated with glucocorticoid replacement therapy for previously diagnosed hypoadrenalism may require an increase in their maintenance or stress doses; this may be especially true for patients treated with cortisone acetate and prednisone. In addition, excessive glucocorticoid therapy may attenuate the growth promoting effects of somatropin in children. Therefore, glucocorticoid replacement therapy should be carefully adjusted in children with concomitant GH and glucocorticoid deficiency to avoid both hypoadrenalism and an inhibitory effect on growth. Also, somatropin administration may alter the clearance of compounds known to be metabolized by CYP450 liver enzymes (eg, corticosteroids). Careful monitoring is advisable when somatropin is administered in combination with other drugs known to be metabolized by CYP450 liver enzymes).
No products indexed under this heading.

Primidone (Limited published data indicate that somatropin treatment increases cytochrome P450 (CYP450)-mediated antipyrine clearance in man. These data suggest that somatropin administration may alter the clearance of compounds known to be metabolized by CYP450 liver enzymes (eg, anticonvulsants). Careful monitoring is advisable when somatropin is administered in combination with other drugs known to be metabolized by CYP450 liver enzymes).
No products indexed under this heading.

Progesterone (Limited published data indicate that somatropin treatment increases cytochrome P450 (CYP450)-mediated antipyrine clearance in man. These data suggest that somatropin administration may alter the clearance of compounds known to be metabolized by CYP450 liver enzymes (eg, corticosteroids, sex steroids, anticonvulsants, cyclosporine). Careful monitoring is advisable when somatropin is administered in combination with other drugs known to be metabolized by CYP450 liver enzymes). Products include:
Crinone 4% **996**
Crinone 8% **996**
Prometrium **3307**

Proguanil Hydrochloride (Limited published data indicate that somatropin treatment increases cytochrome P450

(CYP450)-mediated antipyrine clearance in man. These data suggest that somatropin administration may alter the clearance of compounds known to be metabolized by CYP450 liver enzymes (eg, corticosteroids, sex steroids, anticonvulsants, cyclosporine). Careful monitoring is advisable when somatropin is administered in combination with other drugs known to be metabolized by CYP450 liver enzymes). Products include:

Malarone Pediatric Tablets 1572
Malarone 1572

Propafenone Hydrochloride (Limited published data indicate that somatropin treatment increases cytochrome P450 (CYP450)-mediated antipyrine clearance in man. These data suggest that somatropin administration may alter the clearance of compounds known to be metabolized by CYP450 liver enzymes (eg, corticosteroids, sex steroids, anticonvulsants, cyclosporine). Careful monitoring is advisable when somatropin is administered in combination with other drugs known to be metabolized by CYP450 liver enzymes). Products include:

Rythmol 1648
Rythmol SR 1652

Propoxyphene Hydrochloride (Limited published data indicate that somatropin treatment increases cytochrome P450 (CYP450)-mediated antipyrine clearance in man. These data suggest that somatropin administration may alter the clearance of compounds known to be metabolized by CYP450 liver enzymes (eg, corticosteroids, sex steroids, anticonvulsants, cyclosporine). Careful monitoring is advisable when somatropin is administered in combination with other drugs known to be metabolized by CYP450 liver enzymes).

No products indexed under this heading.

Propoxyphene Napsylate (Limited published data indicate that somatropin treatment increases cytochrome P450 (CYP450)-mediated antipyrine clearance in man. These data suggest that somatropin administration may alter the clearance of compounds known to be metabolized by CYP450 liver enzymes (eg, corticosteroids, sex steroids, anticonvulsants, cyclosporine). Careful monitoring is advisable when somatropin is administered in combination with other drugs known to be metabolized by CYP450 liver enzymes).

No products indexed under this heading.

Propranolol Hydrochloride (Limited published data indicate that somatropin treatment increases cytochrome P450 (CYP450)-mediated antipyrine clearance in man. These data suggest that somatropin administration may alter the clearance of compounds known to be metabolized by CYP450 liver enzymes (eg, corticosteroids, sex steroids, anticonvulsants, cyclosporine). Careful monitoring is advisable when somatropin is administered in combination with other drugs known to be metabolized by CYP450 liver enzymes). Products include:

InnoPran XL 1517

Protriptyline Hydrochloride (Limited published data indicate that somatropin treatment increases cytochrome P450 (CYP450)-mediated antipyrine clearance in man. These data suggest that somatropin administration may alter the clearance of compounds known to be metabolized by CYP450 liver enzymes (eg, corticosteroids, sex steroids, anticonvulsants, cyclosporine). Careful monitoring is advisable when somatropin is administered in combination with other drugs known to be metabolized by CYP450 liver enzymes).

No products indexed under this heading.

Quetiapine Fumarate (Limited published data indicate that somatropin treatment increases cytochrome P450 (CYP450)-mediated antipyrine clearance in man. These data suggest that somatropin administration may alter the clearance of compounds known to be metabolized by CYP450 liver enzymes (eg, corticosteroids, sex steroids, anticonvulsants, cyclosporine). Careful monitoring is advisable when somatropin is administered in combination with other drugs known to be metabolized by CYP450 liver enzymes). Products include:

Seroquel 750
Seroquel XR 759

Quinestrol (In adult women on oral estrogen replacement, a larger dose of somatropin may be required to achieve the defined treatment goal).

No products indexed under this heading.

Quinidine Gluconate (Limited published data indicate that somatropin treatment increases cytochrome P450 (CYP450)-mediated antipyrine clearance in man. These data suggest that somatropin administration may alter the clearance of compounds known to be metabolized by CYP450 liver enzymes (eg, corticosteroids, sex steroids, anticonvulsants, cyclosporine). Careful monitoring is advisable when somatropin is administered in combination with other drugs known to be metabolized by CYP450 liver enzymes).

No products indexed under this heading.

Quinidine Hydrochloride (Limited published data indicate that somatropin treatment increases cytochrome P450 (CYP450)-mediated antipyrine clearance in man. These data suggest that somatropin administration may alter the clearance of compounds known to be metabolized by CYP450 liver enzymes (eg, corticosteroids, sex steroids, anticonvulsants, cyclosporine). Careful monitoring is advisable when somatropin is administered in combination with other drugs known to be metabolized by CYP450 liver enzymes).

No products indexed under this heading.

Quinidine Polygalacturonate (Limited published data indicate that somatropin treatment increases cytochrome P450 (CYP450)-mediated antipyrine clearance in man. These data suggest that somatropin administration may alter the clearance of compounds known to be metabolized by CYP450 liver enzymes (eg, corticosteroids, sex steroids, anticonvulsants, cyclosporine). Careful monitoring is advisable when somatropin is administered in combination with other drugs known to be metabolized by CYP450 liver enzymes).

No products indexed under this heading.

Quinidine Sulfate (Limited published data indicate that somatropin treatment increases cytochrome P450 (CYP450)-mediated antipyrine clearance in man. These data suggest that somatropin administration may alter the clearance of compounds known to be metabolized by CYP450 liver enzymes (eg, corticosteroids, sex steroids, anticonvulsants, cyclosporine). Careful monitoring is advisable when somatropin is administered in combination with other drugs known to be metabolized by CYP450 liver enzymes).

No products indexed under this heading.

Quinine (Limited published data indicate that somatropin treatment increases cytochrome P450 (CYP450)-mediated antipyrine clearance in man. These data suggest that somatropin administration may alter the clearance of compounds known to be metabolized by CYP450 liver enzymes (eg, corticosteroids, sex steroids, anticonvulsants, cyclosporine). Careful monitoring is advisable when somatropin is administered in combination with other drugs known to be metabolized by CYP450 liver enzymes). Products include:

Hyland's Leg Cramps PM with Quinine 3315

Quinine Sulfate (Limited published data indicate that somatropin treatment increases cytochrome P450 (CYP450)-mediated antipyrine clearance in man. These data suggest that somatropin administration may alter the clearance of compounds known to be metabolized by CYP450 liver enzymes (eg, corticosteroids, sex steroids, anticonvulsants, cyclosporine). Careful monitoring is advisable when somatropin is administered in combination with other drugs known to be metabolized by CYP450 liver enzymes).

No products indexed under this heading.

Rabeprazole Sodium (Limited published data indicate that somatropin treatment increases cytochrome P450 (CYP450)-mediated antipyrine clearance in man. These data suggest that somatropin administration may alter the clearance of compounds known to be metabolized by CYP450 liver enzymes (eg, corticosteroids, sex steroids, anticonvulsants, cyclosporine). Careful monitoring is advisable when somatropin is administered in combination with other drugs known to be metabolized by CYP450 liver enzymes). Products include:

Aciphex 1035

Repaglinide (In patients with diabetes mellitus requiring drug therapy, the dose of insulin and/or oral agents may require adjustment when somatropin therapy is initiated).

No products indexed under this heading.

Rifabutin (Limited published data indicate that somatropin treatment increases cytochrome P450 (CYP450)-mediated antipyrine clearance in man. These data suggest that somatropin administration may alter the clearance of compounds known to be metabolized by CYP450 liver enzymes (eg, corticosteroids, sex steroids, anticonvulsants, cyclosporine). Careful monitoring is advisable when somatropin is administered in combination with other drugs known to be metabolized by CYP450 liver enzymes).

No products indexed under this heading.

Riluzole (Limited published data indicate that somatropin treatment increases cytochrome P450 (CYP450)-mediated antipyrine clearance in man. These data suggest that somatropin administration may alter the clearance of compounds known to be metabolized by CYP450 liver enzymes (eg, corticosteroids, sex steroids, anticonvulsants, cyclosporine). Careful monitoring is advisable when somatropin is administered in combination with other drugs known to be metabolized by CYP450 liver enzymes). Products include:

Rilutek 3032

Risperidone (Limited published data indicate that somatropin treatment increases cytochrome P450 (CYP450)-mediated antipyrine clearance in man. These data suggest that somatropin administration may alter the clearance of compounds known to be metabolized by CYP450 liver enzymes (eg, corticosteroids, sex steroids, anticonvulsants, cyclosporine). Careful monitoring is advisable when somatropin is administered in combination with other drugs known to be metabolized by CYP450 liver enzymes). Products include:

Risperdal Consta 2682

Ritonavir (Limited published data indicate that somatropin treatment increases cytochrome P450 (CYP450)-mediated antipyrine clearance in man. These data suggest that somatropin administration may alter the clearance of compounds known to be metabolized by CYP450 liver enzymes (eg, corticosteroids, sex steroids, anticonvulsants, cyclosporine). Careful monitoring is advisable when somatropin is administered in combination with other drugs known to be metabolized by CYP450 liver enzymes). Products include:

Kaletra 458
Norvir 509

Rofecoxib (Limited published data indicate that somatropin treatment increases cytochrome P450 (CYP450)-mediated antipyrine clearance in man. These data suggest that somatropin administration may alter the clearance of compounds known to be metabolized by CYP450 liver enzymes (eg, corticosteroids, sex steroids, anticonvulsants, cyclosporine). Careful monitoring is advisable when somatropin is administered in combination with other drugs known to be metabolized by CYP450 liver enzymes).

No products indexed under this heading.

Ropinirole Hydrochloride (Limited published data indicate that somatropin treatment increases cytochrome P450 (CYP450)-mediated antipyrine clearance in man. These data suggest that somatropin administration may alter the clearance of compounds known to be metabolized by CYP450 liver enzymes (eg, corticosteroids, sex steroids, anticonvulsants, cyclosporine). Careful monitoring is advisable when somatropin is administered in combination with other drugs known to be metabolized by CYP450 liver enzymes). Products include:

Requip 1620
Requip XL 1628

Ropivacaine Hydrochloride (Limited published data indicate that somatropin treatment increases cytochrome P450 (CYP450)-mediated antipyrine clearance in man. These data suggest that somatropin administration may alter the clearance of compounds known to be metabolized by CYP450 liver enzymes (eg, corticosteroids, sex steroids, anticonvulsants, cyclosporine). Careful monitoring is advisable when somatropin is administered in combination with other drugs known to be metabolized by CYP450 liver enzymes).

No products indexed under this heading.

Rosiglitazone (Limited published data indicate that somatropin treatment increases cytochrome P450 (CYP450)-mediated antipyrine clearance in man. These data suggest that somatropin administration may alter the clearance of compounds known to be metabolized by CYP450 liver enzymes (eg, corticosteroids, sex steroids, anticonvulsants, cyclosporine). Careful monitoring is advisable when somatropin is administered in combination with other drugs known to be metabolized by CYP450 liver enzymes).

No products indexed under this heading.

Rosiglitazone Maleate (In patients with diabetes mellitus requiring drug therapy, the dose of insulin and/or oral agents may require adjustment when somatropin therapy is initiated). Products include:

Avandamet 1345
Avandaryl 1356

Avandia 1366

Rosiglitazone/Metformin (Limited published data indicate that somatropin treatment increases cytochrome P450 (CYP450)-mediated antipyrine clearance in man. These data suggest that somatropin administration may alter the clearance of compounds known to be metabolized by CYP450 liver enzymes (eg, corticosteroids, sex steroids, anticonvulsants, cyclosporine). Careful monitoring is advisable when somatropin is administered in combination with other drugs known to be metabolized by CYP450 liver enzymes).
No products indexed under this heading.

Rufinamide (Limited published data indicate that somatropin treatment increases cytochrome P450 (CYP450)-mediated antipyrine clearance in man. These data suggest that somatropin administration may alter the clearance of compounds known to be metabolized by CYP450 liver enzymes (eg, anticonvulsants). Careful monitoring is advisable when somatropin is administered in combination with other drugs known to be metabolized by CYP450 liver enzymes). Products include:
Banzel 1050

Saquinavir (Limited published data indicate that somatropin treatment increases cytochrome P450 (CYP450)-mediated antipyrine clearance in man. These data suggest that somatropin administration may alter the clearance of compounds known to be metabolized by CYP450 liver enzymes (eg, corticosteroids, sex steroids, anticonvulsants, cyclosporine). Careful monitoring is advisable when somatropin is administered in combination with other drugs known to be metabolized by CYP450 liver enzymes).
No products indexed under this heading.

Saquinavir Mesylate (Limited published data indicate that somatropin treatment increases cytochrome P450 (CYP450)-mediated antipyrine clearance in man. These data suggest that somatropin administration may alter the clearance of compounds known to be metabolized by CYP450 liver enzymes (eg, corticosteroids, sex steroids, anticonvulsants, cyclosporine). Careful monitoring is advisable when somatropin is administered in combination with other drugs known to be metabolized by CYP450 liver enzymes).
No products indexed under this heading.

Sertraline Hydrochloride (Limited published data indicate that somatropin treatment increases cytochrome P450 (CYP450)-mediated antipyrine clearance in man. These data suggest that somatropin administration may alter the clearance of compounds known to be metabolized by CYP450 liver enzymes (eg, corticosteroids, sex steroids, anticonvulsants, cyclosporine). Careful monitoring is advisable when somatropin is administered in combination with other drugs known to be metabolized by CYP450 liver enzymes).
No products indexed under this heading.

Sildenafil Citrate (Limited published data indicate that somatropin treatment increases cytochrome P450 (CYP450)-mediated antipyrine clearance in man. These data suggest that somatropin administration may alter the clearance of compounds known to be metabolized by CYP450 liver enzymes (eg, corticosteroids, sex steroids, anticonvulsants, cyclosporine). Careful monitoring is advisable when somatropin is administered in combination with other drugs known to be metabolized by CYP450 liver enzymes).
No products indexed under this heading.

Simvastatin (Limited published data indicate that somatropin treatment increases cytochrome P450 (CYP450)-mediated antipyrine clearance in man. These data suggest that somatropin administration may alter the clearance of compounds known to be metabolized by CYP450 liver enzymes (eg, corticosteroids, sex steroids, anticonvulsants, cyclosporine). Careful monitoring is advisable when somatropin is administered in combination with other drugs known to be metabolized by CYP450 liver enzymes). Products include:
Simcor 524
Vytorin 10/10 .... 2303, 3240
Vytorin 10/20 .... 2303, 3240
Vytorin 10/40 .... 2303, 3240
Vytorin 10/80 .... 2303, 3240
Zocor 2289

Sirolimus (Limited published data indicate that somatropin treatment increases cytochrome P450 (CYP450)-mediated antipyrine clearance in man. These data suggest that somatropin administration may alter the clearance of compounds known to be metabolized by CYP450 liver enzymes (eg, corticosteroids, sex steroids, anticonvulsants, cyclosporine). Careful monitoring is advisable when somatropin is administered in combination with other drugs known to be metabolized by CYP450 liver enzymes). Products include:
Rapamune 3579

Sitagliptin Phosphate (In patients with diabetes mellitus requiring drug therapy, the dose of insulin and/or oral agents may require adjustment when somatropin therapy is initiated). Products include:
Janumet 2188
Januvia 2196

Sulfamethoxazole (Limited published data indicate that somatropin treatment increases cytochrome P450 (CYP450)-mediated antipyrine clearance in man. These data suggest that somatropin administration may alter the clearance of compounds known to be metabolized by CYP450 liver enzymes (eg, corticosteroids, sex steroids, anticonvulsants, cyclosporine). Careful monitoring is advisable when somatropin is administered in combination with other drugs known to be metabolized by CYP450 liver enzymes).
No products indexed under this heading.

Sulindac (Limited published data indicate that somatropin treatment increases cytochrome P450 (CYP450)-mediated antipyrine clearance in man. These data suggest that somatropin administration may alter the clearance of compounds known to be metabolized by CYP450 liver enzymes (eg, corticosteroids, sex steroids, anticonvulsants, cyclosporine). Careful monitoring is advisable when somatropin is administered in combination with other drugs known to be metabolized by CYP450 liver enzymes). Products include:
Clinoril 2098

Suprofen (Limited published data indicate that somatropin treatment increases cytochrome P450 (CYP450)-mediated antipyrine clearance in man. These data suggest that somatropin administration may alter the clearance of compounds known to be metabolized by CYP450 liver enzymes (eg, corticosteroids, sex steroids, anticonvulsants, cyclosporine). Careful monitoring is advisable when somatropin is administered in combination with other drugs known to be metabolized by CYP450 liver enzymes).
No products indexed under this heading.

Tacrine Hydrochloride (Limited published data indicate that somatropin treatment increases cytochrome P450 (CYP450)-mediated antipyrine clearance in man. These data suggest that somatropin administration may alter the clearance of compounds known to be metabolized by CYP450 liver enzymes (eg, corticosteroids, sex steroids, anticonvulsants, cyclosporine). Careful monitoring is advisable when somatropin is administered in combination with other drugs known to be metabolized by CYP450 liver enzymes).
No products indexed under this heading.

Tacrolimus (Limited published data indicate that somatropin treatment increases cytochrome P450 (CYP450)-mediated antipyrine clearance in man. These data suggest that somatropin administration may alter the clearance of compounds known to be metabolized by CYP450 liver enzymes (eg, corticosteroids, sex steroids, anticonvulsants, cyclosporine). Careful monitoring is advisable when somatropin is administered in combination with other drugs known to be metabolized by CYP450 liver enzymes). Products include:
Prograf Capsules 677
Prograf Injection 677
Protopic 685

Tadalafil (Limited published data indicate that somatropin treatment increases cytochrome P450 (CYP450)-mediated antipyrine clearance in man. These data suggest that somatropin administration may alter the clearance of compounds known to be metabolized by CYP450 liver enzymes (eg, corticosteroids, sex steroids, anticonvulsants, cyclosporine). Careful monitoring is advisable when somatropin is administered in combination with other drugs known to be metabolized by CYP450 liver enzymes). Products include:
Adcirca 3461
Cialis 1861

Tamoxifen Citrate (Limited published data indicate that somatropin treatment increases cytochrome P450 (CYP450)-mediated antipyrine clearance in man. These data suggest that somatropin administration may alter the clearance of compounds known to be metabolized by CYP450 liver enzymes (eg, corticosteroids, sex steroids, anticonvulsants, cyclosporine). Careful monitoring is advisable when somatropin is administered in combination with other drugs known to be metabolized by CYP450 liver enzymes).
No products indexed under this heading.

Telmisartan (Limited published data indicate that somatropin treatment increases cytochrome P450 (CYP450)-mediated antipyrine clearance in man. These data suggest that somatropin administration may alter the clearance of compounds known to be metabolized by CYP450 liver enzymes (eg, corticosteroids, sex steroids, anticonvulsants, cyclosporine). Careful monitoring is advisable when somatropin is administered in combination with other drugs known to be metabolized by CYP450 liver enzymes). Products include:
Micardis 887
Micardis HCT 889

Teniposide (Limited published data indicate that somatropin treatment increases cytochrome P450 (CYP450)-mediated antipyrine clearance in man. These data suggest that somatropin administration may alter the clearance of compounds known to be metabolized by CYP450 liver enzymes (eg, corticosteroids, sex steroids, anticonvulsants, cyclosporine). Careful monitoring is advisable when somatropin is administered in combination with other drugs known to be metabolized by CYP450 liver enzymes).
No products indexed under this heading.

Terfenadine (Limited published data indicate that somatropin treatment increases cytochrome P450 (CYP450)-mediated antipyrine clearance in man. These data suggest that somatropin administration may alter the clearance of compounds known to be metabolized by CYP450 liver enzymes (eg, corticosteroids, sex steroids, anticonvulsants, cyclosporine). Careful monitoring is advisable when somatropin is administered in combination with other drugs known to be metabolized by CYP450 liver enzymes).
No products indexed under this heading.

Testosterone (Limited published data indicate that somatropin treatment increases cytochrome P450 (CYP450)-mediated antipyrine clearance in man. These data suggest that somatropin administration may alter the clearance of compounds known to be metabolized by CYP450 liver enzymes (eg, sex steroids). Careful monitoring is advisable when somatropin is administered in combination with other drugs known to be metabolized by CYP450 liver enzymes). Products include:
AndroGel 3456

Testosterone Cypionate (Limited published data indicate that somatropin treatment increases cytochrome P450 (CYP450)-mediated antipyrine clearance in man. These data suggest that somatropin administration may alter the clearance of compounds known to be metabolized by CYP450 liver enzymes (eg, corticosteroids, sex steroids, anticonvulsants, cyclosporine). Careful monitoring is advisable when somatropin is administered in combination with other drugs known to be metabolized by CYP450 liver enzymes).
No products indexed under this heading.

Testosterone Enanthate (Limited published data indicate that somatropin treatment increases cytochrome P450 (CYP450)-mediated antipyrine clearance in man. These data suggest that somatropin administration may alter the clearance of compounds known to be metabolized by CYP450 liver enzymes (eg, corticosteroids, sex steroids, anticonvulsants, cyclosporine). Careful monitoring is advisable when somatropin is administered in combination with other drugs known to be metabolized by CYP450 liver enzymes). Products include:
Delatestryl 1102

Testosterone Propionate (Limited published data indicate that somatropin treatment increases cytochrome P450 (CYP450)-mediated antipyrine clearance in man. These data suggest that somatropin administration may alter the clearance of compounds known to be metabolized by CYP450 liver enzymes (eg, corticosteroids, sex steroids, anticonvulsants, cyclosporine). Careful monitoring is advisable when somatropin is administered in combination with other drugs known to be metabolized by CYP450 liver enzymes).
No products indexed under this heading.

Theophylline (Limited published data indicate that somatropin treatment increases cytochrome P450 (CYP450)-mediated antipyrine clearance in man. These data suggest that somatropin administration may alter the clearance of compounds known to be metabolized by CYP450 liver enzymes (eg, corticosteroids, sex steroids, anticonvulsants, cyclosporine). Careful monitoring is advisable when somatropin is administered in combination with other drugs known to be metabolized by CYP450 liver enzymes).
No products indexed under this heading.

Theophylline Anhydrous (Limited published data indicate that somatropin treatment increases cytochrome P450

(CYP450)-mediated antipyrine clearance in man. These data suggest that somatropin administration may alter the clearance of compounds known to be metabolized by CYP450 liver enzymes (eg, corticosteroids, sex steroids, anticonvulsants, cyclosporine). Careful monitoring is advisable when somatropin is administered in combination with other drugs known to be metabolized by CYP450 liver enzymes). Products include:

Uniphyl 2817

Theophylline Calcium Salicylate (Limited published data indicate that somatropin treatment increases cytochrome P450 (CYP450)-mediated antipyrine clearance in man. These data suggest that somatropin administration may alter the clearance of compounds known to be metabolized by CYP450 liver enzymes (eg, corticosteroids, sex steroids, anticonvulsants, cyclosporine). Careful monitoring is advisable when somatropin is administered in combination with other drugs known to be metabolized by CYP450 liver enzymes).

No products indexed under this heading.

Theophylline Dihydroxypropyl (Glyceryl) (Limited published data indicate that somatropin treatment increases cytochrome P450 (CYP450)-mediated antipyrine clearance in man. These data suggest that somatropin administration may alter the clearance of compounds known to be metabolized by CYP450 liver enzymes (eg, corticosteroids, sex steroids, anticonvulsants, cyclosporine). Careful monitoring is advisable when somatropin is administered in combination with other drugs known to be metabolized by CYP450 liver enzymes).

No products indexed under this heading.

Theophylline Ethylenediamine (Limited published data indicate that somatropin treatment increases cytochrome P450 (CYP450)-mediated antipyrine clearance in man. These data suggest that somatropin administration may alter the clearance of compounds known to be metabolized by CYP450 liver enzymes (eg, corticosteroids, sex steroids, anticonvulsants, cyclosporine). Careful monitoring is advisable when somatropin is administered in combination with other drugs known to be metabolized by CYP450 liver enzymes).

No products indexed under this heading.

Theophylline Sodium Glycinate (Limited published data indicate that somatropin treatment increases cytochrome P450 (CYP450)-mediated antipyrine clearance in man. These data suggest that somatropin administration may alter the clearance of compounds known to be metabolized by CYP450 liver enzymes (eg, corticosteroids, sex steroids, anticonvulsants, cyclosporine). Careful monitoring is advisable when somatropin is administered in combination with other drugs known to be metabolized by CYP450 liver enzymes).

No products indexed under this heading.

Thioridazine (Limited published data indicate that somatropin treatment increases cytochrome P450 (CYP450)-mediated antipyrine clearance in man. These data suggest that somatropin administration may alter the clearance of compounds known to be metabolized by CYP450 liver enzymes (eg, corticosteroids, sex steroids, anticonvulsants, cyclosporine). Careful monitoring is advisable when somatropin is administered in combination with other drugs known to be metabolized by CYP450 liver enzymes).

No products indexed under this heading.

Thioridazine Hydrochloride (Limited published data indicate that somatropin treatment increases cytochrome P450 (CYP450)-mediated antipyrine clearance in man. These data suggest that somatropin administration may alter the clearance of compounds known to be metabolized by CYP450 liver enzymes (eg, corticosteroids, sex steroids, anticonvulsants, cyclosporine). Careful monitoring is advisable when somatropin is administered in combination with other drugs known to be metabolized by CYP450 liver enzymes). Products include:

Thioridazine Hydrochloride 2384

Tiagabine Hydrochloride (Limited published data indicate that somatropin treatment increases cytochrome P450 (CYP450)-mediated antipyrine clearance in man. These data suggest that somatropin administration may alter the clearance of compounds known to be metabolized by CYP450 liver enzymes (eg, anticonvulsants). Careful monitoring is advisable when somatropin is administered in combination with other drugs known to be metabolized by CYP450 liver enzymes). Products include:

Gabitril 972

Timolol Maleate (Limited published data indicate that somatropin treatment increases cytochrome P450 (CYP450)-mediated antipyrine clearance in man. These data suggest that somatropin administration may alter the clearance of compounds known to be metabolized by CYP450 liver enzymes (eg, corticosteroids, sex steroids, anticonvulsants, cyclosporine). Careful monitoring is advisable when somatropin is administered in combination with other drugs known to be metabolized by CYP450 liver enzymes). Products include:

Combigan 601
Dorzolamide Hydrochloride/Timolol Maleate Ophthalmic Solution .... ⊙243
Timoptic in Ocudose .... ⊙231

Tolazamide (In patients with diabetes mellitus requiring drug therapy, the dose of insulin and/or oral agents may require adjustment when somatropin therapy is initiated).

No products indexed under this heading.

Tolbutamide (In patients with diabetes mellitus requiring drug therapy, the dose of insulin and/or oral agents may require adjustment when somatropin therapy is initiated).

No products indexed under this heading.

Tolbutamide Sodium (Limited published data indicate that somatropin treatment increases cytochrome P450 (CYP450)-mediated antipyrine clearance in man. These data suggest that somatropin administration may alter the clearance of compounds known to be metabolized by CYP450 liver enzymes (eg, corticosteroids, sex steroids, anticonvulsants, cyclosporine). Careful monitoring is advisable when somatropin is administered in combination with other drugs known to be metabolized by CYP450 liver enzymes).

No products indexed under this heading.

Tolmetin Sodium (Limited published data indicate that somatropin treatment increases cytochrome P450 (CYP450)-mediated antipyrine clearance in man. These data suggest that somatropin administration may alter the clearance of compounds known to be metabolized by CYP450 liver enzymes (eg, corticosteroids, sex steroids, anticonvulsants, cyclosporine). Careful monitoring is advisable when somatropin is administered in combination with other drugs known to be metabolized by CYP450 liver enzymes).

No products indexed under this heading.

Tolterodine Tartrate (Limited published data indicate that somatropin treatment increases cytochrome P450 (CYP450)-mediated antipyrine clearance in man. These data suggest that somatropin administration may alter the clearance of compounds known to be metabolized by CYP450 liver enzymes (eg, corticosteroids, sex steroids, anticonvulsants, cyclosporine). Careful monitoring is advisable when somatropin is administered in combination with other drugs known to be metabolized by CYP450 liver enzymes).

No products indexed under this heading.

Topiramate (Limited published data indicate that somatropin treatment increases cytochrome P450 (CYP450)-mediated antipyrine clearance in man. These data suggest that somatropin administration may alter the clearance of compounds known to be metabolized by CYP450 liver enzymes (eg, anticonvulsants). Careful monitoring is advisable when somatropin is administered in combination with other drugs known to be metabolized by CYP450 liver enzymes).

No products indexed under this heading.

Torsemide (Limited published data indicate that somatropin treatment increases cytochrome P450 (CYP450)-mediated antipyrine clearance in man. These data suggest that somatropin administration may alter the clearance of compounds known to be metabolized by CYP450 liver enzymes (eg, corticosteroids, sex steroids, anticonvulsants, cyclosporine). Careful monitoring is advisable when somatropin is administered in combination with other drugs known to be metabolized by CYP450 liver enzymes).

No products indexed under this heading.

Tramadol Hydrochloride (Limited published data indicate that somatropin treatment increases cytochrome P450 (CYP450)-mediated antipyrine clearance in man. These data suggest that somatropin administration may alter the clearance of compounds known to be metabolized by CYP450 liver enzymes (eg, corticosteroids, sex steroids, anticonvulsants, cyclosporine). Careful monitoring is advisable when somatropin is administered in combination with other drugs known to be metabolized by CYP450 liver enzymes). Products include:

Ryzolt 2813
Ultram ER 2693

Trazodone Hydrochloride (Limited published data indicate that somatropin treatment increases cytochrome P450 (CYP450)-mediated antipyrine clearance in man. These data suggest that somatropin administration may alter the clearance of compounds known to be metabolized by CYP450 liver enzymes (eg, corticosteroids, sex steroids, anticonvulsants, cyclosporine). Careful monitoring is advisable when somatropin is administered in combination with other drugs known to be metabolized by CYP450 liver enzymes).

No products indexed under this heading.

Tretinoin (Limited published data indicate that somatropin treatment increases cytochrome P450 (CYP450)-mediated antipyrine clearance in man. These data suggest that somatropin administration may alter the clearance of compounds known to be metabolized by CYP450 liver enzymes (eg, corticosteroids, sex steroids, anticonvulsants, cyclosporine). Careful monitoring is advisable when somatropin is administered in combination with other drugs known to be metabolized by CYP450 liver enzymes).

No products indexed under this heading.

Triamcinolone (Somatropin inhibits 11β-hydroxysteroid dehydrogenase type 1 (11βHSD-1) in adipose/hepatic tissue and may significantly impact the metabolism of cortisol and cortisone. Patients treated with glucocorticoid replacement therapy for previously diagnosed hypoadrenalism may require an increase in their maintenance or stress doses; this may be especially true for patients treated with cortisone acetate and prednisone. In addition, excessive glucocorticoid therapy may attenuate the growth promoting effects of somatropin in children. Therefore, glucocorticoid replacement therapy should be carefully adjusted in children with concomitant GH and glucocorticoid deficiency to avoid both hypoadrenalism and an inhibitory effect on growth. Also, somatropin administration may alter the clearance of compounds known to be metabolized by CYP450 liver enzymes (eg, corticosteroids). Careful monitoring is advisable when somatropin is administered in combination with other drugs known to be metabolized by CYP450 liver enzymes).

No products indexed under this heading.

Triamcinolone Acetonide (Somatropin inhibits 11β-hydroxysteroid dehydrogenase type 1 (11βHSD-1) in adipose/hepatic tissue and may significantly impact the metabolism of cortisol and cortisone. Patients treated with glucocorticoid replacement therapy for previously diagnosed hypoadrenalism may require an increase in their maintenance or stress doses; this may be especially true for patients treated with cortisone acetate and prednisone. In addition, excessive glucocorticoid therapy may attenuate the growth promoting effects of somatropin in children. Therefore, glucocorticoid replacement therapy should be carefully adjusted in children with concomitant GH and glucocorticoid deficiency to avoid both hypoadrenalism and an inhibitory effect on growth. Also, somatropin administration may alter the clearance of compounds known to be metabolized by CYP450 liver enzymes (eg, corticosteroids). Careful monitoring is advisable when somatropin is administered in combination with other drugs known to be metabolized by CYP450 liver enzymes). Products include:

Azmacort 408
Nasacort AQ 3019

Triamcinolone Diacetate (Somatropin inhibits 11β-hydroxysteroid dehydrogenase type 1 (11βHSD-1) in adipose/hepatic tissue and may significantly impact the metabolism of cortisol and cortisone. Patients treated with glucocorticoid replacement therapy for previously diagnosed hypoadrenalism may require an increase in their maintenance or stress doses; this may be especially true for patients treated with cortisone acetate and prednisone. In addition, excessive glucocorticoid therapy may attenuate the growth promoting effects of somatropin in children. Therefore, glucocorticoid replacement therapy should be carefully adjusted in children with concomitant GH and glucocorticoid deficiency to avoid both hypoadrenalism and an inhibitory effect on growth. Also, somatropin administration may alter the clearance of compounds known to be metabolized by CYP450 liver enzymes (eg, corticosteroids). Careful monitoring is advisable when somatropin is administered in combination with other drugs known to be metabolized by CYP450 liver enzymes).

No products indexed under this heading.

Triamcinolone Hexacetonide (Somatropin inhibits 11β-hydroxysteroid dehydrogenase type 1 (11βHSD-1) in adipose/hepatic tissue and may significantly impact the metabolism of cortisol and cortisone. Patients treated with glucocorticoid replacement therapy for previously diagnosed hypoadrenalism

may require an increase in their maintenance or stress doses; this may be especially true for patients treated with cortisone acetate and prednisone. In addition, excessive glucocorticoid therapy may attenuate the growth promoting effects of somatropin in children. Therefore, glucocorticoid replacement therapy should be carefully adjusted in children with concomitant GH and glucocorticoid deficiency to avoid both hypoadrenalism and an inhibitory effect on growth. Also, somatropin administration may alter the clearance of compounds known to be metabolized by CYP450 liver enzymes (eg, corticosteroids). Careful monitoring is advisable when somatropin is administered in combination with other drugs known to be metabolized by CYP450 liver enzymes).

No products indexed under this heading.

Triazolam (Limited published data indicate that somatropin treatment increases cytochrome P450 (CYP450)-mediated antipyrine clearance in man. These data suggest that somatropin administration may alter the clearance of compounds known to be metabolized by CYP450 liver enzymes (eg, corticosteroids, sex steroids, anticonvulsants, cyclosporine). Careful monitoring is advisable when somatropin is administered in combination with other drugs known to be metabolized by CYP450 liver enzymes).

No products indexed under this heading.

Trimethadione (Limited published data indicate that somatropin treatment increases cytochrome P450 (CYP450)-mediated antipyrine clearance in man. These data suggest that somatropin administration may alter the clearance of compounds known to be metabolized by CYP450 liver enzymes (eg, anticonvulsants). Careful monitoring is advisable when somatropin is administered in combination with other drugs known to be metabolized by CYP450 liver enzymes).

No products indexed under this heading.

Trimethaphan Camsylate (Limited published data indicate that somatropin treatment increases cytochrome P450 (CYP450)-mediated antipyrine clearance in man. These data suggest that somatropin administration may alter the clearance of compounds known to be metabolized by CYP450 liver enzymes (eg, corticosteroids, sex steroids, anticonvulsants, cyclosporine). Careful monitoring is advisable when somatropin is administered in combination with other drugs known to be metabolized by CYP450 liver enzymes).

No products indexed under this heading.

Trimipramine Maleate (Limited published data indicate that somatropin treatment increases cytochrome P450 (CYP450)-mediated antipyrine clearance in man. These data suggest that somatropin administration may alter the clearance of compounds known to be metabolized by CYP450 liver enzymes (eg, corticosteroids, sex steroids, anticonvulsants, cyclosporine). Careful monitoring is advisable when somatropin is administered in combination with other drugs known to be metabolized by CYP450 liver enzymes).

No products indexed under this heading.

Troglitazone (In patients with diabetes mellitus requiring drug therapy, the dose of insulin and/or oral agents may require adjustment when somatropin therapy is initiated).

No products indexed under this heading.

Trovafloxacin Mesylate (Limited published data indicate that somatropin treatment increases cytochrome P450 (CYP450)-mediated antipyrine clearance in man. These data suggest that somatropin administration may alter the clearance of compounds known to be metabolized by CYP450 liver enzymes (eg, corticosteroids, sex steroids, anticonvulsants, cyclosporine). Careful monitoring is advisable when somatropin is administered in combination with other drugs known to be metabolized by CYP450 liver enzymes).

No products indexed under this heading.

Valdecoxib (Limited published data indicate that somatropin treatment increases cytochrome P450 (CYP450)-mediated antipyrine clearance in man. These data suggest that somatropin administration may alter the clearance of compounds known to be metabolized by CYP450 liver enzymes (eg, corticosteroids, sex steroids, anticonvulsants, cyclosporine). Careful monitoring is advisable when somatropin is administered in combination with other drugs known to be metabolized by CYP450 liver enzymes).

No products indexed under this heading.

Valproate Sodium (Limited published data indicate that somatropin treatment increases cytochrome P450 (CYP450)-mediated antipyrine clearance in man. These data suggest that somatropin administration may alter the clearance of compounds known to be metabolized by CYP450 liver enzymes (eg, anticonvulsants). Careful monitoring is advisable when somatropin is administered in combination with other drugs known to be metabolized by CYP450 liver enzymes).

No products indexed under this heading.

Valproic Acid (Limited published data indicate that somatropin treatment increases cytochrome P450 (CYP450)-mediated antipyrine clearance in man. These data suggest that somatropin administration may alter the clearance of compounds known to be metabolized by CYP450 liver enzymes (eg, anticonvulsants). Careful monitoring is advisable when somatropin is administered in combination with other drugs known to be metabolized by CYP450 liver enzymes).

No products indexed under this heading.

Valsartan (Limited published data indicate that somatropin treatment increases cytochrome P450 (CYP450)-mediated antipyrine clearance in man. These data suggest that somatropin administration may alter the clearance of compounds known to be metabolized by CYP450 liver enzymes (eg, corticosteroids, sex steroids, anticonvulsants, cyclosporine). Careful monitoring is advisable when somatropin is administered in combination with other drugs known to be metabolized by CYP450 liver enzymes). Products include:

Diovan 2413
Diovan HCT 2419
Exforge 2443
Exforge HCT 2449
Valturna 3637

Vardenafil Hydrochloride (Limited published data indicate that somatropin treatment increases cytochrome P450 (CYP450)-mediated antipyrine clearance in man. These data suggest that somatropin administration may alter the clearance of compounds known to be metabolized by CYP450 liver enzymes (eg, corticosteroids, sex steroids, anticonvulsants, cyclosporine). Careful monitoring is advisable when somatropin is administered in combination with other drugs known to be metabolized by CYP450 liver enzymes). Products include:

Levitra 3157

Venlafaxine Hydrochloride (Limited published data indicate that somatropin treatment increases cytochrome P450 (CYP450)-mediated antipyrine clearance in man. These data suggest that somatropin administration may alter the clearance of compounds known to be metabolized by CYP450 liver enzymes (eg, corticosteroids, sex steroids, anticonvulsants, cyclosporine). Careful monitoring is advisable when somatropin is administered in combination with other drugs known to be metabolized by CYP450 liver enzymes). Products include:

Effexor XR 3504
Venlafaxine Hydrochloride Tablets ... 2388

Verapamil Hydrochloride (Limited published data indicate that somatropin treatment increases cytochrome P450 (CYP450)-mediated antipyrine clearance in man. These data suggest that somatropin administration may alter the clearance of compounds known to be metabolized by CYP450 liver enzymes (eg, corticosteroids, sex steroids, anticonvulsants, cyclosporine). Careful monitoring is advisable when somatropin is administered in combination with other drugs known to be metabolized by CYP450 liver enzymes). Products include:

Tarka 534

Vinblastine Sulfate (Limited published data indicate that somatropin treatment increases cytochrome P450 (CYP450)-mediated antipyrine clearance in man. These data suggest that somatropin administration may alter the clearance of compounds known to be metabolized by CYP450 liver enzymes (eg, corticosteroids, sex steroids, anticonvulsants, cyclosporine). Careful monitoring is advisable when somatropin is administered in combination with other drugs known to be metabolized by CYP450 liver enzymes).

No products indexed under this heading.

Vincristine Sulfate (Limited published data indicate that somatropin treatment increases cytochrome P450 (CYP450)-mediated antipyrine clearance in man. These data suggest that somatropin administration may alter the clearance of compounds known to be metabolized by CYP450 liver enzymes (eg, corticosteroids, sex steroids, anticonvulsants, cyclosporine). Careful monitoring is advisable when somatropin is administered in combination with other drugs known to be metabolized by CYP450 liver enzymes).

No products indexed under this heading.

Vitamin A (Limited published data indicate that somatropin treatment increases cytochrome P450 (CYP450)-mediated antipyrine clearance in man. These data suggest that somatropin administration may alter the clearance of compounds known to be metabolized by CYP450 liver enzymes (eg, corticosteroids, sex steroids, anticonvulsants, cyclosporine). Careful monitoring is advisable when somatropin is administered in combination with other drugs known to be metabolized by CYP450 liver enzymes). Products include:

Cardio Basics 3455
Heplive 607
Norwegian Cod Liver Oil 919

Vitamin A Acetate (Limited published data indicate that somatropin treatment increases cytochrome P450 (CYP450)-mediated antipyrine clearance in man. These data suggest that somatropin administration may alter the clearance of compounds known to be metabolized by CYP450 liver enzymes (eg, corticosteroids, sex steroids, anticonvulsants, cyclosporine). Careful monitoring is advisable when somatropin is administered in combination with other drugs known to be metabolized by CYP450 liver enzymes).

No products indexed under this heading.

Voriconazole (Limited published data indicate that somatropin treatment increases cytochrome P450 (CYP450)-mediated antipyrine clearance in man. These data suggest that somatropin administration may alter the clearance of compounds known to be metabolized by CYP450 liver enzymes (eg, corticosteroids, sex steroids, anticonvulsants, cyclosporine). Careful monitoring is advisable when somatropin is administered in combination with other drugs known to be metabolized by CYP450 liver enzymes).

No products indexed under this heading.

Warfarin Sodium (Limited published data indicate that somatropin treatment increases cytochrome P450 (CYP450)-mediated antipyrine clearance in man. These data suggest that somatropin administration may alter the clearance of compounds known to be metabolized by CYP450 liver enzymes (eg, corticosteroids, sex steroids, anticonvulsants, cyclosporine). Careful monitoring is advisable when somatropin is administered in combination with other drugs known to be metabolized by CYP450 liver enzymes).

No products indexed under this heading.

Zafirlukast (Limited published data indicate that somatropin treatment increases cytochrome P450 (CYP450)-mediated antipyrine clearance in man. These data suggest that somatropin administration may alter the clearance of compounds known to be metabolized by CYP450 liver enzymes (eg, corticosteroids, sex steroids, anticonvulsants, cyclosporine). Careful monitoring is advisable when somatropin is administered in combination with other drugs known to be metabolized by CYP450 liver enzymes). Products include:

Accolate 3612

Zileuton (Limited published data indicate that somatropin treatment increases cytochrome P450 (CYP450)-mediated antipyrine clearance in man. These data suggest that somatropin administration may alter the clearance of compounds known to be metabolized by CYP450 liver enzymes (eg, corticosteroids, sex steroids, anticonvulsants, cyclosporine). Careful monitoring is advisable when somatropin is administered in combination with other drugs known to be metabolized by CYP450 liver enzymes).

No products indexed under this heading.

Zolmitriptan (Limited published data indicate that somatropin treatment increases cytochrome P450 (CYP450)-mediated antipyrine clearance in man. These data suggest that somatropin administration may alter the clearance of compounds known to be metabolized by CYP450 liver enzymes (eg, corticosteroids, sex steroids, anticonvulsants, cyclosporine). Careful monitoring is advisable when somatropin is administered in combination with other drugs known to be metabolized by CYP450 liver enzymes). Products include:

Zomig Tablets 773
Zomig Nasal Spray 768
Zomig-ZMT Tablets 773

Zonisamide (Limited published data indicate that somatropin treatment increases cytochrome P450 (CYP450)-mediated antipyrine clearance in man. These data suggest that somatropin administration may alter the clearance of compounds known to be metabolized by CYP450 liver enzymes (eg, anticonvulsants). Careful monitoring is advisable when somatropin is administered in combination with other drugs known to be metabolized by CYP450 liver enzymes). Products include:

Zonegran 1081

Zopiclone (Limited published data indicate that somatropin treatment

increases cytochrome P450 (CYP450)-mediated antipyrine clearance in man. These data suggest that somatropin administration may alter the clearance of compounds known to be metabolized by CYP450 liver enzymes (eg, corticosteroids, sex steroids, anticonvulsants, cyclosporine). Careful monitoring is advisable when somatropin is administered in combination with other drugs known to be metabolized by CYP450 liver enzymes).

No products indexed under this heading.

Food Interactions

Beverages, caffeine-containing (Limited published data indicate that somatropin treatment increases cytochrome P450 (CYP450)-mediated antipyrine clearance in man. These data suggest that somatropin administration may alter the clearance of compounds known to be metabolized by CYP450 liver enzymes (eg, corticosteroids, sex steroids, anticonvulsants, cyclosporine). Careful monitoring is advisable when somatropin is administered in combination with other drugs known to be metabolized by CYP450 liver enzymes).

Food, caffeine-containing (Limited published data indicate that somatropin treatment increases cytochrome P450 (CYP450)-mediated antipyrine clearance in man. These data suggest that somatropin administration may alter the clearance of compounds known to be metabolized by CYP450 liver enzymes (eg, corticosteroids, sex steroids, anticonvulsants, cyclosporine). Careful monitoring is advisable when somatropin is administered in combination with other drugs known to be metabolized by CYP450 liver enzymes).

NOROXIN TABLETS

(Norfloxacin) 2220
May interact with antacids containing aluminum, calcium and magnesium, antipsychotic agents, class 1A antiarrhythmics, class III antiarrhythmics, corticosteroids, drugs that prolong the QT interval, erythromycin, iron containing oral preparations, non-steroidal anti-inflammatory agents, oral anticoagulants, tricyclic antidepressants, xanthines, and certain other agents. Compounds in these categories include:

Alclometasone Dipropionate (The risk of ruptures of the shoulder, hand or Achilles tendons may be increased in patients receiving concomitant corticosteroids, especially in the elderly).

No products indexed under this heading.

Alprazolam (Precaution should be taken in elderly patients when using norfloxacin concomitantly with drugs that can result in prolongation of the QTc interval (eg, Class IA or Class III antiarrhythmics) or in patients with risk factors for torsades de pointes (eg, known QTc prolongation, uncorrected hypokalemia).

No products indexed under this heading.

Aluminum Carbonate (May interfere with absorption, resulting in lower serum and urine levels of norfloxacin; antacids should not be administered concomitantly with, or within 2 hours of, the administration of norfloxacin).

No products indexed under this heading.

Aluminum Hydroxide (May interfere with absorption, resulting in lower serum and urine levels of norfloxacin; antacids should not be administered concomitantly with, or within 2 hours of, the administration of norfloxacin).

No products indexed under this heading.

Aminophylline (Co-administration of quinolone with theophylline has resulted in elevated plasma levels of theophylline resulting in theophylline-related side effects).

No products indexed under this heading.

Amiodarone Hydrochloride (Risk of developing arrhythmias with norfloxacin may be reduced by avoiding concurrent treatment with class III antiarrhythmic agents).

No products indexed under this heading.

Amitriptyline Hydrochloride (Norfloxacin should be used with caution in subjects receiving drugs that affect the QTc interval, such as tricyclic antidepressants).

No products indexed under this heading.

Amoxapine (Norfloxacin should be used with caution in subjects receiving drugs that affect the QTc interval, such as tricyclic antidepressants).

No products indexed under this heading.

Anisindione (Co-administration may enhance the effects of oral anticoagulants).

No products indexed under this heading.

Aripiprazole (Norfloxacin should be used with caution in subjects receiving drugs that affect the QTc interval, such as antipsychotics).

No products indexed under this heading.

Astemizole (Precaution should be taken in elderly patients when using norfloxacin concomitantly with drugs that can result in prolongation of the QTc interval (eg, Class IA or Class III antiarrhythmics) or in patients with risk factors for torsades de pointes (eg, known QTc prolongation, uncorrected hypokalemia)).

No products indexed under this heading.

Beclomethasone Dipropionate (The risk of ruptures of the shoulder, hand or Achilles tendons may be increased in patients receiving concomitant corticosteroids, especially in the elderly). Products include:
Qvar 3398

Beclomethasone Dipropionate Monohydrate (The risk of ruptures of the shoulder, hand or Achilles tendons may be increased in patients receiving concomitant corticosteroids, especially in the elderly). Products include:
Beconase AQ 1386

Betamethasone (The risk of ruptures of the shoulder, hand or Achilles tendons may be increased in patients receiving concomitant corticosteroids, especially in the elderly).

No products indexed under this heading.

Betamethasone Acetate (The risk of ruptures of the shoulder, hand or Achilles tendons may be increased in patients receiving concomitant corticosteroids, especially in the elderly).

No products indexed under this heading.

Betamethasone Benzoate (The risk of ruptures of the shoulder, hand or Achilles tendons may be increased in patients receiving concomitant corticosteroids, especially in the elderly).

No products indexed under this heading.

Betamethasone Dipropionate (The risk of ruptures of the shoulder, hand or Achilles tendons may be increased in patients receiving concomitant corticosteroids, especially in the elderly). Products include:
Diprolene Lotion 0.05% 3108
Diprolene Ointment 0.05% 3109
Diprolene AF Cream 0.05% 3107
Lotrisone 3163

Betamethasone Sodium Phosphate (The risk of ruptures of the shoulder, hand or Achilles tendons may be increased in patients receiving concomitant corticosteroids, especially in the elderly).

No products indexed under this heading.

Betamethasone Valerate (The risk of ruptures of the shoulder, hand or Achilles tendons may be increased in patients receiving concomitant corticosteroids, especially in the elderly). Products include:
Luxíq 3321

Bretylium Tosylate (Risk of developing arrhythmias with norfloxacin may be reduced by avoiding concurrent treatment with class III antiarrhythmic agents).

No products indexed under this heading.

Budesonide (The risk of ruptures of the shoulder, hand or Achilles tendons may be increased in patients receiving concomitant corticosteroids, especially in the elderly). Products include:
Pulmicort Flexhaler 714
Symbicort 80/4.5 720
Symbicort 160/4.5 720

Buspirone Hydrochloride (Precaution should be taken in elderly patients when using norfloxacin concomitantly with drugs that can result in prolongation of the QTc interval (eg, Class IA or Class III antiarrhythmics) or in patients with risk factors for torsades de pointes (eg, known QTc prolongation, uncorrected hypokalemia)).

No products indexed under this heading.

Caffeine (Some quinolones have been shown to interfere with the metabolism of caffeine leading to reduced clearance of caffeine and a prolongation of its plasma half-life, which may lead to accumulation of caffeine in plasma when products containing caffeine are consumed while taking norfloxacin).

No products indexed under this heading.

Calcium Carbonate (May interfere with absorption, resulting in lower serum and urine levels of norfloxacin; antacids should not be administered concomitantly with, or within 2 hours of, the administration of norfloxacin). Products include:
Chelated Mineral 3476
Pepcid Complete 1822
Extra Strength Rolaids Softchews
Vanilla Creme 2045

Celecoxib (The concomitant administration of a non-steroidal anti-inflammatory drug (NSAID) with a quinolone, including norfloxacin, may increase the risk of CNS stimulation and convulsive seizures. Therefore, norfloxacin should be used with caution in individuals receiving NSAIDs concomitantly). Products include:
Celebrex 3272

Chlordiazepoxide (Precaution should be taken in elderly patients when using norfloxacin concomitantly with drugs that can result in prolongation of the QTc interval (eg, Class IA or Class III antiarrhythmics) or in patients with risk factors for torsades de pointes (eg, known QTc prolongation, uncorrected hypokalemia)).

No products indexed under this heading.

Chlordiazepoxide Hydrochloride (Precaution should be taken in elderly patients when using norfloxacin concomitantly with drugs that can result in prolongation of the QTc interval (eg, Class IA or Class III antiarrhythmics) or in patients with risk factors for torsades de pointes (eg, known QTc prolongation, uncorrected hypokalemia)).

No products indexed under this heading.

Chlorpromazine (Precaution should be taken in elderly patients when using norfloxacin concomitantly with drugs that can result in prolongation of the QTc interval (eg, Class IA or Class III antiarrhythmics) or in patients with risk factors for torsades de pointes (eg, known QTc prolongation, uncorrected hypokalemia)).

No products indexed under this heading.

Chlorpromazine Hydrochloride (Precaution should be taken in elderly patients when using norfloxacin concomitantly with drugs that can result in prolongation of the QTc interval (eg, Class IA or Class III antiarrhythmics) or in patients with risk factors for torsades de pointes (eg, known QTc prolongation, uncorrected hypokalemia)).

No products indexed under this heading.

Chlorprothixene (Precaution should be taken in elderly patients when using norfloxacin concomitantly with drugs that can result in prolongation of the QTc interval (eg, Class IA or Class III antiarrhythmics) or in patients with risk factors for torsades de pointes (eg, known QTc prolongation, uncorrected hypokalemia)).

No products indexed under this heading.

Chlorprothixene Hydrochloride (Precaution should be taken in elderly patients when using norfloxacin concomitantly with drugs that can result in prolongation of the QTc interval (eg, Class IA or Class III antiarrhythmics) or in patients with risk factors for torsades de pointes (eg, known QTc prolongation, uncorrected hypokalemia)).

No products indexed under this heading.

Chlorprothixene Lactate (Norfloxacin should be used with caution in subjects receiving drugs that affect the QTc interval, such as antipsychotics).

No products indexed under this heading.

Ciclesonide (The risk of ruptures of the shoulder, hand or Achilles tendons may be increased in patients receiving concomitant corticosteroids, especially in the elderly).

No products indexed under this heading.

Cisapride (Norfloxacin should be used with caution in subjects receiving drugs that affect the QTc interval, such as cisapride).

No products indexed under this heading.

Clomipramine Hydrochloride (Norfloxacin should be used with caution in subjects receiving drugs that affect the QTc interval, such as tricyclic antidepressants).

No products indexed under this heading.

Clorazepate Dipotassium (Precaution should be taken in elderly patients when using norfloxacin concomitantly with drugs that can result in prolongation of the QTc interval (eg, Class IA or Class III antiarrhythmics) or in patients with risk factors for torsades de pointes (eg, known QTc prolongation, uncorrected hypokalemia)).

No products indexed under this heading.

Clozapine (Precaution should be taken in elderly patients when using norfloxacin concomitantly with drugs that can result in prolongation of the QTc interval (eg, Class IA or Class III antiarrhythmics) or in patients with risk factors for torsades de pointes (eg, known QTc prolongation, uncorrected hypokalemia)).

No products indexed under this heading.

Cortisone Acetate (The risk of ruptures of the shoulder, hand or Achilles tendons may be increased in patients receiving concomitant corticosteroids, especially in the elderly).

No products indexed under this heading.

Cyclosporine (Co-administration has resulted in elevated serum levels of cyclosporine). Products include:

(⊙ Described in PDR® for Ophthalmic Medicines)

Desipramine Hydrochloride (Norfloxacin should be used with caution in subjects receiving drugs that affect the QTc interval, such as tricyclic antidepressants).
No products indexed under this heading.

Desoximetasone (The risk of ruptures of the shoulder, hand or Achilles tendons may be increased in patients receiving concomitant corticosteroids, especially in the elderly).
No products indexed under this heading.

Dexamethasone (The risk of ruptures of the shoulder, hand or Achilles tendons may be increased in patients receiving concomitant corticosteroids, especially in the elderly). Products include:

Dexamethasone Acetate (The risk of ruptures of the shoulder, hand or Achilles tendons may be increased in patients receiving concomitant corticosteroids, especially in the elderly).
No products indexed under this heading.

Dexamethasone Phosphate (The risk of ruptures of the shoulder, hand or Achilles tendons may be increased in patients receiving concomitant corticosteroids, especially in the elderly).
No products indexed under this heading.

Dexamethasone Sodium (The risk of ruptures of the shoulder, hand or Achilles tendons may be increased in patients receiving concomitant corticosteroids, especially in the elderly).
No products indexed under this heading.

Dexamethasone Sodium Phosphate (The risk of ruptures of the shoulder, hand or Achilles tendons may be increased in patients receiving concomitant corticosteroids, especially in the elderly).
No products indexed under this heading.

Dexamethasone Sodium Phosphate Injection (The risk of ruptures of the shoulder, hand or Achilles tendons may be increased in patients receiving concomitant corticosteroids, especially in the elderly).
No products indexed under this heading.

Diazepam (Precaution should be taken in elderly patients when using norfloxacin concomitantly with drugs that can result in prolongation of the QTc interval (eg, Class IA or Class III antiarrhythmics) or in patients with risk factors for torsades de pointes (eg, known QTc prolongation, uncorrected hypokalemia)). Products include:

Diclofenac Epolamine (The concomitant administration of a non-steroidal anti-inflammatory drug (NSAID) with a quinolone, including norfloxacin, may increase the risk of CNS stimulation and convulsive seizures. Therefore, norfloxacin should be used with caution in individuals receiving NSAIDs concomitantly). Products include:

Diclofenac Potassium (The concomitant administration of a non-steroidal anti-inflammatory drug (NSAID) with a quinolone, including norfloxacin, may increase the risk of CNS stimulation and convulsive seizures. Therefore, norfloxacin should be used with caution in individuals receiving NSAIDs concomitantly).
No products indexed under this heading.

Diclofenac Sodium (The concomitant administration of a non-steroidal anti-inflammatory drug (NSAID) with a quinolone, including norfloxacin, may increase the risk of CNS stimulation and convulsive seizures. Therefore, norfloxacin should be used with caution in individuals receiving NSAIDs concomitantly).
No products indexed under this heading.

Dicumarol (Co-administration may enhance the effects of oral anticoagulants).
No products indexed under this heading.

Didanosine (Co-administration with Videx, didanosine chewable/buffered tablets or the pediatric powder for oral solution may interfere with absorption resulting in lower serum and urine levels of norfloxacin; this combination should not be administered concomitantly or within 2 hours of administration of norfloxacin).
No products indexed under this heading.

Diflorasone Diacetate (The risk of ruptures of the shoulder, hand or Achilles tendons may be increased in patients receiving concomitant corticosteroids, especially in the elderly).
No products indexed under this heading.

Disopyramide (Risk of developing arrhythmias with norfloxacin may be reduced by avoiding concurrent treatment with class IA antiarrhythmic agents).
No products indexed under this heading.

Disopyramide Phosphate (Risk of developing arrhythmias with norfloxacin may be reduced by avoiding concurrent treatment with class IA antiarrhythmic agents).
No products indexed under this heading.

Dofetilide (Precaution should be taken in elderly patients when using norfloxacin concomitantly with drugs that can result in prolongation of the QTc interval (eg, Class IA or Class III antiarrhythmics) or in patients with risk factors for torsades de pointes (eg, known QTc prolongation, uncorrected hypokalemia)).
No products indexed under this heading.

Doxepin Hydrochloride (Norfloxacin should be used with caution in subjects receiving drugs that affect the QTc interval, such as tricyclic antidepressants).
No products indexed under this heading.

Droperidol (Precaution should be taken in elderly patients when using norfloxacin concomitantly with drugs that can result in prolongation of the QTc interval (eg, Class IA or Class III antiarrhythmics) or in patients with risk factors for torsades de pointes (eg, known QTc prolongation, uncorrected hypokalemia)).
No products indexed under this heading.

Dyphylline (Co-administration of quinolone with theophylline has resulted in elevated plasma levels of theophylline resulting in theophylline-related side effects).
No products indexed under this heading.

Erythromycin (Norfloxacin should be used with caution in subjects receiving drugs that affect the QTc interval, such as erythromycin).
No products indexed under this heading.

Erythromycin, Topical (Norfloxacin should be used with caution in subjects receiving drugs that affect the QTc interval, such as erythromycin).
No products indexed under this heading.

Erythromycin Estolate (Norfloxacin should be used with caution in subjects receiving drugs that affect the QTc interval, such as erythromycin).
No products indexed under this heading.

Erythromycin Ethylsuccinate (Norfloxacin should be used with caution in subjects receiving drugs that affect the QTc interval, such as erythromycin). Products include:

Erythromycin Gluceptate (Norfloxacin should be used with caution in subjects receiving drugs that affect the QTc interval, such as erythromycin).
No products indexed under this heading.

Erythromycin Lactobionate (Norfloxacin should be used with caution in subjects receiving drugs that affect the QTc interval, such as erythromycin).
No products indexed under this heading.

Erythromycin Stearate (Norfloxacin should be used with caution in subjects receiving drugs that affect the QTc interval, such as erythromycin).
No products indexed under this heading.

Etodolac (The concomitant administration of a non-steroidal anti-inflammatory drug (NSAID) with a quinolone, including norfloxacin, may increase the risk of CNS stimulation and convulsive seizures. Therefore, norfloxacin should be used with caution in individuals receiving NSAIDs concomitantly).
No products indexed under this heading.

Fenoprofen Calcium (The concomitant administration of a non-steroidal anti-inflammatory drug (NSAID) with a quinolone, including norfloxacin, may increase the risk of CNS stimulation and convulsive seizures. Therefore, norfloxacin should be used with caution in individuals receiving NSAIDs concomitantly).
No products indexed under this heading.

Ferrous Fumarate (May interfere with absorption, resulting in lower serum and urine levels of norfloxacin; iron-containing products should not be administered concomitantly with, or within 2 hours of, the administration of norfloxacin). Products include:

Ferrous Gluconate (May interfere with absorption, resulting in lower serum and urine levels of norfloxacin; iron-containing products should not be administered concomitantly with, or within 2 hours of, the administration of norfloxacin). Products include:

Ferrous Sulfate (May interfere with absorption, resulting in lower serum and urine levels of norfloxacin; iron-containing products should not be administered concomitantly with, or within 2 hours of, the administration of norfloxacin).
No products indexed under this heading.

Flecainide Acetate (Precaution should be taken in elderly patients when using norfloxacin concomitantly with drugs that can result in prolongation of the QTc interval (eg, Class IA or Class III antiarrhythmics) or in patients with risk factors for torsades de pointes (eg, known QTc prolongation, uncorrected hypokalemia)).
No products indexed under this heading.

Fludrocortisone Acetate (The risk of ruptures of the shoulder, hand or Achilles tendons may be increased in patients receiving concomitant corticosteroids, especially in the elderly).
No products indexed under this heading.

Flumethasone Pivalate (The risk of ruptures of the shoulder, hand or Achilles tendons may be increased in patients receiving concomitant corticosteroids, especially in the elderly).
No products indexed under this heading.

Flunisolide Hemihydrate (The risk of ruptures of the shoulder, hand or Achilles tendons may be increased in patients receiving concomitant corticosteroids, especially in the elderly).
No products indexed under this heading.

Fluphenazine Decanoate (Precaution should be taken in elderly patients when using norfloxacin concomitantly with drugs that can result in prolongation of the QTc interval (eg, Class IA or Class III antiarrhythmics) or in patients with risk factors for torsades de pointes (eg, known QTc prolongation, uncorrected hypokalemia)).
No products indexed under this heading.

Fluphenazine Enanthate (Precaution should be taken in elderly patients when using norfloxacin concomitantly with drugs that can result in prolongation of the QTc interval (eg, Class IA or Class III antiarrhythmics) or in patients with risk factors for torsades de pointes (eg, known QTc prolongation, uncorrected hypokalemia)).
No products indexed under this heading.

Fluphenazine Hydrochloride (Precaution should be taken in elderly patients when using norfloxacin concomitantly with drugs that can result in prolongation of the QTc interval (eg, Class IA or Class III antiarrhythmics) or in patients with risk factors for torsades de pointes (eg, known QTc prolongation, uncorrected hypokalemia)).
No products indexed under this heading.

Flurbiprofen (The concomitant administration of a non-steroidal anti-inflammatory drug (NSAID) with a quinolone, including norfloxacin, may increase the risk of CNS stimulation and convulsive seizures. Therefore, norfloxacin should be used with caution in individuals receiving NSAIDs concomitantly).
No products indexed under this heading.

Fluticasone Furoate (The risk of ruptures of the shoulder, hand or Achilles tendons may be increased in patients receiving concomitant corticosteroids, especially in the elderly). Products include:

Fluticasone Propionate (The risk of ruptures of the shoulder, hand or Achilles tendons may be increased in patients receiving concomitant corticosteroids, especially in the elderly). Products include:

Glyburide (Concomitant administration of norfloxacin with glyburide has rarely resulted in severe hypoglycemia; monitoring of blood glucose is recommended when these agents are co-administered).
No products indexed under this heading.

Haloperidol (Precaution should be taken in elderly patients when using norfloxacin concomitantly with drugs that can result in prolongation of the QTc interval (eg, Class IA or Class III antiarrhythmics) or in patients with risk factors for torsades de pointes (eg, known QTc prolongation, uncorrected hypokalemia)).
No products indexed under this heading.

IMPORTANT NOTE: Always consult each drug listing in the patient's regimen for possible interactions.

Noroxin

Interactions Index

1224

Haloperidol Decanoate (Precaution should be taken in elderly patients when using norfloxacin concomitantly with drugs that can result in prolongation of the QTc interval (eg, Class IA or Class III antiarrhythmics) or in patients with risk factors for torsades de pointes (eg, known QTc prolongation, uncorrected hypokalemia)).
No products indexed under this heading.

Haloperidol Lactate (Precaution should be taken in elderly patients when using norfloxacin concomitantly with drugs that can result in prolongation of the QTc interval (eg, Class IA or Class III antiarrhythmics) or in patients with risk factors for torsades de pointes (eg, known QTc prolongation, uncorrected hypokalemia)).
No products indexed under this heading.

Hydrocortisone (The risk of ruptures of the shoulder, hand or Achilles tendons may be increased in patients receiving concomitant corticosteroids, especially in the elderly).
No products indexed under this heading.

Hydrocortisone (Alcohol) (The risk of ruptures of the shoulder, hand or Achilles tendons may be increased in patients receiving concomitant corticosteroids, especially in the elderly).
No products indexed under this heading.

Hydrocortisone Acetate (The risk of ruptures of the shoulder, hand or Achilles tendons may be increased in patients receiving concomitant corticosteroids, especially in the elderly).
No products indexed under this heading.

Hydrocortisone Butyrate (The risk of ruptures of the shoulder, hand or Achilles tendons may be increased in patients receiving concomitant corticosteroids, especially in the elderly).
No products indexed under this heading.

Hydrocortisone Cypionate (The risk of ruptures of the shoulder, hand or Achilles tendons may be increased in patients receiving concomitant corticosteroids, especially in the elderly).
No products indexed under this heading.

Hydrocortisone Hemisuccinate (The risk of ruptures of the shoulder, hand or Achilles tendons may be increased in patients receiving concomitant corticosteroids, especially in the elderly).
No products indexed under this heading.

Hydrocortisone Probutate (The risk of ruptures of the shoulder, hand or Achilles tendons may be increased in patients receiving concomitant corticosteroids, especially in the elderly).
No products indexed under this heading.

Hydrocortisone Sodium Phosphate (The risk of ruptures of the shoulder, hand or Achilles tendons may be increased in patients receiving concomitant corticosteroids, especially in the elderly).
No products indexed under this heading.

Hydrocortisone Sodium Succinate (The risk of ruptures of the shoulder, hand or Achilles tendons may be increased in patients receiving concomitant corticosteroids, especially in the elderly).
No products indexed under this heading.

Hydrocortisone Valerate (The risk of ruptures of the shoulder, hand or Achilles tendons may be increased in patients receiving concomitant corticosteroids, especially in the elderly).
No products indexed under this heading.

Hydroxyzine Hydrochloride (Precaution should be taken in elderly patients when using norfloxacin concomitantly with drugs that can result in prolongation of the QTc interval (eg, Class IA or Class III antiarrhythmics) or in patients with risk factors for torsades de pointes (eg, known QTc prolongation, uncorrected hypokalemia)).
No products indexed under this heading.

Ibuprofen (The concomitant administration of a non-steroidal anti-inflammatory drug (NSAID) with a quinolone, including norfloxacin, may increase the risk of CNS stimulation and convulsive seizures. Therefore, norfloxacin should be used with caution in individuals receiving NSAIDs concomitantly). Products include:
Motrin IB 2043
Children's Motrin 2044
Children's Motrin Non-Staining Dye-Free 2044
Infants' Motrin 2044
Infants' Motrin Dye-Free 2044
Junior Strength Motrin 2044
Vicoprofen 564

Imipramine Hydrochloride (Norfloxacin should be used with caution in subjects receiving drugs that affect the QTc interval, such as tricyclic antidepressants).
No products indexed under this heading.

Imipramine Pamoate (Norfloxacin should be used with caution in subjects receiving drugs that affect the QTc interval, such as tricyclic antidepressants).
No products indexed under this heading.

Indomethacin (The concomitant administration of a non-steroidal anti-inflammatory drug (NSAID) with a quinolone, including norfloxacin, may increase the risk of CNS stimulation and convulsive seizures. Therefore, norfloxacin should be used with caution in individuals receiving NSAIDs concomitantly). Products include:
Indocin 2167

Indomethacin Sodium Trihydrate (The concomitant administration of a non-steroidal anti-inflammatory drug (NSAID) with a quinolone, including norfloxacin, may increase the risk of CNS stimulation and convulsive seizures. Therefore, norfloxacin should be used with caution in individuals receiving NSAIDs concomitantly). Products include:
Indocin I.V. 2007

Iron (May interfere with absorption, resulting in lower serum and urine levels of norfloxacin; iron-containing products should not be administered concomitantly with, or within 2 hours of, the administration of norfloxacin).
No products indexed under this heading.

Isocarboxazid (Precaution should be taken in elderly patients when using norfloxacin concomitantly with drugs that can result in prolongation of the QTc interval (eg, Class IA or Class III antiarrhythmics) or in patients with risk factors for torsades de pointes (eg, known QTc prolongation, uncorrected hypokalemia)). Products include:
Marplan 3481

Ketoprofen (The concomitant administration of a non-steroidal anti-inflammatory drug (NSAID) with a quinolone, including norfloxacin, may increase the risk of CNS stimulation and convulsive seizures. Therefore, norfloxacin should be used with caution in individuals receiving NSAIDs concomitantly).
No products indexed under this heading.

Ketorolac Tromethamine (The concomitant administration of a non-steroidal anti-inflammatory drug (NSAID) with a quinolone, including norfloxacin, may increase the risk of CNS stimulation and convulsive seizures. Therefore, norfloxacin should be used with caution in individuals receiving NSAIDs concomitantly). Products include:
Acuvail .... ⊙ 209

Lidocaine (Precaution should be taken in elderly patients when using norfloxacin concomitantly with drugs that can result in prolongation of the QTc interval (eg, Class IA or Class III antiarrhythmics) or in patients with risk factors for torsades de pointes (eg, known QTc prolongation, uncorrected hypokalemia)). Products include:
Lidoderm 1107

Lidocaine Hydrochloride (Precaution should be taken in elderly patients when using norfloxacin concomitantly with drugs that can result in prolongation of the QTc interval (eg, Class IA or Class III antiarrhythmics) or in patients with risk factors for torsades de pointes (eg, known QTc prolongation, uncorrected hypokalemia)).
No products indexed under this heading.

Lithium (Norfloxacin should be used with caution in subjects receiving drugs that affect the QTc interval, such as antipsychotics).
No products indexed under this heading.

Lithium Carbonate (Precaution should be taken in elderly patients when using norfloxacin concomitantly with drugs that can result in prolongation of the QTc interval (eg, Class IA or Class III antiarrhythmics) or in patients with risk factors for torsades de pointes (eg, known QTc prolongation, uncorrected hypokalemia)).
No products indexed under this heading.

Lithium Citrate (Precaution should be taken in elderly patients when using norfloxacin concomitantly with drugs that can result in prolongation of the QTc interval (eg, Class IA or Class III antiarrhythmics) or in patients with risk factors for torsades de pointes (eg, known QTc prolongation, uncorrected hypokalemia)).
No products indexed under this heading.

Lorazepam (Precaution should be taken in elderly patients when using norfloxacin concomitantly with drugs that can result in prolongation of the QTc interval (eg, Class IA or Class III antiarrhythmics) or in patients with risk factors for torsades de pointes (eg, known QTc prolongation, uncorrected hypokalemia)).
No products indexed under this heading.

Loxapine Hydrochloride (Precaution should be taken in elderly patients when using norfloxacin concomitantly with drugs that can result in prolongation of the QTc interval (eg, Class IA or Class III antiarrhythmics) or in patients with risk factors for torsades de pointes (eg, known QTc prolongation, uncorrected hypokalemia)).
No products indexed under this heading.

Loxapine Succinate (Precaution should be taken in elderly patients when using norfloxacin concomitantly with drugs that can result in prolongation of the QTc interval (eg, Class IA or Class III antiarrhythmics) or in patients with risk factors for torsades de pointes (eg, known QTc prolongation, uncorrected hypokalemia)).
No products indexed under this heading.

Magaldrate (May interfere with absorption, resulting in lower serum and urine levels of norfloxacin; antacids should not be administered concomitantly with, or within 2 hours of, the administration of norfloxacin).
No products indexed under this heading.

Magnesium Carbonate (May interfere with absorption, resulting in lower serum and urine levels of norfloxacin; antacids should not be administered concomitantly with, or within 2 hours of, the administration of norfloxacin).
No products indexed under this heading.

Magnesium Hydroxide (May interfere with absorption, resulting in lower serum and urine levels of norfloxacin; antacids should not be administered concomitantly with, or within 2 hours of, the administration of norfloxacin). Products include:
Fleet Pedia-Lax Chewable Tablets 1144
Pepcid Complete 1822

Magnesium Oxide (May interfere with absorption, resulting in lower serum and urine levels of norfloxacin; antacids should not be administered concomitantly with, or within 2 hours of, the administration of norfloxacin). Products include:
Beelith 873

Magnesium Trisilicate (May interfere with absorption, resulting in lower serum and urine levels of norfloxacin; antacids should not be administered concomitantly with, or within 2 hours of, the administration of norfloxacin).
No products indexed under this heading.

Maprotiline Hydrochloride (Norfloxacin should be used with caution in subjects receiving drugs that affect the QTc interval, such as tricyclic antidepressants).
No products indexed under this heading.

Meclofenamate Sodium (The concomitant administration of a non-steroidal anti-inflammatory drug (NSAID) with a quinolone, including norfloxacin, may increase the risk of CNS stimulation and convulsive seizures. Therefore, norfloxacin should be used with caution in individuals receiving NSAIDs concomitantly).
No products indexed under this heading.

Mefenamic Acid (The concomitant administration of a non-steroidal anti-inflammatory drug (NSAID) with a quinolone, including norfloxacin, may increase the risk of CNS stimulation and convulsive seizures. Therefore, norfloxacin should be used with caution in individuals receiving NSAIDs concomitantly).
No products indexed under this heading.

Meloxicam (The concomitant administration of a non-steroidal anti-inflammatory drug (NSAID) with a quinolone, including norfloxacin, may increase the risk of CNS stimulation and convulsive seizures. Therefore, norfloxacin should be used with caution in individuals receiving NSAIDs concomitantly).
No products indexed under this heading.

Meprobamate (Precaution should be taken in elderly patients when using norfloxacin concomitantly with drugs that can result in prolongation of the QTc interval (eg, Class IA or Class III antiarrhythmics) or in patients with risk factors for torsades de pointes (eg, known QTc prolongation, uncorrected hypokalemia)).
No products indexed under this heading.

Mesoridazine Besylate (Precaution should be taken in elderly patients when using norfloxacin concomitantly with drugs that can result in prolongation of the QTc interval (eg, Class IA or Class III antiarrhythmics) or in patients with risk factors for torsades de pointes (eg, known QTc prolongation, uncorrected hypokalemia)).
No products indexed under this heading.

Methotrimeprazine (Norfloxacin should be used with caution in subjects receiving drugs that affect the QTc interval, such as antipsychotics).
No products indexed under this heading.

Methylprednisolone (The risk of ruptures of the shoulder, hand or Achilles tendons may be increased in patients receiving concomitant corticosteroids, especially in the elderly).
No products indexed under this heading.

Methylprednisolone Acetate (The risk of ruptures of the shoulder, hand or Achilles tendons may be increased in patients receiving concomitant corticosteroids, especially in the elderly).
No products indexed under this heading.

Methylprednisolone Sodium Succinate (The risk of ruptures of the shoulder, hand or Achilles tendons may be increased in patients receiving concomitant corticosteroids, especially in the elderly).
No products indexed under this heading.

Mexiletine Hydrochloride (Precaution should be taken in elderly patients when using norfloxacin concomitantly with drugs that can result in prolongation of the QTc interval (eg, Class IA or Class III antiarrhythmics) or in patients with risk factors for torsades de pointes (eg, known QTc prolongation, uncorrected hypokalemia)).
No products indexed under this heading.

Midazolam Hydrochloride (Precaution should be taken in elderly patients when using norfloxacin concomitantly with drugs that can result in prolongation of the QTc interval (eg, Class IA or Class III antiarrhythmics) or in patients with risk factors for torsades de pointes (eg, known QTc prolongation, uncorrected hypokalemia)).
No products indexed under this heading.

Molindone Hydrochloride (Precaution should be taken in elderly patients when using norfloxacin concomitantly with drugs that can result in prolongation of the QTc interval (eg, Class IA or Class III antiarrhythmics) or in patients with risk factors for torsades de pointes (eg, known QTc prolongation, uncorrected hypokalemia)). Products include:

Mometasone Furoate (The risk of ruptures of the shoulder, hand or Achilles tendons may be increased in patients receiving concomitant corticosteroids, especially in the elderly). Products include:

Mometasone Furoate Monohydrate (The risk of ruptures of the shoulder, hand or Achilles tendons may be increased in patients receiving concomitant corticosteroids, especially in the elderly). Products include:

Moricizine Hydrochloride (Risk of developing arrhythmias with norfloxacin may be reduced by avoiding concurrent treatment with class IA antiarrhythmic agents).
No products indexed under this heading.

Nabumetone (The concomitant administration of a non-steroidal anti-inflammatory drug (NSAID) with a quinolone, including norfloxacin, may increase the risk of CNS stimulation and convulsive seizures. Therefore, norfloxacin should be used with caution in individuals receiving NSAIDs concomitantly).
No products indexed under this heading.

Naproxen (The concomitant administration of a non-steroidal anti-inflammatory drug (NSAID) with a quinolone, including norfloxacin, may increase the risk of CNS stimulation and convulsive seizures. Therefore, norfloxacin should be used with caution in individuals receiving NSAIDs concomitantly). Products include:

Naproxen Sodium (The concomitant administration of a non-steroidal anti-inflammatory drug (NSAID) with a quinolone, including norfloxacin, may increase the risk of CNS stimulation and convulsive seizures. Therefore, norfloxacin should be used with caution in individuals receiving NSAIDs concomitantly). Products include:

Nitrofurantoin (Nitrofurantoin may antagonize the antibacterial effect of norfloxacin in the urinary tract; concurrent use is not recommended).
No products indexed under this heading.

Nortriptyline Hydrochloride (Norfloxacin should be used with caution in subjects receiving drugs that affect the QTc interval, such as tricyclic antidepressants).
No products indexed under this heading.

Olanzapine (Precaution should be taken in elderly patients when using norfloxacin concomitantly with drugs that can result in prolongation of the QTc interval (eg, Class IA or Class III antiarrhythmics) or in patients with risk factors for torsades de pointes (eg, known QTc prolongation, uncorrected hypokalemia)). Products include:

Oxaprozin (The concomitant administration of a non-steroidal anti-inflammatory drug (NSAID) with a quinolone, including norfloxacin, may increase the risk of CNS stimulation and convulsive seizures. Therefore, norfloxacin should be used with caution in individuals receiving NSAIDs concomitantly).
No products indexed under this heading.

Oxazepam (Precaution should be taken in elderly patients when using norfloxacin concomitantly with drugs that can result in prolongation of the QTc interval (eg, Class IA or Class III antiarrhythmics) or in patients with risk factors for torsades de pointes (eg, known QTc prolongation, uncorrected hypokalemia)).
No products indexed under this heading.

Paliperidone (Norfloxacin should be used with caution in subjects receiving drugs that affect the QTc interval, such as antipsychotics). Products include:

Perphenazine (Precaution should be taken in elderly patients when using norfloxacin concomitantly with drugs that can result in prolongation of the QTc interval (eg, Class IA or Class III antiarrhythmics) or in patients with risk factors for torsades de pointes (eg, known QTc prolongation, uncorrected hypokalemia)).
No products indexed under this heading.

Phenelzine Sulfate (Precaution should be taken in elderly patients when using norfloxacin concomitantly with drugs that can result in prolongation of the QTc interval (eg, Class IA or Class III antiarrhythmics) or in patients with risk factors for torsades de pointes (eg, known QTc prolongation, uncorrected hypokalemia)).
No products indexed under this heading.

Phenylbutazone (The concomitant administration of a non-steroidal anti-inflammatory drug (NSAID) with a quinolone, including norfloxacin, may increase the risk of CNS stimulation and convulsive seizures. Therefore, norfloxacin should be used with caution in individuals receiving NSAIDs concomitantly).
No products indexed under this heading.

Pimozide (Norfloxacin should be used with caution in subjects receiving drugs that affect the QTc interval, such as antipsychotics).
No products indexed under this heading.

Piroxicam (The concomitant administration of a non-steroidal anti-inflammatory drug (NSAID) with a quinolone, including norfloxacin, may increase the risk of CNS stimulation and convulsive seizures. Therefore, norfloxacin should be used with caution in individuals receiving NSAIDs concomitantly).
No products indexed under this heading.

Polysaccharide Iron Complex (May interfere with absorption, resulting in lower serum and urine levels of norfloxacin; iron-containing products should not be administered concomitantly with, or within 2 hours of, the administration of norfloxacin). Products include:

Prazepam (Precaution should be taken in elderly patients when using norfloxacin concomitantly with drugs that can result in prolongation of the QTc interval (eg, Class IA or Class III antiarrhythmics) or in patients with risk factors for torsades de pointes (eg, known QTc prolongation, uncorrected hypokalemia)).
No products indexed under this heading.

Prednisolone (The risk of ruptures of the shoulder, hand or Achilles tendons may be increased in patients receiving concomitant corticosteroids, especially in the elderly).
No products indexed under this heading.

Prednisolone Acetate (The risk of ruptures of the shoulder, hand or Achilles tendons may be increased in patients receiving concomitant corticosteroids, especially in the elderly). Products include:

Prednisolone Sodium Phosphate (The risk of ruptures of the shoulder, hand or Achilles tendons may be increased in patients receiving concomitant corticosteroids, especially in the elderly).
No products indexed under this heading.

Prednisolone Tebutate (The risk of ruptures of the shoulder, hand or Achilles tendons may be increased in patients receiving concomitant corticosteroids, especially in the elderly).
No products indexed under this heading.

Prednisone (The risk of ruptures of the shoulder, hand or Achilles tendons may be increased in patients receiving concomitant corticosteroids, especially in the elderly).
No products indexed under this heading.

Prednisone sodium phosphate (The risk of ruptures of the shoulder, hand or Achilles tendons may be increased in patients receiving concomitant corticosteroids, especially in the elderly).
No products indexed under this heading.

Probenecid (Co-administration with probenecid has resulted in diminished urinary excretion).
No products indexed under this heading.

Procainamide (Risk of developing arrhythmias with norfloxacin may be reduced by avoiding concurrent treatment with class IA antiarrhythmic agents).
No products indexed under this heading.

Procainamide Hydrochloride (Precaution should be taken in elderly patients when using norfloxacin concomitantly with drugs that can result in prolongation of the QTc interval (eg, Class IA or Class III antiarrhythmics) or in patients with risk factors for torsades de pointes (eg, known QTc prolongation, uncorrected hypokalemia)).
No products indexed under this heading.

Prochlorperazine (Precaution should be taken in elderly patients when using norfloxacin concomitantly with drugs that can result in prolongation of the QTc interval (eg, Class IA or Class III antiarrhythmics) or in patients with risk factors for torsades de pointes (eg, known QTc prolongation, uncorrected hypokalemia)).
No products indexed under this heading.

Promethazine Hydrochloride (Precaution should be taken in elderly patients when using norfloxacin concomitantly with drugs that can result in prolongation of the QTc interval (eg, Class IA or Class III antiarrhythmics) or in patients with risk factors for torsades de pointes (eg, known QTc prolongation, uncorrected hypokalemia)).
No products indexed under this heading.

Propafenone Hydrochloride (Precaution should be taken in elderly patients when using norfloxacin concomitantly with drugs that can result in prolongation of the QTc interval (eg, Class IA or Class III antiarrhythmics) or in patients with risk factors for torsades de pointes (eg, known QTc prolongation, uncorrected hypokalemia)). Products include:

Protriptyline Hydrochloride (Norfloxacin should be used with caution in subjects receiving drugs that affect the QTc interval, such as tricyclic antidepressants).
No products indexed under this heading.

Quetiapine Fumarate (Precaution should be taken in elderly patients when using norfloxacin concomitantly with drugs that can result in prolongation of the QTc interval (eg, Class IA or Class III antiarrhythmics) or in patients with risk factors for torsades de pointes (eg, known QTc prolongation, uncorrected hypokalemia)). Products include:

Quinidine (Risk of developing arrhythmias with norfloxacin may be reduced by avoiding concurrent treatment with class IA antiarrhythmic agents).
No products indexed under this heading.

Quinidine Gluconate (Risk of developing arrhythmias with norfloxacin may be reduced by avoiding concurrent treatment with class IA antiarrhythmic agents).
No products indexed under this heading.

Quinidine Hydrochloride (Risk of developing arrhythmias with norfloxacin may be reduced by avoiding concurrent treatment with class IA antiarrhythmic agents).
No products indexed under this heading.

Quinidine Polygalacturonate (Risk of developing arrhythmias with norfloxacin may be reduced by avoiding concurrent treatment with class IA antiarrhythmic agents).
No products indexed under this heading.

IMPORTANT NOTE: Always consult each drug listing in the patient's regimen for possible interactions.

Quinidine Sulfate (Risk of developing arrhythmias with norfloxacin may be reduced by avoiding concurrent treatment with class IA antiarrhythmic agents).
No products indexed under this heading.

Risperidone (Precaution should be taken in elderly patients when using norfloxacin concomitantly with drugs that can result in prolongation of the QTc interval (eg, Class IA or Class III antiarrhythmics) or in patients with risk factors for torsades de pointes (eg, known QTc prolongation, uncorrected hypokalemia)). Products include:
Risperdal Consta 2682

Rofecoxib (The concomitant administration of a non-steroidal anti-inflammatory drug (NSAID) with a quinolone, including norfloxacin, may increase the risk of CNS stimulation and convulsive seizures. Therefore, norfloxacin should be used with caution in individuals receiving NSAIDs concomitantly).
No products indexed under this heading.

Sotalol Hydrochloride (Risk of developing arrhythmias with norfloxacin may be reduced by avoiding concurrent treatment with class III antiarrhythmic agents).
No products indexed under this heading.

Sucralfate (May interfere with absorption, resulting in lower serum and urine levels of norfloxacin; sucralfate should not be administered concomitantly with, or within 2 hours of, the administration of norfloxacin). Products include:
Carafate Suspension 784
Carafate Tablets 785

Sulindac (The concomitant administration of a non-steroidal anti-inflammatory drug (NSAID) with a quinolone, including norfloxacin, may increase the risk of CNS stimulation and convulsive seizures. Therefore, norfloxacin should be used with caution in individuals receiving NSAIDs concomitantly). Products include:
Clinoril 2098

Theophylline (Co-administration of quinolone with theophylline has resulted in elevated plasma levels of theophylline resulting in theophylline-related side effects).
No products indexed under this heading.

Theophylline Anhydrous (Co-administration of quinolone with theophylline has resulted in elevated plasma levels of theophylline resulting in theophylline-related side effects). Products include:
Uniphyl 2817

Theophylline Calcium Salicylate (Co-administration of quinolone with theophylline has resulted in elevated plasma levels of theophylline resulting in theophylline-related side effects).
No products indexed under this heading.

Theophylline Dihydroxypropyl (Glyceryl) (Co-administration of quinolone with theophylline has resulted in elevated plasma levels of theophylline resulting in theophylline-related side effects).
No products indexed under this heading.

Theophylline Ethylenediamine (Co-administration of quinolone with theophylline has resulted in elevated plasma levels of theophylline resulting in theophylline-related side effects).
No products indexed under this heading.

Theophylline Sodium Glycinate (Co-administration of quinolone with theophylline has resulted in elevated plasma levels of theophylline resulting in theophylline-related side effects).
No products indexed under this heading.

Thioridazine Hydrochloride (Precaution should be taken in elderly patients when using norfloxacin concomitantly with drugs that can result in prolongation of the QTc interval (eg, Class IA or Class III antiarrhythmics) or in patients with risk factors for torsades de pointes (eg, known QTc prolongation, uncorrected hypokalemia)). Products include:
Thioridazine Hydrochloride 2384

Thiothixene (Precaution should be taken in elderly patients when using norfloxacin concomitantly with drugs that can result in prolongation of the QTc interval (eg, Class IA or Class III antiarrhythmics) or in patients with risk factors for torsades de pointes (eg, known QTc prolongation, uncorrected hypokalemia)). Products include:
Thiothixene 2386

Tocainide Hydrochloride (Precaution should be taken in elderly patients when using norfloxacin concomitantly with drugs that can result in prolongation of the QTc interval (eg, Class IA or Class III antiarrhythmics) or in patients with risk factors for torsades de pointes (eg, known QTc prolongation, uncorrected hypokalemia)).
No products indexed under this heading.

Tolmetin Sodium (The concomitant administration of a non-steroidal anti-inflammatory drug (NSAID) with a quinolone, including norfloxacin, may increase the risk of CNS stimulation and convulsive seizures. Therefore, norfloxacin should be used with caution in individuals receiving NSAIDs concomitantly).
No products indexed under this heading.

Tranylcypromine Sulfate (Precaution should be taken in elderly patients when using norfloxacin concomitantly with drugs that can result in prolongation of the QTc interval (eg, Class IA or Class III antiarrhythmics) or in patients with risk factors for torsades de pointes (eg, known QTc prolongation, uncorrected hypokalemia)). Products include:
Parnate 1584

Triamcinolone (The risk of ruptures of the shoulder, hand or Achilles tendons may be increased in patients receiving concomitant corticosteroids, especially in the elderly).
No products indexed under this heading.

Triamcinolone Acetonide (The risk of ruptures of the shoulder, hand or Achilles tendons may be increased in patients receiving concomitant corticosteroids, especially in the elderly). Products include:
Azmacort 408
Nasacort AQ 3019

Triamcinolone Diacetate (The risk of ruptures of the shoulder, hand or Achilles tendons may be increased in patients receiving concomitant corticosteroids, especially in the elderly).
No products indexed under this heading.

Triamcinolone Hexacetonide (The risk of ruptures of the shoulder, hand or Achilles tendons may be increased in patients receiving concomitant corticosteroids, especially in the elderly).
No products indexed under this heading.

Trifluoperazine Hydrochloride (Precaution should be taken in elderly patients when using norfloxacin concomitantly with drugs that can result in prolongation of the QTc interval (eg, Class IA or Class III antiarrhythmics) or in patients with risk factors for torsades de pointes (eg, known QTc prolongation, uncorrected hypokalemia)).
No products indexed under this heading.

Trimipramine Maleate (Norfloxacin should be used with caution in subjects receiving drugs that affect the QTc interval, such as tricyclic antidepressants).
No products indexed under this heading.

Valdecoxib (The concomitant administration of a non-steroidal anti-inflammatory drug (NSAID) with a quinolone, including norfloxacin, may increase the risk of CNS stimulation and convulsive seizures. Therefore, norfloxacin should be used with caution in individuals receiving NSAIDs concomitantly).
No products indexed under this heading.

Warfarin Sodium (Co-administration may enhance the effects of oral anticoagulants).
No products indexed under this heading.

Zinc Sulfate (May interfere with absorption, resulting in lower serum and urine levels of norfloxacin; zinc-containing oral products should not be administered concomitantly with, or within 2 hours of, the administration of norfloxacin). Products include:
Heplive 607
Zinc-220 606

Ziprasidone Hydrochloride (Precaution should be taken in elderly patients when using norfloxacin concomitantly with drugs that can result in prolongation of the QTc interval (eg, Class IA or Class III antiarrhythmics) or in patients with risk factors for torsades de pointes (eg, known QTc prolongation, uncorrected hypokalemia)). Products include:
Geodon 2723

Food Interactions

Dairy products (Avoid simultaneous ingestion; administer norfloxacin at least one hour before or two hours after ingestion of milk and/or other dairy products).

Food, unspecified (Co-administration may decrease the absorption of norfloxacin; administer at least one hour before or two hours after a meal).

NORVIR ORAL SOLUTION

(Ritonavir) 509
See Norvir Soft Gelatin Capsules

NORVIR SOFT GELATIN CAPSULES

(Ritonavir) 509
May interact with antiarrhythmics, anticoagulants, anticonvulsants, antidepressant drugs, antihistamines, antineoplastics, antipsychotic agents, beta-blockers, calcium channel blockers, corticosteroids, cytochrome p450 2d6 substrates (selected), cytochrome p450 3a substrates (selected), dexamethasones, drugs that prolong the PR interval, ergot-containing drugs, HMG-CoA reductase inhibitors, hypnotics and sedatives, immunosuppressive agents, insulin, metronidazoles, narcotic analgesics, oral hypoglycemic agents, PDE5 inhibitors, phenytoin, quinidine, selective serotonin reuptake inhibitors, theophyllines, tricyclic antidepressants, and certain other agents. Compounds in these categories include:

Acarbose (New onset diabetes mellitus, exacerbation of pre-existing diabetes mellitus, and hyperglycemia have been reported during postmarketing surveillance in HIV-infected patients receiving protease inhibitor therapy. Some patients required either initiation or dose adjustments of insulin or oral hypoglycemic agents for treatment of these events).
No products indexed under this heading.

Acebutolol Hydrochloride (Co-administration of ritonavir with certain antiarrhythmics may result in potentially serious and/or life-threatening adverse events due to possible effects of ritonavir on the hepatic metabolism of certain drugs. Co-administration of antiarrhythmics, such as disopyramide, lidocaine, mexilitine, with ritonavir may result in increased plasma concentrations of antiarrhythmics. Caution is warranted and therapeutic concentration monitoring is recommended for antiarrhythmics when co-administered with ritonavir, if available).
No products indexed under this heading.

Acrivastine (Co-administration of ritonavir with certain nonsedating antihistamines may result in potentially serious and/or life-threatening adverse events due to possible effects of ritonavir on the hepatic metabolism of certain drugs).
No products indexed under this heading.

Adenosine (Co-administration of ritonavir with certain antiarrhythmics may result in potentially serious and/or life-threatening adverse events due to possible effects of ritonavir on the hepatic metabolism of certain drugs. Co-administration of antiarrhythmics, such as disopyramide, lidocaine, mexilitine, with ritonavir may result in increased plasma concentrations of antiarrhythmics. Caution is warranted and therapeutic concentration monitoring is recommended for antiarrhythmics when co-administered with ritonavir, if available). Products include:
Adenocard 656
Adenoscan 657

Alclometasone Dipropionate (When co-administering ritonavir with some steroids, it is possible that a substantial increase in the concentrations of some steroids may occur. A dose decrease may be needed for steroids, such as dexamethasone, fluticasone, prednisone, when co-administered with ritonavir).
No products indexed under this heading.

Alfentanil Hydrochloride (When co-administering ritonavir with some narcotic analgesics which are partially mediated by CYP2D6 metabolism, it is possible that substantial increases in concentrations of these narcotic analgesics may occur, possibly requiring a dosage reduction).
No products indexed under this heading.

Alfuzosin Hydrochloride (Co-administration of ritonavir and alfuzosin is contraindicated due to potential for serious reactions such as hypotension). Products include:
Uroxatral 3050

Alprazolam (Co-administration of alprazolam with ritonavir resulted in a decrease in AUC and C_{max} of alprazolam by 12% and 16% respectively).
No products indexed under this heading.

Altretamine (Concentrations of vincristine or vinblastine may be increased when co-administered with ritonavir, resulting in the potential for increased adverse events usually associated with these anticancer agents. Consideration should be given to temporarily withholding the ritonavir containing antiretroviral regimen in patients who develop significant hematologic or gastrointestinal side effects when ritonavir is administered concurrently with vincristine or vinblastine. Clinicians should be aware that if the ritonavir containing regimen is withheld for a prolonged period, consideration should be given to altering the regimen to not include a CYP3A or P-gp inhibitor in order to control HIV-1 viral load). Products include:
Hexalen 1066

Aminophylline (Ritonavir is an inhibitor of cytochrome P450 3A (CYP3A) both *in vitro* and *in vivo*. Ritonavir also inhibits CYP2D6 *in vitro*, but to a lesser extent than CYP3A. Co-administration of ritonavir and drugs primarily metabolized by CYP3A or CYP2D6 may result in increased plasma concentrations of other drugs that could increase or prolong its therapeutic and adverse effects. A dosage reduction of the other drug may be necessary).
No products indexed under this heading.

1227 Interactions Index Norvir

Amiodarone Hydrochloride (Co-administration of ritonavir and amiodarone is contraindicated due to potential for serious and/or life threatening reactions such as cardiac arrhythmias).
No products indexed under this heading.

Amitriptyline Hydrochloride (Co-administration of antidepressants, such as nefazodone, selective serotonin reuptake inhibitors (SSRIs), or tricyclics, with ritonavir may result in increased plasma concentrations of antidepressants. A dose decrease may be needed for these drugs when co-administered with ritonavir).
No products indexed under this heading.

Amlodipine Besylate (Co-administration of calcium channel blockers, such as diltiazem, nifedipine, verapamil, with ritonavir may result in increased plasma concentrations of calcium channel blockers. A dose decrease may be needed for these drugs when co-administered with ritonavir. In addition, ritonavir prolongs the PR interval in some patients. The impact on the PR interval of co-administration of ritonavir with other drugs that prolong the PR interval (including calcium channel blockers) has not been evaluated. Co-administration of ritonavir with these drugs should be undertaken with caution, particularly with those drugs metabolized by CYP3A. Clinical monitoring is recommended). Products include:
Azor 1010
Exforge 2443
Exforge HCT 2449

Amoxapine (Co-administration of antidepressants, such as nefazodone, selective serotonin reuptake inhibitors (SSRIs), or tricyclics, with ritonavir may result in increased plasma concentrations of antidepressants. A dose decrease may be needed for these drugs when co-administered with ritonavir).
No products indexed under this heading.

Amphetamine Aspartate (Ritonavir is an inhibitor of cytochrome P450 3A (CYP3A) both *in vitro* and *in vivo*. Ritonavir also inhibits CYP2D6 *in vitro*, but to a lesser extent than CYP3A. Co-administration of ritonavir and drugs primarily metabolized by CYP3A or CYP2D6 may result in increased plasma concentrations of other drugs that could increase or prolong its therapeutic and adverse effects. A dosage reduction of the other drug may be necessary).
No products indexed under this heading.

Amphetamine Aspartate Monohydrate (Ritonavir is an inhibitor of cytochrome P450 3A (CYP3A) both *in vitro* and *in vivo*. Ritonavir also inhibits CYP2D6 *in vitro*, but to a lesser extent than CYP3A. Co-administration of ritonavir and drugs primarily metabolized by CYP3A or CYP2D6 may result in increased plasma concentrations of other drugs that could increase or prolong its therapeutic and adverse effects. A dosage reduction of the other drug may be necessary).
No products indexed under this heading.

Amphetamine Sulfate (Ritonavir is an inhibitor of cytochrome P450 3A (CYP3A) both *in vitro* and *in vivo*. Ritonavir also inhibits CYP2D6 *in vitro*, but to a lesser extent than CYP3A. Co-administration of ritonavir and drugs primarily metabolized by CYP3A or CYP2D6 may result in increased plasma concentrations of other drugs that could increase or prolong its therapeutic and adverse effects. A dosage reduction of the other drug may be necessary).
No products indexed under this heading.

Anastrozole (Concentrations of vincristine or vinblastine may be increased when co-administered with ritonavir, resulting in the potential for increased adverse events usually associated with these anticancer agents. Consideration should be given to temporarily withholding the ritonavir containing antiretroviral regimen in patients who develop significant hematologic or gastrointestinal side effects when ritonavir is administered concurrently with vincristine or vinblastine. Clinicians should be aware that if the ritonavir containing regimen is withheld for a prolonged period, consideration should be given to altering the regimen to not include a CYP3A or P-gp inhibitor in order to control HIV-1 viral load).
No products indexed under this heading.

Anisindione (When co-administering ritonavir with any agent having a narrow therapeutic margin, such as anticoagulants, special attention is warranted).
No products indexed under this heading.

Apomorphine (When co-administering ritonavir with some narcotic analgesics which are partially mediated by CYP2D6 metabolism, it is possible that substantial increases in concentrations of these narcotic analgesics may occur, possibly requiring a dosage reduction).
No products indexed under this heading.

Apomorphine Hydrochloride (When co-administering ritonavir with some narcotic analgesics which are partially mediated by CYP2D6 metabolism, it is possible that substantial increases in concentrations of these narcotic analgesics may occur, possibly requiring a dosage reduction).
No products indexed under this heading.

Aprepitant (Ritonavir is an inhibitor of cytochrome P450 3A (CYP3A) both *in vitro* and *in vivo*. Ritonavir also inhibits CYP2D6 *in vitro*, but to a lesser extent than CYP3A. Co-administration of ritonavir and drugs primarily metabolized by CYP3A or CYP2D6 may result in increased plasma concentrations of other drugs that could increase or prolong its therapeutic and adverse effects. A dosage reduction of the other drug may be necessary). Products include:
Emend 2124

Ardeparin Sodium (When co-administering ritonavir with any agent having a narrow therapeutic margin, such as anticoagulants, special attention is warranted).
No products indexed under this heading.

Aripiprazole (Co-administration of neuroleptics, such as perphenazine, risperidone, and thioridazine, with ritonavir may result in inceased plasma concentrations of neuroleptics. A dose decrease may be needed for these drugs when co-administered with ritonavir).
No products indexed under this heading.

Asparaginase (Concentrations of vincristine or vinblastine may be increased when co-administered with ritonavir, resulting in the potential for increased adverse events usually associated with these anticancer agents. Consideration should be given to temporarily withholding the ritonavir containing antiretroviral regimen in patients who develop significant hematologic or gastrointestinal side effects when ritonavir is administered concurrently with vincristine or vinblastine. Clinicians should be aware that if the ritonavir containing regimen is withheld for a prolonged period, consideration should be given to altering the regimen to not include a CYP3A or P-gp inhibitor in order to control HIV-1 viral load). Products include:
Elspar 2005, 2122

Astemizole (Co-administration of ritonavir and astemizole is contraindicated due to potential for serious and/or life-threatening reactions such as cardiac arrhythmias).
No products indexed under this heading.

Atazanavir (When co-administered with reduced doses of atazanavir and ritonavir, increased concentrations of atazanavir (increased AUC, increased C_{max}, increased C_{min}) may occur. In addition, ritonavir prolongs the PR interval in some patients. The impact on the PR interval of co-administration of ritonavir with other drugs that prolong the PR interval (including atazanavir) has not been evaluated. As a result, co-administration of ritonavir with these drugs should be undertaken with caution, particularly with those drugs metabolized by CYP3A. Clinical monitoring is recommended).
No products indexed under this heading.

Atazanavir Sulfate (When co-administered with reduced doses of atazanavir and ritonavir, increased concentrations of atazanavir (increased AUC, increased C_{max}, increased C_{min}) may occur. In addition, ritonavir prolongs the PR interval in some patients. The impact on the PR interval of co-administration of ritonavir with other drugs that prolong the PR interval (including atazanavir) has not been evaluated. As a result, co-administration of ritonavir with these drugs should be undertaken with caution, particularly with those drugs metabolized by CYP3A. Clinical monitoring is recommended).
No products indexed under this heading.

Atenolol (Co-administration of beta-blockers, such as metoprolol or timolol, with ritonavir, may result in increased plasma concentrations of the β-blocker. Cardiac and neurologic events have been reported with ritonavir when co-administered with β-blockers. A dose decrease may be needed for these drugs when co-administered with ritonavir. In addition, ritonavir prolongs the PR interval in some patients. The impact on the PR interval of co-administration of ritonavir with other drugs that prolong the PR interval (including β-adrenergic blockers) has not been evaluated. As a result, co-administration of ritonavir with these drugs should be undertaken with caution, particularly with those drugs metabolized by CYP3A. Clinical monitoring is recommended).
No products indexed under this heading.

Atomoxetine Hydrochloride (Ritonavir is an inhibitor of cytochrome P450 3A (CYP3A) both *in vitro* and *in vivo*. Ritonavir also inhibits CYP2D6 *in vitro*, but to a lesser extent than CYP3A. Co-administration of ritonavir and drugs primarily metabolized by CYP3A or CYP2D6 may result in increased plasma concentrations of other drugs that could increase or prolong its therapeutic and adverse effects. A dosage reduction of the other drug may be necessary). Products include:
Strattera 1957

Atorvastatin Calcium (Co-administration of atorvastatin with ritonavir may result in increased plasma concentrations of atorvastatin. Caution should be exercised if ritonavir is used concurrently with atorvastatin. The risk of myopathy including rhabdomyolysis may be increased when ritonavir is used in combination with atorvastatin. Use the lowest possible dose of atorvastatin with careful monitoring in combination with ritonavir or consider other HMG-CoA reductase inhibitors such as pravastatin or fluvastatin in combination with ritonavir). Products include:
Lipitor 2703

Atovaquone (Co-administration of atovaquone with ritonavir may result in decreased plasma concentrations of atovaquone. Clinical significance is unknown; however, increase in atovaquone dose may be needed). Products include:
Malarone Pediatric Tablets 1572
Malarone 1572
Mepron Suspension 1576

Azatadine Maleate (Co-administration of ritonavir with certain nonsedating antihistamines may result in potentially serious and/or life-threatening adverse events due to possible effects of ritonavir on the hepatic metabolism of certain drugs).
No products indexed under this heading.

Azathioprine (Co-administration of immunosuppressants, such as cyclosporine, tacrolimus, sirolimus, rapamycin, with ritonavir may result in increased plasma concentrations of immunosuppressants. Therapeutic concentration monitoring is recommended for immunosuppressant agents when co-administered with ritonavir).
No products indexed under this heading.

Basiliximab (Co-administration of immunosuppressants, such as cyclosporine, tacrolimus, sirolimus, rapamycin, with ritonavir may result in increased plasma concentrations of immunosuppressants. Therapeutic concentration monitoring is recommended for immunosuppressant agents when co-administered with ritonavir). Products include:
Simulect 2524

Beclomethasone Dipropionate (When co-administering ritonavir with some steroids, it is possible that a substantial increase in the concentrations of some steroids may occur. A dose decrease may be needed for steroids, such as dexamethasone, fluticasone, prednisone, when co-administered with ritonavir). Products include:
Qvar 3398

Beclomethasone Dipropionate Monohydrate (When co-administering ritonavir with some steroids, it is possible that a substantial increase in the concentrations of some steroids may occur. A dose decrease may be needed for steroids, such as dexamethasone, fluticasone, prednisone, when co-administered with ritonavir). Products include:
Beconase AQ 1386

Bepridil Hydrochloride (Co-administration of ritonavir and bepridil is contraindicated due to potential for serious and/or life threatening reactions such as cardiac arrhythmias).
No products indexed under this heading.

Betamethasone (When co-administering ritonavir with some steroids, it is possible that a substantial increase in the concentrations of some steroids may occur. A dose decrease may be needed for steroids, such as dexamethasone, fluticasone, prednisone, when co-administered with ritonavir).
No products indexed under this heading.

Betamethasone Acetate (When co-administering ritonavir with some steroids, it is possible that a substantial increase in the concentrations of some steroids may occur. A dose decrease may be needed for steroids, such as dexamethasone, fluticasone, prednisone, when co-administered with ritonavir).
No products indexed under this heading.

IMPORTANT NOTE: Always consult each drug listing in the patient's regimen for possible interactions.

Norvir Interactions Index 1228

Betamethasone Benzoate (When co-administering ritonavir with some steroids, it is possible that a substantial increase in the concentrations of some steroids may occur. A dose decrease may be needed for steroids, such as dexamethasone, fluticasone, prednisone, when co-administered with ritonavir).
No products indexed under this heading.

Betamethasone Dipropionate (When co-administering ritonavir with some steroids, it is possible that a substantial increase in the concentrations of some steroids may occur. A dose decrease may be needed for steroids, such as dexamethasone, fluticasone, prednisone, when co-administered with ritonavir). Products include:
Diprolene Lotion 0.05% 3108
Diprolene Ointment 0.05% 3109
Diprolene AF Cream 0.05% 3107
Lotrisone 3163

Betamethasone Sodium Phosphate (When co-administering ritonavir with some steroids, it is possible that a substantial increase in the concentrations of some steroids may occur. A dose decrease may be needed for steroids, such as dexamethasone, fluticasone, prednisone, when co-administered with ritonavir).
No products indexed under this heading.

Betamethasone Valerate (When co-administering ritonavir with some steroids, it is possible that a substantial increase in the concentrations of some steroids may occur. A dose decrease may be needed for steroids, such as dexamethasone, fluticasone, prednisone, when co-administered with ritonavir). Products include:
Luxíq 3321

Betaxolol Hydrochloride (Co-administration of beta-blockers, such as metoprolol or timolol, with ritonavir, may result in increased plasma concentrations of the β-blocker. Cardiac and neurologic events have been reported with ritonavir when co-administered with β-blockers. A dose decrease may be needed for these drugs when co-administered with ritonavir. In addition, ritonavir prolongs the PR interval in some patients. The impact on the PR interval of co-administration of ritonavir with other drugs that prolong the PR interval (including β-adrenergic blockers) has not been evaluated. As a result, co-administration of ritonavir with these drugs should be undertaken with caution, particularly with those drugs metabolized by CYP3A. Clinical monitoring is recommended).
No products indexed under this heading.

Bicalutamide (Concentrations of vincristine or vinblastine may be increased when co-administered with ritonavir, resulting in the potential for increased adverse events usually associated with these anticancer agents. Consideration should be given to temporarily withholding the ritonavir containing antiretroviral regimen in patients who develop significant hematologic or gastrointestinal side effects when ritonavir is administered concurrently with vincristine or vinblastine. Clinicians should be aware that if the ritonavir containing regimen is withheld for a prolonged period, consideration should be given to altering the regimen to not include a CYP3A or P-gp inhibitor in order to control HIV-1 viral load).
No products indexed under this heading.

Bisoprolol Fumarate (Co-administration of beta-blockers, such as metoprolol or timolol, with ritonavir, may result in increased plasma concentrations of the β-blocker. Cardiac and neurologic events have been reported with ritonavir when co-administered with β-blockers. A dose decrease may be needed for these drugs when co-administered with ritonavir. In addition, ritonavir prolongs the PR interval in some patients. The impact on the PR interval of co-administration of ritonavir with other drugs that prolong the PR interval (including β-adrenergic blockers) has not been evaluated. As a result, co-administration of ritonavir with these drugs should be undertaken with caution, particularly with those drugs metabolized by CYP3A. Clinical monitoring is recommended).
No products indexed under this heading.

Bleomycin Sulfate (Concentrations of vincristine or vinblastine may be increased when co-administered with ritonavir, resulting in the potential for increased adverse events usually associated with these anticancer agents. Consideration should be given to temporarily withholding the ritonavir containing antiretroviral regimen in patients who develop significant hematologic or gastrointestinal side effects when ritonavir is administered concurrently with vincristine or vinblastine. Clinicians should be aware that if the ritonavir containing regimen is withheld for a prolonged period, consideration should be given to altering the regimen to not include a CYP3A or P-gp inhibitor in order to control HIV-1 viral load).
No products indexed under this heading.

Bretylium Tosylate (Co-administration of ritonavir with certain antiarrhythmics may result in potentially serious and/or life-threatening adverse events due to possible effects of ritonavir on the hepatic metabolism of certain drugs. Co-administration of antiarrhythmics, such as disopyramide, lidocaine, mexilitine, with ritonavir may result in increased plasma concentrations of antiarrhythmics. Caution is warranted and therapeutic concentration monitoring is recommended for antiarrhythmics when co-administered with ritonavir, if available).
No products indexed under this heading.

Bromocriptine Mesylate (Ritonavir is an inhibitor of cytochrome P450 3A (CYP3A) both *in vitro* and *in vivo*. Ritonavir also inhibits CYP2D6 *in vitro*, but to a lesser extent than CYP3A. Co-administration of ritonavir and drugs primarily metabolized by CYP3A or CYP2D6 may result in increased plasma concentrations of other drugs that could increase or prolong its therapeutic and adverse effects. A dosage reduction of the other drug may be necessary).
No products indexed under this heading.

Bromodiphenhydramine Hydrochloride (Co-administration of ritonavir with certain nonsedating antihistamines may result in potentially serious and/or life-threatening adverse events due to possible effects of ritonavir on the hepatic metabolism of certain drugs).
No products indexed under this heading.

Brompheniramine Maleate (Co-administration of ritonavir with certain nonsedating antihistamines may result in potentially serious and/or life-threatening adverse events due to possible effects of ritonavir on the hepatic metabolism of certain drugs).
No products indexed under this heading.

Budesonide (When co-administering ritonavir with some steroids, it is possible that a substantial increase in the concentrations of some steroids may occur. A dose decrease may be needed for steroids, such as dexamethasone, fluticasone, prednisone, when co-administered with ritonavir). Products include:
Pulmicort Flexhaler 714
Symbicort 80/4.5 720
Symbicort 160/4.5 720

Buprenorphine Hydrochloride (When co-administering ritonavir with some narcotic analgesics which are partially mediated by CYP2D6 metabolism, it is possible that substantial increases in concentrations of these narcotic analgesics may occur, possibly requiring a dosage reduction).
No products indexed under this heading.

Bupropion (Concurrent administration of bupropion with ritonavir may decrease plasma levels of both bupropion and its active metabolite (hydroxybupropion). Patients receiving ritonavir and bupropion concurrently should be monitored for an adequate clinical response to bupropion).
No products indexed under this heading.

Bupropion Hydrochloride (Concurrent administration of bupropion with ritonavir may decrease plasma levels of both bupropion and its active metabolite (hydroxybupropion). Patients receiving ritonavir and bupropion concurrently should be monitored for an adequate clinical response to bupropion). Products include:
Aplenzin 2948
Wellbutrin 1719
Wellbutrin SR 1725
Zyban 1762

Buspirone Hydrochloride (Co-administration of sedative/hypnotics, such as buspirone, with ritonavir may result in increased plasma concentrations of sedative/hypnotics. A dose decrease may be needed for these drugs when co-administered with ritonavir).
No products indexed under this heading.

Busulfan (Concentrations of vincristine or vinblastine may be increased when co-administered with ritonavir, resulting in the potential for increased adverse events usually associated with these anticancer agents. Consideration should be given to temporarily withholding the ritonavir containing antiretroviral regimen in patients who develop significant hematologic or gastrointestinal side effects when ritonavir is administered concurrently with vincristine or vinblastine. Clinicians should be aware that if the ritonavir containing regimen is withheld for a prolonged period, consideration should be given to altering the regimen to not include a CYP3A or P-gp inhibitor in order to control HIV-1 viral load). Products include:
Myleran 1581

Butabarbital (Co-administration of ritonavir with certain sedative hypnotics may result in potentially serious and/or life-threatening adverse events due to possible effects of ritonavir on the hepatic metabolism of certain drugs. Co-administration of sedative/hypnotics such as buspirone, clorazepate, diazepam, estazolam, flurazepam, or zolpidem with ritonavir may result in increased plasma concentrations of sedative/hypnotics. A dose decrease may be needed for these drugs when co-administered with ritonavir).
No products indexed under this heading.

Butabarbital Sodium (Co-administration of ritonavir with certain sedative hypnotics may result in potentially serious and/or life-threatening adverse events due to possible effects of ritonavir on the hepatic metabolism of certain drugs. Co-administration of sedative/hypnotics such as buspirone, clorazepate, diazepam, estazolam, flurazepam, or zolpidem with ritonavir may result in increased plasma concentrations of sedative/hypnotics. A dose decrease may be needed for these drugs when co-administered with ritonavir).
No products indexed under this heading.

Butalbital (Co-administration of ritonavir with certain sedative hypnotics may result in potentially serious and/or life-threatening adverse events due to possible effects of ritonavir on the hepatic metabolism of certain drugs. Co-administration of sedative/hypnotics such as buspirone, clorazepate, diazepam, estazolam, flurazepam, or zolpidem with ritonavir may result in increased plasma concentrations of sedative/hypnotics. A dose decrease may be needed for these drugs when co-administered with ritonavir).
No products indexed under this heading.

Captopril (Ritonavir is an inhibitor of cytochrome P450 3A (CYP3A) both *in vitro* and *in vivo*. Ritonavir also inhibits CYP2D6 *in vitro*, but to a lesser extent than CYP3A. Co-administration of ritonavir and drugs primarily metabolized by CYP3A or CYP2D6 may result in increased plasma concentrations of other drugs that could increase or prolong its therapeutic and adverse effects. A dosage reduction of the other drug may be necessary). Products include:
Captopril 2341

Carbamazepine (Co-administration of carbamazepine with ritonavir may result in increased plasma concentrations of carbamazepine. Use with caution. A dose decrease may be needed for carbamazepine when co-administered with ritonavir and therapeutic concentration monitoring is recommended, if available). Products include:
Carbatrol 3280
Equetro 3477

Carboplatin (Concentrations of vincristine or vinblastine may be increased when co-administered with ritonavir, resulting in the potential for increased adverse events usually associated with these anticancer agents. Consideration should be given to temporarily withholding the ritonavir containing antiretroviral regimen in patients who develop significant hematologic or gastrointestinal side effects when ritonavir is administered concurrently with vincristine or vinblastine. Clinicians should be aware that if the ritonavir containing regimen is withheld for a prolonged period, consideration should be given to altering the regimen to not include a CYP3A or P-gp inhibitor in order to control HIV-1 viral load).
No products indexed under this heading.

Carmustine (BCNU) (Concentrations of vincristine or vinblastine may be increased when co-administered with ritonavir, resulting in the potential for increased adverse events usually associated with these anticancer agents. Consideration should be given to temporarily withholding the ritonavir containing antiretroviral regimen in patients who develop significant hematologic or gastrointestinal side effects when ritonavir is administered concurrently with vincristine or vinblastine. Clinicians should be aware that if the ritonavir containing regimen is withheld for a prolonged period, consideration should be given to altering the regimen to not include a CYP3A or P-gp inhibitor in order to control HIV-1 viral load).
No products indexed under this heading.

Carteolol Hydrochloride (Co-administration of beta-blockers, such as metoprolol or timolol, with ritonavir, may result in increased plasma concentrations of the β-blocker. Cardiac and neurologic events have been reported with ritonavir when co-administered with β-blockers. A dose decrease may be needed for these drugs when co-administered with ritonavir. In addition, ritonavir prolongs the PR interval in some patients. The impact on the PR interval of co-administration of ritonavir with other drugs that prolong the PR interval (including β-adrenergic block-

ers) has not been evaluated. As a result, co-administration of ritonavir with these drugs should be undertaken with caution, particularly with those drugs metabolized by CYP3A. Clinical monitoring is recommended).
No products indexed under this heading.

Carvedilol (Co-administration of beta-blockers, such as metoprolol or timolol, with ritonavir, may result in increased plasma concentrations of the β-blocker. Cardiac and neurologic events have been reported with ritonavir when co-administered with β-blockers. A dose decrease may be needed for these drugs when co-administered with ritonavir. In addition, ritonavir prolongs the PR interval in some patients. The impact on the PR interval of co-administration of ritonavir with other drugs that prolong the PR interval (including β-adrenergic blockers) has not been evaluated. As a result, co-administration of ritonavir with these drugs should be undertaken with caution, particularly with those drugs metabolized by CYP3A. Clinical monitoring is recommended). Products include:
Coreg 1409

Carvedilol Phosphate (Co-administration of beta-blockers, such as metoprolol or timolol, with ritonavir, may result in increased plasma concentrations of the β-blocker. Cardiac and neurologic events have been reported with ritonavir when co-administered with β-blockers. A dose decrease may be needed for these drugs when co-administered with ritonavir. In addition, ritonavir prolongs the PR interval in some patients. The impact on the PR interval of co-administration of ritonavir with other drugs that prolong the PR interval (including β-adrenergic blockers) has not been evaluated. As a result, co-administration of ritonavir with these drugs should be undertaken with caution, particularly with those drugs metabolized by CYP3A. Clinical monitoring is recommended). Products include:
Coreg CR 1416

Cerivastatin Sodium (Caution should be exercised if HIV protease inhibitors, including ritonavir, are used concurrently with HMG-CoA reductase inhibitors that are also metabolized by the CYP3A4 pathway (eg, atorvastatin or cerivastatin). It is possible that a substantial increase of some HMG-CoA reductase inhibitors may occur. The risk of myopathy including rhabdomyolysis may be increased when HIV protease inhibitors, including ritonavir, are used in combination with HMG-CoA reductase inhibitors).
No products indexed under this heading.

Cetirizine Hydrochloride (Co-administration of ritonavir with certain nonsedating antihistamines may result in potentially serious and/or life-threatening adverse events due to possible effects of ritonavir on the hepatic metabolism of certain drugs). Products include:
Zyrtec Allergy 2052
Children's Zyrtec Allergy Syrup 2053
Children's Zyrtec Allergy 2053
Children's Zyrtec Hives Relief 2053
Zyrtec-D Allergy & Congestion 2054

Cevimeline Hydrochloride (Ritonavir is an inhibitor of cytochrome P450 3A (CYP3A) both *in vitro* and *in vivo*. Ritonavir also inhibits CYP2D6 *in vitro*, but to a lesser extent than CYP3A. Co-administration of ritonavir and drugs primarily metabolized by CYP3A or CYP2D6 may result in increased plasma concentrations of other drugs that could increase or prolong its therapeutic and adverse effects. A dosage reduction of the other drug may be necessary). Products include:
Evoxac 1027

Chloral Hydrate (Co-administration of ritonavir with certain sedative hypnotics may result in potentially serious and/or life-threatening adverse events due to possible effects of ritonavir on the hepatic metabolism of certain drugs. Co-administration of sedative/hypnotics such as buspirone, clorazepate, diazepam, estazolam, flurazepam, or zolpidem with ritonavir may result in increased plasma concentrations of sedative/hypnotics. A dose decrease may be needed for these drugs when co-administered with ritonavir).
No products indexed under this heading.

Chlorambucil (Concentrations of vincristine or vinblastine may be increased when co-administered with ritonavir, resulting in the potential for increased adverse events usually associated with these anticancer agents. Consideration should be given to temporarily withholding the ritonavir containing antiretroviral regimen in patients who develop significant hematologic or gastrointestinal side effects when ritonavir is administered concurrently with vincristine or vinblastine. Clinicians should be aware that if the ritonavir containing regimen is withheld for a prolonged period, consideration should be given to altering the regimen to not include a CYP3A or P-gp inhibitor in order to control HIV-1 viral load). Products include:
Leukeran 1557

Chlorpheniramine (Ritonavir is an inhibitor of cytochrome P450 3A (CYP3A) both *in vitro* and *in vivo*. Ritonavir also inhibits CYP2D6 *in vitro*, but to a lesser extent than CYP3A. Co-administration of ritonavir and drugs primarily metabolized by CYP3A or CYP2D6 may result in increased plasma concentrations of other drugs that could increase or prolong its therapeutic and adverse effects. A dosage reduction of the other drug may be necessary).
No products indexed under this heading.

Chlorpheniramine Maleate (Co-administration of ritonavir with certain nonsedating antihistamines may result in potentially serious and/or life-threatening adverse events due to possible effects of ritonavir on the hepatic metabolism of certain drugs).
No products indexed under this heading.

Chlorpheniramine Polistirex (Co-administration of ritonavir with certain nonsedating antihistamines may result in potentially serious and/or life-threatening adverse events due to possible effects of ritonavir on the hepatic metabolism of certain drugs). Products include:
Tussionex 3443

Chlorpheniramine Tannate (Co-administration of ritonavir with certain nonsedating antihistamines may result in potentially serious and/or life-threatening adverse events due to possible effects of ritonavir on the hepatic metabolism of certain drugs).
No products indexed under this heading.

Chlorpromazine (Co-administration of neuroleptics, such as perphenazine, risperidone, and thioridazine, with ritonavir may result in inceased plasma concentrations of neuroleptics. A dose decrease may be needed for these drugs when co-administered with ritonavir).
No products indexed under this heading.

Chlorpromazine Hydrochloride (Co-administration of neuroleptics, such as perphenazine, risperidone, and thioridazine, with ritonavir may result in inceased plasma concentrations of neuroleptics. A dose decrease may be needed for these drugs when co-administered with ritonavir).
No products indexed under this heading.

Chlorpropamide (New onset diabetes mellitus, exacerbation of pre-existing diabetes mellitus, and hyperglycemia have been reported during postmarketing surveillance in HIV-infected patients receiving protease inhibitor therapy. Some patients required either initiation or dose adjustments of insulin or oral hypoglycemic agents for treatment of these events).
No products indexed under this heading.

Chlorprothixene (Co-administration of neuroleptics, such as perphenazine, risperidone, and thioridazine, with ritonavir may result in inceased plasma concentrations of neuroleptics. A dose decrease may be needed for these drugs when co-administered with ritonavir).
No products indexed under this heading.

Chlorprothixene Hydrochloride (Co-administration of neuroleptics, such as perphenazine, risperidone, and thioridazine, with ritonavir may result in inceased plasma concentrations of neuroleptics. A dose decrease may be needed for these drugs when co-administered with ritonavir).
No products indexed under this heading.

Chlorprothixene Lactate (Co-administration of neuroleptics, such as perphenazine, risperidone, and thioridazine, with ritonavir may result in inceased plasma concentrations of neuroleptics. A dose decrease may be needed for these drugs when co-administered with ritonavir).
No products indexed under this heading.

Ciclesonide (When co-administering ritonavir with some steroids, it is possible that a substantial increase in the concentrations of some steroids may occur. A dose decrease may be needed for steroids, such as dexamethasone, fluticasone, prednisone, when co-administered with ritonavir).
No products indexed under this heading.

Cilostazol (Ritonavir is an inhibitor of cytochrome P450 3A (CYP3A) both *in vitro* and *in vivo*. Ritonavir also inhibits CYP2D6 *in vitro*, but to a lesser extent than CYP3A. Co-administration of ritonavir and drugs primarily metabolized by CYP3A or CYP2D6 may result in increased plasma concentrations of other drugs that could increase or prolong its therapeutic and adverse effects. A dosage reduction of the other drug may be necessary).
No products indexed under this heading.

Cisapride (Co-administration of ritonavir and cisapride is contraindicated due to potential for serious and/or life-threatening reactions such as cardiac arrhythmias).
No products indexed under this heading.

Cisplatin (Concentrations of vincristine or vinblastine may be increased when co-administered with ritonavir, resulting in the potential for increased adverse events usually associated with these anticancer agents. Consideration should be given to temporarily withholding the ritonavir containing antiretroviral regimen in patients who develop significant hematologic or gastrointestinal side effects when ritonavir is administered concurrently with vincristine or vinblastine. Clinicians should be aware that if the ritonavir containing regimen is withheld for a prolonged period, consideration should be given to altering the regimen to not include a CYP3A or P-gp inhibitor in order to control HIV-1 viral load).
No products indexed under this heading.

Citalopram Hydrobromide (Co-administration of antidepressants, such as nefazodone, selective serotonin reuptake inhibitors (SSRIs), tricyclics, with ritonavir may result in increased plasma concentrations of antidepressants. A dose decrease may be needed for these drugs when co-administered with ritonavir). Products include:
Celexa 1153

Clarithromycin (Co-administration of clarithromycin with ritonavir may increase clarithromycin concentrations. Co-administration with clarithromycin led to an increase in AUC, C_{max}, and C_{min} of ritonavir by 12%, 15%, and 14%, respectively. Dosage adjustments should be considered for patients with renal impairment. For patients with CL_{CR} 30 to 60 mL/min, the dose of clarithromycin should be reduced by 50%. For patients with $CL_{CR} < 30$ mL/min, the dose of clarithromycin should be decreased by 75%). Products include:
Biaxin/Biaxin XL 412

Clemastine Fumarate (Co-administration of ritonavir with certain nonsedating antihistamines may result in potentially serious and/or life-threatening adverse events due to possible effects of ritonavir on the hepatic metabolism of certain drugs).
No products indexed under this heading.

Clomipramine Hydrochloride (Co-administration of antidepressants, such as nefazodone, selective serotonin reuptake inhibitors (SSRIs), or tricyclics, with ritonavir may result in increased plasma concentrations of antidepressants. A dose decrease may be needed for these drugs when co-administered with ritonavir).
No products indexed under this heading.

Clonazepam (Co-administration of clonazepam with ritonavir may result in increased plasma concentrations of clonazepam. Use with caution. A dose decrease may be needed for clonazepam when co-administered with ritonavir and therapeutic concentration monitoring is recommended, if available). Products include:
Klonopin 2855

Clorazepate Dipotassium (Co-administration of sedative/hypnotics such as clorazepate with ritonavir may result in increased plasma concentrations of sedative/hypnotics. A dose decrease may be needed for these drugs when co-administered with ritonavir).
No products indexed under this heading.

Clozapine (Co-administration of neuroleptics, such as perphenazine, risperidone, and thioridazine, with ritonavir may result in inceased plasma concentrations of neuroleptics. A dose decrease may be needed for these drugs when co-administered with ritonavir).
No products indexed under this heading.

Codeine Phosphate (When co-administering ritonavir with some narcotic analgesics which are partially mediated by CYP2D6 metabolism, it is possible that substantial increases in concentrations of these narcotic analgesics may occur, possibly requiring a dosage reduction). Products include:
Tylenol with Codeine 2691

Codeine Sulfate (When co-administering ritonavir with some narcotic analgesics which are partially mediated by CYP2D6 metabolism, it is possible that substantial increases in concentrations of these narcotic analgesics may occur, possibly requiring a dosage reduction).
No products indexed under this heading.

Cortisone Acetate (When co-administering ritonavir with some steroids, it is possible that a substantial increase in the concentrations of some steroids may occur. A dose decrease may be needed for steroids, such as dexamethasone, fluticasone, prednisone, when co-administered with ritonavir).
No products indexed under this heading.

Cyclobenzaprine Hydrochloride (Ritonavir is an inhibitor of cytochrome P450 3A (CYP3A) both *in vitro* and *in vivo*. Ritonavir also inhibits CYP2D6 *in vitro*, but to a lesser extent than CYP3A. Co-administration of ritonavir and drugs primarily metabolized by CYP3A or CYP2D6 may result in increased plasma concentrations of other drugs that could increase or prolong its therapeutic and adverse effects. A dosage reduction of the other drug may be necessary). Products include:
Amrix **964**

Cyclophosphamide (Concentrations of vincristine or vinblastine may be increased when co-administered with ritonavir, resulting in the potential for increased adverse events usually associated with these anticancer agents. Consideration should be given to temporarily withholding the ritonavir containing antiretroviral regimen in patients who develop significant hematologic or gastrointestinal side effects when ritonavir is administered concurrently with vincristine or vinblastine. Clinicians should be aware that if the ritonavir containing regimen is withheld for a prolonged period, consideration should be given to altering the regimen to not include a CYP3A or P-gp inhibitor in order to control HIV-1 viral load).
No products indexed under this heading.

Cyclosporine (Co-administration of immunosuppressants, such as cyclosporine, with ritonavir may result in increased plasma concentrations of immunosuppressants. Therapeutic concentration monitoring is recommended for immunosuppressant agents when co-administered with ritonavir). Products include:
Gengraf **440**
Neoral Oral Solution **2496**
Neoral Capsules **2496**
Restasis **605**

Cyproheptadine Hydrochloride (Co-administration of ritonavir with certain nonsedating antihistamines may result in potentially serious and/or life-threatening adverse events due to possible effects of ritonavir on the hepatic metabolism of certain drugs).
No products indexed under this heading.

Dacarbazine (Concentrations of vincristine or vinblastine may be increased when co-administered with ritonavir, resulting in the potential for increased adverse events usually associated with these anticancer agents. Consideration should be given to temporarily withholding the ritonavir containing antiretroviral regimen in patients who develop significant hematologic or gastrointestinal side effects when ritonavir is administered concurrently with vincristine or vinblastine. Clinicians should be aware that if the ritonavir containing regimen is withheld for a prolonged period, consideration should be given to altering the regimen to not include a CYP3A or P-gp inhibitor in order to control HIV-1 viral load).
No products indexed under this heading.

Dalteparin Sodium (When co-administering ritonavir with any agent having a narrow therapeutic margin, such as anticoagulants, special attention is warranted). Products include:
Fragmin **1058**

Danaparoid Sodium (When co-administering ritonavir with any agent having a narrow therapeutic margin, such as anticoagulants, special attention is warranted).
No products indexed under this heading.

Darunavir (Co-administration of darunavir with reduced doses of ritonavir may result in increased plasma concentrations of darunavir (increased AUC, increased C_{max}, increased C_{min})).
No products indexed under this heading.

Daunorubicin Citrate (Concentrations of vincristine or vinblastine may be increased when co-administered with ritonavir, resulting in the potential for increased adverse events usually associated with these anticancer agents. Consideration should be given to temporarily withholding the ritonavir containing antiretroviral regimen in patients who develop significant hematologic or gastrointestinal side effects when ritonavir is administered concurrently with vincristine or vinblastine. Clinicians should be aware that if the ritonavir containing regimen is withheld for a prolonged period, consideration should be given to altering the regimen to not include a CYP3A or P-gp inhibitor in order to control HIV-1 viral load).
No products indexed under this heading.

Daunorubicin Hydrochloride (Concentrations of vincristine or vinblastine may be increased when co-administered with ritonavir, resulting in the potential for increased adverse events usually associated with these anticancer agents. Consideration should be given to temporarily withholding the ritonavir containing antiretroviral regimen in patients who develop significant hematologic or gastrointestinal side effects when ritonavir is administered concurrently with vincristine or vinblastine. Clinicians should be aware that if the ritonavir containing regimen is withheld for a prolonged period, consideration should be given to altering the regimen to not include a CYP3A or P-gp inhibitor in order to control HIV-1 viral load).
No products indexed under this heading.

Debrisoquine (Ritonavir is an inhibitor of cytochrome P450 3A (CYP3A) both *in vitro* and *in vivo*. Ritonavir also inhibits CYP2D6 *in vitro*, but to a lesser extent than CYP3A. Co-administration of ritonavir and drugs primarily metabolized by CYP3A or CYP2D6 may result in increased plasma concentrations of other drugs that could increase or prolong its therapeutic and adverse effects. A dosage reduction of the other drug may be necessary).
No products indexed under this heading.

Delavirdine Mesylate (Co-administration of delavirdine with ritonavir may result in increased plasma concentrations of ritonavir (increased AUC, increased C_{max}, increased C_{min}). Appropriate doses of this combination with respect to safety and efficacy have not been established).
No products indexed under this heading.

Denileukin Diftitox (Concentrations of vincristine or vinblastine may be increased when co-administered with ritonavir, resulting in the potential for increased adverse events usually associated with these anticancer agents. Consideration should be given to temporarily withholding the ritonavir containing antiretroviral regimen in patients who develop significant hematologic or gastrointestinal side effects when ritonavir is administered concurrently with vincristine or vinblastine. Clinicians should be aware that if the ritonavir containing regimen is withheld for a prolonged period, consideration should be given to altering the regimen to not include a CYP3A or P-gp inhibitor in order to control HIV-1 viral load). Products include:
Ontak **1068**

Desipramine Hydrochloride (Co-administration of desipramine with ritonavir may increase desipramine concentrations. Dosage reduction and concentration monitoring of desipramine is recommended).
No products indexed under this heading.

Desogestrel (Ritonavir is an inhibitor of cytochrome P450 3A (CYP3A) both *in vitro* and *in vivo*. Ritonavir also inhibits CYP2D6 *in vitro*, but to a lesser extent than CYP3A. Co-administration of ritonavir and drugs primarily metabolized by CYP3A or CYP2D6 may result in increased plasma concentrations of other drugs that could increase or prolong its therapeutic and adverse effects. A dosage reduction of the other drug may be necessary).
No products indexed under this heading.

Desoximetasone (When co-administering ritonavir with some steroids, it is possible that a substantial increase in the concentrations of some steroids may occur. A dose decrease may be needed for steroids, such as dexamethasone, fluticasone, prednisone, when co-administered with ritonavir).
No products indexed under this heading.

Dexamethasone (When co-administering ritonavir with some steroids, it is possible that a substantial increase in the concentrations of some steroids may occur. A dose decrease may be needed for steroids, such as dexamethasone, when co-administered with ritonavir). Products include:
Ciprodex **583**
Ozurdex .... ⊙**223**
Tobramycin and Dexamethasone Ophthalmic Suspension .... ⊙**251**

Dexamethasone Acetate (When co-administering ritonavir with some steroids, it is possible that a substantial increase in the concentrations of some steroids may occur. A dose decrease may be needed for steroids, such as dexamethasone, when co-administered with ritonavir).
No products indexed under this heading.

Dexamethasone Phosphate (When co-administering ritonavir with some steroids, it is possible that a substantial increase in the concentrations of some steroids may occur. A dose decrease may be needed for steroids, such as dexamethasone, when co-administered with ritonavir).
No products indexed under this heading.

Dexamethasone Sodium (When co-administering ritonavir with some steroids, it is possible that a substantial increase in the concentrations of some steroids may occur. A dose decrease may be needed for steroids, such as dexamethasone, when co-administered with ritonavir).
No products indexed under this heading.

Dexamethasone Sodium Phosphate (When co-administering ritonavir with some steroids, it is possible that a substantial increase in the concentrations of some steroids may occur. A dose decrease may be needed for steroids, such as dexamethasone, when co-administered with ritonavir).
No products indexed under this heading.

Dexamethasone Sodium Phosphate Injection (When co-administering ritonavir with some steroids, it is possible that a substantial increase in the concentrations of some steroids may occur. A dose decrease may be needed for steroids, such as dexamethasone, when co-administered with ritonavir).
No products indexed under this heading.

Dexchlorpheniramine Maleate (Co-administration of ritonavir with certain nonsedating antihistamines may result in potentially serious and/or life-threatening adverse events due to possible effects of ritonavir on the hepatic metabolism of certain drugs).
No products indexed under this heading.

Dexfenfluramine Hydrochloride (Ritonavir is an inhibitor of cytochrome P450 3A (CYP3A) both *in vitro* and *in vivo*. Ritonavir also inhibits CYP2D6 *in vitro*, but to a lesser extent than CYP3A. Co-administration of ritonavir and drugs primarily metabolized by CYP3A or CYP2D6 may result in increased plasma concentrations of other drugs that could increase or prolong its therapeutic and adverse effects. A dosage reduction of the other drug may be necessary).
No products indexed under this heading.

Dextromethorphan Hydrobromide (Ritonavir is an inhibitor of cytochrome P450 3A (CYP3A) both *in vitro* and *in vivo*. Ritonavir also inhibits CYP2D6 *in vitro*, but to a lesser extent than CYP3A. Co-administration of ritonavir and drugs primarily metabolized by CYP3A or CYP2D6 may result in increased plasma concentrations of other drugs that could increase or prolong its therapeutic and adverse effects. A dosage reduction of the other drug may be necessary).
No products indexed under this heading.

Dextromethorphan Polistirex (Ritonavir is an inhibitor of cytochrome P450 3A (CYP3A) both *in vitro* and *in vivo*. Ritonavir also inhibits CYP2D6 *in vitro*, but to a lesser extent than CYP3A. Co-administration of ritonavir and drugs primarily metabolized by CYP3A or CYP2D6 may result in increased plasma concentrations of other drugs that could increase or prolong its therapeutic and adverse effects. A dosage reduction of the other drug may be necessary).
No products indexed under this heading.

Dezocine (When co-administering ritonavir with some narcotic analgesics which are partially mediated by CYP2D6 metabolism, it is possible that substantial increases in concentrations of these narcotic analgesics may occur, possibly requiring a dosage reduction).
No products indexed under this heading.

Diazepam (Co-administration of sedative/hypnotics, such as diazepam, with ritonavir may result in increased plasma concentrations of sedative/hypnotics. A dose decrease may be needed for these drugs when co-administered with ritonavir). Products include:
Valium Tablets **2880**

Dicumarol (When co-administering ritonavir with any agent having a narrow therapeutic margin, such as anticoagulants, special attention is warranted).
No products indexed under this heading.

Didanosine (Co-administration of didanosine with ritonavir resulted in a decrease in AUC and C_{max} of didanosine by 13% and 16% respectively. Dosing of didanosine and ritonavir should be separated by 2.5 hours to avoid formulation incompatibility).
No products indexed under this heading.

Diflorasone Diacetate (When co-administering ritonavir with some steroids, it is possible that a substantial increase in the concentrations of some steroids may occur. A dose decrease may be needed for steroids, such as dexamethasone, fluticasone, prednisone, when co-administered with ritonavir).
No products indexed under this heading.

Digoxin (Concomitant administration of ritonavir with digoxin may increase

1231 Interactions Index Norvir

digoxin levels. Caution should be exercised when co-administering ritonavir with digoxin, with appropriate monitoring of serum digoxin levels. In addition, ritonavir prolongs the PR interval in some patients. The impact on the PR interval of co-administration of ritonavir with other drugs that prolong the PR interval (including digoxin) has not been evaluated. As a result, co-administration of ritonavir with these drugs should be undertaken with caution, particularly with those drugs metabolized by CYP3A. Clinical monitoring is recommended). Products include:
Lanoxin Injection 1546
Lanoxin Injection Pediatric 1549
Lanoxin Tablets 1553

Dihydrocodeine Bitartrate (When co-administering ritonavir with some narcotic analgesics which are partially mediated by CYP2D6 metabolism, it is possible that substantial increases in concentrations of these narcotic analgesics may occur, possibly requiring a dosage reduction).
No products indexed under this heading.

Dihydrocodeinone Bitartrate (When co-administering ritonavir with some narcotic analgesics which are partially mediated by CYP2D6 metabolism, it is possible that substantial increases in concentrations of these narcotic analgesics may occur, possibly requiring a dosage reduction).
No products indexed under this heading.

Dihydroergotamine Mesylate (Co-administration of ritonavir and the ergot derivatives dihydroergotamine, ergonovine, ergotamine, or methylergonovine is contraindicated due to potential for serious and/or life-threatening reactions such as acute ergot toxicity characterized by vasospasm and ischemia of the extremities and other tissues including the central nervous system).
No products indexed under this heading.

Diltiazem Hydrochloride (Co-administration of calcium channel blockers, such as diltiazem with ritonavir may result in increased plasma concentrations of calcium channel blockers. A dose decrease may be needed for these drugs when co-administered with ritonavir. In addition, ritonavir prolongs the PR interval in some patients. The impact on the PR interval of co-administration of ritonavir with other drugs that prolong the PR interval (including calcium channel blockers) has not been evaluated. Co-administration of ritonavir with these drugs should be undertaken with caution, particularly with those drugs metabolized by CYP3A. Clinical monitoring is recommended). Products include:
Cardizem LA 423

Diltiazem Maleate (Co-administration of calcium channel blockers, such as diltiazem with ritonavir may result in increased plasma concentrations of calcium channel blockers. A dose decrease may be needed for these drugs when co-administered with ritonavir. In addition, ritonavir prolongs the PR interval in some patients. The impact on the PR interval of co-administration of ritonavir with other drugs that prolong the PR interval (including calcium channel blockers) has not been evaluated. Co-administration of ritonavir with these drugs should be undertaken with caution, particularly with those drugs metabolized by CYP3A. Clinical monitoring is recommended).
No products indexed under this heading.

Diphenhydramine Hydrochloride (Co-administration of ritonavir with certain nonsedating antihistamines may result in potentially serious and/or life-threatening adverse events due to possible effects of ritonavir on the hepatic metabolism of certain drugs). Products include:
Benadryl Allergy Ultratab 2042
Children's Benadryl Allergy Liquid 2042

Diphenylpyraline Hydrochloride (Co-administration of ritonavir with certain nonsedating antihistamines may result in potentially serious and/or life-threatening adverse events due to possible effects of ritonavir on the hepatic metabolism of certain drugs).
No products indexed under this heading.

Disopyramide (Co-administration of antiarrhythmics, such as disopyramide, with ritonavir may result in increased plasma concentrations of antiarrhythmics. Cardiac and neurologic events have been reported with ritonavir when co-administered with disopyramide. Caution is warranted and therapeutic concentration monitoring is recommended for antiarrhythmics when co-administered with ritonavir, if available).
No products indexed under this heading.

Disopyramide Phosphate (Co-administration of antiarrhythmics, such as disopyramide, with ritonavir may result in increased plasma concentrations of antiarrhythmics. Cardiac and neurologic events have been reported with ritonavir when co-administered with disopyramide. Caution is warranted and therapeutic concentration monitoring is recommended for antiarrhythmics when co-administered with ritonavir, if available).
No products indexed under this heading.

Disulfiram (Ritonavir formulations contain alcohol, which can produce disulfiram-like reactions when co-administered with disulfiram or other drugs that produce this reaction).
No products indexed under this heading.

Divalproex Sodium (Co-administration of divalproex with ritonavir may result in decreased plasma concentrations of divalproex. Use with caution. A dose increase may be needed for divalproex when co-administered with ritonavir and therapeutic concentration monitoring is recommended, if available). Products include:
Depakote ER 426

Docetaxel (Concentrations of vincristine or vinblastine may be increased when co-administered with ritonavir, resulting in the potential for increased adverse events usually associated with these anticancer agents. Consideration should be given to temporarily withholding the ritonavir containing antiretroviral regimen in patients who develop significant hematologic or gastrointestinal side effects when ritonavir is administered concurrently with vincristine or vinblastine. Clinicians should be aware that if the ritonavir containing regimen is withheld for a prolonged period, consideration should be given to altering the regimen to not include a CYP3A or P-gp inhibitor in order to control HIV-1 viral load). Products include:
Taxotere 3035

Dofetilide (Co-administration of ritonavir with certain antiarrhythmics may result in potentially serious and/or life-threatening adverse events due to possible effects of ritonavir on the hepatic metabolism of certain drugs. Co-administration of antiarrhythmics, such as disopyramide, lidocaine, mexiletine, with ritonavir may result in increased plasma concentrations of antiarrhythmics. Caution is warranted and therapeutic concentration monitoring is recommended for antiarrhythmics when co-administered with ritonavir, if available).
No products indexed under this heading.

Dolasetron Mesylate (Ritonavir is an inhibitor of cytochrome P450 3A (CYP3A) both *in vitro* and *in vivo*. Ritonavir also inhibits CYP2D6 *in vitro*, but to a lesser extent than CYP3A. Co-administration of ritonavir and drugs primarily metabolized by CYP3A or CYP2D6 may result in increased plasma concentrations of other drugs that could increase or prolong its therapeutic and adverse effects. A dosage reduction of the other drug may be necessary). Products include:
Anzemet Injection 2931
Anzemet Tablets 2934

Donepezil Hydrochloride (Ritonavir is an inhibitor of cytochrome P450 3A (CYP3A) both *in vitro* and *in vivo*. Ritonavir also inhibits CYP2D6 *in vitro*, but to a lesser extent than CYP3A. Co-administration of ritonavir and drugs primarily metabolized by CYP3A or CYP2D6 may result in increased plasma concentrations of other drugs that could increase or prolong its therapeutic and adverse effects. A dosage reduction of the other drug may be necessary). Products include:
Aricept 1045
Aricept ODT 1045

Doxepin Hydrochloride (Co-administration of antidepressants, such as nefazodone, selective serotonin reuptake inhibitors (SSRIs), or tricyclics, with ritonavir may result in increased plasma concentrations of antidepressants. A dose decrease may be needed for these drugs when co-administered with ritonavir).
No products indexed under this heading.

Doxorubicin Hydrochloride (Concentrations of vincristine or vinblastine may be increased when co-administered with ritonavir, resulting in the potential for increased adverse events usually associated with these anticancer agents. Consideration should be given to temporarily withholding the ritonavir containing antiretroviral regimen in patients who develop significant hematologic or gastrointestinal side effects when ritonavir is administered concurrently with vincristine or vinblastine. Clinicians should be aware that if the ritonavir containing regimen is withheld for a prolonged period, consideration should be given to altering the regimen to not include a CYP3A or P-gp inhibitor in order to control HIV-1 viral load).
No products indexed under this heading.

Dronabinol (Co-administration of dronabinol with ritonavir may result in increased plasma concentrations of dronabinol. A dose decrease of dronabinol may be needed when co-administered with ritonavir).
No products indexed under this heading.

Dyphylline (Ritonavir is an inhibitor of cytochrome P450 3A (CYP3A) both *in vitro* and *in vivo*. Ritonavir also inhibits CYP2D6 *in vitro*, but to a lesser extent than CYP3A. Co-administration of ritonavir and drugs primarily metabolized by CYP3A or CYP2D6 may result in increased plasma concentrations of other drugs that could increase or prolong its therapeutic and adverse effects. A dosage reduction of the other drug may be necessary).
No products indexed under this heading.

Encainide Hydrochloride (Ritonavir is an inhibitor of cytochrome P450 3A (CYP3A) both *in vitro* and *in vivo*. Ritonavir also inhibits CYP2D6 *in vitro*, but to a lesser extent than CYP3A. Co-administration of ritonavir and drugs primarily metabolized by CYP3A or CYP2D6 may result in increased plasma concentrations of other drugs that could increase or prolong its therapeutic and adverse effects. A dosage reduction of the other drug may be necessary).
No products indexed under this heading.

Enoxaparin Sodium (When co-administering ritonavir with any agent having a narrow therapeutic margin, such as anticoagulants, special attention is warranted). Products include:
Lovenox 3005

Epirubicin Hydrochloride (Concentrations of vincristine or vinblastine may be increased when co-administered with ritonavir, resulting in the potential for increased adverse events usually associated with these anticancer agents. Consideration should be given to temporarily withholding the ritonavir containing antiretroviral regimen in patients who develop significant hematologic or gastrointestinal side effects when ritonavir is administered concurrently with vincristine or vinblastine. Clinicians should be aware that if the ritonavir containing regimen is withheld for a prolonged period, consideration should be given to altering the regimen to not include a CYP3A or P-gp inhibitor in order to control HIV-1 viral load).
No products indexed under this heading.

Ergonovine Maleate (Co-administration of ritonavir and the ergot derivatives dihydroergotamine, ergonovine, ergotamine, or methylergonovine is contraindicated due to potential for serious and/or life-threatening reactions such as acute ergot toxicity characterized by vasospasm and ischemia of the extremities and other tissues including the central nervous system).
No products indexed under this heading.

Ergotamine Tartrate (Co-administration of ritonavir and the ergot derivatives dihydroergotamine, ergonovine, ergotamine, or methylergonovine is contraindicated due to potential for serious and/or life-threatening reactions such as acute ergot toxicity characterized by vasospasm and ischemia of the extremities and other tissues including the central nervous system).
No products indexed under this heading.

Erythromycin (Ritonavir is an inhibitor of cytochrome P450 3A (CYP3A) both *in vitro* and *in vivo*. Ritonavir also inhibits CYP2D6 *in vitro*, but to a lesser extent than CYP3A. Co-administration of ritonavir and drugs primarily metabolized by CYP3A or CYP2D6 may result in increased plasma concentrations of other drugs that could increase or prolong its therapeutic and adverse effects. A dosage reduction of the other drug may be necessary).
No products indexed under this heading.

Erythromycin Estolate (Ritonavir is an inhibitor of cytochrome P450 3A (CYP3A) both *in vitro* and *in vivo*. Ritonavir also inhibits CYP2D6 *in vitro*, but to a lesser extent than CYP3A. Co-administration of ritonavir and drugs primarily metabolized by CYP3A or CYP2D6 may result in increased plasma concentrations of other drugs that could increase or prolong its therapeutic and adverse effects. A dosage reduction of the other drug may be necessary).
No products indexed under this heading.

Erythromycin Ethylsuccinate (Ritonavir is an inhibitor of cytochrome P450 3A (CYP3A) both *in vitro* and *in vivo*. Ritonavir also inhibits CYP2D6 *in vitro*, but to a lesser extent than CYP3A. Co-administration of ritonavir and drugs primarily metabolized by CYP3A or CYP2D6 may result in increased plasma concentrations of other drugs that could increase or prolong its therapeutic and adverse effects. A dosage reduction of the other drug may be necessary). Products include:

IMPORTANT NOTE: Always consult each drug listing in the patient's regimen for possible interactions.

Erythromycin Gluceptate (Ritonavir is an inhibitor of cytochrome P450 3A (CYP3A) both *in vitro* and *in vivo*. Ritonavir also inhibits CYP2D6 *in vitro*, but to a lesser extent than CYP3A. Co-administration of ritonavir and drugs primarily metabolized by CYP3A or CYP2D6 may result in increased plasma concentrations of other drugs that could increase or prolong its therapeutic and adverse effects. A dosage reduction of the other drug may be necessary).
No products indexed under this heading.

Erythromycin Lactobionate (Ritonavir is an inhibitor of cytochrome P450 3A (CYP3A) both *in vitro* and *in vivo*. Ritonavir also inhibits CYP2D6 *in vitro*, but to a lesser extent than CYP3A. Co-administration of ritonavir and drugs primarily metabolized by CYP3A or CYP2D6 may result in increased plasma concentrations of other drugs that could increase or prolong its therapeutic and adverse effects. A dosage reduction of the other drug may be necessary).
No products indexed under this heading.

Erythromycin Stearate (Ritonavir is an inhibitor of cytochrome P450 3A (CYP3A) both *in vitro* and *in vivo*. Ritonavir also inhibits CYP2D6 *in vitro*, but to a lesser extent than CYP3A. Co-administration of ritonavir and drugs primarily metabolized by CYP3A or CYP2D6 may result in increased plasma concentrations of other drugs that could increase or prolong its therapeutic and adverse effects. A dosage reduction of the other drug may be necessary).
No products indexed under this heading.

Escitalopram Oxalate (Co-administration of antidepressants, such as nefazodone, selective serotonin reuptake inhibitors (SSRIs), tricyclics, with ritonavir may result in increased plasma concentrations of antidepressants. A dose decrease may be needed for these drugs when co-administered with ritonavir). Products include:

Esmolol Hydrochloride (Co-administration of beta-blockers, such as metoprolol or timolol, with ritonavir, may result in increased plasma concentrations of the β-blocker. Cardiac and neurologic events have been reported with ritonavir when co-administered with β-blockers. A dose decrease may be needed for these drugs when co-administered with ritonavir. In addition, ritonavir prolongs the PR interval in some patients. The impact on the PR interval of co-administration of ritonavir with other drugs that prolong the PR interval (including β-adrenergic blockers) has not been evaluated. As a result, co-administration of ritonavir with these drugs should be undertaken with caution, particularly with those drugs metabolized by CYP3A. Clinical monitoring is recommended).
No products indexed under this heading.

Estazolam (Co-administration of sedative/hypnotics, such as estazolam, with ritonavir may result in increased plasma concentrations of sedative/hypnotics. A dose decrease may be needed for these drugs when co-administered with ritonavir).
No products indexed under this heading.

Estramustine Phosphate Sodium (Concentrations of vincristine or vinblastine may be increased when co-administered with ritonavir, resulting in the potential for increased adverse events usually associated with these anticancer agents. Consideration should be given to temporarily withhold-

ing the ritonavir containing antiretroviral regimen in patients who develop significant hematologic or gastrointestinal side effects when ritonavir is administered concurrently with vincristine or vinblastine. Clinicians should be aware that if the ritonavir containing regimen is withheld for a prolonged period, consideration should be given to altering the regimen to not include a CYP3A or P-gp inhibitor in order to control HIV-1 viral load).
No products indexed under this heading.

Estrogen (Ritonavir is an inhibitor of cytochrome P450 3A (CYP3A) both *in vitro* and *in vivo*. Ritonavir also inhibits CYP2D6 *in vitro*, but to a lesser extent than CYP3A. Co-administration of ritonavir and drugs primarily metabolized by CYP3A or CYP2D6 may result in increased plasma concentrations of other drugs that could increase or prolong its therapeutic and adverse effects. A dosage reduction of the other drug may be necessary).
No products indexed under this heading.

Estrogens, Conjugated (Ritonavir is an inhibitor of cytochrome P450 3A (CYP3A) both *in vitro* and *in vivo*. Ritonavir also inhibits CYP2D6 *in vitro*, but to a lesser extent than CYP3A. Co-administration of ritonavir and drugs primarily metabolized by CYP3A or CYP2D6 may result in increased plasma concentrations of other drugs that could increase or prolong its therapeutic and adverse effects. A dosage reduction of the other drug may be necessary). Products include:

Estrogens, Conjugated, Synthetic A (Ritonavir is an inhibitor of cytochrome P450 3A (CYP3A) both *in vitro* and *in vivo*. Ritonavir also inhibits CYP2D6 *in vitro*, but to a lesser extent than CYP3A. Co-administration of ritonavir and drugs primarily metabolized by CYP3A or CYP2D6 may result in increased plasma concentrations of other drugs that could increase or prolong its therapeutic and adverse effects. A dosage reduction of the other drug may be necessary).
No products indexed under this heading.

Estrogens, Esterified (Ritonavir is an inhibitor of cytochrome P450 3A (CYP3A) both *in vitro* and *in vivo*. Ritonavir also inhibits CYP2D6 *in vitro*, but to a lesser extent than CYP3A. Co-administration of ritonavir and drugs primarily metabolized by CYP3A or CYP2D6 may result in increased plasma concentrations of other drugs that could increase or prolong its therapeutic and adverse effects. A dosage reduction of the other drug may be necessary).
No products indexed under this heading.

Ethchlorvynol (Co-administration of ritonavir with certain sedative hypnotics may result in potentially serious and/or life-threatening adverse events due to possible effects of ritonavir on the hepatic metabolism of certain drugs. Co-administration of sedative/hypnotics such as buspirone, clorazepate, diazepam, estazolam, flurazepam, or zolpidem with ritonavir may result in increased plasma concentrations of sedative/hypnotics. A dose decrease may be needed for these drugs when co-administered with ritonavir).
No products indexed under this heading.

Ethinamate (Co-administration of ritonavir with certain sedative hypnotics may result in potentially serious and/or life-threatening adverse events due to possible effects of ritonavir on the hepatic metabolism of certain drugs.

Co-administration of sedative/hypnotics such as buspirone, clorazepate, diazepam, estazolam, flurazepam, or zolpidem with ritonavir may result in increased plasma concentrations of sedative/hypnotics. A dose decrease may be needed for these drugs when co-administered with ritonavir).
No products indexed under this heading.

Ethinyl Estradiol (A pharmacokinetic study demonstrated that the concomitant administration of ritonavir 500 mg q 12h and a fixed-combination oral contraceptive resulted in reductions of the ethinyl estradiol mean C_{max} and mean AUC by 32% and 40%, respectively. Alternate methods of contraception should be considered). Products include:

Ethosuximide (Co-administration of ethosuximide with ritonavir may result in increased plasma concentrations of ethosuximide. Use with caution. A dose decrease may be needed for ethosuximide when co-administered with ritonavir and therapeutic concentration monitoring is recommended, if available).
No products indexed under this heading.

Ethotoin (When co-administering ritonavir with any agent having a narrow therapeutic margin, such as anticonvulsants, special attention is warranted).
No products indexed under this heading.

Ethynodiol Diacetate (Ritonavir is an inhibitor of cytochrome P450 3A (CYP3A) both *in vitro* and *in vivo*. Ritonavir also inhibits CYP2D6 *in vitro*, but to a lesser extent than CYP3A. Co-administration of ritonavir and drugs primarily metabolized by CYP3A or CYP2D6 may result in increased plasma concentrations of other drugs that could increase or prolong its therapeutic and adverse effects. A dosage reduction of the other drug may be necessary).
No products indexed under this heading.

Etoposide (Concentrations of vincristine or vinblastine may be increased when co-administered with ritonavir, resulting in the potential for increased adverse events usually associated with these anticancer agents. Consideration should be given to temporarily withholding the ritonavir containing antiretroviral regimen in patients who develop significant hematologic or gastrointestinal side effects when ritonavir is administered concurrently with vincristine or vinblastine. Clinicians should be aware that if the ritonavir containing regimen is withheld for a prolonged period, consideration should be given to altering the regimen to not include a CYP3A or P-gp inhibitor in order to control HIV-1 viral load).
No products indexed under this heading.

Etoposide Phosphate (Ritonavir is an inhibitor of cytochrome P450 3A (CYP3A) both *in vitro* and *in vivo*. Ritonavir also inhibits CYP2D6 *in vitro*, but to a lesser extent than CYP3A. Co-administration of ritonavir and drugs primarily metabolized by CYP3A or CYP2D6 may result in increased plasma concentrations of other drugs that could increase or prolong its therapeutic and adverse effects. A dosage reduction of the other drug may be necessary).
No products indexed under this heading.

Exemestane (Concentrations of vincristine or vinblastine may be increased

when co-administered with ritonavir, resulting in the potential for increased adverse events usually associated with these anticancer agents. Consideration should be given to temporarily withholding the ritonavir containing antiretroviral regimen in patients who develop significant hematologic or gastrointestinal side effects when ritonavir is administered concurrently with vincristine or vinblastine. Clinicians should be aware that if the ritonavir containing regimen is withheld for a prolonged period, consideration should be given to altering the regimen to not include a CYP3A or P-gp inhibitor in order to control HIV-1 viral load). Products include:

Felbamate (When co-administering ritonavir with any agent having a narrow therapeutic margin, such as anticonvulsants, special attention is warranted).
No products indexed under this heading.

Felodipine (Co-administration of calcium channel blockers, such as diltiazem, nifedipine, verapamil, with ritonavir may result in increased plasma concentrations of calcium channel blockers. A dose decrease may be needed for these drugs when co-administered with ritonavir. In addition, ritonavir prolongs the PR interval in some patients. The impact on the PR interval of co-administration of ritonavir with other drugs that prolong the PR interval (including calcium channel blockers) has not been evaluated. Co-administration of ritonavir with these drugs should be undertaken with caution, particularly with those drugs metabolized by CYP3A. Clinical monitoring is recommended).
No products indexed under this heading.

Fentanyl (When co-administering ritonavir with some narcotic analgesics which are partially mediated by CYP2D6 metabolism, it is possible that substantial increases in concentrations of these narcotic analgesics may occur, possibly requiring a dosage reduction). Products include:

Fentanyl Citrate (When co-administering ritonavir with some narcotic analgesics which are partially mediated by CYP2D6 metabolism, it is possible that substantial increases in concentrations of these narcotic analgesics may occur, possibly requiring a dosage reduction). Products include:

Fexofenadine Hydrochloride (Co-administration of ritonavir with certain nonsedating antihistamines may result in potentially serious and/or life-threatening adverse events due to possible effects of ritonavir on the hepatic metabolism of certain drugs). Products include:

Flecainide Acetate (Co-administration of ritonavir and flecainide is contraindicated due to potential for serious and/or life threatening reactions such as cardiac arrhythmias).
No products indexed under this heading.

Floxuridine (Concentrations of vincristine or vinblastine may be increased when co-administered with ritonavir, resulting in the potential for increased adverse events usually associated with these anticancer agents. Consideration should be given to temporarily withholding the ritonavir containing antiretroviral regimen in patients who develop significant hematologic or gastrointestinal side effects when ritonavir is adminis-

tered concurrently with vincristine or vinblastine. Clinicians should be aware that if the ritonavir containing regimen is withheld for a prolonged period, consideration should be given to altering the regimen to not include a CYP3A or P-gp inhibitor in order to control HIV-1 viral load).
No products indexed under this heading.

Fluconazole (Co-administration of fluconazole with ritonavir resulted in an increase in AUC, C_{max}, and C_{min} of ritonavir by 12%, 15%, and 14%, respectively).
No products indexed under this heading.

Fludrocortisone Acetate (When co-administering ritonavir with some steroids, it is possible that a substantial increase in the concentrations of some steroids may occur. A dose decrease may be needed for steroids, such as dexamethasone, fluticasone, prednisone, when co-administered with ritonavir).
No products indexed under this heading.

Flumethasone Pivalate (When co-administering ritonavir with some steroids, it is possible that a substantial increase in the concentrations of some steroids may occur. A dose decrease may be needed for steroids, such as dexamethasone, fluticasone, prednisone, when co-administered with ritonavir).
No products indexed under this heading.

Flunisolide Hemihydrate (When co-administering ritonavir with some steroids, it is possible that a substantial increase in the concentrations of some steroids may occur. A dose decrease may be needed for steroids, such as dexamethasone, fluticasone, prednisone, when co-administered with ritonavir).
No products indexed under this heading.

Fluorouracil (Concentrations of vincristine or vinblastine may be increased when co-administered with ritonavir, resulting in the potential for increased adverse events usually associated with these anticancer agents. Consideration should be given to temporarily withholding the ritonavir containing antiretroviral regimen in patients who develop significant hematologic or gastrointestinal side effects when ritonavir is administered concurrently with vincristine or vinblastine. Clinicians should be aware that if the ritonavir containing regimen is withheld for a prolonged period, consideration should be given to altering the regimen to not include a CYP3A or P-gp inhibitor in order to control HIV-1 viral load). Products include:
Carac **2966**

Fluoxetine (Co-administration of fluoexetine with ritonavir resulted in an increase in AUC of ritonavir by 19%. Cardiac and neurologic events have been reported with ritonavir when co-administered with fluoxetine. A dose decrease of selective serotonin reuptake inhibitors (SSRIs) may be needed when co-administered with ritonavir).
No products indexed under this heading.

Fluoxetine Hydrochloride (Co-administration of fluoexetine with ritonavir resulted in an increase in AUC of ritonavir by 19%. Cardiac and neurologic events have been reported with ritonavir when co-administered with fluoxetine. A dose decrease of selective serotonin reuptake inhibitors (SSRIs) may be needed when co-administered with ritonavir). Products include:
Prozac Weekly **1941**
Prozac Pulvules **1941**
Symbyax **1965**

Fluphenazine Decanoate (Co-administration of neuroleptics, such as perphenazine, risperidone, and thioridazine, with ritonavir may result in inceased plasma concentrations of neuroleptics. A dose decrease may be needed for these drugs when co-administered with ritonavir).
No products indexed under this heading.

Fluphenazine Enanthate (Co-administration of neuroleptics, such as perphenazine, risperidone, and thioridazine, with ritonavir may result in inceased plasma concentrations of neuroleptics. A dose decrease may be needed for these drugs when co-administered with ritonavir).
No products indexed under this heading.

Fluphenazine Hydrochloride (Co-administration of neuroleptics, such as perphenazine, risperidone, and thioridazine, with ritonavir may result in inceased plasma concentrations of neuroleptics. A dose decrease may be needed for these drugs when co-administered with ritonavir).
No products indexed under this heading.

Flurazepam Hydrochloride (Co-administration of sedative/hypnotics, such as flurazepam, with ritonavir may result in increased plasma concentrations of sedative/hypnotics. A dose decrease may be needed for these drugs when co-administered with ritonavir).
No products indexed under this heading.

Flutamide (Concentrations of vincristine or vinblastine may be increased when co-administered with ritonavir, resulting in the potential for increased adverse events usually associated with these anticancer agents. Consideration should be given to temporarily withholding the ritonavir containing antiretroviral regimen in patients who develop significant hematologic or gastrointestinal side effects when ritonavir is administered concurrently with vincristine or vinblastine. Clinicians should be aware that if the ritonavir containing regimen is withheld for a prolonged period, consideration should be given to altering the regimen to not include a CYP3A or P-gp inhibitor in order to control HIV-1 viral load).
No products indexed under this heading.

Fluticasone Furoate (When co-administering ritonavir with some steroids, it is possible that a substantial increase in the concentrations of some steroids may occur. A dose decrease may be needed for steroids, such as fluticasone, when co-administered with ritonavir). Products include:
Veramyst **1713**

Fluticasone Propionate (A drug interaction study in healthy subjects has shown that ritonavir significantly increases plasma fluticasone propionate exposures, resulting in significantly decreased serum cortisol concentrations. Systemic corticosteroid effects, including Cushing's syndrome and adrenal suppression have been reported during postmarketing use in patients receiving ritonavir and inhaled or intranasally administered fluticasone propionate. Therefore, co-administration of fluticasone propionate and ritonavir is not recommended unless the potential benefit to the patient outweighs the risk of systemic corticosteroid side effects). Products include:
Advair 100/50 .... **1275**
Advair 250/50 .... **1275**
Advair 500/50 .... **1275**
Advair HFA 45/21 .... **1288**
Advair HFA 115/21 .... **1288**
Advair HFA 230/21 .... **1288**
Flonase **1459**
Flovent Diskus **1463**
Flovent HFA **1470**

Fluvastatin Sodium (Caution should be exercised if HIV protease inhibitors, including ritonavir, are used concurrently with HMG-CoA reductase inhibitors that are also metabolized by the CYP3A4 pathway (eg, atorvastatin or cerivastatin). It is possible that a substantial increase of some HMG-CoA reductase inhibitors may occur. The risk of myopathy including rhabdomyolysis may be increased when HIV protease inhibitors, including ritonavir, are used in combination with HMG-CoA reductase inhibitors).
No products indexed under this heading.

Fluvoxamine (Co-administration of antidepressants, such as nefazodone, selective serotonin reuptake inhibitors (SSRIs), tricyclics, with ritonavir may result in increased plasma concentrations of antidepressants. A dose decrease may be needed for these drugs when co-administered with ritonavir).
No products indexed under this heading.

Fluvoxamine Maleate (Co-administration of antidepressants, such as nefazodone, selective serotonin reuptake inhibitors (SSRIs), tricyclics, with ritonavir may result in increased plasma concentrations of antidepressants. A dose decrease may be needed for these drugs when co-administered with ritonavir).
No products indexed under this heading.

Fondaparinux Sodium (When co-administering ritonavir with any agent having a narrow therapeutic margin, such as anticoagulants, special attention is warranted). Products include:
Arixtra **1320**

Formoterol Fumarate (Ritonavir is an inhibitor of cytochrome P450 3A (CYP3A) both *in vitro* and *in vivo*. Ritonavir also inhibits CYP2D6 *in vitro*, but to a lesser extent than CYP3A. Co-administration of ritonavir and drugs primarily metabolized by CYP3A or CYP2D6 may result in increased plasma concentrations of other drugs that could increase or prolong its therapeutic and adverse effects. A dosage reduction of the other drug may be necessary). Products include:
Foradil **3121**
Perforomist **3634**

Fosamprenavir Calcium (Co-administration of fosamprenavir with reduced doses of ritonavir may result in increased plasma concentrations of amprenavir (increased AUC, increased C_{max}, increased C_{min})). Products include:
Lexiva Oral Suspension **1558**
Lexiva **1558**

Fosphenytoin (Co-administration of phenytoin with ritonavir may result in decreased plasma concentrations of phenytoin. Use with caution. A dose increase may be needed for phenytoin when co-administered with ritonavir and therapeutic concentration monitoring is recommended, if available).
No products indexed under this heading.

Fosphenytoin Sodium (Co-administration of phenytoin with ritonavir may result in decreased plasma concentrations of phenytoin. Use with caution. A dose increase may be needed for phenytoin when co-administered with ritonavir and therapeutic concentration monitoring is recommended, if available).
No products indexed under this heading.

Gabapentin (When co-administering ritonavir with any agent having a narrow therapeutic margin, such as anticonvulsants, special attention is warranted).
No products indexed under this heading.

Galantamine Hydrobromide (Ritonavir is an inhibitor of cytochrome P450 3A (CYP3A) both *in vitro* and *in vivo*. Ritonavir also inhibits CYP2D6 *in vitro*, but to a lesser extent than CYP3A. Co-administration of ritonavir and drugs primarily metabolized by CYP3A or CYP2D6 may result in increased plasma concentrations of other drugs that could increase or prolong its therapeutic and adverse effects. A dosage reduction of the other drug may be necessary).
No products indexed under this heading.

Gemcitabine Hydrochloride (Concentrations of vincristine or vinblastine may be increased when co-administered with ritonavir, resulting in the potential for increased adverse events usually associated with these anticancer agents. Consideration should be given to temporarily withholding the ritonavir containing antiretroviral regimen in patients who develop significant hematologic or gastrointestinal side effects when ritonavir is administered concurrently with vincristine or vinblastine. Clinicians should be aware that if the ritonavir containing regimen is withheld for a prolonged period, consideration should be given to altering the regimen to not include a CYP3A or P-gp inhibitor in order to control HIV-1 viral load). Products include:
Gemzar **1900**

Glibenclamide (New onset diabetes mellitus, exacerbation of pre-existing diabetes mellitus, and hyperglycemia have been reported during postmarketing surveillance in HIV-infected patients receiving protease inhibitor therapy. Some patients required either initiation or dose adjustments of insulin or oral hypoglycemic agents for treatment of these events).
No products indexed under this heading.

Glimepiride (New onset diabetes mellitus, exacerbation of pre-existing diabetes mellitus, and hyperglycemia have been reported during postmarketing surveillance in HIV-infected patients receiving protease inhibitor therapy. Some patients required either initiation or dose adjustments of insulin or oral hypoglycemic agents for treatment of these events). Products include:
Avandaryl **1356**
Duetact **3354**

Glipizide (New onset diabetes mellitus, exacerbation of pre-existing diabetes mellitus, and hyperglycemia have been reported during postmarketing surveillance in HIV-infected patients receiving protease inhibitor therapy. Some patients required either initiation or dose adjustments of insulin or oral hypoglycemic agents for treatment of these events).
No products indexed under this heading.

Glutethimide (Co-administration of ritonavir with certain sedative hypnotics may result in potentially serious and/or life-threatening adverse events due to possible effects of ritonavir on the hepatic metabolism of certain drugs. Co-administration of sedative/hypnotics such as buspirone, clorazepate, diazepam, estazolam, flurazepam, or zolpidem with ritonavir may result in increased plasma concentrations of sedative/hypnotics. A dose decrease may be needed for these drugs when co-administered with ritonavir).
No products indexed under this heading.

Glyburide (New onset diabetes mellitus, exacerbation of pre-existing diabetes mellitus, and hyperglycemia have been reported during postmarketing surveillance in HIV-infected patients receiving protease inhibitor therapy. Some patients required either initiation or dose adjustments of insulin or oral hypoglycemic agents for treatment of these events).
No products indexed under this heading.

Haloperidol (Co-administration of neuroleptics, such as perphenazine, risperidone, and thioridazine, with ritonavir may result in inceased plasma concentrations of neuroleptics. A dose decrease may be needed for these drugs when co-administered with ritonavir).
No products indexed under this heading.

Haloperidol Decanoate (Co-administration of neuroleptics, such as perphenazine, risperidone, and thioridazine, with ritonavir may result in inceased plasma concentrations of neuroleptics. A dose decrease may be needed for these drugs when co-administered with ritonavir).
No products indexed under this heading.

Haloperidol Lactate (Co-administration of neuroleptics, such as perphenazine, risperidone, and thioridazine, with ritonavir may result in inceased plasma concentrations of neuroleptics. A dose decrease may be needed for these drugs when co-administered with ritonavir).
No products indexed under this heading.

Heparin Calcium (When co-administering ritonavir with any agent having a narrow therapeutic margin, such as anticoagulants, special attention is warranted).
No products indexed under this heading.

Heparin Sodium (When co-administering ritonavir with any agent having a narrow therapeutic margin, such as anticoagulants, special attention is warranted).
No products indexed under this heading.

Hydrocodone Bitartrate (When co-administering ritonavir with some narcotic analgesics which are partially mediated by CYP2D6 metabolism, it is possible that substantial increases in concentrations of these narcotic analgesics may occur, possibly requiring a dosage reduction). Products include:

Vicodin	560
Vicodin ES	561
Vicodin HP	563
Vicoprofen	564
Zydone	1138

Hydrocodone Polistirex (When co-administering ritonavir with some narcotic analgesics which are partially mediated by CYP2D6 metabolism, it is possible that substantial increases in concentrations of these narcotic analgesics may occur, possibly requiring a dosage reduction). Products include:

Tussionex	3443

Hydrocortisone (When co-administering ritonavir with some steroids, it is possible that a substantial increase in the concentrations of some steroids may occur. A dose decrease may be needed for steroids, such as dexamethasone, fluticasone, prednisone, when co-administered with ritonavir).
No products indexed under this heading.

Hydrocortisone (Alcohol) (When co-administering ritonavir with some steroids, it is possible that a substantial increase in the concentrations of some steroids may occur. A dose decrease may be needed for steroids, such as dexamethasone, fluticasone, prednisone, when co-administered with ritonavir).
No products indexed under this heading.

Hydrocortisone Acetate (When co-administering ritonavir with some steroids, it is possible that a substantial increase in the concentrations of some steroids may occur. A dose decrease may be needed for steroids, such as dexamethasone, fluticasone, prednisone, when co-administered with ritonavir).
No products indexed under this heading.

Hydrocortisone Butyrate (When co-administering ritonavir with some steroids, it is possible that a substantial increase in the concentrations of some steroids may occur. A dose decrease may be needed for steroids, such as dexamethasone, fluticasone, prednisone, when co-administered with ritonavir).
No products indexed under this heading.

Hydrocortisone Cypionate (When co-administering ritonavir with some steroids, it is possible that a substantial increase in the concentrations of some steroids may occur. A dose decrease may be needed for steroids, such as dexamethasone, fluticasone, prednisone, when co-administered with ritonavir).
No products indexed under this heading.

Hydrocortisone Hemisuccinate (When co-administering ritonavir with some steroids, it is possible that a substantial increase in the concentrations of some steroids may occur. A dose decrease may be needed for steroids, such as dexamethasone, fluticasone, prednisone, when co-administered with ritonavir).
No products indexed under this heading.

Hydrocortisone Probutate (When co-administering ritonavir with some steroids, it is possible that a substantial increase in the concentrations of some steroids may occur. A dose decrease may be needed for steroids, such as dexamethasone, fluticasone, prednisone, when co-administered with ritonavir).
No products indexed under this heading.

Hydrocortisone Sodium Phosphate (When co-administering ritonavir with some steroids, it is possible that a substantial increase in the concentrations of some steroids may occur. A dose decrease may be needed for steroids, such as dexamethasone, fluticasone, prednisone, when co-administered with ritonavir).
No products indexed under this heading.

Hydrocortisone Sodium Succinate (When co-administering ritonavir with some steroids, it is possible that a substantial increase in the concentrations of some steroids may occur. A dose decrease may be needed for steroids, such as dexamethasone, fluticasone, prednisone, when co-administered with ritonavir).
No products indexed under this heading.

Hydrocortisone Valerate (When co-administering ritonavir with some steroids, it is possible that a substantial increase in the concentrations of some steroids may occur. A dose decrease may be needed for steroids, such as dexamethasone, fluticasone, prednisone, when co-administered with ritonavir).
No products indexed under this heading.

Hydromorphone (When co-administering ritonavir with some narcotic analgesics which are partially mediated by CYP2D6 metabolism, it is possible that substantial increases in concentrations of these narcotic analgesics may occur, possibly requiring a dosage reduction).
No products indexed under this heading.

Hydromorphone Hydrochloride (When co-administering ritonavir with some narcotic analgesics which are partially mediated by CYP2D6 metabolism, it is possible that substantial increases in concentrations of these narcotic analgesics may occur, possibly requiring a dosage reduction). Products include:

Dilaudid Injection	2800
Dilaudid Oral	2797
Dilaudid Tablets	2797

Dilaudid-HP	2800

Hydroxyurea (Concentrations of vincristine or vinblastine may be increased when co-administered with ritonavir, resulting in the potential for increased adverse events usually associated with these anticancer agents. Consideration should be given to temporarily withholding the ritonavir containing antiretroviral regimen in patients who develop significant hematologic or gastrointestinal side effects when ritonavir is administered concurrently with vincristine or vinblastine. Clinicians should be aware that if the ritonavir containing regimen is withheld for a prolonged period, consideration should be given to altering the regimen to not include a CYP3A or P-gp inhibitor in order to control HIV-1 viral load).
No products indexed under this heading.

Hypericum Perforatum (Concomitant use of ritonavir, and St. John's wort (hypericum perforatum) or products containing St. John's wort is not recommended. Co-administration of protease inhibitors, including ritonavir, with St. John's wort is expected to substantially decrease protease inhibitor concentrations and may result in sub-optimal levels of ritonavir and lead to loss of virologic response and possible resistance to ritonavir or to the class of protease inhibitors). Products include:

Traumeel	1800

Idarubicin Hydrochloride (Concentrations of vincristine or vinblastine may be increased when co-administered with ritonavir, resulting in the potential for increased adverse events usually associated with these anticancer agents. Consideration should be given to temporarily withholding the ritonavir containing antiretroviral regimen in patients who develop significant hematologic or gastrointestinal side effects when ritonavir is administered concurrently with vincristine or vinblastine. Clinicians should be aware that if the ritonavir containing regimen is withheld for a prolonged period, consideration should be given to altering the regimen to not include a CYP3A or P-gp inhibitor in order to control HIV-1 viral load).
No products indexed under this heading.

Ifosfamide (Concentrations of vincristine or vinblastine may be increased when co-administered with ritonavir, resulting in the potential for increased adverse events usually associated with these anticancer agents. Consideration should be given to temporarily withholding the ritonavir containing antiretroviral regimen in patients who develop significant hematologic or gastrointestinal side effects when ritonavir is administered concurrently with vincristine or vinblastine. Clinicians should be aware that if the ritonavir containing regimen is withheld for a prolonged period, consideration should be given to altering the regimen to not include a CYP3A or P-gp inhibitor in order to control HIV-1 viral load).
No products indexed under this heading.

Imipramine Hydrochloride (Co-administration of antidepressants, such as nefazodone, selective serotonin reuptake inhibitors (SSRIs), or tricyclics, with ritonavir may result in increased plasma concentrations of antidepressants. A dose decrease may be needed for these drugs when co-administered with ritonavir).
No products indexed under this heading.

Imipramine Pamoate (Co-administration of antidepressants, such as nefazodone, selective serotonin reuptake inhibitors (SSRIs), or tricyclics, with ritonavir may result in increased plasma concentrations of antidepressants. A dose decrease may be needed for these drugs when co-administered with ritonavir).
No products indexed under this heading.

Indinavir Sulfate (Alterations in concentrations are noted when reduced doses of indinavir are co-administered with ritonavir. Appropriate doses for this combination, with respect to efficacy and safety, have not been established). Products include:

Crixivan	2113

Indoramin Hydrochloride (Ritonavir is an inhibitor of cytochrome P450 3A (CYP3A) both *in vitro* and *in vivo*. Ritonavir also inhibits CYP2D6 *in vitro*, but to a lesser extent than CYP3A. Co-administration of ritonavir and drugs primarily metabolized by CYP3A or CYP2D6 may result in increased plasma concentrations of other drugs that could increase or prolong its therapeutic and adverse effects. A dosage reduction of the other drug may be necessary).
No products indexed under this heading.

Insulin (New onset diabetes mellitus, exacerbation of pre-existing diabetes mellitus, and hyperglycemia have been reported during postmarketing surveillance in HIV-infected patients receiving protease inhibitor therapy. Some patients required either initiation or dose adjustments of insulin or oral hypoglycemic agents for treatment of these events).
No products indexed under this heading.

Insulin, Human, Zinc Suspension (New onset diabetes mellitus, exacerbation of pre-existing diabetes mellitus, and hyperglycemia have been reported during postmarketing surveillance in HIV-infected patients receiving protease inhibitor therapy. Some patients required either initiation or dose adjustments of insulin or oral hypoglycemic agents for treatment of these events).
No products indexed under this heading.

Insulin, Human (rDNA origin) (New onset diabetes mellitus, exacerbation of pre-existing diabetes mellitus, and hyperglycemia have been reported during postmarketing surveillance in HIV-infected patients receiving protease inhibitor therapy. Some patients required either initiation or dose adjustments of insulin or oral hypoglycemic agents for treatment of these events). Products include:

Exubera	2717

Insulin, Human NPH (New onset diabetes mellitus, exacerbation of pre-existing diabetes mellitus, and hyperglycemia have been reported during postmarketing surveillance in HIV-infected patients receiving protease inhibitor therapy. Some patients required either initiation or dose adjustments of insulin or oral hypoglycemic agents for treatment of these events). Products include:

Humulin N Vial	1934

Insulin, Human Regular (New onset diabetes mellitus, exacerbation of pre-existing diabetes mellitus, and hyperglycemia have been reported during postmarketing surveillance in HIV-infected patients receiving protease inhibitor therapy. Some patients required either initiation or dose adjustments of insulin or oral hypoglycemic agents for treatment of these events). Products include:

Humulin R	1937
Humulin R (U-500)	1939

1235 Interactions Index Norvir

Insulin, Human Regular and Human NPH Mixture (New onset diabetes mellitus, exacerbation of pre-existing diabetes mellitus, and hyperglycemia have been reported during postmarketing surveillance in HIV-infected patients receiving protease inhibitor therapy. Some patients required either initiation or dose adjustments of insulin or oral hypoglycemic agents for treatment of these events). Products include:
Humulin 50/50 1930
Humulin 70/30 Vial 1931

Insulin, NPH (New onset diabetes mellitus, exacerbation of pre-existing diabetes mellitus, and hyperglycemia have been reported during postmarketing surveillance in HIV-infected patients receiving protease inhibitor therapy. Some patients required either initiation or dose adjustments of insulin or oral hypoglycemic agents for treatment of these events).
No products indexed under this heading.

Insulin, Regular (New onset diabetes mellitus, exacerbation of pre-existing diabetes mellitus, and hyperglycemia have been reported during postmarketing surveillance in HIV-infected patients receiving protease inhibitor therapy. Some patients required either initiation or dose adjustments of insulin or oral hypoglycemic agents for treatment of these events).
No products indexed under this heading.

Insulin, Regular and NPH mixture (New onset diabetes mellitus, exacerbation of pre-existing diabetes mellitus, and hyperglycemia have been reported during postmarketing surveillance in HIV-infected patients receiving protease inhibitor therapy. Some patients required either initiation or dose adjustments of insulin or oral hypoglycemic agents for treatment of these events).
No products indexed under this heading.

Insulin, Zinc Crystals (New onset diabetes mellitus, exacerbation of pre-existing diabetes mellitus, and hyperglycemia have been reported during postmarketing surveillance in HIV-infected patients receiving protease inhibitor therapy. Some patients required either initiation or dose adjustments of insulin or oral hypoglycemic agents for treatment of these events).
No products indexed under this heading.

Insulin, Zinc Suspension (New onset diabetes mellitus, exacerbation of pre-existing diabetes mellitus, and hyperglycemia have been reported during postmarketing surveillance in HIV-infected patients receiving protease inhibitor therapy. Some patients required either initiation or dose adjustments of insulin or oral hypoglycemic agents for treatment of these events).
No products indexed under this heading.

Insulin Aspart (New onset diabetes mellitus, exacerbation of pre-existing diabetes mellitus, and hyperglycemia have been reported during postmarketing surveillance in HIV-infected patients receiving protease inhibitor therapy. Some patients required either initiation or dose adjustments of insulin or oral hypoglycemic agents for treatment of these events).
No products indexed under this heading.

Insulin Aspart, Human (New onset diabetes mellitus, exacerbation of pre-existing diabetes mellitus, and hyperglycemia have been reported during postmarketing surveillance in HIV-infected patients receiving protease inhibitor therapy. Some patients required either initiation or dose adjustments of insulin or oral hypoglycemic agents for treatment of these events). Products include:
NovoLog Mix 70/30 2581

Insulin Aspart, Human Regular (New onset diabetes mellitus, exacerbation of pre-existing diabetes mellitus, and hyperglycemia have been reported during postmarketing surveillance in HIV-infected patients receiving protease inhibitor therapy. Some patients required either initiation or dose adjustments of insulin or oral hypoglycemic agents for treatment of these events). Products include:
NovoLog 2575

Insulin Aspart Protamine, Human (New onset diabetes mellitus, exacerbation of pre-existing diabetes mellitus, and hyperglycemia have been reported during postmarketing surveillance in HIV-infected patients receiving protease inhibitor therapy. Some patients required either initiation or dose adjustments of insulin or oral hypoglycemic agents for treatment of these events). Products include:
NovoLog Mix 70/30 2581

Insulin Detemir (rDNA Origin) (New onset diabetes mellitus, exacerbation of pre-existing diabetes mellitus, and hyperglycemia have been reported during postmarketing surveillance in HIV-infected patients receiving protease inhibitor therapy. Some patients required either initiation or dose adjustments of insulin or oral hypoglycemic agents for treatment of these events). Products include:
Levemir 2566

Insulin Glargine (New onset diabetes mellitus, exacerbation of pre-existing diabetes mellitus, and hyperglycemia have been reported during postmarketing surveillance in HIV-infected patients receiving protease inhibitor therapy. Some patients required either initiation or dose adjustments of insulin or oral hypoglycemic agents for treatment of these events). Products include:
Lantus 2996

Insulin Glulisine (New onset diabetes mellitus, exacerbation of pre-existing diabetes mellitus, and hyperglycemia have been reported during postmarketing surveillance in HIV-infected patients receiving protease inhibitor therapy. Some patients required either initiation or dose adjustments of insulin or oral hypoglycemic agents for treatment of these events). Products include:
Apidra 2937
Apidra SoloStar 2937

Insulin Lispro, Human (New onset diabetes mellitus, exacerbation of pre-existing diabetes mellitus, and hyperglycemia have been reported during postmarketing surveillance in HIV-infected patients receiving protease inhibitor therapy. Some patients required either initiation or dose adjustments of insulin or oral hypoglycemic agents for treatment of these events). Products include:
Humalog 1910
Humalog Mix 1914
Humalog Mix75/25 1917

Insulin Lispro Protamine, Human (New onset diabetes mellitus, exacerbation of pre-existing diabetes mellitus, and hyperglycemia have been reported during postmarketing surveillance in HIV-infected patients receiving protease inhibitor therapy. Some patients required either initiation or dose adjustments of insulin or oral hypoglycemic agents for treatment of these events). Products include:
Humalog Mix 1914
Humalog Mix75/25 1917

Interferon alfa-2a, Recombinant (Concentrations of vincristine or vinblastine may be increased when co-administered with ritonavir, resulting in the potential for increased adverse events usually associated with these anticancer agents. Consideration should be given to temporarily withholding the ritonavir containing antiretroviral regimen in patients who develop significant hematologic or gastrointestinal side effects when ritonavir is administered concurrently with vincristine or vinblastine. Clinicians should be aware that if the ritonavir containing regimen is withheld for a prolonged period, consideration should be given to altering the regimen to not include a CYP3A or P-gp inhibitor in order to control HIV-1 viral load).
No products indexed under this heading.

Interferon alfa-2b, Recombinant (Concentrations of vincristine or vinblastine may be increased when co-administered with ritonavir, resulting in the potential for increased adverse events usually associated with these anticancer agents. Consideration should be given to temporarily withholding the ritonavir containing antiretroviral regimen in patients who develop significant hematologic or gastrointestinal side effects when ritonavir is administered concurrently with vincristine or vinblastine. Clinicians should be aware that if the ritonavir containing regimen is withheld for a prolonged period, consideration should be given to altering the regimen to not include a CYP3A or P-gp inhibitor in order to control HIV-1 viral load). Products include:
Intron A 3140

Irinotecan Hydrochloride (Concentrations of vincristine or vinblastine may be increased when co-administered with ritonavir, resulting in the potential for increased adverse events usually associated with these anticancer agents. Consideration should be given to temporarily withholding the ritonavir containing antiretroviral regimen in patients who develop significant hematologic or gastrointestinal side effects when ritonavir is administered concurrently with vincristine or vinblastine. Clinicians should be aware that if the ritonavir containing regimen is withheld for a prolonged period, consideration should be given to altering the regimen to not include a CYP3A or P-gp inhibitor in order to control HIV-1 viral load).
No products indexed under this heading.

Isocarboxazid (Co-administration of antidepressants, such as nefazodone, selective serotonin reuptake inhibitors (SSRIs), or tricyclics, with ritonavir may result in increased plasma concentrations of antidepressants. A dose decrease may be needed for these drugs when co-administered with ritonavir). Products include:
Marplan 3481

Isradipine (Co-administration of calcium channel blockers, such as diltiazem, nifedipine, verapamil, with ritonavir may result in increased plasma concentrations of calcium channel blockers. A dose decrease may be needed for these drugs when co-administered with ritonavir. In addition, ritonavir prolongs the PR interval in some patients. The impact on the PR interval of co-administration of ritonavir with other drugs that prolong the PR interval (including calcium channel blockers) has not been evaluated. Co-administration of ritonavir with these drugs should be undertaken with caution, particularly with those drugs metabolized by CYP3A. Clinical monitoring is recommended). Products include:
DynaCirc CR 1432

Itraconazole (Co-administration of itraconazole with ritonavir may result in increased plasma concentrations of itraconazole. High doses of itraconazole (> 200 mg/day) is not recommended).
No products indexed under this heading.

Ketoconazole (Co-administration of ketoconazole with ritonavir may cause an increase in ketoconazole concentrations. Co-administration of ketoconazole with ritonavir led to an increase in AUC and C_{max} of ritonavir by 18% and 10%, respectively. High doses of ketoconazole (> 200 mg/day) is not recommended). Products include:
Extina 3319
Xolegel 3337

Labetalol Hydrochloride (Co-administration of beta-blockers, such as metoprolol or timolol, with ritonavir, may result in increased plasma concentrations of the β-blocker. Cardiac and neurologic events have been reported with ritonavir when co-administered with β-blockers. A dose decrease may be needed for these drugs when co-administered with ritonavir. In addition, ritonavir prolongs the PR interval in some patients. The impact on the PR interval of co-administration of ritonavir with other drugs that prolong the PR interval (including β-adrenergic blockers) has not been evaluated. As a result, co-administration of ritonavir with these drugs should be undertaken with caution, particularly with those drugs metabolized by CYP3A. Clinical monitoring is recommended).
No products indexed under this heading.

Lamotrigine (Co-administration of lamotrigine with ritonavir may result in decreased plasma concentrations of lamotrigine. Use with caution. A dose increase may be needed for lamotrigine when co-administered with ritonavir and therapeutic concentration monitoring is recommended, if available). Products include:
Lamictal 1522
Lamictal ODT 1522
Lamictal XR 1536

Levamisole Hydrochloride (Concentrations of vincristine or vinblastine may be increased when co-administered with ritonavir, resulting in the potential for increased adverse events usually associated with these anticancer agents. Consideration should be given to temporarily withholding the ritonavir containing antiretroviral regimen in patients who develop significant hematologic or gastrointestinal side effects when ritonavir is administered concurrently with vincristine or vinblastine. Clinicians should be aware that if the ritonavir containing regimen is withheld for a prolonged period, consideration should be given to altering the regimen to not include a CYP3A or P-gp inhibitor in order to control HIV-1 viral load).
No products indexed under this heading.

Levetiracetam (When co-administering ritonavir with any agent having a narrow therapeutic margin, such as anticonvulsants, special attention is warranted). Products include:
Keppra XR 3434

Levobunolol Hydrochloride (Co-administration of beta-blockers, such as metoprolol or timolol, with ritonavir, may result in increased plasma concentrations of the β-blocker. Cardiac and neurologic events have been reported with ritonavir when co-administered with β-blockers. A dose decrease may be needed for these drugs when co-administered with ritonavir. In addition, ritonavir prolongs the PR interval in some patients. The impact on the PR interval of co-administration of ritonavir with other drugs that prolong the PR interval (including β-adrenergic blockers) has not been evaluated. As a result, co-administration of ritonavir with these drugs should be undertaken with caution, particularly with those drugs metabolized by CYP3A. Clinical monitoring is recommended).
No products indexed under this heading.

IMPORTANT NOTE: Always consult each drug listing in the patient's regimen for possible interactions.

Levonorgestrel (Ritonavir is an inhibitor of cytochrome P450 3A (CYP3A) both *in vitro* and *in vivo*. Ritonavir also inhibits CYP2D6 *in vitro*, but to a lesser extent than CYP3A. Co-administration of ritonavir and drugs primarily metabolized by CYP3A or CYP2D6 may result in increased plasma concentrations of other drugs that could increase or prolong its therapeutic and adverse effects. A dosage reduction of the other drug may be necessary). Products include:

Climara Pro **847**
LoSeasonique **3407**
Lybrel **3514**
Mirena **854**
Plan B **3416**
Seasonique **3418**

Levorphanol Tartrate (When co-administering ritonavir with some narcotic analgesics which are partially mediated by CYP2D6 metabolism, it is possible that substantial increases in concentrations of these narcotic analgesics may occur, possibly requiring a dosage reduction).
No products indexed under this heading.

Lidocaine (Co-administration of antiarrhythmics, such as disopyramide, lidocaine, mexilitine, with ritonavir may result in increased plasma concentrations of antiarrhythmics. Caution is warranted and therapeutic concentration monitoring is recommended for antiarrhythmics when co-administered with ritonavir, if available). Products include:

Lidoderm **1107**

Lidocaine Base (Co-administration of antiarrhythmics, such as disopyramide, lidocaine, mexilitine, with ritonavir may result in increased plasma concentrations of antiarrhythmics. Caution is warranted and therapeutic concentration monitoring is recommended for antiarrhythmics when co-administered with ritonavir, if available).
No products indexed under this heading.

Lidocaine Hydrochloride (Co-administration of antiarrhythmics, such as disopyramide, lidocaine, mexilitine, with ritonavir may result in increased plasma concentrations of antiarrhythmics. Caution is warranted and therapeutic concentration monitoring is recommended for antiarrhythmics when co-administered with ritonavir, if available).
No products indexed under this heading.

Lithium (Co-administration of neuroleptics, such as perphenazine, risperidone, and thioridazine, with ritonavir may result in inceased plasma concentrations of neuroleptics. A dose decrease may be needed for these drugs when co-administered with ritonavir).
No products indexed under this heading.

Lithium Carbonate (Co-administration of neuroleptics, such as perphenazine, risperidone, and thioridazine, with ritonavir may result in inceased plasma concentrations of neuroleptics. A dose decrease may be needed for these drugs when co-administered with ritonavir).
No products indexed under this heading.

Lithium Citrate (Co-administration of neuroleptics, such as perphenazine, risperidone, and thioridazine, with ritonavir may result in inceased plasma concentrations of neuroleptics. A dose decrease may be needed for these drugs when co-administered with ritonavir).
No products indexed under this heading.

Lomustine (CCNU) (Concentrations of vincristine or vinblastine may be increased when co-administered with ritonavir, resulting in the potential for increased adverse events usually associated with these anticancer agents. Consideration should be given to temporarily withholding the ritonavir containing antiretroviral regimen in patients who develop significant hematologic or gastrointestinal side effects when ritonavir is administered concurrently with vincristine or vinblastine. Clinicians should be aware that if the ritonavir containing regimen is withheld for a prolonged period, consideration should be given to altering the regimen to not include a CYP3A or P-gp inhibitor in order to control HIV-1 viral load).
No products indexed under this heading.

Loratadine (Co-administration of ritonavir with certain nonsedating antihistamines may result in potentially serious and/or life-threatening adverse events due to possible effects of ritonavir on the hepatic metabolism of certain drugs).
No products indexed under this heading.

Lorazepam (Co-administration of ritonavir with certain sedative hypnotics may result in potentially serious and/or life-threatening adverse events due to possible effects of ritonavir on the hepatic metabolism of certain drugs. Co-administration of sedative/hypnotics such as buspirone, clorazepate, diazepam, estazolam, flurazepam, or zolpidem with ritonavir may result in increased plasma concentrations of sedative/hypnotics. A dose decrease may be needed for these drugs when co-administered with ritonavir).
No products indexed under this heading.

Lovastatin (Concomitant use of ritonavir with lovastatin is not recommended. There is the potential for serious reactions, such as the risk of myopathy including rhabdomyolysis, with concomitant use). Products include:

Advicor **402**
Mevacor **2212**

Low Molecular Weight Heparins (When co-administering ritonavir with any agent having a narrow therapeutic margin, such as anticoagulants, special attention is warranted).
No products indexed under this heading.

Loxapine Hydrochloride (Co-administration of neuroleptics, such as perphenazine, risperidone, and thioridazine, with ritonavir may result in inceased plasma concentrations of neuroleptics. A dose decrease may be needed for these drugs when co-administered with ritonavir).
No products indexed under this heading.

Loxapine Succinate (Co-administration of neuroleptics, such as perphenazine, risperidone, and thioridazine, with ritonavir may result in inceased plasma concentrations of neuroleptics. A dose decrease may be needed for these drugs when co-administered with ritonavir).
No products indexed under this heading.

Maprotiline Hydrochloride (Co-administration of antidepressants, such as nefazodone, selective serotonin reuptake inhibitors (SSRIs), or tricyclics, with ritonavir may result in increased plasma concentrations of antidepressants. A dose decrease may be needed for these drugs when co-administered with ritonavir).
No products indexed under this heading.

Maraviroc (Concurrent administration of maraviroc with ritonavir will increase plasma levels of maraviroc. When co-administered, patients should receive 150 mg BID of maraviroc). Products include:

Selzentry **2740**

Mechlorethamine Hydrochloride (Concentrations of vincristine or vinblastine may be increased when co-administered with ritonavir, resulting in the potential for increased adverse events usually associated with these anticancer agents. Consideration should be given to temporarily withholding the ritonavir containing antiretroviral regimen in patients who develop significant hematologic or gastrointestinal side effects when ritonavir is administered concurrently with vincristine or vinblastine. Clinicians should be aware that if the ritonavir containing regimen is withheld for a prolonged period, consideration should be given to altering the regimen to not include a CYP3A or P-gp inhibitor in order to control HIV-1 viral load). Products include:

Mustargen **2010**

Megestrol Acetate (Concentrations of vincristine or vinblastine may be increased when co-administered with ritonavir, resulting in the potential for increased adverse events usually associated with these anticancer agents. Consideration should be given to temporarily withholding the ritonavir containing antiretroviral regimen in patients who develop significant hematologic or gastrointestinal side effects when ritonavir is administered concurrently with vincristine or vinblastine. Clinicians should be aware that if the ritonavir containing regimen is withheld for a prolonged period, consideration should be given to altering the regimen to not include a CYP3A or P-gp inhibitor in order to control HIV-1 viral load). Products include:

Megace ES **2698**

Melphalan (Concentrations of vincristine or vinblastine may be increased when co-administered with ritonavir, resulting in the potential for increased adverse events usually associated with these anticancer agents. Consideration should be given to temporarily withholding the ritonavir containing antiretroviral regimen in patients who develop significant hematologic or gastrointestinal side effects when ritonavir is administered concurrently with vincristine or vinblastine. Clinicians should be aware that if the ritonavir containing regimen is withheld for a prolonged period, consideration should be given to altering the regimen to not include a CYP3A or P-gp inhibitor in order to control HIV-1 viral load). Products include:

Alkeran **1302**

Meperidine Hydrochloride (Co-administration of meperidine with ritonavir may decrease meperidine concentrations and increase normeperidine (metabolite) concentrations. Dosage increase and long-term use of meperidine with ritonavir are not recommended due to the increased concentrations of the metabolite normeperidine which has both analgesic activity and CNS stimulant activity (eg, seizures)).
No products indexed under this heading.

Mephenytoin (When co-administering ritonavir with any agent having a narrow therapeutic margin, such as anticonvulsants, special attention is warranted).
No products indexed under this heading.

Mercaptopurine (Concentrations of vincristine or vinblastine may be increased when co-administered with ritonavir, resulting in the potential for increased adverse events usually associated with these anticancer agents. Consideration should be given to temporarily withholding the ritonavir containing antiretroviral regimen in patients who develop significant hematologic or gastrointestinal side effects when ritonavir is administered concurrently with vincristine or vinblastine. Clinicians should be aware that if the ritonavir containing regimen is withheld for a prolonged period, consideration should be given to altering the regimen to not include a CYP3A or P-gp inhibitor in order to control HIV-1 viral load).
No products indexed under this heading.

Mesoridazine Besylate (Co-administration of neuroleptics, such as perphenazine, risperidone, and thioridazine, with ritonavir may result in increased plasma concentrations of neuroleptics. A dose decrease may be needed for these drugs when co-administered with ritonavir).
No products indexed under this heading.

Mestranol (Ritonavir is an inhibitor of cytochrome P450 3A (CYP3A) both *in vitro* and *in vivo*. Ritonavir also inhibits CYP2D6 *in vitro*, but to a lesser extent than CYP3A. Co-administration of ritonavir and drugs primarily metabolized by CYP3A or CYP2D6 may result in increased plasma concentrations of other drugs that could increase or prolong its therapeutic and adverse effects. A dosage reduction of the other drug may be necessary).
No products indexed under this heading.

Metformin Hydrochloride (New onset diabetes mellitus, exacerbation of pre-existing diabetes mellitus, and hyperglycemia have been reported during postmarketing surveillance in HIV-infected patients receiving protease inhibitor therapy. Some patients required either initiation or dose adjustments of insulin or oral hypoglycemic agents for treatment of these events). Products include:

ActoPlus **3338**
Avandamet **1345**
Janumet **2188**

Methadone Hydrochloride (Co-administration of methadone with ritonavir, may decrease methadone concentrations. Dosage increase of methadone may be considered).
No products indexed under this heading.

Methamphetamine Hydrochloride (Co-administration of methamphetamine with ritonavir may result in increased methamphetamine plasma concentrations. A dose decrease of methamphetamine may be needed when co-administered with ritonavir. Use with caution).
No products indexed under this heading.

Methdilazine Hydrochloride (Co-administration of ritonavir with certain nonsedating antihistamines may result in potentially serious and/or life-threatening adverse events due to possible effects of ritonavir on the hepatic metabolism of certain drugs).
No products indexed under this heading.

Methotrexate (Concentrations of vincristine or vinblastine may be increased when co-administered with ritonavir, resulting in the potential for increased adverse events usually associated with these anticancer agents. Consideration should be given to temporarily withholding the ritonavir containing antiretroviral regimen in patients who develop significant hematologic or gastrointestinal side effects when ritonavir is administered concurrently with vincristine or vinblastine. Clinicians should be aware that if the ritonavir containing regimen is withheld for a prolonged period, consideration should be given to altering the regimen to not include a CYP3A or P-gp inhibitor in order to control HIV-1 viral load).
No products indexed under this heading.

Methotrexate Sodium (Concentrations of vincristine or vinblastine may be increased when co-administered with ritonavir, resulting in the potential for increased adverse events usually associated with these anticancer agents. Consideration should be given to temporarily withholding the ritonavir containing antiretroviral regimen in patients who develop significant hematologic or gastrointestinal side effects when ritonavir is administered concurrently with vincristine or vinblastine. Clinicians

1237 **Interactions Index** **Norvir**

should be aware that if the ritonavir containing regimen is withheld for a prolonged period, consideration should be given to altering the regimen to not include a CYP3A or P-gp inhibitor in order to control HIV-1 viral load).
No products indexed under this heading.

Methotrimeprazine (Co-administration of neuroleptics, such as perphenazine, risperidone, and thioridazine, with ritonavir may result in inceased plasma concentrations of neuroleptics. A dose decrease may be needed for these drugs when co-administered with ritonavir).
No products indexed under this heading.

Methoxyphenamine (Ritonavir is an inhibitor of cytochrome P450 3A (CYP3A) both *in vitro* and *in vivo*. Ritonavir also inhibits CYP2D6 *in vitro*, but to a lesser extent than CYP3A. Co-administration of ritonavir and drugs primarily metabolized by CYP3A or CYP2D6 may result in increased plasma concentrations of other drugs that could increase or prolong its therapeutic and adverse effects. A dosage reduction of the other drug may be necessary).
No products indexed under this heading.

Methsuximide (When co-administering ritonavir with any agent having a narrow therapeutic margin, such as anticonvulsants, special attention is warranted).
No products indexed under this heading.

Methylergonovine Maleate (Co-administration of ritonavir and the ergot derivatives dihydroergotamine, ergonovine, ergotamine, or methylergonovine is contraindicated due to potential for serious and/or life-threatening reactions such as acute ergot toxicity characterized by vasospasm and ischemia of the extremities and other tissues including the central nervous system).
No products indexed under this heading.

Methylprednisolone (When co-administering ritonavir with some steroids, it is possible that a substantial increase in the concentrations of some steroids may occur. A dose decrease may be needed for steroids, such as dexamethasone, fluticasone, prednisone, when co-administered with ritonavir).
No products indexed under this heading.

Methylprednisolone Acetate (When co-administering ritonavir with some steroids, it is possible that a substantial increase in the concentrations of some steroids may occur. A dose decrease may be needed for steroids, such as dexamethasone, fluticasone, prednisone, when co-administered with ritonavir).
No products indexed under this heading.

Methylprednisolone Sodium Succinate (When co-administering ritonavir with some steroids, it is possible that a substantial increase in the concentrations of some steroids may occur. A dose decrease may be needed for steroids, such as dexamethasone, fluticasone, prednisone, when co-administered with ritonavir).
No products indexed under this heading.

Methysergide Maleate (Co-administration of ritonavir and the ergot derivatives dihydroergotamine, ergonovine, ergotamine, or methylergonovine is contraindicated due to potential for serious and/or life-threatening reactions such as acute ergot toxicity characterized by vasospasm and ischemia of the extremities and other tissues including the central nervous system).
No products indexed under this heading.

Metipranolol Hydrochloride (Co-administration of beta-blockers, such as metoprolol or timolol, with ritonavir, may result in increased plasma concentrations of the β-blocker. Cardiac and neurologic events have been reported with ritonavir when co-administered with β-blockers. A dose decrease may be needed for these drugs when co-administered with ritonavir. In addition, ritonavir prolongs the PR interval in some patients. The impact on the PR interval of co-administration of ritonavir with other drugs that prolong the PR interval (including β-adrenergic blockers) has not been evaluated. As a result, co-administration of ritonavir with these drugs should be undertaken with caution, particularly with those drugs metabolized by CYP3A. Clinical monitoring is recommended).
No products indexed under this heading.

Metoprolol Succinate (Co-administration of β-blockers, such as metoprolol, with ritonavir, may result in increased plasma concentrations of the β-blocker. Cardiac and neurologic events have been reported with ritonavir when co-administered with β-blockers. A dose decrease may be needed for these drugs when co-administered with ritonavir. In addition, ritonavir prolongs the PR interval in some patients. The impact on the PR interval of co-administration of ritonavir with other drugs that prolong the PR interval (including β-adrenergic blockers) has not been evaluated. As a result, co-administration of ritonavir with these drugs should be undertaken with caution, particularly with those drugs metabolized by CYP3A. Clinical monitoring is recommended). Products include:
Toprol XL 732

Metoprolol Tartrate (Co-administration of β-blockers, such as metoprolol, with ritonavir, may result in increased plasma concentrations of the β-blocker. Cardiac and neurologic events have been reported with ritonavir when co-administered with β-blockers. A dose decrease may be needed for these drugs when co-administered with ritonavir. In addition, ritonavir prolongs the PR interval in some patients. The impact on the PR interval of co-administration of ritonavir with other drugs that prolong the PR interval (including β-adrenergic blockers) has not been evaluated. As a result, co-administration of ritonavir with these drugs should be undertaken with caution, particularly with those drugs metabolized by CYP3A. Clinical monitoring is recommended).
No products indexed under this heading.

Metronidazole (Ritonavir formulations contain alcohol, which can produce disulfiram-like reactions when co-administered with disulfiram or other drugs that produce this reaction (eg, metronidazole)). Products include:
Pylera 793

Metronidazole Benzoate (Ritonavir formulations contain alcohol, which can produce disulfiram-like reactions when co-administered with disulfiram or other drugs that produce this reaction (eg, metronidazole)).
No products indexed under this heading.

Metronidazole Hydrochloride (Ritonavir formulations contain alcohol, which can produce disulfiram-like reactions when co-administered with disulfiram or other drugs that produce this reaction (eg, metronidazole)).
No products indexed under this heading.

Metronidazole Sodium (Ritonavir formulations contain alcohol, which can produce disulfiram-like reactions when co-administered with disulfiram or other drugs that produce this reaction (eg, metronidazole)).
No products indexed under this heading.

Mexiletine Hydrochloride (Co-administration of antiarrhythmics, such as mexilitine, with ritonavir may result in an increased plasma concentrations of antiarrhythmics. Cardiac and neurologic events have been reported with ritonavir when co-administered with mexiletine. Caution is warranted and therapeutic concentration monitoring is recommended for antiarrhythmics when co-administered with ritonavir, if available).
No products indexed under this heading.

Mibefradil Dihydrochloride (Co-administration of calcium channel blockers, such as diltiazem, nifedipine, verapamil, with ritonavir may result in increased plasma concentrations of calcium channel blockers. A dose decrease may be needed for these drugs when co-administered with ritonavir. In addition, ritonavir prolongs the PR interval in some patients. The impact on the PR interval of co-administration of ritonavir with other drugs that prolong the PR interval (including calcium channel blockers) has not been evaluated. Co-administration of ritonavir with these drugs should be undertaken with caution, particularly with those drugs metabolized by CYP3A. Clinical monitoring is recommended).
No products indexed under this heading.

Midazolam Hydrochloride (Co-administration of ritonavir and midazolam is contraindicated due to potential for serious and/or life-threatening reactions such as prolonged or increased sedation or respiratory depression).
No products indexed under this heading.

Miglitol (New onset diabetes mellitus, exacerbation of pre-existing diabetes mellitus, and hyperglycemia have been reported during postmarketing surveillance in HIV-infected patients receiving protease inhibitor therapy. Some patients required either initiation or dose adjustments of insulin or oral hypoglycemic agents for treatment of these events).
No products indexed under this heading.

Mirtazapine (Co-administration of antidepressants, such as nefazodone, selective serotonin reuptake inhibitors (SSRIs), or tricyclics, with ritonavir may result in increased plasma concentrations of antidepressants. A dose decrease may be needed for these drugs when co-administered with ritonavir). Products include:
Remeron Tablets 3214
RemeronSolTab Tablets 3219

Mitomycin (Mitomycin-C) (Concentrations of vincristine or vinblastine may be increased when co-administered with ritonavir, resulting in the potential for increased adverse events usually associated with these anticancer agents. Consideration should be given to temporarily withholding the ritonavir containing antiretroviral regimen in patients who develop significant hematologic or gastrointestinal side effects when ritonavir is administered concurrently with vincristine or vinblastine. Clinicians should be aware that if the ritonavir containing regimen is withheld for a prolonged period, consideration should be given to altering the regimen to not include a CYP3A or P-gp inhibitor in order to control HIV-1 viral load).
No products indexed under this heading.

Mitotane (Concentrations of vincristine or vinblastine may be increased when co-administered with ritonavir, resulting in the potential for increased adverse events usually associated with these anticancer agents. Consideration should be given to temporarily withholding the ritonavir containing antiretroviral regimen in patients who develop significant hematologic or gastrointestinal side effects when ritonavir is administered concurrently with vincristine or vinblastine. Clinicians should be aware that if the ritonavir containing regimen is withheld for a prolonged period, consideration should be given to altering the regimen to not include a CYP3A or P-gp inhibitor in order to control HIV-1 viral load).
No products indexed under this heading.

Mitoxantrone Hydrochloride (Concentrations of vincristine or vinblastine may be increased when co-administered with ritonavir, resulting in the potential for increased adverse events usually associated with these anticancer agents. Consideration should be given to temporarily withholding the ritonavir containing antiretroviral regimen in patients who develop significant hematologic or gastrointestinal side effects when ritonavir is administered concurrently with vincristine or vinblastine. Clinicians should be aware that if the ritonavir containing regimen is withheld for a prolonged period, consideration should be given to altering the regimen to not include a CYP3A or P-gp inhibitor in order to control HIV-1 viral load). Products include:
Novantrone 1088

Molindone Hydrochloride (Co-administration of neuroleptics, such as perphenazine, risperidone, and thioridazine, with ritonavir may result in inceased plasma concentrations of neuroleptics. A dose decrease may be needed for these drugs when co-administered with ritonavir). Products include:
Moban 1108

Mometasone Furoate (When co-administering ritonavir with some steroids, it is possible that a substantial increase in the concentrations of some steroids may occur. A dose decrease may be needed for steroids, such as dexamethasone, fluticasone, prednisone, when co-administered with ritonavir). Products include:
Asmanex 3058
Elocon Cream 3111
Elocon Lotion 3112
Elocon Ointment 3114

Mometasone Furoate Monohydrate (When co-administering ritonavir with some steroids, it is possible that a substantial increase in the concentrations of some steroids may occur. A dose decrease may be needed for steroids, such as dexamethasone, fluticasone, prednisone, when co-administered with ritonavir). Products include:
Nasonex 3166

Moricizine Hydrochloride (Co-administration of ritonavir with certain antiarrhythmics may result in potentially serious and/or life-threatening adverse events due to possible effects of ritonavir on the hepatic metabolism of certain drugs. Co-administration of antiarrhythmics, such as disopyramide, lidocaine, mexilitine, with ritonavir may result in increased plasma concentrations of antiarrhythmics. Caution is warranted and therapeutic concentration monitoring is recommended for antiarrhythmics when co-administered with ritonavir, if available).
No products indexed under this heading.

Morphine Sulfate (When co-administering ritonavir with some narcotic analgesics which are partially mediated by CYP2D6 metabolism, it is possible that substantial increases in concentrations of these narcotic analgesics may occur, possibly requiring a dosage reduction). Products include:
Avinza 1822
Embeda 1831
MS Contin 2803

IMPORTANT NOTE: Always consult each drug listing in the patient's regimen for possible interactions.

Morphine Sulfate, Liposomal (When co-administering ritonavir with some narcotic analgesics which are partially mediated by CYP2D6 metabolism, it is possible that substantial increases in concentrations of these narcotic analgesics may occur, possibly requiring a dosage reduction).
No products indexed under this heading.

Muromonab-CD3 (Co-administration of immunosuppressants, such as cyclosporine, tacrolimus, sirolimus, rapamycin, with ritonavir may result in increased plasma concentrations of immunosuppressants. Therapeutic concentration monitoring is recommended for immunosuppressant agents when co-administered with ritonavir).
Products include:
Orthoclone OKT3 949

Mycophenolate Mofetil (Co-administration of immunosuppressants, such as cyclosporine, tacrolimus, sirolimus, rapamycin, with ritonavir may result in increased plasma concentrations of immunosuppressants. Therapeutic concentration monitoring is recommended for immunosuppressant agents when co-administered with ritonavir).
No products indexed under this heading.

Nadolol (Co-administration of beta-blockers, such as metoprolol or timolol, with ritonavir, may result in increased plasma concentrations of the β-blocker. Cardiac and neurologic events have been reported with ritonavir when co-administered with β-blockers. A dose decrease may be needed for these drugs when co-administered with ritonavir. In addition, ritonavir prolongs the PR interval in some patients. The impact on the PR interval of co-administration of ritonavir with other drugs that prolong the PR interval (including β-adrenergic blockers) has not been evaluated. As a result, co-administration of ritonavir with these drugs should be undertaken with caution, particularly with those drugs metabolized by CYP3A. Clinical monitoring is recommended). Products include:
Nadolol 2359

Nateglinide (New onset diabetes mellitus, exacerbation of pre-existing diabetes mellitus, and hyperglycemia have been reported during postmarketing surveillance in HIV-infected patients receiving protease inhibitor therapy. Some patients required either initiation or dose adjustments of insulin or oral hypoglycemic agents for treatment of these events).
No products indexed under this heading.

Nebivolol (Co-administration of beta-blockers, such as metoprolol or timolol, with ritonavir, may result in increased plasma concentrations of the β-blocker. Cardiac and neurologic events have been reported with ritonavir when co-administered with β-blockers. A dose decrease may be needed for these drugs when co-administered with ritonavir. In addition, ritonavir prolongs the PR interval in some patients. The impact on the PR interval of co-administration of ritonavir with other drugs that prolong the PR interval (including β-adrenergic blockers) has not been evaluated. As a result, co-administration of ritonavir with these drugs should be undertaken with caution, particularly with those drugs metabolized by CYP3A. Clinical monitoring is recommended). Products include:
Bystolic 1147

Nefazodone Hydrochloride (Co-administration of antidepressants, such as nefazodone, with ritonavir may result in increased plasma concentrations of antidepressants. A dose decrease may be needed for these drugs when co-administered with ritonavir. Cardiac and neurologic events have been reported with ritonavir when co-administered with nefazodone).
No products indexed under this heading.

Nelfinavir Mesylate (Ritonavir is an inhibitor of cytochrome P450 3A (CYP3A) both *in vitro* and *in vivo*. Ritonavir also inhibits CYP2D6 *in vitro*, but to a lesser extent than CYP3A. Co-administration of ritonavir and drugs primarily metabolized by CYP3A or CYP2D6 may result in increased plasma concentrations of other drugs that could increase or prolong its therapeutic and adverse effects. A dosage reduction of the other drug may be necessary).
No products indexed under this heading.

Nicardipine (Co-administration of calcium channel blockers, such as diltiazem, nifedipine, verapamil, with ritonavir may result in increased plasma concentrations of calcium channel blockers. A dose decrease may be needed for these drugs when co-administered with ritonavir. In addition, ritonavir prolongs the PR interval in some patients. The impact on the PR interval of co-administration of ritonavir with other drugs that prolong the PR interval (including calcium channel blockers) has not been evaluated. Co-administration of ritonavir with these drugs should be undertaken with caution, particularly with those drugs metabolized by CYP3A. Clinical monitoring is recommended).
No products indexed under this heading.

Nicardipine Hydrochloride (Co-administration of calcium channel blockers, such as diltiazem, nifedipine, verapamil, with ritonavir may result in increased plasma concentrations of calcium channel blockers. A dose decrease may be needed for these drugs when co-administered with ritonavir. In addition, ritonavir prolongs the PR interval in some patients. The impact on the PR interval of co-administration of ritonavir with other drugs that prolong the PR interval (including calcium channel blockers) has not been evaluated. Co-administration of ritonavir with these drugs should be undertaken with caution, particularly with those drugs metabolized by CYP3A. Clinical monitoring is recommended).
No products indexed under this heading.

Nifedipine (Co-administration of calcium channel blockers, such as nifedipine with ritonavir may result in increased plasma concentrations of calcium channel blockers. A dose decrease may be needed for these drugs when co-administered with ritonavir. In addition, ritonavir prolongs the PR interval in some patients. The impact on the PR interval of co-administration of ritonavir with other drugs that prolong the PR interval (including calcium channel blockers) has not been evaluated. Co-administration of ritonavir with these drugs should be undertaken with caution, particularly with those drugs metabolized by CYP3A. Clinical monitoring is recommended).
No products indexed under this heading.

Nimodipine (Co-administration of calcium channel blockers, such as diltiazem, nifedipine, verapamil, with ritonavir may result in increased plasma concentrations of calcium channel blockers. A dose decrease may be needed for these drugs when co-administered with ritonavir. In addition,

ritonavir prolongs the PR interval in some patients. The impact on the PR interval of co-administration of ritonavir with other drugs that prolong the PR interval (including calcium channel blockers) has not been evaluated. Co-administration of ritonavir with these drugs should be undertaken with caution, particularly with those drugs metabolized by CYP3A. Clinical monitoring is recommended).
No products indexed under this heading.

Nisoldipine (Co-administration of calcium channel blockers, such as diltiazem, nifedipine, verapamil, with ritonavir may result in increased plasma concentrations of calcium channel blockers. A dose decrease may be needed for these drugs when co-administered with ritonavir. In addition, ritonavir prolongs the PR interval in some patients. The impact on the PR interval of co-administration of ritonavir with other drugs that prolong the PR interval (including calcium channel blockers) has not been evaluated. Co-administration of ritonavir with these drugs should be undertaken with caution, particularly with those drugs metabolized by CYP3A. Clinical monitoring is recommended).
No products indexed under this heading.

Norethindrone (Ritonavir is an inhibitor of cytochrome P450 3A (CYP3A) both *in vitro* and *in vivo*. Ritonavir also inhibits CYP2D6 *in vitro*, but to a lesser extent than CYP3A. Co-administration of ritonavir and drugs primarily metabolized by CYP3A or CYP2D6 may result in increased plasma concentrations of other drugs that could increase or prolong its therapeutic and adverse effects. A dosage reduction of the other drug may be necessary). Products include:
Ortho Micronor 2660

Norgestrel (Ritonavir is an inhibitor of cytochrome P450 3A (CYP3A) both *in vitro* and *in vivo*. Ritonavir also inhibits CYP2D6 *in vitro*, but to a lesser extent than CYP3A. Co-administration of ritonavir and drugs primarily metabolized by CYP3A or CYP2D6 may result in increased plasma concentrations of other drugs that could increase or prolong its therapeutic and adverse effects. A dosage reduction of the other drug may be necessary).
No products indexed under this heading.

Nortriptyline Hydrochloride (Co-administration of antidepressants, such as nefazodone, selective serotonin reuptake inhibitors (SSRIs), or tricyclics, with ritonavir may result in increased plasma concentrations of antidepressants. A dose decrease may be needed for these drugs when co-administered with ritonavir).
No products indexed under this heading.

Olanzapine (Co-administration of neuroleptics, such as perphenazine, risperidone, and thioridazine, with ritonavir may result in inceased plasma concentrations of neuroleptics. A dose decrease may be needed for these drugs when co-administered with ritonavir). Products include:
Symbyax 1965
Zyprexa 1984
Zyprexa IntraMuscular 1984
Zyprexa ZYDIS 1984

Omeprazole (Ritonavir is an inhibitor of cytochrome P450 3A (CYP3A) both *in vitro* and *in vivo*. Ritonavir also inhibits CYP2D6 *in vitro*, but to a lesser extent than CYP3A. Co-administration of ritonavir and drugs primarily metabolized by CYP3A or CYP2D6 may result in increased plasma concentrations of other drugs that could increase or pro-

long its therapeutic and adverse effects. A dosage reduction of the other drug may be necessary).
No products indexed under this heading.

Ondansetron (Ritonavir is an inhibitor of cytochrome P450 3A (CYP3A) both *in vitro* and *in vivo*. Ritonavir also inhibits CYP2D6 *in vitro*, but to a lesser extent than CYP3A. Co-administration of ritonavir and drugs primarily metabolized by CYP3A or CYP2D6 may result in increased plasma concentrations of other drugs that could increase or prolong its therapeutic and adverse effects. A dosage reduction of the other drug may be necessary).
No products indexed under this heading.

Ondansetron Hydrochloride (Ritonavir is an inhibitor of cytochrome P450 3A (CYP3A) both *in vitro* and *in vivo*. Ritonavir also inhibits CYP2D6 *in vitro*, but to a lesser extent than CYP3A. Co-administration of ritonavir and drugs primarily metabolized by CYP3A or CYP2D6 may result in increased plasma concentrations of other drugs that could increase or prolong its therapeutic and adverse effects. A dosage reduction of the other drug may be necessary). Products include:
Zofran Injection 1750
Zofran 1756
Zofran ODT 1756

Oxaliplatin (Concentrations of vincristine or vinblastine may be increased when co-administered with ritonavir, resulting in the potential for increased adverse events usually associated with these anticancer agents. Consideration should be given to temporarily withholding the ritonavir containing antiretroviral regimen in patients who develop significant hematologic or gastrointestinal side effects when ritonavir is administered concurrently with vincristine or vinblastine. Clinicians should be aware that if the ritonavir containing regimen is withheld for a prolonged period, consideration should be given to altering the regimen to not include a CYP3A or P-gp inhibitor in order to control HIV-1 viral load). Products include:
Eloxatin 2975

Oxcarbazepine (When co-administering ritonavir with any agent having a narrow therapeutic margin, such as anticonvulsants, special attention is warranted).
No products indexed under this heading.

Oxycodone Hydrochloride (When co-administering ritonavir with some narcotic analgesics which are partially mediated by CYP2D6 metabolism, it is possible that substantial increases in concentrations of these narcotic analgesics may occur, possibly requiring a dosage reduction). Products include:
OxyContin 2807
Percocet 1121
Percodan 1124

Oxycodone Terephthalate (When co-administering ritonavir with some narcotic analgesics which are partially mediated by CYP2D6 metabolism, it is possible that substantial increases in concentrations of these narcotic analgesics may occur, possibly requiring a dosage reduction).
No products indexed under this heading.

Oxymorphone Hydrochloride (When co-administering ritonavir with some narcotic analgesics which are partially mediated by CYP2D6 metabolism, it is possible that substantial increases in concentrations of these narcotic analgesics may occur, possibly requiring a dosage reduction). Products include:
Opana 1110
Opana ER 1114

Paclitaxel (Concentrations of vincristine or vinblastine may be increased

when co-administered with ritonavir, resulting in the potential for increased adverse events usually associated with these anticancer agents. Consideration should be given to temporarily withholding the ritonavir containing antiretroviral regimen in patients who develop significant hematologic or gastrointestinal side effects when ritonavir is administered concurrently with vincristine or vinblastine. Clinicians should be aware that if the ritonavir containing regimen is withheld for a prolonged period, consideration should be given to altering the regimen to not include a CYP3A or P-gp inhibitor in order to control HIV-1 viral load).

No products indexed under this heading.

Paliperidone (Co-administration of neuroleptics, such as perphenazine, risperidone, and thioridazine, with ritonavir may result in inceased plasma concentrations of neuroleptics. A dose decrease may be needed for these drugs when co-administered with ritonavir). Products include:

Invega **2613**
Invega Sustenna **2621**

Paramethadione (When co-administering ritonavir with any agent having a narrow therapeutic margin, such as anticonvulsants, special attention is warranted).

No products indexed under this heading.

Paroxetine (Co-administration of antidepressants, such as nefazodone, selective serotonin reuptake inhibitors (SSRIs), tricyclics, with ritonavir may result in increased plasma concentrations of antidepressants. A dose decrease may be needed for these drugs when co-administered with ritonavir).

No products indexed under this heading.

Paroxetine Hydrochloride (Co-administration of antidepressants, such as nefazodone, selective serotonin reuptake inhibitors (SSRIs), tricyclics, with ritonavir may result in increased plasma concentrations of antidepressants. A dose decrease may be needed for these drugs when co-administered with ritonavir). Products include:

Paroxetine CR **2361**
Paroxetine ER **2371**
Paxil **1586**
Paxil CR **1596**

Paroxetine Mesylate (Co-administration of antidepressants, such as nefazodone, selective serotonin reuptake inhibitors (SSRIs), tricyclics, with ritonavir may result in increased plasma concentrations of antidepressants. A dose decrease may be needed for these drugs when co-administered with ritonavir).

No products indexed under this heading.

Penbutolol Sulfate (Co-administration of beta-blockers, such as metoprolol or timolol, with ritonavir, may result in increased plasma concentrations of the β-blocker. Cardiac and neurologic events have been reported with ritonavir when co-administered with β-blockers. A dose decrease may be needed for these drugs when co-administered with ritonavir. In addition, ritonavir prolongs the PR interval in some patients. The impact on the PR interval of co-administration of ritonavir with other drugs that prolong the PR interval (including β-adrenergic blockers) has not been evaluated. As a result, co-administration of ritonavir with these drugs should be undertaken with caution, particularly with those drugs metabolized by CYP3A. Clinical monitoring is recommended).

No products indexed under this heading.

Perphenazine (Co-administration of neuroleptics, such as perphenazine, with ritonavir may result in increased plasma concentrations of neuroleptics. A dose decrease may be needed for these drugs when co-administered with ritonavir).

No products indexed under this heading.

Phenacemide (When co-administering ritonavir with any agent having a narrow therapeutic margin, such as anticonvulsants, special attention is warranted).

No products indexed under this heading.

Phenelzine Sulfate (Co-administration of antidepressants, such as nefazodone, selective serotonin reuptake inhibitors (SSRIs), or tricyclics, with ritonavir may result in increased plasma concentrations of antidepressants. A dose decrease may be needed for these drugs when co-administered with ritonavir).

No products indexed under this heading.

Phenobarbital (When co-administering ritonavir with any agent having a narrow therapeutic margin, such as anticonvulsants, special attention is warranted). Products include:

Donnatal **2711**

Phenobarbital Sodium (When co-administering ritonavir with any agent having a narrow therapeutic margin, such as anticonvulsants, special attention is warranted).

No products indexed under this heading.

Phensuximide (When co-administering ritonavir with any agent having a narrow therapeutic margin, such as anticonvulsants, special attention is warranted).

No products indexed under this heading.

Phenytoin (Co-administration of phenytoin with ritonavir may result in decreased plasma concentrations of phenytoin. Use with caution. A dose increase may be needed for phenytoin when co-administered with ritonavir and therapeutic concentration monitoring is recommended, if available).

No products indexed under this heading.

Phenytoin Sodium (Co-administration of phenytoin with ritonavir may result in decreased plasma concentrations of phenytoin. Use with caution. A dose increase may be needed for phenytoin when co-administered with ritonavir and therapeutic concentration monitoring is recommended, if available). Products include:

Phenytek Capsules **2380**

Pimozide (Co-administration of ritonavir and pimozide is contraindicated due to the potential for serious and/or life-threatening reactions such as cardiac arrhythmias).

No products indexed under this heading.

Pindolol (Co-administration of beta-blockers, such as metoprolol or timolol, with ritonavir, may result in increased plasma concentrations of the β-blocker. Cardiac and neurologic events have been reported with ritonavir when co-administered with β-blockers. A dose decrease may be needed for these drugs when co-administered with ritonavir. In addition, ritonavir prolongs the PR interval in some patients. The impact on the PR interval of co-administration of ritonavir with other drugs that prolong the PR interval (including β-adrenergic blockers) has not been evaluated. As a result, co-administration of ritonavir with these drugs should be undertaken with caution, particularly with those drugs metabolized by CYP3A. Clinical monitoring is recommended).

No products indexed under this heading.

Pioglitazone Hydrochloride (New onset diabetes mellitus, exacerbation of pre-existing diabetes mellitus, and hyperglycemia have been reported during postmarketing surveillance in HIV-infected patients receiving protease inhibitor therapy. Some patients required either initiation or dose adjustments of insulin or oral hypoglycemic agents for treatment of these events). Products include:

ActoPlus **3338**
Actos **3345**
Duetact **3354**

Pravastatin Sodium (Caution should be exercised if HIV protease inhibitors, including ritonavir, are used concurrently with HMG-CoA reductase inhibitors that are also metabolized by the CYP3A4 pathway (eg, atorvastatin or cerivastatin). It is possible that a substantial increase of some HMG-CoA reductase inhibitors may occur. The risk of myopathy including rhabdomyolysis may be increased when HIV protease inhibitors, including ritonavir, are used in combination with HMG-CoA reductase inhibitors).

No products indexed under this heading.

Prednisolone (When co-administering ritonavir with some steroids, it is possible that a substantial increase in the concentrations of some steroids may occur. A dose decrease may be needed for steroids, such as dexamethasone, fluticasone, prednisone, when co-administered with ritonavir).

No products indexed under this heading.

Prednisolone Acetate (When co-administering ritonavir with some steroids, it is possible that a substantial increase in the concentrations of some steroids may occur. A dose decrease may be needed for steroids, such as dexamethasone, fluticasone, prednisone, when co-administered with ritonavir). Products include:

Blephamide .... ⊙**212**, ⊙**214**
Pred Forte .... ⊙**225**
Pred Mild .... ⊙**230**
Pred-G .... ⊙**226**, ⊙**227**

Prednisolone Sodium Phosphate (When co-administering ritonavir with some steroids, it is possible that a substantial increase in the concentrations of some steroids may occur. A dose decrease may be needed for steroids, such as dexamethasone, fluticasone, prednisone, when co-administered with ritonavir).

No products indexed under this heading.

Prednisolone Tebutate (When co-administering ritonavir with some steroids, it is possible that a substantial increase in the concentrations of some steroids may occur. A dose decrease may be needed for steroids, such as dexamethasone, fluticasone, prednisone, when co-administered with ritonavir).

No products indexed under this heading.

Prednisone (When co-administering ritonavir with some steroids, it is possible that a substantial increase in the concentrations of some steroids may occur. A dose decrease may be needed for steroids such as prednisone when co-administered with ritonavir).

No products indexed under this heading.

Prednisone sodium phosphate (When co-administering ritonavir with some steroids, it is possible that a substantial increase in the concentrations of some steroids may occur. A dose decrease may be needed for steroids such as prednisone when co-administered with ritonavir).

No products indexed under this heading.

Primidone (When co-administering ritonavir with any agent having a narrow therapeutic margin, such as anticonvulsants, special attention is warranted).

No products indexed under this heading.

Procainamide Hydrochloride (Co-administration of ritonavir with certain antiarrhythmics may result in potentially serious and/or life-threatening adverse events due to possible effects of ritonavir on the hepatic metabolism of certain drugs. Co-administration of antiarrhythmics, such as disopyramide, lidocaine, mexilitine, with ritonavir may result in increased plasma concentrations of antiarrhythmics. Caution is warranted and therapeutic concentration monitoring is recommended for antiarrhythmics when co-administered with ritonavir, if available).

No products indexed under this heading.

Procarbazine Hydrochloride (Concentrations of vincristine or vinblastine may be increased when co-administered with ritonavir, resulting in the potential for increased adverse events usually associated with these anticancer agents. Consideration should be given to temporarily withholding the ritonavir containing antiretroviral regimen in patients who develop significant hematologic or gastrointestinal side effects when ritonavir is administered concurrently with vincristine or vinblastine. Clinicians should be aware that if the ritonavir containing regimen is withheld for a prolonged period, consideration should be given to altering the regimen to not include a CYP3A or P-gp inhibitor in order to control HIV-1 viral load).

No products indexed under this heading.

Prochlorperazine (Co-administration of neuroleptics, such as perphenazine, risperidone, and thioridazine, with ritonavir may result in inceased plasma concentrations of neuroleptics. A dose decrease may be needed for these drugs when co-administered with ritonavir).

No products indexed under this heading.

Promethazine Hydrochloride (Co-administration of ritonavir with certain nonsedating antihistamines may result in potentially serious and/or life-threatening adverse events due to possible effects of ritonavir on the hepatic metabolism of certain drugs).

No products indexed under this heading.

Propafenone Hydrochloride (Co-administration of ritonavir and propafenone is contraindicated due to potential for serious and/or life threatening reactions such as cardiac arrhythmias). Products include:

Rythmol **1648**
Rythmol SR **1652**

Propofol (Co-administration of ritonavir with certain sedative hypnotics may result in potentially serious and/or life-threatening adverse events due to possible effects of ritonavir on the hepatic metabolism of certain drugs. Co-administration of sedative/hypnotics such as buspirone, clorazepate, diazepam, estazolam, flurazepam, or zolpidem with ritonavir may result in increased plasma concentrations of sedative/hypnotics. A dose decrease may be needed for these drugs when co-administered with ritonavir).

No products indexed under this heading.

Propoxyphene Hydrochloride (A dose decrease may be needed for propoxyphene when co-administered with ritonavir).

No products indexed under this heading.

Propoxyphene Napsylate (A dose decrease may be needed for propoxyphene when co-administered with ritonavir).

No products indexed under this heading.

Propranolol Hydrochloride (Co-administration of ritonavir with certain antiarrhythmics may result in potentially serious and/or life-threatening adverse events due to possible effects of ritonavir on the hepatic metabolism of certain drugs. Co-administration of antiarrhythmics, such as disopyramide,

lidocaine, mexilitine, with ritonavir may result in increased plasma concentrations of antiarrhythmics. Caution is warranted and therapeutic concentration monitoring is recommended for antiarrhythmics when co-administered with ritonavir, if available). Products include:
InnoPran XL ... **1517**

Protriptyline Hydrochloride (Co-administration of antidepressants, such as nefazodone, selective serotonin reuptake inhibitors (SSRIs), or tricyclics, with ritonavir may result in increased plasma concentrations of antidepressants. A dose decrease may be needed for these drugs when co-administered with ritonavir).
No products indexed under this heading.

Pyrilamine Maleate (Co-administration of ritonavir with certain nonsedating antihistamines may result in potentially serious and/or life-threatening adverse events due to possible effects of ritonavir on the hepatic metabolism of certain drugs).
No products indexed under this heading.

Pyrilamine Tannate (Co-administration of ritonavir with certain nonsedating antihistamines may result in potentially serious and/or life-threatening adverse events due to possible effects of ritonavir on the hepatic metabolism of certain drugs).
No products indexed under this heading.

Quazepam (Co-administration of ritonavir with certain sedative hypnotics may result in potentially serious and/or life-threatening adverse events due to possible effects of ritonavir on the hepatic metabolism of certain drugs. Co-administration of sedative/hypnotics such as buspirone, clorazepate, diazepam, estazolam, flurazepam, or zolpidem with ritonavir may result in increased plasma concentrations of sedative/hypnotics. A dose decrease may be needed for these drugs when co-administered with ritonavir).
No products indexed under this heading.

Quetiapine Fumarate (Co-administration of neuroleptics, such as perphenazine, risperidone, and thioridazine, with ritonavir may result in inceased plasma concentrations of neuroleptics. A dose decrease may be needed for these drugs when co-administered with ritonavir). Products include:
Seroquel ... **750**
Seroquel XR ... **759**

Quinidine (Co-administration of ritonavir and quinidine is contraindicated due to potential for serious and/or life threatening reactions such as cardiac arrhythmias).
No products indexed under this heading.

Quinidine Gluconate (Co-administration of ritonavir and quinidine is contraindicated due to potential for serious and/or life threatening reactions such as cardiac arrhythmias).
No products indexed under this heading.

Quinidine Hydrochloride (Co-administration of ritonavir and quinidine is contraindicated due to potential for serious and/or life threatening reactions such as cardiac arrhythmias).
No products indexed under this heading.

Quinidine Polygalacturonate (Co-administration of ritonavir and quinidine is contraindicated due to potential for serious and/or life threatening reactions such as cardiac arrhythmias).
No products indexed under this heading.

Quinidine Sulfate (Co-administration of ritonavir and quinidine is contraindicated due to potential for serious and/or life threatening reactions such as cardiac arrhythmias).
No products indexed under this heading.

Quinine (Co-administration of quinine with ritonavir may result in increased plasma concentrations of quinine. A dose decrease of quinine may be needed when co-administered with ritonavir). Products include:
Hyland's Leg Cramps PM with Quinine ... **3315**

Quinine Sulfate (Co-administration of quinine with ritonavir may result in increased plasma concentrations of quinine. A dose decrease of quinine may be needed when co-administered with ritonavir).
No products indexed under this heading.

Ramelteon (Co-administration of ritonavir with certain sedative hypnotics may result in potentially serious and/or life-threatening adverse events due to possible effects of ritonavir on the hepatic metabolism of certain drugs. Co-administration of sedative/hypnotics such as buspirone, clorazepate, diazepam, estazolam, flurazepam, or zolpidem with ritonavir may result in increased plasma concentrations of sedative/hypnotics. A dose decrease may be needed for these drugs when co-administered with ritonavir). Products include:
Rozerem ... **3366**

Rapamycin (Co-administration of immunosuppressants, such as rapamycin, with ritonavir may result in increased plasma concentrations of immunosuppressants. Therapeutic concentration monitoring is recommended for immunosuppressant agents when co-administered with ritonavir).
No products indexed under this heading.

Remifentanil Hydrochloride (When co-administering ritonavir with some narcotic analgesics which are partially mediated by CYP2D6 metabolism, it is possible that substantial increases in concentrations of these narcotic analgesics may occur, possibly requiring a dosage reduction).
No products indexed under this heading.

Repaglinide (New onset diabetes mellitus, exacerbation of pre-existing diabetes mellitus, and hyperglycemia have been reported during postmarketing surveillance in HIV-infected patients receiving protease inhibitor therapy. Some patients required either initiation or dose adjustments of insulin or oral hypoglycemic agents for treatment of these events).
No products indexed under this heading.

Rifabutin (Co-administration of rifabutin with ritonavir may result in increased plasma concentrations of rifabutin and rifabutin metabolite. Dosage reduction of rifabutin by at least three-quarters of the usual dose of 300 mg/day is recommended (eg, 150 mg every other day or three times a week). Further dosage reduction may be necessary).
No products indexed under this heading.

Rifampin (Co-administration of rifampin with ritonavir may decrease ritonavir concentrations and may lead to loss of virologic response. Alternate antimycobacterial agents, such as rifabutin, should be considered).
No products indexed under this heading.

Risperidone (Co-administration of neuroleptics, such as risperidone, with ritonavir may result in increased plasma concentrations of neuroleptics. A dose decrease may be needed for these drugs when co-administered with ritonavir). Products include:
Risperdal Consta ... **2682**

Rosiglitazone Maleate (New onset diabetes mellitus, exacerbation of pre-existing diabetes mellitus, and hyperglycemia have been reported during post-marketing surveillance in HIV-infected patients receiving protease inhibitor therapy. Some patients required either initiation or dose adjustments of insulin or oral hypoglycemic agents for treatment of these events). Products include:
Avandamet ... **1345**
Avandaryl ... **1356**
Avandia ... **1366**

Rosuvastatin Calcium (Co-administration of rosuvastatin with ritonavir may result in increased plasma concentrations of rosuvastatin. Use the lowest possible dose of rosuvastatin with careful monitoring in combination with ritonavir). Products include:
Crestor ... **736**

Rufinamide (When co-administering ritonavir with any agent having a narrow therapeutic margin, such as anticonvulsants, special attention is warranted). Products include:
Banzel ... **1050**

Saquinavir (Co-administration of saquinavir with reduced doses of ritonavir may result in increased plasma concentrations of saquinavir (increased AUC, increased C_{max}, increased C_{min}). Saquinavir/ritonavir should not be given together with rifampin, due to the risk of severe hepatotoxicity (presenting as increased hepatic transaminases) if the three drugs are given together. In addition, treatment with ritonavir therapy alone or in combination with saquinavir has resulted in substantial increases in the concentration of total triglycerides and cholesterol).
No products indexed under this heading.

Saquinavir Mesylate (Co-administration of saquinavir with reduced doses of ritonavir may result in increased plasma concentrations of saquinavir (increased AUC, increased C_{max}, increased C_{min}). Saquinavir/ritonavir should not be given together with rifampin, due to the risk of severe hepatotoxicity (presenting as increased hepatic transaminases) if the three drugs are given together. In addition, treatment with ritonavir therapy alone or in combination with saquinavir has resulted in substantial increases in the concentration of total triglycerides and cholesterol).
No products indexed under this heading.

Secobarbital Sodium (Co-administration of ritonavir with certain sedative hypnotics may result in potentially serious and/or life-threatening adverse events due to possible effects of ritonavir on the hepatic metabolism of certain drugs. Co-administration of sedative/hypnotics such as buspirone, clorazepate, diazepam, estazolam, flurazepam, or zolpidem with ritonavir may result in increased plasma concentrations of sedative/hypnotics. A dose decrease may be needed for these drugs when co-administered with ritonavir).
No products indexed under this heading.

Selegiline (Co-administration of antidepressants, such as nefazodone, selective serotonin reuptake inhibitors (SSRIs), or tricyclics, with ritonavir may result in increased plasma concentrations of antidepressants. A dose decrease may be needed for these drugs when co-administered with ritonavir). Products include:
Emsam ... **3623**

Selegiline Hydrochloride (Co-administration of antidepressants, such as nefazodone, selective serotonin reuptake inhibitors (SSRIs), or tricyclics, with ritonavir may result in increased plasma concentrations of antidepressants. A dose decrease may be needed for these drugs when co-administered with ritonavir). Products include:
Eldepryl ... **3312**

Sertraline Hydrochloride (Co-administration of antidepressants, such as nefazodone, selective serotonin reuptake inhibitors (SSRIs), tricyclics, with ritonavir may result in increased plasma concentrations of antidepressants. A dose decrease may be needed for these drugs when co-administered with ritonavir).
No products indexed under this heading.

Sildenafil Citrate (Particular caution should be used when prescribing sildenafil in patients receiving ritonavir. Co-administration of ritonavir with sildenafil is expected to substantially increase sildenafil concentrations (11-fold increase in AUC) and may result in an increase in sildenafil-associated adverse events, including hypotension, syncope, visual changes, and prolonged erection. The starting dose should not, in any case, exceed 25 mg in a 48-hour period in patients receiving concomitant ritonavir therapy).
No products indexed under this heading.

Simvastatin (Concomitant use of ritonavir with simvastatin is not recommended. There is the potential for serious reactions, such as risk of myopathy including rhabdomyolysis, with concomitant use). Products include:
Simcor ... **524**
Vytorin 10/10 ... **2303, 3240**
Vytorin 10/20 ... **2303, 3240**
Vytorin 10/40 ... **2303, 3240**
Vytorin 10/80 ... **2303, 3240**
Zocor ... **2289**

Sirolimus (Co-administration of immunosuppressants, such as sirolimus, with ritonavir may result in increased plasma concentrations of immunosuppressants. Therapeutic concentration monitoring is recommended for immunosuppressant agents when co-administered with ritonavir). Products include:
Rapamune ... **3579**

Sitagliptin Phosphate (New onset diabetes mellitus, exacerbation of pre-existing diabetes mellitus, and hyperglycemia have been reported during post-marketing surveillance in HIV-infected patients receiving protease inhibitor therapy. Some patients required either initiation or dose adjustments of insulin or oral hypoglycemic agents for treatment of these events). Products include:
Janumet ... **2188**
Januvia ... **2196**

Sodium Butabarbital (Co-administration of ritonavir with certain sedative hypnotics may result in potentially serious and/or life-threatening adverse events due to possible effects of ritonavir on the hepatic metabolism of certain drugs. Co-administration of sedative/hypnotics such as buspirone, clorazepate, diazepam, estazolam, flurazepam, or zolpidem with ritonavir may result in increased plasma concentrations of sedative/hypnotics. A dose decrease may be needed for these drugs when co-administered with ritonavir).
No products indexed under this heading.

Sotalol Hydrochloride (Co-administration of ritonavir with certain antiarrhythmics may result in potentially serious and/or life-threatening adverse events due to possible effects of ritonavir on the hepatic metabolism of certain drugs. Co-administration of antiarrhythmics, such as disopyramide, lidocaine, mexilitine, with ritonavir may result in increased plasma concentrations of antiarrhythmics. Caution is warranted and therapeutic concentration monitoring is recommended for antiarrhythmics when co-administered with ritonavir, if available).
No products indexed under this heading.

Streptozocin (Concentrations of vincristine or vinblastine may be increased

when co-administered with ritonavir, resulting in the potential for increased adverse events usually associated with these anticancer agents. Consideration should be given to temporarily withholding the ritonavir containing antiretroviral regimen in patients who develop significant hematologic or gastrointestinal side effects when ritonavir is administered concurrently with vincristine or vinblastine. Clinicians should be aware that if the ritonavir containing regimen is withheld for a prolonged period, consideration should be given to altering the regimen to not include a CYP3A or P-gp inhibitor in order to control HIV-1 viral load).
No products indexed under this heading.

Sufentanil Citrate (When co-administering ritonavir with some narcotic analgesics which are partially mediated by CYP2D6 metabolism, it is possible that substantial increases in concentrations of these narcotic analgesics may occur, possibly requiring a dosage reduction).
No products indexed under this heading.

Sulfamethoxazole (Co-administration of sulfamethoxazole with ritonavir resulted in a decrease in AUC of sulfamethoxazole by 20%).
No products indexed under this heading.

Tacrolimus (Co-administration of immunosuppressants, such as tacrolimus, with ritonavir may result in increased plasma concentrations of immunosuppressants. Therapeutic concentration monitoring is recommended for immunosuppressant agents when co-administered with ritonavir).
Products include:
Prograf Capsules 677
Prograf Injection 677
Protopic 685

Tadalafil (Co-administration of tadalafil with ritonavir may increase the concentrations of tadalafil. Concomitant use resulted in an increase in AUC of tadalafil by 124%. Use tadalafil with caution at reduced doses of no more than 10 mg every 72 hours with increased monitoring for adverse events). Products include:
Adcirca 3461
Cialis 1861

Tamoxifen Citrate (Concentrations of vincristine or vinblastine may be increased when co-administered with ritonavir, resulting in the potential for increased adverse events usually associated with these anticancer agents. Consideration should be given to temporarily withholding the ritonavir containing antiretroviral regimen in patients who develop significant hematologic or gastrointestinal side effects when ritonavir is administered concurrently with vincristine or vinblastine. Clinicians should be aware that if the ritonavir containing regimen is withheld for a prolonged period, consideration should be given to altering the regimen to not include a CYP3A or P-gp inhibitor in order to control HIV-1 viral load).
No products indexed under this heading.

Temazepam (Co-administration of ritonavir with certain sedative hypnotics may result in potentially serious and/or life-threatening adverse events due to possible effects of ritonavir on the hepatic metabolism of certain drugs. Co-administration of sedative/hypnotics such as buspirone, clorazepate, diazepam, estazolam, flurazepam, or zolpidem with ritonavir may result in increased plasma concentrations of sedative/hypnotics. A dose decrease may be needed for these drugs when co-administered with ritonavir).
No products indexed under this heading.

Teniposide (Concentrations of vincristine or vinblastine may be increased when co-administered with ritonavir, resulting in the potential for increased adverse events usually associated with these anticancer agents. Consideration should be given to temporarily withholding the ritonavir containing antiretroviral regimen in patients who develop significant hematologic or gastrointestinal side effects when ritonavir is administered concurrently with vincristine or vinblastine. Clinicians should be aware that if the ritonavir containing regimen is withheld for a prolonged period, consideration should be given to altering the regimen to not include a CYP3A or P-gp inhibitor in order to control HIV-1 viral load).
No products indexed under this heading.

Terfenadine (Co-administration of ritonavir and terfenadine is contraindicated due to potential for serious and/or life-threatening reactions such as cardiac arrhythmias).
No products indexed under this heading.

Testosterone (Ritonavir is an inhibitor of cytochrome P450 3A (CYP3A) both *in vitro* and *in vivo*. Ritonavir also inhibits CYP2D6 *in vitro*, but to a lesser extent than CYP3A. Co-administration of ritonavir and drugs primarily metabolized by CYP3A or CYP2D6 may result in increased plasma concentrations of other drugs that could increase or prolong its therapeutic and adverse effects. A dosage reduction of the other drug may be necessary). Products include:
AndroGel 3456

Testosterone Cypionate (Ritonavir is an inhibitor of cytochrome P450 3A (CYP3A) both *in vitro* and *in vivo*. Ritonavir also inhibits CYP2D6 *in vitro*, but to a lesser extent than CYP3A. Co-administration of ritonavir and drugs primarily metabolized by CYP3A or CYP2D6 may result in increased plasma concentrations of other drugs that could increase or prolong its therapeutic and adverse effects. A dosage reduction of the other drug may be necessary).
No products indexed under this heading.

Testosterone Enanthate (Ritonavir is an inhibitor of cytochrome P450 3A (CYP3A) both *in vitro* and *in vivo*. Ritonavir also inhibits CYP2D6 *in vitro*, but to a lesser extent than CYP3A. Co-administration of ritonavir and drugs primarily metabolized by CYP3A or CYP2D6 may result in increased plasma concentrations of other drugs that could increase or prolong its therapeutic and adverse effects. A dosage reduction of the other drug may be necessary). Products include:
Delatestryl 1102

Testosterone Propionate (Ritonavir is an inhibitor of cytochrome P450 3A (CYP3A) both *in vitro* and *in vivo*. Ritonavir also inhibits CYP2D6 *in vitro*, but to a lesser extent than CYP3A. Co-administration of ritonavir and drugs primarily metabolized by CYP3A or CYP2D6 may result in increased plasma concentrations of other drugs that could increase or prolong its therapeutic and adverse effects. A dosage reduction of the other drug may be necessary).
No products indexed under this heading.

Theophylline (Co-administration of theophylline with ritonavir may result in decreased plasma concentrations of theophylline. Increased dosage of theophylline may be required; therapeutic monitoring should be considered).
No products indexed under this heading.

Theophylline Anhydrous (Co-administration of theophylline with ritonavir may result in decreased plasma concentrations of theophylline. Increased dosage of theophylline may be required; therapeutic monitoring should be considered). Products include:
Uniphyl 2817

Theophylline Calcium Salicylate (Co-administration of theophylline with ritonavir may result in decreased plasma concentrations of theophylline. Increased dosage of theophylline may be required; therapeutic monitoring should be considered).
No products indexed under this heading.

Theophylline Dihydroxypropyl (Glyceryl) (Co-administration of theophylline with ritonavir may result in decreased plasma concentrations of theophylline. Increased dosage of theophylline may be required; therapeutic monitoring should be considered).
No products indexed under this heading.

Theophylline Ethylenediamine (Co-administration of theophylline with ritonavir may result in decreased plasma concentrations of theophylline. Increased dosage of theophylline may be required; therapeutic monitoring should be considered).
No products indexed under this heading.

Theophylline Sodium Glycinate (Co-administration of theophylline with ritonavir may result in decreased plasma concentrations of theophylline. Increased dosage of theophylline may be required; therapeutic monitoring should be considered).
No products indexed under this heading.

Thioguanine (Concentrations of vincristine or vinblastine may be increased when co-administered with ritonavir, resulting in the potential for increased adverse events usually associated with these anticancer agents. Consideration should be given to temporarily withholding the ritonavir containing antiretroviral regimen in patients who develop significant hematologic or gastrointestinal side effects when ritonavir is administered concurrently with vincristine or vinblastine. Clinicians should be aware that if the ritonavir containing regimen is withheld for a prolonged period, consideration should be given to altering the regimen to not include a CYP3A or P-gp inhibitor in order to control HIV-1 viral load). Products include:
Tabloid 1664

Thioridazine (Co-administration of neuroleptics, such as thioridazine, with ritonavir may result in inceased plasma concentrations of neuroleptics. A dose decrease may be needed for these drugs when co-administered with ritonavir).
No products indexed under this heading.

Thioridazine Hydrochloride (Co-administration of neuroleptics, such as thioridazine, with ritonavir may result in inceased plasma concentrations of neuroleptics. A dose decrease may be needed for these drugs when co-administered with ritonavir). Products include:
Thioridazine Hydrochloride 2384

Thiotepa (Concentrations of vincristine or vinblastine may be increased when co-administered with ritonavir, resulting in the potential for increased adverse events usually associated with these anticancer agents. Consideration should be given to temporarily withholding the ritonavir containing antiretroviral regimen in patients who develop significant hematologic or gastrointestinal side effects when ritonavir is administered concurrently with vincristine or vinblastine. Clinicians should be aware that if the ritonavir containing regimen is withheld for a prolonged period, consideration should be given to altering the regimen to not include a CYP3A or P-gp inhibitor in order to control HIV-1 viral load).
No products indexed under this heading.

Thiothixene (Co-administration of neuroleptics, such as perphenazine, risperidone, and thioridazine, with ritonavir may result in inceased plasma concentrations of neuroleptics. A dose decrease may be needed for these drugs when co-administered with ritonavir). Products include:
Thiothixene 2386

Tiagabine Hydrochloride (When co-administering ritonavir with any agent having a narrow therapeutic margin, such as anticonvulsants, special attention is warranted). Products include:
Gabitril 972

Timolol Hemihydrate (Co-administration of β-blockers, such as timolol, with ritonavir, may result in increased plasma concentrations of the β-blocker. Cardiac and neurologic events have been reported with ritonavir when co-administered with β-blockers. A dose decrease may be needed for these drugs when co-administered with ritonavir. In addition, ritonavir prolongs the PR interval in some patients. The impact on the PR interval of co-administration of ritonavir with other drugs that prolong the PR interval (including β-adrenergic blockers) has not been evaluated. As a result, co-administration of ritonavir with these drugs should be undertaken with caution, particularly with those drugs metabolized by CYP3A. Clinical monitoring is recommended). Products include:
Betimol 3490

Timolol Maleate (Co-administration of β-blockers, such as timolol, with ritonavir, may result in increased plasma concentrations of the β-blocker. Cardiac and neurologic events have been reported with ritonavir when co-administered with β-blockers. A dose decrease may be needed for these drugs when co-administered with ritonavir. In addition, ritonavir prolongs the PR interval in some patients. The impact on the PR interval of co-administration of ritonavir with other drugs that prolong the PR interval (including β-adrenergic blockers) has not been evaluated. As a result, co-administration of ritonavir with these drugs should be undertaken with caution, particularly with those drugs metabolized by CYP3A. Clinical monitoring is recommended). Products include:
Combigan 601
Dorzolamide Hydrochloride/Timolol Maleate Ophthalmic Solution .... ⊙ 243
Timoptic in Ocudose .... ⊙ 231

Tinzaparin Sodium (When co-administering ritonavir with any agent having a narrow therapeutic margin, such as anticoagulants, special attention is warranted).
No products indexed under this heading.

Tipranavir (Co-administration of tipranavir with reduced doses of ritonavir may result in increased plasma concentrations of tipranavir (an increase in C_{max}, an increase in AUC, and an increase in C_{min}). Tipranavir co-administered with 200 mg of ritonavir has been associated with reports of clinical hepatitis and hepatic decompensation including some fatalities. Extra vigilance is warranted in patients with chronic hepatitis B or hepatitis C co-infection, as these patients have an increased risk of hepatotoxicity).
No products indexed under this heading.

Tocainide Hydrochloride (Co-administration of ritonavir with certain antiarrhythmics may result in potentially serious and/or life-threatening adverse

IMPORTANT NOTE: Always consult each drug listing in the patient's regimen for possible interactions.

Norvir **Interactions Index** 1242

events due to possible effects of ritonavir on the hepatic metabolism of certain drugs. Co-administration of antiarrhythmics, such as disopyramide, lidocaine, mexilitine, with ritonavir may result in increased plasma concentrations of antiarrhythmics. Caution is warranted and therapeutic concentration monitoring is recommended for antiarrhythmics when co-administered with ritonavir, if available).
No products indexed under this heading.

Tolazamide (New onset diabetes mellitus, exacerbation of pre-existing diabetes mellitus, and hyperglycemia have been reported during postmarketing surveillance in HIV-infected patients receiving protease inhibitor therapy. Some patients required either initiation or dose adjustments of insulin or oral hypoglycemic agents for treatment of these events).
No products indexed under this heading.

Tolbutamide (New onset diabetes mellitus, exacerbation of pre-existing diabetes mellitus, and hyperglycemia have been reported during postmarketing surveillance in HIV-infected patients receiving protease inhibitor therapy. Some patients required either initiation or dose adjustments of insulin or oral hypoglycemic agents for treatment of these events).
No products indexed under this heading.

Tolterodine Tartrate (Ritonavir is an inhibitor of cytochrome P450 3A (CYP3A) both *in vitro* and *in vivo*. Ritonavir also inhibits CYP2D6 *in vitro*, but to a lesser extent than CYP3A. Co-administration of ritonavir and drugs primarily metabolized by CYP3A or CYP2D6 may result in increased plasma concentrations of other drugs that could increase or prolong its therapeutic and adverse effects. A dosage reduction of the other drug may be necessary).
No products indexed under this heading.

Topiramate (When co-administering ritonavir with any agent having a narrow therapeutic margin, such as anticonvulsants, special attention is warranted).
No products indexed under this heading.

Topotecan Hydrochloride (Concentrations of vincristine or vinblastine may be increased when co-administered with ritonavir, resulting in the potential for increased adverse events usually associated with these anticancer agents. Consideration should be given to temporarily withholding the ritonavir containing antiretroviral regimen in patients who develop significant hematologic or gastrointestinal side effects when ritonavir is administered concurrently with vincristine or vinblastine. Clinicians should be aware that if the ritonavir containing regimen is withheld for a prolonged period, consideration should be given to altering the regimen to not include a CYP3A or P-gp inhibitor in order to control HIV-1 viral load). Products include:
Hycamtin 1491
Hycamtin Capsules 1488

Toremifene Citrate (Concentrations of vincristine or vinblastine may be increased when co-administered with ritonavir, resulting in the potential for increased adverse events usually associated with these anticancer agents. Consideration should be given to temporarily withholding the ritonavir containing antiretroviral regimen in patients who develop significant hematologic or gastrointestinal side effects when ritonavir is administered concurrently with vincristine or vinblastine. Clinicians should be aware that if the ritonavir containing regimen is withheld for a prolonged period, consideration should be given to altering the regimen to not include a CYP3A or P-gp inhibitor in order to control HIV-1 viral load).
No products indexed under this heading.

Tramadol Hydrochloride (A dose decrease may be needed for tramadol when co-administered with ritonavir). Products include:
Ryzolt 2813
Ultram ER 2693

Tranylcypromine Sulfate (Co-administration of antidepressants, such as nefazodone, selective serotonin reuptake inhibitors (SSRIs), or tricyclics, with ritonavir may result in increased plasma concentrations of antidepressants. A dose decrease may be needed for these drugs when co-administered with ritonavir). Products include:
Parnate 1584

Trazodone Hydrochloride (Concomitant use of trazodone and ritonavir increases plasma concentrations of trazodone. Adverse events of nausea, dizziness, hypotension and syncope have been observed following co-administration of trazodone and ritonavir. If trazodone is used with a CYP3A4 inhibitor such as ritonavir, the combination should be used with caution and a lower dose of trazodone should be considered).
No products indexed under this heading.

Triamcinolone (When co-administering ritonavir with some steroids, it is possible that a substantial increase in the concentrations of some steroids may occur. A dose decrease may be needed for steroids, such as dexamethasone, fluticasone, prednisone, when co-administered with ritonavir).
No products indexed under this heading.

Triamcinolone Acetonide (When co-administering ritonavir with some steroids, it is possible that a substantial increase in the concentrations of some steroids may occur. A dose decrease may be needed for steroids, such as dexamethasone, fluticasone, prednisone, when co-administered with ritonavir). Products include:
Azmacort 408
Nasacort AQ 3019

Triamcinolone Diacetate (When co-administering ritonavir with some steroids, it is possible that a substantial increase in the concentrations of some steroids may occur. A dose decrease may be needed for steroids, such as dexamethasone, fluticasone, prednisone, when co-administered with ritonavir).
No products indexed under this heading.

Triamcinolone Hexacetonide (When co-administering ritonavir with some steroids, it is possible that a substantial increase in the concentrations of some steroids may occur. A dose decrease may be needed for steroids, such as dexamethasone, fluticasone, prednisone, when co-administered with ritonavir).
No products indexed under this heading.

Triazolam (Co-administration of ritonavir and triazolam is contraindicated due to potential for serious and/or life-threatening reactions such as prolonged or increased sedation or respiratory depression).
No products indexed under this heading.

Trifluoperazine Hydrochloride (Co-administration of neuroleptics, such as perphenazine, risperidone, and thioridazine, with ritonavir may result in inceased plasma concentrations of neuroleptics. A dose decrease may be needed for these drugs when co-administered with ritonavir).
No products indexed under this heading.

Trimeprazine Tartrate (Co-administration of ritonavir with certain nonsedating antihistamines may result in potentially serious and/or life-threatening adverse events due to possible effects of ritonavir on the hepatic metabolism of certain drugs).
No products indexed under this heading.

Trimethadione (When co-administering ritonavir with any agent having a narrow therapeutic margin, such as anticonvulsants, special attention is warranted).
No products indexed under this heading.

Trimethoprim (Co-administration of trimethoprim with ritonavir resulted in an increase in AUC of trimethoprim by 20%).
No products indexed under this heading.

Trimethoprim Hydrochloride (Co-administration of trimethoprim with ritonavir resulted in an increase in AUC of trimethoprim by 20%).
No products indexed under this heading.

Trimethoprim Sulfate (Co-administration of trimethoprim with ritonavir resulted in an increase in AUC of trimethoprim by 20%).
No products indexed under this heading.

Trimipramine Maleate (Co-administration of antidepressants, such as nefazodone, selective serotonin reuptake inhibitors (SSRIs), or tricyclics, with ritonavir may result in increased plasma concentrations of antidepressants. A dose decrease may be needed for these drugs when co-administered with ritonavir).
No products indexed under this heading.

Tripelennamine Hydrochloride (Co-administration of ritonavir with certain nonsedating antihistamines may result in potentially serious and/or life-threatening adverse events due to possible effects of ritonavir on the hepatic metabolism of certain drugs).
No products indexed under this heading.

Triprolidine Hydrochloride (Co-administration of ritonavir with certain nonsedating antihistamines may result in potentially serious and/or life-threatening adverse events due to possible effects of ritonavir on the hepatic metabolism of certain drugs).
No products indexed under this heading.

Troglitazone (New onset diabetes mellitus, exacerbation of pre-existing diabetes mellitus, and hyperglycemia have been reported during postmarketing surveillance in HIV-infected patients receiving protease inhibitor therapy. Some patients required either initiation or dose adjustments of insulin or oral hypoglycemic agents for treatment of these events).
No products indexed under this heading.

Valproate Sodium (When co-administering ritonavir with any agent having a narrow therapeutic margin, such as anticonvulsants, special attention is warranted).
No products indexed under this heading.

Valproic Acid (When co-administering ritonavir with any agent having a narrow therapeutic margin, such as anticonvulsants, special attention is warranted).
No products indexed under this heading.

Valrubicin (Concentrations of vincristine or vinblastine may be increased when co-administered with ritonavir, resulting in the potential for increased adverse events usually associated with these anticancer agents. Consideration should be given to temporarily withholding the ritonavir containing antiretroviral regimen in patients who develop significant hematologic or gastrointestinal side effects when ritonavir is administered concurrently with vincristine or vinblastine. Clinicians should be aware that if the ritonavir containing regimen is withheld for a prolonged period, consideration should be given to altering the regimen to not include a CYP3A or P-gp inhibitor in order to control HIV-1 viral load). Products include:
Valstar 1131

Vardenafil Hydrochloride (Co-administration of vardenafil with ritonavir may result in increased plasma concentrations of vardenafil. Use vardenafil with caution at reduced doses of no more than 2.5 mg every 72 hours with increased monitoring for adverse events). Products include:
Levitra 3157

Venlafaxine Hydrochloride (Co-administration of antidepressants, such as nefazodone, selective serotonin reuptake inhibitors (SSRIs), or tricyclics, with ritonavir may result in increased plasma concentrations of antidepressants. A dose decrease may be needed for these drugs when co-administered with ritonavir). Products include:
Effexor XR 3504
Venlafaxine Hydrochloride Tablets ... 2388

Verapamil Hydrochloride (Co-administration of calcium channel blockers, such as verapamil, with ritonavir may result in increased plasma concentrations of calcium channel blockers. A dose decrease may be needed for these drugs when co-administered with ritonavir. In addition, ritonavir prolongs the PR interval in some patients. The impact on the PR interval of co-administration of ritonavir with other drugs that prolong the PR interval (including calcium channel blockers) has not been evaluated. Co-administration of ritonavir with these drugs should be undertaken with caution, particularly with those drugs metabolized by CYP3A. Clinical monitoring is recommended). Products include:
Tarka 534

Vinblastine Sulfate (Concentrations of vincristine or vinblastine may be increased when co-administered with ritonavir resulting in the potential for increased adverse events usually associated with these anticancer agents. Consideration should be given to temporarily withholding the ritonavir containing antiretroviral regimen in patients who develop significant hematologic or gastrointestinal side effects when ritonavir is administered concurrently with vincristine or vinblastine. Clinicians should be aware that if the ritonavir containing regimen is withheld for a prolonged period, consideration should be given to altering the regimen to not include a CYP3A or P-gp inhibitor in order to control HIV-1 viral load).
No products indexed under this heading.

Vincristine Sulfate (Concentrations of vincristine or vinblastine may be increased when co-administered with ritonavir resulting in the potential for increased adverse events usually associated with these anticancer agents. Consideration should be given to temporarily withholding the ritonavir containing antiretroviral regimen in patients who develop significant hematologic or gastrointestinal side effects when ritonavir is administered concurrently with vincristine or vinblastine. Clinicians should be aware that if the ritonavir containing regimen is withheld for a prolonged period, consideration should be given to altering the regimen to not include a CYP3A or P-gp inhibitor in order to control HIV-1 viral load).
No products indexed under this heading.

Vinorelbine Tartrate (Concentrations of vincristine or vinblastine may be increased when co-administered with ritonavir, resulting in the potential for increased adverse events usually associated with these anticancer agents.

Consideration should be given to temporarily withholding the ritonavir containing antiretroviral regimen in patients who develop significant hematologic or gastrointestinal side effects when ritonavir is administered concurrently with vincristine or vinblastine. Clinicians should be aware that if the ritonavir containing regimen is withheld for a prolonged period, consideration should be given to altering the regimen to not include a CYP3A or P-gp inhibitor in order to control HIV-1 viral load).
   No products indexed under this heading.

Voriconazole (Co-administration of ritonavir and voriconazole is contraindicated due to significant decreases in voriconazole plasma concentrations and may lead to loss of antifungal response).
   No products indexed under this heading.

Warfarin Sodium (Co-administration of warfarin with ritonavir may result in decreased plasma concentrations of warfarin. Initial frequent monitoring of the INR during ritonavir and warfarin co-administration is indicated).
   No products indexed under this heading.

Zaleplon (Co-administration of ritonavir with certain sedative hypnotics may result in potentially serious and/or life-threatening adverse events due to possible effects of ritonavir on the hepatic metabolism of certain drugs. Co-administration of sedative/hypnotics such as buspirone, clorazepate, diazepam, estazolam, flurazepam, or zolpidem with ritonavir may result in increased plasma concentrations of sedative/hypnotics. A dose decrease may be needed for these drugs when co-administered with ritonavir).
   No products indexed under this heading.

Zidovudine (Co-administration of ritonavir with zidovudine led to a decrease in AUC and C_{max} of zidovudine by 25% and 27%, respectively).
Products include:
   Combivir 1404
   Retrovir 1634
   Retrovir IV 1640
   Trizivir 1688

Ziprasidone Hydrochloride (Co-administration of neuroleptics, such as perphenazine, risperidone, and thioridazine, with ritonavir may result in inceased plasma concentrations of neuroleptics. A dose decrease may be needed for these drugs when co-administered with ritonavir). Products include:
   Geodon 2723

Zolpidem Tartrate (Co-administration of sedative/hypnotics, such as zolpidem, with ritonavir may result in increased plasma concentrations of sedative/hypnotics. A dose decrease may be needed for these drugs when co-administered with ritonavir). Products include:
   Ambien 2920
   Ambien CR 2925

Zonisamide (When co-administering ritonavir with any agent having a narrow therapeutic margin, such as anticonvulsants, special attention is warranted). Products include:
   Zonegran 1081

Food Interactions

Food, unspecified (When the oral solution was given under non-fasting conditions, peak ritonavir concentrations decreased 23% and the extent of absorption decreased 7% relative to fasting conditions. Relative to fasting conditions, the extent of absorption of ritonavir from the soft gelatin capsule formulation was 13% higher when administered with a meal).

Meal, unspecified (When the oral solution was given under non-fasting conditions, peak ritonavir concentrations decreased 23% and the extent of absorption decreased 7% relative to fasting conditions. Relative to fasting conditions, the extent of absorption of ritonavir from the soft gelatin capsule formulation was 13% higher when administered with a meal).

NORWEGIAN COD LIVER OIL

(ALA (Alpha-Linolenic Acid), Cod Liver Oil, Docosahexaenoic Acid (DHA), Eicosapentaenoic Acid (EPA), Omega-3 Acids, Vitamin A, Vitamin D, Vitamin E) 919
None cited in PDR database.

NOVANTRONE FOR INJECTION CONCENTRATE

(Mitoxantrone Hydrochloride) 1088
May interact with antineoplastics, and certain other agents. Compounds in these categories include:

Altretamine (Topoisomerase II inhibitors, including mitoxantrone, in combination with other antineoplastic agents, have been associated with the development of acute leukemia). Products include:
   Hexalen 1066

Anastrozole (Topoisomerase II inhibitors, including mitoxantrone, in combination with other antineoplastic agents, have been associated with the development of acute leukemia).
   No products indexed under this heading.

Asparaginase (Topoisomerase II inhibitors, including mitoxantrone, in combination with other antineoplastic agents, have been associated with the development of acute leukemia). Products include:
   Elspar 2005, 2122

Bicalutamide (Topoisomerase II inhibitors, including mitoxantrone, in combination with other antineoplastic agents, have been associated with the development of acute leukemia).
   No products indexed under this heading.

Bleomycin Sulfate (Topoisomerase II inhibitors, including mitoxantrone, in combination with other antineoplastic agents, have been associated with the development of acute leukemia).
   No products indexed under this heading.

Busulfan (Topoisomerase II inhibitors, including mitoxantrone, in combination with other antineoplastic agents, have been associated with the development of acute leukemia). Products include:
   Myleran 1581

Carboplatin (Topoisomerase II inhibitors, including mitoxantrone, in combination with other antineoplastic agents, have been associated with the development of acute leukemia).
   No products indexed under this heading.

Carmustine (BCNU) (Topoisomerase II inhibitors, including mitoxantrone, in combination with other antineoplastic agents, have been associated with the development of acute leukemia).
   No products indexed under this heading.

Chlorambucil (Topoisomerase II inhibitors, including mitoxantrone, in combination with other antineoplastic agents, have been associated with the development of acute leukemia). Products include:
   Leukeran 1557

Cisplatin (Topoisomerase II inhibitors, including mitoxantrone, in combination with other antineoplastic agents, have been associated with the development of acute leukemia).
   No products indexed under this heading.

Cyclophosphamide (Topoisomerase II inhibitors, including mitoxantrone, in combination with other antineoplastic agents, have been associated with the development of acute leukemia).
   No products indexed under this heading.

Cytarabine (In first line comparative trials of mitoxantrone with cytarabine versus daunorubicin with cytarabine in adult patients with previously untreated ANLL, therapy was associated with congestive heart failure in 6.5% of patients on each arm).
   No products indexed under this heading.

Cytarabine Liposome (In first line comparative trials of mitoxantrone with cytarabine versus daunorubicin with cytarabine in adult patients with previously untreated ANLL, therapy was associated with congestive heart failure in 6.5% of patients on each arm).
   No products indexed under this heading.

Dacarbazine (Topoisomerase II inhibitors, including mitoxantrone, in combination with other antineoplastic agents, have been associated with the development of acute leukemia).
   No products indexed under this heading.

Daunorubicin Citrate (Topoisomerase II inhibitors, including mitoxantrone, in combination with other antineoplastic agents, have been associated with the development of acute leukemia).
   No products indexed under this heading.

Daunorubicin Hydrochloride (Topoisomerase II inhibitors, including mitoxantrone, in combination with other antineoplastic agents, have been associated with the development of acute leukemia).
   No products indexed under this heading.

Denileukin Diftitox (Topoisomerase II inhibitors, including mitoxantrone, in combination with other antineoplastic agents, have been associated with the development of acute leukemia). Products include:
   Ontak 1068

Docetaxel (Topoisomerase II inhibitors, including mitoxantrone, in combination with other antineoplastic agents, have been associated with the development of acute leukemia). Products include:
   Taxotere 3035

Doxorubicin Hydrochloride (Topoisomerase II inhibitors, including mitoxantrone, in combination with other antineoplastic agents, have been associated with the development of acute leukemia).
   No products indexed under this heading.

Epirubicin Hydrochloride (Topoisomerase II inhibitors, including mitoxantrone, in combination with other antineoplastic agents, have been associated with the development of acute leukemia).
   No products indexed under this heading.

Estramustine Phosphate Sodium (Topoisomerase II inhibitors, including mitoxantrone, in combination with other antineoplastic agents, have been associated with the development of acute leukemia).
   No products indexed under this heading.

Etoposide (Topoisomerase II inhibitors, including mitoxantrone, in combination with other antineoplastic agents, have been associated with the development of acute leukemia).
   No products indexed under this heading.

Exemestane (Topoisomerase II inhibitors, including mitoxantrone, in combination with other antineoplastic agents, have been associated with the development of acute leukemia). Products include:
   Aromasin 2758

Floxuridine (Topoisomerase II inhibitors, including mitoxantrone, in combination with other antineoplastic agents, have been associated with the development of acute leukemia).
   No products indexed under this heading.

Fluorouracil (Topoisomerase II inhibitors, including mitoxantrone, in combination with other antineoplastic agents, have been associated with the development of acute leukemia). Products include:
   Carac 2966

Flutamide (Topoisomerase II inhibitors, including mitoxantrone, in combination with other antineoplastic agents, have been associated with the development of acute leukemia).
   No products indexed under this heading.

Gemcitabine Hydrochloride (Topoisomerase II inhibitors, including mitoxantrone, in combination with other antineoplastic agents, have been associated with the development of acute leukemia). Products include:
   Gemzar 1900

Hydroxyurea (Topoisomerase II inhibitors, including mitoxantrone, in combination with other antineoplastic agents, have been associated with the development of acute leukemia).
   No products indexed under this heading.

Idarubicin Hydrochloride (Topoisomerase II inhibitors, including mitoxantrone, in combination with other antineoplastic agents, have been associated with the development of acute leukemia).
   No products indexed under this heading.

Ifosfamide (Topoisomerase II inhibitors, including mitoxantrone, in combination with other antineoplastic agents, have been associated with the development of acute leukemia).
   No products indexed under this heading.

Interferon alfa-2a, Recombinant (Topoisomerase II inhibitors, including mitoxantrone, in combination with other antineoplastic agents, have been associated with the development of acute leukemia).
   No products indexed under this heading.

Interferon alfa-2b, Recombinant (Topoisomerase II inhibitors, including mitoxantrone, in combination with other antineoplastic agents, have been associated with the development of acute leukemia). Products include:
   Intron A 3140

Irinotecan Hydrochloride (Topoisomerase II inhibitors, including mitoxantrone, in combination with other antineoplastic agents, have been associated with the development of acute leukemia).
   No products indexed under this heading.

Levamisole Hydrochloride (Topoisomerase II inhibitors, including mitoxantrone, in combination with other antineoplastic agents, have been associated with the development of acute leukemia).
   No products indexed under this heading.

Lomustine (CCNU) (Topoisomerase II inhibitors, including mitoxantrone, in combination with other antineoplastic agents, have been associated with the development of acute leukemia).
   No products indexed under this heading.

Mechlorethamine Hydrochloride (Topoisomerase II inhibitors, including mitoxantrone, in combination with other antineoplastic agents, have been associated with the development of acute leukemia). Products include:
   Mustargen 2010

Megestrol Acetate (Topoisomerase II inhibitors, including mitoxantrone, in combination with other antineoplastic

agents, have been associated with the development of acute leukemia). Products include:
Megace ES 2698

Melphalan (Topoisomerase II inhibitors, including mitoxantrone, in combination with other antineoplastic agents, have been associated with the development of acute leukemia). Products include:
Alkeran 1302

Mercaptopurine (Topoisomerase II inhibitors, including mitoxantrone, in combination with other antineoplastic agents, have been associated with the development of acute leukemia).
No products indexed under this heading.

Methotrexate (Topoisomerase II inhibitors, including mitoxantrone, in combination with other antineoplastic agents, have been associated with the development of acute leukemia).
No products indexed under this heading.

Methotrexate Sodium (Topoisomerase II inhibitors, including mitoxantrone, in combination with other antineoplastic agents, have been associated with the development of acute leukemia).
No products indexed under this heading.

Mitomycin (Mitomycin-C) (Topoisomerase II inhibitors, including mitoxantrone, in combination with other antineoplastic agents, have been associated with the development of acute leukemia).
No products indexed under this heading.

Mitotane (Topoisomerase II inhibitors, including mitoxantrone, in combination with other antineoplastic agents, have been associated with the development of acute leukemia).
No products indexed under this heading.

Oxaliplatin (Topoisomerase II inhibitors, including mitoxantrone, in combination with other antineoplastic agents, have been associated with the development of acute leukemia). Products include:
Eloxatin 2975

Paclitaxel (Topoisomerase II inhibitors, including mitoxantrone, in combination with other antineoplastic agents, have been associated with the development of acute leukemia).
No products indexed under this heading.

Prednisone (In a ramdomized study where dose escalation was required for neutrophil counts greater than 1000/mm^3, grade 4 neutropenia (ANC < 500 /mm^3) was observed in 54% of patients treated with mitoxantrone with low-dose prednisone).
No products indexed under this heading.

Prednisone sodium phosphate (In a ramdomized study where dose escalation was required for neutrophil counts greater than 1000/mm^3, grade 4 neutropenia (ANC < 500 /mm^3) was observed in 54% of patients treated with mitoxantrone with low-dose prednisone).
No products indexed under this heading.

Procarbazine Hydrochloride (Topoisomerase II inhibitors, including mitoxantrone, in combination with other antineoplastic agents, have been associated with the development of acute leukemia).
No products indexed under this heading.

Radiation (Patients with breast cancer who received mitoxantrone concomitantly with other cytotoxic agents and radiotherapy, the cumulative risk of developing treatment-related acute myelogenous leukemia was estimated as 1.1% and 1.6% at 5 and 10 years, respectively. The second largest report involved 449 patients with breast cancer treated with mitoxantrone, usually in combination with radiotherapy and/or other cytotoxic agents).
No products indexed under this heading.

Streptozocin (Topoisomerase II inhibitors, including mitoxantrone, in combination with other antineoplastic agents, have been associated with the development of acute leukemia).
No products indexed under this heading.

Tamoxifen Citrate (Topoisomerase II inhibitors, including mitoxantrone, in combination with other antineoplastic agents, have been associated with the development of acute leukemia).
No products indexed under this heading.

Teniposide (Topoisomerase II inhibitors, including mitoxantrone, in combination with other antineoplastic agents, have been associated with the development of acute leukemia).
No products indexed under this heading.

Thioguanine (Topoisomerase II inhibitors, including mitoxantrone, in combination with other antineoplastic agents, have been associated with the development of acute leukemia). Products include:
Tabloid 1664

Thiotepa (Topoisomerase II inhibitors, including mitoxantrone, in combination with other antineoplastic agents, have been associated with the development of acute leukemia).
No products indexed under this heading.

Topotecan Hydrochloride (Topoisomerase II inhibitors, including mitoxantrone, in combination with other antineoplastic agents, have been associated with the development of acute leukemia). Products include:
Hycamtin 1491
Hycamtin Capsules 1488

Toremifene Citrate (Topoisomerase II inhibitors, including mitoxantrone, in combination with other antineoplastic agents, have been associated with the development of acute leukemia).
No products indexed under this heading.

Valrubicin (Topoisomerase II inhibitors, including mitoxantrone, in combination with other antineoplastic agents, have been associated with the development of acute leukemia). Products include:
Valstar 1131

Vincristine Sulfate (Topoisomerase II inhibitors, including mitoxantrone, in combination with other antineoplastic agents, have been associated with the development of acute leukemia).
No products indexed under this heading.

Vinorelbine Tartrate (Topoisomerase II inhibitors, including mitoxantrone, in combination with other antineoplastic agents, have been associated with the development of acute leukemia).
No products indexed under this heading.

NOVOLOG INJECTION

(Insulin Aspart, Human Regular) 2575

May interact with ACE inhibitors, alcohols, atypical antipsychotics, beta-blockers, corticosteroids, diuretics, drugs that lower serum potassium (selected), epinephrine-containing products, estrogens, fibrates, lithium preparations, monoamine oxidase inhibitors, oral contraceptives, oral hypoglycemic agents, phenothiazines, progestins, salicylates, somatostatin analogs, sulfonamides, sympathomimetics, thyroid preparations, and certain other agents. Compounds in these categories include:

Acarbose (A number of substances affect glucose metabolism and may require insulin dose adjustment and particularly close monitoring. Examples of substances that may increase the blood-glucose-lowering effect of insulin and the susceptibility to hypoglycemia include oral antidiabetic products).
No products indexed under this heading.

Acebutolol Hydrochloride (A number of substances affect glucose metabolism and may require insulin dose adjustment and particularly close monitoring. Examples of substances that may either potentiate or weaken the blood-glucose-lowering effect of insulin include beta-blockers. In addition, under the influence of sympatholytic products, such as β-blockers, the signs of hypoglycemia may be reduced or absent. Early warning symptoms of hypoglycemia may be different or less pronounced under certain conditions, such as use of medications such as β-blockers).
No products indexed under this heading.

Albuterol (A number of substances affect glucose metabolism and may require insulin dose adjustment and particularly close monitoring. Examples of substances that may reduce the blood-glucose-lowering effect of insulin include sympathomimetic agents (eg, epinephrine, salbutamol, terbutaline)).
No products indexed under this heading.

Albuterol Sulfate (A number of substances affect glucose metabolism and may require insulin dose adjustment and particularly close monitoring. Examples of substances that may reduce the blood-glucose-lowering effect of insulin include sympathomimetic agents (eg, epinephrine, salbutamol, terbutaline)). Products include:
ProAir HFA 3393
Proventil HFA 3204
Ventolin HFA 1708

Alclometasone Dipropionate (A number of substances affect glucose metabolism and may require insulin dose adjustment and particularly close monitoring. Examples of substances that may reduce the blood-glucose-lowering effect of insulin include corticosteroids).
No products indexed under this heading.

Amiloride Hydrochloride (A number of substances affect glucose metabolism and may require insulin dose adjustment and particularly close monitoring. Examples of substances that may reduce the blood-glucose-lowering effect of insulin include diuretics).
No products indexed under this heading.

Aripiprazole (A number of substances affect glucose metabolism and may require insulin dose adjustment and particularly close monitoring. Examples of substances that may reduce the blood-glucose-lowering effect of insulin include atypical antipsychotics).
No products indexed under this heading.

Aspirin (A number of substances affect glucose metabolism and may require insulin dose adjustment and particularly close monitoring. Examples of substances that may increase the blood-glucose-lowering effect of insulin and the susceptibility to hypoglycemia include salicylates). Products include:
Aggrenox 880
Bayer Aspirin 829
Percodan 1124
St. Joseph Aspirin 2045

Aspirin, Enteric Coated (A number of substances affect glucose metabolism and may require insulin dose adjustment and particularly close monitoring. Examples of substances that may increase the blood-glucose-lowering effect of insulin and the susceptibility to hypoglycemia include salicylates).
No products indexed under this heading.

Aspirin Buffered (A number of substances affect glucose metabolism and may require insulin dose adjustment and particularly close monitoring. Examples of substances that may increase the blood-glucose-lowering effect of insulin and the susceptibility to hypoglycemia include salicylates).
No products indexed under this heading.

Atenolol (A number of substances affect glucose metabolism and may require insulin dose adjustment and particularly close monitoring. Examples of substances that may either potentiate or weaken the blood-glucose-lowering effect of insulin include beta-blockers. In addition, under the influence of sympatholytic products, such as β-blockers, the signs of hypoglycemia may be reduced or absent. Early warning symptoms of hypoglycemia may be different or less pronounced under certain conditions, such as use of medications such as β-blockers).
No products indexed under this heading.

Beclomethasone Dipropionate (A number of substances affect glucose metabolism and may require insulin dose adjustment and particularly close monitoring. Examples of substances that may reduce the blood-glucose-lowering effect of insulin include corticosteroids). Products include:
Qvar 3398

Beclomethasone Dipropionate Monohydrate (A number of substances affect glucose metabolism and may require insulin dose adjustment and particularly close monitoring. Examples of substances that may reduce the blood-glucose-lowering effect of insulin include corticosteroids). Products include:
Beconase AQ 1386

Benazepril Hydrochloride (A number of substances affect glucose metabolism and may require insulin dose adjustment and particularly close monitoring. Examples of substances that may increase the blood-glucose-lowering effect of insulin and the susceptibility to hypoglycemia include ACE inhibitors).
No products indexed under this heading.

Bendroflumethiazide (A number of substances affect glucose metabolism and may require insulin dose adjustment and particularly close monitoring. Examples of substances that may increase the blood-glucose-lowering effect of insulin and the susceptibility to hypoglycemia include sulfonamide antibiotics).
No products indexed under this heading.

Betamethasone (A number of substances affect glucose metabolism and may require insulin dose adjustment and particularly close monitoring. Examples of substances that may reduce the blood-glucose-lowering effect of insulin include corticosteroids).
No products indexed under this heading.

Betamethasone Acetate (A number of substances affect glucose metabolism and may require insulin dose adjustment and particularly close monitoring. Examples of substances that may reduce the blood-glucose-lowering effect of insulin include corticosteroids).
No products indexed under this heading.

Betamethasone Benzoate (A number of substances affect glucose metabolism and may require insulin dose adjustment and particularly close monitoring. Examples of substances that may reduce the blood-glucose-lowering effect of insulin include corticosteroids).
No products indexed under this heading.

Betamethasone Dipropionate (A number of substances affect glucose metabolism and may require insulin dose adjustment and particularly close monitoring. Examples of substances that may reduce the blood-glucose-lowering effect of insulin include corticosteroids). Products include:
Diprolene Lotion 0.05% 3108
Diprolene Ointment 0.05% 3109
Diprolene AF Cream 0.05% 3107
Lotrisone 3163

Betamethasone Sodium Phosphate (A number of substances affect glucose metabolism and may require insulin dose adjustment and particularly close monitoring. Examples of substances that may reduce the blood-glucose-lowering effect of insulin include corticosteroids).
No products indexed under this heading.

Betamethasone Valerate (A number of substances affect glucose metabolism and may require insulin dose adjustment and particularly close monitoring. Examples of substances that may reduce the blood-glucose-lowering effect of insulin include corticosteroids). Products include:
Luxíq 3321

Betaxolol Hydrochloride (A number of substances affect glucose metabolism and may require insulin dose adjustment and particularly close monitoring. Examples of substances that may either potentiate or weaken the blood-glucose-lowering effect of insulin include beta-blockers. In addition, under the influence of sympatholytic products, such as β-blockers, the signs of hypoglycemia may be reduced or absent. Early warning symptoms of hypoglycemia may be different or less pronounced under certain conditions, such as use of medications such as β-blockers).
No products indexed under this heading.

Bisoprolol Fumarate (A number of substances affect glucose metabolism and may require insulin dose adjustment and particularly close monitoring. Examples of substances that may either potentiate or weaken the blood-glucose-lowering effect of insulin include beta-blockers. In addition, under the influence of sympatholytic products, such as β-blockers, the signs of hypoglycemia may be reduced or absent. Early warning symptoms of hypoglycemia may be different or less pronounced under certain conditions, such as use of medications such as β-blockers).
No products indexed under this heading.

Budesonide (A number of substances affect glucose metabolism and may require insulin dose adjustment and particularly close monitoring. Examples of substances that may reduce the blood-glucose-lowering effect of insulin include corticosteroids). Products include:
Pulmicort Flexhaler 714
Symbicort 80/4.5 720
Symbicort 160/4.5 720

Bumetanide (A number of substances affect glucose metabolism and may require insulin dose adjustment and particularly close monitoring. Examples of substances that may reduce the blood-glucose-lowering effect of insulin include diuretics).
No products indexed under this heading.

Captopril (A number of substances affect glucose metabolism and may require insulin dose adjustment and particularly close monitoring. Examples of substances that may increase the blood-glucose-lowering effect of insulin and the susceptibility to hypoglycemia include ACE inhibitors). Products include:
Captopril 2341

Carteolol Hydrochloride (A number of substances affect glucose metabolism and may require insulin dose adjustment and particularly close monitoring. Examples of substances that may either potentiate or weaken the blood-glucose-lowering effect of insulin include beta-blockers. In addition, under the influence of sympatholytic products, such as β-blockers, the signs of hypoglycemia may be reduced or absent. Early warning symptoms of hypoglycemia may be different or less pronounced under certain conditions, such as use of medications such as β-blockers).
No products indexed under this heading.

Carvedilol (A number of substances affect glucose metabolism and may require insulin dose adjustment and particularly close monitoring. Examples of substances that may either potentiate or weaken the blood-glucose-lowering effect of insulin include beta-blockers. In addition, under the influence of sympatholytic products, such as β-blockers, the signs of hypoglycemia may be reduced or absent. Early warning symptoms of hypoglycemia may be different or less pronounced under certain conditions, such as use of medications such as β-blockers). Products include:
Coreg 1409

Carvedilol Phosphate (A number of substances affect glucose metabolism and may require insulin dose adjustment and particularly close monitoring. Examples of substances that may either potentiate or weaken the blood-glucose-lowering effect of insulin include beta-blockers. In addition, under the influence of sympatholytic products, such as β-blockers, the signs of hypoglycemia may be reduced or absent. Early warning symptoms of hypoglycemia may be different or less pronounced under certain conditions, such as use of medications such as β-blockers). Products include:
Coreg CR 1416

Chlorothiazide (A number of substances affect glucose metabolism and may require insulin dose adjustment and particularly close monitoring. Examples of substances that may increase the blood-glucose-lowering effect of insulin and the susceptibility to hypoglycemia include sulfonamide antibiotics).
No products indexed under this heading.

Chlorothiazide Sodium (A number of substances affect glucose metabolism and may require insulin dose adjustment and particularly close monitoring. Examples of substances that may increase the blood-glucose-lowering effect of insulin and the susceptibility to hypoglycemia include sulfonamide antibiotics). Products include:
Diuril Intravenous 2009

Chlorotrianisene (A number of substances affect glucose metabolism and may require insulin dose adjustment and particularly close monitoring. Examples of substances that may reduce the blood-glucose-lowering effect of insulin include estrogens).
No products indexed under this heading.

Chlorpromazine (A number of substances affect glucose metabolism and may require insulin dose adjustment and particularly close monitoring. Examples of substances that may reduce the blood-glucose-lowering effect of insulin include phenothiazine derivatives).
No products indexed under this heading.

Chlorpromazine Hydrochloride (A number of substances affect glucose metabolism and may require insulin dose adjustment and particularly close monitoring. Examples of substances that may reduce the blood-glucose-lowering effect of insulin include phenothiazine derivatives).
No products indexed under this heading.

Chlorpropamide (A number of substances affect glucose metabolism and may require insulin dose adjustment and particularly close monitoring. Examples of substances that may increase the blood-glucose-lowering effect of insulin and the susceptibility to hypoglycemia include oral antidiabetic products).
No products indexed under this heading.

Chlorthalidone (A number of substances affect glucose metabolism and may require insulin dose adjustment and particularly close monitoring. Examples of substances that may reduce the blood-glucose-lowering effect of insulin include diuretics). Products include:
Clorpres 2344

Choline Magnesium Trisalicylate (A number of substances affect glucose metabolism and may require insulin dose adjustment and particularly close monitoring. Examples of substances that may increase the blood-glucose-lowering effect of insulin and the susceptibility to hypoglycemia include salicylates).
No products indexed under this heading.

Ciclesonide (A number of substances affect glucose metabolism and may require insulin dose adjustment and particularly close monitoring. Examples of substances that may reduce the blood-glucose-lowering effect of insulin include corticosteroids).
No products indexed under this heading.

Clofibrate (A number of substances affect glucose metabolism and may require insulin dose adjustment and particularly close monitoring. Examples of substances that may increase the blood-glucose-lowering effect of insulin and the susceptibility to hypoglycemia include fibrates).
No products indexed under this heading.

Clonidine (A number of substances affect glucose metabolism and may require insulin dose adjustment and particularly close monitoring. Examples of substances that may either potentiate or weaken the blood-glucose-lowering effect of insulin include clonidine. In addition, under the influence of sympatholytic products, such as clonidine, the signs of hypoglycemia may be reduced or absent). Products include:
Catapres-TTS 884

Clonidine Hydrochloride (A number of substances affect glucose metabolism and may require insulin dose adjustment and particularly close monitoring. Examples of substances that may either potentiate or weaken the blood-glucose-lowering effect of insulin include clonidine. In addition, under the influence of sympatholytic products, such as clonidine, the signs of hypoglycemia may be reduced or absent). Products include:
Clorpres 2344

Clozapine (A number of substances affect glucose metabolism and may require insulin dose adjustment and particularly close monitoring. Examples of substances that may reduce the blood-glucose-lowering effect of insulin include atypical antipsychotics).
No products indexed under this heading.

Cortisone Acetate (A number of substances affect glucose metabolism and may require insulin dose adjustment and particularly close monitoring. Examples of substances that may reduce the blood-glucose-lowering effect of insulin include corticosteroids).
No products indexed under this heading.

Danazol (A number of substances affect glucose metabolism and may require insulin dose adjustment and particularly close monitoring. Examples of substances that may reduce the blood-glucose-lowering effect of insulin include danazol).
No products indexed under this heading.

Desogestrel (A number of substances affect glucose metabolism and may require insulin dose adjustment and particularly close monitoring. Examples of substances that may reduce the blood-glucose-lowering effect of insulin include progestogens).
No products indexed under this heading.

Desoximetasone (A number of substances affect glucose metabolism and may require insulin dose adjustment and particularly close monitoring. Examples of substances that may reduce the blood-glucose-lowering effect of insulin include corticosteroids).
No products indexed under this heading.

Dexamethasone (A number of substances affect glucose metabolism and may require insulin dose adjustment and particularly close monitoring. Examples of substances that may reduce the blood-glucose-lowering effect of insulin include corticosteroids). Products include:
Ciprodex 583
Ozurdex .... ⊙ 223
Tobramycin and Dexamethasone Ophthalmic Suspension .... ⊙ 251

Dexamethasone Acetate (A number of substances affect glucose metabolism and may require insulin dose adjustment and particularly close monitoring. Examples of substances that may reduce the blood-glucose-lowering effect of insulin include corticosteroids).
No products indexed under this heading.

Dexamethasone Phosphate (A number of substances affect glucose metabolism and may require insulin dose adjustment and particularly close monitoring. Examples of substances that may reduce the blood-glucose-lowering effect of insulin include corticosteroids).
No products indexed under this heading.

Dexamethasone Sodium (A number of substances affect glucose metabolism and may require insulin dose adjustment and particularly close monitoring. Examples of substances that may reduce the blood-glucose-lowering effect of insulin include corticosteroids).
No products indexed under this heading.

Dexamethasone Sodium Phosphate (A number of substances affect glucose metabolism and may require insulin dose adjustment and particularly close monitoring. Examples of substances that may reduce the blood-glucose-lowering effect of insulin include corticosteroids).
No products indexed under this heading.

IMPORTANT NOTE: Always consult each drug listing in the patient's regimen for possible interactions.

Dexamethasone Sodium Phosphate Injection (A number of substances affect glucose metabolism and may require insulin dose adjustment and particularly close monitoring. Examples of substances that may reduce the blood-glucose-lowering effect of insulin include corticosteroids).
No products indexed under this heading.

Dienestrol (A number of substances affect glucose metabolism and may require insulin dose adjustment and particularly close monitoring. Examples of substances that may reduce the blood-glucose-lowering effect of insulin include estrogens).
No products indexed under this heading.

Diethylstilbestrol (A number of substances affect glucose metabolism and may require insulin dose adjustment and particularly close monitoring. Examples of substances that may reduce the blood-glucose-lowering effect of insulin include estrogens).
No products indexed under this heading.

Diflorasone Diacetate (A number of substances affect glucose metabolism and may require insulin dose adjustment and particularly close monitoring. Examples of substances that may reduce the blood-glucose-lowering effect of insulin include corticosteroids).
No products indexed under this heading.

Diflunisal (A number of substances affect glucose metabolism and may require insulin dose adjustment and particularly close monitoring. Examples of substances that may increase the blood-glucose-lowering effect of insulin and the susceptibility to hypoglycemia include salicylates).
No products indexed under this heading.

Disopyramide (A number of substances affect glucose metabolism and may require insulin dose adjustment and particularly close monitoring. Examples of substances that may increase the blood-glucose-lowering effect of insulin and the susceptibility to hypoglycemia include disopyramide).
No products indexed under this heading.

Disopyramide Phosphate (A number of substances affect glucose metabolism and may require insulin dose adjustment and particularly close monitoring. Examples of substances that may increase the blood-glucose-lowering effect of insulin and the susceptibility to hypoglycemia include disopyramide).
No products indexed under this heading.

Dobutamine Hydrochloride (A number of substances affect glucose metabolism and may require insulin dose adjustment and particularly close monitoring. Examples of substances that may reduce the blood-glucose-lowering effect of insulin include sympathomimetic agents (eg, epinephrine, salbutamol, terbutaline)).
No products indexed under this heading.

Dopamine Hydrochloride (A number of substances affect glucose metabolism and may require insulin dose adjustment and particularly close monitoring. Examples of substances that may reduce the blood-glucose-lowering effect of insulin include sympathomimetic agents (eg, epinephrine, salbutamol, terbutaline)).
No products indexed under this heading.

Enalapril Maleate (A number of substances affect glucose metabolism and may require insulin dose adjustment and particularly close monitoring. Examples of substances that may increase the blood-glucose-lowering effect of insulin and the susceptibility to hypoglycemia include ACE inhibitors).
No products indexed under this heading.

Enalaprilat (A number of substances affect glucose metabolism and may require insulin dose adjustment and particularly close monitoring. Examples of substances that may increase the blood-glucose-lowering effect of insulin and the susceptibility to hypoglycemia include ACE inhibitors).
No products indexed under this heading.

Ephedrine Hydrochloride (A number of substances affect glucose metabolism and may require insulin dose adjustment and particularly close monitoring. Examples of substances that may reduce the blood-glucose-lowering effect of insulin include sympathomimetic agents (eg, epinephrine, salbutamol, terbutaline)).
No products indexed under this heading.

Ephedrine Sulfate (A number of substances affect glucose metabolism and may require insulin dose adjustment and particularly close monitoring. Examples of substances that may reduce the blood-glucose-lowering effect of insulin include sympathomimetic agents (eg, epinephrine, salbutamol, terbutaline)).
No products indexed under this heading.

Ephedrine Tannate (A number of substances affect glucose metabolism and may require insulin dose adjustment and particularly close monitoring. Examples of substances that may reduce the blood-glucose-lowering effect of insulin include sympathomimetic agents (eg, epinephrine, salbutamol, terbutaline)).
No products indexed under this heading.

Epinephrine (A number of substances affect glucose metabolism and may require insulin dose adjustment and particularly close monitoring. Examples of substances that may reduce the blood-glucose-lowering effect of insulin include sympathomimetic agents (eg, epinephrine, salbutamol, terbutaline)). Products include:
EpiPen **3631**
Twinject **3268**

Epinephrine, Racemic (A number of substances affect glucose metabolism and may require insulin dose adjustment and particularly close monitoring. Examples of substances that may reduce the blood-glucose-lowering effect of insulin include sympathomimetic agents, such as epinephrine).
No products indexed under this heading.

Epinephrine Bitartrate (A number of substances affect glucose metabolism and may require insulin dose adjustment and particularly close monitoring. Examples of substances that may reduce the blood-glucose-lowering effect of insulin include sympathomimetic agents (eg, epinephrine, salbutamol, terbutaline)).
No products indexed under this heading.

Epinephrine Hydrochloride (A number of substances affect glucose metabolism and may require insulin dose adjustment and particularly close monitoring. Examples of substances that may reduce the blood-glucose-lowering effect of insulin include sympathomimetic agents (eg, epinephrine, salbutamol, terbutaline)).
No products indexed under this heading.

Esmolol Hydrochloride (A number of substances affect glucose metabolism and may require insulin dose adjustment and particularly close monitoring. Examples of substances that may either potentiate or weaken the blood-glucose-lowering effect of insulin include beta-blockers. In addition, under the influence of sympatholytic products, such as β-blockers, the signs of hypoglycemia may be reduced or absent. Early warning symptoms of hypoglycemia may be different or less pronounced under certain conditions, such as use of medications such as β-blockers).
No products indexed under this heading.

Estradiol (A number of substances affect glucose metabolism and may require insulin dose adjustment and particularly close monitoring. Examples of substances that may reduce the blood-glucose-lowering effect of insulin include estrogens). Products include:
Activella **2561**
Angeliq **831**
Climara **841**
Climara Pro **847**
Divigel **3467**
Estrasorb **1777**
Vagifem **2589**

Estrogens, Conjugated (A number of substances affect glucose metabolism and may require insulin dose adjustment and particularly close monitoring. Examples of substances that may reduce the blood-glucose-lowering effect of insulin include estrogens). Products include:
Premarin Intravenous **3528**
Premarin Tablets **3533**
Premarin Vaginal Cream **3540**
Premphase **3549**
Prempro **3549**

Estrogens, Esterified (A number of substances affect glucose metabolism and may require insulin dose adjustment and particularly close monitoring. Examples of substances that may reduce the blood-glucose-lowering effect of insulin include estrogens).
No products indexed under this heading.

Estropipate (A number of substances affect glucose metabolism and may require insulin dose adjustment and particularly close monitoring. Examples of substances that may reduce the blood-glucose-lowering effect of insulin include estrogens).
No products indexed under this heading.

Ethacrynic Acid (A number of substances affect glucose metabolism and may require insulin dose adjustment and particularly close monitoring. Examples of substances that may reduce the blood-glucose-lowering effect of insulin include diuretics).
No products indexed under this heading.

Ethanol (A number of substances affect glucose metabolism and may require insulin dose adjustment and particularly close monitoring. Examples of substances that may either potentiate or weaken the blood-glucose-lowering effect of insulin include alcohol).
No products indexed under this heading.

Ethinyl Estradiol (A number of substances affect glucose metabolism and may require insulin dose adjustment and particularly close monitoring. Examples of substances that may reduce the blood-glucose-lowering effect of insulin include estrogens). Products include:
LoSeasonique **3407**
Lybrel **3514**
NuvaRing **3181**
Ortho Evra **2648**
Ortho-Cyclen/Ortho Tri-Cyclen **2663**
Ortho Tri-Cyclen Lo Tablets **2673**
Seasonique **3418**
Yaz **864**

Ethyl Alcohol (A number of substances affect glucose metabolism and may require insulin dose adjustment and particularly close monitoring. Examples of substances that may either potentiate or weaken the blood-glucose-lowering effect of insulin include alcohol).
No products indexed under this heading.

Ethynodiol Diacetate (A number of substances affect glucose metabolism and may require insulin dose adjustment and particularly close monitoring. Examples of substances that may reduce the blood-glucose-lowering effect of insulin include progestogens (eg, in oral contraceptives)).
No products indexed under this heading.

Fenofibrate (A number of substances affect glucose metabolism and may require insulin dose adjustment and particularly close monitoring. Examples of substances that may increase the blood-glucose-lowering effect of insulin and the susceptibility to hypoglycemia include fibrates). Products include:
Fenoglide **3263**
Tricor **544**
Trilipix **548**

Fludrocortisone Acetate (A number of substances affect glucose metabolism and may require insulin dose adjustment and particularly close monitoring. Examples of substances that may reduce the blood-glucose-lowering effect of insulin include corticosteroids).
No products indexed under this heading.

Flumethasone Pivalate (A number of substances affect glucose metabolism and may require insulin dose adjustment and particularly close monitoring. Examples of substances that may reduce the blood-glucose-lowering effect of insulin include corticosteroids).
No products indexed under this heading.

Flunisolide Hemihydrate (A number of substances affect glucose metabolism and may require insulin dose adjustment and particularly close monitoring. Examples of substances that may reduce the blood-glucose-lowering effect of insulin include corticosteroids).
No products indexed under this heading.

Fluoxetine (A number of substances affect glucose metabolism and may require insulin dose adjustment and particularly close monitoring. Examples of substances that may increase the blood-glucose-lowering effect of insulin and the susceptibility to hypoglycemia include fluoxetine).
No products indexed under this heading.

Fluoxetine Hydrochloride (A number of substances affect glucose metabolism and may require insulin dose adjustment and particularly close monitoring. Examples of substances that may increase the blood-glucose-lowering effect of insulin and the susceptibility to hypoglycemia include fluoxetine). Products include:
Prozac Weekly **1941**
Prozac Pulvules **1941**
Symbyax **1965**

Fluphenazine Decanoate (A number of substances affect glucose metabolism and may require insulin dose adjustment and particularly close monitoring. Examples of substances that may reduce the blood-glucose-lowering effect of insulin include phenothiazine derivatives).
No products indexed under this heading.

Fluphenazine Enanthate (A number of substances affect glucose metabolism and may require insulin dose adjustment and particularly close monitoring. Examples of substances that may reduce the blood-glucose-lowering effect of insulin include phenothiazine derivatives).
No products indexed under this heading.

Fluphenazine Hydrochloride (A number of substances affect glucose metabolism and may require insulin dose adjustment and particularly close monitoring. Examples of substances that may reduce the blood-glucose-lowering effect of insulin include phenothiazine derivatives).
No products indexed under this heading.

Fluticasone Furoate (A number of substances affect glucose metabolism and may require insulin dose adjustment and particularly close monitoring. Examples of substances that may reduce the blood-glucose-lowering effect of insulin include corticosteroids). Products include:
Veramyst 1713

Fluticasone Propionate (A number of substances affect glucose metabolism and may require insulin dose adjustment and particularly close monitoring. Examples of substances that may reduce the blood-glucose-lowering effect of insulin include corticosteroids). Products include:
Advair 100/50 1275
Advair 250/50 1275
Advair 500/50 1275
Advair HFA 45/21 1288
Advair HFA 115/21 1288
Advair HFA 230/21 1288
Flonase 1459
Flovent Diskus 1463
Flovent HFA 1470

Fosinopril Sodium (A number of substances affect glucose metabolism and may require insulin dose adjustment and particularly close monitoring. Examples of substances that may increase the blood-glucose-lowering effect of insulin and the susceptibility to hypoglycemia include ACE inhibitors).
No products indexed under this heading.

Furosemide (A number of substances affect glucose metabolism and may require insulin dose adjustment and particularly close monitoring. Examples of substances that may reduce the blood-glucose-lowering effect of insulin include diuretics). Products include:
Furosemide 2354

Gemfibrozil (A number of substances affect glucose metabolism and may require insulin dose adjustment and particularly close monitoring. Examples of substances that may increase the blood-glucose-lowering effect of insulin and the susceptibility to hypoglycemia include fibrates).
No products indexed under this heading.

Glibenclamide (A number of substances affect glucose metabolism and may require insulin dose adjustment and particularly close monitoring. Examples of substances that may increase the blood-glucose-lowering effect of insulin and the susceptibility to hypoglycemia include oral antidiabetic products).
No products indexed under this heading.

Glimepiride (A number of substances affect glucose metabolism and may require insulin dose adjustment and particularly close monitoring. Examples of substances that may increase the blood-glucose-lowering effect of insulin and the susceptibility to hypoglycemia include oral antidiabetic products). Products include:
Avandaryl 1356
Duetact 3354

Glipizide (A number of substances affect glucose metabolism and may require insulin dose adjustment and particularly close monitoring. Examples of substances that may increase the blood-glucose-lowering effect of insulin and the susceptibility to hypoglycemia include oral antidiabetic products).
No products indexed under this heading.

Glyburide (A number of substances affect glucose metabolism and may require insulin dose adjustment and particularly close monitoring. Examples of substances that may increase the blood-glucose-lowering effect of insulin and the susceptibility to hypoglycemia include oral antidiabetic products).
No products indexed under this heading.

Guanethidine (A number of substances affect glucose metabolism and may require insulin dose adjustment and particularly close monitoring. Under the influence of sympatholytic products such as guanethidine, the signs of hypoglycemia may be reduced or absent).
No products indexed under this heading.

Guanethidine Monosulfate (A number of substances affect glucose metabolism and may require insulin dose adjustment and particularly close monitoring. Under the influence of sympatholytic products such as guanethidine, the signs of hypoglycemia may be reduced or absent).
No products indexed under this heading.

Guanethidine Sulfate (A number of substances affect glucose metabolism and may require insulin dose adjustment and particularly close monitoring. Under the influence of sympatholytic products such as guanethidine, the signs of hypoglycemia may be reduced or absent).
No products indexed under this heading.

Hydrochlorothiazide (A number of substances affect glucose metabolism and may require insulin dose adjustment and particularly close monitoring. Examples of substances that may increase the blood-glucose-lowering effect of insulin and the susceptibility to hypoglycemia include sulfonamide antibiotics). Products include:
Atacand HCT 700
Avalide 2956
Benicar HCT 1017
Diovan HCT 2419
Dyazide 1429
Exforge HCT 2449
Hyzaar 2162
Hyzaar 100-12.5 2162
Micardis HCT 889
Prinzide 2246
Tekturna HCT 2541
Teveten HCT 541

Hydrocortisone (A number of substances affect glucose metabolism and may require insulin dose adjustment and particularly close monitoring. Examples of substances that may reduce the blood-glucose-lowering effect of insulin include corticosteroids).
No products indexed under this heading.

Hydrocortisone (Alcohol) (A number of substances affect glucose metabolism and may require insulin dose adjustment and particularly close monitoring. Examples of substances that may reduce the blood-glucose-lowering effect of insulin include corticosteroids).
No products indexed under this heading.

Hydrocortisone Acetate (A number of substances affect glucose metabolism and may require insulin dose adjustment and particularly close monitoring. Examples of substances that may reduce the blood-glucose-lowering effect of insulin include corticosteroids).
No products indexed under this heading.

Hydrocortisone Butyrate (A number of substances affect glucose metabolism and may require insulin dose adjustment and particularly close monitoring. Examples of substances that may reduce the blood-glucose-lowering effect of insulin include corticosteroids).
No products indexed under this heading.

Hydrocortisone Cypionate (A number of substances affect glucose metabolism and may require insulin dose adjustment and particularly close monitoring. Examples of substances that may reduce the blood-glucose-lowering effect of insulin include corticosteroids).
No products indexed under this heading.

Hydrocortisone Hemisuccinate (A number of substances affect glucose metabolism and may require insulin dose adjustment and particularly close monitoring. Examples of substances that may reduce the blood-glucose-lowering effect of insulin include corticosteroids).
No products indexed under this heading.

Hydrocortisone Probutate (A number of substances affect glucose metabolism and may require insulin dose adjustment and particularly close monitoring. Examples of substances that may reduce the blood-glucose-lowering effect of insulin include corticosteroids).
No products indexed under this heading.

Hydrocortisone Sodium Phosphate (A number of substances affect glucose metabolism and may require insulin dose adjustment and particularly close monitoring. Examples of substances that may reduce the blood-glucose-lowering effect of insulin include corticosteroids).
No products indexed under this heading.

Hydrocortisone Sodium Succinate (A number of substances affect glucose metabolism and may require insulin dose adjustment and particularly close monitoring. Examples of substances that may reduce the blood-glucose-lowering effect of insulin include corticosteroids).
No products indexed under this heading.

Hydrocortisone Valerate (A number of substances affect glucose metabolism and may require insulin dose adjustment and particularly close monitoring. Examples of substances that may reduce the blood-glucose-lowering effect of insulin include corticosteroids).
No products indexed under this heading.

Hydroflumethiazide (A number of substances affect glucose metabolism and may require insulin dose adjustment and particularly close monitoring. Examples of substances that may increase the blood-glucose-lowering effect of insulin and the susceptibility to hypoglycemia include sulfonamide antibiotics).
No products indexed under this heading.

Indapamide (A number of substances affect glucose metabolism and may require insulin dose adjustment and particularly close monitoring. Examples of substances that may reduce the blood-glucose-lowering effect of insulin include diuretics). Products include:
Indapamide 2356

Isocarboxazid (A number of substances affect glucose metabolism and may require insulin dose adjustment and particularly close monitoring. Examples of substances that may increase the blood-glucose-lowering effect of insulin and the susceptibility to hypoglycemia include monoamine oxidase (MAO) inhibitors). Products include:
Marplan 3481

Isoniazid (A number of substances affect glucose metabolism and may require insulin dose adjustment and particularly close monitoring. Examples of substances that may reduce the blood-glucose-lowering effect of insulin include isoniazid).
No products indexed under this heading.

Isoproterenol Hydrochloride (A number of substances affect glucose metabolism and may require insulin dose adjustment and particularly close monitoring. Examples of substances that may reduce the blood-glucose-lowering effect of insulin include sympathomimetic agents (eg, epinephrine, salbutamol, terbutaline)).
No products indexed under this heading.

Isoproterenol Sulfate (A number of substances affect glucose metabolism and may require insulin dose adjustment and particularly close monitoring. Examples of substances that may reduce the blood-glucose-lowering effect of insulin include sympathomimetic agents (eg, epinephrine, salbutamol, terbutaline)).
No products indexed under this heading.

Labetalol Hydrochloride (A number of substances affect glucose metabolism and may require insulin dose adjustment and particularly close monitoring. Examples of substances that may either potentiate or weaken the blood-glucose-lowering effect of insulin include beta-blockers. In addition, under the influence of sympatholytic products, such as β-blockers, the signs of hypoglycemia may be reduced or absent. Early warning symptoms of hypoglycemia may be different or less pronounced under certain conditions, such as use of medications such as β-blockers).
No products indexed under this heading.

Lanreotide (A number of substances affect glucose metabolism and may require insulin dose adjustment and particularly close monitoring. Somatostatin analog (eg, octreotide) is an example of substances that may increase the blood-glucose-lowering effect and susceptibility to hypoglycemia).
No products indexed under this heading.

Levalbuterol Hydrochloride (A number of substances affect glucose metabolism and may require insulin dose adjustment and particularly close monitoring. Examples of substances that may reduce the blood-glucose-lowering effect of insulin include sympathomimetic agents (eg, epinephrine, salbutamol, terbutaline)).
No products indexed under this heading.

Levobunolol Hydrochloride (A number of substances affect glucose metabolism and may require insulin dose adjustment and particularly close monitoring. Examples of substances that may either potentiate or weaken the blood-glucose-lowering effect of insulin include beta-blockers. In addition, under the influence of sympatholytic products, such as β-blockers, the signs of hypoglycemia may be reduced or absent. Early warning symptoms of hypoglycemia may be different or less pronounced under certain conditions, such as use of medications such as β-blockers).
No products indexed under this heading.

Levonorgestrel (A number of substances affect glucose metabolism and may require insulin dose adjustment and particularly close monitoring. Examples of substances that may reduce the blood-glucose-lowering effect of insulin include progestogens (eg, in oral contraceptives)). Products include:
Climara Pro 847
LoSeasonique 3407
Lybrel 3514
Mirena 854
Plan B 3416
Seasonique 3418

Levothyroxine Sodium (A number of substances affect glucose metabolism and may require insulin dose adjustment and particularly close monitoring. Examples of substances that may reduce the blood-glucose-lowering effect of insulin include thyroid hormones). Products include:
Levoxyl Tablets 1843
Synthroid 529

Liothyronine Sodium (A number of substances affect glucose metabolism and may require insulin dose adjustment and particularly close monitoring. Examples of substances that may

(⊙ Described in PDR® for Ophthalmic Medicines)

1249 **Interactions Index** **NovoLog**

Norepinephrine Bitartrate (A number of substances affect glucose metabolism and may require insulin dose adjustment and particularly close monitoring. Examples of substances that may reduce the blood-glucose-lowering effect of insulin include sympathomimetic agents (eg, epinephrine, salbutamol, terbutaline)).
No products indexed under this heading.

Norepinephrine Hydrochloride (A number of substances affect glucose metabolism and may require insulin dose adjustment and particularly close monitoring. Examples of substances that may reduce the blood-glucose-lowering effect of insulin include sympathomimetic agents, such as epinephrine).
No products indexed under this heading.

Norethindrone (A number of substances affect glucose metabolism and may require insulin dose adjustment and particularly close monitoring. Examples of substances that may reduce the blood-glucose-lowering effect of insulin include progestogens). Products include:
Ortho Micronor **2660**

Norethindrone Acetate (A number of substances affect glucose metabolism and may require insulin dose adjustment and particularly close monitoring. Examples of substances that may reduce the blood-glucose-lowering effect of insulin include progestogens). Products include:
Activella **2561**

Norethynodrel (A number of substances affect glucose metabolism and may require insulin dose adjustment and particularly close monitoring. Examples of substances that may reduce the blood-glucose-lowering effect of insulin include progestogens (eg, in oral contraceptives)).
No products indexed under this heading.

Norgestimate (A number of substances affect glucose metabolism and may require insulin dose adjustment and particularly close monitoring. Examples of substances that may reduce the blood-glucose-lowering effect of insulin include progestogens). Products include:
Ortho-Cyclen/Ortho Tri-Cyclen **2663**
Ortho Tri-Cyclen Lo Tablets **2673**

Norgestrel (A number of substances affect glucose metabolism and may require insulin dose adjustment and particularly close monitoring. Examples of substances that may reduce the blood-glucose-lowering effect of insulin include progestogens (eg, in oral contraceptives)).
No products indexed under this heading.

Octreotide Acetate (A number of substances affect glucose metabolism and may require insulin dose adjustment and particularly close monitoring. Examples of substances that may increase the blood-glucose-lowering effect of insulin and the susceptibility to hypoglycemia include somatostatin analog (eg, octreotide)). Products include:
Sandostatin **2517**
Sandostatin LAR **2519**

Olanzapine (A number of substances affect glucose metabolism and may require insulin dose adjustment and particularly close monitoring. Examples of substances that may reduce the blood-glucose-lowering effect of insulin include atypical antipsychotics). Products include:
Symbyax **1965**
Zyprexa **1984**
Zyprexa IntraMuscular **1984**
Zyprexa ZYDIS **1984**

Pargyline Hydrochloride (A number of substances affect glucose metabolism and may require insulin dose adjustment and particularly close monitoring. Examples of substances that may increase the blood-glucose-lowering effect of insulin and the susceptibility to hypoglycemia include monoamine oxidase (MAO) inhibitors).
No products indexed under this heading.

Penbutolol Sulfate (A number of substances affect glucose metabolism and may require insulin dose adjustment and particularly close monitoring. Examples of substances that may either potentiate or weaken the blood-glucose-lowering effect of insulin include beta-blockers. In addition, under the influence of sympatholytic products, such as β-blockers, the signs of hypoglycemia may be reduced or absent. Early warning symptoms of hypoglycemia may be different or less pronounced under certain conditions, such as use of medications such as β-blockers).
No products indexed under this heading.

Pentamidine Isethionate (A number of substances affect glucose metabolism and may require insulin dose adjustment and particularly close monitoring. Pentamidine may cause hypoglycemia, which may sometimes be followed by hyperglycemia).
No products indexed under this heading.

Perindopril Erbumine (A number of substances affect glucose metabolism and may require insulin dose adjustment and particularly close monitoring. Examples of substances that may increase the blood-glucose-lowering effect of insulin and the susceptibility to hypoglycemia include ACE inhibitors).
No products indexed under this heading.

Perphenazine (A number of substances affect glucose metabolism and may require insulin dose adjustment and particularly close monitoring. Examples of substances that may reduce the blood-glucose-lowering effect of insulin include phenothiazine derivatives).
No products indexed under this heading.

Phenelzine Sulfate (A number of substances affect glucose metabolism and may require insulin dose adjustment and particularly close monitoring. Examples of substances that may increase the blood-glucose-lowering effect of insulin and the susceptibility to hypoglycemia include monoamine oxidase (MAO) inhibitors).
No products indexed under this heading.

Phenothiazine Derivatives (A number of substances affect glucose metabolism and may require insulin dose adjustment and particularly close monitoring. Examples of substances that may reduce the blood-glucose-lowering effect of insulin include phenothiazine derivatives).
No products indexed under this heading.

Phenothiazines (A number of substances affect glucose metabolism and may require insulin dose adjustment and particularly close monitoring. Examples of substances that may reduce the blood-glucose-lowering effect of insulin include phenothiazine derivatives).
No products indexed under this heading.

Phenylephrine Bitartrate (A number of substances affect glucose metabolism and may require insulin dose adjustment and particularly close monitoring. Examples of substances that may reduce the blood-glucose-lowering effect of insulin include sympathomimetic agents (eg, epinephrine, salbutamol, terbutaline)).
No products indexed under this heading.

Phenylephrine Hydrochloride (A number of substances affect glucose metabolism and may require insulin dose adjustment and particularly close monitoring. Examples of substances that may reduce the blood-glucose-lowering effect of insulin include sympathomimetic agents (eg, epinephrine, salbutamol, terbutaline)). Products include:
Sudafed PE Nasal Decongestant **2048**
Children's Sudafed PE Nasal Decongestant **2047**

Phenylephrine Tannate (A number of substances affect glucose metabolism and may require insulin dose adjustment and particularly close monitoring. Examples of substances that may reduce the blood-glucose-lowering effect of insulin include sympathomimetic agents (eg, epinephrine, salbutamol, terbutaline)).
No products indexed under this heading.

Phenylpropanolamine Hydrochloride (A number of substances affect glucose metabolism and may require insulin dose adjustment and particularly close monitoring. Examples of substances that may reduce the blood-glucose-lowering effect of insulin include sympathomimetic agents (eg, epinephrine, salbutamol, terbutaline)).
No products indexed under this heading.

Pindolol (A number of substances affect glucose metabolism and may require insulin dose adjustment and particularly close monitoring. Examples of substances that may either potentiate or weaken the blood-glucose-lowering effect of insulin include beta-blockers. In addition, under the influence of sympatholytic products, such as β-blockers, the signs of hypoglycemia may be reduced or absent. Early warning symptoms of hypoglycemia may be different or less pronounced under certain conditions, such as use of medications such as β-blockers).
No products indexed under this heading.

Pioglitazone Hydrochloride (A number of substances affect glucose metabolism and may require insulin dose adjustment and particularly close monitoring. Examples of substances that may increase the blood-glucose-lowering effect of insulin and the susceptibility to hypoglycemia include oral antidiabetic products). Products include:
ActoPlus **3338**
Actos **3345**
Duetact **3354**

Pirbuterol Acetate (A number of substances affect glucose metabolism and may require insulin dose adjustment and particularly close monitoring. Examples of substances that may reduce the blood-glucose-lowering effect of insulin include sympathomimetic agents (eg, epinephrine, salbutamol, terbutaline)). Products include:
Maxair Autohaler **1782**

Polyestradiol Phosphate (A number of substances affect glucose metabolism and may require insulin dose adjustment and particularly close monitoring. Examples of substances that may reduce the blood-glucose-lowering effect of insulin include estrogens).
No products indexed under this heading.

Polythiazide (A number of substances affect glucose metabolism and may require insulin dose adjustment and particularly close monitoring. Examples of substances that may increase the blood-glucose-lowering effect of insulin and the susceptibility to hypoglycemia include sulfonamide antibiotics).
No products indexed under this heading.

Pramlintide Acetate (A number of substances affect glucose metabolism and may require insulin dose adjustment and particularly close monitoring. Examples of substances that may increase the blood-glucose-lowering effect of insulin and the susceptibility to hypoglycemia include pramlintide). Products include:
Symlin **651**
SymlinPen **651**

Prednisolone (A number of substances affect glucose metabolism and may require insulin dose adjustment and particularly close monitoring. Examples of substances that may reduce the blood-glucose-lowering effect of insulin include corticosteroids).
No products indexed under this heading.

Prednisolone Acetate (A number of substances affect glucose metabolism and may require insulin dose adjustment and particularly close monitoring. Examples of substances that may reduce the blood-glucose-lowering effect of insulin include corticosteroids). Products include:
Blephamide .... ⊙**212**, ⊙**214**
Pred Forte .... ⊙**225**
Pred Mild .... ⊙**230**
Pred-G .... ⊙**226**, ⊙**227**

Prednisolone Sodium Phosphate (A number of substances affect glucose metabolism and may require insulin dose adjustment and particularly close monitoring. Examples of substances that may reduce the blood-glucose-lowering effect of insulin include corticosteroids).
No products indexed under this heading.

Prednisolone Tebutate (A number of substances affect glucose metabolism and may require insulin dose adjustment and particularly close monitoring. Examples of substances that may reduce the blood-glucose-lowering effect of insulin include corticosteroids).
No products indexed under this heading.

Prednisone (A number of substances affect glucose metabolism and may require insulin dose adjustment and particularly close monitoring. Examples of substances that may reduce the blood-glucose-lowering effect of insulin include corticosteroids).
No products indexed under this heading.

Prednisone sodium phosphate (A number of substances affect glucose metabolism and may require insulin dose adjustment and particularly close monitoring. Examples of substances that may reduce the blood-glucose-lowering effect of insulin include corticosteroids).
No products indexed under this heading.

Procarbazine Hydrochloride (A number of substances affect glucose metabolism and may require insulin dose adjustment and particularly close monitoring. Examples of substances that may increase the blood-glucose-lowering effect of insulin and the susceptibility to hypoglycemia include monoamine oxidase (MAO) inhibitors).
No products indexed under this heading.

Prochlorperazine (A number of substances affect glucose metabolism and may require insulin dose adjustment and particularly close monitoring. Examples of substances that may reduce the blood-glucose-lowering effect of insulin include phenothiazine derivatives).
No products indexed under this heading.

Prochlorperazine Edisylate (A number of substances affect glucose metabolism and may require insulin dose adjustment and particularly close monitoring. Examples of substances that may reduce the blood-glucose-lowering effect of insulin include phenothiazine derivatives).
No products indexed under this heading.

IMPORTANT NOTE: Always consult each drug listing in the patient's regimen for possible interactions.

Prochlorperazine Maleate (A number of substances affect glucose metabolism and may require insulin dose adjustment and particularly close monitoring. Examples of substances that may reduce the blood-glucose-lowering effect of insulin include phenothiazine derivatives).
No products indexed under this heading.

Promethazine (A number of substances affect glucose metabolism and may require insulin dose adjustment and particularly close monitoring. Examples of substances that may reduce the blood-glucose-lowering effect of insulin include phenothiazine derivatives).
No products indexed under this heading.

Promethazine Hydrochloride (A number of substances affect glucose metabolism and may require insulin dose adjustment and particularly close monitoring. Examples of substances that may reduce the blood-glucose-lowering effect of insulin include phenothiazine derivatives).
No products indexed under this heading.

Propoxyphene Hydrochloride (A number of substances affect glucose metabolism and may require insulin dose adjustment and particularly close monitoring. Examples of substances that may increase the blood-glucose-lowering effect of insulin and the susceptibility to hypoglycemia include propoxyphene).
No products indexed under this heading.

Propoxyphene Napsylate (A number of substances affect glucose metabolism and may require insulin dose adjustment and particularly close monitoring. Examples of substances that may increase the blood-glucose-lowering effect of insulin and the susceptibility to hypoglycemia include propoxyphene).
No products indexed under this heading.

Propranolol Hydrochloride (A number of substances affect glucose metabolism and may require insulin dose adjustment and particularly close monitoring. Examples of substances that may either potentiate or weaken the blood-glucose-lowering effect of insulin include beta-blockers. In addition, under the influence of sympatholytic products, such as β-blockers, the signs of hypoglycemia may be reduced or absent. Early warning symptoms of hypoglycemia may be different or less pronounced under certain conditions, such as use of medications such as β-blockers). Products include:

Pseudoephedrine Hydrochloride (A number of substances affect glucose metabolism and may require insulin dose adjustment and particularly close monitoring. Examples of substances that may reduce the blood-glucose-lowering effect of insulin include sympathomimetic agents (eg, epinephrine, salbutamol, terbutaline)). Products include:

Pseudoephedrine Sulfate (A number of substances affect glucose metabolism and may require insulin dose adjustment and particularly close monitoring. Examples of substances that may reduce the blood-glucose-lowering effect of insulin include sympathomimetic agents (eg, epinephrine, salbutamol, terbutaline)). Products include:

Quetiapine Fumarate (A number of substances affect glucose metabolism and may require insulin dose adjustment and particularly close monitoring. Examples of substances that may reduce the blood-glucose-lowering effect of insulin include atypical antipsychotics). Products include:

Quinapril Hydrochloride (A number of substances affect glucose metabolism and may require insulin dose adjustment and particularly close monitoring. Examples of substances that may increase the blood-glucose-lowering effect of insulin and the susceptibility to hypoglycemia include ACE inhibitors).
No products indexed under this heading.

Quinestrol (A number of substances affect glucose metabolism and may require insulin dose adjustment and particularly close monitoring. Examples of substances that may reduce the blood-glucose-lowering effect of insulin include estrogens).
No products indexed under this heading.

Ramipril (A number of substances affect glucose metabolism and may require insulin dose adjustment and particularly close monitoring. Examples of substances that may increase the blood-glucose-lowering effect of insulin and the susceptibility to hypoglycemia include ACE inhibitors).
No products indexed under this heading.

Rasagiline Mesylate (A number of substances affect glucose metabolism and may require insulin dose adjustment and particularly close monitoring. Examples of substances that may increase the blood-glucose-lowering effect of insulin and the susceptibility to hypoglycemia include monoamine oxidase (MAO) inhibitors). Products include:

Repaglinide (A number of substances affect glucose metabolism and may require insulin dose adjustment and particularly close monitoring. Examples of substances that may increase the blood-glucose-lowering effect of insulin and the susceptibility to hypoglycemia include oral antidiabetic products).
No products indexed under this heading.

Reserpine (A number of substances affect glucose metabolism and may require insulin dose adjustment and particularly close monitoring. Under the influence of sympatholytic products such as reserpine, the signs of hypoglycemia may be reduced or absent).
No products indexed under this heading.

Risperidone (A number of substances affect glucose metabolism and may require insulin dose adjustment and particularly close monitoring. Examples of substances that may reduce the blood-glucose-lowering effect of insulin include atypical antipsychotics).
Products include:

Rosiglitazone Maleate (A number of substances affect glucose metabolism and may require insulin dose adjustment and particularly close monitoring. Examples of substances that may increase the blood-glucose-lowering effect of insulin and the susceptibility to hypoglycemia include oral antidiabetic products). Products include:

Salbutamol (A number of substances affect glucose metabolism and may require insulin dose adjustment and particularly close monitoring. Examples of substances that may reduce the blood-glucose-lowering effect of insulin include sympathomimetic agents, such as salbutamol).
No products indexed under this heading.

Salmeterol Xinafoate (A number of substances affect glucose metabolism and may require insulin dose adjustment and particularly close monitoring. Examples of substances that may reduce the blood-glucose-lowering effect of insulin include sympathomimetic agents (eg, epinephrine, salbutamol, terbutaline)). Products include:

Salsalate (A number of substances affect glucose metabolism and may require insulin dose adjustment and particularly close monitoring. Examples of substances that may increase the blood-glucose-lowering effect of insulin and the susceptibility to hypoglycemia include salicylates).
No products indexed under this heading.

Selegiline (A number of substances affect glucose metabolism and may require insulin dose adjustment and particularly close monitoring. Examples of substances that may increase the blood-glucose-lowering effect of insulin and the susceptibility to hypoglycemia include monoamine oxidase (MAO) inhibitors). Products include:

Selegiline Hydrochloride (A number of substances affect glucose metabolism and may require insulin dose adjustment and particularly close monitoring. Examples of substances that may increase the blood-glucose-lowering effect of insulin and the susceptibility to hypoglycemia include monoamine oxidase (MAO) inhibitors). Products include:

Sitagliptin Phosphate (A number of substances affect glucose metabolism and may require insulin dose adjustment and particularly close monitoring. Examples of substances that may increase the blood-glucose-lowering effect of insulin and the susceptibility to hypoglycemia include oral antidiabetic products). Products include:

Somatropin (A number of substances affect glucose metabolism and may require insulin dose adjustment and particularly close monitoring. Examples of substances that may reduce the blood-glucose-lowering effect of insulin include somatropin). Products include:

Somatropin (rDNA Origin) (A number of substances affect glucose metabolism and may require insulin dose adjustment and particularly close monitoring. Examples of substances that may reduce the blood-glucose-lowering effect of insulin include somatropin). Products include:

Sotalol Hydrochloride (A number of substances affect glucose metabolism

and may require insulin dose adjustment and particularly close monitoring. Examples of substances that may either potentiate or weaken the blood-glucose-lowering effect of insulin include beta-blockers. In addition, under the influence of sympatholytic products, such as β-blockers, the signs of hypoglycemia may be reduced or absent. Early warning symptoms of hypoglycemia may be different or less pronounced under certain conditions, such as use of medications such as β-blockers).
No products indexed under this heading.

Spirapril Hydrochloride (A number of substances affect glucose metabolism and may require insulin dose adjustment and particularly close monitoring. Examples of substances that may increase the blood-glucose-lowering effect of insulin and the susceptibility to hypoglycemia include ACE inhibitors).
No products indexed under this heading.

Spironolactone (A number of substances affect glucose metabolism and may require insulin dose adjustment and particularly close monitoring. Examples of substances that may reduce the blood-glucose-lowering effect of insulin include diuretics).
No products indexed under this heading.

Sulfacytine (A number of substances affect glucose metabolism and may require insulin dose adjustment and particularly close monitoring. Examples of substances that may increase the blood-glucose-lowering effect of insulin and the susceptibility to hypoglycemia include sulfonamide antibiotics).
No products indexed under this heading.

Sulfamethizole (A number of substances affect glucose metabolism and may require insulin dose adjustment and particularly close monitoring. Examples of substances that may increase the blood-glucose-lowering effect of insulin and the susceptibility to hypoglycemia include sulfonamide antibiotics).
No products indexed under this heading.

Sulfamethoxazole (A number of substances affect glucose metabolism and may require insulin dose adjustment and particularly close monitoring. Examples of substances that may increase the blood-glucose-lowering effect of insulin and the susceptibility to hypoglycemia include sulfonamide antibiotics).
No products indexed under this heading.

Sulfasalazine (A number of substances affect glucose metabolism and may require insulin dose adjustment and particularly close monitoring. Examples of substances that may increase the blood-glucose-lowering effect of insulin and the susceptibility to hypoglycemia include sulfonamide antibiotics).
No products indexed under this heading.

Sulfinpyrazone (A number of substances affect glucose metabolism and may require insulin dose adjustment and particularly close monitoring. Examples of substances that may increase the blood-glucose-lowering effect of insulin and the susceptibility to hypoglycemia include sulfonamide antibiotics).
No products indexed under this heading.

Sulfisoxazole Acetyl (A number of substances affect glucose metabolism and may require insulin dose adjustment and particularly close monitoring. Examples of substances that may increase the blood-glucose-lowering effect of insulin and the susceptibility to hypoglycemia include sulfonamide antibiotics).
No products indexed under this heading.

Sulfisoxazole Diolamine (A number of substances affect glucose metabolism and may require insulin dose adjustment and particularly close monitoring. Examples of substances that may increase the blood-glucose-lowering effect of insulin and the susceptibility to hypoglycemia include sulfonamide antibiotics).

No products indexed under this heading.

Terbutaline Sulfate (A number of substances affect glucose metabolism and may require insulin dose adjustment and particularly close monitoring. Examples of substances that may reduce the blood-glucose-lowering effect of insulin include sympathomimetic agents, such as terbutaline).

No products indexed under this heading.

Thioridazine (A number of substances affect glucose metabolism and may require insulin dose adjustment and particularly close monitoring. Examples of substances that may reduce the blood-glucose-lowering effect of insulin include phenothiazine derivatives).

No products indexed under this heading.

Thioridazine Hydrochloride (A number of substances affect glucose metabolism and may require insulin dose adjustment and particularly close monitoring. Examples of substances that may reduce the blood-glucose-lowering effect of insulin include phenothiazine derivatives). Products include:
Thioridazine Hydrochloride 2384

Thyroglobulin (A number of substances affect glucose metabolism and may require insulin dose adjustment and particularly close monitoring. Examples of substances that may reduce the blood-glucose-lowering effect of insulin include thyroid hormones).

No products indexed under this heading.

Thyroid (A number of substances affect glucose metabolism and may require insulin dose adjustment and particularly close monitoring. Examples of substances that may reduce the blood-glucose-lowering effect of insulin include thyroid hormones). Products include:
Naturethroid 2830

Thyroxine (A number of substances affect glucose metabolism and may require insulin dose adjustment and particularly close monitoring. Examples of substances that may reduce the blood-glucose-lowering effect of insulin include thyroid hormones).

No products indexed under this heading.

Thyroxine Sodium (A number of substances affect glucose metabolism and may require insulin dose adjustment and particularly close monitoring. Examples of substances that may reduce the blood-glucose-lowering effect of insulin include thyroid hormones).

No products indexed under this heading.

Timolol Hemihydrate (A number of substances affect glucose metabolism and may require insulin dose adjustment and particularly close monitoring. Examples of substances that may either potentiate or weaken the blood-glucose-lowering effect of insulin include beta-blockers. In addition, under the influence of sympatholytic products, such as β-blockers, the signs of hypoglycemia may be reduced or absent. Early warning symptoms of hypoglycemia may be different or less pronounced under certain conditions, such as use of medications such as β-blockers). Products include:
Betimol 3490

Timolol Maleate (A number of substances affect glucose metabolism and may require insulin dose adjustment and particularly close monitoring. Examples of substances that may either potentiate or weaken the blood-glucose-

lowering effect of insulin include beta-blockers. In addition, under the influence of sympatholytic products, such as β-blockers, the signs of hypoglycemia may be reduced or absent. Early warning symptoms of hypoglycemia may be different or less pronounced under certain conditions, such as use of medications such as β-blockers). Products include:
Combigan 601
Dorzolamide
Hydrochloride/Timolol Maleate
Ophthalmic Solution.....................⊙243
Timoptic in Ocudose ....⊙231

Tobacco (The pharmacokinetic and pharmacodynamic profiles of all insulins may be altered by the site used for injection and the degree of vascularization of the site. Smoking, temperature, and exercise contribute to variations in blood flow and insulin absorption).

No products indexed under this heading.

Tolazamide (A number of substances affect glucose metabolism and may require insulin dose adjustment and particularly close monitoring. Examples of substances that may increase the blood-glucose-lowering effect of insulin and the susceptibility to hypoglycemia include oral antidiabetic products).

No products indexed under this heading.

Tolbutamide (A number of substances affect glucose metabolism and may require insulin dose adjustment and particularly close monitoring. Examples of substances that may increase the blood-glucose-lowering effect of insulin and the susceptibility to hypoglycemia include oral antidiabetic products).

No products indexed under this heading.

Torsemide (A number of substances affect glucose metabolism and may require insulin dose adjustment and particularly close monitoring. Examples of substances that may reduce the blood-glucose-lowering effect of insulin include diuretics).

No products indexed under this heading.

Trandolapril (A number of substances affect glucose metabolism and may require insulin dose adjustment and particularly close monitoring. Examples of substances that may increase the blood-glucose-lowering effect of insulin and the susceptibility to hypoglycemia include ACE inhibitors). Products include:
Mavik 489
Tarka 534

Tranylcypromine Sulfate (A number of substances affect glucose metabolism and may require insulin dose adjustment and particularly close monitoring. Examples of substances that may increase the blood-glucose-lowering effect of insulin and the susceptibility to hypoglycemia include monoamine oxidase (MAO) inhibitors). Products include:
Parnate 1584

Triamcinolone (A number of substances affect glucose metabolism and may require insulin dose adjustment and particularly close monitoring. Examples of substances that may reduce the blood-glucose-lowering effect of insulin include corticosteroids).

No products indexed under this heading.

Triamcinolone Acetonide (A number of substances affect glucose metabolism and may require insulin dose adjustment and particularly close monitoring. Examples of substances that may reduce the blood-glucose-lowering effect of insulin include corticosteroids). Products include:
Azmacort 408
Nasacort AQ 3019

Triamcinolone Diacetate (A number of substances affect glucose metabolism and may require insulin dose adjustment and particularly close monitoring. Examples of substances that may reduce the blood-glucose-lowering effect of insulin include corticosteroids).

No products indexed under this heading.

Triamcinolone Hexacetonide (A number of substances affect glucose metabolism and may require insulin dose adjustment and particularly close monitoring. Examples of substances that may reduce the blood-glucose-lowering effect of insulin include corticosteroids).

No products indexed under this heading.

Triamterene (A number of substances affect glucose metabolism and may require insulin dose adjustment and particularly close monitoring. Examples of substances that may reduce the blood-glucose-lowering effect of insulin include diuretics). Products include:
Dyazide 1429
Dyrenium 3495

Trifluoperazine Hydrochloride (A number of substances affect glucose metabolism and may require insulin dose adjustment and particularly close monitoring. Examples of substances that may reduce the blood-glucose-lowering effect of insulin include phenothiazine derivatives).

No products indexed under this heading.

Troglitazone (A number of substances affect glucose metabolism and may require insulin dose adjustment and particularly close monitoring. Examples of substances that may increase the blood-glucose-lowering effect of insulin and the susceptibility to hypoglycemia include oral antidiabetic products).

No products indexed under this heading.

Ziprasidone Hydrochloride (A number of substances affect glucose metabolism and may require insulin dose adjustment and particularly close monitoring. Examples of substances that may reduce the blood-glucose-lowering effect of insulin include atypical antipsychotics). Products include:
Geodon 2723

Ziprasidone Mesylate (A number of substances affect glucose metabolism and may require insulin dose adjustment and particularly close monitoring. Examples of substances that may reduce the blood-glucose-lowering effect of insulin include atypical antipsychotics). Products include:
Geodon 2723

Food Interactions

Alcohol (A number of substances affect glucose metabolism and may require insulin dose adjustment and particularly close monitoring. Examples of substances that may either potentiate or weaken the blood-glucose-lowering effect of insulin include alcohol).

Beer, reduced-alcohol (A number of substances affect glucose metabolism and may require insulin dose adjustment and particularly close monitoring. Examples of substances that may either potentiate or weaken the blood-glucose-lowering effect of insulin include alcohol).

Beer, unspecified (A number of substances affect glucose metabolism and may require insulin dose adjustment and particularly close monitoring. Examples of substances that may either potentiate or weaken the blood-glucose-lowering effect of insulin include alcohol).

Food, unspecified (The timing of hypoglycemia usually reflects the time-action profile of the administered insulin formulations. Other factors such as changes in

food intake (eg, amount of food or timing of meals) may also alter the risk of hypoglycemia. As with all insulins, use caution in patients with hypoglycemia unawareness and in patients who may be predisposed to hypoglycemia (eg, patients who are fasting or have erratic food intake)).

Meal, unspecified (The timing of hypoglycemia usually reflects the time-action profile of the administered insulin formulations. Other factors such as changes in food intake (eg, amount of food or timing of meals) may also alter the risk of hypoglycemia. As with all insulins, use caution in patients with hypoglycemia unawareness and in patients who may be predisposed to hypoglycemia (eg, patients who are fasting or have erratic food intake)).

Wine, Chianti (A number of substances affect glucose metabolism and may require insulin dose adjustment and particularly close monitoring. Examples of substances that may either potentiate or weaken the blood-glucose-lowering effect of insulin include alcohol).

Wine, Red (A number of substances affect glucose metabolism and may require insulin dose adjustment and particularly close monitoring. Examples of substances that may either potentiate or weaken the blood-glucose-lowering effect of insulin include alcohol).

Wine, unspecified (A number of substances affect glucose metabolism and may require insulin dose adjustment and particularly close monitoring. Examples of substances that may either potentiate or weaken the blood-glucose-lowering effect of insulin include alcohol).

Wine products (A number of substances affect glucose metabolism and may require insulin dose adjustment and particularly close monitoring. Examples of substances that may either potentiate or weaken the blood-glucose-lowering effect of insulin include alcohol).

NOVOLOG MIX 70/30
(Insulin Aspart, Human, Insulin Aspart Protamine, Human).............................2581
May interact with ACE inhibitors, beta-blockers, corticosteroids, diuretics, estrogens, fibrates, monoamine oxidase inhibitors, oral contraceptives, phenothiazines, progestins, sulfonamides, sympathomimetics, thyroid preparations, and certain other agents. Compounds in these categories include:

Acebutolol Hydrochloride (May potentiate or weaken the blood-glucose-lowering effect of insulin. The signs of hypoglycemia may be reduced or absent).

No products indexed under this heading.

Albuterol (Substances that may reduce the blood-glucose-lowering effect).

No products indexed under this heading.

Albuterol Sulfate (Substances that may reduce the blood-glucose-lowering effect). Products include:
ProAir HFA 3393
Proventil HFA 3204
Ventolin HFA 1708

Alclometasone Dipropionate (Substances that may reduce the blood-glucose-lowering effect).

No products indexed under this heading.

Amiloride Hydrochloride (Substances that may reduce the blood-glucose-lowering effect).

No products indexed under this heading.

Atenolol (May potentiate or weaken the blood-glucose-lowering effect of insulin. The signs of hypoglycemia may be reduced or absent).

No products indexed under this heading.

(⊙ Described in PDR® for Ophthalmic Medicines)

IMPORTANT NOTE: Always consult each drug listing in the patient's regimen for possible interactions.

Prothrombin complex concentrates (Concomitant treatment with aPCCs/PCCs (activated or nonactivated prothrombin complex concentrates) have an increased risk of developing thrombotic events due to circulating tissue factor (TF) or predisposing coagulopathy. The risk of a potential interaction between rFVIIa and coagulation factor concentrates has not been adequately evaluated in preclinical or clinical studies. Simultaneous use of prothrombin complex concentrates or activated prothrombin complex concentrates should be avoided).
No products indexed under this heading.

NOXAFIL ORAL SUSPENSION
(Posaconazole) 3172
May interact with benzodiazepine that are metabolized by CYP3A4, calcium channel blockers, cytochrome p450 3a4 substrates (selected), drugs that prolong the QT interval, ergot-containing drugs, HMG-CoA reductase inhibitors, P-glycoprotein inducers, P-glycoprotein inhibitors, phenytoin, quinidine, statins that are metabolized by CYP3A4, UDP-glucuronosyltransferase (UGT) inducers (selected), vinca alkaloids, and certain other agents. Compounds in these categories include:

Alfentanil Hydrochloride (A clinical study in healthy volunteers indicates that posaconazole is a strong CYP3A4 inhibitor. Therefore, plasma concentrations of drugs predominantly metabolized by CYP3A4 may be increased by posaconazole).
No products indexed under this heading.

Alprazolam (Frequent monitoring of adverse effects of benzodiazepines metabolized by CYP3A4 should be performed and dose reduction of these benzodiazepines should be considered during co-administration with posaconazole).
No products indexed under this heading.

Amiodarone Hydrochloride (Posaconazole should be administered with caution to patients with potentially proarrhythmic conditions and should not be administered with drugs that are known to prolong the QTc interval and are metabolized through CYP3A4).
No products indexed under this heading.

Amitriptyline Hydrochloride (Posaconazole should be administered with caution to patients with potentially proarrhythmic conditions and should not be administered with drugs that are known to prolong the QTc interval and are metabolized through CYP3A4).
No products indexed under this heading.

Amlodipine Besylate (Frequent monitoring for adverse events and toxicity related to calcium channel blockers which are metabolized through CYP3A4 is recommended during co-administration. Dose reduction of calcium channel blockers which are metabolized through CYP3A4 may be needed). Products include:
Azor **1010**
Exforge **2443**
Exforge HCT **2449**

Amoxapine (Posaconazole should be administered with caution to patients with potentially proarrhythmic conditions and should not be administered with drugs that are known to prolong the QTc interval and are metabolized through CYP3A4).
No products indexed under this heading.

Amprenavir (Posaconazole is a substrate for p-glycoprotein (P-gp) efflux. Therefore, inducers of p-glycoprotein may affect posaconazole plasma concentrations).
No products indexed under this heading.

Aprepitant (A clinical study in healthy volunteers indicates that posaconazole is a strong CYP3A4 inhibitor. Therefore, plasma concentrations of drugs predominantly metabolized by CYP3A4 may be increased by posaconazole). Products include:
Emend **2124**

Astemizole (Co-administration of the CYP3A4 substrate astemizole with posaconazole is contraindicated since it may result in increased plasma concentrations of astemizole, leading to QTc prolongation and rare occurrences of torsades de pointes).
No products indexed under this heading.

Atazanavir (Frequent monitoring of adverse effects and toxicity of atazanavir should be performed during co-administration with posaconazole).
No products indexed under this heading.

Atazanavir Sulfate (Frequent monitoring of adverse effects and toxicity of atazanavir should be performed during co-administration with posaconazole).
No products indexed under this heading.

Atenolol (Posaconazole is a substrate for p-glycoprotein (P-gp) efflux. Therefore, inhibitors of p-glycoprotein may affect posaconazole plasma concentrations).
No products indexed under this heading.

Atorvastatin Calcium (It is recommended that dose reduction of statins metabolized through CYP3A4 be considered during co-administration. Increased statin concentrations in plasma can be associated with rhabdomyolysis). Products include:
Lipitor **2703**

Azithromycin Dihydrate (Posaconazole is a substrate for p-glycoprotein (P-gp) efflux. Therefore, inhibitors of p-glycoprotein may affect posaconazole plasma concentrations).
No products indexed under this heading.

Belladonna Ergotamine (A clinical study in healthy volunteers indicates that posaconazole is a strong CYP3A4 inhibitor. Therefore, plasma concentrations of drugs predominantly metabolized by CYP3A4 may be increased by posaconazole).
No products indexed under this heading.

Bepridil Hydrochloride (Frequent monitoring for adverse events and toxicity related to calcium channel blockers which are metabolized through CYP3A4 is recommended during co-administration. Dose reduction of calcium channel blockers which are metabolized through CYP3A4 may be needed).
No products indexed under this heading.

Bretylium Tosylate (Posaconazole should be administered with caution to patients with potentially proarrhythmic conditions and should not be administered with drugs that are known to prolong the QTc interval and are metabolized through CYP3A4).
No products indexed under this heading.

Buspirone Hydrochloride (Posaconazole should be administered with caution to patients with potentially proarrhythmic conditions and should not be administered with drugs that are known to prolong the QTc interval and are metabolized through CYP3A4).
No products indexed under this heading.

Busulfan (A clinical study in healthy volunteers indicates that posaconazole is a strong CYP3A4 inhibitor. Therefore, plasma concentrations of drugs predominantly metabolized by CYP3A4 may be increased by posaconazole). Products include:
Myleran **1581**

Carbamazepine (A clinical study in healthy volunteers indicates that posaconazole is a strong CYP3A4 inhibitor. Therefore, plasma concentrations of drugs predominantly metabolized by CYP3A4 may be increased by posaconazole). Products include:
Carbatrol **3280**
Equetro **3477**

Carvedilol (Posaconazole is a substrate for p-glycoprotein (P-gp) efflux. Therefore, inhibitors of p-glycoprotein may affect posaconazole plasma concentrations). Products include:
Coreg **1409**

Carvedilol Phosphate (Posaconazole is a substrate for p-glycoprotein (P-gp) efflux. Therefore, inhibitors of p-glycoprotein may affect posaconazole plasma concentrations). Products include:
Coreg CR **1416**

Cerivastatin Sodium (A clinical study in healthy volunteers indicates that posaconazole is a strong CYP3A4 inhibitor. Therefore, plasma concentrations of drugs predominantly metabolized by CYP3A4 may be increased by posaconazole).
No products indexed under this heading.

Chlordiazepoxide (Posaconazole should be administered with caution to patients with potentially proarrhythmic conditions and should not be administered with drugs that are known to prolong the QTc interval and are metabolized through CYP3A4).
No products indexed under this heading.

Chlordiazepoxide Hydrochloride (Posaconazole should be administered with caution to patients with potentially proarrhythmic conditions and should not be administered with drugs that are known to prolong the QTc interval and are metabolized through CYP3A4).
No products indexed under this heading.

Chlorpheniramine (A clinical study in healthy volunteers indicates that posaconazole is a strong CYP3A4 inhibitor. Therefore, plasma concentrations of drugs predominantly metabolized by CYP3A4 may be increased by posaconazole).
No products indexed under this heading.

Chlorpheniramine Maleate (A clinical study in healthy volunteers indicates that posaconazole is a strong CYP3A4 inhibitor. Therefore, plasma concentrations of drugs predominantly metabolized by CYP3A4 may be increased by posaconazole).
No products indexed under this heading.

Chlorpheniramine Polistirex (A clinical study in healthy volunteers indicates that posaconazole is a strong CYP3A4 inhibitor. Therefore, plasma concentrations of drugs predominantly metabolized by CYP3A4 may be increased by posaconazole). Products include:
Tussionex **3443**

Chlorpheniramine Tannate (A clinical study in healthy volunteers indicates that posaconazole is a strong CYP3A4 inhibitor. Therefore, plasma concentrations of drugs predominantly metabolized by CYP3A4 may be increased by posaconazole).
No products indexed under this heading.

Chlorpromazine (Posaconazole should be administered with caution to patients with potentially proarrhythmic conditions and should not be administered with drugs that are known to prolong the QTc interval and are metabolized through CYP3A4).
No products indexed under this heading.

Chlorpromazine Hydrochloride (Posaconazole should be administered with caution to patients with potentially proarrhythmic conditions and should not be administered with drugs that are known to prolong the QTc interval and are metabolized through CYP3A4).
No products indexed under this heading.

Chlorprothixene (Posaconazole should be administered with caution to patients with potentially proarrhythmic conditions and should not be administered with drugs that are known to prolong the QTc interval and are metabolized through CYP3A4).
No products indexed under this heading.

Chlorprothixene Hydrochloride (Posaconazole should be administered with caution to patients with potentially proarrhythmic conditions and should not be administered with drugs that are known to prolong the QTc interval and are metabolized through CYP3A4).
No products indexed under this heading.

Cimetidine (Co-administration of cimetidine with posaconazole may result in lower plasma concentrations of posaconazole. Therefore, concomitant use should be avoided unless the benefits outweigh the risks).
No products indexed under this heading.

Cimetidine Hydrochloride (Co-administration of cimetidine with posaconazole may result in lower plasma concentrations of posaconazole. Therefore, concomitant use should be avoided unless the benefits outweigh the risks).
No products indexed under this heading.

Cisapride (Co-administration of the CYP3A4 substrate cisapride with posaconazole is contraindicated since it may result in increased plasma concentrations of cisapride, leading to QTc prolongation and rare occurrences of torsades de pointes).
No products indexed under this heading.

Clarithromycin (A clinical study in healthy volunteers indicates that posaconazole is a strong CYP3A4 inhibitor. Therefore, plasma concentrations of drugs predominantly metabolized by CYP3A4 may be increased by posaconazole). Products include:
Biaxin/Biaxin XL **412**

Clomipramine Hydrochloride (Posaconazole should be administered with caution to patients with potentially proarrhythmic conditions and should not be administered with drugs that are known to prolong the QTc interval and are metabolized through CYP3A4).
No products indexed under this heading.

Clorazepate Dipotassium (Posaconazole should be administered with caution to patients with potentially proarrhythmic conditions and should not be administered with drugs that are known to prolong the QTc interval and are metabolized through CYP3A4).
No products indexed under this heading.

Clotrimazole (Posaconazole is a substrate for p-glycoprotein (P-gp) efflux. Therefore, inducers of p-glycoprotein may affect posaconazole plasma concentrations). Products include:
Lotrisone **3163**

Clotrimazole, Topical (Posaconazole is a substrate for p-glycoprotein (P-gp) efflux. Therefore, inducers of p-glycoprotein may affect posaconazole plasma concentrations).
No products indexed under this heading.

Clozapine (Posaconazole should be administered with caution to patients with potentially proarrhythmic conditions and should not be administered with drugs that are known to prolong the QTc interval and are metabolized through CYP3A4).
No products indexed under this heading.

Cyclosporine (Increased cyclosporine concentrations resulted in cyclosporine dose reductions in heart transplant patients co-administered posaconazole. At initiation of posaconazole treatment, reduce the cyclosporine dose to approximately 3/4 of the original dose. Frequent monitoring of cyclosporine whole blood trough concentrations should be performed during and at discontinuation of posaconazole treatment and the cyclosporine dose adjusted accordingly). Products include:
Gengraf **440**
Neoral Oral Solution **2496**
Neoral Capsules **2496**
Restasis **605**

Desipramine Hydrochloride (Posaconazole should be administered with caution to patients with potentially proarrhythmic conditions and should not be administered with drugs that are known to prolong the QTc interval and are metabolized through CYP3A4).
No products indexed under this heading.

Desogestrel (A clinical study in healthy volunteers indicates that posaconazole is a strong CYP3A4 inhibitor. Therefore, plasma concentrations of drugs predominantly metabolized by CYP3A4 may be increased by posaconazole).
No products indexed under this heading.

Diazepam (Frequent monitoring of adverse effects of benzodiazepines metabolized by CYP3A4 should be performed and dose reduction of these benzodiazepines should be considered during co-administration with posaconazole). Products include:
Valium Tablets **2880**

Digoxin (Increased plasma concentrations of digoxin have been reported in patients receiving digoxin and posaconazole. Therefore, monitoring of digoxin plasma concentrations is recommended during co-administration). Products include:
Lanoxin Injection **1546**
Lanoxin Injection Pediatric **1549**

IMPORTANT NOTE: Always consult each drug listing in the patient's regimen for possible interactions.

Noxafil **Interactions Index** **1256**

Lanoxin Tablets 1553

Dihydroergotamine Mesylate (Co-administration of posaconazole with ergot alkaloids is contraindicated. Posaconazole may increase the plasma concentrations of ergot alkaloids (eg, dihydroergotamine) which may lead to ergotism).
No products indexed under this heading.

Diltiazem Hydrochloride (Frequent monitoring for adverse events and toxicity related to calcium channel blockers which are metabolized through CYP3A4 is recommended during co-administration. Dose reduction of calcium channel blockers which are metabolized through CYP3A4 may be needed).
Products include:
Cardizem LA 423

Diltiazem Maleate (A clinical study in healthy volunteers indicates that posaconazole is a strong CYP3A4 inhibitor. Therefore, plasma concentrations of drugs predominantly metabolized by CYP3A4 may be increased by posaconazole).
No products indexed under this heading.

Dirithromycin (Posaconazole is a substrate for p-glycoprotein (P-gp) efflux. Therefore, inhibitors of p-glycoprotein may affect posaconazole plasma concentrations).
No products indexed under this heading.

Disopyramide (Posaconazole should be administered with caution to patients with potentially proarrhythmic conditions and should not be administered with drugs that are known to prolong the QTc interval and are metabolized through CYP3A4).
No products indexed under this heading.

Disopyramide Phosphate (Posaconazole should be administered with caution to patients with potentially proarrhythmic conditions and should not be administered with drugs that are known to prolong the QTc interval and are metabolized through CYP3A4).
No products indexed under this heading.

Disulfiram (A clinical study in healthy volunteers indicates that posaconazole is a strong CYP3A4 inhibitor. Therefore, plasma concentrations of drugs predominantly metabolized by CYP3A4 may be increased by posaconazole).
No products indexed under this heading.

Dofetilide (Posaconazole should be administered with caution to patients with potentially proarrhythmic conditions and should not be administered with drugs that are known to prolong the QTc interval and are metabolized through CYP3A4).
No products indexed under this heading.

Doxepin Hydrochloride (Posaconazole should be administered with caution to patients with potentially proarrhythmic conditions and should not be administered with drugs that are known to prolong the QTc interval and are metabolized through CYP3A4).
No products indexed under this heading.

Doxorubicin Hydrochloride (A clinical study in healthy volunteers indicates that posaconazole is a strong CYP3A4 inhibitor. Therefore, plasma concentrations of drugs predominantly metabolized by CYP3A4 may be increased by posaconazole).
No products indexed under this heading.

Dronabinol (A clinical study in healthy volunteers indicates that posaconazole is a strong CYP3A4 inhibitor. Therefore, plasma concentrations of drugs predominantly metabolized by CYP3A4 may be increased by posaconazole).
No products indexed under this heading.

Droperidol (Posaconazole should be administered with caution to patients with potentially proarrhythmic conditions and should not be administered with drugs that are known to prolong the QTc interval and are metabolized through CYP3A4).
No products indexed under this heading.

Efavirenz (Co-administration of efavirenz with posaconazole may result in lower plasma concentrations of posaconazole. Avoid concomitant use unless the benefit outweigh the risks).
Products include:
Atripla 906

Elacridar (Posaconazole is a substrate for p-glycoprotein (P-gp) efflux. Therefore, inhibitors of p-glycoprotein may affect posaconazole plasma concentrations).
No products indexed under this heading.

Ergonovine Maleate (Co-administration of posaconazole with ergot alkaloids is contraindicated. Posaconazole may increase the plasma concentrations of ergot alkaloids which may lead to ergotism).
No products indexed under this heading.

Ergotamine Tartrate (Co-administration of posaconazole with ergot alkaloids is contraindicated. Posaconazole may increase the plasma concentrations of ergot alkaloids (eg, ergotamine) which may lead to ergotism).
No products indexed under this heading.

Erythromycin (Posaconazole should be administered with caution to patients with potentially proarrhythmic conditions and should not be administered with drugs that are known to prolong the QTc interval and are metabolized through CYP3A4).
No products indexed under this heading.

Erythromycin, Topical (Posaconazole is a substrate for p-glycoprotein (P-gp) efflux. Therefore, inhibitors of p-glycoprotein may affect posaconazole plasma concentrations).
No products indexed under this heading.

Erythromycin Estolate (Posaconazole should be administered with caution to patients with potentially proarrhythmic conditions and should not be administered with drugs that are known to prolong the QTc interval and are metabolized through CYP3A4).
No products indexed under this heading.

Erythromycin Ethylsuccinate (Posaconazole should be administered with caution to patients with potentially proarrhythmic conditions and should not be administered with drugs that are known to prolong the QTc interval and are metabolized through CYP3A4).
Products include:
E.E.S. 437
EryPed 435

Erythromycin Gluceptate (Posaconazole should be administered with caution to patients with potentially proarrhythmic conditions and should not be administered with drugs that are known to prolong the QTc interval and are metabolized through CYP3A4).
No products indexed under this heading.

Erythromycin Lactobionate (Posaconazole should be administered with caution to patients with potentially proarrhythmic conditions and should not be administered with drugs that are known to prolong the QTc interval and are metabolized through CYP3A4).
No products indexed under this heading.

Erythromycin Stearate (Posaconazole should be administered with caution to patients with potentially proarrhythmic conditions and should not be administered with drugs that are known to prolong the QTc interval and are metabolized through CYP3A4).
No products indexed under this heading.

Esomeprazole Magnesium (Co-administration of esomeperazole with posaconazole may result in lower plasma concentrations of posaconazole. Monitor closely for breakthrough fungal infections if posaconazole is used concomitantly with esomeprazole).
Products include:
Nexium Capsules 704
Nexium Oral Suspension 704

Esomeprazole Sodium (Co-administration of esomeperazole with posaconazole may result in lower plasma concentrations of posaconazole. Monitor closely for breakthrough fungal infections if posaconazole is used concomitantly with esomeprazole).
Products include:
Nexium I.V. 712

Estradiol (A clinical study in healthy volunteers indicates that posaconazole is a strong CYP3A4 inhibitor. Therefore, plasma concentrations of drugs predominantly metabolized by CYP3A4 may be increased by posaconazole).
Products include:
Activella 2561
Angeliq 831
Climara 841
Climara Pro 847
Divigel 3467
Estrasorb 1777
Vagifem 2589

Estradiol Benzoate (A clinical study in healthy volunteers indicates that posaconazole is a strong CYP3A4 inhibitor. Therefore, plasma concentrations of drugs predominantly metabolized by CYP3A4 may be increased by posaconazole).
No products indexed under this heading.

Estradiol Cypionate (A clinical study in healthy volunteers indicates that posaconazole is a strong CYP3A4 inhibitor. Therefore, plasma concentrations of drugs predominantly metabolized by CYP3A4 may be increased by posaconazole).
No products indexed under this heading.

Estradiol Valerate (A clinical study in healthy volunteers indicates that posaconazole is a strong CYP3A4 inhibitor. Therefore, plasma concentrations of drugs predominantly metabolized by CYP3A4 may be increased by posaconazole).
No products indexed under this heading.

Ethinyl Estradiol (A clinical study in healthy volunteers indicates that posaconazole is a strong CYP3A4 inhibitor. Therefore, plasma concentrations of drugs predominantly metabolized by CYP3A4 may be increased by posaconazole). Products include:
LoSeasonique 3407
Lybrel 3514
NuvaRing 3181
Ortho Evra 2648
Ortho-Cyclen/Ortho Tri-Cyclen 2663
Ortho Tri-Cyclen Lo Tablets 2673
Seasonique 3418
Yaz 864

Ethosuximide (A clinical study in healthy volunteers indicates that posaconazole is a strong CYP3A4 inhibitor. Therefore, plasma concentrations of drugs predominantly metabolized by CYP3A4 may be increased by posaconazole).
No products indexed under this heading.

Ethynodiol Diacetate (A clinical study in healthy volunteers indicates that posaconazole is a strong CYP3A4 inhibitor. Therefore, plasma concentrations of drugs predominantly metabolized by CYP3A4 may be increased by posaconazole).
No products indexed under this heading.

Etoposide (A clinical study in healthy volunteers indicates that posaconazole is a strong CYP3A4 inhibitor. Therefore, plasma concentrations of drugs predominantly metabolized by CYP3A4 may be increased by posaconazole).
No products indexed under this heading.

Etoposide Phosphate (A clinical study in healthy volunteers indicates that posaconazole is a strong CYP3A4 inhibitor. Therefore, plasma concentrations of drugs predominantly metabolized by CYP3A4 may be increased by posaconazole).
No products indexed under this heading.

Felodipine (Frequent monitoring for adverse events and toxicity related to calcium channel blockers which are metabolized through CYP3A4 is recommended during co-administration. Dose reduction of calcium channel blockers which are metabolized through CYP3A4 may be needed).
No products indexed under this heading.

Fentanyl (A clinical study in healthy volunteers indicates that posaconazole is a strong CYP3A4 inhibitor. Therefore, plasma concentrations of drugs predominantly metabolized by CYP3A4 may be increased by posaconazole).
Products include:
Duragesic 2604
Fentanyl Transdermal System 2346
Onsolis 2054

Fentanyl Citrate (A clinical study in healthy volunteers indicates that posaconazole is a strong CYP3A4 inhibitor. Therefore, plasma concentrations of drugs predominantly metabolized by CYP3A4 may be increased by posaconazole). Products include:
Fentora 966

Flecainide Acetate (Posaconazole should be administered with caution to patients with potentially proarrhythmic conditions and should not be administered with drugs that are known to prolong the QTc interval and are metabolized through CYP3A4).
No products indexed under this heading.

Fluphenazine Decanoate (Posaconazole should be administered with caution to patients with potentially proarrhythmic conditions and should not be administered with drugs that are known to prolong the QTc interval and are metabolized through CYP3A4).
No products indexed under this heading.

Fluphenazine Enanthate (Posaconazole should be administered with caution to patients with potentially proarrhythmic conditions and should not be administered with drugs that are known to prolong the QTc interval and are metabolized through CYP3A4).
No products indexed under this heading.

Fluphenazine Hydrochloride (Posaconazole should be administered with caution to patients with potentially proarrhythmic conditions and should not be administered with drugs that are known to prolong the QTc interval and are metabolized through CYP3A4).
No products indexed under this heading.

Fluvastatin Sodium (It is recommended that dose reduction of HMG-CoA reductase inhibitors metabolized through CYP3A4 be considered during co-administration. Increased statin concentrations in plasma can be associated with rhabdomyolysis).
No products indexed under this heading.

Fosamprenavir Calcium (Posaconazole is a substrate for p-glycoprotein (P-gp) efflux. Therefore, inducers of p-glycoprotein may affect posaconazole plasma concentrations). Products include:
Lexiva Oral Suspension 1558
Lexiva 1558

Fosphenytoin (Co-administration of phenytoin with posaconazole may result in lower plasma concentrations of posaconazole and increased concentrations of phenytoin. Frequent monitoring of phenytoin concentrations should be performed when co-administered with posaconazole and dose reduction of phenytoin should be considered. Avoid concomitant use unless the benefit outweighs the risks).
No products indexed under this heading.

Fosphenytoin Sodium (Co-administration of phenytoin with posaconazole may result in lower plasma concentrations of posaconazole and increased concentrations of phenytoin. Frequent monitoring of phenytoin concentrations should be performed when co-administered with posaconazole and dose reduction of phenytoin should be considered. Avoid concomitant use unless the benefit outweighs the risks).
No products indexed under this heading.

Glipizide (Posaconazole administration with glipizide does not require a dose adjustment in either drug; however, glucose concentrations decreased in some healthy volunteers administered the combination. Therefore, glucose concentrations should be monitored in accordance with the current standard of care for patients with diabetes when posaconazole is co-administered with glipizide).
No products indexed under this heading.

Halofantrine (Co-administration of the CYP3A4 substrate halofantrine with posaconazole is contraindicated since it may result in increased plasma concentrations of halofantrine, leading to QTc prolongation and rare occurrences of torsades de pointes).
No products indexed under this heading.

Halofantrine Hydrochloride (Co-administration of the CYP3A4 substrate halofantrine with posaconazole is contraindicated since it may result in increased plasma concentrations of halofantrine, leading to QTc prolongation and rare occurrences of torsades de pointes).
No products indexed under this heading.

Haloperidol (Posaconazole should be administered with caution to patients with potentially proarrhythmic conditions and should not be administered with drugs that are known to prolong the QTc interval and are metabolized through CYP3A4).
No products indexed under this heading.

Haloperidol Decanoate (Posaconazole should be administered with caution to patients with potentially proarrhythmic conditions and should not be administered with drugs that are known to prolong the QTc interval and are metabolized through CYP3A4).
No products indexed under this heading.

Haloperidol Lactate (Posaconazole should be administered with caution to patients with potentially proarrhythmic conditions and should not be administered with drugs that are known to prolong the QTc interval and are metabolized through CYP3A4).
No products indexed under this heading.

Hydroxyzine Hydrochloride (Posaconazole should be administered with caution to patients with potentially proarrhythmic conditions and should not be administered with drugs that are known to prolong the QTc interval and are metabolized through CYP3A4).
No products indexed under this heading.

Hypericum (Posaconazole is a substrate for p-glycoprotein (P-gp) efflux. Therefore, inducers of p-glycoprotein may affect posaconazole plasma concentrations).
No products indexed under this heading.

Hypericum Perforatum (Posaconazole is a substrate for p-glycoprotein (P-gp) efflux. Therefore, inducers of p-glycoprotein may affect posaconazole plasma concentrations). Products include:
Traumeel 1800

Imipramine Hydrochloride (Posaconazole should be administered with caution to patients with potentially proarrhythmic conditions and should not be administered with drugs that are known to prolong the QTc interval and are metabolized through CYP3A4).
No products indexed under this heading.

Imipramine Pamoate (Posaconazole should be administered with caution to patients with potentially proarrhythmic conditions and should not be administered with drugs that are known to prolong the QTc interval and are metabolized through CYP3A4).
No products indexed under this heading.

Indinavir Sulfate (A clinical study in healthy volunteers indicates that posaconazole is a strong CYP3A4 inhibitor. Therefore, plasma concentrations of drugs predominantly metabolized by CYP3A4 may be increased by posaconazole). Products include:
Crixivan 2113

Isocarboxazid (Posaconazole should be administered with caution to patients with potentially proarrhythmic conditions and should not be administered with drugs that are known to prolong the QTc interval and are metabolized through CYP3A4). Products include:
Marplan 3481

Isradipine (Frequent monitoring for adverse events and toxicity related to calcium channel blockers which are metabolized through CYP3A4 is recommended during co-administration. Dose reduction of calcium channel blockers which are metabolized through CYP3A4 may be needed). Products include:
DynaCirc CR 1432

Itraconazole (A clinical study in healthy volunteers indicates that posaconazole is a strong CYP3A4 inhibitor. Therefore, plasma concentrations of drugs predominantly metabolized by CYP3A4 may be increased by posaconazole).
No products indexed under this heading.

Ixabepilone (A clinical study in healthy volunteers indicates that posaconazole is a strong CYP3A4 inhibitor. Therefore, plasma concentrations of drugs predominantly metabolized by CYP3A4 may be increased by posaconazole).
No products indexed under this heading.

Ketoconazole (A clinical study in healthy volunteers indicates that posaconazole is a strong CYP3A4 inhibitor. Therefore, plasma concentrations of drugs predominantly metabolized by CYP3A4 may be increased by posaconazole). Products include:
Extina 3319
Xolegel 3337

Levonorgestrel (A clinical study in healthy volunteers indicates that posaconazole is a strong CYP3A4 inhibitor. Therefore, plasma concentrations of drugs predominantly metabolized by CYP3A4 may be increased by posaconazole). Products include:
Climara Pro 847
LoSeasonique 3407
Lybrel 3514
Mirena 854
Plan B 3416
Seasonique 3418

Lidocaine (Posaconazole should be administered with caution to patients with potentially proarrhythmic conditions and should not be administered with drugs that are known to prolong the QTc interval and are metabolized through CYP3A4). Products include:
Lidoderm 1107

Lidocaine Hydrochloride (Posaconazole should be administered with caution to patients with potentially proarrhythmic conditions and should not be administered with drugs that are known to prolong the QTc interval and are metabolized through CYP3A4).
No products indexed under this heading.

Lithium Carbonate (Posaconazole should be administered with caution to patients with potentially proarrhythmic conditions and should not be administered with drugs that are known to prolong the QTc interval and are metabolized through CYP3A4).
No products indexed under this heading.

Lithium Citrate (Posaconazole should be administered with caution to patients with potentially proarrhythmic conditions and should not be administered with drugs that are known to prolong the QTc interval and are metabolized through CYP3A4).
No products indexed under this heading.

Lorazepam (Posaconazole should be administered with caution to patients with potentially proarrhythmic conditions and should not be administered with drugs that are known to prolong the QTc interval and are metabolized through CYP3A4).
No products indexed under this heading.

Lovastatin (It is recommended that dose reduction of statins metabolized through CYP3A4 be considered during co-administration. Increased statin concentrations in plasma can be associated with rhabdomyolysis). Products include:
Advicor 402
Mevacor 2212

Loxapine Hydrochloride (Posaconazole should be administered with caution to patients with potentially proarrhythmic conditions and should not be administered with drugs that are known to prolong the QTc interval and are metabolized through CYP3A4).
No products indexed under this heading.

Loxapine Succinate (Posaconazole should be administered with caution to patients with potentially proarrhythmic conditions and should not be administered with drugs that are known to prolong the QTc interval and are metabolized through CYP3A4).
No products indexed under this heading.

Maprotiline Hydrochloride (Posaconazole should be administered with caution to patients with potentially proarrhythmic conditions and should not be administered with drugs that are known to prolong the QTc interval and are metabolized through CYP3A4).
No products indexed under this heading.

Mephenytoin (Posaconazole is primarily metabolized via UDP glucuronidation (phase 2 enzymes) and is a substrate for p-glycoprotein (P-gp) efflux. Therefore, inhibitors or inducers of these clearance pathways may affect posaconazole plasma concentrations).
No products indexed under this heading.

Meprobamate (Posaconazole should be administered with caution to patients with potentially proarrhythmic conditions and should not be administered with drugs that are known to prolong the QTc interval and are metabolized through CYP3A4).
No products indexed under this heading.

Mesoridazine Besylate (Posaconazole should be administered with caution to patients with potentially proarrhythmic conditions and should not be administered with drugs that are known to prolong the QTc interval and are metabolized through CYP3A4).
No products indexed under this heading.

Mestranol (A clinical study in healthy volunteers indicates that posaconazole is a strong CYP3A4 inhibitor. Therefore, plasma concentrations of drugs predominantly metabolized by CYP3A4 may be increased by posaconazole).
No products indexed under this heading.

Methadone Hydrochloride (A clinical study in healthy volunteers indicates that posaconazole is a strong CYP3A4 inhibitor. Therefore, plasma concentrations of drugs predominantly metabolized by CYP3A4 may be increased by posaconazole).
No products indexed under this heading.

Methylergonovine Maleate (Co-administration of posaconazole with ergot alkaloids is contraindicated. Posaconazole may increase the plasma concentrations of ergot alkaloids which may lead to ergotism).
No products indexed under this heading.

Methysergide Maleate (Co-administration of posaconazole with ergot alkaloids is contraindicated. Posaconazole may increase the plasma concentrations of ergot alkaloids which may lead to ergotism).
No products indexed under this heading.

Metoclopramide Hydrochloride (Co-administration of metoclopramide with posaconazole may result in lower plasma concentrations of posaconazole. Monitor closely for breakthrough of fungal infections if posaconazole is used concomitantly with metoclopramide). Products include:
Metozolv ODT 2901

Mexiletine Hydrochloride (Posaconazole should be administered with caution to patients with potentially proarrhythmic conditions and should not be administered with drugs that are known to prolong the QTc interval and are metabolized through CYP3A4).
No products indexed under this heading.

Mibefradil Dihydrochloride (Frequent monitoring for adverse events and toxicity related to calcium channel blockers which are metabolized through CYP3A4 is recommended during co-administration. Dose reduction of calcium channel blockers which are metabolized through CYP3A4 may be needed).
No products indexed under this heading.

Midazolam Hydrochloride (A clinical study in healthy volunteers indicates that posaconazole is a strong CYP3A4 inhibitor as evidenced by a>5-fold increase in midazolam AUC. Frequent monitoring of adverse effects of benzodiazepines metabolized by CYP3A4 should be performed and dose reduction of these benzodiazepines should be considered during co-administration with posaconazole).
No products indexed under this heading.

Molindone Hydrochloride (Posaconazole should be administered with caution to patients with potentially proarrhythmic conditions and should not be administered with drugs that are known to prolong the QTc interval and are metabolized through CYP3A4). Products include:
Moban 1108

IMPORTANT NOTE: Always consult each drug listing in the patient's regimen for possible interactions.

Noxafil Interactions Index 1258

Nefazodone Hydrochloride (A clinical study in healthy volunteers indicates that posaconazole is a strong CYP3A4 inhibitor. Therefore, plasma concentrations of drugs predominantly metabolized by CYP3A4 may be increased by posaconazole).
No products indexed under this heading.

Nelfinavir Mesylate (A clinical study in healthy volunteers indicates that posaconazole is a strong CYP3A4 inhibitor. Therefore, plasma concentrations of drugs predominantly metabolized by CYP3A4 may be increased by posaconazole).
No products indexed under this heading.

Nicardipine (Frequent monitoring for adverse events and toxicity related to calcium channel blockers which are metabolized through CYP3A4 is recommended during co-administration. Dose reduction of calcium channel blockers which are metabolized through CYP3A4 may be needed).
No products indexed under this heading.

Nicardipine Hydrochloride (Frequent monitoring for adverse events and toxicity related to calcium channel blockers which are metabolized through CYP3A4 is recommended during co-administration. Dose reduction of calcium channel blockers which are metabolized through CYP3A4 may be needed).
No products indexed under this heading.

Nifedipine (Frequent monitoring for adverse events and toxicity related to calcium channel blockers which are metabolized through CYP3A4 is recommended during co-administration. Dose reduction of calcium channel blockers which are metabolized through CYP3A4 may be needed).
No products indexed under this heading.

Nimodipine (Frequent monitoring for adverse events and toxicity related to calcium channel blockers which are metabolized through CYP3A4 is recommended during co-administration. Dose reduction of calcium channel blockers which are metabolized through CYP3A4 may be needed).
No products indexed under this heading.

Nisoldipine (Frequent monitoring for adverse events and toxicity related to calcium channel blockers which are metabolized through CYP3A4 is recommended during co-administration. Dose reduction of calcium channel blockers which are metabolized through CYP3A4 may be needed).
No products indexed under this heading.

Nitrendipine (A clinical study in healthy volunteers indicates that posaconazole is a strong CYP3A4 inhibitor. Therefore, plasma concentrations of drugs predominantly metabolized by CYP3A4 may be increased by posaconazole).
No products indexed under this heading.

Norethindrone (A clinical study in healthy volunteers indicates that posaconazole is a strong CYP3A4 inhibitor. Therefore, plasma concentrations of drugs predominantly metabolized by CYP3A4 may be increased by posaconazole). Products include:
Ortho Micronor 2660

Norethindrone Acetate (A clinical study in healthy volunteers indicates that posaconazole is a strong CYP3A4 inhibitor. Therefore, plasma concentrations of drugs predominantly metabolized by CYP3A4 may be increased by posaconazole). Products include:
Activella 2561

Norgestrel (A clinical study in healthy volunteers indicates that posaconazole is a strong CYP3A4 inhibitor. Therefore, plasma concentrations of drugs predominantly metabolized by CYP3A4 may be increased by posaconazole).
No products indexed under this heading.

Nortriptyline Hydrochloride (Posaconazole should be administered with caution to patients with potentially proarrhythmic conditions and should not be administered with drugs that are known to prolong the QTc interval and are metabolized through CYP3A4).
No products indexed under this heading.

Olanzapine (Posaconazole should be administered with caution to patients with potentially proarrhythmic conditions and should not be administered with drugs that are known to prolong the QTc interval and are metabolized through CYP3A4). Products include:
Symbyax 1965
Zyprexa 1984
Zyprexa IntraMuscular 1984
Zyprexa ZYDIS 1984

Ondansetron (A clinical study in healthy volunteers indicates that posaconazole is a strong CYP3A4 inhibitor. Therefore, plasma concentrations of drugs predominantly metabolized by CYP3A4 may be increased by posaconazole).
No products indexed under this heading.

Ondansetron Hydrochloride (A clinical study in healthy volunteers indicates that posaconazole is a strong CYP3A4 inhibitor. Therefore, plasma concentrations of drugs predominantly metabolized by CYP3A4 may be increased by posaconazole). Products include:
Zofran Injection 1750
Zofran 1756
Zofran ODT 1756

Oxazepam (Posaconazole should be administered with caution to patients with potentially proarrhythmic conditions and should not be administered with drugs that are known to prolong the QTc interval and are metabolized through CYP3A4).
No products indexed under this heading.

Paclitaxel (A clinical study in healthy volunteers indicates that posaconazole is a strong CYP3A4 inhibitor. Therefore, plasma concentrations of drugs predominantly metabolized by CYP3A4 may be increased by posaconazole).
No products indexed under this heading.

Perphenazine (Posaconazole should be administered with caution to patients with potentially proarrhythmic conditions and should not be administered with drugs that are known to prolong the QTc interval and are metabolized through CYP3A4).
No products indexed under this heading.

Phenelzine Sulfate (Posaconazole should be administered with caution to patients with potentially proarrhythmic conditions and should not be administered with drugs that are known to prolong the QTc interval and are metabolized through CYP3A4).
No products indexed under this heading.

Phenobarbital (Posaconazole is primarily metabolized via UDP glucuronidation (phase 2 enzymes) and is a substrate for p-glycoprotein (P-gp) efflux. Therefore, inhibitors or inducers of these clearance pathways may affect posaconazole plasma concentrations). Products include:
Donnatal 2711

Phenobarbital Sodium (Posaconazole is primarily metabolized via UDP glucuronidation (phase 2 enzymes) and is a substrate for p-glycoprotein (P-gp) efflux. Therefore, inhibitors or inducers of these clearance pathways may affect posaconazole plasma concentrations).
No products indexed under this heading.

Phenothiazine Derivatives (Posaconazole is a substrate for p-glycoprotein (P-gp) efflux. Therefore, inducers of p-glycoprotein may affect posaconazole plasma concentrations).
No products indexed under this heading.

Phenothiazines (Posaconazole is a substrate for p-glycoprotein (P-gp) efflux. Therefore, inducers of p-glycoprotein may affect posaconazole plasma concentrations).
No products indexed under this heading.

Phenytoin (Co-administration of phenytoin with posaconazole may result in lower plasma concentrations of posaconazole and increased concentrations of phenytoin. Frequent monitoring of phenytoin concentrations should be performed when co-administered with posaconazole and dose reduction of phenytoin should be considered. Avoid concomitant use unless the benefit outweighs the risks).
No products indexed under this heading.

Phenytoin Sodium (Co-administration of phenytoin with posaconazole may result in lower plasma concentrations of posaconazole and increased concentrations of phenytoin. Frequent monitoring of phenytoin concentrations should be performed when co-administered with posaconazole and dose reduction of phenytoin should be considered. Avoid concomitant use unless the benefit outweighs the risks). Products include:
Phenytek Capsules 2380

Pimozide (Co-administration of the CYP3A4 substrate pimozide with posaconazole is contraindicated since it may result in increased plasma concentrations of pimozide, leading to QTc prolongation and rare occurrences of torsades de pointes).
No products indexed under this heading.

Polyestradiol Phosphate (A clinical study in healthy volunteers indicates that posaconazole is a strong CYP3A4 inhibitor. Therefore, plasma concentrations of drugs predominantly metabolized by CYP3A4 may be increased by posaconazole).
No products indexed under this heading.

Pravastatin Sodium (It is recommended that dose reduction of HMG-CoA reductase inhibitors metabolized through CYP3A4 be considered during co-administration. Increased statin concentrations in plasma can be associated with rhabdomyolysis).
No products indexed under this heading.

Prazepam (Posaconazole should be administered with caution to patients with potentially proarrhythmic conditions and should not be administered with drugs that are known to prolong the QTc interval and are metabolized through CYP3A4).
No products indexed under this heading.

Procainamide Hydrochloride (Posaconazole should be administered with caution to patients with potentially proarrhythmic conditions and should not be administered with drugs that are known to prolong the QTc interval and are metabolized through CYP3A4).
No products indexed under this heading.

Prochlorperazine (Posaconazole should be administered with caution to patients with potentially proarrhythmic conditions and should not be administered with drugs that are known to prolong the QTc interval and are metabolized through CYP3A4).
No products indexed under this heading.

Prochlorperazine Edisylate (Posaconazole is a substrate for p-glycoprotein (P-gp) efflux. Therefore, inducers of p-glycoprotein may affect posaconazole plasma concentrations).
No products indexed under this heading.

Prochlorperazine Maleate (Posaconazole is a substrate for p-glycoprotein (P-gp) efflux. Therefore, inducers of p-glycoprotein may affect posaconazole plasma concentrations).
No products indexed under this heading.

Promethazine (Posaconazole is a substrate for p-glycoprotein (P-gp) efflux. Therefore, inducers of p-glycoprotein may affect posaconazole plasma concentrations).
No products indexed under this heading.

Promethazine Hydrochloride (Posaconazole should be administered with caution to patients with potentially proarrhythmic conditions and should not be administered with drugs that are known to prolong the QTc interval and are metabolized through CYP3A4).
No products indexed under this heading.

Propafenone Hydrochloride (Posaconazole should be administered with caution to patients with potentially proarrhythmic conditions and should not be administered with drugs that are known to prolong the QTc interval and are metabolized through CYP3A4). Products include:
Rythmol 1648
Rythmol SR 1652

Protriptyline Hydrochloride (Posaconazole should be administered with caution to patients with potentially proarrhythmic conditions and should not be administered with drugs that are known to prolong the QTc interval and are metabolized through CYP3A4).
No products indexed under this heading.

Quetiapine Fumarate (Posaconazole should be administered with caution to patients with potentially proarrhythmic conditions and should not be administered with drugs that are known to prolong the QTc interval and are metabolized through CYP3A4). Products include:
Seroquel 750
Seroquel XR 759

Quinidine (Posaconazole should be administered with caution to patients with potentially proarrhythmic conditions and should not be administered with drugs that are known to prolong the QTc interval and are metabolized through CYP3A4).
No products indexed under this heading.

Quinidine Gluconate (Posaconazole should be administered with caution to patients with potentially proarrhythmic conditions and should not be administered with drugs that are known to prolong the QTc interval and are metabolized through CYP3A4).
No products indexed under this heading.

Quinidine Hydrochloride (Posaconazole should be administered with caution to patients with potentially proarrhythmic conditions and should not be administered with drugs that are known to prolong the QTc interval and are metabolized through CYP3A4).
No products indexed under this heading.

Quinidine Polygalacturonate (Posaconazole should be administered with caution to patients with potentially proarrhythmic conditions and should not be administered with drugs that are known to prolong the QTc interval and are metabolized through CYP3A4).
No products indexed under this heading.

Quinidine Sulfate (Posaconazole should be administered with caution to patients with potentially proarrhythmic conditions and should not be administered with drugs that are known to prolong the QTc interval and are metabolized through CYP3A4).

No products indexed under this heading.

Rifabutin (Concomitant use of posaconazole and rifabutin should be avoided unless the benefit to the patient outweighs the risk. However, if concomitant administration is required, frequent monitoring of full blood counts and adverse events due to increased rifabutin levels (eg, uveitis, leukopenia) is recommended).

No products indexed under this heading.

Rifampicin (Posaconazole is a substrate for p-glycoprotein (P-gp) efflux. Therefore, inducers of p-glycoprotein may affect posaconazole plasma concentrations).

No products indexed under this heading.

Rifampin (Posaconazole is a substrate for p-glycoprotein (P-gp) efflux. Therefore, inducers of p-glycoprotein may affect posaconazole plasma concentrations).

No products indexed under this heading.

Risperidone (Posaconazole should be administered with caution to patients with potentially proarrhythmic conditions and should not be administered with drugs that are known to prolong the QTc interval and are metabolized through CYP3A4). Products include:

Ritonavir (Frequent monitoring of adverse effects and toxicity of ritonavir should be performed during co-administration with posaconazole). Products include:

Rosuvastatin Calcium (It is recommended that dose reduction of HMG-CoA reductase inhibitors metabolized through CYP3A4 be considered during co-administration. Increased statin concentrations in plasma can be associated with rhabdomyolysis). Products include:

Saquinavir (A clinical study in healthy volunteers indicates that posaconazole is a strong CYP3A4 inhibitor. Therefore, plasma concentrations of drugs predominantly metabolized by CYP3A4 may be increased by posaconazole).

No products indexed under this heading.

Saquinavir Mesylate (A clinical study in healthy volunteers indicates that posaconazole is a strong CYP3A4 inhibitor. Therefore, plasma concentrations of drugs predominantly metabolized by CYP3A4 may be increased by posaconazole).

No products indexed under this heading.

Sertraline Hydrochloride (A clinical study in healthy volunteers indicates that posaconazole is a strong CYP3A4 inhibitor. Therefore, plasma concentrations of drugs predominantly metabolized by CYP3A4 may be increased by posaconazole).

No products indexed under this heading.

Sildenafil Citrate (A clinical study in healthy volunteers indicates that posaconazole is a strong CYP3A4 inhibitor. Therefore, plasma concentrations of drugs predominantly metabolized by CYP3A4 may be increased by posaconazole).

No products indexed under this heading.

Simvastatin (It is recommended that dose reduction of statins metabolized through CYP3A4 be considered during co-administration. Increased statin concentrations in plasma can be associated with rhabdomyolysis). Products include:

Sirolimus (Co-administration of posaconazole with sirolimus is contraindicated. Concomitant use of a 2 mg single dose of sirolimus with 400 mg bid of posaconazole for 16 days was found to increase the mean C_{max} of sirolimus by 572% and the mean AUC of sirolimus by 788%). Products include:

Tacrolimus (Posaconazole has been shown to increase C_{max} and AUC of tacrolimus significantly. At initiation of posaconazole treatment, reduce the tacrolimus dose to approximately 1/3 of the original dose. Frequent monitoring of tacrolimus whole blood trough concentrations should be performed during and at discontinuation of posaconazole treatment and the tacrolimus dose adjusted accordingly). Products include:

Tadalafil (A clinical study in healthy volunteers indicates that posaconazole is a strong CYP3A4 inhibitor. Therefore, plasma concentrations of drugs predominantly metabolized by CYP3A4 may be increased by posaconazole). Products include:

Tamoxifen Citrate (A clinical study in healthy volunteers indicates that posaconazole is a strong CYP3A4 inhibitor. Therefore, plasma concentrations of drugs predominantly metabolized by CYP3A4 may be increased by posaconazole).

No products indexed under this heading.

Terfenadine (Co-administration of the CYP3A4 substrate terfenadine with posaconazole is contraindicated since it may result in increased plasma concentrations of terfenadine, leading to QTc prolongation and rare occurrences of torsades de pointes).

No products indexed under this heading.

Theophylline (A clinical study in healthy volunteers indicates that posaconazole is a strong CYP3A4 inhibitor. Therefore, plasma concentrations of drugs predominantly metabolized by CYP3A4 may be increased by posaconazole).

No products indexed under this heading.

Theophylline Anhydrous (A clinical study in healthy volunteers indicates that posaconazole is a strong CYP3A4 inhibitor. Therefore, plasma concentrations of drugs predominantly metabolized by CYP3A4 may be increased by posaconazole). Products include:

Theophylline Calcium Salicylate (A clinical study in healthy volunteers indicates that posaconazole is a strong CYP3A4 inhibitor. Therefore, plasma concentrations of drugs predominantly metabolized by CYP3A4 may be increased by posaconazole).

No products indexed under this heading.

Theophylline Dihydroxypropyl (Glyceryl) (A clinical study in healthy volunteers indicates that posaconazole is a strong CYP3A4 inhibitor. Therefore, plasma concentrations of drugs predominantly metabolized by CYP3A4 may be increased by posaconazole).

No products indexed under this heading.

Theophylline Ethylenediamine (A clinical study in healthy volunteers indicates that posaconazole is a strong CYP3A4 inhibitor. Therefore, plasma concentrations of drugs predominantly metabolized by CYP3A4 may be increased by posaconazole).

No products indexed under this heading.

Theophylline Sodium Glycinate (A clinical study in healthy volunteers indicates that posaconazole is a strong CYP3A4 inhibitor. Therefore, plasma concentrations of drugs predominantly metabolized by CYP3A4 may be increased by posaconazole).

No products indexed under this heading.

Thioridazine (Posaconazole is a substrate for p-glycoprotein (P-gp) efflux. Therefore, inducers of p-glycoprotein may affect posaconazole plasma concentrations).

No products indexed under this heading.

Thioridazine Hydrochloride (Posaconazole should be administered with caution to patients with potentially proarrhythmic conditions and should not be administered with drugs that are known to prolong the QTc interval and are metabolized through CYP3A4). Products include:

Thiothixene (Posaconazole should be administered with caution to patients with potentially proarrhythmic conditions and should not be administered with drugs that are known to prolong the QTc interval and are metabolized through CYP3A4). Products include:

Tiagabine Hydrochloride (A clinical study in healthy volunteers indicates that posaconazole is a strong CYP3A4 inhibitor. Therefore, plasma concentrations of drugs predominantly metabolized by CYP3A4 may be increased by posaconazole). Products include:

Tocainide Hydrochloride (Posaconazole should be administered with caution to patients with potentially proarrhythmic conditions and should not be administered with drugs that are known to prolong the QTc interval and are metabolized through CYP3A4).

No products indexed under this heading.

Tolterodine Tartrate (A clinical study in healthy volunteers indicates that posaconazole is a strong CYP3A4 inhibitor. Therefore, plasma concentrations of drugs predominantly metabolized by CYP3A4 may be increased by posaconazole).

No products indexed under this heading.

Tranylcypromine Sulfate (Posaconazole should be administered with caution to patients with potentially proarrhythmic conditions and should not be administered with drugs that are known to prolong the QTc interval and are metabolized through CYP3A4). Products include:

Trazodone Hydrochloride (A clinical study in healthy volunteers indicates that posaconazole is a strong CYP3A4 inhibitor. Therefore, plasma concentrations of drugs predominantly metabolized by CYP3A4 may be increased by posaconazole).

No products indexed under this heading.

Triazolam (Frequent monitoring of adverse effects of benzodiazepines metabolized by CYP3A4 should be performed and dose reduction of these benzodiazepines should be considered during co-administration with posaconazole).

No products indexed under this heading.

Trifluoperazine Hydrochloride (Posaconazole should be administered with caution to patients with potentially proarrhythmic conditions and should not be administered with drugs that are known to prolong the QTc interval and are metabolized through CYP3A4).

No products indexed under this heading.

Trimipramine Maleate (Posaconazole should be administered with caution to patients with potentially proarrhythmic conditions and should not be administered with drugs that are known to prolong the QTc interval and are metabolized through CYP3A4).

No products indexed under this heading.

Troleandomycin (Posaconazole is a substrate for p-glycoprotein (P-gp) efflux. Therefore, inhibitors of p-glycoprotein may affect posaconazole plasma concentrations).

No products indexed under this heading.

Udp-Glucuronosyltransferase (Ugt) Inhibitors (Posaconazole is primarily metabolized via UDP glucuronidation (phase 2 enzymes) and is a substrate for p-glycoprotein (P-gp) efflux. Therefore, inhibitors or inducers of these clearance pathways may affect posaconazole plasma concentrations).

No products indexed under this heading.

Vardenafil Hydrochloride (A clinical study in healthy volunteers indicates that posaconazole is a strong CYP3A4 inhibitor. Therefore, plasma concentrations of drugs predominantly metabolized by CYP3A4 may be increased by posaconazole). Products include:

Verapamil Hydrochloride (Frequent monitoring for adverse events and toxicity related to calcium channel blockers which are metabolized through CYP3A4 is recommended during co-administration. Dose reduction of calcium channel blockers which are metabolized through CYP3A4 may be needed). Products include:

Vinblastine Sulfate (Posaconazole may increase the plasma concentrations of vinca alkaloids (eg, vinblastine) which may lead to neurotoxicity. Therefore, it is recommended that the dose adjustment of the vinca alkaloid be considered).

No products indexed under this heading.

Vincristine Sulfate (Posaconazole may increase the plasma concentrations of vinca alkaloids (eg, vincristine) which may lead to neurotoxicity. Therefore, it is recommended that the dose adjustment of the vinca alkaloid be considered).

No products indexed under this heading.

Vinorelbine Tartrate (Posaconazole may increase the plasma concentrations of vinca alkaloids (eg, vincristine, vinblastine) which may lead to neurotoxicity. Therefore, it is recommended that the dose adjustment of the vinca alkaloid be considered).

No products indexed under this heading.

Warfarin Sodium (A clinical study in healthy volunteers indicates that posaconazole is a strong CYP3A4 inhibitor. Therefore, plasma concentrations of drugs predominantly metabolized by CYP3A4 may be increased by posaconazole).

No products indexed under this heading.

Ziprasidone Hydrochloride (Posaconazole should be administered with caution to patients with potentially proarrhythmic conditions and should not be administered with drugs that are known to prolong the QTc interval and are metabolized through CYP3A4). Products include:

IMPORTANT NOTE: Always consult each drug listing in the patient's regimen for possible interactions.

Nplate Interactions Index 1260

NPLATE FOR SUBCUTANEOUS INJECTION
(Romiplostim) 637
None cited in PDR database.

NUCYNTA TABLETS
(Tapentadol Hydrochloride) 2643
May interact with alcohols, antiemetics, central nervous system depressants, general anesthetics, hypnotics and sedatives, monoamine oxidase inhibitors, narcotic analgesics, phenothiazines, selective serotonin reuptake inhibitors, serotonin and norepinephrine reuptake inhibitors, serotoninergic agents, tranquilizers, tricyclic antidepressants, triptans, and certain other agents. Compounds in these categories include:

Alfentanil Hydrochloride (Patients receiving other opioid agonist analgesics, general anesthetics, phenothiazines, antiemetics, other tranquilizers, sedatives, hypnotics, or other CNS depressants (including alcohol) concomitantly with tapentadol hydrochloride may exhibit an additive CNS depression. Interactive effects resulting in respiratory depression, hypotension, profound sedation, or coma may result if these drugs are taken in combination with tapentadol hydrochloride. When such combined therapy is contemplated, a dose reduction of one or both agents should be considered).
No products indexed under this heading.

Almotriptan Malate (The development of a potentially life-threatening serotonin syndrome may occur with use of Serotonin and Norepinephrine Reuptake Inhibitor (SNRI) products, including tapentadol hydrochloride, particularly with concomitant use of serotonergic drugs such as Selective Serotonin Reuptake Inhibitors (SSRIs), SNRIs, tricyclic antidepressants (TCAs), MAOIs and triptans, and with drugs that impair metabolism of serotonin (including MAOIs). This may occur within the recommended dose. Serotonin syndrome may include mental-status changes, autonomic instability, neuromuscular aberrations and/or gastrointestinal symptoms). Products include:
Axert 2593

Alprazolam (Patients receiving other opioid agonist analgesics, general anesthetics, phenothiazines, antiemetics, other tranquilizers, sedatives, hypnotics, or other CNS depressants (including alcohol) concomitantly with tapentadol hydrochloride may exhibit an additive CNS depression. Interactive effects resulting in respiratory depression, hypotension, profound sedation, or coma may result if these drugs are taken in combination with tapentadol hydrochloride. When such combined therapy is contemplated, a dose reduction of one or both agents should be considered).
No products indexed under this heading.

Amitriptyline Hydrochloride (The development of a potentially life-threatening serotonin syndrome may occur with use of Serotonin and Norepinephrine Reuptake Inhibitor (SNRI) products, including tapentadol hydrochloride, particularly with concomitant use of serotonergic drugs such as Selective Serotonin Reuptake Inhibitors (SSRIs), SNRIs, tricyclic antidepressants (TCAs), MAOIs and triptans, and with drugs that impair metabolism of serotonin (including MAOIs). This may occur within the recommended dose. Serotonin syndrome may include mental-status changes, autonomic instability, neuromuscular aberrations and/or gastrointestinal symptoms).
No products indexed under this heading.

Amobarbital (Patients receiving other opioid agonist analgesics, general anesthetics, phenothiazines, antiemetics, other tranquilizers, sedatives, hypnotics, or other CNS depressants (including alcohol) concomitantly with tapentadol hydrochloride may exhibit an additive CNS depression. Interactive effects resulting in respiratory depression, hypotension, profound sedation, or coma may result if these drugs are taken in combination with tapentadol hydrochloride. When such combined therapy is contemplated, a dose reduction of one or both agents should be considered).
No products indexed under this heading.

Amobarbital Sodium (Patients receiving other opioid agonist analgesics, general anesthetics, phenothiazines, antiemetics, other tranquilizers, sedatives, hypnotics, or other CNS depressants (including alcohol) concomitantly with tapentadol hydrochloride may exhibit an additive CNS depression. Interactive effects resulting in respiratory depression, hypotension, profound sedation, or coma may result if these drugs are taken in combination with tapentadol hydrochloride. When such combined therapy is contemplated, a dose reduction of one or both agents should be considered).
No products indexed under this heading.

Amoxapine (The development of a potentially life-threatening serotonin syndrome may occur with use of Serotonin and Norepinephrine Reuptake Inhibitor (SNRI) products, including tapentadol hydrochloride, particularly with concomitant use of serotonergic drugs such as Selective Serotonin Reuptake Inhibitors (SSRIs), SNRIs, tricyclic antidepressants (TCAs), MAOIs and triptans, and with drugs that impair metabolism of serotonin (including MAOIs). This may occur within the recommended dose. Serotonin syndrome may include mental-status changes, autonomic instability, neuromuscular aberrations and/or gastrointestinal symptoms).
No products indexed under this heading.

Apomorphine (Patients receiving other opioid agonist analgesics, general anesthetics, phenothiazines, antiemetics, other tranquilizers, sedatives, hypnotics, or other CNS depressants (including alcohol) concomitantly with tapentadol hydrochloride may exhibit an additive CNS depression. Interactive effects resulting in respiratory depression, hypotension, profound sedation, or coma may result if these drugs are taken in combination with tapentadol hydrochloride. When such combined therapy is contemplated, a dose reduction of one or both agents should be considered).
No products indexed under this heading.

Apomorphine Hydrochloride (Patients receiving other opioid agonist analgesics, general anesthetics, phenothiazines, antiemetics, other tranquilizers, sedatives, hypnotics, or other CNS depressants (including alcohol) concomitantly with tapentadol hydrochloride may exhibit an additive CNS depression. Interactive effects resulting in respiratory depression, hypotension, profound sedation, or coma may result if these drugs are taken in combination with tapentadol hydrochloride. When such combined therapy is contemplated, a dose reduction of one or both agents should be considered).
No products indexed under this heading.

Aprepitant (Patients receiving other opioid agonist analgesics, general anesthetics, phenothiazines, antiemetics, other tranquilizers, sedatives, hypnotics, or other CNS depressants (including alcohol) concomitantly with tapentadol hydrochloride may exhibit an additive CNS depression. Interactive effects resulting in respiratory depression, hypotension, profound sedation, or coma may result if these drugs are taken in combination with tapentadol hydrochloride. When such combined therapy is contemplated, a dose reduction of one or both agents should be considered). Products include:
Emend 2124

Aprobarbital (Patients receiving other opioid agonist analgesics, general anesthetics, phenothiazines, antiemetics, other tranquilizers, sedatives, hypnotics, or other CNS depressants (including alcohol) concomitantly with tapentadol hydrochloride may exhibit an additive CNS depression. Interactive effects resulting in respiratory depression, hypotension, profound sedation, or coma may result if these drugs are taken in combination with tapentadol hydrochloride. When such combined therapy is contemplated, a dose reduction of one or both agents should be considered).
No products indexed under this heading.

Buprenorphine Hydrochloride (Patients receiving other opioid agonist analgesics, general anesthetics, phenothiazines, antiemetics, other tranquilizers, sedatives, hypnotics, or other CNS depressants (including alcohol) concomitantly with tapentadol hydrochloride may exhibit an additive CNS depression. Interactive effects resulting in respiratory depression, hypotension, profound sedation, or coma may result if these drugs are taken in combination with tapentadol hydrochloride. When such combined therapy is contemplated, a dose reduction of one or both agents should be considered).
No products indexed under this heading.

Buspirone Hydrochloride (Patients receiving other opioid agonist analgesics, general anesthetics, phenothiazines, antiemetics, other tranquilizers, sedatives, hypnotics, or other CNS depressants (including alcohol) concomitantly with tapentadol hydrochloride may exhibit an additive CNS depression. Interactive effects resulting in respiratory depression, hypotension, profound sedation, or coma may result if these drugs are taken in combination with tapentadol hydrochloride. When such combined therapy is contemplated, a dose reduction of one or both agents should be considered).
No products indexed under this heading.

Butabarbital (Patients receiving other opioid agonist analgesics, general anesthetics, phenothiazines, antiemetics, other tranquilizers, sedatives, hypnotics, or other CNS depressants (including alcohol) concomitantly with tapentadol hydrochloride may exhibit an additive CNS depression. Interactive effects resulting in respiratory depression, hypotension, profound sedation, or coma may result if these drugs are taken in combination with tapentadol hydrochloride. When such combined therapy is contemplated, a dose reduction of one or both agents should be considered).
No products indexed under this heading.

Butabarbital Sodium (Patients receiving other opioid agonist analgesics, general anesthetics, phenothiazines, antiemetics, other tranquilizers, sedatives, hypnotics, or other CNS depressants (including alcohol) concomitantly with tapentadol hydrochloride may exhibit an additive CNS depression. Interactive effects resulting in respiratory depression, hypotension, profound sedation, or coma may result if these drugs are taken in combination with tapentadol hydrochloride. When such combined therapy is contemplated, a dose reduction of one or both agents should be considered).
No products indexed under this heading.

Butalbital (Patients receiving other opioid agonist analgesics, general anesthetics, phenothiazines, antiemetics, other tranquilizers, sedatives, hypnotics, or other CNS depressants (including alcohol) concomitantly with tapentadol hydrochloride may exhibit an additive CNS depression. Interactive effects resulting in respiratory depression, hypotension, profound sedation, or coma may result if these drugs are taken in combination with tapentadol hydrochloride. When such combined therapy is contemplated, a dose reduction of one or both agents should be considered).
No products indexed under this heading.

Chloral Hydrate (Patients receiving other opioid agonist analgesics, general anesthetics, phenothiazines, antiemetics, other tranquilizers, sedatives, hypnotics, or other CNS depressants (including alcohol) concomitantly with tapentadol hydrochloride may exhibit an additive CNS depression. Interactive effects resulting in respiratory depression, hypotension, profound sedation, or coma may result if these drugs are taken in combination with tapentadol hydrochloride. When such combined therapy is contemplated, a dose reduction of one or both agents should be considered).
No products indexed under this heading.

Chlordiazepoxide (Patients receiving other opioid agonist analgesics, general anesthetics, phenothiazines, antiemetics, other tranquilizers, sedatives, hypnotics, or other CNS depressants (including alcohol) concomitantly with tapentadol hydrochloride may exhibit an additive CNS depression. Interactive effects resulting in respiratory depression, hypotension, profound sedation, or coma may result if these drugs are taken in combination with tapentadol hydrochloride. When such combined therapy is contemplated, a dose reduction of one or both agents should be considered).
No products indexed under this heading.

Chlordiazepoxide Hydrochloride (Patients receiving other opioid agonist analgesics, general anesthetics, phenothiazines, antiemetics, other tranquilizers, sedatives, hypnotics, or other CNS depressants (including alcohol) concomitantly with tapentadol hydrochloride may exhibit an additive CNS depression. Interactive effects resulting in respiratory depression, hypotension, profound sedation, or coma may result if these drugs are taken in combination with tapentadol hydrochloride. When such combined therapy is contemplated, a dose reduction of one or both agents should be considered).
No products indexed under this heading.

Chlorpromazine (Patients receiving other opioid agonist analgesics, general anesthetics, phenothiazines, antiemetics, other tranquilizers, sedatives, hypnotics, or other CNS depressants (including alcohol) concomitantly with tapentadol hydrochloride may exhibit an additive CNS depression. Interactive effects resulting in respiratory depression, hypotension, profound sedation, or coma may result if these drugs are taken in combination with tapentadol hydrochloride. When such combined therapy is contemplated, a dose reduction of one or both agents should be considered).
No products indexed under this heading.

Chlorpromazine Hydrochloride (Patients receiving other opioid agonist analgesics, general anesthetics, phenothiazines, antiemetics, other tranquiliz-

1261 Interactions Index Nucynta

ers, sedatives, hypnotics, or other CNS depressants (including alcohol) concomitantly with tapentadol hydrochloride may exhibit an additive CNS depression. Interactive effects resulting in respiratory depression, hypotension, profound sedation, or coma may result if these drugs are taken in combination with tapentadol hydrochloride. When such combined therapy is contemplated, a dose reduction of one or both agents should be considered).
No products indexed under this heading.

Chlorprothixene (Patients receiving other opioid agonist analgesics, general anesthetics, phenothiazines, antiemetics, other tranquilizers, sedatives, hypnotics, or other CNS depressants (including alcohol) concomitantly with tapentadol hydrochloride may exhibit an additive CNS depression. Interactive effects resulting in respiratory depression, hypotension, profound sedation, or coma may result if these drugs are taken in combination with tapentadol hydrochloride. When such combined therapy is contemplated, a dose reduction of one or both agents should be considered).
No products indexed under this heading.

Chlorprothixene Hydrochloride (Patients receiving other opioid agonist analgesics, general anesthetics, phenothiazines, antiemetics, other tranquilizers, sedatives, hypnotics, or other CNS depressants (including alcohol) concomitantly with tapentadol hydrochloride may exhibit an additive CNS depression. Interactive effects resulting in respiratory depression, hypotension, profound sedation, or coma may result if these drugs are taken in combination with tapentadol hydrochloride. When such combined therapy is contemplated, a dose reduction of one or both agents should be considered).
No products indexed under this heading.

Chlorprothixene Lactate (Patients receiving other opioid agonist analgesics, general anesthetics, phenothiazines, antiemetics, other tranquilizers, sedatives, hypnotics, or other CNS depressants (including alcohol) concomitantly with tapentadol hydrochloride may exhibit an additive CNS depression. Interactive effects resulting in respiratory depression, hypotension, profound sedation, or coma may result if these drugs are taken in combination with tapentadol hydrochloride. When such combined therapy is contemplated, a dose reduction of one or both agents should be considered).
No products indexed under this heading.

Citalopram Hydrobromide (The development of a potentially life-threatening serotonin syndrome may occur with use of Serotonin and Norepinephrine Reuptake Inhibitor (SNRI) products, including tapentadol hydrochloride, particularly with concomitant use of serotonergic drugs such as Selective Serotonin Reuptake Inhibitors (SSRIs), SNRIs, tricyclic antidepressants (TCAs), MAOIs and triptans, and with drugs that impair metabolism of serotonin (including MAOIs). This may occur within the recommended dose. Serotonin syndrome may include mental-status changes, autonomic instability, neuromuscular aberrations and/or gastrointestinal symptoms). Products include:
Celexa 1153

Clomipramine Hydrochloride (The development of a potentially life-threatening serotonin syndrome may occur with use of Serotonin and Norepinephrine Reuptake Inhibitor (SNRI) products, including tapentadol hydrochloride, particularly with concomitant use of serotonergic drugs such as Selective Serotonin Reuptake Inhibitors (SSRIs), SNRIs, tricyclic antidepressants (TCAs), MAOIs and triptans, and with drugs that impair metabolism of serotonin (including MAOIs). This may occur within the recommended dose. Serotonin syndrome may include mental-status changes, autonomic instability, neuromuscular aberrations and/or gastrointestinal symptoms).
No products indexed under this heading.

Clonazepam (Patients receiving other opioid agonist analgesics, general anesthetics, phenothiazines, antiemetics, other tranquilizers, sedatives, hypnotics, or other CNS depressants (including alcohol) concomitantly with tapentadol hydrochloride may exhibit an additive CNS depression. Interactive effects resulting in respiratory depression, hypotension, profound sedation, or coma may result if these drugs are taken in combination with tapentadol hydrochloride. When such combined therapy is contemplated, a dose reduction of one or both agents should be considered). Products include:
Klonopin 2855

Clorazepate Dipotassium (Patients receiving other opioid agonist analgesics, general anesthetics, phenothiazines, antiemetics, other tranquilizers, sedatives, hypnotics, or other CNS depressants (including alcohol) concomitantly with tapentadol hydrochloride may exhibit an additive CNS depression. Interactive effects resulting in respiratory depression, hypotension, profound sedation, or coma may result if these drugs are taken in combination with tapentadol hydrochloride. When such combined therapy is contemplated, a dose reduction of one or both agents should be considered).
No products indexed under this heading.

Clozapine (Patients receiving other opioid agonist analgesics, general anesthetics, phenothiazines, antiemetics, other tranquilizers, sedatives, hypnotics, or other CNS depressants (including alcohol) concomitantly with tapentadol hydrochloride may exhibit an additive CNS depression. Interactive effects resulting in respiratory depression, hypotension, profound sedation, or coma may result if these drugs are taken in combination with tapentadol hydrochloride. When such combined therapy is contemplated, a dose reduction of one or both agents should be considered).
No products indexed under this heading.

Codeine Phosphate (Patients receiving other opioid agonist analgesics, general anesthetics, phenothiazines, antiemetics, other tranquilizers, sedatives, hypnotics, or other CNS depressants (including alcohol) concomitantly with tapentadol hydrochloride may exhibit an additive CNS depression. Interactive effects resulting in respiratory depression, hypotension, profound sedation, or coma may result if these drugs are taken in combination with tapentadol hydrochloride. When such combined therapy is contemplated, a dose reduction of one or both agents should be considered). Products include:
Tylenol with Codeine 2691

Codeine Sulfate (Patients receiving other opioid agonist analgesics, general anesthetics, phenothiazines, antiemetics, other tranquilizers, sedatives, hypnotics, or other CNS depressants (including alcohol) concomitantly with tapentadol hydrochloride may exhibit an additive CNS depression. Interactive effects resulting in respiratory depression, hypotension, profound sedation, or coma may result if these drugs are taken in combination with tapentadol hydrochloride. When such combined therapy is contemplated, a dose reduction of one or both agents should be considered).
No products indexed under this heading.

Desflurane (Patients receiving other opioid agonist analgesics, general anesthetics, phenothiazines, antiemetics, other tranquilizers, sedatives, hypnotics, or other CNS depressants (including alcohol) concomitantly with tapentadol hydrochloride may exhibit an additive CNS depression. Interactive effects resulting in respiratory depression, hypotension, profound sedation, or coma may result if these drugs are taken in combination with tapentadol hydrochloride. When such combined therapy is contemplated, a dose reduction of one or both agents should be considered).
No products indexed under this heading.

Desipramine Hydrochloride (The development of a potentially life-threatening serotonin syndrome may occur with use of Serotonin and Norepinephrine Reuptake Inhibitor (SNRI) products, including tapentadol hydrochloride, particularly with concomitant use of serotonergic drugs such as Selective Serotonin Reuptake Inhibitors (SSRIs), SNRIs, tricyclic antidepressants (TCAs), MAOIs and triptans, and with drugs that impair metabolism of serotonin (including MAOIs). This may occur within the recommended dose. Serotonin syndrome may include mental-status changes, autonomic instability, neuromuscular aberrations and/or gastrointestinal symptoms).
No products indexed under this heading.

Desvenlafaxine Succinate (The development of a potentially life-threatening serotonin syndrome may occur with use of Serotonin and Norepinephrine Reuptake Inhibitor (SNRI) products, including tapentadol hydrochloride, particularly with concomitant use of serotonergic drugs such as Selective Serotonin Reuptake Inhibitors (SSRIs), SNRIs, tricyclic antidepressants (TCAs), MAOIs and triptans, and with drugs that impair metabolism of serotonin (including MAOIs). This may occur within the recommended dose. Serotonin syndrome may include mental-status changes, autonomic instability, neuromuscular aberrations and/or gastrointestinal symptoms). Products include:
Pristiq 3564

Dezocine (Patients receiving other opioid agonist analgesics, general anesthetics, phenothiazines, antiemetics, other tranquilizers, sedatives, hypnotics, or other CNS depressants (including alcohol) concomitantly with tapentadol hydrochloride may exhibit an additive CNS depression. Interactive effects resulting in respiratory depression, hypotension, profound sedation, or coma may result if these drugs are taken in combination with tapentadol hydrochloride. When such combined therapy is contemplated, a dose reduction of one or both agents should be considered).
No products indexed under this heading.

Diazepam (Patients receiving other opioid agonist analgesics, general anesthetics, phenothiazines, antiemetics, other tranquilizers, sedatives, hypnotics, or other CNS depressants (including alcohol) concomitantly with tapentadol hydrochloride may exhibit an additive CNS depression. Interactive effects resulting in respiratory depression, hypotension, profound sedation, or coma may result if these drugs are taken in combination with tapentadol hydrochloride. When such combined therapy is contemplated, a dose reduction of one or both agents should be considered). Products include:
Valium Tablets 2880

Dihydrocodeine Bitartrate (Patients receiving other opioid agonist analgesics, general anesthetics, phenothiazines, antiemetics, other tranquilizers, sedatives, hypnotics, or other CNS depressants (including alcohol) concomitantly with tapentadol hydrochloride may exhibit an additive CNS depression. Interactive effects resulting in respiratory depression, hypotension, profound sedation, or coma may result if these drugs are taken in combination with tapentadol hydrochloride. When such combined therapy is contemplated, a dose reduction of one or both agents should be considered).
No products indexed under this heading.

Dihydrocodeinone Bitartrate (Patients receiving other opioid agonist analgesics, general anesthetics, phenothiazines, antiemetics, other tranquilizers, sedatives, hypnotics, or other CNS depressants (including alcohol) concomitantly with tapentadol hydrochloride may exhibit an additive CNS depression. Interactive effects resulting in respiratory depression, hypotension, profound sedation, or coma may result if these drugs are taken in combination with tapentadol hydrochloride. When such combined therapy is contemplated, a dose reduction of one or both agents should be considered).
No products indexed under this heading.

Dimenhydrinate (Patients receiving other opioid agonist analgesics, general anesthetics, phenothiazines, antiemetics, other tranquilizers, sedatives, hypnotics, or other CNS depressants (including alcohol) concomitantly with tapentadol hydrochloride may exhibit an additive CNS depression. Interactive effects resulting in respiratory depression, hypotension, profound sedation, or coma may result if these drugs are taken in combination with tapentadol hydrochloride. When such combined therapy is contemplated, a dose reduction of one or both agents should be considered).
No products indexed under this heading.

Diphenhydramine (Patients receiving other opioid agonist analgesics, general anesthetics, phenothiazines, antiemetics, other tranquilizers, sedatives, hypnotics, or other CNS depressants (including alcohol) concomitantly with tapentadol hydrochloride may exhibit an additive CNS depression. Interactive effects resulting in respiratory depression, hypotension, profound sedation, or coma may result if these drugs are taken in combination with tapentadol hydrochloride. When such combined therapy is contemplated, a dose reduction of one or both agents should be considered).
No products indexed under this heading.

Diphenhydramine Hydrochloride (Patients receiving other opioid agonist analgesics, general anesthetics, phenothiazines, antiemetics, other tranquilizers, sedatives, hypnotics, or other CNS depressants (including alcohol) concomitantly with tapentadol hydrochloride may exhibit an additive CNS depression. Interactive effects resulting in respiratory depression, hypotension, profound sedation, or coma may result if these drugs are taken in combination with tapentadol hydrochloride. When such combined therapy is contemplated, a dose reduction of one or both agents should be considered). Products include:
Benadryl Allergy Ultratab 2042
Children's Benadryl Allergy Liquid 2042

Dolasetron Mesylate (Patients receiving other opioid agonist analgesics, general anesthetics, phenothiazines, antiemetics, other tranquilizers, sedatives, hypnotics, or other CNS depressants (including alcohol) concom-

IMPORTANT NOTE: Always consult each drug listing in the patient's regimen for possible interactions.

Nucynta Interactions Index 1262

itantly with tapentadol hydrochloride may exhibit an additive CNS depression. Interactive effects resulting in respiratory depression, hypotension, profound sedation, or coma may result if these drugs are taken in combination with tapentadol hydrochloride. When such combined therapy is contemplated, a dose reduction of one or both agents should be considered). Products include:

Anzemet Injection 2931
Anzemet Tablets 2934

Doxepin Hydrochloride (The development of a potentially life-threatening serotonin syndrome may occur with use of Serotonin and Norepinephrine Reuptake Inhibitor (SNRI) products, including tapentadol hydrochloride, particularly with concomitant use of serotonergic drugs such as Selective Serotonin Reuptake Inhibitors (SSRIs), SNRIs, tricyclic antidepressants (TCAs), MAOIs and triptans, and with drugs that impair metabolism of serotonin (including MAOIs). This may occur within the recommended dose. Serotonin syndrome may include mental-status changes, autonomic instability, neuromuscular aberrations and/or gastrointestinal symptoms).
No products indexed under this heading.

Dronabinol (Patients receiving other opioid agonist analgesics, general anesthetics, phenothiazines, antiemetics, other tranquilizers, sedatives, hypnotics, or other CNS depressants (including alcohol) concomitantly with tapentadol hydrochloride may exhibit an additive CNS depression. Interactive effects resulting in respiratory depression, hypotension, profound sedation, or coma may result if these drugs are taken in combination with tapentadol hydrochloride. When such combined therapy is contemplated, a dose reduction of one or both agents should be considered).
No products indexed under this heading.

Droperidol (Patients receiving other opioid agonist analgesics, general anesthetics, phenothiazines, antiemetics, other tranquilizers, sedatives, hypnotics, or other CNS depressants (including alcohol) concomitantly with tapentadol hydrochloride may exhibit an additive CNS depression. Interactive effects resulting in respiratory depression, hypotension, profound sedation, or coma may result if these drugs are taken in combination with tapentadol hydrochloride. When such combined therapy is contemplated, a dose reduction of one or both agents should be considered).
No products indexed under this heading.

Duloxetine Hydrochloride (The development of a potentially life-threatening serotonin syndrome may occur with use of Serotonin and Norepinephrine Reuptake Inhibitor (SNRI) products, including tapentadol hydrochloride, particularly with concomitant use of serotonergic drugs such as Selective Serotonin Reuptake Inhibitors (SSRIs), SNRIs, tricyclic antidepressants (TCAs), MAOIs and triptans, and with drugs that impair metabolism of serotonin (including MAOIs). This may occur within the recommended dose. Serotonin syndrome may include mental-status changes, autonomic instability, neuromuscular aberrations and/or gastrointestinal symptoms). Products include:

Cymbalta 1871

Eletriptan Hydrobromide (The development of a potentially life-threatening serotonin syndrome may occur with use of Serotonin and Norepinephrine Reuptake Inhibitor (SNRI) products, including tapentadol hydrochloride, particularly with concomitant use of serotonergic drugs such as Selective Serotonin Reuptake Inhibitors (SSRIs), SNRIs, tricyclic antidepressants (TCAs), MAOIs and triptans, and with drugs that impair metabolism of serotonin (including MAOIs). This may occur within the recommended dose. Serotonin syndrome may include mental-status changes, autonomic instability, neuromuscular aberrations and/or gastrointestinal symptoms).
No products indexed under this heading.

Enflurane (Patients receiving other opioid agonist analgesics, general anesthetics, phenothiazines, antiemetics, other tranquilizers, sedatives, hypnotics, or other CNS depressants (including alcohol) concomitantly with tapentadol hydrochloride may exhibit an additive CNS depression. Interactive effects resulting in respiratory depression, hypotension, profound sedation, or coma may result if these drugs are taken in combination with tapentadol hydrochloride. When such combined therapy is contemplated, a dose reduction of one or both agents should be considered).
No products indexed under this heading.

Escitalopram Oxalate (The development of a potentially life-threatening serotonin syndrome may occur with use of Serotonin and Norepinephrine Reuptake Inhibitor (SNRI) products, including tapentadol hydrochloride, particularly with concomitant use of serotonergic drugs such as Selective Serotonin Reuptake Inhibitors (SSRIs), SNRIs, tricyclic antidepressants (TCAs), MAOIs and triptans, and with drugs that impair metabolism of serotonin (including MAOIs). This may occur within the recommended dose. Serotonin syndrome may include mental-status changes, autonomic instability, neuromuscular aberrations and/or gastrointestinal symptoms). Products include:

Lexapro Oral Suspension 1160
Lexapro Tablets 1160

Estazolam (Patients receiving other opioid agonist analgesics, general anesthetics, phenothiazines, antiemetics, other tranquilizers, sedatives, hypnotics, or other CNS depressants (including alcohol) concomitantly with tapentadol hydrochloride may exhibit an additive CNS depression. Interactive effects resulting in respiratory depression, hypotension, profound sedation, or coma may result if these drugs are taken in combination with tapentadol hydrochloride. When such combined therapy is contemplated, a dose reduction of one or both agents should be considered).
No products indexed under this heading.

Ethanol (Patients receiving other opioid agonist analgesics, general anesthetics, phenothiazines, antiemetics, other tranquilizers, sedatives, hypnotics, or other CNS depressants (including alcohol) concomitantly with tapentadol hydrochloride may exhibit an additive CNS depression. Interactive effects resulting in respiratory depression, hypotension, profound sedation, or coma may result if these drugs are taken in combination with tapentadol hydrochloride. When such combined therapy is contemplated, a dose reduction of one or both agents should be considered).
No products indexed under this heading.

Ethchlorvynol (Patients receiving other opioid agonist analgesics, general anesthetics, phenothiazines, antiemetics, other tranquilizers, sedatives, hypnotics, or other CNS depressants (including alcohol) concomitantly with tapentadol hydrochloride may exhibit an additive CNS depression. Interactive effects resulting in respiratory depression, hypotension, profound sedation, or coma may result if these drugs are taken in combination with tapentadol hydrochloride. When such combined therapy is contemplated, a dose reduction of one or both agents should be considered).
No products indexed under this heading.

Ethinamate (Patients receiving other opioid agonist analgesics, general anesthetics, phenothiazines, antiemetics, other tranquilizers, sedatives, hypnotics, or other CNS depressants (including alcohol) concomitantly with tapentadol hydrochloride may exhibit an additive CNS depression. Interactive effects resulting in respiratory depression, hypotension, profound sedation, or coma may result if these drugs are taken in combination with tapentadol hydrochloride. When such combined therapy is contemplated, a dose reduction of one or both agents should be considered).
No products indexed under this heading.

Ethyl Alcohol (Patients receiving other opioid agonist analgesics, general anesthetics, phenothiazines, antiemetics, other tranquilizers, sedatives, hypnotics, or other CNS depressants (including alcohol) concomitantly with tapentadol hydrochloride may exhibit an additive CNS depression. Interactive effects resulting in respiratory depression, hypotension, profound sedation, or coma may result if these drugs are taken in combination with tapentadol hydrochloride. When such combined therapy is contemplated, a dose reduction of one or both agents should be considered).
No products indexed under this heading.

Fat (The AUC and C_{max} increased by 25% and 16%, respectively, when tapentadol hydrochloride was administered after a high-fat, high-calorie breakfast. Tapentadol hydrochloride may be given with or without food).
No products indexed under this heading.

Fentanyl (Patients receiving other opioid agonist analgesics, general anesthetics, phenothiazines, antiemetics, other tranquilizers, sedatives, hypnotics, or other CNS depressants (including alcohol) concomitantly with tapentadol hydrochloride may exhibit an additive CNS depression. Interactive effects resulting in respiratory depression, hypotension, profound sedation, or coma may result if these drugs are taken in combination with tapentadol hydrochloride. When such combined therapy is contemplated, a dose reduction of one or both agents should be considered). Products include:

Duragesic 2604
Fentanyl Transdermal System 2346
Onsolis 2054

Fentanyl Citrate (Patients receiving other opioid agonist analgesics, general anesthetics, phenothiazines, antiemetics, other tranquilizers, sedatives, hypnotics, or other CNS depressants (including alcohol) concomitantly with tapentadol hydrochloride may exhibit an additive CNS depression. Interactive effects resulting in respiratory depression, hypotension, profound sedation, or coma may result if these drugs are taken in combination with tapentadol hydrochloride. When such combined therapy is contemplated, a dose reduction of one or both agents should be considered). Products include:

Fentora 966

Fluoxetine (The development of a potentially life-threatening serotonin syndrome may occur with use of Serotonin and Norepinephrine Reuptake Inhibitor (SNRI) products, including tapentadol hydrochloride, particularly with concomitant use of serotonergic drugs such as Selective Serotonin Reuptake Inhibitors (SSRIs), SNRIs, tricyclic antidepressants (TCAs), MAOIs and triptans, and with drugs that impair metabolism of serotonin (including MAOIs). This may occur within the recommended dose. Serotonin syndrome may include mental-status changes (eg, agitation, hallucinations, coma), autonomic instability (eg, tachycardia, labile blood pressure, hyperthermia), neuromuscular aberrations (eg, hyperreflexia, incoordination) and/or gastrointestinal symptoms (eg, nausea, vomiting, diarrhea)).
No products indexed under this heading.

Fluoxetine Hydrochloride (The development of a potentially life-threatening serotonin syndrome may occur with use of Serotonin and Norepinephrine Reuptake Inhibitor (SNRI) products, including tapentadol hydrochloride, particularly with concomitant use of serotonergic drugs such as Selective Serotonin Reuptake Inhibitors (SSRIs), SNRIs, tricyclic antidepressants (TCAs), MAOIs and triptans, and with drugs that impair metabolism of serotonin (including MAOIs). This may occur within the recommended dose. Serotonin syndrome may include mental-status changes, autonomic instability, neuromuscular aberrations and/or gastrointestinal symptoms). Products include:

Prozac Weekly 1941
Prozac Pulvules 1941
Symbyax 1965

Fluphenazine Decanoate (Patients receiving other opioid agonist analgesics, general anesthetics, phenothiazines, antiemetics, other tranquilizers, sedatives, hypnotics, or other CNS depressants (including alcohol) concomitantly with tapentadol hydrochloride may exhibit an additive CNS depression. Interactive effects resulting in respiratory depression, hypotension, profound sedation, or coma may result if these drugs are taken in combination with tapentadol hydrochloride. When such combined therapy is contemplated, a dose reduction of one or both agents should be considered).
No products indexed under this heading.

Fluphenazine Enanthate (Patients receiving other opioid agonist analgesics, general anesthetics, phenothiazines, antiemetics, other tranquilizers, sedatives, hypnotics, or other CNS depressants (including alcohol) concomitantly with tapentadol hydrochloride may exhibit an additive CNS depression. Interactive effects resulting in respiratory depression, hypotension, profound sedation, or coma may result if these drugs are taken in combination with tapentadol hydrochloride. When such combined therapy is contemplated, a dose reduction of one or both agents should be considered).
No products indexed under this heading.

Fluphenazine Hydrochloride (Patients receiving other opioid agonist analgesics, general anesthetics, phenothiazines, antiemetics, other tranquilizers, sedatives, hypnotics, or other CNS depressants (including alcohol) concomitantly with tapentadol hydrochloride may exhibit an additive CNS depression. Interactive effects resulting in respiratory depression, hypotension, profound sedation, or coma may result if these drugs are taken in combination with tapentadol hydrochloride. When such combined therapy is contemplated, a dose reduction of one or both agents should be considered).
No products indexed under this heading.

Flurazepam Hydrochloride (Patients receiving other opioid agonist analgesics, general anesthetics, phenothiazines, antiemetics, other tranquilizers, sedatives, hypnotics, or other CNS depressants (including alcohol) concomitantly with tapentadol hydrochloride may exhibit an additive CNS depression. Interactive effects resulting in res-

1263 Interactions Index Nucynta

piratory depression, hypotension, profound sedation, or coma may result if these drugs are taken in combination with tapentadol hydrochloride. When such combined therapy is contemplated, a dose reduction of one or both agents should be considered).
No products indexed under this heading.

Fluvoxamine (The development of a potentially life-threatening serotonin syndrome may occur with use of Serotonin and Norepinephrine Reuptake Inhibitor (SNRI) products, including tapentadol hydrochloride, particularly with concomitant use of serotonergic drugs such as Selective Serotonin Reuptake Inhibitors (SSRIs), SNRIs, tricyclic antidepressants (TCAs), MAOIs and triptans, and with drugs that impair metabolism of serotonin (including MAOIs). This may occur within the recommended dose. Serotonin syndrome may include mental-status changes (eg, agitation, hallucinations, coma), autonomic instability (eg, tachycardia, labile blood pressure, hyperthermia), neuromuscular aberrations (eg, hyperreflexia, incoordination) and/or gastrointestinal symptoms (eg, nausea, vomiting, diarrhea)).
No products indexed under this heading.

Fluvoxamine Maleate (The development of a potentially life-threatening serotonin syndrome may occur with use of Serotonin and Norepinephrine Reuptake Inhibitor (SNRI) products, including tapentadol hydrochloride, particularly with concomitant use of serotonergic drugs such as Selective Serotonin Reuptake Inhibitors (SSRIs), SNRIs, tricyclic antidepressants (TCAs), MAOIs and triptans, and with drugs that impair metabolism of serotonin (including MAOIs). This may occur within the recommended dose. Serotonin syndrome may include mental-status changes, autonomic instability, neuromuscular aberrations and/or gastrointestinal symptoms).
No products indexed under this heading.

Frovatriptan Succinate (The development of a potentially life-threatening serotonin syndrome may occur with use of Serotonin and Norepinephrine Reuptake Inhibitor (SNRI) products, including tapentadol hydrochloride, particularly with concomitant use of serotonergic drugs such as Selective Serotonin Reuptake Inhibitors (SSRIs), SNRIs, tricyclic antidepressants (TCAs), MAOIs and triptans, and with drugs that impair metabolism of serotonin (including MAOIs). This may occur within the recommended dose. Serotonin syndrome may include mental-status changes, autonomic instability, neuromuscular aberrations and/or gastrointestinal symptoms). Products include:
Frova 1103

Glutethimide (Patients receiving other opioid agonist analgesics, general anesthetics, phenothiazines, antiemetics, other tranquilizers, sedatives, hypnotics, or other CNS depressants (including alcohol) concomitantly with tapentadol hydrochloride may exhibit an additive CNS depression. Interactive effects resulting in respiratory depression, hypotension, profound sedation, or coma may result if these drugs are taken in combination with tapentadol hydrochloride. When such combined therapy is contemplated, a dose reduction of one or both agents should be considered).
No products indexed under this heading.

Granisetron Hydrochloride (Patients receiving other opioid agonist analgesics, general anesthetics, phenothiazines, antiemetics, other tranquilizers, sedatives, hypnotics, or other CNS depressants (including alcohol) concomitantly with tapentadol hydrochloride may exhibit an additive CNS depression. Interactive effects resulting in respiratory depression, hypotension, profound sedation, or coma may result if these drugs are taken in combination with tapentadol hydrochloride. When such combined therapy is contemplated, a dose reduction of one or both agents should be considered).
No products indexed under this heading.

Halazepam (Patients receiving other opioid agonist analgesics, general anesthetics, phenothiazines, antiemetics, other tranquilizers, sedatives, hypnotics, or other CNS depressants (including alcohol) concomitantly with tapentadol hydrochloride may exhibit an additive CNS depression. Interactive effects resulting in respiratory depression, hypotension, profound sedation, or coma may result if these drugs are taken in combination with tapentadol hydrochloride. When such combined therapy is contemplated, a dose reduction of one or both agents should be considered).
No products indexed under this heading.

Haloperidol (Patients receiving other opioid agonist analgesics, general anesthetics, phenothiazines, antiemetics, other tranquilizers, sedatives, hypnotics, or other CNS depressants (including alcohol) concomitantly with tapentadol hydrochloride may exhibit an additive CNS depression. Interactive effects resulting in respiratory depression, hypotension, profound sedation, or coma may result if these drugs are taken in combination with tapentadol hydrochloride. When such combined therapy is contemplated, a dose reduction of one or both agents should be considered).
No products indexed under this heading.

Haloperidol Decanoate (Patients receiving other opioid agonist analgesics, general anesthetics, phenothiazines, antiemetics, other tranquilizers, sedatives, hypnotics, or other CNS depressants (including alcohol) concomitantly with tapentadol hydrochloride may exhibit an additive CNS depression. Interactive effects resulting in respiratory depression, hypotension, profound sedation, or coma may result if these drugs are taken in combination with tapentadol hydrochloride. When such combined therapy is contemplated, a dose reduction of one or both agents should be considered).
No products indexed under this heading.

Haloperidol Lactate (Patients receiving other opioid agonist analgesics, general anesthetics, phenothiazines, antiemetics, other tranquilizers, sedatives, hypnotics, or other CNS depressants (including alcohol) concomitantly with tapentadol hydrochloride may exhibit an additive CNS depression. Interactive effects resulting in respiratory depression, hypotension, profound sedation, or coma may result if these drugs are taken in combination with tapentadol hydrochloride. When such combined therapy is contemplated, a dose reduction of one or both agents should be considered).
No products indexed under this heading.

Halothane (Patients receiving other opioid agonist analgesics, general anesthetics, phenothiazines, antiemetics, other tranquilizers, sedatives, hypnotics, or other CNS depressants (including alcohol) concomitantly with tapentadol hydrochloride may exhibit an additive CNS depression. Interactive effects resulting in respiratory depression, hypotension, profound sedation, or coma may result if these drugs are taken in combination with tapentadol hydrochloride. When such combined therapy is contemplated, a dose reduction of one or both agents should be considered).
No products indexed under this heading.

Hexobarbital (Patients receiving other opioid agonist analgesics, general anesthetics, phenothiazines, antiemetics, other tranquilizers, sedatives, hypnotics, or other CNS depressants (including alcohol) concomitantly with tapentadol hydrochloride may exhibit an additive CNS depression. Interactive effects resulting in respiratory depression, hypotension, profound sedation, or coma may result if these drugs are taken in combination with tapentadol hydrochloride. When such combined therapy is contemplated, a dose reduction of one or both agents should be considered).
No products indexed under this heading.

Hydrocodone Bitartrate (Patients receiving other opioid agonist analgesics, general anesthetics, phenothiazines, antiemetics, other tranquilizers, sedatives, hypnotics, or other CNS depressants (including alcohol) concomitantly with tapentadol hydrochloride may exhibit an additive CNS depression. Interactive effects resulting in respiratory depression, hypotension, profound sedation, or coma may result if these drugs are taken in combination with tapentadol hydrochloride. When such combined therapy is contemplated, a dose reduction of one or both agents should be considered). Products include:
Vicodin 560
Vicodin ES 561
Vicodin HP 563
Vicoprofen 564
Zydone 1138

Hydrocodone Polistirex (Patients receiving other opioid agonist analgesics, general anesthetics, phenothiazines, antiemetics, other tranquilizers, sedatives, hypnotics, or other CNS depressants (including alcohol) concomitantly with tapentadol hydrochloride may exhibit an additive CNS depression. Interactive effects resulting in respiratory depression, hypotension, profound sedation, or coma may result if these drugs are taken in combination with tapentadol hydrochloride. When such combined therapy is contemplated, a dose reduction of one or both agents should be considered). Products include:
Tussionex 3443

Hydromorphone (Patients receiving other opioid agonist analgesics, general anesthetics, phenothiazines, antiemetics, other tranquilizers, sedatives, hypnotics, or other CNS depressants (including alcohol) concomitantly with tapentadol hydrochloride may exhibit an additive CNS depression. Interactive effects resulting in respiratory depression, hypotension, profound sedation, or coma may result if these drugs are taken in combination with tapentadol hydrochloride. When such combined therapy is contemplated, a dose reduction of one or both agents should be considered).
No products indexed under this heading.

Hydromorphone Hydrochloride (Patients receiving other opioid agonist analgesics, general anesthetics, phenothiazines, antiemetics, other tranquilizers, sedatives, hypnotics, or other CNS depressants (including alcohol) concomitantly with tapentadol hydrochloride may exhibit an additive CNS depression. Interactive effects resulting in respiratory depression, hypotension, profound sedation, or coma may result if these drugs are taken in combination with tapentadol hydrochloride. When such combined therapy is contemplated, a dose reduction of one or both agents should be considered). Products include:
Dilaudid Injection 2800
Dilaudid Oral 2797
Dilaudid Tablets 2797
Dilaudid-HP 2800

Hydroxyzine Hydrochloride (Patients receiving other opioid agonist analgesics, general anesthetics, phenothiazines, antiemetics, other tranquilizers, sedatives, hypnotics, or other CNS depressants (including alcohol) concomitantly with tapentadol hydrochloride may exhibit an additive CNS depression. Interactive effects resulting in respiratory depression, hypotension, profound sedation, or coma may result if these drugs are taken in combination with tapentadol hydrochloride. When such combined therapy is contemplated, a dose reduction of one or both agents should be considered).
No products indexed under this heading.

Imipramine Hydrochloride (The development of a potentially life-threatening serotonin syndrome may occur with use of Serotonin and Norepinephrine Reuptake Inhibitor (SNRI) products, including tapentadol hydrochloride, particularly with concomitant use of serotonergic drugs such as Selective Serotonin Reuptake Inhibitors (SSRIs), SNRIs, tricyclic antidepressants (TCAs), MAOIs and triptans, and with drugs that impair metabolism of serotonin (including MAOIs). This may occur within the recommended dose. Serotonin syndrome may include mental-status changes, autonomic instability, neuromuscular aberrations and/or gastrointestinal symptoms).
No products indexed under this heading.

Imipramine Pamoate (The development of a potentially life-threatening serotonin syndrome may occur with use of Serotonin and Norepinephrine Reuptake Inhibitor (SNRI) products, including tapentadol hydrochloride, particularly with concomitant use of serotonergic drugs such as Selective Serotonin Reuptake Inhibitors (SSRIs), SNRIs, tricyclic antidepressants (TCAs), MAOIs and triptans, and with drugs that impair metabolism of serotonin (including MAOIs). This may occur within the recommended dose. Serotonin syndrome may include mental-status changes, autonomic instability, neuromuscular aberrations and/or gastrointestinal symptoms).
No products indexed under this heading.

Isocarboxazid (Tapentadol hydrochloride is contraindicated in patients who are receiving monoamine oxidase (MAO) inhibitors or who have taken them within the last 14 days due to potential additive effects on norepinephrine levels which may result in adverse cardiovascular events). Products include:
Marplan 3481

Isoflurane (Patients receiving other opioid agonist analgesics, general anesthetics, phenothiazines, antiemetics, other tranquilizers, sedatives, hypnotics, or other CNS depressants (including alcohol) concomitantly with tapentadol hydrochloride may exhibit an additive CNS depression. Interactive effects resulting in respiratory depression, hypotension, profound sedation, or coma may result if these drugs are taken in combination with tapentadol hydrochloride. When such combined therapy is contemplated, a dose reduction of one or both agents should be considered).
No products indexed under this heading.

Ketamine Hydrochloride (Patients receiving other opioid agonist analgesics, general anesthetics, phenothiazines, antiemetics, other tranquilizers, sedatives, hypnotics, or other CNS

IMPORTANT NOTE: Always consult each drug listing in the patient's regimen for possible interactions.

Nucynta Interactions Index 1264

depressants (including alcohol) concomitantly with tapentadol hydrochloride may exhibit an additive CNS depression. Interactive effects resulting in respiratory depression, hypotension, profound sedation, or coma may result if these drugs are taken in combination with tapentadol hydrochloride. When such combined therapy is contemplated, a dose reduction of one or both agents should be considered).
No products indexed under this heading.

Levomethadyl Acetate Hydrochloride (Patients receiving other opioid agonist analgesics, general anesthetics, phenothiazines, antiemetics, other tranquilizers, sedatives, hypnotics, or other CNS depressants (including alcohol) concomitantly with tapentadol hydrochloride may exhibit an additive CNS depression. Interactive effects resulting in respiratory depression, hypotension, profound sedation, or coma may result if these drugs are taken in combination with tapentadol hydrochloride. When such combined therapy is contemplated, a dose reduction of one or both agents should be considered).
No products indexed under this heading.

Levorphanol Tartrate (Patients receiving other opioid agonist analgesics, general anesthetics, phenothiazines, antiemetics, other tranquilizers, sedatives, hypnotics, or other CNS depressants (including alcohol) concomitantly with tapentadol hydrochloride may exhibit an additive CNS depression. Interactive effects resulting in respiratory depression, hypotension, profound sedation, or coma may result if these drugs are taken in combination with tapentadol hydrochloride. When such combined therapy is contemplated, a dose reduction of one or both agents should be considered).
No products indexed under this heading.

Lorazepam (Patients receiving other opioid agonist analgesics, general anesthetics, phenothiazines, antiemetics, other tranquilizers, sedatives, hypnotics, or other CNS depressants (including alcohol) concomitantly with tapentadol hydrochloride may exhibit an additive CNS depression. Interactive effects resulting in respiratory depression, hypotension, profound sedation, or coma may result if these drugs are taken in combination with tapentadol hydrochloride. When such combined therapy is contemplated, a dose reduction of one or both agents should be considered).
No products indexed under this heading.

Loxapine Hydrochloride (Patients receiving other opioid agonist analgesics, general anesthetics, phenothiazines, antiemetics, other tranquilizers, sedatives, hypnotics, or other CNS depressants (including alcohol) concomitantly with tapentadol hydrochloride may exhibit an additive CNS depression. Interactive effects resulting in respiratory depression, hypotension, profound sedation, or coma may result if these drugs are taken in combination with tapentadol hydrochloride. When such combined therapy is contemplated, a dose reduction of one or both agents should be considered).
No products indexed under this heading.

Loxapine Succinate (Patients receiving other opioid agonist analgesics, general anesthetics, phenothiazines, antiemetics, other tranquilizers, sedatives, hypnotics, or other CNS depressants (including alcohol) concomitantly with tapentadol hydrochloride may exhibit an additive CNS depression. Interactive effects resulting in respiratory depression, hypotension, profound sedation, or coma may result if these drugs are taken in combination with tapentadol hydrochloride. When such combined therapy is contemplated, a dose reduction of one or both agents should be considered).
No products indexed under this heading.

Maprotiline Hydrochloride (The development of a potentially life-threatening serotonin syndrome may occur with use of Serotonin and Norepinephrine Reuptake Inhibitor (SNRI) products, including tapentadol hydrochloride, particularly with concomitant use of serotonergic drugs such as Selective Serotonin Reuptake Inhibitors (SSRIs), SNRIs, tricyclic antidepressants (TCAs), MAOIs and triptans, and with drugs that impair metabolism of serotonin (including MAOIs). This may occur within the recommended dose. Serotonin syndrome may include mental-status changes, autonomic instability, neuromuscular aberrations and/or gastrointestinal symptoms).
No products indexed under this heading.

Meclizine Hydrochloride (Patients receiving other opioid agonist analgesics, general anesthetics, phenothiazines, antiemetics, other tranquilizers, sedatives, hypnotics, or other CNS depressants (including alcohol) concomitantly with tapentadol hydrochloride may exhibit an additive CNS depression. Interactive effects resulting in respiratory depression, hypotension, profound sedation, or coma may result if these drugs are taken in combination with tapentadol hydrochloride. When such combined therapy is contemplated, a dose reduction of one or both agents should be considered).
No products indexed under this heading.

Meperidine Hydrochloride (Patients receiving other opioid agonist analgesics, general anesthetics, phenothiazines, antiemetics, other tranquilizers, sedatives, hypnotics, or other CNS depressants (including alcohol) concomitantly with tapentadol hydrochloride may exhibit an additive CNS depression. Interactive effects resulting in respiratory depression, hypotension, profound sedation, or coma may result if these drugs are taken in combination with tapentadol hydrochloride. When such combined therapy is contemplated, a dose reduction of one or both agents should be considered).
No products indexed under this heading.

Mephobarbital (Patients receiving other opioid agonist analgesics, general anesthetics, phenothiazines, antiemetics, other tranquilizers, sedatives, hypnotics, or other CNS depressants (including alcohol) concomitantly with tapentadol hydrochloride may exhibit an additive CNS depression. Interactive effects resulting in respiratory depression, hypotension, profound sedation, or coma may result if these drugs are taken in combination with tapentadol hydrochloride. When such combined therapy is contemplated, a dose reduction of one or both agents should be considered).
No products indexed under this heading.

Meprobamate (Patients receiving other opioid agonist analgesics, general anesthetics, phenothiazines, antiemetics, other tranquilizers, sedatives, hypnotics, or other CNS depressants (including alcohol) concomitantly with tapentadol hydrochloride may exhibit an additive CNS depression. Interactive effects resulting in respiratory depression, hypotension, profound sedation, or coma may result if these drugs are taken in combination with tapentadol hydrochloride. When such combined therapy is contemplated, a dose reduction of one or both agents should be considered).
No products indexed under this heading.

Mesoridazine Besylate (Patients receiving other opioid agonist analgesics, general anesthetics, phenothiazines, antiemetics, other tranquilizers, sedatives, hypnotics, or other CNS depressants (including alcohol) concomitantly with tapentadol hydrochloride may exhibit an additive CNS depression. Interactive effects resulting in respiratory depression, hypotension, profound sedation, or coma may result if these drugs are taken in combination with tapentadol hydrochloride. When such combined therapy is contemplated, a dose reduction of one or both agents should be considered).
No products indexed under this heading.

Methadone Hydrochloride (Patients receiving other opioid agonist analgesics, general anesthetics, phenothiazines, antiemetics, other tranquilizers, sedatives, hypnotics, or other CNS depressants (including alcohol) concomitantly with tapentadol hydrochloride may exhibit an additive CNS depression. Interactive effects resulting in respiratory depression, hypotension, profound sedation, or coma may result if these drugs are taken in combination with tapentadol hydrochloride. When such combined therapy is contemplated, a dose reduction of one or both agents should be considered).
No products indexed under this heading.

Methohexital Sodium (Patients receiving other opioid agonist analgesics, general anesthetics, phenothiazines, antiemetics, other tranquilizers, sedatives, hypnotics, or other CNS depressants (including alcohol) concomitantly with tapentadol hydrochloride may exhibit an additive CNS depression. Interactive effects resulting in respiratory depression, hypotension, profound sedation, or coma may result if these drugs are taken in combination with tapentadol hydrochloride. When such combined therapy is contemplated, a dose reduction of one or both agents should be considered).
No products indexed under this heading.

Methotrimeprazine (Patients receiving other opioid agonist analgesics, general anesthetics, phenothiazines, antiemetics, other tranquilizers, sedatives, hypnotics, or other CNS depressants (including alcohol) concomitantly with tapentadol hydrochloride may exhibit an additive CNS depression. Interactive effects resulting in respiratory depression, hypotension, profound sedation, or coma may result if these drugs are taken in combination with tapentadol hydrochloride. When such combined therapy is contemplated, a dose reduction of one or both agents should be considered).
No products indexed under this heading.

Methoxyflurane (Patients receiving other opioid agonist analgesics, general anesthetics, phenothiazines, antiemetics, other tranquilizers, sedatives, hypnotics, or other CNS depressants (including alcohol) concomitantly with tapentadol hydrochloride may exhibit an additive CNS depression. Interactive effects resulting in respiratory depression, hypotension, profound sedation, or coma may result if these drugs are taken in combination with tapentadol hydrochloride. When such combined therapy is contemplated, a dose reduction of one or both agents should be considered).
No products indexed under this heading.

Metoclopramide Hydrochloride (Patients receiving other opioid agonist analgesics, general anesthetics, phenothiazines, antiemetics, other tranquilizers, sedatives, hypnotics, or other CNS depressants (including alcohol) concomitantly with tapentadol hydrochloride may exhibit an additive CNS depression. Interactive effects resulting in respiratory depression, hypotension, profound sedation, or coma may result if these drugs are taken in combination with tapentadol hydrochloride. When such combined therapy is contemplated, a dose reduction of one or both agents should be considered). Products include:
Metozolv ODT 2901

Midazolam Hydrochloride (Patients receiving other opioid agonist analgesics, general anesthetics, phenothiazines, antiemetics, other tranquilizers, sedatives, hypnotics, or other CNS depressants (including alcohol) concomitantly with tapentadol hydrochloride may exhibit an additive CNS depression. Interactive effects resulting in respiratory depression, hypotension, profound sedation, or coma may result if these drugs are taken in combination with tapentadol hydrochloride. When such combined therapy is contemplated, a dose reduction of one or both agents should be considered).
No products indexed under this heading.

Moclobemide (Tapentadol hydrochloride is contraindicated in patients who are receiving monoamine oxidase (MAO) inhibitors or who have taken them within the last 14 days due to potential additive effects on norepinephrine levels which may result in adverse cardiovascular events).
No products indexed under this heading.

Molindone Hydrochloride (Patients receiving other opioid agonist analgesics, general anesthetics, phenothiazines, antiemetics, other tranquilizers, sedatives, hypnotics, or other CNS depressants (including alcohol) concomitantly with tapentadol hydrochloride may exhibit an additive CNS depression. Interactive effects resulting in respiratory depression, hypotension, profound sedation, or coma may result if these drugs are taken in combination with tapentadol hydrochloride. When such combined therapy is contemplated, a dose reduction of one or both agents should be considered). Products include:
Moban 1108

Morphine Sulfate (Patients receiving other opioid agonist analgesics, general anesthetics, phenothiazines, antiemetics, other tranquilizers, sedatives, hypnotics, or other CNS depressants (including alcohol) concomitantly with tapentadol hydrochloride may exhibit an additive CNS depression. Interactive effects resulting in respiratory depression, hypotension, profound sedation, or coma may result if these drugs are taken in combination with tapentadol hydrochloride. When such combined therapy is contemplated, a dose reduction of one or both agents should be considered). Products include:
Avinza 1822
Embeda 1831
MS Contin 2803

Morphine Sulfate, Liposomal (Patients receiving other opioid agonist analgesics, general anesthetics, phenothiazines, antiemetics, other tranquilizers, sedatives, hypnotics, or other CNS depressants (including alcohol) concomitantly with tapentadol hydrochloride may exhibit an additive CNS depression. Interactive effects resulting in respiratory depression, hypotension, profound sedation, or coma may result if these drugs are taken in combination with tapentadol hydrochloride. When such combined therapy is contemplated, a dose reduction of one or both agents should be considered).
No products indexed under this heading.

Nabilone (Patients receiving other opioid agonist analgesics, general anesthetics, phenothiazines, antiemetics,

other tranquilizers, sedatives, hypnotics, or other CNS depressants (including alcohol) concomitantly with tapentadol hydrochloride may exhibit an additive CNS depression. Interactive effects resulting in respiratory depression, hypotension, profound sedation, or coma may result if these drugs are taken in combination with tapentadol hydrochloride. When such combined therapy is contemplated, a dose reduction of one or both agents should be considered).
No products indexed under this heading.

Naproxen (Naproxen increased the AUC of tapentadol by 17%. This change is not considered clinically relevant and no change in dose is required). Products include:
EC-Naprosyn **2850**
Naprosyn **2850**
Anaprox/Naprosyn **2850**

Naproxen Sodium (Naproxen increased the AUC of tapentadol by 17%. This change is not considered clinically relevant and no change in dose is required). Products include:
Anaprox **2850**
Anaprox DS **2850**
Treximet **1681**

Naratriptan Hydrochloride (The development of a potentially life-threatening serotonin syndrome may occur with use of Serotonin and Norepinephrine Reuptake Inhibitor (SNRI) products, including tapentadol hydrochloride, particularly with concomitant use of serotonergic drugs such as Selective Serotonin Reuptake Inhibitors (SSRIs), SNRIs, tricyclic antidepressants (TCAs), MAOIs and triptans, and with drugs that impair metabolism of serotonin (including MAOIs). This may occur within the recommended dose. Serotonin syndrome may include mental-status changes, autonomic instability, neuromuscular aberrations and/or gastrointestinal symptoms). Products include:
Amerge **1306**

Nefazodone Hydrochloride (The development of a potentially life-threatening serotonin syndrome may occur with use of Serotonin and Norepinephrine Reuptake Inhibitor (SNRI) products, including tapentadol hydrochloride, particularly with concomitant use of serotonergic drugs such as Selective Serotonin Reuptake Inhibitors (SSRIs), SNRIs, tricyclic antidepressants (TCAs), MAOIs and triptans, and with drugs that impair metabolism of serotonin (including MAOIs). This may occur within the recommended dose. Serotonin syndrome may include mental-status changes, autonomic instability, neuromuscular aberrations and/or gastrointestinal symptoms).
No products indexed under this heading.

Nitrous Oxide (Patients receiving other opioid agonist analgesics, general anesthetics, phenothiazines, antiemetics, other tranquilizers, sedatives, hypnotics, or other CNS depressants (including alcohol) concomitantly with tapentadol hydrochloride may exhibit an additive CNS depression. Interactive effects resulting in respiratory depression, hypotension, profound sedation, or coma may result if these drugs are taken in combination with tapentadol hydrochloride. When such combined therapy is contemplated, a dose reduction of one or both agents should be considered).
No products indexed under this heading.

Nortriptyline Hydrochloride (The development of a potentially life-threatening serotonin syndrome may occur with use of Serotonin and Norepinephrine Reuptake Inhibitor (SNRI) products, including tapentadol hydrochloride, particularly with concomitant use of serotonergic drugs such as Selective Serotonin Reuptake Inhibitors (SSRIs), SNRIs, tricyclic antidepressants (TCAs), MAOIs and triptans, and with drugs that impair metabolism of serotonin (including MAOIs). This may occur within the recommended dose. Serotonin syndrome may include mental-status changes, autonomic instability, neuromuscular aberrations and/or gastrointestinal symptoms).
No products indexed under this heading.

Olanzapine (Patients receiving other opioid agonist analgesics, general anesthetics, phenothiazines, antiemetics, other tranquilizers, sedatives, hypnotics, or other CNS depressants (including alcohol) concomitantly with tapentadol hydrochloride may exhibit an additive CNS depression. Interactive effects resulting in respiratory depression, hypotension, profound sedation, or coma may result if these drugs are taken in combination with tapentadol hydrochloride. When such combined therapy is contemplated, a dose reduction of one or both agents should be considered). Products include:
Symbyax **1965**
Zyprexa **1984**
Zyprexa IntraMuscular **1984**
Zyprexa ZYDIS **1984**

Ondansetron (Patients receiving other opioid agonist analgesics, general anesthetics, phenothiazines, antiemetics, other tranquilizers, sedatives, hypnotics, or other CNS depressants (including alcohol) concomitantly with tapentadol hydrochloride may exhibit an additive CNS depression. Interactive effects resulting in respiratory depression, hypotension, profound sedation, or coma may result if these drugs are taken in combination with tapentadol hydrochloride. When such combined therapy is contemplated, a dose reduction of one or both agents should be considered).
No products indexed under this heading.

Ondansetron Hydrochloride (Patients receiving other opioid agonist analgesics, general anesthetics, phenothiazines, antiemetics, other tranquilizers, sedatives, hypnotics, or other CNS depressants (including alcohol) concomitantly with tapentadol hydrochloride may exhibit an additive CNS depression. Interactive effects resulting in respiratory depression, hypotension, profound sedation, or coma may result if these drugs are taken in combination with tapentadol hydrochloride. When such combined therapy is contemplated, a dose reduction of one or both agents should be considered). Products include:
Zofran Injection **1750**
Zofran **1756**
Zofran ODT **1756**

Oxazepam (Patients receiving other opioid agonist analgesics, general anesthetics, phenothiazines, antiemetics, other tranquilizers, sedatives, hypnotics, or other CNS depressants (including alcohol) concomitantly with tapentadol hydrochloride may exhibit an additive CNS depression. Interactive effects resulting in respiratory depression, hypotension, profound sedation, or coma may result if these drugs are taken in combination with tapentadol hydrochloride. When such combined therapy is contemplated, a dose reduction of one or both agents should be considered).
No products indexed under this heading.

Oxycodone Hydrochloride (Patients receiving other opioid agonist analgesics, general anesthetics, phenothiazines, antiemetics, other tranquilizers, sedatives, hypnotics, or other CNS depressants (including alcohol) concomitantly with tapentadol hydrochloride may exhibit an additive CNS depression. Interactive effects resulting in respiratory depression, hypotension, profound sedation, or coma may result if these drugs are taken in combination with tapentadol hydrochloride. When such combined therapy is contemplated, a dose reduction of one or both agents should be considered). Products include:
OxyContin **2807**
Percocet **1121**
Percodan **1124**

Oxycodone Terephthalate (Patients receiving other opioid agonist analgesics, general anesthetics, phenothiazines, antiemetics, other tranquilizers, sedatives, hypnotics, or other CNS depressants (including alcohol) concomitantly with tapentadol hydrochloride may exhibit an additive CNS depression. Interactive effects resulting in respiratory depression, hypotension, profound sedation, or coma may result if these drugs are taken in combination with tapentadol hydrochloride. When such combined therapy is contemplated, a dose reduction of one or both agents should be considered).
No products indexed under this heading.

Oxymorphone Hydrochloride (Patients receiving other opioid agonist analgesics, general anesthetics, phenothiazines, antiemetics, other tranquilizers, sedatives, hypnotics, or other CNS depressants (including alcohol) concomitantly with tapentadol hydrochloride may exhibit an additive CNS depression. Interactive effects resulting in respiratory depression, hypotension, profound sedation, or coma may result if these drugs are taken in combination with tapentadol hydrochloride. When such combined therapy is contemplated, a dose reduction of one or both agents should be considered). Products include:
Opana **1110**
Opana ER **1114**

Palonosetron Hydrochloride (Patients receiving other opioid agonist analgesics, general anesthetics, phenothiazines, antiemetics, other tranquilizers, sedatives, hypnotics, or other CNS depressants (including alcohol) concomitantly with tapentadol hydrochloride may exhibit an additive CNS depression. Interactive effects resulting in respiratory depression, hypotension, profound sedation, or coma may result if these drugs are taken in combination with tapentadol hydrochloride. When such combined therapy is contemplated, a dose reduction of one or both agents should be considered). Products include:
Aloxi **1042**

Pargyline Hydrochloride (Tapentadol hydrochloride is contraindicated in patients who are receiving monoamine oxidase (MAO) inhibitors or who have taken them within the last 14 days due to potential additive effects on norepinephrine levels which may result in adverse cardiovascular events).
No products indexed under this heading.

Paroxetine (The development of a potentially life-threatening serotonin syndrome may occur with use of Serotonin and Norepinephrine Reuptake Inhibitor (SNRI) products, including tapentadol hydrochloride, particularly with concomitant use of serotonergic drugs such as Selective Serotonin Reuptake Inhibitors (SSRIs), SNRIs, tricyclic antidepressants (TCAs), MAOIs and triptans, and with drugs that impair metabolism of serotonin (including MAOIs). This may occur within the recommended dose. Serotonin syndrome may include mental-status changes (eg, agitation, hallucinations, coma), autonomic instability (eg, tachycardia, labile blood pressure, hyperthermia), neuromuscular aberrations (eg, hyperreflexia, incoordination) and/or gastrointestinal symptoms (eg, nausea, vomiting, diarrhea)).
No products indexed under this heading.

Paroxetine Hydrochloride (The development of a potentially life-threatening serotonin syndrome may occur with use of Serotonin and Norepinephrine Reuptake Inhibitor (SNRI) products, including tapentadol hydrochloride, particularly with concomitant use of serotonergic drugs such as Selective Serotonin Reuptake Inhibitors (SSRIs), SNRIs, tricyclic antidepressants (TCAs), MAOIs and triptans, and with drugs that impair metabolism of serotonin (including MAOIs). This may occur within the recommended dose. Serotonin syndrome may include mental-status changes, autonomic instability, neuromuscular aberrations and/or gastrointestinal symptoms). Products include:
Paroxetine CR **2361**
Paroxetine ER **2371**
Paxil **1586**
Paxil CR **1596**

Paroxetine Mesylate (The development of a potentially life-threatening serotonin syndrome may occur with use of Serotonin and Norepinephrine Reuptake Inhibitor (SNRI) products, including tapentadol hydrochloride, particularly with concomitant use of serotonergic drugs such as Selective Serotonin Reuptake Inhibitors (SSRIs), SNRIs, tricyclic antidepressants (TCAs), MAOIs and triptans, and with drugs that impair metabolism of serotonin (including MAOIs). This may occur within the recommended dose. Serotonin syndrome may include mental-status changes (eg, agitation, hallucinations, coma), autonomic instability (eg, tachycardia, labile blood pressure, hyperthermia), neuromuscular aberrations (eg, hyperreflexia, incoordination) and/or gastrointestinal symptoms (eg, nausea, vomiting, diarrhea)).
No products indexed under this heading.

Pentobarbital (Patients receiving other opioid agonist analgesics, general anesthetics, phenothiazines, antiemetics, other tranquilizers, sedatives, hypnotics, or other CNS depressants (including alcohol) concomitantly with tapentadol hydrochloride may exhibit an additive CNS depression. Interactive effects resulting in respiratory depression, hypotension, profound sedation, or coma may result if these drugs are taken in combination with tapentadol hydrochloride. When such combined therapy is contemplated, a dose reduction of one or both agents should be considered).
No products indexed under this heading.

Pentobarbital Sodium (Patients receiving other opioid agonist analgesics, general anesthetics, phenothiazines, antiemetics, other tranquilizers, sedatives, hypnotics, or other CNS depressants (including alcohol) concomitantly with tapentadol hydrochloride may exhibit an additive CNS depression. Interactive effects resulting in respiratory depression, hypotension, profound sedation, or coma may result if these drugs are taken in combination with tapentadol hydrochloride. When such combined therapy is contemplated, a dose reduction of one or both agents should be considered). Products include:
Nembutal **2012**

Perphenazine (Patients receiving other opioid agonist analgesics, general anesthetics, phenothiazines, antiemetics, other tranquilizers, sedatives, hypnotics, or other CNS depressants (including alcohol) concomitantly with tapentadol hydrochloride may exhibit an additive CNS depression. Interactive effects resulting in respiratory depres-

Nucynta Interactions Index 1266

sion, hypotension, profound sedation, or coma may result if these drugs are taken in combination with tapentadol hydrochloride. When such combined therapy is contemplated, a dose reduction of one or both agents should be considered).
No products indexed under this heading.

Phenelzine Sulfate (Tapentadol hydrochloride is contraindicated in patients who are receiving monoamine oxidase (MAO) inhibitors or who have taken them within the last 14 days due to potential additive effects on norepinephrine levels which may result in adverse cardiovascular events).
No products indexed under this heading.

Phenobarbital (Patients receiving other opioid agonist analgesics, general anesthetics, phenothiazines, antiemetics, other tranquilizers, sedatives, hypnotics, or other CNS depressants (including alcohol) concomitantly with tapentadol hydrochloride may exhibit an additive CNS depression. Interactive effects resulting in respiratory depression, hypotension, profound sedation, or coma may result if these drugs are taken in combination with tapentadol hydrochloride. When such combined therapy is contemplated, a dose reduction of one or both agents should be considered). Products include:
Donnatal 2711

Phenobarbital Sodium (Patients receiving other opioid agonist analgesics, general anesthetics, phenothiazines, antiemetics, other tranquilizers, sedatives, hypnotics, or other CNS depressants (including alcohol) concomitantly with tapentadol hydrochloride may exhibit an additive CNS depression. Interactive effects resulting in respiratory depression, hypotension, profound sedation, or coma may result if these drugs are taken in combination with tapentadol hydrochloride. When such combined therapy is contemplated, a dose reduction of one or both agents should be considered).
No products indexed under this heading.

Phenothiazine Derivatives (Patients receiving other opioid agonist analgesics, general anesthetics, phenothiazines, antiemetics, other tranquilizers, sedatives, hypnotics, or other CNS depressants (including alcohol) concomitantly with tapentadol hydrochloride may exhibit an additive CNS depression. Interactive effects resulting in respiratory depression, hypotension, profound sedation, or coma may result if these drugs are taken in combination with tapentadol hydrochloride. When such combined therapy is contemplated, a dose reduction of one or both agents should be considered).
No products indexed under this heading.

Phenothiazines (Patients receiving other opioid agonist analgesics, general anesthetics, phenothiazines, antiemetics, other tranquilizers, sedatives, hypnotics, or other CNS depressants (including alcohol) concomitantly with tapentadol hydrochloride may exhibit an additive CNS depression. Interactive effects resulting in respiratory depression, hypotension, profound sedation, or coma may result if these drugs are taken in combination with tapentadol hydrochloride. When such combined therapy is contemplated, a dose reduction of one or both agents should be considered).
No products indexed under this heading.

Prazepam (Patients receiving other opioid agonist analgesics, general anesthetics, phenothiazines, antiemetics, other tranquilizers, sedatives, hypnotics, or other CNS depressants (including alcohol) concomitantly with tapentadol hydrochloride may exhibit an additive CNS depression. Interactive effects resulting in respiratory depression, hypotension, profound sedation, or coma may result if these drugs are taken in combination with tapentadol hydrochloride. When such combined therapy is contemplated, a dose reduction of one or both agents should be considered).
No products indexed under this heading.

Probenecid (Probenecid increased the AUC of tapentadol 57%. This change is not considered clinically relevant and no change in dose is required).
No products indexed under this heading.

Procarbazine Hydrochloride (Tapentadol hydrochloride is contraindicated in patients who are receiving monoamine oxidase (MAO) inhibitors or who have taken them within the last 14 days due to potential additive effects on norepinephrine levels which may result in adverse cardiovascular events).
No products indexed under this heading.

Prochlorperazine (Patients receiving other opioid agonist analgesics, general anesthetics, phenothiazines, antiemetics, other tranquilizers, sedatives, hypnotics, or other CNS depressants (including alcohol) concomitantly with tapentadol hydrochloride may exhibit an additive CNS depression. Interactive effects resulting in respiratory depression, hypotension, profound sedation, or coma may result if these drugs are taken in combination with tapentadol hydrochloride. When such combined therapy is contemplated, a dose reduction of one or both agents should be considered).
No products indexed under this heading.

Prochlorperazine Edisylate (Patients receiving other opioid agonist analgesics, general anesthetics, phenothiazines, antiemetics, other tranquilizers, sedatives, hypnotics, or other CNS depressants (including alcohol) concomitantly with tapentadol hydrochloride may exhibit an additive CNS depression. Interactive effects resulting in respiratory depression, hypotension, profound sedation, or coma may result if these drugs are taken in combination with tapentadol hydrochloride. When such combined therapy is contemplated, a dose reduction of one or both agents should be considered).
No products indexed under this heading.

Prochlorperazine Maleate (Patients receiving other opioid agonist analgesics, general anesthetics, phenothiazines, antiemetics, other tranquilizers, sedatives, hypnotics, or other CNS depressants (including alcohol) concomitantly with tapentadol hydrochloride may exhibit an additive CNS depression. Interactive effects resulting in respiratory depression, hypotension, profound sedation, or coma may result if these drugs are taken in combination with tapentadol hydrochloride. When such combined therapy is contemplated, a dose reduction of one or both agents should be considered).
No products indexed under this heading.

Promethazine (Patients receiving other opioid agonist analgesics, general anesthetics, phenothiazines, antiemetics, other tranquilizers, sedatives, hypnotics, or other CNS depressants (including alcohol) concomitantly with tapentadol hydrochloride may exhibit an additive CNS depression. Interactive effects resulting in respiratory depression, hypotension, profound sedation, or coma may result if these drugs are taken in combination with tapentadol hydrochloride. When such combined therapy is contemplated, a dose reduction of one or both agents should be considered).
No products indexed under this heading.

Promethazine Hydrochloride (Patients receiving other opioid agonist analgesics, general anesthetics, phenothiazines, antiemetics, other tranquilizers, sedatives, hypnotics, or other CNS depressants (including alcohol) concomitantly with tapentadol hydrochloride may exhibit an additive CNS depression. Interactive effects resulting in respiratory depression, hypotension, profound sedation, or coma may result if these drugs are taken in combination with tapentadol hydrochloride. When such combined therapy is contemplated, a dose reduction of one or both agents should be considered).
No products indexed under this heading.

Propofol (Patients receiving other opioid agonist analgesics, general anesthetics, phenothiazines, antiemetics, other tranquilizers, sedatives, hypnotics, or other CNS depressants (including alcohol) concomitantly with tapentadol hydrochloride may exhibit an additive CNS depression. Interactive effects resulting in respiratory depression, hypotension, profound sedation, or coma may result if these drugs are taken in combination with tapentadol hydrochloride. When such combined therapy is contemplated, a dose reduction of one or both agents should be considered).
No products indexed under this heading.

Propoxyphene Hydrochloride (Patients receiving other opioid agonist analgesics, general anesthetics, phenothiazines, antiemetics, other tranquilizers, sedatives, hypnotics, or other CNS depressants (including alcohol) concomitantly with tapentadol hydrochloride may exhibit an additive CNS depression. Interactive effects resulting in respiratory depression, hypotension, profound sedation, or coma may result if these drugs are taken in combination with tapentadol hydrochloride. When such combined therapy is contemplated, a dose reduction of one or both agents should be considered).
No products indexed under this heading.

Propoxyphene Napsylate (Patients receiving other opioid agonist analgesics, general anesthetics, phenothiazines, antiemetics, other tranquilizers, sedatives, hypnotics, or other CNS depressants (including alcohol) concomitantly with tapentadol hydrochloride may exhibit an additive CNS depression. Interactive effects resulting in respiratory depression, hypotension, profound sedation, or coma may result if these drugs are taken in combination with tapentadol hydrochloride. When such combined therapy is contemplated, a dose reduction of one or both agents should be considered).
No products indexed under this heading.

Protriptyline Hydrochloride (The development of a potentially life-threatening serotonin syndrome may occur with use of Serotonin and Norepinephrine Reuptake Inhibitor (SNRI) products, including tapentadol hydrochloride, particularly with concomitant use of serotonergic drugs such as Selective Serotonin Reuptake Inhibitors (SSRIs), SNRIs, tricyclic antidepressants (TCAs), MAOIs and triptans, and with drugs that impair metabolism of serotonin (including MAOIs). This may occur within the recommended dose. Serotonin syndrome may include mental-status changes, autonomic instability, neuromuscular aberrations and/or gastrointestinal symptoms).
No products indexed under this heading.

Quazepam (Patients receiving other opioid agonist analgesics, general anesthetics, phenothiazines, antiemetics, other tranquilizers, sedatives, hypnotics, or other CNS depressants (including alcohol) concomitantly with tapentadol hydrochloride may exhibit an additive CNS depression. Interactive effects resulting in respiratory depression, hypotension, profound sedation, or coma may result if these drugs are taken in combination with tapentadol hydrochloride. When such combined therapy is contemplated, a dose reduction of one or both agents should be considered).
No products indexed under this heading.

Quetiapine Fumarate (Patients receiving other opioid agonist analgesics, general anesthetics, phenothiazines, antiemetics, other tranquilizers, sedatives, hypnotics, or other CNS depressants (including alcohol) concomitantly with tapentadol hydrochloride may exhibit an additive CNS depression. Interactive effects resulting in respiratory depression, hypotension, profound sedation, or coma may result if these drugs are taken in combination with tapentadol hydrochloride. When such combined therapy is contemplated, a dose reduction of one or both agents should be considered). Products include:
Seroquel 750
Seroquel XR 759

Ramelteon (Patients receiving other opioid agonist analgesics, general anesthetics, phenothiazines, antiemetics, other tranquilizers, sedatives, hypnotics, or other CNS depressants (including alcohol) concomitantly with tapentadol hydrochloride may exhibit an additive CNS depression. Interactive effects resulting in respiratory depression, hypotension, profound sedation, or coma may result if these drugs are taken in combination with tapentadol hydrochloride. When such combined therapy is contemplated, a dose reduction of one or both agents should be considered). Products include:
Rozerem 3366

Rasagiline Mesylate (Tapentadol hydrochloride is contraindicated in patients who are receiving monoamine oxidase (MAO) inhibitors or who have taken them within the last 14 days due to potential additive effects on norepinephrine levels which may result in adverse cardiovascular events).
Products include:
Azilect 3383

Remifentanil Hydrochloride (Patients receiving other opioid agonist analgesics, general anesthetics, phenothiazines, antiemetics, other tranquilizers, sedatives, hypnotics, or other CNS depressants (including alcohol) concomitantly with tapentadol hydrochloride may exhibit an additive CNS depression. Interactive effects resulting in respiratory depression, hypotension, profound sedation, or coma may result if these drugs are taken in combination with tapentadol hydrochloride. When such combined therapy is contemplated, a dose reduction of one or both agents should be considered).
No products indexed under this heading.

Risperidone (Patients receiving other opioid agonist analgesics, general anesthetics, phenothiazines, antiemetics, other tranquilizers, sedatives, hypnotics, or other CNS depressants (including alcohol) concomitantly with tapentadol hydrochloride may exhibit an additive CNS depression. Interactive effects resulting in respiratory depression, hypotension, profound sedation, or coma may result if these drugs are taken in combination with tapentadol hydrochloride. When such combined therapy is contemplated, a dose reduction of one or both agents should be considered). Products include:
Risperdal Consta 2682

Rizatriptan Benzoate (The development of a potentially life-threatening serotonin syndrome may occur with use of Serotonin and Norepinephrine

Reuptake Inhibitor (SNRI) products, including tapentadol hydrochloride, particularly with concomitant use of serotonergic drugs such as Selective Serotonin Reuptake Inhibitors (SSRIs), SNRIs, tricyclic antidepressants (TCAs), MAOIs and triptans, and with drugs that impair metabolism of serotonin (including MAOIs). This may occur within the recommended dose. Serotonin syndrome may include mental-status changes, autonomic instability, neuromuscular aberrations and/or gastrointestinal symptoms). Products include:

Maxalt 2206
Maxalt-MLT 2206

Scopolamine (Patients receiving other opioid agonist analgesics, general anesthetics, phenothiazines, antiemetics, other tranquilizers, sedatives, hypnotics, or other CNS depressants (including alcohol) concomitantly with tapentadol hydrochloride may exhibit an additive CNS depression. Interactive effects resulting in respiratory depression, hypotension, profound sedation, or coma may result if these drugs are taken in combination with tapentadol hydrochloride. When such combined therapy is contemplated, a dose reduction of one or both agents should be considered). Products include:

Transderm Scōp 2397

Scopolamine Hydrobromide (Patients receiving other opioid agonist analgesics, general anesthetics, phenothiazines, antiemetics, other tranquilizers, sedatives, hypnotics, or other CNS depressants (including alcohol) concomitantly with tapentadol hydrochloride may exhibit an additive CNS depression. Interactive effects resulting in respiratory depression, hypotension, profound sedation, or coma may result if these drugs are taken in combination with tapentadol hydrochloride. When such combined therapy is contemplated, a dose reduction of one or both agents should be considered). Products include:

Donnatal 2711

Secobarbital Sodium (Patients receiving other opioid agonist analgesics, general anesthetics, phenothiazines, antiemetics, other tranquilizers, sedatives, hypnotics, or other CNS depressants (including alcohol) concomitantly with tapentadol hydrochloride may exhibit an additive CNS depression. Interactive effects resulting in respiratory depression, hypotension, profound sedation, or coma may result if these drugs are taken in combination with tapentadol hydrochloride. When such combined therapy is contemplated, a dose reduction of one or both agents should be considered).

No products indexed under this heading.

Selegiline (Tapentadol hydrochloride is contraindicated in patients who are receiving monoamine oxidase (MAO) inhibitors or who have taken them within the last 14 days due to potential additive effects on norepinephrine levels which may result in adverse cardiovascular events). Products include:

Emsam 3623

Selegiline Hydrochloride (Tapentadol hydrochloride is contraindicated in patients who are receiving monoamine oxidase (MAO) inhibitors or who have taken them within the last 14 days due to potential additive effects on norepinephrine levels which may result in adverse cardiovascular events). Products include:

Eldepryl 3312

Sertraline Hydrochloride (The development of a potentially life-threatening serotonin syndrome may occur with use of Serotonin and Norepinephrine Reuptake Inhibitor (SNRI) products, including tapentadol hydrochloride, particularly with concomitant use of serotonergic drugs such as Selective Serotonin Reuptake Inhibitors (SSRIs), SNRIs, tricyclic antidepressants (TCAs), MAOIs and triptans, and with drugs that impair metabolism of serotonin (including MAOIs). This may occur within the recommended dose. Serotonin syndrome may include mental-status changes, autonomic instability, neuromuscular aberrations and/or gastrointestinal symptoms).

No products indexed under this heading.

Sevoflurane (Patients receiving other opioid agonist analgesics, general anesthetics, phenothiazines, antiemetics, other tranquilizers, sedatives, hypnotics, or other CNS depressants (including alcohol) concomitantly with tapentadol hydrochloride may exhibit an additive CNS depression. Interactive effects resulting in respiratory depression, hypotension, profound sedation, or coma may result if these drugs are taken in combination with tapentadol hydrochloride. When such combined therapy is contemplated, a dose reduction of one or both agents should be considered). Products include:

Ultane 554

Sodium Butabarbital (Patients receiving other opioid agonist analgesics, general anesthetics, phenothiazines, antiemetics, other tranquilizers, sedatives, hypnotics, or other CNS depressants (including alcohol) concomitantly with tapentadol hydrochloride may exhibit an additive CNS depression. Interactive effects resulting in respiratory depression, hypotension, profound sedation, or coma may result if these drugs are taken in combination with tapentadol hydrochloride. When such combined therapy is contemplated, a dose reduction of one or both agents should be considered).

No products indexed under this heading.

Sodium Oxybate (Patients receiving other opioid agonist analgesics, general anesthetics, phenothiazines, antiemetics, other tranquilizers, sedatives, hypnotics, or other CNS depressants (including alcohol) concomitantly with tapentadol hydrochloride may exhibit an additive CNS depression. Interactive effects resulting in respiratory depression, hypotension, profound sedation, or coma may result if these drugs are taken in combination with tapentadol hydrochloride. When such combined therapy is contemplated, a dose reduction of one or both agents should be considered).

No products indexed under this heading.

Sodium Pentobarbital (Patients receiving other opioid agonist analgesics, general anesthetics, phenothiazines, antiemetics, other tranquilizers, sedatives, hypnotics, or other CNS depressants (including alcohol) concomitantly with tapentadol hydrochloride may exhibit an additive CNS depression. Interactive effects resulting in respiratory depression, hypotension, profound sedation, or coma may result if these drugs are taken in combination with tapentadol hydrochloride. When such combined therapy is contemplated, a dose reduction of one or both agents should be considered).

No products indexed under this heading.

Sufentanil Citrate (Patients receiving other opioid agonist analgesics, general anesthetics, phenothiazines, antiemetics, other tranquilizers, sedatives, hypnotics, or other CNS depressants (including alcohol) concomitantly with tapentadol hydrochloride may exhibit an additive CNS depression. Interactive effects resulting in respiratory depression, hypotension, profound sedation, or coma may result if these drugs are taken in combination with tapentadol hydrochloride. When such combined therapy is contemplated, a dose reduction of one or both agents should be considered).

No products indexed under this heading.

Sumatriptan (The development of a potentially life-threatening serotonin syndrome may occur with use of Serotonin and Norepinephrine Reuptake Inhibitor (SNRI) products, including tapentadol hydrochloride, particularly with concomitant use of serotonergic drugs such as Selective Serotonin Reuptake Inhibitors (SSRIs), SNRIs, tricyclic antidepressants (TCAs), MAOIs and triptans, and with drugs that impair metabolism of serotonin (including MAOIs). This may occur within the recommended dose. Serotonin syndrome may include mental-status changes, autonomic instability, neuromuscular aberrations and/or gastrointestinal symptoms). Products include:

Imitrex Nasal 1503

Sumatriptan Succinate (The development of a potentially life-threatening serotonin syndrome may occur with use of Serotonin and Norepinephrine Reuptake Inhibitor (SNRI) products, including tapentadol hydrochloride, particularly with concomitant use of serotonergic drugs such as Selective Serotonin Reuptake Inhibitors (SSRIs), SNRIs, tricyclic antidepressants (TCAs), MAOIs and triptans, and with drugs that impair metabolism of serotonin (including MAOIs). This may occur within the recommended dose. Serotonin syndrome may include mental-status changes, autonomic instability, neuromuscular aberrations and/or gastrointestinal symptoms). Products include:

Imitrex 1497
Imitrex Tablets 1508
Treximet 1681

Talbutal (Patients receiving other opioid agonist analgesics, general anesthetics, phenothiazines, antiemetics, other tranquilizers, sedatives, hypnotics, or other CNS depressants (including alcohol) concomitantly with tapentadol hydrochloride may exhibit an additive CNS depression. Interactive effects resulting in respiratory depression, hypotension, profound sedation, or coma may result if these drugs are taken in combination with tapentadol hydrochloride. When such combined therapy is contemplated, a dose reduction of one or both agents should be considered).

No products indexed under this heading.

Temazepam (Patients receiving other opioid agonist analgesics, general anesthetics, phenothiazines, antiemetics, other tranquilizers, sedatives, hypnotics, or other CNS depressants (including alcohol) concomitantly with tapentadol hydrochloride may exhibit an additive CNS depression. Interactive effects resulting in respiratory depression, hypotension, profound sedation, or coma may result if these drugs are taken in combination with tapentadol hydrochloride. When such combined therapy is contemplated, a dose reduction of one or both agents should be considered).

No products indexed under this heading.

Thiamylal Sodium (Patients receiving other opioid agonist analgesics, general anesthetics, phenothiazines, antiemetics, other tranquilizers, sedatives, hypnotics, or other CNS depressants (including alcohol) concomitantly with tapentadol hydrochloride may exhibit an additive CNS depression. Interactive effects resulting in respiratory depression, hypotension, profound sedation, or coma may result if these drugs are taken in combination with tapentadol hydrochloride. When such combined therapy is contemplated, a dose reduction of one or both agents should be considered).

No products indexed under this heading.

Thioridazine (Patients receiving other opioid agonist analgesics, general anesthetics, phenothiazines, antiemetics, other tranquilizers, sedatives, hypnotics, or other CNS depressants (including alcohol) concomitantly with tapentadol hydrochloride may exhibit an additive CNS depression. Interactive effects resulting in respiratory depression, hypotension, profound sedation, or coma may result if these drugs are taken in combination with tapentadol hydrochloride. When such combined therapy is contemplated, a dose reduction of one or both agents should be considered).

No products indexed under this heading.

Thioridazine Hydrochloride (Patients receiving other opioid agonist analgesics, general anesthetics, phenothiazines, antiemetics, other tranquilizers, sedatives, hypnotics, or other CNS depressants (including alcohol) concomitantly with tapentadol hydrochloride may exhibit an additive CNS depression. Interactive effects resulting in respiratory depression, hypotension, profound sedation, or coma may result if these drugs are taken in combination with tapentadol hydrochloride. When such combined therapy is contemplated, a dose reduction of one or both agents should be considered). Products include:

Thioridazine Hydrochloride 2384

Thiothixene (Patients receiving other opioid agonist analgesics, general anesthetics, phenothiazines, antiemetics, other tranquilizers, sedatives, hypnotics, or other CNS depressants (including alcohol) concomitantly with tapentadol hydrochloride may exhibit an additive CNS depression. Interactive effects resulting in respiratory depression, hypotension, profound sedation, or coma may result if these drugs are taken in combination with tapentadol hydrochloride. When such combined therapy is contemplated, a dose reduction of one or both agents should be considered). Products include:

Thiothixene 2386

Thiothixene Hydrochloride (Patients receiving other opioid agonist analgesics, general anesthetics, phenothiazines, antiemetics, other tranquilizers, sedatives, hypnotics, or other CNS depressants (including alcohol) concomitantly with tapentadol hydrochloride may exhibit an additive CNS depression. Interactive effects resulting in respiratory depression, hypotension, profound sedation, or coma may result if these drugs are taken in combination with tapentadol hydrochloride. When such combined therapy is contemplated, a dose reduction of one or both agents should be considered).

No products indexed under this heading.

Tranylcypromine Sulfate (Tapentadol hydrochloride is contraindicated in patients who are receiving monoamine oxidase (MAO) inhibitors or who have taken them within the last 14 days due to potential additive effects on norepinephrine levels which may result in adverse cardiovascular events). Products include:

Parnate 1584

Triazolam (Patients receiving other opioid agonist analgesics, general anesthetics, phenothiazines, antiemetics, other tranquilizers, sedatives, hypnotics, or other CNS depressants (including alcohol) concomitantly with tapentadol hydrochloride may exhibit an additive CNS depression. Interactive effects resulting in respiratory depression, hypotension, profound sedation,

IMPORTANT NOTE: Always consult each drug listing in the patient's regimen for possible interactions.

or coma may result if these drugs are taken in combination with tapentadol hydrochloride. When such combined therapy is contemplated, a dose reduction of one or both agents should be considered).

No products indexed under this heading.

Trifluoperazine Hydrochloride (Patients receiving other opioid agonist analgesics, general anesthetics, phenothiazines, antiemetics, other tranquilizers, sedatives, hypnotics, or other CNS depressants (including alcohol) concomitantly with tapentadol hydrochloride may exhibit an additive CNS depression. Interactive effects resulting in respiratory depression, hypotension, profound sedation, or coma may result if these drugs are taken in combination with tapentadol hydrochloride. When such combined therapy is contemplated, a dose reduction of one or both agents should be considered).

No products indexed under this heading.

Trimethobenzamide Hydrochloride (Patients receiving other opioid agonist analgesics, general anesthetics, phenothiazines, antiemetics, other tranquilizers, sedatives, hypnotics, or other CNS depressants (including alcohol) concomitantly with tapentadol hydrochloride may exhibit an additive CNS depression. Interactive effects resulting in respiratory depression, hypotension, profound sedation, or coma may result if these drugs are taken in combination with tapentadol hydrochloride. When such combined therapy is contemplated, a dose reduction of one or both agents should be considered).

No products indexed under this heading.

Trimipramine Maleate (The development of a potentially life-threatening serotonin syndrome may occur with use of Serotonin and Norepinephrine Reuptake Inhibitor (SNRI) products, including tapentadol hydrochloride, particularly with concomitant use of serotonergic drugs such as Selective Serotonin Reuptake Inhibitors (SSRIs), SNRIs, tricyclic antidepressants (TCAs), MAOIs and triptans, and with drugs that impair metabolism of serotonin (including MAOIs). This may occur within the recommended dose. Serotonin syndrome may include mental-status changes, autonomic instability, neuromuscular aberrations and/or gastrointestinal symptoms).

No products indexed under this heading.

Venlafaxine Hydrochloride (The development of a potentially life-threatening serotonin syndrome may occur with use of Serotonin and Norepinephrine Reuptake Inhibitor (SNRI) products, including tapentadol hydrochloride, particularly with concomitant use of serotonergic drugs such as Selective Serotonin Reuptake Inhibitors (SSRIs), SNRIs, tricyclic antidepressants (TCAs), MAOIs and triptans, and with drugs that impair metabolism of serotonin (including MAOIs). This may occur within the recommended dose. Serotonin syndrome may include mental-status changes, autonomic instability, neuromuscular aberrations and/or gastrointestinal symptoms). Products include:

Zaleplon (Patients receiving other opioid agonist analgesics, general anesthetics, phenothiazines, antiemetics, other tranquilizers, sedatives, hypnotics, or other CNS depressants (including alcohol) concomitantly with tapentadol hydrochloride may exhibit an additive CNS depression. Interactive effects resulting in respiratory depression, hypotension, profound sedation, or coma may result if these drugs are taken in combination with tapentadol

hydrochloride. When such combined therapy is contemplated, a dose reduction of one or both agents should be considered).

No products indexed under this heading.

Ziprasidone Hydrochloride (Patients receiving other opioid agonist analgesics, general anesthetics, phenothiazines, antiemetics, other tranquilizers, sedatives, hypnotics, or other CNS depressants (including alcohol) concomitantly with tapentadol hydrochloride may exhibit an additive CNS depression. Interactive effects resulting in respiratory depression, hypotension, profound sedation, or coma may result if these drugs are taken in combination with tapentadol hydrochloride. When such combined therapy is contemplated, a dose reduction of one or both agents should be considered). Products include:

Zolmitriptan (The development of a potentially life-threatening serotonin syndrome may occur with use of Serotonin and Norepinephrine Reuptake Inhibitor (SNRI) products, including tapentadol hydrochloride, particularly with concomitant use of serotonergic drugs such as Selective Serotonin Reuptake Inhibitors (SSRIs), SNRIs, tricyclic antidepressants (TCAs), MAOIs and triptans, and with drugs that impair metabolism of serotonin (including MAOIs). This may occur within the recommended dose. Serotonin syndrome may include mental-status changes, autonomic instability, neuromuscular aberrations and/or gastrointestinal symptoms). Products include:

Zolpidem Tartrate (Patients receiving other opioid agonist analgesics, general anesthetics, phenothiazines, antiemetics, other tranquilizers, sedatives, hypnotics, or other CNS depressants (including alcohol) concomitantly with tapentadol hydrochloride may exhibit an additive CNS depression. Interactive effects resulting in respiratory depression, hypotension, profound sedation, or coma may result if these drugs are taken in combination with tapentadol hydrochloride. When such combined therapy is contemplated, a dose reduction of one or both agents should be considered). Products include:

Food Interactions

Alcohol (Patients receiving other opioid agonist analgesics, general anesthetics, phenothiazines, antiemetics, other tranquilizers, sedatives, hypnotics, or other CNS depressants (including alcohol) concomitantly with tapentadol hydrochloride may exhibit an additive CNS depression. Interactive effects resulting in respiratory depression, hypotension, profound sedation, or coma may result if these drugs are taken in combination with tapentadol hydrochloride. When such combined therapy is contemplated, a dose reduction of one or both agents should be considered).

Beer, reduced-alcohol (Due to its mu-opioid agonist activity, tapentadol hydrochloride may be expected to have additive effects when used in conjunction with alcohol, opioids, or illicit drugs that cause central nervous system depression, respiratory depression, hypotension, and profound sedation, coma or death).

Beer, unspecified (Due to its mu-opioid agonist activity, tapentadol hydrochloride may be expected to have additive effects when used in conjunction with

alcohol, opioids, or illicit drugs that cause central nervous system depression, respiratory depression, hypotension, and profound sedation, coma or death).

Food, unspecified (The AUC and C_{max} increased by 25% and 16%, respectively, when tapentadol hydrochloride was administered after a high-fat, high-calorie breakfast. Tapentadol hydrochloride may be given with or without food).

Meal, unspecified (The AUC and C_{max} increased by 25% and 16%, respectively, when tapentadol hydrochloride was administered after a high-fat, high-calorie breakfast. Tapentadol hydrochloride may be given with or without food).

Wine, Chianti (Due to its mu-opioid agonist activity, tapentadol hydrochloride may be expected to have additive effects when used in conjunction with alcohol, opioids, or illicit drugs that cause central nervous system depression, respiratory depression, hypotension, and profound sedation, coma or death).

Wine, Red (Due to its mu-opioid agonist activity, tapentadol hydrochloride may be expected to have additive effects when used in conjunction with alcohol, opioids, or illicit drugs that cause central nervous system depression, respiratory depression, hypotension, and profound sedation, coma or death).

Wine, unspecified (Due to its mu-opioid agonist activity, tapentadol hydrochloride may be expected to have additive effects when used in conjunction with alcohol, opioids, or illicit drugs that cause central nervous system depression, respiratory depression, hypotension, and profound sedation, coma or death).

Wine products (Due to its mu-opioid agonist activity, tapentadol hydrochloride may be expected to have additive effects when used in conjunction with alcohol, opioids, or illicit drugs that cause central nervous system depression, respiratory depression, hypotension, and profound sedation, coma or death).

NU-IRON 150 CAPSULES
None cited in PDR database.

NUTROPIN FOR INJECTION
May interact with corticosteroids, phenytoin, and certain other agents. Compounds in these categories include:

Alclometasone Dipropionate (Excessive glucocorticoid therapy will inhibit the growth-promoting effect of human growth hormone).

No products indexed under this heading.

Beclomethasone Dipropionate (Excessive glucocorticoid therapy will inhibit the growth-promoting effect of human growth hormone). Products include:

Beclomethasone Dipropionate Monohydrate (Excessive glucocorticoid therapy will inhibit the growth-promoting effect of human growth hormone). Products include:

Betamethasone (Excessive glucocorticoid therapy will inhibit the growth-promoting effect of human growth hormone).

No products indexed under this heading.

Betamethasone Acetate (Excessive glucocorticoid therapy will inhibit the growth-promoting effect of human growth hormone).

No products indexed under this heading.

Betamethasone Benzoate (Excessive glucocorticoid therapy will inhibit the growth-promoting effect of human growth hormone).

No products indexed under this heading.

Betamethasone Dipropionate (Excessive glucocorticoid therapy will inhibit the growth-promoting effect of human growth hormone). Products include:

Betamethasone Sodium Phosphate (Excessive glucocorticoid therapy will inhibit the growth-promoting effect of human growth hormone).

No products indexed under this heading.

Betamethasone Valerate (Excessive glucocorticoid therapy will inhibit the growth-promoting effect of human growth hormone). Products include:

Budesonide (Excessive glucocorticoid therapy will inhibit the growth-promoting effect of human growth hormone). Products include:

Carbamazepine (Limited published data suggests that growth hormone treatment increased CYP450 mediated antipyrine clearance in man; therefore, growth hormone administration may alter the clearance of compounds known to be metabolized by CYP450 liver enzymes, such as anticonvulsanta including carbamazepine). Products include:

Ciclesonide (Excessive glucocorticoid therapy will inhibit the growth-promoting effect of human growth hormone).

No products indexed under this heading.

Cortisone Acetate (Excessive glucocorticoid therapy will inhibit the growth-promoting effect of human growth hormone).

No products indexed under this heading.

Cyclosporine (Limited published data suggests that growth hormone treatment increases CYP450 mediated antipyrine clearance in man, therefore, growth hormone administration may alter the clearance of compounds known to be metabolized by CYP450 liver enzymes, such as cyclosporine). Products include:

Desoximetasone (Excessive glucocorticoid therapy will inhibit the growth-promoting effect of human growth hormone).

No products indexed under this heading.

Dexamethasone (Excessive glucocorticoid therapy will inhibit the growth-promoting effect of human growth hormone). Products include:

Dexamethasone Acetate (Excessive glucocorticoid therapy will inhibit the growth-promoting effect of human growth hormone).

No products indexed under this heading.

Dexamethasone Phosphate (Excessive glucocorticoid therapy will inhibit the growth-promoting effect of human growth hormone).
    No products indexed under this heading.

Dexamethasone Sodium (Excessive glucocorticoid therapy will inhibit the growth-promoting effect of human growth hormone).
    No products indexed under this heading.

Dexamethasone Sodium Phosphate (Excessive glucocorticoid therapy will inhibit the growth-promoting effect of human growth hormone).
    No products indexed under this heading.

Dexamethasone Sodium Phosphate Injection (Excessive glucocorticoid therapy will inhibit the growth-promoting effect of human growth hormone).
    No products indexed under this heading.

Diflorasone Diacetate (Excessive glucocorticoid therapy will inhibit the growth-promoting effect of human growth hormone).
    No products indexed under this heading.

Fludrocortisone Acetate (Excessive glucocorticoid therapy will inhibit the growth-promoting effect of human growth hormone).
    No products indexed under this heading.

Flumethasone Pivalate (Excessive glucocorticoid therapy will inhibit the growth-promoting effect of human growth hormone).
    No products indexed under this heading.

Flunisolide Hemihydrate (Excessive glucocorticoid therapy will inhibit the growth-promoting effect of human growth hormone).
    No products indexed under this heading.

Fluticasone Furoate (Excessive glucocorticoid therapy will inhibit the growth-promoting effect of human growth hormone). Products include:
    Veramyst 1713

Fluticasone Propionate (Excessive glucocorticoid therapy will inhibit the growth-promoting effect of human growth hormone). Products include:
    Advair 100/50 1275
    Advair 250/50 1275
    Advair 500/50 1275
    Advair HFA 45/21 1288
    Advair HFA 115/21 1288
    Advair HFA 230/21 1288
    Flonase 1459
    Flovent Diskus 1463
    Flovent HFA 1470

Fosphenytoin (Limited published data suggests that growth hormone treatment increases CYP450 mediated antipyrine clearance in man; therefore, growth hormone administration may alter the clearance of compounds known to be metabolized by CYP450 liver enzymes, such as anticonvulsants, including phenytoin).
    No products indexed under this heading.

Fosphenytoin Sodium (Limited published data suggests that growth hormone treatment increases CYP450 mediated antipyrine clearance in man; therefore, growth hormone administration may alter the clearance of compounds known to be metabolized by CYP450 liver enzymes, such as anticonvulsants, including phenytoin).
    No products indexed under this heading.

Hydrocortisone (Excessive glucocorticoid therapy will inhibit the growth-promoting effect of human growth hormone).
    No products indexed under this heading.

Hydrocortisone (Alcohol) (Excessive glucocorticoid therapy will inhibit the growth-promoting effect of human growth hormone).
    No products indexed under this heading.

Hydrocortisone Acetate (Excessive glucocorticoid therapy will inhibit the growth-promoting effect of human growth hormone).
    No products indexed under this heading.

Hydrocortisone Butyrate (Excessive glucocorticoid therapy will inhibit the growth-promoting effect of human growth hormone).
    No products indexed under this heading.

Hydrocortisone Cypionate (Excessive glucocorticoid therapy will inhibit the growth-promoting effect of human growth hormone).
    No products indexed under this heading.

Hydrocortisone Hemisuccinate (Excessive glucocorticoid therapy will inhibit the growth-promoting effect of human growth hormone).
    No products indexed under this heading.

Hydrocortisone Probutate (Excessive glucocorticoid therapy will inhibit the growth-promoting effect of human growth hormone).
    No products indexed under this heading.

Hydrocortisone Sodium Phosphate (Excessive glucocorticoid therapy will inhibit the growth-promoting effect of human growth hormone).
    No products indexed under this heading.

Hydrocortisone Sodium Succinate (Excessive glucocorticoid therapy will inhibit the growth-promoting effect of human growth hormone).
    No products indexed under this heading.

Hydrocortisone Valerate (Excessive glucocorticoid therapy will inhibit the growth-promoting effect of human growth hormone).
    No products indexed under this heading.

Methylprednisolone (Excessive glucocorticoid therapy will inhibit the growth-promoting effect of human growth hormone).
    No products indexed under this heading.

Methylprednisolone Acetate (Excessive glucocorticoid therapy will inhibit the growth-promoting effect of human growth hormone).
    No products indexed under this heading.

Methylprednisolone Sodium Succinate (Excessive glucocorticoid therapy will inhibit the growth-promoting effect of human growth hormone).
    No products indexed under this heading.

Mometasone Furoate (Excessive glucocorticoid therapy will inhibit the growth-promoting effect of human growth hormone). Products include:
    Asmanex 3058
    Elocon Cream 3111
    Elocon Lotion 3112
    Elocon Ointment 3114

Mometasone Furoate Monohydrate (Excessive glucocorticoid therapy will inhibit the growth-promoting effect of human growth hormone). Products include:
    Nasonex 3166

Phenytoin (Limited published data suggests that growth hormone treatment increases CYP450 mediated antipyrine clearance in man; therefore, growth hormone administration may alter the clearance of compounds known to be metabolized by CYP450 liver enzymes, such as anticonvulsants, including phenytoin).
    No products indexed under this heading.

Phenytoin Sodium (Limited published data suggests that growth hormone treatment increases CYP450 mediated antipyrine clearance in man; therefore, growth hormone administration may alter the clearance of compounds known to be metabolized by CYP450 liver enzymes, such as anticonvulsants, including phenytoin). Products include:
    Phenytek Capsules 2380

Prednisolone (Excessive glucocorticoid therapy will inhibit the growth-promoting effect of human growth hormone).
    No products indexed under this heading.

Prednisolone Acetate (Excessive glucocorticoid therapy will inhibit the growth-promoting effect of human growth hormone). Products include:
    Blephamide .... ⊙212, ⊙214
    Pred Forte .... ⊙225
    Pred Mild .... ⊙230
    Pred-G .... ⊙226, ⊙227

Prednisolone Sodium Phosphate (Excessive glucocorticoid therapy will inhibit the growth-promoting effect of human growth hormone).
    No products indexed under this heading.

Prednisolone Tebutate (Excessive glucocorticoid therapy will inhibit the growth-promoting effect of human growth hormone).
    No products indexed under this heading.

Prednisone (Excessive glucocorticoid therapy will inhibit the growth-promoting effect of human growth hormone).
    No products indexed under this heading.

Prednisone sodium phosphate (Excessive glucocorticoid therapy will inhibit the growth-promoting effect of human growth hormone).
    No products indexed under this heading.

Triamcinolone (Excessive glucocorticoid therapy will inhibit the growth-promoting effect of human growth hormone).
    No products indexed under this heading.

Triamcinolone Acetonide (Excessive glucocorticoid therapy will inhibit the growth-promoting effect of human growth hormone). Products include:
    Azmacort 408
    Nasacort AQ 3019

Triamcinolone Diacetate (Excessive glucocorticoid therapy will inhibit the growth-promoting effect of human growth hormone).
    No products indexed under this heading.

Triamcinolone Hexacetonide (Excessive glucocorticoid therapy will inhibit the growth-promoting effect of human growth hormone).
    No products indexed under this heading.

NUTROPIN AQ INJECTION
(Somatropin) 1209
See Nutropin for Injection

NUTROPIN AQ NUSPIN INJECTION
(Somatropin) 1209
See Nutropin for Injection

NUTROPIN AQ PEN
(Somatropin) 1209
See Nutropin for Injection

NUTROPIN AQ PEN CARTRIDGE
(Somatropin) 1209
See Nutropin for Injection

NUVARING
(Ethinyl Estradiol, Etonogestrel) 3181
May interact with anticonvulsants, antifungals, barbiturates, cytochrome p450 3a4 inhibitors (selected), hepatic microsomal enzyme inducers, phenytoin, prednisolone, protease inhibitors, theophyllines, and certain other agents. Compounds in these categories include:

Acetaminophen (Acetaminophen may increase plasma ethinyl estradiol levels, possibly by inhibition of conjugation. Also, decreased plasma concentrations of acetaminophen have been noted when administered with oral contraceptives). Products include:

Acetaminophen-containing products (Acetaminophen may increase plasma ethinyl estradiol levels, possibly by inhibition of conjugation. Also, decreased plasma concentrations of acetaminophen have been noted when administered with oral contraceptives).
    No products indexed under this heading.

Acetazolamide (CYP3A4 inhibitors may increase plasma hormone levels).
    No products indexed under this heading.

Acetazolamide Sodium (CYP3A4 inhibitors may increase plasma hormone levels).
    No products indexed under this heading.

Allium sativum (Contraceptive effectiveness may be reduced when hormonal contraceptives are co-administered with some antifungals, anticonvulsants, and other drugs that increase the metabolism of contraceptive steroids. This could result in unintended pregnancy or breakthrough bleeding. Women may need to use an additional contraceptive method when taking such medications).
    No products indexed under this heading.

Aminoglutethimide (Contraceptive effectiveness may be reduced when hormonal contraceptives are co-administered with some antifungals, anticonvulsants, and other drugs that increase the metabolism of contraceptive steroids. This could result in unintended pregnancy or breakthrough bleeding. Women may need to use an additional contraceptive method when taking such medications).
    No products indexed under this heading.

Amiodarone Hydrochloride (CYP3A4 inhibitors may increase plasma hormone levels).
    No products indexed under this heading.

Amobarbital (Contraceptive effectiveness may be reduced when hormonal contraceptives are co-administered with barbiturates. This could result in unintended pregnancy or breakthrough bleeding. Women may need to use an additional contraceptive method when taking such medications).
    No products indexed under this heading.

Amobarbital Sodium (Contraceptive effectiveness may be reduced when hormonal contraceptives are co-administered with barbiturates. This could result in unintended pregnancy or breakthrough bleeding. Women may need to use an additional contraceptive method when taking such medications).
    No products indexed under this heading.

IMPORTANT NOTE: Always consult each drug listing in the patient's regimen for possible interactions.

Amphotericin B (Contraceptive effectiveness may be reduced when hormonal contraceptives are co-administered with some antifungals, anticonvulsants, and other drugs that increase the metabolism of contraceptive steroids. This could result in unintended pregnancy or breakthrough bleeding. Women may need to use an additional contraceptive method when taking such medications).
No products indexed under this heading.

Amphotericin B, liposomal (Contraceptive effectiveness may be reduced when hormonal contraceptives are co-administered with some antifungals, anticonvulsants, and other drugs that increase the metabolism of contraceptive steroids. This could result in unintended pregnancy or breakthrough bleeding. Women may need to use an additional contraceptive method when taking such medications). Products include:
AmBisome 659

Amphotericin B Cholesteryl Sulfate (Contraceptive effectiveness may be reduced when hormonal contraceptives are co-administered with some antifungals, anticonvulsants, and other drugs that increase the metabolism of contraceptive steroids. This could result in unintended pregnancy or breakthrough bleeding. Women may need to use an additional contraceptive method when taking such medications).
No products indexed under this heading.

Amphotericin B Lipid Complex (Contraceptive effectiveness may be reduced when hormonal contraceptives are co-administered with some antifungals, anticonvulsants, and other drugs that increase the metabolism of contraceptive steroids. This could result in unintended pregnancy or breakthrough bleeding. Women may need to use an additional contraceptive method when taking such medications).
No products indexed under this heading.

Amprenavir (Several of the anti-HIV protease inhibitors have been studied with co-administration of oral combination hormonal contraceptives; significant changes (increases and decreases) in the plasma levels of the estrogen and progestin have been noted in some cases. The efficacy and safety of hormonal contraceptive products may be affected with co-administration of anti-HIV protease inhibitors).
No products indexed under this heading.

Anastrozole (CYP3A4 inhibitors may increase plasma hormone levels).
No products indexed under this heading.

Anidulafungin (Contraceptive effectiveness may be reduced when hormonal contraceptives are co-administered with some antifungals, anticonvulsants, and other drugs that increase the metabolism of contraceptive steroids. This could result in unintended pregnancy or breakthrough bleeding. Women may need to use an additional contraceptive method when taking such medications).
No products indexed under this heading.

Aprepitant (Contraceptive effectiveness may be reduced when hormonal contraceptives are co-administered with some antifungals, anticonvulsants, and other drugs that increase the metabolism of contraceptive steroids. This could result in unintended pregnancy or breakthrough bleeding. Women may need to use an additional contraceptive method when taking such medications). Products include:
Emend 2124

Aprobarbital (Contraceptive effectiveness may be reduced when hormonal contraceptives are co-administered with barbiturates. This could result in unintended pregnancy or breakthrough bleeding. Women may need to use an additional contraceptive method when taking such medications).
No products indexed under this heading.

Ascorbic Acid (Ascorbic acid may increase plasma ethinyl estradiol levels, possibly by inhibition of conjugation).
No products indexed under this heading.

Atazanavir (Several of the anti-HIV protease inhibitors have been studied with co-administration of oral combination hormonal contraceptives; significant changes (increases and decreases) in the plasma levels of the estrogen and progestin have been noted in some cases. The efficacy and safety of hormonal contraceptive products may be affected with co-administration of anti-HIV protease inhibitors).
No products indexed under this heading.

Atazanavir Sulfate (Several of the anti-HIV protease inhibitors have been studied with co-administration of oral combination hormonal contraceptives; significant changes (increases and decreases) in the plasma levels of the estrogen and progestin have been noted in some cases. The efficacy and safety of hormonal contraceptive products may be affected with co-administration of anti-HIV protease inhibitors).
No products indexed under this heading.

Atorvastatin Calcium (Co-administration of atorvastatin and certain oral contraceptives containing ethinyl estradiol increase AUC values for ethinyl estradiol by approximately 20%). Products include:
Lipitor 2703

Betamethasone (Contraceptive effectiveness may be reduced when hormonal contraceptives are co-administered with some antifungals, anticonvulsants, and other drugs that increase the metabolism of contraceptive steroids. This could result in unintended pregnancy or breakthrough bleeding. Women may need to use an additional contraceptive method when taking such medications).
No products indexed under this heading.

Betamethasone Sodium Phosphate (Contraceptive effectiveness may be reduced when hormonal contraceptives are co-administered with some antifungals, anticonvulsants, and other drugs that increase the metabolism of contraceptive steroids. This could result in unintended pregnancy or breakthrough bleeding. Women may need to use an additional contraceptive method when taking such medications).
No products indexed under this heading.

Bosentan (Contraceptive effectiveness may be reduced when hormonal contraceptives are co-administered with some antifungals, anticonvulsants, and other drugs that increase the metabolism of contraceptive steroids. This could result in unintended pregnancy or breakthrough bleeding. Women may need to use an additional contraceptive method when taking such medications). Products include:
Tracleer 573

Butabarbital (Contraceptive effectiveness may be reduced when hormonal contraceptives are co-administered with barbiturates. This could result in unintended pregnancy or breakthrough bleeding. Women may need to use an additional contraceptive method when taking such medications).
No products indexed under this heading.

Butabarbital Sodium (Contraceptive effectiveness may be reduced when hormonal contraceptives are co-administered with barbiturates. This could result in unintended pregnancy or breakthrough bleeding. Women may need to use an additional contraceptive method when taking such medications).
No products indexed under this heading.

Butalbital (Contraceptive effectiveness may be reduced when hormonal contraceptives are co-administered with barbiturates. This could result in unintended pregnancy or breakthrough bleeding. Women may need to use an additional contraceptive method when taking such medications).
No products indexed under this heading.

Butoconazole Nitrate (Contraceptive effectiveness may be reduced when hormonal contraceptives are co-administered with some antifungals, anticonvulsants, and other drugs that increase the metabolism of contraceptive steroids. This could result in unintended pregnancy or breakthrough bleeding. Women may need to use an additional contraceptive method when taking such medications).
No products indexed under this heading.

Carbamazepine (Contraceptive effectiveness may be reduced when hormonal contraceptives are co-administered with carbamazepine. This could result in unintended pregnancy or breakthrough bleeding. Women may need to use an additional contraceptive method when taking carbamazepine). Products include:
Carbatrol 3280
Equetro 3477

Caspofungin acetate (Contraceptive effectiveness may be reduced when hormonal contraceptives are co-administered with some antifungals, anticonvulsants, and other drugs that increase the metabolism of contraceptive steroids. This could result in unintended pregnancy or breakthrough bleeding. Women may need to use an additional contraceptive method when taking such medications). Products include:
Cancidas 2088

Chlorpropamide (Contraceptive effectiveness may be reduced when hormonal contraceptives are co-administered with some antifungals, anticonvulsants, and other drugs that increase the metabolism of contraceptive steroids. This could result in unintended pregnancy or breakthrough bleeding. Women may need to use an additional contraceptive method when taking such medications).
No products indexed under this heading.

Cimetidine (CYP3A4 inhibitors may increase plasma hormone levels).
No products indexed under this heading.

Cimetidine Hydrochloride (CYP3A4 inhibitors may increase plasma hormone levels).
No products indexed under this heading.

Ciprofloxacin (Contraceptive effectiveness may be reduced when hormonal contraceptives are co-administered with some antifungals, anticonvulsants, and other drugs that increase the metabolism of contraceptive steroids. This could result in unintended pregnancy or breakthrough bleeding. Women may need to use an additional contraceptive method when taking such medications). Products include:
Cipro I.V. 3082
Cipro 3073
Cipro XR 3091
Ciprodex 583

Ciprofloxacin Hydrochloride (Contraceptive effectiveness may be reduced when hormonal contraceptives are co-administered with some antifungals, anticonvulsants, and other drugs that increase the metabolism of contraceptive steroids. This could result in unintended pregnancy or breakthrough bleeding. Women may need to use an additional contraceptive method when taking such medications). Products include:
Cipro 3073

Cisplatin (Contraceptive effectiveness may be reduced when hormonal contraceptives are co-administered with some antifungals, anticonvulsants, and other drugs that increase the metabolism of contraceptive steroids. This could result in unintended pregnancy or breakthrough bleeding. Women may need to use an additional contraceptive method when taking such medications).
No products indexed under this heading.

Citalopram Hydrobromide (Contraceptive effectiveness may be reduced when hormonal contraceptives are co-administered with some antifungals, anticonvulsants, and other drugs that increase the metabolism of contraceptive steroids. This could result in unintended pregnancy or breakthrough bleeding. Women may need to use an additional contraceptive method when taking such medications). Products include:
Celexa 1153

Clarithromycin (CYP3A4 inhibitors may increase plasma hormone levels). Products include:
Biaxin/Biaxin XL 412

Clofibric Acid (Increased clearance of clofibric acid have been noted when administered with oral contraceptives).
No products indexed under this heading.

Clotrimazole (Contraceptive effectiveness may be reduced when hormonal contraceptives are co-administered with some antifungals, anticonvulsants, and other drugs that increase the metabolism of contraceptive steroids. This could result in unintended pregnancy or breakthrough bleeding. Women may need to use an additional contraceptive method when taking such medications). Products include:
Lotrisone 3163

Clotrimazole, Topical (Contraceptive effectiveness may be reduced when hormonal contraceptives are co-administered with some antifungals, anticonvulsants, and other drugs that increase the metabolism of contraceptive steroids. This could result in unintended pregnancy or breakthrough bleeding. Women may need to use an additional contraceptive method when taking such medications).
No products indexed under this heading.

Conivaptan Hydrochloride (CYP3A4 inhibitors may increase plasma hormone levels). Products include:
Vaprisol 689

Cortisone Acetate (Contraceptive effectiveness may be reduced when hormonal contraceptives are co-administered with some antifungals, anticonvulsants, and other drugs that increase the metabolism of contraceptive steroids. This could result in unintended pregnancy or breakthrough bleeding. Women may need to use an additional contraceptive method when taking such medications).
No products indexed under this heading.

Cyclosporine (Combination hormonal contraceptives containing some synthetic estrogens may inhibit the metabolism of other compounds. Increased plasma concentrations of cyclosporine have been reported with concomitant administration of oral contraceptives). Products include:
Gengraf 440
Neoral Oral Solution 2496
Neoral Capsules 2496

IMPORTANT NOTE: Always consult each drug listing in the patient's regimen for possible interactions.

NuvaRing Interactions Index 1272

Fluconazole (Contraceptive effectiveness may be reduced when hormonal contraceptives are co-administered with some antifungals, anticonvulsants, and other drugs that increase the metabolism of contraceptive steroids. This could result in unintended pregnancy or breakthrough bleeding. Women may need to use an additional contraceptive method when taking such medications).
No products indexed under this heading.

Flucytosine (Contraceptive effectiveness may be reduced when hormonal contraceptives are co-administered with some antifungals, anticonvulsants, and other drugs that increase the metabolism of contraceptive steroids. This could result in unintended pregnancy or breakthrough bleeding. Women may need to use an additional contraceptive method when taking such medications).
No products indexed under this heading.

Fludrocortisone Acetate (Contraceptive effectiveness may be reduced when hormonal contraceptives are co-administered with some antifungals, anticonvulsants, and other drugs that increase the metabolism of contraceptive steroids. This could result in unintended pregnancy or breakthrough bleeding. Women may need to use an additional contraceptive method when taking such medications).
No products indexed under this heading.

Fluoxetine (CYP3A4 inhibitors may increase plasma hormone levels).
No products indexed under this heading.

Fluoxetine Hydrochloride (CYP3A4 inhibitors may increase plasma hormone levels). Products include:
Prozac Weekly 1941
Prozac Pulvules 1941
Symbyax 1965

Fluvoxamine (Contraceptive effectiveness may be reduced when hormonal contraceptives are co-administered with some antifungals, anticonvulsants, and other drugs that increase the metabolism of contraceptive steroids. This could result in unintended pregnancy or breakthrough bleeding. Women may need to use an additional contraceptive method when taking such medications).
No products indexed under this heading.

Fluvoxamine Maleate (Contraceptive effectiveness may be reduced when hormonal contraceptives are co-administered with some antifungals, anticonvulsants, and other drugs that increase the metabolism of contraceptive steroids. This could result in unintended pregnancy or breakthrough bleeding. Women may need to use an additional contraceptive method when taking such medications).
No products indexed under this heading.

Fosamprenavir Calcium (Several of the anti-HIV protease inhibitors have been studied with co-administration of oral combination hormonal contraceptives; significant changes (increases and decreases) in the plasma levels of the estrogen and progestin have been noted in some cases. The efficacy and safety of hormonal contraceptive products may be affected with co-administration of anti-HIV protease inhibitors). Products include:
Lexiva Oral Suspension 1558
Lexiva 1558

Fosphenytoin (Contraceptive effectiveness may be reduced when hormonal contraceptives are co-administered with phenytoin. This could result in unintended pregnancy or breakthrough bleeding. Women may need to use an additional contraceptive method when taking phenytoin).
No products indexed under this heading.

Fosphenytoin Sodium (Contraceptive effectiveness may be reduced when hormonal contraceptives are co-administered with phenytoin. This could result in unintended pregnancy or breakthrough bleeding. Women may need to use an additional contraceptive method when taking phenytoin).
No products indexed under this heading.

Gabapentin (Contraceptive effectiveness may be reduced when hormonal contraceptives are co-administered with some antifungals, anticonvulsants, and other drugs that increase the metabolism of contraceptive steroids. This could result in unintended pregnancy or breakthrough bleeding. Women may need to use an additional contraceptive method when taking such medications).
No products indexed under this heading.

Garlic Extract (Contraceptive effectiveness may be reduced when hormonal contraceptives are co-administered with some antifungals, anticonvulsants, and other drugs that increase the metabolism of contraceptive steroids. This could result in unintended pregnancy or breakthrough bleeding. Women may need to use an additional contraceptive method when taking such medications).
No products indexed under this heading.

Garlic Oil (Contraceptive effectiveness may be reduced when hormonal contraceptives are co-administered with some antifungals, anticonvulsants, and other drugs that increase the metabolism of contraceptive steroids. This could result in unintended pregnancy or breakthrough bleeding. Women may need to use an additional contraceptive method when taking such medications).
No products indexed under this heading.

Glipizide (Contraceptive effectiveness may be reduced when hormonal contraceptives are co-administered with some antifungals, anticonvulsants, and other drugs that increase the metabolism of contraceptive steroids. This could result in unintended pregnancy or breakthrough bleeding. Women may need to use an additional contraceptive method when taking such medications).
No products indexed under this heading.

Glyburide (Contraceptive effectiveness may be reduced when hormonal contraceptives are co-administered with some antifungals, anticonvulsants, and other drugs that increase the metabolism of contraceptive steroids. This could result in unintended pregnancy or breakthrough bleeding. Women may need to use an additional contraceptive method when taking such medications).
No products indexed under this heading.

Griseofulvin (Contraceptive effectiveness may be reduced when hormonal contraceptives are co-administered with griseofulvin. This could result in unintended pregnancy or breakthrough bleeding. Women may need to use an additional contraceptive method when taking griseofulvin).
No products indexed under this heading.

Hepatic Enzyme-Inducing Agents (Contraceptive effectiveness may be reduced when hormonal contraceptives are co-administered with some antifungals, anticonvulsants, and other drugs that increase the metabolism of contraceptive steroids. This could result in unintended pregnancy or breakthrough bleeding. Women may need to use an additional contraceptive method when taking such medications).
No products indexed under this heading.

Hexobarbital (Contraceptive effectiveness may be reduced when hormonal contraceptives are co-administered with barbiturates. This could result in unintended pregnancy or breakthrough bleeding. Women may need to use an additional contraceptive method when taking such medications).
No products indexed under this heading.

Hydrocortisone (Alcohol) (Contraceptive effectiveness may be reduced when hormonal contraceptives are co-administered with some antifungals, anticonvulsants, and other drugs that increase the metabolism of contraceptive steroids. This could result in unintended pregnancy or breakthrough bleeding. Women may need to use an additional contraceptive method when taking such medications).
No products indexed under this heading.

Hydrocortisone Acetate (Contraceptive effectiveness may be reduced when hormonal contraceptives are co-administered with some antifungals, anticonvulsants, and other drugs that increase the metabolism of contraceptive steroids. This could result in unintended pregnancy or breakthrough bleeding. Women may need to use an additional contraceptive method when taking such medications).
No products indexed under this heading.

Hydrocortisone Butyrate (Contraceptive effectiveness may be reduced when hormonal contraceptives are co-administered with some antifungals, anticonvulsants, and other drugs that increase the metabolism of contraceptive steroids. This could result in unintended pregnancy or breakthrough bleeding. Women may need to use an additional contraceptive method when taking such medications).
No products indexed under this heading.

Hydrocortisone Cypionate (Contraceptive effectiveness may be reduced when hormonal contraceptives are co-administered with some antifungals, anticonvulsants, and other drugs that increase the metabolism of contraceptive steroids. This could result in unintended pregnancy or breakthrough bleeding. Women may need to use an additional contraceptive method when taking such medications).
No products indexed under this heading.

Hydrocortisone Hemisuccinate (Contraceptive effectiveness may be reduced when hormonal contraceptives are co-administered with some antifungals, anticonvulsants, and other drugs that increase the metabolism of contraceptive steroids. This could result in unintended pregnancy or breakthrough bleeding. Women may need to use an additional contraceptive method when taking such medications).
No products indexed under this heading.

Hydrocortisone Probutate (Contraceptive effectiveness may be reduced when hormonal contraceptives are co-administered with some antifungals, anticonvulsants, and other drugs that increase the metabolism of contraceptive steroids. This could result in unintended pregnancy or breakthrough bleeding. Women may need to use an additional contraceptive method when taking such medications).
No products indexed under this heading.

Hydrocortisone Sodium Phosphate (Contraceptive effectiveness may be reduced when hormonal contraceptives are co-administered with some antifungals, anticonvulsants, and other drugs that increase the metabolism of contraceptive steroids. This could result in unintended pregnancy or breakthrough bleeding. Women may need to use an additional contraceptive method when taking such medications).
No products indexed under this heading.

Hydrocortisone Sodium Succinate (Contraceptive effectiveness may be reduced when hormonal contraceptives are co-administered with some antifungals, anticonvulsants, and other drugs that increase the metabolism of contraceptive steroids. This could result in unintended pregnancy or breakthrough bleeding. Women may need to use an additional contraceptive method when taking such medications).
No products indexed under this heading.

Hydrocortisone Valerate (Contraceptive effectiveness may be reduced when hormonal contraceptives are co-administered with some antifungals, anticonvulsants, and other drugs that increase the metabolism of contraceptive steroids. This could result in unintended pregnancy or breakthrough bleeding. Women may need to use an additional contraceptive method when taking such medications).
No products indexed under this heading.

Hypericum (Herbal products containing St. John's Wort (hypericum perforatum) may induce hepatic enzymes (cytochrome P450) and p-glycoprotein transporter and may reduce the effectiveness of contraceptive steroids. This may also result in breakthrough bleeding).
No products indexed under this heading.

Hypericum Perforatum (Herbal products containing St. John's Wort (hypericum perforatum) may induce hepatic enzymes (cytochrome P450) and p-glycoprotein transporter and may reduce the effectiveness of contraceptive steroids. This may also result in breakthrough bleeding). Products include:
Traumeel 1800

Imatinib Mesylate (CYP3A4 inhibitors may increase plasma hormone levels). Products include:
Gleevec 2477

Indinavir Sulfate (Several of the anti-HIV protease inhibitors have been studied with co-administration of oral combination hormonal contraceptives; significant changes (increases and decreases) in the plasma levels of the estrogen and progestin have been noted in some cases. The efficacy and safety of hormonal contraceptive products may be affected with co-administration of anti-HIV protease inhibitors). Products include:
Crixivan 2113

Insulin (Contraceptive effectiveness may be reduced when hormonal contraceptives are co-administered with some antifungals, anticonvulsants, and other drugs that increase the metabolism of contraceptive steroids. This could result in unintended pregnancy or breakthrough bleeding. Women may need to use an additional contraceptive method when taking such medications).
No products indexed under this heading.

Insulin, Human, Zinc Suspension (Contraceptive effectiveness may be reduced when hormonal contraceptives are co-administered with some antifungals, anticonvulsants, and other drugs that increase the metabolism of contraceptive steroids. This could result in unintended pregnancy or breakthrough bleeding. Women may need to use an additional contraceptive method when taking such medications).
No products indexed under this heading.

Insulin, Human (rDNA origin) (Contraceptive effectiveness may be reduced when hormonal contraceptives are co-administered with some antifungals, anticonvulsants, and other drugs that increase the metabolism of contraceptive steroids. This could result in unintended pregnancy or breakthrough bleeding. Women may need to use an

IMPORTANT NOTE: Always consult each drug listing in the patient's regimen for possible interactions.

NuvaRing Interactions Index 1274

Metronidazole Hydrochloride (CYP3A4 inhibitors may increase plasma hormone levels).
No products indexed under this heading.

Metronidazole Sodium (CYP3A4 inhibitors may increase plasma hormone levels).
No products indexed under this heading.

Micafungin Sodium (Contraceptive effectiveness may be reduced when hormonal contraceptives are co-administered with some antifungals, anticonvulsants, and other drugs that increase the metabolism of contraceptive steroids. This could result in unintended pregnancy or breakthrough bleeding. Women may need to use an additional contraceptive method when taking such medications). Products include:
Mycamine 670

Miconazole (Co-administration of vaginal miconazole nitrate and NuvaRing increases the serum concentrations of etonogestrel and ethinyl estradiol by up to 40%).
No products indexed under this heading.

Miconazole Nitrate (Co-administration of vaginal miconazole nitrate and NuvaRing increases the serum concentrations of etonogestrel and ethinyl estradiol by up to 40%).
Products include:
Vusion Ointment 3335

Mifepristone (CYP3A4 inhibitors may increase plasma hormone levels).
No products indexed under this heading.

Modafinil (Contraceptive effectiveness may be reduced when hormonal contraceptives are co-administered with modafinil. This could result in unintended pregnancy or breakthrough bleeding. Women may need to use an additional contraceptive method when taking modafinil). Products include:
Provigil 983

Morphine Sulfate (Increased clearance of morphine has been noted when administered with oral contraceptives).
Products include:
Avinza 1822
Embeda 1831
MS Contin 2803

Nafcillin Sodium (Contraceptive effectiveness may be reduced when hormonal contraceptives are co-administered with some antifungals, anticonvulsants, and other drugs that increase the metabolism of contraceptive steroids. This could result in unintended pregnancy or breakthrough bleeding. Women may need to use an additional contraceptive method when taking such medications).
No products indexed under this heading.

Nefazodone Hydrochloride (CYP3A4 inhibitors may increase plasma hormone levels).
No products indexed under this heading.

Nelfinavir Mesylate (Several of the anti-HIV protease inhibitors have been studied with co-administration of oral combination hormonal contraceptives; significant changes (increases and decreases) in the plasma levels of the estrogen and progestin have been noted in some cases. The efficacy and safety of hormonal contraceptive products may be affected with co-administration of anti-HIV protease inhibitors).
No products indexed under this heading.

Nevirapine (Contraceptive effectiveness may be reduced when hormonal contraceptives are co-administered with some antifungals, anticonvulsants, and other drugs that increase the metabolism of contraceptive steroids. This could result in unintended pregnancy or breakthrough bleeding. Women may need to use an additional contraceptive method when taking such medications). Products include:
Viramune Oral Suspension 897
Viramune Tablets 897

Niacin (CYP3A4 inhibitors may increase plasma hormone levels).
Products include:
Advicor 402
Cardio Basics 3455
Niaspan 497
Simcor 524

Niacinamide (CYP3A4 inhibitors may increase plasma hormone levels).
Products include:
CitraNatal 90 DHA Capsules 2332
CitraNatal Assure 2332
CitraNatal Rx 2332
Heplive 607

Niacinamide Hydroiodide (CYP3A4 inhibitors may increase plasma hormone levels).
No products indexed under this heading.

Nicotinamide (CYP3A4 inhibitors may increase plasma hormone levels).
No products indexed under this heading.

Nicotine (Contraceptive effectiveness may be reduced when hormonal contraceptives are co-administered with some antifungals, anticonvulsants, and other drugs that increase the metabolism of contraceptive steroids. This could result in unintended pregnancy or breakthrough bleeding. Women may need to use an additional contraceptive method when taking such medications).
No products indexed under this heading.

Nicotine Polacrilex (Contraceptive effectiveness may be reduced when hormonal contraceptives are co-administered with some antifungals, anticonvulsants, and other drugs that increase the metabolism of contraceptive steroids. This could result in unintended pregnancy or breakthrough bleeding. Women may need to use an additional contraceptive method when taking such medications).
No products indexed under this heading.

Nicotine Salicylate (Contraceptive effectiveness may be reduced when hormonal contraceptives are co-administered with some antifungals, anticonvulsants, and other drugs that increase the metabolism of contraceptive steroids. This could result in unintended pregnancy or breakthrough bleeding. Women may need to use an additional contraceptive method when taking such medications).
No products indexed under this heading.

Nicotine Sulfate (Contraceptive effectiveness may be reduced when hormonal contraceptives are co-administered with some antifungals, anticonvulsants, and other drugs that increase the metabolism of contraceptive steroids. This could result in unintended pregnancy or breakthrough bleeding. Women may need to use an additional contraceptive method when taking such medications).
No products indexed under this heading.

Nifedipine (CYP3A4 inhibitors may increase plasma hormone levels).
No products indexed under this heading.

Norethindrone (Contraceptive effectiveness may be reduced when hormonal contraceptives are co-administered with some antifungals, anticonvulsants, and other drugs that increase the metabolism of contraceptive steroids. This could result in unintended pregnancy or breakthrough bleeding. Women may need to use an additional contraceptive method when taking such medications). Products include:
Ortho Micronor 2660

Norethindrone Acetate (Contraceptive effectiveness may be reduced when hormonal contraceptives are co-administered with some antifungals, anticonvulsants, and other drugs that increase the metabolism of contraceptive steroids. This could result in unintended pregnancy or breakthrough bleeding. Women may need to use an additional contraceptive method when taking such medications). Products include:
Activella 2561

Norfloxacin (CYP3A4 inhibitors may increase plasma hormone levels).
Products include:
Noroxin 2220

Omeprazole (Contraceptive effectiveness may be reduced when hormonal contraceptives are co-administered with some antifungals, anticonvulsants, and other drugs that increase the metabolism of contraceptive steroids. This could result in unintended pregnancy or breakthrough bleeding. Women may need to use an additional contraceptive method when taking such medications).
No products indexed under this heading.

Omeprazole Magnesium (Contraceptive effectiveness may be reduced when hormonal contraceptives are co-administered with some antifungals, anticonvulsants, and other drugs that increase the metabolism of contraceptive steroids. This could result in unintended pregnancy or breakthrough bleeding. Women may need to use an additional contraceptive method when taking such medications).
No products indexed under this heading.

Oxcarbazepine (Contraceptive effectiveness may be reduced when hormonal contraceptives are co-administered with oxcarbazepine. This could result in unintended pregnancy or breakthrough bleeding. Women may need to use an additional contraceptive method when taking oxcarbazepine).
No products indexed under this heading.

Oxiconazole Nitrate (Contraceptive effectiveness may be reduced when hormonal contraceptives are co-administered with some antifungals, anticonvulsants, and other drugs that increase the metabolism of contraceptive steroids. This could result in unintended pregnancy or breakthrough bleeding. Women may need to use an additional contraceptive method when taking such medications).
No products indexed under this heading.

Paramethadione (Contraceptive effectiveness may be reduced when hormonal contraceptives are co-administered with some antifungals, anticonvulsants, and other drugs that increase the metabolism of contraceptive steroids. This could result in unintended pregnancy or breakthrough bleeding. Women may need to use an additional contraceptive method when taking such medications).
No products indexed under this heading.

Paroxetine Hydrochloride (CYP3A4 inhibitors may increase plasma hormone levels). Products include:
Paroxetine CR 2361
Paroxetine ER 2371
Paxil 1586
Paxil CR 1596

Pentobarbital (Contraceptive effectiveness may be reduced when hormonal contraceptives are co-administered with barbiturates. This could result in unintended pregnancy or breakthrough bleeding. Women may need to use an additional contraceptive method when taking such medications).
No products indexed under this heading.

Pentobarbital Sodium (Contraceptive effectiveness may be reduced when hormonal contraceptives are co-administered with barbiturates. This could result in unintended pregnancy or breakthrough bleeding. Women may need to use an additional contraceptive method when taking such medications).
Products include:
Nembutal 2012

Phenacemide (Contraceptive effectiveness may be reduced when hormonal contraceptives are co-administered with some antifungals, anticonvulsants, and other drugs that increase the metabolism of contraceptive steroids. This could result in unintended pregnancy or breakthrough bleeding. Women may need to use an additional contraceptive method when taking such medications).
No products indexed under this heading.

Phenobarbital (Contraceptive effectiveness may be reduced when hormonal contraceptives are co-administered with barbiturates. This could result in unintended pregnancy or breakthrough bleeding. Women may need to use an additional contraceptive method when taking such medications). Products include:
Donnatal 2711

Phenobarbital Sodium (Contraceptive effectiveness may be reduced when hormonal contraceptives are co-administered with barbiturates. This could result in unintended pregnancy or breakthrough bleeding. Women may need to use an additional contraceptive method when taking such medications).
No products indexed under this heading.

Phensuximide (Contraceptive effectiveness may be reduced when hormonal contraceptives are co-administered with some antifungals, anticonvulsants, and other drugs that increase the metabolism of contraceptive steroids. This could result in unintended pregnancy or breakthrough bleeding. Women may need to use an additional contraceptive method when taking such medications).
No products indexed under this heading.

Phenylbutazone (Contraceptive effectiveness may be reduced when hormonal contraceptives are co-administered with phenylbutazone. This could result in unintended pregnancy or breakthrough bleeding. Women may need to use an additional contraceptive method when taking phenylbutazone).
No products indexed under this heading.

Phenytoin (Contraceptive effectiveness may be reduced when hormonal contraceptives are co-administered with phenytoin. This could result in unintended pregnancy or breakthrough bleeding. Women may need to use an additional contraceptive method when taking phenytoin).
No products indexed under this heading.

Phenytoin Sodium (Contraceptive effectiveness may be reduced when hormonal contraceptives are co-administered with phenytoin. This could result in unintended pregnancy or breakthrough bleeding. Women may need to use an additional contraceptive method when taking phenytoin). Products include:
Phenytek Capsules 2380

Posaconazole (Contraceptive effectiveness may be reduced when hormonal contraceptives are co-administered with some antifungals, anticonvulsants, and other drugs that increase the metabolism of contraceptive steroids. This could result in unintended pregnancy or breakthrough bleeding. Women may need to use an additional contraceptive method when taking such medications). Products include:
Noxafil 3172

Prednisolone (Combination hormonal contraceptives containing some synthetic estrogens (eg, ethinyl estradiol) may inhibit the metabolism of other compounds. Increased plasma concentrations of prednisolone have been reported with concomitant administration of oral contraceptives).
No products indexed under this heading.

Prednisolone Acetate (Combination hormonal contraceptives containing some synthetic estrogens (eg, ethinyl estradiol) may inhibit the metabolism of other compounds. Increased plasma concentrations of prednisolone have been reported with concomitant administration of oral contraceptives).
Products include:
Blephamide .... ⊙212, ⊙214
Pred Forte .... ⊙225
Pred Mild .... ⊙230
Pred-G .... ⊙226, ⊙227

Prednisolone Sodium Phosphate (Combination hormonal contraceptives containing some synthetic estrogens (eg, ethinyl estradiol) may inhibit the metabolism of other compounds. Increased plasma concentrations of prednisolone have been reported with concomitant administration of oral contraceptives).
No products indexed under this heading.

Prednisolone Tebutate (Combination hormonal contraceptives containing some synthetic estrogens (eg, ethinyl estradiol) may inhibit the metabolism of other compounds. Increased plasma concentrations of prednisolone have been reported with concomitant administration of oral contraceptives).
No products indexed under this heading.

Prednisone (Contraceptive effectiveness may be reduced when hormonal contraceptives are co-administered with some antifungals, anticonvulsants, and other drugs that increase the metabolism of contraceptive steroids. This could result in unintended pregnancy or breakthrough bleeding. Women may need to use an additional contraceptive method when taking such medications).
No products indexed under this heading.

Prednisone sodium phosphate (Contraceptive effectiveness may be reduced when hormonal contraceptives are co-administered with some antifungals, anticonvulsants, and other drugs that increase the metabolism of contraceptive steroids. This could result in unintended pregnancy or breakthrough bleeding. Women may need to use an additional contraceptive method when taking such medications).
No products indexed under this heading.

Primidone (Contraceptive effectiveness may be reduced when hormonal contraceptives are co-administered with some antifungals, anticonvulsants, and other drugs that increase the metabolism of contraceptive steroids. This could result in unintended pregnancy or breakthrough bleeding. Women may need to use an additional contraceptive method when taking such medications).
No products indexed under this heading.

Propoxyphene Hydrochloride (CYP3A4 inhibitors may increase plasma hormone levels).
No products indexed under this heading.

Propoxyphene Napsylate (CYP3A4 inhibitors may increase plasma hormone levels).
No products indexed under this heading.

Quinidine (CYP3A4 inhibitors may increase plasma hormone levels).
No products indexed under this heading.

Quinidine Hydrochloride (CYP3A4 inhibitors may increase plasma hormone levels).
No products indexed under this heading.

Quinidine Polygalacturonate (CYP3A4 inhibitors may increase plasma hormone levels).
No products indexed under this heading.

Quinidine Sulfate (CYP3A4 inhibitors may increase plasma hormone levels).
No products indexed under this heading.

Quinine (CYP3A4 inhibitors may increase plasma hormone levels).
Products include:
Hyland's Leg Cramps PM with Quinine 3315

Quinine Sulfate (CYP3A4 inhibitors may increase plasma hormone levels).
No products indexed under this heading.

Quinupristin (CYP3A4 inhibitors may increase plasma hormone levels).
No products indexed under this heading.

Ranitidine Bismuth Citrate (CYP3A4 inhibitors may increase plasma hormone levels).
No products indexed under this heading.

Ranitidine Hydrochloride (CYP3A4 inhibitors may increase plasma hormone levels). Products include:
Zantac 1737
Zantac Injection 1732
Zantac Pharmacy 1735

Rifabutin (Contraceptive effectiveness may be reduced when hormonal contraceptives are co-administered with some antifungals, anticonvulsants, and other drugs that increase the metabolism of contraceptive steroids. This could result in unintended pregnancy or breakthrough bleeding. Women may need to use an additional contraceptive method when taking such medications).
No products indexed under this heading.

Rifampicin (Contraceptive effectiveness may be reduced when hormonal contraceptives are co-administered with some antifungals, anticonvulsants, and other drugs that increase the metabolism of contraceptive steroids. This could result in unintended pregnancy or breakthrough bleeding. Women may need to use an additional contraceptive method when taking such medications).
No products indexed under this heading.

Rifampin (Contraceptive effectiveness may be reduced when hormonal contraceptives are co-administered with rifampin. This could result in unintended pregnancy or breakthrough bleeding. Women may need to use an additional contraceptive method when taking rifampin).
No products indexed under this heading.

Rifapentine (Contraceptive effectiveness may be reduced when hormonal contraceptives are co-administered with some antifungals, anticonvulsants, and other drugs that increase the metabolism of contraceptive steroids. This could result in unintended pregnancy or breakthrough bleeding. Women may need to use an additional contraceptive method when taking such medications).
No products indexed under this heading.

Ritonavir (Several of the anti-HIV protease inhibitors have been studied with co-administration of oral combination hormonal contraceptives; significant changes (increases and decreases) in the plasma levels of the estrogen and progestin have been noted in some cases. The efficacy and safety of hormonal contraceptive products may be affected with co-administration of anti-HIV protease inhibitors). Products include:
Kaletra 458
Norvir 509

Rufinamide (Contraceptive effectiveness may be reduced when hormonal contraceptives are co-administered with some antifungals, anticonvulsants, and other drugs that increase the metabolism of contraceptive steroids. This could result in unintended pregnancy or breakthrough bleeding. Women may need to use an additional contraceptive method when taking such medications).
Products include:
Banzel 1050

Salicylic Acid (Increased clearance of salicylic acid has been noted when administered with oral contraceptives).
No products indexed under this heading.

Saquinavir (Several of the anti-HIV protease inhibitors have been studied with co-administration of oral combination hormonal contraceptives; significant changes (increases and decreases) in the plasma levels of the estrogen and progestin have been noted in some cases. The efficacy and safety of hormonal contraceptive products may be affected with co-administration of anti-HIV protease inhibitors).
No products indexed under this heading.

Saquinavir Mesylate (Several of the anti-HIV protease inhibitors have been studied with co-administration of oral combination hormonal contraceptives; significant changes (increases and decreases) in the plasma levels of the estrogen and progestin have been noted in some cases. The efficacy and safety of hormonal contraceptive products may be affected with co-administration of anti-HIV protease inhibitors).
No products indexed under this heading.

Secobarbital Sodium (Contraceptive effectiveness may be reduced when hormonal contraceptives are co-administered with barbiturates. This could result in unintended pregnancy or breakthrough bleeding. Women may need to use an additional contraceptive method when taking such medications).
No products indexed under this heading.

Sertaconazole Nitrate (Contraceptive effectiveness may be reduced when hormonal contraceptives are co-administered with some antifungals, anticonvulsants, and other drugs that increase the metabolism of contraceptive steroids. This could result in unintended pregnancy or breakthrough bleeding. Women may need to use an additional contraceptive method when taking such medications).
No products indexed under this heading.

Sertraline Hydrochloride (CYP3A4 inhibitors may increase plasma hormone levels).
No products indexed under this heading.

Sildenafil Citrate (CYP3A4 inhibitors may increase plasma hormone levels).
No products indexed under this heading.

Sodium Butabarbital (Contraceptive effectiveness may be reduced when hormonal contraceptives are co-administered with barbiturates. This could result in unintended pregnancy or breakthrough bleeding. Women may need to use an additional contraceptive method when taking such medications).
No products indexed under this heading.

Sodium Pentobarbital (Contraceptive effectiveness may be reduced when hormonal contraceptives are co-administered with barbiturates. This could result in unintended pregnancy or breakthrough bleeding. Women may need to use an additional contraceptive method when taking such medications).
No products indexed under this heading.

Telithromycin (CYP3A4 inhibitors may increase plasma hormone levels).
Products include:
Ketek 2991

Temazepam (Increased clearance of temazepam has been noted when administered with oral contraceptives).
No products indexed under this heading.

Terbinafine Hydrochloride (Contraceptive effectiveness may be reduced when hormonal contraceptives are co-administered with some antifungals, anticonvulsants, and other drugs that increase the metabolism of contraceptive steroids. This could result in unintended pregnancy or breakthrough bleeding. Women may need to use an additional contraceptive method when taking such medications).
No products indexed under this heading.

Terconazole (Contraceptive effectiveness may be reduced when hormonal contraceptives are co-administered with some antifungals, anticonvulsants, and other drugs that increase the metabolism of contraceptive steroids. This could result in unintended pregnancy or breakthrough bleeding. Women may need to use an additional contraceptive method when taking such medications).
No products indexed under this heading.

Theophylline (Combination hormonal contraceptives containing some synthetic estrogens may inhibit the metabolism of other compounds. Increased plasma concentrations of theophylline have been reported with concomitant administration of oral contraceptives).
No products indexed under this heading.

Theophylline Anhydrous (Combination hormonal contraceptives containing some synthetic estrogens may inhibit the metabolism of other compounds. Increased plasma concentrations of theophylline have been reported with concomitant administration of oral contraceptives). Products include:
Uniphyl 2817

Theophylline Calcium Salicylate (Combination hormonal contraceptives containing some synthetic estrogens may inhibit the metabolism of other compounds. Increased plasma concentrations of theophylline have been reported with concomitant administration of oral contraceptives).
No products indexed under this heading.

Theophylline Dihydroxypropyl (Glyceryl) (Combination hormonal contraceptives containing some synthetic estrogens may inhibit the metabolism of other compounds. Increased plasma concentrations of theophylline have been reported with concomitant administration of oral contraceptives).
No products indexed under this heading.

Theophylline Ethylenediamine (Combination hormonal contraceptives containing some synthetic estrogens may inhibit the metabolism of other compounds. Increased plasma concentrations of theophylline have been reported with concomitant administration of oral contraceptives).
No products indexed under this heading.

Theophylline Sodium Glycinate (Combination hormonal contraceptives containing some synthetic estrogens may inhibit the metabolism of other compounds. Increased plasma concentrations of theophylline have been reported with concomitant administration of oral contraceptives).
No products indexed under this heading.

Thiamylal Sodium (Contraceptive effectiveness may be reduced when hormonal contraceptives are co-administered with barbiturates. This could result in unintended pregnancy or breakthrough bleeding. Women may need to use an additional contraceptive method when taking such medications).
No products indexed under this heading.

Tiagabine Hydrochloride (Contraceptive effectiveness may be reduced when hormonal contraceptives are co-administered with some antifungals, anticonvulsants, and other drugs that increase the metabolism of contracep-

IMPORTANT NOTE: Always consult each drug listing in the patient's regimen for possible interactions.

NuvaRing Interactions Index 1276

tive steroids. This could result in unintended pregnancy or breakthrough bleeding. Women may need to use an additional contraceptive method when taking such medications). Products include:
Gabitril ... 972

Tipranavir (Several of the anti-HIV protease inhibitors have been studied with co-administration of oral combination hormonal contraceptives; significant changes (increases and decreases) in the plasma levels of the estrogen and progestin have been noted in some cases. The efficacy and safety of hormonal contraceptive products may be affected with co-administration of anti-HIV protease inhibitors).
No products indexed under this heading.

Tobacco (Cigarette smoking increases the risk of serious cardiovascular side effects when combined with oral contraceptives. Women who use combination hormonal contraceptives, including NuvaRing should be strongly advised not to smoke).
No products indexed under this heading.

Tolazamide (Contraceptive effectiveness may be reduced when hormonal contraceptives are co-administered with some antifungals, anticonvulsants, and other drugs that increase the metabolism of contraceptive steroids. This could result in unintended pregnancy or breakthrough bleeding. Women may need to use an additional contraceptive method when taking such medications).
No products indexed under this heading.

Tolbutamide (Contraceptive effectiveness may be reduced when hormonal contraceptives are co-administered with some antifungals, anticonvulsants, and other drugs that increase the metabolism of contraceptive steroids. This could result in unintended pregnancy or breakthrough bleeding. Women may need to use an additional contraceptive method when taking such medications).
No products indexed under this heading.

Topiramate (Contraceptive effectiveness may be reduced when hormonal contraceptives are co-administered with topiramate. This could result in unintended pregnancy or breakthrough bleeding. Women may need to use an additional contraceptive method when taking topiramate).
No products indexed under this heading.

Triamcinolone (Contraceptive effectiveness may be reduced when hormonal contraceptives are co-administered with some antifungals, anticonvulsants, and other drugs that increase the metabolism of contraceptive steroids. This could result in unintended pregnancy or breakthrough bleeding. Women may need to use an additional contraceptive method when taking such medications).
No products indexed under this heading.

Triamcinolone Acetonide (Contraceptive effectiveness may be reduced when hormonal contraceptives are co-administered with some antifungals, anticonvulsants, and other drugs that increase the metabolism of contraceptive steroids. This could result in unintended pregnancy or breakthrough bleeding. Women may need to use an additional contraceptive method when taking such medications). Products include:
Azmacort ... 408
Nasacort AQ ... 3019

Triamcinolone Diacetate (Contraceptive effectiveness may be reduced when hormonal contraceptives are co-administered with some antifungals, anticonvulsants, and other drugs that increase the metabolism of contraceptive steroids. This could result in unintended pregnancy or breakthrough bleeding. Women may need to use an additional contraceptive method when taking such medications).
No products indexed under this heading.

Triamcinolone Hexacetonide (Contraceptive effectiveness may be reduced when hormonal contraceptives are co-administered with some antifungals, anticonvulsants, and other drugs that increase the metabolism of contraceptive steroids. This could result in unintended pregnancy or breakthrough bleeding. Women may need to use an additional contraceptive method when taking such medications).
No products indexed under this heading.

Trimethadione (Contraceptive effectiveness may be reduced when hormonal contraceptives are co-administered with some antifungals, anticonvulsants, and other drugs that increase the metabolism of contraceptive steroids. This could result in unintended pregnancy or breakthrough bleeding. Women may need to use an additional contraceptive method when taking such medications).
No products indexed under this heading.

Troglitazone (Contraceptive effectiveness may be reduced when hormonal contraceptives are co-administered with some antifungals, anticonvulsants, and other drugs that increase the metabolism of contraceptive steroids. This could result in unintended pregnancy or breakthrough bleeding. Women may need to use an additional contraceptive method when taking such medications).
No products indexed under this heading.

Troleandomycin (CYP3A4 inhibitors may increase plasma hormone levels).
No products indexed under this heading.

Valproate Sodium (Contraceptive effectiveness may be reduced when hormonal contraceptives are co-administered with some antifungals, anticonvulsants, and other drugs that increase the metabolism of contraceptive steroids. This could result in unintended pregnancy or breakthrough bleeding. Women may need to use an additional contraceptive method when taking such medications).
No products indexed under this heading.

Valproic Acid (Contraceptive effectiveness may be reduced when hormonal contraceptives are co-administered with some antifungals, anticonvulsants, and other drugs that increase the metabolism of contraceptive steroids. This could result in unintended pregnancy or breakthrough bleeding. Women may need to use an additional contraceptive method when taking such medications).
No products indexed under this heading.

Vardenafil Hydrochloride (CYP3A4 inhibitors may increase plasma hormone levels). Products include:
Levitra ... 3157

Verapamil Hydrochloride (CYP3A4 inhibitors may increase plasma hormone levels). Products include:
Tarka ... 534

Vitamin C (Ascorbic acid may increase plasma ethinyl estradiol levels). Products include:
Bausch & Lomb Ocuvite Adult 50+ ... ⊙238
Bio-C ... 3454
BoneMate Plus ... 3454
Cardio Basics ... 3455
CitraNatal 90 DHA Capsules ... 2332
CitraNatal Assure ... 2332
CitraNatal Rx ... 2332
Ferralet ... 2333
Heplive ... 607
Meili Clear ... 607
MoviPrep Oral Solution ... 2905
PreNexa ... 3473
Proflavanol 90 ... 3476

Voriconazole (Contraceptive effectiveness may be reduced when hormonal contraceptives are co-administered with some antifungals, anticonvulsants, and other drugs that increase the metabolism of contraceptive steroids. This could result in unintended pregnancy or breakthrough bleeding. Women may need to use an additional contraceptive method when taking such medications).
No products indexed under this heading.

Zafirlukast (CYP3A4 inhibitors may increase plasma hormone levels). Products include:
Accolate ... 3612

Zileuton (CYP3A4 inhibitors may increase plasma hormone levels).
No products indexed under this heading.

Zonisamide (Contraceptive effectiveness may be reduced when hormonal contraceptives are co-administered with some antifungals, anticonvulsants, and other drugs that increase the metabolism of contraceptive steroids. This could result in unintended pregnancy or breakthrough bleeding. Women may need to use an additional contraceptive method when taking such medications). Products include:
Zonegran ... 1081

Food Interactions

Broccoli (Contraceptive effectiveness may be reduced when hormonal contraceptives are co-administered with some antifungals, anticonvulsants, and other drugs that increase the metabolism of contraceptive steroids. This could result in unintended pregnancy or breakthrough bleeding. Women may need to use an additional contraceptive method when taking such medications).

Brussel Sprouts (Contraceptive effectiveness may be reduced when hormonal contraceptives are co-administered with some antifungals, anticonvulsants, and other drugs that increase the metabolism of contraceptive steroids. This could result in unintended pregnancy or breakthrough bleeding. Women may need to use an additional contraceptive method when taking such medications).

Charbroiled Food (Contraceptive effectiveness may be reduced when hormonal contraceptives are co-administered with some antifungals, anticonvulsants, and other drugs that increase the metabolism of contraceptive steroids. This could result in unintended pregnancy or breakthrough bleeding. Women may need to use an additional contraceptive method when taking such medications).

Grapefruit (CYP3A4 inhibitors may increase plasma hormone levels).

Grapefruit Juice (CYP3A4 inhibitors may increase plasma hormone levels).

NUVIGIL TABLETS

(Armodafinil) ... 978
May interact with alcohols, cytochrome p450 1a2 substrates (selected), cytochrome p450 2c19 substrates (selected), cytochrome p450 3a4 substrates (selected), drugs affecting hepatic drug metabolizing enzyme systems, oral contraceptives, and certain other agents. Compounds in these categories include:

Acetaminophen (*In vitro* data demonstrated that armodafinil shows a weak inductive response for CYP1A2 and possibly CYP3A activities in a concentration related manner and demonstrated that CYP2C19 activity is reversibly inhibited by armodafinil. However, the effect on CYP1A2 activity was not observed clinically in an interaction study performed with caffeine).
Products include:
Percocet ... 1121
Tylenol ... 2049
Tylenol 8 Hour ... 2049
Extra Strength Tylenol Caplets, Cool Caplets, and EZ Tabs ... 2049
Extra Strength Tylenol Adult Rapid Blast Liquid ... 2049
Extra Strength Tylenol Rapid Release ... 2049
Tylenol with Codeine ... 2691
Tylenol Arthritis Pain Extended Release Geltabs/Caplets ... 2049
Children's Tylenol Suspension Liquid ... 2048
Children's Tylenol Meltaways ... 2048
Tylenol, Infants' Drops ... 2048
Junior Tylenol ... 2048
Vicodin ... 560
Vicodin ES ... 561
Vicodin HP ... 563
Zydone ... 1138

Alatrofloxacin Mesylate (*In vitro* data demonstrated that armodafinil shows a weak inductive response for CYP1A2 and possibly CYP3A activities in a concentration related manner and demonstrated that CYP2C19 activity is reversibly inhibited by armodafinil. However, the effect on CYP1A2 activity was not observed clinically in an interaction study performed with caffeine).
No products indexed under this heading.

Alfentanil Hydrochloride (Chronic administration of armodafinil resulted in moderate induction of CYP3A activity. Hence, the effectiveness of drugs that are substrates for CYP3A enzymes may be reduced after initiation of concurrent administration of armodafinil with midazolam. Dose adjustment may be required).
No products indexed under this heading.

Alprazolam (Chronic administration of armodafinil resulted in moderate induction of CYP3A activity. Hence, the effectiveness of drugs that are substrates for CYP3A enzymes may be reduced after initiation of concurrent administration of armodafinil with midazolam. Dose adjustment may be required).
No products indexed under this heading.

Aminophylline (*In vitro* data demonstrated that armodafinil shows a weak inductive response for CYP1A2 and possibly CYP3A activities in a concentration related manner and demonstrated that CYP2C19 activity is reversibly inhibited by armodafinil. However, the effect on CYP1A2 activity was not observed clinically in an interaction study performed with caffeine).
No products indexed under this heading.

Amiodarone Hydrochloride (Chronic administration of armodafinil resulted in moderate induction of CYP3A activity. Hence, the effectiveness of drugs that are substrates for CYP3A enzymes may be reduced after initiation of concurrent administration of armodafinil with midazolam. Dose adjustment may be required).
No products indexed under this heading.

Amitriptyline Hydrochloride (Administration of armodafinil resulted in moderate inhibition of CYP2C19 activity. Hence, dosage reduction may be required for some drugs that are substrates for CYP2C19 when used concurrently with armodafinil. A 40% increase in exposure was seen upon concomitant administration of armodafinil with omeprazole).
No products indexed under this heading.

IMPORTANT NOTE: Always consult each drug listing in the patient's regimen for possible interactions.

Nuvigil Interactions Index 1278

Cyclobenzaprine (*In vitro* data demonstrated that armodafinil shows a weak inductive response for CYP1A2 and possibly CYP3A activities in a concentration related manner and demonstrated that CYP2C19 activity is reversibly inhibited by armodafinil. However, the effect on CYP1A2 activity was not observed clinically in an interaction study performed with caffeine).
No products indexed under this heading.

Cyclobenzaprine Hydrochloride (*In vitro* data demonstrated that armodafinil shows a weak inductive response for CYP1A2 and possibly CYP3A activities in a concentration related manner and demonstrated that CYP2C19 activity is reversibly inhibited by armodafinil. However, the effect on CYP1A2 activity was not observed clinically in an interaction study performed with caffeine). Products include:
Amrix 964

Cyclophosphamide (Administration of armodafinil resulted in moderate inhibition of CYP2C19 activity. Hence, dosage reduction may be required for some drugs that are substrates for CYP2C19 when used concurrently with armodafinil. A 40% increase in exposure was seen upon concomitant administration of armodafinil with omeprazole).
No products indexed under this heading.

Cyclosporine (The blood levels of cyclosporine may be reduced when used with armodafinil. Monitoring of circulating cyclosporine concentrations and appropriate dosage adjustment for cyclosporine should be considered when these drugs are used concomitantly). Products include:
Gengraf 440
Neoral Oral Solution 2496
Neoral Capsules 2496
Restasis 605

Desipramine Hydrochloride (Administration of armodafinil resulted in moderate inhibition of CYP2C19 activity. Hence, dosage reduction may be required for some drugs that are substrates for CYP2C19 when used concurrently with armodafinil. A 40% increase in exposure was seen upon concomitant administration of armodafinil with omeprazole).
No products indexed under this heading.

Desogestrel (The effectiveness of steroidal contraceptives may be reduced when used with armodafinil and for one month after the discontinuation of therapy. Alternative or concomitant methods of contraception are recommended for patients treated with armodafinil and for one month after discontinuation of treatment of armodafinil).
No products indexed under this heading.

Dextromethorphan (Administration of armodafinil resulted in moderate inhibition of CYP2C19 activity. Hence, dosage reduction may be required for some drugs that are substrates for CYP2C19 when used concurrently with armodafinil. A 40% increase in exposure was seen upon concomitant administration of armodafinil with omeprazole).
No products indexed under this heading.

Dextromethorphan Hydrobromide (Administration of armodafinil resulted in moderate inhibition of CYP2C19 activity. Hence, dosage reduction may be required for some drugs that are substrates for CYP2C19 when used concurrently with armodafinil. A 40% increase in exposure was seen upon concomitant administration of armodafinil with omeprazole).
No products indexed under this heading.

Diazepam (Administration of armodafinil resulted in moderate inhibition of CYP2C19 activity. Hence, dosage reduction may be required for some drugs that are substrates for CYP2C19 when used concurrently with armodafinil. A 40% increase in exposure was seen upon concomitant administration of armodafinil with omeprazole). Products include:
Valium Tablets 2880

Dihydroergotamine Mesylate (Chronic administration of armodafinil resulted in moderate induction of CYP3A activity. Hence, the effectiveness of drugs that are substrates for CYP3A enzymes may be reduced after initiation of concurrent administration of armodafinil with midazolam. Dose adjustment may be required).
No products indexed under this heading.

Diltiazem Hydrochloride (Chronic administration of armodafinil resulted in moderate induction of CYP3A activity. Hence, the effectiveness of drugs that are substrates for CYP3A enzymes may be reduced after initiation of concurrent administration of armodafinil with midazolam. Dose adjustment may be required). Products include:
Cardizem LA 423

Diltiazem Maleate (Chronic administration of armodafinil resulted in moderate induction of CYP3A activity. Hence, the effectiveness of drugs that are substrates for CYP3A enzymes may be reduced after initiation of concurrent administration of armodafinil with midazolam. Dose adjustment may be required).
No products indexed under this heading.

Disopyramide (Chronic administration of armodafinil resulted in moderate induction of CYP3A activity. Hence, the effectiveness of drugs that are substrates for CYP3A enzymes may be reduced after initiation of concurrent administration of armodafinil with midazolam. Dose adjustment may be required).
No products indexed under this heading.

Disopyramide Phosphate (Chronic administration of armodafinil resulted in moderate induction of CYP3A activity. Hence, the effectiveness of drugs that are substrates for CYP3A enzymes may be reduced after initiation of concurrent administration of armodafinil with midazolam. Dose adjustment may be required).
No products indexed under this heading.

Disulfiram (Chronic administration of armodafinil resulted in moderate induction of CYP3A activity. Hence, the effectiveness of drugs that are substrates for CYP3A enzymes may be reduced after initiation of concurrent administration of armodafinil with midazolam. Dose adjustment may be required).
No products indexed under this heading.

Divalproex Sodium (Administration of armodafinil resulted in moderate inhibition of CYP2C19 activity. Hence, dosage reduction may be required for some drugs that are substrates for CYP2C19 when used concurrently with armodafinil. A 40% increase in exposure was seen upon concomitant administration of armodafinil with omeprazole). Products include:
Depakote ER 426

Doxepin Hydrochloride (Administration of armodafinil resulted in moderate inhibition of CYP2C19 activity. Hence, dosage reduction may be required for some drugs that are substrates for CYP2C19 when used concurrently with armodafinil. A 40% increase in exposure was seen upon concomitant administration of armodafinil with omeprazole).
No products indexed under this heading.

Doxorubicin Hydrochloride (Chronic administration of armodafinil resulted in moderate induction of CYP3A activity. Hence, the effectiveness of drugs that are substrates for CYP3A enzymes may be reduced after initiation of concurrent administration of armodafinil with midazolam. Dose adjustment may be required).
No products indexed under this heading.

Dronabinol (Chronic administration of armodafinil resulted in moderate induction of CYP3A activity. Hence, the effectiveness of drugs that are substrates for CYP3A enzymes may be reduced after initiation of concurrent administration of armodafinil with midazolam. Dose adjustment may be required).
No products indexed under this heading.

Enoxacin (*In vitro* data demonstrated that armodafinil shows a weak inductive response for CYP1A2 and possibly CYP3A activities in a concentration related manner and demonstrated that CYP2C19 activity is reversibly inhibited by armodafinil. However, the effect on CYP1A2 activity was not observed clinically in an interaction study performed with caffeine).
No products indexed under this heading.

Ergotamine Tartrate (Chronic administration of armodafinil resulted in moderate induction of CYP3A activity. Hence, the effectiveness of drugs that are substrates for CYP3A enzymes may be reduced after initiation of concurrent administration of armodafinil with midazolam. Dose adjustment may be required).
No products indexed under this heading.

Erythromycin (Chronic administration of armodafinil resulted in moderate induction of CYP3A activity. Hence, the effectiveness of drugs that are substrates for CYP3A enzymes may be reduced after initiation of concurrent administration of armodafinil with midazolam. Dose adjustment may be required).
No products indexed under this heading.

Erythromycin Estolate (Chronic administration of armodafinil resulted in moderate induction of CYP3A activity. Hence, the effectiveness of drugs that are substrates for CYP3A enzymes may be reduced after initiation of concurrent administration of armodafinil with midazolam. Dose adjustment may be required).
No products indexed under this heading.

Erythromycin Ethylsuccinate (Chronic administration of armodafinil resulted in moderate induction of CYP3A activity. Hence, the effectiveness of drugs that are substrates for CYP3A enzymes may be reduced after initiation of concurrent administration of armodafinil with midazolam. Dose adjustment may be required). Products include:
E.E.S. 437
EryPed 435

Erythromycin Gluceptate (Chronic administration of armodafinil resulted in moderate induction of CYP3A activity. Hence, the effectiveness of drugs that are substrates for CYP3A enzymes may be reduced after initiation of concurrent administration of armodafinil with midazolam. Dose adjustment may be required).
No products indexed under this heading.

Erythromycin Lactobionate (Chronic administration of armodafinil resulted in moderate induction of CYP3A activity. Hence, the effectiveness of drugs that are substrates for CYP3A enzymes may be reduced after initiation of concurrent administration of armodafinil with midazolam. Dose adjustment may be required).
No products indexed under this heading.

Erythromycin Stearate (Chronic administration of armodafinil resulted in moderate induction of CYP3A activity. Hence, the effectiveness of drugs that are substrates for CYP3A enzymes may be reduced after initiation of concurrent administration of armodafinil with midazolam. Dose adjustment may be required).
No products indexed under this heading.

Esomeprazole Magnesium (Administration of armodafinil resulted in moderate inhibition of CYP2C19 activity. Hence, dosage reduction may be required for some drugs that are substrates for CYP2C19 when used concurrently with armodafinil. A 40% increase in exposure was seen upon concomitant administration of armodafinil with omeprazole). Products include:
Nexium Capsules 704
Nexium Oral Suspension 704

Esomeprazole Sodium (Administration of armodafinil resulted in moderate inhibition of CYP2C19 activity. Hence, dosage reduction may be required for some drugs that are substrates for CYP2C19 when used concurrently with armodafinil. A 40% increase in exposure was seen upon concomitant administration of armodafinil with omeprazole). Products include:
Nexium I.V. 712

Estradiol (Chronic administration of armodafinil resulted in moderate induction of CYP3A activity. Hence, the effectiveness of drugs that are substrates for CYP3A enzymes may be reduced after initiation of concurrent administration of armodafinil with midazolam. Dose adjustment may be required). Products include:
Activella 2561
Angeliq 831
Climara 841
Climara Pro 847
Divigel 3467
Estrasorb 1777
Vagifem 2589

Estradiol Benzoate (Chronic administration of armodafinil resulted in moderate induction of CYP3A activity. Hence, the effectiveness of drugs that are substrates for CYP3A enzymes may be reduced after initiation of concurrent administration of armodafinil with midazolam. Dose adjustment may be required).
No products indexed under this heading.

Estradiol Cypionate (Chronic administration of armodafinil resulted in moderate induction of CYP3A activity. Hence, the effectiveness of drugs that are substrates for CYP3A enzymes may be reduced after initiation of concurrent administration of armodafinil with midazolam. Dose adjustment may be required).
No products indexed under this heading.

Estradiol Valerate (Chronic administration of armodafinil resulted in moderate induction of CYP3A activity. Hence, the effectiveness of drugs that are substrates for CYP3A enzymes may be reduced after initiation of concurrent administration of armodafinil with midazolam. Dose adjustment may be required).
No products indexed under this heading.

Ethanol (Patients should be advised that the use of armodafinil in combination with alcohol has not been studied. Patients should be advised that it is prudent to avoid alcohol while taking armodafinil).
No products indexed under this heading.

Ethinyl Estradiol (The effectiveness of steroidal contraceptives may be reduced when used with armodafinil and for one month after the discontinuation of therapy. Alternative or concomitant methods of contraception are recom-

1279 Interactions Index Nuvigil

mended for patients treated with armodafinil and for one month after discontinuation of treatment of armodafinil). Products include:
LoSeasonique 3407
Lybrel 3514
NuvaRing 3181
Ortho Evra 2648
Ortho-Cyclen/Ortho Tri-Cyclen 2663
Ortho Tri-Cyclen Lo Tablets 2673
Seasonique 3418
Yaz 864

Ethosuximide (Administration of armodafinil resulted in moderate inhibition of CYP2C19 activity. Hence, dosage reduction may be required for some drugs that are substrates for CYP2C19 when used concurrently with armodafinil. A 40% increase in exposure was seen upon concomitant administration of armodafinil with omeprazole).
No products indexed under this heading.

Ethotoin (Administration of armodafinil resulted in moderate inhibition of CYP2C19 activity. Hence, dosage reduction may be required for some drugs that are substrates for CYP2C19 when used concurrently with armodafinil. A 40% increase in exposure was seen upon concomitant administration of armodafinil with omeprazole).
No products indexed under this heading.

Ethyl Alcohol (Patients should be advised that the use of armodafinil in combination with alcohol has not been studied. Patients should be advised that it is prudent to avoid alcohol while taking armodafinil).
No products indexed under this heading.

Ethynodiol Diacetate (The effectiveness of steroidal contraceptives may be reduced when used with armodafinil and for one month after the discontinuation of therapy. Alternative or concomitant methods of contraception are recommended for patients treated with armodafinil and for one month after discontinuation of treatment of armodafinil).
No products indexed under this heading.

Etoposide (Chronic administration of armodafinil resulted in moderate induction of CYP3A activity. Hence, the effectiveness of drugs that are substrates for CYP3A enzymes may be reduced after initiation of concurrent administration of armodafinil with midazolam. Dose adjustment may be required).
No products indexed under this heading.

Etoposide Phosphate (Chronic administration of armodafinil resulted in moderate induction of CYP3A activity. Hence, the effectiveness of drugs that are substrates for CYP3A enzymes may be reduced after initiation of concurrent administration of armodafinil with midazolam. Dose adjustment may be required).
No products indexed under this heading.

Felbamate (Administration of armodafinil resulted in moderate inhibition of CYP2C19 activity. Hence, dosage reduction may be required for some drugs that are substrates for CYP2C19 when used concurrently with armodafinil. A 40% increase in exposure was seen upon concomitant administration of armodafinil with omeprazole).
No products indexed under this heading.

Felodipine (Chronic administration of armodafinil resulted in moderate induction of CYP3A activity. Hence, the effectiveness of drugs that are substrates for CYP3A enzymes may be reduced after initiation of concurrent administration of armodafinil with midazolam. Dose adjustment may be required).
No products indexed under this heading.

Fentanyl (Chronic administration of armodafinil resulted in moderate induction of CYP3A activity. Hence, the effectiveness of drugs that are substrates for CYP3A enzymes may be reduced after initiation of concurrent administration of armodafinil with midazolam. Dose adjustment may be required). Products include:
Duragesic 2604
Fentanyl Transdermal System 2346
Onsolis 2054

Fentanyl Citrate (Chronic administration of armodafinil resulted in moderate induction of CYP3A activity. Hence, the effectiveness of drugs that are substrates for CYP3A enzymes may be reduced after initiation of concurrent administration of armodafinil with midazolam. Dose adjustment may be required). Products include:
Fentora 966

Flutamide (*In vitro* data demonstrated that armodafinil shows a weak inductive response for CYP1A2 and possibly CYP3A activities in a concentration related manner and demonstrated that CYP2C19 activity is reversibly inhibited by armodafinil. However, the effect on CYP1A2 activity was not observed clinically in an interaction study performed with caffeine).
No products indexed under this heading.

Fluticasone Propionate (*In vitro* data demonstrated that armodafinil shows a weak inductive response for CYP1A2 and possibly CYP3A activities in a concentration related manner and demonstrated that CYP2C19 activity is reversibly inhibited by armodafinil. However, the effect on CYP1A2 activity was not observed clinically in an interaction study performed with caffeine). Products include:
Advair 100/50 1275
Advair 250/50 1275
Advair 500/50 1275
Advair HFA 45/21 1288
Advair HFA 115/21 1288
Advair HFA 230/21 1288
Flonase 1459
Flovent Diskus 1463
Flovent HFA 1470

Fluvoxamine Maleate (*In vitro* data demonstrated that armodafinil shows a weak inductive response for CYP1A2 and possibly CYP3A activities in a concentration related manner and demonstrated that CYP2C19 activity is reversibly inhibited by armodafinil. However, the effect on CYP1A2 activity was not observed clinically in an interaction study performed with caffeine).
No products indexed under this heading.

Formoterol Fumarate (Administration of armodafinil resulted in moderate inhibition of CYP2C19 activity. Hence, dosage reduction may be required for some drugs that are substrates for CYP2C19 when used concurrently with armodafinil. A 40% increase in exposure was seen upon concomitant administration of armodafinil with omeprazole). Products include:
Foradil 3121
Perforomist 3634

Fosphenytoin (Administration of armodafinil resulted in moderate inhibition of CYP2C19 activity. Hence, dosage reduction may be required for some drugs that are substrates for CYP2C19 when used concurrently with armodafinil. A 40% increase in exposure was seen upon concomitant administration of armodafinil with omeprazole).
No products indexed under this heading.

Fosphenytoin Sodium (Administration of armodafinil resulted in moderate inhibition of CYP2C19 activity. Hence, dosage reduction may be required for some drugs that are substrates for CYP2C19 when used concurrently with armodafinil. A 40% increase in exposure was seen upon concomitant administration of armodafinil with omeprazole).
No products indexed under this heading.

Gabapentin (Administration of armodafinil resulted in moderate inhibition of CYP2C19 activity. Hence, dosage reduction may be required for some drugs that are substrates for CYP2C19 when used concurrently with armodafinil. A 40% increase in exposure was seen upon concomitant administration of armodafinil with omeprazole).
No products indexed under this heading.

Grepafloxacin Hydrochloride (*In vitro* data demonstrated that armodafinil shows a weak inductive response for CYP1A2 and possibly CYP3A activities in a concentration related manner and demonstrated that CYP2C19 activity is reversibly inhibited by armodafinil. However, the effect on CYP1A2 activity was not observed clinically in an interaction study performed with caffeine).
No products indexed under this heading.

Haloperidol (Chronic administration of armodafinil resulted in moderate induction of CYP3A activity. Hence, the effectiveness of drugs that are substrates for CYP3A enzymes may be reduced after initiation of concurrent administration of armodafinil with midazolam. Dose adjustment may be required).
No products indexed under this heading.

Haloperidol Decanoate (Chronic administration of armodafinil resulted in moderate induction of CYP3A activity. Hence, the effectiveness of drugs that are substrates for CYP3A enzymes may be reduced after initiation of concurrent administration of armodafinil with midazolam. Dose adjustment may be required).
No products indexed under this heading.

Haloperidol Lactate (Chronic administration of armodafinil resulted in moderate induction of CYP3A activity. Hence, the effectiveness of drugs that are substrates for CYP3A enzymes may be reduced after initiation of concurrent administration of armodafinil with midazolam. Dose adjustment may be required).
No products indexed under this heading.

Imipramine Hydrochloride (Administration of armodafinil resulted in moderate inhibition of CYP2C19 activity. Hence, dosage reduction may be required for some drugs that are substrates for CYP2C19 when used concurrently with armodafinil. A 40% increase in exposure was seen upon concomitant administration of armodafinil with omeprazole).
No products indexed under this heading.

Imipramine Pamoate (Administration of armodafinil resulted in moderate inhibition of CYP2C19 activity. Hence, dosage reduction may be required for some drugs that are substrates for CYP2C19 when used concurrently with armodafinil. A 40% increase in exposure was seen upon concomitant administration of armodafinil with omeprazole).
No products indexed under this heading.

Indinavir Sulfate (Chronic administration of armodafinil resulted in moderate induction of CYP3A activity. Hence, the effectiveness of drugs that are substrates for CYP3A enzymes may be reduced after initiation of concurrent administration of armodafinil with midazolam. Dose adjustment may be required). Products include:
Crixivan 2113

Indomethacin (Administration of armodafinil resulted in moderate inhibition of CYP2C19 activity. Hence, dosage reduction may be required for some drugs that are substrates for CYP2C19 when used concurrently with armodafinil. A 40% increase in exposure was seen upon concomitant administration of armodafinil with omeprazole). Products include:
Indocin 2167

Indomethacin Sodium Trihydrate (Administration of armodafinil resulted in moderate inhibition of CYP2C19 activity. Hence, dosage reduction may be required for some drugs that are substrates for CYP2C19 when used concurrently with armodafinil. A 40% increase in exposure was seen upon concomitant administration of armodafinil with omeprazole). Products include:
Indocin I.V. 2007

Isradipine (Chronic administration of armodafinil resulted in moderate induction of CYP3A activity. Hence, the effectiveness of drugs that are substrates for CYP3A enzymes may be reduced after initiation of concurrent administration of armodafinil with midazolam. Dose adjustment may be required). Products include:
DynaCirc CR 1432

Itraconazole (Chronic administration of armodafinil resulted in moderate induction of CYP3A activity. Hence, the effectiveness of drugs that are substrates for CYP3A enzymes may be reduced after initiation of concurrent administration of armodafinil with midazolam. Dose adjustment may be required).
No products indexed under this heading.

Ixabepilone (Chronic administration of armodafinil resulted in moderate induction of CYP3A activity. Hence, the effectiveness of drugs that are substrates for CYP3A enzymes may be reduced after initiation of concurrent administration of armodafinil with midazolam. Dose adjustment may be required).
No products indexed under this heading.

Ketoconazole (Chronic administration of armodafinil resulted in moderate induction of CYP3A activity. Hence, the effectiveness of drugs that are substrates for CYP3A enzymes may be reduced after initiation of concurrent administration of armodafinil with midazolam. Dose adjustment may be required). Products include:
Extina 3319
Xolegel 3337

Lamotrigine (Administration of armodafinil resulted in moderate inhibition of CYP2C19 activity. Hence, dosage reduction may be required for some drugs that are substrates for CYP2C19 when used concurrently with armodafinil. A 40% increase in exposure was seen upon concomitant administration of armodafinil with omeprazole). Products include:
Lamictal 1522
Lamictal ODT 1522
Lamictal XR 1536

Lansoprazole (Administration of armodafinil resulted in moderate inhibition of CYP2C19 activity. Hence, dosage reduction may be required for some drugs that are substrates for CYP2C19 when used concurrently with armodafinil. A 40% increase in exposure was seen upon concomitant administration of armodafinil with omeprazole).
No products indexed under this heading.

Levetiracetam (Administration of armodafinil resulted in moderate inhibition of CYP2C19 activity. Hence, dosage reduction may be required for some drugs that are substrates for CYP2C19 when used concurrently with armodafinil. A 40% increase in exposure was seen upon concomitant administration of armodafinil with omeprazole). Products include:
Keppra XR 3434

IMPORTANT NOTE: Always consult each drug listing in the patient's regimen for possible interactions.

Nuvigil Interactions Index 1280

Levobupivacaine Hydrochloride (*In vitro* data demonstrated that armodafinil shows a weak inductive response for CYP1A2 and possibly CYP3A activities in a concentration related manner and demonstrated that CYP2C19 activity is reversibly inhibited by armodafinil. However, the effect on CYP1A2 activity was not observed clinically in an interaction study performed with caffeine).
No products indexed under this heading.

Levonorgestrel (The effectiveness of steroidal contraceptives may be reduced when used with armodafinil and for one month after the discontinuation of therapy. Alternative or concomitant methods of contraception are recommended for patients treated with armodafinil and for one month after discontinuation of treatment of armodafinil). Products include:
Climara Pro 847
LoSeasonique 3407
Lybrel 3514
Mirena 854
Plan B 3416
Seasonique 3418

Lidocaine (Chronic administration of armodafinil resulted in moderate induction of CYP3A activity. Hence, the effectiveness of drugs that are substrates for CYP3A enzymes may be reduced after initiation of concurrent administration of armodafinil with midazolam. Dose adjustment may be required). Products include:
Lidoderm 1107

Lidocaine Hydrochloride (Chronic administration of armodafinil resulted in moderate induction of CYP3A activity. Hence, the effectiveness of drugs that are substrates for CYP3A enzymes may be reduced after initiation of concurrent administration of armodafinil with midazolam. Dose adjustment may be required).
No products indexed under this heading.

Lomefloxacin Hydrochloride (*In vitro* data demonstrated that armodafinil shows a weak inductive response for CYP1A2 and possibly CYP3A activities in a concentration related manner and demonstrated that CYP2C19 activity is reversibly inhibited by armodafinil. However, the effect on CYP1A2 activity was not observed clinically in an interaction study performed with caffeine).
No products indexed under this heading.

Lovastatin (Chronic administration of armodafinil resulted in moderate induction of CYP3A activity. Hence, the effectiveness of drugs that are substrates for CYP3A enzymes may be reduced after initiation of concurrent administration of armodafinil with midazolam. Dose adjustment may be required). Products include:
Advicor 402
Mevacor 2212

Maprotiline Hydrochloride (Administration of armodafinil resulted in moderate inhibition of CYP2C19 activity. Hence, dosage reduction may be required for some drugs that are substrates for CYP2C19 when used concurrently with armodafinil. A 40% increase in exposure was seen upon concomitant administration of armodafinil with omeprazole).
No products indexed under this heading.

Mephenytoin (Administration of armodafinil resulted in moderate inhibition of CYP2C19 activity. Hence, dosage reduction may be required for some drugs that are substrates for CYP2C19 when used concurrently with armodafinil. A 40% increase in exposure was seen upon concomitant administration of armodafinil with omeprazole).
No products indexed under this heading.

Mephobarbital (Administration of armodafinil resulted in moderate inhibition of CYP2C19 activity. Hence, dosage reduction may be required for some drugs that are substrates for CYP2C19 when used concurrently with armodafinil. A 40% increase in exposure was seen upon concomitant administration of armodafinil with omeprazole).
No products indexed under this heading.

Meprobamate (Administration of armodafinil resulted in moderate inhibition of CYP2C19 activity. Hence, dosage reduction may be required for some drugs that are substrates for CYP2C19 when used concurrently with armodafinil. A 40% increase in exposure was seen upon concomitant administration of armodafinil with omeprazole).
No products indexed under this heading.

Mestranol (The effectiveness of steroidal contraceptives may be reduced when used with armodafinil and for one month after the discontinuation of therapy. Alternative or concomitant methods of contraception are recommended for patients treated with armodafinil and for one month after discontinuation of treatment of armodafinil).
No products indexed under this heading.

Methadone Hydrochloride (Chronic administration of armodafinil resulted in moderate induction of CYP3A activity. Hence, the effectiveness of drugs that are substrates for CYP3A enzymes may be reduced after initiation of concurrent administration of armodafinil with midazolam. Dose adjustment may be required).
No products indexed under this heading.

Methsuximide (Administration of armodafinil resulted in moderate inhibition of CYP2C19 activity. Hence, dosage reduction may be required for some drugs that are substrates for CYP2C19 when used concurrently with armodafinil. A 40% increase in exposure was seen upon concomitant administration of armodafinil with omeprazole).
No products indexed under this heading.

Mexiletine Hydrochloride (*In vitro* data demonstrated that armodafinil shows a weak inductive response for CYP1A2 and possibly CYP3A activities in a concentration related manner and demonstrated that CYP2C19 activity is reversibly inhibited by armodafinil. However, the effect on CYP1A2 activity was not observed clinically in an interaction study performed with caffeine).
No products indexed under this heading.

Midazolam Hydrochloride (Administration of armodafinil resulted in moderate inhibition of CYP2C19 activity. Hence, dosage reduction may be required for some drugs that are substrates for CYP2C19 when used concurrently with armodafinil. A 40% increase in exposure was seen upon concomitant administration of armodafinil with omeprazole).
No products indexed under this heading.

Mirtazapine (*In vitro* data demonstrated that armodafinil shows a weak inductive response for CYP1A2 and possibly CYP3A activities in a concentration related manner and demonstrated that CYP2C19 activity is reversibly inhibited by armodafinil. However, the effect on CYP1A2 activity was not observed clinically in an interaction study performed with caffeine). Products include:
Remeron Tablets 3214
RemeronSolTab Tablets 3219

Modafinil (Concomitant modafinil or clomipramine did not alter the PK profile of either drug; however, one incident of increased levels of clomipramine and its active metabolite desmethylclomipramine was reported in a patient with narcolepsy during treatment with modafinil). Products include:
Provigil 983

Moxifloxacin Hydrochloride (*In vitro* data demonstrated that armodafinil shows a weak inductive response for CYP1A2 and possibly CYP3A activities in a concentration related manner and demonstrated that CYP2C19 activity is reversibly inhibited by armodafinil. However, the effect on CYP1A2 activity was not observed clinically in an interaction study performed with caffeine). Products include:
Avelox 3064
Vigamox 589

Nafcillin Sodium (*In vitro* data demonstrated that armodafinil shows a weak inductive response for CYP1A2 and possibly CYP3A activities in a concentration related manner and demonstrated that CYP2C19 activity is reversibly inhibited by armodafinil. However, the effect on CYP1A2 activity was not observed clinically in an interaction study performed with caffeine).
No products indexed under this heading.

Naproxen (*In vitro* data demonstrated that armodafinil shows a weak inductive response for CYP1A2 and possibly CYP3A activities in a concentration related manner and demonstrated that CYP2C19 activity is reversibly inhibited by armodafinil. However, the effect on CYP1A2 activity was not observed clinically in an interaction study performed with caffeine). Products include:
EC-Naprosyn 2850
Naprosyn 2850
Anaprox/Naprosyn 2850

Naproxen Sodium (*In vitro* data demonstrated that armodafinil shows a weak inductive response for CYP1A2 and possibly CYP3A activities in a concentration related manner and demonstrated that CYP2C19 activity is reversibly inhibited by armodafinil. However, the effect on CYP1A2 activity was not observed clinically in an interaction study performed with caffeine). Products include:
Anaprox 2850
Anaprox DS 2850
Treximet 1681

Nefazodone Hydrochloride (Chronic administration of armodafinil resulted in moderate induction of CYP3A activity. Hence, the effectiveness of drugs that are substrates for CYP3A enzymes may be reduced after initiation of concurrent administration of armodafinil with midazolam. Dose adjustment may be required).
No products indexed under this heading.

Nelfinavir Mesylate (Administration of armodafinil resulted in moderate inhibition of CYP2C19 activity. Hence, dosage reduction may be required for some drugs that are substrates for CYP2C19 when used concurrently with armodafinil. A 40% increase in exposure was seen upon concomitant administration of armodafinil with omeprazole).
No products indexed under this heading.

Nicardipine (Chronic administration of armodafinil resulted in moderate induction of CYP3A activity. Hence, the effectiveness of drugs that are substrates for CYP3A enzymes may be reduced after initiation of concurrent administration of armodafinil with midazolam. Dose adjustment may be required).
No products indexed under this heading.

Nicardipine Hydrochloride (Chronic administration of armodafinil resulted in moderate induction of CYP3A activity. Hence, the effectiveness of drugs that are substrates for CYP3A enzymes may be reduced after initiation of concurrent administration of armodafinil with midazolam. Dose adjustment may be required).
No products indexed under this heading.

Nicotine Polacrilex (*In vitro* data demonstrated that armodafinil shows a weak inductive response for CYP1A2 and possibly CYP3A activities in a concentration related manner and demonstrated that CYP2C19 activity is reversibly inhibited by armodafinil. However, the effect on CYP1A2 activity was not observed clinically in an interaction study performed with caffeine).
No products indexed under this heading.

Nicotine Salicylate (*In vitro* data demonstrated that armodafinil shows a weak inductive response for CYP1A2 and possibly CYP3A activities in a concentration related manner and demonstrated that CYP2C19 activity is reversibly inhibited by armodafinil. However, the effect on CYP1A2 activity was not observed clinically in an interaction study performed with caffeine).
No products indexed under this heading.

Nicotine Sulfate (*In vitro* data demonstrated that armodafinil shows a weak inductive response for CYP1A2 and possibly CYP3A activities in a concentration related manner and demonstrated that CYP2C19 activity is reversibly inhibited by armodafinil. However, the effect on CYP1A2 activity was not observed clinically in an interaction study performed with caffeine).
No products indexed under this heading.

Nifedipine (Chronic administration of armodafinil resulted in moderate induction of CYP3A activity. Hence, the effectiveness of drugs that are substrates for CYP3A enzymes may be reduced after initiation of concurrent administration of armodafinil with midazolam. Dose adjustment may be required).
No products indexed under this heading.

Nilutamide (Administration of armodafinil resulted in moderate inhibition of CYP2C19 activity. Hence, dosage reduction may be required for some drugs that are substrates for CYP2C19 when used concurrently with armodafinil. A 40% increase in exposure was seen upon concomitant administration of armodafinil with omeprazole).
No products indexed under this heading.

Nimodipine (Chronic administration of armodafinil resulted in moderate induction of CYP3A activity. Hence, the effectiveness of drugs that are substrates for CYP3A enzymes may be reduced after initiation of concurrent administration of armodafinil with midazolam. Dose adjustment may be required).
No products indexed under this heading.

Nisoldipine (Chronic administration of armodafinil resulted in moderate induction of CYP3A activity. Hence, the effectiveness of drugs that are substrates for CYP3A enzymes may be reduced after initiation of concurrent administration of armodafinil with midazolam. Dose adjustment may be required).
No products indexed under this heading.

Nitrendipine (Chronic administration of armodafinil resulted in moderate induction of CYP3A activity. Hence, the effectiveness of drugs that are substrates for CYP3A enzymes may be reduced after initiation of concurrent administration of armodafinil with midazolam. Dose adjustment may be required).
No products indexed under this heading.

Norethindrone (The effectiveness of steroidal contraceptives may be reduced when used with armodafinil and for one month after the discontinuation of therapy. Alternative or concomitant methods of contraception are recommended for patients treated with armodafinil and for one month after discontinuation of treatment of armodafinil). Products include:
Ortho Micronor 2660

Norethindrone Acetate (Chronic administration of armodafinil resulted in moderate induction of CYP3A activity. Hence, the effectiveness of drugs that are substrates for CYP3A enzymes may be reduced after initiation of concurrent administration of armodafinil with midazolam. Dose adjustment may be required). Products include:
Activella 2561

Norethynodrel (The effectiveness of steroidal contraceptives may be reduced when used with armodafinil and for one month after the discontinuation of therapy. Alternative or concomitant methods of contraception are recommended for patients treated with armodafinil and for one month after discontinuation of treatment of armodafinil).
No products indexed under this heading.

Norfloxacin (In vitro data demonstrated that armodafinil shows a weak inductive response for CYP1A2 and possibly CYP3A activities in a concentration related manner and demonstrated that CYP2C19 activity is reversibly inhibited by armodafinil. However, the effect on CYP1A2 activity was not observed clinically in an interaction study performed with caffeine). Products include:
Noroxin 2220

Norgestimate (The effectiveness of steroidal contraceptives may be reduced when used with armodafinil and for one month after the discontinuation of therapy. Alternative or concomitant methods of contraception are recommended for patients treated with armodafinil and for one month after discontinuation of treatment of armodafinil). Products include:
Ortho-Cyclen/Ortho Tri-Cyclen 2663
Ortho Tri-Cyclen Lo Tablets 2673

Norgestrel (The effectiveness of steroidal contraceptives may be reduced when used with armodafinil and for one month after the discontinuation of therapy. Alternative or concomitant methods of contraception are recommended for patients treated with armodafinil and for one month after discontinuation of treatment of armodafinil).
No products indexed under this heading.

Nortriptyline Hydrochloride (Administration of armodafinil resulted in moderate inhibition of CYP2C19 activity. Hence, dosage reduction may be required for some drugs that are substrates for CYP2C19 when used concurrently with armodafinil. A 40% increase in exposure was seen upon concomitant administration of armodafinil with omeprazole).
No products indexed under this heading.

Ofloxacin (In vitro data demonstrated that armodafinil shows a weak inductive response for CYP1A2 and possibly CYP3A activities in a concentration related manner and demonstrated that CYP2C19 activity is reversibly inhibited by armodafinil. However, the effect on CYP1A2 activity was not observed clinically in an interaction study performed with caffeine).
No products indexed under this heading.

Olanzapine (In vitro data demonstrated that armodafinil shows a weak inductive response for CYP1A2 and possibly CYP3A activities in a concentration related manner and demonstrated that CYP2C19 activity is reversibly inhibited by armodafinil. However, the effect on CYP1A2 activity was not observed clinically in an interaction study performed with caffeine). Products include:
Symbyax 1965
Zyprexa 1984
Zyprexa IntraMuscular 1984
Zyprexa ZYDIS 1984

Omeprazole (Administration of armodafinil resulted in moderate inhibition of CYP2C19 activity. Hence, dosage reduction may be required for some drugs that are substrates for CYP2C19 when used concurrently with armodafinil. A 40% increase in exposure was seen upon concomitant administration of armodafinil with omeprazole).
No products indexed under this heading.

Omeprazole Magnesium (Administration of armodafinil resulted in moderate inhibition of CYP2C19 activity. Hence, dosage reduction may be required for some drugs that are substrates for CYP2C19 when used concurrently with armodafinil. A 40% increase in exposure was seen upon concomitant administration of armodafinil with omeprazole).
No products indexed under this heading.

Ondansetron (Chronic administration of armodafinil resulted in moderate induction of CYP3A activity. Hence, the effectiveness of drugs that are substrates for CYP3A enzymes may be reduced after initiation of concurrent administration of armodafinil with midazolam. Dose adjustment may be required).
No products indexed under this heading.

Ondansetron Hydrochloride (Chronic administration of armodafinil resulted in moderate induction of CYP3A activity. Hence, the effectiveness of drugs that are substrates for CYP3A enzymes may be reduced after initiation of concurrent administration of armodafinil with midazolam. Dose adjustment may be required). Products include:
Zofran Injection 1750
Zofran 1756
Zofran ODT 1756

Oxcarbazepine (Administration of armodafinil resulted in moderate inhibition of CYP2C19 activity. Hence, dosage reduction may be required for some drugs that are substrates for CYP2C19 when used concurrently with armodafinil. A 40% increase in exposure was seen upon concomitant administration of armodafinil with omeprazole).
No products indexed under this heading.

Paclitaxel (Chronic administration of armodafinil resulted in moderate induction of CYP3A activity. Hence, the effectiveness of drugs that are substrates for CYP3A enzymes may be reduced after initiation of concurrent administration of armodafinil with midazolam. Dose adjustment may be required).
No products indexed under this heading.

Pantoprazole Sodium (Administration of armodafinil resulted in moderate inhibition of CYP2C19 activity. Hence, dosage reduction may be required for some drugs that are substrates for CYP2C19 when used concurrently with armodafinil. A 40% increase in exposure was seen upon concomitant administration of armodafinil with omeprazole). Products include:
Protonix Tablets 3571
Protonix 3575

Paramethadione (Administration of armodafinil resulted in moderate inhibition of CYP2C19 activity. Hence, dosage reduction may be required for some drugs that are substrates for CYP2C19 when used concurrently with armodafinil. A 40% increase in exposure was seen upon concomitant administration of armodafinil with omeprazole).
No products indexed under this heading.

Pentamidine Isethionate (Administration of armodafinil resulted in moderate inhibition of CYP2C19 activity. Hence, dosage reduction may be required for some drugs that are substrates for CYP2C19 when used concurrently with armodafinil. A 40% increase in exposure was seen upon concomitant administration of armodafinil with omeprazole).
No products indexed under this heading.

Phenacemide (Administration of armodafinil resulted in moderate inhibition of CYP2C19 activity. Hence, dosage reduction may be required for some drugs that are substrates for CYP2C19 when used concurrently with armodafinil. A 40% increase in exposure was seen upon concomitant administration of armodafinil with omeprazole).
No products indexed under this heading.

Phenobarbital (Administration of armodafinil resulted in moderate inhibition of CYP2C19 activity. Hence, dosage reduction may be required for some drugs that are substrates for CYP2C19 when used concurrently with armodafinil. A 40% increase in exposure was seen upon concomitant administration of armodafinil with omeprazole). Products include:
Donnatal 2711

Phenobarbital Sodium (Administration of armodafinil resulted in moderate inhibition of CYP2C19 activity. Hence, dosage reduction may be required for some drugs that are substrates for CYP2C19 when used concurrently with armodafinil. A 40% increase in exposure was seen upon concomitant administration of armodafinil with omeprazole).
No products indexed under this heading.

Phensuximide (Administration of armodafinil resulted in moderate inhibition of CYP2C19 activity. Hence, dosage reduction may be required for some drugs that are substrates for CYP2C19 when used concurrently with armodafinil. A 40% increase in exposure was seen upon concomitant administration of armodafinil with omeprazole).
No products indexed under this heading.

Phenytoin (Administration of armodafinil resulted in moderate inhibition of CYP2C19 activity. Hence, dosage reduction may be required for some drugs that are substrates for CYP2C19 when used concurrently with armodafinil. A 40% increase in exposure was seen upon concomitant administration of armodafinil with omeprazole).
No products indexed under this heading.

Phenytoin Sodium (Administration of armodafinil resulted in moderate inhibition of CYP2C19 activity. Hence, dosage reduction may be required for some drugs that are substrates for CYP2C19 when used concurrently with armodafinil. A 40% increase in exposure was seen upon concomitant administration of armodafinil with omeprazole). Products include:
Phenytek Capsules 2380

Pimozide (Chronic administration of armodafinil resulted in moderate induction of CYP3A activity. Hence, the effectiveness of drugs that are substrates for CYP3A enzymes may be reduced after initiation of concurrent administration of armodafinil with midazolam. Dose adjustment may be required).
No products indexed under this heading.

Polyestradiol Phosphate (Chronic administration of armodafinil resulted in moderate induction of CYP3A activity. Hence, the effectiveness of drugs that are substrates for CYP3A enzymes may be reduced after initiation of concurrent administration of armodafinil with midazolam. Dose adjustment may be required).
No products indexed under this heading.

Primidone (Administration of armodafinil resulted in moderate inhibition of CYP2C19 activity. Hence, dosage reduction may be required for some drugs that are substrates for CYP2C19 when used concurrently with armodafinil. A 40% increase in exposure was seen upon concomitant administration of armodafinil with omeprazole).
No products indexed under this heading.

Progesterone (Administration of armodafinil resulted in moderate inhibition of CYP2C19 activity. Hence, dosage reduction may be required for some drugs that are substrates for CYP2C19 when used concurrently with armodafinil. A 40% increase in exposure was seen upon concomitant administration of armodafinil with omeprazole). Products include:
Crinone 4% 996
Crinone 8% 996
Prometrium 3307

Proguanil Hydrochloride (Administration of armodafinil resulted in moderate inhibition of CYP2C19 activity. Hence, dosage reduction may be required for some drugs that are substrates for CYP2C19 when used concurrently with armodafinil. A 40% increase in exposure was seen upon concomitant administration of armodafinil with omeprazole). Products include:
Malarone Pediatric Tablets 1572
Malarone 1572

Propafenone Hydrochloride (In vitro data demonstrated that armodafinil shows a weak inductive response for CYP1A2 and possibly CYP3A activities in a concentration related manner and demonstrated that CYP2C19 activity is reversibly inhibited by armodafinil. However, the effect on CYP1A2 activity was not observed clinically in an interaction study performed with caffeine). Products include:
Rythmol 1648
Rythmol SR 1652

Propranolol Hydrochloride (Administration of armodafinil resulted in moderate inhibition of CYP2C19 activity. Hence, dosage reduction may be required for some drugs that are substrates for CYP2C19 when used concurrently with armodafinil. A 40% increase in exposure was seen upon concomitant administration of armodafinil with omeprazole). Products include:
InnoPran XL 1517

Protriptyline Hydrochloride (Administration of armodafinil resulted in moderate inhibition of CYP2C19 activity. Hence, dosage reduction may be required for some drugs that are substrates for CYP2C19 when used concurrently with armodafinil. A 40% increase in exposure was seen upon concomitant administration of armodafinil with omeprazole).
No products indexed under this heading.

Quinidine Gluconate (Chronic administration of armodafinil resulted in moderate induction of CYP3A activity. Hence, the effectiveness of drugs that are substrates for CYP3A enzymes may be reduced after initiation of concurrent administration of armodafinil with midazolam. Dose adjustment may be required).
No products indexed under this heading.

Quinidine Polygalacturonate (Chronic administration of armodafinil resulted in moderate induction of CYP3A activity. Hence, the effectiveness of drugs that are substrates for CYP3A enzymes may be reduced after initiation of concurrent administration of armodafinil with midazolam. Dose adjustment may be required).
No products indexed under this heading.

IMPORTANT NOTE: Always consult each drug listing in the patient's regimen for possible interactions.

Nuvigil Interactions Index 1282

Quinidine Sulfate (Chronic administration of armodafinil resulted in moderate induction of CYP3A activity. Hence, the effectiveness of drugs that are substrates for CYP3A enzymes may be reduced after initiation of concurrent administration of armodafinil with midazolam. Dose adjustment may be required).
No products indexed under this heading.

Rabeprazole Sodium (Administration of armodafinil resulted in moderate inhibition of CYP2C19 activity. Hence, dosage reduction may be required for some drugs that are substrates for CYP2C19 when used concurrently with armodafinil. A 40% increase in exposure was seen upon concomitant administration of armodafinil with omeprazole). Products include:
Aciphex 1035

Rifabutin (Chronic administration of armodafinil resulted in moderate induction of CYP3A activity. Hence, the effectiveness of drugs that are substrates for CYP3A enzymes may be reduced after initiation of concurrent administration of armodafinil with midazolam. Dose adjustment may be required).
No products indexed under this heading.

Riluzole (*In vitro* data demonstrated that armodafinil shows a weak inductive response for CYP1A2 and possibly CYP3A activities in a concentration related manner and demonstrated that CYP2C19 activity is reversibly inhibited by armodafinil. However, the effect on CYP1A2 activity was not observed clinically in an interaction study performed with caffeine). Products include:
Rilutek 3032

Ritonavir (Chronic administration of armodafinil resulted in moderate induction of CYP3A activity. Hence, the effectiveness of drugs that are substrates for CYP3A enzymes may be reduced after initiation of concurrent administration of armodafinil with midazolam. Dose adjustment may be required). Products include:
Kaletra 458
Norvir 509

Ropinirole Hydrochloride (*In vitro* data demonstrated that armodafinil shows a weak inductive response for CYP1A2 and possibly CYP3A activities in a concentration related manner and demonstrated that CYP2C19 activity is reversibly inhibited by armodafinil. However, the effect on CYP1A2 activity was not observed clinically in an interaction study performed with caffeine). Products include:
Requip 1620
Requip XL 1628

Ropivacaine Hydrochloride (*In vitro* data demonstrated that armodafinil shows a weak inductive response for CYP1A2 and possibly CYP3A activities in a concentration related manner and demonstrated that CYP2C19 activity is reversibly inhibited by armodafinil. However, the effect on CYP1A2 activity was not observed clinically in an interaction study performed with caffeine).
No products indexed under this heading.

Saquinavir (Chronic administration of armodafinil resulted in moderate induction of CYP3A activity. Hence, the effectiveness of drugs that are substrates for CYP3A enzymes may be reduced after initiation of concurrent administration of armodafinil with midazolam. Dose adjustment may be required).
No products indexed under this heading.

Saquinavir Mesylate (Chronic administration of armodafinil resulted in moderate induction of CYP3A activity. Hence, the effectiveness of drugs that are substrates for CYP3A enzymes may be reduced after initiation of concurrent administration of armodafinil with midazolam. Dose adjustment may be required).
No products indexed under this heading.

Sertraline Hydrochloride (Administration of armodafinil resulted in moderate inhibition of CYP2C19 activity. Hence, dosage reduction may be required for some drugs that are substrates for CYP2C19 when used concurrently with armodafinil. A 40% increase in exposure was seen upon concomitant administration of armodafinil with omeprazole).
No products indexed under this heading.

Sildenafil Citrate (Chronic administration of armodafinil resulted in moderate induction of CYP3A activity. Hence, the effectiveness of drugs that are substrates for CYP3A enzymes may be reduced after initiation of concurrent administration of armodafinil with midazolam. Dose adjustment may be required).
No products indexed under this heading.

Simvastatin (Chronic administration of armodafinil resulted in moderate induction of CYP3A activity. Hence, the effectiveness of drugs that are substrates for CYP3A enzymes may be reduced after initiation of concurrent administration of armodafinil with midazolam. Dose adjustment may be required). Products include:
Simcor 524
Vytorin 10/10 .... 2303, 3240
Vytorin 10/20 .... 2303, 3240
Vytorin 10/40 .... 2303, 3240
Vytorin 10/80 .... 2303, 3240
Zocor 2289

Sirolimus (Chronic administration of armodafinil resulted in moderate induction of CYP3A activity. Hence, the effectiveness of drugs that are substrates for CYP3A enzymes may be reduced after initiation of concurrent administration of armodafinil with midazolam. Dose adjustment may be required). Products include:
Rapamune 3579

Tacrine Hydrochloride (*In vitro* data demonstrated that armodafinil shows a weak inductive response for CYP1A2 and possibly CYP3A activities in a concentration related manner and demonstrated that CYP2C19 activity is reversibly inhibited by armodafinil. However, the effect on CYP1A2 activity was not observed clinically in an interaction study performed with caffeine).
No products indexed under this heading.

Tacrolimus (Chronic administration of armodafinil resulted in moderate induction of CYP3A activity. Hence, the effectiveness of drugs that are substrates for CYP3A enzymes may be reduced after initiation of concurrent administration of armodafinil with midazolam. Dose adjustment may be required). Products include:
Prograf Capsules 677
Prograf Injection 677
Protopic 685

Tadalafil (Chronic administration of armodafinil resulted in moderate induction of CYP3A activity. Hence, the effectiveness of drugs that are substrates for CYP3A enzymes may be reduced after initiation of concurrent administration of armodafinil with midazolam. Dose adjustment may be required). Products include:
Adcirca 3461
Cialis 1861

Tamoxifen Citrate (Chronic administration of armodafinil resulted in moderate induction of CYP3A activity. Hence, the effectiveness of drugs that are substrates for CYP3A enzymes may be reduced after initiation of concurrent administration of armodafinil with midazolam. Dose adjustment may be required).
No products indexed under this heading.

Teniposide (Administration of armodafinil resulted in moderate inhibition of CYP2C19 activity. Hence, dosage reduction may be required for some drugs that are substrates for CYP2C19 when used concurrently with armodafinil. A 40% increase in exposure was seen upon concomitant administration of armodafinil with omeprazole).
No products indexed under this heading.

Terfenadine (Chronic administration of armodafinil resulted in moderate induction of CYP3A activity. Hence, the effectiveness of drugs that are substrates for CYP3A enzymes may be reduced after initiation of concurrent administration of armodafinil with midazolam. Dose adjustment may be required).
No products indexed under this heading.

Theobromine (*In vitro* data demonstrated that armodafinil shows a weak inductive response for CYP1A2 and possibly CYP3A activities in a concentration related manner and demonstrated that CYP2C19 activity is reversibly inhibited by armodafinil. However, the effect on CYP1A2 activity was not observed clinically in an interaction study performed with caffeine).
No products indexed under this heading.

Theophyllinate (Potential interactions with drugs that inhibit, induce, or are metabolized by cytochrome P450 isoenzymes and other hepatic enzymes may be seen when co-administered with armodafinil).
No products indexed under this heading.

Theophylline (Chronic administration of armodafinil resulted in moderate induction of CYP3A activity. Hence, the effectiveness of drugs that are substrates for CYP3A enzymes may be reduced after initiation of concurrent administration of armodafinil with midazolam. Dose adjustment may be required).
No products indexed under this heading.

Theophylline Anhydrous (Chronic administration of armodafinil resulted in moderate induction of CYP3A activity. Hence, the effectiveness of drugs that are substrates for CYP3A enzymes may be reduced after initiation of concurrent administration of armodafinil with midazolam. Dose adjustment may be required). Products include:
Uniphyl 2817

Theophylline Calcium Salicylate (Chronic administration of armodafinil resulted in moderate induction of CYP3A activity. Hence, the effectiveness of drugs that are substrates for CYP3A enzymes may be reduced after initiation of concurrent administration of armodafinil with midazolam. Dose adjustment may be required).
No products indexed under this heading.

Theophylline Dihydroxypropyl (Glyceryl) (Chronic administration of armodafinil resulted in moderate induction of CYP3A activity. Hence, the effectiveness of drugs that are substrates for CYP3A enzymes may be reduced after initiation of concurrent administration of armodafinil with midazolam. Dose adjustment may be required).
No products indexed under this heading.

Theophylline Ethylenediamine (Chronic administration of armodafinil resulted in moderate induction of CYP3A activity. Hence, the effectiveness of drugs that are substrates for CYP3A enzymes may be reduced after initiation of concurrent administration of armodafinil with midazolam. Dose adjustment may be required).
No products indexed under this heading.

Theophylline Sodium Glycinate (Chronic administration of armodafinil resulted in moderate induction of CYP3A activity. Hence, the effectiveness of drugs that are substrates for CYP3A enzymes may be reduced after initiation of concurrent administration of armodafinil with midazolam. Dose adjustment may be required).
No products indexed under this heading.

Thioridazine (Administration of armodafinil resulted in moderate inhibition of CYP2C19 activity. Hence, dosage reduction may be required for some drugs that are substrates for CYP2C19 when used concurrently with armodafinil. A 40% increase in exposure was seen upon concomitant administration of armodafinil with omeprazole).
No products indexed under this heading.

Thioridazine Hydrochloride (Administration of armodafinil resulted in moderate inhibition of CYP2C19 activity. Hence, dosage reduction may be required for some drugs that are substrates for CYP2C19 when used concurrently with armodafinil. A 40% increase in exposure was seen upon concomitant administration of armodafinil with omeprazole). Products include:
Thioridazine Hydrochloride 2384

Tiagabine Hydrochloride (Administration of armodafinil resulted in moderate inhibition of CYP2C19 activity. Hence, dosage reduction may be required for some drugs that are substrates for CYP2C19 when used concurrently with armodafinil. A 40% increase in exposure was seen upon concomitant administration of armodafinil with omeprazole). Products include:
Gabitril 972

Tizanidine (*In vitro* data demonstrated that armodafinil shows a weak inductive response for CYP1A2 and possibly CYP3A activities in a concentration related manner and demonstrated that CYP2C19 activity is reversibly inhibited by armodafinil. However, the effect on CYP1A2 activity was not observed clinically in an interaction study performed with caffeine).
No products indexed under this heading.

Tizanidine Hydrochloride (*In vitro* data demonstrated that armodafinil shows a weak inductive response for CYP1A2 and possibly CYP3A activities in a concentration related manner and demonstrated that CYP2C19 activity is reversibly inhibited by armodafinil. However, the effect on CYP1A2 activity was not observed clinically in an interaction study performed with caffeine).
No products indexed under this heading.

Tolbutamide (Administration of armodafinil resulted in moderate inhibition of CYP2C19 activity. Hence, dosage reduction may be required for some drugs that are substrates for CYP2C19 when used concurrently with armodafinil. A 40% increase in exposure was seen upon concomitant administration of armodafinil with omeprazole).
No products indexed under this heading.

1283 Interactions Index Omnicef

Tolbutamide Sodium (Administration of armodafinil resulted in moderate inhibition of CYP2C19 activity. Hence, dosage reduction may be required for some drugs that are substrates for CYP2C19 when used concurrently with armodafinil. A 40% increase in exposure was seen upon concomitant administration of armodafinil with omeprazole).
No products indexed under this heading.

Tolterodine Tartrate (Chronic administration of armodafinil resulted in moderate induction of CYP3A activity. Hence, the effectiveness of drugs that are substrates for CYP3A enzymes may be reduced after initiation of concurrent administration of armodafinil with midazolam. Dose adjustment may be required).
No products indexed under this heading.

Topiramate (Administration of armodafinil resulted in moderate inhibition of CYP2C19 activity. Hence, dosage reduction may be required for some drugs that are substrates for CYP2C19 when used concurrently with armodafinil. A 40% increase in exposure was seen upon concomitant administration of armodafinil with omeprazole).
No products indexed under this heading.

Trazodone Hydrochloride (Chronic administration of armodafinil resulted in moderate induction of CYP3A activity. Hence, the effectiveness of drugs that are substrates for CYP3A enzymes may be reduced after initiation of concurrent administration of armodafinil with midazolam. Dose adjustment may be required).
No products indexed under this heading.

Triazolam (Chronic administration of armodafinil resulted in moderate induction of CYP3A activity. Hence, the effectiveness of drugs that are substrates for CYP3A enzymes may be reduced after initiation of concurrent administration of armodafinil with midazolam. Dose adjustment may be required).
No products indexed under this heading.

Trimethadione (Administration of armodafinil resulted in moderate inhibition of CYP2C19 activity. Hence, dosage reduction may be required for some drugs that are substrates for CYP2C19 when used concurrently with armodafinil. A 40% increase in exposure was seen upon concomitant administration of armodafinil with omeprazole).
No products indexed under this heading.

Trimethaphan Camsylate (*In vitro* data demonstrated that armodafinil shows a weak inductive response for CYP1A2 and possibly CYP3A activities in a concentration related manner and demonstrated that CYP2C19 activity is reversibly inhibited by armodafinil. However, the effect on CYP1A2 activity was not observed clinically in an interaction study performed with caffeine).
No products indexed under this heading.

Trimipramine Maleate (Administration of armodafinil resulted in moderate inhibition of CYP2C19 activity. Hence, dosage reduction may be required for some drugs that are substrates for CYP2C19 when used concurrently with armodafinil. A 40% increase in exposure was seen upon concomitant administration of armodafinil with omeprazole).
No products indexed under this heading.

Trovafloxacin Mesylate (*In vitro* data demonstrated that armodafinil shows a weak inductive response for CYP1A2 and possibly CYP3A activities in a concentration related manner and demonstrated that CYP2C19 activity is reversibly inhibited by armodafinil. However, the effect on CYP1A2 activity was not observed clinically in an interaction study performed with caffeine).
No products indexed under this heading.

Valproate Sodium (Administration of armodafinil resulted in moderate inhibition of CYP2C19 activity. Hence, dosage reduction may be required for some drugs that are substrates for CYP2C19 when used concurrently with armodafinil. A 40% increase in exposure was seen upon concomitant administration of armodafinil with omeprazole).
No products indexed under this heading.

Valproic Acid (Administration of armodafinil resulted in moderate inhibition of CYP2C19 activity. Hence, dosage reduction may be required for some drugs that are substrates for CYP2C19 when used concurrently with armodafinil. A 40% increase in exposure was seen upon concomitant administration of armodafinil with omeprazole).
No products indexed under this heading.

Vardenafil Hydrochloride (Chronic administration of armodafinil resulted in moderate induction of CYP3A activity. Hence, the effectiveness of drugs that are substrates for CYP3A enzymes may be reduced after initiation of concurrent administration of armodafinil with midazolam. Dose adjustment may be required). Products include:
Levitra 3157

Verapamil Hydrochloride (Chronic administration of armodafinil resulted in moderate induction of CYP3A activity. Hence, the effectiveness of drugs that are substrates for CYP3A enzymes may be reduced after initiation of concurrent administration of armodafinil with midazolam. Dose adjustment may be required). Products include:
Tarka 534

Vinblastine Sulfate (Chronic administration of armodafinil resulted in moderate induction of CYP3A activity. Hence, the effectiveness of drugs that are substrates for CYP3A enzymes may be reduced after initiation of concurrent administration of armodafinil with midazolam. Dose adjustment may be required).
No products indexed under this heading.

Vincristine Sulfate (Chronic administration of armodafinil resulted in moderate induction of CYP3A activity. Hence, the effectiveness of drugs that are substrates for CYP3A enzymes may be reduced after initiation of concurrent administration of armodafinil with midazolam. Dose adjustment may be required).
No products indexed under this heading.

Voriconazole (Administration of armodafinil resulted in moderate inhibition of CYP2C19 activity. Hence, dosage reduction may be required for some drugs that are substrates for CYP2C19 when used concurrently with armodafinil. A 40% increase in exposure was seen upon concomitant administration of armodafinil with omeprazole).
No products indexed under this heading.

Warfarin Sodium (Administration of armodafinil resulted in moderate inhibition of CYP2C19 activity. Hence, dosage reduction may be required for some drugs that are substrates for CYP2C19 when used concurrently with armodafinil. A 40% increase in exposure was seen upon concomitant administration of armodafinil with omeprazole).
No products indexed under this heading.

Zileuton (*In vitro* data demonstrated that armodafinil shows a weak inductive response for CYP1A2 and possibly CYP3A activities in a concentration related manner and demonstrated that CYP2C19 activity is reversibly inhibited by armodafinil. However, the effect on CYP1A2 activity was not observed clinically in an interaction study performed with caffeine).
No products indexed under this heading.

Zolmitriptan (*In vitro* data demonstrated that armodafinil shows a weak inductive response for CYP1A2 and possibly CYP3A activities in a concentration related manner and demonstrated that CYP2C19 activity is reversibly inhibited by armodafinil. However, the effect on CYP1A2 activity was not observed clinically in an interaction study performed with caffeine). Products include:
Zomig Tablets 773
Zomig Nasal Spray 768
Zomig-ZMT Tablets 773

Zonisamide (Administration of armodafinil resulted in moderate inhibition of CYP2C19 activity. Hence, dosage reduction may be required for some drugs that are substrates for CYP2C19 when used concurrently with armodafinil. A 40% increase in exposure was seen upon concomitant administration of armodafinil with omeprazole). Products include:
Zonegran 1081

Food Interactions

Alcohol (Patients should be advised that the use of armodafinil in combination with alcohol has not been studied. Patients should be advised that it is prudent to avoid alcohol while taking armodafinil).

Beer, reduced-alcohol (Patients should be advised that the use of armodafinil in combination with alcohol has not been studied. Patients should be advised that it is prudent to avoid alcohol while taking armodafinil).

Beer, unspecified (Patients should be advised that the use of armodafinil in combination with alcohol has not been studied. Patients should be advised that it is prudent to avoid alcohol while taking armodafinil).

Food, caffeine-containing (*In vitro* data demonstrated that armodafinil shows a weak inductive response for CYP1A2 and possibly CYP3A activities in a concentration related manner and demonstrated that CYP2C19 activity is reversibly inhibited by armodafinil. However, the effect on CYP1A2 activity was not observed clinically in an interaction study performed with caffeine).

Food, unspecified (Although food effect on the bioavailability of armodafinil is considered minimal, food can potentially affect the onset and time course of pharmacologic action of armodafinil. The time to reach peak concentration (T_{max}) may be delayed by approximately 2-4 hours in the fed state).

Meal, unspecified (Although food effect on the bioavailability of armodafinil is considered minimal, food can potentially affect the onset and time course of pharmacologic action of armodafinil. The time to reach peak concentration (T_{max}) may be delayed by approximately 2-4 hours in the fed state).

Wine, Chianti (Patients should be advised that the use of armodafinil in combination with alcohol has not been studied. Patients should be advised that it is prudent to avoid alcohol while taking armodafinil).

Wine, Red (Patients should be advised that the use of armodafinil in combination with alcohol has not been studied. Patients should be advised that it is prudent to avoid alcohol while taking armodafinil).

Wine, unspecified (Patients should be advised that the use of armodafinil in combination with alcohol has not been studied. Patients should be advised that it is prudent to avoid alcohol while taking armodafinil).

Wine products (Patients should be advised that the use of armodafinil in combination with alcohol has not been studied. Patients should be advised that it is prudent to avoid alcohol while taking armodafinil).

NYSTOP TOPICAL POWDER USP

(Nystatin) 2697
None cited in PDR database.

OFORTA TABLETS

(Fludarabine Phosphate) 3023

Pentostatin (The use of fludarabine phosphate in combination with pentostatin is not recommended due to the risk of severe pulmonary toxicity).
No products indexed under this heading.

OLUX FOAM

(Clobetasol Propionate) 3324
None cited in PDR database.

OLUX-E FOAM

(Clobetasol Propionate) 3322
None cited in PDR database.

OMEGALIFE-3 SUPPLEMENTATION

(Docosahexaenoic Acid (DHA), Eicosapentaenoic Acid (EPA), Vitamin E) 3456
None cited in PDR database.

OMNICEF CAPSULES

(Cefdinir) 518
May interact with antacids containing aluminum, calcium and magnesium, iron containing oral preparations, and certain other agents. Compounds in these categories include:

Aluminum Carbonate (Antacids (aluminum- or magnesium-containing) interfere with the absorption of cefdinir; Omnicef should be taken at least 2 hours before or after the antacids).
No products indexed under this heading.

Aluminum Hydroxide (Antacids (aluminum- or magnesium-containing) interfere with the absorption of cefdinir; Omnicef should be taken at least 2 hours before or after the antacids).
No products indexed under this heading.

Calcium Carbonate (Antacids (aluminum- or magnesium-containing) interfere with the absorption of cefdinir; Omnicef should be taken at least 2 hours before or after the antacids). Products include:
Chelated Mineral 3476
Pepcid Complete 1822
Extra Strength Rolaids Softchews Vanilla Creme 2045

Ferrous Fumarate (Iron supplements, including multivitamins that contain iron, interfere with the absorption of cefdinir; Omnicef should be taken at least 2 hours before or after the administration of iron-containing products). Products include:
PreNexa 3473

Ferrous Gluconate (Iron supplements, including multivitamins that contain iron, interfere with the absorption of cefdinir; Omnicef should be taken at least 2 hours before or after the administration of iron-containing products). Products include:
CitraNatal Assure 2332
CitraNatal Rx 2332

Ferrous Sulfate (Iron supplements, including multivitamins that contain iron, interfere with the absorption of cefdinir; Omnicef should be taken at least 2 hours before or after the administration of iron-containing products).
No products indexed under this heading.

IMPORTANT NOTE: Always consult each drug listing in the patient's regimen for possible interactions.

Omnicef Interactions Index 1284

Iron (Iron supplements, including multivitamins that contain iron, interfere with the absorption of cefdinir; Omnicef should be taken at least 2 hours before or after the administration of iron-containing products).
No products indexed under this heading.

Magaldrate (Antacids (aluminum- or magnesium-containing) interfere with the absorption of cefdinir; Omnicef should be taken at least 2 hours before or after the antacids).
No products indexed under this heading.

Magnesium Carbonate (Antacids (aluminum- or magnesium-containing) interfere with the absorption of cefdinir; Omnicef should be taken at least 2 hours before or after the antacids).
No products indexed under this heading.

Magnesium Hydroxide (Antacids (aluminum- or magnesium-containing) interfere with the absorption of cefdinir; Omnicef should be taken at least 2 hours before or after the antacids). Products include:
Fleet Pedia-Lax Chewable Tablets 1144
Pepcid Complete 1822

Magnesium Oxide (Antacids (aluminum- or magnesium-containing) interfere with the absorption of cefdinir; Omnicef should be taken at least 2 hours before or after the antacids). Products include:
Beelith 873

Magnesium Trisilicate (Antacids (aluminum- or magnesium-containing) interfere with the absorption of cefdinir; Omnicef should be taken at least 2 hours before or after the antacids).
No products indexed under this heading.

Polysaccharide Iron Complex (Iron supplements, including multivitamins that contain iron, interfere with the absorption of cefdinir; Omnicef should be taken at least 2 hours before or after the administration of iron-containing products). Products include:
Nu-Iron 150 2321

Probenecid (Inhibits renal excretion of cefdinir, resulting in an approximate doubling in AUC, a 54% increase in peak cefdinir plasma levels, and a 50% prolongation in the apparent elimination).
No products indexed under this heading.

Food Interactions

Food, unspecified (Although C_{max} and AUC of cefdinir absorption from capsules are reduced by 44% and 33%, respectively, when given with a high-fat meal, the magnitude of these reductions is not likely to be clinically significant; therefore, cefdinir may be taken without regard to food).

OMNICEF FOR ORAL SUSPENSION

(Cefdinir) 518
See Omnicef Capsules

ONCASPAR INJECTION

(Pegaspargase) 1139
May interact with anticoagulants, antineoplastics, highly protein bound drugs (selected), non-steroidal anti-inflammatory agents, and certain other agents. Compounds in these categories include:

Altretamine (Potential for unspecified unfavorable interactions). Products include:
Hexalen 1066

Amiodarone Hydrochloride (Depletion of serum proteins by pegaspargase may increase the toxicity of other drugs which are protein bound).
No products indexed under this heading.

Amitriptyline Hydrochloride (Depletion of serum proteins by pegaspargase may increase the toxicity of other drugs which are protein bound).
No products indexed under this heading.

Anastrozole (Potential for unspecified unfavorable interactions).
No products indexed under this heading.

Anisindione (Increased risk of bleeding and/or thrombosis).
No products indexed under this heading.

Ardeparin Sodium (Increased risk of bleeding and/or thrombosis).
No products indexed under this heading.

Asparaginase (Potential for unspecified unfavorable interactions). Products include:
Elspar 2005, 2122

Aspirin (Increased risk of bleeding and/or thrombosis). Products include:
Aggrenox 880
Bayer Aspirin 829
Percodan 1124
St. Joseph Aspirin 2045

Atovaquone (Depletion of serum proteins by pegaspargase may increase the toxicity of other drugs which are protein bound). Products include:
Malarone Pediatric Tablets 1572
Malarone 1572
Mepron Suspension 1576

Bicalutamide (Potential for unspecified unfavorable interactions).
No products indexed under this heading.

Bleomycin Sulfate (Potential for unspecified unfavorable interactions).
No products indexed under this heading.

Busulfan (Potential for unspecified unfavorable interactions). Products include:
Myleran 1581

Carboplatin (Potential for unspecified unfavorable interactions).
No products indexed under this heading.

Carmustine (BCNU) (Potential for unspecified unfavorable interactions).
No products indexed under this heading.

Cefonicid Sodium (Depletion of serum proteins by pegaspargase may increase the toxicity of other drugs which are protein bound).
No products indexed under this heading.

Celecoxib (Depletion of serum proteins by pegaspargase may increase the toxicity of other drugs which are protein bound). Products include:
Celebrex 3272

Celecoxib (Increased risk of bleeding and/or thrombosis). Products include:
Celebrex 3272

Chlorambucil (Potential for unspecified unfavorable interactions). Products include:
Leukeran 1557

Chlordiazepoxide (Depletion of serum proteins by pegaspargase may increase the toxicity of other drugs which are protein bound).
No products indexed under this heading.

Chlordiazepoxide Hydrochloride (Depletion of serum proteins by pegaspargase may increase the toxicity of other drugs which are protein bound).
No products indexed under this heading.

Chlorpromazine (Depletion of serum proteins by pegaspargase may increase the toxicity of other drugs which are protein bound).
No products indexed under this heading.

Chlorpromazine Hydrochloride (Depletion of serum proteins by pegaspargase may increase the toxicity of other drugs which are protein bound).
No products indexed under this heading.

Cisplatin (Potential for unspecified unfavorable interactions).
No products indexed under this heading.

Clomipramine Hydrochloride (Depletion of serum proteins by pegaspargase may increase the toxicity of other drugs which are protein bound).
No products indexed under this heading.

Clozapine (Depletion of serum proteins by pegaspargase may increase the toxicity of other drugs which are protein bound).
No products indexed under this heading.

Cyclophosphamide (Potential for unspecified unfavorable interactions).
No products indexed under this heading.

Cyclosporine (Depletion of serum proteins by pegaspargase may increase the toxicity of other drugs which are protein bound). Products include:
Gengraf 440
Neoral Oral Solution 2496
Neoral Capsules 2496
Restasis 605

Dacarbazine (Potential for unspecified unfavorable interactions).
No products indexed under this heading.

Dalteparin Sodium (Increased risk of bleeding and/or thrombosis). Products include:
Fragmin 1058

Danaparoid Sodium (Increased risk of bleeding and/or thrombosis).
No products indexed under this heading.

Daunorubicin Citrate (Potential for unspecified unfavorable interactions).
No products indexed under this heading.

Daunorubicin Hydrochloride (Potential for unspecified unfavorable interactions).
No products indexed under this heading.

Denileukin Diftitox (Potential for unspecified unfavorable interactions). Products include:
Ontak 1068

Diazepam (Depletion of serum proteins by pegaspargase may increase the toxicity of other drugs which are protein bound). Products include:
Valium Tablets 2880

Diclofenac Epolamine (Increased risk of bleeding and/or thrombosis). Products include:
Flector 1839

Diclofenac Potassium (Depletion of serum proteins by pegaspargase may increase the toxicity of other drugs which are protein bound; increased risk of bleeding and/or thrombosis).
No products indexed under this heading.

Diclofenac Sodium (Depletion of serum proteins by pegaspargase may increase the toxicity of other drugs which are protein bound; increased risk of bleeding and/or thrombosis).
No products indexed under this heading.

Dicumarol (Increased risk of bleeding and/or thrombosis).
No products indexed under this heading.

Digitalis Glycoside Preparations (Depletion of serum proteins by pegaspargase may increase the toxicity of other drugs which are protein bound).
No products indexed under this heading.

Digitalis Lanata (Depletion of serum proteins by pegaspargase may increase the toxicity of other drugs which are protein bound).
No products indexed under this heading.

Digitalis Purpurea (Depletion of serum proteins by pegaspargase may increase the toxicity of other drugs which are protein bound).
No products indexed under this heading.

Dipyridamole (Depletion of serum proteins by pegaspargase may increase the toxicity of other drugs which are protein bound). Products include:
Aggrenox 880

Docetaxel (Potential for unspecified unfavorable interactions). Products include:
Taxotere 3035

Doxorubicin Hydrochloride (Potential for unspecified unfavorable interactions).
No products indexed under this heading.

Enoxaparin Sodium (Increased risk of bleeding and/or thrombosis). Products include:
Lovenox 3005

Epirubicin Hydrochloride (Potential for unspecified unfavorable interactions).
No products indexed under this heading.

Estramustine Phosphate Sodium (Potential for unspecified unfavorable interactions).
No products indexed under this heading.

Etodolac (Increased risk of bleeding and/or thrombosis).
No products indexed under this heading.

Etoposide (Potential for unspecified unfavorable interactions).
No products indexed under this heading.

Exemestane (Potential for unspecified unfavorable interactions). Products include:
Aromasin 2758

Fenoprofen Calcium (Depletion of serum proteins by pegaspargase may increase the toxicity of other drugs which are protein bound; increased risk of bleeding and/or thrombosis).
No products indexed under this heading.

Floxuridine (Potential for unspecified unfavorable interactions).
No products indexed under this heading.

Fluorouracil (Potential for unspecified unfavorable interactions). Products include:
Carac 2966

Flurazepam Hydrochloride (Depletion of serum proteins by pegaspargase may increase the toxicity of other drugs which are protein bound).
No products indexed under this heading.

Flurbiprofen (Depletion of serum proteins by pegaspargase may increase the toxicity of other drugs which are protein bound; increased risk of bleeding and/or thrombosis).
No products indexed under this heading.

Flutamide (Potential for unspecified unfavorable interactions).
No products indexed under this heading.

Fondaparinux Sodium (Increased risk of bleeding and/or thrombosis). Products include:
Arixtra 1320

Gemcitabine Hydrochloride (Potential for unspecified unfavorable interactions). Products include:
Gemzar 1900

Glipizide (Depletion of serum proteins by pegaspargase may increase the toxicity of other drugs which are protein bound).
No products indexed under this heading.

Heparin Calcium (Increased risk of bleeding and/or thrombosis).
No products indexed under this heading.

Heparin Sodium (Increased risk of bleeding and/or thrombosis).
No products indexed under this heading.

Hydroxyurea (Potential for unspecified unfavorable interactions).
No products indexed under this heading.

Ibuprofen (Depletion of serum proteins by pegaspargase may increase the toxicity of other drugs which are protein bound; increased risk of bleeding and/or thrombosis). Products include:
Motrin IB 2043
Children's Motrin 2044
Children's Motrin Non-Staining Dye-Free 2044
Infants' Motrin 2044

Infants' Motrin Dye-Free 2044
Junior Strength Motrin 2044
Vicoprofen 564

Idarubicin Hydrochloride (Potential for unspecified unfavorable interactions).
No products indexed under this heading.

Ifosfamide (Potential for unspecified unfavorable interactions).
No products indexed under this heading.

Imipramine Hydrochloride (Depletion of serum proteins by pegaspargase may increase the toxicity of other drugs which are protein bound).
No products indexed under this heading.

Imipramine Pamoate (Depletion of serum proteins by pegaspargase may increase the toxicity of other drugs which are protein bound).
No products indexed under this heading.

Indomethacin (Depletion of serum proteins by pegaspargase may increase the toxicity of other drugs which are protein bound; increased risk of bleeding and/or thrombosis). Products include:
Indocin 2167

Indomethacin Sodium Trihydrate (Depletion of serum proteins by pegaspargase may increase the toxicity of other drugs which are protein bound; increased risk of bleeding and/or thrombosis). Products include:
Indocin I.V. 2007

Interferon alfa-2a, Recombinant (Potential for unspecified unfavorable interactions).
No products indexed under this heading.

Interferon alfa-2b, Recombinant (Potential for unspecified unfavorable interactions). Products include:
Intron A 3140

Irinotecan Hydrochloride (Potential for unspecified unfavorable interactions).
No products indexed under this heading.

Ketoprofen (Depletion of serum proteins by pegaspargase may increase the toxicity of other drugs which are protein bound; increased risk of bleeding and/or thrombosis).
No products indexed under this heading.

Ketorolac Tromethamine (Depletion of serum proteins by pegaspargase may increase the toxicity of other drugs which are protein bound; increased risk of bleeding and/or thrombosis). Products include:
Acuvail .... ⊙ 209

Levamisole Hydrochloride (Potential for unspecified unfavorable interactions).
No products indexed under this heading.

Lomustine (CCNU) (Potential for unspecified unfavorable interactions).
No products indexed under this heading.

Low Molecular Weight Heparins (Increased risk of bleeding and/or thrombosis).
No products indexed under this heading.

Mechlorethamine Hydrochloride (Potential for unspecified unfavorable interactions). Products include:
Mustargen 2010

Meclofenamate Sodium (Depletion of serum proteins by pegaspargase may increase the toxicity of other drugs which are protein bound; increased risk of bleeding and/or thrombosis).
No products indexed under this heading.

Mefenamic Acid (Depletion of serum proteins by pegaspargase may increase the toxicity of other drugs which are protein bound; increased risk of bleeding and/or thrombosis).
No products indexed under this heading.

Megestrol Acetate (Potential for unspecified unfavorable interactions). Products include:
Megace ES 2698

Meloxicam (Increased risk of bleeding and/or thrombosis).
No products indexed under this heading.

Melphalan (Potential for unspecified unfavorable interactions). Products include:
Alkeran 1302

Mercaptopurine (Potential for unspecified unfavorable interactions).
No products indexed under this heading.

Methotrexate (Potential for unspecified unfavorable interactions).
No products indexed under this heading.

Methotrexate Sodium (Pegaspargase inhibits protein synthesis and cell replication and thus interferes with the action of methotrexate which requires cell replication for its lethal effect; potential for unspecified unfavorable interactions).
No products indexed under this heading.

Midazolam Hydrochloride (Depletion of serum proteins by pegaspargase may increase the toxicity of other drugs which are protein bound).
No products indexed under this heading.

Mitomycin (Mitomycin-C) (Potential for unspecified unfavorable interactions).
No products indexed under this heading.

Mitotane (Potential for unspecified unfavorable interactions).
No products indexed under this heading.

Mitoxantrone Hydrochloride (Potential for unspecified unfavorable interactions). Products include:
Novantrone 1088

Nabumetone (Increased risk of bleeding and/or thrombosis).
No products indexed under this heading.

Naproxen (Depletion of serum proteins by pegaspargase may increase the toxicity of other drugs which are protein bound; increased risk of bleeding and/or thrombosis). Products include:
EC-Naprosyn 2850
Naprosyn 2850
Anaprox/Naprosyn 2850

Naproxen Sodium (Depletion of serum proteins by pegaspargase may increase the toxicity of other drugs which are protein bound; increased risk of bleeding and/or thrombosis). Products include:
Anaprox 2850
Anaprox DS 2850
Treximet 1681

Nortriptyline Hydrochloride (Depletion of serum proteins by pegaspargase may increase the toxicity of other drugs which are protein bound).
No products indexed under this heading.

Oxaliplatin (Potential for unspecified unfavorable interactions). Products include:
Eloxatin 2975

Oxaprozin (Depletion of serum proteins by pegaspargase may increase the toxicity of other drugs which are protein bound; increased risk of bleeding and/or thrombosis).
No products indexed under this heading.

Oxazepam (Depletion of serum proteins by pegaspargase may increase the toxicity of other drugs which are protein bound).
No products indexed under this heading.

Paclitaxel (Potential for unspecified unfavorable interactions).
No products indexed under this heading.

Phenylbutazone (Depletion of serum proteins by pegaspargase may increase the toxicity of other drugs which are protein bound; increased risk of bleeding and/or thrombosis).
No products indexed under this heading.

Piroxicam (Depletion of serum proteins by pegaspargase may increase the toxicity of other drugs which are protein bound; increased risk of bleeding and/or thrombosis).
No products indexed under this heading.

Procarbazine Hydrochloride (Potential for unspecified unfavorable interactions).
No products indexed under this heading.

Propranolol Hydrochloride (Depletion of serum proteins by pegaspargase may increase the toxicity of other drugs which are protein bound). Products include:
InnoPran XL 1517

Rofecoxib (Increased risk of bleeding and/or thrombosis).
No products indexed under this heading.

Streptozocin (Potential for unspecified unfavorable interactions).
No products indexed under this heading.

Sulindac (Depletion of serum proteins by pegaspargase may increase the toxicity of other drugs which are protein bound; increased risk of bleeding and/or thrombosis). Products include:
Clinoril 2098

Tamoxifen Citrate (Potential for unspecified unfavorable interactions).
No products indexed under this heading.

Temazepam (Depletion of serum proteins by pegaspargase may increase the toxicity of other drugs which are protein bound).
No products indexed under this heading.

Teniposide (Potential for unspecified unfavorable interactions).
No products indexed under this heading.

Thioguanine (Potential for unspecified unfavorable interactions). Products include:
Tabloid 1664

Thiotepa (Potential for unspecified unfavorable interactions).
No products indexed under this heading.

Tinzaparin Sodium (Increased risk of bleeding and/or thrombosis).
No products indexed under this heading.

Tolbutamide (Depletion of serum proteins by pegaspargase may increase the toxicity of other drugs which are protein bound).
No products indexed under this heading.

Tolmetin Sodium (Depletion of serum proteins by pegaspargase may increase the toxicity of other drugs which are protein bound; increased risk of bleeding and/or thrombosis).
No products indexed under this heading.

Topotecan Hydrochloride (Potential for unspecified unfavorable interactions). Products include:
Hycamtin 1491
Hycamtin Capsules 1488

Toremifene Citrate (Potential for unspecified unfavorable interactions).
No products indexed under this heading.

Trimipramine Maleate (Depletion of serum proteins by pegaspargase may increase the toxicity of other drugs which are protein bound).
No products indexed under this heading.

Valdecoxib (Increased risk of bleeding and/or thrombosis).
No products indexed under this heading.

Valrubicin (Potential for unspecified unfavorable interactions). Products include:
Valstar 1131

Vincristine Sulfate (Potential for unspecified unfavorable interactions).
No products indexed under this heading.

Vinorelbine Tartrate (Potential for unspecified unfavorable interactions).
No products indexed under this heading.

Warfarin Sodium (Depletion of serum proteins by pegaspargase may increase the toxicity of other drugs which are protein bound; increased risk of bleeding and/or thrombosis).
No products indexed under this heading.

ONGLYZA TABLETS

(Saxagliptin) 3615

May interact with antacids containing aluminum, calcium and magnesium, cytochrome p450 3a inhibitors (selected), cytochrome p450 3a4 inhibitors (selected), cytochrome p450 3a4 inhibitors, potent (selected), erythromycin, sulfonylureas, and certain other agents. Compounds in these categories include:

Acetazolamide (Co-administration of saxagliptin with other moderate CYP3A4/5 inhibitors (eg, amprenavir, aprepitant, erythromycin, fluconazole, fosamprenavir, grapefruit juice, verapamil) may increase plasma concentrations of saxagliptin; however, dosage adjustment is not recommended).
No products indexed under this heading.

Acetazolamide Sodium (Co-administration of saxagliptin with other moderate CYP3A4/5 inhibitors (eg, amprenavir, aprepitant, erythromycin, fluconazole, fosamprenavir, grapefruit juice, verapamil) may increase plasma concentrations of saxagliptin; however, dosage adjustment is not recommended).
No products indexed under this heading.

Aluminum Carbonate (Co-administration of saxagliptin with a liquid containing aluminum/magnesium hydroxide and simethicone decreased the C_{max} of saxagliptin).
No products indexed under this heading.

Aluminum Hydroxide (Co-administration of saxagliptin with a liquid containing aluminum/magnesium hydroxide and simethicone decreased the C_{max} of saxagliptin).
No products indexed under this heading.

Amiodarone Hydrochloride (Co-administration of saxagliptin with other moderate CYP3A4/5 inhibitors (eg, amprenavir, aprepitant, erythromycin, fluconazole, fosamprenavir, grapefruit juice, verapamil) may increase plasma concentrations of saxagliptin; however, dosage adjustment is not recommended).
No products indexed under this heading.

Amprenavir (Co-administration of saxagliptin with other moderate CYP3A4/5 inhibitors (eg, amprenavir, aprepitant, erythromycin, fluconazole, fosamprenavir, grapefruit juice, verapamil) may increase plasma concentrations of saxagliptin; however, dosage adjustment is not recommended).
No products indexed under this heading.

Anastrozole (Co-administration of saxagliptin with other moderate CYP3A4/5 inhibitors (eg, amprenavir, aprepitant, erythromycin, fluconazole, fosamprenavir, grapefruit juice, verapamil) may increase plasma concentrations of saxagliptin; however, dosage adjustment is not recommended).
No products indexed under this heading.

Aprepitant (Co-administration of saxagliptin with other moderate CYP3A4/5 inhibitors (eg, amprenavir, aprepitant, erythromycin, fluconazole, fosamprenavir, grapefruit juice, verapamil) may increase plasma concentrations of saxagliptin; however, dosage adjustment is not recommended). Products include:
Emend 2124

IMPORTANT NOTE: Always consult each drug listing in the patient's regimen for possible interactions.

Atazanavir (Co-administration of saxagliptin with other moderate CYP3A4/5 inhibitors (eg, amprenavir, aprepitant, erythromycin, fluconazole, fosamprenavir, grapefruit juice, verapamil) may increase plasma concentrations of saxagliptin; however, dosage adjustment is not recommended).
No products indexed under this heading.

Atazanavir Sulfate (Co-administration of saxagliptin with other moderate CYP3A4/5 inhibitors (eg, amprenavir, aprepitant, erythromycin, fluconazole, fosamprenavir, grapefruit juice, verapamil) may increase plasma concentrations of saxagliptin; however, dosage adjustment is not recommended).
No products indexed under this heading.

Calcium Carbonate (Co-administration of saxagliptin with a liquid containing aluminum/magnesium hydroxide and simethicone decreased the C_{max} of saxagliptin). Products include:

Chlorpropamide (When used with an insulin secretagogue (sulfonylurea), a lower dose of the insulin secretagogue may be required to reduce the risk of hypoglycemia).
No products indexed under this heading.

Cimetidine (Co-administration of saxagliptin with other moderate CYP3A4/5 inhibitors (eg, amprenavir, aprepitant, erythromycin, fluconazole, fosamprenavir, grapefruit juice, verapamil) may increase plasma concentrations of saxagliptin; however, dosage adjustment is not recommended).
No products indexed under this heading.

Cimetidine Hydrochloride (Co-administration of saxagliptin with other moderate CYP3A4/5 inhibitors (eg, amprenavir, aprepitant, erythromycin, fluconazole, fosamprenavir, grapefruit juice, verapamil) may increase plasma concentrations of saxagliptin; however, dosage adjustment is not recommended).
No products indexed under this heading.

Ciprofloxacin (Co-administration of saxagliptin with other moderate CYP3A4/5 inhibitors (eg, amprenavir, aprepitant, erythromycin, fluconazole, fosamprenavir, grapefruit juice, verapamil) may increase plasma concentrations of saxagliptin; however, dosage adjustment is not recommended). Products include:

Ciprofloxacin Hydrochloride (Co-administration of saxagliptin with other moderate CYP3A4/5 inhibitors (eg, amprenavir, aprepitant, erythromycin, fluconazole, fosamprenavir, grapefruit juice, verapamil) may increase plasma concentrations of saxagliptin; however, dosage adjustment is not recommended). Products include:

Clarithromycin (Co-administration of saxagliptin with other moderate CYP3A4/5 inhibitors (eg, amprenavir, aprepitant, erythromycin, fluconazole, fosamprenavir, grapefruit juice, verapamil) may increase plasma concentrations of saxagliptin; however, dosage adjustment is not recommended). Products include:

Clotrimazole (Co-administration of saxagliptin with other moderate CYP3A4/5 inhibitors (eg, amprenavir, aprepitant, erythromycin, fluconazole, fosamprenavir, grapefruit juice, vera-

pamil) may increase plasma concentrations of saxagliptin; however, dosage adjustment is not recommended). Products include:

Conivaptan Hydrochloride (Co-administration of saxagliptin with other moderate CYP3A4/5 inhibitors (eg, amprenavir, aprepitant, erythromycin, fluconazole, fosamprenavir, grapefruit juice, verapamil) may increase plasma concentrations of saxagliptin; however, dosage adjustment is not recommended). Products include:

Cyclosporine (Co-administration of saxagliptin with other moderate CYP3A4/5 inhibitors (eg, amprenavir, aprepitant, erythromycin, fluconazole, fosamprenavir, grapefruit juice, verapamil) may increase plasma concentrations of saxagliptin; however, dosage adjustment is not recommended). Products include:

Dalfopristin (Co-administration of saxagliptin with other moderate CYP3A4/5 inhibitors (eg, amprenavir, aprepitant, erythromycin, fluconazole, fosamprenavir, grapefruit juice, verapamil) may increase plasma concentrations of saxagliptin; however, dosage adjustment is not recommended).
No products indexed under this heading.

Danazol (Co-administration of saxagliptin with other moderate CYP3A4/5 inhibitors (eg, amprenavir, aprepitant, erythromycin, fluconazole, fosamprenavir, grapefruit juice, verapamil) may increase plasma concentrations of saxagliptin; however, dosage adjustment is not recommended).
No products indexed under this heading.

Darunavir (Co-administration of saxagliptin with other moderate CYP3A4/5 inhibitors (eg, amprenavir, aprepitant, erythromycin, fluconazole, fosamprenavir, grapefruit juice, verapamil) may increase plasma concentrations of saxagliptin; however, dosage adjustment is not recommended).
No products indexed under this heading.

Dasatinib (Co-administration of saxagliptin with other moderate CYP3A4/5 inhibitors (eg, amprenavir, aprepitant, erythromycin, fluconazole, fosamprenavir, grapefruit juice, verapamil) may increase plasma concentrations of saxagliptin; however, dosage adjustment is not recommended).
No products indexed under this heading.

Delavirdine Mesylate (Co-administration of saxagliptin with other moderate CYP3A4/5 inhibitors (eg, amprenavir, aprepitant, erythromycin, fluconazole, fosamprenavir, grapefruit juice, verapamil) may increase plasma concentrations of saxagliptin; however, dosage adjustment is not recommended).
No products indexed under this heading.

Delavirine (Co-administration of saxagliptin with other moderate CYP3A4/5 inhibitors (eg, amprenavir, aprepitant, erythromycin, fluconazole, fosamprenavir, grapefruit juice, verapamil) may increase plasma concentrations of saxagliptin; however, dosage adjustment is not recommended).
No products indexed under this heading.

Desloratadine (Co-administration of saxagliptin with other moderate CYP3A4/5 inhibitors (eg, amprenavir, aprepitant, erythromycin, fluconazole, fosamprenavir, grapefruit juice, verapamil) may increase plasma concentrations of saxagliptin; however, dosage adjustment is not recommended). Products include:

Diltiazem Hydrochloride (Co-administration of saxagliptin with diltiazem may increase the exposure of saxagliptin). Products include:

Diltiazem Maleate (Co-administration of saxagliptin with diltiazem may increase the exposure of saxagliptin).
No products indexed under this heading.

Efavirenz (Co-administration of saxagliptin with other moderate CYP3A4/5 inhibitors (eg, amprenavir, aprepitant, erythromycin, fluconazole, fosamprenavir, grapefruit juice, verapamil) may increase plasma concentrations of saxagliptin; however, dosage adjustment is not recommended). Products include:

Erythromycin (Co-administration of saxagliptin with other moderate CYP3A4/5 inhibitors (eg, amprenavir, aprepitant, erythromycin, fluconazole, fosamprenavir, grapefruit juice, verapamil) may increase plasma concentrations of saxagliptin; however, dosage adjustment is not recommended).
No products indexed under this heading.

Erythromycin, Topical (Co-administration of saxagliptin with other moderate CYP3A4 inhibitor such as erythromycin may increase the plasma concentrations of saxagliptin; however, dosage adjustment is not recommended).
No products indexed under this heading.

Erythromycin Estolate (Co-administration of saxagliptin with other moderate CYP3A4/5 inhibitors (eg, amprenavir, aprepitant, erythromycin, fluconazole, fosamprenavir, grapefruit juice, verapamil) may increase plasma concentrations of saxagliptin; however, dosage adjustment is not recommended).
No products indexed under this heading.

Erythromycin Ethylsuccinate (Co-administration of saxagliptin with other moderate CYP3A4/5 inhibitors (eg, amprenavir, aprepitant, erythromycin, fluconazole, fosamprenavir, grapefruit juice, verapamil) may increase plasma concentrations of saxagliptin; however, dosage adjustment is not recommended). Products include:

Erythromycin Gluceptate (Co-administration of saxagliptin with other moderate CYP3A4/5 inhibitors (eg, amprenavir, aprepitant, erythromycin, fluconazole, fosamprenavir, grapefruit juice, verapamil) may increase plasma concentrations of saxagliptin; however, dosage adjustment is not recommended).
No products indexed under this heading.

Erythromycin Lactobionate (Co-administration of saxagliptin with other moderate CYP3A4/5 inhibitors (eg, amprenavir, aprepitant, erythromycin, fluconazole, fosamprenavir, grapefruit juice, verapamil) may increase plasma concentrations of saxagliptin; however, dosage adjustment is not recommended).
No products indexed under this heading.

Erythromycin Stearate (Co-administration of saxagliptin with other moderate CYP3A4/5 inhibitors (eg, amprenavir, aprepitant, erythromycin, fluconazole, fosamprenavir, grapefruit juice, verapamil) may increase plasma concentrations of saxagliptin; however, dosage adjustment is not recommended).
No products indexed under this heading.

Esomeprazole Magnesium (Co-administration of saxagliptin with other moderate CYP3A4/5 inhibitors (eg, amprenavir, aprepitant, erythromycin, fluconazole, fosamprenavir, grapefruit juice, verapamil) may increase plasma concentrations of saxagliptin; however, dosage adjustment is not recommended). Products include:

Esomeprazole Sodium (Co-administration of saxagliptin with other moderate CYP3A4/5 inhibitors (eg, amprenavir, aprepitant, erythromycin, fluconazole, fosamprenavir, grapefruit juice, verapamil) may increase plasma concentrations of saxagliptin; however, dosage adjustment is not recommended). Products include:

Famotidine (Administration of saxagliptin 3 hours after a single dose of famotidine increased the C_{max} of saxagliptin; however, AUC of saxagliptin was unchanged). Products include:

Fluconazole (Co-administration of saxagliptin with other moderate CYP3A4/5 inhibitors (eg, amprenavir, aprepitant, erythromycin, fluconazole, fosamprenavir, grapefruit juice, verapamil) may increase plasma concentrations of saxagliptin; however, dosage adjustment is not recommended).
No products indexed under this heading.

Fluoxetine (Co-administration of saxagliptin with other moderate CYP3A4/5 inhibitors (eg, amprenavir, aprepitant, erythromycin, fluconazole, fosamprenavir, grapefruit juice, verapamil) may increase plasma concentrations of saxagliptin; however, dosage adjustment is not recommended).
No products indexed under this heading.

Fluoxetine Hydrochloride (Co-administration of saxagliptin with other moderate CYP3A4/5 inhibitors (eg, amprenavir, aprepitant, erythromycin, fluconazole, fosamprenavir, grapefruit juice, verapamil) may increase plasma concentrations of saxagliptin; however, dosage adjustment is not recommended). Products include:

Fluvoxamine Maleate (Co-administration of saxagliptin with other moderate CYP3A4/5 inhibitors (eg, amprenavir, aprepitant, erythromycin, fluconazole, fosamprenavir, grapefruit juice, verapamil) may increase plasma concentrations of saxagliptin; however, dosage adjustment is not recommended).
No products indexed under this heading.

Fosamprenavir Calcium (Co-administration of saxagliptin with other moderate CYP3A4/5 inhibitors (eg, amprenavir, aprepitant, erythromycin, fluconazole, fosamprenavir, grapefruit juice, verapamil) may increase plasma concentrations of saxagliptin; however, dosage adjustment is not recommended). Products include:

Glimepiride (When used with an insulin secretagogue (sulfonylurea), a lower dose of the insulin secretagogue may be required to reduce the risk of hypoglycemia). Products include:

Glipizide (When used with an insulin secretagogue (sulfonylurea), a lower dose of the insulin secretagogue may be required to reduce the risk of hypoglycemia).
No products indexed under this heading.

Glyburide (Co-administration of saxagliptin with glyburide, a CYP2C9 substrate increased the plasma C_{max} of glyburide; however, the AUC of glyburide was unchanged).
No products indexed under this heading.

Imatinib Mesylate (Co-administration of saxagliptin with other moderate CYP3A4/5 inhibitors (eg, amprenavir, aprepitant, erythromycin, fluconazole, fosamprenavir, grapefruit juice, verapamil) may increase plasma concentrations of saxagliptin; however, dosage adjustment is not recommended). Products include:
Gleevec 2477

Indinavir Sulfate (Co-administration of saxagliptin with other moderate CYP3A4/5 inhibitors (eg, amprenavir, aprepitant, erythromycin, fluconazole, fosamprenavir, grapefruit juice, verapamil) may increase plasma concentrations of saxagliptin; however, dosage adjustment is not recommended). Products include:
Crixivan 2113

Isoniazid (Co-administration of saxagliptin with other moderate CYP3A4/5 inhibitors (eg, amprenavir, aprepitant, erythromycin, fluconazole, fosamprenavir, grapefruit juice, verapamil) may increase plasma concentrations of saxagliptin; however, dosage adjustment is not recommended).
No products indexed under this heading.

Itraconazole (Co-administration of saxagliptin with other moderate CYP3A4/5 inhibitors (eg, amprenavir, aprepitant, erythromycin, fluconazole, fosamprenavir, grapefruit juice, verapamil) may increase plasma concentrations of saxagliptin; however, dosage adjustment is not recommended).
No products indexed under this heading.

Ketoconazole (Co-administration of saxagliptin with ketoconazole may increase saxagliptin exposure). Products include:
Extina 3319
Xolegel 3337

Lapatinib (Co-administration of saxagliptin with other moderate CYP3A4/5 inhibitors (eg, amprenavir, aprepitant, erythromycin, fluconazole, fosamprenavir, grapefruit juice, verapamil) may increase plasma concentrations of saxagliptin; however, dosage adjustment is not recommended). Products include:
Tykerb 1698

Lopinavir (Co-administration of saxagliptin with other moderate CYP3A4/5 inhibitors (eg, amprenavir, aprepitant, erythromycin, fluconazole, fosamprenavir, grapefruit juice, verapamil) may increase plasma concentrations of saxagliptin; however, dosage adjustment is not recommended). Products include:
Kaletra 458

Loratadine (Co-administration of saxagliptin with other moderate CYP3A4/5 inhibitors (eg, amprenavir, aprepitant, erythromycin, fluconazole, fosamprenavir, grapefruit juice, verapamil) may increase plasma concentrations of saxagliptin; however, dosage adjustment is not recommended).
No products indexed under this heading.

Magaldrate (Co-administration of saxagliptin with a liquid containing aluminum/magnesium hydroxide and simethicone decreased the C_{max} of saxagliptin).
No products indexed under this heading.

Magnesium Carbonate (Co-administration of saxagliptin with a liquid containing aluminum/magnesium hydroxide and simethicone decreased the C_{max} of saxagliptin).
No products indexed under this heading.

Magnesium Hydroxide (Co-administration of saxagliptin with a liquid containing aluminum/magnesium hydroxide and simethicone decreased the C_{max} of saxagliptin). Products include:
Fleet Pedia-Lax Chewable Tablets 1144
Pepcid Complete 1822

Magnesium Oxide (Co-administration of saxagliptin with a liquid containing aluminum/magnesium hydroxide and simethicone decreased the C_{max} of saxagliptin). Products include:
Beelith 873

Magnesium Trisilicate (Co-administration of saxagliptin with a liquid containing aluminum/magnesium hydroxide and simethicone decreased the C_{max} of saxagliptin).
No products indexed under this heading.

Metformin (Co-administration of saxagliptin with metformin may decrease the C_{max} of saxagliptin; however, the AUC of saxagliptin was unchanged).
No products indexed under this heading.

Metronidazole (Co-administration of saxagliptin with other moderate CYP3A4/5 inhibitors (eg, amprenavir, aprepitant, erythromycin, fluconazole, fosamprenavir, grapefruit juice, verapamil) may increase plasma concentrations of saxagliptin; however, dosage adjustment is not recommended). Products include:
Pylera 793

Metronidazole Benzoate (Co-administration of saxagliptin with other moderate CYP3A4/5 inhibitors (eg, amprenavir, aprepitant, erythromycin, fluconazole, fosamprenavir, grapefruit juice, verapamil) may increase plasma concentrations of saxagliptin; however, dosage adjustment is not recommended).
No products indexed under this heading.

Metronidazole Hydrochloride (Co-administration of saxagliptin with other moderate CYP3A4/5 inhibitors (eg, amprenavir, aprepitant, erythromycin, fluconazole, fosamprenavir, grapefruit juice, verapamil) may increase plasma concentrations of saxagliptin; however, dosage adjustment is not recommended).
No products indexed under this heading.

Metronidazole Sodium (Co-administration of saxagliptin with other moderate CYP3A4/5 inhibitors (eg, amprenavir, aprepitant, erythromycin, fluconazole, fosamprenavir, grapefruit juice, verapamil) may increase plasma concentrations of saxagliptin; however, dosage adjustment is not recommended).
No products indexed under this heading.

Miconazole (Co-administration of saxagliptin with other moderate CYP3A4/5 inhibitors (eg, amprenavir, aprepitant, erythromycin, fluconazole, fosamprenavir, grapefruit juice, verapamil) may increase plasma concentrations of saxagliptin; however, dosage adjustment is not recommended).
No products indexed under this heading.

Miconazole Nitrate (Co-administration of saxagliptin with other moderate CYP3A4/5 inhibitors (eg, amprenavir, aprepitant, erythromycin, fluconazole, fosamprenavir, grapefruit juice, verapamil) may increase plasma concentrations of saxagliptin; however, dosage adjustment is not recommended). Products include:
Vusion Ointment 3335

Mifepristone (Co-administration of saxagliptin with other moderate CYP3A4/5 inhibitors (eg, amprenavir, aprepitant, erythromycin, fluconazole, fosamprenavir, grapefruit juice, verapamil) may increase plasma concentrations of saxagliptin; however, dosage adjustment is not recommended).
No products indexed under this heading.

Nefazodone Hydrochloride (Co-administration of saxagliptin with other moderate CYP3A4/5 inhibitors (eg, amprenavir, aprepitant, erythromycin, fluconazole, fosamprenavir, grapefruit juice, verapamil) may increase plasma concentrations of saxagliptin; however, dosage adjustment is not recommended).
No products indexed under this heading.

Nelfinavir Mesylate (Co-administration of saxagliptin with other moderate CYP3A4/5 inhibitors (eg, amprenavir, aprepitant, erythromycin, fluconazole, fosamprenavir, grapefruit juice, verapamil) may increase plasma concentrations of saxagliptin; however, dosage adjustment is not recommended).
No products indexed under this heading.

Nevirapine (Co-administration of saxagliptin with other moderate CYP3A4/5 inhibitors (eg, amprenavir, aprepitant, erythromycin, fluconazole, fosamprenavir, grapefruit juice, verapamil) may increase plasma concentrations of saxagliptin; however, dosage adjustment is not recommended). Products include:
Viramune Oral Suspension 897
Viramune Tablets 897

Niacin (Co-administration of saxagliptin with other moderate CYP3A4/5 inhibitors (eg, amprenavir, aprepitant, erythromycin, fluconazole, fosamprenavir, grapefruit juice, verapamil) may increase plasma concentrations of saxagliptin; however, dosage adjustment is not recommended). Products include:
Advicor 402
Cardio Basics 3455
Niaspan 497
Simcor 524

Niacinamide (Co-administration of saxagliptin with other moderate CYP3A4/5 inhibitors (eg, amprenavir, aprepitant, erythromycin, fluconazole, fosamprenavir, grapefruit juice, verapamil) may increase plasma concentrations of saxagliptin; however, dosage adjustment is not recommended). Products include:
CitraNatal 90 DHA Capsules 2332
CitraNatal Assure 2332
CitraNatal Rx 2332
Heplive 607

Niacinamide Hydroiodide (Co-administration of saxagliptin with other moderate CYP3A4/5 inhibitors (eg, amprenavir, aprepitant, erythromycin, fluconazole, fosamprenavir, grapefruit juice, verapamil) may increase plasma concentrations of saxagliptin; however, dosage adjustment is not recommended).
No products indexed under this heading.

Nicotinamide (Co-administration of saxagliptin with other moderate CYP3A4/5 inhibitors (eg, amprenavir, aprepitant, erythromycin, fluconazole, fosamprenavir, grapefruit juice, verapamil) may increase plasma concentrations of saxagliptin; however, dosage adjustment is not recommended).
No products indexed under this heading.

Nifedipine (Co-administration of saxagliptin with other moderate CYP3A4/5 inhibitors (eg, amprenavir, aprepitant, erythromycin, fluconazole, fosamprenavir, grapefruit juice, verapamil) may increase plasma concentrations of saxagliptin; however, dosage adjustment is not recommended).
No products indexed under this heading.

Norfloxacin (Co-administration of saxagliptin with other moderate CYP3A4/5 inhibitors (eg, amprenavir, aprepitant, erythromycin, fluconazole, fosamprenavir, grapefruit juice, verapamil) may increase plasma concentrations of saxagliptin; however, dosage adjustment is not recommended). Products include:
Noroxin 2220

Omeprazole (Co-administration of saxagliptin with other moderate CYP3A4/5 inhibitors (eg, amprenavir, aprepitant, erythromycin, fluconazole, fosamprenavir, grapefruit juice, verapamil) may increase plasma concentrations of saxagliptin; however, dosage adjustment is not recommended).
No products indexed under this heading.

Paroxetine Hydrochloride (Co-administration of saxagliptin with other moderate CYP3A4/5 inhibitors (eg, amprenavir, aprepitant, erythromycin, fluconazole, fosamprenavir, grapefruit juice, verapamil) may increase plasma concentrations of saxagliptin; however, dosage adjustment is not recommended). Products include:
Paroxetine CR 2361
Paroxetine ER 2371
Paxil 1586
Paxil CR 1596

Pioglitazone Hydrochloride (Co-administration of saxagliptin with pioglitazone, a CYP2C8 substrate, increased the plasma C_{max} of pioglitazone; however, the AUC was unchanged). Products include:
ActoPlus 3338
Actos 3345
Duetact 3354

Posaconazole (Co-administration of saxagliptin with other moderate CYP3A4/5 inhibitors (eg, amprenavir, aprepitant, erythromycin, fluconazole, fosamprenavir, grapefruit juice, verapamil) may increase plasma concentrations of saxagliptin; however, dosage adjustment is not recommended). Products include:
Noxafil 3172

Propoxyphene Hydrochloride (Co-administration of saxagliptin with other moderate CYP3A4/5 inhibitors (eg, amprenavir, aprepitant, erythromycin, fluconazole, fosamprenavir, grapefruit juice, verapamil) may increase plasma concentrations of saxagliptin; however, dosage adjustment is not recommended).
No products indexed under this heading.

Propoxyphene Napsylate (Co-administration of saxagliptin with other moderate CYP3A4/5 inhibitors (eg, amprenavir, aprepitant, erythromycin, fluconazole, fosamprenavir, grapefruit juice, verapamil) may increase plasma concentrations of saxagliptin; however, dosage adjustment is not recommended).
No products indexed under this heading.

Quinidine (Co-administration of saxagliptin with other moderate CYP3A4/5 inhibitors (eg, amprenavir, aprepitant, erythromycin, fluconazole, fosamprenavir, grapefruit juice, verapamil) may increase plasma concentrations of saxagliptin; however, dosage adjustment is not recommended).
No products indexed under this heading.

IMPORTANT NOTE: Always consult each drug listing in the patient's regimen for possible interactions.

Quinidine Hydrochloride (Co-administration of saxagliptin with other moderate CYP3A4/5 inhibitors (eg, amprenavir, aprepitant, erythromycin, fluconazole, fosamprenavir, grapefruit juice, verapamil) may increase plasma concentrations of saxagliptin; however, dosage adjustment is not recommended).
No products indexed under this heading.

Quinidine Polygalacturonate (Co-administration of saxagliptin with other moderate CYP3A4/5 inhibitors (eg, amprenavir, aprepitant, erythromycin, fluconazole, fosamprenavir, grapefruit juice, verapamil) may increase plasma concentrations of saxagliptin; however, dosage adjustment is not recommended).
No products indexed under this heading.

Quinidine Sulfate (Co-administration of saxagliptin with other moderate CYP3A4/5 inhibitors (eg, amprenavir, aprepitant, erythromycin, fluconazole, fosamprenavir, grapefruit juice, verapamil) may increase plasma concentrations of saxagliptin; however, dosage adjustment is not recommended).
No products indexed under this heading.

Quinine (Co-administration of saxagliptin with other moderate CYP3A4/5 inhibitors (eg, amprenavir, aprepitant, erythromycin, fluconazole, fosamprenavir, grapefruit juice, verapamil) may increase plasma concentrations of saxagliptin; however, dosage adjustment is not recommended). Products include:
Hyland's Leg Cramps PM with Quinine 3315

Quinine Sulfate (Co-administration of saxagliptin with other moderate CYP3A4/5 inhibitors (eg, amprenavir, aprepitant, erythromycin, fluconazole, fosamprenavir, grapefruit juice, verapamil) may increase plasma concentrations of saxagliptin; however, dosage adjustment is not recommended).
No products indexed under this heading.

Quinupristin (Co-administration of saxagliptin with other moderate CYP3A4/5 inhibitors (eg, amprenavir, aprepitant, erythromycin, fluconazole, fosamprenavir, grapefruit juice, verapamil) may increase plasma concentrations of saxagliptin; however, dosage adjustment is not recommended).
No products indexed under this heading.

Ranitidine Bismuth Citrate (Co-administration of saxagliptin with other moderate CYP3A4/5 inhibitors (eg, amprenavir, aprepitant, erythromycin, fluconazole, fosamprenavir, grapefruit juice, verapamil) may increase plasma concentrations of saxagliptin; however, dosage adjustment is not recommended).
No products indexed under this heading.

Ranitidine Hydrochloride (Co-administration of saxagliptin with other moderate CYP3A4/5 inhibitors (eg, amprenavir, aprepitant, erythromycin, fluconazole, fosamprenavir, grapefruit juice, verapamil) may increase plasma concentrations of saxagliptin; however, dosage adjustment is not recommended). Products include:
Zantac 1737
Zantac Injection 1732
Zantac Pharmacy 1735

Rifampin (Rifampin significantly decreased saxagliptin exposure with no change in the area under the time-concentration curve (AUC) of its active metabolite, 5-hydroxy saxagliptin).
No products indexed under this heading.

Ritonavir (Co-administration of saxagliptin with other moderate CYP3A4/5 inhibitors (eg, amprenavir, aprepitant, erythromycin, fluconazole, fosamprenavir, grapefruit juice, verapamil) may increase plasma concentrations of saxagliptin; however, dosage adjustment is not recommended). Products include:
Kaletra 458
Norvir 509

Saquinavir (Co-administration of saxagliptin with other moderate CYP3A4/5 inhibitors (eg, amprenavir, aprepitant, erythromycin, fluconazole, fosamprenavir, grapefruit juice, verapamil) may increase plasma concentrations of saxagliptin; however, dosage adjustment is not recommended).
No products indexed under this heading.

Saquinavir Mesylate (Co-administration of saxagliptin with other moderate CYP3A4/5 inhibitors (eg, amprenavir, aprepitant, erythromycin, fluconazole, fosamprenavir, grapefruit juice, verapamil) may increase plasma concentrations of saxagliptin; however, dosage adjustment is not recommended).
No products indexed under this heading.

Sertraline Hydrochloride (Co-administration of saxagliptin with other moderate CYP3A4/5 inhibitors (eg, amprenavir, aprepitant, erythromycin, fluconazole, fosamprenavir, grapefruit juice, verapamil) may increase plasma concentrations of saxagliptin; however, dosage adjustment is not recommended).
No products indexed under this heading.

Sildenafil Citrate (Co-administration of saxagliptin with other moderate CYP3A4/5 inhibitors (eg, amprenavir, aprepitant, erythromycin, fluconazole, fosamprenavir, grapefruit juice, verapamil) may increase plasma concentrations of saxagliptin; however, dosage adjustment is not recommended).
No products indexed under this heading.

Simvastatin (Co-administration of saxagliptin with simvastatin, a CYP3A4/5 substrate, increased the C_{max} of saxagliptin; however, the AUC of saxagliptin was unchanged). Products include:
Simcor 524
Vytorin 10/10 .... 2303, 3240
Vytorin 10/20 .... 2303, 3240
Vytorin 10/40 .... 2303, 3240
Vytorin 10/80 .... 2303, 3240
Zocor 2289

Telithromycin (Co-administration of saxagliptin with other moderate CYP3A4/5 inhibitors (eg, amprenavir, aprepitant, erythromycin, fluconazole, fosamprenavir, grapefruit juice, verapamil) may increase plasma concentrations of saxagliptin; however, dosage adjustment is not recommended). Products include:
Ketek 2991

Tolazamide (When used with an insulin secretagogue (sulfonylurea), a lower dose of the insulin secretagogue may be required to reduce the risk of hypoglycemia).
No products indexed under this heading.

Tolbutamide (When used with an insulin secretagogue (sulfonylurea), a lower dose of the insulin secretagogue may be required to reduce the risk of hypoglycemia).
No products indexed under this heading.

Troglitazone (Co-administration of saxagliptin with other moderate CYP3A4/5 inhibitors (eg, amprenavir, aprepitant, erythromycin, fluconazole, fosamprenavir, grapefruit juice, verapamil) may increase plasma concentrations of saxagliptin; however, dosage adjustment is not recommended).
No products indexed under this heading.

Troleandomycin (Co-administration of saxagliptin with other moderate CYP3A4/5 inhibitors (eg, amprenavir, aprepitant, erythromycin, fluconazole, fosamprenavir, grapefruit juice, verapamil) may increase plasma concentrations of saxagliptin; however, dosage adjustment is not recommended).
No products indexed under this heading.

Valproate Sodium (Co-administration of saxagliptin with other moderate CYP3A4/5 inhibitors (eg, amprenavir, aprepitant, erythromycin, fluconazole, fosamprenavir, grapefruit juice, verapamil) may increase plasma concentrations of saxagliptin; however, dosage adjustment is not recommended).
No products indexed under this heading.

Vardenafil Hydrochloride (Co-administration of saxagliptin with other moderate CYP3A4/5 inhibitors (eg, amprenavir, aprepitant, erythromycin, fluconazole, fosamprenavir, grapefruit juice, verapamil) may increase plasma concentrations of saxagliptin; however, dosage adjustment is not recommended). Products include:
Levitra 3157

Venlafaxine Hydrochloride (Co-administration of saxagliptin with other moderate CYP3A4/5 inhibitors (eg, amprenavir, aprepitant, erythromycin, fluconazole, fosamprenavir, grapefruit juice, verapamil) may increase plasma concentrations of saxagliptin; however, dosage adjustment is not recommended). Products include:
Effexor XR 3504
Venlafaxine Hydrochloride Tablets ... 2388

Verapamil Hydrochloride (Co-administration of saxagliptin with other moderate CYP3A4/5 inhibitors (eg, amprenavir, aprepitant, erythromycin, fluconazole, fosamprenavir, grapefruit juice, verapamil) may increase plasma concentrations of saxagliptin; however, dosage adjustment is not recommended). Products include:
Tarka 534

Voriconazole (Co-administration of saxagliptin with other moderate CYP3A4/5 inhibitors (eg, amprenavir, aprepitant, erythromycin, fluconazole, fosamprenavir, grapefruit juice, verapamil) may increase plasma concentrations of saxagliptin; however, dosage adjustment is not recommended).
No products indexed under this heading.

Zafirlukast (Co-administration of saxagliptin with other moderate CYP3A4/5 inhibitors (eg, amprenavir, aprepitant, erythromycin, fluconazole, fosamprenavir, grapefruit juice, verapamil) may increase plasma concentrations of saxagliptin; however, dosage adjustment is not recommended). Products include:
Accolate 3612

Zileuton (Co-administration of saxagliptin with other moderate CYP3A4/5 inhibitors (eg, amprenavir, aprepitant, erythromycin, fluconazole, fosamprenavir, grapefruit juice, verapamil) may increase plasma concentrations of saxagliptin; however, dosage adjustment is not recommended).
No products indexed under this heading.

Food Interactions

Grapefruit (Co-administration of saxagliptin with other moderate CYP3A4/5 inhibitors (eg, amprenavir, aprepitant, erythromycin, fluconazole, fosamprenavir, grapefruit juice, verapamil) may increase plasma concentrations of saxagliptin; however, dosage adjustment is not recommended).

Grapefruit Juice (Co-administration of saxagliptin with other moderate CYP3A4/5 inhibitors (eg, amprenavir, aprepitant, erythromycin, fluconazole, fosamprenavir, grapefruit juice, verapamil) may increase plasma concentrations of saxagliptin; however, dosage adjustment is not recommended).

ONSOLIS FILM

(Fentanyl) 2054
May interact with alcohols, barbiturates, central nervous system depressants, cytochrome p450 3a4 inducers (selected), cytochrome p450 3a4 inhibitors (selected), erythromycin, general anesthetics, glucocorticoids, hypnotics and sedatives, monoamine oxidase inhibitors, narcotic analgesics, phenothiazines, phenytoin, protease inhibitors, sedating antihistamines, skeletal muscle relaxants, tranquilizers. Compounds in these categories include:

Acetazolamide (The concomitant use of fentanyl with CYP3A4 inhibitors (eg, indinavir, nelfinavir, ritonavir, clarithromycin, itraconazole, ketoconazole, nefazodone, saquinavir, telithromycin, aprepitant, diltiazem, erythromycin, fluconazole, grapefruit juice, verapamil, or cimetidine) may result in a potentially dangerous increase in fentanyl plasma concentrations).
No products indexed under this heading.

Acetazolamide Sodium (The concomitant use of fentanyl with CYP3A4 inhibitors (eg, indinavir, nelfinavir, ritonavir, clarithromycin, itraconazole, ketoconazole, nefazodone, saquinavir, telithromycin, aprepitant, diltiazem, erythromycin, fluconazole, grapefruit juice, verapamil, or cimetidine) may result in a potentially dangerous increase in fentanyl plasma concentrations).
No products indexed under this heading.

Acrivastine (The concomitant use of fentanyl with other CNS depressants, including other opioids, sedatives or hypnotics, general anesthetics, phenothiazines, tranquilizers, skeletal muscle relaxants, sedating antihistamines, and alcoholic beverages may produce increased depressant effects).
No products indexed under this heading.

Alfentanil Hydrochloride (The concomitant use of fentanyl with other CNS depressants, including other opioids, sedatives or hypnotics, general anesthetics, phenothizines, tranquilizers, skeletal muscle relaxants, sedating antihistamines, and alcoholic beverages may produce increased depressant effects. Patients on concomitant CNS depressants must be monitored for a change in opioid effects. Consideration should be given to adjusting the dose of fentanyl if warranted).
No products indexed under this heading.

Allium sativum (The concomitant use of fentanyl with CYP3A4 inducers (eg, barbiturates, carbamazepine, efavirenz, glucocorticoids, modafinil, nevirapine, oxcarbazepine, phenobarbital, phenytoin, pioglitazone, rifabutin, rifampin, St. John's wort, or troglitazone) may result in a decrease fentanyl plasma concentrations).
No products indexed under this heading.

Alprazolam (The concomitant use of fentanyl with other CNS depressants, including other opioids, sedatives or hypnotics, general anesthetics, phenothizines, tranquilizers, skeletal muscle relaxants, sedating antihistamines, and alcoholic beverages may produce increased depressant effects. Patients on concomitant CNS depressants must be monitored for a change in opioid effects. Consideration should be given to adjusting the dose of fentanyl if warranted).
No products indexed under this heading.

Aminoglutethimide (The concomitant use of fentanyl with CYP3A4 inducers (eg, barbiturates, carbamazepine, efavirenz, glucocorticoids, modafinil, nevirapine, oxcarbazepine, phenobarbital, phenytoin, pioglitazone, rifabutin, rifampin, St. John's wort, or troglitazone) may result in a decrease fentanyl plasma concentrations).
No products indexed under this heading.

Amiodarone Hydrochloride (The concomitant use of fentanyl with CYP3A4 inhibitors (eg, indinavir, nelfinavir, ritonavir, clarithromycin, itraconazole, ketoconazole, nefazodone, saquinavir, telithromycin, aprepitant, diltiazem, erythromycin, fluconazole, grapefruit juice, verapamil, or cimetidine) may result in a potentially dangerous increase in fentanyl plasma concentrations).
No products indexed under this heading.

Amobarbital (The concomitant use of fentanyl with other CNS depressants, including other opioids, sedatives or hypnotics, general anesthetics, phenothizines, tranquilizers, skeletal muscle relaxants, sedating antihistamines, and alcoholic beverages may produce increased depressant effects. Patients on concomitant CNS depressants must be monitored for a change in opioid effects. Consideration should be given to adjusting the dose of fentanyl if warranted).
No products indexed under this heading.

Amobarbital Sodium (The concomitant use of fentanyl with other CNS depressants, including other opioids, sedatives or hypnotics, general anesthetics, phenothizines, tranquilizers, skeletal muscle relaxants, sedating antihistamines, and alcoholic beverages may produce increased depressant effects. Patients on concomitant CNS depressants must be monitored for a change in opioid effects. Consideration should be given to adjusting the dose of fentanyl if warranted).
No products indexed under this heading.

Amprenavir (The concomitant use of fentanyl with CYP3A4 inhibitors (eg, indinavir, nelfinavir, ritonavir, clarithromycin, itraconazole, ketoconazole, nefazodone, saquinavir, telithromycin, aprepitant, diltiazem, erythromycin, fluconazole, grapefruit juice, verapamil, or cimetidine) may result in a potentially dangerous increase in fentanyl plasma concentrations).
No products indexed under this heading.

Anastrozole (The concomitant use of fentanyl with CYP3A4 inhibitors (eg, indinavir, nelfinavir, ritonavir, clarithromycin, itraconazole, ketoconazole, nefazodone, saquinavir, telithromycin, aprepitant, diltiazem, erythromycin, fluconazole, grapefruit juice, verapamil, or cimetidine) may result in a potentially dangerous increase in fentanyl plasma concentrations).
No products indexed under this heading.

Apomorphine (The concomitant use of fentanyl with other CNS depressants, including other opioids may produce increased depressant effects).
No products indexed under this heading.

Apomorphine Hydrochloride (The concomitant use of fentanyl with other CNS depressants, including other opioids may produce increased depressant effects).
No products indexed under this heading.

Aprepitant (The concomitant use of fentanyl with CYP3A4 inducers (eg, barbiturates, carbamazepine, efavirenz, glucocorticoids, modafinil, nevirapine, oxcarbazepine, phenobarbital, phenytoin, pioglitazone, rifabutin, rifampin, St. John's wort, or troglitazone) may result in a decrease fentanyl plasma concentrations). Products include:
Emend 2124

Aprobarbital (The concomitant use of fentanyl with other CNS depressants, including other opioids, sedatives or hypnotics, general anesthetics, phenothizines, tranquilizers, skeletal muscle relaxants, sedating antihistamines, and alcoholic beverages may produce increased depressant effects. Patients on concomitant CNS depressants must be monitored for a change in opioid effects. Consideration should be given to adjusting the dose of fentanyl if warranted).
No products indexed under this heading.

Atazanavir (The concomitant use of fentanyl with CYP3A4 inhibitors (eg, indinavir, nelfinavir, ritonavir, clarithromycin, itraconazole, ketoconazole, nefazodone, saquinavir, telithromycin, aprepitant, diltiazem, erythromycin, fluconazole, grapefruit juice, verapamil, or cimetidine) may result in a potentially dangerous increase in fentanyl plasma concentrations).
No products indexed under this heading.

Atazanavir Sulfate (The concomitant use of fentanyl with CYP3A4 inhibitors (eg, indinavir, nelfinavir, ritonavir, clarithromycin, itraconazole, ketoconazole, nefazodone, saquinavir, telithromycin, aprepitant, diltiazem, erythromycin, fluconazole, grapefruit juice, verapamil, or cimetidine) may result in a potentially dangerous increase in fentanyl plasma concentrations).
No products indexed under this heading.

Atracurium Besylate (The concomitant use of fentanyl with other CNS depressants, including other opioids, sedatives or hypnotics, general anesthetics, phenothiazines, tranquilizers, skeletal muscle relaxants, sedating antihistamines, and alcoholic beverages may produce increased depressant effects).
No products indexed under this heading.

Azatadine Maleate (The concomitant use of fentanyl with other CNS depressants, including other opioids, sedatives or hypnotics, general anesthetics, phenothiazines, tranquilizers, skeletal muscle relaxants, sedating antihistamines, and alcoholic beverages may produce increased depressant effects).
No products indexed under this heading.

Baclofen (The concomitant use of fentanyl with other CNS depressants, including other opioids, sedatives or hypnotics, general anesthetics, phenothiazines, tranquilizers, skeletal muscle relaxants, sedating antihistamines, and alcoholic beverages may produce increased depressant effects).
No products indexed under this heading.

Betamethasone (The concomitant use of fentanyl with CYP3A4 inducers (eg, barbiturates, carbamazepine, efavirenz, glucocorticoids, modafinil, nevirapine, oxcarbazepine, phenobarbital, phenytoin, pioglitazone, rifabutin, rifampin, St. John's wort, or troglitazone) may result in a decrease fentanyl plasma concentrations).
No products indexed under this heading.

Betamethasone Acetate (The concomitant use of fentanyl with CYP3A4 inducers (eg, barbiturates, carbamazepine, efavirenz, glucocorticoids, modafinil, nevirapine, oxcarbazepine, phenobarbital, phenytoin, pioglitazone, rifabutin, rifampin, St. John's wort, or troglitazone) may result in a decrease fentanyl plasma concentrations).
No products indexed under this heading.

Betamethasone Benzoate (The concomitant use of fentanyl with CYP3A4 inducers (eg, barbiturates, carbamazepine, efavirenz, glucocorticoids, modafinil, nevirapine, oxcarbazepine, phenobarbital, phenytoin, pioglitazone, rifabutin, rifampin, St. John's wort, or troglitazone) may result in a decrease fentanyl plasma concentrations).
No products indexed under this heading.

Betamethasone Dipropionate (The concomitant use of fentanyl with CYP3A4 inducers (eg, barbiturates, carbamazepine, efavirenz, glucocorticoids, modafinil, nevirapine, oxcarbazepine, phenobarbital, phenytoin, pioglitazone, rifabutin, rifampin, St. John's wort, or troglitazone) may result in a decrease fentanyl plasma concentrations). Products include:
Diprolene Lotion 0.05% 3108
Diprolene Ointment 0.05% 3109
Diprolene AF Cream 0.05% 3107
Lotrisone 3163

Betamethasone Sodium Phosphate (The concomitant use of fentanyl with CYP3A4 inducers (eg, barbiturates, carbamazepine, efavirenz, glucocorticoids, modafinil, nevirapine, oxcarbazepine, phenobarbital, phenytoin, pioglitazone, rifabutin, rifampin, St. John's wort, or troglitazone) may result in a decrease fentanyl plasma concentrations).
No products indexed under this heading.

Betamethasone Valerate (The concomitant use of fentanyl with CYP3A4 inducers (eg, barbiturates, carbamazepine, efavirenz, glucocorticoids, modafinil, nevirapine, oxcarbazepine, phenobarbital, phenytoin, pioglitazone, rifabutin, rifampin, St. John's wort, or troglitazone) may result in a decrease fentanyl plasma concentrations). Products include:
Luxíq 3321

Bosentan (The concomitant use of fentanyl with CYP3A4 inducers (eg, barbiturates, carbamazepine, efavirenz, glucocorticoids, modafinil, nevirapine, oxcarbazepine, phenobarbital, phenytoin, pioglitazone, rifabutin, rifampin, St. John's wort, or troglitazone) may result in a decrease fentanyl plasma concentrations). Products include:
Tracleer 573

Bromodiphenhydramine Hydrochloride (The concomitant use of fentanyl with other CNS depressants, including other opioids, sedatives or hypnotics, general anesthetics, phenothiazines, tranquilizers, skeletal muscle relaxants, sedating antihistamines, and alcoholic beverages may produce increased depressant effects).
No products indexed under this heading.

Brompheniramine Maleate (The concomitant use of fentanyl with other CNS depressants, including other opioids, sedatives or hypnotics, general anesthetics, phenothiazines, tranquilizers, skeletal muscle relaxants, sedating antihistamines, and alcoholic beverages may produce increased depressant effects).
No products indexed under this heading.

Budesonide (The concomitant use of fentanyl with CYP3A4 inducers (eg, barbiturates, carbamazepine, efavirenz, glucocorticoids, modafinil, nevirapine, oxcarbazepine, phenobarbital, phenytoin, pioglitazone, rifabutin, rifampin, St. John's wort, or troglitazone) may result in a decrease fentanyl plasma concentrations). Products include:
Pulmicort Flexhaler 714
Symbicort 80/4.5 720
Symbicort 160/4.5 720

Buprenorphine Hydrochloride (The concomitant use of fentanyl with other CNS depressants, including other opioids, sedatives or hypnotics, general anesthetics, phenothizines, tranquilizers, skeletal muscle relaxants, sedating antihistamines, and alcoholic beverages may produce increased depressant effects. Patients on concomitant CNS depressants must be monitored for a change in opioid effects. Consideration should be given to adjusting the dose of fentanyl if warranted).
No products indexed under this heading.

Buspirone Hydrochloride (The concomitant use of fentanyl with other CNS depressants, including other opioids, sedatives or hypnotics, general anesthetics, phenothizines, tranquilizers, skeletal muscle relaxants, sedating antihistamines, and alcoholic beverages may produce increased depressant effects. Patients on concomitant CNS depressants must be monitored for a change in opioid effects. Consideration should be given to adjusting the dose of fentanyl if warranted).
No products indexed under this heading.

Butabarbital (The concomitant use of fentanyl with other CNS depressants, including other opioids, sedatives or hypnotics, general anesthetics, phenothizines, tranquilizers, skeletal muscle relaxants, sedating antihistamines, and alcoholic beverages may produce increased depressant effects. Patients on concomitant CNS depressants must be monitored for a change in opioid effects. Consideration should be given to adjusting the dose of fentanyl if warranted).
No products indexed under this heading.

Butabarbital Sodium (The concomitant use of fentanyl with other CNS depressants, including other opioids, sedatives or hypnotics, general anesthetics, phenothizines, tranquilizers, skeletal muscle relaxants, sedating antihistamines, and alcoholic beverages may produce increased depressant effects. Patients on concomitant CNS depressants must be monitored for a change in opioid effects. Consideration should be given to adjusting the dose of fentanyl if warranted).
No products indexed under this heading.

Butalbital (The concomitant use of fentanyl with other CNS depressants, including other opioids, sedatives or hypnotics, general anesthetics, phenothizines, tranquilizers, skeletal muscle relaxants, sedating antihistamines, and alcoholic beverages may produce increased depressant effects. Patients on concomitant CNS depressants must be monitored for a change in opioid effects. Consideration should be given to adjusting the dose of fentanyl if warranted).
No products indexed under this heading.

Carbamazepine (The concomitant use of fentanyl with CYP3A4 inducers (eg, barbiturates, carbamazepine, efavirenz, glucocorticoids, modafinil, nevirapine, oxcarbazepine, phenobarbital, phenytoin, pioglitazone, rifabutin, rifampin, St. John's wort, or troglitazone) may result in a decrease fentanyl plasma concentrations). Products include:
Carbatrol 3280
Equetro 3477

Carisoprodol (The concomitant use of fentanyl with other CNS depressants, including other opioids, sedatives or hypnotics, general anesthetics, phenothiazines, tranquilizers, skeletal muscle relaxants, sedating antihistamines, and alcoholic beverages may produce increased depressant effects).
No products indexed under this heading.

Chloral Hydrate (The concomitant use of fentanyl with other CNS depressants, including other opioids, sedatives or hypnotics, general anesthetics, phenothiazines, tranquilizers, skeletal muscle relaxants, sedating antihistamines, and alcoholic beverages may produce increased depressant effects).
No products indexed under this heading.

Chlordiazepoxide (The concomitant use of fentanyl with other CNS depressants, including other opioids, sedatives or hypnotics, general anesthetics, phenothizines, tranquilizers, skeletal muscle relaxants, sedating antihistamines, and alcoholic beverages may produce increased depressant effects. Patients on concomitant CNS depressants must be monitored for a change in opioid effects. Consideration should be given to adjusting the dose of fentanyl if warranted).
No products indexed under this heading.

Chlordiazepoxide Hydrochloride (The concomitant use of fentanyl with other CNS depressants, including other opioids, sedatives or hypnotics, general anesthetics, phenothizines, tranquilizers, skeletal muscle relaxants, sedating antihistamines, and alcoholic beverages may produce increased depressant effects. Patients on concomitant CNS depressants must be monitored for a change in opioid effects. Consideration should be given to adjusting the dose of fentanyl if warranted).
No products indexed under this heading.

Chlorpheniramine Maleate (The concomitant use of fentanyl with other CNS depressants, including other opioids, sedatives or hypnotics, general anesthetics, phenothiazines, tranquilizers, skeletal muscle relaxants, sedating antihistamines, and alcoholic beverages may produce increased depressant effects).
No products indexed under this heading.

Chlorpheniramine Polistirex (The concomitant use of fentanyl with other CNS depressants, including other opioids, sedatives or hypnotics, general anesthetics, phenothiazines, tranquilizers, skeletal muscle relaxants, sedating antihistamines, and alcoholic beverages may produce increased depressant effects). Products include:
Tussionex 3443

Chlorpheniramine Tannate (The concomitant use of fentanyl with other CNS depressants, including other opioids, sedatives or hypnotics, general anesthetics, phenothiazines, tranquilizers, skeletal muscle relaxants, sedating antihistamines, and alcoholic beverages may produce increased depressant effects).
No products indexed under this heading.

Chlorpromazine (The concomitant use of fentanyl with other CNS depressants, including other opioids, sedatives or hypnotics, general anesthetics, phenothizines, tranquilizers, skeletal muscle relaxants, sedating antihistamines, and alcoholic beverages may produce increased depressant effects. Patients on concomitant CNS depressants must be monitored for a change in opioid effects. Consideration should be given to adjusting the dose of fentanyl if warranted).
No products indexed under this heading.

Chlorpromazine Hydrochloride (The concomitant use of fentanyl with other CNS depressants, including other opioids, sedatives or hypnotics, general anesthetics, phenothizines, tranquilizers, skeletal muscle relaxants, sedating antihistamines, and alcoholic beverages may produce increased depressant effects. Patients on concomitant CNS depressants must be monitored for a change in opioid effects. Consideration should be given to adjusting the dose of fentanyl if warranted).
No products indexed under this heading.

Chlorprothixene (The concomitant use of fentanyl with other CNS depressants, including other opioids, sedatives or hypnotics, general anesthetics, phenothizines, tranquilizers, skeletal muscle relaxants, sedating antihistamines, and alcoholic beverages may produce increased depressant effects. Patients on concomitant CNS depressants must be monitored for a change in opioid effects. Consideration should be given to adjusting the dose of fentanyl if warranted).
No products indexed under this heading.

Chlorprothixene Hydrochloride (The concomitant use of fentanyl with other CNS depressants, including other opioids, sedatives or hypnotics, general anesthetics, phenothizines, tranquilizers, skeletal muscle relaxants, sedating antihistamines, and alcoholic beverages may produce increased depressant effects. Patients on concomitant CNS depressants must be monitored for a change in opioid effects. Consideration should be given to adjusting the dose of fentanyl if warranted).
No products indexed under this heading.

Chlorprothixene Lactate (The concomitant use of fentanyl with other CNS depressants, including other opioids, sedatives or hypnotics, general anesthetics, phenothizines, tranquilizers, skeletal muscle relaxants, sedating antihistamines, and alcoholic beverages may produce increased depressant effects. Patients on concomitant CNS depressants must be monitored for a change in opioid effects. Consideration should be given to adjusting the dose of fentanyl if warranted).
No products indexed under this heading.

Chlorzoxazone (The concomitant use of fentanyl with other CNS depressants, including other opioids, sedatives or hypnotics, general anesthetics, phenothiazines, tranquilizers, skeletal muscle relaxants, sedating antihistamines, and alcoholic beverages may produce increased depressant effects).
No products indexed under this heading.

Cimetidine (The concomitant use of fentanyl with CYP3A4 inhibitors (eg, indinavir, nelfinavir, ritonavir, clarithromycin, itraconazole, ketoconazole, nefazodone, saquinavir, telithromycin, aprepitant, diltiazem, erythromycin, fluconazole, grapefruit juice, verapamil, or cimetidine) may result in a potentially dangerous increase in fentanyl plasma concentrations).
No products indexed under this heading.

Cimetidine Hydrochloride (The concomitant use of fentanyl with CYP3A4 inhibitors (eg, indinavir, nelfinavir, ritonavir, clarithromycin, itraconazole, ketoconazole, nefazodone, saquinavir, telithromycin, aprepitant, diltiazem, erythromycin, fluconazole, grapefruit juice, verapamil, or cimetidine) may result in a potentially dangerous increase in fentanyl plasma concentrations).
No products indexed under this heading.

Ciprofloxacin (The concomitant use of fentanyl with CYP3A4 inducers (eg, barbiturates, carbamazepine, efavirenz, glucocorticoids, modafinil, nevirapine, oxcarbazepine, phenobarbital, phenytoin, pioglitazone, rifabutin, rifampin, St. John's wort, or troglitazone) may result in a decrease fentanyl plasma concentrations). Products include:
Cipro I.V. 3082
Cipro 3073
Cipro XR 3091
Ciprodex 583

Ciprofloxacin Hydrochloride (The concomitant use of fentanyl with CYP3A4 inducers (eg, barbiturates, carbamazepine, efavirenz, glucocorticoids, modafinil, nevirapine, oxcarbazepine, phenobarbital, phenytoin, pioglitazone, rifabutin, rifampin, St. John's wort, or troglitazone) may result in a decrease fentanyl plasma concentrations). Products include:
Cipro 3073

Cisatracurium Besylate (The concomitant use of fentanyl with other CNS depressants, including other opioids, sedatives or hypnotics, general anesthetics, phenothiazines, tranquilizers, skeletal muscle relaxants, sedating antihistamines, and alcoholic beverages may produce increased depressant effects). Products include:
Nimbex 503

Cisplatin (The concomitant use of fentanyl with CYP3A4 inducers (eg, barbiturates, carbamazepine, efavirenz, glucocorticoids, modafinil, nevirapine, oxcarbazepine, phenobarbital, phenytoin, pioglitazone, rifabutin, rifampin, St. John's wort, or troglitazone) may result in a decrease fentanyl plasma concentrations).
No products indexed under this heading.

Clarithromycin (The concomitant use of fentanyl with CYP3A4 inhibitors (eg, indinavir, nelfinavir, ritonavir, clarithromycin, itraconazole, ketoconazole, nefazodone, saquinavir, telithromycin, aprepitant, diltiazem, erythromycin, fluconazole, grapefruit juice, verapamil, or cimetidine) may result in a potentially dangerous increase in fentanyl plasma concentrations). Products include:
Biaxin/Biaxin XL 412

Clemastine Fumarate (The concomitant use of fentanyl with other CNS depressants, including other opioids, sedatives or hypnotics, general anesthetics, phenothizines, tranquilizers, skeletal muscle relaxants, sedating antihistamines, and alcoholic beverages may produce increased depressant effects).
No products indexed under this heading.

Clonazepam (The concomitant use of fentanyl with other CNS depressants, including other opioids, sedatives or hypnotics, general anesthetics, phenothizines, tranquilizers, skeletal muscle relaxants, sedating antihistamines, and alcoholic beverages may produce increased depressant effects. Patients on concomitant CNS depressants must be monitored for a change in opioid effects. Consideration should be given to adjusting the dose of fentanyl if warranted). Products include:
Klonopin 2855

Clorazepate Dipotassium (The concomitant use of fentanyl with other CNS depressants, including other opioids, sedatives or hypnotics, general anesthetics, phenothizines, tranquilizers, skeletal muscle relaxants, sedating antihistamines, and alcoholic beverages may produce increased depressant effects. Patients on concomitant CNS depressants must be monitored for a change in opioid effects. Consideration should be given to adjusting the dose of fentanyl if warranted).
No products indexed under this heading.

Clotrimazole (The concomitant use of fentanyl with CYP3A4 inhibitors (eg, indinavir, nelfinavir, ritonavir, clarithromycin, itraconazole, ketoconazole, nefazodone, saquinavir, telithromycin, aprepitant, diltiazem, erythromycin, fluconazole, grapefruit juice, verapamil, or cimetidine) may result in a potentially dangerous increase in fentanyl plasma concentrations). Products include:
Lotrisone 3163

Clozapine (The concomitant use of fentanyl with other CNS depressants, including other opioids, sedatives or hypnotics, general anesthetics, phenothizines, tranquilizers, skeletal muscle relaxants, sedating antihistamines, and alcoholic beverages may produce increased depressant effects. Patients on concomitant CNS depressants must be monitored for a change in opioid effects. Consideration should be given to adjusting the dose of fentanyl if warranted).
No products indexed under this heading.

Codeine Phosphate (The concomitant use of fentanyl with other CNS depressants, including other opioids, sedatives or hypnotics, general anesthetics, phenothizines, tranquilizers, skeletal muscle relaxants, sedating antihistamines, and alcoholic beverages may produce increased depressant effects. Patients on concomitant CNS depressants must be monitored for a change in opioid effects. Consideration should be given to adjusting the dose of fentanyl if warranted). Products include:
Tylenol with Codeine 2691

Codeine Sulfate (The concomitant use of fentanyl with other CNS depressants, including other opioids, sedatives or hypnotics, general anesthetics, phenothizines, tranquilizers, skeletal muscle relaxants, sedating antihistamines, and alcoholic beverages may produce increased depressant effects. Patients on concomitant CNS depressants must be monitored for a change in opioid effects. Consideration should be given to adjusting the dose of fentanyl if warranted).
No products indexed under this heading.

Conivaptan Hydrochloride (The concomitant use of fentanyl with CYP3A4 inhibitors (eg, indinavir, nelfinavir, ritonavir, clarithromycin, itraconazole, ketoconazole, nefazodone, saquinavir, telithromycin, aprepitant, diltiazem, erythromycin, fluconazole, grapefruit juice, verapamil, or cimetidine) may result in a potentially dangerous increase in fentanyl plasma concentrations). Products include:
Vaprisol 689

Cortisone Acetate (The concomitant use of fentanyl with CYP3A4 inducers (eg, barbiturates, carbamazepine, efavirenz, glucocorticoids, modafinil, nevirapine, oxcarbazepine, phenobarbital, phenytoin, pioglitazone, rifabutin, rifampin, St. John's wort, or troglitazone) may result in a decrease fentanyl plasma concentrations).
No products indexed under this heading.

Cyclobenzaprine Hydrochloride (The concomitant use of fentanyl with other CNS depressants, including other opioids, sedatives or hypnotics, general anesthetics, phenothiazines, tranquilizers, skeletal muscle relaxants, sedating antihistamines, and alcoholic beverages may produce increased depressant effects). Products include:
Amrix 964

Cyclosporine (The concomitant use of fentanyl with CYP3A4 inhibitors (eg, indinavir, nelfinavir, ritonavir, clarithromycin, itraconazole, ketoconazole, nefazodone, saquinavir, telithromycin, aprepitant, diltiazem, erythromycin, fluconazole, grapefruit juice, verapamil, or cimetidine) may result in a potentially dangerous increase in fentanyl plasma concentrations). Products include:
Gengraf 440
Neoral Oral Solution 2496
Neoral Capsules 2496
Restasis 605

(⊙ Described in PDR® for Ophthalmic Medicines)

1291 Interactions Index Onsolis

Cyproheptadine Hydrochloride (The concomitant use of fentanyl with other CNS depressants, including other opioids, sedatives or hypnotics, general anesthetics, phenothiazines, tranquilizers, skeletal muscle relaxants, sedating antihistamines, and alcoholic beverages may produce increased depressant effects).
No products indexed under this heading.

Dalfopristin (The concomitant use of fentanyl with CYP3A4 inhibitors (eg, indinavir, nelfinavir, ritonavir, clarithromycin, itraconazole, ketoconazole, nefazodone, saquinavir, telithromycin, aprepitant, diltiazem, erythromycin, fluconazole, grapefruit juice, verapamil, or cimetidine) may result in a potentially dangerous increase in fentanyl plasma concentrations).
No products indexed under this heading.

Danazol (The concomitant use of fentanyl with CYP3A4 inhibitors (eg, indinavir, nelfinavir, ritonavir, clarithromycin, itraconazole, ketoconazole, nefazodone, saquinavir, telithromycin, aprepitant, diltiazem, erythromycin, fluconazole, grapefruit juice, verapamil, or cimetidine) may result in a potentially dangerous increase in fentanyl plasma concentrations).
No products indexed under this heading.

Dantrolene Sodium (The concomitant use of fentanyl with other CNS depressants, including other opioids, sedatives or hypnotics, general anesthetics, phenothiazines, tranquilizers, skeletal muscle relaxants, sedating antihistamines, and alcoholic beverages may produce increased depressant effects).
No products indexed under this heading.

Darunavir (The concomitant use of fentanyl with CYP3A4 inhibitors (eg, indinavir, nelfinavir, ritonavir, clarithromycin, itraconazole, ketoconazole, nefazodone, saquinavir, telithromycin, aprepitant, diltiazem, erythromycin, fluconazole, grapefruit juice, verapamil, or cimetidine) may result in a potentially dangerous increase in fentanyl plasma concentrations).
No products indexed under this heading.

Dasatinib (The concomitant use of fentanyl with CYP3A4 inhibitors (eg, indinavir, nelfinavir, ritonavir, clarithromycin, itraconazole, ketoconazole, nefazodone, saquinavir, telithromycin, aprepitant, diltiazem, erythromycin, fluconazole, grapefruit juice, verapamil, or cimetidine) may result in a potentially dangerous increase in fentanyl plasma concentrations).
No products indexed under this heading.

Delavirdine Mesylate (The concomitant use of fentanyl with CYP3A4 inhibitors (eg, indinavir, nelfinavir, ritonavir, clarithromycin, itraconazole, ketoconazole, nefazodone, saquinavir, telithromycin, aprepitant, diltiazem, erythromycin, fluconazole, grapefruit juice, verapamil, or cimetidine) may result in a potentially dangerous increase in fentanyl plasma concentrations).
No products indexed under this heading.

Delavirine (The concomitant use of fentanyl with CYP3A4 inhibitors (eg, indinavir, nelfinavir, ritonavir, clarithromycin, itraconazole, ketoconazole, nefazodone, saquinavir, telithromycin, aprepitant, diltiazem, erythromycin, fluconazole, grapefruit juice, verapamil, or cimetidine) may result in a potentially dangerous increase in fentanyl plasma concentrations).
No products indexed under this heading.

Desflurane (The concomitant use of fentanyl with other CNS depressants, including other opioids, sedatives or hypnotics, general anesthetics, phenothiazines, tranquilizers, skeletal muscle relaxants, sedating antihistamines, and alcoholic beverages may produce increased depressant effects. Patients on concomitant CNS depressants must be monitored for a change in opioid effects. Consideration should be given to adjusting the dose of fentanyl if warranted).
No products indexed under this heading.

Desloratadine (The concomitant use of fentanyl with CYP3A4 inhibitors (eg, indinavir, nelfinavir, ritonavir, clarithromycin, itraconazole, ketoconazole, nefazodone, saquinavir, telithromycin, aprepitant, diltiazem, erythromycin, fluconazole, grapefruit juice, verapamil, or cimetidine) may result in a potentially dangerous increase in fentanyl plasma concentrations). Products include:
Clarinex Syrup 3098
Clarinex 3098
Clarinex Reditabs 3098
Clarinex-D 12-Hour 3101
Clarinex-D 3104

Dexamethasone (The concomitant use of fentanyl with CYP3A4 inducers (eg, barbiturates, carbamazepine, efavirenz, glucocorticoids, modafinil, nevirapine, oxcarbazepine, phenobarbital, phenytoin, pioglitazone, rifabutin, rifampin, St. John's wort, or troglitazone) may result in a decrease fentanyl plasma concentrations). Products include:
Ciprodex 583
Ozurdex .... ⊙ 223
Tobramycin and Dexamethasone Ophthalmic Suspension .... ⊙ 251

Dexamethasone Acetate (The concomitant use of fentanyl with CYP3A4 inducers (eg, barbiturates, carbamazepine, efavirenz, glucocorticoids, modafinil, nevirapine, oxcarbazepine, phenobarbital, phenytoin, pioglitazone, rifabutin, rifampin, St. John's wort, or troglitazone) may result in a decrease fentanyl plasma concentrations).
No products indexed under this heading.

Dexamethasone Phosphate (The concomitant use of fentanyl with CYP3A4 inducers (eg, barbiturates, carbamazepine, efavirenz, glucocorticoids, modafinil, nevirapine, oxcarbazepine, phenobarbital, phenytoin, pioglitazone, rifabutin, rifampin, St. John's wort, or troglitazone) may result in a decrease fentanyl plasma concentrations).
No products indexed under this heading.

Dexamethasone Sodium (The concomitant use of fentanyl with CYP3A4 inducers (eg, barbiturates, carbamazepine, efavirenz, glucocorticoids, modafinil, nevirapine, oxcarbazepine, phenobarbital, phenytoin, pioglitazone, rifabutin, rifampin, St. John's wort, or troglitazone) may result in a decrease fentanyl plasma concentrations).
No products indexed under this heading.

Dexamethasone Sodium Phosphate (The concomitant use of fentanyl with CYP3A4 inducers (eg, barbiturates, carbamazepine, efavirenz, glucocorticoids, modafinil, nevirapine, oxcarbazepine, phenobarbital, phenytoin, pioglitazone, rifabutin, rifampin, St. John's wort, or troglitazone) may result in a decrease fentanyl plasma concentrations).
No products indexed under this heading.

Dexamethasone Sodium Phosphate Injection (The concomitant use of fentanyl with CYP3A4 inducers (eg, barbiturates, carbamazepine, efavirenz, glucocorticoids, modafinil, nevirapine, oxcarbazepine, phenobarbital, phenytoin, pioglitazone, rifabutin, rifampin, St. John's wort, or troglitazone) may result in a decrease fentanyl plasma concentrations).
No products indexed under this heading.

Dexchlorpheniramine Maleate (The concomitant use of fentanyl with other CNS depressants, including other opioids, sedatives or hypnotics, general anesthetics, phenothiazines, tranquilizers, skeletal muscle relaxants, sedating antihistamines, and alcoholic beverages may produce increased depressant effects).
No products indexed under this heading.

Dezocine (The concomitant use of fentanyl with other CNS depressants, including other opioids, sedatives or hypnotics, general anesthetics, phenothizines, tranquilizers, skeletal muscle relaxants, sedating antihistamines, and alcoholic beverages may produce increased depressant effects. Patients on concomitant CNS depressants must be monitored for a change in opioid effects. Consideration should be given to adjusting the dose of fentanyl if warranted).
No products indexed under this heading.

Diazepam (The concomitant use of fentanyl with other CNS depressants, including other opioids, sedatives or hypnotics, general anesthetics, phenothizines, tranquilizers, skeletal muscle relaxants, sedating antihistamines, and alcoholic beverages may produce increased depressant effects. Patients on concomitant CNS depressants must be monitored for a change in opioid effects. Consideration should be given to adjusting the dose of fentanyl if warranted). Products include:
Valium Tablets 2880

Dihydrocodeine Bitartrate (The concomitant use of fentanyl with other CNS depressants, including other opioids may produce increased depressant effects).
No products indexed under this heading.

Dihydrocodeinone Bitartrate (The concomitant use of fentanyl with other CNS depressants, including other opioids may produce increased depressant effects).
No products indexed under this heading.

Diltiazem Hydrochloride (The concomitant use of fentanyl with CYP3A4 inhibitors (eg, indinavir, nelfinavir, ritonavir, clarithromycin, itraconazole, ketoconazole, nefazodone, saquinavir, telithromycin, aprepitant, diltiazem, erythromycin, fluconazole, grapefruit juice, verapamil, or cimetidine) may result in a potentially dangerous increase in fentanyl plasma concentrations). Products include:
Cardizem LA 423

Diltiazem Maleate (The concomitant use of fentanyl with CYP3A4 inhibitors (eg, indinavir, nelfinavir, ritonavir, clarithromycin, itraconazole, ketoconazole, nefazodone, saquinavir, telithromycin, aprepitant, diltiazem, erythromycin, fluconazole, grapefruit juice, verapamil, or cimetidine) may result in a potentially dangerous increase in fentanyl plasma concentrations).
No products indexed under this heading.

Diphenhydramine Hydrochloride (The concomitant use of fentanyl with other CNS depressants, including other opioids, sedatives or hypnotics, general anesthetics, phenothiazines, tranquilizers, skeletal muscle relaxants, sedating antihistamines, and alcoholic beverages may produce increased depressant effects). Products include:
Benadryl Allergy Ultratab 2042
Children's Benadryl Allergy Liquid 2042

Diphenylpyraline Hydrochloride (The concomitant use of fentanyl with other CNS depressants, including other opioids, sedatives or hypnotics, general anesthetics, phenothiazines, tranquilizers, skeletal muscle relaxants, sedating antihistamines, and alcoholic beverages may produce increased depressant effects).
No products indexed under this heading.

Doxacurium Chloride (The concomitant use of fentanyl with other CNS depressants, including other opioids, sedatives or hypnotics, general anesthetics, phenothiazines, tranquilizers, skeletal muscle relaxants, sedating antihistamines, and alcoholic beverages may produce increased depressant effects).
No products indexed under this heading.

Doxorubicin Hydrochloride (The concomitant use of fentanyl with CYP3A4 inducers (eg, barbiturates, carbamazepine, efavirenz, glucocorticoids, modafinil, nevirapine, oxcarbazepine, phenobarbital, phenytoin, pioglitazone, rifabutin, rifampin, St. John's wort, or troglitazone) may result in a decrease fentanyl plasma concentrations).
No products indexed under this heading.

Droperidol (The concomitant use of fentanyl with other CNS depressants, including other opioids, sedatives or hypnotics, general anesthetics, phenothizines, tranquilizers, skeletal muscle relaxants, sedating antihistamines, and alcoholic beverages may produce increased depressant effects. Patients on concomitant CNS depressants must be monitored for a change in opioid effects. Consideration should be given to adjusting the dose of fentanyl if warranted).
No products indexed under this heading.

d-Tubocurarine (The concomitant use of fentanyl with other CNS depressants, including other opioids, sedatives or hypnotics, general anesthetics, phenothiazines, tranquilizers, skeletal muscle relaxants, sedating antihistamines, and alcoholic beverages may produce increased depressant effects).
No products indexed under this heading.

Efavirenz (The concomitant use of fentanyl with CYP3A4 inducers (eg, barbiturates, carbamazepine, efavirenz, glucocorticoids, modafinil, nevirapine, oxcarbazepine, phenobarbital, phenytoin, pioglitazone, rifabutin, rifampin, St. John's wort, or troglitazone) may result in a decrease fentanyl plasma concentrations). Products include:
Atripla 906

Enflurane (The concomitant use of fentanyl with other CNS depressants, including other opioids, sedatives or hypnotics, general anesthetics, phenothizines, tranquilizers, skeletal muscle relaxants, sedating antihistamines, and alcoholic beverages may produce increased depressant effects. Patients on concomitant CNS depressants must be monitored for a change in opioid effects. Consideration should be given to adjusting the dose of fentanyl if warranted).
No products indexed under this heading.

Erythromycin (The concomitant use of fentanyl with CYP3A4 inhibitors (eg, indinavir, nelfinavir, ritonavir, clarithromycin, itraconazole, ketoconazole, nefazodone, saquinavir, telithromycin, aprepitant, diltiazem, erythromycin, fluconazole, grapefruit juice, verapamil, or cimetidine) may result in a potentially dangerous increase in fentanyl plasma concentrations).
No products indexed under this heading.

IMPORTANT NOTE: Always consult each drug listing in the patient's regimen for possible interactions.

Erythromycin, Topical (The concomitant use of fentanyl with CYP3A4 inhibitors (eg, erythromycin) may result in a potentially dangerous increase in fentanyl plasma concentrations).

No products indexed under this heading.

Erythromycin Estolate (The concomitant use of fentanyl with CYP3A4 inhibitors (eg, indinavir, nelfinavir, ritonavir, clarithromycin, itraconazole, ketoconazole, nefazodone, saquinavir, telithromycin, aprepitant, diltiazem, erythromycin, fluconazole, grapefruit juice, verapamil, or cimetidine) may result in a potentially dangerous increase in fentanyl plasma concentrations).

No products indexed under this heading.

Erythromycin Ethylsuccinate (The concomitant use of fentanyl with CYP3A4 inhibitors (eg, indinavir, nelfinavir, ritonavir, clarithromycin, itraconazole, ketoconazole, nefazodone, saquinavir, telithromycin, aprepitant, diltiazem, erythromycin, fluconazole, grapefruit juice, verapamil, or cimetidine) may result in a potentially dangerous increase in fentanyl plasma concentrations). Products include:

E.E.S. 437
EryPed 435

Erythromycin Gluceptate (The concomitant use of fentanyl with CYP3A4 inhibitors (eg, indinavir, nelfinavir, ritonavir, clarithromycin, itraconazole, ketoconazole, nefazodone, saquinavir, telithromycin, aprepitant, diltiazem, erythromycin, fluconazole, grapefruit juice, verapamil, or cimetidine) may result in a potentially dangerous increase in fentanyl plasma concentrations).

No products indexed under this heading.

Erythromycin Lactobionate (The concomitant use of fentanyl with CYP3A4 inhibitors (eg, indinavir, nelfinavir, ritonavir, clarithromycin, itraconazole, ketoconazole, nefazodone, saquinavir, telithromycin, aprepitant, diltiazem, erythromycin, fluconazole, grapefruit juice, verapamil, or cimetidine) may result in a potentially dangerous increase in fentanyl plasma concentrations).

No products indexed under this heading.

Erythromycin Stearate (The concomitant use of fentanyl with CYP3A4 inhibitors (eg, indinavir, nelfinavir, ritonavir, clarithromycin, itraconazole, ketoconazole, nefazodone, saquinavir, telithromycin, aprepitant, diltiazem, erythromycin, fluconazole, grapefruit juice, verapamil, or cimetidine) may result in a potentially dangerous increase in fentanyl plasma concentrations).

No products indexed under this heading.

Esomeprazole Magnesium (The concomitant use of fentanyl with CYP3A4 inhibitors (eg, indinavir, nelfinavir, ritonavir, clarithromycin, itraconazole, ketoconazole, nefazodone, saquinavir, telithromycin, aprepitant, diltiazem, erythromycin, fluconazole, grapefruit juice, verapamil, or cimetidine) may result in a potentially dangerous increase in fentanyl plasma concentrations). Products include:

Nexium Capsules 704
Nexium Oral Suspension 704

Esomeprazole Sodium (The concomitant use of fentanyl with CYP3A4 inhibitors (eg, indinavir, nelfinavir, ritonavir, clarithromycin, itraconazole, ketoconazole, nefazodone, saquinavir, telithromycin, aprepitant, diltiazem, erythromycin, fluconazole, grapefruit juice, verapamil, or cimetidine) may result in a potentially dangerous increase in fentanyl plasma concentrations). Products include:

Nexium I.V. 712

Estazolam (The concomitant use of fentanyl with other CNS depressants, including other opioids, sedatives or hypnotics, general anesthetics, phenothizines, tranquilizers, skeletal muscle relaxants, sedating antihistamines, and alcoholic beverages may produce increased depressant effects. Patients on concomitant CNS depressants must be monitored for a change in opioid effects. Consideration should be given to adjusting the dose of fentanyl if warranted).

No products indexed under this heading.

Ethanol (The concomitant use of fentanyl with other CNS depressants, including other opioids, sedatives or hypnotics, general anesthetics, phenothizines, tranquilizers, skeletal muscle relaxants, sedating antihistamines, and alcoholic beverages may produce increased depressant effects. Patients on concomitant CNS depressants must be monitored for a change in opioid effects. Consideration should be given to adjusting the dose of fentanyl if warranted).

No products indexed under this heading.

Ethchlorvynol (The concomitant use of fentanyl with other CNS depressants, including other opioids, sedatives or hypnotics, general anesthetics, phenothizines, tranquilizers, skeletal muscle relaxants, sedating antihistamines, and alcoholic beverages may produce increased depressant effects. Patients on concomitant CNS depressants must be monitored for a change in opioid effects. Consideration should be given to adjusting the dose of fentanyl if warranted).

No products indexed under this heading.

Ethinamate (The concomitant use of fentanyl with other CNS depressants, including other opioids, sedatives or hypnotics, general anesthetics, phenothizines, tranquilizers, skeletal muscle relaxants, sedating antihistamines, and alcoholic beverages may produce increased depressant effects. Patients on concomitant CNS depressants must be monitored for a change in opioid effects. Consideration should be given to adjusting the dose of fentanyl if warranted).

No products indexed under this heading.

Ethosuximide (The concomitant use of fentanyl with CYP3A4 inducers (eg, barbiturates, carbamazepine, efavirenz, glucocorticoids, modafinil, nevirapine, oxcarbazepine, phenobarbital, phenytoin, pioglitazone, rifabutin, rifampin, St. John's wort, or troglitazone) may result in a decrease fentanyl plasma concentrations).

No products indexed under this heading.

Ethyl Alcohol (The concomitant use of fentanyl with other CNS depressants, including other opioids, sedatives or hypnotics, general anesthetics, phenothizines, tranquilizers, skeletal muscle relaxants, sedating antihistamines, and alcoholic beverages may produce increased depressant effects. Patients on concomitant CNS depressants must be monitored for a change in opioid effects. Consideration should be given to adjusting the dose of fentanyl if warranted).

No products indexed under this heading.

Felbamate (The concomitant use of fentanyl with CYP3A4 inducers (eg, barbiturates, carbamazepine, efavirenz, glucocorticoids, modafinil, nevirapine, oxcarbazepine, phenobarbital, phenytoin, pioglitazone, rifabutin, rifampin, St. John's wort, or troglitazone) may result in a decrease fentanyl plasma concentrations).

No products indexed under this heading.

Fentanyl Citrate (The concomitant use of fentanyl with other CNS depres-

sants, including other opioids, sedatives or hypnotics, general anesthetics, phenothizines, tranquilizers, skeletal muscle relaxants, sedating antihistamines, and alcoholic beverages may produce increased depressant effects. Patients on concomitant CNS depressants must be monitored for a change in opioid effects. Consideration should be given to adjusting the dose of fentanyl if warranted). Products include:

Fentora 966

Fluconazole (The concomitant use of fentanyl with CYP3A4 inhibitors (eg, indinavir, nelfinavir, ritonavir, clarithromycin, itraconazole, ketoconazole, nefazodone, saquinavir, telithromycin, aprepitant, diltiazem, erythromycin, fluconazole, grapefruit juice, verapamil, or cimetidine) may result in a potentially dangerous increase in fentanyl plasma concentrations).

No products indexed under this heading.

Fludrocortisone Acetate (The concomitant use of fentanyl with CYP3A4 inducers (eg, barbiturates, carbamazepine, efavirenz, glucocorticoids, modafinil, nevirapine, oxcarbazepine, phenobarbital, phenytoin, pioglitazone, rifabutin, rifampin, St. John's wort, or troglitazone) may result in a decrease fentanyl plasma concentrations).

No products indexed under this heading.

Fluoxetine (The concomitant use of fentanyl with CYP3A4 inhibitors (eg, indinavir, nelfinavir, ritonavir, clarithromycin, itraconazole, ketoconazole, nefazodone, saquinavir, telithromycin, aprepitant, diltiazem, erythromycin, fluconazole, grapefruit juice, verapamil, or cimetidine) may result in a potentially dangerous increase in fentanyl plasma concentrations).

No products indexed under this heading.

Fluoxetine Hydrochloride (The concomitant use of fentanyl with CYP3A4 inhibitors (eg, indinavir, nelfinavir, ritonavir, clarithromycin, itraconazole, ketoconazole, nefazodone, saquinavir, telithromycin, aprepitant, diltiazem, erythromycin, fluconazole, grapefruit juice, verapamil, or cimetidine) may result in a potentially dangerous increase in fentanyl plasma concentrations). Products include:

Prozac Weekly 1941
Prozac Pulvules 1941
Symbyax 1965

Fluphenazine Decanoate (The concomitant use of fentanyl with other CNS depressants, including other opioids, sedatives or hypnotics, general anesthetics, phenothizines, tranquilizers, skeletal muscle relaxants, sedating antihistamines, and alcoholic beverages may produce increased depressant effects. Patients on concomitant CNS depressants must be monitored for a change in opioid effects. Consideration should be given to adjusting the dose of fentanyl if warranted).

No products indexed under this heading.

Fluphenazine Enanthate (The concomitant use of fentanyl with other CNS depressants, including other opioids, sedatives or hypnotics, general anesthetics, phenothizines, tranquilizers, skeletal muscle relaxants, sedating antihistamines, and alcoholic beverages may produce increased depressant effects. Patients on concomitant CNS depressants must be monitored for a change in opioid effects. Consideration should be given to adjusting the dose of fentanyl if warranted).

No products indexed under this heading.

Fluphenazine Hydrochloride (The concomitant use of fentanyl with other CNS depressants, including other opioids, sedatives or hypnotics, general anesthetics, phenothizines, tranquilizers, skeletal muscle relaxants, sedating antihistamines, and alcoholic beverages

may produce increased depressant effects. Patients on concomitant CNS depressants must be monitored for a change in opioid effects. Consideration should be given to adjusting the dose of fentanyl if warranted).

No products indexed under this heading.

Flurazepam Hydrochloride (The concomitant use of fentanyl with other CNS depressants, including other opioids, sedatives or hypnotics, general anesthetics, phenothizines, tranquilizers, skeletal muscle relaxants, sedating antihistamines, and alcoholic beverages may produce increased depressant effects. Patients on concomitant CNS depressants must be monitored for a change in opioid effects. Consideration should be given to adjusting the dose of fentanyl if warranted).

No products indexed under this heading.

Fluvoxamine Maleate (The concomitant use of fentanyl with CYP3A4 inhibitors (eg, indinavir, nelfinavir, ritonavir, clarithromycin, itraconazole, ketoconazole, nefazodone, saquinavir, telithromycin, aprepitant, diltiazem, erythromycin, fluconazole, grapefruit juice, verapamil, or cimetidine) may result in a potentially dangerous increase in fentanyl plasma concentrations).

No products indexed under this heading.

Fosamprenavir Calcium (The concomitant use of fentanyl with CYP3A4 inhibitors (eg, indinavir, nelfinavir, ritonavir, clarithromycin, itraconazole, ketoconazole, nefazodone, saquinavir, telithromycin, aprepitant, diltiazem, erythromycin, fluconazole, grapefruit juice, verapamil, or cimetidine) may result in a potentially dangerous increase in fentanyl plasma concentrations). Products include:

Lexiva Oral Suspension 1558
Lexiva 1558

Fosphenytoin (The concomitant use of fentanyl with CYP3A4 inducers (eg, phenytoin) may result in a decrease fentanyl plasma concentrations).

No products indexed under this heading.

Fosphenytoin Sodium (The concomitant use of fentanyl with CYP3A4 inducers (eg, barbiturates, carbamazepine, efavirenz, glucocorticoids, modafinil, nevirapine, oxcarbazepine, phenobarbital, phenytoin, pioglitazone, rifabutin, rifampin, St. John's wort, or troglitazone) may result in a decrease fentanyl plasma concentrations).

No products indexed under this heading.

Gallamine (The concomitant use of fentanyl with other CNS depressants, including other opioids, sedatives or hypnotics, general anesthetics, phenothiazines, tranquilizers, skeletal muscle relaxants, sedating antihistamines, and alcoholic beverages may produce increased depressant effects).

No products indexed under this heading.

Gallamine Triethiodide (The concomitant use of fentanyl with other CNS depressants, including other opioids, sedatives or hypnotics, general anesthetics, phenothiazines, tranquilizers, skeletal muscle relaxants, sedating antihistamines, and alcoholic beverages may produce increased depressant effects).

No products indexed under this heading.

Garlic Extract (The concomitant use of fentanyl with CYP3A4 inducers (eg, barbiturates, carbamazepine, efavirenz, glucocorticoids, modafinil, nevirapine, oxcarbazepine, phenobarbital, phenytoin, pioglitazone, rifabutin, rifampin, St. John's wort, or troglitazone) may result in a decrease fentanyl plasma concentrations).

No products indexed under this heading.

Garlic Oil (The concomitant use of fentanyl with CYP3A4 inducers (eg, barbiturates, carbamazepine, efavirenz, glucocorticoids, modafinil, nevirapine, oxcarbazepine, phenobarbital, phenytoin, pioglitazone, rifabutin, rifampin, St. John's wort, or troglitazone) may result in a decrease fentanyl plasma concentrations).
No products indexed under this heading.

Glutethimide (The concomitant use of fentanyl with other CNS depressants, including other opioids, sedatives or hypnotics, general anesthetics, phenothizines, tranquilizers, skeletal muscle relaxants, sedating antihistamines, and alcoholic beverages may produce increased depressant effects. Patients on concomitant CNS depressants must be monitored for a change in opioid effects. Consideration should be given to adjusting the dose of fentanyl if warranted).
No products indexed under this heading.

Halazepam (The concomitant use of fentanyl with other CNS depressants, including other opioids, sedatives or hypnotics, general anesthetics, phenothizines, tranquilizers, skeletal muscle relaxants, sedating antihistamines, and alcoholic beverages may produce increased depressant effects. Patients on concomitant CNS depressants must be monitored for a change in opioid effects. Consideration should be given to adjusting the dose of fentanyl if warranted).
No products indexed under this heading.

Haloperidol (The concomitant use of fentanyl with other CNS depressants, including other opioids, sedatives or hypnotics, general anesthetics, phenothizines, tranquilizers, skeletal muscle relaxants, sedating antihistamines, and alcoholic beverages may produce increased depressant effects. Patients on concomitant CNS depressants must be monitored for a change in opioid effects. Consideration should be given to adjusting the dose of fentanyl if warranted).
No products indexed under this heading.

Haloperidol Decanoate (The concomitant use of fentanyl with other CNS depressants, including other opioids, sedatives or hypnotics, general anesthetics, phenothizines, tranquilizers, skeletal muscle relaxants, sedating antihistamines, and alcoholic beverages may produce increased depressant effects. Patients on concomitant CNS depressants must be monitored for a change in opioid effects. Consideration should be given to adjusting the dose of fentanyl if warranted).
No products indexed under this heading.

Haloperidol Lactate (The concomitant use of fentanyl with other CNS depressants, including other opioids, sedatives or hypnotics, general anesthetics, phenothizines, tranquilizers, skeletal muscle relaxants, sedating antihistamines, and alcoholic beverages may produce increased depressant effects. Patients on concomitant CNS depressants must be monitored for a change in opioid effects. Consideration should be given to adjusting the dose of fentanyl if warranted).
No products indexed under this heading.

Halothane (The concomitant use of fentanyl with other CNS depressants, including other opioids, sedatives or hypnotics, general anesthetics, phenothiazines, tranquilizers, skeletal muscle relaxants, sedating antihistamines, and alcoholic beverages may produce increased depressant effects).
No products indexed under this heading.

Hexobarbital (The concomitant use of fentanyl with other CNS depressants, including other opioids, sedatives or hypnotics, general anesthetics, phenothizines, tranquilizers, skeletal muscle relaxants, sedating antihistamines, and alcoholic beverages may produce increased depressant effects. Patients on concomitant CNS depressants must be monitored for a change in opioid effects. Consideration should be given to adjusting the dose of fentanyl if warranted).
No products indexed under this heading.

Hydrocodone Bitartrate (The concomitant use of fentanyl with other CNS depressants, including other opioids, sedatives or hypnotics, general anesthetics, phenothizines, tranquilizers, skeletal muscle relaxants, sedating antihistamines, and alcoholic beverages may produce increased depressant effects. Patients on concomitant CNS depressants must be monitored for a change in opioid effects. Consideration should be given to adjusting the dose of fentanyl if warranted). Products include:
Vicodin 560
Vicodin ES 561
Vicodin HP 563
Vicoprofen 564
Zydone 1138

Hydrocodone Polistirex (The concomitant use of fentanyl with other CNS depressants, including other opioids, sedatives or hypnotics, general anesthetics, phenothizines, tranquilizers, skeletal muscle relaxants, sedating antihistamines, and alcoholic beverages may produce increased depressant effects. Patients on concomitant CNS depressants must be monitored for a change in opioid effects. Consideration should be given to adjusting the dose of fentanyl if warranted). Products include:
Tussionex 3443

Hydrocortisone (The concomitant use of fentanyl with CYP3A4 inducers (eg, barbiturates, carbamazepine, efavirenz, glucocorticoids, modafinil, nevirapine, oxcarbazepine, phenobarbital, phenytoin, pioglitazone, rifabutin, rifampin, St. John's wort, or troglitazone) may result in a decrease fentanyl plasma concentrations).
No products indexed under this heading.

Hydrocortisone (Alcohol) (The concomitant use of fentanyl with CYP3A4 inducers (eg, barbiturates, carbamazepine, efavirenz, glucocorticoids, modafinil, nevirapine, oxcarbazepine, phenobarbital, phenytoin, pioglitazone, rifabutin, rifampin, St. John's wort, or troglitazone) may result in a decrease fentanyl plasma concentrations).
No products indexed under this heading.

Hydrocortisone Acetate (The concomitant use of fentanyl with CYP3A4 inducers (eg, barbiturates, carbamazepine, efavirenz, glucocorticoids, modafinil, nevirapine, oxcarbazepine, phenobarbital, phenytoin, pioglitazone, rifabutin, rifampin, St. John's wort, or troglitazone) may result in a decrease fentanyl plasma concentrations).
No products indexed under this heading.

Hydrocortisone Butyrate (The concomitant use of fentanyl with CYP3A4 inducers (eg, barbiturates, carbamazepine, efavirenz, glucocorticoids, modafinil, nevirapine, oxcarbazepine, phenobarbital, phenytoin, pioglitazone, rifabutin, rifampin, St. John's wort, or troglitazone) may result in a decrease fentanyl plasma concentrations).
No products indexed under this heading.

Hydrocortisone Cypionate (The concomitant use of fentanyl with CYP3A4 inducers (eg, barbiturates, carbamazepine, efavirenz, glucocorticoids, modafinil, nevirapine, oxcarbazepine, phenobarbital, phenytoin, pioglitazone, rifabutin, rifampin, St. John's wort, or troglitazone) may result in a decrease fentanyl plasma concentrations).
No products indexed under this heading.

Hydrocortisone Hemisuccinate (The concomitant use of fentanyl with CYP3A4 inducers (eg, barbiturates, carbamazepine, efavirenz, glucocorticoids, modafinil, nevirapine, oxcarbazepine, phenobarbital, phenytoin, pioglitazone, rifabutin, rifampin, St. John's wort, or troglitazone) may result in a decrease fentanyl plasma concentrations).
No products indexed under this heading.

Hydrocortisone Probutate (The concomitant use of fentanyl with CYP3A4 inducers (eg, barbiturates, carbamazepine, efavirenz, glucocorticoids, modafinil, nevirapine, oxcarbazepine, phenobarbital, phenytoin, pioglitazone, rifabutin, rifampin, St. John's wort, or troglitazone) may result in a decrease fentanyl plasma concentrations).
No products indexed under this heading.

Hydrocortisone Sodium Phosphate (The concomitant use of fentanyl with CYP3A4 inducers (eg, barbiturates, carbamazepine, efavirenz, glucocorticoids, modafinil, nevirapine, oxcarbazepine, phenobarbital, phenytoin, pioglitazone, rifabutin, rifampin, St. John's wort, or troglitazone) may result in a decrease fentanyl plasma concentrations).
No products indexed under this heading.

Hydrocortisone Sodium Succinate (The concomitant use of fentanyl with CYP3A4 inducers (eg, barbiturates, carbamazepine, efavirenz, glucocorticoids, modafinil, nevirapine, oxcarbazepine, phenobarbital, phenytoin, pioglitazone, rifabutin, rifampin, St. John's wort, or troglitazone) may result in a decrease fentanyl plasma concentrations).
No products indexed under this heading.

Hydrocortisone Valerate (The concomitant use of fentanyl with CYP3A4 inducers (eg, barbiturates, carbamazepine, efavirenz, glucocorticoids, modafinil, nevirapine, oxcarbazepine, phenobarbital, phenytoin, pioglitazone, rifabutin, rifampin, St. John's wort, or troglitazone) may result in a decrease fentanyl plasma concentrations).
No products indexed under this heading.

Hydromorphone (The concomitant use of fentanyl with other CNS depressants, including other opioids, sedatives or hypnotics, general anesthetics, phenothizines, tranquilizers, skeletal muscle relaxants, sedating antihistamines, and alcoholic beverages may produce increased depressant effects. Patients on concomitant CNS depressants must be monitored for a change in opioid effects. Consideration should be given to adjusting the dose of fentanyl if warranted).
No products indexed under this heading.

Hydromorphone Hydrochloride (The concomitant use of fentanyl with other CNS depressants, including other opioids, sedatives or hypnotics, general anesthetics, phenothizines, tranquilizers, skeletal muscle relaxants, sedating antihistamines, and alcoholic beverages may produce increased depressant effects. Patients on concomitant CNS depressants must be monitored for a change in opioid effects. Consideration should be given to adjusting the dose of fentanyl if warranted). Products include:
Dilaudid Injection 2800
Dilaudid Oral 2797
Dilaudid Tablets 2797
Dilaudid-HP 2800

Hydroxyzine Hydrochloride (The concomitant use of fentanyl with other CNS depressants, including other opioids, sedatives or hypnotics, general anesthetics, phenothizines, tranquilizers, skeletal muscle relaxants, sedating antihistamines, and alcoholic beverages may produce increased depressant effects. Patients on concomitant CNS depressants must be monitored for a change in opioid effects. Consideration should be given to adjusting the dose of fentanyl if warranted).
No products indexed under this heading.

Hypericum (The concomitant use of fentanyl with CYP3A4 inducers (eg, barbiturates, carbamazepine, efavirenz, glucocorticoids, modafinil, nevirapine, oxcarbazepine, phenobarbital, phenytoin, pioglitazone, rifabutin, rifampin, St. John's wort, or troglitazone) may result in a decrease fentanyl plasma concentrations).
No products indexed under this heading.

Hypericum Perforatum (The concomitant use of fentanyl with CYP3A4 inducers (eg, barbiturates, carbamazepine, efavirenz, glucocorticoids, modafinil, nevirapine, oxcarbazepine, phenobarbital, phenytoin, pioglitazone, rifabutin, rifampin, St. John's wort, or troglitazone) may result in a decrease fentanyl plasma concentrations). Products include:
Traumeel 1800

Imatinib Mesylate (The concomitant use of fentanyl with CYP3A4 inhibitors (eg, indinavir, nelfinavir, ritonavir, clarithromycin, itraconazole, ketoconazole, nefazodone, saquinavir, telithromycin, aprepitant, diltiazem, erythromycin, fluconazole, grapefruit juice, verapamil, or cimetidine) may result in a potentially dangerous increase in fentanyl plasma concentrations). Products include:
Gleevec 2477

Indinavir Sulfate (The concomitant use of fentanyl with CYP3A4 inhibitors (eg, indinavir, nelfinavir, ritonavir, clarithromycin, itraconazole, ketoconazole, nefazodone, saquinavir, telithromycin, aprepitant, diltiazem, erythromycin, fluconazole, grapefruit juice, verapamil, or cimetidine) may result in a potentially dangerous increase in fentanyl plasma concentrations). Products include:
Crixivan 2113

Isocarboxazid (Fentanyl is not recommended in patients who have received MAO inhibitors within 14 days because severe and unpredictable potentiation by MAO inhibitors has been reported with opioid analgesics). Products include:
Marplan 3481

Isoflurane (The concomitant use of fentanyl with other CNS depressants, including other opioids, sedatives or hypnotics, general anesthetics, phenothizines, tranquilizers, skeletal muscle relaxants, sedating antihistamines, and alcoholic beverages may produce increased depressant effects. Patients on concomitant CNS depressants must be monitored for a change in opioid effects. Consideration should be given to adjusting the dose of fentanyl if warranted).
No products indexed under this heading.

Isoniazid (The concomitant use of fentanyl with CYP3A4 inhibitors (eg, indinavir, nelfinavir, ritonavir, clarithromycin, itraconazole, ketoconazole, nefazodone, saquinavir, telithromycin, aprepitant, diltiazem, erythromycin, fluconazole, grapefruit juice, verapamil, or cimetidine) may result in a potentially dangerous increase in fentanyl plasma concentrations).
No products indexed under this heading.

Itraconazole (The concomitant use of fentanyl with CYP3A4 inhibitors (eg, indinavir, nelfinavir, ritonavir, clarithromycin, itraconazole, ketoconazole, nefazodone, saquinavir, telithromycin, aprepitant, diltiazem, erythromycin, fluconazole, grapefruit juice, verapamil, or cimetidine) may result in a potentially dangerous increase in fentanyl plasma concentrations).
No products indexed under this heading.

Ketamine Hydrochloride (The concomitant use of fentanyl with other CNS depressants, including other opioids, sedatives or hypnotics, general anesthetics, phenothizines, tranquilizers, skeletal muscle relaxants, sedating antihistamines, and alcoholic beverages may produce increased depressant effects. Patients on concomitant CNS depressants must be monitored for a change in opioid effects. Consideration should be given to adjusting the dose of fentanyl if warranted).
No products indexed under this heading.

Ketoconazole (The concomitant use of fentanyl with CYP3A4 inhibitors (eg, indinavir, nelfinavir, ritonavir, clarithromycin, itraconazole, ketoconazole, nefazodone, saquinavir, telithromycin, aprepitant, diltiazem, erythromycin, fluconazole, grapefruit juice, verapamil, or cimetidine) may result in a potentially dangerous increase in fentanyl plasma concentrations). Products include:
Extina 3319
Xolegel 3337

Lapatinib (The concomitant use of fentanyl with CYP3A4 inhibitors (eg, indinavir, nelfinavir, ritonavir, clarithromycin, itraconazole, ketoconazole, nefazodone, saquinavir, telithromycin, aprepitant, diltiazem, erythromycin, fluconazole, grapefruit juice, verapamil, or cimetidine) may result in a potentially dangerous increase in fentanyl plasma concentrations). Products include:
Tykerb 1698

Levomethadyl Acetate Hydrochloride (The concomitant use of fentanyl with other CNS depressants, including other opioids, sedatives or hypnotics, general anesthetics, phenothizines, tranquilizers, skeletal muscle relaxants, sedating antihistamines, and alcoholic beverages may produce increased depressant effects. Patients on concomitant CNS depressants must be monitored for a change in opioid effects. Consideration should be given to adjusting the dose of fentanyl if warranted).
No products indexed under this heading.

Levorphanol Tartrate (The concomitant use of fentanyl with other CNS depressants, including other opioids, sedatives or hypnotics, general anesthetics, phenothizines, tranquilizers, skeletal muscle relaxants, sedating antihistamines, and alcoholic beverages may produce increased depressant effects. Patients on concomitant CNS depressants must be monitored for a change in opioid effects. Consideration should be given to adjusting the dose of fentanyl if warranted).
No products indexed under this heading.

Lopinavir (The concomitant use of fentanyl with CYP3A4 inhibitors (eg, indinavir, nelfinavir, ritonavir, clarithromycin, itraconazole, ketoconazole, nefazodone, saquinavir, telithromycin, aprepitant, diltiazem, erythromycin, fluconazole, grapefruit juice, verapamil, or cimetidine) may result in a potentially dangerous increase in fentanyl plasma concentrations). Products include:
Kaletra 458

Loratadine (The concomitant use of fentanyl with CYP3A4 inhibitors (eg, indinavir, nelfinavir, ritonavir, clarithromycin, itraconazole, ketoconazole, nefazodone, saquinavir, telithromycin, aprepitant, diltiazem, erythromycin, fluconazole, grapefruit juice, verapamil, or cimetidine) may result in a potentially dangerous increase in fentanyl plasma concentrations).
No products indexed under this heading.

Lorazepam (The concomitant use of fentanyl with other CNS depressants, including other opioids, sedatives or hypnotics, general anesthetics, phenothizines, tranquilizers, skeletal muscle relaxants, sedating antihistamines, and alcoholic beverages may produce increased depressant effects. Patients on concomitant CNS depressants must be monitored for a change in opioid effects. Consideration should be given to adjusting the dose of fentanyl if warranted).
No products indexed under this heading.

Loxapine Hydrochloride (The concomitant use of fentanyl with other CNS depressants, including other opioids, sedatives or hypnotics, general anesthetics, phenothizines, tranquilizers, skeletal muscle relaxants, sedating antihistamines, and alcoholic beverages may produce increased depressant effects. Patients on concomitant CNS depressants must be monitored for a change in opioid effects. Consideration should be given to adjusting the dose of fentanyl if warranted).
No products indexed under this heading.

Loxapine Succinate (The concomitant use of fentanyl with other CNS depressants, including other opioids, sedatives or hypnotics, general anesthetics, phenothizines, tranquilizers, skeletal muscle relaxants, sedating antihistamines, and alcoholic beverages may produce increased depressant effects. Patients on concomitant CNS depressants must be monitored for a change in opioid effects. Consideration should be given to adjusting the dose of fentanyl if warranted).
No products indexed under this heading.

Meperidine Hydrochloride (The concomitant use of fentanyl with other CNS depressants, including other opioids, sedatives or hypnotics, general anesthetics, phenothizines, tranquilizers, skeletal muscle relaxants, sedating antihistamines, and alcoholic beverages may produce increased depressant effects. Patients on concomitant CNS depressants must be monitored for a change in opioid effects. Consideration should be given to adjusting the dose of fentanyl if warranted).
No products indexed under this heading.

Mephenytoin (The concomitant use of fentanyl with CYP3A4 inducers (eg, barbiturates, carbamazepine, efavirenz, glucocorticoids, modafinil, nevirapine, oxcarbazepine, phenobarbital, phenytoin, pioglitazone, rifabutin, rifampin, St. John's wort, or troglitazone) may result in a decrease fentanyl plasma concentrations).
No products indexed under this heading.

Mephobarbital (The concomitant use of fentanyl with other CNS depressants, including other opioids, sedatives or hypnotics, general anesthetics, phenothizines, tranquilizers, skeletal muscle relaxants, sedating antihistamines, and alcoholic beverages may produce increased depressant effects. Patients on concomitant CNS depressants must be monitored for a change in opioid effects. Consideration should be given to adjusting the dose of fentanyl if warranted).
No products indexed under this heading.

Meprobamate (The concomitant use of fentanyl with other CNS depressants, including other opioids, sedatives or hypnotics, general anesthetics, phenothizines, tranquilizers, skeletal muscle relaxants, sedating antihistamines, and alcoholic beverages may produce increased depressant effects. Patients on concomitant CNS depressants must be monitored for a change in opioid effects. Consideration should be given to adjusting the dose of fentanyl if warranted).
No products indexed under this heading.

Mesoridazine Besylate (The concomitant use of fentanyl with other CNS depressants, including other opioids, sedatives or hypnotics, general anesthetics, phenothizines, tranquilizers, skeletal muscle relaxants, sedating antihistamines, and alcoholic beverages may produce increased depressant effects. Patients on concomitant CNS depressants must be monitored for a change in opioid effects. Consideration should be given to adjusting the dose of fentanyl if warranted).
No products indexed under this heading.

Metaxalone (The concomitant use of fentanyl with other CNS depressants, including other opioids, sedatives or hypnotics, general anesthetics, phenothiazines, tranquilizers, skeletal muscle relaxants, sedating antihistamines, and alcoholic beverages may produce increased depressant effects). Products include:
Skelaxin 1848

Methadone Hydrochloride (The concomitant use of fentanyl with other CNS depressants, including other opioids, sedatives or hypnotics, general anesthetics, phenothizines, tranquilizers, skeletal muscle relaxants, sedating antihistamines, and alcoholic beverages may produce increased depressant effects. Patients on concomitant CNS depressants must be monitored for a change in opioid effects. Consideration should be given to adjusting the dose of fentanyl if warranted).
No products indexed under this heading.

Methdilazine Hydrochloride (The concomitant use of fentanyl with other CNS depressants, including other opioids, sedatives or hypnotics, general anesthetics, phenothiazines, tranquilizers, skeletal muscle relaxants, sedating antihistamines, and alcoholic beverages may produce increased depressant effects).
No products indexed under this heading.

Methocarbamol (The concomitant use of fentanyl with other CNS depressants, including other opioids, sedatives or hypnotics, general anesthetics, phenothiazines, tranquilizers, skeletal muscle relaxants, sedating antihistamines, and alcoholic beverages may produce increased depressant effects).
No products indexed under this heading.

Methohexital Sodium (The concomitant use of fentanyl with other CNS depressants, including other opioids, sedatives or hypnotics, general anesthetics, phenothizines, tranquilizers, skeletal muscle relaxants, sedating antihistamines, and alcoholic beverages may produce increased depressant effects. Patients on concomitant CNS depressants must be monitored for a change in opioid effects. Consideration should be given to adjusting the dose of fentanyl if warranted).
No products indexed under this heading.

Methotrimeprazine (The concomitant use of fentanyl with other CNS depressants, including other opioids, sedatives or hypnotics, general anesthetics, phenothizines, tranquilizers, skeletal muscle relaxants, sedating antihistamines, and alcoholic beverages may produce increased depressant effects. Patients on concomitant CNS depressants must be monitored for a change in opioid effects. Consideration should be given to adjusting the dose of fentanyl if warranted).
No products indexed under this heading.

Methoxyflurane (The concomitant use of fentanyl with other CNS depressants, including other opioids, sedatives or hypnotics, general anesthetics, phenothizines, tranquilizers, skeletal muscle relaxants, sedating antihistamines, and alcoholic beverages may produce increased depressant effects. Patients on concomitant CNS depressants must be monitored for a change in opioid effects. Consideration should be given to adjusting the dose of fentanyl if warranted).
No products indexed under this heading.

Methsuximide (The concomitant use of fentanyl with CYP3A4 inducers (eg, barbiturates, carbamazepine, efavirenz, glucocorticoids, modafinil, nevirapine, oxcarbazepine, phenobarbital, phenytoin, pioglitazone, rifabutin, rifampin, St. John's wort, or troglitazone) may result in a decrease fentanyl plasma concentrations).
No products indexed under this heading.

Methylprednisolone (The concomitant use of fentanyl with CYP3A4 inducers (eg, barbiturates, carbamazepine, efavirenz, glucocorticoids, modafinil, nevirapine, oxcarbazepine, phenobarbital, phenytoin, pioglitazone, rifabutin, rifampin, St. John's wort, or troglitazone) may result in a decrease fentanyl plasma concentrations).
No products indexed under this heading.

Methylprednisolone Acetate (The concomitant use of fentanyl with CYP3A4 inducers (eg, barbiturates, carbamazepine, efavirenz, glucocorticoids, modafinil, nevirapine, oxcarbazepine, phenobarbital, phenytoin, pioglitazone, rifabutin, rifampin, St. John's wort, or troglitazone) may result in a decrease fentanyl plasma concentrations).
No products indexed under this heading.

Methylprednisolone Sodium Succinate (The concomitant use of fentanyl with CYP3A4 inducers (eg, barbiturates, carbamazepine, efavirenz, glucocorticoids, modafinil, nevirapine, oxcarbazepine, phenobarbital, phenytoin, pioglitazone, rifabutin, rifampin, St. John's wort, or troglitazone) may result in a decrease fentanyl plasma concentrations).
No products indexed under this heading.

Metocurine Iodide (The concomitant use of fentanyl with other CNS depressants, including other opioids, sedatives or hypnotics, general anesthetics, phenothiazines, tranquilizers, skeletal muscle relaxants, sedating antihistamines, and alcoholic beverages may produce increased depressant effects).
No products indexed under this heading.

Metronidazole (The concomitant use of fentanyl with CYP3A4 inhibitors (eg, indinavir, nelfinavir, ritonavir, clarithromycin, itraconazole, ketoconazole, nefazodone, saquinavir, telithromycin, aprepitant, diltiazem, erythromycin, fluconazole, grapefruit juice, verapamil, or cimetidine) may result in a potentially dangerous increase in fentanyl plasma concentrations). Products include:
Pylera 793

1295 Interactions Index Onsolis

Metronidazole Benzoate (The concomitant use of fentanyl with CYP3A4 inhibitors (eg, indinavir, nelfinavir, ritonavir, clarithromycin, itraconazole, ketoconazole, nefazodone, saquinavir, telithromycin, aprepitant, diltiazem, erythromycin, fluconazole, grapefruit juice, verapamil, or cimetidine) may result in a potentially dangerous increase in fentanyl plasma concentrations).
No products indexed under this heading.

Metronidazole Hydrochloride (The concomitant use of fentanyl with CYP3A4 inhibitors (eg, indinavir, nelfinavir, ritonavir, clarithromycin, itraconazole, ketoconazole, nefazodone, saquinavir, telithromycin, aprepitant, diltiazem, erythromycin, fluconazole, grapefruit juice, verapamil, or cimetidine) may result in a potentially dangerous increase in fentanyl plasma concentrations).
No products indexed under this heading.

Metronidazole Sodium (The concomitant use of fentanyl with CYP3A4 inhibitors (eg, indinavir, nelfinavir, ritonavir, clarithromycin, itraconazole, ketoconazole, nefazodone, saquinavir, telithromycin, aprepitant, diltiazem, erythromycin, fluconazole, grapefruit juice, verapamil, or cimetidine) may result in a potentially dangerous increase in fentanyl plasma concentrations).
No products indexed under this heading.

Miconazole (The concomitant use of fentanyl with CYP3A4 inhibitors (eg, indinavir, nelfinavir, ritonavir, clarithromycin, itraconazole, ketoconazole, nefazodone, saquinavir, telithromycin, aprepitant, diltiazem, erythromycin, fluconazole, grapefruit juice, verapamil, or cimetidine) may result in a potentially dangerous increase in fentanyl plasma concentrations).
No products indexed under this heading.

Miconazole Nitrate (The concomitant use of fentanyl with CYP3A4 inhibitors (eg, indinavir, nelfinavir, ritonavir, clarithromycin, itraconazole, ketoconazole, nefazodone, saquinavir, telithromycin, aprepitant, diltiazem, erythromycin, fluconazole, grapefruit juice, verapamil, or cimetidine) may result in a potentially dangerous increase in fentanyl plasma concentrations). Products include:
Vusion Ointment 3335

Midazolam Hydrochloride (The concomitant use of fentanyl with other CNS depressants, including other opioids, sedatives or hypnotics, general anesthetics, phenothizines, tranquilizers, skeletal muscle relaxants, sedating antihistamines, and alcoholic beverages may produce increased depressant effects. Patients on concomitant CNS depressants must be monitored for a change in opioid effects. Consideration should be given to adjusting the dose of fentanyl if warranted).
No products indexed under this heading.

Mifepristone (The concomitant use of fentanyl with CYP3A4 inhibitors (eg, indinavir, nelfinavir, ritonavir, clarithromycin, itraconazole, ketoconazole, nefazodone, saquinavir, telithromycin, aprepitant, diltiazem, erythromycin, fluconazole, grapefruit juice, verapamil, or cimetidine) may result in a potentially dangerous increase in fentanyl plasma concentrations).
No products indexed under this heading.

Mivacurium Chloride (The concomitant use of fentanyl with other CNS depressants, including other opioids, sedatives or hypnotics, general anesthetics, phenothiazines, tranquilizers, skeletal muscle relaxants, sedating antihistamines, and alcoholic beverages may produce increased depressant effects).
No products indexed under this heading.

Moclobemide (Fentanyl is not recommended in patients who have received MAO inhibitors within 14 days because severe and unpredictable potentiation by MAO inhibitors has been reported with opioid analgesics).
No products indexed under this heading.

Modafinil (The concomitant use of fentanyl with CYP3A4 inducers (eg, barbiturates, carbamazepine, efavirenz, glucocorticoids, modafinil, nevirapine, oxcarbazepine, phenobarbital, phenytoin, pioglitazone, rifabutin, rifampin, St. John's wort, or troglitazone) may result in a decrease fentanyl plasma concentrations). Products include:
Provigil 983

Molindone Hydrochloride (The concomitant use of fentanyl with other CNS depressants, including other opioids, sedatives or hypnotics, general anesthetics, phenothizines, tranquilizers, skeletal muscle relaxants, sedating antihistamines, and alcoholic beverages may produce increased depressant effects. Patients on concomitant CNS depressants must be monitored for a change in opioid effects. Consideration should be given to adjusting the dose of fentanyl if warranted). Products include:
Moban 1108

Morphine Sulfate (The concomitant use of fentanyl with other CNS depressants, including other opioids, sedatives or hypnotics, general anesthetics, phenothizines, tranquilizers, skeletal muscle relaxants, sedating antihistamines, and alcoholic beverages may produce increased depressant effects. Patients on concomitant CNS depressants must be monitored for a change in opioid effects. Consideration should be given to adjusting the dose of fentanyl if warranted). Products include:
Avinza 1822
Embeda 1831
MS Contin 2803

Morphine Sulfate, Liposomal (The concomitant use of fentanyl with other CNS depressants, including other opioids, sedatives or hypnotics, general anesthetics, phenothizines, tranquilizers, skeletal muscle relaxants, sedating antihistamines, and alcoholic beverages may produce increased depressant effects. Patients on concomitant CNS depressants must be monitored for a change in opioid effects. Consideration should be given to adjusting the dose of fentanyl if warranted).
No products indexed under this heading.

Nafcillin Sodium (The concomitant use of fentanyl with CYP3A4 inducers (eg, barbiturates, carbamazepine, efavirenz, glucocorticoids, modafinil, nevirapine, oxcarbazepine, phenobarbital, phenytoin, pioglitazone, rifabutin, rifampin, St. John's wort, or troglitazone) may result in a decrease fentanyl plasma concentrations).
No products indexed under this heading.

Nefazodone Hydrochloride (The concomitant use of fentanyl with CYP3A4 inhibitors (eg, indinavir, nelfinavir, ritonavir, clarithromycin, itraconazole, ketoconazole, nefazodone, saquinavir, telithromycin, aprepitant, diltiazem, erythromycin, fluconazole, grapefruit juice, verapamil, or cimetidine) may result in a potentially dangerous increase in fentanyl plasma concentrations).
No products indexed under this heading.

Nelfinavir Mesylate (The concomitant use of fentanyl with CYP3A4 inhibitors (eg, indinavir, nelfinavir, ritonavir, clarithromycin, itraconazole, ketoconazole, nefazodone, saquinavir, telithromycin, aprepitant, diltiazem, erythromycin, fluconazole, grapefruit juice, verapamil, or cimetidine) may result in a potentially dangerous increase in fentanyl plasma concentrations).
No products indexed under this heading.

Nevirapine (The concomitant use of fentanyl with CYP3A4 inducers (eg, barbiturates, carbamazepine, efavirenz, glucocorticoids, modafinil, nevirapine, oxcarbazepine, phenobarbital, phenytoin, pioglitazone, rifabutin, rifampin, St. John's wort, or troglitazone) may result in a decrease fentanyl plasma concentrations). Products include:
Viramune Oral Suspension 897
Viramune Tablets 897

Niacin (The concomitant use of fentanyl with CYP3A4 inhibitors (eg, indinavir, nelfinavir, ritonavir, clarithromycin, itraconazole, ketoconazole, nefazodone, saquinavir, telithromycin, aprepitant, diltiazem, erythromycin, fluconazole, grapefruit juice, verapamil, or cimetidine) may result in a potentially dangerous increase in fentanyl plasma concentrations). Products include:
Advicor 402
Cardio Basics 3455
Niaspan 497
Simcor 524

Niacinamide (The concomitant use of fentanyl with CYP3A4 inhibitors (eg, indinavir, nelfinavir, ritonavir, clarithromycin, itraconazole, ketoconazole, nefazodone, saquinavir, telithromycin, aprepitant, diltiazem, erythromycin, fluconazole, grapefruit juice, verapamil, or cimetidine) may result in a potentially dangerous increase in fentanyl plasma concentrations). Products include:
CitraNatal 90 DHA Capsules 2332
CitraNatal Assure 2332
CitraNatal Rx 2332
Heplive 607

Niacinamide Hydroiodide (The concomitant use of fentanyl with CYP3A4 inhibitors (eg, indinavir, nelfinavir, ritonavir, clarithromycin, itraconazole, ketoconazole, nefazodone, saquinavir, telithromycin, aprepitant, diltiazem, erythromycin, fluconazole, grapefruit juice, verapamil, or cimetidine) may result in a potentially dangerous increase in fentanyl plasma concentrations).
No products indexed under this heading.

Nicotinamide (The concomitant use of fentanyl with CYP3A4 inhibitors (eg, indinavir, nelfinavir, ritonavir, clarithromycin, itraconazole, ketoconazole, nefazodone, saquinavir, telithromycin, aprepitant, diltiazem, erythromycin, fluconazole, grapefruit juice, verapamil, or cimetidine) may result in a potentially dangerous increase in fentanyl plasma concentrations).
No products indexed under this heading.

Nifedipine (The concomitant use of fentanyl with CYP3A4 inhibitors (eg, indinavir, nelfinavir, ritonavir, clarithromycin, itraconazole, ketoconazole, nefazodone, saquinavir, telithromycin, aprepitant, diltiazem, erythromycin, fluconazole, grapefruit juice, verapamil, or cimetidine) may result in a potentially dangerous increase in fentanyl plasma concentrations).
No products indexed under this heading.

Nitrous Oxide (The concomitant use of fentanyl with other CNS depressants, including other opioids, sedatives or hypnotics, general anesthetics, phenothiazines, tranquilizers, skeletal muscle relaxants, sedating antihistamines, and alcoholic beverages may produce increased depressant effects).
No products indexed under this heading.

Norfloxacin (The concomitant use of fentanyl with CYP3A4 inhibitors (eg, indinavir, nelfinavir, ritonavir, clarithromycin, itraconazole, ketoconazole, nefazodone, saquinavir, telithromycin, aprepitant, diltiazem, erythromycin, fluconazole, grapefruit juice, verapamil, or cimetidine) may result in a potentially dangerous increase in fentanyl plasma concentrations). Products include:
Noroxin 2220

Olanzapine (The concomitant use of fentanyl with other CNS depressants, including other opioids, sedatives or hypnotics, general anesthetics, phenothizines, tranquilizers, skeletal muscle relaxants, sedating antihistamines, and alcoholic beverages may produce increased depressant effects. Patients on concomitant CNS depressants must be monitored for a change in opioid effects. Consideration should be given to adjusting the dose of fentanyl if warranted). Products include:
Symbyax 1965
Zyprexa 1984
Zyprexa IntraMuscular 1984
Zyprexa ZYDIS 1984

Omeprazole (The concomitant use of fentanyl with CYP3A4 inhibitors (eg, indinavir, nelfinavir, ritonavir, clarithromycin, itraconazole, ketoconazole, nefazodone, saquinavir, telithromycin, aprepitant, diltiazem, erythromycin, fluconazole, grapefruit juice, verapamil, or cimetidine) may result in a potentially dangerous increase in fentanyl plasma concentrations).
No products indexed under this heading.

Orphenadrine Citrate (The concomitant use of fentanyl with other CNS depressants, including other opioids, sedatives or hypnotics, general anesthetics, phenothiazines, tranquilizers, skeletal muscle relaxants, sedating antihistamines, and alcoholic beverages may produce increased depressant effects).
No products indexed under this heading.

Oxazepam (The concomitant use of fentanyl with other CNS depressants, including other opioids, sedatives or hypnotics, general anesthetics, phenothizines, tranquilizers, skeletal muscle relaxants, sedating antihistamines, and alcoholic beverages may produce increased depressant effects. Patients on concomitant CNS depressants must be monitored for a change in opioid effects. Consideration should be given to adjusting the dose of fentanyl if warranted).
No products indexed under this heading.

Oxcarbazepine (The concomitant use of fentanyl with CYP3A4 inducers (eg, barbiturates, carbamazepine, efavirenz, glucocorticoids, modafinil, nevirapine, oxcarbazepine, phenobarbital, phenytoin, pioglitazone, rifabutin, rifampin, St. John's wort, or troglitazone) may result in a decrease fentanyl plasma concentrations).
No products indexed under this heading.

Oxycodone Hydrochloride (The concomitant use of fentanyl with other CNS depressants, including other opioids, sedatives or hypnotics, general anesthetics, phenothizines, tranquilizers, skeletal muscle relaxants, sedating antihistamines, and alcoholic beverages may produce increased depressant effects. Patients on concomitant CNS depressants must be monitored for a

IMPORTANT NOTE: Always consult each drug listing in the patient's regimen for possible interactions.

change in opioid effects. Consideration should be given to adjusting the dose of fentanyl if warranted). Products include:
OxyContin 2807
Percocet 1121
Percodan 1124

Oxycodone Terephthalate (The concomitant use of fentanyl with other CNS depressants, including other opioids, sedatives or hypnotics, general anesthetics, phenothizines, tranquilizers, skeletal muscle relaxants, sedating antihistamines, and alcoholic beverages may produce increased depressant effects. Patients on concomitant CNS depressants must be monitored for a change in opioid effects. Consideration should be given to adjusting the dose of fentanyl if warranted).
No products indexed under this heading.

Oxymorphone Hydrochloride (The concomitant use of fentanyl with other CNS depressants, including other opioids, sedatives or hypnotics, general anesthetics, phenothizines, tranquilizers, skeletal muscle relaxants, sedating antihistamines, and alcoholic beverages may produce increased depressant effects. Patients on concomitant CNS depressants must be monitored for a change in opioid effects. Consideration should be given to adjusting the dose of fentanyl if warranted). Products include:
Opana 1110
Opana ER 1114

Pancuronium Bromide (The concomitant use of fentanyl with other CNS depressants, including other opioids, sedatives or hypnotics, general anesthetics, phenothiazines, tranquilizers, skeletal muscle relaxants, sedating antihistamines, and alcoholic beverages may produce increased depressant effects).
No products indexed under this heading.

Pargyline Hydrochloride (Fentanyl is not recommended in patients who have received MAO inhibitors within 14 days because severe and unpredictable potentiation by MAO inhibitors has been reported with opioid analgesics).
No products indexed under this heading.

Paroxetine Hydrochloride (The concomitant use of fentanyl with CYP3A4 inhibitors (eg, indinavir, nelfinavir, ritonavir, clarithromycin, itraconazole, ketoconazole, nefazodone, saquinavir, telithromycin, aprepitant, diltiazem, erythromycin, fluconazole, grapefruit juice, verapamil, or cimetidine) may result in a potentially dangerous increase in fentanyl plasma concentrations). Products include:
Paroxetine CR 2361
Paroxetine ER 2371
Paxil 1586
Paxil CR 1596

Pentobarbital (The concomitant use of fentanyl with other CNS depressants, including other opioids, sedatives or hypnotics, general anesthetics, phenothizines, tranquilizers, skeletal muscle relaxants, sedating antihistamines, and alcoholic beverages may produce increased depressant effects. Patients on concomitant CNS depressants must be monitored for a change in opioid effects. Consideration should be given to adjusting the dose of fentanyl if warranted).
No products indexed under this heading.

Pentobarbital Sodium (The concomitant use of fentanyl with other CNS depressants, including other opioids, sedatives or hypnotics, general anesthetics, phenothizines, tranquilizers, skeletal muscle relaxants, sedating antihistamines, and alcoholic beverages may produce increased depressant effects. Patients on concomitant CNS depressants must be monitored for a change in opioid effects. Consideration should be given to adjusting the dose of fentanyl if warranted). Products include:
Nembutal 2012

Perphenazine (The concomitant use of fentanyl with other CNS depressants, including other opioids, sedatives or hypnotics, general anesthetics, phenothizines, tranquilizers, skeletal muscle relaxants, sedating antihistamines, and alcoholic beverages may produce increased depressant effects. Patients on concomitant CNS depressants must be monitored for a change in opioid effects. Consideration should be given to adjusting the dose of fentanyl if warranted).
No products indexed under this heading.

Phenelzine Sulfate (Fentanyl is not recommended in patients who have received MAO inhibitors within 14 days because severe and unpredictable potentiation by MAO inhibitors has been reported with opioid analgesics).
No products indexed under this heading.

Phenobarbital (The concomitant use of fentanyl with other CNS depressants, including other opioids, sedatives or hypnotics, general anesthetics, phenothizines, tranquilizers, skeletal muscle relaxants, sedating antihistamines, and alcoholic beverages may produce increased depressant effects. Patients on concomitant CNS depressants must be monitored for a change in opioid effects. Consideration should be given to adjusting the dose of fentanyl if warranted). Products include:
Donnatal 2711

Phenobarbital Sodium (The concomitant use of fentanyl with other CNS depressants, including other opioids, sedatives or hypnotics, general anesthetics, phenothizines, tranquilizers, skeletal muscle relaxants, sedating antihistamines, and alcoholic beverages may produce increased depressant effects. Patients on concomitant CNS depressants must be monitored for a change in opioid effects. Consideration should be given to adjusting the dose of fentanyl if warranted).
No products indexed under this heading.

Phenothiazine Derivatives (The concomitant use of fentanyl with other CNS depressants, including other opioids, sedatives or hypnotics, general anesthetics, phenothiazines, tranquilizers, skeletal muscle relaxants, sedating antihistamines, and alcoholic beverages may produce increased depressant effects).
No products indexed under this heading.

Phenothiazines (The concomitant use of fentanyl with other CNS depressants, including other opioids, sedatives or hypnotics, general anesthetics, phenothiazines, tranquilizers, skeletal muscle relaxants, sedating antihistamines, and alcoholic beverages may produce increased depressant effects).
No products indexed under this heading.

Phenytoin (The concomitant use of fentanyl with CYP3A4 inducers (eg, barbiturates, carbamazepine, efavirenz, glucocorticoids, modafinil, nevirapine, oxcarbazepine, phenobarbital, phenytoin, pioglitazone, rifabutin, rifampin, St. John's wort, or troglitazone) may result in a decrease fentanyl plasma concentrations).
No products indexed under this heading.

Phenytoin Sodium (The concomitant use of fentanyl with CYP3A4 inducers (eg, barbiturates, carbamazepine, efavirenz, glucocorticoids, modafinil, nevirapine, oxcarbazepine, phenobarbital, phenytoin, pioglitazone, rifabutin, rifampin, St. John's wort, or troglitazone) may result in a decrease fentanyl plasma concentrations). Products include:
Phenytek Capsules 2380

Pipecuronium Bromide (The concomitant use of fentanyl with other CNS depressants, including other opioids, sedatives or hypnotics, general anesthetics, phenothizines, tranquilizers, skeletal muscle relaxants, sedating antihistamines, and alcoholic beverages may produce increased depressant effects).
No products indexed under this heading.

Posaconazole (The concomitant use of fentanyl with CYP3A4 inhibitors (eg, indinavir, nelfinavir, ritonavir, clarithromycin, itraconazole, ketoconazole, nefazodone, saquinavir, telithromycin, aprepitant, diltiazem, erythromycin, fluconazole, grapefruit juice, verapamil, or cimetidine) may result in a potentially dangerous increase in fentanyl plasma concentrations). Products include:
Noxafil 3172

Prazepam (The concomitant use of fentanyl with other CNS depressants, including other opioids, sedatives or hypnotics, general anesthetics, phenothizines, tranquilizers, skeletal muscle relaxants, sedating antihistamines, and alcoholic beverages may produce increased depressant effects. Patients on concomitant CNS depressants must be monitored for a change in opioid effects. Consideration should be given to adjusting the dose of fentanyl if warranted).
No products indexed under this heading.

Prednisolone (The concomitant use of fentanyl with CYP3A4 inducers (eg, barbiturates, carbamazepine, efavirenz, glucocorticoids, modafinil, nevirapine, oxcarbazepine, phenobarbital, phenytoin, pioglitazone, rifabutin, rifampin, St. John's wort, or troglitazone) may result in a decrease fentanyl plasma concentrations).
No products indexed under this heading.

Prednisolone Acetate (The concomitant use of fentanyl with CYP3A4 inducers (eg, barbiturates, carbamazepine, efavirenz, glucocorticoids, modafinil, nevirapine, oxcarbazepine, phenobarbital, phenytoin, pioglitazone, rifabutin, rifampin, St. John's wort, or troglitazone) may result in a decrease fentanyl plasma concentrations). Products include:
Blephamide .... ⊙212, ⊙214
Pred Forte .... ⊙225
Pred Mild .... ⊙230
Pred-G .... ⊙226, ⊙227

Prednisolone Sodium Phosphate (The concomitant use of fentanyl with CYP3A4 inducers (eg, barbiturates, carbamazepine, efavirenz, glucocorticoids, modafinil, nevirapine, oxcarbazepine, phenobarbital, phenytoin, pioglitazone, rifabutin, rifampin, St. John's wort, or troglitazone) may result in a decrease fentanyl plasma concentrations).
No products indexed under this heading.

Prednisolone Tebutate (The concomitant use of fentanyl with CYP3A4 inducers (eg, barbiturates, carbamazepine, efavirenz, glucocorticoids, modafinil, nevirapine, oxcarbazepine, phenobarbital, phenytoin, pioglitazone, rifabutin, rifampin, St. John's wort, or troglitazone) may result in a decrease fentanyl plasma concentrations).
No products indexed under this heading.

Prednisone (The concomitant use of fentanyl with CYP3A4 inducers (eg, barbiturates, carbamazepine, efavirenz, glucocorticoids, modafinil, nevirapine, oxcarbazepine, phenobarbital, phenytoin, pioglitazone, rifabutin, rifampin, St. John's wort, or troglitazone) may result in a decrease fentanyl plasma concentrations).
No products indexed under this heading.

Prednisone sodium phosphate (The concomitant use of fentanyl with CYP3A4 inducers (eg, barbiturates, carbamazepine, efavirenz, glucocorticoids, modafinil, nevirapine, oxcarbazepine, phenobarbital, phenytoin, pioglitazone, rifabutin, rifampin, St. John's wort, or troglitazone) may result in a decrease fentanyl plasma concentrations).
No products indexed under this heading.

Primidone (The concomitant use of fentanyl with CYP3A4 inducers (eg, barbiturates, carbamazepine, efavirenz, glucocorticoids, modafinil, nevirapine, oxcarbazepine, phenobarbital, phenytoin, pioglitazone, rifabutin, rifampin, St. John's wort, or troglitazone) may result in a decrease fentanyl plasma concentrations).
No products indexed under this heading.

Procarbazine Hydrochloride (Fentanyl is not recommended in patients who have received MAO inhibitors within 14 days because severe and unpredictable potentiation by MAO inhibitors has been reported with opioid analgesics).
No products indexed under this heading.

Prochlorperazine (The concomitant use of fentanyl with other CNS depressants, including other opioids, sedatives or hypnotics, general anesthetics, phenothizines, tranquilizers, skeletal muscle relaxants, sedating antihistamines, and alcoholic beverages may produce increased depressant effects. Patients on concomitant CNS depressants must be monitored for a change in opioid effects. Consideration should be given to adjusting the dose of fentanyl if warranted).
No products indexed under this heading.

Prochlorperazine Edisylate (The concomitant use of fentanyl with other CNS depressants, including other opioids, sedatives or hypnotics, general anesthetics, phenothizines, tranquilizers, skeletal muscle relaxants, sedating antihistamines, and alcoholic beverages may produce increased depressant effects. Patients on concomitant CNS depressants must be monitored for a change in opioid effects. Consideration should be given to adjusting the dose of fentanyl if warranted).
No products indexed under this heading.

Prochlorperazine Maleate (The concomitant use of fentanyl with other CNS depressants, including other opioids, sedatives or hypnotics, general anesthetics, phenothizines, tranquilizers, skeletal muscle relaxants, sedating antihistamines, and alcoholic beverages may produce increased depressant effects. Patients on concomitant CNS depressants must be monitored for a change in opioid effects. Consideration should be given to adjusting the dose of fentanyl if warranted).
No products indexed under this heading.

Promethazine (The concomitant use of fentanyl with other CNS depressants, including other opioids, sedatives or hypnotics, general anesthetics, phenothizines, tranquilizers, skeletal muscle relaxants, sedating antihistamines, and alcoholic beverages may produce increased depressant effects. Patients on concomitant CNS depressants must be monitored for a change in opioid effects. Consideration should be given to adjusting the dose of fentanyl if warranted).
No products indexed under this heading.

Promethazine Hydrochloride (The concomitant use of fentanyl with other CNS depressants, including other opioids, sedatives or hypnotics, general anesthetics, phenothizines, tranquilizers, skeletal muscle relaxants, sedating antihistamines, and alcoholic beverages may produce increased depressant

effects. Patients on concomitant CNS depressants must be monitored for a change in opioid effects. Consideration should be given to adjusting the dose of fentanyl if warranted).
No products indexed under this heading.

Propofol (The concomitant use of fentanyl with other CNS depressants, including other opioids, sedatives or hypnotics, general anesthetics, phenothizines, tranquilizers, skeletal muscle relaxants, sedating antihistamines, and alcoholic beverages may produce increased depressant effects. Patients on concomitant CNS depressants must be monitored for a change in opioid effects. Consideration should be given to adjusting the dose of fentanyl if warranted).
No products indexed under this heading.

Propoxyphene Hydrochloride (The concomitant use of fentanyl with other CNS depressants, including other opioids, sedatives or hypnotics, general anesthetics, phenothizines, tranquilizers, skeletal muscle relaxants, sedating antihistamines, and alcoholic beverages may produce increased depressant effects. Patients on concomitant CNS depressants must be monitored for a change in opioid effects. Consideration should be given to adjusting the dose of fentanyl if warranted).
No products indexed under this heading.

Propoxyphene Napsylate (The concomitant use of fentanyl with other CNS depressants, including other opioids, sedatives or hypnotics, general anesthetics, phenothizines, tranquilizers, skeletal muscle relaxants, sedating antihistamines, and alcoholic beverages may produce increased depressant effects. Patients on concomitant CNS depressants must be monitored for a change in opioid effects. Consideration should be given to adjusting the dose of fentanyl if warranted).
No products indexed under this heading.

Pyrilamine Maleate (The concomitant use of fentanyl with other CNS depressants, including other opioids, sedatives or hypnotics, general anesthetics, phenothiazines, tranquilizers, skeletal muscle relaxants, sedating antihistamines, and alcoholic beverages may produce increased depressant effects).
No products indexed under this heading.

Pyrilamine Tannate (The concomitant use of fentanyl with other CNS depressants, including other opioids, sedatives or hypnotics, general anesthetics, phenothiazines, tranquilizers, skeletal muscle relaxants, sedating antihistamines, and alcoholic beverages may produce increased depressant effects).
No products indexed under this heading.

Quazepam (The concomitant use of fentanyl with other CNS depressants, including other opioids, sedatives or hypnotics, general anesthetics, phenothizines, tranquilizers, skeletal muscle relaxants, sedating antihistamines, and alcoholic beverages may produce increased depressant effects. Patients on concomitant CNS depressants must be monitored for a change in opioid effects. Consideration should be given to adjusting the dose of fentanyl if warranted).
No products indexed under this heading.

Quetiapine Fumarate (The concomitant use of fentanyl with other CNS depressants, including other opioids, sedatives or hypnotics, general anesthetics, phenothizines, tranquilizers, skeletal muscle relaxants, sedating antihistamines, and alcoholic beverages may produce increased depressant effects. Patients on concomitant CNS depressants must be monitored for a change in opioid effects. Consideration should be given to adjusting the dose of fentanyl if warranted). Products include:
Seroquel **750**
Seroquel XR **759**

Quinidine (The concomitant use of fentanyl with CYP3A4 inhibitors (eg, indinavir, nelfinavir, ritonavir, clarithromycin, itraconazole, ketoconazole, nefazodone, saquinavir, telithromycin, aprepitant, diltiazem, erythromycin, fluconazole, grapefruit juice, verapamil, or cimetidine) may result in a potentially dangerous increase in fentanyl plasma concentrations).
No products indexed under this heading.

Quinidine Hydrochloride (The concomitant use of fentanyl with CYP3A4 inhibitors (eg, indinavir, nelfinavir, ritonavir, clarithromycin, itraconazole, ketoconazole, nefazodone, saquinavir, telithromycin, aprepitant, diltiazem, erythromycin, fluconazole, grapefruit juice, verapamil, or cimetidine) may result in a potentially dangerous increase in fentanyl plasma concentrations).
No products indexed under this heading.

Quinidine Polygalacturonate (The concomitant use of fentanyl with CYP3A4 inhibitors (eg, indinavir, nelfinavir, ritonavir, clarithromycin, itraconazole, ketoconazole, nefazodone, saquinavir, telithromycin, aprepitant, diltiazem, erythromycin, fluconazole, grapefruit juice, verapamil, or cimetidine) may result in a potentially dangerous increase in fentanyl plasma concentrations).
No products indexed under this heading.

Quinidine Sulfate (The concomitant use of fentanyl with CYP3A4 inhibitors (eg, indinavir, nelfinavir, ritonavir, clarithromycin, itraconazole, ketoconazole, nefazodone, saquinavir, telithromycin, aprepitant, diltiazem, erythromycin, fluconazole, grapefruit juice, verapamil, or cimetidine) may result in a potentially dangerous increase in fentanyl plasma concentrations).
No products indexed under this heading.

Quinine (The concomitant use of fentanyl with CYP3A4 inhibitors (eg, indinavir, nelfinavir, ritonavir, clarithromycin, itraconazole, ketoconazole, nefazodone, saquinavir, telithromycin, aprepitant, diltiazem, erythromycin, fluconazole, grapefruit juice, verapamil, or cimetidine) may result in a potentially dangerous increase in fentanyl plasma concentrations). Products include:
Hyland's Leg Cramps PM with Quinine **3315**

Quinine Sulfate (The concomitant use of fentanyl with CYP3A4 inhibitors (eg, indinavir, nelfinavir, ritonavir, clarithromycin, itraconazole, ketoconazole, nefazodone, saquinavir, telithromycin, aprepitant, diltiazem, erythromycin, fluconazole, grapefruit juice, verapamil, or cimetidine) may result in a potentially dangerous increase in fentanyl plasma concentrations).
No products indexed under this heading.

Quinupristin (The concomitant use of fentanyl with CYP3A4 inhibitors (eg, indinavir, nelfinavir, ritonavir, clarithromycin, itraconazole, ketoconazole, nefazodone, saquinavir, telithromycin, aprepitant, diltiazem, erythromycin, fluconazole, grapefruit juice, verapamil, or cimetidine) may result in a potentially dangerous increase in fentanyl plasma concentrations).
No products indexed under this heading.

Ramelteon (The concomitant use of fentanyl with other CNS depressants, including other opioids, sedatives or hypnotics, general anesthetics, phenothiazines, tranquilizers, skeletal muscle relaxants, sedating antihistamines, and alcoholic beverages may produce increased depressant effects). Products include:
Rozerem **3366**

Ranitidine Bismuth Citrate (The concomitant use of fentanyl with CYP3A4 inhibitors (eg, indinavir, nelfinavir, ritonavir, clarithromycin, itraconazole, ketoconazole, nefazodone, saquinavir, telithromycin, aprepitant, diltiazem, erythromycin, fluconazole, grapefruit juice, verapamil, or cimetidine) may result in a potentially dangerous increase in fentanyl plasma concentrations).
No products indexed under this heading.

Ranitidine Hydrochloride (The concomitant use of fentanyl with CYP3A4 inhibitors (eg, indinavir, nelfinavir, ritonavir, clarithromycin, itraconazole, ketoconazole, nefazodone, saquinavir, telithromycin, aprepitant, diltiazem, erythromycin, fluconazole, grapefruit juice, verapamil, or cimetidine) may result in a potentially dangerous increase in fentanyl plasma concentrations). Products include:
Zantac **1737**
Zantac Injection **1732**
Zantac Pharmacy **1735**

Rapacuronium Bromide (The concomitant use of fentanyl with other CNS depressants, including other opioids, sedatives or hypnotics, general anesthetics, phenothiazines, tranquilizers, skeletal muscle relaxants, sedating antihistamines, and alcoholic beverages may produce increased depressant effects).
No products indexed under this heading.

Rasagiline Mesylate (Fentanyl is not recommended in patients who have received MAO inhibitors within 14 days because severe and unpredictable potentiation by MAO inhibitors has been reported with opioid analgesics). Products include:
Azilect **3383**

Remifentanil Hydrochloride (The concomitant use of fentanyl with other CNS depressants, including other opioids, sedatives or hypnotics, general anesthetics, phenothizines, tranquilizers, skeletal muscle relaxants, sedating antihistamines, and alcoholic beverages may produce increased depressant effects. Patients on concomitant CNS depressants must be monitored for a change in opioid effects. Consideration should be given to adjusting the dose of fentanyl if warranted).
No products indexed under this heading.

Rifabutin (The concomitant use of fentanyl with CYP3A4 inducers (eg, barbiturates, carbamazepine, efavirenz, glucocorticoids, modafinil, nevirapine, oxcarbazepine, phenobarbital, phenytoin, pioglitazone, rifabutin, rifampin, St. John's wort, or troglitazone) may result in a decrease fentanyl plasma concentrations).
No products indexed under this heading.

Rifampicin (The concomitant use of fentanyl with CYP3A4 inducers (eg, barbiturates, carbamazepine, efavirenz, glucocorticoids, modafinil, nevirapine, oxcarbazepine, phenobarbital, phenytoin, pioglitazone, rifabutin, rifampin, St. John's wort, or troglitazone) may result in a decrease fentanyl plasma concentrations).
No products indexed under this heading.

Rifampin (The concomitant use of fentanyl with CYP3A4 inducers (eg, barbiturates, carbamazepine, efavirenz, glucocorticoids, modafinil, nevirapine, oxcarbazepine, phenobarbital, phenytoin, pioglitazone, rifabutin, rifampin, St. John's wort, or troglitazone) may result in a decrease fentanyl plasma concentrations).
No products indexed under this heading.

Rifapentine (The concomitant use of fentanyl with CYP3A4 inducers (eg, barbiturates, carbamazepine, efavirenz, glucocorticoids, modafinil, nevirapine, oxcarbazepine, phenobarbital, phenytoin, pioglitazone, rifabutin, rifampin, St. John's wort, or troglitazone) may result in a decrease fentanyl plasma concentrations).
No products indexed under this heading.

Risperidone (The concomitant use of fentanyl with other CNS depressants, including other opioids, sedatives or hypnotics, general anesthetics, phenothizines, tranquilizers, skeletal muscle relaxants, sedating antihistamines, and alcoholic beverages may produce increased depressant effects. Patients on concomitant CNS depressants must be monitored for a change in opioid effects. Consideration should be given to adjusting the dose of fentanyl if warranted). Products include:
Risperdal Consta **2682**

Ritonavir (The concomitant use of fentanyl with CYP3A4 inhibitors (eg, indinavir, nelfinavir, ritonavir, clarithromycin, itraconazole, ketoconazole, nefazodone, saquinavir, telithromycin, aprepitant, diltiazem, erythromycin, fluconazole, grapefruit juice, verapamil, or cimetidine) may result in a potentially dangerous increase in fentanyl plasma concentrations). Products include:
Kaletra **458**
Norvir **509**

Rocuronium Bromide (The concomitant use of fentanyl with other CNS depressants, including other opioids, sedatives or hypnotics, general anesthetics, phenothiazines, tranquilizers, skeletal muscle relaxants, sedating antihistamines, and alcoholic beverages may produce increased depressant effects). Products include:
Zemuron **3249**

Saquinavir (The concomitant use of fentanyl with CYP3A4 inhibitors (eg, indinavir, nelfinavir, ritonavir, clarithromycin, itraconazole, ketoconazole, nefazodone, saquinavir, telithromycin, aprepitant, diltiazem, erythromycin, fluconazole, grapefruit juice, verapamil, or cimetidine) may result in a potentially dangerous increase in fentanyl plasma concentrations).
No products indexed under this heading.

Saquinavir Mesylate (The concomitant use of fentanyl with CYP3A4 inhibitors (eg, indinavir, nelfinavir, ritonavir, clarithromycin, itraconazole, ketoconazole, nefazodone, saquinavir, telithromycin, aprepitant, diltiazem, erythromycin, fluconazole, grapefruit juice, verapamil, or cimetidine) may result in a potentially dangerous increase in fentanyl plasma concentrations).
No products indexed under this heading.

Secobarbital Sodium (The concomitant use of fentanyl with other CNS depressants, including other opioids, sedatives or hypnotics, general anesthetics, phenothizines, tranquilizers, skeletal muscle relaxants, sedating antihistamines, and alcoholic beverages may produce increased depressant effects. Patients on concomitant CNS depressants must be monitored for a change in opioid effects. Consideration should be given to adjusting the dose of fentanyl if warranted).
No products indexed under this heading.

Selegiline (Fentanyl is not recommended in patients who have received MAO inhibitors within 14 days because severe and unpredictable potentiation by MAO inhibitors has been reported with opioid analgesics). Products include:
Emsam **3623**

Selegiline Hydrochloride (Fentanyl is not recommended in patients who

have received MAO inhibitors within 14 days because severe and unpredictable potentiation by MAO inhibitors has been reported with opioid analgesics). Products include:
Eldepryl 3312

Sertraline Hydrochloride (The concomitant use of fentanyl with CYP3A4 inhibitors (eg, indinavir, nelfinavir, ritonavir, clarithromycin, itraconazole, ketoconazole, nefazodone, saquinavir, telithromycin, aprepitant, diltiazem, erythromycin, fluconazole, grapefruit juice, verapamil, or cimetidine) may result in a potentially dangerous increase in fentanyl plasma concentrations).
No products indexed under this heading.

Sevoflurane (The concomitant use of fentanyl with other CNS depressants, including other opioids, sedatives or hypnotics, general anesthetics, phenothizines, tranquilizers, skeletal muscle relaxants, sedating antihistamines, and alcoholic beverages may produce increased depressant effects. Patients on concomitant CNS depressants must be monitored for a change in opioid effects. Consideration should be given to adjusting the dose of fentanyl if warranted). Products include:
Ultane 554

Sildenafil Citrate (The concomitant use of fentanyl with CYP3A4 inhibitors (eg, indinavir, nelfinavir, ritonavir, clarithromycin, itraconazole, ketoconazole, nefazodone, saquinavir, telithromycin, aprepitant, diltiazem, erythromycin, fluconazole, grapefruit juice, verapamil, or cimetidine) may result in a potentially dangerous increase in fentanyl plasma concentrations).
No products indexed under this heading.

Sodium Butabarbital (The concomitant use of fentanyl with other CNS depressants, including other opioids, sedatives or hypnotics, general anesthetics, phenothizines, tranquilizers, skeletal muscle relaxants, sedating antihistamines, and alcoholic beverages may produce increased depressant effects. Patients on concomitant CNS depressants must be monitored for a change in opioid effects. Consideration should be given to adjusting the dose of fentanyl if warranted).
No products indexed under this heading.

Sodium Oxybate (The concomitant use of fentanyl with other CNS depressants, including other opioids, sedatives or hypnotics, general anesthetics, phenothizines, tranquilizers, skeletal muscle relaxants, sedating antihistamines, and alcoholic beverages may produce increased depressant effects. Patients on concomitant CNS depressants must be monitored for a change in opioid effects. Consideration should be given to adjusting the dose of fentanyl if warranted).
No products indexed under this heading.

Sodium Pentobarbital (The concomitant use of fentanyl with other CNS depressants, including other opioids, sedatives or hypnotics, general anesthetics, phenothizines, tranquilizers, skeletal muscle relaxants, sedating antihistamines, and alcoholic beverages may produce increased depressant effects. Patients on concomitant CNS depressants must be monitored for a change in opioid effects. Consideration should be given to adjusting the dose of fentanyl if warranted).
No products indexed under this heading.

Succinylcholine Chloride (The concomitant use of fentanyl with other CNS depressants, including other opioids, sedatives or hypnotics, general anesthetics, phenothiazines, tranquilizers, skeletal muscle relaxants, sedating antihistamines, and alcoholic beverages may produce increased depressant effects).
No products indexed under this heading.

Sufentanil Citrate (The concomitant use of fentanyl with other CNS depressants, including other opioids, sedatives or hypnotics, general anesthetics, phenothizines, tranquilizers, skeletal muscle relaxants, sedating antihistamines, and alcoholic beverages may produce increased depressant effects. Patients on concomitant CNS depressants must be monitored for a change in opioid effects. Consideration should be given to adjusting the dose of fentanyl if warranted).
No products indexed under this heading.

Sulfinpyrazone (The concomitant use of fentanyl with CYP3A4 inducers (eg, barbiturates, carbamazepine, efavirenz, glucocorticoids, modafinil, nevirapine, oxcarbazepine, phenobarbital, phenytoin, pioglitazone, rifabutin, rifampin, St. John's wort, or troglitazone) may result in a decrease fentanyl plasma concentrations).
No products indexed under this heading.

Talbutal (The concomitant use of fentanyl with other CNS depressants, including other opioids, sedatives or hypnotics, general anesthetics, phenothizines, tranquilizers, skeletal muscle relaxants, sedating antihistamines, and alcoholic beverages may produce increased depressant effects. Patients on concomitant CNS depressants must be monitored for a change in opioid effects. Consideration should be given to adjusting the dose of fentanyl if warranted).
No products indexed under this heading.

Telithromycin (The concomitant use of fentanyl with CYP3A4 inhibitors (eg, indinavir, nelfinavir, ritonavir, clarithromycin, itraconazole, ketoconazole, nefazodone, saquinavir, telithromycin, aprepitant, diltiazem, erythromycin, fluconazole, grapefruit juice, verapamil, or cimetidine) may result in a potentially dangerous increase in fentanyl plasma concentrations). Products include:
Ketek 2991

Temazepam (The concomitant use of fentanyl with other CNS depressants, including other opioids, sedatives or hypnotics, general anesthetics, phenothizines, tranquilizers, skeletal muscle relaxants, sedating antihistamines, and alcoholic beverages may produce increased depressant effects. Patients on concomitant CNS depressants must be monitored for a change in opioid effects. Consideration should be given to adjusting the dose of fentanyl if warranted).
No products indexed under this heading.

Theophyllinate (The concomitant use of fentanyl with CYP3A4 inducers (eg, barbiturates, carbamazepine, efavirenz, glucocorticoids, modafinil, nevirapine, oxcarbazepine, phenobarbital, phenytoin, pioglitazone, rifabutin, rifampin, St. John's wort, or troglitazone) may result in a decrease fentanyl plasma concentrations).
No products indexed under this heading.

Theophylline (The concomitant use of fentanyl with CYP3A4 inducers (eg, barbiturates, carbamazepine, efavirenz, glucocorticoids, modafinil, nevirapine, oxcarbazepine, phenobarbital, phenytoin, pioglitazone, rifabutin, rifampin, St. John's wort, or troglitazone) may result in a decrease fentanyl plasma concentrations).
No products indexed under this heading.

Theophylline Anhydrous (The concomitant use of fentanyl with CYP3A4 inducers (eg, barbiturates, carbamazepine, efavirenz, glucocorticoids, modafinil, nevirapine, oxcarbazepine, phenobarbital, phenytoin, pioglitazone, rifabutin, rifampin, St. John's wort, or troglitazone) may result in a decrease fentanyl plasma concentrations). Products include:
Uniphyl 2817

Theophylline Calcium Salicylate (The concomitant use of fentanyl with CYP3A4 inducers (eg, barbiturates, carbamazepine, efavirenz, glucocorticoids, modafinil, nevirapine, oxcarbazepine, phenobarbital, phenytoin, pioglitazone, rifabutin, rifampin, St. John's wort, or troglitazone) may result in a decrease fentanyl plasma concentrations).
No products indexed under this heading.

Theophylline Dihydroxypropyl (Glyceryl) (The concomitant use of fentanyl with CYP3A4 inducers (eg, barbiturates, carbamazepine, efavirenz, glucocorticoids, modafinil, nevirapine, oxcarbazepine, phenobarbital, phenytoin, pioglitazone, rifabutin, rifampin, St. John's wort, or troglitazone) may result in a decrease fentanyl plasma concentrations).
No products indexed under this heading.

Theophylline Ethylenediamine (The concomitant use of fentanyl with CYP3A4 inducers (eg, barbiturates, carbamazepine, efavirenz, glucocorticoids, modafinil, nevirapine, oxcarbazepine, phenobarbital, phenytoin, pioglitazone, rifabutin, rifampin, St. John's wort, or troglitazone) may result in a decrease fentanyl plasma concentrations).
No products indexed under this heading.

Theophylline Sodium Glycinate (The concomitant use of fentanyl with CYP3A4 inducers (eg, barbiturates, carbamazepine, efavirenz, glucocorticoids, modafinil, nevirapine, oxcarbazepine, phenobarbital, phenytoin, pioglitazone, rifabutin, rifampin, St. John's wort, or troglitazone) may result in a decrease fentanyl plasma concentrations).
No products indexed under this heading.

Thiamylal Sodium (The concomitant use of fentanyl with other CNS depressants, including other opioids, sedatives or hypnotics, general anesthetics, phenothizines, tranquilizers, skeletal muscle relaxants, sedating antihistamines, and alcoholic beverages may produce increased depressant effects. Patients on concomitant CNS depressants must be monitored for a change in opioid effects. Consideration should be given to adjusting the dose of fentanyl if warranted).
No products indexed under this heading.

Thioridazine (The concomitant use of fentanyl with other CNS depressants, including other opioids, sedatives or hypnotics, general anesthetics, phenothizines, tranquilizers, skeletal muscle relaxants, sedating antihistamines, and alcoholic beverages may produce increased depressant effects. Patients on concomitant CNS depressants must be monitored for a change in opioid effects. Consideration should be given to adjusting the dose of fentanyl if warranted).
No products indexed under this heading.

Thioridazine Hydrochloride (The concomitant use of fentanyl with other CNS depressants, including other opioids, sedatives or hypnotics, general anesthetics, phenothizines, tranquilizers, skeletal muscle relaxants, sedating antihistamines, and alcoholic beverages may produce increased depressant effects. Patients on concomitant CNS depressants must be monitored for a change in opioid effects. Consideration should be given to adjusting the dose of fentanyl if warranted). Products include:
Thioridazine Hydrochloride 2384

Thiothixene (The concomitant use of fentanyl with other CNS depressants, including other opioids, sedatives or hypnotics, general anesthetics, phenothizines, tranquilizers, skeletal muscle relaxants, sedating antihistamines, and alcoholic beverages may produce increased depressant effects. Patients on concomitant CNS depressants must be monitored for a change in opioid effects. Consideration should be given to adjusting the dose of fentanyl if warranted). Products include:
Thiothixene 2386

Thiothixene Hydrochloride (The concomitant use of fentanyl with other CNS depressants, including other opioids, sedatives or hypnotics, general anesthetics, phenothizines, tranquilizers, skeletal muscle relaxants, sedating antihistamines, and alcoholic beverages may produce increased depressant effects. Patients on concomitant CNS depressants must be monitored for a change in opioid effects. Consideration should be given to adjusting the dose of fentanyl if warranted).
No products indexed under this heading.

Tipranavir (Concomitant use with inhibitors of the cytochrome P450 3A4 (CYP3A4) isoform (eg, certain protease inhibitors) may increase fentanyl levels, resulting in increased depressant effects).
No products indexed under this heading.

Tizanidine (The concomitant use of fentanyl with other CNS depressants, including other opioids, sedatives or hypnotics, general anesthetics, phenothiazines, tranquilizers, skeletal muscle relaxants, sedating antihistamines, and alcoholic beverages may produce increased depressant effects).
No products indexed under this heading.

Tizanidine Hydrochloride (The concomitant use of fentanyl with other CNS depressants, including other opioids, sedatives or hypnotics, general anesthetics, phenothiazines, tranquilizers, skeletal muscle relaxants, sedating antihistamines, and alcoholic beverages may produce increased depressant effects).
No products indexed under this heading.

Tranylcypromine Sulfate (Fentanyl is not recommended in patients who have received MAO inhibitors within 14 days because severe and unpredictable potentiation by MAO inhibitors has been reported with opioid analgesics). Products include:
Parnate 1584

Triamcinolone (The concomitant use of fentanyl with CYP3A4 inducers (eg, barbiturates, carbamazepine, efavirenz, glucocorticoids, modafinil, nevirapine, oxcarbazepine, phenobarbital, phenytoin, pioglitazone, rifabutin, rifampin, St. John's wort, or troglitazone) may result in a decrease fentanyl plasma concentrations).
No products indexed under this heading.

Triamcinolone Acetonide (The concomitant use of fentanyl with CYP3A4 inducers (eg, barbiturates, carbamazepine, efavirenz, glucocorticoids, modafinil, nevirapine, oxcarbazepine, phenobarbital, phenytoin, pioglitazone, rifabutin, rifampin, St. John's wort, or troglitazone) may result in a decrease fentanyl plasma concentrations). Products include:
Azmacort 408
Nasacort AQ 3019

Triamcinolone Diacetate (The concomitant use of fentanyl with CYP3A4 inducers (eg, barbiturates, carbamazepine, efavirenz, glucocorticoids, modafinil, nevirapine, oxcarbazepine, phenobarbital, phenytoin, pioglitazone, rifabutin, rifampin, St. John's wort, or troglitazone) may result in a decrease fentanyl plasma concentrations).
No products indexed under this heading.

Triamcinolone Hexacetonide (The concomitant use of fentanyl with CYP3A4 inducers (eg, barbiturates, carbamazepine, efavirenz, glucocorticoids, modafinil, nevirapine, oxcarbazepine, phenobarbital, phenytoin, pioglitazone, rifabutin, rifampin, St. John's wort, or troglitazone) may result in a decrease fentanyl plasma concentrations).
No products indexed under this heading.

Triazolam (The concomitant use of fentanyl with other CNS depressants, including other opioids, sedatives or hypnotics, general anesthetics, phenothizines, tranquilizers, skeletal muscle relaxants, sedating antihistamines, and alcoholic beverages may produce increased depressant effects. Patients on concomitant CNS depressants must be monitored for a change in opioid effects. Consideration should be given to adjusting the dose of fentanyl if warranted).
No products indexed under this heading.

Trifluoperazine Hydrochloride (The concomitant use of fentanyl with other CNS depressants, including other opioids, sedatives or hypnotics, general anesthetics, phenothizines, tranquilizers, skeletal muscle relaxants, sedating antihistamines, and alcoholic beverages may produce increased depressant effects. Patients on concomitant CNS depressants must be monitored for a change in opioid effects. Consideration should be given to adjusting the dose of fentanyl if warranted).
No products indexed under this heading.

Trimeprazine Tartrate (The concomitant use of fentanyl with other CNS depressants, including other opioids, sedatives or hypnotics, general anesthetics, phenothiazines, tranquilizers, skeletal muscle relaxants, sedating antihistamines, and alcoholic beverages may produce increased depressant effects).
No products indexed under this heading.

Tripelennamine Hydrochloride (The concomitant use of fentanyl with other CNS depressants, including other opioids, sedatives or hypnotics, general anesthetics, phenothiazines, tranquilizers, skeletal muscle relaxants, sedating antihistamines, and alcoholic beverages may produce increased depressant effects).
No products indexed under this heading.

Triprolidine Hydrochloride (The concomitant use of fentanyl with other CNS depressants, including other opioids, sedatives or hypnotics, general anesthetics, phenothiazines, tranquilizers, skeletal muscle relaxants, sedating antihistamines, and alcoholic beverages may produce increased depressant effects).
No products indexed under this heading.

Troglitazone (The concomitant use of fentanyl with CYP3A4 inducers (eg, barbiturates, carbamazepine, efavirenz, glucocorticoids, modafinil, nevirapine, oxcarbazepine, phenobarbital, phenytoin, pioglitazone, rifabutin, rifampin, St. John's wort, or troglitazone) may result in a decrease fentanyl plasma concentrations).
No products indexed under this heading.

Troleandomycin (The concomitant use of fentanyl with CYP3A4 inhibitors (eg, indinavir, nelfinavir, ritonavir, clarithromycin, itraconazole, ketoconazole, nefazodone, saquinavir, telithromycin, aprepitant, diltiazem, erythromycin, fluconazole, grapefruit juice, verapamil, or cimetidine) may result in a potentially dangerous increase in fentanyl plasma concentrations).
No products indexed under this heading.

Tubocurarine Chloride (The concomitant use of fentanyl with other CNS depressants, including other opioids, sedatives or hypnotics, general anesthetics, phenothiazines, tranquilizers, skeletal muscle relaxants, sedating antihistamines, and alcoholic beverages may produce increased depressant effects).
No products indexed under this heading.

Valproate Sodium (The concomitant use of fentanyl with CYP3A4 inhibitors (eg, indinavir, nelfinavir, ritonavir, clarithromycin, itraconazole, ketoconazole, nefazodone, saquinavir, telithromycin, aprepitant, diltiazem, erythromycin, fluconazole, grapefruit juice, verapamil, or cimetidine) may result in a potentially dangerous increase in fentanyl plasma concentrations).
No products indexed under this heading.

Vardenafil Hydrochloride (The concomitant use of fentanyl with CYP3A4 inhibitors (eg, indinavir, nelfinavir, ritonavir, clarithromycin, itraconazole, ketoconazole, nefazodone, saquinavir, telithromycin, aprepitant, diltiazem, erythromycin, fluconazole, grapefruit juice, verapamil, or cimetidine) may result in a potentially dangerous increase in fentanyl plasma concentrations). Products include:
Levitra 3157

Vecuronium Bromide (The concomitant use of fentanyl with other CNS depressants, including other opioids, sedatives or hypnotics, general anesthetics, phenothiazines, tranquilizers, skeletal muscle relaxants, sedating antihistamines, and alcoholic beverages may produce increased depressant effects).
No products indexed under this heading.

Verapamil Hydrochloride (The concomitant use of fentanyl with CYP3A4 inhibitors (eg, indinavir, nelfinavir, ritonavir, clarithromycin, itraconazole, ketoconazole, nefazodone, saquinavir, telithromycin, aprepitant, diltiazem, erythromycin, fluconazole, grapefruit juice, verapamil, or cimetidine) may result in a potentially dangerous increase in fentanyl plasma concentrations). Products include:
Tarka 534

Voriconazole (The concomitant use of fentanyl with CYP3A4 inhibitors (eg, indinavir, nelfinavir, ritonavir, clarithromycin, itraconazole, ketoconazole, nefazodone, saquinavir, telithromycin, aprepitant, diltiazem, erythromycin, fluconazole, grapefruit juice, verapamil, or cimetidine) may result in a potentially dangerous increase in fentanyl plasma concentrations).
No products indexed under this heading.

Zafirlukast (The concomitant use of fentanyl with CYP3A4 inhibitors (eg, indinavir, nelfinavir, ritonavir, clarithromycin, itraconazole, ketoconazole, nefazodone, saquinavir, telithromycin, aprepitant, diltiazem, erythromycin, fluconazole, grapefruit juice, verapamil, or cimetidine) may result in a potentially dangerous increase in fentanyl plasma concentrations). Products include:
Accolate 3612

Zaleplon (The concomitant use of fentanyl with other CNS depressants, including other opioids, sedatives or hypnotics, general anesthetics, phenothizines, tranquilizers, skeletal muscle relaxants, sedating antihistamines, and alcoholic beverages may produce increased depressant effects. Patients on concomitant CNS depressants must be monitored for a change in opioid effects. Consideration should be given to adjusting the dose of fentanyl if warranted).
No products indexed under this heading.

Zileuton (The concomitant use of fentanyl with CYP3A4 inhibitors (eg, indinavir, nelfinavir, ritonavir, clarithromycin, itraconazole, ketoconazole, nefazodone, saquinavir, telithromycin, aprepitant, diltiazem, erythromycin, fluconazole, grapefruit juice, verapamil, or cimetidine) may result in a potentially dangerous increase in fentanyl plasma concentrations).
No products indexed under this heading.

Ziprasidone Hydrochloride (The concomitant use of fentanyl with other CNS depressants, including other opioids, sedatives or hypnotics, general anesthetics, phenothizines, tranquilizers, skeletal muscle relaxants, sedating antihistamines, and alcoholic beverages may produce increased depressant effects. Patients on concomitant CNS depressants must be monitored for a change in opioid effects. Consideration should be given to adjusting the dose of fentanyl if warranted). Products include:
Geodon 2723

Zolpidem Tartrate (The concomitant use of fentanyl with other CNS depressants, including other opioids, sedatives or hypnotics, general anesthetics, phenothizines, tranquilizers, skeletal muscle relaxants, sedating antihistamines, and alcoholic beverages may produce increased depressant effects. Patients on concomitant CNS depressants must be monitored for a change in opioid effects. Consideration should be given to adjusting the dose of fentanyl if warranted). Products include:
Ambien 2920
Ambien CR 2925

Food Interactions

Alcohol (The concomitant use of fentanyl with other CNS depressants, including other opioids, sedatives or hypnotics, general anesthetics, phenothizines, tranquilizers, skeletal muscle relaxants, sedating antihistamines, and alcoholic beverages may produce increased depressant effects. Patients on concomitant CNS depressants must be monitored for a change in opioid effects. Consideration should be given to adjusting the dose of fentanyl if warranted).

Beer, reduced-alcohol (The concomitant use of fentanyl with other CNS depressants, including other opioids, sedatives or hypnotics, general anesthetics, phenothiazines, tranquilizers, skeletal muscle relaxants, sedating antihistamines, and alcoholic beverages may produce increased depressant effects).

Beer, unspecified (The concomitant use of fentanyl with other CNS depressants, including other opioids, sedatives or hypnotics, general anesthetics, phenothiazines, tranquilizers, skeletal muscle relaxants, sedating antihistamines, and alcoholic beverages may produce increased depressant effects).

Grapefruit (The concomitant use of fentanyl with CYP3A4 inhibitors (eg, indinavir, nelfinavir, ritonavir, clarithromycin, itraconazole, ketoconazole, nefazodone, saquinavir, telithromycin, aprepitant, diltiazem, erythromycin, fluconazole, grapefruit juice, verapamil, or cimetidine) may result in a potentially dangerous increase in fentanyl plasma concentrations).

Grapefruit Juice (The concomitant use of fentanyl with CYP3A4 inhibitors (eg, indinavir, nelfinavir, ritonavir, clarithromycin, itraconazole, ketoconazole, nefazodone, saquinavir, telithromycin, aprepitant, diltiazem, erythromycin, fluconazole, grapefruit juice, verapamil, or cimetidine) may result in a potentially dangerous increase in fentanyl plasma concentrations).

Wine, Chianti (The concomitant use of fentanyl with other CNS depressants, including other opioids, sedatives or hypnotics, general anesthetics, phenothiazines, tranquilizers, skeletal muscle relaxants, sedating antihistamines, and alcoholic beverages may produce increased depressant effects).

Wine, Red (The concomitant use of fentanyl with other CNS depressants, including other opioids, sedatives or hypnotics, general anesthetics, phenothiazines, tranquilizers, skeletal muscle relaxants, sedating antihistamines, and alcoholic beverages may produce increased depressant effects).

Wine, unspecified (The concomitant use of fentanyl with other CNS depressants, including other opioids, sedatives or hypnotics, general anesthetics, phenothiazines, tranquilizers, skeletal muscle relaxants, sedating antihistamines, and alcoholic beverages may produce increased depressant effects).

Wine products (The concomitant use of fentanyl with other CNS depressants, including other opioids, sedatives or hypnotics, general anesthetics, phenothiazines, tranquilizers, skeletal muscle relaxants, sedating antihistamines, and alcoholic beverages may produce increased depressant effects).

ONTAK VIALS

(Denileukin Diftitox) 1068
None cited in PDR database.

OPANA TABLETS

(Oxymorphone Hydrochloride) 1110
May interact with alcohols, anesthetics, anticholinergics, central nervous system depressants, hypnotics and sedatives, mixed agonist/antagonist opioid analgesics, monoamine oxidase inhibitors, narcotic analgesics, phenothiazines, tranquilizers, and certain other agents. Compounds in these categories include:

Alfentanil Hydrochloride (The concomitant use of other CNS depressants including sedatives, hypnotics, tranquilizers, general anesthetics, phenothiazines, other opioids, and alcohol may produce additive CNS depressant effects. Additive effects resulting in respiratory depression, hypotension, profound sedation or coma may result if these drugs are taken in combination with the usual doses of oxymorphone hydrochloride).
No products indexed under this heading.

Alprazolam (The concomitant use of other CNS depressants including sedatives, hypnotics, tranquilizers, general anesthetics, phenothiazines, other opioids, and alcohol may produce additive CNS depressant effects. Additive effects resulting in respiratory depression, hypotension, profound sedation or coma may result if these drugs are taken in combination with the usual doses of oxymorphone hydrochloride).
No products indexed under this heading.

Amobarbital (The concomitant use of other CNS depressants including sedatives, hypnotics, tranquilizers, general anesthetics, phenothiazines, other opioids, and alcohol may produce additive CNS depressant effects. Additive effects resulting in respiratory depres-

IMPORTANT NOTE: Always consult each drug listing in the patient's regimen for possible interactions.

sion, hypotension, profound sedation or coma may result if these drugs are taken in combination with the usual dose of oxymorphone hydrochloride).

No products indexed under this heading.

Amobarbital Sodium (The concomitant use of other CNS depressants including sedatives, hypnotics, tranquilizers, general anesthetics, phenothiazines, other opioids, and alcohol may produce additive CNS depressant effects. Additive effects resulting in respiratory depression, hypotension, profound sedation or coma may result if these drugs are taken in combination with the usual dose of oxymorphone hydrochloride).

No products indexed under this heading.

Apomorphine (The concomitant use of other CNS depressants including sedatives, hypnotics, tranquilizers, general anesthetics, phenothiazines, other opioids, and alcohol may produce additive CNS depressant effects. Additive effects resulting in respiratory depression, hypotension, profound sedation or coma may result if these drugs are taken in combination with the usual doses of oxymorphone hydrochloride).

No products indexed under this heading.

Apomorphine Hydrochloride (The concomitant use of other CNS depressants including sedatives, hypnotics, tranquilizers, general anesthetics, phenothiazines, other opioids, and alcohol may produce additive CNS depressant effects. Additive effects resulting in respiratory depression, hypotension, profound sedation or coma may result if these drugs are taken in combination with the usual doses of oxymorphone hydrochloride).

No products indexed under this heading.

Aprobarbital (The concomitant use of other CNS depressants including sedatives, hypnotics, tranquilizers, general anesthetics, phenothiazines, other opioids, and alcohol may produce additive CNS depressant effects. Additive effects resulting in respiratory depression, hypotension, profound sedation or coma may result if these drugs are taken in combination with the usual dose of oxymorphone hydrochloride).

No products indexed under this heading.

Articaine Hydrochloride (The concomitant use of other CNS depressants including sedatives, hypnotics, tranquilizers, general anesthetics, phenothiazines, other opioids, and alcohol may produce additive CNS depressant effects. Additive effects resulting in respiratory depression, hypotension, profound sedation or coma may result if these drugs are taken in combination with the usual doses of oxymorphone hydrochloride).

No products indexed under this heading.

Atropine Sulfate (Anticholinergics or other medications with anticholinergic activity when used concurrently with opioid analgesics may result in increased risk of urinary retention and/or severe constipation, which may lead to paralytic ileus). Products include:
Donnatal 2711

Belladonna Alkaloids (Anticholinergics or other medications with anticholinergic activity when used concurrently with opioid analgesics may result in increased risk of urinary retention and/or severe constipation, which may lead to paralytic ileus). Products include:
Hyland's Teething Tablets 3316

Benzocaine (The concomitant use of other CNS depressants including sedatives, hypnotics, tranquilizers, general anesthetics, phenothiazines, other opioids, and alcohol may produce additive CNS depressant effects. Additive effects resulting in respiratory depres-

---

sion, hypotension, profound sedation or coma may result if these drugs are taken in combination with the usual doses of oxymorphone hydrochloride).

No products indexed under this heading.

Benztropine Mesylate (Anticholinergics or other medications with anticholinergic activity when used concurrently with opioid analgesics may result in increased risk of urinary retention and/or severe constipation, which may lead to paralytic ileus).

No products indexed under this heading.

Biperiden Hydrochloride (Anticholinergics or other medications with anticholinergic activity when used concurrently with opioid analgesics may result in increased risk of urinary retention and/or severe constipation, which may lead to paralytic ileus).

No products indexed under this heading.

Bupivacaine Hydrochloride (The concomitant use of other CNS depressants including sedatives, hypnotics, tranquilizers, general anesthetics, phenothiazines, other opioids, and alcohol may produce additive CNS depressant effects. Additive effects resulting in respiratory depression, hypotension, profound sedation or coma may result if these drugs are taken in combination with the usual doses of oxymorphone hydrochloride).

No products indexed under this heading.

Buprenorphine Hydrochloride (The concomitant use of other CNS depressants including sedatives, hypnotics, tranquilizers, general anesthetics, phenothiazines, other opioids, and alcohol may produce additive CNS depressant effects. Additive effects resulting in respiratory depression, hypotension, profound sedation or coma may result if these drugs are taken in combination with the usual doses of oxymorphone hydrochloride).

No products indexed under this heading.

Buspirone Hydrochloride (The concomitant use of other CNS depressants including sedatives, hypnotics, tranquilizers, general anesthetics, phenothiazines, other opioids, and alcohol may produce additive CNS depressant effects. Additive effects resulting in respiratory depression, hypotension, profound sedation or coma may result if these drugs are taken in combination with the usual doses of oxymorphone hydrochloride).

No products indexed under this heading.

Butabarbital (The concomitant use of other CNS depressants including sedatives, hypnotics, tranquilizers, general anesthetics, phenothiazines, other opioids, and alcohol may produce additive CNS depressant effects. Additive effects resulting in respiratory depression, hypotension, profound sedation or coma may result if these drugs are taken in combination with the usual doses of oxymorphone hydrochloride).

No products indexed under this heading.

Butabarbital Sodium (The concomitant use of other CNS depressants including sedatives, hypnotics, tranquilizers, general anesthetics, phenothiazines, other opioids, and alcohol may produce additive CNS depressant effects. Additive effects resulting in respiratory depression, hypotension, profound sedation or coma may result if these drugs are taken in combination with the usual doses of oxymorphone hydrochloride).

No products indexed under this heading.

Butalbital (The concomitant use of other CNS depressants including sedatives, hypnotics, tranquilizers, general anesthetics, phenothiazines, other opioids, and alcohol may produce additive CNS depressant effects. Additive effects resulting in respiratory depres-

---

sion, hypotension, profound sedation or coma may result if these drugs are taken in combination with the usual doses of oxymorphone hydrochloride).

No products indexed under this heading.

Butorphanol Tartrate (Agonist/antagonist analgesics should not be administered to patients who have received or are receiving a course of therapy with pure opioid agonist analgesic, such as oxymorphone hydrochloride. In this situation, mixed agonist/antagonist analgesics may reduce the analgesic effect of oxymorphone hydrochloride and/or may precipitate withdrawal symptoms).

No products indexed under this heading.

Chloral Hydrate (The concomitant use of other CNS depressants including sedatives, hypnotics, tranquilizers, general anesthetics, phenothiazines, other opioids, and alcohol may produce additive CNS depressant effects. Additive effects resulting in respiratory depression, hypotension, profound sedation or coma may result if these drugs are taken in combination with the usual doses of oxymorphone hydrochloride).

No products indexed under this heading.

Chlordiazepoxide (The concomitant use of other CNS depressants including sedatives, hypnotics, tranquilizers, general anesthetics, phenothiazines, other opioids, and alcohol may produce additive CNS depressant effects. Additive effects resulting in respiratory depression, hypotension, profound sedation or coma may result if these drugs are taken in combination with the usual doses of oxymorphone hydrochloride).

No products indexed under this heading.

Chlordiazepoxide Hydrochloride (The concomitant use of other CNS depressants including sedatives, hypnotics, tranquilizers, general anesthetics, phenothiazines, other opioids, and alcohol may produce additive CNS depressant effects. Additive effects resulting in respiratory depression, hypotension, profound sedation or coma may result if these drugs are taken in combination with the usual doses of oxymorphone hydrochloride).

No products indexed under this heading.

Chloroprocaine Hydrochloride (The concomitant use of other CNS depressants including sedatives, hypnotics, tranquilizers, general anesthetics, phenothiazines, other opioids, and alcohol may produce additive CNS depressant effects. Additive effects resulting in respiratory depression, hypotension, profound sedation or coma may result if these drugs are taken in combination with the usual doses of oxymorphone hydrochloride).

No products indexed under this heading.

Chlorpromazine (The concomitant use of other CNS depressants including sedatives, hypnotics, tranquilizers, general anesthetics, phenothiazines, other opioids, and alcohol may produce additive CNS depressant effects. Additive effects resulting in respiratory depression, hypotension, profound sedation or coma may result if these drugs are taken in combination with the usual doses of oxymorphone hydrochloride).

No products indexed under this heading.

Chlorpromazine Hydrochloride (The concomitant use of other CNS depressants including sedatives, hypnotics, tranquilizers, general anesthetics, phenothiazines, other opioids, and alcohol may produce additive CNS depressant effects. Additive effects resulting in respiratory depression, hypotension, profound sedation or coma may result if these drugs are taken in combination with the usual doses of oxymorphone hydrochloride).

No products indexed under this heading.

Chlorprothixene (The concomitant use of other CNS depressants including sedatives, hypnotics, tranquilizers, general anesthetics, phenothiazines, other opioids, and alcohol may produce additive CNS depressant effects. Additive effects resulting in respiratory depression, hypotension, profound sedation or coma may result if these drugs are taken in combination with the usual doses of oxymorphone hydrochloride).

No products indexed under this heading.

Chlorprothixene Hydrochloride (The concomitant use of other CNS depressants including sedatives, hypnotics, tranquilizers, general anesthetics, phenothiazines, other opioids, and alcohol may produce additive CNS depressant effects. Additive effects resulting in respiratory depression, hypotension, profound sedation or coma may result if these drugs are taken in combination with the usual doses of oxymorphone hydrochloride).

No products indexed under this heading.

Chlorprothixene Lactate (The concomitant use of other CNS depressants including sedatives, hypnotics, tranquilizers, general anesthetics, phenothiazines, other opioids, and alcohol may produce additive CNS depressant effects. Additive effects resulting in respiratory depression, hypotension, profound sedation or coma may result if these drugs are taken in combination with the usual doses of oxymorphone hydrochloride).

No products indexed under this heading.

Clidinium Bromide (Anticholinergics or other medications with anticholinergic activity when used concurrently with opioid analgesics may result in increased risk of urinary retention and/or severe constipation, which may lead to paralytic ileus).

No products indexed under this heading.

Clonazepam (The concomitant use of other CNS depressants including sedatives, hypnotics, tranquilizers, general anesthetics, phenothiazines, other opioids, and alcohol may produce additive CNS depressant effects. Additive effects resulting in respiratory depression, hypotension, profound sedation or coma may result if these drugs are taken in combination with the usual dose of oxymorphone hydrochloride). Products include:
Klonopin 2855

Clorazepate Dipotassium (The concomitant use of other CNS depressants including sedatives, hypnotics, tranquilizers, general anesthetics, phenothiazines, other opioids, and alcohol may produce additive CNS depressant effects. Additive effects resulting in respiratory depression, hypotension, profound sedation or coma may result if these drugs are taken in combination with the usual doses of oxymorphone hydrochloride).

No products indexed under this heading.

Clozapine (The concomitant use of other CNS depressants including sedatives, hypnotics, tranquilizers, general anesthetics, phenothiazines, other opioids, and alcohol may produce additive CNS depressant effects. Additive effects resulting in respiratory depression, hypotension, profound sedation or coma may result if these drugs are taken in combination with the usual dose of oxymorphone hydrochloride).

No products indexed under this heading.

Cocaine Hydrochloride (The concomitant use of other CNS depressants including sedatives, hypnotics, tranquilizers, general anesthetics, phenothiazines, other opioids, and alcohol may produce additive CNS depressant effects. Additive effects resulting in respiratory depression, hypotension, pro-

1301 Interactions Index Opana

found sedation or coma may result if these drugs are taken in combination with the usual doses of oxymorphone hydrochloride).
No products indexed under this heading.

Codeine Phosphate (The concomitant use of other CNS depressants including sedatives, hypnotics, tranquilizers, general anesthetics, phenothiazines, other opioids, and alcohol may produce additive CNS depressant effects. Additive effects resulting in respiratory depression, hypotension, profound sedation or coma may result if these drugs are taken in combination with the usual doses of oxymorphone hydrochloride). Products include:
Tylenol with Codeine 2691

Codeine Sulfate (The concomitant use of other CNS depressants including sedatives, hypnotics, tranquilizers, general anesthetics, phenothiazines, other opioids, and alcohol may produce additive CNS depressant effects. Additive effects resulting in respiratory depression, hypotension, profound sedation or coma may result if these drugs are taken in combination with the usual doses of oxymorphone hydrochloride).
No products indexed under this heading.

Desflurane (The concomitant use of other CNS depressants including sedatives, hypnotics, tranquilizers, general anesthetics, phenothiazines, other opioids, and alcohol may produce additive CNS depressant effects. Additive effects resulting in respiratory depression, hypotension, profound sedation or coma may result if these drugs are taken in combination with the usual dose of oxymorphone hydrochloride).
No products indexed under this heading.

Dezocine (The concomitant use of other CNS depressants including sedatives, hypnotics, tranquilizers, general anesthetics, phenothiazines, other opioids, and alcohol may produce additive CNS depressant effects. Additive effects resulting in respiratory depression, hypotension, profound sedation or coma may result if these drugs are taken in combination with the usual doses of oxymorphone hydrochloride).
No products indexed under this heading.

Diazepam (The concomitant use of other CNS depressants including sedatives, hypnotics, tranquilizers, general anesthetics, phenothiazines, other opioids, and alcohol may produce additive CNS depressant effects. Additive effects resulting in respiratory depression, hypotension, profound sedation or coma may result if these drugs are taken in combination with the usual doses of oxymorphone hydrochloride). Products include:
Valium Tablets 2880

Dibucaine (The concomitant use of other CNS depressants including sedatives, hypnotics, tranquilizers, general anesthetics, phenothiazines, other opioids, and alcohol may produce additive CNS depressant effects. Additive effects resulting in respiratory depression, hypotension, profound sedation or coma may result if these drugs are taken in combination with the usual doses of oxymorphone hydrochloride).
No products indexed under this heading.

Dibucaine Hydrochloride (The concomitant use of other CNS depressants including sedatives, hypnotics, tranquilizers, general anesthetics, phenothiazines, other opioids, and alcohol may produce additive CNS depressant effects. Additive effects resulting in respiratory depression, hypotension, profound sedation or coma may result if these drugs are taken in combination with the usual doses of oxymorphone hydrochloride).
No products indexed under this heading.

Dicyclomine Hydrochloride (Anticholinergics or other medications with anticholinergic activity when used concurrently with opioid analgesics may result in increased risk of urinary retention and/or severe constipation, which may lead to paralytic ileus). Products include:
Bentyl Capsules 780
Bentyl Injection 780
Bentyl Syrup 780
Bentyl Tablets 780

Dihydrocodeine Bitartrate (The concomitant use of other CNS depressants including sedatives, hypnotics, tranquilizers, general anesthetics, phenothiazines, other opioids, and alcohol may produce additive CNS depressant effects. Additive effects resulting in respiratory depression, hypotension, profound sedation or coma may result if these drugs are taken in combination with the usual doses of oxymorphone hydrochloride).
No products indexed under this heading.

Dihydrocodeinone Bitartrate (The concomitant use of other CNS depressants including sedatives, hypnotics, tranquilizers, general anesthetics, phenothiazines, other opioids, and alcohol may produce additive CNS depressant effects. Additive effects resulting in respiratory depression, hypotension, profound sedation or coma may result if these drugs are taken in combination with the usual doses of oxymorphone hydrochloride).
No products indexed under this heading.

Droperidol (The concomitant use of other CNS depressants including sedatives, hypnotics, tranquilizers, general anesthetics, phenothiazines, other opioids, and alcohol may produce additive CNS depressant effects. Additive effects resulting in respiratory depression, hypotension, profound sedation or coma may result if these drugs are taken in combination with the usual doses of oxymorphone hydrochloride).
No products indexed under this heading.

Enflurane (The concomitant use of other CNS depressants including sedatives, hypnotics, tranquilizers, general anesthetics, phenothiazines, other opioids, and alcohol may produce additive CNS depressant effects. Additive effects resulting in respiratory depression, hypotension, profound sedation or coma may result if these drugs are taken in combination with the usual doses of oxymorphone hydrochloride).
No products indexed under this heading.

Estazolam (The concomitant use of other CNS depressants including sedatives, hypnotics, tranquilizers, general anesthetics, phenothiazines, other opioids, and alcohol may produce additive CNS depressant effects. Additive effects resulting in respiratory depression, hypotension, profound sedation or coma may result if these drugs are taken in combination with the usual doses of oxymorphone hydrochloride).
No products indexed under this heading.

Ethanol (The concomitant use of other CNS depressants including sedatives, hypnotics, tranquilizers, general anesthetics, phenothiazines, other opioids, and alcohol may produce additive CNS depressant effects. Additive effects resulting in respiratory depression, hypotension, profound sedation or coma may result if these drugs are taken in combination with the usual dose of oxymorphone hydrochloride).
No products indexed under this heading.

Ethchlorvynol (The concomitant use of other CNS depressants including sedatives, hypnotics, tranquilizers, general anesthetics, phenothiazines, other opioids, and alcohol may produce additive CNS depressant effects. Additive effects resulting in respiratory depression, hypotension, profound sedation or coma may result if these drugs are taken in combination with the usual doses of oxymorphone hydrochloride).
No products indexed under this heading.

Ethinamate (The concomitant use of other CNS depressants including sedatives, hypnotics, tranquilizers, general anesthetics, phenothiazines, other opioids, and alcohol may produce additive CNS depressant effects. Additive effects resulting in respiratory depression, hypotension, profound sedation or coma may result if these drugs are taken in combination with the usual doses of oxymorphone hydrochloride).
No products indexed under this heading.

Ethyl Alcohol (The concomitant use of other CNS depressants including sedatives, hypnotics, tranquilizers, general anesthetics, phenothiazines, other opioids, and alcohol may produce additive CNS depressant effects. Additive effects resulting in respiratory depression, hypotension, profound sedation or coma may result if these drugs are taken in combination with the usual dose of oxymorphone hydrochloride).
No products indexed under this heading.

Etidocaine Hydrochloride (The concomitant use of other CNS depressants including sedatives, hypnotics, tranquilizers, general anesthetics, phenothiazines, other opioids, and alcohol may produce additive CNS depressant effects. Additive effects resulting in respiratory depression, hypotension, profound sedation or coma may result if these drugs are taken in combination with the usual doses of oxymorphone hydrochloride).
No products indexed under this heading.

Fentanyl (The concomitant use of other CNS depressants including sedatives, hypnotics, tranquilizers, general anesthetics, phenothiazines, other opioids, and alcohol may produce additive CNS depressant effects. Additive effects resulting in respiratory depression, hypotension, profound sedation or coma may result if these drugs are taken in combination with the usual doses of oxymorphone hydrochloride). Products include:
Duragesic 2604
Fentanyl Transdermal System 2346
Onsolis 2054

Fentanyl Citrate (The concomitant use of other CNS depressants including sedatives, hypnotics, tranquilizers, general anesthetics, phenothiazines, other opioids, and alcohol may produce additive CNS depressant effects. Additive effects resulting in respiratory depression, hypotension, profound sedation or coma may result if these drugs are taken in combination with the usual doses of oxymorphone hydrochloride). Products include:
Fentora 966

Fluphenazine Decanoate (The concomitant use of other CNS depressants including sedatives, hypnotics, tranquilizers, general anesthetics, phenothiazines, other opioids, and alcohol may produce additive CNS depressant effects. Additive effects resulting in respiratory depression, hypotension, profound sedation or coma may result if these drugs are taken in combination with the usual doses of oxymorphone hydrochloride).
No products indexed under this heading.

Fluphenazine Enanthate (The concomitant use of other CNS depressants including sedatives, hypnotics, tranquilizers, general anesthetics, phenothiazines, other opioids, and alcohol may produce additive CNS depressant effects. Additive effects resulting in respiratory depression, hypotension, profound sedation or coma may result if these drugs are taken in combination with the usual doses of oxymorphone hydrochloride).
No products indexed under this heading.

Fluphenazine Hydrochloride (The concomitant use of other CNS depressants including sedatives, hypnotics, tranquilizers, general anesthetics, phenothiazines, other opioids, and alcohol may produce additive CNS depressant effects. Additive effects resulting in respiratory depression, hypotension, profound sedation or coma may result if these drugs are taken in combination with the usual doses of oxymorphone hydrochloride).
No products indexed under this heading.

Flurazepam Hydrochloride (The concomitant use of other CNS depressants including sedatives, hypnotics, tranquilizers, general anesthetics, phenothiazines, other opioids, and alcohol may produce additive CNS depressant effects. Additive effects resulting in respiratory depression, hypotension, profound sedation or coma may result if these drugs are taken in combination with the usual doses of oxymorphone hydrochloride).
No products indexed under this heading.

Glutethimide (The concomitant use of other CNS depressants including sedatives, hypnotics, tranquilizers, general anesthetics, phenothiazines, other opioids, and alcohol may produce additive CNS depressant effects. Additive effects resulting in respiratory depression, hypotension, profound sedation or coma may result if these drugs are taken in combination with the usual doses of oxymorphone hydrochloride).
No products indexed under this heading.

Glycopyrrolate (Anticholinergics or other medications with anticholinergic activity when used concurrently with opioid analgesics may result in increased risk of urinary retention and/or severe constipation, which may lead to paralytic ileus).
No products indexed under this heading.

Halazepam (The concomitant use of other CNS depressants including sedatives, hypnotics, tranquilizers, general anesthetics, phenothiazines, other opioids, and alcohol may produce additive CNS depressant effects. Additive effects resulting in respiratory depression, hypotension, profound sedation or coma may result if these drugs are taken in combination with the usual dose of oxymorphone hydrochloride).
No products indexed under this heading.

Haloperidol (The concomitant use of other CNS depressants including sedatives, hypnotics, tranquilizers, general anesthetics, phenothiazines, other opioids, and alcohol may produce additive CNS depressant effects. Additive effects resulting in respiratory depression, hypotension, profound sedation or coma may result if these drugs are taken in combination with the usual doses of oxymorphone hydrochloride).
No products indexed under this heading.

Haloperidol Decanoate (The concomitant use of other CNS depressants including sedatives, hypnotics, tranquilizers, general anesthetics, phenothiazines, other opioids, and alcohol may produce additive CNS depressant effects. Additive effects resulting in respiratory depression, hypotension, profound sedation or coma may result if these drugs are taken in combination with the usual doses of oxymorphone hydrochloride).
No products indexed under this heading.

Haloperidol Lactate (The concomitant use of other CNS depressants including sedatives, hypnotics, tranquilizers, general anesthetics, phenothia-

IMPORTANT NOTE: Always consult each drug listing in the patient's regimen for possible interactions.

zines, other opioids, and alcohol may produce additive CNS depressant effects. Additive effects resulting in respiratory depression, hypotension, profound sedation or coma may result if these drugs are taken in combination with the usual dose of oxymorphone hydrochloride).

No products indexed under this heading.

Halothane (The concomitant use of other CNS depressants including sedatives, hypnotics, tranquilizers, general anesthetics, phenothiazines, other opioids, and alcohol may produce additive CNS depressant effects. Additive effects resulting in respiratory depression, hypotension, profound sedation or coma may result if these drugs are taken in combination with the usual doses of oxymorphone hydrochloride).

No products indexed under this heading.

Hexobarbital (The concomitant use of other CNS depressants including sedatives, hypnotics, tranquilizers, general anesthetics, phenothiazines, other opioids, and alcohol may produce additive CNS depressant effects. Additive effects resulting in respiratory depression, hypotension, profound sedation or coma may result if these drugs are taken in combination with the usual dose of oxymorphone hydrochloride).

No products indexed under this heading.

Hydrocodone Bitartrate (The concomitant use of other CNS depressants including sedatives, hypnotics, tranquilizers, general anesthetics, phenothiazines, other opioids, and alcohol may produce additive CNS depressant effects. Additive effects resulting in respiratory depression, hypotension, profound sedation or coma may result if these drugs are taken in combination with the usual doses of oxymorphone hydrochloride). Products include:

Vicodin	560
Vicodin ES	561
Vicodin HP	563
Vicoprofen	564
Zydone	1138

Hydrocodone Polistirex (The concomitant use of other CNS depressants including sedatives, hypnotics, tranquilizers, general anesthetics, phenothiazines, other opioids, and alcohol may produce additive CNS depressant effects. Additive effects resulting in respiratory depression, hypotension, profound sedation or coma may result if these drugs are taken in combination with the usual doses of oxymorphone hydrochloride). Products include:

Tussionex 3443

Hydromorphone (The concomitant use of other CNS depressants including sedatives, hypnotics, tranquilizers, general anesthetics, phenothiazines, other opioids, and alcohol may produce additive CNS depressant effects. Additive effects resulting in respiratory depression, hypotension, profound sedation or coma may result if these drugs are taken in combination with the usual doses of oxymorphone hydrochloride).

No products indexed under this heading.

Hydromorphone Hydrochloride (The concomitant use of other CNS depressants including sedatives, hypnotics, tranquilizers, general anesthetics, phenothiazines, other opioids, and alcohol may produce additive CNS depressant effects. Additive effects resulting in respiratory depression, hypotension, profound sedation or coma may result if these drugs are taken in combination with the usual doses of oxymorphone hydrochloride). Products include:

Dilaudid Injection	2800
Dilaudid Oral	2797
Dilaudid Tablets	2797
Dilaudid-HP	2800

Hydroxyzine Hydrochloride (The concomitant use of other CNS depressants including sedatives, hypnotics, tranquilizers, general anesthetics, phenothiazines, other opioids, and alcohol may produce additive CNS depressant effects. Additive effects resulting in respiratory depression, hypotension, profound sedation or coma may result if these drugs are taken in combination with the usual doses of oxymorphone hydrochloride).

No products indexed under this heading.

Hyoscyamine (Anticholinergics or other medications with anticholinergic activity when used concurrently with opioid analgesics may result in increased risk of urinary retention and/or severe constipation, which may lead to paralytic ileus).

No products indexed under this heading.

Hyoscyamine Sulfate (Anticholinergics or other medications with anticholinergic activity when used concurrently with opioid analgesics may result in increased risk of urinary retention and/or severe constipation, which may lead to paralytic ileus). Products include:

Donnatal 2711

Ipratropium Bromide (Anticholinergics or other medications with anticholinergic activity when used concurrently with opioid analgesics may result in increased risk of urinary retention and/or severe constipation, which may lead to paralytic ileus).

No products indexed under this heading.

Isocarboxazid (No specific interaction between oxymorphone and monoamine oxidase inhibitors has been observed, but caution in the use of any opioid in patients taking this class of drugs is appropriate). Products include:

Marplan 3481

Isoflurane (The concomitant use of other CNS depressants including sedatives, hypnotics, tranquilizers, general anesthetics, phenothiazines, other opioids, and alcohol may produce additive CNS depressant effects. Additive effects resulting in respiratory depression, hypotension, profound sedation or coma may result if these drugs are taken in combination with the usual doses of oxymorphone hydrochloride).

No products indexed under this heading.

Ketamine Hydrochloride (The concomitant use of other CNS depressants including sedatives, hypnotics, tranquilizers, general anesthetics, phenothiazines, other opioids, and alcohol may produce additive CNS depressant effects. Additive effects resulting in respiratory depression, hypotension, profound sedation or coma may result if these drugs are taken in combination with the usual doses of oxymorphone hydrochloride).

No products indexed under this heading.

Levobupivacaine Hydrochloride (The concomitant use of other CNS depressants including sedatives, hypnotics, tranquilizers, general anesthetics, phenothiazines, other opioids, and alcohol may produce additive CNS depressant effects. Additive effects resulting in respiratory depression, hypotension, profound sedation or coma may result if these drugs are taken in combination with the usual doses of oxymorphone hydrochloride).

No products indexed under this heading.

Levomethadyl Acetate Hydrochloride (The concomitant use of other CNS depressants including sedatives, hypnotics, tranquilizers, general anesthetics, phenothiazines, other opioids, and alcohol may produce additive CNS depressant effects. Additive effects resulting in respiratory depression, hypotension, profound sedation or

coma may result if these drugs are taken in combination with the usual dose of oxymorphone hydrochloride).

No products indexed under this heading.

Levorphanol Tartrate (The concomitant use of other CNS depressants including sedatives, hypnotics, tranquilizers, general anesthetics, phenothiazines, other opioids, and alcohol may produce additive CNS depressant effects. Additive effects resulting in respiratory depression, hypotension, profound sedation or coma may result if these drugs are taken in combination with the usual doses of oxymorphone hydrochloride).

No products indexed under this heading.

Lidocaine (The concomitant use of other CNS depressants including sedatives, hypnotics, tranquilizers, general anesthetics, phenothiazines, other opioids, and alcohol may produce additive CNS depressant effects. Additive effects resulting in respiratory depression, hypotension, profound sedation or coma may result if these drugs are taken in combination with the usual doses of oxymorphone hydrochloride). Products include:

Lidoderm 1107

Lidocaine Base (The concomitant use of other CNS depressants including sedatives, hypnotics, tranquilizers, general anesthetics, phenothiazines, other opioids, and alcohol may produce additive CNS depressant effects. Additive effects resulting in respiratory depression, hypotension, profound sedation or coma may result if these drugs are taken in combination with the usual doses of oxymorphone hydrochloride).

No products indexed under this heading.

Lidocaine Hydrochloride (The concomitant use of other CNS depressants including sedatives, hypnotics, tranquilizers, general anesthetics, phenothiazines, other opioids, and alcohol may produce additive CNS depressant effects. Additive effects resulting in respiratory depression, hypotension, profound sedation or coma may result if these drugs are taken in combination with the usual doses of oxymorphone hydrochloride).

No products indexed under this heading.

Lorazepam (The concomitant use of other CNS depressants including sedatives, hypnotics, tranquilizers, general anesthetics, phenothiazines, other opioids, and alcohol may produce additive CNS depressant effects. Additive effects resulting in respiratory depression, hypotension, profound sedation or coma may result if these drugs are taken in combination with the usual doses of oxymorphone hydrochloride).

No products indexed under this heading.

Loxapine Hydrochloride (The concomitant use of other CNS depressants including sedatives, hypnotics, tranquilizers, general anesthetics, phenothiazines, other opioids, and alcohol may produce additive CNS depressant effects. Additive effects resulting in respiratory depression, hypotension, profound sedation or coma may result if these drugs are taken in combination with the usual doses of oxymorphone hydrochloride).

No products indexed under this heading.

Loxapine Succinate (The concomitant use of other CNS depressants including sedatives, hypnotics, tranquilizers, general anesthetics, phenothiazines, other opioids, and alcohol may produce additive CNS depressant effects. Additive effects resulting in respiratory depression, hypotension, profound sedation or coma may result if these drugs are taken in combination with the usual doses of oxymorphone hydrochloride).

No products indexed under this heading.

Mepenzolate Bromide (Anticholinergics or other medications with anticholinergic activity when used concurrently with opioid analgesics may result in increased risk of urinary retention and/or severe constipation, which may lead to paralytic ileus).

No products indexed under this heading.

Meperidine Hydrochloride (The concomitant use of other CNS depressants including sedatives, hypnotics, tranquilizers, general anesthetics, phenothiazines, other opioids, and alcohol may produce additive CNS depressant effects. Additive effects resulting in respiratory depression, hypotension, profound sedation or coma may result if these drugs are taken in combination with the usual doses of oxymorphone hydrochloride).

No products indexed under this heading.

Mephobarbital (The concomitant use of other CNS depressants including sedatives, hypnotics, tranquilizers, general anesthetics, phenothiazines, other opioids, and alcohol may produce additive CNS depressant effects. Additive effects resulting in respiratory depression, hypotension, profound sedation or coma may result if these drugs are taken in combination with the usual dose of oxymorphone hydrochloride).

No products indexed under this heading.

Mepivacaine Hydrochloride (The concomitant use of other CNS depressants including sedatives, hypnotics, tranquilizers, general anesthetics, phenothiazines, other opioids, and alcohol may produce additive CNS depressant effects. Additive effects resulting in respiratory depression, hypotension, profound sedation or coma may result if these drugs are taken in combination with the usual doses of oxymorphone hydrochloride).

No products indexed under this heading.

Meprobamate (The concomitant use of other CNS depressants including sedatives, hypnotics, tranquilizers, general anesthetics, phenothiazines, other opioids, and alcohol may produce additive CNS depressant effects. Additive effects resulting in respiratory depression, hypotension, profound sedation or coma may result if these drugs are taken in combination with the usual doses of oxymorphone hydrochloride).

No products indexed under this heading.

Mesoridazine Besylate (The concomitant use of other CNS depressants including sedatives, hypnotics, tranquilizers, general anesthetics, phenothiazines, other opioids, and alcohol may produce additive CNS depressant effects. Additive effects resulting in respiratory depression, hypotension, profound sedation or coma may result if these drugs are taken in combination with the usual doses of oxymorphone hydrochloride).

No products indexed under this heading.

Methadone Hydrochloride (The concomitant use of other CNS depressants including sedatives, hypnotics, tranquilizers, general anesthetics, phenothiazines, other opioids, and alcohol may produce additive CNS depressant effects. Additive effects resulting in respiratory depression, hypotension, profound sedation or coma may result if these drugs are taken in combination with the usual doses of oxymorphone hydrochloride).

No products indexed under this heading.

Methohexital Sodium (The concomitant use of other CNS depressants including sedatives, hypnotics, tranquilizers, general anesthetics, phenothiazines, other opioids, and alcohol may produce additive CNS depressant effects. Additive effects resulting in respiratory depression, hypotension, pro-

1303 **Interactions Index** **Opana**

found sedation or coma may result if these drugs are taken in combination with the usual doses of oxymorphone hydrochloride).
No products indexed under this heading.

Methotrimeprazine (The concomitant use of other CNS depressants including sedatives, hypnotics, tranquilizers, general anesthetics, phenothiazines, other opioids, and alcohol may produce additive CNS depressant effects. Additive effects resulting in respiratory depression, hypotension, profound sedation or coma may result if these drugs are taken in combination with the usual doses of oxymorphone hydrochloride).
No products indexed under this heading.

Methoxyflurane (The concomitant use of other CNS depressants including sedatives, hypnotics, tranquilizers, general anesthetics, phenothiazines, other opioids, and alcohol may produce additive CNS depressant effects. Additive effects resulting in respiratory depression, hypotension, profound sedation or coma may result if these drugs are taken in combination with the usual dose of oxymorphone hydrochloride).
No products indexed under this heading.

Midazolam Hydrochloride (The concomitant use of other CNS depressants including sedatives, hypnotics, tranquilizers, general anesthetics, phenothiazines, other opioids, and alcohol may produce additive CNS depressant effects. Additive effects resulting in respiratory depression, hypotension, profound sedation or coma may result if these drugs are taken in combination with the usual doses of oxymorphone hydrochloride).
No products indexed under this heading.

Moclobemide (No specific interaction between oxymorphone and monoamine oxidase inhibitors has been observed, but caution in the use of any opioid in patients taking this class of drugs is appropriate).
No products indexed under this heading.

Molindone Hydrochloride (The concomitant use of other CNS depressants including sedatives, hypnotics, tranquilizers, general anesthetics, phenothiazines, other opioids, and alcohol may produce additive CNS depressant effects. Additive effects resulting in respiratory depression, hypotension, profound sedation or coma may result if these drugs are taken in combination with the usual doses of oxymorphone hydrochloride). Products include:
Moban 1108

Morphine Sulfate (The concomitant use of other CNS depressants including sedatives, hypnotics, tranquilizers, general anesthetics, phenothiazines, other opioids, and alcohol may produce additive CNS depressant effects. Additive effects resulting in respiratory depression, hypotension, profound sedation or coma may result if these drugs are taken in combination with the usual doses of oxymorphone hydrochloride). Products include:
Avinza 1822
Embeda 1831
MS Contin 2803

Morphine Sulfate, Liposomal (The concomitant use of other CNS depressants including sedatives, hypnotics, tranquilizers, general anesthetics, phenothiazines, other opioids, and alcohol may produce additive CNS depressant effects. Additive effects resulting in respiratory depression, hypotension, profound sedation or coma may result if these drugs are taken in combination with the usual doses of oxymorphone hydrochloride).
No products indexed under this heading.

Nalbuphine Hydrochloride (Agonist/antagonist analgesics should not be administered to patients who have received or are receiving a course of therapy with pure opioid agonist analgesic, such as oxymorphone hydrochloride. In this situation, mixed agonist/antagonist analgesics may reduce the analgesic effect of oxymorphone hydrochloride and/or may precipitate withdrawal symptoms).
No products indexed under this heading.

Olanzapine (The concomitant use of other CNS depressants including sedatives, hypnotics, tranquilizers, general anesthetics, phenothiazines, other opioids, and alcohol may produce additive CNS depressant effects. Additive effects resulting in respiratory depression, hypotension, profound sedation or coma may result if these drugs are taken in combination with the usual dose of oxymorphone hydrochloride). Products include:
Symbyax 1965
Zyprexa 1984
Zyprexa IntraMuscular 1984
Zyprexa ZYDIS 1984

Oxazepam (The concomitant use of other CNS depressants including sedatives, hypnotics, tranquilizers, general anesthetics, phenothiazines, other opioids, and alcohol may produce additive CNS depressant effects. Additive effects resulting in respiratory depression, hypotension, profound sedation or coma may result if these drugs are taken in combination with the usual doses of oxymorphone hydrochloride).
No products indexed under this heading.

Oxybutynin Chloride (Anticholinergics or other medications with anticholinergic activity when used concurrently with opioid analgesics may result in increased risk of urinary retention and/or severe constipation, which may lead to paralytic ileus).
No products indexed under this heading.

Oxycodone Hydrochloride (The concomitant use of other CNS depressants including sedatives, hypnotics, tranquilizers, general anesthetics, phenothiazines, other opioids, and alcohol may produce additive CNS depressant effects. Additive effects resulting in respiratory depression, hypotension, profound sedation or coma may result if these drugs are taken in combination with the usual doses of oxymorphone hydrochloride). Products include:
OxyContin 2807
Percocet 1121
Percodan 1124

Oxycodone Terephthalate (The concomitant use of other CNS depressants including sedatives, hypnotics, tranquilizers, general anesthetics, phenothiazines, other opioids, and alcohol may produce additive CNS depressant effects. Additive effects resulting in respiratory depression, hypotension, profound sedation or coma may result if these drugs are taken in combination with the usual doses of oxymorphone hydrochloride).
No products indexed under this heading.

Pargyline Hydrochloride (No specific interaction between oxymorphone and monoamine oxidase inhibitors has been observed, but caution in the use of any opioid in patients taking this class of drugs is appropriate).
No products indexed under this heading.

Pentazocine Hydrochloride (Agonist/antagonist analgesics should not be administered to patients who have received or are receiving a course of therapy with pure opioid agonist analgesic, such as oxymorphone hydrochloride. In this situation, mixed agonist/antagonist analgesics may reduce the analgesic effect of oxymorphone hydrochloride and/or may precipitate withdrawal symptoms).
No products indexed under this heading.

Pentazocine Lactate (Agonist/antagonist analgesics should not be administered to patients who have received or are receiving a course of therapy with pure opioid agonist analgesic, such as oxymorphone hydrochloride. In this situation, mixed agonist/antagonist analgesics may reduce the analgesic effect of oxymorphone hydrochloride and/or may precipitate withdrawal symptoms).
No products indexed under this heading.

Pentobarbital (The concomitant use of other CNS depressants including sedatives, hypnotics, tranquilizers, general anesthetics, phenothiazines, other opioids, and alcohol may produce additive CNS depressant effects. Additive effects resulting in respiratory depression, hypotension, profound sedation or coma may result if these drugs are taken in combination with the usual dose of oxymorphone hydrochloride).
No products indexed under this heading.

Pentobarbital Sodium (The concomitant use of other CNS depressants including sedatives, hypnotics, tranquilizers, general anesthetics, phenothiazines, other opioids, and alcohol may produce additive CNS depressant effects. Additive effects resulting in respiratory depression, hypotension, profound sedation or coma may result if these drugs are taken in combination with the usual dose of oxymorphone hydrochloride). Products include:
Nembutal 2012

Perphenazine (The concomitant use of other CNS depressants including sedatives, hypnotics, tranquilizers, general anesthetics, phenothiazines, other opioids, and alcohol may produce additive CNS depressant effects. Additive effects resulting in respiratory depression, hypotension, profound sedation or coma may result if these drugs are taken in combination with the usual doses of oxymorphone hydrochloride).
No products indexed under this heading.

Phenelzine Sulfate (No specific interaction between oxymorphone and monoamine oxidase inhibitors has been observed, but caution in the use of any opioid in patients taking this class of drugs is appropriate).
No products indexed under this heading.

Phenobarbital (The concomitant use of other CNS depressants including sedatives, hypnotics, tranquilizers, general anesthetics, phenothiazines, other opioids, and alcohol may produce additive CNS depressant effects. Additive effects resulting in respiratory depression, hypotension, profound sedation or coma may result if these drugs are taken in combination with the usual dose of oxymorphone hydrochloride). Products include:
Donnatal 2711

Phenobarbital Sodium (The concomitant use of other CNS depressants including sedatives, hypnotics, tranquilizers, general anesthetics, phenothiazines, other opioids, and alcohol may produce additive CNS depressant effects. Additive effects resulting in respiratory depression, hypotension, profound sedation or coma may result if these drugs are taken in combination with the usual dose of oxymorphone hydrochloride).
No products indexed under this heading.

Phenothiazine Derivatives (The concomitant use of other CNS depressants including sedatives, hypnotics, tranquilizers, general anesthetics, phenothiazines, other opioids, and alcohol may produce additive CNS depressant effects. Additive effects resulting in respiratory depression, hypotension, profound sedation or coma may result if these drugs are taken in combination with the usual doses of oxymorphone hydrochloride).
No products indexed under this heading.

Phenothiazines (The concomitant use of other CNS depressants including sedatives, hypnotics, tranquilizers, general anesthetics, phenothiazines, other opioids, and alcohol may produce additive CNS depressant effects. Additive effects resulting in respiratory depression, hypotension, profound sedation or coma may result if these drugs are taken in combination with the usual doses of oxymorphone hydrochloride).
No products indexed under this heading.

Prazepam (The concomitant use of other CNS depressants including sedatives, hypnotics, tranquilizers, general anesthetics, phenothiazines, other opioids, and alcohol may produce additive CNS depressant effects. Additive effects resulting in respiratory depression, hypotension, profound sedation or coma may result if these drugs are taken in combination with the usual doses of oxymorphone hydrochloride).
No products indexed under this heading.

Prilocaine (The concomitant use of other CNS depressants including sedatives, hypnotics, tranquilizers, general anesthetics, phenothiazines, other opioids, and alcohol may produce additive CNS depressant effects. Additive effects resulting in respiratory depression, hypotension, profound sedation or coma may result if these drugs are taken in combination with the usual doses of oxymorphone hydrochloride).
No products indexed under this heading.

Prilocaine Hydrochloride (The concomitant use of other CNS depressants including sedatives, hypnotics, tranquilizers, general anesthetics, phenothiazines, other opioids, and alcohol may produce additive CNS depressant effects. Additive effects resulting in respiratory depression, hypotension, profound sedation or coma may result if these drugs are taken in combination with the usual doses of oxymorphone hydrochloride).
No products indexed under this heading.

Procaine (The concomitant use of other CNS depressants including sedatives, hypnotics, tranquilizers, general anesthetics, phenothiazines, other opioids, and alcohol may produce additive CNS depressant effects. Additive effects resulting in respiratory depression, hypotension, profound sedation or coma may result if these drugs are taken in combination with the usual doses of oxymorphone hydrochloride).
No products indexed under this heading.

Procaine Hydrochloride (The concomitant use of other CNS depressants including sedatives, hypnotics, tranquilizers, general anesthetics, phenothiazines, other opioids, and alcohol may produce additive CNS depressant effects. Additive effects resulting in respiratory depression, hypotension, profound sedation or coma may result if these drugs are taken in combination with the usual doses of oxymorphone hydrochloride).
No products indexed under this heading.

IMPORTANT NOTE: Always consult each drug listing in the patient's regimen for possible interactions.

Opana Interactions Index 1304

Procarbazine Hydrochloride (No specific interaction between oxymorphone and monoamine oxidase inhibitors has been observed, but caution in the use of any opioid in patients taking this class of drugs is appropriate).
No products indexed under this heading.

Prochlorperazine (The concomitant use of other CNS depressants including sedatives, hypnotics, tranquilizers, general anesthetics, phenothiazines, other opioids, and alcohol may produce additive CNS depressant effects. Additive effects resulting in respiratory depression, hypotension, profound sedation or coma may result if these drugs are taken in combination with the usual doses of oxymorphone hydrochloride).
No products indexed under this heading.

Prochlorperazine Edisylate (The concomitant use of other CNS depressants including sedatives, hypnotics, tranquilizers, general anesthetics, phenothiazines, other opioids, and alcohol may produce additive CNS depressant effects. Additive effects resulting in respiratory depression, hypotension, profound sedation or coma may result if these drugs are taken in combination with the usual doses of oxymorphone hydrochloride).
No products indexed under this heading.

Prochlorperazine Maleate (The concomitant use of other CNS depressants including sedatives, hypnotics, tranquilizers, general anesthetics, phenothiazines, other opioids, and alcohol may produce additive CNS depressant effects. Additive effects resulting in respiratory depression, hypotension, profound sedation or coma may result if these drugs are taken in combination with the usual doses of oxymorphone hydrochloride).
No products indexed under this heading.

Procyclidine Hydrochloride (Anticholinergics or other medications with anticholinergic activity when used concurrently with opioid analgesics may result in increased risk of urinary retention and/or severe constipation, which may lead to paralytic ileus).
No products indexed under this heading.

Promethazine (The concomitant use of other CNS depressants including sedatives, hypnotics, tranquilizers, general anesthetics, phenothiazines, other opioids, and alcohol may produce additive CNS depressant effects. Additive effects resulting in respiratory depression, hypotension, profound sedation or coma may result if these drugs are taken in combination with the usual doses of oxymorphone hydrochloride).
No products indexed under this heading.

Promethazine Hydrochloride (The concomitant use of other CNS depressants including sedatives, hypnotics, tranquilizers, general anesthetics, phenothiazines, other opioids, and alcohol may produce additive CNS depressant effects. Additive effects resulting in respiratory depression, hypotension, profound sedation or coma may result if these drugs are taken in combination with the usual doses of oxymorphone hydrochloride).
No products indexed under this heading.

Propantheline Bromide (Anticholinergics or other medications with anticholinergic activity when used concurrently with opioid analgesics may result in increased risk of urinary retention and/or severe constipation, which may lead to paralytic ileus).
No products indexed under this heading.

Proparacaine Hydrochloride (The concomitant use of other CNS depressants including sedatives, hypnotics, tranquilizers, general anesthetics, phenothiazines, other opioids, and alcohol may produce additive CNS depressant effects. Additive effects resulting in respiratory depression, hypotension, profound sedation or coma may result if these drugs are taken in combination with the usual doses of oxymorphone hydrochloride).
No products indexed under this heading.

Propofol (The concomitant use of other CNS depressants including sedatives, hypnotics, tranquilizers, general anesthetics, phenothiazines, other opioids, and alcohol may produce additive CNS depressant effects. Additive effects resulting in respiratory depression, hypotension, profound sedation or coma may result if these drugs are taken in combination with the usual doses of oxymorphone hydrochloride).
No products indexed under this heading.

Propoxyphene Hydrochloride (The concomitant use of other CNS depressants including sedatives, hypnotics, tranquilizers, general anesthetics, phenothiazines, other opioids, and alcohol may produce additive CNS depressant effects. Additive effects resulting in respiratory depression, hypotension, profound sedation or coma may result if these drugs are taken in combination with the usual doses of oxymorphone hydrochloride).
No products indexed under this heading.

Propoxyphene Napsylate (The concomitant use of other CNS depressants including sedatives, hypnotics, tranquilizers, general anesthetics, phenothiazines, other opioids, and alcohol may produce additive CNS depressant effects. Additive effects resulting in respiratory depression, hypotension, profound sedation or coma may result if these drugs are taken in combination with the usual doses of oxymorphone hydrochloride).
No products indexed under this heading.

Quazepam (The concomitant use of other CNS depressants including sedatives, hypnotics, tranquilizers, general anesthetics, phenothiazines, other opioids, and alcohol may produce additive CNS depressant effects. Additive effects resulting in respiratory depression, hypotension, profound sedation or coma may result if these drugs are taken in combination with the usual doses of oxymorphone hydrochloride).
No products indexed under this heading.

Quetiapine Fumarate (The concomitant use of other CNS depressants including sedatives, hypnotics, tranquilizers, general anesthetics, phenothiazines, other opioids, and alcohol may produce additive CNS depressant effects. Additive effects resulting in respiratory depression, hypotension, profound sedation or coma may result if these drugs are taken in combination with the usual dose of oxymorphone hydrochloride). Products include:
Seroquel 750
Seroquel XR 759

Ramelteon (The concomitant use of other CNS depressants including sedatives, hypnotics, tranquilizers, general anesthetics, phenothiazines, other opioids, and alcohol may produce additive CNS depressant effects. Additive effects resulting in respiratory depression, hypotension, profound sedation or coma may result if these drugs are taken in combination with the usual doses of oxymorphone hydrochloride). Products include:
Rozerem 3366

Rasagiline Mesylate (No specific interaction between oxymorphone and monoamine oxidase inhibitors has been observed, but caution in the use of any opioid in patients taking this class of drugs is appropriate). Products include:
Azilect 3383

Remifentanil Hydrochloride (The concomitant use of other CNS depressants including sedatives, hypnotics, tranquilizers, general anesthetics, phenothiazines, other opioids, and alcohol may produce additive CNS depressant effects. Additive effects resulting in respiratory depression, hypotension, profound sedation or coma may result if these drugs are taken in combination with the usual doses of oxymorphone hydrochloride).
No products indexed under this heading.

Risperidone (The concomitant use of other CNS depressants including sedatives, hypnotics, tranquilizers, general anesthetics, phenothiazines, other opioids, and alcohol may produce additive CNS depressant effects. Additive effects resulting in respiratory depression, hypotension, profound sedation or coma may result if these drugs are taken in combination with the usual dose of oxymorphone hydrochloride). Products include:
Risperdal Consta 2682

Ropivacaine Hydrochloride (The concomitant use of other CNS depressants including sedatives, hypnotics, tranquilizers, general anesthetics, phenothiazines, other opioids, and alcohol may produce additive CNS depressant effects. Additive effects resulting in respiratory depression, hypotension, profound sedation or coma may result if these drugs are taken in combination with the usual doses of oxymorphone hydrochloride).
No products indexed under this heading.

Scopolamine (Anticholinergics or other medications with anticholinergic activity when used concurrently with opioid analgesics may result in increased risk of urinary retention and/or severe constipation, which may lead to paralytic ileus). Products include:
Transderm Scōp 2397

Scopolamine Hydrobromide (Anticholinergics or other medications with anticholinergic activity when used concurrently with opioid analgesics may result in increased risk of urinary retention and/or severe constipation, which may lead to paralytic ileus). Products include:
Donnatal 2711

Secobarbital Sodium (The concomitant use of other CNS depressants including sedatives, hypnotics, tranquilizers, general anesthetics, phenothiazines, other opioids, and alcohol may produce additive CNS depressant effects. Additive effects resulting in respiratory depression, hypotension, profound sedation or coma may result if these drugs are taken in combination with the usual doses of oxymorphone hydrochloride).
No products indexed under this heading.

Selegiline (No specific interaction between oxymorphone and monoamine oxidase inhibitors has been observed, but caution in the use of any opioid in patients taking this class of drugs is appropriate). Products include:
Emsam 3623

Selegiline Hydrochloride (No specific interaction between oxymorphone and monoamine oxidase inhibitors has been observed, but caution in the use of any opioid in patients taking this class of drugs is appropriate). Products include:
Eldepryl 3312

Sevoflurane (The concomitant use of other CNS depressants including sedatives, hypnotics, tranquilizers, general anesthetics, phenothiazines, other opioids, and alcohol may produce additive CNS depressant effects. Additive effects resulting in respiratory depression, hypotension, profound sedation or coma may result if these drugs are taken in combination with the usual dose of oxymorphone hydrochloride). Products include:
Ultane 554

Sodium Butabarbital (The concomitant use of other CNS depressants including sedatives, hypnotics, tranquilizers, general anesthetics, phenothiazines, other opioids, and alcohol may produce additive CNS depressant effects. Additive effects resulting in respiratory depression, hypotension, profound sedation or coma may result if these drugs are taken in combination with the usual doses of oxymorphone hydrochloride).
No products indexed under this heading.

Sodium Oxybate (The concomitant use of other CNS depressants including sedatives, hypnotics, tranquilizers, general anesthetics, phenothiazines, other opioids, and alcohol may produce additive CNS depressant effects. Additive effects resulting in respiratory depression, hypotension, profound sedation or coma may result if these drugs are taken in combination with the usual dose of oxymorphone hydrochloride).
No products indexed under this heading.

Sodium Pentobarbital (The concomitant use of other CNS depressants including sedatives, hypnotics, tranquilizers, general anesthetics, phenothiazines, other opioids, and alcohol may produce additive CNS depressant effects. Additive effects resulting in respiratory depression, hypotension, profound sedation or coma may result if these drugs are taken in combination with the usual dose of oxymorphone hydrochloride).
No products indexed under this heading.

Sufentanil Citrate (The concomitant use of other CNS depressants including sedatives, hypnotics, tranquilizers, general anesthetics, phenothiazines, other opioids, and alcohol may produce additive CNS depressant effects. Additive effects resulting in respiratory depression, hypotension, profound sedation or coma may result if these drugs are taken in combination with the usual doses of oxymorphone hydrochloride).
No products indexed under this heading.

Talbutal (The concomitant use of other CNS depressants including sedatives, hypnotics, tranquilizers, general anesthetics, phenothiazines, other opioids, and alcohol may produce additive CNS depressant effects. Additive effects resulting in respiratory depression, hypotension, profound sedation or coma may result if these drugs are taken in combination with the usual dose of oxymorphone hydrochloride).
No products indexed under this heading.

Temazepam (The concomitant use of other CNS depressants including sedatives, hypnotics, tranquilizers, general anesthetics, phenothiazines, other opioids, and alcohol may produce additive CNS depressant effects. Additive effects resulting in respiratory depression, hypotension, profound sedation or coma may result if these drugs are taken in combination with the usual doses of oxymorphone hydrochloride).
No products indexed under this heading.

Tetracaine (The concomitant use of other CNS depressants including sedatives, hypnotics, tranquilizers, general anesthetics, phenothiazines, other opioids, and alcohol may produce additive CNS depressant effects. Additive effects resulting in respiratory depression, hypotension, profound sedation or coma may result if these drugs are taken in combination with the usual doses of oxymorphone hydrochloride).
No products indexed under this heading.

Tetracaine Hydrochloride (The concomitant use of other CNS depressants including sedatives, hypnotics, tranquilizers, general anesthetics, phenothiazines, other opioids, and alcohol may produce additive CNS depressant effects. Additive effects resulting in respiratory depression, hypotension, profound sedation or coma may result if these drugs are taken in combination with the usual doses of oxymorphone hydrochloride).
No products indexed under this heading.

Thiamylal Sodium (The concomitant use of other CNS depressants including sedatives, hypnotics, tranquilizers, general anesthetics, phenothiazines, other opioids, and alcohol may produce additive CNS depressant effects. Additive effects resulting in respiratory depression, hypotension, profound sedation or coma may result if these drugs are taken in combination with the usual doses of oxymorphone hydrochloride).
No products indexed under this heading.

Thioridazine (The concomitant use of other CNS depressants including sedatives, hypnotics, tranquilizers, general anesthetics, phenothiazines, other opioids, and alcohol may produce additive CNS depressant effects. Additive effects resulting in respiratory depression, hypotension, profound sedation or coma may result if these drugs are taken in combination with the usual doses of oxymorphone hydrochloride).
No products indexed under this heading.

Thioridazine Hydrochloride (The concomitant use of other CNS depressants including sedatives, hypnotics, tranquilizers, general anesthetics, phenothiazines, other opioids, and alcohol may produce additive CNS depressant effects. Additive effects resulting in respiratory depression, hypotension, profound sedation or coma may result if these drugs are taken in combination with the usual doses of oxymorphone hydrochloride). Products include:
Thioridazine Hydrochloride 2384

Thiothixene (The concomitant use of other CNS depressants including sedatives, hypnotics, tranquilizers, general anesthetics, phenothiazines, other opioids, and alcohol may produce additive CNS depressant effects. Additive effects resulting in respiratory depression, hypotension, profound sedation or coma may result if these drugs are taken in combination with the usual doses of oxymorphone hydrochloride). Products include:
Thiothixene 2386

Thiothixene Hydrochloride (The concomitant use of other CNS depressants including sedatives, hypnotics, tranquilizers, general anesthetics, phenothiazines, other opioids, and alcohol may produce additive CNS depressant effects. Additive effects resulting in respiratory depression, hypotension, profound sedation or coma may result if these drugs are taken in combination with the usual dose of oxymorphone hydrochloride).
No products indexed under this heading.

Tolterodine Tartrate (Anticholinergics or other medications with anticholinergic activity when used concurrently with opioid analgesics may result in increased risk of urinary retention and/or severe constipation, which may lead to paralytic ileus).
No products indexed under this heading.

Tranylcypromine Sulfate (No specific interaction between oxymorphone and monoamine oxidase inhibitors has been observed, but caution in the use of any opioid in patients taking this class of drugs is appropriate). Products include:
Parnate 1584

Triazolam (The concomitant use of other CNS depressants including sedatives, hypnotics, tranquilizers, general anesthetics, phenothiazines, other opioids, and alcohol may produce additive CNS depressant effects. Additive effects resulting in respiratory depression, hypotension, profound sedation or coma may result if these drugs are taken in combination with the usual doses of oxymorphone hydrochloride).
No products indexed under this heading.

Tridihexethyl Chloride (Anticholinergics or other medications with anticholinergic activity when used concurrently with opioid analgesics may result in increased risk of urinary retention and/or severe constipation, which may lead to paralytic ileus).
No products indexed under this heading.

Trifluoperazine Hydrochloride (The concomitant use of other CNS depressants including sedatives, hypnotics, tranquilizers, general anesthetics, phenothiazines, other opioids, and alcohol may produce additive CNS depressant effects. Additive effects resulting in respiratory depression, hypotension, profound sedation or coma may result if these drugs are taken in combination with the usual doses of oxymorphone hydrochloride).
No products indexed under this heading.

Trihexyphenidyl Hydrochloride (Anticholinergics or other medications with anticholinergic activity when used concurrently with opioid analgesics may result in increased risk of urinary retention and/or severe constipation, which may lead to paralytic ileus).
No products indexed under this heading.

Zaleplon (The concomitant use of other CNS depressants including sedatives, hypnotics, tranquilizers, general anesthetics, phenothiazines, other opioids, and alcohol may produce additive CNS depressant effects. Additive effects resulting in respiratory depression, hypotension, profound sedation or coma may result if these drugs are taken in combination with the usual doses of oxymorphone hydrochloride).
No products indexed under this heading.

Ziprasidone Hydrochloride (The concomitant use of other CNS depressants including sedatives, hypnotics, tranquilizers, general anesthetics, phenothiazines, other opioids, and alcohol may produce additive CNS depressant effects. Additive effects resulting in respiratory depression, hypotension, profound sedation or coma may result if these drugs are taken in combination with the usual dose of oxymorphone hydrochloride). Products include:
Geodon 2723

Zolpidem Tartrate (The concomitant use of other CNS depressants including sedatives, hypnotics, tranquilizers, general anesthetics, phenothiazines, other opioids, and alcohol may produce additive CNS depressant effects. Additive effects resulting in respiratory depression, hypotension, profound sedation or coma may result if these drugs are taken in combination with the usual doses of oxymorphone hydrochloride). Products include:
Ambien 2920
Ambien CR 2925

Food Interactions

Alcohol (The concomitant use of other CNS depressants including sedatives, hypnotics, tranquilizers, general anesthetics, phenothiazines, other opioids, and alcohol may produce additive CNS depressant effects. Additive effects resulting in respiratory depression, hypotension, profound sedation or coma may result if these drugs are taken in combination with the usual dose of oxymorphone hydrochloride).

Beer, reduced-alcohol (The concomitant use of other CNS depressants including sedatives, hypnotics, tranquilizers, general anesthetics, phenothiazines, other opioids, and alcohol may produce additive CNS depressant effects. Additive effects resulting in respiratory depression, hypotension, profound sedation or coma may result if these drugs are taken in combination with the usual doses of oxymorphone hydrochloride).

Beer, unspecified (The concomitant use of other CNS depressants including sedatives, hypnotics, tranquilizers, general anesthetics, phenothiazines, other opioids, and alcohol may produce additive CNS depressant effects. Additive effects resulting in respiratory depression, hypotension, profound sedation or coma may result if these drugs are taken in combination with the usual doses of oxymorphone hydrochloride).

Wine, Chianti (The concomitant use of other CNS depressants including sedatives, hypnotics, tranquilizers, general anesthetics, phenothiazines, other opioids, and alcohol may produce additive CNS depressant effects. Additive effects resulting in respiratory depression, hypotension, profound sedation or coma may result if these drugs are taken in combination with the usual doses of oxymorphone hydrochloride).

Wine, Red (The concomitant use of other CNS depressants including sedatives, hypnotics, tranquilizers, general anesthetics, phenothiazines, other opioids, and alcohol may produce additive CNS depressant effects. Additive effects resulting in respiratory depression, hypotension, profound sedation or coma may result if these drugs are taken in combination with the usual doses of oxymorphone hydrochloride).

Wine, unspecified (The concomitant use of other CNS depressants including sedatives, hypnotics, tranquilizers, general anesthetics, phenothiazines, other opioids, and alcohol may produce additive CNS depressant effects. Additive effects resulting in respiratory depression, hypotension, profound sedation or coma may result if these drugs are taken in combination with the usual doses of oxymorphone hydrochloride).

Wine products (The concomitant use of other CNS depressants including sedatives, hypnotics, tranquilizers, general anesthetics, phenothiazines, other opioids, and alcohol may produce additive CNS depressant effects. Additive effects resulting in respiratory depression, hypotension, profound sedation or coma may result if these drugs are taken in combination with the usual doses of oxymorphone hydrochloride).

OPANA ER TABLETS

(Oxymorphone Hydrochloride) 1114
See Opana Tablets

OPTIPRANOLOL OPHTHALMIC SOLUTION 0.3%

(Metipranolol) .... ⊙249
May interact with adrenergic augmenting psychotropics, beta-blockers, calcium channel blockers, cardiac glycosides, and certain other agents. Compounds in these categories include:

Acebutolol Hydrochloride (Co-administration with oral beta blockers may result in additive effects or systemic beta blockade).
No products indexed under this heading.

Amlodipine Besylate (Co-administration with oral or intravenous calcium channel antagonists may result in possible precipitation of left ventricular failure and hypotension). Products include:
Azor 1010
Exforge 2443
Exforge HCT 2449

Atenolol (Co-administration with oral beta blockers may result in additive effects or systemic beta blockade).
No products indexed under this heading.

Bepridil Hydrochloride (Co-administration with oral or intravenous calcium channel antagonists may result in possible precipitation of left ventricular failure and hypotension).
No products indexed under this heading.

Betaxolol Hydrochloride (Co-administration with oral beta blockers may result in additive effects or systemic beta blockade).
No products indexed under this heading.

Bisoprolol Fumarate (Co-administration with oral beta blockers may result in additive effects or systemic beta blockade).
No products indexed under this heading.

Carteolol Hydrochloride (Co-administration with oral beta blockers may result in additive effects or systemic beta blockade).
No products indexed under this heading.

Carvedilol (Co-administration with oral beta blockers may result in additive effects or systemic beta blockade). Products include:
Coreg 1409

Carvedilol Phosphate (Co-administration with oral beta blockers may result in additive effects or systemic beta blockade). Products include:
Coreg CR 1416

Deserpidine (Possible additive effects and production of hypotension and/or bradycardia when beta blocker is concurrently used with catecholamine-depleting drugs).
No products indexed under this heading.

Deslanoside (Concomitant use of beta blockers with digitalis and calcium channel blockers may result in additive effects in prolonging atrioventricular conduction time).
No products indexed under this heading.

Digitalis Glycoside Preparations (Concomitant use of beta blockers with digitalis and calcium channel blockers may result in additive effects in prolonging atrioventricular conduction time).
No products indexed under this heading.

Digitalis Lanata (Concomitant use of beta blockers with digitalis and calcium channel blockers may result in additive effects in prolonging atrioventricular conduction time).
No products indexed under this heading.

Digitalis Purpurea (Concomitant use of beta blockers with digitalis and calcium channel blockers may result in additive effects in prolonging atrioventricular conduction time).
No products indexed under this heading.

Digitoxin (Concomitant use of beta blockers with digitalis and calcium channel blockers may result in additive effects in prolonging atrioventricular conduction time).
No products indexed under this heading.

Digoxin (Concomitant use of beta blockers with digitalis and calcium channel blockers may result in additive effects in prolonging atrioventricular conduction time). Products include:
Lanoxin Injection 1546
Lanoxin Injection Pediatric 1549
Lanoxin Tablets 1553

Diltiazem Hydrochloride (Co-administration with oral or intravenous

calcium channel antagonists may result in possible precipitation of left ventricular failure and hypotension). Products include:

Cardizem LA 423

Epinephrine (Concurrent use in patients with history of atopy or severe anaphylactic reaction to allergens may be unresponsive to the usual doses of epinephrine used to treat anaphylactic reaction). Products include:

EpiPen 3631
Twinject 3268

Epinephrine Hydrochloride (Concurrent use in patients with history of atopy or severe anaphylactic reaction to allergens may be unresponsive to the usual doses of epinephrine used to treat anaphylactic reaction).

No products indexed under this heading.

Esmolol Hydrochloride (Co-administration with oral beta blockers may result in additive effects or systemic beta blockade).

No products indexed under this heading.

Felodipine (Co-administration with oral or intravenous calcium channel antagonists may result in possible precipitation of left ventricular failure and hypotension).

No products indexed under this heading.

Isocarboxazid (Exercise caution when used concurrently with adrenergic psychotropic drugs). Products include:

Marplan 3481

Isradipine (Co-administration with oral or intravenous calcium channel antagonists may result in possible precipitation of left ventricular failure and hypotension). Products include:

DynaCirc CR 1432

Labetalol Hydrochloride (Co-administration with oral beta blockers may result in additive effects or systemic beta blockade).

No products indexed under this heading.

Levobunolol Hydrochloride (Co-administration with oral beta blockers may result in additive effects or systemic beta blockade).

No products indexed under this heading.

Metipranolol Hydrochloride (Co-administration with oral beta blockers may result in additive effects or systemic beta blockade).

No products indexed under this heading.

Metoprolol Succinate (Co-administration with oral beta blockers may result in additive effects or systemic beta blockade). Products include:

Toprol XL 732

Metoprolol Tartrate (Co-administration with oral beta blockers may result in additive effects or systemic beta blockade).

No products indexed under this heading.

Mibefradil Dihydrochloride (Co-administration with oral or intravenous calcium channel antagonists may result in possible precipitation of left ventricular failure and hypotension).

No products indexed under this heading.

Nadolol (Co-administration with oral beta blockers may result in additive effects or systemic beta blockade). Products include:

Nadolol 2359

Nebivolol (Co-administration with oral beta blockers may result in additive effects or systemic beta blockade). Products include:

Bystolic 1147

Nicardipine (Co-administration with oral or intravenous calcium channel antagonists may result in possible precipitation of left ventricular failure and hypotension).

No products indexed under this heading.

Nicardipine Hydrochloride (Co-administration with oral or intravenous calcium channel antagonists may result in possible precipitation of left ventricular failure and hypotension).

No products indexed under this heading.

Nifedipine (Co-administration with oral or intravenous calcium channel antagonists may result in possible precipitation of left ventricular failure and hypotension).

No products indexed under this heading.

Nimodipine (Co-administration with oral or intravenous calcium channel antagonists may result in possible precipitation of left ventricular failure and hypotension).

No products indexed under this heading.

Nisoldipine (Co-administration with oral or intravenous calcium channel antagonists may result in possible precipitation of left ventricular failure and hypotension).

No products indexed under this heading.

Pargyline Hydrochloride (Exercise caution when used concurrently with adrenergic psychotropic drugs).

No products indexed under this heading.

Penbutolol Sulfate (Co-administration with oral beta blockers may result in additive effects or systemic beta blockade).

No products indexed under this heading.

Phenelzine Sulfate (Exercise caution when used concurrently with adrenergic psychotropic drugs).

No products indexed under this heading.

Pindolol (Co-administration with oral beta blockers may result in additive effects or systemic beta blockade).

No products indexed under this heading.

Propranolol Hydrochloride (Co-administration with oral beta blockers may result in additive effects or systemic beta blockade). Products include:

InnoPran XL 1517

Rauwolfia Serpentina (Possible additive effects and production of hypotension and/or bradycardia when beta blocker is concurrently used with catecholamine-depleting drugs).

No products indexed under this heading.

Rescinnamine (Possible additive effects and production of hypotension and/or bradycardia when beta blocker is concurrently used with catecholamine-depleting drugs).

No products indexed under this heading.

Reserpine (Possible additive effects and production of hypotension and/or bradycardia when beta blocker is concurrently used with catecholamine-depleting drugs).

No products indexed under this heading.

Sotalol Hydrochloride (Co-administration with oral beta blockers may result in additive effects or systemic beta blockade).

No products indexed under this heading.

Timolol Hemihydrate (Co-administration with oral beta blockers may result in additive effects or systemic beta blockade). Products include:

Betimol 3490

Timolol Maleate (Co-administration with oral beta blockers may result in additive effects or systemic beta blockade). Products include:

Combigan 601
Dorzolamide
Hydrochloride/Timolol Maleate
Ophthalmic Solution .... ⊙243
Timoptic in Ocudose .... ⊙231

Tranylcypromine Sulfate (Exercise caution when used concurrently with adrenergic psychotropic drugs). Products include:

Parnate 1584

Verapamil Hydrochloride (Co-administration with oral or intravenous calcium channel antagonists may result in possible precipitation of left ventricular failure and hypotension). Products include:

Tarka 534

ORTHO EVRA TRANSDERMAL SYSTEM

(Ethinyl Estradiol, Norelgestromin) 2648
May interact with ampicillins, antibiotics, barbiturates, cytochrome p450 3a4 inducers (selected), cytochrome p450 3a4 inhibitors (selected), cytochrome p450 inducers (selected), drugs which undergo biotransformation by cytochrome p-450 mixed function oxidase, hepatic microsomal enzyme inducers, phenytoin, prednisolone, protease inhibitors, tetracyclines, theophyllines, and certain other agents. Compounds in these categories include:

Acarbose (Although norelgestromin and its metabolites inhibit a variety of P450 enzymes in human liver microsomes, the clinical consequence of such an interaction on the levels of other concomitant medications is likely to be insignificant. Under the recommended dosing regimen, the *in vivo* concentrations of norelgestromin and its metabolites, even at the peak serum levels, are relatively low compared to the inhibitory constant (Ki) (based on results of *in vitro* studies)).

No products indexed under this heading.

Acetaminophen (Concomitant use with acetaminophen may increase plasma ethinyl estradiol levels, possibly by inhibition of conjugation. In addition, decreased plasma concentrations of acetaminophen have been noted when acetaminophen was administered with oral contraceptives). Products include:

Percocet 1121
Tylenol 2049
Tylenol 8 Hour 2049
Extra Strength Tylenol Caplets,
Cool Caplets, and EZ Tabs 2049
Extra Strength Tylenol Adult Rapid
Blast Liquid........................ 2049
Extra Strength Tylenol Rapid
Release 2049
Tylenol with Codeine 2691
Tylenol Arthritis Pain Extended
Release Geltabs/Caplets 2049
Children's Tylenol Suspension
Liquid............................... 2048
Chlidren's Tylenol Meltaways 2048
Tylenol, Infants' Drops 2048
Junior Tylenol 2048
Vicodin 560
Vicodin ES 561
Vicodin HP 563
Zydone 1138

Acetaminophen-containing products (Concomitant use with acetaminophen may increase plasma ethinyl estradiol levels, possibly by inhibition of conjugation. In addition, decreased plasma concentrations of acetaminophen have been noted when acetaminophen was administered with oral contraceptives).

No products indexed under this heading.

Acetazolamide (CYP3A4 inhibitors, such as itraconazole or ketoconazole, may increase plasma hormone levels).

No products indexed under this heading.

Acetazolamide Sodium (CYP3A4 inhibitors, such as itraconazole or ketoconazole, may increase plasma hormone levels).

No products indexed under this heading.

Alatrofloxacin Mesylate (There have been reports of pregnancy while taking hormonal contraceptives and antibiotics, but clinical pharmacokinetic studies have not shown consistent effects of antibiotics on plasma concentrations of synthetic steroids. The metabolism of hormonal contraceptives may be influ-

enced by various drugs. Of potential clinical importance are drugs that interrupt entero-hepatic recirculation of estrogen (eg, certain antibiotics). Literature suggests possible interactions with the concomitant use of hormonal contraceptives and ampicillin or tetracycline).

No products indexed under this heading.

Alfentanil Hydrochloride (Although norelgestromin and its metabolites inhibit a variety of P450 enzymes in human liver microsomes, the clinical consequence of such an interaction on the levels of other concomitant medications is likely to be insignificant. Under the recommended dosing regimen, the *in vivo* concentrations of norelgestromin and its metabolites, even at the peak serum levels, are relatively low compared to the inhibitory constant (Ki) (based on results of *in vitro* studies)).

No products indexed under this heading.

Allium cepa (If a woman on hormonal contraceptives takes a drug or herbal product that induces enzymes, including CYP3A4, that metabolize contraceptive hormones, counsel her to use additional contraception or a different method of contraception. Drugs or herbal products that induce such enzymes may decrease the plasma concentrations of contraceptive hormones, and may decrease the effectiveness of hormonal contraceptives or increase breakthrough bleeding). Products include:

Hyland's Cold 'N Cough 3314
Mederma 2319
Mederma for Kids 2319

Allium sativum (If a woman on hormonal contraceptives takes a drug or herbal product that induces enzymes, including CYP3A4, that metabolize contraceptive hormones, counsel her to use additional contraception or a different method of contraception. Drugs or herbal products that induce such enzymes may decrease the plasma concentrations of contraceptive hormones, and may decrease the effectiveness of hormonal contraceptives or increase breakthrough bleeding).

No products indexed under this heading.

Allium schoenoprasum (If a woman on hormonal contraceptives takes a drug or herbal product that induces enzymes, including CYP3A4, that metabolize contraceptive hormones, counsel her to use additional contraception or a different method of contraception. Drugs or herbal products that induce such enzymes may decrease the plasma concentrations of contraceptive hormones, and may decrease the effectiveness of hormonal contraceptives or increase breakthrough bleeding).

No products indexed under this heading.

Allium ursinum (If a woman on hormonal contraceptives takes a drug or herbal product that induces enzymes, including CYP3A4, that metabolize contraceptive hormones, counsel her to use additional contraception or a different method of contraception. Drugs or herbal products that induce such enzymes may decrease the plasma concentrations of contraceptive hormones, and may decrease the effectiveness of hormonal contraceptives or increase breakthrough bleeding).

No products indexed under this heading.

Alprazolam (Although norelgestromin and its metabolites inhibit a variety of P450 enzymes in human liver microsomes, the clinical consequence of such an interaction on the levels of other concomitant medications is likely to be insignificant. Under the recommended dosing regimen, the *in vivo* concentrations of norelgestromin and its metabolites, even at the peak serum

levels, are relatively low compared to the inhibitory constant (Ki) (based on results of *in vitro* studies)).
No products indexed under this heading.

Amikacin Sulfate (There have been reports of pregnancy while taking hormonal contraceptives and antibiotics, but clinical pharmacokinetic studies have not shown consistent effects of antibiotics on plasma concentrations of synthetic steroids. The metabolism of hormonal contraceptives may be influenced by various drugs. Of potential clinical importance are drugs that interrupt entero-hepatic recirculation of estrogen (eg, certain antibiotics). Literature suggests possible interactions with the concomitant use of hormonal contraceptives and ampicillin or tetracycline).
No products indexed under this heading.

Aminoglutethimide (If a woman on hormonal contraceptives takes a drug or herbal product that induces enzymes, including CYP3A4, that metabolize contraceptive hormones, counsel her to use additional contraception or a different method of contraception. Drugs or herbal products that induce such enzymes may decrease the plasma concentrations of contraceptive hormones, and may decrease the effectiveness of hormonal contraceptives or increase breakthrough bleeding).
No products indexed under this heading.

Aminophylline (Although norelgestromin and its metabolites inhibit a variety of P450 enzymes in human liver microsomes, the clinical consequence of such an interaction on the levels of other concomitant medications is likely to be insignificant. Under the recommended dosing regimen, the *in vivo* concentrations of norelgestromin and its metabolites, even at the peak serum levels, are relatively low compared to the inhibitory constant (Ki) (based on results of *in vitro* studies)).
No products indexed under this heading.

Amiodarone Hydrochloride (CYP3A4 inhibitors, such as itraconazole or ketoconazole, may increase plasma hormone levels).
No products indexed under this heading.

Amitriptyline Hydrochloride (Although norelgestromin and its metabolites inhibit a variety of P450 enzymes in human liver microsomes, the clinical consequence of such an interaction on the levels of other concomitant medications is likely to be insignificant. Under the recommended dosing regimen, the *in vivo* concentrations of norelgestromin and its metabolites, even at the peak serum levels, are relatively low compared to the inhibitory constant (Ki) (based on results of *in vitro* studies)).
No products indexed under this heading.

Amlodipine Besylate (Although norelgestromin and its metabolites inhibit a variety of P450 enzymes in human liver microsomes, the clinical consequence of such an interaction on the levels of other concomitant medications is likely to be insignificant. Under the recommended dosing regimen, the *in vivo* concentrations of norelgestromin and its metabolites, even at the peak serum levels, are relatively low compared to the inhibitory constant (Ki) (based on results of *in vitro* studies)). Products include:
Azor **1010**
Exforge **2443**
Exforge HCT **2449**

Amobarbital (Concomitant use with barbiturates may decrease the plasma concentrations of hormonal contraceptives, and may decrease the effectiveness of hormonal contraceptives or increase breakthrough bleeding. Patients who are concomitantly using barbiturates should be counseled to use additional contraception or a different method of contraception).
No products indexed under this heading.

Amobarbital Sodium (Concomitant use with barbiturates may decrease the plasma concentrations of hormonal contraceptives, and may decrease the effectiveness of hormonal contraceptives or increase breakthrough bleeding. Patients who are concomitantly using barbiturates should be counseled to use additional contraception or a different method of contraception).
No products indexed under this heading.

Amoxapine (Although norelgestromin and its metabolites inhibit a variety of P450 enzymes in human liver microsomes, the clinical consequence of such an interaction on the levels of other concomitant medications is likely to be insignificant. Under the recommended dosing regimen, the *in vivo* concentrations of norelgestromin and its metabolites, even at the peak serum levels, are relatively low compared to the inhibitory constant (Ki) (based on results of *in vitro* studies)).
No products indexed under this heading.

Amoxicillin (There have been reports of pregnancy while taking hormonal contraceptives and antibiotics, but clinical pharmacokinetic studies have not shown consistent effects of antibiotics on plasma concentrations of synthetic steroids. The metabolism of hormonal contraceptives may be influenced by various drugs. Of potential clinical importance are drugs that interrupt entero-hepatic recirculation of estrogen (eg, certain antibiotics). Literature suggests possible interactions with the concomitant use of hormonal contraceptives and ampicillin or tetracycline). Products include:
Amoxil Capsules **1311**
Amoxil Chewable Tablets **1311**
Amoxil **1311**
Amoxil Powder **1311**
Augmentin **1331**
Augmentin Tablets **1335**
Augmentin ES-600 .... **1338**
Augmentin XR **1342**
Moxatag **2321**

Amoxicillin Trihydrate (There have been reports of pregnancy while taking hormonal contraceptives and antibiotics, but clinical pharmacokinetic studies have not shown consistent effects of antibiotics on plasma concentrations of synthetic steroids. The metabolism of hormonal contraceptives may be influenced by various drugs. Of potential clinical importance are drugs that interrupt entero-hepatic recirculation of estrogen (eg, certain antibiotics). Literature suggests possible interactions with the concomitant use of hormonal contraceptives and ampicillin or tetracycline).
No products indexed under this heading.

Amphetamine Aspartate (Although norelgestromin and its metabolites inhibit a variety of P450 enzymes in human liver microsomes, the clinical consequence of such an interaction on the levels of other concomitant medications is likely to be insignificant. Under the recommended dosing regimen, the *in vivo* concentrations of norelgestromin and its metabolites, even at the peak serum levels, are relatively low compared to the inhibitory constant (Ki) (based on results of *in vitro* studies)).
No products indexed under this heading.

Amphetamine Aspartate Monohydrate (Although norelgestromin and its metabolites inhibit a variety of P450 enzymes in human liver microsomes, the clinical consequence of such an interaction on the levels of other concomitant medications is likely to be insignificant. Under the recommended dosing regimen, the *in vivo* concentrations of norelgestromin and its metabolites, even at the peak serum levels, are relatively low compared to the inhibitory constant (Ki) (based on results of *in vitro* studies)).
No products indexed under this heading.

Amphetamine Sulfate (Although norelgestromin and its metabolites inhibit a variety of P450 enzymes in human liver microsomes, the clinical consequence of such an interaction on the levels of other concomitant medications is likely to be insignificant. Under the recommended dosing regimen, the *in vivo* concentrations of norelgestromin and its metabolites, even at the peak serum levels, are relatively low compared to the inhibitory constant (Ki) (based on results of *in vitro* studies)).
No products indexed under this heading.

Ampicillin (There have been reports of pregnancy while taking hormonal contraceptives and antibiotics, but clinical pharmacokinetic studies have not shown consistent effects of antibiotics on plasma concentrations of synthetic steroids. The metabolism of hormonal contraceptives may be influenced by various drugs. Of potential clinical importance are drugs that interrupt entero-hepatic recirculation of estrogen (eg, certain antibiotics). Literature suggests possible interactions with the concomitant use of hormonal contraceptives and ampicillin or tetracycline).
No products indexed under this heading.

Ampicillin Sodium (There have been reports of pregnancy while taking hormonal contraceptives and antibiotics, but clinical pharmacokinetic studies have not shown consistent effects of antibiotics on plasma concentrations of synthetic steroids. The metabolism of hormonal contraceptives may be influenced by various drugs. Of potential clinical importance are drugs that interrupt entero-hepatic recirculation of estrogen (eg, certain antibiotics). Literature suggests possible interactions with the concomitant use of hormonal contraceptives and ampicillin or tetracycline).
No products indexed under this heading.

Ampicillin Trihydrate (There have been reports of pregnancy while taking hormonal contraceptives and antibiotics, but clinical pharmacokinetic studies have not shown consistent effects of antibiotics on plasma concentrations of synthetic steroids. The metabolism of hormonal contraceptives may be influenced by various drugs. Of potential clinical importance are drugs that interrupt entero-hepatic recirculation of estrogen (eg, certain antibiotics). Literature suggests possible interactions with the concomitant use of hormonal contraceptives and ampicillin or tetracycline).
No products indexed under this heading.

Amprenavir (Significant changes (increase or decrease) in the plasma levels of the estrogen and progestin have been noted in some cases of co-administration of HIV protease inhibitors).
No products indexed under this heading.

Anagrelide Hydrochloride (Although norelgestromin and its metabolites inhibit a variety of P450 enzymes in human liver microsomes, the clinical consequence of such an interaction on the levels of other concomitant medications is likely to be insignificant. Under the recommended dosing regimen, the *in vivo* concentrations of norelgestromin and its metabolites, even at the peak serum levels, are relatively low compared to the inhibitory constant (Ki) (based on results of *in vitro* studies)).
No products indexed under this heading.

Anastrozole (CYP3A4 inhibitors, such as itraconazole or ketoconazole, may increase plasma hormone levels).
No products indexed under this heading.

Antibiotics, non-penicillin, unspecified (There have been reports of pregnancy while taking hormonal contraceptives and antibiotics, but clinical pharmacokinetic studies have not shown consistent effects of antibiotics on plasma concentrations of synthetic steroids. The metabolism of hormonal contraceptives may be influenced by various drugs. Of potential clinical importance are drugs that interrupt entero-hepatic recirculation of estrogen (eg, certain antibiotics). Literature suggests possible interactions with the concomitant use of hormonal contraceptives and ampicillin or tetracycline).
No products indexed under this heading.

Aprepitant (If a woman on hormonal contraceptives takes a drug or herbal product that induces enzymes, including CYP3A4, that metabolize contraceptive hormones, counsel her to use additional contraception or a different method of contraception. Drugs or herbal products that induce such enzymes may decrease the plasma concentrations of contraceptive hormones, and may decrease the effectiveness of hormonal contraceptives or increase breakthrough bleeding). Products include:
Emend **2124**

Aprobarbital (Concomitant use with barbiturates may decrease the plasma concentrations of hormonal contraceptives, and may decrease the effectiveness of hormonal contraceptives or increase breakthrough bleeding. Patients who are concomitantly using barbiturates should be counseled to use additional contraception or a different method of contraception).
No products indexed under this heading.

Astemizole (Although norelgestromin and its metabolites inhibit a variety of P450 enzymes in human liver microsomes, the clinical consequence of such an interaction on the levels of other concomitant medications is likely to be insignificant. Under the recommended dosing regimen, the *in vivo* concentrations of norelgestromin and its metabolites, even at the peak serum levels, are relatively low compared to the inhibitory constant (Ki) (based on results of *in vitro* studies)).
No products indexed under this heading.

Atazanavir (Significant changes (increase or decrease) in the plasma levels of the estrogen and progestin have been noted in some cases of co-administration of HIV protease inhibitors).
No products indexed under this heading.

Atazanavir Sulfate (Significant changes (increase or decrease) in the plasma levels of the estrogen and progestin have been noted in some cases of co-administration of HIV protease inhibitors).
No products indexed under this heading.

Atomoxetine Hydrochloride (Although norelgestromin and its metabolites inhibit a variety of P450 enzymes in human liver microsomes, the clinical consequence of such an interaction on the levels of other concomitant medications is likely to be insignificant. Under the recommended dosing regimen, the *in vivo* concentrations of norelgestromin

Ortho Evra | Interactions Index | 1308

and its metabolites, even at the peak serum levels, are relatively low compared to the inhibitory constant (Ki) (based on results of *in vitro* studies)). Products include:
Strattera 1957

Atorvastatin Calcium (Co-administration of atorvastatin and certain oral contraceptives containing ethinyl estradiol increased AUC values for ethinyl estradiol by approximately 20%). Products include:
Lipitor 2703

Azithromycin Dihydrate (There have been reports of pregnancy while taking hormonal contraceptives and antibiotics, but clinical pharmacokinetic studies have not shown consistent effects of antibiotics on plasma concentrations of synthetic steroids. The metabolism of hormonal contraceptives may be influenced by various drugs. Of potential clinical importance are drugs that interrupt entero-hepatic recirculation of estrogen (eg, certain antibiotics). Literature suggests possible interactions with the concomitant use of hormonal contraceptives and ampicillin or tetracycline).
No products indexed under this heading.

Azlocillin Sodium (There have been reports of pregnancy while taking hormonal contraceptives and antibiotics, but clinical pharmacokinetic studies have not shown consistent effects of antibiotics on plasma concentrations of synthetic steroids. The metabolism of hormonal contraceptives may be influenced by various drugs. Of potential clinical importance are drugs that interrupt entero-hepatic recirculation of estrogen (eg, certain antibiotics). Literature suggests possible interactions with the concomitant use of hormonal contraceptives and ampicillin or tetracycline).
No products indexed under this heading.

Aztreonam (There have been reports of pregnancy while taking hormonal contraceptives and antibiotics, but clinical pharmacokinetic studies have not shown consistent effects of antibiotics on plasma concentrations of synthetic steroids. The metabolism of hormonal contraceptives may be influenced by various drugs. Of potential clinical importance are drugs that interrupt entero-hepatic recirculation of estrogen (eg, certain antibiotics). Literature suggests possible interactions with the concomitant use of hormonal contraceptives and ampicillin or tetracycline).
No products indexed under this heading.

Bacampicillin Hydrochloride (There have been reports of pregnancy while taking hormonal contraceptives and antibiotics, but clinical pharmacokinetic studies have not shown consistent effects of antibiotics on plasma concentrations of synthetic steroids. The metabolism of hormonal contraceptives may be influenced by various drugs. Of potential clinical importance are drugs that interrupt entero-hepatic recirculation of estrogen (eg, certain antibiotics). Literature suggests possible interactions with the concomitant use of hormonal contraceptives and ampicillin or tetracycline).
No products indexed under this heading.

Belladonna Ergotamine (Although norelgestromin and its metabolites inhibit a variety of P450 enzymes in human liver microsomes, the clinical consequence of such an interaction on the levels of other concomitant medications is likely to be insignificant. Under the recommended dosing regimen, the *in vivo* concentrations of norelgestromin and its metabolites, even at the peak serum levels, are relatively low compared to the inhibitory constant (Ki) (based on results of *in vitro* studies)).
No products indexed under this heading.

Benzphetamine Hydrochloride (Although norelgestromin and its metabolites inhibit a variety of P450 enzymes in human liver microsomes, the clinical consequence of such an interaction on the levels of other concomitant medications is likely to be insignificant. Under the recommended dosing regimen, the *in vivo* concentrations of norelgestromin and its metabolites, even at the peak serum levels, are relatively low compared to the inhibitory constant (Ki) (based on results of *in vitro* studies)).
No products indexed under this heading.

Betamethasone (If a woman on hormonal contraceptives takes a drug or herbal product that induces enzymes, including CYP3A4, that metabolize contraceptive hormones, counsel her to use additional contraception or a different method of contraception. Drugs or herbal products that induce such enzymes may decrease the plasma concentrations of contraceptive hormones, and may decrease the effectiveness of hormonal contraceptives or increase breakthrough bleeding).
No products indexed under this heading.

Betamethasone Acetate (If a woman on hormonal contraceptives takes a drug or herbal product that induces enzymes, including CYP3A4, that metabolize contraceptive hormones, counsel her to use additional contraception or a different method of contraception. Drugs or herbal products that induce such enzymes may decrease the plasma concentrations of contraceptive hormones, and may decrease the effectiveness of hormonal contraceptives or increase breakthrough bleeding).
No products indexed under this heading.

Betamethasone Benzoate (If a woman on hormonal contraceptives takes a drug or herbal product that induces enzymes, including CYP3A4, that metabolize contraceptive hormones, counsel her to use additional contraception or a different method of contraception. Drugs or herbal products that induce such enzymes may decrease the plasma concentrations of contraceptive hormones, and may decrease the effectiveness of hormonal contraceptives or increase breakthrough bleeding).
No products indexed under this heading.

Betamethasone Dipropionate (If a woman on hormonal contraceptives takes a drug or herbal product that induces enzymes, including CYP3A4, that metabolize contraceptive hormones, counsel her to use additional contraception or a different method of contraception. Drugs or herbal products that induce such enzymes may decrease the plasma concentrations of contraceptive hormones, and may decrease the effectiveness of hormonal contraceptives or increase breakthrough bleeding). Products include:
Diprolene Lotion 0.05% 3108
Diprolene Ointment 0.05% 3109
Diprolene AF Cream 0.05% 3107
Lotrisone 3163

Betamethasone Sodium Phosphate (If a woman on hormonal contraceptives takes a drug or herbal product that induces enzymes, including CYP3A4, that metabolize contraceptive hormones, counsel her to use additional contraception or a different method of contraception. Drugs or herbal products that induce such enzymes may decrease the plasma concentrations of contraceptive hormones, and may decrease the effectiveness of hormonal contraceptives or increase breakthrough bleeding).
No products indexed under this heading.

Betamethasone Valerate (If a woman on hormonal contraceptives takes a drug or herbal product that induces enzymes, including CYP3A4, that metabolize contraceptive hormones, counsel her to use additional contraception or a different method of contraception. Drugs or herbal products that induce such enzymes may decrease the plasma concentrations of contraceptive hormones, and may decrease the effectiveness of hormonal contraceptives or increase breakthrough bleeding). Products include:
Luxíq 3321

Bisoprolol Fumarate (Although norelgestromin and its metabolites inhibit a variety of P450 enzymes in human liver microsomes, the clinical consequence of such an interaction on the levels of other concomitant medications is likely to be insignificant. Under the recommended dosing regimen, the *in vivo* concentrations of norelgestromin and its metabolites, even at the peak serum levels, are relatively low compared to the inhibitory constant (Ki) (based on results of *in vitro* studies)).
No products indexed under this heading.

Bosentan (Concomitant use with bosentan may decrease the plasma concentrations of hormonal contraceptives, and may decrease the effectiveness of hormonal contraceptives or increase breakthrough bleeding. Patients who are concomitantly using bosentan, should be counseled to use additional contraception or a different method of contraception). Products include:
Tracleer 573

Bromocriptine Mesylate (Although norelgestromin and its metabolites inhibit a variety of P450 enzymes in human liver microsomes, the clinical consequence of such an interaction on the levels of other concomitant medications is likely to be insignificant. Under the recommended dosing regimen, the *in vivo* concentrations of norelgestromin and its metabolites, even at the peak serum levels, are relatively low compared to the inhibitory constant (Ki) (based on results of *in vitro* studies)).
No products indexed under this heading.

Buspirone Hydrochloride (Although norelgestromin and its metabolites inhibit a variety of P450 enzymes in human liver microsomes, the clinical consequence of such an interaction on the levels of other concomitant medications is likely to be insignificant. Under the recommended dosing regimen, the *in vivo* concentrations of norelgestromin and its metabolites, even at the peak serum levels, are relatively low compared to the inhibitory constant (Ki) (based on results of *in vitro* studies)).
No products indexed under this heading.

Busulfan (Although norelgestromin and its metabolites inhibit a variety of P450 enzymes in human liver microsomes, the clinical consequence of such an interaction on the levels of other concomitant medications is likely to be insignificant. Under the recommended dosing regimen, the *in vivo* concentrations of norelgestromin and its metabolites, even at the peak serum levels, are relatively low compared to the inhibitory constant (Ki) (based on results of *in vitro* studies)). Products include:
Myleran 1581

Butabarbital (Concomitant use with barbiturates may decrease the plasma concentrations of hormonal contraceptives, and may decrease the effectiveness of hormonal contraceptives or increase breakthrough bleeding. Patients who are concomitantly using barbiturates should be counseled to use additional contraception or a different method of contraception).
No products indexed under this heading.

Butabarbital Sodium (Concomitant use with barbiturates may decrease the plasma concentrations of hormonal contraceptives, and may decrease the effectiveness of hormonal contraceptives or increase breakthrough bleeding. Patients who are concomitantly using barbiturates should be counseled to use additional contraception or a different method of contraception).
No products indexed under this heading.

Butalbital (Concomitant use with barbiturates may decrease the plasma concentrations of hormonal contraceptives, and may decrease the effectiveness of hormonal contraceptives or increase breakthrough bleeding. Patients who are concomitantly using barbiturates should be counseled to use additional contraception or a different method of contraception).
No products indexed under this heading.

Caffeine (Although norelgestromin and its metabolites inhibit a variety of P450 enzymes in human liver microsomes, the clinical consequence of such an interaction on the levels of other concomitant medications is likely to be insignificant. Under the recommended dosing regimen, the *in vivo* concentrations of norelgestromin and its metabolites, even at the peak serum levels, are relatively low compared to the inhibitory constant (Ki) (based on results of *in vitro* studies)).
No products indexed under this heading.

Caffeine Anhydrous (Although norelgestromin and its metabolites inhibit a variety of P450 enzymes in human liver microsomes, the clinical consequence of such an interaction on the levels of other concomitant medications is likely to be insignificant. Under the recommended dosing regimen, the *in vivo* concentrations of norelgestromin and its metabolites, even at the peak serum levels, are relatively low compared to the inhibitory constant (Ki) (based on results of *in vitro* studies)).
No products indexed under this heading.

Caffeine Citrate (Although norelgestromin and its metabolites inhibit a variety of P450 enzymes in human liver microsomes, the clinical consequence of such an interaction on the levels of other concomitant medications is likely to be insignificant. Under the recommended dosing regimen, the *in vivo* concentrations of norelgestromin and its metabolites, even at the peak serum levels, are relatively low compared to the inhibitory constant (Ki) (based on results of *in vitro* studies)).
No products indexed under this heading.

Caffeine-containing medications (Although norelgestromin and its metabolites inhibit a variety of P450 enzymes in human liver microsomes, the clinical consequence of such an interaction on the levels of other concomitant medications is likely to be insignificant. Under the recommended dosing regimen, the *in vivo* concentrations of norelgestromin and its metabolites, even at the peak serum levels, are relatively low compared to the inhibitory constant (Ki) (based on results of *in vitro* studies)).
No products indexed under this heading.

Caffeine Sodium Benzoate (Although norelgestromin and its metabolites inhibit a variety of P450 enzymes

1309 Interactions Index Ortho Evra

in human liver microsomes, the clinical consequence of such an interaction on the levels of other concomitant medications is likely to be insignificant. Under the recommended dosing regimen, the *in vivo* concentrations of norelgestromin and its metabolites, even at the peak serum levels, are relatively low compared to the inhibitory constant (Ki) (based on results of *in vitro* studies)).
No products indexed under this heading.

Candesartan Cilexetil (Although norelgestromin and its metabolites inhibit a variety of P450 enzymes in human liver microsomes, the clinical consequence of such an interaction on the levels of other concomitant medications is likely to be insignificant. Under the recommended dosing regimen, the *in vivo* concentrations of norelgestromin and its metabolites, even at the peak serum levels, are relatively low compared to the inhibitory constant (Ki) (based on results of *in vitro* studies)).
Products include:
Atacand 697
Atacand HCT 700

Captopril (Although norelgestromin and its metabolites inhibit a variety of P450 enzymes in human liver microsomes, the clinical consequence of such an interaction on the levels of other concomitant medications is likely to be insignificant. Under the recommended dosing regimen, the *in vivo* concentrations of norelgestromin and its metabolites, even at the peak serum levels, are relatively low compared to the inhibitory constant (Ki) (based on results of *in vitro* studies)). Products include:
Captopril 2341

Carbamazepine (Concomitant use with carbamazepine may decrease the plasma concentrations of hormonal contraceptives, and may decrease the effectiveness of hormonal contraceptives or increase breakthrough bleeding. Patients who are concomitantly using carbamazepine, should be counseled to use additional contraception or a different method of contraception).
Products include:
Carbatrol 3280
Equetro 3477

Carbenicillin Disodium (There have been reports of pregnancy while taking hormonal contraceptives and antibiotics, but clinical pharmacokinetic studies have not shown consistent effects of antibiotics on plasma concentrations of synthetic steroids. The metabolism of hormonal contraceptives may be influenced by various drugs. Of potential clinical importance are drugs that interrupt entero-hepatic recirculation of estrogen (eg, certain antibiotics). Literature suggests possible interactions with the concomitant use of hormonal contraceptives and ampicillin or tetracycline).
No products indexed under this heading.

Carbenicillin Indanyl Sodium (There have been reports of pregnancy while taking hormonal contraceptives and antibiotics, but clinical pharmacokinetic studies have not shown consistent effects of antibiotics on plasma concentrations of synthetic steroids. The metabolism of hormonal contraceptives may be influenced by various drugs. Of potential clinical importance are drugs that interrupt entero-hepatic recirculation of estrogen (eg, certain antibiotics). Literature suggests possible interactions with the concomitant use of hormonal contraceptives and ampicillin or tetracycline).
No products indexed under this heading.

Carisoprodol (Although norelgestromin and its metabolites inhibit a variety of P450 enzymes in human liver microsomes, the clinical consequence of such an interaction on the levels of other concomitant medications is likely to be insignificant. Under the recommended dosing regimen, the *in vivo* concentrations of norelgestromin and its metabolites, even at the peak serum levels, are relatively low compared to the inhibitory constant (Ki) (based on results of *in vitro* studies)).
No products indexed under this heading.

Carvedilol (Although norelgestromin and its metabolites inhibit a variety of P450 enzymes in human liver microsomes, the clinical consequence of such an interaction on the levels of other concomitant medications is likely to be insignificant. Under the recommended dosing regimen, the *in vivo* concentrations of norelgestromin and its metabolites, even at the peak serum levels, are relatively low compared to the inhibitory constant (Ki) (based on results of *in vitro* studies)). Products include:
Coreg 1409

Cefaclor (There have been reports of pregnancy while taking hormonal contraceptives and antibiotics, but clinical pharmacokinetic studies have not shown consistent effects of antibiotics on plasma concentrations of synthetic steroids. The metabolism of hormonal contraceptives may be influenced by various drugs. Of potential clinical importance are drugs that interrupt entero-hepatic recirculation of estrogen (eg, certain antibiotics). Literature suggests possible interactions with the concomitant use of hormonal contraceptives and ampicillin or tetracycline).
No products indexed under this heading.

Cefadroxil (There have been reports of pregnancy while taking hormonal contraceptives and antibiotics, but clinical pharmacokinetic studies have not shown consistent effects of antibiotics on plasma concentrations of synthetic steroids. The metabolism of hormonal contraceptives may be influenced by various drugs. Of potential clinical importance are drugs that interrupt entero-hepatic recirculation of estrogen (eg, certain antibiotics). Literature suggests possible interactions with the concomitant use of hormonal contraceptives and ampicillin or tetracycline).
No products indexed under this heading.

Cefamandole Nafate (There have been reports of pregnancy while taking hormonal contraceptives and antibiotics, but clinical pharmacokinetic studies have not shown consistent effects of antibiotics on plasma concentrations of synthetic steroids. The metabolism of hormonal contraceptives may be influenced by various drugs. Of potential clinical importance are drugs that interrupt entero-hepatic recirculation of estrogen (eg, certain antibiotics). Literature suggests possible interactions with the concomitant use of hormonal contraceptives and ampicillin or tetracycline).
No products indexed under this heading.

Cefazolin Sodium (There have been reports of pregnancy while taking hormonal contraceptives and antibiotics, but clinical pharmacokinetic studies have not shown consistent effects of antibiotics on plasma concentrations of synthetic steroids. The metabolism of hormonal contraceptives may be influenced by various drugs. Of potential clinical importance are drugs that interrupt entero-hepatic recirculation of estrogen (eg, certain antibiotics). Literature suggests possible interactions with the concomitant use of hormonal contraceptives and ampicillin or tetracycline).
No products indexed under this heading.

Cefixime (There have been reports of pregnancy while taking hormonal contraceptives and antibiotics, but clinical pharmacokinetic studies have not shown consistent effects of antibiotics on plasma concentrations of synthetic steroids. The metabolism of hormonal contraceptives may be influenced by various drugs. Of potential clinical importance are drugs that interrupt entero-hepatic recirculation of estrogen (eg, certain antibiotics). Literature suggests possible interactions with the concomitant use of hormonal contraceptives and ampicillin or tetracycline).
Products include:
Suprax for Oral Suspension 2038
Suprax Tablets 2038

Cefmetazole Sodium (There have been reports of pregnancy while taking hormonal contraceptives and antibiotics, but clinical pharmacokinetic studies have not shown consistent effects of antibiotics on plasma concentrations of synthetic steroids. The metabolism of hormonal contraceptives may be influenced by various drugs. Of potential clinical importance are drugs that interrupt entero-hepatic recirculation of estrogen (eg, certain antibiotics). Literature suggests possible interactions with the concomitant use of hormonal contraceptives and ampicillin or tetracycline).
No products indexed under this heading.

Cefonicid Sodium (There have been reports of pregnancy while taking hormonal contraceptives and antibiotics, but clinical pharmacokinetic studies have not shown consistent effects of antibiotics on plasma concentrations of synthetic steroids. The metabolism of hormonal contraceptives may be influenced by various drugs. Of potential clinical importance are drugs that interrupt entero-hepatic recirculation of estrogen (eg, certain antibiotics). Literature suggests possible interactions with the concomitant use of hormonal contraceptives and ampicillin or tetracycline).
No products indexed under this heading.

Cefoperazone Sodium (There have been reports of pregnancy while taking hormonal contraceptives and antibiotics, but clinical pharmacokinetic studies have not shown consistent effects of antibiotics on plasma concentrations of synthetic steroids. The metabolism of hormonal contraceptives may be influenced by various drugs. Of potential clinical importance are drugs that interrupt entero-hepatic recirculation of estrogen (eg, certain antibiotics). Literature suggests possible interactions with the concomitant use of hormonal contraceptives and ampicillin or tetracycline).
No products indexed under this heading.

Ceforanide (There have been reports of pregnancy while taking hormonal contraceptives and antibiotics, but clinical pharmacokinetic studies have not shown consistent effects of antibiotics on plasma concentrations of synthetic steroids. The metabolism of hormonal contraceptives may be influenced by various drugs. Of potential clinical importance are drugs that interrupt entero-hepatic recirculation of estrogen (eg, certain antibiotics). Literature suggests possible interactions with the concomitant use of hormonal contraceptives and ampicillin or tetracycline).
No products indexed under this heading.

Cefotaxime Sodium (There have been reports of pregnancy while taking hormonal contraceptives and antibiotics, but clinical pharmacokinetic studies have not shown consistent effects of antibiotics on plasma concentrations of synthetic steroids. The metabolism of hormonal contraceptives may be influenced by various drugs. Of potential clinical importance are drugs that interrupt entero-hepatic recirculation of estrogen (eg, certain antibiotics). Literature suggests possible interactions with the concomitant use of hormonal contraceptives and ampicillin or tetracycline).
No products indexed under this heading.

Cefotetan (There have been reports of pregnancy while taking hormonal contraceptives and antibiotics, but clinical pharmacokinetic studies have not shown consistent effects of antibiotics on plasma concentrations of synthetic steroids. The metabolism of hormonal contraceptives may be influenced by various drugs. Of potential clinical importance are drugs that interrupt entero-hepatic recirculation of estrogen (eg, certain antibiotics). Literature suggests possible interactions with the concomitant use of hormonal contraceptives and ampicillin or tetracycline).
No products indexed under this heading.

Cefoxitin Sodium (There have been reports of pregnancy while taking hormonal contraceptives and antibiotics, but clinical pharmacokinetic studies have not shown consistent effects of antibiotics on plasma concentrations of synthetic steroids. The metabolism of hormonal contraceptives may be influenced by various drugs. Of potential clinical importance are drugs that interrupt entero-hepatic recirculation of estrogen (eg, certain antibiotics). Literature suggests possible interactions with the concomitant use of hormonal contraceptives and ampicillin or tetracycline).
No products indexed under this heading.

Cefpodoxime Proxetil (There have been reports of pregnancy while taking hormonal contraceptives and antibiotics, but clinical pharmacokinetic studies have not shown consistent effects of antibiotics on plasma concentrations of synthetic steroids. The metabolism of hormonal contraceptives may be influenced by various drugs. Of potential clinical importance are drugs that interrupt entero-hepatic recirculation of estrogen (eg, certain antibiotics). Literature suggests possible interactions with the concomitant use of hormonal contraceptives and ampicillin or tetracycline).
No products indexed under this heading.

Cefprozil (There have been reports of pregnancy while taking hormonal contraceptives and antibiotics, but clinical pharmacokinetic studies have not shown consistent effects of antibiotics on plasma concentrations of synthetic steroids. The metabolism of hormonal contraceptives may be influenced by various drugs. Of potential clinical importance are drugs that interrupt entero-hepatic recirculation of estrogen (eg, certain antibiotics). Literature suggests possible interactions with the concomitant use of hormonal contraceptives and ampicillin or tetracycline).
No products indexed under this heading.

Ceftazidime (There have been reports of pregnancy while taking hormonal contraceptives and antibiotics, but clinical pharmacokinetic studies have not shown consistent effects of antibiotics on plasma concentrations of synthetic steroids. The metabolism of hormonal contraceptives may be influenced by various drugs. Of potential clinical importance are drugs that interrupt entero-hepatic recirculation of estrogen (eg, certain antibiotics). Literature suggests possible interactions with the concomitant use of hormonal contraceptives and ampicillin or tetracycline).
Products include:
Fortaz 1481

Ceftizoxime Sodium (There have been reports of pregnancy while taking hormonal contraceptives and antibiot-

IMPORTANT NOTE: Always consult each drug listing in the patient's regimen for possible interactions.

Ortho Evra Interactions Index 1310

ics, but clinical pharmacokinetic studies have not shown consistent effects of antibiotics on plasma concentrations of synthetic steroids. The metabolism of hormonal contraceptives may be influenced by various drugs. Of potential clinical importance are drugs that interrupt entero-hepatic recirculation of estrogen (eg, certain antibiotics). Literature suggests possible interactions with the concomitant use of hormonal contraceptives and ampicillin or tetracycline).
No products indexed under this heading.

Ceftriaxone Sodium (There have been reports of pregnancy while taking hormonal contraceptives and antibiotics, but clinical pharmacokinetic studies have not shown consistent effects of antibiotics on plasma concentrations of synthetic steroids. The metabolism of hormonal contraceptives may be influenced by various drugs. Of potential clinical importance are drugs that interrupt entero-hepatic recirculation of estrogen (eg, certain antibiotics). Literature suggests possible interactions with the concomitant use of hormonal contraceptives and ampicillin or tetracycline). Products include:
Rocephin 2859

Cefuroxime Axetil (There have been reports of pregnancy while taking hormonal contraceptives and antibiotics, but clinical pharmacokinetic studies have not shown consistent effects of antibiotics on plasma concentrations of synthetic steroids. The metabolism of hormonal contraceptives may be influenced by various drugs. Of potential clinical importance are drugs that interrupt entero-hepatic recirculation of estrogen (eg, certain antibiotics). Literature suggests possible interactions with the concomitant use of hormonal contraceptives and ampicillin or tetracycline). Products include:
Ceftin 1399

Cefuroxime Sodium (There have been reports of pregnancy while taking hormonal contraceptives and antibiotics, but clinical pharmacokinetic studies have not shown consistent effects of antibiotics on plasma concentrations of synthetic steroids. The metabolism of hormonal contraceptives may be influenced by various drugs. Of potential clinical importance are drugs that interrupt entero-hepatic recirculation of estrogen (eg, certain antibiotics). Literature suggests possible interactions with the concomitant use of hormonal contraceptives and ampicillin or tetracycline).
No products indexed under this heading.

Celecoxib (Although norelgestromin and its metabolites inhibit a variety of P450 enzymes in human liver microsomes, the clinical consequence of such an interaction on the levels of other concomitant medications is likely to be insignificant. Under the recommended dosing regimen, the *in vivo* concentrations of norelgestromin and its metabolites, even at the peak serum levels, are relatively low compared to the inhibitory constant (Ki) (based on results of *in vitro* studies)). Products include:
Celebrex 3272

Cephalexin (There have been reports of pregnancy while taking hormonal contraceptives and antibiotics, but clinical pharmacokinetic studies have not shown consistent effects of antibiotics on plasma concentrations of synthetic steroids. The metabolism of hormonal contraceptives may be influenced by various drugs. Of potential clinical importance are drugs that interrupt entero-hepatic recirculation of estrogen (eg, certain antibiotics). Literature suggests possible interactions with the concomitant use of hormonal contraceptives and ampicillin or tetracycline).
No products indexed under this heading.

Cephalothin Sodium (There have been reports of pregnancy while taking hormonal contraceptives and antibiotics, but clinical pharmacokinetic studies have not shown consistent effects of antibiotics on plasma concentrations of synthetic steroids. The metabolism of hormonal contraceptives may be influenced by various drugs. Of potential clinical importance are drugs that interrupt entero-hepatic recirculation of estrogen (eg, certain antibiotics). Literature suggests possible interactions with the concomitant use of hormonal contraceptives and ampicillin or tetracycline).
No products indexed under this heading.

Cephapirin Sodium (There have been reports of pregnancy while taking hormonal contraceptives and antibiotics, but clinical pharmacokinetic studies have not shown consistent effects of antibiotics on plasma concentrations of synthetic steroids. The metabolism of hormonal contraceptives may be influenced by various drugs. Of potential clinical importance are drugs that interrupt entero-hepatic recirculation of estrogen (eg, certain antibiotics). Literature suggests possible interactions with the concomitant use of hormonal contraceptives and ampicillin or tetracycline).
No products indexed under this heading.

Cephradine (There have been reports of pregnancy while taking hormonal contraceptives and antibiotics, but clinical pharmacokinetic studies have not shown consistent effects of antibiotics on plasma concentrations of synthetic steroids. The metabolism of hormonal contraceptives may be influenced by various drugs. Of potential clinical importance are drugs that interrupt entero-hepatic recirculation of estrogen (eg, certain antibiotics). Literature suggests possible interactions with the concomitant use of hormonal contraceptives and ampicillin or tetracycline).
No products indexed under this heading.

Cerivastatin Sodium (Although norelgestromin and its metabolites inhibit a variety of P450 enzymes in human liver microsomes, the clinical consequence of such an interaction on the levels of other concomitant medications is likely to be insignificant. Under the recommended dosing regimen, the *in vivo* concentrations of norelgestromin and its metabolites, even at the peak serum levels, are relatively low compared to the inhibitory constant (Ki) (based on results of *in vitro* studies)).
No products indexed under this heading.

Cevimeline Hydrochloride (Although norelgestromin and its metabolites inhibit a variety of P450 enzymes in human liver microsomes, the clinical consequence of such an interaction on the levels of other concomitant medications is likely to be insignificant. Under the recommended dosing regimen, the *in vivo* concentrations of norelgestromin and its metabolites, even at the peak serum levels, are relatively low compared to the inhibitory constant (Ki) (based on results of *in vitro* studies)). Products include:
Evoxac 1027

Chloramphenicol (There have been reports of pregnancy while taking hormonal contraceptives and antibiotics, but clinical pharmacokinetic studies have not shown consistent effects of antibiotics on plasma concentrations of synthetic steroids. The metabolism of hormonal contraceptives may be influenced by various drugs. Of potential clinical importance are drugs that interrupt entero-hepatic recirculation of estrogen (eg, certain antibiotics). Literature suggests possible interactions with the concomitant use of hormonal contraceptives and ampicillin or tetracycline).
No products indexed under this heading.

Chloramphenicol Palmitate (There have been reports of pregnancy while taking hormonal contraceptives and antibiotics, but clinical pharmacokinetic studies have not shown consistent effects of antibiotics on plasma concentrations of synthetic steroids. The metabolism of hormonal contraceptives may be influenced by various drugs. Of potential clinical importance are drugs that interrupt entero-hepatic recirculation of estrogen (eg, certain antibiotics). Literature suggests possible interactions with the concomitant use of hormonal contraceptives and ampicillin or tetracycline).
No products indexed under this heading.

Chloramphenicol Sodium Succinate (There have been reports of pregnancy while taking hormonal contraceptives and antibiotics, but clinical pharmacokinetic studies have not shown consistent effects of antibiotics on plasma concentrations of synthetic steroids. The metabolism of hormonal contraceptives may be influenced by various drugs. Of potential clinical importance are drugs that interrupt entero-hepatic recirculation of estrogen (eg, certain antibiotics). Literature suggests possible interactions with the concomitant use of hormonal contraceptives and ampicillin or tetracycline).
No products indexed under this heading.

Chlordiazepoxide (Although norelgestromin and its metabolites inhibit a variety of P450 enzymes in human liver microsomes, the clinical consequence of such an interaction on the levels of other concomitant medications is likely to be insignificant. Under the recommended dosing regimen, the *in vivo* concentrations of norelgestromin and its metabolites, even at the peak serum levels, are relatively low compared to the inhibitory constant (Ki) (based on results of *in vitro* studies)).
No products indexed under this heading.

Chlordiazepoxide Hydrochloride (Although norelgestromin and its metabolites inhibit a variety of P450 enzymes in human liver microsomes, the clinical consequence of such an interaction on the levels of other concomitant medications is likely to be insignificant. Under the recommended dosing regimen, the *in vivo* concentrations of norelgestromin and its metabolites, even at the peak serum levels, are relatively low compared to the inhibitory constant (Ki) (based on results of *in vitro* studies)).
No products indexed under this heading.

Chlorpheniramine (Although norelgestromin and its metabolites inhibit a variety of P450 enzymes in human liver microsomes, the clinical consequence of such an interaction on the levels of other concomitant medications is likely to be insignificant. Under the recommended dosing regimen, the *in vivo* concentrations of norelgestromin and its metabolites, even at the peak serum levels, are relatively low compared to the inhibitory constant (Ki) (based on results of *in vitro* studies)).
No products indexed under this heading.

Chlorpheniramine Maleate (Although norelgestromin and its metabolites inhibit a variety of P450 enzymes in human liver microsomes, the clinical consequence of such an interaction on the levels of other concomitant medications is likely to be insignificant. Under the recommended dosing regimen, the *in vivo* concentrations of norelgestromin and its metabolites, even at the peak serum levels, are relatively low compared to the inhibitory constant (Ki) (based on results of *in vitro* studies)).
No products indexed under this heading.

Chlorpheniramine Polistirex (Although norelgestromin and its metabolites inhibit a variety of P450 enzymes in human liver microsomes, the clinical consequence of such an interaction on the levels of other concomitant medications is likely to be insignificant. Under the recommended dosing regimen, the *in vivo* concentrations of norelgestromin and its metabolites, even at the peak serum levels, are relatively low compared to the inhibitory constant (Ki) (based on results of *in vitro* studies)). Products include:
Tussionex 3443

Chlorpheniramine Tannate (Although norelgestromin and its metabolites inhibit a variety of P450 enzymes in human liver microsomes, the clinical consequence of such an interaction on the levels of other concomitant medications is likely to be insignificant. Under the recommended dosing regimen, the *in vivo* concentrations of norelgestromin and its metabolites, even at the peak serum levels, are relatively low compared to the inhibitory constant (Ki) (based on results of *in vitro* studies)).
No products indexed under this heading.

Chlorpromazine (Although norelgestromin and its metabolites inhibit a variety of P450 enzymes in human liver microsomes, the clinical consequence of such an interaction on the levels of other concomitant medications is likely to be insignificant. Under the recommended dosing regimen, the *in vivo* concentrations of norelgestromin and its metabolites, even at the peak serum levels, are relatively low compared to the inhibitory constant (Ki) (based on results of *in vitro* studies)).
No products indexed under this heading.

Chlorpromazine Hydrochloride (Although norelgestromin and its metabolites inhibit a variety of P450 enzymes in human liver microsomes, the clinical consequence of such an interaction on the levels of other concomitant medications is likely to be insignificant. Under the recommended dosing regimen, the *in vivo* concentrations of norelgestromin and its metabolites, even at the peak serum levels, are relatively low compared to the inhibitory constant (Ki) (based on results of *in vitro* studies)).
No products indexed under this heading.

Chlorpropamide (If a woman on hormonal contraceptives takes a drug or herbal product that induces enzymes, including CYP3A4, that metabolize contraceptive hormones, counsel her to use additional contraception or a different method of contraception. Drugs or herbal products that induce such enzymes may decrease the plasma concentrations of contraceptive hormones, and may decrease the effectiveness of hormonal contraceptives or increase breakthrough bleeding).
No products indexed under this heading.

Cilastatin Sodium (There have been reports of pregnancy while taking hormonal contraceptives and antibiotics, but clinical pharmacokinetic studies have not shown consistent effects of antibiotics on plasma concentrations of synthetic steroids. The metabolism of hormonal contraceptives may be influenced by various drugs. Of potential clinical importance are drugs that interrupt entero-hepatic recirculation of estrogen (eg, certain antibiotics). Literature suggests possible interactions with the concomitant use of hormonal contraceptives and ampicillin or tetracycline). Products include:
Primaxin I.M. 2232

1311 Interactions Index Ortho Evra

Primaxin I.V. 2235

Cilostazol (Although norelgestromin and its metabolites inhibit a variety of P450 enzymes in human liver microsomes, the clinical consequence of such an interaction on the levels of other concomitant medications is likely to be insignificant. Under the recommended dosing regimen, the *in vivo* concentrations of norelgestromin and its metabolites, even at the peak serum levels, are relatively low compared to the inhibitory constant (Ki) (based on results of *in vitro* studies)).
No products indexed under this heading.

Cimetidine (CYP3A4 inhibitors, such as itraconazole or ketoconazole, may increase plasma hormone levels).
No products indexed under this heading.

Cimetidine Hydrochloride (CYP3A4 inhibitors, such as itraconazole or ketoconazole, may increase plasma hormone levels).
No products indexed under this heading.

Ciprofloxacin (If a woman on hormonal contraceptives takes a drug or herbal product that induces enzymes, including CYP3A4, that metabolize contraceptive hormones, counsel her to use additional contraception or a different method of contraception. Drugs or herbal products that induce such enzymes may decrease the plasma concentrations of contraceptive hormones, and may decrease the effectiveness of hormonal contraceptives or increase breakthrough bleeding). Products include:
Cipro I.V. 3082
Cipro 3073
Cipro XR 3091
Ciprodex 583

Ciprofloxacin Hydrochloride (If a woman on hormonal contraceptives takes a drug or herbal product that induces enzymes, including CYP3A4, that metabolize contraceptive hormones, counsel her to use additional contraception or a different method of contraception. Drugs or herbal products that induce such enzymes may decrease the plasma concentrations of contraceptive hormones, and may decrease the effectiveness of hormonal contraceptives or increase breakthrough bleeding). Products include:
Cipro 3073

Cisapride (Although norelgestromin and its metabolites inhibit a variety of P450 enzymes in human liver microsomes, the clinical consequence of such an interaction on the levels of other concomitant medications is likely to be insignificant. Under the recommended dosing regimen, the *in vivo* concentrations of norelgestromin and its metabolites, even at the peak serum levels, are relatively low compared to the inhibitory constant (Ki) (based on results of *in vitro* studies)).
No products indexed under this heading.

Cisplatin (If a woman on hormonal contraceptives takes a drug or herbal product that induces enzymes, including CYP3A4, that metabolize contraceptive hormones, counsel her to use additional contraception or a different method of contraception. Drugs or herbal products that induce such enzymes may decrease the plasma concentrations of contraceptive hormones, and may decrease the effectiveness of hormonal contraceptives or increase breakthrough bleeding).
No products indexed under this heading.

Citalopram Hydrobromide (If a woman on hormonal contraceptives takes a drug or herbal product that induces enzymes, including CYP3A4, that metabolize contraceptive hormones, counsel her to use additional contraception or a different method of contraception. Drugs or herbal products that induce such enzymes may decrease the plasma concentrations of contraceptive hormones, and may decrease the effectiveness of hormonal contraceptives or increase breakthrough bleeding). Products include:
Celexa 1153

Clarithromycin (CYP3A4 inhibitors, such as itraconazole or ketoconazole, may increase plasma hormone levels). Products include:
Biaxin/Biaxin XL 412

Clofibric Acid (Increased clearance of clofibric acid has been noted when administered concomitantly with oral contraceptives).
No products indexed under this heading.

Clomipramine Hydrochloride (Although norelgestromin and its metabolites inhibit a variety of P450 enzymes in human liver microsomes, the clinical consequence of such an interaction on the levels of other concomitant medications is likely to be insignificant. Under the recommended dosing regimen, the *in vivo* concentrations of norelgestromin and its metabolites, even at the peak serum levels, are relatively low compared to the inhibitory constant (Ki) (based on results of *in vitro* studies)).
No products indexed under this heading.

Clopidogrel Bisulfate (Although norelgestromin and its metabolites inhibit a variety of P450 enzymes in human liver microsomes, the clinical consequence of such an interaction on the levels of other concomitant medications is likely to be insignificant. Under the recommended dosing regimen, the *in vivo* concentrations of norelgestromin and its metabolites, even at the peak serum levels, are relatively low compared to the inhibitory constant (Ki) (based on results of *in vitro* studies)). Products include:
Plavix 3027

Clopidogrel Hydrogen Sulfate (Although norelgestromin and its metabolites inhibit a variety of P450 enzymes in human liver microsomes, the clinical consequence of such an interaction on the levels of other concomitant medications is likely to be insignificant. Under the recommended dosing regimen, the *in vivo* concentrations of norelgestromin and its metabolites, even at the peak serum levels, are relatively low compared to the inhibitory constant (Ki) (based on results of *in vitro* studies)).
No products indexed under this heading.

Clotrimazole (CYP3A4 inhibitors, such as itraconazole or ketoconazole, may increase plasma hormone levels). Products include:
Lotrisone 3163

Cloxacillin (There have been reports of pregnancy while taking hormonal contraceptives and antibiotics, but clinical pharmacokinetic studies have not shown consistent effects of antibiotics on plasma concentrations of synthetic steroids. The metabolism of hormonal contraceptives may be influenced by various drugs. Of potential clinical importance are drugs that interrupt entero-hepatic recirculation of estrogen (eg, certain antibiotics). Literature suggests possible interactions with the concomitant use of hormonal contraceptives and ampicillin or tetracycline).
No products indexed under this heading.

Cloxacillin Sodium (There have been reports of pregnancy while taking hormonal contraceptives and antibiotics, but clinical pharmacokinetic studies have not shown consistent effects of antibiotics on plasma concentrations of synthetic steroids. The metabolism of hormonal contraceptives may be influenced by various drugs. Of potential clinical importance are drugs that interrupt entero-hepatic recirculation of estrogen (eg, certain antibiotics). Literature suggests possible interactions with the concomitant use of hormonal contraceptives and ampicillin or tetracycline).
No products indexed under this heading.

Cloxacillin Sodium Monohydrate (There have been reports of pregnancy while taking hormonal contraceptives and antibiotics, but clinical pharmacokinetic studies have not shown consistent effects of antibiotics on plasma concentrations of synthetic steroids. The metabolism of hormonal contraceptives may be influenced by various drugs. Of potential clinical importance are drugs that interrupt entero-hepatic recirculation of estrogen (eg, certain antibiotics). Literature suggests possible interactions with the concomitant use of hormonal contraceptives and ampicillin or tetracycline).
No products indexed under this heading.

Clozapine (Although norelgestromin and its metabolites inhibit a variety of P450 enzymes in human liver microsomes, the clinical consequence of such an interaction on the levels of other concomitant medications is likely to be insignificant. Under the recommended dosing regimen, the *in vivo* concentrations of norelgestromin and its metabolites, even at the peak serum levels, are relatively low compared to the inhibitory constant (Ki) (based on results of *in vitro* studies)).
No products indexed under this heading.

Codeine Phosphate (Although norelgestromin and its metabolites inhibit a variety of P450 enzymes in human liver microsomes, the clinical consequence of such an interaction on the levels of other concomitant medications is likely to be insignificant. Under the recommended dosing regimen, the *in vivo* concentrations of norelgestromin and its metabolites, even at the peak serum levels, are relatively low compared to the inhibitory constant (Ki) (based on results of *in vitro* studies)). Products include:
Tylenol with Codeine 2691

Codeine Sulfate (Although norelgestromin and its metabolites inhibit a variety of P450 enzymes in human liver microsomes, the clinical consequence of such an interaction on the levels of other concomitant medications is likely to be insignificant. Under the recommended dosing regimen, the *in vivo* concentrations of norelgestromin and its metabolites, even at the peak serum levels, are relatively low compared to the inhibitory constant (Ki) (based on results of *in vitro* studies)).
No products indexed under this heading.

Conivaptan Hydrochloride (CYP3A4 inhibitors, such as itraconazole or ketoconazole, may increase plasma hormone levels). Products include:
Vaprisol 689

Cortisone Acetate (If a woman on hormonal contraceptives takes a drug or herbal product that induces enzymes, including CYP3A4, that metabolize contraceptive hormones, counsel her to use additional contraception or a different method of contraception. Drugs or herbal products that induce such enzymes may decrease the plasma concentrations of contraceptive hormones, and may decrease the effectiveness of hormonal contraceptives or increase breakthrough bleeding).
No products indexed under this heading.

Cyclobenzaprine (Although norelgestromin and its metabolites inhibit a variety of P450 enzymes in human liver microsomes, the clinical consequence of such an interaction on the levels of other concomitant medications is likely to be insignificant. Under the recommended dosing regimen, the *in vivo* concentrations of norelgestromin and its metabolites, even at the peak serum levels, are relatively low compared to the inhibitory constant (Ki) (based on results of *in vitro* studies)).
No products indexed under this heading.

Cyclobenzaprine Hydrochloride (Although norelgestromin and its metabolites inhibit a variety of P450 enzymes in human liver microsomes, the clinical consequence of such an interaction on the levels of other concomitant medications is likely to be insignificant. Under the recommended dosing regimen, the *in vivo* concentrations of norelgestromin and its metabolites, even at the peak serum levels, are relatively low compared to the inhibitory constant (Ki) (based on results of *in vitro* studies)). Products include:
Amrix 964

Cyclophosphamide (Although norelgestromin and its metabolites inhibit a variety of P450 enzymes in human liver microsomes, the clinical consequence of such an interaction on the levels of other concomitant medications is likely to be insignificant. Under the recommended dosing regimen, the *in vivo* concentrations of norelgestromin and its metabolites, even at the peak serum levels, are relatively low compared to the inhibitory constant (Ki) (based on results of *in vitro* studies)).
No products indexed under this heading.

Cyclosporine (Increased plasma concentrations of cyclosporine have been reported with concomitant administration of oral contraceptives). Products include:
Gengraf 440
Neoral Oral Solution 2496
Neoral Capsules 2496
Restasis 605

Dalfopristin (CYP3A4 inhibitors, such as itraconazole or ketoconazole, may increase plasma hormone levels).
No products indexed under this heading.

Danazol (CYP3A4 inhibitors, such as itraconazole or ketoconazole, may increase plasma hormone levels).
No products indexed under this heading.

Darunavir (Significant changes (increase or decrease) in the plasma levels of the estrogen and progestin have been noted in some cases of co-administration of HIV protease inhibitors).
No products indexed under this heading.

Dasatinib (CYP3A4 inhibitors, such as itraconazole or ketoconazole, may increase plasma hormone levels).
No products indexed under this heading.

Daunorubicin Hydrochloride (There have been reports of pregnancy while taking hormonal contraceptives and antibiotics, but clinical pharmacokinetic studies have not shown consistent effects of antibiotics on plasma concentrations of synthetic steroids. The metabolism of hormonal contraceptives may be influenced by various drugs. Of potential clinical importance are drugs that interrupt entero-hepatic recirculation of estrogen (eg, certain antibiotics). Literature suggests possible interactions with the concomitant use of hormonal contraceptives and ampicillin or tetracycline).
No products indexed under this heading.

Delavirdine Mesylate (CYP3A4 inhibitors, such as itraconazole or ketoconazole, may increase plasma hormone levels).
No products indexed under this heading.

Delavirine (CYP3A4 inhibitors, such as itraconazole or ketoconazole, may increase plasma hormone levels).
No products indexed under this heading.

IMPORTANT NOTE: Always consult each drug listing in the patient's regimen for possible interactions.

Ortho Evra Interactions Index 1312

Demeclocycline Hydrochloride (There have been reports of pregnancy while taking hormonal contraceptives and antibiotics, but clinical pharmacokinetic studies have not shown consistent effects of antibiotics on plasma concentrations of synthetic steroids. The metabolism of hormonal contraceptives may be influenced by various drugs. Of potential clinical importance are drugs that interrupt entero-hepatic recirculation of estrogen (eg, certain antibiotics). Literature suggests possible interactions with the concomitant use of hormonal contraceptives and ampicillin or tetracycline).
No products indexed under this heading.

Desipramine Hydrochloride (Although norelgestromin and its metabolites inhibit a variety of P450 enzymes in human liver microsomes, the clinical consequence of such an interaction on the levels of other concomitant medications is likely to be insignificant. Under the recommended dosing regimen, the *in vivo* concentrations of norelgestromin and its metabolites, even at the peak serum levels, are relatively low compared to the inhibitory constant (Ki) (based on results of *in vitro* studies)).
No products indexed under this heading.

Desloratadine (CYP3A4 inhibitors, such as itraconazole or ketoconazole, may increase plasma hormone levels). Products include:
Clarinex Syrup 3098
Clarinex 3098
Clarinex Reditabs 3098
Clarinex-D 12-Hour 3101
Clarinex-D 3104

Desogestrel (Although norelgestromin and its metabolites inhibit a variety of P450 enzymes in human liver microsomes, the clinical consequence of such an interaction on the levels of other concomitant medications is likely to be insignificant. Under the recommended dosing regimen, the *in vivo* concentrations of norelgestromin and its metabolites, even at the peak serum levels, are relatively low compared to the inhibitory constant (Ki) (based on results of *in vitro* studies)).
No products indexed under this heading.

Dexamethasone (If a woman on hormonal contraceptives takes a drug or herbal product that induces enzymes, including CYP3A4, that metabolize contraceptive hormones, counsel her to use additional contraception or a different method of contraception. Drugs or herbal products that induce such enzymes may decrease the plasma concentrations of contraceptive hormones, and may decrease the effectiveness of hormonal contraceptives or increase breakthrough bleeding). Products include:
Ciprodex 583
Ozurdex .... ⊙223
Tobramycin and Dexamethasone Ophthalmic Suspension .... ⊙251

Dexamethasone Acetate (If a woman on hormonal contraceptives takes a drug or herbal product that induces enzymes, including CYP3A4, that metabolize contraceptive hormones, counsel her to use additional contraception or a different method of contraception. Drugs or herbal products that induce such enzymes may decrease the plasma concentrations of contraceptive hormones, and may decrease the effectiveness of hormonal contraceptives or increase breakthrough bleeding).
No products indexed under this heading.

Dexamethasone Phosphate (If a woman on hormonal contraceptives takes a drug or herbal product that induces enzymes, including CYP3A4, that metabolize contraceptive hormones, counsel her to use additional contraception or a different method of contraception. Drugs or herbal products that induce such enzymes may decrease the plasma concentrations of contraceptive hormones, and may decrease the effectiveness of hormonal contraceptives or increase breakthrough bleeding).
No products indexed under this heading.

Dexamethasone Sodium (If a woman on hormonal contraceptives takes a drug or herbal product that induces enzymes, including CYP3A4, that metabolize contraceptive hormones, counsel her to use additional contraception or a different method of contraception. Drugs or herbal products that induce such enzymes may decrease the plasma concentrations of contraceptive hormones, and may decrease the effectiveness of hormonal contraceptives or increase breakthrough bleeding).
No products indexed under this heading.

Dexamethasone Sodium Phosphate (If a woman on hormonal contraceptives takes a drug or herbal product that induces enzymes, including CYP3A4, that metabolize contraceptive hormones, counsel her to use additional contraception or a different method of contraception. Drugs or herbal products that induce such enzymes may decrease the plasma concentrations of contraceptive hormones, and may decrease the effectiveness of hormonal contraceptives or increase breakthrough bleeding).
No products indexed under this heading.

Dexamethasone Sodium Phosphate Injection (If a woman on hormonal contraceptives takes a drug or herbal product that induces enzymes, including CYP3A4, that metabolize contraceptive hormones, counsel her to use additional contraception or a different method of contraception. Drugs or herbal products that induce such enzymes may decrease the plasma concentrations of contraceptive hormones, and may decrease the effectiveness of hormonal contraceptives or increase breakthrough bleeding).
No products indexed under this heading.

Dexfenfluramine Hydrochloride (Although norelgestromin and its metabolites inhibit a variety of P450 enzymes in human liver microsomes, the clinical consequence of such an interaction on the levels of other concomitant medications is likely to be insignificant. Under the recommended dosing regimen, the *in vivo* concentrations of norelgestromin and its metabolites, even at the peak serum levels, are relatively low compared to the inhibitory constant (Ki) (based on results of *in vitro* studies)).
No products indexed under this heading.

Dextromethorphan (Although norelgestromin and its metabolites inhibit a variety of P450 enzymes in human liver microsomes, the clinical consequence of such an interaction on the levels of other concomitant medications is likely to be insignificant. Under the recommended dosing regimen, the *in vivo* concentrations of norelgestromin and its metabolites, even at the peak serum levels, are relatively low compared to the inhibitory constant (Ki) (based on results of *in vitro* studies)).
No products indexed under this heading.

Dextromethorphan Hydrobromide (Although norelgestromin and its metabolites inhibit a variety of P450 enzymes in human liver microsomes, the clinical consequence of such an interaction on the levels of other concomitant medications is likely to be insignificant. Under the recommended dosing regimen, the *in vivo* concentrations of norelgestromin and its metabolites, even at the peak serum levels, are relatively low compared to the inhibitory constant (Ki) (based on results of *in vitro* studies)).
No products indexed under this heading.

Dextromethorphan Polistirex (Although norelgestromin and its metabolites inhibit a variety of P450 enzymes in human liver microsomes, the clinical consequence of such an interaction on the levels of other concomitant medications is likely to be insignificant. Under the recommended dosing regimen, the *in vivo* concentrations of norelgestromin and its metabolites, even at the peak serum levels, are relatively low compared to the inhibitory constant (Ki) (based on results of *in vitro* studies)).
No products indexed under this heading.

Diazepam (Although norelgestromin and its metabolites inhibit a variety of P450 enzymes in human liver microsomes, the clinical consequence of such an interaction on the levels of other concomitant medications is likely to be insignificant. Under the recommended dosing regimen, the *in vivo* concentrations of norelgestromin and its metabolites, even at the peak serum levels, are relatively low compared to the inhibitory constant (Ki) (based on results of *in vitro* studies)). Products include:
Valium Tablets 2880

Diclofenac Potassium (Although norelgestromin and its metabolites inhibit a variety of P450 enzymes in human liver microsomes, the clinical consequence of such an interaction on the levels of other concomitant medications is likely to be insignificant. Under the recommended dosing regimen, the *in vivo* concentrations of norelgestromin and its metabolites, even at the peak serum levels, are relatively low compared to the inhibitory constant (Ki) (based on results of *in vitro* studies)).
No products indexed under this heading.

Diclofenac Sodium (Although norelgestromin and its metabolites inhibit a variety of P450 enzymes in human liver microsomes, the clinical consequence of such an interaction on the levels of other concomitant medications is likely to be insignificant. Under the recommended dosing regimen, the *in vivo* concentrations of norelgestromin and its metabolites, even at the peak serum levels, are relatively low compared to the inhibitory constant (Ki) (based on results of *in vitro* studies)).
No products indexed under this heading.

Dicloxacillin (There have been reports of pregnancy while taking hormonal contraceptives and antibiotics, but clinical pharmacokinetic studies have not shown consistent effects of antibiotics on plasma concentrations of synthetic steroids. The metabolism of hormonal contraceptives may be influenced by various drugs. Of potential clinical importance are drugs that interrupt entero-hepatic recirculation of estrogen (eg, certain antibiotics). Literature suggests possible interactions with the concomitant use of hormonal contraceptives and ampicillin or tetracycline).
No products indexed under this heading.

Dicloxacillin Sodium (There have been reports of pregnancy while taking hormonal contraceptives and antibiotics, but clinical pharmacokinetic studies have not shown consistent effects of antibiotics on plasma concentrations of synthetic steroids. The metabolism of hormonal contraceptives may be influenced by various drugs. Of potential clinical importance are drugs that interrupt entero-hepatic recirculation of estrogen (eg, certain antibiotics). Literature suggests possible interactions with the concomitant use of hormonal contraceptives and ampicillin or tetracycline).
No products indexed under this heading.

Dihydroergotamine Mesylate (Although norelgestromin and its metabolites inhibit a variety of P450 enzymes in human liver microsomes, the clinical consequence of such an interaction on the levels of other concomitant medications is likely to be insignificant. Under the recommended dosing regimen, the *in vivo* concentrations of norelgestromin and its metabolites, even at the peak serum levels, are relatively low compared to the inhibitory constant (Ki) (based on results of *in vitro* studies)).
No products indexed under this heading.

Diltiazem Hydrochloride (If a woman on hormonal contraceptives takes a drug or herbal product that induces enzymes, including CYP3A4, that metabolize contraceptive hormones, counsel her to use additional contraception or a different method of contraception. Drugs or herbal products that induce such enzymes may decrease the plasma concentrations of contraceptive hormones, and may decrease the effectiveness of hormonal contraceptives or increase breakthrough bleeding). Products include:
Cardizem LA 423

Diltiazem Maleate (If a woman on hormonal contraceptives takes a drug or herbal product that induces enzymes, including CYP3A4, that metabolize contraceptive hormones, counsel her to use additional contraception or a different method of contraception. Drugs or herbal products that induce such enzymes may decrease the plasma concentrations of contraceptive hormones, and may decrease the effectiveness of hormonal contraceptives or increase breakthrough bleeding).
No products indexed under this heading.

Dirithromycin (There have been reports of pregnancy while taking hormonal contraceptives and antibiotics, but clinical pharmacokinetic studies have not shown consistent effects of antibiotics on plasma concentrations of synthetic steroids. The metabolism of hormonal contraceptives may be influenced by various drugs. Of potential clinical importance are drugs that interrupt entero-hepatic recirculation of estrogen (eg, certain antibiotics). Literature suggests possible interactions with the concomitant use of hormonal contraceptives and ampicillin or tetracycline).
No products indexed under this heading.

Disodium Carbenicillin (There have been reports of pregnancy while taking hormonal contraceptives and antibiotics, but clinical pharmacokinetic studies have not shown consistent effects of antibiotics on plasma concentrations of synthetic steroids. The metabolism of hormonal contraceptives may be influenced by various drugs. Of potential clinical importance are drugs that interrupt entero-hepatic recirculation of estrogen (eg, certain antibiotics). Literature suggests possible interactions with the concomitant use of hormonal contraceptives and ampicillin or tetracycline).
No products indexed under this heading.

Disopyramide (Although norelgestromin and its metabolites inhibit a variety of P450 enzymes in human liver microsomes, the clinical consequence of such an interaction on the levels of other concomitant medications is likely to be insignificant. Under the recommended dosing regimen, the *in vivo* concentrations of norelgestromin and its metabolites, even at the peak serum

levels, are relatively low compared to the inhibitory constant (Ki) (based on results of *in vitro* studies)).
No products indexed under this heading.

Disopyramide Phosphate (Although norelgestromin and its metabolites inhibit a variety of P450 enzymes in human liver microsomes, the clinical consequence of such an interaction on the levels of other concomitant medications is likely to be insignificant. Under the recommended dosing regimen, the *in vivo* concentrations of norelgestromin and its metabolites, even at the peak serum levels, are relatively low compared to the inhibitory constant (Ki) (based on results of *in vitro* studies)).
No products indexed under this heading.

Disulfiram (Although norelgestromin and its metabolites inhibit a variety of P450 enzymes in human liver microsomes, the clinical consequence of such an interaction on the levels of other concomitant medications is likely to be insignificant. Under the recommended dosing regimen, the *in vivo* concentrations of norelgestromin and its metabolites, even at the peak serum levels, are relatively low compared to the inhibitory constant (Ki) (based on results of *in vitro* studies)).
No products indexed under this heading.

Divalproex Sodium (Although norelgestromin and its metabolites inhibit a variety of P450 enzymes in human liver microsomes, the clinical consequence of such an interaction on the levels of other concomitant medications is likely to be insignificant. Under the recommended dosing regimen, the *in vivo* concentrations of norelgestromin and its metabolites, even at the peak serum levels, are relatively low compared to the inhibitory constant (Ki) (based on results of *in vitro* studies)). Products include:
Depakote ER **426**

Docetaxel (Although norelgestromin and its metabolites inhibit a variety of P450 enzymes in human liver microsomes, the clinical consequence of such an interaction on the levels of other concomitant medications is likely to be insignificant. Under the recommended dosing regimen, the *in vivo* concentrations of norelgestromin and its metabolites, even at the peak serum levels, are relatively low compared to the inhibitory constant (Ki) (based on results of *in vitro* studies)). Products include:
Taxotere **3035**

Dolasetron Mesylate (Although norelgestromin and its metabolites inhibit a variety of P450 enzymes in human liver microsomes, the clinical consequence of such an interaction on the levels of other concomitant medications is likely to be insignificant. Under the recommended dosing regimen, the *in vivo* concentrations of norelgestromin and its metabolites, even at the peak serum levels, are relatively low compared to the inhibitory constant (Ki) (based on results of *in vitro* studies)). Products include:
Anzemet Injection **2931**
Anzemet Tablets **2934**

Donepezil Hydrochloride (Although norelgestromin and its metabolites inhibit a variety of P450 enzymes in human liver microsomes, the clinical consequence of such an interaction on the levels of other concomitant medications is likely to be insignificant. Under the recommended dosing regimen, the *in vivo* concentrations of norelgestromin and its metabolites, even at the peak serum levels, are relatively low compared to the inhibitory constant (Ki) (based on results of *in vitro* studies)). Products include:
Aricept **1045**
Aricept ODT **1045**

Doxepin Hydrochloride (Although norelgestromin and its metabolites inhibit a variety of P450 enzymes in human liver microsomes, the clinical consequence of such an interaction on the levels of other concomitant medications is likely to be insignificant. Under the recommended dosing regimen, the *in vivo* concentrations of norelgestromin and its metabolites, even at the peak serum levels, are relatively low compared to the inhibitory constant (Ki) (based on results of *in vitro* studies)).
No products indexed under this heading.

Doxorubicin Hydrochloride (If a woman on hormonal contraceptives takes a drug or herbal product that induces enzymes, including CYP3A4, that metabolize contraceptive hormones, counsel her to use additional contraception or a different method of contraception. Drugs or herbal products that induce such enzymes may decrease the plasma concentrations of contraceptive hormones, and may decrease the effectiveness of hormonal contraceptives or increase breakthrough bleeding).
No products indexed under this heading.

Doxycycline (There have been reports of pregnancy while taking hormonal contraceptives and antibiotics, but clinical pharmacokinetic studies have not shown consistent effects of antibiotics on plasma concentrations of synthetic steroids. The metabolism of hormonal contraceptives may be influenced by various drugs. Of potential clinical importance are drugs that interrupt entero-hepatic recirculation of estrogen (eg, certain antibiotics). Literature suggests possible interactions with the concomitant use of hormonal contraceptives and ampicillin or tetracycline).
No products indexed under this heading.

Doxycycline Calcium (There have been reports of pregnancy while taking hormonal contraceptives and antibiotics, but clinical pharmacokinetic studies have not shown consistent effects of antibiotics on plasma concentrations of synthetic steroids. The metabolism of hormonal contraceptives may be influenced by various drugs. Of potential clinical importance are drugs that interrupt entero-hepatic recirculation of estrogen (eg, certain antibiotics). Literature suggests possible interactions with the concomitant use of hormonal contraceptives and ampicillin or tetracycline).
No products indexed under this heading.

Doxycycline Hyclate (There have been reports of pregnancy while taking hormonal contraceptives and antibiotics, but clinical pharmacokinetic studies have not shown consistent effects of antibiotics on plasma concentrations of synthetic steroids. The metabolism of hormonal contraceptives may be influenced by various drugs. Of potential clinical importance are drugs that interrupt entero-hepatic recirculation of estrogen (eg, certain antibiotics). Literature suggests possible interactions with the concomitant use of hormonal contraceptives and ampicillin or tetracycline).
No products indexed under this heading.

Doxycycline Monohydrate (There have been reports of pregnancy while taking hormonal contraceptives and antibiotics, but clinical pharmacokinetic studies have not shown consistent effects of antibiotics on plasma concentrations of synthetic steroids. The metabolism of hormonal contraceptives may be influenced by various drugs. Of potential clinical importance are drugs that interrupt entero-hepatic recirculation of estrogen (eg, certain antibiotics). Literature suggests possible interactions with the concomitant use of hormonal contraceptives and ampicillin or tetracycline).
No products indexed under this heading.

Dronabinol (Although norelgestromin and its metabolites inhibit a variety of P450 enzymes in human liver microsomes, the clinical consequence of such an interaction on the levels of other concomitant medications is likely to be insignificant. Under the recommended dosing regimen, the *in vivo* concentrations of norelgestromin and its metabolites, even at the peak serum levels, are relatively low compared to the inhibitory constant (Ki) (based on results of *in vitro* studies)).
No products indexed under this heading.

Drugs that Undergo Biotransformation by Cytochrome P-450 Mixed Function Oxidase (Although norelgestromin and its metabolites inhibit a variety of P450 enzymes in human liver microsomes, the clinical consequence of such an interaction on the levels of other concomitant medications is likely to be insignificant. Under the recommended dosing regimen, the *in vivo* concentrations of norelgestromin and its metabolites, even at the peak serum levels, are relatively low compared to the inhibitory constant (Ki) (based on results of *in vitro* studies)).
No products indexed under this heading.

Dyphylline (Although norelgestromin and its metabolites inhibit a variety of P450 enzymes in human liver microsomes, the clinical consequence of such an interaction on the levels of other concomitant medications is likely to be insignificant. Under the recommended dosing regimen, the *in vivo* concentrations of norelgestromin and its metabolites, even at the peak serum levels, are relatively low compared to the inhibitory constant (Ki) (based on results of *in vitro* studies)).
No products indexed under this heading.

Efavirenz (If a woman on hormonal contraceptives takes a drug or herbal product that induces enzymes, including CYP3A4, that metabolize contraceptive hormones, counsel her to use additional contraception or a different method of contraception. Drugs or herbal products that induce such enzymes may decrease the plasma concentrations of contraceptive hormones, and may decrease the effectiveness of hormonal contraceptives or increase breakthrough bleeding). Products include:
Atripla **906**

Encainide Hydrochloride (Although norelgestromin and its metabolites inhibit a variety of P450 enzymes in human liver microsomes, the clinical consequence of such an interaction on the levels of other concomitant medications is likely to be insignificant. Under the recommended dosing regimen, the *in vivo* concentrations of norelgestromin and its metabolites, even at the peak serum levels, are relatively low compared to the inhibitory constant (Ki) (based on results of *in vitro* studies)).
No products indexed under this heading.

Enoxacin (There have been reports of pregnancy while taking hormonal contraceptives and antibiotics, but clinical pharmacokinetic studies have not shown consistent effects of antibiotics on plasma concentrations of synthetic steroids. The metabolism of hormonal contraceptives may be influenced by various drugs. Of potential clinical importance are drugs that interrupt entero-hepatic recirculation of estrogen (eg, certain antibiotics). Literature suggests possible interactions with the concomitant use of hormonal contraceptives and ampicillin or tetracycline).
No products indexed under this heading.

Epirubicin Hydrochloride (There have been reports of pregnancy while taking hormonal contraceptives and antibiotics, but clinical pharmacokinetic studies have not shown consistent effects of antibiotics on plasma concentrations of synthetic steroids. The metabolism of hormonal contraceptives may be influenced by various drugs. Of potential clinical importance are drugs that interrupt entero-hepatic recirculation of estrogen (eg, certain antibiotics). Literature suggests possible interactions with the concomitant use of hormonal contraceptives and ampicillin or tetracycline).
No products indexed under this heading.

Eprosartan Mesylate (Although norelgestromin and its metabolites inhibit a variety of P450 enzymes in human liver microsomes, the clinical consequence of such an interaction on the levels of other concomitant medications is likely to be insignificant. Under the recommended dosing regimen, the *in vivo* concentrations of norelgestromin and its metabolites, even at the peak serum levels, are relatively low compared to the inhibitory constant (Ki) (based on results of *in vitro* studies)). Products include:
Teveten **538**
Teveten HCT **541**

Ergotamine Tartrate (Although norelgestromin and its metabolites inhibit a variety of P450 enzymes in human liver microsomes, the clinical consequence of such an interaction on the levels of other concomitant medications is likely to be insignificant. Under the recommended dosing regimen, the *in vivo* concentrations of norelgestromin and its metabolites, even at the peak serum levels, are relatively low compared to the inhibitory constant (Ki) (based on results of *in vitro* studies)).
No products indexed under this heading.

Erythromycin (If a woman on hormonal contraceptives takes a drug or herbal product that induces enzymes, including CYP3A4, that metabolize contraceptive hormones, counsel her to use additional contraception or a different method of contraception. Drugs or herbal products that induce such enzymes may decrease the plasma concentrations of contraceptive hormones, and may decrease the effectiveness of hormonal contraceptives or increase breakthrough bleeding).
No products indexed under this heading.

Erythromycin, Topical (If a woman on hormonal contraceptives takes a drug or herbal product that induces enzymes, including CYP3A4, that metabolize contraceptive hormones, counsel her to use additional contraception or a different method of contraception. Drugs or herbal products that induce such enzymes may decrease the plasma concentrations of contraceptive hormones, and may decrease the effectiveness of hormonal contraceptives or increase breakthrough bleeding).
No products indexed under this heading.

Erythromycin Estolate (If a woman on hormonal contraceptives takes a drug or herbal product that induces enzymes, including CYP3A4, that metabolize contraceptive hormones, counsel her to use additional contraception or a different method of contraception. Drugs or herbal products that induce such enzymes may decrease the plasma concentrations of contraceptive hormones, and may decrease the effectiveness of hormonal contraceptives or increase breakthrough bleeding).
No products indexed under this heading.

Ortho Evra Interactions Index 1314

Erythromycin Ethylsuccinate (If a woman on hormonal contraceptives takes a drug or herbal product that induces enzymes, including CYP3A4, that metabolize contraceptive hormones, counsel her to use additional contraception or a different method of contraception. Drugs or herbal products that induce such enzymes may decrease the plasma concentrations of contraceptive hormones, and may decrease the effectiveness of hormonal contraceptives or increase breakthrough bleeding). Products include:

E.E.S. 437
EryPed 435

Erythromycin Gluceptate (If a woman on hormonal contraceptives takes a drug or herbal product that induces enzymes, including CYP3A4, that metabolize contraceptive hormones, counsel her to use additional contraception or a different method of contraception. Drugs or herbal products that induce such enzymes may decrease the plasma concentrations of contraceptive hormones, and may decrease the effectiveness of hormonal contraceptives or increase breakthrough bleeding).

No products indexed under this heading.

Erythromycin Lactobionate (If a woman on hormonal contraceptives takes a drug or herbal product that induces enzymes, including CYP3A4, that metabolize contraceptive hormones, counsel her to use additional contraception or a different method of contraception. Drugs or herbal products that induce such enzymes may decrease the plasma concentrations of contraceptive hormones, and may decrease the effectiveness of hormonal contraceptives or increase breakthrough bleeding).

No products indexed under this heading.

Erythromycin Stearate (If a woman on hormonal contraceptives takes a drug or herbal product that induces enzymes, including CYP3A4, that metabolize contraceptive hormones, counsel her to use additional contraception or a different method of contraception. Drugs or herbal products that induce such enzymes may decrease the plasma concentrations of contraceptive hormones, and may decrease the effectiveness of hormonal contraceptives or increase breakthrough bleeding).

No products indexed under this heading.

Escitalopram Oxalate (If a woman on hormonal contraceptives takes a drug or herbal product that induces enzymes, including CYP3A4, that metabolize contraceptive hormones, counsel her to use additional contraception or a different method of contraception. Drugs or herbal products that induce such enzymes may decrease the plasma concentrations of contraceptive hormones, and may decrease the effectiveness of hormonal contraceptives or increase breakthrough bleeding). Products include:

Lexapro Oral Suspension 1160
Lexapro Tablets 1160

Esomeprazole Magnesium (If a woman on hormonal contraceptives takes a drug or herbal product that induces enzymes, including CYP3A4, that metabolize contraceptive hormones, counsel her to use additional contraception or a different method of contraception. Drugs or herbal products that induce such enzymes may decrease the plasma concentrations of contraceptive hormones, and may decrease the effectiveness of hormonal contraceptives or increase breakthrough bleeding). Products include:

Nexium Capsules 704
Nexium Oral Suspension 704

Esomeprazole Sodium (If a woman on hormonal contraceptives takes a drug or herbal product that induces enzymes, including CYP3A4, that metabolize contraceptive hormones, counsel her to use additional contraception or a different method of contraception. Drugs or herbal products that induce such enzymes may decrease the plasma concentrations of contraceptive hormones, and may decrease the effectiveness of hormonal contraceptives or increase breakthrough bleeding). Products include:

Nexium I.V. 712

Estradiol (Although norelgestromin and its metabolites inhibit a variety of P450 enzymes in human liver microsomes, the clinical consequence of such an interaction on the levels of other concomitant medications is likely to be insignificant. Under the recommended dosing regimen, the *in vivo* concentrations of norelgestromin and its metabolites, even at the peak serum levels, are relatively low compared to the inhibitory constant (Ki) (based on results of *in vitro* studies)). Products include:

Activella 2561
Angeliq 831
Climara 841
Climara Pro 847
Divigel 3467
Estrasorb 1777
Vagifem 2589

Estradiol Benzoate (Although norelgestromin and its metabolites inhibit a variety of P450 enzymes in human liver microsomes, the clinical consequence of such an interaction on the levels of other concomitant medications is likely to be insignificant. Under the recommended dosing regimen, the *in vivo* concentrations of norelgestromin and its metabolites, even at the peak serum levels, are relatively low compared to the inhibitory constant (Ki) (based on results of *in vitro* studies)).

No products indexed under this heading.

Estradiol Cypionate (Although norelgestromin and its metabolites inhibit a variety of P450 enzymes in human liver microsomes, the clinical consequence of such an interaction on the levels of other concomitant medications is likely to be insignificant. Under the recommended dosing regimen, the *in vivo* concentrations of norelgestromin and its metabolites, even at the peak serum levels, are relatively low compared to the inhibitory constant (Ki) (based on results of *in vitro* studies)).

No products indexed under this heading.

Estradiol Valerate (Although norelgestromin and its metabolites inhibit a variety of P450 enzymes in human liver microsomes, the clinical consequence of such an interaction on the levels of other concomitant medications is likely to be insignificant. Under the recommended dosing regimen, the *in vivo* concentrations of norelgestromin and its metabolites, even at the peak serum levels, are relatively low compared to the inhibitory constant (Ki) (based on results of *in vitro* studies)).

No products indexed under this heading.

Estrogen (Although norelgestromin and its metabolites inhibit a variety of P450 enzymes in human liver microsomes, the clinical consequence of such an interaction on the levels of other concomitant medications is likely to be insignificant. Under the recommended dosing regimen, the *in vivo* concentrations of norelgestromin and its metabolites, even at the peak serum levels, are relatively low compared to the inhibitory constant (Ki) (based on results of *in vitro* studies)).

No products indexed under this heading.

Estrogens, Conjugated (Although norelgestromin and its metabolites inhibit a variety of P450 enzymes in human liver microsomes, the clinical consequence of such an interaction on the levels of other concomitant medications is likely to be insignificant. Under the recommended dosing regimen, the *in vivo* concentrations of norelgestromin and its metabolites, even at the peak serum levels, are relatively low compared to the inhibitory constant (Ki) (based on results of *in vitro* studies)). Products include:

Premarin Intravenous 3528
Premarin Tablets 3533
Premarin Vaginal Cream 3540
Premphase 3549
Prempro 3549

Estrogens, Conjugated, Synthetic A (Although norelgestromin and its metabolites inhibit a variety of P450 enzymes in human liver microsomes, the clinical consequence of such an interaction on the levels of other concomitant medications is likely to be insignificant. Under the recommended dosing regimen, the *in vivo* concentrations of norelgestromin and its metabolites, even at the peak serum levels, are relatively low compared to the inhibitory constant (Ki) (based on results of *in vitro* studies)).

No products indexed under this heading.

Estrogens, Esterified (Although norelgestromin and its metabolites inhibit a variety of P450 enzymes in human liver microsomes, the clinical consequence of such an interaction on the levels of other concomitant medications is likely to be insignificant. Under the recommended dosing regimen, the *in vivo* concentrations of norelgestromin and its metabolites, even at the peak serum levels, are relatively low compared to the inhibitory constant (Ki) (based on results of *in vitro* studies)).

No products indexed under this heading.

Ethanol (If a woman on hormonal contraceptives takes a drug or herbal product that induces enzymes, including CYP3A4, that metabolize contraceptive hormones, counsel her to use additional contraception or a different method of contraception. Drugs or herbal products that induce such enzymes may decrease the plasma concentrations of contraceptive hormones, and may decrease the effectiveness of hormonal contraceptives or increase breakthrough bleeding).

No products indexed under this heading.

Ethosuximide (If a woman on hormonal contraceptives takes a drug or herbal product that induces enzymes, including CYP3A4, that metabolize contraceptive hormones, counsel her to use additional contraception or a different method of contraception. Drugs or herbal products that induce such enzymes may decrease the plasma concentrations of contraceptive hormones, and may decrease the effectiveness of hormonal contraceptives or increase breakthrough bleeding).

No products indexed under this heading.

Ethotoin (Although norelgestromin and its metabolites inhibit a variety of P450 enzymes in human liver microsomes, the clinical consequence of such an interaction on the levels of other concomitant medications is likely to be insignificant. Under the recommended dosing regimen, the *in vivo* concentrations of norelgestromin and its metabolites, even at the peak serum levels, are relatively low compared to the inhibitory constant (Ki) (based on results of *in vitro* studies)).

No products indexed under this heading.

Ethyl Alcohol (If a woman on hormonal contraceptives takes a drug or herbal product that induces enzymes, including CYP3A4, that metabolize contraceptive hormones, counsel her to use additional contraception or a different method of contraception. Drugs or herbal products that induce such enzymes may decrease the plasma concentrations of contraceptive hormones, and may decrease the effectiveness of hormonal contraceptives or increase breakthrough bleeding).

No products indexed under this heading.

Ethynodiol Diacetate (Although norelgestromin and its metabolites inhibit a variety of P450 enzymes in human liver microsomes, the clinical consequence of such an interaction on the levels of other concomitant medications is likely to be insignificant. Under the recommended dosing regimen, the *in vivo* concentrations of norelgestromin and its metabolites, even at the peak serum levels, are relatively low compared to the inhibitory constant (Ki) (based on results of *in vitro* studies)).

No products indexed under this heading.

Etodolac (Although norelgestromin and its metabolites inhibit a variety of P450 enzymes in human liver microsomes, the clinical consequence of such an interaction on the levels of other concomitant medications is likely to be insignificant. Under the recommended dosing regimen, the *in vivo* concentrations of norelgestromin and its metabolites, even at the peak serum levels, are relatively low compared to the inhibitory constant (Ki) (based on results of *in vitro* studies)).

No products indexed under this heading.

Etoposide (Although norelgestromin and its metabolites inhibit a variety of P450 enzymes in human liver microsomes, the clinical consequence of such an interaction on the levels of other concomitant medications is likely to be insignificant. Under the recommended dosing regimen, the *in vivo* concentrations of norelgestromin and its metabolites, even at the peak serum levels, are relatively low compared to the inhibitory constant (Ki) (based on results of *in vitro* studies)).

No products indexed under this heading.

Etoposide Phosphate (Although norelgestromin and its metabolites inhibit a variety of P450 enzymes in human liver microsomes, the clinical consequence of such an interaction on the levels of other concomitant medications is likely to be insignificant. Under the recommended dosing regimen, the *in vivo* concentrations of norelgestromin and its metabolites, even at the peak serum levels, are relatively low compared to the inhibitory constant (Ki) (based on results of *in vitro* studies)).

No products indexed under this heading.

Felbamate (Concomitant use with felbamate may decrease the plasma concentrations of hormonal contraceptives, and may decrease the effectiveness of hormonal contraceptives or increase breakthrough bleeding. Patients who are concomitantly using felbamate should be counseled to use additional contraception or a different method of contraception).

No products indexed under this heading.

Felodipine (Although norelgestromin and its metabolites inhibit a variety of P450 enzymes in human liver microsomes, the clinical consequence of such an interaction on the levels of other concomitant medications is likely to be insignificant. Under the recommended dosing regimen, the *in vivo* concentrations of norelgestromin and its metabolites, even at the peak serum levels, are relatively low compared to the inhibitory constant (Ki) (based on results of *in vitro* studies)).

No products indexed under this heading.

Fenoprofen Calcium (Although norelgestromin and its metabolites inhibit a variety of P450 enzymes in human liver

microsomes, the clinical consequence of such an interaction on the levels of other concomitant medications is likely to be insignificant. Under the recommended dosing regimen, the *in vivo* concentrations of norelgestromin and its metabolites, even at the peak serum levels, are relatively low compared to the inhibitory constant (Ki) (based on results of *in vitro* studies)).
No products indexed under this heading.

Fentanyl (Although norelgestromin and its metabolites inhibit a variety of P450 enzymes in human liver microsomes, the clinical consequence of such an interaction on the levels of other concomitant medications is likely to be insignificant. Under the recommended dosing regimen, the *in vivo* concentrations of norelgestromin and its metabolites, even at the peak serum levels, are relatively low compared to the inhibitory constant (Ki) (based on results of *in vitro* studies)). Products include:
Duragesic 2604
Fentanyl Transdermal System 2346
Onsolis 2054

Fentanyl Citrate (Although norelgestromin and its metabolites inhibit a variety of P450 enzymes in human liver microsomes, the clinical consequence of such an interaction on the levels of other concomitant medications is likely to be insignificant. Under the recommended dosing regimen, the *in vivo* concentrations of norelgestromin and its metabolites, even at the peak serum levels, are relatively low compared to the inhibitory constant (Ki) (based on results of *in vitro* studies)). Products include:
Fentora 966

Flecainide Acetate (Although norelgestromin and its metabolites inhibit a variety of P450 enzymes in human liver microsomes, the clinical consequence of such an interaction on the levels of other concomitant medications is likely to be insignificant. Under the recommended dosing regimen, the *in vivo* concentrations of norelgestromin and its metabolites, even at the peak serum levels, are relatively low compared to the inhibitory constant (Ki) (based on results of *in vitro* studies)).
No products indexed under this heading.

Fluconazole (CYP3A4 inhibitors, such as itraconazole or ketoconazole, may increase plasma hormone levels).
No products indexed under this heading.

Fludrocortisone Acetate (If a woman on hormonal contraceptives takes a drug or herbal product that induces enzymes, including CYP3A4, that metabolize contraceptive hormones, counsel her to use additional contraception or a different method of contraception. Drugs or herbal products that induce such enzymes may decrease the plasma concentrations of contraceptive hormones, and may decrease the effectiveness of hormonal contraceptives or increase breakthrough bleeding).
No products indexed under this heading.

Fluoxetine (CYP3A4 inhibitors, such as itraconazole or ketoconazole, may increase plasma hormone levels).
No products indexed under this heading.

Fluoxetine Hydrochloride (CYP3A4 inhibitors, such as itraconazole or ketoconazole, may increase plasma hormone levels). Products include:
Prozac Weekly 1941
Prozac Pulvules 1941
Symbyax 1965

Fluphenazine Decanoate (Although norelgestromin and its metabolites inhibit a variety of P450 enzymes in human liver microsomes, the clinical consequence of such an interaction on the levels of other concomitant medications is likely to be insignificant. Under the recommended dosing regimen, the *in vivo* concentrations of norelgestromin and its metabolites, even at the peak serum levels, are relatively low compared to the inhibitory constant (Ki) (based on results of *in vitro* studies)).
No products indexed under this heading.

Fluphenazine Enanthate (Although norelgestromin and its metabolites inhibit a variety of P450 enzymes in human liver microsomes, the clinical consequence of such an interaction on the levels of other concomitant medications is likely to be insignificant. Under the recommended dosing regimen, the *in vivo* concentrations of norelgestromin and its metabolites, even at the peak serum levels, are relatively low compared to the inhibitory constant (Ki) (based on results of *in vitro* studies)).
No products indexed under this heading.

Fluphenazine Hydrochloride (Although norelgestromin and its metabolites inhibit a variety of P450 enzymes in human liver microsomes, the clinical consequence of such an interaction on the levels of other concomitant medications is likely to be insignificant. Under the recommended dosing regimen, the *in vivo* concentrations of norelgestromin and its metabolites, even at the peak serum levels, are relatively low compared to the inhibitory constant (Ki) (based on results of *in vitro* studies)).
No products indexed under this heading.

Flurbiprofen (Although norelgestromin and its metabolites inhibit a variety of P450 enzymes in human liver microsomes, the clinical consequence of such an interaction on the levels of other concomitant medications is likely to be insignificant. Under the recommended dosing regimen, the *in vivo* concentrations of norelgestromin and its metabolites, even at the peak serum levels, are relatively low compared to the inhibitory constant (Ki) (based on results of *in vitro* studies)).
No products indexed under this heading.

Flurbiprofen Sodium (Although norelgestromin and its metabolites inhibit a variety of P450 enzymes in human liver microsomes, the clinical consequence of such an interaction on the levels of other concomitant medications is likely to be insignificant. Under the recommended dosing regimen, the *in vivo* concentrations of norelgestromin and its metabolites, even at the peak serum levels, are relatively low compared to the inhibitory constant (Ki) (based on results of *in vitro* studies)).
No products indexed under this heading.

Flutamide (Although norelgestromin and its metabolites inhibit a variety of P450 enzymes in human liver microsomes, the clinical consequence of such an interaction on the levels of other concomitant medications is likely to be insignificant. Under the recommended dosing regimen, the *in vivo* concentrations of norelgestromin and its metabolites, even at the peak serum levels, are relatively low compared to the inhibitory constant (Ki) (based on results of *in vitro* studies)).
No products indexed under this heading.

Fluticasone Propionate (Although norelgestromin and its metabolites inhibit a variety of P450 enzymes in human liver microsomes, the clinical consequence of such an interaction on the levels of other concomitant medications is likely to be insignificant. Under the recommended dosing regimen, the *in vivo* concentrations of norelgestromin and its metabolites, even at the peak serum levels, are relatively low compared to the inhibitory constant (Ki) (based on results of *in vitro* studies)). Products include:
Advair 100/50 1275
Advair 250/50 1275
Advair 500/50 1275
Advair HFA 45/21 1288
Advair HFA 115/21 1288
Advair HFA 230/21 1288
Flonase 1459
Flovent Diskus 1463
Flovent HFA 1470

Fluvastatin Sodium (Although norelgestromin and its metabolites inhibit a variety of P450 enzymes in human liver microsomes, the clinical consequence of such an interaction on the levels of other concomitant medications is likely to be insignificant. Under the recommended dosing regimen, the *in vivo* concentrations of norelgestromin and its metabolites, even at the peak serum levels, are relatively low compared to the inhibitory constant (Ki) (based on results of *in vitro* studies)).
No products indexed under this heading.

Fluvoxamine (If a woman on hormonal contraceptives takes a drug or herbal product that induces enzymes, including CYP3A4, that metabolize contraceptive hormones, counsel her to use additional contraception or a different method of contraception. Drugs or herbal products that induce such enzymes may decrease the plasma concentrations of contraceptive hormones, and may decrease the effectiveness of hormonal contraceptives or increase breakthrough bleeding).
No products indexed under this heading.

Fluvoxamine Maleate (If a woman on hormonal contraceptives takes a drug or herbal product that induces enzymes, including CYP3A4, that metabolize contraceptive hormones, counsel her to use additional contraception or a different method of contraception. Drugs or herbal products that induce such enzymes may decrease the plasma concentrations of contraceptive hormones, and may decrease the effectiveness of hormonal contraceptives or increase breakthrough bleeding).
No products indexed under this heading.

Formoterol Fumarate (Although norelgestromin and its metabolites inhibit a variety of P450 enzymes in human liver microsomes, the clinical consequence of such an interaction on the levels of other concomitant medications is likely to be insignificant. Under the recommended dosing regimen, the *in vivo* concentrations of norelgestromin and its metabolites, even at the peak serum levels, are relatively low compared to the inhibitory constant (Ki) (based on results of *in vitro* studies)). Products include:
Foradil 3121
Perforomist 3634

Fosamprenavir Calcium (Significant changes (increase or decrease) in the plasma levels of the estrogen and progestin have been noted in some cases of co-administration of HIV protease inhibitors). Products include:
Lexiva Oral Suspension 1558
Lexiva 1558

Fosphenytoin (Concomitant use with phenytoin may decrease the plasma concentrations of hormonal contraceptives, and may decrease the effectiveness of hormonal contraceptives or increase breakthrough bleeding. Patients who are concomitantly using phenytoin should be counseled to use additional contraception or a different method of contraception).
No products indexed under this heading.

Fosphenytoin Sodium (Concomitant use with phenytoin may decrease the plasma concentrations of hormonal contraceptives, and may decrease the effectiveness of hormonal contraceptives or increase breakthrough bleeding. Patients who are concomitantly using phenytoin should be counseled to use additional contraception or a different method of contraception).
No products indexed under this heading.

Gabapentin (Although norelgestromin and its metabolites inhibit a variety of P450 enzymes in human liver microsomes, the clinical consequence of such an interaction on the levels of other concomitant medications is likely to be insignificant. Under the recommended dosing regimen, the *in vivo* concentrations of norelgestromin and its metabolites, even at the peak serum levels, are relatively low compared to the inhibitory constant (Ki) (based on results of *in vitro* studies)).
No products indexed under this heading.

Galantamine Hydrobromide (Although norelgestromin and its metabolites inhibit a variety of P450 enzymes in human liver microsomes, the clinical consequence of such an interaction on the levels of other concomitant medications is likely to be insignificant. Under the recommended dosing regimen, the *in vivo* concentrations of norelgestromin and its metabolites, even at the peak serum levels, are relatively low compared to the inhibitory constant (Ki) (based on results of *in vitro* studies)).
No products indexed under this heading.

Garlic Extract (If a woman on hormonal contraceptives takes a drug or herbal product that induces enzymes, including CYP3A4, that metabolize contraceptive hormones, counsel her to use additional contraception or a different method of contraception. Drugs or herbal products that induce such enzymes may decrease the plasma concentrations of contraceptive hormones, and may decrease the effectiveness of hormonal contraceptives or increase breakthrough bleeding).
No products indexed under this heading.

Garlic Oil (If a woman on hormonal contraceptives takes a drug or herbal product that induces enzymes, including CYP3A4, that metabolize contraceptive hormones, counsel her to use additional contraception or a different method of contraception. Drugs or herbal products that induce such enzymes may decrease the plasma concentrations of contraceptive hormones, and may decrease the effectiveness of hormonal contraceptives or increase breakthrough bleeding).
No products indexed under this heading.

Gatifloxacin (There have been reports of pregnancy while taking hormonal contraceptives and antibiotics, but clinical pharmacokinetic studies have not shown consistent effects of antibiotics on plasma concentrations of synthetic steroids. The metabolism of hormonal contraceptives may be influenced by various drugs. Of potential clinical importance are drugs that interrupt entero-hepatic recirculation of estrogen (eg, certain antibiotics). Literature suggests possible interactions with the concomitant use of hormonal contraceptives and ampicillin or tetracycline).
No products indexed under this heading.

Gemifloxacin Mesylate (There have been reports of pregnancy while taking hormonal contraceptives and antibiotics, but clinical pharmacokinetic studies have not shown consistent effects of antibiotics on plasma concentrations of synthetic steroids. The metabolism of hormonal contraceptives may be influenced by various drugs. Of potential

clinical importance are drugs that interrupt entero-hepatic recirculation of estrogen (eg, certain antibiotics). Literature suggests possible interactions with the concomitant use of hormonal contraceptives and ampicillin or tetracycline).
No products indexed under this heading.

Gentamicin Sulfate (There have been reports of pregnancy while taking hormonal contraceptives and antibiotics, but clinical pharmacokinetic studies have not shown consistent effects of antibiotics on plasma concentrations of synthetic steroids. The metabolism of hormonal contraceptives may be influenced by various drugs. Of potential clinical importance are drugs that interrupt entero-hepatic recirculation of estrogen (eg, certain antibiotics). Literature suggests possible interactions with the concomitant use of hormonal contraceptives and ampicillin or tetracycline). Products include:
Pred-G .... ⊙226, ⊙227

Glimepiride (Although norelgestromin and its metabolites inhibit a variety of P450 enzymes in human liver microsomes, the clinical consequence of such an interaction on the levels of other concomitant medications is likely to be insignificant. Under the recommended dosing regimen, the *in vivo* concentrations of norelgestromin and its metabolites, even at the peak serum levels, are relatively low compared to the inhibitory constant (Ki) (based on results of *in vitro* studies)). Products include:
Avandaryl **1356**
Duetact **3354**

Glipizide (If a woman on hormonal contraceptives takes a drug or herbal product that induces enzymes, including CYP3A4, that metabolize contraceptive hormones, counsel her to use additional contraception or a different method of contraception. Drugs or herbal products that induce such enzymes may decrease the plasma concentrations of contraceptive hormones, and may decrease the effectiveness of hormonal contraceptives or increase breakthrough bleeding).
No products indexed under this heading.

Glyburide (If a woman on hormonal contraceptives takes a drug or herbal product that induces enzymes, including CYP3A4, that metabolize contraceptive hormones, counsel her to use additional contraception or a different method of contraception. Drugs or herbal products that induce such enzymes may decrease the plasma concentrations of contraceptive hormones, and may decrease the effectiveness of hormonal contraceptives or increase breakthrough bleeding).
No products indexed under this heading.

Grepafloxacin Hydrochloride (There have been reports of pregnancy while taking hormonal contraceptives and antibiotics, but clinical pharmacokinetic studies have not shown consistent effects of antibiotics on plasma concentrations of synthetic steroids. The metabolism of hormonal contraceptives may be influenced by various drugs. Of potential clinical importance are drugs that interrupt entero-hepatic recirculation of estrogen (eg, certain antibiotics). Literature suggests possible interactions with the concomitant use of hormonal contraceptives and ampicillin or tetracycline).
No products indexed under this heading.

Griseofulvin (Concomitant use with griseofulvin may decrease the plasma concentrations of hormonal contraceptives, and may decrease the effectiveness of hormonal contraceptives or increase breakthrough bleeding. Patients who are concomitantly using griseofulvin, should be counseled to use additional contraception or a different method of contraception).
No products indexed under this heading.

Haloperidol (Although norelgestromin and its metabolites inhibit a variety of P450 enzymes in human liver microsomes, the clinical consequence of such an interaction on the levels of other concomitant medications is likely to be insignificant. Under the recommended dosing regimen, the *in vivo* concentrations of norelgestromin and its metabolites, even at the peak serum levels, are relatively low compared to the inhibitory constant (Ki) (based on results of *in vitro* studies)).
No products indexed under this heading.

Haloperidol Decanoate (Although norelgestromin and its metabolites inhibit a variety of P450 enzymes in human liver microsomes, the clinical consequence of such an interaction on the levels of other concomitant medications is likely to be insignificant. Under the recommended dosing regimen, the *in vivo* concentrations of norelgestromin and its metabolites, even at the peak serum levels, are relatively low compared to the inhibitory constant (Ki) (based on results of *in vitro* studies)).
No products indexed under this heading.

Haloperidol Lactate (Although norelgestromin and its metabolites inhibit a variety of P450 enzymes in human liver microsomes, the clinical consequence of such an interaction on the levels of other concomitant medications is likely to be insignificant. Under the recommended dosing regimen, the *in vivo* concentrations of norelgestromin and its metabolites, even at the peak serum levels, are relatively low compared to the inhibitory constant (Ki) (based on results of *in vitro* studies)).
No products indexed under this heading.

Hepatic Enzyme-Inducing Agents (If a woman on hormonal contraceptives takes a drug or herbal product that induces enzymes, including CYP3A4, that metabolize contraceptive hormones, counsel her to use additional contraception or a different method of contraception. Drugs or herbal products that induce such enzymes may decrease the plasma concentrations of contraceptive hormones, and may decrease the effectiveness of hormonal contraceptives or increase breakthrough bleeding).
No products indexed under this heading.

Hexobarbital (Concomitant use with barbiturates may decrease the plasma concentrations of hormonal contraceptives, and may decrease the effectiveness of hormonal contraceptives or increase breakthrough bleeding. Patients who are concomitantly using barbiturates should be counseled to use additional contraception or a different method of contraception).
No products indexed under this heading.

Hydrocodone Bitartrate (Although norelgestromin and its metabolites inhibit a variety of P450 enzymes in human liver microsomes, the clinical consequence of such an interaction on the levels of other concomitant medications is likely to be insignificant. Under the recommended dosing regimen, the *in vivo* concentrations of norelgestromin and its metabolites, even at the peak serum levels, are relatively low compared to the inhibitory constant (Ki) (based on results of *in vitro* studies)). Products include:
Vicodin **560**
Vicodin ES **561**
Vicodin HP **563**
Vicoprofen **564**
Zydone **1138**

Hydrocortisone (If a woman on hormonal contraceptives takes a drug or herbal product that induces enzymes, including CYP3A4, that metabolize contraceptive hormones, counsel her to use additional contraception or a different method of contraception. Drugs or herbal products that induce such enzymes may decrease the plasma concentrations of contraceptive hormones, and may decrease the effectiveness of hormonal contraceptives or increase breakthrough bleeding).
No products indexed under this heading.

Hydrocortisone (Alcohol) (If a woman on hormonal contraceptives takes a drug or herbal product that induces enzymes, including CYP3A4, that metabolize contraceptive hormones, counsel her to use additional contraception or a different method of contraception. Drugs or herbal products that induce such enzymes may decrease the plasma concentrations of contraceptive hormones, and may decrease the effectiveness of hormonal contraceptives or increase breakthrough bleeding).
No products indexed under this heading.

Hydrocortisone Acetate (If a woman on hormonal contraceptives takes a drug or herbal product that induces enzymes, including CYP3A4, that metabolize contraceptive hormones, counsel her to use additional contraception or a different method of contraception. Drugs or herbal products that induce such enzymes may decrease the plasma concentrations of contraceptive hormones, and may decrease the effectiveness of hormonal contraceptives or increase breakthrough bleeding).
No products indexed under this heading.

Hydrocortisone Butyrate (If a woman on hormonal contraceptives takes a drug or herbal product that induces enzymes, including CYP3A4, that metabolize contraceptive hormones, counsel her to use additional contraception or a different method of contraception. Drugs or herbal products that induce such enzymes may decrease the plasma concentrations of contraceptive hormones, and may decrease the effectiveness of hormonal contraceptives or increase breakthrough bleeding).
No products indexed under this heading.

Hydrocortisone Cypionate (If a woman on hormonal contraceptives takes a drug or herbal product that induces enzymes, including CYP3A4, that metabolize contraceptive hormones, counsel her to use additional contraception or a different method of contraception. Drugs or herbal products that induce such enzymes may decrease the plasma concentrations of contraceptive hormones, and may decrease the effectiveness of hormonal contraceptives or increase breakthrough bleeding).
No products indexed under this heading.

Hydrocortisone Hemisuccinate (If a woman on hormonal contraceptives takes a drug or herbal product that induces enzymes, including CYP3A4, that metabolize contraceptive hormones, counsel her to use additional contraception or a different method of contraception. Drugs or herbal products that induce such enzymes may decrease the plasma concentrations of contraceptive hormones, and may decrease the effectiveness of hormonal contraceptives or increase breakthrough bleeding).
No products indexed under this heading.

Hydrocortisone Probutate (If a woman on hormonal contraceptives takes a drug or herbal product that induces enzymes, including CYP3A4, that metabolize contraceptive hormones, counsel her to use additional contraception or a different method of contraception. Drugs or herbal products that induce such enzymes may decrease the plasma concentrations of contraceptive hormones, and may decrease the effectiveness of hormonal contraceptives or increase breakthrough bleeding).
No products indexed under this heading.

Hydrocortisone Sodium Phosphate (If a woman on hormonal contraceptives takes a drug or herbal product that induces enzymes, including CYP3A4, that metabolize contraceptive hormones, counsel her to use additional contraception or a different method of contraception. Drugs or herbal products that induce such enzymes may decrease the plasma concentrations of contraceptive hormones, and may decrease the effectiveness of hormonal contraceptives or increase breakthrough bleeding).
No products indexed under this heading.

Hydrocortisone Sodium Succinate (If a woman on hormonal contraceptives takes a drug or herbal product that induces enzymes, including CYP3A4, that metabolize contraceptive hormones, counsel her to use additional contraception or a different method of contraception. Drugs or herbal products that induce such enzymes may decrease the plasma concentrations of contraceptive hormones, and may decrease the effectiveness of hormonal contraceptives or increase breakthrough bleeding).
No products indexed under this heading.

Hydrocortisone Valerate (If a woman on hormonal contraceptives takes a drug or herbal product that induces enzymes, including CYP3A4, that metabolize contraceptive hormones, counsel her to use additional contraception or a different method of contraception. Drugs or herbal products that induce such enzymes may decrease the plasma concentrations of contraceptive hormones, and may decrease the effectiveness of hormonal contraceptives or increase breakthrough bleeding).
No products indexed under this heading.

Hypericum (If a woman on hormonal contraceptives takes a drug or herbal product that induces enzymes, including CYP3A4, that metabolize contraceptive hormones, counsel her to use additional contraception or a different method of contraception. Drugs or herbal products that induce such enzymes may decrease the plasma concentrations of contraceptive hormones, and may decrease the effectiveness of hormonal contraceptives or increase breakthrough bleeding).
No products indexed under this heading.

Hypericum Perforatum (Concomitant use with St. John's wort may decrease the plasma concentrations of hormonal contraceptives, and may decrease the effectiveness of hormonal contraceptives or increase breakthrough bleeding. Patients who are concomitantly using St. John's wort, should be counseled to use additional contraception or a different method of contraception). Products include:
Traumeel **1800**

Ibuprofen (Although norelgestromin and its metabolites inhibit a variety of P450 enzymes in human liver microsomes, the clinical consequence of such an interaction on the levels of other concomitant medications is likely to be insignificant. Under the recommended dosing regimen, the *in vivo* concentrations of norelgestromin and its metabolites, even at the peak serum

1317 Interactions Index Ortho Evra

levels, are relatively low compared to the inhibitory constant (Ki) (based on results of *in vitro* studies)). Products include:
Motrin IB 2043
Children's Motrin 2044
Children's Motrin Non-Staining Dye-Free 2044
Infants' Motrin 2044
Infants' Motrin Dye-Free 2044
Junior Strength Motrin 2044
Vicoprofen 564

Idarubicin Hydrochloride (There have been reports of pregnancy while taking hormonal contraceptives and antibiotics, but clinical pharmacokinetic studies have not shown consistent effects of antibiotics on plasma concentrations of synthetic steroids. The metabolism of hormonal contraceptives may be influenced by various drugs. Of potential clinical importance are drugs that interrupt entero-hepatic recirculation of estrogen (eg, certain antibiotics). Literature suggests possible interactions with the concomitant use of hormonal contraceptives and ampicillin or tetracycline).
No products indexed under this heading.

Imatinib Mesylate (CYP3A4 inhibitors, such as itraconazole or ketoconazole, may increase plasma hormone levels). Products include:
Gleevec 2477

Imipenem (There have been reports of pregnancy while taking hormonal contraceptives and antibiotics, but clinical pharmacokinetic studies have not shown consistent effects of antibiotics on plasma concentrations of synthetic steroids. The metabolism of hormonal contraceptives may be influenced by various drugs. Of potential clinical importance are drugs that interrupt entero-hepatic recirculation of estrogen (eg, certain antibiotics). Literature suggests possible interactions with the concomitant use of hormonal contraceptives and ampicillin or tetracycline). Products include:
Primaxin I.M. 2232
Primaxin I.V. 2235

Imipramine Hydrochloride (Although norelgestromin and its metabolites inhibit a variety of P450 enzymes in human liver microsomes, the clinical consequence of such an interaction on the levels of other concomitant medications is likely to be insignificant. Under the recommended dosing regimen, the *in vivo* concentrations of norelgestromin and its metabolites, even at the peak serum levels, are relatively low compared to the inhibitory constant (Ki) (based on results of *in vitro* studies)).
No products indexed under this heading.

Imipramine Pamoate (Although norelgestromin and its metabolites inhibit a variety of P450 enzymes in human liver microsomes, the clinical consequence of such an interaction on the levels of other concomitant medications is likely to be insignificant. Under the recommended dosing regimen, the *in vivo* concentrations of norelgestromin and its metabolites, even at the peak serum levels, are relatively low compared to the inhibitory constant (Ki) (based on results of *in vitro* studies)).
No products indexed under this heading.

Indinavir Sulfate (Significant changes (increase or decrease) in the plasma levels of the estrogen and progestin have been noted in some cases of co-administration of HIV protease inhibitors). Products include:
Crixivan 2113

Indomethacin (Although norelgestromin and its metabolites inhibit a variety of P450 enzymes in human liver microsomes, the clinical consequence of such an interaction on the levels of other concomitant medications is likely to be insignificant. Under the recommended dosing regimen, the *in vivo* concentrations of norelgestromin and its metabolites, even at the peak serum levels, are relatively low compared to the inhibitory constant (Ki) (based on results of *in vitro* studies)). Products include:
Indocin 2167

Indomethacin Sodium Trihydrate (Although norelgestromin and its metabolites inhibit a variety of P450 enzymes in human liver microsomes, the clinical consequence of such an interaction on the levels of other concomitant medications is likely to be insignificant. Under the recommended dosing regimen, the *in vivo* concentrations of norelgestromin and its metabolites, even at the peak serum levels, are relatively low compared to the inhibitory constant (Ki) (based on results of *in vitro* studies)). Products include:
Indocin I.V. 2007

Indoramin Hydrochloride (Although norelgestromin and its metabolites inhibit a variety of P450 enzymes in human liver microsomes, the clinical consequence of such an interaction on the levels of other concomitant medications is likely to be insignificant. Under the recommended dosing regimen, the *in vivo* concentrations of norelgestromin and its metabolites, even at the peak serum levels, are relatively low compared to the inhibitory constant (Ki) (based on results of *in vitro* studies)).
No products indexed under this heading.

Insulin (If a woman on hormonal contraceptives takes a drug or herbal product that induces enzymes, including CYP3A4, that metabolize contraceptive hormones, counsel her to use additional contraception or a different method of contraception. Drugs or herbal products that induce such enzymes may decrease the plasma concentrations of contraceptive hormones, and may decrease the effectiveness of hormonal contraceptives or increase breakthrough bleeding).
No products indexed under this heading.

Insulin, Human, Zinc Suspension (If a woman on hormonal contraceptives takes a drug or herbal product that induces enzymes, including CYP3A4, that metabolize contraceptive hormones, counsel her to use additional contraception or a different method of contraception. Drugs or herbal products that induce such enzymes may decrease the plasma concentrations of contraceptive hormones, and may decrease the effectiveness of hormonal contraceptives or increase breakthrough bleeding).
No products indexed under this heading.

Insulin, Human (rDNA origin) (If a woman on hormonal contraceptives takes a drug or herbal product that induces enzymes, including CYP3A4, that metabolize contraceptive hormones, counsel her to use additional contraception or a different method of contraception. Drugs or herbal products that induce such enzymes may decrease the plasma concentrations of contraceptive hormones, and may decrease the effectiveness of hormonal contraceptives or increase breakthrough bleeding). Products include:
Exubera 2717

Insulin, Human NPH (If a woman on hormonal contraceptives takes a drug or herbal product that induces enzymes, including CYP3A4, that metabolize contraceptive hormones, counsel her to use additional contraception or a different method of contraception. Drugs or herbal products that induce such enzymes may decrease the plasma concentrations of contraceptive hormones, and may decrease the effectiveness of hormonal contraceptives or increase breakthrough bleeding). Products include:
Humulin N Vial 1934

Insulin, Human Regular (If a woman on hormonal contraceptives takes a drug or herbal product that induces enzymes, including CYP3A4, that metabolize contraceptive hormones, counsel her to use additional contraception or a different method of contraception. Drugs or herbal products that induce such enzymes may decrease the plasma concentrations of contraceptive hormones, and may decrease the effectiveness of hormonal contraceptives or increase breakthrough bleeding). Products include:
Humulin R 1937
Humulin R (U-500) 1939

Insulin, Human Regular and Human NPH Mixture (If a woman on hormonal contraceptives takes a drug or herbal product that induces enzymes, including CYP3A4, that metabolize contraceptive hormones, counsel her to use additional contraception or a different method of contraception. Drugs or herbal products that induce such enzymes may decrease the plasma concentrations of contraceptive hormones, and may decrease the effectiveness of hormonal contraceptives or increase breakthrough bleeding). Products include:
Humulin 50/50 1930
Humulin 70/30 Vial 1931

Insulin, NPH (If a woman on hormonal contraceptives takes a drug or herbal product that induces enzymes, including CYP3A4, that metabolize contraceptive hormones, counsel her to use additional contraception or a different method of contraception. Drugs or herbal products that induce such enzymes may decrease the plasma concentrations of contraceptive hormones, and may decrease the effectiveness of hormonal contraceptives or increase breakthrough bleeding).
No products indexed under this heading.

Insulin, Regular (If a woman on hormonal contraceptives takes a drug or herbal product that induces enzymes, including CYP3A4, that metabolize contraceptive hormones, counsel her to use additional contraception or a different method of contraception. Drugs or herbal products that induce such enzymes may decrease the plasma concentrations of contraceptive hormones, and may decrease the effectiveness of hormonal contraceptives or increase breakthrough bleeding).
No products indexed under this heading.

Insulin, Regular and NPH mixture (If a woman on hormonal contraceptives takes a drug or herbal product that induces enzymes, including CYP3A4, that metabolize contraceptive hormones, counsel her to use additional contraception or a different method of contraception. Drugs or herbal products that induce such enzymes may decrease the plasma concentrations of contraceptive hormones, and may decrease the effectiveness of hormonal contraceptives or increase breakthrough bleeding).
No products indexed under this heading.

Insulin, Zinc Crystals (If a woman on hormonal contraceptives takes a drug or herbal product that induces enzymes, including CYP3A4, that metabolize contraceptive hormones, counsel her to use additional contraception or a different method of contraception. Drugs or herbal products that induce such enzymes may decrease the plasma concentrations of contraceptive hormones, and may decrease the effectiveness of hormonal contraceptives or increase breakthrough bleeding).
No products indexed under this heading.

Insulin, Zinc Suspension (If a woman on hormonal contraceptives takes a drug or herbal product that induces enzymes, including CYP3A4, that metabolize contraceptive hormones, counsel her to use additional contraception or a different method of contraception. Drugs or herbal products that induce such enzymes may decrease the plasma concentrations of contraceptive hormones, and may decrease the effectiveness of hormonal contraceptives or increase breakthrough bleeding).
No products indexed under this heading.

Insulin Aspart (If a woman on hormonal contraceptives takes a drug or herbal product that induces enzymes, including CYP3A4, that metabolize contraceptive hormones, counsel her to use additional contraception or a different method of contraception. Drugs or herbal products that induce such enzymes may decrease the plasma concentrations of contraceptive hormones, and may decrease the effectiveness of hormonal contraceptives or increase breakthrough bleeding).
No products indexed under this heading.

Insulin Aspart, Human (If a woman on hormonal contraceptives takes a drug or herbal product that induces enzymes, including CYP3A4, that metabolize contraceptive hormones, counsel her to use additional contraception or a different method of contraception. Drugs or herbal products that induce such enzymes may decrease the plasma concentrations of contraceptive hormones, and may decrease the effectiveness of hormonal contraceptives or increase breakthrough bleeding). Products include:
NovoLog Mix 70/30 2581

Insulin Aspart, Human Regular (If a woman on hormonal contraceptives takes a drug or herbal product that induces enzymes, including CYP3A4, that metabolize contraceptive hormones, counsel her to use additional contraception or a different method of contraception. Drugs or herbal products that induce such enzymes may decrease the plasma concentrations of contraceptive hormones, and may decrease the effectiveness of hormonal contraceptives or increase breakthrough bleeding). Products include:
NovoLog 2575

Insulin Aspart Protamine, Human (If a woman on hormonal contraceptives takes a drug or herbal product that induces enzymes, including CYP3A4, that metabolize contraceptive hormones, counsel her to use additional contraception or a different method of contraception. Drugs or herbal products that induce such enzymes may decrease the plasma concentrations of contraceptive hormones, and may decrease the effectiveness of hormonal contraceptives or increase breakthrough bleeding). Products include:
NovoLog Mix 70/30 2581

Insulin Detemir (rDNA Origin) (If a woman on hormonal contraceptives takes a drug or herbal product that induces enzymes, including CYP3A4, that metabolize contraceptive hormones, counsel her to use additional contraception or a different method of contraception. Drugs or herbal products that induce such enzymes may decrease the plasma concentrations of contraceptive hormones, and may decrease the effectiveness of hormonal contraceptives or increase breakthrough bleeding). Products include:
Levemir 2566

IMPORTANT NOTE: Always consult each drug listing in the patient's regimen for possible interactions.

Ortho Evra Interactions Index 1318

Insulin Glargine (If a woman on hormonal contraceptives takes a drug or herbal product that induces enzymes, including CYP3A4, that metabolize contraceptive hormones, counsel her to use additional contraception or a different method of contraception. Drugs or herbal products that induce such enzymes may decrease the plasma concentrations of contraceptive hormones, and may decrease the effectiveness of hormonal contraceptives or increase breakthrough bleeding). Products include:

Lantus 2996

Insulin Glulisine (If a woman on hormonal contraceptives takes a drug or herbal product that induces enzymes, including CYP3A4, that metabolize contraceptive hormones, counsel her to use additional contraception or a different method of contraception. Drugs or herbal products that induce such enzymes may decrease the plasma concentrations of contraceptive hormones, and may decrease the effectiveness of hormonal contraceptives or increase breakthrough bleeding). Products include:

Apidra 2937
Apidra SoloStar 2937

Insulin Lispro, Human (If a woman on hormonal contraceptives takes a drug or herbal product that induces enzymes, including CYP3A4, that metabolize contraceptive hormones, counsel her to use additional contraception or a different method of contraception. Drugs or herbal products that induce such enzymes may decrease the plasma concentrations of contraceptive hormones, and may decrease the effectiveness of hormonal contraceptives or increase breakthrough bleeding). Products include:

Humalog 1910
Humalog Mix 1914
Humalog Mix75/25 1917

Insulin Lispro Protamine, Human (If a woman on hormonal contraceptives takes a drug or herbal product that induces enzymes, including CYP3A4, that metabolize contraceptive hormones, counsel her to use additional contraception or a different method of contraception. Drugs or herbal products that induce such enzymes may decrease the plasma concentrations of contraceptive hormones, and may decrease the effectiveness of hormonal contraceptives or increase breakthrough bleeding). Products include:

Humalog Mix 1914
Humalog Mix75/25 1917

Irbesartan (Although norelgestromin and its metabolites inhibit a variety of P450 enzymes in human liver microsomes, the clinical consequence of such an interaction on the levels of other concomitant medications is likely to be insignificant. Under the recommended dosing regimen, the *in vivo* concentrations of norelgestromin and its metabolites, even at the peak serum levels, are relatively low compared to the inhibitory constant (Ki) (based on results of *in vitro* studies)). Products include:

Avalide 2956
Avapro 2962

Isoniazid (CYP3A4 inhibitors, such as itraconazole or ketoconazole, may increase plasma hormone levels).
No products indexed under this heading.

Isotretinoin (Although norelgestromin and its metabolites inhibit a variety of P450 enzymes in human liver microsomes, the clinical consequence of such an interaction on the levels of other concomitant medications is likely to be insignificant. Under the recommended dosing regimen, the *in vivo* concentrations of norelgestromin and its metabolites, even at the peak serum levels, are relatively low compared to the inhibitory constant (Ki) (based on results of *in vitro* studies)). Products include:

Accutane 2832

Isradipine (Although norelgestromin and its metabolites inhibit a variety of P450 enzymes in human liver microsomes, the clinical consequence of such an interaction on the levels of other concomitant medications is likely to be insignificant. Under the recommended dosing regimen, the *in vivo* concentrations of norelgestromin and its metabolites, even at the peak serum levels, are relatively low compared to the inhibitory constant (Ki) (based on results of *in vitro* studies)). Products include:

DynaCirc CR 1432

Itraconazole (CYP3A4 inhibitors, such as itraconazole, may increase plasma hormone levels).
No products indexed under this heading.

Ixabepilone (Although norelgestromin and its metabolites inhibit a variety of P450 enzymes in human liver microsomes, the clinical consequence of such an interaction on the levels of other concomitant medications is likely to be insignificant. Under the recommended dosing regimen, the *in vivo* concentrations of norelgestromin and its metabolites, even at the peak serum levels, are relatively low compared to the inhibitory constant (Ki) (based on results of *in vitro* studies)).
No products indexed under this heading.

Kanamycin Sulfate (There have been reports of pregnancy while taking hormonal contraceptives and antibiotics, but clinical pharmacokinetic studies have not shown consistent effects of antibiotics on plasma concentrations of synthetic steroids. The metabolism of hormonal contraceptives may be influenced by various drugs. Of potential clinical importance are drugs that interrupt entero-hepatic recirculation of estrogen (eg, certain antibiotics). Literature suggests possible interactions with the concomitant use of hormonal contraceptives and ampicillin or tetracycline).
No products indexed under this heading.

Ketoconazole (CYP3A4 inhibitors, such as ketoconazole, may increase plasma hormone levels). Products include:

Extina 3319
Xolegel 3337

Ketoprofen (Although norelgestromin and its metabolites inhibit a variety of P450 enzymes in human liver microsomes, the clinical consequence of such an interaction on the levels of other concomitant medications is likely to be insignificant. Under the recommended dosing regimen, the *in vivo* concentrations of norelgestromin and its metabolites, even at the peak serum levels, are relatively low compared to the inhibitory constant (Ki) (based on results of *in vitro* studies)).
No products indexed under this heading.

Ketorolac Tromethamine (Although norelgestromin and its metabolites inhibit a variety of P450 enzymes in human liver microsomes, the clinical consequence of such an interaction on the levels of other concomitant medications is likely to be insignificant. Under the recommended dosing regimen, the *in vivo* concentrations of norelgestromin and its metabolites, even at the peak serum levels, are relatively low compared to the inhibitory constant (Ki) (based on results of *in vitro* studies)). Products include:

Acuvail .... ⊙209

Labetalol Hydrochloride (Although norelgestromin and its metabolites inhibit a variety of P450 enzymes in human liver microsomes, the clinical consequence of such an interaction on the levels of other concomitant medications is likely to be insignificant. Under the recommended dosing regimen, the *in vivo* concentrations of norelgestromin and its metabolites, even at the peak serum levels, are relatively low compared to the inhibitory constant (Ki) (based on results of *in vitro* studies)).
No products indexed under this heading.

Lamotrigine (Combined hormonal contraceptives have been shown to significantly decrease plasma concentrations of lamotrigine when co-administered likely due to induction of lamotrigine glucuronidation. This may reduce seizure control; therefore, dosage adjustments of lamotrigine may be necessary). Products include:

Lamictal 1522
Lamictal ODT 1522
Lamictal XR 1536

Lansoprazole (If a woman on hormonal contraceptives takes a drug or herbal product that induces enzymes, including CYP3A4, that metabolize contraceptive hormones, counsel her to use additional contraception or a different method of contraception. Drugs or herbal products that induce such enzymes may decrease the plasma concentrations of contraceptive hormones, and may decrease the effectiveness of hormonal contraceptives or increase breakthrough bleeding).
No products indexed under this heading.

Lapatinib (CYP3A4 inhibitors, such as itraconazole or ketoconazole, may increase plasma hormone levels). Products include:

Tykerb 1698

Levetiracetam (Although norelgestromin and its metabolites inhibit a variety of P450 enzymes in human liver microsomes, the clinical consequence of such an interaction on the levels of other concomitant medications is likely to be insignificant. Under the recommended dosing regimen, the *in vivo* concentrations of norelgestromin and its metabolites, even at the peak serum levels, are relatively low compared to the inhibitory constant (Ki) (based on results of *in vitro* studies)). Products include:

Keppra XR 3434

Levobupivacaine Hydrochloride (Although norelgestromin and its metabolites inhibit a variety of P450 enzymes in human liver microsomes, the clinical consequence of such an interaction on the levels of other concomitant medications is likely to be insignificant. Under the recommended dosing regimen, the *in vivo* concentrations of norelgestromin and its metabolites, even at the peak serum levels, are relatively low compared to the inhibitory constant (Ki) (based on results of *in vitro* studies)).
No products indexed under this heading.

Levofloxacin (There have been reports of pregnancy while taking hormonal contraceptives and antibiotics, but clinical pharmacokinetic studies have not shown consistent effects of antibiotics on plasma concentrations of synthetic steroids. The metabolism of hormonal contraceptives may be influenced by various drugs. Of potential clinical importance are drugs that interrupt entero-hepatic recirculation of estrogen (eg, certain antibiotics). Literature suggests possible interactions with the concomitant use of hormonal contraceptives and ampicillin or tetracycline). Products include:

Iquix 3492
Levaquin 2629
Levaquin in 5% Dextrose 2629
Quixin 3493

Levonorgestrel (Although norelgestromin and its metabolites inhibit a variety of P450 enzymes in human liver microsomes, the clinical consequence of such an interaction on the levels of other concomitant medications is likely to be insignificant. Under the recommended dosing regimen, the *in vivo* concentrations of norelgestromin and its metabolites, even at the peak serum levels, are relatively low compared to the inhibitory constant (Ki) (based on results of *in vitro* studies)). Products include:

Climara Pro 847
LoSeasonique 3407
Lybrel 3514
Mirena 854
Plan B 3416
Seasonique 3418

Lidocaine (Although norelgestromin and its metabolites inhibit a variety of P450 enzymes in human liver microsomes, the clinical consequence of such an interaction on the levels of other concomitant medications is likely to be insignificant. Under the recommended dosing regimen, the *in vivo* concentrations of norelgestromin and its metabolites, even at the peak serum levels, are relatively low compared to the inhibitory constant (Ki) (based on results of *in vitro* studies)). Products include:

Lidoderm 1107

Lidocaine Base (Although norelgestromin and its metabolites inhibit a variety of P450 enzymes in human liver microsomes, the clinical consequence of such an interaction on the levels of other concomitant medications is likely to be insignificant. Under the recommended dosing regimen, the *in vivo* concentrations of norelgestromin and its metabolites, even at the peak serum levels, are relatively low compared to the inhibitory constant (Ki) (based on results of *in vitro* studies)).
No products indexed under this heading.

Lidocaine Hydrochloride (Although norelgestromin and its metabolites inhibit a variety of P450 enzymes in human liver microsomes, the clinical consequence of such an interaction on the levels of other concomitant medications is likely to be insignificant. Under the recommended dosing regimen, the *in vivo* concentrations of norelgestromin and its metabolites, even at the peak serum levels, are relatively low compared to the inhibitory constant (Ki) (based on results of *in vitro* studies)).
No products indexed under this heading.

Lomefloxacin Hydrochloride (There have been reports of pregnancy while taking hormonal contraceptives and antibiotics, but clinical pharmacokinetic studies have not shown consistent effects of antibiotics on plasma concentrations of synthetic steroids. The metabolism of hormonal contraceptives may be influenced by various drugs. Of potential clinical importance are drugs that interrupt entero-hepatic recirculation of estrogen (eg, certain antibiotics). Literature suggests possible interactions with the concomitant use of hormonal contraceptives and ampicillin or tetracycline).
No products indexed under this heading.

Lopinavir (Significant changes (increase or decrease) in the plasma levels of the estrogen and progestin have been noted in some cases of co-administration of HIV protease inhibitors). Products include:

Kaletra 458

Loracarbef (There have been reports of pregnancy while taking hormonal contraceptives and antibiotics, but clinical pharmacokinetic studies have not

1319 Interactions Index Ortho Evra

shown consistent effects of antibiotics on plasma concentrations of synthetic steroids. The metabolism of hormonal contraceptives may be influenced by various drugs. Of potential clinical importance are drugs that interrupt entero-hepatic recirculation of estrogen (eg, certain antibiotics). Literature suggests possible interactions with the concomitant use of hormonal contraceptives and ampicillin or tetracycline).
No products indexed under this heading.

Loratadine (CYP3A4 inhibitors, such as itraconazole or ketoconazole, may increase plasma hormone levels).
No products indexed under this heading.

Losartan Potassium (Although norelgestromin and its metabolites inhibit a variety of P450 enzymes in human liver microsomes, the clinical consequence of such an interaction on the levels of other concomitant medications is likely to be insignificant. Under the recommended dosing regimen, the *in vivo* concentrations of norelgestromin and its metabolites, even at the peak serum levels, are relatively low compared to the inhibitory constant (Ki) (based on results of *in vitro* studies)). Products include:
Cozaar 2106
Hyzaar 2162
Hyzaar 100-12.5 2162

Lovastatin (Although norelgestromin and its metabolites inhibit a variety of P450 enzymes in human liver microsomes, the clinical consequence of such an interaction on the levels of other concomitant medications is likely to be insignificant. Under the recommended dosing regimen, the *in vivo* concentrations of norelgestromin and its metabolites, even at the peak serum levels, are relatively low compared to the inhibitory constant (Ki) (based on results of *in vitro* studies)). Products include:
Advicor 402
Mevacor 2212

Maprotiline Hydrochloride (Although norelgestromin and its metabolites inhibit a variety of P450 enzymes in human liver microsomes, the clinical consequence of such an interaction on the levels of other concomitant medications is likely to be insignificant. Under the recommended dosing regimen, the *in vivo* concentrations of norelgestromin and its metabolites, even at the peak serum levels, are relatively low compared to the inhibitory constant (Ki) (based on results of *in vitro* studies)).
No products indexed under this heading.

Meclofenamate Sodium (Although norelgestromin and its metabolites inhibit a variety of P450 enzymes in human liver microsomes, the clinical consequence of such an interaction on the levels of other concomitant medications is likely to be insignificant. Under the recommended dosing regimen, the *in vivo* concentrations of norelgestromin and its metabolites, even at the peak serum levels, are relatively low compared to the inhibitory constant (Ki) (based on results of *in vitro* studies)).
No products indexed under this heading.

Mefenamic Acid (Although norelgestromin and its metabolites inhibit a variety of P450 enzymes in human liver microsomes, the clinical consequence of such an interaction on the levels of other concomitant medications is likely to be insignificant. Under the recommended dosing regimen, the *in vivo* concentrations of norelgestromin and its metabolites, even at the peak serum levels, are relatively low compared to the inhibitory constant (Ki) (based on results of *in vitro* studies)).
No products indexed under this heading.

Meloxicam (Although norelgestromin and its metabolites inhibit a variety of P450 enzymes in human liver microsomes, the clinical consequence of such an interaction on the levels of other concomitant medications is likely to be insignificant. Under the recommended dosing regimen, the *in vivo* concentrations of norelgestromin and its metabolites, even at the peak serum levels, are relatively low compared to the inhibitory constant (Ki) (based on results of *in vitro* studies)).
No products indexed under this heading.

Meperidine Hydrochloride (Although norelgestromin and its metabolites inhibit a variety of P450 enzymes in human liver microsomes, the clinical consequence of such an interaction on the levels of other concomitant medications is likely to be insignificant. Under the recommended dosing regimen, the *in vivo* concentrations of norelgestromin and its metabolites, even at the peak serum levels, are relatively low compared to the inhibitory constant (Ki) (based on results of *in vitro* studies)).
No products indexed under this heading.

Mephenytoin (If a woman on hormonal contraceptives takes a drug or herbal product that induces enzymes, including CYP3A4, that metabolize contraceptive hormones, counsel her to use additional contraception or a different method of contraception. Drugs or herbal products that induce such enzymes may decrease the plasma concentrations of contraceptive hormones, and may decrease the effectiveness of hormonal contraceptives or increase breakthrough bleeding).
No products indexed under this heading.

Mephobarbital (Concomitant use with barbiturates may decrease the plasma concentrations of hormonal contraceptives, and may decrease the effectiveness of hormonal contraceptives or increase breakthrough bleeding. Patients who are concomitantly using barbiturates should be counseled to use additional contraception or a different method of contraception).
No products indexed under this heading.

Meprobamate (Although norelgestromin and its metabolites inhibit a variety of P450 enzymes in human liver microsomes, the clinical consequence of such an interaction on the levels of other concomitant medications is likely to be insignificant. Under the recommended dosing regimen, the *in vivo* concentrations of norelgestromin and its metabolites, even at the peak serum levels, are relatively low compared to the inhibitory constant (Ki) (based on results of *in vitro* studies)).
No products indexed under this heading.

Mestranol (Although norelgestromin and its metabolites inhibit a variety of P450 enzymes in human liver microsomes, the clinical consequence of such an interaction on the levels of other concomitant medications is likely to be insignificant. Under the recommended dosing regimen, the *in vivo* concentrations of norelgestromin and its metabolites, even at the peak serum levels, are relatively low compared to the inhibitory constant (Ki) (based on results of *in vitro* studies)).
No products indexed under this heading.

Metformin Hydrochloride (Although norelgestromin and its metabolites inhibit a variety of P450 enzymes in human liver microsomes, the clinical consequence of such an interaction on the levels of other concomitant medications is likely to be insignificant. Under the recommended dosing regimen, the *in vivo* concentrations of norelgestromin and its metabolites, even at the peak serum levels, are relatively low compared to the inhibitory constant (Ki) (based on results of *in vitro* studies)). Products include:
ActoPlus 3338
Avandamet 1345
Janumet 2188

Methacycline Hydrochloride (There have been reports of pregnancy while taking hormonal contraceptives and antibiotics, but clinical pharmacokinetic studies have not shown consistent effects of antibiotics on plasma concentrations of synthetic steroids. The metabolism of hormonal contraceptives may be influenced by various drugs. Of potential clinical importance are drugs that interrupt entero-hepatic recirculation of estrogen (eg, certain antibiotics). Literature suggests possible interactions with the concomitant use of hormonal contraceptives and ampicillin or tetracycline).
No products indexed under this heading.

Methadone Hydrochloride (Although norelgestromin and its metabolites inhibit a variety of P450 enzymes in human liver microsomes, the clinical consequence of such an interaction on the levels of other concomitant medications is likely to be insignificant. Under the recommended dosing regimen, the *in vivo* concentrations of norelgestromin and its metabolites, even at the peak serum levels, are relatively low compared to the inhibitory constant (Ki) (based on results of *in vitro* studies)).
No products indexed under this heading.

Methamphetamine Hydrochloride (Although norelgestromin and its metabolites inhibit a variety of P450 enzymes in human liver microsomes, the clinical consequence of such an interaction on the levels of other concomitant medications is likely to be insignificant. Under the recommended dosing regimen, the *in vivo* concentrations of norelgestromin and its metabolites, even at the peak serum levels, are relatively low compared to the inhibitory constant (Ki) (based on results of *in vitro* studies)).
No products indexed under this heading.

Methicillin Sodium (There have been reports of pregnancy while taking hormonal contraceptives and antibiotics, but clinical pharmacokinetic studies have not shown consistent effects of antibiotics on plasma concentrations of synthetic steroids. The metabolism of hormonal contraceptives may be influenced by various drugs. Of potential clinical importance are drugs that interrupt entero-hepatic recirculation of estrogen (eg, certain antibiotics). Literature suggests possible interactions with the concomitant use of hormonal contraceptives and ampicillin or tetracycline).
No products indexed under this heading.

Methsuximide (If a woman on hormonal contraceptives takes a drug or herbal product that induces enzymes, including CYP3A4, that metabolize contraceptive hormones, counsel her to use additional contraception or a different method of contraception. Drugs or herbal products that induce such enzymes may decrease the plasma concentrations of contraceptive hormones, and may decrease the effectiveness of hormonal contraceptives or increase breakthrough bleeding).
No products indexed under this heading.

Methylprednisolone (If a woman on hormonal contraceptives takes a drug or herbal product that induces enzymes, including CYP3A4, that metabolize contraceptive hormones, counsel her to use additional contraception or a different method of contraception. Drugs or herbal products that induce such enzymes may decrease the plasma concentrations of contraceptive hormones, and may decrease the effectiveness of hormonal contraceptives or increase breakthrough bleeding).
No products indexed under this heading.

Methylprednisolone Acetate (If a woman on hormonal contraceptives takes a drug or herbal product that induces enzymes, including CYP3A4, that metabolize contraceptive hormones, counsel her to use additional contraception or a different method of contraception. Drugs or herbal products that induce such enzymes may decrease the plasma concentrations of contraceptive hormones, and may decrease the effectiveness of hormonal contraceptives or increase breakthrough bleeding).
No products indexed under this heading.

Methylprednisolone Sodium Succinate (If a woman on hormonal contraceptives takes a drug or herbal product that induces enzymes, including CYP3A4, that metabolize contraceptive hormones, counsel her to use additional contraception or a different method of contraception. Drugs or herbal products that induce such enzymes may decrease the plasma concentrations of contraceptive hormones, and may decrease the effectiveness of hormonal contraceptives or increase breakthrough bleeding).
No products indexed under this heading.

Metoprolol Succinate (Although norelgestromin and its metabolites inhibit a variety of P450 enzymes in human liver microsomes, the clinical consequence of such an interaction on the levels of other concomitant medications is likely to be insignificant. Under the recommended dosing regimen, the *in vivo* concentrations of norelgestromin and its metabolites, even at the peak serum levels, are relatively low compared to the inhibitory constant (Ki) (based on results of *in vitro* studies)). Products include:
Toprol XL 732

Metoprolol Tartrate (Although norelgestromin and its metabolites inhibit a variety of P450 enzymes in human liver microsomes, the clinical consequence of such an interaction on the levels of other concomitant medications is likely to be insignificant. Under the recommended dosing regimen, the *in vivo* concentrations of norelgestromin and its metabolites, even at the peak serum levels, are relatively low compared to the inhibitory constant (Ki) (based on results of *in vitro* studies)).
No products indexed under this heading.

Metronidazole (CYP3A4 inhibitors, such as itraconazole or ketoconazole, may increase plasma hormone levels). Products include:
Pylera 793

Metronidazole Benzoate (CYP3A4 inhibitors, such as itraconazole or ketoconazole, may increase plasma hormone levels).
No products indexed under this heading.

Metronidazole Hydrochloride (CYP3A4 inhibitors, such as itraconazole or ketoconazole, may increase plasma hormone levels).
No products indexed under this heading.

Metronidazole Sodium (CYP3A4 inhibitors, such as itraconazole or ketoconazole, may increase plasma hormone levels).
No products indexed under this heading.

Mexiletine Hydrochloride (Although norelgestromin and its metabolites inhibit a variety of P450 enzymes in human liver microsomes, the clinical consequence of such an interaction on the levels of other concomitant medications is likely to be insignificant. Under the recommended dosing regimen, the *in vivo* concentrations of norelgestromin and its metabolites, even at the peak

IMPORTANT NOTE: Always consult each drug listing in the patient's regimen for possible interactions.

(⊙ Described in PDR® for Ophthalmic Medicines)

1321 Interactions Index Ortho Evra

Nifedipine (CYP3A4 inhibitors, such as itraconazole or ketoconazole, may increase plasma hormone levels).
No products indexed under this heading.

Nilutamide (Although norelgestromin and its metabolites inhibit a variety of P450 enzymes in human liver microsomes, the clinical consequence of such an interaction on the levels of other concomitant medications is likely to be insignificant. Under the recommended dosing regimen, the *in vivo* concentrations of norelgestromin and its metabolites, even at the peak serum levels, are relatively low compared to the inhibitory constant (Ki) (based on results of *in vitro* studies)).
No products indexed under this heading.

Nimodipine (Although norelgestromin and its metabolites inhibit a variety of P450 enzymes in human liver microsomes, the clinical consequence of such an interaction on the levels of other concomitant medications is likely to be insignificant. Under the recommended dosing regimen, the *in vivo* concentrations of norelgestromin and its metabolites, even at the peak serum levels, are relatively low compared to the inhibitory constant (Ki) (based on results of *in vitro* studies)).
No products indexed under this heading.

Nisoldipine (Although norelgestromin and its metabolites inhibit a variety of P450 enzymes in human liver microsomes, the clinical consequence of such an interaction on the levels of other concomitant medications is likely to be insignificant. Under the recommended dosing regimen, the *in vivo* concentrations of norelgestromin and its metabolites, even at the peak serum levels, are relatively low compared to the inhibitory constant (Ki) (based on results of *in vitro* studies)).
No products indexed under this heading.

Nitrendipine (Although norelgestromin and its metabolites inhibit a variety of P450 enzymes in human liver microsomes, the clinical consequence of such an interaction on the levels of other concomitant medications is likely to be insignificant. Under the recommended dosing regimen, the *in vivo* concentrations of norelgestromin and its metabolites, even at the peak serum levels, are relatively low compared to the inhibitory constant (Ki) (based on results of *in vitro* studies)).
No products indexed under this heading.

Norethindrone (If a woman on hormonal contraceptives takes a drug or herbal product that induces enzymes, including CYP3A4, that metabolize contraceptive hormones, counsel her to use additional contraception or a different method of contraception. Drugs or herbal products that induce such enzymes may decrease the plasma concentrations of contraceptive hormones, and may decrease the effectiveness of hormonal contraceptives or increase breakthrough bleeding). Products include:
Ortho Micronor 2660

Norethindrone Acetate (If a woman on hormonal contraceptives takes a drug or herbal product that induces enzymes, including CYP3A4, that metabolize contraceptive hormones, counsel her to use additional contraception or a different method of contraception. Drugs or herbal products that induce such enzymes may decrease the plasma concentrations of contraceptive hormones, and may decrease the effectiveness of hormonal contraceptives or increase breakthrough bleeding).
Products include:
Activella 2561

Norfloxacin (CYP3A4 inhibitors, such as itraconazole or ketoconazole, may increase plasma hormone levels).
Products include:
Noroxin 2220

Norgestrel (Although norelgestromin and its metabolites inhibit a variety of P450 enzymes in human liver microsomes, the clinical consequence of such an interaction on the levels of other concomitant medications is likely to be insignificant. Under the recommended dosing regimen, the *in vivo* concentrations of norelgestromin and its metabolites, even at the peak serum levels, are relatively low compared to the inhibitory constant (Ki) (based on results of *in vitro* studies)).
No products indexed under this heading.

Nortriptyline Hydrochloride (Although norelgestromin and its metabolites inhibit a variety of P450 enzymes in human liver microsomes, the clinical consequence of such an interaction on the levels of other concomitant medications is likely to be insignificant. Under the recommended dosing regimen, the *in vivo* concentrations of norelgestromin and its metabolites, even at the peak serum levels, are relatively low compared to the inhibitory constant (Ki) (based on results of *in vitro* studies)).
No products indexed under this heading.

Ofloxacin (There have been reports of pregnancy while taking hormonal contraceptives and antibiotics, but clinical pharmacokinetic studies have not shown consistent effects of antibiotics on plasma concentrations of synthetic steroids. The metabolism of hormonal contraceptives may be influenced by various drugs. Of potential clinical importance are drugs that interrupt entero-hepatic recirculation of estrogen (eg, certain antibiotics). Literature suggests possible interactions with the concomitant use of hormonal contraceptives and ampicillin or tetracycline).
No products indexed under this heading.

Olanzapine (Although norelgestromin and its metabolites inhibit a variety of P450 enzymes in human liver microsomes, the clinical consequence of such an interaction on the levels of other concomitant medications is likely to be insignificant. Under the recommended dosing regimen, the *in vivo* concentrations of norelgestromin and its metabolites, even at the peak serum levels, are relatively low compared to the inhibitory constant (Ki) (based on results of *in vitro* studies)). Products include:
Symbyax 1965
Zyprexa 1984
Zyprexa IntraMuscular 1984
Zyprexa ZYDIS 1984

Omeprazole (If a woman on hormonal contraceptives takes a drug or herbal product that induces enzymes, including CYP3A4, that metabolize contraceptive hormones, counsel her to use additional contraception or a different method of contraception. Drugs or herbal products that induce such enzymes may decrease the plasma concentrations of contraceptive hormones, and may decrease the effectiveness of hormonal contraceptives or increase breakthrough bleeding).
No products indexed under this heading.

Omeprazole Magnesium (If a woman on hormonal contraceptives takes a drug or herbal product that induces enzymes, including CYP3A4, that metabolize contraceptive hormones, counsel her to use additional contraception or a different method of contraception. Drugs or herbal products that induce such enzymes may decrease the plasma concentrations of contraceptive hormones, and may decrease the effectiveness of hormonal contraceptives or increase breakthrough bleeding).
No products indexed under this heading.

Ondansetron (Although norelgestromin and its metabolites inhibit a variety of P450 enzymes in human liver microsomes, the clinical consequence of such an interaction on the levels of other concomitant medications is likely to be insignificant. Under the recommended dosing regimen, the *in vivo* concentrations of norelgestromin and its metabolites, even at the peak serum levels, are relatively low compared to the inhibitory constant (Ki) (based on results of *in vitro* studies)).
No products indexed under this heading.

Ondansetron Hydrochloride (Although norelgestromin and its metabolites inhibit a variety of P450 enzymes in human liver microsomes, the clinical consequence of such an interaction on the levels of other concomitant medications is likely to be insignificant. Under the recommended dosing regimen, the *in vivo* concentrations of norelgestromin and its metabolites, even at the peak serum levels, are relatively low compared to the inhibitory constant (Ki) (based on results of *in vitro* studies)).
Products include:
Zofran Injection 1750
Zofran 1756
Zofran ODT 1756

Oxacillin (There have been reports of pregnancy while taking hormonal contraceptives and antibiotics, but clinical pharmacokinetic studies have not shown consistent effects of antibiotics on plasma concentrations of synthetic steroids. The metabolism of hormonal contraceptives may be influenced by various drugs. Of potential clinical importance are drugs that interrupt entero-hepatic recirculation of estrogen (eg, certain antibiotics). Literature suggests possible interactions with the concomitant use of hormonal contraceptives and ampicillin or tetracycline).
No products indexed under this heading.

Oxacillin Sodium (There have been reports of pregnancy while taking hormonal contraceptives and antibiotics, but clinical pharmacokinetic studies have not shown consistent effects of antibiotics on plasma concentrations of synthetic steroids. The metabolism of hormonal contraceptives may be influenced by various drugs. Of potential clinical importance are drugs that interrupt entero-hepatic recirculation of estrogen (eg, certain antibiotics). Literature suggests possible interactions with the concomitant use of hormonal contraceptives and ampicillin or tetracycline).
No products indexed under this heading.

Oxaprozin (Although norelgestromin and its metabolites inhibit a variety of P450 enzymes in human liver microsomes, the clinical consequence of such an interaction on the levels of other concomitant medications is likely to be insignificant. Under the recommended dosing regimen, the *in vivo* concentrations of norelgestromin and its metabolites, even at the peak serum levels, are relatively low compared to the inhibitory constant (Ki) (based on results of *in vitro* studies)).
No products indexed under this heading.

Oxcarbazepine (Concomitant use with oxcarbazepine may decrease the plasma concentrations of hormonal contraceptives, and may decrease the effectiveness of hormonal contraceptives or increase breakthrough bleeding. Patients who are concomitantly using oxcarbazepine, should be counseled to use additional contraception or a different method of contraception).
No products indexed under this heading.

Oxycodone Hydrochloride (Although norelgestromin and its metabolites inhibit a variety of P450 enzymes in human liver microsomes, the clinical consequence of such an interaction on the levels of other concomitant medications is likely to be insignificant. Under the recommended dosing regimen, the *in vivo* concentrations of norelgestromin and its metabolites, even at the peak serum levels, are relatively low compared to the inhibitory constant (Ki) (based on results of *in vitro* studies)).
Products include:
OxyContin 2807
Percocet 1121
Percodan 1124

Oxytetracycline (There have been reports of pregnancy while taking hormonal contraceptives and antibiotics, but clinical pharmacokinetic studies have not shown consistent effects of antibiotics on plasma concentrations of synthetic steroids. The metabolism of hormonal contraceptives may be influenced by various drugs. Of potential clinical importance are drugs that interrupt entero-hepatic recirculation of estrogen (eg, certain antibiotics). Literature suggests possible interactions with the concomitant use of hormonal contraceptives and ampicillin or tetracycline).
No products indexed under this heading.

Oxytetracycline Hydrochloride (There have been reports of pregnancy while taking hormonal contraceptives and antibiotics, but clinical pharmacokinetic studies have not shown consistent effects of antibiotics on plasma concentrations of synthetic steroids. The metabolism of hormonal contraceptives may be influenced by various drugs. Of potential clinical importance are drugs that interrupt entero-hepatic recirculation of estrogen (eg, certain antibiotics). Literature suggests possible interactions with the concomitant use of hormonal contraceptives and ampicillin or tetracycline).
No products indexed under this heading.

Paclitaxel (Although norelgestromin and its metabolites inhibit a variety of P450 enzymes in human liver microsomes, the clinical consequence of such an interaction on the levels of other concomitant medications is likely to be insignificant. Under the recommended dosing regimen, the *in vivo* concentrations of norelgestromin and its metabolites, even at the peak serum levels, are relatively low compared to the inhibitory constant (Ki) (based on results of *in vitro* studies)).
No products indexed under this heading.

Pantoprazole Sodium (Although norelgestromin and its metabolites inhibit a variety of P450 enzymes in human liver microsomes, the clinical consequence of such an interaction on the levels of other concomitant medications is likely to be insignificant. Under the recommended dosing regimen, the *in vivo* concentrations of norelgestromin and its metabolites, even at the peak serum levels, are relatively low compared to the inhibitory constant (Ki) (based on results of *in vitro* studies)).
Products include:
Protonix Tablets 3571
Protonix 3575

Paramethadione (Although norelgestromin and its metabolites inhibit a variety of P450 enzymes in human liver microsomes, the clinical consequence of such an interaction on the levels of other concomitant medications is likely to be insignificant. Under the recommended dosing regimen, the *in vivo* concentrations of norelgestromin and its metabolites, even at the peak serum

IMPORTANT NOTE: Always consult each drug listing in the patient's regimen for possible interactions.

levels, are relatively low compared to the inhibitory constant (Ki) (based on results of *in vitro* studies)).
No products indexed under this heading.

Paroxetine Hydrochloride (CYP3A4 inhibitors, such as itraconazole or ketoconazole, may increase plasma hormone levels). Products include:
Paroxetine CR **2361**
Paroxetine ER **2371**
Paxil **1586**
Paxil CR **1596**

Penicillin, Potassium Phenoxymethyl (There have been reports of pregnancy while taking hormonal contraceptives and antibiotics, but clinical pharmacokinetic studies have not shown consistent effects of antibiotics on plasma concentrations of synthetic steroids. The metabolism of hormonal contraceptives may be influenced by various drugs. Of potential clinical importance are drugs that interrupt entero-hepatic recirculation of estrogen (eg, certain antibiotics). Literature suggests possible interactions with the concomitant use of hormonal contraceptives and ampicillin or tetracycline).
No products indexed under this heading.

Penicillin G Benzathine (There have been reports of pregnancy while taking hormonal contraceptives and antibiotics, but clinical pharmacokinetic studies have not shown consistent effects of antibiotics on plasma concentrations of synthetic steroids. The metabolism of hormonal contraceptives may be influenced by various drugs. Of potential clinical importance are drugs that interrupt entero-hepatic recirculation of estrogen (eg, certain antibiotics). Literature suggests possible interactions with the concomitant use of hormonal contraceptives and ampicillin or tetracycline). Products include:
Bicillin C-R Injectable Suspension **1826**
Bicillin L-A **1828**

Penicillin G Dibenzylethyenediamine (There have been reports of pregnancy while taking hormonal contraceptives and antibiotics, but clinical pharmacokinetic studies have not shown consistent effects of antibiotics on plasma concentrations of synthetic steroids. The metabolism of hormonal contraceptives may be influenced by various drugs. Of potential clinical importance are drugs that interrupt entero-hepatic recirculation of estrogen (eg, certain antibiotics). Literature suggests possible interactions with the concomitant use of hormonal contraceptives and ampicillin or tetracycline).
No products indexed under this heading.

Penicillin G Potassium (There have been reports of pregnancy while taking hormonal contraceptives and antibiotics, but clinical pharmacokinetic studies have not shown consistent effects of antibiotics on plasma concentrations of synthetic steroids. The metabolism of hormonal contraceptives may be influenced by various drugs. Of potential clinical importance are drugs that interrupt entero-hepatic recirculation of estrogen (eg, certain antibiotics). Literature suggests possible interactions with the concomitant use of hormonal contraceptives and ampicillin or tetracycline).
No products indexed under this heading.

Penicillin G Procaine (There have been reports of pregnancy while taking hormonal contraceptives and antibiotics, but clinical pharmacokinetic studies have not shown consistent effects of antibiotics on plasma concentrations of synthetic steroids. The metabolism of hormonal contraceptives may be influenced by various drugs. Of potential clinical importance are drugs that interrupt entero-hepatic recirculation of estrogen (eg, certain antibiotics). Literature suggests possible interactions with the concomitant use of hormonal contraceptives and ampicillin or tetracycline). Products include:
Bicillin C-R Injectable Suspension **1826**
Bicillin L-A **1828**

Penicillin G Sodium (There have been reports of pregnancy while taking hormonal contraceptives and antibiotics, but clinical pharmacokinetic studies have not shown consistent effects of antibiotics on plasma concentrations of synthetic steroids. The metabolism of hormonal contraceptives may be influenced by various drugs. Of potential clinical importance are drugs that interrupt entero-hepatic recirculation of estrogen (eg, certain antibiotics). Literature suggests possible interactions with the concomitant use of hormonal contraceptives and ampicillin or tetracycline).
No products indexed under this heading.

Penicillin V (There have been reports of pregnancy while taking hormonal contraceptives and antibiotics, but clinical pharmacokinetic studies have not shown consistent effects of antibiotics on plasma concentrations of synthetic steroids. The metabolism of hormonal contraceptives may be influenced by various drugs. Of potential clinical importance are drugs that interrupt entero-hepatic recirculation of estrogen (eg, certain antibiotics). Literature suggests possible interactions with the concomitant use of hormonal contraceptives and ampicillin or tetracycline).
No products indexed under this heading.

Penicillin V Potassium (There have been reports of pregnancy while taking hormonal contraceptives and antibiotics, but clinical pharmacokinetic studies have not shown consistent effects of antibiotics on plasma concentrations of synthetic steroids. The metabolism of hormonal contraceptives may be influenced by various drugs. Of potential clinical importance are drugs that interrupt entero-hepatic recirculation of estrogen (eg, certain antibiotics). Literature suggests possible interactions with the concomitant use of hormonal contraceptives and ampicillin or tetracycline).
No products indexed under this heading.

Penicillins (There have been reports of pregnancy while taking hormonal contraceptives and antibiotics, but clinical pharmacokinetic studies have not shown consistent effects of antibiotics on plasma concentrations of synthetic steroids. The metabolism of hormonal contraceptives may be influenced by various drugs. Of potential clinical importance are drugs that interrupt entero-hepatic recirculation of estrogen (eg, certain antibiotics). Literature suggests possible interactions with the concomitant use of hormonal contraceptives and ampicillin or tetracycline).
No products indexed under this heading.

Pentamidine Isethionate (Although norelgestromin and its metabolites inhibit a variety of P450 enzymes in human liver microsomes, the clinical consequence of such an interaction on the levels of other concomitant medications is likely to be insignificant. Under the recommended dosing regimen, the *in vivo* concentrations of norelgestromin and its metabolites, even at the peak serum levels, are relatively low compared to the inhibitory constant (Ki) (based on results of *in vitro* studies)).
No products indexed under this heading.

Pentobarbital (Concomitant use with barbiturates may decrease the plasma concentrations of hormonal contraceptives, and may decrease the effectiveness of hormonal contraceptives or increase breakthrough bleeding. Patients who are concomitantly using barbiturates should be counseled to use additional contraception or a different method of contraception).
No products indexed under this heading.

Pentobarbital Sodium (Concomitant use with barbiturates may decrease the plasma concentrations of hormonal contraceptives, and may decrease the effectiveness of hormonal contraceptives or increase breakthrough bleeding. Patients who are concomitantly using barbiturates should be counseled to use additional contraception or a different method of contraception). Products include:
Nembutal **2012**

Phenacemide (Although norelgestromin and its metabolites inhibit a variety of P450 enzymes in human liver microsomes, the clinical consequence of such an interaction on the levels of other concomitant medications is likely to be insignificant. Under the recommended dosing regimen, the *in vivo* concentrations of norelgestromin and its metabolites, even at the peak serum levels, are relatively low compared to the inhibitory constant (Ki) (based on results of *in vitro* studies)).
No products indexed under this heading.

Phenobarbital (Concomitant use with barbiturates may decrease the plasma concentrations of hormonal contraceptives, and may decrease the effectiveness of hormonal contraceptives or increase breakthrough bleeding. Patients who are concomitantly using barbiturates should be counseled to use additional contraception or a different method of contraception). Products include:
Donnatal **2711**

Phenobarbital Sodium (Concomitant use with barbiturates may decrease the plasma concentrations of hormonal contraceptives, and may decrease the effectiveness of hormonal contraceptives or increase breakthrough bleeding. Patients who are concomitantly using barbiturates should be counseled to use additional contraception or a different method of contraception).
No products indexed under this heading.

Phensuximide (Although norelgestromin and its metabolites inhibit a variety of P450 enzymes in human liver microsomes, the clinical consequence of such an interaction on the levels of other concomitant medications is likely to be insignificant. Under the recommended dosing regimen, the *in vivo* concentrations of norelgestromin and its metabolites, even at the peak serum levels, are relatively low compared to the inhibitory constant (Ki) (based on results of *in vitro* studies)).
No products indexed under this heading.

Phenylbutazone (If a woman on hormonal contraceptives takes a drug or herbal product that induces enzymes, including CYP3A4, that metabolize contraceptive hormones, counsel her to use additional contraception or a different method of contraception. Drugs or herbal products that induce such enzymes may decrease the plasma concentrations of contraceptive hormones, and may decrease the effectiveness of hormonal contraceptives or increase breakthrough bleeding).
No products indexed under this heading.

Phenytoin (Concomitant use with phenytoin may decrease the plasma concentrations of hormonal contraceptives, and may decrease the effectiveness of hormonal contraceptives or increase breakthrough bleeding. Patients who are concomitantly using phenytoin should be counseled to use additional contraception or a different method of contraception).
No products indexed under this heading.

Phenytoin Sodium (Concomitant use with phenytoin may decrease the plasma concentrations of hormonal contraceptives, and may decrease the effectiveness of hormonal contraceptives or increase breakthrough bleeding. Patients who are concomitantly using phenytoin should be counseled to use additional contraception or a different method of contraception). Products include:
Phenytek Capsules **2380**

Pimozide (Although norelgestromin and its metabolites inhibit a variety of P450 enzymes in human liver microsomes, the clinical consequence of such an interaction on the levels of other concomitant medications is likely to be insignificant. Under the recommended dosing regimen, the *in vivo* concentrations of norelgestromin and its metabolites, even at the peak serum levels, are relatively low compared to the inhibitory constant (Ki) (based on results of *in vitro* studies)).
No products indexed under this heading.

Pindolol (Although norelgestromin and its metabolites inhibit a variety of P450 enzymes in human liver microsomes, the clinical consequence of such an interaction on the levels of other concomitant medications is likely to be insignificant. Under the recommended dosing regimen, the *in vivo* concentrations of norelgestromin and its metabolites, even at the peak serum levels, are relatively low compared to the inhibitory constant (Ki) (based on results of *in vitro* studies)).
No products indexed under this heading.

Pioglitazone Hydrochloride (Although norelgestromin and its metabolites inhibit a variety of P450 enzymes in human liver microsomes, the clinical consequence of such an interaction on the levels of other concomitant medications is likely to be insignificant. Under the recommended dosing regimen, the *in vivo* concentrations of norelgestromin and its metabolites, even at the peak serum levels, are relatively low compared to the inhibitory constant (Ki) (based on results of *in vitro* studies)). Products include:
ActoPlus **3338**
Actos **3345**
Duetact **3354**

Piperacillin Sodium (There have been reports of pregnancy while taking hormonal contraceptives and antibiotics, but clinical pharmacokinetic studies have not shown consistent effects of antibiotics on plasma concentrations of synthetic steroids. The metabolism of hormonal contraceptives may be influenced by various drugs. Of potential clinical importance are drugs that interrupt entero-hepatic recirculation of estrogen (eg, certain antibiotics). Literature suggests possible interactions with the concomitant use of hormonal contraceptives and ampicillin or tetracycline). Products include:
Zosyn **3607**

Piroxicam (Although norelgestromin and its metabolites inhibit a variety of P450 enzymes in human liver microsomes, the clinical consequence of such an interaction on the levels of other concomitant medications is likely to be insignificant. Under the recommended dosing regimen, the *in vivo*

concentrations of norelgestromin and its metabolites, even at the peak serum levels, are relatively low compared to the inhibitory constant (Ki) (based on results of *in vitro* studies)).
No products indexed under this heading.

Polyestradiol Phosphate (Although norelgestromin and its metabolites inhibit a variety of P450 enzymes in human liver microsomes, the clinical consequence of such an interaction on the levels of other concomitant medications is likely to be insignificant. Under the recommended dosing regimen, the *in vivo* concentrations of norelgestromin and its metabolites, even at the peak serum levels, are relatively low compared to the inhibitory constant (Ki) (based on results of *in vitro* studies)).
No products indexed under this heading.

Posaconazole (CYP3A4 inhibitors, such as itraconazole or ketoconazole, may increase plasma hormone levels).
Products include:
Noxafil 3172

Prednisolone (If a woman on hormonal contraceptives takes a drug or herbal product that induces enzymes, including CYP3A4, that metabolize contraceptive hormones, counsel her to use additional contraception or a different method of contraception. Drugs or herbal products that induce such enzymes may decrease the plasma concentrations of contraceptive hormones, and may decrease the effectiveness of hormonal contraceptives or increase breakthrough bleeding).
No products indexed under this heading.

Prednisolone Acetate (If a woman on hormonal contraceptives takes a drug or herbal product that induces enzymes, including CYP3A4, that metabolize contraceptive hormones, counsel her to use additional contraception or a different method of contraception. Drugs or herbal products that induce such enzymes may decrease the plasma concentrations of contraceptive hormones, and may decrease the effectiveness of hormonal contraceptives or increase breakthrough bleeding).
Products include:
Blephamide .... ⊙212, ⊙214
Pred Forte .... ⊙225
Pred Mild .... ⊙230
Pred-G .... ⊙226, ⊙227

Prednisolone Sodium Phosphate (If a woman on hormonal contraceptives takes a drug or herbal product that induces enzymes, including CYP3A4, that metabolize contraceptive hormones, counsel her to use additional contraception or a different method of contraception. Drugs or herbal products that induce such enzymes may decrease the plasma concentrations of contraceptive hormones, and may decrease the effectiveness of hormonal contraceptives or increase breakthrough bleeding).
No products indexed under this heading.

Prednisolone Tebutate (If a woman on hormonal contraceptives takes a drug or herbal product that induces enzymes, including CYP3A4, that metabolize contraceptive hormones, counsel her to use additional contraception or a different method of contraception. Drugs or herbal products that induce such enzymes may decrease the plasma concentrations of contraceptive hormones, and may decrease the effectiveness of hormonal contraceptives or increase breakthrough bleeding).
No products indexed under this heading.

Prednisone (If a woman on hormonal contraceptives takes a drug or herbal product that induces enzymes, including CYP3A4, that metabolize contraceptive hormones, counsel her to use additional contraception or a different method of contraception. Drugs or herbal products that induce such enzymes may decrease the plasma concentrations of contraceptive hormones, and may decrease the effectiveness of hormonal contraceptives or increase breakthrough bleeding).
No products indexed under this heading.

Prednisone sodium phosphate (If a woman on hormonal contraceptives takes a drug or herbal product that induces enzymes, including CYP3A4, that metabolize contraceptive hormones, counsel her to use additional contraception or a different method of contraception. Drugs or herbal products that induce such enzymes may decrease the plasma concentrations of contraceptive hormones, and may decrease the effectiveness of hormonal contraceptives or increase breakthrough bleeding).
No products indexed under this heading.

Primidone (If a woman on hormonal contraceptives takes a drug or herbal product that induces enzymes, including CYP3A4, that metabolize contraceptive hormones, counsel her to use additional contraception or a different method of contraception. Drugs or herbal products that induce such enzymes may decrease the plasma concentrations of contraceptive hormones, and may decrease the effectiveness of hormonal contraceptives or increase breakthrough bleeding).
No products indexed under this heading.

Progesterone (Although norelgestromin and its metabolites inhibit a variety of P450 enzymes in human liver microsomes, the clinical consequence of such an interaction on the levels of other concomitant medications is likely to be insignificant. Under the recommended dosing regimen, the *in vivo* concentrations of norelgestromin and its metabolites, even at the peak serum levels, are relatively low compared to the inhibitory constant (Ki) (based on results of *in vitro* studies)). Products include:
Crinone 4% 996
Crinone 8% 996
Prometrium 3307

Proguanil Hydrochloride (Although norelgestromin and its metabolites inhibit a variety of P450 enzymes in human liver microsomes, the clinical consequence of such an interaction on the levels of other concomitant medications is likely to be insignificant. Under the recommended dosing regimen, the *in vivo* concentrations of norelgestromin and its metabolites, even at the peak serum levels, are relatively low compared to the inhibitory constant (Ki) (based on results of *in vitro* studies)).
Products include:
Malarone Pediatric Tablets 1572
Malarone 1572

Propafenone Hydrochloride (Although norelgestromin and its metabolites inhibit a variety of P450 enzymes in human liver microsomes, the clinical consequence of such an interaction on the levels of other concomitant medications is likely to be insignificant. Under the recommended dosing regimen, the *in vivo* concentrations of norelgestromin and its metabolites, even at the peak serum levels, are relatively low compared to the inhibitory constant (Ki) (based on results of *in vitro* studies)).
Products include:
Rythmol 1648
Rythmol SR 1652

Propoxyphene Hydrochloride (CYP3A4 inhibitors, such as itraconazole or ketoconazole, may increase plasma hormone levels).
No products indexed under this heading.

Propoxyphene Napsylate (CYP3A4 inhibitors, such as itraconazole or ketoconazole, may increase plasma hormone levels).
No products indexed under this heading.

Propranolol Hydrochloride (Although norelgestromin and its metabolites inhibit a variety of P450 enzymes in human liver microsomes, the clinical consequence of such an interaction on the levels of other concomitant medications is likely to be insignificant. Under the recommended dosing regimen, the *in vivo* concentrations of norelgestromin and its metabolites, even at the peak serum levels, are relatively low compared to the inhibitory constant (Ki) (based on results of *in vitro* studies)).
Products include:
InnoPran XL 1517

Protriptyline Hydrochloride (Although norelgestromin and its metabolites inhibit a variety of P450 enzymes in human liver microsomes, the clinical consequence of such an interaction on the levels of other concomitant medications is likely to be insignificant. Under the recommended dosing regimen, the *in vivo* concentrations of norelgestromin and its metabolites, even at the peak serum levels, are relatively low compared to the inhibitory constant (Ki) (based on results of *in vitro* studies)).
No products indexed under this heading.

Quetiapine Fumarate (Although norelgestromin and its metabolites inhibit a variety of P450 enzymes in human liver microsomes, the clinical consequence of such an interaction on the levels of other concomitant medications is likely to be insignificant. Under the recommended dosing regimen, the *in vivo* concentrations of norelgestromin and its metabolites, even at the peak serum levels, are relatively low compared to the inhibitory constant (Ki) (based on results of *in vitro* studies)).
Products include:
Seroquel 750
Seroquel XR 759

Quinidine (CYP3A4 inhibitors, such as itraconazole or ketoconazole, may increase plasma hormone levels).
No products indexed under this heading.

Quinidine Gluconate (Although norelgestromin and its metabolites inhibit a variety of P450 enzymes in human liver microsomes, the clinical consequence of such an interaction on the levels of other concomitant medications is likely to be insignificant. Under the recommended dosing regimen, the *in vivo* concentrations of norelgestromin and its metabolites, even at the peak serum levels, are relatively low compared to the inhibitory constant (Ki) (based on results of *in vitro* studies)).
No products indexed under this heading.

Quinidine Hydrochloride (CYP3A4 inhibitors, such as itraconazole or ketoconazole, may increase plasma hormone levels).
No products indexed under this heading.

Quinidine Polygalacturonate (CYP3A4 inhibitors, such as itraconazole or ketoconazole, may increase plasma hormone levels).
No products indexed under this heading.

Quinidine Sulfate (CYP3A4 inhibitors, such as itraconazole or ketoconazole, may increase plasma hormone levels).
No products indexed under this heading.

Quinine (CYP3A4 inhibitors, such as itraconazole or ketoconazole, may increase plasma hormone levels).
Products include:
Hyland's Leg Cramps PM with Quinine 3315

Quinine Sulfate (CYP3A4 inhibitors, such as itraconazole or ketoconazole, may increase plasma hormone levels).
No products indexed under this heading.

Quinupristin (CYP3A4 inhibitors, such as itraconazole or ketoconazole, may increase plasma hormone levels).
No products indexed under this heading.

Rabeprazole Sodium (Although norelgestromin and its metabolites inhibit a variety of P450 enzymes in human liver microsomes, the clinical consequence of such an interaction on the levels of other concomitant medications is likely to be insignificant. Under the recommended dosing regimen, the *in vivo* concentrations of norelgestromin and its metabolites, even at the peak serum levels, are relatively low compared to the inhibitory constant (Ki) (based on results of *in vitro* studies)).
Products include:
Aciphex 1035

Ranitidine Bismuth Citrate (CYP3A4 inhibitors, such as itraconazole or ketoconazole, may increase plasma hormone levels).
No products indexed under this heading.

Ranitidine Hydrochloride (CYP3A4 inhibitors, such as itraconazole or ketoconazole, may increase plasma hormone levels). Products include:
Zantac 1737
Zantac Injection 1732
Zantac Pharmacy 1735

Repaglinide (Although norelgestromin and its metabolites inhibit a variety of P450 enzymes in human liver microsomes, the clinical consequence of such an interaction on the levels of other concomitant medications is likely to be insignificant. Under the recommended dosing regimen, the *in vivo* concentrations of norelgestromin and its metabolites, even at the peak serum levels, are relatively low compared to the inhibitory constant (Ki) (based on results of *in vitro* studies)).
No products indexed under this heading.

Rifabutin (If a woman on hormonal contraceptives takes a drug or herbal product that induces enzymes, including CYP3A4, that metabolize contraceptive hormones, counsel her to use additional contraception or a different method of contraception. Drugs or herbal products that induce such enzymes may decrease the plasma concentrations of contraceptive hormones, and may decrease the effectiveness of hormonal contraceptives or increase breakthrough bleeding).
No products indexed under this heading.

Rifampicin (If a woman on hormonal contraceptives takes a drug or herbal product that induces enzymes, including CYP3A4, that metabolize contraceptive hormones, counsel her to use additional contraception or a different method of contraception. Drugs or herbal products that induce such enzymes may decrease the plasma concentrations of contraceptive hormones, and may decrease the effectiveness of hormonal contraceptives or increase breakthrough bleeding).
No products indexed under this heading.

Rifampin (Concomitant use with rifampin may decrease the plasma concentrations of hormonal contraceptives, and may decrease the effectiveness of hormonal contraceptives or increase breakthrough bleeding. Patients who are concomitantly using rifampin should be counseled to use additional contraception or a different method of contraception).
No products indexed under this heading.

Rifapentine (If a woman on hormonal contraceptives takes a drug or herbal product that induces enzymes, including CYP3A4, that metabolize contraceptive hormones, counsel her to use additional contraception or a different method of contraception. Drugs or herbal products that induce such

IMPORTANT NOTE: Always consult each drug listing in the patient's regimen for possible interactions.

enzymes may decrease the plasma concentrations of contraceptive hormones, and may decrease the effectiveness of hormonal contraceptives or increase breakthrough bleeding).

No products indexed under this heading.

Riluzole (Although norelgestromin and its metabolites inhibit a variety of P450 enzymes in human liver microsomes, the clinical consequence of such an interaction on the levels of other concomitant medications is likely to be insignificant. Under the recommended dosing regimen, the *in vivo* concentrations of norelgestromin and its metabolites, even at the peak serum levels, are relatively low compared to the inhibitory constant (Ki) (based on results of *in vitro* studies). Products include:

Rilutek 3032

Risperidone (Although norelgestromin and its metabolites inhibit a variety of P450 enzymes in human liver microsomes, the clinical consequence of such an interaction on the levels of other concomitant medications is likely to be insignificant. Under the recommended dosing regimen, the *in vivo* concentrations of norelgestromin and its metabolites, even at the peak serum levels, are relatively low compared to the inhibitory constant (Ki) (based on results of *in vitro* studies). Products include:

Risperdal Consta 2682

Ritonavir (If a woman on hormonal contraceptives takes a drug or herbal product that induces enzymes, including CYP3A4, that metabolize contraceptive hormones, counsel her to use additional contraception or a different method of contraception. Drugs or herbal products that induce such enzymes may decrease the plasma concentrations of contraceptive hormones, and may decrease the effectiveness of hormonal contraceptives or increase breakthrough bleeding). Products include:

Kaletra 458
Norvir 509

Rofecoxib (Although norelgestromin and its metabolites inhibit a variety of P450 enzymes in human liver microsomes, the clinical consequence of such an interaction on the levels of other concomitant medications is likely to be insignificant. Under the recommended dosing regimen, the *in vivo* concentrations of norelgestromin and its metabolites, even at the peak serum levels, are relatively low compared to the inhibitory constant (Ki) (based on results of *in vitro* studies).

No products indexed under this heading.

Ropinirole Hydrochloride (Although norelgestromin and its metabolites inhibit a variety of P450 enzymes in human liver microsomes, the clinical consequence of such an interaction on the levels of other concomitant medications is likely to be insignificant. Under the recommended dosing regimen, the *in vivo* concentrations of norelgestromin and its metabolites, even at the peak serum levels, are relatively low compared to the inhibitory constant (Ki) (based on results of *in vitro* studies). Products include:

Requip 1620
Requip XL 1628

Ropivacaine Hydrochloride (Although norelgestromin and its metabolites inhibit a variety of P450 enzymes in human liver microsomes, the clinical consequence of such an interaction on the levels of other concomitant medications is likely to be insignificant. Under the recommended dosing regimen, the *in vivo* concentrations of norelgestromin and its metabolites, even at the peak

serum levels, are relatively low compared to the inhibitory constant (Ki) (based on results of *in vitro* studies).

No products indexed under this heading.

Rosiglitazone (Although norelgestromin and its metabolites inhibit a variety of P450 enzymes in human liver microsomes, the clinical consequence of such an interaction on the levels of other concomitant medications is likely to be insignificant. Under the recommended dosing regimen, the *in vivo* concentrations of norelgestromin and its metabolites, even at the peak serum levels, are relatively low compared to the inhibitory constant (Ki) (based on results of *in vitro* studies).

No products indexed under this heading.

Rosiglitazone Maleate (Although norelgestromin and its metabolites inhibit a variety of P450 enzymes in human liver microsomes, the clinical consequence of such an interaction on the levels of other concomitant medications is likely to be insignificant. Under the recommended dosing regimen, the *in vivo* concentrations of norelgestromin and its metabolites, even at the peak serum levels, are relatively low compared to the inhibitory constant (Ki) (based on results of *in vitro* studies). Products include:

Avandamet 1345
Avandaryl 1356
Avandia 1366

Rosiglitazone/Metformin (Although norelgestromin and its metabolites inhibit a variety of P450 enzymes in human liver microsomes, the clinical consequence of such an interaction on the levels of other concomitant medications is likely to be insignificant. Under the recommended dosing regimen, the *in vivo* concentrations of norelgestromin and its metabolites, even at the peak serum levels, are relatively low compared to the inhibitory constant (Ki) (based on results of *in vitro* studies).

No products indexed under this heading.

Salicylic Acid (Increased clearance of salicylic acid has been noted when concomitantly administered with oral contraceptives).

No products indexed under this heading.

Saquinavir (Significant changes (increase or decrease) in the plasma levels of the estrogen and progestin have been noted in some cases of co-administration of HIV protease inhibitors).

No products indexed under this heading.

Saquinavir Mesylate (Significant changes (increase or decrease) in the plasma levels of the estrogen and progestin have been noted in some cases of co-administration of HIV protease inhibitors).

No products indexed under this heading.

Secobarbital Sodium (Concomitant use with barbiturates may decrease the plasma concentrations of hormonal contraceptives, and may decrease the effectiveness of hormonal contraceptives or increase breakthrough bleeding. Patients who are concomitantly using barbiturates should be counseled to use additional contraception or a different method of contraception).

No products indexed under this heading.

Sertraline Hydrochloride (CYP3A4 inhibitors, such as itraconazole or ketoconazole, may increase plasma hormone levels).

No products indexed under this heading.

Sildenafil Citrate (CYP3A4 inhibitors, such as itraconazole or ketoconazole, may increase plasma hormone levels).

No products indexed under this heading.

Simvastatin (Although norelgestromin and its metabolites inhibit a variety of P450 enzymes in human liver

microsomes, the clinical consequence of such an interaction on the levels of other concomitant medications is likely to be insignificant. Under the recommended dosing regimen, the *in vivo* concentrations of norelgestromin and its metabolites, even at the peak serum levels, are relatively low compared to the inhibitory constant (Ki) (based on results of *in vitro* studies)). Products include:

Simcor 524
Vytorin 10/10 .... 2303, 3240
Vytorin 10/20 .... 2303, 3240
Vytorin 10/40 .... 2303, 3240
Vytorin 10/80 .... 2303, 3240
Zocor 2289

Sirolimus (Although norelgestromin and its metabolites inhibit a variety of P450 enzymes in human liver microsomes, the clinical consequence of such an interaction on the levels of other concomitant medications is likely to be insignificant. Under the recommended dosing regimen, the *in vivo* concentrations of norelgestromin and its metabolites, even at the peak serum levels, are relatively low compared to the inhibitory constant (Ki) (based on results of *in vitro* studies)). Products include:

Rapamune 3579

Sodium Butabarbital (Concomitant use with barbiturates may decrease the plasma concentrations of hormonal contraceptives, and may decrease the effectiveness of hormonal contraceptives or increase breakthrough bleeding. Patients who are concomitantly using barbiturates should be counseled to use additional contraception or a different method of contraception).

No products indexed under this heading.

Sodium Cloxacillin Monohydrate (There have been reports of pregnancy while taking hormonal contraceptives and antibiotics, but clinical pharmacokinetic studies have not shown consistent effects of antibiotics on plasma concentrations of synthetic steroids. The metabolism of hormonal contraceptives may be influenced by various drugs. Of potential clinical importance are drugs that interrupt entero-hepatic recirculation of estrogen (eg, certain antibiotics). Literature suggests possible interactions with the concomitant use of hormonal contraceptives and ampicillin or tetracycline).

No products indexed under this heading.

Sodium Pentobarbital (Concomitant use with barbiturates may decrease the plasma concentrations of hormonal contraceptives, and may decrease the effectiveness of hormonal contraceptives or increase breakthrough bleeding. Patients who are concomitantly using barbiturates should be counseled to use additional contraception or a different method of contraception).

No products indexed under this heading.

Sparfloxacin (There have been reports of pregnancy while taking hormonal contraceptives and antibiotics, but clinical pharmacokinetic studies have not shown consistent effects of antibiotics on plasma concentrations of synthetic steroids. The metabolism of hormonal contraceptives may be influenced by various drugs. Of potential clinical importance are drugs that interrupt entero-hepatic recirculation of estrogen (eg, certain antibiotics). Literature suggests possible interactions with the concomitant use of hormonal contraceptives and ampicillin or tetracycline).

No products indexed under this heading.

Streptomycin Sulfate (There have been reports of pregnancy while taking hormonal contraceptives and antibiotics, but clinical pharmacokinetic studies have not shown consistent effects of

antibiotics on plasma concentrations of synthetic steroids. The metabolism of hormonal contraceptives may be influenced by various drugs. Of potential clinical importance are drugs that interrupt entero-hepatic recirculation of estrogen (eg, certain antibiotics). Literature suggests possible interactions with the concomitant use of hormonal contraceptives and ampicillin or tetracycline).

No products indexed under this heading.

Sulfamethizole (There have been reports of pregnancy while taking hormonal contraceptives and antibiotics, but clinical pharmacokinetic studies have not shown consistent effects of antibiotics on plasma concentrations of synthetic steroids. The metabolism of hormonal contraceptives may be influenced by various drugs. Of potential clinical importance are drugs that interrupt entero-hepatic recirculation of estrogen (eg, certain antibiotics). Literature suggests possible interactions with the concomitant use of hormonal contraceptives and ampicillin or tetracycline).

No products indexed under this heading.

Sulfamethoxazole (There have been reports of pregnancy while taking hormonal contraceptives and antibiotics, but clinical pharmacokinetic studies have not shown consistent effects of antibiotics on plasma concentrations of synthetic steroids. The metabolism of hormonal contraceptives may be influenced by various drugs. Of potential clinical importance are drugs that interrupt entero-hepatic recirculation of estrogen (eg, certain antibiotics). Literature suggests possible interactions with the concomitant use of hormonal contraceptives and ampicillin or tetracycline).

No products indexed under this heading.

Sulfinpyrazone (If a woman on hormonal contraceptives takes a drug or herbal product that induces enzymes, including CYP3A4, that metabolize contraceptive hormones, counsel her to use additional contraception or a different method of contraception. Drugs or herbal products that induce such enzymes may decrease the plasma concentrations of contraceptive hormones, and may decrease the effectiveness of hormonal contraceptives or increase breakthrough bleeding).

No products indexed under this heading.

Sulfisoxazole Acetyl (There have been reports of pregnancy while taking hormonal contraceptives and antibiotics, but clinical pharmacokinetic studies have not shown consistent effects of antibiotics on plasma concentrations of synthetic steroids. The metabolism of hormonal contraceptives may be influenced by various drugs. Of potential clinical importance are drugs that interrupt entero-hepatic recirculation of estrogen (eg, certain antibiotics). Literature suggests possible interactions with the concomitant use of hormonal contraceptives and ampicillin or tetracycline).

No products indexed under this heading.

Sulfisoxazole Diolamine (There have been reports of pregnancy while taking hormonal contraceptives and antibiotics, but clinical pharmacokinetic studies have not shown consistent effects of antibiotics on plasma concentrations of synthetic steroids. The metabolism of hormonal contraceptives may be influenced by various drugs. Of potential clinical importance are drugs that interrupt entero-hepatic recirculation of estrogen (eg, certain antibiotics). Literature suggests possible interac-

1325 Interactions Index Ortho Evra

tions with the concomitant use of hormonal contraceptives and ampicillin or tetracycline).
No products indexed under this heading.

Sulindac (Although norelgestromin and its metabolites inhibit a variety of P450 enzymes in human liver microsomes, the clinical consequence of such an interaction on the levels of other concomitant medications is likely to be insignificant. Under the recommended dosing regimen, the *in vivo* concentrations of norelgestromin and its metabolites, even at the peak serum levels, are relatively low compared to the inhibitory constant (Ki) (based on results of *in vitro* studies)). Products include:
Clinoril **2098**

Suprofen (Although norelgestromin and its metabolites inhibit a variety of P450 enzymes in human liver microsomes, the clinical consequence of such an interaction on the levels of other concomitant medications is likely to be insignificant. Under the recommended dosing regimen, the *in vivo* concentrations of norelgestromin and its metabolites, even at the peak serum levels, are relatively low compared to the inhibitory constant (Ki) (based on results of *in vitro* studies)).
No products indexed under this heading.

Tacrine Hydrochloride (Although norelgestromin and its metabolites inhibit a variety of P450 enzymes in human liver microsomes, the clinical consequence of such an interaction on the levels of other concomitant medications is likely to be insignificant. Under the recommended dosing regimen, the *in vivo* concentrations of norelgestromin and its metabolites, even at the peak serum levels, are relatively low compared to the inhibitory constant (Ki) (based on results of *in vitro* studies)).
No products indexed under this heading.

Tacrolimus (Although norelgestromin and its metabolites inhibit a variety of P450 enzymes in human liver microsomes, the clinical consequence of such an interaction on the levels of other concomitant medications is likely to be insignificant. Under the recommended dosing regimen, the *in vivo* concentrations of norelgestromin and its metabolites, even at the peak serum levels, are relatively low compared to the inhibitory constant (Ki) (based on results of *in vitro* studies)). Products include:
Prograf Capsules **677**
Prograf Injection **677**
Protopic **685**

Tadalafil (Although norelgestromin and its metabolites inhibit a variety of P450 enzymes in human liver microsomes, the clinical consequence of such an interaction on the levels of other concomitant medications is likely to be insignificant. Under the recommended dosing regimen, the *in vivo* concentrations of norelgestromin and its metabolites, even at the peak serum levels, are relatively low compared to the inhibitory constant (Ki) (based on results of *in vitro* studies)). Products include:
Adcirca **3461**
Cialis **1861**

Tamoxifen Citrate (Although norelgestromin and its metabolites inhibit a variety of P450 enzymes in human liver microsomes, the clinical consequence of such an interaction on the levels of other concomitant medications is likely to be insignificant. Under the recommended dosing regimen, the *in vivo* concentrations of norelgestromin and its metabolites, even at the peak serum levels, are relatively low compared to the inhibitory constant (Ki) (based on results of *in vitro* studies)).
No products indexed under this heading.

Telithromycin (CYP3A4 inhibitors, such as itraconazole or ketoconazole, may increase plasma hormone levels). Products include:
Ketek **2991**

Telmisartan (Although norelgestromin and its metabolites inhibit a variety of P450 enzymes in human liver microsomes, the clinical consequence of such an interaction on the levels of other concomitant medications is likely to be insignificant. Under the recommended dosing regimen, the *in vivo* concentrations of norelgestromin and its metabolites, even at the peak serum levels, are relatively low compared to the inhibitory constant (Ki) (based on results of *in vitro* studies)). Products include:
Micardis **887**
Micardis HCT **889**

Temazepam (Increased clearance of temazepam has been noted when administered concomitantly with oral contraceptives).
No products indexed under this heading.

Teniposide (Although norelgestromin and its metabolites inhibit a variety of P450 enzymes in human liver microsomes, the clinical consequence of such an interaction on the levels of other concomitant medications is likely to be insignificant. Under the recommended dosing regimen, the *in vivo* concentrations of norelgestromin and its metabolites, even at the peak serum levels, are relatively low compared to the inhibitory constant (Ki) (based on results of *in vitro* studies)).
No products indexed under this heading.

Terfenadine (Although norelgestromin and its metabolites inhibit a variety of P450 enzymes in human liver microsomes, the clinical consequence of such an interaction on the levels of other concomitant medications is likely to be insignificant. Under the recommended dosing regimen, the *in vivo* concentrations of norelgestromin and its metabolites, even at the peak serum levels, are relatively low compared to the inhibitory constant (Ki) (based on results of *in vitro* studies)).
No products indexed under this heading.

Testosterone (Although norelgestromin and its metabolites inhibit a variety of P450 enzymes in human liver microsomes, the clinical consequence of such an interaction on the levels of other concomitant medications is likely to be insignificant. Under the recommended dosing regimen, the *in vivo* concentrations of norelgestromin and its metabolites, even at the peak serum levels, are relatively low compared to the inhibitory constant (Ki) (based on results of *in vitro* studies)). Products include:
AndroGel **3456**

Testosterone Cypionate (Although norelgestromin and its metabolites inhibit a variety of P450 enzymes in human liver microsomes, the clinical consequence of such an interaction on the levels of other concomitant medications is likely to be insignificant. Under the recommended dosing regimen, the *in vivo* concentrations of norelgestromin and its metabolites, even at the peak serum levels, are relatively low compared to the inhibitory constant (Ki) (based on results of *in vitro* studies)).
No products indexed under this heading.

Testosterone Enanthate (Although norelgestromin and its metabolites inhibit a variety of P450 enzymes in human liver microsomes, the clinical consequence of such an interaction on the levels of other concomitant medications is likely to be insignificant. Under the recommended dosing regimen, the *in vivo* concentrations of norelgestromin and its metabolites, even at the peak serum levels, are relatively low compared to the inhibitory constant (Ki) (based on results of *in vitro* studies)). Products include:
Delatestryl **1102**

Testosterone Propionate (Although norelgestromin and its metabolites inhibit a variety of P450 enzymes in human liver microsomes, the clinical consequence of such an interaction on the levels of other concomitant medications is likely to be insignificant. Under the recommended dosing regimen, the *in vivo* concentrations of norelgestromin and its metabolites, even at the peak serum levels, are relatively low compared to the inhibitory constant (Ki) (based on results of *in vitro* studies)).
No products indexed under this heading.

Tetracycline Hydrochloride (There have been reports of pregnancy while taking hormonal contraceptives and antibiotics, but clinical pharmacokinetic studies have not shown consistent effects of antibiotics on plasma concentrations of synthetic steroids. The metabolism of hormonal contraceptives may be influenced by various drugs. Of potential clinical importance are drugs that interrupt entero-hepatic recirculation of estrogen (eg, certain antibiotics). Literature suggests possible interactions with the concomitant use of hormonal contraceptives and ampicillin or tetracycline). Products include:
Pylera **793**

Tetracycline Phosphate Complex (There have been reports of pregnancy while taking hormonal contraceptives and antibiotics, but clinical pharmacokinetic studies have not shown consistent effects of antibiotics on plasma concentrations of synthetic steroids. The metabolism of hormonal contraceptives may be influenced by various drugs. Of potential clinical importance are drugs that interrupt entero-hepatic recirculation of estrogen (eg, certain antibiotics). Literature suggests possible interactions with the concomitant use of hormonal contraceptives and ampicillin or tetracycline).
No products indexed under this heading.

Theophyllinate (If a woman on hormonal contraceptives takes a drug or herbal product that induces enzymes, including CYP3A4, that metabolize contraceptive hormones, counsel her to use additional contraception or a different method of contraception. Drugs or herbal products that induce such enzymes may decrease the plasma concentrations of contraceptive hormones, and may decrease the effectiveness of hormonal contraceptives or increase breakthrough bleeding).
No products indexed under this heading.

Theophylline (If a woman on hormonal contraceptives takes a drug or herbal product that induces enzymes, including CYP3A4, that metabolize contraceptive hormones, counsel her to use additional contraception or a different method of contraception. Drugs or herbal products that induce such enzymes may decrease the plasma concentrations of contraceptive hormones, and may decrease the effectiveness of hormonal contraceptives or increase breakthrough bleeding).
No products indexed under this heading.

Theophylline Anhydrous (If a woman on hormonal contraceptives takes a drug or herbal product that induces enzymes, including CYP3A4, that metabolize contraceptive hormones, counsel her to use additional contraception or a different method of contraception. Drugs or herbal products that induce such enzymes may decrease the plasma concentrations of contraceptive hormones, and may decrease the effectiveness of hormonal contraceptives or increase breakthrough bleeding). Products include:
Uniphyl **2817**

Theophylline Calcium Salicylate (If a woman on hormonal contraceptives takes a drug or herbal product that induces enzymes, including CYP3A4, that metabolize contraceptive hormones, counsel her to use additional contraception or a different method of contraception. Drugs or herbal products that induce such enzymes may decrease the plasma concentrations of contraceptive hormones, and may decrease the effectiveness of hormonal contraceptives or increase breakthrough bleeding).
No products indexed under this heading.

Theophylline Dihydroxypropyl (Glyceryl) (If a woman on hormonal contraceptives takes a drug or herbal product that induces enzymes, including CYP3A4, that metabolize contraceptive hormones, counsel her to use additional contraception or a different method of contraception. Drugs or herbal products that induce such enzymes may decrease the plasma concentrations of contraceptive hormones, and may decrease the effectiveness of hormonal contraceptives or increase breakthrough bleeding).
No products indexed under this heading.

Theophylline Ethylenediamine (If a woman on hormonal contraceptives takes a drug or herbal product that induces enzymes, including CYP3A4, that metabolize contraceptive hormones, counsel her to use additional contraception or a different method of contraception. Drugs or herbal products that induce such enzymes may decrease the plasma concentrations of contraceptive hormones, and may decrease the effectiveness of hormonal contraceptives or increase breakthrough bleeding).
No products indexed under this heading.

Theophylline Sodium Glycinate (If a woman on hormonal contraceptives takes a drug or herbal product that induces enzymes, including CYP3A4, that metabolize contraceptive hormones, counsel her to use additional contraception or a different method of contraception. Drugs or herbal products that induce such enzymes may decrease the plasma concentrations of contraceptive hormones, and may decrease the effectiveness of hormonal contraceptives or increase breakthrough bleeding).
No products indexed under this heading.

Thiamylal Sodium (Concomitant use with barbiturates may decrease the plasma concentrations of hormonal contraceptives, and may decrease the effectiveness of hormonal contraceptives or increase breakthrough bleeding. Patients who are concomitantly using barbiturates should be counseled to use additional contraception or a different method of contraception).
No products indexed under this heading.

Thioridazine (Although norelgestromin and its metabolites inhibit a variety of P450 enzymes in human liver microsomes, the clinical consequence of such an interaction on the levels of other concomitant medications is likely to be insignificant. Under the recommended dosing regimen, the *in vivo* concentrations of norelgestromin and its metabolites, even at the peak serum levels, are relatively low compared to the inhibitory constant (Ki) (based on results of *in vitro* studies)).
No products indexed under this heading.

Thioridazine Hydrochloride (Although norelgestromin and its metabolites inhibit a variety of P450 enzymes

IMPORTANT NOTE: Always consult each drug listing in the patient's regimen for possible interactions.

Ortho Evra | Interactions Index | 1326

in human liver microsomes, the clinical consequence of such an interaction on the levels of other concomitant medications is likely to be insignificant. Under the recommended dosing regimen, the *in vivo* concentrations of norelgestromin and its metabolites, even at the peak serum levels, are relatively low compared to the inhibitory constant (Ki) (based on results of *in vitro* studies)). Products include:
Thioridazine Hydrochloride 2384

Tiagabine Hydrochloride (Although norelgestromin and its metabolites inhibit a variety of P450 enzymes in human liver microsomes, the clinical consequence of such an interaction on the levels of other concomitant medications is likely to be insignificant. Under the recommended dosing regimen, the *in vivo* concentrations of norelgestromin and its metabolites, even at the peak serum levels, are relatively low compared to the inhibitory constant (Ki) (based on results of *in vitro* studies)). Products include:
Gabitril 972

Ticarcillin Disodium (There have been reports of pregnancy while taking hormonal contraceptives and antibiotics, but clinical pharmacokinetic studies have not shown consistent effects of antibiotics on plasma concentrations of synthetic steroids. The metabolism of hormonal contraceptives may be influenced by various drugs. Of potential clinical importance are drugs that interrupt entero-hepatic recirculation of estrogen (eg, certain antibiotics). Literature suggests possible interactions with the concomitant use of hormonal contraceptives and ampicillin or tetracycline). Products include:
Timentin ADD-Vantage 1670
Timentin Galaxy 1674
Timentin 1666
Timentin Pharmacy 1678

Timolol Maleate (Although norelgestromin and its metabolites inhibit a variety of P450 enzymes in human liver microsomes, the clinical consequence of such an interaction on the levels of other concomitant medications is likely to be insignificant. Under the recommended dosing regimen, the *in vivo* concentrations of norelgestromin and its metabolites, even at the peak serum levels, are relatively low compared to the inhibitory constant (Ki) (based on results of *in vitro* studies)). Products include:
Combigan 601
Dorzolamide Hydrochloride/Timolol Maleate Ophthalmic Solution .... ⊙243
Timoptic in Ocudose .... ⊙231

Tipranavir (Significant changes (increase or decrease) in the plasma levels of the estrogen and progestin have been noted in some cases of co-administration of HIV protease inhibitors).
No products indexed under this heading.

Tobacco (Cigarette smoking increases the risk of serious cardiovascular side effects from hormonal contraceptive use. Women who use hormonal contraceptives, including Ortho Evra, should be strongly advised not to smoke).
No products indexed under this heading.

Tobramycin (There have been reports of pregnancy while taking hormonal contraceptives and antibiotics, but clinical pharmacokinetic studies have not shown consistent effects of antibiotics on plasma concentrations of synthetic steroids. The metabolism of hormonal contraceptives may be influenced by various drugs. Of potential clinical importance are drugs that interrupt entero-hepatic recirculation of estrogen (eg, certain antibiotics). Literature suggests possible interactions with the concomitant use of hormonal contraceptives and ampicillin or tetracycline). Products include:
Tobi Nebulizer 2546
Tobramycin and Dexamethasone Ophthalmic Suspension .... ⊙251
Zylet .... ⊙252

Tobramycin Sulfate (There have been reports of pregnancy while taking hormonal contraceptives and antibiotics, but clinical pharmacokinetic studies have not shown consistent effects of antibiotics on plasma concentrations of synthetic steroids. The metabolism of hormonal contraceptives may be influenced by various drugs. Of potential clinical importance are drugs that interrupt entero-hepatic recirculation of estrogen (eg, certain antibiotics). Literature suggests possible interactions with the concomitant use of hormonal contraceptives and ampicillin or tetracycline).
No products indexed under this heading.

Tolazamide (If a woman on hormonal contraceptives takes a drug or herbal product that induces enzymes, including CYP3A4, that metabolize contraceptive hormones, counsel her to use additional contraception or a different method of contraception. Drugs or herbal products that induce such enzymes may decrease the plasma concentrations of contraceptive hormones, and may decrease the effectiveness of hormonal contraceptives or increase breakthrough bleeding).
No products indexed under this heading.

Tolbutamide (If a woman on hormonal contraceptives takes a drug or herbal product that induces enzymes, including CYP3A4, that metabolize contraceptive hormones, counsel her to use additional contraception or a different method of contraception. Drugs or herbal products that induce such enzymes may decrease the plasma concentrations of contraceptive hormones, and may decrease the effectiveness of hormonal contraceptives or increase breakthrough bleeding).
No products indexed under this heading.

Tolbutamide Sodium (Although norelgestromin and its metabolites inhibit a variety of P450 enzymes in human liver microsomes, the clinical consequence of such an interaction on the levels of other concomitant medications is likely to be insignificant. Under the recommended dosing regimen, the *in vivo* concentrations of norelgestromin and its metabolites, even at the peak serum levels, are relatively low compared to the inhibitory constant (Ki) (based on results of *in vitro* studies)).
No products indexed under this heading.

Tolmetin Sodium (Although norelgestromin and its metabolites inhibit a variety of P450 enzymes in human liver microsomes, the clinical consequence of such an interaction on the levels of other concomitant medications is likely to be insignificant. Under the recommended dosing regimen, the *in vivo* concentrations of norelgestromin and its metabolites, even at the peak serum levels, are relatively low compared to the inhibitory constant (Ki) (based on results of *in vitro* studies)).
No products indexed under this heading.

Tolterodine Tartrate (Although norelgestromin and its metabolites inhibit a variety of P450 enzymes in human liver microsomes, the clinical consequence of such an interaction on the levels of other concomitant medications is likely to be insignificant. Under the recommended dosing regimen, the *in vivo* concentrations of norelgestromin and its metabolites, even at the peak serum levels, are relatively low compared to the inhibitory constant (Ki) (based on results of *in vitro* studies)).
No products indexed under this heading.

Topiramate (Concomitant use with topiramate may decrease the plasma concentrations of hormonal contraceptives, and may decrease the effectiveness of hormonal contraceptives or increase breakthrough bleeding. Patients who are concomitantly using topiramate should be counseled to use additional contraception or a different method of contraception).
No products indexed under this heading.

Torsemide (Although norelgestromin and its metabolites inhibit a variety of P450 enzymes in human liver microsomes, the clinical consequence of such an interaction on the levels of other concomitant medications is likely to be insignificant. Under the recommended dosing regimen, the *in vivo* concentrations of norelgestromin and its metabolites, even at the peak serum levels, are relatively low compared to the inhibitory constant (Ki) (based on results of *in vitro* studies)).
No products indexed under this heading.

Tramadol Hydrochloride (Although norelgestromin and its metabolites inhibit a variety of P450 enzymes in human liver microsomes, the clinical consequence of such an interaction on the levels of other concomitant medications is likely to be insignificant. Under the recommended dosing regimen, the *in vivo* concentrations of norelgestromin and its metabolites, even at the peak serum levels, are relatively low compared to the inhibitory constant (Ki) (based on results of *in vitro* studies)). Products include:
Ryzolt 2813
Ultram ER 2693

Trazodone Hydrochloride (Although norelgestromin and its metabolites inhibit a variety of P450 enzymes in human liver microsomes, the clinical consequence of such an interaction on the levels of other concomitant medications is likely to be insignificant. Under the recommended dosing regimen, the *in vivo* concentrations of norelgestromin and its metabolites, even at the peak serum levels, are relatively low compared to the inhibitory constant (Ki) (based on results of *in vitro* studies)).
No products indexed under this heading.

Tretinoin (Although norelgestromin and its metabolites inhibit a variety of P450 enzymes in human liver microsomes, the clinical consequence of such an interaction on the levels of other concomitant medications is likely to be insignificant. Under the recommended dosing regimen, the *in vivo* concentrations of norelgestromin and its metabolites, even at the peak serum levels, are relatively low compared to the inhibitory constant (Ki) (based on results of *in vitro* studies)).
No products indexed under this heading.

Triamcinolone (If a woman on hormonal contraceptives takes a drug or herbal product that induces enzymes, including CYP3A4, that metabolize contraceptive hormones, counsel her to use additional contraception or a different method of contraception. Drugs or herbal products that induce such enzymes may decrease the plasma concentrations of contraceptive hormones, and may decrease the effectiveness of hormonal contraceptives or increase breakthrough bleeding).
No products indexed under this heading.

Triamcinolone Acetonide (If a woman on hormonal contraceptives takes a drug or herbal product that induces enzymes, including CYP3A4, that metabolize contraceptive hormones, counsel her to use additional contraception or a different method of contraception. Drugs or herbal products that induce such enzymes may decrease the plasma concentrations of contraceptive hormones, and may decrease the effectiveness of hormonal contraceptives or increase breakthrough bleeding). Products include:
Azmacort 408
Nasacort AQ 3019

Triamcinolone Diacetate (If a woman on hormonal contraceptives takes a drug or herbal product that induces enzymes, including CYP3A4, that metabolize contraceptive hormones, counsel her to use additional contraception or a different method of contraception. Drugs or herbal products that induce such enzymes may decrease the plasma concentrations of contraceptive hormones, and may decrease the effectiveness of hormonal contraceptives or increase breakthrough bleeding).
No products indexed under this heading.

Triamcinolone Hexacetonide (If a woman on hormonal contraceptives takes a drug or herbal product that induces enzymes, including CYP3A4, that metabolize contraceptive hormones, counsel her to use additional contraception or a different method of contraception. Drugs or herbal products that induce such enzymes may decrease the plasma concentrations of contraceptive hormones, and may decrease the effectiveness of hormonal contraceptives or increase breakthrough bleeding).
No products indexed under this heading.

Triazolam (Although norelgestromin and its metabolites inhibit a variety of P450 enzymes in human liver microsomes, the clinical consequence of such an interaction on the levels of other concomitant medications is likely to be insignificant. Under the recommended dosing regimen, the *in vivo* concentrations of norelgestromin and its metabolites, even at the peak serum levels, are relatively low compared to the inhibitory constant (Ki) (based on results of *in vitro* studies)).
No products indexed under this heading.

Trimethadione (Although norelgestromin and its metabolites inhibit a variety of P450 enzymes in human liver microsomes, the clinical consequence of such an interaction on the levels of other concomitant medications is likely to be insignificant. Under the recommended dosing regimen, the *in vivo* concentrations of norelgestromin and its metabolites, even at the peak serum levels, are relatively low compared to the inhibitory constant (Ki) (based on results of *in vitro* studies)).
No products indexed under this heading.

Trimethaphan Camsylate (Although norelgestromin and its metabolites inhibit a variety of P450 enzymes in human liver microsomes, the clinical consequence of such an interaction on the levels of other concomitant medications is likely to be insignificant. Under the recommended dosing regimen, the *in vivo* concentrations of norelgestromin and its metabolites, even at the peak serum levels, are relatively low compared to the inhibitory constant (Ki) (based on results of *in vitro* studies)).
No products indexed under this heading.

Trimipramine Maleate (Although norelgestromin and its metabolites inhibit a variety of P450 enzymes in human liver microsomes, the clinical consequence of such an interaction on the levels of other concomitant medications is likely to be insignificant. Under the recommended dosing regimen, the *in vivo* concentrations of norelgestromin and its metabolites, even at the peak

(⊙ Described in PDR® for Ophthalmic Medicines)

serum levels, are relatively low compared to the inhibitory constant (Ki) (based on results of *in vitro* studies)).
No products indexed under this heading.

Troglitazone (If a woman on hormonal contraceptives takes a drug or herbal product that induces enzymes, including CYP3A4, that metabolize contraceptive hormones, counsel her to use additional contraception or a different method of contraception. Drugs or herbal products that induce such enzymes may decrease the plasma concentrations of contraceptive hormones, and may decrease the effectiveness of hormonal contraceptives or increase breakthrough bleeding).
No products indexed under this heading.

Troleandomycin (CYP3A4 inhibitors, such as itraconazole or ketoconazole, may increase plasma hormone levels).
No products indexed under this heading.

Trovafloxacin Mesylate (There have been reports of pregnancy while taking hormonal contraceptives and antibiotics, but clinical pharmacokinetic studies have not shown consistent effects of antibiotics on plasma concentrations of synthetic steroids. The metabolism of hormonal contraceptives may be influenced by various drugs. Of potential clinical importance are drugs that interrupt entero-hepatic recirculation of estrogen (eg, certain antibiotics). Literature suggests possible interactions with the concomitant use of hormonal contraceptives and ampicillin or tetracycline).
No products indexed under this heading.

Valdecoxib (Although norelgestromin and its metabolites inhibit a variety of P450 enzymes in human liver microsomes, the clinical consequence of such an interaction on the levels of other concomitant medications is likely to be insignificant. Under the recommended dosing regimen, the *in vivo* concentrations of norelgestromin and its metabolites, even at the peak serum levels, are relatively low compared to the inhibitory constant (Ki) (based on results of *in vitro* studies)).
No products indexed under this heading.

Valproate Sodium (CYP3A4 inhibitors, such as itraconazole or ketoconazole, may increase plasma hormone levels).
No products indexed under this heading.

Valproic Acid (Although norelgestromin and its metabolites inhibit a variety of P450 enzymes in human liver microsomes, the clinical consequence of such an interaction on the levels of other concomitant medications is likely to be insignificant. Under the recommended dosing regimen, the *in vivo* concentrations of norelgestromin and its metabolites, even at the peak serum levels, are relatively low compared to the inhibitory constant (Ki) (based on results of *in vitro* studies)).
No products indexed under this heading.

Valsartan (Although norelgestromin and its metabolites inhibit a variety of P450 enzymes in human liver microsomes, the clinical consequence of such an interaction on the levels of other concomitant medications is likely to be insignificant. Under the recommended dosing regimen, the *in vivo* concentrations of norelgestromin and its metabolites, even at the peak serum levels, are relatively low compared to the inhibitory constant (Ki) (based on results of *in vitro* studies)). Products include:
Diovan **2413**
Diovan HCT **2419**
Exforge **2443**
Exforge HCT **2449**
Valturna **3637**

Vardenafil Hydrochloride (CYP3A4 inhibitors, such as itraconazole or ketoconazole, may increase plasma hormone levels). Products include:
Levitra **3157**

Venlafaxine Hydrochloride (Although norelgestromin and its metabolites inhibit a variety of P450 enzymes in human liver microsomes, the clinical consequence of such an interaction on the levels of other concomitant medications is likely to be insignificant. Under the recommended dosing regimen, the *in vivo* concentrations of norelgestromin and its metabolites, even at the peak serum levels, are relatively low compared to the inhibitory constant (Ki) (based on results of *in vitro* studies)). Products include:
Effexor XR **3504**
Venlafaxine Hydrochloride Tablets ... **2388**

Verapamil Hydrochloride (CYP3A4 inhibitors, such as itraconazole or ketoconazole, may increase plasma hormone levels). Products include:
Tarka **534**

Vinblastine Sulfate (Although norelgestromin and its metabolites inhibit a variety of P450 enzymes in human liver microsomes, the clinical consequence of such an interaction on the levels of other concomitant medications is likely to be insignificant. Under the recommended dosing regimen, the *in vivo* concentrations of norelgestromin and its metabolites, even at the peak serum levels, are relatively low compared to the inhibitory constant (Ki) (based on results of *in vitro* studies)).
No products indexed under this heading.

Vincristine Sulfate (Although norelgestromin and its metabolites inhibit a variety of P450 enzymes in human liver microsomes, the clinical consequence of such an interaction on the levels of other concomitant medications is likely to be insignificant. Under the recommended dosing regimen, the *in vivo* concentrations of norelgestromin and its metabolites, even at the peak serum levels, are relatively low compared to the inhibitory constant (Ki) (based on results of *in vitro* studies)).
No products indexed under this heading.

Vitamin A (Although norelgestromin and its metabolites inhibit a variety of P450 enzymes in human liver microsomes, the clinical consequence of such an interaction on the levels of other concomitant medications is likely to be insignificant. Under the recommended dosing regimen, the *in vivo* concentrations of norelgestromin and its metabolites, even at the peak serum levels, are relatively low compared to the inhibitory constant (Ki) (based on results of *in vitro* studies)). Products include:
Cardio Basics **3455**
Heplive **607**
Norwegian Cod Liver Oil **919**

Vitamin A Acetate (Although norelgestromin and its metabolites inhibit a variety of P450 enzymes in human liver microsomes, the clinical consequence of such an interaction on the levels of other concomitant medications is likely to be insignificant. Under the recommended dosing regimen, the *in vivo* concentrations of norelgestromin and its metabolites, even at the peak serum levels, are relatively low compared to the inhibitory constant (Ki) (based on results of *in vitro* studies)).
No products indexed under this heading.

Vitamin C (Ascorbic acid may increase plasma ethinyl estradiol levels, possibly by inhibition of conjugation). Products include:
Bausch & Lomb Ocuvite Adult 50+ .... ⊙ **238**
Bio-C **3454**
BoneMate Plus **3454**
Cardio Basics **3455**
CitraNatal 90 DHA Capsules **2332**
CitraNatal Assure **2332**
CitraNatal Rx **2332**
Ferralet **2333**
Heplive **607**
Meili Clear **607**
MoviPrep Oral Solution **2905**
PreNexa **3473**
Proflavanol 90 .... **3476**

Voriconazole (CYP3A4 inhibitors, such as itraconazole or ketoconazole, may increase plasma hormone levels).
No products indexed under this heading.

Warfarin Sodium (Although norelgestromin and its metabolites inhibit a variety of P450 enzymes in human liver microsomes, the clinical consequence of such an interaction on the levels of other concomitant medications is likely to be insignificant. Under the recommended dosing regimen, the *in vivo* concentrations of norelgestromin and its metabolites, even at the peak serum levels, are relatively low compared to the inhibitory constant (Ki) (based on results of *in vitro* studies)).
No products indexed under this heading.

Zafirlukast (CYP3A4 inhibitors, such as itraconazole or ketoconazole, may increase plasma hormone levels). Products include:
Accolate **3612**

Zileuton (CYP3A4 inhibitors, such as itraconazole or ketoconazole, may increase plasma hormone levels).
No products indexed under this heading.

Zolmitriptan (Although norelgestromin and its metabolites inhibit a variety of P450 enzymes in human liver microsomes, the clinical consequence of such an interaction on the levels of other concomitant medications is likely to be insignificant. Under the recommended dosing regimen, the *in vivo* concentrations of norelgestromin and its metabolites, even at the peak serum levels, are relatively low compared to the inhibitory constant (Ki) (based on results of *in vitro* studies)). Products include:
Zomig Tablets **773**
Zomig Nasal Spray **768**
Zomig-ZMT Tablets **773**

Zonisamide (Although norelgestromin and its metabolites inhibit a variety of P450 enzymes in human liver microsomes, the clinical consequence of such an interaction on the levels of other concomitant medications is likely to be insignificant. Under the recommended dosing regimen, the *in vivo* concentrations of norelgestromin and its metabolites, even at the peak serum levels, are relatively low compared to the inhibitory constant (Ki) (based on results of *in vitro* studies)). Products include:
Zonegran **1081**

Zopiclone (Although norelgestromin and its metabolites inhibit a variety of P450 enzymes in human liver microsomes, the clinical consequence of such an interaction on the levels of other concomitant medications is likely to be insignificant. Under the recommended dosing regimen, the *in vivo* concentrations of norelgestromin and its metabolites, even at the peak serum levels, are relatively low compared to the inhibitory constant (Ki) (based on results of *in vitro* studies)).
No products indexed under this heading.

Food Interactions

Beverages, caffeine-containing (Although norelgestromin and its metabolites inhibit a variety of P450 enzymes in human liver microsomes, the clinical consequence of such an interaction on the levels of other concomitant medications is likely to be insignificant. Under the recommended dosing regimen, the *in vivo* concentrations of norelgestromin and its metabolites, even at the peak serum levels, are relatively low compared to the inhibitory constant (Ki) (based on results of *in vitro* studies)).

Broccoli (If a woman on hormonal contraceptives takes a drug or herbal product that induces enzymes, including CYP3A4, that metabolize contraceptive hormones, counsel her to use additional contraception or a different method of contraception. Drugs or herbal products that induce such enzymes may decrease the plasma concentrations of contraceptive hormones, and may decrease the effectiveness of hormonal contraceptives or increase breakthrough bleeding).

Brussel Sprouts (If a woman on hormonal contraceptives takes a drug or herbal product that induces enzymes, including CYP3A4, that metabolize contraceptive hormones, counsel her to use additional contraception or a different method of contraception. Drugs or herbal products that induce such enzymes may decrease the plasma concentrations of contraceptive hormones, and may decrease the effectiveness of hormonal contraceptives or increase breakthrough bleeding).

Charbroiled Food (If a woman on hormonal contraceptives takes a drug or herbal product that induces enzymes, including CYP3A4, that metabolize contraceptive hormones, counsel her to use additional contraception or a different method of contraception. Drugs or herbal products that induce such enzymes may decrease the plasma concentrations of contraceptive hormones, and may decrease the effectiveness of hormonal contraceptives or increase breakthrough bleeding).

Food, caffeine-containing (Although norelgestromin and its metabolites inhibit a variety of P450 enzymes in human liver microsomes, the clinical consequence of such an interaction on the levels of other concomitant medications is likely to be insignificant. Under the recommended dosing regimen, the *in vivo* concentrations of norelgestromin and its metabolites, even at the peak serum levels, are relatively low compared to the inhibitory constant (Ki) (based on results of *in vitro* studies)).

Grapefruit (CYP3A4 inhibitors, such as itraconazole or ketoconazole, may increase plasma hormone levels).

Grapefruit Juice (CYP3A4 inhibitors, such as itraconazole or ketoconazole, may increase plasma hormone levels).

ORTHO MICRONOR TABLETS

(Norethindrone) **2660**
May interact with barbiturates, hepatic microsomal enzyme inducers, phenytoin, and certain other agents. Compounds in these categories include:

Allium sativum (The effectiveness of progestin-only pills is reduced by hepatic enzyme-inducing drugs such as the anticonvulsants phenytoin, carbamazepine, and barbiturates, and the antituberculosis drug rifampin).
No products indexed under this heading.

Aminoglutethimide (The effectiveness of progestin-only pills is reduced by hepatic enzyme-inducing drugs such as the anticonvulsants phenytoin, carbamazepine, and barbiturates, and the antituberculosis drug rifampin).
No products indexed under this heading.

IMPORTANT NOTE: Always consult each drug listing in the patient's regimen for possible interactions.

Amobarbital (The effectiveness of progestin-only pills is reduced by hepatic enzyme-inducing drugs such as the anticonvulsants phenytoin, carbamazepine, and barbiturates).
No products indexed under this heading.

Amobarbital Sodium (The effectiveness of progestin-only pills is reduced by hepatic enzyme-inducing drugs such as the anticonvulsants phenytoin, carbamazepine, and barbiturates).
No products indexed under this heading.

Aprepitant (The effectiveness of progestin-only pills is reduced by hepatic enzyme-inducing drugs such as the anticonvulsants phenytoin, carbamazepine, and barbiturates, and the antituberculosis drug rifampin). Products include:
Emend 2124

Aprobarbital (The effectiveness of progestin-only pills is reduced by hepatic enzyme-inducing drugs such as the anticonvulsants phenytoin, carbamazepine, and barbiturates).
No products indexed under this heading.

Betamethasone (The effectiveness of progestin-only pills is reduced by hepatic enzyme-inducing drugs such as the anticonvulsants phenytoin, carbamazepine, and barbiturates, and the antituberculosis drug rifampin).
No products indexed under this heading.

Betamethasone Sodium Phosphate (The effectiveness of progestin-only pills is reduced by hepatic enzyme-inducing drugs such as the anticonvulsants phenytoin, carbamazepine, and barbiturates, and the antituberculosis drug rifampin).
No products indexed under this heading.

Bosentan (Concurrent use of bosentan and norethindrone containing products may result in decreased concentration of these contraceptive hormones thereby increasing the risk of unintended pregnancy and unscheduled bleeding). Products include:
Tracleer 573

Butabarbital (The effectiveness of progestin-only pills is reduced by hepatic enzyme-inducing drugs such as the anticonvulsants phenytoin, carbamazepine, and barbiturates).
No products indexed under this heading.

Butabarbital Sodium (The effectiveness of progestin-only pills is reduced by hepatic enzyme-inducing drugs such as the anticonvulsants phenytoin, carbamazepine, and barbiturates).
No products indexed under this heading.

Butalbital (The effectiveness of progestin-only pills is reduced by hepatic enzyme-inducing drugs such as the anticonvulsants phenytoin, carbamazepine, and barbiturates).
No products indexed under this heading.

Carbamazepine (The effectiveness of progestin-only pills is reduced by hepatic enzyme-inducing drugs such as the anticonvulsant carbamazepine). Products include:
Carbatrol 3280
Equetro 3477

Chlorpropamide (The effectiveness of progestin-only pills is reduced by hepatic enzyme-inducing drugs such as the anticonvulsants phenytoin, carbamazepine, and barbiturates, and the antituberculosis drug rifampin).
No products indexed under this heading.

Ciprofloxacin (The effectiveness of progestin-only pills is reduced by hepatic enzyme-inducing drugs such as the anticonvulsants phenytoin, carbamazepine, and barbiturates, and the antituberculosis drug rifampin). Products include:
Cipro I.V. 3082
Cipro 3073
Cipro XR 3091
Ciprodex 583

Ciprofloxacin Hydrochloride (The effectiveness of progestin-only pills is reduced by hepatic enzyme-inducing drugs such as the anticonvulsants phenytoin, carbamazepine, and barbiturates, and the antituberculosis drug rifampin). Products include:
Cipro 3073

Cisplatin (The effectiveness of progestin-only pills is reduced by hepatic enzyme-inducing drugs such as the anticonvulsants phenytoin, carbamazepine, and barbiturates, and the antituberculosis drug rifampin).
No products indexed under this heading.

Citalopram Hydrobromide (The effectiveness of progestin-only pills is reduced by hepatic enzyme-inducing drugs such as the anticonvulsants phenytoin, carbamazepine, and barbiturates, and the antituberculosis drug rifampin). Products include:
Celexa 1153

Cortisone Acetate (The effectiveness of progestin-only pills is reduced by hepatic enzyme-inducing drugs such as the anticonvulsants phenytoin, carbamazepine, and barbiturates, and the antituberculosis drug rifampin).
No products indexed under this heading.

Dexamethasone (The effectiveness of progestin-only pills is reduced by hepatic enzyme-inducing drugs such as the anticonvulsants phenytoin, carbamazepine, and barbiturates, and the antituberculosis drug rifampin). Products include:
Ciprodex 583
Ozurdex .... ⊙ 223
Tobramycin and Dexamethasone Ophthalmic Suspension .... ⊙ 251

Dexamethasone Acetate (The effectiveness of progestin-only pills is reduced by hepatic enzyme-inducing drugs such as the anticonvulsants phenytoin, carbamazepine, and barbiturates, and the antituberculosis drug rifampin).
No products indexed under this heading.

Dexamethasone Phosphate (The effectiveness of progestin-only pills is reduced by hepatic enzyme-inducing drugs such as the anticonvulsants phenytoin, carbamazepine, and barbiturates, and the antituberculosis drug rifampin).
No products indexed under this heading.

Dexamethasone Sodium (The effectiveness of progestin-only pills is reduced by hepatic enzyme-inducing drugs such as the anticonvulsants phenytoin, carbamazepine, and barbiturates, and the antituberculosis drug rifampin).
No products indexed under this heading.

Dexamethasone Sodium Phosphate (The effectiveness of progestin-only pills is reduced by hepatic enzyme-inducing drugs such as the anticonvulsants phenytoin, carbamazepine, and barbiturates, and the antituberculosis drug rifampin).
No products indexed under this heading.

Diltiazem Hydrochloride (The effectiveness of progestin-only pills is reduced by hepatic enzyme-inducing drugs such as the anticonvulsants phenytoin, carbamazepine, and barbiturates, and the antituberculosis drug rifampin). Products include:
Cardizem LA 423

Diltiazem Maleate (The effectiveness of progestin-only pills is reduced by hepatic enzyme-inducing drugs such as the anticonvulsants phenytoin, carbamazepine, and barbiturates, and the antituberculosis drug rifampin).
No products indexed under this heading.

Doxorubicin Hydrochloride (The effectiveness of progestin-only pills is reduced by hepatic enzyme-inducing drugs such as the anticonvulsants phenytoin, carbamazepine, and barbiturates, and the antituberculosis drug rifampin).
No products indexed under this heading.

Efavirenz (The effectiveness of progestin-only pills is reduced by hepatic enzyme-inducing drugs such as the anticonvulsants phenytoin, carbamazepine, and barbiturates, and the antituberculosis drug rifampin). Products include:
Atripla 906

Erythromycin (The effectiveness of progestin-only pills is reduced by hepatic enzyme-inducing drugs such as the anticonvulsants phenytoin, carbamazepine, and barbiturates, and the antituberculosis drug rifampin).
No products indexed under this heading.

Erythromycin, Topical (The effectiveness of progestin-only pills is reduced by hepatic enzyme-inducing drugs such as the anticonvulsants phenytoin, carbamazepine, and barbiturates, and the antituberculosis drug rifampin).
No products indexed under this heading.

Erythromycin Estolate (The effectiveness of progestin-only pills is reduced by hepatic enzyme-inducing drugs such as the anticonvulsants phenytoin, carbamazepine, and barbiturates, and the antituberculosis drug rifampin).
No products indexed under this heading.

Erythromycin Ethylsuccinate (The effectiveness of progestin-only pills is reduced by hepatic enzyme-inducing drugs such as the anticonvulsants phenytoin, carbamazepine, and barbiturates, and the antituberculosis drug rifampin). Products include:
E.E.S. 437
EryPed 435

Erythromycin Gluceptate (The effectiveness of progestin-only pills is reduced by hepatic enzyme-inducing drugs such as the anticonvulsants phenytoin, carbamazepine, and barbiturates, and the antituberculosis drug rifampin).
No products indexed under this heading.

Erythromycin Lactobionate (The effectiveness of progestin-only pills is reduced by hepatic enzyme-inducing drugs such as the anticonvulsants phenytoin, carbamazepine, and barbiturates, and the antituberculosis drug rifampin).
No products indexed under this heading.

Erythromycin Stearate (The effectiveness of progestin-only pills is reduced by hepatic enzyme-inducing drugs such as the anticonvulsants phenytoin, carbamazepine, and barbiturates, and the antituberculosis drug rifampin).
No products indexed under this heading.

Escitalopram Oxalate (The effectiveness of progestin-only pills is reduced by hepatic enzyme-inducing drugs such as the anticonvulsants phenytoin, carbamazepine, and barbiturates, and the antituberculosis drug rifampin). Products include:
Lexapro Oral Suspension 1160
Lexapro Tablets 1160

Esomeprazole Magnesium (The effectiveness of progestin-only pills is reduced by hepatic enzyme-inducing drugs such as the anticonvulsants phenytoin, carbamazepine, and barbiturates, and the antituberculosis drug rifampin). Products include:
Nexium Capsules 704
Nexium Oral Suspension 704

Esomeprazole Sodium (The effectiveness of progestin-only pills is reduced by hepatic enzyme-inducing drugs such as the anticonvulsants phenytoin, carbamazepine, and barbiturates, and the antituberculosis drug rifampin). Products include:
Nexium I.V. 712

Ethanol (The effectiveness of progestin-only pills is reduced by hepatic enzyme-inducing drugs such as the anticonvulsants phenytoin, carbamazepine, and barbiturates, and the antituberculosis drug rifampin).
No products indexed under this heading.

Ethosuximide (The effectiveness of progestin-only pills is reduced by hepatic enzyme-inducing drugs such as the anticonvulsants phenytoin, carbamazepine, and barbiturates, and the antituberculosis drug rifampin).
No products indexed under this heading.

Ethyl Alcohol (The effectiveness of progestin-only pills is reduced by hepatic enzyme-inducing drugs such as the anticonvulsants phenytoin, carbamazepine, and barbiturates, and the antituberculosis drug rifampin).
No products indexed under this heading.

Felbamate (The effectiveness of progestin-only pills is reduced by hepatic enzyme-inducing drugs such as the anticonvulsants phenytoin, carbamazepine, and barbiturates, and the antituberculosis drug rifampin).
No products indexed under this heading.

Fludrocortisone Acetate (The effectiveness of progestin-only pills is reduced by hepatic enzyme-inducing drugs such as the anticonvulsants phenytoin, carbamazepine, and barbiturates, and the antituberculosis drug rifampin).
No products indexed under this heading.

Fluvoxamine (The effectiveness of progestin-only pills is reduced by hepatic enzyme-inducing drugs such as the anticonvulsants phenytoin, carbamazepine, and barbiturates, and the antituberculosis drug rifampin).
No products indexed under this heading.

Fluvoxamine Maleate (The effectiveness of progestin-only pills is reduced by hepatic enzyme-inducing drugs such as the anticonvulsants phenytoin, carbamazepine, and barbiturates, and the antituberculosis drug rifampin).
No products indexed under this heading.

Fosphenytoin (The effectiveness of progestin-only pills is reduced by hepatic enzyme-inducing drugs such as the anticonvulsant phenytoin).
No products indexed under this heading.

Fosphenytoin Sodium (The effectiveness of progestin-only pills is reduced by hepatic enzyme-inducing drugs such as the anticonvulsant phenytoin).
No products indexed under this heading.

Garlic Extract (The effectiveness of progestin-only pills is reduced by hepatic enzyme-inducing drugs such as the anticonvulsants phenytoin, carbamazepine, and barbiturates, and the antituberculosis drug rifampin).
No products indexed under this heading.

Garlic Oil (The effectiveness of progestin-only pills is reduced by hepatic enzyme-inducing drugs such as the anticonvulsants phenytoin, carbamazepine, and barbiturates, and the antituberculosis drug rifampin).
No products indexed under this heading.

Glipizide (The effectiveness of progestin-only pills is reduced by hepatic enzyme-inducing drugs such as the anticonvulsants phenytoin, carbamazepine, and barbiturates, and the antituberculosis drug rifampin).
No products indexed under this heading.

Glyburide (The effectiveness of progestin-only pills is reduced by hepatic enzyme-inducing drugs such as the anticonvulsants phenytoin, carbamazepine, and barbiturates, and the antituberculosis drug rifampin).
No products indexed under this heading.

(⊙ Described in PDR® for Ophthalmic Medicines)

Hepatic Enzyme-Inducing Agents (The effectiveness of progestin-only pills is reduced by hepatic enzyme-inducing drugs such as the anticonvulsants phenytoin, carbamazepine, and barbiturates, and the antituberculosis drug rifampin).
No products indexed under this heading.

Hexobarbital (The effectiveness of progestin-only pills is reduced by hepatic enzyme-inducing drugs such as the anticonvulsants phenytoin, carbamazepine, and barbiturates).
No products indexed under this heading.

Hydrocortisone (Alcohol) (The effectiveness of progestin-only pills is reduced by hepatic enzyme-inducing drugs such as the anticonvulsants phenytoin, carbamazepine, and barbiturates, and the antituberculosis drug rifampin).
No products indexed under this heading.

Hydrocortisone Acetate (The effectiveness of progestin-only pills is reduced by hepatic enzyme-inducing drugs such as the anticonvulsants phenytoin, carbamazepine, and barbiturates, and the antituberculosis drug rifampin).
No products indexed under this heading.

Hydrocortisone Butyrate (The effectiveness of progestin-only pills is reduced by hepatic enzyme-inducing drugs such as the anticonvulsants phenytoin, carbamazepine, and barbiturates, and the antituberculosis drug rifampin).
No products indexed under this heading.

Hydrocortisone Cypionate (The effectiveness of progestin-only pills is reduced by hepatic enzyme-inducing drugs such as the anticonvulsants phenytoin, carbamazepine, and barbiturates, and the antituberculosis drug rifampin).
No products indexed under this heading.

Hydrocortisone Hemisuccinate (The effectiveness of progestin-only pills is reduced by hepatic enzyme-inducing drugs such as the anticonvulsants phenytoin, carbamazepine, and barbiturates, and the antituberculosis drug rifampin).
No products indexed under this heading.

Hydrocortisone Probutate (The effectiveness of progestin-only pills is reduced by hepatic enzyme-inducing drugs such as the anticonvulsants phenytoin, carbamazepine, and barbiturates, and the antituberculosis drug rifampin).
No products indexed under this heading.

Hydrocortisone Sodium Phosphate (The effectiveness of progestin-only pills is reduced by hepatic enzyme-inducing drugs such as the anticonvulsants phenytoin, carbamazepine, and barbiturates, and the antituberculosis drug rifampin).
No products indexed under this heading.

Hydrocortisone Sodium Succinate (The effectiveness of progestin-only pills is reduced by hepatic enzyme-inducing drugs such as the anticonvulsants phenytoin, carbamazepine, and barbiturates, and the antituberculosis drug rifampin).
No products indexed under this heading.

Hydrocortisone Valerate (The effectiveness of progestin-only pills is reduced by hepatic enzyme-inducing drugs such as the anticonvulsants phenytoin, carbamazepine, and barbiturates, and the antituberculosis drug rifampin).
No products indexed under this heading.

Hypericum (The effectiveness of progestin-only pills is reduced by hepatic enzyme-inducing drugs such as the anticonvulsants phenytoin, carbamazepine, and barbiturates, and the antituberculosis drug rifampin).
No products indexed under this heading.

Hypericum Perforatum (Herbal products containing St. John's Wort (hypericum perforatum) may induce hepatic enzymes (cytochrome P450) and p-glycoprotein transporter and may reduce the effectiveness of contraceptive steroids. This may also result in breakthrough bleeding). Products include:
Traumeel 1800

Insulin (The effectiveness of progestin-only pills is reduced by hepatic enzyme-inducing drugs such as the anticonvulsants phenytoin, carbamazepine, and barbiturates, and the antituberculosis drug rifampin).
No products indexed under this heading.

Insulin, Human, Zinc Suspension (The effectiveness of progestin-only pills is reduced by hepatic enzyme-inducing drugs such as the anticonvulsants phenytoin, carbamazepine, and barbiturates, and the antituberculosis drug rifampin).
No products indexed under this heading.

Insulin, Human (rDNA origin) (The effectiveness of progestin-only pills is reduced by hepatic enzyme-inducing drugs such as the anticonvulsants phenytoin, carbamazepine, and barbiturates, and the antituberculosis drug rifampin). Products include:
Exubera 2717

Insulin, Human NPH (The effectiveness of progestin-only pills is reduced by hepatic enzyme-inducing drugs such as the anticonvulsants phenytoin, carbamazepine, and barbiturates, and the antituberculosis drug rifampin). Products include:
Humulin N Vial 1934

Insulin, Human Regular (The effectiveness of progestin-only pills is reduced by hepatic enzyme-inducing drugs such as the anticonvulsants phenytoin, carbamazepine, and barbiturates, and the antituberculosis drug rifampin). Products include:
Humulin R 1937
Humulin R (U-500) 1939

Insulin, Human Regular and Human NPH Mixture (The effectiveness of progestin-only pills is reduced by hepatic enzyme-inducing drugs such as the anticonvulsants phenytoin, carbamazepine, and barbiturates, and the antituberculosis drug rifampin). Products include:
Humulin 50/50 1930
Humulin 70/30 Vial 1931

Insulin, NPH (The effectiveness of progestin-only pills is reduced by hepatic enzyme-inducing drugs such as the anticonvulsants phenytoin, carbamazepine, and barbiturates, and the antituberculosis drug rifampin).
No products indexed under this heading.

Insulin, Regular (The effectiveness of progestin-only pills is reduced by hepatic enzyme-inducing drugs such as the anticonvulsants phenytoin, carbamazepine, and barbiturates, and the antituberculosis drug rifampin).
No products indexed under this heading.

Insulin, Regular and NPH mixture (The effectiveness of progestin-only pills is reduced by hepatic enzyme-inducing drugs such as the anticonvulsants phenytoin, carbamazepine, and barbiturates, and the antituberculosis drug rifampin).
No products indexed under this heading.

Insulin, Zinc Crystals (The effectiveness of progestin-only pills is reduced by hepatic enzyme-inducing drugs such as the anticonvulsants phenytoin, carbamazepine, and barbiturates, and the antituberculosis drug rifampin).
No products indexed under this heading.

Insulin, Zinc Suspension (The effectiveness of progestin-only pills is reduced by hepatic enzyme-inducing drugs such as the anticonvulsants phenytoin, carbamazepine, and barbiturates, and the antituberculosis drug rifampin).
No products indexed under this heading.

Insulin Aspart (The effectiveness of progestin-only pills is reduced by hepatic enzyme-inducing drugs such as the anticonvulsants phenytoin, carbamazepine, and barbiturates, and the antituberculosis drug rifampin).
No products indexed under this heading.

Insulin Aspart, Human (The effectiveness of progestin-only pills is reduced by hepatic enzyme-inducing drugs such as the anticonvulsants phenytoin, carbamazepine, and barbiturates, and the antituberculosis drug rifampin). Products include:
NovoLog Mix 70/30 2581

Insulin Aspart, Human Regular (The effectiveness of progestin-only pills is reduced by hepatic enzyme-inducing drugs such as the anticonvulsants phenytoin, carbamazepine, and barbiturates, and the antituberculosis drug rifampin). Products include:
NovoLog 2575

Insulin Aspart Protamine, Human (The effectiveness of progestin-only pills is reduced by hepatic enzyme-inducing drugs such as the anticonvulsants phenytoin, carbamazepine, and barbiturates, and the antituberculosis drug rifampin). Products include:
NovoLog Mix 70/30 2581

Insulin Detemir (rDNA Origin) (The effectiveness of progestin-only pills is reduced by hepatic enzyme-inducing drugs such as the anticonvulsants phenytoin, carbamazepine, and barbiturates, and the antituberculosis drug rifampin). Products include:
Levemir 2566

Insulin Glargine (The effectiveness of progestin-only pills is reduced by hepatic enzyme-inducing drugs such as the anticonvulsants phenytoin, carbamazepine, and barbiturates, and the antituberculosis drug rifampin). Products include:
Lantus 2996

Insulin Glulisine (The effectiveness of progestin-only pills is reduced by hepatic enzyme-inducing drugs such as the anticonvulsants phenytoin, carbamazepine, and barbiturates, and the antituberculosis drug rifampin). Products include:
Apidra 2937
Apidra SoloStar 2937

Insulin Lispro, Human (The effectiveness of progestin-only pills is reduced by hepatic enzyme-inducing drugs such as the anticonvulsants phenytoin, carbamazepine, and barbiturates, and the antituberculosis drug rifampin). Products include:
Humalog 1910
Humalog Mix 1914
Humalog Mix75/25 1917

Insulin Lispro Protamine, Human (The effectiveness of progestin-only pills is reduced by hepatic enzyme-inducing drugs such as the anticonvulsants phenytoin, carbamazepine, and barbiturates, and the antituberculosis drug rifampin). Products include:
Humalog Mix 1914
Humalog Mix75/25 1917

Lansoprazole (The effectiveness of progestin-only pills is reduced by hepatic enzyme-inducing drugs such as the anticonvulsants phenytoin, carbamazepine, and barbiturates, and the antituberculosis drug rifampin).
No products indexed under this heading.

Mephenytoin (The effectiveness of progestin-only pills is reduced by hepatic enzyme-inducing drugs such as the anticonvulsants phenytoin, carbamazepine, and barbiturates, and the antituberculosis drug rifampin).
No products indexed under this heading.

Mephobarbital (The effectiveness of progestin-only pills is reduced by hepatic enzyme-inducing drugs such as the anticonvulsants phenytoin, carbamazepine, and barbiturates).
No products indexed under this heading.

Methsuximide (The effectiveness of progestin-only pills is reduced by hepatic enzyme-inducing drugs such as the anticonvulsants phenytoin, carbamazepine, and barbiturates, and the antituberculosis drug rifampin).
No products indexed under this heading.

Methylprednisolone (The effectiveness of progestin-only pills is reduced by hepatic enzyme-inducing drugs such as the anticonvulsants phenytoin, carbamazepine, and barbiturates, and the antituberculosis drug rifampin).
No products indexed under this heading.

Methylprednisolone Acetate (The effectiveness of progestin-only pills is reduced by hepatic enzyme-inducing drugs such as the anticonvulsants phenytoin, carbamazepine, and barbiturates, and the antituberculosis drug rifampin).
No products indexed under this heading.

Methylprednisolone Sodium Succinate (The effectiveness of progestin-only pills is reduced by hepatic enzyme-inducing drugs such as the anticonvulsants phenytoin, carbamazepine, and barbiturates, and the antituberculosis drug rifampin).
No products indexed under this heading.

Modafinil (The effectiveness of progestin-only pills is reduced by hepatic enzyme-inducing drugs such as the anticonvulsants phenytoin, carbamazepine, and barbiturates, and the antituberculosis drug rifampin). Products include:
Provigil 983

Nafcillin Sodium (The effectiveness of progestin-only pills is reduced by hepatic enzyme-inducing drugs such as the anticonvulsants phenytoin, carbamazepine, and barbiturates, and the antituberculosis drug rifampin).
No products indexed under this heading.

Nevirapine (The effectiveness of progestin-only pills is reduced by hepatic enzyme-inducing drugs such as the anticonvulsants phenytoin, carbamazepine, and barbiturates, and the antituberculosis drug rifampin). Products include:
Viramune Oral Suspension 897
Viramune Tablets 897

Nicotine (The effectiveness of progestin-only pills is reduced by hepatic enzyme-inducing drugs such as the anticonvulsants phenytoin, carbamazepine, and barbiturates, and the antituberculosis drug rifampin).
No products indexed under this heading.

Nicotine Polacrilex (The effectiveness of progestin-only pills is reduced by hepatic enzyme-inducing drugs such as the anticonvulsants phenytoin, carbamazepine, and barbiturates, and the antituberculosis drug rifampin).
No products indexed under this heading.

Nicotine Salicylate (The effectiveness of progestin-only pills is reduced by hepatic enzyme-inducing drugs such as the anticonvulsants phenytoin, carbamazepine, and barbiturates, and the antituberculosis drug rifampin).
No products indexed under this heading.

Nicotine Sulfate (The effectiveness of progestin-only pills is reduced by hepatic enzyme-inducing drugs such as the anticonvulsants phenytoin, carbamazepine, and barbiturates, and the antituberculosis drug rifampin).
No products indexed under this heading.

Norethindrone Acetate (The effectiveness of progestin-only pills is reduced by hepatic enzyme-inducing

drugs such as the anticonvulsants phenytoin, carbamazepine, and barbiturates, and the antituberculosis drug rifampin). Products include:
Activella 2561

Omeprazole (The effectiveness of progestin-only pills is reduced by hepatic enzyme-inducing drugs such as the anticonvulsants phenytoin, carbamazepine, and barbiturates, and the antituberculosis drug rifampin).
No products indexed under this heading.

Omeprazole Magnesium (The effectiveness of progestin-only pills is reduced by hepatic enzyme-inducing drugs such as the anticonvulsants phenytoin, carbamazepine, and barbiturates, and the antituberculosis drug rifampin).
No products indexed under this heading.

Oxcarbazepine (The effectiveness of progestin-only pills is reduced by hepatic enzyme-inducing drugs such as the anticonvulsants phenytoin, carbamazepine, and barbiturates, and the antituberculosis drug rifampin).
No products indexed under this heading.

Pentobarbital (The effectiveness of progestin-only pills is reduced by hepatic enzyme-inducing drugs such as the anticonvulsants phenytoin, carbamazepine, and barbiturates).
No products indexed under this heading.

Pentobarbital Sodium (The effectiveness of progestin-only pills is reduced by hepatic enzyme-inducing drugs such as the anticonvulsants phenytoin, carbamazepine, and barbiturates). Products include:
Nembutal 2012

Phenobarbital (The effectiveness of progestin-only pills is reduced by hepatic enzyme-inducing drugs such as the anticonvulsants phenytoin, carbamazepine, and barbiturates). Products include:
Donnatal 2711

Phenobarbital Sodium (The effectiveness of progestin-only pills is reduced by hepatic enzyme-inducing drugs such as the anticonvulsants phenytoin, carbamazepine, and barbiturates).
No products indexed under this heading.

Phenylbutazone (The effectiveness of progestin-only pills is reduced by hepatic enzyme-inducing drugs such as the anticonvulsants phenytoin, carbamazepine, and barbiturates, and the antituberculosis drug rifampin).
No products indexed under this heading.

Phenytoin (The effectiveness of progestin-only pills is reduced by hepatic enzyme-inducing drugs such as the anticonvulsant phenytoin).
No products indexed under this heading.

Phenytoin Sodium (The effectiveness of progestin-only pills is reduced by hepatic enzyme-inducing drugs such as the anticonvulsant phenytoin). Products include:
Phenytek Capsules 2380

Prednisolone (The effectiveness of progestin-only pills is reduced by hepatic enzyme-inducing drugs such as the anticonvulsants phenytoin, carbamazepine, and barbiturates, and the antituberculosis drug rifampin).
No products indexed under this heading.

Prednisolone Acetate (The effectiveness of progestin-only pills is reduced by hepatic enzyme-inducing drugs such as the anticonvulsants phenytoin, carbamazepine, and barbiturates, and the antituberculosis drug rifampin).
Products include:
Blephamide .... ⊙212, ⊙214
Pred Forte .... ⊙225
Pred Mild .... ⊙230
Pred-G .... ⊙226, ⊙227

Prednisolone Sodium Phosphate (The effectiveness of progestin-only pills is reduced by hepatic enzyme-inducing drugs such as the anticonvulsants phenytoin, carbamazepine, and barbiturates, and the antituberculosis drug rifampin).
No products indexed under this heading.

Prednisolone Tebutate (The effectiveness of progestin-only pills is reduced by hepatic enzyme-inducing drugs such as the anticonvulsants phenytoin, carbamazepine, and barbiturates, and the antituberculosis drug rifampin).
No products indexed under this heading.

Prednisone (The effectiveness of progestin-only pills is reduced by hepatic enzyme-inducing drugs such as the anticonvulsants phenytoin, carbamazepine, and barbiturates, and the antituberculosis drug rifampin).
No products indexed under this heading.

Prednisone sodium phosphate (The effectiveness of progestin-only pills is reduced by hepatic enzyme-inducing drugs such as the anticonvulsants phenytoin, carbamazepine, and barbiturates, and the antituberculosis drug rifampin).
No products indexed under this heading.

Primidone (The effectiveness of progestin-only pills is reduced by hepatic enzyme-inducing drugs such as the anticonvulsants phenytoin, carbamazepine, and barbiturates, and the antituberculosis drug rifampin).
No products indexed under this heading.

Rifabutin (The effectiveness of progestin-only pills is reduced by hepatic enzyme-inducing drugs such as the anticonvulsants phenytoin, carbamazepine, and barbiturates, and the antituberculosis drug rifampin).
No products indexed under this heading.

Rifampicin (The effectiveness of progestin-only pills is reduced by hepatic enzyme-inducing drugs such as the anticonvulsants phenytoin, carbamazepine, and barbiturates, and the antituberculosis drug rifampin).
No products indexed under this heading.

Rifampin (The effectiveness of progestin-only pills is reduced by hepatic enzyme-inducing drugs such as the antituberculosis drug rifampin).
No products indexed under this heading.

Rifapentine (The effectiveness of progestin-only pills is reduced by hepatic enzyme-inducing drugs such as the anticonvulsants phenytoin, carbamazepine, and barbiturates, and the antituberculosis drug rifampin).
No products indexed under this heading.

Ritonavir (The effectiveness of progestin-only pills is reduced by hepatic enzyme-inducing drugs such as the anticonvulsants phenytoin, carbamazepine, and barbiturates, and the antituberculosis drug rifampin). Products include:
Kaletra 458
Norvir 509

Secobarbital Sodium (The effectiveness of progestin-only pills is reduced by hepatic enzyme-inducing drugs such as the anticonvulsants phenytoin, carbamazepine, and barbiturates).
No products indexed under this heading.

Sodium Butabarbital (The effectiveness of progestin-only pills is reduced by hepatic enzyme-inducing drugs such as the anticonvulsants phenytoin, carbamazepine, and barbiturates).
No products indexed under this heading.

Sodium Pentobarbital (The effectiveness of progestin-only pills is reduced by hepatic enzyme-inducing drugs such as the anticonvulsants phenytoin, carbamazepine, and barbiturates).
No products indexed under this heading.

Theophylline (The effectiveness of progestin-only pills is reduced by hepatic enzyme-inducing drugs such as the anticonvulsants phenytoin, carbamazepine, and barbiturates, and the antituberculosis drug rifampin).
No products indexed under this heading.

Theophylline Anhydrous (The effectiveness of progestin-only pills is reduced by hepatic enzyme-inducing drugs such as the anticonvulsants phenytoin, carbamazepine, and barbiturates, and the antituberculosis drug rifampin). Products include:
Uniphyl 2817

Theophylline Calcium Salicylate (The effectiveness of progestin-only pills is reduced by hepatic enzyme-inducing drugs such as the anticonvulsants phenytoin, carbamazepine, and barbiturates, and the antituberculosis drug rifampin).
No products indexed under this heading.

Theophylline Dihydroxypropyl (Glyceryl) (The effectiveness of progestin-only pills is reduced by hepatic enzyme-inducing drugs such as the anticonvulsants phenytoin, carbamazepine, and barbiturates, and the antituberculosis drug rifampin).
No products indexed under this heading.

Theophylline Ethylenediamine (The effectiveness of progestin-only pills is reduced by hepatic enzyme-inducing drugs such as the anticonvulsants phenytoin, carbamazepine, and barbiturates, and the antituberculosis drug rifampin).
No products indexed under this heading.

Theophylline Sodium Glycinate (The effectiveness of progestin-only pills is reduced by hepatic enzyme-inducing drugs such as the anticonvulsants phenytoin, carbamazepine, and barbiturates, and the antituberculosis drug rifampin).
No products indexed under this heading.

Thiamylal Sodium (The effectiveness of progestin-only pills is reduced by hepatic enzyme-inducing drugs such as the anticonvulsants phenytoin, carbamazepine, and barbiturates).
No products indexed under this heading.

Tobacco (Cigarette smoking increases the risk of serious cardiovascular disease. Women who use oral contraceptives should be strongly advised not to smoke).
No products indexed under this heading.

Tolazamide (The effectiveness of progestin-only pills is reduced by hepatic enzyme-inducing drugs such as the anticonvulsants phenytoin, carbamazepine, and barbiturates, and the antituberculosis drug rifampin).
No products indexed under this heading.

Tolbutamide (The effectiveness of progestin-only pills is reduced by hepatic enzyme-inducing drugs such as the anticonvulsants phenytoin, carbamazepine, and barbiturates, and the antituberculosis drug rifampin).
No products indexed under this heading.

Triamcinolone (The effectiveness of progestin-only pills is reduced by hepatic enzyme-inducing drugs such as the anticonvulsants phenytoin, carbamazepine, and barbiturates, and the antituberculosis drug rifampin).
No products indexed under this heading.

Triamcinolone Acetonide (The effectiveness of progestin-only pills is reduced by hepatic enzyme-inducing drugs such as the anticonvulsants phenytoin, carbamazepine, and barbiturates, and the antituberculosis drug rifampin). Products include:
Azmacort 408
Nasacort AQ 3019

Triamcinolone Diacetate (The effectiveness of progestin-only pills is reduced by hepatic enzyme-inducing drugs such as the anticonvulsants phenytoin, carbamazepine, and barbiturates, and the antituberculosis drug rifampin).
No products indexed under this heading.

Triamcinolone Hexacetonide (The effectiveness of progestin-only pills is reduced by hepatic enzyme-inducing drugs such as the anticonvulsants phenytoin, carbamazepine, and barbiturates, and the antituberculosis drug rifampin).
No products indexed under this heading.

Troglitazone (The effectiveness of progestin-only pills is reduced by hepatic enzyme-inducing drugs such as the anticonvulsants phenytoin, carbamazepine, and barbiturates, and the antituberculosis drug rifampin).
No products indexed under this heading.

Food Interactions

Broccoli (The effectiveness of progestin-only pills is reduced by hepatic enzyme-inducing drugs such as the anticonvulsants phenytoin, carbamazepine, and barbiturates, and the antituberculosis drug rifampin).

Brussel Sprouts (The effectiveness of progestin-only pills is reduced by hepatic enzyme-inducing drugs such as the anticonvulsants phenytoin, carbamazepine, and barbiturates, and the antituberculosis drug rifampin).

Charbroiled Food (The effectiveness of progestin-only pills is reduced by hepatic enzyme-inducing drugs such as the anticonvulsants phenytoin, carbamazepine, and barbiturates, and the antituberculosis drug rifampin).

ORTHO TRI-CYCLEN TABLETS

(Ethinyl Estradiol, Norgestimate) 2663
See Ortho-Cyclen Tablets

ORTHO TRI-CYCLEN LO TABLETS

(Ethinyl Estradiol, Norgestimate) 2673

May interact with ampicillins, antibiotics, anticonvulsants, barbiturates, cytochrome p450 3a4 inhibitors (selected), hepatic microsomal enzyme inducers, phenytoin, prednisolone, protease inhibitors, tetracyclines, theophyllines, and certain other agents. Compounds in these categories include:

Acetaminophen (Acetaminophen may increase plasma ethinyl estradiol levels, possibly by inhibition of conjugation. Concomitant use may also decrease plasma concentrations of acetaminophen). Products include:
Percocet 1121
Tylenol 2049
Tylenol 8 Hour 2049
Extra Strength Tylenol Caplets, Cool Caplets, and EZ Tabs 2049
Extra Strength Tylenol Adult Rapid Blast Liquid 2049
Extra Strength Tylenol Rapid Release 2049
Tylenol with Codeine 2691
Tylenol Arthritis Pain Extended Release Geltabs/Caplets 2049
Children's Tylenol Suspension Liquid 2048
Chlidren's Tylenol Meltaways 2048
Tylenol, Infants' Drops 2048
Junior Tylenol 2048
Vicodin 560
Vicodin ES 561
Vicodin HP 563
Zydone 1138

Acetaminophen-containing products (Acetaminophen may increase plasma ethinyl estradiol levels, possibly by inhibition of conjugation. Concomitant use may also decrease plasma concentrations of acetaminophen).
No products indexed under this heading.

Acetazolamide (CYP3A4 inhibitors such as itraconazole or ketoconazole may increase plasma hormone levels).
No products indexed under this heading.

Acetazolamide Sodium (CYP3A4 inhibitors such as itraconazole or ketoconazole may increase plasma hormone levels).
No products indexed under this heading.

Alatrofloxacin Mesylate (Contraceptive effectiveness may be reduced when hormonal contraceptives are co-administered with antibiotics, anticonvulsants, and other drugs that increase the metabolism of contraceptive steroids. This could result in unintended pregnancy or breakthrough bleeding).
No products indexed under this heading.

Allium sativum (Contraceptive effectiveness may be reduced when hormonal contraceptives are co-administered with antibiotics, anticonvulsants, and other drugs that increase the metabolism of contraceptive steroids. This could result in unintended pregnancy or breakthrough bleeding).
No products indexed under this heading.

Amikacin Sulfate (Contraceptive effectiveness may be reduced when hormonal contraceptives are co-administered with antibiotics, anticonvulsants, and other drugs that increase the metabolism of contraceptive steroids. This could result in unintended pregnancy or breakthrough bleeding).
No products indexed under this heading.

Aminoglutethimide (Contraceptive effectiveness may be reduced when hormonal contraceptives are co-administered with antibiotics, anticonvulsants, and other drugs that increase the metabolism of contraceptive steroids. This could result in unintended pregnancy or breakthrough bleeding).
No products indexed under this heading.

Amiodarone Hydrochloride (CYP3A4 inhibitors such as itraconazole or ketoconazole may increase plasma hormone levels).
No products indexed under this heading.

Amobarbital (Contraceptive effectiveness may be reduced when hormonal contraceptives are co-administered with barbiturates. This could result in unintended pregnancy or breakthrough bleeding).
No products indexed under this heading.

Amobarbital Sodium (Contraceptive effectiveness may be reduced when hormonal contraceptives are co-administered with barbiturates. This could result in unintended pregnancy or breakthrough bleeding).
No products indexed under this heading.

Amoxicillin (Contraceptive effectiveness may be reduced when hormonal contraceptives are co-administered with antibiotics, anticonvulsants, and other drugs that increase the metabolism of contraceptive steroids. This could result in unintended pregnancy or breakthrough bleeding). Products include:

Amoxicillin Trihydrate (Contraceptive effectiveness may be reduced when hormonal contraceptives are co-administered with antibiotics, anticonvulsants, and other drugs that increase the metabolism of contraceptive steroids. This could result in unintended pregnancy or breakthrough bleeding).
No products indexed under this heading.

Ampicillin (Several cases of contraceptive failure and breakthrough bleeding have been reported in the literature with concomitant administration of antibiotics such as ampicillin and tetracyclines. However, clinical pharmacology studies investigating drug interaction between combined oral contraceptives and these antibiotics have reported inconsistent results).
No products indexed under this heading.

Ampicillin Sodium (Several cases of contraceptive failure and breakthrough bleeding have been reported in the literature with concomitant administration of antibiotics such as ampicillin and tetracyclines. However, clinical pharmacology studies investigating drug interaction between combined oral contraceptives and these antibiotics have reported inconsistent results).
No products indexed under this heading.

Ampicillin Trihydrate (Several cases of contraceptive failure and breakthrough bleeding have been reported in the literature with concomitant administration of antibiotics such as ampicillin and tetracyclines. However, clinical pharmacology studies investigating drug interaction between combined oral contraceptives and these antibiotics have reported inconsistent results).
No products indexed under this heading.

Amprenavir (Several of the anti-HIV protease inhibitors have been studied with co-administration of oral combination hormonal contraceptives; significant changes (increase and decrease) in the plasma levels of the estrogen and progestin have been noted in some cases. The safety and efficacy of oral contraceptive products may be affected with co-administration of anti-HIV protease inhibitors).
No products indexed under this heading.

Anastrozole (CYP3A4 inhibitors such as itraconazole or ketoconazole may increase plasma hormone levels).
No products indexed under this heading.

Antibiotics, non-penicillin, unspecified (Contraceptive effectiveness may be reduced when hormonal contraceptives are co-administered with antibiotics, anticonvulsants, and other drugs that increase the metabolism of contraceptive steroids. This could result in unintended pregnancy or breakthrough bleeding).
No products indexed under this heading.

Aprepitant (CYP3A4 inhibitors such as itraconazole or ketoconazole may increase plasma hormone levels). Products include:

Aprobarbital (Contraceptive effectiveness may be reduced when hormonal contraceptives are co-administered with barbiturates. This could result in unintended pregnancy or breakthrough bleeding).
No products indexed under this heading.

Atazanavir (Several of the anti-HIV protease inhibitors have been studied with co-administration of oral combination hormonal contraceptives; significant changes (increase and decrease) in the plasma levels of the estrogen and progestin have been noted in some cases. The safety and efficacy of oral contraceptive products may be affected with co-administration of anti-HIV protease inhibitors).
No products indexed under this heading.

Atazanavir Sulfate (Several of the anti-HIV protease inhibitors have been studied with co-administration of oral combination hormonal contraceptives; significant changes (increase and decrease) in the plasma levels of the estrogen and progestin have been noted in some cases. The safety and efficacy of oral contraceptive products may be affected with co-administration of anti-HIV protease inhibitors).
No products indexed under this heading.

Atorvastatin Calcium (Co-administration of atorvastatin and certain oral contraceptives containing ethinyl estradiol increase AUC values for ethinyl estradiol by approximately 20%). Products include:

Azithromycin Dihydrate (Contraceptive effectiveness may be reduced when hormonal contraceptives are co-administered with antibiotics, anticonvulsants, and other drugs that increase the metabolism of contraceptive steroids. This could result in unintended pregnancy or breakthrough bleeding).
No products indexed under this heading.

Azlocillin Sodium (Contraceptive effectiveness may be reduced when hormonal contraceptives are co-administered with antibiotics, anticonvulsants, and other drugs that increase the metabolism of contraceptive steroids. This could result in unintended pregnancy or breakthrough bleeding).
No products indexed under this heading.

Aztreonam (Contraceptive effectiveness may be reduced when hormonal contraceptives are co-administered with antibiotics, anticonvulsants, and other drugs that increase the metabolism of contraceptive steroids. This could result in unintended pregnancy or breakthrough bleeding).
No products indexed under this heading.

Bacampicillin Hydrochloride (Several cases of contraceptive failure and breakthrough bleeding have been reported in the literature with concomitant administration of antibiotics such as ampicillin and tetracyclines. However, clinical pharmacology studies investigating drug interaction between combined oral contraceptives and these antibiotics have reported inconsistent results).
No products indexed under this heading.

Betamethasone (Contraceptive effectiveness may be reduced when hormonal contraceptives are co-administered with antibiotics, anticonvulsants, and other drugs that increase the metabolism of contraceptive steroids. This could result in unintended pregnancy or breakthrough bleeding).
No products indexed under this heading.

Betamethasone Sodium Phosphate (Contraceptive effectiveness may be reduced when hormonal contraceptives are co-administered with antibiotics, anticonvulsants, and other drugs that increase the metabolism of contraceptive steroids. This could result in unintended pregnancy or breakthrough bleeding).
No products indexed under this heading.

Bosentan (Contraceptive effectiveness may be reduced when hormonal contraceptives are co-administered with antibiotics, anticonvulsants, and other drugs that increase the metabolism of contraceptive steroids. This could result in unintended pregnancy or breakthrough bleeding). Products include:

Butabarbital (Contraceptive effectiveness may be reduced when hormonal contraceptives are co-administered with barbiturates. This could result in unintended pregnancy or breakthrough bleeding).
No products indexed under this heading.

Butabarbital Sodium (Contraceptive effectiveness may be reduced when hormonal contraceptives are co-administered with barbiturates. This could result in unintended pregnancy or breakthrough bleeding).
No products indexed under this heading.

Butalbital (Contraceptive effectiveness may be reduced when hormonal contraceptives are co-administered with barbiturates. This could result in unintended pregnancy or breakthrough bleeding).
No products indexed under this heading.

Carbamazepine (Contraceptive effectiveness may be reduced when hormonal contraceptives are co-administered with carbamazepine. This could result in unintended pregnancy or breakthrough bleeding). Products include:

Carbenicillin Disodium (Contraceptive effectiveness may be reduced when hormonal contraceptives are co-administered with antibiotics, anticonvulsants, and other drugs that increase the metabolism of contraceptive steroids. This could result in unintended pregnancy or breakthrough bleeding).
No products indexed under this heading.

Carbenicillin Indanyl Sodium (Contraceptive effectiveness may be reduced when hormonal contraceptives are co-administered with antibiotics, anticonvulsants, and other drugs that increase the metabolism of contraceptive steroids. This could result in unintended pregnancy or breakthrough bleeding).
No products indexed under this heading.

Cefaclor (Contraceptive effectiveness may be reduced when hormonal contraceptives are co-administered with antibiotics, anticonvulsants, and other drugs that increase the metabolism of contraceptive steroids. This could result in unintended pregnancy or breakthrough bleeding).
No products indexed under this heading.

Cefadroxil (Contraceptive effectiveness may be reduced when hormonal contraceptives are co-administered with antibiotics, anticonvulsants, and other drugs that increase the metabolism of contraceptive steroids. This could result in unintended pregnancy or breakthrough bleeding).
No products indexed under this heading.

Cefamandole Nafate (Contraceptive effectiveness may be reduced when hormonal contraceptives are co-administered with antibiotics, anticonvulsants, and other drugs that increase the metabolism of contraceptive steroids. This could result in unintended pregnancy or breakthrough bleeding).
No products indexed under this heading.

Cefazolin Sodium (Contraceptive effectiveness may be reduced when hormonal contraceptives are co-administered with antibiotics, anticonvulsants, and other drugs that increase the metabolism of contraceptive steroids. This could result in unintended pregnancy or breakthrough bleeding).
No products indexed under this heading.

Cefixime (Contraceptive effectiveness may be reduced when hormonal contraceptives are co-administered with antibiotics, anticonvulsants, and other drugs that increase the metabolism of contra-

ceptive steroids. This could result in unintended pregnancy or breakthrough bleeding). Products include:

Cefmetazole Sodium (Contraceptive effectiveness may be reduced when hormonal contraceptives are co-administered with antibiotics, anticonvulsants, and other drugs that increase the metabolism of contraceptive steroids. This could result in unintended pregnancy or breakthrough bleeding).
No products indexed under this heading.

Cefonicid Sodium (Contraceptive effectiveness may be reduced when hormonal contraceptives are co-administered with antibiotics, anticonvulsants, and other drugs that increase the metabolism of contraceptive steroids. This could result in unintended pregnancy or breakthrough bleeding).
No products indexed under this heading.

Cefoperazone Sodium (Contraceptive effectiveness may be reduced when hormonal contraceptives are co-administered with antibiotics, anticonvulsants, and other drugs that increase the metabolism of contraceptive steroids. This could result in unintended pregnancy or breakthrough bleeding).
No products indexed under this heading.

Ceforanide (Contraceptive effectiveness may be reduced when hormonal contraceptives are co-administered with antibiotics, anticonvulsants, and other drugs that increase the metabolism of contraceptive steroids. This could result in unintended pregnancy or breakthrough bleeding).
No products indexed under this heading.

Cefotaxime Sodium (Contraceptive effectiveness may be reduced when hormonal contraceptives are co-administered with antibiotics, anticonvulsants, and other drugs that increase the metabolism of contraceptive steroids. This could result in unintended pregnancy or breakthrough bleeding).
No products indexed under this heading.

Cefotetan (Contraceptive effectiveness may be reduced when hormonal contraceptives are co-administered with antibiotics, anticonvulsants, and other drugs that increase the metabolism of contraceptive steroids. This could result in unintended pregnancy or breakthrough bleeding).
No products indexed under this heading.

Cefoxitin Sodium (Contraceptive effectiveness may be reduced when hormonal contraceptives are co-administered with antibiotics, anticonvulsants, and other drugs that increase the metabolism of contraceptive steroids. This could result in unintended pregnancy or breakthrough bleeding).
No products indexed under this heading.

Cefpodoxime Proxetil (Contraceptive effectiveness may be reduced when hormonal contraceptives are co-administered with antibiotics, anticonvulsants, and other drugs that increase the metabolism of contraceptive steroids. This could result in unintended pregnancy or breakthrough bleeding).
No products indexed under this heading.

Cefprozil (Contraceptive effectiveness may be reduced when hormonal contraceptives are co-administered with antibiotics, anticonvulsants, and other drugs that increase the metabolism of contraceptive steroids. This could result in unintended pregnancy or breakthrough bleeding).
No products indexed under this heading.

Ceftazidime (Contraceptive effectiveness may be reduced when hormonal contraceptives are co-administered with antibiotics, anticonvulsants, and other drugs that increase the metabolism of

contraceptive steroids. This could result in unintended pregnancy or breakthrough bleeding). Products include:

Ceftizoxime Sodium (Contraceptive effectiveness may be reduced when hormonal contraceptives are co-administered with antibiotics, anticonvulsants, and other drugs that increase the metabolism of contraceptive steroids. This could result in unintended pregnancy or breakthrough bleeding).
No products indexed under this heading.

Ceftriaxone Sodium (Contraceptive effectiveness may be reduced when hormonal contraceptives are co-administered with antibiotics, anticonvulsants, and other drugs that increase the metabolism of contraceptive steroids. This could result in unintended pregnancy or breakthrough bleeding). Products include:

Cefuroxime Axetil (Contraceptive effectiveness may be reduced when hormonal contraceptives are co-administered with antibiotics, anticonvulsants, and other drugs that increase the metabolism of contraceptive steroids. This could result in unintended pregnancy or breakthrough bleeding). Products include:

Cefuroxime Sodium (Contraceptive effectiveness may be reduced when hormonal contraceptives are co-administered with antibiotics, anticonvulsants, and other drugs that increase the metabolism of contraceptive steroids. This could result in unintended pregnancy or breakthrough bleeding).
No products indexed under this heading.

Cephalexin (Contraceptive effectiveness may be reduced when hormonal contraceptives are co-administered with antibiotics, anticonvulsants, and other drugs that increase the metabolism of contraceptive steroids. This could result in unintended pregnancy or breakthrough bleeding).
No products indexed under this heading.

Cephalothin Sodium (Contraceptive effectiveness may be reduced when hormonal contraceptives are co-administered with antibiotics, anticonvulsants, and other drugs that increase the metabolism of contraceptive steroids. This could result in unintended pregnancy or breakthrough bleeding).
No products indexed under this heading.

Cephapirin Sodium (Contraceptive effectiveness may be reduced when hormonal contraceptives are co-administered with antibiotics, anticonvulsants, and other drugs that increase the metabolism of contraceptive steroids. This could result in unintended pregnancy or breakthrough bleeding).
No products indexed under this heading.

Cephradine (Contraceptive effectiveness may be reduced when hormonal contraceptives are co-administered with antibiotics, anticonvulsants, and other drugs that increase the metabolism of contraceptive steroids. This could result in unintended pregnancy or breakthrough bleeding).
No products indexed under this heading.

Chloramphenicol (Contraceptive effectiveness may be reduced when hormonal contraceptives are co-administered with antibiotics, anticonvulsants, and other drugs that increase the metabolism of contraceptive steroids. This could result in unintended pregnancy or breakthrough bleeding).
No products indexed under this heading.

Chloramphenicol Palmitate (Contraceptive effectiveness may be reduced when hormonal contraceptives are co-administered with antibiotics, anticonvulsants, and other drugs that increase the metabolism of contraceptive steroids. This could result in unintended pregnancy or breakthrough bleeding).
No products indexed under this heading.

Chloramphenicol Sodium Succinate (Contraceptive effectiveness may be reduced when hormonal contraceptives are co-administered with antibiotics, anticonvulsants, and other drugs that increase the metabolism of contraceptive steroids. This could result in unintended pregnancy or breakthrough bleeding).
No products indexed under this heading.

Chlorpropamide (Contraceptive effectiveness may be reduced when hormonal contraceptives are co-administered with antibiotics, anticonvulsants, and other drugs that increase the metabolism of contraceptive steroids. This could result in unintended pregnancy or breakthrough bleeding).
No products indexed under this heading.

Cilastatin Sodium (Contraceptive effectiveness may be reduced when hormonal contraceptives are co-administered with antibiotics, anticonvulsants, and other drugs that increase the metabolism of contraceptive steroids. This could result in unintended pregnancy or breakthrough bleeding). Products include:

Cimetidine (CYP3A4 inhibitors such as itraconazole or ketoconazole may increase plasma hormone levels).
No products indexed under this heading.

Cimetidine Hydrochloride (CYP3A4 inhibitors such as itraconazole or ketoconazole may increase plasma hormone levels).
No products indexed under this heading.

Ciprofloxacin (Contraceptive effectiveness may be reduced when hormonal contraceptives are co-administered with antibiotics, anticonvulsants, and other drugs that increase the metabolism of contraceptive steroids. This could result in unintended pregnancy or breakthrough bleeding). Products include:

Ciprofloxacin Hydrochloride (Contraceptive effectiveness may be reduced when hormonal contraceptives are co-administered with antibiotics, anticonvulsants, and other drugs that increase the metabolism of contraceptive steroids. This could result in unintended pregnancy or breakthrough bleeding). Products include:

Cisplatin (Contraceptive effectiveness may be reduced when hormonal contraceptives are co-administered with antibiotics, anticonvulsants, and other drugs that increase the metabolism of contraceptive steroids. This could result in unintended pregnancy or breakthrough bleeding).
No products indexed under this heading.

Citalopram Hydrobromide (Contraceptive effectiveness may be reduced when hormonal contraceptives are co-administered with antibiotics, anticonvulsants, and other drugs that increase the metabolism of contraceptive steroids. This could result in unintended pregnancy or breakthrough bleeding). Products include:

Clarithromycin (Contraceptive effectiveness may be reduced when hormonal contraceptives are co-administered with antibiotics, anticonvulsants, and other drugs that increase the metabolism of contraceptive steroids. This could result in unintended pregnancy or breakthrough bleeding). Products include:

Clofibric Acid (Increased clearance of clofibric acid, due to induction of conjugation, has been noted when concomitantly administered with oral contraceptives).
No products indexed under this heading.

Clotrimazole (Contraceptive effectiveness may be reduced when hormonal contraceptives are co-administered with antibiotics, anticonvulsants, and other drugs that increase the metabolism of contraceptive steroids. This could result in unintended pregnancy or breakthrough bleeding). Products include:

Cloxacillin (Contraceptive effectiveness may be reduced when hormonal contraceptives are co-administered with antibiotics, anticonvulsants, and other drugs that increase the metabolism of contraceptive steroids. This could result in unintended pregnancy or breakthrough bleeding).
No products indexed under this heading.

Cloxacillin Sodium (Contraceptive effectiveness may be reduced when hormonal contraceptives are co-administered with antibiotics, anticonvulsants, and other drugs that increase the metabolism of contraceptive steroids. This could result in unintended pregnancy or breakthrough bleeding).
No products indexed under this heading.

Cloxacillin Sodium Monohydrate (Contraceptive effectiveness may be reduced when hormonal contraceptives are co-administered with antibiotics, anticonvulsants, and other drugs that increase the metabolism of contraceptive steroids. This could result in unintended pregnancy or breakthrough bleeding).
No products indexed under this heading.

Conivaptan Hydrochloride (CYP3A4 inhibitors such as itraconazole or ketoconazole may increase plasma hormone levels). Products include:

Cortisone Acetate (Contraceptive effectiveness may be reduced when hormonal contraceptives are co-administered with antibiotics, anticonvulsants, and other drugs that increase the metabolism of contraceptive steroids. This could result in unintended pregnancy or breakthrough bleeding).
No products indexed under this heading.

Cyclosporine (Combination hormonal contraceptives containing some synthetic estrogens (eg, ethinyl estradiol) may inhibit the metabolism of other compounds. Increased plasma concentrations of cyclosporine has been reported with concomitant administration of oral contraceptives). Products include:

Dalfopristin (CYP3A4 inhibitors such as itraconazole or ketoconazole may increase plasma hormone levels).
No products indexed under this heading.

Danazol (CYP3A4 inhibitors such as itraconazole or ketoconazole may increase plasma hormone levels).
No products indexed under this heading.

Darunavir (Several of the anti-HIV protease inhibitors have been studied with co-administration of oral combination

hormonal contraceptives; significant changes (increase and decrease) in the plasma levels of the estrogen and progestin have been noted in some cases. The safety and efficacy of oral contraceptive products may be affected with co-administration of anti-HIV protease inhibitors).

No products indexed under this heading.

Dasatinib (CYP3A4 inhibitors such as itraconazole or ketoconazole may increase plasma hormone levels).

No products indexed under this heading.

Daunorubicin Hydrochloride (Contraceptive effectiveness may be reduced when hormonal contraceptives are co-administered with antibiotics, anticonvulsants, and other drugs that increase the metabolism of contraceptive steroids. This could result in unintended pregnancy or breakthrough bleeding).

No products indexed under this heading.

Delavirdine Mesylate (CYP3A4 inhibitors such as itraconazole or ketoconazole may increase plasma hormone levels).

No products indexed under this heading.

Delavirine (CYP3A4 inhibitors such as itraconazole or ketoconazole may increase plasma hormone levels).

No products indexed under this heading.

Demeclocycline Hydrochloride (Several cases of contraceptive failure and breakthrough bleeding have been reported in the literature with concomitant administration of antibiotics such as ampicillin and tetracyclines. However, clinical pharmacology studies investigating drug interaction between combined oral contraceptives and these antibiotics have reported inconsistent results).

No products indexed under this heading.

Desloratadine (CYP3A4 inhibitors such as itraconazole or ketoconazole may increase plasma hormone levels). Products include:

Dexamethasone (Contraceptive effectiveness may be reduced when hormonal contraceptives are co-administered with antibiotics, anticonvulsants, and other drugs that increase the metabolism of contraceptive steroids. This could result in unintended pregnancy or breakthrough bleeding). Products include:

Dexamethasone Acetate (Contraceptive effectiveness may be reduced when hormonal contraceptives are co-administered with antibiotics, anticonvulsants, and other drugs that increase the metabolism of contraceptive steroids. This could result in unintended pregnancy or breakthrough bleeding).

No products indexed under this heading.

Dexamethasone Phosphate (Contraceptive effectiveness may be reduced when hormonal contraceptives are co-administered with antibiotics, anticonvulsants, and other drugs that increase the metabolism of contraceptive steroids. This could result in unintended pregnancy or breakthrough bleeding).

No products indexed under this heading.

Dexamethasone Sodium (Contraceptive effectiveness may be reduced when hormonal contraceptives are co-administered with antibiotics, anticonvulsants, and other drugs that increase the metabolism of contraceptive steroids. This could result in unintended pregnancy or breakthrough bleeding).

No products indexed under this heading.

Dexamethasone Sodium Phosphate (Contraceptive effectiveness may be reduced when hormonal contraceptives are co-administered with antibiotics, anticonvulsants, and other drugs that increase the metabolism of contraceptive steroids. This could result in unintended pregnancy or breakthrough bleeding).

No products indexed under this heading.

Dicloxacillin (Contraceptive effectiveness may be reduced when hormonal contraceptives are co-administered with antibiotics, anticonvulsants, and other drugs that increase the metabolism of contraceptive steroids. This could result in unintended pregnancy or breakthrough bleeding).

No products indexed under this heading.

Dicloxacillin Sodium (Contraceptive effectiveness may be reduced when hormonal contraceptives are co-administered with antibiotics, anticonvulsants, and other drugs that increase the metabolism of contraceptive steroids. This could result in unintended pregnancy or breakthrough bleeding).

No products indexed under this heading.

Diltiazem Hydrochloride (CYP3A4 inhibitors such as itraconazole or ketoconazole may increase plasma hormone levels). Products include:

Diltiazem Maleate (CYP3A4 inhibitors such as itraconazole or ketoconazole may increase plasma hormone levels).

No products indexed under this heading.

Dirithromycin (Contraceptive effectiveness may be reduced when hormonal contraceptives are co-administered with antibiotics, anticonvulsants, and other drugs that increase the metabolism of contraceptive steroids. This could result in unintended pregnancy or breakthrough bleeding).

No products indexed under this heading.

Disodium Carbenicillin (Contraceptive effectiveness may be reduced when hormonal contraceptives are co-administered with antibiotics, anticonvulsants, and other drugs that increase the metabolism of contraceptive steroids. This could result in unintended pregnancy or breakthrough bleeding).

No products indexed under this heading.

Divalproex Sodium (Contraceptive effectiveness may be reduced when hormonal contraceptives are co-administered with antibiotics, anticonvulsants, and other drugs that increase the metabolism of contraceptive steroids. This could result in unintended pregnancy or breakthrough bleeding). Products include:

Doxorubicin Hydrochloride (Contraceptive effectiveness may be reduced when hormonal contraceptives are co-administered with antibiotics, anticonvulsants, and other drugs that increase the metabolism of contraceptive steroids. This could result in unintended pregnancy or breakthrough bleeding).

No products indexed under this heading.

Doxycycline (Several cases of contraceptive failure and breakthrough bleeding have been reported in the literature with concomitant administration of antibiotics such as ampicillin and tetracyclines. However, clinical pharmacology studies investigating drug interaction between combined oral contraceptives and these antibiotics have reported inconsistent results).

No products indexed under this heading.

Doxycycline Calcium (Several cases of contraceptive failure and breakthrough bleeding have been reported in the literature with concomitant administration of antibiotics such as ampicillin and tetracyclines. However, clinical pharmacology studies investigating drug interaction between combined oral contraceptives and these antibiotics have reported inconsistent results).

No products indexed under this heading.

Doxycycline Hyclate (Several cases of contraceptive failure and breakthrough bleeding have been reported in the literature with concomitant administration of antibiotics such as ampicillin and tetracyclines. However, clinical pharmacology studies investigating drug interaction between combined oral contraceptives and these antibiotics have reported inconsistent results).

No products indexed under this heading.

Doxycycline Monohydrate (Several cases of contraceptive failure and breakthrough bleeding have been reported in the literature with concomitant administration of antibiotics such as ampicillin and tetracyclines. However, clinical pharmacology studies investigating drug interaction between combined oral contraceptives and these antibiotics have reported inconsistent results).

No products indexed under this heading.

Efavirenz (CYP3A4 inhibitors such as itraconazole or ketoconazole may increase plasma hormone levels). Products include:

Enoxacin (Contraceptive effectiveness may be reduced when hormonal contraceptives are co-administered with antibiotics, anticonvulsants, and other drugs that increase the metabolism of contraceptive steroids. This could result in unintended pregnancy or breakthrough bleeding).

No products indexed under this heading.

Epirubicin Hydrochloride (Contraceptive effectiveness may be reduced when hormonal contraceptives are co-administered with antibiotics, anticonvulsants, and other drugs that increase the metabolism of contraceptive steroids. This could result in unintended pregnancy or breakthrough bleeding).

No products indexed under this heading.

Erythromycin (Contraceptive effectiveness may be reduced when hormonal contraceptives are co-administered with antibiotics, anticonvulsants, and other drugs that increase the metabolism of contraceptive steroids. This could result in unintended pregnancy or breakthrough bleeding).

No products indexed under this heading.

Erythromycin, Topical (Contraceptive effectiveness may be reduced when hormonal contraceptives are co-administered with antibiotics, anticonvulsants, and other drugs that increase the metabolism of contraceptive steroids. This could result in unintended pregnancy or breakthrough bleeding).

No products indexed under this heading.

Erythromycin Estolate (Contraceptive effectiveness may be reduced when hormonal contraceptives are co-administered with antibiotics, anticonvulsants, and other drugs that increase the metabolism of contraceptive steroids. This could result in unintended pregnancy or breakthrough bleeding).

No products indexed under this heading.

Erythromycin Ethylsuccinate (Contraceptive effectiveness may be reduced when hormonal contraceptives are co-administered with antibiotics, anticonvulsants, and other drugs that increase the metabolism of contraceptive steroids. This could result in unintended pregnancy or breakthrough bleeding). Products include:

Erythromycin Gluceptate (Contraceptive effectiveness may be reduced when hormonal contraceptives are co-administered with antibiotics, anticonvulsants, and other drugs that increase the metabolism of contraceptive steroids. This could result in unintended pregnancy or breakthrough bleeding).

No products indexed under this heading.

Erythromycin Lactobionate (Contraceptive effectiveness may be reduced when hormonal contraceptives are co-administered with antibiotics, anticonvulsants, and other drugs that increase the metabolism of contraceptive steroids. This could result in unintended pregnancy or breakthrough bleeding).

No products indexed under this heading.

Erythromycin Stearate (Contraceptive effectiveness may be reduced when hormonal contraceptives are co-administered with antibiotics, anticonvulsants, and other drugs that increase the metabolism of contraceptive steroids. This could result in unintended pregnancy or breakthrough bleeding).

No products indexed under this heading.

Escitalopram Oxalate (Contraceptive effectiveness may be reduced when hormonal contraceptives are co-administered with antibiotics, anticonvulsants, and other drugs that increase the metabolism of contraceptive steroids. This could result in unintended pregnancy or breakthrough bleeding). Products include:

Esomeprazole Magnesium (CYP3A4 inhibitors such as itraconazole or ketoconazole may increase plasma hormone levels). Products include:

Esomeprazole Sodium (CYP3A4 inhibitors such as itraconazole or ketoconazole may increase plasma hormone levels). Products include:

Ethanol (Contraceptive effectiveness may be reduced when hormonal contraceptives are co-administered with antibiotics, anticonvulsants, and other drugs that increase the metabolism of contraceptive steroids. This could result in unintended pregnancy or breakthrough bleeding).

No products indexed under this heading.

Ethosuximide (Contraceptive effectiveness may be reduced when hormonal contraceptives are co-administered with antibiotics, anticonvulsants, and other drugs that increase the metabolism of contraceptive steroids. This could result in unintended pregnancy or breakthrough bleeding).

No products indexed under this heading.

IMPORTANT NOTE: Always consult each drug listing in the patient's regimen for possible interactions.

Ethotoin (Contraceptive effectiveness may be reduced when hormonal contraceptives are co-administered with antibiotics, anticonvulsants, and other drugs that increase the metabolism of contraceptive steroids. This could result in unintended pregnancy or breakthrough bleeding).
No products indexed under this heading.

Ethyl Alcohol (Contraceptive effectiveness may be reduced when hormonal contraceptives are co-administered with antibiotics, anticonvulsants, and other drugs that increase the metabolism of contraceptive steroids. This could result in unintended pregnancy or breakthrough bleeding).
No products indexed under this heading.

Felbamate (Contraceptive effectiveness may be reduced when hormonal contraceptives are co-administered with felbamate. This could result in unintended pregnancy or breakthrough bleeding).
No products indexed under this heading.

Fluconazole (CYP3A4 inhibitors such as itraconazole or ketoconazole may increase plasma hormone levels).
No products indexed under this heading.

Fludrocortisone Acetate (Contraceptive effectiveness may be reduced when hormonal contraceptives are co-administered with antibiotics, anticonvulsants, and other drugs that increase the metabolism of contraceptive steroids. This could result in unintended pregnancy or breakthrough bleeding).
No products indexed under this heading.

Fluoxetine (CYP3A4 inhibitors such as itraconazole or ketoconazole may increase plasma hormone levels).
No products indexed under this heading.

Fluoxetine Hydrochloride (CYP3A4 inhibitors such as itraconazole or ketoconazole may increase plasma hormone levels). Products include:
Prozac Weekly 1941
Prozac Pulvules 1941
Symbyax 1965

Fluvoxamine (Contraceptive effectiveness may be reduced when hormonal contraceptives are co-administered with antibiotics, anticonvulsants, and other drugs that increase the metabolism of contraceptive steroids. This could result in unintended pregnancy or breakthrough bleeding).
No products indexed under this heading.

Fluvoxamine Maleate (CYP3A4 inhibitors such as itraconazole or ketoconazole may increase plasma hormone levels).
No products indexed under this heading.

Fosamprenavir Calcium (Several of the anti-HIV protease inhibitors have been studied with co-administration of oral combination hormonal contraceptives; significant changes (increase and decrease) in the plasma levels of the estrogen and progestin have been noted in some cases. The safety and efficacy of oral contraceptive products may be affected with co-administration of anti-HIV protease inhibitors). Products include:
Lexiva Oral Suspension 1558
Lexiva 1558

Fosphenytoin (Contraceptive effectiveness may be reduced when hormonal contraceptives are co-administered with phenytoin. This could result in unintended pregnancy or breakthrough bleeding).
No products indexed under this heading.

Fosphenytoin Sodium (Contraceptive effectiveness may be reduced when hormonal contraceptives are co-administered with phenytoin. This could result in unintended pregnancy or breakthrough bleeding).
No products indexed under this heading.

Gabapentin (Contraceptive effectiveness may be reduced when hormonal contraceptives are co-administered with antibiotics, anticonvulsants, and other drugs that increase the metabolism of contraceptive steroids. This could result in unintended pregnancy or breakthrough bleeding).
No products indexed under this heading.

Garlic Extract (Contraceptive effectiveness may be reduced when hormonal contraceptives are co-administered with antibiotics, anticonvulsants, and other drugs that increase the metabolism of contraceptive steroids. This could result in unintended pregnancy or breakthrough bleeding).
No products indexed under this heading.

Garlic Oil (Contraceptive effectiveness may be reduced when hormonal contraceptives are co-administered with antibiotics, anticonvulsants, and other drugs that increase the metabolism of contraceptive steroids. This could result in unintended pregnancy or breakthrough bleeding).
No products indexed under this heading.

Gatifloxacin (Contraceptive effectiveness may be reduced when hormonal contraceptives are co-administered with antibiotics, anticonvulsants, and other drugs that increase the metabolism of contraceptive steroids. This could result in unintended pregnancy or breakthrough bleeding).
No products indexed under this heading.

Gemifloxacin Mesylate (Contraceptive effectiveness may be reduced when hormonal contraceptives are co-administered with antibiotics, anticonvulsants, and other drugs that increase the metabolism of contraceptive steroids. This could result in unintended pregnancy or breakthrough bleeding).
No products indexed under this heading.

Gentamicin Sulfate (Contraceptive effectiveness may be reduced when hormonal contraceptives are co-administered with antibiotics, anticonvulsants, and other drugs that increase the metabolism of contraceptive steroids. This could result in unintended pregnancy or breakthrough bleeding). Products include:
Pred-G .... ☉ 226, ☉ 227

Glipizide (Contraceptive effectiveness may be reduced when hormonal contraceptives are co-administered with antibiotics, anticonvulsants, and other drugs that increase the metabolism of contraceptive steroids. This could result in unintended pregnancy or breakthrough bleeding).
No products indexed under this heading.

Glyburide (Contraceptive effectiveness may be reduced when hormonal contraceptives are co-administered with antibiotics, anticonvulsants, and other drugs that increase the metabolism of contraceptive steroids. This could result in unintended pregnancy or breakthrough bleeding).
No products indexed under this heading.

Grepafloxacin Hydrochloride (Contraceptive effectiveness may be reduced when hormonal contraceptives are co-administered with antibiotics, anticonvulsants, and other drugs that increase the metabolism of contraceptive steroids. This could result in unintended pregnancy or breakthrough bleeding).
No products indexed under this heading.

Griseofulvin (Contraceptive effectiveness may be reduced when hormonal contraceptives are co-administered with griseofulvin. This could result in unintended pregnancy or breakthrough bleeding).
No products indexed under this heading.

Hepatic Enzyme-Inducing Agents (Contraceptive effectiveness may be reduced when hormonal contraceptives are co-administered with antibiotics, anticonvulsants, and other drugs that increase the metabolism of contraceptive steroids. This could result in unintended pregnancy or breakthrough bleeding).
No products indexed under this heading.

Hexobarbital (Contraceptive effectiveness may be reduced when hormonal contraceptives are co-administered with barbiturates. This could result in unintended pregnancy or breakthrough bleeding).
No products indexed under this heading.

Hydrocortisone (Alcohol) (Contraceptive effectiveness may be reduced when hormonal contraceptives are co-administered with antibiotics, anticonvulsants, and other drugs that increase the metabolism of contraceptive steroids. This could result in unintended pregnancy or breakthrough bleeding).
No products indexed under this heading.

Hydrocortisone Acetate (Contraceptive effectiveness may be reduced when hormonal contraceptives are co-administered with antibiotics, anticonvulsants, and other drugs that increase the metabolism of contraceptive steroids. This could result in unintended pregnancy or breakthrough bleeding).
No products indexed under this heading.

Hydrocortisone Butyrate (Contraceptive effectiveness may be reduced when hormonal contraceptives are co-administered with antibiotics, anticonvulsants, and other drugs that increase the metabolism of contraceptive steroids. This could result in unintended pregnancy or breakthrough bleeding).
No products indexed under this heading.

Hydrocortisone Cypionate (Contraceptive effectiveness may be reduced when hormonal contraceptives are co-administered with antibiotics, anticonvulsants, and other drugs that increase the metabolism of contraceptive steroids. This could result in unintended pregnancy or breakthrough bleeding).
No products indexed under this heading.

Hydrocortisone Hemisuccinate (Contraceptive effectiveness may be reduced when hormonal contraceptives are co-administered with antibiotics, anticonvulsants, and other drugs that increase the metabolism of contraceptive steroids. This could result in unintended pregnancy or breakthrough bleeding).
No products indexed under this heading.

Hydrocortisone Probutate (Contraceptive effectiveness may be reduced when hormonal contraceptives are co-administered with antibiotics, anticonvulsants, and other drugs that increase the metabolism of contraceptive steroids. This could result in unintended pregnancy or breakthrough bleeding).
No products indexed under this heading.

Hydrocortisone Sodium Phosphate (Contraceptive effectiveness may be reduced when hormonal contraceptives are co-administered with antibiotics, anticonvulsants, and other drugs that increase the metabolism of contraceptive steroids. This could result in unintended pregnancy or breakthrough bleeding).
No products indexed under this heading.

Hydrocortisone Sodium Succinate (Contraceptive effectiveness may be reduced when hormonal contraceptives are co-administered with antibiotics, anticonvulsants, and other drugs that increase the metabolism of contraceptive steroids. This could result in unintended pregnancy or breakthrough bleeding).
No products indexed under this heading.

Hydrocortisone Valerate (Contraceptive effectiveness may be reduced when hormonal contraceptives are co-administered with antibiotics, anticonvulsants, and other drugs that increase the metabolism of contraceptive steroids. This could result in unintended pregnancy or breakthrough bleeding).
No products indexed under this heading.

Hypericum (Contraceptive effectiveness may be reduced when hormonal contraceptives are co-administered with antibiotics, anticonvulsants, and other drugs that increase the metabolism of contraceptive steroids. This could result in unintended pregnancy or breakthrough bleeding).
No products indexed under this heading.

Hypericum Perforatum (Herbal products containing St. John's Wort (hypericum perforatum) may induce hepatic enzymes (cytochrome P450) and p-glycoprotein transporter and may reduce the effectiveness of contraceptive steroids. This may also result in breakthrough bleeding). Products include:
Traumeel 1800

Idarubicin Hydrochloride (Contraceptive effectiveness may be reduced when hormonal contraceptives are co-administered with antibiotics, anticonvulsants, and other drugs that increase the metabolism of contraceptive steroids. This could result in unintended pregnancy or breakthrough bleeding).
No products indexed under this heading.

Imatinib Mesylate (CYP3A4 inhibitors such as itraconazole or ketoconazole may increase plasma hormone levels). Products include:
Gleevec 2477

Imipenem (Contraceptive effectiveness may be reduced when hormonal contraceptives are co-administered with antibiotics, anticonvulsants, and other drugs that increase the metabolism of contraceptive steroids. This could result in unintended pregnancy or breakthrough bleeding). Products include:
Primaxin I.M. 2232
Primaxin I.V. 2235

Indinavir Sulfate (Several of the anti-HIV protease inhibitors have been studied with co-administration of oral combination hormonal contraceptives; significant changes (increase and decrease) in the plasma levels of the estrogen and progestin have been noted in some cases. The safety and efficacy of oral contraceptive products may be affected with co-administration of anti-HIV protease inhibitors). Products include:
Crixivan 2113

Insulin (Contraceptive effectiveness may be reduced when hormonal contraceptives are co-administered with antibiotics, anticonvulsants, and other drugs that increase the metabolism of contraceptive steroids. This could result in unintended pregnancy or breakthrough bleeding).
No products indexed under this heading.

Insulin, Human, Zinc Suspension (Contraceptive effectiveness may be reduced when hormonal contraceptives are co-administered with antibiotics, anticonvulsants, and other drugs that increase the metabolism of contraceptive steroids. This could result in unintended pregnancy or breakthrough bleeding).
No products indexed under this heading.

Insulin, Human (rDNA origin) (Contraceptive effectiveness may be reduced when hormonal contraceptives are co-administered with antibiotics, anticonvulsants, and other drugs that increase the metabolism of contracep-

1335 Interactions Index Ortho Tri-Cyclen Lo

tive steroids. This could result in unintended pregnancy or breakthrough bleeding). Products include:
Exubera ... 2717

Insulin, Human NPH (Contraceptive effectiveness may be reduced when hormonal contraceptives are co-administered with antibiotics, anticonvulsants, and other drugs that increase the metabolism of contraceptive steroids. This could result in unintended pregnancy or breakthrough bleeding). Products include:
Humulin N Vial ... 1934

Insulin, Human Regular (Contraceptive effectiveness may be reduced when hormonal contraceptives are co-administered with antibiotics, anticonvulsants, and other drugs that increase the metabolism of contraceptive steroids. This could result in unintended pregnancy or breakthrough bleeding). Products include:
Humulin R ... 1937
Humulin R (U-500) ... 1939

Insulin, Human Regular and Human NPH Mixture (Contraceptive effectiveness may be reduced when hormonal contraceptives are co-administered with antibiotics, anticonvulsants, and other drugs that increase the metabolism of contraceptive steroids. This could result in unintended pregnancy or breakthrough bleeding). Products include:
Humulin 50/50 ... 1930
Humulin 70/30 Vial ... 1931

Insulin, NPH (Contraceptive effectiveness may be reduced when hormonal contraceptives are co-administered with antibiotics, anticonvulsants, and other drugs that increase the metabolism of contraceptive steroids. This could result in unintended pregnancy or breakthrough bleeding).
No products indexed under this heading.

Insulin, Regular (Contraceptive effectiveness may be reduced when hormonal contraceptives are co-administered with antibiotics, anticonvulsants, and other drugs that increase the metabolism of contraceptive steroids. This could result in unintended pregnancy or breakthrough bleeding).
No products indexed under this heading.

Insulin, Regular and NPH mixture (Contraceptive effectiveness may be reduced when hormonal contraceptives are co-administered with antibiotics, anticonvulsants, and other drugs that increase the metabolism of contraceptive steroids. This could result in unintended pregnancy or breakthrough bleeding).
No products indexed under this heading.

Insulin, Zinc Crystals (Contraceptive effectiveness may be reduced when hormonal contraceptives are co-administered with antibiotics, anticonvulsants, and other drugs that increase the metabolism of contraceptive steroids. This could result in unintended pregnancy or breakthrough bleeding).
No products indexed under this heading.

Insulin, Zinc Suspension (Contraceptive effectiveness may be reduced when hormonal contraceptives are co-administered with antibiotics, anticonvulsants, and other drugs that increase the metabolism of contraceptive steroids. This could result in unintended pregnancy or breakthrough bleeding).
No products indexed under this heading.

Insulin Aspart (Contraceptive effectiveness may be reduced when hormonal contraceptives are co-administered with antibiotics, anticonvulsants, and other drugs that increase the metabolism of contraceptive steroids. This could result in unintended pregnancy or breakthrough bleeding).
No products indexed under this heading.

Insulin Aspart, Human (Contraceptive effectiveness may be reduced when hormonal contraceptives are co-administered with antibiotics, anticonvulsants, and other drugs that increase the metabolism of contraceptive steroids. This could result in unintended pregnancy or breakthrough bleeding). Products include:
NovoLog Mix 70/30 ... 2581

Insulin Aspart, Human Regular (Contraceptive effectiveness may be reduced when hormonal contraceptives are co-administered with antibiotics, anticonvulsants, and other drugs that increase the metabolism of contraceptive steroids. This could result in unintended pregnancy or breakthrough bleeding). Products include:
NovoLog ... 2575

Insulin Aspart Protamine, Human (Contraceptive effectiveness may be reduced when hormonal contraceptives are co-administered with antibiotics, anticonvulsants, and other drugs that increase the metabolism of contraceptive steroids. This could result in unintended pregnancy or breakthrough bleeding). Products include:
NovoLog Mix 70/30 ... 2581

Insulin Detemir (rDNA Origin) (Contraceptive effectiveness may be reduced when hormonal contraceptives are co-administered with antibiotics, anticonvulsants, and other drugs that increase the metabolism of contraceptive steroids. This could result in unintended pregnancy or breakthrough bleeding). Products include:
Levemir ... 2566

Insulin Glargine (Contraceptive effectiveness may be reduced when hormonal contraceptives are co-administered with antibiotics, anticonvulsants, and other drugs that increase the metabolism of contraceptive steroids. This could result in unintended pregnancy or breakthrough bleeding). Products include:
Lantus ... 2996

Insulin Glulisine (Contraceptive effectiveness may be reduced when hormonal contraceptives are co-administered with antibiotics, anticonvulsants, and other drugs that increase the metabolism of contraceptive steroids. This could result in unintended pregnancy or breakthrough bleeding). Products include:
Apidra ... 2937
Apidra SoloStar ... 2937

Insulin Lispro, Human (Contraceptive effectiveness may be reduced when hormonal contraceptives are co-administered with antibiotics, anticonvulsants, and other drugs that increase the metabolism of contraceptive steroids. This could result in unintended pregnancy or breakthrough bleeding). Products include:
Humalog ... 1910
Humalog Mix ... 1914
Humalog Mix75/25 ... 1917

Insulin Lispro Protamine, Human (Contraceptive effectiveness may be reduced when hormonal contraceptives are co-administered with antibiotics, anticonvulsants, and other drugs that increase the metabolism of contraceptive steroids. This could result in unintended pregnancy or breakthrough bleeding). Products include:
Humalog Mix ... 1914
Humalog Mix75/25 ... 1917

Isoniazid (CYP3A4 inhibitors such as itraconazole or ketoconazole may increase plasma hormone levels).
No products indexed under this heading.

Itraconazole (CYP3A4 inhibitors such as itraconazole or ketoconazole may increase plasma hormone levels).
No products indexed under this heading.

Kanamycin Sulfate (Contraceptive effectiveness may be reduced when hormonal contraceptives are co-administered with antibiotics, anticonvulsants, and other drugs that increase the metabolism of contraceptive steroids. This could result in unintended pregnancy or breakthrough bleeding).
No products indexed under this heading.

Ketoconazole (CYP3A4 inhibitors such as itraconazole or ketoconazole may increase plasma hormone levels). Products include:
Extina ... 3319
Xolegel ... 3337

Lamotrigine (Combined hormonal contraceptives have been shown to significantly decrease plasma concentrations of lamotrigine when co-administered, due to induction of lamotrigine glucuronidation. This may reduce seizure control; therefore, dosage adjustments of lamotrigine may be necessary). Products include:
Lamictal ... 1522
Lamictal ODT ... 1522
Lamictal XR ... 1536

Lansoprazole (Contraceptive effectiveness may be reduced when hormonal contraceptives are co-administered with antibiotics, anticonvulsants, and other drugs that increase the metabolism of contraceptive steroids. This could result in unintended pregnancy or breakthrough bleeding).
No products indexed under this heading.

Lapatinib (CYP3A4 inhibitors such as itraconazole or ketoconazole may increase plasma hormone levels). Products include:
Tykerb ... 1698

Levetiracetam (Contraceptive effectiveness may be reduced when hormonal contraceptives are co-administered with antibiotics, anticonvulsants, and other drugs that increase the metabolism of contraceptive steroids. This could result in unintended pregnancy or breakthrough bleeding). Products include:
Keppra XR ... 3434

Levofloxacin (Contraceptive effectiveness may be reduced when hormonal contraceptives are co-administered with antibiotics, anticonvulsants, and other drugs that increase the metabolism of contraceptive steroids. This could result in unintended pregnancy or breakthrough bleeding). Products include:
Iquix ... 3492
Levaquin ... 2629
Levaquin in 5% Dextrose ... 2629
Quixin ... 3493

Lomefloxacin Hydrochloride (Contraceptive effectiveness may be reduced when hormonal contraceptives are co-administered with antibiotics, anticonvulsants, and other drugs that increase the metabolism of contraceptive steroids. This could result in unintended pregnancy or breakthrough bleeding).
No products indexed under this heading.

Lopinavir (Several of the anti-HIV protease inhibitors have been studied with co-administration of oral combination hormonal contraceptives; significant changes (increase and decrease) in the plasma levels of the estrogen and progestin have been noted in some cases. The safety and efficacy of oral contraceptive products may be affected with co-administration of anti-HIV protease inhibitors). Products include:
Kaletra ... 458

Loracarbef (Contraceptive effectiveness may be reduced when hormonal contraceptives are co-administered with antibiotics, anticonvulsants, and other drugs that increase the metabolism of contraceptive steroids. This could result in unintended pregnancy or breakthrough bleeding).
No products indexed under this heading.

Loratadine (CYP3A4 inhibitors such as itraconazole or ketoconazole may increase plasma hormone levels).
No products indexed under this heading.

Mephenytoin (Contraceptive effectiveness may be reduced when hormonal contraceptives are co-administered with antibiotics, anticonvulsants, and other drugs that increase the metabolism of contraceptive steroids. This could result in unintended pregnancy or breakthrough bleeding).
No products indexed under this heading.

Mephobarbital (Contraceptive effectiveness may be reduced when hormonal contraceptives are co-administered with barbiturates. This could result in unintended pregnancy or breakthrough bleeding).
No products indexed under this heading.

Methacycline Hydrochloride (Several cases of contraceptive failure and breakthrough bleeding have been reported in the literature with concomitant administration of antibiotics such as ampicillin and tetracyclines. However, clinical pharmacology studies investigating drug interaction between combined oral contraceptives and these antibiotics have reported inconsistent results).
No products indexed under this heading.

Methicillin Sodium (Contraceptive effectiveness may be reduced when hormonal contraceptives are co-administered with antibiotics, anticonvulsants, and other drugs that increase the metabolism of contraceptive steroids. This could result in unintended pregnancy or breakthrough bleeding).
No products indexed under this heading.

Methsuximide (Contraceptive effectiveness may be reduced when hormonal contraceptives are co-administered with antibiotics, anticonvulsants, and other drugs that increase the metabolism of contraceptive steroids. This could result in unintended pregnancy or breakthrough bleeding).
No products indexed under this heading.

Methylprednisolone (Contraceptive effectiveness may be reduced when hormonal contraceptives are co-administered with antibiotics, anticonvulsants, and other drugs that increase the metabolism of contraceptive steroids. This could result in unintended pregnancy or breakthrough bleeding).
No products indexed under this heading.

Methylprednisolone Acetate (Contraceptive effectiveness may be reduced when hormonal contraceptives are co-administered with antibiotics, anticonvulsants, and other drugs that increase the metabolism of contraceptive steroids. This could result in unintended pregnancy or breakthrough bleeding).
No products indexed under this heading.

Methylprednisolone Sodium Succinate (Contraceptive effectiveness may be reduced when hormonal contraceptives are co-administered with antibiotics, anticonvulsants, and other drugs that increase the metabolism of contraceptive steroids. This could result in unintended pregnancy or breakthrough bleeding).
No products indexed under this heading.

Metronidazole (CYP3A4 inhibitors such as itraconazole or ketoconazole may increase plasma hormone levels). Products include:

IMPORTANT NOTE: Always consult each drug listing in the patient's regimen for possible interactions.

Ortho Tri-Cyclen Lo Interactions Index 1336

Pylera 793

Metronidazole Benzoate (CYP3A4 inhibitors such as itraconazole or ketoconazole may increase plasma hormone levels).
No products indexed under this heading.

Metronidazole Hydrochloride (CYP3A4 inhibitors such as itraconazole or ketoconazole may increase plasma hormone levels).
No products indexed under this heading.

Metronidazole Sodium (CYP3A4 inhibitors such as itraconazole or ketoconazole may increase plasma hormone levels).
No products indexed under this heading.

Mezlocillin Sodium (Contraceptive effectiveness may be reduced when hormonal contraceptives are co-administered with antibiotics, anticonvulsants, and other drugs that increase the metabolism of contraceptive steroids. This could result in unintended pregnancy or breakthrough bleeding).
No products indexed under this heading.

Miconazole (CYP3A4 inhibitors such as itraconazole or ketoconazole may increase plasma hormone levels).
No products indexed under this heading.

Miconazole Nitrate (CYP3A4 inhibitors such as itraconazole or ketoconazole may increase plasma hormone levels). Products include:
Vusion Ointment 3335

Mifepristone (CYP3A4 inhibitors such as itraconazole or ketoconazole may increase plasma hormone levels).
No products indexed under this heading.

Minocycline Hydrochloride (Several cases of contraceptive failure and breakthrough bleeding have been reported in the literature with concomitant administration of antibiotics such as ampicillin and tetracyclines. However, clinical pharmacology studies investigating drug interaction between combined oral contraceptives and these antibiotics have reported inconsistent results). Products include:
Solodyn 2073

Modafinil (Contraceptive effectiveness may be reduced when hormonal contraceptives are co-administered with antibiotics, anticonvulsants, and other drugs that increase the metabolism of contraceptive steroids. This could result in unintended pregnancy or breakthrough bleeding). Products include:
Provigil 983

Morphine Sulfate (Increased clearance of morphine, due to induction of conjugation, has been noted when concomitantly administered with oral contraceptives). Products include:
Avinza 1822
Embeda 1831
MS Contin 2803

Moxifloxacin Hydrochloride (Contraceptive effectiveness may be reduced when hormonal contraceptives are co-administered with antibiotics, anticonvulsants, and other drugs that increase the metabolism of contraceptive steroids. This could result in unintended pregnancy or breakthrough bleeding). Products include:
Avelox 3064
Vigamox 589

Nafcillin Sodium (Contraceptive effectiveness may be reduced when hormonal contraceptives are co-administered with antibiotics, anticonvulsants, and other drugs that increase the metabolism of contraceptive steroids. This could result in unintended pregnancy or breakthrough bleeding).
No products indexed under this heading.

Nefazodone Hydrochloride (CYP3A4 inhibitors such as itraconazole or ketoconazole may increase plasma hormone levels).
No products indexed under this heading.

Nelfinavir Mesylate (Several of the anti-HIV protease inhibitors have been studied with co-administration of oral combination hormonal contraceptives; significant changes (increase and decrease) in the plasma levels of the estrogen and progestin have been noted in some cases. The safety and efficacy of oral contraceptive products may be affected with co-administration of anti-HIV protease inhibitors).
No products indexed under this heading.

Nevirapine (CYP3A4 inhibitors such as itraconazole or ketoconazole may increase plasma hormone levels). Products include:
Viramune Oral Suspension 897
Viramune Tablets 897

Niacin (CYP3A4 inhibitors such as itraconazole or ketoconazole may increase plasma hormone levels). Products include:
Advicor 402
Cardio Basics 3455
Niaspan 497
Simcor 524

Niacinamide (CYP3A4 inhibitors such as itraconazole or ketoconazole may increase plasma hormone levels). Products include:
CitraNatal 90 DHA Capsules 2332
CitraNatal Assure 2332
CitraNatal Rx 2332
Heplive 607

Niacinamide Hydroiodide (CYP3A4 inhibitors such as itraconazole or ketoconazole may increase plasma hormone levels).
No products indexed under this heading.

Nicotinamide (CYP3A4 inhibitors such as itraconazole or ketoconazole may increase plasma hormone levels).
No products indexed under this heading.

Nicotine (Contraceptive effectiveness may be reduced when hormonal contraceptives are co-administered with antibiotics, anticonvulsants, and other drugs that increase the metabolism of contraceptive steroids. This could result in unintended pregnancy or breakthrough bleeding).
No products indexed under this heading.

Nicotine Polacrilex (Contraceptive effectiveness may be reduced when hormonal contraceptives are co-administered with antibiotics, anticonvulsants, and other drugs that increase the metabolism of contraceptive steroids. This could result in unintended pregnancy or breakthrough bleeding).
No products indexed under this heading.

Nicotine Salicylate (Contraceptive effectiveness may be reduced when hormonal contraceptives are co-administered with antibiotics, anticonvulsants, and other drugs that increase the metabolism of contraceptive steroids. This could result in unintended pregnancy or breakthrough bleeding).
No products indexed under this heading.

Nicotine Sulfate (Contraceptive effectiveness may be reduced when hormonal contraceptives are co-administered with antibiotics, anticonvulsants, and other drugs that increase the metabolism of contraceptive steroids. This could result in unintended pregnancy or breakthrough bleeding).
No products indexed under this heading.

Nifedipine (CYP3A4 inhibitors such as itraconazole or ketoconazole may increase plasma hormone levels).
No products indexed under this heading.

Norethindrone (Contraceptive effectiveness may be reduced when hormonal contraceptives are co-administered with antibiotics, anticonvulsants, and other drugs that increase the metabolism of contraceptive steroids. This could result in unintended pregnancy or breakthrough bleeding). Products include:
Ortho Micronor 2660

Norethindrone Acetate (Contraceptive effectiveness may be reduced when hormonal contraceptives are co-administered with antibiotics, anticonvulsants, and other drugs that increase the metabolism of contraceptive steroids. This could result in unintended pregnancy or breakthrough bleeding). Products include:
Activella 2561

Norfloxacin (Contraceptive effectiveness may be reduced when hormonal contraceptives are co-administered with antibiotics, anticonvulsants, and other drugs that increase the metabolism of contraceptive steroids. This could result in unintended pregnancy or breakthrough bleeding). Products include:
Noroxin 2220

Ofloxacin (Contraceptive effectiveness may be reduced when hormonal contraceptives are co-administered with antibiotics, anticonvulsants, and other drugs that increase the metabolism of contraceptive steroids. This could result in unintended pregnancy or breakthrough bleeding).
No products indexed under this heading.

Omeprazole (CYP3A4 inhibitors such as itraconazole or ketoconazole may increase plasma hormone levels).
No products indexed under this heading.

Omeprazole Magnesium (Contraceptive effectiveness may be reduced when hormonal contraceptives are co-administered with antibiotics, anticonvulsants, and other drugs that increase the metabolism of contraceptive steroids. This could result in unintended pregnancy or breakthrough bleeding).
No products indexed under this heading.

Oxacillin (Contraceptive effectiveness may be reduced when hormonal contraceptives are co-administered with antibiotics, anticonvulsants, and other drugs that increase the metabolism of contraceptive steroids. This could result in unintended pregnancy or breakthrough bleeding).
No products indexed under this heading.

Oxacillin Sodium (Contraceptive effectiveness may be reduced when hormonal contraceptives are co-administered with antibiotics, anticonvulsants, and other drugs that increase the metabolism of contraceptive steroids. This could result in unintended pregnancy or breakthrough bleeding).
No products indexed under this heading.

Oxcarbazepine (Contraceptive effectiveness may be reduced when hormonal contraceptives are co-administered with oxcarbazepine. This could result in unintended pregnancy or breakthrough bleeding).
No products indexed under this heading.

Oxytetracycline (Several cases of contraceptive failure and breakthrough bleeding have been reported in the literature with concomitant administration of antibiotics such as ampicillin and tetracyclines. However, clinical pharmacology studies investigating drug interaction between combined oral contraceptives and these antibiotics have reported inconsistent results).
No products indexed under this heading.

Oxytetracycline Hydrochloride (Several cases of contraceptive failure and breakthrough bleeding have been reported in the literature with concomitant administration of antibiotics such as ampicillin and tetracyclines. However, clinical pharmacology studies investigating drug interaction between combined oral contraceptives and these antibiotics have reported inconsistent results).
No products indexed under this heading.

Paramethadione (Contraceptive effectiveness may be reduced when hormonal contraceptives are co-administered with antibiotics, anticonvulsants, and other drugs that increase the metabolism of contraceptive steroids. This could result in unintended pregnancy or breakthrough bleeding).
No products indexed under this heading.

Paroxetine Hydrochloride (CYP3A4 inhibitors such as itraconazole or ketoconazole may increase plasma hormone levels). Products include:
Paroxetine CR 2361
Paroxetine ER 2371
Paxil 1586
Paxil CR 1596

Penicillin, Potassium Phenoxymethyl (Contraceptive effectiveness may be reduced when hormonal contraceptives are co-administered with antibiotics, anticonvulsants, and other drugs that increase the metabolism of contraceptive steroids. This could result in unintended pregnancy or breakthrough bleeding).
No products indexed under this heading.

Penicillin G Benzathine (Contraceptive effectiveness may be reduced when hormonal contraceptives are co-administered with antibiotics, anticonvulsants, and other drugs that increase the metabolism of contraceptive steroids. This could result in unintended pregnancy or breakthrough bleeding). Products include:
Bicillin C-R Injectable Suspension 1826
Bicillin L-A 1828

Penicillin G Dibenzylethyenediamine (Contraceptive effectiveness may be reduced when hormonal contraceptives are co-administered with antibiotics, anticonvulsants, and other drugs that increase the metabolism of contraceptive steroids. This could result in unintended pregnancy or breakthrough bleeding).
No products indexed under this heading.

Penicillin G Potassium (Contraceptive effectiveness may be reduced when hormonal contraceptives are co-administered with antibiotics, anticonvulsants, and other drugs that increase the metabolism of contraceptive steroids. This could result in unintended pregnancy or breakthrough bleeding).
No products indexed under this heading.

Penicillin G Procaine (Contraceptive effectiveness may be reduced when hormonal contraceptives are co-administered with antibiotics, anticonvulsants, and other drugs that increase the metabolism of contraceptive steroids. This could result in unintended pregnancy or breakthrough bleeding). Products include:
Bicillin C-R Injectable Suspension 1826
Bicillin L-A 1828

Penicillin G Sodium (Contraceptive effectiveness may be reduced when hormonal contraceptives are co-administered with antibiotics, anticonvulsants, and other drugs that increase the metabolism of contraceptive steroids. This could result in unintended pregnancy or breakthrough bleeding).
No products indexed under this heading.

Penicillin V (Contraceptive effectiveness may be reduced when hormonal contraceptives are co-administered with antibiotics, anticonvulsants, and other drugs that increase the metabolism of contraceptive steroids. This could result in unintended pregnancy or breakthrough bleeding).
No products indexed under this heading.

Penicillin V Potassium (Contraceptive effectiveness may be reduced when hormonal contraceptives are co-administered with antibiotics, anticonvulsants, and other drugs that increase the metabolism of contraceptive steroids. This could result in unintended pregnancy or breakthrough bleeding).
No products indexed under this heading.

Penicillins (Contraceptive effectiveness may be reduced when hormonal contraceptives are co-administered with antibiotics, anticonvulsants, and other drugs that increase the metabolism of contraceptive steroids. This could result in unintended pregnancy or breakthrough bleeding).
No products indexed under this heading.

Pentobarbital (Contraceptive effectiveness may be reduced when hormonal contraceptives are co-administered with barbiturates. This could result in unintended pregnancy or breakthrough bleeding).
No products indexed under this heading.

Pentobarbital Sodium (Contraceptive effectiveness may be reduced when hormonal contraceptives are co-administered with barbiturates. This could result in unintended pregnancy or breakthrough bleeding). Products include:
Nembutal 2012

Phenacemide (Contraceptive effectiveness may be reduced when hormonal contraceptives are co-administered with antibiotics, anticonvulsants, and other drugs that increase the metabolism of contraceptive steroids. This could result in unintended pregnancy or breakthrough bleeding).
No products indexed under this heading.

Phenobarbital (Contraceptive effectiveness may be reduced when hormonal contraceptives are co-administered with barbiturates. This could result in unintended pregnancy or breakthrough bleeding). Products include:
Donnatal 2711

Phenobarbital Sodium (Contraceptive effectiveness may be reduced when hormonal contraceptives are co-administered with barbiturates. This could result in unintended pregnancy or breakthrough bleeding).
No products indexed under this heading.

Phensuximide (Contraceptive effectiveness may be reduced when hormonal contraceptives are co-administered with antibiotics, anticonvulsants, and other drugs that increase the metabolism of contraceptive steroids. This could result in unintended pregnancy or breakthrough bleeding).
No products indexed under this heading.

Phenylbutazone (Contraceptive effectiveness may be reduced when hormonal contraceptives are co-administered with phenylbutazone. This could result in unintended pregnancy or breakthrough bleeding).
No products indexed under this heading.

Phenytoin (Contraceptive effectiveness may be reduced when hormonal contraceptives are co-administered with phenytoin. This could result in unintended pregnancy or breakthrough bleeding).
No products indexed under this heading.

Phenytoin Sodium (Contraceptive effectiveness may be reduced when hormonal contraceptives are co-

administered with phenytoin. This could result in unintended pregnancy or breakthrough bleeding). Products include:
Phenytek Capsules 2380

Piperacillin Sodium (Contraceptive effectiveness may be reduced when hormonal contraceptives are co-administered with antibiotics, anticonvulsants, and other drugs that increase the metabolism of contraceptive steroids. This could result in unintended pregnancy or breakthrough bleeding). Products include:
Zosyn 3607

Posaconazole (CYP3A4 inhibitors such as itraconazole or ketoconazole may increase plasma hormone levels). Products include:
Noxafil 3172

Prednisolone (Combination hormonal contraceptives containing some synthetic estrogens (eg, ethinyl estradiol) may inhibit the metabolism of other compounds. Increased plasma concentrations of prednisolone has been reported with concomitant administration of oral contraceptives).
No products indexed under this heading.

Prednisolone Acetate (Combination hormonal contraceptives containing some synthetic estrogens (eg, ethinyl estradiol) may inhibit the metabolism of other compounds. Increased plasma concentrations of prednisolone has been reported with concomitant administration of oral contraceptives). Products include:
Blephamide ....⊙212, ⊙214
Pred Forte ....⊙225
Pred Mild ....⊙230
Pred-G ....⊙226, ⊙227

Prednisolone Sodium Phosphate (Combination hormonal contraceptives containing some synthetic estrogens (eg, ethinyl estradiol) may inhibit the metabolism of other compounds. Increased plasma concentrations of prednisolone has been reported with concomitant administration of oral contraceptives).
No products indexed under this heading.

Prednisolone Tebutate (Combination hormonal contraceptives containing some synthetic estrogens (eg, ethinyl estradiol) may inhibit the metabolism of other compounds. Increased plasma concentrations of prednisolone has been reported with concomitant administration of oral contraceptives).
No products indexed under this heading.

Prednisone (Contraceptive effectiveness may be reduced when hormonal contraceptives are co-administered with antibiotics, anticonvulsants, and other drugs that increase the metabolism of contraceptive steroids. This could result in unintended pregnancy or breakthrough bleeding).
No products indexed under this heading.

Prednisone sodium phosphate (Contraceptive effectiveness may be reduced when hormonal contraceptives are co-administered with antibiotics, anticonvulsants, and other drugs that increase the metabolism of contraceptive steroids. This could result in unintended pregnancy or breakthrough bleeding).
No products indexed under this heading.

Primidone (Contraceptive effectiveness may be reduced when hormonal contraceptives are co-administered with antibiotics, anticonvulsants, and other drugs that increase the metabolism of contraceptive steroids. This could result in unintended pregnancy or breakthrough bleeding).
No products indexed under this heading.

Propoxyphene Hydrochloride (CYP3A4 inhibitors such as itraconazole or ketoconazole may increase plasma hormone levels).
No products indexed under this heading.

Propoxyphene Napsylate (CYP3A4 inhibitors such as itraconazole or ketoconazole may increase plasma hormone levels).
No products indexed under this heading.

Quinidine (CYP3A4 inhibitors such as itraconazole or ketoconazole may increase plasma hormone levels).
No products indexed under this heading.

Quinidine Hydrochloride (CYP3A4 inhibitors such as itraconazole or ketoconazole may increase plasma hormone levels).
No products indexed under this heading.

Quinidine Polygalacturonate (CYP3A4 inhibitors such as itraconazole or ketoconazole may increase plasma hormone levels).
No products indexed under this heading.

Quinidine Sulfate (CYP3A4 inhibitors such as itraconazole or ketoconazole may increase plasma hormone levels).
No products indexed under this heading.

Quinine (CYP3A4 inhibitors such as itraconazole or ketoconazole may increase plasma hormone levels). Products include:
Hyland's Leg Cramps PM with
Quinine 3315

Quinine Sulfate (CYP3A4 inhibitors such as itraconazole or ketoconazole may increase plasma hormone levels).
No products indexed under this heading.

Quinupristin (CYP3A4 inhibitors such as itraconazole or ketoconazole may increase plasma hormone levels).
No products indexed under this heading.

Ranitidine Bismuth Citrate (CYP3A4 inhibitors such as itraconazole or ketoconazole may increase plasma hormone levels).
No products indexed under this heading.

Ranitidine Hydrochloride (CYP3A4 inhibitors such as itraconazole or ketoconazole may increase plasma hormone levels). Products include:
Zantac 1737
Zantac Injection 1732
Zantac Pharmacy 1735

Rifabutin (Contraceptive effectiveness may be reduced when hormonal contraceptives are co-administered with antibiotics, anticonvulsants, and other drugs that increase the metabolism of contraceptive steroids. This could result in unintended pregnancy or breakthrough bleeding).
No products indexed under this heading.

Rifampicin (Contraceptive effectiveness may be reduced when hormonal contraceptives are co-administered with antibiotics, anticonvulsants, and other drugs that increase the metabolism of contraceptive steroids. This could result in unintended pregnancy or breakthrough bleeding).
No products indexed under this heading.

Rifampin (Contraceptive effectiveness may be reduced when hormonal contraceptives are co-administered with rifampin. This could result in unintended pregnancy or breakthrough bleeding).
No products indexed under this heading.

Rifapentine (Contraceptive effectiveness may be reduced when hormonal contraceptives are co-administered with antibiotics, anticonvulsants, and other drugs that increase the metabolism of contraceptive steroids. This could result in unintended pregnancy or breakthrough bleeding).
No products indexed under this heading.

Ritonavir (Several of the anti-HIV protease inhibitors have been studied with

co-administration of oral combination hormonal contraceptives; significant changes (increase and decrease) in the plasma levels of the estrogen and progestin have been noted in some cases. The safety and efficacy of oral contraceptive products may be affected with co-administration of anti-HIV protease inhibitors). Products include:
Kaletra 458
Norvir 509

Rufinamide (Contraceptive effectiveness may be reduced when hormonal contraceptives are co-administered with antibiotics, anticonvulsants, and other drugs that increase the metabolism of contraceptive steroids. This could result in unintended pregnancy or breakthrough bleeding). Products include:
Banzel 1050

Salicylic Acid (Increased clearance of salicylic acid, due to induction of conjugation, has been noted when concomitantly administered with oral contraceptives).
No products indexed under this heading.

Saquinavir (Several of the anti-HIV protease inhibitors have been studied with co-administration of oral combination hormonal contraceptives; significant changes (increase and decrease) in the plasma levels of the estrogen and progestin have been noted in some cases. The safety and efficacy of oral contraceptive products may be affected with co-administration of anti-HIV protease inhibitors).
No products indexed under this heading.

Saquinavir Mesylate (Several of the anti-HIV protease inhibitors have been studied with co-administration of oral combination hormonal contraceptives; significant changes (increase and decrease) in the plasma levels of the estrogen and progestin have been noted in some cases. The safety and efficacy of oral contraceptive products may be affected with co-administration of anti-HIV protease inhibitors).
No products indexed under this heading.

Secobarbital Sodium (Contraceptive effectiveness may be reduced when hormonal contraceptives are co-administered with barbiturates. This could result in unintended pregnancy or breakthrough bleeding).
No products indexed under this heading.

Sertraline Hydrochloride (CYP3A4 inhibitors such as itraconazole or ketoconazole may increase plasma hormone levels).
No products indexed under this heading.

Sildenafil Citrate (CYP3A4 inhibitors such as itraconazole or ketoconazole may increase plasma hormone levels).
No products indexed under this heading.

Sodium Butabarbital (Contraceptive effectiveness may be reduced when hormonal contraceptives are co-administered with barbiturates. This could result in unintended pregnancy or breakthrough bleeding).
No products indexed under this heading.

Sodium Cloxacillin Monohydrate (Contraceptive effectiveness may be reduced when hormonal contraceptives are co-administered with antibiotics, anticonvulsants, and other drugs that increase the metabolism of contraceptive steroids. This could result in unintended pregnancy or breakthrough bleeding).
No products indexed under this heading.

Sodium Pentobarbital (Contraceptive effectiveness may be reduced when hormonal contraceptives are co-administered with barbiturates. This could result in unintended pregnancy or breakthrough bleeding).
No products indexed under this heading.

IMPORTANT NOTE: Always consult each drug listing in the patient's regimen for possible interactions.

Ortho Tri-Cyclen Lo — Interactions Index — 1338

Sparfloxacin (Contraceptive effectiveness may be reduced when hormonal contraceptives are co-administered with antibiotics, anticonvulsants, and other drugs that increase the metabolism of contraceptive steroids. This could result in unintended pregnancy or breakthrough bleeding).
No products indexed under this heading.

Streptomycin Sulfate (Contraceptive effectiveness may be reduced when hormonal contraceptives are co-administered with antibiotics, anticonvulsants, and other drugs that increase the metabolism of contraceptive steroids. This could result in unintended pregnancy or breakthrough bleeding).
No products indexed under this heading.

Sulfamethizole (Contraceptive effectiveness may be reduced when hormonal contraceptives are co-administered with antibiotics, anticonvulsants, and other drugs that increase the metabolism of contraceptive steroids. This could result in unintended pregnancy or breakthrough bleeding).
No products indexed under this heading.

Sulfamethoxazole (Contraceptive effectiveness may be reduced when hormonal contraceptives are co-administered with antibiotics, anticonvulsants, and other drugs that increase the metabolism of contraceptive steroids. This could result in unintended pregnancy or breakthrough bleeding).
No products indexed under this heading.

Sulfisoxazole Acetyl (Contraceptive effectiveness may be reduced when hormonal contraceptives are co-administered with antibiotics, anticonvulsants, and other drugs that increase the metabolism of contraceptive steroids. This could result in unintended pregnancy or breakthrough bleeding).
No products indexed under this heading.

Sulfisoxazole Diolamine (Contraceptive effectiveness may be reduced when hormonal contraceptives are co-administered with antibiotics, anticonvulsants, and other drugs that increase the metabolism of contraceptive steroids. This could result in unintended pregnancy or breakthrough bleeding).
No products indexed under this heading.

Telithromycin (CYP3A4 inhibitors such as itraconazole or ketoconazole may increase plasma hormone levels). Products include:
Ketek 2991

Temazepam (Increased clearance of temazepam, due to induction of conjugation, has been noted when concomitantly administered with oral contraceptives).
No products indexed under this heading.

Tetracycline Hydrochloride (Several cases of contraceptive failure and breakthrough bleeding have been reported in the literature with concomitant administration of antibiotics such as ampicillin and tetracyclines. However, clinical pharmacology studies investigating drug interaction between combined oral contraceptives and these antibiotics have reported inconsistent results). Products include:
Pylera 793

Tetracycline Phosphate Complex (Several cases of contraceptive failure and breakthrough bleeding have been reported in the literature with concomitant administration of antibiotics such as ampicillin and tetracyclines. However, clinical pharmacology studies investigating drug interaction between combined oral contraceptives and these antibiotics have reported inconsistent results).
No products indexed under this heading.

Theophylline (Combination hormonal contraceptives containing some synthetic estrogens (eg, ethinyl estradiol) may inhibit the metabolism of other compounds. Increased plasma concentrations of theophylline has been reported with concomitant administration of oral contraceptives).
No products indexed under this heading.

Theophylline Anhydrous (Combination hormonal contraceptives containing some synthetic estrogens (eg, ethinyl estradiol) may inhibit the metabolism of other compounds. Increased plasma concentrations of theophylline has been reported with concomitant administration of oral contraceptives). Products include:
Uniphyl 2817

Theophylline Calcium Salicylate (Combination hormonal contraceptives containing some synthetic estrogens (eg, ethinyl estradiol) may inhibit the metabolism of other compounds. Increased plasma concentrations of theophylline has been reported with concomitant administration of oral contraceptives).
No products indexed under this heading.

Theophylline Dihydroxypropyl (Glyceryl) (Combination hormonal contraceptives containing some synthetic estrogens (eg, ethinyl estradiol) may inhibit the metabolism of other compounds. Increased plasma concentrations of theophylline has been reported with concomitant administration of oral contraceptives).
No products indexed under this heading.

Theophylline Ethylenediamine (Combination hormonal contraceptives containing some synthetic estrogens (eg, ethinyl estradiol) may inhibit the metabolism of other compounds. Increased plasma concentrations of theophylline has been reported with concomitant administration of oral contraceptives).
No products indexed under this heading.

Theophylline Sodium Glycinate (Combination hormonal contraceptives containing some synthetic estrogens (eg, ethinyl estradiol) may inhibit the metabolism of other compounds. Increased plasma concentrations of theophylline has been reported with concomitant administration of oral contraceptives).
No products indexed under this heading.

Thiamylal Sodium (Contraceptive effectiveness may be reduced when hormonal contraceptives are co-administered with barbiturates. This could result in unintended pregnancy or breakthrough bleeding).
No products indexed under this heading.

Tiagabine Hydrochloride (Contraceptive effectiveness may be reduced when hormonal contraceptives are co-administered with antibiotics, anticonvulsants, and other drugs that increase the metabolism of contraceptive steroids. This could result in unintended pregnancy or breakthrough bleeding). Products include:
Gabitril 972

Ticarcillin Disodium (Contraceptive effectiveness may be reduced when hormonal contraceptives are co-administered with antibiotics, anticonvulsants, and other drugs that increase the metabolism of contraceptive steroids. This could result in unintended pregnancy or breakthrough bleeding). Products include:
Timentin ADD-Vantage 1670
Timentin Galaxy 1674
Timentin 1666
Timentin Pharmacy 1678

Tipranavir (Several of the anti-HIV protease inhibitors have been studied with co-administration of oral combination hormonal contraceptives; significant changes (increase and decrease) in the plasma levels of the estrogen and progestin have been noted in some cases. The safety and efficacy of oral contraceptive products may be affected with co-administration of anti-HIV protease inhibitors).
No products indexed under this heading.

Tobacco (Cigarette smoking increases the risk of serious cardiovascular side effects from oral contraceptive use. Women who use oral contraceptives should be strongly advised not to smoke).
No products indexed under this heading.

Tobramycin (Contraceptive effectiveness may be reduced when hormonal contraceptives are co-administered with antibiotics, anticonvulsants, and other drugs that increase the metabolism of contraceptive steroids. This could result in unintended pregnancy or breakthrough bleeding). Products include:
Tobi Nebulizer 2546
Tobramycin and Dexamethasone Ophthalmic Suspension .... ⊙ 251
Zylet .... ⊙ 252

Tobramycin Sulfate (Contraceptive effectiveness may be reduced when hormonal contraceptives are co-administered with antibiotics, anticonvulsants, and other drugs that increase the metabolism of contraceptive steroids. This could result in unintended pregnancy or breakthrough bleeding).
No products indexed under this heading.

Tolazamide (Contraceptive effectiveness may be reduced when hormonal contraceptives are co-administered with antibiotics, anticonvulsants, and other drugs that increase the metabolism of contraceptive steroids. This could result in unintended pregnancy or breakthrough bleeding).
No products indexed under this heading.

Tolbutamide (Contraceptive effectiveness may be reduced when hormonal contraceptives are co-administered with antibiotics, anticonvulsants, and other drugs that increase the metabolism of contraceptive steroids. This could result in unintended pregnancy or breakthrough bleeding).
No products indexed under this heading.

Topiramate (Contraceptive effectiveness may be reduced when hormonal contraceptives are co-administered with topiramate. This could result in unintended pregnancy or breakthrough bleeding).
No products indexed under this heading.

Triamcinolone (Contraceptive effectiveness may be reduced when hormonal contraceptives are co-administered with antibiotics, anticonvulsants, and other drugs that increase the metabolism of contraceptive steroids. This could result in unintended pregnancy or breakthrough bleeding).
No products indexed under this heading.

Triamcinolone Acetonide (Contraceptive effectiveness may be reduced when hormonal contraceptives are co-administered with antibiotics, anticonvulsants, and other drugs that increase the metabolism of contraceptive steroids. This could result in unintended pregnancy or breakthrough bleeding). Products include:
Azmacort 408
Nasacort AQ 3019

Triamcinolone Diacetate (Contraceptive effectiveness may be reduced when hormonal contraceptives are co-administered with antibiotics, anticonvulsants, and other drugs that increase the metabolism of contraceptive steroids. This could result in unintended pregnancy or breakthrough bleeding).
No products indexed under this heading.

Triamcinolone Hexacetonide (Contraceptive effectiveness may be reduced when hormonal contraceptives are co-administered with antibiotics, anticonvulsants, and other drugs that increase the metabolism of contraceptive steroids. This could result in unintended pregnancy or breakthrough bleeding).
No products indexed under this heading.

Trimethadione (Contraceptive effectiveness may be reduced when hormonal contraceptives are co-administered with antibiotics, anticonvulsants, and other drugs that increase the metabolism of contraceptive steroids. This could result in unintended pregnancy or breakthrough bleeding).
No products indexed under this heading.

Troglitazone (CYP3A4 inhibitors such as itraconazole or ketoconazole may increase plasma hormone levels).
No products indexed under this heading.

Troleandomycin (Contraceptive effectiveness may be reduced when hormonal contraceptives are co-administered with antibiotics, anticonvulsants, and other drugs that increase the metabolism of contraceptive steroids. This could result in unintended pregnancy or breakthrough bleeding).
No products indexed under this heading.

Trovafloxacin Mesylate (Contraceptive effectiveness may be reduced when hormonal contraceptives are co-administered with antibiotics, anticonvulsants, and other drugs that increase the metabolism of contraceptive steroids. This could result in unintended pregnancy or breakthrough bleeding).
No products indexed under this heading.

Valproate Sodium (Contraceptive effectiveness may be reduced when hormonal contraceptives are co-administered with antibiotics, anticonvulsants, and other drugs that increase the metabolism of contraceptive steroids. This could result in unintended pregnancy or breakthrough bleeding).
No products indexed under this heading.

Valproic Acid (Contraceptive effectiveness may be reduced when hormonal contraceptives are co-administered with antibiotics, anticonvulsants, and other drugs that increase the metabolism of contraceptive steroids. This could result in unintended pregnancy or breakthrough bleeding).
No products indexed under this heading.

Vardenafil Hydrochloride (CYP3A4 inhibitors such as itraconazole or ketoconazole may increase plasma hormone levels). Products include:
Levitra 3157

Verapamil Hydrochloride (CYP3A4 inhibitors such as itraconazole or ketoconazole may increase plasma hormone levels). Products include:
Tarka 534

Vitamin C (Ascorbic acid may increase plasma ethinyl estradiol levels, possibly by inhibition of conjugation). Products include:
Bausch & Lomb Ocuvite Adult 50+ .... ⊙ 238
Bio-C 3454
BoneMate Plus 3454
Cardio Basics 3455
CitraNatal 90 DHA Capsules 2332
CitraNatal Assure 2332
CitraNatal Rx 2332
Ferralet 2333
Heplive 607
Meili Clear 607
MoviPrep Oral Solution 2905
PreNexa 3473
Proflavanol 90 3476

Voriconazole (CYP3A4 inhibitors such as itraconazole or ketoconazole may increase plasma hormone levels).
No products indexed under this heading.

Zafirlukast (CYP3A4 inhibitors such as itraconazole or ketoconazole may increase plasma hormone levels). Products include:
Accolate 3612

Zileuton (CYP3A4 inhibitors such as itraconazole or ketoconazole may increase plasma hormone levels).
No products indexed under this heading.

Zonisamide (Contraceptive effectiveness may be reduced when hormonal contraceptives are co-administered with antibiotics, anticonvulsants, and other drugs that increase the metabolism of contraceptive steroids. This could result in unintended pregnancy or breakthrough bleeding). Products include:
Zonegran 1081

Food Interactions

Broccoli (Contraceptive effectiveness may be reduced when hormonal contraceptives are co-administered with antibiotics, anticonvulsants, and other drugs that increase the metabolism of contraceptive steroids. This could result in unintended pregnancy or breakthrough bleeding).

Brussel Sprouts (Contraceptive effectiveness may be reduced when hormonal contraceptives are co-administered with antibiotics, anticonvulsants, and other drugs that increase the metabolism of contraceptive steroids. This could result in unintended pregnancy or breakthrough bleeding).

Charbroiled Food (Contraceptive effectiveness may be reduced when hormonal contraceptives are co-administered with antibiotics, anticonvulsants, and other drugs that increase the metabolism of contraceptive steroids. This could result in unintended pregnancy or breakthrough bleeding).

Grapefruit (CYP3A4 inhibitors such as itraconazole or ketoconazole may increase plasma hormone levels).

Grapefruit Juice (CYP3A4 inhibitors such as itraconazole or ketoconazole may increase plasma hormone levels).

ORTHOCLONE OKT3 STERILE SOLUTION

(Muromonab-CD3) 949
May interact with corticosteroids, and certain other agents. Compounds in these categories include:

Alclometasone Dipropionate (Psychosis and infection have been reported in patients treated with corticosteroids alone and in conjunction with muromonab-CD3).
No products indexed under this heading.

Azathioprine (Infection or malignancies have been reported with azathioprine alone and in conjunction with muromonab-CD3).
No products indexed under this heading.

Beclomethasone Dipropionate (Psychosis and infection have been reported in patients treated with corticosteroids alone and in conjunction with muromonab-CD3). Products include:
Qvar 3398

Beclomethasone Dipropionate Monohydrate (Psychosis and infection have been reported in patients treated with corticosteroids alone and in conjunction with muromonab-CD3). Products include:
Beconase AQ 1386

Betamethasone (Psychosis and infection have been reported in patients treated with corticosteroids alone and in conjunction with muromonab-CD3).
No products indexed under this heading.

Betamethasone Acetate (Psychosis and infection have been reported in patients treated with corticosteroids alone and in conjunction with muromonab-CD3).
No products indexed under this heading.

Betamethasone Benzoate (Psychosis and infection have been reported in patients treated with corticosteroids alone and in conjunction with muromonab-CD3).
No products indexed under this heading.

Betamethasone Dipropionate (Psychosis and infection have been reported in patients treated with corticosteroids alone and in conjunction with muromonab-CD3). Products include:
Diprolene Lotion 0.05% 3108
Diprolene Ointment 0.05% 3109
Diprolene AF Cream 0.05% 3107
Lotrisone 3163

Betamethasone Sodium Phosphate (Psychosis and infection have been reported in patients treated with corticosteroids alone and in conjunction with muromonab-CD3).
No products indexed under this heading.

Betamethasone Valerate (Psychosis and infection have been reported in patients treated with corticosteroids alone and in conjunction with muromonab-CD3). Products include:
Luxíq 3321

Budesonide (Psychosis and infection have been reported in patients treated with corticosteroids alone and in conjunction with muromonab-CD3). Products include:
Pulmicort Flexhaler 714
Symbicort 80/4.5 720
Symbicort 160/4.5 720

Ciclesonide (Psychosis and infection have been reported in patients treated with corticosteroids alone and in conjunction with muromonab-CD3).
No products indexed under this heading.

Cortisone Acetate (Psychosis and infection have been reported in patients treated with corticosteroids alone and in conjunction with muromonab-CD3).
No products indexed under this heading.

Cyclosporine (Seizures, encephalopathy, infections, malignancies, and thrombotic events have been reported in patients receiving cyclosporine alone and in conjunction with muromonab-CD3). Products include:
Gengraf 440
Neoral Oral Solution 2496
Neoral Capsules 2496
Restasis 605

Desoximetasone (Psychosis and infection have been reported in patients treated with corticosteroids alone and in conjunction with muromonab-CD3).
No products indexed under this heading.

Dexamethasone (Psychosis and infection have been reported in patients treated with corticosteroids alone and in conjunction with muromonab-CD3). Products include:
Ciprodex 583
Ozurdex .... ⊙ 223
Tobramycin and Dexamethasone Ophthalmic Suspension .... ⊙ 251

Dexamethasone Acetate (Psychosis and infection have been reported in patients treated with corticosteroids alone and in conjunction with muromonab-CD3).
No products indexed under this heading.

Dexamethasone Phosphate (Psychosis and infection have been reported in patients treated with corticosteroids alone and in conjunction with muromonab-CD3).
No products indexed under this heading.

Dexamethasone Sodium (Psychosis and infection have been reported in patients treated with corticosteroids alone and in conjunction with muromonab-CD3).
No products indexed under this heading.

Dexamethasone Sodium Phosphate (Psychosis and infection have been reported in patients treated with corticosteroids alone and in conjunction with muromonab-CD3).
No products indexed under this heading.

Dexamethasone Sodium Phosphate Injection (Psychosis and infection have been reported in patients treated with corticosteroids alone and in conjunction with muromonab-CD3).
No products indexed under this heading.

Diflorasone Diacetate (Psychosis and infection have been reported in patients treated with corticosteroids alone and in conjunction with muromonab-CD3).
No products indexed under this heading.

Fludrocortisone Acetate (Psychosis and infection have been reported in patients treated with corticosteroids alone and in conjunction with muromonab-CD3).
No products indexed under this heading.

Flumethasone Pivalate (Psychosis and infection have been reported in patients treated with corticosteroids alone and in conjunction with muromonab-CD3).
No products indexed under this heading.

Flunisolide Hemihydrate (Psychosis and infection have been reported in patients treated with corticosteroids alone and in conjunction with muromonab-CD3).
No products indexed under this heading.

Fluticasone Furoate (Psychosis and infection have been reported in patients treated with corticosteroids alone and in conjunction with muromonab-CD3). Products include:
Veramyst 1713

Fluticasone Propionate (Psychosis and infection have been reported in patients treated with corticosteroids alone and in conjunction with muromonab-CD3). Products include:
Advair 100/50 1275
Advair 250/50 1275
Advair 500/50 1275
Advair HFA 45/21 1288
Advair HFA 115/21 1288
Advair HFA 230/21 1288
Flonase 1459
Flovent Diskus 1463
Flovent HFA 1470

Hydrocortisone (Psychosis and infection have been reported in patients treated with corticosteroids alone and in conjunction with muromonab-CD3).
No products indexed under this heading.

Hydrocortisone (Alcohol) (Psychosis and infection have been reported in patients treated with corticosteroids alone and in conjunction with muromonab-CD3).
No products indexed under this heading.

Hydrocortisone Acetate (Psychosis and infection have been reported in patients treated with corticosteroids alone and in conjunction with muromonab-CD3).
No products indexed under this heading.

Hydrocortisone Butyrate (Psychosis and infection have been reported in patients treated with corticosteroids alone and in conjunction with muromonab-CD3).
No products indexed under this heading.

Hydrocortisone Cypionate (Psychosis and infection have been reported in patients treated with corticosteroids alone and in conjunction with muromonab-CD3).
No products indexed under this heading.

Hydrocortisone Hemisuccinate (Psychosis and infection have been reported in patients treated with corticosteroids alone and in conjunction with muromonab-CD3).
No products indexed under this heading.

Hydrocortisone Probutate (Psychosis and infection have been reported in patients treated with corticosteroids alone and in conjunction with muromonab-CD3).
No products indexed under this heading.

Hydrocortisone Sodium Phosphate (Psychosis and infection have been reported in patients treated with corticosteroids alone and in conjunction with muromonab-CD3).
No products indexed under this heading.

Hydrocortisone Sodium Succinate (Psychosis and infection have been reported in patients treated with corticosteroids alone and in conjunction with muromonab-CD3).
No products indexed under this heading.

Hydrocortisone Valerate (Psychosis and infection have been reported in patients treated with corticosteroids alone and in conjunction with muromonab-CD3).
No products indexed under this heading.

Indomethacin (Encephalopathy and other CNS effects have been reported in patients treated with indomethacin alone and in conjunction with muromonab-CD3). Products include:
Indocin 2167

Indomethacin Sodium Trihydrate (Encephalopathy and other CNS effects have been reported in patients treated with indomethacin alone and in conjunction with muromonab-CD3). Products include:
Indocin I.V. 2007

Methylprednisolone (Psychosis and infection have been reported in patients treated with corticosteroids alone and in conjunction with muromonab-CD3).
No products indexed under this heading.

Methylprednisolone Acetate (Psychosis and infection have been reported in patients treated with corticosteroids alone and in conjunction with muromonab-CD3).
No products indexed under this heading.

Methylprednisolone Sodium Succinate (Psychosis and infection have been reported in patients treated with corticosteroids alone and in conjunction with muromonab-CD3).
No products indexed under this heading.

Mometasone Furoate (Psychosis and infection have been reported in patients treated with corticosteroids alone and in conjunction with muromonab-CD3). Products include:
Asmanex 3058
Elocon Cream 3111
Elocon Lotion 3112
Elocon Ointment 3114

Mometasone Furoate Monohydrate (Psychosis and infection have been reported in patients treated with corticosteroids alone and in conjunction with muromonab-CD3). Products include:
Nasonex 3166

Prednisolone (Psychosis and infection have been reported in patients treated with corticosteroids alone and in conjunction with muromonab-CD3).
No products indexed under this heading.

Prednisolone Acetate (Psychosis and infection have been reported in

patients treated with corticosteroids alone and in conjunction with muromonab-CD3). Products include:

Prednisolone Sodium Phosphate (Psychosis and infection have been reported in patients treated with corticosteroids alone and in conjunction with muromonab-CD3).
No products indexed under this heading.

Prednisolone Tebutate (Psychosis and infection have been reported in patients treated with corticosteroids alone and in conjunction with muromonab-CD3).
No products indexed under this heading.

Prednisone (Psychosis and infection have been reported in patients treated with corticosteroids alone and in conjunction with muromonab-CD3).
No products indexed under this heading.

Prednisone sodium phosphate (Psychosis and infection have been reported in patients treated with corticosteroids alone and in conjunction with muromonab-CD3).
No products indexed under this heading.

Triamcinolone (Psychosis and infection have been reported in patients treated with corticosteroids alone and in conjunction with muromonab-CD3).
No products indexed under this heading.

Triamcinolone Acetonide (Psychosis and infection have been reported in patients treated with corticosteroids alone and in conjunction with muromonab-CD3). Products include:

Triamcinolone Diacetate (Psychosis and infection have been reported in patients treated with corticosteroids alone and in conjunction with muromonab-CD3).
No products indexed under this heading.

Triamcinolone Hexacetonide (Psychosis and infection have been reported in patients treated with corticosteroids alone and in conjunction with muromonab-CD3).
No products indexed under this heading.

ORTHO-CYCLEN TABLETS

(Ethinyl Estradiol, Norgestimate) 2663
May interact with antibiotics, anticonvulsants, barbiturates, cytochrome p450 3a4 inhibitors (selected), hepatic microsomal enzyme inducers, phenytoin, prednisolone, protease inhibitors, theophyllines, and certain other agents. Compounds in these categories include:

Acetaminophen (Acetaminophen may increase plasma ethinyl estradiol levels, possibly by inhibition of conjugation. Concomitant use may also decrease plasma concentrations of acetaminophen). Products include:

Acetaminophen-containing products (Acetaminophen may increase plasma ethinyl estradiol levels, possibly by inhibition of conjugation. Concomitant use may also decrease plasma concentrations of acetaminophen).
No products indexed under this heading.

Acetazolamide (CYP3A4 inhibitors, such as itraconazole or ketoconazole, may increase plasma hormone levels).
No products indexed under this heading.

Acetazolamide Sodium (CYP3A4 inhibitors, such as itraconazole or ketoconazole, may increase plasma hormone levels).
No products indexed under this heading.

Alatrofloxacin Mesylate (Contraceptive effectiveness may be reduced when hormonal contraceptives are co-administered with antibiotics, anticonvulsants, and other drugs that increase the metabolism of contraceptive steroids. This could result in unintended pregnancy or breakthrough bleeding).
No products indexed under this heading.

Allium sativum (Contraceptive effectiveness may be reduced when hormonal contraceptives are co-administered with antibiotics, anticonvulsants, and other drugs that increase the metabolism of contraceptive steroids. This could result in unintended pregnancy or breakthrough bleeding).
No products indexed under this heading.

Amikacin Sulfate (Contraceptive effectiveness may be reduced when hormonal contraceptives are co-administered with antibiotics, anticonvulsants, and other drugs that increase the metabolism of contraceptive steroids. This could result in unintended pregnancy or breakthrough bleeding).
No products indexed under this heading.

Aminoglutethimide (Contraceptive effectiveness may be reduced when hormonal contraceptives are co-administered with antibiotics, anticonvulsants, and other drugs that increase the metabolism of contraceptive steroids. This could result in unintended pregnancy or breakthrough bleeding).
No products indexed under this heading.

Amiodarone Hydrochloride (CYP3A4 inhibitors, such as itraconazole or ketoconazole, may increase plasma hormone levels).
No products indexed under this heading.

Amobarbital (Contraceptive effectiveness may be reduced when hormonal contraceptives are co-administered with barbiturates. This could result in unintended pregnancy or breakthrough bleeding).
No products indexed under this heading.

Amobarbital Sodium (Contraceptive effectiveness may be reduced when hormonal contraceptives are co-administered with barbiturates. This could result in unintended pregnancy or breakthrough bleeding).
No products indexed under this heading.

Amoxicillin (Contraceptive effectiveness may be reduced when hormonal contraceptives are co-administered with antibiotics, anticonvulsants, and other drugs that increase the metabolism of contraceptive steroids. This could result in unintended pregnancy or breakthrough bleeding). Products include:

Amoxicillin Trihydrate (Contraceptive effectiveness may be reduced when hormonal contraceptives are co-administered with antibiotics, anticonvulsants, and other drugs that increase the metabolism of contraceptive steroids. This could result in unintended pregnancy or breakthrough bleeding).
No products indexed under this heading.

Ampicillin (Contraceptive effectiveness may be reduced when hormonal contraceptives are co-administered with antibiotics, anticonvulsants, and other drugs that increase the metabolism of contraceptive steroids. This could result in unintended pregnancy or breakthrough bleeding).
No products indexed under this heading.

Ampicillin Sodium (Contraceptive effectiveness may be reduced when hormonal contraceptives are co-administered with antibiotics, anticonvulsants, and other drugs that increase the metabolism of contraceptive steroids. This could result in unintended pregnancy or breakthrough bleeding).
No products indexed under this heading.

Ampicillin Trihydrate (Contraceptive effectiveness may be reduced when hormonal contraceptives are co-administered with antibiotics, anticonvulsants, and other drugs that increase the metabolism of contraceptive steroids. This could result in unintended pregnancy or breakthrough bleeding).
No products indexed under this heading.

Amprenavir (Several of the anti-HIV protease inhibitors have been studied with co-administration of oral combination hormonal contraceptives; significant changes (increase and decrease) in the plasma levels of the estrogen and progestin have been noted in some cases. The safety and efficacy of oral contraceptive products may be affected with co-administration of anti-HIV protease inhibitors).
No products indexed under this heading.

Anastrozole (CYP3A4 inhibitors, such as itraconazole or ketoconazole, may increase plasma hormone levels).
No products indexed under this heading.

Antibiotics, non-penicillin, unspecified (Contraceptive effectiveness may be reduced when hormonal contraceptives are co-administered with antibiotics, anticonvulsants, and other drugs that increase the metabolism of contraceptive steroids. This could result in unintended pregnancy or breakthrough bleeding).
No products indexed under this heading.

Aprepitant (CYP3A4 inhibitors, such as itraconazole or ketoconazole, may increase plasma hormone levels). Products include:

Aprobarbital (Contraceptive effectiveness may be reduced when hormonal contraceptives are co-administered with barbiturates. This could result in unintended pregnancy or breakthrough bleeding).
No products indexed under this heading.

Atazanavir (Several of the anti-HIV protease inhibitors have been studied with co-administration of oral combination hormonal contraceptives; significant changes (increase and decrease) in the plasma levels of the estrogen and progestin have been noted in some cases. The safety and efficacy of oral contraceptive products may be affected with co-administration of anti-HIV protease inhibitors).
No products indexed under this heading.

Atazanavir Sulfate (Several of the anti-HIV protease inhibitors have been studied with co-administration of oral combination hormonal contraceptives; significant changes (increase and

decrease) in the plasma levels of the estrogen and progestin have been noted in some cases. The safety and efficacy of oral contraceptive products may be affected with co-administration of anti-HIV protease inhibitors).
No products indexed under this heading.

Atorvastatin Calcium (Co-administration of atorvastatin and certain oral contraceptives containing ethinyl estradiol increase AUC values for ethinyl estradiol by approximately 20%). Products include:

Azithromycin Dihydrate (Contraceptive effectiveness may be reduced when hormonal contraceptives are co-administered with antibiotics, anticonvulsants, and other drugs that increase the metabolism of contraceptive steroids. This could result in unintended pregnancy or breakthrough bleeding).
No products indexed under this heading.

Azlocillin Sodium (Contraceptive effectiveness may be reduced when hormonal contraceptives are co-administered with antibiotics, anticonvulsants, and other drugs that increase the metabolism of contraceptive steroids. This could result in unintended pregnancy or breakthrough bleeding).
No products indexed under this heading.

Aztreonam (Contraceptive effectiveness may be reduced when hormonal contraceptives are co-administered with antibiotics, anticonvulsants, and other drugs that increase the metabolism of contraceptive steroids. This could result in unintended pregnancy or breakthrough bleeding).
No products indexed under this heading.

Bacampicillin Hydrochloride (Contraceptive effectiveness may be reduced when hormonal contraceptives are co-administered with antibiotics, anticonvulsants, and other drugs that increase the metabolism of contraceptive steroids. This could result in unintended pregnancy or breakthrough bleeding).
No products indexed under this heading.

Betamethasone (Contraceptive effectiveness may be reduced when hormonal contraceptives are co-administered with antibiotics, anticonvulsants, and other drugs that increase the metabolism of contraceptive steroids. This could result in unintended pregnancy or breakthrough bleeding).
No products indexed under this heading.

Betamethasone Sodium Phosphate (Contraceptive effectiveness may be reduced when hormonal contraceptives are co-administered with antibiotics, anticonvulsants, and other drugs that increase the metabolism of contraceptive steroids. This could result in unintended pregnancy or breakthrough bleeding).
No products indexed under this heading.

Bosentan (Contraceptive effectiveness may be reduced when hormonal contraceptives are co-administered with bosentan. This could result in unintended pregnancy or breakthrough bleeding). Products include:

Butabarbital (Contraceptive effectiveness may be reduced when hormonal contraceptives are co-administered with barbiturates. This could result in unintended pregnancy or breakthrough bleeding).
No products indexed under this heading.

Butabarbital Sodium (Contraceptive effectiveness may be reduced when hormonal contraceptives are co-administered with barbiturates. This could result in unintended pregnancy or breakthrough bleeding).
No products indexed under this heading.

Butalbital (Contraceptive effectiveness may be reduced when hormonal contraceptives are co-administered with barbiturates. This could result in unintended pregnancy or breakthrough bleeding).
No products indexed under this heading.

Carbamazepine (Contraceptive effectiveness may be reduced when hormonal contraceptives are co-administered with carbamazepine. This could result in unintended pregnancy or breakthrough bleeding). Products include:
Carbatrol 3280
Equetro 3477

Carbenicillin Disodium (Contraceptive effectiveness may be reduced when hormonal contraceptives are co-administered with antibiotics, anticonvulsants, and other drugs that increase the metabolism of contraceptive steroids. This could result in unintended pregnancy or breakthrough bleeding).
No products indexed under this heading.

Carbenicillin Indanyl Sodium (Contraceptive effectiveness may be reduced when hormonal contraceptives are co-administered with antibiotics, anticonvulsants, and other drugs that increase the metabolism of contraceptive steroids. This could result in unintended pregnancy or breakthrough bleeding).
No products indexed under this heading.

Cefaclor (Contraceptive effectiveness may be reduced when hormonal contraceptives are co-administered with antibiotics, anticonvulsants, and other drugs that increase the metabolism of contraceptive steroids. This could result in unintended pregnancy or breakthrough bleeding).
No products indexed under this heading.

Cefadroxil (Contraceptive effectiveness may be reduced when hormonal contraceptives are co-administered with antibiotics, anticonvulsants, and other drugs that increase the metabolism of contraceptive steroids. This could result in unintended pregnancy or breakthrough bleeding).
No products indexed under this heading.

Cefamandole Nafate (Contraceptive effectiveness may be reduced when hormonal contraceptives are co-administered with antibiotics, anticonvulsants, and other drugs that increase the metabolism of contraceptive steroids. This could result in unintended pregnancy or breakthrough bleeding).
No products indexed under this heading.

Cefazolin Sodium (Contraceptive effectiveness may be reduced when hormonal contraceptives are co-administered with antibiotics, anticonvulsants, and other drugs that increase the metabolism of contraceptive steroids. This could result in unintended pregnancy or breakthrough bleeding).
No products indexed under this heading.

Cefixime (Contraceptive effectiveness may be reduced when hormonal contraceptives are co-administered with antibiotics, anticonvulsants, and other drugs that increase the metabolism of contraceptive steroids. This could result in unintended pregnancy or breakthrough bleeding). Products include:
Suprax for Oral Suspension 2038
Suprax Tablets 2038

Cefmetazole Sodium (Contraceptive effectiveness may be reduced when hormonal contraceptives are co-administered with antibiotics, anticonvulsants, and other drugs that increase the metabolism of contraceptive steroids. This could result in unintended pregnancy or breakthrough bleeding).
No products indexed under this heading.

Cefonicid Sodium (Contraceptive effectiveness may be reduced when hormonal contraceptives are co-administered with antibiotics, anticonvulsants, and other drugs that increase the metabolism of contraceptive steroids. This could result in unintended pregnancy or breakthrough bleeding).
No products indexed under this heading.

Cefoperazone Sodium (Contraceptive effectiveness may be reduced when hormonal contraceptives are co-administered with antibiotics, anticonvulsants, and other drugs that increase the metabolism of contraceptive steroids. This could result in unintended pregnancy or breakthrough bleeding).
No products indexed under this heading.

Ceforanide (Contraceptive effectiveness may be reduced when hormonal contraceptives are co-administered with antibiotics, anticonvulsants, and other drugs that increase the metabolism of contraceptive steroids. This could result in unintended pregnancy or breakthrough bleeding).
No products indexed under this heading.

Cefotaxime Sodium (Contraceptive effectiveness may be reduced when hormonal contraceptives are co-administered with antibiotics, anticonvulsants, and other drugs that increase the metabolism of contraceptive steroids. This could result in unintended pregnancy or breakthrough bleeding).
No products indexed under this heading.

Cefotetan (Contraceptive effectiveness may be reduced when hormonal contraceptives are co-administered with antibiotics, anticonvulsants, and other drugs that increase the metabolism of contraceptive steroids. This could result in unintended pregnancy or breakthrough bleeding).
No products indexed under this heading.

Cefoxitin Sodium (Contraceptive effectiveness may be reduced when hormonal contraceptives are co-administered with antibiotics, anticonvulsants, and other drugs that increase the metabolism of contraceptive steroids. This could result in unintended pregnancy or breakthrough bleeding).
No products indexed under this heading.

Cefpodoxime Proxetil (Contraceptive effectiveness may be reduced when hormonal contraceptives are co-administered with antibiotics, anticonvulsants, and other drugs that increase the metabolism of contraceptive steroids. This could result in unintended pregnancy or breakthrough bleeding).
No products indexed under this heading.

Cefprozil (Contraceptive effectiveness may be reduced when hormonal contraceptives are co-administered with antibiotics, anticonvulsants, and other drugs that increase the metabolism of contraceptive steroids. This could result in unintended pregnancy or breakthrough bleeding).
No products indexed under this heading.

Ceftazidime (Contraceptive effectiveness may be reduced when hormonal contraceptives are co-administered with antibiotics, anticonvulsants, and other drugs that increase the metabolism of contraceptive steroids. This could result in unintended pregnancy or breakthrough bleeding). Products include:
Fortaz 1481

Ceftizoxime Sodium (Contraceptive effectiveness may be reduced when hormonal contraceptives are co-administered with antibiotics, anticonvulsants, and other drugs that increase the metabolism of contraceptive steroids. This could result in unintended pregnancy or breakthrough bleeding).
No products indexed under this heading.

Ceftriaxone Sodium (Contraceptive effectiveness may be reduced when hormonal contraceptives are co-administered with antibiotics, anticonvulsants, and other drugs that increase the metabolism of contraceptive steroids. This could result in unintended pregnancy or breakthrough bleeding). Products include:
Rocephin 2859

Cefuroxime Axetil (Contraceptive effectiveness may be reduced when hormonal contraceptives are co-administered with antibiotics, anticonvulsants, and other drugs that increase the metabolism of contraceptive steroids. This could result in unintended pregnancy or breakthrough bleeding). Products include:
Ceftin 1399

Cefuroxime Sodium (Contraceptive effectiveness may be reduced when hormonal contraceptives are co-administered with antibiotics, anticonvulsants, and other drugs that increase the metabolism of contraceptive steroids. This could result in unintended pregnancy or breakthrough bleeding).
No products indexed under this heading.

Cephalexin (Contraceptive effectiveness may be reduced when hormonal contraceptives are co-administered with antibiotics, anticonvulsants, and other drugs that increase the metabolism of contraceptive steroids. This could result in unintended pregnancy or breakthrough bleeding).
No products indexed under this heading.

Cephalothin Sodium (Contraceptive effectiveness may be reduced when hormonal contraceptives are co-administered with antibiotics, anticonvulsants, and other drugs that increase the metabolism of contraceptive steroids. This could result in unintended pregnancy or breakthrough bleeding).
No products indexed under this heading.

Cephapirin Sodium (Contraceptive effectiveness may be reduced when hormonal contraceptives are co-administered with antibiotics, anticonvulsants, and other drugs that increase the metabolism of contraceptive steroids. This could result in unintended pregnancy or breakthrough bleeding).
No products indexed under this heading.

Cephradine (Contraceptive effectiveness may be reduced when hormonal contraceptives are co-administered with antibiotics, anticonvulsants, and other drugs that increase the metabolism of contraceptive steroids. This could result in unintended pregnancy or breakthrough bleeding).
No products indexed under this heading.

Chloramphenicol (Contraceptive effectiveness may be reduced when hormonal contraceptives are co-administered with antibiotics, anticonvulsants, and other drugs that increase the metabolism of contraceptive steroids. This could result in unintended pregnancy or breakthrough bleeding).
No products indexed under this heading.

Chloramphenicol Palmitate (Contraceptive effectiveness may be reduced when hormonal contraceptives are co-administered with antibiotics, anticonvulsants, and other drugs that increase the metabolism of contraceptive steroids. This could result in unintended pregnancy or breakthrough bleeding).
No products indexed under this heading.

Chloramphenicol Sodium Succinate (Contraceptive effectiveness may be reduced when hormonal contraceptives are co-administered with antibiotics, anticonvulsants, and other drugs that increase the metabolism of contraceptive steroids. This could result in unintended pregnancy or breakthrough bleeding).
No products indexed under this heading.

Chlorpropamide (Contraceptive effectiveness may be reduced when hormonal contraceptives are co-administered with antibiotics, anticonvulsants, and other drugs that increase the metabolism of contraceptive steroids. This could result in unintended pregnancy or breakthrough bleeding).
No products indexed under this heading.

Cilastatin Sodium (Contraceptive effectiveness may be reduced when hormonal contraceptives are co-administered with antibiotics, anticonvulsants, and other drugs that increase the metabolism of contraceptive steroids. This could result in unintended pregnancy or breakthrough bleeding). Products include:
Primaxin I.M. 2232
Primaxin I.V. 2235

Cimetidine (CYP3A4 inhibitors, such as itraconazole or ketoconazole, may increase plasma hormone levels).
No products indexed under this heading.

Cimetidine Hydrochloride (CYP3A4 inhibitors, such as itraconazole or ketoconazole, may increase plasma hormone levels).
No products indexed under this heading.

Ciprofloxacin (Contraceptive effectiveness may be reduced when hormonal contraceptives are co-administered with antibiotics, anticonvulsants, and other drugs that increase the metabolism of contraceptive steroids. This could result in unintended pregnancy or breakthrough bleeding). Products include:
Cipro I.V. 3082
Cipro 3073
Cipro XR 3091
Ciprodex 583

Ciprofloxacin Hydrochloride (Contraceptive effectiveness may be reduced when hormonal contraceptives are co-administered with antibiotics, anticonvulsants, and other drugs that increase the metabolism of contraceptive steroids. This could result in unintended pregnancy or breakthrough bleeding). Products include:
Cipro 3073

Cisplatin (Contraceptive effectiveness may be reduced when hormonal contraceptives are co-administered with antibiotics, anticonvulsants, and other drugs that increase the metabolism of contraceptive steroids. This could result in unintended pregnancy or breakthrough bleeding).
No products indexed under this heading.

Citalopram Hydrobromide (Contraceptive effectiveness may be reduced when hormonal contraceptives are co-administered with antibiotics, anticonvulsants, and other drugs that increase the metabolism of contraceptive steroids. This could result in unintended pregnancy or breakthrough bleeding). Products include:
Celexa 1153

Clarithromycin (Contraceptive effectiveness may be reduced when hormonal contraceptives are co-administered with antibiotics, anticonvulsants, and other drugs that increase the metabolism of contraceptive steroids. This could result in unintended pregnancy or breakthrough bleeding). Products include:
Biaxin/Biaxin XL 412

IMPORTANT NOTE: Always consult each drug listing in the patient's regimen for possible interactions.

Ortho-Cyclen Interactions Index 1342

Clofibric Acid (Increased clearance of clofibric acid, due to induction of conjugation, has been noted when concomitantly administered with oral contraceptives).
No products indexed under this heading.

Clotrimazole (Contraceptive effectiveness may be reduced when hormonal contraceptives are co-administered with antibiotics, anticonvulsants, and other drugs that increase the metabolism of contraceptive steroids. This could result in unintended pregnancy or breakthrough bleeding). Products include:
Lotrisone 3163

Cloxacillin (Contraceptive effectiveness may be reduced when hormonal contraceptives are co-administered with antibiotics, anticonvulsants, and other drugs that increase the metabolism of contraceptive steroids. This could result in unintended pregnancy or breakthrough bleeding).
No products indexed under this heading.

Cloxacillin Sodium (Contraceptive effectiveness may be reduced when hormonal contraceptives are co-administered with antibiotics, anticonvulsants, and other drugs that increase the metabolism of contraceptive steroids. This could result in unintended pregnancy or breakthrough bleeding).
No products indexed under this heading.

Cloxacillin Sodium Monohydrate (Contraceptive effectiveness may be reduced when hormonal contraceptives are co-administered with antibiotics, anticonvulsants, and other drugs that increase the metabolism of contraceptive steroids. This could result in unintended pregnancy or breakthrough bleeding).
No products indexed under this heading.

Conivaptan Hydrochloride (CYP3A4 inhibitors, such as itraconazole or ketoconazole, may increase plasma hormone levels). Products include:
Vaprisol 689

Cortisone Acetate (Contraceptive effectiveness may be reduced when hormonal contraceptives are co-administered with antibiotics, anticonvulsants, and other drugs that increase the metabolism of contraceptive steroids. This could result in unintended pregnancy or breakthrough bleeding).
No products indexed under this heading.

Cyclosporine (Combination hormonal contraceptives containing some synthetic estrogens (eg, ethinyl estradiol) may inhibit the metabolism of other compounds. Increased plasma concentrations of cyclosporine has been reported with concomitant administration of oral contraceptives). Products include:
Gengraf 440
Neoral Oral Solution 2496
Neoral Capsules 2496
Restasis 605

Dalfopristin (CYP3A4 inhibitors, such as itraconazole or ketoconazole, may increase plasma hormone levels).
No products indexed under this heading.

Danazol (CYP3A4 inhibitors, such as itraconazole or ketoconazole, may increase plasma hormone levels).
No products indexed under this heading.

Darunavir (Several of the anti-HIV protease inhibitors have been studied with co-administration of oral combination hormonal contraceptives; significant changes (increase and decrease) in the plasma levels of the estrogen and progestin have been noted in some cases. The safety and efficacy of oral contraceptive products may be affected with co-administration of anti-HIV protease inhibitors).
No products indexed under this heading.

Dasatinib (CYP3A4 inhibitors, such as itraconazole or ketoconazole, may increase plasma hormone levels).
No products indexed under this heading.

Daunorubicin Hydrochloride (Contraceptive effectiveness may be reduced when hormonal contraceptives are co-administered with antibiotics, anticonvulsants, and other drugs that increase the metabolism of contraceptive steroids. This could result in unintended pregnancy or breakthrough bleeding).
No products indexed under this heading.

Delavirdine Mesylate (CYP3A4 inhibitors, such as itraconazole or ketoconazole, may increase plasma hormone levels).
No products indexed under this heading.

Delavirine (CYP3A4 inhibitors, such as itraconazole or ketoconazole, may increase plasma hormone levels).
No products indexed under this heading.

Demeclocycline Hydrochloride (Contraceptive effectiveness may be reduced when hormonal contraceptives are co-administered with antibiotics, anticonvulsants, and other drugs that increase the metabolism of contraceptive steroids. This could result in unintended pregnancy or breakthrough bleeding).
No products indexed under this heading.

Desloratadine (CYP3A4 inhibitors, such as itraconazole or ketoconazole, may increase plasma hormone levels). Products include:
Clarinex Syrup 3098
Clarinex 3098
Clarinex Reditabs 3098
Clarinex-D 12-Hour 3101
Clarinex-D 3104

Dexamethasone (Contraceptive effectiveness may be reduced when hormonal contraceptives are co-administered with antibiotics, anticonvulsants, and other drugs that increase the metabolism of contraceptive steroids. This could result in unintended pregnancy or breakthrough bleeding). Products include:
Ciprodex 583
Ozurdex .... ⊙ 223
Tobramycin and Dexamethasone Ophthalmic Suspension .... ⊙ 251

Dexamethasone Acetate (Contraceptive effectiveness may be reduced when hormonal contraceptives are co-administered with antibiotics, anticonvulsants, and other drugs that increase the metabolism of contraceptive steroids. This could result in unintended pregnancy or breakthrough bleeding).
No products indexed under this heading.

Dexamethasone Phosphate (Contraceptive effectiveness may be reduced when hormonal contraceptives are co-administered with antibiotics, anticonvulsants, and other drugs that increase the metabolism of contraceptive steroids. This could result in unintended pregnancy or breakthrough bleeding).
No products indexed under this heading.

Dexamethasone Sodium (Contraceptive effectiveness may be reduced when hormonal contraceptives are co-administered with antibiotics, anticonvulsants, and other drugs that increase the metabolism of contraceptive steroids. This could result in unintended pregnancy or breakthrough bleeding).
No products indexed under this heading.

Dexamethasone Sodium Phosphate (Contraceptive effectiveness may be reduced when hormonal contraceptives are co-administered with antibiotics, anticonvulsants, and other drugs that increase the metabolism of contraceptive steroids. This could result in unintended pregnancy or breakthrough bleeding).
No products indexed under this heading.

Dicloxacillin (Contraceptive effectiveness may be reduced when hormonal contraceptives are co-administered with antibiotics, anticonvulsants, and other drugs that increase the metabolism of contraceptive steroids. This could result in unintended pregnancy or breakthrough bleeding).
No products indexed under this heading.

Dicloxacillin Sodium (Contraceptive effectiveness may be reduced when hormonal contraceptives are co-administered with antibiotics, anticonvulsants, and other drugs that increase the metabolism of contraceptive steroids. This could result in unintended pregnancy or breakthrough bleeding).
No products indexed under this heading.

Diltiazem Hydrochloride (CYP3A4 inhibitors, such as itraconazole or ketoconazole, may increase plasma hormone levels). Products include:
Cardizem LA 423

Diltiazem Maleate (CYP3A4 inhibitors, such as itraconazole or ketoconazole, may increase plasma hormone levels).
No products indexed under this heading.

Dirithromycin (Contraceptive effectiveness may be reduced when hormonal contraceptives are co-administered with antibiotics, anticonvulsants, and other drugs that increase the metabolism of contraceptive steroids. This could result in unintended pregnancy or breakthrough bleeding).
No products indexed under this heading.

Disodium Carbenicillin (Contraceptive effectiveness may be reduced when hormonal contraceptives are co-administered with antibiotics, anticonvulsants, and other drugs that increase the metabolism of contraceptive steroids. This could result in unintended pregnancy or breakthrough bleeding).
No products indexed under this heading.

Divalproex Sodium (Contraceptive effectiveness may be reduced when hormonal contraceptives are co-administered with antibiotics, anticonvulsants, and other drugs that increase the metabolism of contraceptive steroids. This could result in unintended pregnancy or breakthrough bleeding). Products include:
Depakote ER 426

Doxorubicin Hydrochloride (Contraceptive effectiveness may be reduced when hormonal contraceptives are co-administered with antibiotics, anticonvulsants, and other drugs that increase the metabolism of contraceptive steroids. This could result in unintended pregnancy or breakthrough bleeding).
No products indexed under this heading.

Doxycycline Calcium (Contraceptive effectiveness may be reduced when hormonal contraceptives are co-administered with antibiotics, anticonvulsants, and other drugs that increase the metabolism of contraceptive steroids. This could result in unintended pregnancy or breakthrough bleeding).
No products indexed under this heading.

Doxycycline Hyclate (Contraceptive effectiveness may be reduced when hormonal contraceptives are co-administered with antibiotics, anticonvulsants, and other drugs that increase the metabolism of contraceptive steroids. This could result in unintended pregnancy or breakthrough bleeding).
No products indexed under this heading.

Doxycycline Monohydrate (Contraceptive effectiveness may be reduced when hormonal contraceptives are co-administered with antibiotics, anticonvulsants, and other drugs that increase the metabolism of contraceptive steroids. This could result in unintended pregnancy or breakthrough bleeding).
No products indexed under this heading.

Efavirenz (CYP3A4 inhibitors, such as itraconazole or ketoconazole, may increase plasma hormone levels). Products include:
Atripla 906

Enoxacin (Contraceptive effectiveness may be reduced when hormonal contraceptives are co-administered with antibiotics, anticonvulsants, and other drugs that increase the metabolism of contraceptive steroids. This could result in unintended pregnancy or breakthrough bleeding).
No products indexed under this heading.

Epirubicin Hydrochloride (Contraceptive effectiveness may be reduced when hormonal contraceptives are co-administered with antibiotics, anticonvulsants, and other drugs that increase the metabolism of contraceptive steroids. This could result in unintended pregnancy or breakthrough bleeding).
No products indexed under this heading.

Erythromycin (Contraceptive effectiveness may be reduced when hormonal contraceptives are co-administered with antibiotics, anticonvulsants, and other drugs that increase the metabolism of contraceptive steroids. This could result in unintended pregnancy or breakthrough bleeding).
No products indexed under this heading.

Erythromycin, Topical (Contraceptive effectiveness may be reduced when hormonal contraceptives are co-administered with antibiotics, anticonvulsants, and other drugs that increase the metabolism of contraceptive steroids. This could result in unintended pregnancy or breakthrough bleeding).
No products indexed under this heading.

Erythromycin Estolate (Contraceptive effectiveness may be reduced when hormonal contraceptives are co-administered with antibiotics, anticonvulsants, and other drugs that increase the metabolism of contraceptive steroids. This could result in unintended pregnancy or breakthrough bleeding).
No products indexed under this heading.

Erythromycin Ethylsuccinate (Contraceptive effectiveness may be reduced when hormonal contraceptives are co-administered with antibiotics, anticonvulsants, and other drugs that increase the metabolism of contraceptive steroids. This could result in unintended pregnancy or breakthrough bleeding). Products include:
E.E.S. 437
EryPed 435

Erythromycin Gluceptate (Contraceptive effectiveness may be reduced when hormonal contraceptives are co-administered with antibiotics, anticonvulsants, and other drugs that increase the metabolism of contraceptive steroids. This could result in unintended pregnancy or breakthrough bleeding).
No products indexed under this heading.

(⊙ Described in PDR® for Ophthalmic Medicines)

Erythromycin Lactobionate (Contraceptive effectiveness may be reduced when hormonal contraceptives are co-administered with antibiotics, anticonvulsants, and other drugs that increase the metabolism of contraceptive steroids. This could result in unintended pregnancy or breakthrough bleeding).
No products indexed under this heading.

Erythromycin Stearate (Contraceptive effectiveness may be reduced when hormonal contraceptives are co-administered with antibiotics, anticonvulsants, and other drugs that increase the metabolism of contraceptive steroids. This could result in unintended pregnancy or breakthrough bleeding).
No products indexed under this heading.

Escitalopram Oxalate (Contraceptive effectiveness may be reduced when hormonal contraceptives are co-administered with antibiotics, anticonvulsants, and other drugs that increase the metabolism of contraceptive steroids. This could result in unintended pregnancy or breakthrough bleeding). Products include:
Lexapro Oral Suspension 1160
Lexapro Tablets 1160

Esomeprazole Magnesium (CYP3A4 inhibitors, such as itraconazole or ketoconazole, may increase plasma hormone levels). Products include:
Nexium Capsules 704
Nexium Oral Suspension 704

Esomeprazole Sodium (CYP3A4 inhibitors, such as itraconazole or ketoconazole, may increase plasma hormone levels). Products include:
Nexium I.V. 712

Ethanol (Contraceptive effectiveness may be reduced when hormonal contraceptives are co-administered with antibiotics, anticonvulsants, and other drugs that increase the metabolism of contraceptive steroids. This could result in unintended pregnancy or breakthrough bleeding).
No products indexed under this heading.

Ethosuximide (Contraceptive effectiveness may be reduced when hormonal contraceptives are co-administered with antibiotics, anticonvulsants, and other drugs that increase the metabolism of contraceptive steroids. This could result in unintended pregnancy or breakthrough bleeding).
No products indexed under this heading.

Ethotoin (Contraceptive effectiveness may be reduced when hormonal contraceptives are co-administered with antibiotics, anticonvulsants, and other drugs that increase the metabolism of contraceptive steroids. This could result in unintended pregnancy or breakthrough bleeding).
No products indexed under this heading.

Ethyl Alcohol (Contraceptive effectiveness may be reduced when hormonal contraceptives are co-administered with antibiotics, anticonvulsants, and other drugs that increase the metabolism of contraceptive steroids. This could result in unintended pregnancy or breakthrough bleeding).
No products indexed under this heading.

Felbamate (Contraceptive effectiveness may be reduced when hormonal contraceptives are co-administered with felbamate. This could result in unintended pregnancy or breakthrough bleeding).
No products indexed under this heading.

Fluconazole (CYP3A4 inhibitors, such as itraconazole or ketoconazole, may increase plasma hormone levels).
No products indexed under this heading.

Fludrocortisone Acetate (Contraceptive effectiveness may be reduced when hormonal contraceptives are co-administered with antibiotics, anticonvulsants, and other drugs that increase the metabolism of contraceptive steroids. This could result in unintended pregnancy or breakthrough bleeding).
No products indexed under this heading.

Fluoxetine (CYP3A4 inhibitors, such as itraconazole or ketoconazole, may increase plasma hormone levels).
No products indexed under this heading.

Fluoxetine Hydrochloride (CYP3A4 inhibitors, such as itraconazole or ketoconazole, may increase plasma hormone levels). Products include:
Prozac Weekly 1941
Prozac Pulvules 1941
Symbyax 1965

Fluvoxamine (Contraceptive effectiveness may be reduced when hormonal contraceptives are co-administered with antibiotics, anticonvulsants, and other drugs that increase the metabolism of contraceptive steroids. This could result in unintended pregnancy or breakthrough bleeding).
No products indexed under this heading.

Fluvoxamine Maleate (CYP3A4 inhibitors, such as itraconazole or ketoconazole, may increase plasma hormone levels).
No products indexed under this heading.

Fosamprenavir Calcium (Several of the anti-HIV protease inhibitors have been studied with co-administration of oral combination hormonal contraceptives; significant changes (increase and decrease) in the plasma levels of the estrogen and progestin have been noted in some cases. The safety and efficacy of oral contraceptive products may be affected with co-administration of anti-HIV protease inhibitors). Products include:
Lexiva Oral Suspension 1558
Lexiva 1558

Fosphenytoin (Contraceptive effectiveness may be reduced when hormonal contraceptives are co-administered with phenytoin. This could result in unintended pregnancy or breakthrough bleeding).
No products indexed under this heading.

Fosphenytoin Sodium (Contraceptive effectiveness may be reduced when hormonal contraceptives are co-administered with phenytoin. This could result in unintended pregnancy or breakthrough bleeding).
No products indexed under this heading.

Gabapentin (Contraceptive effectiveness may be reduced when hormonal contraceptives are co-administered with antibiotics, anticonvulsants, and other drugs that increase the metabolism of contraceptive steroids. This could result in unintended pregnancy or breakthrough bleeding).
No products indexed under this heading.

Garlic Extract (Contraceptive effectiveness may be reduced when hormonal contraceptives are co-administered with antibiotics, anticonvulsants, and other drugs that increase the metabolism of contraceptive steroids. This could result in unintended pregnancy or breakthrough bleeding).
No products indexed under this heading.

Garlic Oil (Contraceptive effectiveness may be reduced when hormonal contraceptives are co-administered with antibiotics, anticonvulsants, and other drugs that increase the metabolism of contraceptive steroids. This could result in unintended pregnancy or breakthrough bleeding).
No products indexed under this heading.

Gatifloxacin (Contraceptive effectiveness may be reduced when hormonal contraceptives are co-administered with antibiotics, anticonvulsants, and other drugs that increase the metabolism of contraceptive steroids. This could result in unintended pregnancy or breakthrough bleeding).
No products indexed under this heading.

Gemifloxacin Mesylate (Contraceptive effectiveness may be reduced when hormonal contraceptives are co-administered with antibiotics, anticonvulsants, and other drugs that increase the metabolism of contraceptive steroids. This could result in unintended pregnancy or breakthrough bleeding).
No products indexed under this heading.

Gentamicin Sulfate (Contraceptive effectiveness may be reduced when hormonal contraceptives are co-administered with antibiotics, anticonvulsants, and other drugs that increase the metabolism of contraceptive steroids. This could result in unintended pregnancy or breakthrough bleeding). Products include:
Pred-G .... ⊙226, ⊙227

Glipizide (Contraceptive effectiveness may be reduced when hormonal contraceptives are co-administered with antibiotics, anticonvulsants, and other drugs that increase the metabolism of contraceptive steroids. This could result in unintended pregnancy or breakthrough bleeding).
No products indexed under this heading.

Glyburide (Contraceptive effectiveness may be reduced when hormonal contraceptives are co-administered with antibiotics, anticonvulsants, and other drugs that increase the metabolism of contraceptive steroids. This could result in unintended pregnancy or breakthrough bleeding).
No products indexed under this heading.

Grepafloxacin Hydrochloride (Contraceptive effectiveness may be reduced when hormonal contraceptives are co-administered with antibiotics, anticonvulsants, and other drugs that increase the metabolism of contraceptive steroids. This could result in unintended pregnancy or breakthrough bleeding).
No products indexed under this heading.

Griseofulvin (Contraceptive effectiveness may be reduced when hormonal contraceptives are co-administered with griseofulvin. This could result in unintended pregnancy or breakthrough bleeding).
No products indexed under this heading.

Hepatic Enzyme-Inducing Agents (Contraceptive effectiveness may be reduced when hormonal contraceptives are co-administered with antibiotics, anticonvulsants, and other drugs that increase the metabolism of contraceptive steroids. This could result in unintended pregnancy or breakthrough bleeding).
No products indexed under this heading.

Hexobarbital (Contraceptive effectiveness may be reduced when hormonal contraceptives are co-administered with barbiturates. This could result in unintended pregnancy or breakthrough bleeding).
No products indexed under this heading.

Hydrocortisone (Alcohol) (Contraceptive effectiveness may be reduced when hormonal contraceptives are co-administered with antibiotics, anticonvulsants, and other drugs that increase the metabolism of contraceptive steroids. This could result in unintended pregnancy or breakthrough bleeding).
No products indexed under this heading.

Hydrocortisone Acetate (Contraceptive effectiveness may be reduced when hormonal contraceptives are co-administered with antibiotics, anticonvulsants, and other drugs that increase the metabolism of contraceptive steroids. This could result in unintended pregnancy or breakthrough bleeding).
No products indexed under this heading.

Hydrocortisone Butyrate (Contraceptive effectiveness may be reduced when hormonal contraceptives are co-administered with antibiotics, anticonvulsants, and other drugs that increase the metabolism of contraceptive steroids. This could result in unintended pregnancy or breakthrough bleeding).
No products indexed under this heading.

Hydrocortisone Cypionate (Contraceptive effectiveness may be reduced when hormonal contraceptives are co-administered with antibiotics, anticonvulsants, and other drugs that increase the metabolism of contraceptive steroids. This could result in unintended pregnancy or breakthrough bleeding).
No products indexed under this heading.

Hydrocortisone Hemisuccinate (Contraceptive effectiveness may be reduced when hormonal contraceptives are co-administered with antibiotics, anticonvulsants, and other drugs that increase the metabolism of contraceptive steroids. This could result in unintended pregnancy or breakthrough bleeding).
No products indexed under this heading.

Hydrocortisone Probutate (Contraceptive effectiveness may be reduced when hormonal contraceptives are co-administered with antibiotics, anticonvulsants, and other drugs that increase the metabolism of contraceptive steroids. This could result in unintended pregnancy or breakthrough bleeding).
No products indexed under this heading.

Hydrocortisone Sodium Phosphate (Contraceptive effectiveness may be reduced when hormonal contraceptives are co-administered with antibiotics, anticonvulsants, and other drugs that increase the metabolism of contraceptive steroids. This could result in unintended pregnancy or breakthrough bleeding).
No products indexed under this heading.

Hydrocortisone Sodium Succinate (Contraceptive effectiveness may be reduced when hormonal contraceptives are co-administered with antibiotics, anticonvulsants, and other drugs that increase the metabolism of contraceptive steroids. This could result in unintended pregnancy or breakthrough bleeding).
No products indexed under this heading.

Hydrocortisone Valerate (Contraceptive effectiveness may be reduced when hormonal contraceptives are co-administered with antibiotics, anticonvulsants, and other drugs that increase the metabolism of contraceptive steroids. This could result in unintended pregnancy or breakthrough bleeding).
No products indexed under this heading.

Hypericum (Contraceptive effectiveness may be reduced when hormonal contraceptives are co-administered with antibiotics, anticonvulsants, and other drugs that increase the metabolism of contraceptive steroids. This could result in unintended pregnancy or breakthrough bleeding).
No products indexed under this heading.

Hypericum Perforatum (Herbal products containing St. John's Wort (hypericum perforatum) may induce hepatic enzymes (cytochrome P450) and p-glycoprotein transporter and may reduce the effectiveness of contracep-

(☉ Described in PDR® for Ophthalmic Medicines)

1345 Interactions Index Ortho-Cyclen

Methacycline Hydrochloride (Contraceptive effectiveness may be reduced when hormonal contraceptives are co-administered with antibiotics, anticonvulsants, and other drugs that increase the metabolism of contraceptive steroids. This could result in unintended pregnancy or breakthrough bleeding).
No products indexed under this heading.

Methicillin Sodium (Contraceptive effectiveness may be reduced when hormonal contraceptives are co-administered with antibiotics, anticonvulsants, and other drugs that increase the metabolism of contraceptive steroids. This could result in unintended pregnancy or breakthrough bleeding).
No products indexed under this heading.

Methsuximide (Contraceptive effectiveness may be reduced when hormonal contraceptives are co-administered with antibiotics, anticonvulsants, and other drugs that increase the metabolism of contraceptive steroids. This could result in unintended pregnancy or breakthrough bleeding).
No products indexed under this heading.

Methylprednisolone (Contraceptive effectiveness may be reduced when hormonal contraceptives are co-administered with antibiotics, anticonvulsants, and other drugs that increase the metabolism of contraceptive steroids. This could result in unintended pregnancy or breakthrough bleeding).
No products indexed under this heading.

Methylprednisolone Acetate (Contraceptive effectiveness may be reduced when hormonal contraceptives are co-administered with antibiotics, anticonvulsants, and other drugs that increase the metabolism of contraceptive steroids. This could result in unintended pregnancy or breakthrough bleeding).
No products indexed under this heading.

Methylprednisolone Sodium Succinate (Contraceptive effectiveness may be reduced when hormonal contraceptives are co-administered with antibiotics, anticonvulsants, and other drugs that increase the metabolism of contraceptive steroids. This could result in unintended pregnancy or breakthrough bleeding).
No products indexed under this heading.

Metronidazole (CYP3A4 inhibitors, such as itraconazole or ketoconazole, may increase plasma hormone levels). Products include:
Pylera 793

Metronidazole Benzoate (CYP3A4 inhibitors, such as itraconazole or ketoconazole, may increase plasma hormone levels).
No products indexed under this heading.

Metronidazole Hydrochloride (CYP3A4 inhibitors, such as itraconazole or ketoconazole, may increase plasma hormone levels).
No products indexed under this heading.

Metronidazole Sodium (CYP3A4 inhibitors, such as itraconazole or ketoconazole, may increase plasma hormone levels).
No products indexed under this heading.

Mezlocillin Sodium (Contraceptive effectiveness may be reduced when hormonal contraceptives are co-administered with antibiotics, anticonvulsants, and other drugs that increase the metabolism of contraceptive steroids. This could result in unintended pregnancy or breakthrough bleeding).
No products indexed under this heading.

Miconazole (CYP3A4 inhibitors, such as itraconazole or ketoconazole, may increase plasma hormone levels).
No products indexed under this heading.

Miconazole Nitrate (CYP3A4 inhibitors, such as itraconazole or ketoconazole, may increase plasma hormone levels). Products include:
Vusion Ointment 3335

Mifepristone (CYP3A4 inhibitors, such as itraconazole or ketoconazole, may increase plasma hormone levels).
No products indexed under this heading.

Minocycline Hydrochloride (Contraceptive effectiveness may be reduced when hormonal contraceptives are co-administered with antibiotics, anticonvulsants, and other drugs that increase the metabolism of contraceptive steroids. This could result in unintended pregnancy or breakthrough bleeding). Products include:
Solodyn 2073

Modafinil (Contraceptive effectiveness may be reduced when hormonal contraceptives are co-administered with antibiotics, anticonvulsants, and other drugs that increase the metabolism of contraceptive steroids. This could result in unintended pregnancy or breakthrough bleeding). Products include:
Provigil 983

Morphine Sulfate (Increased clearance of morphine, due to induction of conjugation, has been noted when concomitantly administered with oral contraceptives). Products include:
Avinza 1822
Embeda 1831
MS Contin 2803

Moxifloxacin Hydrochloride (Contraceptive effectiveness may be reduced when hormonal contraceptives are co-administered with antibiotics, anticonvulsants, and other drugs that increase the metabolism of contraceptive steroids. This could result in unintended pregnancy or breakthrough bleeding). Products include:
Avelox 3064
Vigamox 589

Nafcillin Sodium (Contraceptive effectiveness may be reduced when hormonal contraceptives are co-administered with antibiotics, anticonvulsants, and other drugs that increase the metabolism of contraceptive steroids. This could result in unintended pregnancy or breakthrough bleeding).
No products indexed under this heading.

Nefazodone Hydrochloride (CYP3A4 inhibitors, such as itraconazole or ketoconazole, may increase plasma hormone levels).
No products indexed under this heading.

Nelfinavir Mesylate (Several of the anti-HIV protease inhibitors have been studied with co-administration of oral combination hormonal contraceptives; significant changes (increase and decrease) in the plasma levels of the estrogen and progestin have been noted in some cases. The safety and efficacy of oral contraceptive products may be affected with co-administration of anti-HIV protease inhibitors).
No products indexed under this heading.

Nevirapine (CYP3A4 inhibitors, such as itraconazole or ketoconazole, may increase plasma hormone levels). Products include:
Viramune Oral Suspension 897
Viramune Tablets 897

Niacin (CYP3A4 inhibitors, such as itraconazole or ketoconazole, may increase plasma hormone levels). Products include:
Advicor 402
Cardio Basics 3455
Niaspan 497
Simcor 524

Niacinamide (CYP3A4 inhibitors, such as itraconazole or ketoconazole, may increase plasma hormone levels). Products include:
CitraNatal 90 DHA Capsules 2332
CitraNatal Assure 2332
CitraNatal Rx 2332
Heplive 607

Niacinamide Hydroiodide (CYP3A4 inhibitors, such as itraconazole or ketoconazole, may increase plasma hormone levels).
No products indexed under this heading.

Nicotinamide (CYP3A4 inhibitors, such as itraconazole or ketoconazole, may increase plasma hormone levels).
No products indexed under this heading.

Nicotine (Contraceptive effectiveness may be reduced when hormonal contraceptives are co-administered with antibiotics, anticonvulsants, and other drugs that increase the metabolism of contraceptive steroids. This could result in unintended pregnancy or breakthrough bleeding).
No products indexed under this heading.

Nicotine Polacrilex (Contraceptive effectiveness may be reduced when hormonal contraceptives are co-administered with antibiotics, anticonvulsants, and other drugs that increase the metabolism of contraceptive steroids. This could result in unintended pregnancy or breakthrough bleeding).
No products indexed under this heading.

Nicotine Salicylate (Contraceptive effectiveness may be reduced when hormonal contraceptives are co-administered with antibiotics, anticonvulsants, and other drugs that increase the metabolism of contraceptive steroids. This could result in unintended pregnancy or breakthrough bleeding).
No products indexed under this heading.

Nicotine Sulfate (Contraceptive effectiveness may be reduced when hormonal contraceptives are co-administered with antibiotics, anticonvulsants, and other drugs that increase the metabolism of contraceptive steroids. This could result in unintended pregnancy or breakthrough bleeding).
No products indexed under this heading.

Nifedipine (CYP3A4 inhibitors, such as itraconazole or ketoconazole, may increase plasma hormone levels).
No products indexed under this heading.

Norethindrone (Contraceptive effectiveness may be reduced when hormonal contraceptives are co-administered with antibiotics, anticonvulsants, and other drugs that increase the metabolism of contraceptive steroids. This could result in unintended pregnancy or breakthrough bleeding). Products include:
Ortho Micronor 2660

Norethindrone Acetate (Contraceptive effectiveness may be reduced when hormonal contraceptives are co-administered with antibiotics, anticonvulsants, and other drugs that increase the metabolism of contraceptive steroids. This could result in unintended pregnancy or breakthrough bleeding). Products include:
Activella 2561

Norfloxacin (Contraceptive effectiveness may be reduced when hormonal contraceptives are co-administered with antibiotics, anticonvulsants, and other drugs that increase the metabolism of contraceptive steroids. This could result in unintended pregnancy or breakthrough bleeding). Products include:
Noroxin 2220

Ofloxacin (Contraceptive effectiveness may be reduced when hormonal contraceptives are co-administered with antibiotics, anticonvulsants, and other drugs that increase the metabolism of contraceptive steroids. This could result in unintended pregnancy or breakthrough bleeding).
No products indexed under this heading.

Omeprazole (CYP3A4 inhibitors, such as itraconazole or ketoconazole, may increase plasma hormone levels).
No products indexed under this heading.

Omeprazole Magnesium (Contraceptive effectiveness may be reduced when hormonal contraceptives are co-administered with antibiotics, anticonvulsants, and other drugs that increase the metabolism of contraceptive steroids. This could result in unintended pregnancy or breakthrough bleeding).
No products indexed under this heading.

Oxacillin (Contraceptive effectiveness may be reduced when hormonal contraceptives are co-administered with antibiotics, anticonvulsants, and other drugs that increase the metabolism of contraceptive steroids. This could result in unintended pregnancy or breakthrough bleeding).
No products indexed under this heading.

Oxacillin Sodium (Contraceptive effectiveness may be reduced when hormonal contraceptives are co-administered with antibiotics, anticonvulsants, and other drugs that increase the metabolism of contraceptive steroids. This could result in unintended pregnancy or breakthrough bleeding).
No products indexed under this heading.

Oxcarbazepine (Contraceptive effectiveness may be reduced when hormonal contraceptives are co-administered with oxcarbazepine. This could result in unintended pregnancy or breakthrough bleeding).
No products indexed under this heading.

Oxytetracycline Hydrochloride (Contraceptive effectiveness may be reduced when hormonal contraceptives are co-administered with antibiotics, anticonvulsants, and other drugs that increase the metabolism of contraceptive steroids. This could result in unintended pregnancy or breakthrough bleeding).
No products indexed under this heading.

Paramethadione (Contraceptive effectiveness may be reduced when hormonal contraceptives are co-administered with antibiotics, anticonvulsants, and other drugs that increase the metabolism of contraceptive steroids. This could result in unintended pregnancy or breakthrough bleeding).
No products indexed under this heading.

Paroxetine Hydrochloride (CYP3A4 inhibitors, such as itraconazole or ketoconazole, may increase plasma hormone levels). Products include:
Paroxetine CR 2361
Paroxetine ER 2371
Paxil 1586
Paxil CR 1596

Penicillin, Potassium Phenoxymethyl (Contraceptive effectiveness may be reduced when hormonal contraceptives are co-administered with antibiotics, anticonvulsants, and other drugs that increase the metabolism of contraceptive steroids. This could result in unintended pregnancy or breakthrough bleeding).
No products indexed under this heading.

Penicillin G Benzathine (Contraceptive effectiveness may be reduced when hormonal contraceptives are co-administered with antibiotics, anticonvulsants, and other drugs that increase the metabolism of contraceptive steroids. This could result in unintended pregnancy or breakthrough bleeding). Products include:
Bicillin C-R Injectable Suspension 1826
Bicillin L-A 1828

IMPORTANT NOTE: Always consult each drug listing in the patient's regimen for possible interactions.

Penicillin G Dibenzylethyenedi-amine (Contraceptive effectiveness may be reduced when hormonal contraceptives are co-administered with antibiotics, anticonvulsants, and other drugs that increase the metabolism of contraceptive steroids. This could result in unintended pregnancy or breakthrough bleeding).
 No products indexed under this heading.

Penicillin G Potassium (Contraceptive effectiveness may be reduced when hormonal contraceptives are co-administered with antibiotics, anticonvulsants, and other drugs that increase the metabolism of contraceptive steroids. This could result in unintended pregnancy or breakthrough bleeding).
 No products indexed under this heading.

Penicillin G Procaine (Contraceptive effectiveness may be reduced when hormonal contraceptives are co-administered with antibiotics, anticonvulsants, and other drugs that increase the metabolism of contraceptive steroids. This could result in unintended pregnancy or breakthrough bleeding). Products include:

Penicillin G Sodium (Contraceptive effectiveness may be reduced when hormonal contraceptives are co-administered with antibiotics, anticonvulsants, and other drugs that increase the metabolism of contraceptive steroids. This could result in unintended pregnancy or breakthrough bleeding).
 No products indexed under this heading.

Penicillin V (Contraceptive effectiveness may be reduced when hormonal contraceptives are co-administered with antibiotics, anticonvulsants, and other drugs that increase the metabolism of contraceptive steroids. This could result in unintended pregnancy or breakthrough bleeding).
 No products indexed under this heading.

Penicillin V Potassium (Contraceptive effectiveness may be reduced when hormonal contraceptives are co-administered with antibiotics, anticonvulsants, and other drugs that increase the metabolism of contraceptive steroids. This could result in unintended pregnancy or breakthrough bleeding).
 No products indexed under this heading.

Penicillins (Contraceptive effectiveness may be reduced when hormonal contraceptives are co-administered with antibiotics, anticonvulsants, and other drugs that increase the metabolism of contraceptive steroids. This could result in unintended pregnancy or breakthrough bleeding).
 No products indexed under this heading.

Pentobarbital (Contraceptive effectiveness may be reduced when hormonal contraceptives are co-administered with barbiturates. This could result in unintended pregnancy or breakthrough bleeding).
 No products indexed under this heading.

Pentobarbital Sodium (Contraceptive effectiveness may be reduced when hormonal contraceptives are co-administered with barbiturates. This could result in unintended pregnancy or breakthrough bleeding). Products include:

Phenacemide (Contraceptive effectiveness may be reduced when hormonal contraceptives are co-administered with antibiotics, anticonvulsants, and other drugs that increase the metabolism of contraceptive steroids. This could result in unintended pregnancy or breakthrough bleeding).
 No products indexed under this heading.

Phenobarbital (Contraceptive effectiveness may be reduced when hormonal contraceptives are co-administered with barbiturates. This could result in unintended pregnancy or breakthrough bleeding). Products include:

Phenobarbital Sodium (Contraceptive effectiveness may be reduced when hormonal contraceptives are co-administered with barbiturates. This could result in unintended pregnancy or breakthrough bleeding).
 No products indexed under this heading.

Phensuximide (Contraceptive effectiveness may be reduced when hormonal contraceptives are co-administered with antibiotics, anticonvulsants, and other drugs that increase the metabolism of contraceptive steroids. This could result in unintended pregnancy or breakthrough bleeding).
 No products indexed under this heading.

Phenylbutazone (Contraceptive effectiveness may be reduced when hormonal contraceptives are co-administered with phenylbutazone. This could result in unintended pregnancy or breakthrough bleeding).
 No products indexed under this heading.

Phenytoin (Contraceptive effectiveness may be reduced when hormonal contraceptives are co-administered with phenytoin. This could result in unintended pregnancy or breakthrough bleeding).
 No products indexed under this heading.

Phenytoin Sodium (Contraceptive effectiveness may be reduced when hormonal contraceptives are co-administered with phenytoin. This could result in unintended pregnancy or breakthrough bleeding). Products include:

Piperacillin Sodium (Contraceptive effectiveness may be reduced when hormonal contraceptives are co-administered with antibiotics, anticonvulsants, and other drugs that increase the metabolism of contraceptive steroids. This could result in unintended pregnancy or breakthrough bleeding). Products include:

Posaconazole (CYP3A4 inhibitors, such as itraconazole or ketoconazole, may increase plasma hormone levels). Products include:

Prednisolone (Combination hormonal contraceptives containing some synthetic estrogens (eg, ethinyl estradiol) may inhibit the metabolism of other compounds. Increased plasma concentrations of prednisolone has been reported with concomitant administration of oral contraceptives).
 No products indexed under this heading.

Prednisolone Acetate (Combination hormonal contraceptives containing some synthetic estrogens (eg, ethinyl estradiol) may inhibit the metabolism of other compounds. Increased plasma concentrations of prednisolone has been reported with concomitant administration of oral contraceptives). Products include:

Prednisolone Sodium Phosphate (Combination hormonal contraceptives containing some synthetic estrogens (eg, ethinyl estradiol) may inhibit the metabolism of other compounds. Increased plasma concentrations of prednisolone has been reported with concomitant administration of oral contraceptives).
 No products indexed under this heading.

Prednisolone Tebutate (Combination hormonal contraceptives containing some synthetic estrogens (eg, ethinyl estradiol) may inhibit the metabolism of other compounds. Increased plasma concentrations of prednisolone has been reported with concomitant administration of oral contraceptives).
 No products indexed under this heading.

Prednisone (Contraceptive effectiveness may be reduced when hormonal contraceptives are co-administered with antibiotics, anticonvulsants, and other drugs that increase the metabolism of contraceptive steroids. This could result in unintended pregnancy or breakthrough bleeding).
 No products indexed under this heading.

Prednisone sodium phosphate (Contraceptive effectiveness may be reduced when hormonal contraceptives are co-administered with antibiotics, anticonvulsants, and other drugs that increase the metabolism of contraceptive steroids. This could result in unintended pregnancy or breakthrough bleeding).
 No products indexed under this heading.

Primidone (Contraceptive effectiveness may be reduced when hormonal contraceptives are co-administered with antibiotics, anticonvulsants, and other drugs that increase the metabolism of contraceptive steroids. This could result in unintended pregnancy or breakthrough bleeding).
 No products indexed under this heading.

Propoxyphene Hydrochloride (CYP3A4 inhibitors, such as itraconazole or ketoconazole, may increase plasma hormone levels).
 No products indexed under this heading.

Propoxyphene Napsylate (CYP3A4 inhibitors, such as itraconazole or ketoconazole, may increase plasma hormone levels).
 No products indexed under this heading.

Quinidine (CYP3A4 inhibitors, such as itraconazole or ketoconazole, may increase plasma hormone levels).
 No products indexed under this heading.

Quinidine Hydrochloride (CYP3A4 inhibitors, such as itraconazole or ketoconazole, may increase plasma hormone levels).
 No products indexed under this heading.

Quinidine Polygalacturonate (CYP3A4 inhibitors, such as itraconazole or ketoconazole, may increase plasma hormone levels).
 No products indexed under this heading.

Quinidine Sulfate (CYP3A4 inhibitors, such as itraconazole or ketoconazole, may increase plasma hormone levels).
 No products indexed under this heading.

Quinine (CYP3A4 inhibitors, such as itraconazole or ketoconazole, may increase plasma hormone levels). Products include:

Quinine Sulfate (CYP3A4 inhibitors, such as itraconazole or ketoconazole, may increase plasma hormone levels).
 No products indexed under this heading.

Quinupristin (CYP3A4 inhibitors, such as itraconazole or ketoconazole, may increase plasma hormone levels).
 No products indexed under this heading.

Ranitidine Bismuth Citrate (CYP3A4 inhibitors, such as itraconazole or ketoconazole, may increase plasma hormone levels).
 No products indexed under this heading.

Ranitidine Hydrochloride (CYP3A4 inhibitors, such as itraconazole or ketoconazole, may increase plasma hormone levels). Products include:

Rifabutin (Contraceptive effectiveness may be reduced when hormonal contraceptives are co-administered with antibiotics, anticonvulsants, and other drugs that increase the metabolism of contraceptive steroids. This could result in unintended pregnancy or breakthrough bleeding).
 No products indexed under this heading.

Rifampicin (Contraceptive effectiveness may be reduced when hormonal contraceptives are co-administered with antibiotics, anticonvulsants, and other drugs that increase the metabolism of contraceptive steroids. This could result in unintended pregnancy or breakthrough bleeding).
 No products indexed under this heading.

Rifampin (Contraceptive effectiveness may be reduced when hormonal contraceptives are co-administered with rifampin. This could result in unintended pregnancy or breakthrough bleeding).
 No products indexed under this heading.

Rifapentine (Contraceptive effectiveness may be reduced when hormonal contraceptives are co-administered with antibiotics, anticonvulsants, and other drugs that increase the metabolism of contraceptive steroids. This could result in unintended pregnancy or breakthrough bleeding).
 No products indexed under this heading.

Ritonavir (Several of the anti-HIV protease inhibitors have been studied with co-administration of oral combination hormonal contraceptives; significant changes (increase and decrease) in the plasma levels of the estrogen and progestin have been noted in some cases. The safety and efficacy of oral contraceptive products may be affected with co-administration of anti-HIV protease inhibitors). Products include:

Rufinamide (Contraceptive effectiveness may be reduced when hormonal contraceptives are co-administered with antibiotics, anticonvulsants, and other drugs that increase the metabolism of contraceptive steroids. This could result in unintended pregnancy or breakthrough bleeding). Products include:

Salicylic Acid (Increased clearance of salicylic acid, due to induction of conjugation, has been noted in some concomitantly administered with oral contraceptives).
 No products indexed under this heading.

Saquinavir (Several of the anti-HIV protease inhibitors have been studied with co-administration of oral combination hormonal contraceptives; significant changes (increase and decrease) in the plasma levels of the estrogen and progestin have been noted in some cases. The safety and efficacy of oral contraceptive products may be affected with co-administration of anti-HIV protease inhibitors).
 No products indexed under this heading.

Saquinavir Mesylate (Several of the anti-HIV protease inhibitors have been studied with co-administration of oral combination hormonal contraceptives; significant changes (increase and decrease) in the plasma levels of the estrogen and progestin have been noted in some cases. The safety and efficacy of oral contraceptive products may be affected with co-administration of anti-HIV protease inhibitors).
 No products indexed under this heading.

(⊙ Described in PDR® for Ophthalmic Medicines)

1347 Interactions Index Ortho-Cyclen

Secobarbital Sodium (Contraceptive effectiveness may be reduced when hormonal contraceptives are co-administered with barbiturates. This could result in unintended pregnancy or breakthrough bleeding).
No products indexed under this heading.

Sertraline Hydrochloride (CYP3A4 inhibitors, such as itraconazole or ketoconazole, may increase plasma hormone levels).
No products indexed under this heading.

Sildenafil Citrate (CYP3A4 inhibitors, such as itraconazole or ketoconazole, may increase plasma hormone levels).
No products indexed under this heading.

Sodium Butabarbital (Contraceptive effectiveness may be reduced when hormonal contraceptives are co-administered with barbiturates. This could result in unintended pregnancy or breakthrough bleeding).
No products indexed under this heading.

Sodium Cloxacillin Monohydrate (Contraceptive effectiveness may be reduced when hormonal contraceptives are co-administered with antibiotics, anticonvulsants, and other drugs that increase the metabolism of contraceptive steroids. This could result in unintended pregnancy or breakthrough bleeding).
No products indexed under this heading.

Sodium Pentobarbital (Contraceptive effectiveness may be reduced when hormonal contraceptives are co-administered with barbiturates. This could result in unintended pregnancy or breakthrough bleeding).
No products indexed under this heading.

Sparfloxacin (Contraceptive effectiveness may be reduced when hormonal contraceptives are co-administered with antibiotics, anticonvulsants, and other drugs that increase the metabolism of contraceptive steroids. This could result in unintended pregnancy or breakthrough bleeding).
No products indexed under this heading.

Streptomycin Sulfate (Contraceptive effectiveness may be reduced when hormonal contraceptives are co-administered with antibiotics, anticonvulsants, and other drugs that increase the metabolism of contraceptive steroids. This could result in unintended pregnancy or breakthrough bleeding).
No products indexed under this heading.

Sulfamethizole (Contraceptive effectiveness may be reduced when hormonal contraceptives are co-administered with antibiotics, anticonvulsants, and other drugs that increase the metabolism of contraceptive steroids. This could result in unintended pregnancy or breakthrough bleeding).
No products indexed under this heading.

Sulfamethoxazole (Contraceptive effectiveness may be reduced when hormonal contraceptives are co-administered with antibiotics, anticonvulsants, and other drugs that increase the metabolism of contraceptive steroids. This could result in unintended pregnancy or breakthrough bleeding).
No products indexed under this heading.

Sulfisoxazole Acetyl (Contraceptive effectiveness may be reduced when hormonal contraceptives are co-administered with antibiotics, anticonvulsants, and other drugs that increase the metabolism of contraceptive steroids. This could result in unintended pregnancy or breakthrough bleeding).
No products indexed under this heading.

Sulfisoxazole Diolamine (Contraceptive effectiveness may be reduced when hormonal contraceptives are co-administered with antibiotics, anticonvulsants, and other drugs that increase the metabolism of contraceptive steroids. This could result in unintended pregnancy or breakthrough bleeding).
No products indexed under this heading.

Telithromycin (CYP3A4 inhibitors, such as itraconazole or ketoconazole, may increase plasma hormone levels). Products include:
Ketek 2991

Temazepam (Increased clearance of temazepam, due to induction of conjugation, has been noted when concomitantly administered with oral contraceptives).
No products indexed under this heading.

Tetracycline Hydrochloride (Contraceptive effectiveness may be reduced when hormonal contraceptives are co-administered with antibiotics, anticonvulsants, and other drugs that increase the metabolism of contraceptive steroids. This could result in unintended pregnancy or breakthrough bleeding). Products include:
Pylera 793

Theophylline (Combination hormonal contraceptives containing some synthetic estrogens (eg, ethinyl estradiol) may inhibit the metabolism of other compounds. Increased plasma concentrations of theophylline has been reported with concomitant administration of oral contraceptives).
No products indexed under this heading.

Theophylline Anhydrous (Combination hormonal contraceptives containing some synthetic estrogens (eg, ethinyl estradiol) may inhibit the metabolism of other compounds. Increased plasma concentrations of theophylline has been reported with concomitant administration of oral contraceptives). Products include:
Uniphyl 2817

Theophylline Calcium Salicylate (Combination hormonal contraceptives containing some synthetic estrogens (eg, ethinyl estradiol) may inhibit the metabolism of other compounds. Increased plasma concentrations of theophylline has been reported with concomitant administration of oral contraceptives).
No products indexed under this heading.

Theophylline Dihydroxypropyl (Glyceryl) (Combination hormonal contraceptives containing some synthetic estrogens (eg, ethinyl estradiol) may inhibit the metabolism of other compounds. Increased plasma concentrations of theophylline has been reported with concomitant administration of oral contraceptives).
No products indexed under this heading.

Theophylline Ethylenediamine (Combination hormonal contraceptives containing some synthetic estrogens (eg, ethinyl estradiol) may inhibit the metabolism of other compounds. Increased plasma concentrations of theophylline has been reported with concomitant administration of oral contraceptives).
No products indexed under this heading.

Theophylline Sodium Glycinate (Combination hormonal contraceptives containing some synthetic estrogens (eg, ethinyl estradiol) may inhibit the metabolism of other compounds. Increased plasma concentrations of theophylline has been reported with concomitant administration of oral contraceptives).
No products indexed under this heading.

Thiamylal Sodium (Contraceptive effectiveness may be reduced when hormonal contraceptives are co-administered with barbiturates. This could result in unintended pregnancy or breakthrough bleeding).
No products indexed under this heading.

Tiagabine Hydrochloride (Contraceptive effectiveness may be reduced when hormonal contraceptives are co-administered with antibiotics, anticonvulsants, and other drugs that increase the metabolism of contraceptive steroids. This could result in unintended pregnancy or breakthrough bleeding). Products include:
Gabitril 972

Ticarcillin Disodium (Contraceptive effectiveness may be reduced when hormonal contraceptives are co-administered with antibiotics, anticonvulsants, and other drugs that increase the metabolism of contraceptive steroids. This could result in unintended pregnancy or breakthrough bleeding). Products include:
Timentin ADD-Vantage 1670
Timentin Galaxy 1674
Timentin 1666
Timentin Pharmacy 1678

Tipranavir (Several of the anti-HIV protease inhibitors have been studied with co-administration of oral combination hormonal contraceptives; significant changes (increase and decrease) in the plasma levels of the estrogen and progestin have been noted in some cases. The safety and efficacy of oral contraceptive products may be affected with co-administration of anti-HIV protease inhibitors).
No products indexed under this heading.

Tobacco (Cigarette smoking increases the risk of serious cardiovascular side effects from oral contraceptive use. Women who use oral contraceptives should be strongly advised not to smoke).
No products indexed under this heading.

Tobramycin (Contraceptive effectiveness may be reduced when hormonal contraceptives are co-administered with antibiotics, anticonvulsants, and other drugs that increase the metabolism of contraceptive steroids. This could result in unintended pregnancy or breakthrough bleeding). Products include:
Tobi Nebulizer 2546
Tobramycin and Dexamethasone Ophthalmic Suspension .... ⊙ 251
Zylet .... ⊙ 252

Tobramycin Sulfate (Contraceptive effectiveness may be reduced when hormonal contraceptives are co-administered with antibiotics, anticonvulsants, and other drugs that increase the metabolism of contraceptive steroids. This could result in unintended pregnancy or breakthrough bleeding).
No products indexed under this heading.

Tolazamide (Contraceptive effectiveness may be reduced when hormonal contraceptives are co-administered with antibiotics, anticonvulsants, and other drugs that increase the metabolism of contraceptive steroids. This could result in unintended pregnancy or breakthrough bleeding).
No products indexed under this heading.

Tolbutamide (Contraceptive effectiveness may be reduced when hormonal contraceptives are co-administered with antibiotics, anticonvulsants, and other drugs that increase the metabolism of contraceptive steroids. This could result in unintended pregnancy or breakthrough bleeding).
No products indexed under this heading.

Topiramate (Contraceptive effectiveness may be reduced when hormonal contraceptives are co-administered with topiramate. This could result in unintended pregnancy or breakthrough bleeding).
No products indexed under this heading.

Triamcinolone (Contraceptive effectiveness may be reduced when hormonal contraceptives are co-administered with antibiotics, anticonvulsants, and other drugs that increase the metabolism of contraceptive steroids. This could result in unintended pregnancy or breakthrough bleeding).
No products indexed under this heading.

Triamcinolone Acetonide (Contraceptive effectiveness may be reduced when hormonal contraceptives are co-administered with antibiotics, anticonvulsants, and other drugs that increase the metabolism of contraceptive steroids. This could result in unintended pregnancy or breakthrough bleeding). Products include:
Azmacort 408
Nasacort AQ 3019

Triamcinolone Diacetate (Contraceptive effectiveness may be reduced when hormonal contraceptives are co-administered with antibiotics, anticonvulsants, and other drugs that increase the metabolism of contraceptive steroids. This could result in unintended pregnancy or breakthrough bleeding).
No products indexed under this heading.

Triamcinolone Hexacetonide (Contraceptive effectiveness may be reduced when hormonal contraceptives are co-administered with antibiotics, anticonvulsants, and other drugs that increase the metabolism of contraceptive steroids. This could result in unintended pregnancy or breakthrough bleeding).
No products indexed under this heading.

Trimethadione (Contraceptive effectiveness may be reduced when hormonal contraceptives are co-administered with antibiotics, anticonvulsants, and other drugs that increase the metabolism of contraceptive steroids. This could result in unintended pregnancy or breakthrough bleeding).
No products indexed under this heading.

Troglitazone (CYP3A4 inhibitors, such as itraconazole or ketoconazole, may increase plasma hormone levels).
No products indexed under this heading.

Troleandomycin (Contraceptive effectiveness may be reduced when hormonal contraceptives are co-administered with antibiotics, anticonvulsants, and other drugs that increase the metabolism of contraceptive steroids. This could result in unintended pregnancy or breakthrough bleeding).
No products indexed under this heading.

Trovafloxacin Mesylate (Contraceptive effectiveness may be reduced when hormonal contraceptives are co-administered with antibiotics, anticonvulsants, and other drugs that increase the metabolism of contraceptive steroids. This could result in unintended pregnancy or breakthrough bleeding).
No products indexed under this heading.

Valproate Sodium (Contraceptive effectiveness may be reduced when hormonal contraceptives are co-administered with antibiotics, anticonvulsants, and other drugs that increase the metabolism of contraceptive steroids. This could result in unintended pregnancy or breakthrough bleeding).
No products indexed under this heading.

IMPORTANT NOTE: Always consult each drug listing in the patient's regimen for possible interactions.

Ortho-Cyclen Interactions Index 1348

Valproic Acid (Contraceptive effectiveness may be reduced when hormonal contraceptives are co-administered with antibiotics, anticonvulsants, and other drugs that increase the metabolism of contraceptive steroids. This could result in unintended pregnancy or breakthrough bleeding).
No products indexed under this heading.

Vardenafil Hydrochloride (CYP3A4 inhibitors, such as itraconazole or ketoconazole, may increase plasma hormone levels). Products include:
Levitra 3157

Verapamil Hydrochloride (CYP3A4 inhibitors, such as itraconazole or ketoconazole, may increase plasma hormone levels). Products include:
Tarka 534

Vitamin C (Ascorbic acid may increase plasma ethinyl estradiol levels, possibly by inhibition of conjugation). Products include:
Bausch & Lomb Ocuvite Adult 50+ .... ⊙238
Bio-C 3454
BoneMate Plus 3454
Cardio Basics 3455
CitraNatal 90 DHA Capsules 2332
CitraNatal Assure 2332
CitraNatal Rx 2332
Ferralet 2333
Heplive 607
Meili Clear 607
MoviPrep Oral Solution 2905
PreNexa 3473
Proflavanol 90 3476

Voriconazole (CYP3A4 inhibitors, such as itraconazole or ketoconazole, may increase plasma hormone levels).
No products indexed under this heading.

Zafirlukast (CYP3A4 inhibitors, such as itraconazole or ketoconazole, may increase plasma hormone levels). Products include:
Accolate 3612

Zileuton (CYP3A4 inhibitors, such as itraconazole or ketoconazole, may increase plasma hormone levels).
No products indexed under this heading.

Zonisamide (Contraceptive effectiveness may be reduced when hormonal contraceptives are co-administered with antibiotics, anticonvulsants, and other drugs that increase the metabolism of contraceptive steroids. This could result in unintended pregnancy or breakthrough bleeding). Products include:
Zonegran 1081

Food Interactions

Broccoli (Contraceptive effectiveness may be reduced when hormonal contraceptives are co-administered with antibiotics, anticonvulsants, and other drugs that increase the metabolism of contraceptive steroids. This could result in unintended pregnancy or breakthrough bleeding).

Brussel Sprouts (Contraceptive effectiveness may be reduced when hormonal contraceptives are co-administered with antibiotics, anticonvulsants, and other drugs that increase the metabolism of contraceptive steroids. This could result in unintended pregnancy or breakthrough bleeding).

Charbroiled Food (Contraceptive effectiveness may be reduced when hormonal contraceptives are co-administered with antibiotics, anticonvulsants, and other drugs that increase the metabolism of contraceptive steroids. This could result in unintended pregnancy or breakthrough bleeding).

Grapefruit (CYP3A4 inhibitors, such as itraconazole or ketoconazole, may increase plasma hormone levels).

Grapefruit Juice (CYP3A4 inhibitors, such as itraconazole or ketoconazole, may increase plasma hormone levels).

OSMOPREP TABLETS

(Sodium Phosphate) 2907

May interact with ACE inhibitors, alcohols, angiotensin-II receptor antagonists, benzodiazepines, diuretics, drugs that prolong the QT interval, drugs which lower seizure threshold, non-steroidal anti-inflammatory agents, tricyclic antidepressants, and certain other agents. Compounds in these categories include:

Alprazolam (Prolongation of the QT interval has been observed in some patients who were dosed with sodium phosphate colon preparations. Sodium phosphate should be used with caution in patients who are taking medications known to prolong the QT interval, since serious complications may occur).
No products indexed under this heading.

Amiloride Hydrochloride (Caution with use if taking concomitant medications that may effect electrolyte levels (such as diuretics). Dehydration from purgation may be exacerbated by the use of diuretics. In addition, patients that are at increased risk of acute phosphate nephropathy may include those using medicines that affect renal perfusion or function (such as diuretics)).
No products indexed under this heading.

Amiodarone Hydrochloride (Prolongation of the QT interval has been observed in some patients who were dosed with sodium phosphate colon preparations. Sodium phosphate should be used with caution in patients who are taking medications known to prolong the QT interval, since serious complications may occur).
No products indexed under this heading.

Amitriptyline Hydrochloride (Prolongation of the QT interval has been observed in some patients who were dosed with sodium phosphate colon preparations. Sodium phosphate should be used with caution in patients who are taking medications known to prolong the QT interval, since serious complications may occur).
No products indexed under this heading.

Amoxapine (Prolongation of the QT interval has been observed in some patients who were dosed with sodium phosphate colon preparations. Sodium phosphate should be used with caution in patients who are taking medications known to prolong the QT interval, since serious complications may occur).
No products indexed under this heading.

Astemizole (Prolongation of the QT interval has been observed in some patients who were dosed with sodium phosphate colon preparations. Sodium phosphate should be used with caution in patients who are taking medications known to prolong the QT interval, since serious complications may occur).
No products indexed under this heading.

Benazepril Hydrochloride (Patients at increased risk of acute phosphate nephropathy may include those using medicines that affect renal perfusion or function (such as angiotensin converting enzyme [ACE] inhibitors)).
No products indexed under this heading.

Bendroflumethiazide (Caution with use if taking concomitant medications that may effect electrolyte levels (such as diuretics). Dehydration from purgation may be exacerbated by the use of diuretics. In addition, patients that are at increased risk of acute phosphate nephropathy may include those using medicines that affect renal perfusion or function (such as diuretics)).
No products indexed under this heading.

Bretylium Tosylate (Prolongation of the QT interval has been observed in some patients who were dosed with sodium phosphate colon preparations. Sodium phosphate should be used with caution in patients who are taking medications known to prolong the QT interval, since serious complications may occur).
No products indexed under this heading.

Bumetanide (Caution with use if taking concomitant medications that may effect electrolyte levels (such as diuretics). Dehydration from purgation may be exacerbated by the use of diuretics. In addition, patients that are at increased risk of acute phosphate nephropathy may include those using medicines that affect renal perfusion or function (such as diuretics)).
No products indexed under this heading.

Buspirone Hydrochloride (Prolongation of the QT interval has been observed in some patients who were dosed with sodium phosphate colon preparations. Sodium phosphate should be used with caution in patients who are taking medications known to prolong the QT interval, since serious complications may occur).
No products indexed under this heading.

Candesartan Cilexetil (Patients at increased risk of acute phosphate nephropathy may include those using medicines that affect renal perfusion or function (such as angiotensin receptor blockers [ARBs])). Products include:
Atacand 697
Atacand HCT 700

Captopril (Patients at increased risk of acute phosphate nephropathy may include those using medicines that affect renal perfusion or function (such as angiotensin converting enzyme [ACE] inhibitors)). Products include:
Captopril 2341

Celecoxib (Patients at increased risk of acute phosphate nephropathy may include those using medicines that affect renal perfusion or function (possibly with nonsteroidal anti-inflammatory drugs [NSAIDs])). Products include:
Celebrex 3272

Chlordiazepoxide (Prolongation of the QT interval has been observed in some patients who were dosed with sodium phosphate colon preparations. Sodium phosphate should be used with caution in patients who are taking medications known to prolong the QT interval, since serious complications may occur).
No products indexed under this heading.

Chlordiazepoxide Hydrochloride (Prolongation of the QT interval has been observed in some patients who were dosed with sodium phosphate colon preparations. Sodium phosphate should be used with caution in patients who are taking medications known to prolong the QT interval, since serious complications may occur).
No products indexed under this heading.

Chlorothiazide (Caution with use if taking concomitant medications that may effect electrolyte levels (such as diuretics). Dehydration from purgation may be exacerbated by the use of diuretics. In addition, patients that are at increased risk of acute phosphate nephropathy may include those using medicines that affect renal perfusion or function (such as diuretics)).
No products indexed under this heading.

Chlorothiazide Sodium (Caution with use if taking concomitant medications that may effect electrolyte levels (such as diuretics). Dehydration from purgation may be exacerbated by the use of diuretics. In addition, patients that are at increased risk of acute phosphate nephropathy may include those using medicines that affect renal perfusion or function (such as diuretics)). Products include:
Diuril Intravenous 2009

Chlorpromazine (Prolongation of the QT interval has been observed in some patients who were dosed with sodium phosphate colon preparations. Sodium phosphate should be used with caution in patients who are taking medications known to prolong the QT interval, since serious complications may occur).
No products indexed under this heading.

Chlorpromazine Hydrochloride (Prolongation of the QT interval has been observed in some patients who were dosed with sodium phosphate colon preparations. Sodium phosphate should be used with caution in patients who are taking medications known to prolong the QT interval, since serious complications may occur).
No products indexed under this heading.

Chlorprothixene (Prolongation of the QT interval has been observed in some patients who were dosed with sodium phosphate colon preparations. Sodium phosphate should be used with caution in patients who are taking medications known to prolong the QT interval, since serious complications may occur).
No products indexed under this heading.

Chlorprothixene Hydrochloride (Prolongation of the QT interval has been observed in some patients who were dosed with sodium phosphate colon preparations. Sodium phosphate should be used with caution in patients who are taking medications known to prolong the QT interval, since serious complications may occur).
No products indexed under this heading.

Chlorthalidone (Caution with use if taking concomitant medications that may effect electrolyte levels (such as diuretics). Dehydration from purgation may be exacerbated by the use of diuretics. In addition, patients that are at increased risk of acute phosphate nephropathy may include those using medicines that affect renal perfusion or function (such as diuretics)). Products include:
Clorpres 2344

Clomipramine Hydrochloride (Prolongation of the QT interval has been observed in some patients who were dosed with sodium phosphate colon preparations. Sodium phosphate should be used with caution in patients who are taking medications known to prolong the QT interval, since serious complications may occur).
No products indexed under this heading.

Clorazepate Dipotassium (Prolongation of the QT interval has been observed in some patients who were dosed with sodium phosphate colon preparations. Sodium phosphate should be used with caution in patients who are taking medications known to prolong the QT interval, since serious complications may occur).
No products indexed under this heading.

Clozapine (Prolongation of the QT interval has been observed in some patients who were dosed with sodium phosphate colon preparations. Sodium phosphate should be used with caution in patients who are taking medications known to prolong the QT interval, since serious complications may occur).
No products indexed under this heading.

(⊙ Described in PDR® for Ophthalmic Medicines)

1349 Interactions Index OsmoPrep

Desipramine Hydrochloride (Prolongation of the QT interval has been observed in some patients who were dosed with sodium phosphate colon preparations. Sodium phosphate should be used with caution in patients who are taking medications known to prolong the QT interval, since serious complications may occur).
No products indexed under this heading.

Diazepam (Prolongation of the QT interval has been observed in some patients who were dosed with sodium phosphate colon preparations. Sodium phosphate should be used with caution in patients who are taking medications known to prolong the QT interval, since serious complications may occur). Products include:
Valium Tablets 2880

Diclofenac Epolamine (Patients at increased risk of acute phosphate nephropathy may include those using medicines that affect renal perfusion or function (possibly with nonsteroidal anti-inflammatory drugs [NSAIDs])). Products include:
Flector 1839

Diclofenac Potassium (Patients at increased risk of acute phosphate nephropathy may include those using medicines that affect renal perfusion or function (possibly with nonsteroidal anti-inflammatory drugs [NSAIDs])).
No products indexed under this heading.

Diclofenac Sodium (Patients at increased risk of acute phosphate nephropathy may include those using medicines that affect renal perfusion or function (possibly with nonsteroidal anti-inflammatory drugs [NSAIDs])).
No products indexed under this heading.

Disopyramide (Prolongation of the QT interval has been observed in some patients who were dosed with sodium phosphate colon preparations. Sodium phosphate should be used with caution in patients who are taking medications known to prolong the QT interval, since serious complications may occur).
No products indexed under this heading.

Disopyramide Phosphate (Prolongation of the QT interval has been observed in some patients who were dosed with sodium phosphate colon preparations. Sodium phosphate should be used with caution in patients who are taking medications known to prolong the QT interval, since serious complications may occur).
No products indexed under this heading.

Dofetilide (Prolongation of the QT interval has been observed in some patients who were dosed with sodium phosphate colon preparations. Sodium phosphate should be used with caution in patients who are taking medications known to prolong the QT interval, since serious complications may occur).
No products indexed under this heading.

Doxepin Hydrochloride (Prolongation of the QT interval has been observed in some patients who were dosed with sodium phosphate colon preparations. Sodium phosphate should be used with caution in patients who are taking medications known to prolong the QT interval, since serious complications may occur).
No products indexed under this heading.

Droperidol (Prolongation of the QT interval has been observed in some patients who were dosed with sodium phosphate colon preparations. Sodium phosphate should be used with caution in patients who are taking medications known to prolong the QT interval, since serious complications may occur).
No products indexed under this heading.

Drugs, Oral, unspecified (Medications administered in close proximity to sodium phosphate tablets may not be absorbed from the gastrointestinal tract due to the rapid intestinal peristalsis and watery diarrhea induced by the purgative agent).
No products indexed under this heading.

Drugs, unspecified (Medications administered in close proximity to sodium phosphate tablets may not be absorbed from the gastrointestinal tract due to the rapid intestinal peristalsis and watery diarrhea induced by the purgative agent).
No products indexed under this heading.

Enalapril Maleate (Patients at increased risk of acute phosphate nephropathy may include those using medicines that affect renal perfusion or function (such as angiotensin converting enzyme [ACE] inhibitors)).
No products indexed under this heading.

Enalaprilat (Patients at increased risk of acute phosphate nephropathy may include those using medicines that affect renal perfusion or function (such as angiotensin converting enzyme [ACE] inhibitors)).
No products indexed under this heading.

Eprosartan Mesylate (Patients at increased risk of acute phosphate nephropathy may include those using medicines that affect renal perfusion or function (such as angiotensin receptor blockers [ARBs])). Products include:
Teveten 538
Teveten HCT 541

Erythromycin (Prolongation of the QT interval has been observed in some patients who were dosed with sodium phosphate colon preparations. Sodium phosphate should be used with caution in patients who are taking medications known to prolong the QT interval, since serious complications may occur).
No products indexed under this heading.

Erythromycin Estolate (Prolongation of the QT interval has been observed in some patients who were dosed with sodium phosphate colon preparations. Sodium phosphate should be used with caution in patients who are taking medications known to prolong the QT interval, since serious complications may occur).
No products indexed under this heading.

Erythromycin Ethylsuccinate (Prolongation of the QT interval has been observed in some patients who were dosed with sodium phosphate colon preparations. Sodium phosphate should be used with caution in patients who are taking medications known to prolong the QT interval, since serious complications may occur). Products include:
E.E.S. 437
EryPed 435

Erythromycin Gluceptate (Prolongation of the QT interval has been observed in some patients who were dosed with sodium phosphate colon preparations. Sodium phosphate should be used with caution in patients who are taking medications known to prolong the QT interval, since serious complications may occur).
No products indexed under this heading.

Erythromycin Lactobionate (Prolongation of the QT interval has been observed in some patients who were dosed with sodium phosphate colon preparations. Sodium phosphate should be used with caution in patients who are taking medications known to prolong the QT interval, since serious complications may occur).
No products indexed under this heading.

Erythromycin Stearate (Prolongation of the QT interval has been observed in some patients who were dosed with sodium phosphate colon preparations. Sodium phosphate should be used with caution in patients who are taking medications known to prolong the QT interval, since serious complications may occur).
No products indexed under this heading.

Estazolam (There have been rare reports of generalized tonic-clonic seizures and/or loss of consciousness associated with use of sodium phosphate products in patients with no prior history of seizures. Sodium phosphate should be used with caution in patients at higher risk of seizure, such as those withdrawing from benzodiazepines).
No products indexed under this heading.

Ethacrynic Acid (Caution with use if taking concomitant medications that may effect electrolyte levels (such as diuretics). Dehydration from purgation may be exacerbated by the use of diuretics. In addition, patients that are at increased risk of acute phosphate nephropathy may include those using medicines that affect renal perfusion or function (such as diuretics)).
No products indexed under this heading.

Ethanol (There have been rare reports of generalized tonic-clonic seizures and/or loss of consciousness associated with use of sodium phosphate products in patients with no prior history of seizures. Sodium phosphate should be used with caution in patients at higher risk of seizure, such as those withdrawing from alcohol).
No products indexed under this heading.

Ethyl Alcohol (There have been rare reports of generalized tonic-clonic seizures and/or loss of consciousness associated with use of sodium phosphate products in patients with no prior history of seizures. Sodium phosphate should be used with caution in patients at higher risk of seizure, such as those withdrawing from alcohol).
No products indexed under this heading.

Etodolac (Patients at increased risk of acute phosphate nephropathy may include those using medicines that affect renal perfusion or function (possibly with nonsteroidal anti-inflammatory drugs [NSAIDs])).
No products indexed under this heading.

Fenoprofen Calcium (Patients at increased risk of acute phosphate nephropathy may include those using medicines that affect renal perfusion or function (possibly with nonsteroidal anti-inflammatory drugs [NSAIDs])).
No products indexed under this heading.

Flecainide Acetate (Prolongation of the QT interval has been observed in some patients who were dosed with sodium phosphate colon preparations. Sodium phosphate should be used with caution in patients who are taking medications known to prolong the QT interval, since serious complications may occur).
No products indexed under this heading.

Fluoxetine Hydrochloride (There have been rare reports of generalized tonic-clonic seizures and/or loss of consciousness associated with use of sodium phosphate products in patients with no prior history of seizures. Sodium phosphate should be used with caution in patients at higher risk of seizure, such as those using concomitant medications that lower the seizure threshold). Products include:
Prozac Weekly 1941
Prozac Pulvules 1941
Symbyax 1965

Fluphenazine Decanoate (Prolongation of the QT interval has been observed in some patients who were dosed with sodium phosphate colon preparations. Sodium phosphate should be used with caution in patients who are taking medications known to prolong the QT interval, since serious complications may occur).
No products indexed under this heading.

Fluphenazine Enanthate (Prolongation of the QT interval has been observed in some patients who were dosed with sodium phosphate colon preparations. Sodium phosphate should be used with caution in patients who are taking medications known to prolong the QT interval, since serious complications may occur).
No products indexed under this heading.

Fluphenazine Hydrochloride (Prolongation of the QT interval has been observed in some patients who were dosed with sodium phosphate colon preparations. Sodium phosphate should be used with caution in patients who are taking medications known to prolong the QT interval, since serious complications may occur).
No products indexed under this heading.

Flurazepam Hydrochloride (There have been rare reports of generalized tonic-clonic seizures and/or loss of consciousness associated with use of sodium phosphate products in patients with no prior history of seizures. Sodium phosphate should be used with caution in patients at higher risk of seizure, such as those withdrawing from benzodiazepines).
No products indexed under this heading.

Flurbiprofen (Patients at increased risk of acute phosphate nephropathy may include those using medicines that affect renal perfusion or function (possibly with nonsteroidal anti-inflammatory drugs [NSAIDs])).
No products indexed under this heading.

Fosinopril Sodium (Patients at increased risk of acute phosphate nephropathy may include those using medicines that affect renal perfusion or function (such as angiotensin converting enzyme [ACE] inhibitors)).
No products indexed under this heading.

Furosemide (Caution with use if taking concomitant medications that may effect electrolyte levels (such as diuretics). Dehydration from purgation may be exacerbated by the use of diuretics. In addition, patients that are at increased risk of acute phosphate nephropathy may include those using medicines that affect renal perfusion or function (such as diuretics)). Products include:
Furosemide 2354

Halazepam (There have been rare reports of generalized tonic-clonic seizures and/or loss of consciousness associated with use of sodium phosphate products in patients with no prior history of seizures. Sodium phosphate should be used with caution in patients at higher risk of seizure, such as those withdrawing from benzodiazepines).
No products indexed under this heading.

Haloperidol (Prolongation of the QT interval has been observed in some patients who were dosed with sodium phosphate colon preparations. Sodium phosphate should be used with caution in patients who are taking medications known to prolong the QT interval, since serious complications may occur).
No products indexed under this heading.

IMPORTANT NOTE: Always consult each drug listing in the patient's regimen for possible interactions.

OsmoPrep Interactions Index 1350

Haloperidol Decanoate (Prolongation of the QT interval has been observed in some patients who were dosed with sodium phosphate colon preparations. Sodium phosphate should be used with caution in patients who are taking medications known to prolong the QT interval, since serious complications may occur).
No products indexed under this heading.

Haloperidol Lactate (Prolongation of the QT interval has been observed in some patients who were dosed with sodium phosphate colon preparations. Sodium phosphate should be used with caution in patients who are taking medications known to prolong the QT interval, since serious complications may occur).
No products indexed under this heading.

Hydrochlorothiazide (Caution with use if taking concomitant medications that may effect electrolyte levels (such as diuretics). Dehydration from purgation may be exacerbated by the use of diuretics. In addition, patients that are at increased risk of acute phosphate nephropathy may include those using medicines that affect renal perfusion or function (such as diuretics)). Products include:
Atacand HCT 700
Avalide 2956
Benicar HCT 1017
Diovan HCT 2419
Dyazide 1429
Exforge HCT 2449
Hyzaar 2162
Hyzaar 100-12.5 2162
Micardis HCT 889
Prinzide 2246
Tekturna HCT 2541
Teveten HCT 541

Hydroflumethiazide (Caution with use if taking concomitant medications that may effect electrolyte levels (such as diuretics). Dehydration from purgation may be exacerbated by the use of diuretics. In addition, patients that are at increased risk of acute phosphate nephropathy may include those using medicines that affect renal perfusion or function (such as diuretics)).
No products indexed under this heading.

Hydroxyzine Hydrochloride (Prolongation of the QT interval has been observed in some patients who were dosed with sodium phosphate colon preparations. Sodium phosphate should be used with caution in patients who are taking medications known to prolong the QT interval, since serious complications may occur).
No products indexed under this heading.

Ibuprofen (Patients at increased risk of acute phosphate nephropathy may include those using medicines that affect renal perfusion or function (possibly with nonsteroidal anti-inflammatory drugs [NSAIDs])). Products include:
Motrin IB 2043
Children's Motrin 2044
Children's Motrin Non-Staining Dye-Free 2044
Infants' Motrin 2044
Infants' Motrin Dye-Free 2044
Junior Strength Motrin 2044
Vicoprofen 564

Imipramine Hydrochloride (Prolongation of the QT interval has been observed in some patients who were dosed with sodium phosphate colon preparations. Sodium phosphate should be used with caution in patients who are taking medications known to prolong the QT interval, since serious complications may occur).
No products indexed under this heading.

Imipramine Pamoate (Prolongation of the QT interval has been observed in some patients who were dosed with sodium phosphate colon preparations. Sodium phosphate should be used with caution in patients who are taking medications known to prolong the QT interval, since serious complications may occur).
No products indexed under this heading.

Indapamide (Caution with use if taking concomitant medications that may effect electrolyte levels (such as diuretics). Dehydration from purgation may be exacerbated by the use of diuretics. In addition, patients that are at increased risk of acute phosphate nephropathy may include those using medicines that affect renal perfusion or function (such as diuretics)). Products include:
Indapamide 2356

Indomethacin (Patients at increased risk of acute phosphate nephropathy may include those using medicines that affect renal perfusion or function (possibly with nonsteroidal anti-inflammatory drugs [NSAIDs])). Products include:
Indocin 2167

Indomethacin Sodium Trihydrate (Patients at increased risk of acute phosphate nephropathy may include those using medicines that affect renal perfusion or function (possibly with nonsteroidal anti-inflammatory drugs [NSAIDs])). Products include:
Indocin I.V. 2007

Irbesartan (Patients at increased risk of acute phosphate nephropathy may include those using medicines that affect renal perfusion or function (such as angiotensin receptor blockers [ARBs])). Products include:
Avalide 2956
Avapro 2962

Isocarboxazid (Prolongation of the QT interval has been observed in some patients who were dosed with sodium phosphate colon preparations. Sodium phosphate should be used with caution in patients who are taking medications known to prolong the QT interval, since serious complications may occur). Products include:
Marplan 3481

Ketoprofen (Patients at increased risk of acute phosphate nephropathy may include those using medicines that affect renal perfusion or function (possibly with nonsteroidal anti-inflammatory drugs [NSAIDs])).
No products indexed under this heading.

Ketorolac Tromethamine (Patients at increased risk of acute phosphate nephropathy may include those using medicines that affect renal perfusion or function (possibly with nonsteroidal anti-inflammatory drugs [NSAIDs])). Products include:
Acuvail .... ⊙ 209

Lidocaine (Prolongation of the QT interval has been observed in some patients who were dosed with sodium phosphate colon preparations. Sodium phosphate should be used with caution in patients who are taking medications known to prolong the QT interval, since serious complications may occur). Products include:
Lidoderm 1107

Lidocaine Hydrochloride (Prolongation of the QT interval has been observed in some patients who were dosed with sodium phosphate colon preparations. Sodium phosphate should be used with caution in patients who are taking medications known to prolong the QT interval, since serious complications may occur).
No products indexed under this heading.

Lisinopril (Patients at increased risk of acute phosphate nephropathy may include those using medicines that affect renal perfusion or function (such as angiotensin converting enzyme [ACE] inhibitors)). Products include:
Prinivil 2241
Prinzide 2246

Lithium Carbonate (Prolongation of the QT interval has been observed in some patients who were dosed with sodium phosphate colon preparations. Sodium phosphate should be used with caution in patients who are taking medications known to prolong the QT interval, since serious complications may occur).
No products indexed under this heading.

Lithium Citrate (Prolongation of the QT interval has been observed in some patients who were dosed with sodium phosphate colon preparations. Sodium phosphate should be used with caution in patients who are taking medications known to prolong the QT interval, since serious complications may occur).
No products indexed under this heading.

Lorazepam (Prolongation of the QT interval has been observed in some patients who were dosed with sodium phosphate colon preparations. Sodium phosphate should be used with caution in patients who are taking medications known to prolong the QT interval, since serious complications may occur).
No products indexed under this heading.

Losartan Potassium (Patients at increased risk of acute phosphate nephropathy may include those using medicines that affect renal perfusion or function (such as angiotensin receptor blockers [ARBs])). Products include:
Cozaar 2106
Hyzaar 2162
Hyzaar 100-12.5 2162

Loxapine Hydrochloride (Prolongation of the QT interval has been observed in some patients who were dosed with sodium phosphate colon preparations. Sodium phosphate should be used with caution in patients who are taking medications known to prolong the QT interval, since serious complications may occur).
No products indexed under this heading.

Loxapine Succinate (Prolongation of the QT interval has been observed in some patients who were dosed with sodium phosphate colon preparations. Sodium phosphate should be used with caution in patients who are taking medications known to prolong the QT interval, since serious complications may occur).
No products indexed under this heading.

Maprotiline Hydrochloride (Prolongation of the QT interval has been observed in some patients who were dosed with sodium phosphate colon preparations. Sodium phosphate should be used with caution in patients who are taking medications known to prolong the QT interval, since serious complications may occur).
No products indexed under this heading.

Meclofenamate Sodium (Patients at increased risk of acute phosphate nephropathy may include those using medicines that affect renal perfusion or function (possibly with nonsteroidal anti-inflammatory drugs [NSAIDs])).
No products indexed under this heading.

Mefenamic Acid (Patients at increased risk of acute phosphate nephropathy may include those using medicines that affect renal perfusion or function (possibly with nonsteroidal anti-inflammatory drugs [NSAIDs])).
No products indexed under this heading.

Meloxicam (Patients at increased risk of acute phosphate nephropathy may include those using medicines that affect renal perfusion or function (possibly with nonsteroidal anti-inflammatory drugs [NSAIDs])).
No products indexed under this heading.

Meprobamate (Prolongation of the QT interval has been observed in some patients who were dosed with sodium phosphate colon preparations. Sodium phosphate should be used with caution in patients who are taking medications known to prolong the QT interval, since serious complications may occur).
No products indexed under this heading.

Mesoridazine Besylate (Prolongation of the QT interval has been observed in some patients who were dosed with sodium phosphate colon preparations. Sodium phosphate should be used with caution in patients who are taking medications known to prolong the QT interval, since serious complications may occur).
No products indexed under this heading.

Methyclothiazide (Caution with use if taking concomitant medications that may effect electrolyte levels (such as diuretics). Dehydration from purgation may be exacerbated by the use of diuretics. In addition, patients that are at increased risk of acute phosphate nephropathy may include those using medicines that affect renal perfusion or function (such as diuretics)).
No products indexed under this heading.

Metolazone (Caution with use if taking concomitant medications that may effect electrolyte levels (such as diuretics). Dehydration from purgation may be exacerbated by the use of diuretics. In addition, patients that are at increased risk of acute phosphate nephropathy may include those using medicines that affect renal perfusion or function (such as diuretics)).
No products indexed under this heading.

Mexiletine Hydrochloride (Prolongation of the QT interval has been observed in some patients who were dosed with sodium phosphate colon preparations. Sodium phosphate should be used with caution in patients who are taking medications known to prolong the QT interval, since serious complications may occur).
No products indexed under this heading.

Midazolam Hydrochloride (Prolongation of the QT interval has been observed in some patients who were dosed with sodium phosphate colon preparations. Sodium phosphate should be used with caution in patients who are taking medications known to prolong the QT interval, since serious complications may occur).
No products indexed under this heading.

Moexipril Hydrochloride (Patients at increased risk of acute phosphate nephropathy may include those using medicines that affect renal perfusion or function (such as angiotensin converting enzyme [ACE] inhibitors)).
No products indexed under this heading.

Molindone Hydrochloride (Prolongation of the QT interval has been observed in some patients who were dosed with sodium phosphate colon preparations. Sodium phosphate should be used with caution in patients who are taking medications known to prolong the QT interval, since serious complications may occur). Products include:
Moban 1108

Nabumetone (Patients at increased risk of acute phosphate nephropathy may include those using medicines that affect renal perfusion or function (possibly with nonsteroidal anti-inflammatory drugs [NSAIDs])).
No products indexed under this heading.

1351 **Interactions Index** **OsmoPrep**

Naproxen (Patients at increased risk of acute phosphate nephropathy may include those using medicines that affect renal perfusion or function (possibly with nonsteroidal anti-inflammatory drugs [NSAIDs])). Products include:
EC-Naprosyn ... **2850**
Naprosyn ... **2850**
Anaprox/Naprosyn ... **2850**

Naproxen Sodium (Patients at increased risk of acute phosphate nephropathy may include those using medicines that affect renal perfusion or function (possibly with nonsteroidal anti-inflammatory drugs [NSAIDs])). Products include:
Anaprox ... **2850**
Anaprox DS ... **2850**
Treximet ... **1681**

Nortriptyline Hydrochloride (Prolongation of the QT interval has been observed in some patients who were dosed with sodium phosphate colon preparations. Sodium phosphate should be used with caution in patients who are taking medications known to prolong the QT interval, since serious complications may occur).
No products indexed under this heading.

Olanzapine (Prolongation of the QT interval has been observed in some patients who were dosed with sodium phosphate colon preparations. Sodium phosphate should be used with caution in patients who are taking medications known to prolong the QT interval, since serious complications may occur). Products include:
Symbyax ... **1965**
Zyprexa ... **1984**
Zyprexa IntraMuscular ... **1984**
Zyprexa ZYDIS ... **1984**

Oral Medications, unspecified (Medications administered in close proximity to sodium phosphate tablets may not be absorbed from the gastrointestinal tract due to the rapid intestinal peristalsis and watery diarrhea induced by the purgative agent).
No products indexed under this heading.

Oxaprozin (Patients at increased risk of acute phosphate nephropathy may include those using medicines that affect renal perfusion or function (possibly with nonsteroidal anti-inflammatory drugs [NSAIDs])).
No products indexed under this heading.

Oxazepam (Prolongation of the QT interval has been observed in some patients who were dosed with sodium phosphate colon preparations. Sodium phosphate should be used with caution in patients who are taking medications known to prolong the QT interval, since serious complications may occur).
No products indexed under this heading.

Perindopril Erbumine (Patients at increased risk of acute phosphate nephropathy may include those using medicines that affect renal perfusion or function (such as angiotensin converting enzyme [ACE] inhibitors)).
No products indexed under this heading.

Perphenazine (Prolongation of the QT interval has been observed in some patients who were dosed with sodium phosphate colon preparations. Sodium phosphate should be used with caution in patients who are taking medications known to prolong the QT interval, since serious complications may occur).
No products indexed under this heading.

Phenelzine Sulfate (Prolongation of the QT interval has been observed in some patients who were dosed with sodium phosphate colon preparations. Sodium phosphate should be used with caution in patients who are taking medications known to prolong the QT interval, since serious complications may occur).
No products indexed under this heading.

Phenylbutazone (Patients at increased risk of acute phosphate nephropathy may include those using medicines that affect renal perfusion or function (possibly with nonsteroidal anti-inflammatory drugs [NSAIDs])).
No products indexed under this heading.

Piroxicam (Patients at increased risk of acute phosphate nephropathy may include those using medicines that affect renal perfusion or function (possibly with nonsteroidal anti-inflammatory drugs [NSAIDs])).
No products indexed under this heading.

Polythiazide (Caution with use if taking concomitant medications that may effect electrolyte levels (such as diuretics). Dehydration from purgation may be exacerbated by the use of diuretics. In addition, patients that are at increased risk of acute phosphate nephropathy may include those using medicines that affect renal perfusion or function (such as diuretics)).
No products indexed under this heading.

Prazepam (Prolongation of the QT interval has been observed in some patients who were dosed with sodium phosphate colon preparations. Sodium phosphate should be used with caution in patients who are taking medications known to prolong the QT interval, since serious complications may occur).
No products indexed under this heading.

Procainamide Hydrochloride (Prolongation of the QT interval has been observed in some patients who were dosed with sodium phosphate colon preparations. Sodium phosphate should be used with caution in patients who are taking medications known to prolong the QT interval, since serious complications may occur).
No products indexed under this heading.

Prochlorperazine (Prolongation of the QT interval has been observed in some patients who were dosed with sodium phosphate colon preparations. Sodium phosphate should be used with caution in patients who are taking medications known to prolong the QT interval, since serious complications may occur).
No products indexed under this heading.

Promethazine Hydrochloride (Prolongation of the QT interval has been observed in some patients who were dosed with sodium phosphate colon preparations. Sodium phosphate should be used with caution in patients who are taking medications known to prolong the QT interval, since serious complications may occur).
No products indexed under this heading.

Propafenone Hydrochloride (Prolongation of the QT interval has been observed in some patients who were dosed with sodium phosphate colon preparations. Sodium phosphate should be used with caution in patients who are taking medications known to prolong the QT interval, since serious complications may occur). Products include:
Rythmol ... **1648**
Rythmol SR ... **1652**

Protriptyline Hydrochloride (Prolongation of the QT interval has been observed in some patients who were dosed with sodium phosphate colon preparations. Sodium phosphate should be used with caution in patients who are taking medications known to prolong the QT interval, since serious complications may occur).
No products indexed under this heading.

Quazepam (There have been rare reports of generalized tonic-clonic seizures and/or loss of consciousness associated with use of sodium phosphate products in patients with no prior history of seizures. Sodium phosphate should be used with caution in patients at higher risk of seizure, such as those withdrawing from benzodiazepines).
No products indexed under this heading.

Quetiapine Fumarate (Prolongation of the QT interval has been observed in some patients who were dosed with sodium phosphate colon preparations. Sodium phosphate should be used with caution in patients who are taking medications known to prolong the QT interval, since serious complications may occur). Products include:
Seroquel ... **750**
Seroquel XR ... **759**

Quinapril Hydrochloride (Patients at increased risk of acute phosphate nephropathy may include those using medicines that affect renal perfusion or function (such as angiotensin converting enzyme [ACE] inhibitors)).
No products indexed under this heading.

Quinidine (Prolongation of the QT interval has been observed in some patients who were dosed with sodium phosphate colon preparations. Sodium phosphate should be used with caution in patients who are taking medications known to prolong the QT interval, since serious complications may occur).
No products indexed under this heading.

Quinidine Gluconate (Prolongation of the QT interval has been observed in some patients who were dosed with sodium phosphate colon preparations. Sodium phosphate should be used with caution in patients who are taking medications known to prolong the QT interval, since serious complications may occur).
No products indexed under this heading.

Quinidine Hydrochloride (Prolongation of the QT interval has been observed in some patients who were dosed with sodium phosphate colon preparations. Sodium phosphate should be used with caution in patients who are taking medications known to prolong the QT interval, since serious complications may occur).
No products indexed under this heading.

Quinidine Polygalacturonate (Prolongation of the QT interval has been observed in some patients who were dosed with sodium phosphate colon preparations. Sodium phosphate should be used with caution in patients who are taking medications known to prolong the QT interval, since serious complications may occur).
No products indexed under this heading.

Quinidine Sulfate (Prolongation of the QT interval has been observed in some patients who were dosed with sodium phosphate colon preparations. Sodium phosphate should be used with caution in patients who are taking medications known to prolong the QT interval, since serious complications may occur).
No products indexed under this heading.

Ramipril (Patients at increased risk of acute phosphate nephropathy may include those using medicines that affect renal perfusion or function (such as angiotensin converting enzyme [ACE] inhibitors)).
No products indexed under this heading.

Risperidone (Prolongation of the QT interval has been observed in some patients who were dosed with sodium phosphate colon preparations. Sodium phosphate should be used with caution in patients who are taking medications known to prolong the QT interval, since serious complications may occur). Products include:
Risperdal Consta ... **2682**

Rofecoxib (Patients at increased risk of acute phosphate nephropathy may include those using medicines that affect renal perfusion or function (possibly with nonsteroidal anti-inflammatory drugs [NSAIDs])).
No products indexed under this heading.

Spirapril Hydrochloride (Patients at increased risk of acute phosphate nephropathy may include those using medicines that affect renal perfusion or function (such as angiotensin converting enzyme [ACE] inhibitors)).
No products indexed under this heading.

Spironolactone (Caution with use if taking concomitant medications that may effect electrolyte levels (such as diuretics). Dehydration from purgation may be exacerbated by the use of diuretics. In addition, patients that are at increased risk of acute phosphate nephropathy may include those using medicines that affect renal perfusion or function (such as diuretics)).
No products indexed under this heading.

Sulindac (Patients at increased risk of acute phosphate nephropathy may include those using medicines that affect renal perfusion or function (possibly with nonsteroidal anti-inflammatory drugs [NSAIDs])). Products include:
Clinoril ... **2098**

Telmisartan (Patients at increased risk of acute phosphate nephropathy may include those using medicines that affect renal perfusion or function (such as angiotensin receptor blockers [ARBs])). Products include:
Micardis ... **887**
Micardis HCT ... **889**

Temazepam (There have been rare reports of generalized tonic-clonic seizures and/or loss of consciousness associated with use of sodium phosphate products in patients with no prior history of seizures. Sodium phosphate should be used with caution in patients at higher risk of seizure, such as those withdrawing from benzodiazepines).
No products indexed under this heading.

Thioridazine Hydrochloride (Prolongation of the QT interval has been observed in some patients who were dosed with sodium phosphate colon preparations. Sodium phosphate should be used with caution in patients who are taking medications known to prolong the QT interval, since serious complications may occur). Products include:
Thioridazine Hydrochloride ... **2384**

Thiothixene (Prolongation of the QT interval has been observed in some patients who were dosed with sodium phosphate colon preparations. Sodium phosphate should be used with caution in patients who are taking medications known to prolong the QT interval, since serious complications may occur). Products include:
Thiothixene ... **2386**

Tocainide Hydrochloride (Prolongation of the QT interval has been observed in some patients who were dosed with sodium phosphate colon preparations. Sodium phosphate should be used with caution in patients who are taking medications known to prolong the QT interval, since serious complications may occur).
No products indexed under this heading.

Tolmetin Sodium (Patients at increased risk of acute phosphate nephropathy may include those using medicines that affect renal perfusion or function (possibly with nonsteroidal anti-inflammatory drugs [NSAIDs])).
No products indexed under this heading.

IMPORTANT NOTE: Always consult each drug listing in the patient's regimen for possible interactions.

Torsemide (Caution with use if taking concomitant medications that may effect electrolyte levels (such as diuretics). Dehydration from purgation may be exacerbated by the use of diuretics. In addition, patients that are at increased risk of acute phosphate nephropathy may include those using medicines that affect renal perfusion or function (such as diuretics)).
No products indexed under this heading.

Trandolapril (Patients at increased risk of acute phosphate nephropathy may include those using medicines that affect renal perfusion or function (such as angiotensin converting enzyme [ACE] inhibitors)). Products include:
Mavik 489
Tarka 534

Tranylcypromine Sulfate (Prolongation of the QT interval has been observed in some patients who were dosed with sodium phosphate colon preparations. Sodium phosphate should be used with caution in patients who are taking medications known to prolong the QT interval, since serious complications may occur). Products include:
Parnate 1584

Trazodone Hydrochloride (There have been rare reports of generalized tonic-clonic seizures and/or loss of consciousness associated with use of sodium phosphate products in patients with no prior history of seizures. Sodium phosphate should be used with caution in patients at higher risk of seizure, such as those using concomitant medications that lower the seizure threshold).
No products indexed under this heading.

Triamterene (Caution with use if taking concomitant medications that may effect electrolyte levels (such as diuretics). Dehydration from purgation may be exacerbated by the use of diuretics. In addition, patients that are at increased risk of acute phosphate nephropathy may include those using medicines that affect renal perfusion or function (such as diuretics)). Products include:
Dyazide 1429
Dyrenium 3495

Triazolam (There have been rare reports of generalized tonic-clonic seizures and/or loss of consciousness associated with use of sodium phosphate products in patients with no prior history of seizures. Sodium phosphate should be used with caution in patients at higher risk of seizure, such as those withdrawing from benzodiazepines).
No products indexed under this heading.

Trifluoperazine Hydrochloride (Prolongation of the QT interval has been observed in some patients who were dosed with sodium phosphate colon preparations. Sodium phosphate should be used with caution in patients who are taking medications known to prolong the QT interval, since serious complications may occur).
No products indexed under this heading.

Trimipramine Maleate (Prolongation of the QT interval has been observed in some patients who were dosed with sodium phosphate colon preparations. Sodium phosphate should be used with caution in patients who are taking medications known to prolong the QT interval, since serious complications may occur).
No products indexed under this heading.

Valdecoxib (Patients at increased risk of acute phosphate nephropathy may include those using medicines that affect renal perfusion or function (possibly with nonsteroidal anti-inflammatory drugs [NSAIDs])).
No products indexed under this heading.

Valsartan (Patients at increased risk of acute phosphate nephropathy may include those using medicines that affect renal perfusion or function (such as angiotensin receptor blockers [ARBs])). Products include:
Diovan 2413
Diovan HCT 2419
Exforge 2443
Exforge HCT 2449
Valturna 3637

Ziprasidone Hydrochloride (Prolongation of the QT interval has been observed in some patients who were dosed with sodium phosphate colon preparations. Sodium phosphate should be used with caution in patients who are taking medications known to prolong the QT interval, since serious complications may occur). Products include:
Geodon 2723

Food Interactions

Alcohol (There have been rare reports of generalized tonic-clonic seizures and/or loss of consciousness associated with use of sodium phosphate products in patients with no prior history of seizures. Sodium phosphate should be used with caution in patients at higher risk of seizure, such as those withdrawing from alcohol).

Beer, reduced-alcohol (There have been rare reports of generalized tonic-clonic seizures and/or loss of consciousness associated with use of sodium phosphate products in patients with no prior history of seizures. Sodium phosphate should be used with caution in patients at higher risk of seizure, such as those withdrawing from alcohol).

Beer, unspecified (There have been rare reports of generalized tonic-clonic seizures and/or loss of consciousness associated with use of sodium phosphate products in patients with no prior history of seizures. Sodium phosphate should be used with caution in patients at higher risk of seizure, such as those withdrawing from alcohol).

Wine, Chianti (There have been rare reports of generalized tonic-clonic seizures and/or loss of consciousness associated with use of sodium phosphate products in patients with no prior history of seizures. Sodium phosphate should be used with caution in patients at higher risk of seizure, such as those withdrawing from alcohol).

Wine, Red (There have been rare reports of generalized tonic-clonic seizures and/or loss of consciousness associated with use of sodium phosphate products in patients with no prior history of seizures. Sodium phosphate should be used with caution in patients at higher risk of seizure, such as those withdrawing from alcohol).

Wine, unspecified (There have been rare reports of generalized tonic-clonic seizures and/or loss of consciousness associated with use of sodium phosphate products in patients with no prior history of seizures. Sodium phosphate should be used with caution in patients at higher risk of seizure, such as those withdrawing from alcohol).

Wine products (There have been rare reports of generalized tonic-clonic seizures and/or loss of consciousness associated with use of sodium phosphate products in patients with no prior history of seizures. Sodium phosphate should be used with caution in patients at higher risk of seizure, such as those withdrawing from alcohol).

OXYCONTIN TABLETS

(Oxycodone Hydrochloride) 2807
May interact with alcohols, antiemetics, central nervous system depressants, cytochrome p450 2d6 inhibitors (selected), general anesthetics, hypnotics and sedatives, mixed agonist/antagonist opioid analgesics, monoamine oxidase inhibitors, phenothiazines, quinidine, skeletal muscle relaxants, tranquilizers, tricyclic antidepressants, and certain other agents. Compounds in these categories include:

Alfentanil Hydrochloride (Oxycodone, like all opioid analgesics, should be started at 1/3 to 1/2 of the usual dosage in patients who are concurrently receiving other central nervous system depressants including sedatives or hypnotics, general anesthetics, phenothiazines, centrally acting anti-emetics, tranquilizers, and alcohol because respiratory depression, hypotension, and profound sedation or coma may result).
No products indexed under this heading.

Alprazolam (Oxycodone like all opioid analgesics, should be started at 1/3 to 1/2 of the usual dosage in patients who are concurrently receiving other central nervous system depressants including tranquilizers because respiratory depression, hypotension, and profound sedation or coma may result).
No products indexed under this heading.

Amiodarone Hydrochloride (Oxycodone is metabolized in part to oxymorphone via cytochrome P450 2D6. While this pathway may be blocked by a variety of drugs (eg, certain cardiovascular drugs including amiodarone), such blockade has not yet been shown to be of clinical significance with this agent. Clinicians should be aware of this possible interaction, however).
No products indexed under this heading.

Amitriptyline Hydrochloride (Oxycodone is metabolized in part to oxymorphone via cytochrome P450 2D6. While this pathway may be blocked by a variety of drugs (eg, polycyclic antidepressants), such blockade has not yet been shown to be of clinical significance with this agent. Clinicians should be aware of this possible interaction).
No products indexed under this heading.

Amobarbital (Oxycodone, like all opioid analgesics, should be started at 1/3 to 1/2 of the usual dosage in patients who are concurrently receiving other central nervous system depressants including sedatives or hypnotics, general anesthetics, phenothiazines, centrally acting anti-emetics, tranquilizers, and alcohol because respiratory depression, hypotension, and profound sedation or coma may result).
No products indexed under this heading.

Amobarbital Sodium (Oxycodone, like all opioid analgesics, should be started at 1/3 to 1/2 of the usual dosage in patients who are concurrently receiving other central nervous system depressants including sedatives or hypnotics, general anesthetics, phenothiazines, centrally acting anti-emetics, tranquilizers, and alcohol because respiratory depression, hypotension, and profound sedation or coma may result).
No products indexed under this heading.

Amoxapine (Oxycodone is metabolized in part to oxymorphone via cytochrome P450 2D6. While this pathway may be blocked by a variety of drugs (eg, polycyclic antidepressants), such blockade has not yet been shown to be of clinical significance with this agent. Clinicians should be aware of this possible interaction).
No products indexed under this heading.

Aprepitant (Oxycodone, like all opioid analgesics, should be started at 1/3 to 1/2 of the usual dosage in patients who are concurrently receiving other central nervous system depressants including centrally acting anti-emetics because respiratory depression, hypotension, and profound sedation or coma may result). Products include:
Emend 2124

Aprobarbital (Oxycodone, like all opioid analgesics, should be started at 1/3 to 1/2 of the usual dosage in patients who are concurrently receiving other central nervous system depressants including sedatives or hypnotics, general anesthetics, phenothiazines, centrally acting anti-emetics, tranquilizers, and alcohol because respiratory depression, hypotension, and profound sedation or coma may result).
No products indexed under this heading.

Atracurium Besylate (Opioid analgesics, including oxycodone, may enhance the neuromuscular blocking action of skeletal muscle relaxants and produce an increased degree of respiratory depression).
No products indexed under this heading.

Baclofen (Opioid analgesics, including oxycodone, may enhance the neuromuscular blocking action of skeletal muscle relaxants and produce an increased degree of respiratory depression).
No products indexed under this heading.

Buprenorphine Hydrochloride (Agonist/antagonist analgesics (ie, pentazocine, nalbuphine, and butorphanol) should be administered with caution to a patient who has received or is receiving a course of therapy with a pure opioid agonist analgesic such as oxycodone. In this situation, mixed agonist/antagonist analgesics may reduce the analgesic effect of oxycodone and/or may precipitate withdrawal symptoms in these patients).
No products indexed under this heading.

Bupropion Hydrochloride (Oxycodone is metabolized in part to oxymorphone via cytochrome P450 2D6. While this pathway may be blocked by a variety of drugs (eg, certain cardiovascular drugs including amiodarone and quinidine as well as polycyclic antidepressants), such blockade has not yet been shown to be of clinical significance with this agent. Clinicians should be aware of this possible interaction, however). Products include:
Aplenzin 2948
Wellbutrin 1719
Wellbutrin SR 1725
Zyban 1762

Buspirone Hydrochloride (Oxycodone like all opioid analgesics, should be started at 1/3 to 1/2 of the usual dosage in patients who are concurrently receiving other central nervous system depressants including tranquilizers because respiratory depression, hypotension, and profound sedation or coma may result).
No products indexed under this heading.

Butabarbital (Oxycodone, like all opioid analgesics, should be started at 1/3 to 1/2 of the usual dosage in patients who are concurrently receiving other central nervous system depressants including sedatives or hypnotics because respiratory depression, hypotension, and profound sedation or coma may result).
No products indexed under this heading.

Butabarbital Sodium (Oxycodone, like all opioid analgesics, should be started at 1/3 to 1/2 of the usual dosage in patients who are concurrently receiving other central nervous system depressants including sedatives or hypnotics because respiratory depression, hypotension, and profound sedation or coma may result).
No products indexed under this heading.

Butalbital (Oxycodone, like all opioid analgesics, should be started at 1/3 to 1/2 of the usual dosage in patients who are concurrently receiving other central nervous system depressants including sedatives or hypnotics because respiratory depression, hypotension, and profound sedation or coma may result).

No products indexed under this heading.

Butorphanol Tartrate (Agonist/antagonist analgesics (ie, pentazocine, nalbuphine, and butorphanol) should be administered with caution to a patient who has received or is receiving a course of therapy with a pure opioid agonist analgesic such as oxycodone. In this situation, mixed agonist/antagonist analgesics may reduce the analgesic effect of oxycodone and/or may precipitate withdrawal symptoms in these patients).

No products indexed under this heading.

Carisoprodol (Opioid analgesics, including oxycodone, may enhance the neuromuscular blocking action of skeletal muscle relaxants and produce an increased degree of respiratory depression).

No products indexed under this heading.

Celecoxib (Oxycodone is metabolized in part to oxymorphone via cytochrome P450 2D6. While this pathway may be blocked by a variety of drugs (eg, certain cardiovascular drugs including amiodarone and quinidine as well as polycyclic antidepressants), such blockade has not yet been shown to be of clinical significance with this agent. Clinicians should be aware of this possible interaction, however). Products include:
Celebrex 3272

Chloral Hydrate (Oxycodone, like all opioid analgesics, should be started at 1/3 to 1/2 of the usual dosage in patients who are concurrently receiving other central nervous system depressants including sedatives or hypnotics because respiratory depression, hypotension, and profound sedation or coma may result).

No products indexed under this heading.

Chlordiazepoxide (Oxycodone like all opioid analgesics, should be started at 1/3 to 1/2 of the usual dosage in patients who are concurrently receiving other central nervous system depressants including tranquilizers because respiratory depression, hypotension, and profound sedation or coma may result).

No products indexed under this heading.

Chlordiazepoxide Hydrochloride (Oxycodone like all opioid analgesics, should be started at 1/3 to 1/2 of the usual dosage in patients who are concurrently receiving other central nervous system depressants including tranquilizers because respiratory depression, hypotension, and profound sedation or coma may result).

No products indexed under this heading.

Chloroquine (Oxycodone is metabolized in part to oxymorphone via cytochrome P450 2D6. While this pathway may be blocked by a variety of drugs (eg, certain cardiovascular drugs including amiodarone and quinidine as well as polycyclic antidepressants), such blockade has not yet been shown to be of clinical significance with this agent. Clinicians should be aware of this possible interaction, however).

No products indexed under this heading.

Chloroquine Hydrochloride (Oxycodone is metabolized in part to oxymorphone via cytochrome P450 2D6. While this pathway may be blocked by a variety of drugs (eg, certain cardiovascular drugs including amiodarone and quinidine as well as polycyclic antidepressants), such blockade has not yet been

shown to be of clinical significance with this agent. Clinicians should be aware of this possible interaction, however).

No products indexed under this heading.

Chloroquine Phosphate (Oxycodone is metabolized in part to oxymorphone via cytochrome P450 2D6. While this pathway may be blocked by a variety of drugs (eg, certain cardiovascular drugs including amiodarone and quinidine as well as polycyclic antidepressants), such blockade has not yet been shown to be of clinical significance with this agent. Clinicians should be aware of this possible interaction, however).

No products indexed under this heading.

Chlorpheniramine (Oxycodone is metabolized in part to oxymorphone via cytochrome P450 2D6. While this pathway may be blocked by a variety of drugs (eg, certain cardiovascular drugs including amiodarone and quinidine as well as polycyclic antidepressants), such blockade has not yet been shown to be of clinical significance with this agent. Clinicians should be aware of this possible interaction, however).

No products indexed under this heading.

Chlorpheniramine Maleate (Oxycodone is metabolized in part to oxymorphone via cytochrome P450 2D6. While this pathway may be blocked by a variety of drugs (eg, certain cardiovascular drugs including amiodarone and quinidine as well as polycyclic antidepressants), such blockade has not yet been shown to be of clinical significance with this agent. Clinicians should be aware of this possible interaction, however).

No products indexed under this heading.

Chlorpheniramine Polistirex (Oxycodone is metabolized in part to oxymorphone via cytochrome P450 2D6. While this pathway may be blocked by a variety of drugs (eg, certain cardiovascular drugs including amiodarone and quinidine as well as polycyclic antidepressants), such blockade has not yet been shown to be of clinical significance with this agent. Clinicians should be aware of this possible interaction, however). Products include:
Tussionex 3443

Chlorpheniramine Tannate (Oxycodone is metabolized in part to oxymorphone via cytochrome P450 2D6. While this pathway may be blocked by a variety of drugs (eg, certain cardiovascular drugs including amiodarone and quinidine as well as polycyclic antidepressants), such blockade has not yet been shown to be of clinical significance with this agent. Clinicians should be aware of this possible interaction, however).

No products indexed under this heading.

Chlorpromazine (Oxycodone, like all opioid analgesics, should be started at 1/3 to 1/2 of the usual dosage in patients who are concurrently receiving other central nervous system depressants including phenothiazines because respiratory depression, hypotension, and profound sedation or coma may result).

No products indexed under this heading.

Chlorpromazine Hydrochloride (Oxycodone, like all opioid analgesics, should be started at 1/3 to 1/2 of the usual dosage in patients who are concurrently receiving other central nervous system depressants including phenothiazines because respiratory depression, hypotension, and profound sedation or coma may result).

No products indexed under this heading.

Chlorprothixene (Oxycodone like all opioid analgesics, should be started at 1/3 to 1/2 of the usual dosage in patients who are concurrently receiving other central nervous system depressants including tranquilizers because respiratory depression, hypotension, and profound sedation or coma may result).

No products indexed under this heading.

Chlorprothixene Hydrochloride (Oxycodone like all opioid analgesics, should be started at 1/3 to 1/2 of the usual dosage in patients who are concurrently receiving other central nervous system depressants including tranquilizers because respiratory depression, hypotension, and profound sedation or coma may result).

No products indexed under this heading.

Chlorprothixene Lactate (Oxycodone like all opioid analgesics, should be started at 1/3 to 1/2 of the usual dosage in patients who are concurrently receiving other central nervous system depressants including tranquilizers because respiratory depression, hypotension, and profound sedation or coma may result).

No products indexed under this heading.

Chlorzoxazone (Opioid analgesics, including oxycodone, may enhance the neuromuscular blocking action of skeletal muscle relaxants and produce an increased degree of respiratory depression).

No products indexed under this heading.

Cimetidine (Oxycodone is metabolized in part to oxymorphone via cytochrome P450 2D6. While this pathway may be blocked by a variety of drugs (eg, certain cardiovascular drugs including amiodarone and quinidine as well as polycyclic antidepressants), such blockade has not yet been shown to be of clinical significance with this agent. Clinicians should be aware of this possible interaction, however).

No products indexed under this heading.

Cimetidine Hydrochloride (Oxycodone is metabolized in part to oxymorphone via cytochrome P450 2D6. While this pathway may be blocked by a variety of drugs (eg, certain cardiovascular drugs including amiodarone and quinidine as well as polycyclic antidepressants), such blockade has not yet been shown to be of clinical significance with this agent. Clinicians should be aware of this possible interaction, however).

No products indexed under this heading.

Cisatracurium Besylate (Opioid analgesics, including oxycodone, may enhance the neuromuscular blocking action of skeletal muscle relaxants and produce an increased degree of respiratory depression). Products include:
Nimbex 503

Citalopram Hydrobromide (Oxycodone is metabolized in part to oxymorphone via cytochrome P450 2D6. While this pathway may be blocked by a variety of drugs (eg, certain cardiovascular drugs including amiodarone and quinidine as well as polycyclic antidepressants), such blockade has not yet been shown to be of clinical significance with this agent. Clinicians should be aware of this possible interaction, however). Products include:
Celexa 1153

Clomipramine Hydrochloride (Oxycodone is metabolized in part to oxymorphone via cytochrome P450 2D6. While this pathway may be blocked by a variety of drugs (eg, polycyclic antidepressants), such blockade has not yet been shown to be of clinical significance with this agent. Clinicians should be aware of this possible interaction).

No products indexed under this heading.

Clonazepam (Oxycodone, like all opioid analgesics, should be started at 1/3 to 1/2 of the usual dosage in patients who are concurrently receiving other central nervous system depressants including sedatives or hypnotics, general anesthetics, phenothiazines, centrally acting anti-emetics, tranquilizers, and alcohol because respiratory depression, hypotension, and profound sedation or coma may result). Products include:
Klonopin 2855

Clorazepate Dipotassium (Oxycodone like all opioid analgesics, should be started at 1/3 to 1/2 of the usual dosage in patients who are concurrently receiving other central nervous system depressants including tranquilizers because respiratory depression, hypotension, and profound sedation or coma may result).

No products indexed under this heading.

Clozapine (Oxycodone, like all opioid analgesics, should be started at 1/3 to 1/2 of the usual dosage in patients who are concurrently receiving other central nervous system depressants including sedatives or hypnotics, general anesthetics, phenothiazines, centrally acting anti-emetics, tranquilizers, and alcohol because respiratory depression, hypotension, and profound sedation or coma may result).

No products indexed under this heading.

Cocaine Hydrochloride (Oxycodone is metabolized in part to oxymorphone via cytochrome P450 2D6. While this pathway may be blocked by a variety of drugs (eg, certain cardiovascular drugs including amiodarone and quinidine as well as polycyclic antidepressants), such blockade has not yet been shown to be of clinical significance with this agent. Clinicians should be aware of this possible interaction, however).

No products indexed under this heading.

Codeine Phosphate (Oxycodone, like all opioid analgesics, should be started at 1/3 to 1/2 of the usual dosage in patients who are concurrently receiving other central nervous system depressants including sedatives or hypnotics, general anesthetics, phenothiazines, centrally acting anti-emetics, tranquilizers, and alcohol because respiratory depression, hypotension, and profound sedation or coma may result). Products include:
Tylenol with Codeine 2691

Codeine Sulfate (Oxycodone, like all opioid analgesics, should be started at 1/3 to 1/2 of the usual dosage in patients who are concurrently receiving other central nervous system depressants including sedatives or hypnotics, general anesthetics, phenothiazines, centrally acting anti-emetics, tranquilizers, and alcohol because respiratory depression, hypotension, and profound sedation or coma may result).

No products indexed under this heading.

Cyclobenzaprine Hydrochloride (Opioid analgesics, including oxycodone, may enhance the neuromuscular blocking action of skeletal muscle relaxants and produce an increased degree of respiratory depression). Products include:
Amrix 964

Dantrolene Sodium (Opioid analgesics, including oxycodone, may enhance the neuromuscular blocking action of skeletal muscle relaxants and produce an increased degree of respiratory depression).

No products indexed under this heading.

IMPORTANT NOTE: Always consult each drug listing in the patient's regimen for possible interactions.

OxyContin Interactions Index 1354

Desflurane (Oxycodone, like all opioid analgesics, should be started at 1/3 to 1/2 of the usual dosage in patients who are concurrently receiving other central nervous system depressants including general anesthetics because respiratory depression, hypotension, and profound sedation or coma may result).
No products indexed under this heading.

Desipramine Hydrochloride (Oxycodone is metabolized in part to oxymorphone via cytochrome P450 2D6. While this pathway may be blocked by a variety of drugs (eg, polycyclic antidepressants), such blockade has not yet been shown to be of clinical significance with this agent. Clinicians should be aware of this possible interaction).
No products indexed under this heading.

Dezocine (Oxycodone, like all opioid analgesics, should be started at 1/3 to 1/2 of the usual dosage in patients who are concurrently receiving other central nervous system depressants including sedatives or hypnotics, general anesthetics, phenothiazines, centrally acting anti-emetics, tranquilizers, and alcohol because respiratory depression, hypotension, and profound sedation or coma may result).
No products indexed under this heading.

Diazepam (Oxycodone like all opioid analgesics, should be started at 1/3 to 1/2 of the usual dosage in patients who are concurrently receiving other central nervous system depressants including tranquilizers because respiratory depression, hypotension, and profound sedation or coma may result). Products include:
Valium Tablets **2880**

Dimenhydrinate (Oxycodone, like all opioid analgesics, should be started at 1/3 to 1/2 of the usual dosage in patients who are concurrently receiving other central nervous system depressants including centrally acting anti-emetics because respiratory depression, hypotension, and profound sedation or coma may result).
No products indexed under this heading.

Diphenhydramine (Oxycodone, like all opioid analgesics, should be started at 1/3 to 1/2 of the usual dosage in patients who are concurrently receiving other central nervous system depressants including centrally acting anti-emetics because respiratory depression, hypotension, and profound sedation or coma may result).
No products indexed under this heading.

Diphenhydramine Hydrochloride (Oxycodone, like all opioid analgesics, should be started at 1/3 to 1/2 of the usual dosage in patients who are concurrently receiving other central nervous system depressants including centrally acting anti-emetics because respiratory depression, hypotension, and profound sedation or coma may result). Products include:
Benadryl Allergy Ultratab **2042**
Children's Benadryl Allergy Liquid **2042**

Dolasetron Mesylate (Oxycodone, like all opioid analgesics, should be started at 1/3 to 1/2 of the usual dosage in patients who are concurrently receiving other central nervous system depressants including centrally acting anti-emetics because respiratory depression, hypotension, and profound sedation or coma may result). Products include:
Anzemet Injection **2931**
Anzemet Tablets **2934**

Doxacurium Chloride (Opioid analgesics, including oxycodone, may enhance the neuromuscular blocking action of skeletal muscle relaxants and produce an increased degree of respiratory depression).
No products indexed under this heading.

Doxepin Hydrochloride (Oxycodone is metabolized in part to oxymorphone via cytochrome P450 2D6. While this pathway may be blocked by a variety of drugs (eg, polycyclic antidepressants), such blockade has not yet been shown to be of clinical significance with this agent. Clinicians should be aware of this possible interaction).
No products indexed under this heading.

Dronabinol (Oxycodone, like all opioid analgesics, should be started at 1/3 to 1/2 of the usual dosage in patients who are concurrently receiving other central nervous system depressants including centrally acting anti-emetics because respiratory depression, hypotension, and profound sedation or coma may result).
No products indexed under this heading.

Droperidol (Oxycodone, like all opioid analgesics, should be started at 1/3 to 1/2 of the usual dosage in patients who are concurrently receiving other central nervous system depressants including centrally acting anti-emetics because respiratory depression, hypotension, and profound sedation or coma may result).
No products indexed under this heading.

d-Tubocurarine (Opioid analgesics, including oxycodone, may enhance the neuromuscular blocking action of skeletal muscle relaxants and produce an increased degree of respiratory depression).
No products indexed under this heading.

Enflurane (Oxycodone, like all opioid analgesics, should be started at 1/3 to 1/2 of the usual dosage in patients who are concurrently receiving other central nervous system depressants including general anesthetics because respiratory depression, hypotension, and profound sedation or coma may result).
No products indexed under this heading.

Escitalopram Oxalate (Oxycodone is metabolized in part to oxymorphone via cytochrome P450 2D6. While this pathway may be blocked by a variety of drugs (eg, certain cardiovascular drugs including amiodarone and quinidine as well as polycyclic antidepressants), such blockade has not yet been shown to be of clinical significance with this agent. Clinicians should be aware of this possible interaction, however). Products include:
Lexapro Oral Suspension **1160**
Lexapro Tablets **1160**

Estazolam (Oxycodone, like all opioid analgesics, should be started at 1/3 to 1/2 of the usual dosage in patients who are concurrently receiving other central nervous system depressants including sedatives or hypnotics because respiratory depression, hypotension, and profound sedation or coma may result).
No products indexed under this heading.

Ethanol (Oxycodone, like all opioid analgesics, should be started at 1/3 to 1/2 of the usual dosage in patients who are concurrently receiving other central nervous system depressants including alcohol because respiratory depression, hypotension, and profound sedation or coma may result).
No products indexed under this heading.

Ethchlorvynol (Oxycodone, like all opioid analgesics, should be started at 1/3 to 1/2 of the usual dosage in patients who are concurrently receiving other central nervous system depressants including sedatives or hypnotics because respiratory depression, hypotension, and profound sedation or coma may result).
No products indexed under this heading.

Ethinamate (Oxycodone, like all opioid analgesics, should be started at 1/3 to 1/2 of the usual dosage in patients who are concurrently receiving other central nervous system depressants including sedatives or hypnotics because respiratory depression, hypotension, and profound sedation or coma may result).
No products indexed under this heading.

Ethyl Alcohol (Oxycodone, like all opioid analgesics, should be started at 1/3 to 1/2 of the usual dosage in patients who are concurrently receiving other central nervous system depressants including alcohol because respiratory depression, hypotension, and profound sedation or coma may result).
No products indexed under this heading.

Fat (The peak plasma concentration of oxycodone increased by 25% when oxycodone was administered with a high-fat meal).
No products indexed under this heading.

Fentanyl (Oxycodone, like all opioid analgesics, should be started at 1/3 to 1/2 of the usual dosage in patients who are concurrently receiving other central nervous system depressants including sedatives or hypnotics, general anesthetics, phenothiazines, centrally acting anti-emetics, tranquilizers, and alcohol because respiratory depression, hypotension, and profound sedation or coma may result). Products include:
Duragesic **2604**
Fentanyl Transdermal System **2346**
Onsolis **2054**

Fentanyl Citrate (Oxycodone, like all opioid analgesics, should be started at 1/3 to 1/2 of the usual dosage in patients who are concurrently receiving other central nervous system depressants including sedatives or hypnotics, general anesthetics, phenothiazines, centrally acting anti-emetics, tranquilizers, and alcohol because respiratory depression, hypotension, and profound sedation or coma may result). Products include:
Fentora **966**

Fluoxetine (Oxycodone is metabolized in part to oxymorphone via cytochrome P450 2D6. While this pathway may be blocked by a variety of drugs (eg, certain cardiovascular drugs including amiodarone and quinidine as well as polycyclic antidepressants), such blockade has not yet been shown to be of clinical significance with this agent. Clinicians should be aware of this possible interaction, however).
No products indexed under this heading.

Fluoxetine Hydrochloride (Oxycodone is metabolized in part to oxymorphone via cytochrome P450 2D6. While this pathway may be blocked by a variety of drugs (eg, certain cardiovascular drugs including amiodarone and quinidine as well as polycyclic antidepressants), such blockade has not yet been shown to be of clinical significance with this agent. Clinicians should be aware of this possible interaction, however). Products include:
Prozac Weekly **1941**
Prozac Pulvules **1941**
Symbyax **1965**

Fluphenazine Decanoate (Oxycodone, like all opioid analgesics, should be started at 1/3 to 1/2 of the usual dosage in patients who are concurrently receiving other central nervous system depressants including phenothiazines because respiratory depression, hypotension, and profound sedation or coma may result).
No products indexed under this heading.

Fluphenazine Enanthate (Oxycodone, like all opioid analgesics, should be started at 1/3 to 1/2 of the usual dosage in patients who are concurrently receiving other central nervous system depressants including phenothiazines because respiratory depression, hypotension, and profound sedation or coma may result).
No products indexed under this heading.

Fluphenazine Hydrochloride (Oxycodone, like all opioid analgesics, should be started at 1/3 to 1/2 of the usual dosage in patients who are concurrently receiving other central nervous system depressants including phenothiazines because respiratory depression, hypotension, and profound sedation or coma may result).
No products indexed under this heading.

Flurazepam Hydrochloride (Oxycodone, like all opioid analgesics, should be started at 1/3 to 1/2 of the usual dosage in patients who are concurrently receiving other central nervous system depressants including sedatives or hypnotics because respiratory depression, hypotension, and profound sedation or coma may result).
No products indexed under this heading.

Fluvoxamine Maleate (Oxycodone is metabolized in part to oxymorphone via cytochrome P450 2D6. While this pathway may be blocked by a variety of drugs (eg, certain cardiovascular drugs including amiodarone and quinidine as well as polycyclic antidepressants), such blockade has not yet been shown to be of clinical significance with this agent. Clinicians should be aware of this possible interaction, however).
No products indexed under this heading.

Gallamine (Opioid analgesics, including oxycodone, may enhance the neuromuscular blocking action of skeletal muscle relaxants and produce an increased degree of respiratory depression).
No products indexed under this heading.

Gallamine Triethiodide (Opioid analgesics, including oxycodone, may enhance the neuromuscular blocking action of skeletal muscle relaxants and produce an increased degree of respiratory depression).
No products indexed under this heading.

Glutethimide (Oxycodone, like all opioid analgesics, should be started at 1/3 to 1/2 of the usual dosage in patients who are concurrently receiving other central nervous system depressants including sedatives or hypnotics because respiratory depression, hypotension, and profound sedation or coma may result).
No products indexed under this heading.

Granisetron Hydrochloride (Oxycodone, like all opioid analgesics, should be started at 1/3 to 1/2 of the usual dosage in patients who are concurrently receiving other central nervous system depressants including centrally acting anti-emetics because respiratory depression, hypotension, and profound sedation or coma may result).
No products indexed under this heading.

Halazepam (Oxycodone, like all opioid analgesics, should be started at 1/3 to 1/2 of the usual dosage in patients who are concurrently receiving other central nervous system depressants including sedatives or hypnotics, general anesthetics, phenothiazines, centrally acting anti-emetics, tranquilizers, and alcohol because respiratory depression, hypotension, and profound sedation or coma may result).
No products indexed under this heading.

Halofantrine Hydrochloride (Oxycodone is metabolized in part to oxymorphone via cytochrome P450 2D6. While

this pathway may be blocked by a variety of drugs (eg, certain cardiovascular drugs including amiodarone and quinidine as well as polycyclic antidepressants), such blockade has not yet been shown to be of clinical significance with this agent. Clinicians should be aware of this possible interaction, however).
No products indexed under this heading.

Haloperidol (Oxycodone like all opioid analgesics, should be started at 1/3 to 1/2 of the usual dosage in patients who are concurrently receiving other central nervous system depressants including tranquilizers because respiratory depression, hypotension, and profound sedation or coma may result).
No products indexed under this heading.

Haloperidol Decanoate (Oxycodone like all opioid analgesics, should be started at 1/3 to 1/2 of the usual dosage in patients who are concurrently receiving other central nervous system depressants including tranquilizers because respiratory depression, hypotension, and profound sedation or coma may result).
No products indexed under this heading.

Haloperidol Lactate (Oxycodone, like all opioid analgesics, should be started at 1/3 to 1/2 of the usual dosage in patients who are concurrently receiving other central nervous system depressants including sedatives or hypnotics, general anesthetics, phenothiazines, centrally acting anti-emetics, tranquilizers, and alcohol because respiratory depression, hypotension, and profound sedation or coma may result).
No products indexed under this heading.

Halothane (Oxycodone, like all opioid analgesics, should be started at 1/3 to 1/2 of the usual dosage in patients who are concurrently receiving other central nervous system depressants including general anesthetics because respiratory depression, hypotension, and profound sedation or coma may result).
No products indexed under this heading.

Hexobarbital (Oxycodone, like all opioid analgesics, should be started at 1/3 to 1/2 of the usual dosage in patients who are concurrently receiving other central nervous system depressants including sedatives or hypnotics, general anesthetics, phenothiazines, centrally acting anti-emetics, tranquilizers, and alcohol because respiratory depression, hypotension, and profound sedation or coma may result).
No products indexed under this heading.

Hydrocodone Bitartrate (Oxycodone, like all opioid analgesics, should be started at 1/3 to 1/2 of the usual dosage in patients who are concurrently receiving other central nervous system depressants including sedatives or hypnotics, general anesthetics, phenothiazines, centrally acting anti-emetics, tranquilizers, and alcohol because respiratory depression, hypotension, and profound sedation or coma may result). Products include:
Vicodin	560
Vicodin ES	561
Vicodin HP	563
Vicoprofen	564
Zydone	1138

Hydrocodone Polistirex (Oxycodone, like all opioid analgesics, should be started at 1/3 to 1/2 of the usual dosage in patients who are concurrently receiving other central nervous system depressants including sedatives or hypnotics, general anesthetics, phenothiazines, centrally acting anti-emetics, tranquilizers, and alcohol because respiratory depression, hypotension, and profound sedation or coma may result). Products include:
Tussionex	3443

Hydromorphone (Oxycodone, like all opioid analgesics, should be started at 1/3 to 1/2 of the usual dosage in patients who are concurrently receiving other central nervous system depressants including sedatives or hypnotics, general anesthetics, phenothiazines, centrally acting anti-emetics, tranquilizers, and alcohol because respiratory depression, hypotension, and profound sedation or coma may result).
No products indexed under this heading.

Hydromorphone Hydrochloride (Oxycodone, like all opioid analgesics, should be started at 1/3 to 1/2 of the usual dosage in patients who are concurrently receiving other central nervous system depressants including sedatives or hypnotics, general anesthetics, phenothiazines, centrally acting anti-emetics, tranquilizers, and alcohol because respiratory depression, hypotension, and profound sedation or coma may result). Products include:
Dilaudid Injection	2800
Dilaudid Oral	2797
Dilaudid Tablets	2797
Dilaudid-HP	2800

Hydroxychloroquine Sulfate (Oxycodone is metabolized in part to oxymorphone via cytochrome P450 2D6. While this pathway may be blocked by a variety of drugs (eg, certain cardiovascular drugs including amiodarone and quinidine as well as polycyclic antidepressants, such blockade has not yet been shown to be of clinical significance with this agent. Clinicians should be aware of this possible interaction, however).
No products indexed under this heading.

Hydroxyzine Hydrochloride (Oxycodone, like all opioid analgesics, should be started at 1/3 to 1/2 of the usual dosage in patients who are concurrently receiving other central nervous system depressants including centrally acting anti-emetics because respiratory depression, hypotension, and profound sedation or coma may result).
No products indexed under this heading.

Imatinib Mesylate (Oxycodone is metabolized in part to oxymorphone via cytochrome P450 2D6. While this pathway may be blocked by a variety of drugs (eg, certain cardiovascular drugs including amiodarone and quinidine as well as polycyclic antidepressants), such blockade has not yet been shown to be of clinical significance with this agent. Clinicians should be aware of this possible interaction, however).
Products include:
Gleevec	2477

Imipramine Hydrochloride (Oxycodone is metabolized in part to oxymorphone via cytochrome P450 2D6. While this pathway may be blocked by a variety of drugs (eg, polycyclic antidepressants), such blockade has not yet been shown to be of clinical significance with this agent. Clinicians should be aware of this possible interaction).
No products indexed under this heading.

Imipramine Pamoate (Oxycodone is metabolized in part to oxymorphone via cytochrome P450 2D6. While this pathway may be blocked by a variety of drugs (eg, polycyclic antidepressants), such blockade has not yet been shown to be of clinical significance with this agent. Clinicians should be aware of this possible interaction).
No products indexed under this heading.

Isocarboxazid (No specific interaction between oxycodone and monoamine oxidase inhibitors has been observed, but caution in the use of any opioid in patients taking this class of drugs is appropriate). Products include:
Marplan	3481

Isoflurane (Oxycodone, like all opioid analgesics, should be started at 1/3 to 1/2 of the usual dosage in patients who are concurrently receiving other central nervous system depressants including general anesthetics because respiratory depression, hypotension, and profound sedation or coma may result).
No products indexed under this heading.

Ketamine Hydrochloride (Oxycodone, like all opioid analgesics, should be started at 1/3 to 1/2 of the usual dosage in patients who are concurrently receiving other central nervous system depressants including general anesthetics because respiratory depression, hypotension, and profound sedation or coma may result).
No products indexed under this heading.

Levomethadyl Acetate Hydrochloride (Oxycodone, like all opioid analgesics, should be started at 1/3 to 1/2 of the usual dosage in patients who are concurrently receiving other central nervous system depressants including sedatives or hypnotics, general anesthetics, phenothiazines, centrally acting anti-emetics, tranquilizers, and alcohol because respiratory depression, hypotension, and profound sedation or coma may result).
No products indexed under this heading.

Levorphanol Tartrate (Oxycodone, like all opioid analgesics, should be started at 1/3 to 1/2 of the usual dosage in patients who are concurrently receiving other central nervous system depressants including sedatives or hypnotics, general anesthetics, phenothiazines, centrally acting anti-emetics, tranquilizers, and alcohol because respiratory depression, hypotension, and profound sedation or coma may result).
No products indexed under this heading.

Lorazepam (Oxycodone, like all opioid analgesics, should be started at 1/3 to 1/2 of the usual dosage in patients who are concurrently receiving other central nervous system depressants including sedatives or hypnotics because respiratory depression, hypotension, and profound sedation or coma may result).
No products indexed under this heading.

Loxapine Hydrochloride (Oxycodone like all opioid analgesics, should be started at 1/3 to 1/2 of the usual dosage in patients who are concurrently receiving other central nervous system depressants including tranquilizers because respiratory depression, hypotension, and profound sedation or coma may result).
No products indexed under this heading.

Loxapine Succinate (Oxycodone like all opioid analgesics, should be started at 1/3 to 1/2 of the usual dosage in patients who are concurrently receiving other central nervous system depressants including tranquilizers because respiratory depression, hypotension, and profound sedation or coma may result).
No products indexed under this heading.

Maprotiline Hydrochloride (Oxycodone is metabolized in part to oxymorphone via cytochrome P450 2D6. While this pathway may be blocked by a variety of drugs (eg, polycyclic antidepressants), such blockade has not yet been shown to be of clinical significance with this agent. Clinicians should be aware of this possible interaction).
No products indexed under this heading.

Meclizine Hydrochloride (Oxycodone, like all opioid analgesics, should be started at 1/3 to 1/2 of the usual dosage in patients who are concurrently receiving other central nervous system depressants including centrally acting anti-emetics because respiratory depression, hypotension, and profound sedation or coma may result).
No products indexed under this heading.

Meperidine Hydrochloride (Oxycodone, like all opioid analgesics, should be started at 1/3 to 1/2 of the usual dosage in patients who are concurrently receiving other central nervous system depressants including sedatives or hypnotics, general anesthetics, phenothiazines, centrally acting anti-emetics, tranquilizers, and alcohol because respiratory depression, hypotension, and profound sedation or coma may result).
No products indexed under this heading.

Mephobarbital (Oxycodone, like all opioid analgesics, should be started at 1/3 to 1/2 of the usual dosage in patients who are concurrently receiving other central nervous system depressants including sedatives or hypnotics, general anesthetics, phenothiazines, centrally acting anti-emetics, tranquilizers, and alcohol because respiratory depression, hypotension, and profound sedation or coma may result).
No products indexed under this heading.

Meprobamate (Oxycodone like all opioid analgesics, should be started at 1/3 to 1/2 of the usual dosage in patients who are concurrently receiving other central nervous system depressants including tranquilizers because respiratory depression, hypotension, and profound sedation or coma may result).
No products indexed under this heading.

Mesoridazine Besylate (Oxycodone, like all opioid analgesics, should be started at 1/3 to 1/2 of the usual dosage in patients who are concurrently receiving other central nervous system depressants including phenothiazines because respiratory depression, hypotension, and profound sedation or coma may result).
No products indexed under this heading.

Metaxalone (Opioid analgesics, including oxycodone, may enhance the neuromuscular blocking action of skeletal muscle relaxants and produce an increased degree of respiratory depression). Products include:
Skelaxin	1848

Methadone Hydrochloride (Oxycodone, like all opioid analgesics, should be started at 1/3 to 1/2 of the usual dosage in patients who are concurrently receiving other central nervous system depressants including sedatives or hypnotics, general anesthetics, phenothiazines, centrally acting anti-emetics, tranquilizers, and alcohol because respiratory depression, hypotension, and profound sedation or coma may result).
No products indexed under this heading.

Methocarbamol (Opioid analgesics, including oxycodone, may enhance the neuromuscular blocking action of skeletal muscle relaxants and produce an increased degree of respiratory depression).
No products indexed under this heading.

Methohexital Sodium (Oxycodone, like all opioid analgesics, should be started at 1/3 to 1/2 of the usual dosage in patients who are concurrently receiving other central nervous system depressants including general anesthetics because respiratory depression, hypotension, and profound sedation or coma may result).
No products indexed under this heading.

IMPORTANT NOTE: Always consult each drug listing in the patient's regimen for possible interactions.

OxyContin Interactions Index 1356

Methotrimeprazine (Oxycodone, like all opioid analgesics, should be started at 1/3 to 1/2 of the usual dosage in patients who are concurrently receiving other central nervous system depressants including phenothiazines because respiratory depression, hypotension, and profound sedation or coma may result).
No products indexed under this heading.

Methoxyflurane (Oxycodone, like all opioid analgesics, should be started at 1/3 to 1/2 of the usual dosage in patients who are concurrently receiving other central nervous system depressants including general anesthetics because respiratory depression, hypotension, and profound sedation or coma may result).
No products indexed under this heading.

Metoclopramide Hydrochloride (Oxycodone, like all opioid analgesics, should be started at 1/3 to 1/2 of the usual dosage in patients who are concurrently receiving other central nervous system depressants including centrally acting anti-emetics because respiratory depression, hypotension, and profound sedation or coma may result). Products include:
Metozolv ODT **2901**

Metocurine Iodide (Opioid analgesics, including oxycodone, may enhance the neuromuscular blocking action of skeletal muscle relaxants and produce an increased degree of respiratory depression).
No products indexed under this heading.

Mibefradil Dihydrochloride (Oxycodone is metabolized in part to oxymorphone via cytochrome P450 2D6. While this pathway may be blocked by a variety of drugs (eg, certain cardiovascular drugs including amiodarone and quinidine as well as polycyclic antidepressants), such blockade has not yet been shown to be of clinical significance with this agent. Clinicians should be aware of this possible interaction, however).
No products indexed under this heading.

Midazolam Hydrochloride (Oxycodone, like all opioid analgesics, should be started at 1/3 to 1/2 of the usual dosage in patients who are concurrently receiving other central nervous system depressants including sedatives or hypnotics because respiratory depression, hypotension, and profound sedation or coma may result).
No products indexed under this heading.

Mirtazapine (Oxycodone is metabolized in part to oxymorphone via cytochrome P450 2D6. While this pathway may be blocked by a variety of drugs (eg, polycyclic antidepressants), such blockade has not yet been shown to be of clinical significance with this agent. Clinicians should be aware of this possible interaction). Products include:
Remeron Tablets **3214**
RemeronSolTab Tablets **3219**

Mivacurium Chloride (Opioid analgesics, including oxycodone, may enhance the neuromuscular blocking action of skeletal muscle relaxants and produce an increased degree of respiratory depression).
No products indexed under this heading.

Moclobemide (No specific interaction between oxycodone and monoamine oxidase inhibitors has been observed, but caution in the use of any opioid in patients taking this class of drugs is appropriate).
No products indexed under this heading.

Molindone Hydrochloride (Oxycodone like all opioid analgesics, should be started at 1/3 to 1/2 of the usual dosage in patients who are concurrently receiving other central nervous system depressants including tranquilizers because respiratory depression, hypotension, and profound sedation or coma may result). Products include:
Moban **1108**

Morphine Sulfate (Oxycodone, like all opioid analgesics, should be started at 1/3 to 1/2 of the usual dosage in patients who are concurrently receiving other central nervous system depressants including sedatives or hypnotics, general anesthetics, phenothiazines, centrally acting anti-emetics, tranquilizers, and alcohol because respiratory depression, hypotension, and profound sedation or coma may result). Products include:
Avinza **1822**
Embeda **1831**
MS Contin **2803**

Morphine Sulfate, Liposomal (Oxycodone, like all opioid analgesics, should be started at 1/3 to 1/2 of the usual dosage in patients who are concurrently receiving other central nervous system depressants including sedatives or hypnotics, general anesthetics, phenothiazines, centrally acting anti-emetics, tranquilizers, and alcohol because respiratory depression, hypotension, and profound sedation or coma may result).
No products indexed under this heading.

Nabilone (Oxycodone, like all opioid analgesics, should be started at 1/3 to 1/2 of the usual dosage in patients who are concurrently receiving other central nervous system depressants including centrally acting anti-emetics because respiratory depression, hypotension, and profound sedation or coma may result).
No products indexed under this heading.

Nalbuphine Hydrochloride (Agonist/antagonist analgesics (ie, pentazocine, nalbuphine, and butorphanol) should be administered with caution to a patient who has received or is receiving a course of therapy with a pure opioid agonist analgesic such as oxycodone. In this situation, mixed agonist/antagonist analgesics may reduce the analgesic effect of oxycodone and/or may precipitate withdrawal symptoms in these patients).
No products indexed under this heading.

Nitrous Oxide (Oxycodone, like all opioid analgesics, should be started at 1/3 to 1/2 of the usual dosage in patients who are concurrently receiving other central nervous system depressants including general anesthetics because respiratory depression, hypotension, and profound sedation or coma may result).
No products indexed under this heading.

Nortriptyline Hydrochloride (Oxycodone is metabolized in part to oxymorphone via cytochrome P450 2D6. While this pathway may be blocked by a variety of drugs (eg, polycyclic antidepressants), such blockade has not yet been shown to be of clinical significance with this agent. Clinicians should be aware of this possible interaction).
No products indexed under this heading.

Olanzapine (Oxycodone, like all opioid analgesics, should be started at 1/3 to 1/2 of the usual dosage in patients who are concurrently receiving other central nervous system depressants including sedatives or hypnotics, general anesthetics, phenothiazines, centrally acting anti-emetics, tranquilizers, and alcohol because respiratory depression, hypotension, and profound sedation or coma may result). Products include:
Symbyax **1965**
Zyprexa **1984**
Zyprexa IntraMuscular **1984**
Zyprexa ZYDIS **1984**

Ondansetron (Oxycodone, like all opioid analgesics, should be started at 1/3 to 1/2 of the usual dosage in patients who are concurrently receiving other central nervous system depressants including centrally acting anti-emetics because respiratory depression, hypotension, and profound sedation or coma may result).
No products indexed under this heading.

Ondansetron Hydrochloride (Oxycodone, like all opioid analgesics, should be started at 1/3 to 1/2 of the usual dosage in patients who are concurrently receiving other central nervous system depressants including centrally acting anti-emetics because respiratory depression, hypotension, and profound sedation or coma may result). Products include:
Zofran Injection **1750**
Zofran **1756**
Zofran ODT **1756**

Orphenadrine Citrate (Opioid analgesics, including oxycodone, may enhance the neuromuscular blocking action of skeletal muscle relaxants and produce an increased degree of respiratory depression).
No products indexed under this heading.

Oxazepam (Oxycodone like all opioid analgesics, should be started at 1/3 to 1/2 of the usual dosage in patients who are concurrently receiving other central nervous system depressants including tranquilizers because respiratory depression, hypotension, and profound sedation or coma may result).
No products indexed under this heading.

Oxycodone Terephthalate (Oxycodone, like all opioid analgesics, should be started at 1/3 to 1/2 of the usual dosage in patients who are concurrently receiving other central nervous system depressants including sedatives or hypnotics, general anesthetics, phenothiazines, centrally acting anti-emetics, tranquilizers, and alcohol because respiratory depression, hypotension, and profound sedation or coma may result).
No products indexed under this heading.

Oxymorphone Hydrochloride (Oxycodone, like all opioid analgesics, should be started at 1/3 to 1/2 of the usual dosage in patients who are concurrently receiving other central nervous system depressants including sedatives or hypnotics, general anesthetics, phenothiazines, centrally acting anti-emetics, tranquilizers, and alcohol because respiratory depression, hypotension, and profound sedation or coma may result). Products include:
Opana **1110**
Opana ER **1114**

Palonosetron Hydrochloride (Oxycodone, like all opioid analgesics, should be started at 1/3 to 1/2 of the usual dosage in patients who are concurrently receiving other central nervous system depressants including centrally acting anti-emetics because respiratory depression, hypotension, and profound sedation or coma may result). Products include:
Aloxi **1042**

Pancuronium Bromide (Opioid analgesics, including oxycodone, may enhance the neuromuscular blocking action of skeletal muscle relaxants and produce an increased degree of respiratory depression).
No products indexed under this heading.

Pargyline Hydrochloride (No specific interaction between oxycodone and monoamine oxidase inhibitors has been observed, but caution in the use of any opioid in patients taking this class of drugs is appropriate).
No products indexed under this heading.

Paroxetine Hydrochloride (Oxycodone is metabolized in part to oxymorphone via cytochrome P450 2D6. While this pathway may be blocked by a variety of drugs (eg, certain cardiovascular drugs including amiodarone and quinidine as well as polycyclic antidepressants), such blockade has not yet been shown to be of clinical significance with this agent. Clinicians should be aware of this possible interaction, however). Products include:
Paroxetine CR **2361**
Paroxetine ER **2371**
Paxil **1586**
Paxil CR **1596**

Pentazocine Hydrochloride (Agonist/antagonist analgesics (ie, pentazocine, nalbuphine, and butorphanol) should be administered with caution to a patient who has received or is receiving a course of therapy with a pure opioid agonist analgesic such as oxycodone. In this situation, mixed agonist/antagonist analgesics may reduce the analgesic effect of oxycodone and/or may precipitate withdrawal symptoms in these patients).
No products indexed under this heading.

Pentazocine Lactate (Agonist/antagonist analgesics (ie, pentazocine, nalbuphine, and butorphanol) should be administered with caution to a patient who has received or is receiving a course of therapy with a pure opioid agonist analgesic such as oxycodone. In this situation, mixed agonist/antagonist analgesics may reduce the analgesic effect of oxycodone and/or may precipitate withdrawal symptoms in these patients).
No products indexed under this heading.

Pentobarbital (Oxycodone, like all opioid analgesics, should be started at 1/3 to 1/2 of the usual dosage in patients who are concurrently receiving other central nervous system depressants including sedatives or hypnotics, general anesthetics, phenothiazines, centrally acting anti-emetics, tranquilizers, and alcohol because respiratory depression, hypotension, and profound sedation or coma may result).
No products indexed under this heading.

Pentobarbital Sodium (Oxycodone, like all opioid analgesics, should be started at 1/3 to 1/2 of the usual dosage in patients who are concurrently receiving other central nervous system depressants including sedatives or hypnotics, general anesthetics, phenothiazines, centrally acting anti-emetics, tranquilizers, and alcohol because respiratory depression, hypotension, and profound sedation or coma may result). Products include:
Nembutal **2012**

Perphenazine (Oxycodone, like all opioid analgesics, should be started at 1/3 to 1/2 of the usual dosage in patients who are concurrently receiving other central nervous system depressants including phenothiazines because respiratory depression, hypotension, and profound sedation or coma may result).
No products indexed under this heading.

Phenelzine Sulfate (No specific interaction between oxycodone and monoamine oxidase inhibitors has been observed, but caution in the use of any opioid in patients taking this class of drugs is appropriate).
No products indexed under this heading.

Phenobarbital (Oxycodone, like all opioid analgesics, should be started at 1/3 to 1/2 of the usual dosage in patients who are concurrently receiving other central nervous system depressants including sedatives or hypnotics, general anesthetics, phenothiazines, centrally acting anti-emetics, tranquilizers, and alcohol because respiratory

(☉ Described in PDR® for Ophthalmic Medicines)

depression, hypotension, and profound sedation or coma may result). Products include:

Donnatal 2711

Phenobarbital Sodium (Oxycodone, like all opioid analgesics, should be started at 1/3 to 1/2 of the usual dosage in patients who are concurrently receiving other central nervous system depressants including sedatives or hypnotics, general anesthetics, phenothiazines, centrally acting anti-emetics, tranquilizers, and alcohol because respiratory depression, hypotension, and profound sedation or coma may result).

No products indexed under this heading.

Phenothiazine Derivatives (Oxycodone, like all opioid analgesics, should be started at 1/3 to 1/2 of the usual dosage in patients who are concurrently receiving other central nervous system depressants including phenothiazines because respiratory depression, hypotension, and profound sedation or coma may result).

No products indexed under this heading.

Phenothiazines (Oxycodone, like all opioid analgesics, should be started at 1/3 to 1/2 of the usual dosage in patients who are concurrently receiving other central nervous system depressants including phenothiazines because respiratory depression, hypotension, and profound sedation or coma may result).

No products indexed under this heading.

Pipecuronium Bromide (Opioid analgesics, including oxycodone, may enhance the neuromuscular blocking action of skeletal muscle relaxants and produce an increased degree of respiratory depression).

No products indexed under this heading.

Prazepam (Oxycodone like all opioid analgesics, should be started at 1/3 to 1/2 of the usual dosage in patients who are concurrently receiving other central nervous system depressants including tranquilizers because respiratory depression, hypotension, and profound sedation or coma may result).

No products indexed under this heading.

Procarbazine Hydrochloride (No specific interaction between oxycodone and monoamine oxidase inhibitors has been observed, but caution in the use of any opioid in patients taking this class of drugs is appropriate).

No products indexed under this heading.

Prochlorperazine (Oxycodone, like all opioid analgesics, should be started at 1/3 to 1/2 of the usual dosage in patients who are concurrently receiving other central nervous system depressants including phenothiazines because respiratory depression, hypotension, and profound sedation or coma may result).

No products indexed under this heading.

Prochlorperazine Edisylate (Oxycodone, like all opioid analgesics, should be started at 1/3 to 1/2 of the usual dosage in patients who are concurrently receiving other central nervous system depressants including phenothiazines because respiratory depression, hypotension, and profound sedation or coma may result).

No products indexed under this heading.

Prochlorperazine Maleate (Oxycodone, like all opioid analgesics, should be started at 1/3 to 1/2 of the usual dosage in patients who are concurrently receiving other central nervous system depressants including phenothiazines because respiratory depression, hypotension, and profound sedation or coma may result).

No products indexed under this heading.

Promethazine (Oxycodone, like all opioid analgesics, should be started at 1/3 to 1/2 of the usual dosage in patients who are concurrently receiving other central nervous system depressants including phenothiazines because respiratory depression, hypotension, and profound sedation or coma may result).

No products indexed under this heading.

Promethazine Hydrochloride (Oxycodone, like all opioid analgesics, should be started at 1/3 to 1/2 of the usual dosage in patients who are concurrently receiving other central nervous system depressants including phenothiazines because respiratory depression, hypotension, and profound sedation or coma may result).

No products indexed under this heading.

Propafenone Hydrochloride (Oxycodone is metabolized in part to oxymorphone via cytochrome P450 2D6. While this pathway may be blocked by a variety of drugs (eg, certain cardiovascular drugs including amiodarone and quinidine as well as polycyclic antidepressants), such blockade has not yet been shown to be of clinical significance with this agent. Clinicians should be aware of this possible interaction, however). Products include:

Rythmol 1648
Rythmol SR 1652

Propofol (Oxycodone, like all opioid analgesics, should be started at 1/3 to 1/2 of the usual dosage in patients who are concurrently receiving other central nervous system depressants including sedatives or hypnotics because respiratory depression, hypotension, and profound sedation or coma may result).

No products indexed under this heading.

Propoxyphene Hydrochloride (Oxycodone, like all opioid analgesics, should be started at 1/3 to 1/2 of the usual dosage in patients who are concurrently receiving other central nervous system depressants including sedatives or hypnotics, general anesthetics, phenothiazines, centrally acting anti-emetics, tranquilizers, and alcohol because respiratory depression, hypotension, and profound sedation or coma may result).

No products indexed under this heading.

Propoxyphene Napsylate (Oxycodone, like all opioid analgesics, should be started at 1/3 to 1/2 of the usual dosage in patients who are concurrently receiving other central nervous system depressants including sedatives or hypnotics, general anesthetics, phenothiazines, centrally acting anti-emetics, tranquilizers, and alcohol because respiratory depression, hypotension, and profound sedation or coma may result).

No products indexed under this heading.

Protriptyline Hydrochloride (Oxycodone is metabolized in part to oxymorphone via cytochrome P450 2D6. While this pathway may be blocked by a variety of drugs (eg, polycyclic antidepressants), such blockade has not yet been shown to be of clinical significance with this agent. Clinicians should be aware of this possible interaction).

No products indexed under this heading.

Quazepam (Oxycodone, like all opioid analgesics, should be started at 1/3 to 1/2 of the usual dosage in patients who are concurrently receiving other central nervous system depressants including sedatives or hypnotics because respiratory depression, hypotension, and profound sedation or coma may result).

No products indexed under this heading.

Quetiapine Fumarate (Oxycodone, like all opioid analgesics, should be started at 1/3 to 1/2 of the usual dosage in patients who are concurrently

receiving other central nervous system depressants including sedatives or hypnotics, general anesthetics, phenothiazines, centrally acting anti-emetics, tranquilizers, and alcohol because respiratory depression, hypotension, and profound sedation or coma may result). Products include:

Seroquel 750
Seroquel XR 759

Quinacrine Hydrochloride (Oxycodone is metabolized in part to oxymorphone via cytochrome P450 2D6. While this pathway may be blocked by a variety of drugs (eg, certain cardiovascular drugs including amiodarone and quinidine as well as polycyclic antidepressants), such blockade has not yet been shown to be of clinical significance with this agent. Clinicians should be aware of this possible interaction, however).

No products indexed under this heading.

Quinidine (Oxycodone is metabolized in part to oxymorphone via cytochrome P450 2D6. While this pathway may be blocked by a variety of drugs (eg, certain cardiovascular drugs including quinidine), such blockade has not yet been shown to be of clinical significance with this agent. Clinicians should be aware of this possible interaction, however).

No products indexed under this heading.

Quinidine Gluconate (Oxycodone is metabolized in part to oxymorphone via cytochrome P450 2D6. While this pathway may be blocked by a variety of drugs (eg, certain cardiovascular drugs including quinidine), such blockade has not yet been shown to be of clinical significance with this agent. Clinicians should be aware of this possible interaction, however).

No products indexed under this heading.

Quinidine Hydrochloride (Oxycodone is metabolized in part to oxymorphone via cytochrome P450 2D6. While this pathway may be blocked by a variety of drugs (eg, certain cardiovascular drugs including quinidine), such blockade has not yet been shown to be of clinical significance with this agent. Clinicians should be aware of this possible interaction, however).

No products indexed under this heading.

Quinidine Polygalacturonate (Oxycodone is metabolized in part to oxymorphone via cytochrome P450 2D6. While this pathway may be blocked by a variety of drugs (eg, certain cardiovascular drugs including quinidine), such blockade has not yet been shown to be of clinical significance with this agent. Clinicians should be aware of this possible interaction, however).

No products indexed under this heading.

Quinidine Sulfate (Oxycodone is metabolized in part to oxymorphone via cytochrome P450 2D6. While this pathway may be blocked by a variety of drugs (eg, certain cardiovascular drugs including quinidine), such blockade has not yet been shown to be of clinical significance with this agent. Clinicians should be aware of this possible interaction, however).

No products indexed under this heading.

Ramelteon (Oxycodone, like all opioid analgesics, should be started at 1/3 to 1/2 of the usual dosage in patients who are concurrently receiving other central nervous system depressants including sedatives or hypnotics because respiratory depression, hypotension, and profound sedation or coma may result). Products include:

Rozerem 3366

Ranitidine Bismuth Citrate (Oxycodone is metabolized in part to oxymorphone via cytochrome P450 2D6. While this pathway may be blocked by a variety of drugs (eg, certain cardiovascular drugs including amiodarone and quini-

dine as well as polycyclic antidepressants), such blockade has not yet been shown to be of clinical significance with this agent. Clinicians should be aware of this possible interaction, however).

No products indexed under this heading.

Ranitidine Hydrochloride (Oxycodone is metabolized in part to oxymorphone via cytochrome P450 2D6. While this pathway may be blocked by a variety of drugs (eg, certain cardiovascular drugs including amiodarone and quinidine as well as polycyclic antidepressants), such blockade has not yet been shown to be of clinical significance with this agent. Clinicians should be aware of this possible interaction, however). Products include:

Zantac 1737
Zantac Injection 1732
Zantac Pharmacy 1735

Rapacuronium Bromide (Opioid analgesics, including oxycodone, may enhance the neuromuscular blocking action of skeletal muscle relaxants and produce an increased degree of respiratory depression).

No products indexed under this heading.

Rasagiline Mesylate (No specific interaction between oxycodone and monoamine oxidase inhibitors has been observed, but caution in the use of any opioid in patients taking this class of drugs is appropriate). Products include:

Azilect 3383

Remifentanil Hydrochloride (Oxycodone, like all opioid analgesics, should be started at 1/3 to 1/2 of the usual dosage in patients who are concurrently receiving other central nervous system depressants including sedatives or hypnotics, general anesthetics, phenothiazines, centrally acting anti-emetics, tranquilizers, and alcohol because respiratory depression, hypotension, and profound sedation or coma may result).

No products indexed under this heading.

Risperidone (Oxycodone, like all opioid analgesics, should be started at 1/3 to 1/2 of the usual dosage in patients who are concurrently receiving other central nervous system depressants including sedatives or hypnotics, general anesthetics, phenothiazines, centrally acting anti-emetics, tranquilizers, and alcohol because respiratory depression, hypotension, and profound sedation or coma may result). Products include:

Risperdal Consta 2682

Ritonavir (Oxycodone is metabolized in part to oxymorphone via cytochrome P450 2D6. While this pathway may be blocked by a variety of drugs (eg, certain cardiovascular drugs including amiodarone and quinidine as well as polycyclic antidepressants), such blockade has not yet been shown to be of clinical significance with this agent. Clinicians should be aware of this possible interaction, however). Products include:

Kaletra 458
Norvir 509

Rocuronium Bromide (Opioid analgesics, including oxycodone, may enhance the neuromuscular blocking action of skeletal muscle relaxants and produce an increased degree of respiratory depression). Products include:

Zemuron 3249

Scopolamine (Oxycodone, like all opioid analgesics, should be started at 1/3 to 1/2 of the usual dosage in patients who are concurrently receiving other central nervous system depressants including centrally acting anti-emetics because respiratory depression, hypotension, and profound sedation or coma may result). Products include:

Transderm Scōp 2397

IMPORTANT NOTE: Always consult each drug listing in the patient's regimen for possible interactions.

Scopolamine Hydrobromide (Oxycodone, like all opioid analgesics, should be started at 1/3 to 1/2 of the usual dosage in patients who are concurrently receiving other central nervous system depressants including centrally acting anti-emetics because respiratory depression, hypotension, and profound sedation or coma may result). Products include:
Donnatal 2711

Secobarbital Sodium (Oxycodone, like all opioid analgesics, should be started at 1/3 to 1/2 of the usual dosage in patients who are concurrently receiving other central nervous system depressants including sedatives or hypnotics because respiratory depression, hypotension, and profound sedation or coma may result).
No products indexed under this heading.

Selegiline (No specific interaction between oxycodone and monoamine oxidase inhibitors has been observed, but caution in the use of any opioid in patients taking this class of drugs is appropriate). Products include:
Emsam 3623

Selegiline Hydrochloride (No specific interaction between oxycodone and monoamine oxidase inhibitors has been observed, but caution in the use of any opioid in patients taking this class of drugs is appropriate). Products include:
Eldepryl 3312

Sertraline Hydrochloride (Oxycodone is metabolized in part to oxymorphone via cytochrome P450 2D6. While this pathway may be blocked by a variety of drugs (eg, certain cardiovascular drugs including amiodarone and quinidine as well as polycyclic antidepressants), such blockade has not yet been shown to be of clinical significance with this agent. Clinicians should be aware of this possible interaction, however).
No products indexed under this heading.

Sevoflurane (Oxycodone, like all opioid analgesics, should be started at 1/3 to 1/2 of the usual dosage in patients who are concurrently receiving other central nervous system depressants including general anesthetics because respiratory depression, hypotension, and profound sedation or coma may result). Products include:
Ultane 554

Sildenafil Citrate (Oxycodone is metabolized in part to oxymorphone via cytochrome P450 2D6. While this pathway may be blocked by a variety of drugs (eg, certain cardiovascular drugs including amiodarone and quinidine as well as polycyclic antidepressants), such blockade has not yet been shown to be of clinical significance with this agent. Clinicians should be aware of this possible interaction, however).
No products indexed under this heading.

Sodium Butabarbital (Oxycodone, like all opioid analgesics, should be started at 1/3 to 1/2 of the usual dosage in patients who are concurrently receiving other central nervous system depressants including sedatives or hypnotics because respiratory depression, hypotension, and profound sedation or coma may result).
No products indexed under this heading.

Sodium Oxybate (Oxycodone, like all opioid analgesics, should be started at 1/3 to 1/2 of the usual dosage in patients who are concurrently receiving other central nervous system depressants including sedatives or hypnotics, general anesthetics, phenothiazines, centrally acting anti-emetics, tranquilizers, and alcohol because respiratory depression, hypotension, and profound sedation or coma may result).
No products indexed under this heading.

Sodium Pentobarbital (Oxycodone, like all opioid analgesics, should be started at 1/3 to 1/2 of the usual dosage in patients who are concurrently receiving other central nervous system depressants including sedatives or hypnotics, general anesthetics, phenothiazines, centrally acting anti-emetics, tranquilizers, and alcohol because respiratory depression, hypotension, and profound sedation or coma may result).
No products indexed under this heading.

Succinylcholine Chloride (Opioid analgesics, including oxycodone, may enhance the neuromuscular blocking action of skeletal muscle relaxants and produce an increased degree of respiratory depression).
No products indexed under this heading.

Sufentanil Citrate (Oxycodone, like all opioid analgesics, should be started at 1/3 to 1/2 of the usual dosage in patients who are concurrently receiving other central nervous system depressants including sedatives or hypnotics, general anesthetics, phenothiazines, centrally acting anti-emetics, tranquilizers, and alcohol because respiratory depression, hypotension, and profound sedation or coma may result).
No products indexed under this heading.

Talbutal (Oxycodone, like all opioid analgesics, should be started at 1/3 to 1/2 of the usual dosage in patients who are concurrently receiving other central nervous system depressants including sedatives or hypnotics, general anesthetics, phenothiazines, centrally acting anti-emetics, tranquilizers, and alcohol because respiratory depression, hypotension, and profound sedation or coma may result).
No products indexed under this heading.

Temazepam (Oxycodone, like all opioid analgesics, should be started at 1/3 to 1/2 of the usual dosage in patients who are concurrently receiving other central nervous system depressants including sedatives or hypnotics because respiratory depression, hypotension, and profound sedation or coma may result).
No products indexed under this heading.

Terbinafine Hydrochloride (Oxycodone is metabolized in part to oxymorphone via cytochrome P450 2D6. While this pathway may be blocked by a variety of drugs (eg, certain cardiovascular drugs including amiodarone and quinidine as well as polycyclic antidepressants), such blockade has not yet been shown to be of clinical significance with this agent. Clinicians should be aware of this possible interaction, however).
No products indexed under this heading.

Thiamylal Sodium (Oxycodone, like all opioid analgesics, should be started at 1/3 to 1/2 of the usual dosage in patients who are concurrently receiving other central nervous system depressants including sedatives or hypnotics, general anesthetics, phenothiazines, centrally acting anti-emetics, tranquilizers, and alcohol because respiratory depression, hypotension, and profound sedation or coma may result).
No products indexed under this heading.

Thioridazine (Oxycodone, like all opioid analgesics, should be started at 1/3 to 1/2 of the usual dosage in patients who are concurrently receiving other central nervous system depressants including phenothiazines because respiratory depression, hypotension, and profound sedation or coma may result).
No products indexed under this heading.

Thioridazine Hydrochloride (Oxycodone, like all opioid analgesics, should be started at 1/3 to 1/2 of the usual dosage in patients who are concurrently

receiving other central nervous system depressants including phenothiazines because respiratory depression, hypotension, and profound sedation or coma may result). Products include:
Thioridazine Hydrochloride 2384

Thiothixene (Oxycodone like all opioid analgesics, should be started at 1/3 to 1/2 of the usual dosage in patients who are concurrently receiving other central nervous system depressants including tranquilizers because respiratory depression, hypotension, and profound sedation or coma may result). Products include:
Thiothixene 2386

Thiothixene Hydrochloride (Oxycodone, like all opioid analgesics, should be started at 1/3 to 1/2 of the usual dosage in patients who are concurrently receiving other central nervous system depressants including sedatives or hypnotics, general anesthetics, phenothiazines, centrally acting anti-emetics, tranquilizers, and alcohol because respiratory depression, hypotension, and profound sedation or coma may result).
No products indexed under this heading.

Tizanidine (Opioid analgesics, including oxycodone, may enhance the neuromuscular blocking action of skeletal muscle relaxants and produce an increased degree of respiratory depression).
No products indexed under this heading.

Tizanidine Hydrochloride (Opioid analgesics, including oxycodone, may enhance the neuromuscular blocking action of skeletal muscle relaxants and produce an increased degree of respiratory depression).
No products indexed under this heading.

Tranylcypromine Sulfate (No specific interaction between oxycodone and monoamine oxidase inhibitors has been observed, but caution in the use of any opioid in patients taking this class of drugs is appropriate). Products include:
Parnate 1584

Triazolam (Oxycodone, like all opioid analgesics, should be started at 1/3 to 1/2 of the usual dosage in patients who are concurrently receiving other central nervous system depressants including sedatives or hypnotics because respiratory depression, hypotension, and profound sedation or coma may result).
No products indexed under this heading.

Trifluoperazine Hydrochloride (Oxycodone, like all opioid analgesics, should be started at 1/3 to 1/2 of the usual dosage in patients who are concurrently receiving other central nervous system depressants including phenothiazines because respiratory depression, hypotension, and profound sedation or coma may result).
No products indexed under this heading.

Trimethobenzamide Hydrochloride (Oxycodone, like all opioid analgesics, should be started at 1/3 to 1/2 of the usual dosage in patients who are concurrently receiving other central nervous system depressants including centrally acting anti-emetics because respiratory depression, hypotension, and profound sedation or coma may result).
No products indexed under this heading.

Trimipramine Maleate (Oxycodone is metabolized in part to oxymorphone via cytochrome P450 2D6. While this pathway may be blocked by a variety of drugs (eg, polycyclic antidepressants), such blockade has not yet been shown to be of clinical significance with this agent. Clinicians should be aware of this possible interaction).
No products indexed under this heading.

Tubocurarine Chloride (Opioid analgesics, including oxycodone, may enhance the neuromuscular blocking action of skeletal muscle relaxants and produce an increased degree of respiratory depression).
No products indexed under this heading.

Vardenafil Hydrochloride (Oxycodone is metabolized in part to oxymorphone via cytochrome P450 2D6. While this pathway may be blocked by a variety of drugs (eg, certain cardiovascular drugs including amiodarone and quinidine as well as polycyclic antidepressants), such blockade has not yet been shown to be of clinical significance with this agent. Clinicians should be aware of this possible interaction, however). Products include:
Levitra 3157

Vecuronium Bromide (Opioid analgesics, including oxycodone, may enhance the neuromuscular blocking action of skeletal muscle relaxants and produce an increased degree of respiratory depression).
No products indexed under this heading.

Zaleplon (Oxycodone, like all opioid analgesics, should be started at 1/3 to 1/2 of the usual dosage in patients who are concurrently receiving other central nervous system depressants including sedatives or hypnotics because respiratory depression, hypotension, and profound sedation or coma may result).
No products indexed under this heading.

Ziprasidone Hydrochloride (Oxycodone, like all opioid analgesics, should be started at 1/3 to 1/2 of the usual dosage in patients who are concurrently receiving other central nervous system depressants including sedatives or hypnotics, general anesthetics, phenothiazines, centrally acting anti-emetics, tranquilizers, and alcohol because respiratory depression, hypotension, and profound sedation or coma may result). Products include:
Geodon 2723

Zolpidem Tartrate (Oxycodone, like all opioid analgesics, should be started at 1/3 to 1/2 of the usual dosage in patients who are concurrently receiving other central nervous system depressants including sedatives or hypnotics because respiratory depression, hypotension, and profound sedation or coma may result). Products include:
Ambien 2920
Ambien CR 2925

Food Interactions

Alcohol (Oxycodone, like all opioid analgesics, should be started at 1/3 to 1/2 of the usual dosage in patients who are concurrently receiving other central nervous system depressants including alcohol because respiratory depression, hypotension, and profound sedation or coma may result).

Beer, reduced-alcohol (Oxycodone, like all opioid analgesics, should be started at 1/3 to 1/2 of the usual dosage in patients who are concurrently receiving other central nervous system depressants including alcohol because respiratory depression, hypotension, and profound sedation or coma may result).

Beer, unspecified (Oxycodone, like all opioid analgesics, should be started at 1/3 to 1/2 of the usual dosage in patients who are concurrently receiving other central nervous system depressants including alcohol because respiratory depression, hypotension, and profound sedation or coma may result).

Food, unspecified (The peak plasma concentration of oxycodone increased by 25% when oxycodone was administered with a high-fat meal).

(⊙ Described in PDR® for Ophthalmic Medicines)

Meal, unspecified (The peak plasma concentration of oxycodone increased by 25% when oxycodone was administered with a high-fat meal).

Wine, Chianti (Oxycodone, like all opioid analgesics, should be started at 1/3 to 1/2 of the usual dosage in patients who are concurrently receiving other central nervous system depressants including alcohol because respiratory depression, hypotension, and profound sedation or coma may result).

Wine, Red (Oxycodone, like all opioid analgesics, should be started at 1/3 to 1/2 of the usual dosage in patients who are concurrently receiving other central nervous system depressants including alcohol because respiratory depression, hypotension, and profound sedation or coma may result).

Wine, unspecified (Oxycodone, like all opioid analgesics, should be started at 1/3 to 1/2 of the usual dosage in patients who are concurrently receiving other central nervous system depressants including alcohol because respiratory depression, hypotension, and profound sedation or coma may result).

Wine products (Oxycodone, like all opioid analgesics, should be started at 1/3 to 1/2 of the usual dosage in patients who are concurrently receiving other central nervous system depressants including alcohol because respiratory depression, hypotension, and profound sedation or coma may result).

OZURDEX INTRAVITREAL IMPLANT

(Dexamethasone) ....⊙223
None cited in PDR database.

PANHEMATIN FOR INJECTION

(Hemin) 2016
May interact with barbiturates, estrogens, oral anticoagulants. Compounds in these categories include:

Amobarbital (Hemin inhibits the enzyme delta-aminolevulinic acid synthetase; concurrent use with drugs that increase the activity of delta-aminolevulinic acid synthetase, such as barbiturates, should be avoided).
  No products indexed under this heading.

Amobarbital Sodium (Hemin inhibits the enzyme delta-aminolevulinic acid synthetase; concurrent use with drugs that increase the activity of delta-aminolevulinic acid synthetase, such as barbiturates, should be avoided).
  No products indexed under this heading.

Anisindione (Hemin exhibits transient, mild anticoagulant effects, therefore, concurrent anticoagulant therapy should be avoided).
  No products indexed under this heading.

Aprobarbital (Hemin inhibits the enzyme delta-aminolevulinic acid synthetase; concurrent use with drugs that increase the activity of delta-aminolevulinic acid synthetase, such as barbiturates, should be avoided).
  No products indexed under this heading.

Butabarbital (Hemin inhibits the enzyme delta-aminolevulinic acid synthetase; concurrent use with drugs that increase the activity of delta-aminolevulinic acid synthetase, such as barbiturates, should be avoided).
  No products indexed under this heading.

Butabarbital Sodium (Hemin inhibits the enzyme delta-aminolevulinic acid synthetase; concurrent use with drugs that increase the activity of delta-aminolevulinic acid synthetase, such as barbiturates, should be avoided).
  No products indexed under this heading.

Butalbital (Hemin inhibits the enzyme delta-aminolevulinic acid synthetase; concurrent use with drugs that increase the activity of delta-aminolevulinic acid synthetase, such as barbiturates, should be avoided).
  No products indexed under this heading.

Chlorotrianisene (Hemin inhibits the enzyme delta-aminolevulinic acid synthetase; concurrent use with drugs that increase the activity of delta-aminolevulinic acid synthetase, such as estrogens, should be avoided).
  No products indexed under this heading.

Dicumarol (Hemin exhibits transient, mild anticoagulant effects, therefore, concurrent anticoagulant therapy should be avoided).
  No products indexed under this heading.

Dienestrol (Hemin inhibits the enzyme delta-aminolevulinic acid synthetase; concurrent use with drugs that increase the activity of delta-aminolevulinic acid synthetase, such as estrogens, should be avoided).
  No products indexed under this heading.

Diethylstilbestrol (Hemin inhibits the enzyme delta-aminolevulinic acid synthetase; concurrent use with drugs that increase the activity of delta-aminolevulinic acid synthetase, such as estrogens, should be avoided).
  No products indexed under this heading.

Estradiol (Hemin inhibits the enzyme delta-aminolevulinic acid synthetase; concurrent use with drugs that increase the activity of delta-aminolevulinic acid synthetase, such as estrogens, should be avoided). Products include:

Estrogens, Conjugated (Hemin inhibits the enzyme delta-aminolevulinic acid synthetase; concurrent use with drugs that increase the activity of delta-aminolevulinic acid synthetase, such as estrogens, should be avoided). Products include:

Estrogens, Esterified (Hemin inhibits the enzyme delta-aminolevulinic acid synthetase; concurrent use with drugs that increase the activity of delta-aminolevulinic acid synthetase, such as estrogens, should be avoided).
  No products indexed under this heading.

Estropipate (Hemin inhibits the enzyme delta-aminolevulinic acid synthetase; concurrent use with drugs that increase the activity of delta-aminolevulinic acid synthetase, such as estrogens, should be avoided).
  No products indexed under this heading.

Ethinyl Estradiol (Hemin inhibits the enzyme delta-aminolevulinic acid synthetase; concurrent use with drugs that increase the activity of delta-aminolevulinic acid synthetase, such as estrogens, should be avoided). Products include:

Hexobarbital (Hemin inhibits the enzyme delta-aminolevulinic acid synthetase; concurrent use with drugs that increase the activity of delta-aminolevulinic acid synthetase, such as barbiturates, should be avoided).
  No products indexed under this heading.

Mephobarbital (Hemin inhibits the enzyme delta-aminolevulinic acid synthetase; concurrent use with drugs that increase the activity of delta-aminolevulinic acid synthetase, such as barbiturates, should be avoided).
  No products indexed under this heading.

Pentobarbital (Hemin inhibits the enzyme delta-aminolevulinic acid synthetase; concurrent use with drugs that increase the activity of delta-aminolevulinic acid synthetase, such as barbiturates, should be avoided).
  No products indexed under this heading.

Pentobarbital Sodium (Hemin inhibits the enzyme delta-aminolevulinic acid synthetase; concurrent use with drugs that increase the activity of delta-aminolevulinic acid synthetase, such as barbiturates, should be avoided).
Products include:

Phenobarbital (Hemin inhibits the enzyme delta-aminolevulinic acid synthetase; concurrent use with drugs that increase the activity of delta-aminolevulinic acid synthetase, such as barbiturates, should be avoided).
Products include:

Phenobarbital Sodium (Hemin inhibits the enzyme delta-aminolevulinic acid synthetase; concurrent use with drugs that increase the activity of delta-aminolevulinic acid synthetase, such as barbiturates, should be avoided).
  No products indexed under this heading.

Polyestradiol Phosphate (Hemin inhibits the enzyme delta-aminolevulinic acid synthetase; concurrent use with drugs that increase the activity of delta-aminolevulinic acid synthetase, such as estrogens, should be avoided).
  No products indexed under this heading.

Quinestrol (Hemin inhibits the enzyme delta-aminolevulinic acid synthetase; concurrent use with drugs that increase the activity of delta-aminolevulinic acid synthetase, such as estrogens, should be avoided).
  No products indexed under this heading.

Secobarbital Sodium (Hemin inhibits the enzyme delta-aminolevulinic acid synthetase; concurrent use with drugs that increase the activity of delta-aminolevulinic acid synthetase, such as barbiturates, should be avoided).
  No products indexed under this heading.

Sodium Butabarbital (Hemin inhibits the enzyme delta-aminolevulinic acid synthetase; concurrent use with drugs that increase the activity of delta-aminolevulinic acid synthetase, such as barbiturates, should be avoided).
  No products indexed under this heading.

Sodium Pentobarbital (Hemin inhibits the enzyme delta-aminolevulinic acid synthetase; concurrent use with drugs that increase the activity of delta-aminolevulinic acid synthetase, such as barbiturates, should be avoided).
  No products indexed under this heading.

Thiamylal Sodium (Hemin inhibits the enzyme delta-aminolevulinic acid synthetase; concurrent use with drugs that increase the activity of delta-aminolevulinic acid synthetase, such as barbiturates, should be avoided).
  No products indexed under this heading.

Warfarin Sodium (Hemin exhibits transient, mild anticoagulant effects, therefore, concurrent anticoagulant therapy should be avoided).
  No products indexed under this heading.

PANRETIN GEL 0.1%

(Alitretinoin) 1070

DEET (N,N-diethyl-m-toluamide) (Avoid DEET (N,N-diethyl-m-toluamide) containing products (eg, insect repellent). Alitretinoin may increase DEET toxicity).
  No products indexed under this heading.

PARAGARD T 380A INTRAUTERINE COPPER CONTRACEPTIVE

(Copper, Intrauterine) 3412
None cited in PDR database.

PARNATE TABLETS

(Tranylcypromine Sulfate) 1584
May interact with alcohols, amphetamines, anorexiants, anticholinergic-type antiparkinsonism drugs, antihypertensives, central nervous system depressants, dibenzazepines, general anesthetics, insulin, local anesthetics, monoamine oxidase inhibitors, narcotic analgesics, oral hypoglycemic agents, phenothiazines, selective serotonin reuptake inhibitors, serotonin and norepinephrine reuptake inhibitors, spinal and peridural anesthetics, sympathomimetics, and certain other agents. Compounds in these categories include:

Acarbose (Some MAO inhibitors have contributed to hypoglycemic episodes in diabetic patients receiving oral hypoglycemic agents. Therefore, tranylcypromine should be used with caution in diabetics using oral hypoglycemic agents).
  No products indexed under this heading.

Acebutolol Hydrochloride (Concomitant use with hypotensive agents is contraindicated. A marked potentiating effect on hypotensive agents has been reported).
  No products indexed under this heading.

Albuterol (Tranylcypromine is contraindicated in combination with sympathomimetics. During therapy with tranylcypromine, it appears that certain patients are particularly vulnerable to the effects of sympathomimetics when the activity of certain enzymes is inhibited. Use of sympathomimetics may precipitate hypertension, headache, and related symptoms).
  No products indexed under this heading.

Albuterol Sulfate (Tranylcypromine is contraindicated in combination with sympathomimetics. During therapy with tranylcypromine, it appears that certain patients are particularly vulnerable to the effects of sympathomimetics when the activity of certain enzymes is inhibited. Use of sympathomimetics may precipitate hypertension, headache, and related symptoms). Products include:

Alfentanil Hydrochloride (Concomitant use with some central nervous system depressants, such as narcotics, is contraindicated. A marked potentiating effect on narcotics has been reported).
  No products indexed under this heading.

Aliskiren (Concomitant use with hypotensive agents is contraindicated. A marked potentiating effect on hypotensive agents has been reported).
Products include:

Alprazolam (Concomitant use with some central nervous system depressants is contraindicated. A marked potentiating effect on some central nervous depressants has been reported).
  No products indexed under this heading.

Amitriptyline Hydrochloride (Tranylcypromine is contraindicated in combi-

nation with or in rapid succession with dibenzazepine-related entities. Hypertensive crises or severe convulsive seizures may occur in patients receiving such combinations. In patients being transferred to tranylcypromine from a dibenzazepine-related entity, allow a medication free interval of at least a week, then initiate tranylcypromine using half the normal starting dosage for at least the first week of therapy. Similarly, at least a week should elapse between the discontinuance of tranylcypromine and the administration of a dibenzazepine-related entity or the re-administration of tranylcypromine).
No products indexed under this heading.

Amlodipine Besylate (Concomitant use with hypotensive agents is contraindicated. A marked potentiating effect on hypotensive agents has been reported). Products include:

Amobarbital (Concomitant use with some central nervous system depressants is contraindicated. A marked potentiating effect on some central nervous depressants has been reported).
No products indexed under this heading.

Amobarbital Sodium (Concomitant use with some central nervous system depressants is contraindicated. A marked potentiating effect on some central nervous depressants has been reported).
No products indexed under this heading.

Amoxapine (Tranylcypromine is contraindicated in combination with or in rapid succession with dibenzazepine-related entities. Hypertensive crises or severe convulsive seizures may occur in patients receiving such combinations. In patients being transferred to tranylcypromine from a dibenzazepine-related entity, allow a medication free interval of at least a week, then initiate tranylcypromine using half the normal starting dosage for at least the first week of therapy. Similarly, at least a week should elapse between the discontinuance of tranylcypromine and the administration of a dibenzazepine-related entity or the re-administration of tranylcypromine).
No products indexed under this heading.

Amphetamine Aspartate (Tranylcypromine is contraindicated in combination with sympathomimetics, including weight reducing preparations that contain vasoconstrictors. During therapy with tranylcypromine, it appears with certain patients are particularly vunerable to the effects of sympathomimetics when the activity of certain enzymes is inhibited).
No products indexed under this heading.

Amphetamine Aspartate Monohydrate (Tranylcypromine is contraindicated in combination with sympathomimetics, including weight reducing preparations that contain vasoconstrictors. During therapy with tranylcypromine, it appears with certain patients are particularly vunerable to the effects of sympathomimetics when the activity of certain enzymes is inhibited).
No products indexed under this heading.

Amphetamine Resins (Tranylcypromine is contraindicated in combination with sympathmimetics including amphetamines).
No products indexed under this heading.

Amphetamine Sulfate (Tranylcypromine is contraindicated in combination with sympathmimetics including amphetamines).
No products indexed under this heading.

Apomorphine (Concomitant use with some central nervous system depressants, such as narcotics, is contraindicated. A marked potentiating effect on narcotics has been reported).
No products indexed under this heading.

Apomorphine Hydrochloride (Concomitant use with some central nervous system depressants, such as narcotics, is contraindicated. A marked potentiating effect on narcotics has been reported).
No products indexed under this heading.

Aprobarbital (Concomitant use with some central nervous system depressants is contraindicated. A marked potentiating effect on some central nervous depressants has been reported).
No products indexed under this heading.

Articaine Hydrochloride (Tranylcypromine is contraindicated in patients undergoing elective surgery. Patients should not be given local anesthesia containing sympathomimetic vasoconstrictors. The possible combined hypotensive effects of tranylcypromine and spinal anesthesia should be kept in mind. Tranylcypromine should be discontinued at least 10 days prior to elective surgery).
No products indexed under this heading.

Atenolol (Concomitant use with hypotensive agents is contraindicated. A marked potentiating effect on hypotensive agents has been reported).
No products indexed under this heading.

Benazepril Hydrochloride (Concomitant use with hypotensive agents is contraindicated. A marked potentiating effect on hypotensive agents has been reported).
No products indexed under this heading.

Bendroflumethiazide (Concomitant use with hypotensive agents is contraindicated. A marked potentiating effect on hypotensive agents has been reported).
No products indexed under this heading.

Benzphetamine Hydrochloride (Tranylcypromine is contraindicated in combination with sympathomimetics, including weight reducing preparations that contain vasoconstrictors. During therapy with tranylcypromine, it appears with certain patients are particularly vunerable to the effects of sympathomimetics when the activity of certain enzymes is inhibited).
No products indexed under this heading.

Benztropine Mesylate (Antiparkinsonism drugs should be used with caution in patients receiving tranylcypromine since severe reactions have been reported).
No products indexed under this heading.

Betaxolol Hydrochloride (Concomitant use with hypotensive agents is contraindicated. A marked potentiating effect on hypotensive agents has been reported).
No products indexed under this heading.

Biperiden Hydrochloride (Antiparkinsonism drugs should be used with caution in patients receiving tranylcypromine since severe reactions have been reported).
No products indexed under this heading.

Bisoprolol Fumarate (Concomitant use with hypotensive agents is contraindicated. A marked potentiating effect on hypotensive agents has been reported).
No products indexed under this heading.

Bupivacaine Hydrochloride (Tranylcypromine is contraindicated in patients undergoing elective surgery. Patients should not be given local anesthesia containing sympathomimetic vasoconstrictors. The possible combined hypotensive effects of tranylcypromine and spinal anesthesia should be kept in mind. Tranylcypromine should be discontinued at least 10 days prior to elective surgery).
No products indexed under this heading.

Buprenorphine Hydrochloride (Concomitant use with some central nervous system depressants, such as narcotics, is contraindicated. A marked potentiating effect on narcotics has been reported).
No products indexed under this heading.

Bupropion Hydrochloride (Tranylcypromine is contraindicated in combination with bupropion. At least 14 days should elapse between discontinuation of a MAO inhibitor and initiation of treatment with bupropion). Products include:

Buspirone Hydrochloride (Tranylcypromine is contraindicated in combination with buspirone. Tranylcypromine should not be used in combination with buspirone since several cases of elevated blood pressure have been reported in patients taking MAO inhibitors who were then given buspirone. At least 10 days should elapse between the discontinuation of tranylcypromine and the initiation of buspirone).
No products indexed under this heading.

Butabarbital (Concomitant use with some central nervous system depressants is contraindicated. A marked potentiating effect on some central nervous depressants has been reported).
No products indexed under this heading.

Butabarbital Sodium (Concomitant use with some central nervous system depressants is contraindicated. A marked potentiating effect on some central nervous depressants has been reported).
No products indexed under this heading.

Butalbital (Concomitant use with some central nervous system depressants is contraindicated. A marked potentiating effect on some central nervous depressants has been reported).
No products indexed under this heading.

Caffeine (Excessive use of caffeine in any form is contraindicated).
No products indexed under this heading.

Caffeine Anhydrous (Excessive use of caffeine in any form is contraindicated).
No products indexed under this heading.

Caffeine Citrate (Excessive use of caffeine in any form is contraindicated).
No products indexed under this heading.

Candesartan Cilexetil (Concomitant use with hypotensive agents is contraindicated. A marked potentiating effect on hypotensive agents has been reported). Products include:

Captopril (Concomitant use with hypotensive agents is contraindicated. A marked potentiating effect on hypotensive agents has been reported). Products include:

Carbamazepine (Tranylcypromine is contraindicated in combination with or in rapid succession with dibenzazepine-related entities. Hypertensive crises or severe convulsive seizures may occur in patients receiving such combinations. In patients being transferred to tranylcypromine from a dibenzazepine-related

entity, allow a medication free interval of at least a week, then initiate tranylcypromine using half the normal starting dosage for at least the first week of therapy. Similarly, at least a week should elapse between the discontinuance of tranylcypromine and the administration of a dibenzazepine-related entity or the re-administration of tranylcypromine). Products include:

Carteolol Hydrochloride (Concomitant use with hypotensive agents is contraindicated. A marked potentiating effect on hypotensive agents has been reported).
No products indexed under this heading.

Carvedilol (Concomitant use with hypotensive agents is contraindicated. A marked potentiating effect on hypotensive agents has been reported). Products include:

Carvedilol Phosphate (Concomitant use with hypotensive agents is contraindicated. A marked potentiating effect on hypotensive agents has been reported). Products include:

Chlordiazepoxide (Concomitant use with some central nervous system depressants is contraindicated. A marked potentiating effect on some central nervous depressants has been reported).
No products indexed under this heading.

Chlordiazepoxide Hydrochloride (Concomitant use with some central nervous system depressants is contraindicated. A marked potentiating effect on some central nervous depressants has been reported).
No products indexed under this heading.

Chloroprocaine Hydrochloride (Tranylcypromine is contraindicated in patients undergoing elective surgery. Patients should not be given local anesthesia containing sympathomimetic vasoconstrictors. The possible combined hypotensive effects of tranylcypromine and spinal anesthesia should be kept in mind. Tranylcypromine should be discontinued at least 10 days prior to elective surgery).
No products indexed under this heading.

Chlorothiazide (Concomitant use with hypotensive agents is contraindicated. A marked potentiating effect on hypotensive agents has been reported).
No products indexed under this heading.

Chlorothiazide Sodium (Concomitant use with hypotensive agents is contraindicated. A marked potentiating effect on hypotensive agents has been reported). Products include:

Chlorpromazine (Concomitant use with some central nervous system depressants is contraindicated. A marked potentiating effect on some central nervous depressants has been reported).
No products indexed under this heading.

Chlorpromazine Hydrochloride (Concomitant use with some central nervous system depressants is contraindicated. A marked potentiating effect on some central nervous depressants has been reported).
No products indexed under this heading.

Chlorpropamide (Some MAO inhibitors have contributed to hypoglycemic episodes in diabetic patients receiving oral hypoglycemic agents. Therefore, tranylcypromine should be used with caution in diabetics using oral hypoglycemic agents).
No products indexed under this heading.

1361 Interactions Index Parnate

Chlorprothixene (Concomitant use with some central nervous system depressants is contraindicated. A marked potentiating effect on some central nervous depressants has been reported).
No products indexed under this heading.

Chlorprothixene Hydrochloride (Concomitant use with some central nervous system depressants is contraindicated. A marked potentiating effect on some central nervous depressants has been reported).
No products indexed under this heading.

Chlorprothixene Lactate (Concomitant use with some central nervous system depressants is contraindicated. A marked potentiating effect on some central nervous depressants has been reported).
No products indexed under this heading.

Chlorthalidone (Concomitant use with hypotensive agents is contraindicated. A marked potentiating effect on hypotensive agents has been reported). Products include:
Clorpres 2344

Citalopram Hydrobromide (Tranylcypromine is contraindicated in combination with selective serotonin reuptake inhibitors (SSRIs). There have been reports of serious, sometimes fatal reactions in patients receiving a SSRI in combination with a MAO inhibitor, and it patients who have recently discontinued a SSRI and are then started on a MAO inhibitor. Some cases presented with features resembling neuroleptic malignant syndrome. Therefore, SSRIs should not be used in combination with a MAO inhibitor, or within 14 days of discontinuing therapy with a MAO inhibitor). Products include:
Celexa 1153

Clomipramine Hydrochloride (Tranylcypromine is contraindicated in combination with or in rapid succession with dibenzazepine-related entities. Hypertensive crises or severe convulsive seizures may occur in patients receiving such combinations. In patients being transferred to tranylcypromine from a dibenzazepine-related entity, allow a medication free interval of at least a week, then initiate tranylcypromine using half the normal starting dosage for at least the first week of therapy. Similarly, at least a week should elapse between the discontinuance of tranylcypromine and the administration of a dibenzazepine-related entity or the re-administration of tranylcypromine).
No products indexed under this heading.

Clonazepam (Concomitant use with some central nervous system depressants is contraindicated. A marked potentiating effect on some central nervous depressants has been reported). Products include:
Klonopin 2855

Clonidine (Concomitant use with hypotensive agents is contraindicated. A marked potentiating effect on hypotensive agents has been reported). Products include:
Catapres-TTS 884

Clonidine Hydrochloride (Concomitant use with hypotensive agents is contraindicated. A marked potentiating effect on hypotensive agents has been reported). Products include:
Clorpres 2344

Clorazepate Dipotassium (Concomitant use with some central nervous system depressants is contraindicated. A marked potentiating effect on some central nervous depressants has been reported).
No products indexed under this heading.

Clozapine (Tranylcypromine is contraindicated in combination with or in rapid succession with dibenzazepine-related entities. Hypertensive crises or severe convulsive seizures may occur in patients receiving such combinations. In patients being transferred to tranylcypromine from a dibenzazepine-related entity, allow a medication free interval of at least a week, then initiate tranylcypromine using half the normal starting dosage for at least the first week of therapy. Similarly, at least a week should elapse between the discontinuance of tranylcypromine and the administration of a dibenzazepine-related entity or the re-administration of tranylcypromine).
No products indexed under this heading.

Cocaine Hydrochloride (Concomitant use with cocaine is contraindicated).
No products indexed under this heading.

Codeine Phosphate (Concomitant use with some central nervous system depressants, such as narcotics, is contraindicated. A marked potentiating effect on narcotics has been reported). Products include:
Tylenol with Codeine 2691

Codeine Sulfate (Concomitant use with some central nervous system depressants, such as narcotics, is contraindicated. A marked potentiating effect on narcotics has been reported).
No products indexed under this heading.

Cyclobenzaprine Hydrochloride (Tranylcypromine is contraindicated in combination with or in rapid succession with dibenzazepine-related entities. Hypertensive crises or severe convulsive seizures may occur in patients receiving such combinations. In patients being transferred to tranylcypromine from a dibenzazepine-related entity, allow a medication free interval of at least a week, then initiate tranylcypromine using half the normal starting dosage for at least the first week of therapy. Similarly, at least a week should elapse between the discontinuance of tranylcypromine and the administration of a dibenzazepine-related entity or the re-administration of tranylcypromine). Products include:
Amrix 964

Deserpidine (Concomitant use with hypotensive agents is contraindicated. A marked potentiating effect on hypotensive agents has been reported).
No products indexed under this heading.

Desflurane (Concomitant use with some central nervous system depressants is contraindicated. A marked potentiating effect on some central nervous depressants has been reported).
No products indexed under this heading.

Desipramine Hydrochloride (Tranylcypromine is contraindicated in combination with or in rapid succession with dibenzazepine-related entities. Hypertensive crises or severe convulsive seizures may occur in patients receiving such combinations. In patients being transferred to tranylcypromine from a dibenzazepine-related entity, allow a medication free interval of at least a week, then initiate tranylcypromine using half the normal starting dosage for at least the first week of therapy. Similarly, at least a week should elapse between the discontinuance of tranylcypromine and the administration of a dibenzazepine-related entity or the re-administration of tranylcypromine).
No products indexed under this heading.

Desvenlafaxine Succinate (Tranylcypromine is contraindicated in combination with selective norepinephrine reuptake inhibitors (SNRIs). There have been reports of serious, sometimes fatal reactions in patients receiving a SNRI in combination with a MAO inhibitor, and it patients who have recently discontinued a SNRI and are then started on a MAO inhibitor. Some cases presented with features resembling neuroleptic malignant syndrome. Therefore, SNRIs should not be used in combination with a MAO inhibitor, or within 14 days of discontinuing therapy with a MAO inhibitor. At least one week should be allowed after stopping a SNRI before starting a MAO inhibitor). Products include:
Pristiq 3564

Dexfenfluramine Hydrochloride (Tranylcypromine is contraindicated in combination with sympathomimetics, including weight reducing preparations that contain vasoconstrictors. During therapy with tranylcypromine, it appears with certain patients are particularly vunerable to the effects of sympathomimetics when the activity of certain enzymes is inhibited).
No products indexed under this heading.

Dextroamphetamine (Tranylcypromine is contraindicated in combination with sympathomimetics, including weight reducing preparations that contain vasoconstrictors. During therapy with tranylcypromine, it appears with certain patients are particularly vunerable to the effects of sympathomimetics when the activity of certain enzymes is inhibited).
No products indexed under this heading.

Dextroamphetamine Saccharate (Tranylcypromine is contraindicated in combination with sympathomimetics, including weight reducing preparations that contain vasoconstrictors. During therapy with tranylcypromine, it appears with certain patients are particularly vunerable to the effects of sympathomimetics when the activity of certain enzymes is inhibited).
No products indexed under this heading.

Dextroamphetamine Sulfate (Tranylcypromine is contraindicated in combination with sympathmimetics including amphetamines). Products include:
Dexedrine 1425

Dextromethorphan Hydrobromide (Tranylcypromine is contraindicated in combination with dextromethorphan. The combination of MAO inhibitors and dextromethorphan has been reported to cause brief episodes of psychosis or bizarre behavior).
No products indexed under this heading.

Dextromethorphan Polistirex (Tranylcypromine is contraindicated in combination with dextromethorphan. The combination of MAO inhibitors and dextromethorphan has been reported to cause brief episodes of psychosis or bizarre behavior).
No products indexed under this heading.

Dextromethorphan Tannate (Tranylcypromine is contradindicated in combination with dextromethorphan. The combination of MAO inhibitors and dextromethorphan has been reported to cause brief episodes of psychosis or bizarre behavior).
No products indexed under this heading.

Dezocine (Concomitant use with some central nervous system depressants, such as narcotics, is contraindicated. A marked potentiating effect on narcotics has been reported).
No products indexed under this heading.

Diazepam (Concomitant use with some central nervous system depressants is contraindicated. A marked potentiating effect on some central nervous depressants has been reported). Products include:
Valium Tablets 2880

Diazoxide (Concomitant use with hypotensive agents is contraindicated. A marked potentiating effect on hypotensive agents has been reported). Products include:
Proglycem 1179
Proglycem Suspension 1179

Diethylpropion Hydrochloride (Tranylcypromine is contraindicated in combination with sympathomimetics, including weight reducing preparations that contain vasoconstrictors. During therapy with tranylcypromine, it appears with certain patients are particularly vunerable to the effects of sympathomimetics when the activity of certain enzymes is inhibited).
No products indexed under this heading.

Dihydrocodeine Bitartrate (Concomitant use with some central nervous system depressants, such as narcotics, is contraindicated. A marked potentiating effect on narcotics has been reported).
No products indexed under this heading.

Dihydrocodeinone Bitartrate (Concomitant use with some central nervous system depressants, such as narcotics, is contraindicated. A marked potentiating effect on narcotics has been reported).
No products indexed under this heading.

Diltiazem Hydrochloride (Concomitant use with hypotensive agents is contraindicated. A marked potentiating effect on hypotensive agents has been reported). Products include:
Cardizem LA 423

Diltiazem Maleate (Concomitant use with hypotensive agents is contraindicated. A marked potentiating effect on hypotensive agents has been reported).
No products indexed under this heading.

Diphenhydramine (Anti-parkinsonism drugs should be used with caution in patients receiving tranylcypromine since severe reactions have been reported).
No products indexed under this heading.

Diphenhydramine Hydrochloride (Anti-parkinsonism drugs should be used with caution in patients receiving tranylcypromine since severe reactions have been reported). Products include:
Benadryl Allergy Ultratab 2042
Children's Benadryl Allergy Liquid 2042

Disulfiram (Tranylcypromine should be administered with caution to patients receiving disulfiram).
No products indexed under this heading.

Dobutamine Hydrochloride (Tranylcypromine is contraindicated in combination with sympathomimetics. During therapy with tranylcypromine, it appears that certain patients are particularly vulnerable to the effects of sympathomimetics when the activity of certain enzymes is inhibited. Use of sympathomimetics may precipitate hypertension, headache, and related symptoms).
No products indexed under this heading.

Dopamine Hydrochloride (Tranylcypromine is contraindicated in combination with dopamine. Use of dopamine with tranylcypromine may precipitate hypertension, headache, and related symptoms).
No products indexed under this heading.

Doxazosin Mesylate (Concomitant use with hypotensive agents is contraindicated. A marked potentiating effect on hypotensive agents has been reported).
No products indexed under this heading.

Doxepin Hydrochloride (Tranylcypromine is contraindicated in combination with or in rapid succession with dibenzazepine-related entities. Hypertensive crises or severe convulsive seizures may occur in patients receiving such combinations. In patients being transferred to tranylcypromine from a dibenzazepine-related entity, allow a medication free interval of at least a week, then initiate tranylcypromine using half the normal starting dosage for at least the first week of therapy.

IMPORTANT NOTE: Always consult each drug listing in the patient's regimen for possible interactions.

Similarly, at least a week should elapse between the discontinuance of tranylcypromine and the administration of a dibenzazepine-related entity or the readministration of tranylcypromine).
No products indexed under this heading.

Droperidol (Concomitant use with some central nervous system depressants is contraindicated. A marked potentiating effect on some central nervous depressants has been reported).
No products indexed under this heading.

Duloxetine Hydrochloride (Tranylcypromine is contraindicated in combination with selective norepinephrine reuptake inhibitors (SNRIs). There have been reports of serious, sometimes fatal reactions in patients receiving a SNRI in combination with a MAO inhibitor, and it patients who have recently discontinued a SNRI and are then started on a MAO inhibitor. Some cases presented with features resembling neuroleptic malignant syndrome. Therefore, SNRIs should not be used in combination with a MAO inhibitor, or within 14 days of discontinuing therapy with a MAO inhibitor. At least one week should be allowed after stopping a SNRI before starting a MAO inhibitor). Products include:
Cymbalta 1871

Enalapril Maleate (Concomitant use with hypotensive agents is contraindicated. A marked potentiating effect on hypotensive agents has been reported).
No products indexed under this heading.

Enalaprilat (Concomitant use with hypotensive agents is contraindicated. A marked potentiating effect on hypotensive agents has been reported).
No products indexed under this heading.

Enflurane (Concomitant use with some central nervous system depressants is contraindicated. A marked potentiating effect on some central nervous depressants has been reported).
No products indexed under this heading.

Ephedrine Hydrochloride (Tranylcypromine is contraindicated in combination with sympathomimetics. During therapy with tranylcypromine, it appears that certain patients are particularly vulnerable to the effects of sympathomimetics when the activity of certain enzymes is inhibited. Use of sympathomimetics may precipitate hypertension, headache, and related symptoms).
No products indexed under this heading.

Ephedrine Sulfate (Tranylcypromine is contraindicated in combination with sympathomimetics. During therapy with tranylcypromine, it appears that certain patients are particularly vulnerable to the effects of sympathomimetics when the activity of certain enzymes is inhibited. Use of sympathomimetics may precipitate hypertension, headache, and related symptoms).
No products indexed under this heading.

Ephedrine Tannate (Tranylcypromine is contraindicated in combination with sympathomimetics. During therapy with tranylcypromine, it appears that certain patients are particularly vulnerable to the effects of sympathomimetics when the activity of certain enzymes is inhibited. Use of sympathomimetics may precipitate hypertension, headache, and related symptoms).
No products indexed under this heading.

Epinephrine (Tranylcypromine is contraindicated in combination with sympathomimetics. During therapy with tranylcypromine, it appears that certain patients are particularly vulnerable to the effects of sympathomimetics when the activity of certain enzymes is inhibited. Use of sympathomimetics may precipitate hypertension, headache, and related symptoms). Products include:
EpiPen 3631
Twinject 3268

Epinephrine Bitartrate (Tranylcypromine is contraindicated in combination with sympathomimetics. During therapy with tranylcypromine, it appears that certain patients are particularly vulnerable to the effects of sympathomimetics when the activity of certain enzymes is inhibited. Use of sympathomimetics may precipitate hypertension, headache, and related symptoms).
No products indexed under this heading.

Epinephrine Hydrochloride (Tranylcypromine is contraindicated in combination with sympathomimetics. During therapy with tranylcypromine, it appears that certain patients are particularly vulnerable to the effects of sympathomimetics when the activity of certain enzymes is inhibited. Use of sympathomimetics may precipitate hypertension, headache, and related symptoms).
No products indexed under this heading.

Eprosartan Mesylate (Concomitant use with hypotensive agents is contraindicated. A marked potentiating effect on hypotensive agents has been reported). Products include:
Teveten 538
Teveten HCT 541

Escitalopram Oxalate (Tranylcypromine is contraindicated in combination with selective serotonin reuptake inhibitors (SSRIs). There have been reports of serious, sometimes fatal reactions in patients receiving a SSRI in combination with a MAO inhibitor, and it patients who have recently discontinued a SSRI and are then started on a MAO inhibitor. Some cases presented with features resembling neuroleptic malignant syndrome. Therefore, SSRIs should not be used in combination with a MAO inhibitor, or within 14 days of discontinuing therapy with a MAO inhibitor). Products include:
Lexapro Oral Suspension 1160
Lexapro Tablets 1160

Esmolol Hydrochloride (Concomitant use with hypotensive agents is contraindicated. A marked potentiating effect on hypotensive agents has been reported).
No products indexed under this heading.

Estazolam (Concomitant use with some central nervous system depressants is contraindicated. A marked potentiating effect on some central nervous depressants has been reported).
No products indexed under this heading.

Ethanol (Concomitant use with some central nervous system depressants, such as alcohol, is contraindicated. A marked potentiating effect on alcohol has been reported).
No products indexed under this heading.

Ethchlorvynol (Concomitant use with some central nervous system depressants is contraindicated. A marked potentiating effect on some central nervous depressants has been reported).
No products indexed under this heading.

Ethinamate (Concomitant use with some central nervous system depressants is contraindicated. A marked potentiating effect on some central nervous depressants has been reported).
No products indexed under this heading.

Ethyl Alcohol (Concomitant use with some central nervous system depressants, such as alcohol, is contraindicated. A marked potentiating effect on alcohol has been reported).
No products indexed under this heading.

Etidocaine Hydrochloride (Tranylcypromine is contraindicated in patients undergoing elective surgery. Patients should not be given local anesthesia containing sympathomimetic vasoconstrictors. The possible combined hypotensive effects of tranylcypromine and spinal anesthesia should be kept in mind. Tranylcypromine should be discontinued at least 10 days prior to elective surgery).
No products indexed under this heading.

Felodipine (Concomitant use with hypotensive agents is contraindicated. A marked potentiating effect on hypotensive agents has been reported).
No products indexed under this heading.

Fenfluramine Hydrochloride (Tranylcypromine is contraindicated in combination with sympathomimetics, including weight reducing preparations that contain vasoconstrictors. During therapy with tranylcypromine, it appears with certain patients are particularly vunerable to the effects of sympathomimetics when the activity of certain enzymes is inhibited).
No products indexed under this heading.

Fentanyl (Concomitant use with some central nervous system depressants, such as narcotics, is contraindicated. A marked potentiating effect on narcotics has been reported). Products include:
Duragesic 2604
Fentanyl Transdermal System 2346
Onsolis 2054

Fentanyl Citrate (Concomitant use with some central nervous system depressants, such as narcotics, is contraindicated. A marked potentiating effect on narcotics has been reported). Products include:
Fentora 966

Fluoxetine (Tranylcypromine is contraindicated in combination with selective serotonin reuptake inhibitors (SSRIs). There have been reports of serious, sometimes fatal reactions in patients receiving a SSRI (eg, fluoxetine) in combination with an MAO inhibitor, and in patients who have recently discontinued a SSRI and are then started on a MAO inhibitor. Some cases presented with features resembling neuroleptic malignant syndrome. Therefore, SSRIs should not be used in combination with a MAO inhibitor, or within 14 days of discontinuing therapy with a MAO inhibitor. Since fluoxetine and its major metabolite have very long elmination half-lives, at least 5 weeks should be allowed after stopping fluoxetine before starting before starting a MAO inhibitor).
No products indexed under this heading.

Fluoxetine Hydrochloride (Tranylcypromine is contraindicated in combination with selective serotonin reuptake inhibitors (SSRIs). There have been reports of serious, sometimes fatal reactions in patients receiving a SSRI (eg, fluoxetine) in combination with an MAO inhibitor, and in patients who have recently discontinued a SSRI and are then started on a MAO inhibitor. Some cases presented with features resembling neuroleptic malignant syndrome. Therefore, SSRIs should not be used in combination with a MAO inhibitor, or within14 days of discontinuing therapy with a MAO inhibitor. Since fluoxetine and its major metabolite have very long elmination half-lives, at least 5 weeks should be allowed after stopping fluoxetine before starting before starting a MAO inhibitor). Products include:
Prozac Weekly 1941
Prozac Pulvules 1941
Symbyax 1965

Fluphenazine Decanoate (Concomitant use with some central nervous system depressants is contraindicated. A marked potentiating effect on some central nervous depressants has been reported).
No products indexed under this heading.

Fluphenazine Enanthate (Concomitant use with some central nervous system depressants is contraindicated. A marked potentiating effect on some central nervous depressants has been reported).
No products indexed under this heading.

Fluphenazine Hydrochloride (Concomitant use with some central nervous system depressants is contraindicated. A marked potentiating effect on some central nervous depressants has been reported).
No products indexed under this heading.

Flurazepam Hydrochloride (Concomitant use with some central nervous system depressants is contraindicated. A marked potentiating effect on some central nervous depressants has been reported).
No products indexed under this heading.

Fluvoxamine (Tranylcypromine is contraindicated in combination with selective serotonin reuptake inhibitors (SSRIs). There have been reports of serious, sometimes fatal reactions in patients receiving a SSRI in combination with a MAO inhibitor, and it patients who have recently discontinued a SSRI and are then started on a MAO inhibitor. Some cases presented with features resembling neuroleptic malignant syndrome. Therefore, SSRIs should not be used in combination with a MAO inhibitor, or within 14 days of discontinuing therapy with a MAO inhibitor).
No products indexed under this heading.

Fluvoxamine Maleate (Tranylcypromine is contraindicated in combination with selective serotonin reuptake inhibitors (SSRIs). There have been reports of serious, sometimes fatal reactions in patients receiving a SSRI in combination with a MAO inhibitor, and it patients who have recently discontinued a SSRI and are then started on a MAO inhibitor. Some cases presented with features resembling neuroleptic malignant syndrome. Therefore, SSRIs should not be used in combination with a MAO inhibitor, or within 14 days of discontinuing therapy with a MAO inhibitor).
No products indexed under this heading.

Fosinopril Sodium (Concomitant use with hypotensive agents is contraindicated. A marked potentiating effect on hypotensive agents has been reported).
No products indexed under this heading.

Furazolidone (Concurrent use with another MAO inhibitor may result in hypertensive crises or severe convulsive seizures; concurrent and/or sequential use is contraindicated).
No products indexed under this heading.

Furosemide (Concomitant use with hypotensive agents is contraindicated. A marked potentiating effect on hypotensive agents has been reported). Products include:
Furosemide 2354

Glibenclamide (Some MAO inhibitors have contributed to hypoglycemic episodes in diabetic patients receiving oral hypoglycemic agents. Therefore, tranylcypromine should be used with caution in diabetics using oral hypoglycemic agents).
No products indexed under this heading.

Glimepiride (Some MAO inhibitors have contributed to hypoglycemic episodes in diabetic patients receiving oral hypoglycemic agents. Therefore, tranyl-

cypromine should be used with caution in diabetics using oral hypoglycemic agents). Products include:

Glipizide (Some MAO inhibitors have contributed to hypoglycemic episodes in diabetic patients receiving oral hypoglycemic agents. Therefore, tranylcypromine should be used with caution in diabetics using oral hypoglycemic agents).

No products indexed under this heading.

Glutethimide (Concomitant use with some central nervous system depressants is contraindicated. A marked potentiating effect on some central nervous depressants has been reported).

No products indexed under this heading.

Glyburide (Some MAO inhibitors have contributed to hypoglycemic episodes in diabetic patients receiving oral hypoglycemic agents. Therefore, tranylcypromine should be used with caution in diabetics using oral hypoglycemic agents).

No products indexed under this heading.

Guanabenz Acetate (Concomitant use with hypotensive agents is contraindicated. A marked potentiating effect on hypotensive agents has been reported).

No products indexed under this heading.

Guanethidine (Concomitant use with hypotensive agents is contraindicated. A marked potentiating effect on hypotensive agents has been reported).

No products indexed under this heading.

Guanethidine Monosulfate (Tranylcypromine is contraindicated in combination with guanethidine. Use of guanethidine with tranylcypromine may preciptate hypertension, headache, and related symptoms).

No products indexed under this heading.

Guanethidine Sulfate (Concomitant use with hypotensive agents is contraindicated. A marked potentiating effect on hypotensive agents has been reported).

No products indexed under this heading.

Halazepam (Concomitant use with some central nervous system depressants is contraindicated. A marked potentiating effect on some central nervous depressants has been reported).

No products indexed under this heading.

Haloperidol (Concomitant use with some central nervous system depressants is contraindicated. A marked potentiating effect on some central nervous depressants has been reported).

No products indexed under this heading.

Haloperidol Decanoate (Concomitant use with some central nervous system depressants is contraindicated. A marked potentiating effect on some central nervous depressants has been reported).

No products indexed under this heading.

Haloperidol Lactate (Concomitant use with some central nervous system depressants is contraindicated. A marked potentiating effect on some central nervous depressants has been reported).

No products indexed under this heading.

Halothane (Tranylcypromine is contraindicated in patients undergoing elective surgery. Patients taking tranylcypromine should not undergo elective surgery requiring general anesthesia. Tranylcypromine should be discontinued at least 10 days prior to elective surgery).

No products indexed under this heading.

Hexobarbital (Concomitant use with some central nervous system depressants is contraindicated. A marked potentiating effect on some central nervous depressants has been reported).

No products indexed under this heading.

Hydralazine Hydrochloride (Concomitant use with hypotensive agents is contraindicated. A marked potentiating effect on hypotensive agents has been reported).

No products indexed under this heading.

Hydrochlorothiazide (Concomitant use with hypotensive agents is contraindicated. A marked potentiating effect on hypotensive agents has been reported). Products include:

Hydrocodone Bitartrate (Concomitant use with some central nervous system depressants, such as narcotics, is contraindicated. A marked potentiating effect on narcotics has been reported). Products include:

Hydrocodone Polistirex (Concomitant use with some central nervous system depressants, such as narcotics, is contraindicated. A marked potentiating effect on narcotics has been reported). Products include:

Hydroflumethiazide (Concomitant use with hypotensive agents is contraindicated. A marked potentiating effect on hypotensive agents has been reported).

No products indexed under this heading.

Hydromorphone (Concomitant use with some central nervous system depressants, such as narcotics, is contraindicated. A marked potentiating effect on narcotics has been reported).

No products indexed under this heading.

Hydromorphone Hydrochloride (Concomitant use with some central nervous system depressants, such as narcotics, is contraindicated. A marked potentiating effect on narcotics has been reported). Products include:

Hydroxyamphetamine Hydrobromide (Tranylcypromine is contraindicated in combination with sympathomimetics, including weight reducing preparations that contain vasoconstrictors. During therapy with tranylcypromine, it appears with certain patients are particularly vunerable to the effects of sympathomimetics when the activity of certain enzymes is inhibited).

No products indexed under this heading.

Hydroxyzine Hydrochloride (Concomitant use with some central nervous system depressants is contraindicated. A marked potentiating effect on some central nervous depressants has been reported).

No products indexed under this heading.

Imipramine Hydrochloride (Tranylcypromine is contraindicated in combination with or in rapid succession with dibenzazepine-related entities. Hypertensive crises or severe convulsive sei-

zures may occur in patients receiving such combinations. In patients being transferred to tranylcypromine from a dibenzazepine-related entity, allow a medication free interval of at least a week, then initiate tranylcypromine using half the normal starting dosage for at least the first week of therapy. Similarly, at least a week should elapse between the discontinuance of tranylcypromine and the administration of a dibenzazepine-related entity or the re-administration of tranylcypromine).

No products indexed under this heading.

Imipramine Pamoate (Tranylcypromine is contraindicated in combination with or in rapid succession with dibenzazepine-related entities. Hypertensive crises or severe convulsive seizures may occur in patients receiving such combinations. In patients being transferred to tranylcypromine from a dibenzazepine-related entity, allow a medication free interval of at least a week, then initiate tranylcypromine using half the normal starting dosage for at least the first week of therapy. Similarly, at least a week should elapse between the discontinuance of tranylcypromine and the administration of a dibenzazepine-related entity or the re-administration of tranylcypromine).

No products indexed under this heading.

Indapamide (Concomitant use with hypotensive agents is contraindicated. A marked potentiating effect on hypotensive agents has been reported). Products include:

Insulin (Some MAO inhibitors have contributed to hypoglycemic episodes in diabetic patients receiving insulin. Therefore, tranylcypromine should be used with caution in diabetics using insulin).

No products indexed under this heading.

Insulin, Human, Zinc Suspension (Some MAO inhibitors have contributed to hypoglycemic episodes in diabetic patients receiving insulin. Therefore, tranylcypromine should be used with caution in diabetics using insulin).

No products indexed under this heading.

Insulin, Human (rDNA origin) (Some MAO inhibitors have contributed to hypoglycemic episodes in diabetic patients receiving insulin. Therefore, tranylcypromine should be used with caution in diabetics using insulin). Products include:

Insulin, Human NPH (Some MAO inhibitors have contributed to hypoglycemic episodes in diabetic patients receiving insulin. Therefore, tranylcypromine should be used with caution in diabetics using insulin). Products include:

Insulin, Human Regular (Some MAO inhibitors have contributed to hypoglycemic episodes in diabetic patients receiving insulin. Therefore, tranylcypromine should be used with caution in diabetics using insulin). Products include:

Insulin, Human Regular and Human NPH Mixture (Some MAO inhibitors have contributed to hypoglycemic episodes in diabetic patients receiving insulin. Therefore, tranylcypromine should be used with caution in diabetics using insulin). Products include:

Insulin, NPH (Some MAO inhibitors have contributed to hypoglycemic episodes in diabetic patients receiving insulin. Therefore, tranylcypromine should be used with caution in diabetics using insulin).

No products indexed under this heading.

Insulin, Regular (Some MAO inhibitors have contributed to hypoglycemic episodes in diabetic patients receiving insulin. Therefore, tranylcypromine should be used with caution in diabetics using insulin).

No products indexed under this heading.

Insulin, Regular and NPH mixture (Some MAO inhibitors have contributed to hypoglycemic episodes in diabetic patients receiving insulin. Therefore, tranylcypromine should be used with caution in diabetics using insulin).

No products indexed under this heading.

Insulin, Zinc Crystals (Some MAO inhibitors have contributed to hypoglycemic episodes in diabetic patients receiving insulin. Therefore, tranylcypromine should be used with caution in diabetics using insulin).

No products indexed under this heading.

Insulin, Zinc Suspension (Some MAO inhibitors have contributed to hypoglycemic episodes in diabetic patients receiving insulin. Therefore, tranylcypromine should be used with caution in diabetics using insulin).

No products indexed under this heading.

Insulin Aspart (Some MAO inhibitors have contributed to hypoglycemic episodes in diabetic patients receiving insulin. Therefore, tranylcypromine should be used with caution in diabetics using insulin).

No products indexed under this heading.

Insulin Aspart, Human (Some MAO inhibitors have contributed to hypoglycemic episodes in diabetic patients receiving insulin. Therefore, tranylcypromine should be used with caution in diabetics using insulin). Products include:

Insulin Aspart, Human Regular (Some MAO inhibitors have contributed to hypoglycemic episodes in diabetic patients receiving insulin. Therefore, tranylcypromine should be used with caution in diabetics using insulin). Products include:

Insulin Aspart Protamine, Human (Some MAO inhibitors have contributed to hypoglycemic episodes in diabetic patients receiving insulin. Therefore, tranylcypromine should be used with caution in diabetics using insulin). Products include:

Insulin Detemir (rDNA Origin) (Some MAO inhibitors have contributed to hypoglycemic episodes in diabetic patients receiving insulin. Therefore, tranylcypromine should be used with caution in diabetics using insulin). Products include:

Insulin Glargine (Some MAO inhibitors have contributed to hypoglycemic episodes in diabetic patients receiving insulin. Therefore, tranylcypromine should be used with caution in diabetics using insulin). Products include:

Insulin Glulisine (Some MAO inhibitors have contributed to hypoglycemic episodes in diabetic patients receiving insulin. Therefore, tranylcypromine should be used with caution in diabetics using insulin). Products include:

Insulin Lispro, Human (Some MAO inhibitors have contributed to hypogly-

Parnate Interactions Index 1364

cemic episodes in diabetic patients receiving insulin. Therefore, tranylcypromine should be used with caution in diabetics using insulin). Products include:
Humalog 1910
Humalog Mix 1914
Humalog Mix75/25 1917

Insulin Lispro Protamine, Human (Some MAO inhibitors have contributed to hypoglycemic episodes in diabetic patients receiving insulin. Therefore, tranylcypromine should be used with caution in diabetics using insulin). Products include:
Humalog Mix 1914
Humalog Mix75/25 1917

Irbesartan (Concomitant use with hypotensive agents is contraindicated. A marked potentiating effect on hypotensive agents has been reported). Products include:
Avalide 2956
Avapro 2962

Isocarboxazid (Concurrent use with another MAO inhibitor may result in hypertensive crises or severe convulsive seizures; concurrent and/or sequential use is contraindicated). Products include:
Marplan 3481

Isoflurane (Concomitant use with some central nervous system depressants is contraindicated. A marked potentiating effect on some central nervous depressants has been reported).
No products indexed under this heading.

Isoproterenol Hydrochloride (Tranylcypromine is contraindicated in combination with sympathomimetics. During therapy with tranylcypromine, it appears that certain patients are particularly vulnerable to the effects of sympathomimetics when the activity of certain enzymes is inhibited. Use of sympathomimetics may precipitate hypertension, headache, and related symptoms).
No products indexed under this heading.

Isoproterenol Sulfate (Tranylcypromine is contraindicated in combination with sympathomimetics. During therapy with tranylcypromine, it appears that certain patients are particularly vulnerable to the effects of sympathomimetics when the activity of certain enzymes is inhibited. Use of sympathomimetics may precipitate hypertension, headache, and related symptoms).
No products indexed under this heading.

Isradipine (Concomitant use with hypotensive agents is contraindicated. A marked potentiating effect on hypotensive agents has been reported). Products include:
DynaCirc CR 1432

Ketamine Hydrochloride (Concomitant use with some central nervous system depressants is contraindicated. A marked potentiating effect on some central nervous depressants has been reported).
No products indexed under this heading.

Labetalol Hydrochloride (Concomitant use with hypotensive agents is contraindicated. A marked potentiating effect on hypotensive agents has been reported).
No products indexed under this heading.

Levalbuterol Hydrochloride (Tranylcypromine is contraindicated in combination with sympathomimetics. During therapy with tranylcypromine, it appears that certain patients are particularly vulnerable to the effects of sympathomimetics when the activity of certain enzymes is inhibited. Use of sympathomimetics may precipitate hypertension, headache, and related symptoms).
No products indexed under this heading.

Levobupivacaine Hydrochloride (Tranylcypromine is contraindicated in patients undergoing elective surgery. Patients should not be given local anesthesia containing sympathomimetic vasoconstrictors. The possible combined hypotensive effects of tranylcypromine and spinal anesthesia should be kept in mind. Tranylcypromine should be discontinued at least 10 days prior to elective surgery).
No products indexed under this heading.

Levodopa (Tranylcypromine is contraindicated in combination with levodopa. Use of levodopa with tranylcypromine may precipitate hypertension, headache, and related symptoms). Products include:
Stalevo 2526

Levomethadyl Acetate Hydrochloride (Concomitant use with some central nervous system depressants is contraindicated. A marked potentiating effect on some central nervous depressants has been reported).
No products indexed under this heading.

Levorphanol Tartrate (Concomitant use with some central nervous system depressants, such as narcotics, is contraindicated. A marked potentiating effect on narcotics has been reported).
No products indexed under this heading.

Lidocaine Hydrochloride (Tranylcypromine is contraindicated in patients undergoing elective surgery. Patients should not be given local anesthesia containing sympathomimetic vasoconstrictors. The possible combined hypotensive effects of tranylcypromine and spinal anesthesia should be kept in mind. Tranylcypromine should be discontinued at least 10 days prior to elective surgery).
No products indexed under this heading.

Lisinopril (Concomitant use with hypotensive agents is contraindicated. A marked potentiating effect on hypotensive agents has been reported). Products include:
Prinivil 2241
Prinzide 2246

Lorazepam (Concomitant use with some central nervous system depressants is contraindicated. A marked potentiating effect on some central nervous depressants has been reported).
No products indexed under this heading.

Losartan Potassium (Concomitant use with hypotensive agents is contraindicated. A marked potentiating effect on hypotensive agents has been reported). Products include:
Cozaar 2106
Hyzaar 2162
Hyzaar 100-12.5 2162

Loxapine Hydrochloride (Concomitant use with some central nervous system depressants is contraindicated. A marked potentiating effect on some central nervous depressants has been reported).
No products indexed under this heading.

Loxapine Succinate (Concomitant use with some central nervous system depressants is contraindicated. A marked potentiating effect on some central nervous depressants has been reported).
No products indexed under this heading.

Maprotiline Hydrochloride (Tranylcypromine is contraindicated in combination with or in rapid succession with dibenzazepine-related entities. Hypertensive crises or severe convulsive seizures may occur in patients receiving such combinations. In patients being transferred to tranylcypromine from a dibenzazepine-related entity, allow a medication free interval of at least a week, then initiate tranylcypromine using half the normal starting dosage for at least the first week of therapy. Similarly, at least a week should elapse between the discontinuance of tranylcypromine and the administration of a dibenzazepine-related entity or the re-administration of tranylcypromine).
No products indexed under this heading.

Mazindol (Tranylcypromine is contraindicated in combination with sympathomimetics, including weight reducing preparations that contain vasoconstrictors. During therapy with tranylcypromine, it appears with certain patients are particularly vunerable to the effects of sympathomimetics when the activity of certain enzymes is inhibited).
No products indexed under this heading.

Mecamylamine Hydrochloride (Concomitant use with hypotensive agents is contraindicated. A marked potentiating effect on hypotensive agents has been reported).
No products indexed under this heading.

Meperidine Hydrochloride (Tranylcypromine is contraindicated in combination with meperidine. Do not use meperidine in combination with MAO inhibitors or within two or three weeks following MAO inhibitor therapy. Serious reactions have been precipitated with concomitant use. It is thought that these reactions may be mediated by accumulation of 5-HT (serotonin) consquent to MAO inhibition).
No products indexed under this heading.

Mephobarbital (Concomitant use with some central nervous system depressants is contraindicated. A marked potentiating effect on some central nervous depressants has been reported).
No products indexed under this heading.

Mepivacaine Hydrochloride (Tranylcypromine is contraindicated in patients undergoing elective surgery. Patients should not be given local anesthesia containing sympathomimetic vasoconstrictors. The possible combined hypotensive effects of tranylcypromine and spinal anesthesia should be kept in mind. Tranylcypromine should be discontinued at least 10 days prior to elective surgery).
No products indexed under this heading.

Meprobamate (Concomitant use with some central nervous system depressants is contraindicated. A marked potentiating effect on some central nervous depressants has been reported).
No products indexed under this heading.

Mesoridazine Besylate (Concomitant use with some central nervous system depressants is contraindicated. A marked potentiating effect on some central nervous depressants has been reported).
No products indexed under this heading.

Metaproterenol Sulfate (Tranylcypromine is contraindicated in combination with sympathomimetics. During therapy with tranylcypromine, it appears that certain patients are particularly vulnerable to the effects of sympathomimetics when the activity of certain enzymes is inhibited. Use of sympathomimetics may precipitate hypertension, headache, and related symptoms).
No products indexed under this heading.

Metaraminol Bitartrate (Tranylcypromine is contraindicated in combination with sympathomimetics. During therapy with tranylcypromine, it appears that certain patients are particularly vulnerable to the effects of sympathomimetics when the activity of certain enzymes is inhibited. Use of sympathomimetics may precipitate hypertension, headache, and related symptoms).
No products indexed under this heading.

Metformin Hydrochloride (Some MAO inhibitors have contributed to hypoglycemic episodes in diabetic patients receiving oral hypoglycemic agents. Therefore, tranylcypromine should be used with caution in diabetics using oral hypoglycemic agents). Products include:
ActoPlus 3338
Avandamet 1345
Janumet 2188

Methadone Hydrochloride (Concomitant use with some central nervous system depressants, such as narcotics, is contraindicated. A marked potentiating effect on narcotics has been reported).
No products indexed under this heading.

Methamphetamine Hydrochloride (Tranylcypromine is contraindicated in combination with sympathmimetics including amphetamines).
No products indexed under this heading.

Methohexital Sodium (Concomitant use with some central nervous system depressants is contraindicated. A marked potentiating effect on some central nervous depressants has been reported).
No products indexed under this heading.

Methotrimeprazine (Concomitant use with some central nervous system depressants is contraindicated. A marked potentiating effect on some central nervous depressants has been reported).
No products indexed under this heading.

Methoxamine Hydrochloride (Tranylcypromine is contraindicated in combination with sympathomimetics. During therapy with tranylcypromine, it appears that certain patients are particularly vulnerable to the effects of sympathomimetics when the activity of certain enzymes is inhibited. Use of sympathomimetics may precipitate hypertension, headache, and related symptoms).
No products indexed under this heading.

Methoxyflurane (Concomitant use with some central nervous system depressants is contraindicated. A marked potentiating effect on some central nervous depressants has been reported).
No products indexed under this heading.

Methyclothiazide (Concomitant use with hypotensive agents is contraindicated. A marked potentiating effect on hypotensive agents has been reported).
No products indexed under this heading.

Methyldopa (Tranylcypromine is contraindicated in combination with methyldopa. Use of methyldopa with tranylcypromine may precipitate hypertension, headache, and related symptoms).
No products indexed under this heading.

Methyldopate Hydrochloride (Concurrent and/or sequential use is contraindicated; combination therapy may precipitate hypertension, headache and related symptoms).
No products indexed under this heading.

Metolazone (Concomitant use with hypotensive agents is contraindicated. A marked potentiating effect on hypotensive agents has been reported).
No products indexed under this heading.

Metoprolol Succinate (Concomitant use with hypotensive agents is contraindicated. A marked potentiating effect on hypotensive agents has been reported). Products include:
Toprol XL 732

Metoprolol Tartrate (Concomitant use with hypotensive agents is contraindicated. A marked potentiating effect on hypotensive agents has been reported).
No products indexed under this heading.

Metyrosine (Concomitant use with hypotensive agents is contraindicated. A marked potentiating effect on hypotensive agents has been reported).
No products indexed under this heading.

1365 **Interactions Index** **Parnate**

Mibefradil Dihydrochloride (Concomitant use with hypotensive agents is contraindicated. A marked potentiating effect on hypotensive agents has been reported).
No products indexed under this heading.

Midazolam Hydrochloride (Concomitant use with some central nervous system depressants is contraindicated. A marked potentiating effect on some central nervous depressants has been reported).
No products indexed under this heading.

Miglitol (Some MAO inhibitors have contributed to hypoglycemic episodes in diabetic patients receiving oral hypoglycemic agents. Therefore, tranylcypromine should be used with caution in diabetics using oral hypoglycemic agents).
No products indexed under this heading.

Minoxidil (Concomitant use with hypotensive agents is contraindicated. A marked potentiating effect on hypotensive agents has been reported).
No products indexed under this heading.

Moclobemide (Concurrent use with another MAO inhibitor may result in hypertensive crises or severe convulsive seizures; concurrent and/or sequential use is contraindicated).
No products indexed under this heading.

Moexipril Hydrochloride (Concomitant use with hypotensive agents is contraindicated. A marked potentiating effect on hypotensive agents has been reported).
No products indexed under this heading.

Molindone Hydrochloride (Concomitant use with some central nervous system depressants is contraindicated. A marked potentiating effect on some central nervous depressants has been reported). Products include:
Moban 1108

Morphine Sulfate (Concomitant use with some central nervous system depressants, such as narcotics, is contraindicated. A marked potentiating effect on narcotics has been reported). Products include:
Avinza 1822
Embeda 1831
MS Contin 2803

Morphine Sulfate, Liposomal (Concomitant use with some central nervous system depressants, such as narcotics, is contraindicated. A marked potentiating effect on narcotics has been reported).
No products indexed under this heading.

Nadolol (Concomitant use with hypotensive agents is contraindicated. A marked potentiating effect on hypotensive agents has been reported). Products include:
Nadolol 2359

Nateglinide (Some MAO inhibitors have contributed to hypoglycemic episodes in diabetic patients receiving oral hypoglycemic agents. Therefore, tranylcypromine should be used with caution in diabetics using oral hypoglycemic agents).
No products indexed under this heading.

Nebivolol (Concomitant use with hypotensive agents is contraindicated. A marked potentiating effect on hypotensive agents has been reported). Products include:
Bystolic 1147

Nefazodone Hydrochloride (Tranylcypromine is contraindicated in combination with selective norepinephrine reuptake inhibitors (SNRIs). There have been reports of serious, sometimes fatal reactions in patients receiving a SNRI in combination with a MAO inhibitor, and it patients who have recently discontinued a SNRI and are then started on a MAO inhibitor. Some cases presented with features resembling neuroleptic malignant syndrome. Therefore, SNRIs should not be used in combination with a MAO inhibitor, or within 14 days of discontinuing therapy with a MAO inhibitor. At least one week should be allowed after stopping a SNRI before starting a MAO inhibitor).
No products indexed under this heading.

Nicardipine Hydrochloride (Concomitant use with hypotensive agents is contraindicated. A marked potentiating effect on hypotensive agents has been reported).
No products indexed under this heading.

Nifedipine (Concomitant use with hypotensive agents is contraindicated. A marked potentiating effect on hypotensive agents has been reported).
No products indexed under this heading.

Nisoldipine (Concomitant use with hypotensive agents is contraindicated. A marked potentiating effect on hypotensive agents has been reported).
No products indexed under this heading.

Nitroglycerin (Concomitant use with hypotensive agents is contraindicated. A marked potentiating effect on hypotensive agents has been reported). Products include:
Nitro-Dur 3170
Nitrolingual 3266

Nitrous Oxide (Tranylcypromine is contraindicated in patients undergoing elective surgery. Patients taking tranylcypromine should not undergo elective surgery requiring general anesthesia. Tranylcypromine should be discontinued at least 10 days prior to elective surgery).
No products indexed under this heading.

Norepinephrine Bitartrate (Tranylcypromine is contraindicated in combination with sympathomimetics. During therapy with tranylcypromine, it appears that certain patients are particularly vulnerable to the effects of sympathomimetics when the activity of certain enzymes is inhibited. Use of sympathomimetics may precipitate hypertension, headache, and related symptoms).
No products indexed under this heading.

Nortriptyline Hydrochloride (Tranylcypromine is contraindicated in combination with or in rapid succession with dibenzazepine-related entities. Hypertensive crises or severe convulsive seizures may occur in patients receiving such combinations. In patients being transferred to tranylcypromine from a dibenzazepine-related entity, allow a medication free interval of at least a week, then initiate tranylcypromine using half the normal starting dosage for at least the first week of therapy. Similarly, at least a week should elapse between the discontinuance of tranylcypromine and the administration of a dibenzazepine-related entity or the re-administration of tranylcypromine).
No products indexed under this heading.

Olanzapine (Concomitant use with some central nervous system depressants is contraindicated. A marked potentiating effect on some central nervous depressants has been reported). Products include:
Symbyax 1965
Zyprexa 1984
Zyprexa IntraMuscular 1984
Zyprexa ZYDIS 1984

Oxazepam (Concomitant use with some central nervous system depressants is contraindicated. A marked potentiating effect on some central nervous depressants has been reported).
No products indexed under this heading.

Oxycodone Hydrochloride (Concomitant use with some central nervous system depressants, such as narcotics, is contraindicated. A marked potentiating effect on narcotics has been reported). Products include:
OxyContin 2807
Percocet 1121
Percodan 1124

Oxycodone Terephthalate (Concomitant use with some central nervous system depressants, such as narcotics, is contraindicated. A marked potentiating effect on narcotics has been reported).
No products indexed under this heading.

Oxymorphone Hydrochloride (Concomitant use with some central nervous system depressants, such as narcotics, is contraindicated. A marked potentiating effect on narcotics has been reported). Products include:
Opana 1110
Opana ER 1114

Pargyline Hydrochloride (Concurrent use with another MAO inhibitor may result in hypertensive crises or severe convulsive seizures; concurrent and/or sequential use is contraindicated).
No products indexed under this heading.

Paroxetine (Tranylcypromine is contraindicated in combination with selective serotonin reuptake inhibitors (SSRIs). There have been reports of serious, sometimes fatal reactions in patients receiving a SSRI in combination with a MAO inhibitor, and in patients who have recently discontinued a SSRI and are then started on a MAO inhibitor. Some cases presented with features resembling neuroleptic malignant syndrome. Therefore, SSRIs should not be used in combination with an MAO inhibitor, or within 14 days of discontinuing therapy with a MAO inhibitor. At least 2 weeks should be allowed after stopping paroxetine before starting a MAO inhibitor).
No products indexed under this heading.

Paroxetine Hydrochloride (Tranylcypromine is contraindicated in combination with selective serotonin reuptake inhibitors (SSRIs). There have been reports of serious, sometimes fatal reactions in patients receiving a SSRI in combination with a MAO inhibitor, and in patients who have recently discontinued a SSRI and are then started on a MAO inhibitor. Some cases presented with features resembling neuroleptic malignant syndrome. Therefore, SSRIs should not be used in combination with an MAO inhibitor, or within 14 days of discontinuing therapy with a MAO inhibitor. At least 2 weeks should be allowed after stopping paroxetine before starting a MAO inhibitor). Products include:
Paroxetine CR 2361
Paroxetine ER 2371
Paxil 1586
Paxil CR 1596

Paroxetine Mesylate (Tranylcypromine is contraindicated in combination with selective serotonin reuptake inhibitors (SSRIs). There have been reports of serious, sometimes fatal reactions in patients receiving a SSRI in combination with a MAO inhibitor, and in patients who have recently discontinued a SSRI and are then started on a MAO inhibitor. Some cases presented with features resembling neuroleptic malignant syndrome. Therefore, SSRIs should not be used in combination with an MAO inhibitor, or within 14 days of discontinuing therapy with a MAO inhibitor. At least 2 weeks should be allowed after stopping paroxetine before starting a MAO inhibitor).
No products indexed under this heading.

Penbutolol Sulfate (Concomitant use with hypotensive agents is contraindicated. A marked potentiating effect on hypotensive agents has been reported).
No products indexed under this heading.

Pentobarbital (Concomitant use with some central nervous system depressants is contraindicated. A marked potentiating effect on some central nervous depressants has been reported).
No products indexed under this heading.

Pentobarbital Sodium (Concomitant use with some central nervous system depressants is contraindicated. A marked potentiating effect on some central nervous depressants has been reported). Products include:
Nembutal 2012

Perindopril Erbumine (Concomitant use with hypotensive agents is contraindicated. A marked potentiating effect on hypotensive agents has been reported).
No products indexed under this heading.

Perphenazine (Concomitant use with some central nervous system depressants is contraindicated. A marked potentiating effect on some central nervous depressants has been reported).
No products indexed under this heading.

Phendimetrazine Tartrate (Tranylcypromine is contraindicated in combination with sympathomimetics, including weight reducing preparations that contain vasoconstrictors. During therapy with tranylcypromine, it appears with certain patients are particularly vunerable to the effects of sympathomimetics when the activity of certain enzymes is inhibited).
No products indexed under this heading.

Phenelzine Sulfate (Concurrent use with another MAO inhibitor may result in hypertensive crises or severe convulsive seizures; concurrent and/or sequential use is contraindicated).
No products indexed under this heading.

Phenmetrazine Hydrochloride (Tranylcypromine is contraindicated in combination with sympathomimetics, including weight reducing preparations that contain vasoconstrictors. During therapy with tranylcypromine, it appears with certain patients are particularly vunerable to the effects of sympathomimetics when the activity of certain enzymes is inhibited).
No products indexed under this heading.

Phenobarbital (Concomitant use with some central nervous system depressants is contraindicated. A marked potentiating effect on some central nervous depressants has been reported). Products include:
Donnatal 2711

Phenobarbital Sodium (Concomitant use with some central nervous system depressants is contraindicated. A marked potentiating effect on some central nervous depressants has been reported).
No products indexed under this heading.

Phenothiazine Derivatives (When tranylcypromine is combined with those phenothiazine derivatives or other compounds known to cause hypotension, the possibility of additive hypotensive effects should be considered).
No products indexed under this heading.

Phenothiazines (When tranylcypromine is combined with those phenothiazine derivatives or other compounds known to cause hypotension, the possibility of additive hypotensive effects should be considered).
No products indexed under this heading.

Phenoxybenzamine Hydrochloride (Concomitant use with hypotensive agents is contraindicated. A marked potentiating effect on hypotensive agents has been reported). Products include:
Dibenzyline 3495

Parnate | Interactions Index | 1366

Phentolamine Mesylate (Concomitant use with hypotensive agents is contraindicated. A marked potentiating effect on hypotensive agents has been reported).
No products indexed under this heading.

Phenylephrine Bitartrate (Tranylcypromine is contraindicated in combination with sympathomimetics. During therapy with tranylcypromine, it appears that certain patients are particularly vulnerable to the effects of sympathomimetics when the activity of certain enzymes is inhibited. Use of sympathomimetics may precipitate hypertension, headache, and related symptoms).
No products indexed under this heading.

Phenylephrine Hydrochloride (Tranylcypromine is contraindicated in combination with sympathomimetics. During therapy with tranylcypromine, it appears that certain patients are particularly vulnerable to the effects of sympathomimetics when the activity of certain enzymes is inhibited. Use of sympathomimetics may precipitate hypertension, headache, and related symptoms). Products include:
Sudafed PE Nasal Decongestant **2048**
Children's Sudafed PE Nasal Decongestant **2047**

Phenylephrine Tannate (Tranylcypromine is contraindicated in combination with sympathomimetics. During therapy with tranylcypromine, it appears that certain patients are particularly vulnerable to the effects of sympathomimetics when the activity of certain enzymes is inhibited. Use of sympathomimetics may precipitate hypertension, headache, and related symptoms).
No products indexed under this heading.

Phenylpropanolamine Hydrochloride (Tranylcypromine is contraindicated in combination with sympathomimetics. During therapy with tranylcypromine, it appears that certain patients are particularly vulnerable to the effects of sympathomimetics when the activity of certain enzymes is inhibited. Use of sympathomimetics may precipitate hypertension, headache, and related symptoms).
No products indexed under this heading.

Pindolol (Concomitant use with hypotensive agents is contraindicated. A marked potentiating effect on hypotensive agents has been reported).
No products indexed under this heading.

Pioglitazone Hydrochloride (Some MAO inhibitors have contributed to hypoglycemic episodes in diabetic patients receiving oral hypoglycemic agents. Therefore, tranylcypromine should be used with caution in diabetics using oral hypoglycemic agents). Products include:
ActoPlus **3338**
Actos **3345**
Duetact **3354**

Pirbuterol Acetate (Tranylcypromine is contraindicated in combination with sympathomimetics. During therapy with tranylcypromine, it appears that certain patients are particularly vulnerable to the effects of sympathomimetics when the activity of certain enzymes is inhibited. Use of sympathomimetics may precipitate hypertension, headache, and related symptoms). Products include:
Maxair Autohaler **1782**

Polythiazide (Concomitant use with hypotensive agents is contraindicated. A marked potentiating effect on hypotensive agents has been reported).
No products indexed under this heading.

Prazepam (Concomitant use with some central nervous system depressants is contraindicated. A marked potentiating effect on some central nervous depressants has been reported).
No products indexed under this heading.

Prazosin Hydrochloride (Concomitant use with hypotensive agents is contraindicated. A marked potentiating effect on hypotensive agents has been reported).
No products indexed under this heading.

Procaine Hydrochloride (Tranylcypromine is contraindicated in patients undergoing elective surgery. Patients should not be given local anesthesia containing sympathomimetic vasoconstrictors. The possible combined hypotensive effects of tranylcypromine and spinal anesthesia should be kept in mind. Tranylcypromine should be discontinued at least 10 days prior to elective surgery).
No products indexed under this heading.

Procarbazine Hydrochloride (Concurrent use with another MAO inhibitor may result in hypertensive crises or severe convulsive seizures; concurrent and/or sequential use is contraindicated).
No products indexed under this heading.

Prochlorperazine (Concomitant use with some central nervous system depressants is contraindicated. A marked potentiating effect on some central nervous depressants has been reported).
No products indexed under this heading.

Prochlorperazine Edisylate (Concomitant use with some central nervous system depressants is contraindicated. A marked potentiating effect on some central nervous depressants has been reported).
No products indexed under this heading.

Prochlorperazine Maleate (Concomitant use with some central nervous system depressants is contraindicated. A marked potentiating effect on some central nervous depressants has been reported).
No products indexed under this heading.

Procyclidine Hydrochloride (Antiparkinsonism drugs should be used with caution in patients receiving tranylcypromine since severe reactions have been reported).
No products indexed under this heading.

Promethazine (Concomitant use with some central nervous system depressants is contraindicated. A marked potentiating effect on some central nervous depressants has been reported).
No products indexed under this heading.

Promethazine Hydrochloride (Concomitant use with some central nervous system depressants is contraindicated. A marked potentiating effect on some central nervous depressants has been reported).
No products indexed under this heading.

Propofol (Concomitant use with some central nervous system depressants is contraindicated. A marked potentiating effect on some central nervous depressants has been reported).
No products indexed under this heading.

Propoxyphene Hydrochloride (Concomitant use with some central nervous system depressants, such as narcotics, is contraindicated. A marked potentiating effect on narcotics has been reported).
No products indexed under this heading.

Propoxyphene Napsylate (Concomitant use with some central nervous system depressants, such as narcotics, is contraindicated. A marked potentiating effect on narcotics has been reported).
No products indexed under this heading.

Propranolol Hydrochloride (Concomitant use with hypotensive agents is contraindicated. A marked potentiating effect on hypotensive agents has been reported). Products include:
InnoPran XL **1517**

Protein Preparations (Tranylcypromine is contraindicated in combination foods with a high tyramine content. Hypertensive crises have sometimes occurred during therapy with tranylcypromine after ingestion of foods with a high tyramine content. In general, the patient should avoid protein foods in which aging or protein breakdown is used to increase flavor).
No products indexed under this heading.

Protriptyline Hydrochloride (Tranylcypromine is contraindicated in combination with or in rapid succession with dibenzazepine-related entities. Hypertensive crises or severe convulsive seizures may occur in patients receiving such combinations. In patients being transferred to tranylcypromine from a dibenzazepine-related entity, allow a medication free interval of at least a week, then initiate tranylcypromine using half the normal starting dosage for at least the first week of therapy. Similarly, at least a week should elapse between the discontinuance of tranylcypromine and the administration of a dibenzazepine-related entity or the re-administration of tranylcypromine).
No products indexed under this heading.

Pseudoephedrine Hydrochloride (Tranylcypromine is contraindicated in combination with sympathomimetics. During therapy with tranylcypromine, it appears that certain patients are particularly vulnerable to the effects of sympathomimetics when the activity of certain enzymes is inhibited. Use of sympathomimetics may precipitate hypertension, headache, and related symptoms). Products include:
Allegra-D **2915**
Allegra-D 24 ..... **2918**
Sudafed 12 Hour Nasal Decongestant Non-Drowsy **2048**
Sudafed 24 Hour **2048**
Sudafed Nasal Decongestant **2047**
Children's Sudafed Nasal Decongestant Liquid **2047**
Zyrtec-D Allergy & Congestion **2054**

Pseudoephedrine Sulfate (Tranylcypromine is contraindicated in combination with sympathomimetics. During therapy with tranylcypromine, it appears that certain patients are particularly vulnerable to the effects of sympathomimetics when the activity of certain enzymes is inhibited. Use of sympathomimetics may precipitate hypertension, headache, and related symptoms). Products include:
Clarinex-D 12-Hour **3101**
Clarinex-D **3104**

Quazepam (Concomitant use with some central nervous system depressants is contraindicated. A marked potentiating effect on some central nervous depressants has been reported).
No products indexed under this heading.

Quetiapine Fumarate (Concomitant use with some central nervous system depressants is contraindicated. A marked potentiating effect on some central nervous depressants has been reported). Products include:
Seroquel **750**
Seroquel XR **759**

Quinapril Hydrochloride (Concomitant use with hypotensive agents is contraindicated. A marked potentiating effect on hypotensive agents has been reported).
No products indexed under this heading.

Ramipril (Concomitant use with hypotensive agents is contraindicated. A marked potentiating effect on hypotensive agents has been reported).
No products indexed under this heading.

Rasagiline Mesylate (Concurrent use with another MAO inhibitor may result in hypertensive crises or severe convulsive seizures; concurrent and/or sequential use is contraindicated). Products include:
Azilect **3383**

Rauwolfia Serpentina (Concomitant use with hypotensive agents is contraindicated. A marked potentiating effect on hypotensive agents has been reported).
No products indexed under this heading.

Remifentanil Hydrochloride (Concomitant use with some central nervous system depressants, such as narcotics, is contraindicated. A marked potentiating effect on narcotics has been reported).
No products indexed under this heading.

Repaglinide (Some MAO inhibitors have contributed to hypoglycemic episodes in diabetic patients receiving oral hypoglycemic agents. Therefore, tranylcypromine should be used with caution in diabetics using oral hypoglycemic agents).
No products indexed under this heading.

Rescinnamine (Concomitant use with hypotensive agents is contraindicated. A marked potentiating effect on hypotensive agents has been reported).
No products indexed under this heading.

Reserpine (Tranylcypromine is contraindicated in combination with reserpine. User of reserpine with tranylcypromine may precipitate hypertension, headache, and related symptoms).
No products indexed under this heading.

Risperidone (Concomitant use with some central nervous system depressants is contraindicated. A marked potentiating effect on some central nervous depressants has been reported). Products include:
Risperdal Consta **2682**

Rosiglitazone Maleate (Some MAO inhibitors have contributed to hypoglycemic episodes in diabetic patients receiving oral hypoglycemic agents. Therefore, tranylcypromine should be used with caution in diabetics using oral hypoglycemic agents). Products include:
Avandamet **1345**
Avandaryl **1356**
Avandia **1366**

Salmeterol Xinafoate (Tranylcypromine is contraindicated in combination with sympathomimetics. During therapy with tranylcypromine, it appears that certain patients are particularly vulnerable to the effects of sympathomimetics when the activity of certain enzymes is inhibited. Use of sympathomimetics may precipitate hypertension, headache, and related symptoms). Products include:
Advair 100/50 ..... **1275**
Advair 250/50 ..... **1275**
Advair 500/50 ..... **1275**
Advair HFA 45/21 ..... **1288**
Advair HFA 115/21 ..... **1288**
Advair HFA 230/21 ..... **1288**
Serevent Diskus **1656**

Secobarbital Sodium (Concomitant use with some central nervous system depressants is contraindicated. A marked potentiating effect on some central nervous depressants has been reported).
No products indexed under this heading.

Selegiline (Concurrent use with another MAO inhibitor may result in hyperten-

1367 Interactions Index Parnate

sive crises or severe convulsive seizures; concurrent and/or sequential use is contraindicated). Products include:
Emsam 3623

Selegiline Hydrochloride (Concurrent use with another MAO inhibitor may result in hypertensive crises or severe convulsive seizures; concurrent and/or sequential use is contraindicated). Products include:
Eldepryl 3312

Sertraline Hydrochloride (Tranylcypromine is contraindicated in combination with selective serotonin reuptake inhibitors (SSRIs). There have been reports of serious, sometimes fatal reactions in patients receiving a SSRI, in combination with a MAO inhibitor, and in patients who have recently discontinued a SSRI and are then started on a MAO inhibitor. Some cases presented with features resembling neuroleptic malignant syndrome. Therefore, SSRIs should not be used in combination with an MAO inhibitor, or within 14 days of discontinuing therapy with a MAO inhibitor. At least 2 weeks should be allowed after stopping paroxetine before starting a MAO inhibitor).
No products indexed under this heading.

Sevoflurane (Concomitant use with some central nervous system depressants is contraindicated. A marked potentiating effect on some central nervous depressants has been reported). Products include:
Ultane 554

Sibutramine Hydrochloride Monohydrate (Tranylcypromine is contraindicated in combination with sympathomimetics, including weight reducing preparations that contain vasoconstrictors. During therapy with tranylcypromine, it appears with certain patients are particularly vunerable to the effects of sympathomimetics when the activity of certain enzymes is inhibited). Products include:
Meridia 492

Sitagliptin Phosphate (Some MAO inhibitors have contributed to hypoglycemic episodes in diabetic patients receiving oral hypoglycemic agents. Therefore, tranylcypromine should be used with caution in diabetics using oral hypoglycemic agents). Products include:
Janumet 2188
Januvia 2196

Sodium Butabarbital (Concomitant use with some central nervous system depressants is contraindicated. A marked potentiating effect on some central nervous depressants has been reported).
No products indexed under this heading.

Sodium Nitroprusside (Concomitant use with hypotensive agents is contraindicated. A marked potentiating effect on hypotensive agents has been reported).
No products indexed under this heading.

Sodium Oxybate (Concomitant use with some central nervous system depressants is contraindicated. A marked potentiating effect on some central nervous depressants has been reported).
No products indexed under this heading.

Sodium Pentobarbital (Concomitant use with some central nervous system depressants is contraindicated. A marked potentiating effect on some central nervous depressants has been reported).
No products indexed under this heading.

Sotalol Hydrochloride (Concomitant use with hypotensive agents is contraindicated. A marked potentiating effect on hypotensive agents has been reported).
No products indexed under this heading.

Spirapril Hydrochloride (Concomitant use with hypotensive agents is contraindicated. A marked potentiating effect on hypotensive agents has been reported).
No products indexed under this heading.

Sufentanil Citrate (Concomitant use with some central nervous system depressants, such as narcotics, is contraindicated. A marked potentiating effect on narcotics has been reported).
No products indexed under this heading.

Talbutal (Concomitant use with some central nervous system depressants is contraindicated. A marked potentiating effect on some central nervous depressants has been reported).
No products indexed under this heading.

Telmisartan (Concomitant use with hypotensive agents is contraindicated. A marked potentiating effect on hypotensive agents has been reported). Products include:
Micardis 887
Micardis HCT 889

Temazepam (Concomitant use with some central nervous system depressants is contraindicated. A marked potentiating effect on some central nervous depressants has been reported).
No products indexed under this heading.

Terazosin Hydrochloride (Concomitant use with hypotensive agents is contraindicated. A marked potentiating effect on hypotensive agents has been reported).
No products indexed under this heading.

Terbutaline Sulfate (Tranylcypromine is contraindicated in combination with sympathomimetics. During therapy with tranylcypromine, it appears that certain patients are particularly vulnerable to the effects of sympathomimetics when the activity of certain enzymes is inhibited. Use of sympathomimetics may precipitate hypertension, headache, and related symptoms).
No products indexed under this heading.

Tetracaine Hydrochloride (Tranylcypromine is contraindicated in patients undergoing elective surgery. Patients should not be given local anesthesia containing sympathomimetic vasoconstrictors. The possible combined hypotensive effects of tranylcypromine and spinal anesthesia should be kept in mind. Tranylcypromine should be discontinued at least 10 days prior to elective surgery).
No products indexed under this heading.

Thiamylal Sodium (Concomitant use with some central nervous system depressants is contraindicated. A marked potentiating effect on some central nervous depressants has been reported).
No products indexed under this heading.

Thioridazine (Concomitant use with some central nervous system depressants is contraindicated. A marked potentiating effect on some central nervous depressants has been reported).
No products indexed under this heading.

Thioridazine Hydrochloride (Concomitant use with some central nervous system depressants is contraindicated. A marked potentiating effect on some central nervous depressants has been reported). Products include:
Thioridazine Hydrochloride 2384

Thiothixene (Concomitant use with some central nervous system depressants is contraindicated. A marked potentiating effect on some central nervous depressants has been reported). Products include:
Thiothixene 2386

Thiothixene Hydrochloride (Concomitant use with some central nervous system depressants is contraindicated. A marked potentiating effect on some central nervous depressants has been reported).
No products indexed under this heading.

Timolol Maleate (Concomitant use with hypotensive agents is contraindicated. A marked potentiating effect on hypotensive agents has been reported). Products include:
Combigan 601
Dorzolamide Hydrochloride/Timolol Maleate Ophthalmic Solution .... ⊙243
Timoptic in Ocudose .... ⊙231

Tolazamide (Some MAO inhibitors have contributed to hypoglycemic episodes in diabetic patients receiving oral hypoglycemic agents. Therefore, tranylcypromine should be used with caution in diabetics using oral hypoglycemic agents).
No products indexed under this heading.

Tolbutamide (Some MAO inhibitors have contributed to hypoglycemic episodes in diabetic patients receiving oral hypoglycemic agents. Therefore, tranylcypromine should be used with caution in diabetics using oral hypoglycemic agents).
No products indexed under this heading.

Torsemide (Concomitant use with hypotensive agents is contraindicated. A marked potentiating effect on hypotensive agents has been reported).
No products indexed under this heading.

Trandolapril (Concomitant use with hypotensive agents is contraindicated. A marked potentiating effect on hypotensive agents has been reported). Products include:
Mavik 489
Tarka 534

Triazolam (Concomitant use with some central nervous system depressants is contraindicated. A marked potentiating effect on some central nervous depressants has been reported).
No products indexed under this heading.

Tridihexethyl Chloride (Anti-parkinsonism drugs should be used with caution in patients receiving tranylcypromine since severe reactions have been reported).
No products indexed under this heading.

Trifluoperazine Hydrochloride (Concomitant use with some central nervous system depressants is contraindicated. A marked potentiating effect on some central nervous depressants has been reported).
No products indexed under this heading.

Trihexyphenidyl Hydrochloride (Anti-parkinsonism drugs should be used with caution in patients receiving tranylcypromine since severe reactions have been reported).
No products indexed under this heading.

Trimethaphan Camsylate (Concomitant use with hypotensive agents is contraindicated. A marked potentiating effect on hypotensive agents has been reported).
No products indexed under this heading.

Trimipramine Maleate (Tranylcypromine is contraindicated in combination with or in rapid succession with dibenzazepine-related entities. Hypertensive crises or severe convulsive seizures may occur in patients receiving such combinations. In patients being transferred to tranylcypromine from a dibenzazepine-related entity, allow a medication free interval of at least a week, then initiate tranylcypromine using half the normal starting dosage for at least the first week of therapy. Similarly, at least a week should elapse between the discontinuance of tranylcypromine and the administration of a dibenzazepine-related entity or the re-administration of tranylcypromine).
No products indexed under this heading.

Troglitazone (Some MAO inhibitors have contributed to hypoglycemic episodes in diabetic patients receiving oral hypoglycemic agents. Therefore, tranylcypromine should be used with caution in diabetics using oral hypoglycemic agents).
No products indexed under this heading.

Tryptophan (Tranylcypromine is contraindicated in combination with tryptophan. Use of tryptophan with tranylcypromine may precipitate hypertension, headache, and related symptoms. The combination of MAO inhibitors and tryptophan has been reported to cause behavioral and neurological syndromes, including disorientation, confusion, amnesia, delirium, agitation, hypomanic signs, ataxia, myoclonus, hyperreflexia, shivering, ocular oscillations, and Babinski's signs).
No products indexed under this heading.

L-Tryptophan (Concurrent and/or sequential use is contraindicated; combination therapy may precipitate hypertension, disorientation, memory impairment, other neurologic and behavioral changes, headache and related symptoms).
No products indexed under this heading.

Tyramine (Tranylcypromine is contraindicated in foods with a high tyramine content. Hypertensive crises have sometimes occurred during therapy with tranylcypromine after ingestion of foods with high tyramine content).
No products indexed under this heading.

Valsartan (Concomitant use with hypotensive agents is contraindicated. A marked potentiating effect on hypotensive agents has been reported). Products include:
Diovan 2413
Diovan HCT 2419
Exforge 2443
Exforge HCT 2449
Valturna 3637

Venlafaxine Hydrochloride (Tranylcypromine is contraindicated in combination with selective norepinephrine reuptake inhibitors (SNRIs). There have been reports of serious, sometimes fatal reactions in patients receiving a SNRI in combination with a MAO inhibitor, and it patients who have recently discontinued a SNRI and are then started on a MAO inhibitor. Some cases presented with features resembling neuroleptic malignant syndrome. Therefore, SNRIs should not be used in combination with a MAO inhibitor, or within 14 days of discontinuing therapy with a MAO inhibitor. At least one week should be allowed after stopping a SNRI before starting a MAO inhibitor). Products include:
Effexor XR 3504
Venlafaxine Hydrochloride Tablets 2388

Verapamil Hydrochloride (Concomitant use with hypotensive agents is contraindicated. A marked potentiating effect on hypotensive agents has been reported). Products include:
Tarka 534

Zaleplon (Concomitant use with some central nervous system depressants is contraindicated. A marked potentiating effect on some central nervous depressants has been reported).
No products indexed under this heading.

Ziprasidone Hydrochloride (Concomitant use with some central nervous system depressants is contraindicated. A marked potentiating effect on some central nervous depressants has been reported). Products include:
Geodon 2723

IMPORTANT NOTE: Always consult each drug listing in the patient's regimen for possible interactions.

Zolpidem Tartrate (Concomitant use with some central nervous system depressants is contraindicated. A marked potentiating effect on some central nervous depressants has been reported). Products include:

Ambien 2920
Ambien CR 2925

Food Interactions

Alcohol (Concomitant use with some central nervous system depressants, such as alcohol, is contraindicated. A marked potentiating effect on alcohol has been reported).

Anchovies (Tranylcypromine is contraindicated in combination with foods with a high tyramine content. Hypertensive crises have sometimes occurred during therapy with tranylcypromine after ingestion of foods with a high tyramine content. In particular, patients should be instructed not to take foods, such as anchovies).

Avocados (Tranylcypromine is contraindicated in combination with foods with a high tyramine content. Hypertensive crises have sometimes occurred during therapy with tranylcypromine after ingestion of foods with a high tyramine content. In particular, patients should be instructed not to take foods, such as avocados).

Bananas (Tranylcypromine is contraindicated in combination with foods with a high tyramine content. Hypertensive crises have sometimes occurred during therapy with tranylcypromine after ingestion of foods with a high tyramine content. In particular, patients should be instructed not to take foods, such as bananas).

Beans, broad (Tranylcypromine is contraindicated in combination with foods with a high tyramine content. Hypertensive crises have sometimes occurred during therapy with tranylcypromine after ingestion of food with a high tyramine content. In particular, patients should be instructed not to take foods, such as the pods of broad beans).

Beans, Fava (Tranylcypromine is contraindicated in combination with foods with a high tyramine content. Hypertensive crises have sometimes occurred during therapy with tranylcypromine after ingestion of food with a high tyramine content. In particular, patients should be instructed not to take foods, such as the pods of broad beans (fava beans)).

Beer, alcohol-free (Tranylcypromine is contraindicated in combination with foods with a high tyramine content. Hypertensive crises have sometimes occurred during therapy with tranylcypromine after ingestion of foods with a high tyramine content. In particular, patients should be instructed not to take foods, such as beer (including non-alcoholic beer)).

Beer, reduced-alcohol (Tranylcypromine is contraindicated in combination with foods with a high tyramine content. Hypertensive crises have sometimes occurred during therapy with tranylcypromine after ingestion of foods with a high tyramine content. In particular, patients should be instructed not to take foods, such as beer (including non-alcoholic beer)).

Beer, unspecified (Tranylcypromine is contraindicated in combination with foods with a high tyramine content. Hypertensive crises have sometimes occurred during therapy with tranylcypromine after ingestion of foods with a high tyramine content. In particular, patients should be instructed not to take foods, such as beer (including non-alcoholic beer)).

Beverages, caffeine-containing (Concomitant use with excessive use of caffeine in any form is contraindicated).

Caviar (Tranylcypromine is contraindicated in combination with foods with a high tyramine content. Hypertensive crises have sometimes occurred during therapy with tranylcypromine after ingestion of foods with a high tyramine content. In particular, patients should be instructed not to take foods, such as caviar).

Cheese, aged (Tranylcypromine is contraindicated in combination with cheese with a high tyramine content. Hypertensive crises have sometimes occurred during therapy with tranylcypromine after ingestion of foods with a high tyramine content. In particular, patients should be instructed not to take foods, such as cheese (particularly strong or aged varieties)).

Cheese, strong, unpasteurized (Tranylcypromine is contraindicated in combination with cheese with a high tyramine content. Hypertensive crises have sometimes occurred during therapy with tranylcypromine after ingestion of foods with a high tyramine content. In particular, patients should be instructed not to take foods, such as cheese (particularly strong or aged varieties)).

Cheese, unspecified (Tranylcypromine is contraindicated in combination with cheese with a high tyramine content. Hypertensive crises have sometimes occurred during therapy with tranylcypromine after ingestion of foods with a high tyramine content. In particular, patients should be instructed not to take foods, such as cheese (particularly strong or aged varieties)).

Chocolate (Tranylcypromine is contraindicated in combination with foods with a high tyramine content. Hypertensive crises have sometimes occurred during therapy with tranylcypromine after ingestion of foods with a high tyramine content. In particular, patients should be instructed not to take foods, such as chocolate).

Cream, sour (Tranylcypromine is contraindicated in combination with foods with a high tyramine content. Hypertensive crises have sometimes occurred during therapy with tranylcypromine after ingestion of foods with a high tyramine content. In particular, patients should be instructed not to take foods, such as sour cream).

Figs, canned (Tranylcypromine is contradindicated in combination with foods with a high tyramine content. Hypertensive crises have sometimes occurred during therapy with tranylcypromine after ingestion of foods with a high tyramine content. In particular, patients should be instructed not to take foods, such as canned figs).

Food with high concentration of tyramine (Tranylcypromine is contraindicated in foods with a high tyramine content. Hypertensive crises have sometimes occurred during therapy with tranylcypromine after ingestion of foods with a high tyramine content).

Fruits, dried (Tranylcypromine is contraindicated in combination with foods with a high tyramine content. Hypertensive crises have sometimes occurred during therapy with tranylcypromine after ingestion of foods with a high tyramine content. In particular, patients should be instructed not to take foods, such as dried fruits).

Fruits, overripe (Tranylcypromine is contraindicated in combination with foods with a high tyramine content. Hypertensive crises have sometimes occurred during therapy with tranylcypromine after ingestion of foods with a high tyramine content. In particular, patients should be instructed not to take foods, such as overripe fruit).

Herring, pickled (Tranylcypromine is contraindicated in combination with foods with a high tyramine content. Hypertensive crises have sometimes occurred during therapy with tranylcypromine after ingestion of foods with a high tyramine content. In particular, patients should be instructed not to take foods, such as pickled herring).

Liqueurs (Tranylcypromine is contraindicated in combination with cheese with a high tyramine content. Hypertensive crises have sometimes occurred during therapy with tranylcypromine after ingestion of foods with a high tyramine content. In particular, patients should be instructed not to take foods, such as liqueurs).

Liver (Tranylcypromine is contraindicated in combination with foods with a high tyramine content. Hypertensive crises have sometimes occurred during therapy with tranylcypromine after ingestion of foods with a high tyramine content. In particular, patients should be instructed not to take foods, such as liver).

Meat extracts (Tranylcypromine is contraindicated in combination with foods with a high tyramine content. Hypertensive crises have sometimes occurred during therapy with tranylcypromine after ingestion of food with a high tyramine content. In particular, patients should be instructed not to take foods, such as meat extracts).

Meat prepared with tenderizers (Tranylcypromine is contraindicated in combination with foods with a high tyramine content. Hypertensive crises have sometimes occurred during therapy with tranylcypromine after ingestion of food with a high tyramine content. In particular, patients should be instructed not to take foods, such as meat prepared with tenderizers).

Prunes (Tranylcypromine is contraindicated in combination with foods with a high tyramine content. Hypertensive crises have sometimes occurred during therapy with tranylcypromine after ingestion of foods with a high tyramine content. In particular, patients should be instructed not to take foods, such as dried fruits (eg, prunes)).

Raisins (Tranylcypromine is contraindicated in combination with foods with a high tyramine content. Hypertensive crises have sometimes occurred during therapy with tranylcypromine after ingestion of foods with a high tyramine content. In particular, patients should be instructed not to take foods, such as fruits (eg, raisins)).

Raspberries (Tranylcypromine is contraindicated in combination with foods with a high tyramine content. Hypertensive crises have sometimes occurred during therapy with tranylcypromine after ingestion of foods with a high tyramine content. In particular, patients should be instructed not to take foods, such as raspberries).

Sauerkraut (Tranylcypromine is contraindicated in combination with foods with a high tyramine content. Hypertensive crises have sometimes occurred during therapy with tranylcypromine after ingestion of food with a high tyramine content. In particular, patients should be instructed not to take foods, such as sauerkraut).

Sherry (Tranylcypromine is contradindicated in combination with foods with a high tyramine content. Hypertensive crises have sometimes occurred during therapy with tranylcypromine after ingestion of foods with a high tyramine content. In particular, patients should be instructed not to take foods, such as sherry).

Soy Sauce (Tranylcypromine is contraindicated in combination with foods with a high tyramine content. Hypertensive crises have sometimes occurred during therapy with tranylcypromine after ingestion of food with a high tyramine content. In particular, patients should be instructed not to take foods, such as soy sauce).

Wine, Chianti (Tranylcypromine is contraindicated in combination with foods with a high tyramine content. Hypertensive crises have sometimes occurred during therapy with tranylcypromine after ingestion of foods with a high tyramine content. In particular, patients should be instructed not to take foods, such as Chianti wine).

Wine, Red (Concomitant use with some central nervous system depressants, such as alcohol, is contraindicated. A marked potentiating effect on alcohol has been reported).

Wine, unspecified (Concomitant use with some central nervous system depressants, such as alcohol, is contraindicated. A marked potentiating effect on alcohol has been reported).

Wine products (Concomitant use with some central nervous system depressants, such as alcohol, is contraindicated. A marked potentiating effect on alcohol has been reported).

Yeast Extract (Tranylcypromine is contraindicated in combination with foods with a high tyramine content. Hypertensive crises have sometimes occurred during therapy with tranylcypromine after ingestion of food with a high tyramine content. In particular, patients should be instructed not to take foods, such as yeast extracts).

Yogurt (Tranylcypromine is contraindicated in combination with foods with a high tyramine content. Hypertensive crises have sometimes occurred during therapy with tranylcypromine after ingestion of food with a high tyramine content. In particular, patients should be instructed not to take foods, such as yogurt).

PAROXETINE HYDROCHLORIDE CONTROLLED-RELEASE TABLETS

(Paroxetine Hydrochloride) 2361

May interact with alcohols, aspirin-acetylsalicylic acid, cytochrome p450 2d6 substrates (selected), highly protein bound drugs (selected), monoamine oxidase inhibitors, non-steroidal anti-inflammatory agents, selective serotonin reuptake inhibitors, serotonin and norepinephrine reuptake inhibitors, tricyclic antidepressants, and certain other agents. Compounds in these categories include:

Amiodarone Hydrochloride (Because paroxetine is highly bound to plasma protein, administration of parox-

etine hydrochloride controlled-release tablets to a patient taking another drug that is highly protein bound may cause increased free concentrations of the other drug, potentially resulting in adverse events. Conversely, adverse effects could result from displacement of paroxetine by other highly bound drugs).

No products indexed under this heading.

Amitriptyline Hydrochloride (Caution is indicated in the co-administration of TCAs with paroxetine hydrochloride controlled-release tablets, because paroxetine may inhibit TCA metabolism. Plasma TCA concentrations may need to be monitored, and the dose of TCA may need to be reduced, if a TCA is co-administered with paroxetine hydrochloride controlled-release tablets).

No products indexed under this heading.

Amoxapine (Caution is indicated in the co-administration of TCAs with paroxetine hydrochloride controlled-release tablets, because paroxetine may inhibit TCA metabolism. Plasma TCA concentrations may need to be monitored, and the dose of TCA may need to be reduced, if a TCA is co-administered with paroxetine hydrochloride controlled-release tablets).

No products indexed under this heading.

Amphetamine Aspartate (Many drugs, including most drugs effective in the treatment of major depressive disorder (paroxetine, other SSRIs, and many tricyclics), are metabolized by the cytochrome P450 isozyme CYP2D6. Like other agents that are metabolized by CYP2D6, paroxetine may significantly inhibit the activity of this isozyme. Therefore, co-administration of paroxetine hydrochloride controlled-release tablets with other drugs that are metabolized by this isozyme, including certain drugs effective in the treatment of major depressive disorder (eg, nortriptyline, amitriptyline, imipramine, desipramine, and fluoxetine), phenothiazines, risperidone, tamoxifen, and Type 1C antiarrhythmics (eg, propafenone, flecainide, and encainide), or that inhibit this enzyme (eg, quinidine), should be approached with caution).

No products indexed under this heading.

Amphetamine Aspartate Monohydrate (Many drugs, including most drugs effective in the treatment of major depressive disorder (paroxetine, other SSRIs, and many tricyclics), are metabolized by the cytochrome P450 isozyme CYP2D6. Like other agents that are metabolized by CYP2D6, paroxetine may significantly inhibit the activity of this isozyme. Therefore, co-administration of paroxetine hydrochloride controlled-release tablets with other drugs that are metabolized by this isozyme, including certain drugs effective in the treatment of major depressive disorder (eg, nortriptyline, amitriptyline, imipramine, desipramine, and fluoxetine), phenothiazines, risperidone, tamoxifen, and Type 1C antiarrhythmics (eg, propafenone, flecainide, and encainide), or that inhibit this enzyme (eg, quinidine), should be approached with caution).

No products indexed under this heading.

Amphetamine Sulfate (Many drugs, including most drugs effective in the treatment of major depressive disorder (paroxetine, other SSRIs, and many tricyclics), are metabolized by the cytochrome P450 isozyme CYP2D6. Like other agents that are metabolized by CYP2D6, paroxetine may significantly inhibit the activity of this isozyme. Therefore, co-administration of paroxetine hydrochloride controlled-release tablets with other drugs that are metabolized by this isozyme, including certain drugs effective in the treatment of major

depressive disorder (eg, nortriptyline, amitriptyline, imipramine, desipramine, and fluoxetine), phenothiazines, risperidone, tamoxifen, and Type 1C antiarrhythmics (eg, propafenone, flecainide, and encainide), or that inhibit this enzyme (eg, quinidine), should be approached with caution).

No products indexed under this heading.

Aspirin (Caution about the concomitant use of aspirin since combined use of psychotropic drugs that interfere with serotonin reuptake and these agents has been associated with an increased risk of bleeding). Products include:

Aspirin, Enteric Coated (Caution about the concomitant use of aspirin since combined use of psychotropic drugs that interfere with serotonin reuptake and these agents has been associated with an increased risk of bleeding).

No products indexed under this heading.

Aspirin Buffered (Caution about the concomitant use of aspirin since combined use of psychotropic drugs that interfere with serotonin reuptake and these agents has been associated with an increased risk of bleeding).

No products indexed under this heading.

Atomoxetine Hydrochloride (Many drugs, including most drugs effective in the treatment of major depressive disorder (paroxetine, other SSRIs, and many tricyclics), are metabolized by the cytochrome P450 isozyme CYP2D6. Like other agents that are metabolized by CYP2D6, paroxetine may significantly inhibit the activity of this isozyme. Therefore, co-administration of paroxetine hydrochloride controlled-release tablets with other drugs that are metabolized by this isozyme, including certain drugs effective in the treatment of major depressive disorder (eg, nortriptyline, amitriptyline, imipramine, desipramine, and fluoxetine), phenothiazines, risperidone, tamoxifen, and Type 1C antiarrhythmics (eg, propafenone, flecainide, and encainide), or that inhibit this enzyme (eg, quinidine), should be approached with caution). Products include:

Atovaquone (Because paroxetine is highly bound to plasma protein, administration of paroxetine hydrochloride controlled-release tablets to a patient taking another drug that is highly protein bound may cause increased free concentrations of the other drug, potentially resulting in adverse events. Conversely, adverse effects could result from displacement of paroxetine by other highly bound drugs). Products include:

Bisoprolol Fumarate (Many drugs, including most drugs effective in the treatment of major depressive disorder (paroxetine, other SSRIs, and many tricyclics), are metabolized by the cytochrome P450 isozyme CYP2D6. Like other agents that are metabolized by CYP2D6, paroxetine may significantly inhibit the activity of this isozyme. Therefore, co-administration of paroxetine hydrochloride controlled-release tablets with other drugs that are metabolized by this isozyme, including certain drugs effective in the treatment of major depressive disorder (eg, nortriptyline, amitriptyline, imipramine, desipramine, and fluoxetine), phenothiazines, risperidone, tamoxifen, and Type 1C antiarrhythmics (eg, propafenone, flecainide,

and encainide), or that inhibit this enzyme (eg, quinidine), should be approached with caution).

No products indexed under this heading.

Captopril (Many drugs, including most drugs effective in the treatment of major depressive disorder (paroxetine, other SSRIs, and many tricyclics), are metabolized by the cytochrome P450 isozyme CYP2D6. Like other agents that are metabolized by CYP2D6, paroxetine may significantly inhibit the activity of this isozyme. Therefore, co-administration of paroxetine hydrochloride controlled-release tablets with other drugs that are metabolized by this isozyme, including certain drugs effective in the treatment of major depressive disorder (eg, nortriptyline, amitriptyline, imipramine, desipramine, and fluoxetine), phenothiazines, risperidone, tamoxifen, and Type 1C antiarrhythmics (eg, propafenone, flecainide, and encainide), or that inhibit this enzyme (eg, quinidine), should be approached with caution). Products include:

Carvedilol (Many drugs, including most drugs effective in the treatment of major depressive disorder (paroxetine, other SSRIs, and many tricyclics), are metabolized by the cytochrome P450 isozyme CYP2D6. Like other agents that are metabolized by CYP2D6, paroxetine may significantly inhibit the activity of this isozyme. Therefore, co-administration of paroxetine hydrochloride controlled-release tablets with other drugs that are metabolized by this isozyme, including certain drugs effective in the treatment of major depressive disorder (eg, nortriptyline, amitriptyline, imipramine, desipramine, and fluoxetine), phenothiazines, risperidone, tamoxifen, and Type 1C antiarrhythmics (eg, propafenone, flecainide, and encainide), or that inhibit this enzyme (eg, quinidine), should be approached with caution). Products include:

Cefonicid Sodium (Because paroxetine is highly bound to plasma protein, administration of paroxetine hydrochloride controlled-release tablets to a patient taking another drug that is highly protein bound may cause increased free concentrations of the other drug, potentially resulting in adverse events. Conversely, adverse effects could result from displacement of paroxetine by other highly bound drugs).

No products indexed under this heading.

Celecoxib (Caution about the concomitant use of NSAIDs since combined use of psychotropic drugs that interfere with serotonin reuptake and these agents has been associated with an increased risk of bleeding). Products include:

Cevimeline Hydrochloride (Many drugs, including most drugs effective in the treatment of major depressive disorder (paroxetine, other SSRIs, and many tricyclics), are metabolized by the cytochrome P450 isozyme CYP2D6. Like other agents that are metabolized by CYP2D6, paroxetine may significantly inhibit the activity of this isozyme. Therefore, co-administration of paroxetine hydrochloride controlled-release tablets with other drugs that are metabolized by this isozyme, including certain drugs effective in the treatment of major depressive disorder (eg, nortriptyline, amitriptyline, imipramine, desipramine, and fluoxetine), phenothiazines, risperidone, tamoxifen, and Type 1C antiarrhythmics (eg, propafenone, flecainide, and encainide), or that inhibit this enzyme (eg, quinidine), should be approached with caution). Products include:

Chlordiazepoxide (Because paroxetine is highly bound to plasma protein, administration of paroxetine hydrochloride controlled-release tablets to a patient taking another drug that is highly protein bound may cause increased free concentrations of the other drug, potentially resulting in adverse events. Conversely, adverse effects could result from displacement of paroxetine by other highly bound drugs).

No products indexed under this heading.

Chlordiazepoxide Hydrochloride (Because paroxetine is highly bound to plasma protein, administration of paroxetine hydrochloride controlled-release tablets to a patient taking another drug that is highly protein bound may cause increased free concentrations of the other drug, potentially resulting in adverse events. Conversely, adverse effects could result from displacement of paroxetine by other highly bound drugs).

No products indexed under this heading.

Chlorpromazine (Many drugs, including most drugs effective in the treatment of major depressive disorder (paroxetine, other SSRIs, and many tricyclics), are metabolized by the cytochrome P450 isozyme CYP2D6. Like other agents that are metabolized by CYP2D6, paroxetine may significantly inhibit the activity of this isozyme. Therefore, co-administration of paroxetine hydrochloride controlled-release tablets with other drugs that are metabolized by this isozyme, including certain drugs effective in the treatment of major depressive disorder (eg, nortriptyline, amitriptyline, imipramine, desipramine, and fluoxetine), phenothiazines, risperidone, tamoxifen, and Type 1C antiarrhythmics (eg, propafenone, flecainide, and encainide), or that inhibit this enzyme (eg, quinidine), should be approached with caution).

No products indexed under this heading.

Chlorpromazine Hydrochloride (Many drugs, including most drugs effective in the treatment of major depressive disorder (paroxetine, other SSRIs, and many tricyclics), are metabolized by the cytochrome P450 isozyme CYP2D6. Like other agents that are metabolized by CYP2D6, paroxetine may significantly inhibit the activity of this isozyme. Therefore, co-administration of paroxetine hydrochloride controlled-release tablets with other drugs that are metabolized by this isozyme, including certain drugs effective in the treatment of major depressive disorder (eg, nortriptyline, amitriptyline, imipramine, desipramine, and fluoxetine), phenothiazines, risperidone, tamoxifen, and Type 1C antiarrhythmics (eg, propafenone, flecainide, and encainide), or that inhibit this enzyme (eg, quinidine), should be approached with caution).

No products indexed under this heading.

Chlorpropamide (Many drugs, including most drugs effective in the treatment of major depressive disorder (paroxetine, other SSRIs, and many tricyclics), are metabolized by the cytochrome P450 isozyme CYP2D6. Like other agents that are metabolized by CYP2D6, paroxetine may significantly inhibit the activity of this isozyme. Therefore, co-administration of paroxetine hydrochloride controlled-release tablets with other drugs that are metabolized by this isozyme, including certain drugs effective in the treatment of major depressive disorder (eg, nortriptyline, amitriptyline, imipramine, desipramine, and fluoxetine), phenothiazines, risperidone, tamoxifen, and Type 1C antiarrhythmics (eg, propafenone, flecainide,

---

IMPORTANT NOTE: Always consult each drug listing in the patient's regimen for possible interactions.

and encainide), or that inhibit this enzyme (eg, quinidine), should be approached with caution).

No products indexed under this heading.

Cimetidine Hydrochloride (Cimetidine inhibits many cytochrome P450 (oxidative) enzymes. Therefore, when these drugs are administered concurrently, dosage adjustment of paroxetine hydrochloride controlled-release tablets after the starting dose should be guided by clinical effect).

No products indexed under this heading.

Citalopram Hydrobromide (Based on the mechanism of action of SSRIs, caution is advised when paroxetine hydrochloride controlled-release tablets are co-administered with other drugs that may affect the serotonergic neurotransmitter systems). Products include:

Clomipramine Hydrochloride (Caution is indicated in the co-administration of TCAs with paroxetine hydrochloride controlled-release tablets, because paroxetine may inhibit TCA metabolism. Plasma TCA concentrations may need to be monitored, and the dose of TCA may need to be reduced, if a TCA is co-administered with paroxetine hydrochloride controlled-release tablets).

No products indexed under this heading.

Clozapine (Many drugs, including most drugs effective in the treatment of major depressive disorder (paroxetine, other SSRIs, and many tricyclics), are metabolized by the cytochrome P450 isozyme CYP2D6. Like other agents that are metabolized by CYP2D6, paroxetine may significantly inhibit the activity of this isozyme.Therefore, co-administration of paroxetine hydrochloride controlled-release tablets with other drugs that are metabolized by this isozyme, including certain drugs effective in the treatment of major depressive disorder (eg, nortriptyline, amitriptyline, imipramine, desipramine, and fluoxetine), phenothiazines, risperidone, tamoxifen, and Type 1C antiarrhythmics (eg, propafenone, flecainide, and encainide), or that inhibit this enzyme (eg, quinidine), should be approached with caution).

No products indexed under this heading.

Codeine Phosphate (Many drugs, including most drugs effective in the treatment of major depressive disorder (paroxetine, other SSRIs, and many tricyclics), are metabolized by the cytochrome P450 isozyme CYP2D6. Like other agents that are metabolized by CYP2D6, paroxetine may significantly inhibit the activity of this isozyme.Therefore, co-administration of paroxetine hydrochloride controlled-release tablets with other drugs that are metabolized by this isozyme, including certain drugs effective in the treatment of major depressive disorder (eg, nortriptyline, amitriptyline, imipramine, desipramine, and fluoxetine), phenothiazines, risperidone, tamoxifen, and Type 1C antiarrhythmics (eg, propafenone, flecainide, and encainide), or that inhibit this enzyme (eg, quinidine), should be approached with caution). Products include:

Codeine Sulfate (Many drugs, including most drugs effective in the treatment of major depressive disorder (paroxetine, other SSRIs, and many tricyclics), are metabolized by the cytochrome P450 isozyme CYP2D6. Like other agents that are metabolized by CYP2D6, paroxetine may significantly inhibit the activity of this isozyme.Therefore, co-administration of paroxetine hydrochloride controlled-release tablets with other drugs that are metabolized by this isozyme, including certain drugs effective in the treatment of major

depressive disorder (eg, nortriptyline, amitriptyline, imipramine, desipramine, and fluoxetine), phenothiazines, risperidone, tamoxifen, and Type 1C antiarrhythmics (eg, propafenone, flecainide, and encainide), or that inhibit this enzyme (eg, quinidine), should be approached with caution).

No products indexed under this heading.

Cyclobenzaprine Hydrochloride (Many drugs, including most drugs effective in the treatment of major depressive disorder (paroxetine, other SSRIs, and many tricyclics), are metabolized by the cytochrome P450 isozyme CYP2D6. Like other agents that are metabolized by CYP2D6, paroxetine may significantly inhibit the activity of this isozyme.Therefore, co-administration of paroxetine hydrochloride controlled-release tablets with other drugs that are metabolized by this isozyme, including certain drugs effective in the treatment of major depressive disorder (eg, nortriptyline, amitriptyline, imipramine, desipramine, and fluoxetine), phenothiazines, risperidone, tamoxifen, and Type 1C antiarrhythmics (eg, propafenone, flecainide, and encainide), or that inhibit this enzyme (eg, quinidine), should be approached with caution). Products include:

Cyclosporine (Because paroxetine is highly bound to plasma protein, administration of paroxetine hydrochloride controlled-release tablets to a patient taking another drug that is highly protein bound may cause increased free concentrations of the other drug, potentially resulting in adverse events. Conversely, adverse effects could result from displacement of paroxetine by other highly bound drugs). Products include:

Debrisoquine (Many drugs, including most drugs effective in the treatment of major depressive disorder (paroxetine, other SSRIs, and many tricyclics), are metabolized by the cytochrome P450 isozyme CYP2D6. Like other agents that are metabolized by CYP2D6, paroxetine may significantly inhibit the activity of this isozyme.Therefore, co-administration of paroxetine hydrochloride controlled-release tablets with other drugs that are metabolized by this isozyme, including certain drugs effective in the treatment of major depressive disorder (eg, nortriptyline, amitriptyline, imipramine, desipramine, and fluoxetine), phenothiazines, risperidone, tamoxifen, and Type 1C antiarrhythmics (eg, propafenone, flecainide, and encainide), or that inhibit this enzyme (eg, quinidine), should be approached with caution).

No products indexed under this heading.

Desipramine Hydrochloride (Caution is indicated in the co-administration of TCAs with paroxetine hydrochloride controlled-release tablets, because paroxetine may inhibit TCA metabolism. Plasma TCA concentrations may need to be monitored, and the dose of TCA may need to be reduced, if a TCA is co-administered with paroxetine hydrochloride controlled-release tablets).

No products indexed under this heading.

Desvenlafaxine Succinate (Based on the mechanism of action of SNRIs, caution is advised when paroxetine hydrochloride controlled-release tablets are co-administered with other drugs that may affect the serotonergic neurotransmitter systems). Products include:

Dexfenfluramine Hydrochloride (Many drugs, including most drugs

effective in the treatment of major depressive disorder (paroxetine, other SSRIs, and many tricyclics), are metabolized by the cytochrome P450 isozyme CYP2D6. Like other agents that are metabolized by CYP2D6, paroxetine may significantly inhibit the activity of this isozyme.Therefore, co-administration of paroxetine hydrochloride controlled-release tablets with other drugs that are metabolized by this isozyme, including certain drugs effective in the treatment of major depressive disorder (eg, nortriptyline, amitriptyline, imipramine, desipramine, and fluoxetine), phenothiazines, risperidone, tamoxifen, and Type 1C antiarrhythmics (eg, propafenone, flecainide, and encainide), or that inhibit this enzyme (eg, quinidine), should be approached with caution).

No products indexed under this heading.

Dextromethorphan Hydrobromide (Many drugs, including most drugs effective in the treatment of major depressive disorder (paroxetine, other SSRIs, and many tricyclics), are metabolized by the cytochrome P450 isozyme CYP2D6. Like other agents that are metabolized by CYP2D6, paroxetine may significantly inhibit the activity of this isozyme.Therefore, co-administration of paroxetine hydrochloride controlled-release tablets with other drugs that are metabolized by this isozyme, including certain drugs effective in the treatment of major depressive disorder (eg, nortriptyline, amitriptyline, imipramine, desipramine, and fluoxetine), phenothiazines, risperidone, tamoxifen, and Type 1C antiarrhythmics (eg, propafenone, flecainide, and encainide), or that inhibit this enzyme (eg, quinidine), should be approached with caution).

No products indexed under this heading.

Dextromethorphan Polistirex (Many drugs, including most drugs effective in the treatment of major depressive disorder (paroxetine, other SSRIs, and many tricyclics), are metabolized by the cytochrome P450 isozyme CYP2D6. Like other agents that are metabolized by CYP2D6, paroxetine may significantly inhibit the activity of this isozyme.Therefore, co-administration of paroxetine hydrochloride controlled-release tablets with other drugs that are metabolized by this isozyme, including certain drugs effective in the treatment of major depressive disorder (eg, nortriptyline, amitriptyline, imipramine, desipramine, and fluoxetine), phenothiazines, risperidone, tamoxifen, and Type 1C antiarrhythmics (eg, propafenone, flecainide, and encainide), or that inhibit this enzyme (eg, quinidine), should be approached with caution).

No products indexed under this heading.

Diazepam (Because paroxetine is highly bound to plasma protein, administration of paroxetine hydrochloride controlled-release tablets to a patient taking another drug that is highly protein bound may cause increased free concentrations of the other drug, potentially resulting in adverse events. Conversely, adverse effects could result from displacement of paroxetine by other highly bound drugs). Products include:

Diclofenac Epolamine (Caution about the concomitant use of NSAIDs since combined use of psychotropic drugs that interfere with serotonin reuptake and these agents has been associated with an increased risk of bleeding). Products include:

Diclofenac Potassium (Caution about the concomitant use of NSAIDs since combined use of psychotropic drugs that interfere with serotonin reuptake and these agents has been associated with an increased risk of bleeding).

No products indexed under this heading.

Diclofenac Sodium (Caution about the concomitant use of NSAIDs since combined use of psychotropic drugs that interfere with serotonin reuptake and these agents has been associated with an increased risk of bleeding).

No products indexed under this heading.

Digitalis Glycoside Preparations (Because paroxetine is highly bound to plasma protein, administration of paroxetine hydrochloride controlled-release tablets to a patient taking another drug that is highly protein bound may cause increased free concentrations of the other drug, potentially resulting in adverse events. Conversely, adverse effects could result from displacement of paroxetine by other highly bound drugs).

No products indexed under this heading.

Digitalis Lanata (Because paroxetine is highly bound to plasma protein, administration of paroxetine hydrochloride controlled-release tablets to a patient taking another drug that is highly protein bound may cause increased free concentrations of the other drug, potentially resulting in adverse events. Conversely, adverse effects could result from displacement of paroxetine by other highly bound drugs).

No products indexed under this heading.

Digitalis Purpurea (Because paroxetine is highly bound to plasma protein, administration of paroxetine hydrochloride controlled-release tablets to a patient taking another drug that is highly protein bound may cause increased free concentrations of the other drug, potentially resulting in adverse events. Conversely, adverse effects could result from displacement of paroxetine by other highly bound drugs).

No products indexed under this heading.

Digoxin (The steady-state pharmacokinetics of paroxetine was not altered when administered with digoxin at steady state. Mean digoxin AUC at steady state decreased by 15% in the presence of paroxetine. Since there is little clinical experience, the concurrent administration of paroxetine hydrochloride controlled-release tablets and digoxin should be undertaken with caution). Products include:

Digoxin Immune Fab (Ovine) (The steady-state pharmacokinetics of paroxetine was not altered when administered with digoxin at steady state. Mean digoxin AUC at steady state decreased by 15% in the presence of paroxetine. Since there is little clinical experience, the concurrent administration of paroxetine hydrochloride controlled-release tablets and digoxin should be undertaken with caution). Products include:

Dipyridamole (Because paroxetine is highly bound to plasma protein, administration of paroxetine hydrochloride controlled-release tablets to a patient taking another drug that is highly protein bound may cause increased free concentrations of the other drug, potentially resulting in adverse events. Conversely, adverse effects could result from displacement of paroxetine by other highly bound drugs). Products include:

(⊙ Described in PDR® for Ophthalmic Medicines)

1371 Interactions Index Paroxetine CR

Dolasetron Mesylate (Many drugs, including most drugs effective in the treatment of major depressive disorder (paroxetine, other SSRIs, and many tricyclics), are metabolized by the cytochrome P450 isozyme CYP2D6. Like other agents that are metabolized by CYP2D6, paroxetine may significantly inhibit the activity of this isozyme.Therefore, co-administration of paroxetine hydrochloride controlled-release tablets with other drugs that are metabolized by this isozyme, including certain drugs effective in the treatment of major depressive disorder (eg, nortriptyline, amitriptyline, imipramine, desipramine, and fluoxetine), phenothiazines, risperidone, tamoxifen, and Type 1C antiarrhythmics (eg, propafenone, flecainide, and encainide), or that inhibit this enzyme (eg, quinidine), should be approached with caution). Products include:

Anzemet Injection **2931**
Anzemet Tablets **2934**

Donepezil Hydrochloride (Many drugs, including most drugs effective in the treatment of major depressive disorder (paroxetine, other SSRIs, and many tricyclics), are metabolized by the cytochrome P450 isozyme CYP2D6. Like other agents that are metabolized by CYP2D6, paroxetine may significantly inhibit the activity of this isozyme.Therefore, co-administration of paroxetine hydrochloride controlled-release tablets with other drugs that are metabolized by this isozyme, including certain drugs effective in the treatment of major depressive disorder (eg, nortriptyline, amitriptyline, imipramine, desipramine, and fluoxetine), phenothiazines, risperidone, tamoxifen, and Type 1C antiarrhythmics (eg, propafenone, flecainide, and encainide), or that inhibit this enzyme (eg, quinidine), should be approached with caution). Products include:

Aricept **1045**
Aricept ODT **1045**

Doxepin Hydrochloride (Caution is indicated in the co-administration of TCAs with paroxetine hydrochloride controlled-release tablets, because paroxetine may inhibit TCA metabolism. Plasma TCA concentrations may need to be monitored, and the dose of TCA may need to be reduced, if a TCA is co-administered with paroxetine hydrochloride controlled-release tablets).
No products indexed under this heading.

Duloxetine Hydrochloride (Based on the mechanism of action of SNRIs, caution is advised when paroxetine hydrochloride controlled-release tablets are co-administered with other drugs that may affect the serotonergic neurotransmitter systems). Products include:

Cymbalta **1871**

Encainide Hydrochloride (Many drugs, including most drugs effective in the treatment of major depressive disorder (paroxetine, other SSRIs, and many tricyclics), are metabolized by the cytochrome P450 isozyme CYP2D6. Like other agents that are metabolized by CYP2D6, paroxetine may significantly inhibit the activity of this isozyme.Therefore, co-administration of paroxetine hydrochloride controlled-release tablets with other drugs that are metabolized by this isozyme, including certain drugs effective in the treatment of major depressive disorder (eg, nortriptyline, amitriptyline, imipramine, desipramine, and fluoxetine), phenothiazines, risperidone, tamoxifen, and Type 1C antiarrhythmics (eg, propafenone, flecainide, and encainide), or that inhibit this enzyme (eg, quinidine), should be approached with caution).
No products indexed under this heading.

Escitalopram Oxalate (Based on the mechanism of action of SSRIs, caution is advised when paroxetine hydrochloride controlled-release tablets are co-administered with other drugs that may affect the serotonergic neurotransmitter systems). Products include:

Lexapro Oral Suspension **1160**
Lexapro Tablets **1160**

Ethanol (Avoid alcohol while taking paroxetine hydrochloride controlled-release tablets).
No products indexed under this heading.

Ethyl Alcohol (Avoid alcohol while taking paroxetine hydrochloride controlled-release tablets).
No products indexed under this heading.

Etodolac (Caution about the concomitant use of NSAIDs since combined use of psychotropic drugs that interfere with serotonin reuptake and these agents has been associated with an increased risk of bleeding).
No products indexed under this heading.

Fenoprofen Calcium (Caution about the concomitant use of NSAIDs since combined use of psychotropic drugs that interfere with serotonin reuptake and these agents has been associated with an increased risk of bleeding).
No products indexed under this heading.

Fentanyl (Many drugs, including most drugs effective in the treatment of major depressive disorder (paroxetine, other SSRIs, and many tricyclics), are metabolized by the cytochrome P450 isozyme CYP2D6. Like other agents that are metabolized by CYP2D6, paroxetine may significantly inhibit the activity of this isozyme.Therefore, co-administration of paroxetine hydrochloride controlled-release tablets with other drugs that are metabolized by this isozyme, including certain drugs effective in the treatment of major depressive disorder (eg, nortriptyline, amitriptyline, imipramine, desipramine, and fluoxetine), phenothiazines, risperidone, tamoxifen, and Type 1C antiarrhythmics (eg, propafenone, flecainide, and encainide), or that inhibit this enzyme (eg, quinidine), should be approached with caution). Products include:

Duragesic **2604**
Fentanyl Transdermal System **2346**
Onsolis **2054**

Fentanyl Citrate (Many drugs, including most drugs effective in the treatment of major depressive disorder (paroxetine, other SSRIs, and many tricyclics), are metabolized by the cytochrome P450 isozyme CYP2D6. Like other agents that are metabolized by CYP2D6, paroxetine may significantly inhibit the activity of this isozyme.Therefore, co-administration of paroxetine hydrochloride controlled-release tablets with other drugs that are metabolized by this isozyme, including certain drugs effective in the treatment of major depressive disorder (eg, nortriptyline, amitriptyline, imipramine, desipramine, and fluoxetine), phenothiazines, risperidone, tamoxifen, and Type 1C antiarrhythmics (eg, propafenone, flecainide, and encainide), or that inhibit this enzyme (eg, quinidine), should be approached with caution). Products include:

Fentora **966**

Flecainide Acetate (Many drugs, including most drugs effective in the treatment of major depressive disorder (paroxetine, other SSRIs, and many tricyclics), are metabolized by the cytochrome P450 isozyme CYP2D6. Like other agents that are metabolized by CYP2D6, paroxetine may significantly inhibit the activity of this isozyme.Therefore, co-administration of paroxetine hydrochloride controlled-release tablets with other drugs that are metabolized by this isozyme, including certain drugs effective in the treatment of major depressive disorder (eg, nortriptyline, amitriptyline, imipramine, desipramine, and fluoxetine), phenothiazines, risperidone, tamoxifen, and Type 1C antiarrhythmics (eg, propafenone, flecainide, and encainide), or that inhibit this enzyme (eg, quinidine), should be approached with caution).
No products indexed under this heading.

Fluoxetine (Based on the mechanism of action of SSRIs, caution is advised when paroxetine hydrochloride controlled-release tablets are co-administered with other drugs that may affect the serotonergic neurotransmitter systems).
No products indexed under this heading.

Fluoxetine Hydrochloride (Based on the mechanism of action of SSRIs, caution is advised when paroxetine hydrochloride controlled-release tablets are co-administered with other drugs that may affect the serotonergic neurotransmitter systems). Products include:

Prozac Weekly **1941**
Prozac Pulvules **1941**
Symbyax **1965**

Fluphenazine Decanoate (Many drugs, including most drugs effective in the treatment of major depressive disorder (paroxetine, other SSRIs, and many tricyclics), are metabolized by the cytochrome P450 isozyme CYP2D6. Like other agents that are metabolized by CYP2D6, paroxetine may significantly inhibit the activity of this isozyme.Therefore, co-administration of paroxetine hydrochloride controlled-release tablets with other drugs that are metabolized by this isozyme, including certain drugs effective in the treatment of major depressive disorder (eg, nortriptyline, amitriptyline, imipramine, desipramine, and fluoxetine), phenothiazines, risperidone, tamoxifen, and Type 1C antiarrhythmics (eg, propafenone, flecainide, and encainide), or that inhibit this enzyme (eg, quinidine), should be approached with caution).
No products indexed under this heading.

Fluphenazine Enanthate (Many drugs, including most drugs effective in the treatment of major depressive disorder (paroxetine, other SSRIs, and many tricyclics), are metabolized by the cytochrome P450 isozyme CYP2D6. Like other agents that are metabolized by CYP2D6, paroxetine may significantly inhibit the activity of this isozyme.Therefore, co-administration of paroxetine hydrochloride controlled-release tablets with other drugs that are metabolized by this isozyme, including certain drugs effective in the treatment of major depressive disorder (eg, nortriptyline, amitriptyline, imipramine, desipramine, and fluoxetine), phenothiazines, risperidone, tamoxifen, and Type 1C antiarrhythmics (eg, propafenone, flecainide, and encainide), or that inhibit this enzyme (eg, quinidine), should be approached with caution).
No products indexed under this heading.

Fluphenazine Hydrochloride (Many drugs, including most drugs effective in the treatment of major depressive disorder (paroxetine, other SSRIs, and many tricyclics), are metabolized by the cytochrome P450 isozyme CYP2D6. Like other agents that are metabolized by CYP2D6, paroxetine may significantly inhibit the activity of this isozyme.Therefore, co-administration of paroxetine hydrochloride controlled-release tablets with other drugs that are metabolized by this isozyme, including certain drugs effective in the treatment of major depressive disorder (eg, nortriptyline, amitriptyline, imipramine, desipramine, and fluoxetine), phenothiazines, risperidone, tamoxifen, and Type 1C antiarrhythmics (eg, propafenone, flecainide, and encainide), or that inhibit this enzyme (eg, quinidine), should be approached with caution).
No products indexed under this heading.

Flurazepam Hydrochloride (Because paroxetine is highly bound to plasma protein, administration of paroxetine hydrochloride controlled-release tablets to a patient taking another drug that is highly protein bound may cause increased free concentrations of the other drug, potentially resulting in adverse events. Conversely, adverse effects could result from displacement of paroxetine by other highly bound drugs).
No products indexed under this heading.

Flurbiprofen (Caution about the concomitant use of NSAIDs since combined use of psychotropic drugs that interfere with serotonin reuptake and these agents has been associated with an increased risk of bleeding).
No products indexed under this heading.

Fluvoxamine (Based on the mechanism of action of SSRIs, caution is advised when paroxetine hydrochloride controlled-release tablets are co-administered with other drugs that may affect the serotonergic neurotransmitter systems).
No products indexed under this heading.

Fluvoxamine Maleate (Based on the mechanism of action of SSRIs, caution is advised when paroxetine hydrochloride controlled-release tablets are co-administered with other drugs that may affect the serotonergic neurotransmitter systems).
No products indexed under this heading.

Formoterol Fumarate (Many drugs, including most drugs effective in the treatment of major depressive disorder (paroxetine, other SSRIs, and many tricyclics), are metabolized by the cytochrome P450 isozyme CYP2D6. Like other agents that are metabolized by CYP2D6, paroxetine may significantly inhibit the activity of this isozyme.Therefore, co-administration of paroxetine hydrochloride controlled-release tablets with other drugs that are metabolized by this isozyme, including certain drugs effective in the treatment of major depressive disorder (eg, nortriptyline, amitriptyline, imipramine, desipramine, and fluoxetine), phenothiazines, risperidone, tamoxifen, and Type 1C antiarrhythmics (eg, propafenone, flecainide, and encainide), or that inhibit this enzyme (eg, quinidine), should be approached with caution). Products include:

Foradil **3121**
Perforomist **3634**

Fosamprenavir Calcium (Co-administration of fosamprenavir with paroxetine significantly decreased plasma levels of paroxetine. Any dose adjustment should be guided by clinical effect). Products include:

Lexiva Oral Suspension **1558**
Lexiva **1558**

Galantamine Hydrobromide (Many drugs, including most drugs effective in the treatment of major depressive disorder (paroxetine, other SSRIs, and many tricyclics), are metabolized by the cytochrome P450 isozyme CYP2D6. Like other agents that are metabolized by CYP2D6, paroxetine may significantly inhibit the activity of this isozyme.Therefore, co-administration of paroxetine hydrochloride controlled-release tablets with other drugs that are metabolized by this isozyme, including certain drugs effective in the treatment of major depressive disorder (eg, nortriptyline, amitriptyline, imipramine, desipramine, and fluoxetine), phenothiazines, risperidone, tamoxifen, and Type 1C antiarrhythmics (eg, propafenone, flecainide,

and encainide), or that inhibit this enzyme (eg, quinidine), should be approached with caution).
No products indexed under this heading.

Glipizide (Because paroxetine is highly bound to plasma protein, administration of paroxetine hydrochloride controlled-release tablets to a patient taking another drug that is highly protein bound may cause increased free concentrations of the other drug, potentially resulting in adverse events. Conversely, adverse effects could result from displacement of paroxetine by other highly bound drugs).
No products indexed under this heading.

Haloperidol (Many drugs, including most drugs effective in the treatment of major depressive disorder (paroxetine, other SSRIs, and many tricyclics), are metabolized by the cytochrome P450 isozyme CYP2D6. Like other agents that are metabolized by CYP2D6, paroxetine may significantly inhibit the activity of this isozyme. Therefore, co-administration of paroxetine hydrochloride controlled-release tablets with other drugs that are metabolized by this isozyme, including certain drugs effective in the treatment of major depressive disorder (eg, nortriptyline, amitriptyline, imipramine, desipramine, and fluoxetine), phenothiazines, risperidone, tamoxifen, and Type 1C antiarrhythmics (eg, propafenone, flecainide, and encainide), or that inhibit this enzyme (eg, quinidine), should be approached with caution).
No products indexed under this heading.

Haloperidol Decanoate (Many drugs, including most drugs effective in the treatment of major depressive disorder (paroxetine, other SSRIs, and many tricyclics), are metabolized by the cytochrome P450 isozyme CYP2D6. Like other agents that are metabolized by CYP2D6, paroxetine may significantly inhibit the activity of this isozyme. Therefore, co-administration of paroxetine hydrochloride controlled-release tablets with other drugs that are metabolized by this isozyme, including certain drugs effective in the treatment of major depressive disorder (eg, nortriptyline, amitriptyline, imipramine, desipramine, and fluoxetine), phenothiazines, risperidone, tamoxifen, and Type 1C antiarrhythmics (eg, propafenone, flecainide, and encainide), or that inhibit this enzyme (eg, quinidine), should be approached with caution).
No products indexed under this heading.

Hydrocodone Bitartrate (Many drugs, including most drugs effective in the treatment of major depressive disorder (paroxetine, other SSRIs, and many tricyclics), are metabolized by the cytochrome P450 isozyme CYP2D6. Like other agents that are metabolized by CYP2D6, paroxetine may significantly inhibit the activity of this isozyme. Therefore, co-administration of paroxetine hydrochloride controlled-release tablets with other drugs that are metabolized by this isozyme, including certain drugs effective in the treatment of major depressive disorder (eg, nortriptyline, amitriptyline, imipramine, desipramine, and fluoxetine), phenothiazines, risperidone, tamoxifen, and Type 1C antiarrhythmics (eg, propafenone, flecainide, and encainide), or that inhibit this enzyme (eg, quinidine), should be approached with caution). Products include:
Vicodin **560**
Vicodin ES **561**
Vicodin HP **563**
Vicoprofen **564**
Zydone **1138**

Hypericum (Caution is advised when paroxetine hydrochloride controlled-release tablets are co-administered with other drugs that may affect the serotonergic neurotransmitter systems, such as St. John's Wort).
No products indexed under this heading.

Ibuprofen (Caution about the concomitant use of NSAIDs since combined use of psychotropic drugs that interfere with serotonin reuptake and these agents has been associated with an increased risk of bleeding). Products include:
Motrin IB **2043**
Children's Motrin **2044**
Children's Motrin Non-Staining Dye-Free **2044**
Infants' Motrin **2044**
Infants' Motrin Dye-Free **2044**
Junior Strength Motrin **2044**
Vicoprofen **564**

Imipramine Hydrochloride (Caution is indicated in the co-administration of TCAs with paroxetine hydrochloride controlled-release tablets, because paroxetine may inhibit TCA metabolism. Plasma TCA concentrations may need to be monitored, and the dose of TCA may need to be reduced, if a TCA is co-administered with paroxetine hydrochloride controlled-release tablets).
No products indexed under this heading.

Imipramine Pamoate (Caution is indicated in the co-administration of TCAs with paroxetine hydrochloride controlled-release tablets, because paroxetine may inhibit TCA metabolism. Plasma TCA concentrations may need to be monitored, and the dose of TCA may need to be reduced, if a TCA is co-administered with paroxetine hydrochloride controlled-release tablets).
No products indexed under this heading.

Indomethacin (Caution about the concomitant use of NSAIDs since combined use of psychotropic drugs that interfere with serotonin reuptake and these agents has been associated with an increased risk of bleeding). Products include:
Indocin **2167**

Indomethacin Sodium Trihydrate (Caution about the concomitant use of NSAIDs since combined use of psychotropic drugs that interfere with serotonin reuptake and these agents has been associated with an increased risk of bleeding). Products include:
Indocin I.V. **2007**

Indoramin Hydrochloride (Many drugs, including most drugs effective in the treatment of major depressive disorder (paroxetine, other SSRIs, and many tricyclics), are metabolized by the cytochrome P450 isozyme CYP2D6. Like other agents that are metabolized by CYP2D6, paroxetine may significantly inhibit the activity of this isozyme. Therefore, co-administration of paroxetine hydrochloride controlled-release tablets with other drugs that are metabolized by this isozyme, including certain drugs effective in the treatment of major depressive disorder (eg, nortriptyline, amitriptyline, imipramine, desipramine, and fluoxetine), phenothiazines, risperidone, tamoxifen, and Type 1C antiarrhythmics (eg, propafenone, flecainide, and encainide), or that inhibit this enzyme (eg, quinidine), should be approached with caution).
No products indexed under this heading.

Isocarboxazid (Concomitant use in patients taking either monoamine oxidase inhibitors (MAOIs), including linezolid, an antibiotic which is a reversible non-selective MAOI, or thioridazine is contraindicated). Products include:
Marplan **3481**

Ketoprofen (Caution about the concomitant use of NSAIDs since combined use of psychotropic drugs that interfere with serotonin reuptake and these agents has been associated with an increased risk of bleeding).
No products indexed under this heading.

Ketorolac Tromethamine (Caution about the concomitant use of NSAIDs since combined use of psychotropic drugs that interfere with serotonin reuptake and these agents has been associated with an increased risk of bleeding). Products include:
Acuvail .... ⊙**209**

Labetalol Hydrochloride (Many drugs, including most drugs effective in the treatment of major depressive disorder (paroxetine, other SSRIs, and many tricyclics), are metabolized by the cytochrome P450 isozyme CYP2D6. Like other agents that are metabolized by CYP2D6, paroxetine may significantly inhibit the activity of this isozyme. Therefore, co-administration of paroxetine hydrochloride controlled-release tablets with other drugs that are metabolized by this isozyme, including certain drugs effective in the treatment of major depressive disorder (eg, nortriptyline, amitriptyline, imipramine, desipramine, and fluoxetine), phenothiazines, risperidone, tamoxifen, and Type 1C antiarrhythmics (eg, propafenone, flecainide, and encainide), or that inhibit this enzyme (eg, quinidine), should be approached with caution).
No products indexed under this heading.

Lidocaine (Many drugs, including most drugs effective in the treatment of major depressive disorder (paroxetine, other SSRIs, and many tricyclics), are metabolized by the cytochrome P450 isozyme CYP2D6. Like other agents that are metabolized by CYP2D6, paroxetine may significantly inhibit the activity of this isozyme. Therefore, co-administration of paroxetine hydrochloride controlled-release tablets with other drugs that are metabolized by this isozyme, including certain drugs effective in the treatment of major depressive disorder (eg, nortriptyline, amitriptyline, imipramine, desipramine, and fluoxetine), phenothiazines, risperidone, tamoxifen, and Type 1C antiarrhythmics (eg, propafenone, flecainide, and encainide), or that inhibit this enzyme (eg, quinidine), should be approached with caution). Products include:
Lidoderm **1107**

Lidocaine Hydrochloride (Many drugs, including most drugs effective in the treatment of major depressive disorder (paroxetine, other SSRIs, and many tricyclics), are metabolized by the cytochrome P450 isozyme CYP2D6. Like other agents that are metabolized by CYP2D6, paroxetine may significantly inhibit the activity of this isozyme. Therefore, co-administration of paroxetine hydrochloride controlled-release tablets with other drugs that are metabolized by this isozyme, including certain drugs effective in the treatment of major depressive disorder (eg, nortriptyline, amitriptyline, imipramine, desipramine, and fluoxetine), phenothiazines, risperidone, tamoxifen, and Type 1C antiarrhythmics (eg, propafenone, flecainide, and encainide), or that inhibit this enzyme (eg, quinidine), should be approached with caution).
No products indexed under this heading.

Linezolid (Concomitant use in patients taking either monoamine oxidase inhibitors (MAOIs), including linezolid, an antibiotic which is a reversible non-selective MAOI, or thioridazine is contraindicated). Products include:
Zyvox **2769**

Lithium (Caution is advised when paroxetine hydrochloride controlled-release tablets are co-administered with other drugs that may affect the serotonergic neurotransmitter systems, such as lithium).
No products indexed under this heading.

Maprotiline Hydrochloride (Caution is indicated in the co-administration of TCAs with paroxetine hydrochloride controlled-release tablets, because paroxetine may inhibit TCA metabolism. Plasma TCA concentrations may need to be monitored, and the dose of TCA may need to be reduced, if a TCA is co-administered with paroxetine hydrochloride controlled-release tablets).
No products indexed under this heading.

Meclofenamate Sodium (Caution about the concomitant use of NSAIDs since combined use of psychotropic drugs that interfere with serotonin reuptake and these agents has been associated with an increased risk of bleeding).
No products indexed under this heading.

Mefenamic Acid (Caution about the concomitant use of NSAIDs since combined use of psychotropic drugs that interfere with serotonin reuptake and these agents has been associated with an increased risk of bleeding).
No products indexed under this heading.

Meloxicam (Caution about the concomitant use of NSAIDs since combined use of psychotropic drugs that interfere with serotonin reuptake and these agents has been associated with an increased risk of bleeding).
No products indexed under this heading.

Meperidine Hydrochloride (Many drugs, including most drugs effective in the treatment of major depressive disorder (paroxetine, other SSRIs, and many tricyclics), are metabolized by the cytochrome P450 isozyme CYP2D6. Like other agents that are metabolized by CYP2D6, paroxetine may significantly inhibit the activity of this isozyme. Therefore, co-administration of paroxetine hydrochloride controlled-release tablets with other drugs that are metabolized by this isozyme, including certain drugs effective in the treatment of major depressive disorder (eg, nortriptyline, amitriptyline, imipramine, desipramine, and fluoxetine), phenothiazines, risperidone, tamoxifen, and Type 1C antiarrhythmics (eg, propafenone, flecainide, and encainide), or that inhibit this enzyme (eg, quinidine), should be approached with caution).
No products indexed under this heading.

Methadone Hydrochloride (Many drugs, including most drugs effective in the treatment of major depressive disorder (paroxetine, other SSRIs, and many tricyclics), are metabolized by the cytochrome P450 isozyme CYP2D6. Like other agents that are metabolized by CYP2D6, paroxetine may significantly inhibit the activity of this isozyme. Therefore, co-administration of paroxetine hydrochloride controlled-release tablets with other drugs that are metabolized by this isozyme, including certain drugs effective in the treatment of major depressive disorder (eg, nortriptyline, amitriptyline, imipramine, desipramine, and fluoxetine), phenothiazines, risperidone, tamoxifen, and Type 1C antiarrhythmics (eg, propafenone, flecainide, and encainide), or that inhibit this enzyme (eg, quinidine), should be approached with caution).
No products indexed under this heading.

Methamphetamine Hydrochloride (Many drugs, including most drugs effective in the treatment of major depressive disorder (paroxetine, other SSRIs, and many tricyclics), are metabolized by the cytochrome P450 iso-

zyme CYP2D6. Like other agents that are metabolized by CYP2D6, paroxetine may significantly inhibit the activity of this isozyme.Therefore, co-administration of paroxetine hydrochloride controlled-release tablets with other drugs that are metabolized by this isozyme, including certain drugs effective in the treatment of major depressive disorder (eg, nortriptyline, amitriptyline, imipramine, desipramine, and fluoxetine), phenothiazines, risperidone, tamoxifen, and Type 1C antiarrhythmics (eg, propafenone, flecainide, and encainide), or that inhibit this enzyme (eg, quinidine), should be approached with caution).

No products indexed under this heading.

Methoxyphenamine (Many drugs, including most drugs effective in the treatment of major depressive disorder (paroxetine, other SSRIs, and many tricyclics), are metabolized by the cytochrome P450 isozyme CYP2D6. Like other agents that are metabolized by CYP2D6, paroxetine may significantly inhibit the activity of this isozyme.Therefore, co-administration of paroxetine hydrochloride controlled-release tablets with other drugs that are metabolized by this isozyme, including certain drugs effective in the treatment of major depressive disorder (eg, nortriptyline, amitriptyline, imipramine, desipramine, and fluoxetine), phenothiazines, risperidone, tamoxifen, and Type 1C antiarrhythmics (eg, propafenone, flecainide, and encainide), or that inhibit this enzyme (eg, quinidine), should be approached with caution).

No products indexed under this heading.

Metoprolol Succinate (Many drugs, including most drugs effective in the treatment of major depressive disorder (paroxetine, other SSRIs, and many tricyclics), are metabolized by the cytochrome P450 isozyme CYP2D6. Like other agents that are metabolized by CYP2D6, paroxetine may significantly inhibit the activity of this isozyme.Therefore, co-administration of paroxetine hydrochloride controlled-release tablets with other drugs that are metabolized by this isozyme, including certain drugs effective in the treatment of major depressive disorder (eg, nortriptyline, amitriptyline, imipramine, desipramine, and fluoxetine), phenothiazines, risperidone, tamoxifen, and Type 1C antiarrhythmics (eg, propafenone, flecainide, and encainide), or that inhibit this enzyme (eg, quinidine), should be approached with caution). Products include:

Toprol XL **732**

Metoprolol Tartrate (Many drugs, including most drugs effective in the treatment of major depressive disorder (paroxetine, other SSRIs, and many tricyclics), are metabolized by the cytochrome P450 isozyme CYP2D6. Like other agents that are metabolized by CYP2D6, paroxetine may significantly inhibit the activity of this isozyme.Therefore, co-administration of paroxetine hydrochloride controlled-release tablets with other drugs that are metabolized by this isozyme, including certain drugs effective in the treatment of major depressive disorder (eg, nortriptyline, amitriptyline, imipramine, desipramine, and fluoxetine), phenothiazines, risperidone, tamoxifen, and Type 1C antiarrhythmics (eg, propafenone, flecainide, and encainide), or that inhibit this enzyme (eg, quinidine), should be approached with caution).

No products indexed under this heading.

Mexiletine Hydrochloride (Many drugs, including most drugs effective in the treatment of major depressive disorder (paroxetine, other SSRIs, and many tricyclics), are metabolized by the cytochrome P450 isozyme CYP2D6. Like other agents that are metabolized by CYP2D6, paroxetine may significantly inhibit the activity of this isozyme.Therefore, co-administration of paroxetine hydrochloride controlled-release tablets with other drugs that are metabolized by this isozyme, including certain drugs effective in the treatment of major depressive disorder (eg, nortriptyline, amitriptyline, imipramine, desipramine, and fluoxetine), phenothiazines, risperidone, tamoxifen, and Type 1C antiarrhythmics (eg, propafenone, flecainide, and encainide), or that inhibit this enzyme (eg, quinidine), should be approached with caution).

No products indexed under this heading.

Midazolam Hydrochloride (Because paroxetine is highly bound to plasma protein, administration of paroxetine hydrochloride controlled-release tablets to a patient taking another drug that is highly protein bound may cause increased free concentrations of the other drug, potentially resulting in adverse events. Conversely, adverse effects could result from displacement of paroxetine by other highly bound drugs).

No products indexed under this heading.

Mirtazapine (Many drugs, including most drugs effective in the treatment of major depressive disorder (paroxetine, other SSRIs, and many tricyclics), are metabolized by the cytochrome P450 isozyme CYP2D6. Like other agents that are metabolized by CYP2D6, paroxetine may significantly inhibit the activity of this isozyme.Therefore, co-administration of paroxetine hydrochloride controlled-release tablets with other drugs that are metabolized by this isozyme, including certain drugs effective in the treatment of major depressive disorder (eg, nortriptyline, amitriptyline, imipramine, desipramine, and fluoxetine), phenothiazines, risperidone, tamoxifen, and Type 1C antiarrhythmics (eg, propafenone, flecainide, and encainide), or that inhibit this enzyme (eg, quinidine), should be approached with caution). Products include:

Remeron Tablets **3214**
RemeronSolTab Tablets **3219**

Moclobemide (Concomitant use in patients taking either monoamine oxidase inhibitors (MAOIs), including linezolid, an antibiotic which is a reversible non-selective MAOI, or thioridazine is contraindicated).

No products indexed under this heading.

Morphine Sulfate (Many drugs, including most drugs effective in the treatment of major depressive disorder (paroxetine, other SSRIs, and many tricyclics), are metabolized by the cytochrome P450 isozyme CYP2D6. Like other agents that are metabolized by CYP2D6, paroxetine may significantly inhibit the activity of this isozyme.Therefore, co-administration of paroxetine hydrochloride controlled-release tablets with other drugs that are metabolized by this isozyme, including certain drugs effective in the treatment of major depressive disorder (eg, nortriptyline, amitriptyline, imipramine, desipramine, and fluoxetine), phenothiazines, risperidone, tamoxifen, and Type 1C antiarrhythmics (eg, propafenone, flecainide, and encainide), or that inhibit this enzyme (eg, quinidine), should be approached with caution). Products include:

Avinza **1822**
Embeda **1831**
MS Contin **2803**

Nabumetone (Caution about the concomitant use of NSAIDs since combined use of psychotropic drugs that interfere with serotonin reuptake and these agents has been associated with an increased risk of bleeding).

No products indexed under this heading.

Naproxen (Caution about the concomitant use of NSAIDs since combined use of psychotropic drugs that interfere with serotonin reuptake and these agents has been associated with an increased risk of bleeding). Products include:

EC-Naprosyn **2850**
Naprosyn **2850**
Anaprox/Naprosyn **2850**

Naproxen Sodium (Caution about the concomitant use of NSAIDs since combined use of psychotropic drugs that interfere with serotonin reuptake and these agents has been associated with an increased risk of bleeding). Products include:

Anaprox **2850**
Anaprox DS **2850**
Treximet **1681**

Nefazodone Hydrochloride (Based on the mechanism of action of SNRIs, caution is advised when paroxetine hydrochloride controlled-release tablets are co-administered with other drugs that may affect the serotonergic neurotransmitter systems).

No products indexed under this heading.

Nelfinavir Mesylate (Many drugs, including most drugs effective in the treatment of major depressive disorder (paroxetine, other SSRIs, and many tricyclics), are metabolized by the cytochrome P450 isozyme CYP2D6. Like other agents that are metabolized by CYP2D6, paroxetine may significantly inhibit the activity of this isozyme.Therefore, co-administration of paroxetine hydrochloride controlled-release tablets with other drugs that are metabolized by this isozyme, including certain drugs effective in the treatment of major depressive disorder (eg, nortriptyline, amitriptyline, imipramine, desipramine, and fluoxetine), phenothiazines, risperidone, tamoxifen, and Type 1C antiarrhythmics (eg, propafenone, flecainide, and encainide), or that inhibit this enzyme (eg, quinidine), should be approached with caution).

No products indexed under this heading.

Nortriptyline Hydrochloride (Caution is indicated in the co-administration of TCAs with paroxetine hydrochloride controlled-release tablets, because paroxetine may inhibit TCA metabolism. Plasma TCA concentrations may need to be monitored, and the dose of TCA may need to be reduced, if a TCA is co-administered with paroxetine hydrochloride controlled-release tablets).

No products indexed under this heading.

Olanzapine (Many drugs, including most drugs effective in the treatment of major depressive disorder (paroxetine, other SSRIs, and many tricyclics), are metabolized by the cytochrome P450 isozyme CYP2D6. Like other agents that are metabolized by CYP2D6, paroxetine may significantly inhibit the activity of this isozyme.Therefore, co-administration of paroxetine hydrochloride controlled-release tablets with other drugs that are metabolized by this isozyme, including certain drugs effective in the treatment of major depressive disorder (eg, nortriptyline, amitriptyline, imipramine, desipramine, and fluoxetine), phenothiazines, risperidone, tamoxifen, and Type 1C antiarrhythmics (eg, propafenone, flecainide, and encainide), or that inhibit this enzyme (eg, quinidine), should be approached with caution). Products include:

Symbyax **1965**
Zyprexa **1984**
Zyprexa IntraMuscular **1984**
Zyprexa ZYDIS **1984**

Omeprazole (Many drugs, including most drugs effective in the treatment of major depressive disorder (paroxetine, other SSRIs, and many tricyclics), are metabolized by the cytochrome P450 isozyme CYP2D6. Like other agents that are metabolized by CYP2D6, paroxetine may significantly inhibit the activity of this isozyme.Therefore, co-administration of paroxetine hydrochloride controlled-release tablets with other drugs that are metabolized by this isozyme, including certain drugs effective in the treatment of major depressive disorder (eg, nortriptyline, amitriptyline, imipramine, desipramine, and fluoxetine), phenothiazines, risperidone, tamoxifen, and Type 1C antiarrhythmics (eg, propafenone, flecainide, and encainide), or that inhibit this enzyme (eg, quinidine), should be approached with caution).

No products indexed under this heading.

Ondansetron (Many drugs, including most drugs effective in the treatment of major depressive disorder (paroxetine, other SSRIs, and many tricyclics), are metabolized by the cytochrome P450 isozyme CYP2D6. Like other agents that are metabolized by CYP2D6, paroxetine may significantly inhibit the activity of this isozyme.Therefore, co-administration of paroxetine hydrochloride controlled-release tablets with other drugs that are metabolized by this isozyme, including certain drugs effective in the treatment of major depressive disorder (eg, nortriptyline, amitriptyline, imipramine, desipramine, and fluoxetine), phenothiazines, risperidone, tamoxifen, and Type 1C antiarrhythmics (eg, propafenone, flecainide, and encainide), or that inhibit this enzyme (eg, quinidine), should be approached with caution).

No products indexed under this heading.

Ondansetron Hydrochloride (Many drugs, including most drugs effective in the treatment of major depressive disorder (paroxetine, other SSRIs, and many tricyclics), are metabolized by the cytochrome P450 isozyme CYP2D6. Like other agents that are metabolized by CYP2D6, paroxetine may significantly inhibit the activity of this isozyme.Therefore, co-administration of paroxetine hydrochloride controlled-release tablets with other drugs that are metabolized by this isozyme, including certain drugs effective in the treatment of major depressive disorder (eg, nortriptyline, amitriptyline, imipramine, desipramine, and fluoxetine), phenothiazines, risperidone, tamoxifen, and Type 1C antiarrhythmics (eg, propafenone, flecainide, and encainide), or that inhibit this enzyme (eg, quinidine), should be approached with caution). Products include:

Zofran Injection **1750**
Zofran **1756**
Zofran ODT **1756**

Oxaprozin (Caution about the concomitant use of NSAIDs since combined use of psychotropic drugs that interfere with serotonin reuptake and these agents has been associated with an increased risk of bleeding).

No products indexed under this heading.

Oxazepam (Because paroxetine is highly bound to plasma protein, administration of paroxetine hydrochloride controlled-release tablets to a patient taking another drug that is highly protein bound may cause increased free concentrations of the other drug, potentially resulting in adverse events. Conversely, adverse effects could result from displacement of paroxetine by other highly bound drugs).

No products indexed under this heading.

Oxycodone Hydrochloride (Many drugs, including most drugs effective in the treatment of major depressive disorder (paroxetine, other SSRIs, and many tricyclics), are metabolized by the cytochrome P450 isozyme CYP2D6. Like other agents that are metabolized by CYP2D6, paroxetine may significantly inhibit the activity of this isozyme. There-fore, co-administration of paroxetine hydrochloride controlled-release tablets with other drugs that are metabolized by this isozyme, including certain drugs effective in the treatment of major depressive disorder (eg, nortriptyline, amitriptyline, imipramine, desipramine, and fluoxetine), phenothiazines, risperidone, tamoxifen, and Type 1C antiarrhythmics (eg, propafenone, flecainide, and encainide), or that inhibit this enzyme (eg, quinidine), should be approached with caution). Products include:

OxyContin 2807
Percocet 1121
Percodan 1124

Paclitaxel (Many drugs, including most drugs effective in the treatment of major depressive disorder (paroxetine, other SSRIs, and many tricyclics), are metabolized by the cytochrome P450 isozyme CYP2D6. Like other agents that are metabolized by CYP2D6, paroxetine may significantly inhibit the activity of this isozyme. Therefore, co-administration of paroxetine hydrochloride controlled-release tablets with other drugs that are metabolized by this isozyme, including certain drugs effective in the treatment of major depressive disorder (eg, nortriptyline, amitriptyline, imipramine, desipramine, and fluoxetine), phenothiazines, risperidone, tamoxifen, and Type 1C antiarrhythmics (eg, propafenone, flecainide, and encainide), or that inhibit this enzyme (eg, quinidine), should be approached with caution).
No products indexed under this heading.

Pargyline Hydrochloride (Concomitant use in patients taking either monoamine oxidase inhibitors (MAOIs), including linezolid, an antibiotic which is a reversible non-selective MAOI, or thioridazine is contraindicated).
No products indexed under this heading.

Paroxetine (Based on the mechanism of action of SSRIs, caution is advised when paroxetine hydrochloride controlled-release tablets are co-administered with other drugs that may affect the serotonergic neurotransmitter systems).
No products indexed under this heading.

Paroxetine Mesylate (Based on the mechanism of action of SSRIs, caution is advised when paroxetine hydrochloride controlled-release tablets are co-administered with other drugs that may affect the serotonergic neurotransmitter systems).
No products indexed under this heading.

Phenelzine Sulfate (Concomitant use in patients taking either monoamine oxidase inhibitors (MAOIs), including linezolid, an antibiotic which is a reversible non-selective MAOI, or thioridazine is contraindicated).
No products indexed under this heading.

Phenobarbital (Phenobarbital induces many cytochrome P450 (oxidative) enzymes. When a single oral 30-mg dose of immediate-release paroxetine was administered at phenobarbital steady state (100 mg once daily for 14 days), paroxetine AUC and T1/2 were reduced (by an average of 25% and 38%, respectively) compared to paroxetine administered alone). Products include:

Donnatal 2711

Phenylbutazone (Caution about the concomitant use of NSAIDs since combined use of psychotropic drugs that interfere with serotonin reuptake and these agents has been associated with an increased risk of bleeding).
No products indexed under this heading.

Phenytoin (When a single oral 30-mg dose of immediate-release paroxetine was administered at phenytoin steady state (300 mg once daily for 14 days), paroxetine AUC and T1/2 were reduced (by an average of 50% and 35%, respectively) compared to immediate-release paroxetine administered alone. In a separate study, when a single oral 300-mg dose of phenytoin was administered at paroxetine steady state (30 mg once daily for 14 days), phenytoin AUC was slightly reduced (12% on average) compared to phenytoin administered alone).
No products indexed under this heading.

Phenytoin Sodium (When a single oral 30-mg dose of immediate-release paroxetine was administered at phenytoin steady state (300 mg once daily for 14 days), paroxetine AUC and T1/2 were reduced (by an average of 50% and 35%, respectively) compared to immediate-release paroxetine administered alone. In a separate study, when a single oral 300-mg dose of phenytoin was administered at paroxetine steady state (30 mg once daily for 14 days), phenytoin AUC was slightly reduced (12% on average) compared to phenytoin administered alone). Products include:

Phenytek Capsules 2380

Pimozide (Concomitant use in patients taking pimozide is contraindicated).
No products indexed under this heading.

Pindolol (Many drugs, including most drugs effective in the treatment of major depressive disorder (paroxetine, other SSRIs, and many tricyclics), are metabolized by the cytochrome P450 isozyme CYP2D6. Like other agents that are metabolized by CYP2D6, paroxetine may significantly inhibit the activity of this isozyme. Therefore, co-administration of paroxetine hydrochloride controlled-release tablets with other drugs that are metabolized by this isozyme, including certain drugs effective in the treatment of major depressive disorder (eg, nortriptyline, amitriptyline, imipramine, desipramine, and fluoxetine), phenothiazines, risperidone, tamoxifen, and Type 1C antiarrhythmics (eg, propafenone, flecainide, and encainide), or that inhibit this enzyme (eg, quinidine), should be approached with caution).
No products indexed under this heading.

Piroxicam (Caution about the concomitant use of NSAIDs since combined use of psychotropic drugs that interfere with serotonin reuptake and these agents has been associated with an increased risk of bleeding).
No products indexed under this heading.

Procarbazine Hydrochloride (Concomitant use in patients taking either monoamine oxidase inhibitors (MAOIs), including linezolid, an antibiotic which is a reversible non-selective MAOI, or thioridazine is contraindicated).
No products indexed under this heading.

Procyclidine Hydrochloride (Daily oral dosing of immediate-release paroxetine (30 mg once daily) increased steady-state AUC0-24, Cmax, and Cmin values of procyclidine (5 mg oral once daily) by 35%, 37%, and 67%, respectively, compared to procyclidine alone at steady state. If anticholinergic effects are seen, the dose of procyclidine should be reduced).
No products indexed under this heading.

Propafenone Hydrochloride (Many drugs, including most drugs effective in the treatment of major depressive disorder (paroxetine, other SSRIs, and many tricyclics), are metabolized by the cytochrome P450 isozyme CYP2D6. Like other agents that are metabolized by CYP2D6, paroxetine may significantly inhibit the activity of this isozyme. Therefore, co-administration of paroxetine hydrochloride controlled-release tablets with other drugs that are metabolized by this isozyme, including certain drugs effective in the treatment of major depressive disorder (eg, nortriptyline, amitriptyline, imipramine, desipramine, and fluoxetine), phenothiazines, risperidone, tamoxifen, and Type 1C antiarrhythmics (eg, propafenone, flecainide, and encainide), or that inhibit this enzyme (eg, quinidine), should be approached with caution). Products include:

Rythmol 1648
Rythmol SR 1652

Propoxyphene Hydrochloride (Many drugs, including most drugs effective in the treatment of major depressive disorder (paroxetine, other SSRIs, and many tricyclics), are metabolized by the cytochrome P450 isozyme CYP2D6. Like other agents that are metabolized by CYP2D6, paroxetine may significantly inhibit the activity of this isozyme. Therefore, co-administration of paroxetine hydrochloride controlled-release tablets with other drugs that are metabolized by this isozyme, including certain drugs effective in the treatment of major depressive disorder (eg, nortriptyline, amitriptyline, imipramine, desipramine, and fluoxetine), phenothiazines, risperidone, tamoxifen, and Type 1C antiarrhythmics (eg, propafenone, flecainide, and encainide), or that inhibit this enzyme (eg, quinidine), should be approached with caution).
No products indexed under this heading.

Propoxyphene Napsylate (Many drugs, including most drugs effective in the treatment of major depressive disorder (paroxetine, other SSRIs, and many tricyclics), are metabolized by the cytochrome P450 isozyme CYP2D6. Like other agents that are metabolized by CYP2D6, paroxetine may significantly inhibit the activity of this isozyme. Therefore, co-administration of paroxetine hydrochloride controlled-release tablets with other drugs that are metabolized by this isozyme, including certain drugs effective in the treatment of major depressive disorder (eg, nortriptyline, amitriptyline, imipramine, desipramine, and fluoxetine), phenothiazines, risperidone, tamoxifen, and Type 1C antiarrhythmics (eg, propafenone, flecainide, and encainide), or that inhibit this enzyme (eg, quinidine), should be approached with caution).
No products indexed under this heading.

Propranolol Hydrochloride (Many drugs, including most drugs effective in the treatment of major depressive disorder (paroxetine, other SSRIs, and many tricyclics), are metabolized by the cytochrome P450 isozyme CYP2D6. Like other agents that are metabolized by CYP2D6, paroxetine may significantly inhibit the activity of this isozyme. Therefore, co-administration of paroxetine hydrochloride controlled-release tablets with other drugs that are metabolized by this isozyme, including certain drugs effective in the treatment of major depressive disorder (eg, nortriptyline, amitriptyline, imipramine, desipramine, and fluoxetine), phenothiazines, risperidone, tamoxifen, and Type 1C antiarrhythmics (eg, propafenone, flecainide, and encainide), or that inhibit this

enzyme (eg, quinidine), should be approached with caution). Products include:

InnoPran XL 1517

Protriptyline Hydrochloride (Caution is indicated in the co-administration of TCAs with paroxetine hydrochloride controlled-release tablets, because paroxetine may inhibit TCA metabolism. Plasma TCA concentrations may need to be monitored, and the dose of TCA may need to be reduced, if a TCA is co-administered with paroxetine hydrochloride controlled-release tablets).
No products indexed under this heading.

Quetiapine Fumarate (Many drugs, including most drugs effective in the treatment of major depressive disorder (paroxetine, other SSRIs, and many tricyclics), are metabolized by the cytochrome P450 isozyme CYP2D6. Like other agents that are metabolized by CYP2D6, paroxetine may significantly inhibit the activity of this isozyme. Therefore, co-administration of paroxetine hydrochloride controlled-release tablets with other drugs that are metabolized by this isozyme, including certain drugs effective in the treatment of major depressive disorder (eg, nortriptyline, amitriptyline, imipramine, desipramine, and fluoxetine), phenothiazines, risperidone, tamoxifen, and Type 1C antiarrhythmics (eg, propafenone, flecainide, and encainide), or that inhibit this enzyme (eg, quinidine), should be approached with caution). Products include:

Seroquel 750
Seroquel XR 759

Quinidine Gluconate (Many drugs, including most drugs effective in the treatment of major depressive disorder (paroxetine, other SSRIs, and many tricyclics), are metabolized by the cytochrome P450 isozyme CYP2D6. Like other agents that are metabolized by CYP2D6, paroxetine may significantly inhibit the activity of this isozyme. Therefore, co-administration of paroxetine hydrochloride controlled-release tablets with other drugs that are metabolized by this isozyme, including certain drugs effective in the treatment of major depressive disorder (eg, nortriptyline, amitriptyline, imipramine, desipramine, and fluoxetine), phenothiazines, risperidone, tamoxifen, and Type 1C antiarrhythmics (eg, propafenone, flecainide, and encainide), or that inhibit this enzyme (eg, quinidine), should be approached with caution).
No products indexed under this heading.

Quinidine Hydrochloride (Many drugs, including most drugs effective in the treatment of major depressive disorder (paroxetine, other SSRIs, and many tricyclics), are metabolized by the cytochrome P450 isozyme CYP2D6. Like other agents that are metabolized by CYP2D6, paroxetine may significantly inhibit the activity of this isozyme. Therefore, co-administration of paroxetine hydrochloride controlled-release tablets with other drugs that are metabolized by this isozyme, including certain drugs effective in the treatment of major depressive disorder (eg, nortriptyline, amitriptyline, imipramine, desipramine, and fluoxetine), phenothiazines, risperidone, tamoxifen, and Type 1C antiarrhythmics (eg, propafenone, flecainide, and encainide), or that inhibit this enzyme (eg, quinidine), should be approached with caution).
No products indexed under this heading.

Quinidine Polygalacturonate (Many drugs, including most drugs effective in the treatment of major depressive disorder (paroxetine, other SSRIs, and many tricyclics), are metabolized by the cytochrome P450 isozyme CYP2D6. Like other agents that are metabolized by

CYP2D6, paroxetine may significantly inhibit the activity of this isozyme. Therefore, co-administration of paroxetine hydrochloride controlled-release tablets with other drugs that are metabolized by this isozyme, including certain drugs effective in the treatment of major depressive disorder (eg, nortriptyline, amitriptyline, imipramine, desipramine, and fluoxetine), phenothiazines, risperidone, tamoxifen, and Type 1C antiarrhythmics (eg, propafenone, flecainide, and encainide), or that inhibit this enzyme (eg, quinidine), should be approached with caution).

No products indexed under this heading.

Quinidine Sulfate (Many drugs, including most drugs effective in the treatment of major depressive disorder (paroxetine, other SSRIs, and many tricyclics), are metabolized by the cytochrome P450 isozyme CYP2D6. Like other agents that are metabolized by CYP2D6, paroxetine may significantly inhibit the activity of this isozyme. Therefore, co-administration of paroxetine hydrochloride controlled-release tablets with other drugs that are metabolized by this isozyme, including certain drugs effective in the treatment of major depressive disorder (eg, nortriptyline, amitriptyline, imipramine, desipramine, and fluoxetine), phenothiazines, risperidone, tamoxifen, and Type 1C antiarrhythmics (eg, propafenone, flecainide, and encainide), or that inhibit this enzyme (eg, quinidine), should be approached with caution).

No products indexed under this heading.

Rasagiline Mesylate (Concomitant use in patients taking either monoamine oxidase inhibitors (MAOIs), including linezolid, an antibiotic which is a reversible non-selective MAOI, or thioridazine is contraindicated). Products include:

Azilect 3383

Risperidone (Many drugs, including most drugs effective in the treatment of major depressive disorder (paroxetine, other SSRIs, and many tricyclics), are metabolized by the cytochrome P450 isozyme CYP2D6. Like other agents that are metabolized by CYP2D6, paroxetine may significantly inhibit the activity of this isozyme. Therefore, co-administration of paroxetine hydrochloride controlled-release tablets with other drugs that are metabolized by this isozyme, including certain drugs effective in the treatment of major depressive disorder (eg, nortriptyline, amitriptyline, imipramine, desipramine, and fluoxetine), phenothiazines, risperidone, tamoxifen, and Type 1C antiarrhythmics (eg, propafenone, flecainide, and encainide), or that inhibit this enzyme (eg, quinidine), should be approached with caution). Products include:

Risperdal Consta 2682

Ritonavir (Co-administration of ritonavir with paroxetine significantly decreased plasma levels of paroxetine. Any dose adjustment should be guided by clinical effect). Products include:

Kaletra 458
Norvir 509

Rofecoxib (Caution about the concomitant use of NSAIDs since combined use of psychotropic drugs that interfere with serotonin reuptake and these agents has been associated with an increased risk of bleeding).

No products indexed under this heading.

Selegiline (Concomitant use in patients taking either monoamine oxidase inhibitors (MAOIs), including linezolid, an antibiotic which is a reversible non-selective MAOI, or thioridazine is contraindicated). Products include:

Emsam 3623

Selegiline Hydrochloride (Concomitant use in patients taking either monoamine oxidase inhibitors (MAOIs), includ-

ing linezolid, an antibiotic which is a reversible non-selective MAOI, or thioridazine is contraindicated). Products include:

Eldepryl 3312

Sertraline Hydrochloride (Based on the mechanism of action of SSRIs, caution is advised when paroxetine hydrochloride controlled-release tablets are co-administered with other drugs that may affect the serotonergic neurotransmitter systems).

No products indexed under this heading.

Sulindac (Caution about the concomitant use of NSAIDs since combined use of psychotropic drugs that interfere with serotonin reuptake and these agents has been associated with an increased risk of bleeding). Products include:

Clinoril 2098

Tamoxifen Citrate (Many drugs, including most drugs effective in the treatment of major depressive disorder (paroxetine, other SSRIs, and many tricyclics), are metabolized by the cytochrome P450 isozyme CYP2D6. Like other agents that are metabolized by CYP2D6, paroxetine may significantly inhibit the activity of this isozyme. Therefore, co-administration of paroxetine hydrochloride controlled-release tablets with other drugs that are metabolized by this isozyme, including certain drugs effective in the treatment of major depressive disorder (eg, nortriptyline, amitriptyline, imipramine, desipramine, and fluoxetine), phenothiazines, risperidone, tamoxifen, and Type 1C antiarrhythmics (eg, propafenone, flecainide, and encainide), or that inhibit this enzyme (eg, quinidine), should be approached with caution).

No products indexed under this heading.

Temazepam (Because paroxetine is highly bound to plasma protein, administration of paroxetine hydrochloride controlled-release tablets to a patient taking another drug that is highly protein bound may cause increased free concentrations of the other drug, potentially resulting in adverse events. Conversely, adverse effects could result from displacement of paroxetine by other highly bound drugs).

No products indexed under this heading.

Teniposide (Many drugs, including most drugs effective in the treatment of major depressive disorder (paroxetine, other SSRIs, and many tricyclics), are metabolized by the cytochrome P450 isozyme CYP2D6. Like other agents that are metabolized by CYP2D6, paroxetine may significantly inhibit the activity of this isozyme. Therefore, co-administration of paroxetine hydrochloride controlled-release tablets with other drugs that are metabolized by this isozyme, including certain drugs effective in the treatment of major depressive disorder (eg, nortriptyline, amitriptyline, imipramine, desipramine, and fluoxetine), phenothiazines, risperidone, tamoxifen, and Type 1C antiarrhythmics (eg, propafenone, flecainide, and encainide), or that inhibit this enzyme (eg, quinidine), should be approached with caution).

No products indexed under this heading.

Testosterone (Many drugs, including most drugs effective in the treatment of major depressive disorder (paroxetine, other SSRIs, and many tricyclics), are metabolized by the cytochrome P450 isozyme CYP2D6. Like other agents that are metabolized by CYP2D6, paroxetine may significantly inhibit the activity of this isozyme. Therefore, co-administration of paroxetine hydrochloride controlled-release tablets with other drugs that are metabolized by this isozyme, including certain drugs effective in the treatment of major depressive disorder (eg, nortriptyline, amitriptyline,

imipramine, desipramine, and fluoxetine), phenothiazines, risperidone, tamoxifen, and Type 1C antiarrhythmics (eg, propafenone, flecainide, and encainide), or that inhibit this enzyme (eg, quinidine), should be approached with caution). Products include:

AndroGel 3456

Testosterone Cypionate (Many drugs, including most drugs effective in the treatment of major depressive disorder (paroxetine, other SSRIs, and many tricyclics), are metabolized by the cytochrome P450 isozyme CYP2D6. Like other agents that are metabolized by CYP2D6, paroxetine may significantly inhibit the activity of this isozyme. Therefore, co-administration of paroxetine hydrochloride controlled-release tablets with other drugs that are metabolized by this isozyme, including certain drugs effective in the treatment of major depressive disorder (eg, nortriptyline, amitriptyline, imipramine, desipramine, and fluoxetine), phenothiazines, risperidone, tamoxifen, and Type 1C antiarrhythmics (eg, propafenone, flecainide, and encainide), or that inhibit this enzyme (eg, quinidine), should be approached with caution).

No products indexed under this heading.

Testosterone Enanthate (Many drugs, including most drugs effective in the treatment of major depressive disorder (paroxetine, other SSRIs, and many tricyclics), are metabolized by the cytochrome P450 isozyme CYP2D6. Like other agents that are metabolized by CYP2D6, paroxetine may significantly inhibit the activity of this isozyme. Therefore, co-administration of paroxetine hydrochloride controlled-release tablets with other drugs that are metabolized by this isozyme, including certain drugs effective in the treatment of major depressive disorder (eg, nortriptyline, amitriptyline, imipramine, desipramine, and fluoxetine), phenothiazines, risperidone, tamoxifen, and Type 1C antiarrhythmics (eg, propafenone, flecainide, and encainide), or that inhibit this enzyme (eg, quinidine), should be approached with caution). Products include:

Delatestryl 1102

Testosterone Propionate (Many drugs, including most drugs effective in the treatment of major depressive disorder (paroxetine, other SSRIs, and many tricyclics), are metabolized by the cytochrome P450 isozyme CYP2D6. Like other agents that are metabolized by CYP2D6, paroxetine may significantly inhibit the activity of this isozyme. Therefore, co-administration of paroxetine hydrochloride controlled-release tablets with other drugs that are metabolized by this isozyme, including certain drugs effective in the treatment of major depressive disorder (eg, nortriptyline, amitriptyline, imipramine, desipramine, and fluoxetine), phenothiazines, risperidone, tamoxifen, and Type 1C antiarrhythmics (eg, propafenone, flecainide, and encainide), or that inhibit this enzyme (eg, quinidine), should be approached with caution).

No products indexed under this heading.

Thioridazine (Concomitant use in patients taking either monoamine oxidase inhibitors (MAOIs), including linezolid, an antibiotic which is a reversible non-selective MAOI, or thioridazine is contraindicated).

No products indexed under this heading.

Thioridazine Hydrochloride (Concomitant use in patients taking either monoamine oxidase inhibitors (MAOIs), including linezolid, an antibiotic which is a reversible non-selective MAOI, or thioridazine is contraindicated). Products include:

Thioridazine Hydrochloride 2384

Timolol Maleate (Many drugs, including most drugs effective in the treatment of major depressive disorder (paroxetine, other SSRIs, and many tricyclics), are metabolized by the cytochrome P450 isozyme CYP2D6. Like other agents that are metabolized by CYP2D6, paroxetine may significantly inhibit the activity of this isozyme. Therefore, co-administration of paroxetine hydrochloride controlled-release tablets with other drugs that are metabolized by this isozyme, including certain drugs effective in the treatment of major depressive disorder (eg, nortriptyline, amitriptyline, imipramine, desipramine, and fluoxetine), phenothiazines, risperidone, tamoxifen, and Type 1C antiarrhythmics (eg, propafenone, flecainide, and encainide), or that inhibit this enzyme (eg, quinidine), should be approached with caution). Products include:

Combigan 601
Dorzolamide
    Hydrochloride/Timolol Maleate
    Ophthalmic Solution .... ⊙243
Timoptic in Ocudose .... ⊙231

Tolbutamide (Because paroxetine is highly bound to plasma protein, administration of paroxetine hydrochloride controlled-release tablets to a patient taking another drug that is highly protein bound may cause increased free concentrations of the other drug, potentially resulting in adverse events. Conversely, adverse effects could result from displacement of paroxetine by other highly bound drugs).

No products indexed under this heading.

Tolmetin Sodium (Caution about the concomitant use of NSAIDs since combined use of psychotropic drugs that interfere with serotonin reuptake and these agents has been associated with an increased risk of bleeding).

No products indexed under this heading.

Tolterodine Tartrate (Many drugs, including most drugs effective in the treatment of major depressive disorder (paroxetine, other SSRIs, and many tricyclics), are metabolized by the cytochrome P450 isozyme CYP2D6. Like other agents that are metabolized by CYP2D6, paroxetine may significantly inhibit the activity of this isozyme. Therefore, co-administration of paroxetine hydrochloride controlled-release tablets with other drugs that are metabolized by this isozyme, including certain drugs effective in the treatment of major depressive disorder (eg, nortriptyline, amitriptyline, imipramine, desipramine, and fluoxetine), phenothiazines, risperidone, tamoxifen, and Type 1C antiarrhythmics (eg, propafenone, flecainide, and encainide), or that inhibit this enzyme (eg, quinidine), should be approached with caution).

No products indexed under this heading.

Tramadol Hydrochloride (Caution is advised when paroxetine hydrochloride controlled-release tablets are co-administered with other drugs that may affect the serotonergic neurotransmitter systems, such as tramadol). Products include:

Ryzolt 2813
Ultram ER 2693

Tranylcypromine Sulfate (Concomitant use in patients taking either monoamine oxidase inhibitors (MAOIs), including linezolid, an antibiotic which is a reversible non-selective MAOI, or thioridazine is contraindicated). Products include:

Parnate 1584

Trazodone Hydrochloride (Many drugs, including most drugs effective in the treatment of major depressive disorder (paroxetine, other SSRIs, and many tricyclics), are metabolized by the cytochrome P450 isozyme CYP2D6. Like

other agents that are metabolized by CYP2D6, paroxetine may significantly inhibit the activity of this isozyme. Therefore, co-administration of paroxetine hydrochloride controlled-release tablets with other drugs that are metabolized by this isozyme, including certain drugs effective in the treatment of major depressive disorder (eg, nortriptyline, amitriptyline, imipramine, desipramine, and fluoxetine), phenothiazines, risperidone, tamoxifen, and Type 1C antiarrhythmics (eg, propafenone, flecainide, and encainide), or that inhibit this enzyme (eg, quinidine), should be approached with caution). No products indexed under this heading.

Triazolam (Many drugs, including most drugs effective in the treatment of major depressive disorder (paroxetine, other SSRIs, and many tricyclics), are metabolized by the cytochrome P450 isozyme CYP2D6. Like other agents that are metabolized by CYP2D6, paroxetine may significantly inhibit the activity of this isozyme. Therefore, co-administration of paroxetine hydrochloride controlled-release tablets with other drugs that are metabolized by this isozyme, including certain drugs effective in the treatment of major depressive disorder (eg, nortriptyline, amitriptyline, imipramine, desipramine, and fluoxetine), phenothiazines, risperidone, tamoxifen, and Type 1C antiarrhythmics (eg, propafenone, flecainide, and encainide), or that inhibit this enzyme (eg, quinidine), should be approached with caution). No products indexed under this heading.

Trimipramine Maleate (Caution is indicated in the co-administration of TCAs with paroxetine hydrochloride controlled-release tablets, because paroxetine may inhibit TCA metabolism. Plasma TCA concentrations may need to be monitored, and the dose of TCA may need to be reduced, if a TCA is co-administered with paroxetine hydrochloride controlled-release tablets). No products indexed under this heading.

Tryptophan (Adverse experiences, consisting primarily of headache, nausea, sweating, and dizziness, have been reported when tryptophan was administered to patients taking immediate release paroxetine. Consequently, concomitant use of paroxetine hydrochloride controlled-release tablets with tryptophan is not recommended). No products indexed under this heading.

Valdecoxib (Caution about the concomitant use of NSAIDs since combined use of psychotropic drugs that interfere with serotonin reuptake and these agents has been associated with an increased risk of bleeding). No products indexed under this heading.

Venlafaxine Hydrochloride (Based on the mechanism of action of SNRIs, caution is advised when paroxetine hydrochloride controlled-release tablets are co-administered with other drugs that may affect the serotonergic neurotransmitter systems). Products include:
Effexor XR 3504
Venlafaxine Hydrochloride Tablets ... 2388

Vinblastine Sulfate (Many drugs, including most drugs effective in the treatment of major depressive disorder (paroxetine, other SSRIs, and many tricyclics), are metabolized by the cytochrome P450 isozyme CYP2D6. Like other agents that are metabolized by CYP2D6, paroxetine may significantly inhibit the activity of this isozyme. Therefore, co-administration of paroxetine hydrochloride controlled-release tablets with other drugs that are metabolized by this isozyme, including certain drugs effective in the treatment of major depressive disorder (eg, nortriptyline, amitriptyline, imipramine, desipramine,

and fluoxetine), phenothiazines, risperidone, tamoxifen, and Type 1C antiarrhythmics (eg, propafenone, flecainide, and encainide), or that inhibit this enzyme (eg, quinidine), should be approached with caution). No products indexed under this heading.

Warfarin Sodium (Caution about the concomitant use of warfarin since combined use of psychotropic drugs that interfere with serotonin reuptake and these agents has been associated with an increased risk of bleeding). No products indexed under this heading.

Zonisamide (Many drugs, including most drugs effective in the treatment of major depressive disorder (paroxetine, other SSRIs, and many tricyclics), are metabolized by the cytochrome P450 isozyme CYP2D6. Like other agents that are metabolized by CYP2D6, paroxetine may significantly inhibit the activity of this isozyme. Therefore, co-administration of paroxetine hydrochloride controlled-release tablets with other drugs that are metabolized by this isozyme, including certain drugs effective in the treatment of major depressive disorder (eg, nortriptyline, amitriptyline, imipramine, desipramine, and fluoxetine), phenothiazines, risperidone, tamoxifen, and Type 1C antiarrhythmics (eg, propafenone, flecainide, and encainide), or that inhibit this enzyme (eg, quinidine), should be approached with caution). Products include:
Zonegran 1081

Food Interactions

Alcohol (Avoid alcohol while taking paroxetine hydrochloride controlled-release tablets).

Beer, reduced-alcohol (Avoid alcohol while taking paroxetine hydrochloride controlled-release tablets).

Beer, unspecified (Avoid alcohol while taking paroxetine hydrochloride controlled-release tablets).

Wine, Chianti (Avoid alcohol while taking paroxetine hydrochloride controlled-release tablets).

Wine, Red (Avoid alcohol while taking paroxetine hydrochloride controlled-release tablets).

Wine, unspecified (Avoid alcohol while taking paroxetine hydrochloride controlled-release tablets).

Wine products (Avoid alcohol while taking paroxetine hydrochloride controlled-release tablets).

PAROXETINE HYDROCHLORIDE EXTENDED-RELEASE TABLETS

(Paroxetine Hydrochloride) 2371
May interact with alcohols, aspirin-acetylsalicylic acid, cytochrome p450 2d6 substrates (selected), highly protein bound drugs (selected), monoamine oxidase inhibitors, non-steroidal anti-inflammatory agents, selective serotonin reuptake inhibitors, serotonin and norepinephrine reuptake inhibitors, tricyclic antidepressants, and certain other agents. Compounds in these categories include:

Amiodarone Hydrochloride

(Because paroxetine is highly bound to plasma protein, administration of paroxetine hydrochloride controlled-release tablets to a patient taking another drug that is highly protein bound may cause increased free concentrations of the other drug, potentially resulting in adverse events. Conversely, adverse effects could result from displacement of paroxetine by other highly bound drugs). No products indexed under this heading.

Amitriptyline Hydrochloride (Caution is indicated in the co-administration of TCAs with paroxetine hydrochloride controlled-release tablets, because paroxetine may inhibit TCA metabolism. Plasma TCA concentrations may need to be monitored, and the dose of TCA may need to be reduced, if a TCA is co-administered with paroxetine hydrochloride controlled-release tablets). No products indexed under this heading.

Amoxapine (Caution is indicated in the co-administration of TCAs with paroxetine hydrochloride controlled-release tablets, because paroxetine may inhibit TCA metabolism. Plasma TCA concentrations may need to be monitored, and the dose of TCA may need to be reduced, if a TCA is co-administered with paroxetine hydrochloride controlled-release tablets). No products indexed under this heading.

Amphetamine Aspartate (Concomitant use in patients taking either monoamine oxidase inhibitors (MAOIs), including linezolid, an antibiotic which is a reversible non-selective MAOI, or thioridazine is contraindicated). No products indexed under this heading.

Amphetamine Aspartate Monohydrate (Concomitant use in patients taking either monoamine oxidase inhibitors (MAOIs), including linezolid, an antibiotic which is a reversible non-selective MAOI, or thioridazine is contraindicated). No products indexed under this heading.

Amphetamine Sulfate (Concomitant use in patients taking either monoamine oxidase inhibitors (MAOIs), including linezolid, an antibiotic which is a reversible non-selective MAOI, or thioridazine is contraindicated). No products indexed under this heading.

Aspirin (Caution about the concomitant use of aspirin since combined use of psychotropic drugs that interfere with serotonin reuptake and these agents has been associated with an increased risk of bleeding). Products include:
Aggrenox 880
Bayer Aspirin 829
Percodan 1124
St. Joseph Aspirin 2045

Aspirin, Enteric Coated (Caution about the concomitant use of aspirin since combined use of psychotropic drugs that interfere with serotonin reuptake and these agents has been associated with an increased risk of bleeding). No products indexed under this heading.

Aspirin Buffered (Caution about the concomitant use of aspirin since combined use of psychotropic drugs that interfere with serotonin reuptake and these agents has been associated with an increased risk of bleeding). No products indexed under this heading.

Atomoxetine Hydrochloride (Concomitant use in patients taking either monoamine oxidase inhibitors (MAOIs), including linezolid, an antibiotic which is a reversible non-selective MAOI, or thioridazine is contraindicated). Products include:
Strattera 1957

Atovaquone (Because paroxetine is highly bound to plasma protein, administration of paroxetine hydrochloride controlled-release tablets to a patient taking another drug that is highly protein bound may cause increased free concentrations of the other drug, potentially resulting in adverse events. Conversely, adverse effects could result from displacement of paroxetine by other highly bound drugs). Products include:
Malarone Pediatric Tablets 1572
Malarone 1572

Mepron Suspension 1576

Bisoprolol Fumarate (Concomitant use in patients taking either monoamine oxidase inhibitors (MAOIs), including linezolid, an antibiotic which is a reversible non-selective MAOI, or thioridazine is contraindicated). No products indexed under this heading.

Captopril (Concomitant use in patients taking either monoamine oxidase inhibitors (MAOIs), including linezolid, an antibiotic which is a reversible non-selective MAOI, or thioridazine is contraindicated). Products include:
Captopril 2341

Carvedilol (Concomitant use in patients taking either monoamine oxidase inhibitors (MAOIs), including linezolid, an antibiotic which is a reversible non-selective MAOI, or thioridazine is contraindicated). Products include:
Coreg 1409

Cefonicid Sodium (Because paroxetine is highly bound to plasma protein, administration of paroxetine hydrochloride controlled-release tablets to a patient taking another drug that is highly protein bound may cause increased free concentrations of the other drug, potentially resulting in adverse events. Conversely, adverse effects could result from displacement of paroxetine by other highly bound drugs). No products indexed under this heading.

Celecoxib (Caution about the concomitant use of NSAIDs since combined use of psychotropic drugs that interfere with serotonin reuptake and these agents has been associated with an increased risk of bleeding). Products include:
Celebrex 3272

Cevimeline Hydrochloride (Concomitant use in patients taking either monoamine oxidase inhibitors (MAOIs), including linezolid, an antibiotic which is a reversible non-selective MAOI, or thioridazine is contraindicated). Products include:
Evoxac 1027

Chlordiazepoxide (Because paroxetine is highly bound to plasma protein, administration of paroxetine hydrochloride controlled-release tablets to a patient taking another drug that is highly protein bound may cause increased free concentrations of the other drug, potentially resulting in adverse events. Conversely, adverse effects could result from displacement of paroxetine by other highly bound drugs). No products indexed under this heading.

Chlordiazepoxide Hydrochloride (Because paroxetine is highly bound to plasma protein, administration of paroxetine hydrochloride controlled-release tablets to a patient taking another drug that is highly protein bound may cause increased free concentrations of the other drug, potentially resulting in adverse events. Conversely, adverse effects could result from displacement of paroxetine by other highly bound drugs). No products indexed under this heading.

Chlorpromazine (Concomitant use in patients taking either monoamine oxidase inhibitors (MAOIs), including linezolid, an antibiotic which is a reversible non-selective MAOI, or thioridazine is contraindicated). No products indexed under this heading.

Chlorpromazine Hydrochloride (Concomitant use in patients taking either monoamine oxidase inhibitors (MAOIs), including linezolid, an antibiotic which is a reversible non-selective MAOI, or thioridazine is contraindicated). No products indexed under this heading.

1377 Interactions Index Paroxetine ER

Chlorpropamide (Concomitant use in patients taking either monoamine oxidase inhibitors (MAOIs), including linezolid, an antibiotic which is a reversible non-selective MAOI, or thioridazine is contraindicated).
No products indexed under this heading.

Cimetidine Hydrochloride (Cimetidine inhibits many cytochrome P450 (oxidative) enzymes. Therefore, when these drugs are administered concurrently, dosage adjustment of paroxetine hydrochloride controlled-release tablets after the starting dose should be guided by clinical effect).
No products indexed under this heading.

Citalopram Hydrobromide (Based on the mechanism of action of SSRIs, caution is advised when paroxetine hydrochloride controlled-release tablets are co-administered with other drugs that may affect the serotonergic neurotransmitter systems). Products include:
Celexa ... 1153

Clomipramine Hydrochloride (Caution is indicated in the co-administration of TCAs with paroxetine hydrochloride controlled-release tablets, because paroxetine may inhibit TCA metabolism. Plasma TCA concentrations may need to be monitored, and the dose of TCA may need to be reduced, if a TCA is co-administered with paroxetine hydrochloride controlled-release tablets).
No products indexed under this heading.

Clozapine (Concomitant use in patients taking either monoamine oxidase inhibitors (MAOIs), including linezolid, an antibiotic which is a reversible non-selective MAOI, or thioridazine is contraindicated).
No products indexed under this heading.

Codeine Phosphate (Concomitant use in patients taking either monoamine oxidase inhibitors (MAOIs), including linezolid, an antibiotic which is a reversible non-selective MAOI, or thioridazine is contraindicated). Products include:
Tylenol with Codeine ... 2691

Codeine Sulfate (Concomitant use in patients taking either monoamine oxidase inhibitors (MAOIs), including linezolid, an antibiotic which is a reversible non-selective MAOI, or thioridazine is contraindicated).
No products indexed under this heading.

Cyclobenzaprine Hydrochloride (Concomitant use in patients taking either monoamine oxidase inhibitors (MAOIs), including linezolid, an antibiotic which is a reversible non-selective MAOI, or thioridazine is contraindicated). Products include:
Amrix ... 964

Cyclosporine (Because paroxetine is highly bound to plasma protein, administration of paroxetine hydrochloride controlled-release tablets to a patient taking another drug that is highly protein bound may cause increased free concentrations of the other drug, potentially resulting in adverse events. Conversely, adverse effects could result from displacement of paroxetine by other highly bound drugs). Products include:
Gengraf ... 440
Neoral Oral Solution ... 2496
Neoral Capsules ... 2496
Restasis ... 605

Debrisoquine (Concomitant use in patients taking either monoamine oxidase inhibitors (MAOIs), including linezolid, an antibiotic which is a reversible non-selective MAOI, or thioridazine is contraindicated).
No products indexed under this heading.

Desipramine Hydrochloride (Caution is indicated in the co-administration of TCAs with paroxetine hydrochloride controlled-release tablets, because paroxetine may inhibit TCA metabolism. Plasma TCA concentrations may need to be monitored, and the dose of TCA may need to be reduced, if a TCA is co-administered with paroxetine hydrochloride controlled-release tablets).
No products indexed under this heading.

Desvenlafaxine Succinate (Based on the mechanism of action of SNRIs, caution is advised when paroxetine hydrochloride controlled-release tablets are co-administered with other drugs that may affect the serotonergic neurotransmitter systems). Products include:
Pristiq ... 3564

Dexfenfluramine Hydrochloride (Concomitant use in patients taking either monoamine oxidase inhibitors (MAOIs), including linezolid, an antibiotic which is a reversible non-selective MAOI, or thioridazine is contraindicated).
No products indexed under this heading.

Dextromethorphan Hydrobromide (Concomitant use in patients taking either monoamine oxidase inhibitors (MAOIs), including linezolid, an antibiotic which is a reversible non-selective MAOI, or thioridazine is contraindicated).
No products indexed under this heading.

Dextromethorphan Polistirex (Concomitant use in patients taking either monoamine oxidase inhibitors (MAOIs), including linezolid, an antibiotic which is a reversible non-selective MAOI, or thioridazine is contraindicated).
No products indexed under this heading.

Diazepam (Because paroxetine is highly bound to plasma protein, administration of paroxetine hydrochloride controlled-release tablets to a patient taking another drug that is highly protein bound may cause increased free concentrations of the other drug, potentially resulting in adverse events. Conversely, adverse effects could result from displacement of paroxetine by other highly bound drugs). Products include:
Valium Tablets ... 2880

Diclofenac Epolamine (Caution about the concomitant use of NSAIDs since combined use of psychotropic drugs that interfere with serotonin reuptake and these agents has been associated with an increased risk of bleeding). Products include:
Flector ... 1839

Diclofenac Potassium (Caution about the concomitant use of NSAIDs since combined use of psychotropic drugs that interfere with serotonin reuptake and these agents has been associated with an increased risk of bleeding).
No products indexed under this heading.

Diclofenac Sodium (Caution about the concomitant use of NSAIDs since combined use of psychotropic drugs that interfere with serotonin reuptake and these agents has been associated with an increased risk of bleeding).
No products indexed under this heading.

Digitalis Glycoside Preparations (Because paroxetine is highly bound to plasma protein, administration of paroxetine hydrochloride controlled-release tablets to a patient taking another drug that is highly protein bound may cause increased free concentrations of the other drug, potentially resulting in adverse events. Conversely, adverse effects could result from displacement of paroxetine by other highly bound drugs).
No products indexed under this heading.

Digitalis Lanata (Because paroxetine is highly bound to plasma protein, administration of paroxetine hydrochloride controlled-release tablets to a patient taking another drug that is highly protein bound may cause increased free concentrations of the other drug, potentially resulting in adverse events. Conversely, adverse effects could result from displacement of paroxetine by other highly bound drugs).
No products indexed under this heading.

Digitalis Purpurea (Because paroxetine is highly bound to plasma protein, administration of paroxetine hydrochloride controlled-release tablets to a patient taking another drug that is highly protein bound may cause increased free concentrations of the other drug, potentially resulting in adverse events. Conversely, adverse effects could result from displacement of paroxetine by other highly bound drugs).
No products indexed under this heading.

Digoxin (The steady-state pharmacokinetics of paroxetine was not altered when administered with digoxin at steady state. Mean digoxin AUC at steady state decreased by 15% in the presence of paroxetine. Since there is little clinical experience, the concurrent administration of paroxetine hydrochloride controlled-release tablets and digoxin should be undertaken with caution). Products include:
Lanoxin Injection ... 1546
Lanoxin Injection Pediatric ... 1549
Lanoxin Tablets ... 1553

Digoxin Immune Fab (Ovine) (The steady-state pharmacokinetics of paroxetine was not altered when administered with digoxin at steady state. Mean digoxin AUC at steady state decreased by 15% in the presence of paroxetine. Since there is little clinical experience, the concurrent administration of paroxetine hydrochloride controlled-release tablets and digoxin should be undertaken with caution). Products include:
Digibind ... 1427

Dipyridamole (Because paroxetine is highly bound to plasma protein, administration of paroxetine hydrochloride controlled-release tablets to a patient taking another drug that is highly protein bound may cause increased free concentrations of the other drug, potentially resulting in adverse events. Conversely, adverse effects could result from displacement of paroxetine by other highly bound drugs). Products include:
Aggrenox ... 880

Dolasetron Mesylate (Concomitant use in patients taking either monoamine oxidase inhibitors (MAOIs), including linezolid, an antibiotic which is a reversible non-selective MAOI, or thioridazine is contraindicated). Products include:
Anzemet Injection ... 2931
Anzemet Tablets ... 2934

Donepezil Hydrochloride (Concomitant use in patients taking either monoamine oxidase inhibitors (MAOIs), including linezolid, an antibiotic which is a reversible non-selective MAOI, or thioridazine is contraindicated). Products include:
Aricept ... 1045
Aricept ODT ... 1045

Doxepin Hydrochloride (Caution is indicated in the co-administration of TCAs with paroxetine hydrochloride controlled-release tablets, because paroxetine may inhibit TCA metabolism. Plasma TCA concentrations may need to be monitored, and the dose of TCA may need to be reduced, if a TCA is co-administered with paroxetine hydrochloride controlled-release tablets).
No products indexed under this heading.

Duloxetine Hydrochloride (Based on the mechanism of action of SNRIs, caution is advised when paroxetine hydrochloride controlled-release tablets are co-administered with other drugs that may affect the serotonergic neurotransmitter systems). Products include:
Cymbalta ... 1871

Encainide Hydrochloride (Concomitant use in patients taking either monoamine oxidase inhibitors (MAOIs), including linezolid, an antibiotic which is a reversible non-selective MAOI, or thioridazine is contraindicated).
No products indexed under this heading.

Escitalopram Oxalate (Based on the mechanism of action of SSRIs, caution is advised when paroxetine hydrochloride controlled-release tablets are co-administered with other drugs that may affect the serotonergic neurotransmitter systems). Products include:
Lexapro Oral Suspension ... 1160
Lexapro Tablets ... 1160

Ethanol (Avoid alcohol while taking paroxetine hydrochloride controlled-release tablets).
No products indexed under this heading.

Ethyl Alcohol (Avoid alcohol while taking paroxetine hydrochloride controlled-release tablets).
No products indexed under this heading.

Etodolac (Caution about the concomitant use of NSAIDs since combined use of psychotropic drugs that interfere with serotonin reuptake and these agents has been associated with an increased risk of bleeding).
No products indexed under this heading.

Fenoprofen Calcium (Caution about the concomitant use of NSAIDs since combined use of psychotropic drugs that interfere with serotonin reuptake and these agents has been associated with an increased risk of bleeding).
No products indexed under this heading.

Fentanyl (Concomitant use in patients taking either monoamine oxidase inhibitors (MAOIs), including linezolid, an antibiotic which is a reversible non-selective MAOI, or thioridazine is contraindicated). Products include:
Duragesic ... 2604
Fentanyl Transdermal System ... 2346
Onsolis ... 2054

Fentanyl Citrate (Concomitant use in patients taking either monoamine oxidase inhibitors (MAOIs), including linezolid, an antibiotic which is a reversible non-selective MAOI, or thioridazine is contraindicated). Products include:
Fentora ... 966

Flecainide Acetate (Concomitant use in patients taking either monoamine oxidase inhibitors (MAOIs), including linezolid, an antibiotic which is a reversible non-selective MAOI, or thioridazine is contraindicated).
No products indexed under this heading.

Fluoxetine (Based on the mechanism of action of SSRIs, caution is advised when paroxetine hydrochloride controlled-release tablets are co-administered with other drugs that may affect the serotonergic neurotransmitter systems).
No products indexed under this heading.

Fluoxetine Hydrochloride (Based on the mechanism of action of SSRIs, caution is advised when paroxetine hydrochloride controlled-release tablets are co-administered with other drugs that may affect the serotonergic neurotransmitter systems). Products include:
Prozac Weekly ... 1941
Prozac Pulvules ... 1941
Symbyax ... 1965

IMPORTANT NOTE: Always consult each drug listing in the patient's regimen for possible interactions.

Paroxetine ER **Interactions Index** **1378**

Fluphenazine Decanoate (Concomitant use in patients taking either monoamine oxidase inhibitors (MAOIs), including linezolid, an antibiotic which is a reversible non-selective MAOI, or thioridazine is contraindicated).
No products indexed under this heading.

Fluphenazine Enanthate (Concomitant use in patients taking either monoamine oxidase inhibitors (MAOIs), including linezolid, an antibiotic which is a reversible non-selective MAOI, or thioridazine is contraindicated).
No products indexed under this heading.

Fluphenazine Hydrochloride (Concomitant use in patients taking either monoamine oxidase inhibitors (MAOIs), including linezolid, an antibiotic which is a reversible non-selective MAOI, or thioridazine is contraindicated).
No products indexed under this heading.

Flurazepam Hydrochloride (Because paroxetine is highly bound to plasma protein, administration of paroxetine hydrochloride controlled-release tablets to a patient taking another drug that is highly protein bound may cause increased free concentrations of the other drug, potentially resulting in adverse events. Conversely, adverse effects could result from displacement of paroxetine by other highly bound drugs).
No products indexed under this heading.

Flurbiprofen (Caution about the concomitant use of NSAIDs since combined use of psychotropic drugs that interfere with serotonin reuptake and these agents has been associated with an increased risk of bleeding).
No products indexed under this heading.

Fluvoxamine (Based on the mechanism of action of SSRIs, caution is advised when paroxetine hydrochloride controlled-release tablets are co-administered with other drugs that may affect the serotonergic neurotransmitter systems).
No products indexed under this heading.

Fluvoxamine Maleate (Based on the mechanism of action of SSRIs, caution is advised when paroxetine hydrochloride controlled-release tablets are co-administered with other drugs that may affect the serotonergic neurotransmitter systems).
No products indexed under this heading.

Formoterol Fumarate (Concomitant use in patients taking either monoamine oxidase inhibitors (MAOIs), including linezolid, an antibiotic which is a reversible non-selective MAOI, or thioridazine is contraindicated). Products include:
Foradil 3121
Perforomist 3634

Fosamprenavir Calcium (Co-administration of fosamprenavir with paroxetine significantly decreased plasma levels of paroxetine. Any dose adjustment should be guided by clinical effect). Products include:
Lexiva Oral Suspension 1558
Lexiva 1558

Galantamine Hydrobromide (Concomitant use in patients taking either monoamine oxidase inhibitors (MAOIs), including linezolid, an antibiotic which is a reversible non-selective MAOI, or thioridazine is contraindicated).
No products indexed under this heading.

Glipizide (Because paroxetine is highly bound to plasma protein, administration of paroxetine hydrochloride controlled-release tablets to a patient taking another drug that is highly protein bound may cause increased free concentrations of the other drug, potentially resulting in adverse events. Conversely, adverse effects could result from displacement of paroxetine by other highly bound drugs).
No products indexed under this heading.

Haloperidol (Concomitant use in patients taking either monoamine oxidase inhibitors (MAOIs), including linezolid, an antibiotic which is a reversible non-selective MAOI, or thioridazine is contraindicated).
No products indexed under this heading.

Haloperidol Decanoate (Concomitant use in patients taking either monoamine oxidase inhibitors (MAOIs), including linezolid, an antibiotic which is a reversible non-selective MAOI, or thioridazine is contraindicated).
No products indexed under this heading.

Hydrocodone Bitartrate (Concomitant use in patients taking either monoamine oxidase inhibitors (MAOIs), including linezolid, an antibiotic which is a reversible non-selective MAOI, or thioridazine is contraindicated). Products include:
Vicodin 560
Vicodin ES 561
Vicodin HP 563
Vicoprofen 564
Zydone 1138

Hypericum (Caution is advised when paroxetine hydrochloride controlled-release tablets are co-administered with other drugs that may affect the serotonergic neurotransmitter systems, such as St. John's Wort).
No products indexed under this heading.

Ibuprofen (Caution about the concomitant use of NSAIDs since combined use of psychotropic drugs that interfere with serotonin reuptake and these agents has been associated with an increased risk of bleeding). Products include:
Motrin IB 2043
Children's Motrin 2044
Children's Motrin Non-Staining Dye-Free 2044
Infants' Motrin 2044
Infants' Motrin Dye-Free 2044
Junior Strength Motrin 2044
Vicoprofen 564

Imipramine Hydrochloride (Caution is indicated in the co-administration of TCAs with paroxetine hydrochloride controlled-release tablets, because paroxetine may inhibit TCA metabolism. Plasma TCA concentrations may need to be monitored, and the dose of TCA may need to be reduced, if a TCA is co-administered with paroxetine hydrochloride controlled-release tablets).
No products indexed under this heading.

Imipramine Pamoate (Caution is indicated in the co-administration of TCAs with paroxetine hydrochloride controlled-release tablets, because paroxetine may inhibit TCA metabolism. Plasma TCA concentrations may need to be monitored, and the dose of TCA may need to be reduced, if a TCA is co-administered with paroxetine hydrochloride controlled-release tablets).
No products indexed under this heading.

Indomethacin (Caution about the concomitant use of NSAIDs since combined use of psychotropic drugs that interfere with serotonin reuptake and these agents has been associated with an increased risk of bleeding). Products include:
Indocin 2167

Indomethacin Sodium Trihydrate (Caution about the concomitant use of NSAIDs since combined use of psychotropic drugs that interfere with serotonin reuptake and these agents has been associated with an increased risk of bleeding). Products include:
Indocin I.V. 2007

Indoramin Hydrochloride (Concomitant use in patients taking either monoamine oxidase inhibitors (MAOIs), including linezolid, an antibiotic which is a reversible non-selective MAOI, or thioridazine is contraindicated).
No products indexed under this heading.

Isocarboxazid (Concomitant use in patients taking either monoamine oxidase inhibitors (MAOIs), including linezolid, an antibiotic which is a reversible non-selective MAOI, or thioridazine is contraindicated). Products include:
Marplan 3481

Ketoprofen (Caution about the concomitant use of NSAIDs since combined use of psychotropic drugs that interfere with serotonin reuptake and these agents has been associated with an increased risk of bleeding).
No products indexed under this heading.

Ketorolac Tromethamine (Caution about the concomitant use of NSAIDs since combined use of psychotropic drugs that interfere with serotonin reuptake and these agents has been associated with an increased risk of bleeding). Products include:
Acuvail .... ⊙ 209

Labetalol Hydrochloride (Concomitant use in patients taking either monoamine oxidase inhibitors (MAOIs), including linezolid, an antibiotic which is a reversible non-selective MAOI, or thioridazine is contraindicated).
No products indexed under this heading.

Lidocaine (Concomitant use in patients taking either monoamine oxidase inhibitors (MAOIs), including linezolid, an antibiotic which is a reversible non-selective MAOI, or thioridazine is contraindicated). Products include:
Lidoderm 1107

Lidocaine Hydrochloride (Concomitant use in patients taking either monoamine oxidase inhibitors (MAOIs), including linezolid, an antibiotic which is a reversible non-selective MAOI, or thioridazine is contraindicated).
No products indexed under this heading.

Linezolid (Concomitant use in patients taking either monoamine oxidase inhibitors (MAOIs), including linezolid, an antibiotic which is a reversible non-selective MAOI, or thioridazine is contraindicated)). Products include:
Zyvox 2769

Lithium (Caution is advised when Paroxetine Hydrochloride Controlled-Release Tablets are co-administered with other drugs that may affect the serotonergic neurotransmitter systems, such as lithium).
No products indexed under this heading.

Maprotiline Hydrochloride (Caution is indicated in the co-administration of TCAs with paroxetine hydrochloride controlled-release tablets, because paroxetine may inhibit TCA metabolism. Plasma TCA concentrations may need to be monitored, and the dose of TCA may need to be reduced, if a TCA is co-administered with paroxetine hydrochloride controlled-release tablets).
No products indexed under this heading.

Meclofenamate Sodium (Caution about the concomitant use of NSAIDs since combined use of psychotropic drugs that interfere with serotonin reuptake and these agents has been associated with an increased risk of bleeding).
No products indexed under this heading.

Mefenamic Acid (Caution about the concomitant use of NSAIDs since combined use of psychotropic drugs that interfere with serotonin reuptake and these agents has been associated with an increased risk of bleeding).
No products indexed under this heading.

Meloxicam (Caution about the concomitant use of NSAIDs since combined use of psychotropic drugs that interfere with serotonin reuptake and these agents has been associated with an increased risk of bleeding).
No products indexed under this heading.

Meperidine Hydrochloride (Concomitant use in patients taking either monoamine oxidase inhibitors (MAOIs), including linezolid, an antibiotic which is a reversible non-selective MAOI, or thioridazine is contraindicated).
No products indexed under this heading.

Methadone Hydrochloride (Concomitant use in patients taking either monoamine oxidase inhibitors (MAOIs), including linezolid, an antibiotic which is a reversible non-selective MAOI, or thioridazine is contraindicated).
No products indexed under this heading.

Methamphetamine Hydrochloride (Concomitant use in patients taking either monoamine oxidase inhibitors (MAOIs), including linezolid, an antibiotic which is a reversible non-selective MAOI, or thioridazine is contraindicated).
No products indexed under this heading.

Methoxyphenamine (Concomitant use in patients taking either monoamine oxidase inhibitors (MAOIs), including linezolid, an antibiotic which is a reversible non-selective MAOI, or thioridazine is contraindicated).
No products indexed under this heading.

Metoprolol Succinate (Concomitant use in patients taking either monoamine oxidase inhibitors (MAOIs), including linezolid, an antibiotic which is a reversible non-selective MAOI, or thioridazine is contraindicated). Products include:
Toprol XL 732

Metoprolol Tartrate (Concomitant use in patients taking either monoamine oxidase inhibitors (MAOIs), including linezolid, an antibiotic which is a reversible non-selective MAOI, or thioridazine is contraindicated).
No products indexed under this heading.

Mexiletine Hydrochloride (Concomitant use in patients taking either monoamine oxidase inhibitors (MAOIs), including linezolid, an antibiotic which is a reversible non-selective MAOI, or thioridazine is contraindicated).
No products indexed under this heading.

Midazolam Hydrochloride (Because paroxetine is highly bound to plasma protein, administration of paroxetine hydrochloride controlled-release tablets to a patient taking another drug that is highly protein bound may cause increased free concentrations of the other drug, potentially resulting in adverse events. Conversely, adverse effects could result from displacement of paroxetine by other highly bound drugs).
No products indexed under this heading.

Mirtazapine (Concomitant use in patients taking either monoamine oxidase inhibitors (MAOIs), including linezolid, an antibiotic which is a reversible non-selective MAOI, or thioridazine is contraindicated). Products include:
Remeron Tablets 3214
RemeronSolTab Tablets 3219

Moclobemide (Concomitant use in patients taking either monoamine oxidase inhibitors (MAOIs), including linezolid, an antibiotic which is a reversible non-selective MAOI, or thioridazine is contraindicated).
No products indexed under this heading.

Morphine Sulfate (Concomitant use in patients taking either monoamine oxidase inhibitors (MAOIs), including linezolid, an antibiotic which is a reversible non-selective MAOI, or thioridazine is contraindicated). Products include:
Avinza 1822
Embeda 1831
MS Contin 2803

(⊙ Described in PDR® for Ophthalmic Medicines)

1379 **Interactions Index** **Paroxetine ER**

Nabumetone (Caution about the concomitant use of NSAIDs since combined use of psychotropic drugs that interfere with serotonin reuptake and these agents has been associated with an increased risk of bleeding).
No products indexed under this heading.

Naproxen (Caution about the concomitant use of NSAIDs since combined use of psychotropic drugs that interfere with serotonin reuptake and these agents has been associated with an increased risk of bleeding). Products include:
EC-Naprosyn 2850
Naprosyn 2850
Anaprox/Naprosyn 2850

Naproxen Sodium (Caution about the concomitant use of NSAIDs since combined use of psychotropic drugs that interfere with serotonin reuptake and these agents has been associated with an increased risk of bleeding). Products include:
Anaprox 2850
Anaprox DS 2850
Treximet 1681

Nefazodone Hydrochloride (Based on the mechanism of action of SNRIs, caution is advised when paroxetine hydrochloride controlled-release tablets are co-administered with other drugs that may affect the serotonergic neurotransmitter systems).
No products indexed under this heading.

Nelfinavir Mesylate (Concomitant use in patients taking either monoamine oxidase inhibitors (MAOIs), including linezolid, an antibiotic which is a reversible non-selective MAOI, or thioridazine is contraindicated).
No products indexed under this heading.

Nortriptyline Hydrochloride (Caution is indicated in the co-administration of TCAs with paroxetine hydrochloride controlled-release tablets, because paroxetine may inhibit TCA metabolism. Plasma TCA concentrations may need to be monitored, and the dose of TCA may need to be reduced, if a TCA is co-administered with paroxetine hydrochloride controlled-release tablets).
No products indexed under this heading.

Olanzapine (Concomitant use in patients taking either monoamine oxidase inhibitors (MAOIs), including linezolid, an antibiotic which is a reversible non-selective MAOI, or thioridazine is contraindicated). Products include:
Symbyax 1965
Zyprexa 1984
Zyprexa IntraMuscular 1984
Zyprexa ZYDIS 1984

Omeprazole (Concomitant use in patients taking either monoamine oxidase inhibitors (MAOIs), including linezolid, an antibiotic which is a reversible non-selective MAOI, or thioridazine is contraindicated).
No products indexed under this heading.

Ondansetron (Concomitant use in patients taking either monoamine oxidase inhibitors (MAOIs), including linezolid, an antibiotic which is a reversible non-selective MAOI, or thioridazine is contraindicated).
No products indexed under this heading.

Ondansetron Hydrochloride (Concomitant use in patients taking either monoamine oxidase inhibitors (MAOIs), including linezolid, an antibiotic which is a reversible non-selective MAOI, or thioridazine is contraindicated). Products include:
Zofran Injection 1750
Zofran 1756
Zofran ODT 1756

Oxaprozin (Caution about the concomitant use of NSAIDs since combined use of psychotropic drugs that interfere with serotonin reuptake and these agents has been associated with an increased risk of bleeding).
No products indexed under this heading.

Oxazepam (Because paroxetine is highly bound to plasma protein, administration of paroxetine hydrochloride controlled-release tablets to a patient taking another drug that is highly protein bound may cause increased free concentrations of the other drug, potentially resulting in adverse events. Conversely, adverse effects could result from displacement of paroxetine by other highly bound drugs).
No products indexed under this heading.

Oxycodone Hydrochloride (Concomitant use in patients taking either monoamine oxidase inhibitors (MAOIs), including linezolid, an antibiotic which is a reversible non-selective MAOI, or thioridazine is contraindicated). Products include:
OxyContin 2807
Percocet 1121
Percodan 1124

Paclitaxel (Concomitant use in patients taking either monoamine oxidase inhibitors (MAOIs), including linezolid, an antibiotic which is a reversible non-selective MAOI, or thioridazine is contraindicated).
No products indexed under this heading.

Pargyline Hydrochloride (Concomitant use in patients taking either monoamine oxidase inhibitors (MAOIs), including linezolid, an antibiotic which is a reversible non-selective MAOI, or thioridazine is contraindicated).
No products indexed under this heading.

Paroxetine (Based on the mechanism of action of SSRIs, caution is advised when paroxetine hydrochloride controlled-release tablets are co-administered with other drugs that may affect the serotonergic neurotransmitter systems).
No products indexed under this heading.

Paroxetine Mesylate (Based on the mechanism of action of SSRIs, caution is advised when paroxetine hydrochloride controlled-release tablets are co-administered with other drugs that may affect the serotonergic neurotransmitter systems).
No products indexed under this heading.

Phenelzine Sulfate (Concomitant use in patients taking either monoamine oxidase inhibitors (MAOIs), including linezolid, an antibiotic which is a reversible non-selective MAOI, or thioridazine is contraindicated).
No products indexed under this heading.

Phenobarbital (Phenobarbital induces many cytochrome P450 (oxidative) enzymes. When a single oral 30-mg dose of immediate-release paroxetine was administered at phenobarbital steady state (100 mg once daily for 14 days), paroxetine AUC and T1/2 were reduced (by an average of 25% and 38%, respectively) compared to paroxetine administered alone). Products include:
Donnatal 2711

Phenylbutazone (Caution about the concomitant use of NSAIDs since combined use of psychotropic drugs that interfere with serotonin reuptake and these agents has been associated with an increased risk of bleeding).
No products indexed under this heading.

Phenytoin (When a single oral 30-mg dose of immediate-release paroxetine was administered at phenytoin steady state (300 mg once daily for 14 days), paroxetine AUC and T1/2 were reduced (by an average of 50% and 35%, respectively) compared to immediate-release paroxetine administered alone. In a separate study, when a single oral 300-mg dose of phenytoin was administered at paroxetine steady state (30 mg once daily for 14 days), phenytoin AUC was slightly reduced (12% on average) compared to phenytoin administered alone).
No products indexed under this heading.

Phenytoin Sodium (When a single oral 30-mg dose of immediate-release paroxetine was administered at phenytoin steady state (300 mg once daily for 14 days), paroxetine AUC and T1/2 were reduced (by an average of 50% and 35%, respectively) compared to immediate-release paroxetine administered alone. In a separate study, when a single oral 300-mg dose of phenytoin was administered at paroxetine steady state (30 mg once daily for 14 days), phenytoin AUC was slightly reduced (12% on average) compared to phenytoin administered alone). Products include:
Phenytek Capsules 2380

Pimozide (Concomitant use in patients taking pimozide is contraindicated).
No products indexed under this heading.

Pindolol (Concomitant use in patients taking either monoamine oxidase inhibitors (MAOIs), including linezolid, an antibiotic which is a reversible non-selective MAOI, or thioridazine is contraindicated).
No products indexed under this heading.

Piroxicam (Caution about the concomitant use of NSAIDs since combined use of psychotropic drugs that interfere with serotonin reuptake and these agents has been associated with an increased risk of bleeding).
No products indexed under this heading.

Procarbazine Hydrochloride (Concomitant use in patients taking either monoamine oxidase inhibitors (MAOIs), including linezolid, an antibiotic which is a reversible non-selective MAOI, or thioridazine is contraindicated).
No products indexed under this heading.

Procyclidine Hydrochloride (Daily oral dosing of immediate-release paroxetine (30 mg once daily) increased steady-state AUC0- 24, C_{max}, and C_{min} values of procyclidine (5 mg oral once daily) by 35%, 37%, and 67%, respectively, compared to procyclidine alone at steady state. If anticholinergic effects are seen, the dose of procyclidine should be reduced).
No products indexed under this heading.

Propafenone Hydrochloride (Concomitant use in patients taking either monoamine oxidase inhibitors (MAOIs), including linezolid, an antibiotic which is a reversible non-selective MAOI, or thioridazine is contraindicated). Products include:
Rythmol 1648
Rythmol SR 1652

Propoxyphene Hydrochloride (Concomitant use in patients taking either monoamine oxidase inhibitors (MAOIs), including linezolid, an antibiotic which is a reversible non-selective MAOI, or thioridazine is contraindicated).
No products indexed under this heading.

Propoxyphene Napsylate (Concomitant use in patients taking either monoamine oxidase inhibitors (MAOIs), including linezolid, an antibiotic which is a reversible non-selective MAOI, or thioridazine is contraindicated).
No products indexed under this heading.

Propranolol Hydrochloride (Concomitant use in patients taking either monoamine oxidase inhibitors (MAOIs), including linezolid, an antibiotic which is a reversible non-selective MAOI, or thioridazine is contraindicated). Products include:
InnoPran XL 1517

Protriptyline Hydrochloride (Caution is indicated in the co-administration of TCAs with paroxetine hydrochloride controlled-release tablets, because paroxetine may inhibit TCA metabolism. Plasma TCA concentrations may need to be monitored, and the dose of TCA may need to be reduced, if a TCA is co-administered with paroxetine hydrochloride controlled-release tablets).
No products indexed under this heading.

Quetiapine Fumarate (Concomitant use in patients taking either monoamine oxidase inhibitors (MAOIs), including linezolid, an antibiotic which is a reversible non-selective MAOI, or thioridazine is contraindicated). Products include:
Seroquel 750
Seroquel XR 759

Quinidine Gluconate (Concomitant use in patients taking either monoamine oxidase inhibitors (MAOIs), including linezolid, an antibiotic which is a reversible non-selective MAOI, or thioridazine is contraindicated).
No products indexed under this heading.

Quinidine Hydrochloride (Concomitant use in patients taking either monoamine oxidase inhibitors (MAOIs), including linezolid, an antibiotic which is a reversible non-selective MAOI, or thioridazine is contraindicated).
No products indexed under this heading.

Quinidine Polygalacturonate (Concomitant use in patients taking either monoamine oxidase inhibitors (MAOIs), including linezolid, an antibiotic which is a reversible non-selective MAOI, or thioridazine is contraindicated).
No products indexed under this heading.

Quinidine Sulfate (Concomitant use in patients taking either monoamine oxidase inhibitors (MAOIs), including linezolid, an antibiotic which is a reversible non-selective MAOI, or thioridazine is contraindicated).
No products indexed under this heading.

Rasagiline Mesylate (Concomitant use in patients taking either monoamine oxidase inhibitors (MAOIs), including linezolid, an antibiotic which is a reversible non-selective MAOI, or thioridazine is contraindicated). Products include:
Azilect 3383

Risperidone (Concomitant use in patients taking either monoamine oxidase inhibitors (MAOIs), including linezolid, an antibiotic which is a reversible non-selective MAOI, or thioridazine is contraindicated). Products include:
Risperdal Consta 2682

Ritonavir (Co-administration of ritonavir with paroxetine significantly decreased plasma levels of paroxetine. Any dose adjustment should be guided by clinical effect). Products include:
Kaletra 458
Norvir 509

Rofecoxib (Caution about the concomitant use of NSAIDs since combined use of psychotropic drugs that interfere with serotonin reuptake and these agents has been associated with an increased risk of bleeding).
No products indexed under this heading.

Selegiline (Concomitant use in patients taking either monoamine oxidase inhibitors (MAOIs), including linezolid, an antibiotic which is a reversible non-selective MAOI, or thioridazine is contraindicated). Products include:
Emsam 3623

Selegiline Hydrochloride (Concomitant use in patients taking either monoamine oxidase inhibitors (MAOIs), including linezolid, an antibiotic which is a reversible non-selective MAOI, or thioridazine is contraindicated). Products include:
Eldepryl 3312

IMPORTANT NOTE: Always consult each drug listing in the patient's regimen for possible interactions.

Sertraline Hydrochloride (Based on the mechanism of action of SSRIs, caution is advised when paroxetine hydrochloride controlled-release tablets are co-administered with other drugs that may affect the serotonergic neurotransmitter systems).
No products indexed under this heading.

Sulindac (Caution about the concomitant use of NSAIDs since combined use of psychotropic drugs that interfere with serotonin reuptake and these agents has been associated with an increased risk of bleeding). Products include:
Clinoril 2098

Tamoxifen Citrate (Concomitant use in patients taking either monoamine oxidase inhibitors (MAOIs), including linezolid, an antibiotic which is a reversible non-selective MAOI, or thioridazine is contraindicated).
No products indexed under this heading.

Temazepam (Because paroxetine is highly bound to plasma protein, administration of paroxetine hydrochloride controlled-release tablets to a patient taking another drug that is highly protein bound may cause increased free concentrations of the other drug, potentially resulting in adverse events. Conversely, adverse effects could result from displacement of paroxetine by other highly bound drugs).
No products indexed under this heading.

Teniposide (Concomitant use in patients taking either monoamine oxidase inhibitors (MAOIs), including linezolid, an antibiotic which is a reversible non-selective MAOI, or thioridazine is contraindicated).
No products indexed under this heading.

Testosterone (Concomitant use in patients taking either monoamine oxidase inhibitors (MAOIs), including linezolid, an antibiotic which is a reversible non-selective MAOI, or thioridazine is contraindicated). Products include:
AndroGel 3456

Testosterone Cypionate (Concomitant use in patients taking either monoamine oxidase inhibitors (MAOIs), including linezolid, an antibiotic which is a reversible non-selective MAOI, or thioridazine is contraindicated).
No products indexed under this heading.

Testosterone Enanthate (Concomitant use in patients taking either monoamine oxidase inhibitors (MAOIs), including linezolid, an antibiotic which is a reversible non-selective MAOI, or thioridazine is contraindicated). Products include:
Delatestryl 1102

Testosterone Propionate (Concomitant use in patients taking either monoamine oxidase inhibitors (MAOIs), including linezolid, an antibiotic which is a reversible non-selective MAOI, or thioridazine is contraindicated).
No products indexed under this heading.

Thioridazine (Concomitant use in patients taking either monoamine oxidase inhibitors (MAOIs), including linezolid, an antibiotic which is a reversible non-selective MAOI, or thioridazine is contraindicated).
No products indexed under this heading.

Thioridazine Hydrochloride (Concomitant use in patients taking either monoamine oxidase inhibitors (MAOIs), including linezolid, an antibiotic which is a reversible non-selective MAOI, or thioridazine is contraindicated). Products include:
Thioridazine Hydrochloride 2384

Timolol Maleate (Concomitant use in patients taking either monoamine oxidase inhibitors (MAOIs), including linezolid, an antibiotic which is a reversible non-selective MAOI, or thioridazine is contraindicated). Products include:

Combigan 601
Dorzolamide
  Hydrochloride/Timolol Maleate
  Ophthalmic Solution.....................⊙243
Timoptic in Ocudose ....⊙231

Tolbutamide (Because paroxetine is highly bound to plasma protein, administration of paroxetine hydrochloride controlled-release tablets to a patient taking another drug that is highly protein-bound may cause increased free concentrations of the other drug, potentially resulting in adverse events. Conversely, adverse effects could result from displacement of paroxetine by other highly bound drugs).
No products indexed under this heading.

Tolmetin Sodium (Caution about the concomitant use of NSAIDs since combined use of psychotropic drugs that interfere with serotonin reuptake and these agents has been associated with an increased risk of bleeding).
No products indexed under this heading.

Tolterodine Tartrate (Concomitant use in patients taking either monoamine oxidase inhibitors (MAOIs), including linezolid, an antibiotic which is a reversible non-selective MAOI, or thioridazine is contraindicated).
No products indexed under this heading.

Tramadol Hydrochloride (Caution is advised when Paroxetine Hydrochloride Controlled-Release Tablets are co-administered with other drugs that may affect the serotonergic neurotransmitter systems, such as tramadol). Products include:
Ryzolt 2813
Ultram ER 2693

Tranylcypromine Sulfate (Concomitant use in patients taking either monoamine oxidase inhibitors (MAOIs), including linezolid, an antibiotic which is a reversible non-selective MAOI, or thioridazine is contraindicated). Products include:
Parnate 1584

Trazodone Hydrochloride (Concomitant use in patients taking either monoamine oxidase inhibitors (MAOIs), including linezolid, an antibiotic which is a reversible non-selective MAOI, or thioridazine is contraindicated).
No products indexed under this heading.

Triazolam (Concomitant use in patients taking either monoamine oxidase inhibitors (MAOIs), including linezolid, an antibiotic which is a reversible non-selective MAOI, or thioridazine is contraindicated).
No products indexed under this heading.

Trimipramine Maleate (Caution is indicated in the co-administration of TCAs with paroxetine hydrochloride controlled-release tablets, because paroxetine may inhibit TCA metabolism. Plasma TCA concentrations may need to be monitored, and the dose of TCA may need to be reduced, if a TCA is co-administered with paroxetine hydrochloride controlled-release tablets).
No products indexed under this heading.

Tryptophan (Adverse experiences, consisting primarily of headache, nausea, sweating, and dizziness, have been reported when tryptophan was administered to patients taking immediate release paroxetine. Consequently, concomitant use of paroxetine hydrochloride controlled-release tablets with tryptophan is not recommended).
No products indexed under this heading.

Valdecoxib (Caution about the concomitant use of NSAIDs since combined use of psychotropic drugs that interfere with serotonin reuptake and these agents has been associated with an increased risk of bleeding).
No products indexed under this heading.

Venlafaxine Hydrochloride (Based on the mechanism of action of SNRIs,

caution is advised when paroxetine hydrochloride controlled-release tablets are co-administered with other drugs that may affect the serotonergic neurotransmitter systems). Products include:
Effexor XR 3504
Venlafaxine Hydrochloride Tablets ... 2388

Vinblastine Sulfate (Concomitant use in patients taking either monoamine oxidase inhibitors (MAOIs), including linezolid, an antibiotic which is a reversible non-selective MAOI, or thioridazine is contraindicated).
No products indexed under this heading.

Warfarin Sodium (Caution about the concomitant use of warfarin since combined use of psychotropic drugs that interfere with serotonin reuptake and these agents has been associated with an increased risk of bleeding).
No products indexed under this heading.

Zonisamide (Concomitant use in patients taking either monoamine oxidase inhibitors (MAOIs), including linezolid, an antibiotic which is a reversible non-selective MAOI, or thioridazine is contraindicated). Products include:
Zonegran 1081

Food Interactions

Alcohol (Avoid alcohol while taking paroxetine hydrochloride controlled-release tablets).

Beer, reduced-alcohol (Avoid alcohol while taking paroxetine hydrochloride controlled-release tablets).

Beer, unspecified (Avoid alcohol while taking paroxetine hydrochloride controlled-release tablets).

Wine, Chianti (Avoid alcohol while taking paroxetine hydrochloride controlled-release tablets).

Wine, Red (Avoid alcohol while taking paroxetine hydrochloride controlled-release tablets).

Wine, unspecified (Avoid alcohol while taking paroxetine hydrochloride controlled-release tablets).

Wine products (Avoid alcohol while taking paroxetine hydrochloride controlled-release tablets).

PASER GRANULES

(Aminosalicylic Acid) 1820

Digoxin (Potential for reduced digoxin levels). Products include:
Lanoxin Injection 1546
Lanoxin Injection Pediatric 1549
Lanoxin Tablets 1553

Isoniazid (Concurrent use with a rapidly available form of aminosalicylic acid has been reported to produce a 20% reduction in the acetylation of INH; the lower serum levels produced by delayed release preparation will result in a reduced effect on the acetylation of INH).
No products indexed under this heading.

Rifampin (May block the absorption of rifampin; PASER granules do not contain excipient that blocks the absorption).
No products indexed under this heading.

Vitamin B12 (Reduced absorption of vitamin B12 with clinically significant erythrocyte abnormalities developing after depletion). Products include:
Animi-3 2711
Authia 3497
Bevitamel 3497
Cardio Basics 3455
Divista 3474
Ferralet 2333
Heplive 607
Nascobal 2700

PATADAY OPHTHALMIC SOLUTION

(Olopatadine Hydrochloride) 584
None cited in PDR database.

PATANASE NASAL SPRAY

(Olopatadine Hydrochloride) 585
May interact with alcohols, central nervous system depressants. Compounds in these categories include:

Alfentanil Hydrochloride (Concurrent use of olopatadine nasal spray with other central nervous system depressants should be avoided because additional reductions in alertness and additional impairment of central nervous system performance may occur).
No products indexed under this heading.

Alprazolam (Concurrent use of olopatadine nasal spray with other central nervous system depressants should be avoided because additional reductions in alertness and additional impairment of central nervous system performance may occur).
No products indexed under this heading.

Amobarbital (Concurrent use of olopatadine nasal spray with other central nervous system depressants should be avoided because additional reductions in alertness and additional impairment of central nervous system performance may occur).
No products indexed under this heading.

Amobarbital Sodium (Concurrent use of olopatadine nasal spray with other central nervous system depressants should be avoided because additional reductions in alertness and additional impairment of central nervous system performance may occur).
No products indexed under this heading.

Aprobarbital (Concurrent use of olopatadine nasal spray with other central nervous system depressants should be avoided because additional reductions in alertness and additional impairment of central nervous system performance may occur).
No products indexed under this heading.

Buprenorphine Hydrochloride (Concurrent use of olopatadine nasal spray with other central nervous system depressants should be avoided because additional reductions in alertness and additional impairment of central nervous system performance may occur).
No products indexed under this heading.

Buspirone Hydrochloride (Concurrent use of olopatadine nasal spray with other central nervous system depressants should be avoided because additional reductions in alertness and additional impairment of central nervous system performance may occur).
No products indexed under this heading.

Butabarbital (Concurrent use of olopatadine nasal spray with other central nervous system depressants should be avoided because additional reductions in alertness and additional impairment of central nervous system performance may occur).
No products indexed under this heading.

Butabarbital Sodium (Concurrent use of olopatadine nasal spray with other central nervous system depressants should be avoided because additional reductions in alertness and additional impairment of central nervous system performance may occur).
No products indexed under this heading.

Butalbital (Concurrent use of olopatadine nasal spray with other central nervous system depressants should be avoided because additional reductions in alertness and additional impairment of central nervous system performance may occur).
No products indexed under this heading.

1381 Interactions Index Patanase

Chlordiazepoxide (Concurrent use of olopatadine nasal spray with other central nervous system depressants should be avoided because additional reductions in alertness and additional impairment of central nervous system performance may occur).
No products indexed under this heading.

Chlordiazepoxide Hydrochloride (Concurrent use of olopatadine nasal spray with other central nervous system depressants should be avoided because additional reductions in alertness and additional impairment of central nervous system performance may occur).
No products indexed under this heading.

Chlorpromazine (Concurrent use of olopatadine nasal spray with other central nervous system depressants should be avoided because additional reductions in alertness and additional impairment of central nervous system performance may occur).
No products indexed under this heading.

Chlorpromazine Hydrochloride (Concurrent use of olopatadine nasal spray with other central nervous system depressants should be avoided because additional reductions in alertness and additional impairment of central nervous system performance may occur).
No products indexed under this heading.

Chlorprothixene (Concurrent use of olopatadine nasal spray with other central nervous system depressants should be avoided because additional reductions in alertness and additional impairment of central nervous system performance may occur).
No products indexed under this heading.

Chlorprothixene Hydrochloride (Concurrent use of olopatadine nasal spray with other central nervous system depressants should be avoided because additional reductions in alertness and additional impairment of central nervous system performance may occur).
No products indexed under this heading.

Chlorprothixene Lactate (Concurrent use of olopatadine nasal spray with other central nervous system depressants should be avoided because additional reductions in alertness and additional impairment of central nervous system performance may occur).
No products indexed under this heading.

Clonazepam (Concurrent use of olopatadine nasal spray with other central nervous system depressants should be avoided because additional reductions in alertness and additional impairment of central nervous system performance may occur). Products include:
Klonopin 2855

Clorazepate Dipotassium (Concurrent use of olopatadine nasal spray with other central nervous system depressants should be avoided because additional reductions in alertness and additional impairment of central nervous system performance may occur).
No products indexed under this heading.

Clozapine (Concurrent use of olopatadine nasal spray with other central nervous system depressants should be avoided because additional reductions in alertness and additional impairment of central nervous system performance may occur).
No products indexed under this heading.

Codeine Phosphate (Concurrent use of olopatadine nasal spray with other central nervous system depressants should be avoided because additional reductions in alertness and additional impairment of central nervous system performance may occur). Products include:
Tylenol with Codeine 2691

Codeine Sulfate (Concurrent use of olopatadine nasal spray with other central nervous system depressants should be avoided because additional reductions in alertness and additional impairment of central nervous system performance may occur).
No products indexed under this heading.

Desflurane (Concurrent use of olopatadine nasal spray with other central nervous system depressants should be avoided because additional reductions in alertness and additional impairment of central nervous system performance may occur).
No products indexed under this heading.

Dezocine (Concurrent use of olopatadine nasal spray with other central nervous system depressants should be avoided because additional reductions in alertness and additional impairment of central nervous system performance may occur).
No products indexed under this heading.

Diazepam (Concurrent use of olopatadine nasal spray with other central nervous system depressants should be avoided because additional reductions in alertness and additional impairment of central nervous system performance may occur). Products include:
Valium Tablets 2880

Droperidol (Concurrent use of olopatadine nasal spray with other central nervous system depressants should be avoided because additional reductions in alertness and additional impairment of central nervous system performance may occur).
No products indexed under this heading.

Enflurane (Concurrent use of olopatadine nasal spray with other central nervous system depressants should be avoided because additional reductions in alertness and additional impairment of central nervous system performance may occur).
No products indexed under this heading.

Estazolam (Concurrent use of olopatadine nasal spray with other central nervous system depressants should be avoided because additional reductions in alertness and additional impairment of central nervous system performance may occur).
No products indexed under this heading.

Ethanol (Concurrent use of olopatadine nasal spray with other central nervous system depressants should be avoided because additional reductions in alertness and additional impairment of central nervous system performance may occur).
No products indexed under this heading.

Ethchlorvynol (Concurrent use of olopatadine nasal spray with other central nervous system depressants should be avoided because additional reductions in alertness and additional impairment of central nervous system performance may occur).
No products indexed under this heading.

Ethinamate (Concurrent use of olopatadine nasal spray with other central nervous system depressants should be avoided because additional reductions in alertness and additional impairment of central nervous system performance may occur).
No products indexed under this heading.

Ethyl Alcohol (Concurrent use of olopatadine nasal spray with other central nervous system depressants should be avoided because additional reductions in alertness and additional impairment of central nervous system performance may occur).
No products indexed under this heading.

Fentanyl (Concurrent use of olopatadine nasal spray with other central nervous system depressants should be avoided because additional reductions in alertness and additional impairment of central nervous system performance may occur). Products include:
Duragesic 2604
Fentanyl Transdermal System 2346
Onsolis 2054

Fentanyl Citrate (Concurrent use of olopatadine nasal spray with other central nervous system depressants should be avoided because additional reductions in alertness and additional impairment of central nervous system performance may occur). Products include:
Fentora 966

Fluphenazine Decanoate (Concurrent use of olopatadine nasal spray with other central nervous system depressants should be avoided because additional reductions in alertness and additional impairment of central nervous system performance may occur).
No products indexed under this heading.

Fluphenazine Enanthate (Concurrent use of olopatadine nasal spray with other central nervous system depressants should be avoided because additional reductions in alertness and additional impairment of central nervous system performance may occur).
No products indexed under this heading.

Fluphenazine Hydrochloride (Concurrent use of olopatadine nasal spray with other central nervous system depressants should be avoided because additional reductions in alertness and additional impairment of central nervous system performance may occur).
No products indexed under this heading.

Flurazepam Hydrochloride (Concurrent use of olopatadine nasal spray with other central nervous system depressants should be avoided because additional reductions in alertness and additional impairment of central nervous system performance may occur).
No products indexed under this heading.

Glutethimide (Concurrent use of olopatadine nasal spray with other central nervous system depressants should be avoided because additional reductions in alertness and additional impairment of central nervous system performance may occur).
No products indexed under this heading.

Halazepam (Concurrent use of olopatadine nasal spray with other central nervous system depressants should be avoided because additional reductions in alertness and additional impairment of central nervous system performance may occur).
No products indexed under this heading.

Haloperidol (Concurrent use of olopatadine nasal spray with other central nervous system depressants should be avoided because additional reductions in alertness and additional impairment of central nervous system performance may occur).
No products indexed under this heading.

Haloperidol Decanoate (Concurrent use of olopatadine nasal spray with other central nervous system depressants should be avoided because additional reductions in alertness and additional impairment of central nervous system performance may occur).
No products indexed under this heading.

Haloperidol Lactate (Concurrent use of olopatadine nasal spray with other central nervous system depressants should be avoided because additional reductions in alertness and additional impairment of central nervous system performance may occur).
No products indexed under this heading.

Hexobarbital (Concurrent use of olopatadine nasal spray with other central nervous system depressants should be avoided because additional reductions in alertness and additional impairment of central nervous system performance may occur).
No products indexed under this heading.

Hydrocodone Bitartrate (Concurrent use of olopatadine nasal spray with other central nervous system depressants should be avoided because additional reductions in alertness and additional impairment of central nervous system performance may occur). Products include:
Vicodin 560
Vicodin ES 561
Vicodin HP 563
Vicoprofen 564
Zydone 1138

Hydrocodone Polistirex (Concurrent use of olopatadine nasal spray with other central nervous system depressants should be avoided because additional reductions in alertness and additional impairment of central nervous system performance may occur). Products include:
Tussionex 3443

Hydromorphone (Concurrent use of olopatadine nasal spray with other central nervous system depressants should be avoided because additional reductions in alertness and additional impairment of central nervous system performance may occur).
No products indexed under this heading.

Hydromorphone Hydrochloride (Concurrent use of olopatadine nasal spray with other central nervous system depressants should be avoided because additional reductions in alertness and additional impairment of central nervous system performance may occur). Products include:
Dilaudid Injection 2800
Dilaudid Oral 2797
Dilaudid Tablets 2797
Dilaudid-HP 2800

Hydroxyzine Hydrochloride (Concurrent use of olopatadine nasal spray with other central nervous system depressants should be avoided because additional reductions in alertness and additional impairment of central nervous system performance may occur).
No products indexed under this heading.

Isoflurane (Concurrent use of olopatadine nasal spray with other central nervous system depressants should be avoided because additional reductions in alertness and additional impairment of central nervous system performance may occur).
No products indexed under this heading.

Ketamine Hydrochloride (Concurrent use of olopatadine nasal spray with other central nervous system depressants should be avoided because additional reductions in alertness and additional impairment of central nervous system performance may occur).
No products indexed under this heading.

Levomethadyl Acetate Hydrochloride (Concurrent use of olopatadine nasal spray with other central nervous system depressants should be avoided because additional reductions in alertness and additional impairment of central nervous system performance may occur).
No products indexed under this heading.

Levorphanol Tartrate (Concurrent use of olopatadine nasal spray with other central nervous system depressants should be avoided because additional reductions in alertness and additional impairment of central nervous system performance may occur).
No products indexed under this heading.

IMPORTANT NOTE: Always consult each drug listing in the patient's regimen for possible interactions.

(☉ Described in PDR® for Ophthalmic Medicines)

Sufentanil Citrate (Concurrent use of olopatadine nasal spray with other central nervous system depressants should be avoided because additional reductions in alertness and additional impairment of central nervous system performance may occur).
No products indexed under this heading.

Talbutal (Concurrent use of olopatadine nasal spray with other central nervous system depressants should be avoided because additional reductions in alertness and additional impairment of central nervous system performance may occur).
No products indexed under this heading.

Temazepam (Concurrent use of olopatadine nasal spray with other central nervous system depressants should be avoided because additional reductions in alertness and additional impairment of central nervous system performance may occur).
No products indexed under this heading.

Thiamylal Sodium (Concurrent use of olopatadine nasal spray with other central nervous system depressants should be avoided because additional reductions in alertness and additional impairment of central nervous system performance may occur).
No products indexed under this heading.

Thioridazine (Concurrent use of olopatadine nasal spray with other central nervous system depressants should be avoided because additional reductions in alertness and additional impairment of central nervous system performance may occur).
No products indexed under this heading.

Thioridazine Hydrochloride (Concurrent use of olopatadine nasal spray with other central nervous system depressants should be avoided because additional reductions in alertness and additional impairment of central nervous system performance may occur). Products include:
Thioridazine Hydrochloride 2384

Thiothixene (Concurrent use of olopatadine nasal spray with other central nervous system depressants should be avoided because additional reductions in alertness and additional impairment of central nervous system performance may occur). Products include:
Thiothixene 2386

Thiothixene Hydrochloride (Concurrent use of olopatadine nasal spray with other central nervous system depressants should be avoided because additional reductions in alertness and additional impairment of central nervous system performance may occur).
No products indexed under this heading.

Triazolam (Concurrent use of olopatadine nasal spray with other central nervous system depressants should be avoided because additional reductions in alertness and additional impairment of central nervous system performance may occur).
No products indexed under this heading.

Trifluoperazine Hydrochloride (Concurrent use of olopatadine nasal spray with other central nervous system depressants should be avoided because additional reductions in alertness and additional impairment of central nervous system performance may occur).
No products indexed under this heading.

Zaleplon (Concurrent use of olopatadine nasal spray with other central nervous system depressants should be avoided because additional reductions in alertness and additional impairment of central nervous system performance may occur).
No products indexed under this heading.

Ziprasidone Hydrochloride (Concurrent use of olopatadine nasal spray with other central nervous system depressants should be avoided because additional reductions in alertness and additional impairment of central nervous system performance may occur). Products include:
Geodon 2723

Zolpidem Tartrate (Concurrent use of olopatadine nasal spray with other central nervous system depressants should be avoided because additional reductions in alertness and additional impairment of central nervous system performance may occur). Products include:
Ambien 2920
Ambien CR 2925

Food Interactions

Alcohol (Concurrent use of olopatadine nasal spray with other central nervous system depressants should be avoided because additional reductions in alertness and additional impairment of central nervous system performance may occur).

Beer, reduced-alcohol (Concurrent use of olopatadine nasal spray with alcohol should be avoided because additional reductions in alertness and additional impairment of central nervous system performance may occur).

Beer, unspecified (Concurrent use of olopatadine nasal spray with alcohol should be avoided because additional reductions in alertness and additional impairment of central nervous system performance may occur).

Wine, Chianti (Concurrent use of olopatadine nasal spray with alcohol should be avoided because additional reductions in alertness and additional impairment of central nervous system performance may occur).

Wine, Red (Concurrent use of olopatadine nasal spray with alcohol should be avoided because additional reductions in alertness and additional impairment of central nervous system performance may occur).

Wine, unspecified (Concurrent use of olopatadine nasal spray with alcohol should be avoided because additional reductions in alertness and additional impairment of central nervous system performance may occur).

Wine products (Concurrent use of olopatadine nasal spray with alcohol should be avoided because additional reductions in alertness and additional impairment of central nervous system performance may occur).

PAXIL ORAL SUSPENSION
(Paroxetine Hydrochloride) 1586
See Paxil Tablets

PAXIL TABLETS
(Paroxetine Hydrochloride) 1586
May interact with 5HT1-receptor agonists, alcohols, anticoagulants, antipsychotic agents, aspirin-acetylsalicylic acid, class IC antiarrhythmics, cytochrome p450 2d6 inhibitors (selected), cytochrome p450 2d6 substrates (selected), diuretics, dopamine antagonists, drugs affecting hepatic drug metabolizing enzyme systems, highly protein bound drugs (selected), lithium preparations, monoamine oxidase inhibitors, non-steroidal anti-inflammatory agents, oral anticoagulants, phenothiazines, phenytoin, quinidine, selective serotonin reuptake inhibitors, serotonin and norepinephrine reuptake inhibitors, serotoninergic agents, theophyllines, tricyclic antidepressants, triptans, and certain other agents. Compounds in these categories include:

Almotriptan Malate (The development of a potentially life-threatening

serotonin syndrome or Neuroleptic Malignant Syndrome (NMS)-like reactions have been reported with paroxetine alone, but particularly, with concomitant use of serotonergic drugs (including triptans). Patients should be monitored for the emergence of serotonin syndrome or NMS-like signs and symptoms. Treatment with paroxetine and any concomitant serotonergic agent should be discontinued immediately if any signs or symptoms of serotonin syndrome or NMS-like signs and symptoms occur and supportive symptomatic treatment should be initiated. If concomitant use of paroxetine with a triptan is clinically warranted, careful observation of the patient is advised, particularly during treatment initiation and dose increases). Products include:
Axert 2593

Amiloride Hydrochloride (Hyponatremia may occur as a result of treatment with paroxetine. Patients taking diuretics may be at greater risk).
No products indexed under this heading.

Amiodarone Hydrochloride (Because paroxetine is highly bound to plasma protein, administration of paroxetine to a patient taking another drug that is highly protein bound may cause increased free concentrations of the other drug, potentially resulting in adverse events. Conversely, adverse effects could result from displacement of paroxetine by other highly bound drugs).
No products indexed under this heading.

Amitriptyline Hydrochloride (Caution is indicated in the co-administration of tricyclic antidepressants (TCAs) with paroxetine, because paroxetine may inhibit TCA metabolism. Plasma TCA concentrations may need to be monitored, and the dose of TCA may need to be reduced if a TCA is co-administered with paroxetine).
No products indexed under this heading.

Amoxapine (Caution is indicated in the co-administration of tricyclic antidepressants (TCAs) with paroxetine, because paroxetine may inhibit TCA metabolism. Plasma TCA concentrations may need to be monitored, and the dose of TCA may need to be reduced if a TCA is co-administered with paroxetine).
No products indexed under this heading.

Amphetamine Aspartate (Paroxetine is metabolized by CYP2D6. Like other agents that are metabolized by CYP2D6, paroxetine may significantly inhibit the activity of this isoenzyme. Co-administration of paroxetine with other drugs that are metabolized by CYP2D6 should be approached with caution and may require lower doses than usually prescribed for either paroxetine or the other drug metabolized by CYP2D6).
No products indexed under this heading.

Amphetamine Aspartate Monohydrate (Paroxetine is metabolized by CYP2D6. Like other agents that are metabolized by CYP2D6, paroxetine may significantly inhibit the activity of this isoenzyme. Co-administration of paroxetine with other drugs that are metabolized by CYP2D6 should be approached with caution and may require lower doses than usually prescribed for either paroxetine or the other drug metabolized by CYP2D6).
No products indexed under this heading.

Amphetamine Sulfate (Paroxetine is metabolized by CYP2D6. Like other agents that are metabolized by CYP2D6, paroxetine may significantly inhibit the activity of this isoenzyme. Co-administration of paroxetine with other drugs that are metabolized by CYP2D6 should be approached with caution and may require lower doses

than usually prescribed for either paroxetine or the other drug metabolized by CYP2D6).
No products indexed under this heading.

Anisindione (Paroxetine may increase the risk of bleeding events, including upper gastrointestinal bleeding. Concomitant use of paroxetine with anticoagulants may increase this risk).
No products indexed under this heading.

Ardeparin Sodium (Concomitant use of paroxetine with drugs affecting coagulation, may increase the risk of bleeding including upper gastrointestinal bleeding).
No products indexed under this heading.

Aripiprazole (The development of a potentially life-threatening serotonin syndrome or Neuroleptic Malignant Syndrome (NMS)-like reactions have been reported with paroxetine alone, but particularly with concomitant use of antipsychotic agents. Patients should be monitored for the emergence of serotonin syndrome or NMS-like signs and symptoms. Treatment with paroxetine and any concomitant antipsychotic should be discontinued immediately if any signs or symptoms of serotonin syndrome or NMS-like signs or symptoms occur and supportive symptomatic treatment should be initiated).
No products indexed under this heading.

Aspirin (Paroxetine may increase the risk of bleeding events, including upper gastrointestinal bleeding. Concomitant use of paroxetine with aspirin may increase this risk). Products include:
Aggrenox 880
Bayer Aspirin 829
Percodan 1124
St. Joseph Aspirin 2045

Aspirin, Enteric Coated (Paroxetine may increase the risk of bleeding events, including upper gastrointestinal bleeding. Concomitant use of paroxetine with aspirin may increase this risk).
No products indexed under this heading.

Aspirin Buffered (Paroxetine may increase the risk of bleeding events, including upper gastrointestinal bleeding. Concomitant use of paroxetine with aspirin may increase this risk).
No products indexed under this heading.

Atomoxetine Hydrochloride (Paroxetine is metabolized by CYP2D6. Like other agents that are metabolized by CYP2D6, paroxetine may significantly inhibit the activity of this isoenzyme. Concomitant use of paroxetine with atomoxetine has resulted in increases in steady state atomoxetine AUC values that were 6- to 8-fold greater and in atomoxetine C_{max} values that were 3- to 4-fold greater than when atomoxetine was given alone. Dosage adjustment of atomoxetine may be necessary and it is recommended that atomoxetine be initiated at a reduced dose when it is given with paroxetine). Products include:
Strattera 1957

Atovaquone (Because paroxetine is highly bound to plasma protein, administration of paroxetine to a patient taking another drug that is highly protein bound may cause increased free concentrations of the other drug, potentially resulting in adverse events. Conversely, adverse effects could result from displacement of paroxetine by other highly bound drugs). Products include:
Malarone Pediatric Tablets 1572
Malarone 1572
Mepron Suspension 1576

Bendroflumethiazide (Hyponatremia may occur as a result of treatment with paroxetine. Patients taking diuretics may be at greater risk).
No products indexed under this heading.

Bisoprolol Fumarate (Paroxetine is metabolized by CYP2D6. Like other

Paxil Interactions Index 1384

agents that are metabolized by CYP2D6, paroxetine may significantly inhibit the activity of this isoenzyme. Co-administration of paroxetine with other drugs that are metabolized by CYP2D6 should be approached with caution and may require lower doses than usually prescribed for either paroxetine or the other drug metabolized by CYP2D6).
No products indexed under this heading.

Bumetanide (Hyponatremia may occur as a result of treatment with paroxetine. Patients taking diuretics may be at greater risk).
No products indexed under this heading.

Bupropion Hydrochloride (Co-administration of paroxetine with drugs that inhibit CYP2D6 should be approached with caution). Products include:
Aplenzin **2948**
Wellbutrin **1719**
Wellbutrin SR **1725**
Zyban **1762**

Captopril (Paroxetine is metabolized by CYP2D6. Like other agents that are metabolized by CYP2D6, paroxetine may significantly inhibit the activity of this isoenzyme. Co-administration of paroxetine with other drugs that are metabolized by CYP2D6 should be approached with caution and may require lower doses than usually prescribed for either paroxetine or the other drug metabolized by CYP2D6). Products include:
Captopril **2341**

Carbamazepine (The metabolism and pharmacokinetics of paroxetine may be affected by the induction or inhibition of drug metabolizing enzymes). Products include:
Carbatrol **3280**
Equetro **3477**

Carvedilol (Paroxetine is metabolized by CYP2D6. Like other agents that are metabolized by CYP2D6, paroxetine may significantly inhibit the activity of this isoenzyme. Co-administration of paroxetine with other drugs that are metabolized by CYP2D6 should be approached with caution and may require lower doses than usually prescribed for either paroxetine or the other drug metabolized by CYP2D6). Products include:
Coreg **1409**

Cefonicid Sodium (Because paroxetine is highly bound to plasma protein, administration of paroxetine to a patient taking another drug that is highly protein bound may cause increased free concentrations of the other drug, potentially resulting in adverse events. Conversely, adverse effects could result from displacement of paroxetine by other highly bound drugs).
No products indexed under this heading.

Celecoxib (Paroxetine may increase the risk of bleeding events, including upper gastrointestinal bleeding. Concomitant use of paroxetine with NSAIDs may increase this risk). Products include:
Celebrex **3272**

Cevimeline Hydrochloride (Paroxetine is metabolized by CYP2D6. Like other agents that are metabolized by CYP2D6, paroxetine may significantly inhibit the activity of this isoenzyme. Co-administration of paroxetine with other drugs that are metabolized by CYP2D6 should be approached with caution and may require lower doses than usually prescribed for either paroxetine or the other drug metabolized by CYP2D6). Products include:
Evoxac **1027**

Chlordiazepoxide (Because paroxetine is highly bound to plasma protein, administration of paroxetine to a patient taking another drug that is highly protein bound may cause increased free concentrations of the other drug, potentially resulting in adverse events. Conversely, adverse effects could result from displacement of paroxetine by other highly bound drugs).
No products indexed under this heading.

Chlordiazepoxide Hydrochloride (Because paroxetine is highly bound to plasma protein, administration of paroxetine to a patient taking another drug that is highly protein bound may cause increased free concentrations of the other drug, potentially resulting in adverse events. Conversely, adverse effects could result from displacement of paroxetine by other highly bound drugs).
No products indexed under this heading.

Chloroquine (Co-administration of paroxetine with drugs that inhibit CYP2D6 should be approached with caution).
No products indexed under this heading.

Chloroquine Hydrochloride (Co-administration of paroxetine with drugs that inhibit CYP2D6 should be approached with caution).
No products indexed under this heading.

Chloroquine Phosphate (Co-administration of paroxetine with drugs that inhibit CYP2D6 should be approached with caution).
No products indexed under this heading.

Chlorothiazide (Hyponatremia may occur as a result of treatment with paroxetine. Patients taking diuretics may be at greater risk).
No products indexed under this heading.

Chlorothiazide Sodium (Hyponatremia may occur as a result of treatment with paroxetine. Patients taking diuretics may be at greater risk). Products include:
Diuril Intravenous **2009**

Chlorpheniramine (Co-administration of paroxetine with drugs that inhibit CYP2D6 should be approached with caution).
No products indexed under this heading.

Chlorpheniramine Maleate (Co-administration of paroxetine with drugs that inhibit CYP2D6 should be approached with caution).
No products indexed under this heading.

Chlorpheniramine Polistirex (Co-administration of paroxetine with drugs that inhibit CYP2D6 should be approached with caution). Products include:
Tussionex **3443**

Chlorpheniramine Tannate (Co-administration of paroxetine with drugs that inhibit CYP2D6 should be approached with caution).
No products indexed under this heading.

Chlorpromazine (Paroxetine is metabolized by CYP2D6. Like other agents that are metabolized by CYP2D6, paroxetine may significantly inhibit the activity of this isoenzyme. Co-administration of paroxetine with other drugs that are metabolized by CYP2D6, such as phentothiazines, should be approached with caution and lower doses than usual may need to be prescribed for paroxetine or the phenothiazine).
No products indexed under this heading.

Chlorpromazine Hydrochloride (Paroxetine is metabolized by CYP2D6. Like other agents that are metabolized by CYP2D6, paroxetine may significantly inhibit the activity of this isoenzyme. Co-administration of paroxetine with other drugs that are metabolized by CYP2D6, such as phentothiazines, should be approached with caution and lower doses than usual may need to be prescribed for paroxetine or the phenothiazine).
No products indexed under this heading.

Chlorpropamide (Paroxetine is metabolized by CYP2D6. Like other agents that are metabolized by CYP2D6, paroxetine may significantly inhibit the activity of this isoenzyme. Co-administration of paroxetine with other drugs that are metabolized by CYP2D6 should be approached with caution and may require lower doses than usually prescribed for either paroxetine or the other drug metabolized by CYP2D6).
No products indexed under this heading.

Chlorprothixene (The development of a potentially life-threatening serotonin syndrome or Neuroleptic Malignant Syndrome (NMS)-like reactions have been reported with paroxetine alone, but particularly with concomitant use of antipsychotic agents. Patients should be monitored for the emergence of serotonin syndrome or NMS-like signs and symptoms. Treatment with paroxetine and any concomitant antipsychotic should be discontinued immediately if any signs or symptoms of serotonin syndrome or NMS-like signs or symptoms occur and supportive symptomatic treatment should be initiated).
No products indexed under this heading.

Chlorprothixene Hydrochloride (The development of a potentially life-threatening serotonin syndrome or Neuroleptic Malignant Syndrome (NMS)-like reactions have been reported with paroxetine alone, but particularly with concomitant use of antipsychotic agents. Patients should be monitored for the emergence of serotonin syndrome or NMS-like signs and symptoms. Treatment with paroxetine and any concomitant antipsychotic should be discontinued immediately if any signs or symptoms of serotonin syndrome or NMS-like signs or symptoms occur and supportive symptomatic treatment should be initiated).
No products indexed under this heading.

Chlorprothixene Lactate (The development of a potentially life-threatening serotonin syndrome or Neuroleptic Malignant Syndrome (NMS)-like reactions have been reported with paroxetine alone, but particularly with concomitant use of antipsychotic agents. Patients should be monitored for the emergence of serotonin syndrome or NMS-like signs and symptoms. Treatment with paroxetine and any concomitant antipsychotic should be discontinued immediately if any signs or symptoms of serotonin syndrome or NMS-like signs or symptoms occur and supportive symptomatic treatment should be initiated).
No products indexed under this heading.

Chlorthalidone (Hyponatremia may occur as a result of treatment with paroxetine. Patients taking diuretics may be at greater risk). Products include:
Clorpres **2344**

Cimetidine (Cimetidine inhibits many cytochrome P_{450} (oxidative) enzymes. In a study where paroxetine (30 mg once daily) was dosed orally for 4 weeks, steady-state plasma concentrations of paroxetine were increased by approximately 50% during co-administration with oral cimetidine (300 mg three times daily) for the final week. Therefore, when these drugs are administered concurrently, dosage adjustment of paroxetine after the 20 mg starting dose should be guided by clinical effect).
No products indexed under this heading.

Cimetidine Hydrochloride (Cimetidine inhibits many cytochrome P_{450} (oxidative) enzymes. In a study where paroxetine (30 mg once daily) was dosed orally for 4 weeks, steady-state plasma concentrations of paroxetine were increased by approximately 50% during co-administration with oral cimetidine (300 mg three times daily) for the final week. Therefore, when these drugs are administered concurrently, dosage adjustment of paroxetine after the 20 mg starting dose should be guided by clinical effect).
No products indexed under this heading.

Citalopram Hydrobromide (The development of a potentially life-threatening serotonin syndrome or Neuroleptic Malignant Syndrome (NMS)-like reactions have been reported with paroxetine alone, but particularly, with concomitant use of serotonergic drugs. The concomitant use of paroxetine with other SSRIs is not recommended). Products include:
Celexa **1153**

Clomipramine Hydrochloride (Caution is indicated in the co-administration of tricyclic antidepressants (TCAs) with paroxetine, because paroxetine may inhibit TCA metabolism. Plasma TCA concentrations may need to be monitored, and the dose of TCA may need to be reduced if a TCA is co-administered with paroxetine).
No products indexed under this heading.

Clozapine (The development of a potentially life-threatening serotonin syndrome or Neuroleptic Malignant Syndrome (NMS)-like reactions have been reported with paroxetine alone, but particularly with concomitant use of antipsychotic agents. Patients should be monitored for the emergence of serotonin syndrome or NMS-like signs and symptoms. Treatment with paroxetine and any concomitant antipsychotic should be discontinued immediately if any signs or symptoms of serotonin syndrome or NMS-like signs or symptoms occur and supportive symptomatic treatment should be initiated).
No products indexed under this heading.

Cocaine Hydrochloride (Co-administration of paroxetine with drugs that inhibit CYP2D6 should be approached with caution).
No products indexed under this heading.

Codeine Phosphate (Paroxetine is metabolized by CYP2D6. Like other agents that are metabolized by CYP2D6, paroxetine may significantly inhibit the activity of this isoenzyme. Co-administration of paroxetine with other drugs that are metabolized by CYP2D6 should be approached with caution and may require lower doses than usually prescribed for either paroxetine or the other drug metabolized by CYP2D6). Products include:
Tylenol with Codeine **2691**

Codeine Sulfate (Paroxetine is metabolized by CYP2D6. Like other agents that are metabolized by CYP2D6, paroxetine may significantly inhibit the activity of this isoenzyme. Co-administration of paroxetine with other drugs that are metabolized by CYP2D6 should be approached with caution and may require lower doses than usually prescribed for either paroxetine or the other drug metabolized by CYP2D6).
No products indexed under this heading.

Cyclobenzaprine Hydrochloride (Paroxetine is metabolized by CYP2D6. Like other agents that are metabolized by CYP2D6, paroxetine may significantly inhibit the activity of this isoenzyme. Co-administration of paroxetine with other drugs that are metabolized by CYP2D6 should be approached with

caution and may require lower doses than usually prescribed for either paroxetine or the other drug metabolized by CYP2D6). Products include:

Cyclosporine (Because paroxetine is highly bound to plasma protein, administration of paroxetine to a patient taking another drug that is highly protein bound may cause increased free concentrations of the other drug, potentially resulting in adverse events. Conversely, adverse effects could result from displacement of paroxetine by other highly bound drugs). Products include:

Dalteparin Sodium (Concomitant use of paroxetine with drugs affecting coagulation, may increase the risk of bleeding including upper gastrointestinal bleeding). Products include:

Danaparoid Sodium (Concomitant use of paroxetine with drugs affecting coagulation, may increase the risk of bleeding including upper gastrointestinal bleeding).

No products indexed under this heading.

Debrisoquine (Paroxetine is metabolized by CYP2D6. Like other agents that are metabolized by CYP2D6, paroxetine may significantly inhibit the activity of this isoenzyme. Co-administration of paroxetine with other drugs that are metabolized by CYP2D6 should be approached with caution and may require lower doses than usually prescribed for either paroxetine or the other drug metabolized by CYP2D6).

No products indexed under this heading.

Desipramine Hydrochloride (Paroxetine is metabolized by CYP2D6. Like other agents that are metabolized by CYP2D6, paroxetine may significantly inhibit the activity of this isoenzyme. In one study, daily dosing of paroxetine (20 mg once daily) under steady-state conditions increased single dose desipramine (100 mg) C_{max}, AUC, and $T_{1/2}$ by an average of approximately 2-, 5-, and 3-fold, respectively. Co-administration of paroxetine with other drugs that are metabolized by CYP2D6, such as desipramine, should be approached with caution. If co-administered, plasma concentrations of desipramine may need to be monitored and a lower dose of paroxetine or desipramine may be required).

No products indexed under this heading.

Desvenlafaxine Succinate (The development of a potentially life-threatening serotonin syndrome or Neuroleptic Malignant Syndrome (NMS)-like reactions have been reported with paroxetine alone, but particularly, with concomitant use of serotonergic drugs. The concomitant use of paroxetine with SNRIs is not recommended). Products include:

Dexfenfluramine Hydrochloride (Paroxetine is metabolized by CYP2D6. Like other agents that are metabolized by CYP2D6, paroxetine may significantly inhibit the activity of this isoenzyme. Co-administration of paroxetine with other drugs that are metabolized by CYP2D6 should be approached with caution and may require lower doses than usually prescribed for either paroxetine or the other drug metabolized by CYP2D6).

No products indexed under this heading.

Dextromethorphan Hydrobromide (Paroxetine is metabolized by CYP2D6. Like other agents that are metabolized by CYP2D6, paroxetine may significant-

ly inhibit the activity of this isoenzyme. Co-administration of paroxetine with other drugs that are metabolized by CYP2D6 should be approached with caution and may require lower doses than usually prescribed for either paroxetine or the other drug metabolized by CYP2D6).

No products indexed under this heading.

Dextromethorphan Polistirex (Paroxetine is metabolized by CYP2D6. Like other agents that are metabolized by CYP2D6, paroxetine may significantly inhibit the activity of this isoenzyme. Co-administration of paroxetine with other drugs that are metabolized by CYP2D6 should be approached with caution and may require lower doses than usually prescribed for either paroxetine or the other drug metabolized by CYP2D6).

No products indexed under this heading.

Diazepam (Because paroxetine is highly bound to plasma protein, administration of paroxetine to a patient taking another drug that is highly protein bound may cause increased free concentrations of the other drug, potentially resulting in adverse events. Conversely, adverse effects could result from displacement of paroxetine by other highly bound drugs). Products include:

Diclofenac Epolamine (Paroxetine may increase the risk of bleeding events, including upper gastrointestinal bleeding. Concomitant use of paroxetine with NSAIDs may increase this risk). Products include:

Diclofenac Potassium (Paroxetine may increase the risk of bleeding events, including upper gastrointestinal bleeding. Concomitant use of paroxetine with NSAIDs may increase this risk).

No products indexed under this heading.

Diclofenac Sodium (Paroxetine may increase the risk of bleeding events, including upper gastrointestinal bleeding. Concomitant use of paroxetine with NSAIDs may increase this risk).

No products indexed under this heading.

Dicumarol (Paroxetine may increase the risk of bleeding events, including upper gastrointestinal bleeding. Concomitant use of paroxetine with anticoagulants may increase this risk).

No products indexed under this heading.

Digitalis Glycoside Preparations (Because paroxetine is highly bound to plasma protein, administration of paroxetine to a patient taking another drug that is highly protein bound may cause increased free concentrations of the other drug, potentially resulting in adverse events. Conversely, adverse effects could result from displacement of paroxetine by other highly bound drugs).

No products indexed under this heading.

Digitalis Lanata (Because paroxetine is highly bound to plasma protein, administration of paroxetine to a patient taking another drug that is highly protein bound may cause increased free concentrations of the other drug, potentially resulting in adverse events. Conversely, adverse effects could result from displacement of paroxetine by other highly bound drugs).

No products indexed under this heading.

Digitalis Purpurea (Because paroxetine is highly bound to plasma protein, administration of paroxetine to a patient taking another drug that is highly protein bound may cause increased free concentrations of the other drug, potentially resulting in adverse events. Conversely, adverse effects could result from displacement of paroxetine by other highly bound drugs).

No products indexed under this heading.

Digoxin (The steady-state pharmacokinetics of paroxetine was not altered when administered with digoxin at steady state. Mean digoxin AUC at steady state decreased by 15% in the presence of paroxetine. Since there is little clinical experience, the concurrent administration of paroxetine and digoxin should be undertaken with caution). Products include:

Diphenhydramine (Co-administration of paroxetine with drugs that inhibit CYP2D6 should be approached with caution).

No products indexed under this heading.

Diphenhydramine Hydrochloride (Co-administration of paroxetine with drugs that inhibit CYP2D6 should be approached with caution). Products include:

Dipyridamole (Because paroxetine is highly bound to plasma protein, administration of paroxetine to a patient taking another drug that is highly protein bound may cause increased free concentrations of the other drug, potentially resulting in adverse events. Conversely, adverse effects could result from displacement of paroxetine by other highly bound drugs). Products include:

Dolasetron Mesylate (Paroxetine is metabolized by CYP2D6. Like other agents that are metabolized by CYP2D6, paroxetine may significantly inhibit the activity of this isoenzyme. Co-administration of paroxetine with other drugs that are metabolized by CYP2D6 should be approached with caution and may require lower doses than usually prescribed for either paroxetine or the other drug metabolized by CYP2D6). Products include:

Donepezil Hydrochloride (Paroxetine is metabolized by CYP2D6. Like other agents that are metabolized by CYP2D6, paroxetine may significantly inhibit the activity of this isoenzyme. Co-administration of paroxetine with other drugs that are metabolized by CYP2D6 should be approached with caution and may require lower doses than usually prescribed for either paroxetine or the other drug metabolized by CYP2D6). Products include:

Doxepin Hydrochloride (Caution is indicated in the co-administration of tricyclic antidepressants (TCAs) with paroxetine, because paroxetine may inhibit TCA metabolism. Plasma TCA concentrations may need to be monitored, and the dose of TCA may need to be reduced if a TCA is co-administered with paroxetine).

No products indexed under this heading.

Duloxetine Hydrochloride (The development of a potentially life-threatening serotonin syndrome or Neuroleptic Malignant Syndrome (NMS)-like reactions have been reported with paroxetine alone, but particularly, with con-

comitant use of serotonergic drugs. The concomitant use of paroxetine with SNRIs is not recommended). Products include:

Eletriptan Hydrobromide (The development of a potentially life-threatening serotonin syndrome or Neuroleptic Malignant Syndrome (NMS)-like reactions have been reported with paroxetine alone, but particularly, with concomitant use of serotonergic drugs (including triptans). Patients should be monitored for the emergence of serotonin syndrome or NMS-like signs and symptoms. Treatment with paroxetine and any concomitant serotonergic agent should be discontinued immediately if any signs or symptoms of serotonin syndrome or NMS-like signs and symptoms occur and supportive symptomatic treatment should be initiated. If concomitant use of paroxetine with a triptan is clinically warranted, careful observation of the patient is advised, particularly during treatment initiation and dose increases).

No products indexed under this heading.

Encainide Hydrochloride (Co-administration of paroxetine with other drugs which are metabolized by CYP2D6, including Type 1C antiarrhythmics (eg, propafenone, flecainide, encainide), should be approached with caution).

No products indexed under this heading.

Enoxaparin Sodium (Concomitant use of paroxetine with drugs affecting coagulation, may increase the risk of bleeding including upper gastrointestinal bleeding). Products include:

Erythromycin (The metabolism and pharmacokinetics of paroxetine may be affected by the induction or inhibition of drug metabolizing enzymes).

No products indexed under this heading.

Erythromycin Estolate (The metabolism and pharmacokinetics of paroxetine may be affected by the induction or inhibition of drug metabolizing enzymes).

No products indexed under this heading.

Erythromycin Ethylsuccinate (The metabolism and pharmacokinetics of paroxetine may be affected by the induction or inhibition of drug metabolizing enzymes). Products include:

Erythromycin Gluceptate (The metabolism and pharmacokinetics of paroxetine may be affected by the induction or inhibition of drug metabolizing enzymes).

No products indexed under this heading.

Erythromycin Lactobionate (The metabolism and pharmacokinetics of paroxetine may be affected by the induction or inhibition of drug metabolizing enzymes).

No products indexed under this heading.

Erythromycin Stearate (The metabolism and pharmacokinetics of paroxetine may be affected by the induction or inhibition of drug metabolizing enzymes).

No products indexed under this heading.

Escitalopram Oxalate (The development of a potentially life-threatening serotonin syndrome or Neuroleptic Malignant Syndrome (NMS)-like reactions have been reported with paroxetine alone, but particularly, with concomitant use of serotonergic drugs. The concomitant use of paroxetine with other SSRIs is not recommended). Products include:

Ethacrynic Acid (Hyponatremia may occur as a result of treatment with paroxetine. Patients taking diuretics may be at greater risk).
No products indexed under this heading.

Ethanol (Although paroxetine has not been shown to increase the impairment of mental and motor skills caused by alcohol, patients should be advised to avoid alcohol while taking paroxetine).
No products indexed under this heading.

Ethyl Alcohol (Although paroxetine has not been shown to increase the impairment of mental and motor skills caused by alcohol, patients should be advised to avoid alcohol while taking paroxetine).
No products indexed under this heading.

Etodolac (Paroxetine may increase the risk of bleeding events, including upper gastrointestinal bleeding. Concomitant use of paroxetine with NSAIDs may increase this risk).
No products indexed under this heading.

Fenoprofen Calcium (Paroxetine may increase the risk of bleeding events, including upper gastrointestinal bleeding. Concomitant use of paroxetine with NSAIDs may increase this risk).
No products indexed under this heading.

Fentanyl (Paroxetine is metabolized by CYP2D6. Like other agents that are metabolized by CYP2D6, paroxetine may significantly inhibit the activity of this isoenzyme. Co-administration of paroxetine with other drugs that are metabolized by CYP2D6 should be approached with caution and may require lower doses than usually prescribed for either paroxetine or the other drug metabolized by CYP2D6). Products include:
Duragesic 2604
Fentanyl Transdermal System 2346
Onsolis 2054

Fentanyl Citrate (Paroxetine is metabolized by CYP2D6. Like other agents that are metabolized by CYP2D6, paroxetine may significantly inhibit the activity of this isoenzyme. Co-administration of paroxetine with other drugs that are metabolized by CYP2D6 should be approached with caution and may require lower doses than usually prescribed for either paroxetine or the other drug metabolized by CYP2D6). Products include:
Fentora 966

Flecainide Acetate (Co-administration of paroxetine with other drugs which are metabolized by CYP2D6, including Type 1C antiarrhythmics (eg, propafenone, flecainide, encainide), should be approached with caution).
No products indexed under this heading.

Fluoxetine (The development of a potentially life-threatening serotonin syndrome or Neuroleptic Malignant Syndrome (NMS)-like reactions have been reported with paroxetine alone, but particularly, with concomitant use of serotonergic drugs. The concomitant use of paroxetine with other SSRIs is not recommended).
No products indexed under this heading.

Fluoxetine Hydrochloride (The development of a potentially life-threatening serotonin syndrome or Neuroleptic Malignant Syndrome (NMS)-like reactions have been reported with paroxetine alone, but particularly, with concomitant use of serotonergic drugs. The concomitant use of paroxetine with other SSRIs is not recommended). Products include:
Prozac Weekly 1941
Prozac Pulvules 1941
Symbyax 1965

Fluphenazine Decanoate (Paroxetine is metabolized by CYP2D6. Like

other agents that are metabolized by CYP2D6, paroxetine may significantly inhibit the activity of this isoenzyme. Co-administration of paroxetine with other drugs that are metabolized by CYP2D6, such as phentothiazines, should be approached with caution and lower doses than usual may need to be prescribed for paroxetine or the phenothiazine).
No products indexed under this heading.

Fluphenazine Enanthate (Paroxetine is metabolized by CYP2D6. Like other agents that are metabolized by CYP2D6, paroxetine may significantly inhibit the activity of this isoenzyme. Co-administration of paroxetine with other drugs that are metabolized by CYP2D6, such as phentothiazines, should be approached with caution and lower doses than usual may need to be prescribed for paroxetine or the phenothiazine).
No products indexed under this heading.

Fluphenazine Hydrochloride (Paroxetine is metabolized by CYP2D6. Like other agents that are metabolized by CYP2D6, paroxetine may significantly inhibit the activity of this isoenzyme. Co-administration of paroxetine with other drugs that are metabolized by CYP2D6, such as phentothiazines, should be approached with caution and lower doses than usual may need to be prescribed for paroxetine or the phenothiazine).
No products indexed under this heading.

Flurazepam Hydrochloride (Because paroxetine is highly bound to plasma protein, administration of paroxetine to a patient taking another drug that is highly protein bound may cause increased free concentrations of the other drug, potentially resulting in adverse events. Conversely, adverse effects could result from displacement of paroxetine by other highly bound drugs).
No products indexed under this heading.

Flurbiprofen (Paroxetine may increase the risk of bleeding events, including upper gastrointestinal bleeding. Concomitant use of paroxetine with NSAIDs may increase this risk).
No products indexed under this heading.

Fluvoxamine (The development of a potentially life-threatening serotonin syndrome or Neuroleptic Malignant Syndrome (NMS)-like reactions have been reported with paroxetine alone, but particularly, with concomitant use of serotonergic drugs. The concomitant use of paroxetine with other SSRIs is not recommended).
No products indexed under this heading.

Fluvoxamine Maleate (The development of a potentially life-threatening serotonin syndrome or Neuroleptic Malignant Syndrome (NMS)-like reactions have been reported with paroxetine alone, but particularly, with concomitant use of serotonergic drugs. The concomitant use of paroxetine with other SSRIs is not recommended).
No products indexed under this heading.

Fondaparinux Sodium (Concomitant use of paroxetine with drugs affecting coagulation, may increase the risk of bleeding including upper gastrointestinal bleeding). Products include:
Arixtra 1320

Formoterol Fumarate (Paroxetine is metabolized by CYP2D6. Like other agents that are metabolized by CYP2D6, paroxetine may significantly inhibit the activity of this isoenzyme. Co-administration of paroxetine with other drugs that are metabolized by CYP2D6 should be approached with caution and may require lower doses

than usually prescribed for either paroxetine or the other drug metabolized by CYP2D6). Products include:
Foradil 3121
Perforomist 3634

Fosamprenavir Calcium (Co-administration of fosamprenavir with paroxetine significantly decreased plasma levels of paroxetine. Any dose adjustment should be guided by clinical effect (tolerability and efficacy)). Products include:
Lexiva Oral Suspension 1558
Lexiva 1558

Fosphenytoin (When a single oral 30 mg dose of paroxetine was administered at phenytoin steady state (300 mg once daily for 14 days), paroxetine AUC and $t_{1/2}$ were reduced (by an average of 50% and 35%, respectively) compared to paroxetine administered alone. Since both drugs exhibit nonlinear pharmacokinetics, the above study may not address the case where two drugs are being chronically dosed. There has been a case report of an elevated phenytoin level after 4 weeks of paroxetine and phenytoin co-administration. No initial dosage adjustments are considered necessary when these drugs are co-administered; any subsequent adjustment should be guided by clinical effect).
No products indexed under this heading.

Fosphenytoin Sodium (When a single oral 30 mg dose of paroxetine was administered at phenytoin steady state (300 mg once daily for 14 days), paroxetine AUC and $t_{1/2}$ were reduced (by an average of 50% and 35%, respectively) compared to paroxetine administered alone. Since both drugs exhibit nonlinear pharmacokinetics, the above study may not address the case where two drugs are being chronically dosed. There has been a case report of an elevated phenytoin level after 4 weeks of paroxetine and phenytoin co-administration. No initial dosage adjustments are considered necessary when these drugs are co-administered; any subsequent adjustment should be guided by clinical effect).
No products indexed under this heading.

Frovatriptan Succinate (The development of a potentially life-threatening serotonin syndrome or Neuroleptic Malignant Syndrome (NMS)-like reactions have been reported with paroxetine alone, but particularly, with concomitant use of serotonergic drugs (including triptans). Patients should be monitored for the emergence of serotonin syndrome or NMS-like signs and symptoms. Treatment with paroxetine and any concomitant serotonergic agent should be discontinued immediately if any signs or symptoms of serotonin syndrome or NMS-like signs and symptoms occur and supportive symptomatic treatment should be initiated. If concomitant use of paroxetine with a triptan is clinically warranted, careful observation of the patient is advised, particularly during treatment initiation and dose increases). Products include:
Frova 1103

Furosemide (Hyponatremia may occur as a result of treatment with paroxetine. Patients taking diuretics may be at greater risk). Products include:
Furosemide 2354

Galantamine Hydrobromide (Paroxetine is metabolized by CYP2D6. Like other agents that are metabolized by CYP2D6, paroxetine may significantly inhibit the activity of this isoenzyme. Co-administration of paroxetine with other drugs that are metabolized by CYP2D6 should be approached with caution and may require lower doses

than usually prescribed for either paroxetine or the other drug metabolized by CYP2D6).
No products indexed under this heading.

Glipizide (Because paroxetine is highly bound to plasma protein, administration of paroxetine to a patient taking another drug that is highly protein bound may cause increased free concentrations of the other drug, potentially resulting in adverse events. Conversely, adverse effects could result from displacement of paroxetine by other highly bound drugs).
No products indexed under this heading.

Halofantrine Hydrochloride (Co-administration of paroxetine with drugs that inhibit CYP2D6 should be approached with caution).
No products indexed under this heading.

Haloperidol (The development of a potentially life-threatening serotonin syndrome or Neuroleptic Malignant Syndrome (NMS)-like reactions have been reported with paroxetine alone, but particularly with concomitant use of antipsychotic agents. Patients should be monitored for the emergence of serotonin syndrome or NMS-like signs and symptoms. Treatment with paroxetine and any concomitant antipsychotic should be discontinued immediately if any signs or symptoms of serotonin syndrome or NMS-like signs or symptoms occur and supportive symptomatic treatment should be initiated).
No products indexed under this heading.

Haloperidol Decanoate (The development of a potentially life-threatening serotonin syndrome or Neuroleptic Malignant Syndrome (NMS)-like reactions have been reported with paroxetine alone, but particularly with concomitant use of antipsychotic agents. Patients should be monitored for the emergence of serotonin syndrome or NMS-like signs and symptoms. Treatment with paroxetine and any concomitant antipsychotic should be discontinued immediately if any signs or symptoms of serotonin syndrome or NMS-like signs or symptoms occur and supportive symptomatic treatment should be initiated).
No products indexed under this heading.

Haloperidol Lactate (The development of a potentially life-threatening serotonin syndrome or Neuroleptic Malignant Syndrome (NMS)-like reactions have been reported with paroxetine alone, but particularly with concomitant use of antipsychotic agents. Patients should be monitored for the emergence of serotonin syndrome or NMS-like signs and symptoms. Treatment with paroxetine and any concomitant antipsychotic should be discontinued immediately if any signs or symptoms of serotonin syndrome or NMS-like signs or symptoms occur and supportive symptomatic treatment should be initiated).
No products indexed under this heading.

Heparin Calcium (Concomitant use of paroxetine with drugs affecting coagulation, may increase the risk of bleeding including upper gastrointestinal bleeding).
No products indexed under this heading.

Heparin Sodium (Concomitant use of paroxetine with drugs affecting coagulation, may increase the risk of bleeding including upper gastrointestinal bleeding).
No products indexed under this heading.

Hydrochlorothiazide (Hyponatremia may occur as a result of treatment with paroxetine. Patients taking diuretics may be at greater risk). Products include:
Atacand HCT 700

Hydrocodone Bitartrate (Paroxetine is metabolized by CYP2D6. Like other agents that are metabolized by CYP2D6, paroxetine may significantly inhibit the activity of this isoenzyme. Co-administration of paroxetine with other drugs that are metabolized by CYP2D6 should be approached with caution and may require lower doses than usually prescribed for either paroxetine or the other drug metabolized by CYP2D6). Products include:

Hydroflumethiazide (Hyponatremia may occur as a result of treatment with paroxetine. Patients taking diuretics may be at greater risk).
No products indexed under this heading.

Hydroxychloroquine Sulfate (Co-administration of paroxetine with drugs that inhibit CYP2D6 should be approached with caution).
No products indexed under this heading.

Hypericum (Based on the mechanism of action of paroxetine and the potential for serotonin syndrome, caution is advised when paroxetine hydrochloride is co-administered with other drugs or agents that may affect the serotonergic neurotransmitter systems, such as St. John's Wort).
No products indexed under this heading.

Hypericum Perforatum (Based on the mechanism of action of paroxetine and the potential for serotonin syndrome, caution is advised when paroxetine hydrochloride is co-administered with other drugs or agents that may affect the serotonergic neurotransmitter systems, such as St. John's Wort). Products include:

Ibuprofen (Paroxetine may increase the risk of bleeding events, including upper gastrointestinal bleeding. Concomitant use of paroxetine with NSAIDs may increase this risk). Products include:

Imatinib Mesylate (Co-administration of paroxetine with drugs that inhibit CYP2D6 should be approached with caution). Products include:

Imipramine Hydrochloride (Caution is indicated in the co-administration of tricyclic antidepressants (TCAs) with paroxetine, because paroxetine may inhibit TCA metabolism. Plasma TCA concentrations may need to be monitored, and the dose of a TCA may need to be reduced if a TCA is co-administered with paroxetine).
No products indexed under this heading.

Imipramine Pamoate (Caution is indicated in the co-administration of tricyclic antidepressants (TCAs) with paroxetine, because paroxetine may inhibit TCA metabolism. Plasma TCA concentrations may need to be monitored, and the dose of TCA may need to be reduced if a TCA is co-administered with paroxetine).
No products indexed under this heading.

Indapamide (Hyponatremia may occur as a result of treatment with paroxetine. Patients taking diuretics may be at greater risk). Products include:

Indomethacin (Paroxetine may increase the risk of bleeding events, including upper gastrointestinal bleeding. Concomitant use of paroxetine with NSAIDs may increase this risk). Products include:

Indomethacin Sodium Trihydrate (Paroxetine may increase the risk of bleeding events, including upper gastrointestinal bleeding. Concomitant use of paroxetine with NSAIDs may increase this risk). Products include:

Indoramin Hydrochloride (Paroxetine is metabolized by CYP2D6. Like other agents that are metabolized by CYP2D6, paroxetine may significantly inhibit the activity of this isoenzyme. Co-administration of paroxetine with other drugs that are metabolized by CYP2D6 should be approached with caution and may require lower doses than usually prescribed for either paroxetine or the other drug metabolized by CYP2D6).
No products indexed under this heading.

Isocarboxazid (Concomitant use of paroxetine in patients taking monoamine oxidase inhibitors (MAOIs) is contraindicated. In patients receiving another serotonin reuptake inhibitor drug in combination with a MAOI, there have been reports of serious, sometimes fatal, reactions. These reactions have also been reported in patients who have recently discontinued that drug and have been started on an MAOI. Some cases presented with features resembling neuroleptic malignant syndrome. While there are no human data showing such an interaction with paroxetine, limited animal data on the effects of combined use of paroxetine and MAOIs suggest that these drugs may act synergistically to elevate blood pressure and evoke behavioral excitation. Therefore, it is recommended that paroxetine not be used in combination with an MAOI, or within 14 days of discontinuing treatment with an MAOI. At least 2 weeks should be allowed after stopping paroxetine before starting an MAOI). Products include:

Ketoprofen (Paroxetine may increase the risk of bleeding events, including upper gastrointestinal bleeding. Concomitant use of paroxetine with NSAIDs may increase this risk).
No products indexed under this heading.

Ketorolac Tromethamine (Paroxetine may increase the risk of bleeding events, including upper gastrointestinal bleeding. Concomitant use of paroxetine with NSAIDs may increase this risk). Products include:

Labetalol Hydrochloride (Paroxetine is metabolized by CYP2D6. Like other agents that are metabolized by CYP2D6, paroxetine may significantly inhibit the activity of this isoenzyme. Co-administration of paroxetine with other drugs that are metabolized by CYP2D6 should be approached with caution and may require lower doses

than usually prescribed for either paroxetine or the other drug metabolized by CYP2D6).
No products indexed under this heading.

Lidocaine (Paroxetine is metabolized by CYP2D6. Like other agents that are metabolized by CYP2D6, paroxetine may significantly inhibit the activity of this isoenzyme. Co-administration of paroxetine with other drugs that are metabolized by CYP2D6 should be approached with caution and may require lower doses than usually prescribed for either paroxetine or the other drug metabolized by CYP2D6). Products include:

Lidocaine Hydrochloride (Paroxetine is metabolized by CYP2D6. Like other agents that are metabolized by CYP2D6, paroxetine may significantly inhibit the activity of this isoenzyme. Co-administration of paroxetine with other drugs that are metabolized by CYP2D6 should be approached with caution and may require lower doses than usually prescribed for either paroxetine or the other drug metabolized by CYP2D6).
No products indexed under this heading.

Linezolid (Concomitant use of paroxetine in patients taking monoamine oxidase inhibitors (MAOIs), including linezolid, an antibiotic which is a reversible non-selective MAOI is contraindicated. In patients receiving another serotonin reuptake inhibitor drug in combination with a MAOI, there have been reports of serious, sometimes fatal, reactions. These reactions have also been reported in patients who have recently discontinued that drug and have been started on an MAOI. Some cases presented with features resembling neuroleptic malignant syndrome. While there are no human data showing such an interaction with paroxetine, limited animal data on the effects of combined use of paroxetine and MAOIs suggest that these drugs may act synergistically to elevate blood pressure and evoke behavioral excitation. Therefore, it is recommended that paroxetine not be used in combination with an MAOI (including linezolid), or within 14 days of discontinuing treatment with an MAOI. At least 2 weeks should be allowed after stopping paroxetine before starting an MAOI). Products include:

Lithium (A multiple-dose study with paroxetine has shown that there is no pharmacokinetic interaction between paroxetine and lithium carbonate. However, due to the potential for serotonin syndrome, caution is advised when paroxetine is co-administered with lithium).
No products indexed under this heading.

Lithium Carbonate (A multiple-dose study with paroxetine has shown that there is no pharmacokinetic interaction between paroxetine and lithium carbonate. However, due to the potential for serotonin syndrome, caution is advised when paroxetine is co-administered with lithium).
No products indexed under this heading.

Lithium Citrate (A multiple-dose study with paroxetine has shown that there is no pharmacokinetic interaction between paroxetine and lithium carbonate. However, due to the potential for serotonin syndrome, caution is advised when paroxetine is co-administered with lithium).
No products indexed under this heading.

Low Molecular Weight Heparins (Concomitant use of paroxetine with drugs affecting coagulation, may increase the risk of bleeding including upper gastrointestinal bleeding).
No products indexed under this heading.

Loxapine Hydrochloride (The development of a potentially life-threatening serotonin syndrome or Neuroleptic Malignant Syndrome (NMS)-like reactions have been reported with paroxetine alone, but particularly with concomitant use of antipsychotic agents. Patients should be monitored for the emergence of serotonin syndrome or NMS-like signs and symptoms. Treatment with paroxetine and any concomitant antipsychotic should be discontinued immediately if any signs or symptoms of serotonin syndrome or NMS-like signs or symptoms occur and supportive symptomatic treatment should be initiated).
No products indexed under this heading.

Loxapine Succinate (The development of a potentially life-threatening serotonin syndrome or Neuroleptic Malignant Syndrome (NMS)-like reactions have been reported with paroxetine alone, but particularly with concomitant use of antipsychotic agents. Patients should be monitored for the emergence of serotonin syndrome or NMS-like signs and symptoms. Treatment with paroxetine and any concomitant antipsychotic should be discontinued immediately if any signs or symptoms of serotonin syndrome or NMS-like signs or symptoms occur and supportive symptomatic treatment should be initiated).
No products indexed under this heading.

Maprotiline Hydrochloride (Caution is indicated in the co-administration of tricyclic antidepressants (TCAs) with paroxetine, because paroxetine may inhibit TCA metabolism. Plasma TCA concentrations may need to be monitored, and the dose of TCA may need to be reduced if a TCA is co-administered with paroxetine).
No products indexed under this heading.

Meclofenamate Sodium (Paroxetine may increase the risk of bleeding events, including upper gastrointestinal bleeding. Concomitant use of paroxetine with NSAIDs may increase this risk).
No products indexed under this heading.

Mefenamic Acid (Paroxetine may increase the risk of bleeding events, including upper gastrointestinal bleeding. Concomitant use of paroxetine with NSAIDs may increase this risk).
No products indexed under this heading.

Meloxicam (Paroxetine may increase the risk of bleeding events, including upper gastrointestinal bleeding. Concomitant use of paroxetine with NSAIDs may increase this risk).
No products indexed under this heading.

Meperidine Hydrochloride (Paroxetine is metabolized by CYP2D6. Like other agents that are metabolized by CYP2D6, paroxetine may significantly inhibit the activity of this isoenzyme. Co-administration of paroxetine with other drugs that are metabolized by CYP2D6 should be approached with caution and may require lower doses than usually prescribed for either paroxetine or the other drug metabolized by CYP2D6).
No products indexed under this heading.

Mesoridazine Besylate (Paroxetine is metabolized by CYP2D6. Like other agents that are metabolized by CYP2D6, paroxetine may significantly inhibit the activity of this isoenzyme. Co-administration of paroxetine with other drugs that are metabolized by CYP2D6, such as phenothiazines, should be approached with caution and lower doses than usual may need to be prescribed for paroxetine or the phenothiazine).
No products indexed under this heading.

Methadone Hydrochloride (Paroxetine is metabolized by CYP2D6. Like

Paxil Interactions Index 1388

other agents that are metabolized by CYP2D6, paroxetine may significantly inhibit the activity of this isoenzyme. Co-administration of paroxetine with other drugs that are metabolized by CYP2D6 should be approached with caution and may require lower doses than usually prescribed for either paroxetine or the other drug metabolized by CYP2D6).

No products indexed under this heading.

Methamphetamine Hydrochloride (Paroxetine is metabolized by CYP2D6. Like other agents that are metabolized by CYP2D6, paroxetine may significantly inhibit the activity of this isoenzyme. Co-administration of paroxetine with other drugs that are metabolized by CYP2D6 should be approached with caution and may require lower doses than usually prescribed for either paroxetine or the other drug metabolized by CYP2D6).

No products indexed under this heading.

Methotrimeprazine (Paroxetine is metabolized by CYP2D6. Like other agents that are metabolized by CYP2D6, paroxetine may significantly inhibit the activity of this isoenzyme. Co-administration of paroxetine with other drugs that are metabolized by CYP2D6, such as phentothiazines, should be approached with caution and lower doses than usual may need to be prescribed for paroxetine or the phenothiazine).

No products indexed under this heading.

Methoxyphenamine (Paroxetine is metabolized by CYP2D6. Like other agents that are metabolized by CYP2D6, paroxetine may significantly inhibit the activity of this isoenzyme. Co-administration of paroxetine with other drugs that are metabolized by CYP2D6 should be approached with caution and may require lower doses than usually prescribed for either paroxetine or the other drug metabolized by CYP2D6).

No products indexed under this heading.

Methyclothiazide (Hyponatremia may occur as a result of treatment with paroxetine. Patients taking diuretics may be at greater risk).

No products indexed under this heading.

Metoclopramide Hydrochloride (The development of a potentially life-threatening serotonin syndrome or Neuroleptic Malignant Syndrome (NMS)-like reactions have been reported with paroxetine alone, but particularly with concomitant use of antidopaminergic agents. Patients should be monitored for the emergence of serotonin syndrome or NMS-like signs and symptoms. Treatment with paroxetine and any concomitant antidopaminergic agent should be discontinued immediately if any signs or symptoms of serotonin syndrome or NMS-like signs and symptoms occur and supportive symptomatic treatment should be initiated). Products include:

Metozolv ODT **2901**

Metolazone (Hyponatremia may occur as a result of treatment with paroxetine. Patients taking diuretics may be at greater risk).

No products indexed under this heading.

Metoprolol Succinate (There has been a case report of severe hypotension when paroxetine was added to chronic metoprolol treatment). Products include:

Toprol XL **732**

Metoprolol Tartrate (There has been a case report of severe hypotension when paroxetine was added to chronic metoprolol treatment).

No products indexed under this heading.

Mexiletine Hydrochloride (Paroxetine is metabolized by CYP2D6. Like other agents that are metabolized by CYP2D6, paroxetine may significantly inhibit the activity of this isoenzyme. Co-administration of paroxetine with other drugs that are metabolized by CYP2D6 should be approached with caution and may require lower doses than usually prescribed for either paroxetine or the other drug metabolized by CYP2D6).

No products indexed under this heading.

Mibefradil Dihydrochloride (Co-administration of paroxetine with drugs that inhibit CYP2D6 should be approached with caution).

No products indexed under this heading.

Midazolam Hydrochloride (Because paroxetine is highly bound to plasma protein, administration of paroxetine to a patient taking another drug that is highly protein bound may cause increased free concentrations of the other drug, potentially resulting in adverse events. Conversely, adverse effects could result from displacement of paroxetine by other highly bound drugs).

No products indexed under this heading.

Mirtazapine (Paroxetine is metabolized by CYP2D6. Like other agents that are metabolized by CYP2D6, paroxetine may significantly inhibit the activity of this isoenzyme. Co-administration of paroxetine with other drugs that are metabolized by CYP2D6 should be approached with caution and may require lower doses than usually prescribed for either paroxetine or the other drug metabolized by CYP2D6). Products include:

Remeron Tablets **3214**
RemeronSolTab Tablets **3219**

Moclobemide (Concomitant use of paroxetine in patients taking monoamine oxidase inhibitors (MAOIs) is contraindicated. In patients receiving another serotonin reuptake inhibitor drug in combination with a MAOI, there have been reports of serious, sometimes fatal, reactions. These reactions have also been reported in patients who have recently discontinued that drug and have been started on an MAOI. Some cases presented with features resembling neuroleptic malignant syndrome. While there are no human data showing such an interaction with paroxetine, limited animal data on the effects of combined use of paroxetine and MAOIs suggest that these drugs may act synergistically to elevate blood pressure and evoke behavioral excitation. Therefore, it is recommended that paroxetine not be used in combination with an MAOI, or within 14 days of discontinuing treatment with an MAOI. At least 2 weeks should be allowed after stopping paroxetine before starting an MAOI).

No products indexed under this heading.

Molindone Hydrochloride (The development of a potentially life-threatening serotonin syndrome or Neuroleptic Malignant Syndrome (NMS)-like reactions have been reported with paroxetine alone, but particularly with concomitant use of antipsychotic agents. Patients should be monitored for the emergence of serotonin syndrome or NMS-like signs and symptoms. Treatment with paroxetine and any concomitant antipsychotic should be discontinued immediately if any signs or symptoms of serotonin syndrome or NMS-like signs or symptoms occur and supportive symptomatic treatment should be initiated). Products include:

Moban **1108**

Morphine Sulfate (Paroxetine is metabolized by CYP2D6. Like other agents that are metabolized by CYP2D6, paroxetine may significantly inhibit the activity of this isoenzyme. Co-administration of paroxetine with other drugs that are metabolized by CYP2D6 should be approached with caution and may require lower doses than usually prescribed for either paroxetine or the other drug metabolized by CYP2D6). Products include:

Avinza **1822**
Embeda **1831**
MS Contin **2803**

Nabumetone (Paroxetine may increase the risk of bleeding events, including upper gastrointestinal bleeding. Concomitant use of paroxetine with NSAIDs may increase this risk).

No products indexed under this heading.

Naproxen (Paroxetine may increase the risk of bleeding events, including upper gastrointestinal bleeding. Concomitant use of paroxetine with NSAIDs may increase this risk). Products include:

EC-Naprosyn **2850**
Naprosyn **2850**
Anaprox/Naprosyn **2850**

Naproxen Sodium (Paroxetine may increase the risk of bleeding events, including upper gastrointestinal bleeding. Concomitant use of paroxetine with NSAIDs may increase this risk). Products include:

Anaprox **2850**
Anaprox DS **2850**
Treximet **1681**

Naratriptan Hydrochloride (The development of a potentially life-threatening serotonin syndrome or Neuroleptic Malignant Syndrome (NMS)-like reactions have been reported with paroxetine alone, but particularly, with concomitant use of serotonergic drugs (including triptans). Patients should be monitored for the emergence of serotonin syndrome or NMS-like signs and symptoms. Treatment with paroxetine and any concomitant serotonergic agent should be discontinued immediately if any signs or symptoms of serotonin syndrome or NMS-like signs and symptoms occur and supportive symptomatic treatment should be initiated. If concomitant use of paroxetine with a triptan is clinically warranted, careful observation of the patient is advised, particularly during treatment initiation and dose increases). Products include:

Amerge **1306**

Nefazodone Hydrochloride (The development of a potentially life-threatening serotonin syndrome or Neuroleptic Malignant Syndrome (NMS)-like reactions have been reported with paroxetine alone, but particularly, with concomitant use of serotonergic drugs. The concomitant use of paroxetine with SNRIs is not recommended).

No products indexed under this heading.

Nelfinavir Mesylate (Paroxetine is metabolized by CYP2D6. Like other agents that are metabolized by CYP2D6, paroxetine may significantly inhibit the activity of this isoenzyme. Co-administration of paroxetine with other drugs that are metabolized by CYP2D6 should be approached with caution and may require lower doses than usually prescribed for either paroxetine or the other drug metabolized by CYP2D6).

No products indexed under this heading.

Nortriptyline Hydrochloride (Caution is indicated in the co-administration of tricyclic antidepressants (TCAs) with paroxetine, because paroxetine may inhibit TCA metabolism. Plasma TCA concentrations may need to be monitored, and the dose of TCA may need to be reduced if a TCA is co-administered with paroxetine).

No products indexed under this heading.

Olanzapine (The development of a potentially life-threatening serotonin syndrome or Neuroleptic Malignant Syndrome (NMS)-like reactions have been reported with paroxetine alone, but particularly with concomitant use of antipsychotic agents. Patients should be monitored for the emergence of serotonin syndrome or NMS-like signs and symptoms. Treatment with paroxetine and any concomitant antipsychotic should be discontinued immediately if any signs or symptoms of serotonin syndrome or NMS-like signs or symptoms occur and supportive symptomatic treatment should be initiated). Products include:

Symbyax **1965**
Zyprexa **1984**
Zyprexa IntraMuscular **1984**
Zyprexa ZYDIS **1984**

Omeprazole (Paroxetine is metabolized by CYP2D6. Like other agents that are metabolized by CYP2D6, paroxetine may significantly inhibit the activity of this isoenzyme. Co-administration of paroxetine with other drugs that are metabolized by CYP2D6 should be approached with caution and may require lower doses than usually prescribed for either paroxetine or the other drug metabolized by CYP2D6).

No products indexed under this heading.

Ondansetron (Paroxetine is metabolized by CYP2D6. Like other agents that are metabolized by CYP2D6, paroxetine may significantly inhibit the activity of this isoenzyme. Co-administration of paroxetine with other drugs that are metabolized by CYP2D6 should be approached with caution and may require lower doses than usually prescribed for either paroxetine or the other drug metabolized by CYP2D6).

No products indexed under this heading.

Ondansetron Hydrochloride (Paroxetine is metabolized by CYP2D6. Like other agents that are metabolized by CYP2D6, paroxetine may significantly inhibit the activity of this isoenzyme. Co-administration of paroxetine with other drugs that are metabolized by CYP2D6 should be approached with caution and may require lower doses than usually prescribed for either paroxetine or the other drug metabolized by CYP2D6). Products include:

Zofran Injection **1750**
Zofran **1756**
Zofran ODT **1756**

Oxaprozin (Paroxetine may increase the risk of bleeding events, including upper gastrointestinal bleeding. Concomitant use of paroxetine with NSAIDs may increase this risk).

No products indexed under this heading.

Oxazepam (Because paroxetine is highly bound to plasma protein, administration of paroxetine to a patient taking another drug that is highly protein bound may cause increased free concentrations of the other drug, potentially resulting in adverse events. Conversely, adverse effects could result from displacement of paroxetine by other highly bound drugs).

No products indexed under this heading.

Oxycodone Hydrochloride (Paroxetine is metabolized by CYP2D6. Like other agents that are metabolized by CYP2D6, paroxetine may significantly inhibit the activity of this isoenzyme. Co-administration of paroxetine with other drugs that are metabolized by CYP2D6 should be approached with caution and may require lower doses than usually prescribed for either paroxetine or the other drug metabolized by CYP2D6). Products include:

OxyContin **2807**
Percocet **1121**
Percodan **1124**

Paclitaxel (Paroxetine is metabolized by CYP2D6. Like other agents that are metabolized by CYP2D6, paroxetine

1389 Interactions Index Paxil

may significantly inhibit the activity of this isoenzyme. Co-administration of paroxetine with other drugs that are metabolized by CYP2D6 should be approached with caution and may require lower doses than usually prescribed for either paroxetine or the other drug metabolized by CYP2D6).
No products indexed under this heading.

Paliperidone (The development of a potentially life-threatening serotonin syndrome or Neuroleptic Malignant Syndrome (NMS)-like reactions have been reported with paroxetine alone, but particularly with concomitant use of antipsychotic agents. Patients should be monitored for the emergence of serotonin syndrome or NMS-like signs and symptoms. Treatment with paroxetine and any concomitant antipsychotic should be discontinued immediately if any signs or symptoms of serotonin syndrome or NMS-like signs or symptoms occur and supportive symptomatic treatment should be initiated).
Products include:
Invega 2613
Invega Sustenna 2621

Pargyline Hydrochloride (Concomitant use of paroxetine in patients taking monoamine oxidase inhibitors (MAOIs) is contraindicated. In patients receiving another serotonin reuptake inhibitor drug in combination with a MAOI, there have been reports of serious, sometimes fatal, reactions. These reactions have also been reported in patients who have recently discontinued that drug and have been started on an MAOI. Some cases presented with features resembling neuroleptic malignant syndrome. While there are no human data showing such an interaction with paroxetine, limited animal data on the effects of combined use of paroxetine and MAOIs suggest that these drugs may act synergistically to elevate blood pressure and evoke behavioral excitation. Therefore, it is recommended that paroxetine not be used in combination with an MAOI, or within 14 days of discontinuing treatment with an MAOI. At least 2 weeks should be allowed after stopping paroxetine before starting an MAOI).
No products indexed under this heading.

Paroxetine (The development of a potentially life-threatening serotonin syndrome or Neuroleptic Malignant Syndrome (NMS)-like reactions have been reported with paroxetine alone, but particularly, with concomitant use of serotonergic drugs. The concomitant use of paroxetine with other SSRIs is not recommended).
No products indexed under this heading.

Paroxetine Mesylate (The development of a potentially life-threatening serotonin syndrome or Neuroleptic Malignant Syndrome (NMS)-like reactions have been reported with paroxetine alone, but particularly, with concomitant use of serotonergic drugs. The concomitant use of paroxetine with other SSRIs is not recommended).
No products indexed under this heading.

Perphenazine (Paroxetine is metabolized by CYP2D6. Like other agents that are metabolized by CYP2D6, paroxetine may significantly inhibit the activity of this isoenzyme. Co-administration of paroxetine with other drugs that are metabolized by CYP2D6, such as phenothiazines, should be approached with caution and lower doses than usual may need to be prescribed for paroxetine or the phenothiazine).
No products indexed under this heading.

Phenelzine Sulfate (Concomitant use of paroxetine in patients taking monoamine oxidase inhibitors (MAOIs) is contraindicated. In patients receiving another serotonin reuptake inhibitor drug in combination with a MAOI, there have been reports of serious, sometimes fatal, reactions. These reactions have also been reported in patients who have recently discontinued that drug and have been started on an MAOI. Some cases presented with features resembling neuroleptic malignant syndrome. While there are no human data showing such an interaction with paroxetine, limited animal data on the effects of combined use of paroxetine and MAOIs suggest that these drugs may act synergistically to elevate blood pressure and evoke behavioral excitation. Therefore, it is recommended that paroxetine not be used in combination with an MAOI, or within 14 days of discontinuing treatment with an MAOI. At least 2 weeks should be allowed after stopping paroxetine before starting an MAOI).
No products indexed under this heading.

Phenobarbital (Phenobarbital induces many cytochrome P_{450} (oxidative) enzymes. When a single oral 30-mg dose of paroxetine was administered at phenobarbital steady state (100 mg once daily for 14 days), paroxetine AUC and $T_{1/2}$ were reduced (by an average of 25% and 38%, respectively) compared to paroxetine administered alone. Since paroxetine exhibits nonlinear pharmacokinetics, the results of this study may not address the case where the 2 drugs are both being chronically dosed. No initial dosage adjustment of paroxetine is considered necessary when co-administered with phenobarbital; any subsequent adjustment should be guided by clinical effect). Products include:
Donnatal 2711

Phenobarbital Sodium (Phenobarbital induces many cytochrome P_{450} (oxidative) enzymes. When a single oral 30-mg dose of paroxetine was administered at phenobarbital steady state (100 mg once daily for 14 days), paroxetine AUC and $T_{1/2}$ were reduced (by an average of 25% and 38%, respectively) compared to paroxetine administered alone. Since paroxetine exhibits nonlinear pharmacokinetics, the results of this study may not address the case where the 2 drugs are both being chronically dosed. No initial dosage adjustment of paroxetine is considered necessary when co-administered with phenobarbital; any subsequent adjustment should be guided by clinical effect).
No products indexed under this heading.

Phenothiazine Derivatives (Paroxetine is metabolized by CYP2D6. Like other agents that are metabolized by CYP2D6, paroxetine may significantly inhibit the activity of this isoenzyme. Co-administration of paroxetine with other drugs that are metabolized by CYP2D6, such as phenothiazines, should be approached with caution and lower doses than usual may need to be prescribed for paroxetine or the phenothiazine).
No products indexed under this heading.

Phenothiazines (Paroxetine is metabolized by CYP2D6. Like other agents that are metabolized by CYP2D6, paroxetine may significantly inhibit the activity of this isoenzyme. Co-administration of paroxetine with other drugs that are metabolized by CYP2D6, such as phenothiazines, should be approached with caution and lower doses than usual may need to be prescribed for paroxetine or the phenothiazine).
No products indexed under this heading.

Phenylbutazone (Paroxetine may increase the risk of bleeding events, including upper gastrointestinal bleeding. Concomitant use of paroxetine with NSAIDs may increase this risk).
No products indexed under this heading.

Phenytoin (When a single oral 30 mg dose of paroxetine was administered at phenytoin steady state (300 mg once daily for 14 days), paroxetine AUC and $t_{1/2}$ were reduced (by an average of 50% and 35%, respectively) compared to paroxetine administered alone. Since both drugs exhibit nonlinear pharmacokinetics, the above study may not address the case where two drugs are being chronically dosed. There has been a case report of an elevated phenytoin level after 4 weeks of paroxetine and phenytoin co-administration. No initial dosage adjustments are considered necessary when these drugs are co-administered; any subsequent adjustment should be guided by clinical effect).
No products indexed under this heading.

Phenytoin Sodium (When a single oral 30 mg dose of paroxetine was administered at phenytoin steady state (300 mg once daily for 14 days), paroxetine AUC and $t_{1/2}$ were reduced (by an average of 50% and 35%, respectively) compared to paroxetine administered alone. Since both drugs exhibit nonlinear pharmacokinetics, the above study may not address the case where two drugs are being chronically dosed. There has been a case report of an elevated phenytoin level after 4 weeks of paroxetine and phenytoin co-administration. No initial dosage adjustments are considered necessary when these drugs are co-administered; any subsequent adjustment should be guided by clinical effect). Products include:
Phenytek Capsules 2380

Pimozide (Concomitant use in patients taking pimozide is contraindicated. In a study of healthy volunteers, after paroxetine was titrated to 60 mg daily, co-administration of a single dose of 2 mg pimozide was associated with mean increases in pimozide AUC of 151% and C_{max} of 62%, compared to pimozide administered alone. The increase in pimozide AUC and C_{max} is due to the CYP2D6 inhibitory properties of paroxetine. Due to the narrow therapeutic index of pimozide and its known ability to prolong the QT interval, concomitant use of pimozide and paroxetine is contraindicated).
No products indexed under this heading.

Pindolol (Paroxetine is metabolized by CYP2D6. Like other agents that are metabolized by CYP2D6, paroxetine may significantly inhibit the activity of this isoenzyme. Co-administration of paroxetine with other drugs that are metabolized by CYP2D6 should be approached with caution and may require lower doses than usually prescribed for either paroxetine or the other drug metabolized by CYP2D6).
No products indexed under this heading.

Piroxicam (Paroxetine may increase the risk of bleeding events, including upper gastrointestinal bleeding. Concomitant use of paroxetine with NSAIDs may increase this risk).
No products indexed under this heading.

Polythiazide (Hyponatremia may occur as a result of treatment with paroxetine. Patients taking diuretics may be at greater risk).
No products indexed under this heading.

Procarbazine Hydrochloride (Concomitant use of paroxetine in patients taking monoamine oxidase inhibitors (MAOIs) is contraindicated. In patients receiving another serotonin reuptake inhibitor drug in combination with a MAOI, there have been reports of serious, sometimes fatal, reactions. These reactions have also been reported in patients who have recently discontinued that drug and have been started on an MAOI. Some cases presented with features resembling neuroleptic malignant syndrome. While there are no human data showing such an interaction with paroxetine, limited animal data on the effects of combined use of paroxetine and MAOIs suggest that these drugs may act synergistically to elevate blood pressure and evoke behavioral excitation. Therefore, it is recommended that paroxetine not be used in combination with an MAOI, or within 14 days of discontinuing treatment with an MAOI. At least 2 weeks should be allowed after stopping paroxetine before starting an MAOI).
No products indexed under this heading.

Prochlorperazine (Paroxetine is metabolized by CYP2D6. Like other agents that are metabolized by CYP2D6, paroxetine may significantly inhibit the activity of this isoenzyme. Co-administration of paroxetine with other drugs that are metabolized by CYP2D6, such as phentothiazines, should be approached with caution and lower doses than usual may need to be prescribed for paroxetine or the phenothiazine).
No products indexed under this heading.

Prochlorperazine Edisylate (Paroxetine is metabolized by CYP2D6. Like other agents that are metabolized by CYP2D6, paroxetine may significantly inhibit the activity of this isoenzyme. Co-administration of paroxetine with other drugs that are metabolized by CYP2D6, such as phentothiazines, should be approached with caution and lower doses than usual may need to be prescribed for paroxetine or the phenothiazine).
No products indexed under this heading.

Prochlorperazine Maleate (Paroxetine is metabolized by CYP2D6. Like other agents that are metabolized by CYP2D6, paroxetine may significantly inhibit the activity of this isoenzyme. Co-administration of paroxetine with other drugs that are metabolized by CYP2D6, such as phentothiazines, should be approached with caution and lower doses than usual may need to be prescribed for paroxetine or the phenothiazine).
No products indexed under this heading.

Procyclidine Hydrochloride (Daily oral dosing of paroxetine (30 mg once daily) increased steady-state AUC, C_{max}, and C_{min} values of procyclidine (5 mg oral once daily) by 35%, 37%, and 67%, respectively, compared to procyclidine alone at steady state. If anticholinergic effects are seen, the dose of procyclidine should be reduced).
No products indexed under this heading.

Promethazine (Paroxetine is metabolized by CYP2D6. Like other agents that are metabolized by CYP2D6, paroxetine may significantly inhibit the activity of this isoenzyme. Co-administration of paroxetine with other drugs that are metabolized by CYP2D6, such as phentothiazines, should be approached with caution and lower doses than usual may need to be prescribed for paroxetine or the phenothiazine).
No products indexed under this heading.

Promethazine Hydrochloride (Paroxetine is metabolized by CYP2D6. Like other agents that are metabolized by CYP2D6, paroxetine may significantly inhibit the activity of this isoenzyme. Co-administration of paroxetine with other drugs that are metabolized by CYP2D6, such as phentothiazines, should be approached with caution and lower doses than usual may need to be prescribed for paroxetine or the phenothiazine).
No products indexed under this heading.

Propafenone Hydrochloride (Co-administration of paroxetine with other drugs which are metabolized by

IMPORTANT NOTE: Always consult each drug listing in the patient's regimen for possible interactions.

CYP2D6, including Type 1C antiarrhythmics (eg, propafenone, flecainide, encainide), should be approached with caution). Products include:

Propoxyphene Hydrochloride (Paroxetine is metabolized by CYP2D6. Like other agents that are metabolized by CYP2D6, paroxetine may significantly inhibit the activity of this isoenzyme. Co-administration of paroxetine with other drugs that are metabolized by CYP2D6 should be approached with caution and may require lower doses than usually prescribed for either paroxetine or the other drug metabolized by CYP2D6).

No products indexed under this heading.

Propoxyphene Napsylate (Paroxetine is metabolized by CYP2D6. Like other agents that are metabolized by CYP2D6, paroxetine may significantly inhibit the activity of this isoenzyme. Co-administration of paroxetine with other drugs that are metabolized by CYP2D6 should be approached with caution and may require lower doses than usually prescribed for either paroxetine or the other drug metabolized by CYP2D6).

No products indexed under this heading.

Propranolol Hydrochloride (Because paroxetine is highly bound to plasma protein, administration of paroxetine to a patient taking another drug that is highly protein bound may cause increased free concentrations of the other drug, potentially resulting in adverse events. Conversely, adverse effects could result from displacement of paroxetine by other highly bound drugs). Products include:

Protriptyline Hydrochloride (Caution is indicated in the co-administration of tricyclic antidepressants (TCAs) with paroxetine, because paroxetine may inhibit TCA metabolism. Plasma TCA concentrations may need to be monitored, and the dose of TCA may need to be reduced if a TCA is co-administered with paroxetine).

No products indexed under this heading.

Quetiapine Fumarate (The development of a potentially life-threatening serotonin syndrome or Neuroleptic Malignant Syndrome (NMS)-like reactions have been reported with paroxetine alone, but particularly with concomitant use of antipsychotic agents. Patients should be monitored for the emergence of serotonin syndrome or NMS-like signs and symptoms. Treatment with paroxetine and any concomitant antipsychotic should be discontinued immediately if any signs or symptoms of serotonin syndrome or NMS-like signs or symptoms occur and supportive symptomatic treatment should be initiated). Products include:

Quinacrine Hydrochloride (Co-administration of paroxetine with drugs that inhibit CYP2D6 should be approached with caution).

No products indexed under this heading.

Quinidine (Co-administration of paroxetine with drugs that inhibit CYP2D6 (eg, quinidine) should be approached with caution).

No products indexed under this heading.

Quinidine Gluconate (Co-administration of paroxetine with drugs that inhibit CYP2D6 (eg, quinidine) should be approached with caution).

No products indexed under this heading.

Quinidine Hydrochloride (Co-administration of paroxetine with drugs that inhibit CYP2D6 (eg, quinidine) should be approached with caution).

No products indexed under this heading.

Quinidine Polygalacturonate (Co-administration of paroxetine with drugs that inhibit CYP2D6 (eg, quinidine) should be approached with caution).

No products indexed under this heading.

Quinidine Sulfate (Co-administration of paroxetine with drugs that inhibit CYP2D6 (eg, quinidine) should be approached with caution).

No products indexed under this heading.

Ranitidine Bismuth Citrate (Co-administration of paroxetine with drugs that inhibit CYP2D6 should be approached with caution).

No products indexed under this heading.

Ranitidine Hydrochloride (Co-administration of paroxetine with drugs that inhibit CYP2D6 should be approached with caution). Products include:

Rasagiline Mesylate (Concomitant use of paroxetine in patients taking monoamine oxidase inhibitors (MAOIs) is contraindicated. In patients receiving another serotonin reuptake inhibitor drug in combination with a MAOI, there have been reports of serious, sometimes fatal, reactions. These reactions have also been reported in patients who have recently discontinued that drug and have been started on an MAOI. Some cases presented with features resembling neuroleptic malignant syndrome. While there are no human data showing such an interaction with paroxetine, limited animal data on the effects of combined use of paroxetine and MAOIs suggest that these drugs may act synergistically to elevate blood pressure and evoke behavioral excitation. Therefore, it is recommended that paroxetine not be used in combination with an MAOI, or within 14 days of discontinuing treatment with an MAOI. At least 2 weeks should be allowed after stopping paroxetine before starting an MAOI). Products include:

Risperidone (Paroxetine is metabolized by CYP2D6. Like other agents that are metabolized by CYP2D6, paroxetine may significantly inhibit the activity of this isoenzyme. Concomitant use of paroxetine with risperidone, a CYP2D6 substrate showed in one study to increase the mean plasma concentrations of risperidone approximately 4-fold, decreased 9-hydroxyrisperidone concentrations approximately 10%, and increased concentrations of the active moiety (the sum of risperidone plus 9-hydroxyrisperidone) approximately 1.4-fold. Therefore, concomitant use with other drugs metabolized by CYP2D6, such as risperidone, should be used with caution). Products include:

Ritonavir (Co-administration of ritonavir with paroxetine significantly decreased plasma levels of paroxetine. Any dose adjustment should be guided by clinical effect (tolerability and efficacy)). Products include:

Rizatriptan Benzoate (The development of a potentially life-threatening serotonin syndrome or Neuroleptic Malignant Syndrome (NMS)-like reactions have been reported with paroxetine alone, but particularly, with concomitant use of serotonergic drugs (including triptans). Patients should be monitored for the emergence of serotonin syndrome or NMS-like signs and symptoms. Treatment with paroxetine and any concomitant serotonergic agent should be discontinued immediately if any signs or symptoms of serotonin syndrome or NMS-like signs and symptoms occur and supportive symptomatic treatment should be initiated. If concomitant use of paroxetine with a triptan is clinically warranted, careful observation of the patient is advised, particularly during treatment initiation and dose increases). Products include:

Rofecoxib (Paroxetine may increase the risk of bleeding events, including upper gastrointestinal bleeding. Concomitant use of paroxetine with NSAIDs may increase this risk).

No products indexed under this heading.

Selegiline (Concomitant use of paroxetine in patients taking monoamine oxidase inhibitors (MAOIs) is contraindicated. In patients receiving another serotonin reuptake inhibitor drug in combination with a MAOI, there have been reports of serious, sometimes fatal, reactions. These reactions have also been reported in patients who have recently discontinued that drug and have been started on an MAOI. Some cases presented with features resembling neuroleptic malignant syndrome. While there are no human data showing such an interaction with paroxetine, limited animal data on the effects of combined use of paroxetine and MAOIs suggest that these drugs may act synergistically to elevate blood pressure and evoke behavioral excitation. Therefore, it is recommended that paroxetine not be used in combination with an MAOI, or within 14 days of discontinuing treatment with an MAOI. At least 2 weeks should be allowed after stopping paroxetine before starting an MAOI). Products include:

Selegiline Hydrochloride (Concomitant use of paroxetine in patients taking monoamine oxidase inhibitors (MAOIs) is contraindicated. In patients receiving another serotonin reuptake inhibitor drug in combination with a MAOI, there have been reports of serious, sometimes fatal, reactions. These reactions have also been reported in patients who have recently discontinued that drug and have been started on an MAOI. Some cases presented with features resembling neuroleptic malignant syndrome. While there are no human data showing such an interaction with paroxetine, limited animal data on the effects of combined use of paroxetine and MAOIs suggest that these drugs may act synergistically to elevate blood pressure and evoke behavioral excitation. Therefore, it is recommended that paroxetine not be used in combination with an MAOI, or within 14 days of discontinuing treatment with an MAOI. At least 2 weeks should be allowed after stopping paroxetine before starting an MAOI). Products include:

Sertraline Hydrochloride (The development of a potentially life-threatening serotonin syndrome or Neuroleptic Malignant Syndrome (NMS)-like reactions have been reported with paroxetine alone, but particularly, with concomitant use of serotonergic drugs. The concomitant use of paroxetine with other SSRIs is not recommended).

No products indexed under this heading.

Sildenafil Citrate (Co-administration of paroxetine with drugs that inhibit CYP2D6 should be approached with caution).

No products indexed under this heading.

Spironolactone (Hyponatremia may occur as a result of treatment with paroxetine. Patients taking diuretics may be at greater risk).

No products indexed under this heading.

Sulindac (Paroxetine may increase the risk of bleeding events, including upper gastrointestinal bleeding. Concomitant use of paroxetine with NSAIDs may increase this risk). Products include:

Sumatriptan (The development of a potentially life-threatening serotonin syndrome or Neuroleptic Malignant Syndrome (NMS)-like reactions have been reported with paroxetine alone, but particularly, with concomitant use of serotonergic drugs (including triptans). Patients should be monitored for the emergence of serotonin syndrome or NMS-like signs and symptoms. Treatment with paroxetine and any concomitant serotonergic agent should be discontinued immediately if any signs or symptoms of serotonin syndrome or NMS-like signs and symptoms occur and supportive symptomatic treatment should be initiated. If concomitant use of paroxetine with a triptan is clinically warranted, careful observation of the patient is advised, particularly during treatment initiation and dose increases). Products include:

Sumatriptan Succinate (The development of a potentially life-threatening serotonin syndrome or Neuroleptic Malignant Syndrome (NMS)-like reactions have been reported with paroxetine alone, but particularly, with concomitant use of serotonergic drugs (including triptans). Patients should be monitored for the emergence of serotonin syndrome or NMS-like signs and symptoms. Treatment with paroxetine and any concomitant serotonergic agent should be discontinued immediately if any signs or symptoms of serotonin syndrome or NMS-like signs and symptoms occur and supportive symptomatic treatment should be initiated. If concomitant use of paroxetine with a triptan is clinically warranted, careful observation of the patient is advised, particularly during treatment initiation and dose increases). Products include:

Tamoxifen Citrate (Tamoxifen is a pro-drug requiring metabolic activation by CYP2D6. Inhibition of CYP2D6 by paroxetine may lead to reduced plasma concentrations of an active metabolite and hence reduced efficacy of tamoxifen).

No products indexed under this heading.

Temazepam (Because paroxetine is highly bound to plasma protein, administration of paroxetine to a patient taking another drug that is highly protein bound may cause increased free concentrations of the other drug, potentially resulting in adverse events. Conversely, adverse effects could result from displacement of paroxetine by other highly bound drugs).

No products indexed under this heading.

Teniposide (Paroxetine is metabolized by CYP2D6. Like other agents that are metabolized by CYP2D6, paroxetine may significantly inhibit the activity of this isoenzyme. Co-administration of paroxetine with other drugs that are metabolized by CYP2D6 should be approached with caution and may require lower doses than usually prescribed for either paroxetine or the other drug metabolized by CYP2D6).

No products indexed under this heading.

Terbinafine Hydrochloride (Co-administration of paroxetine with drugs that inhibit CYP2D6 should be approached with caution).
No products indexed under this heading.

Testosterone (Paroxetine is metabolized by CYP2D6. Like other agents that are metabolized by CYP2D6, paroxetine may significantly inhibit the activity of this isoenzyme. Co-administration of paroxetine with other drugs that are metabolized by CYP2D6 should be approached with caution and may require lower doses than usually prescribed for either paroxetine or the other drug metabolized by CYP2D6). Products include:
AndroGel 3456

Testosterone Cypionate (Paroxetine is metabolized by CYP2D6. Like other agents that are metabolized by CYP2D6, paroxetine may significantly inhibit the activity of this isoenzyme. Co-administration of paroxetine with other drugs that are metabolized by CYP2D6 should be approached with caution and may require lower doses than usually prescribed for either paroxetine or the other drug metabolized by CYP2D6).
No products indexed under this heading.

Testosterone Enanthate (Paroxetine is metabolized by CYP2D6. Like other agents that are metabolized by CYP2D6, paroxetine may significantly inhibit the activity of this isoenzyme. Co-administration of paroxetine with other drugs that are metabolized by CYP2D6 should be approached with caution and may require lower doses than usually prescribed for either paroxetine or the other drug metabolized by CYP2D6). Products include:
Delatestryl 1102

Testosterone Propionate (Paroxetine is metabolized by CYP2D6. Like other agents that are metabolized by CYP2D6, paroxetine may significantly inhibit the activity of this isoenzyme. Co-administration of paroxetine with other drugs that are metabolized by CYP2D6 should be approached with caution and may require lower doses than usually prescribed for either paroxetine or the other drug metabolized by CYP2D6).
No products indexed under this heading.

Theophyllinate (The metabolism and pharmacokinetics of paroxetine may be affected by the induction or inhibition of drug metabolizing enzymes).
No products indexed under this heading.

Theophylline (Reports of elevated theophylline levels associated with treatment with paroxetine have been reported. While this interaction has not been formally studied, it is recommended that theophylline levels be monitored when these drugs are concurrently administered).
No products indexed under this heading.

Theophylline Anhydrous (Reports of elevated theophylline levels associated with treatment with paroxetine have been reported. While this interaction has not been formally studied, it is recommended that theophylline levels be monitored when these drugs are concurrently administered). Products include:
Uniphyl 2817

Theophylline Calcium Salicylate (Reports of elevated theophylline levels associated with treatment with paroxetine have been reported. While this interaction has not been formally studied, it is recommended that theophylline levels be monitored when these drugs are concurrently administered).
No products indexed under this heading.

Theophylline Dihydroxypropyl (Glyceryl) (Reports of elevated theophylline levels associated with treatment with paroxetine have been reported. While this interaction has not been formally studied, it is recommended that theophylline levels be monitored when these drugs are concurrently administered).
No products indexed under this heading.

Theophylline Ethylenediamine (Reports of elevated theophylline levels associated with treatment with paroxetine have been reported. While this interaction has not been formally studied, it is recommended that theophylline levels be monitored when these drugs are concurrently administered).
No products indexed under this heading.

Theophylline Sodium Glycinate (Reports of elevated theophylline levels associated with treatment with paroxetine have been reported. While this interaction has not been formally studied, it is recommended that theophylline levels be monitored when these drugs are concurrently administered).
No products indexed under this heading.

Thioridazine (Concomitant use in patients taking thioridazine is contraindicated. Thioridazine administration alone produces prolongation of the QTc interval, which is associated with serious ventricular arrhythmias, such as torsade de pointes-type arrhythmias, and sudden death. This effect appears to be dose related. An *in vivo* study suggests that drugs which inhibit CYP2D6, such as paroxetine, will elevate plasma levels of thioridazine. Therefore, it is recommended that paroxetine not be used in combination with thioridazine).
No products indexed under this heading.

Thioridazine Hydrochloride (Concomitant use in patients taking thioridazine is contraindicated. Thioridazine administration alone produces prolongation of the QTc interval, which is associated with serious ventricular arrhythmias, such as torsade de pointes-type arrhythmias, and sudden death. This effect appears to be dose related. An *in vivo* study suggests that drugs which inhibit CYP2D6, such as paroxetine, will elevate plasma levels of thioridazine. Therefore, it is recommended that paroxetine not be used in combination with thioridazine). Products include:
Thioridazine Hydrochloride 2384

Thiothixene (The development of a potentially life-threatening serotonin syndrome or Neuroleptic Malignant Syndrome (NMS)-like reactions have been reported with paroxetine alone, but particularly with concomitant use of antipsychotic agents. Patients should be monitored for the emergence of serotonin syndrome or NMS-like signs and symptoms. Treatment with paroxetine and any concomitant antipsychotic should be discontinued immediately if any signs or symptoms of serotonin syndrome or NMS-like signs or symptoms occur and supportive symptomatic treatment should be initiated). Products include:
Thiothixene 2386

Timolol Maleate (Paroxetine is metabolized by CYP2D6. Like other agents that are metabolized by CYP2D6, paroxetine may significantly inhibit the activity of this isoenzyme. Co-administration of paroxetine with other drugs that are metabolized by CYP2D6 should be approached with caution and may require lower doses than usually prescribed for either paroxetine or the other drug metabolized by CYP2D6). Products include:
Combigan 601

Dorzolamide Hydrochloride/Timolol Maleate
Ophthalmic Solution.................... ☉243
Timoptic in Ocudose .... ☉231

Tinzaparin Sodium (Concomitant use of paroxetine with drugs affecting coagulation, may increase the risk of bleeding including upper gastrointestinal bleeding).
No products indexed under this heading.

Tolbutamide (Because paroxetine is highly bound to plasma protein, administration of paroxetine to a patient taking another drug that is highly protein bound may cause increased free concentrations of the other drug, potentially resulting in adverse events. Conversely, adverse effects could result from displacement of paroxetine by other highly bound drugs).
No products indexed under this heading.

Tolmetin Sodium (Paroxetine may increase the risk of bleeding events, including upper gastrointestinal bleeding. Concomitant use of paroxetine with NSAIDs may increase this risk).
No products indexed under this heading.

Tolterodine Tartrate (Paroxetine is metabolized by CYP2D6. Like other agents that are metabolized by CYP2D6, paroxetine may significantly inhibit the activity of this isoenzyme. Co-administration of paroxetine with other drugs that are metabolized by CYP2D6 should be approached with caution and may require lower doses than usually prescribed for either paroxetine or the other drug metabolized by CYP2D6).
No products indexed under this heading.

Torsemide (Hyponatremia may occur as a result of treatment with paroxetine. Patients taking diuretics may be at greater risk).
No products indexed under this heading.

Tramadol Hydrochloride (Based on the mechanism of action of paroxetine and the potential for serotonin syndrome, caution is advised when paroxetine hydrochloride is co-administered with other drugs or agents that may affect the serotonergic neurotransmitter systems, such as tramadol). Products include:
Ryzolt 2813
Ultram ER 2693

Tranylcypromine Sulfate (Concomitant use of paroxetine in patients taking monoamine oxidase inhibitors (MAOIs) is contraindicated. In patients receiving another serotonin reuptake inhibitor drug in combination with a MAOI, there have been reports of serious, sometimes fatal, reactions. These reactions have also been reported in patients who have recently discontinued that drug and have been started on an MAOI. Some cases presented with features resembling neuroleptic malignant syndrome. While there are no human data showing such an interaction with paroxetine, limited animal data on the effects of combined use of paroxetine and MAOIs suggest that these drugs may act synergistically to elevate blood pressure and evoke behavioral excitation. Therefore, it is recommended that paroxetine not be used in combination with an MAOI, or within 14 days of discontinuing treatment with an MAOI. At least 2 weeks should be allowed after stopping paroxetine before starting an MAOI). Products include:
Parnate 1584

Trazodone Hydrochloride (Paroxetine is metabolized by CYP2D6. Like other agents that are metabolized by CYP2D6, paroxetine may significantly inhibit the activity of this isoenzyme. Co-administration of paroxetine with other drugs that are metabolized by CYP2D6 should be approached with

caution and may require lower doses than usually prescribed for either paroxetine or the other drug metabolized by CYP2D6).
No products indexed under this heading.

Triamterene (Hyponatremia may occur as a result of treatment with paroxetine. Patients taking diuretics may be at greater risk). Products include:
Dyazide 1429
Dyrenium 3495

Triazolam (Paroxetine is metabolized by CYP2D6. Like other agents that are metabolized by CYP2D6, paroxetine may significantly inhibit the activity of this isoenzyme. Co-administration of paroxetine with other drugs that are metabolized by CYP2D6 should be approached with caution and may require lower doses than usually prescribed for either paroxetine or the other drug metabolized by CYP2D6).
No products indexed under this heading.

Trifluoperazine Hydrochloride (Paroxetine is metabolized by CYP2D6. Like other agents that are metabolized by CYP2D6, paroxetine may significantly inhibit the activity of this isoenzyme. Co-administration of paroxetine with other drugs that are metabolized by CYP2D6, such as phenothiazines, should be approached with caution and lower doses than usual may need to be prescribed for paroxetine or the phenothiazine).
No products indexed under this heading.

Trimipramine Maleate (Caution is indicated in the co-administration of tricyclic antidepressants (TCAs) with paroxetine, because paroxetine may inhibit TCA metabolism. Plasma TCA concentrations may need to be monitored, and the dose of TCA may need to be reduced if a TCA is co-administered with paroxetine).
No products indexed under this heading.

Tryptophan (As with other serotonin reuptake inhibitors, an interaction between paroxetine and tryptophan may occur when they are co-administered. Adverse experiences, consisting primarily of headache, nausea, sweating, and dizziness, have been reported when tryptophan was administered to patients taking paroxetine. Consequently, concomitant use of paroxetine with serotonin precursors such as tryptophan, is not recommended).
No products indexed under this heading.

Valdecoxib (Paroxetine may increase the risk of bleeding events, including upper gastrointestinal bleeding. Concomitant use of paroxetine with NSAIDs may increase this risk).
No products indexed under this heading.

Vardenafil Hydrochloride (Co-administration of paroxetine with drugs that inhibit CYP2D6 should be approached with caution). Products include:
Levitra 3157

Venlafaxine Hydrochloride (The development of a potentially life-threatening serotonin syndrome or Neuroleptic Malignant Syndrome (NMS)-like reactions have been reported with paroxetine alone, but particularly, with concomitant use of serotonergic drugs. The concomitant use of paroxetine with SNRIs is not recommended). Products include:
Effexor XR 3504
Venlafaxine Hydrochloride Tablets ... 2388

Vinblastine Sulfate (Paroxetine is metabolized by CYP2D6. Like other agents that are metabolized by CYP2D6, paroxetine may significantly inhibit the activity of this isoenzyme. Co-administration of paroxetine with other drugs that are metabolized by CYP2D6 should be approached with caution and may require lower doses

---

IMPORTANT NOTE: Always consult each drug listing in the patient's regimen for possible interactions.

than usually prescribed for either paroxetine or the other drug metabolized by CYP2D6).

No products indexed under this heading.

Warfarin Sodium (Altered anticoagulant effects, including increased bleeding, have been reported when SSRIs or SNRIs are co-administered with warfarin. Patients receiving warfarin therapy should be carefully monitored when paroxetine is initiated or discontinued).

No products indexed under this heading.

Ziprasidone Hydrochloride (The development of a potentially life-threatening serotonin syndrome or Neuroleptic Malignant Syndrome (NMS)-like reactions have been reported with paroxetine alone, but particularly with concomitant use of antipsychotic agents. Patients should be monitored for the emergence of serotonin syndrome or NMS-like signs and symptoms. Treatment with paroxetine and any concomitant antipsychotic should be discontinued immediately if any signs or symptoms of serotonin syndrome or NMS-like signs or symptoms occur and supportive symptomatic treatment should be initiated). Products include:

Geodon 2723

Zolmitriptan (The development of a potentially life-threatening serotonin syndrome or Neuroleptic Malignant Syndrome (NMS)-like reactions have been reported with paroxetine alone, but particularly, with concomitant use of serotonergic drugs (including triptans). Patients should be monitored for the emergence of serotonin syndrome or NMS-like signs and symptoms. Treatment with paroxetine and any concomitant serotonergic agent should be discontinued immediately if any signs or symptoms of serotonin syndrome or NMS-like signs and symptoms occur and supportive symptomatic treatment should be initiated. If concomitant use of paroxetine with a triptan is clinically warranted, careful observation of the patient is advised, particularly during treatment initiation and dose increases). Products include:

Zomig Tablets 773
Zomig Nasal Spray 768
Zomig-ZMT Tablets 773

Zonisamide (Paroxetine is metabolized by CYP2D6. Like other agents that are metabolized by CYP2D6, paroxetine may significantly inhibit the activity of this isoenzyme. Co-administration of paroxetine with other drugs that are metabolized by CYP2D6 should be approached with caution and may require lower doses than usually prescribed for either paroxetine or the other drug metabolized by CYP2D6). Products include:

Zonegran 1081

Food Interactions

Alcohol (Although paroxetine has not been shown to increase the impairment of mental and motor skills caused by alcohol, patients should be advised to avoid alcohol while taking paroxetine).

Beer, reduced-alcohol (Although paroxetine has not been shown to increase the impairment of mental and motor skills caused by alcohol, patients should be advised to avoid alcohol while taking paroxetine).

Beer, unspecified (Although paroxetine has not been shown to increase the impairment of mental and motor skills caused by alcohol, patients should be advised to avoid alcohol while taking paroxetine).

Food, unspecified (The effects of food on the bioavailability of paroxetine were studied in subjects administered a single dose with and without food. AUC was only slightly increased (6%) when drug

was administered with food but the C_{max} was 29% greater, while the time to reach peak plasma concentration decreased from 6.4 hours post-dosing to 4.9 hours; paroxetine may be administered with or without food).

Meal, unspecified (The effects of food on the bioavailability of paroxetine were studied in subjects administered a single dose with and without food. AUC was only slightly increased (6%) when drug was administered with food but the C_{max} was 29% greater, while the time to reach peak plasma concentration decreased from 6.4 hours post-dosing to 4.9 hours; paroxetine may be administered with or without food).

Wine, Chianti (Although paroxetine has not been shown to increase the impairment of mental and motor skills caused by alcohol, patients should be advised to avoid alcohol while taking paroxetine).

Wine, Red (Although paroxetine has not been shown to increase the impairment of mental and motor skills caused by alcohol, patients should be advised to avoid alcohol while taking paroxetine).

Wine, unspecified (Although paroxetine has not been shown to increase the impairment of mental and motor skills caused by alcohol, patients should be advised to avoid alcohol while taking paroxetine).

Wine products (Although paroxetine has not been shown to increase the impairment of mental and motor skills caused by alcohol, patients should be advised to avoid alcohol while taking paroxetine).

PAXIL CR CONTROLLED-RELEASE TABLETS

(Paroxetine Hydrochloride) 1596
May interact with 5HT1-receptor agonists, alcohols, anticoagulants, antipsychotic agents, aspirin-acetylsalicylic acid, class IC antiarrhythmics, cytochrome p450 2d6 inhibitors (selected), cytochrome p450 2d6 substrates (selected), diuretics, dopamine antagonists, drugs affecting hepatic drug metabolizing enzyme systems, highly protein bound drugs (selected), lithium preparations, monoamine oxidase inhibitors, non-steroidal anti-inflammatory agents, oral anticoagulants, phenothiazines, phenytoin, quinidine, selective serotonin reuptake inhibitors, serotonin and norepinephrine reuptake inhibitors, serotoninergic agents, theophyllines, tricyclic antidepressants, triptans, and certain other agents. Compounds in these categories include:

Almotriptan Malate (The development of a potentially life-threatening serotonin syndrome or Neuroleptic Malignant Syndrome (NMS)-like reactions have been reported with paroxetine alone, but particularly, with concomitant use of serotonergic drugs (including triptans). Patients should be monitored for the emergence of serotonin syndrome or NMS-like signs and symptoms. Treatment with paroxetine and any concomitant serotonergic agent should be discontinued immediately if any signs or symptoms of serotonin syndrome or NMS-like signs and symptoms occur and supportive symptomatic treatment should be initiated. If concomitant use of paroxetine with a triptan is clinically warranted, careful observation of the patient is advised, particularly during treatment initiation and dose increases). Products include:

Axert... 2593

Amiloride Hydrochloride (Hyponatremia may occur as a result of treatment with paroxetine. Patients taking diuretics may be at greater risk).

No products indexed under this heading.

Amiodarone Hydrochloride (Because paroxetine is highly bound to plasma protein, administration of paroxetine to a patient taking another drug that is highly protein bound may cause increased free concentrations of the other drug, potentially resulting in adverse events. Conversely, adverse effects could result from displacement of paroxetine by other highly bound drugs).

No products indexed under this heading.

Amitriptyline Hydrochloride (Caution is indicated in the co-administration of tricyclic antidepressants (TCAs) with paroxetine, because paroxetine may inhibit TCA metabolism. Plasma TCA concentrations may need to be monitored, and the dose of TCA may need to be reduced if a TCA is co-administered with paroxetine).

No products indexed under this heading.

Amoxapine (Caution is indicated in the co-administration of tricyclic antidepressants (TCAs) with paroxetine, because paroxetine may inhibit TCA metabolism. Plasma TCA concentrations may need to be monitored, and the dose of TCA may need to be reduced if a TCA is co-administered with paroxetine).

No products indexed under this heading.

Amphetamine Aspartate (Paroxetine is metabolized by CYP2D6. Like other agents that are metabolized by CYP2D6, paroxetine may significantly inhibit the activity of this isoenzyme. Co-administration of paroxetine with other drugs that are metabolized by CYP2D6 should be approached with caution and may require lower doses than usually prescribed for either paroxetine or the other drug metabolized by CYP2D6).

No products indexed under this heading.

Amphetamine Aspartate Monohydrate (Paroxetine is metabolized by CYP2D6. Like other agents that are metabolized by CYP2D6, paroxetine may significantly inhibit the activity of this isoenzyme. Co-administration of paroxetine with other drugs that are metabolized by CYP2D6 should be approached with caution and may require lower doses than usually prescribed for either paroxetine or the other drug metabolized by CYP2D6).

No products indexed under this heading.

Amphetamine Sulfate (Paroxetine is metabolized by CYP2D6. Like other agents that are metabolized by CYP2D6, paroxetine may significantly inhibit the activity of this isoenzyme. Co-administration of paroxetine with other drugs that are metabolized by CYP2D6 should be approached with caution and may require lower doses than usually prescribed for either paroxetine or the other drug metabolized by CYP2D6).

No products indexed under this heading.

Anisindione (Concomitant use of paroxetine with drugs affecting coagulation may increase the risk of bleeding including upper gastrointestinal bleeding).

No products indexed under this heading.

Ardeparin Sodium (Paroxetine may increase the risk of bleeding events, including upper gastrointestinal bleeding. Concomitant use of paroxetine with anticoagulants may increase this risk).

No products indexed under this heading.

Aripiprazole (The development of a potentially life-threatening serotonin syndrome or Neuroleptic Malignant Syndrome (NMS)-like reactions have been reported with paroxetine alone, but particularly with concomitant use of antipsychotic agents. Patients should be monitored for the emergence of serotonin syndrome or NMS-like signs and symptoms. Treatment with paroxetine and any concomitant antipsychotic

should be discontinued immediately if any signs or symptoms of serotonin syndrome or NMS-like signs or symptoms occur and supportive symptomatic treatment should be initiated).

No products indexed under this heading.

Aspirin (Paroxetine may increase the risk of bleeding events, including upper gastrointestinal bleeding. Concomitant use of paroxetine with aspirin may increase this risk). Products include:

Aggrenox 880
Bayer Aspirin 829
Percodan 1124
St. Joseph Aspirin 2045

Aspirin, Enteric Coated (Paroxetine may increase the risk of bleeding events, including upper gastrointestinal bleeding. Concomitant use of paroxetine with aspirin may increase this risk).

No products indexed under this heading.

Aspirin Buffered (Paroxetine may increase the risk of bleeding events, including upper gastrointestinal bleeding. Concomitant use of paroxetine with aspirin may increase this risk).

No products indexed under this heading.

Atomoxetine Hydrochloride (Paroxetine is metabolized by CYP2D6. Like other agents that are metabolized by CYP2D6, paroxetine may significantly inhibit the activity of this isoenzyme. Concomitant use of paroxetine with atomoxetine has resulted in increases in steady state atomoxetine AUC values that were 6- to 8-fold greater and in atomoxetine C_{max} values that were 3- to 4-fold greater than when atomoxetine was given alone. Dosage adjustment of atomoxetine may be necessary and it is recommended that atomoxetine be initiated at a reduced dose when it is given with paroxetine). Products include:

Strattera 1957

Atovaquone (Because paroxetine is highly bound to plasma protein, administration of paroxetine to a patient taking another drug that is highly protein bound may cause increased free concentrations of the other drug, potentially resulting in adverse events. Conversely, adverse effects could result from displacement of paroxetine by other highly bound drugs). Products include:

Malarone Pediatric Tablets 1572
Malarone 1572
Mepron Suspension 1576

Bendroflumethiazide (Hyponatremia may occur as a result of treatment with paroxetine. Patients taking diuretics may be at greater risk).

No products indexed under this heading.

Bisoprolol Fumarate (Paroxetine is metabolized by CYP2D6. Like other agents that are metabolized by CYP2D6, paroxetine may significantly inhibit the activity of this isoenzyme. Co-administration of paroxetine with other drugs that are metabolized by CYP2D6 should be approached with caution and may require lower doses than usually prescribed for either paroxetine or the other drug metabolized by CYP2D6).

No products indexed under this heading.

Bumetanide (Hyponatremia may occur as a result of treatment with paroxetine. Patients taking diuretics may be at greater risk).

No products indexed under this heading.

Bupropion Hydrochloride (Co-administration of paroxetine with drugs that inhibit CYP2D6 should be approached with caution). Products include:

Aplenzin 2948
Wellbutrin 1719
Wellbutrin SR 1725
Zyban 1762

Captopril (Paroxetine is metabolized by CYP2D6. Like other agents that are metabolized by CYP2D6, paroxetine may significantly inhibit the activity of this isoenzyme. Co-administration of paroxetine with other drugs that are metabolized by CYP2D6 should be approached with caution and may require lower doses than usually prescribed for either paroxetine or the other drug metabolized by CYP2D6). Products include:
Captopril 2341

Carbamazepine (The metabolism and pharmacokinetics of paroxetine may be affected by the induction or inhibition of drug metabolizing enzymes). Products include:
Carbatrol 3280
Equetro 3477

Carvedilol (Paroxetine is metabolized by CYP2D6. Like other agents that are metabolized by CYP2D6, paroxetine may significantly inhibit the activity of this isoenzyme. Co-administration of paroxetine with other drugs that are metabolized by CYP2D6 should be approached with caution and may require lower doses than usually prescribed for either paroxetine or the other drug metabolized by CYP2D6). Products include:
Coreg 1409

Cefonicid Sodium (Because paroxetine is highly bound to plasma protein, administration of paroxetine to a patient taking another drug that is highly protein bound may cause increased free concentrations of the other drug, potentially resulting in adverse events. Conversely, adverse effects could result from displacement of paroxetine by other highly bound drugs).
No products indexed under this heading.

Celecoxib (Paroxetine may increase the risk of bleeding events, including upper gastrointestinal bleeding. Concomitant use of paroxetine with NSAIDs may increase this risk). Products include:
Celebrex 3272

Cevimeline Hydrochloride (Paroxetine is metabolized by CYP2D6. Like other agents that are metabolized by CYP2D6, paroxetine may significantly inhibit the activity of this isoenzyme. Co-administration of paroxetine with other drugs that are metabolized by CYP2D6 should be approached with caution and may require lower doses than usually prescribed for either paroxetine or the other drug metabolized by CYP2D6). Products include:
Evoxac 1027

Chlordiazepoxide (Because paroxetine is highly bound to plasma protein, administration of paroxetine to a patient taking another drug that is highly protein bound may cause increased free concentrations of the other drug, potentially resulting in adverse events. Conversely, adverse effects could result from displacement of paroxetine by other highly bound drugs).
No products indexed under this heading.

Chlordiazepoxide Hydrochloride (Because paroxetine is highly bound to plasma protein, administration of paroxetine to a patient taking another drug that is highly protein bound may cause increased free concentrations of the other drug, potentially resulting in adverse events. Conversely, adverse effects could result from displacement of paroxetine by other highly bound drugs).
No products indexed under this heading.

Chloroquine (Co-administration of paroxetine with drugs that inhibit CYP2D6 should be approached with caution).
No products indexed under this heading.

Chloroquine Hydrochloride (Co-administration of paroxetine with drugs that inhibit CYP2D6 should be approached with caution).
No products indexed under this heading.

Chloroquine Phosphate (Co-administration of paroxetine with drugs that inhibit CYP2D6 should be approached with caution).
No products indexed under this heading.

Chlorothiazide (Hyponatremia may occur as a result of treatment with paroxetine. Patients taking diuretics may be at greater risk).
No products indexed under this heading.

Chlorothiazide Sodium (Hyponatremia may occur as a result of treatment with paroxetine. Patients taking diuretics may be at greater risk). Products include:
Diuril Intravenous 2009

Chlorpheniramine (Co-administration of paroxetine with drugs that inhibit CYP2D6 should be approached with caution).
No products indexed under this heading.

Chlorpheniramine Maleate (Co-administration of paroxetine with drugs that inhibit CYP2D6 should be approached with caution).
No products indexed under this heading.

Chlorpheniramine Polistirex (Co-administration of paroxetine with drugs that inhibit CYP2D6 should be approached with caution). Products include:
Tussionex 3443

Chlorpheniramine Tannate (Co-administration of paroxetine with drugs that inhibit CYP2D6 should be approached with caution).
No products indexed under this heading.

Chlorpromazine (Paroxetine is metabolized by CYP2D6. Like other agents that are metabolized by CYP2D6, paroxetine may significantly inhibit the activity of this isoenzyme. Co-administration of paroxetine with other drugs that are metabolized by CYP2D6, such as phenothiazines, should be approached with caution and lower doses than usual may need to be prescribed for paroxetine or the phenothiazine).
No products indexed under this heading.

Chlorpromazine Hydrochloride (Paroxetine is metabolized by CYP2D6. Like other agents that are metabolized by CYP2D6, paroxetine may significantly inhibit the activity of this isoenzyme. Co-administration of paroxetine with other drugs that are metabolized by CYP2D6, such as phenothiazines, should be approached with caution and lower doses than usual may need to be prescribed for paroxetine or the phenothiazine).
No products indexed under this heading.

Chlorpropamide (Paroxetine is metabolized by CYP2D6. Like other agents that are metabolized by CYP2D6, paroxetine may significantly inhibit the activity of this isoenzyme. Co-administration of paroxetine with other drugs that are metabolized by CYP2D6 should be approached with caution and may require lower doses than usually prescribed for either paroxetine or the other drug metabolized by CYP2D6).
No products indexed under this heading.

Chlorprothixene (The development of a potentially life-threatening serotonin syndrome or Neuroleptic Malignant Syndrome (NMS)-like reactions have been reported with paroxetine alone, but particularly with concomitant use of antipsychotic agents. Patients should be monitored for the emergence of serotonin syndrome or NMS-like signs and symptoms. Treatment with paroxetine

and any concomitant antipsychotic should be discontinued immediately if any signs or symptoms of serotonin syndrome or NMS-like signs or symptoms occur and supportive symptomatic treatment should be initiated).
No products indexed under this heading.

Chlorprothixene Hydrochloride (The development of a potentially life-threatening serotonin syndrome or Neuroleptic Malignant Syndrome (NMS)-like reactions have been reported with paroxetine alone, but particularly with concomitant use of antipsychotic agents. Patients should be monitored for the emergence of serotonin syndrome or NMS-like signs and symptoms. Treatment with paroxetine and any concomitant antipsychotic should be discontinued immediately if any signs or symptoms of serotonin syndrome or NMS-like signs or symptoms occur and supportive symptomatic treatment should be initiated).
No products indexed under this heading.

Chlorprothixene Lactate (The development of a potentially life-threatening serotonin syndrome or Neuroleptic Malignant Syndrome (NMS)-like reactions have been reported with paroxetine alone, but particularly with concomitant use of antipsychotic agents. Patients should be monitored for the emergence of serotonin syndrome or NMS-like signs and symptoms. Treatment with paroxetine and any concomitant antipsychotic should be discontinued immediately if any signs or symptoms of serotonin syndrome or NMS-like signs or symptoms occur and supportive symptomatic treatment should be initiated).
No products indexed under this heading.

Chlorthalidone (Hyponatremia may occur as a result of treatment with paroxetine. Patients taking diuretics may be at greater risk). Products include:
Clorpres 2344

Cimetidine (Cimetidine inhibits many cytochrome P$_{450}$ (oxidative) enzymes. In a study where immediate-release paroxetine (30 mg once daily) was dosed orally for 4 weeks, steady-state plasma concentrations of paroxetine were increased by approximately 50% during co-administration with oral cimetidine (300 mg three times daily) for the final week. Therefore, when these drugs are administered concurrently, dosage adjustment of paroxetine controlled release after the starting dose should be guided by clinical effect).
No products indexed under this heading.

Cimetidine Hydrochloride (Cimetidine inhibits many cytochrome P$_{450}$ (oxidative) enzymes. In a study where immediate-release paroxetine (30 mg once daily) was dosed orally for 4 weeks, steady-state plasma concentrations of paroxetine were increased by approximately 50% during co-administration with oral cimetidine (300 mg three times daily) for the final week. Therefore, when these drugs are administered concurrently, dosage adjustment of paroxetine controlled release after the starting dose should be guided by clinical effect).
No products indexed under this heading.

Citalopram Hydrobromide (The development of a potentially life-threatening serotonin syndrome or Neuroleptic Malignant Syndrome (NMS)-like reactions have been reported with paroxetine alone, but particularly, with concomitant use of serotonergic drugs. The concomitant use of paroxetine with other SSRIs is not recommended). Products include:
Celexa 1153

Clomipramine Hydrochloride (Caution is indicated in the co-administration of tricyclic antidepressants (TCAs) with paroxetine, because paroxetine may inhibit TCA metabolism. Plasma TCA concentrations may need to be monitored, and the dose of TCA may need to be reduced if a TCA is co-administered with paroxetine).
No products indexed under this heading.

Clozapine (The development of a potentially life-threatening serotonin syndrome or Neuroleptic Malignant Syndrome (NMS)-like reactions have been reported with paroxetine alone, but particularly with concomitant use of antipsychotic agents. Patients should be monitored for the emergence of serotonin syndrome or NMS-like signs and symptoms. Treatment with paroxetine and any concomitant antipsychotic should be discontinued immediately if any signs or symptoms of serotonin syndrome or NMS-like signs or symptoms occur and supportive symptomatic treatment should be initiated).
No products indexed under this heading.

Cocaine Hydrochloride (Co-administration of paroxetine with drugs that inhibit CYP2D6 should be approached with caution).
No products indexed under this heading.

Codeine Phosphate (Paroxetine is metabolized by CYP2D6. Like other agents that are metabolized by CYP2D6, paroxetine may significantly inhibit the activity of this isoenzyme. Co-administration of paroxetine with other drugs that are metabolized by CYP2D6 should be approached with caution and may require lower doses than usually prescribed for either paroxetine or the other drug metabolized by CYP2D6). Products include:
Tylenol with Codeine 2691

Codeine Sulfate (Paroxetine is metabolized by CYP2D6. Like other agents that are metabolized by CYP2D6, paroxetine may significantly inhibit the activity of this isoenzyme. Co-administration of paroxetine with other drugs that are metabolized by CYP2D6 should be approached with caution and may require lower doses than usually prescribed for either paroxetine or the other drug metabolized by CYP2D6).
No products indexed under this heading.

Cyclobenzaprine Hydrochloride (Paroxetine is metabolized by CYP2D6. Like other agents that are metabolized by CYP2D6, paroxetine may significantly inhibit the activity of this isoenzyme. Co-administration of paroxetine with other drugs that are metabolized by CYP2D6 should be approached with caution and may require lower doses than usually prescribed for either paroxetine or the other drug metabolized by CYP2D6). Products include:
Amrix 964

Cyclosporine (Because paroxetine is highly bound to plasma protein, administration of paroxetine to a patient taking another drug that is highly protein bound may cause increased free concentrations of the other drug, potentially resulting in adverse events. Conversely, adverse effects could result from displacement of paroxetine by other highly bound drugs). Products include:
Gengraf 440
Neoral Oral Solution 2496
Neoral Capsules 2496
Restasis 605

Dalteparin Sodium (Paroxetine may increase the risk of bleeding events, including upper gastrointestinal bleeding. Concomitant use of paroxetine with anticoagulants may increase this risk). Products include:

IMPORTANT NOTE: Always consult each drug listing in the patient's regimen for possible interactions.

Paxil CR Interactions Index 1394

Fragmin 1058

Danaparoid Sodium (Paroxetine may increase the risk of bleeding events, including upper gastrointestinal bleeding. Concomitant use of paroxetine with anticoagulants may increase this risk).
No products indexed under this heading.

Debrisoquine (Paroxetine is metabolized by CYP2D6. Like other agents that are metabolized by CYP2D6, paroxetine may significantly inhibit the activity of this isoenzyme. Co-administration of paroxetine with other drugs that are metabolized by CYP2D6 should be approached with caution and may require lower doses than usually prescribed for either paroxetine or the other drug metabolized by CYP2D6).
No products indexed under this heading.

Desipramine Hydrochloride (Paroxetine inhibits CYP2D6. Like other agents that are metabolized by CYP2D6, paroxetine may significantly inhibit the activity of this isoenzyme. In one study, daily dosing of immediate-release paroxetine (20 mg once daily) under steady-state conditions increased single dose desipramine (100 mg) C_{max}, AUC, and $T_{1/2}$ by an average of approximately 2-, 5-, and 3-fold, respectively. Co-administration of paroxetine with other drugs that are metabolized by CYP2D6, such as desipramine, should be approached with caution. If co-administered, plasma concentrations of desipramine may need to be monitored and a lower dose of paroxetine or desipramine may be required).
No products indexed under this heading.

Desvenlafaxine Succinate (The development of a potentially life-threatening serotonin syndrome or Neuroleptic Malignant Syndrome (NMS)-like reactions have been reported with paroxetine alone, but particularly, with concomitant use of serotonergic drugs. The concomitant use of paroxetine with SNRIs is not recommended). Products include:
Pristiq 3564

Dexfenfluramine Hydrochloride (Paroxetine is metabolized by CYP2D6. Like other agents that are metabolized by CYP2D6, paroxetine may significantly inhibit the activity of this isoenzyme. Co-administration of paroxetine with other drugs that are metabolized by CYP2D6 should be approached with caution and may require lower doses than usually prescribed for either paroxetine or the other drug metabolized by CYP2D6).
No products indexed under this heading.

Dextromethorphan Hydrobromide (Paroxetine is metabolized by CYP2D6. Like other agents that are metabolized by CYP2D6, paroxetine may significantly inhibit the activity of this isoenzyme. Co-administration of paroxetine with other drugs that are metabolized by CYP2D6 should be approached with caution and may require lower doses than usually prescribed for either paroxetine or the other drug metabolized by CYP2D6).
No products indexed under this heading.

Dextromethorphan Polistirex (Paroxetine is metabolized by CYP2D6. Like other agents that are metabolized by CYP2D6, paroxetine may significantly inhibit the activity of this isoenzyme. Co-administration of paroxetine with other drugs that are metabolized by CYP2D6 should be approached with caution and may require lower doses than usually prescribed for either paroxetine or the other drug metabolized by CYP2D6).
No products indexed under this heading.

Diazepam (Because paroxetine is highly bound to plasma protein, administration of paroxetine to a patient taking another drug that is highly protein bound may cause increased free concentrations of the other drug, potentially resulting in adverse events. Conversely, adverse effects could result from displacement of paroxetine by other highly bound drugs). Products include:
Valium Tablets 2880

Diclofenac Epolamine (Paroxetine may increase the risk of bleeding events, including upper gastrointestinal bleeding. Concomitant use of paroxetine with NSAIDs may increase this risk). Products include:
Flector 1839

Diclofenac Potassium (Paroxetine may increase the risk of bleeding events, including upper gastrointestinal bleeding. Concomitant use of paroxetine with NSAIDs may increase this risk).
No products indexed under this heading.

Diclofenac Sodium (Paroxetine may increase the risk of bleeding events, including upper gastrointestinal bleeding. Concomitant use of paroxetine with NSAIDs may increase this risk).
No products indexed under this heading.

Dicumarol (Concomitant use of paroxetine with drugs affecting coagulation may increase the risk of bleeding including upper gastrointestinal bleeding).
No products indexed under this heading.

Digitalis Glycoside Preparations (Because paroxetine is highly bound to plasma protein, administration of paroxetine to a patient taking another drug that is highly protein bound may cause increased free concentrations of the other drug, potentially resulting in adverse events. Conversely, adverse effects could result from displacement of paroxetine by other highly bound drugs).
No products indexed under this heading.

Digitalis Lanata (Because paroxetine is highly bound to plasma protein, administration of paroxetine to a patient taking another drug that is highly protein bound may cause increased free concentrations of the other drug, potentially resulting in adverse events. Conversely, adverse effects could result from displacement of paroxetine by other highly bound drugs).
No products indexed under this heading.

Digitalis Purpurea (Because paroxetine is highly bound to plasma protein, administration of paroxetine to a patient taking another drug that is highly protein bound may cause increased free concentrations of the other drug, potentially resulting in adverse events. Conversely, adverse effects could result from displacement of paroxetine by other highly bound drugs).
No products indexed under this heading.

Digoxin (The steady-state pharmacokinetics of paroxetine was not altered when administered with digoxin at steady state. Mean digoxin AUC at steady state decreased by 15% in the presence of paroxetine. Since there is little clinical experience, the concurrent administration of paroxetine and digoxin should be undertaken with caution). Products include:
Lanoxin Injection 1546
Lanoxin Injection Pediatric 1549
Lanoxin Tablets 1553

Diphenhydramine (Co-administration of paroxetine with drugs that inhibit CYP2D6 should be approached with caution).
No products indexed under this heading.

Diphenhydramine Hydrochloride (Co-administration of paroxetine with drugs that inhibit CYP2D6 should be approached with caution). Products include:
Benadryl Allergy Ultratab 2042
Children's Benadryl Allergy Liquid 2042

Dipyridamole (Because paroxetine is highly bound to plasma protein, administration of paroxetine to a patient taking another drug that is highly protein bound may cause increased free concentrations of the other drug, potentially resulting in adverse events. Conversely, adverse effects could result from displacement of paroxetine by other highly bound drugs). Products include:
Aggrenox 880

Dolasetron Mesylate (Paroxetine is metabolized by CYP2D6. Like other agents that are metabolized by CYP2D6, paroxetine may significantly inhibit the activity of this isoenzyme. Co-administration of paroxetine with other drugs that are metabolized by CYP2D6 should be approached with caution and may require lower doses than usually prescribed for either paroxetine or the other drug metabolized by CYP2D6). Products include:
Anzemet Injection 2931
Anzemet Tablets 2934

Donepezil Hydrochloride (Paroxetine is metabolized by CYP2D6. Like other agents that are metabolized by CYP2D6, paroxetine may significantly inhibit the activity of this isoenzyme. Co-administration of paroxetine with other drugs that are metabolized by CYP2D6 should be approached with caution and may require lower doses than usually prescribed for either paroxetine or the other drug metabolized by CYP2D6). Products include:
Aricept 1045
Aricept ODT 1045

Doxepin Hydrochloride (Caution is indicated in the co-administration of tricyclic antidepressants (TCAs) with paroxetine, because paroxetine may inhibit TCA metabolism. Plasma TCA concentrations may need to be monitored, and the dose of TCA may need to be reduced if a TCA is co-administered with paroxetine).
No products indexed under this heading.

Duloxetine Hydrochloride (The development of a potentially life-threatening serotonin syndrome or Neuroleptic Malignant Syndrome (NMS)-like reactions have been reported with paroxetine alone, but particularly, with concomitant use of serotonergic drugs. The concomitant use of paroxetine with SNRIs is not recommended). Products include:
Cymbalta 1871

Eletriptan Hydrobromide (The development of a potentially life-threatening serotonin syndrome or Neuroleptic Malignant Syndrome (NMS)-like reactions have been reported with paroxetine alone, but particularly, with concomitant use of serotonergic drugs (including triptans). Patients should be monitored for the emergence of serotonin syndrome or NMS-like signs and symptoms. Treatment with paroxetine and any concomitant serotonergic agent should be discontinued immediately if any signs or symptoms of serotonin syndrome or NMS-like signs and symptoms occur and supportive symptomatic treatment should be initiated. If concomitant use of paroxetine with a triptan is clinically warranted, careful observation of the patient is advised, particularly during treatment initiation and dose increases).
No products indexed under this heading.

Encainide Hydrochloride (Co-administration of paroxetine with other drugs which are metabolized by CYP2D6, including Type 1C antiarrhythmics (eg, propafenone, flecainide, encainide), should be approached with caution).
No products indexed under this heading.

Enoxaparin Sodium (Paroxetine may increase the risk of bleeding events, including upper gastrointestinal bleeding. Concomitant use of paroxetine with anticoagulants may increase this risk). Products include:
Lovenox 3005

Erythromycin (The metabolism and pharmacokinetics of paroxetine may be affected by the induction or inhibition of drug metabolizing enzymes).
No products indexed under this heading.

Erythromycin Estolate (The metabolism and pharmacokinetics of paroxetine may be affected by the induction or inhibition of drug metabolizing enzymes).
No products indexed under this heading.

Erythromycin Ethylsuccinate (The metabolism and pharmacokinetics of paroxetine may be affected by the induction or inhibition of drug metabolizing enzymes). Products include:
E.E.S. 437
EryPed 435

Erythromycin Gluceptate (The metabolism and pharmacokinetics of paroxetine may be affected by the induction or inhibition of drug metabolizing enzymes).
No products indexed under this heading.

Erythromycin Lactobionate (The metabolism and pharmacokinetics of paroxetine may be affected by the induction or inhibition of drug metabolizing enzymes).
No products indexed under this heading.

Erythromycin Stearate (The metabolism and pharmacokinetics of paroxetine may be affected by the induction or inhibition of drug metabolizing enzymes).
No products indexed under this heading.

Escitalopram Oxalate (The development of a potentially life-threatening serotonin syndrome or Neuroleptic Malignant Syndrome (NMS)-like reactions have been reported with paroxetine alone, but particularly, with concomitant use of serotonergic drugs. The concomitant use of paroxetine with other SSRIs is not recommended). Products include:
Lexapro Oral Suspension 1160
Lexapro Tablets 1160

Ethacrynic Acid (Hyponatremia may occur as a result of treatment with paroxetine. Patients taking diuretics may be at greater risk).
No products indexed under this heading.

Ethanol (Although paroxetine has not been shown to increase the impairment of mental and motor skills caused by alcohol, patients should be advised to avoid alcohol while taking paroxetine).
No products indexed under this heading.

Ethyl Alcohol (Although paroxetine has not been shown to increase the impairment of mental and motor skills caused by alcohol, patients should be advised to avoid alcohol while taking paroxetine).
No products indexed under this heading.

Etodolac (Paroxetine may increase the risk of bleeding events, including upper gastrointestinal bleeding. Concomitant use of paroxetine with NSAIDs may increase this risk).
No products indexed under this heading.

Fenoprofen Calcium (Paroxetine may increase the risk of bleeding events, including upper gastrointestinal bleeding. Concomitant use of paroxetine with NSAIDs may increase this risk).
No products indexed under this heading.

Fentanyl (Paroxetine is metabolized by CYP2D6. Like other agents that are metabolized by CYP2D6, paroxetine may significantly inhibit the activity of this isoenzyme. Co-administration of

paroxetine with other drugs that are metabolized by CYP2D6 should be approached with caution and may require lower doses than usually prescribed for either paroxetine or the other drug metabolized by CYP2D6). Products include:

Fentanyl Citrate (Paroxetine is metabolized by CYP2D6. Like other agents that are metabolized by CYP2D6, paroxetine may significantly inhibit the activity of this isoenzyme. Co-administration of paroxetine with other drugs that are metabolized by CYP2D6 should be approached with caution and may require lower doses than usually prescribed for either paroxetine or the other drug metabolized by CYP2D6). Products include:

Flecainide Acetate (Co-administration of paroxetine with other drugs which are metabolized by CYP2D6, including Type 1C antiarrhythmics (eg, propafenone, flecainide, encainide), should be approached with caution).

No products indexed under this heading.

Fluoxetine (The development of a potentially life-threatening serotonin syndrome or Neuroleptic Malignant Syndrome (NMS)-like reactions have been reported with paroxetine alone, but particularly, with concomitant use of serotonergic drugs. The concomitant use of paroxetine with other SSRIs is not recommended).

No products indexed under this heading.

Fluoxetine Hydrochloride (The development of a potentially life-threatening serotonin syndrome or Neuroleptic Malignant Syndrome (NMS)-like reactions have been reported with paroxetine alone, but particularly, with concomitant use of serotonergic drugs. The concomitant use of paroxetine with other SSRIs is not recommended). Products include:

Fluphenazine Decanoate (Paroxetine is metabolized by CYP2D6. Like other agents that are metabolized by CYP2D6, paroxetine may significantly inhibit the activity of this isoenzyme. Co-administration of paroxetine with other drugs that are metabolized by CYP2D6, such as phentothiazines, should be approached with caution and lower doses than usual may need to be prescribed for paroxetine or the phenothiazine).

No products indexed under this heading.

Fluphenazine Enanthate (Paroxetine is metabolized by CYP2D6. Like other agents that are metabolized by CYP2D6, paroxetine may significantly inhibit the activity of this isoenzyme. Co-administration of paroxetine with other drugs that are metabolized by CYP2D6, such as phentothiazines, should be approached with caution and lower doses than usual may need to be prescribed for paroxetine or the phenothiazine).

No products indexed under this heading.

Fluphenazine Hydrochloride (Paroxetine is metabolized by CYP2D6. Like other agents that are metabolized by CYP2D6, paroxetine may significantly inhibit the activity of this isoenzyme. Co-administration of paroxetine with other drugs that are metabolized by CYP2D6, such as phentothiazines, should be approached with caution and lower doses than usual may need to be prescribed for paroxetine or the phenothiazine).

No products indexed under this heading.

Flurazepam Hydrochloride (Because paroxetine is highly bound to plasma protein, administration of paroxetine to a patient taking another drug that is highly protein bound may cause increased free concentrations of the other drug, potentially resulting in adverse events. Conversely, adverse effects could result from displacement of paroxetine by other highly bound drugs).

No products indexed under this heading.

Flurbiprofen (Paroxetine may increase the risk of bleeding events, including upper gastrointestinal bleeding. Concomitant use of paroxetine with NSAIDs may increase this risk).

No products indexed under this heading.

Fluvoxamine (The development of a potentially life-threatening serotonin syndrome or Neuroleptic Malignant Syndrome (NMS)-like reactions have been reported with paroxetine alone, but particularly, with concomitant use of serotonergic drugs. The concomitant use of paroxetine with other SSRIs is not recommended).

No products indexed under this heading.

Fluvoxamine Maleate (The development of a potentially life-threatening serotonin syndrome or Neuroleptic Malignant Syndrome (NMS)-like reactions have been reported with paroxetine alone, but particularly, with concomitant use of serotonergic drugs. The concomitant use of paroxetine with other SSRIs is not recommended).

No products indexed under this heading.

Fondaparinux Sodium (Paroxetine may increase the risk of bleeding events, including upper gastrointestinal bleeding. Concomitant use of paroxetine with anticoagulants may increase this risk). Products include:

Formoterol Fumarate (Paroxetine is metabolized by CYP2D6. Like other agents that are metabolized by CYP2D6, paroxetine may significantly inhibit the activity of this isoenzyme. Co-administration of paroxetine with other drugs that are metabolized by CYP2D6 should be approached with caution and may require lower doses than usually prescribed for either paroxetine or the other drug metabolized by CYP2D6). Products include:

Fosamprenavir Calcium (Co-administration of fosamprenavir with paroxetine significantly decreased plasma levels of paroxetine. Any dose adjustment should be guided by clinical effect (tolerability and efficacy)). Products include:

Fosphenytoin (When a single oral 30 mg dose of immediate-release paroxetine was administered at phenytoin steady state (300 mg once daily for 14 days), paroxetine AUC and $T_{1/2}$ were reduced (by an average of 50% and 35%, respectively) compared to paroxetine administered alone. Since both drugs exhibit nonlinear pharmacokinetics, the above study may not address the case where two drugs are being chronically dosed. There has been a case report of an elevated phenytoin level after 4 weeks of immediate-release paroxetine and phenytoin co-administration. No initial dosage adjustments are considered necessary when paroxetine controlled release is co-administered with phenytoin; any subsequent adjustment should be guided by clinical effect).

No products indexed under this heading.

Fosphenytoin Sodium (When a single oral 30 mg dose of immediate-

release paroxetine was administered at phenytoin steady state (300 mg once daily for 14 days), paroxetine AUC and $T_{1/2}$ were reduced (by an average of 50% and 35%, respectively) compared to paroxetine administered alone. Since both drugs exhibit nonlinear pharmacokinetics, the above study may not address the case where two drugs are being chronically dosed. There has been a case report of an elevated phenytoin level after 4 weeks of immediate-release paroxetine and phenytoin co-administration. No initial dosage adjustments are considered necessary when paroxetine controlled release is co-administered with phenytoin; any subsequent adjustment should be guided by clinical effect).

No products indexed under this heading.

Frovatriptan Succinate (The development of a potentially life-threatening serotonin syndrome or Neuroleptic Malignant Syndrome (NMS)-like reactions have been reported with paroxetine alone, but particularly, with concomitant use of serotonergic drugs (including triptans). Patients should be monitored for the emergence of serotonin syndrome or NMS-like signs and symptoms. Treatment with paroxetine and any concomitant serotonergic agent should be discontinued immediately if any signs or symptoms of serotonin syndrome or NMS-like signs and symptoms occur and supportive symptomatic treatment should be initiated. If concomitant use of paroxetine with a triptan is clinically warranted, careful observation of the patient is advised, particularly during treatment initiation and dose increases). Products include:

Furosemide (Hyponatremia may occur as a result of treatment with paroxetine. Patients taking diuretics may be at greater risk). Products include:

Galantamine Hydrobromide (Paroxetine is metabolized by CYP2D6. Like other agents that are metabolized by CYP2D6, paroxetine may significantly inhibit the activity of this isoenzyme. Co-administration of paroxetine with other drugs that are metabolized by CYP2D6 should be approached with caution and may require lower doses than usually prescribed for either paroxetine or the other drug metabolized by CYP2D6).

No products indexed under this heading.

Glipizide (Because paroxetine is highly bound to plasma protein, administration of paroxetine to a patient taking another drug that is highly protein bound may cause increased free concentrations of the other drug, potentially resulting in adverse events. Conversely, adverse effects could result from displacement of paroxetine by other highly bound drugs).

No products indexed under this heading.

Halofantrine Hydrochloride (Co-administration of paroxetine with drugs that inhibit CYP2D6 should be approached with caution).

No products indexed under this heading.

Haloperidol (The development of a potentially life-threatening serotonin syndrome or Neuroleptic Malignant Syndrome (NMS)-like reactions have been reported with paroxetine alone, but particularly with concomitant use of antipsychotic agents. Patients should be monitored for the emergence of serotonin syndrome or NMS-like signs and symptoms. Treatment with paroxetine and any concomitant antipsychotic should be discontinued immediately if any signs or symptoms of serotonin

syndrome or NMS-like signs or symptoms occur and supportive symptomatic treatment should be initiated).

No products indexed under this heading.

Haloperidol Decanoate (The development of a potentially life-threatening serotonin syndrome or Neuroleptic Malignant Syndrome (NMS)-like reactions have been reported with paroxetine alone, but particularly with concomitant use of antipsychotic agents. Patients should be monitored for the emergence of serotonin syndrome or NMS-like signs and symptoms. Treatment with paroxetine and any concomitant antipsychotic should be discontinued immediately if any signs or symptoms of serotonin syndrome or NMS-like signs or symptoms occur and supportive symptomatic treatment should be initiated).

No products indexed under this heading.

Haloperidol Lactate (The development of a potentially life-threatening serotonin syndrome or Neuroleptic Malignant Syndrome (NMS)-like reactions have been reported with paroxetine alone, but particularly with concomitant use of antipsychotic agents. Patients should be monitored for the emergence of serotonin syndrome or NMS-like signs and symptoms. Treatment with paroxetine and any concomitant antipsychotic should be discontinued immediately if any signs or symptoms of serotonin syndrome or NMS-like signs or symptoms occur and supportive symptomatic treatment should be initiated).

No products indexed under this heading.

Heparin Calcium (Paroxetine may increase the risk of bleeding events, including upper gastrointestinal bleeding. Concomitant use of paroxetine with anticoagulants may increase this risk).

No products indexed under this heading.

Heparin Sodium (Paroxetine may increase the risk of bleeding events, including upper gastrointestinal bleeding. Concomitant use of paroxetine with anticoagulants may increase this risk).

No products indexed under this heading.

Hydrochlorothiazide (Hyponatremia may occur as a result of treatment with paroxetine. Patients taking diuretics may be at greater risk). Products include:

Hydrocodone Bitartrate (Paroxetine is metabolized by CYP2D6. Like other agents that are metabolized by CYP2D6, paroxetine may significantly inhibit the activity of this isoenzyme. Co-administration of paroxetine with other drugs that are metabolized by CYP2D6 should be approached with caution and may require lower doses than usually prescribed for either paroxetine or the other drug metabolized by CYP2D6). Products include:

Hydroflumethiazide (Hyponatremia may occur as a result of treatment with paroxetine. Patients taking diuretics may be at greater risk).

No products indexed under this heading.

Hydroxychloroquine Sulfate (Co-administration of paroxetine with drugs that inhibit CYP2D6 should be approached with caution).
No products indexed under this heading.

Hypericum (Based on the mechanism of action of paroxetine and the potential for serotonin syndrome, caution is advised when paroxetine hydrochloride is co-administered with other drugs or agents that may affect the serotonergic neurotransmitter systems, such as St. John's Wort).
No products indexed under this heading.

Hypericum Perforatum (Based on the mechanism of action of paroxetine and the potential for serotonin syndrome, caution is advised when paroxetine hydrochloride is co-administered with other drugs or agents that may affect the serotonergic neurotransmitter systems, such as St. John's Wort). Products include:
Traumeel 1800

Ibuprofen (Paroxetine may increase the risk of bleeding events, including upper gastrointestinal bleeding. Concomitant use of paroxetine with NSAIDs may increase this risk). Products include:
Motrin IB 2043
Children's Motrin 2044
Children's Motrin Non-Staining Dye-Free 2044
Infants' Motrin 2044
Infants' Motrin Dye-Free 2044
Junior Strength Motrin 2044
Vicoprofen 564

Imatinib Mesylate (Co-administration of paroxetine with drugs that inhibit CYP2D6 should be approached with caution). Products include:
Gleevec 2477

Imipramine Hydrochloride (Caution is indicated in the co-administration of tricyclic antidepressants (TCAs) with paroxetine, because paroxetine may inhibit TCA metabolism. Plasma TCA concentrations may need to be monitored, and the dose of TCA may need to be reduced if a TCA is co-administered with paroxetine).
No products indexed under this heading.

Imipramine Pamoate (Caution is indicated in the co-administration of tricyclic antidepressants (TCAs) with paroxetine, because paroxetine may inhibit TCA metabolism. Plasma TCA concentrations may need to be monitored, and the dose of TCA may need to be reduced if a TCA is co-administered with paroxetine).
No products indexed under this heading.

Indapamide (Hyponatremia may occur as a result of treatment with paroxetine. Patients taking diuretics may be at greater risk). Products include:
Indapamide 2356

Indomethacin (Paroxetine may increase the risk of bleeding events, including upper gastrointestinal bleeding. Concomitant use of paroxetine with NSAIDs may increase this risk). Products include:
Indocin 2167

Indomethacin Sodium Trihydrate (Paroxetine may increase the risk of bleeding events, including upper gastrointestinal bleeding. Concomitant use of paroxetine with NSAIDs may increase this risk). Products include:
Indocin I.V. 2007

Indoramin Hydrochloride (Paroxetine is metabolized by CYP2D6. Like other agents that are metabolized by CYP2D6, paroxetine may significantly inhibit the activity of this isoenzyme. Co-administration of paroxetine with other drugs that are metabolized by CYP2D6 should be approached with caution and may require lower doses than usually prescribed for either paroxetine or the other drug metabolized by CYP2D6).
No products indexed under this heading.

Isocarboxazid (Concomitant use in patients taking monoamine oxidase inhibitors (MAOIs), is contraindicated. In patients receiving another serotonin reuptake inhibitor drug in combination with an MAOI, there have been reports of serious, sometimes fatal reactions. These reactions have also been reported in patients who have recently discontinued that drug and have been started on an MAOI. Some cases presented with features resembling neuroleptic malignant syndrome. While there are no human data showing such an interaction with paroxetine hydrochloride, limited animal data on the effects of combined use of paroxetine and MAOIs suggest that these drugs may act synergistically to elevate blood pressure and evoke behavioral excitation. Therefore, it is recommended that paroxetine not be used in combination with an MAOI, or within 14 days of discontinuing treatment with an MAOI. At least 2 weeks should be allowed after stopping paroxetine before starting an MAOI). Products include:
Marplan 3481

Ketoprofen (Paroxetine may increase the risk of bleeding events, including upper gastrointestinal bleeding. Concomitant use of paroxetine with NSAIDs may increase this risk).
No products indexed under this heading.

Ketorolac Tromethamine (Paroxetine may increase the risk of bleeding events, including upper gastrointestinal bleeding. Concomitant use of paroxetine with NSAIDs may increase this risk). Products include:
Acuvail .... ⊙ 209

Labetalol Hydrochloride (Paroxetine is metabolized by CYP2D6. Like other agents that are metabolized by CYP2D6, paroxetine may significantly inhibit the activity of this isoenzyme. Co-administration of paroxetine with other drugs that are metabolized by CYP2D6 should be approached with caution and may require lower doses than usually prescribed for either paroxetine or the other drug metabolized by CYP2D6).
No products indexed under this heading.

Lidocaine (Paroxetine is metabolized by CYP2D6. Like other agents that are metabolized by CYP2D6, paroxetine may significantly inhibit the activity of this isoenzyme. Co-administration of paroxetine with other drugs that are metabolized by CYP2D6 should be approached with caution and may require lower doses than usually prescribed for either paroxetine or the other drug metabolized by CYP2D6). Products include:
Lidoderm 1107

Lidocaine Hydrochloride (Paroxetine is metabolized by CYP2D6. Like other agents that are metabolized by CYP2D6, paroxetine may significantly inhibit the activity of this isoenzyme. Co-administration of paroxetine with other drugs that are metabolized by CYP2D6 should be approached with caution and may require lower doses than usually prescribed for either paroxetine or the other drug metabolized by CYP2D6).
No products indexed under this heading.

Linezolid (Concomitant use in patients taking monoamine oxidase inhibitors (MAOIs), including linezolid, an antibiotic which is a reversible non-selective MAOI is contraindicated. In patients receiving another serotonin reuptake inhibitor drug in combination with an MAOI, there have been reports of serious, sometimes fatal reactions. These reactions have also been reported in patients who have recently discontinued that drug and have been started on an MAOI. Some cases presented with features resembling neuroleptic malignant syndrome. While there are no human data showing such an interaction with paroxetine hydrochloride, limited animal data on the effects of combined use of paroxetine and MAOIs suggest that these drugs may act synergistically to elevate blood pressure and evoke behavioral excitation. Therefore, it is recommended that paroxetine not be used in combination with an MAOI (including linezolid), or within 14 days of discontinuing treatment with an MAOI. At least 2 weeks should be allowed after stopping paroxetine before starting an MAOI). Products include:
Zyvox 2769

Lithium (A multiple-dose study with paroxetine has shown that there is no pharmacokinetic interaction between paroxetine and lithium carbonate. However, due to the potential for serotonin syndrome, caution is advised when paroxetine is co-administered with lithium).
No products indexed under this heading.

Lithium Carbonate (A multiple-dose study with paroxetine has shown that there is no pharmacokinetic interaction between paroxetine and lithium carbonate. However, due to the potential for serotonin syndrome, caution is advised when paroxetine is co-administered with lithium).
No products indexed under this heading.

Lithium Citrate (A multiple-dose study with paroxetine has shown that there is no pharmacokinetic interaction between paroxetine and lithium carbonate. However, due to the potential for serotonin syndrome, caution is advised when paroxetine is co-administered with lithium).
No products indexed under this heading.

Low Molecular Weight Heparins (Paroxetine may increase the risk of bleeding events, including upper gastrointestinal bleeding. Concomitant use of paroxetine with anticoagulants may increase this risk).
No products indexed under this heading.

Loxapine Hydrochloride (The development of a potentially life-threatening serotonin syndrome or Neuroleptic Malignant Syndrome (NMS)-like reactions have been reported with paroxetine alone, but particularly with concomitant use of antipsychotic agents. Patients should be monitored for the emergence of serotonin syndrome or NMS-like signs and symptoms. Treatment with paroxetine and any concomitant antipsychotic should be discontinued immediately if any signs or symptoms of serotonin syndrome or NMS-like signs or symptoms occur and supportive symptomatic treatment should be initiated).
No products indexed under this heading.

Loxapine Succinate (The development of a potentially life-threatening serotonin syndrome or Neuroleptic Malignant Syndrome (NMS)-like reactions have been reported with paroxetine alone, but particularly with concomitant use of antipsychotic agents. Patients should be monitored for the emergence of serotonin syndrome or NMS-like signs and symptoms. Treatment with paroxetine and any concomitant antipsychotic should be discontinued immediately if any signs or symptoms of serotonin syndrome or NMS-like signs or symptoms occur and supportive symptomatic treatment should be initiated).
No products indexed under this heading.

Maprotiline Hydrochloride (Caution is indicated in the co-administration of tricyclic antidepressants (TCAs) with paroxetine, because paroxetine may inhibit TCA metabolism. Plasma TCA concentrations may need to be monitored, and the dose of TCA may need to be reduced if a TCA is co-administered with paroxetine).
No products indexed under this heading.

Meclofenamate Sodium (Paroxetine may increase the risk of bleeding events, including upper gastrointestinal bleeding. Concomitant use of paroxetine with NSAIDs may increase this risk).
No products indexed under this heading.

Mefenamic Acid (Paroxetine may increase the risk of bleeding events, including upper gastrointestinal bleeding. Concomitant use of paroxetine with NSAIDs may increase this risk).
No products indexed under this heading.

Meloxicam (Paroxetine may increase the risk of bleeding events, including upper gastrointestinal bleeding. Concomitant use of paroxetine with NSAIDs may increase this risk).
No products indexed under this heading.

Meperidine Hydrochloride (Paroxetine is metabolized by CYP2D6. Like other agents that are metabolized by CYP2D6, paroxetine may significantly inhibit the activity of this isoenzyme. Co-administration of paroxetine with other drugs that are metabolized by CYP2D6 should be approached with caution and may require lower doses than usually prescribed for either paroxetine or the other drug metabolized by CYP2D6).
No products indexed under this heading.

Mesoridazine Besylate (Paroxetine is metabolized by CYP2D6. Like other agents that are metabolized by CYP2D6, paroxetine may significantly inhibit the activity of this isoenzyme. Co-administration of paroxetine with other drugs that are metabolized by CYP2D6, such as phentothiazines, should be approached with caution and lower doses than usual may need to be prescribed for paroxetine or the phenothiazine).
No products indexed under this heading.

Methadone Hydrochloride (Paroxetine is metabolized by CYP2D6. Like other agents that are metabolized by CYP2D6, paroxetine may significantly inhibit the activity of this isoenzyme. Co-administration of paroxetine with other drugs that are metabolized by CYP2D6 should be approached with caution and may require lower doses than usually prescribed for either paroxetine or the other drug metabolized by CYP2D6).
No products indexed under this heading.

Methamphetamine Hydrochloride (Paroxetine is metabolized by CYP2D6. Like other agents that are metabolized by CYP2D6, paroxetine may significantly inhibit the activity of this isoenzyme. Co-administration of paroxetine with other drugs that are metabolized by CYP2D6 should be approached with caution and may require lower doses than usually prescribed for either paroxetine or the other drug metabolized by CYP2D6).
No products indexed under this heading.

Methotrimeprazine (Paroxetine is metabolized by CYP2D6. Like other agents that are metabolized by CYP2D6, paroxetine may significantly inhibit the activity of this isoenzyme. Co-administration of paroxetine with other drugs that are metabolized by CYP2D6, such as phentothiazines, should be approached with caution and

1397 Interactions Index Paxil CR

lower doses than usual may need to be prescribed for paroxetine or the phenothiazine).
No products indexed under this heading.

Methoxyphenamine (Paroxetine is metabolized by CYP2D6. Like other agents that are metabolized by CYP2D6, paroxetine may significantly inhibit the activity of this isoenzyme. Co-administration of paroxetine with other drugs that are metabolized by CYP2D6 should be approached with caution and may require lower doses than usually prescribed for either paroxetine or the other drug metabolized by CYP2D6).
No products indexed under this heading.

Methyclothiazide (Hyponatremia may occur as a result of treatment with paroxetine. Patients taking diuretics may be at greater risk).
No products indexed under this heading.

Metoclopramide Hydrochloride (The development of a potentially life-threatening serotonin syndrome or Neuroleptic Malignant Syndrome (NMS)-like reactions have been reported with paroxetine alone, but particularly with concomitant use of antidopaminergic agents. Patients should be monitored for the emergence of serotonin syndrome or NMS-like signs and symptoms. Treatment with paroxetine and any concomitant antidopaminergic agent should be discontinued immediately if any signs or symptoms of serotonin syndrome or NMS-like signs and symptoms occur and supportive symptomatic treatment should be initiated). Products include:
Metozolv ODT 2901

Metolazone (Hyponatremia may occur as a result of treatment with paroxetine. Patients taking diuretics may be at greater risk).
No products indexed under this heading.

Metoprolol Succinate (There has been a case report of severe hypotension when immediate-release paroxetine was added to chronic metoprolol treatment). Products include:
Toprol XL 732

Metoprolol Tartrate (There has been a case report of severe hypotension when immediate-release paroxetine was added to chronic metoprolol treatment).
No products indexed under this heading.

Mexiletine Hydrochloride (Paroxetine is metabolized by CYP2D6. Like other agents that are metabolized by CYP2D6, paroxetine may significantly inhibit the activity of this isoenzyme. Co-administration of paroxetine with other drugs that are metabolized by CYP2D6 should be approached with caution and may require lower doses than usually prescribed for either paroxetine or the other drug metabolized by CYP2D6).
No products indexed under this heading.

Mibefradil Dihydrochloride (Co-administration of paroxetine with drugs that inhibit CYP2D6 should be approached with caution).
No products indexed under this heading.

Midazolam Hydrochloride (Because paroxetine is highly bound to plasma protein, administration of paroxetine to a patient taking another drug that is highly protein bound may cause increased free concentrations of the other drug, potentially resulting in adverse events. Conversely, adverse effects could result from displacement of paroxetine by other highly bound drugs).
No products indexed under this heading.

Mirtazapine (Paroxetine is metabolized by CYP2D6. Like other agents that are metabolized by CYP2D6, paroxetine may significantly inhibit the activity of this isoenzyme. Co-administration of paroxetine with other drugs that are metabolized by CYP2D6 should be approached with caution and may require lower doses than usually prescribed for either paroxetine or the other drug metabolized by CYP2D6). Products include:
Remeron Tablets 3214
RemeronSolTab Tablets 3219

Moclobemide (Concomitant use in patients taking monoamine oxidase inhibitors (MAOIs), is contraindicated. In patients receiving another serotonin reuptake inhibitor drug in combination with an MAOI, there have been reports of serious, sometimes fatal reactions. These reactions have also been reported in patients who have recently discontinued that drug and have been started on an MAOI. Some cases presented with features resembling neuroleptic malignant syndrome. While there are no human data showing such an interaction with paroxetine hydrochloride, limited animal data on the effects of combined use of paroxetine and MAOIs suggest that these drugs may act synergistically to elevate blood pressure and evoke behavioral excitation. Therefore, it is recommended that paroxetine not be used in combination with an MAOI, or within 14 days of discontinuing treatment with an MAOI. At least 2 weeks should be allowed after stopping paroxetine before starting an MAOI).
No products indexed under this heading.

Molindone Hydrochloride (The development of a potentially life-threatening serotonin syndrome or Neuroleptic Malignant Syndrome (NMS)-like reactions have been reported with paroxetine alone, but particularly with concomitant use of antipsychotic agents. Patients should be monitored for the emergence of serotonin syndrome or NMS-like signs and symptoms. Treatment with paroxetine and any concomitant antipsychotic should be discontinued immediately if any signs or symptoms of serotonin syndrome or NMS-like signs or symptoms occur and supportive symptomatic treatment should be initiated). Products include:
Moban 1108

Morphine Sulfate (Paroxetine is metabolized by CYP2D6. Like other agents that are metabolized by CYP2D6, paroxetine may significantly inhibit the activity of this isoenzyme. Co-administration of paroxetine with other drugs that are metabolized by CYP2D6 should be approached with caution and may require lower doses than usually prescribed for either paroxetine or the other drug metabolized by CYP2D6). Products include:
Avinza 1822
Embeda 1831
MS Contin 2803

Nabumetone (Paroxetine may increase the risk of bleeding events, including upper gastrointestinal bleeding. Concomitant use of paroxetine with NSAIDs may increase this risk).
No products indexed under this heading.

Naproxen (Paroxetine may increase the risk of bleeding events, including upper gastrointestinal bleeding. Concomitant use of paroxetine with NSAIDs may increase this risk). Products include:
EC-Naprosyn 2850
Naprosyn 2850
Anaprox/Naprosyn 2850

Naproxen Sodium (Paroxetine may increase the risk of bleeding events, including upper gastrointestinal bleeding. Concomitant use of paroxetine with NSAIDs may increase this risk). Products include:
Anaprox 2850
Anaprox DS 2850
Treximet 1681

Naratriptan Hydrochloride (The development of a potentially life-threatening serotonin syndrome or Neuroleptic Malignant Syndrome (NMS)-like reactions have been reported with paroxetine alone, but particularly, with concomitant use of serotonergic drugs (including triptans). Patients should be monitored for the emergence of serotonin syndrome or NMS-like signs and symptoms. Treatment with paroxetine and any concomitant serotonergic agent should be discontinued immediately if any signs or symptoms of serotonin syndrome or NMS-like signs and symptoms occur and supportive symptomatic treatment should be initiated. If concomitant use of paroxetine with a triptan is clinically warranted, careful observation of the patient is advised, particularly during treatment initiation and dose increases). Products include:
Amerge 1306

Nefazodone Hydrochloride (The development of a potentially life-threatening serotonin syndrome or Neuroleptic Malignant Syndrome (NMS)-like reactions have been reported with paroxetine alone, but particularly, with concomitant use of serotonergic drugs. The concomitant use of paroxetine with SNRIs is not recommended).
No products indexed under this heading.

Nelfinavir Mesylate (Paroxetine is metabolized by CYP2D6. Like other agents that are metabolized by CYP2D6, paroxetine may significantly inhibit the activity of this isoenzyme. Co-administration of paroxetine with other drugs that are metabolized by CYP2D6 should be approached with caution and may require lower doses than usually prescribed for either paroxetine or the other drug metabolized by CYP2D6).
No products indexed under this heading.

Nortriptyline Hydrochloride (Caution is indicated in the co-administration of tricyclic antidepressants (TCAs) with paroxetine, because paroxetine may inhibit TCA metabolism. Plasma TCA concentrations may need to be monitored, and the dose of TCA may need to be reduced if a TCA is co-administered with paroxetine).
No products indexed under this heading.

Olanzapine (The development of a potentially life-threatening serotonin syndrome or Neuroleptic Malignant Syndrome (NMS)-like reactions have been reported with paroxetine alone, but particularly with concomitant use of antipsychotic agents. Patients should be monitored for the emergence of serotonin syndrome or NMS-like signs and symptoms. Treatment with paroxetine and any concomitant antipsychotic should be discontinued immediately if any signs or symptoms of serotonin syndrome or NMS-like signs or symptoms occur and supportive symptomatic treatment should be initiated). Products include:
Symbyax 1965
Zyprexa 1984
Zyprexa IntraMuscular 1984
Zyprexa ZYDIS 1984

Omeprazole (Paroxetine is metabolized by CYP2D6. Like other agents that are metabolized by CYP2D6, paroxetine may significantly inhibit the activity of this isoenzyme. Co-administration of paroxetine with other drugs that are metabolized by CYP2D6 should be approached with caution and may require lower doses than usually prescribed for either paroxetine or the other drug metabolized by CYP2D6).
No products indexed under this heading.

Ondansetron (Paroxetine is metabolized by CYP2D6. Like other agents that are metabolized by CYP2D6, paroxetine may significantly inhibit the activity of this isoenzyme. Co-administration of paroxetine with other drugs that are metabolized by CYP2D6 should be approached with caution and may require lower doses than usually prescribed for either paroxetine or the other drug metabolized by CYP2D6).
No products indexed under this heading.

Ondansetron Hydrochloride (Paroxetine is metabolized by CYP2D6. Like other agents that are metabolized by CYP2D6, paroxetine may significantly inhibit the activity of this isoenzyme. Co-administration of paroxetine with other drugs that are metabolized by CYP2D6 should be approached with caution and may require lower doses than usually prescribed for either paroxetine or the other drug metabolized by CYP2D6). Products include:
Zofran Injection 1750
Zofran 1756
Zofran ODT 1756

Oxaprozin (Paroxetine may increase the risk of bleeding events, including upper gastrointestinal bleeding. Concomitant use of paroxetine with NSAIDs may increase this risk).
No products indexed under this heading.

Oxazepam (Because paroxetine is highly bound to plasma protein, administration of paroxetine to a patient taking another drug that is highly protein bound may cause increased free concentrations of the other drug, potentially resulting in adverse events. Conversely, adverse effects could result from displacement of paroxetine by other highly bound drugs).
No products indexed under this heading.

Oxycodone Hydrochloride (Paroxetine is metabolized by CYP2D6. Like other agents that are metabolized by CYP2D6, paroxetine may significantly inhibit the activity of this isoenzyme. Co-administration of paroxetine with other drugs that are metabolized by CYP2D6 should be approached with caution and may require lower doses than usually prescribed for either paroxetine or the other drug metabolized by CYP2D6). Products include:
OxyContin 2807
Percocet 1121
Percodan 1124

Paclitaxel (Paroxetine is metabolized by CYP2D6. Like other agents that are metabolized by CYP2D6, paroxetine may significantly inhibit the activity of this isoenzyme. Co-administration of paroxetine with other drugs that are metabolized by CYP2D6 should be approached with caution and may require lower doses than usually prescribed for either paroxetine or the other drug metabolized by CYP2D6).
No products indexed under this heading.

Paliperidone (The development of a potentially life-threatening serotonin syndrome or Neuroleptic Malignant Syndrome (NMS)-like reactions have been reported with paroxetine alone, but particularly with concomitant use of antipsychotic agents. Patients should be monitored for the emergence of serotonin syndrome or NMS-like signs and symptoms. Treatment with paroxetine and any concomitant antipsychotic should be discontinued immediately if any signs or symptoms of serotonin syndrome or NMS-like signs or symptoms occur and supportive symptomatic treatment should be initiated). Products include:
Invega 2613
Invega Sustenna 2621

Pargyline Hydrochloride (Concomitant use in patients taking monoamine oxidase inhibitors (MAOIs), is contraindicated. In patients receiving another serotonin reuptake inhibitor drug in combi-

IMPORTANT NOTE: Always consult each drug listing in the patient's regimen for possible interactions.

nation with an MAOI, there have been reports of serious, sometimes fatal reactions. These reactions have also been reported in patients who have recently discontinued that drug and have been started on an MAOI. Some cases presented with features resembling neuroleptic malignant syndrome. While there are no human data showing such an interaction with paroxetine hydrochloride, limited animal data on the effects of combined use of paroxetine and MAOIs suggest that these drugs may act synergistically to elevate blood pressure and evoke behavioral excitation. Therefore, it is recommended that paroxetine not be used in combination with an MAOI, or within 14 days of discontinuing treatment with an MAOI. At least 2 weeks should be allowed after stopping paroxetine before starting an MAOI).

No products indexed under this heading.

Paroxetine (The development of a potentially life-threatening serotonin syndrome or Neuroleptic Malignant Syndrome (NMS)-like reactions have been reported with paroxetine alone, but particularly, with concomitant use of serotonergic drugs. The concomitant use of paroxetine with other SSRIs is not recommended).

No products indexed under this heading.

Paroxetine Mesylate (The development of a potentially life-threatening serotonin syndrome or Neuroleptic Malignant Syndrome (NMS)-like reactions have been reported with paroxetine alone, but particularly, with concomitant use of serotonergic drugs. The concomitant use of paroxetine with other SSRIs is not recommended).

No products indexed under this heading.

Perphenazine (Paroxetine is metabolized by CYP2D6. Like other agents that are metabolized by CYP2D6, paroxetine may significantly inhibit the activity of this isoenzyme. Co-administration of paroxetine with other drugs that are metabolized by CYP2D6, such as phentothiazines, should be approached with caution and lower doses than usual may need to be prescribed for paroxetine or the phenothiazine).

No products indexed under this heading.

Phenelzine Sulfate (Concomitant use in patients taking monoamine oxidase inhibitors (MAOIs), is contraindicated. In patients receiving another serotonin reuptake inhibitor drug in combination with an MAOI, there have been reports of serious, sometimes fatal reactions. These reactions have also been reported in patients who have recently discontinued that drug and have been started on an MAOI. Some cases presented with features resembling neuroleptic malignant syndrome. While there are no human data showing such an interaction with paroxetine hydrochloride, limited animal data on the effects of combined use of paroxetine and MAOIs suggest that these drugs may act synergistically to elevate blood pressure and evoke behavioral excitation. Therefore, it is recommended that paroxetine not be used in combination with an MAOI, or within 14 days of discontinuing treatment with an MAOI. At least 2 weeks should be allowed after stopping paroxetine before starting an MAOI).

No products indexed under this heading.

Phenobarbital (Phenobarbital induces many cytochrome P_{450} (oxidative) enzymes. When a single oral 30 mg dose of immediate-release paroxetine was administered at phenobarbital steady state (100 mg once daily for 14 days), paroxetine AUC and $T_{1/2}$ were reduced (by an average of 25% and 38%, respectively) compared to paroxetine administered alone. Since paroxetine exhibits nonlinear pharmacokinetics,

the results of this study may not address the case where the 2 drugs are both being chronically dosed. No initial dosage adjustment of paroxetine controlled release is considered necessary when co-administered with phenobarbital; any subsequent adjustment should be guided by clinical effect). Products include:

Donnatal 2711

Phenobarbital Sodium (Phenobarbital induces many cytochrome P_{450} (oxidative) enzymes. When a single oral 30 mg dose of immediate-release paroxetine was administered at phenobarbital steady state (100 mg once daily for 14 days), paroxetine AUC and T1/2 were reduced (by an average of 25% and 38%, respectively) compared to paroxetine administered alone. Since paroxetine exhibits nonlinear pharmacokinetics, the results of this study may not address the case where the 2 drugs are both being chronically dosed. No initial dosage adjustment of paroxetine controlled release is considered necessary when co-administered with phenobarbital; any subsequent adjustment should be guided by clinical effect).

No products indexed under this heading.

Phenothiazine Derivatives (Paroxetine is metabolized by CYP2D6. Like other agents that are metabolized by CYP2D6, paroxetine may significantly inhibit the activity of this isoenzyme. Co-administration of paroxetine with other drugs that are metabolized by CYP2D6, such as phentothiazines, should be approached with caution and lower doses than usual may need to be prescribed for paroxetine or the phenothiazine).

No products indexed under this heading.

Phenothiazines (Paroxetine is metabolized by CYP2D6. Like other agents that are metabolized by CYP2D6, paroxetine may significantly inhibit the activity of this isoenzyme. Co-administration of paroxetine with other drugs that are metabolized by CYP2D6, such as phentothiazines, should be approached with caution and lower doses than usual may need to be prescribed for paroxetine or the phenothiazine).

No products indexed under this heading.

Phenylbutazone (Paroxetine may increase the risk of bleeding events, including upper gastrointestinal bleeding. Concomitant use of paroxetine with NSAIDs may increase this risk).

No products indexed under this heading.

Phenytoin (When a single oral 30 mg dose of immediate-release paroxetine was administered at phenytoin steady state (300 mg once daily for 14 days), paroxetine AUC and $T_{1/2}$ were reduced (by an average of 50% and 35%, respectively) compared to paroxetine administered alone. Since both drugs exhibit nonlinear pharmacokinetics, the above study may not address the case where two drugs are being chronically dosed. There has been a case report of an elevated phenytoin level after 4 weeks of immediate-release paroxetine and phenytoin co-administration. No initial dosage adjustments are considered necessary when paroxetine controlled release is co-administered with phenytoin; any subsequent adjustment should be guided by clinical effect).

No products indexed under this heading.

Phenytoin Sodium (When a single oral 30 mg dose of immediate-release paroxetine was administered at phenytoin steady state (300 mg once daily for 14 days), paroxetine AUC and T1/2 were reduced (by an average of 50% and 35%, respectively) compared to paroxetine administered alone. Since both drugs exhibit nonlinear pharmacokinetics, the above study may not address the case where two drugs are

being chronically dosed. There has been a case report of an elevated phenytoin level after 4 weeks of immediate-release paroxetine and phenytoin co-administration. No initial dosage adjustments are considered necessary when paroxetine controlled release is co-administered with phenytoin; any subsequent adjustment should be guided by clinical effect). Products include:

Phenytek Capsules 2380

Pimozide (Concomitant use in patients taking pimozide is contraindicated. In a study of healthy volunteers, after immediate release paroxetine was titrated to 60 mg daily, co-administration of a single dose of 2 mg pimozide was associated with mean increases in pimozide AUC of 151% and C_{max} of 62%, compared to pimozide administered alone. The increase in pimozide AUC and C_{max} is due to the CYP2D6 inhibitory properties of paroxetine. Due to the narrow therapeutic index of pimozide and its known ability to prolong the QT interval, concomitant use of pimozide and paroxetine is contraindicated).

No products indexed under this heading.

Pindolol (Paroxetine is metabolized by CYP2D6. Like other agents that are metabolized by CYP2D6, paroxetine may significantly inhibit the activity of this isoenzyme. Co-administration of paroxetine with other drugs that are metabolized by CYP2D6 should be approached with caution and may require lower doses than usually prescribed for either paroxetine or the other drug metabolized by CYP2D6).

No products indexed under this heading.

Piroxicam (Paroxetine may increase the risk of bleeding events, including upper gastrointestinal bleeding. Concomitant use of paroxetine with NSAIDs may increase this risk).

No products indexed under this heading.

Polythiazide (Hyponatremia may occur as a result of treatment with paroxetine. Patients taking diuretics may be at greater risk).

No products indexed under this heading.

Procarbazine Hydrochloride (Concomitant use in patients taking monoamine oxidase inhibitors (MAOIs), is contraindicated. In patients receiving another serotonin reuptake inhibitor drug in combination with an MAOI, there have been reports of serious, sometimes fatal reactions. These reactions have also been reported in patients who have recently discontinued that drug and have been started on an MAOI. Some cases presented with features resembling neuroleptic malignant syndrome. While there are no human data showing such an interaction with paroxetine hydrochloride, limited animal data on the effects of combined use of paroxetine and MAOIs suggest that these drugs may act synergistically to elevate blood pressure and evoke behavioral excitation. Therefore, it is recommended that paroxetine not be used in combination with an MAOI, or within 14 days of discontinuing treatment with an MAOI. At least 2 weeks should be allowed after stopping paroxetine before starting an MAOI).

No products indexed under this heading.

Prochlorperazine (Paroxetine is metabolized by CYP2D6. Like other agents that are metabolized by CYP2D6, paroxetine may significantly inhibit the activity of this isoenzyme. Co-administration of paroxetine with other drugs that are metabolized by CYP2D6, such as phentothiazines, should be approached with caution and lower doses than usual may need to be prescribed for paroxetine or the phenothiazine).

No products indexed under this heading.

Prochlorperazine Edisylate (Paroxetine is metabolized by CYP2D6. Like other agents that are metabolized by CYP2D6, paroxetine may significantly inhibit the activity of this isoenzyme. Co-administration of paroxetine with other drugs that are metabolized by CYP2D6, such as phentothiazines, should be approached with caution and lower doses than usual may need to be prescribed for paroxetine or the phenothiazine).

No products indexed under this heading.

Prochlorperazine Maleate (Paroxetine is metabolized by CYP2D6. Like other agents that are metabolized by CYP2D6, paroxetine may significantly inhibit the activity of this isoenzyme. Co-administration of paroxetine with other drugs that are metabolized by CYP2D6, such as phentothiazines, should be approached with caution and lower doses than usual may need to be prescribed for paroxetine or the phenothiazine).

No products indexed under this heading.

Procyclidine Hydrochloride (Daily oral dosing of immediate-release paroxetine (30 mg once daily) increased steady-state AUC, C_{max}, and C_{min} values of procyclidine (5 mg oral once daily) by 35%, 37%, and 67%, respectively, compared to procyclidine alone at steady state. If anticholinergic effects are seen, the dose of procyclidine should be reduced).

No products indexed under this heading.

Promethazine (Paroxetine is metabolized by CYP2D6. Like other agents that are metabolized by CYP2D6, paroxetine may significantly inhibit the activity of this isoenzyme. Co-administration of paroxetine with other drugs that are metabolized by CYP2D6, such as phentothiazines, should be approached with caution and lower doses than usual may need to be prescribed for paroxetine or the phenothiazine).

No products indexed under this heading.

Promethazine Hydrochloride (Paroxetine is metabolized by CYP2D6. Like other agents that are metabolized by CYP2D6, paroxetine may significantly inhibit the activity of this isoenzyme. Co-administration of paroxetine with other drugs that are metabolized by CYP2D6, such as phentothiazines, should be approached with caution and lower doses than usual may need to be prescribed for paroxetine or the phenothiazine).

No products indexed under this heading.

Propafenone Hydrochloride (Co-administration of paroxetine with other drugs which are metabolized by CYP2D6, including Type 1C antiarrhythmics (eg, propafenone, flecainide, encainide), should be approached with caution). Products include:

Rythmol 1648
Rythmol SR 1652

Propoxyphene Hydrochloride (Paroxetine is metabolized by CYP2D6. Like other agents that are metabolized by CYP2D6, paroxetine may significantly inhibit the activity of this isoenzyme. Co-administration of paroxetine with other drugs that are metabolized by CYP2D6 should be approached with caution and may require lower doses than usually prescribed for either paroxetine or the other drug metabolized by CYP2D6).

No products indexed under this heading.

Propoxyphene Napsylate (Paroxetine is metabolized by CYP2D6. Like other agents that are metabolized by CYP2D6, paroxetine may significantly inhibit the activity of this isoenzyme. Co-administration of paroxetine with other drugs that are metabolized by CYP2D6 should be approached with

caution and may require lower doses than usually prescribed for either paroxetine or the other drug metabolized by CYP2D6).

No products indexed under this heading.

Propranolol Hydrochloride (Because paroxetine is highly bound to plasma protein, administration of paroxetine to a patient taking another drug that is highly protein bound may cause increased free concentrations of the other drug, potentially resulting in adverse events. Conversely, adverse effects could result from displacement of paroxetine by other highly bound drugs). Products include:

InnoPran XL 1517

Protriptyline Hydrochloride (Caution is indicated in the co-administration of tricyclic antidepressants (TCAs) with paroxetine, because paroxetine may inhibit TCA metabolism. Plasma TCA concentrations may need to be monitored, and the dose of TCA may need to be reduced if a TCA is co-administered with paroxetine).

No products indexed under this heading.

Quetiapine Fumarate (The development of a potentially life-threatening serotonin syndrome or Neuroleptic Malignant Syndrome (NMS)-like reactions have been reported with paroxetine alone, but particularly with concomitant use of antipsychotic agents. Patients should be monitored for the emergence of serotonin syndrome or NMS-like signs and symptoms. Treatment with paroxetine and any concomitant antipsychotic should be discontinued immediately if any signs or symptoms of serotonin syndrome or NMS-like signs or symptoms occur and supportive symptomatic treatment should be initiated). Products include:

Seroquel 750
Seroquel XR 759

Quinacrine Hydrochloride (Co-administration of paroxetine with drugs that inhibit CYP2D6 should be approached with caution).

No products indexed under this heading.

Quinidine (Co-administration of paroxetine with drugs that inhibit CYP2D6 (eg, quinidine) should be approached with caution).

No products indexed under this heading.

Quinidine Gluconate (Co-administration of paroxetine with drugs that inhibit CYP2D6 (eg, quinidine) should be approached with caution).

No products indexed under this heading.

Quinidine Hydrochloride (Co-administration of paroxetine with drugs that inhibit CYP2D6 (eg, quinidine) should be approached with caution).

No products indexed under this heading.

Quinidine Polygalacturonate (Co-administration of paroxetine with drugs that inhibit CYP2D6 (eg, quinidine) should be approached with caution).

No products indexed under this heading.

Quinidine Sulfate (Co-administration of paroxetine with drugs that inhibit CYP2D6 (eg, quinidine) should be approached with caution).

No products indexed under this heading.

Ranitidine Bismuth Citrate (Co-administration of paroxetine with drugs that inhibit CYP2D6 should be approached with caution).

No products indexed under this heading.

Ranitidine Hydrochloride (Co-administration of paroxetine with drugs that inhibit CYP2D6 should be approached with caution). Products include:

Zantac 1737
Zantac Injection 1732
Zantac Pharmacy 1735

Rasagiline Mesylate (Concomitant use in patients taking monoamine oxi-

dase inhibitors (MAOIs), is contraindicated. In patients receiving another serotonin reuptake inhibitor drug in combination with an MAOI, there have been reports of serious, sometimes fatal reactions. These reactions have also been reported in patients who have recently discontinued that drug and have been started on an MAOI. Some cases presented with features resembling neuroleptic malignant syndrome. While there are no human data showing such an interaction with paroxetine hydrochloride, limited animal data on the effects of combined use of paroxetine and MAOIs suggest that these drugs may act synergistically to elevate blood pressure and evoke behavioral excitation. Therefore, it is recommended that paroxetine not be used in combination with an MAOI, or within 14 days of discontinuing treatment with an MAOI. At least 2 weeks should be allowed after stopping paroxetine before starting an MAOI). Products include:

Azilect 3383

Risperidone (Paroxetine is metabolized by CYP2D6. Like other agents that are metabolized by CYP2D6, paroxetine may significantly inhibit the activity of this isoenzyme. Concomitant use of paroxetine with risperidone, a CYP2D6 substrate showed in one study to increase the mean plasma concentrations of risperidone approximately 4-fold, decreased 9-hydroxyrisperidone concentrations approximately 10%, and increased concentrations of the active moiety (the sum of risperidone plus 9-hydroxyrisperidone) approximately 1.4-fold. Therefore, concomitant use with other drugs metabolized by CYP2D6, such as risperidone, should be used with caution). Products include:

Risperdal Consta 2682

Ritonavir (Co-administration of ritonavir with paroxetine significantly decreased plasma levels of paroxetine. Any dose adjustment should be guided by clinical effect (tolerability and efficacy)). Products include:

Kaletra 458
Norvir 509

Rizatriptan Benzoate (The development of a potentially life-threatening serotonin syndrome or Neuroleptic Malignant Syndrome (NMS)-like reactions have been reported with paroxetine alone, but particularly, with concomitant use of serotonergic drugs (including triptans). Patients should be monitored for the emergence of serotonin syndrome or NMS-like signs and symptoms. Treatment with paroxetine and any concomitant serotonergic agent should be discontinued immediately if any signs or symptoms of serotonin syndrome or NMS-like signs and symptoms occur and supportive symptomatic treatment should be initiated. If concomitant use of paroxetine with a triptan is clinically warranted, careful observation of the patient is advised, particularly during treatment initiation and dose increases). Products include:

Maxalt 2206
Maxalt-MLT 2206

Rofecoxib (Paroxetine may increase the risk of bleeding events, including upper gastrointestinal bleeding. Concomitant use of paroxetine with NSAIDs may increase this risk).

No products indexed under this heading.

Selegiline (Concomitant use in patients taking monoamine oxidase inhibitors (MAOIs), is contraindicated. In patients receiving another serotonin reuptake inhibitor drug in combination with an MAOI, there have been reports of serious, sometimes fatal reactions. These reactions have also been reported in patients who have recently discontinued that drug and have been started

on an MAOI. Some cases presented with features resembling neuroleptic malignant syndrome. While there are no human data showing such an interaction with paroxetine hydrochloride, limited animal data on the effects of combined use of paroxetine and MAOIs suggest that these drugs may act synergistically to elevate blood pressure and evoke behavioral excitation. Therefore, it is recommended that paroxetine not be used in combination with an MAOI, or within 14 days of discontinuing treatment with an MAOI. At least 2 weeks should be allowed after stopping paroxetine before starting an MAOI). Products include:

Emsam 3623

Selegiline Hydrochloride (Concomitant use in patients taking monoamine oxidase inhibitors (MAOIs), is contraindicated. In patients receiving another serotonin reuptake inhibitor drug in combination with an MAOI, there have been reports of serious, sometimes fatal reactions. These reactions have also been reported in patients who have recently discontinued that drug and have been started on an MAOI. Some cases presented with features resembling neuroleptic malignant syndrome. While there are no human data showing such an interaction with paroxetine hydrochloride, limited animal data on the effects of combined use of paroxetine and MAOIs suggest that these drugs may act synergistically to elevate blood pressure and evoke behavioral excitation. Therefore, it is recommended that paroxetine not be used in combination with an MAOI, or within 14 days of discontinuing treatment with an MAOI. At least 2 weeks should be allowed after stopping paroxetine before starting an MAOI). Products include:

Eldepryl 3312

Sertraline Hydrochloride (The development of a potentially life-threatening serotonin syndrome or Neuroleptic Malignant Syndrome (NMS)-like reactions have been reported with paroxetine alone, but particularly, with concomitant use of serotonergic drugs. The concomitant use of paroxetine with other SSRIs is not recommended).

No products indexed under this heading.

Sildenafil Citrate (Co-administration of paroxetine with drugs that inhibit CYP2D6 should be approached with caution).

No products indexed under this heading.

Spironolactone (Hyponatremia may occur as a result of treatment with paroxetine. Patients taking diuretics may be at greater risk).

No products indexed under this heading.

Sulindac (Paroxetine may increase the risk of bleeding events, including upper gastrointestinal bleeding. Concomitant use of paroxetine with NSAIDs may increase this risk). Products include:

Clinoril 2098

Sumatriptan (The development of a potentially life-threatening serotonin syndrome or Neuroleptic Malignant Syndrome (NMS)-like reactions have been reported with paroxetine alone, but particularly, with concomitant use of serotonergic drugs (including triptans). Patients should be monitored for the emergence of serotonin syndrome or NMS-like signs and symptoms. Treatment with paroxetine and any concomitant serotonergic agent should be discontinued immediately if any signs or symptoms of serotonin syndrome or NMS-like signs and symptoms occur and supportive symptomatic treatment should be initiated. If concomitant use of paroxetine with a triptan is clinically warranted, careful observation of the

patient is advised, particularly during treatment initiation and dose increases). Products include:

Imitrex Nasal 1503

Sumatriptan Succinate (The development of a potentially life-threatening serotonin syndrome or Neuroleptic Malignant Syndrome (NMS)-like reactions have been reported with paroxetine alone, but particularly, with concomitant use of serotonergic drugs (including triptans). Patients should be monitored for the emergence of serotonin syndrome or NMS-like signs and symptoms. Treatment with paroxetine and any concomitant serotonergic agent should be discontinued immediately if any signs or symptoms of serotonin syndrome or NMS-like signs and symptoms occur and supportive symptomatic treatment should be initiated. If concomitant use of paroxetine with a triptan is clinically warranted, careful observation of the patient is advised, particularly during treatment initiation and dose increases). Products include:

Imitrex 1497
Imitrex Tablets 1508
Treximet 1681

Tamoxifen Citrate (Tamoxifen is a pro-drug requiring metabolic activation by CYP2D6. Inhibition of CYP2D6 by paroxetine may lead to reduced plasma concentrations of an active metabolite and hence reduced efficacy of tamoxifen).

No products indexed under this heading.

Temazepam (Because paroxetine is highly bound to plasma protein, administration of paroxetine to a patient taking another drug that is highly protein bound may cause increased free concentrations of the other drug, potentially resulting in adverse events. Conversely, adverse effects could result from displacement of paroxetine by other highly bound drugs).

No products indexed under this heading.

Teniposide (Paroxetine is metabolized by CYP2D6. Like other agents that are metabolized by CYP2D6, paroxetine may significantly inhibit the activity of this isoenzyme. Co-administration of paroxetine with other drugs that are metabolized by CYP2D6 should be approached with caution and may require lower doses than usually prescribed for either paroxetine or the other drug metabolized by CYP2D6).

No products indexed under this heading.

Terbinafine Hydrochloride (Co-administration of paroxetine with drugs that inhibit CYP2D6 should be approached with caution).

No products indexed under this heading.

Testosterone (Paroxetine is metabolized by CYP2D6. Like other agents that are metabolized by CYP2D6, paroxetine may significantly inhibit the activity of this isoenzyme. Co-administration of paroxetine with other drugs that are metabolized by CYP2D6 should be approached with caution and may require lower doses than usually prescribed for either paroxetine or the other drug metabolized by CYP2D6). Products include:

AndroGel 3456

Testosterone Cypionate (Paroxetine is metabolized by CYP2D6. Like other agents that are metabolized by CYP2D6, paroxetine may significantly inhibit the activity of this isoenzyme. Co-administration of paroxetine with other drugs that are metabolized by CYP2D6 should be approached with caution and may require lower doses than usually prescribed for either paroxetine or the other drug metabolized by CYP2D6).

No products indexed under this heading.

IMPORTANT NOTE: Always consult each drug listing in the patient's regimen for possible interactions.

Testosterone Enanthate (Paroxetine is metabolized by CYP2D6. Like other agents that are metabolized by CYP2D6, paroxetine may significantly inhibit the activity of this isoenzyme. Co-administration of paroxetine with other drugs that are metabolized by CYP2D6 should be approached with caution and may require lower doses than usually prescribed for either parox-etine or the other drug metabolized by CYP2D6). Products include:

Testosterone Propionate (Paroxet-ine is metabolized by CYP2D6. Like other agents that are metabolized by CYP2D6, paroxetine may significantly inhibit the activity of this isoenzyme. Co-administration of paroxetine with other drugs that are metabolized by CYP2D6 should be approached with caution and may require lower doses than usually prescribed for either parox-etine or the other drug metabolized by CYP2D6).
No products indexed under this heading.

Theophyllinate (The metabolism and pharmacokinetics of paroxetine may be affected by the induction or inhibition of drug metabolizing enzymes).
No products indexed under this heading.

Theophylline (Reports of elevated theophylline levels associated with treat-ment with immediate-release paroxetine have been reported. While this interac-tion has not been formally studied, it is recommended that theophylline levels be monitored when these drugs are concurrently administered).
No products indexed under this heading.

Theophylline Anhydrous (Reports of elevated theophylline levels associated with treatment with immediate-release paroxetine have been reported. While this interaction has not been formally studied, it is recommended that theo-phylline levels be monitored when these drugs are concurrently administered). Products include:

Theophylline Calcium Salicylate (Reports of elevated theophylline levels associated with treatment with immediate-release paroxetine have been reported. While this interaction has not been formally studied, it is rec-ommended that theophylline levels be monitored when these drugs are con-currently administered).
No products indexed under this heading.

Theophylline Dihydroxypropyl (Glyceryl) (Reports of elevated theo-phylline levels associated with treat-ment with immediate-release paroxetine have been reported. While this interac-tion has not been formally studied, it is recommended that theophylline levels be monitored when these drugs are concurrently administered).
No products indexed under this heading.

Theophylline Ethylenediamine (Reports of elevated theophylline levels associated with treatment with immediate-release paroxetine have been reported. While this interaction has not been formally studied, it is rec-ommended that theophylline levels be monitored when these drugs are con-currently administered).
No products indexed under this heading.

Theophylline Sodium Glycinate (Reports of elevated theophylline levels associated with treatment with immediate-release paroxetine have been reported. While this interaction has not been formally studied, it is rec-ommended that theophylline levels be monitored when these drugs are con-currently administered).
No products indexed under this heading.

Thioridazine (Concomitant use in patients taking thioridazine is contraindi-cated. Thioridazine administration alone produces prolongation of the QTc inter-val, which is associated with serious ventricular arrhythmias, such as tor-sade de pointes-type arrhythmias, and sudden death. This effect appears to be dose related. An *in vivo* study suggests that drugs which inhibit CYP2D6, such as paroxetine, will elevate plasma levels of thioridazine. Therefore, it is recom-mended that paroxetine not be used in combination with thioridazine).
No products indexed under this heading.

Thioridazine Hydrochloride (Con-comitant use in patients taking thiorida-zine is contraindicated. Thioridazine administration alone produces prolonga-tion of the QTc interval, which is associ-ated with serious ventricular arrhyth-mias, such as torsade de pointes-type arrhythmias, and sudden death. This effect appears to be dose related. An *in vivo* study suggests that drugs which inhibit CYP2D6, such as paroxetine, will elevate plasma levels of thioridazine. Therefore, it is recommended that par-oxetine not be used in combination with thioridazine). Products include:

Thiothixene (The development of a potentially life-threatening serotonin syndrome or Neuroleptic Malignant Syn-drome (NMS)-like reactions have been reported with paroxetine alone, but par-ticularly with concomitant use of anti-psychotic agents. Patients should be monitored for the emergence of seroto-nin syndrome or NMS-like signs and symptoms. Treatment with paroxetine and any concomitant antipsychotic should be discontinued immediately if any signs or symptoms of serotonin syndrome or NMS-like signs or symp-toms occur and supportive symptomat-ic treatment should be initiated). Products include:

Timolol Maleate (Paroxetine is metabolized by CYP2D6. Like other agents that are metabolized by CYP2D6, paroxetine may significantly inhibit the activity of this isoenzyme. Co-administration of paroxetine with other drugs that are metabolized by CYP2D6 should be approached with caution and may require lower doses than usually prescribed for either parox-etine or the other drug metabolized by CYP2D6). Products include:

Tinzaparin Sodium (Paroxetine may increase the risk of bleeding events, including upper gastrointestinal bleed-ing. Concomitant use of paroxetine with anticoagulants may increase this risk).
No products indexed under this heading.

Tolbutamide (Because paroxetine is highly bound to plasma protein, admin-istration of paroxetine to a patient tak-ing another drug that is highly protein bound may cause increased free con-centrations of the other drug, potential-ly resulting in adverse events. Con-versely, adverse effects could result from displacement of paroxetine by other highly bound drugs).
No products indexed under this heading.

Tolmetin Sodium (Paroxetine may increase the risk of bleeding events, including upper gastrointestinal bleed-ing. Concomitant use of paroxetine with NSAIDs may increase this risk).
No products indexed under this heading.

Tolterodine Tartrate (Paroxetine is metabolized by CYP2D6. Like other agents that are metabolized by CYP2D6, paroxetine may significantly inhibit the activity of this isoenzyme. Co-administration of paroxetine with other drugs that are metabolized by CYP2D6 should be approached with caution and may require lower doses than usually prescribed for either parox-etine or the other drug metabolized by CYP2D6).
No products indexed under this heading.

Torsemide (Hyponatremia may occur as a result of treatment with paroxetine. Patients taking diuretics may be at greater risk).
No products indexed under this heading.

Tramadol Hydrochloride (Based on the mechanism of action of paroxetine and the potential for serotonin syn-drome, caution is advised when parox-etine hydrochloride is co-administered with other drugs or agents that may affect the serotonergic neurotransmitter systems, such as tramadol). Products include:

Tranylcypromine Sulfate (Concomi-tant use in patients taking monoamine oxidase inhibitors (MAOIs), is contraindi-cated. In patients receiving another ser-otonin reuptake inhibitor drug in combi-nation with an MAOI, there have been reports of serious, sometimes fatal reactions. These reactions have also been reported in patients who have recently discontinued that drug and have been started on an MAOI. Some cases presented with features resem-bling neuroleptic malignant syndrome. While there are no human data showing such an interaction with paroxetine hydrochloride, limited animal data on the effects of combined use of paroxet-ine and MAOIs suggest that these drugs may act synergistically to elevate blood pressure and evoke behavioral excita-tion. Therefore, it is recommended that paroxetine not be used in combination with an MAOI, or within 14 days of dis-continuing treatment with an MAOI. At least 2 weeks should be allowed after stopping paroxetine before starting an MAOI). Products include:

Trazodone Hydrochloride (Paroxet-ine is metabolized by CYP2D6. Like other agents that are metabolized by CYP2D6, paroxetine may significantly inhibit the activity of this isoenzyme. Co-administration of paroxetine with other drugs that are metabolized by CYP2D6 should be approached with caution and may require lower doses than usually prescribed for either parox-etine or the other drug metabolized by CYP2D6).
No products indexed under this heading.

Triamterene (Hyponatremia may occur as a result of treatment with par-oxetine. Patients taking diuretics may be at greater risk). Products include:

Triazolam (Paroxetine is metabolized by CYP2D6. Like other agents that are metabolized by CYP2D6, paroxetine may significantly inhibit the activity of this isoenzyme. Co-administration of paroxetine with other drugs that are metabolized by CYP2D6 should be approached with caution and may require lower doses than usually pre-scribed for either paroxetine or the oth-er drug metabolized by CYP2D6).
No products indexed under this heading.

Trifluoperazine Hydrochloride (Par-oxetine is metabolized by CYP2D6. Like other agents that are metabolized by CYP2D6, paroxetine may significantly inhibit the activity of this isoenzyme. Co-administration of paroxetine with other drugs that are metabolized by CYP2D6, such as phentothiazines, should be approached with caution and

other drugs that are metabolized by CYP2D6 should be approached with caution and may require lower doses than usually prescribed for either parox-etine or the other drug metabolized by CYP2D6).
No products indexed under this heading.

lower doses than usual may need to be prescribed for paroxetine or the pheno-thiazine).
No products indexed under this heading.

Trimipramine Maleate (Caution is indicated in the co-administration of tricyclic antidepressants (TCAs) with paroxetine, because paroxetine may inhibit TCA metabolism. Plasma TCA concentrations may need to be moni-tored, and the dose of TCA may need to be reduced if a TCA is co-administered with paroxetine).
No products indexed under this heading.

Tryptophan (As with other serotonin reuptake inhibitors, an interaction between paroxetine and tryptophan may occur when they are co-administered. Adverse experiences, consisting primar-ily of headache, nausea, sweating, and dizziness, have been reported when tryptophan was administered to patients taking immediate-release par-oxetine. Consequently, concomitant use of controlled release paroxetine with serotonin precursors, such as trypto-phan, is not recommended).
No products indexed under this heading.

Valdecoxib (Paroxetine may increase the risk of bleeding events, including upper gastrointestinal bleeding. Con-comitant use of paroxetine with NSAIDs may increase this risk).
No products indexed under this heading.

Vardenafil Hydrochloride (Co-administration of paroxetine with drugs that inhibit CYP2D6 should be approached with caution). Products include:

Venlafaxine Hydrochloride (The development of a potentially life-threatening serotonin syndrome or Neu-roleptic Malignant Syndrome (NMS)-like reactions have been reported with par-oxetine alone, but particularly, with con-comitant use of serotonergic drugs. The concomitant use of paroxetine with SNRIs is not recommended). Products include:

Vinblastine Sulfate (Paroxetine is metabolized by CYP2D6. Like other agents that are metabolized by CYP2D6, paroxetine may significantly inhibit the activity of this isoenzyme. Co-administration of paroxetine with other drugs that are metabolized by CYP2D6 should be approached with caution and may require lower doses than usually prescribed for either parox-etine or the other drug metabolized by CYP2D6).
No products indexed under this heading.

Warfarin Sodium (Altered anticoagu-lant effects, including increased bleed-ing, have been reported when SSRIs or SNRIs are co-administered with warfa-rin. Patients receiving warfarin therapy should be carefully monitored when par-oxetine is initiated or discontinued).
No products indexed under this heading.

Ziprasidone Hydrochloride (The development of a potentially life-threatening serotonin syndrome or Neu-roleptic Malignant Syndrome (NMS)-like reactions have been reported with par-oxetine alone, but particularly with con-comitant use of antipsychotic agents. Patients should be monitored for the emergence of serotonin syndrome or NMS-like signs and symptoms. Treat-ment with paroxetine and any concomi-tant antipsychotic should be discontin-ued immediately if any signs or symptoms of serotonin syndrome or NMS-like signs or symptoms occur and supportive symptomatic treatment should be initiated). Products include:

(⊙ Described in PDR® for Ophthalmic Medicines)

Zolmitriptan (The development of a potentially life-threatening serotonin syndrome or Neuroleptic Malignant Syndrome (NMS)-like reactions have been reported with paroxetine alone, but particularly, with concomitant use of serotonergic drugs (including triptans). Patients should be monitored for the emergence of serotonin syndrome or NMS-like signs and symptoms. Treatment with paroxetine and any concomitant serotonergic agent should be discontinued immediately if any signs or symptoms of serotonin syndrome or NMS-like signs and symptoms occur and supportive symptomatic treatment should be initiated. If concomitant use of paroxetine with a triptan is clinically warranted, careful observation of the patient is advised, particularly during treatment initiation and dose increases). Products include:
- Zomig Tablets 773
- Zomig Nasal Spray 768
- Zomig-ZMT Tablets 773

Zonisamide (Paroxetine is metabolized by CYP2D6. Like other agents that are metabolized by CYP2D6, paroxetine may significantly inhibit the activity of this isoenzyme. Co-administration of paroxetine with other drugs that are metabolized by CYP2D6 should be approached with caution and may require lower doses than usually prescribed for either paroxetine or the other drug metabolized by CYP2D6). Products include:
- Zonegran 1081

Food Interactions

Alcohol (Although paroxetine has not been shown to increase the impairment of mental and motor skills caused by alcohol, patients should be advised to avoid alcohol while taking paroxetine).

Beer, reduced-alcohol (Although paroxetine has not been shown to increase the impairment of mental and motor skills caused by alcohol, patients should be advised to avoid alcohol while taking paroxetine).

Beer, unspecified (Although paroxetine has not been shown to increase the impairment of mental and motor skills caused by alcohol, patients should be advised to avoid alcohol while taking paroxetine).

Wine, Chianti (Although paroxetine has not been shown to increase the impairment of mental and motor skills caused by alcohol, patients should be advised to avoid alcohol while taking paroxetine).

Wine, Red (Although paroxetine has not been shown to increase the impairment of mental and motor skills caused by alcohol, patients should be advised to avoid alcohol while taking paroxetine).

Wine, unspecified (Although paroxetine has not been shown to increase the impairment of mental and motor skills caused by alcohol, patients should be advised to avoid alcohol while taking paroxetine).

Wine products (Although paroxetine has not been shown to increase the impairment of mental and motor skills caused by alcohol, patients should be advised to avoid alcohol while taking paroxetine).

PEDIARIX VACCINE

(Diphtheria & Tetanus Toxoids and Acellular Pertussis Vaccine Adsorbed, Hepatitis B Vaccine, Recombinant, Poliovirus Vaccine Inactivated) 1606

May interact with alkylating agents, anticoagulants, antimetabolites, corticosteroids, cytotoxic drugs, immunosuppressive agents, and certain other agents. Compounds in these categories include:

Alclometasone Dipropionate (Immunosuppressive therapies, including corticosteroids (used in greater than physiologic doses), may reduce the immune response to vaccine).
No products indexed under this heading.

Anisindione (Pediarix should be given with caution in children with bleeding disorders, such as hemophilia or thrombocytopenia, and in children on anticoagulant therapy, with steps taken to avoid the risk of hematoma following the injection).
No products indexed under this heading.

Ardeparin Sodium (Pediarix should be given with caution in children with bleeding disorders, such as hemophilia or thrombocytopenia, and in children on anticoagulant therapy, with steps taken to avoid the risk of hematoma following the injection).
No products indexed under this heading.

Azathioprine (Immunosuppressive therapies, including irradiation, antimetabolites, alkylating agents, cytotoxic drugs, and corticosteroids (used in greater than physiologic doses), may reduce the immune response to vaccine).
No products indexed under this heading.

Basiliximab (Immunosuppressive therapies, including irradiation, antimetabolites, alkylating agents, cytotoxic drugs, and corticosteroids (used in greater than physiologic doses), may reduce the immune response to vaccine). Products include:
- Simulect 2524

Beclomethasone Dipropionate (Immunosuppressive therapies, including corticosteroids (used in greater than physiologic doses), may reduce the immune response to vaccine). Products include:
- Qvar 3398

Beclomethasone Dipropionate Monohydrate (Immunosuppressive therapies, including corticosteroids (used in greater than physiologic doses), may reduce the immune response to vaccine). Products include:
- Beconase AQ 1386

Betamethasone (Immunosuppressive therapies, including corticosteroids (used in greater than physiologic doses), may reduce the immune response to vaccine).
No products indexed under this heading.

Betamethasone Acetate (Immunosuppressive therapies, including corticosteroids (used in greater than physiologic doses), may reduce the immune response to vaccine).
No products indexed under this heading.

Betamethasone Benzoate (Immunosuppressive therapies, including corticosteroids (used in greater than physiologic doses), may reduce the immune response to vaccine).
No products indexed under this heading.

Betamethasone Dipropionate (Immunosuppressive therapies, including corticosteroids (used in greater than physiologic doses), may reduce the immune response to vaccine). Products include:
- Diprolene Lotion 0.05% 3108
- Diprolene Ointment 0.05% 3109
- Diprolene AF Cream 0.05% 3107
- Lotrisone 3163

Betamethasone Sodium Phosphate (Immunosuppressive therapies, including corticosteroids (used in greater than physiologic doses), may reduce the immune response to vaccine).
No products indexed under this heading.

Betamethasone Valerate (Immunosuppressive therapies, including corticosteroids (used in greater than physiologic doses), may reduce the immune response to vaccine). Products include:
- Luxiq 3321

Bleomycin Sulfate (Immunosuppressive therapies, including cytotoxic drugs, may reduce the immune response to vaccine).
No products indexed under this heading.

Budesonide (Immunosuppressive therapies, including corticosteroids (used in greater than physiologic doses), may reduce the immune response to vaccine). Products include:
- Pulmicort Flexhaler 714
- Symbicort 80/4.5 720
- Symbicort 160/4.5 720

Busulfan (Immunosuppressive therapies, including alkylating agents, may reduce the immune response to vaccine). Products include:
- Myleran 1581

Capecitabine (Immunosuppressive therapies, including antimetabolites, may reduce the immune response to vaccine). Products include:
- Xeloda 2882

Carmustine (BCNU) (Immunosuppressive therapies, including alkylating agents, may reduce the immune response to vaccine).
No products indexed under this heading.

Chlorambucil (Immunosuppressive therapies, including alkylating agents, may reduce the immune response to vaccine). Products include:
- Leukeran 1557

Ciclesonide (Immunosuppressive therapies, including corticosteroids (used in greater than physiologic doses), may reduce the immune response to vaccine).
No products indexed under this heading.

Cladribine (Immunosuppressive therapies, including antimetabolites, may reduce the immune response to vaccine). Products include:
- Leustatin 946

Cortisone Acetate (Immunosuppressive therapies, including corticosteroids (used in greater than physiologic doses), may reduce the immune response to vaccine).
No products indexed under this heading.

Cyclophosphamide (Immunosuppressive therapies, including alkylating agents, may reduce the immune response to vaccine).
No products indexed under this heading.

Cyclosporine (Immunosuppressive therapies, including irradiation, antimetabolites, alkylating agents, cytotoxic drugs, and corticosteroids (used in greater than physiologic doses), may reduce the immune response to vaccine). Products include:
- Gengraf 440
- Neoral Oral Solution 2496
- Neoral Capsules 2496
- Restasis 605

Cytarabine (Immunosuppressive therapies, including antimetabolites, may reduce the immune response to vaccine).
No products indexed under this heading.

Dacarbazine (Immunosuppressive therapies, including alkylating agents, may reduce the immune response to vaccine).
No products indexed under this heading.

Dalteparin Sodium (Pediarix should be given with caution in children with bleeding disorders, such as hemophilia or thrombocytopenia, and in children on anticoagulant therapy, with steps taken to avoid the risk of hematoma following the injection). Products include:
- Fragmin 1058

Danaparoid Sodium (Pediarix should be given with caution in children with bleeding disorders, such as hemophilia or thrombocytopenia, and in children on anticoagulant therapy, with steps taken to avoid the risk of hematoma following the injection).
No products indexed under this heading.

Daunorubicin Hydrochloride (Immunosuppressive therapies, including cytotoxic drugs, may reduce the immune response to vaccine).
No products indexed under this heading.

Desoximetasone (Immunosuppressive therapies, including corticosteroids (used in greater than physiologic doses), may reduce the immune response to vaccine).
No products indexed under this heading.

Dexamethasone (Immunosuppressive therapies, including corticosteroids (used in greater than physiologic doses), may reduce the immune response to vaccine). Products include:
- Ciprodex 583
- Ozurdex .... ⊙223
- Tobramycin and Dexamethasone Ophthalmic Suspension .... ⊙251

Dexamethasone Acetate (Immunosuppressive therapies, including corticosteroids (used in greater than physiologic doses), may reduce the immune response to vaccine).
No products indexed under this heading.

Dexamethasone Phosphate (Immunosuppressive therapies, including corticosteroids (used in greater than physiologic doses), may reduce the immune response to vaccine).
No products indexed under this heading.

Dexamethasone Sodium (Immunosuppressive therapies, including corticosteroids (used in greater than physiologic doses), may reduce the immune response to vaccine).
No products indexed under this heading.

Dexamethasone Sodium Phosphate (Immunosuppressive therapies, including corticosteroids (used in greater than physiologic doses), may reduce the immune response to vaccine).
No products indexed under this heading.

Dexamethasone Sodium Phosphate Injection (Immunosuppressive therapies, including corticosteroids (used in greater than physiologic doses), may reduce the immune response to vaccine).
No products indexed under this heading.

Dicumarol (Pediarix should be given with caution in children with bleeding disorders, such as hemophilia or thrombocytopenia, and in children on anticoagulant therapy, with steps taken to avoid the risk of hematoma following the injection).
No products indexed under this heading.

Diflorasone Diacetate (Immunosuppressive therapies, including corticosteroids (used in greater than physiologic doses), may reduce the immune response to vaccine).
No products indexed under this heading.

Doxorubicin Hydrochloride (Immunosuppressive therapies, including cytotoxic drugs, may reduce the immune response to vaccine).
No products indexed under this heading.

Enoxaparin Sodium (Pediarix should be given with caution in children with bleeding disorders, such as hemophilia or thrombocytopenia, and in children on anticoagulant therapy, with steps taken to avoid the risk of hematoma following the injection). Products include:
- Lovenox 3005

Epirubicin Hydrochloride (Immunosuppressive therapies, including cytotoxic drugs, may reduce the immune response to vaccine).
No products indexed under this heading.

IMPORTANT NOTE: Always consult each drug listing in the patient's regimen for possible interactions.

Pediarix Interactions Index 1402

Floxuridine (Immunosuppressive therapies, including antimetabolites, may reduce the immune response to vaccine).
No products indexed under this heading.

Fludarabine Phosphate (Immunosuppressive therapies, including antimetabolites, may reduce the immune response to vaccine). Products include:
Oforta 3023

Fludrocortisone Acetate (Immunosuppressive therapies, including corticosteroids (used in greater than physiologic doses), may reduce the immune response to vaccine).
No products indexed under this heading.

Flumethasone Pivalate (Immunosuppressive therapies, including corticosteroids (used in greater than physiologic doses), may reduce the immune response to vaccine).
No products indexed under this heading.

Flunisolide Hemihydrate (Immunosuppressive therapies, including corticosteroids (used in greater than physiologic doses), may reduce the immune response to vaccine).
No products indexed under this heading.

Fluorouracil (Immunosuppressive therapies, including antimetabolites, may reduce the immune response to vaccine). Products include:
Carac 2966

Fluticasone Furoate (Immunosuppressive therapies, including corticosteroids (used in greater than physiologic doses), may reduce the immune response to vaccine). Products include:
Veramyst 1713

Fluticasone Propionate (Immunosuppressive therapies, including corticosteroids (used in greater than physiologic doses), may reduce the immune response to vaccine). Products include:
Advair 100/50 1275
Advair 250/50 1275
Advair 500/50 1275
Advair HFA 45/21 1288
Advair HFA 115/21 1288
Advair HFA 230/21 1288
Flonase 1459
Flovent Diskus 1463
Flovent HFA 1470

Fondaparinux Sodium (Pediarix should be given with caution in children with bleeding disorders, such as hemophilia or thrombocytopenia, and in children on anticoagulant therapy, with steps taken to avoid the risk of hematoma following the injection). Products include:
Arixtra 1320

Gemcitabine Hydrochloride (Immunosuppressive therapies, including antimetabolites, may reduce the immune response to vaccine). Products include:
Gemzar 1900

Heparin Calcium (Pediarix should be given with caution in children with bleeding disorders, such as hemophilia or thrombocytopenia, and in children on anticoagulant therapy, with steps taken to avoid the risk of hematoma following the injection).
No products indexed under this heading.

Heparin Sodium (Pediarix should be given with caution in children with bleeding disorders, such as hemophilia or thrombocytopenia, and in children on anticoagulant therapy, with steps taken to avoid the risk of hematoma following the injection).
No products indexed under this heading.

Hydrocortisone (Immunosuppressive therapies, including corticosteroids (used in greater than physiologic doses), may reduce the immune response to vaccine).
No products indexed under this heading.

Hydrocortisone (Alcohol) (Immunosuppressive therapies, including corticosteroids (used in greater than physiologic doses), may reduce the immune response to vaccine).
No products indexed under this heading.

Hydrocortisone Acetate (Immunosuppressive therapies, including corticosteroids (used in greater than physiologic doses), may reduce the immune response to vaccine).
No products indexed under this heading.

Hydrocortisone Butyrate (Immunosuppressive therapies, including corticosteroids (used in greater than physiologic doses), may reduce the immune response to vaccine).
No products indexed under this heading.

Hydrocortisone Cypionate (Immunosuppressive therapies, including corticosteroids (used in greater than physiologic doses), may reduce the immune response to vaccine).
No products indexed under this heading.

Hydrocortisone Hemisuccinate (Immunosuppressive therapies, including corticosteroids (used in greater than physiologic doses), may reduce the immune response to vaccine).
No products indexed under this heading.

Hydrocortisone Probutate (Immunosuppressive therapies, including corticosteroids (used in greater than physiologic doses), may reduce the immune response to vaccine).
No products indexed under this heading.

Hydrocortisone Sodium Phosphate (Immunosuppressive therapies, including corticosteroids (used in greater than physiologic doses), may reduce the immune response to vaccine).
No products indexed under this heading.

Hydrocortisone Sodium Succinate (Immunosuppressive therapies, including corticosteroids (used in greater than physiologic doses), may reduce the immune response to vaccine).
No products indexed under this heading.

Hydrocortisone Valerate (Immunosuppressive therapies, including corticosteroids (used in greater than physiologic doses), may reduce the immune response to vaccine).
No products indexed under this heading.

Hydroxyurea (Immunosuppressive therapies, including cytotoxic drugs, may reduce the immune response to vaccine).
No products indexed under this heading.

Lomustine (CCNU) (Immunosuppressive therapies, including alkylating agents, may reduce the immune response to vaccine).
No products indexed under this heading.

Low Molecular Weight Heparins (Pediarix should be given with caution in children with bleeding disorders, such as hemophilia or thrombocytopenia, and in children on anticoagulant therapy, with steps taken to avoid the risk of hematoma following the injection).
No products indexed under this heading.

Mechlorethamine Hydrochloride (Immunosuppressive therapies, including alkylating agents, may reduce the immune response to vaccine). Products include:
Mustargen 2010

Melphalan (Immunosuppressive therapies, including alkylating agents, may reduce the immune response to vaccine). Products include:
Alkeran 1302

Mercaptopurine (Immunosuppressive therapies, including antimetabolites, may reduce the immune response to vaccine).
No products indexed under this heading.

Methotrexate (Immunosuppressive therapies, including antimetabolites, may reduce the immune response to vaccine).
No products indexed under this heading.

Methotrexate Sodium (Immunosuppressive therapies, including antimetabolites, may reduce the immune response to vaccine).
No products indexed under this heading.

Methylprednisolone (Immunosuppressive therapies, including corticosteroids (used in greater than physiologic doses), may reduce the immune response to vaccine).
No products indexed under this heading.

Methylprednisolone Acetate (Immunosuppressive therapies, including corticosteroids (used in greater than physiologic doses), may reduce the immune response to vaccine).
No products indexed under this heading.

Methylprednisolone Sodium Succinate (Immunosuppressive therapies, including corticosteroids (used in greater than physiologic doses), may reduce the immune response to vaccine).
No products indexed under this heading.

Mitotane (Immunosuppressive therapies, including cytotoxic drugs, may reduce the immune response to vaccine).
No products indexed under this heading.

Mitoxantrone Hydrochloride (Immunosuppressive therapies, including cytotoxic drugs, may reduce the immune response to vaccine). Products include:
Novantrone 1088

Mometasone Furoate (Immunosuppressive therapies, including corticosteroids (used in greater than physiologic doses), may reduce the immune response to vaccine). Products include:
Asmanex 3058
Elocon Cream 3111
Elocon Lotion 3112
Elocon Ointment 3114

Mometasone Furoate Monohydrate (Immunosuppressive therapies, including corticosteroids (used in greater than physiologic doses), may reduce the immune response to vaccine). Products include:
Nasonex 3166

Muromonab-CD3 (Immunosuppressive therapies, including irradiation, antimetabolites, alkylating agents, cytotoxic drugs, and corticosteroids (used in greater than physiologic doses), may reduce the immune response to vaccine). Products include:
Orthoclone OKT3 949

Mycophenolate Mofetil (Immunosuppressive therapies, including irradiation, antimetabolites, alkylating agents, cytotoxic drugs, and corticosteroids (used in greater than physiologic doses), may reduce the immune response to vaccine).
No products indexed under this heading.

Pentostatin (Immunosuppressive therapies, including antimetabolites, may reduce the immune response to vaccine).
No products indexed under this heading.

Prednisolone (Immunosuppressive therapies, including corticosteroids (used in greater than physiologic doses), may reduce the immune response to vaccine).
No products indexed under this heading.

Prednisolone Acetate (Immunosuppressive therapies, including corticosteroids (used in greater than physiologic doses), may reduce the immune response to vaccine). Products include:
Blephamide .... ⊙212, ⊙214
Pred Forte .... ⊙225
Pred Mild .... ⊙230
Pred-G .... ⊙226, ⊙227

Prednisolone Sodium Phosphate (Immunosuppressive therapies, including corticosteroids (used in greater than physiologic doses), may reduce the immune response to vaccine).
No products indexed under this heading.

Prednisolone Tebutate (Immunosuppressive therapies, including corticosteroids (used in greater than physiologic doses), may reduce the immune response to vaccine).
No products indexed under this heading.

Prednisone (Immunosuppressive therapies, including corticosteroids (used in greater than physiologic doses), may reduce the immune response to vaccine).
No products indexed under this heading.

Prednisone sodium phosphate (Immunosuppressive therapies, including corticosteroids (used in greater than physiologic doses), may reduce the immune response to vaccine).
No products indexed under this heading.

Procarbazine Hydrochloride (Immunosuppressive therapies, including cytotoxic drugs, may reduce the immune response to vaccine).
No products indexed under this heading.

Radiation (Immunosuppressive therapies, including irradiation, may reduce the immune response to vaccines).
No products indexed under this heading.

Rapamycin (Immunosuppressive therapies, including irradiation, antimetabolites, alkylating agents, cytotoxic drugs, and corticosteroids (used in greater than physiologic doses), may reduce the immune response to vaccine).
No products indexed under this heading.

Sirolimus (Immunosuppressive therapies, including irradiation, antimetabolites, alkylating agents, cytotoxic drugs, and corticosteroids (used in greater than physiologic doses), may reduce the immune response to vaccine). Products include:
Rapamune 3579

Tacrolimus (Immunosuppressive therapies, including irradiation, antimetabolites, alkylating agents, cytotoxic drugs, and corticosteroids (used in greater than physiologic doses), may reduce the immune response to vaccine). Products include:
Prograf Capsules 677
Prograf Injection 677
Protopic 685

Tamoxifen Citrate (Immunosuppressive therapies, including cytotoxic drugs, may reduce the immune response to vaccine).
No products indexed under this heading.

Thioguanine (Immunosuppressive therapies, including antimetabolites, may reduce the immune response to vaccine). Products include:
Tabloid 1664

Thiotepa (Immunosuppressive therapies, including alkylating agents, may reduce the immune response to vaccine).
No products indexed under this heading.

Tinzaparin Sodium (Pediarix should be given with caution in children with bleeding disorders, such as hemophilia or thrombocytopenia, and in children on anticoagulant therapy, with steps taken to avoid the risk of hematoma following the injection).
No products indexed under this heading.

Triamcinolone (Immunosuppressive therapies, including corticosteroids (used in greater than physiologic doses), may reduce the immune response to vaccine).
No products indexed under this heading.

Triamcinolone Acetonide (Immunosuppressive therapies, including corticosteroids (used in greater than physio-

logic doses), may reduce the immune response to vaccine). Products include:

Triamcinolone Diacetate (Immunosuppressive therapies, including corticosteroids (used in greater than physiologic doses), may reduce the immune response to vaccine).

No products indexed under this heading.

Triamcinolone Hexacetonide (Immunosuppressive therapies, including corticosteroids (used in greater than physiologic doses), may reduce the immune response to vaccine).

No products indexed under this heading.

Vinblastine Sulfate (Immunosuppressive therapies, including cytotoxic drugs, may reduce the immune response to vaccine).

No products indexed under this heading.

Vincristine Sulfate (Immunosuppressive therapies, including cytotoxic drugs, may reduce the immune response to vaccine).

No products indexed under this heading.

Vinorelbine Tartrate (Immunosuppressive therapies, including cytotoxic drugs, may reduce the immune response to vaccine).

No products indexed under this heading.

Warfarin Sodium (Pediarix should be given with caution in children with bleeding disorders, such as hemophilia or thrombocytopenia, and in children on anticoagulant therapy, with steps taken to avoid the risk of hematoma following the injection).

No products indexed under this heading.

LIQUID PEDVAXHIB

None cited in PDR database.

PEGINTRON POWDER FOR INJECTION

May interact with cytochrome p450 2c8 substrates (selected), cytochrome p450 2c9 substrates (selected), cytochrome p450 2d6 substrates (selected), nucleoside/nucleotide analogue reverse transcriptase inhibitors, phenytoin, and certain other agents. Compounds in these categories include:

Abacavir Sulfate (Hepatic decompensation (some fatal) has occurred in cirrhotic HIV/HCV co-infected patients receiving combination antiretroviral therapy for HIV and interferon alpha and ribavirin. Adding treatment with alpha interferons alone or in combination with ribavirin may increase the risk in this patient subset. Patients receiving interferon with ribavirin and nucleoside reverse transcriptase inhibitors (NRTIs) should be closely monitored for treatment-associated toxicities, especially hepatic decompensation andanemia. Discontinuationof NRTIs should be considered as medically appropriate. Dose reduction or discontinuation of interferon, ribavirin, or both should also be considered if worsening clinical toxicities are observed, including hepatic decompensation). Products include:

Acarbose (When administering peginterferon alfa-2b with medications metabolized by CYP2C8/9 (eg, warfarin and phenytoin), the therapeutic effect of these substrates may be decreased. Concomitant use with peginterferon alfa-2b treatment resulted in a 28% (mean) increase in a measure of CYP2C8/9 activity).

No products indexed under this heading.

Adefovir dipivoxil (Hepatic decompensation (some fatal) has occurred in cirrhotic HIV/HCV co-infected patients receiving combination antiretroviral therapy for HIV and interferon alpha and ribavirin. Adding treatment with alpha interferons alone or in combination with ribavirin may increase the risk in this patient subset. Patients receiving interferon with ribavirin and nucleoside reverse transcriptase inhibitors (NRTIs) should be closely monitored for treatment-associated toxicities, especially hepatic decompensation andanemia. Discontinuationof NRTIs should be considered as medically appropriate. Dose reduction or discontinuation of interferon, ribavirin, or both should also be considered if worsening clinical toxicities are observed, including hepatic decompensation). Products include:

Amiodarone Hydrochloride (When administering peginterferon alfa-2b with medications metabolized by CYP2C8/9 (eg, warfarin and phenytoin), the therapeutic effect of these substrates may be decreased. Concomitant use with peginterferon alfa-2b treatment resulted in a 28% (mean) increase in a measure of CYP2C8/9 activity).

No products indexed under this heading.

Amitriptyline Hydrochloride (When administering peginterferon alfa-2b with medications metabolized by CYP2C8/9 (eg, warfarin and phenytoin), the therapeutic effect of these substrates may be decreased. Concomitant use with peginterferon alfa-2b treatment resulted in a 28% (mean) increase in a measure of CYP2C8/9 activity).

No products indexed under this heading.

Amoxapine (When administering peginterferon alfa-2b with medications metabolized by CYP2C8/9 (eg, warfarin and phenytoin), the therapeutic effect of these substrates may be decreased. Concomitant use with peginterferon alfa-2b treatment resulted in a 28% (mean) increase in a measure of CYP2C8/9 activity).

No products indexed under this heading.

Amphetamine Aspartate (When administering peginterferon alfa-2b with medications metabolized by CYP2D6 (eg, flecainide), the therapeutic effect of this substrate may be decreased. Peginterferon alfa-2b treatment resulted in a 66% (mean) increase in a measure of CYP2D6 activity).

No products indexed under this heading.

Amphetamine Aspartate Monohydrate (When administering peginterferon alfa-2b with medications metabolized by CYP2D6 (eg, flecainide), the therapeutic effect of this substrate may be decreased. Peginterferon alfa-2b treatment resulted in a 66% (mean) increase in a measure of CYP2D6 activity).

No products indexed under this heading.

Amphetamine Sulfate (When administering peginterferon alfa-2b with medications metabolized by CYP2D6 (eg, flecainide), the therapeutic effect of this substrate may be decreased. Peginterferon alfa-2b treatment resulted in a 66% (mean) increase in a measure of CYP2D6 activity).

No products indexed under this heading.

Atomoxetine Hydrochloride (When administering peginterferon alfa-2b with medications metabolized by CYP2D6 (eg, flecainide), the therapeutic effect of this substrate may be decreased. Peginterferon alfa-2b treatment resulted in a 66% (mean) increase in a measure of CYP2D6 activity). Products include:

Benzphetamine Hydrochloride (When administering peginterferon alfa-2b with medications metabolized by CYP2C8/9 (eg, warfarin and phenytoin), the therapeutic effect of these substrates may be decreased. Concomitant use with peginterferon alfa-2b treatment resulted in a 28% (mean) increase in a measure of CYP2C8/9 activity).

No products indexed under this heading.

Bisoprolol Fumarate (When administering peginterferon alfa-2b with medications metabolized by CYP2D6 (eg, flecainide), the therapeutic effect of this substrate may be decreased. Peginterferon alfa-2b treatment resulted in a 66% (mean) increase in a measure of CYP2D6 activity).

No products indexed under this heading.

Candesartan Cilexetil (When administering peginterferon alfa-2b with medications metabolized by CYP2C8/9 (eg, warfarin and phenytoin), the therapeutic effect of these substrates may be decreased. Concomitant use with peginterferon alfa-2b treatment resulted in a 28% (mean) increase in a measure of CYP2C8/9 activity). Products include:

Captopril (When administering peginterferon alfa-2b with medications metabolized by CYP2D6 (eg, flecainide), the therapeutic effect of this substrate may be decreased. Peginterferon alfa-2b treatment resulted in a 66% (mean) increase in a measure of CYP2D6 activity). Products include:

Carbamazepine (When administering peginterferon alfa-2b with medications metabolized by CYP2C8/9 (eg, warfarin and phenytoin), the therapeutic effect of these substrates may be decreased. Concomitant use with peginterferon alfa-2b treatment resulted in a 28% (mean) increase in a measure of CYP2C8/9 activity). Products include:

Carvedilol (When administering peginterferon alfa-2b with medications metabolized by CYP2C8/9 (eg, warfarin and phenytoin), the therapeutic effect of these substrates may be decreased. Concomitant use with peginterferon alfa-2b treatment resulted in a 28% (mean) increase in a measure of CYP2C8/9 activity). Products include:

Celecoxib (When administering peginterferon alfa-2b with medications metabolized by CYP2C8/9 (eg, warfarin and phenytoin), the therapeutic effect of these substrates may be decreased. Concomitant use with peginterferon alfa-2b treatment resulted in a 28% (mean) increase in a measure of CYP2C8/9 activity). Products include:

Cevimeline Hydrochloride (When administering peginterferon alfa-2b with medications metabolized by CYP2D6 (eg, flecainide), the therapeutic effect of this substrate may be decreased. Peginterferon alfa-2b treatment resulted in a 66% (mean) increase in a measure of CYP2D6 activity). Products include:

Chlorpromazine (When administering peginterferon alfa-2b with medications metabolized by CYP2D6 (eg, flecainide), the therapeutic effect of this substrate may be decreased. Peginterferon alfa-2b treatment resulted in a 66% (mean) increase in a measure of CYP2D6 activity).

No products indexed under this heading.

Chlorpromazine Hydrochloride (When administering peginterferon alfa-2b with medications metabolized by CYP2D6 (eg, flecainide), the therapeutic effect of this substrate may be decreased. Peginterferon alfa-2b treatment resulted in a 66% (mean) increase in a measure of CYP2D6 activity).

No products indexed under this heading.

Chlorpropamide (When administering peginterferon alfa-2b with medications metabolized by CYP2C8/9 (eg, warfarin and phenytoin), the therapeutic effect of these substrates may be decreased. Concomitant use with peginterferon alfa-2b treatment resulted in a 28% (mean) increase in a measure of CYP2C8/9 activity).

No products indexed under this heading.

Clomipramine Hydrochloride (When administering peginterferon alfa-2b with medications metabolized by CYP2C8/9 (eg, warfarin and phenytoin), the therapeutic effect of these substrates may be decreased. Concomitant use with peginterferon alfa-2b treatment resulted in a 28% (mean) increase in a measure of CYP2C8/9 activity).

No products indexed under this heading.

Clozapine (When administering peginterferon alfa-2b with medications metabolized by CYP2D6 (eg, flecainide), the therapeutic effect of this substrate may be decreased. Peginterferon alfa-2b treatment resulted in a 66% (mean) increase in a measure of CYP2D6 activity).

No products indexed under this heading.

Codeine Phosphate (When administering peginterferon alfa-2b with medications metabolized by CYP2D6 (eg, flecainide), the therapeutic effect of this substrate may be decreased. Peginterferon alfa-2b treatment resulted in a 66% (mean) increase in a measure of CYP2D6 activity). Products include:

Codeine Sulfate (When administering peginterferon alfa-2b with medications metabolized by CYP2D6 (eg, flecainide), the therapeutic effect of this substrate may be decreased. Peginterferon alfa-2b treatment resulted in a 66% (mean) increase in a measure of CYP2D6 activity).

No products indexed under this heading.

Cyclobenzaprine Hydrochloride (When administering peginterferon alfa-2b with medications metabolized by CYP2D6 (eg, flecainide), the therapeutic effect of this substrate may be decreased. Peginterferon alfa-2b treatment resulted in a 66% (mean) increase in a measure of CYP2D6 activity). Products include:

Debrisoquine (When administering peginterferon alfa-2b with medications metabolized by CYP2D6 (eg, flecainide), the therapeutic effect of this substrate may be decreased. Peginterferon alfa-2b treatment resulted in a 66% (mean) increase in a measure of CYP2D6 activity).

No products indexed under this heading.

Desipramine Hydrochloride (When administering peginterferon alfa-2b with medications metabolized by CYP2C8/9 (eg, warfarin and phenytoin), the therapeutic effect of these substrates may be decreased. Concomitant use with peginterferon alfa-2b treatment resulted in a 28% (mean) increase in a measure of CYP2C8/9 activity).

No products indexed under this heading.

Desogestrel (When administering peginterferon alfa-2b with medications metabolized by CYP2C8/9 (eg, warfarin and phenytoin), the therapeutic effect of these substrates may be decreased. Concomitant use with peginterferon alfa-2b treatment resulted in a 28% (mean) increase in a measure of CYP2C8/9 activity).
No products indexed under this heading.

Dexfenfluramine Hydrochloride (When administering peginterferon alfa-2b with medications metabolized by CYP2D6 (eg, flecainide), the therapeutic effect of this substrate may be decreased. Peginterferon alfa-2b treatment resulted in a 66% (mean) increase in a measure of CYP2D6 activity).
No products indexed under this heading.

Dextromethorphan (When administering peginterferon alfa-2b with medications metabolized by CYP2C8/9 (eg, warfarin and phenytoin), the therapeutic effect of these substrates may be decreased. Concomitant use with peginterferon alfa-2b treatment resulted in a 28% (mean) increase in a measure of CYP2C8/9 activity).
No products indexed under this heading.

Dextromethorphan Hydrobromide (When administering peginterferon alfa-2b with medications metabolized by CYP2D6 (eg, flecainide), the therapeutic effect of this substrate may be decreased. Peginterferon alfa-2b treatment resulted in a 66% (mean) increase in a measure of CYP2D6 activity).
No products indexed under this heading.

Dextromethorphan Polistirex (When administering peginterferon alfa-2b with medications metabolized by CYP2D6 (eg, flecainide), the therapeutic effect of this substrate may be decreased. Peginterferon alfa-2b treatment resulted in a 66% (mean) increase in a measure of CYP2D6 activity).
No products indexed under this heading.

Diazepam (When administering peginterferon alfa-2b with medications metabolized by CYP2C8/9 (eg, warfarin and phenytoin), the therapeutic effect of these substrates may be decreased. Concomitant use with peginterferon alfa-2b treatment resulted in a 28% (mean) increase in a measure of CYP2C8/9 activity). Products include:
Valium Tablets **2880**

Diclofenac Potassium (When administering peginterferon alfa-2b with medications metabolized by CYP2C8/9 (eg, warfarin and phenytoin), the therapeutic effect of these substrates may be decreased. Concomitant use with peginterferon alfa-2b treatment resulted in a 28% (mean) increase in a measure of CYP2C8/9 activity).
No products indexed under this heading.

Diclofenac Sodium (When administering peginterferon alfa-2b with medications metabolized by CYP2C8/9 (eg, warfarin and phenytoin), the therapeutic effect of these substrates may be decreased. Concomitant use with peginterferon alfa-2b treatment resulted in a 28% (mean) increase in a measure of CYP2C8/9 activity).
No products indexed under this heading.

Didanosine (Hepatic decompensation (some fatal) has occurred in cirrhotic HIV/HCV co-infected patients receiving combination antiretroviral therapy for HIV and interferon alpha and ribavirin. Adding treatment with alpha interferons alone or in combination with ribavirin may increase the risk in this patient subset. Patients receiving interferon with ribavirin and nucleoside reverse transcriptase inhibitors (NRTIs) should be closely monitored for treamtent-associated toxicities, especially hepatic decompensation andanemia. Discontinuationof NRTIs should be considered as medically appropriate. Dose reduction or discontinuation of interferon, ribavirin, or both should also be considered if worsening clinical toxicities are observed, including hepatic decompensation).
No products indexed under this heading.

Docetaxel (When administering peginterferon alfa-2b with medications metabolized by CYP2C8/9 (eg, warfarin and phenytoin), the therapeutic effect of these substrates may be decreased. Concomitant use with peginterferon alfa-2b treatment resulted in a 28% (mean) increase in a measure of CYP2C8/9 activity). Products include:
Taxotere **3035**

Dolasetron Mesylate (When administering peginterferon alfa-2b with medications metabolized by CYP2D6 (eg, flecainide), the therapeutic effect of this substrate may be decreased. Peginterferon alfa-2b treatment resulted in a 66% (mean) increase in a measure of CYP2D6 activity). Products include:
Anzemet Injection **2931**
Anzemet Tablets **2934**

Donepezil Hydrochloride (When administering peginterferon alfa-2b with medications metabolized by CYP2D6 (eg, flecainide), the therapeutic effect of this substrate may be decreased. Peginterferon alfa-2b treatment resulted in a 66% (mean) increase in a measure of CYP2D6 activity). Products include:
Aricept **1045**
Aricept ODT **1045**

Doxepin Hydrochloride (When administering peginterferon alfa-2b with medications metabolized by CYP2C8/9 (eg, warfarin and phenytoin), the therapeutic effect of these substrates may be decreased. Concomitant use with peginterferon alfa-2b treatment resulted in a 28% (mean) increase in a measure of CYP2C8/9 activity).
No products indexed under this heading.

Dronabinol (When administering peginterferon alfa-2b with medications metabolized by CYP2C8/9 (eg, warfarin and phenytoin), the therapeutic effect of these substrates may be decreased. Concomitant use with peginterferon alfa-2b treatment resulted in a 28% (mean) increase in a measure of CYP2C8/9 activity).
No products indexed under this heading.

Emtricitabine (Hepatic decompensation (some fatal) has occurred in cirrhotic HIV/HCV co-infected patients receiving combination antiretroviral therapy for HIV and interferon alpha and ribavirin. Adding treatment with alpha interferons alone or in combination with ribavirin may increase the risk in this patient subset. Patients receiving interferon with ribavirin and nucleoside reverse transcriptase inhibitors (NRTIs) should be closely monitored for treamtent-associated toxicities, especially hepatic decompensation andanemia. Discontinuationof NRTIs should be considered as medically appropriate. Dose reduction or discontinuation of interferon, ribavirin, or both should also be considered if worsening clinical toxicities are observed, including hepatic decompensation). Products include:
Atripla **906**
Emtriva **1238**
Emtriva Oral Solution **1238**
Truvada **1258**

Encainide Hydrochloride (When administering peginterferon alfa-2b with medications metabolized by CYP2D6 (eg, flecainide), the therapeutic effect of this substrate may be decreased. Peginterferon alfa-2b treatment resulted in a 66% (mean) increase in a measure of CYP2D6 activity).
No products indexed under this heading.

Eprosartan Mesylate (When administering peginterferon alfa-2b with medications metabolized by CYP2C8/9 (eg, warfarin and phenytoin), the therapeutic effect of these substrates may be decreased. Concomitant use with peginterferon alfa-2b treatment resulted in a 28% (mean) increase in a measure of CYP2C8/9 activity). Products include:
Teveten **538**
Teveten HCT **541**

Etodolac (When administering peginterferon alfa-2b with medications metabolized by CYP2C8/9 (eg, warfarin and phenytoin), the therapeutic effect of these substrates may be decreased. Concomitant use with peginterferon alfa-2b treatment resulted in a 28% (mean) increase in a measure of CYP2C8/9 activity).
No products indexed under this heading.

Fenoprofen Calcium (When administering peginterferon alfa-2b with medications metabolized by CYP2C8/9 (eg, warfarin and phenytoin), the therapeutic effect of these substrates may be decreased. Concomitant use with peginterferon alfa-2b treatment resulted in a 28% (mean) increase in a measure of CYP2C8/9 activity).
No products indexed under this heading.

Fentanyl (When administering peginterferon alfa-2b with medications metabolized by CYP2D6 (eg, flecainide), the therapeutic effect of this substrate may be decreased. Peginterferon alfa-2b treatment resulted in a 66% (mean) increase in a measure of CYP2D6 activity). Products include:
Duragesic **2604**
Fentanyl Transdermal System **2346**
Onsolis **2054**

Fentanyl Citrate (When administering peginterferon alfa-2b with medications metabolized by CYP2D6 (eg, flecainide), the therapeutic effect of this substrate may be decreased. Peginterferon alfa-2b treatment resulted in a 66% (mean) increase in a measure of CYP2D6 activity). Products include:
Fentora **966**

Flecainide Acetate (When administering peginterferon alfa-2b with medications metabolized by CYP2D6 (eg, flecainide), the therapeutic effect of this substrate may be decreased. Concomitant use with peginterferon alfa-2b treatment resulted in a 66% (mean) increase in a measure of CYP2D6 activity).
No products indexed under this heading.

Fluoxetine (When administering peginterferon alfa-2b with medications metabolized by CYP2D6 (eg, flecainide), the therapeutic effect of this substrate may be decreased. Peginterferon alfa-2b treatment resulted in a 66% (mean) increase in a measure of CYP2D6 activity).
No products indexed under this heading.

Fluoxetine Hydrochloride (When administering peginterferon alfa-2b with medications metabolized by CYP2C8/9 (eg, warfarin and phenytoin), the therapeutic effect of these substrates may be decreased. Concomitant use with peginterferon alfa-2b treatment resulted in a 28% (mean) increase in a measure of CYP2C8/9 activity). Products include:
Prozac Weekly **1941**
Prozac Pulvules **1941**
Symbyax **1965**

Fluphenazine Decanoate (When administering peginterferon alfa-2b with medications metabolized by CYP2D6 (eg, flecainide), the therapeutic effect of this substrate may be decreased. Peginterferon alfa-2b treatment resulted in a 66% (mean) increase in a measure of CYP2D6 activity).
No products indexed under this heading.

Fluphenazine Enanthate (When administering peginterferon alfa-2b with medications metabolized by CYP2D6 (eg, flecainide), the therapeutic effect of this substrate may be decreased. Peginterferon alfa-2b treatment resulted in a 66% (mean) increase in a measure of CYP2D6 activity).
No products indexed under this heading.

Fluphenazine Hydrochloride (When administering peginterferon alfa-2b with medications metabolized by CYP2D6 (eg, flecainide), the therapeutic effect of this substrate may be decreased. Peginterferon alfa-2b treatment resulted in a 66% (mean) increase in a measure of CYP2D6 activity).
No products indexed under this heading.

Flurbiprofen (When administering peginterferon alfa-2b with medications metabolized by CYP2C8/9 (eg, warfarin and phenytoin), the therapeutic effect of these substrates may be decreased. Concomitant use with peginterferon alfa-2b treatment resulted in a 28% (mean) increase in a measure of CYP2C8/9 activity).
No products indexed under this heading.

Flurbiprofen Sodium (When administering peginterferon alfa-2b with medications metabolized by CYP2C8/9 (eg, warfarin and phenytoin), the therapeutic effect of these substrates may be decreased. Concomitant use with peginterferon alfa-2b treatment resulted in a 28% (mean) increase in a measure of CYP2C8/9 activity).
No products indexed under this heading.

Fluvastatin Sodium (When administering peginterferon alfa-2b with medications metabolized by CYP2C8/9 (eg, warfarin and phenytoin), the therapeutic effect of these substrates may be decreased. Concomitant use with peginterferon alfa-2b treatment resulted in a 28% (mean) increase in a measure of CYP2C8/9 activity).
No products indexed under this heading.

Fluvoxamine Maleate (When administering peginterferon alfa-2b with medications metabolized by CYP2D6 (eg, flecainide), the therapeutic effect of this substrate may be decreased. Peginterferon alfa-2b treatment resulted in a 66% (mean) increase in a measure of CYP2D6 activity).
No products indexed under this heading.

Formoterol Fumarate (When administering peginterferon alfa-2b with medications metabolized by CYP2D6 (eg, flecainide), the therapeutic effect of this substrate may be decreased. Peginterferon alfa-2b treatment resulted in a 66% (mean) increase in a measure of CYP2D6 activity). Products include:
Foradil **3121**
Perforomist **3634**

Fosphenytoin (When administering peginterferon alfa-2b with medications metabolized by CYP2C8/9 (eg, warfarin and phenytoin), the therapeutic effect of these substrates may be decreased. Peginterferon alfa-2b treatment resulted in a 28% (mean) increase in a measure of CYP2C8/9 activity).
No products indexed under this heading.

Fosphenytoin Sodium (When administering peginterferon alfa-2b with medications metabolized by CYP2C8/9 (eg, warfarin and phenytoin), the therapeutic effect of these substrates may be decreased. Peginterferon alfa-2b treatment resulted in a 28% (mean) increase in a measure of CYP2C8/9 activity).
No products indexed under this heading.

Galantamine Hydrobromide (When administering peginterferon alfa-2b with medications metabolized by CYP2D6 (eg, flecainide), the therapeutic effect of this substrate may be decreased. Peginterferon alfa-2b treatment resulted in a 66% (mean) increase in a measure of CYP2D6 activity).

No products indexed under this heading.

Glimepiride (When administering peginterferon alfa-2b with medications metabolized by CYP2C8/9 (eg, warfarin and phenytoin), the therapeutic effect of these substrates may be decreased. Concomitant use with peginterferon alfa-2b treatment resulted in a 28% (mean) increase in a measure of CYP2C8/9 activity). Products include:

Avandaryl 1356
Duetact 3354

Glipizide (When administering peginterferon alfa-2b with medications metabolized by CYP2C8/9 (eg, warfarin and phenytoin), the therapeutic effect of these substrates may be decreased. Concomitant use with peginterferon alfa-2b treatment resulted in a 28% (mean) increase in a measure of CYP2C8/9 activity).

No products indexed under this heading.

Haloperidol (When administering peginterferon alfa-2b with medications metabolized by CYP2D6 (eg, flecainide), the therapeutic effect of this substrate may be decreased. Peginterferon alfa-2b treatment resulted in a 66% (mean) increase in a measure of CYP2D6 activity).

No products indexed under this heading.

Haloperidol Decanoate (When administering peginterferon alfa-2b with medications metabolized by CYP2D6 (eg, flecainide), the therapeutic effect of this substrate may be decreased. Peginterferon alfa-2b treatment resulted in a 66% (mean) increase in a measure of CYP2D6 activity).

No products indexed under this heading.

Hydrocodone Bitartrate (When administering peginterferon alfa-2b with medications metabolized by CYP2D6 (eg, flecainide), the therapeutic effect of this substrate may be decreased. Peginterferon alfa-2b treatment resulted in a 66% (mean) increase in a measure of CYP2D6 activity). Products include:

Vicodin 560
Vicodin ES 561
Vicodin HP 563
Vicoprofen 564
Zydone 1138

Ibuprofen (When administering peginterferon alfa-2b with medications metabolized by CYP2C8/9 (eg, warfarin and phenytoin), the therapeutic effect of these substrates may be decreased. Concomitant use with peginterferon alfa-2b treatment resulted in a 28% (mean) increase in a measure of CYP2C8/9 activity). Products include:

Motrin IB 2043
Children's Motrin 2044
Children's Motrin Non-Staining
   Dye-Free 2044
Infants' Motrin 2044
Infants' Motrin Dye-Free 2044
Junior Strength Motrin 2044
Vicoprofen 564

Imipramine Hydrochloride (When administering peginterferon alfa-2b with medications metabolized by CYP2C8/9 (eg, warfarin and phenytoin), the therapeutic effect of these substrates may be decreased. Concomitant use with peginterferon alfa-2b treatment resulted in a 28% (mean) increase in a measure of CYP2C8/9 activity).

No products indexed under this heading.

Imipramine Pamoate (When administering peginterferon alfa-2b with medications metabolized by CYP2C8/9 (eg, warfarin and phenytoin), the therapeutic effect of these substrates may be decreased. Concomitant use with peginterferon alfa-2b treatment resulted in a 28% (mean) increase in a measure of CYP2C8/9 activity).

No products indexed under this heading.

Indomethacin (When administering peginterferon alfa-2b with medications metabolized by CYP2C8/9 (eg, warfarin and phenytoin), the therapeutic effect of these substrates may be decreased. Concomitant use with peginterferon alfa-2b treatment resulted in a 28% (mean) increase in a measure of CYP2C8/9 activity). Products include:

Indocin 2167

Indomethacin Sodium Trihydrate (When administering peginterferon alfa-2b with medications metabolized by CYP2C8/9 (eg, warfarin and phenytoin), the therapeutic effect of these substrates may be decreased. Concomitant use with peginterferon alfa-2b treatment resulted in a 28% (mean) increase in a measure of CYP2C8/9 activity). Products include:

Indocin I.V. 2007

Indoramin Hydrochloride (When administering peginterferon alfa-2b with medications metabolized by CYP2D6 (eg, flecainide), the therapeutic effect of this substrate may be decreased. Peginterferon alfa-2b treatment resulted in a 66% (mean) increase in a measure of CYP2D6 activity).

No products indexed under this heading.

Irbesartan (When administering peginterferon alfa-2b with medications metabolized by CYP2C8/9 (eg, warfarin and phenytoin), the therapeutic effect of these substrates may be decreased. Concomitant use with peginterferon alfa-2b treatment resulted in a 28% (mean) increase in a measure of CYP2C8/9 activity). Products include:

Avalide 2956
Avapro 2962

Isotretinoin (When administering peginterferon alfa-2b with medications metabolized by CYP2C8/9 (eg, warfarin and phenytoin), the therapeutic effect of these substrates may be decreased. Concomitant use with peginterferon alfa-2b treatment resulted in a 28% (mean) increase in a measure of CYP2C8/9 activity). Products include:

Accutane 2832

Ketoprofen (When administering peginterferon alfa-2b with medications metabolized by CYP2C8/9 (eg, warfarin and phenytoin), the therapeutic effect of these substrates may be decreased. Concomitant use with peginterferon alfa-2b treatment resulted in a 28% (mean) increase in a measure of CYP2C8/9 activity).

No products indexed under this heading.

Ketorolac Tromethamine (When administering peginterferon alfa-2b with medications metabolized by CYP2C8/9 (eg, warfarin and phenytoin), the therapeutic effect of these substrates may be decreased. Concomitant use with peginterferon alfa-2b treatment resulted in a 28% (mean) increase in a measure of CYP2C8/9 activity). Products include:

Acuvail .... ⊙209

Labetalol Hydrochloride (When administering peginterferon alfa-2b with medications metabolized by CYP2D6 (eg, flecainide), the therapeutic effect of this substrate may be decreased. Peginterferon alfa-2b treatment resulted in a 66% (mean) increase in a measure of CYP2D6 activity).

No products indexed under this heading.

Lamivudine (Hepatic decompensation (some fatal) has occurred in cirrhotic HIV/HCV co-infected patients receiving combination antiretroviral therapy for HIV and interferon alpha and ribavirin. Adding treatment with alpha interferons alone or in combination with ribavirin may increase the risk in this patient subset. Patients receiving interferon with ribavirin and nucleoside reverse transcriptase inhibitors (NRTIs) should be closely monitored for treamtent-associated toxicities, especially hepatic decompensation andanemia. Discontinuationof NRTIs should be considered as medically appropriate. Dose reduction or discontinuation of interferon, ribavirin, or both should also be considered if worsening clinical toxicities are observed, including hepatic decompensation). Products include:

Combivir 1404
Epivir 1437
Epivir-HBV 1443
Epzicom 1448
Trizivir 1688

Lansoprazole (When administering peginterferon alfa-2b with medications metabolized by CYP2C8/9 (eg, warfarin and phenytoin), the therapeutic effect of these substrates may be decreased. Concomitant use with peginterferon alfa-2b treatment resulted in a 28% (mean) increase in a measure of CYP2C8/9 activity).

No products indexed under this heading.

Lidocaine (When administering peginterferon alfa-2b with medications metabolized by CYP2D6 (eg, flecainide), the therapeutic effect of this substrate may be decreased. Peginterferon alfa-2b treatment resulted in a 66% (mean) increase in a measure of CYP2D6 activity). Products include:

Lidoderm 1107

Lidocaine Hydrochloride (When administering peginterferon alfa-2b with medications metabolized by CYP2D6 (eg, flecainide), the therapeutic effect of this substrate may be decreased. Peginterferon alfa-2b treatment resulted in a 66% (mean) increase in a measure of CYP2D6 activity).

No products indexed under this heading.

Losartan Potassium (When administering peginterferon alfa-2b with medications metabolized by CYP2C8/9 (eg, warfarin and phenytoin), the therapeutic effect of these substrates may be decreased. Concomitant use with peginterferon alfa-2b treatment resulted in a 28% (mean) increase in a measure of CYP2C8/9 activity). Products include:

Cozaar 2106
Hyzaar 2162
Hyzaar 100-12.5 2162

Maprotiline Hydrochloride (When administering peginterferon alfa-2b with medications metabolized by CYP2C8/9 (eg, warfarin and phenytoin), the therapeutic effect of these substrates may be decreased. Concomitant use with peginterferon alfa-2b treatment resulted in a 28% (mean) increase in a measure of CYP2C8/9 activity).

No products indexed under this heading.

Meclofenamate Sodium (When administering peginterferon alfa-2b with medications metabolized by CYP2C8/9 (eg, warfarin and phenytoin), the therapeutic effect of these substrates may be decreased. Concomitant use with peginterferon alfa-2b treatment resulted in a 28% (mean) increase in a measure of CYP2C8/9 activity).

No products indexed under this heading.

Mefenamic Acid (When administering peginterferon alfa-2b with medications metabolized by CYP2C8/9 (eg, warfarin and phenytoin), the therapeutic effect of these substrates may be decreased. Concomitant use with peginterferon alfa-2b treatment resulted in a 28% (mean) increase in a measure of CYP2C8/9 activity).

No products indexed under this heading.

Meloxicam (When administering peginterferon alfa-2b with medications metabolized by CYP2C8/9 (eg, warfarin and phenytoin), the therapeutic effect of these substrates may be decreased. Concomitant use with peginterferon alfa-2b treatment resulted in a 28% (mean) increase in a measure of CYP2C8/9 activity).

No products indexed under this heading.

Meperidine Hydrochloride (When administering peginterferon alfa-2b with medications metabolized by CYP2D6 (eg, flecainide), the therapeutic effect of this substrate may be decreased. Peginterferon alfa-2b treatment resulted in a 66% (mean) increase in a measure of CYP2D6 activity).

No products indexed under this heading.

Mephobarbital (When administering peginterferon alfa-2b with medications metabolized by CYP2C8/9 (eg, warfarin and phenytoin), the therapeutic effect of these substrates may be decreased. Concomitant use with peginterferon alfa-2b treatment resulted in a 28% (mean) increase in a measure of CYP2C8/9 activity).

No products indexed under this heading.

Metformin Hydrochloride (When administering peginterferon alfa-2b with medications metabolized by CYP2C8/9 (eg, warfarin and phenytoin), the therapeutic effect of these substrates may be decreased. Concomitant use with peginterferon alfa-2b treatment resulted in a 28% (mean) increase in a measure of CYP2C8/9 activity). Products include:

ActoPlus 3338
Avandamet 1345
Janumet 2188

Methadone Hydrochloride (Peginterferon alfa-2b may increase methadone concentrations. Patients should be monitored for the signs and symptoms of increased narcotic effect. The pharmacokinetics of concomitant administration of methadone and peginterferon alfa-2b were evaluated in 18 peginterferon alfa-2b-naive chronice hepatitis C subjects receiving 1.5 mcg/kg peginterfern alfa-2b SC weekly. All subjects were on stable methadone maintenance therapy. Mean methadone AUC was approximately 16% higher after 4 weeks of peginterferon alfa-2b treatment as compared to baseline. In subjects, methadone AUC was approximately 16% higher after 4 weeks of peginterferon alfa-2b treatment. In 2 subjects, methadone AUC was approximately doube after 4 weeks of peginterferon alfa-2b treatment).

No products indexed under this heading.

Methamphetamine Hydrochloride (When administering peginterferon alfa-2b with medications metabolized by CYP2D6 (eg, flecainide), the therapeutic effect of this substrate may be decreased. Peginterferon alfa-2b treatment resulted in a 66% (mean) increase in a measure of CYP2D6 activity).

No products indexed under this heading.

Methoxyphenamine (When administering peginterferon alfa-2b with medications metabolized by CYP2D6 (eg, flecainide), the therapeutic effect of this substrate may be decreased. Peginterferon alfa-2b treatment resulted in a 66% (mean) increase in a measure of CYP2D6 activity).

No products indexed under this heading.

IMPORTANT NOTE: Always consult each drug listing in the patient's regimen for possible interactions.

PegIntron Interactions Index 1406

Metoprolol Succinate (When administering peginterferon alfa-2b with medications metabolized by CYP2D6 (eg, flecainide), the therapeutic effect of this substrate may be decreased. Peginterferon alfa-2b treatment resulted in a 66% (mean) increase in a measure of CYP2D6 activity). Products include:
Toprol XL 732

Metoprolol Tartrate (When administering peginterferon alfa-2b with medications metabolized by CYP2D6 (eg, flecainide), the therapeutic effect of this substrate may be decreased. Peginterferon alfa-2b treatment resulted in a 66% (mean) increase in a measure of CYP2D6 activity).
No products indexed under this heading.

Mexiletine Hydrochloride (When administering peginterferon alfa-2b with medications metabolized by CYP2D6 (eg, flecainide), the therapeutic effect of this substrate may be decreased. Peginterferon alfa-2b treatment resulted in a 66% (mean) increase in a measure of CYP2D6 activity).
No products indexed under this heading.

Miglitol (When administering peginterferon alfa-2b with medications metabolized by CYP2C8/9 (eg, warfarin and phenytoin), the therapeutic effect of these substrates may be decreased. Concomitant use with peginterferon alfa-2b treatment resulted in a 28% (mean) increase in a measure of CYP2C8/9 activity).
No products indexed under this heading.

Mirtazapine (When administering peginterferon alfa-2b with medications metabolized by CYP2C8/9 (eg, warfarin and phenytoin), the therapeutic effect of these substrates may be decreased. Concomitant use with peginterferon alfa-2b treatment resulted in a 28% (mean) increase in a measure of CYP2C8/9 activity). Products include:
Remeron Tablets 3214
RemeronSolTab Tablets 3219

Montelukast Sodium (When administering peginterferon alfa-2b with medications metabolized by CYP2C8/9 (eg, warfarin and phenytoin), the therapeutic effect of these substrates may be decreased. Concomitant use with peginterferon alfa-2b treatment resulted in a 28% (mean) increase in a measure of CYP2C8/9 activity). Products include:
Singulair 2270

Morphine Sulfate (When administering peginterferon alfa-2b with medications metabolized by CYP2D6 (eg, flecainide), the therapeutic effect of this substrate may be decreased. Peginterferon alfa-2b treatment resulted in a 66% (mean) increase in a measure of CYP2D6 activity). Products include:
Avinza 1822
Embeda 1831
MS Contin 2803

Nabumetone (When administering peginterferon alfa-2b with medications metabolized by CYP2C8/9 (eg, warfarin and phenytoin), the therapeutic effect of these substrates may be decreased. Concomitant use with peginterferon alfa-2b treatment resulted in a 28% (mean) increase in a measure of CYP2C8/9 activity).
No products indexed under this heading.

Naproxen (When administering peginterferon alfa-2b with medications metabolized by CYP2C8/9 (eg, warfarin and phenytoin), the therapeutic effect of these substrates may be decreased. Concomitant use with peginterferon alfa-2b treatment resulted in a 28% (mean) increase in a measure of CYP2C8/9 activity). Products include:
EC-Naprosyn 2850
Naprosyn 2850
Anaprox/Naprosyn 2850

Naproxen Sodium (When administering peginterferon alfa-2b with medications metabolized by CYP2C8/9 (eg, warfarin and phenytoin), the therapeutic effect of these substrates may be decreased. Concomitant use with peginterferon alfa-2b treatment resulted in a 28% (mean) increase in a measure of CYP2C8/9 activity). Products include:
Anaprox 2850
Anaprox DS 2850
Treximet 1681

Nateglinide (When administering peginterferon alfa-2b with medications metabolized by CYP2C8/9 (eg, warfarin and phenytoin), the therapeutic effect of these substrates may be decreased. Concomitant use with peginterferon alfa-2b treatment resulted in a 28% (mean) increase in a measure of CYP2C8/9 activity).
No products indexed under this heading.

Nelfinavir Mesylate (When administering peginterferon alfa-2b with medications metabolized by CYP2D6 (eg, flecainide), the therapeutic effect of this substrate may be decreased. Peginterferon alfa-2b treatment resulted in a 66% (mean) increase in a measure of CYP2D6 activity).
No products indexed under this heading.

Nifedipine (When administering peginterferon alfa-2b with medications metabolized by CYP2C8/9 (eg, warfarin and phenytoin), the therapeutic effect of these substrates may be decreased. Concomitant use with peginterferon alfa-2b treatment resulted in a 28% (mean) increase in a measure of CYP2C8/9 activity).
No products indexed under this heading.

Nortriptyline Hydrochloride (When administering peginterferon alfa-2b with medications metabolized by CYP2C8/9 (eg, warfarin and phenytoin), the therapeutic effect of these substrates may be decreased. Concomitant use with peginterferon alfa-2b treatment resulted in a 28% (mean) increase in a measure of CYP2C8/9 activity).
No products indexed under this heading.

Olanzapine (When administering peginterferon alfa-2b with medications metabolized by CYP2D6 (eg, flecainide), the therapeutic effect of this substrate may be decreased. Peginterferon alfa-2b treatment resulted in a 66% (mean) increase in a measure of CYP2D6 activity). Products include:
Symbyax 1965
Zyprexa 1984
Zyprexa IntraMuscular 1984
Zyprexa ZYDIS 1984

Omeprazole (When administering peginterferon alfa-2b with medications metabolized by CYP2C8/9 (eg, warfarin and phenytoin), the therapeutic effect of these substrates may be decreased. Concomitant use with peginterferon alfa-2b treatment resulted in a 28% (mean) increase in a measure of CYP2C8/9 activity).
No products indexed under this heading.

Ondansetron (When administering peginterferon alfa-2b with medications metabolized by CYP2D6 (eg, flecainide), the therapeutic effect of this substrate may be decreased. Peginterferon alfa-2b treatment resulted in a 66% (mean) increase in a measure of CYP2D6 activity).
No products indexed under this heading.

Ondansetron Hydrochloride (When administering peginterferon alfa-2b with medications metabolized by CYP2D6 (eg, flecainide), the therapeutic effect of this substrate may be decreased. Peginterferon alfa-2b treatment resulted in a 66% (mean) increase in a measure of CYP2D6 activity). Products include:
Zofran Injection 1750
Zofran 1756
Zofran ODT 1756

Oxaprozin (When administering peginterferon alfa-2b with medications metabolized by CYP2C8/9 (eg, warfarin and phenytoin), the therapeutic effect of these substrates may be decreased. Concomitant use with peginterferon alfa-2b treatment resulted in a 28% (mean) increase in a measure of CYP2C8/9 activity).
No products indexed under this heading.

Oxycodone Hydrochloride (When administering peginterferon alfa-2b with medications metabolized by CYP2D6 (eg, flecainide), the therapeutic effect of this substrate may be decreased. Peginterferon alfa-2b treatment resulted in a 66% (mean) increase in a measure of CYP2D6 activity). Products include:
OxyContin 2807
Percocet 1121
Percodan 1124

Paclitaxel (When administering peginterferon alfa-2b with medications metabolized by CYP2C8/9 (eg, warfarin and phenytoin), the therapeutic effect of these substrates may be decreased. Concomitant use with peginterferon alfa-2b treatment resulted in a 28% (mean) increase in a measure of CYP2C8/9 activity).
No products indexed under this heading.

Paroxetine Hydrochloride (When administering peginterferon alfa-2b with medications metabolized by CYP2D6 (eg, flecainide), the therapeutic effect of this substrate may be decreased. Peginterferon alfa-2b treatment resulted in a 66% (mean) increase in a measure of CYP2D6 activity). Products include:
Paroxetine CR 2361
Paroxetine ER 2371
Paxil 1586
Paxil CR 1596

Phenylbutazone (When administering peginterferon alfa-2b with medications metabolized by CYP2C8/9 (eg, warfarin and phenytoin), the therapeutic effect of these substrates may be decreased. Concomitant use with peginterferon alfa-2b treatment resulted in a 28% (mean) increase in a measure of CYP2C8/9 activity).
No products indexed under this heading.

Phenytoin (When administering peginterferon alfa-2b with medications metabolized by CYP2C8/9 (eg, warfarin and phenytoin), the therapeutic effect of these substrates may be decreased. Peginterferon alfa-2b treatment resulted in a 28% (mean) increase in a measure of CYP2C8/9 activity).
No products indexed under this heading.

Phenytoin Sodium (When administering peginterferon alfa-2b with medications metabolized by CYP2C8/9 (eg, warfarin and phenytoin), the therapeutic effect of these substrates may be decreased. Peginterferon alfa-2b treatment resulted in a 28% (mean) increase in a measure of CYP2C8/9 activity). Products include:
Phenytek Capsules 2380

Pindolol (When administering peginterferon alfa-2b with medications metabolized by CYP2D6 (eg, flecainide), the therapeutic effect of this substrate may be decreased. Peginterferon alfa-2b treatment resulted in a 66% (mean) increase in a measure of CYP2D6 activity).
No products indexed under this heading.

Pioglitazone Hydrochloride (When administering peginterferon alfa-2b with medications metabolized by CYP2C8/9 (eg, warfarin and phenytoin), the therapeutic effect of these substrates may be decreased. Concomitant use with peginterferon alfa-2b treatment resulted in a 28% (mean) increase in a measure of CYP2C8/9 activity). Products include:
ActoPlus 3338
Actos 3345
Duetact 3354

Piroxicam (When administering peginterferon alfa-2b with medications metabolized by CYP2C8/9 (eg, warfarin and phenytoin), the therapeutic effect of these substrates may be decreased. Concomitant use with peginterferon alfa-2b treatment resulted in a 28% (mean) increase in a measure of CYP2C8/9 activity).
No products indexed under this heading.

Propafenone Hydrochloride (When administering peginterferon alfa-2b with medications metabolized by CYP2D6 (eg, flecainide), the therapeutic effect of this substrate may be decreased. Peginterferon alfa-2b treatment resulted in a 66% (mean) increase in a measure of CYP2D6 activity). Products include:
Rythmol 1648
Rythmol SR 1652

Propoxyphene Hydrochloride (When administering peginterferon alfa-2b with medications metabolized by CYP2D6 (eg, flecainide), the therapeutic effect of this substrate may be decreased. Peginterferon alfa-2b treatment resulted in a 66% (mean) increase in a measure of CYP2D6 activity).
No products indexed under this heading.

Propoxyphene Napsylate (When administering peginterferon alfa-2b with medications metabolized by CYP2D6 (eg, flecainide), the therapeutic effect of this substrate may be decreased. Peginterferon alfa-2b treatment resulted in a 66% (mean) increase in a measure of CYP2D6 activity).
No products indexed under this heading.

Propranolol Hydrochloride (When administering peginterferon alfa-2b with medications metabolized by CYP2D6 (eg, flecainide), the therapeutic effect of this substrate may be decreased. Peginterferon alfa-2b treatment resulted in a 66% (mean) increase in a measure of CYP2D6 activity). Products include:
InnoPran XL 1517

Protriptyline Hydrochloride (When administering peginterferon alfa-2b with medications metabolized by CYP2C8/9 (eg, warfarin and phenytoin), the therapeutic effect of these substrates may be decreased. Concomitant use with peginterferon alfa-2b treatment resulted in a 28% (mean) increase in a measure of CYP2C8/9 activity).
No products indexed under this heading.

Quetiapine Fumarate (When administering peginterferon alfa-2b with medications metabolized by CYP2D6 (eg, flecainide), the therapeutic effect of this substrate may be decreased. Peginterferon alfa-2b treatment resulted in a 66% (mean) increase in a measure of CYP2D6 activity). Products include:
Seroquel 750
Seroquel XR 759

Quinidine Gluconate (When administering peginterferon alfa-2b with medications metabolized by CYP2D6 (eg, flecainide), the therapeutic effect of this substrate may be decreased. Peginterferon alfa-2b treatment resulted in a 66% (mean) increase in a measure of CYP2D6 activity).
No products indexed under this heading.

Quinidine Hydrochloride (When administering peginterferon alfa-2b with medications metabolized by CYP2D6 (eg, flecainide), the therapeutic effect of this substrate may be decreased. Peginterferon alfa-2b treatment resulted in a 66% (mean) increase in a measure of CYP2D6 activity).
No products indexed under this heading.

Quinidine Polygalacturonate (When administering peginterferon alfa-2b with medications metabolized by CYP2D6 (eg, flecainide), the therapeutic effect of this substrate may be decreased. Peginterferon alfa-2b treatment resulted in a 66% (mean) increase in a measure of CYP2D6 activity).

No products indexed under this heading.

Quinidine Sulfate (When administering peginterferon alfa-2b with medications metabolized by CYP2D6 (eg, flecainide), the therapeutic effect of this substrate may be decreased. Peginterferon alfa-2b treatment resulted in a 66% (mean) increase in a measure of CYP2D6 activity).

No products indexed under this heading.

Repaglinide (When administering peginterferon alfa-2b with medications metabolized by CYP2C8/9 (eg, warfarin and phenytoin), the therapeutic effect of these substrates may be decreased. Concomitant use with peginterferon alfa-2b treatment resulted in a 28% (mean) increase in a measure of CYP2C8/9 activity).

No products indexed under this heading.

Ribavirin (Hepatic decompensation (some fatal) has occurred in cirrhotic HIV/HCV co-infected patients receiving combination antiretoviral therapy for HIV and interferon alpha and ribavirin. Adding treatment with alpha interferons alone or in combination with ribavirin may increase the risk in this patient subset). Products include:

Rebetol 3207

Risperidone (When administering peginterferon alfa-2b with medications metabolized by CYP2D6 (eg, flecainide), the therapeutic effect of this substrate may be decreased. Peginterferon alfa-2b treatment resulted in a 66% (mean) increase in a measure of CYP2D6 activity). Products include:

Risperdal Consta 2682

Ritonavir (When administering peginterferon alfa-2b with medications metabolized by CYP2D6 (eg, flecainide), the therapeutic effect of this substrate may be decreased. Peginterferon alfa-2b treatment resulted in a 66% (mean) increase in a measure of CYP2D6 activity). Products include:

Kaletra 458
Norvir 509

Rofecoxib (When administering peginterferon alfa-2b with medications metabolized by CYP2C8/9 (eg, warfarin and phenytoin), the therapeutic effect of these substrates may be decreased. Concomitant use with peginterferon alfa-2b treatment resulted in a 28% (mean) increase in a measure of CYP2C8/9 activity).

No products indexed under this heading.

Rosiglitazone Maleate (When administering peginterferon alfa-2b with medications metabolized by CYP2C8/9 (eg, warfarin and phenytoin), the therapeutic effect of these substrates may be decreased. Concomitant use with peginterferon alfa-2b treatment resulted in a 28% (mean) increase in a measure of CYP2C8/9 activity). Products include:

Avandamet 1345
Avandaryl 1356
Avandia 1366

Rosiglitazone/Metformin (When administering peginterferon alfa-2b with medications metabolized by CYP2C8/9 (eg, warfarin and phenytoin), the therapeutic effect of these substrates may be decreased. Concomitant use with peginterferon alfa-2b treatment resulted in a 28% (mean) increase in a measure of CYP2C8/9 activity).

No products indexed under this heading.

Sildenafil Citrate (When administering peginterferon alfa-2b with medications metabolized by CYP2C8/9 (eg, warfarin and phenytoin), the therapeutic effect of these substrates may be decreased. Concomitant use with peginterferon alfa-2b treatment resulted in a 28% (mean) increase in a measure of CYP2C8/9 activity).

No products indexed under this heading.

Stavudine (Hepatic decompensation (some fatal) has occurred in cirrhotic HIV/HCV co-infected patients receiving combination antiretroviral therapy for HIV and interferon alpha and ribavirin. Adding treatment with alpha interferons alone or in combination with ribavirin may increase the risk in this patient subset. Patients receiving interferon with ribavirin and nucleoside reverse transcriptase inhibitors (NRTIs) should be closely monitored for treamtent-associated toxicities, especially hepatic decompensation andanemia. Discontinuationof NRTIs should be considered as medically appropriate. Dose reduction or discontinuation of interferon, ribavirin, or both should also be considered if worsening clinical toxicities are observed, including hepatic decompensation).

No products indexed under this heading.

Sulfamethoxazole (When administering peginterferon alfa-2b with medications metabolized by CYP2C8/9 (eg, warfarin and phenytoin), the therapeutic effect of these substrates may be decreased. Concomitant use with peginterferon alfa-2b treatment resulted in a 28% (mean) increase in a measure of CYP2C8/9 activity).

No products indexed under this heading.

Sulindac (When administering peginterferon alfa-2b with medications metabolized by CYP2C8/9 (eg, warfarin and phenytoin), the therapeutic effect of these substrates may be decreased. Concomitant use with peginterferon alfa-2b treatment resulted in a 28% (mean) increase in a measure of CYP2C8/9 activity). Products include:

Clinoril 2098

Suprofen (When administering peginterferon alfa-2b with medications metabolized by CYP2C8/9 (eg, warfarin and phenytoin), the therapeutic effect of these substrates may be decreased. Concomitant use with peginterferon alfa-2b treatment resulted in a 28% (mean) increase in a measure of CYP2C8/9 activity).

No products indexed under this heading.

Tamoxifen Citrate (When administering peginterferon alfa-2b with medications metabolized by CYP2C8/9 (eg, warfarin and phenytoin), the therapeutic effect of these substrates may be decreased. Concomitant use with peginterferon alfa-2b treatment resulted in a 28% (mean) increase in a measure of CYP2C8/9 activity).

No products indexed under this heading.

Telmisartan (When administering peginterferon alfa-2b with medications metabolized by CYP2C8/9 (eg, warfarin and phenytoin), the therapeutic effect of these substrates may be decreased. Concomitant use with peginterferon alfa-2b treatment resulted in a 28% (mean) increase in a measure of CYP2C8/9 activity). Products include:

Micardis 887
Micardis HCT 889

Teniposide (When administering peginterferon alfa-2b with medications metabolized by CYP2D6 (eg, flecainide), the therapeutic effect of this substrate may be decreased. Peginterferon alfa-2b treatment resulted in a 66% (mean) increase in a measure of CYP2D6 activity).

No products indexed under this heading.

Tenofovir Disoproxil Fumarate (Hepatic decompensation (some fatal) has occurred in cirrhotic HIV/HCV co-infected patients receiving combination antiretroviral therapy for HIV and interferon alpha and ribavirin. Adding treatment with alpha interferons alone or in combination with ribavirin may increase the risk in this patient subset. Patients receiving interferon with ribavirin and nucleoside reverse transcriptase inhibitors (NRTIs) should be closely monitored for treamtent-associated toxicities, especially hepatic decompensation andanemia. Discontinuationof NRTIs should be considered as medically appropriate. Dose reduction or discontinuation of interferon, ribavirin, or both should also be considered if worsening clinical toxicities are observed, including hepatic decompensation). Products include:

Atripla 906
Truvada 1258
Viread 1266

Testosterone (When administering peginterferon alfa-2b with medications metabolized by CYP2D6 (eg, flecainide), the therapeutic effect of this substrate may be decreased. Peginterferon alfa-2b treatment resulted in a 66% (mean) increase in a measure of CYP2D6 activity). Products include:

AndroGel 3456

Testosterone Cypionate (When administering peginterferon alfa-2b with medications metabolized by CYP2D6 (eg, flecainide), the therapeutic effect of this substrate may be decreased. Peginterferon alfa-2b treatment resulted in a 66% (mean) increase in a measure of CYP2D6 activity).

No products indexed under this heading.

Testosterone Enanthate (When administering peginterferon alfa-2b with medications metabolized by CYP2D6 (eg, flecainide), the therapeutic effect of this substrate may be decreased. Peginterferon alfa-2b treatment resulted in a 66% (mean) increase in a measure of CYP2D6 activity). Products include:

Delatestryl 1102

Testosterone Propionate (When administering peginterferon alfa-2b with medications metabolized by CYP2D6 (eg, flecainide), the therapeutic effect of this substrate may be decreased. Peginterferon alfa-2b treatment resulted in a 66% (mean) increase in a measure of CYP2D6 activity).

No products indexed under this heading.

Thioridazine (When administering peginterferon alfa-2b with medications metabolized by CYP2D6 (eg, flecainide), the therapeutic effect of this substrate may be decreased. Peginterferon alfa-2b treatment resulted in a 66% (mean) increase in a measure of CYP2D6 activity).

No products indexed under this heading.

Thioridazine Hydrochloride (When administering peginterferon alfa-2b with medications metabolized by CYP2D6 (eg, flecainide), the therapeutic effect of this substrate may be decreased. Peginterferon alfa-2b treatment resulted in a 66% (mean) increase in a measure of CYP2D6 activity). Products include:

Thioridazine Hydrochloride 2384

Timolol Maleate (When administering peginterferon alfa-2b with medications metabolized by CYP2D6 (eg, flecainide), the therapeutic effect of this substrate may be decreased. Peginterferon alfa-2b treatment resulted in a 66% (mean) increase in a measure of CYP2D6 activity). Products include:

Combigan 601
Dorzolamide
  Hydrochloride/Timolol Maleate
  Ophthalmic Solution .... ⊙243
Timoptic in Ocudose .... ⊙231

Tolazamide (When administering peginterferon alfa-2b with medications metabolized by CYP2C8/9 (eg, warfarin and phenytoin), the therapeutic effect of these substrates may be decreased. Concomitant use with peginterferon alfa-2b treatment resulted in a 28% (mean) increase in a measure of CYP2C8/9 activity).

No products indexed under this heading.

Tolbutamide (When administering peginterferon alfa-2b with medications metabolized by CYP2C8/9 (eg, warfarin and phenytoin), the therapeutic effect of these substrates may be decreased. Concomitant use with peginterferon alfa-2b treatment resulted in a 28% (mean) increase in a measure of CYP2C8/9 activity).

No products indexed under this heading.

Tolbutamide Sodium (When administering peginterferon alfa-2b with medications metabolized by CYP2C8/9 (eg, warfarin and phenytoin), the therapeutic effect of these substrates may be decreased. Concomitant use with peginterferon alfa-2b treatment resulted in a 28% (mean) increase in a measure of CYP2C8/9 activity).

No products indexed under this heading.

Tolmetin Sodium (When administering peginterferon alfa-2b with medications metabolized by CYP2C8/9 (eg, warfarin and phenytoin), the therapeutic effect of these substrates may be decreased. Concomitant use with peginterferon alfa-2b treatment resulted in a 28% (mean) increase in a measure of CYP2C8/9 activity).

No products indexed under this heading.

Tolterodine Tartrate (When administering peginterferon alfa-2b with medications metabolized by CYP2D6 (eg, flecainide), the therapeutic effect of this substrate may be decreased. Peginterferon alfa-2b treatment resulted in a 66% (mean) increase in a measure of CYP2D6 activity).

No products indexed under this heading.

Torsemide (When administering peginterferon alfa-2b with medications metabolized by CYP2C8/9 (eg, warfarin and phenytoin), the therapeutic effect of these substrates may be decreased. Concomitant use with peginterferon alfa-2b treatment resulted in a 28% (mean) increase in a measure of CYP2C8/9 activity).

No products indexed under this heading.

Tramadol Hydrochloride (When administering peginterferon alfa-2b with medications metabolized by CYP2D6 (eg, flecainide), the therapeutic effect of this substrate may be decreased. Peginterferon alfa-2b treatment resulted in a 66% (mean) increase in a measure of CYP2D6 activity). Products include:

Ryzolt 2813
Ultram ER 2693

Trazodone Hydrochloride (When administering peginterferon alfa-2b with medications metabolized by CYP2D6 (eg, flecainide), the therapeutic effect of this substrate may be decreased. Peginterferon alfa-2b treatment resulted in a 66% (mean) increase in a measure of CYP2D6 activity).

No products indexed under this heading.

Tretinoin (When administering peginterferon alfa-2b with medications metabolized by CYP2C8/9 (eg, warfarin and phenytoin), the therapeutic effect of these substrates may be decreased. Concomitant use with peginterferon alfa-2b treatment resulted in a 28% (mean) increase in a measure of CYP2C8/9 activity).

No products indexed under this heading.

IMPORTANT NOTE: Always consult each drug listing in the patient's regimen for possible interactions.

Triazolam (When administering peginterferon alfa-2b with medications metabolized by CYP2D6 (eg, flecainide), the therapeutic effect of this substrate may be decreased. Peginterferon alfa-2b treatment resulted in a 66% (mean) increase in a measure of CYP2D6 activity).
No products indexed under this heading.

Trimipramine Maleate (When administering peginterferon alfa-2b with medications metabolized by CYP2C8/9 (eg, warfarin and phenytoin), the therapeutic effect of these substrates may be decreased. Concomitant use with peginterferon alfa-2b treatment resulted in a 28% (mean) increase in a measure of CYP2C8/9 activity).
No products indexed under this heading.

Troglitazone (When administering peginterferon alfa-2b with medications metabolized by CYP2C8/9 (eg, warfarin and phenytoin), the therapeutic effect of these substrates may be decreased. Concomitant use with peginterferon alfa-2b treatment resulted in a 28% (mean) increase in a measure of CYP2C8/9 activity).
No products indexed under this heading.

Valdecoxib (When administering peginterferon alfa-2b with medications metabolized by CYP2C8/9 (eg, warfarin and phenytoin), the therapeutic effect of these substrates may be decreased. Concomitant use with peginterferon alfa-2b treatment resulted in a 28% (mean) increase in a measure of CYP2C8/9 activity).
No products indexed under this heading.

Valsartan (When administering peginterferon alfa-2b with medications metabolized by CYP2C8/9 (eg, warfarin and phenytoin), the therapeutic effect of these substrates may be decreased. Concomitant use with peginterferon alfa-2b treatment resulted in a 28% (mean) increase in a measure of CYP2C8/9 activity). Products include:

Vardenafil Hydrochloride (When administering peginterferon alfa-2b with medications metabolized by CYP2C8/9 (eg, warfarin and phenytoin), the therapeutic effect of these substrates may be decreased. Concomitant use with peginterferon alfa-2b treatment resulted in a 28% (mean) increase in a measure of CYP2C8/9 activity). Products include:

Venlafaxine Hydrochloride (When administering peginterferon alfa-2b with medications metabolized by CYP2D6 (eg, flecainide), the therapeutic effect of this substrate may be decreased. Peginterferon alfa-2b treatment resulted in a 66% (mean) increase in a measure of CYP2D6 activity). Products include:

Verapamil Hydrochloride (When administering peginterferon alfa-2b with medications metabolized by CYP2C8/9 (eg, warfarin and phenytoin), the therapeutic effect of these substrates may be decreased. Concomitant use with peginterferon alfa-2b treatment resulted in a 28% (mean) increase in a measure of CYP2C8/9 activity). Products include:

Vinblastine Sulfate (When administering peginterferon alfa-2b with medications metabolized by CYP2D6 (eg, flecainide), the therapeutic effect of this substrate may be decreased. Peginterferon alfa-2b treatment resulted in a 66% (mean) increase in a measure of CYP2D6 activity).
No products indexed under this heading.

Vitamin A (When administering peginterferon alfa-2b with medications metabolized by CYP2C8/9 (eg, warfarin and phenytoin), the therapeutic effect of these substrates may be decreased. Concomitant use with peginterferon alfa-2b treatment resulted in a 28% (mean) increase in a measure of CYP2C8/9 activity). Products include:

Vitamin A Acetate (When administering peginterferon alfa-2b with medications metabolized by CYP2C8/9 (eg, warfarin and phenytoin), the therapeutic effect of these substrates may be decreased. Concomitant use with peginterferon alfa-2b treatment resulted in a 28% (mean) increase in a measure of CYP2C8/9 activity).
No products indexed under this heading.

Voriconazole (When administering peginterferon alfa-2b with medications metabolized by CYP2C8/9 (eg, warfarin and phenytoin), the therapeutic effect of these substrates may be decreased. Concomitant use with peginterferon alfa-2b treatment resulted in a 28% (mean) increase in a measure of CYP2C8/9 activity).
No products indexed under this heading.

Warfarin Sodium (When administering peginterferon alfa-2b with medications metabolized by CYP2C8/9 (eg, warfarin and phenytoin), the therapeutic effect of these substrates may be decreased. Peginterferon alfa-2b treatment resulted in a 28% (mean) increase in a measure of CYP2C8/9 activity).
No products indexed under this heading.

Zafirlukast (When administering peginterferon alfa-2b with medications metabolized by CYP2C8/9 (eg, warfarin and phenytoin), the therapeutic effect of these substrates may be decreased. Concomitant use with peginterferon alfa-2b treatment resulted in a 28% (mean) increase in a measure of CYP2C8/9 activity). Products include:

Zalcitabine (Hepatic decompensation (some fatal) has occurred in cirrhotic HIV/HCV co-infected patients receiving combination antiretroviral therapy for HIV and interferon alpha and ribavirin. Adding treatment with alpha interferons alone or in combination with ribavirin may increase the risk in this patient subset. Patients receiving interferon with ribavirin and nucleoside reverse transcriptase inhibitors (NRTIs) should be closely monitored for treatment-associated toxicities, especially hepatic decompensation andanemia. Discontinuationof NRTIs should be considered as medically appropriate. Dose reduction or discontinuation of interferon, ribavirin, or both should also be considered if worsening clinical toxicities are observed, including hepatic decompensation).
No products indexed under this heading.

Zidovudine (HIV/HCV co-infected subjects who were administered zidovudine in combination with pegylated interferon alpha and ribavirin developed severe neutropenia (ANC<500) and severe anemia (hemoglobin <8g/dL) more frequently than similiar subjects not receiving zidovudine). Products include:

Zileuton (When administering peginterferon alfa-2b with medications metabolized by CYP2C8/9 (eg, warfarin and phenytoin), the therapeutic effect of these substrates may be decreased. Concomitant use with peginterferon alfa-2b treatment resulted in a 28% (mean) increase in a measure of CYP2C8/9 activity).
No products indexed under this heading.

Zonisamide (When administering peginterferon alfa-2b with medications metabolized by CYP2D6 (eg, flecainide), the therapeutic effect of this substrate may be decreased. Peginterferon alfa-2b treatment resulted in a 66% (mean) increase in a measure of CYP2D6 activity). Products include:

Zopiclone (When administering peginterferon alfa-2b with medications metabolized by CYP2C8/9 (eg, warfarin and phenytoin), the therapeutic effect of these substrates may be decreased. Concomitant use with peginterferon alfa-2b treatment resulted in a 28% (mean) increase in a measure of CYP2C8/9 activity).
No products indexed under this heading.

PENTASA CAPSULES

None cited in PDR database.

PEPCID TABLETS

May interact with antacids, and certain other agents. Compounds in these categories include:

Aluminum Carbonate (Bioavailability may be slightly decreased by antacids).
No products indexed under this heading.

Aluminum Hydroxide (Bioavailability may be slightly decreased by antacids).
No products indexed under this heading.

Calcium Carbonate (Bioavailability may be slightly decreased by antacids). Products include:

Magaldrate (Bioavailability may be slightly decreased by antacids).
No products indexed under this heading.

Magnesium Carbonate (Bioavailability may be slightly decreased by antacids).
No products indexed under this heading.

Magnesium Hydroxide (Bioavailability may be slightly decreased by antacids). Products include:

Magnesium Oxide (Bioavailability may be slightly decreased by antacids). Products include:

Magnesium Trisilicate (Bioavailability may be slightly decreased by antacids).
No products indexed under this heading.

Sodium Bicarbonate (Bioavailability may be slightly decreased by antacids).
No products indexed under this heading.

Food Interactions

Food, unspecified (Bioavailability may be slightly increased by antacids).

ORIGINAL STRENGTH PEPCID AC GELCAPS

None cited in PDR database.

ORIGINAL STRENGTH PEPCID AC TABLETS

None cited in PDR database.

MAXIMUM STRENGTH PEPCID AC TABLETS

None cited in PDR database.

PEPCID COMPLETE CHEWABLE TABLETS

Prescription Drugs, unspecified (Antacids contained in Pepcid Complete may interact with certain prescription drugs).
No products indexed under this heading.

PERCOCET TABLETS

May interact with alcohols, anticholinergics, central nervous system depressants, general anesthetics, hypnotics and sedatives, loop diuretics, mixed agonist/antagonist opioid analgesics, monoamine oxidase inhibitors, narcotic analgesics, oral contraceptives, phenothiazines, skeletal muscle relaxants, tranquilizers, tricyclic antidepressants, vasodilators, and certain other agents. Compounds in these categories include:

Alfentanil Hydrochloride (Additive CNS depression; dose of one or both agents should be reduced).
No products indexed under this heading.

Alprazolam (Additive CNS depression; dose of one or both agents should be reduced).
No products indexed under this heading.

Amitriptyline Hydrochloride (Increased effect of antidepressant or oxycodone).
No products indexed under this heading.

Amobarbital (Additive CNS depression; dose of one or both agents should be reduced).
No products indexed under this heading.

Amobarbital Sodium (Additive CNS depression; dose of one or both agents should be reduced).
No products indexed under this heading.

Amoxapine (Increased effect of antidepressant or oxycodone).
No products indexed under this heading.

Amyl Nitrite (Oxycodone may cause severe hypotension after concurrent administration with drugs which compromise vasomotor tone).
No products indexed under this heading.

Apomorphine (Additive CNS depression; dose of one or both agents should be reduced).
No products indexed under this heading.

Apomorphine Hydrochloride (Additive CNS depression; dose of one or both agents should be reduced).
No products indexed under this heading.

Aprobarbital (Additive CNS depression; dose of one or both agents should be reduced).
No products indexed under this heading.

Atracurium Besylate (Opioid analgesics may enhance the neuromuscular-blocking action of skeletal muscle relaxants and produce an increase in the degree of respiratory depression).
No products indexed under this heading.

Atropine Sulfate (May produce paralytic ileus). Products include:

Baclofen (Opioid analgesics may enhance the neuromuscular-blocking action of skeletal muscle relaxants and produce an increase in the degree of respiratory depression).
No products indexed under this heading.

Belladonna Alkaloids (May produce paralytic ileus). Products include:

Benztropine Mesylate (May produce paralytic ileus).
No products indexed under this heading.

Biperiden Hydrochloride (May produce paralytic ileus).
No products indexed under this heading.

Bumetanide (The effects of loop diuretics may be decreased).
No products indexed under this heading.

Buprenorphine Hydrochloride (Additive CNS depression; dose of one or both agents should be reduced).
No products indexed under this heading.

Buspirone Hydrochloride (Additive CNS depression; dose of one or both agents should be reduced).
No products indexed under this heading.

Butabarbital (Additive CNS depression; dose of one or both agents should be reduced).
No products indexed under this heading.

Butabarbital Sodium (Additive CNS depression; dose of one or both agents should be reduced).
No products indexed under this heading.

Butalbital (Additive CNS depression; dose of one or both agents should be reduced).
No products indexed under this heading.

Butorphanol Tartrate (Mixed agonist/antagonist analgesics may reduce the analgesic effect of oxycodone and/or may precipitate withdrawal symptoms in these patients).
No products indexed under this heading.

Carisoprodol (Opioid analgesics may enhance the neuromuscular-blocking action of skeletal muscle relaxants and produce an increase in the degree of respiratory depression).
No products indexed under this heading.

Chloral Hydrate (Additive CNS depression; dose of one or both agents should be reduced).
No products indexed under this heading.

Chlordiazepoxide (Additive CNS depression; dose of one or both agents should be reduced).
No products indexed under this heading.

Chlordiazepoxide Hydrochloride (Additive CNS depression; dose of one or both agents should be reduced).
No products indexed under this heading.

Chlorpromazine (Additive CNS depression; dose of one or both agents should be reduced).
No products indexed under this heading.

Chlorpromazine Hydrochloride (Additive CNS depression; dose of one or both agents should be reduced).
No products indexed under this heading.

Chlorprothixene (Additive CNS depression; dose of one or both agents should be reduced).
No products indexed under this heading.

Chlorprothixene Hydrochloride (Additive CNS depression; dose of one or both agents should be reduced).
No products indexed under this heading.

Chlorprothixene Lactate (Additive CNS depression; dose of one or both agents should be reduced).
No products indexed under this heading.

Chlorzoxazone (Opioid analgesics may enhance the neuromuscular-blocking action of skeletal muscle relaxants and produce an increase in the degree of respiratory depression).
No products indexed under this heading.

Cisatracurium Besylate (Opioid analgesics may enhance the neuromuscular-blocking action of skeletal muscle relaxants and produce an increase in the degree of respiratory depression). Products include:

Clidinium Bromide (May produce paralytic ileus).
No products indexed under this heading.

Clomipramine Hydrochloride (Increased effect of antidepressant or oxycodone).
No products indexed under this heading.

Clonazepam (Additive CNS depression; dose of one or both agents should be reduced). Products include:

Clorazepate Dipotassium (Additive CNS depression; dose of one or both agents should be reduced).
No products indexed under this heading.

Clozapine (Additive CNS depression; dose of one or both agents should be reduced).
No products indexed under this heading.

Codeine Phosphate (Additive CNS depression; dose of one or both agents should be reduced). Products include:

Codeine Sulfate (Additive CNS depression; dose of one or both agents should be reduced).
No products indexed under this heading.

Cyclobenzaprine Hydrochloride (Opioid analgesics may enhance the neuromuscular-blocking action of skeletal muscle relaxants and produce an increase in the degree of respiratory depression). Products include:

Dantrolene Sodium (Opioid analgesics may enhance the neuromuscular-blocking action of skeletal muscle relaxants and produce an increase in the degree of respiratory depression).
No products indexed under this heading.

Desflurane (Additive CNS depression; dose of one or both agents should be reduced).
No products indexed under this heading.

Desipramine Hydrochloride (Increased effect of antidepressant or oxycodone).
No products indexed under this heading.

Desogestrel (Increase in glucoronidation resulting in increased plasma clearance and a decreased half-life of acetaminophen).
No products indexed under this heading.

Dezocine (Additive CNS depression; dose of one or both agents should be reduced).
No products indexed under this heading.

Diazepam (Additive CNS depression; dose of one or both agents should be reduced). Products include:

Diazoxide (Oxycodone may cause severe hypotension after concurrent administration with drugs which compromise vasomotor tone). Products include:

Dicyclomine Hydrochloride (May produce paralytic ileus). Products include:

Dihydrocodeine Bitartrate (Additive CNS depression; dose of one or both agents should be reduced).
No products indexed under this heading.

Dihydrocodeinone Bitartrate (Additive CNS depression; dose of one or both agents should be reduced).
No products indexed under this heading.

Doxacurium Chloride (Opioid analgesics may enhance the neuromuscular-blocking action of skeletal muscle relaxants and produce an increase in the degree of respiratory depression).
No products indexed under this heading.

Doxepin Hydrochloride (Increased effect of antidepressant or oxycodone).
No products indexed under this heading.

Droperidol (Additive CNS depression; dose of one or both agents should be reduced).
No products indexed under this heading.

d-Tubocurarine (Opioid analgesics may enhance the neuromuscular-blocking action of skeletal muscle relaxants and produce an increase in the degree of respiratory depression).
No products indexed under this heading.

Enflurane (Additive CNS depression; dose of one or both agents should be reduced).
No products indexed under this heading.

Epoprostenol Sodium (Oxycodone may cause severe hypotension after concurrent administration with drugs which compromise vasomotor tone). Products include:

Estazolam (Additive CNS depression; dose of one or both agents should be reduced).
No products indexed under this heading.

Ethacrynic Acid (The effects of loop diuretics may be decreased).
No products indexed under this heading.

Ethanol (Additive CNS depression; dose of one or both agents should be reduced).
No products indexed under this heading.

Ethaverine Hydrochloride (Oxycodone may cause severe hypotension after concurrent administration with drugs which compromise vasomotor tone).
No products indexed under this heading.

Ethchlorvynol (Additive CNS depression; dose of one or both agents should be reduced).
No products indexed under this heading.

Ethinamate (Additive CNS depression; dose of one or both agents should be reduced).
No products indexed under this heading.

Ethinyl Estradiol (Increase in glucoronidation resulting in increased plasma clearance and a decreased half-life of acetaminophen). Products include:

Ethopropazine Hydrochloride (May produce paralytic ileus).
No products indexed under this heading.

Ethyl Alcohol (Additive CNS depression; dose of one or both agents should be reduced).
No products indexed under this heading.

Ethynodiol Diacetate (Increase in glucoronidation resulting in increased plasma clearance and a decreased half-life of acetaminophen).
No products indexed under this heading.

Fentanyl (Additive CNS depression; dose of one or both agents should be reduced). Products include:

Fentanyl Citrate (Additive CNS depression; dose of one or both agents should be reduced). Products include:

Fluphenazine Decanoate (Additive CNS depression; dose of one or both agents should be reduced).
No products indexed under this heading.

Fluphenazine Enanthate (Additive CNS depression; dose of one or both agents should be reduced).
No products indexed under this heading.

Fluphenazine Hydrochloride (Additive CNS depression; dose of one or both agents should be reduced).
No products indexed under this heading.

Flurazepam Hydrochloride (Additive CNS depression; dose of one or both agents should be reduced).
No products indexed under this heading.

Furosemide (The effects of loop diuretics may be decreased). Products include:

Gallamine (Opioid analgesics may enhance the neuromuscular-blocking action of skeletal muscle relaxants and produce an increase in the degree of respiratory depression).
No products indexed under this heading.

Gallamine Triethiodide (Opioid analgesics may enhance the neuromuscular-blocking action of skeletal muscle relaxants and produce an increase in the degree of respiratory depression).
No products indexed under this heading.

Glutethimide (Additive CNS depression; dose of one or both agents should be reduced).
No products indexed under this heading.

Glycopyrrolate (May produce paralytic ileus).
No products indexed under this heading.

Halazepam (Additive CNS depression; dose of one or both agents should be reduced).
No products indexed under this heading.

Haloperidol (Additive CNS depression; dose of one or both agents should be reduced).
No products indexed under this heading.

Haloperidol Decanoate (Additive CNS depression; dose of one or both agents should be reduced).
No products indexed under this heading.

Haloperidol Lactate (Additive CNS depression; dose of one or both agents should be reduced).
No products indexed under this heading.

Halothane (Additive CNS depression; dose of one or both agents should be reduced).
No products indexed under this heading.

Hexobarbital (Additive CNS depression; dose of one or both agents should be reduced).
No products indexed under this heading.

Hydralazine Hydrochloride (Oxycodone may cause severe hypotension after concurrent administration with drugs which compromise vasomotor tone).
No products indexed under this heading.

Hydrocodone Bitartrate (Additive CNS depression; dose of one or both agents should be reduced). Products include:

Hydrocodone Polistirex (Additive CNS depression; dose of one or both agents should be reduced). Products include:

IMPORTANT NOTE: Always consult each drug listing in the patient's regimen for possible interactions.

Percocet | Interactions Index | 1410

Hydromorphone (Additive CNS depression; dose of one or both agents should be reduced).
No products indexed under this heading.

Hydromorphone Hydrochloride (Additive CNS depression; dose of one or both agents should be reduced). Products include:
Dilaudid Injection ... 2800
Dilaudid Oral ... 2797
Dilaudid Tablets ... 2797
Dilaudid-HP ... 2800

Hydroxyzine Hydrochloride (Additive CNS depression; dose of one or both agents should be reduced).
No products indexed under this heading.

Hyoscyamine (May produce paralytic ileus).
No products indexed under this heading.

Hyoscyamine Sulfate (May produce paralytic ileus). Products include:
Donnatal ... 2711

Imipramine Hydrochloride (Increased effect of antidepressant or oxycodone).
No products indexed under this heading.

Imipramine Pamoate (Increased effect of antidepressant or oxycodone).
No products indexed under this heading.

Ipratropium Bromide (May produce paralytic ileus).
No products indexed under this heading.

Isocarboxazid (Increased effect of either oxycodone or MAO inhibitor). Products include:
Marplan ... 3481

Isoflurane (Additive CNS depression; dose of one or both agents should be reduced).
No products indexed under this heading.

Isosorbide Dinitrate (Oxycodone may cause severe hypotension after concurrent administration with drugs which compromise vasomotor tone).
No products indexed under this heading.

Isosorbide Mononitrate (Oxycodone may cause severe hypotension after concurrent administration with drugs which compromise vasomotor tone).
No products indexed under this heading.

Isoxsuprine Hydrochloride (Oxycodone may cause severe hypotension after concurrent administration with drugs which compromise vasomotor tone).
No products indexed under this heading.

Ketamine Hydrochloride (Additive CNS depression; dose of one or both agents should be reduced).
No products indexed under this heading.

Lamotrigine (Serum lamotigrine concentrations may be reduced, producing a decrease in therapeutic effects). Products include:
Lamictal ... 1522
Lamictal ODT ... 1522
Lamictal XR ... 1536

Levomethadyl Acetate Hydrochloride (Additive CNS depression; dose of one or both agents should be reduced).
No products indexed under this heading.

Levonorgestrel (Increase in glucoronidation resulting in increased plasma clearance and a decreased half-life of acetaminophen). Products include:
Climara Pro ... 847
LoSeasonique ... 3407
Lybrel ... 3514
Mirena ... 854
Plan B ... 3416
Seasonique ... 3418

Levorphanol Tartrate (Additive CNS depression; dose of one or both agents should be reduced).
No products indexed under this heading.

Lorazepam (Additive CNS depression; dose of one or both agents should be reduced).
No products indexed under this heading.

Loxapine Hydrochloride (Additive CNS depression; dose of one or both agents should be reduced).
No products indexed under this heading.

Loxapine Succinate (Additive CNS depression; dose of one or both agents should be reduced).
No products indexed under this heading.

Maprotiline Hydrochloride (Increased effect of antidepressant or oxycodone).
No products indexed under this heading.

Mepenzolate Bromide (May produce paralytic ileus).
No products indexed under this heading.

Meperidine Hydrochloride (Additive CNS depression; dose of one or both agents should be reduced).
No products indexed under this heading.

Mephobarbital (Additive CNS depression; dose of one or both agents should be reduced).
No products indexed under this heading.

Meprobamate (Additive CNS depression; dose of one or both agents should be reduced).
No products indexed under this heading.

Mesoridazine Besylate (Additive CNS depression; dose of one or both agents should be reduced).
No products indexed under this heading.

Mestranol (Increase in glucoronidation resulting in increased plasma clearance and a decreased half-life of acetaminophen).
No products indexed under this heading.

Metaxalone (Opioid analgesics may enhance the neuromuscular-blocking action of skeletal muscle relaxants and produce an increase in the degree of respiratory depression). Products include:
Skelaxin ... 1848

Methadone Hydrochloride (Additive CNS depression; dose of one or both agents should be reduced).
No products indexed under this heading.

Methocarbamol (Opioid analgesics may enhance the neuromuscular-blocking action of skeletal muscle relaxants and produce an increase in the degree of respiratory depression).
No products indexed under this heading.

Methohexital Sodium (Additive CNS depression; dose of one or both agents should be reduced).
No products indexed under this heading.

Methotrimeprazine (Additive CNS depression; dose of one or both agents should be reduced).
No products indexed under this heading.

Methoxyflurane (Additive CNS depression; dose of one or both agents should be reduced).
No products indexed under this heading.

Metocurine Iodide (Opioid analgesics may enhance the neuromuscular-blocking action of skeletal muscle relaxants and produce an increase in the degree of respiratory depression).
No products indexed under this heading.

Midazolam Hydrochloride (Additive CNS depression; dose of one or both agents should be reduced).
No products indexed under this heading.

Minoxidil (Oxycodone may cause severe hypotension after concurrent administration with drugs which compromise vasomotor tone).
No products indexed under this heading.

Mivacurium Chloride (Opioid analgesics may enhance the neuromuscular-blocking action of skeletal muscle relaxants and produce an increase in the degree of respiratory depression).
No products indexed under this heading.

Moclobemide (Increased effect of either oxycodone or MAO inhibitor).
No products indexed under this heading.

Molindone Hydrochloride (Additive CNS depression; dose of one or both agents should be reduced). Products include:
Moban ... 1108

Morphine Sulfate (Additive CNS depression; dose of one or both agents should be reduced). Products include:
Avinza ... 1822
Embeda ... 1831
MS Contin ... 2803

Morphine Sulfate, Liposomal (Additive CNS depression; dose of one or both agents should be reduced).
No products indexed under this heading.

Nalbuphine Hydrochloride (Mixed agonist/antagonist analgesics may reduce the analgesic effect of oxycodone and/or may precipitate withdrawal symptoms in these patients).
No products indexed under this heading.

Nitroglycerin (Oxycodone may cause severe hypotension after concurrent administration with drugs which compromise vasomotor tone). Products include:
Nitro-Dur ... 3170
Nitrolingual ... 3266

Nitroglycerin, long-acting formulations (Oxycodone may cause severe hypotension after concurrent administration with drugs which compromise vasomotor tone).
No products indexed under this heading.

Nitroglycerin Intravenous (Oxycodone may cause severe hypotension after concurrent administration with drugs which compromise vasomotor tone).
No products indexed under this heading.

Nitrous Oxide (Additive CNS depression; dose of one or both agents should be reduced).
No products indexed under this heading.

Norethindrone (Increase in glucoronidation resulting in increased plasma clearance and a decreased half-life of acetaminophen). Products include:
Ortho Micronor ... 2660

Norethynodrel (Increase in glucoronidation resulting in increased plasma clearance and a decreased half-life of acetaminophen).
No products indexed under this heading.

Norgestimate (Increase in glucoronidation resulting in increased plasma clearance and a decreased half-life of acetaminophen). Products include:
Ortho-Cyclen/Ortho Tri-Cyclen ... 2663
Ortho Tri-Cyclen Lo Tablets ... 2673

Norgestrel (Increase in glucoronidation resulting in increased plasma clearance and a decreased half-life of acetaminophen).
No products indexed under this heading.

Nortriptyline Hydrochloride (Increased effect of antidepressant or oxycodone).
No products indexed under this heading.

Olanzapine (Additive CNS depression; dose of one or both agents should be reduced). Products include:
Symbyax ... 1965
Zyprexa ... 1984
Zyprexa IntraMuscular ... 1984
Zyprexa ZYDIS ... 1984

Orphenadrine Citrate (Opioid analgesics may enhance the neuromuscular-blocking action of skeletal muscle relaxants and produce an increase in the degree of respiratory depression).
No products indexed under this heading.

Oxazepam (Additive CNS depression; dose of one or both agents should be reduced; increased effect of antidepressant).
No products indexed under this heading.

Oxybutynin Chloride (May produce paralytic ileus).
No products indexed under this heading.

Oxycodone Terephthalate (Additive CNS depression; dose of one or both agents should be reduced).
No products indexed under this heading.

Oxymorphone Hydrochloride (Additive CNS depression; dose of one or both agents should be reduced). Products include:
Opana ... 1110
Opana ER ... 1114

Oxyphenonium Bromide (May produce paralytic ileus).
No products indexed under this heading.

Pancuronium Bromide (Opioid analgesics may enhance the neuromuscular-blocking action of skeletal muscle relaxants and produce an increase in the degree of respiratory depression).
No products indexed under this heading.

Papaverine (Oxycodone may cause severe hypotension after concurrent administration with drugs which compromise vasomotor tone).
No products indexed under this heading.

Papaverine Hydrochloride (Oxycodone may cause severe hypotension after concurrent administration with drugs which compromise vasomotor tone).
No products indexed under this heading.

Pargyline Hydrochloride (Increased effect of either oxycodone or MAO inhibitor).
No products indexed under this heading.

Pentazocine Hydrochloride (Mixed agonist/antagonist analgesics may reduce the analgesic effect of oxycodone and/or may precipitate withdrawal symptoms in these patients).
No products indexed under this heading.

Pentazocine Lactate (Mixed agonist/antagonist analgesics may reduce the analgesic effect of oxycodone and/or may precipitate withdrawal symptoms in these patients).
No products indexed under this heading.

Pentobarbital (Additive CNS depression; dose of one or both agents should be reduced).
No products indexed under this heading.

Pentobarbital Sodium (Additive CNS depression; dose of one or both agents should be reduced). Products include:
Nembutal ... 2012

Perphenazine (Additive CNS depression; dose of one or both agents should be reduced).
No products indexed under this heading.

Phenelzine Sulfate (Increased effect of either oxycodone or MAO inhibitor).
No products indexed under this heading.

Phenobarbital (Additive CNS depression; dose of one or both agents should be reduced). Products include:
Donnatal ... 2711

Phenobarbital Sodium (Additive CNS depression; dose of one or both agents should be reduced).
No products indexed under this heading.

Phenothiazine Derivatives (Additive CNS depression; dose of one or both agents should be reduced).
No products indexed under this heading.

Phenothiazines (Additive CNS depression; dose of one or both agents should be reduced).
No products indexed under this heading.

Pipecuronium Bromide (Opioid analgesics may enhance the neuromuscular-blocking action of skeletal muscle relaxants and produce an increase in the degree of respiratory depression).
No products indexed under this heading.

Prazepam (Additive CNS depression; dose of one or both agents should be reduced).
No products indexed under this heading.

Probenecid (Probenicid may increase the therapeutic effectiveness of acetaminophen slightly).
No products indexed under this heading.

Procarbazine Hydrochloride (Increased effect of either oxycodone or MAO inhibitor).
No products indexed under this heading.

Prochlorperazine (Additive CNS depression; dose of one or both agents should be reduced).
No products indexed under this heading.

Prochlorperazine Edisylate (Additive CNS depression; dose of one or both agents should be reduced).
No products indexed under this heading.

Prochlorperazine Maleate (Additive CNS depression; dose of one or both agents should be reduced).
No products indexed under this heading.

Procyclidine Hydrochloride (May produce paralytic ileus).
No products indexed under this heading.

Promethazine (Additive CNS depression; dose of one or both agents should be reduced).
No products indexed under this heading.

Promethazine Hydrochloride (Additive CNS depression; dose of one or both agents should be reduced).
No products indexed under this heading.

Propantheline Bromide (May produce paralytic ileus).
No products indexed under this heading.

Propofol (Additive CNS depression; dose of one or both agents should be reduced).
No products indexed under this heading.

Propoxyphene Hydrochloride (Additive CNS depression; dose of one or both agents should be reduced).
No products indexed under this heading.

Propoxyphene Napsylate (Additive CNS depression; dose of one or both agents should be reduced).
No products indexed under this heading.

Propranolol (Propanolol appears to inhibit the enzyme system responsible for the metabolism of acetaminophen. Therefore, the pharmacologic effects of acetaminophen may be increased).
No products indexed under this heading.

Protriptyline Hydrochloride (Increased effect of antidepressant or oxycodone).
No products indexed under this heading.

Quazepam (Additive CNS depression; dose of one or both agents should be reduced).
No products indexed under this heading.

Quetiapine Fumarate (Additive CNS depression; dose of one or both agents should be reduced). Products include:
Seroquel 750
Seroquel XR 759

Ramelteon (Additive CNS depression; dose of one or both agents should be reduced). Products include:
Rozerem 3366

Rapacuronium Bromide (Opioid analgesics may enhance the neuromuscular-blocking action of skeletal muscle relaxants and produce an increase in the degree of respiratory depression).
No products indexed under this heading.

Rasagiline Mesylate (Increased effect of either oxycodone or MAO inhibitor). Products include:
Azilect 3383

Remifentanil Hydrochloride (Additive CNS depression; dose of one or both agents should be reduced).
No products indexed under this heading.

Risperidone (Additive CNS depression; dose of one or both agents should be reduced). Products include:
Risperdal Consta 2682

Rocuronium Bromide (Opioid analgesics may enhance the neuromuscular-blocking action of skeletal muscle relaxants and produce an increase in the degree of respiratory depression). Products include:
Zemuron 3249

Scopolamine (May produce paralytic ileus). Products include:
Transderm Scōp 2397

Scopolamine Hydrobromide (May produce paralytic ileus). Products include:
Donnatal 2711

Secobarbital Sodium (Additive CNS depression; dose of one or both agents should be reduced).
No products indexed under this heading.

Selegiline (Increased effect of either oxycodone or MAO inhibitor). Products include:
Emsam 3623

Selegiline Hydrochloride (Increased effect of either oxycodone or MAO inhibitor). Products include:
Eldepryl 3312

Sevoflurane (Additive CNS depression; dose of one or both agents should be reduced). Products include:
Ultane 554

Sodium Butabarbital (Additive CNS depression; dose of one or both agents should be reduced).
No products indexed under this heading.

Sodium Oxybate (Additive CNS depression; dose of one or both agents should be reduced).
No products indexed under this heading.

Sodium Pentobarbital (Additive CNS depression; dose of one or both agents should be reduced).
No products indexed under this heading.

Succinylcholine Chloride (Opioid analgesics may enhance the neuromuscular-blocking action of skeletal muscle relaxants and produce an increase in the degree of respiratory depression).
No products indexed under this heading.

Sufentanil Citrate (Additive CNS depression; dose of one or both agents should be reduced).
No products indexed under this heading.

Talbutal (Additive CNS depression; dose of one or both agents should be reduced).
No products indexed under this heading.

Temazepam (Additive CNS depression; dose of one or both agents should be reduced).
No products indexed under this heading.

Thiamylal Sodium (Additive CNS depression; dose of one or both agents should be reduced).
No products indexed under this heading.

Thioridazine (Additive CNS depression; dose of one or both agents should be reduced).
No products indexed under this heading.

Thioridazine Hydrochloride (Additive CNS depression; dose of one or both agents should be reduced). Products include:
Thioridazine Hydrochloride 2384

Thiothixene (Additive CNS depression; dose of one or both agents should be reduced). Products include:
Thiothixene 2386

Thiothixene Hydrochloride (Additive CNS depression; dose of one or both agents should be reduced).
No products indexed under this heading.

Tizanidine (Opioid analgesics may enhance the neuromuscular-blocking action of skeletal muscle relaxants and produce an increase in the degree of respiratory depression).
No products indexed under this heading.

Tizanidine Hydrochloride (Opioid analgesics may enhance the neuromuscular-blocking action of skeletal muscle relaxants and produce an increase in the degree of respiratory depression).
No products indexed under this heading.

Tolazoline Hydrochloride (Oxycodone may cause severe hypotension after concurrent administration with drugs which compromise vasomotor tone).
No products indexed under this heading.

Tolterodine Tartrate (May produce paralytic ileus).
No products indexed under this heading.

Torsemide (The effects of loop diuretics may be decreased).
No products indexed under this heading.

Tranylcypromine Sulfate (Increased effect of either oxycodone or MAO inhibitor). Products include:
Parnate 1584

Triazolam (Additive CNS depression; dose of one or both agents should be reduced).
No products indexed under this heading.

Tridihexethyl Chloride (May produce paralytic ileus).
No products indexed under this heading.

Trifluoperazine Hydrochloride (Additive CNS depression; dose of one or both agents should be reduced).
No products indexed under this heading.

Trihexyphenidyl Hydrochloride (May produce paralytic ileus).
No products indexed under this heading.

Trimipramine Maleate (Increased effect of antidepressant or oxycodone).
No products indexed under this heading.

Tubocurarine Chloride (Opioid analgesics may enhance the neuromuscular-blocking action of skeletal muscle relaxants and produce an increase in the degree of respiratory depression).
No products indexed under this heading.

Vecuronium Bromide (Opioid analgesics may enhance the neuromuscular-blocking action of skeletal muscle relaxants and produce an increase in the degree of respiratory depression).
No products indexed under this heading.

Zaleplon (Additive CNS depression; dose of one or both agents should be reduced).
No products indexed under this heading.

Zidovudine (The pharmacologic effects of zidovudine may be decreased because of enhanced non-hepatic or renal clearance of zidovudine). Products include:
Combivir 1404
Retrovir 1634
Retrovir IV 1640
Trizivir 1688

Ziprasidone Hydrochloride (Additive CNS depression; dose of one or both agents should be reduced). Products include:
Geodon 2723

Zolpidem Tartrate (Additive CNS depression; dose of one or both agents should be reduced). Products include:
Ambien 2920
Ambien CR 2925

Food Interactions

Alcohol (Additive CNS depression; dose of one or both agents should be reduced).

Beer, reduced-alcohol (Additive CNS depression).

Beer, unspecified (Additive CNS depression).

Wine, Chianti (Additive CNS depression).

Wine, Red (Additive CNS depression).

Wine, unspecified (Additive CNS depression).

Wine products (Additive CNS depression).

PERCODAN TABLETS

(Aspirin, Oxycodone Hydrochloride) 1124
May interact with ACE inhibitors, alcohols, anticoagulants, anticonvulsants, antigout agents, beta-blockers, central nervous system depressants, diuretics, general anesthetics, hypnotics and sedatives, mixed agonist/antagonist opioid analgesics, narcotic analgesics, non-steroidal anti-inflammatory agents, oral hypoglycemic agents, phenothiazines, skeletal muscle relaxants, tranquilizers, and certain other agents. Compounds in these categories include:

Acarbose (Aspirin may increase the serum glucose-lowering action of insulin and sulfonylureas leading to hypoglycemia).
No products indexed under this heading.

Acebutolol Hydrochloride (The hypotensive effects of beta blockers may be diminished by concomitant administration of aspirin).
No products indexed under this heading.

Acetazolamide (Concurrent use of acetazolamide can lead to high serum levels of acetazolamide and toxicity).
No products indexed under this heading.

Acetazolamide Sodium (Concurrent use of acetazolamide can lead to high serum levels of acetazolamide and toxicity).
No products indexed under this heading.

Alfentanil Hydrochloride (Additive CNS depression).
No products indexed under this heading.

Allopurinol (Salicylates antagonize the uricosuric action of uricosuric agents).
No products indexed under this heading.

Alprazolam (Additive CNS depression).
No products indexed under this heading.

Amiloride Hydrochloride (The effectiveness of diuretics in patients with underlying renal or cardiovascular disease may be diminished by the concomitant administration of aspirin).
No products indexed under this heading.

Amobarbital (Additive CNS depression).
No products indexed under this heading.

Amobarbital Sodium (Additive CNS depression).
No products indexed under this heading.

Anisindione (Enhanced effect of anticoagulant).
No products indexed under this heading.

Apomorphine (Additive CNS depression).
No products indexed under this heading.

Percodan Interactions Index 1412

Apomorphine Hydrochloride (Additive CNS depression).
No products indexed under this heading.

Aprobarbital (Additive CNS depression).
No products indexed under this heading.

Ardeparin Sodium (Enhanced effect of anticoagulant).
No products indexed under this heading.

Atenolol (The hypotensive effects of beta blockers may be diminished by concomitant administration of aspirin).
No products indexed under this heading.

Atracurium Besylate (Opioid analgesics may enhance the neuromuscular-blocking action of skeletal muscle relaxants and produce an increase in the degree of respiratory depression).
No products indexed under this heading.

Baclofen (Opioid analgesics may enhance the neuromuscular-blocking action of skeletal muscle relaxants and produce an increase in the degree of respiratory depression).
No products indexed under this heading.

Benazepril Hydrochloride (Reports suggested that NSAIDs may diminish the hyponatremic and hypotensive effect of ACE inhibitors).
No products indexed under this heading.

Bendroflumethiazide (The effectiveness of diuretics in patients with underlying renal or cardiovascular disease may by diminished by the concomitant administration of aspirin).
No products indexed under this heading.

Betaxolol Hydrochloride (The hypotensive effects of beta blockers may be diminished by concomitant administration of aspirin).
No products indexed under this heading.

Bisoprolol Fumarate (The hypotensive effects of beta blockers may be diminished by concomitant administration of aspirin).
No products indexed under this heading.

Bumetanide (The effectiveness of diuretics in patients with underlying renal or cardiovascular disease may by diminished by the concomitant administration of aspirin).
No products indexed under this heading.

Buprenorphine Hydrochloride (Additive CNS depression).
No products indexed under this heading.

Buspirone Hydrochloride (Additive CNS depression).
No products indexed under this heading.

Butabarbital (Additive CNS depression).
No products indexed under this heading.

Butabarbital Sodium (Additive CNS depression).
No products indexed under this heading.

Butalbital (Additive CNS depression).
No products indexed under this heading.

Butorphanol Tartrate (Agonist/antagonist analgesics may reduce the analgesic effect of oxycodone or may precipitate withdrawal symptoms).
No products indexed under this heading.

Captopril (Reports suggested that NSAIDs may diminish the hyponatremic and hypotensive effect of ACE inhibitors). Products include:
Captopril 2341

Carbamazepine (Salicylate can displace protein-bound phenytoin and valproic acid, leading to a decrease in the total concentration of phenytoin and an increase in serum valproic acid levels). Products include:
Carbatrol 3280
Equetro 3477

Carisoprodol (Opioid analgesics may enhance the neuromuscular-blocking action of skeletal muscle relaxants and produce an increase in the degree of respiratory depression).
No products indexed under this heading.

Carteolol Hydrochloride (The hypotensive effects of beta blockers may be diminished by concomitant administration of aspirin).
No products indexed under this heading.

Carvedilol (The hypotensive effects of beta blockers may be diminished by concomitant administration of aspirin). Products include:
Coreg 1409

Carvedilol Phosphate (The hypotensive effects of beta blockers may be diminished by concomitant administration of aspirin). Products include:
Coreg CR 1416

Celecoxib (The concurrent use of aspirin with other NSAIDs should be avoided because this may increase bleeding or lead to decreased renal function). Products include:
Celebrex 3272

Chloral Hydrate (Additive CNS depression).
No products indexed under this heading.

Chlordiazepoxide (Additive CNS depression).
No products indexed under this heading.

Chlordiazepoxide Hydrochloride (Additive CNS depression).
No products indexed under this heading.

Chlorothiazide (The effectiveness of diuretics in patients with underlying renal or cardiovascular disease may by diminished by the concomitant administration of aspirin).
No products indexed under this heading.

Chlorothiazide Sodium (The effectiveness of diuretics in patients with underlying renal or cardiovascular disease may by diminished by the concomitant administration of aspirin). Products include:
Diuril Intravenous 2009

Chlorpromazine (Additive CNS depression).
No products indexed under this heading.

Chlorpromazine Hydrochloride (Additive CNS depression).
No products indexed under this heading.

Chlorpropamide (Aspirin may increase the serum glucose-lowering action of insulin and sulfonylureas leading to hypoglycemia).
No products indexed under this heading.

Chlorprothixene (Additive CNS depression).
No products indexed under this heading.

Chlorprothixene Hydrochloride (Additive CNS depression).
No products indexed under this heading.

Chlorprothixene Lactate (Additive CNS depression).
No products indexed under this heading.

Chlorthalidone (The effectiveness of diuretics in patients with underlying renal or cardiovascular disease may by diminished by the concomitant administration of aspirin). Products include:
Clorpres 2344

Chlorzoxazone (Opioid analgesics may enhance the neuromuscular-blocking action of skeletal muscle relaxants and produce an increase in the degree of respiratory depression).
No products indexed under this heading.

Cisatracurium Besylate (Opioid analgesics may enhance the neuromuscular-blocking action of skeletal muscle relaxants and produce an increase in the degree of respiratory depression). Products include:
Nimbex 503

Clonazepam (Additive CNS depression). Products include:
Klonopin 2855

Clorazepate Dipotassium (Additive CNS depression).
No products indexed under this heading.

Clozapine (Additive CNS depression).
No products indexed under this heading.

Codeine Phosphate (Additive CNS depression). Products include:
Tylenol with Codeine 2691

Codeine Sulfate (Additive CNS depression).
No products indexed under this heading.

Colchicine (Salicylates antagonize the uricosuric action of uricosuric agents).
No products indexed under this heading.

Cyclobenzaprine Hydrochloride (Opioid analgesics may enhance the neuromuscular-blocking action of skeletal muscle relaxants and produce an increase in the degree of respiratory depression). Products include:
Amrix 964

Dalteparin Sodium (Enhanced effect of anticoagulant). Products include:
Fragmin 1058

Danaparoid Sodium (Enhanced effect of anticoagulant).
No products indexed under this heading.

Dantrolene Sodium (Opioid analgesics may enhance the neuromuscular-blocking action of skeletal muscle relaxants and produce an increase in the degree of respiratory depression).
No products indexed under this heading.

Desflurane (Additive CNS depression).
No products indexed under this heading.

Dezocine (Additive CNS depression).
No products indexed under this heading.

Diazepam (Additive CNS depression). Products include:
Valium Tablets 2880

Diclofenac Epolamine (The concurrent use of aspirin with other NSAIDs should be avoided because this may increase bleeding or lead to decreased renal function). Products include:
Flector 1839

Diclofenac Potassium (The concurrent use of aspirin with other NSAIDs should be avoided because this may increase bleeding or lead to decreased renal function).
No products indexed under this heading.

Diclofenac Sodium (The concurrent use of aspirin with other NSAIDs should be avoided because this may increase bleeding or lead to decreased renal function).
No products indexed under this heading.

Dicumarol (Enhanced effect of anticoagulant).
No products indexed under this heading.

Dihydrocodeine Bitartrate (Additive CNS depression).
No products indexed under this heading.

Dihydrocodeinone Bitartrate (Additive CNS depression).
No products indexed under this heading.

Divalproex Sodium (Salicylate can displace protein-bound phenytoin and valproic acid, leading to a decrease in the total concentration of phenytoin and an increase in serum valproic acid levels). Products include:
Depakote ER 426

Doxacurium Chloride (Opioid analgesics may enhance the neuromuscular-blocking action of skeletal muscle relaxants and produce an increase in the degree of respiratory depression).
No products indexed under this heading.

Droperidol (Additive CNS depression).
No products indexed under this heading.

d-Tubocurarine (Opioid analgesics may enhance the neuromuscular-blocking action of skeletal muscle relaxants and produce an increase in the degree of respiratory depression).
No products indexed under this heading.

Enalapril Maleate (Reports suggested that NSAIDs may diminish the hyponatremic and hypotensive effect of ACE inhibitors).
No products indexed under this heading.

Enalaprilat (Reports suggested that NSAIDs may diminish the hyponatremic and hypotensive effect of ACE inhibitors).
No products indexed under this heading.

Enflurane (Additive CNS depression).
No products indexed under this heading.

Enoxaparin Sodium (Enhanced effect of anticoagulant). Products include:
Lovenox 3005

Esmolol Hydrochloride (The hypotensive effects of beta blockers may be diminished by concomitant administration of aspirin).
No products indexed under this heading.

Estazolam (Additive CNS depression).
No products indexed under this heading.

Ethacrynic Acid (The effectiveness of diuretics in patients with underlying renal or cardiovascular disease may by diminished by the concomitant administration of aspirin).
No products indexed under this heading.

Ethanol (Additive CNS depression).
No products indexed under this heading.

Ethchlorvynol (Additive CNS depression).
No products indexed under this heading.

Ethinamate (Additive CNS depression).
No products indexed under this heading.

Ethosuximide (Salicylate can displace protein-bound phenytoin and valproic acid, leading to a decrease in the total concentration of phenytoin and an increase in serum valproic acid levels).
No products indexed under this heading.

Ethotoin (Salicylate can displace protein-bound phenytoin and valproic acid, leading to a decrease in the total concentration of phenytoin and an increase in serum valproic acid levels).
No products indexed under this heading.

Ethyl Alcohol (Additive CNS depression).
No products indexed under this heading.

Etodolac (The concurrent use of aspirin with other NSAIDs should be avoided because this may increase bleeding or lead to decreased renal function).
No products indexed under this heading.

Febuxostat (Salicylates antagonize the uricosuric action of uricosuric agents). Products include:
Uloric 3370

Felbamate (Salicylate can displace protein-bound phenytoin and valproic acid, leading to a decrease in the total concentration of phenytoin and an increase in serum valproic acid levels).
No products indexed under this heading.

Fenoprofen Calcium (The concurrent use of aspirin with other NSAIDs should be avoided because this may increase bleeding or lead to decreased renal function).
No products indexed under this heading.

Fentanyl (Additive CNS depression). Products include:
Duragesic 2604
Fentanyl Transdermal System 2346
Onsolis 2054

Fentanyl Citrate (Additive CNS depression). Products include:
Fentora 966

1413 Interactions Index Percodan

Fluphenazine Decanoate (Additive CNS depression).
No products indexed under this heading.

Fluphenazine Enanthate (Additive CNS depression).
No products indexed under this heading.

Fluphenazine Hydrochloride (Additive CNS depression).
No products indexed under this heading.

Flurazepam Hydrochloride (Additive CNS depression).
No products indexed under this heading.

Flurbiprofen (The concurrent use of aspirin with other NSAIDs should be avoided because this may increase bleeding or lead to decreased renal function).
No products indexed under this heading.

Fondaparinux Sodium (Enhanced effect of anticoagulant). Products include:
Arixtra 1320

Fosinopril Sodium (Reports suggested that NSAIDs may diminish the hyponatremic and hypotensive effect of ACE inhibitors).
No products indexed under this heading.

Fosphenytoin (Salicylate can displace protein-bound phenytoin and valproic acid, leading to a decrease in the total concentration of phenytoin and an increase in serum valproic acid levels).
No products indexed under this heading.

Fosphenytoin Sodium (Salicylate can displace protein-bound phenytoin and valproic acid, leading to a decrease in the total concentration of phenytoin and an increase in serum valproic acid levels).
No products indexed under this heading.

Furosemide (The effectiveness of diuretics in patients with underlying renal or cardiovascular disease may by diminished by the concomitant administration of aspirin). Products include:
Furosemide 2354

Gabapentin (Salicylate can displace protein-bound phenytoin and valproic acid, leading to a decrease in the total concentration of phenytoin and an increase in serum valproic acid levels).
No products indexed under this heading.

Gallamine (Opioid analgesics may enhance the neuromuscular-blocking action of skeletal muscle relaxants and produce an increase in the degree of respiratory depression).
No products indexed under this heading.

Gallamine Triethiodide (Opioid analgesics may enhance the neuromuscular-blocking action of skeletal muscle relaxants and produce an increase in the degree of respiratory depression).
No products indexed under this heading.

Glibenclamide (Aspirin may increase the serum glucose-lowering action of insulin and sulfonylureas leading to hypoglycemia).
No products indexed under this heading.

Glimepiride (Aspirin may increase the serum glucose-lowering action of insulin and sulfonylureas leading to hypoglycemia). Products include:
Avandaryl 1356
Duetact 3354

Glipizide (Aspirin may increase the serum glucose-lowering action of insulin and sulfonylureas leading to hypoglycemia).
No products indexed under this heading.

Glutethimide (Additive CNS depression).
No products indexed under this heading.

Glyburide (Aspirin may increase the serum glucose-lowering action of insulin and sulfonylureas leading to hypoglycemia).
No products indexed under this heading.

Halazepam (Additive CNS depression).
No products indexed under this heading.

Haloperidol (Additive CNS depression).
No products indexed under this heading.

Haloperidol Decanoate (Additive CNS depression).
No products indexed under this heading.

Haloperidol Lactate (Additive CNS depression).
No products indexed under this heading.

Halothane (Additive CNS depression).
No products indexed under this heading.

Heparin Calcium (Enhanced effect of anticoagulant).
No products indexed under this heading.

Heparin Sodium (Enhanced effect of anticoagulant).
No products indexed under this heading.

Hexobarbital (Additive CNS depression).
No products indexed under this heading.

Hydrochlorothiazide (The effectiveness of diuretics in patients with underlying renal or cardiovascular disease may by diminished by the concomitant administration of aspirin). Products include:
Atacand HCT 700
Avalide 2956
Benicar HCT 1017
Diovan HCT 2419
Dyazide 1429
Exforge HCT 2449
Hyzaar 2162
Hyzaar 100-12.5 2162
Micardis HCT 889
Prinzide 2246
Tekturna HCT 2541
Teveten HCT 541

Hydrocodone Bitartrate (Additive CNS depression). Products include:
Vicodin 560
Vicodin ES 561
Vicodin HP 563
Vicoprofen 564
Zydone 1138

Hydrocodone Polistirex (Additive CNS depression). Products include:
Tussionex 3443

Hydroflumethiazide (The effectiveness of diuretics in patients with underlying renal or cardiovascular disease may by diminished by the concomitant administration of aspirin).
No products indexed under this heading.

Hydromorphone (Additive CNS depression).
No products indexed under this heading.

Hydromorphone Hydrochloride (Additive CNS depression). Products include:
Dilaudid Injection 2800
Dilaudid Oral 2797
Dilaudid Tablets 2797
Dilaudid-HP 2800

Hydroxyzine Hydrochloride (Additive CNS depression).
No products indexed under this heading.

Ibuprofen (The concurrent use of aspirin with other NSAIDs should be avoided because this may increase bleeding or lead to decreased renal function). Products include:
Motrin IB 2043
Children's Motrin 2044
Children's Motrin Non-Staining Dye-Free 2044
Infants' Motrin 2044
Infants' Motrin Dye-Free 2044
Junior Strength Motrin 2044
Vicoprofen 564

Indapamide (The effectiveness of diuretics in patients with underlying renal or cardiovascular disease may by diminished by the concomitant administration of aspirin). Products include:
Indapamide 2356

Indomethacin (The concurrent use of aspirin with other NSAIDs should be avoided because this may increase bleeding or lead to decreased renal function). Products include:
Indocin 2167

Indomethacin Sodium Trihydrate (The concurrent use of aspirin with other NSAIDs should be avoided because this may increase bleeding or lead to decreased renal function). Products include:
Indocin I.V. 2007

Isoflurane (Additive CNS depression).
No products indexed under this heading.

Ketamine Hydrochloride (Additive CNS depression).
No products indexed under this heading.

Ketoprofen (The concurrent use of aspirin with other NSAIDs should be avoided because this may increase bleeding or lead to decreased renal function).
No products indexed under this heading.

Ketorolac Tromethamine (The concurrent use of aspirin with other NSAIDs should be avoided because this may increase bleeding or lead to decreased renal function). Products include:
Acuvail .... ⊙ 209

Labetalol Hydrochloride (The hypotensive effects of beta blockers may be diminished by concomitant administration of aspirin).
No products indexed under this heading.

Lamotrigine (Salicylate can displace protein-bound phenytoin and valproic acid, leading to a decrease in the total concentration of phenytoin and an increase in serum valproic acid levels). Products include:
Lamictal 1522
Lamictal ODT 1522
Lamictal XR 1536

Levetiracetam (Salicylate can displace protein-bound phenytoin and valproic acid, leading to a decrease in the total concentration of phenytoin and an increase in serum valproic acid levels). Products include:
Keppra XR 3434

Levobunolol Hydrochloride (The hypotensive effects of beta blockers may be diminished by concomitant administration of aspirin).
No products indexed under this heading.

Levomethadyl Acetate Hydrochloride (Additive CNS depression).
No products indexed under this heading.

Levorphanol Tartrate (Additive CNS depression).
No products indexed under this heading.

Lisinopril (Reports suggested that NSAIDs may diminish the hyponatremic and hypotensive effect of ACE inhibitors). Products include:
Prinivil 2241
Prinzide 2246

Lorazepam (Additive CNS depression).
No products indexed under this heading.

Low Molecular Weight Heparins (Enhanced effect of anticoagulant).
No products indexed under this heading.

Loxapine Hydrochloride (Additive CNS depression).
No products indexed under this heading.

Loxapine Succinate (Additive CNS depression).
No products indexed under this heading.

Meclofenamate Sodium (The concurrent use of aspirin with other NSAIDs should be avoided because this may increase bleeding or lead to decreased renal function).
No products indexed under this heading.

Mefenamic Acid (The concurrent use of aspirin with other NSAIDs should be avoided because this may increase bleeding or lead to decreased renal function).
No products indexed under this heading.

Meloxicam (The concurrent use of aspirin with other NSAIDs should be avoided because this may increase bleeding or lead to decreased renal function).
No products indexed under this heading.

Meperidine Hydrochloride (Additive CNS depression).
No products indexed under this heading.

Mephenytoin (Salicylate can displace protein-bound phenytoin and valproic acid, leading to a decrease in the total concentration of phenytoin and an increase in serum valproic acid levels).
No products indexed under this heading.

Mephobarbital (Additive CNS depression).
No products indexed under this heading.

Meprobamate (Additive CNS depression).
No products indexed under this heading.

Mesoridazine Besylate (Additive CNS depression).
No products indexed under this heading.

Metaxalone (Opioid analgesics may enhance the neuromuscular-blocking action of skeletal muscle relaxants and produce an increase in the degree of respiratory depression). Products include:
Skelaxin 1848

Metformin Hydrochloride (Aspirin may increase the serum glucose-lowering action of insulin and sulfonylureas leading to hypoglycemia). Products include:
ActoPlus 3338
Avandamet 1345
Janumet 2188

Methadone Hydrochloride (Additive CNS depression).
No products indexed under this heading.

Methocarbamol (Opioid analgesics may enhance the neuromuscular-blocking action of skeletal muscle relaxants and produce an increase in the degree of respiratory depression).
No products indexed under this heading.

Methohexital Sodium (Additive CNS depression).
No products indexed under this heading.

Methotrexate (Salicylate can inhibit renal clearance of methotrexate, leading to bone marrow toxicity, especially in the elderly or renal impaired).
No products indexed under this heading.

Methotrexate Sodium (Salicylate can inhibit renal clearance of methotrexate, leading to bone marrow toxicity, especially in the elderly or renal impaired).
No products indexed under this heading.

Methotrimeprazine (Additive CNS depression).
No products indexed under this heading.

Methoxyflurane (Additive CNS depression).
No products indexed under this heading.

Methsuximide (Salicylate can displace protein-bound phenytoin and valproic acid, leading to a decrease in the total concentration of phenytoin and an increase in serum valproic acid levels).
No products indexed under this heading.

Methyclothiazide (The effectiveness of diuretics in patients with underlying renal or cardiovascular disease may by diminished by the concomitant administration of aspirin).
No products indexed under this heading.

IMPORTANT NOTE: Always consult each drug listing in the patient's regimen for possible interactions.

(⊙ Described in PDR® for Ophthalmic Medicines)

Rufinamide (Salicylate can displace protein-bound phenytoin and valproic acid, leading to a decrease in the total concentration of phenytoin and an increase in serum valproic acid levels). Products include:

Secobarbital Sodium (Additive CNS depression).
No products indexed under this heading.

Sevoflurane (Additive CNS depression). Products include:

Sitagliptin Phosphate (Aspirin may increase the serum glucose-lowering action of insulin and sulfonylureas leading to hypoglycemia). Products include:

Sodium Butabarbital (Additive CNS depression).
No products indexed under this heading.

Sodium Oxybate (Additive CNS depression).
No products indexed under this heading.

Sodium Pentobarbital (Additive CNS depression).
No products indexed under this heading.

Sotalol Hydrochloride (The hypotensive effects of beta blockers may be diminished by concomitant administration of aspirin).
No products indexed under this heading.

Spirapril Hydrochloride (Reports suggested that NSAIDs may diminish the hyponatremic and hypotensive effect of ACE inhibitors).
No products indexed under this heading.

Spironolactone (The effectiveness of diuretics in patients with underlying renal or cardiovascular disease may by diminished by the concomitant administration of aspirin).
No products indexed under this heading.

Succinylcholine Chloride (Opioid analgesics may enhance the neuromuscular-blocking action of skeletal muscle relaxants and produce an increase in the degree of respiratory depression).
No products indexed under this heading.

Sufentanil Citrate (Additive CNS depression).
No products indexed under this heading.

Sulfinpyrazone (Aspirin may inhibit the uricosuric effects).
No products indexed under this heading.

Sulindac (The concurrent use of aspirin with other NSAIDs should be avoided because this may increase bleeding or lead to decreased renal function). Products include:

Talbutal (Additive CNS depression).
No products indexed under this heading.

Temazepam (Additive CNS depression).
No products indexed under this heading.

Thiamylal Sodium (Additive CNS depression).
No products indexed under this heading.

Thioridazine (Additive CNS depression).
No products indexed under this heading.

Thioridazine Hydrochloride (Additive CNS depression). Products include:

Thiothixene (Additive CNS depression). Products include:

Thiothixene Hydrochloride (Additive CNS depression).
No products indexed under this heading.

Tiagabine Hydrochloride (Salicylate can displace protein-bound phenytoin and valproic acid, leading to a decrease

in the total concentration of phenytoin and an increase in serum valproic acid levels). Products include:

Timolol Hemihydrate (The hypotensive effects of beta blockers may be diminished by concomitant administration of aspirin). Products include:

Timolol Maleate (The hypotensive effects of beta blockers may be diminished by concomitant administration of aspirin). Products include:

Tinzaparin Sodium (Enhanced effect of anticoagulant).
No products indexed under this heading.

Tizanidine (Opioid analgesics may enhance the neuromuscular-blocking action of skeletal muscle relaxants and produce an increase in the degree of respiratory depression).
No products indexed under this heading.

Tizanidine Hydrochloride (Opioid analgesics may enhance the neuromuscular-blocking action of skeletal muscle relaxants and produce an increase in the degree of respiratory depression).
No products indexed under this heading.

Tolazamide (Aspirin may increase the serum glucose-lowering action of insulin and sulfonylureas leading to hypoglycemia).
No products indexed under this heading.

Tolbutamide (Aspirin may increase the serum glucose-lowering action of insulin and sulfonylureas leading to hypoglycemia).
No products indexed under this heading.

Tolmetin Sodium (The concurrent use of aspirin with other NSAIDs should be avoided because this may increase bleeding or lead to decreased renal function).
No products indexed under this heading.

Topiramate (Salicylate can displace protein-bound phenytoin and valproic acid, leading to a decrease in the total concentration of phenytoin and an increase in serum valproic acid levels).
No products indexed under this heading.

Torsemide (The effectiveness of diuretics in patients with underlying renal or cardiovascular disease may by diminished by the concomitant administration of aspirin).
No products indexed under this heading.

Trandolapril (Reports suggested that NSAIDs may diminish the hyponatremic and hypotensive effect of ACE inhibitors). Products include:

Triamterene (The effectiveness of diuretics in patients with underlying renal or cardiovascular disease may by diminished by the concomitant administration of aspirin). Products include:

Triazolam (Additive CNS depression).
No products indexed under this heading.

Trifluoperazine Hydrochloride (Additive CNS depression).
No products indexed under this heading.

Trimethadione (Salicylate can displace protein-bound phenytoin and valproic acid, leading to a decrease in the total concentration of phenytoin and an increase in serum valproic acid levels).
No products indexed under this heading.

Troglitazone (Aspirin may increase the serum glucose-lowering action of insulin and sulfonylureas leading to hypoglycemia).
No products indexed under this heading.

Tubocurarine Chloride (Opioid analgesics may enhance the neuromuscular-blocking action of skeletal muscle relaxants and produce an increase in the degree of respiratory depression).
No products indexed under this heading.

Valdecoxib (The concurrent use of aspirin with other NSAIDs should be avoided because this may increase bleeding or lead to decreased renal function).
No products indexed under this heading.

Valproate Sodium (Salicylate can displace protein-bound phenytoin and valproic acid, leading to a decrease in the total concentration of phenytoin and an increase in serum valproic acid levels).
No products indexed under this heading.

Valproic Acid (Salicylate can displace protein-bound phenytoin and valproic acid, leading to a decrease in the total concentration of phenytoin and an increase in serum valproic acid levels).
No products indexed under this heading.

Vecuronium Bromide (Opioid analgesics may enhance the neuromuscular-blocking action of skeletal muscle relaxants and produce an increase in the degree of respiratory depression).
No products indexed under this heading.

Warfarin Sodium (Enhanced effect of anticoagulant).
No products indexed under this heading.

Zaleplon (Additive CNS depression).
No products indexed under this heading.

Ziprasidone Hydrochloride (Additive CNS depression). Products include:

Zolpidem Tartrate (Additive CNS depression). Products include:

Zonisamide (Salicylate can displace protein-bound phenytoin and valproic acid, leading to a decrease in the total concentration of phenytoin and an increase in serum valproic acid levels). Products include:

Food Interactions

Alcohol (Additive CNS depression).

Beer, reduced-alcohol (Additive CNS depression).

Beer, unspecified (Additive CNS depression).

Wine, Chianti (Additive CNS depression).

Wine, Red (Additive CNS depression).

Wine, unspecified (Additive CNS depression).

Wine products (Additive CNS depression).

PERFOROMIST INHALATION SOLUTION

May interact with alpha adrenergic stimulants, beta-adrenergic stimulating agents, beta-blockers, corticosteroids, diuretics, drugs that prolong the QT interval, loop diuretics, monoamine oxidase inhibitors, nonpotassium-sparing diuretics, sympathomimetics, thiazides, tricyclic antidepressants, xanthines. Compounds in these categories include:

Acebutolol Hydrochloride (Beta-adrenergic receptor antagonists (beta-blockers) and formoterol may inhibit the effect of each other when administered concurrently. Beta-blockers not only block the therapeutic effects of beta-agonists, but may produce severe bronchospasm in COPD patients. Therefore, patients with COPD should not normally be treated with beta-blockers).
No products indexed under this heading.

Albuterol (Co-administration with additional adrenergic drugs may potentiate the sympathetic effects of formoterol).
No products indexed under this heading.

Albuterol Sulfate (Co-administration with additional adrenergic drugs may potentiate the sympathetic effects of formoterol). Products include:

Alclometasone Dipropionate (Concomitant treatment with steroids may potentiate any hypokalemic effect of adrenergic agonists).
No products indexed under this heading.

Alprazolam (Formoterol, as with other beta2-agonists, should be administered with extreme caution to patients being treated with drugs known to prolong the QTc interval because the effect of adrenergic agonists on the cardiovascular system may be potentiated by these agents. Drugs that are known to prolong the QTc interval have an increased risk of ventricular arrhythmias).
No products indexed under this heading.

Amiloride Hydrochloride (Concomitant treatment with diuretics may potentiate any hypokalemic effect of adrenergic agonists).
No products indexed under this heading.

Aminophylline (Concomitant treatment with xanthine derivatives may potentiate any hypokalemic effect of adrenergic agonists).
No products indexed under this heading.

Amiodarone Hydrochloride (Formoterol, as with other beta2-agonists, should be administered with extreme caution to patients being treated with drugs known to prolong the QTc interval because the effect of adrenergic agonists on the cardiovascular system may be potentiated by these agents. Drugs that are known to prolong the QTc interval have an increased risk of ventricular arrhythmias).
No products indexed under this heading.

Amitriptyline Hydrochloride (Formoterol, as with other beta2-agonists, should be administered with extreme caution to patients being treated with tricyclic antidepressants because the effect of adrenergic agonists on the cardiovascular system may be potentiated by these agents).
No products indexed under this heading.

Amoxapine (Formoterol, as with other beta2-agonists, should be administered with extreme caution to patients being treated with tricyclic antidepressants because the effect of adrenergic agonists on the cardiovascular system may be potentiated by these agents).
No products indexed under this heading.

Astemizole (Formoterol, as with other beta2-agonists, should be administered with extreme caution to patients being treated with drugs known to prolong the QTc interval because the effect of adrenergic agonists on the cardiovascular system may be potentiated by these agents. Drugs that are known to prolong the QTc interval have an increased risk of ventricular arrhythmias).
No products indexed under this heading.

IMPORTANT NOTE: Always consult each drug listing in the patient's regimen for possible interactions.

Atenolol (Beta-adrenergic receptor antagonists (beta-blockers) and formoterol may inhibit the effect of each other when administered concurrently. Beta-blockers not only block the therapeutic effects of beta-agonists, but may produce severe bronchospasm in COPD patients. Therefore, patients with COPD should not normally be treated with beta-blockers).
    No products indexed under this heading.

Beclomethasone Dipropionate (Concomitant treatment with steroids may potentiate any hypokalemic effect of adrenergic agonists). Products include:
    Qvar 3398

Beclomethasone Dipropionate Monohydrate (Concomitant treatment with steroids may potentiate any hypokalemic effect of adrenergic agonists). Products include:
    Beconase AQ 1386

Bendroflumethiazide (The ECG changes and/or hypokalemia that may result from the administration of non-potassium sparing diuretics (such as loop or thiazide diuretics) can be acutely worsened by beta-agonists, especially when the recommended dose of the beta-agonist is exceeded).
    No products indexed under this heading.

Betamethasone (Concomitant treatment with steroids may potentiate any hypokalemic effect of adrenergic agonists).
    No products indexed under this heading.

Betamethasone Acetate (Concomitant treatment with steroids may potentiate any hypokalemic effect of adrenergic agonists).
    No products indexed under this heading.

Betamethasone Benzoate (Concomitant treatment with steroids may potentiate any hypokalemic effect of adrenergic agonists).
    No products indexed under this heading.

Betamethasone Dipropionate (Concomitant treatment with steroids may potentiate any hypokalemic effect of adrenergic agonists). Products include:
    Diprolene Lotion 0.05% 3108
    Diprolene Ointment 0.05% 3109
    Diprolene AF Cream 0.05% 3107
    Lotrisone 3163

Betamethasone Sodium Phosphate (Concomitant treatment with steroids may potentiate any hypokalemic effect of adrenergic agonists).
    No products indexed under this heading.

Betamethasone Valerate (Concomitant treatment with steroids may potentiate any hypokalemic effect of adrenergic agonists). Products include:
    Luxiq 3321

Betaxolol Hydrochloride (Beta-adrenergic receptor antagonists (beta-blockers) and formoterol may inhibit the effect of each other when administered concurrently. Beta-blockers not only block the therapeutic effects of beta-agonists, but may produce severe bronchospasm in COPD patients. Therefore, patients with COPD should not normally be treated with beta-blockers).
    No products indexed under this heading.

Bisoprolol Fumarate (Beta-adrenergic receptor antagonists (beta-blockers) and formoterol may inhibit the effect of each other when administered concurrently. Beta-blockers not only block the therapeutic effects of beta-agonists, but may produce severe bronchospasm in COPD patients. Therefore, patients with COPD should not normally be treated with beta-blockers).
    No products indexed under this heading.

Bitolterol Mesylate (If additional adrenergic drugs are to be administered by any route, they should be used with caution because the sympathetic effects of formoterol may be potentiated).
    No products indexed under this heading.

Bretylium Tosylate (Formoterol, as with other beta2-agonists, should be administered with extreme caution to patients being treated with drugs known to prolong the QTc interval because the effect of adrenergic agonists on the cardiovascular system may be potentiated by these agents. Drugs that are known to prolong the QTc interval have an increased risk of ventricular arrhythmias).
    No products indexed under this heading.

Budesonide (Concomitant treatment with steroids may potentiate any hypokalemic effect of adrenergic agonists). Products include:
    Pulmicort Flexhaler **714**
    Symbicort 80/4.5 .... **720**
    Symbicort 160/4.5 .... **720**

Bumetanide (The ECG changes and/or hypokalemia that may result from the administration of non-potassium sparing diuretics (such as loop or thiazide diuretics) can be acutely worsened by beta-agonists, especially when the recommended dose of the beta-agonist is exceeded).
    No products indexed under this heading.

Buspirone Hydrochloride (Formoterol, as with other beta2-agonists, should be administered with extreme caution to patients being treated with drugs known to prolong the QTc interval because the effect of adrenergic agonists on the cardiovascular system may be potentiated by these agents. Drugs that are known to prolong the QTc interval have an increased risk of ventricular arrhythmias).
    No products indexed under this heading.

Carteolol Hydrochloride (Beta-adrenergic receptor antagonists (beta-blockers) and formoterol may inhibit the effect of each other when administered concurrently. Beta-blockers not only block the therapeutic effects of beta-agonists, but may produce severe bronchospasm in COPD patients. Therefore, patients with COPD should not normally be treated with beta-blockers).
    No products indexed under this heading.

Carvedilol (Beta-adrenergic receptor antagonists (beta-blockers) and formoterol may inhibit the effect of each other when administered concurrently. Beta-blockers not only block the therapeutic effects of beta-agonists, but may produce severe bronchospasm in COPD patients. Therefore, patients with COPD should not normally be treated with beta-blockers). Products include:
    Coreg 1409

Carvedilol Phosphate (Beta-adrenergic receptor antagonists (beta-blockers) and formoterol may inhibit the effect of each other when administered concurrently. Beta-blockers not only block the therapeutic effects of beta-agonists, but may produce severe bronchospasm in COPD patients. Therefore, patients with COPD should not normally be treated with beta-blockers). Products include:
    Coreg CR 1416

Chlordiazepoxide (Formoterol, as with other beta2-agonists, should be administered with extreme caution to patients being treated with drugs known to prolong the QTc interval because the effect of adrenergic agonists on the cardiovascular system may be potentiated by these agents. Drugs that are known to prolong the QTc interval have an increased risk of ventricular arrhythmias).
    No products indexed under this heading.

Chlordiazepoxide Hydrochloride (Formoterol, as with other beta2-agonists, should be administered with extreme caution to patients being treated with drugs known to prolong the QTc interval because the effect of adrenergic agonists on the cardiovascular system may be potentiated by these agents. Drugs that are known to prolong the QTc interval have an increased risk of ventricular arrhythmias).
    No products indexed under this heading.

Chlorothiazide (The ECG changes and/or hypokalemia that may result from the administration of non-potassium sparing diuretics (such as loop or thiazide diuretics) can be acutely worsened by beta-agonists, especially when the recommended dose of the beta-agonist is exceeded).
    No products indexed under this heading.

Chlorothiazide Sodium (The ECG changes and/or hypokalemia that may result from the administration of non-potassium sparing diuretics (such as loop or thiazide diuretics) can be acutely worsened by beta-agonists, especially when the recommended dose of the beta-agonist is exceeded). Products include:
    Diuril Intravenous 2009

Chlorpromazine (Formoterol, as with other beta2-agonists, should be administered with extreme caution to patients being treated with drugs known to prolong the QTc interval because the effect of adrenergic agonists on the cardiovascular system may be potentiated by these agents. Drugs that are known to prolong the QTc interval have an increased risk of ventricular arrhythmias).
    No products indexed under this heading.

Chlorpromazine Hydrochloride (Formoterol, as with other beta2-agonists, should be administered with extreme caution to patients being treated with drugs known to prolong the QTc interval because the effect of adrenergic agonists on the cardiovascular system may be potentiated by these agents. Drugs that are known to prolong the QTc interval have an increased risk of ventricular arrhythmias).
    No products indexed under this heading.

Chlorprothixene (Formoterol, as with other beta2-agonists, should be administered with extreme caution to patients being treated with drugs known to prolong the QTc interval because the effect of adrenergic agonists on the cardiovascular system may be potentiated by these agents. Drugs that are known to prolong the QTc interval have an increased risk of ventricular arrhythmias).
    No products indexed under this heading.

Chlorprothixene Hydrochloride (Formoterol, as with other beta2-agonists, should be administered with extreme caution to patients being treated with drugs known to prolong the QTc interval because the effect of adrenergic agonists on the cardiovascular system may be potentiated by these agents. Drugs that are known to prolong the QTc interval have an increased risk of ventricular arrhythmias).
    No products indexed under this heading.

Chlorthalidone (Concomitant treatment with diuretics may potentiate any hypokalemic effect of adrenergic agonists). Products include:
    Clorpres 2344

Ciclesonide (Concomitant treatment with steroids may potentiate any hypokalemic effect of adrenergic agonists).
    No products indexed under this heading.

Clomipramine Hydrochloride (Formoterol, as with other beta2-agonists, should be administered with extreme caution to patients being treated with tricyclic antidepressants because the effect of adrenergic agonists on the cardiovascular system may be potentiated by these agents).
    No products indexed under this heading.

Clorazepate Dipotassium (Formoterol, as with other beta2-agonists, should be administered with extreme caution to patients being treated with drugs known to prolong the QTc interval because the effect of adrenergic agonists on the cardiovascular system may be potentiated by these agents. Drugs that are known to prolong the QTc interval have an increased risk of ventricular arrhythmias).
    No products indexed under this heading.

Clozapine (Formoterol, as with other beta2-agonists, should be administered with extreme caution to patients being treated with drugs known to prolong the QTc interval because the effect of adrenergic agonists on the cardiovascular system may be potentiated by these agents. Drugs that are known to prolong the QTc interval have an increased risk of ventricular arrhythmias).
    No products indexed under this heading.

Cortisone Acetate (Concomitant treatment with steroids may potentiate any hypokalemic effect of adrenergic agonists).
    No products indexed under this heading.

Desipramine Hydrochloride (Formoterol, as with other beta2-agonists, should be administered with extreme caution to patients being treated with tricyclic antidepressants because the effect of adrenergic agonists on the cardiovascular system may be potentiated by these agents).
    No products indexed under this heading.

Desoximetasone (Concomitant treatment with steroids may potentiate any hypokalemic effect of adrenergic agonists).
    No products indexed under this heading.

Dexamethasone (Concomitant treatment with steroids may potentiate any hypokalemic effect of adrenergic agonists). Products include:
    Ciprodex **583**
    Ozurdex ....⊙**223**
    Tobramycin and Dexamethasone
      Ophthalmic Suspension ....⊙**251**

Dexamethasone Acetate (Concomitant treatment with steroids may potentiate any hypokalemic effect of adrenergic agonists).
    No products indexed under this heading.

Dexamethasone Phosphate (Concomitant treatment with steroids may potentiate any hypokalemic effect of adrenergic agonists).
    No products indexed under this heading.

Dexamethasone Sodium (Concomitant treatment with steroids may potentiate any hypokalemic effect of adrenergic agonists).
    No products indexed under this heading.

Dexamethasone Sodium Phosphate (Concomitant treatment with steroids may potentiate any hypokalemic effect of adrenergic agonists).
    No products indexed under this heading.

Dexamethasone Sodium Phosphate Injection (Concomitant treatment with steroids may potentiate any hypokalemic effect of adrenergic agonists).
    No products indexed under this heading.

Diazepam (Formoterol, as with other beta2-agonists, should be administered with extreme caution to patients being treated with drugs known to prolong the QTc interval because the effect of

1417 **Interactions Index** **Performist**

adrenergic agonists on the cardiovascular system may be potentiated by these agents. Drugs that are known to prolong the QTc interval have an increased risk of ventricular arrhythmias). Products include:
Valium Tablets **2880**

Diflorasone Diacetate (Concomitant treatment with steroids may potentiate any hypokalemic effect of adrenergic agonists).
No products indexed under this heading.

Disopyramide (Formoterol, as with other beta2-agonists, should be administered with extreme caution to patients being treated with drugs known to prolong the QTc interval because the effect of adrenergic agonists on the cardiovascular system may be potentiated by these agents. Drugs that are known to prolong the QTc interval have an increased risk of ventricular arrhythmias).
No products indexed under this heading.

Disopyramide Phosphate (Formoterol, as with other beta2-agonists, should be administered with extreme caution to patients being treated with drugs known to prolong the QTc interval because the effect of adrenergic agonists on the cardiovascular system may be potentiated by these agents. Drugs that are known to prolong the QTc interval have an increased risk of ventricular arrhythmias).
No products indexed under this heading.

Dobutamine (If additional adrenergic drugs are to be administered by any route, they should be used with caution because the sympathetic effects of formoterol may be potentiated).
No products indexed under this heading.

Dobutamine Hydrochloride (Co-administration with additional adrenergic drugs may potentiate the sympathetic effects of formoterol).
No products indexed under this heading.

Dofetilide (Formoterol, as with other beta2-agonists, should be administered with extreme caution to patients being treated with drugs known to prolong the QTc interval because the effect of adrenergic agonists on the cardiovascular system may be potentiated by these agents. Drugs that are known to prolong the QTc interval have an increased risk of ventricular arrhythmias).
No products indexed under this heading.

Dopamine Hydrochloride (Co-administration with additional adrenergic drugs may potentiate the sympathetic effects of formoterol).
No products indexed under this heading.

Doxepin Hydrochloride (Formoterol, as with other beta2-agonists, should be administered with extreme caution to patients being treated with tricyclic antidepressants because the effect of adrenergic agonists on the cardiovascular system may be potentiated by these agents).
No products indexed under this heading.

Droperidol (Formoterol, as with other beta2-agonists, should be administered with extreme caution to patients being treated with drugs known to prolong the QTc interval because the effect of adrenergic agonists on the cardiovascular system may be potentiated by these agents. Drugs that are known to prolong the QTc interval have an increased risk of ventricular arrhythmias).
No products indexed under this heading.

Dyphylline (Concomitant treatment with xanthine derivatives may potentiate any hypokalemic effect of adrenergic agonists).
No products indexed under this heading.

Ephedrine Hydrochloride (Co-administration with additional adrenergic drugs may potentiate the sympathetic effects of formoterol).
No products indexed under this heading.

Ephedrine Sulfate (Co-administration with additional adrenergic drugs may potentiate the sympathetic effects of formoterol).
No products indexed under this heading.

Ephedrine Tannate (Co-administration with additional adrenergic drugs may potentiate the sympathetic effects of formoterol).
No products indexed under this heading.

Epinephrine (Co-administration with additional adrenergic drugs may potentiate the sympathetic effects of formoterol). Products include:
EpiPen **3631**
Twinject **3268**

Epinephrine Bitartrate (Co-administration with additional adrenergic drugs may potentiate the sympathetic effects of formoterol).
No products indexed under this heading.

Epinephrine Hydrochloride (Co-administration with additional adrenergic drugs may potentiate the sympathetic effects of formoterol).
No products indexed under this heading.

Erythromycin (Formoterol, as with other beta2-agonists, should be administered with extreme caution to patients being treated with drugs known to prolong the QTc interval because the effect of adrenergic agonists on the cardiovascular system may be potentiated by these agents. Drugs that are known to prolong the QTc interval have an increased risk of ventricular arrhythmias).
No products indexed under this heading.

Erythromycin Estolate (Formoterol, as with other beta2-agonists, should be administered with extreme caution to patients being treated with drugs known to prolong the QTc interval because the effect of adrenergic agonists on the cardiovascular system may be potentiated by these agents. Drugs that are known to prolong the QTc interval have an increased risk of ventricular arrhythmias).
No products indexed under this heading.

Erythromycin Ethylsuccinate (Formoterol, as with other beta2-agonists, should be administered with extreme caution to patients being treated with drugs known to prolong the QTc interval because the effect of adrenergic agonists on the cardiovascular system may be potentiated by these agents. Drugs that are known to prolong the QTc interval have an increased risk of ventricular arrhythmias). Products include:
E.E.S. **437**
EryPed **435**

Erythromycin Gluceptate (Formoterol, as with other beta2-agonists, should be administered with extreme caution to patients being treated with drugs known to prolong the QTc interval because the effect of adrenergic agonists on the cardiovascular system may be potentiated by these agents. Drugs that are known to prolong the QTc interval have an increased risk of ventricular arrhythmias).
No products indexed under this heading.

Erythromycin Lactobionate (Formoterol, as with other beta2-agonists, should be administered with extreme caution to patients being treated with drugs known to prolong the QTc interval because the effect of adrenergic agonists on the cardiovascular system may be potentiated by these agents. Drugs that are known to prolong the QTc interval have an increased risk of ventricular arrhythmias).
No products indexed under this heading.

Erythromycin Stearate (Formoterol, as with other beta2-agonists, should be administered with extreme caution to patients being treated with drugs known to prolong the QTc interval because the effect of adrenergic agonists on the cardiovascular system may be potentiated by these agents. Drugs that are known to prolong the QTc interval have an increased risk of ventricular arrhythmias).
No products indexed under this heading.

Esmolol Hydrochloride (Beta-adrenergic receptor antagonists (beta-blockers) and formoterol may inhibit the effect of each other when administered concurrently. Beta-blockers not only block the therapeutic effects of beta-agonists, but may produce severe bronchospasm in COPD patients. Therefore, patients with COPD should not normally be treated with beta-blockers).
No products indexed under this heading.

Ethacrynic Acid (The ECG changes and/or hypokalemia that may result from the administration of non-potassium sparing diuretics (such as loop or thiazide diuretics) can be acutely worsened by beta-agonists, especially when the recommended dose of the beta-agonist is exceeded).
No products indexed under this heading.

Flecainide Acetate (Formoterol, as with other beta2-agonists, should be administered with extreme caution to patients being treated with drugs known to prolong the QTc interval because the effect of adrenergic agonists on the cardiovascular system may be potentiated by these agents. Drugs that are known to prolong the QTc interval have an increased risk of ventricular arrhythmias).
No products indexed under this heading.

Fludrocortisone Acetate (Concomitant treatment with steroids may potentiate any hypokalemic effect of adrenergic agonists).
No products indexed under this heading.

Flumethasone Pivalate (Concomitant treatment with steroids may potentiate any hypokalemic effect of adrenergic agonists).
No products indexed under this heading.

Flunisolide Hemihydrate (Concomitant treatment with steroids may potentiate any hypokalemic effect of adrenergic agonists).
No products indexed under this heading.

Fluphenazine Decanoate (Formoterol, as with other beta2-agonists, should be administered with extreme caution to patients being treated with drugs known to prolong the QTc interval because the effect of adrenergic agonists on the cardiovascular system may be potentiated by these agents. Drugs that are known to prolong the QTc interval have an increased risk of ventricular arrhythmias).
No products indexed under this heading.

Fluphenazine Enanthate (Formoterol, as with other beta2-agonists, should be administered with extreme caution to patients being treated with drugs known to prolong the QTc interval because the effect of adrenergic agonists on the cardiovascular system may be potentiated by these agents. Drugs that are known to prolong the QTc interval have an increased risk of ventricular arrhythmias).
No products indexed under this heading.

Fluphenazine Hydrochloride (Formoterol, as with other beta2-agonists, should be administered with extreme caution to patients being treated with drugs known to prolong the QTc interval because the effect of adrenergic agonists on the cardiovascular system may be potentiated by these agents. Drugs that are known to prolong the QTc interval have an increased risk of ventricular arrhythmias).
No products indexed under this heading.

Fluticasone Furoate (Concomitant treatment with steroids may potentiate any hypokalemic effect of adrenergic agonists). Products include:
Veramyst **1713**

Fluticasone Propionate (Concomitant treatment with steroids may potentiate any hypokalemic effect of adrenergic agonists). Products include:
Advair 100/50 .... **1275**
Advair 250/50 .... **1275**
Advair 500/50 .... **1275**
Advair HFA 45/21 .... **1288**
Advair HFA 115/21 .... **1288**
Advair HFA 230/21 .... **1288**
Flonase **1459**
Flovent Diskus **1463**
Flovent HFA **1470**

Furosemide (The ECG changes and/or hypokalemia that may result from the administration of non-potassium sparing diuretics (such as loop or thiazide diuretics) can be acutely worsened by beta-agonists, especially when the recommended dose of the beta-agonist is exceeded). Products include:
Furosemide **2354**

Haloperidol (Formoterol, as with other beta2-agonists, should be administered with extreme caution to patients being treated with drugs known to prolong the QTc interval because the effect of adrenergic agonists on the cardiovascular system may be potentiated by these agents. Drugs that are known to prolong the QTc interval have an increased risk of ventricular arrhythmias).
No products indexed under this heading.

Haloperidol Decanoate (Formoterol, as with other beta2-agonists, should be administered with extreme caution to patients being treated with drugs known to prolong the QTc interval because the effect of adrenergic agonists on the cardiovascular system may be potentiated by these agents. Drugs that are known to prolong the QTc interval have an increased risk of ventricular arrhythmias).
No products indexed under this heading.

Haloperidol Lactate (Formoterol, as with other beta2-agonists, should be administered with extreme caution to patients being treated with drugs known to prolong the QTc interval because the effect of adrenergic agonists on the cardiovascular system may be potentiated by these agents. Drugs that are known to prolong the QTc interval have an increased risk of ventricular arrhythmias).
No products indexed under this heading.

Hydrochlorothiazide (The ECG changes and/or hypokalemia that may result from the administration of non-potassium sparing diuretics (such as loop or thiazide diuretics) can be acutely worsened by beta-agonists, especially when the recommended dose of the beta-agonist is exceeded). Products include:
Atacand HCT **700**
Avalide **2956**
Benicar HCT **1017**
Diovan HCT **2419**
Dyazide **1429**
Exforge HCT **2449**
Hyzaar **2162**
Hyzaar 100-12.5 .... **2162**
Micardis HCT **889**
Prinzide **2246**
Tekturna HCT **2541**
Teveten HCT **541**

Hydrocortisone (Concomitant treatment with steroids may potentiate any hypokalemic effect of adrenergic agonists).
No products indexed under this heading.

IMPORTANT NOTE: Always consult each drug listing in the patient's regimen for possible interactions.

Hydrocortisone (Alcohol) (Concomitant treatment with steroids may potentiate any hypokalemic effect of adrenergic agonists).

No products indexed under this heading.

Hydrocortisone Acetate (Concomitant treatment with steroids may potentiate any hypokalemic effect of adrenergic agonists).

No products indexed under this heading.

Hydrocortisone Butyrate (Concomitant treatment with steroids may potentiate any hypokalemic effect of adrenergic agonists).

No products indexed under this heading.

Hydrocortisone Cypionate (Concomitant treatment with steroids may potentiate any hypokalemic effect of adrenergic agonists).

No products indexed under this heading.

Hydrocortisone Hemisuccinate (Concomitant treatment with steroids may potentiate any hypokalemic effect of adrenergic agonists).

No products indexed under this heading.

Hydrocortisone Probutate (Concomitant treatment with steroids may potentiate any hypokalemic effect of adrenergic agonists).

No products indexed under this heading.

Hydrocortisone Sodium Phosphate (Concomitant treatment with steroids may potentiate any hypokalemic effect of adrenergic agonists).

No products indexed under this heading.

Hydrocortisone Sodium Succinate (Concomitant treatment with steroids may potentiate any hypokalemic effect of adrenergic agonists).

No products indexed under this heading.

Hydrocortisone Valerate (Concomitant treatment with steroids may potentiate any hypokalemic effect of adrenergic agonists).

No products indexed under this heading.

Hydroflumethiazide (The ECG changes and/or hypokalemia that may result from the administration of non-potassium sparing diuretics (such as loop or thiazide diuretics) can be acutely worsened by beta-agonists, especially when the recommended dose of the beta-agonist is exceeded).

No products indexed under this heading.

Hydroxyzine Hydrochloride (Formoterol, as with other beta2-agonists, should be administered with extreme caution to patients being treated with drugs known to prolong the QTc interval because the effect of adrenergic agonists on the cardiovascular system may be potentiated by these agents. Drugs that are known to prolong the QTc interval have an increased risk of ventricular arrhythmias).

No products indexed under this heading.

Imipramine Hydrochloride (Formoterol, as with other beta2-agonists, should be administered with extreme caution to patients being treated with tricyclic antidepressants because the effect of adrenergic agonists on the cardiovascular system may be potentiated by these agents).

No products indexed under this heading.

Imipramine Pamoate (Formoterol, as with other beta2-agonists, should be administered with extreme caution to patients being treated with tricyclic antidepressants because the effect of adrenergic agonists on the cardiovascular system may be potentiated by these agents).

No products indexed under this heading.

Indapamide (Concomitant treatment with diuretics may potentiate any hypokalemic effect of adrenergic agonists).
Products include:
Indapamide 2356

Isocarboxazid (Formoterol, as with other beta2-agonists, should be administered with extreme caution to patients being treated with monoamine oxidase inhibitors because the effect of adrenergic agonists on the cardiovascular system may be potentiated by these agents). Products include:
Marplan 3481

Isoetharine (If additional adrenergic drugs are to be administered by any route, they should be used with caution because the sympathetic effects of formoterol may be potentiated).

No products indexed under this heading.

Isoproterenol Hydrochloride (Co-administration with additional adrenergic drugs may potentiate the sympathetic effects of formoterol).

No products indexed under this heading.

Isoproterenol Sulfate (Co-administration with additional adrenergic drugs may potentiate the sympathetic effects of formoterol).

No products indexed under this heading.

Labetalol Hydrochloride (Beta-adrenergic receptor antagonists (beta-blockers) and formoterol may inhibit the effect of each other when administered concurrently. Beta-blockers not only block the therapeutic effects of beta-agonists, but may produce severe bronchospasm in COPD patients. Therefore, patients with COPD should not normally be treated with beta-blockers).

No products indexed under this heading.

Levalbuterol Hydrochloride (Co-administration with additional adrenergic drugs may potentiate the sympathetic effects of formoterol).

No products indexed under this heading.

Levobunolol Hydrochloride (Beta-adrenergic receptor antagonists (beta-blockers) and formoterol may inhibit the effect of each other when administered concurrently. Beta-blockers not only block the therapeutic effects of beta-agonists, but may produce severe bronchospasm in COPD patients. Therefore, patients with COPD should not normally be treated with beta-blockers).

No products indexed under this heading.

Lidocaine (Formoterol, as with other beta2-agonists, should be administered with extreme caution to patients being treated with drugs known to prolong the QTc interval because the effect of adrenergic agonists on the cardiovascular system may be potentiated by these agents. Drugs that are known to prolong the QTc interval have an increased risk of ventricular arrhythmias).
Products include:
Lidoderm 1107

Lidocaine Hydrochloride (Formoterol, as with other beta2-agonists, should be administered with extreme caution to patients being treated with drugs known to prolong the QTc interval because the effect of adrenergic agonists on the cardiovascular system may be potentiated by these agents. Drugs that are known to prolong the QTc interval have an increased risk of ventricular arrhythmias).

No products indexed under this heading.

Lithium Carbonate (Formoterol, as with other beta2-agonists, should be administered with extreme caution to patients being treated with drugs known to prolong the QTc interval because the effect of adrenergic agonists on the cardiovascular system may be potentiated by these agents. Drugs that are known to prolong the QTc interval have an increased risk of ventricular arrhythmias).

No products indexed under this heading.

Lithium Citrate (Formoterol, as with other beta2-agonists, should be administered with extreme caution to patients being treated with drugs known to prolong the QTc interval because the effect of adrenergic agonists on the cardiovascular system may be potentiated by these agents. Drugs that are known to prolong the QTc interval have an increased risk of ventricular arrhythmias).

No products indexed under this heading.

Lorazepam (Formoterol, as with other beta2-agonists, should be administered with extreme caution to patients being treated with drugs known to prolong the QTc interval because the effect of adrenergic agonists on the cardiovascular system may be potentiated by these agents. Drugs that are known to prolong the QTc interval have an increased risk of ventricular arrhythmias).

No products indexed under this heading.

Loxapine Hydrochloride (Formoterol, as with other beta2-agonists, should be administered with extreme caution to patients being treated with drugs known to prolong the QTc interval because the effect of adrenergic agonists on the cardiovascular system may be potentiated by these agents. Drugs that are known to prolong the QTc interval have an increased risk of ventricular arrhythmias).

No products indexed under this heading.

Loxapine Succinate (Formoterol, as with other beta2-agonists, should be administered with extreme caution to patients being treated with drugs known to prolong the QTc interval because the effect of adrenergic agonists on the cardiovascular system may be potentiated by these agents. Drugs that are known to prolong the QTc interval have an increased risk of ventricular arrhythmias).

No products indexed under this heading.

Maprotiline Hydrochloride (Formoterol, as with other beta2-agonists, should be administered with extreme caution to patients being treated with tricyclic antidepressants because the effect of adrenergic agonists on the cardiovascular system may be potentiated by these agents).

No products indexed under this heading.

Meprobamate (Formoterol, as with other beta2-agonists, should be administered with extreme caution to patients being treated with drugs known to prolong the QTc interval because the effect of adrenergic agonists on the cardiovascular system may be potentiated by these agents. Drugs that are known to prolong the QTc interval have an increased risk of ventricular arrhythmias).

No products indexed under this heading.

Mesoridazine Besylate (Formoterol, as with other beta2-agonists, should be administered with extreme caution to patients being treated with drugs known to prolong the QTc interval because the effect of adrenergic agonists on the cardiovascular system may be potentiated by these agents. Drugs that are known to prolong the QTc interval have an increased risk of ventricular arrhythmias).

No products indexed under this heading.

Metaproterenol Sulfate (Co-administration with additional adrenergic drugs may potentiate the sympathetic effects of formoterol).

No products indexed under this heading.

Metaraminol Bitartrate (Co-administration with additional adrenergic drugs may potentiate the sympathetic effects of formoterol).

No products indexed under this heading.

Methoxamine Hydrochloride (Co-administration with additional adrenergic drugs may potentiate the sympathetic effects of formoterol).

No products indexed under this heading.

Methyclothiazide (The ECG changes and/or hypokalemia that may result from the administration of non-potassium sparing diuretics (such as loop or thiazide diuretics) can be acutely worsened by beta-agonists, especially when the recommended dose of the beta-agonist is exceeded).

No products indexed under this heading.

Methylprednisolone (Concomitant treatment with steroids may potentiate any hypokalemic effect of adrenergic agonists).

No products indexed under this heading.

Methylprednisolone Acetate (Concomitant treatment with steroids may potentiate any hypokalemic effect of adrenergic agonists).

No products indexed under this heading.

Methylprednisolone Sodium Succinate (Concomitant treatment with steroids may potentiate any hypokalemic effect of adrenergic agonists).

No products indexed under this heading.

Metipranolol Hydrochloride (Beta-adrenergic receptor antagonists (beta-blockers) and formoterol may inhibit the effect of each other when administered concurrently. Beta-blockers not only block the therapeutic effects of beta-agonists, but may produce severe bronchospasm in COPD patients. Therefore, patients with COPD should not normally be treated with beta-blockers).

No products indexed under this heading.

Metolazone (Concomitant treatment with diuretics may potentiate any hypokalemic effect of adrenergic agonists).

No products indexed under this heading.

Metoprolol Succinate (Beta-adrenergic receptor antagonists (beta-blockers) and formoterol may inhibit the effect of each other when administered concurrently. Beta-blockers not only block the therapeutic effects of beta-agonists, but may produce severe bronchospasm in COPD patients. Therefore, patients with COPD should not normally be treated with beta-blockers). Products include:
Toprol XL 732

Metoprolol Tartrate (Beta-adrenergic receptor antagonists (beta-blockers) and formoterol may inhibit the effect of each other when administered concurrently. Beta-blockers not only block the therapeutic effects of beta-agonists, but may produce severe bronchospasm in COPD patients. Therefore, patients with COPD should not normally be treated with beta-blockers).

No products indexed under this heading.

Mexiletine Hydrochloride (Formoterol, as with other beta2-agonists, should be administered with extreme caution to patients being treated with drugs known to prolong the QTc interval because the effect of adrenergic agonists on the cardiovascular system may be potentiated by these agents. Drugs that are known to prolong the QTc interval have an increased risk of ventricular arrhythmias).

No products indexed under this heading.

Midazolam Hydrochloride (Formoterol, as with other beta2-agonists, should be administered with extreme caution to patients being treated with drugs known to prolong the QTc interval because the effect of adrenergic agonists on the cardiovascular system may be potentiated by these agents. Drugs that are known to prolong the QTc interval have an increased risk of ventricular arrhythmias).

No products indexed under this heading.

1419 Interactions Index Performomist

Moclobemide (Formoterol, as with other beta2-agonists, should be administered with extreme caution to patients being treated with monoamine oxidase inhibitors because the effect of adrenergic agonists on the cardiovascular system may be potentiated by these agents).
No products indexed under this heading.

Molindone Hydrochloride (Formoterol, as with other beta2-agonists, should be administered with extreme caution to patients being treated with drugs known to prolong the QTc interval because the effect of adrenergic agonists on the cardiovascular system may be potentiated by these agents. Drugs that are known to prolong the QTc interval have an increased risk of ventricular arrhythmias). Products include:
Moban **1108**

Mometasone Furoate (Concomitant treatment with steroids may potentiate any hypokalemic effect of adrenergic agonists). Products include:
Asmanex **3058**
Elocon Cream **3111**
Elocon Lotion **3112**
Elocon Ointment **3114**

Mometasone Furoate Monohydrate (Concomitant treatment with steroids may potentiate any hypokalemic effect of adrenergic agonists). Products include:
Nasonex **3166**

Nadolol (Beta-adrenergic receptor antagonists (beta-blockers) and formoterol may inhibit the effect of each other when administered concurrently. Beta-blockers not only block the therapeutic effects of beta-agonists, but may produce severe bronchospasm in COPD patients. Therefore, patients with COPD should not normally be treated with beta-blockers). Products include:
Nadolol **2359**

Naphazoline Hydrochloride (If additional adrenergic drugs are to be administered by any route, they should be used with caution because the sympathetic effects of formoterol may be potentiated). Products include:
Visine-A .... ⊙ **257**

Nebivolol (Beta-adrenergic receptor antagonists (beta-blockers) and formoterol may inhibit the effect of each other when administered concurrently. Beta-blockers not only block the therapeutic effects of beta-agonists, but may produce severe bronchospasm in COPD patients. Therefore, patients with COPD should not normally be treated with beta-blockers). Products include:
Bystolic **1147**

Norepinephrine Bitartrate (Co-administration with additional adrenergic drugs may potentiate the sympathetic effects of formoterol).
No products indexed under this heading.

Nortriptyline Hydrochloride (Formoterol, as with other beta2-agonists, should be administered with extreme caution to patients being treated with tricyclic antidepressants because the effect of adrenergic agonists on the cardiovascular system may be potentiated by these agents).
No products indexed under this heading.

Olanzapine (Formoterol, as with other beta2-agonists, should be administered with extreme caution to patients being treated with drugs known to prolong the QTc interval because the effect of adrenergic agonists on the cardiovascular system may be potentiated by these agents. Drugs that are known to prolong the QTc interval have an increased risk of ventricular arrhythmias). Products include:
Symbyax **1965**
Zyprexa **1984**
Zyprexa IntraMuscular **1984**
Zyprexa ZYDIS **1984**

Oxazepam (Formoterol, as with other beta2-agonists, should be administered with extreme caution to patients being treated with drugs known to prolong the QTc interval because the effect of adrenergic agonists on the cardiovascular system may be potentiated by these agents. Drugs that are known to prolong the QTc interval have an increased risk of ventricular arrhythmias).
No products indexed under this heading.

Oxymetazoline Hydrochloride (If additional adrenergic drugs are to be administered by any route, they should be used with caution because the sympathetic effects of formoterol may be potentiated). Products include:
Sudafed OM Sinus Congestion **2048**

Pargyline Hydrochloride (Formoterol, as with other beta2-agonists, should be administered with extreme caution to patients being treated with monoamine oxidase inhibitors because the effect of adrenergic agonists on the cardiovascular system may be potentiated by these agents).
No products indexed under this heading.

Penbutolol Sulfate (Beta-adrenergic receptor antagonists (beta-blockers) and formoterol may inhibit the effect of each other when administered concurrently. Beta-blockers not only block the therapeutic effects of beta-agonists, but may produce severe bronchospasm in COPD patients. Therefore, patients with COPD should not normally be treated with beta-blockers).
No products indexed under this heading.

Perphenazine (Formoterol, as with other beta2-agonists, should be administered with extreme caution to patients being treated with drugs known to prolong the QTc interval because the effect of adrenergic agonists on the cardiovascular system may be potentiated by these agents. Drugs that are known to prolong the QTc interval have an increased risk of ventricular arrhythmias).
No products indexed under this heading.

Phenelzine Sulfate (Formoterol, as with other beta2-agonists, should be administered with extreme caution to patients being treated with monoamine oxidase inhibitors because the effect of adrenergic agonists on the cardiovascular system may be potentiated by these agents).
No products indexed under this heading.

Phenylephrine Bitartrate (Co-administration with additional adrenergic drugs may potentiate the sympathetic effects of formoterol).
No products indexed under this heading.

Phenylephrine Hydrochloride (Co-administration with additional adrenergic drugs may potentiate the sympathetic effects of formoterol). Products include:
Sudafed PE Nasal Decongestant **2048**
Children's Sudafed PE Nasal Decongestant **2047**

Phenylephrine Tannate (Co-administration with additional adrenergic drugs may potentiate the sympathetic effects of formoterol).
No products indexed under this heading.

Phenylpropanolamine Hydrochloride (Co-administration with additional adrenergic drugs may potentiate the sympathetic effects of formoterol).
No products indexed under this heading.

Pindolol (Beta-adrenergic receptor antagonists (beta-blockers) and formoterol may inhibit the effect of each other when administered concurrently. Beta-blockers not only block the therapeutic effects of beta-agonists, but may produce severe bronchospasm in COPD patients. Therefore, patients with COPD should not normally be treated with beta-blockers).
No products indexed under this heading.

Pirbuterol Acetate (Co-administration with additional adrenergic drugs may potentiate the sympathetic effects of formoterol). Products include:
Maxair Autohaler **1782**

Polythiazide (The ECG changes and/or hypokalemia that may result from the administration of non-potassium sparing diuretics (such as loop or thiazide diuretics) can be acutely worsened by beta-agonists, especially when the recommended dose of the beta-agonist is exceeded).
No products indexed under this heading.

Prazepam (Formoterol, as with other beta2-agonists, should be administered with extreme caution to patients being treated with drugs known to prolong the QTc interval because the effect of adrenergic agonists on the cardiovascular system may be potentiated by these agents. Drugs that are known to prolong the QTc interval have an increased risk of ventricular arrhythmias).
No products indexed under this heading.

Prednisolone (Concomitant treatment with steroids may potentiate any hypokalemic effect of adrenergic agonists).
No products indexed under this heading.

Prednisolone Acetate (Concomitant treatment with steroids may potentiate any hypokalemic effect of adrenergic agonists). Products include:
Blephamide .... ⊙ **212**, ⊙ **214**
Pred Forte .... ⊙ **225**
Pred Mild .... ⊙ **230**
Pred-G .... ⊙ **226**, ⊙ **227**

Prednisolone Sodium Phosphate (Concomitant treatment with steroids may potentiate any hypokalemic effect of adrenergic agonists).
No products indexed under this heading.

Prednisolone Tebutate (Concomitant treatment with steroids may potentiate any hypokalemic effect of adrenergic agonists).
No products indexed under this heading.

Prednisone (Concomitant treatment with steroids may potentiate any hypokalemic effect of adrenergic agonists).
No products indexed under this heading.

Prednisone sodium phosphate (Concomitant treatment with steroids may potentiate any hypokalemic effect of adrenergic agonists).
No products indexed under this heading.

Procainamide Hydrochloride (Formoterol, as with other beta2-agonists, should be administered with extreme caution to patients being treated with drugs known to prolong the QTc interval because the effect of adrenergic agonists on the cardiovascular system may be potentiated by these agents. Drugs that are known to prolong the QTc interval have an increased risk of ventricular arrhythmias).
No products indexed under this heading.

Procarbazine Hydrochloride (Formoterol, as with other beta2-agonists, should be administered with extreme caution to patients being treated with monoamine oxidase inhibitors because the effect of adrenergic agonists on the cardiovascular system may be potentiated by these agents).
No products indexed under this heading.

Prochlorperazine (Formoterol, as with other beta2-agonists, should be administered with extreme caution to patients being treated with drugs known to prolong the QTc interval because the effect of adrenergic agonists on the cardiovascular system may be potentiated by these agents. Drugs that are known to prolong the QTc interval have an increased risk of ventricular arrhythmias).
No products indexed under this heading.

Promethazine Hydrochloride (Formoterol, as with other beta2-agonists, should be administered with extreme caution to patients being treated with drugs known to prolong the QTc interval because the effect of adrenergic agonists on the cardiovascular system may be potentiated by these agents. Drugs that are known to prolong the QTc interval have an increased risk of ventricular arrhythmias).
No products indexed under this heading.

Propafenone Hydrochloride (Formoterol, as with other beta2-agonists, should be administered with extreme caution to patients being treated with drugs known to prolong the QTc interval because the effect of adrenergic agonists on the cardiovascular system may be potentiated by these agents. Drugs that are known to prolong the QTc interval have an increased risk of ventricular arrhythmias). Products include:
Rythmol **1648**
Rythmol SR **1652**

Propranolol Hydrochloride (Beta-adrenergic receptor antagonists (beta-blockers) and formoterol may inhibit the effect of each other when administered concurrently. Beta-blockers not only block the therapeutic effects of beta-agonists, but may produce severe bronchospasm in COPD patients. Therefore, patients with COPD should not normally be treated with beta-blockers). Products include:
InnoPran XL **1517**

Protriptyline Hydrochloride (Formoterol, as with other beta2-agonists, should be administered with extreme caution to patients being treated with tricyclic antidepressants because the effect of adrenergic agonists on the cardiovascular system may be potentiated by these agents).
No products indexed under this heading.

Pseudoephedrine Hydrochloride (Co-administration with additional adrenergic drugs may potentiate the sympathetic effects of formoterol). Products include:
Allegra-D **2915**
Allegra-D 24 .... **2918**
Sudafed 12 Hour Nasal Decongestant Non-Drowsy **2048**
Sudafed 24 Hour **2048**
Sudafed Nasal Decongestant **2047**
Children's Sudafed Nasal Decongestant Liquid **2047**
Zyrtec-D Allergy & Congestion **2054**

Pseudoephedrine Sulfate (Co-administration with additional adrenergic drugs may potentiate the sympathetic effects of formoterol). Products include:
Clarinex-D 12-Hour **3101**
Clarinex-D **3104**

Quetiapine Fumarate (Formoterol, as with other beta2-agonists, should be administered with extreme caution to patients being treated with drugs known to prolong the QTc interval because the effect of adrenergic agonists on the cardiovascular system may be potentiated by these agents. Drugs that are known to prolong the QTc interval have an increased risk of ventricular arrhythmias). Products include:
Seroquel **750**
Seroquel XR **759**

IMPORTANT NOTE: Always consult each drug listing in the patient's regimen for possible interactions.

Perforomist Interactions Index 1420

Quinidine (Formoterol, as with other beta2-agonists, should be administered with extreme caution to patients being treated with drugs known to prolong the QTc interval because the effect of adrenergic agonists on the cardiovascular system may be potentiated by these agents. Drugs that are known to prolong the QTc interval have an increased risk of ventricular arrhythmias).
No products indexed under this heading.

Quinidine Gluconate (Formoterol, as with other beta2-agonists, should be administered with extreme caution to patients being treated with drugs known to prolong the QTc interval because the effect of adrenergic agonists on the cardiovascular system may be potentiated by these agents. Drugs that are known to prolong the QTc interval have an increased risk of ventricular arrhythmias).
No products indexed under this heading.

Quinidine Hydrochloride (Formoterol, as with other beta2-agonists, should be administered with extreme caution to patients being treated with drugs known to prolong the QTc interval because the effect of adrenergic agonists on the cardiovascular system may be potentiated by these agents. Drugs that are known to prolong the QTc interval have an increased risk of ventricular arrhythmias).
No products indexed under this heading.

Quinidine Polygalacturonate (Formoterol, as with other beta2-agonists, should be administered with extreme caution to patients being treated with drugs known to prolong the QTc interval because the effect of adrenergic agonists on the cardiovascular system may be potentiated by these agents. Drugs that are known to prolong the QTc interval have an increased risk of ventricular arrhythmias).
No products indexed under this heading.

Quinidine Sulfate (Formoterol, as with other beta2-agonists, should be administered with extreme caution to patients being treated with drugs known to prolong the QTc interval because the effect of adrenergic agonists on the cardiovascular system may be potentiated by these agents. Drugs that are known to prolong the QTc interval have an increased risk of ventricular arrhythmias).
No products indexed under this heading.

Rasagiline Mesylate (Formoterol, as with other beta2-agonists, should be administered with extreme caution to patients being treated with monoamine oxidase inhibitors because the effect of adrenergic agonists on the cardiovascular system may be potentiated by these agents). Products include:
Azilect 3383

Risperidone (Formoterol, as with other beta2-agonists, should be administered with extreme caution to patients being treated with drugs known to prolong the QTc interval because the effect of adrenergic agonists on the cardiovascular system may be potentiated by these agents. Drugs that are known to prolong the QTc interval have an increased risk of ventricular arrhythmias). Products include:
Risperdal Consta 2682

Salmeterol Xinafoate (Coadministration with additional adrenergic drugs may potentiate the sympathetic effects of formoterol). Products include:
Advair 100/50 1275
Advair 250/50 1275
Advair 500/50 1275
Advair HFA 45/21 1288
Advair HFA 115/21 1288
Advair HFA 230/21 1288
Serevent Diskus 1656

Selegiline (Formoterol, as with other beta2-agonists, should be administered with extreme caution to patients being treated with monoamine oxidase inhibitors because the effect of adrenergic agonists on the cardiovascular system may be potentiated by these agents). Products include:
Emsam 3623

Selegiline Hydrochloride (Formoterol, as with other beta2-agonists, should be administered with extreme caution to patients being treated with monoamine oxidase inhibitors because the effect of adrenergic agonists on the cardiovascular system may be potentiated by these agents). Products include:
Eldepryl 3312

Sotalol Hydrochloride (Beta-adrenergic receptor antagonists (beta-blockers) and formoterol may inhibit the effect of each other when administered concurrently. Beta-blockers not only block the therapeutic effects of beta-agonists, but may produce severe bronchospasm in COPD patients. Therefore, patients with COPD should not normally be treated with beta-blockers).
No products indexed under this heading.

Spironolactone (Concomitant treatment with diuretics may potentiate any hypokalemic effect of adrenergic agonists).
No products indexed under this heading.

Terbutaline Sulfate (Coadministration with additional adrenergic drugs may potentiate the sympathetic effects of formoterol).
No products indexed under this heading.

Tetrahydrozoline Hydrochloride (If additional adrenergic drugs are to be administered by any route, they should be used with caution because the sympathetic effects of formoterol may be potentiated).
No products indexed under this heading.

Theophylline (Concomitant treatment with xanthine derivatives may potentiate any hypokalemic effect of adrenergic agonists).
No products indexed under this heading.

Theophylline Anhydrous (Concomitant treatment with xanthine derivatives may potentiate any hypokalemic effect of adrenergic agonists). Products include:
Uniphyl 2817

Theophylline Calcium Salicylate (Concomitant treatment with xanthine derivatives may potentiate any hypokalemic effect of adrenergic agonists).
No products indexed under this heading.

Theophylline Dihydroxypropyl (Glyceryl) (Concomitant treatment with xanthine derivatives may potentiate any hypokalemic effect of adrenergic agonists).
No products indexed under this heading.

Theophylline Ethylenediamine (Concomitant treatment with xanthine derivatives may potentiate any hypokalemic effect of adrenergic agonists).
No products indexed under this heading.

Theophylline Sodium Glycinate (Concomitant treatment with xanthine derivatives may potentiate any hypokalemic effect of adrenergic agonists).
No products indexed under this heading.

Thioridazine Hydrochloride (Formoterol, as with other beta2-agonists, should be administered with extreme caution to patients being treated with drugs known to prolong the QTc interval because the effect of adrenergic agonists on the cardiovascular system may be potentiated by these agents. Drugs that are known to prolong the QTc interval have an increased risk of ventricular arrhythmias). Products include:
Thioridazine Hydrochloride 2384

Thiothixene (Formoterol, as with other beta2-agonists, should be administered with extreme caution to patients being treated with drugs known to prolong the QTc interval because the effect of adrenergic agonists on the cardiovascular system may be potentiated by these agents. Drugs that are known to prolong the QTc interval have an increased risk of ventricular arrhythmias). Products include:
Thiothixene 2386

Timolol Hemihydrate (Beta-adrenergic receptor antagonists (beta-blockers) and formoterol may inhibit the effect of each other when administered concurrently. Beta-blockers not only block the therapeutic effects of beta-agonists, but may produce severe bronchospasm in COPD patients. Therefore, patients with COPD should not normally be treated with beta-blockers). Products include:
Betimol 3490

Timolol Maleate (Beta-adrenergic receptor antagonists (beta-blockers) and formoterol may inhibit the effect of each other when administered concurrently. Beta-blockers not only block the therapeutic effects of beta-agonists, but may produce severe bronchospasm in COPD patients. Therefore, patients with COPD should not normally be treated with beta-blockers). Products include:
Combigan 601
Dorzolamide Hydrochloride/Timolol Maleate Ophthalmic Solution .... ⊙243
Timoptic in Ocudose .... ⊙231

Tocainide Hydrochloride (Formoterol, as with other beta2-agonists, should be administered with extreme caution to patients being treated with drugs known to prolong the QTc interval because the effect of adrenergic agonists on the cardiovascular system may be potentiated by these agents. Drugs that are known to prolong the QTc interval have an increased risk of ventricular arrhythmias).
No products indexed under this heading.

Torsemide (The ECG changes and/or hypokalemia that may result from the administration of non-potassium sparing diuretics (such as loop or thiazide diuretics) can be acutely worsened by beta-agonists, especially when the recommended dose of the beta-agonist is exceeded).
No products indexed under this heading.

Tranylcypromine Sulfate (Formoterol, as with other beta2-agonists, should be administered with extreme caution to patients being treated with monoamine oxidase inhibitors because the effect of adrenergic agonists on the cardiovascular system may be potentiated by these agents). Products include:
Parnate 1584

Triamcinolone (Concomitant treatment with steroids may potentiate any hypokalemic effect of adrenergic agonists).
No products indexed under this heading.

Triamcinolone Acetonide (Concomitant treatment with steroids may potentiate any hypokalemic effect of adrenergic agonists). Products include:
Azmacort 408
Nasacort AQ 3019

Triamcinolone Diacetate (Concomitant treatment with steroids may potentiate any hypokalemic effect of adrenergic agonists).
No products indexed under this heading.

Triamcinolone Hexacetonide (Concomitant treatment with steroids may potentiate any hypokalemic effect of adrenergic agonists).
No products indexed under this heading.

Triamterene (Concomitant treatment with diuretics may potentiate any hypokalemic effect of adrenergic agonists). Products include:
Dyazide 1429
Dyrenium 3495

Trifluoperazine Hydrochloride (Formoterol, as with other beta2-agonists, should be administered with extreme caution to patients being treated with drugs known to prolong the QTc interval because the effect of adrenergic agonists on the cardiovascular system may be potentiated by these agents. Drugs that are known to prolong the QTc interval have an increased risk of ventricular arrhythmias).
No products indexed under this heading.

Trimipramine Maleate (Formoterol, as with other beta2-agonists, should be administered with extreme caution to patients being treated with tricyclic antidepressants because the effect of adrenergic agonists on the cardiovascular system may be potentiated by these agents).
No products indexed under this heading.

Ziprasidone Hydrochloride (Formoterol, as with other beta2-agonists, should be administered with extreme caution to patients being treated with drugs known to prolong the QTc interval because the effect of adrenergic agonists on the cardiovascular system may be potentiated by these agents. Drugs that are known to prolong the QTc interval have an increased risk of ventricular arrhythmias). Products include:
Geodon 2723

PHENYTEK CAPSULES

(Phenytoin Sodium) 2380
May interact with alcohols, barbiturates, chloramphenicol, corticosteroids, doxycycline, estrogens, histamine H2-receptor antagonists, oral anticoagulants, oral contraceptives, phenothiazines, quinidine, salicylates, succinimides, sulfonamides, theophyllines, tricyclic antidepressants, valproate, and certain other agents. Compounds in these categories include:

Alclometasone Dipropionate (Phenytoin impairs the efficacy of corticosteroids).
No products indexed under this heading.

Amiodarone Hydrochloride (Coadministration of amiodarone with phenytoin may increase phenytoin serum levels).
No products indexed under this heading.

Amitriptyline Hydrochloride (Although not a true drug interaction, co-administration of tricyclic antidepressants with phenytoin may precipitate seizures in susceptible patients and phenytoin dosage may need to be adjusted).
No products indexed under this heading.

Amobarbital (Caution should be exercised if using structurally similar compounds (eg, barbiturates) in patients who have exhibited hypersensitivity to phenytoin or other hydantoins).
No products indexed under this heading.

Amobarbital Sodium (Caution should be exercised if using structurally similar compounds (eg, barbiturates) in patients who have exhibited hypersensitivity to phenytoin or other hydantoins).
No products indexed under this heading.

Amoxapine (Although not a true drug interaction, co-administration of tricyclic antidepressants with phenytoin may precipitate seizures in susceptible patients and phenytoin dosage may need to be adjusted).
No products indexed under this heading.

Anisindione (Phenytoin impairs the efficacy of coumarin anticoagulants).
No products indexed under this heading.

Famotidine (Co-administration of H2-antagonists with phenytoin may increase phenytoin serum levels). Products include:

Fludrocortisone Acetate (Phenytoin impairs the efficacy of corticosteroids).
No products indexed under this heading.

Flumethasone Pivalate (Phenytoin impairs the efficacy of corticosteroids).
No products indexed under this heading.

Flunisolide Hemihydrate (Phenytoin impairs the efficacy of corticosteroids).
No products indexed under this heading.

Fluphenazine Decanoate (Co-administration of phenothiazines with phenytoin may increase phenytoin serum levels).
No products indexed under this heading.

Fluphenazine Enanthate (Co-administration of phenothiazines with phenytoin may increase phenytoin serum levels).
No products indexed under this heading.

Fluphenazine Hydrochloride (Co-administration of phenothiazines with phenytoin may increase phenytoin serum levels).
No products indexed under this heading.

Fluticasone Furoate (Phenytoin impairs the efficacy of corticosteroids). Products include:

Fluticasone Propionate (Phenytoin impairs the efficacy of corticosteroids). Products include:

Furosemide (Phenytoin impairs the efficacy of furosemide). Products include:

Glipizide (Co-administration of sulfonamides with phenytoin may increase phenytoin serum levels).
No products indexed under this heading.

Glyburide (Co-administration of sulfonamides with phenytoin may increase phenytoin serum levels).
No products indexed under this heading.

Halothane (Co-administration of halothane with phenytoin may increase phenytoin serum levels).
No products indexed under this heading.

Hexobarbital (Caution should be exercised if using structurally similar compounds (eg, barbiturates) in patients who have exhibited hypersensitivity to phenytoin or other hydantoins).
No products indexed under this heading.

Hydrochlorothiazide (Co-administration of sulfonamides with phenytoin may increase phenytoin serum levels). Products include:

Hydrocortisone (Phenytoin impairs the efficacy of corticosteroids).
No products indexed under this heading.

Hydrocortisone (Alcohol) (Phenytoin impairs the efficacy of corticosteroids).
No products indexed under this heading.

Hydrocortisone Acetate (Phenytoin impairs the efficacy of corticosteroids).
No products indexed under this heading.

Hydrocortisone Butyrate (Phenytoin impairs the efficacy of corticosteroids).
No products indexed under this heading.

Hydrocortisone Cypionate (Phenytoin impairs the efficacy of corticosteroids).
No products indexed under this heading.

Hydrocortisone Hemisuccinate (Phenytoin impairs the efficacy of corticosteroids).
No products indexed under this heading.

Hydrocortisone Probutate (Phenytoin impairs the efficacy of corticosteroids).
No products indexed under this heading.

Hydrocortisone Sodium Phosphate (Phenytoin impairs the efficacy of corticosteroids).
No products indexed under this heading.

Hydrocortisone Sodium Succinate (Phenytoin impairs the efficacy of corticosteroids).
No products indexed under this heading.

Hydrocortisone Valerate (Phenytoin impairs the efficacy of corticosteroids).
No products indexed under this heading.

Hydroflumethiazide (Co-administration of sulfonamides with phenytoin may increase phenytoin serum levels).
No products indexed under this heading.

Imipramine Hydrochloride (Although not a true drug interaction, co-administration of tricyclic antidepressants with phenytoin may precipitate seizures in susceptible patients and phenytoin dosage may need to be adjusted).
No products indexed under this heading.

Imipramine Pamoate (Although not a true drug interaction, co-administration of tricyclic antidepressants with phenytoin may precipitate seizures in susceptible patients and phenytoin dosage may need to be adjusted).
No products indexed under this heading.

Isoniazid (Co-administration of isoniazid with phenytoin may increase phenytoin serum levels).
No products indexed under this heading.

Levonorgestrel (Phenytoin impairs the efficacy of oral contraceptives). Products include:

Magnesium Salicylate (Co-administration of salicylates with phenytoin may increase phenytoin serum levels).
No products indexed under this heading.

Maprotiline Hydrochloride (Although not a true drug interaction, co-administration of tricyclic antidepressants with phenytoin may precipitate seizures in susceptible patients and phenytoin dosage may need to be adjusted).
No products indexed under this heading.

Mephobarbital (Caution should be exercised if using structurally similar compounds (eg, barbiturates) in patients who have exhibited hypersensitivity to phenytoin or other hydantoins).
No products indexed under this heading.

Mesoridazine Besylate (Co-administration of phenothiazines with phenytoin may increase phenytoin serum levels).
No products indexed under this heading.

Mestranol (Phenytoin impairs the efficacy of oral contraceptives).
No products indexed under this heading.

Methotrimeprazine (Co-administration of phenothiazines with phenytoin may increase phenytoin serum levels).
No products indexed under this heading.

Methsuximide (Co-administration of succinamides with phenytoin may increase phenytoin serum levels. Caution should be exercised if using structurally similar compounds (eg, succinimides) in patients who have exhibited hypersensitivity to phenytoin or other hydantoins).
No products indexed under this heading.

Methyclothiazide (Co-administration of sulfonamides with phenytoin may increase phenytoin serum levels).
No products indexed under this heading.

Methylphenidate Hydrochloride (Co-administration of methylphenidate with phenytoin may increase phenytoin serum levels). Products include:

Methylprednisolone (Phenytoin impairs the efficacy of corticosteroids).
No products indexed under this heading.

Methylprednisolone Acetate (Phenytoin impairs the efficacy of corticosteroids).
No products indexed under this heading.

Methylprednisolone Sodium Succinate (Phenytoin impairs the efficacy of corticosteroids).
No products indexed under this heading.

Molindone Hydrochloride (Molindone hydrochloride (ie, Moban) contains calcium ions which interfere with the absorption of phenytoin). Products include:

Mometasone Furoate (Phenytoin impairs the efficacy of corticosteroids). Products include:

Mometasone Furoate Monohydrate (Phenytoin impairs the efficacy of corticosteroids). Products include:

Nizatidine (Co-administration of H2-antagonists with phenytoin may increase phenytoin serum levels). Products include:

Norethindrone (Phenytoin impairs the efficacy of oral contraceptives). Products include:

Norethynodrel (Phenytoin impairs the efficacy of oral contraceptives).
No products indexed under this heading.

Norgestimate (Phenytoin impairs the efficacy of oral contraceptives). Products include:

Norgestrel (Phenytoin impairs the efficacy of oral contraceptives).
No products indexed under this heading.

Nortriptyline Hydrochloride (Although not a true drug interaction, co-administration of tricyclic antidepressants with phenytoin may precipitate seizures in susceptible patients and phenytoin dosage may need to be adjusted).
No products indexed under this heading.

Paramethadione (Caution should be exercised if using structurally similar compounds (eg, oxazolidinediones) in patients who have exhibited hypersensitivity to phenytoin or other hydantoins).
No products indexed under this heading.

Pentobarbital (Caution should be exercised if using structurally similar compounds (eg, barbiturates) in patients who have exhibited hypersensitivity to phenytoin or other hydantoins).
No products indexed under this heading.

Pentobarbital Sodium (Caution should be exercised if using structurally similar compounds (eg, barbiturates) in patients who have exhibited hypersensitivity to phenytoin or other hydantoins). Products include:

Perphenazine (Co-administration of phenothiazines with phenytoin may increase phenytoin serum levels).
No products indexed under this heading.

Phenobarbital (Co-administration of phenobarbital with phenytoin may either increase or decrease phenytoin serum levels. Caution should be exercised if using structurally similar compounds (eg, barbiturates) in patients who have exhibited hypersensitivity to phenytoin or other hydantoins). Products include:

Phenobarbital Sodium (Co-administration of phenobarbital with phenytoin may either increase or decrease phenytoin serum levels. Caution should be exercised if using structurally similar compounds (eg, barbiturates) in patients who have exhibited hypersensitivity to phenytoin or other hydantoins).
No products indexed under this heading.

Phenothiazine Derivatives (Co-administration of phenothiazines with phenytoin may increase phenytoin serum levels).
No products indexed under this heading.

Phenothiazines (Co-administration of phenothiazines with phenytoin may increase phenytoin serum levels).
No products indexed under this heading.

Phensuximide (Co-administration of succinamides with phenytoin may increase phenytoin serum levels. Caution should be exercised if using structurally similar compounds (eg, succinimides) in patients who have exhibited hypersensitivity to phenytoin or other hydantoins).
No products indexed under this heading.

Phenylbutazone (Co-administration of phenylbutazone with phenytoin may increase phenytoin serum levels).
No products indexed under this heading.

Polyestradiol Phosphate (Co-administration of estrogens with phenytoin may increase phenytoin serum levels; phenytoin impairs the efficacy of estrogens).
No products indexed under this heading.

Polythiazide (Co-administration of sulfonamides with phenytoin may increase phenytoin serum levels).
No products indexed under this heading.

Prednisolone (Phenytoin impairs the efficacy of corticosteroids).
No products indexed under this heading.

Prednisolone Acetate (Phenytoin impairs the efficacy of corticosteroids). Products include:

Prednisolone Sodium Phosphate (Phenytoin impairs the efficacy of corticosteroids).
No products indexed under this heading.

Prednisolone Tebutate (Phenytoin impairs the efficacy of corticosteroids).
No products indexed under this heading.

Prednisone (Phenytoin impairs the efficacy of corticosteroids).
No products indexed under this heading.

Prednisone sodium phosphate (Phenytoin impairs the efficacy of corticosteroids).
No products indexed under this heading.

Prochlorperazine (Co-administration of phenothiazines with phenytoin may increase phenytoin serum levels).
No products indexed under this heading.

Prochlorperazine Edisylate (Co-administration of phenothiazines with phenytoin may increase phenytoin serum levels).
No products indexed under this heading.

Prochlorperazine Maleate (Co-administration of phenothiazines with phenytoin may increase phenytoin serum levels).
No products indexed under this heading.

Promethazine (Co-administration of phenothiazines with phenytoin may increase phenytoin serum levels).
No products indexed under this heading.

Promethazine Hydrochloride (Co-administration of phenothiazines with phenytoin may increase phenytoin serum levels).
No products indexed under this heading.

Protriptyline Hydrochloride (Although not a true drug interaction, co-administration of tricyclic antidepressants with phenytoin may precipitate seizures in susceptible patients and phenytoin dosage may need to be adjusted).
No products indexed under this heading.

Quinestrol (Co-administration of estrogens with phenytoin may increase phenytoin serum levels; phenytoin impairs the efficacy of estrogens).
No products indexed under this heading.

Quinidine (Phenytoin impairs the efficacy of quinidine).
No products indexed under this heading.

Quinidine Gluconate (Phenytoin impairs the efficacy of quinidine).
No products indexed under this heading.

Quinidine Hydrochloride (Phenytoin impairs the efficacy of quinidine).
No products indexed under this heading.

Quinidine Polygalacturonate (Phenytoin impairs the efficacy of quinidine).
No products indexed under this heading.

Quinidine Sulfate (Phenytoin impairs the efficacy of quinidine).
No products indexed under this heading.

Ranitidine Bismuth Citrate (Co-administration of H2-antagonists with phenytoin may increase phenytoin serum levels).
No products indexed under this heading.

Ranitidine Hydrochloride (Co-administration of H2-antagonists with phenytoin may increase phenytoin serum levels). Products include:

Reserpine (Co-administration of reserpine with phenytoin may decrease phenytoin serum levels).
No products indexed under this heading.

Rifampin (Co-administration of rifampin with phenytoin impairs the efficacy of rifampin).
No products indexed under this heading.

Salsalate (Co-administration of salicylates with phenytoin may increase phenytoin serum levels).
No products indexed under this heading.

Secobarbital Sodium (Caution should be exercised if using structurally similar compounds (eg, barbiturates) in patients who have exhibited hypersensitivity to phenytoin or other hydantoins).
No products indexed under this heading.

Sodium Butabarbital (Caution should be exercised if using structurally similar compounds (eg, barbiturates) in patients who have exhibited hypersensitivity to phenytoin or other hydantoins).
No products indexed under this heading.

Sodium Pentobarbital (Caution should be exercised if using structurally similar compounds (eg, barbiturates) in patients who have exhibited hypersensitivity to phenytoin or other hydantoins).
No products indexed under this heading.

Sucralfate (Co-administration of sucralfate with phenytoin may decrease phenytoin serum levels). Products include:

Sulfacytine (Co-administration of sulfonamides with phenytoin may increase phenytoin serum levels).
No products indexed under this heading.

Sulfamethizole (Co-administration of sulfonamides with phenytoin may increase phenytoin serum levels).
No products indexed under this heading.

Sulfamethoxazole (Co-administration of sulfonamides with phenytoin may increase phenytoin serum levels).
No products indexed under this heading.

Sulfasalazine (Co-administration of sulfonamides with phenytoin may increase phenytoin serum levels).
No products indexed under this heading.

Sulfinpyrazone (Co-administration of sulfonamides with phenytoin may increase phenytoin serum levels).
No products indexed under this heading.

Sulfisoxazole Acetyl (Co-administration of sulfonamides with phenytoin may increase phenytoin serum levels).
No products indexed under this heading.

Sulfisoxazole Diolamine (Co-administration of sulfonamides with phenytoin may increase phenytoin serum levels).
No products indexed under this heading.

Theophylline (Phenytoin impairs the efficacy of theophylline).
No products indexed under this heading.

Theophylline Anhydrous (Phenytoin impairs the efficacy of theophylline). Products include:

Theophylline Calcium Salicylate (Phenytoin impairs the efficacy of theophylline).
No products indexed under this heading.

Theophylline Dihydroxypropyl (Glyceryl) (Phenytoin impairs the efficacy of theophylline).
No products indexed under this heading.

Theophylline Ethylenediamine (Phenytoin impairs the efficacy of theophylline).
No products indexed under this heading.

Theophylline Sodium Glycinate (Phenytoin impairs the efficacy of theophylline).
No products indexed under this heading.

Thiamylal Sodium (Caution should be exercised if using structurally similar compounds (eg, barbiturates) in patients who have exhibited hypersensitivity to phenytoin or other hydantoins).
No products indexed under this heading.

Thioridazine (Co-administration of phenothiazines with phenytoin may increase phenytoin serum levels).
No products indexed under this heading.

Thioridazine Hydrochloride (Co-administration of phenothiazines with phenytoin may increase phenytoin serum levels). Products include:

Tolazamide (Co-administration of sulfonamides with phenytoin may increase phenytoin serum levels).
No products indexed under this heading.

Tolbutamide (Co-administration of tolbutamide with phenytoin may increase phenytoin serum levels).
No products indexed under this heading.

Trazodone Hydrochloride (Co-administration of trazodone. with phenytoin may increase phenytoin serum levels).
No products indexed under this heading.

Triamcinolone (Phenytoin impairs the efficacy of corticosteroids).
No products indexed under this heading.

Triamcinolone Acetonide (Phenytoin impairs the efficacy of corticosteroids). Products include:

Triamcinolone Diacetate (Phenytoin impairs the efficacy of corticosteroids).
No products indexed under this heading.

Triamcinolone Hexacetonide (Phenytoin impairs the efficacy of corticosteroids).
No products indexed under this heading.

Trifluoperazine Hydrochloride (Co-administration of phenothiazines with phenytoin may increase phenytoin serum levels).
No products indexed under this heading.

Trimethadione (Caution should be exercised if using structurally similar compounds (eg, oxazolidinediones) in patients who have exhibited hypersensitivity to phenytoin or other hydantoins).
No products indexed under this heading.

Trimipramine Maleate (Although not a true drug interaction, co-administration of tricyclic antidepressants with phenytoin may precipitate seizures in susceptible patients and phenytoin dosage may need to be adjusted).
No products indexed under this heading.

Valproate Sodium (Co-administration of sodium valproate with phenytoin may either increase or decrease phenytoin serum levels. Similarly, the effect of phenytoin on sodium valproate serum levels is unpredictable).
No products indexed under this heading.

Valproic Acid (Co-administration of valproic acid with phenytoin may either increase or decrease phenytoin serum levels. Similarly, the effect of phenytoin on valproic acid serum levels is unpredictable).
No products indexed under this heading.

Vitamin D (Phenytoin impairs the efficacy of vitamin D). Products include:

Warfarin Sodium (Phenytoin impairs the efficacy of coumarin anticoagulants).
No products indexed under this heading.

Food Interactions

Alcohol (Acute alcohol intake with phenytoin may increase phenytoin serum levels; chronic alcohol abuse with phenytoin may decrease phenytoin serum levels).

Beer, reduced-alcohol (Acute alcohol intake with phenytoin may increase phenytoin serum levels; chronic alcohol abuse with phenytoin may decrease phenytoin serum levels).

Beer, unspecified (Acute alcohol intake with phenytoin may increase phenytoin serum levels; chronic alcohol abuse with phenytoin may decrease phenytoin serum levels).

Wine, Chianti (Acute alcohol intake with phenytoin may increase phenytoin serum levels; chronic alcohol abuse with phenytoin may decrease phenytoin serum levels).

Wine, Red (Acute alcohol intake with phenytoin may increase phenytoin serum levels; chronic alcohol abuse with phenytoin may decrease phenytoin serum levels).

Wine, unspecified (Acute alcohol intake with phenytoin may increase phenytoin serum levels; chronic alcohol abuse with phenytoin may decrease phenytoin serum levels).

Wine products (Acute alcohol intake with phenytoin may increase phenytoin serum levels; chronic alcohol abuse with phenytoin may decrease phenytoin serum levels).

PHOTOFRIN FOR INJECTION

(Porfimer Sodium) 786
May interact with alcohols, anticoagulants, calcium channel blockers, drugs known to be photosensitizers, fluoroquinolone antibiotics, glucocorticoids, inhibitors of endogenous prostaglandin synthesis, phenothiazines, platelet inhibitors, sulfonamides, sulfonylureas, tetracyclines, thiazides, vasodilators, and certain other agents. Compounds in these categories include:

Abciximab (Drugs that decrease platelet aggregation could decrease the efficacy of photodynamic therapy (PDT)). Products include:

Acetazolamide (Concomitant use of porfimer with other photosensitizing agents (eg, tetracyclines, sulfonamides, phenothiazines, sulfonylurea hypoglycemic agents, thiazide diuretics, griseofulvin, and fluoroquinolones) could increase the risk of photosensitivity reaction).
No products indexed under this heading.

Acitretin (Concomitant use of porfimer with other photosensitizing agents (eg, tetracyclines, sulfonamides, phenothiazines, sulfonylurea hypoglycemic agents, thiazide diuretics, griseofulvin, and fluoroquinolones) could increase the risk of photosensitivity reaction). Products include:

Alatrofloxacin Mesylate (Concomitant use of porfimer with other photosensitizing agents (eg, fluoroquinolones) could increase the risk of photosensitivity reaction).
No products indexed under this heading.

Allopurinol (Preclinical data also suggest that allopurinol could interfere with porfimer photodynamic therapy (PDT)).
No products indexed under this heading.

Amlodipine Besylate (Preclinical data suggest that calcium channel blockers could interfere with porfimer photodynamic therapy (PDT)). Products include:

Amyl Nitrite (Drugs that decrease vasoconstriction could decrease the efficacy of photodynamic therapy (PDT)).
No products indexed under this heading.

Anisindione (Drugs that decrease clotting could decrease the efficacy of photodynamic therapy (PDT)).
No products indexed under this heading.

IMPORTANT NOTE: Always consult each drug listing in the patient's regimen for possible interactions.

Anthralin (Concomitant use of porfimer with other photosensitizing agents (eg, tetracyclines, sulfonamides, phenothiazines, sulfonylurea hypoglycemic agents, thiazide diuretics, griseofulvin, and fluoroquinolones) could increase the risk of photosensitivity reaction).
No products indexed under this heading.

Ardeparin Sodium (Drugs that decrease clotting could decrease the efficacy of photodynamic therapy (PDT)).
No products indexed under this heading.

Aspirin (Preclinical data suggest that some prostaglandin synthesis inhibitors could interfere with porfimer photodynamic therapy (PDT)). Products include:
Aggrenox 880
Bayer Aspirin 829
Percodan 1124
St. Joseph Aspirin 2045

Aspirin, Enteric Coated (Drugs that decrease platelet aggregation could decrease the efficacy of photodynamic therapy (PDT)).
No products indexed under this heading.

Aspirin Buffered (Drugs that decrease platelet aggregation could decrease the efficacy of photodynamic therapy (PDT)).
No products indexed under this heading.

Azlocillin Sodium (Drugs that decrease platelet aggregation could decrease the efficacy of photodynamic therapy (PDT)).
No products indexed under this heading.

Bendroflumethiazide (Concomitant use of porfimer with other photosensitizing agents (eg, sulfonamides) could increase the risk of photosensitivity reaction).
No products indexed under this heading.

Bepridil Hydrochloride (Preclinical data suggest that calcium channel blockers could interfere with porfimer photodynamic therapy (PDT)).
No products indexed under this heading.

Beta-Carotene (Compounds that quench active oxygen species or scavenge radicals, such as β-carotene, would be expected to decrease photodynamic therapy (PDT) activity). Products include:
Cardio Basics 3455
Meili Clear 607

Betamethasone Acetate (Glucocorticoid hormones given before or concomitant with photodynamic therapy (PDT) may decrease the efficacy of the treatment).
No products indexed under this heading.

Betamethasone Sodium Phosphate (Glucocorticoid hormones given before or concomitant with photodynamic therapy (PDT) may decrease the efficacy of the treatment).
No products indexed under this heading.

Budesonide (Glucocorticoid hormones given before or concomitant with photodynamic therapy (PDT) may decrease the efficacy of the treatment). Products include:
Pulmicort Flexhaler 714
Symbicort 80/4.5 720
Symbicort 160/4.5 720

Carbenicillin Indanyl Sodium (Drugs that decrease platelet aggregation could decrease the efficacy of photodynamic therapy (PDT)).
No products indexed under this heading.

Celecoxib (Preclinical data suggest that some prostaglandin synthesis inhibitors could interfere with porfimer photodynamic therapy (PDT)). Products include:
Celebrex 3272

Chlorothiazide (Concomitant use of porfimer with other photosensitizing agents (eg, sulfonamides) could increase the risk of photosensitivity reaction).
No products indexed under this heading.

Chlorothiazide Sodium (Concomitant use of porfimer with other photosensitizing agents (eg, sulfonamides) could increase the risk of photosensitivity reaction). Products include:
Diuril Intravenous 2009

Chlorpromazine (Concomitant use of porfimer with other photosensitizing agents (eg, phenothiazines) could increase the risk of photosensitivity reaction).
No products indexed under this heading.

Chlorpromazine Hydrochloride (Concomitant use of porfimer with other photosensitizing agents (eg, phenothiazines) could increase the risk of photosensitivity reaction).
No products indexed under this heading.

Chlorpropamide (Concomitant use of porfimer with other photosensitizing agents (eg, sulfonamides) could increase the risk of photosensitivity reaction).
No products indexed under this heading.

Choline Magnesium Trisalicylate (Drugs that decrease platelet aggregation could decrease the efficacy of photodynamic therapy (PDT)).
No products indexed under this heading.

Ciprofloxacin (Concomitant use of porfimer with other photosensitizing agents (eg, fluoroquinolones) could increase the risk of photosensitivity reaction). Products include:
Cipro I.V. 3082
Cipro 3073
Cipro XR 3091
Ciprodex 583

Ciprofloxacin Hydrochloride (Concomitant use of porfimer with other photosensitizing agents (eg, fluoroquinolones) could increase the risk of photosensitivity reaction). Products include:
Cipro 3073

Clopidogrel Bisulfate (Drugs that decrease platelet aggregation could decrease the efficacy of photodynamic therapy (PDT)). Products include:
Plavix 3027

Coal Tar (Concomitant use of porfimer with other photosensitizing agents (eg, tetracyclines, sulfonamides, phenothiazines, sulfonylurea hypoglycemic agents, thiazide diuretics, griseofulvin, and fluoroquinolones) could increase the risk of photosensitivity reaction).
No products indexed under this heading.

Cortisone Acetate (Glucocorticoid hormones given before or concomitant with photodynamic therapy (PDT) may decrease the efficacy of the treatment).
No products indexed under this heading.

Dalteparin Sodium (Drugs that decrease clotting could decrease the efficacy of photodynamic therapy (PDT)). Products include:
Fragmin 1058

Danaparoid Sodium (Drugs that decrease clotting could decrease the efficacy of photodynamic therapy (PDT)).
No products indexed under this heading.

Demeclocycline Hydrochloride (Concomitant use of porfimer with other photosensitizing agents (eg, tetracyclines) could increase the risk of photosensitivity reaction).
No products indexed under this heading.

Dexamethasone (Glucocorticoid hormones given before or concomitant with photodynamic therapy (PDT) may decrease the efficacy of the treatment). Products include:

Ciprodex 583
Ozurdex .... ⊙223
Tobramycin and Dexamethasone
Ophthalmic Suspension .... ⊙251

Dexamethasone Acetate (Glucocorticoid hormones given before or concomitant with photodynamic therapy (PDT) may decrease the efficacy of the treatment).
No products indexed under this heading.

Dexamethasone Sodium Phosphate (Glucocorticoid hormones given before or concomitant with photodynamic therapy (PDT) may decrease the efficacy of the treatment).
No products indexed under this heading.

Dextran (Drugs that decrease platelet aggregation could decrease the efficacy of photodynamic therapy (PDT)).
No products indexed under this heading.

Dextran 40 (Drugs that decrease platelet aggregation could decrease the efficacy of photodynamic therapy (PDT)).
No products indexed under this heading.

Dextran 70 (Drugs that decrease platelet aggregation could decrease the efficacy of photodynamic therapy (PDT)).
No products indexed under this heading.

Dextran I (Drugs that decrease platelet aggregation could decrease the efficacy of photodynamic therapy (PDT)).
No products indexed under this heading.

Dextrans (Low Molecular Weight) (Drugs that decrease platelet aggregation could decrease the efficacy of photodynamic therapy (PDT)).
No products indexed under this heading.

Diazoxide (Drugs that decrease vasoconstriction could decrease the efficacy of photodynamic therapy (PDT)). Products include:
Proglycem 1179
Proglycem Suspension 1179

Diclofenac Potassium (Preclinical data suggest that some prostaglandin synthesis inhibitors could interfere with porfimer photodynamic therapy (PDT)).
No products indexed under this heading.

Diclofenac Sodium (Preclinical data suggest that some prostaglandin synthesis inhibitors could interfere with porfimer photodynamic therapy (PDT)).
No products indexed under this heading.

Dicumarol (Drugs that decrease clotting could decrease the efficacy of photodynamic therapy (PDT)).
No products indexed under this heading.

Diflunisal (Drugs that decrease platelet aggregation could decrease the efficacy of photodynamic therapy (PDT)).
No products indexed under this heading.

Diltiazem Hydrochloride (Preclinical data suggest that calcium channel blockers could interfere with porfimer photodynamic therapy (PDT)). Products include:
Cardizem LA 423

Dimethyl Sulfoxide (Compounds that quench active oxygen species or scavenge radicals, such as dimethyl sulfoxide, would be expected to decrease photodynamic therapy (PDT) activity).
No products indexed under this heading.

Dipyridamole (Drugs that decrease platelet aggregation could decrease the efficacy of photodynamic therapy (PDT)). Products include:
Aggrenox 880

Doxycycline (Concomitant use of porfimer with other photosensitizing agents (eg, tetracyclines) could increase the risk of photosensitivity reaction).
No products indexed under this heading.

Doxycycline Calcium (Concomitant use of porfimer with other photosensitizing agents (eg, tetracyclines) could increase the risk of photosensitivity reaction).
No products indexed under this heading.

Doxycycline Hyclate (Concomitant use of porfimer with other photosensitizing agents (eg, tetracyclines) could increase the risk of photosensitivity reaction).
No products indexed under this heading.

Doxycycline Monohydrate (Concomitant use of porfimer with other photosensitizing agents (eg, tetracyclines) could increase the risk of photosensitivity reaction).
No products indexed under this heading.

Enoxacin (Concomitant use of porfimer with other photosensitizing agents (eg, fluoroquinolones) could increase the risk of photosensitivity reaction).
No products indexed under this heading.

Enoxaparin Sodium (Drugs that decrease clotting could decrease the efficacy of photodynamic therapy (PDT)). Products include:
Lovenox 3005

Epoprostenol Sodium (Drugs that decrease vasoconstriction could decrease the efficacy of photodynamic therapy (PDT)). Products include:
Flolan 1453

Eptifibatide (Drugs that decrease platelet aggregation could decrease the efficacy of photodynamic therapy (PDT)). Products include:
Integrilin 3135

Ethanol (Compounds that quench active oxygen species or scavenge radicals, such as ethanol would be expected to decrease photodynamic therapy (PDT) activity).
No products indexed under this heading.

Ethaverine Hydrochloride (Drugs that decrease vasoconstriction could decrease the efficacy of photodynamic therapy (PDT)).
No products indexed under this heading.

Ethyl Alcohol (Compounds that quench active oxygen species or scavenge radicals, such as ethanol would be expected to decrease photodynamic therapy (PDT) activity).
No products indexed under this heading.

Felodipine (Preclinical data suggest that calcium channel blockers could interfere with porfimer photodynamic therapy (PDT)).
No products indexed under this heading.

Fenoprofen Calcium (Preclinical data suggest that some prostaglandin synthesis inhibitors could interfere with porfimer photodynamic therapy (PDT)).
No products indexed under this heading.

Fludrocortisone Acetate (Glucocorticoid hormones given before or concomitant with photodynamic therapy (PDT) may decrease the efficacy of the treatment).
No products indexed under this heading.

Fluphenazine Decanoate (Concomitant use of porfimer with other photosensitizing agents (eg, phenothiazines) could increase the risk of photosensitivity reaction).
No products indexed under this heading.

Fluphenazine Enanthate (Concomitant use of porfimer with other photosensitizing agents (eg, phenothiazines) could increase the risk of photosensitivity reaction).
No products indexed under this heading.

Fluphenazine Hydrochloride (Concomitant use of porfimer with other photosensitizing agents (eg, phenothiazines) could increase the risk of photosensitivity reaction).
No products indexed under this heading.

(⊙ Described in PDR® for Ophthalmic Medicines)

1425 Interactions Index Photofrin

Flurbiprofen (Preclinical data suggest that some prostaglandin synthesis inhibitors could interfere with porfimer photodynamic therapy (PDT)).
No products indexed under this heading.

Fondaparinux Sodium (Drugs that decrease clotting could decrease the efficacy of photodynamic therapy (PDT)). Products include:
Arixtra 1320

Formate (Compounds that quench active oxygen species or scavenge radicals, such as formate, would be expected to decrease photodynamic therapy (PDT) activity).
No products indexed under this heading.

Furosemide (Concomitant use of porfimer with other photosensitizing agents (eg, tetracyclines, sulfonamides, phenothiazines, sulfonylurea hypoglycemic agents, thiazide diuretics, griseofulvin, and fluoroquinolones) could increase the risk of photosensitivity reaction). Products include:
Furosemide 2354

Gatifloxacin (Concomitant use of porfimer with other photosensitizing agents (eg, fluoroquinolones) could increase the risk of photosensitivity reaction).
No products indexed under this heading.

Glimepiride (Concomitant use of porfimer with other photosensitizing agents (eg, sulfonylurea hypoglycemic agents) could increase the risk of photosensitivity reaction). Products include:
Avandaryl 1356
Duetact 3354

Glipizide (Concomitant use of porfimer with other photosensitizing agents (eg, sulfonamides) could increase the risk of photosensitivity reaction).
No products indexed under this heading.

Glyburide (Concomitant use of porfimer with other photosensitizing agents (eg, sulfonamides) could increase the risk of photosensitivity reaction).
No products indexed under this heading.

Grepafloxacin Hydrochloride (Concomitant use of porfimer with other photosensitizing agents (eg, fluoroquinolones) could increase the risk of photosensitivity reaction).
No products indexed under this heading.

Griseofulvin (Concomitant use of porfimer with other photosensitizing agents (eg, griseofulvin) could increase the risk of photosensitivity reaction).
No products indexed under this heading.

Heparin Calcium (Drugs that decrease clotting could decrease the efficacy of photodynamic therapy (PDT)).
No products indexed under this heading.

Heparin Sodium (Drugs that decrease clotting could decrease the efficacy of photodynamic therapy (PDT)).
No products indexed under this heading.

Hydralazine Hydrochloride (Drugs that decrease vasoconstriction could decrease the efficacy of photodynamic therapy (PDT)).
No products indexed under this heading.

Hydrochlorothiazide (Concomitant use of porfimer with other photosensitizing agents (eg, sulfonamides) could increase the risk of photosensitivity reaction). Products include:
Atacand HCT 700
Avalide 2956
Benicar HCT 1017
Diovan HCT 2419
Dyazide 1429
Exforge HCT 2449
Hyzaar 2162
Hyzaar 100-12.5 2162
Micardis HCT 889
Prinzide 2246
Tekturna HCT 2541
Teveten HCT 541

Hydrocortisone (Glucocorticoid hormones given before or concomitant with photodynamic therapy (PDT) may decrease the efficacy of the treatment).
No products indexed under this heading.

Hydrocortisone Acetate (Glucocorticoid hormones given before or concomitant with photodynamic therapy (PDT) may decrease the efficacy of the treatment).
No products indexed under this heading.

Hydrocortisone Sodium Phosphate (Glucocorticoid hormones given before or concomitant with photodynamic therapy (PDT) may decrease the efficacy of the treatment).
No products indexed under this heading.

Hydrocortisone Sodium Succinate (Glucocorticoid hormones given before or concomitant with photodynamic therapy (PDT) may decrease the efficacy of the treatment).
No products indexed under this heading.

Hydroflumethiazide (Concomitant use of porfimer with other photosensitizing agents (eg, sulfonamides) could increase the risk of photosensitivity reaction).
No products indexed under this heading.

Hydroxychloroquine Sulfate (Drugs that decrease platelet aggregation could decrease the efficacy of photodynamic therapy (PDT)).
No products indexed under this heading.

Ibuprofen (Preclinical data suggest that some prostaglandin synthesis inhibitors could interfere with porfimer photodynamic therapy (PDT)). Products include:
Motrin IB 2043
Children's Motrin 2044
Children's Motrin Non-Staining Dye-Free 2044
Infants' Motrin 2044
Infants' Motrin Dye-Free 2044
Junior Strength Motrin 2044
Vicoprofen 564

Indomethacin (Preclinical data suggest that some prostaglandin synthesis inhibitors could interfere with porfimer photodynamic therapy (PDT)). Products include:
Indocin 2167

Indomethacin Sodium Trihydrate (Preclinical data suggest that some prostaglandin synthesis inhibitors could interfere with porfimer photodynamic therapy (PDT)). Products include:
Indocin I.V. 2007

Isosorbide Dinitrate (Drugs that decrease vasoconstriction could decrease the efficacy of photodynamic therapy (PDT)).
No products indexed under this heading.

Isosorbide Mononitrate (Drugs that decrease vasoconstriction could decrease the efficacy of photodynamic therapy (PDT)).
No products indexed under this heading.

Isoxsuprine Hydrochloride (Drugs that decrease vasoconstriction could decrease the efficacy of photodynamic therapy (PDT)).
No products indexed under this heading.

Isradipine (Preclinical data suggest that calcium channel blockers could interfere with porfimer photodynamic therapy (PDT)). Products include:
DynaCirc CR 1432

Ketoprofen (Preclinical data suggest that some prostaglandin synthesis inhibitors could interfere with porfimer photodynamic therapy (PDT)).
No products indexed under this heading.

Levofloxacin (Concomitant use of porfimer with other photosensitizing agents (eg, fluoroquinolones) could increase the risk of photosensitivity reaction). Products include:
Iquix 3492
Levaquin 2629
Levaquin in 5% Dextrose 2629
Quixin 3493

Lomefloxacin Hydrochloride (Concomitant use of porfimer with other photosensitizing agents (eg, fluoroquinolones) could increase the risk of photosensitivity reaction).
No products indexed under this heading.

Low Molecular Weight Heparins (Drugs that decrease clotting could decrease the efficacy of photodynamic therapy (PDT)).
No products indexed under this heading.

Magnesium Salicylate (Drugs that decrease platelet aggregation could decrease the efficacy of photodynamic therapy (PDT)).
No products indexed under this heading.

Mannitol (Compounds that quench active oxygen species or scavenge radicals, such as mannitol, would be expected to decrease photodynamic therapy (PDT) activity).
No products indexed under this heading.

Meclofenamate Sodium (Preclinical data suggest that some prostaglandin synthesis inhibitors could interfere with porfimer photodynamic therapy (PDT)).
No products indexed under this heading.

Mefenamic Acid (Preclinical data suggest that some prostaglandin synthesis inhibitors could interfere with porfimer photodynamic therapy (PDT)).
No products indexed under this heading.

Mesoridazine Besylate (Concomitant use of porfimer with other photosensitizing agents (eg, phenothiazines) could increase the risk of photosensitivity reaction).
No products indexed under this heading.

Metabromsalan (Concomitant use of porfimer with other photosensitizing agents (eg, tetracyclines, sulfonamides, phenothiazines, sulfonylurea hypoglycemic agents, thiazide diuretics, griseofulvin, and fluoroquinolones) could increase the risk of photosensitivity reaction).
No products indexed under this heading.

Methacycline Hydrochloride (Concomitant use of porfimer with other photosensitizing agents (eg, tetracyclines) could increase the risk of photosensitivity reaction).
No products indexed under this heading.

Methotrimeprazine (Concomitant use of porfimer with other photosensitizing agents (eg, phenothiazines) could increase the risk of photosensitivity reaction).
No products indexed under this heading.

Methyclothiazide (Concomitant use of porfimer with other photosensitizing agents (eg, sulfonamides) could increase the risk of photosensitivity reaction).
No products indexed under this heading.

Methylprednisolone Acetate (Glucocorticoid hormones given before or concomitant with photodynamic therapy (PDT) may decrease the efficacy of the treatment).
No products indexed under this heading.

Methylprednisolone Sodium Succinate (Glucocorticoid hormones given before or concomitant with photodynamic therapy (PDT) may decrease the efficacy of the treatment).
No products indexed under this heading.

Mezlocillin Sodium (Drugs that decrease platelet aggregation could decrease the efficacy of photodynamic therapy (PDT)).
No products indexed under this heading.

Mibefradil Dihydrochloride (Preclinical data suggest that calcium channel blockers could interfere with porfimer photodynamic therapy (PDT)).
No products indexed under this heading.

Minocycline Hydrochloride (Concomitant use of porfimer with other photosensitizing agents (eg, tetracyclines) could increase the risk of photosensitivity reaction). Products include:
Solodyn 2073

Minoxidil (Drugs that decrease vasoconstriction could decrease the efficacy of photodynamic therapy (PDT)).
No products indexed under this heading.

Moxifloxacin Hydrochloride (Concomitant use of porfimer with other photosensitizing agents (eg, fluoroquinolones) could increase the risk of photosensitivity reaction). Products include:
Avelox 3064
Vigamox 589

Nafcillin Sodium (Drugs that decrease platelet aggregation could decrease the efficacy of photodynamic therapy (PDT)).
No products indexed under this heading.

Nalidixic Acid (Concomitant use of porfimer with other photosensitizing agents (eg, tetracyclines, sulfonamides, phenothiazines, sulfonylurea hypoglycemic agents, thiazide diuretics, griseofulvin, and fluoroquinolones) could increase the risk of photosensitivity reaction).
No products indexed under this heading.

Naproxen (Preclinical data suggest that some prostaglandin synthesis inhibitors could interfere with porfimer photodynamic therapy (PDT)). Products include:
EC-Naprosyn 2850
Naprosyn 2850
Anaprox/Naprosyn 2850

Naproxen Sodium (Preclinical data suggest that some prostaglandin synthesis inhibitors could interfere with porfimer photodynamic therapy (PDT)). Products include:
Anaprox 2850
Anaprox DS 2850
Treximet 1681

Nicardipine (Preclinical data suggest that calcium channel blockers could interfere with porfimer photodynamic therapy (PDT)).
No products indexed under this heading.

Nicardipine Hydrochloride (Preclinical data suggest that calcium channel blockers could interfere with porfimer photodynamic therapy (PDT)).
No products indexed under this heading.

Nifedipine (Preclinical data suggest that calcium channel blockers could interfere with porfimer photodynamic therapy (PDT)).
No products indexed under this heading.

Nimodipine (Preclinical data suggest that calcium channel blockers could interfere with porfimer photodynamic therapy (PDT)).
No products indexed under this heading.

Nisoldipine (Preclinical data suggest that calcium channel blockers could interfere with porfimer photodynamic therapy (PDT)).
No products indexed under this heading.

Nitroglycerin (Drugs that decrease vasoconstriction could decrease the efficacy of photodynamic therapy (PDT)). Products include:
Nitro-Dur 3170
Nitrolingual 3266

Nitroglycerin, long-acting formulations (Drugs that decrease vasoconstriction could decrease the efficacy of photodynamic therapy (PDT)).
No products indexed under this heading.

IMPORTANT NOTE: Always consult each drug listing in the patient's regimen for possible interactions.

Photofrin **Interactions Index** 1426

Nitroglycerin Intravenous (Drugs that decrease vasoconstriction could decrease the efficacy of photodynamic therapy (PDT)).
No products indexed under this heading.

Norfloxacin (Concomitant use of porfimer with other photosensitizing agents (eg, fluoroquinolones) could increase the risk of photosensitivity reaction). Products include:
Noroxin **2220**

Ofloxacin (Concomitant use of porfimer with other photosensitizing agents (eg, fluoroquinolones) could increase the risk of photosensitivity reaction).
No products indexed under this heading.

Oxytetracycline (Concomitant use of porfimer with other photosensitizing agents (eg, tetracyclines) could increase the risk of photosensitivity reaction).
No products indexed under this heading.

Oxytetracycline Hydrochloride (Concomitant use of porfimer with other photosensitizing agents (eg, tetracyclines) could increase the risk of photosensitivity reaction).
No products indexed under this heading.

Papaverine (Drugs that decrease vasoconstriction could decrease the efficacy of photodynamic therapy (PDT)).
No products indexed under this heading.

Papaverine Hydrochloride (Drugs that decrease vasoconstriction could decrease the efficacy of photodynamic therapy (PDT)).
No products indexed under this heading.

Penicillin G Benzathine (Drugs that decrease platelet aggregation could decrease the efficacy of photodynamic therapy (PDT)). Products include:
Bicillin C-R Injectable Suspension **1826**
Bicillin L-A **1828**

Penicillin G Procaine (Drugs that decrease platelet aggregation could decrease the efficacy of photodynamic therapy (PDT)). Products include:
Bicillin C-R Injectable Suspension **1826**
Bicillin L-A **1828**

Perphenazine (Concomitant use of porfimer with other photosensitizing agents (eg, phenothiazines) could increase the risk of photosensitivity reaction).
No products indexed under this heading.

Phenothiazine Derivatives (Concomitant use of porfimer with other photosensitizing agents (eg, phenothiazines) could increase the risk of photosensitivity reaction).
No products indexed under this heading.

Phenothiazines (Concomitant use of porfimer with other photosensitizing agents (eg, phenothiazines) could increase the risk of photosensitivity reaction).
No products indexed under this heading.

Phenylbutazone (Preclinical data suggest that some prostaglandin synthesis inhibitors could interfere with porfimer photodynamic therapy (PDT)).
No products indexed under this heading.

Piroxicam (Preclinical data suggest that some prostaglandin synthesis inhibitors could interfere with porfimer photodynamic therapy (PDT)).
No products indexed under this heading.

Polythiazide (Concomitant use of porfimer with other photosensitizing agents (eg, sulfonamides) could increase the risk of photosensitivity reaction).
No products indexed under this heading.

Prednisolone Acetate (Glucocorticoid hormones given before or concomitant with photodynamic therapy (PDT) may decrease the efficacy of the treatment). Products include:
Blephamide .... ⊙**212**, ⊙**214**
Pred Forte .... ⊙**225**
Pred Mild .... ⊙**230**
Pred-G .... ⊙**226**, ⊙**227**

Prednisolone Sodium Phosphate (Glucocorticoid hormones given before or concomitant with photodynamic therapy (PDT) may decrease the efficacy of the treatment).
No products indexed under this heading.

Prednisolone Tebutate (Glucocorticoid hormones given before or concomitant with photodynamic therapy (PDT) may decrease the efficacy of the treatment).
No products indexed under this heading.

Prednisone (Glucocorticoid hormones given before or concomitant with photodynamic therapy (PDT) may decrease the efficacy of the treatment).
No products indexed under this heading.

Prochlorperazine (Concomitant use of porfimer with other photosensitizing agents (eg, phenothiazines) could increase the risk of photosensitivity reaction).
No products indexed under this heading.

Prochlorperazine Edisylate (Concomitant use of porfimer with other photosensitizing agents (eg, phenothiazines) could increase the risk of photosensitivity reaction).
No products indexed under this heading.

Prochlorperazine Maleate (Concomitant use of porfimer with other photosensitizing agents (eg, phenothiazines) could increase the risk of photosensitivity reaction).
No products indexed under this heading.

Promethazine (Concomitant use of porfimer with other photosensitizing agents (eg, phenothiazines) could increase the risk of photosensitivity reaction).
No products indexed under this heading.

Promethazine Hydrochloride (Concomitant use of porfimer with other photosensitizing agents (eg, phenothiazines) could increase the risk of photosensitivity reaction).
No products indexed under this heading.

Salsalate (Drugs that decrease platelet aggregation could decrease the efficacy of photodynamic therapy (PDT)).
No products indexed under this heading.

Sulfacytine (Concomitant use of porfimer with other photosensitizing agents (eg, sulfonamides) could increase the risk of photosensitivity reaction).
No products indexed under this heading.

Sulfamethizole (Concomitant use of porfimer with other photosensitizing agents (eg, sulfonamides) could increase the risk of photosensitivity reaction).
No products indexed under this heading.

Sulfamethoxazole (Concomitant use of porfimer with other photosensitizing agents (eg, sulfonamides) could increase the risk of photosensitivity reaction).
No products indexed under this heading.

Sulfasalazine (Concomitant use of porfimer with other photosensitizing agents (eg, sulfonamides) could increase the risk of photosensitivity reaction).
No products indexed under this heading.

Sulfinpyrazone (Concomitant use of porfimer with other photosensitizing agents (eg, sulfonamides) could increase the risk of photosensitivity reaction).
No products indexed under this heading.

Sulfisoxazole Acetyl (Concomitant use of porfimer with other photosensitizing agents (eg, sulfonamides) could increase the risk of photosensitivity reaction).
No products indexed under this heading.

Sulfisoxazole Diolamine (Concomitant use of porfimer with other photosensitizing agents (eg, sulfonamides) could increase the risk of photosensitivity reaction).
No products indexed under this heading.

Sulindac (Preclinical data suggest that some prostaglandin synthesis inhibitors could interfere with porfimer photodynamic therapy (PDT)). Products include:
Clinoril **2098**

Tetrachlorosalicylanilide (Concomitant use of porfimer with other photosensitizing agents (eg, tetracyclines, sulfonamides, phenothiazines, sulfonylurea hypoglycemic agents, thiazide diuretics, griseofulvin, and fluoroquinolones) could increase the risk of photosensitivity reaction).
No products indexed under this heading.

Tetracycline Hydrochloride (Concomitant use of porfimer with other photosensitizing agents (eg, tetracyclines) could increase the risk of photosensitivity reaction). Products include:
Pylera **793**

Tetracycline Phosphate Complex (Concomitant use of porfimer with other photosensitizing agents (eg, tetracyclines) could increase the risk of photosensitivity reaction).
No products indexed under this heading.

Thioridazine (Concomitant use of porfimer with other photosensitizing agents (eg, phenothiazines) could increase the risk of photosensitivity reaction).
No products indexed under this heading.

Thioridazine Hydrochloride (Concomitant use of porfimer with other photosensitizing agents (eg, phenothiazines) could increase the risk of photosensitivity reaction). Products include:
Thioridazine Hydrochloride **2384**

Ticarcillin Disodium (Drugs that decrease platelet aggregation could decrease the efficacy of photodynamic therapy (PDT)). Products include:
Timentin ADD-Vantage **1670**
Timentin Galaxy **1674**
Timentin **1666**
Timentin Pharmacy **1678**

Ticlopidine Hydrochloride (Drugs that decrease platelet aggregation could decrease the efficacy of photodynamic therapy (PDT)).
No products indexed under this heading.

Tinzaparin Sodium (Drugs that decrease clotting could decrease the efficacy of photodynamic therapy (PDT)).
No products indexed under this heading.

Tirofiban Hydrochloride (Drugs that decrease platelet aggregation could decrease the efficacy of photodynamic therapy (PDT)).
No products indexed under this heading.

Tolazamide (Concomitant use of porfimer with other photosensitizing agents (eg, sulfonamides) could increase the risk of photosensitivity reaction).
No products indexed under this heading.

Tolazoline Hydrochloride (Drugs that decrease vasoconstriction could decrease the efficacy of photodynamic therapy (PDT)).
No products indexed under this heading.

Tolbutamide (Concomitant use of porfimer with other photosensitizing agents (eg, sulfonamides) could increase the risk of photosensitivity reaction).
No products indexed under this heading.

Tolmetin Sodium (Preclinical data suggest that some prostaglandin synthesis inhibitors could interfere with porfimer photodynamic therapy (PDT)).
No products indexed under this heading.

Triamcinolone (Glucocorticoid hormones given before or concomitant with photodynamic therapy (PDT) may decrease the efficacy of the treatment).
No products indexed under this heading.

Triamcinolone Acetonide (Glucocorticoid hormones given before or concomitant with photodynamic therapy (PDT) may decrease the efficacy of the treatment). Products include:
Azmacort **408**
Nasacort AQ **3019**

Triamcinolone Diacetate (Glucocorticoid hormones given before or concomitant with photodynamic therapy (PDT) may decrease the efficacy of the treatment).
No products indexed under this heading.

Triamcinolone Hexacetonide (Glucocorticoid hormones given before or concomitant with photodynamic therapy (PDT) may decrease the efficacy of the treatment).
No products indexed under this heading.

Trifluoperazine Hydrochloride (Concomitant use of porfimer with other photosensitizing agents (eg, phenothiazines) could increase the risk of photosensitivity reaction).
No products indexed under this heading.

Trovafloxacin Mesylate (Concomitant use of porfimer with other photosensitizing agents (eg, fluoroquinolones) could increase the risk of photosensitivity reaction).
No products indexed under this heading.

Verapamil Hydrochloride (Preclinical data suggest that calcium channel blockers could interfere with porfimer photodynamic therapy (PDT)). Products include:
Tarka **534**

Warfarin Sodium (Drugs that decrease clotting could decrease the efficacy of photodynamic therapy (PDT)).
No products indexed under this heading.

Food Interactions

Alcohol (Drugs that decrease vasoconstriction could decrease the efficacy of photodynamic therapy (PDT)).

Beer, reduced-alcohol (Compounds that quench active oxygen species or scavenge radicals, such as ethanol would be expected to decrease photodynamic therapy (PDT) activity).

Beer, unspecified (Compounds that quench active oxygen species or scavenge radicals, such as ethanol would be expected to decrease photodynamic therapy (PDT) activity).

Wine, Chianti (Compounds that quench active oxygen species or scavenge radicals, such as ethanol would be expected to decrease photodynamic therapy (PDT) activity).

Wine, Red (Compounds that quench active oxygen species or scavenge radicals, such as ethanol would be expected to decrease photodynamic therapy (PDT) activity).

Wine, unspecified (Compounds that quench active oxygen species or scavenge radicals, such as ethanol would be expected to decrease photodynamic therapy (PDT) activity).

Wine products (Compounds that quench active oxygen species or scavenge radicals, such as ethanol would be expected to decrease photodynamic therapy (PDT) activity).

PLAN B ONE-STEP TABLETS

(Levonorgestrel) **3416**
May interact with barbiturates, cytochrome p450 3a4 inducers (selected),

cytochrome p450 inducers (selected), Non-nucleoside reverse transcriptase inhibitors, phenytoin, protease inhibitors, and certain other agents. Compounds in these categories include:

Allium cepa (Drugs or herbal products that induce enzymes, including CYP3A4, that metabolize progestins may decrease the plasma concentrations of progestins, and may decrease the effectiveness of progestin-only pills. Some drugs or herbal products that may decrease the effectiveness of progestin-only pills include barbiturates, bosentan, carbamazepine, felbamate, griseofulvin, oxcarbazepine, phenytoin, rifampin, St. John's wort, topiramate). Products include:

Hyland's Cold 'N Cough	3314
Mederma	2319
Mederma for Kids	2319

Allium sativum (Drugs or herbal products that induce enzymes, including CYP3A4, that metabolize progestins may decrease the plasma concentrations of progestins, and may decrease the effectiveness of progestin-only pills. Some drugs or herbal products that may decrease the effectiveness of progestin-only pills include barbiturates, bosentan, carbamazepine, felbamate, griseofulvin, oxcarbazepine, phenytoin, rifampin, St. John's wort, topiramate).
No products indexed under this heading.

Allium schoenoprasum (Drugs or herbal products that induce enzymes, including CYP3A4, that metabolize progestins may decrease the plasma concentrations of progestins, and may decrease the effectiveness of progestin-only pills. Some drugs or herbal products that may decrease the effectiveness of progestin-only pills include barbiturates, bosentan, carbamazepine, felbamate, griseofulvin, oxcarbazepine, phenytoin, rifampin, St. John's wort, topiramate).
No products indexed under this heading.

Allium ursinum (Drugs or herbal products that induce enzymes, including CYP3A4, that metabolize progestins may decrease the plasma concentrations of progestins, and may decrease the effectiveness of progestin-only pills. Some drugs or herbal products that may decrease the effectiveness of progestin-only pills include barbiturates, bosentan, carbamazepine, felbamate, griseofulvin, oxcarbazepine, phenytoin, rifampin, St. John's wort, topiramate).
No products indexed under this heading.

Aminoglutethimide (Drugs or herbal products that induce enzymes, including CYP3A4, that metabolize progestins may decrease the plasma concentrations of progestins, and may decrease the effectiveness of progestin-only pills. Some drugs or herbal products that may decrease the effectiveness of progestin-only pills include barbiturates, bosentan, carbamazepine, felbamate, griseofulvin, oxcarbazepine, phenytoin, rifampin, St. John's wort, topiramate).
No products indexed under this heading.

Amobarbital (Drugs or herbal products that induce enzymes, including CYP3A4, that metabolize progestins may decrease the plasma concentrations of progestins, and may decrease the effectiveness of progestin-only pills. Some drugs or herbal products that may decrease the effectiveness of progestin-only pills include barbiturates).
No products indexed under this heading.

Amobarbital Sodium (Drugs or herbal products that induce enzymes, including CYP3A4, that metabolize progestins may decrease the plasma concentrations of progestins, and may decrease the effectiveness of progestin-only pills. Some drugs or herbal products that may decrease the effectiveness of progestin-only pills include barbiturates).
No products indexed under this heading.

Amprenavir (Significant changes (increase or decrease) in the plasma levels of the progestin have been noted in some cases of co-administration of levonorgestrel with HIV protease inhibitors).
No products indexed under this heading.

Aprepitant (Drugs or herbal products that induce enzymes, including CYP3A4, that metabolize progestins may decrease the plasma concentrations of progestins, and may decrease the effectiveness of progestin-only pills. Some drugs or herbal products that may decrease the effectiveness of progestin-only pills include barbiturates, bosentan, carbamazepine, felbamate, griseofulvin, oxcarbazepine, phenytoin, rifampin, St. John's wort, topiramate). Products include:

Emend	2124

Aprobarbital (Drugs or herbal products that induce enzymes, including CYP3A4, that metabolize progestins may decrease the plasma concentrations of progestins, and may decrease the effectiveness of progestin-only pills. Some drugs or herbal products that may decrease the effectiveness of progestin-only pills include barbiturates).
No products indexed under this heading.

Atazanavir (Significant changes (increase or decrease) in the plasma levels of the progestin have been noted in some cases of co-administration of levonorgestrel with HIV protease inhibitors).
No products indexed under this heading.

Atazanavir Sulfate (Significant changes (increase or decrease) in the plasma levels of the progestin have been noted in some cases of co-administration of levonorgestrel with HIV protease inhibitors).
No products indexed under this heading.

Betamethasone (Drugs or herbal products that induce enzymes, including CYP3A4, that metabolize progestins may decrease the plasma concentrations of progestins, and may decrease the effectiveness of progestin-only pills. Some drugs or herbal products that may decrease the effectiveness of progestin-only pills include barbiturates, bosentan, carbamazepine, felbamate, griseofulvin, oxcarbazepine, phenytoin, rifampin, St. John's wort, topiramate).
No products indexed under this heading.

Betamethasone Acetate (Drugs or herbal products that induce enzymes, including CYP3A4, that metabolize progestins may decrease the plasma concentrations of progestins, and may decrease the effectiveness of progestin-only pills. Some drugs or herbal products that may decrease the effectiveness of progestin-only pills include barbiturates, bosentan, carbamazepine, felbamate, griseofulvin, oxcarbazepine, phenytoin, rifampin, St. John's wort, topiramate).
No products indexed under this heading.

Betamethasone Benzoate (Drugs or herbal products that induce enzymes, including CYP3A4, that metabolize progestins may decrease the plasma concentrations of progestins, and may decrease the effectiveness of progestin-only pills. Some drugs or herbal products that

may decrease the effectiveness of progestin-only pills include barbiturates, bosentan, carbamazepine, felbamate, griseofulvin, oxcarbazepine, phenytoin, rifampin, St. John's wort, topiramate).
No products indexed under this heading.

Betamethasone Dipropionate (Drugs or herbal products that induce enzymes, including CYP3A4, that metabolize progestins may decrease the plasma concentrations of progestins, and may decrease the effectiveness of progestin-only pills. Some drugs or herbal products that may decrease the effectiveness of progestin-only pills include barbiturates, bosentan, carbamazepine, felbamate, griseofulvin, oxcarbazepine, phenytoin, rifampin, St. John's wort, topiramate). Products include:

Diprolene Lotion 0.05%	3108
Diprolene Ointment 0.05%	3109
Diprolene AF Cream 0.05%	3107
Lotrisone	3163

Betamethasone Sodium Phosphate (Drugs or herbal products that induce enzymes, including CYP3A4, that metabolize progestins may decrease the plasma concentrations of progestins, and may decrease the effectiveness of progestin-only pills. Some drugs or herbal products that may decrease the effectiveness of progestin-only pills include barbiturates, bosentan, carbamazepine, felbamate, griseofulvin, oxcarbazepine, phenytoin, rifampin, St. John's wort, topiramate).
No products indexed under this heading.

Betamethasone Valerate (Drugs or herbal products that induce enzymes, including CYP3A4, that metabolize progestins may decrease the plasma concentrations of progestins, and may decrease the effectiveness of progestin-only pills. Some drugs or herbal products that may decrease the effectiveness of progestin-only pills include barbiturates, bosentan, carbamazepine, felbamate, griseofulvin, oxcarbazepine, phenytoin, rifampin, St. John's wort, topiramate). Products include:

Luxíq	3321

Bosentan (Drugs or herbal products that induce enzymes, including CYP3A4, that metabolize progestins may decrease the plasma concentrations of progestins, and may decrease the effectiveness of progestin-only pills. Some drugs or herbal products that may decrease the effectiveness of progestin-only pills include bosentan). Products include:

Tracleer	573

Butabarbital (Drugs or herbal products that induce enzymes, including CYP3A4, that metabolize progestins may decrease the plasma concentrations of progestins, and may decrease the effectiveness of progestin-only pills. Some drugs or herbal products that may decrease the effectiveness of progestin-only pills include barbiturates).
No products indexed under this heading.

Butabarbital Sodium (Drugs or herbal products that induce enzymes, including CYP3A4, that metabolize progestins may decrease the plasma concentrations of progestins, and may decrease the effectiveness of progestin-only pills. Some drugs or herbal products that may decrease the effectiveness of progestin-only pills include barbiturates).
No products indexed under this heading.

Butalbital (Drugs or herbal products that induce enzymes, including CYP3A4, that metabolize progestins may decrease the plasma concentrations of progestins, and may decrease the effectiveness of progestin-only pills. Some drugs or herbal products that may decrease the effectiveness of progestin-only pills include barbiturates).
No products indexed under this heading.

Carbamazepine (Drugs or herbal products that induce enzymes, including CYP3A4, that metabolize progestins may decrease the plasma concentrations of progestins, and may decrease the effectiveness of progestin-only pills. Some drugs or herbal products that may decrease the effectiveness of progestin-only pills include carbamazepine). Products include:

Carbatrol	3280
Equetro	3477

Ciprofloxacin (Drugs or herbal products that induce enzymes, including CYP3A4, that metabolize progestins may decrease the plasma concentrations of progestins, and may decrease the effectiveness of progestin-only pills. Some drugs or herbal products that may decrease the effectiveness of progestin-only pills include barbiturates, bosentan, carbamazepine, felbamate, griseofulvin, oxcarbazepine, phenytoin, rifampin, St. John's wort, topiramate). Products include:

Cipro I.V.	3082
Cipro	3073
Cipro XR	3091
Ciprodex	583

Ciprofloxacin Hydrochloride (Drugs or herbal products that induce enzymes, including CYP3A4, that metabolize progestins may decrease the plasma concentrations of progestins, and may decrease the effectiveness of progestin-only pills. Some drugs or herbal products that may decrease the effectiveness of progestin-only pills include barbiturates, bosentan, carbamazepine, felbamate, griseofulvin, oxcarbazepine, phenytoin, rifampin, St. John's wort, topiramate). Products include:

Cipro	3073

Cisplatin (Drugs or herbal products that induce enzymes, including CYP3A4, that metabolize progestins may decrease the plasma concentrations of progestins, and may decrease the effectiveness of progestin-only pills. Some drugs or herbal products that may decrease the effectiveness of progestin-only pills include barbiturates, bosentan, carbamazepine, felbamate, griseofulvin, oxcarbazepine, phenytoin, rifampin, St. John's wort, topiramate).
No products indexed under this heading.

Citalopram Hydrobromide (Drugs or herbal products that induce enzymes, including CYP3A4, that metabolize progestins may decrease the plasma concentrations of progestins, and may decrease the effectiveness of progestin-only pills. Some drugs or herbal products that may decrease the effectiveness of progestin-only pills include barbiturates, bosentan, carbamazepine, felbamate, griseofulvin, oxcarbazepine, phenytoin, rifampin, St. John's wort, topiramate). Products include:

Celexa	1153

Cortisone Acetate (Drugs or herbal products that induce enzymes, including CYP3A4, that metabolize progestins may decrease the plasma concentrations of progestins, and may decrease the effectiveness of progestin-only pills. Some drugs or herbal products that may decrease the effectiveness of progestin-only pills include barbiturates,

Plan B Interactions Index 1428

bosentan, carbamazepine, felbamate, griseofulvin, oxcarbazepine, phenytoin, rifampin, St. John's wort, topiramate).
No products indexed under this heading.

Darunavir (Significant changes (increase or decrease) in the plasma levels of the progestin have been noted in some cases of co-administration of levonorgestrel with HIV protease inhibitors).
No products indexed under this heading.

Delavirdine Mesylate (Significant changes (increase or decrease) in the plasma levels of the progestin have been noted in some cases of co-administration of levonorgestrel with non-nucleoside reverse transcriptase inhibitors).
No products indexed under this heading.

Dexamethasone (Drugs or herbal products that induce enzymes, including CYP3A4, that metabolize progestins may decrease the plasma concentrations of progestins, and may decrease the effectiveness of progestin-only pills. Some drugs or herbal products that may decrease the effectiveness of progestin-only pills include barbiturates, bosentan, carbamazepine, felbamate, griseofulvin, oxcarbazepine, phenytoin, rifampin, St. John's wort, topiramate).
Products include:
Ciprodex 583
Ozurdex .... ⊙223
Tobramycin and Dexamethasone Ophthalmic Suspension .... ⊙251

Dexamethasone Acetate (Drugs or herbal products that induce enzymes, including CYP3A4, that metabolize progestins may decrease the plasma concentrations of progestins, and may decrease the effectiveness of progestin-only pills. Some drugs or herbal products that may decrease the effectiveness of progestin-only pills include barbiturates, bosentan, carbamazepine, felbamate, griseofulvin, oxcarbazepine, phenytoin, rifampin, St. John's wort, topiramate).
No products indexed under this heading.

Dexamethasone Phosphate (Drugs or herbal products that induce enzymes, including CYP3A4, that metabolize progestins may decrease the plasma concentrations of progestins, and may decrease the effectiveness of progestin-only pills. Some drugs or herbal products that may decrease the effectiveness of progestin-only pills include barbiturates, bosentan, carbamazepine, felbamate, griseofulvin, oxcarbazepine, phenytoin, rifampin, St. John's wort, topiramate).
No products indexed under this heading.

Dexamethasone Sodium (Drugs or herbal products that induce enzymes, including CYP3A4, that metabolize progestins may decrease the plasma concentrations of progestins, and may decrease the effectiveness of progestin-only pills. Some drugs or herbal products that may decrease the effectiveness of progestin-only pills include barbiturates, bosentan, carbamazepine, felbamate, griseofulvin, oxcarbazepine, phenytoin, rifampin, St. John's wort, topiramate).
No products indexed under this heading.

Dexamethasone Sodium Phosphate (Drugs or herbal products that induce enzymes, including CYP3A4, that metabolize progestins may decrease the plasma concentrations of progestins, and may decrease the effectiveness of progestin-only pills. Some drugs or herbal products that may decrease the effectiveness of progestin-only pills include barbiturates, bosentan, carbamazepine, felbamate, griseofulvin, oxcarbazepine, phenytoin, rifampin, St. John's wort, topiramate).
No products indexed under this heading.

Dexamethasone Sodium Phosphate Injection (Drugs or herbal products that induce enzymes, including CYP3A4, that metabolize progestins may decrease the plasma concentrations of progestins, and may decrease the effectiveness of progestin-only pills. Some drugs or herbal products that may decrease the effectiveness of progestin-only pills include barbiturates, bosentan, carbamazepine, felbamate, griseofulvin, oxcarbazepine, phenytoin, rifampin, St. John's wort, topiramate).
No products indexed under this heading.

Diltiazem Hydrochloride (Drugs or herbal products that induce enzymes, including CYP3A4, that metabolize progestins may decrease the plasma concentrations of progestins, and may decrease the effectiveness of progestin-only pills. Some drugs or herbal products that may decrease the effectiveness of progestin-only pills include barbiturates, bosentan, carbamazepine, felbamate, griseofulvin, oxcarbazepine, phenytoin, rifampin, St. John's wort, topiramate). Products include:
Cardizem LA 423

Diltiazem Maleate (Drugs or herbal products that induce enzymes, including CYP3A4, that metabolize progestins may decrease the plasma concentrations of progestins, and may decrease the effectiveness of progestin-only pills. Some drugs or herbal products that may decrease the effectiveness of progestin-only pills include barbiturates, bosentan, carbamazepine, felbamate, griseofulvin, oxcarbazepine, phenytoin, rifampin, St. John's wort, topiramate).
No products indexed under this heading.

Doxorubicin Hydrochloride (Drugs or herbal products that induce enzymes, including CYP3A4, that metabolize progestins may decrease the plasma concentrations of progestins, and may decrease the effectiveness of progestin-only pills. Some drugs or herbal products that may decrease the effectiveness of progestin-only pills include barbiturates, bosentan, carbamazepine, felbamate, griseofulvin, oxcarbazepine, phenytoin, rifampin, St. John's wort, topiramate).
No products indexed under this heading.

Efavirenz (Drugs or herbal products that induce enzymes, including CYP3A4, that metabolize progestins may decrease the plasma concentrations of progestins, and may decrease the effectiveness of progestin-only pills. Some drugs or herbal products that may decrease the effectiveness of progestin-only pills include barbiturates, bosentan, carbamazepine, felbamate, griseofulvin, oxcarbazepine, phenytoin, rifampin, St. John's wort, topiramate).
Products include:
Atripla 906

Erythromycin (Drugs or herbal products that induce enzymes, including CYP3A4, that metabolize progestins may decrease the plasma concentrations of progestins, and may decrease the effectiveness of progestin-only pills. Some drugs or herbal products that may decrease the effectiveness of progestin-only pills include barbiturates, bosentan, carbamazepine, felbamate, griseofulvin, oxcarbazepine, phenytoin, rifampin, St. John's wort, topiramate).
No products indexed under this heading.

Erythromycin, Topical (Drugs or herbal products that induce enzymes, including CYP3A4, that metabolize progestins may decrease the plasma concentrations of progestins, and may decrease the effectiveness of progestin-only pills. Some drugs or herbal products that may decrease the effectiveness of progestin-only pills include barbiturates, bosentan, carbamazepine, felbamate, griseofulvin, oxcarbazepine, phenytoin, rifampin, St. John's wort, topiramate).
No products indexed under this heading.

Erythromycin Estolate (Drugs or herbal products that induce enzymes, including CYP3A4, that metabolize progestins may decrease the plasma concentrations of progestins, and may decrease the effectiveness of progestin-only pills. Some drugs or herbal products that may decrease the effectiveness of progestin-only pills include barbiturates, bosentan, carbamazepine, felbamate, griseofulvin, oxcarbazepine, phenytoin, rifampin, St. John's wort, topiramate).
No products indexed under this heading.

Erythromycin Ethylsuccinate (Drugs or herbal products that induce enzymes, including CYP3A4, that metabolize progestins may decrease the plasma concentrations of progestins, and may decrease the effectiveness of progestin-only pills. Some drugs or herbal products that may decrease the effectiveness of progestin-only pills include barbiturates, bosentan, carbamazepine, felbamate, griseofulvin, oxcarbazepine, phenytoin, rifampin, St. John's wort, topiramate).
Products include:
E.E.S. 437
EryPed 435

Erythromycin Gluceptate (Drugs or herbal products that induce enzymes, including CYP3A4, that metabolize progestins may decrease the plasma concentrations of progestins, and may decrease the effectiveness of progestin-only pills. Some drugs or herbal products that may decrease the effectiveness of progestin-only pills include barbiturates, bosentan, carbamazepine, felbamate, griseofulvin, oxcarbazepine, phenytoin, rifampin, St. John's wort, topiramate).
No products indexed under this heading.

Erythromycin Lactobionate (Drugs or herbal products that induce enzymes, including CYP3A4, that metabolize progestins may decrease the plasma concentrations of progestins, and may decrease the effectiveness of progestin-only pills. Some drugs or herbal products that may decrease the effectiveness of progestin-only pills include barbiturates, bosentan, carbamazepine, felbamate, griseofulvin, oxcarbazepine, phenytoin, rifampin, St. John's wort, topiramate).
No products indexed under this heading.

Erythromycin Stearate (Drugs or herbal products that induce enzymes, including CYP3A4, that metabolize progestins may decrease the plasma concentrations of progestins, and may decrease the effectiveness of progestin-only pills. Some drugs or herbal products that may decrease the effectiveness of progestin-only pills include barbiturates, bosentan, carbamazepine, felbamate, griseofulvin, oxcarbazepine, phenytoin, rifampin, St. John's wort, topiramate).
No products indexed under this heading.

Escitalopram Oxalate (Drugs or herbal products that induce enzymes, including CYP3A4, that metabolize progestins may decrease the plasma concentrations of progestins, and may decrease the effectiveness of progestin-only pills. Some drugs or herbal products that may decrease the effectiveness of progestin-only pills include barbiturates, bosentan, carbamazepine, felbamate, griseofulvin, oxcarbazepine, phenytoin, rifampin, St. John's wort, topiramate). Products include:
Lexapro Oral Suspension 1160
Lexapro Tablets 1160

Esomeprazole Magnesium (Drugs or herbal products that induce enzymes, including CYP3A4, that metabolize progestins may decrease the plasma concentrations of progestins, and may decrease the effectiveness of progestin-only pills. Some drugs or herbal products that may decrease the effectiveness of progestin-only pills include barbiturates, bosentan, carbamazepine, felbamate, griseofulvin, oxcarbazepine, phenytoin, rifampin, St. John's wort, topiramate).
Products include:
Nexium Capsules 704
Nexium Oral Suspension 704

Esomeprazole Sodium (Drugs or herbal products that induce enzymes, including CYP3A4, that metabolize progestins may decrease the plasma concentrations of progestins, and may decrease the effectiveness of progestin-only pills. Some drugs or herbal products that may decrease the effectiveness of progestin-only pills include barbiturates, bosentan, carbamazepine, felbamate, griseofulvin, oxcarbazepine, phenytoin, rifampin, St. John's wort, topiramate). Products include:
Nexium I.V. 712

Ethanol (Drugs or herbal products that induce enzymes, including CYP3A4, that metabolize progestins may decrease the plasma concentrations of progestins, and may decrease the effectiveness of progestin-only pills. Some drugs or herbal products that may decrease the effectiveness of progestin-only pills include barbiturates, bosentan, carbamazepine, felbamate, griseofulvin, oxcarbazepine, phenytoin, rifampin, St. John's wort, topiramate).
No products indexed under this heading.

Ethosuximide (Drugs or herbal products that induce enzymes, including CYP3A4, that metabolize progestins may decrease the plasma concentrations of progestins, and may decrease the effectiveness of progestin-only pills. Some drugs or herbal products that may decrease the effectiveness of progestin-only pills include barbiturates, bosentan, carbamazepine, felbamate, griseofulvin, oxcarbazepine, phenytoin, rifampin, St. John's wort, topiramate).
No products indexed under this heading.

Etravirine (Significant changes (increase or decrease) in the plasma levels of the progestin have been noted in some cases of co-administration of levonorgestrel with non-nucleoside reverse transcriptase inhibitors).
No products indexed under this heading.

Felbamate (Drugs or herbal products that induce enzymes, including CYP3A4, that metabolize progestins may decrease the plasma concentrations of progestins, and may decrease the effectiveness of progestin-only pills. Some drugs or herbal products that may decrease the effectiveness of progestin-only pills include felbamate).
No products indexed under this heading.

Fludrocortisone Acetate (Drugs or herbal products that induce enzymes, including CYP3A4, that metabolize progestins may decrease the plasma concentrations of progestins, and may decrease the effectiveness of progestin-only pills. Some drugs or herbal products that may decrease the effectiveness of progestin-only pills include barbiturates, bosentan, carbamazepine, felbamate, griseofulvin, oxcarbazepine, phenytoin, rifampin, St. John's wort, topiramate).
No products indexed under this heading.

Fluvoxamine (Drugs or herbal products that induce enzymes, including CYP3A4, that metabolize progestins may decrease the plasma concentra-

(⊙ Described in PDR® for Ophthalmic Medicines)

1429 Interactions Index Plan B

tions of progestins, and may decrease the effectiveness of progestin-only pills. Some drugs or herbal products that may decrease the effectiveness of progestin-only pills include barbiturates, bosentan, carbamazepine, felbamate, griseofulvin, oxcarbazepine, phenytoin, rifampin, St. John's wort, topiramate).
No products indexed under this heading.

Fluvoxamine Maleate (Drugs or herbal products that induce enzymes, including CYP3A4, that metabolize progestins may decrease the plasma concentrations of progestins, and may decrease the effectiveness of progestin-only pills. Some drugs or herbal products that may decrease the effectiveness of progestin-only pills include barbiturates, bosentan, carbamazepine, felbamate, griseofulvin, oxcarbazepine, phenytoin, rifampin, St. John's wort, topiramate).
No products indexed under this heading.

Fosamprenavir Calcium (Significant changes (increase or decrease) in the plasma levels of the progestin have been noted in some cases of co-administration of levonorgestrel with HIV protease inhibitors). Products include:
Lexiva Oral Suspension 1558
Lexiva 1558

Fosphenytoin (Drugs or herbal products that induce enzymes, including CYP3A4, that metabolize progestins may decrease the plasma concentrations of progestins, and may decrease the effectiveness of progestin-only pills. Some drugs or herbal products that may decrease the effectiveness of progestin-only pills include phenytoin).
No products indexed under this heading.

Fosphenytoin Sodium (Drugs or herbal products that induce enzymes, including CYP3A4, that metabolize progestins may decrease the plasma concentrations of progestins, and may decrease the effectiveness of progestin-only pills. Some drugs or herbal products that may decrease the effectiveness of progestin-only pills include phenytoin).
No products indexed under this heading.

Garlic Extract (Drugs or herbal products that induce enzymes, including CYP3A4, that metabolize progestins may decrease the plasma concentrations of progestins, and may decrease the effectiveness of progestin-only pills. Some drugs or herbal products that may decrease the effectiveness of progestin-only pills include barbiturates, bosentan, carbamazepine, felbamate, griseofulvin, oxcarbazepine, phenytoin, rifampin, St. John's wort, topiramate).
No products indexed under this heading.

Garlic Oil (Drugs or herbal products that induce enzymes, including CYP3A4, that metabolize progestins may decrease the plasma concentrations of progestins, and may decrease the effectiveness of progestin-only pills. Some drugs or herbal products that may decrease the effectiveness of progestin-only pills include barbiturates, bosentan, carbamazepine, felbamate, griseofulvin, oxcarbazepine, phenytoin, rifampin, St. John's wort, topiramate).
No products indexed under this heading.

Griseofulvin (Drugs or herbal products that induce enzymes, including CYP3A4, that metabolize progestins may decrease the plasma concentrations of progestins, and may decrease the effectiveness of progestin-only pills. Some drugs or herbal products that may decrease the effectiveness of progestin-only pills include griseofulvin).
No products indexed under this heading.

Hexobarbital (Drugs or herbal products that induce enzymes, including CYP3A4, that metabolize progestins may decrease the plasma concentrations of progestins, and may decrease the effectiveness of progestin-only pills. Some drugs or herbal products that may decrease the effectiveness of progestin-only pills include barbiturates).
No products indexed under this heading.

Hydrocortisone (Drugs or herbal products that induce enzymes, including CYP3A4, that metabolize progestins may decrease the plasma concentrations of progestins, and may decrease the effectiveness of progestin-only pills. Some drugs or herbal products that may decrease the effectiveness of progestin-only pills include barbiturates, bosentan, carbamazepine, felbamate, griseofulvin, oxcarbazepine, phenytoin, rifampin, St. John's wort, topiramate).
No products indexed under this heading.

Hydrocortisone (Alcohol) (Drugs or herbal products that induce enzymes, including CYP3A4, that metabolize progestins may decrease the plasma concentrations of progestins, and may decrease the effectiveness of progestin-only pills. Some drugs or herbal products that may decrease the effectiveness of progestin-only pills include barbiturates, bosentan, carbamazepine, felbamate, griseofulvin, oxcarbazepine, phenytoin, rifampin, St. John's wort, topiramate).
No products indexed under this heading.

Hydrocortisone Acetate (Drugs or herbal products that induce enzymes, including CYP3A4, that metabolize progestins may decrease the plasma concentrations of progestins, and may decrease the effectiveness of progestin-only pills. Some drugs or herbal products that may decrease the effectiveness of progestin-only pills include barbiturates, bosentan, carbamazepine, felbamate, griseofulvin, oxcarbazepine, phenytoin, rifampin, St. John's wort, topiramate).
No products indexed under this heading.

Hydrocortisone Butyrate (Drugs or herbal products that induce enzymes, including CYP3A4, that metabolize progestins may decrease the plasma concentrations of progestins, and may decrease the effectiveness of progestin-only pills. Some drugs or herbal products that may decrease the effectiveness of progestin-only pills include barbiturates, bosentan, carbamazepine, felbamate, griseofulvin, oxcarbazepine, phenytoin, rifampin, St. John's wort, topiramate).
No products indexed under this heading.

Hydrocortisone Cypionate (Drugs or herbal products that induce enzymes, including CYP3A4, that metabolize progestins may decrease the plasma concentrations of progestins, and may decrease the effectiveness of progestin-only pills. Some drugs or herbal products that may decrease the effectiveness of progestin-only pills include barbiturates, bosentan, carbamazepine, felbamate, griseofulvin, oxcarbazepine, phenytoin, rifampin, St. John's wort, topiramate).
No products indexed under this heading.

Hydrocortisone Hemisuccinate (Drugs or herbal products that induce enzymes, including CYP3A4, that metabolize progestins may decrease the plasma concentrations of progestins, and may decrease the effectiveness of progestin-only pills. Some drugs or herbal products that may decrease the effectiveness of progestin-only pills include barbiturates, bosentan, carbamazepine, felbamate, griseofulvin, oxcarbazepine, phenytoin, rifampin, St. John's wort, topiramate).
No products indexed under this heading.

Hydrocortisone Probutate (Drugs or herbal products that induce enzymes, including CYP3A4, that metabolize progestins may decrease the plasma concentrations of progestins, and may decrease the effectiveness of progestin-only pills. Some drugs or herbal products that may decrease the effectiveness of progestin-only pills include barbiturates, bosentan, carbamazepine, felbamate, griseofulvin, oxcarbazepine, phenytoin, rifampin, St. John's wort, topiramate).
No products indexed under this heading.

Hydrocortisone Sodium Phosphate (Drugs or herbal products that induce enzymes, including CYP3A4, that metabolize progestins may decrease the plasma concentrations of progestins, and may decrease the effectiveness of progestin-only pills. Some drugs or herbal products that may decrease the effectiveness of progestin-only pills include barbiturates, bosentan, carbamazepine, felbamate, griseofulvin, oxcarbazepine, phenytoin, rifampin, St. John's wort, topiramate).
No products indexed under this heading.

Hydrocortisone Sodium Succinate (Drugs or herbal products that induce enzymes, including CYP3A4, that metabolize progestins may decrease the plasma concentrations of progestins, and may decrease the effectiveness of progestin-only pills. Some drugs or herbal products that may decrease the effectiveness of progestin-only pills include barbiturates, bosentan, carbamazepine, felbamate, griseofulvin, oxcarbazepine, phenytoin, rifampin, St. John's wort, topiramate).
No products indexed under this heading.

Hydrocortisone Valerate (Drugs or herbal products that induce enzymes, including CYP3A4, that metabolize progestins may decrease the plasma concentrations of progestins, and may decrease the effectiveness of progestin-only pills. Some drugs or herbal products that may decrease the effectiveness of progestin-only pills include barbiturates, bosentan, carbamazepine, felbamate, griseofulvin, oxcarbazepine, phenytoin, rifampin, St. John's wort, topiramate).
No products indexed under this heading.

Hypericum (Drugs or herbal products that induce enzymes, including CYP3A4, that metabolize progestins may decrease the plasma concentrations of progestins, and may decrease the effectiveness of progestin-only pills. Some drugs or herbal products that may decrease the effectiveness of progestin-only pills include barbiturates, bosentan, carbamazepine, felbamate, griseofulvin, oxcarbazepine, phenytoin, rifampin, St. John's wort, topiramate).
No products indexed under this heading.

Hypericum Perforatum (Drugs or herbal products that induce enzymes, including CYP3A4, that metabolize progestins may decrease the plasma concentrations of progestins, and may decrease the effectiveness of progestin-only pills. Some drugs or herbal products that may decrease the effectiveness of progestin-only pills include St. John's wort). Products include:
Traumeel 1800

Indinavir Sulfate (Significant changes (increase or decrease) in the plasma levels of the progestin have been noted in some cases of co-administration of levonorgestrel with HIV protease inhibitors). Products include:
Crixivan 2113

Insulin (Drugs or herbal products that induce enzymes, including CYP3A4, that metabolize progestins may decrease the plasma concentrations of progestins, and may decrease the effectiveness of progestin-only pills. Some drugs or herbal products that may decrease the effectiveness of progestin-only pills include barbiturates, bosentan, carbamazepine, felbamate, griseofulvin, oxcarbazepine, phenytoin, rifampin, St. John's wort, topiramate).
No products indexed under this heading.

Insulin, Human, Zinc Suspension (Drugs or herbal products that induce enzymes, including CYP3A4, that metabolize progestins may decrease the plasma concentrations of progestins, and may decrease the effectiveness of progestin-only pills. Some drugs or herbal products that may decrease the effectiveness of progestin-only pills include barbiturates, bosentan, carbamazepine, felbamate, griseofulvin, oxcarbazepine, phenytoin, rifampin, St. John's wort, topiramate).
No products indexed under this heading.

Insulin, Human (rDNA origin) (Drugs or herbal products that induce enzymes, including CYP3A4, that metabolize progestins may decrease the plasma concentrations of progestins, and may decrease the effectiveness of progestin-only pills. Some drugs or herbal products that may decrease the effectiveness of progestin-only pills include barbiturates, bosentan, carbamazepine, felbamate, griseofulvin, oxcarbazepine, phenytoin, rifampin, St. John's wort, topiramate). Products include:
Exubera 2717

Insulin, Human NPH (Drugs or herbal products that induce enzymes, including CYP3A4, that metabolize progestins may decrease the plasma concentrations of progestins, and may decrease the effectiveness of progestin-only pills. Some drugs or herbal products that may decrease the effectiveness of progestin-only pills include barbiturates, bosentan, carbamazepine, felbamate, griseofulvin, oxcarbazepine, phenytoin, rifampin, St. John's wort, topiramate). Products include:
Humulin N Vial 1934

Insulin, Human Regular (Drugs or herbal products that induce enzymes, including CYP3A4, that metabolize progestins may decrease the plasma concentrations of progestins, and may decrease the effectiveness of progestin-only pills. Some drugs or herbal products that may decrease the effectiveness of progestin-only pills include barbiturates, bosentan, carbamazepine, felbamate, griseofulvin, oxcarbazepine, phenytoin, rifampin, St. John's wort, topiramate). Products include:
Humulin R 1937
Humulin R (U-500) 1939

Insulin, Human Regular and Human NPH Mixture (Drugs or herbal products that induce enzymes, including CYP3A4, that metabolize progestins may decrease the plasma concentrations of progestins, and may decrease the effectiveness of progestin-only pills. Some drugs or herbal products that may decrease the effectiveness of progestin-only pills include barbiturates, bosentan, carbamazepine, felbamate, griseofulvin, oxcarbazepine, phenytoin, rifampin, St. John's wort, topiramate). Products include:
Humulin 50/50 1930
Humulin 70/30 Vial 1931

Insulin, NPH (Drugs or herbal products that induce enzymes, including CYP3A4, that metabolize progestins may decrease the plasma concentrations of progestins, and may decrease

IMPORTANT NOTE: Always consult each drug listing in the patient's regimen for possible interactions.

the effectiveness of progestin-only pills. Some drugs or herbal products that may decrease the effectiveness of progestin-only pills include barbiturates, bosentan, carbamazepine, felbamate, griseofulvin, oxcarbazepine, phenytoin, rifampin, St. John's wort, topiramate).

No products indexed under this heading.

Insulin, Regular (Drugs or herbal products that induce enzymes, including CYP3A4, that metabolize progestins may decrease the plasma concentrations of progestins, and may decrease the effectiveness of progestin-only pills. Some drugs or herbal products that may decrease the effectiveness of progestin-only pills include barbiturates, bosentan, carbamazepine, felbamate, griseofulvin, oxcarbazepine, phenytoin, rifampin, St. John's wort, topiramate).

No products indexed under this heading.

Insulin, Regular and NPH mixture (Drugs or herbal products that induce enzymes, including CYP3A4, that metabolize progestins may decrease the plasma concentrations of progestins, and may decrease the effectiveness of progestin-only pills. Some drugs or herbal products that may decrease the effectiveness of progestin-only pills include barbiturates, bosentan, carbamazepine, felbamate, griseofulvin, oxcarbazepine, phenytoin, rifampin, St. John's wort, topiramate).

No products indexed under this heading.

Insulin, Zinc Crystals (Drugs or herbal products that induce enzymes, including CYP3A4, that metabolize progestins may decrease the plasma concentrations of progestins, and may decrease the effectiveness of progestin-only pills. Some drugs or herbal products that may decrease the effectiveness of progestin-only pills include barbiturates, bosentan, carbamazepine, felbamate, griseofulvin, oxcarbazepine, phenytoin, rifampin, St. John's wort, topiramate).

No products indexed under this heading.

Insulin, Zinc Suspension (Drugs or herbal products that induce enzymes, including CYP3A4, that metabolize progestins may decrease the plasma concentrations of progestins, and may decrease the effectiveness of progestin-only pills. Some drugs or herbal products that may decrease the effectiveness of progestin-only pills include barbiturates, bosentan, carbamazepine, felbamate, griseofulvin, oxcarbazepine, phenytoin, rifampin, St. John's wort, topiramate).

No products indexed under this heading.

Insulin Aspart (Drugs or herbal products that induce enzymes, including CYP3A4, that metabolize progestins may decrease the plasma concentrations of progestins, and may decrease the effectiveness of progestin-only pills. Some drugs or herbal products that may decrease the effectiveness of progestin-only pills include barbiturates, bosentan, carbamazepine, felbamate, griseofulvin, oxcarbazepine, phenytoin, rifampin, St. John's wort, topiramate).

No products indexed under this heading.

Insulin Aspart, Human (Drugs or herbal products that induce enzymes, including CYP3A4, that metabolize progestins may decrease the plasma concentrations of progestins, and may decrease the effectiveness of progestin-only pills. Some drugs or herbal products that may decrease the effectiveness of progestin-only pills include barbiturates, bosentan, carbamazepine, felbamate, griseofulvin, oxcarbazepine, phenytoin, rifampin, St. John's wort, topiramate). Products include:
NovoLog Mix 70/30 2581

Insulin Aspart, Human Regular (Drugs or herbal products that induce

enzymes, including CYP3A4, that metabolize progestins may decrease the plasma concentrations of progestins, and may decrease the effectiveness of progestin-only pills. Some drugs or herbal products that may decrease the effectiveness of progestin-only pills include barbiturates, bosentan, carbamazepine, felbamate, griseofulvin, oxcarbazepine, phenytoin, rifampin, St. John's wort, topiramate). Products include:
NovoLog 2575

Insulin Aspart Protamine, Human (Drugs or herbal products that induce enzymes, including CYP3A4, that metabolize progestins may decrease the plasma concentrations of progestins, and may decrease the effectiveness of progestin-only pills. Some drugs or herbal products that may decrease the effectiveness of progestin-only pills include barbiturates, bosentan, carbamazepine, felbamate, griseofulvin, oxcarbazepine, phenytoin, rifampin, St. John's wort, topiramate). Products include:
NovoLog Mix 70/30 2581

Insulin Detemir (rDNA Origin) (Drugs or herbal products that induce enzymes, including CYP3A4, that metabolize progestins may decrease the plasma concentrations of progestins, and may decrease the effectiveness of progestin-only pills. Some drugs or herbal products that may decrease the effectiveness of progestin-only pills include barbiturates, bosentan, carbamazepine, felbamate, griseofulvin, oxcarbazepine, phenytoin, rifampin, St. John's wort, topiramate). Products include:
Levemir 2566

Insulin Glargine (Drugs or herbal products that induce enzymes, including CYP3A4, that metabolize progestins may decrease the plasma concentrations of progestins, and may decrease the effectiveness of progestin-only pills. Some drugs or herbal products that may decrease the effectiveness of progestin-only pills include barbiturates, bosentan, carbamazepine, felbamate, griseofulvin, oxcarbazepine, phenytoin, rifampin, St. John's wort, topiramate). Products include:
Lantus 2996

Insulin Glulisine (Drugs or herbal products that induce enzymes, including CYP3A4, that metabolize progestins may decrease the plasma concentrations of progestins, and may decrease the effectiveness of progestin-only pills. Some drugs or herbal products that may decrease the effectiveness of progestin-only pills include barbiturates, bosentan, carbamazepine, felbamate, griseofulvin, oxcarbazepine, phenytoin, rifampin, St. John's wort, topiramate). Products include:
Apidra 2937
Apidra SoloStar 2937

Insulin Lispro, Human (Drugs or herbal products that induce enzymes, including CYP3A4, that metabolize progestins may decrease the plasma concentrations of progestins, and may decrease the effectiveness of progestin-only pills. Some drugs or herbal products that may decrease the effectiveness of progestin-only pills include barbiturates, bosentan, carbamazepine, felbamate, griseofulvin, oxcarbazepine, phenytoin, rifampin, St. John's wort, topiramate). Products include:
Humalog 1910
Humalog Mix 1914
Humalog Mix75/25 1917

Insulin Lispro Protamine, Human (Drugs or herbal products that induce enzymes, including CYP3A4, that metabolize progestins may decrease

the plasma concentrations of progestins, and may decrease the effectiveness of progestin-only pills. Some drugs or herbal products that may decrease the effectiveness of progestin-only pills include barbiturates, bosentan, carbamazepine, felbamate, griseofulvin, oxcarbazepine, phenytoin, rifampin, St. John's wort, topiramate). Products include:
Humalog Mix 1914
Humalog Mix75/25 1917

Lansoprazole (Drugs or herbal products that induce enzymes, including CYP3A4, that metabolize progestins may decrease the plasma concentrations of progestins, and may decrease the effectiveness of progestin-only pills. Some drugs or herbal products that may decrease the effectiveness of progestin-only pills include barbiturates, bosentan, carbamazepine, felbamate, griseofulvin, oxcarbazepine, phenytoin, rifampin, St. John's wort, topiramate).

No products indexed under this heading.

Lopinavir (Significant changes (increase or decrease) in the plasma levels of the progestin have been noted in some cases of co-administration of levonorgestrel with HIV protease inhibitors). Products include:
Kaletra **458**

Mephenytoin (Drugs or herbal products that induce enzymes, including CYP3A4, that metabolize progestins may decrease the plasma concentrations of progestins, and may decrease the effectiveness of progestin-only pills. Some drugs or herbal products that may decrease the effectiveness of progestin-only pills include barbiturates, bosentan, carbamazepine, felbamate, griseofulvin, oxcarbazepine, phenytoin, rifampin, St. John's wort, topiramate).

No products indexed under this heading.

Mephobarbital (Drugs or herbal products that induce enzymes, including CYP3A4, that metabolize progestins may decrease the plasma concentrations of progestins, and may decrease the effectiveness of progestin-only pills. Some drugs or herbal products that may decrease the effectiveness of progestin-only pills include barbiturates).

No products indexed under this heading.

Methsuximide (Drugs or herbal products that induce enzymes, including CYP3A4, that metabolize progestins may decrease the plasma concentrations of progestins, and may decrease the effectiveness of progestin-only pills. Some drugs or herbal products that may decrease the effectiveness of progestin-only pills include barbiturates, bosentan, carbamazepine, felbamate, griseofulvin, oxcarbazepine, phenytoin, rifampin, St. John's wort, topiramate).

No products indexed under this heading.

Methylprednisolone (Drugs or herbal products that induce enzymes, including CYP3A4, that metabolize progestins may decrease the plasma concentrations of progestins, and may decrease the effectiveness of progestin-only pills. Some drugs or herbal products that may decrease the effectiveness of progestin-only pills include barbiturates, bosentan, carbamazepine, felbamate, griseofulvin, oxcarbazepine, phenytoin, rifampin, St. John's wort, topiramate).

No products indexed under this heading.

Methylprednisolone Acetate (Drugs or herbal products that induce enzymes, including CYP3A4, that metabolize progestins may decrease the plasma concentrations of progestins, and may decrease the effectiveness of progestin-only pills. Some drugs or herbal products that may decrease the effectiveness of progestin-only pills include barbiturates,

bosentan, carbamazepine, felbamate, griseofulvin, oxcarbazepine, phenytoin, rifampin, St. John's wort, topiramate).

No products indexed under this heading.

Methylprednisolone Sodium Succinate (Drugs or herbal products that induce enzymes, including CYP3A4, that metabolize progestins may decrease the plasma concentrations of progestins, and may decrease the effectiveness of progestin-only pills. Some drugs or herbal products that may decrease the effectiveness of progestin-only pills include barbiturates, bosentan, carbamazepine, felbamate, griseofulvin, oxcarbazepine, phenytoin, rifampin, St. John's wort, topiramate).

No products indexed under this heading.

Modafinil (Drugs or herbal products that induce enzymes, including CYP3A4, that metabolize progestins may decrease the plasma concentrations of progestins, and may decrease the effectiveness of progestin-only pills. Some drugs or herbal products that may decrease the effectiveness of progestin-only pills include barbiturates, bosentan, carbamazepine, felbamate, griseofulvin, oxcarbazepine, phenytoin, rifampin, St. John's wort, topiramate). Products include:
Provigil **983**

Nafcillin Sodium (Drugs or herbal products that induce enzymes, including CYP3A4, that metabolize progestins may decrease the plasma concentrations of progestins, and may decrease the effectiveness of progestin-only pills. Some drugs or herbal products that may decrease the effectiveness of progestin-only pills include barbiturates, bosentan, carbamazepine, felbamate, griseofulvin, oxcarbazepine, phenytoin, rifampin, St. John's wort, topiramate).

No products indexed under this heading.

Nelfinavir Mesylate (Significant changes (increase or decrease) in the plasma levels of the progestin have been noted in some cases of co-administration of levonorgestrel with HIV protease inhibitors).

No products indexed under this heading.

Nevirapine (Drugs or herbal products that induce enzymes, including CYP3A4, that metabolize progestins may decrease the plasma concentrations of progestins, and may decrease the effectiveness of progestin-only pills. Some drugs or herbal products that may decrease the effectiveness of progestin-only pills include barbiturates, bosentan, carbamazepine, felbamate, griseofulvin, oxcarbazepine, phenytoin, rifampin, St. John's wort, topiramate). Products include:
Viramune Oral Suspension **897**
Viramune Tablets **897**

Nicotine (Drugs or herbal products that induce enzymes, including CYP3A4, that metabolize progestins may decrease the plasma concentrations of progestins, and may decrease the effectiveness of progestin-only pills. Some drugs or herbal products that may decrease the effectiveness of progestin-only pills include barbiturates, bosentan, carbamazepine, felbamate, griseofulvin, oxcarbazepine, phenytoin, rifampin, St. John's wort, topiramate).

No products indexed under this heading.

Nicotine Polacrilex (Drugs or herbal products that induce enzymes, including CYP3A4, that metabolize progestins may decrease the plasma concentrations of progestins, and may decrease the effectiveness of progestin-only pills. Some drugs or herbal products that may decrease the effectiveness of progestin-only pills include barbiturates, bosentan, carbamazepine, felbamate, griseofulvin, oxcarbazepine, phenytoin, rifampin, St. John's wort, topiramate).

No products indexed under this heading.

Nicotine Salicylate (Drugs or herbal products that induce enzymes, including CYP3A4, that metabolize progestins may decrease the plasma concentrations of progestins, and may decrease the effectiveness of progestin-only pills. Some drugs or herbal products that may decrease the effectiveness of progestin-only pills include barbiturates, bosentan, carbamazepine, felbamate, griseofulvin, oxcarbazepine, phenytoin, rifampin, St. John's wort, topiramate).
No products indexed under this heading.

Nicotine Sulfate (Drugs or herbal products that induce enzymes, including CYP3A4, that metabolize progestins may decrease the plasma concentrations of progestins, and may decrease the effectiveness of progestin-only pills. Some drugs or herbal products that may decrease the effectiveness of progestin-only pills include barbiturates, bosentan, carbamazepine, felbamate, griseofulvin, oxcarbazepine, phenytoin, rifampin, St. John's wort, topiramate).
No products indexed under this heading.

Norethindrone (Drugs or herbal products that induce enzymes, including CYP3A4, that metabolize progestins may decrease the plasma concentrations of progestins, and may decrease the effectiveness of progestin-only pills. Some drugs or herbal products that may decrease the effectiveness of progestin-only pills include barbiturates, bosentan, carbamazepine, felbamate, griseofulvin, oxcarbazepine, phenytoin, rifampin, St. John's wort, topiramate). Products include:
Ortho Micronor 2660

Norethindrone Acetate (Drugs or herbal products that induce enzymes, including CYP3A4, that metabolize progestins may decrease the plasma concentrations of progestins, and may decrease the effectiveness of progestin-only pills. Some drugs or herbal products that may decrease the effectiveness of progestin-only pills include barbiturates, bosentan, carbamazepine, felbamate, griseofulvin, oxcarbazepine, phenytoin, rifampin, St. John's wort, topiramate). Products include:
Activella 2561

Omeprazole (Drugs or herbal products that induce enzymes, including CYP3A4, that metabolize progestins may decrease the plasma concentrations of progestins, and may decrease the effectiveness of progestin-only pills. Some drugs or herbal products that may decrease the effectiveness of progestin-only pills include barbiturates, bosentan, carbamazepine, felbamate, griseofulvin, oxcarbazepine, phenytoin, rifampin, St. John's wort, topiramate).
No products indexed under this heading.

Omeprazole Magnesium (Drugs or herbal products that induce enzymes, including CYP3A4, that metabolize progestins may decrease the plasma concentrations of progestins, and may decrease the effectiveness of progestin-only pills. Some drugs or herbal products that may decrease the effectiveness of progestin-only pills include barbiturates, bosentan, carbamazepine, felbamate, griseofulvin, oxcarbazepine, phenytoin, rifampin, St. John's wort, topiramate).
No products indexed under this heading.

Oxcarbazepine (Drugs or herbal products that induce enzymes, including CYP3A4, that metabolize progestins may decrease the plasma concentrations of progestins, and may decrease the effectiveness of progestin-only pills. Some drugs or herbal products that may decrease the effectiveness of progestin-only pills include oxcarbazepine).
No products indexed under this heading.

Pentobarbital (Drugs or herbal products that induce enzymes, including CYP3A4, that metabolize progestins may decrease the plasma concentrations of progestins, and may decrease the effectiveness of progestin-only pills. Some drugs or herbal products that may decrease the effectiveness of progestin-only pills include barbiturates).
No products indexed under this heading.

Pentobarbital Sodium (Drugs or herbal products that induce enzymes, including CYP3A4, that metabolize progestins may decrease the plasma concentrations of progestins, and may decrease the effectiveness of progestin-only pills. Some drugs or herbal products that may decrease the effectiveness of progestin-only pills include barbiturates). Products include:
Nembutal 2012

Phenobarbital (Drugs or herbal products that induce enzymes, including CYP3A4, that metabolize progestins may decrease the plasma concentrations of progestins, and may decrease the effectiveness of progestin-only pills. Some drugs or herbal products that may decrease the effectiveness of progestin-only pills include barbiturates). Products include:
Donnatal 2711

Phenobarbital Sodium (Drugs or herbal products that induce enzymes, including CYP3A4, that metabolize progestins may decrease the plasma concentrations of progestins, and may decrease the effectiveness of progestin-only pills. Some drugs or herbal products that may decrease the effectiveness of progestin-only pills include barbiturates).
No products indexed under this heading.

Phenytoin (Drugs or herbal products that induce enzymes, including CYP3A4, that metabolize progestins may decrease the plasma concentrations of progestins, and may decrease the effectiveness of progestin-only pills. Some drugs or herbal products that may decrease the effectiveness of progestin-only pills include phenytoin).
No products indexed under this heading.

Phenytoin Sodium (Drugs or herbal products that induce enzymes, including CYP3A4, that metabolize progestins may decrease the plasma concentrations of progestins, and may decrease the effectiveness of progestin-only pills. Some drugs or herbal products that may decrease the effectiveness of progestin-only pills include phenytoin). Products include:
Phenytek Capsules 2380

Prednisolone (Drugs or herbal products that induce enzymes, including CYP3A4, that metabolize progestins may decrease the plasma concentrations of progestins, and may decrease the effectiveness of progestin-only pills. Some drugs or herbal products that may decrease the effectiveness of progestin-only pills include barbiturates, bosentan, carbamazepine, felbamate, griseofulvin, oxcarbazepine, phenytoin, rifampin, St. John's wort, topiramate).
No products indexed under this heading.

Prednisolone Acetate (Drugs or herbal products that induce enzymes, including CYP3A4, that metabolize progestins may decrease the plasma concentrations of progestins, and may decrease the effectiveness of progestin-only pills. Some drugs or herbal products that may decrease the effectiveness of progestin-only pills include barbiturates, bosentan, carbamazepine, felbamate, griseofulvin, oxcarbazepine, phenytoin, rifampin, St. John's wort, topiramate). Products include:

Blephamide .... ⊙212, ⊙214
Pred Forte .... ⊙225
Pred Mild .... ⊙230
Pred-G .... ⊙226, ⊙227

Prednisolone Sodium Phosphate (Drugs or herbal products that induce enzymes, including CYP3A4, that metabolize progestins may decrease the plasma concentrations of progestins, and may decrease the effectiveness of progestin-only pills. Some drugs or herbal products that may decrease the effectiveness of progestin-only pills include barbiturates, bosentan, carbamazepine, felbamate, griseofulvin, oxcarbazepine, phenytoin, rifampin, St. John's wort, topiramate).
No products indexed under this heading.

Prednisolone Tebutate (Drugs or herbal products that induce enzymes, including CYP3A4, that metabolize progestins may decrease the plasma concentrations of progestins, and may decrease the effectiveness of progestin-only pills. Some drugs or herbal products that may decrease the effectiveness of progestin-only pills include barbiturates, bosentan, carbamazepine, felbamate, griseofulvin, oxcarbazepine, phenytoin, rifampin, St. John's wort, topiramate).
No products indexed under this heading.

Prednisone (Drugs or herbal products that induce enzymes, including CYP3A4, that metabolize progestins may decrease the plasma concentrations of progestins, and may decrease the effectiveness of progestin-only pills. Some drugs or herbal products that may decrease the effectiveness of progestin-only pills include barbiturates, bosentan, carbamazepine, felbamate, griseofulvin, oxcarbazepine, phenytoin, rifampin, St. John's wort, topiramate).
No products indexed under this heading.

Prednisone sodium phosphate (Drugs or herbal products that induce enzymes, including CYP3A4, that metabolize progestins may decrease the plasma concentrations of progestins, and may decrease the effectiveness of progestin-only pills. Some drugs or herbal products that may decrease the effectiveness of progestin-only pills include barbiturates, bosentan, carbamazepine, felbamate, griseofulvin, oxcarbazepine, phenytoin, rifampin, St. John's wort, topiramate).
No products indexed under this heading.

Primidone (Drugs or herbal products that induce enzymes, including CYP3A4, that metabolize progestins may decrease the plasma concentrations of progestins, and may decrease the effectiveness of progestin-only pills. Some drugs or herbal products that may decrease the effectiveness of progestin-only pills include barbiturates, bosentan, carbamazepine, felbamate, griseofulvin, oxcarbazepine, phenytoin, rifampin, St. John's wort, topiramate).
No products indexed under this heading.

Rifabutin (Drugs or herbal products that induce enzymes, including CYP3A4, that metabolize progestins may decrease the plasma concentrations of progestins, and may decrease the effectiveness of progestin-only pills. Some drugs or herbal products that may decrease the effectiveness of progestin-only pills include barbiturates, bosentan, carbamazepine, felbamate, griseofulvin, oxcarbazepine, phenytoin, rifampin, St. John's wort, topiramate).
No products indexed under this heading.

Rifampicin (Drugs or herbal products that induce enzymes, including CYP3A4, that metabolize progestins may decrease the plasma concentrations of progestins, and may decrease the effectiveness of progestin-only pills. Some drugs or herbal products that

may decrease the effectiveness of progestin-only pills include barbiturates, bosentan, carbamazepine, felbamate, griseofulvin, oxcarbazepine, phenytoin, rifampin, St. John's wort, topiramate).
No products indexed under this heading.

Rifampin (Drugs or herbal products that induce enzymes, including CYP3A4, that metabolize progestins may decrease the plasma concentrations of progestins, and may decrease the effectiveness of progestin-only pills. Some drugs or herbal products that may decrease the effectiveness of progestin-only pills include rifampin).
No products indexed under this heading.

Rifapentine (Drugs or herbal products that induce enzymes, including CYP3A4, that metabolize progestins may decrease the plasma concentrations of progestins, and may decrease the effectiveness of progestin-only pills. Some drugs or herbal products that may decrease the effectiveness of progestin-only pills include barbiturates, bosentan, carbamazepine, felbamate, griseofulvin, oxcarbazepine, phenytoin, rifampin, St. John's wort, topiramate).
No products indexed under this heading.

Ritonavir (Drugs or herbal products that induce enzymes, including CYP3A4, that metabolize progestins may decrease the plasma concentrations of progestins, and may decrease the effectiveness of progestin-only pills. Some drugs or herbal products that may decrease the effectiveness of progestin-only pills include barbiturates, bosentan, carbamazepine, felbamate, griseofulvin, oxcarbazepine, phenytoin, rifampin, St. John's wort, topiramate). Products include:
Kaletra 458
Norvir 509

Saquinavir (Significant changes (increase or decrease) in the plasma levels of the progestin have been noted in some cases of co-administration of levonorgestrel with HIV protease inhibitors).
No products indexed under this heading.

Saquinavir Mesylate (Significant changes (increase or decrease) in the plasma levels of the progestin have been noted in some cases of co-administration of levonorgestrel with HIV protease inhibitors).
No products indexed under this heading.

Secobarbital Sodium (Drugs or herbal products that induce enzymes, including CYP3A4, that metabolize progestins may decrease the plasma concentrations of progestins, and may decrease the effectiveness of progestin-only pills. Some drugs or herbal products that may decrease the effectiveness of progestin-only pills include barbiturates).
No products indexed under this heading.

Sodium Butabarbital (Drugs or herbal products that induce enzymes, including CYP3A4, that metabolize progestins may decrease the plasma concentrations of progestins, and may decrease the effectiveness of progestin-only pills. Some drugs or herbal products that may decrease the effectiveness of progestin-only pills include barbiturates).
No products indexed under this heading.

Sodium Pentobarbital (Drugs or herbal products that induce enzymes, including CYP3A4, that metabolize progestins may decrease the plasma concentrations of progestins, and may decrease the effectiveness of progestin-only pills. Some drugs or herbal products that may decrease the effectiveness of progestin-only pills include barbiturates).
No products indexed under this heading.

IMPORTANT NOTE: Always consult each drug listing in the patient's regimen for possible interactions.

Sulfinpyrazone (Drugs or herbal products that induce enzymes, including CYP3A4, that metabolize progestins may decrease the plasma concentrations of progestins, and may decrease the effectiveness of progestin-only pills. Some drugs or herbal products that may decrease the effectiveness of progestin-only pills include barbiturates, bosentan, carbamazepine, felbamate, griseofulvin, oxcarbazepine, phenytoin, rifampin, St. John's wort, topiramate).
No products indexed under this heading.

Theophyllinate (Drugs or herbal products that induce enzymes, including CYP3A4, that metabolize progestins may decrease the plasma concentrations of progestins, and may decrease the effectiveness of progestin-only pills. Some drugs or herbal products that may decrease the effectiveness of progestin-only pills include barbiturates, bosentan, carbamazepine, felbamate, griseofulvin, oxcarbazepine, phenytoin, rifampin, St. John's wort, topiramate).
No products indexed under this heading.

Theophylline (Drugs or herbal products that induce enzymes, including CYP3A4, that metabolize progestins may decrease the plasma concentrations of progestins, and may decrease the effectiveness of progestin-only pills. Some drugs or herbal products that may decrease the effectiveness of progestin-only pills include barbiturates, bosentan, carbamazepine, felbamate, griseofulvin, oxcarbazepine, phenytoin, rifampin, St. John's wort, topiramate).
No products indexed under this heading.

Theophylline Anhydrous (Drugs or herbal products that induce enzymes, including CYP3A4, that metabolize progestins may decrease the plasma concentrations of progestins, and may decrease the effectiveness of progestin-only pills. Some drugs or herbal products that may decrease the effectiveness of progestin-only pills include barbiturates, bosentan, carbamazepine, felbamate, griseofulvin, oxcarbazepine, phenytoin, rifampin, St. John's wort, topiramate). Products include:
Uniphyl 2817

Theophylline Calcium Salicylate (Drugs or herbal products that induce enzymes, including CYP3A4, that metabolize progestins may decrease the plasma concentrations of progestins, and may decrease the effectiveness of progestin-only pills. Some drugs or herbal products that may decrease the effectiveness of progestin-only pills include barbiturates, bosentan, carbamazepine, felbamate, griseofulvin, oxcarbazepine, phenytoin, rifampin, St. John's wort, topiramate).
No products indexed under this heading.

Theophylline Dihydroxypropyl (Glyceryl) (Drugs or herbal products that induce enzymes, including CYP3A4, that metabolize progestins may decrease the plasma concentrations of progestins, and may decrease the effectiveness of progestin-only pills. Some drugs or herbal products that may decrease the effectiveness of progestin-only pills include barbiturates, bosentan, carbamazepine, felbamate, griseofulvin, oxcarbazepine, phenytoin, rifampin, St. John's wort, topiramate).
No products indexed under this heading.

Theophylline Ethylenediamine (Drugs or herbal products that induce enzymes, including CYP3A4, that metabolize progestins may decrease the plasma concentrations of progestins, and may decrease the effectiveness of progestin-only pills. Some drugs or herbal products that may decrease the effectiveness of progestin-only pills include barbiturates,

bosentan, carbamazepine, felbamate, griseofulvin, oxcarbazepine, phenytoin, rifampin, St. John's wort, topiramate).
No products indexed under this heading.

Theophylline Sodium Glycinate (Drugs or herbal products that induce enzymes, including CYP3A4, that metabolize progestins may decrease the plasma concentrations of progestins, and may decrease the effectiveness of progestin-only pills. Some drugs or herbal products that may decrease the effectiveness of progestin-only pills include barbiturates, bosentan, carbamazepine, felbamate, griseofulvin, oxcarbazepine, phenytoin, rifampin, St. John's wort, topiramate).
No products indexed under this heading.

Thiamylal Sodium (Drugs or herbal products that induce enzymes, including CYP3A4, that metabolize progestins may decrease the plasma concentrations of progestins, and may decrease the effectiveness of progestin-only pills. Some drugs or herbal products that may decrease the effectiveness of progestin-only pills include barbiturates).
No products indexed under this heading.

Tipranavir (Significant changes (increase or decrease) in the plasma levels of the progestin have been noted in some cases of co-administration of levonorgestrel with HIV protease inhibitors).
No products indexed under this heading.

Tobacco (Drugs or herbal products that induce enzymes, including CYP3A4, that metabolize progestins may decrease the plasma concentrations of progestins, and may decrease the effectiveness of progestin-only pills. Some drugs or herbal products that may decrease the effectiveness of progestin-only pills include barbiturates, bosentan, carbamazepine, felbamate, griseofulvin, oxcarbazepine, phenytoin, rifampin, St. John's wort, topiramate).
No products indexed under this heading.

Topiramate (Drugs or herbal products that induce enzymes, including CYP3A4, that metabolize progestins may decrease the plasma concentrations of progestins, and may decrease the effectiveness of progestin-only pills. Some drugs or herbal products that may decrease the effectiveness of progestin-only pills include topiramate).
No products indexed under this heading.

Triamcinolone (Drugs or herbal products that induce enzymes, including CYP3A4, that metabolize progestins may decrease the plasma concentrations of progestins, and may decrease the effectiveness of progestin-only pills. Some drugs or herbal products that may decrease the effectiveness of progestin-only pills include barbiturates, bosentan, carbamazepine, felbamate, griseofulvin, oxcarbazepine, phenytoin, rifampin, St. John's wort, topiramate).
No products indexed under this heading.

Triamcinolone Acetonide (Drugs or herbal products that induce enzymes, including CYP3A4, that metabolize progestins may decrease the plasma concentrations of progestins, and may decrease the effectiveness of progestin-only pills. Some drugs or herbal products that may decrease the effectiveness of progestin-only pills include barbiturates, bosentan, carbamazepine, felbamate, griseofulvin, oxcarbazepine, phenytoin, rifampin, St. John's wort, topiramate). Products include:
Azmacort 408
Nasacort AQ 3019

Triamcinolone Diacetate (Drugs or herbal products that induce enzymes, including CYP3A4, that metabolize progestins may decrease the plasma

concentrations of progestins, and may decrease the effectiveness of progestin-only pills. Some drugs or herbal products that may decrease the effectiveness of progestin-only pills include barbiturates, bosentan, carbamazepine, felbamate, griseofulvin, oxcarbazepine, phenytoin, rifampin, St. John's wort, topiramate).
No products indexed under this heading.

Triamcinolone Hexacetonide (Drugs or herbal products that induce enzymes, including CYP3A4, that metabolize progestins may decrease the plasma concentrations of progestins, and may decrease the effectiveness of progestin-only pills. Some drugs or herbal products that may decrease the effectiveness of progestin-only pills include barbiturates, bosentan, carbamazepine, felbamate, griseofulvin, oxcarbazepine, phenytoin, rifampin, St. John's wort, topiramate).
No products indexed under this heading.

Troglitazone (Drugs or herbal products that induce enzymes, including CYP3A4, that metabolize progestins may decrease the plasma concentrations of progestins, and may decrease the effectiveness of progestin-only pills. Some drugs or herbal products that may decrease the effectiveness of progestin-only pills include barbiturates, bosentan, carbamazepine, felbamate, griseofulvin, oxcarbazepine, phenytoin, rifampin, St. John's wort, topiramate).
No products indexed under this heading.

Food Interactions

Broccoli (Drugs or herbal products that induce enzymes, including CYP3A4, that metabolize progestins may decrease the plasma concentrations of progestins, and may decrease the effectiveness of progestin-only pills. Some drugs or herbal products that may decrease the effectiveness of progestin-only pills include barbiturates, bosentan, carbamazepine, felbamate, griseofulvin, oxcarbazepine, phenytoin, rifampin, St. John's wort, topiramate).

Brussel Sprouts (Drugs or herbal products that induce enzymes, including CYP3A4, that metabolize progestins may decrease the plasma concentrations of progestins, and may decrease the effectiveness of progestin-only pills. Some drugs or herbal products that may decrease the effectiveness of progestin-only pills include barbiturates, bosentan, carbamazepine, felbamate, griseofulvin, oxcarbazepine, phenytoin, rifampin, St. John's wort, topiramate).

Charbroiled Food (Drugs or herbal products that induce enzymes, including CYP3A4, that metabolize progestins may decrease the plasma concentrations of progestins, and may decrease the effectiveness of progestin-only pills. Some drugs or herbal products that may decrease the effectiveness of progestin-only pills include barbiturates, bosentan, carbamazepine, felbamate, griseofulvin, oxcarbazepine, phenytoin, rifampin, St. John's wort, topiramate).

PLAVIX TABLETS
(Clopidogrel Bisulfate) 3027
May interact with aspirin-acetylsalicylic acid, cytochrome p450 2c19 inhibitors (selected), non-steroidal anti-inflammatory agents, phenytoin, and certain other agents. Compounds in these categories include:

Aspirin (Aspirin did not modify the clopidogrel-mediated inhibition of ADP-induced platelet aggregation. Concomitant administration of 500 mg of aspirin twice a day for 1 day did not significantly increase the prolongation of bleeding time induced by clopidogrel. Clopi-

dogrel potentiated the effect of aspirin on collagen induced platelet aggregation. Clopidogrel and aspirin have been administered together for up to one year). Products include:
Aggrenox 880
Bayer Aspirin 829
Percodan 1124
St. Joseph Aspirin 2045

Aspirin, Enteric Coated (Aspirin did not modify the clopidogrel-mediated inhibition of ADP-induced platelet aggregation. Concomitant administration of 500 mg of aspirin twice a day for 1 day did not significantly increase the prolongation of bleeding time induced by clopidogrel. Clopidogrel potentiated the effect of aspirin on collagen induced platelet aggregation. Clopidogrel and aspirin have been administered together for up to one year).
No products indexed under this heading.

Aspirin Buffered (Aspirin did not modify the clopidogrel-mediated inhibition of ADP-induced platelet aggregation. Concomitant administration of 500 mg of aspirin twice a day for 1 day did not significantly increase the prolongation of bleeding time induced by clopidogrel. Clopidogrel potentiated the effect of aspirin on collagen induced platelet aggregation. Clopidogrel and aspirin have been administered together for up to one year).
No products indexed under this heading.

Celecoxib (In healthy volunteers receiving naproxen, concomitant administration of clopidogrel was associated with increased occult gastrointestinal blood loss. At high concentrations *in vitro*, clopidogrel inhibits P450 (2C9). Accordingly, clopidogrel may interfere with the metabolism of many non-steroidal anti-inflammatory agents, but there is no data with which to predict the magnitude of this interaction. NSAIDs and clopidogrel should be co-administered with caution). Products include:
Celebrex 3272

Cimetidine (Since clopidogrel is metabolized to its active metabolite by CYP2C19, use of drugs that inhibit the activity of this enzyme would be expected to result in reduced drug levels of the active metabolite of clopidogrel and a reduction in clinical efficacy. Concomitant use of drugs that inhibit CYP2C19 should be discouraged).
No products indexed under this heading.

Cimetidine Hydrochloride (Since clopidogrel is metabolized to its active metabolite by CYP2C19, use of drugs that inhibit the activity of this enzyme would be expected to result in reduced drug levels of the active metabolite of clopidogrel and a reduction in clinical efficacy. Concomitant use of drugs that inhibit CYP2C19 should be discouraged).
No products indexed under this heading.

Citalopram Hydrobromide (Since clopidogrel is metabolized to its active metabolite by CYP2C19, use of drugs that inhibit the activity of this enzyme would be expected to result in reduced drug levels of the active metabolite of clopidogrel and a reduction in clinical efficacy. Concomitant use of drugs that inhibit CYP2C19 should be discouraged). Products include:
Celexa 1153

1433 Interactions Index Plavix

Delavirdine Mesylate (Since clopidogrel is metabolized to its active metabolite by CYP2C19, use of drugs that inhibit the activity of this enzyme would be expected to result in reduced drug levels of the active metabolite of clopidogrel and a reduction in clinical efficacy. Concomitant use of drugs that inhibit CYP2C19 should be discouraged).
No products indexed under this heading.

Desogestrel (Since clopidogrel is metabolized to its active metabolite by CYP2C19, use of drugs that inhibit the activity of this enzyme would be expected to result in reduced drug levels of the active metabolite of clopidogrel and a reduction in clinical efficacy. Concomitant use of drugs that inhibit CYP2C19 should be discouraged).
No products indexed under this heading.

Diclofenac Epolamine (In healthy volunteers receiving naproxen, concomitant administration of clopidogrel was associated with increased occult gastrointestinal blood loss. At high concentrations *in vitro*, clopidogrel inhibits P450 (2C9). Accordingly, clopidogrel may interfere with the metabolism of many non-steroidal anti-inflammatory agents, but there is no data with which to predict the magnitude of this interaction. NSAIDs and clopidogrel should be co-administered with caution). Products include:
Flector 1839

Diclofenac Potassium (In healthy volunteers receiving naproxen, concomitant administration of clopidogrel was associated with increased occult gastrointestinal blood loss. At high concentrations *in vitro*, clopidogrel inhibits P450 (2C9). Accordingly, clopidogrel may interfere with the metabolism of many non-steroidal anti-inflammatory agents, but there is no data with which to predict the magnitude of this interaction. NSAIDs and clopidogrel should be co-administered with caution).
No products indexed under this heading.

Diclofenac Sodium (In healthy volunteers receiving naproxen, concomitant administration of clopidogrel was associated with increased occult gastrointestinal blood loss. At high concentrations *in vitro*, clopidogrel inhibits P450 (2C9). Accordingly, clopidogrel may interfere with the metabolism of many non-steroidal anti-inflammatory agents, but there is no data with which to predict the magnitude of this interaction. NSAIDs and clopidogrel should be co-administered with caution).
No products indexed under this heading.

Efavirenz (Since clopidogrel is metabolized to its active metabolite by CYP2C19, use of drugs that inhibit the activity of this enzyme would be expected to result in reduced drug levels of the active metabolite of clopidogrel and a reduction in clinical efficacy. Concomitant use of drugs that inhibit CYP2C19 should be discouraged). Products include:
Atripla 906

Ethinyl Estradiol (Since clopidogrel is metabolized to its active metabolite by CYP2C19, use of drugs that inhibit the activity of this enzyme would be expected to result in reduced drug levels of the active metabolite of clopidogrel and a reduction in clinical efficacy. Concomitant use of drugs that inhibit CYP2C19 should be discouraged). Products include:
LoSeasonique 3407
Lybrel 3514
NuvaRing 3181
Ortho Evra 2648
Ortho-Cyclen/Ortho Tri-Cyclen 2663
Ortho Tri-Cyclen Lo Tablets 2673
Seasonique 3418
Yaz 864

Ethynodiol Diacetate (Since clopidogrel is metabolized to its active metabolite by CYP2C19, use of drugs that inhibit the activity of this enzyme would be expected to result in reduced drug levels of the active metabolite of clopidogrel and a reduction in clinical efficacy. Concomitant use of drugs that inhibit CYP2C19 should be discouraged).
No products indexed under this heading.

Etodolac (In healthy volunteers receiving naproxen, concomitant administration of clopidogrel was associated with increased occult gastrointestinal blood loss. At high concentrations *in vitro*, clopidogrel inhibits P450 (2C9). Accordingly, clopidogrel may interfere with the metabolism of many non-steroidal anti-inflammatory agents, but there is no data with which to predict the magnitude of this interaction. NSAIDs and clopidogrel should be co-administered with caution).
No products indexed under this heading.

Felbamate (Since clopidogrel is metabolized to its active metabolite by CYP2C19, use of drugs that inhibit the activity of this enzyme would be expected to result in reduced drug levels of the active metabolite of clopidogrel and a reduction in clinical efficacy. Concomitant use of drugs that inhibit CYP2C19 should be discouraged).
No products indexed under this heading.

Fenoprofen Calcium (In healthy volunteers receiving naproxen, concomitant administration of clopidogrel was associated with increased occult gastrointestinal blood loss. At high concentrations *in vitro*, clopidogrel inhibits P450 (2C9). Accordingly, clopidogrel may interfere with the metabolism of many non-steroidal anti-inflammatory agents, but there is no data with which to predict the magnitude of this interaction. NSAIDs and clopidogrel should be co-administered with caution).
No products indexed under this heading.

Fluoxetine (Since clopidogrel is metabolized to its active metabolite by CYP2C19, use of drugs that inhibit the activity of this enzyme would be expected to result in reduced drug levels of the active metabolite of clopidogrel and a reduction in clinical efficacy. Concomitant use of drugs that inhibit CYP2C19 should be discouraged).
No products indexed under this heading.

Fluoxetine Hydrochloride (Since clopidogrel is metabolized to its active metabolite by CYP2C19, use of drugs that inhibit the activity of this enzyme would be expected to result in reduced drug levels of the active metabolite of clopidogrel and a reduction in clinical efficacy. Concomitant use of drugs that inhibit CYP2C19 should be discouraged). Products include:
Prozac Weekly 1941
Prozac Pulvules 1941
Symbyax 1965

Flurbiprofen (In healthy volunteers receiving naproxen, concomitant administration of clopidogrel was associated with increased occult gastrointestinal blood loss. At high concentrations *in vitro*, clopidogrel inhibits P450 (2C9). Accordingly, clopidogrel may interfere with the metabolism of many non-steroidal anti-inflammatory agents, but there is no data with which to predict the magnitude of this interaction. NSAIDs and clopidogrel should be co-administered with caution).
No products indexed under this heading.

Fluvastatin Sodium (At high concentrations *in vitro*, clopidogrel inhibits P450 (2C9). Accordingly, clopidogrel may interfere with the metabolism of fluvastatin but there is no data with which to predict the magnitude of this interaction. Caution should be used when this drug is co-administered with clopidogrel).
No products indexed under this heading.

Fluvoxamine (Since clopidogrel is metabolized to its active metabolite by CYP2C19, use of drugs that inhibit the activity of this enzyme would be expected to result in reduced drug levels of the active metabolite of clopidogrel and a reduction in clinical efficacy. Concomitant use of drugs that inhibit CYP2C19 should be discouraged).
No products indexed under this heading.

Fluvoxamine Maleate (Since clopidogrel is metabolized to its active metabolite by CYP2C19, use of drugs that inhibit the activity of this enzyme would be expected to result in reduced drug levels of the active metabolite of clopidogrel and a reduction in clinical efficacy. Concomitant use of drugs that inhibit CYP2C19 should be discouraged).
No products indexed under this heading.

Fosphenytoin (At high concentrations *in vitro*, clopidogrel inhibits P450 (2C9). Accordingly, clopidogrel may interfere with the metabolism of phenytoin but there is no data with which to predict the magnitude of this interaction. Caution should be used when this drug is co-administered with clopidogrel).
No products indexed under this heading.

Fosphenytoin Sodium (At high concentrations *in vitro*, clopidogrel inhibits P450 (2C9). Accordingly, clopidogrel may interfere with the metabolism of phenytoin but there is no data with which to predict the magnitude of this interaction. Caution should be used when this drug is co-administered with clopidogrel).
No products indexed under this heading.

Ibuprofen (In healthy volunteers receiving naproxen, concomitant administration of clopidogrel was associated with increased occult gastrointestinal blood loss. At high concentrations *in vitro*, clopidogrel inhibits P450 (2C9). Accordingly, clopidogrel may interfere with the metabolism of many non-steroidal anti-inflammatory agents, but there is no data with which to predict the magnitude of this interaction. NSAIDs and clopidogrel should be co-administered with caution). Products include:
Motrin IB 2043
Children's Motrin 2044
Children's Motrin Non-Staining Dye-Free 2044
Infants' Motrin 2044
Infants' Motrin Dye-Free 2044
Junior Strength Motrin 2044
Vicoprofen 564

Indomethacin (In healthy volunteers receiving naproxen, concomitant administration of clopidogrel was associated with increased occult gastrointestinal blood loss. At high concentrations *in vitro*, clopidogrel inhibits P450 (2C9). Accordingly, clopidogrel may interfere with the metabolism of many non-steroidal anti-inflammatory agents, but there is no data with which to predict the magnitude of this interaction. NSAIDs and clopidogrel should be co-administered with caution). Products include:
Indocin 2167

Indomethacin Sodium Trihydrate (In healthy volunteers receiving naproxen, concomitant administration of clopidogrel was associated with increased occult gastrointestinal blood loss. At high concentrations *in vitro*, clopidogrel inhibits P450 (2C9). Accordingly, clopidogrel may interfere with the metabolism of many non-steroidal anti-inflammatory agents, but there is no data with which to predict the magnitude of this interaction. NSAIDs and clopidogrel should be co-administered with caution). Products include:
Indocin I.V. 2007

Isoniazid (Since clopidogrel is metabolized to its active metabolite by CYP2C19, use of drugs that inhibit the activity of this enzyme would be expected to result in reduced drug levels of the active metabolite of clopidogrel and a reduction in clinical efficacy. Concomitant use of drugs that inhibit CYP2C19 should be discouraged).
No products indexed under this heading.

Ketoconazole (Since clopidogrel is metabolized to its active metabolite by CYP2C19, use of drugs that inhibit the activity of this enzyme would be expected to result in reduced drug levels of the active metabolite of clopidogrel and a reduction in clinical efficacy. Concomitant use of drugs that inhibit CYP2C19 should be discouraged). Products include:
Extina 3319
Xolegel 3337

Ketoprofen (In healthy volunteers receiving naproxen, concomitant administration of clopidogrel was associated with increased occult gastrointestinal blood loss. At high concentrations *in vitro*, clopidogrel inhibits P450 (2C9). Accordingly, clopidogrel may interfere with the metabolism of many non-steroidal anti-inflammatory agents, but there is no data with which to predict the magnitude of this interaction. NSAIDs and clopidogrel should be co-administered with caution).
No products indexed under this heading.

Ketorolac Tromethamine (In healthy volunteers receiving naproxen, concomitant administration of clopidogrel was associated with increased occult gastrointestinal blood loss. At high concentrations *in vitro*, clopidogrel inhibits P450 (2C9). Accordingly, clopidogrel may interfere with the metabolism of many non-steroidal anti-inflammatory agents, but there is no data with which to predict the magnitude of this interaction. NSAIDs and clopidogrel should be co-administered with caution). Products include:
Acuvail .... ⊙ 209

Lansoprazole (Since clopidogrel is metabolized to its active metabolite by CYP2C19, use of drugs that inhibit the activity of this enzyme would be expected to result in reduced drug levels of the active metabolite of clopidogrel and a reduction in clinical efficacy. Concomitant use of drugs that inhibit CYP2C19 should be discouraged).
No products indexed under this heading.

Letrozole (Since clopidogrel is metabolized to its active metabolite by CYP2C19, use of drugs that inhibit the activity of this enzyme would be expected to result in reduced drug levels of the active metabolite of clopidogrel and a reduction in clinical efficacy. Concomitant use of drugs that inhibit CYP2C19 should be discouraged). Products include:
Femara 2466

Levonorgestrel (Since clopidogrel is metabolized to its active metabolite by CYP2C19, use of drugs that inhibit the activity of this enzyme would be expected to result in reduced drug levels of the active metabolite of clopidogrel and a reduction in clinical effica-

IMPORTANT NOTE: Always consult each drug listing in the patient's regimen for possible interactions.

Plavix Interactions Index 1434

cy. Concomitant use of drugs that inhibit CYP2C19 should be discouraged). Products include:
Climara Pro 847
LoSeasonique 3407
Lybrel 3514
Mirena 854
Plan B 3416
Seasonique 3418

Meclofenamate Sodium (In healthy volunteers receiving naproxen, concomitant administration of clopidogrel was associated with increased occult gastrointestinal blood loss. At high concentrations *in vitro*, clopidogrel inhibits P450 (2C9). Accordingly, clopidogrel may interfere with the metabolism of many non-steroidal anti-inflammatory agents, but there is no data with which to predict the magnitude of this interaction. NSAIDs and clopidogrel should be co-administered with caution).
No products indexed under this heading.

Mefenamic Acid (In healthy volunteers receiving naproxen, concomitant administration of clopidogrel was associated with increased occult gastrointestinal blood loss. At high concentrations *in vitro*, clopidogrel inhibits P450 (2C9). Accordingly, clopidogrel may interfere with the metabolism of many non-steroidal anti-inflammatory agents, but there is no data with which to predict the magnitude of this interaction. NSAIDs and clopidogrel should be co-administered with caution).
No products indexed under this heading.

Meloxicam (In healthy volunteers receiving naproxen, concomitant administration of clopidogrel was associated with increased occult gastrointestinal blood loss. At high concentrations *in vitro*, clopidogrel inhibits P450 (2C9). Accordingly, clopidogrel may interfere with the metabolism of many non-steroidal anti-inflammatory agents, but there is no data with which to predict the magnitude of this interaction. NSAIDs and clopidogrel should be co-administered with caution).
No products indexed under this heading.

Mestranol (Since clopidogrel is metabolized to its active metabolite by CYP2C19, use of drugs that inhibit the activity of this enzyme would be expected to result in reduced drug levels of the active metabolite of clopidogrel and a reduction in clinical efficacy. Concomitant use of drugs that inhibit CYP2C19 should be discouraged).
No products indexed under this heading.

Modafinil (Since clopidogrel is metabolized to its active metabolite by CYP2C19, use of drugs that inhibit the activity of this enzyme would be expected to result in reduced drug levels of the active metabolite of clopidogrel and a reduction in clinical efficacy. Concomitant use of drugs that inhibit CYP2C19 should be discouraged). Products include:
Provigil 983

Nabumetone (In healthy volunteers receiving naproxen, concomitant administration of clopidogrel was associated with increased occult gastrointestinal blood loss. At high concentrations *in vitro*, clopidogrel inhibits P450 (2C9). Accordingly, clopidogrel may interfere with the metabolism of many non-steroidal anti-inflammatory agents, but there is no data with which to predict the magnitude of this interaction. NSAIDs and clopidogrel should be co-administered with caution).
No products indexed under this heading.

Naproxen (In healthy volunteers receiving naproxen, concomitant administration of clopidogrel was associated with increased occult gastrointestinal blood loss. At high concentrations *in vitro*, clopidogrel inhibits P450 (2C9). Accordingly, clopidogrel may interfere with the metabolism of many non-steroidal anti-inflammatory agents, but there is no data with which to predict the magnitude of this interaction. NSAIDs and clopidogrel should be co-administered with caution). Products include:
EC-Naprosyn 2850
Naprosyn 2850
Anaprox/Naprosyn 2850

Naproxen Sodium (In healthy volunteers receiving naproxen, concomitant administration of clopidogrel was associated with increased occult gastrointestinal blood loss. At high concentrations *in vitro*, clopidogrel inhibits P450 (2C9). Accordingly, clopidogrel may interfere with the metabolism of many non-steroidal anti-inflammatory agents, but there is no data with which to predict the magnitude of this interaction. NSAIDs and clopidogrel should be co-administered with caution). Products include:
Anaprox 2850
Anaprox DS 2850
Treximet 1681

Norethindrone (Since clopidogrel is metabolized to its active metabolite by CYP2C19, use of drugs that inhibit the activity of this enzyme would be expected to result in reduced drug levels of the active metabolite of clopidogrel and a reduction in clinical efficacy. Concomitant use of drugs that inhibit CYP2C19 should be discouraged). Products include:
Ortho Micronor 2660

Norethynodrel (Since clopidogrel is metabolized to its active metabolite by CYP2C19, use of drugs that inhibit the activity of this enzyme would be expected to result in reduced drug levels of the active metabolite of clopidogrel and a reduction in clinical efficacy. Concomitant use of drugs that inhibit CYP2C19 should be discouraged).
No products indexed under this heading.

Norgestimate (Since clopidogrel is metabolized to its active metabolite by CYP2C19, use of drugs that inhibit the activity of this enzyme would be expected to result in reduced drug levels of the active metabolite of clopidogrel and a reduction in clinical efficacy. Concomitant use of drugs that inhibit CYP2C19 should be discouraged). Products include:
Ortho-Cyclen/Ortho Tri-Cyclen 2663
Ortho Tri-Cyclen Lo Tablets 2673

Norgestrel (Since clopidogrel is metabolized to its active metabolite by CYP2C19, use of drugs that inhibit the activity of this enzyme would be expected to result in reduced drug levels of the active metabolite of clopidogrel and a reduction in clinical efficacy. Concomitant use of drugs that inhibit CYP2C19 should be discouraged).
No products indexed under this heading.

Omeprazole (Since clopidogrel is metabolized to its active metabolite by CYP2C19, use of drugs that inhibit the activity of this enzyme would be expected to result in reduced drug levels of the active metabolite of clopidogrel and a reduction in clinical efficacy. Concomitant use of drugs that inhibit CYP2C19 (eg, omeprazole) should be discouraged).
No products indexed under this heading.

Omeprazole Magnesium (Since clopidogrel is metabolized to its active metabolite by CYP2C19, use of drugs that inhibit the activity of this enzyme would be expected to result in reduced drug levels of the active metabolite of clopidogrel and a reduction in clinical efficacy. Concomitant use of drugs that inhibit CYP2C19 (eg, omeprazole) should be discouraged).
No products indexed under this heading.

Oxaprozin (In healthy volunteers receiving naproxen, concomitant administration of clopidogrel was associated with increased occult gastrointestinal blood loss. At high concentrations *in vitro*, clopidogrel inhibits P450 (2C9). Accordingly, clopidogrel may interfere with the metabolism of many non-steroidal anti-inflammatory agents, but there is no data with which to predict the magnitude of this interaction. NSAIDs and clopidogrel should be co-administered with caution).
No products indexed under this heading.

Oxcarbazepine (Since clopidogrel is metabolized to its active metabolite by CYP2C19, use of drugs that inhibit the activity of this enzyme would be expected to result in reduced drug levels of the active metabolite of clopidogrel and a reduction in clinical efficacy. Concomitant use of drugs that inhibit CYP2C19 should be discouraged).
No products indexed under this heading.

Paroxetine Hydrochloride (Since clopidogrel is metabolized to its active metabolite by CYP2C19, use of drugs that inhibit the activity of this enzyme would be expected to result in reduced drug levels of the active metabolite of clopidogrel and a reduction in clinical efficacy. Concomitant use of drugs that inhibit CYP2C19 should be discouraged). Products include:
Paroxetine CR 2361
Paroxetine ER 2371
Paxil 1586
Paxil CR 1596

Phenylbutazone (In healthy volunteers receiving naproxen, concomitant administration of clopidogrel was associated with increased occult gastrointestinal blood loss. At high concentrations *in vitro*, clopidogrel inhibits P450 (2C9). Accordingly, clopidogrel may interfere with the metabolism of many non-steroidal anti-inflammatory agents, but there is no data with which to predict the magnitude of this interaction. NSAIDs and clopidogrel should be co-administered with caution).
No products indexed under this heading.

Phenytoin (At high concentrations *in vitro*, clopidogrel inhibits P450 (2C9). Accordingly, clopidogrel may interfere with the metabolism of phenytoin but there is no data with which to predict the magnitude of this interaction. Caution should be used when this drug is co-administered with clopidogrel).
No products indexed under this heading.

Phenytoin Sodium (At high concentrations *in vitro*, clopidogrel inhibits P450 (2C9). Accordingly, clopidogrel may interfere with the metabolism of phenytoin but there is no data with which to predict the magnitude of this interaction. Caution should be used when this drug is co-administered with clopidogrel). Products include:
Phenytek Capsules 2380

Piroxicam (In healthy volunteers receiving naproxen, concomitant administration of clopidogrel was associated with increased occult gastrointestinal blood loss. At high concentrations *in vitro*, clopidogrel inhibits P450 (2C9). Accordingly, clopidogrel may interfere with the metabolism of many non-steroidal anti-inflammatory agents, but there is no data with which to predict the magnitude of this interaction. NSAIDs and clopidogrel should be co-administered with caution).
No products indexed under this heading.

Quinidine (Since clopidogrel is metabolized to its active metabolite by CYP2C19, use of drugs that inhibit the activity of this enzyme would be expected to result in reduced drug levels of the active metabolite of clopidogrel and a reduction in clinical efficacy. Concomitant use of drugs that inhibit CYP2C19 should be discouraged).
No products indexed under this heading.

Quinidine Gluconate (Since clopidogrel is metabolized to its active metabolite by CYP2C19, use of drugs that inhibit the activity of this enzyme would be expected to result in reduced drug levels of the active metabolite of clopidogrel and a reduction in clinical efficacy. Concomitant use of drugs that inhibit CYP2C19 should be discouraged).
No products indexed under this heading.

Quinidine Hydrochloride (Since clopidogrel is metabolized to its active metabolite by CYP2C19, use of drugs that inhibit the activity of this enzyme would be expected to result in reduced drug levels of the active metabolite of clopidogrel and a reduction in clinical efficacy. Concomitant use of drugs that inhibit CYP2C19 should be discouraged).
No products indexed under this heading.

Quinidine Polygalacturonate (Since clopidogrel is metabolized to its active metabolite by CYP2C19, use of drugs that inhibit the activity of this enzyme would be expected to result in reduced drug levels of the active metabolite of clopidogrel and a reduction in clinical efficacy. Concomitant use of drugs that inhibit CYP2C19 should be discouraged).
No products indexed under this heading.

Quinidine Sulfate (Since clopidogrel is metabolized to its active metabolite by CYP2C19, use of drugs that inhibit the activity of this enzyme would be expected to result in reduced drug levels of the active metabolite of clopidogrel and a reduction in clinical efficacy. Concomitant use of drugs that inhibit CYP2C19 should be discouraged).
No products indexed under this heading.

Ritonavir (Since clopidogrel is metabolized to its active metabolite by CYP2C19, use of drugs that inhibit the activity of this enzyme would be expected to result in reduced drug levels of the active metabolite of clopidogrel and a reduction in clinical efficacy. Concomitant use of drugs that inhibit CYP2C19 should be discouraged). Products include:
Kaletra 458
Norvir 509

Rofecoxib (In healthy volunteers receiving naproxen, concomitant administration of clopidogrel was associated with increased occult gastrointestinal blood loss. At high concentrations *in vitro*, clopidogrel inhibits P450 (2C9). Accordingly, clopidogrel may interfere with the metabolism of many non-steroidal anti-inflammatory agents, but there is no data with which to predict the magnitude of this interaction. NSAIDs and clopidogrel should be co-administered with caution).
No products indexed under this heading.

Sertraline Hydrochloride (Since clopidogrel is metabolized to its active metabolite by CYP2C19, use of drugs that inhibit the activity of this enzyme would be expected to result in reduced drug levels of the active metabolite of clopidogrel and a reduction in clinical efficacy. Concomitant use of drugs that inhibit CYP2C19 should be discouraged).
No products indexed under this heading.

Sildenafil Citrate (Since clopidogrel is metabolized to its active metabolite by CYP2C19, use of drugs that inhibit the activity of this enzyme would be expected to result in reduced drug levels of the active metabolite of clopidogrel and a reduction in clinical efficacy. Concomitant use of drugs that inhibit CYP2C19 should be discouraged).
No products indexed under this heading.

Sulfaphenazole (Since clopidogrel is metabolized to its active metabolite by CYP2C19, use of drugs that inhibit the activity of this enzyme would be expected to result in reduced drug levels of the active metabolite of clopidogrel and a reduction in clinical efficacy. Concomitant use of drugs that inhibit CYP2C19 should be discouraged).
No products indexed under this heading.

Sulindac (In healthy volunteers receiving naproxen, concomitant administration of clopidogrel was associated with increased occult gastrointestinal blood loss. At high concentrations in vitro, clopidogrel inhibits P450 (2C9). Accordingly, clopidogrel may interfere with the metabolism of many non-steroidal anti-inflammatory agents, but there is no data with which to predict the magnitude of this interaction. NSAIDs and clopidogrel should be co-administered with caution). Products include:
Clinoril 2098

Tamoxifen Citrate (At high concentrations in vitro, clopidogrel inhibits P450 (2C9). Accordingly, clopidogrel may interfere with the metabolism of tamoxifen but there is no data with which to predict the magnitude of this interaction. Caution should be used when this drug is co-administered with clopidogrel).
No products indexed under this heading.

Telmisartan (Since clopidogrel is metabolized to its active metabolite by CYP2C19, use of drugs that inhibit the activity of this enzyme would be expected to result in reduced drug levels of the active metabolite of clopidogrel and a reduction in clinical efficacy. Concomitant use of drugs that inhibit CYP2C19 should be discouraged). Products include:
Micardis 887
Micardis HCT 889

Ticlopidine Hydrochloride (Since clopidogrel is metabolized to its active metabolite by CYP2C19, use of drugs that inhibit the activity of this enzyme would be expected to result in reduced drug levels of the active metabolite of clopidogrel and a reduction in clinical efficacy. Concomitant use of drugs that inhibit CYP2C19 should be discouraged).
No products indexed under this heading.

Tolbutamide (At high concentrations in vitro, clopidogrel inhibits P450 (2C9). Accordingly, clopidogrel may interfere with the metabolism of tolbutamide but there is no data with which to predict the magnitude of this interaction. Caution should be used when this drug is co-administered with clopidogrel).
No products indexed under this heading.

Tolbutamide Sodium (At high concentrations in vitro, clopidogrel inhibits P450 (2C9). Accordingly, clopidogrel may interfere with the metabolism of tolbutamide but there is no data with which to predict the magnitude of this interaction. Caution should be used when this drug is co-administered with clopidogrel).
No products indexed under this heading.

Tolmetin Sodium (In healthy volunteers receiving naproxen, concomitant administration of clopidogrel was associated with increased occult gastrointestinal blood loss. At high concentrations in vitro, clopidogrel inhibits P450 (2C9). Accordingly, clopidogrel may interfere with the metabolism of many non-steroidal anti-inflammatory agents, but there is no data with which to predict the magnitude of this interaction. NSAIDs and clopidogrel should be co-administered with caution).
No products indexed under this heading.

Topiramate (Since clopidogrel is metabolized to its active metabolite by CYP2C19, use of drugs that inhibit the activity of this enzyme would be expected to result in reduced drug levels of the active metabolite of clopidogrel and a reduction in clinical efficacy. Concomitant use of drugs that inhibit CYP2C19 should be discouraged).
No products indexed under this heading.

Torsemide (At high concentrations in vitro, clopidogrel inhibits P450 (2C9). Accordingly, clopidogrel may interfere with the metabolism of torsemide but there is no data with which to predict the magnitude of this interaction. Caution should be used when this drug is co-administered with clopidogrel).
No products indexed under this heading.

Tranylcypromine Sulfate (Since clopidogrel is metabolized to its active metabolite by CYP2C19, use of drugs that inhibit the activity of this enzyme would be expected to result in reduced drug levels of the active metabolite of clopidogrel and a reduction in clinical efficacy. Concomitant use of drugs that inhibit CYP2C19 should be discouraged). Products include:
Parnate 1584

Valdecoxib (In healthy volunteers receiving naproxen, concomitant administration of clopidogrel was associated with increased occult gastrointestinal blood loss. At high concentrations in vitro, clopidogrel inhibits P450 (2C9). Accordingly, clopidogrel may interfere with the metabolism of many non-steroidal anti-inflammatory agents, but there is no data with which to predict the magnitude of this interaction. NSAIDs and clopidogrel should be co-administered with caution).
No products indexed under this heading.

Vardenafil Hydrochloride (Since clopidogrel is metabolized to its active metabolite by CYP2C19, use of drugs that inhibit the activity of this enzyme would be expected to result in reduced drug levels of the active metabolite of clopidogrel and a reduction in clinical efficacy. Concomitant use of drugs that inhibit CYP2C19 should be discouraged). Products include:
Levitra 3157

Voriconazole (Since clopidogrel is metabolized to its active metabolite by CYP2C19, use of drugs that inhibit the activity of this enzyme would be expected to result in reduced drug levels of the active metabolite of clopidogrel and a reduction in clinical efficacy. Concomitant use of drugs that inhibit CYP2C19 should be discouraged).
No products indexed under this heading.

Warfarin Sodium (Because of the increased risk of bleeding, the concomitant administration of warfarin with clopidogrel should be undertaken with caution. At high concentrations in vitro, clopidogrel inhibits P450 (2C9). Accordingly, clopidogrel may interfere with the metabolism of warfarin but there is no data with which to predict the magnitude of this interaction. Caution should be used when this drug is co-administered with clopidogrel).
No products indexed under this heading.

PNEUMOVAX 23
(Pneumococcal Vaccine, Polyvalent) 2230
May interact with immunosuppressive agents. Compounds in these categories include:

Azathioprine (Co-administration of vaccine in patients receiving immunosuppressive therapy may not result in expected serum antibody response; potential impairment of future immune responses to pneumoccocal antigens may occur. Pneumococcal vaccination should be administered at least two weeks prior to the initiation of immunosuppressive therapy).
No products indexed under this heading.

Basiliximab (Co-administration of vaccine in patients receiving immunosuppressive therapy may not result in expected serum antibody response; potential impairment of future immune responses to pneumoccocal antigens may occur. Pneumococcal vaccination should be administered at least two weeks prior to the initiation of immunosuppressive therapy). Products include:
Simulect 2524

Cyclosporine (Co-administration of vaccine in patients receiving immunosuppressive therapy may not result in expected serum antibody response; potential impairment of future immune responses to pneumoccocal antigens may occur. Pneumococcal vaccination should be administered at least two weeks prior to the initiation of immunosuppressive therapy). Products include:
Gengraf 440
Neoral Oral Solution 2496
Neoral Capsules 2496
Restasis 605

Muromonab-CD3 (Co-administration of vaccine in patients receiving immunosuppressive therapy may not result in expected serum antibody response; potential impairment of future immune responses to pneumoccocal antigens may occur. Pneumococcal vaccination should be administered at least two weeks prior to the initiation of immunosuppressive therapy). Products include:
Orthoclone OKT3 949

Mycophenolate Mofetil (Co-administration of vaccine in patients receiving immunosuppressive therapy may not result in expected serum antibody response; potential impairment of future immune responses to pneumoccocal antigens may occur. Pneumococcal vaccination should be administered at least two weeks prior to the initiation of immunosuppressive therapy).
No products indexed under this heading.

Rapamycin (Co-administration of vaccine in patients receiving immunosuppressive therapy may not result in expected serum antibody response; potential impairment of future immune responses to pneumoccocal antigens may occur. Pneumococcal vaccination should be administered at least two weeks prior to the initiation of immunosuppressive therapy).
No products indexed under this heading.

Sirolimus (Co-administration of vaccine in patients receiving immunosuppressive therapy may not result in expected serum antibody response;

potential impairment of future immune responses to pneumoccocal antigens may occur. Pneumococcal vaccination should be administered at least two weeks prior to the initiation of immunosuppressive therapy). Products include:
Rapamune 3579

Tacrolimus (Co-administration of vaccine in patients receiving immunosuppressive therapy may not result in expected serum antibody response; potential impairment of future immune responses to pneumoccocal antigens may occur. Pneumococcal vaccination should be administered at least two weeks prior to the initiation of immunosuppressive therapy). Products include:
Prograf Capsules 677
Prograf Injection 677
Protopic 685

POTABA CAPSULES
(Aminobenzoate Potassium) 1769
May interact with sulfonamides. Compounds in these categories include:

Bendroflumethiazide (Co-administration with sulfonamides is contraindicated).
No products indexed under this heading.

Chlorothiazide (Co-administration with sulfonamides is contraindicated).
No products indexed under this heading.

Chlorothiazide Sodium (Co-administration with sulfonamides is contraindicated). Products include:
Diuril Intravenous 2009

Chlorpropamide (Co-administration with sulfonamides is contraindicated).
No products indexed under this heading.

Glipizide (Co-administration with sulfonamides is contraindicated).
No products indexed under this heading.

Glyburide (Co-administration with sulfonamides is contraindicated).
No products indexed under this heading.

Hydrochlorothiazide (Co-administration with sulfonamides is contraindicated). Products include:
Atacand HCT 700
Avalide 2956
Benicar HCT 1017
Diovan HCT 2419
Dyazide 1429
Exforge HCT 2449
Hyzaar 2162
Hyzaar 100-12.5 2162
Micardis HCT 889
Prinzide 2246
Tekturna HCT 2541
Teveten HCT 541

Hydroflumethiazide (Co-administration with sulfonamides is contraindicated).
No products indexed under this heading.

Methyclothiazide (Co-administration with sulfonamides is contraindicated).
No products indexed under this heading.

Polythiazide (Co-administration with sulfonamides is contraindicated).
No products indexed under this heading.

Sulfacytine (Co-administration with sulfonamides is contraindicated).
No products indexed under this heading.

Sulfamethizole (Co-administration with sulfonamides is contraindicated).
No products indexed under this heading.

Sulfamethoxazole (Co-administration with sulfonamides is contraindicated).
No products indexed under this heading.

Sulfasalazine (Co-administration with sulfonamides is contraindicated).
No products indexed under this heading.

Sulfinpyrazone (Co-administration with sulfonamides is contraindicated).
No products indexed under this heading.

Sulfisoxazole Acetyl (Co-administration with sulfonamides is contraindicated).
No products indexed under this heading.

Sulfisoxazole Diolamine (Co-administration with sulfonamides is contraindicated).
No products indexed under this heading.

Tolazamide (Co-administration with sulfonamides is contraindicated).
No products indexed under this heading.

Tolbutamide (Co-administration with sulfonamides is contraindicated).
No products indexed under this heading.

POTABA TABLETS
(Aminobenzoate Potassium) 1769
See Potaba Capsules

PRED FORTE OPHTHALMIC SUSPENSION
(Prednisolone Acetate) .... ⊙225
None cited in PDR database.

PRED MILD OPHTHALMIC SUSPENSION
(Prednisolone Acetate) .... ⊙230
None cited in PDR database.

PRED-G OPHTHALMIC OINTMENT
(Gentamicin Sulfate, Prednisolone Acetate)... ⊙226
None cited in PDR database.

PRED-G OPHTHALMIC SUSPENSION
(Gentamicin Sulfate, Prednisolone Acetate)... ⊙227
None cited in PDR database.

PREMARIN INTRAVENOUS
(Estrogens, Conjugated) 3528
See Premarin Tablets

PREMARIN TABLETS
(Estrogens, Conjugated) 3533
May interact with cytochrome p450 3a4 inducers (selected), cytochrome p450 3a4 inhibitors (selected), and certain other agents. Compounds in these categories include:

Acetazolamide (Co-administration of inhibitors of CYP3A4 with estrogens may affect estrogen drug metabolism. Inhibitors of CYP3A4 may increase plasma concentrations of estrogens and may result in side effects).
No products indexed under this heading.

Acetazolamide Sodium (Co-administration of inhibitors of CYP3A4 with estrogens may affect estrogen drug metabolism. Inhibitors of CYP3A4 may increase plasma concentrations of estrogens and may result in side effects).
No products indexed under this heading.

Allium sativum (Co-administration of inducers of CYP3A4 with estrogens may affect estrogen drug metabolism. Inducers of CYP3A4 may reduce plasma concentrations of estrogens, possibly resulting in a decrease in therapeutic effects and/or changes in the uterine bleeding profile).
No products indexed under this heading.

Aminoglutethimide (Co-administration of inducers of CYP3A4 with estrogens may affect estrogen drug metabolism. Inducers of CYP3A4 may reduce plasma concentrations of estrogens, possibly resulting in a decrease in therapeutic effects and/or changes in the uterine bleeding profile).
No products indexed under this heading.

Amiodarone Hydrochloride (Co-administration of inhibitors of CYP3A4 with estrogens may affect estrogen drug metabolism. Inhibitors of CYP3A4 may increase plasma concentrations of estrogens and may result in side effects).
No products indexed under this heading.

Amprenavir (Co-administration of inhibitors of CYP3A4 with estrogens may affect estrogen drug metabolism. Inhibitors of CYP3A4 may increase plasma concentrations of estrogens and may result in side effects).
No products indexed under this heading.

Anastrozole (Co-administration of inhibitors of CYP3A4 with estrogens may affect estrogen drug metabolism. Inhibitors of CYP3A4 may increase plasma concentrations of estrogens and may result in side effects).
No products indexed under this heading.

Aprepitant (Co-administration of inducers of CYP3A4 with estrogens may affect estrogen drug metabolism. Inducers of CYP3A4 may reduce plasma concentrations of estrogens, possibly resulting in a decrease in therapeutic effects and/or changes in the uterine bleeding profile). Products include:
Emend 2124

Atazanavir (Co-administration of inhibitors of CYP3A4 with estrogens may affect estrogen drug metabolism. Inhibitors of CYP3A4 may increase plasma concentrations of estrogens and may result in side effects).
No products indexed under this heading.

Atazanavir Sulfate (Co-administration of inhibitors of CYP3A4 with estrogens may affect estrogen drug metabolism. Inhibitors of CYP3A4 may increase plasma concentrations of estrogens and may result in side effects).
No products indexed under this heading.

Betamethasone (Co-administration of inducers of CYP3A4 with estrogens may affect estrogen drug metabolism. Inducers of CYP3A4 may reduce plasma concentrations of estrogens, possibly resulting in a decrease in therapeutic effects and/or changes in the uterine bleeding profile).
No products indexed under this heading.

Betamethasone Acetate (Co-administration of inducers of CYP3A4 with estrogens may affect estrogen drug metabolism. Inducers of CYP3A4 may reduce plasma concentrations of estrogens, possibly resulting in a decrease in therapeutic effects and/or changes in the uterine bleeding profile).
No products indexed under this heading.

Betamethasone Benzoate (Co-administration of inducers of CYP3A4 with estrogens may affect estrogen drug metabolism. Inducers of CYP3A4 may reduce plasma concentrations of estrogens, possibly resulting in a decrease in therapeutic effects and/or changes in the uterine bleeding profile).
No products indexed under this heading.

Betamethasone Dipropionate (Co-administration of inducers of CYP3A4 with estrogens may affect estrogen drug metabolism. Inducers of CYP3A4 may reduce plasma concentrations of estrogens, possibly resulting in a decrease in therapeutic effects and/or changes in the uterine bleeding profile). Products include:
Diprolene Lotion 0.05% 3108
Diprolene Ointment 0.05% 3109
Diprolene AF Cream 0.05% 3107
Lotrisone 3163

Betamethasone Sodium Phosphate (Co-administration of inducers of CYP3A4 with estrogens may affect estrogen drug metabolism. Inducers of CYP3A4 may reduce plasma concentrations of estrogens, possibly resulting in a decrease in therapeutic effects and/or changes in the uterine bleeding profile).
No products indexed under this heading.

Betamethasone Valerate (Co-administration of inducers of CYP3A4 with estrogens may affect estrogen drug metabolism. Inducers of CYP3A4 may reduce plasma concentrations of estrogens, possibly resulting in a decrease in therapeutic effects and/or changes in the uterine bleeding profile). Products include:
Luxiq 3321

Bosentan (Co-administration of inducers of CYP3A4 with estrogens may affect estrogen drug metabolism. Inducers of CYP3A4 may reduce plasma concentrations of estrogens, possibly resulting in a decrease in therapeutic effects and/or changes in the uterine bleeding profile). Products include:
Tracleer 573

Carbamazepine (Co-administration of inducers of CYP3A4 with estrogens may affect estrogen drug metabolism. Inducers of CYP3A4 may reduce plasma concentrations of estrogens, possibly resulting in a decrease in therapeutic effects and/or changes in the uterine bleeding profile). Products include:
Carbatrol 3280
Equetro 3477

Cimetidine (Co-administration of inhibitors of CYP3A4 with estrogens may affect estrogen drug metabolism. Inhibitors of CYP3A4 may increase plasma concentrations of estrogens and may result in side effects).
No products indexed under this heading.

Cimetidine Hydrochloride (Co-administration of inhibitors of CYP3A4 with estrogens may affect estrogen drug metabolism. Inhibitors of CYP3A4 may increase plasma concentrations of estrogens and may result in side effects).
No products indexed under this heading.

Ciprofloxacin (Co-administration of inducers of CYP3A4 with estrogens may affect estrogen drug metabolism. Inducers of CYP3A4 may reduce plasma concentrations of estrogens, possibly resulting in a decrease in therapeutic effects and/or changes in the uterine bleeding profile). Products include:
Cipro I.V. 3082
Cipro 3073
Cipro XR 3091
Ciprodex 583

Ciprofloxacin Hydrochloride (Co-administration of inducers of CYP3A4 with estrogens may affect estrogen drug metabolism. Inducers of CYP3A4 may reduce plasma concentrations of estrogens, possibly resulting in a decrease in therapeutic effects and/or changes in the uterine bleeding profile). Products include:
Cipro 3073

Cisplatin (Co-administration of inducers of CYP3A4 with estrogens may affect estrogen drug metabolism. Inducers of CYP3A4 may reduce plasma concentrations of estrogens, possibly resulting in a decrease in therapeutic effects and/or changes in the uterine bleeding profile).
No products indexed under this heading.

Clarithromycin (Co-administration of inhibitors of CYP3A4 with estrogens may affect estrogen drug metabolism. Inhibitors of CYP3A4 may increase plas-

ma concentrations of estrogens and may result in side effects). Products include:
Biaxin/Biaxin XL 412

Clotrimazole (Co-administration of inhibitors of CYP3A4 with estrogens may affect estrogen drug metabolism. Inhibitors of CYP3A4 may increase plasma concentrations of estrogens and may result in side effects). Products include:
Lotrisone 3163

Conivaptan Hydrochloride (Co-administration of inhibitors of CYP3A4 with estrogens may affect estrogen drug metabolism. Inhibitors of CYP3A4 may increase plasma concentrations of estrogens and may result in side effects). Products include:
Vaprisol 689

Cortisone Acetate (Co-administration of inducers of CYP3A4 with estrogens may affect estrogen drug metabolism. Inducers of CYP3A4 may reduce plasma concentrations of estrogens, possibly resulting in a decrease in therapeutic effects and/or changes in the uterine bleeding profile).
No products indexed under this heading.

Cyclosporine (Co-administration of inhibitors of CYP3A4 with estrogens may affect estrogen drug metabolism. Inhibitors of CYP3A4 may increase plasma concentrations of estrogens and may result in side effects). Products include:
Gengraf 440
Neoral Oral Solution 2496
Neoral Capsules 2496
Restasis 605

Dalfopristin (Co-administration of inhibitors of CYP3A4 with estrogens may affect estrogen drug metabolism. Inhibitors of CYP3A4 may increase plasma concentrations of estrogens and may result in side effects).
No products indexed under this heading.

Danazol (Co-administration of inhibitors of CYP3A4 with estrogens may affect estrogen drug metabolism. Inhibitors of CYP3A4 may increase plasma concentrations of estrogens and may result in side effects).
No products indexed under this heading.

Darunavir (Co-administration of inhibitors of CYP3A4 with estrogens may affect estrogen drug metabolism. Inhibitors of CYP3A4 may increase plasma concentrations of estrogens and may result in side effects).
No products indexed under this heading.

Dasatinib (Co-administration of inhibitors of CYP3A4 with estrogens may affect estrogen drug metabolism. Inhibitors of CYP3A4 may increase plasma concentrations of estrogens and may result in side effects).
No products indexed under this heading.

Delavirdine Mesylate (Co-administration of inhibitors of CYP3A4 with estrogens may affect estrogen drug metabolism. Inhibitors of CYP3A4 may increase plasma concentrations of estrogens and may result in side effects).
No products indexed under this heading.

Delavirine (Co-administration of inhibitors of CYP3A4 with estrogens may affect estrogen drug metabolism. Inhibitors of CYP3A4 may increase plasma concentrations of estrogens and may result in side effects).
No products indexed under this heading.

Desloratadine (Co-administration of inhibitors of CYP3A4 with estrogens may affect estrogen drug metabolism. Inhibitors of CYP3A4 may increase plasma concentrations of estrogens and may result in side effects). Products include:
Clarinex Syrup 3098

(⊙ Described in PDR® for Ophthalmic Medicines)

Dexamethasone (Co-administration of inducers of CYP3A4 with estrogens may affect estrogen drug metabolism. Inducers of CYP3A4 may reduce plasma concentrations of estrogens, possibly resulting in a decrease in therapeutic effects and/or changes in the uterine bleeding profile). Products include:

Dexamethasone Acetate (Co-administration of inducers of CYP3A4 with estrogens may affect estrogen drug metabolism. Inducers of CYP3A4 may reduce plasma concentrations of estrogens, possibly resulting in a decrease in therapeutic effects and/or changes in the uterine bleeding profile).
No products indexed under this heading.

Dexamethasone Phosphate (Co-administration of inducers of CYP3A4 with estrogens may affect estrogen drug metabolism. Inducers of CYP3A4 may reduce plasma concentrations of estrogens, possibly resulting in a decrease in therapeutic effects and/or changes in the uterine bleeding profile).
No products indexed under this heading.

Dexamethasone Sodium (Co-administration of inducers of CYP3A4 with estrogens may affect estrogen drug metabolism. Inducers of CYP3A4 may reduce plasma concentrations of estrogens, possibly resulting in a decrease in therapeutic effects and/or changes in the uterine bleeding profile).
No products indexed under this heading.

Dexamethasone Sodium Phosphate (Co-administration of inducers of CYP3A4 with estrogens may affect estrogen drug metabolism. Inducers of CYP3A4 may reduce plasma concentrations of estrogens, possibly resulting in a decrease in therapeutic effects and/or changes in the uterine bleeding profile).
No products indexed under this heading.

Dexamethasone Sodium Phosphate Injection (Co-administration of inducers of CYP3A4 with estrogens may affect estrogen drug metabolism. Inducers of CYP3A4 may reduce plasma concentrations of estrogens, possibly resulting in a decrease in therapeutic effects and/or changes in the uterine bleeding profile).
No products indexed under this heading.

Diltiazem Hydrochloride (Co-administration of inhibitors of CYP3A4 with estrogens may affect estrogen drug metabolism. Inhibitors of CYP3A4 may increase plasma concentrations of estrogens and may result in side effects). Products include:

Diltiazem Maleate (Co-administration of inhibitors of CYP3A4 with estrogens may affect estrogen drug metabolism. Inhibitors of CYP3A4 may increase plasma concentrations of estrogens and may result in side effects).
No products indexed under this heading.

Doxorubicin Hydrochloride (Co-administration of inducers of CYP3A4 with estrogens may affect estrogen drug metabolism. Inducers of CYP3A4 may reduce plasma concentrations of estrogens, possibly resulting in a decrease in therapeutic effects and/or changes in the uterine bleeding profile).
No products indexed under this heading.

Efavirenz (Co-administration of inducers of CYP3A4 with estrogens may affect estrogen drug metabolism. Inducers of CYP3A4 may reduce plasma con-

centrations of estrogens, possibly resulting in a decrease in therapeutic effects and/or changes in the uterine bleeding profile). Products include:

Erythromycin (Co-administration of inhibitors of CYP3A4 with estrogens may affect estrogen drug metabolism. Inhibitors of CYP3A4 may increase plasma concentrations of estrogens and may result in side effects).
No products indexed under this heading.

Erythromycin Estolate (Co-administration of inhibitors of CYP3A4 with estrogens may affect estrogen drug metabolism. Inhibitors of CYP3A4 may increase plasma concentrations of estrogens and may result in side effects).
No products indexed under this heading.

Erythromycin Ethylsuccinate (Co-administration of inhibitors of CYP3A4 with estrogens may affect estrogen drug metabolism. Inhibitors of CYP3A4 may increase plasma concentrations of estrogens and may result in side effects). Products include:

Erythromycin Gluceptate (Co-administration of inhibitors of CYP3A4 with estrogens may affect estrogen drug metabolism. Inhibitors of CYP3A4 may increase plasma concentrations of estrogens and may result in side effects).
No products indexed under this heading.

Erythromycin Lactobionate (Co-administration of inhibitors of CYP3A4 with estrogens may affect estrogen drug metabolism. Inhibitors of CYP3A4 may increase plasma concentrations of estrogens and may result in side effects).
No products indexed under this heading.

Erythromycin Stearate (Co-administration of inhibitors of CYP3A4 with estrogens may affect estrogen drug metabolism. Inhibitors of CYP3A4 may increase plasma concentrations of estrogens and may result in side effects).
No products indexed under this heading.

Esomeprazole Magnesium (Co-administration of inhibitors of CYP3A4 with estrogens may affect estrogen drug metabolism. Inhibitors of CYP3A4 may increase plasma concentrations of estrogens and may result in side effects). Products include:

Esomeprazole Sodium (Co-administration of inhibitors of CYP3A4 with estrogens may affect estrogen drug metabolism. Inhibitors of CYP3A4 may increase plasma concentrations of estrogens and may result in side effects). Products include:

Ethosuximide (Co-administration of inducers of CYP3A4 with estrogens may affect estrogen drug metabolism. Inducers of CYP3A4 may reduce plasma concentrations of estrogens, possibly resulting in a decrease in therapeutic effects and/or changes in the uterine bleeding profile).
No products indexed under this heading.

Felbamate (Co-administration of inducers of CYP3A4 with estrogens may affect estrogen drug metabolism. Inducers of CYP3A4 may reduce plasma concentrations of estrogens, possibly resulting in a decrease in therapeutic effects and/or changes in the uterine bleeding profile).
No products indexed under this heading.

Fluconazole (Co-administration of inhibitors of CYP3A4 with estrogens may affect estrogen drug metabolism. Inhibitors of CYP3A4 may increase plasma concentrations of estrogens and may result in side effects).
No products indexed under this heading.

Fludrocortisone Acetate (Co-administration of inducers of CYP3A4 with estrogens may affect estrogen drug metabolism. Inducers of CYP3A4 may reduce plasma concentrations of estrogens, possibly resulting in a decrease in therapeutic effects and/or changes in the uterine bleeding profile).
No products indexed under this heading.

Fluoxetine (Co-administration of inhibitors of CYP3A4 with estrogens may affect estrogen drug metabolism. Inhibitors of CYP3A4 may increase plasma concentrations of estrogens and may result in side effects).
No products indexed under this heading.

Fluoxetine Hydrochloride (Co-administration of inhibitors of CYP3A4 with estrogens may affect estrogen drug metabolism. Inhibitors of CYP3A4 may increase plasma concentrations of estrogens and may result in side effects). Products include:

Fluvoxamine Maleate (Co-administration of inhibitors of CYP3A4 with estrogens may affect estrogen drug metabolism. Inhibitors of CYP3A4 may increase plasma concentrations of estrogens and may result in side effects).
No products indexed under this heading.

Fosamprenavir Calcium (Co-administration of inhibitors of CYP3A4 with estrogens may affect estrogen drug metabolism. Inhibitors of CYP3A4 may increase plasma concentrations of estrogens and may result in side effects). Products include:

Fosphenytoin Sodium (Co-administration of inducers of CYP3A4 with estrogens may affect estrogen drug metabolism. Inducers of CYP3A4 may reduce plasma concentrations of estrogens, possibly resulting in a decrease in therapeutic effects and/or changes in the uterine bleeding profile).
No products indexed under this heading.

Garlic Extract (Co-administration of inducers of CYP3A4 with estrogens may affect estrogen drug metabolism. Inducers of CYP3A4 may reduce plasma concentrations of estrogens, possibly resulting in a decrease in therapeutic effects and/or changes in the uterine bleeding profile).
No products indexed under this heading.

Garlic Oil (Co-administration of inducers of CYP3A4 with estrogens may affect estrogen drug metabolism. Inducers of CYP3A4 may reduce plasma concentrations of estrogens, possibly resulting in a decrease in therapeutic effects and/or changes in the uterine bleeding profile).
No products indexed under this heading.

Hydrocortisone (Co-administration of inducers of CYP3A4 with estrogens may affect estrogen drug metabolism. Inducers of CYP3A4 may reduce plasma concentrations of estrogens, possibly resulting in a decrease in therapeutic effects and/or changes in the uterine bleeding profile).
No products indexed under this heading.

Hydrocortisone (Alcohol) (Co-administration of inducers of CYP3A4 with estrogens may affect estrogen drug metabolism. Inducers of CYP3A4 may reduce plasma concentrations of estrogens, possibly resulting in a decrease in therapeutic effects and/or changes in the uterine bleeding profile).
No products indexed under this heading.

Hydrocortisone Acetate (Co-administration of inducers of CYP3A4 with estrogens may affect estrogen drug metabolism. Inducers of CYP3A4 may reduce plasma concentrations of estrogens, possibly resulting in a decrease in therapeutic effects and/or changes in the uterine bleeding profile).
No products indexed under this heading.

Hydrocortisone Butyrate (Co-administration of inducers of CYP3A4 with estrogens may affect estrogen drug metabolism. Inducers of CYP3A4 may reduce plasma concentrations of estrogens, possibly resulting in a decrease in therapeutic effects and/or changes in the uterine bleeding profile).
No products indexed under this heading.

Hydrocortisone Cypionate (Co-administration of inducers of CYP3A4 with estrogens may affect estrogen drug metabolism. Inducers of CYP3A4 may reduce plasma concentrations of estrogens, possibly resulting in a decrease in therapeutic effects and/or changes in the uterine bleeding profile).
No products indexed under this heading.

Hydrocortisone Hemisuccinate (Co-administration of inducers of CYP3A4 with estrogens may affect estrogen drug metabolism. Inducers of CYP3A4 may reduce plasma concentrations of estrogens, possibly resulting in a decrease in therapeutic effects and/or changes in the uterine bleeding profile).
No products indexed under this heading.

Hydrocortisone Probutate (Co-administration of inducers of CYP3A4 with estrogens may affect estrogen drug metabolism. Inducers of CYP3A4 may reduce plasma concentrations of estrogens, possibly resulting in a decrease in therapeutic effects and/or changes in the uterine bleeding profile).
No products indexed under this heading.

Hydrocortisone Sodium Phosphate (Co-administration of inducers of CYP3A4 with estrogens may affect estrogen drug metabolism. Inducers of CYP3A4 may reduce plasma concentrations of estrogens, possibly resulting in a decrease in therapeutic effects and/or changes in the uterine bleeding profile).
No products indexed under this heading.

Hydrocortisone Sodium Succinate (Co-administration of inducers of CYP3A4 with estrogens may affect estrogen drug metabolism. Inducers of CYP3A4 may reduce plasma concentrations of estrogens, possibly resulting in a decrease in therapeutic effects and/or changes in the uterine bleeding profile).
No products indexed under this heading.

Hydrocortisone Valerate (Co-administration of inducers of CYP3A4 with estrogens may affect estrogen drug metabolism. Inducers of CYP3A4 may reduce plasma concentrations of estrogens, possibly resulting in a decrease in therapeutic effects and/or changes in the uterine bleeding profile).
No products indexed under this heading.

IMPORTANT NOTE: Always consult each drug listing in the patient's regimen for possible interactions.

Premarin Tablets Interactions Index 1438

Hypericum (Co-administration of inducers of CYP3A4 with estrogens may affect estrogen drug metabolism. Inducers of CYP3A4 may reduce plasma concentrations of estrogens, possibly resulting in a decrease in therapeutic effects and/or changes in the uterine bleeding profile).
No products indexed under this heading.

Hypericum Perforatum (Co-administration of inducers of CYP3A4 with estrogens may affect estrogen drug metabolism. Inducers of CYP3A4 may reduce plasma concentrations of estrogens, possibly resulting in a decrease in therapeutic effects and/or changes in the uterine bleeding profile). Products include:
Traumeel 1800

Imatinib Mesylate (Co-administration of inhibitors of CYP3A4 with estrogens may affect estrogen drug metabolism. Inhibitors of CYP3A4 may increase plasma concentrations of estrogens and may result in side effects). Products include:
Gleevec 2477

Indinavir Sulfate (Co-administration of inhibitors of CYP3A4 with estrogens may affect estrogen drug metabolism. Inhibitors of CYP3A4 may increase plasma concentrations of estrogens and may result in side effects). Products include:
Crixivan 2113

Isoniazid (Co-administration of inhibitors of CYP3A4 with estrogens may affect estrogen drug metabolism. Inhibitors of CYP3A4 may increase plasma concentrations of estrogens and may result in side effects).
No products indexed under this heading.

Itraconazole (Co-administration of inhibitors of CYP3A4 with estrogens may affect estrogen drug metabolism. Inhibitors of CYP3A4 may increase plasma concentrations of estrogens and may result in side effects).
No products indexed under this heading.

Ketoconazole (Co-administration of inhibitors of CYP3A4 with estrogens may affect estrogen drug metabolism. Inhibitors of CYP3A4 may increase plasma concentrations of estrogens and may result in side effects). Products include:
Extina 3319
Xolegel 3337

Lapatinib (Co-administration of inhibitors of CYP3A4 with estrogens may affect estrogen drug metabolism. Inhibitors of CYP3A4 may increase plasma concentrations of estrogens and may result in side effects). Products include:
Tykerb 1698

Lopinavir (Co-administration of inhibitors of CYP3A4 with estrogens may affect estrogen drug metabolism. Inhibitors of CYP3A4 may increase plasma concentrations of estrogens and may result in side effects). Products include:
Kaletra 458

Loratadine (Co-administration of inhibitors of CYP3A4 with estrogens may affect estrogen drug metabolism. Inhibitors of CYP3A4 may increase plasma concentrations of estrogens and may result in side effects).
No products indexed under this heading.

Mephenytoin (Co-administration of inducers of CYP3A4 with estrogens may affect estrogen drug metabolism. Inducers of CYP3A4 may reduce plasma concentrations of estrogens, possibly resulting in a decrease in therapeutic effects and/or changes in the uterine bleeding profile).
No products indexed under this heading.

Methsuximide (Co-administration of inducers of CYP3A4 with estrogens may affect estrogen drug metabolism. Inducers of CYP3A4 may reduce plasma concentrations of estrogens, possibly resulting in a decrease in therapeutic effects and/or changes in the uterine bleeding profile).
No products indexed under this heading.

Methylprednisolone (Co-administration of inducers of CYP3A4 with estrogens may affect estrogen drug metabolism. Inducers of CYP3A4 may reduce plasma concentrations of estrogens, possibly resulting in a decrease in therapeutic effects and/or changes in the uterine bleeding profile).
No products indexed under this heading.

Methylprednisolone Acetate (Co-administration of inducers of CYP3A4 with estrogens may affect estrogen drug metabolism. Inducers of CYP3A4 may reduce plasma concentrations of estrogens, possibly resulting in a decrease in therapeutic effects and/or changes in the uterine bleeding profile).
No products indexed under this heading.

Methylprednisolone Sodium Succinate (Co-administration of inducers of CYP3A4 with estrogens may affect estrogen drug metabolism. Inducers of CYP3A4 may reduce plasma concentrations of estrogens, possibly resulting in a decrease in therapeutic effects and/or changes in the uterine bleeding profile).
No products indexed under this heading.

Metronidazole (Co-administration of inhibitors of CYP3A4 with estrogens may affect estrogen drug metabolism. Inhibitors of CYP3A4 may increase plasma concentrations of estrogens and may result in side effects). Products include:
Pylera 793

Metronidazole Benzoate (Co-administration of inhibitors of CYP3A4 with estrogens may affect estrogen drug metabolism. Inhibitors of CYP3A4 may increase plasma concentrations of estrogens and may result in side effects).
No products indexed under this heading.

Metronidazole Hydrochloride (Co-administration of inhibitors of CYP3A4 with estrogens may affect estrogen drug metabolism. Inhibitors of CYP3A4 may increase plasma concentrations of estrogens and may result in side effects).
No products indexed under this heading.

Metronidazole Sodium (Co-administration of inhibitors of CYP3A4 with estrogens may affect estrogen drug metabolism. Inhibitors of CYP3A4 may increase plasma concentrations of estrogens and may result in side effects).
No products indexed under this heading.

Miconazole (Co-administration of inhibitors of CYP3A4 with estrogens may affect estrogen drug metabolism. Inhibitors of CYP3A4 may increase plasma concentrations of estrogens and may result in side effects).
No products indexed under this heading.

Miconazole Nitrate (Co-administration of inhibitors of CYP3A4 with estrogens may affect estrogen drug metabolism. Inhibitors of CYP3A4 may increase plasma concentrations of estrogens and may result in side effects). Products include:
Vusion Ointment 3335

Mifepristone (Co-administration of inhibitors of CYP3A4 with estrogens may affect estrogen drug metabolism. Inhibitors of CYP3A4 may increase plasma concentrations of estrogens and may result in side effects).
No products indexed under this heading.

Modafinil (Co-administration of inducers of CYP3A4 with estrogens may affect estrogen drug metabolism. Inducers of CYP3A4 may reduce plasma concentrations of estrogens, possibly resulting in a decrease in therapeutic effects and/or changes in the uterine bleeding profile). Products include:
Provigil 983

Nafcillin Sodium (Co-administration of inducers of CYP3A4 with estrogens may affect estrogen drug metabolism. Inducers of CYP3A4 may reduce plasma concentrations of estrogens, possibly resulting in a decrease in therapeutic effects and/or changes in the uterine bleeding profile).
No products indexed under this heading.

Nefazodone Hydrochloride (Co-administration of inhibitors of CYP3A4 with estrogens may affect estrogen drug metabolism. Inhibitors of CYP3A4 may increase plasma concentrations of estrogens and may result in side effects).
No products indexed under this heading.

Nelfinavir Mesylate (Co-administration of inhibitors of CYP3A4 with estrogens may affect estrogen drug metabolism. Inhibitors of CYP3A4 may increase plasma concentrations of estrogens and may result in side effects).
No products indexed under this heading.

Nevirapine (Co-administration of inducers of CYP3A4 with estrogens may affect estrogen drug metabolism. Inducers of CYP3A4 may reduce plasma concentrations of estrogens, possibly resulting in a decrease in therapeutic effects and/or changes in the uterine bleeding profile). Products include:
Viramune Oral Suspension 897
Viramune Tablets 897

Niacin (Co-administration of inhibitors of CYP3A4 with estrogens may affect estrogen drug metabolism. Inhibitors of CYP3A4 may increase plasma concentrations of estrogens and may result in side effects). Products include:
Advicor 402
Cardio Basics 3455
Niaspan 497
Simcor 524

Niacinamide (Co-administration of inhibitors of CYP3A4 with estrogens may affect estrogen drug metabolism. Inhibitors of CYP3A4 may increase plasma concentrations of estrogens and may result in side effects). Products include:
CitraNatal 90 DHA Capsules 2332
CitraNatal Assure 2332
CitraNatal Rx 2332
Heplive 607

Niacinamide Hydroiodide (Co-administration of inhibitors of CYP3A4 with estrogens may affect estrogen drug metabolism. Inhibitors of CYP3A4 may increase plasma concentrations of estrogens and may result in side effects).
No products indexed under this heading.

Nicotinamide (Co-administration of inhibitors of CYP3A4 with estrogens may affect estrogen drug metabolism. Inhibitors of CYP3A4 may increase plasma concentrations of estrogens and may result in side effects).
No products indexed under this heading.

Nifedipine (Co-administration of inhibitors of CYP3A4 with estrogens may affect estrogen drug metabolism. Inhibitors of CYP3A4 may increase plasma concentrations of estrogens and may result in side effects).
No products indexed under this heading.

Norfloxacin (Co-administration of inhibitors of CYP3A4 with estrogens may affect estrogen drug metabolism. Inhibitors of CYP3A4 may increase plasma concentrations of estrogens and may result in side effects). Products include:
Noroxin 2220

Omeprazole (Co-administration of inhibitors of CYP3A4 with estrogens may affect estrogen drug metabolism. Inhibitors of CYP3A4 may increase plasma concentrations of estrogens and may result in side effects).
No products indexed under this heading.

Oxcarbazepine (Co-administration of inducers of CYP3A4 with estrogens may affect estrogen drug metabolism. Inducers of CYP3A4 may reduce plasma concentrations of estrogens, possibly resulting in a decrease in therapeutic effects and/or changes in the uterine bleeding profile).
No products indexed under this heading.

Paroxetine Hydrochloride (Co-administration of inhibitors of CYP3A4 with estrogens may affect estrogen drug metabolism. Inhibitors of CYP3A4 may increase plasma concentrations of estrogens and may result in side effects). Products include:
Paroxetine CR 2361
Paroxetine ER 2371
Paxil 1586
Paxil CR 1596

Phenobarbital (Co-administration of inducers of CYP3A4 with estrogens may affect estrogen drug metabolism. Inducers of CYP3A4 may reduce plasma concentrations of estrogens, possibly resulting in a decrease in therapeutic effects and/or changes in the uterine bleeding profile). Products include:
Donnatal 2711

Phenobarbital Sodium (Co-administration of inducers of CYP3A4 with estrogens may affect estrogen drug metabolism. Inducers of CYP3A4 may reduce plasma concentrations of estrogens, possibly resulting in a decrease in therapeutic effects and/or changes in the uterine bleeding profile).
No products indexed under this heading.

Phenytoin (Co-administration of inducers of CYP3A4 with estrogens may affect estrogen drug metabolism. Inducers of CYP3A4 may reduce plasma concentrations of estrogens, possibly resulting in a decrease in therapeutic effects and/or changes in the uterine bleeding profile).
No products indexed under this heading.

Phenytoin Sodium (Co-administration of inducers of CYP3A4 with estrogens may affect estrogen drug metabolism. Inducers of CYP3A4 may reduce plasma concentrations of estrogens, possibly resulting in a decrease in therapeutic effects and/or changes in the uterine bleeding profile). Products include:
Phenytek Capsules 2380

Posaconazole (Co-administration of inhibitors of CYP3A4 with estrogens may affect estrogen drug metabolism. Inhibitors of CYP3A4 may increase plasma concentrations of estrogens and may result in side effects). Products include:
Noxafil 3172

Prednisolone (Co-administration of inducers of CYP3A4 with estrogens may affect estrogen drug metabolism. Inducers of CYP3A4 may reduce plasma concentrations of estrogens, possibly resulting in a decrease in therapeutic effects and/or changes in the uterine bleeding profile).
No products indexed under this heading.

Prednisolone Acetate (Co-administration of inducers of CYP3A4 with estrogens may affect estrogen drug metabolism. Inducers of CYP3A4 may reduce plasma concentrations of estrogens, possibly resulting in a

decrease in therapeutic effects and/or changes in the uterine bleeding profile). Products include:

Prednisolone Sodium Phosphate (Co-administration of inducers of CYP3A4 with estrogens may affect estrogen drug metabolism. Inducers of CYP3A4 may reduce plasma concentrations of estrogens, possibly resulting in a decrease in therapeutic effects and/or changes in the uterine bleeding profile).
No products indexed under this heading.

Prednisolone Tebutate (Co-administration of inducers of CYP3A4 with estrogens may affect estrogen drug metabolism. Inducers of CYP3A4 may reduce plasma concentrations of estrogens, possibly resulting in a decrease in therapeutic effects and/or changes in the uterine bleeding profile).
No products indexed under this heading.

Prednisone (Co-administration of inducers of CYP3A4 with estrogens may affect estrogen drug metabolism. Inducers of CYP3A4 may reduce plasma concentrations of estrogens, possibly resulting in a decrease in therapeutic effects and/or changes in the uterine bleeding profile).
No products indexed under this heading.

Prednisone sodium phosphate (Co-administration of inducers of CYP3A4 with estrogens may affect estrogen drug metabolism. Inducers of CYP3A4 may reduce plasma concentrations of estrogens, possibly resulting in a decrease in therapeutic effects and/or changes in the uterine bleeding profile).
No products indexed under this heading.

Primidone (Co-administration of inducers of CYP3A4 with estrogens may affect estrogen drug metabolism. Inducers of CYP3A4 may reduce plasma concentrations of estrogens, possibly resulting in a dᴀecrease in therapeutic effects and/or changes in the uterine bleeding profile).
No products indexed under this heading.

Propoxyphene Hydrochloride (Co-administration of inhibitors of CYP3A4 with estrogens may affect estrogen drug metabolism. Inhibitors of CYP3A4 may increase plasma concentrations of estrogens and may result in side effects).
No products indexed under this heading.

Propoxyphene Napsylate (Co-administration of inhibitors of CYP3A4 with estrogens may affect estrogen drug metabolism. Inhibitors of CYP3A4 may increase plasma concentrations of estrogens and may result in side effects).
No products indexed under this heading.

Quinidine (Co-administration of inhibitors of CYP3A4 with estrogens may affect estrogen drug metabolism. Inhibitors of CYP3A4 may increase plasma concentrations of estrogens and may result in side effects).
No products indexed under this heading.

Quinidine Hydrochloride (Co-administration of inhibitors of CYP3A4 with estrogens may affect estrogen drug metabolism. Inhibitors of CYP3A4 may increase plasma concentrations of estrogens and may result in side effects).
No products indexed under this heading.

Quinidine Polygalacturonate (Co-administration of inhibitors of CYP3A4 with estrogens may affect estrogen drug metabolism. Inhibitors of CYP3A4 may increase plasma concentrations of estrogens and may result in side effects).
No products indexed under this heading.

Quinidine Sulfate (Co-administration of inhibitors of CYP3A4 with estrogens may affect estrogen drug metabolism. Inhibitors of CYP3A4 may increase plasma concentrations of estrogens and may result in side effects).
No products indexed under this heading.

Quinine (Co-administration of inhibitors of CYP3A4 with estrogens may affect estrogen drug metabolism. Inhibitors of CYP3A4 may increase plasma concentrations of estrogens and may result in side effects). Products include:

Quinine Sulfate (Co-administration of inhibitors of CYP3A4 with estrogens may affect estrogen drug metabolism. Inhibitors of CYP3A4 may increase plasma concentrations of estrogens and may result in side effects).
No products indexed under this heading.

Quinupristin (Co-administration of inhibitors of CYP3A4 with estrogens may affect estrogen drug metabolism. Inhibitors of CYP3A4 may increase plasma concentrations of estrogens and may result in side effects).
No products indexed under this heading.

Ranitidine Bismuth Citrate (Co-administration of inhibitors of CYP3A4 with estrogens may affect estrogen drug metabolism. Inhibitors of CYP3A4 may increase plasma concentrations of estrogens and may result in side effects).
No products indexed under this heading.

Ranitidine Hydrochloride (Co-administration of inhibitors of CYP3A4 with estrogens may affect estrogen drug metabolism. Inhibitors of CYP3A4 may increase plasma concentrations of estrogens and may result in side effects). Products include:

Rifabutin (Co-administration of inducers of CYP3A4 with estrogens may affect estrogen drug metabolism. Inducers of CYP3A4 may reduce plasma concentrations of estrogens, possibly resulting in a decrease in therapeutic effects and/or changes in the uterine bleeding profile).
No products indexed under this heading.

Rifampicin (Co-administration of inducers of CYP3A4 with estrogens may affect estrogen drug metabolism. Inducers of CYP3A4 may reduce plasma concentrations of estrogens, possibly resulting in a decrease in therapeutic effects and/or changes in the uterine bleeding profile).
No products indexed under this heading.

Rifampin (Co-administration of inducers of CYP3A4 with estrogens may affect estrogen drug metabolism. Inducers of CYP3A4 may reduce plasma concentrations of estrogens, possibly resulting in a decrease in therapeutic effects and/or changes in the uterine bleeding profile).
No products indexed under this heading.

Rifapentine (Co-administration of inducers of CYP3A4 with estrogens may affect estrogen drug metabolism. Inducers of CYP3A4 may reduce plasma concentrations of estrogens, possibly resulting in a decrease in therapeutic effects and/or changes in the uterine bleeding profile).
No products indexed under this heading.

Ritonavir (Co-administration of inhibitors of CYP3A4 with estrogens may affect estrogen drug metabolism. Inhibitors of CYP3A4 may increase plasma concentrations of estrogens and may result in side effects). Products include:

Saquinavir (Co-administration of inhibitors of CYP3A4 with estrogens may affect estrogen drug metabolism. Inhibitors of CYP3A4 may increase plasma concentrations of estrogens and may result in side effects).
No products indexed under this heading.

Saquinavir Mesylate (Co-administration of inhibitors of CYP3A4 with estrogens may affect estrogen drug metabolism. Inhibitors of CYP3A4 may increase plasma concentrations of estrogens and may result in side effects).
No products indexed under this heading.

Sertraline Hydrochloride (Co-administration of inhibitors of CYP3A4 with estrogens may affect estrogen drug metabolism. Inhibitors of CYP3A4 may increase plasma concentrations of estrogens and may result in side effects).
No products indexed under this heading.

Sildenafil Citrate (Co-administration of inhibitors of CYP3A4 with estrogens may affect estrogen drug metabolism. Inhibitors of CYP3A4 may increase plasma concentrations of estrogens and may result in side effects).
No products indexed under this heading.

Sulfinpyrazone (Co-administration of inducers of CYP3A4 with estrogens may affect estrogen drug metabolism. Inducers of CYP3A4 may reduce plasma concentrations of estrogens, possibly resulting in a decrease in therapeutic effects and/or changes in the uterine bleeding profile).
No products indexed under this heading.

Telithromycin (Co-administration of inhibitors of CYP3A4 with estrogens may affect estrogen drug metabolism. Inhibitors of CYP3A4 may increase plasma concentrations of estrogens and may result in side effects). Products include:

Theophyllinate (Co-administration of inducers of CYP3A4 with estrogens may affect estrogen drug metabolism. Inducers of CYP3A4 may reduce plasma concentrations of estrogens, possibly resulting in a decrease in therapeutic effects and/or changes in the uterine bleeding profile).
No products indexed under this heading.

Theophylline (Co-administration of inducers of CYP3A4 with estrogens may affect estrogen drug metabolism. Inducers of CYP3A4 may reduce plasma concentrations of estrogens, possibly resulting in a decrease in therapeutic effects and/or changes in the uterine bleeding profile).
No products indexed under this heading.

Theophylline Anhydrous (Co-administration of inducers of CYP3A4 with estrogens may affect estrogen drug metabolism. Inducers of CYP3A4 may reduce plasma concentrations of estrogens, possibly resulting in a decrease in therapeutic effects and/or changes in the uterine bleeding profile). Products include:

Theophylline Calcium Salicylate (Co-administration of inducers of CYP3A4 with estrogens may affect estrogen drug metabolism. Inducers of CYP3A4 may reduce plasma concentrations of estrogens, possibly resulting in a decrease in therapeutic effects and/or changes in the uterine bleeding profile).
No products indexed under this heading.

Theophylline Dihydroxypropyl (Glyceryl) (Co-administration of inducers of CYP3A4 with estrogens may affect estrogen drug metabolism. Inducers of CYP3A4 may reduce plasma concentrations of estrogens, possibly resulting in a decrease in therapeutic effects and/or changes in the uterine bleeding profile).
No products indexed under this heading.

Theophylline Ethylenediamine (Co-administration of inducers of CYP3A4 with estrogens may affect estrogen drug metabolism. Inducers of CYP3A4 may reduce plasma concentrations of estrogens, possibly resulting in a decrease in therapeutic effects and/or changes in the uterine bleeding profile).
No products indexed under this heading.

Theophylline Sodium Glycinate (Co-administration of inducers of CYP3A4 with estrogens may affect estrogen drug metabolism. Inducers of CYP3A4 may reduce plasma concentrations of estrogens, possibly resulting in a decrease in therapeutic effects and/or changes in the uterine bleeding profile).
No products indexed under this heading.

Triamcinolone (Co-administration of inducers of CYP3A4 with estrogens may affect estrogen drug metabolism. Inducers of CYP3A4 may reduce plasma concentrations of estrogens, possibly resulting in a decrease in therapeutic effects and/or changes in the uterine bleeding profile).
No products indexed under this heading.

Triamcinolone Acetonide (Co-administration of inducers of CYP3A4 with estrogens may affect estrogen drug metabolism. Inducers of CYP3A4 may reduce plasma concentrations of estrogens, possibly resulting in a decrease in therapeutic effects and/or changes in the uterine bleeding profile). Products include:

Triamcinolone Diacetate (Co-administration of inducers of CYP3A4 with estrogens may affect estrogen drug metabolism. Inducers of CYP3A4 may reduce plasma concentrations of estrogens, possibly resulting in a decrease in therapeutic effects and/or changes in the uterine bleeding profile).
No products indexed under this heading.

Triamcinolone Hexacetonide (Co-administration of inducers of CYP3A4 with estrogens may affect estrogen drug metabolism. Inducers of CYP3A4 may reduce plasma concentrations of estrogens, possibly resulting in a decrease in therapeutic effects and/or changes in the uterine bleeding profile).
No products indexed under this heading.

Troglitazone (Co-administration of inducers of CYP3A4 with estrogens may affect estrogen drug metabolism. Inducers of CYP3A4 may reduce plasma concentrations of estrogens, possibly resulting in a decrease in therapeutic effects and/or changes in the uterine bleeding profile).
No products indexed under this heading.

Troleandomycin (Co-administration of inhibitors of CYP3A4 with estrogens may affect estrogen drug metabolism. Inhibitors of CYP3A4 may increase plasma concentrations of estrogens and may result in side effects).
No products indexed under this heading.

Valproate Sodium (Co-administration of inhibitors of CYP3A4 with estrogens may affect estrogen drug metabolism. Inhibitors of CYP3A4 may increase plasma concentrations of estrogens and may result in side effects).
No products indexed under this heading.

Vardenafil Hydrochloride (Co-administration of inhibitors of CYP3A4

Premarin Tablets Interactions Index 1440

with estrogens may affect estrogen drug metabolism. Inhibitors of CYP3A4 may increase plasma concentrations of estrogens and may result in side effects). Products include:
Levitra 3157

Verapamil Hydrochloride (Co-administration of inhibitors of CYP3A4 with estrogens may affect estrogen drug metabolism. Inhibitors of CYP3A4 may increase plasma concentrations of estrogens and may result in side effects). Products include:
Tarka 534

Voriconazole (Co-administration of inhibitors of CYP3A4 with estrogens may affect estrogen drug metabolism. Inhibitors of CYP3A4 may increase plasma concentrations of estrogens and may result in side effects).
No products indexed under this heading.

Zafirlukast (Co-administration of inhibitors of CYP3A4 with estrogens may affect estrogen drug metabolism. Inhibitors of CYP3A4 may increase plasma concentrations of estrogens and may result in side effects). Products include:
Accolate 3612

Zileuton (Co-administration of inhibitors of CYP3A4 with estrogens may affect estrogen drug metabolism. Inhibitors of CYP3A4 may increase plasma concentrations of estrogens and may result in side effects).
No products indexed under this heading.

Food Interactions

Grapefruit (Co-administration of inhibitors of CYP3A4 with estrogens may affect estrogen drug metabolism. Inhibitors of CYP3A4 may increase plasma concentrations of estrogens and may result in side effects).

Grapefruit Juice (Co-administration of grapefruit juice with estrogens may increase plasma concentrations of estrogens and may result in side effects).

PREMARIN VAGINAL CREAM

(Estrogens, Conjugated) 3540
May interact with cytochrome p450 3a4 inducers (selected), cytochrome p450 3a4 inhibitors (selected), erythromycin, and certain other agents. Compounds in these categories include:

Acetazolamide (Inhibitors of CYP3A4 may affect estrogen drug metabolism. Inhibitors of CYP3A4, such as erythromycin, clarithromycin, ketoconazole, itraconazole, ritonavir and grapefruit juice, may increase plasma concentrations of estrogens and may result in side effects).
No products indexed under this heading.

Acetazolamide Sodium (Inhibitors of CYP3A4 may affect estrogen drug metabolism. Inhibitors of CYP3A4, such as erythromycin, clarithromycin, ketoconazole, itraconazole, ritonavir and grapefruit juice, may increase plasma concentrations of estrogens and may result in side effects).
No products indexed under this heading.

Allium sativum (Inducers of CYP3A4 may affect estrogen drug metabolism. Inducers of CYP3A4, such as St. John's Wort (Hypericum perforatum) preparations, phenobarbital, carbamazepine, and rifampin, may reduce plasma concentrations of estrogens, possibly resulting in a decrease in therapeutic effects and/or changes in the uterine bleeding profile).
No products indexed under this heading.

Aminoglutethimide (Inducers of CYP3A4 may affect estrogen drug metabolism. Inducers of CYP3A4, such as St. John's Wort (Hypericum perforatum) preparations, phenobarbital, carbamazepine, and rifampin, may reduce plasma concentrations of estrogens, possibly resulting in a decrease in therapeutic effects and/or changes in the uterine bleeding profile).
No products indexed under this heading.

Amiodarone Hydrochloride (Inhibitors of CYP3A4 may affect estrogen drug metabolism. Inhibitors of CYP3A4, such as erythromycin, clarithromycin, ketoconazole, itraconazole, ritonavir and grapefruit juice, may increase plasma concentrations of estrogens and may result in side effects).
No products indexed under this heading.

Amprenavir (Inhibitors of CYP3A4 may affect estrogen drug metabolism. Inhibitors of CYP3A4, such as erythromycin, clarithromycin, ketoconazole, itraconazole, ritonavir and grapefruit juice, may increase plasma concentrations of estrogens and may result in side effects).
No products indexed under this heading.

Anastrozole (Inhibitors of CYP3A4 may affect estrogen drug metabolism. Inhibitors of CYP3A4, such as erythromycin, clarithromycin, ketoconazole, itraconazole, ritonavir and grapefruit juice, may increase plasma concentrations of estrogens and may result in side effects).
No products indexed under this heading.

Aprepitant (Inducers of CYP3A4 may affect estrogen drug metabolism. Inducers of CYP3A4, such as St. John's Wort (Hypericum perforatum) preparations, phenobarbital, carbamazepine, and rifampin, may reduce plasma concentrations of estrogens, possibly resulting in a decrease in therapeutic effects and/or changes in the uterine bleeding profile). Products include:
Emend 2124

Atazanavir (Inhibitors of CYP3A4 may affect estrogen drug metabolism. Inhibitors of CYP3A4, such as erythromycin, clarithromycin, ketoconazole, itraconazole, ritonavir and grapefruit juice, may increase plasma concentrations of estrogens and may result in side effects).
No products indexed under this heading.

Atazanavir Sulfate (Inhibitors of CYP3A4 may affect estrogen drug metabolism. Inhibitors of CYP3A4, such as erythromycin, clarithromycin, ketoconazole, itraconazole, ritonavir and grapefruit juice, may increase plasma concentrations of estrogens and may result in side effects).
No products indexed under this heading.

Betamethasone (Inducers of CYP3A4 may affect estrogen drug metabolism. Inducers of CYP3A4, such as St. John's Wort (Hypericum perforatum) preparations, phenobarbital, carbamazepine, and rifampin, may reduce plasma concentrations of estrogens, possibly resulting in a decrease in therapeutic effects and/or changes in the uterine bleeding profile).
No products indexed under this heading.

Betamethasone Acetate (Inducers of CYP3A4 may affect estrogen drug metabolism. Inducers of CYP3A4, such as St. John's Wort (Hypericum perforatum) preparations, phenobarbital, carbamazepine, and rifampin, may reduce plasma concentrations of estrogens, possibly resulting in a decrease in therapeutic effects and/or changes in the uterine bleeding profile).
No products indexed under this heading.

Betamethasone Benzoate (Inducers of CYP3A4 may affect estrogen drug metabolism. Inducers of CYP3A4, such as St. John's Wort (Hypericum perforatum) preparations, phenobarbital, carbamazepine, and rifampin, may reduce plasma concentrations of estrogens, possibly resulting in a decrease in therapeutic effects and/or changes in the uterine bleeding profile).
No products indexed under this heading.

Betamethasone Dipropionate (Inducers of CYP3A4 may affect estrogen drug metabolism. Inducers of CYP3A4, such as St. John's Wort (Hypericum perforatum) preparations, phenobarbital, carbamazepine, and rifampin, may reduce plasma concentrations of estrogens, possibly resulting in a decrease in therapeutic effects and/or changes in the uterine bleeding profile). Products include:
Diprolene Lotion 0.05% 3108
Diprolene Ointment 0.05% 3109
Diprolene AF Cream 0.05% 3107
Lotrisone 3163

Betamethasone Sodium Phosphate (Inducers of CYP3A4 may affect estrogen drug metabolism. Inducers of CYP3A4, such as St. John's Wort (Hypericum perforatum) preparations, phenobarbital, carbamazepine, and rifampin, may reduce plasma concentrations of estrogens, possibly resulting in a decrease in therapeutic effects and/or changes in the uterine bleeding profile).
No products indexed under this heading.

Betamethasone Valerate (Inducers of CYP3A4 may affect estrogen drug metabolism. Inducers of CYP3A4, such as St. John's Wort (Hypericum perforatum) preparations, phenobarbital, carbamazepine, and rifampin, may reduce plasma concentrations of estrogens, possibly resulting in a decrease in therapeutic effects and/or changes in the uterine bleeding profile). Products include:
Luxíq 3321

Bosentan (Inducers of CYP3A4 may affect estrogen drug metabolism. Inducers of CYP3A4, such as St. John's Wort (Hypericum perforatum) preparations, phenobarbital, carbamazepine, and rifampin, may reduce plasma concentrations of estrogens, possibly resulting in a decrease in therapeutic effects and/or changes in the uterine bleeding profile). Products include:
Tracleer 573

Carbamazepine (Inducers of CYP3A4 may affect estrogen drug metabolism. Inducers of CYP3A4, such as carbamzepine, may reduce plasma concentrations of estrogens, possibly resulting in a decrease in therapeutic effects and/or changes in the uterine bleeding profile). Products include:
Carbatrol 3280
Equetro 3477

Cimetidine (Inhibitors of CYP3A4 may affect estrogen drug metabolism. Inhibitors of CYP3A4, such as erythromycin, clarithromycin, ketoconazole, itraconazole, ritonavir and grapefruit juice, may increase plasma concentrations of estrogens and may result in side effects).
No products indexed under this heading.

Cimetidine Hydrochloride (Inhibitors of CYP3A4 may affect estrogen drug metabolism. Inhibitors of CYP3A4, such as erythromycin, clarithromycin, ketoconazole, itraconazole, ritonavir and grapefruit juice, may increase plasma concentrations of estrogens and may result in side effects).
No products indexed under this heading.

Ciprofloxacin (Inducers of CYP3A4 may affect estrogen drug metabolism. Inducers of CYP3A4, such as St. John's Wort (Hypericum perforatum) preparations, phenobarbital, carbamazepine, and rifampin, may reduce plasma concentrations of estrogens, possibly resulting in a decrease in therapeutic effects and/or changes in the uterine bleeding profile). Products include:
Cipro I.V. 3082
Cipro 3073
Cipro XR 3091
Ciprodex 583

Ciprofloxacin Hydrochloride (Inducers of CYP3A4 may affect estrogen drug metabolism. Inducers of CYP3A4, such as St. John's Wort (Hypericum perforatum) preparations, phenobarbital, carbamazepine, and rifampin, may reduce plasma concentrations of estrogens, possibly resulting in a decrease in therapeutic effects and/or changes in the uterine bleeding profile). Products include:
Cipro 3073

Cisplatin (Inducers of CYP3A4 may affect estrogen drug metabolism. Inducers of CYP3A4, such as St. John's Wort (Hypericum perforatum) preparations, phenobarbital, carbamazepine, and rifampin, may reduce plasma concentrations of estrogens, possibly resulting in a decrease in therapeutic effects and/or changes in the uterine bleeding profile).
No products indexed under this heading.

Clarithromycin (Inhibitors of CYP3A4 may affect estrogen drug metabolism. Inhibitors of CYP3A4, such as clarithromycin, may increase plasma concentrations of estrogens and may result in side effects). Products include:
Biaxin/Biaxin XL 412

Clotrimazole (Inhibitors of CYP3A4 may affect estrogen drug metabolism. Inhibitors of CYP3A4, such as erythromycin, clarithromycin, ketoconazole, itraconazole, ritonavir and grapefruit juice, may increase plasma concentrations of estrogens and may result in side effects). Products include:
Lotrisone 3163

Conivaptan Hydrochloride (Inhibitors of CYP3A4 may affect estrogen drug metabolism. Inhibitors of CYP3A4, such as erythromycin, clarithromycin, ketoconazole, itraconazole, ritonavir and grapefruit juice, may increase plasma concentrations of estrogens and may result in side effects). Products include:
Vaprisol 689

Cortisone Acetate (Inducers of CYP3A4 may affect estrogen drug metabolism. Inducers of CYP3A4, such as St. John's Wort (Hypericum perforatum) preparations, phenobarbital, carbamazepine, and rifampin, may reduce plasma concentrations of estrogens, possibly resulting in a decrease in therapeutic effects and/or changes in the uterine bleeding profile).
No products indexed under this heading.

Cyclosporine (Inhibitors of CYP3A4 may affect estrogen drug metabolism. Inhibitors of CYP3A4, such as erythromycin, clarithromycin, ketoconazole, itraconazole, ritonavir and grapefruit juice, may increase plasma concentrations of estrogens and may result in side effects). Products include:
Gengraf 440
Neoral Oral Solution 2496
Neoral Capsules 2496
Restasis 605

Dalfopristin (Inhibitors of CYP3A4 may affect estrogen drug metabolism. Inhibitors of CYP3A4, such as erythromycin, clarithromycin, ketoconazole, itraconazole, ritonavir and grapefruit juice, may increase plasma concentrations of estrogens and may result in side effects).
No products indexed under this heading.

Danazol (Inhibitors of CYP3A4 may affect estrogen drug metabolism. Inhibitors of CYP3A4, such as erythromycin, clarithromycin, ketoconazole, itraconazole, ritonavir and grapefruit juice, may increase plasma concentrations of estrogens and may result in side effects).
No products indexed under this heading.

Darunavir (Inhibitors of CYP3A4 may affect estrogen drug metabolism. Inhibitors of CYP3A4, such as erythromycin, clarithromycin, ketoconazole, itraconazole, ritonavir and grapefruit juice, may increase plasma concentrations of estrogens and may result in side effects).
No products indexed under this heading.

Dasatinib (Inhibitors of CYP3A4 may affect estrogen drug metabolism. Inhibitors of CYP3A4, such as erythromycin, clarithromycin, ketoconazole, itraconazole, ritonavir and grapefruit juice, may increase plasma concentrations of estrogens and may result in side effects).
No products indexed under this heading.

Delavirdine Mesylate (Inhibitors of CYP3A4 may affect estrogen drug metabolism. Inhibitors of CYP3A4, such as erythromycin, clarithromycin, ketoconazole, itraconazole, ritonavir and grapefruit juice, may increase plasma concentrations of estrogens and may result in side effects).
No products indexed under this heading.

Delavirine (Inhibitors of CYP3A4 may affect estrogen drug metabolism. Inhibitors of CYP3A4, such as erythromycin, clarithromycin, ketoconazole, itraconazole, ritonavir and grapefruit juice, may increase plasma concentrations of estrogens and may result in side effects).
No products indexed under this heading.

Desloratadine (Inhibitors of CYP3A4 may affect estrogen drug metabolism. Inhibitors of CYP3A4, such as erythromycin, clarithromycin, ketoconazole, itraconazole, ritonavir and grapefruit juice, may increase plasma concentrations of estrogens and may result in side effects). Products include:

Dexamethasone (Inducers of CYP3A4 may affect estrogen drug metabolism. Inducers of CYP3A4, such as St. John's Wort (Hypericum perforatum) preparations, phenobarbital, carbamazepine, and rifampin, may reduce plasma concentrations of estrogens, possibly resulting in a decrease in therapeutic effects and/or changes in the uterine bleeding profile). Products include:

Dexamethasone Acetate (Inducers of CYP3A4 may affect estrogen drug metabolism. Inducers of CYP3A4, such as St. John's Wort (Hypericum perforatum) preparations, phenobarbital, carbamazepine, and rifampin, may reduce plasma concentrations of estrogens, possibly resulting in a decrease in therapeutic effects and/or changes in the uterine bleeding profile).
No products indexed under this heading.

Dexamethasone Phosphate (Inducers of CYP3A4 may affect estrogen drug metabolism. Inducers of CYP3A4, such as St. John's Wort (Hypericum perforatum) preparations, phenobarbital, carbamazepine, and rifampin, may reduce plasma concentrations of estrogens, possibly resulting in a decrease in therapeutic effects and/or changes in the uterine bleeding profile).
No products indexed under this heading.

Dexamethasone Sodium (Inducers of CYP3A4 may affect estrogen drug metabolism. Inducers of CYP3A4, such as St. John's Wort (Hypericum perforatum) preparations, phenobarbital, carbamazepine, and rifampin, may reduce plasma concentrations of estrogens, possibly resulting in a decrease in therapeutic effects and/or changes in the uterine bleeding profile).
No products indexed under this heading.

Dexamethasone Sodium Phosphate (Inducers of CYP3A4 may affect estrogen drug metabolism. Inducers of CYP3A4, such as St. John's Wort (Hypericum perforatum) preparations, phenobarbital, carbamazepine, and rifampin, may reduce plasma concentrations of estrogens, possibly resulting in a decrease in therapeutic effects and/or changes in the uterine bleeding profile).
No products indexed under this heading.

Dexamethasone Sodium Phosphate Injection (Inducers of CYP3A4 may affect estrogen drug metabolism. Inducers of CYP3A4, such as St. John's Wort (Hypericum perforatum) preparations, phenobarbital, carbamazepine, and rifampin, may reduce plasma concentrations of estrogens, possibly resulting in a decrease in therapeutic effects and/or changes in the uterine bleeding profile).
No products indexed under this heading.

Diltiazem Hydrochloride (Inhibitors of CYP3A4 may affect estrogen drug metabolism. Inhibitors of CYP3A4, such as erythromycin, clarithromycin, ketoconazole, itraconazole, ritonavir and grapefruit juice, may increase plasma concentrations of estrogens and may result in side effects). Products include:

Diltiazem Maleate (Inhibitors of CYP3A4 may affect estrogen drug metabolism. Inhibitors of CYP3A4, such as erythromycin, clarithromycin, ketoconazole, itraconazole, ritonavir and grapefruit juice, may increase plasma concentrations of estrogens and may result in side effects).
No products indexed under this heading.

Doxorubicin Hydrochloride (Inducers of CYP3A4 may affect estrogen drug metabolism. Inducers of CYP3A4, such as St. John's Wort (Hypericum perforatum) preparations, phenobarbital, carbamazepine, and rifampin, may reduce plasma concentrations of estrogens, possibly resulting in a decrease in therapeutic effects and/or changes in the uterine bleeding profile).
No products indexed under this heading.

Efavirenz (Inducers of CYP3A4 may affect estrogen drug metabolism. Inducers of CYP3A4, such as St. John's Wort (Hypericum perforatum) preparations, phenobarbital, carbamazepine, and rifampin, may reduce plasma concentrations of estrogens, possibly resulting in a decrease in therapeutic effects and/or changes in the uterine bleeding profile). Products include:

Erythromycin (Inhibitors of CYP3A4 may affect estrogen drug metabolism. Inhibitors of CYP3A4, such as erythromycin may increase plasma concentrations of estrogens and may result in side effects).
No products indexed under this heading.

Erythromycin, Topical (Inhibitors of CYP3A4 may affect estrogen drug metabolism. Inhibitors of CYP3A4, such as erythromycin may increase plasma concentrations of estrogens and may result in side effects).
No products indexed under this heading.

Erythromycin Estolate (Inhibitors of CYP3A4 may affect estrogen drug metabolism. Inhibitors of CYP3A4, such as erythromycin may increase plasma concentrations of estrogens and may result in side effects).
No products indexed under this heading.

Erythromycin Ethylsuccinate (Inhibitors of CYP3A4 may affect estrogen drug metabolism. Inhibitors of CYP3A4, such as erythromycin may increase plasma concentrations of estrogens and may result in side effects). Products include:

Erythromycin Gluceptate (Inhibitors of CYP3A4 may affect estrogen drug metabolism. Inhibitors of CYP3A4, such as erythromycin may increase plasma concentrations of estrogens and may result in side effects).
No products indexed under this heading.

Erythromycin Lactobionate (Inhibitors of CYP3A4 may affect estrogen drug metabolism. Inhibitors of CYP3A4, such as erythromycin may increase plasma concentrations of estrogens and may result in side effects).
No products indexed under this heading.

Erythromycin Stearate (Inhibitors of CYP3A4 may affect estrogen drug metabolism. Inhibitors of CYP3A4, such as erythromycin may increase plasma concentrations of estrogens and may result in side effects).
No products indexed under this heading.

Esomeprazole Magnesium (Inhibitors of CYP3A4 may affect estrogen drug metabolism. Inhibitors of CYP3A4, such as erythromycin, clarithromycin, ketoconazole, itraconazole, ritonavir and grapefruit juice, may increase plasma concentrations of estrogens and may result in side effects). Products include:

Esomeprazole Sodium (Inhibitors of CYP3A4 may affect estrogen drug metabolism. Inhibitors of CYP3A4, such as erythromycin, clarithromycin, ketoconazole, itraconazole, ritonavir and grapefruit juice, may increase plasma concentrations of estrogens and may result in side effects). Products include:

Ethosuximide (Inducers of CYP3A4 may affect estrogen drug metabolism. Inducers of CYP3A4, such as St. John's Wort (Hypericum perforatum) preparations, phenobarbital, carbamazepine, and rifampin, may reduce plasma concentrations of estrogens, possibly resulting in a decrease in therapeutic effects and/or changes in the uterine bleeding profile).
No products indexed under this heading.

Felbamate (Inducers of CYP3A4 may affect estrogen drug metabolism. Inducers of CYP3A4, such as St. John's Wort (Hypericum perforatum) preparations, phenobarbital, carbamazepine, and rifampin, may reduce plasma concentrations of estrogens, possibly resulting in a decrease in therapeutic effects and/or changes in the uterine bleeding profile).
No products indexed under this heading.

Fluconazole (Inhibitors of CYP3A4 may affect estrogen drug metabolism. Inhibitors of CYP3A4, such as erythromycin, clarithromycin, ketoconazole, itraconazole, ritonavir and grapefruit juice, may increase plasma concentrations of estrogens and may result in side effects).
No products indexed under this heading.

Fludrocortisone Acetate (Inducers of CYP3A4 may affect estrogen drug metabolism. Inducers of CYP3A4, such as St. John's Wort (Hypericum perforatum) preparations, phenobarbital, carbamazepine, and rifampin, may reduce plasma concentrations of estrogens, possibly resulting in a decrease in therapeutic effects and/or changes in the uterine bleeding profile).
No products indexed under this heading.

Fluoxetine (Inhibitors of CYP3A4 may affect estrogen drug metabolism. Inhibitors of CYP3A4, such as erythromycin, clarithromycin, ketoconazole, itraconazole, ritonavir and grapefruit juice, may increase plasma concentrations of estrogens and may result in side effects).
No products indexed under this heading.

Fluoxetine Hydrochloride (Inhibitors of CYP3A4 may affect estrogen drug metabolism. Inhibitors of CYP3A4, such as erythromycin, clarithromycin, ketoconazole, itraconazole, ritonavir and grapefruit juice, may increase plasma concentrations of estrogens and may result in side effects). Products include:

Fluvoxamine Maleate (Inhibitors of CYP3A4 may affect estrogen drug metabolism. Inhibitors of CYP3A4, such as erythromycin, clarithromycin, ketoconazole, itraconazole, ritonavir and grapefruit juice, may increase plasma concentrations of estrogens and may result in side effects).
No products indexed under this heading.

Fosamprenavir Calcium (Inhibitors of CYP3A4 may affect estrogen drug metabolism. Inhibitors of CYP3A4, such as erythromycin, clarithromycin, ketoconazole, itraconazole, ritonavir and grapefruit juice, may increase plasma concentrations of estrogens and may result in side effects). Products include:

Fosphenytoin Sodium (Inducers of CYP3A4 may affect estrogen drug metabolism. Inducers of CYP3A4, such as St. John's Wort (Hypericum perforatum) preparations, phenobarbital, carbamazepine, and rifampin, may reduce plasma concentrations of estrogens, possibly resulting in a decrease in therapeutic effects and/or changes in the uterine bleeding profile).
No products indexed under this heading.

Garlic Extract (Inducers of CYP3A4 may affect estrogen drug metabolism. Inducers of CYP3A4, such as St. John's Wort (Hypericum perforatum) preparations, phenobarbital, carbamazepine, and rifampin, may reduce plasma concentrations of estrogens, possibly resulting in a decrease in therapeutic effects and/or changes in the uterine bleeding profile).
No products indexed under this heading.

IMPORTANT NOTE: Always consult each drug listing in the patient's regimen for possible interactions.

Garlic Oil (Inducers of CYP3A4 may affect estrogen drug metabolism. Inducers of CYP3A4, such as St. John's Wort (Hypericum perforatum) preparations, phenobarbital, carbamazepine, and rifampin, may reduce plasma concentrations of estrogens, possibly resulting in a decrease in therapeutic effects and/or changes in the uterine bleeding profile).
No products indexed under this heading.

Hydrocortisone (Inducers of CYP3A4 may affect estrogen drug metabolism. Inducers of CYP3A4, such as St. John's Wort (Hypericum perforatum) preparations, phenobarbital, carbamazepine, and rifampin, may reduce plasma concentrations of estrogens, possibly resulting in a decrease in therapeutic effects and/or changes in the uterine bleeding profile).
No products indexed under this heading.

Hydrocortisone (Alcohol) (Inducers of CYP3A4 may affect estrogen drug metabolism. Inducers of CYP3A4, such as St. John's Wort (Hypericum perforatum) preparations, phenobarbital, carbamazepine, and rifampin, may reduce plasma concentrations of estrogens, possibly resulting in a decrease in therapeutic effects and/or changes in the uterine bleeding profile).
No products indexed under this heading.

Hydrocortisone Acetate (Inducers of CYP3A4 may affect estrogen drug metabolism. Inducers of CYP3A4, such as St. John's Wort (Hypericum perforatum) preparations, phenobarbital, carbamazepine, and rifampin, may reduce plasma concentrations of estrogens, possibly resulting in a decrease in therapeutic effects and/or changes in the uterine bleeding profile).
No products indexed under this heading.

Hydrocortisone Butyrate (Inducers of CYP3A4 may affect estrogen drug metabolism. Inducers of CYP3A4, such as St. John's Wort (Hypericum perforatum) preparations, phenobarbital, carbamazepine, and rifampin, may reduce plasma concentrations of estrogens, possibly resulting in a decrease in therapeutic effects and/or changes in the uterine bleeding profile).
No products indexed under this heading.

Hydrocortisone Cypionate (Inducers of CYP3A4 may affect estrogen drug metabolism. Inducers of CYP3A4, such as St. John's Wort (Hypericum perforatum) preparations, phenobarbital, carbamazepine, and rifampin, may reduce plasma concentrations of estrogens, possibly resulting in a decrease in therapeutic effects and/or changes in the uterine bleeding profile).
No products indexed under this heading.

Hydrocortisone Hemisuccinate (Inducers of CYP3A4 may affect estrogen drug metabolism. Inducers of CYP3A4, such as St. John's Wort (Hypericum perforatum) preparations, phenobarbital, carbamazepine, and rifampin, may reduce plasma concentrations of estrogens, possibly resulting in a decrease in therapeutic effects and/or changes in the uterine bleeding profile).
No products indexed under this heading.

Hydrocortisone Probutate (Inducers of CYP3A4 may affect estrogen drug metabolism. Inducers of CYP3A4, such as St. John's Wort (Hypericum perforatum) preparations, phenobarbital, carbamazepine, and rifampin, may reduce plasma concentrations of estrogens, possibly resulting in a decrease in therapeutic effects and/or changes in the uterine bleeding profile).
No products indexed under this heading.

Hydrocortisone Sodium Phosphate (Inducers of CYP3A4 may affect estrogen drug metabolism. Inducers of CYP3A4, such as St. John's Wort (Hypericum perforatum) preparations, phenobarbital, carbamazepine, and rifampin, may reduce plasma concentrations of estrogens, possibly resulting in a decrease in therapeutic effects and/or changes in the uterine bleeding profile).
No products indexed under this heading.

Hydrocortisone Sodium Succinate (Inducers of CYP3A4 may affect estrogen drug metabolism. Inducers of CYP3A4, such as St. John's Wort (Hypericum perforatum) preparations, phenobarbital, carbamazepine, and rifampin, may reduce plasma concentrations of estrogens, possibly resulting in a decrease in therapeutic effects and/or changes in the uterine bleeding profile).
No products indexed under this heading.

Hydrocortisone Valerate (Inducers of CYP3A4 may affect estrogen drug metabolism. Inducers of CYP3A4, such as St. John's Wort (Hypericum perforatum) preparations, phenobarbital, carbamazepine, and rifampin, may reduce plasma concentrations of estrogens, possibly resulting in a decrease in therapeutic effects and/or changes in the uterine bleeding profile).
No products indexed under this heading.

Hypericum (Inducers of CYP3A4 may affect estrogen drug metabolism. Inducers of CYP3A4, such as St. John's Wort (Hypericum perforatum) preparations, phenobarbital, carbamazepine, and rifampin, may reduce plasma concentrations of estrogens, possibly resulting in a decrease in therapeutic effects and/or changes in the uterine bleeding profile).
No products indexed under this heading.

Hypericum Perforatum (Inducers of CYP3A4 may affect estrogen drug metabolism. Inducers of CYP3A4, such as St. John's Wort (Hypericum perforatum), may reduce plasma concentrations of estrogens, possibly resulting in a decrease in therapeutic effects and/or changes in the uterine bleeding profile). Products include:
Traumeel 1800

Imatinib Mesylate (Inhibitors of CYP3A4 may affect estrogen drug metabolism. Inhibitors of CYP3A4, such as erythromycin, clarithromycin, ketoconazole, itraconazole, ritonavir and grapefruit juice, may increase plasma concentrations of estrogens and may result in side effects). Products include:
Gleevec 2477

Indinavir Sulfate (Inhibitors of CYP3A4 may affect estrogen drug metabolism. Inhibitors of CYP3A4, such as erythromycin, clarithromycin, ketoconazole, itraconazole, ritonavir and grapefruit juice, may increase plasma concentrations of estrogens and may result in side effects). Products include:
Crixivan 2113

Isoniazid (Inhibitors of CYP3A4 may affect estrogen drug metabolism. Inhibitors of CYP3A4, such as erythromycin, clarithromycin, ketoconazole, itraconazole, ritonavir and grapefruit juice, may increase plasma concentrations of estrogens and may result in side effects).
No products indexed under this heading.

Itraconazole (Inhibitors of CYP3A4 may affect estrogen drug metabolism. Inhibitors of CYP3A4, such as erythromycin, clarithromycin, ketoconazole, itraconazole, ritonavir and grapefruit juice, may increase plasma concentrations of estrogens and may result in side effects).
No products indexed under this heading.

Ketoconazole (Inhibitors of CYP3A4 may affect estrogen drug metabolism. Inhibitors of CYP3A4, such as erythromycin, clarithromycin, ketoconazole, itraconazole, ritonavir and grapefruit juice, may increase plasma concentrations of estrogens and may result in side effects). Products include:
Extina 3319
Xolegel 3337

Lapatinib (Inhibitors of CYP3A4 may affect estrogen drug metabolism. Inhibitors of CYP3A4, such as erythromycin, clarithromycin, ketoconazole, itraconazole, ritonavir and grapefruit juice, may increase plasma concentrations of estrogens and may result in side effects). Products include:
Tykerb 1698

Lopinavir (Inhibitors of CYP3A4 may affect estrogen drug metabolism. Inhibitors of CYP3A4, such as erythromycin, clarithromycin, ketoconazole, itraconazole, ritonavir and grapefruit juice, may increase plasma concentrations of estrogens and may result in side effects). Products include:
Kaletra 458

Loratadine (Inhibitors of CYP3A4 may affect estrogen drug metabolism. Inhibitors of CYP3A4, such as erythromycin, clarithromycin, ketoconazole, itraconazole, ritonavir and grapefruit juice, may increase plasma concentrations of estrogens and may result in side effects).
No products indexed under this heading.

Mephenytoin (Inducers of CYP3A4 may affect estrogen drug metabolism. Inducers of CYP3A4, such as St. John's Wort (Hypericum perforatum) preparations, phenobarbital, carbamazepine, and rifampin, may reduce plasma concentrations of estrogens, possibly resulting in a decrease in therapeutic effects and/or changes in the uterine bleeding profile).
No products indexed under this heading.

Methsuximide (Inducers of CYP3A4 may affect estrogen drug metabolism. Inducers of CYP3A4, such as St. John's Wort (Hypericum perforatum) preparations, phenobarbital, carbamazepine, and rifampin, may reduce plasma concentrations of estrogens, possibly resulting in a decrease in therapeutic effects and/or changes in the uterine bleeding profile).
No products indexed under this heading.

Methylprednisolone (Inducers of CYP3A4 may affect estrogen drug metabolism. Inducers of CYP3A4, such as St. John's Wort (Hypericum perforatum) preparations, phenobarbital, carbamazepine, and rifampin, may reduce plasma concentrations of estrogens, possibly resulting in a decrease in therapeutic effects and/or changes in the uterine bleeding profile).
No products indexed under this heading.

Methylprednisolone Acetate (Inducers of CYP3A4 may affect estrogen drug metabolism. Inducers of CYP3A4, such as St. John's Wort (Hypericum perforatum) preparations, phenobarbital, carbamazepine, and rifampin, may reduce plasma concentrations of estrogens, possibly resulting in a decrease in therapeutic effects and/or changes in the uterine bleeding profile).
No products indexed under this heading.

Methylprednisolone Sodium Succinate (Inducers of CYP3A4 may affect estrogen drug metabolism. Inducers of CYP3A4, such as St. John's Wort (Hypericum perforatum) preparations, phenobarbital, carbamazepine, and rifampin, may reduce plasma concentrations of estrogens, possibly resulting in a decrease in therapeutic effects and/or changes in the uterine bleeding profile).
No products indexed under this heading.

Metronidazole (Inhibitors of CYP3A4 may affect estrogen drug metabolism. Inhibitors of CYP3A4, such as erythromycin, clarithromycin, ketoconazole, itraconazole, ritonavir and grapefruit juice, may increase plasma concentrations of estrogens and may result in side effects). Products include:
Pylera 793

Metronidazole Benzoate (Inhibitors of CYP3A4 may affect estrogen drug metabolism. Inhibitors of CYP3A4, such as erythromycin, clarithromycin, ketoconazole, itraconazole, ritonavir and grapefruit juice, may increase plasma concentrations of estrogens and may result in side effects).
No products indexed under this heading.

Metronidazole Hydrochloride (Inhibitors of CYP3A4 may affect estrogen drug metabolism. Inhibitors of CYP3A4, such as erythromycin, clarithromycin, ketoconazole, itraconazole, ritonavir and grapefruit juice, may increase plasma concentrations of estrogens and may result in side effects).
No products indexed under this heading.

Metronidazole Sodium (Inhibitors of CYP3A4 may affect estrogen drug metabolism. Inhibitors of CYP3A4, such as erythromycin, clarithromycin, ketoconazole, itraconazole, ritonavir and grapefruit juice, may increase plasma concentrations of estrogens and may result in side effects).
No products indexed under this heading.

Miconazole (Inhibitors of CYP3A4 may affect estrogen drug metabolism. Inhibitors of CYP3A4, such as erythromycin, clarithromycin, ketoconazole, itraconazole, ritonavir and grapefruit juice, may increase plasma concentrations of estrogens and may result in side effects).
No products indexed under this heading.

Miconazole Nitrate (Inhibitors of CYP3A4 may affect estrogen drug metabolism. Inhibitors of CYP3A4, such as erythromycin, clarithromycin, ketoconazole, itraconazole, ritonavir and grapefruit juice, may increase plasma concentrations of estrogens and may result in side effects). Products include:
Vusion Ointment 3335

Mifepristone (Inhibitors of CYP3A4 may affect estrogen drug metabolism. Inhibitors of CYP3A4, such as erythromycin, clarithromycin, ketoconazole, itraconazole, ritonavir and grapefruit juice, may increase plasma concentrations of estrogens and may result in side effects).
No products indexed under this heading.

Modafinil (Inducers of CYP3A4 may affect estrogen drug metabolism. Inducers of CYP3A4, such as St. John's Wort (Hypericum perforatum) preparations, phenobarbital, carbamazepine, and rifampin, may reduce plasma concentrations of estrogens, possibly resulting in a decrease in therapeutic effects and/or changes in the uterine bleeding profile). Products include:
Provigil 983

Nafcillin Sodium (Inducers of CYP3A4 may affect estrogen drug metabolism. Inducers of CYP3A4, such as St. John's Wort (Hypericum perforatum) preparations, phenobarbital, carbamazepine, and rifampin, may reduce plasma concentrations of estrogens, possibly resulting in a decrease in therapeutic effects and/or changes in the uterine bleeding profile).
No products indexed under this heading.

Nefazodone Hydrochloride (Inhibitors of CYP3A4 may affect estrogen drug metabolism. Inhibitors of CYP3A4, such as erythromycin, clarithromycin, ketoconazole, itraconazole, ritonavir and grapefruit juice, may increase plasma concentrations of estrogens and may result in side effects).
No products indexed under this heading.

Nelfinavir Mesylate (Inhibitors of CYP3A4 may affect estrogen drug metabolism. Inhibitors of CYP3A4, such as erythromycin, clarithromycin, ketoconazole, itraconazole, ritonavir and grapefruit juice, may increase plasma concentrations of estrogens and may result in side effects).
No products indexed under this heading.

Nevirapine (Inducers of CYP3A4 may affect estrogen drug metabolism. Inducers of CYP3A4, such as St. John's Wort (Hypericum perforatum) preparations, phenobarbital, carbamazepine, and rifampin, may reduce plasma concentrations of estrogens, possibly resulting in a decrease in therapeutic effects and/or changes in the uterine bleeding profile). Products include:

Niacin (Inhibitors of CYP3A4 may affect estrogen drug metabolism. Inhibitors of CYP3A4, such as erythromycin, clarithromycin, ketoconazole, itraconazole, ritonavir and grapefruit juice, may increase plasma concentrations of estrogens and may result in side effects). Products include:

Niacinamide (Inhibitors of CYP3A4 may affect estrogen drug metabolism. Inhibitors of CYP3A4, such as erythromycin, clarithromycin, ketoconazole, itraconazole, ritonavir and grapefruit juice, may increase plasma concentrations of estrogens and may result in side effects). Products include:

Niacinamide Hydroiodide (Inhibitors of CYP3A4 may affect estrogen drug metabolism. Inhibitors of CYP3A4, such as erythromycin, clarithromycin, ketoconazole, itraconazole, ritonavir and grapefruit juice, may increase plasma concentrations of estrogens and may result in side effects).
No products indexed under this heading.

Nicotinamide (Inhibitors of CYP3A4 may affect estrogen drug metabolism. Inhibitors of CYP3A4, such as erythromycin, clarithromycin, ketoconazole, itraconazole, ritonavir and grapefruit juice, may increase plasma concentrations of estrogens and may result in side effects).
No products indexed under this heading.

Nifedipine (Inhibitors of CYP3A4 may affect estrogen drug metabolism. Inhibitors of CYP3A4, such as erythromycin, clarithromycin, ketoconazole, itraconazole, ritonavir and grapefruit juice, may increase plasma concentrations of estrogens and may result in side effects).
No products indexed under this heading.

Norfloxacin (Inhibitors of CYP3A4 may affect estrogen drug metabolism. Inhibitors of CYP3A4, such as erythromycin, clarithromycin, ketoconazole, itraconazole, ritonavir and grapefruit juice, may increase plasma concentrations of estrogens and may result in side effects). Products include:

Omeprazole (Inhibitors of CYP3A4 may affect estrogen drug metabolism. Inhibitors of CYP3A4, such as erythromycin, clarithromycin, ketoconazole, itraconazole, ritonavir and grapefruit juice, may increase plasma concentrations of estrogens and may result in side effects).
No products indexed under this heading.

Oxcarbazepine (Inducers of CYP3A4 may affect estrogen drug metabolism. Inducers of CYP3A4, such as St. John's Wort (Hypericum perforatum) preparations, phenobarbital, carbamazepine, and rifampin, may reduce plasma concentrations of estrogens, possibly resulting in a decrease in therapeutic effects and/or changes in the uterine bleeding profile).
No products indexed under this heading.

Paroxetine Hydrochloride (Inhibitors of CYP3A4 may affect estrogen drug metabolism. Inhibitors of CYP3A4, such as erythromycin, clarithromycin, ketoconazole, itraconazole, ritonavir and grapefruit juice, may increase plasma concentrations of estrogens and may result in side effects). Products include:

Phenobarbital (Inducers of CYP3A4 may affect estrogen drug metabolism. Inducers of CYP3A4, such as phenobarbital, may reduce plasma concentrations of estrogens, possibly resulting in a decrease in therapeutic effects and/or changes in the uterine bleeding profile). Products include:

Phenobarbital Sodium (Inducers of CYP3A4 may affect estrogen drug metabolism. Inducers of CYP3A4, such as phenobarbital, may reduce plasma concentrations of estrogens, possibly resulting in a decrease in therapeutic effects and/or changes in the uterine bleeding profile).
No products indexed under this heading.

Phenytoin (Inducers of CYP3A4 may affect estrogen drug metabolism. Inducers of CYP3A4, such as St. John's Wort (Hypericum perforatum) preparations, phenobarbital, carbamazepine, and rifampin, may reduce plasma concentrations of estrogens, possibly resulting in a decrease in therapeutic effects and/or changes in the uterine bleeding profile).
No products indexed under this heading.

Phenytoin Sodium (Inducers of CYP3A4 may affect estrogen drug metabolism. Inducers of CYP3A4, such as St. John's Wort (Hypericum perforatum) preparations, phenobarbital, carbamazepine, and rifampin, may reduce plasma concentrations of estrogens, possibly resulting in a decrease in therapeutic effects and/or changes in the uterine bleeding profile). Products include:

Posaconazole (Inhibitors of CYP3A4 may affect estrogen drug metabolism. Inhibitors of CYP3A4, such as erythromycin, clarithromycin, ketoconazole, itraconazole, ritonavir and grapefruit juice, may increase plasma concentrations of estrogens and may result in side effects). Products include:

Prednisolone (Inducers of CYP3A4 may affect estrogen drug metabolism. Inducers of CYP3A4, such as St. John's Wort (Hypericum perforatum) preparations, phenobarbital, carbamazepine, and rifampin, may reduce plasma concentrations of estrogens, possibly resulting in a decrease in therapeutic effects and/or changes in the uterine bleeding profile).
No products indexed under this heading.

Prednisolone Acetate (Inducers of CYP3A4 may affect estrogen drug metabolism. Inducers of CYP3A4, such as St. John's Wort (Hypericum perforatum) preparations, phenobarbital, carbamazepine, and rifampin, may reduce plasma concentrations of estrogens, possibly resulting in a decrease in therapeutic effects and/or changes in the uterine bleeding profile). Products include:

Prednisolone Sodium Phosphate (Inducers of CYP3A4 may affect estrogen drug metabolism. Inducers of CYP3A4, such as St. John's Wort (Hypericum perforatum) preparations, phenobarbital, carbamazepine, and rifampin, may reduce plasma concentrations of estrogens, possibly resulting in a decrease in therapeutic effects and/or changes in the uterine bleeding profile).
No products indexed under this heading.

Prednisolone Tebutate (Inducers of CYP3A4 may affect estrogen drug metabolism. Inducers of CYP3A4, such as St. John's Wort (Hypericum perforatum) preparations, phenobarbital, carbamazepine, and rifampin, may reduce plasma concentrations of estrogens, possibly resulting in a decrease in therapeutic effects and/or changes in the uterine bleeding profile).
No products indexed under this heading.

Prednisone (Inducers of CYP3A4 may affect estrogen drug metabolism. Inducers of CYP3A4, such as St. John's Wort (Hypericum perforatum) preparations, phenobarbital, carbamazepine, and rifampin, may reduce plasma concentrations of estrogens, possibly resulting in a decrease in therapeutic effects and/or changes in the uterine bleeding profile).
No products indexed under this heading.

Prednisone sodium phosphate (Inducers of CYP3A4 may affect estrogen drug metabolism. Inducers of CYP3A4, such as St. John's Wort (Hypericum perforatum) preparations, phenobarbital, carbamazepine, and rifampin, may reduce plasma concentrations of estrogens, possibly resulting in a decrease in therapeutic effects and/or changes in the uterine bleeding profile).
No products indexed under this heading.

Primidone (Inducers of CYP3A4 may affect estrogen drug metabolism. Inducers of CYP3A4, such as St. John's Wort (Hypericum perforatum) preparations, phenobarbital, carbamazepine, and rifampin, may reduce plasma concentrations of estrogens, possibly resulting in a decrease in therapeutic effects and/or changes in the uterine bleeding profile).
No products indexed under this heading.

Propoxyphene Hydrochloride (Inhibitors of CYP3A4 may affect estrogen drug metabolism. Inhibitors of CYP3A4, such as erythromycin, clarithromycin, ketoconazole, itraconazole, ritonavir and grapefruit juice, may increase plasma concentrations of estrogens and may result in side effects).
No products indexed under this heading.

Propoxyphene Napsylate (Inhibitors of CYP3A4 may affect estrogen drug metabolism. Inhibitors of CYP3A4, such as erythromycin, clarithromycin, ketoconazole, itraconazole, ritonavir and grapefruit juice, may increase plasma concentrations of estrogens and may result in side effects).
No products indexed under this heading.

Quinidine (Inhibitors of CYP3A4 may affect estrogen drug metabolism. Inhibitors of CYP3A4, such as erythromycin, clarithromycin, ketoconazole, itraconazole, ritonavir and grapefruit juice, may increase plasma concentrations of estrogens and may result in side effects).
No products indexed under this heading.

Quinidine Hydrochloride (Inhibitors of CYP3A4 may affect estrogen drug metabolism. Inhibitors of CYP3A4, such as erythromycin, clarithromycin, ketoconazole, itraconazole, ritonavir and grapefruit juice, may increase plasma concentrations of estrogens and may result in side effects).
No products indexed under this heading.

Quinidine Polygalacturonate (Inhibitors of CYP3A4 may affect estrogen drug metabolism. Inhibitors of CYP3A4, such as erythromycin, clarithromycin, ketoconazole, itraconazole, ritonavir and grapefruit juice, may increase plasma concentrations of estrogens and may result in side effects).
No products indexed under this heading.

Quinidine Sulfate (Inhibitors of CYP3A4 may affect estrogen drug metabolism. Inhibitors of CYP3A4, such as erythromycin, clarithromycin, ketoconazole, itraconazole, ritonavir and grapefruit juice, may increase plasma concentrations of estrogens and may result in side effects).
No products indexed under this heading.

Quinine (Inhibitors of CYP3A4 may affect estrogen drug metabolism. Inhibitors of CYP3A4, such as erythromycin, clarithromycin, ketoconazole, itraconazole, ritonavir and grapefruit juice, may increase plasma concentrations of estrogens and may result in side effects). Products include:

Quinine Sulfate (Inhibitors of CYP3A4 may affect estrogen drug metabolism. Inhibitors of CYP3A4, such as erythromycin, clarithromycin, ketoconazole, itraconazole, ritonavir and grapefruit juice, may increase plasma concentrations of estrogens and may result in side effects).
No products indexed under this heading.

Quinupristin (Inhibitors of CYP3A4 may affect estrogen drug metabolism. Inhibitors of CYP3A4, such as erythromycin, clarithromycin, ketoconazole, itraconazole, ritonavir and grapefruit juice, may increase plasma concentrations of estrogens and may result in side effects).
No products indexed under this heading.

Ranitidine Bismuth Citrate (Inhibitors of CYP3A4 may affect estrogen drug metabolism. Inhibitors of CYP3A4, such as erythromycin, clarithromycin, ketoconazole, itraconazole, ritonavir and grapefruit juice, may increase plasma concentrations of estrogens and may result in side effects).
No products indexed under this heading.

Ranitidine Hydrochloride (Inhibitors of CYP3A4 may affect estrogen drug metabolism. Inhibitors of CYP3A4, such as erythromycin, clarithromycin, ketoconazole, itraconazole, ritonavir and grapefruit juice, may increase plasma concentrations of estrogens and may result in side effects). Products include:
Zantac 1737
Zantac Injection 1732
Zantac Pharmacy 1735

Rifabutin (Inducers of CYP3A4 may affect estrogen drug metabolism. Inducers of CYP3A4, such as St. John's Wort (Hypericum perforatum) preparations, phenobarbital, carbamazepine, and rifampin, may reduce plasma concentrations of estrogens, possibly resulting in a decrease in therapeutic effects and/or changes in the uterine bleeding profile).
No products indexed under this heading.

Rifampicin (Inducers of CYP3A4 may affect estrogen drug metabolism. Inducers of CYP3A4, such as St. John's Wort (Hypericum perforatum) preparations, phenobarbital, carbamazepine, and rifampin, may reduce plasma concentrations of estrogens, possibly resulting in a decrease in therapeutic effects and/or changes in the uterine bleeding profile).
No products indexed under this heading.

Rifampin (Inducers of CYP3A4 may affect estrogen drug metabolism. Inducers of CYP3A4, such as rifampin, may reduce plasma concentrations of estrogens, possibly resulting in a decrease in therapeutic effects and/or changes in the uterine bleeding profile).
No products indexed under this heading.

Rifapentine (Inducers of CYP3A4 may affect estrogen drug metabolism. Inducers of CYP3A4, such as St. John's Wort (Hypericum perforatum) preparations, phenobarbital, carbamazepine, and rifampin, may reduce plasma concentrations of estrogens, possibly resulting in a decrease in therapeutic effects and/or changes in the uterine bleeding profile).
No products indexed under this heading.

Ritonavir (Inhibitors of CYP3A4 may affect estrogen drug metabolism. Inhibitors of CYP3A4, such as ritonavir, may increase plasma concentrations of estrogens and may result in side effects). Products include:
Kaletra 458
Norvir 509

Saquinavir (Inhibitors of CYP3A4 may affect estrogen drug metabolism. Inhibitors of CYP3A4, such as erythromycin, clarithromycin, ketoconazole, itraconazole, ritonavir and grapefruit juice, may increase plasma concentrations of estrogens and may result in side effects).
No products indexed under this heading.

Saquinavir Mesylate (Inhibitors of CYP3A4 may affect estrogen drug metabolism. Inhibitors of CYP3A4, such as erythromycin, clarithromycin, ketoconazole, itraconazole, ritonavir and grapefruit juice, may increase plasma concentrations of estrogens and may result in side effects).
No products indexed under this heading.

Sertraline Hydrochloride (Inhibitors of CYP3A4 may affect estrogen drug metabolism. Inhibitors of CYP3A4, such as erythromycin, clarithromycin, ketoconazole, itraconazole, ritonavir and grapefruit juice, may increase plasma concentrations of estrogens and may result in side effects).
No products indexed under this heading.

Sildenafil Citrate (Inhibitors of CYP3A4 may affect estrogen drug metabolism. Inhibitors of CYP3A4, such as erythromycin, clarithromycin, ketoconazole, itraconazole, ritonavir and grapefruit juice, may increase plasma concentrations of estrogens and may result in side effects).
No products indexed under this heading.

Sulfinpyrazone (Inducers of CYP3A4 may affect estrogen drug metabolism. Inducers of CYP3A4, such as St. John's Wort (Hypericum perforatum) preparations, phenobarbital, carbamazepine, and rifampin, may reduce plasma concentrations of estrogens, possibly resulting in a decrease in therapeutic effects and/or changes in the uterine bleeding profile).
No products indexed under this heading.

Telithromycin (Inhibitors of CYP3A4 may affect estrogen drug metabolism. Inhibitors of CYP3A4, such as erythromycin, clarithromycin, ketoconazole, itraconazole, ritonavir and grapefruit juice, may increase plasma concentrations of estrogens and may result in side effects). Products include:
Ketek 2991

Theophyllinate (Inducers of CYP3A4 may affect estrogen drug metabolism. Inducers of CYP3A4, such as St. John's Wort (Hypericum perforatum) preparations, phenobarbital, carbamazepine, and rifampin, may reduce plasma concentrations of estrogens, possibly resulting in a decrease in therapeutic effects and/or changes in the uterine bleeding profile).
No products indexed under this heading.

Theophylline (Inducers of CYP3A4 may affect estrogen drug metabolism. Inducers of CYP3A4, such as St. John's Wort (Hypericum perforatum) preparations, phenobarbital, carbamazepine, and rifampin, may reduce plasma concentrations of estrogens, possibly resulting in a decrease in therapeutic effects and/or changes in the uterine bleeding profile).
No products indexed under this heading.

Theophylline Anhydrous (Inducers of CYP3A4 may affect estrogen drug metabolism. Inducers of CYP3A4, such as St. John's Wort (Hypericum perforatum) preparations, phenobarbital, carbamazepine, and rifampin, may reduce plasma concentrations of estrogens, possibly resulting in a decrease in therapeutic effects and/or changes in the uterine bleeding profile). Products include:
Uniphyl 2817

Theophylline Calcium Salicylate (Inducers of CYP3A4 may affect estrogen drug metabolism. Inducers of CYP3A4, such as St. John's Wort (Hypericum perforatum) preparations, phenobarbital, carbamazepine, and rifampin, may reduce plasma concentrations of estrogens, possibly resulting in a decrease in therapeutic effects and/or changes in the uterine bleeding profile).
No products indexed under this heading.

Theophylline Dihydroxypropyl (Glyceryl) (Inducers of CYP3A4 may affect estrogen drug metabolism. Inducers of CYP3A4, such as St. John's Wort (Hypericum perforatum) preparations, phenobarbital, carbamazepine, and rifampin, may reduce plasma concentrations of estrogens, possibly resulting in a decrease in therapeutic effects and/or changes in the uterine bleeding profile).
No products indexed under this heading.

Theophylline Ethylenediamine (Inducers of CYP3A4 may affect estrogen drug metabolism. Inducers of CYP3A4, such as St. John's Wort (Hypericum perforatum) preparations, phenobarbital, carbamazepine, and rifampin, may reduce plasma concentrations of estrogens, possibly resulting in a decrease in therapeutic effects and/or changes in the uterine bleeding profile).
No products indexed under this heading.

Theophylline Sodium Glycinate (Inducers of CYP3A4 may affect estrogen drug metabolism. Inducers of CYP3A4, such as St. John's Wort (Hypericum perforatum) preparations, phenobarbital, carbamazepine, and rifampin, may reduce plasma concentrations of estrogens, possibly resulting in a decrease in therapeutic effects and/or changes in the uterine bleeding profile).
No products indexed under this heading.

Triamcinolone (Inducers of CYP3A4 may affect estrogen drug metabolism. Inducers of CYP3A4, such as St. John's Wort (Hypericum perforatum) preparations, phenobarbital, carbamazepine, and rifampin, may reduce plasma concentrations of estrogens, possibly resulting in a decrease in therapeutic effects and/or changes in the uterine bleeding profile).
No products indexed under this heading.

Triamcinolone Acetonide (Inducers of CYP3A4 may affect estrogen drug metabolism. Inducers of CYP3A4, such as St. John's Wort (Hypericum perforatum) preparations, phenobarbital, carbamazepine, and rifampin, may reduce plasma concentrations of estrogens, possibly resulting in a decrease in therapeutic effects and/or changes in the uterine bleeding profile). Products include:
Azmacort 408
Nasacort AQ 3019

Triamcinolone Diacetate (Inducers of CYP3A4 may affect estrogen drug metabolism. Inducers of CYP3A4, such as St. John's Wort (Hypericum perforatum) preparations, phenobarbital, carbamazepine, and rifampin, may reduce plasma concentrations of estrogens, possibly resulting in a decrease in therapeutic effects and/or changes in the uterine bleeding profile).
No products indexed under this heading.

Triamcinolone Hexacetonide (Inducers of CYP3A4 may affect estrogen drug metabolism. Inducers of CYP3A4, such as St. John's Wort (Hypericum perforatum) preparations, phenobarbital, carbamazepine, and rifampin, may reduce plasma concentrations of estrogens, possibly resulting in a decrease in therapeutic effects and/or changes in the uterine bleeding profile).
No products indexed under this heading.

Troglitazone (Inducers of CYP3A4 may affect estrogen drug metabolism. Inducers of CYP3A4, such as St. John's Wort (Hypericum perforatum) preparations, phenobarbital, carbamazepine, and rifampin, may reduce plasma concentrations of estrogens, possibly resulting in a decrease in therapeutic effects and/or changes in the uterine bleeding profile).
No products indexed under this heading.

Troleandomycin (Inhibitors of CYP3A4 may affect estrogen drug metabolism. Inhibitors of CYP3A4, such as erythromycin, clarithromycin, ketoconazole, itraconazole, ritonavir and grapefruit juice, may increase plasma concentrations of estrogens and may result in side effects).
No products indexed under this heading.

Valproate Sodium (Inhibitors of CYP3A4 may affect estrogen drug metabolism. Inhibitors of CYP3A4, such as erythromycin, clarithromycin, ketoconazole, itraconazole, ritonavir and grapefruit juice, may increase plasma concentrations of estrogens and may result in side effects).
No products indexed under this heading.

Vardenafil Hydrochloride (Inhibitors of CYP3A4 may affect estrogen drug metabolism. Inhibitors of CYP3A4, such as erythromycin, clarithromycin, ketoconazole, itraconazole, ritonavir and grapefruit juice, may increase plasma concentrations of estrogens and may result in side effects). Products include:
Levitra 3157

Verapamil Hydrochloride (Inhibitors of CYP3A4 may affect estrogen drug metabolism. Inhibitors of CYP3A4, such as erythromycin, clarithromycin, ketoconazole, itraconazole, ritonavir and grapefruit juice, may increase plasma concentrations of estrogens and may result in side effects). Products include:
Tarka 534

Voriconazole (Inhibitors of CYP3A4 may affect estrogen drug metabolism. Inhibitors of CYP3A4, such as erythromycin, clarithromycin, ketoconazole, itraconazole, ritonavir and grapefruit juice, may increase plasma concentrations of estrogens and may result in side effects).
No products indexed under this heading.

Zafirlukast (Inhibitors of CYP3A4 may affect estrogen drug metabolism. Inhibitors of CYP3A4, such as erythromycin, clarithromycin, ketoconazole, itraconazole, ritonavir and grapefruit juice, may increase plasma concentrations of estrogens and may result in side effects). Products include:
Accolate 3612

Zileuton (Inhibitors of CYP3A4 may affect estrogen drug metabolism. Inhibitors of CYP3A4, such as erythromycin, clarithromycin, ketoconazole, itraconazole, ritonavir and grapefruit juice, may increase plasma concentrations of estrogens and may result in side effects).
No products indexed under this heading.

Food Interactions

Grapefruit (Inhibitors of CYP3A4 may affect estrogen drug metabolism. Inhibitors of CYP3A4, such as erythromycin, clarithromycin, ketoconazole, itraconazole, ritonavir and grapefruit juice, may increase plasma concentrations of estrogens and may result in side effects).

Grapefruit Juice (Inhibitors of CYP3A4 may affect estrogen drug metabolism. Inhibitors of CYP3A4, such as grapefruit juice, may increase plasma concentrations of estrogens and may result in side effects).

PREMPHASE TABLETS
(Estrogens, Conjugated, Medroxyprogesterone Acetate)............ **3549**
May interact with cytochrome p450 3a4 inducers (selected), cytochrome p450 3a4 inhibitors (selected), erythromycin, thyroid preparations, and certain other agents. Compounds in these categories include:

Acetazolamide (Inhibitors of CYP3A4, such as erythromycin, clarithromycin, ketoconazole, itraconazole, ritonavir and grapefruit juice, may increase plasma concentrations of estrogens and may result in side effects).
No products indexed under this heading.

Acetazolamide Sodium (Inhibitors of CYP3A4, such as erythromycin, clarithromycin, ketoconazole, itraconazole, ritonavir and grapefruit juice, may increase plasma concentrations of estrogens and may result in side effects).
No products indexed under this heading.

Allium sativum (Inducers of CYP3A4, such as St. John's Wort preparations (Hypericum perforatum), phenobarbital, carbamazepine, and rifampin, may reduce plasma concentrations of estrogens, possibly resulting in a decrease in therapeutic effects and/or changes in the uterine bleeding profile).
No products indexed under this heading.

Aminoglutethimide (Aminoglutethimide administered concomitantly with medroxyprogesterone acetate (MPA) may significantly depress the bioavailability of MPA).
No products indexed under this heading.

Amiodarone Hydrochloride (Inhibitors of CYP3A4, such as erythromycin, clarithromycin, ketoconazole, itraconazole, ritonavir and grapefruit juice, may increase plasma concentrations of estrogens and may result in side effects).
No products indexed under this heading.

Amprenavir (Inhibitors of CYP3A4, such as erythromycin, clarithromycin, ketoconazole, itraconazole, ritonavir and grapefruit juice, may increase plasma concentrations of estrogens and may result in side effects).
No products indexed under this heading.

Anastrozole (Inhibitors of CYP3A4, such as erythromycin, clarithromycin, ketoconazole, itraconazole, ritonavir and grapefruit juice, may increase plasma concentrations of estrogens and may result in side effects).
No products indexed under this heading.

Aprepitant (Inhibitors of CYP3A4, such as erythromycin, clarithromycin, ketoconazole, itraconazole, ritonavir and grapefruit juice, may increase plasma concentrations of estrogens and may result in side effects). Products include:
Emend 2124

Atazanavir (Inhibitors of CYP3A4, such as erythromycin, clarithromycin, ketoconazole, itraconazole, ritonavir and grapefruit juice, may increase plasma concentrations of estrogens and may result in side effects).
No products indexed under this heading.

Atazanavir Sulfate (Inhibitors of CYP3A4, such as erythromycin, clarithromycin, ketoconazole, itraconazole, ritonavir and grapefruit juice, may increase plasma concentrations of estrogens and may result in side effects).
No products indexed under this heading.

Betamethasone (Inducers of CYP3A4, such as St. John's Wort preparations (Hypericum perforatum), phenobarbital, carbamazepine, and rifampin, may reduce plasma concentrations of estrogens, possibly resulting in a decrease in therapeutic effects and/or changes in the uterine bleeding profile).
No products indexed under this heading.

Betamethasone Acetate (Inducers of CYP3A4, such as St. John's Wort preparations (Hypericum perforatum), phenobarbital, carbamazepine, and rifampin, may reduce plasma concentrations of estrogens, possibly resulting in a decrease in therapeutic effects and/or changes in the uterine bleeding profile).
No products indexed under this heading.

Betamethasone Benzoate (Inducers of CYP3A4, such as St. John's Wort preparations (Hypericum perforatum), phenobarbital, carbamazepine, and rifampin, may reduce plasma concentrations of estrogens, possibly resulting in a decrease in therapeutic effects and/or changes in the uterine bleeding profile).
No products indexed under this heading.

Betamethasone Dipropionate (Inducers of CYP3A4, such as St. John's Wort preparations (Hypericum perforatum), phenobarbital, carbamazepine, and rifampin, may reduce plasma concentrations of estrogens, possibly resulting in a decrease in therapeutic effects and/or changes in the uterine bleeding profile). Products include:
Diprolene Lotion 0.05% 3108
Diprolene Ointment 0.05% 3109
Diprolene AF Cream 0.05% 3107
Lotrisone 3163

Betamethasone Sodium Phosphate (Inducers of CYP3A4, such as St. John's Wort preparations (Hypericum perforatum), phenobarbital, carbamazepine, and rifampin, may reduce plasma concentrations of estrogens, possibly resulting in a decrease in therapeutic effects and/or changes in the uterine bleeding profile).
No products indexed under this heading.

Betamethasone Valerate (Inducers of CYP3A4, such as St. John's Wort preparations (Hypericum perforatum), phenobarbital, carbamazepine, and rifampin, may reduce plasma concentrations of estrogens, possibly resulting in a decrease in therapeutic effects and/or changes in the uterine bleeding profile). Products include:
Luxíq 3321

Bosentan (Inducers of CYP3A4, such as St. John's Wort preparations (Hypericum perforatum), phenobarbital, carbamazepine, and rifampin, may reduce plasma concentrations of estrogens, possibly resulting in a decrease in therapeutic effects and/or changes in the uterine bleeding profile). Products include:
Tracleer 573

Carbamazepine (Inducers of CYP3A4, such as carbamazepine, may reduce plasma concentrations of estrogens, possibly resulting in a decrease in therapeutic effects and/or changes in the uterine bleeding profile). Products include:
Carbatrol 3280
Equetro 3477

Cimetidine (Inhibitors of CYP3A4, such as erythromycin, clarithromycin, ketoconazole, itraconazole, ritonavir and grapefruit juice, may increase plasma concentrations of estrogens and may result in side effects).
No products indexed under this heading.

Cimetidine Hydrochloride (Inhibitors of CYP3A4, such as erythromycin, clarithromycin, ketoconazole, itraconazole, ritonavir and grapefruit juice, may increase plasma concentrations of estrogens and may result in side effects).
No products indexed under this heading.

Ciprofloxacin (Inhibitors of CYP3A4, such as erythromycin, clarithromycin, ketoconazole, itraconazole, ritonavir and grapefruit juice, may increase plasma concentrations of estrogens and may result in side effects). Products include:
Cipro I.V. 3082
Cipro 3073
Cipro XR 3091
Ciprodex 583

Ciprofloxacin Hydrochloride (Inducers of CYP3A4, such as St. John's Wort preparations (Hypericum perforatum), phenobarbital, carbamazepine, and rifampin, may reduce plasma concentrations of estrogens, possibly resulting in a decrease in therapeutic effects and/or changes in the uterine bleeding profile). Products include:
Cipro 3073

Cisplatin (Inducers of CYP3A4, such as St. John's Wort preparations (Hypericum perforatum), phenobarbital, carbamazepine, and rifampin, may reduce plasma concentrations of estrogens, possibly resulting in a decrease in therapeutic effects and/or changes in the uterine bleeding profile).
No products indexed under this heading.

Clarithromycin (Inhibitors of CYP3A4, such as clarithromycin, may increase plasma concentrations of estrogens and may result in side effects). Products include:
Biaxin/Biaxin XL 412

Clotrimazole (Inhibitors of CYP3A4, such as erythromycin, clarithromycin, ketoconazole, itraconazole, ritonavir and grapefruit juice, may increase plasma concentrations of estrogens and may result in side effects). Products include:
Lotrisone 3163

Conivaptan Hydrochloride (Inhibitors of CYP3A4, such as erythromycin, clarithromycin, ketoconazole, itraconazole, ritonavir and grapefruit juice, may increase plasma concentrations of estrogens and may result in side effects). Products include:
Vaprisol 689

Cortisone Acetate (Inducers of CYP3A4, such as St. John's Wort preparations (Hypericum perforatum), phenobarbital, carbamazepine, and rifampin, may reduce plasma concentrations of estrogens, possibly resulting in a decrease in therapeutic effects and/or changes in the uterine bleeding profile).
No products indexed under this heading.

Cyclosporine (Inhibitors of CYP3A4, such as erythromycin, clarithromycin, ketoconazole, itraconazole, ritonavir and grapefruit juice, may increase plasma concentrations of estrogens and may result in side effects). Products include:
Gengraf 440
Neoral Oral Solution 2496
Neoral Capsules 2496
Restasis 605

Dalfopristin (Inhibitors of CYP3A4, such as erythromycin, clarithromycin, ketoconazole, itraconazole, ritonavir and grapefruit juice, may increase plasma concentrations of estrogens and may result in side effects).
No products indexed under this heading.

Danazol (Inhibitors of CYP3A4, such as erythromycin, clarithromycin, ketoconazole, itraconazole, ritonavir and grapefruit juice, may increase plasma concentrations of estrogens and may result in side effects).
No products indexed under this heading.

Darunavir (Inhibitors of CYP3A4, such as erythromycin, clarithromycin, ketoconazole, itraconazole, ritonavir and grapefruit juice, may increase plasma concentrations of estrogens and may result in side effects).
No products indexed under this heading.

Dasatinib (Inhibitors of CYP3A4, such as erythromycin, clarithromycin, ketoconazole, itraconazole, ritonavir and grapefruit juice, may increase plasma concentrations of estrogens and may result in side effects).
No products indexed under this heading.

Delavirdine Mesylate (Inhibitors of CYP3A4, such as erythromycin, clarithromycin, ketoconazole, itraconazole, ritonavir and grapefruit juice, may increase plasma concentrations of estrogens and may result in side effects).
No products indexed under this heading.

Delavirine (Inhibitors of CYP3A4, such as erythromycin, clarithromycin, ketoconazole, itraconazole, ritonavir and grapefruit juice, may increase plasma concentrations of estrogens and may result in side effects).
No products indexed under this heading.

Desloratadine (Inhibitors of CYP3A4, such as erythromycin, clarithromycin, ketoconazole, itraconazole, ritonavir and grapefruit juice, may increase plasma concentrations of estrogens and may result in side effects). Products include:
Clarinex Syrup 3098
Clarinex 3098
Clarinex Reditabs 3098
Clarinex-D 12-Hour 3101
Clarinex-D 3104

Dexamethasone (Inducers of CYP3A4, such as St. John's Wort preparations (Hypericum perforatum), phenobarbital, carbamazepine, and rifampin, may reduce plasma concentrations of estrogens, possibly resulting in a decrease in therapeutic effects and/or changes in the uterine bleeding profile). Products include:
Ciprodex 583
Ozurdex ....⊙223
Tobramycin and Dexamethasone
Ophthalmic Suspension ....⊙251

Dexamethasone Acetate (Inducers of CYP3A4, such as St. John's Wort preparations (Hypericum perforatum), phenobarbital, carbamazepine, and rifampin, may reduce plasma concentrations of estrogens, possibly resulting in a decrease in therapeutic effects and/or changes in the uterine bleeding profile).
No products indexed under this heading.

Dexamethasone Phosphate (Inducers of CYP3A4, such as St. John's Wort preparations (Hypericum perforatum), phenobarbital, carbamazepine, and rifampin, may reduce plasma concentrations of estrogens, possibly resulting in a decrease in therapeutic effects and/or changes in the uterine bleeding profile).
No products indexed under this heading.

Dexamethasone Sodium (Inducers of CYP3A4, such as St. John's Wort preparations (Hypericum perforatum), phenobarbital, carbamazepine, and rifampin, may reduce plasma concentrations of estrogens, possibly resulting in a decrease in therapeutic effects and/or changes in the uterine bleeding profile).
No products indexed under this heading.

IMPORTANT NOTE: Always consult each drug listing in the patient's regimen for possible interactions.

Premphase Interactions Index 1446

Dexamethasone Sodium Phosphate (Inducers of CYP3A4, such as St. John's Wort preparations (Hypericum perforatum), phenobarbital, carbamazepine, and rifampin, may reduce plasma concentrations of estrogens, possibly resulting in a decrease in therapeutic effects and/or changes in the uterine bleeding profile).
No products indexed under this heading.

Dexamethasone Sodium Phosphate Injection (Inducers of CYP3A4, such as St. John's Wort preparations (Hypericum perforatum), phenobarbital, carbamazepine, and rifampin, may reduce plasma concentrations of estrogens, possibly resulting in a decrease in therapeutic effects and/or changes in the uterine bleeding profile).
No products indexed under this heading.

Diltiazem Hydrochloride (Inhibitors of CYP3A4, such as erythromycin, clarithromycin, ketoconazole, itraconazole, ritonavir and grapefruit juice, may increase plasma concentrations of estrogens and may result in side effects). Products include:
Cardizem LA 423

Diltiazem Maleate (Inhibitors of CYP3A4, such as erythromycin, clarithromycin, ketoconazole, itraconazole, ritonavir and grapefruit juice, may increase plasma concentrations of estrogens and may result in side effects).
No products indexed under this heading.

Doxorubicin Hydrochloride (Inducers of CYP3A4, such as St. John's Wort preparations (Hypericum perforatum), phenobarbital, carbamazepine, and rifampin, may reduce plasma concentrations of estrogens, possibly resulting in a decrease in therapeutic effects and/or changes in the uterine bleeding profile).
No products indexed under this heading.

Efavirenz (Inhibitors of CYP3A4, such as erythromycin, clarithromycin, ketoconazole, itraconazole, ritonavir and grapefruit juice, may increase plasma concentrations of estrogens and may result in side effects). Products include:
Atripla 906

Erythromycin (Inhibitors of CYP3A4, such as erythromycin, may increase plasma concentrations of estrogens and may result in side effects).
No products indexed under this heading.

Erythromycin, Topical (Inhibitors of CYP3A4, such as erythromycin, may increase plasma concentrations of estrogens and may result in side effects).
No products indexed under this heading.

Erythromycin Estolate (Inhibitors of CYP3A4, such as erythromycin, may increase plasma concentrations of estrogens and may result in side effects).
No products indexed under this heading.

Erythromycin Ethylsuccinate (Inhibitors of CYP3A4, such as erythromycin, may increase plasma concentrations of estrogens and may result in side effects). Products include:
E.E.S. 437
EryPed 435

Erythromycin Gluceptate (Inhibitors of CYP3A4, such as erythromycin, may increase plasma concentrations of estrogens and may result in side effects).
No products indexed under this heading.

Erythromycin Lactobionate (Inhibitors of CYP3A4, such as erythromycin, may increase plasma concentrations of estrogens and may result in side effects).
No products indexed under this heading.

Erythromycin Stearate (Inhibitors of CYP3A4, such as erythromycin, may increase plasma concentrations of estrogens and may result in side effects).
No products indexed under this heading.

Esomeprazole Magnesium (Inhibitors of CYP3A4, such as erythromycin, clarithromycin, ketoconazole, itraconazole, ritonavir and grapefruit juice, may increase plasma concentrations of estrogens and may result in side effects). Products include:
Nexium Capsules 704
Nexium Oral Suspension 704

Esomeprazole Sodium (Inhibitors of CYP3A4, such as erythromycin, clarithromycin, ketoconazole, itraconazole, ritonavir and grapefruit juice, may increase plasma concentrations of estrogens and may result in side effects). Products include:
Nexium I.V. 712

Ethosuximide (Inducers of CYP3A4, such as St. John's Wort preparations (Hypericum perforatum), phenobarbital, carbamazepine, and rifampin, may reduce plasma concentrations of estrogens, possibly resulting in a decrease in therapeutic effects and/or changes in the uterine bleeding profile).
No products indexed under this heading.

Fat (Single dose studies in healthy, postmenopausal women were conducted to investigate any potential drug interaction when PREMPHASE is administered with a high fat breakfast. Administration with food decreased the C_{max} of total estrone by 18% to 34% and increased total equilin C_{max} by 38% compared to the fasting state, with no other effect on the rate or extent of absorption of other conjugated or unconjugated estrogens. Administration with food approximately doubles MPA C_{max} and increases MPA AUC by approximately 20% to 30%).
No products indexed under this heading.

Felbamate (Inducers of CYP3A4, such as St. John's Wort preparations (Hypericum perforatum), phenobarbital, carbamazepine, and rifampin, may reduce plasma concentrations of estrogens, possibly resulting in a decrease in therapeutic effects and/or changes in the uterine bleeding profile).
No products indexed under this heading.

Fluconazole (Inhibitors of CYP3A4, such as erythromycin, clarithromycin, ketoconazole, itraconazole, ritonavir and grapefruit juice, may increase plasma concentrations of estrogens and may result in side effects).
No products indexed under this heading.

Fludrocortisone Acetate (Inducers of CYP3A4, such as St. John's Wort preparations (Hypericum perforatum), phenobarbital, carbamazepine, and rifampin, may reduce plasma concentrations of estrogens, possibly resulting in a decrease in therapeutic effects and/or changes in the uterine bleeding profile).
No products indexed under this heading.

Fluoxetine (Inhibitors of CYP3A4, such as erythromycin, clarithromycin, ketoconazole, itraconazole, ritonavir and grapefruit juice, may increase plasma concentrations of estrogens and may result in side effects).
No products indexed under this heading.

Fluoxetine Hydrochloride (Inhibitors of CYP3A4, such as erythromycin, clarithromycin, ketoconazole, itraconazole, ritonavir and grapefruit juice, may increase plasma concentrations of estrogens and may result in side effects). Products include:
Prozac Weekly 1941
Prozac Pulvules 1941
Symbyax 1965

Fluvoxamine Maleate (Inhibitors of CYP3A4, such as erythromycin, clarithromycin, ketoconazole, itraconazole, ritonavir and grapefruit juice, may increase plasma concentrations of estrogens and may result in side effects).
No products indexed under this heading.

Fosamprenavir Calcium (Inhibitors of CYP3A4, such as erythromycin, clarithromycin, ketoconazole, itraconazole, ritonavir and grapefruit juice, may increase plasma concentrations of estrogens and may result in side effects). Products include:
Lexiva Oral Suspension 1558
Lexiva 1558

Fosphenytoin Sodium (Inducers of CYP3A4, such as St. John's Wort preparations (Hypericum perforatum), phenobarbital, carbamazepine, and rifampin, may reduce plasma concentrations of estrogens, possibly resulting in a decrease in therapeutic effects and/or changes in the uterine bleeding profile).
No products indexed under this heading.

Garlic Extract (Inducers of CYP3A4, such as St. John's Wort preparations (Hypericum perforatum), phenobarbital, carbamazepine, and rifampin, may reduce plasma concentrations of estrogens, possibly resulting in a decrease in therapeutic effects and/or changes in the uterine bleeding profile).
No products indexed under this heading.

Garlic Oil (Inducers of CYP3A4, such as St. John's Wort preparations (Hypericum perforatum), phenobarbital, carbamazepine, and rifampin, may reduce plasma concentrations of estrogens, possibly resulting in a decrease in therapeutic effects and/or changes in the uterine bleeding profile).
No products indexed under this heading.

Hydrocortisone (Inducers of CYP3A4, such as St. John's Wort preparations (Hypericum perforatum), phenobarbital, carbamazepine, and rifampin, may reduce plasma concentrations of estrogens, possibly resulting in a decrease in therapeutic effects and/or changes in the uterine bleeding profile).
No products indexed under this heading.

Hydrocortisone (Alcohol) (Inducers of CYP3A4, such as St. John's Wort preparations (Hypericum perforatum), phenobarbital, carbamazepine, and rifampin, may reduce plasma concentrations of estrogens, possibly resulting in a decrease in therapeutic effects and/or changes in the uterine bleeding profile).
No products indexed under this heading.

Hydrocortisone Acetate (Inducers of CYP3A4, such as St. John's Wort preparations (Hypericum perforatum), phenobarbital, carbamazepine, and rifampin, may reduce plasma concentrations of estrogens, possibly resulting in a decrease in therapeutic effects and/or changes in the uterine bleeding profile).
No products indexed under this heading.

Hydrocortisone Butyrate (Inducers of CYP3A4, such as St. John's Wort preparations (Hypericum perforatum), phenobarbital, carbamazepine, and rifampin, may reduce plasma concentrations of estrogens, possibly resulting in a decrease in therapeutic effects and/or changes in the uterine bleeding profile).
No products indexed under this heading.

Hydrocortisone Cypionate (Inducers of CYP3A4, such as St. John's Wort preparations (Hypericum perforatum), phenobarbital, carbamazepine, and rifampin, may reduce plasma concentrations of estrogens, possibly resulting in a decrease in therapeutic effects and/or changes in the uterine bleeding profile).
No products indexed under this heading.

Hydrocortisone Hemisuccinate (Inducers of CYP3A4, such as St. John's Wort preparations (Hypericum perforatum), phenobarbital, carbamazepine, and rifampin, may reduce plasma concentrations of estrogens, possibly resulting in a decrease in therapeutic effects and/or changes in the uterine bleeding profile).
No products indexed under this heading.

Hydrocortisone Probutate (Inducers of CYP3A4, such as St. John's Wort preparations (Hypericum perforatum), phenobarbital, carbamazepine, and rifampin, may reduce plasma concentrations of estrogens, possibly resulting in a decrease in therapeutic effects and/or changes in the uterine bleeding profile).
No products indexed under this heading.

Hydrocortisone Sodium Phosphate (Inducers of CYP3A4, such as St. John's Wort preparations (Hypericum perforatum), phenobarbital, carbamazepine, and rifampin, may reduce plasma concentrations of estrogens, possibly resulting in a decrease in therapeutic effects and/or changes in the uterine bleeding profile).
No products indexed under this heading.

Hydrocortisone Sodium Succinate (Inducers of CYP3A4, such as St. John's Wort preparations (Hypericum perforatum), phenobarbital, carbamazepine, and rifampin, may reduce plasma concentrations of estrogens, possibly resulting in a decrease in therapeutic effects and/or changes in the uterine bleeding profile).
No products indexed under this heading.

Hydrocortisone Valerate (Inducers of CYP3A4, such as St. John's Wort preparations (Hypericum perforatum), phenobarbital, carbamazepine, and rifampin, may reduce plasma concentrations of estrogens, possibly resulting in a decrease in therapeutic effects and/or changes in the uterine bleeding profile).
No products indexed under this heading.

Hypericum (Inducers of CYP3A4, such as St. John's Wort preparations (Hypericum perforatum), phenobarbital, carbamazepine, and rifampin, may reduce plasma concentrations of estrogens, possibly resulting in a decrease in therapeutic effects and/or changes in the uterine bleeding profile).
No products indexed under this heading.

Hypericum Perforatum (Inducers of CYP3A4, such as St. John's Wort preparations (Hypericum perforatum), may reduce plasma concentrations of estrogens, possibly resulting in a decrease in therapeutic effects and/or changes in the uterine bleeding profile). Products include:
Traumeel 1800

Imatinib Mesylate (Inhibitors of CYP3A4, such as erythromycin, clarithromycin, ketoconazole, itraconazole, ritonavir and grapefruit juice, may increase plasma concentrations of estrogens and may result in side effects). Products include:
Gleevec 2477

Indinavir Sulfate (Inhibitors of CYP3A4, such as erythromycin, clarithromycin, ketoconazole, itraconazole, ritonavir and grapefruit juice, may

increase plasma concentrations of estrogens and may result in side effects). Products include:

Isoniazid (Inhibitors of CYP3A4, such as erythromycin, clarithromycin, ketoconazole, itraconazole, ritonavir and grapefruit juice, may increase plasma concentrations of estrogens and may result in side effects).

No products indexed under this heading.

Itraconazole (Inhibitors of CYP3A4, such as itraconazole, may increase plasma concentrations of estrogens and may result in side effects).

No products indexed under this heading.

Ketoconazole (Inhibitors of CYP3A4, such as ketoconazole, may increase plasma concentrations of estrogens and may result in side effects). Products include:

Lapatinib (Inhibitors of CYP3A4, such as erythromycin, clarithromycin, ketoconazole, itraconazole, ritonavir and grapefruit juice, may increase plasma concentrations of estrogens and may result in side effects). Products include:

Levothyroxine Sodium (Estrogen administration leads to increased thyroid-binding globulin (TBG) levels. Patients with normal thyroid function can compensate for the increased TBG by making more thyroid hormone, thus maintaining free T4 and T3 serum concentrations in the normal range. Patients dependent on thyroid hormone replacement therapy who are also receiving estrogens may require increased doses of their thyroid replacement therapy. These patients should have their thyroid function monitored in order to maintain their free thyroid hormone levels in an acceptable range). Products include:

Liothyronine Sodium (Estrogen administration leads to increased thyroid-binding globulin (TBG) levels. Patients with normal thyroid function can compensate for the increased TBG by making more thyroid hormone, thus maintaining free T4 and T3 serum concentrations in the normal range. Patients dependent on thyroid hormone replacement therapy who are also receiving estrogens may require increased doses of their thyroid replacement therapy. These patients should have their thyroid function monitored in order to maintain their free thyroid hormone levels in an acceptable range). Products include:

Liotrix (Estrogen administration leads to increased thyroid-binding globulin (TBG) levels. Patients with normal thyroid function can compensate for the increased TBG by making more thyroid hormone, thus maintaining free T4 and T3 serum concentrations in the normal range. Patients dependent on thyroid hormone replacement therapy who are also receiving estrogens may require increased doses of their thyroid replacement therapy. These patients should have their thyroid function monitored in order to maintain their free thyroid hormone levels in an acceptable range).

No products indexed under this heading.

Lopinavir (Inhibitors of CYP3A4, such as erythromycin, clarithromycin, ketoconazole, itraconazole, ritonavir and grapefruit juice, may increase plasma concentrations of estrogens and may result in side effects). Products include:

Loratadine (Inhibitors of CYP3A4, such as erythromycin, clarithromycin, ketoconazole, itraconazole, ritonavir and grapefruit juice, may increase plasma concentrations of estrogens and may result in side effects).

No products indexed under this heading.

Mephenytoin (Inducers of CYP3A4, such as St. John's Wort preparations (Hypericum perforatum), phenobarbital, carbamazepine, and rifampin, may reduce plasma concentrations of estrogens, possibly resulting in a decrease in therapeutic effects and/or changes in the uterine bleeding profile).

No products indexed under this heading.

Methsuximide (Inducers of CYP3A4, such as St. John's Wort preparations (Hypericum perforatum), phenobarbital, carbamazepine, and rifampin, may reduce plasma concentrations of estrogens, possibly resulting in a decrease in therapeutic effects and/or changes in the uterine bleeding profile).

No products indexed under this heading.

Methylprednisolone (Inducers of CYP3A4, such as St. John's Wort preparations (Hypericum perforatum), phenobarbital, carbamazepine, and rifampin, may reduce plasma concentrations of estrogens, possibly resulting in a decrease in therapeutic effects and/or changes in the uterine bleeding profile).

No products indexed under this heading.

Methylprednisolone Acetate (Inducers of CYP3A4, such as St. John's Wort preparations (Hypericum perforatum), phenobarbital, carbamazepine, and rifampin, may reduce plasma concentrations of estrogens, possibly resulting in a decrease in therapeutic effects and/or changes in the uterine bleeding profile).

No products indexed under this heading.

Methylprednisolone Sodium Succinate (Inducers of CYP3A4, such as St. John's Wort preparations (Hypericum perforatum), phenobarbital, carbamazepine, and rifampin, may reduce plasma concentrations of estrogens, possibly resulting in a decrease in therapeutic effects and/or changes in the uterine bleeding profile).

No products indexed under this heading.

Metronidazole (Inhibitors of CYP3A4, such as erythromycin, clarithromycin, ketoconazole, itraconazole, ritonavir and grapefruit juice, may increase plasma concentrations of estrogens and may result in side effects). Products include:

Metronidazole Benzoate (Inhibitors of CYP3A4, such as erythromycin, clarithromycin, ketoconazole, itraconazole, ritonavir and grapefruit juice, may increase plasma concentrations of estrogens and may result in side effects).

No products indexed under this heading.

Metronidazole Hydrochloride (Inhibitors of CYP3A4, such as erythromycin, clarithromycin, ketoconazole, itraconazole, ritonavir and grapefruit juice, may increase plasma concentrations of estrogens and may result in side effects).

No products indexed under this heading.

Metronidazole Sodium (Inhibitors of CYP3A4, such as erythromycin, clarithromycin, ketoconazole, itraconazole, ritonavir and grapefruit juice, may increase plasma concentrations of estrogens and may result in side effects).

No products indexed under this heading.

Miconazole (Inhibitors of CYP3A4, such as erythromycin, clarithromycin, ketoconazole, itraconazole, ritonavir and grapefruit juice, may increase plasma concentrations of estrogens and may result in side effects).

No products indexed under this heading.

Miconazole Nitrate (Inhibitors of CYP3A4, such as erythromycin, clarithromycin, ketoconazole, itraconazole, ritonavir and grapefruit juice, may increase plasma concentrations of estrogens and may result in side effects). Products include:

Mifepristone (Inhibitors of CYP3A4, such as erythromycin, clarithromycin, ketoconazole, itraconazole, ritonavir and grapefruit juice, may increase plasma concentrations of estrogens and may result in side effects).

No products indexed under this heading.

Modafinil (Inducers of CYP3A4, such as St. John's Wort preparations (Hypericum perforatum), phenobarbital, carbamazepine, and rifampin, may reduce plasma concentrations of estrogens, possibly resulting in a decrease in therapeutic effects and/or changes in the uterine bleeding profile). Products include:

Nafcillin Sodium (Inducers of CYP3A4, such as St. John's Wort preparations (Hypericum perforatum), phenobarbital, carbamazepine, and rifampin, may reduce plasma concentrations of estrogens, possibly resulting in a decrease in therapeutic effects and/or changes in the uterine bleeding profile).

No products indexed under this heading.

Nefazodone Hydrochloride (Inhibitors of CYP3A4, such as erythromycin, clarithromycin, ketoconazole, itraconazole, ritonavir and grapefruit juice, may increase plasma concentrations of estrogens and may result in side effects).

No products indexed under this heading.

Nelfinavir Mesylate (Inhibitors of CYP3A4, such as erythromycin, clarithromycin, ketoconazole, itraconazole, ritonavir and grapefruit juice, may increase plasma concentrations of estrogens and may result in side effects).

No products indexed under this heading.

Nevirapine (Inhibitors of CYP3A4, such as erythromycin, clarithromycin, ketoconazole, itraconazole, ritonavir and grapefruit juice, may increase plasma concentrations of estrogens and may result in side effects). Products include:

Niacin (Inhibitors of CYP3A4, such as erythromycin, clarithromycin, ketoconazole, itraconazole, ritonavir and grapefruit juice, may increase plasma concentrations of estrogens and may result in side effects). Products include:

Niacinamide (Inhibitors of CYP3A4, such as erythromycin, clarithromycin, ketoconazole, itraconazole, ritonavir and grapefruit juice, may increase plasma concentrations of estrogens and may result in side effects). Products include:

Niacinamide Hydroiodide (Inhibitors of CYP3A4, such as erythromycin, clarithromycin, ketoconazole, itraconazole, ritonavir and grapefruit juice, may increase plasma concentrations of estrogens and may result in side effects).

No products indexed under this heading.

Nicotinamide (Inhibitors of CYP3A4, such as erythromycin, clarithromycin, ketoconazole, itraconazole, ritonavir and grapefruit juice, may increase plasma concentrations of estrogens and may result in side effects).

No products indexed under this heading.

Nifedipine (Inhibitors of CYP3A4, such as erythromycin, clarithromycin, ketoconazole, itraconazole, ritonavir and grapefruit juice, may increase plasma concentrations of estrogens and may result in side effects).

No products indexed under this heading.

Norfloxacin (Inhibitors of CYP3A4, such as erythromycin, clarithromycin, ketoconazole, itraconazole, ritonavir and grapefruit juice, may increase plasma concentrations of estrogens and may result in side effects). Products include:

Omeprazole (Inhibitors of CYP3A4, such as erythromycin, clarithromycin, ketoconazole, itraconazole, ritonavir and grapefruit juice, may increase plasma concentrations of estrogens and may result in side effects).

No products indexed under this heading.

Oxcarbazepine (Inducers of CYP3A4, such as St. John's Wort preparations (Hypericum perforatum), phenobarbital, carbamazepine, and rifampin, may reduce plasma concentrations of estrogens, possibly resulting in a decrease in therapeutic effects and/or changes in the uterine bleeding profile).

No products indexed under this heading.

Paroxetine Hydrochloride (Inhibitors of CYP3A4, such as erythromycin, clarithromycin, ketoconazole, itraconazole, ritonavir and grapefruit juice, may increase plasma concentrations of estrogens and may result in side effects). Products include:

Phenobarbital (Inducers of CYP3A4, such as phenobarbital, may reduce plasma concentrations of estrogens, possibly resulting in a decrease in therapeutic effects and/or changes in the uterine bleeding profile). Products include:

Phenobarbital Sodium (Inducers of CYP3A4, such as phenobarbital, may reduce plasma concentrations of estrogens, possibly resulting in a decrease in therapeutic effects and/or changes in the uterine bleeding profile).

No products indexed under this heading.

Phenytoin (Inducers of CYP3A4, such as St. John's Wort preparations (Hypericum perforatum), phenobarbital, carbamazepine, and rifampin, may reduce plasma concentrations of estrogens, possibly resulting in a decrease in therapeutic effects and/or changes in the uterine bleeding profile).

No products indexed under this heading.

Phenytoin Sodium (Inducers of CYP3A4, such as St. John's Wort preparations (Hypericum perforatum), phenobarbital, carbamazepine, and rifampin, may reduce plasma concentrations of estrogens, possibly resulting in a decrease in therapeutic effects and/or changes in the uterine bleeding profile). Products include:

IMPORTANT NOTE: Always consult each drug listing in the patient's regimen for possible interactions.

Posaconazole (Inhibitors of CYP3A4, such as erythromycin, clarithromycin, ketoconazole, itraconazole, ritonavir and grapefruit juice, may increase plasma concentrations of estrogens and may result in side effects). Products include:
　Noxafil 3172

Prednisolone (Inducers of CYP3A4, such as St. John's Wort preparations (Hypericum perforatum), phenobarbital, carbamazepine, and rifampin, may reduce plasma concentrations of estrogens, possibly resulting in a decrease in therapeutic effects and/or changes in the uterine bleeding profile).
　No products indexed under this heading.

Prednisolone Acetate (Inducers of CYP3A4, such as St. John's Wort preparations (Hypericum perforatum), phenobarbital, carbamazepine, and rifampin, may reduce plasma concentrations of estrogens, possibly resulting in a decrease in therapeutic effects and/or changes in the uterine bleeding profile). Products include:
　Blephamide .... ⊙212, ⊙214
　Pred Forte .... ⊙225
　Pred Mild .... ⊙230
　Pred-G .... ⊙226, ⊙227

Prednisolone Sodium Phosphate (Inducers of CYP3A4, such as St. John's Wort preparations (Hypericum perforatum), phenobarbital, carbamazepine, and rifampin, may reduce plasma concentrations of estrogens, possibly resulting in a decrease in therapeutic effects and/or changes in the uterine bleeding profile).
　No products indexed under this heading.

Prednisolone Tebutate (Inducers of CYP3A4, such as St. John's Wort preparations (Hypericum perforatum), phenobarbital, carbamazepine, and rifampin, may reduce plasma concentrations of estrogens, possibly resulting in a decrease in therapeutic effects and/or changes in the uterine bleeding profile).
　No products indexed under this heading.

Prednisone (Inducers of CYP3A4, such as St. John's Wort preparations (Hypericum perforatum), phenobarbital, carbamazepine, and rifampin, may reduce plasma concentrations of estrogens, possibly resulting in a decrease in therapeutic effects and/or changes in the uterine bleeding profile).
　No products indexed under this heading.

Prednisone sodium phosphate (Inducers of CYP3A4, such as St. John's Wort preparations (Hypericum perforatum), phenobarbital, carbamazepine, and rifampin, may reduce plasma concentrations of estrogens, possibly resulting in a decrease in therapeutic effects and/or changes in the uterine bleeding profile).
　No products indexed under this heading.

Primidone (Inducers of CYP3A4, such as St. John's Wort preparations (Hypericum perforatum), phenobarbital, carbamazepine, and rifampin, may reduce plasma concentrations of estrogens, possibly resulting in a decrease in therapeutic effects and/or changes in the uterine bleeding profile).
　No products indexed under this heading.

Propoxyphene Hydrochloride (Inhibitors of CYP3A4, such as erythromycin, clarithromycin, ketoconazole, itraconazole, ritonavir and grapefruit juice, may increase plasma concentrations of estrogens and may result in side effects).
　No products indexed under this heading.

Propoxyphene Napsylate (Inhibitors of CYP3A4, such as erythromycin, clarithromycin, ketoconazole, itraconazole, ritonavir and grapefruit juice, may increase plasma concentrations of estrogens and may result in side effects).
　No products indexed under this heading.

Quinidine (Inhibitors of CYP3A4, such as erythromycin, clarithromycin, ketoconazole, itraconazole, ritonavir and grapefruit juice, may increase plasma concentrations of estrogens and may result in side effects).
　No products indexed under this heading.

Quinidine Hydrochloride (Inhibitors of CYP3A4, such as erythromycin, clarithromycin, ketoconazole, itraconazole, ritonavir and grapefruit juice, may increase plasma concentrations of estrogens and may result in side effects).
　No products indexed under this heading.

Quinidine Polygalacturonate (Inhibitors of CYP3A4, such as erythromycin, clarithromycin, ketoconazole, itraconazole, ritonavir and grapefruit juice, may increase plasma concentrations of estrogens and may result in side effects).
　No products indexed under this heading.

Quinidine Sulfate (Inhibitors of CYP3A4, such as erythromycin, clarithromycin, ketoconazole, itraconazole, ritonavir and grapefruit juice, may increase plasma concentrations of estrogens and may result in side effects).
　No products indexed under this heading.

Quinine (Inhibitors of CYP3A4, such as erythromycin, clarithromycin, ketoconazole, itraconazole, ritonavir and grapefruit juice, may increase plasma concentrations of estrogens and may result in side effects). Products include:
　Hyland's Leg Cramps PM with Quinine 3315

Quinine Sulfate (Inhibitors of CYP3A4, such as erythromycin, clarithromycin, ketoconazole, itraconazole, ritonavir and grapefruit juice, may increase plasma concentrations of estrogens and may result in side effects).
　No products indexed under this heading.

Quinupristin (Inhibitors of CYP3A4, such as erythromycin, clarithromycin, ketoconazole, itraconazole, ritonavir and grapefruit juice, may increase plasma concentrations of estrogens and may result in side effects).
　No products indexed under this heading.

Ranitidine Bismuth Citrate (Inhibitors of CYP3A4, such as erythromycin, clarithromycin, ketoconazole, itraconazole, ritonavir and grapefruit juice, may increase plasma concentrations of estrogens and may result in side effects).
　No products indexed under this heading.

Ranitidine Hydrochloride (Inhibitors of CYP3A4, such as erythromycin, clarithromycin, ketoconazole, itraconazole, ritonavir and grapefruit juice, may increase plasma concentrations of estrogens and may result in side effects). Products include:
　Zantac 1737
　Zantac Injection 1732
　Zantac Pharmacy 1735

Rifabutin (Inducers of CYP3A4, such as St. John's Wort preparations (Hypericum perforatum), phenobarbital, carbamazepine, and rifampin, may reduce plasma concentrations of estrogens, possibly resulting in a decrease in therapeutic effects and/or changes in the uterine bleeding profile).
　No products indexed under this heading.

Rifampicin (Inducers of CYP3A4, such as St. John's Wort preparations (Hypericum perforatum), phenobarbital, carbamazepine, and rifampin, may reduce plasma concentrations of estrogens, possibly resulting in a decrease in therapeutic effects and/or changes in the uterine bleeding profile).
　No products indexed under this heading.

Rifampin (Inducers of CYP3A4, such as rifampin, may reduce plasma concentrations of estrogens, possibly resulting in a decrease in therapeutic effects and/or changes in the uterine bleeding profile).
　No products indexed under this heading.

Rifapentine (Inducers of CYP3A4, such as St. John's Wort preparations (Hypericum perforatum), phenobarbital, carbamazepine, and rifampin, may reduce plasma concentrations of estrogens, possibly resulting in a decrease in therapeutic effects and/or changes in the uterine bleeding profile).
　No products indexed under this heading.

Ritonavir (Inhibitors of CYP3A4, such as ritonavir, may increase plasma concentrations of estrogens and may result in side effects). Products include:
　Kaletra 458
　Norvir 509

Saquinavir (Inhibitors of CYP3A4, such as erythromycin, clarithromycin, ketoconazole, itraconazole, ritonavir and grapefruit juice, may increase plasma concentrations of estrogens and may result in side effects).
　No products indexed under this heading.

Saquinavir Mesylate (Inhibitors of CYP3A4, such as erythromycin, clarithromycin, ketoconazole, itraconazole, ritonavir and grapefruit juice, may increase plasma concentrations of estrogens and may result in side effects).
　No products indexed under this heading.

Sertraline Hydrochloride (Inhibitors of CYP3A4, such as erythromycin, clarithromycin, ketoconazole, itraconazole, ritonavir and grapefruit juice, may increase plasma concentrations of estrogens and may result in side effects).
　No products indexed under this heading.

Sildenafil Citrate (Inhibitors of CYP3A4, such as erythromycin, clarithromycin, ketoconazole, itraconazole, ritonavir and grapefruit juice, may increase plasma concentrations of estrogens and may result in side effects).
　No products indexed under this heading.

Sulfinpyrazone (Inducers of CYP3A4, such as St. John's Wort preparations (Hypericum perforatum), phenobarbital, carbamazepine, and rifampin, may reduce plasma concentrations of estrogens, possibly resulting in a decrease in therapeutic effects and/or changes in the uterine bleeding profile).
　No products indexed under this heading.

Telithromycin (Inhibitors of CYP3A4, such as erythromycin, clarithromycin, ketoconazole, itraconazole, ritonavir and grapefruit juice, may increase plasma concentrations of estrogens and may result in side effects). Products include:
　Ketek 2991

Theophyllinate (Inducers of CYP3A4, such as St. John's Wort preparations (Hypericum perforatum), phenobarbital, carbamazepine, and rifampin, may reduce plasma concentrations of estrogens, possibly resulting in a decrease in therapeutic effects and/or changes in the uterine bleeding profile).
　No products indexed under this heading.

Theophylline (Inducers of CYP3A4, such as St. John's Wort preparations (Hypericum perforatum), phenobarbital, carbamazepine, and rifampin, may reduce plasma concentrations of estrogens, possibly resulting in a decrease in therapeutic effects and/or changes in the uterine bleeding profile).
　No products indexed under this heading.

Theophylline Anhydrous (Inducers of CYP3A4, such as St. John's Wort preparations (Hypericum perforatum), phenobarbital, carbamazepine, and rifampin, may reduce plasma concentrations of estrogens, possibly resulting in a decrease in therapeutic effects and/or changes in the uterine bleeding profile). Products include:
　Uniphyl 2817

Theophylline Calcium Salicylate (Inducers of CYP3A4, such as St. John's Wort preparations (Hypericum perforatum), phenobarbital, carbamazepine, and rifampin, may reduce plasma concentrations of estrogens, possibly resulting in a decrease in therapeutic effects and/or changes in the uterine bleeding profile).
　No products indexed under this heading.

Theophylline Dihydroxypropyl (Glyceryl) (Inducers of CYP3A4, such as St. John's Wort preparations (Hypericum perforatum), phenobarbital, carbamazepine, and rifampin, may reduce plasma concentrations of estrogens, possibly resulting in a decrease in therapeutic effects and/or changes in the uterine bleeding profile).
　No products indexed under this heading.

Theophylline Ethylenediamine (Inducers of CYP3A4, such as St. John's Wort preparations (Hypericum perforatum), phenobarbital, carbamazepine, and rifampin, may reduce plasma concentrations of estrogens, possibly resulting in a decrease in therapeutic effects and/or changes in the uterine bleeding profile).
　No products indexed under this heading.

Theophylline Sodium Glycinate (Inducers of CYP3A4, such as St. John's Wort preparations (Hypericum perforatum), phenobarbital, carbamazepine, and rifampin, may reduce plasma concentrations of estrogens, possibly resulting in a decrease in therapeutic effects and/or changes in the uterine bleeding profile).
　No products indexed under this heading.

Thyroglobulin (Estrogen administration leads to increased thyroid-binding globulin (TBG) levels. Patients with normal thyroid function can compensate for the increased TBG by making more thyroid hormone, thus maintaining free T4 and T3 serum concentrations in the normal range. Patients dependent on thyroid hormone replacement therapy who are also receiving estrogens may require increased doses of their thyroid replacement therapy. These patients should have their thyroid function monitored in order to maintain their free thyroid hormone levels in an acceptable range).
　No products indexed under this heading.

Thyroid (Estrogen administration leads to increased thyroid-binding globulin (TBG) levels. Patients with normal thyroid function can compensate for the increased TBG by making more thyroid hormone, thus maintaining free T4 and T3 serum concentrations in the normal range. Patients dependent on thyroid hormone replacement therapy who are also receiving estrogens may require increased doses of their thyroid replacement therapy. These patients should have their thyroid function monitored in order to maintain their free thyroid hormone levels in an acceptable range). Products include:

1449 Interactions Index Prempro

Naturethroid 2830

Thyroxine (Estrogen administration leads to increased thyroid-binding globulin (TBG) levels. Patients with normal thyroid function can compensate for the increased TBG by making more thyroid hormone, thus maintaining free T4 and T3 serum concentrations in the normal range. Patients dependent on thyroid hormone replacement therapy who are also receiving estrogens may require increased doses of their thyroid replacement therapy. These patients should have their thyroid function monitored in order to maintain their free thyroid hormone levels in an acceptable range).
No products indexed under this heading.

Thyroxine Sodium (Estrogen administration leads to increased thyroid-binding globulin (TBG) levels. Patients with normal thyroid function can compensate for the increased TBG by making more thyroid hormone, thus maintaining free T4 and T3 serum concentrations in the normal range. Patients dependent on thyroid hormone replacement therapy who are also receiving estrogens may require increased doses of their thyroid replacement therapy. These patients should have their thyroid function monitored in order to maintain their free thyroid hormone levels in an acceptable range).
No products indexed under this heading.

Triamcinolone (Inducers of CYP3A4, such as St. John's Wort preparations (Hypericum perforatum), phenobarbital, carbamazepine, and rifampin, may reduce plasma concentrations of estrogens, possibly resulting in a decrease in therapeutic effects and/or changes in the uterine bleeding profile).
No products indexed under this heading.

Triamcinolone Acetonide (Inducers of CYP3A4, such as St. John's Wort preparations (Hypericum perforatum), phenobarbital, carbamazepine, and rifampin, may reduce plasma concentrations of estrogens, possibly resulting in a decrease in therapeutic effects and/or changes in the uterine bleeding profile). Products include:
Azmacort 408
Nasacort AQ 3019

Triamcinolone Diacetate (Inducers of CYP3A4, such as St. John's Wort preparations (Hypericum perforatum), phenobarbital, carbamazepine, and rifampin, may reduce plasma concentrations of estrogens, possibly resulting in a decrease in therapeutic effects and/or changes in the uterine bleeding profile).
No products indexed under this heading.

Triamcinolone Hexacetonide (Inducers of CYP3A4, such as St. John's Wort preparations (Hypericum perforatum), phenobarbital, carbamazepine, and rifampin, may reduce plasma concentrations of estrogens, possibly resulting in a decrease in therapeutic effects and/or changes in the uterine bleeding profile).
No products indexed under this heading.

Troglitazone (Inhibitors of CYP3A4, such as erythromycin, clarithromycin, ketoconazole, itraconazole, ritonavir and grapefruit juice, may increase plasma concentrations of estrogens and may result in side effects).
No products indexed under this heading.

Troleandomycin (Inhibitors of CYP3A4, such as erythromycin, clarithromycin, ketoconazole, itraconazole, ritonavir and grapefruit juice, may increase plasma concentrations of estrogens and may result in side effects).
No products indexed under this heading.

Valproate Sodium (Inhibitors of CYP3A4, such as erythromycin, clarithromycin, ketoconazole, itraconazole, ritonavir and grapefruit juice, may increase plasma concentrations of estrogens and may result in side effects).
No products indexed under this heading.

Vardenafil Hydrochloride (Inhibitors of CYP3A4, such as erythromycin, clarithromycin, ketoconazole, itraconazole, ritonavir and grapefruit juice, may increase plasma concentrations of estrogens and may result in side effects). Products include:
Levitra 3157

Verapamil Hydrochloride (Inhibitors of CYP3A4, such as erythromycin, clarithromycin, ketoconazole, itraconazole, ritonavir and grapefruit juice, may increase plasma concentrations of estrogens and may result in side effects). Products include:
Tarka 534

Voriconazole (Inhibitors of CYP3A4, such as erythromycin, clarithromycin, ketoconazole, itraconazole, ritonavir and grapefruit juice, may increase plasma concentrations of estrogens and may result in side effects).
No products indexed under this heading.

Zafirlukast (Inhibitors of CYP3A4, such as erythromycin, clarithromycin, ketoconazole, itraconazole, ritonavir and grapefruit juice, may increase plasma concentrations of estrogens and may result in side effects). Products include:
Accolate 3612

Zileuton (Inhibitors of CYP3A4, such as erythromycin, clarithromycin, ketoconazole, itraconazole, ritonavir and grapefruit juice, may increase plasma concentrations of estrogens and may result in side effects).
No products indexed under this heading.

Food Interactions

Food, unspecified (Single dose studies in healthy, postmenopausal women were conducted to investigate any potential drug interaction when PREMPHASE is administered with a high fat breakfast. Administration with food decreased the C_{max} of total estrone by 18% to 34% and increased total equilin C_{max} by 38% compared to the fasting state, with no other effect on the rate or extent of absorption of other conjugated or unconjugated estrogens. Administration with food approximately doubles MPA C_{max} and increases MPA AUC by approximately 20% to 30%).

Grapefruit (Inhibitors of CYP3A4, such as grapefruit juice, may increase plasma concentrations of estrogens and may result in side effects).

Grapefruit Juice (Inhibitors of CYP3A4, such as grapefruit juice, may increase plasma concentrations of estrogens and may result in side effects).

Meal, unspecified (Single dose studies in healthy, postmenopausal women were conducted to investigate any potential drug interaction when PREMPHASE is administered with a high fat breakfast. Administration with food decreased the C_{max} of total estrone by 18% to 34% and increased total equilin C_{max} by 38% compared to the fasting state, with no other effect on the rate or extent of absorption of other conjugated or unconjugated estrogens. Administration with food approximately doubles MPA C_{max} and increases MPA AUC by approximately 20% to 30%).

PREMPRO TABLETS

(Estrogens, Conjugated, Medroxyprogesterone Acetate) 3549

May interact with cytochrome p450 3a4 inducers (selected), cytochrome p450 3a4 inhibitors (selected), erythromycin, thyroid preparations, and certain other agents. Compounds in these categories include:

Acetazolamide (Inhibitors of CYP3A4, such as erythromycin, clarithromycin, ketoconazole, itraconazole, ritonavir and grapefruit juice, may increase plasma concentrations of estrogens and may result in side effects).
No products indexed under this heading.

Acetazolamide Sodium (Inhibitors of CYP3A4, such as erythromycin, clarithromycin, ketoconazole, itraconazole, ritonavir and grapefruit juice, may increase plasma concentrations of estrogens and may result in side effects).
No products indexed under this heading.

Allium sativum (Inducers of CYP3A4, such as St. John's Wort preparations (Hypericum perforatum), phenobarbital, carbamazepine, and rifampin, may reduce plasma concentrations of estrogens, possibly resulting in a decrease in therapeutic effects and/or changes in the uterine bleeding profile).
No products indexed under this heading.

Aminoglutethimide (Aminoglutethimide administered concomitantly with medroxyprogesterone acetate (MPA) may significantly depress the bioavailability of MPA).
No products indexed under this heading.

Amiodarone Hydrochloride (Inhibitors of CYP3A4, such as erythromycin, clarithromycin, ketoconazole, itraconazole, ritonavir and grapefruit juice, may increase plasma concentrations of estrogens and may result in side effects).
No products indexed under this heading.

Amprenavir (Inhibitors of CYP3A4, such as erythromycin, clarithromycin, ketoconazole, itraconazole, ritonavir and grapefruit juice, may increase plasma concentrations of estrogens and may result in side effects).
No products indexed under this heading.

Anastrozole (Inhibitors of CYP3A4, such as erythromycin, clarithromycin, ketoconazole, itraconazole, ritonavir and grapefruit juice, may increase plasma concentrations of estrogens and may result in side effects).
No products indexed under this heading.

Aprepitant (Inhibitors of CYP3A4, such as erythromycin, clarithromycin, ketoconazole, itraconazole, ritonavir and grapefruit juice, may increase plasma concentrations of estrogens and may result in side effects). Products include:
Emend 2124

Atazanavir (Inhibitors of CYP3A4, such as erythromycin, clarithromycin, ketoconazole, itraconazole, ritonavir and grapefruit juice, may increase plasma concentrations of estrogens and may result in side effects).
No products indexed under this heading.

Atazanavir Sulfate (Inhibitors of CYP3A4, such as erythromycin, clarithromycin, ketoconazole, itraconazole, ritonavir and grapefruit juice, may increase plasma concentrations of estrogens and may result in side effects).
No products indexed under this heading.

Betamethasone (Inducers of CYP3A4, such as St. John's Wort preparations (Hypericum perforatum), phenobarbital, carbamazepine, and rifampin, may reduce plasma concentrations of estrogens, possibly resulting in a decrease in therapeutic effects and/or changes in the uterine bleeding profile).
No products indexed under this heading.

Betamethasone Acetate (Inducers of CYP3A4, such as St. John's Wort preparations (Hypericum perforatum), phenobarbital, carbamazepine, and rifampin, may reduce plasma concentrations of estrogens, possibly resulting in a decrease in therapeutic effects and/or changes in the uterine bleeding profile).
No products indexed under this heading.

Betamethasone Benzoate (Inducers of CYP3A4, such as St. John's Wort preparations (Hypericum perforatum), phenobarbital, carbamazepine, and rifampin, may reduce plasma concentrations of estrogens, possibly resulting in a decrease in therapeutic effects and/or changes in the uterine bleeding profile).
No products indexed under this heading.

Betamethasone Dipropionate (Inducers of CYP3A4, such as St. John's Wort preparations (Hypericum perforatum), phenobarbital, carbamazepine, and rifampin, may reduce plasma concentrations of estrogens, possibly resulting in a decrease in therapeutic effects and/or changes in the uterine bleeding profile). Products include:
Diprolene Lotion 0.05% 3108
Diprolene Ointment 0.05% 3109
Diprolene AF Cream 0.05% 3107
Lotrisone 3163

Betamethasone Sodium Phosphate (Inducers of CYP3A4, such as St. John's Wort preparations (Hypericum perforatum), phenobarbital, carbamazepine, and rifampin, may reduce plasma concentrations of estrogens, possibly resulting in a decrease in therapeutic effects and/or changes in the uterine bleeding profile).
No products indexed under this heading.

Betamethasone Valerate (Inducers of CYP3A4, such as St. John's Wort preparations (Hypericum perforatum), phenobarbital, carbamazepine, and rifampin, may reduce plasma concentrations of estrogens, possibly resulting in a decrease in therapeutic effects and/or changes in the uterine bleeding profile). Products include:
Luxíq 3321

Bosentan (Inducers of CYP3A4, such as St. John's Wort preparations (Hypericum perforatum), phenobarbital, carbamazepine, and rifampin, may reduce plasma concentrations of estrogens, possibly resulting in a decrease in therapeutic effects and/or changes in the uterine bleeding profile). Products include:
Tracleer 573

Carbamazepine (Inducers of CYP3A4, such as carbamazepine, may reduce plasma concentrations of estrogens, possibly resulting in a decrease in therapeutic effects and/or changes in the uterine bleeding profile). Products include:
Carbatrol 3280
Equetro 3477

Cimetidine (Inhibitors of CYP3A4, such as erythromycin, clarithromycin, ketoconazole, itraconazole, ritonavir and grapefruit juice, may increase plasma concentrations of estrogens and may result in side effects).
No products indexed under this heading.

Cimetidine Hydrochloride (Inhibitors of CYP3A4, such as erythromycin, clarithromycin, ketoconazole, itraconazole, ritonavir and grapefruit juice, may increase plasma concentrations of estrogens and may result in side effects).
No products indexed under this heading.

Ciprofloxacin (Inhibitors of CYP3A4, such as erythromycin, clarithromycin, ketoconazole, itraconazole, ritonavir and grapefruit juice, may increase plas-

IMPORTANT NOTE: Always consult each drug listing in the patient's regimen for possible interactions.

ma concentrations of estrogens and may result in side effects). Products include:

Ciprofloxacin Hydrochloride (Inducers of CYP3A4, such as St. John's Wort preparations (Hypericum perforatum), phenobarbital, carbamazepine, and rifampin, may reduce plasma concentrations of estrogens, possibly resulting in a decrease in therapeutic effects and/or changes in the uterine bleeding profile). Products include:

Cisplatin (Inducers of CYP3A4, such as St. John's Wort preparations (Hypericum perforatum), phenobarbital, carbamazepine, and rifampin, may reduce plasma concentrations of estrogens, possibly resulting in a decrease in therapeutic effects and/or changes in the uterine bleeding profile).

No products indexed under this heading.

Clarithromycin (Inhibitors of CYP3A4, such as clarithromycin, may increase plasma concentrations of estrogens and may result in side effects). Products include:

Clotrimazole (Inhibitors of CYP3A4, such as erythromycin, clarithromycin, ketoconazole, itraconazole, ritonavir and grapefruit juice, may increase plasma concentrations of estrogens and may result in side effects). Products include:

Conivaptan Hydrochloride (Inhibitors of CYP3A4, such as erythromycin, clarithromycin, ketoconazole, itraconazole, ritonavir and grapefruit juice, may increase plasma concentrations of estrogens and may result in side effects). Products include:

Cortisone Acetate (Inducers of CYP3A4, such as St. John's Wort preparations (Hypericum perforatum), phenobarbital, carbamazepine, and rifampin, may reduce plasma concentrations of estrogens, possibly resulting in a decrease in therapeutic effects and/or changes in the uterine bleeding profile).

No products indexed under this heading.

Cyclosporine (Inhibitors of CYP3A4, such as erythromycin, clarithromycin, ketoconazole, itraconazole, ritonavir and grapefruit juice, may increase plasma concentrations of estrogens and may result in side effects). Products include:

Dalfopristin (Inhibitors of CYP3A4, such as erythromycin, clarithromycin, ketoconazole, itraconazole, ritonavir and grapefruit juice, may increase plasma concentrations of estrogens and may result in side effects).

No products indexed under this heading.

Danazol (Inhibitors of CYP3A4, such as erythromycin, clarithromycin, ketoconazole, itraconazole, ritonavir and grapefruit juice, may increase plasma concentrations of estrogens and may result in side effects).

No products indexed under this heading.

Darunavir (Inhibitors of CYP3A4, such as erythromycin, clarithromycin, ketoconazole, itraconazole, ritonavir and grapefruit juice, may increase plasma concentrations of estrogens and may result in side effects).

No products indexed under this heading.

Dasatinib (Inhibitors of CYP3A4, such as erythromycin, clarithromycin, ketoconazole, itraconazole, ritonavir and grapefruit juice, may increase plasma concentrations of estrogens and may result in side effects).

No products indexed under this heading.

Delavirdine Mesylate (Inhibitors of CYP3A4, such as erythromycin, clarithromycin, ketoconazole, itraconazole, ritonavir and grapefruit juice, may increase plasma concentrations of estrogens and may result in side effects).

No products indexed under this heading.

Delavirine (Inhibitors of CYP3A4, such as erythromycin, clarithromycin, ketoconazole, itraconazole, ritonavir and grapefruit juice, may increase plasma concentrations of estrogens and may result in side effects).

No products indexed under this heading.

Desloratadine (Inhibitors of CYP3A4, such as erythromycin, clarithromycin, ketoconazole, itraconazole, ritonavir and grapefruit juice, may increase plasma concentrations of estrogens and may result in side effects). Products include:

Dexamethasone (Inducers of CYP3A4, such as St. John's Wort preparations (Hypericum perforatum), phenobarbital, carbamazepine, and rifampin, may reduce plasma concentrations of estrogens, possibly resulting in a decrease in therapeutic effects and/or changes in the uterine bleeding profile). Products include:

Dexamethasone Acetate (Inducers of CYP3A4, such as St. John's Wort preparations (Hypericum perforatum), phenobarbital, carbamazepine, and rifampin, may reduce plasma concentrations of estrogens, possibly resulting in a decrease in therapeutic effects and/or changes in the uterine bleeding profile).

No products indexed under this heading.

Dexamethasone Phosphate (Inducers of CYP3A4, such as St. John's Wort preparations (Hypericum perforatum), phenobarbital, carbamazepine, and rifampin, may reduce plasma concentrations of estrogens, possibly resulting in a decrease in therapeutic effects and/or changes in the uterine bleeding profile).

No products indexed under this heading.

Dexamethasone Sodium (Inducers of CYP3A4, such as St. John's Wort preparations (Hypericum perforatum), phenobarbital, carbamazepine, and rifampin, may reduce plasma concentrations of estrogens, possibly resulting in a decrease in therapeutic effects and/or changes in the uterine bleeding profile).

No products indexed under this heading.

Dexamethasone Sodium Phosphate (Inducers of CYP3A4, such as St. John's Wort preparations (Hypericum perforatum), phenobarbital, carbamazepine, and rifampin, may reduce plasma concentrations of estrogens, possibly resulting in a decrease in therapeutic effects and/or changes in the uterine bleeding profile).

No products indexed under this heading.

Dexamethasone Sodium Phosphate Injection (Inducers of CYP3A4, such as St. John's Wort preparations (Hypericum perforatum), phenobarbital, carbamazepine, and rifampin, may reduce plasma concentrations of estrogens, possibly resulting in a decrease in therapeutic effects and/or changes in the uterine bleeding profile).

No products indexed under this heading.

Diltiazem Hydrochloride (Inhibitors of CYP3A4, such as erythromycin, clarithromycin, ketoconazole, itraconazole, ritonavir and grapefruit juice, may increase plasma concentrations of estrogens and may result in side effects). Products include:

Diltiazem Maleate (Inhibitors of CYP3A4, such as erythromycin, clarithromycin, ketoconazole, itraconazole, ritonavir and grapefruit juice, may increase plasma concentrations of estrogens and may result in side effects).

No products indexed under this heading.

Doxorubicin Hydrochloride (Inducers of CYP3A4, such as St. John's Wort preparations (Hypericum perforatum), phenobarbital, carbamazepine, and rifampin, may reduce plasma concentrations of estrogens, possibly resulting in a decrease in therapeutic effects and/or changes in the uterine bleeding profile).

No products indexed under this heading.

Efavirenz (Inhibitors of CYP3A4, such as erythromycin, clarithromycin, ketoconazole, itraconazole, ritonavir and grapefruit juice, may increase plasma concentrations of estrogens and may result in side effects). Products include:

Erythromycin (Inhibitors of CYP3A4, such as erythromycin, may increase plasma concentrations of estrogens and may result in side effects).

No products indexed under this heading.

Erythromycin, Topical (Inhibitors of CYP3A4, such as erythromycin, may increase plasma concentrations of estrogens and may result in side effects).

No products indexed under this heading.

Erythromycin Estolate (Inhibitors of CYP3A4, such as erythromycin, may increase plasma concentrations of estrogens and may result in side effects).

No products indexed under this heading.

Erythromycin Ethylsuccinate (Inhibitors of CYP3A4, such as erythromycin, may increase plasma concentrations of estrogens and may result in side effects). Products include:

Erythromycin Gluceptate (Inhibitors of CYP3A4, such as erythromycin, may increase plasma concentrations of estrogens and may result in side effects).

No products indexed under this heading.

Erythromycin Lactobionate (Inhibitors of CYP3A4, such as erythromycin, may increase plasma concentrations of estrogens and may result in side effects).

No products indexed under this heading.

Erythromycin Stearate (Inhibitors of CYP3A4, such as erythromycin, may increase plasma concentrations of estrogens and may result in side effects).

No products indexed under this heading.

Esomeprazole Magnesium (Inhibitors of CYP3A4, such as erythromycin, clarithromycin, ketoconazole, itraconazole, ritonavir and grapefruit juice, may

increase plasma concentrations of estrogens and may result in side effects). Products include:

Esomeprazole Sodium (Inhibitors of CYP3A4, such as erythromycin, clarithromycin, ketoconazole, itraconazole, ritonavir and grapefruit juice, may increase plasma concentrations of estrogens and may result in side effects). Products include:

Ethosuximide (Inducers of CYP3A4, such as St. John's Wort preparations (Hypericum perforatum), phenobarbital, carbamazepine, and rifampin, may reduce plasma concentrations of estrogens, possibly resulting in a decrease in therapeutic effects and/or changes in the uterine bleeding profile).

No products indexed under this heading.

Fat (Single dose studies in healthy, postmenopausal women were conducted to investigate any potential drug interaction when PREMPRO is administered with a high fat breakfast. Administration with food decreased the C_{max} of total estrone by 18% to 34% and increased total equilin C_{max} by 38% compared to the fasting state, with no other effect on the rate or extent of absorption of other conjugated or unconjugated estrogens. Administration with food approximately doubles MPA C_{max} and increases MPA AUC by approximately 20% to 30%).

No products indexed under this heading.

Felbamate (Inducers of CYP3A4, such as St. John's Wort preparations (Hypericum perforatum), phenobarbital, carbamazepine, and rifampin, may reduce plasma concentrations of estrogens, possibly resulting in a decrease in therapeutic effects and/or changes in the uterine bleeding profile).

No products indexed under this heading.

Fluconazole (Inhibitors of CYP3A4, such as erythromycin, clarithromycin, ketoconazole, itraconazole, ritonavir and grapefruit juice, may increase plasma concentrations of estrogens and may result in side effects).

No products indexed under this heading.

Fludrocortisone Acetate (Inducers of CYP3A4, such as St. John's Wort preparations (Hypericum perforatum), phenobarbital, carbamazepine, and rifampin, may reduce plasma concentrations of estrogens, possibly resulting in a decrease in therapeutic effects and/or changes in the uterine bleeding profile).

No products indexed under this heading.

Fluoxetine (Inhibitors of CYP3A4, such as erythromycin, clarithromycin, ketoconazole, itraconazole, ritonavir and grapefruit juice, may increase plasma concentrations of estrogens and may result in side effects).

No products indexed under this heading.

Fluoxetine Hydrochloride (Inhibitors of CYP3A4, such as erythromycin, clarithromycin, ketoconazole, itraconazole, ritonavir and grapefruit juice, may increase plasma concentrations of estrogens and may result in side effects). Products include:

Fluvoxamine Maleate (Inhibitors of CYP3A4, such as erythromycin, clarithromycin, ketoconazole, itraconazole, ritonavir and grapefruit juice, may increase plasma concentrations of estrogens and may result in side effects).

No products indexed under this heading.

Fosamprenavir Calcium (Inhibitors of CYP3A4, such as erythromycin, clarithromycin, ketoconazole, itracona-

IMPORTANT NOTE: Always consult each drug listing in the patient's regimen for possible interactions.

Mifepristone (Inhibitors of CYP3A4, such as erythromycin, clarithromycin, ketoconazole, itraconazole, ritonavir and grapefruit juice, may increase plasma concentrations of estrogens and may result in side effects).
No products indexed under this heading.

Modafinil (Inducers of CYP3A4, such as St. John's Wort preparations (Hypericum perforatum), phenobarbital, carbamazepine, and rifampin, may reduce plasma concentrations of estrogens, possibly resulting in a decrease in therapeutic effects and/or changes in the uterine bleeding profile). Products include:
Provigil 983

Nafcillin Sodium (Inducers of CYP3A4, such as St. John's Wort preparations (Hypericum perforatum), phenobarbital, carbamazepine, and rifampin, may reduce plasma concentrations of estrogens, possibly resulting in a decrease in therapeutic effects and/or changes in the uterine bleeding profile).
No products indexed under this heading.

Nefazodone Hydrochloride (Inhibitors of CYP3A4, such as erythromycin, clarithromycin, ketoconazole, itraconazole, ritonavir and grapefruit juice, may increase plasma concentrations of estrogens and may result in side effects).
No products indexed under this heading.

Nelfinavir Mesylate (Inhibitors of CYP3A4, such as erythromycin, clarithromycin, ketoconazole, itraconazole, ritonavir and grapefruit juice, may increase plasma concentrations of estrogens and may result in side effects).
No products indexed under this heading.

Nevirapine (Inhibitors of CYP3A4, such as erythromycin, clarithromycin, ketoconazole, itraconazole, ritonavir and grapefruit juice, may increase plasma concentrations of estrogens and may result in side effects). Products include:
Viramune Oral Suspension 897
Viramune Tablets 897

Niacin (Inhibitors of CYP3A4, such as erythromycin, clarithromycin, ketoconazole, itraconazole, ritonavir and grapefruit juice, may increase plasma concentrations of estrogens and may result in side effects). Products include:
Advicor 402
Cardio Basics 3455
Niaspan 497
Simcor 524

Niacinamide (Inhibitors of CYP3A4, such as erythromycin, clarithromycin, ketoconazole, itraconazole, ritonavir and grapefruit juice, may increase plasma concentrations of estrogens and may result in side effects). Products include:
CitraNatal 90 DHA Capsules 2332
CitraNatal Assure 2332
CitraNatal Rx 2332
Heplive 607

Niacinamide Hydroiodide (Inhibitors of CYP3A4, such as erythromycin, clarithromycin, ketoconazole, itraconazole, ritonavir and grapefruit juice, may increase plasma concentrations of estrogens and may result in side effects).
No products indexed under this heading.

Nicotinamide (Inhibitors of CYP3A4, such as erythromycin, clarithromycin, ketoconazole, itraconazole, ritonavir and grapefruit juice, may increase plasma concentrations of estrogens and may result in side effects).
No products indexed under this heading.

Nifedipine (Inhibitors of CYP3A4, such as erythromycin, clarithromycin, ketoconazole, itraconazole, ritonavir and grapefruit juice, may increase plasma concentrations of estrogens and may result in side effects).
No products indexed under this heading.

Norfloxacin (Inhibitors of CYP3A4, such as erythromycin, clarithromycin, ketoconazole, itraconazole, ritonavir and grapefruit juice, may increase plasma concentrations of estrogens and may result in side effects). Products include:
Noroxin 2220

Omeprazole (Inhibitors of CYP3A4, such as erythromycin, clarithromycin, ketoconazole, itraconazole, ritonavir and grapefruit juice, may increase plasma concentrations of estrogens and may result in side effects).
No products indexed under this heading.

Oxcarbazepine (Inducers of CYP3A4, such as St. John's Wort preparations (Hypericum perforatum), phenobarbital, carbamazepine, and rifampin, may reduce plasma concentrations of estrogens, possibly resulting in a decrease in therapeutic effects and/or changes in the uterine bleeding profile).
No products indexed under this heading.

Paroxetine Hydrochloride (Inhibitors of CYP3A4, such as erythromycin, clarithromycin, ketoconazole, itraconazole, ritonavir and grapefruit juice, may increase plasma concentrations of estrogens and may result in side effects). Products include:
Paroxetine CR 2361
Paroxetine ER 2371
Paxil 1586
Paxil CR 1596

Phenobarbital (Inducers of CYP3A4, such as phenobarbital, may reduce plasma concentrations of estrogens, possibly resulting in a decrease in therapeutic effects and/or changes in the uterine bleeding profile). Products include:
Donnatal 2711

Phenobarbital Sodium (Inducers of CYP3A4, such as phenobarbital, may reduce plasma concentrations of estrogens, possibly resulting in a decrease in therapeutic effects and/or changes in the uterine bleeding profile).
No products indexed under this heading.

Phenytoin (Inducers of CYP3A4, such as St. John's Wort preparations (Hypericum perforatum), phenobarbital, carbamazepine, and rifampin, may reduce plasma concentrations of estrogens, possibly resulting in a decrease in therapeutic effects and/or changes in the uterine bleeding profile).
No products indexed under this heading.

Phenytoin Sodium (Inducers of CYP3A4, such as St. John's Wort preparations (Hypericum perforatum), phenobarbital, carbamazepine, and rifampin, may reduce plasma concentrations of estrogens, possibly resulting in a decrease in therapeutic effects and/or changes in the uterine bleeding profile). Products include:
Phenytek Capsules 2380

Posaconazole (Inhibitors of CYP3A4, such as erythromycin, clarithromycin, ketoconazole, itraconazole, ritonavir and grapefruit juice, may increase plasma concentrations of estrogens and may result in side effects). Products include:
Noxafil 3172

Prednisolone (Inducers of CYP3A4, such as St. John's Wort preparations (Hypericum perforatum), phenobarbital, carbamazepine, and rifampin, may reduce plasma concentrations of estrogens, possibly resulting in a decrease in therapeutic effects and/or changes in the uterine bleeding profile).
No products indexed under this heading.

Prednisolone Acetate (Inducers of CYP3A4, such as St. John's Wort preparations (Hypericum perforatum), phenobarbital, carbamazepine, and rifampin, may reduce plasma concentrations of estrogens, possibly resulting in a decrease in therapeutic effects and/or changes in the uterine bleeding profile). Products include:
Blephamide .... ⊙212, ⊙214
Pred Forte .... ⊙225
Pred Mild .... ⊙230
Pred-G .... ⊙226, ⊙227

Prednisolone Sodium Phosphate (Inducers of CYP3A4, such as St. John's Wort preparations (Hypericum perforatum), phenobarbital, carbamazepine, and rifampin, may reduce plasma concentrations of estrogens, possibly resulting in a decrease in therapeutic effects and/or changes in the uterine bleeding profile).
No products indexed under this heading.

Prednisolone Tebutate (Inducers of CYP3A4, such as St. John's Wort preparations (Hypericum perforatum), phenobarbital, carbamazepine, and rifampin, may reduce plasma concentrations of estrogens, possibly resulting in a decrease in therapeutic effects and/or changes in the uterine bleeding profile).
No products indexed under this heading.

Prednisone (Inducers of CYP3A4, such as St. John's Wort preparations (Hypericum perforatum), phenobarbital, carbamazepine, and rifampin, may reduce plasma concentrations of estrogens, possibly resulting in a decrease in therapeutic effects and/or changes in the uterine bleeding profile).
No products indexed under this heading.

Prednisone sodium phosphate (Inducers of CYP3A4, such as St. John's Wort preparations (Hypericum perforatum), phenobarbital, carbamazepine, and rifampin, may reduce plasma concentrations of estrogens, possibly resulting in a decrease in therapeutic effects and/or changes in the uterine bleeding profile).
No products indexed under this heading.

Primidone (Inducers of CYP3A4, such as St. John's Wort preparations (Hypericum perforatum), phenobarbital, carbamazepine, and rifampin, may reduce plasma concentrations of estrogens, possibly resulting in a decrease in therapeutic effects and/or changes in the uterine bleeding profile).
No products indexed under this heading.

Propoxyphene Hydrochloride (Inhibitors of CYP3A4, such as erythromycin, clarithromycin, ketoconazole, itraconazole, ritonavir and grapefruit juice, may increase plasma concentrations of estrogens and may result in side effects).
No products indexed under this heading.

Propoxyphene Napsylate (Inhibitors of CYP3A4, such as erythromycin, clarithromycin, ketoconazole, itraconazole, ritonavir and grapefruit juice, may increase plasma concentrations of estrogens and may result in side effects).
No products indexed under this heading.

Quinidine (Inhibitors of CYP3A4, such as erythromycin, clarithromycin, ketoconazole, itraconazole, ritonavir and grapefruit juice, may increase plasma concentrations of estrogens and may result in side effects).
No products indexed under this heading.

Quinidine Hydrochloride (Inhibitors of CYP3A4, such as erythromycin, clarithromycin, ketoconazole, itraconazole, ritonavir and grapefruit juice, may increase plasma concentrations of estrogens and may result in side effects).
No products indexed under this heading.

Quinidine Polygalacturonate (Inhibitors of CYP3A4, such as erythromycin, clarithromycin, ketoconazole, itraconazole, ritonavir and grapefruit juice, may increase plasma concentrations of estrogens and may result in side effects).
No products indexed under this heading.

Quinidine Sulfate (Inhibitors of CYP3A4, such as erythromycin, clarithromycin, ketoconazole, itraconazole, ritonavir and grapefruit juice, may increase plasma concentrations of estrogens and may result in side effects).
No products indexed under this heading.

Quinine (Inhibitors of CYP3A4, such as erythromycin, clarithromycin, ketoconazole, itraconazole, ritonavir and grapefruit juice, may increase plasma concentrations of estrogens and may result in side effects). Products include:
Hyland's Leg Cramps PM with Quinine 3315

Quinine Sulfate (Inhibitors of CYP3A4, such as erythromycin, clarithromycin, ketoconazole, itraconazole, ritonavir and grapefruit juice, may increase plasma concentrations of estrogens and may result in side effects).
No products indexed under this heading.

Quinupristin (Inhibitors of CYP3A4, such as erythromycin, clarithromycin, ketoconazole, itraconazole, ritonavir and grapefruit juice, may increase plasma concentrations of estrogens and may result in side effects).
No products indexed under this heading.

Ranitidine Bismuth Citrate (Inhibitors of CYP3A4, such as erythromycin, clarithromycin, ketoconazole, itraconazole, ritonavir and grapefruit juice, may increase plasma concentrations of estrogens and may result in side effects).
No products indexed under this heading.

Ranitidine Hydrochloride (Inhibitors of CYP3A4, such as erythromycin, clarithromycin, ketoconazole, itraconazole, ritonavir and grapefruit juice, may increase plasma concentrations of estrogens and may result in side effects). Products include:
Zantac 1737
Zantac Injection 1732
Zantac Pharmacy 1735

Rifabutin (Inducers of CYP3A4, such as St. John's Wort preparations (Hypericum perforatum), phenobarbital, carbamazepine, and rifampin, may reduce plasma concentrations of estrogens, possibly resulting in a decrease in therapeutic effects and/or changes in the uterine bleeding profile).
No products indexed under this heading.

Rifampicin (Inducers of CYP3A4, such as St. John's Wort preparations (Hypericum perforatum), phenobarbital, carbamazepine, and rifampin, may reduce plasma concentrations of estrogens, possibly resulting in a decrease in therapeutic effects and/or changes in the uterine bleeding profile).
No products indexed under this heading.

Rifampin (Inducers of CYP3A4, such as rifampin, may reduce plasma concentrations of estrogens, possibly resulting in a decrease in therapeutic effects and/or changes in the uterine bleeding profile).
No products indexed under this heading.

Rifapentine (Inducers of CYP3A4, such as St. John's Wort preparations (Hypericum perforatum), phenobarbital, carbamazepine, and rifampin, may reduce plasma concentrations of estrogens, possibly resulting in a decrease in therapeutic effects and/or changes in the uterine bleeding profile).
No products indexed under this heading.

Ritonavir (Inhibitors of CYP3A4, such as ritonavir, may increase plasma concentrations of estrogens and may result in side effects). Products include:
Kaletra 458
Norvir 509

Saquinavir (Inhibitors of CYP3A4, such as erythromycin, clarithromycin, ketoconazole, itraconazole, ritonavir and grapefruit juice, may increase plasma concentrations of estrogens and may result in side effects).
No products indexed under this heading.

Saquinavir Mesylate (Inhibitors of CYP3A4, such as erythromycin, clarithromycin, ketoconazole, itraconazole, ritonavir and grapefruit juice, may increase plasma concentrations of estrogens and may result in side effects).
No products indexed under this heading.

Sertraline Hydrochloride (Inhibitors of CYP3A4, such as erythromycin, clarithromycin, ketoconazole, itraconazole, ritonavir and grapefruit juice, may increase plasma concentrations of estrogens and may result in side effects).
No products indexed under this heading.

Sildenafil Citrate (Inhibitors of CYP3A4, such as erythromycin, clarithromycin, ketoconazole, itraconazole, ritonavir and grapefruit juice, may increase plasma concentrations of estrogens and may result in side effects).
No products indexed under this heading.

Sulfinpyrazone (Inducers of CYP3A4, such as St. John's Wort preparations (Hypericum perforatum), phenobarbital, carbamazepine, and rifampin, may reduce plasma concentrations of estrogens, possibly resulting in a decrease in therapeutic effects and/or changes in the uterine bleeding profile).
No products indexed under this heading.

Telithromycin (Inhibitors of CYP3A4, such as erythromycin, clarithromycin, ketoconazole, itraconazole, ritonavir and grapefruit juice, may increase plasma concentrations of estrogens and may result in side effects). Products include:
Ketek 2991

Theophyllinate (Inducers of CYP3A4, such as St. John's Wort preparations (Hypericum perforatum), phenobarbital, carbamazepine, and rifampin, may reduce plasma concentrations of estrogens, possibly resulting in a decrease in therapeutic effects and/or changes in the uterine bleeding profile).
No products indexed under this heading.

Theophylline (Inducers of CYP3A4, such as St. John's Wort preparations (Hypericum perforatum), phenobarbital, carbamazepine, and rifampin, may reduce plasma concentrations of estrogens, possibly resulting in a decrease in therapeutic effects and/or changes in the uterine bleeding profile).
No products indexed under this heading.

Theophylline Anhydrous (Inducers of CYP3A4, such as St. John's Wort preparations (Hypericum perforatum), phenobarbital, carbamazepine, and rifampin, may reduce plasma concentrations of estrogens, possibly resulting in a decrease in therapeutic effects and/or changes in the uterine bleeding profile). Products include:
Uniphyl 2817

Theophylline Calcium Salicylate (Inducers of CYP3A4, such as St. John's Wort preparations (Hypericum perforatum), phenobarbital, carbamazepine, and rifampin, may reduce plasma concentrations of estrogens, possibly resulting in a decrease in therapeutic effects and/or changes in the uterine bleeding profile).
No products indexed under this heading.

Theophylline Dihydroxypropyl (Glyceryl) (Inducers of CYP3A4, such as St. John's Wort preparations (Hypericum perforatum), phenobarbital, carbamazepine, and rifampin, may reduce plasma concentrations of estrogens, possibly resulting in a decrease in therapeutic effects and/or changes in the uterine bleeding profile).
No products indexed under this heading.

Theophylline Ethylenediamine (Inducers of CYP3A4, such as St. John's Wort preparations (Hypericum perforatum), phenobarbital, carbamazepine, and rifampin, may reduce plasma concentrations of estrogens, possibly resulting in a decrease in therapeutic effects and/or changes in the uterine bleeding profile).
No products indexed under this heading.

Theophylline Sodium Glycinate (Inducers of CYP3A4, such as St. John's Wort preparations (Hypericum perforatum), phenobarbital, carbamazepine, and rifampin, may reduce plasma concentrations of estrogens, possibly resulting in a decrease in therapeutic effects and/or changes in the uterine bleeding profile).
No products indexed under this heading.

Thyroglobulin (Estrogen administration leads to increased thyroid-binding globulin (TBG) levels. Patients with normal thyroid function can compensate for the increased TBG by making more thyroid hormone, thus maintaining free T4 and T3 serum concentrations in the normal range. Patients dependent on thyroid hormone replacement therapy who are also receiving estrogens may require increased doses of their thyroid replacement therapy. These patients should have their thyroid function monitored in order to maintain their free thyroid hormone levels in an acceptable range).
No products indexed under this heading.

Thyroid (Estrogen administration leads to increased thyroid-binding globulin (TBG) levels. Patients with normal thyroid function can compensate for the increased TBG by making more thyroid hormone, thus maintaining free T4 and T3 serum concentrations in the normal range. Patients dependent on thyroid hormone replacement therapy who are also receiving estrogens may require increased doses of their thyroid replacement therapy. These patients should have their thyroid function monitored in order to maintain their free thyroid hormone levels in an acceptable range). Products include:
Naturethroid 2830

Thyroxine (Estrogen administration leads to increased thyroid-binding globulin (TBG) levels. Patients with normal thyroid function can compensate for the increased TBG by making more thyroid hormone, thus maintaining free T4 and T3 serum concentrations in the normal range. Patients dependent on thyroid hormone replacement therapy who are also receiving estrogens may require increased doses of their thyroid replacement therapy. These patients should have their thyroid function monitored in order to maintain their free thyroid hormone levels in an acceptable range).
No products indexed under this heading.

Thyroxine Sodium (Estrogen administration leads to increased thyroid-binding globulin (TBG) levels. Patients with normal thyroid function can compensate for the increased TBG by making more thyroid hormone, thus maintaining free T4 and T3 serum concentrations in the normal range. Patients dependent on thyroid hormone replacement therapy who are also receiving estrogens may require increased doses of their thyroid replacement therapy. These patients should have their thyroid function monitored in order to maintain their free thyroid hormone levels in an acceptable range).
No products indexed under this heading.

Triamcinolone (Inducers of CYP3A4, such as St. John's Wort preparations (Hypericum perforatum), phenobarbital, carbamazepine, and rifampin, may reduce plasma concentrations of estrogens, possibly resulting in a decrease in therapeutic effects and/or changes in the uterine bleeding profile).
No products indexed under this heading.

Triamcinolone Acetonide (Inducers of CYP3A4, such as St. John's Wort preparations (Hypericum perforatum), phenobarbital, carbamazepine, and rifampin, may reduce plasma concentrations of estrogens, possibly resulting in a decrease in therapeutic effects and/or changes in the uterine bleeding profile). Products include:
Azmacort 408
Nasacort AQ 3019

Triamcinolone Diacetate (Inducers of CYP3A4, such as St. John's Wort preparations (Hypericum perforatum), phenobarbital, carbamazepine, and rifampin, may reduce plasma concentrations of estrogens, possibly resulting in a decrease in therapeutic effects and/or changes in the uterine bleeding profile).
No products indexed under this heading.

Triamcinolone Hexacetonide (Inducers of CYP3A4, such as St. John's Wort preparations (Hypericum perforatum), phenobarbital, carbamazepine, and rifampin, may reduce plasma concentrations of estrogens, possibly resulting in a decrease in therapeutic effects and/or changes in the uterine bleeding profile).
No products indexed under this heading.

Troglitazone (Inhibitors of CYP3A4, such as erythromycin, clarithromycin, ketoconazole, itraconazole, ritonavir and grapefruit juice, may increase plasma concentrations of estrogens and may result in side effects).
No products indexed under this heading.

Troleandomycin (Inhibitors of CYP3A4, such as erythromycin, clarithromycin, ketoconazole, itraconazole, ritonavir and grapefruit juice, may increase plasma concentrations of estrogens and may result in side effects).
No products indexed under this heading.

Valproate Sodium (Inhibitors of CYP3A4, such as erythromycin, clarithromycin, ketoconazole, itraconazole, ritonavir and grapefruit juice, may increase plasma concentrations of estrogens and may result in side effects).
No products indexed under this heading.

Vardenafil Hydrochloride (Inhibitors of CYP3A4, such as erythromycin, clarithromycin, ketoconazole, itraconazole, ritonavir and grapefruit juice, may increase plasma concentrations of estrogens and may result in side effects). Products include:
Levitra 3157

Verapamil Hydrochloride (Inhibitors of CYP3A4, such as erythromycin, clarithromycin, ketoconazole, itracona-

zole, ritonavir and grapefruit juice, may increase plasma concentrations of estrogens and may result in side effects). Products include:
Tarka 534

Voriconazole (Inhibitors of CYP3A4, such as erythromycin, clarithromycin, ketoconazole, itraconazole, ritonavir and grapefruit juice, may increase plasma concentrations of estrogens and may result in side effects).
No products indexed under this heading.

Zafirlukast (Inhibitors of CYP3A4, such as erythromycin, clarithromycin, ketoconazole, itraconazole, ritonavir and grapefruit juice, may increase plasma concentrations of estrogens and may result in side effects). Products include:
Accolate 3612

Zileuton (Inhibitors of CYP3A4, such as erythromycin, clarithromycin, ketoconazole, itraconazole, ritonavir and grapefruit juice, may increase plasma concentrations of estrogens and may result in side effects).
No products indexed under this heading.

Food Interactions

Food, unspecified (Single dose studies in healthy, postmenopausal women were conducted to investigate any potential drug interaction when PREMPRO is administered with a high fat breakfast. Administration with food decreased the C_{max} of total estrone by 18% to 34% and increased total equilin C_{max} by 38% compared to the fasting state, with no other effect on the rate or extent of absorption of other conjugated or unconjugated estrogens. Administration with food approximately doubles MPA C_{max} and increases MPA AUC by approximately 20% to 30%).

Grapefruit (Inhibitors of CYP3A4, such as grapefruit juice, may increase plasma concentrations of estrogens and may result in side effects).

Grapefruit Juice (Inhibitors of CYP3A4, such as grapefruit juice, may increase plasma concentrations of estrogens and may result in side effects).

Meal, unspecified (Single dose studies in healthy, postmenopausal women were conducted to investigate any potential drug interaction when PREMPRO is administered with a high fat breakfast. Administration with food decreased the C_{max} of total estrone by 18% to 34% and increased total equilin C_{max} by 38% compared to the fasting state, with no other effect on the rate or extent of absorption of other conjugated or unconjugated estrogens. Administration with food approximately doubles MPA C_{max} and increases MPA AUC by approximately 20% to 30%).

PRENEXA CAPSULES

(Docosahexaenoic Acid (DHA), Docusate Sodium, Ferrous Fumarate, Folic Acid, Tribasic Calcium Phosphate, Vitamin B6, Vitamin C, Vitamin D3, Vitamin E) 3473
May interact with anticoagulants, and certain other agents. Compounds in these categories include:

Anisindione (Ingestion of more than 3 grams of omega-3 fatty acids per day has shown to have potential antithrombotic effects including increased bleeding time and INR. Administration of omega-3 fatty acids should be avoided in patients on anticoagulants).
No products indexed under this heading.

IMPORTANT NOTE: Always consult each drug listing in the patient's regimen for possible interactions.

(⊙ Described in PDR® for Ophthalmic Medicines)

1455 Interactions Index Prevnar

Dexamethasone Sodium (Children receiving therapy with immunosuppressive agents (large amounts of corticosteroids, antimetabolites, alkylating agents, cytotoxic agents) may not respond optimally to active immunization).
No products indexed under this heading.

Dexamethasone Sodium Phosphate (Children receiving therapy with immunosuppressive agents (large amounts of corticosteroids, antimetabolites, alkylating agents, cytotoxic agents) may not respond optimally to active immunization).
No products indexed under this heading.

Dexamethasone Sodium Phosphate Injection (Children receiving therapy with immunosuppressive agents (large amounts of corticosteroids, antimetabolites, alkylating agents, cytotoxic agents) may not respond optimally to active immunization).
No products indexed under this heading.

Dicumarol (As with other intramuscular injections, Prevnar should be given with caution to children on anticoagulant therapy).
No products indexed under this heading.

Diflorasone Diacetate (Children receiving therapy with immunosuppressive agents (large amounts of corticosteroids, antimetabolites, alkylating agents, cytotoxic agents) may not respond optimally to active immunization).
No products indexed under this heading.

Doxorubicin Hydrochloride (Children receiving therapy with immunosuppressive agents (large amounts of corticosteroids, antimetabolites, alkylating agents, cytotoxic agents) may not respond optimally to active immunization).
No products indexed under this heading.

Enoxaparin Sodium (As with other intramuscular injections, Prevnar should be given with caution to children on anticoagulant therapy). Products include:
Lovenox 3005

Epirubicin Hydrochloride (Children receiving therapy with immunosuppressive agents (large amounts of corticosteroids, antimetabolites, alkylating agents, cytotoxic agents) may not respond optimally to active immunization).
No products indexed under this heading.

Floxuridine (Children receiving therapy with immunosuppressive agents (large amounts of corticosteroids, antimetabolites, alkylating agents, cytotoxic agents) may not respond optimally to active immunization).
No products indexed under this heading.

Fludarabine Phosphate (Children receiving therapy with immunosuppressive agents (large amounts of corticosteroids, antimetabolites, alkylating agents, cytotoxic agents) may not respond optimally to active immunization). Products include:
Oforta 3023

Fludrocortisone Acetate (Children receiving therapy with immunosuppressive agents (large amounts of corticosteroids, antimetabolites, alkylating agents, cytotoxic agents) may not respond optimally to active immunization).
No products indexed under this heading.

Flumethasone Pivalate (Children receiving therapy with immunosuppressive agents (large amounts of corticosteroids, antimetabolites, alkylating agents, cytotoxic agents) may not respond optimally to active immunization).
No products indexed under this heading.

Flunisolide Hemihydrate (Children receiving therapy with immunosuppressive agents (large amounts of corticosteroids, antimetabolites, alkylating agents, cytotoxic agents) may not respond optimally to active immunization).
No products indexed under this heading.

Fluorouracil (Children receiving therapy with immunosuppressive agents (large amounts of corticosteroids, antimetabolites, alkylating agents, cytotoxic agents) may not respond optimally to active immunization). Products include:
Carac 2966

Fluticasone Furoate (Children receiving therapy with immunosuppressive agents (large amounts of corticosteroids, antimetabolites, alkylating agents, cytotoxic agents) may not respond optimally to active immunization). Products include:
Veramyst 1713

Fluticasone Propionate (Children receiving therapy with immunosuppressive agents (large amounts of corticosteroids, antimetabolites, alkylating agents, cytotoxic agents) may not respond optimally to active immunization). Products include:
Advair 100/50 1275
Advair 250/50 1275
Advair 500/50 1275
Advair HFA 45/21 1288
Advair HFA 115/21 1288
Advair HFA 230/21 1288
Flonase 1459
Flovent Diskus 1463
Flovent HFA 1470

Fondaparinux Sodium (As with other intramuscular injections, Prevnar should be given with caution to children on anticoagulant therapy). Products include:
Arixtra 1320

Gemcitabine Hydrochloride (Children receiving therapy with immunosuppressive agents (large amounts of corticosteroids, antimetabolites, alkylating agents, cytotoxic agents) may not respond optimally to active immunization). Products include:
Gemzar 1900

Heparin Calcium (As with other intramuscular injections, Prevnar should be given with caution to children on anticoagulant therapy).
No products indexed under this heading.

Heparin Sodium (As with other intramuscular injections, Prevnar should be given with caution to children on anticoagulant therapy).
No products indexed under this heading.

Hydrocortisone (Children receiving therapy with immunosuppressive agents (large amounts of corticosteroids, antimetabolites, alkylating agents, cytotoxic agents) may not respond optimally to active immunization).
No products indexed under this heading.

Hydrocortisone (Alcohol) (Children receiving therapy with immunosuppressive agents (large amounts of corticosteroids, antimetabolites, alkylating agents, cytotoxic agents) may not respond optimally to active immunization).
No products indexed under this heading.

Hydrocortisone Acetate (Children receiving therapy with immunosuppressive agents (large amounts of corticosteroids, antimetabolites, alkylating agents, cytotoxic agents) may not respond optimally to active immunization).
No products indexed under this heading.

Hydrocortisone Butyrate (Children receiving therapy with immunosuppressive agents (large amounts of corticosteroids, antimetabolites, alkylating agents, cytotoxic agents) may not respond optimally to active immunization).
No products indexed under this heading.

Hydrocortisone Cypionate (Children receiving therapy with immunosuppressive agents (large amounts of corticosteroids, antimetabolites, alkylating agents, cytotoxic agents) may not respond optimally to active immunization).
No products indexed under this heading.

Hydrocortisone Hemisuccinate (Children receiving therapy with immunosuppressive agents (large amounts of corticosteroids, antimetabolites, alkylating agents, cytotoxic agents) may not respond optimally to active immunization).
No products indexed under this heading.

Hydrocortisone Probutate (Children receiving therapy with immunosuppressive agents (large amounts of corticosteroids, antimetabolites, alkylating agents, cytotoxic agents) may not respond optimally to active immunization).
No products indexed under this heading.

Hydrocortisone Sodium Phosphate (Children receiving therapy with immunosuppressive agents (large amounts of corticosteroids, antimetabolites, alkylating agents, cytotoxic agents) may not respond optimally to active immunization).
No products indexed under this heading.

Hydrocortisone Sodium Succinate (Children receiving therapy with immunosuppressive agents (large amounts of corticosteroids, antimetabolites, alkylating agents, cytotoxic agents) may not respond optimally to active immunization).
No products indexed under this heading.

Hydrocortisone Valerate (Children receiving therapy with immunosuppressive agents (large amounts of corticosteroids, antimetabolites, alkylating agents, cytotoxic agents) may not respond optimally to active immunization).
No products indexed under this heading.

Hydroxyurea (Children receiving therapy with immunosuppressive agents (large amounts of corticosteroids, antimetabolites, alkylating agents, cytotoxic agents) may not respond optimally to active immunization).
No products indexed under this heading.

Lomustine (CCNU) (Children receiving therapy with immunosuppressive agents (large amounts of corticosteroids, antimetabolites, alkylating agents, cytotoxic agents) may not respond optimally to active immunization).
No products indexed under this heading.

Low Molecular Weight Heparins (As with other intramuscular injections, Prevnar should be given with caution to children on anticoagulant therapy).
No products indexed under this heading.

Mechlorethamine Hydrochloride (Children receiving therapy with immunosuppressive agents (large amounts of corticosteroids, antimetabolites, alkylating agents, cytotoxic agents) may not respond optimally to active immunization). Products include:
Mustargen 2010

Melphalan (Children receiving therapy with immunosuppressive agents (large amounts of corticosteroids, antimetabolites, alkylating agents, cytotoxic agents) may not respond optimally to active immunization). Products include:
Alkeran 1302

Mercaptopurine (Children receiving therapy with immunosuppressive agents (large amounts of corticosteroids, antimetabolites, alkylating agents, cytotoxic agents) may not respond optimally to active immunization).
No products indexed under this heading.

Methotrexate (Children receiving therapy with immunosuppressive agents (large amounts of corticosteroids, antimetabolites, alkylating agents, cytotoxic agents) may not respond optimally to active immunization).
No products indexed under this heading.

Methotrexate Sodium (Children receiving therapy with immunosuppressive agents (large amounts of corticosteroids, antimetabolites, alkylating agents, cytotoxic agents) may not respond optimally to active immunization).
No products indexed under this heading.

Methylprednisolone (Children receiving therapy with immunosuppressive agents (large amounts of corticosteroids, antimetabolites, alkylating agents, cytotoxic agents) may not respond optimally to active immunization).
No products indexed under this heading.

Methylprednisolone Acetate (Children receiving therapy with immunosuppressive agents (large amounts of corticosteroids, antimetabolites, alkylating agents, cytotoxic agents) may not respond optimally to active immunization).
No products indexed under this heading.

Methylprednisolone Sodium Succinate (Children receiving therapy with immunosuppressive agents (large amounts of corticosteroids, antimetabolites, alkylating agents, cytotoxic agents) may not respond optimally to active immunization).
No products indexed under this heading.

Mitotane (Children receiving therapy with immunosuppressive agents (large amounts of corticosteroids, antimetabolites, alkylating agents, cytotoxic agents) may not respond optimally to active immunization).
No products indexed under this heading.

Mitoxantrone Hydrochloride (Children receiving therapy with immunosuppressive agents (large amounts of corticosteroids, antimetabolites, alkylating agents, cytotoxic agents) may not respond optimally to active immunization). Products include:
Novantrone 1088

Mometasone Furoate (Children receiving therapy with immunosuppressive agents (large amounts of corticosteroids, antimetabolites, alkylating agents, cytotoxic agents) may not respond optimally to active immunization). Products include:
Asmanex 3058
Elocon Cream 3111
Elocon Lotion 3112
Elocon Ointment 3114

Mometasone Furoate Monohydrate (Children receiving therapy with immunosuppressive agents (large amounts of corticosteroids, antimetabolites, alkylating agents, cytotoxic agents) may not respond optimally to active immunization). Products include:
Nasonex 3166

Muromonab-CD3 (Children receiving therapy with immunosuppressive agents (large amounts of corticosteroids, antimetabolites, alkylating agents, cytotoxic agents) may not respond optimally to active immunization). Products include:
Orthoclone OKT3 949

IMPORTANT NOTE: Always consult each drug listing in the patient's regimen for possible interactions.

Mycophenolate Mofetil (Children receiving therapy with immunosuppressive agents (large amounts of corticosteroids, antimetabolites, alkylating agents, cytotoxic agents) may not respond optimally to active immunization).
No products indexed under this heading.

Pentostatin (Children receiving therapy with immunosuppressive agents (large amounts of corticosteroids, antimetabolites, alkylating agents, cytotoxic agents) may not respond optimally to active immunization).
No products indexed under this heading.

Prednisolone (Children receiving therapy with immunosuppressive agents (large amounts of corticosteroids, antimetabolites, alkylating agents, cytotoxic agents) may not respond optimally to active immunization).
No products indexed under this heading.

Prednisolone Acetate (Children receiving therapy with immunosuppressive agents (large amounts of corticosteroids, antimetabolites, alkylating agents, cytotoxic agents) may not respond optimally to active immunization). Products include:
Blephamide .... ⊙212, ⊙214
Pred Forte .... ⊙225
Pred Mild .... ⊙230
Pred-G .... ⊙226, ⊙227

Prednisolone Sodium Phosphate (Children receiving therapy with immunosuppressive agents (large amounts of corticosteroids, antimetabolites, alkylating agents, cytotoxic agents) may not respond optimally to active immunization).
No products indexed under this heading.

Prednisolone Tebutate (Children receiving therapy with immunosuppressive agents (large amounts of corticosteroids, antimetabolites, alkylating agents, cytotoxic agents) may not respond optimally to active immunization).
No products indexed under this heading.

Prednisone (Children receiving therapy with immunosuppressive agents (large amounts of corticosteroids, antimetabolites, alkylating agents, cytotoxic agents) may not respond optimally to active immunization).
No products indexed under this heading.

Prednisone sodium phosphate (Children receiving therapy with immunosuppressive agents (large amounts of corticosteroids, antimetabolites, alkylating agents, cytotoxic agents) may not respond optimally to active immunization).
No products indexed under this heading.

Procarbazine Hydrochloride (Children receiving therapy with immunosuppressive agents (large amounts of corticosteroids, antimetabolites, alkylating agents, cytotoxic agents) may not respond optimally to active immunization).
No products indexed under this heading.

Radiation (Children with impaired immune responsiveness, whether due to the use of immunosuppressive therapy (including irradiation, corticosteroids, antimetabolites, alkylating agents, and cytotoxic agents), a genetic defect, HIV infection, or other causes, may have reduced antibody response to active immunization).
No products indexed under this heading.

Rapamycin (Children receiving therapy with immunosuppressive agents (large amounts of corticosteroids, antimetabolites, alkylating agents, cytotoxic agents) may not respond optimally to active immunization).
No products indexed under this heading.

Sirolimus (Children receiving therapy with immunosuppressive agents (large

amounts of corticosteroids, antimetabolites, alkylating agents, cytotoxic agents) may not respond optimally to active immunization). Products include:
Rapamune 3579

Tacrolimus (Children receiving therapy with immunosuppressive agents (large amounts of corticosteroids, antimetabolites, alkylating agents, cytotoxic agents) may not respond optimally to active immunization). Products include:
Prograf Capsules 677
Prograf Injection 677
Protopic 685

Tamoxifen Citrate (Children receiving therapy with immunosuppressive agents (large amounts of corticosteroids, antimetabolites, alkylating agents, cytotoxic agents) may not respond optimally to active immunization).
No products indexed under this heading.

Thioguanine (Children receiving therapy with immunosuppressive agents (large amounts of corticosteroids, antimetabolites, alkylating agents, cytotoxic agents) may not respond optimally to active immunization). Products include:
Tabloid 1664

Thiotepa (Children receiving therapy with immunosuppressive agents (large amounts of corticosteroids, antimetabolites, alkylating agents, cytotoxic agents) may not respond optimally to active immunization).
No products indexed under this heading.

Tinzaparin Sodium (As with other intramuscular injections, Prevnar should be given with caution to children on anticoagulant therapy).
No products indexed under this heading.

Triamcinolone (Children receiving therapy with immunosuppressive agents (large amounts of corticosteroids, antimetabolites, alkylating agents, cytotoxic agents) may not respond optimally to active immunization).
No products indexed under this heading.

Triamcinolone Acetonide (Children receiving therapy with immunosuppressive agents (large amounts of corticosteroids, antimetabolites, alkylating agents, cytotoxic agents) may not respond optimally to active immunization). Products include:
Azmacort 408
Nasacort AQ 3019

Triamcinolone Diacetate (Children receiving therapy with immunosuppressive agents (large amounts of corticosteroids, antimetabolites, alkylating agents, cytotoxic agents) may not respond optimally to active immunization).
No products indexed under this heading.

Triamcinolone Hexacetonide (Children receiving therapy with immunosuppressive agents (large amounts of corticosteroids, antimetabolites, alkylating agents, cytotoxic agents) may not respond optimally to active immunization).
No products indexed under this heading.

Vinblastine Sulfate (Children receiving therapy with immunosuppressive agents (large amounts of corticosteroids, antimetabolites, alkylating agents, cytotoxic agents) may not respond optimally to active immunization).
No products indexed under this heading.

Vincristine Sulfate (Children receiving therapy with immunosuppressive agents (large amounts of corticosteroids, antimetabolites, alkylating agents, cytotoxic agents) may not respond optimally to active immunization).
No products indexed under this heading.

Vinorelbine Tartrate (Children receiving therapy with immunosuppressive agents (large amounts of corticosteroids, antimetabolites, alkylating agents, cytotoxic agents) may not respond optimally to active immunization).
No products indexed under this heading.

Warfarin Sodium (As with other intramuscular injections, Prevnar should be given with caution to children on anticoagulant therapy).
No products indexed under this heading.

PRIMAXIN I.M.
(Cilastatin Sodium, Imipenem) 2232
May interact with local anesthetics, valproate, and certain other agents. Compounds in these categories include:

Articaine Hydrochloride (Due to the use of lidocaine hydrochloride diluent, this product is contraindicated in patients with a known hypersensitivity to local anesthetics of the amide type).
No products indexed under this heading.

Bupivacaine Hydrochloride (Due to the use of lidocaine hydrochloride diluent, this product is contraindicated in patients with a known hypersensitivity to local anesthetics of the amide type).
No products indexed under this heading.

Chloroprocaine Hydrochloride (Due to the use of lidocaine hydrochloride diluent, this product is contraindicated in patients with a known hypersensitivity to local anesthetics of the amide type).
No products indexed under this heading.

Cocaine Hydrochloride (Due to the use of lidocaine hydrochloride diluent, this product is contraindicated in patients with a known hypersensitivity to local anesthetics of the amide type).
No products indexed under this heading.

Divalproex Sodium (Carbapenems, including imipenem, may reduce serum valproic acid concentrations to subtherapeutic levels, resulting in loss of seizure control. Serum valproic acid concentrations should be monitored frequently after initiating carbapenem therapy. Alternative antibacterial or anticonvulsant therapy should be considered if serum valproic acid concentrations drop below the therapeutic range or a seizure occurs). Products include:
Depakote ER 426

Etidocaine Hydrochloride (Due to the use of lidocaine hydrochloride diluent, this product is contraindicated in patients with a known hypersensitivity to local anesthetics of the amide type).
No products indexed under this heading.

Levobupivacaine Hydrochloride (Due to the use of lidocaine hydrochloride diluent, this product is contraindicated in patients with a known hypersensitivity to local anesthetics of the amide type).
No products indexed under this heading.

Lidocaine Hydrochloride (Due to the use of lidocaine hydrochloride diluent, this product is contraindicated in patients with a known hypersensitivity to local anesthetics of the amide type).
No products indexed under this heading.

Mepivacaine Hydrochloride (Due to the use of lidocaine hydrochloride diluent, this product is contraindicated in patients with a known hypersensitivity to local anesthetics of the amide type).
No products indexed under this heading.

Probenecid (Since concomitant administration of Primaxin and probenecid results in only minimal increases in plasma levels of imipenem and plasma half-life, it is not recommended that probenecid be given with Primaxin).
No products indexed under this heading.

Procaine Hydrochloride (Due to the use of lidocaine hydrochloride diluent, this product is contraindicated in patients with a known hypersensitivity to local anesthetics of the amide type).
No products indexed under this heading.

Tetracaine Hydrochloride (Due to the use of lidocaine hydrochloride diluent, this product is contraindicated in patients with a known hypersensitivity to local anesthetics of the amide type).
No products indexed under this heading.

Valproate Sodium (Carbapenems, including imipenem, may reduce serum valproic acid concentrations to subtherapeutic levels, resulting in loss of seizure control. Serum valproic acid concentrations should be monitored frequently after initiating carbapenem therapy. Alternative antibacterial or anticonvulsant therapy should be considered if serum valproic acid concentrations drop below the therapeutic range or a seizure occurs).
No products indexed under this heading.

Valproic Acid (Carbapenems, including imipenem, may reduce serum valproic acid concentrations to subtherapeutic levels, resulting in loss of seizure control. Serum valproic acid concentrations should be monitored frequently after initiating carbapenem therapy. Alternative antibacterial or anticonvulsant therapy should be considered if serum valproic acid concentrations drop below the therapeutic range or a seizure occurs).
No products indexed under this heading.

PRIMAXIN I.V.
(Cilastatin Sodium, Imipenem) 2235
May interact with valproate, and certain other agents. Compounds in these categories include:

Divalproex Sodium (Carbapenems, including imipenem, may reduce serum valproic acid concentrations to subtherapeutic levels, resulting in loss of seizure control. Serum valproic acid concentrations should be monitored frequently after initiating carbapenem therapy. Alternative antibacterial or anticonvulsant therapy should be considered if serum valproic acid concentrations drop below the therapeutic range or a seizure occurs). Products include:
Depakote ER 426

Ganciclovir Sodium (Generalized seizures have been reported in patients who received ganciclovir and Primaxin. These drugs should not be used concomitantly unless the potential benefits outweigh the risks).
No products indexed under this heading.

Probenecid (Since concomitant administration of Primaxin and probenecid results in only minimal increases in plasma levels of imipenem and plasma half-life, it is not recommended that probenecid be given with Primaxin).
No products indexed under this heading.

Valproate Sodium (Carbapenems, including imipenem, may reduce serum valproic acid concentrations to subtherapeutic levels, resulting in loss of seizure control. Serum valproic acid concentrations should be monitored frequently after initiating carbapenem therapy. Alternative antibacterial or anticonvulsant therapy should be considered if serum valproic acid concentrations drop below the therapeutic range or a seizure occurs).
No products indexed under this heading.

Valproic Acid (Carbapenems, including imipenem, may reduce serum valproic acid concentrations to subtherapeutic levels, resulting in loss of seizure control. Serum valproic acid concentrations should be monitored frequently after initiating carbapenem therapy.

(⊙ Described in PDR® for Ophthalmic Medicines)

1457 Interactions Index Prinivil

Alternative antibacterial or anticonvulsant therapy should be considered if serum valproic acid concentrations drop below the therapeutic range or a seizure occurs).
No products indexed under this heading.

PRINIVIL TABLETS
(Lisinopril) 2241
May interact with diuretics, insulin, lithium preparations, non-steroidal anti-inflammatory agents, oral hypoglycemic agents, potassium preparations, potassium sparing diuretics, thiazides, and certain other agents. Compounds in these categories include:

Acarbose (Epidemiological studies have suggested that concomitant administration of ACE inhibitors and antidiabetic medicines (insulins, oral hypoglycemic agents) may cause an increased blood-glucose-lowering effect with risk of hypoglycemia. This phenomenon appeared to be more likely to occur during the first weeks of combined treatment and in patients with renal impairment. In diabetic patients treated with oral antidiabetic agents or insulin, glycemic control should be closely monitored for hypoglycemia, especially during the first month of treatment with an ACE inhibitor).
No products indexed under this heading.

Amiloride Hydrochloride (Use of lisinopril with potassium-sparing diuretics (such as spironolactone, triamterene or amiloride), potassium supplements or potassium-containing salt substitutes may lead to significant increases in serum potassium. Therefore, if concomitant use of these agents is indicated because of demonstrated hypokalemia, they should be used with caution and with frequent monitoring of serum potassium. Potassium-sparing agents should generally not be used in patients with heart failure who are receiving lisinopril).
No products indexed under this heading.

Bendroflumethiazide (Thiazide-induced potassium loss attenuated; possibility of excessive reduction in blood pressure).
No products indexed under this heading.

Bumetanide (Possibility of excessive reduction in blood pressure).
No products indexed under this heading.

Celecoxib (Reports suggest that NSAIDs, including selective COX-2 inhibitors, may diminish the antihypertensive effect of ACE inhibitors, including lisinopril. This interaction should be given consideration in patients taking NSAIDs or selective COX-2 inhibitors concomitantly with ACE inhibitors. In some patients with compromised renal function who are being treated with NSAIDs, including selective COX-2 inhibitors, the co-administration of angiotensin II receptor antagonists or ACE inhibitors, may result in further deterioration of renal function, including possible acute renal failure. These effects are usually reversible. Therefore, monitor effects on blood pressure and renal fuction when administering the combination, especially in the elderly). Products include:
Celebrex 3272

Chlorothiazide (Thiazide-induced potassium loss attenuated; possibility of excessive reduction in blood pressure).
No products indexed under this heading.

Chlorothiazide Sodium (Thiazide-induced potassium loss attenuated; possibility of excessive reduction in blood pressure). Products include:
Diuril Intravenous 2009

Chlorpropamide (Epidemiological studies have suggested that concomitant administration of ACE inhibitors and antidiabetic medicines (insulins, oral hypoglycemic agents) may cause an increased blood-glucose-lowering effect with risk of hypoglycemia. This phenomenon appeared to be more likely to occur during the first weeks of combined treatment and in patients with renal impairment. In diabetic patients treated with oral antidiabetic agents or insulin, glycemic control should be closely monitored for hypoglycemia, especially during the first month of treatment with an ACE inhibitor).
No products indexed under this heading.

Chlorthalidone (Possibility of excessive reduction in blood pressure). Products include:
Clorpres 2344

Diclofenac Epolamine (Reports suggest that NSAIDs, including selective COX-2 inhibitors, may diminish the antihypertensive effect of ACE inhibitors, including lisinopril. This interaction should be given consideration in patients taking NSAIDs or selective COX-2 inhibitors concomitantly with ACE inhibitors. In some patients with compromised renal function who are being treated with NSAIDs, including selective COX-2 inhibitors, the co-administration of angiotensin II receptor antagonists or ACE inhibitors, may result in further deterioration of renal function, including possible acute renal failure. These effects are usually reversible. Therefore, monitor effects on blood pressure and renal fuction when administering the combination, especially in the elderly). Products include:
Flector 1839

Diclofenac Potassium (Reports suggest that NSAIDs, including selective COX-2 inhibitors, may diminish the antihypertensive effect of ACE inhibitors, including lisinopril. This interaction should be given consideration in patients taking NSAIDs or selective COX-2 inhibitors concomitantly with ACE inhibitors. In some patients with compromised renal function who are being treated with NSAIDs, including selective COX-2 inhibitors, the co-administration of angiotensin II receptor antagonists or ACE inhibitors, may result in further deterioration of renal function, including possible acute renal failure. These effects are usually reversible. Therefore, monitor effects on blood pressure and renal fuction when administering the combination, especially in the elderly).
No products indexed under this heading.

Diclofenac Sodium (Reports suggest that NSAIDs, including selective COX-2 inhibitors, may diminish the antihypertensive effect of ACE inhibitors, including lisinopril. This interaction should be given consideration in patients taking NSAIDs or selective COX-2 inhibitors concomitantly with ACE inhibitors. In some patients with compromised renal function who are being treated with NSAIDs, including selective COX-2 inhibitors, the co-administration of angiotensin II receptor antagonists or ACE inhibitors, may result in further deterioration of renal function, including possible acute renal failure. These effects are usually reversible. Therefore, monitor effects on blood pressure and renal fuction when administering the combination, especially in the elderly).
No products indexed under this heading.

Eplerenone (Use of lisinopril with potassium-sparing diuretics (such as spironolactone, triamterene or amiloride), potassium supplements or potassium-containing salt substitutes may lead to significant increases in serum potassium. Therefore, if concomitant use of these agents is indicated because of demonstrated hypokalemia, they should be used with caution and with frequent monitoring of serum potassium. Potassium-sparing agents should generally not be used in patients with heart failure who are receiving lisinopril).
No products indexed under this heading.

Ethacrynic Acid (Possibility of excessive reduction in blood pressure).
No products indexed under this heading.

Etodolac (Reports suggest that NSAIDs, including selective COX-2 inhibitors, may diminish the antihypertensive effect of ACE inhibitors, including lisinopril. This interaction should be given consideration in patients taking NSAIDs or selective COX-2 inhibitors concomitantly with ACE inhibitors. In some patients with compromised renal function who are being treated with NSAIDs, including selective COX-2 inhibitors, the co-administration of angiotensin II receptor antagonists or ACE inhibitors, may result in further deterioration of renal function, including possible acute renal failure. These effects are usually reversible. Therefore, monitor effects on blood pressure and renal fuction when administering the combination, especially in the elderly).
No products indexed under this heading.

Fenoprofen Calcium (Reports suggest that NSAIDs, including selective COX-2 inhibitors, may diminish the antihypertensive effect of ACE inhibitors, including lisinopril. This interaction should be given consideration in patients taking NSAIDs or selective COX-2 inhibitors concomitantly with ACE inhibitors. In some patients with compromised renal function who are being treated with NSAIDs, including selective COX-2 inhibitors, the co-administration of angiotensin II receptor antagonists or ACE inhibitors, may result in further deterioration of renal function, including possible acute renal failure. These effects are usually reversible. Therefore, monitor effects on blood pressure and renal fuction when administering the combination, especially in the elderly).
No products indexed under this heading.

Flurbiprofen (Reports suggest that NSAIDs, including selective COX-2 inhibitors, may diminish the antihypertensive effect of ACE inhibitors, including lisinopril. This interaction should be given consideration in patients taking NSAIDs or selective COX-2 inhibitors concomitantly with ACE inhibitors. In some patients with compromised renal function who are being treated with NSAIDs, including selective COX-2 inhibitors, the co-administration of angiotensin II receptor antagonists or ACE inhibitors, may result in further deterioration of renal function, including possible acute renal failure. These effects are usually reversible. Therefore, monitor effects on blood pressure and renal fuction when administering the combination, especially in the elderly).
No products indexed under this heading.

Furosemide (Possibility of excessive reduction in blood pressure). Products include:
Furosemide 2354

Glibenclamide (Epidemiological studies have suggested that concomitant administration of ACE inhibitors and antidiabetic medicines (insulins, oral hypoglycemic agents) may cause an increased blood-glucose-lowering effect with risk of hypoglycemia. This phenomenon appeared to be more likely to occur during the first weeks of combined treatment and in patients with renal impairment. In diabetic patients treated with oral antidiabetic agents or insulin, glycemic control should be closely monitored for hypoglycemia, especially during the first month of treatment with an ACE inhibitor).
No products indexed under this heading.

Glimepiride (Epidemiological studies have suggested that concomitant administration of ACE inhibitors and antidiabetic medicines (insulins, oral hypoglycemic agents) may cause an increased blood-glucose-lowering effect with risk of hypoglycemia. This phenomenon appeared to be more likely to occur during the first weeks of combined treatment and in patients with renal impairment. In diabetic patients treated with oral antidiabetic agents or insulin, glycemic control should be closely monitored for hypoglycemia, especially during the first month of treatment with an ACE inhibitor). Products include:
Avandaryl 1356
Duetact 3354

Glipizide (Epidemiological studies have suggested that concomitant administration of ACE inhibitors and antidiabetic medicines (insulins, oral hypoglycemic agents) may cause an increased blood-glucose-lowering effect with risk of hypoglycemia. This phenomenon appeared to be more likely to occur during the first weeks of combined treatment and in patients with renal impairment. In diabetic patients treated with oral antidiabetic agents or insulin, glycemic control should be closely monitored for hypoglycemia, especially during the first month of treatment with an ACE inhibitor).
No products indexed under this heading.

Glyburide (Epidemiological studies have suggested that concomitant administration of ACE inhibitors and antidiabetic medicines (insulins, oral hypoglycemic agents) may cause an increased blood-glucose-lowering effect with risk of hypoglycemia. This phenomenon appeared to be more likely to occur during the first weeks of combined treatment and in patients with renal impairment. In diabetic patients treated with oral antidiabetic agents or insulin, glycemic control should be closely monitored for hypoglycemia, especially during the first month of treatment with an ACE inhibitor).
No products indexed under this heading.

Gold Sodium Thiomalate (Nitroid reactions (symptoms include facial flushing, nausea, vomiting and hypotension) have been reported rarely in patients on therapy with injectable gold and concomitant ACE inhibitor therapy including lisinopril).
No products indexed under this heading.

Gold Therapy (Nitroid reactions (symptoms include facial flushing, nausea, vomiting and hypotension) have been reported rarely in patients on therapy with injectable gold and concomitant ACE inhibitor therapy including lisinopril).
No products indexed under this heading.

Hydrochlorothiazide (Thiazide-induced potassium loss attenuated; possibility of excessive reduction in blood pressure). Products include:
Atacand HCT 700
Avalide 2956
Benicar HCT 1017
Diovan HCT 2419
Dyazide 1429
Exforge HCT 2449
Hyzaar 2162
Hyzaar 100-12.5 2162
Micardis HCT 889
Prinzide 2246
Tekturna HCT 2541
Teveten HCT 541

IMPORTANT NOTE: Always consult each drug listing in the patient's regimen for possible interactions.

Prinivil Interactions Index 1458

Hydroflumethiazide (Thiazide-induced potassium loss attenuated; possibility of excessive reduction in blood pressure).
No products indexed under this heading.

Ibuprofen (Reports suggest that NSAIDs, including selective COX-2 inhibitors, may diminish the antihypertensive effect of ACE inhibitors, including lisinopril. This interaction should be given consideration in patients taking NSAIDs or selective COX-2 inhibitors concomitantly with ACE inhibitors. In some patients with compromised renal function who are being treated with NSAIDs, including selective COX-2 inhibitors, the co-administration of angiotensin II receptor antagonists or ACE inhibitors, may result in further deterioration of renal function, including possible acute renal failure. These effects are usually reversible. Therefore, monitor effects on blood pressure and renal fuction when administering the combination, especially in the elderly). Products include:
Motrin IB 2043
Children's Motrin 2044
Children's Motrin Non-Staining Dye-Free 2044
Infants' Motrin 2044
Infants' Motrin Dye-Free 2044
Junior Strength Motrin 2044
Vicoprofen 564

Indapamide (Possibility of excessive reduction in blood pressure). Products include:
Indapamide 2356

Indomethacin (Co-administration in some patients with compromised renal function who are being treated with NSAIDs may result in a further deterioration of renal function. In a study, the use of indomethacin was associated with a reduced antihypertensive effect, although the difference between lisinopril alone to lisinopril given concomitantly with indomethacin was not significant). Products include:
Indocin 2167

Indomethacin Sodium Trihydrate (Reports suggest that NSAIDs, including selective COX-2 inhibitors, may diminish the antihypertensive effect of ACE inhibitors, including lisinopril. This interaction should be given consideration in patients taking NSAIDs or selective COX-2 inhibitors concomitantly with ACE inhibitors. In some patients with compromised renal function who are being treated with NSAIDs, including selective COX-2 inhibitors, the co-administration of angiotensin II receptor antagonists or ACE inhibitors, may result in further deterioration of renal function, including possible acute renal failure. These effects are usually reversible. Therefore, monitor effects on blood pressure and renal fuction when administering the combination, especially in the elderly). Products include:
Indocin I.V. 2007

Insulin (Epidemiological studies have suggested that concomitant administration of ACE inhibitors and antidiabetic medicines (insulins, oral hypoglycemic agents) may cause an increased blood-glucose-lowering effect with risk of hypoglycemia. This phenomenon appeared to be more likely to occur during the first weeks of combined treatment and in patients with renal impairment. In diabetic patients treated with oral antidiabetic agents or insulin, glycemic control should be closely monitored for hypoglycemia, especially during the first month of treatment with an ACE inhibitor).
No products indexed under this heading.

Insulin, Human, Zinc Suspension (Epidemiological studies have suggested that concomitant administration of ACE inhibitors and antidiabetic medicines (insulins, oral hypoglycemic agents) may cause an increased blood-glucose-lowering effect with risk of hypoglycemia. This phenomenon appeared to be more likely to occur during the first weeks of combined treatment and in patients with renal impairment. In diabetic patients treated with oral antidiabetic agents or insulin, glycemic control should be closely monitored for hypoglycemia, especially during the first month of treatment with an ACE inhibitor).
No products indexed under this heading.

Insulin, Human (rDNA origin) (Epidemiological studies have suggested that concomitant administration of ACE inhibitors and antidiabetic medicines (insulins, oral hypoglycemic agents) may cause an increased blood-glucose-lowering effect with risk of hypoglycemia. This phenomenon appeared to be more likely to occur during the first weeks of combined treatment and in patients with renal impairment. In diabetic patients treated with oral antidiabetic agents or insulin, glycemic control should be closely monitored for hypoglycemia, especially during the first month of treatment with an ACE inhibitor). Products include:
Exubera 2717

Insulin, Human NPH (Epidemiological studies have suggested that concomitant administration of ACE inhibitors and antidiabetic medicines (insulins, oral hypoglycemic agents) may cause an increased blood-glucose-lowering effect with risk of hypoglycemia. This phenomenon appeared to be more likely to occur during the first weeks of combined treatment and in patients with renal impairment. In diabetic patients treated with oral antidiabetic agents or insulin, glycemic control should be closely monitored for hypoglycemia, especially during the first month of treatment with an ACE inhibitor). Products include:
Humulin N Vial 1934

Insulin, Human Regular (Epidemiological studies have suggested that concomitant administration of ACE inhibitors and antidiabetic medicines (insulins, oral hypoglycemic agents) may cause an increased blood-glucose-lowering effect with risk of hypoglycemia. This phenomenon appeared to be more likely to occur during the first weeks of combined treatment and in patients with renal impairment. In diabetic patients treated with oral antidiabetic agents or insulin, glycemic control should be closely monitored for hypoglycemia, especially during the first month of treatment with an ACE inhibitor). Products include:
Humulin R 1937
Humulin R (U-500) 1939

Insulin, Human Regular and Human NPH Mixture (Epidemiological studies have suggested that concomitant administration of ACE inhibitors and antidiabetic medicines (insulins, oral hypoglycemic agents) may cause an increased blood-glucose-lowering effect with risk of hypoglycemia. This phenomenon appeared to be more likely to occur during the first weeks of combined treatment and in patients with renal impairment. In diabetic patients treated with oral antidiabetic agents or insulin, glycemic control should be closely monitored for hypoglycemia, especially during the first month of treatment with an ACE inhibitor). Products include:
Humulin 50/50 1930
Humulin 70/30 Vial 1931

Insulin, NPH (Epidemiological studies have suggested that concomitant administration of ACE inhibitors and antidiabetic medicines (insulins, oral hypoglycemic agents) may cause an increased blood-glucose-lowering effect with risk of hypoglycemia. This phenomenon appeared to be more likely to occur during the first weeks of combined treatment and in patients with renal impairment. In diabetic patients treated with oral antidiabetic agents or insulin, glycemic control should be closely monitored for hypoglycemia, especially during the first month of treatment with an ACE inhibitor).
No products indexed under this heading.

Insulin, Regular (Epidemiological studies have suggested that concomitant administration of ACE inhibitors and antidiabetic medicines (insulins, oral hypoglycemic agents) may cause an increased blood-glucose-lowering effect with risk of hypoglycemia. This phenomenon appeared to be more likely to occur during the first weeks of combined treatment and in patients with renal impairment. In diabetic patients treated with oral antidiabetic agents or insulin, glycemic control should be closely monitored for hypoglycemia, especially during the first month of treatment with an ACE inhibitor).
No products indexed under this heading.

Insulin, Regular and NPH mixture (Epidemiological studies have suggested that concomitant administration of ACE inhibitors and antidiabetic medicines (insulins, oral hypoglycemic agents) may cause an increased blood-glucose-lowering effect with risk of hypoglycemia. This phenomenon appeared to be more likely to occur during the first weeks of combined treatment and in patients with renal impairment. In diabetic patients treated with oral antidiabetic agents or insulin, glycemic control should be closely monitored for hypoglycemia, especially during the first month of treatment with an ACE inhibitor).
No products indexed under this heading.

Insulin, Zinc Crystals (Epidemiological studies have suggested that concomitant administration of ACE inhibitors and antidiabetic medicines (insulins, oral hypoglycemic agents) may cause an increased blood-glucose-lowering effect with risk of hypoglycemia. This phenomenon appeared to be more likely to occur during the first weeks of combined treatment and in patients with renal impairment. In diabetic patients treated with oral antidiabetic agents or insulin, glycemic control should be closely monitored for hypoglycemia, especially during the first month of treatment with an ACE inhibitor).
No products indexed under this heading.

Insulin, Zinc Suspension (Epidemiological studies have suggested that concomitant administration of ACE inhibitors and antidiabetic medicines (insulins, oral hypoglycemic agents) may cause an increased blood-glucose-lowering effect with risk of hypoglycemia. This phenomenon appeared to be more likely to occur during the first weeks of combined treatment and in patients with renal impairment. In diabetic patients treated with oral antidiabetic agents or insulin, glycemic control should be closely monitored for hypoglycemia, especially during the first month of treatment with an ACE inhibitor).
No products indexed under this heading.

Insulin Aspart (Epidemiological studies have suggested that concomitant administration of ACE inhibitors and antidiabetic medicines (insulins, oral hypoglycemic agents) may cause an increased blood-glucose-lowering effect with risk of hypoglycemia. This phenomenon appeared to be more likely to occur during the first weeks of combined treatment and in patients with renal impairment. In diabetic patients treated with oral antidiabetic agents or insulin, glycemic control should be closely monitored for hypoglycemia, especially during the first month of treatment with an ACE inhibitor).
No products indexed under this heading.

Insulin Aspart, Human (Epidemiological studies have suggested that concomitant administration of ACE inhibitors and antidiabetic medicines (insulins, oral hypoglycemic agents) may cause an increased blood-glucose-lowering effect with risk of hypoglycemia. This phenomenon appeared to be more likely to occur during the first weeks of combined treatment and in patients with renal impairment. In diabetic patients treated with oral antidiabetic agents or insulin, glycemic control should be closely monitored for hypoglycemia, especially during the first month of treatment with an ACE inhibitor). Products include:
NovoLog Mix 70/30 2581

Insulin Aspart, Human Regular (Epidemiological studies have suggested that concomitant administration of ACE inhibitors and antidiabetic medicines (insulins, oral hypoglycemic agents) may cause an increased blood-glucose-lowering effect with risk of hypoglycemia. This phenomenon appeared to be more likely to occur during the first weeks of combined treatment and in patients with renal impairment. In diabetic patients treated with oral antidiabetic agents or insulin, glycemic control should be closely monitored for hypoglycemia, especially during the first month of treatment with an ACE inhibitor). Products include:
NovoLog 2575

Insulin Aspart Protamine, Human (Epidemiological studies have suggested that concomitant administration of ACE inhibitors and antidiabetic medicines (insulins, oral hypoglycemic agents) may cause an increased blood-glucose-lowering effect with risk of hypoglycemia. This phenomenon appeared to be more likely to occur during the first weeks of combined treatment and in patients with renal impairment. In diabetic patients treated with oral antidiabetic agents or insulin, glycemic control should be closely monitored for hypoglycemia, especially during the first month of treatment with an ACE inhibitor). Products include:
NovoLog Mix 70/30 2581

Insulin Detemir (rDNA Origin) (Epidemiological studies have suggested that concomitant administration of ACE inhibitors and antidiabetic medicines (insulins, oral hypoglycemic agents) may cause an increased blood-glucose-lowering effect with risk of hypoglycemia. This phenomenon appeared to be more likely to occur during the first weeks of combined treatment and in patients with renal impairment. In diabetic patients treated with oral antidiabetic agents or insulin, glycemic control should be closely monitored for hypoglycemia, especially during the first month of treatment with an ACE inhibitor). Products include:
Levemir 2566

Insulin Glargine (Epidemiological studies have suggested that concomitant administration of ACE inhibitors and antidiabetic medicines (insulins, oral hypoglycemic agents) may cause an increased blood-glucose-lowering effect with risk of hypoglycemia. This phenomenon appeared to be more likely to occur during the first weeks of combined treatment and in patients with renal impairment. In diabetic patients treated with oral antidiabetic agents or insulin, glycemic control should be

closely monitored for hypoglycemia, especially during the first month of treatment with an ACE inhibitor). Products include:
Lantus 2996

Insulin Glulisine (Epidemiological studies have suggested that concomitant administration of ACE inhibitors and antidiabetic medicines (insulins, oral hypoglycemic agents) may cause an increased blood-glucose-lowering effect with risk of hypoglycemia. This phenomenon appeared to be more likely to occur during the first weeks of combined treatment and in patients with renal impairment. In diabetic patients treated with oral antidiabetic agents or insulin, glycemic control should be closely monitored for hypoglycemia, especially during the first month of treatment with an ACE inhibitor). Products include:
Apidra 2937
Apidra SoloStar 2937

Insulin Lispro, Human (Epidemiological studies have suggested that concomitant administration of ACE inhibitors and antidiabetic medicines (insulins, oral hypoglycemic agents) may cause an increased blood-glucose-lowering effect with risk of hypoglycemia. This phenomenon appeared to be more likely to occur during the first weeks of combined treatment and in patients with renal impairment. In diabetic patients treated with oral antidiabetic agents or insulin, glycemic control should be closely monitored for hypoglycemia, especially during the first month of treatment with an ACE inhibitor). Products include:
Humalog 1910
Humalog Mix 1914
Humalog Mix75/25 1917

Insulin Lispro Protamine, Human (Epidemiological studies have suggested that concomitant administration of ACE inhibitors and antidiabetic medicines (insulins, oral hypoglycemic agents) may cause an increased blood-glucose-lowering effect with risk of hypoglycemia. This phenomenon appeared to be more likely to occur during the first weeks of combined treatment and in patients with renal impairment. In diabetic patients treated with oral antidiabetic agents or insulin, glycemic control should be closely monitored for hypoglycemia, especially during the first month of treatment with an ACE inhibitor). Products include:
Humalog Mix 1914
Humalog Mix75/25 1917

Ketoprofen (Reports suggest that NSAIDs, including selective COX-2 inhibitors, may diminish the antihypertensive effect of ACE inhibitors, including lisinopril. This interaction should be given consideration in patients taking NSAIDs or selective COX-2 inhibitors concomitantly with ACE inhibitors. In some patients with compromised renal function who are being treated with NSAIDs, including selective COX-2 inhibitors, the co-administration of angiotensin II receptor antagonists or ACE inhibitors, may result in further deterioration of renal function, including possible acute renal failure. These effects are usually reversible. Therefore, monitor effects on blood pressure and renal fuction when administering the combination, especially in the elderly).
No products indexed under this heading.

Ketorolac Tromethamine (Reports suggest that NSAIDs, including selective COX-2 inhibitors, may diminish the antihypertensive effect of ACE inhibitors, including lisinopril. This interaction should be given consideration in patients taking NSAIDs or selective COX-2 inhibitors concomitantly with ACE

inhibitors. In some patients with compromised renal function who are being treated with NSAIDs, including selective COX-2 inhibitors, the co-administration of angiotensin II receptor antagonists or ACE inhibitors, may result in further deterioration of renal function, including possible acute renal failure. These effects are usually reversible. Therefore, monitor effects on blood pressure and renal fuction when administering the combination, especially in the elderly). Products include:
Acuvail .... ⊙209

Lithium (Potential for reversible lithium toxicity; frequent monitoring of lithium levels is recommended).
No products indexed under this heading.

Lithium Carbonate (Potential for reversible lithium toxicity; frequent monitoring of lithium levels is recommended).
No products indexed under this heading.

Lithium Citrate (Potential for reversible lithium toxicity; frequent monitoring of lithium levels is recommended).
No products indexed under this heading.

Meclofenamate Sodium (Reports suggest that NSAIDs, including selective COX-2 inhibitors, may diminish the antihypertensive effect of ACE inhibitors, including lisinopril. This interaction should be given consideration in patients taking NSAIDs or selective COX-2 inhibitors concomitantly with ACE inhibitors. In some patients with compromised renal function who are being treated with NSAIDs, including selective COX-2 inhibitors, the co-administration of angiotensin II receptor antagonists or ACE inhibitors, may result in further deterioration of renal function, including possible acute renal failure. These effects are usually reversible. Therefore, monitor effects on blood pressure and renal fuction when administering the combination, especially in the elderly).
No products indexed under this heading.

Mefenamic Acid (Reports suggest that NSAIDs, including selective COX-2 inhibitors, may diminish the antihypertensive effect of ACE inhibitors, including lisinopril. This interaction should be given consideration in patients taking NSAIDs or selective COX-2 inhibitors concomitantly with ACE inhibitors. In some patients with compromised renal function who are being treated with NSAIDs, including selective COX-2 inhibitors, the co-administration of angiotensin II receptor antagonists or ACE inhibitors, may result in further deterioration of renal function, including possible acute renal failure. These effects are usually reversible. Therefore, monitor effects on blood pressure and renal fuction when administering the combination, especially in the elderly).
No products indexed under this heading.

Meloxicam (Reports suggest that NSAIDs, including selective COX-2 inhibitors, may diminish the antihypertensive effect of ACE inhibitors, including lisinopril. This interaction should be given consideration in patients taking NSAIDs or selective COX-2 inhibitors concomitantly with ACE inhibitors. In some patients with compromised renal function who are being treated with NSAIDs, including selective COX-2 inhibitors, the co-administration of angiotensin II receptor antagonists or ACE inhibitors, may result in further deterioration of renal function, including possible acute renal failure. These effects are usually reversible. Therefore, monitor effects on blood pressure and renal fuction when administering the combination, especially in the elderly).
No products indexed under this heading.

Metformin Hydrochloride (Epidemiological studies have suggested that concomitant administration of ACE inhibitors and antidiabetic medicines (insulins, oral hypoglycemic agents) may cause an increased blood-glucose-lowering effect with risk of hypoglycemia. This phenomenon appeared to be more likely to occur during the first weeks of combined treatment and in patients with renal impairment. In diabetic patients treated with oral antidiabetic agents or insulin, glycemic control should be closely monitored for hypoglycemia, especially during the first month of treatment with an ACE inhibitor). Products include:
ActoPlus 3338
Avandamet 1345
Janumet 2188

Methyclothiazide (Thiazide-induced potassium loss attenuated; possibility of excessive reduction in blood pressure).
No products indexed under this heading.

Metolazone (Possibility of excessive reduction in blood pressure).
No products indexed under this heading.

Miglitol (Epidemiological studies have suggested that concomitant administration of ACE inhibitors and antidiabetic medicines (insulins, oral hypoglycemic agents) may cause an increased blood-glucose-lowering effect with risk of hypoglycemia. This phenomenon appeared to be more likely to occur during the first weeks of combined treatment and in patients with renal impairment. In diabetic patients treated with oral antidiabetic agents or insulin, glycemic control should be closely monitored for hypoglycemia, especially during the first month of treatment with an ACE inhibitor).
No products indexed under this heading.

Nabumetone (Reports suggest that NSAIDs, including selective COX-2 inhibitors, may diminish the antihypertensive effect of ACE inhibitors, including lisinopril. This interaction should be given consideration in patients taking NSAIDs or selective COX-2 inhibitors concomitantly with ACE inhibitors. In some patients with compromised renal function who are being treated with NSAIDs, including selective COX-2 inhibitors, the co-administration of angiotensin II receptor antagonists or ACE inhibitors, may result in further deterioration of renal function, including possible acute renal failure. These effects are usually reversible. Therefore, monitor effects on blood pressure and renal fuction when administering the combination, especially in the elderly).
No products indexed under this heading.

Naproxen (Reports suggest that NSAIDs, including selective COX-2 inhibitors, may diminish the antihypertensive effect of ACE inhibitors, including lisinopril. This interaction should be given consideration in patients taking NSAIDs or selective COX-2 inhibitors concomitantly with ACE inhibitors. In some patients with compromised renal function who are being treated with NSAIDs, including selective COX-2 inhibitors, the co-administration of angiotensin II receptor antagonists or ACE inhibitors, may result in further deterioration of renal function, including possible acute renal failure. These effects are usually reversible. Therefore, monitor effects on blood pressure and renal fuction when administering the combination, especially in the elderly). Products include:
EC-Naprosyn 2850
Naprosyn 2850
Anaprox/Naprosyn 2850

Naproxen Sodium (Reports suggest that NSAIDs, including selective COX-2

inhibitors, may diminish the antihypertensive effect of ACE inhibitors, including lisinopril. This interaction should be given consideration in patients taking NSAIDs or selective COX-2 inhibitors concomitantly with ACE inhibitors. In some patients with compromised renal function who are being treated with NSAIDs, including selective COX-2 inhibitors, the co-administration of angiotensin II receptor antagonists or ACE inhibitors, may result in further deterioration of renal function, including possible acute renal failure. These effects are usually reversible. Therefore, monitor effects on blood pressure and renal fuction when administering the combination, especially in the elderly). Products include:
Anaprox 2850
Anaprox DS 2850
Treximet 1681

Nateglinide (Epidemiological studies have suggested that concomitant administration of ACE inhibitors and antidiabetic medicines (insulins, oral hypoglycemic agents) may cause an increased blood-glucose-lowering effect with risk of hypoglycemia. This phenomenon appeared to be more likely to occur during the first weeks of combined treatment and in patients with renal impairment. In diabetic patients treated with oral antidiabetic agents or insulin, glycemic control should be closely monitored for hypoglycemia, especially during the first month of treatment with an ACE inhibitor).
No products indexed under this heading.

Oxaprozin (Reports suggest that NSAIDs, including selective COX-2 inhibitors, may diminish the antihypertensive effect of ACE inhibitors, including lisinopril. This interaction should be given consideration in patients taking NSAIDs or selective COX-2 inhibitors concomitantly with ACE inhibitors. In some patients with compromised renal function who are being treated with NSAIDs, including selective COX-2 inhibitors, the co-administration of angiotensin II receptor antagonists or ACE inhibitors, may result in further deterioration of renal function, including possible acute renal failure. These effects are usually reversible. Therefore, monitor effects on blood pressure and renal fuction when administering the combination, especially in the elderly).
No products indexed under this heading.

Phenylbutazone (Reports suggest that NSAIDs, including selective COX-2 inhibitors, may diminish the antihypertensive effect of ACE inhibitors, including lisinopril. This interaction should be given consideration in patients taking NSAIDs or selective COX-2 inhibitors concomitantly with ACE inhibitors. In some patients with compromised renal function who are being treated with NSAIDs, including selective COX-2 inhibitors, the co-administration of angiotensin II receptor antagonists or ACE inhibitors, may result in further deterioration of renal function, including possible acute renal failure. These effects are usually reversible. Therefore, monitor effects on blood pressure and renal fuction when administering the combination, especially in the elderly).
No products indexed under this heading.

Pioglitazone Hydrochloride (Epidemiological studies have suggested that concomitant administration of ACE inhibitors and antidiabetic medicines (insulins, oral hypoglycemic agents) may cause an increased blood-glucose-lowering effect with risk of hypoglycemia. This phenomenon appeared to be more likely to occur during the first weeks of combined treatment and in

patients with renal impairment. In diabetic patients treated with oral antidiabetic agents or insulin, glycemic control should be closely monitored for hypoglycemia, especially during the first month of treatment with an ACE inhibitor). Products include:

ActoPlus 3338
Actos 3345
Duetact 3354

Piroxicam (Reports suggest that NSAIDs, including selective COX-2 inhibitors, may diminish the antihypertensive effect of ACE inhibitors, including lisinopril. This interaction should be given consideration in patients taking NSAIDs or selective COX-2 inhibitors concomitantly with ACE inhibitors. In some patients with compromised renal function who are being treated with NSAIDs, including selective COX-2 inhibitors, the co-administration of angiotensin II receptor antagonists or ACE inhibitors, may result in further deterioration of renal function, including possible acute renal failure. These effects are usually reversible. Therefore, monitor effects on blood pressure and renal fuction when administering the combination, especially in the elderly).

No products indexed under this heading.

Polythiazide (Thiazide-induced potassium loss attenuated; possibility of excessive reduction in blood pressure).

No products indexed under this heading.

Potassium Acid Phosphate (Use of lisinopril with potassium-sparing diuretics (such as spironolactone, triamterene or amiloride), potassium supplements or potassium-containing salt substitutes may lead to significant increases in serum potassium. Therefore, if concomitant use of these agents is indicated because of demonstrated hypokalemia, they should be used with caution and with frequent monitoring of serum potassium. Potassium-sparing agents should generally not be used in patients with heart failure who are receiving lisinopril). Products include:

K-Phos Original 874

Potassium Bicarbonate (Use of lisinopril with potassium-sparing diuretics (such as spironolactone, triamterene or amiloride), potassium supplements or potassium-containing salt substitutes may lead to significant increases in serum potassium. Therefore, if concomitant use of these agents is indicated because of demonstrated hypokalemia, they should be used with caution and with frequent monitoring of serum potassium. Potassium-sparing agents should generally not be used in patients with heart failure who are receiving lisinopril).

No products indexed under this heading.

Potassium Chloride (Use of lisinopril with potassium-sparing diuretics (such as spironolactone, triamterene or amiloride), potassium supplements or potassium-containing salt substitutes may lead to significant increases in serum potassium. Therefore, if concomitant use of these agents is indicated because of demonstrated hypokalemia, they should be used with caution and with frequent monitoring of serum potassium. Potassium-sparing agents should generally not be used in patients with heart failure who are receiving lisinopril). Products include:

MoviPrep Oral Solution 2905

Potassium Citrate (Use of lisinopril with potassium-sparing diuretics (such as spironolactone, triamterene or amiloride), potassium supplements or potassium-containing salt substitutes may lead to significant increases in serum potassium. Therefore, if concomitant use of these agents is indicated because of demonstrated hypokalemia, they should be used with caution and with frequent monitoring of serum potassium. Potassium-sparing agents should generally not be used in patients with heart failure who are receiving lisinopril). Products include:

Urocit-K 2333

Potassium Gluconate (Use of lisinopril with potassium-sparing diuretics (such as spironolactone, triamterene or amiloride), potassium supplements or potassium-containing salt substitutes may lead to significant increases in serum potassium. Therefore, if concomitant use of these agents is indicated because of demonstrated hypokalemia, they should be used with caution and with frequent monitoring of serum potassium. Potassium-sparing agents should generally not be used in patients with heart failure who are receiving lisinopril).

No products indexed under this heading.

Potassium Phosphate (Use of lisinopril with potassium-sparing diuretics (such as spironolactone, triamterene or amiloride), potassium supplements or potassium-containing salt substitutes may lead to significant increases in serum potassium. Therefore, if concomitant use of these agents is indicated because of demonstrated hypokalemia, they should be used with caution and with frequent monitoring of serum potassium. Potassium-sparing agents should generally not be used in patients with heart failure who are receiving lisinopril). Products include:

K-Phos Neutral 873

Repaglinide (Epidemiological studies have suggested that concomitant administration of ACE inhibitors and antidiabetic medicines (insulins, oral hypoglycemic agents) may cause an increased blood-glucose-lowering effect with risk of hypoglycemia. This phenomenon appeared to be more likely to occur during the first weeks of combined treatment and in patients with renal impairment. In diabetic patients treated with oral antidiabetic agents or insulin, glycemic control should be closely monitored for hypoglycemia, especially during the first month of treatment with an ACE inhibitor).

No products indexed under this heading.

Rofecoxib (Reports suggest that NSAIDs, including selective COX-2 inhibitors, may diminish the antihypertensive effect of ACE inhibitors, including lisinopril. This interaction should be given consideration in patients taking NSAIDs or selective COX-2 inhibitors concomitantly with ACE inhibitors. In some patients with compromised renal function who are being treated with NSAIDs, including selective COX-2 inhibitors, the co-administration of angiotensin II receptor antagonists or ACE inhibitors, may result in further deterioration of renal function, including possible acute renal failure. These effects are usually reversible. Therefore, monitor effects on blood pressure and renal fuction when administering the combination, especially in the elderly).

No products indexed under this heading.

Rosiglitazone Maleate (Epidemiological studies have suggested that concomitant administration of ACE inhibitors and antidiabetic medicines (insulins, oral hypoglycemic agents) may cause an increased blood-glucose-lowering effect with risk of hypoglycemia. This phenomenon appeared to be more likely to occur during the first weeks of combined treatment and in patients with renal impairment. In diabetic patients treated with oral antidiabetic agents or insulin, glycemic control should be closely monitored for hypoglycemia, especially during the first month of treatment with an ACE inhibitor). Products include:

Avandamet 1345
Avandaryl 1356
Avandia 1366

Sitagliptin Phosphate (Epidemiological studies have suggested that concomitant administration of ACE inhibitors and antidiabetic medicines (insulins, oral hypoglycemic agents) may cause an increased blood-glucose-lowering effect with risk of hypoglycemia. This phenomenon appeared to be more likely to occur during the first weeks of combined treatment and in patients with renal impairment. In diabetic patients treated with oral antidiabetic agents or insulin, glycemic control should be closely monitored for hypoglycemia, especially during the first month of treatment with an ACE inhibitor). Products include:

Janumet 2188
Januvia 2196

Spironolactone (Use of lisinopril with potassium-sparing diuretics (such as spironolactone, triamterene or amiloride), potassium supplements or potassium-containing salt substitutes may lead to significant increases in serum potassium. Therefore, if concomitant use of these agents is indicated because of demonstrated hypokalemia, they should be used with caution and with frequent monitoring of serum potassium. Potassium-sparing agents should generally not be used in patients with heart failure who are receiving lisinopril).

No products indexed under this heading.

Sulindac (Reports suggest that NSAIDs, including selective COX-2 inhibitors, may diminish the antihypertensive effect of ACE inhibitors, including lisinopril. This interaction should be given consideration in patients taking NSAIDs or selective COX-2 inhibitors concomitantly with ACE inhibitors. In some patients with compromised renal function who are being treated with NSAIDs, including selective COX-2 inhibitors, the co-administration of angiotensin II receptor antagonists or ACE inhibitors, may result in further deterioration of renal function, including possible acute renal failure. These effects are usually reversible. Therefore, monitor effects on blood pressure and renal fuction when administering the combination, especially in the elderly). Products include:

Clinoril 2098

Tolazamide (Epidemiological studies have suggested that concomitant administration of ACE inhibitors and antidiabetic medicines (insulins, oral hypoglycemic agents) may cause an increased blood-glucose-lowering effect with risk of hypoglycemia. This phenomenon appeared to be more likely to occur during the first weeks of combined treatment and in patients with renal impairment. In diabetic patients treated with oral antidiabetic agents or insulin, glycemic control should be closely monitored for hypoglycemia, especially during the first month of treatment with an ACE inhibitor).

No products indexed under this heading.

Tolbutamide (Epidemiological studies have suggested that concomitant administration of ACE inhibitors and antidiabetic medicines (insulins, oral hypoglycemic agents) may cause an increased blood-glucose-lowering effect with risk of hypoglycemia. This phenomenon appeared to be more likely to occur during the first weeks of combined treatment and in patients with renal impairment. In diabetic patients treated with oral antidiabetic agents or insulin, glycemic control should be closely monitored for hypoglycemia, especially during the first month of treatment with an ACE inhibitor).

No products indexed under this heading.

Tolmetin Sodium (Reports suggest that NSAIDs, including selective COX-2 inhibitors, may diminish the antihypertensive effect of ACE inhibitors, including lisinopril. This interaction should be given consideration in patients taking NSAIDs or selective COX-2 inhibitors concomitantly with ACE inhibitors. In some patients with compromised renal function who are being treated with NSAIDs, including selective COX-2 inhibitors, the co-administration of angiotensin II receptor antagonists or ACE inhibitors, may result in further deterioration of renal function, including possible acute renal failure. These effects are usually reversible. Therefore, monitor effects on blood pressure and renal fuction when administering the combination, especially in the elderly).

No products indexed under this heading.

Torsemide (Possibility of excessive reduction in blood pressure).

No products indexed under this heading.

Triamterene (Use of lisinopril with potassium-sparing diuretics (such as spironolactone, triamterene or amiloride), potassium supplements or potassium-containing salt substitutes may lead to significant increases in serum potassium. Therefore, if concomitant use of these agents is indicated because of demonstrated hypokalemia, they should be used with caution and with frequent monitoring of serum potassium. Potassium-sparing agents should generally not be used in patients with heart failure who are receiving lisinopril). Products include:

Dyazide 1429
Dyrenium 3495

Troglitazone (Epidemiological studies have suggested that concomitant administration of ACE inhibitors and antidiabetic medicines (insulins, oral hypoglycemic agents) may cause an increased blood-glucose-lowering effect with risk of hypoglycemia. This phenomenon appeared to be more likely to occur during the first weeks of combined treatment and in patients with renal impairment. In diabetic patients treated with oral antidiabetic agents or insulin, glycemic control should be closely monitored for hypoglycemia, especially during the first month of treatment with an ACE inhibitor).

No products indexed under this heading.

Valdecoxib (Reports suggest that NSAIDs, including selective COX-2 inhibitors, may diminish the antihypertensive effect of ACE inhibitors, including lisinopril. This interaction should be given consideration in patients taking NSAIDs or selective COX-2 inhibitors concomitantly with ACE inhibitors. In some patients with compromised renal function who are being treated with NSAIDs, including selective COX-2 inhibitors, the co-administration of angiotensin II receptor antagonists or ACE inhibitors, may result in further deterioration of renal function, including possible acute renal failure. These effects are usually reversible. Therefore, monitor effects on blood pressure and renal fuction when administering the combination, especially in the elderly).

No products indexed under this heading.

Food Interactions

Salt Substitutes, Potassium-Containing (Use of lisinopril with potassium-sparing diuretics (such as spironolactone, triamterene or amiloride), potassium supplements or potassium-containing salt substitutes

(⊙ Described in PDR® for Ophthalmic Medicines)

1461 Interactions Index Prinzide

may lead to significant increases in serum potassium. Therefore, if concomitant use of these agents is indicated because of demonstrated hypokalemia, they should be used with caution and with frequent monitoring of serum potassium. Potassium-sparing agents should generally not be used in patients with heart failure who are receiving lisinopril).

PRINZIDE TABLETS
(Hydrochlorothiazide, Lisinopril) 2246
May interact with alcohols, antihypertensives, barbiturates, cardiac glycosides, corticosteroids, diuretics, insulin, lithium preparations, narcotic analgesics, non-steroidal anti-inflammatory agents, nondepolarizing neuromuscular blocking agents, oral hypoglycemic agents, potassium preparations, potassium sparing diuretics, and certain other agents. Compounds in these categories include:

Acarbose (Hyperglycemia may occur with thiazide diuretics; dosage adjustment of oral hypoglycemic agents may be required).
No products indexed under this heading.

Acebutolol Hydrochloride (Co-administration of thiazide and other antihypertensive agents can lead to additive effect or potentiation).
No products indexed under this heading.

ACTH (Co-administration of thiazide diuretics with ACTH intensifies electrolyte depletion, particularly potassium).
No products indexed under this heading.

Alclometasone Dipropionate (Co-administration of thiazide diuretics with corticosteroids intensifies electrolyte depletion, particularly potassium).
No products indexed under this heading.

Alfentanil Hydrochloride (Co-administration of thiazide and narcotics may potentiate orthostatic hypotension).
No products indexed under this heading.

Aliskiren (Co-administration of thiazide and other antihypertensive agents can lead to additive effect or potentiation). Products include:
Tekturna 2538
Tekturna HCT 2541
Valturna 3637

Amiloride Hydrochloride (Risk factors for the development of hyperkalemia include the concomitant use of potassium-sparing diuretics, potassium supplements and/or potassium-containing salt substitutes. Hyperkalemia can cause serious, sometimes fatal, arrhythmias. Prinzide should be used cautiously, if at all, with these agents and with frequent monitoring of serum potassium).
No products indexed under this heading.

Amlodipine Besylate (Co-administration of thiazide and other antihypertensive agents can lead to additive effect or potentiation). Products include:
Azor 1010
Exforge 2443
Exforge HCT 2449

Amobarbital (Co-administration of thiazide and barbiturates may potentiate orthostatic hypotension).
No products indexed under this heading.

Amobarbital Sodium (Co-administration of thiazide and barbiturates may potentiate orthostatic hypotension).
No products indexed under this heading.

Apomorphine (Co-administration of thiazide and narcotics may potentiate orthostatic hypotension).
No products indexed under this heading.

Apomorphine Hydrochloride (Co-administration of thiazide and narcotics may potentiate orthostatic hypotension).
No products indexed under this heading.

Aprobarbital (Co-administration of thiazide and barbiturates may potentiate orthostatic hypotension).
No products indexed under this heading.

Atenolol (Co-administration of thiazide and other antihypertensive agents can lead to additive effect or potentiation).
No products indexed under this heading.

Atracurium Besylate (Co-administration with nondepolarizing skeletal muscle relaxants may result in possible increased responsiveness to the muscle relaxant).
No products indexed under this heading.

Beclomethasone Dipropionate (Co-administration of thiazide diuretics with corticosteroids intensifies electrolyte depletion, particularly potassium). Products include:
Qvar 3398

Beclomethasone Dipropionate Monohydrate (Co-administration of thiazide diuretics with corticosteroids intensifies electrolyte depletion, particularly potassium). Products include:
Beconase AQ 1386

Benazepril Hydrochloride (Co-administration of thiazide and other antihypertensive agents can lead to additive effect or potentiation).
No products indexed under this heading.

Bendroflumethiazide (Co-administration of lisinopril in patients on diuretics, especially those in whom diuretic therapy was recently instituted, may occasionally experience excessive hypotension; antihypertensive effects of lisinopril are augmented by antihypertensive agents that cause renin release).
No products indexed under this heading.

Betamethasone (Co-administration of thiazide diuretics with corticosteroids intensifies electrolyte depletion, particularly potassium).
No products indexed under this heading.

Betamethasone Acetate (Co-administration of thiazide diuretics with corticosteroids intensifies electrolyte depletion, particularly potassium).
No products indexed under this heading.

Betamethasone Benzoate (Co-administration of thiazide diuretics with corticosteroids intensifies electrolyte depletion, particularly potassium).
No products indexed under this heading.

Betamethasone Dipropionate (Co-administration of thiazide diuretics with corticosteroids intensifies electrolyte depletion, particularly potassium). Products include:
Diprolene Lotion 0.05% 3108
Diprolene Ointment 0.05% 3109
Diprolene AF Cream 0.05% 3107
Lotrisone 3163

Betamethasone Sodium Phosphate (Co-administration of thiazide diuretics with corticosteroids intensifies electrolyte depletion, particularly potassium).
No products indexed under this heading.

Betamethasone Valerate (Co-administration of thiazide diuretics with corticosteroids intensifies electrolyte depletion, particularly potassium). Products include:
Luxíq 3321

Betaxolol Hydrochloride (Co-administration of thiazide and other antihypertensive agents can lead to additive effect or potentiation).
No products indexed under this heading.

Bisoprolol Fumarate (Co-administration of thiazide and other antihypertensive agents can lead to additive effect or potentiation).
No products indexed under this heading.

Budesonide (Co-administration of thiazide diuretics with corticosteroids intensifies electrolyte depletion, particularly potassium). Products include:
Pulmicort Flexhaler 714
Symbicort 80/4.5 720
Symbicort 160/4.5 720

Bumetanide (Co-administration of lisinopril in patients on diuretics, especially those in whom diuretic therapy was recently instituted, may occasionally experience excessive hypotension; antihypertensive effects of lisinopril are augmented by antihypertensive agents that cause renin release).
No products indexed under this heading.

Buprenorphine Hydrochloride (Co-administration of thiazide and narcotics may potentiate orthostatic hypotension).
No products indexed under this heading.

Butabarbital (Co-administration of thiazide and barbiturates may potentiate orthostatic hypotension).
No products indexed under this heading.

Butabarbital Sodium (Co-administration of thiazide and barbiturates may potentiate orthostatic hypotension).
No products indexed under this heading.

Butalbital (Co-administration of thiazide and barbiturates may potentiate orthostatic hypotension).
No products indexed under this heading.

Candesartan Cilexetil (Co-administration of thiazide and other antihypertensive agents can lead to additive effect or potentiation). Products include:
Atacand 697
Atacand HCT 700

Captopril (Co-administration of thiazide and other antihypertensive agents can lead to additive effect or potentiation). Products include:
Captopril 2341

Carteolol Hydrochloride (Co-administration of thiazide and other antihypertensive agents can lead to additive effect or potentiation).
No products indexed under this heading.

Carvedilol (Co-administration of thiazide and other antihypertensive agents can lead to additive effect or potentiation). Products include:
Coreg 1409

Carvedilol Phosphate (Co-administration of thiazide and other antihypertensive agents can lead to additive effect or potentiation). Products include:
Coreg CR 1416

Celecoxib (Reports suggest that NSAIDs, including selective COX-2 inhibitors, may diminish the antihypertensive effect of ACE inhibitors, including lisinopril. This interaction should be given consideration in patients taking NSAIDs or selective COX-2 inhibitors concomitantly with ACE inhibitors. In some patients with compromised renal function who are being treated with NSAIDs, including selective COX-2 inhibitors, the co-administration of angiotensin II receptor antagonists or ACE inhibitors, may result in further deterioration of renal function, including possible acute renal failure. These effects are usually reversible. Therefore, monitor effects on blood pressure and renal fuction when administering the combination, especially in the elderly). Products include:
Celebrex 3272

Chlorothiazide (Co-administration of lisinopril in patients on diuretics, especially those in whom diuretic therapy was recently instituted, may occasionally experience excessive hypotension; antihypertensive effects of lisinopril are augmented by antihypertensive agents that cause renin release).
No products indexed under this heading.

Chlorothiazide Sodium (Co-administration of lisinopril in patients on diuretics, especially those in whom diuretic therapy was recently instituted, may occasionally experience excessive hypotension; antihypertensive effects of lisinopril are augmented by antihypertensive agents that cause renin release). Products include:
Diuril Intravenous 2009

Chlorpropamide (Hyperglycemia may occur with thiazide diuretics; dosage adjustment of oral hypoglycemic agents may be required).
No products indexed under this heading.

Chlorthalidone (Co-administration of lisinopril in patients on diuretics, especially those in whom diuretic therapy was recently instituted, may occasionally experience excessive hypotension; antihypertensive effects of lisinopril are augmented by antihypertensive agents that cause renin release). Products include:
Clorpres 2344

Cholestyramine (Absorption of hydrochlorothiazide is impaired in the presence of anionic exchange resins; these resins bind the hydrochlorothiazide and reduce its absorption from GI tract).
No products indexed under this heading.

Ciclesonide (Co-administration of thiazide diuretics with corticosteroids intensifies electrolyte depletion, particularly potassium).
No products indexed under this heading.

Cisatracurium Besylate (Co-administration with nondepolarizing skeletal muscle relaxants may result in possible increased responsiveness to the muscle relaxant). Products include:
Nimbex 503

Clonidine (Co-administration of thiazide and other antihypertensive agents can lead to additive effect or potentiation). Products include:
Catapres-TTS 884

Clonidine Hydrochloride (Co-administration of thiazide and other antihypertensive agents can lead to additive effect or potentiation). Products include:
Clorpres 2344

Codeine Phosphate (Co-administration of thiazide and narcotics may potentiate orthostatic hypotension). Products include:
Tylenol with Codeine 2691

Codeine Sulfate (Co-administration of thiazide and narcotics may potentiate orthostatic hypotension).
No products indexed under this heading.

Colestipol Hydrochloride (Absorption of hydrochlorothiazide is impaired in the presence of anionic exchange resins; these resins bind the hydrochlorothiazide and reduce its absorption from GI tract).
No products indexed under this heading.

Cortisone Acetate (Co-administration of thiazide diuretics with corticosteroids intensifies electrolyte depletion, particularly potassium).
No products indexed under this heading.

Deserpidine (Co-administration of thiazide and other antihypertensive agents can lead to additive effect or potentiation).
No products indexed under this heading.

IMPORTANT NOTE: Always consult each drug listing in the patient's regimen for possible interactions.

Prinzide Interactions Index 1462

Deslanoside (Hypokalemia induced by thiazide diuretics may cause cardiac arrhythmia and may also sensitize or exaggerate the response to the heart to the toxic effects of digitalis, such as ventricular irritability).
No products indexed under this heading.

Desoximetasone (Co-administration of thiazide diuretics with corticosteroids intensifies electrolyte depletion, particularly potassium).
No products indexed under this heading.

Dexamethasone (Co-administration of thiazide diuretics with corticosteroids intensifies electrolyte depletion, particularly potassium). Products include:
Ciprodex 583
Ozurdex .... ⊙223
Tobramycin and Dexamethasone Ophthalmic Suspension .... ⊙251

Dexamethasone Acetate (Co-administration of thiazide diuretics with corticosteroids intensifies electrolyte depletion, particularly potassium).
No products indexed under this heading.

Dexamethasone Phosphate (Co-administration of thiazide diuretics with corticosteroids intensifies electrolyte depletion, particularly potassium).
No products indexed under this heading.

Dexamethasone Sodium (Co-administration of thiazide diuretics with corticosteroids intensifies electrolyte depletion, particularly potassium).
No products indexed under this heading.

Dexamethasone Sodium Phosphate (Co-administration of thiazide diuretics with corticosteroids intensifies electrolyte depletion, particularly potassium).
No products indexed under this heading.

Dexamethasone Sodium Phosphate Injection (Co-administration of thiazide diuretics with corticosteroids intensifies electrolyte depletion, particularly potassium).
No products indexed under this heading.

Dezocine (Co-administration of thiazide and narcotics may potentiate orthostatic hypotension).
No products indexed under this heading.

Diazoxide (Co-administration of thiazide and other antihypertensive agents can lead to additive effect or potentiation). Products include:
Proglycem 1179
Proglycem Suspension 1179

Diclofenac Epolamine (Reports suggest that NSAIDs, including selective COX-2 inhibitors, may diminish the antihypertensive effect of ACE inhibitors, including lisinopril. This interaction should be given consideration in patients taking NSAIDs or selective COX-2 inhibitors concomitantly with ACE inhibitors. In some patients with compromised renal function who are being treated with NSAIDs, including selective COX-2 inhibitors, the co-administration of angiotensin II receptor antagonists or ACE inhibitors, may result in further deterioration of renal function, including possible acute renal failure. These effects are usually reversible. Therefore, monitor effects on blood pressure and renal fuction when administering the combination, especially in the elderly). Products include:
Flector 1839

Diclofenac Potassium (Reports suggest that NSAIDs, including selective COX-2 inhibitors, may diminish the antihypertensive effect of ACE inhibitors, including lisinopril. This interaction should be given consideration in patients taking NSAIDs or selective COX-2 inhibitors concomitantly with ACE inhibitors. In some patients with compromised renal function who are being treated with NSAIDs, including selective COX-2 inhibitors, the co-administration of angiotensin II receptor antagonists or ACE inhibitors, may result in further deterioration of renal function, including possible acute renal failure. These effects are usually reversible. Therefore, monitor effects on blood pressure and renal fuction when administering the combination, especially in the elderly).
No products indexed under this heading.

Diclofenac Sodium (Reports suggest that NSAIDs, including selective COX-2 inhibitors, may diminish the antihypertensive effect of ACE inhibitors, including lisinopril. This interaction should be given consideration in patients taking NSAIDs or selective COX-2 inhibitors concomitantly with ACE inhibitors. In some patients with compromised renal function who are being treated with NSAIDs, including selective COX-2 inhibitors, the co-administration of angiotensin II receptor antagonists or ACE inhibitors, may result in further deterioration of renal function, including possible acute renal failure. These effects are usually reversible. Therefore, monitor effects on blood pressure and renal fuction when administering the combination, especially in the elderly).
No products indexed under this heading.

Diflorasone Diacetate (Co-administration of thiazide diuretics with corticosteroids intensifies electrolyte depletion, particularly potassium).
No products indexed under this heading.

Digitalis Glycoside Preparations (Hypokalemia induced by thiazide diuretics may cause cardiac arrhythmia and may also sensitize or exaggerate the response to the heart to the toxic effects of digitalis, such as ventricular irritability).
No products indexed under this heading.

Digitalis Lanata (Hypokalemia induced by thiazide diuretics may cause cardiac arrhythmia and may also sensitize or exaggerate the response to the heart to the toxic effects of digitalis, such as ventricular irritability).
No products indexed under this heading.

Digitalis Purpurea (Hypokalemia induced by thiazide diuretics may cause cardiac arrhythmia and may also sensitize or exaggerate the response to the heart to the toxic effects of digitalis, such as ventricular irritability).
No products indexed under this heading.

Digitoxin (Hypokalemia induced by thiazide diuretics may cause cardiac arrhythmia and may also sensitize or exaggerate the response to the heart to the toxic effects of digitalis, such as ventricular irritability).
No products indexed under this heading.

Digoxin (Hypokalemia induced by thiazide diuretics may cause cardiac arrhythmia and may also sensitize or exaggerate the response to the heart to the toxic effects of digitalis, such as ventricular irritability). Products include:
Lanoxin Injection 1546
Lanoxin Injection Pediatric 1549
Lanoxin Tablets 1553

Dihydrocodeine Bitartrate (Co-administration of thiazide and narcotics may potentiate orthostatic hypotension).
No products indexed under this heading.

Dihydrocodeinone Bitartrate (Co-administration of thiazide and narcotics may potentiate orthostatic hypotension).
No products indexed under this heading.

Diltiazem Hydrochloride (Co-administration of thiazide and other antihypertensive agents can lead to additive effect or potentiation). Products include:
Cardizem LA 423

Diltiazem Maleate (Co-administration of thiazide and other antihypertensive agents can lead to additive effect or potentiation).
No products indexed under this heading.

Doxacurium Chloride (Co-administration with nondepolarizing skeletal muscle relaxants may result in possible increased responsiveness to the muscle relaxant).
No products indexed under this heading.

Doxazosin Mesylate (Co-administration of thiazide and other antihypertensive agents can lead to additive effect or potentiation).
No products indexed under this heading.

d-Tubocurarine (Co-administration with nondepolarizing skeletal muscle relaxants may result in possible increased responsiveness to the muscle relaxant).
No products indexed under this heading.

Enalapril Maleate (Co-administration of thiazide and other antihypertensive agents can lead to additive effect or potentiation).
No products indexed under this heading.

Enalaprilat (Co-administration of thiazide and other antihypertensive agents can lead to additive effect or potentiation).
No products indexed under this heading.

Eplerenone (Use of lisinopril with potassium-sparing diuretics (such as spironolactone, triamterene or amiloride), potassium supplements or potassium-containing salt substitutes may lead to significant increases in serum potassium. Therefore, if concomitant use of these agents is indicated because of demonstrated hypokalemia, they should be used with caution and with frequent monitoring of serum potassium. Potassium-sparing agents should generally not be used in patients with heart failure who are receiving lisinopril).
No products indexed under this heading.

Eprosartan Mesylate (Co-administration of thiazide and other antihypertensive agents can lead to additive effect or potentiation). Products include:
Teveten 538
Teveten HCT 541

Esmolol Hydrochloride (Co-administration of thiazide and other antihypertensive agents can lead to additive effect or potentiation).
No products indexed under this heading.

Ethacrynic Acid (Co-administration of lisinopril in patients on diuretics, especially those in whom diuretic therapy was recently instituted, may occasionally experience excessive hypotension; antihypertensive effects of lisinopril are augmented by antihypertensive agents that cause renin release).
No products indexed under this heading.

Ethanol (Co-administration of thiazide and alcohol may potentiate orthostatic hypotension).
No products indexed under this heading.

Ethyl Alcohol (Co-administration of thiazide and alcohol may potentiate orthostatic hypotension).
No products indexed under this heading.

Etodolac (Reports suggest that NSAIDs, including selective COX-2 inhibitors, may diminish the antihypertensive effect of ACE inhibitors, including lisinopril. This interaction should be given consideration in patients taking NSAIDs or selective COX-2 inhibitors concomitantly with ACE inhibitors. In some patients with compromised renal function who are being treated with NSAIDs, including selective COX-2 inhibitors, the co-administration of angiotensin II receptor antagonists or ACE inhibitors, may result in further deterioration of renal function, including possible acute renal failure. These effects are usually reversible. Therefore, monitor effects on blood pressure and renal fuction when administering the combination, especially in the elderly).
No products indexed under this heading.

Felodipine (Co-administration of thiazide and other antihypertensive agents can lead to additive effect or potentiation).
No products indexed under this heading.

Fenoprofen Calcium (Reports suggest that NSAIDs, including selective COX-2 inhibitors, may diminish the antihypertensive effect of ACE inhibitors, including lisinopril. This interaction should be given consideration in patients taking NSAIDs or selective COX-2 inhibitors concomitantly with ACE inhibitors. In some patients with compromised renal function who are being treated with NSAIDs, including selective COX-2 inhibitors, the co-administration of angiotensin II receptor antagonists or ACE inhibitors, may result in further deterioration of renal function, including possible acute renal failure. These effects are usually reversible. Therefore, monitor effects on blood pressure and renal fuction when administering the combination, especially in the elderly).
No products indexed under this heading.

Fentanyl (Co-administration of thiazide and narcotics may potentiate orthostatic hypotension). Products include:
Duragesic 2604
Fentanyl Transdermal System 2346
Onsolis 2054

Fentanyl Citrate (Co-administration of thiazide and narcotics may potentiate orthostatic hypotension). Products include:
Fentora 966

Fludrocortisone Acetate (Co-administration of thiazide diuretics with corticosteroids intensifies electrolyte depletion, particularly potassium).
No products indexed under this heading.

Flumethasone Pivalate (Co-administration of thiazide diuretics with corticosteroids intensifies electrolyte depletion, particularly potassium).
No products indexed under this heading.

Flunisolide Hemihydrate (Co-administration of thiazide diuretics with corticosteroids intensifies electrolyte depletion, particularly potassium).
No products indexed under this heading.

Flurbiprofen (Reports suggest that NSAIDs, including selective COX-2 inhibitors, may diminish the antihypertensive effect of ACE inhibitors, including lisinopril. This interaction should be given consideration in patients taking NSAIDs or selective COX-2 inhibitors concomitantly with ACE inhibitors. In some patients with compromised renal function who are being treated with NSAIDs, including selective COX-2 inhibitors, the co-administration of angiotensin II receptor antagonists or ACE inhibitors, may result in further deterioration of renal function, including possible acute renal failure. These effects are usually reversible. Therefore, monitor effects on blood pressure and renal fuction when administering the combination, especially in the elderly).
No products indexed under this heading.

Fluticasone Furoate (Co-administration of thiazide diuretics with corticosteroids intensifies electrolyte depletion, particularly potassium). Products include:
Veramyst 1713

(⊙ Described in PDR® for Ophthalmic Medicines)

Prinzide Interactions Index 1464

Humalog Mix75/25 1917

Irbesartan (Co-administration of thiazide and other antihypertensive agents can lead to additive effect or potentiation). Products include:
Avalide 2956
Avapro 2962

Isradipine (Co-administration of thiazide and other antihypertensive agents can lead to additive effect or potentiation). Products include:
DynaCirc CR 1432

Ketoprofen (Reports suggest that NSAIDs, including selective COX-2 inhibitors, may diminish the antihypertensive effect of ACE inhibitors, including lisinopril. This interaction should be given consideration in patients taking NSAIDs or selective COX-2 inhibitors concomitantly with ACE inhibitors. In some patients with compromised renal function who are being treated with NSAIDs, including selective COX-2 inhibitors, the co-administration of angiotensin II receptor antagonists or ACE inhibitors, may result in further deterioration of renal function, including possible acute renal failure. These effects are usually reversible. Therefore, monitor effects on blood pressure and renal fuction when administering the combination, especially in the elderly).
No products indexed under this heading.

Ketorolac Tromethamine (Reports suggest that NSAIDs, including selective COX-2 inhibitors, may diminish the antihypertensive effect of ACE inhibitors, including lisinopril. This interaction should be given consideration in patients taking NSAIDs or selective COX-2 inhibitors concomitantly with ACE inhibitors. In some patients with compromised renal function who are being treated with NSAIDs, including selective COX-2 inhibitors, the co-administration of angiotensin II receptor antagonists or ACE inhibitors, may result in further deterioration of renal function, including possible acute renal failure. These effects are usually reversible. Therefore, monitor effects on blood pressure and renal fuction when administering the combination, especially in the elderly). Products include:
Acuvail .... ⊙ 209

Labetalol Hydrochloride (Co-administration of thiazide and other antihypertensive agents can lead to additive effect or potentiation).
No products indexed under this heading.

Levorphanol Tartrate (Co-administration of thiazide and narcotics may potentiate orthostatic hypotension).
No products indexed under this heading.

Lithium (Co-administration of lithium with drugs that cause elimination of sodium, including ACE inhibitors, can lead to lithium toxicity; diuretics can reduce renal clearance of lithium and add a high risk of lithium toxicity).
No products indexed under this heading.

Lithium Carbonate (Co-administration of lithium with drugs that cause elimination of sodium, including ACE inhibitors, can lead to lithium toxicity; diuretics can reduce renal clearance of lithium and add a high risk of lithium toxicity).
No products indexed under this heading.

Lithium Citrate (Co-administration of lithium with drugs that cause elimination of sodium, including ACE inhibitors, can lead to lithium toxicity; diuretics can reduce renal clearance of lithium and add a high risk of lithium toxicity).
No products indexed under this heading.

Losartan Potassium (Co-administration of thiazide and other antihypertensive agents can lead to additive effect or potentiation). Products include:
Cozaar 2106
Hyzaar 2162
Hyzaar 100-12.5 2162

Mecamylamine Hydrochloride (Co-administration of thiazide and other antihypertensive agents can lead to additive effect or potentiation).
No products indexed under this heading.

Meclofenamate Sodium (Reports suggest that NSAIDs, including selective COX-2 inhibitors, may diminish the antihypertensive effect of ACE inhibitors, including lisinopril. This interaction should be given consideration in patients taking NSAIDs or selective COX-2 inhibitors concomitantly with ACE inhibitors. In some patients with compromised renal function who are being treated with NSAIDs, including selective COX-2 inhibitors, the co-administration of angiotensin II receptor antagonists or ACE inhibitors, may result in further deterioration of renal function, including possible acute renal failure. These effects are usually reversible. Therefore, monitor effects on blood pressure and renal fuction when administering the combination, especially in the elderly).
No products indexed under this heading.

Mefenamic Acid (Reports suggest that NSAIDs, including selective COX-2 inhibitors, may diminish the antihypertensive effect of ACE inhibitors, including lisinopril. This interaction should be given consideration in patients taking NSAIDs or selective COX-2 inhibitors concomitantly with ACE inhibitors. In some patients with compromised renal function who are being treated with NSAIDs, including selective COX-2 inhibitors, the co-administration of angiotensin II receptor antagonists or ACE inhibitors, may result in further deterioration of renal function, including possible acute renal failure. These effects are usually reversible. Therefore, monitor effects on blood pressure and renal fuction when administering the combination, especially in the elderly).
No products indexed under this heading.

Meloxicam (Reports suggest that NSAIDs, including selective COX-2 inhibitors, may diminish the antihypertensive effect of ACE inhibitors, including lisinopril. This interaction should be given consideration in patients taking NSAIDs or selective COX-2 inhibitors concomitantly with ACE inhibitors. In some patients with compromised renal function who are being treated with NSAIDs, including selective COX-2 inhibitors, the co-administration of angiotensin II receptor antagonists or ACE inhibitors, may result in further deterioration of renal function, including possible acute renal failure. These effects are usually reversible. Therefore, monitor effects on blood pressure and renal fuction when administering the combination, especially in the elderly).
No products indexed under this heading.

Meperidine Hydrochloride (Co-administration of thiazide and narcotics may potentiate orthostatic hypotension).
No products indexed under this heading.

Mephobarbital (Co-administration of thiazide and barbiturates may potentiate orthostatic hypotension).
No products indexed under this heading.

Metformin Hydrochloride (Hyperglycemia may occur with thiazide diuretics; dosage adjustment of oral hypoglycemic agents may be required). Products include:
ActoPlus 3338
Avandamet 1345
Janumet 2188

Methadone Hydrochloride (Co-administration of thiazide and narcotics may potentiate orthostatic hypotension).
No products indexed under this heading.

Methyclothiazide (Co-administration of lisinopril in patients on diuretics, especially those in whom diuretic therapy was recently instituted, may occasionally experience excessive hypotension; antihypertensive effects of lisinopril are augmented by antihypertensive agents that cause renin release).
No products indexed under this heading.

Methyldopa (Co-administration of thiazide and other antihypertensive agents can lead to additive effect or potentiation).
No products indexed under this heading.

Methyldopate Hydrochloride (Co-administration of thiazide and other antihypertensive agents can lead to additive effect or potentiation).
No products indexed under this heading.

Methylprednisolone (Co-administration of thiazide diuretics with corticosteroids intensifies electrolyte depletion, particularly potassium).
No products indexed under this heading.

Methylprednisolone Acetate (Co-administration of thiazide diuretics with corticosteroids intensifies electrolyte depletion, particularly potassium).
No products indexed under this heading.

Methylprednisolone Sodium Succinate (Co-administration of thiazide diuretics with corticosteroids intensifies electrolyte depletion, particularly potassium).
No products indexed under this heading.

Metocurine Iodide (Co-administration with nondepolarizing skeletal muscle relaxants may result in possible increased responsiveness to the muscle relaxant).
No products indexed under this heading.

Metolazone (Co-administration of lisinopril in patients on diuretics, especially those in whom diuretic therapy was recently instituted, may occasionally experience excessive hypotension; antihypertensive effects of lisinopril are augmented by antihypertensive agents that cause renin release).
No products indexed under this heading.

Metoprolol Succinate (Co-administration of thiazide and other antihypertensive agents can lead to additive effect or potentiation). Products include:
Toprol XL 732

Metoprolol Tartrate (Co-administration of thiazide and other antihypertensive agents can lead to additive effect or potentiation).
No products indexed under this heading.

Metyrosine (Co-administration of thiazide and other antihypertensive agents can lead to additive effect or potentiation).
No products indexed under this heading.

Mibefradil Dihydrochloride (Co-administration of thiazide and other antihypertensive agents can lead to additive effect or potentiation).
No products indexed under this heading.

Miglitol (Hyperglycemia may occur with thiazide diuretics; dosage adjustment of oral hypoglycemic agents may be required).
No products indexed under this heading.

Minoxidil (Co-administration of thiazide and other antihypertensive agents can lead to additive effect or potentiation).
No products indexed under this heading.

Mivacurium Chloride (Co-administration with nondepolarizing skeletal muscle relaxants may result in possible increased responsiveness to the muscle relaxant).
No products indexed under this heading.

Moexipril Hydrochloride (Co-administration of thiazide and other antihypertensive agents can lead to additive effect or potentiation).
No products indexed under this heading.

Mometasone Furoate (Co-administration of thiazide diuretics with corticosteroids intensifies electrolyte depletion, particularly potassium). Products include:
Asmanex 3058
Elocon Cream 3111
Elocon Lotion 3112
Elocon Ointment 3114

Mometasone Furoate Monohydrate (Co-administration of thiazide diuretics with corticosteroids intensifies electrolyte depletion, particularly potassium). Products include:
Nasonex 3166

Morphine Sulfate (Co-administration of thiazide and narcotics may potentiate orthostatic hypotension). Products include:
Avinza 1822
Embeda 1831
MS Contin 2803

Morphine Sulfate, Liposomal (Co-administration of thiazide and narcotics may potentiate orthostatic hypotension).
No products indexed under this heading.

Nabumetone (Reports suggest that NSAIDs, including selective COX-2 inhibitors, may diminish the antihypertensive effect of ACE inhibitors, including lisinopril. This interaction should be given consideration in patients taking NSAIDs or selective COX-2 inhibitors concomitantly with ACE inhibitors. In some patients with compromised renal function who are being treated with NSAIDs, including selective COX-2 inhibitors, the co-administration of angiotensin II receptor antagonists or ACE inhibitors, may result in further deterioration of renal function, including possible acute renal failure. These effects are usually reversible. Therefore, monitor effects on blood pressure and renal fuction when administering the combination, especially in the elderly).
No products indexed under this heading.

Nadolol (Co-administration of thiazide and other antihypertensive agents can lead to additive effect or potentiation). Products include:
Nadolol 2359

Naproxen (Reports suggest that NSAIDs, including selective COX-2 inhibitors, may diminish the antihypertensive effect of ACE inhibitors, including lisinopril. This interaction should be given consideration in patients taking NSAIDs or selective COX-2 inhibitors concomitantly with ACE inhibitors. In some patients with compromised renal function who are being treated with NSAIDs, including selective COX-2 inhibitors, the co-administration of angiotensin II receptor antagonists or ACE inhibitors, may result in further deterioration of renal function, including possible acute renal failure. These effects are usually reversible. Therefore, monitor effects on blood pressure and renal fuction when administering the combination, especially in the elderly). Products include:
EC-Naprosyn 2850
Naprosyn 2850
Anaprox/Naprosyn 2850

Naproxen Sodium (Reports suggest that NSAIDs, including selective COX-2 inhibitors, may diminish the antihyper-

tensive effect of ACE inhibitors, including lisinopril. This interaction should be given consideration in patients taking NSAIDs or selective COX-2 inhibitors concomitantly with ACE inhibitors. In some patients with compromised renal function who are being treated with NSAIDs, including selective COX-2 inhibitors, the co-administration of angiotensin II receptor antagonists or ACE inhibitors, may result in further deterioration of renal function, including possible acute renal failure. These effects are usually reversible. Therefore, monitor effects on blood pressure and renal fuction when administering the combination, especially in the elderly). Products include:

Nateglinide (Hyperglycemia may occur with thiazide diuretics; dosage adjustment of oral hypoglycemic agents may be required).
No products indexed under this heading.

Nebivolol (Co-administration of thiazide and other antihypertensive agents can lead to additive effect or potentiation). Products include:

Nicardipine Hydrochloride (Co-administration of thiazide and other antihypertensive agents can lead to additive effect or potentiation).
No products indexed under this heading.

Nifedipine (Co-administration of thiazide and other antihypertensive agents can lead to additive effect or potentiation).
No products indexed under this heading.

Nisoldipine (Co-administration of thiazide and other antihypertensive agents can lead to additive effect or potentiation).
No products indexed under this heading.

Nitroglycerin (Co-administration of thiazide and other antihypertensive agents can lead to additive effect or potentiation). Products include:

Norepinephrine Bitartrate (Possible decreased response to pressor amines but not sufficient to preclude pressor amine use).
No products indexed under this heading.

Oxaprozin (Reports suggest that NSAIDs, including selective COX-2 inhibitors, may diminish the antihypertensive effect of ACE inhibitors, including lisinopril. This interaction should be given consideration in patients taking NSAIDs or selective COX-2 inhibitors concomitantly with ACE inhibitors. In some patients with compromised renal function who are being treated with NSAIDs, including selective COX-2 inhibitors, the co-administration of angiotensin II receptor antagonists or ACE inhibitors, may result in further deterioration of renal function, including possible acute renal failure. These effects are usually reversible. Therefore, monitor effects on blood pressure and renal fuction when administering the combination, especially in the elderly).
No products indexed under this heading.

Oxycodone Hydrochloride (Co-administration of thiazide and narcotics may potentiate orthostatic hypotension). Products include:

Oxycodone Terephthalate (Co-administration of thiazide and narcotics may potentiate orthostatic hypotension).
No products indexed under this heading.

Oxymorphone Hydrochloride (Co-administration of thiazide and narcotics may potentiate orthostatic hypotension). Products include:

Pancuronium Bromide (Co-administration with nondepolarizing skeletal muscle relaxants may result in possible increased responsiveness to the muscle relaxant).
No products indexed under this heading.

Penbutolol Sulfate (Co-administration of thiazide and other antihypertensive agents can lead to additive effect or potentiation).
No products indexed under this heading.

Pentobarbital (Co-administration of thiazide and barbiturates may potentiate orthostatic hypotension).
No products indexed under this heading.

Pentobarbital Sodium (Co-administration of thiazide and barbiturates may potentiate orthostatic hypotension). Products include:

Perindopril Erbumine (Co-administration of thiazide and other antihypertensive agents can lead to additive effect or potentiation).
No products indexed under this heading.

Phenobarbital (Co-administration of thiazide and barbiturates may potentiate orthostatic hypotension). Products include:

Phenobarbital Sodium (Co-administration of thiazide and barbiturates may potentiate orthostatic hypotension).
No products indexed under this heading.

Phenoxybenzamine Hydrochloride (Co-administration of thiazide and other antihypertensive agents can lead to additive effect or potentiation). Products include:

Phentolamine Mesylate (Co-administration of thiazide and other antihypertensive agents can lead to additive effect or potentiation).
No products indexed under this heading.

Phenylbutazone (Reports suggest that NSAIDs, including selective COX-2 inhibitors, may diminish the antihypertensive effect of ACE inhibitors, including lisinopril. This interaction should be given consideration in patients taking NSAIDs or selective COX-2 inhibitors concomitantly with ACE inhibitors. In some patients with compromised renal function who are being treated with NSAIDs, including selective COX-2 inhibitors, the co-administration of angiotensin II receptor antagonists or ACE inhibitors, may result in further deterioration of renal function, including possible acute renal failure. These effects are usually reversible. Therefore, monitor effects on blood pressure and renal fuction when administering the combination, especially in the elderly).
No products indexed under this heading.

Pindolol (Co-administration of thiazide and other antihypertensive agents can lead to additive effect or potentiation).
No products indexed under this heading.

Pioglitazone Hydrochloride (Hyperglycemia may occur with thiazide diuretics; dosage adjustment of oral hypoglycemic agents may be required). Products include:

Pipecuronium Bromide (Co-administration with nondepolarizing skeletal muscle relaxants may result in possible increased responsiveness to the muscle relaxant).
No products indexed under this heading.

Piroxicam (Reports suggest that NSAIDs, including selective COX-2 inhibitors, may diminish the antihypertensive effect of ACE inhibitors, including lisinopril. This interaction should be given consideration in patients taking NSAIDs or selective COX-2 inhibitors concomitantly with ACE inhibitors. In some patients with compromised renal function who are being treated with NSAIDs, including selective COX-2 inhibitors, the co-administration of angiotensin II receptor antagonists or ACE inhibitors, may result in further deterioration of renal function, including possible acute renal failure. These effects are usually reversible. Therefore, monitor effects on blood pressure and renal fuction when administering the combination, especially in the elderly).
No products indexed under this heading.

Polythiazide (Co-administration of lisinopril in patients on diuretics, especially those in whom diuretic therapy was recently instituted, may occasionally experience excessive hypotension; antihypertensive effects of lisinopril are augmented by antihypertensive agents that cause renin release).
No products indexed under this heading.

Potassium Acid Phosphate (Risk factors for the development of hyperkalemia include the concomitant use of potassium-sparing diuretics, potassium supplements and/or potassium-containing salt substitutes. Hyperkalemia can cause serious, sometimes fatal, arrhythmias. Prinzide should be used cautiously, if at all, with these agents and with frequent monitoring of serum potassium). Products include:

Potassium Bicarbonate (Risk factors for the development of hyperkalemia include the concomitant use of potassium-sparing diuretics, potassium supplements and/or potassium-containing salt substitutes. Hyperkalemia can cause serious, sometimes fatal, arrhythmias. Prinzide should be used cautiously, if at all, with these agents and with frequent monitoring of serum potassium).
No products indexed under this heading.

Potassium Chloride (Risk factors for the development of hyperkalemia include the concomitant use of potassium-sparing diuretics, potassium supplements and/or potassium-containing salt substitutes. Hyperkalemia can cause serious, sometimes fatal, arrhythmias. Prinzide should be used cautiously, if at all, with these agents and with frequent monitoring of serum potassium). Products include:

Potassium Citrate (Risk factors for the development of hyperkalemia include the concomitant use of potassium-sparing diuretics, potassium supplements and/or potassium-containing salt substitutes. Hyperkalemia can cause serious, sometimes fatal, arrhythmias. Prinzide should be used cautiously, if at all, with these agents and with frequent monitoring of serum potassium). Products include:

Potassium Gluconate (Risk factors for the development of hyperkalemia include the concomitant use of potassium-sparing diuretics, potassium supplements and/or potassium-containing salt substitutes. Hyperkalemia can cause serious, sometimes fatal, arrhythmias. Prinzide should be used cautiously, if at all, with these agents and with frequent monitoring of serum potassium).
No products indexed under this heading.

Potassium Phosphate (Risk factors for the development of hyperkalemia include the concomitant use of potassium-sparing diuretics, potassium supplements and/or potassium-containing salt substitutes. Hyperkalemia can cause serious, sometimes fatal, arrhythmias. Prinzide should be used cautiously, if at all, with these agents and with frequent monitoring of serum potassium). Products include:

Prazosin Hydrochloride (Co-administration of thiazide and other antihypertensive agents can lead to additive effect or potentiation).
No products indexed under this heading.

Prednisolone (Co-administration of thiazide diuretics with corticosteroids intensifies electrolyte depletion, particularly potassium).
No products indexed under this heading.

Prednisolone Acetate (Co-administration of thiazide diuretics with corticosteroids intensifies electrolyte depletion, particularly potassium). Products include:

Prednisolone Sodium Phosphate (Co-administration of thiazide diuretics with corticosteroids intensifies electrolyte depletion, particularly potassium).
No products indexed under this heading.

Prednisolone Tebutate (Co-administration of thiazide diuretics with corticosteroids intensifies electrolyte depletion, particularly potassium).
No products indexed under this heading.

Prednisone (Co-administration of thiazide diuretics with corticosteroids intensifies electrolyte depletion, particularly potassium).
No products indexed under this heading.

Prednisone sodium phosphate (Co-administration of thiazide diuretics with corticosteroids intensifies electrolyte depletion, particularly potassium).
No products indexed under this heading.

Propoxyphene Hydrochloride (Co-administration of thiazide and narcotics may potentiate orthostatic hypotension).
No products indexed under this heading.

Propoxyphene Napsylate (Co-administration of thiazide and narcotics may potentiate orthostatic hypotension).
No products indexed under this heading.

Propranolol Hydrochloride (Co-administration of thiazide and other antihypertensive agents can lead to additive effect or potentiation). Products include:

Quinapril Hydrochloride (Co-administration of thiazide and other antihypertensive agents can lead to additive effect or potentiation).
No products indexed under this heading.

Ramipril (Co-administration of thiazide and other antihypertensive agents can lead to additive effect or potentiation).
No products indexed under this heading.

Prinzide | Interactions Index | 1466

Rapacuronium Bromide (Co-administration with nondepolarizing skeletal muscle relaxants may result in possible increased responsiveness to the muscle relaxant).
No products indexed under this heading.

Rauwolfia Serpentina (Co-administration of thiazide and other antihypertensive agents can lead to additive effect or potentiation).
No products indexed under this heading.

Remifentanil Hydrochloride (Co-administration of thiazide and narcotics may potentiate orthostatic hypotension).
No products indexed under this heading.

Repaglinide (Hyperglycemia may occur with thiazide diuretics; dosage adjustment of oral hypoglycemic agents may be required).
No products indexed under this heading.

Rescinnamine (Co-administration of thiazide and other antihypertensive agents can lead to additive effect or potentiation).
No products indexed under this heading.

Reserpine (Co-administration of thiazide and other antihypertensive agents can lead to additive effect or potentiation).
No products indexed under this heading.

Rocuronium Bromide (Co-administration with nondepolarizing skeletal muscle relaxants may result in possible increased responsiveness to the muscle relaxant). Products include:
Zemuron 3249

Rofecoxib (Reports suggest that NSAIDs, including selective COX-2 inhibitors, may diminish the antihypertensive effect of ACE inhibitors, including lisinopril. This interaction should be given consideration in patients taking NSAIDs or selective COX-2 inhibitors concomitantly with ACE inhibitors. In some patients with compromised renal function who are being treated with NSAIDs, including selective COX-2 inhibitors, the co-administration of angiotensin II receptor antagonists or ACE inhibitors, may result in further deterioration of renal function, including possible acute renal failure. These effects are usually reversible. Therefore, monitor effects on blood pressure and renal fuction when administering the combination, especially in the elderly).
No products indexed under this heading.

Rosiglitazone Maleate (Hyperglycemia may occur with thiazide diuretics; dosage adjustment of oral hypoglycemic agents may be required). Products include:
Avandamet 1345
Avandaryl 1356
Avandia 1366

Secobarbital Sodium (Co-administration of thiazide and barbiturates may potentiate orthostatic hypotension).
No products indexed under this heading.

Sitagliptin Phosphate (Hyperglycemia may occur with thiazide diuretics; dosage adjustment of oral hypoglycemic agents may be required). Products include:
Janumet 2188
Januvia 2196

Sodium Butabarbital (Co-administration of thiazide and barbiturates may potentiate orthostatic hypotension).
No products indexed under this heading.

Sodium Nitroprusside (Co-administration of thiazide and other antihypertensive agents can lead to additive effect or potentiation).
No products indexed under this heading.

Sodium Pentobarbital (Co-administration of thiazide and barbiturates may potentiate orthostatic hypotension).
No products indexed under this heading.

Sotalol Hydrochloride (Co-administration of thiazide and other antihypertensive agents can lead to additive effect or potentiation).
No products indexed under this heading.

Spirapril Hydrochloride (Co-administration of thiazide and other antihypertensive agents can lead to additive effect or potentiation).
No products indexed under this heading.

Spironolactone (Risk factors for the development of hyperkalemia include the concomitant use of potassium-sparing diuretics, potassium supplements and/or potassium-containing salt substitutes. Hyperkalemia can cause serious, sometimes fatal, arrhythmias. Prinzide should be used cautiously, if at all, with these agents and with frequent monitoring of serum potassium).
No products indexed under this heading.

Sufentanil Citrate (Co-administration of thiazide and narcotics may potentiate orthostatic hypotension).
No products indexed under this heading.

Sulindac (Reports suggest that NSAIDs, including selective COX-2 inhibitors, may diminish the antihypertensive effect of ACE inhibitors, including lisinopril. This interaction should be given consideration in patients taking NSAIDs or selective COX-2 inhibitors concomitantly with ACE inhibitors. In some patients with compromised renal function who are being treated with NSAIDs, including selective COX-2 inhibitors, the co-administration of angiotensin II receptor antagonists or ACE inhibitors, may result in further deterioration of renal function, including possible acute renal failure. These effects are usually reversible. Therefore, monitor effects on blood pressure and renal fuction when administering the combination, especially in the elderly). Products include:
Clinoril 2098

Telmisartan (Co-administration of thiazide and other antihypertensive agents can lead to additive effect or potentiation). Products include:
Micardis 887
Micardis HCT 889

Terazosin Hydrochloride (Co-administration of thiazide and other antihypertensive agents can lead to additive effect or potentiation).
No products indexed under this heading.

Thiamylal Sodium (Co-administration of thiazide and barbiturates may potentiate orthostatic hypotension).
No products indexed under this heading.

Timolol Maleate (Co-administration of thiazide and other antihypertensive agents can lead to additive effect or potentiation). Products include:
Combigan 601
Dorzolamide Hydrochloride/Timolol Maleate Ophthalmic Solution .... ⊙243
Timoptic in Ocudose .... ⊙231

Tolazamide (Hyperglycemia may occur with thiazide diuretics; dosage adjustment of oral hypoglycemic agents may be required).
No products indexed under this heading.

Tolbutamide (Hyperglycemia may occur with thiazide diuretics; dosage adjustment of oral hypoglycemic agents may be required).
No products indexed under this heading.

Tolmetin Sodium (Reports suggest that NSAIDs, including selective COX-2 inhibitors, may diminish the antihypertensive effect of ACE inhibitors, including lisinopril. This interaction should be given consideration in patients taking NSAIDs or selective COX-2 inhibitors concomitantly with ACE inhibitors. In some patients with compromised renal function who are being treated with NSAIDs, including selective COX-2 inhibitors, the co-administration of angiotensin II receptor antagonists or ACE inhibitors, may result in further deterioration of renal function, including possible acute renal failure. These effects are usually reversible. Therefore, monitor effects on blood pressure and renal fuction when administering the combination, especially in the elderly).
No products indexed under this heading.

Torsemide (Co-administration of lisinopril in patients on diuretics, especially those in whom diuretic therapy was recently instituted, may occasionally experience excessive hypotension; antihypertensive effects of lisinopril are augmented by antihypertensive agents that cause renin release).
No products indexed under this heading.

Trandolapril (Co-administration of thiazide and other antihypertensive agents can lead to additive effect or potentiation). Products include:
Mavik 489
Tarka 534

Triamcinolone (Co-administration of thiazide diuretics with corticosteroids intensifies electrolyte depletion, particularly potassium).
No products indexed under this heading.

Triamcinolone Acetonide (Co-administration of thiazide diuretics with corticosteroids intensifies electrolyte depletion, particularly potassium). Products include:
Azmacort 408
Nasacort AQ 3019

Triamcinolone Diacetate (Co-administration of thiazide diuretics with corticosteroids intensifies electrolyte depletion, particularly potassium).
No products indexed under this heading.

Triamcinolone Hexacetonide (Co-administration of thiazide diuretics with corticosteroids intensifies electrolyte depletion, particularly potassium).
No products indexed under this heading.

Triamterene (Risk factors for the development of hyperkalemia include the concomitant use of potassium-sparing diuretics, potassium supplements and/or potassium-containing salt substitutes. Hyperkalemia can cause serious, sometimes fatal, arrhythmias. Prinzide should be used cautiously, if at all, with these agents and with frequent monitoring of serum potassium). Products include:
Dyazide 1429
Dyrenium 3495

Trimethaphan Camsylate (Co-administration of thiazide and other antihypertensive agents can lead to additive effect or potentiation).
No products indexed under this heading.

Troglitazone (Hyperglycemia may occur with thiazide diuretics; dosage adjustment of oral hypoglycemic agents may be required).
No products indexed under this heading.

Tubocurarine Chloride (Co-administration with nondepolarizing skeletal muscle relaxants may result in possible increased responsiveness to the muscle relaxant).
No products indexed under this heading.

Valdecoxib (Reports suggest that NSAIDs, including selective COX-2 inhibitors, may diminish the antihypertensive effect of ACE inhibitors, including lisinopril. This interaction should be given consideration in patients taking NSAIDs or selective COX-2 inhibitors concomitantly with ACE inhibitors. In some patients with compromised renal function who are being treated with NSAIDs, including selective COX-2 inhibitors, the co-administration of angiotensin II receptor antagonists or ACE inhibitors, may result in further deterioration of renal function, including possible acute renal failure. These effects are usually reversible. Therefore, monitor effects on blood pressure and renal fuction when administering the combination, especially in the elderly).
No products indexed under this heading.

Valsartan (Co-administration of thiazide and other antihypertensive agents can lead to additive effect or potentiation). Products include:
Diovan 2413
Diovan HCT 2419
Exforge 2443
Exforge HCT 2449
Valturna 3637

Vecuronium Bromide (Co-administration with nondepolarizing skeletal muscle relaxants may result in possible increased responsiveness to the muscle relaxant).
No products indexed under this heading.

Verapamil Hydrochloride (Co-administration of thiazide and other antihypertensive agents can lead to additive effect or potentiation). Products include:
Tarka 534

Food Interactions

Alcohol (Co-administration of thiazide and alcohol may potentiate orthostatic hypotension).

Beer, reduced-alcohol (Co-administration of thiazide and alcohol may potentiate orthostatic hypotension).

Beer, unspecified (Co-administration of thiazide and alcohol may potentiate orthostatic hypotension).

Salt Substitutes, Potassium-Containing (Risk factors for the development of hyperkalemia include the concomitant use of potassium-sparing diuretics, potassium supplements and/or potassium-containing salt substitutes. Hyperkalemia can cause serious, sometimes, fatal, arrhythmias. Prinzide should be used cautiously, if at all, with these agents and with frequent monitoring of serum potassium).

Wine, Chianti (Co-administration of thiazide and alcohol may potentiate orthostatic hypotension).

Wine, Red (Co-administration of thiazide and alcohol may potentiate orthostatic hypotension).

Wine, unspecified (Co-administration of thiazide and alcohol may potentiate orthostatic hypotension).

Wine products (Co-administration of thiazide and alcohol may potentiate orthostatic hypotension).

PRISTIQ EXTENDED-RELEASE TABLETS

(Desvenlafaxine Succinate) 3564

May interact with alcohols, aspirin-acetylsalicylic acid, central nervous system depressants, central nervous system stimulants, cytochrome p450 2d6 substrates (selected), cytochrome p450 3a4 inhibitors (selected), cytochrome p450 3a4 substrates (selected), monoamine oxidase inhibitors, non-steroidal anti-inflammatory agents, selective serotonin reuptake inhibitors, serotonin and norepinephrine reuptake inhibitors, triptans, and certain other agents. Compounds in these categories include:

5-hydroxytryptophan (Concomitant use of desvenlafaxine with serotonin precursors (such as tryptophan supplements) is not recommended).
No products indexed under this heading.

Acetazolamide (CYP3A4 is a minor pathway for the metabolism of desvenlafaxine. In a clinical study, ketoconazole (200 mg b.i.d.) increased the area under the concentration vs. time curve AUC of desvenlafaxine (400 mg single dose) by about 43% and C_{max} by about 8%. Concomitant use of desvenlafaxine with potent inhibitors of CYP3A4 may result in higher concentrations of desvenlafaxine).
No products indexed under this heading.

Acetazolamide Sodium (CYP3A4 is a minor pathway for the metabolism of desvenlafaxine. In a clinical study, ketoconazole (200 mg b.i.d.) increased the area under the concentration vs. time curve AUC of desvenlafaxine (400 mg single dose) by about 43% and C_{max} by about 8%. Concomitant use of desvenlafaxine with potent inhibitors of CYP3A4 may result in higher concentrations of desvenlafaxine).
No products indexed under this heading.

Alfentanil Hydrochloride (Caution is advised when desvenlafaxine is taken in combination with other CNS-active drugs).
No products indexed under this heading.

Almotriptan Malate (The development of potentially life-threatening serotonin syndrome may occur when desvenlafaxine is used concomitantly with triptans. Serotonin syndrome symptoms may include mental status changes, autonomic instability, neuromuscular aberrations, and/or gastrointestinal symptoms. If concomitant treatment with desvenlafaxine and a triptan is clinically warranted, careful observation of the patient is advised, particularly during treatment initiation and dose increases). Products include:
Axert 2593

Alprazolam (Caution is advised when desvenlafaxine is taken in combination with other CNS-active drugs).
No products indexed under this heading.

Amiodarone Hydrochloride (CYP3A4 is a minor pathway for the metabolism of desvenlafaxine. In a clinical study, ketoconazole (200 mg b.i.d.) increased the area under the concentration vs. time curve AUC of desvenlafaxine (400 mg single dose) by about 43% and C_{max} by about 8%. Concomitant use of desvenlafaxine with potent inhibitors of CYP3A4 may result in higher concentrations of desvenlafaxine).
No products indexed under this heading.

Amitriptyline Hydrochloride (Concomitant use of desvenlafaxine with a drug metabolized by CYP2D6 can result in higher concentrations of that drug).
No products indexed under this heading.

Amlodipine Besylate (Concomitant use of desvenlafaxine with a drug metabolized by CYP3A4 can result in lower exposures to that drug). Products include:
Azor 1010
Exforge 2443
Exforge HCT 2449

Amobarbital (Caution is advised when desvenlafaxine is taken in combination with other CNS-active drugs).
No products indexed under this heading.

Amobarbital Sodium (Caution is advised when desvenlafaxine is taken in combination with other CNS-active drugs).
No products indexed under this heading.

Amphetamine Aspartate (Caution is advised when desvenlafaxine is taken in combination with other CNS-active drugs).
No products indexed under this heading.

Amphetamine Aspartate Monohydrate (Caution is advised when desvenlafaxine is taken in combination with other CNS-active drugs).
No products indexed under this heading.

Amphetamine Resins (Caution is advised when desvenlafaxine is taken in combination with other CNS-active drugs).
No products indexed under this heading.

Amphetamine Sulfate (Caution is advised when desvenlafaxine is taken in combination with other CNS-active drugs).
No products indexed under this heading.

Amprenavir (CYP3A4 is a minor pathway for the metabolism of desvenlafaxine. In a clinical study, ketoconazole (200 mg b.i.d.) increased the area under the concentration vs. time curve AUC of desvenlafaxine (400 mg single dose) by about 43% and C_{max} by about 8%. Concomitant use of desvenlafaxine with potent inhibitors of CYP3A4 may result in higher concentrations of desvenlafaxine).
No products indexed under this heading.

Anastrozole (CYP3A4 is a minor pathway for the metabolism of desvenlafaxine. In a clinical study, ketoconazole (200 mg b.i.d.) increased the area under the concentration vs. time curve AUC of desvenlafaxine (400 mg single dose) by about 43% and C_{max} by about 8%. Concomitant use of desvenlafaxine with potent inhibitors of CYP3A4 may result in higher concentrations of desvenlafaxine).
No products indexed under this heading.

Aprepitant (CYP3A4 is a minor pathway for the metabolism of desvenlafaxine. In a clinical study, ketoconazole (200 mg b.i.d.) increased the area under the concentration vs. time curve AUC of desvenlafaxine (400 mg single dose) by about 43% and C_{max} by about 8%. Concomitant use of desvenlafaxine with potent inhibitors of CYP3A4 may result in higher concentrations of desvenlafaxine). Products include:
Emend 2124

Aprobarbital (Caution is advised when desvenlafaxine is taken in combination with other CNS-active drugs).
No products indexed under this heading.

Aspirin (Studies have shown that concurrent use of aspirin may potentiate the risk of upper GI bleeding. Patients should be cautioned about the concomitant use of desvenlafaxine with aspirin). Products include:
Aggrenox 880
Bayer Aspirin 829
Percodan 1124
St. Joseph Aspirin 2045

Aspirin, Enteric Coated (Studies have shown that concurrent use of aspirin may potentiate the risk of upper GI bleeding. Patients should be cautioned about the concomitant use of desvenlafaxine with aspirin).
No products indexed under this heading.

Aspirin Buffered (Studies have shown that concurrent use of aspirin may potentiate the risk of upper GI bleeding. Patients should be cautioned about the concomitant use of desvenlafaxine with aspirin).
No products indexed under this heading.

Astemizole (Concomitant use of desvenlafaxine with a drug metabolized by CYP3A4 can result in lower exposures to that drug).
No products indexed under this heading.

Atazanavir (CYP3A4 is a minor pathway for the metabolism of desvenlafax-

ine. In a clinical study, ketoconazole (200 mg b.i.d.) increased the area under the concentration vs. time curve AUC of desvenlafaxine (400 mg single dose) by about 43% and C_{max} by about 8%. Concomitant use of desvenlafaxine with potent inhibitors of CYP3A4 may result in higher concentrations of desvenlafaxine).
No products indexed under this heading.

Atazanavir Sulfate (CYP3A4 is a minor pathway for the metabolism of desvenlafaxine. In a clinical study, ketoconazole (200 mg b.i.d.) increased the area under the concentration vs. time curve AUC of desvenlafaxine (400 mg single dose) by about 43% and C_{max} by about 8%. Concomitant use of desvenlafaxine with potent inhibitors of CYP3A4 may result in higher concentrations of desvenlafaxine).
No products indexed under this heading.

Atomoxetine Hydrochloride (Concomitant use of desvenlafaxine with a drug metabolized by CYP2D6 can result in higher concentrations of that drug). Products include:
Strattera 1957

Atorvastatin Calcium (Concomitant use of desvenlafaxine with a drug metabolized by CYP3A4 can result in lower exposures to that drug). Products include:
Lipitor 2703

Belladonna Ergotamine (Concomitant use of desvenlafaxine with a drug metabolized by CYP3A4 can result in lower exposures to that drug).
No products indexed under this heading.

Bisoprolol Fumarate (Concomitant use of desvenlafaxine with a drug metabolized by CYP2D6 can result in higher concentrations of that drug).
No products indexed under this heading.

Buprenorphine Hydrochloride (Caution is advised when desvenlafaxine is taken in combination with other CNS-active drugs).
No products indexed under this heading.

Buspirone Hydrochloride (Caution is advised when desvenlafaxine is taken in combination with other CNS-active drugs).
No products indexed under this heading.

Busulfan (Concomitant use of desvenlafaxine with a drug metabolized by CYP3A4 can result in lower exposures to that drug). Products include:
Myleran 1581

Butabarbital (Caution is advised when desvenlafaxine is taken in combination with other CNS-active drugs).
No products indexed under this heading.

Butabarbital Sodium (Caution is advised when desvenlafaxine is taken in combination with other CNS-active drugs).
No products indexed under this heading.

Butalbital (Caution is advised when desvenlafaxine is taken in combination with other CNS-active drugs).
No products indexed under this heading.

Captopril (Concomitant use of desvenlafaxine with a drug metabolized by CYP2D6 can result in higher concentrations of that drug). Products include:
Captopril 2341

Carbamazepine (Concomitant use of desvenlafaxine with a drug metabolized by CYP3A4 can result in lower exposures to that drug). Products include:
Carbatrol 3280
Equetro 3477

Carvedilol (Concomitant use of desvenlafaxine with a drug metabolized by CYP2D6 can result in higher concentrations of that drug). Products include:
Coreg 1409

Celecoxib (Studies have shown that concurrent use of an NSAID may poten-

tiate the risk of upper GI bleeding. Patients should be cautioned about the concomitant use of desvenlafaxine with NSAIDs). Products include:
Celebrex 3272

Cerivastatin Sodium (Concomitant use of desvenlafaxine with a drug metabolized by CYP3A4 can result in lower exposures to that drug).
No products indexed under this heading.

Cevimeline Hydrochloride (Concomitant use of desvenlafaxine with a drug metabolized by CYP2D6 can result in higher concentrations of that drug). Products include:
Evoxac 1027

Chlordiazepoxide (Caution is advised when desvenlafaxine is taken in combination with other CNS-active drugs).
No products indexed under this heading.

Chlordiazepoxide Hydrochloride (Caution is advised when desvenlafaxine is taken in combination with other CNS-active drugs).
No products indexed under this heading.

Chlorpheniramine (Concomitant use of desvenlafaxine with a drug metabolized by CYP3A4 can result in lower exposures to that drug).
No products indexed under this heading.

Chlorpheniramine Maleate (Concomitant use of desvenlafaxine with a drug metabolized by CYP3A4 can result in lower exposures to that drug).
No products indexed under this heading.

Chlorpheniramine Polistirex (Concomitant use of desvenlafaxine with a drug metabolized by CYP3A4 can result in lower exposures to that drug). Products include:
Tussionex 3443

Chlorpheniramine Tannate (Concomitant use of desvenlafaxine with a drug metabolized by CYP3A4 can result in lower exposures to that drug).
No products indexed under this heading.

Chlorpromazine (Caution is advised when desvenlafaxine is taken in combination with other CNS-active drugs).
No products indexed under this heading.

Chlorpromazine Hydrochloride (Caution is advised when desvenlafaxine is taken in combination with other CNS-active drugs).
No products indexed under this heading.

Chlorpropamide (Concomitant use of desvenlafaxine with a drug metabolized by CYP2D6 can result in higher concentrations of that drug).
No products indexed under this heading.

Chlorprothixene (Caution is advised when desvenlafaxine is taken in combination with other CNS-active drugs).
No products indexed under this heading.

Chlorprothixene Hydrochloride (Caution is advised when desvenlafaxine is taken in combination with other CNS-active drugs).
No products indexed under this heading.

Chlorprothixene Lactate (Caution is advised when desvenlafaxine is taken in combination with other CNS-active drugs).
No products indexed under this heading.

Cimetidine (CYP3A4 is a minor pathway for the metabolism of desvenlafaxine. In a clinical study, ketoconazole (200 mg b.i.d.) increased the area under the concentration vs. time curve AUC of desvenlafaxine (400 mg single dose) by about 43% and C_{max} by about 8%. Concomitant use of desvenlafaxine with potent inhibitors of CYP3A4 may result in higher concentrations of desvenlafaxine).
No products indexed under this heading.

Cimetidine Hydrochloride (CYP3A4 is a minor pathway for the metabolism of desvenlafaxine. In a clinical study,

ketoconazole (200 mg b.i.d.) increased the area under the concentration vs. time curve AUC of desvenlafaxine (400 mg single dose) by about 43% and C_{max} by about 8%. Concomitant use of desvenlafaxine with potent inhibitors of CYP3A4 may result in higher concentrations of desvenlafaxine).
No products indexed under this heading.

Ciprofloxacin (CYP3A4 is a minor pathway for the metabolism of desvenlafaxine. In a clinical study, ketoconazole (200 mg b.i.d.) increased the area under the concentration vs. time curve AUC of desvenlafaxine (400 mg single dose) by about 43% and C_{max} by about 8%. Concomitant use of desvenlafaxine with potent inhibitors of CYP3A4 may result in higher concentrations of desvenlafaxine). Products include:
Cipro I.V. **3082**
Cipro **3073**
Cipro XR **3091**
Ciprodex **583**

Cisapride (Concomitant use of desvenlafaxine with a drug metabolized by CYP3A4 can result in lower exposures to that drug).
No products indexed under this heading.

Citalopram Hydrobromide (The development of potentially life-threatening serotonin syndrome may occur when desvenlafaxine is used concomitantly with SSRIs. Serotonin syndrome symptoms may include mental status changes, autonomic instability, neuromuscular aberrations, and/or gastrointestinal symptoms. If concomitant treatment with desvenlafaxine and an SSRI is clinically warranted, careful observation of the patient is advised, particularly during treatment initiation and dose increases). Products include:
Celexa **1153**

Clarithromycin (CYP3A4 is a minor pathway for the metabolism of desvenlafaxine. In a clinical study, ketoconazole (200 mg b.i.d.) increased the area under the concentration vs. time curve AUC of desvenlafaxine (400 mg single dose) by about 43% and C_{max} by about 8%. Concomitant use of desvenlafaxine with potent inhibitors of CYP3A4 may result in higher concentrations of desvenlafaxine). Products include:
Biaxin/Biaxin XL **412**

Clomipramine Hydrochloride (Concomitant use of desvenlafaxine with a drug metabolized by CYP2D6 can result in higher concentrations of that drug).
No products indexed under this heading.

Clonazepam (Caution is advised when desvenlafaxine is taken in combination with other CNS-active drugs). Products include:
Klonopin **2855**

Clorazepate Dipotassium (Caution is advised when desvenlafaxine is taken in combination with other CNS-active drugs).
No products indexed under this heading.

Clotrimazole (CYP3A4 is a minor pathway for the metabolism of desvenlafaxine. In a clinical study, ketoconazole (200 mg b.i.d.) increased the area under the concentration vs. time curve AUC of desvenlafaxine (400 mg single dose) by about 43% and C_{max} by about 8%. Concomitant use of desvenlafaxine with potent inhibitors of CYP3A4 may result in higher concentrations of desvenlafaxine). Products include:
Lotrisone **3163**

Clozapine (Caution is advised when desvenlafaxine is taken in combination with other CNS-active drugs).
No products indexed under this heading.

Codeine Phosphate (Caution is advised when desvenlafaxine is taken in combination with other CNS-active drugs). Products include:
Tylenol with Codeine **2691**

Codeine Sulfate (Caution is advised when desvenlafaxine is taken in combination with other CNS-active drugs).
No products indexed under this heading.

Conivaptan Hydrochloride (CYP3A4 is a minor pathway for the metabolism of desvenlafaxine. In a clinical study, ketoconazole (200 mg b.i.d.) increased the area under the concentration vs. time curve AUC of desvenlafaxine (400 mg single dose) by about 43% and C_{max} by about 8%. Concomitant use of desvenlafaxine with potent inhibitors of CYP3A4 may result in higher concentrations of desvenlafaxine). Products include:
Vaprisol **689**

Cyclobenzaprine Hydrochloride (Concomitant use of desvenlafaxine with a drug metabolized by CYP2D6 can result in higher concentrations of that drug). Products include:
Amrix **964**

Cyclosporine (CYP3A4 is a minor pathway for the metabolism of desvenlafaxine. In a clinical study, ketoconazole (200 mg b.i.d.) increased the area under the concentration vs. time curve AUC of desvenlafaxine (400 mg single dose) by about 43% and C_{max} by about 8%. Concomitant use of desvenlafaxine with potent inhibitors of CYP3A4 may result in higher concentrations of desvenlafaxine). Products include:
Gengraf **440**
Neoral Oral Solution **2496**
Neoral Capsules **2496**
Restasis **605**

Dalfopristin (CYP3A4 is a minor pathway for the metabolism of desvenlafaxine. In a clinical study, ketoconazole (200 mg b.i.d.) increased the area under the concentration vs. time curve AUC of desvenlafaxine (400 mg single dose) by about 43% and C_{max} by about 8%. Concomitant use of desvenlafaxine with potent inhibitors of CYP3A4 may result in higher concentrations of desvenlafaxine).
No products indexed under this heading.

Danazol (CYP3A4 is a minor pathway for the metabolism of desvenlafaxine. In a clinical study, ketoconazole (200 mg b.i.d.) increased the area under the concentration vs. time curve AUC of desvenlafaxine (400 mg single dose) by about 43% and C_{max} by about 8%. Concomitant use of desvenlafaxine with potent inhibitors of CYP3A4 may result in higher concentrations of desvenlafaxine).
No products indexed under this heading.

Darunavir (CYP3A4 is a minor pathway for the metabolism of desvenlafaxine. In a clinical study, ketoconazole (200 mg b.i.d.) increased the area under the concentration vs. time curve AUC of desvenlafaxine (400 mg single dose) by about 43% and C_{max} by about 8%. Concomitant use of desvenlafaxine with potent inhibitors of CYP3A4 may result in higher concentrations of desvenlafaxine).
No products indexed under this heading.

Dasatinib (CYP3A4 is a minor pathway for the metabolism of desvenlafaxine. In a clinical study, ketoconazole (200 mg b.i.d.) increased the area under the concentration vs. time curve AUC of desvenlafaxine (400 mg single dose) by about 43% and C_{max} by about 8%. Concomitant use of desvenlafaxine with potent inhibitors of CYP3A4 may result in higher concentrations of desvenlafaxine).
No products indexed under this heading.

Debrisoquine (Concomitant use of desvenlafaxine with a drug metabolized by CYP2D6 can result in higher concentrations of that drug).
No products indexed under this heading.

Delavirdine Mesylate (CYP3A4 is a minor pathway for the metabolism of desvenlafaxine. In a clinical study, ketoconazole (200 mg b.i.d.) increased the area under the concentration vs. time curve AUC of desvenlafaxine (400 mg single dose) by about 43% and C_{max} by about 8%. Concomitant use of desvenlafaxine with potent inhibitors of CYP3A4 may result in higher concentrations of desvenlafaxine).
No products indexed under this heading.

Delavirine (CYP3A4 is a minor pathway for the metabolism of desvenlafaxine. In a clinical study, ketoconazole (200 mg b.i.d.) increased the area under the concentration vs. time curve AUC of desvenlafaxine (400 mg single dose) by about 43% and C_{max} by about 8%. Concomitant use of desvenlafaxine with potent inhibitors of CYP3A4 may result in higher concentrations of desvenlafaxine).
No products indexed under this heading.

Desflurane (Caution is advised when desvenlafaxine is taken in combination with other CNS-active drugs).
No products indexed under this heading.

Desipramine Hydrochloride (When desvenlafaxine succinate was administered at a dose of 100 mg daily in conjunction with a single 50 mg dose of desipramine, the C_{max} and AUC of desipramine increased approximately 25% and 17%, respectively. When 400 mg (8 times the recommended 50 mg dose) was administered, the C_{max} and AUC of desipramine increased approximately 50% and 90%, respectively).
No products indexed under this heading.

Desloratadine (CYP3A4 is a minor pathway for the metabolism of desvenlafaxine. In a clinical study, ketoconazole (200 mg b.i.d.) increased the area under the concentration vs. time curve AUC of desvenlafaxine (400 mg single dose) by about 43% and C_{max} by about 8%. Concomitant use of desvenlafaxine with potent inhibitors of CYP3A4 may result in higher concentrations of desvenlafaxine). Products include:
Clarinex Syrup **3098**
Clarinex **3098**
Clarinex Reditabs **3098**
Clarinex-D 12-Hour **3101**
Clarinex-D **3104**

Desogestrel (Concomitant use of desvenlafaxine with a drug metabolized by CYP3A4 can result in lower exposures to that drug).
No products indexed under this heading.

Dexfenfluramine Hydrochloride (Concomitant use of desvenlafaxine with a drug metabolized by CYP2D6 can result in higher concentrations of that drug).
No products indexed under this heading.

Dexmethylphenidate Hydrochloride (Caution is advised when desvenlafaxine is taken in combination with other CNS-active drugs). Products include:
Focalin XR **2472**

Dextroamphetamine (Caution is advised when desvenlafaxine is taken in combination with other CNS-active drugs).
No products indexed under this heading.

Dextroamphetamine Saccharate (Caution is advised when desvenlafaxine is taken in combination with other CNS-active drugs).
No products indexed under this heading.

Dextroamphetamine Sulfate (Caution is advised when desvenlafaxine is taken in combination with other CNS-active drugs). Products include:
Dexedrine **1425**

Dextromethorphan Hydrobromide (Concomitant use of desvenlafaxine with a drug metabolized by CYP2D6 can result in higher concentrations of that drug).
No products indexed under this heading.

Dextromethorphan Polistirex (Concomitant use of desvenlafaxine with a drug metabolized by CYP2D6 can result in higher concentrations of that drug).
No products indexed under this heading.

Dezocine (Caution is advised when desvenlafaxine is taken in combination with other CNS-active drugs).
No products indexed under this heading.

Diazepam (Caution is advised when desvenlafaxine is taken in combination with other CNS-active drugs). Products include:
Valium Tablets **2880**

Diclofenac Epolamine (Studies have shown that concurrent use of an NSAID may potentiate the risk of upper GI bleeding. Patients should be cautioned about the concomitant use of desvenlafaxine with NSAIDs). Products include:
Flector **1839**

Diclofenac Potassium (Studies have shown that concurrent use of an NSAID may potentiate the risk of upper GI bleeding. Patients should be cautioned about the concomitant use of desvenlafaxine with NSAIDs).
No products indexed under this heading.

Diclofenac Sodium (Studies have shown that concurrent use of an NSAID may potentiate the risk of upper GI bleeding. Patients should be cautioned about the concomitant use of desvenlafaxine with NSAIDs).
No products indexed under this heading.

Dihydroergotamine Mesylate (Concomitant use of desvenlafaxine with a drug metabolized by CYP3A4 can result in lower exposures to that drug).
No products indexed under this heading.

Diltiazem Hydrochloride (CYP3A4 is a minor pathway for the metabolism of desvenlafaxine. In a clinical study, ketoconazole (200 mg b.i.d.) increased the area under the concentration vs. time curve AUC of desvenlafaxine (400 mg single dose) by about 43% and C_{max} by about 8%. Concomitant use of desvenlafaxine with potent inhibitors of CYP3A4 may result in higher concentrations of desvenlafaxine). Products include:
Cardizem LA **423**

Diltiazem Maleate (CYP3A4 is a minor pathway for the metabolism of desvenlafaxine. In a clinical study, ketoconazole (200 mg b.i.d.) increased the area under the concentration vs. time curve AUC of desvenlafaxine (400 mg single dose) by about 43% and C_{max} by about 8%. Concomitant use of desvenlafaxine with potent inhibitors of CYP3A4 may result in higher concentrations of desvenlafaxine).
No products indexed under this heading.

Disopyramide (Concomitant use of desvenlafaxine with a drug metabolized by CYP3A4 can result in lower exposures to that drug).
No products indexed under this heading.

Disopyramide Phosphate (Concomitant use of desvenlafaxine with a drug metabolized by CYP3A4 can result in lower exposures to that drug).
No products indexed under this heading.

Disulfiram (Concomitant use of desvenlafaxine with a drug metabolized by CYP3A4 can result in lower exposures to that drug).
No products indexed under this heading.

Dolasetron Mesylate (Concomitant use of desvenlafaxine with a drug metabolized by CYP2D6 can result in higher concentrations of that drug). Products include:

Donepezil Hydrochloride (Concomitant use of desvenlafaxine with a drug metabolized by CYP2D6 can result in higher concentrations of that drug). Products include:

Doxepin Hydrochloride (Concomitant use of desvenlafaxine with a drug metabolized by CYP2D6 can result in higher concentrations of that drug).
No products indexed under this heading.

Doxorubicin Hydrochloride (Concomitant use of desvenlafaxine with a drug metabolized by CYP3A4 can result in lower exposures to that drug).
No products indexed under this heading.

Dronabinol (Concomitant use of desvenlafaxine with a drug metabolized by CYP3A4 can result in lower exposures to that drug).
No products indexed under this heading.

Droperidol (Caution is advised when desvenlafaxine is taken in combination with other CNS-active drugs).
No products indexed under this heading.

Duloxetine Hydrochloride (The development of potentially life-threatening serotonin syndrome may occur when desvenlafaxine is used concomitantly with other SNRIs. Serotonin syndrome symptoms may include mental status changes, autonomic instability, neuromuscular aberrations, and/or gastrointestinal symptoms. If concomitant treatment with desvenlafaxine and another SNRI is clinically warranted, careful observation of the patient is advised, particularly during treatment initiation and dose increases). Products include:

Efavirenz (CYP3A4 is a minor pathway for the metabolism of desvenlafaxine. In a clinical study, ketoconazole (200 mg b.i.d.) increased the area under the concentration vs. time curve AUC of desvenlafaxine (400 mg single dose) by about 43% and C_{max} by about 8%. Concomitant use of desvenlafaxine with potent inhibitors of CYP3A4 may result in higher concentrations of desvenlafaxine). Products include:

Eletriptan Hydrobromide (The development of potentially life-threatening serotonin syndrome may occur when desvenlafaxine is used concomitantly with triptans. Serotonin syndrome symptoms may include mental status changes, autonomic instability, neuromuscular aberrations, and/or gastrointestinal symptoms. If concomitant treatment with desvenlafaxine and a triptan is clinically warranted, careful observation of the patient is advised, particularly during treatment initiation and dose increases).
No products indexed under this heading.

Encainide Hydrochloride (Concomitant use of desvenlafaxine with a drug metabolized by CYP2D6 can result in higher concentrations of that drug).
No products indexed under this heading.

Enflurane (Caution is advised when desvenlafaxine is taken in combination with other CNS-active drugs).
No products indexed under this heading.

Ergotamine Tartrate (Concomitant use of desvenlafaxine with a drug metabolized by CYP3A4 can result in lower exposures to that drug).
No products indexed under this heading.

Erythromycin (CYP3A4 is a minor pathway for the metabolism of desvenlafaxine. In a clinical study, ketoconazole (200 mg b.i.d.) increased the area under the concentration vs. time curve AUC of desvenlafaxine (400 mg single dose) by about 43% and C_{max} by about 8%. Concomitant use of desvenlafaxine with potent inhibitors of CYP3A4 may result in higher concentrations of desvenlafaxine).
No products indexed under this heading.

Erythromycin Estolate (CYP3A4 is a minor pathway for the metabolism of desvenlafaxine. In a clinical study, ketoconazole (200 mg b.i.d.) increased the area under the concentration vs. time curve AUC of desvenlafaxine (400 mg single dose) by about 43% and C_{max} by about 8%. Concomitant use of desvenlafaxine with potent inhibitors of CYP3A4 may result in higher concentrations of desvenlafaxine).
No products indexed under this heading.

Erythromycin Ethylsuccinate (CYP3A4 is a minor pathway for the metabolism of desvenlafaxine. In a clinical study, ketoconazole (200 mg b.i.d.) increased the area under the concentration vs. time curve AUC of desvenlafaxine (400 mg single dose) by about 43% and C_{max} by about 8%. Concomitant use of desvenlafaxine with potent inhibitors of CYP3A4 may result in higher concentrations of desvenlafaxine). Products include:

Erythromycin Gluceptate (CYP3A4 is a minor pathway for the metabolism of desvenlafaxine. In a clinical study, ketoconazole (200 mg b.i.d.) increased the area under the concentration vs. time curve AUC of desvenlafaxine (400 mg single dose) by about 43% and C_{max} by about 8%. Concomitant use of desvenlafaxine with potent inhibitors of CYP3A4 may result in higher concentrations of desvenlafaxine).
No products indexed under this heading.

Erythromycin Lactobionate (CYP3A4 is a minor pathway for the metabolism of desvenlafaxine. In a clinical study, ketoconazole (200 mg b.i.d.) increased the area under the concentration vs. time curve AUC of desvenlafaxine (400 mg single dose) by about 43% and C_{max} by about 8%. Concomitant use of desvenlafaxine with potent inhibitors of CYP3A4 may result in higher concentrations of desvenlafaxine).
No products indexed under this heading.

Erythromycin Stearate (CYP3A4 is a minor pathway for the metabolism of desvenlafaxine. In a clinical study, ketoconazole (200 mg b.i.d.) increased the area under the concentration vs. time curve AUC of desvenlafaxine (400 mg single dose) by about 43% and C_{max} by about 8%. Concomitant use of desvenlafaxine with potent inhibitors of CYP3A4 may result in higher concentrations of desvenlafaxine).
No products indexed under this heading.

Escitalopram Oxalate (The development of potentially life-threatening serotonin syndrome may occur when desvenlafaxine is used concomitantly with SSRIs. Serotonin syndrome symptoms may include mental status changes, autonomic instability, neuromuscular aberrations, and/or gastrointestinal symptoms. If concomitant treatment with desvenlafaxine and an SSRI is clinically warranted, careful observation of the patient is advised, particularly during treatment initiation and dose increases). Products include:

Esomeprazole Magnesium (CYP3A4 is a minor pathway for the metabolism of desvenlafaxine. In a clinical study, ketoconazole (200 mg b.i.d.) increased the area under the concentration vs. time curve AUC of desvenlafaxine (400 mg single dose) by about 43% and C_{max} by about 8%. Concomitant

use of desvenlafaxine with potent inhibitors of CYP3A4 may result in higher concentrations of desvenlafaxine). Products include:

Esomeprazole Sodium (CYP3A4 is a minor pathway for the metabolism of desvenlafaxine. In a clinical study, ketoconazole (200 mg b.i.d.) increased the area under the concentration vs. time curve AUC of desvenlafaxine (400 mg single dose) by about 43% and C_{max} by about 8%. Concomitant use of desvenlafaxine with potent inhibitors of CYP3A4 may result in higher concentrations of desvenlafaxine). Products include:

Estazolam (Caution is advised when desvenlafaxine is taken in combination with other CNS-active drugs).
No products indexed under this heading.

Estradiol (Concomitant use of desvenlafaxine with a drug metabolized by CYP3A4 can result in lower exposures to that drug). Products include:

Estradiol Benzoate (Concomitant use of desvenlafaxine with a drug metabolized by CYP3A4 can result in lower exposures to that drug).
No products indexed under this heading.

Estradiol Cypionate (Concomitant use of desvenlafaxine with a drug metabolized by CYP3A4 can result in lower exposures to that drug).
No products indexed under this heading.

Estradiol Valerate (Concomitant use of desvenlafaxine with a drug metabolized by CYP3A4 can result in lower exposures to that drug).
No products indexed under this heading.

Ethanol (A clinical study has shown that desvenlafaxine does not increase the impairment of mental and motor skills caused by ethanol. However, patients should be advised to avoid alcohol consumption while taking desvenlafaxine).
No products indexed under this heading.

Ethchlorvynol (Caution is advised when desvenlafaxine is taken in combination with other CNS-active drugs).
No products indexed under this heading.

Ethinamate (Caution is advised when desvenlafaxine is taken in combination with other CNS-active drugs).
No products indexed under this heading.

Ethinyl Estradiol (Concomitant use of desvenlafaxine with a drug metabolized by CYP3A4 can result in lower exposures to that drug). Products include:

Ethosuximide (Concomitant use of desvenlafaxine with a drug metabolized by CYP3A4 can result in lower exposures to that drug).
No products indexed under this heading.

Ethyl Alcohol (Caution is advised when desvenlafaxine is taken in combination with other CNS-active drugs).
No products indexed under this heading.

Ethynodiol Diacetate (Concomitant use of desvenlafaxine with a drug metabolized by CYP3A4 can result in lower exposures to that drug).
No products indexed under this heading.

Etodolac (Studies have shown that concurrent use of an NSAID may potentiate the risk of upper GI bleeding. Patients should be cautioned about the concomitant use of desvenlafaxine with NSAIDs).
No products indexed under this heading.

Etoposide (Concomitant use of desvenlafaxine with a drug metabolized by CYP3A4 can result in lower exposures to that drug).
No products indexed under this heading.

Etoposide Phosphate (Concomitant use of desvenlafaxine with a drug metabolized by CYP3A4 can result in lower exposures to that drug).
No products indexed under this heading.

Felodipine (Concomitant use of desvenlafaxine with a drug metabolized by CYP3A4 can result in lower exposures to that drug).
No products indexed under this heading.

Fenoprofen Calcium (Studies have shown that concurrent use of an NSAID may potentiate the risk of upper GI bleeding. Patients should be cautioned about the concomitant use of desvenlafaxine with NSAIDs).
No products indexed under this heading.

Fentanyl (Caution is advised when desvenlafaxine is taken in combination with other CNS-active drugs). Products include:

Fentanyl Citrate (Caution is advised when desvenlafaxine is taken in combination with other CNS-active drugs). Products include:

Flecainide Acetate (Concomitant use of desvenlafaxine with a drug metabolized by CYP2D6 can result in higher concentrations of that drug).
No products indexed under this heading.

Fluconazole (CYP3A4 is a minor pathway for the metabolism of desvenlafaxine. In a clinical study, ketoconazole (200 mg b.i.d.) increased the area under the concentration vs. time curve AUC of desvenlafaxine (400 mg single dose) by about 43% and C_{max} by about 8%. Concomitant use of desvenlafaxine with potent inhibitors of CYP3A4 may result in higher concentrations of desvenlafaxine).
No products indexed under this heading.

Fluoxetine (The development of potentially life-threatening serotonin syndrome may occur when desvenlafaxine is used concomitantly with SSRIs. Serotonin syndrome symptoms may include mental status changes, autonomic instability, neuromuscular aberrations, and/or gastrointestinal symptoms. If concomitant treatment with desvenlafaxine and an SSRI is clinically warranted, careful observation of the patient is advised, particularly during treatment initiation and dose increases).
No products indexed under this heading.

Fluoxetine Hydrochloride (The development of potentially life-threatening serotonin syndrome may occur when desvenlafaxine is used concomitantly with SSRIs. Serotonin syndrome symptoms may include mental status changes, autonomic instability, neuromuscular aberrations, and/or gastrointestinal symptoms. If concomitant treatment with desvenlafaxine and an SSRI is clinically warranted, careful observation of the patient is advised, particularly during treatment initiation and dose increases). Products include:

IMPORTANT NOTE: Always consult each drug listing in the patient's regimen for possible interactions.

IMPORTANT NOTE: Always consult each drug listing in the patient's regimen for possible interactions.

lafaxine with potent inhibitors of CYP3A4 may result in higher concentrations of desvenlafaxine).

No products indexed under this heading.

Nevirapine (CYP3A4 is a minor pathway for the metabolism of desvenlafaxine. In a clinical study, ketoconazole (200 mg b.i.d.) increased the area under the concentration vs. time curve AUC of desvenlafaxine (400 mg single dose) by about 43% and C_{max} by about 8%. Concomitant use of desvenlafaxine with potent inhibitors of CYP3A4 may result in higher concentrations of desvenlafaxine). Products include:

Viramune Oral Suspension 897
Viramune Tablets 897

Niacin (CYP3A4 is a minor pathway for the metabolism of desvenlafaxine. In a clinical study, ketoconazole (200 mg b.i.d.) increased the area under the concentration vs. time curve AUC of desvenlafaxine (400 mg single dose) by about 43% and C_{max} by about 8%. Concomitant use of desvenlafaxine with potent inhibitors of CYP3A4 may result in higher concentrations of desvenlafaxine). Products include:

Advicor 402
Cardio Basics 3455
Niaspan 497
Simcor 524

Niacinamide (CYP3A4 is a minor pathway for the metabolism of desvenlafaxine. In a clinical study, ketoconazole (200 mg b.i.d.) increased the area under the concentration vs. time curve AUC of desvenlafaxine (400 mg single dose) by about 43% and C_{max} by about 8%. Concomitant use of desvenlafaxine with potent inhibitors of CYP3A4 may result in higher concentrations of desvenlafaxine). Products include:

CitraNatal 90 DHA Capsules 2332
CitraNatal Assure 2332
CitraNatal Rx 2332
Heplive 607

Niacinamide Hydroiodide (CYP3A4 is a minor pathway for the metabolism of desvenlafaxine. In a clinical study, ketoconazole (200 mg b.i.d.) increased the area under the concentration vs. time curve AUC of desvenlafaxine (400 mg single dose) by about 43% and C_{max} by about 8%. Concomitant use of desvenlafaxine with potent inhibitors of CYP3A4 may result in higher concentrations of desvenlafaxine).

No products indexed under this heading.

Nicardipine (Concomitant use of desvenlafaxine with a drug metabolized by CYP3A4 can result in lower exposures to that drug).

No products indexed under this heading.

Nicardipine Hydrochloride (Concomitant use of desvenlafaxine with a drug metabolized by CYP3A4 can result in lower exposures to that drug).

No products indexed under this heading.

Nicotinamide (CYP3A4 is a minor pathway for the metabolism of desvenlafaxine. In a clinical study, ketoconazole (200 mg b.i.d.) increased the area under the concentration vs. time curve AUC of desvenlafaxine (400 mg single dose) by about 43% and C_{max} by about 8%. Concomitant use of desvenlafaxine with potent inhibitors of CYP3A4 may result in higher concentrations of desvenlafaxine).

No products indexed under this heading.

Nifedipine (CYP3A4 is a minor pathway for the metabolism of desvenlafaxine. In a clinical study, ketoconazole (200 mg b.i.d.) increased the area under the concentration vs. time curve AUC of desvenlafaxine (400 mg single dose) by about 43% and C_{max} by about 8%. Concomitant use of desvenlafaxine with potent inhibitors of CYP3A4 may result in higher concentrations of desvenlafaxine).

No products indexed under this heading.

Nimodipine (Concomitant use of desvenlafaxine with a drug metabolized by CYP3A4 can result in lower exposures to that drug).

No products indexed under this heading.

Nisoldipine (Concomitant use of desvenlafaxine with a drug metabolized by CYP3A4 can result in lower exposures to that drug).

No products indexed under this heading.

Nitrendipine (Concomitant use of desvenlafaxine with a drug metabolized by CYP3A4 can result in lower exposures to that drug).

No products indexed under this heading.

Norethindrone (Concomitant use of desvenlafaxine with a drug metabolized by CYP3A4 can result in lower exposures to that drug). Products include:

Ortho Micronor 2660

Norethindrone Acetate (Concomitant use of desvenlafaxine with a drug metabolized by CYP3A4 can result in lower exposures to that drug). Products include:

Activella 2561

Norfloxacin (CYP3A4 is a minor pathway for the metabolism of desvenlafaxine. In a clinical study, ketoconazole (200 mg b.i.d.) increased the area under the concentration vs. time curve AUC of desvenlafaxine (400 mg single dose) by about 43% and C_{max} by about 8%. Concomitant use of desvenlafaxine with potent inhibitors of CYP3A4 may result in higher concentrations of desvenlafaxine). Products include:

Noroxin 2220

Norgestrel (Concomitant use of desvenlafaxine with a drug metabolized by CYP3A4 can result in lower exposures to that drug).

No products indexed under this heading.

Nortriptyline Hydrochloride (Concomitant use of desvenlafaxine with a drug metabolized by CYP2D6 can result in higher concentrations of that drug).

No products indexed under this heading.

Olanzapine (Caution is advised when desvenlafaxine is taken in combination with other CNS-active drugs). Products include:

Symbyax 1965
Zyprexa 1984
Zyprexa IntraMuscular 1984
Zyprexa ZYDIS 1984

Omeprazole (CYP3A4 is a minor pathway for the metabolism of desvenlafaxine. In a clinical study, ketoconazole (200 mg b.i.d.) increased the area under the concentration vs. time curve AUC of desvenlafaxine (400 mg single dose) by about 43% and C_{max} by about 8%. Concomitant use of desvenlafaxine with potent inhibitors of CYP3A4 may result in higher concentrations of desvenlafaxine).

No products indexed under this heading.

Ondansetron (Concomitant use of desvenlafaxine with a drug metabolized by CYP2D6 can result in higher concentrations of that drug).

No products indexed under this heading.

Ondansetron Hydrochloride (Concomitant use of desvenlafaxine with a drug metabolized by CYP2D6 can result in higher concentrations of that drug). Products include:

Zofran Injection 1750
Zofran 1756
Zofran ODT 1756

Oxaprozin (Studies have shown that concurrent use of an NSAID may potentiate the risk of upper GI bleeding. Patients should be cautioned about the concomitant use of desvenlafaxine with NSAIDs).

No products indexed under this heading.

Oxazepam (Caution is advised when desvenlafaxine is taken in combination with other CNS-active drugs).

No products indexed under this heading.

Oxycodone Hydrochloride (Caution is advised when desvenlafaxine is taken in combination with other CNS-active drugs). Products include:

OxyContin 2807
Percocet 1121
Percodan 1124

Oxycodone Terephthalate (Caution is advised when desvenlafaxine is taken in combination with other CNS-active drugs).

No products indexed under this heading.

Oxymorphone Hydrochloride (Caution is advised when desvenlafaxine is taken in combination with other CNS-active drugs). Products include:

Opana 1110
Opana ER 1114

Paclitaxel (Concomitant use of desvenlafaxine with a drug metabolized by CYP2D6 can result in higher concentrations of that drug).

No products indexed under this heading.

Pargyline Hydrochloride (Desvenlafaxine must not be used concomitantly in patients taking monoamine oxidase inhibitors (MAOIs) or in patients who have taken MAOIs in the preceding 14 days due to the risk of serious, sometimes fatal, drug interactions with an SNRI. These interactions have been associated with symptoms that include tremor, myoclonus, diaphoresis, nausea, vomiting, flushing, dizziness, hyperthermia with features resembling neuroleptic malignant syndrome, seizures, rigidity, autonomic instability with possible rapid fluctuations of vital signs, and mental status changes. Based on the half-life of desvenlafaxine, at least 7 days should be allowed after stopping desvenlafaxine before starting an MAOI).

No products indexed under this heading.

Paroxetine (The development of potentially life-threatening serotonin syndrome may occur when desvenlafaxine is used concomitantly with SSRIs. Serotonin syndrome symptoms may include mental status changes, autonomic instability, neuromuscular aberrations, and/or gastrointestinal symptoms. If concomitant treatment with desvenlafaxine and an SSRI is clinically warranted, careful observation of the patient is advised, particularly during treatment initiation and dose increases).

No products indexed under this heading.

Paroxetine Hydrochloride (The development of potentially life-threatening serotonin syndrome may occur when desvenlafaxine is used concomitantly with SSRIs. Serotonin syndrome symptoms may include mental status changes, autonomic instability, neuromuscular aberrations, and/or gastrointestinal symptoms. If concomitant treatment with desvenlafaxine and an SSRI is clinically warranted, careful observation of the patient is advised, particularly during treatment initiation and dose increases). Products include:

Paroxetine CR 2361
Paroxetine ER 2371
Paxil 1586
Paxil CR 1596

Paroxetine Mesylate (The development of potentially life-threatening serotonin syndrome may occur when desvenlafaxine is used concomitantly with SSRIs. Serotonin syndrome symptoms may include mental status changes, autonomic instability, neuromuscular aberrations, and/or gastrointestinal symptoms. If concomitant treatment with desvenlafaxine and an SSRI is clinically warranted, careful observation of

the patient is advised, particularly during treatment initiation and dose increases).

No products indexed under this heading.

Pemoline (Caution is advised when desvenlafaxine is taken in combination with other CNS-active drugs).

No products indexed under this heading.

Pentobarbital (Caution is advised when desvenlafaxine is taken in combination with other CNS-active drugs).

No products indexed under this heading.

Pentobarbital Sodium (Caution is advised when desvenlafaxine is taken in combination with other CNS-active drugs). Products include:

Nembutal 2012

Perphenazine (Caution is advised when desvenlafaxine is taken in combination with other CNS-active drugs).

No products indexed under this heading.

Phenelzine Sulfate (Desvenlafaxine must not be used concomitantly in patients taking monoamine oxidase inhibitors (MAOIs) or in patients who have taken MAOIs in the preceding 14 days due to the risk of serious, sometimes fatal, drug interactions with an SNRI. These interactions have been associated with symptoms that include tremor, myoclonus, diaphoresis, nausea, vomiting, flushing, dizziness, hyperthermia with features resembling neuroleptic malignant syndrome, seizures, rigidity, autonomic instability with possible rapid fluctuations of vital signs, and mental status changes. Based on the half-life of desvenlafaxine, at least 7 days should be allowed after stopping desvenlafaxine before starting an MAOI).

No products indexed under this heading.

Phenobarbital (Caution is advised when desvenlafaxine is taken in combination with other CNS-active drugs). Products include:

Donnatal 2711

Phenobarbital Sodium (Caution is advised when desvenlafaxine is taken in combination with other CNS-active drugs).

No products indexed under this heading.

Phenylbutazone (Studies have shown that concurrent use of an NSAID may potentiate the risk of upper GI bleeding. Patients should be cautioned about the concomitant use of desvenlafaxine with NSAIDs).

No products indexed under this heading.

Pimozide (Concomitant use of desvenlafaxine with a drug metabolized by CYP3A4 can result in lower exposures to that drug).

No products indexed under this heading.

Pindolol (Concomitant use of desvenlafaxine with a drug metabolized by CYP2D6 can result in higher concentrations of that drug).

No products indexed under this heading.

Piroxicam (Studies have shown that concurrent use of an NSAID may potentiate the risk of upper GI bleeding. Patients should be cautioned about the concomitant use of desvenlafaxine with NSAIDs).

No products indexed under this heading.

Polyestradiol Phosphate (Concomitant use of desvenlafaxine with a drug metabolized by CYP3A4 can result in lower exposures to that drug).

No products indexed under this heading.

Posaconazole (CYP3A4 is a minor pathway for the metabolism of desvenlafaxine. In a clinical study, ketoconazole (200 mg b.i.d.) increased the area under the concentration vs. time curve AUC of desvenlafaxine (400 mg single dose) by about 43% and C_{max} by about 8%. Concomitant use of desvenlafaxine

1473 Interactions Index Pristiq

with potent inhibitors of CYP3A4 may result in higher concentrations of desvenlafaxine). Products include:
Noxafil 3172

Prazepam (Caution is advised when desvenlafaxine is taken in combination with other CNS-active drugs).
No products indexed under this heading.

Procarbazine Hydrochloride (Desvenlafaxine must not be used concomitantly in patients taking monoamine oxidase inhibitors (MAOIs) or in patients who have taken MAOIs in the preceding 14 days due to the risk of serious, sometimes fatal, drug interactions with an SNRI. These interactions have been associated with symptoms that include tremor, myoclonus, diaphoresis, nausea, vomiting, flushing, dizziness, hyperthermia with features resembling neuroleptic malignant syndrome, seizures, rigidity, autonomic instability with possible rapid fluctuations of vital signs, and mental status changes. Based on the half-life of desvenlafaxine, at least 7 days should be allowed after stopping desvenlafaxine before starting an MAOI).
No products indexed under this heading.

Prochlorperazine (Caution is advised when desvenlafaxine is taken in combination with other CNS-active drugs).
No products indexed under this heading.

Prochlorperazine Edisylate (Caution is advised when desvenlafaxine is taken in combination with other CNS-active drugs).
No products indexed under this heading.

Prochlorperazine Maleate (Caution is advised when desvenlafaxine is taken in combination with other CNS-active drugs).
No products indexed under this heading.

Promethazine (Caution is advised when desvenlafaxine is taken in combination with other CNS-active drugs).
No products indexed under this heading.

Promethazine Hydrochloride (Caution is advised when desvenlafaxine is taken in combination with other CNS-active drugs).
No products indexed under this heading.

Propafenone Hydrochloride (Concomitant use of desvenlafaxine with a drug metabolized by CYP2D6 can result in higher concentrations of that drug). Products include:
Rythmol 1648
Rythmol SR 1652

Propofol (Caution is advised when desvenlafaxine is taken in combination with other CNS-active drugs).
No products indexed under this heading.

Propoxyphene Hydrochloride (Caution is advised when desvenlafaxine is taken in combination with other CNS-active drugs).
No products indexed under this heading.

Propoxyphene Napsylate (Caution is advised when desvenlafaxine is taken in combination with other CNS-active drugs).
No products indexed under this heading.

Propranolol Hydrochloride (Concomitant use of desvenlafaxine with a drug metabolized by CYP2D6 can result in higher concentrations of that drug). Products include:
InnoPran XL 1517

Quazepam (Caution is advised when desvenlafaxine is taken in combination with other CNS-active drugs).
No products indexed under this heading.

Quetiapine Fumarate (Caution is advised when desvenlafaxine is taken in combination with other CNS-active drugs). Products include:
Seroquel 750
Seroquel XR 759

Quinidine (CYP3A4 is a minor pathway for the metabolism of desvenlafaxine. In a clinical study, ketoconazole (200 mg b.i.d.) increased the area under the concentration vs. time curve AUC of desvenlafaxine (400 mg single dose) by about 43% and C_{max} by about 8%. Concomitant use of desvenlafaxine with potent inhibitors of CYP3A4 may result in higher concentrations of desvenlafaxine).
No products indexed under this heading.

Quinidine Gluconate (Concomitant use of desvenlafaxine with a drug metabolized by CYP2D6 can result in higher concentrations of that drug).
No products indexed under this heading.

Quinidine Hydrochloride (CYP3A4 is a minor pathway for the metabolism of desvenlafaxine. In a clinical study, ketoconazole (200 mg b.i.d.) increased the area under the concentration vs. time curve AUC of desvenlafaxine (400 mg single dose) by about 43% and C_{max} by about 8%. Concomitant use of desvenlafaxine with potent inhibitors of CYP3A4 may result in higher concentrations of desvenlafaxine).
No products indexed under this heading.

Quinidine Polygalacturonate (CYP3A4 is a minor pathway for the metabolism of desvenlafaxine. In a clinical study, ketoconazole (200 mg b.i.d.) increased the area under the concentration vs. time curve AUC of desvenlafaxine (400 mg single dose) by about 43% and C_{max} by about 8%. Concomitant use of desvenlafaxine with potent inhibitors of CYP3A4 may result in higher concentrations of desvenlafaxine).
No products indexed under this heading.

Quinidine Sulfate (CYP3A4 is a minor pathway for the metabolism of desvenlafaxine. In a clinical study, ketoconazole (200 mg b.i.d.) increased the area under the concentration vs. time curve AUC of desvenlafaxine (400 mg single dose) by about 43% and C_{max} by about 8%. Concomitant use of desvenlafaxine with potent inhibitors of CYP3A4 may result in higher concentrations of desvenlafaxine).
No products indexed under this heading.

Quinine (CYP3A4 is a minor pathway for the metabolism of desvenlafaxine. In a clinical study, ketoconazole (200 mg b.i.d.) increased the area under the concentration vs. time curve AUC of desvenlafaxine (400 mg single dose) by about 43% and C_{max} by about 8%. Concomitant use of desvenlafaxine with potent inhibitors of CYP3A4 may result in higher concentrations of desvenlafaxine). Products include:
Hyland's Leg Cramps PM with Quinine 3315

Quinine Sulfate (CYP3A4 is a minor pathway for the metabolism of desvenlafaxine. In a clinical study, ketoconazole (200 mg b.i.d.) increased the area under the concentration vs. time curve AUC of desvenlafaxine (400 mg single dose) by about 43% and C_{max} by about 8%. Concomitant use of desvenlafaxine with potent inhibitors of CYP3A4 may result in higher concentrations of desvenlafaxine).
No products indexed under this heading.

Quinupristin (CYP3A4 is a minor pathway for the metabolism of desvenlafaxine. In a clinical study, ketoconazole (200 mg b.i.d.) increased the area under the concentration vs. time curve AUC of desvenlafaxine (400 mg single dose) by about 43% and C_{max} by about 8%. Concomitant use of desvenlafaxine with potent inhibitors of CYP3A4 may result in higher concentrations of desvenlafaxine).
No products indexed under this heading.

Ranitidine Bismuth Citrate (CYP3A4 is a minor pathway for the metabolism of desvenlafaxine. In a clinical study, ketoconazole (200 mg b.i.d.) increased the area under the concentration vs. time curve AUC of desvenlafaxine (400 mg single dose) by about 43% and C_{max} by about 8%. Concomitant use of desvenlafaxine with potent inhibitors of CYP3A4 may result in higher concentrations of desvenlafaxine).
No products indexed under this heading.

Ranitidine Hydrochloride (CYP3A4 is a minor pathway for the metabolism of desvenlafaxine. In a clinical study, ketoconazole (200 mg b.i.d.) increased the area under the concentration vs. time curve AUC of desvenlafaxine (400 mg single dose) by about 43% and C_{max} by about 8%. Concomitant use of desvenlafaxine with potent inhibitors of CYP3A4 may result in higher concentrations of desvenlafaxine). Products include:
Zantac 1737
Zantac Injection 1732
Zantac Pharmacy 1735

Rasagiline Mesylate (Desvenlafaxine must not be used concomitantly in patients taking monoamine oxidase inhibitors (MAOIs) or in patients who have taken MAOIs in the preceding 14 days due to the risk of serious, sometimes fatal, drug interactions with an SNRI. These interactions have been associated with symptoms that include tremor, myoclonus, diaphoresis, nausea, vomiting, flushing, dizziness, hyperthermia with features resembling neuroleptic malignant syndrome, seizures, rigidity, autonomic instability with possible rapid fluctuations of vital signs, and mental status changes. Based on the half-life of desvenlafaxine, at least 7 days should be allowed after stopping desvenlafaxine before starting an MAOI). Products include:
Azilect 3383

Remifentanil Hydrochloride (Caution is advised when desvenlafaxine is taken in combination with other CNS-active drugs).
No products indexed under this heading.

Rifabutin (Concomitant use of desvenlafaxine with a drug metabolized by CYP3A4 can result in lower exposures to that drug).
No products indexed under this heading.

Risperidone (Caution is advised when desvenlafaxine is taken in combination with other CNS-active drugs). Products include:
Risperdal Consta 2682

Ritonavir (CYP3A4 is a minor pathway for the metabolism of desvenlafaxine. In a clinical study, ketoconazole (200 mg b.i.d.) increased the area under the concentration vs. time curve AUC of desvenlafaxine (400 mg single dose) by about 43% and C_{max} by about 8%. Concomitant use of desvenlafaxine with potent inhibitors of CYP3A4 may result in higher concentrations of desvenlafaxine). Products include:
Kaletra 458
Norvir 509

Rizatriptan Benzoate (The development of potentially life-threatening serotonin syndrome may occur when desvenlafaxine is used concomitantly with triptans. Serotonin syndrome symptoms may include mental status changes, autonomic instability, neuromuscular aberrations, and/or gastrointestinal symptoms. If concomitant treatment with desvenlafaxine and a triptan is clinically warranted, careful observation of the patient is advised, particularly during treatment initiation and dose increases). Products include:
Maxalt 2206
Maxalt-MLT 2206

Rofecoxib (Studies have shown that concurrent use of an NSAID may potentiate the risk of upper GI bleeding. Patients should be cautioned about the concomitant use of desvenlafaxine with NSAIDs).
No products indexed under this heading.

Saquinavir (CYP3A4 is a minor pathway for the metabolism of desvenlafaxine. In a clinical study, ketoconazole (200 mg b.i.d.) increased the area under the concentration vs. time curve AUC of desvenlafaxine (400 mg single dose) by about 43% and C_{max} by about 8%. Concomitant use of desvenlafaxine with potent inhibitors of CYP3A4 may result in higher concentrations of desvenlafaxine).
No products indexed under this heading.

Saquinavir Mesylate (CYP3A4 is a minor pathway for the metabolism of desvenlafaxine. In a clinical study, ketoconazole (200 mg b.i.d.) increased the area under the concentration vs. time curve AUC of desvenlafaxine (400 mg single dose) by about 43% and C_{max} by about 8%. Concomitant use of desvenlafaxine with potent inhibitors of CYP3A4 may result in higher concentrations of desvenlafaxine).
No products indexed under this heading.

Secobarbital Sodium (Caution is advised when desvenlafaxine is taken in combination with other CNS-active drugs).
No products indexed under this heading.

Selegiline (Desvenlafaxine must not be used concomitantly in patients taking monoamine oxidase inhibitors (MAOIs) or in patients who have taken MAOIs in the preceding 14 days due to the risk of serious, sometimes fatal, drug interactions with an SNRI. These interactions have been associated with symptoms that include tremor, myoclonus, diaphoresis, nausea, vomiting, flushing, dizziness, hyperthermia with features resembling neuroleptic malignant syndrome, seizures, rigidity, autonomic instability with possible rapid fluctuations of vital signs, and mental status changes. Based on the half-life of desvenlafaxine, at least 7 days should be allowed after stopping desvenlafaxine before starting an MAOI). Products include:
Emsam 3623

Selegiline Hydrochloride (Desvenlafaxine must not be used concomitantly in patients taking monoamine oxidase inhibitors (MAOIs) or in patients who have taken MAOIs in the preceding 14 days due to the risk of serious, sometimes fatal, drug interactions with an SNRI. These interactions have been associated with symptoms that include tremor, myoclonus, diaphoresis, nausea, vomiting, flushing, dizziness, hyperthermia with features resembling neuroleptic malignant syndrome, seizures, rigidity, autonomic instability with possible rapid fluctuations of vital signs, and mental status changes. Based on the half-life of desvenlafaxine, at least 7 days should be allowed after stopping desvenlafaxine before starting an MAOI). Products include:
Eldepryl 3312

Sertraline Hydrochloride (The development of potentially life-threatening serotonin syndrome may occur when desvenlafaxine is used concomitantly with SSRIs. Serotonin syndrome symptoms may include mental status changes, autonomic instability, neuromuscular aberrations, and/or gastrointestinal symptoms. If concomitant treatment with desvenlafaxine and an SSRI is clinically warranted, careful observation of the patient is advised, particularly during treatment initiation and dose increases).
No products indexed under this heading.

IMPORTANT NOTE: Always consult each drug listing in the patient's regimen for possible interactions.

1475 Interactions Index ProAir

tal status changes, autonomic instability, neuromuscular aberrations, and/or gastrointestinal symptoms. If concomitant treatment with desvenlafaxine and another SNRI is clinically warranted, careful observation of the patient is advised, particularly during treatment initiation and dose increases). Products include:
Effexor XR ... **3504**
Venlafaxine Hydrochloride Tablets ... **2388**

Verapamil Hydrochloride (CYP3A4 is a minor pathway for the metabolism of desvenlafaxine. In a clinical study, ketoconazole (200 mg b.i.d.) increased the area under the concentration vs. time curve AUC of desvenlafaxine (400 mg single dose) by about 43% and C_{max} by about 8%. Concomitant use of desvenlafaxine with potent inhibitors of CYP3A4 may result in higher concentrations of desvenlafaxine). Products include:
Tarka ... **534**

Vinblastine Sulfate (Concomitant use of desvenlafaxine with a drug metabolized by CYP2D6 can result in higher concentrations of that drug).
No products indexed under this heading.

Vincristine Sulfate (Concomitant use of desvenlafaxine with a drug metabolized by CYP3A4 can result in lower exposures to that drug).
No products indexed under this heading.

Voriconazole (CYP3A4 is a minor pathway for the metabolism of desvenlafaxine. In a clinical study, ketoconazole (200 mg b.i.d.) increased the area under the concentration vs. time curve AUC of desvenlafaxine (400 mg single dose) by about 43% and C_{max} by about 8%. Concomitant use of desvenlafaxine with potent inhibitors of CYP3A4 may result in higher concentrations of desvenlafaxine).
No products indexed under this heading.

Warfarin Sodium (Altered anticoagulant effects, including increased bleeding, have been reported when SNRIs are co-administered with warfarin. Patients receiving warfarin therapy should be carefully monitored when desvenlafaxine is initiated or discontinued).
No products indexed under this heading.

Zafirlukast (CYP3A4 is a minor pathway for the metabolism of desvenlafaxine. In a clinical study, ketoconazole (200 mg b.i.d.) increased the area under the concentration vs. time curve AUC of desvenlafaxine (400 mg single dose) by about 43% and C_{max} by about 8%. Concomitant use of desvenlafaxine with potent inhibitors of CYP3A4 may result in higher concentrations of desvenlafaxine). Products include:
Accolate ... **3612**

Zaleplon (Caution is advised when desvenlafaxine is taken in combination with other CNS-active drugs).
No products indexed under this heading.

Zileuton (CYP3A4 is a minor pathway for the metabolism of desvenlafaxine. In a clinical study, ketoconazole (200 mg b.i.d.) increased the area under the concentration vs. time curve AUC of desvenlafaxine (400 mg single dose) by about 43% and C_{max} by about 8%. Concomitant use of desvenlafaxine with potent inhibitors of CYP3A4 may result in higher concentrations of desvenlafaxine).
No products indexed under this heading.

Ziprasidone Hydrochloride (Caution is advised when desvenlafaxine is taken in combination with other CNS-active drugs). Products include:
Geodon ... **2723**

Zolmitriptan (The development of potentially life-threatening serotonin syndrome may occur when desvenlafaxine is used concomitantly with triptans. Serotonin syndrome symptoms may include mental status changes, autonomic instability, neuromuscular aberrations, and/or gastrointestinal symptoms. If concomitant treatment with desvenlafaxine and a triptan is clinically warranted, careful observation of the patient is advised, particularly during treatment initiation and dose increases). Products include:
Zomig Tablets ... **773**
Zomig Nasal Spray ... **768**
Zomig-ZMT Tablets ... **773**

Zolpidem Tartrate (Caution is advised when desvenlafaxine is taken in combination with other CNS-active drugs). Products include:
Ambien ... **2920**
Ambien CR ... **2925**

Zonisamide (Concomitant use of desvenlafaxine with a drug metabolized by CYP2D6 can result in higher concentrations of that drug). Products include:
Zonegran ... **1081**

Food Interactions

Alcohol (Caution is advised when desvenlafaxine is taken in combination with other CNS-active drugs).

Beer, reduced-alcohol (A clinical study has shown that desvenlafaxine does not increase the impairment of mental and motor skills caused by ethanol. However, patients should be advised to avoid alcohol consumption while taking desvenlafaxine).

Beer, unspecified (A clinical study has shown that desvenlafaxine does not increase the impairment of mental and motor skills caused by ethanol. However, patients should be advised to avoid alcohol consumption while taking desvenlafaxine).

Grapefruit (CYP3A4 is a minor pathway for the metabolism of desvenlafaxine. In a clinical study, ketoconazole (200 mg b.i.d.) increased the area under the concentration vs. time curve AUC of desvenlafaxine (400 mg single dose) by about 43% and C_{max} by about 8%. Concomitant use of desvenlafaxine with potent inhibitors of CYP3A4 may result in higher concentrations of desvenlafaxine).

Grapefruit Juice (CYP3A4 is a minor pathway for the metabolism of desvenlafaxine. In a clinical study, ketoconazole (200 mg b.i.d.) increased the area under the concentration vs. time curve AUC of desvenlafaxine (400 mg single dose) by about 43% and C_{max} by about 8%. Concomitant use of desvenlafaxine with potent inhibitors of CYP3A4 may result in higher concentrations of desvenlafaxine).

Wine, Chianti (A clinical study has shown that desvenlafaxine does not increase the impairment of mental and motor skills caused by ethanol. However, patients should be advised to avoid alcohol consumption while taking desvenlafaxine).

Wine, Red (A clinical study has shown that desvenlafaxine does not increase the impairment of mental and motor skills caused by ethanol. However, patients should be advised to avoid alcohol consumption while taking desvenlafaxine).

Wine, unspecified (A clinical study has shown that desvenlafaxine does not increase the impairment of mental and motor skills caused by ethanol. However, patients should be advised to avoid alcohol consumption while taking desvenlafaxine).

Wine products (A clinical study has shown that desvenlafaxine does not increase the impairment of mental and motor skills caused by ethanol. However, patients should be advised to avoid alcohol consumption while taking desvenlafaxine).

PROAIR HFA INHALATION AEROSOL

(Albuterol Sulfate) ... **3393**

May interact with alpha adrenergic stimulants, beta-adrenergic stimulating agents, beta-blockers, loop diuretics, monoamine oxidase inhibitors, nonpotassium-sparing diuretics, sympathomimetic aerosol bronchodilators, thiazides, tricyclic antidepressants, and certain other agents. Compounds in these categories include:

Acebutolol Hydrochloride (β-adrenergic-receptor blocking agents not only block the pulmonary effect of β-agonists, such as albuterol sulfate, but may produce severe bronchospasm in asthmatic patients. Therefore, patients with asthma should not normally be treated with β-blockers. However, under certain circumstances, (eg, as prophylaxis after myocardial infarction), there may be no acceptable alternatives to the use of β-adrenergic-blocking agents in patients with asthma. In this setting, cardioselective β-blockers should be considered, although they should be administered with caution).
No products indexed under this heading.

Albuterol (Other short-acting sympathomimetic aerosol bronchodilators should not be used concomitantly with albuterol sulfate. If additional adrenergic drugs are to be administered by any route, they should be used with caution to avoid deleterious cardiovascular effects).
No products indexed under this heading.

Amitriptyline Hydrochloride (Albuterol sulfate should be administered with extreme caution to patients being treated with monoamine oxidase inhibitors or tricyclic antidepressants, or within 2 weeks of discontinuation of such agents, because the action of albuterol on the cardiovascular system may be potentiated).
No products indexed under this heading.

Amoxapine (Albuterol sulfate should be administered with extreme caution to patients being treated with monoamine oxidase inhibitors or tricyclic antidepressants, or within 2 weeks of discontinuation of such agents, because the action of albuterol on the cardiovascular system may be potentiated).
No products indexed under this heading.

Atenolol (β-adrenergic-receptor blocking agents not only block the pulmonary effect of β-agonists, such as albuterol sulfate, but may produce severe bronchospasm in asthmatic patients. Therefore, patients with asthma should not normally be treated with β-blockers. However, under certain circumstances, (eg, as prophylaxis after myocardial infarction), there may be no acceptable alternatives to the use of β-adrenergic-blocking agents in patients with asthma. In this setting, cardioselective β-blockers should be considered, although they should be administered with caution).
No products indexed under this heading.

Bendroflumethiazide (The ECG changes and/or hypokalemia which may result from the administration of non-potassium sparing diuretics (such as loop or thiazide diuretics) can be acutely worsened by β-agonists, especially when the recommended dose of β-agonist is exceeded. Although the clinical significance of these effects is not known, caution is advised in the co-administration of β-agonists with non-potassium sparing diuretics).
No products indexed under this heading.

Betaxolol Hydrochloride (β-adrenergic-receptor blocking agents not only block the pulmonary effect of β-agonists, such as albuterol sulfate, but may produce severe bronchospasm in asthmatic patients. Therefore, patients with asthma should not normally be treated with β-blockers. However, under certain circumstances, (eg, as prophylaxis after myocardial infarction), there may be no acceptable alternatives to the use of β-adrenergic-blocking agents in patients with asthma. In this setting, cardioselective β-blockers should be considered, although they should be administered with caution).
No products indexed under this heading.

Bisoprolol Fumarate (β-adrenergic-receptor blocking agents not only block the pulmonary effect of β-agonists, such as albuterol sulfate, but may produce severe bronchospasm in asthmatic patients. Therefore, patients with asthma should not normally be treated with β-blockers. However, under certain circumstances, (eg, as prophylaxis after myocardial infarction), there may be no acceptable alternatives to the use of β-adrenergic-blocking agents in patients with asthma. In this setting, cardioselective β-blockers should be considered, although they should be administered with caution).
No products indexed under this heading.

Bitolterol Mesylate (Other short-acting sympathomimetic aerosol bronchodilators should not be used concomitantly with albuterol sulfate. If additional adrenergic drugs are to be administered by any route, they should be used with caution to avoid deleterious cardiovascular effects).
No products indexed under this heading.

Bumetanide (The ECG changes and/or hypokalemia which may result from the administration of non-potassium sparing diuretics (such as loop or thiazide diuretics) can be acutely worsened by β-agonists, especially when the recommended dose of β-agonist is exceeded. Although the clinical significance of these effects is not known, caution is advised in the co-administration of β-agonists with non-potassium sparing diuretics).
No products indexed under this heading.

Carteolol Hydrochloride (β-adrenergic-receptor blocking agents not only block the pulmonary effect of β-agonists, such as albuterol sulfate, but may produce severe bronchospasm in asthmatic patients. Therefore, patients with asthma should not normally be treated with β-blockers. However, under certain circumstances, (eg, as prophylaxis after myocardial infarction), there may be no acceptable alternatives to the use of β-adrenergic-blocking agents in patients with asthma. In this setting, cardioselective β-blockers should be considered, although they should be administered with caution).
No products indexed under this heading.

Carvedilol (β-adrenergic-receptor blocking agents not only block the pulmonary effect of β-agonists, such as albuterol sulfate, but may produce severe bronchospasm in asthmatic patients. Therefore, patients with asthma should not normally be treated with β-blockers. However, under certain circumstances, (eg, as prophylaxis after myocardial infarction), there may be no acceptable alternatives to the use of β-adrenergic-blocking agents in patients with asthma. In this setting, cardioselective β-blockers should be considered, although they should be administered with caution). Products include:
Coreg ... **1409**

Carvedilol Phosphate (β-adrenergic-receptor blocking agents not only block the pulmonary effect of β-agonists, such as albuterol sulfate, but may produce severe bronchospasm in asthmat-

IMPORTANT NOTE: Always consult each drug listing in the patient's regimen for possible interactions.

ProAir Interactions Index 1476

ic patients. Therefore, patients with asthma should not normally be treated with β-blockers. However, under certain circumstances, (eg, as prophylaxis after myocardial infarction), there may be no acceptable alternatives to the use of β-adrenergic-blocking agents in patients with asthma. In this setting, cardioselective β-blockers should be considered, although they should be administered with caution). Products include:

Coreg CR 1416

Chlorothiazide (The ECG changes and/or hypokalemia which may result from the administration of non-potassium sparing diuretics (such as loop or thiazide diuretics) can be acutely worsened by β-agonists, especially when the recommended dose of β-agonist is exceeded. Although the clinical significance of these effects is not known, caution is advised in the co-administration of β-agonists with non-potassium sparing diuretics).

No products indexed under this heading.

Chlorothiazide Sodium (The ECG changes and/or hypokalemia which may result from the administration of non-potassium sparing diuretics (such as loop or thiazide diuretics) can be acutely worsened by β-agonists, especially when the recommended dose of β-agonist is exceeded. Although the clinical significance of these effects is not known, caution is advised in the co-administration of β-agonists with non-potassium sparing diuretics). Products include:

Diuril Intravenous 2009

Clomipramine Hydrochloride (Albuterol sulfate should be administered with extreme caution to patients being treated with monoamine oxidase inhibitors or tricyclic antidepressants, or within 2 weeks of discontinuation of such agents, because the action of albuterol on the cardiovascular system may be potentiated).

No products indexed under this heading.

Desipramine Hydrochloride (Albuterol sulfate should be administered with extreme caution to patients being treated with monoamine oxidase inhibitors or tricyclic antidepressants, or within 2 weeks of discontinuation of such agents, because the action of albuterol on the cardiovascular system may be potentiated).

No products indexed under this heading.

Digoxin (Mean decreases of 16% and 22% in serum digoxin levels were demonstrated after single dose intravenous and oral administration of albuterol, respectively, to normal volunteers who had received digoxin for 10 days. The clinical significance of these findings for patients with obstructive airway disease who are receiving albuterol and digoxin on a chronic basis is unclear. Nevertheless, it would be prudent to carefully evaluate the serum digoxin levels in patients who are currently receiving digoxin and albuterol sulfate). Products include:

Lanoxin Injection 1546
Lanoxin Injection Pediatric 1549
Lanoxin Tablets 1553

Dobutamine (If additional adrenergic drugs are to be administered by any route, they should be used with caution to avoid deleterious cardiovascular effects).

No products indexed under this heading.

Dobutamine Hydrochloride (If additional adrenergic drugs are to be administered by any route, they should be used with caution to avoid deleterious cardiovascular effects).

No products indexed under this heading.

Doxepin Hydrochloride (Albuterol sulfate should be administered with extreme caution to patients being treated with monoamine oxidase inhibitors or tricyclic antidepressants, or within 2 weeks of discontinuation of such agents, because the action of albuterol on the cardiovascular system may be potentiated).

No products indexed under this heading.

Ephedrine Hydrochloride (If additional adrenergic drugs are to be administered by any route, they should be used with caution to avoid deleterious cardiovascular effects).

No products indexed under this heading.

Ephedrine Sulfate (If additional adrenergic drugs are to be administered by any route, they should be used with caution to avoid deleterious cardiovascular effects).

No products indexed under this heading.

Ephedrine Tannate (If additional adrenergic drugs are to be administered by any route, they should be used with caution to avoid deleterious cardiovascular effects).

No products indexed under this heading.

Epinephrine (If additional adrenergic drugs are to be administered by any route, they should be used with caution to avoid deleterious cardiovascular effects). Products include:

EpiPen 3631
Twinject 3268

Epinephrine Hydrochloride (If additional adrenergic drugs are to be administered by any route, they should be used with caution to avoid deleterious cardiovascular effects).

No products indexed under this heading.

Esmolol Hydrochloride (β-adrenergic-receptor blocking agents not only block the pulmonary effect of β-agonists, such as albuterol sulfate, but may produce severe bronchospasm in asthmatic patients. Therefore, patients with asthma should not normally be treated with β-blockers. However, under certain circumstances, (eg, as prophylaxis after myocardial infarction), there may be no acceptable alternatives to the use of β-adrenergic-blocking agents in patients with asthma. In this setting, cardioselective β-blockers should be considered, although they should be administered with caution).

No products indexed under this heading.

Ethacrynic Acid (The ECG changes and/or hypokalemia which may result from the administration of non-potassium sparing diuretics (such as loop or thiazide diuretics) can be acutely worsened by β-agonists, especially when the recommended dose of β-agonist is exceeded. Although the clinical significance of these effects is not known, caution is advised in the co-administration of β-agonists with non-potassium sparing diuretics).

No products indexed under this heading.

Furosemide (The ECG changes and/or hypokalemia which may result from the administration of non-potassium sparing diuretics (such as loop or thiazide diuretics) can be acutely worsened by β-agonists, especially when the recommended dose of β-agonist is exceeded. Although the clinical significance of these effects is not known, caution is advised in the co-administration of β-agonists with non-potassium sparing diuretics). Products include:

Furosemide 2354

Hydrochlorothiazide (The ECG changes and/or hypokalemia which may result from the administration of non-potassium sparing diuretics (such as loop or thiazide diuretics) can be acutely worsened by β-agonists, especially when the recommended dose of β-agonist is exceeded. Although the clinical significance of these effects is not known, caution is advised in the co-administration of β-agonists with non-potassium sparing diuretics). Products include:

Atacand HCT 700
Avalide 2956
Benicar HCT 1017
Diovan HCT 2419
Dyazide 1429
Exforge HCT 2449
Hyzaar 2162
Hyzaar 100-12.5 2162
Micardis HCT 889
Prinzide 2246
Tekturna HCT 2541
Teveten HCT 541

Hydroflumethiazide (The ECG changes and/or hypokalemia which may result from the administration of non-potassium sparing diuretics (such as loop or thiazide diuretics) can be acutely worsened by β-agonists, especially when the recommended dose of β-agonist is exceeded. Although the clinical significance of these effects is not known, caution is advised in the co-administration of β-agonists with non-potassium sparing diuretics).

No products indexed under this heading.

Imipramine Hydrochloride (Albuterol sulfate should be administered with extreme caution to patients being treated with monoamine oxidase inhibitors or tricyclic antidepressants, or within 2 weeks of discontinuation of such agents, because the action of albuterol on the cardiovascular system may be potentiated).

No products indexed under this heading.

Imipramine Pamoate (Albuterol sulfate should be administered with extreme caution to patients being treated with monoamine oxidase inhibitors or tricyclic antidepressants, or within 2 weeks of discontinuation of such agents, because the action of albuterol on the cardiovascular system may be potentiated).

No products indexed under this heading.

Isocarboxazid (Albuterol sulfate should be administered with extreme caution to patients being treated with monoamine oxidase inhibitors or tricyclic antidepressants, or within 2 weeks of discontinuation of such agents, because the action of albuterol on the cardiovascular system may be potentiated). Products include:

Marplan 3481

Isoetharine (Other short-acting sympathomimetic aerosol bronchodilators should not be used concomitantly with albuterol sulfate. If additional adrenergic drugs are to be administered by any route, they should be used with caution to avoid deleterious cardiovascular effects).

No products indexed under this heading.

Isoproterenol Hydrochloride (Other short-acting sympathomimetic aerosol bronchodilators should not be used concomitantly with albuterol sulfate. If additional adrenergic drugs are to be administered by any route, they should be used with caution to avoid deleterious cardiovascular effects).

No products indexed under this heading.

Isoproterenol Sulfate (If additional adrenergic drugs are to be administered by any route, they should be used with caution to avoid deleterious cardiovascular effects).

No products indexed under this heading.

Labetalol Hydrochloride (β-adrenergic-receptor blocking agents not only block the pulmonary effect of β-agonists, such as albuterol sulfate, but may produce severe bronchospasm in asthmatic patients. Therefore, patients with asthma should not normally be treated with β-blockers. However, under certain circumstances, (eg, as prophylaxis after myocardial infarction), there may be no acceptable alternatives to the use of β-adrenergic-blocking agents in patients with asthma. In this setting, cardioselective β-blockers should be considered, although they should be administered with caution).

No products indexed under this heading.

Levalbuterol Hydrochloride (Other short-acting sympathomimetic aerosol bronchodilators should not be used concomitantly with albuterol sulfate. If additional adrenergic drugs are to be administered by any route, they should be used with caution to avoid deleterious cardiovascular effects).

No products indexed under this heading.

Levobunolol Hydrochloride (β-adrenergic-receptor blocking agents not only block the pulmonary effect of β-agonists, such as albuterol sulfate, but may produce severe bronchospasm in asthmatic patients. Therefore, patients with asthma should not normally be treated with β-blockers. However, under certain circumstances, (eg, as prophylaxis after myocardial infarction), there may be no acceptable alternatives to the use of β-adrenergic-blocking agents in patients with asthma. In this setting, cardioselective β-blockers should be considered, although they should be administered with caution).

No products indexed under this heading.

Maprotiline Hydrochloride (Albuterol sulfate should be administered with extreme caution to patients being treated with monoamine oxidase inhibitors or tricyclic antidepressants, or within 2 weeks of discontinuation of such agents, because the action of albuterol on the cardiovascular system may be potentiated).

No products indexed under this heading.

Metaproterenol Sulfate (Other short-acting sympathomimetic aerosol bronchodilators should not be used concomitantly with albuterol sulfate. If additional adrenergic drugs are to be administered by any route, they should be used with caution to avoid deleterious cardiovascular effects).

No products indexed under this heading.

Methyclothiazide (The ECG changes and/or hypokalemia which may result from the administration of non-potassium sparing diuretics (such as loop or thiazide diuretics) can be acutely worsened by β-agonists, especially when the recommended dose of β-agonist is exceeded. Although the clinical significance of these effects is not known, caution is advised in the co-administration of β-agonists with non-potassium sparing diuretics).

No products indexed under this heading.

Metipranolol Hydrochloride (β-adrenergic-receptor blocking agents not only block the pulmonary effect of β-agonists, such as albuterol sulfate, but may produce severe bronchospasm in asthmatic patients. Therefore, patients with asthma should not normally be treated with β-blockers. However, under certain circumstances, (eg, as prophylaxis after myocardial infarction), there may be no acceptable alternatives to the use of β-adrenergic-blocking agents in patients with asthma. In this setting, cardioselective β-blockers should be considered, although they should be administered with caution).

No products indexed under this heading.

Metoprolol Succinate (β-adrenergic-receptor blocking agents not only block the pulmonary effect of β-agonists, such as albuterol sulfate, but may produce severe bronchospasm in asthmatic patients. Therefore, patients with asthma should not normally be treated

with β-blockers. However, under certain circumstances, (eg, as prophylaxis after myocardial infarction), there may be no acceptable alternatives to the use of β-adrenergic-blocking agents in patients with asthma. In this setting, cardioselective β-blockers should be considered, although they should be administered with caution). Products include:

Toprol XL 732

Metoprolol Tartrate (β-adrenergic-receptor blocking agents not only block the pulmonary effect of β-agonists, such as albuterol sulfate, but may produce severe bronchospasm in asthmatic patients. Therefore, patients with asthma should not normally be treated with β-blockers. However, under certain circumstances, (eg, as prophylaxis after myocardial infarction), there may be no acceptable alternatives to the use of β-adrenergic-blocking agents in patients with asthma. In this setting, cardioselective β-blockers should be considered, although they should be administered with caution).

No products indexed under this heading.

Moclobemide (Albuterol sulfate should be administered with extreme caution to patients being treated with monoamine oxidase inhibitors or tricyclic antidepressants, or within 2 weeks of discontinuation of such agents, because the action of albuterol on the cardiovascular system may be potentiated).

No products indexed under this heading.

Nadolol (β-adrenergic-receptor blocking agents not only block the pulmonary effect of β-agonists, such as albuterol sulfate, but may produce severe bronchospasm in asthmatic patients. Therefore, patients with asthma should not normally be treated with β-blockers. However, under certain circumstances, (eg, as prophylaxis after myocardial infarction), there may be no acceptable alternatives to the use of β-adrenergic-blocking agents in patients with asthma. In this setting, cardioselective β-blockers should be considered, although they should be administered with caution). Products include:

Nadolol 2359

Naphazoline Hydrochloride (If additional adrenergic drugs are to be administered by any route, they should be used with caution to avoid deleterious cardiovascular effects). Products include:

Visine-A .... ☉257

Nebivolol (β-adrenergic-receptor blocking agents not only block the pulmonary effect of β-agonists, such as albuterol sulfate, but may produce severe bronchospasm in asthmatic patients. Therefore, patients with asthma should not normally be treated with β-blockers. However, under certain circumstances, (eg, as prophylaxis after myocardial infarction), there may be no acceptable alternatives to the use of β-adrenergic-blocking agents in patients with asthma. In this setting, cardioselective β-blockers should be considered, although they should be administered with caution). Products include:

Bystolic 1147

Nortriptyline Hydrochloride (Albuterol sulfate should be administered with extreme caution to patients being treated with monoamine oxidase inhibitors or tricyclic antidepressants, or within 2 weeks of discontinuation of such agents, because the action of albuterol on the cardiovascular system may be potentiated).

No products indexed under this heading.

Oxymetazoline Hydrochloride (If additional adrenergic drugs are to be administered by any route, they should

be used with caution to avoid deleterious cardiovascular effects). Products include:

Sudafed OM Sinus Congestion 2048

Pargyline Hydrochloride (Albuterol sulfate should be administered with extreme caution to patients being treated with monoamine oxidase inhibitors or tricyclic antidepressants, or within 2 weeks of discontinuation of such agents, because the action of albuterol on the cardiovascular system may be potentiated).

No products indexed under this heading.

Penbutolol Sulfate (β-adrenergic-receptor blocking agents not only block the pulmonary effect of β-agonists, such as albuterol sulfate, but may produce severe bronchospasm in asthmatic patients. Therefore, patients with asthma should not normally be treated with β-blockers. However, under certain circumstances, (eg, as prophylaxis after myocardial infarction), there may be no acceptable alternatives to the use of β-adrenergic-blocking agents in patients with asthma. In this setting, cardioselective β-blockers should be considered, although they should be administered with caution).

No products indexed under this heading.

Phenelzine Sulfate (Albuterol sulfate should be administered with extreme caution to patients being treated with monoamine oxidase inhibitors or tricyclic antidepressants, or within 2 weeks of discontinuation of such agents, because the action of albuterol on the cardiovascular system may be potentiated).

No products indexed under this heading.

Phenylephrine Hydrochloride (If additional adrenergic drugs are to be administered by any route, they should be used with caution to avoid deleterious cardiovascular effects). Products include:

Sudafed PE Nasal Decongestant 2048
Children's Sudafed PE Nasal
 Decongestant 2047

Phenylpropanolamine Hydrochloride (If additional adrenergic drugs are to be administered by any route, they should be used with caution to avoid deleterious cardiovascular effects).

No products indexed under this heading.

Pindolol (β-adrenergic-receptor blocking agents not only block the pulmonary effect of β-agonists, such as albuterol sulfate, but may produce severe bronchospasm in asthmatic patients. Therefore, patients with asthma should not normally be treated with β-blockers. However, under certain circumstances, (eg, as prophylaxis after myocardial infarction), there may be no acceptable alternatives to the use of β-adrenergic-blocking agents in patients with asthma. In this setting, cardioselective β-blockers should be considered, although they should be administered with caution).

No products indexed under this heading.

Pirbuterol Acetate (Other short-acting sympathomimetic aerosol bronchodilators should not be used concomitantly with albuterol sulfate. If additional adrenergic drugs are to be administered by any route, they should be used with caution to avoid deleterious cardiovascular effects). Products include:

Maxair Autohaler 1782

Polythiazide (The ECG changes and/or hypokalemia which may result from the administration of non-potassium sparing diuretics (such as loop or thiazide diuretics) can be acutely worsened by β-agonists, especially when the recommended dose of β-agonist is exceeded. Although the clinical significance of these effects is not known,

caution is advised in the co-administration of β-agonists with non-potassium sparing diuretics).

No products indexed under this heading.

Procarbazine Hydrochloride (Albuterol sulfate should be administered with extreme caution to patients being treated with monoamine oxidase inhibitors or tricyclic antidepressants, or within 2 weeks of discontinuation of such agents, because the action of albuterol on the cardiovascular system may be potentiated).

No products indexed under this heading.

Propranolol Hydrochloride (β-adrenergic-receptor blocking agents not only block the pulmonary effect of β-agonists, such as albuterol sulfate, but may produce severe bronchospasm in asthmatic patients. Therefore, patients with asthma should not normally be treated with β-blockers. However, under certain circumstances, (eg, as prophylaxis after myocardial infarction), there may be no acceptable alternatives to the use of β-adrenergic-blocking agents in patients with asthma. In this setting, cardioselective β-blockers should be considered, although they should be administered with caution). Products include:

InnoPran XL 1517

Protriptyline Hydrochloride (Albuterol sulfate should be administered with extreme caution to patients being treated with monoamine oxidase inhibitors or tricyclic antidepressants, or within 2 weeks of discontinuation of such agents, because the action of albuterol on the cardiovascular system may be potentiated).

No products indexed under this heading.

Pseudoephedrine Hydrochloride (If additional adrenergic drugs are to be administered by any route, they should be used with caution to avoid deleterious cardiovascular effects). Products include:

Allegra-D 2915
Allegra-D 24 2918
Sudafed 12 Hour Nasal
 Decongestant Non-Drowsy 2048
Sudafed 24 Hour 2048
Sudafed Nasal Decongestant 2047
Children's Sudafed Nasal
 Decongestant Liquid 2047
Zyrtec-D Allergy & Congestion 2054

Rasagiline Mesylate (Albuterol sulfate should be administered with extreme caution to patients being treated with monoamine oxidase inhibitors or tricyclic antidepressants, or within 2 weeks of discontinuation of such agents, because the action of albuterol on the cardiovascular system may be potentiated). Products include:

Azilect 3383

Salmeterol Xinafoate (Other short-acting sympathomimetic aerosol bronchodilators should not be used concomitantly with albuterol sulfate. If additional adrenergic drugs are to be administered by any route, they should be used with caution to avoid deleterious cardiovascular effects). Products include:

Advair 100/50 1275
Advair 250/50 1275
Advair 500/50 1275
Advair HFA 45/21 1288
Advair HFA 115/21 1288
Advair HFA 230/21 1288
Serevent Diskus 1656

Selegiline (Albuterol sulfate should be administered with extreme caution to patients being treated with monoamine oxidase inhibitors or tricyclic antidepressants, or within 2 weeks of discontinuation of such agents, because the action of albuterol on the cardiovascular system may be potentiated). Products include:

Emsam 3623

Selegiline Hydrochloride (Albuterol sulfate should be administered with extreme caution to patients being treated with monoamine oxidase inhibitors or tricyclic antidepressants, or within 2 weeks of discontinuation of such agents, because the action of albuterol on the cardiovascular system may be potentiated). Products include:

Eldepryl 3312

Sotalol Hydrochloride (β-adrenergic-receptor blocking agents not only block the pulmonary effect of β-agonists, such as albuterol sulfate, but may produce severe bronchospasm in asthmatic patients. Therefore, patients with asthma should not normally be treated with β-blockers. However, under certain circumstances, (eg, as prophylaxis after myocardial infarction), there may be no acceptable alternatives to the use of β-adrenergic-blocking agents in patients with asthma. In this setting, cardioselective β-blockers should be considered, although they should be administered with caution).

No products indexed under this heading.

Terbutaline Sulfate (Other short-acting sympathomimetic aerosol bronchodilators should not be used concomitantly with albuterol sulfate. If additional adrenergic drugs are to be administered by any route, they should be used with caution to avoid deleterious cardiovascular effects).

No products indexed under this heading.

Tetrahydrozoline Hydrochloride (If additional adrenergic drugs are to be administered by any route, they should be used with caution to avoid deleterious cardiovascular effects).

No products indexed under this heading.

Timolol Hemihydrate (β-adrenergic-receptor blocking agents not only block the pulmonary effect of β-agonists, such as albuterol sulfate, but may produce severe bronchospasm in asthmatic patients. Therefore, patients with asthma should not normally be treated with β-blockers. However, under certain circumstances, (eg, as prophylaxis after myocardial infarction), there may be no acceptable alternatives to the use of β-adrenergic-blocking agents in patients with asthma. In this setting, cardioselective β-blockers should be considered, although they should be administered with caution). Products include:

Betimol 3490

Timolol Maleate (β-adrenergic-receptor blocking agents not only block the pulmonary effect of β-agonists, such as albuterol sulfate, but may produce severe bronchospasm in asthmatic patients. Therefore, patients with asthma should not normally be treated with β-blockers. However, under certain circumstances, (eg, as prophylaxis after myocardial infarction), there may be no acceptable alternatives to the use of β-adrenergic-blocking agents in patients with asthma. In this setting, cardioselective β-blockers should be considered, although they should be administered with caution). Products include:

Combigan 601
Dorzolamide
 Hydrochloride/Timolol Maleate
 Ophthalmic Solution .... ☉243
Timoptic in Ocudose .... ☉231

Torsemide (The ECG changes and/or hypokalemia which may result from the administration of non-potassium sparing diuretics (such as loop or thiazide diuretics) can be acutely worsened by β-agonists, especially when the recommended dose of β-agonist is exceeded. Although the clinical significance of these effects is not known, caution is advised in the co-administration of β-agonists with non-potassium sparing diuretics).

No products indexed under this heading.

IMPORTANT NOTE: Always consult each drug listing in the patient's regimen for possible interactions.

ProAir Interactions Index 1478

Tranylcypromine Sulfate (Albuterol sulfate should be administered with extreme caution to patients being treated with monoamine oxidase inhibitors or tricyclic antidepressants, or within 2 weeks of discontinuation of such agents, because the action of albuterol on the cardiovascular system may be potentiated). Products include:
Parnate 1584

Trimipramine Maleate (Albuterol sulfate should be administered with extreme caution to patients being treated with monoamine oxidase inhibitors or tricyclic antidepressants, or within 2 weeks of discontinuation of such agents, because the action of albuterol on the cardiovascular system may be potentiated).
No products indexed under this heading.

PROCOSA II TABLETS
(Calcium Ascorbate, Glucosamine Sulfate, Herbals with Vitamins & Minerals, Manganese, Silicone) 3476
None cited in PDR database.

PROCRIT FOR INJECTION
(Epoetin Alfa) 954
None cited in PDR database.

PROFILNINE SD
(Factor IX Complex) 1797
None cited in PDR database.

PROFLAVANOL 90 TABLETS
(Calcium Ascorbate, Vitamin C, Vitis Vinifera) 3476
None cited in PDR database.

PROGLYCEM CAPSULES
(Diazoxide) 1179
May interact with diuretics, highly protein bound drugs (selected), thiazides, and certain other agents. Compounds in these categories include:

Amiloride Hydrochloride (The concomitant administration of commonly used diuretics may potentiate the hyperglycemic effects of diazoxide).
No products indexed under this heading.

Amiodarone Hydrochloride (Since diazoxide is highly bound to serum proteins, it may displace other substances which are also bound to protein, resulting in higher blood levels of these substances).
No products indexed under this heading.

Amitriptyline Hydrochloride (Since diazoxide is highly bound to serum proteins, it may displace other substances which are also bound to protein, resulting in higher blood levels of these substances).
No products indexed under this heading.

Atovaquone (Since diazoxide is highly bound to serum proteins, it may displace other substances which are also bound to protein, resulting in higher blood levels of these substances). Products include:
Malarone Pediatric Tablets 1572
Malarone 1572
Mepron Suspension 1576

Bendroflumethiazide (The concomitant administration of thiazides may potentiate the hyperglycemic and hyperuricemic effects of diazoxide).
No products indexed under this heading.

Bumetanide (The concomitant administration of commonly used diuretics may potentiate the hyperglycemic effects of diazoxide).
No products indexed under this heading.

Cefonicid Sodium (Since diazoxide is highly bound to serum proteins, it may displace other substances which are also bound to protein, resulting in higher blood levels of these substances).
No products indexed under this heading.

Celecoxib (Since diazoxide is highly bound to serum proteins, it may displace other substances which are also bound to protein, resulting in higher blood levels of these substances). Products include:
Celebrex 3272

Chlordiazepoxide (Since diazoxide is highly bound to serum proteins, it may displace other substances which are also bound to protein, resulting in higher blood levels of these substances).
No products indexed under this heading.

Chlordiazepoxide Hydrochloride (Since diazoxide is highly bound to serum proteins, it may displace other substances which are also bound to protein, resulting in higher blood levels of these substances).
No products indexed under this heading.

Chlorothiazide (The concomitant administration of thiazides may potentiate the hyperglycemic and hyperuricemic effects of diazoxide).
No products indexed under this heading.

Chlorothiazide Sodium (The concomitant administration of thiazides may potentiate the hyperglycemic and hyperuricemic effects of diazoxide). Products include:
Diuril Intravenous 2009

Chlorpromazine (Since diazoxide is highly bound to serum proteins, it may displace other substances which are also bound to protein, resulting in higher blood levels of these substances).
No products indexed under this heading.

Chlorpromazine Hydrochloride (Since diazoxide is highly bound to serum proteins, it may displace other substances which are also bound to protein, resulting in higher blood levels of these substances).
No products indexed under this heading.

Chlorthalidone (The concomitant administration of commonly used diuretics may potentiate the hyperglycemic effects of diazoxide). Products include:
Clorpres 2344

Clomipramine Hydrochloride (Since diazoxide is highly bound to serum proteins, it may displace other substances which are also bound to protein, resulting in higher blood levels of these substances).
No products indexed under this heading.

Clozapine (Since diazoxide is highly bound to serum proteins, it may displace other substances which are also bound to protein, resulting in higher blood levels of these substances).
No products indexed under this heading.

Cyclosporine (Since diazoxide is highly bound to serum proteins, it may displace other substances which are also bound to protein, resulting in higher blood levels of these substances). Products include:
Gengraf 440
Neoral Oral Solution 2496
Neoral Capsules 2496
Restasis 605

Diazepam (Since diazoxide is highly bound to serum proteins, it may displace other substances which are also bound to protein, resulting in higher blood levels of these substances). Products include:
Valium Tablets 2880

Diclofenac Potassium (Since diazoxide is highly bound to serum proteins, it may displace other substances which are also bound to protein, resulting in higher blood levels of these substances).
No products indexed under this heading.

Diclofenac Sodium (Since diazoxide is highly bound to serum proteins, it may displace other substances which are also bound to protein, resulting in higher blood levels of these substances).
No products indexed under this heading.

Digitalis Glycoside Preparations (Since diazoxide is highly bound to serum proteins, it may displace other substances which are also bound to protein, resulting in higher blood levels of these substances).
No products indexed under this heading.

Digitalis Lanata (Since diazoxide is highly bound to serum proteins, it may displace other substances which are also bound to protein, resulting in higher blood levels of these substances).
No products indexed under this heading.

Digitalis Purpurea (Since diazoxide is highly bound to serum proteins, it may displace other substances which are also bound to protein, resulting in higher blood levels of these substances).
No products indexed under this heading.

Diphenylhydantoin (Concomitant administration of oral diazoxide and diphenylhydantoin may result in a loss of seizure control).
No products indexed under this heading.

Diphenylhydantoin Sodium (Concomitant administration of oral diazoxide and diphenylhydantoin may result in a loss of seizure control).
No products indexed under this heading.

Dipyridamole (Since diazoxide is highly bound to serum proteins, it may displace other substances which are also bound to protein, resulting in higher blood levels of these substances). Products include:
Aggrenox 880

Ethacrynic Acid (The concomitant administration of commonly used diuretics may potentiate the hyperglycemic effects of diazoxide).
No products indexed under this heading.

Fenoprofen Calcium (Since diazoxide is highly bound to serum proteins, it may displace other substances which are also bound to protein, resulting in higher blood levels of these substances).
No products indexed under this heading.

Flurazepam Hydrochloride (Since diazoxide is highly bound to serum proteins, it may displace other substances which are also bound to protein, resulting in higher blood levels of these substances).
No products indexed under this heading.

Flurbiprofen (Since diazoxide is highly bound to serum proteins, it may displace other substances which are also bound to protein, resulting in higher blood levels of these substances).
No products indexed under this heading.

Furosemide (The concomitant administration of commonly used diuretics may potentiate the hyperglycemic effects of diazoxide). Products include:
Furosemide 2354

Glipizide (Since diazoxide is highly bound to serum proteins, it may displace other substances which are also bound to protein, resulting in higher blood levels of these substances).
No products indexed under this heading.

Hydrochlorothiazide (The concomitant administration of thiazides may potentiate the hyperglycemic and hyperuricemic effects of diazoxide). Products include:
Atacand HCT 700
Avalide 2956
Benicar HCT 1017
Diovan HCT 2419
Dyazide 1429
Exforge HCT 2449
Hyzaar 2162
Hyzaar 100-12.5 2162
Micardis HCT 889
Prinzide 2246
Tekturna HCT 2541
Teveten HCT 541

Hydroflumethiazide (The concomitant administration of thiazides may potentiate the hyperglycemic and hyperuricemic effects of diazoxide).
No products indexed under this heading.

Ibuprofen (Since diazoxide is highly bound to serum proteins, it may displace other substances which are also bound to protein, resulting in higher blood levels of these substances). Products include:
Motrin IB 2043
Children's Motrin 2044
Children's Motrin Non-Staining Dye-Free 2044
Infants' Motrin 2044
Infants' Motrin Dye-Free 2044
Junior Strength Motrin 2044
Vicoprofen 564

Imipramine Hydrochloride (Since diazoxide is highly bound to serum proteins, it may displace other substances which are also bound to protein, resulting in higher blood levels of these substances).
No products indexed under this heading.

Imipramine Pamoate (Since diazoxide is highly bound to serum proteins, it may displace other substances which are also bound to protein, resulting in higher blood levels of these substances).
No products indexed under this heading.

Indapamide (The concomitant administration of commonly used diuretics may potentiate the hyperglycemic effects of diazoxide). Products include:
Indapamide 2356

Indomethacin (Since diazoxide is highly bound to serum proteins, it may displace other substances which are also bound to protein, resulting in higher blood levels of these substances). Products include:
Indocin 2167

Indomethacin Sodium Trihydrate (Since diazoxide is highly bound to serum proteins, it may displace other substances which are also bound to protein, resulting in higher blood levels of these substances). Products include:
Indocin I.V. 2007

Ketoprofen (Since diazoxide is highly bound to serum proteins, it may displace other substances which are also bound to protein, resulting in higher blood levels of these substances).
No products indexed under this heading.

Ketorolac Tromethamine (Since diazoxide is highly bound to serum proteins, it may displace other substances which are also bound to protein, resulting in higher blood levels of these substances). Products include:
Acuvail .... ⊙209

Meclofenamate Sodium (Since diazoxide is highly bound to serum proteins, it may displace other substances which are also bound to protein, resulting in higher blood levels of these substances).
No products indexed under this heading.

Mefenamic Acid (Since diazoxide is highly bound to serum proteins, it may displace other substances which are also bound to protein, resulting in higher blood levels of these substances).
No products indexed under this heading.

Methyclothiazide (The concomitant administration of thiazides may potentiate the hyperglycemic and hyperuricemic effects of diazoxide).
No products indexed under this heading.

Metolazone (The concomitant administration of commonly used diuretics may potentiate the hyperglycemic effects of diazoxide).
No products indexed under this heading.

Midazolam Hydrochloride (Since diazoxide is highly bound to serum proteins, it may displace other substances which are also bound to protein, resulting in higher blood levels of these substances).
No products indexed under this heading.

Naproxen (Since diazoxide is highly bound to serum proteins, it may displace other substances which are also bound to protein, resulting in higher blood levels of these substances). Products include:
EC-Naprosyn 2850
Naprosyn 2850
Anaprox/Naprosyn 2850

Naproxen Sodium (Since diazoxide is highly bound to serum proteins, it may displace other substances which are also bound to protein, resulting in higher blood levels of these substances). Products include:
Anaprox 2850
Anaprox DS 2850
Treximet 1681

Nortriptyline Hydrochloride (Since diazoxide is highly bound to serum proteins, it may displace other substances which are also bound to protein, resulting in higher blood levels of these substances).
No products indexed under this heading.

Oxaprozin (Since diazoxide is highly bound to serum proteins, it may displace other substances which are also bound to protein, resulting in higher blood levels of these substances).
No products indexed under this heading.

Oxazepam (Since diazoxide is highly bound to serum proteins, it may displace other substances which are also bound to protein, resulting in higher blood levels of these substances).
No products indexed under this heading.

Phenylbutazone (Since diazoxide is highly bound to serum proteins, it may displace other substances which are also bound to protein, resulting in higher blood levels of these substances).
No products indexed under this heading.

Piroxicam (Since diazoxide is highly bound to serum proteins, it may displace other substances which are also bound to protein, resulting in higher blood levels of these substances).
No products indexed under this heading.

Polythiazide (The concomitant administration of thiazides may potentiate the hyperglycemic and hyperuricemic effects of diazoxide).
No products indexed under this heading.

Propranolol Hydrochloride (Since diazoxide is highly bound to serum proteins, it may displace other substances which are also bound to protein, resulting in higher blood levels of these substances). Products include:
InnoPran XL 1517

Spironolactone (The concomitant administration of commonly used diuretics may potentiate the hyperglycemic effects of diazoxide).
No products indexed under this heading.

Sulindac (Since diazoxide is highly bound to serum proteins, it may displace other substances which are also bound to protein, resulting in higher blood levels of these substances). Products include:
Clinoril 2098

Temazepam (Since diazoxide is highly bound to serum proteins, it may displace other substances which are also bound to protein, resulting in higher blood levels of these substances).
No products indexed under this heading.

Tolbutamide (Since diazoxide is highly bound to serum proteins, it may displace other substances which are also bound to protein, resulting in higher blood levels of these substances).
No products indexed under this heading.

Tolmetin Sodium (Since diazoxide is highly bound to serum proteins, it may displace other substances which are also bound to protein, resulting in higher blood levels of these substances).
No products indexed under this heading.

Torsemide (The concomitant administration of commonly used diuretics may potentiate the hyperglycemic effects of diazoxide).
No products indexed under this heading.

Triamterene (The concomitant administration of commonly used diuretics may potentiate the hyperglycemic effects of diazoxide). Products include:
Dyazide 1429
Dyrenium 3495

Trimipramine Maleate (Since diazoxide is highly bound to serum proteins, it may displace other substances which are also bound to protein, resulting in higher blood levels of these substances).
No products indexed under this heading.

Warfarin Sodium (Since diazoxide is highly bound to serum proteins, it may displace other substances which are also bound to protein, resulting in higher blood levels of these substances).
No products indexed under this heading.

PROGLYCEM SUSPENSION

(Diazoxide) 1179
See Proglycem Capsules

PROGRAF CAPSULES

(Tacrolimus) 677
May interact with aminoglycosides, amphotericins, calcium channel blockers, chloramphenicol, cytochrome p450 3a inducers (selected), cytochrome p450 3a inhibitors (selected), cytochrome p450 3a substrates (selected), erythromycin, immunosuppressive agents, killed/inactivated vaccines, methylprednisolone, nephrotoxic agents, phenytoin, potassium sparing diuretics, protease inhibitors, vaccines, live, and certain other agents. Compounds in these categories include:

Abacavir Sulfate (Tacrolimus can cause nephrotoxicity, particularly when used in high doses. Due to the potential for additive or synergistic impairment of renal function, care should be taken when administering tacrolimus with drugs that may be associated with renal dysfunction. These include, but are not limited to, aminoglycosides, amphotericin B, and cisplatin). Products include:
Epzicom 1448
Trizivir 1688
Ziagen 1740

Acyclovir (Tacrolimus can cause nephrotoxicity, particularly when used in high doses. Due to the potential for additive or synergistic impairment of renal function, care should be taken when administering tacrolimus with drugs that may be associated with renal dysfunction. These include, but are not limited to, aminoglycosides, amphotericin B, and cisplatin). Products include:
Zovirax 1760

Acyclovir Sodium (Tacrolimus can cause nephrotoxicity, particularly when used in high doses. Due to the potential for additive or synergistic impairment of renal function, care should be taken when administering tacrolimus with drugs that may be associated with renal dysfunction. These include, but are not limited to, aminoglycosides, amphotericin B, and cisplatin).
No products indexed under this heading.

Alatrofloxacin Mesylate (Tacrolimus can cause nephrotoxicity, particularly when used in high doses. Due to the potential for additive or synergistic impairment of renal function, care should be taken when administering tacrolimus with drugs that may be associated with renal dysfunction. These include, but are not limited to, aminoglycosides, amphotericin B, and cisplatin).
No products indexed under this heading.

Aldesleukin (Tacrolimus can cause nephrotoxicity, particularly when used in high doses. Due to the potential for additive or synergistic impairment of renal function, care should be taken when administering tacrolimus with drugs that may be associated with renal dysfunction. These include, but are not limited to, aminoglycosides, amphotericin B, and cisplatin). Products include:
Proleukin 2504

Alfentanil Hydrochloride (Care should be exercised when drugs that are metabolized by CYP3A (eg, nelfinavir, ritonavir) are administered concomitantly with tacrolimus).
No products indexed under this heading.

Allium sativum (Since tacrolimus is metabolized mainly by the CYP3A enzyme systems, drugs known to induce these enzyme systems may result in an increased metabolism of tacrolimus or decreased bioavailability as indicated by decreased whole blood or plasma concentrations. Monitoring of blood concentrations and appropriate dosage adjustments are essential when such drugs are used concomitantly).
No products indexed under this heading.

Alprazolam (Care should be exercised when drugs that are metabolized by CYP3A (eg, nelfinavir, ritonavir) are administered concomitantly with tacrolimus).
No products indexed under this heading.

Aluminum Hydroxide (In a single-dose crossover study in healthy volunteers, co-administration of tacrolimus and magnesium-aluminum-hydroxide resulted in a 21% increase in the mean tacrolimus AUC and a 10% decrease in the mean tacrolimus C_{max} relative to tacrolimus administration alone).
No products indexed under this heading.

Amikacin Sulfate (Due to the potential for additive or synergistic impairment of renal function, care should be taken when administering tacrolimus with drugs that may be associated with renal dysfunction. These include, but are not limited to, aminoglycosides, amphotericin B, and cisplatin).
No products indexed under this heading.

Amiloride Hydrochloride (Since tacrolimus may cause hyperkalemia, potassium-sparing diuretics should be avoided).
No products indexed under this heading.

Aminophylline (Care should be exercised when drugs that are metabolized by CYP3A (eg, nelfinavir, ritonavir) are administered concomitantly with tacrolimus).
No products indexed under this heading.

Amiodarone Hydrochloride (Since tacrolimus is metabolized mainly by the CYP3A enzyme systems, substances known to inhibit these enzymes may decrease the metabolism or increase bioavailability of tacrolimus as indicated by increased whole blood or plasma concentrations. Monitoring of blood concentrations and appropriate dosage adjustments are essential when such drugs are used concomitantly).
No products indexed under this heading.

Amitriptyline Hydrochloride (Care should be exercised when drugs that are metabolized by CYP3A (eg, nelfinavir, ritonavir) are administered concomitantly with tacrolimus).
No products indexed under this heading.

Amlodipine Besylate (While calcium-channel blocking agents can be effective in treating tacrolimus-associated hypertension, care should be taken since interference with tacrolimus metabolism may require a dosage reduction). Products include:
Azor 1010
Exforge 2443
Exforge HCT 2449

Amoxicillin (Tacrolimus can cause nephrotoxicity, particularly when used in high doses. Due to the potential for additive or synergistic impairment of renal function, care should be taken when administering tacrolimus with drugs that may be associated with renal dysfunction. These include, but are not limited to, aminoglycosides, amphotericin B, and cisplatin). Products include:
Amoxil Capsules 1311
Amoxil Chewable Tablets 1311
Amoxil 1311
Amoxil Powder 1311
Augmentin 1331
Augmentin Tablets 1335
Augmentin ES-600 1338
Augmentin XR 1342
Moxatag 2321

Amoxicillin Trihydrate (Tacrolimus can cause nephrotoxicity, particularly when used in high doses. Due to the potential for additive or synergistic impairment of renal function, care should be taken when administering tacrolimus with drugs that may be associated with renal dysfunction. These include, but are not limited to, aminoglycosides, amphotericin B, and cisplatin).
No products indexed under this heading.

Amphotericin B (Due to the potential for additive or synergistic impairment of renal function, care should be taken when administering tacrolimus with drugs that may be associated with renal dysfunction. These include, but are not limited to, aminoglycosides, amphotericin B, and cisplatin).
No products indexed under this heading.

Amphotericin B, liposomal (Due to the potential for additive or synergistic impairment of renal function, care should be taken when administering tacrolimus with drugs that may be associated with renal dysfunction. These include, but are not limited to, aminoglycosides, amphotericin B, and cisplatin). Products include:
AmBisome 659

Amphotericin B Cholesteryl Sulfate (Due to the potential for additive or synergistic impairment of renal function, care should be taken when administering tacrolimus with drugs that may be associated with renal dysfunction. These include, but are not limited to, aminoglycosides, amphotericin B, and cisplatin).
No products indexed under this heading.

Prograf Interactions Index 1480

Amphotericin B Lipid Complex (Due to the potential for additive or synergistic impairment of renal function, care should be taken when administering tacrolimus with drugs that may be associated with renal dysfunction. These include, but are not limited to, aminoglycosides, amphotericin B, and cisplatin).
No products indexed under this heading.

Ampicillin (Tacrolimus can cause nephrotoxicity, particularly when used in high doses. Due to the potential for additive or synergistic impairment of renal function, care should be taken when administering tacrolimus with drugs that may be associated with renal dysfunction. These include, but are not limited to, aminoglycosides, amphotericin B, and cisplatin).
No products indexed under this heading.

Ampicillin Sodium (Tacrolimus can cause nephrotoxicity, particularly when used in high doses. Due to the potential for additive or synergistic impairment of renal function, care should be taken when administering tacrolimus with drugs that may be associated with renal dysfunction. These include, but are not limited to, aminoglycosides, amphotericin B, and cisplatin).
No products indexed under this heading.

Ampicillin Trihydrate (Tacrolimus can cause nephrotoxicity, particularly when used in high doses. Due to the potential for additive or synergistic impairment of renal function, care should be taken when administering tacrolimus with drugs that may be associated with renal dysfunction. These include, but are not limited to, aminoglycosides, amphotericin B, and cisplatin).
No products indexed under this heading.

Amprenavir (Co-administration of protease inhibitors with tacrolimus may increase tacrolimus blood concentrations).
No products indexed under this heading.

Aprepitant (Since tacrolimus is metabolized mainly by the CYP3A enzyme systems, drugs known to induce these enzyme systems may result in an increased metabolism of tacrolimus or decreased bioavailability as indicated by decreased whole blood or plasma concentrations. Monitoring of blood concentrations and appropriate dosage adjustments are essential when such drugs are used concomitantly). Products include:
Emend 2124

Aspirin (Tacrolimus can cause nephrotoxicity, particularly when used in high doses. Due to the potential for additive or synergistic impairment of renal function, care should be taken when administering tacrolimus with drugs that may be associated with renal dysfunction. These include, but are not limited to, aminoglycosides, amphotericin B, and cisplatin). Products include:
Aggrenox 880
Bayer Aspirin 829
Percodan 1124
St. Joseph Aspirin 2045

Astemizole (Care should be exercised when drugs that are metabolized by CYP3A (eg, nelfinavir, ritonavir) are administered concomitantly with tacrolimus).
No products indexed under this heading.

Atazanavir (Co-administration of protease inhibitors with tacrolimus may increase tacrolimus blood concentrations).
No products indexed under this heading.

Atazanavir Sulfate (Co-administration of protease inhibitors with tacrolimus may increase tacrolimus blood concentrations).
No products indexed under this heading.

Atorvastatin Calcium (Tacrolimus can cause nephrotoxicity, particularly when used in high doses. Due to the potential for additive or synergistic impairment of renal function, care should be taken when administering tacrolimus with drugs that may be associated with renal dysfunction. These include, but are not limited to, aminoglycosides, amphotericin B, and cisplatin). Products include:
Lipitor 2703

Azathioprine (Because of the danger of oversuppression of the immune system, which can increase susceptibility to infection, combination immunosuppressant therapy should be used with caution).
No products indexed under this heading.

Azithromycin Dihydrate (Tacrolimus can cause nephrotoxicity, particularly when used in high doses. Due to the potential for additive or synergistic impairment of renal function, care should be taken when administering tacrolimus with drugs that may be associated with renal dysfunction. These include, but are not limited to, aminoglycosides, amphotericin B, and cisplatin).
No products indexed under this heading.

Azlocillin Sodium (Tacrolimus can cause nephrotoxicity, particularly when used in high doses. Due to the potential for additive or synergistic impairment of renal function, care should be taken when administering tacrolimus with drugs that may be associated with renal dysfunction. These include, but are not limited to, aminoglycosides, amphotericin B, and cisplatin).
No products indexed under this heading.

Aztreonam (Tacrolimus can cause nephrotoxicity, particularly when used in high doses. Due to the potential for additive or synergistic impairment of renal function, care should be taken when administering tacrolimus with drugs that may be associated with renal dysfunction. These include, but are not limited to, aminoglycosides, amphotericin B, and cisplatin).
No products indexed under this heading.

Bacampicillin Hydrochloride (Tacrolimus can cause nephrotoxicity, particularly when used in high doses. Due to the potential for additive or synergistic impairment of renal function, care should be taken when administering tacrolimus with drugs that may be associated with renal dysfunction. These include, but are not limited to, aminoglycosides, amphotericin B, and cisplatin).
No products indexed under this heading.

Bacitracin (Tacrolimus can cause nephrotoxicity, particularly when used in high doses. Due to the potential for additive or synergistic impairment of renal function, care should be taken when administering tacrolimus with drugs that may be associated with renal dysfunction. These include, but are not limited to, aminoglycosides, amphotericin B, and cisplatin).
No products indexed under this heading.

Bacitracin Zinc (Tacrolimus can cause nephrotoxicity, particularly when used in high doses. Due to the potential for additive or synergistic impairment of renal function, care should be taken when administering tacrolimus with drugs that may be associated with renal dysfunction. These include, but are not limited to, aminoglycosides, amphotericin B, and cisplatin).
No products indexed under this heading.

Balsalazide Disodium (Tacrolimus can cause nephrotoxicity, particularly when used in high doses. Due to the potential for additive or synergistic impairment of renal function, care should be taken when administering tacrolimus with drugs that may be associated with renal dysfunction. These include, but are not limited to, aminoglycosides, amphotericin B, and cisplatin).
No products indexed under this heading.

Basiliximab (Because of the danger of oversuppression of the immune system, which can increase susceptibility to infection, combination immunosuppressant therapy should be used with caution). Products include:
Simulect 2524

BCG Vaccine (Immunosuppressants may affect vaccination. Therefore, during treatment with tacrolimus, vaccination may be less effective. The use of live vaccines should be avoided; live vaccines may include, but are not limited to, measles, mumps, rubella, oral polio, BCG, yellow fever, and TY 21a typhoid).
No products indexed under this heading.

Benazepril Hydrochloride (Tacrolimus can cause nephrotoxicity, particularly when used in high doses. Due to the potential for additive or synergistic impairment of renal function, care should be taken when administering tacrolimus with drugs that may be associated with renal dysfunction. These include, but are not limited to, aminoglycosides, amphotericin B, and cisplatin).
No products indexed under this heading.

Bendroflumethiazide (Tacrolimus can cause nephrotoxicity, particularly when used in high doses. Due to the potential for additive or synergistic impairment of renal function, care should be taken when administering tacrolimus with drugs that may be associated with renal dysfunction. These include, but are not limited to, aminoglycosides, amphotericin B, and cisplatin).
No products indexed under this heading.

Bepridil Hydrochloride (While calcium-channel blocking agents can be effective in treating tacrolimus-associated hypertension, care should be taken since interference with tacrolimus metabolism may require a dosage reduction).
No products indexed under this heading.

Bromocriptine Mesylate (Co-administration of bromocriptine with tacrolimus may increase tacrolimus blood concentrations).
No products indexed under this heading.

Buspirone Hydrochloride (Care should be exercised when drugs that are metabolized by CYP3A (eg, nelfinavir, ritonavir) are administered concomitantly with tacrolimus).
No products indexed under this heading.

Busulfan (Care should be exercised when drugs that are metabolized by CYP3A (eg, nelfinavir, ritonavir) are administered concomitantly with tacrolimus). Products include:
Myleran 1581

Caffeine (Tacrolimus can cause nephrotoxicity, particularly when used in high doses. Due to the potential for additive or synergistic impairment of renal function, care should be taken when administering tacrolimus with drugs that may be associated with renal dysfunction. These include, but are not limited to, aminoglycosides, amphotericin B, and cisplatin).
No products indexed under this heading.

Captopril (Tacrolimus can cause nephrotoxicity, particularly when used in high doses. Due to the potential for additive or synergistic impairment of renal function, care should be taken when administering tacrolimus with drugs that may be associated with renal dysfunction. These include, but are not limited to, aminoglycosides, amphotericin B, and cisplatin). Products include:
Captopril 2341

Carbamazepine (Co-administration of carbamazepine with tacrolimus may decrease tacrolimus blood concentrations). Products include:
Carbatrol 3280
Equetro 3477

Carbenicillin Disodium (Tacrolimus can cause nephrotoxicity, particularly when used in high doses. Due to the potential for additive or synergistic impairment of renal function, care should be taken when administering tacrolimus with drugs that may be associated with renal dysfunction. These include, but are not limited to, aminoglycosides, amphotericin B, and cisplatin).
No products indexed under this heading.

Carbenicillin Indanyl Sodium (Tacrolimus can cause nephrotoxicity, particularly when used in high doses. Due to the potential for additive or synergistic impairment of renal function, care should be taken when administering tacrolimus with drugs that may be associated with renal dysfunction. These include, but are not limited to, aminoglycosides, amphotericin B, and cisplatin).
No products indexed under this heading.

Carboplatin (Tacrolimus can cause nephrotoxicity, particularly when used in high doses. Due to the potential for additive or synergistic impairment of renal function, care should be taken when administering tacrolimus with drugs that may be associated with renal dysfunction. These include, but are not limited to, aminoglycosides, amphotericin B, and cisplatin).
No products indexed under this heading.

Carmustine (BCNU) (Tacrolimus can cause nephrotoxicity, particularly when used in high doses. Due to the potential for additive or synergistic impairment of renal function, care should be taken when administering tacrolimus with drugs that may be associated with renal dysfunction. These include, but are not limited to, aminoglycosides, amphotericin B, and cisplatin).
No products indexed under this heading.

Caspofungin acetate (Co-administration of caspofungin with tacrolimus may decrease tacrolimus blood concentrations). Products include:
Cancidas 2088

Cefaclor (Tacrolimus can cause nephrotoxicity, particularly when used in high doses. Due to the potential for additive or synergistic impairment of renal function, care should be taken when administering tacrolimus with drugs that may be associated with renal dysfunction. These include, but are not limited to, aminoglycosides, amphotericin B, and cisplatin).
No products indexed under this heading.

Cefadroxil (Tacrolimus can cause nephrotoxicity, particularly when used in high doses. Due to the potential for additive or synergistic impairment of renal function, care should be taken when administering tacrolimus with drugs that may be associated with renal dysfunction. These include, but are not limited to, aminoglycosides, amphotericin B, and cisplatin).
No products indexed under this heading.

1481 Interactions Index Prograf

Cefamandole Nafate (Tacrolimus can cause nephrotoxicity, particularly when used in high doses. Due to the potential for additive or synergistic impairment of renal function, care should be taken when administering tacrolimus with drugs that may be associated with renal dysfunction. These include, but are not limited to, aminoglycosides, amphotericin B, and cisplatin).
No products indexed under this heading.

Cefazolin Sodium (Tacrolimus can cause nephrotoxicity, particularly when used in high doses. Due to the potential for additive or synergistic impairment of renal function, care should be taken when administering tacrolimus with drugs that may be associated with renal dysfunction. These include, but are not limited to, aminoglycosides, amphotericin B, and cisplatin).
No products indexed under this heading.

Cefdinir (Tacrolimus can cause nephrotoxicity, particularly when used in high doses. Due to the potential for additive or synergistic impairment of renal function, care should be taken when administering tacrolimus with drugs that may be associated with renal dysfunction. These include, but are not limited to, aminoglycosides, amphotericin B, and cisplatin). Products include:
Omnicef Capsules 518
Omnicef Oral Suspension 518

Cefepime Hydrochloride (Tacrolimus can cause nephrotoxicity, particularly when used in high doses. Due to the potential for additive or synergistic impairment of renal function, care should be taken when administering tacrolimus with drugs that may be associated with renal dysfunction. These include, but are not limited to, aminoglycosides, amphotericin B, and cisplatin).
No products indexed under this heading.

Cefixime (Tacrolimus can cause nephrotoxicity, particularly when used in high doses. Due to the potential for additive or synergistic impairment of renal function, care should be taken when administering tacrolimus with drugs that may be associated with renal dysfunction. These include, but are not limited to, aminoglycosides, amphotericin B, and cisplatin). Products include:
Suprax for Oral Suspension 2038
Suprax Tablets 2038

Cefmetazole Sodium (Tacrolimus can cause nephrotoxicity, particularly when used in high doses. Due to the potential for additive or synergistic impairment of renal function, care should be taken when administering tacrolimus with drugs that may be associated with renal dysfunction. These include, but are not limited to, aminoglycosides, amphotericin B, and cisplatin).
No products indexed under this heading.

Cefonicid Sodium (Tacrolimus can cause nephrotoxicity, particularly when used in high doses. Due to the potential for additive or synergistic impairment of renal function, care should be taken when administering tacrolimus with drugs that may be associated with renal dysfunction. These include, but are not limited to, aminoglycosides, amphotericin B, and cisplatin).
No products indexed under this heading.

Cefoperazone Sodium (Tacrolimus can cause nephrotoxicity, particularly when used in high doses. Due to the potential for additive or synergistic impairment of renal function, care should be taken when administering tacrolimus with drugs that may be associated with renal dysfunction. These include, but are not limited to, aminoglycosides, amphotericin B, and cisplatin).
No products indexed under this heading.

Ceforanide (Tacrolimus can cause nephrotoxicity, particularly when used in high doses. Due to the potential for additive or synergistic impairment of renal function, care should be taken when administering tacrolimus with drugs that may be associated with renal dysfunction. These include, but are not limited to, aminoglycosides, amphotericin B, and cisplatin).
No products indexed under this heading.

Cefotaxime Sodium (Tacrolimus can cause nephrotoxicity, particularly when used in high doses. Due to the potential for additive or synergistic impairment of renal function, care should be taken when administering tacrolimus with drugs that may be associated with renal dysfunction. These include, but are not limited to, aminoglycosides, amphotericin B, and cisplatin).
No products indexed under this heading.

Cefotetan (Tacrolimus can cause nephrotoxicity, particularly when used in high doses. Due to the potential for additive or synergistic impairment of renal function, care should be taken when administering tacrolimus with drugs that may be associated with renal dysfunction. These include, but are not limited to, aminoglycosides, amphotericin B, and cisplatin).
No products indexed under this heading.

Cefoxitin Sodium (Tacrolimus can cause nephrotoxicity, particularly when used in high doses. Due to the potential for additive or synergistic impairment of renal function, care should be taken when administering tacrolimus with drugs that may be associated with renal dysfunction. These include, but are not limited to, aminoglycosides, amphotericin B, and cisplatin).
No products indexed under this heading.

Cefpodoxime Proxetil (Tacrolimus can cause nephrotoxicity, particularly when used in high doses. Due to the potential for additive or synergistic impairment of renal function, care should be taken when administering tacrolimus with drugs that may be associated with renal dysfunction. These include, but are not limited to, aminoglycosides, amphotericin B, and cisplatin).
No products indexed under this heading.

Cefprozil (Tacrolimus can cause nephrotoxicity, particularly when used in high doses. Due to the potential for additive or synergistic impairment of renal function, care should be taken when administering tacrolimus with drugs that may be associated with renal dysfunction. These include, but are not limited to, aminoglycosides, amphotericin B, and cisplatin).
No products indexed under this heading.

Ceftazidime (Tacrolimus can cause nephrotoxicity, particularly when used in high doses. Due to the potential for additive or synergistic impairment of renal function, care should be taken when administering tacrolimus with drugs that may be associated with renal dysfunction. These include, but are not limited to, aminoglycosides, amphotericin B, and cisplatin). Products include:
Fortaz 1481

Ceftizoxime Sodium (Tacrolimus can cause nephrotoxicity, particularly when used in high doses. Due to the potential for additive or synergistic impairment of renal function, care should be taken when administering tacrolimus with drugs that may be associated with renal dysfunction. These include, but are not limited to, aminoglycosides, amphotericin B, and cisplatin).
No products indexed under this heading.

Ceftriaxone Sodium (Tacrolimus can cause nephrotoxicity, particularly when used in high doses. Due to the potential for additive or synergistic impairment of renal function, care should be taken when administering tacrolimus with drugs that may be associated with renal dysfunction. These include, but are not limited to, aminoglycosides, amphotericin B, and cisplatin). Products include:
Rocephin 2859

Cefuroxime Axetil (Tacrolimus can cause nephrotoxicity, particularly when used in high doses. Due to the potential for additive or synergistic impairment of renal function, care should be taken when administering tacrolimus with drugs that may be associated with renal dysfunction. These include, but are not limited to, aminoglycosides, amphotericin B, and cisplatin). Products include:
Ceftin 1399

Cefuroxime Sodium (Tacrolimus can cause nephrotoxicity, particularly when used in high doses. Due to the potential for additive or synergistic impairment of renal function, care should be taken when administering tacrolimus with drugs that may be associated with renal dysfunction. These include, but are not limited to, aminoglycosides, amphotericin B, and cisplatin).
No products indexed under this heading.

Celecoxib (Tacrolimus can cause nephrotoxicity, particularly when used in high doses. Due to the potential for additive or synergistic impairment of renal function, care should be taken when administering tacrolimus with drugs that may be associated with renal dysfunction. These include, but are not limited to, aminoglycosides, amphotericin B, and cisplatin). Products include:
Celebrex 3272

Cephalexin (Tacrolimus can cause nephrotoxicity, particularly when used in high doses. Due to the potential for additive or synergistic impairment of renal function, care should be taken when administering tacrolimus with drugs that may be associated with renal dysfunction. These include, but are not limited to, aminoglycosides, amphotericin B, and cisplatin).
No products indexed under this heading.

Cephalothin Sodium (Tacrolimus can cause nephrotoxicity, particularly when used in high doses. Due to the potential for additive or synergistic impairment of renal function, care should be taken when administering tacrolimus with drugs that may be associated with renal dysfunction. These include, but are not limited to, aminoglycosides, amphotericin B, and cisplatin).
No products indexed under this heading.

Cephapirin Sodium (Tacrolimus can cause nephrotoxicity, particularly when used in high doses. Due to the potential for additive or synergistic impairment of renal function, care should be taken when administering tacrolimus with drugs that may be associated with renal dysfunction. These include, but are not limited to, aminoglycosides, amphotericin B, and cisplatin).
No products indexed under this heading.

Cephradine (Tacrolimus can cause nephrotoxicity, particularly when used in high doses. Due to the potential for additive or synergistic impairment of renal function, care should be taken when administering tacrolimus with drugs that may be associated with renal dysfunction. These include, but are not limited to, aminoglycosides, amphotericin B, and cisplatin).
No products indexed under this heading.

Cerivastatin Sodium (Tacrolimus can cause nephrotoxicity, particularly when used in high doses. Due to the potential for additive or synergistic impairment of renal function, care should be taken when administering tacrolimus with drugs that may be associated with renal dysfunction. These include, but are not limited to, aminoglycosides, amphotericin B, and cisplatin).
No products indexed under this heading.

Chloramphenicol (Co-administration of chloramphenicol with tacrolimus may increase tacrolimus blood concentrations).
No products indexed under this heading.

Chloramphenicol Palmitate (Co-administration of chloramphenicol with tacrolimus may increase tacrolimus blood concentrations).
No products indexed under this heading.

Chloramphenicol Sodium Succinate (Co-administration of chloramphenicol with tacrolimus may increase tacrolimus blood concentrations).
No products indexed under this heading.

Chlorothiazide (Tacrolimus can cause nephrotoxicity, particularly when used in high doses. Due to the potential for additive or synergistic impairment of renal function, care should be taken when administering tacrolimus with drugs that may be associated with renal dysfunction. These include, but are not limited to, aminoglycosides, amphotericin B, and cisplatin).
No products indexed under this heading.

Chlorothiazide Sodium (Tacrolimus can cause nephrotoxicity, particularly when used in high doses. Due to the potential for additive or synergistic impairment of renal function, care should be taken when administering tacrolimus with drugs that may be associated with renal dysfunction. These include, but are not limited to, aminoglycosides, amphotericin B, and cisplatin). Products include:
Diuril Intravenous 2009

Chlorpheniramine (Care should be exercised when drugs that are metabolized by CYP3A (eg, nelfinavir, ritonavir) are administered concomitantly with tacrolimus).
No products indexed under this heading.

Chlorpheniramine Maleate (Care should be exercised when drugs that are metabolized by CYP3A (eg, nelfinavir, ritonavir) are administered concomitantly with tacrolimus).
No products indexed under this heading.

Chlorpheniramine Polistirex (Care should be exercised when drugs that are metabolized by CYP3A (eg, nelfinavir, ritonavir) are administered concomitantly with tacrolimus). Products include:
Tussionex 3443

Chlorpheniramine Tannate (Care should be exercised when drugs that are metabolized by CYP3A (eg, nelfinavir, ritonavir) are administered concomitantly with tacrolimus).
No products indexed under this heading.

Chlorpropamide (Tacrolimus can cause nephrotoxicity, particularly when used in high doses. Due to the potential for additive or synergistic impairment of renal function, care should be taken when administering tacrolimus with drugs that may be associated with renal dysfunction. These include, but are not limited to, aminoglycosides, amphotericin B, and cisplatin).
No products indexed under this heading.

IMPORTANT NOTE: Always consult each drug listing in the patient's regimen for possible interactions.

Cidofovir (Tacrolimus can cause nephrotoxicity, particularly when used in high doses. Due to the potential for additive or synergistic impairment of renal function, care should be taken when administering tacrolimus with drugs that may be associated with renal dysfunction. These include, but are not limited to, aminoglycosides, amphotericin B, and cisplatin).
No products indexed under this heading.

Cilastatin Sodium (Tacrolimus can cause nephrotoxicity, particularly when used in high doses. Due to the potential for additive or synergistic impairment of renal function, care should be taken when administering tacrolimus with drugs that may be associated with renal dysfunction. These include, but are not limited to, aminoglycosides, amphotericin B, and cisplatin). Products include:
Primaxin I.M. 2232
Primaxin I.V. 2235

Cilostazol (Care should be exercised when drugs that are metabolized by CYP3A (eg, nelfinavir, ritonavir) are administered concomitantly with tacrolimus).
No products indexed under this heading.

Cimetidine (Co-administration of cimetidine with tacrolimus may increase tacrolimus blood concentrations).
No products indexed under this heading.

Cimetidine Hydrochloride (Co-administration of cimetidine with tacrolimus may increase tacrolimus blood concentrations).
No products indexed under this heading.

Ciprofloxacin (Since tacrolimus is metabolized mainly by the CYP3A enzyme systems, substances known to inhibit these enzymes may decrease the metabolism or increase bioavailability of tacrolimus as indicated by increased whole blood or plasma concentrations. Monitoring of blood concentrations and appropriate dosage adjustments are essential when such drugs are used concomitantly). Products include:
Cipro I.V. 3082
Cipro 3073
Cipro XR 3091
Ciprodex 583

Ciprofloxacin Hydrochloride (Since tacrolimus is metabolized mainly by the CYP3A enzyme systems, substances known to inhibit these enzymes may decrease the metabolism or increase bioavailability of tacrolimus as indicated by increased whole blood or plasma concentrations. Monitoring of blood concentrations and appropriate dosage adjustments are essential when such drugs are used concomitantly). Products include:
Cipro 3073

Cisapride (Co-administration of cisapride with tacrolimus may increase tacrolimus blood concentrations).
No products indexed under this heading.

Cisplatin (Due to the potential for additive or synergistic impairment of renal function, care should be taken when administering tacrolimus with drugs that may be associated with renal dysfunction. These include, but are not limited to, aminoglycosides, amphotericin B, and cisplatin).
No products indexed under this heading.

Cladribine (Tacrolimus can cause nephrotoxicity, particularly when used in high doses. Due to the potential for additive or synergistic impairment of renal function, care should be taken when administering tacrolimus with drugs that may be associated with renal dysfunction. These include, but are not limited to, aminoglycosides, amphotericin B, and cisplatin). Products include:
Leustatin 946

Clarithromycin (Co-administration of clarithromycin with tacrolimus may increase tacrolimus blood concentrations). Products include:
Biaxin/Biaxin XL 412

Clotrimazole (Co-administration of clotrimazole with tacrolimus may increase tacrolimus blood concentrations). Products include:
Lotrisone 3163

Clotrimazole, Topical (Co-administration of clotrimazole with tacrolimus may increase tacrolimus blood concentrations).
No products indexed under this heading.

Clozapine (Tacrolimus can cause nephrotoxicity, particularly when used in high doses. Due to the potential for additive or synergistic impairment of renal function, care should be taken when administering tacrolimus with drugs that may be associated with renal dysfunction. These include, but are not limited to, aminoglycosides, amphotericin B, and cisplatin).
No products indexed under this heading.

Colistimethate Sodium (Tacrolimus can cause nephrotoxicity, particularly when used in high doses. Due to the potential for additive or synergistic impairment of renal function, care should be taken when administering tacrolimus with drugs that may be associated with renal dysfunction. These include, but are not limited to, aminoglycosides, amphotericin B, and cisplatin).
No products indexed under this heading.

Colistin Sulfate (Tacrolimus can cause nephrotoxicity, particularly when used in high doses. Due to the potential for additive or synergistic impairment of renal function, care should be taken when administering tacrolimus with drugs that may be associated with renal dysfunction. These include, but are not limited to, aminoglycosides, amphotericin B, and cisplatin).
No products indexed under this heading.

Cyclophosphamide (Tacrolimus can cause nephrotoxicity, particularly when used in high doses. Due to the potential for additive or synergistic impairment of renal function, care should be taken when administering tacrolimus with drugs that may be associated with renal dysfunction. These include, but are not limited to, aminoglycosides, amphotericin B, and cisplatin).
No products indexed under this heading.

Cyclosporine (Co-administration of cyclosporine with tacrolimus may increase tacrolimus blood concentrations. Initial clinical experience with the co-administration of tacrolimus and cyclosporine resulted in additive/synergistic nephrotoxicity. Tacrolimus should not be used simultaneously with cyclosporine. Tacrolimus or cyclosporine should be discontinued at least 24 hours before initiating the other. In the presence of elevated tacrolimus or cyclosporine concentrations, dosing with the other drug usually should be further delayed). Products include:
Gengraf 440
Neoral Oral Solution 2496
Neoral Capsules 2496
Restasis 605

Cytarabine (Tacrolimus can cause nephrotoxicity, particularly when used in high doses. Due to the potential for additive or synergistic impairment of renal function, care should be taken when administering tacrolimus with drugs that may be associated with renal dysfunction. These include, but are not limited to, aminoglycosides, amphotericin B, and cisplatin).
No products indexed under this heading.

Cytarabine Liposome (Tacrolimus can cause nephrotoxicity, particularly when used in high doses. Due to the potential for additive or synergistic impairment of renal function, care should be taken when administering tacrolimus with drugs that may be associated with renal dysfunction. These include, but are not limited to, aminoglycosides, amphotericin B, and cisplatin).
No products indexed under this heading.

Danazol (Co-administration of danazol with tacrolimus may increase tacrolimus blood concentrations).
No products indexed under this heading.

Darunavir (Co-administration of protease inhibitors with tacrolimus may increase tacrolimus blood concentrations).
No products indexed under this heading.

Delavirdine Mesylate (Tacrolimus can cause nephrotoxicity, particularly when used in high doses. Due to the potential for additive or synergistic impairment of renal function, care should be taken when administering tacrolimus with drugs that may be associated with renal dysfunction. These include, but are not limited to, aminoglycosides, amphotericin B, and cisplatin).
No products indexed under this heading.

Desogestrel (Care should be exercised when drugs that are metabolized by CYP3A (eg, nelfinavir, ritonavir) are administered concomitantly with tacrolimus).
No products indexed under this heading.

Dexamethasone (Since tacrolimus is metabolized mainly by the CYP3A enzyme systems, drugs known to induce these enzyme systems may result in an increased metabolism of tacrolimus or decreased bioavailability as indicated by decreased whole blood or plasma concentrations. Monitoring of blood concentrations and appropriate dosage adjustments are essential when such drugs are used concomitantly). Products include:
Ciprodex 583
Ozurdex .... ⊙223
Tobramycin and Dexamethasone
Ophthalmic Suspension .... ⊙251

Dexamethasone Acetate (Care should be exercised when drugs that are metabolized by CYP3A (eg, nelfinavir, ritonavir) are administered concomitantly with tacrolimus).
No products indexed under this heading.

Dexamethasone Phosphate (Care should be exercised when drugs that are metabolized by CYP3A (eg, nelfinavir, ritonavir) are administered concomitantly with tacrolimus).
No products indexed under this heading.

Dexamethasone Sodium (Care should be exercised when drugs that are metabolized by CYP3A (eg, nelfinavir, ritonavir) are administered concomitantly with tacrolimus).
No products indexed under this heading.

Dexamethasone Sodium Phosphate (Care should be exercised when drugs that are metabolized by CYP3A (eg, nelfinavir, ritonavir) are administered concomitantly with tacrolimus).
No products indexed under this heading.

Diatrizoate Meglumine (Tacrolimus can cause nephrotoxicity, particularly when used in high doses. Due to the potential for additive or synergistic impairment of renal function, care should be taken when administering tacrolimus with drugs that may be associated with renal dysfunction. These include, but are not limited to, aminoglycosides, amphotericin B, and cisplatin).
No products indexed under this heading.

Diatrizoate Sodium (Tacrolimus can cause nephrotoxicity, particularly when used in high doses. Due to the potential for additive or synergistic impairment of renal function, care should be taken when administering tacrolimus with drugs that may be associated with renal dysfunction. These include, but are not limited to, aminoglycosides, amphotericin B, and cisplatin).
No products indexed under this heading.

Diazepam (Care should be exercised when drugs that are metabolized by CYP3A (eg, nelfinavir, ritonavir) are administered concomitantly with tacrolimus). Products include:
Valium Tablets 2880

Diclofenac Potassium (Tacrolimus can cause nephrotoxicity, particularly when used in high doses. Due to the potential for additive or synergistic impairment of renal function, care should be taken when administering tacrolimus with drugs that may be associated with renal dysfunction. These include, but are not limited to, aminoglycosides, amphotericin B, and cisplatin).
No products indexed under this heading.

Diclofenac Sodium (Tacrolimus can cause nephrotoxicity, particularly when used in high doses. Due to the potential for additive or synergistic impairment of renal function, care should be taken when administering tacrolimus with drugs that may be associated with renal dysfunction. These include, but are not limited to, aminoglycosides, amphotericin B, and cisplatin).
No products indexed under this heading.

Dicloxacillin Sodium (Tacrolimus can cause nephrotoxicity, particularly when used in high doses. Due to the potential for additive or synergistic impairment of renal function, care should be taken when administering tacrolimus with drugs that may be associated with renal dysfunction. These include, but are not limited to, aminoglycosides, amphotericin B, and cisplatin).
No products indexed under this heading.

Didanosine (Tacrolimus can cause nephrotoxicity, particularly when used in high doses. Due to the potential for additive or synergistic impairment of renal function, care should be taken when administering tacrolimus with drugs that may be associated with renal dysfunction. These include, but are not limited to, aminoglycosides, amphotericin B, and cisplatin).
No products indexed under this heading.

Dihydroergotamine Mesylate (Care should be exercised when drugs that are metabolized by CYP3A (eg, nelfinavir, ritonavir) are administered concomitantly with tacrolimus).
No products indexed under this heading.

Dihydrostreptomycin (Due to the potential for additive or synergistic impairment of renal function, care should be taken when administering tacrolimus with drugs that may be associated with renal dysfunction. These include, but are not limited to, aminoglycosides, amphotericin B, and cisplatin).
No products indexed under this heading.

Diltiazem Hydrochloride (Co-administration of diltiazem with tacrolimus may increase tacrolimus blood concentrations). Products include:
Cardizem LA 423

Diltiazem Maleate (Co-administration of diltiazem with tacrolimus may increase tacrolimus blood concentrations).
No products indexed under this heading.

(⊙ Described in PDR® for Ophthalmic Medicines)

Diphtheria & Tetanus Toxoids and Acellular Pertussis Vaccine Adsorbed, Hepatitis B (recombinant) and Inactivated Poliovirus Vaccine Combined (Immunosuppressants may affect vaccination. Therefore, during treatment with tacrolimus, vaccination may be less effective).
No products indexed under this heading.

Disopyramide Phosphate (Care should be exercised when drugs that are metabolized by CYP3A (eg, nelfinavir, ritonavir) are administered concomitantly with tacrolimus).
No products indexed under this heading.

Doxorubicin Hydrochloride (Care should be exercised when drugs that are metabolized by CYP3A (eg, nelfinavir, ritonavir) are administered concomitantly with tacrolimus).
No products indexed under this heading.

Dronabinol (Care should be exercised when drugs that are metabolized by CYP3A (eg, nelfinavir, ritonavir) are administered concomitantly with tacrolimus).
No products indexed under this heading.

Dyphylline (Care should be exercised when drugs that are metabolized by CYP3A (eg, nelfinavir, ritonavir) are administered concomitantly with tacrolimus).
No products indexed under this heading.

Efavirenz (Tacrolimus can cause nephrotoxicity, particularly when used in high doses. Due to the potential for additive or synergistic impairment of renal function, care should be taken when administering tacrolimus with drugs that may be associated with renal dysfunction. These include, but are not limited to, aminoglycosides, amphotericin B, and cisplatin). Products include:
Atripla 906

Emtricitabine (Tacrolimus can cause nephrotoxicity, particularly when used in high doses. Due to the potential for additive or synergistic impairment of renal function, care should be taken when administering tacrolimus with drugs that may be associated with renal dysfunction. These include, but are not limited to, aminoglycosides, amphotericin B, and cisplatin). Products include:

Enalapril Maleate (Tacrolimus can cause nephrotoxicity, particularly when used in high doses. Due to the potential for additive or synergistic impairment of renal function, care should be taken when administering tacrolimus with drugs that may be associated with renal dysfunction. These include, but are not limited to, aminoglycosides, amphotericin B, and cisplatin).
No products indexed under this heading.

Enalaprilat (Tacrolimus can cause nephrotoxicity, particularly when used in high doses. Due to the potential for additive or synergistic impairment of renal function, care should be taken when administering tacrolimus with drugs that may be associated with renal dysfunction. These include, but are not limited to, aminoglycosides, amphotericin B, and cisplatin).
No products indexed under this heading.

Enfuvirtide (Tacrolimus can cause nephrotoxicity, particularly when used in high doses. Due to the potential for additive or synergistic impairment of renal function, care should be taken when administering tacrolimus with drugs that may be associated with renal dysfunction. These include, but are not limited to, aminoglycosides, amphotericin B, and cisplatin).
No products indexed under this heading.

Ergotamine Tartrate (Care should be exercised when drugs that are metabolized by CYP3A (eg, nelfinavir, ritonavir) are administered concomitantly with tacrolimus).
No products indexed under this heading.

Erythromycin (Co-administration of erythromycin with tacrolimus may increase tacrolimus blood concentrations).
No products indexed under this heading.

Erythromycin, Topical (Co-administration of erythromycin with tacrolimus may increase tacrolimus blood concentrations).
No products indexed under this heading.

Erythromycin Estolate (Co-administration of erythromycin with tacrolimus may increase tacrolimus blood concentrations).
No products indexed under this heading.

Erythromycin Ethylsuccinate (Co-administration of erythromycin with tacrolimus may increase tacrolimus blood concentrations). Products include:

Erythromycin Gluceptate (Co-administration of erythromycin with tacrolimus may increase tacrolimus blood concentrations).
No products indexed under this heading.

Erythromycin Lactobionate (Co-administration of erythromycin with tacrolimus may increase tacrolimus blood concentrations).
No products indexed under this heading.

Erythromycin Stearate (Co-administration of erythromycin with tacrolimus may increase tacrolimus blood concentrations).
No products indexed under this heading.

Estrogen (Care should be exercised when drugs that are metabolized by CYP3A (eg, nelfinavir, ritonavir) are administered concomitantly with tacrolimus).
No products indexed under this heading.

Estrogens, Conjugated (Care should be exercised when drugs that are metabolized by CYP3A (eg, nelfinavir, ritonavir) are administered concomitantly with tacrolimus). Products include:

Estrogens, Conjugated, Synthetic A (Care should be exercised when drugs that are metabolized by CYP3A (eg, nelfinavir, ritonavir) are administered concomitantly with tacrolimus).
No products indexed under this heading.

Estrogens, Esterified (Care should be exercised when drugs that are metabolized by CYP3A (eg, nelfinavir, ritonavir) are administered concomitantly with tacrolimus).
No products indexed under this heading.

Ethinyl Estradiol (Co-administration of ethinyl estradiol with tacrolimus may increase tacrolimus blood concentrations). Products include:

Ethiodized Oil (Tacrolimus can cause nephrotoxicity, particularly when used in high doses. Due to the potential for additive or synergistic impairment of renal function, care should be taken when administering tacrolimus with drugs that may be associated with renal dysfunction. These include, but are not limited to, aminoglycosides, amphotericin B, and cisplatin).
No products indexed under this heading.

Ethosuximide (Since tacrolimus is metabolized mainly by the CYP3A enzyme systems, drugs known to induce these enzyme systems may result in an increased metabolism of tacrolimus or decreased bioavailability as indicated by decreased whole blood or plasma concentrations. Monitoring of blood concentrations and appropriate dosage adjustments are essential when such drugs are used concomitantly).
No products indexed under this heading.

Ethynodiol Diacetate (Care should be exercised when drugs that are metabolized by CYP3A (eg, nelfinavir, ritonavir) are administered concomitantly with tacrolimus).
No products indexed under this heading.

Etodolac (Tacrolimus can cause nephrotoxicity, particularly when used in high doses. Due to the potential for additive or synergistic impairment of renal function, care should be taken when administering tacrolimus with drugs that may be associated with renal dysfunction. These include, but are not limited to, aminoglycosides, amphotericin B, and cisplatin).
No products indexed under this heading.

Etoposide (Care should be exercised when drugs that are metabolized by CYP3A (eg, nelfinavir, ritonavir) are administered concomitantly with tacrolimus).
No products indexed under this heading.

Etoposide Phosphate (Care should be exercised when drugs that are metabolized by CYP3A (eg, nelfinavir, ritonavir) are administered concomitantly with tacrolimus).
No products indexed under this heading.

Fat (The rate and extent of tacrolimus absorption were greatest under fasted conditions. The presence and composition of food decreased both the rate and extent of tacrolimus absorption. The effect was most pronounced with a high-fat meal (848 kcal, 46% fat): mean AUC and C_{max} were decreased 37% and 77%, respectively; T_{max} was lengthened 5-fold. A high-carbohydrate meal (668 kcal, 85% carbohydrate) decreased mean AUC and mean C_{max} by 28% and 65%, respectively. The time of the meal also affected tacrolimus bioavailability. When given immediately following the meal, mean C_{max} was reduced 71%, and mean AUC was reduced 39%, relative to the fasted condition. When administered 1.5 hours following the meal, mean C_{max} was reduced 63%, and mean AUC was reduced 39%, relative to the fasted condition).
No products indexed under this heading.

Felodipine (While calcium-channel blocking agents can be effective in treating tacrolimus-associated hypertension, care should be taken since interference with tacrolimus metabolism may require a dosage reduction).
No products indexed under this heading.

Fenoprofen Calcium (Tacrolimus can cause nephrotoxicity, particularly when used in high doses. Due to the potential for additive or synergistic impairment of renal function, care should be taken when administering tacrolimus with drugs that may be associated with renal dysfunction. These include, but are not limited to, aminoglycosides, amphotericin B, and cisplatin).
No products indexed under this heading.

Fentanyl (Care should be exercised when drugs that are metabolized by CYP3A (eg, nelfinavir, ritonavir) are administered concomitantly with tacrolimus). Products include:

Fentanyl Citrate (Care should be exercised when drugs that are metabolized by CYP3A (eg, nelfinavir, ritonavir) are administered concomitantly with tacrolimus). Products include:

Filgrastim (Tacrolimus can cause nephrotoxicity, particularly when used in high doses. Due to the potential for additive or synergistic impairment of renal function, care should be taken when administering tacrolimus with drugs that may be associated with renal dysfunction. These include, but are not limited to, aminoglycosides, amphotericin B, and cisplatin). Products include:

Fluconazole (Co-administration of fluconazole with tacrolimus may increase tacrolimus blood concentrations).
No products indexed under this heading.

Fluorouracil (Tacrolimus can cause nephrotoxicity, particularly when used in high doses. Due to the potential for additive or synergistic impairment of renal function, care should be taken when administering tacrolimus with drugs that may be associated with renal dysfunction. These include, but are not limited to, aminoglycosides, amphotericin B, and cisplatin). Products include:

Fluoxetine (Since tacrolimus is metabolized mainly by the CYP3A enzyme systems, substances known to inhibit these enzymes may decrease the metabolism or increase bioavailability of tacrolimus as indicated by increased whole blood or plasma concentrations. Monitoring of blood concentrations and appropriate dosage adjustments are essential when such drugs are used concomitantly).
No products indexed under this heading.

Fluoxetine Hydrochloride (Since tacrolimus is metabolized mainly by the CYP3A enzyme systems, substances known to inhibit these enzymes may decrease the metabolism or increase bioavailability of tacrolimus as indicated by increased whole blood or plasma concentrations. Monitoring of blood concentrations and appropriate dosage adjustments are essential when such drugs are used concomitantly). Products include:

Flurbiprofen (Tacrolimus can cause nephrotoxicity, particularly when used in high doses. Due to the potential for additive or synergistic impairment of renal function, care should be taken when administering tacrolimus with drugs that may be associated with renal dysfunction. These include, but are not limited to, aminoglycosides, amphotericin B, and cisplatin).
No products indexed under this heading.

Fluvastatin Sodium (Tacrolimus can cause nephrotoxicity, particularly when used in high doses. Due to the potential for additive or synergistic impairment of renal function, care should be taken when administering tacrolimus with drugs that may be associated with renal dysfunction. These include, but are not limited to, aminoglycosides, amphotericin B, and cisplatin).
No products indexed under this heading.

Fluvoxamine Maleate (Since tacrolimus is metabolized mainly by the CYP3A enzyme systems, substances known to inhibit these enzymes may decrease the metabolism or increase bioavailability of tacrolimus as indicated by increased whole blood or plasma concentrations. Monitoring of blood concentrations and appropriate dosage adjustments are essential when such drugs are used concomitantly).
No products indexed under this heading.

Fosamprenavir Calcium (Co-administration of protease inhibitors with tacrolimus may increase tacrolimus blood concentrations). Products include:
Lexiva Oral Suspension 1558
Lexiva 1558

Foscarnet Sodium (Tacrolimus can cause nephrotoxicity, particularly when used in high doses. Due to the potential for additive or synergistic impairment of renal function, care should be taken when administering tacrolimus with drugs that may be associated with renal dysfunction. These include, but are not limited to, aminoglycosides, amphotericin B, and cisplatin).
No products indexed under this heading.

Fosinopril Sodium (Tacrolimus can cause nephrotoxicity, particularly when used in high doses. Due to the potential for additive or synergistic impairment of renal function, care should be taken when administering tacrolimus with drugs that may be associated with renal dysfunction. These include, but are not limited to, aminoglycosides, amphotericin B, and cisplatin).
No products indexed under this heading.

Fosphenytoin (Tacrolimus may affect the pharmacokinetics of other drugs (eg, phenytoin) and increase their concentration. Co-administration of phenytoin with tacrolimus may decrease tacrolimus blood concentrations).
No products indexed under this heading.

Fosphenytoin Sodium (Tacrolimus may affect the pharmacokinetics of other drugs (eg, phenytoin) and increase their concentration. Co-administration of phenytoin with tacrolimus may decrease tacrolimus blood concentrations).
No products indexed under this heading.

Furosemide (Tacrolimus can cause nephrotoxicity, particularly when used in high doses. Due to the potential for additive or synergistic impairment of renal function, care should be taken when administering tacrolimus with drugs that may be associated with renal dysfunction. These include, but are not limited to, aminoglycosides, amphotericin B, and cisplatin). Products include:
Furosemide 2354

Gadopentetate Dimeglumine (Tacrolimus can cause nephrotoxicity, particularly when used in high doses. Due to the potential for additive or synergistic impairment of renal function, care should be taken when administering tacrolimus with drugs that may be associated with renal dysfunction. These include, but are not limited to, aminoglycosides, amphotericin B, and cisplatin).
No products indexed under this heading.

Ganciclovir (Care should be exercised when drugs that are nephrotoxic (eg, ganciclovir) are administered concomitantly with tacrolimus).
No products indexed under this heading.

Ganciclovir Sodium (Care should be exercised when drugs that are nephrotoxic (eg, ganciclovir) are administered concomitantly with tacrolimus).
No products indexed under this heading.

Gentamicin (Due to the potential for additive or synergistic impairment of renal function, care should be taken when administering tacrolimus with drugs that may be associated with renal dysfunction. These include, but are not limited to, aminoglycosides, amphotericin B, and cisplatin).
No products indexed under this heading.

Gentamicin Sulfate (Due to the potential for additive or synergistic impairment of renal function, care should be taken when administering tacrolimus with drugs that may be associated with renal dysfunction. These include, but are not limited to, aminoglycosides, amphotericin B, and cisplatin). Products include:
Pred-G .... ⊙226, ⊙227

Glipizide (Tacrolimus can cause nephrotoxicity, particularly when used in high doses. Due to the potential for additive or synergistic impairment of renal function, care should be taken when administering tacrolimus with drugs that may be associated with renal dysfunction. These include, but are not limited to, aminoglycosides, amphotericin B, and cisplatin).
No products indexed under this heading.

Globulin, Immune (Human) (Tacrolimus can cause nephrotoxicity, particularly when used in high doses. Due to the potential for additive or synergistic impairment of renal function, care should be taken when administering tacrolimus with drugs that may be associated with renal dysfunction. These include, but are not limited to, aminoglycosides, amphotericin B, and cisplatin). Products include:

Glyburide (Tacrolimus can cause nephrotoxicity, particularly when used in high doses. Due to the potential for additive or synergistic impairment of renal function, care should be taken when administering tacrolimus with drugs that may be associated with renal dysfunction. These include, but are not limited to, aminoglycosides, amphotericin B, and cisplatin).
No products indexed under this heading.

Gold Therapy (Tacrolimus can cause nephrotoxicity, particularly when used in high doses. Due to the potential for additive or synergistic impairment of renal function, care should be taken when administering tacrolimus with drugs that may be associated with renal dysfunction. These include, but are not limited to, aminoglycosides, amphotericin B, and cisplatin).
No products indexed under this heading.

Haloperidol (Care should be exercised when drugs that are metabolized by CYP3A (eg, nelfinavir, ritonavir) are administered concomitantly with tacrolimus).
No products indexed under this heading.

Haloperidol Decanoate (Care should be exercised when drugs that are metabolized by CYP3A (eg, nelfinavir, ritonavir) are administered concomitantly with tacrolimus).
No products indexed under this heading.

Hepatitis A Vaccine, Inactivated (Immunosuppressants may affect vaccination. Therefore, during treatment with tacrolimus, vaccination may be less effective). Products include:
Havrix 1485

Twinrix 1694
Vaqta 2281

HMG-CoA Reductase Inhibitors (Tacrolimus can cause nephrotoxicity, particularly when used in high doses. Due to the potential for additive or synergistic impairment of renal function, care should be taken when administering tacrolimus with drugs that may be associated with renal dysfunction. These include, but are not limited to, aminoglycosides, amphotericin B, and cisplatin).
No products indexed under this heading.

Hydrochlorothiazide (Tacrolimus can cause nephrotoxicity, particularly when used in high doses. Due to the potential for additive or synergistic impairment of renal function, care should be taken when administering tacrolimus with drugs that may be associated with renal dysfunction. These include, but are not limited to, aminoglycosides, amphotericin B, and cisplatin). Products include:
Atacand HCT 700
Avalide 2956
Benicar HCT 1017
Diovan HCT 2419
Dyazide 1429
Exforge HCT 2449
Hyzaar 2162
Hyzaar 100-12.5 2162
Micardis HCT 889
Prinzide 2246
Tekturna HCT 2541
Teveten HCT 541

Hydroflumethiazide (Tacrolimus can cause nephrotoxicity, particularly when used in high doses. Due to the potential for additive or synergistic impairment of renal function, care should be taken when administering tacrolimus with drugs that may be associated with renal dysfunction. These include, but are not limited to, aminoglycosides, amphotericin B, and cisplatin).
No products indexed under this heading.

Hypericum Perforatum (St. John's Wort (hypericum perforatum) induces CYP3A4 and P-glycoprotein. Since tacrolimus is a substrate for CYP3A4, there is the potential that the use of St. John's Wort in patients receiving tacrolimus could result in reduced tacrolimus levels). Products include:
Traumeel 1800

Ibuprofen (Tacrolimus can cause nephrotoxicity, particularly when used in high doses. Due to the potential for additive or synergistic impairment of renal function, care should be taken when administering tacrolimus with drugs that may be associated with renal dysfunction. These include, but are not limited to, aminoglycosides, amphotericin B, and cisplatin). Products include:
Motrin IB 2043
Children's Motrin 2044
Children's Motrin Non-Staining
Dye-Free 2044
Infants' Motrin 2044
Infants' Motrin Dye-Free 2044
Junior Strength Motrin 2044
Vicoprofen 564

Idarubicin Hydrochloride (Tacrolimus can cause nephrotoxicity, particularly when used in high doses. Due to the potential for additive or synergistic impairment of renal function, care should be taken when administering tacrolimus with drugs that may be associated with renal dysfunction. These include, but are not limited to, aminoglycosides, amphotericin B, and cisplatin).
No products indexed under this heading.

Ifosfamide (Tacrolimus can cause nephrotoxicity, particularly when used in high doses. Due to the potential for additive or synergistic impairment of renal function, care should be taken when administering tacrolimus with drugs that may be associated with renal dysfunction. These include, but are not limited to, aminoglycosides, amphotericin B, and cisplatin).
No products indexed under this heading.

Imipenem (Tacrolimus can cause nephrotoxicity, particularly when used in high doses. Due to the potential for additive or synergistic impairment of renal function, care should be taken when administering tacrolimus with drugs that may be associated with renal dysfunction. These include, but are not limited to, aminoglycosides, amphotericin B, and cisplatin). Products include:
Primaxin I.M. 2232
Primaxin I.V. 2235

Imipramine Hydrochloride (Care should be exercised when drugs that are metabolized by CYP3A (eg, nelfinavir, ritonavir) are administered concomitantly with tacrolimus).
No products indexed under this heading.

Imipramine Pamoate (Care should be exercised when drugs that are metabolized by CYP3A (eg, nelfinavir, ritonavir) are administered concomitantly with tacrolimus).
No products indexed under this heading.

Immune Globulin Intravenous (Human) (Tacrolimus can cause nephrotoxicity, particularly when used in high doses. Due to the potential for additive or synergistic impairment of renal function, care should be taken when administering tacrolimus with drugs that may be associated with renal dysfunction. These include, but are not limited to, aminoglycosides, amphotericin B, and cisplatin). Products include:
Flebogamma 5% DIF 1794
Gammagard 812, 815
Gamunex 3374

Indinavir Sulfate (Co-administration of protease inhibitors with tacrolimus may increase tacrolimus blood concentrations). Products include:
Crixivan 2113

Indomethacin (Tacrolimus can cause nephrotoxicity, particularly when used in high doses. Due to the potential for additive or synergistic impairment of renal function, care should be taken when administering tacrolimus with drugs that may be associated with renal dysfunction. These include, but are not limited to, aminoglycosides, amphotericin B, and cisplatin). Products include:
Indocin 2167

Indomethacin Sodium Trihydrate (Tacrolimus can cause nephrotoxicity, particularly when used in high doses. Due to the potential for additive or synergistic impairment of renal function, care should be taken when administering tacrolimus with drugs that may be associated with renal dysfunction. These include, but are not limited to, aminoglycosides, amphotericin B, and cisplatin). Products include:
Indocin I.V. 2007

Influenza Vaccine, Live Attenuated (Immunosuppressants may affect vaccination. Therefore, during treatment with tacrolimus, vaccination may be less effective. The use of live vaccines should be avoided; live vaccines may include, but are not limited to, measles, mumps, rubella, oral polio, BCG, yellow fever, and TY 21a typhoid).
No products indexed under this heading.

Influenza Virus Vaccine (Immunosuppressants may affect vaccination. Therefore, during treatment with tacrolimus, vaccination may be less effective). Products include:

1485 Interactions Index Prograf

Fluarix 1476
Flulaval 1479

Influenza Virus Vaccine Live, Intranasal (Immunosuppressants may affect vaccination. Therefore, during treatment with tacrolimus, vaccination may be less effective. The use of live vaccines should be avoided; live vaccines may include, but are not limited to, measles, mumps, rubella, oral polio, BCG, yellow fever, and TY 21a typhoid). Products include:
FluMist 2078

Interferon Beta-1b (Tacrolimus can cause nephrotoxicity, particularly when used in high doses. Due to the potential for additive or synergistic impairment of renal function, care should be taken when administering tacrolimus with drugs that may be associated with renal dysfunction. These include, but are not limited to, aminoglycosides, amphotericin B, and cisplatin). Products include:
Betaseron 836
Extavia 2459

Interleuken-2 (Tacrolimus can cause nephrotoxicity, particularly when used in high doses. Due to the potential for additive or synergistic impairment of renal function, care should be taken when administering tacrolimus with drugs that may be associated with renal dysfunction. These include, but are not limited to, aminoglycosides, amphotericin B, and cisplatin).
No products indexed under this heading.

Iodamide Meglumine (Tacrolimus can cause nephrotoxicity, particularly when used in high doses. Due to the potential for additive or synergistic impairment of renal function, care should be taken when administering tacrolimus with drugs that may be associated with renal dysfunction. These include, but are not limited to, aminoglycosides, amphotericin B, and cisplatin).
No products indexed under this heading.

Iohexol (Tacrolimus can cause nephrotoxicity, particularly when used in high doses. Due to the potential for additive or synergistic impairment of renal function, care should be taken when administering tacrolimus with drugs that may be associated with renal dysfunction. These include, but are not limited to, aminoglycosides, amphotericin B, and cisplatin).
No products indexed under this heading.

Iopamidol (Tacrolimus can cause nephrotoxicity, particularly when used in high doses. Due to the potential for additive or synergistic impairment of renal function, care should be taken when administering tacrolimus with drugs that may be associated with renal dysfunction. These include, but are not limited to, aminoglycosides, amphotericin B, and cisplatin).
No products indexed under this heading.

Iopanoic Acid (Tacrolimus can cause nephrotoxicity, particularly when used in high doses. Due to the potential for additive or synergistic impairment of renal function, care should be taken when administering tacrolimus with drugs that may be associated with renal dysfunction. These include, but are not limited to, aminoglycosides, amphotericin B, and cisplatin).
No products indexed under this heading.

Iothalamate Meglumine (Tacrolimus can cause nephrotoxicity, particularly when used in high doses. Due to the potential for additive or synergistic impairment of renal function, care should be taken when administering tacrolimus with drugs that may be associated with renal dysfunction. These include, but are not limited to, aminoglycosides, amphotericin B, and cisplatin).
No products indexed under this heading.

Ioxaglate Meglumine (Tacrolimus can cause nephrotoxicity, particularly when used in high doses. Due to the potential for additive or synergistic impairment of renal function, care should be taken when administering tacrolimus with drugs that may be associated with renal dysfunction. These include, but are not limited to, aminoglycosides, amphotericin B, and cisplatin).
No products indexed under this heading.

Ioxaglate Sodium (Tacrolimus can cause nephrotoxicity, particularly when used in high doses. Due to the potential for additive or synergistic impairment of renal function, care should be taken when administering tacrolimus with drugs that may be associated with renal dysfunction. These include, but are not limited to, aminoglycosides, amphotericin B, and cisplatin).
No products indexed under this heading.

Isoniazid (Since tacrolimus is metabolized mainly by the CYP3A enzyme systems, substances known to inhibit these enzymes may decrease the metabolism or increase bioavailability of tacrolimus as indicated by increased whole blood or plasma concentrations. Monitoring of blood concentrations and appropriate dosage adjustments are essential when such drugs are used concomitantly).
No products indexed under this heading.

Isradipine (While calcium-channel blocking agents can be effective in treating tacrolimus-associated hypertension, care should be taken since interference with tacrolimus metabolism may require a dosage reduction). Products include:
DynaCirc CR 1432

Itraconazole (Co-administration of itraconazole with tacrolimus may increase tacrolimus blood concentrations).
No products indexed under this heading.

Japanese Encephalitis Vaccine Inactivated (Immunosuppressants may affect vaccination. Therefore, during treatment with tacrolimus, vaccination may be less effective).
No products indexed under this heading.

Kanamycin Sulfate (Due to the potential for additive or synergistic impairment of renal function, care should be taken when administering tacrolimus with drugs that may be associated with renal dysfunction. These include, but are not limited to, aminoglycosides, amphotericin B, and cisplatin).
No products indexed under this heading.

Ketoconazole (In a study of 6 normal volunteers, a significant increase in tacrolimus oral bioavailability (14±5% vs. 30±8%) was observed with concomitant ketoconazole administration (200 mg). The apparent oral clearance of tacrolimus during ketoconazole administration was significantly decreased compared to tacrolimus alone (0.430±0.129 L/hr/kg vs. 0.148±0.043 L/hr/kg). Overall, IV clearance of tacrolimus was not significantly changed by ketoconazole co-administration, although it was highly variable between patients). Products include:
Extina 3319
Xolegel 3337

Ketoprofen (Tacrolimus can cause nephrotoxicity, particularly when used in high doses. Due to the potential for additive or synergistic impairment of renal function, care should be taken when administering tacrolimus with drugs that may be associated with renal dysfunction. These include, but are not limited to, aminoglycosides, amphotericin B, and cisplatin).
No products indexed under this heading.

Ketorolac Tromethamine (Tacrolimus can cause nephrotoxicity, particularly when used in high doses. Due to the potential for additive or synergistic impairment of renal function, care should be taken when administering tacrolimus with drugs that may be associated with renal dysfunction. These include, but are not limited to, aminoglycosides, amphotericin B, and cisplatin). Products include:
Acuvail .... ⊙209

Lamium album (Tacrolimus can cause nephrotoxicity, particularly when used in high doses. Due to the potential for additive or synergistic impairment of renal function, care should be taken when administering tacrolimus with drugs that may be associated with renal dysfunction. These include, but are not limited to, aminoglycosides, amphotericin B, and cisplatin).
No products indexed under this heading.

Lansoprazole (Lansoprazole (CYP2C19, CYP3A4 substrate) may potentially inhibit CYP3A4-mediated metabolism of tacrolimus and thereby substantially increase tacrolimus whole blood concentrations, especially in transplant patients who are intermediate or poor CYP2C19 metabolizers, as compared to those patients who are efficient CYP2C19 metabolizers).
No products indexed under this heading.

Levonorgestrel (Care should be exercised when drugs that are metabolized by CYP3A (eg, nelfinavir, ritonavir) are administered concomitantly with tacrolimus). Products include:
Climara Pro 847
LoSeasonique 3407
Lybrel 3514
Mirena 854
Plan B 3416
Seasonique 3418

Lidocaine (Care should be exercised when drugs that are metabolized by CYP3A (eg, nelfinavir, ritonavir) are administered concomitantly with tacrolimus). Products include:
Lidoderm 1107

Lidocaine Hydrochloride (Care should be exercised when drugs that are metabolized by CYP3A (eg, nelfinavir, ritonavir) are administered concomitantly with tacrolimus).
No products indexed under this heading.

Lisinopril (Tacrolimus can cause nephrotoxicity, particularly when used in high doses. Due to the potential for additive or synergistic impairment of renal function, care should be taken when administering tacrolimus with drugs that may be associated with renal dysfunction. These include, but are not limited to, aminoglycosides, amphotericin B, and cisplatin). Products include:
Prinivil 2241
Prinzide 2246

Lithium (Tacrolimus can cause nephrotoxicity, particularly when used in high doses. Due to the potential for additive or synergistic impairment of renal function, care should be taken when administering tacrolimus with drugs that may be associated with renal dysfunction. These include, but are not limited to, aminoglycosides, amphotericin B, and cisplatin).
No products indexed under this heading.

Lithium Carbonate (Tacrolimus can cause nephrotoxicity, particularly when used in high doses. Due to the potential for additive or synergistic impairment of renal function, care should be taken when administering tacrolimus with drugs that may be associated with renal dysfunction. These include, but are not limited to, aminoglycosides, amphotericin B, and cisplatin).
No products indexed under this heading.

Lithium Citrate (Tacrolimus can cause nephrotoxicity, particularly when used in high doses. Due to the potential for additive or synergistic impairment of renal function, care should be taken when administering tacrolimus with drugs that may be associated with renal dysfunction. These include, but are not limited to, aminoglycosides, amphotericin B, and cisplatin).
No products indexed under this heading.

Lopinavir (Co-administration of protease inhibitors with tacrolimus may increase tacrolimus blood concentrations). Products include:
Kaletra 458

Loracarbef (Tacrolimus can cause nephrotoxicity, particularly when used in high doses. Due to the potential for additive or synergistic impairment of renal function, care should be taken when administering tacrolimus with drugs that may be associated with renal dysfunction. These include, but are not limited to, aminoglycosides, amphotericin B, and cisplatin).
No products indexed under this heading.

Lovastatin (Tacrolimus can cause nephrotoxicity, particularly when used in high doses. Due to the potential for additive or synergistic impairment of renal function, care should be taken when administering tacrolimus with drugs that may be associated with renal dysfunction. These include, but are not limited to, aminoglycosides, amphotericin B, and cisplatin). Products include:
Advicor 402
Mevacor 2212

Magnesium Hydroxide (In a single-dose crossover study in healthy volunteers, co-administration of tacrolimus and magnesium-aluminum-hydroxide resulted in a 21% increase in the mean tacrolimus AUC and a 10% decrease in the mean tacrolimus C_{max} relative to tacrolimus administration alone). Products include:
Fleet Pedia-Lax Chewable Tablets 1144
Pepcid Complete 1822

Measles, Mumps, Rubella and Varicella Virus Vaccine Live (Immunosuppressants may affect vaccination. Therefore, during treatment with tacrolimus, vaccination may be less effective. The use of live vaccines should be avoided; live vaccines may include, but are not limited to, measles, mumps, rubella, oral polio, BCG, yellow fever, and TY 21a typhoid). Products include:
ProQuad 2254

Measles, Mumps & Rubella Virus Vaccine, Live (Immunosuppressants may affect vaccination. Therefore, during treatment with tacrolimus, vaccination may be less effective. The use of live vaccines should be avoided; live vaccines may include, but are not limited to, measles, mumps, rubella, oral polio, BCG, yellow fever, and TY 21a typhoid). Products include:
M-M-R II 2203
ProQuad 2254

Measles & Rubella Virus Vaccine Live (Immunosuppressants may affect vaccination. Therefore, during treatment with tacrolimus, vaccination may be less effective. The use of live vaccines should be avoided; live vaccines may include, but are not limited to, measles, mumps, rubella, oral polio, BCG, yellow fever, and TY 21a typhoid).
No products indexed under this heading.

Measles Virus Vaccine Live (Immunosuppressants may affect vaccination. Therefore, during treatment with tacrolimus, vaccination may be less effective. The use of live vaccines should be avoided; live vaccines may include, but are not limited to, measles, mumps, rubella, oral polio, BCG, yellow fever, and TY 21a typhoid). Products include:

IMPORTANT NOTE: Always consult each drug listing in the patient's regimen for possible interactions.

Prograf Interactions Index 1486

Attenuvax 2086

Meclofenamate Sodium (Tacrolimus can cause nephrotoxicity, particularly when used in high doses. Due to the potential for additive or synergistic impairment of renal function, care should be taken when administering tacrolimus with drugs that may be associated with renal dysfunction. These include, but are not limited to, aminoglycosides, amphotericin B, and cisplatin).
No products indexed under this heading.

Mefenamic Acid (Tacrolimus can cause nephrotoxicity, particularly when used in high doses. Due to the potential for additive or synergistic impairment of renal function, care should be taken when administering tacrolimus with drugs that may be associated with renal dysfunction. These include, but are not limited to, aminoglycosides, amphotericin B, and cisplatin).
No products indexed under this heading.

Meloxicam (Tacrolimus can cause nephrotoxicity, particularly when used in high doses. Due to the potential for additive or synergistic impairment of renal function, care should be taken when administering tacrolimus with drugs that may be associated with renal dysfunction. These include, but are not limited to, aminoglycosides, amphotericin B, and cisplatin).
No products indexed under this heading.

Melphalan Hydrochloride (Tacrolimus can cause nephrotoxicity, particularly when used in high doses. Due to the potential for additive or synergistic impairment of renal function, care should be taken when administering tacrolimus with drugs that may be associated with renal dysfunction. These include, but are not limited to, aminoglycosides, amphotericin B, and cisplatin). Products include:
Alkeran for Injection 1300

Mesalamine (Tacrolimus can cause nephrotoxicity, particularly when used in high doses. Due to the potential for additive or synergistic impairment of renal function, care should be taken when administering tacrolimus with drugs that may be associated with renal dysfunction. These include, but are not limited to, aminoglycosides, amphotericin B, and cisplatin). Products include:
Apriso 2899
Asacol 2786
Asacol HD 2787
Canasa 782
Lialda 3295
Pentasa 3297

Mestranol (Care should be exercised when drugs that are metabolized by CYP3A (eg, nelfinavir, ritonavir) are administered concomitantly with tacrolimus).
No products indexed under this heading.

Methadone Hydrochloride (Care should be exercised when drugs that are metabolized by CYP3A (eg, nelfinavir, ritonavir) are administered concomitantly with tacrolimus).
No products indexed under this heading.

Methimazole (Tacrolimus can cause nephrotoxicity, particularly when used in high doses. Due to the potential for additive or synergistic impairment of renal function, care should be taken when administering tacrolimus with drugs that may be associated with renal dysfunction. These include, but are not limited to, aminoglycosides, amphotericin B, and cisplatin).
No products indexed under this heading.

Methotrexate (Tacrolimus can cause nephrotoxicity, particularly when used in high doses. Due to the potential for additive or synergistic impairment of renal function, care should be taken when administering tacrolimus with drugs that may be associated with renal dysfunction. These include, but are not limited to, aminoglycosides, amphotericin B, and cisplatin).
No products indexed under this heading.

Methotrexate Sodium (Tacrolimus can cause nephrotoxicity, particularly when used in high doses. Due to the potential for additive or synergistic impairment of renal function, care should be taken when administering tacrolimus with drugs that may be associated with renal dysfunction. These include, but are not limited to, aminoglycosides, amphotericin B, and cisplatin).
No products indexed under this heading.

Methyclothiazide (Tacrolimus can cause nephrotoxicity, particularly when used in high doses. Due to the potential for additive or synergistic impairment of renal function, care should be taken when administering tacrolimus with drugs that may be associated with renal dysfunction. These include, but are not limited to, aminoglycosides, amphotericin B, and cisplatin).
No products indexed under this heading.

Methylprednisolone (Co-administration of methylprednisolone with tacrolimus may increase tacrolimus blood concentrations).
No products indexed under this heading.

Methylprednisolone Acetate (Co-administration of methylprednisolone with tacrolimus may increase tacrolimus blood concentrations).
No products indexed under this heading.

Methylprednisolone Sodium Succinate (Co-administration of methylprednisolone with tacrolimus may increase tacrolimus blood concentrations).
No products indexed under this heading.

Metoclopramide Hydrochloride (Co-administration of metoclopramide with tacrolimus may increase tacrolimus blood concentrations). Products include:
Metozolv ODT 2901

Metronidazole (Since tacrolimus is metabolized mainly by the CYP3A enzyme systems, substances known to inhibit these enzymes may decrease the metabolism or increase bioavailability of tacrolimus as indicated by increased whole blood or plasma concentrations. Monitoring of blood concentrations and appropriate dosage adjustments are essential when such drugs are used concomitantly). Products include:
Pylera 793

Metronidazole Benzoate (Since tacrolimus is metabolized mainly by the CYP3A enzyme systems, substances known to inhibit these enzymes may decrease the metabolism or increase bioavailability of tacrolimus as indicated by increased whole blood or plasma concentrations. Monitoring of blood concentrations and appropriate dosage adjustments are essential when such drugs are used concomitantly).
No products indexed under this heading.

Metronidazole Hydrochloride (Since tacrolimus is metabolized mainly by the CYP3A enzyme systems, substances known to inhibit these enzymes may decrease the metabolism or increase bioavailability of tacrolimus as indicated by increased whole blood or plasma concentrations. Monitoring of blood concentrations and appropriate dosage adjustments are essential when such drugs are used concomitantly).
No products indexed under this heading.

Mezlocillin Sodium (Tacrolimus can cause nephrotoxicity, particularly when used in high doses. Due to the potential for additive or synergistic impairment of renal function, care should be taken when administering tacrolimus with drugs that may be associated with renal dysfunction. These include, but are not limited to, aminoglycosides, amphotericin B, and cisplatin).
No products indexed under this heading.

Mibefradil Dihydrochloride (While calcium-channel blocking agents can be effective in treating tacrolimus-associated hypertension, care should be taken since interference with tacrolimus metabolism may require a dosage reduction).
No products indexed under this heading.

Miconazole (Since tacrolimus is metabolized mainly by the CYP3A enzyme systems, substances known to inhibit these enzymes may decrease the metabolism or increase bioavailability of tacrolimus as indicated by increased whole blood or plasma concentrations. Monitoring of blood concentrations and appropriate dosage adjustments are essential when such drugs are used concomitantly).
No products indexed under this heading.

Midazolam Hydrochloride (Care should be exercised when drugs that are metabolized by CYP3A (eg, nelfinavir, ritonavir) are administered concomitantly with tacrolimus).
No products indexed under this heading.

Minocycline Hydrochloride (Tacrolimus can cause nephrotoxicity, particularly when used in high doses. Due to the potential for additive or synergistic impairment of renal function, care should be taken when administering tacrolimus with drugs that may be associated with renal dysfunction. These include, but are not limited to, aminoglycosides, amphotericin B, and cisplatin). Products include:
Solodyn 2073

Mitomycin (Mitomycin-C) (Tacrolimus can cause nephrotoxicity, particularly when used in high doses. Due to the potential for additive or synergistic impairment of renal function, care should be taken when administering tacrolimus with drugs that may be associated with renal dysfunction. These include, but are not limited to, aminoglycosides, amphotericin B, and cisplatin).
No products indexed under this heading.

Modafinil (Since tacrolimus is metabolized mainly by the CYP3A enzyme systems, drugs known to induce these enzyme systems may result in an increased metabolism of tacrolimus or decreased bioavailability as indicated by decreased whole blood or plasma concentrations. Monitoring of blood concentrations and appropriate dosage adjustments are essential when such drugs are used concomitantly). Products include:
Provigil 983

Moexipril Hydrochloride (Tacrolimus can cause nephrotoxicity, particularly when used in high doses. Due to the potential for additive or synergistic impairment of renal function, care should be taken when administering tacrolimus with drugs that may be associated with renal dysfunction. These include, but are not limited to, aminoglycosides, amphotericin B, and cisplatin).
No products indexed under this heading.

Mumps Virus Vaccine, Live (Immunosuppressants may affect vaccination. Therefore, during treatment with tacrolimus, vaccination may be less effective. The use of live vaccines should be avoided; live vaccines may include, but are not limited to, measles, mumps, rubella, oral polio, BCG, yellow fever, and TY 21a typhoid). Products include:
Mumpsvax 2218

Muromonab-CD3 (Tacrolimus can cause nephrotoxicity, particularly when used in high doses. Due to the potential for additive or synergistic impairment of renal function, care should be taken when administering tacrolimus with drugs that may be associated with renal dysfunction. These include, but are not limited to, aminoglycosides, amphotericin B, and cisplatin). Products include:
Orthoclone OKT3 949

Mycophenolate Mofetil (At a given mycophenolate mofetil (MMF) dose, mycophenolic acid (MPA) exposure is higher with tacrolimus co-administration than with cyclosporine co-administration due to the differences in the interruption of the enterohepatic recirculation of MPA. Clinicians should be aware that there is also a potential for increased MPA exposure after crossover from cyclosporine to tacrolimus in patients concomitantly receiving MMF or MPA).
No products indexed under this heading.

Mycophenolic Acid (At a given mycophenolate mofetil (MMF) dose, mycophenolic acid (MPA) exposure is higher with tacrolimus co-administration than with cyclosporine co-administration due to the differences in the interruption of the enterohepatic recirculation of MPA. Clinicians should be aware that there is also a potential for increased MPA exposure after crossover from cyclosporine to tacrolimus in patients concomitantly receiving MMF or MPA). Products include:
Myfortic 2491

Nabumetone (Tacrolimus can cause nephrotoxicity, particularly when used in high doses. Due to the potential for additive or synergistic impairment of renal function, care should be taken when administering tacrolimus with drugs that may be associated with renal dysfunction. These include, but are not limited to, aminoglycosides, amphotericin B, and cisplatin).
No products indexed under this heading.

Nafcillin Sodium (Tacrolimus can cause nephrotoxicity, particularly when used in high doses. Due to the potential for additive or synergistic impairment of renal function, care should be taken when administering tacrolimus with drugs that may be associated with renal dysfunction. These include, but are not limited to, aminoglycosides, amphotericin B, and cisplatin).
No products indexed under this heading.

Naproxen (Tacrolimus can cause nephrotoxicity, particularly when used in high doses. Due to the potential for additive or synergistic impairment of renal function, care should be taken when administering tacrolimus with drugs that may be associated with renal dysfunction. These include, but are not limited to, aminoglycosides, amphotericin B, and cisplatin). Products include:
EC-Naprosyn 2850
Naprosyn 2850
Anaprox/Naprosyn 2850

Naproxen Sodium (Tacrolimus can cause nephrotoxicity, particularly when used in high doses. Due to the potential for additive or synergistic impairment of renal function, care should be taken when administering tacrolimus with drugs that may be associated with renal dysfunction. These include, but are not limited to, aminoglycosides, amphotericin B, and cisplatin). Products include:
Anaprox 2850
Anaprox DS 2850
Treximet 1681

Nefazodone Hydrochloride (Co-administration of nefazodone with tacrolimus may increase tacrolimus blood concentrations).
No products indexed under this heading.

Nelfinavir Mesylate (Care should be exercised when drugs that are metabolized by CYP3A (eg, nelfinavir, ritonavir) are administered concomitantly with tacrolimus. Co-administration of tacrolimus with nelfinavir increased blood concentrations of tacrolimus significantly and, as a result, a reduction in the tacrolimus dose by an average of 16-fold was needed to maintain mean trough tacrolimus blood concentrations of 9.7 ng/mL. Thus, frequent monitoring of tacrolimus blood concentrations and appropriate dosage adjustments are essential when nelfinavir is used concomitantly).
No products indexed under this heading.

Neomycin (Due to the potential for additive or synergistic impairment of renal function, care should be taken when administering tacrolimus with drugs that may be associated with renal dysfunction. These include, but are not limited to, aminoglycosides, amphotericin B, and cisplatin).
No products indexed under this heading.

Neomycin, oral (Due to the potential for additive or synergistic impairment of renal function, care should be taken when administering tacrolimus with drugs that may be associated with renal dysfunction. These include, but are not limited to, aminoglycosides, amphotericin B, and cisplatin).
No products indexed under this heading.

Neomycin Sulfate (Due to the potential for additive or synergistic impairment of renal function, care should be taken when administering tacrolimus with drugs that may be associated with renal dysfunction. These include, but are not limited to, aminoglycosides, amphotericin B, and cisplatin).
No products indexed under this heading.

Nevirapine (Tacrolimus can cause nephrotoxicity, particularly when used in high doses. Due to the potential for additive or synergistic impairment of renal function, care should be taken when administering tacrolimus with drugs that may be associated with renal dysfunction. These include, but are not limited to, aminoglycosides, amphotericin B, and cisplatin). Products include:
Viramune Oral Suspension 897
Viramune Tablets 897

Nicardipine (Co-administration of nicardipine with tacrolimus may increase tacrolimus blood concentrations).
No products indexed under this heading.

Nicardipine Hydrochloride (Co-administration of nicardipine with tacrolimus may increase tacrolimus blood concentrations).
No products indexed under this heading.

Nifedipine (Co-administration of nifedipine with tacrolimus may increase tacrolimus blood concentrations).
No products indexed under this heading.

Nimodipine (While calcium-channel blocking agents can be effective in treating tacrolimus-associated hypertension, care should be taken since interference with tacrolimus metabolism may require a dosage reduction).
No products indexed under this heading.

Nisoldipine (While calcium-channel blocking agents can be effective in treating tacrolimus-associated hypertension, care should be taken since interference with tacrolimus metabolism may require a dosage reduction).
No products indexed under this heading.

Norethindrone (Care should be exercised when drugs that are metabolized by CYP3A (eg, nelfinavir, ritonavir) are administered concomitantly with tacrolimus). Products include:
Ortho Micronor 2660

Norfloxacin (Tacrolimus can cause nephrotoxicity, particularly when used in high doses. Due to the potential for additive or synergistic impairment of renal function, care should be taken when administering tacrolimus with drugs that may be associated with renal dysfunction. These include, but are not limited to, aminoglycosides, amphotericin B, and cisplatin). Products include:
Noroxin 2220

Norgestrel (Care should be exercised when drugs that are metabolized by CYP3A (eg, nelfinavir, ritonavir) are administered concomitantly with tacrolimus).
No products indexed under this heading.

Olsalazine Sodium (Tacrolimus can cause nephrotoxicity, particularly when used in high doses. Due to the potential for additive or synergistic impairment of renal function, care should be taken when administering tacrolimus with drugs that may be associated with renal dysfunction. These include, but are not limited to, aminoglycosides, amphotericin B, and cisplatin).
No products indexed under this heading.

Omeprazole (Co-administration of omeprazole with tacrolimus may increase tacrolimus blood concentrations).
No products indexed under this heading.

Omeprazole Magnesium (Co-administration of omeprazole with tacrolimus may increase tacrolimus blood concentrations).
No products indexed under this heading.

Ondansetron Hydrochloride (Care should be exercised when drugs that are metabolized by CYP3A (eg, nelfinavir, ritonavir) are administered concomitantly with tacrolimus). Products include:
Zofran Injection 1750
Zofran 1756
Zofran ODT 1756

Oxaprozin (Tacrolimus can cause nephrotoxicity, particularly when used in high doses. Due to the potential for additive or synergistic impairment of renal function, care should be taken when administering tacrolimus with drugs that may be associated with renal dysfunction. These include, but are not limited to, aminoglycosides, amphotericin B, and cisplatin).
No products indexed under this heading.

Paclitaxel (Care should be exercised when drugs that are metabolized by CYP3A (eg, nelfinavir, ritonavir) are administered concomitantly with tacrolimus).
No products indexed under this heading.

Pamidronate Disodium (Tacrolimus can cause nephrotoxicity, particularly when used in high doses. Due to the potential for additive or synergistic impairment of renal function, care should be taken when administering tacrolimus with drugs that may be associated with renal dysfunction. These include, but are not limited to, aminoglycosides, amphotericin B, and cisplatin).
No products indexed under this heading.

Paroxetine Hydrochloride (Tacrolimus can cause nephrotoxicity, particularly when used in high doses. Due to the potential for additive or synergistic impairment of renal function, care should be taken when administering tacrolimus with drugs that may be associated with renal dysfunction. These include, but are not limited to, aminoglycosides, amphotericin B, and cisplatin). Products include:
Paroxetine CR 2361

Paroxetine ER 2371
Paxil 1586
Paxil CR 1596

Penicillamine (Tacrolimus can cause nephrotoxicity, particularly when used in high doses. Due to the potential for additive or synergistic impairment of renal function, care should be taken when administering tacrolimus with drugs that may be associated with renal dysfunction. These include, but are not limited to, aminoglycosides, amphotericin B, and cisplatin).
No products indexed under this heading.

Penicillin G Benzathine (Tacrolimus can cause nephrotoxicity, particularly when used in high doses. Due to the potential for additive or synergistic impairment of renal function, care should be taken when administering tacrolimus with drugs that may be associated with renal dysfunction. These include, but are not limited to, aminoglycosides, amphotericin B, and cisplatin). Products include:
Bicillin C-R Injectable Suspension 1826
Bicillin L-A 1828

Penicillin G Potassium (Tacrolimus can cause nephrotoxicity, particularly when used in high doses. Due to the potential for additive or synergistic impairment of renal function, care should be taken when administering tacrolimus with drugs that may be associated with renal dysfunction. These include, but are not limited to, aminoglycosides, amphotericin B, and cisplatin).
No products indexed under this heading.

Penicillin G Procaine (Tacrolimus can cause nephrotoxicity, particularly when used in high doses. Due to the potential for additive or synergistic impairment of renal function, care should be taken when administering tacrolimus with drugs that may be associated with renal dysfunction. These include, but are not limited to, aminoglycosides, amphotericin B, and cisplatin). Products include:
Bicillin C-R Injectable Suspension 1826
Bicillin L-A 1828

Penicillin G Sodium (Tacrolimus can cause nephrotoxicity, particularly when used in high doses. Due to the potential for additive or synergistic impairment of renal function, care should be taken when administering tacrolimus with drugs that may be associated with renal dysfunction. These include, but are not limited to, aminoglycosides, amphotericin B, and cisplatin).
No products indexed under this heading.

Penicillin V Potassium (Tacrolimus can cause nephrotoxicity, particularly when used in high doses. Due to the potential for additive or synergistic impairment of renal function, care should be taken when administering tacrolimus with drugs that may be associated with renal dysfunction. These include, but are not limited to, aminoglycosides, amphotericin B, and cisplatin).
No products indexed under this heading.

Pentamidine Isethionate (Tacrolimus can cause nephrotoxicity, particularly when used in high doses. Due to the potential for additive or synergistic impairment of renal function, care should be taken when administering tacrolimus with drugs that may be associated with renal dysfunction. These include, but are not limited to, aminoglycosides, amphotericin B, and cisplatin).
No products indexed under this heading.

Perindopril Erbumine (Tacrolimus can cause nephrotoxicity, particularly when used in high doses. Due to the potential for additive or synergistic impairment of renal function, care should be taken when administering tacrolimus with drugs that may be associated with renal dysfunction. These include, but are not limited to, aminoglycosides, amphotericin B, and cisplatin).
No products indexed under this heading.

Phenobarbital (Co-administration of phenobarbital with tacrolimus may decrease tacrolimus blood concentrations). Products include:
Donnatal 2711

Phenobarbital Sodium (Co-administration of phenobarbital with tacrolimus may decrease tacrolimus blood concentrations).
No products indexed under this heading.

Phenylbutazone (Tacrolimus can cause nephrotoxicity, particularly when used in high doses. Due to the potential for additive or synergistic impairment of renal function, care should be taken when administering tacrolimus with drugs that may be associated with renal dysfunction. These include, but are not limited to, aminoglycosides, amphotericin B, and cisplatin).
No products indexed under this heading.

Phenytoin (Tacrolimus may affect the pharmacokinetics of other drugs (eg, phenytoin) and increase their concentration. Co-administration of phenytoin with tacrolimus may decrease tacrolimus blood concentrations).
No products indexed under this heading.

Phenytoin Sodium (Tacrolimus may affect the pharmacokinetics of other drugs (eg, phenytoin) and increase their concentration. Co-administration of phenytoin with tacrolimus may decrease tacrolimus blood concentrations). Products include:
Phenytek Capsules 2380

Pimozide (Care should be exercised when drugs that are metabolized by CYP3A (eg, nelfinavir, ritonavir) are administered concomitantly with tacrolimus).
No products indexed under this heading.

Piroxicam (Tacrolimus can cause nephrotoxicity, particularly when used in high doses. Due to the potential for additive or synergistic impairment of renal function, care should be taken when administering tacrolimus with drugs that may be associated with renal dysfunction. These include, but are not limited to, aminoglycosides, amphotericin B, and cisplatin).
No products indexed under this heading.

Plicamycin (Tacrolimus can cause nephrotoxicity, particularly when used in high doses. Due to the potential for additive or synergistic impairment of renal function, care should be taken when administering tacrolimus with drugs that may be associated with renal dysfunction. These include, but are not limited to, aminoglycosides, amphotericin B, and cisplatin).
No products indexed under this heading.

Pneumococcal vaccine, diphtheria conjugate (Immunosuppressants may affect vaccination. Therefore, during treatment with tacrolimus, vaccination may be less effective). Products include:
Prevnar 3557

Pneumococcal Vaccine, Polyvalent (Immunosuppressants may affect vaccination. Therefore, during treatment with tacrolimus, vaccination may be less effective). Products include:
Pneumovax 23 2230

IMPORTANT NOTE: Always consult each drug listing in the patient's regimen for possible interactions.

Poliovirus Vaccine, Live, Oral, Trivalent, Types 1,2,3 (Sabin) (Immunosuppressants may affect vaccination. Therefore, during treatment with tacrolimus, vaccination may be less effective. The use of live vaccines should be avoided; live vaccines may include, but are not limited to, measles, mumps, rubella, oral polio, BCG, yellow fever, and TY 21a typhoid).
No products indexed under this heading.

Poliovirus Vaccine Inactivated (Immunosuppressants may affect vaccination. Therefore, during treatment with tacrolimus, vaccination may be less effective). Products include:
Pediarix 1606

Polymyxin (Tacrolimus can cause nephrotoxicity, particularly when used in high doses. Due to the potential for additive or synergistic impairment of renal function, care should be taken when administering tacrolimus with drugs that may be associated with renal dysfunction. These include, but are not limited to, aminoglycosides, amphotericin B, and cisplatin).
No products indexed under this heading.

Polymyxin B Sulfate (Tacrolimus can cause nephrotoxicity, particularly when used in high doses. Due to the potential for additive or synergistic impairment of renal function, care should be taken when administering tacrolimus with drugs that may be associated with renal dysfunction. These include, but are not limited to, aminoglycosides, amphotericin B, and cisplatin).
No products indexed under this heading.

Polythiazide (Tacrolimus can cause nephrotoxicity, particularly when used in high doses. Due to the potential for additive or synergistic impairment of renal function, care should be taken when administering tacrolimus with drugs that may be associated with renal dysfunction. These include, but are not limited to, aminoglycosides, amphotericin B, and cisplatin).
No products indexed under this heading.

Pravastatin Sodium (Tacrolimus can cause nephrotoxicity, particularly when used in high doses. Due to the potential for additive or synergistic impairment of renal function, care should be taken when administering tacrolimus with drugs that may be associated with renal dysfunction. These include, but are not limited to, aminoglycosides, amphotericin B, and cisplatin).
No products indexed under this heading.

Quinapril Hydrochloride (Tacrolimus can cause nephrotoxicity, particularly when used in high doses. Due to the potential for additive or synergistic impairment of renal function, care should be taken when administering tacrolimus with drugs that may be associated with renal dysfunction. These include, but are not limited to, aminoglycosides, amphotericin B, and cisplatin).
No products indexed under this heading.

Quinidine Gluconate (Care should be exercised when drugs that are metabolized by CYP3A (eg, nelfinavir, ritonavir) are administered concomitantly with tacrolimus).
No products indexed under this heading.

Quinidine Polygalacturonate (Care should be exercised when drugs that are metabolized by CYP3A (eg, nelfinavir, ritonavir) are administered concomitantly with tacrolimus).
No products indexed under this heading.

Quinidine Sulfate (Care should be exercised when drugs that are metabolized by CYP3A (eg, nelfinavir, ritonavir) are administered concomitantly with tacrolimus).
No products indexed under this heading.

Quinine (Since tacrolimus is metabolized mainly by the CYP3A enzyme systems, substances known to inhibit these enzymes may decrease the metabolism or increase bioavailability of tacrolimus as indicated by increased whole blood or plasma concentrations. Monitoring of blood concentrations and appropriate dosage adjustments are essential when such drugs are used concomitantly). Products include:
Hyland's Leg Cramps PM with Quinine 3315

Quinine Sulfate (Since tacrolimus is metabolized mainly by the CYP3A enzyme systems, substances known to inhibit these enzymes may decrease the metabolism or increase bioavailability of tacrolimus as indicated by increased whole blood or plasma concentrations. Monitoring of blood concentrations and appropriate dosage adjustments are essential when such drugs are used concomitantly).
No products indexed under this heading.

Rabeprazole Sodium (Tacrolimus can cause nephrotoxicity, particularly when used in high doses. Due to the potential for additive or synergistic impairment of renal function, care should be taken when administering tacrolimus with drugs that may be associated with renal dysfunction. These include, but are not limited to, aminoglycosides, amphotericin B, and cisplatin). Products include:
Aciphex 1035

Ramipril (Tacrolimus can cause nephrotoxicity, particularly when used in high doses. Due to the potential for additive or synergistic impairment of renal function, care should be taken when administering tacrolimus with drugs that may be associated with renal dysfunction. These include, but are not limited to, aminoglycosides, amphotericin B, and cisplatin).
No products indexed under this heading.

Rapamycin (Because of the danger of oversuppression of the immune system, which can increase susceptibility to infection, combination immunosuppressant therapy should be used with caution).
No products indexed under this heading.

Rifabutin (Co-administration of rifabutin with tacrolimus may decrease tacrolimus blood concentrations).
No products indexed under this heading.

Rifampicin (Since tacrolimus is metabolized mainly by the CYP3A enzyme systems, drugs known to induce these enzyme systems may result in an increased metabolism of tacrolimus or decreased bioavailability as indicated by decreased whole blood or plasma concentrations. Monitoring of blood concentrations and appropriate dosage adjustments are essential when such drugs are used concomitantly).
No products indexed under this heading.

Rifampin (In a study of 6 normal volunteers, a significant decrease in tacrolimus oral bioavailability ($14\pm6\%$ vs. $7\pm3\%$) was observed with concomitant rifampin administration (600 mg). In addition, there was a significant increase in tacrolimus clearance (0.036 ± 0.008 L/hr/kg vs. 0.053 ± 0.010 L/hr/kg) with concomitant rifampin administration).
No products indexed under this heading.

Rifapentine (Since tacrolimus is metabolized mainly by the CYP3A enzyme systems, drugs known to induce these enzyme systems may result in an increased metabolism of tacrolimus or decreased bioavailability as indicated by decreased whole blood or plasma concentrations. Monitoring of blood concentrations and appropriate dosage adjustments are essential when such drugs are used concomitantly).
No products indexed under this heading.

Riluzole (Tacrolimus can cause nephrotoxicity, particularly when used in high doses. Due to the potential for additive or synergistic impairment of renal function, care should be taken when administering tacrolimus with drugs that may be associated with renal dysfunction. These include, but are not limited to, aminoglycosides, amphotericin B, and cisplatin). Products include:
Rilutek 3032

Ritonavir (Care should be exercised when drugs that are metabolized by CYP3A (eg, nelfinavir, ritonavir) are administered concomitantly with tacrolimus. Co-administration of protease inhibitors with tacrolimus may increase tacrolimus blood concentrations). Products include:
Kaletra 458
Norvir 509

Rofecoxib (Tacrolimus can cause nephrotoxicity, particularly when used in high doses. Due to the potential for additive or synergistic impairment of renal function, care should be taken when administering tacrolimus with drugs that may be associated with renal dysfunction. These include, but are not limited to, aminoglycosides, amphotericin B, and cisplatin).
No products indexed under this heading.

Rotavirus Vaccine, Live, Oral, Tetravalent (Immunosuppressants may affect vaccination. Therefore, during treatment with tacrolimus, vaccination may be less effective. The use of live vaccines should be avoided; live vaccines may include, but are not limited to, measles, mumps, rubella, oral polio, BCG, yellow fever, and TY 21a typhoid).
No products indexed under this heading.

Rubella & Mumps Virus Vaccine Live (Immunosuppressants may affect vaccination. Therefore, during treatment with tacrolimus, vaccination may be less effective. The use of live vaccines should be avoided; live vaccines may include, but are not limited to, measles, mumps, rubella, oral polio, BCG, yellow fever, and TY 21a typhoid).
No products indexed under this heading.

Rubella Virus Vaccine Live (Immunosuppressants may affect vaccination. Therefore, during treatment with tacrolimus, vaccination may be less effective. The use of live vaccines should be avoided; live vaccines may include, but are not limited to, measles, mumps, rubella, oral polio, BCG, yellow fever, and TY 21a typhoid). Products include:
Meruvax II 2210

Saquinavir (Co-administration of protease inhibitors with tacrolimus may increase tacrolimus blood concentrations).
No products indexed under this heading.

Saquinavir Mesylate (Co-administration of protease inhibitors with tacrolimus may increase tacrolimus blood concentrations).
No products indexed under this heading.

Sertraline Hydrochloride (Since tacrolimus is metabolized mainly by the CYP3A enzyme systems, substances known to inhibit these enzymes may decrease the metabolism or increase bioavailability of tacrolimus as indicated by increased whole blood or plasma concentrations. Monitoring of blood concentrations and appropriate dosage adjustments are essential when such drugs are used concomitantly).
No products indexed under this heading.

Sibutramine Hydrochloride Monohydrate (Tacrolimus can cause nephrotoxicity, particularly when used in high doses. Due to the potential for additive or synergistic impairment of renal function, care should be taken when administering tacrolimus with drugs that may be associated with renal dysfunction. These include, but are not limited to, aminoglycosides, amphotericin B, and cisplatin). Products include:
Meridia 492

Sildenafil Citrate (Care should be exercised when drugs that are metabolized by CYP3A (eg, nelfinavir, ritonavir) are administered concomitantly with tacrolimus).
No products indexed under this heading.

Simvastatin (Tacrolimus can cause nephrotoxicity, particularly when used in high doses. Due to the potential for additive or synergistic impairment of renal function, care should be taken when administering tacrolimus with drugs that may be associated with renal dysfunction. These include, but are not limited to, aminoglycosides, amphotericin B, and cisplatin). Products include:
Simcor 524
Vytorin 10/10 .... 2303, 3240
Vytorin 10/20 .... 2303, 3240
Vytorin 10/40 .... 2303, 3240
Vytorin 10/80 .... 2303, 3240
Zocor 2289

Sirolimus (The use of full-dose tacrolimus with sirolimus (2 mg per day) in heart transplant recipients was associated with increased risk of wound healing complications, renal function impairment, and insulin-dependent post-transplant diabetes mellitus, and is not recommended. Following co-administration of tacrolimus and sirolimus (2 or 5 mg/day) in stable renal transplant patients, mean tacrolimus $AUC_{0\text{-}12}$ and C_{min} decreased approximately by 30% relative to tacrolimus alone. Mean tacrolimus $AUC_{0\text{-}12}$ and C_{min} following co-administration of 1 mg/day of sirolimus decreased approximately 3% and 11%, respectively. The safety and efficacy of tacrolimus used in combination with sirolimus for the prevention of graft rejection has not been established and is not recommended). Products include:
Rapamune 3579

Smallpox Vaccine (Immunosuppressants may affect vaccination. Therefore, during treatment with tacrolimus, vaccination may be less effective. The use of live vaccines should be avoided; live vaccines may include, but are not limited to, measles, mumps, rubella, oral polio, BCG, yellow fever, and TY 21a typhoid).
No products indexed under this heading.

Spirapril Hydrochloride (Tacrolimus can cause nephrotoxicity, particularly when used in high doses. Due to the potential for additive or synergistic impairment of renal function, care should be taken when administering tacrolimus with drugs that may be associated with renal dysfunction. These include, but are not limited to, aminoglycosides, amphotericin B, and cisplatin).
No products indexed under this heading.

Spironolactone (Since tacrolimus may cause hyperkalemia, potassium-sparing diuretics should be avoided).
No products indexed under this heading.

Stavudine (Tacrolimus can cause nephrotoxicity, particularly when used in high doses. Due to the potential for additive or synergistic impairment of renal function, care should be taken when administering tacrolimus with drugs that may be associated with renal dysfunction. These include, but are not limited to, aminoglycosides, amphotericin B, and cisplatin).
No products indexed under this heading.

Streptomycin Sulfate (Due to the potential for additive or synergistic impairment of renal function, care should be taken when administering tacrolimus with drugs that may be associated with renal dysfunction. These include, but are not limited to, aminoglycosides, amphotericin B, and cisplatin).
No products indexed under this heading.

Streptozocin (Tacrolimus can cause nephrotoxicity, particularly when used in high doses. Due to the potential for additive or synergistic impairment of renal function, care should be taken when administering tacrolimus with drugs that may be associated with renal dysfunction. These include, but are not limited to, aminoglycosides, amphotericin B, and cisplatin).
No products indexed under this heading.

Sulfacytine (Tacrolimus can cause nephrotoxicity, particularly when used in high doses. Due to the potential for additive or synergistic impairment of renal function, care should be taken when administering tacrolimus with drugs that may be associated with renal dysfunction. These include, but are not limited to, aminoglycosides, amphotericin B, and cisplatin).
No products indexed under this heading.

Sulfamethizole (Tacrolimus can cause nephrotoxicity, particularly when used in high doses. Due to the potential for additive or synergistic impairment of renal function, care should be taken when administering tacrolimus with drugs that may be associated with renal dysfunction. These include, but are not limited to, aminoglycosides, amphotericin B, and cisplatin).
No products indexed under this heading.

Sulfamethoxazole (Tacrolimus can cause nephrotoxicity, particularly when used in high doses. Due to the potential for additive or synergistic impairment of renal function, care should be taken when administering tacrolimus with drugs that may be associated with renal dysfunction. These include, but are not limited to, aminoglycosides, amphotericin B, and cisplatin).
No products indexed under this heading.

Sulfasalazine (Tacrolimus can cause nephrotoxicity, particularly when used in high doses. Due to the potential for additive or synergistic impairment of renal function, care should be taken when administering tacrolimus with drugs that may be associated with renal dysfunction. These include, but are not limited to, aminoglycosides, amphotericin B, and cisplatin).
No products indexed under this heading.

Sulfinpyrazone (Tacrolimus can cause nephrotoxicity, particularly when used in high doses. Due to the potential for additive or synergistic impairment of renal function, care should be taken when administering tacrolimus with drugs that may be associated with renal dysfunction. These include, but are not limited to, aminoglycosides, amphotericin B, and cisplatin).
No products indexed under this heading.

Sulfisoxazole Acetyl (Tacrolimus can cause nephrotoxicity, particularly when used in high doses. Due to the potential for additive or synergistic impairment of renal function, care should be taken when administering tacrolimus with drugs that may be associated with renal dysfunction. These include, but are not limited to, aminoglycosides, amphotericin B, and cisplatin).
No products indexed under this heading.

Sulfisoxazole Diolamine (Tacrolimus can cause nephrotoxicity, particularly when used in high doses. Due to the potential for additive or synergistic impairment of renal function, care should be taken when administering tacrolimus with drugs that may be associated with renal dysfunction. These include, but are not limited to, aminoglycosides, amphotericin B, and cisplatin).
No products indexed under this heading.

Sulindac (Tacrolimus can cause nephrotoxicity, particularly when used in high doses. Due to the potential for additive or synergistic impairment of renal function, care should be taken when administering tacrolimus with drugs that may be associated with renal dysfunction. These include, but are not limited to, aminoglycosides, amphotericin B, and cisplatin). Products include:
Clinoril 2098

Tamoxifen Citrate (Care should be exercised when drugs that are metabolized by CYP3A (eg, nelfinavir, ritonavir) are administered concomitantly with tacrolimus).
No products indexed under this heading.

Tenofovir Disoproxil Fumarate (Tacrolimus can cause nephrotoxicity, particularly when used in high doses. Due to the potential for additive or synergistic impairment of renal function, care should be taken when administering tacrolimus with drugs that may be associated with renal dysfunction. These include, but are not limited to, aminoglycosides, amphotericin B, and cisplatin). Products include:
Atripla 906
Truvada 1258
Viread 1266

Terfenadine (Care should be exercised when drugs that are metabolized by CYP3A (eg, nelfinavir, ritonavir) are administered concomitantly with tacrolimus).
No products indexed under this heading.

Testosterone (Care should be exercised when drugs that are metabolized by CYP3A (eg, nelfinavir, ritonavir) are administered concomitantly with tacrolimus). Products include:
AndroGel 3456

Testosterone Cypionate (Care should be exercised when drugs that are metabolized by CYP3A (eg, nelfinavir, ritonavir) are administered concomitantly with tacrolimus).
No products indexed under this heading.

Testosterone Enanthate (Care should be exercised when drugs that are metabolized by CYP3A (eg, nelfinavir, ritonavir) are administered concomitantly with tacrolimus). Products include:
Delatestryl 1102

Testosterone Propionate (Care should be exercised when drugs that are metabolized by CYP3A (eg, nelfinavir, ritonavir) are administered concomitantly with tacrolimus).
No products indexed under this heading.

Theophylline (Care should be exercised when drugs that are metabolized by CYP3A (eg, nelfinavir, ritonavir) are administered concomitantly with tacrolimus).
No products indexed under this heading.

Theophylline Anhydrous (Care should be exercised when drugs that are metabolized by CYP3A (eg, nelfinavir, ritonavir) are administered concomitantly with tacrolimus). Products include:
Uniphyl 2817

Theophylline Calcium Salicylate (Care should be exercised when drugs that are metabolized by CYP3A (eg, nelfinavir, ritonavir) are administered concomitantly with tacrolimus).
No products indexed under this heading.

Theophylline Sodium Glycinate (Care should be exercised when drugs that are metabolized by CYP3A (eg, nelfinavir, ritonavir) are administered concomitantly with tacrolimus).
No products indexed under this heading.

Thioguanine (Tacrolimus can cause nephrotoxicity, particularly when used in high doses. Due to the potential for additive or synergistic impairment of renal function, care should be taken when administering tacrolimus with drugs that may be associated with renal dysfunction. These include, but are not limited to, aminoglycosides, amphotericin B, and cisplatin). Products include:
Tabloid 1664

Tiagabine Hydrochloride (Care should be exercised when drugs that are metabolized by CYP3A (eg, nelfinavir, ritonavir) are administered concomitantly with tacrolimus). Products include:
Gabitril 972

Ticarcillin Disodium (Tacrolimus can cause nephrotoxicity, particularly when used in high doses. Due to the potential for additive or synergistic impairment of renal function, care should be taken when administering tacrolimus with drugs that may be associated with renal dysfunction. These include, but are not limited to, aminoglycosides, amphotericin B, and cisplatin). Products include:
Timentin ADD-Vantage 1670
Timentin Galaxy 1674
Timentin 1666
Timentin Pharmacy 1678

Tipranavir (Co-administration of protease inhibitors with tacrolimus may increase tacrolimus blood concentrations).
No products indexed under this heading.

Tobramycin (Due to the potential for additive or synergistic impairment of renal function, care should be taken when administering tacrolimus with drugs that may be associated with renal dysfunction. These include, but are not limited to, aminoglycosides, amphotericin B, and cisplatin). Products include:
Tobi Nebulizer 2546
Tobramycin and Dexamethasone
  Ophthalmic Suspension .... ⊙251
Zylet .... ⊙252

Tobramycin Sulfate (Due to the potential for additive or synergistic impairment of renal function, care should be taken when administering tacrolimus with drugs that may be associated with renal dysfunction. These include, but are not limited to, aminoglycosides, amphotericin B, and cisplatin).
No products indexed under this heading.

Tolazamide (Tacrolimus can cause nephrotoxicity, particularly when used in high doses. Due to the potential for additive or synergistic impairment of renal function, care should be taken when administering tacrolimus with drugs that may be associated with renal dysfunction. These include, but are not limited to, aminoglycosides, amphotericin B, and cisplatin).
No products indexed under this heading.

Tolbutamide (Tacrolimus can cause nephrotoxicity, particularly when used in high doses. Due to the potential for additive or synergistic impairment of renal function, care should be taken when administering tacrolimus with drugs that may be associated with renal dysfunction. These include, but are not limited to, aminoglycosides, amphotericin B, and cisplatin).
No products indexed under this heading.

Tolmetin Sodium (Tacrolimus can cause nephrotoxicity, particularly when used in high doses. Due to the potential for additive or synergistic impairment of renal function, care should be taken when administering tacrolimus with drugs that may be associated with renal dysfunction. These include, but are not limited to, aminoglycosides, amphotericin B, and cisplatin).
No products indexed under this heading.

Tolterodine Tartrate (Care should be exercised when drugs that are metabolized by CYP3A (eg, nelfinavir, ritonavir) are administered concomitantly with tacrolimus).
No products indexed under this heading.

Trandolapril (Tacrolimus can cause nephrotoxicity, particularly when used in high doses. Due to the potential for additive or synergistic impairment of renal function, care should be taken when administering tacrolimus with drugs that may be associated with renal dysfunction. These include, but are not limited to, aminoglycosides, amphotericin B, and cisplatin). Products include:
Mavik 489
Tarka 534

Trazodone Hydrochloride (Care should be exercised when drugs that are metabolized by CYP3A (eg, nelfinavir, ritonavir) are administered concomitantly with tacrolimus).
No products indexed under this heading.

Triamterene (Since tacrolimus may cause hyperkalemia, potassium-sparing diuretics should be avoided). Products include:
Dyazide 1429
Dyrenium 3495

Triazolam (Care should be exercised when drugs that are metabolized by CYP3A (eg, nelfinavir, ritonavir) are administered concomitantly with tacrolimus).
No products indexed under this heading.

Trimethadione (Tacrolimus can cause nephrotoxicity, particularly when used in high doses. Due to the potential for additive or synergistic impairment of renal function, care should be taken when administering tacrolimus with drugs that may be associated with renal dysfunction. These include, but are not limited to, aminoglycosides, amphotericin B, and cisplatin).
No products indexed under this heading.

Troleandomycin (Co-administration of troleandomycin with tacrolimus may increase tacrolimus blood concentrations).
No products indexed under this heading.

Trovafloxacin Mesylate (Tacrolimus can cause nephrotoxicity, particularly when used in high doses. Due to the potential for additive or synergistic impairment of renal function, care should be taken when administering tacrolimus with drugs that may be associated with renal dysfunction. These include, but are not limited to, aminoglycosides, amphotericin B, and cisplatin).
No products indexed under this heading.

Typhoid Vaccine (Immunosuppressants may affect vaccination. Therefore, during treatment with tacrolimus, vaccination may be less effective. The use of live vaccines should be avoided; live vaccines may include, but are not limited to, measles, mumps, rubella, oral polio, BCG, yellow fever, and TY 21a typhoid).
No products indexed under this heading.

IMPORTANT NOTE: Always consult each drug listing in the patient's regimen for possible interactions.

Tyropanoate Sodium (Tacrolimus can cause nephrotoxicity, particularly when used in high doses. Due to the potential for additive or synergistic impairment of renal function, care should be taken when administering tacrolimus with drugs that may be associated with renal dysfunction. These include, but are not limited to, aminoglycosides, amphotericin B, and cisplatin).
No products indexed under this heading.

Ultraviolet radiation (As with other immunosuppressive agents, owing to the potential risk of malignant skin changes, exposure to sunlight and ultraviolet (UV) light should be limited by wearing protective clothing and using a sunscreen with a high protection factor).
No products indexed under this heading.

Valacyclovir Hydrochloride (Tacrolimus can cause nephrotoxicity, particularly when used in high doses. Due to the potential for additive or synergistic impairment of renal function, care should be taken when administering tacrolimus with drugs that may be associated with renal dysfunction. These include, but are not limited to, aminoglycosides, amphotericin B, and cisplatin). Products include:
Valtrex 1702

Valdecoxib (Tacrolimus can cause nephrotoxicity, particularly when used in high doses. Due to the potential for additive or synergistic impairment of renal function, care should be taken when administering tacrolimus with drugs that may be associated with renal dysfunction. These include, but are not limited to, aminoglycosides, amphotericin B, and cisplatin).
No products indexed under this heading.

Vancomycin Hydrochloride (Tacrolimus can cause nephrotoxicity, particularly when used in high doses. Due to the potential for additive or synergistic impairment of renal function, care should be taken when administering tacrolimus with drugs that may be associated with renal dysfunction. These include, but are not limited to, aminoglycosides, amphotericin B, and cisplatin).
No products indexed under this heading.

Varicella Virus Vaccine, Live (Immunosuppressants may affect vaccination. Therefore, during treatment with tacrolimus, vaccination may be less effective. The use of live vaccines should be avoided; live vaccines may include, but are not limited to, measles, mumps, rubella, oral polio, BCG, yellow fever, and TY 21a typhoid). Products include:
Varivax 2285

Venlafaxine Hydrochloride (Since tacrolimus is metabolized mainly by the CYP3A enzyme systems, substances known to inhibit these enzymes may decrease the metabolism or increase bioavailability of tacrolimus as indicated by increased whole blood or plasma concentrations. Monitoring of blood concentrations and appropriate dosage adjustments are essential when such drugs are used concomitantly). Products include:
Effexor XR 3504
Venlafaxine Hydrochloride Tablets ... 2388

Verapamil Hydrochloride (Co-administration of verapamil with tacrolimus may increase tacrolimus blood concentrations). Products include:
Tarka 534

Vinblastine Sulfate (Care should be exercised when drugs that are metabolized by CYP3A (eg, nelfinavir, ritonavir) are administered concomitantly with tacrolimus).
No products indexed under this heading.

Vincristine Sulfate (Care should be exercised when drugs that are metabolized by CYP3A (eg, nelfinavir, ritonavir) are administered concomitantly with tacrolimus).
No products indexed under this heading.

Voriconazole (Co-administration of voriconazole with tacrolimus may increase tacrolimus blood concentrations).
No products indexed under this heading.

Warfarin Sodium (Care should be exercised when drugs that are metabolized by CYP3A (eg, nelfinavir, ritonavir) are administered concomitantly with tacrolimus).
No products indexed under this heading.

Yellow Fever Vaccine (Immunosuppressants may affect vaccination. Therefore, during treatment with tacrolimus, vaccination may be less effective. The use of live vaccines should be avoided; live vaccines may include, but are not limited to, measles, mumps, rubella, oral polio, BCG, yellow fever, and TY 21a typhoid).
No products indexed under this heading.

Zafirlukast (Since tacrolimus is metabolized mainly by the CYP3A enzyme systems, substances known to inhibit these enzymes may decrease the metabolism or increase bioavailability of tacrolimus as indicated by increased whole blood or plasma concentrations. Monitoring of blood concentrations and appropriate dosage adjustments are essential when such drugs are used concomitantly). Products include:
Accolate 3612

Zalcitabine (Tacrolimus can cause nephrotoxicity, particularly when used in high doses. Due to the potential for additive or synergistic impairment of renal function, care should be taken when administering tacrolimus with drugs that may be associated with renal dysfunction. These include, but are not limited to, aminoglycosides, amphotericin B, and cisplatin).
No products indexed under this heading.

Zidovudine (Tacrolimus can cause nephrotoxicity, particularly when used in high doses. Due to the potential for additive or synergistic impairment of renal function, care should be taken when administering tacrolimus with drugs that may be associated with renal dysfunction. These include, but are not limited to, aminoglycosides, amphotericin B, and cisplatin). Products include:
Combivir 1404
Retrovir 1634
Retrovir IV 1640
Trizivir 1688

Zileuton (Since tacrolimus is metabolized mainly by the CYP3A enzyme systems, substances known to inhibit these enzymes may decrease the metabolism or increase bioavailability of tacrolimus as indicated by increased whole blood or plasma concentrations. Monitoring of blood concentrations and appropriate dosage adjustments are essential when such drugs are used concomitantly).
No products indexed under this heading.

Zoledronic Acid (Tacrolimus can cause nephrotoxicity, particularly when used in high doses. Due to the potential for additive or synergistic impairment of renal function, care should be taken when administering tacrolimus with drugs that may be associated with renal dysfunction. These include, but are not limited to, aminoglycosides, amphotericin B, and cisplatin). Products include:
Reclast 2509
Zometa 2554

Zoster Vaccine Live (Immunosuppressants may affect vaccination. Therefore, during treatment with tacrolimus, vaccination may be less effective.

The use of live vaccines should be avoided; live vaccines may include, but are not limited to, measles, mumps, rubella, oral polio, BCG, yellow fever, and TY 21a typhoid). Products include:
Zostavax 2299

Food Interactions

Food, unspecified (The rate and extent of tacrolimus absorption were greatest under fasted conditions. The presence and composition of food decreased both the rate and extent of tacrolimus absorption. The effect was most pronounced with a high-fat meal (848 kcal, 46% fat): mean AUC and C_{max} were decreased 37% and 77%, respectively; T_{max} was lengthened 5-fold. A high-carbohydrate meal (668 kcal, 85% carbohydrate) decreased mean AUC and mean C_{max} by 28% and 65%, respectively. The time of the meal also affected tacrolimus bioavailability. When given immediately following the meal, mean C_{max} was reduced 71%, and mean AUC was reduced 39%, relative to the fasted condition. When administered 1.5 hours following the meal, mean C_{max} was reduced 63%, and mean AUC was reduced 39%, relative to the fasted condition).

Grapefruit (Grapefruit juice affects CYP3A-mediated metabolism and should be avoided during therapy with tacrolimus. Co-administered grapefruit juice has been reported to increase tacrolimus blood trough concentrations in liver transplant patients).

Grapefruit Juice (Grapefruit juice affects CYP3A-mediated metabolism and should be avoided during therapy with tacrolimus. Co-administered grapefruit juice has been reported to increase tacrolimus blood trough concentrations in liver transplant patients).

Meal, unspecified (The rate and extent of tacrolimus absorption were greatest under fasted conditions. The presence and composition of food decreased both the rate and extent of tacrolimus absorption. The effect was most pronounced with a high-fat meal (848 kcal, 46% fat): mean AUC and C_{max} were decreased 37% and 77%, respectively; T_{max} was lengthened 5-fold. A high-carbohydrate meal (668 kcal, 85% carbohydrate) decreased mean AUC and mean C_{max} by 28% and 65%, respectively. The time of the meal also affected tacrolimus bioavailability. When given immediately following the meal, mean C_{max} was reduced 71%, and mean AUC was reduced 39%, relative to the fasted condition. When administered 1.5 hours following the meal, mean C_{max} was reduced 63%, and mean AUC was reduced 39%, relative to the fasted condition).

PROGRAF INJECTION
(Tacrolimus) 677
See Prograf Capsules

PROLASTIN
(Alpha1-Proteinase Inhibitor (Human)) ... 3382
None cited in PDR database.

PROLEUKIN FOR INJECTION
(Aldesleukin) 2504
May interact with agents associated with myelosuppression, aminoglycosides, antiemetics, antihypertensives, antineoplastics, beta-blockers, cardiotoxic drugs, cytotoxic drugs, glucocorticoids, hepatotoxic drugs, hypnotics and sedatives, narcotic analgesics, nephrotoxic agents, parenteral analgesics, psychotropics, radiographic iodinated contrast media, tranquilizers, and certain other agents. Compounds in these categories include:

Abacavir Sulfate (Concurrent administration of drugs possessing nephrotoxic effects with aldesleukin may increase the potential for nephrotoxicity). Products include:
Epzicom 1448
Trizivir 1688
Ziagen 1740

Acebutolol Hydrochloride (Beta-blockers may potentiate the hypotension seen with aldesleukin).
No products indexed under this heading.

Acyclovir (Concurrent administration of drugs possessing nephrotoxic effects with aldesleukin may increase the potential for nephrotoxicity). Products include:
Zovirax 1760

Acyclovir Sodium (Concurrent administration of drugs possessing nephrotoxic effects with aldesleukin may increase the potential for nephrotoxicity).
No products indexed under this heading.

Alatrofloxacin Mesylate (Concurrent administration of drugs possessing nephrotoxic effects with aldesleukin may increase the potential for nephrotoxicity).
No products indexed under this heading.

Alfentanil Hydrochloride (Aldesleukin may affect central nervous function. Therefore, interactions could occur following concomitant administration of narcotics).
No products indexed under this heading.

Aliskiren (Concurrent use with antihypertensive drugs may potentiate the hypotension seen with aldesleukin). Products include:
Tekturna 2538
Tekturna HCT 2541
Valturna 3637

Alprazolam (Aldesleukin may affect central nervous function. Therefore, interactions could occur following concomitant administration of psychotropic drugs).
No products indexed under this heading.

Altretamine (Concurrent administration of drugs possessing myelotoxic effects with aldesleukin may increase the potential for myelotoxicity). Products include:
Hexalen 1066

Amikacin Sulfate (Concurrent administration of drugs possessing nephrotoxic effects with aldesleukin may increase the potential for nephrotoxicity).
No products indexed under this heading.

Amiodarone Hydrochloride (Concurrent administration of drugs possessing hepatotoxic effects with aldesleukin may increase toxicity in the liver).
No products indexed under this heading.

Amitriptyline Hydrochloride (Aldesleukin may affect central nervous function. Therefore, interactions could occur following concomitant administration of psychotropic drugs).
No products indexed under this heading.

Amlodipine Besylate (Concurrent use with antihypertensive drugs may potentiate the hypotension seen with aldesleukin). Products include:
Azor 1010
Exforge 2443
Exforge HCT 2449

Amoxapine (Aldesleukin may affect central nervous function. Therefore, interactions could occur following concomitant administration of psychotropic drugs).
No products indexed under this heading.

Amoxicillin (Concurrent administration of drugs possessing nephrotoxic effects with aldesleukin may increase the potential for nephrotoxicity). Products include:

1491 Interactions Index Proleukin

Amoxil Capsules 1311
Amoxil Chewable Tablets 1311
Amoxil 1311
Amoxil Powder 1311
Augmentin 1331
Augmentin Tablets 1335
Augmentin ES-600 1338
Augmentin XR 1342
Moxatag 2321

Amoxicillin Trihydrate (Concurrent administration of drugs possessing nephrotoxic effects with aldesleukin may increase the potential for nephrotoxicity).
No products indexed under this heading.

Amphetamine Aspartate (Concurrent administration of drugs possessing cardiotoxic effects with aldesleukin may increase toxicity in the cardiovascular systems).
No products indexed under this heading.

Amphetamine Aspartate Monohydrate (Concurrent administration of drugs possessing cardiotoxic effects with aldesleukin may increase toxicity in the cardiovascular systems).
No products indexed under this heading.

Amphetamine Resins (Concurrent administration of drugs possessing cardiotoxic effects with aldesleukin may increase toxicity in the cardiovascular systems).
No products indexed under this heading.

Amphetamine Sulfate (Concurrent administration of drugs possessing cardiotoxic effects with aldesleukin may increase toxicity in the cardiovascular systems).
No products indexed under this heading.

Amphotericin B (Concurrent administration of drugs possessing nephrotoxic effects with aldesleukin may increase the potential for nephrotoxicity).
No products indexed under this heading.

Amphotericin B, liposomal (Concurrent administration of drugs possessing nephrotoxic effects with aldesleukin may increase the potential for nephrotoxicity). Products include:
AmBisome 659

Amphotericin B Cholesteryl Sulfate (Concurrent administration of drugs possessing nephrotoxic effects with aldesleukin may increase the potential for nephrotoxicity).
No products indexed under this heading.

Amphotericin B Lipid Complex (Concurrent administration of drugs possessing nephrotoxic effects with aldesleukin may increase the potential for nephrotoxicity).
No products indexed under this heading.

Ampicillin (Concurrent administration of drugs possessing nephrotoxic effects with aldesleukin may increase the potential for nephrotoxicity).
No products indexed under this heading.

Ampicillin Sodium (Concurrent administration of drugs possessing nephrotoxic effects with aldesleukin may increase the potential for nephrotoxicity).
No products indexed under this heading.

Ampicillin Trihydrate (Concurrent administration of drugs possessing nephrotoxic effects with aldesleukin may increase the potential for nephrotoxicity).
No products indexed under this heading.

Amprenavir (Concurrent administration of drugs possessing nephrotoxic effects with aldesleukin may increase the potential for nephrotoxicity).
No products indexed under this heading.

Anastrozole (Hypersensitivity reactions have been reported in patients receiving combination regimens containing sequential high dose aldesleukin and antineoplastic agents. These reactions consisted of erythema, pruritus, and hypotension and occurred within hours of administration of chemotherapy. These events required medical intervention in some patients).
No products indexed under this heading.

Apomorphine (Aldesleukin may affect central nervous function. Therefore, interactions could occur following concomitant administration of narcotics).
No products indexed under this heading.

Apomorphine Hydrochloride (Aldesleukin may affect central nervous function. Therefore, interactions could occur following concomitant administration of narcotics).
No products indexed under this heading.

Aprepitant (Aldesleukin may affect central nervous function. Therefore, interactions could occur following concomitant administration of antiemetics). Products include:
Emend 2124

Asparaginase (Concurrent administration of drugs possessing hepatotoxic effects with aldesleukin may increase the potential for hepatotoxicity). Products include:
Elspar 2005, 2122

Aspirin (Concurrent administration of drugs possessing nephrotoxic effects with aldesleukin may increase the potential for nephrotoxicity). Products include:
Aggrenox 880
Bayer Aspirin 829
Percodan 1124
St. Joseph Aspirin 2045

Atazanavir (Concurrent administration of drugs possessing nephrotoxic effects with aldesleukin may increase the potential for nephrotoxicity).
No products indexed under this heading.

Atazanavir Sulfate (Concurrent administration of drugs possessing hepatotoxic effects with aldesleukin may increase toxicity in the liver).
No products indexed under this heading.

Atenolol (Beta-blockers may potentiate the hypotension seen with aldesleukin).
No products indexed under this heading.

Atorvastatin Calcium (Concurrent administration of drugs possessing nephrotoxic effects with aldesleukin may increase the potential for nephrotoxicity). Products include:
Lipitor 2703

Azathioprine (Concurrent administration of drugs possessing hepatotoxic effects with aldesleukin may increase toxicity in the liver).
No products indexed under this heading.

Azathioprine Sodium (Concurrent administration of drugs possessing hepatotoxic effects with aldesleukin may increase toxicity in the liver).
No products indexed under this heading.

Azithromycin Dihydrate (Concurrent administration of drugs possessing nephrotoxic effects with aldesleukin may increase the potential for nephrotoxicity).
No products indexed under this heading.

Azlocillin Sodium (Concurrent administration of drugs possessing nephrotoxic effects with aldesleukin may increase the potential for nephrotoxicity).
No products indexed under this heading.

Aztreonam (Concurrent administration of drugs possessing nephrotoxic effects with aldesleukin may increase the potential for nephrotoxicity).
No products indexed under this heading.

Bacampicillin Hydrochloride (Concurrent administration of drugs possessing nephrotoxic effects with aldesleukin may increase the potential for nephrotoxicity).
No products indexed under this heading.

Bacitracin (Concurrent administration of drugs possessing nephrotoxic effects with aldesleukin may increase the potential for nephrotoxicity).
No products indexed under this heading.

Bacitracin Zinc (Concurrent administration of drugs possessing nephrotoxic effects with aldesleukin may increase the potential for nephrotoxicity).
No products indexed under this heading.

Balsalazide Disodium (Concurrent administration of drugs possessing nephrotoxic effects with aldesleukin may increase the potential for nephrotoxicity).
No products indexed under this heading.

Benazepril Hydrochloride (Concurrent administration of drugs possessing nephrotoxic effects with aldesleukin may increase the potential for nephrotoxicity).
No products indexed under this heading.

Bendroflumethiazide (Concurrent administration of drugs possessing nephrotoxic effects with aldesleukin may increase the potential for nephrotoxicity).
No products indexed under this heading.

Betamethasone Acetate (Although glucocorticoids have been shown to reduce aldesleukin-induced side effects including fever, renal insufficiency, hyperbilirubinemia, confusion, and dyspnea, concomitant administration of these agents with aldesleukin may reduce the antitumor effectiveness of aldesleukin and thus should be avoided).
No products indexed under this heading.

Betamethasone Sodium Phosphate (Although glucocorticoids have been shown to reduce aldesleukin-induced side effects including fever, renal insufficiency, hyperbilirubinemia, confusion, and dyspnea, concomitant administration of these agents with aldesleukin may reduce the antitumor effectiveness of aldesleukin and thus should be avoided).
No products indexed under this heading.

Betaxolol Hydrochloride (Beta-blockers may potentiate the hypotension seen with aldesleukin).
No products indexed under this heading.

Bicalutamide (Hypersensitivity reactions have been reported in patients receiving combination regimens containing sequential high dose aldesleukin and antineoplastic agents. These reactions consisted of erythema, pruritus, and hypotension and occurred within hours of administration of chemotherapy. These events required medical intervention in some patients).
No products indexed under this heading.

Bisoprolol Fumarate (Beta-blockers may potentiate the hypotension seen with aldesleukin).
No products indexed under this heading.

Bleomycin Sulfate (Concurrent administration of drugs possessing myelotoxic effects with aldesleukin may increase the potential for myelotoxicity).
No products indexed under this heading.

Budesonide (Although glucocorticoids have been shown to reduce aldesleukin-induced side effects including fever, renal insufficiency, hyperbilirubinemia, confusion, and dyspnea, concomitant administration of these agents with aldesleukin may reduce the antitumor effectiveness of aldesleukin and thus should be avoided). Products include:
Pulmicort Flexhaler 714
Symbicort 80/4.5 720
Symbicort 160/4.5 720

Buprenorphine Hydrochloride (Aldesleukin may affect central nervous function. Therefore, interactions could occur following concomitant administration of narcotics).
No products indexed under this heading.

Bupropion (Concurrent administration of drugs possessing hepatotoxic effects with aldesleukin may increase toxicity in the liver).
No products indexed under this heading.

Bupropion Hydrochloride (Concurrent administration of drugs possessing hepatotoxic effects with aldesleukin may increase toxicity in the liver). Products include:
Aplenzin 2948
Wellbutrin 1719
Wellbutrin SR 1725
Zyban 1762

Buspirone Hydrochloride (Aldesleukin may affect central nervous function. Therefore, interactions could occur following concomitant administration of psychotropic drugs).
No products indexed under this heading.

Busulfan (Concurrent administration of drugs possessing myelotoxic effects with aldesleukin may increase the potential for myelotoxicity). Products include:
Myleran 1581

Butabarbital (Aldesleukin may affect central nervous function. Therefore, interactions could occur following concomitant administration of psychotropic drugs).
No products indexed under this heading.

Butabarbital Sodium (Aldesleukin may affect central nervous function. Therefore, interactions could occur following concomitant administration of psychotropic drugs).
No products indexed under this heading.

Butalbital (Aldesleukin may affect central nervous function. Therefore, interactions could occur following concomitant administration of psychotropic drugs).
No products indexed under this heading.

Butorphanol Tartrate (Aldesleukin may affect central nervous function. Therefore, interactions could occur following concomitant administration of analgesics).
No products indexed under this heading.

Caffeine (Concurrent administration of drugs possessing nephrotoxic effects with aldesleukin may increase the potential for nephrotoxicity).
No products indexed under this heading.

Candesartan Cilexetil (Concurrent use with antihypertensive drugs may potentiate the hypotension seen with aldesleukin). Products include:
Atacand 697
Atacand HCT 700

Captopril (Concurrent administration of drugs possessing nephrotoxic effects with aldesleukin may increase the potential for nephrotoxicity). Products include:
Captopril 2341

Carbamazepine (Concurrent administration of drugs possessing hepatotoxic effects with aldesleukin may increase toxicity in the liver). Products include:
Carbatrol 3280
Equetro 3477

Carbenicillin Disodium (Concurrent administration of drugs possessing nephrotoxic effects with aldesleukin may increase the potential for nephrotoxicity).
No products indexed under this heading.

IMPORTANT NOTE: Always consult each drug listing in the patient's regimen for possible interactions.

Proleukin Interactions Index 1492

Carbenicillin Indanyl Sodium (Concurrent administration of drugs possessing nephrotoxic effects with aldesleukin may increase the potential for nephrotoxicity).
No products indexed under this heading.

Carboplatin (Concurrent administration of drugs possessing nephrotoxic effects with aldesleukin may increase the potential for nephrotoxicity).
No products indexed under this heading.

Carmustine (BCNU) (Concurrent administration of drugs possessing nephrotoxic effects with aldesleukin may increase the potential for nephrotoxicity).
No products indexed under this heading.

Carteolol Hydrochloride (Beta-blockers may potentiate the hypotension seen with aldesleukin).
No products indexed under this heading.

Carvedilol (Beta-blockers may potentiate the hypotension seen with aldesleukin). Products include:
Coreg 1409

Carvedilol Phosphate (Beta-blockers may potentiate the hypotension seen with aldesleukin). Products include:
Coreg CR 1416

Cefaclor (Concurrent administration of drugs possessing nephrotoxic effects with aldesleukin may increase the potential for nephrotoxicity).
No products indexed under this heading.

Cefadroxil (Concurrent administration of drugs possessing nephrotoxic effects with aldesleukin may increase the potential for nephrotoxicity).
No products indexed under this heading.

Cefamandole Nafate (Concurrent administration of drugs possessing nephrotoxic effects with aldesleukin may increase the potential for nephrotoxicity).
No products indexed under this heading.

Cefazolin Sodium (Concurrent administration of drugs possessing nephrotoxic effects with aldesleukin may increase the potential for nephrotoxicity).
No products indexed under this heading.

Cefdinir (Concurrent administration of drugs possessing nephrotoxic effects with aldesleukin may increase the potential for nephrotoxicity). Products include:
Omnicef Capsules 518
Omnicef Oral Suspension 518

Cefepime Hydrochloride (Concurrent administration of drugs possessing nephrotoxic effects with aldesleukin may increase the potential for nephrotoxicity).
No products indexed under this heading.

Cefixime (Concurrent administration of drugs possessing nephrotoxic effects with aldesleukin may increase the potential for nephrotoxicity).
Products include:
Suprax for Oral Suspension 2038
Suprax Tablets 2038

Cefmetazole Sodium (Concurrent administration of drugs possessing nephrotoxic effects with aldesleukin may increase the potential for nephrotoxicity).
No products indexed under this heading.

Cefonicid Sodium (Concurrent administration of drugs possessing nephrotoxic effects with aldesleukin may increase the potential for nephrotoxicity).
No products indexed under this heading.

Cefoperazone Sodium (Concurrent administration of drugs possessing nephrotoxic effects with aldesleukin may increase the potential for nephrotoxicity).
No products indexed under this heading.

Ceforanide (Concurrent administration of drugs possessing nephrotoxic effects with aldesleukin may increase the potential for nephrotoxicity).
No products indexed under this heading.

Cefotaxime Sodium (Concurrent administration of drugs possessing nephrotoxic effects with aldesleukin may increase the potential for nephrotoxicity).
No products indexed under this heading.

Cefotetan (Concurrent administration of drugs possessing nephrotoxic effects with aldesleukin may increase the potential for nephrotoxicity).
No products indexed under this heading.

Cefoxitin Sodium (Concurrent administration of drugs possessing nephrotoxic effects with aldesleukin may increase the potential for nephrotoxicity).
No products indexed under this heading.

Cefpodoxime Proxetil (Concurrent administration of drugs possessing nephrotoxic effects with aldesleukin may increase the potential for nephrotoxicity).
No products indexed under this heading.

Cefprozil (Concurrent administration of drugs possessing nephrotoxic effects with aldesleukin may increase the potential for nephrotoxicity).
No products indexed under this heading.

Ceftazidime (Concurrent administration of drugs possessing nephrotoxic effects with aldesleukin may increase the potential for nephrotoxicity).
Products include:
Fortaz 1481

Ceftizoxime Sodium (Concurrent administration of drugs possessing nephrotoxic effects with aldesleukin may increase the potential for nephrotoxicity).
No products indexed under this heading.

Ceftriaxone Sodium (Concurrent administration of drugs possessing nephrotoxic effects with aldesleukin may increase the potential for nephrotoxicity). Products include:
Rocephin 2859

Cefuroxime Axetil (Concurrent administration of drugs possessing nephrotoxic effects with aldesleukin may increase the potential for nephrotoxicity). Products include:
Ceftin 1399

Cefuroxime Sodium (Concurrent administration of drugs possessing nephrotoxic effects with aldesleukin may increase the potential for nephrotoxicity).
No products indexed under this heading.

Celecoxib (Concurrent administration of drugs possessing nephrotoxic effects with aldesleukin may increase the potential for nephrotoxicity).
Products include:
Celebrex 3272

Cephalexin (Concurrent administration of drugs possessing nephrotoxic effects with aldesleukin may increase the potential for nephrotoxicity).
No products indexed under this heading.

Cephalothin Sodium (Concurrent administration of drugs possessing nephrotoxic effects with aldesleukin may increase the potential for nephrotoxicity).
No products indexed under this heading.

Cephapirin Sodium (Concurrent administration of drugs possessing nephrotoxic effects with aldesleukin may increase the potential for nephrotoxicity).
No products indexed under this heading.

Cephradine (Concurrent administration of drugs possessing nephrotoxic effects with aldesleukin may increase the potential for nephrotoxicity).
No products indexed under this heading.

Cerivastatin Sodium (Concurrent administration of drugs possessing nephrotoxic effects with aldesleukin may increase the potential for nephrotoxicity).
No products indexed under this heading.

Chloral Hydrate (Aldesleukin may affect central nervous function. Therefore, interactions could occur following concomitant administration of psychotropic drugs).
No products indexed under this heading.

Chlorambucil (Concurrent administration of drugs possessing myelotoxic effects with aldesleukin may increase the potential for myelotoxicity).
Products include:
Leukeran 1557

Chloramphenicol (Concurrent administration of drugs possessing myelotoxic effects with aldesleukin may increase the potential for myelotoxicity).
No products indexed under this heading.

Chloramphenicol Palmitate (Concurrent administration of drugs possessing myelotoxic effects with aldesleukin may increase the potential for myelotoxicity).
No products indexed under this heading.

Chloramphenicol Sodium Succinate (Concurrent administration of drugs possessing myelotoxic effects with aldesleukin may increase the potential for myelotoxicity).
No products indexed under this heading.

Chlordiazepoxide (Aldesleukin may affect central nervous function. Therefore, interactions could occur following concomitant administration of psychotropic drugs).
No products indexed under this heading.

Chlordiazepoxide Hydrochloride (Aldesleukin may affect central nervous function. Therefore, interactions could occur following concomitant administration of psychotropic drugs).
No products indexed under this heading.

Chlorothiazide (Concurrent administration of drugs possessing nephrotoxic effects with aldesleukin may increase the potential for nephrotoxicity).
No products indexed under this heading.

Chlorothiazide Sodium (Concurrent administration of drugs possessing nephrotoxic effects with aldesleukin may increase the potential for nephrotoxicity). Products include:
Diuril Intravenous 2009

Chlorpromazine (Aldesleukin may affect central nervous function. Therefore, interactions could occur following concomitant administration of psychotropic drugs).
No products indexed under this heading.

Chlorpromazine Hydrochloride (Aldesleukin may affect central nervous function. Therefore, interactions could occur following concomitant administration of psychotropic drugs).
No products indexed under this heading.

Chlorpropamide (Concurrent administration of drugs possessing nephrotoxic effects with aldesleukin may increase the potential for nephrotoxicity).
No products indexed under this heading.

Chlorprothixene (Aldesleukin may affect central nervous function. Therefore, interactions could occur following concomitant administration of psychotropic drugs).
No products indexed under this heading.

Chlorprothixene Hydrochloride (Aldesleukin may affect central nervous function. Therefore, interactions could occur following concomitant administration of psychotropic drugs).
No products indexed under this heading.

Chlorprothixene Lactate (Aldesleukin may affect central nervous function. Therefore, interactions could occur following concomitant administration of tranquilizers).
No products indexed under this heading.

Chlorthalidone (Concurrent use with antihypertensive drugs may potentiate the hypotension seen with aldesleukin).
Products include:
Clorpres 2344

Cidofovir (Concurrent administration of drugs possessing nephrotoxic effects with aldesleukin may increase the potential for nephrotoxicity).
No products indexed under this heading.

Cilastatin Sodium (Concurrent administration of drugs possessing nephrotoxic effects with aldesleukin may increase the potential for nephrotoxicity). Products include:
Primaxin I.M. 2232
Primaxin I.V. 2235

Cimetidine (Concurrent administration of drugs possessing nephrotoxic effects with aldesleukin may increase the potential for nephrotoxicity).
No products indexed under this heading.

Cimetidine Hydrochloride (Concurrent administration of drugs possessing nephrotoxic effects with aldesleukin may increase the potential for nephrotoxicity).
No products indexed under this heading.

Cisplatin (Hypersensitivity reactions have been reported in patients receiving combination regimens containing sequential high dose aldesleukin and antineoplastic agents, specifically cisplatin. These reactions consisted of erythema, pruritis, and hypotension and occurred within hours of administration of chemotherapy. These events required medical intervention in some patients).
No products indexed under this heading.

Cladribine (Concurrent administration of drugs possessing nephrotoxic effects with aldesleukin may increase the potential for nephrotoxicity).
Products include:
Leustatin 946

Clomipramine Hydrochloride (Concurrent administration of drugs possessing hepatotoxic effects with aldesleukin may increase toxicity in the liver).
No products indexed under this heading.

Clonidine (Concurrent use with antihypertensive drugs may potentiate the hypotension seen with aldesleukin).
Products include:
Catapres-TTS 884

Clonidine Hydrochloride (Aldesleukin may affect central nervous function. Therefore, interactions could occur following concomitant administration of analgesics). Products include:
Clorpres 2344

Clorazepate Dipotassium (Aldesleukin may affect central nervous function. Therefore, interactions could occur following concomitant administration of psychotropic drugs).
No products indexed under this heading.

Cloxacillin (Concurrent administration of drugs possessing hepatotoxic effects with aldesleukin may increase toxicity in the liver).
No products indexed under this heading.

Cloxacillin Sodium (Concurrent administration of drugs possessing hepatotoxic effects with aldesleukin may increase toxicity in the liver).
No products indexed under this heading.

Cloxacillin Sodium Monohydrate (Concurrent administration of drugs possessing hepatotoxic effects with aldesleukin may increase toxicity in the liver).
No products indexed under this heading.

Clozapine (Aldesleukin may affect central nervous function. Therefore, interactions could occur following concomitant administration of psychotropic drugs).
No products indexed under this heading.

Cocaine Hydrochloride (Concurrent administration of drugs possessing cardiotoxic effects with aldesleukin may increase toxicity in the cardiovascular systems).
No products indexed under this heading.

Codeine Phosphate (Aldesleukin may affect central nervous function. Therefore, interactions could occur following concomitant administration of narcotics). Products include:
Tylenol with Codeine 2691

Codeine Sulfate (Aldesleukin may affect central nervous function. Therefore, interactions could occur following concomitant administration of narcotics).
No products indexed under this heading.

Colistimethate Sodium (Concurrent administration of drugs possessing nephrotoxic effects with aldesleukin may increase the potential for nephrotoxicity).
No products indexed under this heading.

Colistin Sulfate (Concurrent administration of drugs possessing nephrotoxic effects with aldesleukin may increase the potential for nephrotoxicity).
No products indexed under this heading.

Cortisone Acetate (Although glucocorticoids have been shown to reduce aldesleukin-induced side effects including fever, renal insufficiency, hyperbilirubinemia, confusion, and dyspnea, concomitant administration of these agents with aldesleukin may reduce the antitumor effectiveness of aldesleukin and thus should be avoided).
No products indexed under this heading.

Cyclophosphamide (Concurrent administration of drugs possessing nephrotoxic effects with aldesleukin may increase the potential for nephrotoxicity).
No products indexed under this heading.

Cyclosporine (Concurrent administration of drugs possessing nephrotoxic effects with aldesleukin may increase the potential for nephrotoxicity). Products include:
Gengraf 440
Neoral Oral Solution 2496
Neoral Capsules 2496
Restasis 605

Cytarabine (Concurrent administration of drugs possessing nephrotoxic effects with aldesleukin may increase the potential for nephrotoxicity).
No products indexed under this heading.

Cytarabine Liposome (Concurrent administration of drugs possessing nephrotoxic effects with aldesleukin may increase the potential for nephrotoxicity).
No products indexed under this heading.

Dacarbazine (Hypersensitivity reactions have been reported in patients receiving combination regimens containing sequential high dose aldesleukin and antineoplastic agents, specifically dacarbazine. These reactions consisted of erythema, pruritis, and hypotension and occurred within hours of administration of chemotherapy. These events required medical intervention in some patients).
No products indexed under this heading.

Darunavir (Concurrent administration of drugs possessing hepatotoxic effects with aldesleukin may increase toxicity in the liver).
No products indexed under this heading.

Daunorubicin Citrate (Hypersensitivity reactions have been reported in patients receiving combination regimens containing sequential high dose aldesleukin and antineoplastic agents. These reactions consisted of erythema, pruritus, and hypotension and occurred within hours of administration of chemotherapy. These events required medical intervention in some patients).
No products indexed under this heading.

Daunorubicin Citrate Liposome (Concurrent administration of drugs possessing myelotoxic effects with aldesleukin may increase the potential for myelotoxicity).
No products indexed under this heading.

Daunorubicin Hydrochloride (Concurrent administration of drugs possessing myelotoxic effects with aldesleukin may increase the potential for myelotoxicity).
No products indexed under this heading.

Delavirdine Mesylate (Concurrent administration of drugs possessing nephrotoxic effects with aldesleukin may increase the potential for nephrotoxicity).
No products indexed under this heading.

Demeclocycline Hydrochloride (Concurrent administration of drugs possessing hepatotoxic effects with aldesleukin may increase toxicity in the liver).
No products indexed under this heading.

Denileukin Diftitox (Hypersensitivity reactions have been reported in patients receiving combination regimens containing sequential high dose aldesleukin and antineoplastic agents. These reactions consisted of erythema, pruritus, and hypotension and occurred within hours of administration of chemotherapy. These events required medical intervention in some patients). Products include:
Ontak 1068

Deserpidine (Concurrent use with antihypertensive drugs may potentiate the hypotension seen with aldesleukin).
No products indexed under this heading.

Desipramine Hydrochloride (Aldesleukin may affect central nervous function. Therefore, interactions could occur following concomitant administration of psychotropic drugs).
No products indexed under this heading.

Dexamethasone (Although glucocorticoids have been shown to reduce aldesleukin-induced side effects including fever, renal insufficiency, hyperbilirubinemia, confusion, and dyspnea, concomitant administration of these agents with aldesleukin may reduce the antitumor effectiveness of aldesleukin and thus should be avoided). Products include:
Ciprodex 583
Ozurdex .... ⊙223
Tobramycin and Dexamethasone
Ophthalmic Suspension .... ⊙251

Dexamethasone Acetate (Although glucocorticoids have been shown to reduce aldesleukin-induced side effects including fever, renal insufficiency, hyperbilirubinemia, confusion, and dyspnea, concomitant administration of these agents with aldesleukin may reduce the antitumor effectiveness of aldesleukin and thus should be avoided).
No products indexed under this heading.

Dexamethasone Sodium Phosphate (Although glucocorticoids have been shown to reduce aldesleukin-induced side effects including fever, renal insufficiency, hyperbilirubinemia, confusion, and dyspnea, concomitant administration of these agents with aldesleukin may reduce the antitumor effectiveness of aldesleukin and thus should be avoided).
No products indexed under this heading.

Dexrazoxane (Concurrent administration of drugs possessing myelotoxic effects with aldesleukin may increase the potential for myelotoxicity).
No products indexed under this heading.

Dextroamphetamine (Concurrent administration of drugs possessing cardiotoxic effects with aldesleukin may increase toxicity in the cardiovascular systems).
No products indexed under this heading.

Dextroamphetamine Saccharate (Concurrent administration of drugs possessing cardiotoxic effects with aldesleukin may increase toxicity in the cardiovascular systems).
No products indexed under this heading.

Dextroamphetamine Sulfate (Concurrent administration of drugs possessing cardiotoxic effects with aldesleukin may increase toxicity in the cardiovascular systems). Products include:
Dexedrine 1425

Dezocine (Aldesleukin may affect central nervous function. Therefore, interactions could occur following concomitant administration of narcotics).
No products indexed under this heading.

Diatrizoate Meglumine (Concurrent administration of drugs possessing nephrotoxic effects with aldesleukin may increase the potential for nephrotoxicity).
No products indexed under this heading.

Diatrizoate Sodium (Concurrent administration of drugs possessing nephrotoxic effects with aldesleukin may increase the potential for nephrotoxicity).
No products indexed under this heading.

Diazepam (Aldesleukin may affect central nervous function. Therefore, interactions could occur following concomitant administration of psychotropic drugs). Products include:
Valium Tablets 2880

Diazoxide (Concurrent use with antihypertensive drugs may potentiate the hypotension seen with aldesleukin). Products include:
Proglycem 1179
Proglycem Suspension 1179

Diclofenac Epolamine (Concurrent administration of drugs possessing hepatotoxic effects with aldesleukin may increase toxicity in the liver). Products include:
Flector 1839

Diclofenac Potassium (Concurrent administration of drugs possessing nephrotoxic effects with aldesleukin may increase the potential for nephrotoxicity).
No products indexed under this heading.

Diclofenac Sodium (Concurrent administration of drugs possessing nephrotoxic effects with aldesleukin may increase the potential for nephrotoxicity).
No products indexed under this heading.

Dicloxacillin (Concurrent administration of drugs possessing hepatotoxic effects with aldesleukin may increase toxicity in the liver).
No products indexed under this heading.

Dicloxacillin Sodium (Concurrent administration of drugs possessing nephrotoxic effects with aldesleukin may increase the potential for nephrotoxicity).
No products indexed under this heading.

Didanosine (Concurrent administration of drugs possessing nephrotoxic effects with aldesleukin may increase the potential for nephrotoxicity).
No products indexed under this heading.

Digitalis Glycoside Preparations (Concurrent administration of drugs possessing cardiotoxic effects with aldesleukin may increase toxicity in the cardiovascular systems).
No products indexed under this heading.

Digitalis Lanata (Concurrent administration of drugs possessing cardiotoxic effects with aldesleukin may increase toxicity in the cardiovascular systems).
No products indexed under this heading.

Digitalis Purpurea (Concurrent administration of drugs possessing cardiotoxic effects with aldesleukin may increase toxicity in the cardiovascular systems).
No products indexed under this heading.

Digitoxin (Concurrent administration of drugs possessing cardiotoxic effects with aldesleukin may increase toxicity in the cardiovascular systems).
No products indexed under this heading.

Digoxin (Concurrent administration of drugs possessing cardiotoxic effects with aldesleukin may increase toxicity in the cardiovascular systems). Products include:
Lanoxin Injection 1546
Lanoxin Injection Pediatric 1549
Lanoxin Tablets 1553

Dihydrocodeine Bitartrate (Aldesleukin may affect central nervous function. Therefore, interactions could occur following concomitant administration of narcotics).
No products indexed under this heading.

Dihydrocodeinone Bitartrate (Aldesleukin may affect central nervous function. Therefore, interactions could occur following concomitant administration of narcotics).
No products indexed under this heading.

Dihydrostreptomycin (Concurrent administration of drugs possessing nephrotoxic effects with aldesleukin may increase the potential for nephrotoxicity).
No products indexed under this heading.

Diltiazem Hydrochloride (Concurrent use with antihypertensive drugs may potentiate the hypotension seen with aldesleukin). Products include:
Cardizem LA 423

Diltiazem Maleate (Concurrent use with antihypertensive drugs may potentiate the hypotension seen with aldesleukin).
No products indexed under this heading.

Dimenhydrinate (Aldesleukin may affect central nervous function. Therefore, interactions could occur following concomitant administration of antiemetics).
No products indexed under this heading.

IMPORTANT NOTE: Always consult each drug listing in the patient's regimen for possible interactions.

1495 Interactions Index Proleukin

myelotoxic effects with aldesleukin may increase the potential for myelotoxicity). Products include:
Oforta 3023

Fludrocortisone Acetate (Although glucocorticoids have been shown to reduce aldesleukin-induced side effects including fever, renal insufficiency, hyperbilirubinemia, confusion, and dyspnea, concomitant administration of these agents with aldesleukin may reduce the antitumor effectiveness of aldesleukin and thus should be avoided).
No products indexed under this heading.

Fluorouracil (Concurrent administration of drugs possessing nephrotoxic effects with aldesleukin may increase the potential for nephrotoxicity). Products include:
Carac 2966

Fluphenazine Decanoate (Aldesleukin may affect central nervous function. Therefore, interactions could occur following concomitant administration of psychotropic drugs).
No products indexed under this heading.

Fluphenazine Enanthate (Aldesleukin may affect central nervous function. Therefore, interactions could occur following concomitant administration of psychotropic drugs).
No products indexed under this heading.

Fluphenazine Hydrochloride (Aldesleukin may affect central nervous function. Therefore, interactions could occur following concomitant administration of psychotropic drugs).
No products indexed under this heading.

Flurazepam Hydrochloride (Aldesleukin may affect central nervous function. Therefore, interactions could occur following concomitant administration of psychotropic drugs).
No products indexed under this heading.

Flurbiprofen (Concurrent administration of drugs possessing nephrotoxic effects with aldesleukin may increase the potential for nephrotoxicity).
No products indexed under this heading.

Flurbiprofen Sodium (Concurrent administration of drugs possessing hepatotoxic effects with aldesleukin may increase toxicity in the liver).
No products indexed under this heading.

Flutamide (Hypersensitivity reactions have been reported in patients receiving combination regimens containing sequential high dose aldesleukin and antineoplastic agents. These reactions consisted of erythema, pruritus, and hypotension and occurred within hours of administration of chemotherapy. These events required medical intervention in some patients).
No products indexed under this heading.

Fluvastatin Sodium (Concurrent administration of drugs possessing nephrotoxic effects with aldesleukin may increase the potential for nephrotoxicity).
No products indexed under this heading.

Fosamprenavir Calcium (Concurrent administration of drugs possessing hepatotoxic effects with aldesleukin may increase toxicity in the liver). Products include:
Lexiva Oral Suspension 1558
Lexiva 1558

Foscarnet Sodium (Concurrent administration of drugs possessing nephrotoxic effects with aldesleukin may increase the potential for nephrotoxicity).
No products indexed under this heading.

Fosinopril Sodium (Concurrent administration of drugs possessing nephrotoxic effects with aldesleukin may increase the potential for nephrotoxicity).
No products indexed under this heading.

Fosphenytoin (Concurrent administration of drugs possessing hepatotoxic effects with aldesleukin may increase toxicity in the liver).
No products indexed under this heading.

Fosphenytoin Sodium (Concurrent administration of drugs possessing hepatotoxic effects with aldesleukin may increase toxicity in the liver).
No products indexed under this heading.

Furosemide (Concurrent administration of drugs possessing nephrotoxic effects with aldesleukin may increase the potential for nephrotoxicity). Products include:
Furosemide 2354

Gadopentetate Dimeglumine (Concurrent administration of drugs possessing nephrotoxic effects with aldesleukin may increase the potential for nephrotoxicity).
No products indexed under this heading.

Gemcitabine Hydrochloride (Concurrent administration of drugs possessing myelotoxic effects with aldesleukin may increase the potential for myelotoxicity). Products include:
Gemzar 1900

Gemfibrozil (Concurrent administration of drugs possessing hepatotoxic effects with aldesleukin may increase toxicity in the liver).
No products indexed under this heading.

Gemtuzumab Ozogamicin (Concurrent administration of drugs possessing myelotoxic effects with aldesleukin may increase the potential for myelotoxicity). Products include:
Mylotarg 3524

Gentamicin (Concurrent administration of drugs possessing nephrotoxic effects with aldesleukin may increase the potential for nephrotoxicity).
No products indexed under this heading.

Gentamicin Sulfate (Concurrent administration of drugs possessing nephrotoxic effects with aldesleukin may increase the potential for nephrotoxicity). Products include:
Pred-G .... ⊙226, ⊙227

Glimepiride (Concurrent administration of drugs possessing hepatotoxic effects with aldesleukin may increase toxicity in the liver). Products include:
Avandaryl 1356
Duetact 3354

Glipizide (Concurrent administration of drugs possessing nephrotoxic effects with aldesleukin may increase the potential for nephrotoxicity).
No products indexed under this heading.

Globulin, Immune (Human) (Concurrent administration of drugs possessing nephrotoxic effects with aldesleukin may increase the potential for nephrotoxicity). Products include:

Glutethimide (Aldesleukin may affect central nervous function. Therefore, interactions could occur following concomitant administration of psychotropic drugs).
No products indexed under this heading.

Glyburide (Concurrent administration of drugs possessing nephrotoxic effects with aldesleukin may increase the potential for nephrotoxicity).
No products indexed under this heading.

Gold Therapy (Concurrent administration of drugs possessing nephrotoxic effects with aldesleukin may increase the potential for nephrotoxicity).
No products indexed under this heading.

Granisetron Hydrochloride (Aldesleukin may affect central nervous function. Therefore, interactions could occur following concomitant administration of antiemetics).
No products indexed under this heading.

Griseofulvin (Concurrent administration of drugs possessing hepatotoxic effects with aldesleukin may increase toxicity in the liver).
No products indexed under this heading.

Guanabenz Acetate (Concurrent use with antihypertensive drugs may potentiate the hypotension seen with aldesleukin).
No products indexed under this heading.

Guanethidine (Concurrent use with antihypertensive drugs may potentiate the hypotension seen with aldesleukin).
No products indexed under this heading.

Guanethidine Monosulfate (Concurrent use with antihypertensive drugs may potentiate the hypotension seen with aldesleukin).
No products indexed under this heading.

Guanethidine Sulfate (Concurrent use with antihypertensive drugs may potentiate the hypotension seen with aldesleukin).
No products indexed under this heading.

Haloperidol (Aldesleukin may affect central nervous function. Therefore, interactions could occur following concomitant administration of psychotropic drugs).
No products indexed under this heading.

Haloperidol Decanoate (Aldesleukin may affect central nervous function. Therefore, interactions could occur following concomitant administration of psychotropic drugs).
No products indexed under this heading.

Halothane (Concurrent administration of drugs possessing hepatotoxic effects with aldesleukin may increase toxicity in the liver).
No products indexed under this heading.

Heparin (Concurrent administration of drugs possessing hepatotoxic effects with aldesleukin may increase toxicity in the liver).
No products indexed under this heading.

Heparin Calcium (Concurrent administration of drugs possessing hepatotoxic effects with aldesleukin may increase toxicity in the liver).
No products indexed under this heading.

Heparin Sodium (Concurrent administration of drugs possessing hepatotoxic effects with aldesleukin may increase toxicity in the liver).
No products indexed under this heading.

HMG-CoA Reductase Inhibitors (Concurrent administration of drugs possessing nephrotoxic effects with aldesleukin may increase the potential for nephrotoxicity).
No products indexed under this heading.

Hydralazine (Concurrent administration of drugs possessing hepatotoxic effects with aldesleukin may increase toxicity in the liver).
No products indexed under this heading.

Hydralazine Hydrochloride (Concurrent use with antihypertensive drugs may potentiate the hypotension seen with aldesleukin).
No products indexed under this heading.

Hydrochlorothiazide (Concurrent administration of drugs possessing nephrotoxic effects with aldesleukin may increase the potential for nephrotoxicity). Products include:
Atacand HCT 700
Avalide 2956
Benicar HCT 1017
Diovan HCT 2419
Dyazide 1429
Exforge HCT 2449
Hyzaar 2162
Hyzaar 100-12.5 2162
Micardis HCT 889
Prinzide 2246
Tekturna HCT 2541
Teveten HCT 541

Hydrochlorothiazide Hydrochloride (Concurrent administration of drugs possessing hepatotoxic effects with aldesleukin may increase toxicity in the liver).
No products indexed under this heading.

Hydrocodone Bitartrate (Aldesleukin may affect central nervous function. Therefore, interactions could occur following concomitant administration of narcotics). Products include:
Vicodin 560
Vicodin ES 561
Vicodin HP 563
Vicoprofen 564
Zydone 1138

Hydrocodone Polistirex (Aldesleukin may affect central nervous function. Therefore, interactions could occur following concomitant administration of narcotics). Products include:
Tussionex 3443

Hydrocortisone (Although glucocorticoids have been shown to reduce aldesleukin-induced side effects including fever, renal insufficiency, hyperbilirubinemia, confusion, and dyspnea, concomitant administration of these agents with aldesleukin may reduce the antitumor effectiveness of aldesleukin and thus should be avoided).
No products indexed under this heading.

Hydrocortisone Acetate (Although glucocorticoids have been shown to reduce aldesleukin-induced side effects including fever, renal insufficiency, hyperbilirubinemia, confusion, and dyspnea, concomitant administration of these agents with aldesleukin may reduce the antitumor effectiveness of aldesleukin and thus should be avoided).
No products indexed under this heading.

Hydrocortisone Sodium Phosphate (Although glucocorticoids have been shown to reduce aldesleukin-induced side effects including fever, renal insufficiency, hyperbilirubinemia, confusion, and dyspnea, concomitant administration of these agents with aldesleukin may reduce the antitumor effectiveness of aldesleukin and thus should be avoided).
No products indexed under this heading.

Hydrocortisone Sodium Succinate (Although glucocorticoids have been shown to reduce aldesleukin-induced side effects including fever, renal insufficiency, hyperbilirubinemia, confusion, and dyspnea, concomitant administration of these agents with aldesleukin may reduce the antitumor effectiveness of aldesleukin and thus should be avoided).
No products indexed under this heading.

Hydroflumethiazide (Concurrent administration of drugs possessing nephrotoxic effects with aldesleukin may increase the potential for nephrotoxicity).
No products indexed under this heading.

Hydromorphone (Aldesleukin may affect central nervous function. Therefore, interactions could occur following concomitant administration of narcotics).
No products indexed under this heading.

Hydromorphone Hydrochloride (Aldesleukin may affect central nervous function. Therefore, interactions could occur following concomitant administration of narcotics). Products include:
Dilaudid Injection 2800
Dilaudid Oral 2797
Dilaudid Tablets 2797
Dilaudid-HP 2800

Hydroxyurea (Concurrent administration of drugs possessing myelotoxic effects with aldesleukin may increase the potential for myelotoxicity).
No products indexed under this heading.

IMPORTANT NOTE: Always consult each drug listing in the patient's regimen for possible interactions.

Proleukin **Interactions Index** **1496**

Hydroxyzine Hydrochloride (Aldesleukin may affect central nervous function. Therefore, interactions could occur following concomitant administration of psychotropic drugs).
No products indexed under this heading.

Ibuprofen (Concurrent administration of drugs possessing nephrotoxic effects with aldesleukin may increase the potential for nephrotoxicity).
Products include:
- Motrin IB 2043
- Children's Motrin 2044
- Children's Motrin Non-Staining Dye-Free 2044
- Infants' Motrin 2044
- Infants' Motrin Dye-Free 2044
- Junior Strength Motrin 2044
- Vicoprofen 564

Idarubicin Hydrochloride (Concurrent administration of drugs possessing nephrotoxic effects with aldesleukin may increase the potential for nephrotoxicity).
No products indexed under this heading.

Ifosfamide (Concurrent administration of drugs possessing nephrotoxic effects with aldesleukin may increase the potential for nephrotoxicity).
No products indexed under this heading.

Imatinib Mesylate (Concurrent administration of drugs possessing hepatotoxic effects with aldesleukin may increase toxicity in the liver). Products include:
- Gleevec 2477

Imipenem (Concurrent administration of drugs possessing nephrotoxic effects with aldesleukin may increase the potential for nephrotoxicity).
Products include:
- Primaxin I.M. 2232
- Primaxin I.V. 2235

Imipramine Hydrochloride (Aldesleukin may affect central nervous function. Therefore, interactions could occur following concomitant administration of psychotropic drugs).
No products indexed under this heading.

Imipramine Pamoate (Aldesleukin may affect central nervous function. Therefore, interactions could occur following concomitant administration of psychotropic drugs).
No products indexed under this heading.

Immune Globulin Intravenous (Human) (Concurrent administration of drugs possessing nephrotoxic effects with aldesleukin may increase the potential for nephrotoxicity). Products include:
- Flebogamma 5% DIF 1794
- Gammagard 812, 815
- Gamunex 3374

Indapamide (Concurrent use with antihypertensive drugs may potentiate the hypotension seen with aldesleukin).
Products include:
- Indapamide 2356

Indinavir Sulfate (Concurrent administration of drugs possessing nephrotoxic effects with aldesleukin may increase the potential for nephrotoxicity). Products include:
- Crixivan 2113

Indomethacin (Concurrent administration of drugs possessing nephrotoxic effects with aldesleukin may increase the potential for nephrotoxicity).
Products include:
- Indocin 2167

Indomethacin Sodium Trihydrate (Concurrent administration of drugs possessing nephrotoxic effects with aldesleukin may increase the potential for nephrotoxicity). Products include:
- Indocin I.V. 2007

Interferon alfa-2a, Recombinant (Myocardial injury and severe rhabdomyolysis appear to be increased with concurrent use of aldesleukin and interferon-alfa. Also, hypersensitivity reactions have been reported in patients receiving combination regimens containing sequential high dose aldesleukin and interferon-alfa. These reactions consisted of erythema, pruritus, and hypotension and occurred within hours of administration of chemotherapy. In addition, exacerbation of the initial presentation of a number of autoimmune and inflammatory disorders has been observed following concurrent use of interferon-alfa and aldesleukin, including crescentic IgA glomerulonephritis, oculo-bulbar myasthenia gravis, inflammatory arthritis, thyroiditis, bullous pemphigoid, and Stevens-Johnson syndrome).
No products indexed under this heading.

Interferon alfa-2b, Recombinant (Myocardial injury and severe rhabdomyolysis appear to be increased with concurrent use of aldesleukin and interferon-alfa. Also, hypersensitivity reactions have been reported in patients receiving combination regimens containing sequential high dose aldesleukin and interferon-alfa. These reactions consisted of erythema, pruritus, and hypotension and occurred within hours of administration of chemotherapy. In addition, exacerbation of the initial presentation of a number of autoimmune and inflammatory disorders has been observed following concurrent use of interferon-alfa and aldesleukin, including crescentic IgA glomerulonephritis, oculo-bulbar myasthenia gravis, inflammatory arthritis, thyroiditis, bullous pemphigoid, and Stevens-Johnson syndrome). Products include:
- Intron A 3140

Interferon Beta-1a (Concurrent administration of drugs possessing hepatotoxic effects with aldesleukin may increase toxicity in the liver). Products include:
- Rebif 1096

Interferon Beta-1b (Concurrent administration of drugs possessing nephrotoxic effects with aldesleukin may increase the potential for nephrotoxicity). Products include:
- Betaseron 836
- Extavia 2459

Interleuken-2 (Concurrent administration of drugs possessing nephrotoxic effects with aldesleukin may increase the potential for nephrotoxicity).
No products indexed under this heading.

Iodamide Meglumine (Concurrent administration of drugs possessing nephrotoxic effects with aldesleukin may increase the potential for nephrotoxicity).
No products indexed under this heading.

Iohexol (Concurrent administration of drugs possessing nephrotoxic effects with aldesleukin may increase the potential for nephrotoxicity).
No products indexed under this heading.

Iopamidol (Concurrent administration of drugs possessing nephrotoxic effects with aldesleukin may increase the potential for nephrotoxicity).
No products indexed under this heading.

Iopanoic Acid (Concurrent administration of drugs possessing nephrotoxic effects with aldesleukin may increase the potential for nephrotoxicity).
No products indexed under this heading.

Iothalamate Meglumine (Concurrent administration of drugs possessing nephrotoxic effects with aldesleukin may increase the potential for nephrotoxicity).
No products indexed under this heading.

Ioxaglate Meglumine (Concurrent administration of drugs possessing nephrotoxic effects with aldesleukin may increase the potential for nephrotoxicity).
No products indexed under this heading.

Ioxaglate Sodium (Concurrent administration of drugs possessing nephrotoxic effects with aldesleukin may increase the potential for nephrotoxicity).
No products indexed under this heading.

Irbesartan (Concurrent use with antihypertensive drugs may potentiate the hypotension seen with aldesleukin).
Products include:
- Avalide 2956
- Avapro 2962

Irinotecan Hydrochloride (Concurrent administration of drugs possessing myelotoxic effects with aldesleukin may increase the potential for myelotoxicity).
No products indexed under this heading.

Isocarboxazid (Aldesleukin may affect central nervous function. Therefore, interactions could occur following concomitant administration of psychotropic drugs). Products include:
- Marplan 3481

Isoniazid (Concurrent administration of drugs possessing cardiotoxic effects with aldesleukin may increase toxicity in the cardiovascular systems).
No products indexed under this heading.

Isotretinoin (Concurrent administration of drugs possessing hepatotoxic effects with aldesleukin may increase toxicity in the liver). Products include:
- Accutane 2832

Isradipine (Concurrent use with antihypertensive drugs may potentiate the hypotension seen with aldesleukin).
Products include:
- DynaCirc CR 1432

Itraconazole (Concurrent administration of drugs possessing hepatotoxic effects with aldesleukin may increase toxicity in the liver).
No products indexed under this heading.

Kanamycin Sulfate (Concurrent administration of drugs possessing nephrotoxic effects with aldesleukin may increase the potential for nephrotoxicity).
No products indexed under this heading.

Ketoconazole (Concurrent administration of drugs possessing hepatotoxic effects with aldesleukin may increase toxicity in the liver). Products include:
- Extina 3319
- Xolegel 3337

Ketoprofen (Concurrent administration of drugs possessing nephrotoxic effects with aldesleukin may increase the potential for nephrotoxicity).
No products indexed under this heading.

Ketorolac Tromethamine (Concurrent administration of drugs possessing nephrotoxic effects with aldesleukin may increase the potential for nephrotoxicity). Products include:
- Acuvail .... ⊙209

Labetalol Hydrochloride (Beta-blockers may potentiate the hypotension seen with aldesleukin).
No products indexed under this heading.

Lamium album (Concurrent administration of drugs possessing nephrotoxic effects with aldesleukin may increase the potential for nephrotoxicity).
No products indexed under this heading.

Leflunomide (Concurrent administration of drugs possessing hepatotoxic effects with aldesleukin may increase toxicity in the liver).
No products indexed under this heading.

Levamisole Hydrochloride (Hypersensitivity reactions have been reported in patients receiving combination regimens containing sequential high dose aldesleukin and antineoplastic agents. These reactions consisted of erythema, pruritus, and hypotension and occurred within hours of administration of chemotherapy. These events required medical intervention in some patients).
No products indexed under this heading.

Levobunolol Hydrochloride (Beta-blockers may potentiate the hypotension seen with aldesleukin).
No products indexed under this heading.

Levorphanol Tartrate (Aldesleukin may affect central nervous function. Therefore, interactions could occur following concomitant administration of narcotics).
No products indexed under this heading.

Lidocaine Hydrochloride (Concurrent administration of drugs possessing cardiotoxic effects with aldesleukin may increase toxicity in the cardiovascular systems).
No products indexed under this heading.

Lisinopril (Concurrent administration of drugs possessing nephrotoxic effects with aldesleukin may increase the potential for nephrotoxicity).
Products include:
- Prinivil 2241
- Prinzide 2246

Lithium (Concurrent administration of drugs possessing nephrotoxic effects with aldesleukin may increase the potential for nephrotoxicity).
No products indexed under this heading.

Lithium Carbonate (Aldesleukin may affect central nervous function. Therefore, interactions could occur following concomitant administration of psychotropic drugs).
No products indexed under this heading.

Lithium Citrate (Aldesleukin may affect central nervous function. Therefore, interactions could occur following concomitant administration of psychotropic drugs).
No products indexed under this heading.

Lomustine (CCNU) (Hypersensitivity reactions have been reported in patients receiving combination regimens containing sequential high dose aldesleukin and antineoplastic agents. These reactions consisted of erythema, pruritus, and hypotension and occurred within hours of administration of chemotherapy. These events required medical intervention in some patients).
No products indexed under this heading.

Lopinavir (Concurrent administration of drugs possessing nephrotoxic effects with aldesleukin may increase the potential for nephrotoxicity).
Products include:
- Kaletra 458

Loracarbef (Concurrent administration of drugs possessing nephrotoxic effects with aldesleukin may increase the potential for nephrotoxicity).
No products indexed under this heading.

Lorazepam (Aldesleukin may affect central nervous function. Therefore, interactions could occur following concomitant administration of psychotropic drugs).
No products indexed under this heading.

Losartan Potassium (Concurrent use with antihypertensive drugs may potentiate the hypotension seen with aldesleukin). Products include:
- Cozaar 2106
- Hyzaar 2162
- Hyzaar 100-12.5 2162

Lovastatin (Concurrent administration of drugs possessing nephrotoxic

effects with aldesleukin may increase the potential for nephrotoxicity).
Products include:

Loxapine Hydrochloride (Aldesleukin may affect central nervous function. Therefore, interactions could occur following concomitant administration of psychotropic drugs).
No products indexed under this heading.

Loxapine Succinate (Aldesleukin may affect central nervous function. Therefore, interactions could occur following concomitant administration of psychotropic drugs).
No products indexed under this heading.

Maprotiline Hydrochloride (Aldesleukin may affect central nervous function. Therefore, interactions could occur following concomitant administration of psychotropic drugs).
No products indexed under this heading.

Maraviroc (Concurrent administration of drugs possessing hepatotoxic effects with aldesleukin may increase toxicity in the liver). Products include:

Mecamylamine Hydrochloride (Concurrent use with antihypertensive drugs may potentiate the hypotension seen with aldesleukin).
No products indexed under this heading.

Mechlorethamine Hydrochloride (Hypersensitivity reactions have been reported in patients receiving combination regimens containing sequential high dose aldesleukin and antineoplastic agents. These reactions consisted of erythema, pruritus, and hypotension and occurred within hours of administration of chemotherapy. These events required medical intervention in some patients). Products include:

Meclizine Hydrochloride (Aldesleukin may affect central nervous function. Therefore, interactions could occur following concomitant administration of antiemetics).
No products indexed under this heading.

Meclofenamate Sodium (Concurrent administration of drugs possessing nephrotoxic effects with aldesleukin may increase the potential for nephrotoxicity).
No products indexed under this heading.

Mefenamic Acid (Concurrent administration of drugs possessing nephrotoxic effects with aldesleukin may increase the potential for nephrotoxicity).
No products indexed under this heading.

Megestrol Acetate (Hypersensitivity reactions have been reported in patients receiving combination regimens containing sequential high dose aldesleukin and antineoplastic agents. These reactions consisted of erythema, pruritus, and hypotension and occurred within hours of administration of chemotherapy. These events required medical intervention in some patients). Products include:

Meloxicam (Concurrent administration of drugs possessing nephrotoxic effects with aldesleukin may increase the potential for nephrotoxicity).
No products indexed under this heading.

Melphalan (Hypersensitivity reactions have been reported in patients receiving combination regimens containing sequential high dose aldesleukin and antineoplastic agents. These reactions consisted of erythema, pruritus, and hypotension and occurred within hours of administration of chemotherapy. These events required medical intervention in some patients). Products include:

Melphalan Hydrochloride (Concurrent administration of drugs possessing nephrotoxic effects with aldesleukin may increase the potential for nephrotoxicity). Products include:

Meperidine Hydrochloride (Aldesleukin may affect central nervous function. Therefore, interactions could occur following concomitant administration of narcotics).
No products indexed under this heading.

Mephenytoin (Concurrent administration of drugs possessing hepatotoxic effects with aldesleukin may increase toxicity in the liver).
No products indexed under this heading.

Meprobamate (Aldesleukin may affect central nervous function. Therefore, interactions could occur following concomitant administration of psychotropic drugs).
No products indexed under this heading.

Mercaptopurine (Concurrent administration of drugs possessing myelotoxic effects with aldesleukin may increase the potential for myelotoxicity).
No products indexed under this heading.

Mesalamine (Concurrent administration of drugs possessing nephrotoxic effects with aldesleukin may increase the potential for nephrotoxicity). Products include:

Mesoridazine Besylate (Aldesleukin may affect central nervous function. Therefore, interactions could occur following concomitant administration of psychotropic drugs).
No products indexed under this heading.

Methacycline Hydrochloride (Concurrent administration of drugs possessing hepatotoxic effects with aldesleukin may increase toxicity in the liver).
No products indexed under this heading.

Methadone Hydrochloride (Aldesleukin may affect central nervous function. Therefore, interactions could occur following concomitant administration of narcotics).
No products indexed under this heading.

Methamphetamine Hydrochloride (Concurrent administration of drugs possessing cardiotoxic effects with aldesleukin may increase toxicity in the cardiovascular systems).
No products indexed under this heading.

Methicillin Sodium (Concurrent administration of drugs possessing hepatotoxic effects with aldesleukin may increase toxicity in the liver).
No products indexed under this heading.

Methimazole (Concurrent administration of drugs possessing nephrotoxic effects with aldesleukin may increase the potential for nephrotoxicity).
No products indexed under this heading.

Methotrexate (Concurrent administration of drugs possessing hepatotoxic effects with aldesleukin may increase the potential for hepatotoxicity).
No products indexed under this heading.

Methotrexate Sodium (Concurrent administration of drugs possessing nephrotoxic effects with aldesleukin may increase the potential for nephrotoxicity).
No products indexed under this heading.

Methyclothiazide (Concurrent administration of drugs possessing nephrotoxic effects with aldesleukin may increase the potential for nephrotoxicity).
No products indexed under this heading.

Methyldopa (Concurrent use with antihypertensive drugs may potentiate the hypotension seen with aldesleukin).
No products indexed under this heading.

Methyldopate Hydrochloride (Concurrent use with antihypertensive drugs may potentiate the hypotension seen with aldesleukin).
No products indexed under this heading.

Methylprednisolone Acetate (Although glucocorticoids have been shown to reduce aldesleukin-induced side effects including fever, renal insufficiency, hyperbilirubinemia, confusion, and dyspnea, concomitant administration of these agents with aldesleukin may reduce the antitumor effectiveness of aldesleukin and thus should be avoided).
No products indexed under this heading.

Methylprednisolone Sodium Succinate (Although glucocorticoids have been shown to reduce aldesleukin-induced side effects including fever, renal insufficiency, hyperbilirubinemia, confusion, and dyspnea, concomitant administration of these agents with aldesleukin may reduce the antitumor effectiveness of aldesleukin and thus should be avoided).
No products indexed under this heading.

Metipranolol Hydrochloride (Beta-blockers may potentiate the hypotension seen with aldesleukin).
No products indexed under this heading.

Metoclopramide Hydrochloride (Aldesleukin may affect central nervous function. Therefore, interactions could occur following concomitant administration of antiemetics). Products include:

Metolazone (Concurrent use with antihypertensive drugs may potentiate the hypotension seen with aldesleukin).
No products indexed under this heading.

Metoprolol Succinate (Beta-blockers may potentiate the hypotension seen with aldesleukin). Products include:

Metoprolol Tartrate (Beta-blockers may potentiate the hypotension seen with aldesleukin).
No products indexed under this heading.

Metyrosine (Concurrent use with antihypertensive drugs may potentiate the hypotension seen with aldesleukin).
No products indexed under this heading.

Mezlocillin Sodium (Concurrent administration of drugs possessing nephrotoxic effects with aldesleukin may increase the potential for nephrotoxicity).
No products indexed under this heading.

Mibefradil Dihydrochloride (Concurrent use with antihypertensive drugs may potentiate the hypotension seen with aldesleukin).
No products indexed under this heading.

Midazolam Hydrochloride (Aldesleukin may affect central nervous function. Therefore, interactions could occur following concomitant administration of psychotropic drugs).
No products indexed under this heading.

Minocycline Hydrochloride (Concurrent administration of drugs possessing nephrotoxic effects with aldesleukin may increase the potential for nephrotoxicity). Products include:

Minoxidil (Concurrent use with antihypertensive drugs may potentiate the hypotension seen with aldesleukin).
No products indexed under this heading.

Mitomycin (Mitomycin-C) (Concurrent administration of drugs possessing nephrotoxic effects with aldesleukin may increase the potential for nephrotoxicity).
No products indexed under this heading.

Mitotane (Concurrent administration of drugs possessing myelotoxic effects with aldesleukin may increase the potential for myelotoxicity).
No products indexed under this heading.

Mitoxantrone Hydrochloride (Concurrent administration of drugs possessing myelotoxic effects with aldesleukin may increase the potential for myelotoxicity). Products include:

Moexipril Hydrochloride (Concurrent administration of drugs possessing nephrotoxic effects with aldesleukin may increase the potential for nephrotoxicity).
No products indexed under this heading.

Molindone Hydrochloride (Aldesleukin may affect central nervous function. Therefore, interactions could occur following concomitant administration of psychotropic drugs). Products include:

Morphine Sulfate (Aldesleukin may affect central nervous function. Therefore, interactions could occur following concomitant administration of narcotics). Products include:

Morphine Sulfate, Liposomal (Aldesleukin may affect central nervous function. Therefore, interactions could occur following concomitant administration of narcotics).
No products indexed under this heading.

Muromonab-CD3 (Concurrent administration of drugs possessing nephrotoxic effects with aldesleukin may increase the potential for nephrotoxicity). Products include:

Nabilone (Aldesleukin may affect central nervous function. Therefore, interactions could occur following concomitant administration of antiemetics).
No products indexed under this heading.

Nabumetone (Concurrent administration of drugs possessing nephrotoxic effects with aldesleukin may increase the potential for nephrotoxicity).
No products indexed under this heading.

Nadolol (Beta-blockers may potentiate the hypotension seen with aldesleukin). Products include:

Nafcillin Sodium (Concurrent administration of drugs possessing nephrotoxic effects with aldesleukin may increase the potential for nephrotoxicity).
No products indexed under this heading.

Nalbuphine Hydrochloride (Aldesleukin may affect central nervous function. Therefore, interactions could occur following concomitant administration of analgesics).
No products indexed under this heading.

Naproxen (Concurrent administration of drugs possessing nephrotoxic effects with aldesleukin may increase the potential for nephrotoxicity). Products include:

Naproxen Sodium (Concurrent administration of drugs possessing nephrotoxic effects with aldesleukin may increase the potential for nephrotoxicity). Products include:

(⊙ Described in PDR® for Ophthalmic Medicines)

1499 **Interactions Index** **Proleukin**

Phenelzine Sulfate (Aldesleukin may affect central nervous function. Therefore, interactions could occur following concomitant administration of psychotropic drugs).
No products indexed under this heading.

Phenoxybenzamine Hydrochloride (Concurrent use with antihypertensive drugs may potentiate the hypotension seen with aldesleukin). Products include:
Dibenzyline 3495

Phentolamine Mesylate (Concurrent use with antihypertensive drugs may potentiate the hypotension seen with aldesleukin).
No products indexed under this heading.

Phenylbutazone (Concurrent administration of drugs possessing nephrotoxic effects with aldesleukin may increase the potential for nephrotoxicity).
No products indexed under this heading.

Phenytoin (Concurrent administration of drugs possessing hepatotoxic effects with aldesleukin may increase toxicity in the liver).
No products indexed under this heading.

Phenytoin Sodium (Concurrent administration of drugs possessing hepatotoxic effects with aldesleukin may increase toxicity in the liver). Products include:
Phenytek Capsules 2380

Pindolol (Beta-blockers may potentiate the hypotension seen with aldesleukin).
No products indexed under this heading.

Pioglitazone Hydrochloride (Concurrent administration of drugs possessing hepatotoxic effects with aldesleukin may increase toxicity in the liver). Products include:
ActoPlus 3338
Actos 3345
Duetact 3354

Piperacillin Sodium (Concurrent administration of drugs possessing hepatotoxic effects with aldesleukin may increase toxicity in the liver). Products include:
Zosyn 3607

Piroxicam (Concurrent administration of drugs possessing nephrotoxic effects with aldesleukin may increase the potential for nephrotoxicity).
No products indexed under this heading.

Plicamycin (Concurrent administration of drugs possessing nephrotoxic effects with aldesleukin may increase the potential for nephrotoxicity).
No products indexed under this heading.

Polymyxin (Concurrent administration of drugs possessing nephrotoxic effects with aldesleukin may increase the potential for nephrotoxicity).
No products indexed under this heading.

Polymyxin B Sulfate (Concurrent administration of drugs possessing nephrotoxic effects with aldesleukin may increase the potential for nephrotoxicity).
No products indexed under this heading.

Polythiazide (Concurrent administration of drugs possessing nephrotoxic effects with aldesleukin may increase the potential for nephrotoxicity).
No products indexed under this heading.

Pravastatin Sodium (Concurrent administration of drugs possessing nephrotoxic effects with aldesleukin may increase the potential for nephrotoxicity).
No products indexed under this heading.

Prazepam (Aldesleukin may affect central nervous function. Therefore, interactions could occur following concomitant administration of psychotropic drugs).
No products indexed under this heading.

Prazosin Hydrochloride (Concurrent use with antihypertensive drugs may potentiate the hypotension seen with aldesleukin).
No products indexed under this heading.

Prednisolone Acetate (Although glucocorticoids have been shown to reduce aldesleukin-induced side effects including fever, renal insufficiency, hyperbilirubinemia, confusion, and dyspnea, concomitant administration of these agents with aldesleukin may reduce the antitumor effectiveness of aldesleukin and thus should be avoided). Products include:
Blephamide .... ⊙212, ⊙214
Pred Forte .... ⊙225
Pred Mild .... ⊙230
Pred-G .... ⊙226, ⊙227

Prednisolone Sodium Phosphate (Although glucocorticoids have been shown to reduce aldesleukin-induced side effects including fever, renal insufficiency, hyperbilirubinemia, confusion, and dyspnea, concomitant administration of these agents with aldesleukin may reduce the antitumor effectiveness of aldesleukin and thus should be avoided).
No products indexed under this heading.

Prednisolone Tebutate (Although glucocorticoids have been shown to reduce aldesleukin-induced side effects including fever, renal insufficiency, hyperbilirubinemia, confusion, and dyspnea, concomitant administration of these agents with aldesleukin may reduce the antitumor effectiveness of aldesleukin and thus should be avoided).
No products indexed under this heading.

Prednisone (Although glucocorticoids have been shown to reduce aldesleukin-induced side effects including fever, renal insufficiency, hyperbilirubinemia, confusion, and dyspnea, concomitant administration of these agents with aldesleukin may reduce the antitumor effectiveness of aldesleukin and thus should be avoided).
No products indexed under this heading.

Procainamide (Concurrent administration of drugs possessing cardiotoxic effects with aldesleukin may increase toxicity in the cardiovascular systems).
No products indexed under this heading.

Procainamide Hydrochloride (Concurrent administration of drugs possessing cardiotoxic effects with aldesleukin may increase toxicity in the cardiovascular systems).
No products indexed under this heading.

Procarbazine Hydrochloride (Concurrent administration of drugs possessing myelotoxic effects with aldesleukin may increase the potential for myelotoxicity).
No products indexed under this heading.

Prochlorperazine (Aldesleukin may affect central nervous function. Therefore, interactions could occur following concomitant administration of psychotropic drugs).
No products indexed under this heading.

Prochlorperazine Edisylate (Aldesleukin may affect central nervous function. Therefore, interactions could occur following concomitant administration of antiemetics).
No products indexed under this heading.

Prochlorperazine Maleate (Aldesleukin may affect central nervous function. Therefore, interactions could occur following concomitant administration of antiemetics).
No products indexed under this heading.

Promethazine (Aldesleukin may affect central nervous function. Therefore, interactions could occur following concomitant administration of antiemetics).
No products indexed under this heading.

Promethazine Hydrochloride (Aldesleukin may affect central nervous function. Therefore, interactions could occur following concomitant administration of psychotropic drugs).
No products indexed under this heading.

Propafenone Hydrochloride (Concurrent administration of drugs possessing cardiotoxic effects with aldesleukin may increase toxicity in the cardiovascular systems). Products include:
Rythmol 1648
Rythmol SR 1652

Propofol (Aldesleukin may affect central nervous function. Therefore, interactions could occur following concomitant administration of psychotropic drugs).
No products indexed under this heading.

Propoxyphene Hydrochloride (Aldesleukin may affect central nervous function. Therefore, interactions could occur following concomitant administration of narcotics).
No products indexed under this heading.

Propoxyphene Napsylate (Aldesleukin may affect central nervous function. Therefore, interactions could occur following concomitant administration of narcotics).
No products indexed under this heading.

Propranolol Hydrochloride (Beta-blockers may potentiate the hypotension seen with aldesleukin). Products include:
InnoPran XL 1517

Propylthiouracil (Concurrent administration of drugs possessing hepatotoxic effects with aldesleukin may increase toxicity in the liver).
No products indexed under this heading.

Protriptyline Hydrochloride (Aldesleukin may affect central nervous function. Therefore, interactions could occur following concomitant administration of psychotropic drugs).
No products indexed under this heading.

Quazepam (Aldesleukin may affect central nervous function. Therefore, interactions could occur following concomitant administration of psychotropic drugs).
No products indexed under this heading.

Quetiapine Fumarate (Aldesleukin may affect central nervous function. Therefore, interactions could occur following concomitant administration of psychotropic drugs). Products include:
Seroquel 750
Seroquel XR 759

Quinapril Hydrochloride (Concurrent administration of drugs possessing nephrotoxic effects with aldesleukin may increase the potential for nephrotoxicity).
No products indexed under this heading.

Rabeprazole Sodium (Concurrent administration of drugs possessing nephrotoxic effects with aldesleukin may increase the potential for nephrotoxicity). Products include:
Aciphex 1035

Ramelteon (Aldesleukin may affect central nervous function. Therefore, interactions could occur following concomitant administration of psychotropic drugs). Products include:
Rozerem 3366

Ramipril (Concurrent administration of drugs possessing nephrotoxic effects with aldesleukin may increase the potential for nephrotoxicity).
No products indexed under this heading.

Rauwolfia Serpentina (Concurrent use with antihypertensive drugs may potentiate the hypotension seen with aldesleukin).
No products indexed under this heading.

Remifentanil Hydrochloride (Aldesleukin may affect central nervous function. Therefore, interactions could occur following concomitant administration of narcotics).
No products indexed under this heading.

Rescinnamine (Concurrent use with antihypertensive drugs may potentiate the hypotension seen with aldesleukin).
No products indexed under this heading.

Reserpine (Concurrent use with antihypertensive drugs may potentiate the hypotension seen with aldesleukin).
No products indexed under this heading.

Rifampin (Concurrent administration of drugs possessing nephrotoxic effects with aldesleukin may increase the potential for nephrotoxicity).
No products indexed under this heading.

Riluzole (Concurrent administration of drugs possessing nephrotoxic effects with aldesleukin may increase the potential for nephrotoxicity). Products include:
Rilutek 3032

Risperidone (Aldesleukin may affect central nervous function. Therefore, interactions could occur following concomitant administration of psychotropic drugs). Products include:
Risperdal Consta 2682

Ritonavir (Concurrent administration of drugs possessing nephrotoxic effects with aldesleukin may increase the potential for nephrotoxicity). Products include:
Kaletra 458
Norvir 509

Rofecoxib (Concurrent administration of drugs possessing nephrotoxic effects with aldesleukin may increase the potential for nephrotoxicity).
No products indexed under this heading.

Rosuvastatin Calcium (Concurrent administration of drugs possessing hepatotoxic effects with aldesleukin may increase toxicity in the liver). Products include:
Crestor 736

Saquinavir (Concurrent administration of drugs possessing nephrotoxic effects with aldesleukin may increase the potential for nephrotoxicity).
No products indexed under this heading.

Saquinavir Mesylate (Concurrent administration of drugs possessing hepatotoxic effects with aldesleukin may increase toxicity in the liver).
No products indexed under this heading.

Scopolamine (Aldesleukin may affect central nervous function. Therefore, interactions could occur following concomitant administration of antiemetics). Products include:
Transderm Scōp 2397

Scopolamine Hydrobromide (Aldesleukin may affect central nervous function. Therefore, interactions could occur following concomitant administration of antiemetics). Products include:
Donnatal 2711

Secobarbital Sodium (Aldesleukin may affect central nervous function. Therefore, interactions could occur following concomitant administration of psychotropic drugs).
No products indexed under this heading.

Sibutramine Hydrochloride Monohydrate (Concurrent administration of drugs possessing nephrotoxic effects with aldesleukin may increase the potential for nephrotoxicity). Products include:
Meridia 492

Simvastatin (Concurrent administration of drugs possessing nephrotoxic effects with aldesleukin may increase the potential for nephrotoxicity). Products include:

IMPORTANT NOTE: Always consult each drug listing in the patient's regimen for possible interactions.

Proleukin Interactions Index 1500

Simcor 524
Vytorin 10/10 .... 2303, 3240
Vytorin 10/20 .... 2303, 3240
Vytorin 10/40 .... 2303, 3240
Vytorin 10/80 .... 2303, 3240
Zocor 2289

Sodium Butabarbital (Aldesleukin may affect central nervous function. Therefore, interactions could occur following concomitant administration of psychotropic drugs).
No products indexed under this heading.

Sodium Cloxacillin Monohydrate (Concurrent administration of drugs possessing hepatotoxic effects with aldesleukin may increase toxicity in the liver).
No products indexed under this heading.

Sodium Nitroprusside (Concurrent use with antihypertensive drugs may potentiate the hypotension seen with aldesleukin).
No products indexed under this heading.

Sotalol Hydrochloride (Beta-blockers may potentiate the hypotension seen with aldesleukin).
No products indexed under this heading.

Spirapril Hydrochloride (Concurrent administration of drugs possessing nephrotoxic effects with aldesleukin may increase the potential for nephrotoxicity).
No products indexed under this heading.

Statins (Concurrent administration of drugs possessing hepatotoxic effects with aldesleukin may increase toxicity in the liver).
No products indexed under this heading.

Stavudine (Concurrent administration of drugs possessing nephrotoxic effects with aldesleukin may increase the potential for nephrotoxicity).
No products indexed under this heading.

Streptomycin Sulfate (Concurrent administration of drugs possessing nephrotoxic effects with aldesleukin may increase the potential for nephrotoxicity).
No products indexed under this heading.

Streptozocin (Concurrent administration of drugs possessing nephrotoxic effects with aldesleukin may increase the potential for nephrotoxicity).
No products indexed under this heading.

Sufentanil Citrate (Aldesleukin may affect central nervous function. Therefore, interactions could occur following concomitant administration of narcotics).
No products indexed under this heading.

Sulfacytine (Concurrent administration of drugs possessing nephrotoxic effects with aldesleukin may increase the potential for nephrotoxicity).
No products indexed under this heading.

Sulfamethizole (Concurrent administration of drugs possessing nephrotoxic effects with aldesleukin may increase the potential for nephrotoxicity).
No products indexed under this heading.

Sulfamethoxazole (Concurrent administration of drugs possessing nephrotoxic effects with aldesleukin may increase the potential for nephrotoxicity).
No products indexed under this heading.

Sulfasalazine (Concurrent administration of drugs possessing nephrotoxic effects with aldesleukin may increase the potential for nephrotoxicity).
No products indexed under this heading.

Sulfinpyrazone (Concurrent administration of drugs possessing nephrotoxic effects with aldesleukin may increase the potential for nephrotoxicity).
No products indexed under this heading.

Sulfisoxazole Acetyl (Concurrent administration of drugs possessing nephrotoxic effects with aldesleukin may increase the potential for nephrotoxicity).
No products indexed under this heading.

Sulfisoxazole Diolamine (Concurrent administration of drugs possessing nephrotoxic effects with aldesleukin may increase the potential for nephrotoxicity).
No products indexed under this heading.

Sulindac (Concurrent administration of drugs possessing nephrotoxic effects with aldesleukin may increase the potential for nephrotoxicity). Products include:
Clinoril 2098

Tacrine Hydrochloride (Concurrent administration of drugs possessing hepatotoxic effects with aldesleukin may increase toxicity in the liver).
No products indexed under this heading.

Tacrolimus (Concurrent administration of drugs possessing nephrotoxic effects with aldesleukin may increase the potential for nephrotoxicity).
Products include:
Prograf Capsules 677
Prograf Injection 677
Protopic 685

Tamoxifen Citrate (Hypersensitivity reactions have been reported in patients receiving combination regimens containing sequential high dose aldesleukin and antineoplastic agents, specifically tamoxifen. These reactions consisted of erythema, pruritis, and hypotension and occurred within hours of administration of chemotherapy. These events required medical intervention in some patients).
No products indexed under this heading.

Telithromycin (Concurrent administration of drugs possessing hepatotoxic effects with aldesleukin may increase toxicity in the liver). Products include:
Ketek 2991

Telmisartan (Concurrent use with antihypertensive drugs may potentiate the hypotension seen with aldesleukin).
Products include:
Micardis 887
Micardis HCT 889

Temazepam (Aldesleukin may affect central nervous function. Therefore, interactions could occur following concomitant administration of psychotropic drugs).
No products indexed under this heading.

Temozolomide (Concurrent administration of drugs possessing myelotoxic effects with aldesleukin may increase the potential for myelotoxicity).
Products include:
Temodar 3230
Temodar Injection 3230

Teniposide (Hypersensitivity reactions have been reported in patients receiving combination regimens containing sequential high dose aldesleukin and antineoplastic agents. These reactions consisted of erythema, pruritus, and hypotension and occurred within hours of administration of chemotherapy. These events required medical intervention in some patients).
No products indexed under this heading.

Tenofovir Disoproxil Fumarate (Concurrent administration of drugs possessing nephrotoxic effects with aldesleukin may increase the potential for nephrotoxicity). Products include:
Atripla 906
Truvada 1258
Viread 1266

Terazosin Hydrochloride (Concurrent use with antihypertensive drugs may potentiate the hypotension seen with aldesleukin).
No products indexed under this heading.

Tetracycline Hydrochloride (Concurrent administration of drugs possessing hepatotoxic effects with aldesleukin may increase toxicity in the liver). Products include:
Pylera 793

Tetracycline Phosphate Complex (Concurrent administration of drugs possessing hepatotoxic effects with aldesleukin may increase toxicity in the liver).
No products indexed under this heading.

Thiazide Diuretics (Concurrent administration of drugs possessing hepatotoxic effects with aldesleukin may increase toxicity in the liver).
No products indexed under this heading.

Thiazides (Concurrent administration of drugs possessing hepatotoxic effects with aldesleukin may increase toxicity in the liver).
No products indexed under this heading.

Thioguanine (Concurrent administration of drugs possessing nephrotoxic effects with aldesleukin may increase the potential for nephrotoxicity).
Products include:
Tabloid 1664

Thioridazine Hydrochloride (Aldesleukin may affect central nervous function. Therefore, interactions could occur following concomitant administration of psychotropic drugs). Products include:
Thioridazine Hydrochloride 2384

Thiotepa (Hypersensitivity reactions have been reported in patients receiving combination regimens containing sequential high dose aldesleukin and antineoplastic agents. These reactions consisted of erythema, pruritus, and hypotension and occurred within hours of administration of chemotherapy. These events required medical intervention in some patients).
No products indexed under this heading.

Thiothixene (Aldesleukin may affect central nervous function. Therefore, interactions could occur following concomitant administration of psychotropic drugs). Products include:
Thiothixene 2386

Ticarcillin Disodium (Concurrent administration of drugs possessing nephrotoxic effects with aldesleukin may increase the potential for nephrotoxicity). Products include:
Timentin ADD-Vantage 1670
Timentin Galaxy 1674
Timentin 1666
Timentin Pharmacy 1678

Timolol Hemihydrate (Beta-blockers may potentiate the hypotension seen with aldesleukin). Products include:
Betimol 3490

Timolol Maleate (Beta-blockers may potentiate the hypotension seen with aldesleukin). Products include:
Combigan 601
Dorzolamide Hydrochloride/Timolol Maleate Ophthalmic Solution .... ⊙ 243
Timoptic in Ocudose .... ⊙ 231

Tipranavir (Concurrent administration of drugs possessing hepatotoxic effects with aldesleukin may increase toxicity in the liver).
No products indexed under this heading.

Tobramycin (Concurrent administration of drugs possessing nephrotoxic effects with aldesleukin may increase the potential for nephrotoxicity).
Products include:
Tobi Nebulizer 2546
Tobramycin and Dexamethasone Ophthalmic Suspension .... ⊙ 251
Zylet .... ⊙ 252

Tobramycin Sulfate (Concurrent administration of drugs possessing nephrotoxic effects with aldesleukin may increase the potential for nephrotoxicity).
No products indexed under this heading.

Tolazamide (Concurrent administration of drugs possessing nephrotoxic effects with aldesleukin may increase the potential for nephrotoxicity).
No products indexed under this heading.

Tolbutamide (Concurrent administration of drugs possessing nephrotoxic effects with aldesleukin may increase the potential for nephrotoxicity).
No products indexed under this heading.

Tolbutamide Sodium (Concurrent administration of drugs possessing hepatotoxic effects with aldesleukin may increase toxicity in the liver).
No products indexed under this heading.

Tolmetin Sodium (Concurrent administration of drugs possessing nephrotoxic effects with aldesleukin may increase the potential for nephrotoxicity).
No products indexed under this heading.

Topotecan Hydrochloride (Hypersensitivity reactions have been reported in patients receiving combination regimens containing sequential high dose aldesleukin and antineoplastic agents. These reactions consisted of erythema, pruritus, and hypotension and occurred within hours of administration of chemotherapy. These events required medical intervention in some patients). Products include:
Hycamtin 1491
Hycamtin Capsules 1488

Toremifene Citrate (Hypersensitivity reactions have been reported in patients receiving combination regimens containing sequential high dose aldesleukin and antineoplastic agents. These reactions consisted of erythema, pruritus, and hypotension and occurred within hours of administration of chemotherapy. These events required medical intervention in some patients).
No products indexed under this heading.

Torsemide (Concurrent use with antihypertensive drugs may potentiate the hypotension seen with aldesleukin).
No products indexed under this heading.

Trandolapril (Concurrent administration of drugs possessing nephrotoxic effects with aldesleukin may increase the potential for nephrotoxicity).
Products include:
Mavik 489
Tarka 534

Tranylcypromine Sulfate (Aldesleukin may affect central nervous function. Therefore, interactions could occur following concomitant administration of psychotropic drugs). Products include:
Parnate 1584

Triamcinolone (Although glucocorticoids have been shown to reduce aldesleukin-induced side effects including fever, renal insufficiency, hyperbilirubinemia, confusion, and dyspnea, concomitant administration of these agents with aldesleukin may reduce the antitumor effectiveness of aldesleukin and thus should be avoided).
No products indexed under this heading.

Triamcinolone Acetonide (Although glucocorticoids have been shown to reduce aldesleukin-induced side effects including fever, renal insufficiency, hyperbilirubinemia, confusion, and dyspnea, concomitant administration of these agents with aldesleukin may reduce the antitumor effectiveness of aldesleukin and thus should be avoided). Products include:
Azmacort 408
Nasacort AQ 3019

(⊙ Described in PDR® for Ophthalmic Medicines)

Triamcinolone Diacetate (Although glucocorticoids have been shown to reduce aldesleukin-induced side effects including fever, renal insufficiency, hyperbilirubinemia, confusion, and dyspnea, concomitant administration of these agents with aldesleukin may reduce the antitumor effectiveness of aldesleukin and thus should be avoided).
  No products indexed under this heading.

Triamcinolone Hexacetonide (Although glucocorticoids have been shown to reduce aldesleukin-induced side effects including fever, renal insufficiency, hyperbilirubinemia, confusion, and dyspnea, concomitant administration of these agents with aldesleukin may reduce the antitumor effectiveness of aldesleukin and thus should be avoided).
  No products indexed under this heading.

Triamterene (Concurrent administration of drugs possessing nephrotoxic effects with aldesleukin may increase the potential for nephrotoxicity). Products include:

Triazolam (Aldesleukin may affect central nervous function. Therefore, interactions could occur following concomitant administration of psychotropic drugs).
  No products indexed under this heading.

Trifluoperazine Hydrochloride (Aldesleukin may affect central nervous function. Therefore, interactions could occur following concomitant administration of psychotropic drugs).
  No products indexed under this heading.

Trimethadione (Concurrent administration of drugs possessing nephrotoxic effects with aldesleukin may increase the potential for nephrotoxicity).
  No products indexed under this heading.

Trimethaphan Camsylate (Concurrent use with antihypertensive drugs may potentiate the hypotension seen with aldesleukin).
  No products indexed under this heading.

Trimethobenzamide Hydrochloride (Aldesleukin may affect central nervous function. Therefore, interactions could occur following concomitant administration of antiemetics).
  No products indexed under this heading.

Trimethoprim (Concurrent administration of drugs possessing hepatotoxic effects with aldesleukin may increase toxicity in the liver).
  No products indexed under this heading.

Trimethoprim Hydrochloride (Concurrent administration of drugs possessing hepatotoxic effects with aldesleukin may increase toxicity in the liver).
  No products indexed under this heading.

Trimethoprim Sulfate (Concurrent administration of drugs possessing hepatotoxic effects with aldesleukin may increase toxicity in the liver).
  No products indexed under this heading.

Trimipramine Maleate (Aldesleukin may affect central nervous function. Therefore, interactions could occur following concomitant administration of psychotropic drugs).
  No products indexed under this heading.

Trovafloxacin Mesylate (Concurrent administration of drugs possessing nephrotoxic effects with aldesleukin may increase the potential for nephrotoxicity).
  No products indexed under this heading.

Tyropanoate Sodium (Concurrent administration of drugs possessing nephrotoxic effects with aldesleukin may increase the potential for nephrotoxicity).
  No products indexed under this heading.

Valacyclovir Hydrochloride (Concurrent administration of drugs possessing nephrotoxic effects with aldesleukin may increase the potential for nephrotoxicity). Products include:

Valdecoxib (Concurrent administration of drugs possessing nephrotoxic effects with aldesleukin may increase the potential for nephrotoxicity).
  No products indexed under this heading.

Valproate Sodium (Concurrent administration of drugs possessing hepatotoxic effects with aldesleukin may increase toxicity in the liver).
  No products indexed under this heading.

Valproic Acid (Concurrent administration of drugs possessing hepatotoxic effects with aldesleukin may increase toxicity in the liver).
  No products indexed under this heading.

Valrubicin (Hypersensitivity reactions have been reported in patients receiving combination regimens containing sequential high dose aldesleukin and antineoplastic agents. These reactions consisted of erythema, pruritus, and hypotension and occurred within hours of administration of chemotherapy. These events required medical intervention in some patients). Products include:

Valsartan (Concurrent use with antihypertensive drugs may potentiate the hypotension seen with aldesleukin). Products include:

Vancomycin Hydrochloride (Concurrent administration of drugs possessing nephrotoxic effects with aldesleukin may increase the potential for nephrotoxicity).
  No products indexed under this heading.

Verapamil Hydrochloride (Concurrent use with antihypertensive drugs may potentiate the hypotension seen with aldesleukin). Products include:

Vinblastine Sulfate (Concurrent administration of drugs possessing myelotoxic effects with aldesleukin may increase the potential for myelotoxicity).
  No products indexed under this heading.

Vincristine Sulfate (Concurrent administration of drugs possessing myelotoxic effects with aldesleukin may increase the potential for myelotoxicity).
  No products indexed under this heading.

Vinorelbine Tartrate (Concurrent administration of drugs possessing myelotoxic effects with aldesleukin may increase the potential for myelotoxicity).
  No products indexed under this heading.

Voriconazole (Concurrent administration of drugs possessing nephrotoxic effects with aldesleukin may increase the potential for nephrotoxicity).
  No products indexed under this heading.

Zalcitabine (Concurrent administration of drugs possessing nephrotoxic effects with aldesleukin may increase the potential for nephrotoxicity).
  No products indexed under this heading.

Zaleplon (Aldesleukin may affect central nervous function. Therefore, interactions could occur following concomitant administration of psychotropic drugs).
  No products indexed under this heading.

Zidovudine (Concurrent administration of drugs possessing nephrotoxic effects with aldesleukin may increase the potential for nephrotoxicity). Products include:

Ziprasidone Hydrochloride (Aldesleukin may affect central nervous function. Therefore, interactions could occur following concomitant administration of psychotropic drugs). Products include:

Zoledronic Acid (Concurrent administration of drugs possessing nephrotoxic effects with aldesleukin may increase the potential for nephrotoxicity). Products include:

Zolpidem Tartrate (Aldesleukin may affect central nervous function. Therefore, interactions could occur following concomitant administration of psychotropic drugs). Products include:

PROMACTA TABLETS

May interact with antacids, antacids containing aluminum, calcium and magnesium, calcium preparations, cations, cytochrome p450 1a2 inducers (selected), cytochrome p450 1a2 inhibitors (selected), cytochrome p450 1a2 substrates (selected), cytochrome p450 2c8 inducers (selected), cytochrome p450 2c8 inhibitors (selected), cytochrome p450 2c8 substrates (selected), iron containing oral preparations, iron salts, narcotic analgesics, non-steroidal anti-inflammatory agents, organic anion transporting polypeptide substrates, UDP-glucuronosyltransferase (UGT) 1A1 substrates (selected), and certain other agents. Compounds in these categories include:

Acetaminophen (In vitro studies demonstrate that eltrombopag is an inhibitor of UGT1A1, UGT1A3, UGT1A4, UGT1A6, UGT1A9, UGT2B7, and UGT2B15, enzymes involved in the metabolism of multiple drugs, such as acetaminophen, narcotics, and nonsteroidal anti-inflammatory drugs (NSAIDs). The significance of this inhibition on the potential for increased systemic exposure of drugs that are substrates of these UGTs following co-administration with eltrombopag has not been evaluated in clinical studies. Monitor patients closely for signs or symptoms of excessive exposure to these drugs when concomitantly administered with eltrombopag). Products include:

Acetaminophen-containing products (In vitro studies demonstrate that eltrombopag is an inhibitor of UGT1A1, UGT1A3, UGT1A4, UGT1A6, UGT1A9, UGT2B7, and UGT2B15, enzymes involved in the metabolism of multiple drugs, such as acetaminophen, narcotics, and nonsteroidal anti-inflammatory drugs (NSAIDs). The significance of this inhibition on the potential for increased systemic exposure of drugs that are substrates of these UGTs following co-

administration with eltrombopag has not been evaluated in clinical studies. Monitor patients closely for signs or symptoms of excessive exposure to these drugs when concomitantly administered with eltrombopag).
  No products indexed under this heading.

Alatrofloxacin Mesylate (In vitro studies demonstrate that CYP1A2 and CYP2C8 are involved in the oxidative metabolism of eltrombopag. The significance of co-administration of eltrombopag with moderate or strong inhibitors of CYP 1A2 (eg, ciprofloxacin, fluvoxamine) and CYP 2C8 (eg, gemfibrozil, trimethoprim) on the systemic exposure of eltrombopag has not been established in clinical studies. Monitor patients for signs and symptoms of excessive eltrombopag exposure when eltrombopag is administered concomitantly with these moderate or strong inhibitors of CYP1A2 or CYP2C8).
  No products indexed under this heading.

Alfentanil Hydrochloride (Studies demonstrate that eltrombopag is an inhibitor of UGT1A1, UGT1A3, UGT1A4, UGT1A6, UGT1A9, UGT2B7, and UGT2B15, enzymes involved in the metabolism of multiple drugs, such as acetaminophen, narcotics, and nonsteroidal anti-inflammatory drugs (NSAIDs). Monitor patients closely for signs of symptoms of excessive exposure to these drugs when concomitantly administered with eltrombopag).
  No products indexed under this heading.

Aluminum Acetate (Eltrombopag chelates polyvalent cations (such as iron, calcium, aluminum, magnesium, selenium, and zinc) in foods, mineral supplements, and antacids. In a clinical study, administration of eltrombopag with a polyvalent cation-containing antacid (1,524 mg aluminum hydroxide, 1,425 mg magnesium carbonate, and sodium alginate) decreased plasma eltrombopag systemic exposure by approximately 70%. Eltrombopag must not be taken within 4 hours of any medications or products containing polyvalent cations such as antacids, dairy products, and mineral supplements to avoid significant reduction in eltrombopag absorption due to chelation).
  No products indexed under this heading.

Aluminum Carbonate (Eltrombopag chelates polyvalent cations (such as iron, calcium, aluminum, magnesium, selenium, and zinc) in foods, mineral supplements, and antacids. In a clinical study, administration of eltrombopag with a polyvalent cation-containing antacid (1,524 mg aluminum hydroxide, 1,425 mg magnesium carbonate, and sodium alginate) decreased plasma eltrombopag systemic exposure by approximately 70%. Eltrombopag must not be taken within 4 hours of any medications or products containing polyvalent cations such as antacids, dairy products, and mineral supplements to avoid significant reduction in eltrombopag absorption due to chelation).
  No products indexed under this heading.

Aluminum Chlorhydroxide (Eltrombopag chelates polyvalent cations (such as iron, calcium, aluminum, magnesium, selenium, and zinc) in foods, mineral supplements, and antacids. In a clinical study, administration of eltrombopag with a polyvalent cation-containing antacid (1,524 mg aluminum hydroxide, 1,425 mg magnesium carbonate, and sodium alginate) decreased plasma eltrombopag systemic exposure by approximately 70%. Eltrombopag must not be taken within 4 hours of any medications or products containing polyvalent cations such as antacids, dairy products, and mineral supple-

ments to avoid significant reduction in eltrombopag absorption due to chelation).
No products indexed under this heading.

Aluminum Chloride (Eltrombopag chelates polyvalent cations (such as iron, calcium, aluminum, magnesium, selenium, and zinc) in foods, mineral supplements, and antacids. In a clinical study, administration of eltrombopag with a polyvalent cation-containing antacid (1,524 mg aluminum hydroxide, 1,425 mg magnesium carbonate, and sodium alginate) decreased plasma eltrombopag systemic exposure by approximately 70%. Eltrombopag must not be taken within 4 hours of any medications or products containing polyvalent cations such as antacids, dairy products, and mineral supplements to avoid significant reduction in eltrombopag absorption due to chelation).
No products indexed under this heading.

Aluminum Chlorohydrate (Eltrombopag chelates polyvalent cations (such as iron, calcium, aluminum, magnesium, selenium, and zinc) in foods, mineral supplements, and antacids. In a clinical study, administration of eltrombopag with a polyvalent cation-containing antacid (1,524 mg aluminum hydroxide, 1,425 mg magnesium carbonate, and sodium alginate) decreased plasma eltrombopag systemic exposure by approximately 70%. Eltrombopag must not be taken within 4 hours of any medications or products containing polyvalent cations such as antacids, dairy products, and mineral supplements to avoid significant reduction in eltrombopag absorption due to chelation).
No products indexed under this heading.

Aluminum Glycinate (Eltrombopag chelates polyvalent cations (such as iron, calcium, aluminum, magnesium, selenium, and zinc) in foods, mineral supplements, and antacids. In a clinical study, administration of eltrombopag with a polyvalent cation-containing antacid (1,524 mg aluminum hydroxide, 1,425 mg magnesium carbonate, and sodium alginate) decreased plasma eltrombopag systemic exposure by approximately 70%. Eltrombopag must not be taken within 4 hours of any medications or products containing polyvalent cations such as antacids, dairy products, and mineral supplements to avoid significant reduction in eltrombopag absorption due to chelation).
No products indexed under this heading.

Aluminum Hydroxide (Eltrombopag chelates polyvalent cations (such as iron, calcium, aluminum, magnesium, selenium, and zinc) in foods, mineral supplements, and antacids. In a clinical study, administration of eltrombopag with a polyvalent cation-containing antacid (1,524 mg aluminum hydroxide, 1,425 mg magnesium carbonate, and sodium alginate) decreased plasma eltrombopag systemic exposure by approximately 70%. Eltrombopag must not be taken within 4 hours of any medications or products containing polyvalent cations such as antacids, dairy products, and mineral supplements to avoid significant reduction in eltrombopag absorption due to chelation).
No products indexed under this heading.

Aluminum Hydroxide Preparations (Eltrombopag chelates polyvalent cations (such as iron, calcium, aluminum, magnesium, selenium, and zinc) in foods, mineral supplements, and antacids. In a clinical study, administration of eltrombopag with a polyvalent cation-containing antacid (1,524 mg aluminum hydroxide, 1,425 mg magnesium carbonate, and sodium alginate) decreased plasma eltrombopag systemic exposure by approximately 70%. Eltrombopag must not be taken within 4 hours of any medications or products containing polyvalent cations such as antacids, dairy products, and mineral supplements to avoid significant reduction in eltrombopag absorption due to chelation).
No products indexed under this heading.

Aluminum Sulfate (Eltrombopag chelates polyvalent cations (such as iron, calcium, aluminum, magnesium, selenium, and zinc) in foods, mineral supplements, and antacids. In a clinical study, administration of eltrombopag with a polyvalent cation-containing antacid (1,524 mg aluminum hydroxide, 1,425 mg magnesium carbonate, and sodium alginate) decreased plasma eltrombopag systemic exposure by approximately 70%. Eltrombopag must not be taken within 4 hours of any medications or products containing polyvalent cations such as antacids, dairy products, and mineral supplements to avoid significant reduction in eltrombopag absorption due to chelation).
No products indexed under this heading.

Aminophylline (*In vitro* studies demonstrate that CYP1A2 and CYP2C8 are involved in the oxidative metabolism of eltrombopag. The significance of co-administration of eltrombopag with other substrates of these CYP enzymes on the systemic exposure of eltrombopag has not been established in clinical studies. Monitor patients for signs and symptoms of excessive eltrombopag exposure when eltrombopag is administered concomitantly with these drugs).
No products indexed under this heading.

Amiodarone Hydrochloride (*In vitro* studies demonstrate that CYP1A2 and CYP2C8 are involved in the oxidative metabolism of eltrombopag. The significance of co-administration of eltrombopag with moderate or strong inhibitors of CYP 1A2 (eg, ciprofloxacin, fluvoxamine) and CYP 2C8 (eg, gemfibrozil, trimethoprim) on the systemic exposure of eltrombopag has not been established in clinical studies. Monitor patients for signs and symptoms of excessive eltrombopag exposure when eltrombopag is administered concomitantly with these moderate or strong inhibitors of CYP1A2 or CYP2C8).
No products indexed under this heading.

Amitriptyline Hydrochloride (*In vitro* studies demonstrate that CYP1A2 and CYP2C8 are involved in the oxidative metabolism of eltrombopag. The significance of co-administration of eltrombopag with other substrates of these CYP enzymes on the systemic exposure of eltrombopag has not been established in clinical studies. Monitor patients for signs and symptoms of excessive eltrombopag exposure when eltrombopag is administered concomitantly with these drugs).
No products indexed under this heading.

Amoxapine (*In vitro* studies demonstrate that CYP1A2 and CYP2C8 are involved in the oxidative metabolism of eltrombopag. The significance of co-administration of eltrombopag with other substrates of these CYP enzymes on the systemic exposure of eltrombopag has not been established in clinical studies. Monitor patients for signs and symptoms of excessive eltrombopag exposure when eltrombopag is administered concomitantly with these drugs).
No products indexed under this heading.

Anagrelide Hydrochloride (*In vitro* studies demonstrate that CYP1A2 and CYP2C8 are involved in the oxidative metabolism of eltrombopag. The significance of co-administration of eltrombopag with other substrates of these CYP enzymes on the systemic exposure of eltrombopag has not been established in clinical studies. Monitor patients for signs and symptoms of excessive eltrombopag exposure when eltrombopag is administered concomitantly with these drugs).
No products indexed under this heading.

Anastrozole (*In vitro* studies demonstrate that CYP1A2 and CYP2C8 are involved in the oxidative metabolism of eltrombopag. The significance of co-administration of eltrombopag with moderate or strong inhibitors of CYP 1A2 (eg, ciprofloxacin, fluvoxamine) and CYP 2C8 (eg, gemfibrozil, trimethoprim) on the systemic exposure of eltrombopag has not been established in clinical studies. Monitor patients for signs and symptoms of excessive eltrombopag exposure when eltrombopag is administered concomitantly with these moderate or strong inhibitors of CYP1A2 or CYP2C8).
No products indexed under this heading.

Apomorphine (Studies demonstrate that eltrombopag is an inhibitor of UGT1A1, UGT1A3, UGT1A4, UGT1A6, UGT1A9, UGT2B7, and UGT2B15, enzymes involved in the metabolism of multiple drugs, such as acetaminophen, narcotics, and nonsteroidal anti-inflammatory drugs (NSAIDs). Monitor patients closely for signs of symptoms of excessive exposure to these drugs when concomitantly administered with eltrombopag).
No products indexed under this heading.

Apomorphine Hydrochloride (Studies demonstrate that eltrombopag is an inhibitor of UGT1A1, UGT1A3, UGT1A4, UGT1A6, UGT1A9, UGT2B7, and UGT2B15, enzymes involved in the metabolism of multiple drugs, such as acetaminophen, narcotics, and nonsteroidal anti-inflammatory drugs (NSAIDs). Monitor patients closely for signs of symptoms of excessive exposure to these drugs when concomitantly administered with eltrombopag).
No products indexed under this heading.

Atorvastatin Calcium (*In vitro* studies demonstrate that eltrombopag is an inhibitor of the organic anion transporting polypeptide OATP1B1 and can increase the systemic exposure of other drugs that are substrates of this transporter (eg, benzylpenicillin, atorvastatin, fluvastatin, pravastatin, rosuvastatin, methotrexate, nateglinide, repaglinide, rifampin). Monitor patients closely for signs and symptoms of excessive exposure to the drugs that are substrates of OATP1B1 and consider reduction of the dose of these drugs). Products include:
Lipitor **2703**

Benzphetamine Hydrochloride (*In vitro* studies demonstrate that CYP1A2 and CYP2C8 are involved in the oxidative metabolism of eltrombopag. The significance of co-administration of eltrombopag with other substrates of these CYP enzymes on the systemic exposure of eltrombopag has not been established in clinical studies. Monitor patients for signs and symptoms of excessive eltrombopag exposure when eltrombopag is administered concomitantly with these drugs).
No products indexed under this heading.

Buprenorphine Hydrochloride (Studies demonstrate that eltrombopag is an inhibitor of UGT1A1, UGT1A3, UGT1A4, UGT1A6, UGT1A9, UGT2B7, and UGT2B15, enzymes involved in the metabolism of multiple drugs, such as acetaminophen, narcotics, and nonsteroidal anti-inflammatory drugs (NSAIDs). Monitor patients closely for signs of symptoms of excessive exposure to these drugs when concomitantly administered with eltrombopag).
No products indexed under this heading.

Caffeine (*In vitro* studies demonstrate that CYP1A2 and CYP2C8 are involved in the oxidative metabolism of eltrombopag. The significance of co-administration of eltrombopag with other substrates of these CYP enzymes on the systemic exposure of eltrombopag has not been established in clinical studies. Monitor patients for signs and symptoms of excessive eltrombopag exposure when eltrombopag is administered concomitantly with these drugs).
No products indexed under this heading.

Caffeine Anhydrous (*In vitro* studies demonstrate that CYP1A2 and CYP2C8 are involved in the oxidative metabolism of eltrombopag. The significance of co-administration of eltrombopag with other substrates of these CYP enzymes on the systemic exposure of eltrombopag has not been established in clinical studies. Monitor patients for signs and symptoms of excessive eltrombopag exposure when eltrombopag is administered concomitantly with these drugs).
No products indexed under this heading.

Caffeine Citrate (*In vitro* studies demonstrate that CYP1A2 and CYP2C8 are involved in the oxidative metabolism of eltrombopag. The significance of co-administration of eltrombopag with other substrates of these CYP enzymes on the systemic exposure of eltrombopag has not been established in clinical studies. Monitor patients for signs and symptoms of excessive eltrombopag exposure when eltrombopag is administered concomitantly with these drugs).
No products indexed under this heading.

Caffeine-containing medications (*In vitro* studies demonstrate that CYP1A2 and CYP2C8 are involved in the oxidative metabolism of eltrombopag. The significance of co-administration of eltrombopag with other substrates of these CYP enzymes on the systemic exposure of eltrombopag has not been established in clinical studies. Monitor patients for signs and symptoms of excessive eltrombopag exposure when eltrombopag is administered concomitantly with these drugs).
No products indexed under this heading.

Caffeine Sodium Benzoate (*In vitro* studies demonstrate that CYP1A2 and CYP2C8 are involved in the oxidative metabolism of eltrombopag. The significance of co-administration of eltrombopag with other substrates of these CYP enzymes on the systemic exposure of eltrombopag has not been established in clinical studies. Monitor patients for signs and symptoms of excessive eltrombopag exposure when eltrombopag is administered concomitantly with these drugs).
No products indexed under this heading.

Calcium (Eltrombopag chelates polyvalent cations (such as iron, calcium, aluminum, magnesium, selenium, and zinc) in foods, mineral supplements, and antacids. In a clinical study, administration of eltrombopag with a polyvalent cation-containing antacid (1,524 mg aluminum hydroxide, 1,425 mg magnesium carbonate, and sodium alginate) decreased plasma eltrombopag systemic exposure by approximately 70%. Eltrombopag must not be taken within 4 hours of any medications or products containing polyvalent cations such as antacids, dairy products, and mineral supplements to avoid significant reduction in eltrombopag absorption due to chelation). Products include:
BoneMate Plus **3454**
Cardio Basics **3455**
Chelated Mineral **3476**
CitraNatal 90 DHA Capsules **2332**
CitraNatal Harmony **2332**

Calcium (Oyster Shell) (Eltrombopag chelates polyvalent cations (such as iron, calcium, aluminum, magnesium, selenium, and zinc) in foods, mineral supplements, and antacids. In a clinical study, administration of eltrombopag with a polyvalent cation-containing antacid (1,524 mg aluminum hydroxide, 1,425 mg magnesium carbonate, and sodium alginate) decreased plasma eltrombopag systemic exposure by approximately 70%. Eltrombopag must not be taken within 4 hours of any medications or products containing polyvalent cations such as antacids, dairy products, and mineral supplements to avoid significant reduction in eltrombopag absorption due to chelation).
No products indexed under this heading.

Calcium Acetate (Eltrombopag chelates polyvalent cations (such as iron, calcium, aluminum, magnesium, selenium, and zinc) in foods, mineral supplements, and antacids. In a clinical study, administration of eltrombopag with a polyvalent cation-containing antacid (1,524 mg aluminum hydroxide, 1,425 mg magnesium carbonate, and sodium alginate) decreased plasma eltrombopag systemic exposure by approximately 70%. Eltrombopag must not be taken within 4 hours of any medications or products containing polyvalent cations such as antacids, dairy products, and mineral supplements to avoid significant reduction in eltrombopag absorption due to chelation).
No products indexed under this heading.

Calcium Ascorbate (Eltrombopag chelates polyvalent cations (such as iron, calcium, aluminum, magnesium, selenium, and zinc) in foods, mineral supplements, and antacids. In a clinical study, administration of eltrombopag with a polyvalent cation-containing antacid (1,524 mg aluminum hydroxide, 1,425 mg magnesium carbonate, and sodium alginate) decreased plasma eltrombopag systemic exposure by approximately 70%. Eltrombopag must not be taken within 4 hours of any medications or products containing polyvalent cations such as antacids, dairy products, and mineral supplements to avoid significant reduction in eltrombopag absorption due to chelation).
Products include:
Bio-C 3454
Procosa II 3476
Proflavanol 90 3476

Calcium Carbaspirin (Eltrombopag chelates polyvalent cations (such as iron, calcium, aluminum, magnesium, selenium, and zinc) in foods, mineral supplements, and antacids. In a clinical study, administration of eltrombopag with a polyvalent cation-containing antacid (1,524 mg aluminum hydroxide, 1,425 mg magnesium carbonate, and sodium alginate) decreased plasma eltrombopag systemic exposure by approximately 70%. Eltrombopag must not be taken within 4 hours of any medications or products containing polyvalent cations such as antacids, dairy products, and mineral supplements to avoid significant reduction in eltrombopag absorption due to chelation).
No products indexed under this heading.

Calcium Carbonate (Eltrombopag chelates polyvalent cations (such as iron, calcium, aluminum, magnesium, selenium, and zinc) in foods, mineral supplements, and antacids. In a clinical study, administration of eltrombopag with a polyvalent cation-containing antacid (1,524 mg aluminum hydroxide, 1,425 mg magnesium carbonate, and sodium alginate) decreased plasma eltrombopag systemic exposure by approximately 70%. Eltrombopag must not be taken within 4 hours of any medications or products containing polyvalent cations such as antacids, dairy products, and mineral supplements to avoid significant reduction in eltrombopag absorption due to chelation).
Products include:
Chelated Mineral 3476
Pepcid Complete 1822
Extra Strength Rolaids Softchews Vanilla Creme 2045

Calcium Carbonate, Precipitated (Eltrombopag chelates polyvalent cations (such as iron, calcium, aluminum, magnesium, selenium, and zinc) in foods, mineral supplements, and antacids. In a clinical study, administration of eltrombopag with a polyvalent cation-containing antacid (1,524 mg aluminum hydroxide, 1,425 mg magnesium carbonate, and sodium alginate) decreased plasma eltrombopag systemic exposure by approximately 70%. Eltrombopag must not be taken within 4 hours of any medications or products containing polyvalent cations such as antacids, dairy products, and mineral supplements to avoid significant reduction in eltrombopag absorption due to chelation).
No products indexed under this heading.

Calcium Caseinate (Eltrombopag chelates polyvalent cations (such as iron, calcium, aluminum, magnesium, selenium, and zinc) in foods, mineral supplements, and antacids. In a clinical study, administration of eltrombopag with a polyvalent cation-containing antacid (1,524 mg aluminum hydroxide, 1,425 mg magnesium carbonate, and sodium alginate) decreased plasma eltrombopag systemic exposure by approximately 70%. Eltrombopag must not be taken within 4 hours of any medications or products containing polyvalent cations such as antacids, dairy products, and mineral supplements to avoid significant reduction in eltrombopag absorption due to chelation).
No products indexed under this heading.

Calcium Chloride (Eltrombopag chelates polyvalent cations (such as iron, calcium, aluminum, magnesium, selenium, and zinc) in foods, mineral supplements, and antacids. In a clinical study, administration of eltrombopag with a polyvalent cation-containing antacid (1,524 mg aluminum hydroxide, 1,425 mg magnesium carbonate, and sodium alginate) decreased plasma eltrombopag systemic exposure by approximately 70%. Eltrombopag must not be taken within 4 hours of any medications or products containing polyvalent cations such as antacids, dairy products, and mineral supplements to avoid significant reduction in eltrombopag absorption due to chelation).
No products indexed under this heading.

Calcium Citrate (Eltrombopag chelates polyvalent cations (such as iron, calcium, aluminum, magnesium, selenium, and zinc) in foods, mineral supplements, and antacids. In a clinical study, administration of eltrombopag with a polyvalent cation-containing antacid (1,524 mg aluminum hydroxide, 1,425 mg magnesium carbonate, and sodium alginate) decreased plasma eltrombopag systemic exposure by approximately 70%. Eltrombopag must not be taken within 4 hours of any medications or products containing polyvalent cations such as antacids, dairy products, and mineral supplements to avoid significant reduction in eltrombopag absorption due to chelation).
Products include:
Active Calcium 3476
Chelated Mineral 3476
CitraNatal 90 DHA Capsules 2332
CitraNatal Assure 2332
CitraNatal Harmony 2332
CitraNatal Rx 2332

Calcium Disodium Edetate (Eltrombopag chelates polyvalent cations (such as iron, calcium, aluminum, magnesium, selenium, and zinc) in foods, mineral supplements, and antacids. In a clinical study, administration of eltrombopag with a polyvalent cation-containing antacid (1,524 mg aluminum hydroxide, 1,425 mg magnesium carbonate, and sodium alginate) decreased plasma eltrombopag systemic exposure by approximately 70%. Eltrombopag must not be taken within 4 hours of any medications or products containing polyvalent cations such as antacids, dairy products, and mineral supplements to avoid significant reduction in eltrombopag absorption due to chelation).
No products indexed under this heading.

Calcium Glubionate (Eltrombopag chelates polyvalent cations (such as iron, calcium, aluminum, magnesium, selenium, and zinc) in foods, mineral supplements, and antacids. In a clinical study, administration of eltrombopag with a polyvalent cation-containing antacid (1,524 mg aluminum hydroxide, 1,425 mg magnesium carbonate, and sodium alginate) decreased plasma eltrombopag systemic exposure by approximately 70%. Eltrombopag must not be taken within 4 hours of any medications or products containing polyvalent cations such as antacids, dairy products, and mineral supplements to avoid significant reduction in eltrombopag absorption due to chelation).
No products indexed under this heading.

Calcium Gluconate (Eltrombopag chelates polyvalent cations (such as iron, calcium, aluminum, magnesium, selenium, and zinc) in foods, mineral supplements, and antacids. In a clinical study, administration of eltrombopag with a polyvalent cation-containing antacid (1,524 mg aluminum hydroxide, 1,425 mg magnesium carbonate, and sodium alginate) decreased plasma eltrombopag systemic exposure by approximately 70%. Eltrombopag must not be taken within 4 hours of any medications or products containing polyvalent cations such as antacids, dairy products, and mineral supplements to avoid significant reduction in eltrombopag absorption due to chelation).
No products indexed under this heading.

Calcium Glycerophosphate (Eltrombopag chelates polyvalent cations (such as iron, calcium, aluminum, magnesium, selenium, and zinc) in foods, mineral supplements, and antacids. In a clinical study, administration of eltrombopag with a polyvalent cation-containing antacid (1,524 mg aluminum hydroxide, 1,425 mg magnesium carbonate, and sodium alginate) decreased plasma eltrombopag systemic exposure by approximately 70%. Eltrombopag must not be taken within 4 hours of any medications or products containing polyvalent cations such as antacids, dairy products, and mineral supplements to avoid significant reduction in eltrombopag absorption due to chelation).
No products indexed under this heading.

Calcium Iodide (Eltrombopag chelates polyvalent cations (such as iron, calcium, aluminum, magnesium, selenium, and zinc) in foods, mineral supplements, and antacids. In a clinical study, administration of eltrombopag with a polyvalent cation-containing antacid (1,524 mg aluminum hydroxide, 1,425 mg magnesium carbonate, and sodium alginate) decreased plasma eltrombopag systemic exposure by approximately 70%. Eltrombopag must not be taken within 4 hours of any medications or products containing polyvalent cations such as antacids, dairy products, and mineral supplements to avoid significant reduction in eltrombopag absorption due to chelation).
No products indexed under this heading.

Calcium Lactate (Eltrombopag chelates polyvalent cations (such as iron, calcium, aluminum, magnesium, selenium, and zinc) in foods, mineral supplements, and antacids. In a clinical study, administration of eltrombopag with a polyvalent cation-containing antacid (1,524 mg aluminum hydroxide, 1,425 mg magnesium carbonate, and sodium alginate) decreased plasma eltrombopag systemic exposure by approximately 70%. Eltrombopag must not be taken within 4 hours of any medications or products containing polyvalent cations such as antacids, dairy products, and mineral supplements to avoid significant reduction in eltrombopag absorption due to chelation).
No products indexed under this heading.

Calcium Levulinate (Eltrombopag chelates polyvalent cations (such as iron, calcium, aluminum, magnesium, selenium, and zinc) in foods, mineral supplements, and antacids. In a clinical study, administration of eltrombopag with a polyvalent cation-containing antacid (1,524 mg aluminum hydroxide, 1,425 mg magnesium carbonate, and sodium alginate) decreased plasma eltrombopag systemic exposure by approximately 70%. Eltrombopag must not be taken within 4 hours of any medications or products containing polyvalent cations such as antacids, dairy products, and mineral supplements to avoid significant reduction in eltrombopag absorption due to chelation).
No products indexed under this heading.

Calcium Pantothenate (Eltrombopag chelates polyvalent cations (such as iron, calcium, aluminum, magnesium, selenium, and zinc) in foods, mineral supplements, and antacids. In a clinical study, administration of eltrombopag with a polyvalent cation-containing antacid (1,524 mg aluminum hydroxide, 1,425 mg magnesium carbonate, and sodium alginate) decreased plasma eltrombopag systemic exposure by approximately 70%. Eltrombopag must not be taken within 4 hours of any medications or products containing polyvalent cations such as antacids, dairy products, and mineral supplements to avoid significant reduction in eltrombopag absorption due to chelation). Products include:
Cardio Basics 3455

Calcium Phosphate (Eltrombopag chelates polyvalent cations (such as iron, calcium, aluminum, magnesium, selenium, and zinc) in foods, mineral supplements, and antacids. In a clinical study, administration of eltrombopag with a polyvalent cation-containing antacid (1,524 mg aluminum hydroxide, 1,425 mg magnesium carbonate, and sodium alginate) decreased plasma eltrombopag systemic exposure by approximately 70%. Eltrombopag must not be taken within 4 hours of any medications or products containing polyvalent cations such as antacids, dairy products, and mineral supplements to avoid significant reduction in eltrombopag absorption due to chelation).
No products indexed under this heading.

Calcium Phosphate, Dibasic (Eltrombopag chelates polyvalent cations (such as iron, calcium, aluminum, magnesium, selenium, and zinc) in foods, mineral supplements, and antacids. In a clinical study, administration of eltrombopag with a polyvalent cation-containing antacid (1,524 mg aluminum hydroxide, 1,425 mg magnesium carbonate, and sodium alginate) decreased plasma eltrombopag systemic exposure by approximately 70%. Eltrombopag

must not be taken within 4 hours of any medications or products containing polyvalent cations such as antacids, dairy products, and mineral supplements to avoid significant reduction in eltrombopag absorption due to chelation).

No products indexed under this heading.

Calcium Phosphate, Tribasic (Eltrombopag chelates polyvalent cations (such as iron, calcium, aluminum, magnesium, selenium, and zinc) in foods, mineral supplements, and antacids. In a clinical study, administration of eltrombopag with a polyvalent cation-containing antacid (1,524 mg aluminum hydroxide, 1,425 mg magnesium carbonate, and sodium alginate) decreased plasma eltrombopag systemic exposure by approximately 70%. Eltrombopag must not be taken within 4 hours of any medications or products containing polyvalent cations such as antacids, dairy products, and mineral supplements to avoid significant reduction in eltrombopag absorption due to chelation).

No products indexed under this heading.

Calcium Phosphorus Preparations (Eltrombopag chelates polyvalent cations (such as iron, calcium, aluminum, magnesium, selenium, and zinc) in foods, mineral supplements, and antacids. In a clinical study, administration of eltrombopag with a polyvalent cation-containing antacid (1,524 mg aluminum hydroxide, 1,425 mg magnesium carbonate, and sodium alginate) decreased plasma eltrombopag systemic exposure by approximately 70%. Eltrombopag must not be taken within 4 hours of any medications or products containing polyvalent cations such as antacids, dairy products, and mineral supplements to avoid significant reduction in eltrombopag absorption due to chelation).

No products indexed under this heading.

Calcium Polycarbophil (Eltrombopag chelates polyvalent cations (such as iron, calcium, aluminum, magnesium, selenium, and zinc) in foods, mineral supplements, and antacids. In a clinical study, administration of eltrombopag with a polyvalent cation-containing antacid (1,524 mg aluminum hydroxide, 1,425 mg magnesium carbonate, and sodium alginate) decreased plasma eltrombopag systemic exposure by approximately 70%. Eltrombopag must not be taken within 4 hours of any medications or products containing polyvalent cations such as antacids, dairy products, and mineral supplements to avoid significant reduction in eltrombopag absorption due to chelation).

No products indexed under this heading.

Calcium Salts (Eltrombopag chelates polyvalent cations (such as iron, calcium, aluminum, magnesium, selenium, and zinc) in foods, mineral supplements, and antacids. In a clinical study, administration of eltrombopag with a polyvalent cation-containing antacid (1,524 mg aluminum hydroxide, 1,425 mg magnesium carbonate, and sodium alginate) decreased plasma eltrombopag systemic exposure by approximately 70%. Eltrombopag must not be taken within 4 hours of any medications or products containing polyvalent cations such as antacids, dairy products, and mineral supplements to avoid significant reduction in eltrombopag absorption due to chelation).

No products indexed under this heading.

Calcium Sodium Alginate Fiber (Eltrombopag chelates polyvalent cations (such as iron, calcium, aluminum, magnesium, selenium, and zinc) in foods, mineral supplements, and antacids. In a clinical study, administration of

eltrombopag with a polyvalent cation-containing antacid (1,524 mg aluminum hydroxide, 1,425 mg magnesium carbonate, and sodium alginate) decreased plasma eltrombopag systemic exposure by approximately 70%. Eltrombopag must not be taken within 4 hours of any medications or products containing polyvalent cations such as antacids, dairy products, and mineral supplements to avoid significant reduction in eltrombopag absorption due to chelation).

No products indexed under this heading.

Calcium Undecylenate (Eltrombopag chelates polyvalent cations (such as iron, calcium, aluminum, magnesium, selenium, and zinc) in foods, mineral supplements, and antacids. In a clinical study, administration of eltrombopag with a polyvalent cation-containing antacid (1,524 mg aluminum hydroxide, 1,425 mg magnesium carbonate, and sodium alginate) decreased plasma eltrombopag systemic exposure by approximately 70%. Eltrombopag must not be taken within 4 hours of any medications or products containing polyvalent cations such as antacids, dairy products, and mineral supplements to avoid significant reduction in eltrombopag absorption due to chelation).

No products indexed under this heading.

Carbamazepine (In vitro studies demonstrate that CYP1A2 and CYP2C8 are involved in the oxidative metabolism of eltrombopag. The significance of co-administration of eltrombopag with inducers of CYP 1A2 (eg, tobacco, omeprazole) and CYP 2C8 (eg, rifampin) on the systemic exposure of eltrombopag has not been established in clinical studies. Monitor patients for signs and symptoms of excessive eltrombopag exposure when eltrombopag is administered concomitantly with these drugs). Products include:

Carbatrol	3280
Equetro	3477

Celecoxib (Studies demonstrate that eltrombopag is an inhibitor of UGT1A1, UGT1A3, UGT1A4, UGT1A6, UGT1A9, UGT2B7, and UGT2B15, enzymes involved in the metabolism of multiple drugs, such as acetaminophen, narcotics, and nonsteroidal anti-inflammatory drugs (NSAIDs). Monitor patients closely for signs of symptoms of excessive exposure to these drugs when concomitantly administered with eltrombopag). Products include:

Celebrex	3272

Chlordiazepoxide (In vitro studies demonstrate that CYP1A2 and CYP2C8 are involved in the oxidative metabolism of eltrombopag. The significance of co-administration of eltrombopag with other substrates of these CYP enzymes on the systemic exposure of eltrombopag has not been established in clinical studies. Monitor patients for signs and symptoms of excessive eltrombopag exposure when eltrombopag is administered concomitantly with these drugs).

No products indexed under this heading.

Chlordiazepoxide Hydrochloride (In vitro studies demonstrate that CYP1A2 and CYP2C8 are involved in the oxidative metabolism of eltrombopag. The significance of co-administration of eltrombopag with other substrates of these CYP enzymes on the systemic exposure of eltrombopag has not been established in clinical studies. Monitor patients for signs and symptoms of excessive eltrombopag exposure when eltrombopag is administered concomitantly with these drugs).

No products indexed under this heading.

Cimetidine (In vitro studies demonstrate that CYP1A2 and CYP2C8 are

involved in the oxidative metabolism of eltrombopag. The significance of co-administration of eltrombopag with moderate or strong inhibitors of CYP 1A2 (eg, ciprofloxacin, fluvoxamine) and CYP 2C8 (eg, gemfibrozil, trimethoprim) on the systemic exposure of eltrombopag has not been established in clinical studies. Monitor patients for signs and symptoms of excessive eltrombopag exposure when eltrombopag is administered concomitantly with these moderate or strong inhibitors of CYP1A2 or CYP2C8).

No products indexed under this heading.

Cimetidine Hydrochloride (In vitro studies demonstrate that CYP1A2 and CYP2C8 are involved in the oxidative metabolism of eltrombopag. The significance of co-administration of eltrombopag with moderate or strong inhibitors of CYP 1A2 (eg, ciprofloxacin, fluvoxamine) and CYP 2C8 (eg, gemfibrozil, trimethoprim) on the systemic exposure of eltrombopag has not been established in clinical studies. Monitor patients for signs and symptoms of excessive eltrombopag exposure when eltrombopag is administered concomitantly with these moderate or strong inhibitors of CYP1A2 or CYP2C8).

No products indexed under this heading.

Ciprofloxacin (In vitro studies demonstrate that CYP1A2 and CYP2C8 are involved in the oxidative metabolism of eltrombopag. The significance of co-administration of eltrombopag with moderate or strong inhibitors of CYP 1A2 (eg, ciprofloxacin, fluvoxamine) and CYP 2C8 (eg, gemfibrozil, trimethoprim) on the systemic exposure of eltrombopag has not been established in clinical studies. Monitor patients for signs and symptoms of excessive eltrombopag exposure when eltrombopag is administered concomitantly with these moderate or strong inhibitors of CYP1A2 or CYP2C8). Products include:

Cipro I.V.	3082
Cipro	3073
Cipro XR	3091
Ciprodex	583

Ciprofloxacin Hydrochloride (In vitro studies demonstrate that CYP1A2 and CYP2C8 are involved in the oxidative metabolism of eltrombopag. The significance of co-administration of eltrombopag with moderate or strong inhibitors of CYP 1A2 (eg, ciprofloxacin, fluvoxamine) and CYP 2C8 (eg, gemfibrozil, trimethoprim) on the systemic exposure of eltrombopag has not been established in clinical studies. Monitor patients for signs and symptoms of excessive eltrombopag exposure when eltrombopag is administered concomitantly with these moderate or strong inhibitors of CYP1A2 or CYP2C8). Products include:

Cipro	3073

Citalopram Hydrobromide (In vitro studies demonstrate that CYP1A2 and CYP2C8 are involved in the oxidative metabolism of eltrombopag. The significance of co-administration of eltrombopag with inducers of CYP 1A2 (eg, tobacco, omeprazole) and CYP 2C8 (eg, rifampin) on the systemic exposure of eltrombopag has not been established in clinical studies. Monitor patients for signs and symptoms of excessive eltrombopag exposure when eltrombopag is administered concomitantly with these drugs). Products include:

Celexa	1153

Clarithromycin (In vitro studies demonstrate that CYP1A2 and CYP2C8 are involved in the oxidative metabolism of eltrombopag. The significance of co-administration of eltrombopag with moderate or strong inhibitors of CYP 1A2 (eg, ciprofloxacin, fluvoxamine) and

CYP 2C8 (eg, gemfibrozil, trimethoprim) on the systemic exposure of eltrombopag has not been established in clinical studies. Monitor patients for signs and symptoms of excessive eltrombopag exposure when eltrombopag is administered concomitantly with these moderate or strong inhibitors of CYP1A2 or CYP2C8). Products include:

Biaxin/Biaxin XL	412

Clomipramine Hydrochloride (In vitro studies demonstrate that CYP1A2 and CYP2C8 are involved in the oxidative metabolism of eltrombopag. The significance of co-administration of eltrombopag with other substrates of these CYP enzymes on the systemic exposure of eltrombopag has not been established in clinical studies. Monitor patients for signs and symptoms of excessive eltrombopag exposure when eltrombopag is administered concomitantly with these drugs).

No products indexed under this heading.

Clopidogrel Bisulfate (In vitro studies demonstrate that CYP1A2 and CYP2C8 are involved in the oxidative metabolism of eltrombopag. The significance of co-administration of eltrombopag with other substrates of these CYP enzymes on the systemic exposure of eltrombopag has not been established in clinical studies. Monitor patients for signs and symptoms of excessive eltrombopag exposure when eltrombopag is administered concomitantly with these drugs). Products include:

Plavix	3027

Clozapine (In vitro studies demonstrate that CYP1A2 and CYP2C8 are involved in the oxidative metabolism of eltrombopag. The significance of co-administration of eltrombopag with other substrates of these CYP enzymes on the systemic exposure of eltrombopag has not been established in clinical studies. Monitor patients for signs and symptoms of excessive eltrombopag exposure when eltrombopag is administered concomitantly with these drugs).

No products indexed under this heading.

Codeine Phosphate (Studies demonstrate that eltrombopag is an inhibitor of UGT1A1, UGT1A3, UGT1A4, UGT1A6, UGT1A9, UGT2B7, and UGT2B15, enzymes involved in the metabolism of multiple drugs, such as acetaminophen, narcotics, and nonsteroidal anti-inflammatory drugs (NSAIDs). Monitor patients closely for signs of symptoms of excessive exposure to these drugs when concomitantly administered with eltrombopag). Products include:

Tylenol with Codeine	2691

Codeine Sulfate (Studies demonstrate that eltrombopag is an inhibitor of UGT1A1, UGT1A3, UGT1A4, UGT1A6, UGT1A9, UGT2B7, and UGT2B15, enzymes involved in the metabolism of multiple drugs, such as acetaminophen, narcotics, and nonsteroidal anti-inflammatory drugs (NSAIDs). Monitor patients closely for signs of symptoms of excessive exposure to these drugs when concomitantly administered with eltrombopag).

No products indexed under this heading.

Cyclobenzaprine (In vitro studies demonstrate that CYP1A2 and CYP2C8 are involved in the oxidative metabolism of eltrombopag. The significance of co-administration of eltrombopag with other substrates of these CYP enzymes on the systemic exposure of eltrombopag has not been established in clinical studies. Monitor patients for signs and symptoms of excessive eltrombopag exposure when eltrombopag is administered concomitantly with these drugs).

No products indexed under this heading.

Cyclobenzaprine Hydrochloride (*In vitro* studies demonstrate that CYP1A2 and CYP2C8 are involved in the oxidative metabolism of eltrombopag. The significance of co-administration of eltrombopag with other substrates of these CYP enzymes on the systemic exposure of eltrombopag has not been established in clinical studies. Monitor patients for signs and symptoms of excessive eltrombopag exposure when eltrombopag is administered concomitantly with these drugs). Products include:

Amrix 964

Desipramine Hydrochloride (*In vitro* studies demonstrate that CYP1A2 and CYP2C8 are involved in the oxidative metabolism of eltrombopag. The significance of co-administration of eltrombopag with other substrates of these CYP enzymes on the systemic exposure of eltrombopag has not been established in clinical studies. Monitor patients for signs and symptoms of excessive eltrombopag exposure when eltrombopag is administered concomitantly with these drugs).

No products indexed under this heading.

Desogestrel (*In vitro* studies demonstrate that CYP1A2 and CYP2C8 are involved in the oxidative metabolism of eltrombopag. The significance of co-administration of eltrombopag with moderate or strong inhibitors of CYP 1A2 (eg, ciprofloxacin, fluvoxamine) and CYP 2C8 (eg, gemfibrozil, trimethoprim) on the systemic exposure of eltrombopag has not been established in clinical studies. Monitor patients for signs and symptoms of excessive eltrombopag exposure when eltrombopag is administered concomitantly with these moderate or strong inhibitors of CYP1A2 or CYP2C8).

No products indexed under this heading.

Dezocine (Studies demonstrate that eltrombopag is an inhibitor of UGT1A1, UGT1A3, UGT1A4, UGT1A6, UGT1A9, UGT2B7, and UGT2B15, enzymes involved in the metabolism of multiple drugs, such as acetaminophen, narcotics, and nonsteroidal anti-inflammatory drugs (NSAIDs). Monitor patients closely for signs of symptoms of excessive exposure to these drugs when concomitantly administered with eltrombopag).

No products indexed under this heading.

Diazepam (*In vitro* studies demonstrate that CYP1A2 and CYP2C8 are involved in the oxidative metabolism of eltrombopag. The significance of co-administration of eltrombopag with other substrates of these CYP enzymes on the systemic exposure of eltrombopag has not been established in clinical studies. Monitor patients for signs and symptoms of excessive eltrombopag exposure when eltrombopag is administered concomitantly with these drugs). Products include:

Valium Tablets 2880

Diclofenac Epolamine (Studies demonstrate that eltrombopag is an inhibitor of UGT1A1, UGT1A3, UGT1A4, UGT1A6, UGT1A9, UGT2B7, and UGT2B15, enzymes involved in the metabolism of multiple drugs, such as acetaminophen, narcotics, and nonsteroidal anti-inflammatory drugs (NSAIDs). Monitor patients closely for signs of symptoms of excessive exposure to these drugs when concomitantly administered with eltrombopag). Products include:

Flector 1839

Diclofenac Potassium (Studies demonstrate that eltrombopag is an inhibitor of UGT1A1, UGT1A3, UGT1A4, UGT1A6, UGT1A9, UGT2B7, and UGT2B15, enzymes involved in the metabolism of multiple drugs, such as acetaminophen, narcotics, and nonsteroidal anti-inflammatory drugs (NSAIDs). Monitor patients closely for signs of symptoms of excessive exposure to these drugs when concomitantly administered with eltrombopag).

No products indexed under this heading.

Diclofenac Sodium (Studies demonstrate that eltrombopag is an inhibitor of UGT1A1, UGT1A3, UGT1A4, UGT1A6, UGT1A9, UGT2B7, and UGT2B15, enzymes involved in the metabolism of multiple drugs, such as acetaminophen, narcotics, and nonsteroidal anti-inflammatory drugs (NSAIDs). Monitor patients closely for signs of symptoms of excessive exposure to these drugs when concomitantly administered with eltrombopag).

No products indexed under this heading.

Dihydrocodeine Bitartrate (Studies demonstrate that eltrombopag is an inhibitor of UGT1A1, UGT1A3, UGT1A4, UGT1A6, UGT1A9, UGT2B7, and UGT2B15, enzymes involved in the metabolism of multiple drugs, such as acetaminophen, narcotics, and nonsteroidal anti-inflammatory drugs (NSAIDs). Monitor patients closely for signs of symptoms of excessive exposure to these drugs when concomitantly administered with eltrombopag).

No products indexed under this heading.

Dihydrocodeinone Bitartrate (Studies demonstrate that eltrombopag is an inhibitor of UGT1A1, UGT1A3, UGT1A4, UGT1A6, UGT1A9, UGT2B7, and UGT2B15, enzymes involved in the metabolism of multiple drugs, such as acetaminophen, narcotics, and nonsteroidal anti-inflammatory drugs (NSAIDs). Monitor patients closely for signs of symptoms of excessive exposure to these drugs when concomitantly administered with eltrombopag).

No products indexed under this heading.

Diltiazem Hydrochloride (*In vitro* studies demonstrate that CYP1A2 and CYP2C8 are involved in the oxidative metabolism of eltrombopag. The significance of co-administration of eltrombopag with inducers of CYP 1A2 (eg, tobacco, omeprazole) and CYP 2C8 (eg, rifampin) on the systemic exposure of eltrombopag has not been established in clinical studies. Monitor patients for signs and symptoms of excessive eltrombopag exposure when eltrombopag is administered concomitantly with these drugs). Products include:

Cardizem LA 423

Diltiazem Maleate (*In vitro* studies demonstrate that CYP1A2 and CYP2C8 are involved in the oxidative metabolism of eltrombopag. The significance of co-administration of eltrombopag with inducers of CYP 1A2 (eg, tobacco, omeprazole) and CYP 2C8 (eg, rifampin) on the systemic exposure of eltrombopag has not been established in clinical studies. Monitor patients for signs and symptoms of excessive eltrombopag exposure when eltrombopag is administered concomitantly with these drugs).

No products indexed under this heading.

Docetaxel (*In vitro* studies demonstrate that CYP1A2 and CYP2C8 are involved in the oxidative metabolism of eltrombopag. The significance of co-administration of eltrombopag with other substrates of these CYP enzymes on the systemic exposure of eltrombopag has not been established in clinical studies. Monitor patients for signs and symptoms of excessive eltrombopag exposure when eltrombopag is administered concomitantly with these drugs). Products include:

Taxotere 3035

Doxepin Hydrochloride (*In vitro* studies demonstrate that CYP1A2 and CYP2C8 are involved in the oxidative metabolism of eltrombopag. The significance of co-administration of eltrombopag with other substrates of these CYP enzymes on the systemic exposure of eltrombopag has not been established in clinical studies. Monitor patients for signs and symptoms of excessive eltrombopag exposure when eltrombopag is administered concomitantly with these drugs).

No products indexed under this heading.

Enoxacin (*In vitro* studies demonstrate that CYP1A2 and CYP2C8 are involved in the oxidative metabolism of eltrombopag. The significance of co-administration of eltrombopag with moderate or strong inhibitors of CYP 1A2 (eg, ciprofloxacin, fluvoxamine) and CYP 2C8 (eg, gemfibrozil, trimethoprim) on the systemic exposure of eltrombopag has not been established in clinical studies. Monitor patients for signs and symptoms of excessive eltrombopag exposure when eltrombopag is administered concomitantly with these moderate or strong inhibitors of CYP1A2 or CYP2C8).

No products indexed under this heading.

Erythromycin (*In vitro* studies demonstrate that CYP1A2 and CYP2C8 are involved in the oxidative metabolism of eltrombopag. The significance of co-administration of eltrombopag with inducers of CYP 1A2 (eg, tobacco, omeprazole) and CYP 2C8 (eg, rifampin) on the systemic exposure of eltrombopag has not been established in clinical studies. Monitor patients for signs and symptoms of excessive eltrombopag exposure when eltrombopag is administered concomitantly with these drugs).

No products indexed under this heading.

Erythromycin, Topical (*In vitro* studies demonstrate that CYP1A2 and CYP2C8 are involved in the oxidative metabolism of eltrombopag. The significance of co-administration of eltrombopag with inducers of CYP 1A2 (eg, tobacco, omeprazole) and CYP 2C8 (eg, rifampin) on the systemic exposure of eltrombopag has not been established in clinical studies. Monitor patients for signs and symptoms of excessive eltrombopag exposure when eltrombopag is administered concomitantly with these drugs).

No products indexed under this heading.

Erythromycin Estolate (*In vitro* studies demonstrate that CYP1A2 and CYP2C8 are involved in the oxidative metabolism of eltrombopag. The significance of co-administration of eltrombopag with inducers of CYP 1A2 (eg, tobacco, omeprazole) and CYP 2C8 (eg, rifampin) on the systemic exposure of eltrombopag has not been established in clinical studies. Monitor patients for signs and symptoms of excessive eltrombopag exposure when eltrombopag is administered concomitantly with these drugs).

No products indexed under this heading.

Erythromycin Ethylsuccinate (*In vitro* studies demonstrate that CYP1A2 and CYP2C8 are involved in the oxidative metabolism of eltrombopag. The significance of co-administration of eltrombopag with inducers of CYP 1A2 (eg, tobacco, omeprazole) and CYP 2C8 (eg, rifampin) on the systemic exposure of eltrombopag has not been established in clinical studies. Monitor patients for signs and symptoms of excessive eltrombopag exposure when eltrombopag is administered concomitantly with these drugs). Products include:

E.E.S. 437

EryPed 435

Erythromycin Gluceptate (*In vitro* studies demonstrate that CYP1A2 and CYP2C8 are involved in the oxidative metabolism of eltrombopag. The significance of co-administration of eltrombopag with inducers of CYP 1A2 (eg, tobacco, omeprazole) and CYP 2C8 (eg, rifampin) on the systemic exposure of eltrombopag has not been established in clinical studies. Monitor patients for signs and symptoms of excessive eltrombopag exposure when eltrombopag is administered concomitantly with these drugs).

No products indexed under this heading.

Erythromycin Lactobionate (*In vitro* studies demonstrate that CYP1A2 and CYP2C8 are involved in the oxidative metabolism of eltrombopag. The significance of co-administration of eltrombopag with inducers of CYP 1A2 (eg, tobacco, omeprazole) and CYP 2C8 (eg, rifampin) on the systemic exposure of eltrombopag has not been established in clinical studies. Monitor patients for signs and symptoms of excessive eltrombopag exposure when eltrombopag is administered concomitantly with these drugs).

No products indexed under this heading.

Erythromycin Stearate (*In vitro* studies demonstrate that CYP1A2 and CYP2C8 are involved in the oxidative metabolism of eltrombopag. The significance of co-administration of eltrombopag with inducers of CYP 1A2 (eg, tobacco, omeprazole) and CYP 2C8 (eg, rifampin) on the systemic exposure of eltrombopag has not been established in clinical studies. Monitor patients for signs and symptoms of excessive eltrombopag exposure when eltrombopag is administered concomitantly with these drugs).

No products indexed under this heading.

Escitalopram Oxalate (*In vitro* studies demonstrate that CYP1A2 and CYP2C8 are involved in the oxidative metabolism of eltrombopag. The significance of co-administration of eltrombopag with inducers of CYP 1A2 (eg, tobacco, omeprazole) and CYP 2C8 (eg, rifampin) on the systemic exposure of eltrombopag has not been established in clinical studies. Monitor patients for signs and symptoms of excessive eltrombopag exposure when eltrombopag is administered concomitantly with these drugs). Products include:

Lexapro Oral Suspension 1160

Lexapro Tablets 1160

Esomeprazole Magnesium (*In vitro* studies demonstrate that CYP1A2 and CYP2C8 are involved in the oxidative metabolism of eltrombopag. The significance of co-administration of eltrombopag with moderate or strong inhibitors of CYP 1A2 (eg, ciprofloxacin, fluvoxamine) and CYP 2C8 (eg, gemfibrozil, trimethoprim) on the systemic exposure of eltrombopag has not been established in clinical studies. Monitor patients for signs and symptoms of excessive eltrombopag exposure when eltrombopag is administered concomitantly with these moderate or strong inhibitors of CYP1A2 or CYP2C8). Products include:

Nexium Capsules 704

Nexium Oral Suspension 704

Esomeprazole Sodium (*In vitro* studies demonstrate that CYP1A2 and CYP2C8 are involved in the oxidative metabolism of eltrombopag. The significance of co-administration of eltrombopag with moderate or strong inhibitors of CYP 1A2 (eg, ciprofloxacin, fluvoxamine) and CYP 2C8 (eg, gemfibrozil, trimethoprim) on the systemic exposure of eltrombopag has not been established in clinical studies. Monitor patients for signs and symptoms of excessive eltrombopag exposure when eltrombopag is administered concomi-

tantly with these moderate or strong inhibitors of CYP1A2 or CYP2C8). Products include:

Nexium I.V. 712

Estradiol (*In vitro* studies demonstrate that eltrombopag is an inhibitor of UGT1A1, UGT1A3, UGT1A4, UGT1A6, UGT1A9, UGT2B7, and UGT2B15, enzymes involved in the metabolism of multiple drugs, such as acetaminophen, narcotics, and nonsteroidal anti-inflammatory drugs (NSAIDs). The significance of this inhibition on the potential for increased systemic exposure of drugs that are substrates of these UGTs following co-administration with eltrombopag has not been evaluated in clinical studies. Monitor patients closely for signs or symptoms of excessive exposure to these drugs when concomitantly administered with eltrombopag). Products include:

Activella 2561
Angeliq 831
Climara 841
Climara Pro 847
Divigel 3467
Estrasorb 1777
Vagifem 2589

Estradiol Acetate (*In vitro* studies demonstrate that eltrombopag is an inhibitor of UGT1A1, UGT1A3, UGT1A4, UGT1A6, UGT1A9, UGT2B7, and UGT2B15, enzymes involved in the metabolism of multiple drugs, such as acetaminophen, narcotics, and nonsteroidal anti-inflammatory drugs (NSAIDs). The significance of this inhibition on the potential for increased systemic exposure of drugs that are substrates of these UGTs following co-administration with eltrombopag has not been evaluated in clinical studies. Monitor patients closely for signs or symptoms of excessive exposure to these drugs when concomitantly administered with eltrombopag).

No products indexed under this heading.

Estradiol Benzoate (*In vitro* studies demonstrate that eltrombopag is an inhibitor of UGT1A1, UGT1A3, UGT1A4, UGT1A6, UGT1A9, UGT2B7, and UGT2B15, enzymes involved in the metabolism of multiple drugs, such as acetaminophen, narcotics, and nonsteroidal anti-inflammatory drugs (NSAIDs). The significance of this inhibition on the potential for increased systemic exposure of drugs that are substrates of these UGTs following co-administration with eltrombopag has not been evaluated in clinical studies. Monitor patients closely for signs or symptoms of excessive exposure to these drugs when concomitantly administered with eltrombopag).

No products indexed under this heading.

Estradiol Cypionate (*In vitro* studies demonstrate that eltrombopag is an inhibitor of UGT1A1, UGT1A3, UGT1A4, UGT1A6, UGT1A9, UGT2B7, and UGT2B15, enzymes involved in the metabolism of multiple drugs, such as acetaminophen, narcotics, and nonsteroidal anti-inflammatory drugs (NSAIDs). The significance of this inhibition on the potential for increased systemic exposure of drugs that are substrates of these UGTs following co-administration with eltrombopag has not been evaluated in clinical studies. Monitor patients closely for signs or symptoms of excessive exposure to these drugs when concomitantly administered with eltrombopag).

No products indexed under this heading.

Estradiol Valerate (*In vitro* studies demonstrate that eltrombopag is an inhibitor of UGT1A1, UGT1A3, UGT1A4, UGT1A6, UGT1A9, UGT2B7, and UGT2B15, enzymes involved in the metabolism of multiple drugs, such as acetaminophen, narcotics, and nonste-

roidal anti-inflammatory drugs (NSAIDs). The significance of this inhibition on the potential for increased systemic exposure of drugs that are substrates of these UGTs following co-administration with eltrombopag has not been evaluated in clinical studies. Monitor patients closely for signs or symptoms of excessive exposure to these drugs when concomitantly administered with eltrombopag).

No products indexed under this heading.

Ethinyl Estradiol (*In vitro* studies demonstrate that eltrombopag is an inhibitor of UGT1A1, UGT1A3, UGT1A4, UGT1A6, UGT1A9, UGT2B7, and UGT2B15, enzymes involved in the metabolism of multiple drugs, such as acetaminophen, narcotics, and nonsteroidal anti-inflammatory drugs (NSAIDs). The significance of this inhibition on the potential for increased systemic exposure of drugs that are substrates of these UGTs following co-administration with eltrombopag has not been evaluated in clinical studies. Monitor patients closely for signs or symptoms of excessive exposure to these drugs when concomitantly administered with eltrombopag). Products include:

LoSeasonique 3407
Lybrel 3514
NuvaRing 3181
Ortho Evra 2648
Ortho-Cyclen/Ortho Tri-Cyclen 2663
Ortho Tri-Cyclen Lo Tablets 2673
Seasonique 3418
Yaz 864

Etodolac (Studies demonstrate that eltrombopag is an inhibitor of UGT1A1, UGT1A3, UGT1A4, UGT1A6, UGT1A9, UGT2B7, and UGT2B15, enzymes involved in the metabolism of multiple drugs, such as acetaminophen, narcotics, and nonsteroidal anti-inflammatory drugs (NSAIDs). Monitor patients closely for signs of symptoms of excessive exposure to these drugs when concomitantly administered with eltrombopag).

No products indexed under this heading.

Etoposide (*In vitro* studies demonstrate that eltrombopag is an inhibitor of UGT1A1, UGT1A3, UGT1A4, UGT1A6, UGT1A9, UGT2B7, and UGT2B15, enzymes involved in the metabolism of multiple drugs, such as acetaminophen, narcotics, and nonsteroidal anti-inflammatory drugs (NSAIDs). The significance of this inhibition on the potential for increased systemic exposure of drugs that are substrates of these UGTs following co-administration with eltrombopag has not been evaluated in clinical studies. Monitor patients closely for signs or symptoms of excessive exposure to these drugs when concomitantly administered with eltrombopag).

No products indexed under this heading.

Etoposide Phosphate (*In vitro* studies demonstrate that eltrombopag is an inhibitor of UGT1A1, UGT1A3, UGT1A4, UGT1A6, UGT1A9, UGT2B7, and UGT2B15, enzymes involved in the metabolism of multiple drugs, such as acetaminophen, narcotics, and nonsteroidal anti-inflammatory drugs (NSAIDs). The significance of this inhibition on the potential for increased systemic exposure of drugs that are substrates of these UGTs following co-administration with eltrombopag has not been evaluated in clinical studies. Monitor patients closely for signs or symptoms of excessive exposure to these drugs when concomitantly administered with eltrombopag).

No products indexed under this heading.

Fenoprofen Calcium (Studies demonstrate that eltrombopag is an inhibitor of UGT1A1, UGT1A3, UGT1A4, UGT1A6, UGT1A9, UGT2B7, and UGT2B15, enzymes involved in the

metabolism of multiple drugs, such as acetaminophen, narcotics, and nonsteroidal anti-inflammatory drugs (NSAIDs). Monitor patients closely for signs of symptoms of excessive exposure to these drugs when concomitantly administered with eltrombopag).

No products indexed under this heading.

Fentanyl (Studies demonstrate that eltrombopag is an inhibitor of UGT1A1, UGT1A3, UGT1A4, UGT1A6, UGT1A9, UGT2B7, and UGT2B15, enzymes involved in the metabolism of multiple drugs, such as acetaminophen, narcotics, and nonsteroidal anti-inflammatory drugs (NSAIDs). Monitor patients closely for signs of symptoms of excessive exposure to these drugs when concomitantly administered with eltrombopag). Products include:

Duragesic 2604
Fentanyl Transdermal System 2346
Onsolis 2054

Fentanyl Citrate (Studies demonstrate that eltrombopag is an inhibitor of UGT1A1, UGT1A3, UGT1A4, UGT1A6, UGT1A9, UGT2B7, and UGT2B15, enzymes involved in the metabolism of multiple drugs, such as acetaminophen, narcotics, and nonsteroidal anti-inflammatory drugs (NSAIDs). Monitor patients closely for signs of symptoms of excessive exposure to these drugs when concomitantly administered with eltrombopag). Products include:

Fentora 966

Ferrous Fumarate (Eltrombopag chelates polyvalent cations (such as iron, calcium, aluminum, magnesium, selenium, and zinc) in foods, mineral supplements, and antacids. In a clinical study, administration of eltrombopag with a polyvalent cation-containing antacid (1,524 mg aluminum hydroxide, 1,425 mg magnesium carbonate, and sodium alginate) decreased plasma eltrombopag systemic exposure by approximately 70%. Eltrombopag must not be taken within 4 hours of any medications or products containing polyvalent cations such as antacids, dairy products, and mineral supplements to avoid significant reduction in eltrombopag absorption due to chelation). Products include:

PreNexa 3473

Ferrous Gluconate (Eltrombopag chelates polyvalent cations (such as iron, calcium, aluminum, magnesium, selenium, and zinc) in foods, mineral supplements, and antacids. In a clinical study, administration of eltrombopag with a polyvalent cation-containing antacid (1,524 mg aluminum hydroxide, 1,425 mg magnesium carbonate, and sodium alginate) decreased plasma eltrombopag systemic exposure by approximately 70%. Eltrombopag must not be taken within 4 hours of any medications or products containing polyvalent cations such as antacids, dairy products, and mineral supplements to avoid significant reduction in eltrombopag absorption due to chelation). Products include:

CitraNatal Assure 2332
CitraNatal Rx 2332

Ferrous Sulfate (Eltrombopag chelates polyvalent cations (such as iron, calcium, aluminum, magnesium, selenium, and zinc) in foods, mineral supplements, and antacids. In a clinical study, administration of eltrombopag with a polyvalent cation-containing antacid (1,524 mg aluminum hydroxide, 1,425 mg magnesium carbonate, and sodium alginate) decreased plasma eltrombopag systemic exposure by approximately 70%. Eltrombopag must not be taken within 4 hours of any medications or products containing polyvalent cations such as antacids, dairy

products, and mineral supplements to avoid significant reduction in eltrombopag absorption due to chelation).

No products indexed under this heading.

Flurbiprofen (Studies demonstrate that eltrombopag is an inhibitor of UGT1A1, UGT1A3, UGT1A4, UGT1A6, UGT1A9, UGT2B7, and UGT2B15, enzymes involved in the metabolism of multiple drugs, such as acetaminophen, narcotics, and nonsteroidal anti-inflammatory drugs (NSAIDs). Monitor patients closely for signs of symptoms of excessive exposure to these drugs when concomitantly administered with eltrombopag).

No products indexed under this heading.

Flutamide (*In vitro* studies demonstrate that CYP1A2 and CYP2C8 are involved in the oxidative metabolism of eltrombopag. The significance of co-administration of eltrombopag with other substrates of these CYP enzymes on the systemic exposure of eltrombopag has not been established in clinical studies. Monitor patients for signs and symptoms of excessive eltrombopag exposure when eltrombopag is administered concomitantly with these drugs).

No products indexed under this heading.

Fluticasone Propionate (*In vitro* studies demonstrate that CYP1A2 and CYP2C8 are involved in the oxidative metabolism of eltrombopag. The significance of co-administration of eltrombopag with other substrates of these CYP enzymes on the systemic exposure of eltrombopag has not been established in clinical studies. Monitor patients for signs and symptoms of excessive eltrombopag exposure when eltrombopag is administered concomitantly with these drugs). Products include:

Advair 100/50 1275
Advair 250/50 1275
Advair 500/50 1275
Advair HFA 45/21 1288
Advair HFA 115/21 1288
Advair HFA 230/21 1288
Flonase 1459
Flovent Diskus 1463
Flovent HFA 1470

Fluvastatin Sodium (*In vitro* studies demonstrate that eltrombopag is an inhibitor of the organic anion transporting polypeptide OATP1B1 and can increase the systemic exposure of other drugs that are substrates of this transporter (eg, benzylpenicillin, atorvastatin, fluvastatin, pravastatin, rosuvastatin, methotrexate, nateglinide, repaglinide, rifampin). Monitor patients closely for signs and symptoms of excessive exposure to the drugs that are substrates of OATP1B1 and consider reduction of the dose of these drugs).

No products indexed under this heading.

Fluvoxamine (*In vitro* studies demonstrate that CYP1A2 and CYP2C8 are involved in the oxidative metabolism of eltrombopag. The significance of co-administration of eltrombopag with moderate or strong inhibitors of CYP 1A2 (eg, ciprofloxacin, fluvoxamine) and CYP 2C8 (eg, gemfibrozil, trimethoprim) on the systemic exposure of eltrombopag has not been established in clinical studies. Monitor patients for signs and symptoms of excessive eltrombopag exposure when eltrombopag is administered concomitantly with these moderate or strong inhibitors of CYP1A2 or CYP2C8).

No products indexed under this heading.

Fluvoxamine Maleate (*In vitro* studies demonstrate that CYP1A2 and CYP2C8 are involved in the oxidative metabolism of eltrombopag. The significance of co-administration of eltrombopag with moderate or strong inhibitors of CYP 1A2 (eg, ciprofloxacin,

1507 Interactions Index Promacta

fluvoxamine) and CYP 2C8 (eg, gemfibrozil, trimethoprim) on the systemic exposure of eltrombopag has not been established in clinical studies. Monitor patients for signs and symptoms of excessive eltrombopag exposure when eltrombopag is administered concomitantly with these moderate or strong inhibitors of CYP1A2 or CYP2C8).
No products indexed under this heading.

Gatifloxacin (*In vitro* studies demonstrate that CYP1A2 and CYP2C8 are involved in the oxidative metabolism of eltrombopag. The significance of co-administration of eltrombopag with moderate or strong inhibitors of CYP 1A2 (eg, ciprofloxacin, fluvoxamine) and CYP 2C8 (eg, gemfibrozil, trimethoprim) on the systemic exposure of eltrombopag has not been established in clinical studies. Monitor patients for signs and symptoms of excessive eltrombopag exposure when eltrombopag is administered concomitantly with these moderate or strong inhibitors of CYP1A2 or CYP2C8).
No products indexed under this heading.

Gemfibrozil (*In vitro* studies demonstrate that CYP1A2 and CYP2C8 are involved in the oxidative metabolism of eltrombopag. The significance of co-administration of eltrombopag with moderate or strong inhibitors of CYP 1A2 (eg, ciprofloxacin, fluvoxamine) and CYP 2C8 (eg, gemfibrozil, trimethoprim) on the systemic exposure of eltrombopag has not been established in clinical studies. Monitor patients for signs and symptoms of excessive eltrombopag exposure when eltrombopag is administered concomitantly with these moderate or strong inhibitors of CYP1A2 or CYP2C8).
No products indexed under this heading.

Gemifloxacin Mesylate (*In vitro* studies demonstrate that CYP1A2 and CYP2C8 are involved in the oxidative metabolism of eltrombopag. The significance of co-administration of eltrombopag with moderate or strong inhibitors of CYP 1A2 (eg, ciprofloxacin, fluvoxamine) and CYP 2C8 (eg, gemfibrozil, trimethoprim) on the systemic exposure of eltrombopag has not been established in clinical studies. Monitor patients for signs and symptoms of excessive eltrombopag exposure when eltrombopag is administered concomitantly with these moderate or strong inhibitors of CYP1A2 or CYP2C8).
No products indexed under this heading.

Grepafloxacin Hydrochloride (*In vitro* studies demonstrate that CYP1A2 and CYP2C8 are involved in the oxidative metabolism of eltrombopag. The significance of co-administration of eltrombopag with moderate or strong inhibitors of CYP 1A2 (eg, ciprofloxacin, fluvoxamine) and CYP 2C8 (eg, gemfibrozil, trimethoprim) on the systemic exposure of eltrombopag has not been established in clinical studies. Monitor patients for signs and symptoms of excessive eltrombopag exposure when eltrombopag is administered concomitantly with these moderate or strong inhibitors of CYP1A2 or CYP2C8).
No products indexed under this heading.

Haloperidol (*In vitro* studies demonstrate that CYP1A2 and CYP2C8 are involved in the oxidative metabolism of eltrombopag. The significance of co-administration of eltrombopag with other substrates of these CYP enzymes on the systemic exposure of eltrombopag has not been established in clinical studies. Monitor patients for signs and symptoms of excessive eltrombopag exposure when eltrombopag is administered concomitantly with these drugs).
No products indexed under this heading.

Haloperidol Decanoate (*In vitro* studies demonstrate that CYP1A2 and CYP2C8 are involved in the oxidative metabolism of eltrombopag. The significance of co-administration of eltrombopag with other substrates of these CYP enzymes on the systemic exposure of eltrombopag has not been established in clinical studies. Monitor patients for signs and symptoms of excessive eltrombopag exposure when eltrombopag is administered concomitantly with these drugs).
No products indexed under this heading.

Haloperidol Lactate (*In vitro* studies demonstrate that CYP1A2 and CYP2C8 are involved in the oxidative metabolism of eltrombopag. The significance of co-administration of eltrombopag with other substrates of these CYP enzymes on the systemic exposure of eltrombopag has not been established in clinical studies. Monitor patients for signs and symptoms of excessive eltrombopag exposure when eltrombopag is administered concomitantly with these drugs).
No products indexed under this heading.

Hydrocodone Bitartrate (Studies demonstrate that eltrombopag is an inhibitor of UGT1A1, UGT1A3, UGT1A4, UGT1A6, UGT1A9, UGT2B7, and UGT2B15, enzymes involved in the metabolism of multiple drugs, such as acetaminophen, narcotics, and nonsteroidal anti-inflammatory drugs (NSAIDs). Monitor patients closely for signs of symptoms of excessive exposure to these drugs when concomitantly administered with eltrombopag). Products include:
Vicodin 560
Vicodin ES 561
Vicodin HP 563
Vicoprofen 564
Zydone 1138

Hydrocodone Polistirex (Studies demonstrate that eltrombopag is an inhibitor of UGT1A1, UGT1A3, UGT1A4, UGT1A6, UGT1A9, UGT2B7, and UGT2B15, enzymes involved in the metabolism of multiple drugs, such as acetaminophen, narcotics, and nonsteroidal anti-inflammatory drugs (NSAIDs). Monitor patients closely for signs of symptoms of excessive exposure to these drugs when concomitantly administered with eltrombopag). Products include:
Tussionex 3443

Hydromorphone (Studies demonstrate that eltrombopag is an inhibitor of UGT1A1, UGT1A3, UGT1A4, UGT1A6, UGT1A9, UGT2B7, and UGT2B15, enzymes involved in the metabolism of multiple drugs, such as acetaminophen, narcotics, and nonsteroidal anti-inflammatory drugs (NSAIDs). Monitor patients closely for signs of symptoms of excessive exposure to these drugs when concomitantly administered with eltrombopag).
No products indexed under this heading.

Hydromorphone Hydrochloride (Studies demonstrate that eltrombopag is an inhibitor of UGT1A1, UGT1A3, UGT1A4, UGT1A6, UGT1A9, UGT2B7, and UGT2B15, enzymes involved in the metabolism of multiple drugs, such as acetaminophen, narcotics, and nonsteroidal anti-inflammatory drugs (NSAIDs). Monitor patients closely for signs of symptoms of excessive exposure to these drugs when concomitantly administered with eltrombopag). Products include:
Dilaudid Injection 2800
Dilaudid Oral 2797
Dilaudid Tablets 2797
Dilaudid-HP 2800

Hypericum (*In vitro* studies demonstrate that CYP1A2 and CYP2C8 are involved in the oxidative metabolism of eltrombopag. The significance of co-administration of eltrombopag with inducers of CYP 1A2 (eg, tobacco, omeprazole) and CYP 2C8 (eg, rifampin) on the systemic exposure of eltrombopag has not been established in clinical studies. Monitor patients for signs and symptoms of excessive eltrombopag exposure when eltrombopag is administered concomitantly with these drugs).
No products indexed under this heading.

Hypericum Perforatum (*In vitro* studies demonstrate that CYP1A2 and CYP2C8 are involved in the oxidative metabolism of eltrombopag. The significance of co-administration of eltrombopag with inducers of CYP 1A2 (eg, tobacco, omeprazole) and CYP 2C8 (eg, rifampin) on the systemic exposure of eltrombopag has not been established in clinical studies. Monitor patients for signs and symptoms of excessive eltrombopag exposure when eltrombopag is administered concomitantly with these drugs). Products include:
Traumeel 1800

Ibuprofen (Studies demonstrate that eltrombopag is an inhibitor of UGT1A1, UGT1A3, UGT1A4, UGT1A6, UGT1A9, UGT2B7, and UGT2B15, enzymes involved in the metabolism of multiple drugs, such as acetaminophen, narcotics, and nonsteroidal anti-inflammatory drugs (NSAIDs). Monitor patients closely for signs of symptoms of excessive exposure to these drugs when concomitantly administered with eltrombopag). Products include:
Motrin IB 2043
Children's Motrin 2044
Children's Motrin Non-Staining Dye-Free 2044
Infants' Motrin 2044
Infants' Motrin Dye-Free 2044
Junior Strength Motrin 2044
Vicoprofen 564

Imipramine Hydrochloride (*In vitro* studies demonstrate that CYP1A2 and CYP2C8 are involved in the oxidative metabolism of eltrombopag. The significance of co-administration of eltrombopag with other substrates of these CYP enzymes on the systemic exposure of eltrombopag has not been established in clinical studies. Monitor patients for signs and symptoms of excessive eltrombopag exposure when eltrombopag is administered concomitantly with these drugs).
No products indexed under this heading.

Imipramine Pamoate (*In vitro* studies demonstrate that CYP1A2 and CYP2C8 are involved in the oxidative metabolism of eltrombopag. The significance of co-administration of eltrombopag with other substrates of these CYP enzymes on the systemic exposure of eltrombopag has not been established in clinical studies. Monitor patients for signs and symptoms of excessive eltrombopag exposure when eltrombopag is administered concomitantly with these drugs).
No products indexed under this heading.

Indomethacin (Studies demonstrate that eltrombopag is an inhibitor of UGT1A1, UGT1A3, UGT1A4, UGT1A6, UGT1A9, UGT2B7, and UGT2B15, enzymes involved in the metabolism of multiple drugs, such as acetaminophen, narcotics, and nonsteroidal anti-inflammatory drugs (NSAIDs). Monitor patients closely for signs of symptoms of excessive exposure to these drugs when concomitantly administered with eltrombopag). Products include:
Indocin 2167

Indomethacin Sodium Trihydrate (Studies demonstrate that eltrombopag is an inhibitor of UGT1A1, UGT1A3, UGT1A4, UGT1A6, UGT1A9, UGT2B7, and UGT2B15, enzymes involved in the metabolism of multiple drugs, such as acetaminophen, narcotics, and nonsteroidal anti-inflammatory drugs (NSAIDs). Monitor patients closely for signs of symptoms of excessive exposure to these drugs when concomitantly administered with eltrombopag). Products include:
Indocin I.V. 2007

Insulin (*In vitro* studies demonstrate that CYP1A2 and CYP2C8 are involved in the oxidative metabolism of eltrombopag. The significance of co-administration of eltrombopag with inducers of CYP 1A2 (eg, tobacco, omeprazole) and CYP 2C8 (eg, rifampin) on the systemic exposure of eltrombopag has not been established in clinical studies. Monitor patients for signs and symptoms of excessive eltrombopag exposure when eltrombopag is administered concomitantly with these drugs).
No products indexed under this heading.

Insulin, Human, Zinc Suspension (*In vitro* studies demonstrate that CYP1A2 and CYP2C8 are involved in the oxidative metabolism of eltrombopag. The significance of co-administration of eltrombopag with inducers of CYP 1A2 (eg, tobacco, omeprazole) and CYP 2C8 (eg, rifampin) on the systemic exposure of eltrombopag has not been established in clinical studies. Monitor patients for signs and symptoms of excessive eltrombopag exposure when eltrombopag is administered concomitantly with these drugs).
No products indexed under this heading.

Insulin, Human (rDNA origin) (*In vitro* studies demonstrate that CYP1A2 and CYP2C8 are involved in the oxidative metabolism of eltrombopag. The significance of co-administration of eltrombopag with inducers of CYP 1A2 (eg, tobacco, omeprazole) and CYP 2C8 (eg, rifampin) on the systemic exposure of eltrombopag has not been established in clinical studies. Monitor patients for signs and symptoms of excessive eltrombopag exposure when eltrombopag is administered concomitantly with these drugs). Products include:
Exubera 2717

Insulin, Human NPH (*In vitro* studies demonstrate that CYP1A2 and CYP2C8 are involved in the oxidative metabolism of eltrombopag. The significance of co-administration of eltrombopag with inducers of CYP 1A2 (eg, tobacco, omeprazole) and CYP 2C8 (eg, rifampin) on the systemic exposure of eltrombopag has not been established in clinical studies. Monitor patients for signs and symptoms of excessive eltrombopag exposure when eltrombopag is administered concomitantly with these drugs). Products include:
Humulin N Vial 1934

Insulin, Human Regular (*In vitro* studies demonstrate that CYP1A2 and CYP2C8 are involved in the oxidative metabolism of eltrombopag. The significance of co-administration of eltrombopag with inducers of CYP 1A2 (eg, tobacco, omeprazole) and CYP 2C8 (eg, rifampin) on the systemic exposure of eltrombopag has not been established in clinical studies. Monitor patients for signs and symptoms of excessive eltrombopag exposure when eltrombopag is administered concomitantly with these drugs). Products include:
Humulin R 1937
Humulin R (U-500) 1939

Insulin, Human Regular and Human NPH Mixture (*In vitro* studies demonstrate that CYP1A2 and CYP2C8 are involved in the oxidative metabolism of eltrombopag. The significance of co-administration of eltrombopag with

IMPORTANT NOTE: Always consult each drug listing in the patient's regimen for possible interactions.

inducers of CYP 1A2 (eg, tobacco, omeprazole) and CYP 2C8 (eg, rifampin) on the systemic exposure of eltrombopag has not been established in clinical studies. Monitor patients for signs and symptoms of excessive eltrombopag exposure when eltrombopag is administered concomitantly with these drugs). Products include:
Humulin 50/50 1930
Humulin 70/30 Vial 1931

Insulin, NPH (*In vitro* studies demonstrate that CYP1A2 and CYP2C8 are involved in the oxidative metabolism of eltrombopag. The significance of co-administration of eltrombopag with inducers of CYP 1A2 (eg, tobacco, omeprazole) and CYP 2C8 (eg, rifampin) on the systemic exposure of eltrombopag has not been established in clinical studies. Monitor patients for signs and symptoms of excessive eltrombopag exposure when eltrombopag is administered concomitantly with these drugs).
No products indexed under this heading.

Insulin, Regular (*In vitro* studies demonstrate that CYP1A2 and CYP2C8 are involved in the oxidative metabolism of eltrombopag. The significance of co-administration of eltrombopag with inducers of CYP 1A2 (eg, tobacco, omeprazole) and CYP 2C8 (eg, rifampin) on the systemic exposure of eltrombopag has not been established in clinical studies. Monitor patients for signs and symptoms of excessive eltrombopag exposure when eltrombopag is administered concomitantly with these drugs).
No products indexed under this heading.

Insulin, Regular and NPH mixture (*In vitro* studies demonstrate that CYP1A2 and CYP2C8 are involved in the oxidative metabolism of eltrombopag. The significance of co-administration of eltrombopag with inducers of CYP 1A2 (eg, tobacco, omeprazole) and CYP 2C8 (eg, rifampin) on the systemic exposure of eltrombopag has not been established in clinical studies. Monitor patients for signs and symptoms of excessive eltrombopag exposure when eltrombopag is administered concomitantly with these drugs).
No products indexed under this heading.

Insulin, Zinc Crystals (*In vitro* studies demonstrate that CYP1A2 and CYP2C8 are involved in the oxidative metabolism of eltrombopag. The significance of co-administration of eltrombopag with inducers of CYP 1A2 (eg, tobacco, omeprazole) and CYP 2C8 (eg, rifampin) on the systemic exposure of eltrombopag has not been established in clinical studies. Monitor patients for signs and symptoms of excessive eltrombopag exposure when eltrombopag is administered concomitantly with these drugs).
No products indexed under this heading.

Insulin, Zinc Suspension (*In vitro* studies demonstrate that CYP1A2 and CYP2C8 are involved in the oxidative metabolism of eltrombopag. The significance of co-administration of eltrombopag with inducers of CYP 1A2 (eg, tobacco, omeprazole) and CYP 2C8 (eg, rifampin) on the systemic exposure of eltrombopag has not been established in clinical studies. Monitor patients for signs and symptoms of excessive eltrombopag exposure when eltrombopag is administered concomitantly with these drugs).
No products indexed under this heading.

Insulin Aspart (*In vitro* studies demonstrate that CYP1A2 and CYP2C8 are involved in the oxidative metabolism of eltrombopag. The significance of co-administration of eltrombopag with inducers of CYP 1A2 (eg, tobacco, omeprazole) and CYP 2C8 (eg, rifampin) on the systemic exposure of eltrombopag has not been established in clinical studies. Monitor patients for signs and symptoms of excessive eltrombopag exposure when eltrombopag is administered concomitantly with these drugs).
No products indexed under this heading.

Insulin Aspart, Human (*In vitro* studies demonstrate that CYP1A2 and CYP2C8 are involved in the oxidative metabolism of eltrombopag. The significance of co-administration of eltrombopag with inducers of CYP 1A2 (eg, tobacco, omeprazole) and CYP 2C8 (eg, rifampin) on the systemic exposure of eltrombopag has not been established in clinical studies. Monitor patients for signs and symptoms of excessive eltrombopag exposure when eltrombopag is administered concomitantly with these drugs). Products include:
NovoLog Mix 70/30 2581

Insulin Aspart, Human Regular (*In vitro* studies demonstrate that CYP1A2 and CYP2C8 are involved in the oxidative metabolism of eltrombopag. The significance of co-administration of eltrombopag with inducers of CYP 1A2 (eg, tobacco, omeprazole) and CYP 2C8 (eg, rifampin) on the systemic exposure of eltrombopag has not been established in clinical studies. Monitor patients for signs and symptoms of excessive eltrombopag exposure when eltrombopag is administered concomitantly with these drugs). Products include:
NovoLog 2575

Insulin Aspart Protamine, Human (*In vitro* studies demonstrate that CYP1A2 and CYP2C8 are involved in the oxidative metabolism of eltrombopag. The significance of co-administration of eltrombopag with inducers of CYP 1A2 (eg, tobacco, omeprazole) and CYP 2C8 (eg, rifampin) on the systemic exposure of eltrombopag has not been established in clinical studies. Monitor patients for signs and symptoms of excessive eltrombopag exposure when eltrombopag is administered concomitantly with these drugs). Products include:
NovoLog Mix 70/30 2581

Insulin Detemir (rDNA Origin) (*In vitro* studies demonstrate that CYP1A2 and CYP2C8 are involved in the oxidative metabolism of eltrombopag. The significance of co-administration of eltrombopag with inducers of CYP 1A2 (eg, tobacco, omeprazole) and CYP 2C8 (eg, rifampin) on the systemic exposure of eltrombopag has not been established in clinical studies. Monitor patients for signs and symptoms of excessive eltrombopag exposure when eltrombopag is administered concomitantly with these drugs). Products include:
Levemir 2566

Insulin Glargine (*In vitro* studies demonstrate that CYP1A2 and CYP2C8 are involved in the oxidative metabolism of eltrombopag. The significance of co-administration of eltrombopag with inducers of CYP 1A2 (eg, tobacco, omeprazole) and CYP 2C8 (eg, rifampin) on the systemic exposure of eltrombopag has not been established in clinical studies. Monitor patients for signs and symptoms of excessive eltrombopag exposure when eltrombopag is administered concomitantly with these drugs). Products include:
Lantus 2996

Insulin Glulisine (*In vitro* studies demonstrate that CYP1A2 and CYP2C8 are involved in the oxidative metabolism of eltrombopag. The significance of co-administration of eltrombopag with inducers of CYP 1A2 (eg, tobacco, omeprazole) and CYP 2C8 (eg, rifampin) on the systemic exposure of eltrombopag has not been established in clinical studies. Monitor patients for signs and symptoms of excessive eltrombopag exposure when eltrombopag is administered concomitantly with these drugs). Products include:
Apidra 2937
Apidra SoloStar 2937

Insulin Lispro, Human (*In vitro* studies demonstrate that CYP1A2 and CYP2C8 are involved in the oxidative metabolism of eltrombopag. The significance of co-administration of eltrombopag with inducers of CYP 1A2 (eg, tobacco, omeprazole) and CYP 2C8 (eg, rifampin) on the systemic exposure of eltrombopag has not been established in clinical studies. Monitor patients for signs and symptoms of excessive eltrombopag exposure when eltrombopag is administered concomitantly with these drugs). Products include:
Humalog 1910
Humalog Mix 1914
Humalog Mix75/25 1917

Insulin Lispro Protamine, Human (*In vitro* studies demonstrate that CYP1A2 and CYP2C8 are involved in the oxidative metabolism of eltrombopag. The significance of co-administration of eltrombopag with inducers of CYP 1A2 (eg, tobacco, omeprazole) and CYP 2C8 (eg, rifampin) on the systemic exposure of eltrombopag has not been established in clinical studies. Monitor patients for signs and symptoms of excessive eltrombopag exposure when eltrombopag is administered concomitantly with these drugs). Products include:
Humalog Mix 1914
Humalog Mix75/25 1917

Irinotecan Hydrochloride (*In vitro* studies demonstrate that eltrombopag is an inhibitor of UGT1A1, UGT1A3, UGT1A4, UGT1A6, UGT1A9, UGT2B7, and UGT2B15, enzymes involved in the metabolism of multiple drugs, such as acetaminophen, narcotics, and nonsteroidal anti-inflammatory drugs (NSAIDs). The significance of this inhibition on the potential for increased systemic exposure of drugs that are substrates of these UGTs following co-administration with eltrombopag has not been evaluated in clinical studies. Monitor patients closely for signs or symptoms of excessive exposure to these drugs when concomitantly administered with eltrombopag).
No products indexed under this heading.

Iron (Eltrombopag chelates polyvalent cations (such as iron, calcium, aluminum, magnesium, selenium, and zinc) in foods, mineral supplements, and antacids. In a clinical study, administration of eltrombopag with a polyvalent cation-containing antacid (1,524 mg aluminum hydroxide, 1,425 mg magnesium carbonate, and sodium alginate) decreased plasma eltrombopag systemic exposure by approximately 70%. Eltrombopag must not be taken within 4 hours of any medications or products containing polyvalent cations such as antacids, dairy products, and mineral supplements to avoid significant reduction in eltrombopag absorption due to chelation).
No products indexed under this heading.

Iron, Peptonized (Eltrombopag chelates polyvalent cations (such as iron, calcium, aluminum, magnesium, selenium, and zinc) in foods, mineral supplements, and antacids. In a clinical study, administration of eltrombopag with a polyvalent cation-containing antacid (1,524 mg aluminum hydroxide, 1,425 mg magnesium carbonate, and sodium alginate) decreased plasma eltrombopag systemic exposure by approximately 70%. Eltrombopag must not be taken within 4 hours of any medications or products containing polyvalent cations such as antacids, dairy products, and mineral supplements to avoid significant reduction in eltrombopag absorption due to chelation).
No products indexed under this heading.

Iron & Ammonium Citrate (Eltrombopag chelates polyvalent cations (such as iron, calcium, aluminum, magnesium, selenium, and zinc) in foods, mineral supplements, and antacids. In a clinical study, administration of eltrombopag with a polyvalent cation-containing antacid (1,524 mg aluminum hydroxide, 1,425 mg magnesium carbonate, and sodium alginate) decreased plasma eltrombopag systemic exposure by approximately 70%. Eltrombopag must not be taken within 4 hours of any medications or products containing polyvalent cations such as antacids, dairy products, and mineral supplements to avoid significant reduction in eltrombopag absorption due to chelation).
No products indexed under this heading.

Iron Cacodylate (Eltrombopag chelates polyvalent cations (such as iron, calcium, aluminum, magnesium, selenium, and zinc) in foods, mineral supplements, and antacids. In a clinical study, administration of eltrombopag with a polyvalent cation-containing antacid (1,524 mg aluminum hydroxide, 1,425 mg magnesium carbonate, and sodium alginate) decreased plasma eltrombopag systemic exposure by approximately 70%. Eltrombopag must not be taken within 4 hours of any medications or products containing polyvalent cations such as antacids, dairy products, and mineral supplements to avoid significant reduction in eltrombopag absorption due to chelation).
No products indexed under this heading.

Iron Carbonyl (Eltrombopag chelates polyvalent cations (such as iron, calcium, aluminum, magnesium, selenium, and zinc) in foods, mineral supplements, and antacids. In a clinical study, administration of eltrombopag with a polyvalent cation-containing antacid (1,524 mg aluminum hydroxide, 1,425 mg magnesium carbonate, and sodium alginate) decreased plasma eltrombopag systemic exposure by approximately 70%. Eltrombopag must not be taken within 4 hours of any medications or products containing polyvalent cations such as antacids, dairy products, and mineral supplements to avoid significant reduction in eltrombopag absorption due to chelation). Products include:
CitraNatal 90 DHA Capsules 2332
CitraNatal Assure 2332
CitraNatal Harmony 2332
CitraNatal Rx 2332
Ferralet 2333

Iron Dextran (Eltrombopag chelates polyvalent cations (such as iron, calcium, aluminum, magnesium, selenium, and zinc) in foods, mineral supplements, and antacids. In a clinical study, administration of eltrombopag with a polyvalent cation-containing antacid (1,524 mg aluminum hydroxide, 1,425 mg magnesium carbonate, and sodium alginate) decreased plasma eltrombopag systemic exposure by approximately 70%. Eltrombopag must not be taken within 4 hours of any medications or products containing polyvalent cations such as antacids, dairy products, and mineral supplements to avoid significant reduction in eltrombopag absorption due to chelation).
No products indexed under this heading.

Iron Polysaccharide Complex (Eltrombopag chelates polyvalent cations (such as iron, calcium, aluminum, magnesium, selenium, and zinc) in foods, mineral supplements, and antacids. In a clinical study, administration of eltrombopag with a polyvalent cation-containing antacid (1,524 mg aluminum hydroxide, 1,425 mg magnesium carbonate, and sodium alginate) decreased plasma eltrombopag systemic exposure by approximately 70%. Eltrombopag must not be taken within 4 hours of any medications or products containing polyvalent cations such as antacids, dairy products, and mineral supplements to avoid significant reduction in eltrombopag absorption due to chelation).

No products indexed under this heading.

Iron Sucrose (Eltrombopag chelates polyvalent cations (such as iron, calcium, aluminum, magnesium, selenium, and zinc) in foods, mineral supplements, and antacids. In a clinical study, administration of eltrombopag with a polyvalent cation-containing antacid (1,524 mg aluminum hydroxide, 1,425 mg magnesium carbonate, and sodium alginate) decreased plasma eltrombopag systemic exposure by approximately 70%. Eltrombopag must not be taken within 4 hours of any medications or products containing polyvalent cations such as antacids, dairy products, and mineral supplements to avoid significant reduction in eltrombopag absorption due to chelation).

No products indexed under this heading.

Iron Supplements (Eltrombopag chelates polyvalent cations (such as iron, calcium, aluminum, magnesium, selenium, and zinc) in foods, mineral supplements, and antacids. In a clinical study, administration of eltrombopag with a polyvalent cation-containing antacid (1,524 mg aluminum hydroxide, 1,425 mg magnesium carbonate, and sodium alginate) decreased plasma eltrombopag systemic exposure by approximately 70%. Eltrombopag must not be taken within 4 hours of any medications or products containing polyvalent cations such as antacids, dairy products, and mineral supplements to avoid significant reduction in eltrombopag absorption due to chelation).

No products indexed under this heading.

Isoniazid (In vitro studies demonstrate that CYP1A2 and CYP2C8 are involved in the oxidative metabolism of eltrombopag. The significance of co-administration of eltrombopag with moderate or strong inhibitors of CYP 1A2 (eg, ciprofloxacin, fluvoxamine) and CYP 2C8 (eg, gemfibrozil, trimethoprim) on the systemic exposure of eltrombopag has not been established in clinical studies. Monitor patients for signs and symptoms of excessive eltrombopag exposure when eltrombopag is administered concomitantly with these moderate or strong inhibitors of CYP1A2 or CYP2C8).

No products indexed under this heading.

Isotretinoin (In vitro studies demonstrate that CYP1A2 and CYP2C8 are involved in the oxidative metabolism of eltrombopag. The significance of co-administration of eltrombopag with other substrates of these CYP enzymes on the systemic exposure of eltrombopag has not been established in clinical studies. Monitor patients for signs and symptoms of excessive eltrombopag exposure when eltrombopag is administered concomitantly with these drugs). Products include:

Accutane 2832

Ketoconazole (In vitro studies demonstrate that CYP1A2 and CYP2C8 are involved in the oxidative metabolism of eltrombopag. The significance of co-

administration of eltrombopag with moderate or strong inhibitors of CYP 1A2 (eg, ciprofloxacin, fluvoxamine) and CYP 2C8 (eg, gemfibrozil, trimethoprim) on the systemic exposure of eltrombopag has not been established in clinical studies. Monitor patients for signs and symptoms of excessive eltrombopag exposure when eltrombopag is administered concomitantly with these moderate or strong inhibitors of CYP1A2 or CYP2C8). Products include:

Extina 3319
Xolegel 3337

Ketoprofen (Studies demonstrate that eltrombopag is an inhibitor of UGT1A1, UGT1A3, UGT1A4, UGT1A6, UGT1A9, UGT2B7, and UGT2B15, enzymes involved in the metabolism of multiple drugs, such as acetaminophen, narcotics, and nonsteroidal anti-inflammatory drugs (NSAIDs). Monitor patients closely for signs of symptoms of excessive exposure to these drugs when concomitantly administered with eltrombopag).

No products indexed under this heading.

Ketorolac Tromethamine (Studies demonstrate that eltrombopag is an inhibitor of UGT1A1, UGT1A3, UGT1A4, UGT1A6, UGT1A9, UGT2B7, and UGT2B15, enzymes involved in the metabolism of multiple drugs, such as acetaminophen, narcotics, and nonsteroidal anti-inflammatory drugs (NSAIDs). Monitor patients closely for signs of symptoms of excessive exposure to these drugs when concomitantly administered with eltrombopag). Products include:

Acuvail .... ⊙ 209

Lansoprazole (In vitro studies demonstrate that CYP1A2 and CYP2C8 are involved in the oxidative metabolism of eltrombopag. The significance of co-administration of eltrombopag with inducers of CYP 1A2 (eg, tobacco, omeprazole) and CYP 2C8 (eg, rifampin) on the systemic exposure of eltrombopag has not been established in clinical studies. Monitor patients for signs and symptoms of excessive eltrombopag exposure when eltrombopag is administered concomitantly with these drugs).

No products indexed under this heading.

Levobupivacaine Hydrochloride (In vitro studies demonstrate that CYP1A2 and CYP2C8 are involved in the oxidative metabolism of eltrombopag. The significance of co-administration of eltrombopag with other substrates of these CYP enzymes on the systemic exposure of eltrombopag has not been established in clinical studies. Monitor patients for signs and symptoms of excessive eltrombopag exposure when eltrombopag is administered concomitantly with these drugs).

No products indexed under this heading.

Levofloxacin (In vitro studies demonstrate that CYP1A2 and CYP2C8 are involved in the oxidative metabolism of eltrombopag. The significance of co-administration of eltrombopag with moderate or strong inhibitors of CYP 1A2 (eg, ciprofloxacin, fluvoxamine) and CYP 2C8 (eg, gemfibrozil, trimethoprim) on the systemic exposure of eltrombopag has not been established in clinical studies. Monitor patients for signs and symptoms of excessive eltrombopag exposure when eltrombopag is administered concomitantly with these moderate or strong inhibitors of CYP1A2 or CYP2C8). Products include:

Iquix 3492
Levaquin 2629
Levaquin in 5% Dextrose 2629
Quixin 3493

Levonorgestrel (In vitro studies demonstrate that CYP1A2 and CYP2C8 are involved in the oxidative metabolism of eltrombopag. The significance of co-

administration of eltrombopag with moderate or strong inhibitors of CYP 1A2 (eg, ciprofloxacin, fluvoxamine) and CYP 2C8 (eg, gemfibrozil, trimethoprim) on the systemic exposure of eltrombopag has not been established in clinical studies. Monitor patients for signs and symptoms of excessive eltrombopag exposure when eltrombopag is administered concomitantly with these moderate or strong inhibitors of CYP1A2 or CYP2C8). Products include:

Climara Pro 847
LoSeasonique 3407
Lybrel 3514
Mirena 854
Plan B 3416
Seasonique 3418

Levorphanol Tartrate (Studies demonstrate that eltrombopag is an inhibitor of UGT1A1, UGT1A3, UGT1A4, UGT1A6, UGT1A9, UGT2B7, and UGT2B15, enzymes involved in the metabolism of multiple drugs, such as acetaminophen, narcotics, and nonsteroidal anti-inflammatory drugs (NSAIDs). Monitor patients closely for signs of symptoms of excessive exposure to these drugs when concomitantly administered with eltrombopag).

No products indexed under this heading.

Lomefloxacin Hydrochloride (In vitro studies demonstrate that CYP1A2 and CYP2C8 are involved in the oxidative metabolism of eltrombopag. The significance of co-administration of eltrombopag with moderate or strong inhibitors of CYP 1A2 (eg, ciprofloxacin, fluvoxamine) and CYP 2C8 (eg, gemfibrozil, trimethoprim) on the systemic exposure of eltrombopag has not been established in clinical studies. Monitor patients for signs and symptoms of excessive eltrombopag exposure when eltrombopag is administered concomitantly with these moderate or strong inhibitors of CYP1A2 or CYP2C8).

No products indexed under this heading.

Magaldrate (Eltrombopag chelates polyvalent cations (such as iron, calcium, aluminum, magnesium, selenium, and zinc) in foods, mineral supplements, and antacids. In a clinical study, administration of eltrombopag with a polyvalent cation-containing antacid (1,524 mg aluminum hydroxide, 1,425 mg magnesium carbonate, and sodium alginate) decreased plasma eltrombopag systemic exposure by approximately 70%. Eltrombopag must not be taken within 4 hours of any medications or products containing polyvalent cations such as antacids, dairy products, and mineral supplements to avoid significant reduction in eltrombopag absorption due to chelation).

No products indexed under this heading.

Magnesium (Eltrombopag chelates polyvalent cations (such as iron, calcium, aluminum, magnesium, selenium, and zinc) in foods, mineral supplements, and antacids. In a clinical study, administration of eltrombopag with a polyvalent cation-containing antacid (1,524 mg aluminum hydroxide, 1,425 mg magnesium carbonate, and sodium alginate) decreased plasma eltrombopag systemic exposure by approximately 70%. Eltrombopag must not be taken within 4 hours of any medications or products containing polyvalent cations such as antacids, dairy products, and mineral supplements to avoid significant reduction in eltrombopag absorption due to chelation). Products include:

BoneMate Plus 3454
Cardio Basics 3455
Chelated Mineral 3476

Magnesium Aluminum Silicate (Eltrombopag chelates polyvalent cations (such as iron, calcium, aluminum, magnesium, selenium, and zinc) in

foods, mineral supplements, and antacids. In a clinical study, administration of eltrombopag with a polyvalent cation-containing antacid (1,524 mg aluminum hydroxide, 1,425 mg magnesium carbonate, and sodium alginate) decreased plasma eltrombopag systemic exposure by approximately 70%. Eltrombopag must not be taken within 4 hours of any medications or products containing polyvalent cations such as antacids, dairy products, and mineral supplements to avoid significant reduction in eltrombopag absorption due to chelation).

No products indexed under this heading.

Magnesium Carbonate (Eltrombopag chelates polyvalent cations (such as iron, calcium, aluminum, magnesium, selenium, and zinc) in foods, mineral supplements, and antacids. In a clinical study, administration of eltrombopag with a polyvalent cation-containing antacid (1,524 mg aluminum hydroxide, 1,425 mg magnesium carbonate, and sodium alginate) decreased plasma eltrombopag systemic exposure by approximately 70%. Eltrombopag must not be taken within 4 hours of any medications or products containing polyvalent cations such as antacids, dairy products, and mineral supplements to avoid significant reduction in eltrombopag absorption due to chelation).

No products indexed under this heading.

Magnesium Chloride (Eltrombopag chelates polyvalent cations (such as iron, calcium, aluminum, magnesium, selenium, and zinc) in foods, mineral supplements, and antacids. In a clinical study, administration of eltrombopag with a polyvalent cation-containing antacid (1,524 mg aluminum hydroxide, 1,425 mg magnesium carbonate, and sodium alginate) decreased plasma eltrombopag systemic exposure by approximately 70%. Eltrombopag must not be taken within 4 hours of any medications or products containing polyvalent cations such as antacids, dairy products, and mineral supplements to avoid significant reduction in eltrombopag absorption due to chelation).

No products indexed under this heading.

Magnesium Citrate (Eltrombopag chelates polyvalent cations (such as iron, calcium, aluminum, magnesium, selenium, and zinc) in foods, mineral supplements, and antacids. In a clinical study, administration of eltrombopag with a polyvalent cation-containing antacid (1,524 mg aluminum hydroxide, 1,425 mg magnesium carbonate, and sodium alginate) decreased plasma eltrombopag systemic exposure by approximately 70%. Eltrombopag must not be taken within 4 hours of any medications or products containing polyvalent cations such as antacids, dairy products, and mineral supplements to avoid significant reduction in eltrombopag absorption due to chelation). Products include:

Chelated Mineral 3476

Magnesium Gluconate (Eltrombopag chelates polyvalent cations, such as iron, calcium, aluminum, magnesium, selenium, and zinc in foods, mineral supplements, and atacids. Eltrombopag must not be taken within four hours of any medications or products containing polyvalent cations, such as antacids, dairy products, and mineral supplements to avoid significant reduction in eltrombopag absorption due chelation).

No products indexed under this heading.

Magnesium Hydroxide (Eltrombopag chelates polyvalent cations (such as iron, calcium, aluminum, magnesium, selenium, and zinc) in foods, mineral supplements, and antacids. In a

clinical study, administration of eltrombopag with a polyvalent cation-containing antacid (1,524 mg aluminum hydroxide, 1,425 mg magnesium carbonate, and sodium alginate) decreased plasma eltrombopag systemic exposure by approximately 70%. Eltrombopag must not be taken within 4 hours of any medications or products containing polyvalent cations such as antacids, dairy products, and mineral supplements to avoid significant reduction in eltrombopag absorption due to chelation). Products include:

Fleet Pedia-Lax Chewable Tablets 1144
Pepcid Complete 1822

Magnesium Lactate (Eltrombopag chelates polyvalent cations (such as iron, calcium, aluminum, magnesium, selenium, and zinc) in foods, mineral supplements, and antacids. In a clinical study, administration of eltrombopag with a polyvalent cation-containing antacid (1,524 mg aluminum hydroxide, 1,425 mg magnesium carbonate, and sodium alginate) decreased plasma eltrombopag systemic exposure by approximately 70%. Eltrombopag must not be taken within 4 hours of any medications or products containing polyvalent cations such as antacids, dairy products, and mineral supplements to avoid significant reduction in eltrombopag absorption due to chelation).
No products indexed under this heading.

Magnesium Oxide (Eltrombopag chelates polyvalent cations, such as iron, calcium, aluminum, magnesium, selenium, and zinc in foods, mineral supplements, and atacids. Eltrombopag must not be taken within four hours of any medications or products containing polyvalent cations, such as antacids, dairy products, and mineral supplements to avoid significant reduction in eltrombopag absorption due to chelation). Products include:

Beelith 873

Magnesium Salicylate (Eltrombopag chelates polyvalent cations (such as iron, calcium, aluminum, magnesium, selenium, and zinc) in foods, mineral supplements, and antacids. In a clinical study, administration of eltrombopag with a polyvalent cation-containing antacid (1,524 mg aluminum hydroxide, 1,425 mg magnesium carbonate, and sodium alginate) decreased plasma eltrombopag systemic exposure by approximately 70%. Eltrombopag must not be taken within 4 hours of any medications or products containing polyvalent cations such as antacids, dairy products, and mineral supplements to avoid significant reduction in eltrombopag absorption due to chelation).
No products indexed under this heading.

Magnesium Salicylate Tetrahydrate (Eltrombopag chelates polyvalent cations (such as iron, calcium, aluminum, magnesium, selenium, and zinc) in foods, mineral supplements, and antacids. In a clinical study, administration of eltrombopag with a polyvalent cation-containing antacid (1,524 mg aluminum hydroxide, 1,425 mg magnesium carbonate, and sodium alginate) decreased plasma eltrombopag systemic exposure by approximately 70%. Eltrombopag must not be taken within 4 hours of any medications or products containing polyvalent cations such as antacids, dairy products, and mineral supplements to avoid significant reduction in eltrombopag absorption due to chelation).
No products indexed under this heading.

Magnesium Salts (Eltrombopag chelates polyvalent cations (such as iron, calcium, aluminum, magnesium, selenium, and zinc) in foods, mineral supplements, and antacids. In a clinical study, administration of eltrombopag with a

polyvalent cation-containing antacid (1,524 mg aluminum hydroxide, 1,425 mg magnesium carbonate, and sodium alginate) decreased plasma eltrombopag systemic exposure by approximately 70%. Eltrombopag must not be taken within 4 hours of any medications or products containing polyvalent cations such as antacids, dairy products, and mineral supplements to avoid significant reduction in eltrombopag absorption due to chelation).
No products indexed under this heading.

Magnesium Sulfate (Eltrombopag chelates polyvalent cations (such as iron, calcium, aluminum, magnesium, selenium, and zinc) in foods, mineral supplements, and antacids. In a clinical study, administration of eltrombopag with a polyvalent cation-containing antacid (1,524 mg aluminum hydroxide, 1,425 mg magnesium carbonate, and sodium alginate) decreased plasma eltrombopag systemic exposure by approximately 70%. Eltrombopag must not be taken within 4 hours of any medications or products containing polyvalent cations such as antacids, dairy products, and mineral supplements to avoid significant reduction in eltrombopag absorption due to chelation).
No products indexed under this heading.

Magnesium Trisilicate (Eltrombopag chelates polyvalent cations (such as iron, calcium, aluminum, magnesium, selenium, and zinc) in foods, mineral supplements, and antacids. In a clinical study, administration of eltrombopag with a polyvalent cation-containing antacid (1,524 mg aluminum hydroxide, 1,425 mg magnesium carbonate, and sodium alginate) decreased plasma eltrombopag systemic exposure by approximately 70%. Eltrombopag must not be taken within 4 hours of any medications or products containing polyvalent cations such as antacids, dairy products, and mineral supplements to avoid significant reduction in eltrombopag absorption due to chelation).
No products indexed under this heading.

Maprotiline Hydrochloride (In vitro studies demonstrate that CYP1A2 and CYP2C8 are involved in the oxidative metabolism of eltrombopag. The significance of co-administration of eltrombopag with other substrates of these CYP enzymes on the systemic exposure of eltrombopag has not been established in clinical studies. Monitor patients for signs and symptoms of excessive eltrombopag exposure when eltrombopag is administered concomitantly with these drugs).
No products indexed under this heading.

Meclofenamate Sodium (Studies demonstrate that eltrombopag is an inhibitor of UGT1A1, UGT1A3, UGT1A4, UGT1A6, UGT1A9, UGT2B7, and UGT2B15, enzymes involved in the metabolism of multiple drugs, such as acetaminophen, narcotics, and nonsteroidal anti-inflammatory drugs (NSAIDs). Monitor patients closely for signs of symptoms of excessive exposure to these drugs when concomitantly administered with eltrombopag).
No products indexed under this heading.

Mefenamic Acid (Studies demonstrate that eltrombopag is an inhibitor of UGT1A1, UGT1A3, UGT1A4, UGT1A6, UGT1A9, UGT2B7, and UGT2B15, enzymes involved in the metabolism of multiple drugs, such as acetaminophen, narcotics, and nonsteroidal anti-inflammatory drugs (NSAIDs). Monitor patients closely for signs of symptoms of excessive exposure to these drugs when concomitantly administered with eltrombopag).
No products indexed under this heading.

Meloxicam (Studies demonstrate that eltrombopag is an inhibitor of UGT1A1,

UGT1A3, UGT1A4, UGT1A6, UGT1A9, UGT2B7, and UGT2B15, enzymes involved in the metabolism of multiple drugs, such as acetaminophen, narcotics, and nonsteroidal anti-inflammatory drugs (NSAIDs). Monitor patients closely for signs of symptoms of excessive exposure to these drugs when concomitantly administered with eltrombopag).
No products indexed under this heading.

Meperidine Hydrochloride (Studies demonstrate that eltrombopag is an inhibitor of UGT1A1, UGT1A3, UGT1A4, UGT1A6, UGT1A9, UGT2B7, and UGT2B15, enzymes involved in the metabolism of multiple drugs, such as acetaminophen, narcotics, and nonsteroidal anti-inflammatory drugs (NSAIDs). Monitor patients closely for signs of symptoms of excessive exposure to these drugs when concomitantly administered with eltrombopag).
No products indexed under this heading.

Mephobarbital (In vitro studies demonstrate that CYP1A2 and CYP2C8 are involved in the oxidative metabolism of eltrombopag. The significance of co-administration of eltrombopag with other substrates of these CYP enzymes on the systemic exposure of eltrombopag has not been established in clinical studies. Monitor patients for signs and symptoms of excessive eltrombopag exposure when eltrombopag is administered concomitantly with these drugs).
No products indexed under this heading.

Mestranol (In vitro studies demonstrate that CYP1A2 and CYP2C8 are involved in the oxidative metabolism of eltrombopag. The significance of co-administration of eltrombopag with moderate or strong inhibitors of CYP 1A2 (eg, ciprofloxacin, fluvoxamine) and CYP 2C8 (eg, gemfibrozil, trimethoprim) on the systemic exposure of eltrombopag has not been established in clinical studies. Monitor patients for signs and symptoms of excessive eltrombopag exposure when eltrombopag is administered concomitantly with these moderate or strong inhibitors of CYP1A2 or CYP2C8).
No products indexed under this heading.

Methadone Hydrochloride (Studies demonstrate that eltrombopag is an inhibitor of UGT1A1, UGT1A3, UGT1A4, UGT1A6, UGT1A9, UGT2B7, and UGT2B15, enzymes involved in the metabolism of multiple drugs, such as acetaminophen, narcotics, and nonsteroidal anti-inflammatory drugs (NSAIDs). Monitor patients closely for signs of symptoms of excessive exposure to these drugs when concomitantly administered with eltrombopag).
No products indexed under this heading.

Methotrexate (In vitro studies demonstrate that eltrombopag is an inhibitor of the organic anion transporting polypeptide OATP1B1 and can increase the systemic exposure of other drugs that are substrates of this transporter (eg, benzylpenicillin, atorvastatin, fluvastatin, pravastatin, rosuvastatin, methotrexate, nateglinide, repaglinide, rifampin). Monitor patients closely for signs and symptoms of excessive exposure to the drugs that are substrates of OATP1B1 and consider reduction of the dose of these drugs).
No products indexed under this heading.

Methotrexate Sodium (In vitro studies demonstrate that eltrombopag is an inhibitor of the organic anion transporting polypeptide OATP1B1 and can increase the systemic exposure of other drugs that are substrates of this transporter (eg, benzylpenicillin, atorvastatin, fluvastatin, pravastatin, rosuvastatin, methotrexate, nateglinide, repaglinide, rifampin). Monitor patients closely for signs and symptoms of excessive exposure to the drugs that

are substrates of OATP1B1 and consider reduction of the dose of these drugs).
No products indexed under this heading.

Methoxsalen (In vitro studies demonstrate that CYP1A2 and CYP2C8 are involved in the oxidative metabolism of eltrombopag. The significance of co-administration of eltrombopag with moderate or strong inhibitors of CYP 1A2 (eg, ciprofloxacin, fluvoxamine) and CYP 2C8 (eg, gemfibrozil, trimethoprim) on the systemic exposure of eltrombopag has not been established in clinical studies. Monitor patients for signs and symptoms of excessive eltrombopag exposure when eltrombopag is administered concomitantly with these moderate or strong inhibitors of CYP1A2 or CYP2C8).
No products indexed under this heading.

Mexiletine Hydrochloride (In vitro studies demonstrate that CYP1A2 and CYP2C8 are involved in the oxidative metabolism of eltrombopag. The significance of co-administration of eltrombopag with moderate or strong inhibitors of CYP 1A2 (eg, ciprofloxacin, fluvoxamine) and CYP 2C8 (eg, gemfibrozil, trimethoprim) on the systemic exposure of eltrombopag has not been established in clinical studies. Monitor patients for signs and symptoms of excessive eltrombopag exposure when eltrombopag is administered concomitantly with these moderate or strong inhibitors of CYP1A2 or CYP2C8).
No products indexed under this heading.

Mibefradil Dihydrochloride (In vitro studies demonstrate that CYP1A2 and CYP2C8 are involved in the oxidative metabolism of eltrombopag. The significance of co-administration of eltrombopag with moderate or strong inhibitors of CYP 1A2 (eg, ciprofloxacin, fluvoxamine) and CYP 2C8 (eg, gemfibrozil, trimethoprim) on the systemic exposure of eltrombopag has not been established in clinical studies. Monitor patients for signs and symptoms of excessive eltrombopag exposure when eltrombopag is administered concomitantly with these moderate or strong inhibitors of CYP1A2 or CYP2C8).
No products indexed under this heading.

Mineral Supplements (Eltrombopag chelates polyvalent cations (such as iron, calcium, aluminum, magnesium, selenium, and zinc) in foods, mineral supplements, and antacids. In a clinical study, administration of eltrombopag with a polyvalent cation-containing antacid (1,524 mg aluminum hydroxide, 1,425 mg magnesium carbonate, and sodium alginate) decreased plasma eltrombopag systemic exposure by approximately 70%. Eltrombopag must not be taken within 4 hours of any medications or products containing polyvalent cations such as antacids, dairy products, and mineral supplements to avoid significant reduction in eltrombopag absorption due to chelation).
No products indexed under this heading.

Mirtazapine (In vitro studies demonstrate that CYP1A2 and CYP2C8 are involved in the oxidative metabolism of eltrombopag. The significance of co-administration of eltrombopag with other substrates of these CYP enzymes on the systemic exposure of eltrombopag has not been established in clinical studies. Monitor patients for signs and symptoms of excessive eltrombopag exposure when eltrombopag is administered concomitantly with these drugs). Products include:

Remeron Tablets ....,....... 3214
RemeronSolTab Tablets 3219

Morphine Sulfate (Studies demonstrate that eltrombopag is an inhibitor of UGT1A1, UGT1A3, UGT1A4, UGT1A6, UGT1A9, UGT2B7, and

UGT2B15, enzymes involved in the metabolism of multiple drugs, such as acetaminophen, narcotics, and nonsteroidal anti-inflammatory drugs (NSAIDs). Monitor patients closely for signs of symptoms of excessive exposure to these drugs when concomitantly administered with eltrombopag). Products include:

Avinza 1822
Embeda 1831
MS Contin 2803

Morphine Sulfate, Liposomal (Studies demonstrate that eltrombopag is an inhibitor of UGT1A1, UGT1A3, UGT1A4, UGT1A6, UGT1A9, UGT2B7, and UGT2B15, enzymes involved in the metabolism of multiple drugs, such as acetaminophen, narcotics, and nonsteroidal anti-inflammatory drugs (NSAIDs). Monitor patients closely for signs of symptoms of excessive exposure to these drugs when concomitantly administered with eltrombopag).
No products indexed under this heading.

Moxifloxacin Hydrochloride (*In vitro* studies demonstrate that CYP1A2 and CYP2C8 are involved in the oxidative metabolism of eltrombopag. The significance of co-administration of eltrombopag with moderate or strong inhibitors of CYP 1A2 (eg, ciprofloxacin, fluvoxamine) and CYP 2C8 (eg, gemfibrozil, trimethoprim) on the systemic exposure of eltrombopag has not been established in clinical studies. Monitor patients for signs and symptoms of excessive eltrombopag exposure when eltrombopag is administered concomitantly with these moderate or strong inhibitors of CYP1A2 or CYP2C8). Products include:

Avelox 3064
Vigamox 589

Nabumetone (Studies demonstrate that eltrombopag is an inhibitor of UGT1A1, UGT1A3, UGT1A4, UGT1A6, UGT1A9, UGT2B7, and UGT2B15, enzymes involved in the metabolism of multiple drugs, such as acetaminophen, narcotics, and nonsteroidal anti-inflammatory drugs (NSAIDs). Monitor patients closely for signs of symptoms of excessive exposure to these drugs when concomitantly administered with eltrombopag).
No products indexed under this heading.

Nafcillin Sodium (*In vitro* studies demonstrate that CYP1A2 and CYP2C8 are involved in the oxidative metabolism of eltrombopag. The significance of co-administration of eltrombopag with inducers of CYP 1A2 (eg, tobacco, omeprazole) and CYP 2C8 (eg, rifampin) on the systemic exposure of eltrombopag has not been established in clinical studies. Monitor patients for signs and symptoms of excessive eltrombopag exposure when eltrombopag is administered concomitantly with these drugs).
No products indexed under this heading.

Nalidixic Acid (*In vitro* studies demonstrate that CYP1A2 and CYP2C8 are involved in the oxidative metabolism of eltrombopag. The significance of co-administration of eltrombopag with moderate or strong inhibitors of CYP 1A2 (eg, ciprofloxacin, fluvoxamine) and CYP 2C8 (eg, gemfibrozil, trimethoprim) on the systemic exposure of eltrombopag has not been established in clinical studies. Monitor patients for signs and symptoms of excessive eltrombopag exposure when eltrombopag is administered concomitantly with these moderate or strong inhibitors of CYP1A2 or CYP2C8).
No products indexed under this heading.

Naproxen (Studies demonstrate that eltrombopag is an inhibitor of UGT1A1, UGT1A3, UGT1A4, UGT1A6, UGT1A9, UGT2B7, and UGT2B15, enzymes involved in the metabolism of multiple drugs, such as acetaminophen, narcotics, and nonsteroidal anti-inflammatory drugs (NSAIDs). Monitor patients closely for signs of symptoms of excessive exposure to these drugs when concomitantly administered with eltrombopag). Products include:

EC-Naprosyn 2850
Naprosyn 2850
Anaprox/Naprosyn 2850

Naproxen Sodium (Studies demonstrate that eltrombopag is an inhibitor of UGT1A1, UGT1A3, UGT1A4, UGT1A6, UGT1A9, UGT2B7, and UGT2B15, enzymes involved in the metabolism of multiple drugs, such as acetaminophen, narcotics, and nonsteroidal anti-inflammatory drugs (NSAIDs). Monitor patients closely for signs of symptoms of excessive exposure to these drugs when concomitantly administered with eltrombopag). Products include:

Anaprox 2850
Anaprox DS 2850
Treximet 1681

Nateglinide (*In vitro* studies demonstrate that eltrombopag is an inhibitor of the organic anion transporting polypeptide OATP1B1 and can increase the systemic exposure of other drugs that are substrates of this transporter (eg, benzylpenicillin, atorvastatin, fluvastatin, pravastatin, rosuvastatin, methotrexate, nateglinide, repaglinide, rifampin). Monitor patients closely for signs and symptoms of excessive exposure to the drugs that are substrates of OATP1B1 and consider reduction of the dose of these drugs).
No products indexed under this heading.

Nicardipine (*In vitro* studies demonstrate that CYP1A2 and CYP2C8 are involved in the oxidative metabolism of eltrombopag. The significance of co-administration of eltrombopag with moderate or strong inhibitors of CYP 1A2 (eg, ciprofloxacin, fluvoxamine) and CYP 2C8 (eg, gemfibrozil, trimethoprim) on the systemic exposure of eltrombopag has not been established in clinical studies. Monitor patients for signs and symptoms of excessive eltrombopag exposure when eltrombopag is administered concomitantly with these moderate or strong inhibitors of CYP1A2 or CYP2C8).
No products indexed under this heading.

Nicardipine Hydrochloride (*In vitro* studies demonstrate that CYP1A2 and CYP2C8 are involved in the oxidative metabolism of eltrombopag. The significance of co-administration of eltrombopag with moderate or strong inhibitors of CYP 1A2 (eg, ciprofloxacin, fluvoxamine) and CYP 2C8 (eg, gemfibrozil, trimethoprim) on the systemic exposure of eltrombopag has not been established in clinical studies. Monitor patients for signs and symptoms of excessive eltrombopag exposure when eltrombopag is administered concomitantly with these moderate or strong inhibitors of CYP1A2 or CYP2C8).
No products indexed under this heading.

Nicotine (*In vitro* studies demonstrate that CYP1A2 and CYP2C8 are involved in the oxidative metabolism of eltrombopag. The significance of co-administration of eltrombopag with inducers of CYP 1A2 (eg, tobacco, omeprazole) and CYP 2C8 (eg, rifampin) on the systemic exposure of eltrombopag has not been established in clinical studies. Monitor patients for signs and symptoms of excessive eltrombopag exposure when eltrombopag is administered concomitantly with these drugs).
No products indexed under this heading.

Nicotine Polacrilex (*In vitro* studies demonstrate that CYP1A2 and CYP2C8 are involved in the oxidative metabolism of eltrombopag. The significance of co-administration of eltrombopag with inducers of CYP 1A2 (eg, tobacco, omeprazole) and CYP 2C8 (eg, rifampin) on the systemic exposure of eltrombopag has not been established in clinical studies. Monitor patients for signs and symptoms of excessive eltrombopag exposure when eltrombopag is administered concomitantly with these drugs).
No products indexed under this heading.

Nicotine Salicylate (*In vitro* studies demonstrate that CYP1A2 and CYP2C8 are involved in the oxidative metabolism of eltrombopag. The significance of co-administration of eltrombopag with inducers of CYP 1A2 (eg, tobacco, omeprazole) and CYP 2C8 (eg, rifampin) on the systemic exposure of eltrombopag has not been established in clinical studies. Monitor patients for signs and symptoms of excessive eltrombopag exposure when eltrombopag is administered concomitantly with these drugs).
No products indexed under this heading.

Nicotine Sulfate (*In vitro* studies demonstrate that CYP1A2 and CYP2C8 are involved in the oxidative metabolism of eltrombopag. The significance of co-administration of eltrombopag with inducers of CYP 1A2 (eg, tobacco, omeprazole) and CYP 2C8 (eg, rifampin) on the systemic exposure of eltrombopag has not been established in clinical studies. Monitor patients for signs and symptoms of excessive eltrombopag exposure when eltrombopag is administered concomitantly with these drugs).
No products indexed under this heading.

Norethindrone (*In vitro* studies demonstrate that CYP1A2 and CYP2C8 are involved in the oxidative metabolism of eltrombopag. The significance of co-administration of eltrombopag with moderate or strong inhibitors of CYP 1A2 (eg, ciprofloxacin, fluvoxamine) and CYP 2C8 (eg, gemfibrozil, trimethoprim) on the systemic exposure of eltrombopag has not been established in clinical studies. Monitor patients for signs and symptoms of excessive eltrombopag exposure when eltrombopag is administered concomitantly with these moderate or strong inhibitors of CYP1A2 or CYP2C8). Products include:

Ortho Micronor 2660

Norethindrone Acetate (*In vitro* studies demonstrate that CYP1A2 and CYP2C8 are involved in the oxidative metabolism of eltrombopag. The significance of co-administration of eltrombopag with moderate or strong inhibitors of CYP 1A2 (eg, ciprofloxacin, fluvoxamine) and CYP 2C8 (eg, gemfibrozil, trimethoprim) on the systemic exposure of eltrombopag has not been established in clinical studies. Monitor patients for signs and symptoms of excessive eltrombopag exposure when eltrombopag is administered concomitantly with these moderate or strong inhibitors of CYP1A2 or CYP2C8). Products include:

Activella 2561

Norfloxacin (*In vitro* studies demonstrate that CYP1A2 and CYP2C8 are involved in the oxidative metabolism of eltrombopag. The significance of co-administration of eltrombopag with moderate or strong inhibitors of CYP 1A2 (eg, ciprofloxacin, fluvoxamine) and CYP 2C8 (eg, gemfibrozil, trimethoprim) on the systemic exposure of eltrombopag has not been established in clinical studies. Monitor patients for signs and symptoms of excessive eltrombopag exposure when eltrombopag is administered concomitantly with these moderate or strong inhibitors of CYP1A2 or CYP2C8). Products include:

Noroxin 2220

Norgestrel (*In vitro* studies demonstrate that CYP1A2 and CYP2C8 are involved in the oxidative metabolism of eltrombopag. The significance of co-administration of eltrombopag with moderate or strong inhibitors of CYP 1A2 (eg, ciprofloxacin, fluvoxamine) and CYP 2C8 (eg, gemfibrozil, trimethoprim) on the systemic exposure of eltrombopag has not been established in clinical studies. Monitor patients for signs and symptoms of excessive eltrombopag exposure when eltrombopag is administered concomitantly with these moderate or strong inhibitors of CYP1A2 or CYP2C8).
No products indexed under this heading.

Nortriptyline Hydrochloride (*In vitro* studies demonstrate that CYP1A2 and CYP2C8 are involved in the oxidative metabolism of eltrombopag. The significance of co-administration of eltrombopag with other substrates of these CYP enzymes on the systemic exposure of eltrombopag has not been established in clinical studies. Monitor patients for signs and symptoms of excessive eltrombopag exposure when eltrombopag is administered concomitantly with these drugs).
No products indexed under this heading.

Ofloxacin (*In vitro* studies demonstrate that CYP1A2 and CYP2C8 are involved in the oxidative metabolism of eltrombopag. The significance of co-administration of eltrombopag with moderate or strong inhibitors of CYP 1A2 (eg, ciprofloxacin, fluvoxamine) and CYP 2C8 (eg, gemfibrozil, trimethoprim) on the systemic exposure of eltrombopag has not been established in clinical studies. Monitor patients for signs and symptoms of excessive eltrombopag exposure when eltrombopag is administered concomitantly with these moderate or strong inhibitors of CYP1A2 or CYP2C8).
No products indexed under this heading.

Olanzapine (*In vitro* studies demonstrate that CYP1A2 and CYP2C8 are involved in the oxidative metabolism of eltrombopag. The significance of co-administration of eltrombopag with other substrates of these CYP enzymes on the systemic exposure of eltrombopag has not been established in clinical studies. Monitor patients for signs and symptoms of excessive eltrombopag exposure when eltrombopag is administered concomitantly with these drugs). Products include:

Symbyax 1965
Zyprexa 1984
Zyprexa IntraMuscular 1984
Zyprexa ZYDIS 1984

Omeprazole (*In vitro* studies demonstrate that CYP1A2 and CYP2C8 are involved in the oxidative metabolism of eltrombopag. The significance of co-administration of eltrombopag with moderate or strong inhibitors of CYP 1A2 (eg, ciprofloxacin, fluvoxamine) and CYP 2C8 (eg, gemfibrozil, trimethoprim) on the systemic exposure of eltrombopag has not been established in clinical studies. Monitor patients for signs and symptoms of excessive eltrombopag exposure when eltrombopag is administered concomitantly with these moderate or strong inhibitors of CYP1A2 or CYP2C8).
No products indexed under this heading.

Omeprazole Magnesium (*In vitro* studies demonstrate that CYP1A2 and CYP2C8 are involved in the oxidative metabolism of eltrombopag. The significance of co-administration of eltrombopag with moderate or strong inhibitors of CYP 1A2 (eg, ciprofloxacin, fluvoxamine) and CYP 2C8 (eg, gemfi-

brozil, trimethoprim) on the systemic exposure of eltrombopag has not been established in clinical studies. Monitor patients for signs and symptoms of excessive eltrombopag exposure when eltrombopag is administered concomitantly with these moderate or strong inhibitors of CYP1A2 or CYP2C8).
No products indexed under this heading.

Ondansetron (*In vitro* studies demonstrate that CYP1A2 and CYP2C8 are involved in the oxidative metabolism of eltrombopag. The significance of co-administration of eltrombopag with other substrates of these CYP enzymes on the systemic exposure of eltrombopag has not been established in clinical studies. Monitor patients for signs and symptoms of excessive eltrombopag exposure when eltrombopag is administered concomitantly with these drugs).
No products indexed under this heading.

Ondansetron Hydrochloride (*In vitro* studies demonstrate that CYP1A2 and CYP2C8 are involved in the oxidative metabolism of eltrombopag. The significance of co-administration of eltrombopag with other substrates of these CYP enzymes on the systemic exposure of eltrombopag has not been established in clinical studies. Monitor patients for signs and symptoms of excessive eltrombopag exposure when eltrombopag is administered concomitantly with these drugs). Products include:
Zofran Injection ... 1750
Zofran ... 1756
Zofran ODT ... 1756

Oxaprozin (Studies demonstrate that eltrombopag is an inhibitor of UGT1A1, UGT1A3, UGT1A4, UGT1A6, UGT1A9, UGT2B7, and UGT2B15, enzymes involved in the metabolism of multiple drugs, such as acetaminophen, narcotics, and nonsteroidal anti-inflammatory drugs (NSAIDs). Monitor patients closely for signs of symptoms of excessive exposure to these drugs when concomitantly administered with eltrombopag).
No products indexed under this heading.

Oxycodone Hydrochloride (Studies demonstrate that eltrombopag is an inhibitor of UGT1A1, UGT1A3, UGT1A4, UGT1A6, UGT1A9, UGT2B7, and UGT2B15, enzymes involved in the metabolism of multiple drugs, such as acetaminophen, narcotics, and nonsteroidal anti-inflammatory drugs (NSAIDs). Monitor patients closely for signs of symptoms of excessive exposure to these drugs when concomitantly administered with eltrombopag). Products include:
OxyContin ... 2807
Percocet ... 1121
Percodan ... 1124

Oxycodone Terephthalate (Studies demonstrate that eltrombopag is an inhibitor of UGT1A1, UGT1A3, UGT1A4, UGT1A6, UGT1A9, UGT2B7, and UGT2B15, enzymes involved in the metabolism of multiple drugs, such as acetaminophen, narcotics, and nonsteroidal anti-inflammatory drugs (NSAIDs). Monitor patients closely for signs of symptoms of excessive exposure to these drugs when concomitantly administered with eltrombopag).
No products indexed under this heading.

Oxymorphone Hydrochloride (Studies demonstrate that eltrombopag is an inhibitor of UGT1A1, UGT1A3, UGT1A4, UGT1A6, UGT1A9, UGT2B7, and UGT2B15, enzymes involved in the metabolism of multiple drugs, such as acetaminophen, narcotics, and nonsteroidal anti-inflammatory drugs (NSAIDs). Monitor patients closely for signs of symptoms of excessive exposure to these drugs when concomitantly administered with eltrombopag). Products include:
Opana ... 1110
Opana ER ... 1114

Paclitaxel (*In vitro* studies demonstrate that CYP1A2 and CYP2C8 are involved in the oxidative metabolism of eltrombopag. The significance of co-administration of eltrombopag with other substrates of these CYP enzymes on the systemic exposure of eltrombopag has not been established in clinical studies. Monitor patients for signs and symptoms of excessive eltrombopag exposure when eltrombopag is administered concomitantly with these drugs).
No products indexed under this heading.

Paroxetine (*In vitro* studies demonstrate that CYP1A2 and CYP2C8 are involved in the oxidative metabolism of eltrombopag. The significance of co-administration of eltrombopag with moderate or strong inhibitors of CYP 1A2 (eg, ciprofloxacin, fluvoxamine) and CYP 2C8 (eg, gemfibrozil, trimethoprim) on the systemic exposure of eltrombopag has not been established in clinical studies. Monitor patients for signs and symptoms of excessive eltrombopag exposure when eltrombopag is administered concomitantly with these moderate or strong inhibitors of CYP1A2 or CYP2C8).
No products indexed under this heading.

Paroxetine Hydrochloride (*In vitro* studies demonstrate that CYP1A2 and CYP2C8 are involved in the oxidative metabolism of eltrombopag. The significance of co-administration of eltrombopag with moderate or strong inhibitors of CYP 1A2 (eg, ciprofloxacin, fluvoxamine) and CYP 2C8 (eg, gemfibrozil, trimethoprim) on the systemic exposure of eltrombopag has not been established in clinical studies. Monitor patients for signs and symptoms of excessive eltrombopag exposure when eltrombopag is administered concomitantly with these moderate or strong inhibitors of CYP1A2 or CYP2C8). Products include:
Paroxetine CR ... 2361
Paroxetine ER ... 2371
Paxil ... 1586
Paxil CR ... 1596

Paroxetine Mesylate (*In vitro* studies demonstrate that CYP1A2 and CYP2C8 are involved in the oxidative metabolism of eltrombopag. The significance of co-administration of eltrombopag with moderate or strong inhibitors of CYP 1A2 (eg, ciprofloxacin, fluvoxamine) and CYP 2C8 (eg, gemfibrozil, trimethoprim) on the systemic exposure of eltrombopag has not been established in clinical studies. Monitor patients for signs and symptoms of excessive eltrombopag exposure when eltrombopag is administered concomitantly with these moderate or strong inhibitors of CYP1A2 or CYP2C8).
No products indexed under this heading.

Phenobarbital (*In vitro* studies demonstrate that CYP1A2 and CYP2C8 are involved in the oxidative metabolism of eltrombopag. The significance of co-administration of eltrombopag with inducers of CYP 1A2 (eg, tobacco, omeprazole) and CYP 2C8 (eg, rifampin) on the systemic exposure of eltrombopag has not been established in clinical studies. Monitor patients for signs and symptoms of excessive eltrombopag exposure when eltrombopag is administered concomitantly with these drugs). Products include:
Donnatal ... 2711

Phenobarbital Sodium (*In vitro* studies demonstrate that CYP1A2 and CYP2C8 are involved in the oxidative metabolism of eltrombopag. The significance of co-administration of eltrombopag with inducers of CYP 1A2 (eg, tobacco, omeprazole) and CYP 2C8 (eg, rifampin) on the systemic exposure of eltrombopag has not been established in clinical studies. Monitor patients for signs and symptoms of excessive eltrombopag exposure when eltrombopag is administered concomitantly with these drugs).
No products indexed under this heading.

Phenylbutazone (Studies demonstrate that eltrombopag is an inhibitor of UGT1A1, UGT1A3, UGT1A4, UGT1A6, UGT1A9, UGT2B7, and UGT2B15, enzymes involved in the metabolism of multiple drugs, such as acetaminophen, narcotics, and nonsteroidal anti-inflammatory drugs (NSAIDs). Monitor patients closely for signs of symptoms of excessive exposure to these drugs when concomitantly administered with eltrombopag).
No products indexed under this heading.

Phenytoin (*In vitro* studies demonstrate that CYP1A2 and CYP2C8 are involved in the oxidative metabolism of eltrombopag. The significance of co-administration of eltrombopag with inducers of CYP 1A2 (eg, tobacco, omeprazole) and CYP 2C8 (eg, rifampin) on the systemic exposure of eltrombopag has not been established in clinical studies. Monitor patients for signs and symptoms of excessive eltrombopag exposure when eltrombopag is administered concomitantly with these drugs).
No products indexed under this heading.

Phenytoin Sodium (*In vitro* studies demonstrate that CYP1A2 and CYP2C8 are involved in the oxidative metabolism of eltrombopag. The significance of co-administration of eltrombopag with inducers of CYP 1A2 (eg, tobacco, omeprazole) and CYP 2C8 (eg, rifampin) on the systemic exposure of eltrombopag has not been established in clinical studies. Monitor patients for signs and symptoms of excessive eltrombopag exposure when eltrombopag is administered concomitantly with these drugs). Products include:
Phenytek Capsules ... 2380

Pioglitazone Hydrochloride (*In vitro* studies demonstrate that CYP1A2 and CYP2C8 are involved in the oxidative metabolism of eltrombopag. The significance of co-administration of eltrombopag with other substrates of these CYP enzymes on the systemic exposure of eltrombopag has not been established in clinical studies. Monitor patients for signs and symptoms of excessive eltrombopag exposure when eltrombopag is administered concomitantly with these drugs). Products include:
ActoPlus ... 3338
Actos ... 3345
Duetact ... 3354

Piroxicam (Studies demonstrate that eltrombopag is an inhibitor of UGT1A1, UGT1A3, UGT1A4, UGT1A6, UGT1A9, UGT2B7, and UGT2B15, enzymes involved in the metabolism of multiple drugs, such as acetaminophen, narcotics, and nonsteroidal anti-inflammatory drugs (NSAIDs). Monitor patients closely for signs of symptoms of excessive exposure to these drugs when concomitantly administered with eltrombopag).
No products indexed under this heading.

Polysaccharide Iron Complex (Eltrombopag chelates polyvalent cations (such as iron, calcium, aluminum, magnesium, selenium, and zinc) in foods, mineral supplements, and antacids. In a clinical study, administration of eltrombopag with a polyvalent cation-containing antacid (1,524 mg aluminum hydroxide, 1,425 mg magnesium carbonate, and sodium alginate) decreased plasma eltrombopag systemic exposure by approximately 70%. Eltrombopag must not be taken within 4 hours of any medications or products containing polyvalent cations such as antacids, dairy products, and mineral supplements to avoid significant reduction in eltrombopag absorption due to chelation). Products include:
Nu-Iron 150 ... 2321

Pravastatin Sodium (*In vitro* studies demonstrate that eltrombopag is an inhibitor of the organic anion transporting polypeptide OATP1B1 and can increase the systemic exposure of other drugs that are substrates of this transporter (eg, benzylpenicillin, atorvastatin, fluvastatin, pravastatin, rosuvastatin, methotrexate, nateglinide, repaglinide, rifampin). Monitor patients closely for signs and symptoms of excessive exposure to the drugs that are substrates of OATP1B1 and consider reduction of the dose of these drugs).
No products indexed under this heading.

Primidone (*In vitro* studies demonstrate that CYP1A2 and CYP2C8 are involved in the oxidative metabolism of eltrombopag. The significance of co-administration of eltrombopag with inducers of CYP 1A2 (eg, tobacco, omeprazole) and CYP 2C8 (eg, rifampin) on the systemic exposure of eltrombopag has not been established in clinical studies. Monitor patients for signs and symptoms of excessive eltrombopag exposure when eltrombopag is administered concomitantly with these drugs).
No products indexed under this heading.

Propafenone Hydrochloride (*In vitro* studies demonstrate that CYP1A2 and CYP2C8 are involved in the oxidative metabolism of eltrombopag. The significance of co-administration of eltrombopag with other substrates of these CYP enzymes on the systemic exposure of eltrombopag has not been established in clinical studies. Monitor patients for signs and symptoms of excessive eltrombopag exposure when eltrombopag is administered concomitantly with these drugs). Products include:
Rythmol ... 1648
Rythmol SR ... 1652

Propoxyphene Hydrochloride (Studies demonstrate that eltrombopag is an inhibitor of UGT1A1, UGT1A3, UGT1A4, UGT1A6, UGT1A9, UGT2B7, and UGT2B15, enzymes involved in the metabolism of multiple drugs, such as acetaminophen, narcotics, and nonsteroidal anti-inflammatory drugs (NSAIDs). Monitor patients closely for signs of symptoms of excessive exposure to these drugs when concomitantly administered with eltrombopag).
No products indexed under this heading.

Propoxyphene Napsylate (Studies demonstrate that eltrombopag is an inhibitor of UGT1A1, UGT1A3, UGT1A4, UGT1A6, UGT1A9, UGT2B7, and UGT2B15, enzymes involved in the metabolism of multiple drugs, such as acetaminophen, narcotics, and nonsteroidal anti-inflammatory drugs (NSAIDs). Monitor patients closely for signs of symptoms of excessive exposure to these drugs when concomitantly administered with eltrombopag).
No products indexed under this heading.

Propranolol Hydrochloride (*In vitro* studies demonstrate that CYP1A2 and CYP2C8 are involved in the oxidative metabolism of eltrombopag. The significance of co-administration of eltrombopag with other substrates of these CYP enzymes on the systemic exposure of eltrombopag has not been established in clinical studies. Monitor patients for signs and symptoms of excessive eltrombopag exposure when eltrombopag is administered concomitantly with these drugs). Products include:

InnoPran XL 1517

Protriptyline Hydrochloride (*In vitro* studies demonstrate that CYP1A2 and CYP2C8 are involved in the oxidative metabolism of eltrombopag. The significance of co-administration of eltrombopag with other substrates of these CYP enzymes on the systemic exposure of eltrombopag has not been established in clinical studies. Monitor patients for signs and symptoms of excessive eltrombopag exposure when eltrombopag is administered concomitantly with these drugs).
No products indexed under this heading.

Quercetin (*In vitro* studies demonstrate that CYP1A2 and CYP2C8 are involved in the oxidative metabolism of eltrombopag. The significance of co-administration of eltrombopag with moderate or strong inhibitors of CYP 1A2 (eg, ciprofloxacin, fluvoxamine) and CYP 2C8 (eg, gemfibrozil, trimethoprim) on the systemic exposure of eltrombopag has not been established in clinical studies. Monitor patients for signs and symptoms of excessive eltrombopag exposure when eltrombopag is administered concomitantly with these moderate or strong inhibitors of CYP1A2 or CYP2C8).
No products indexed under this heading.

Ranitidine Bismuth Citrate (*In vitro* studies demonstrate that CYP1A2 and CYP2C8 are involved in the oxidative metabolism of eltrombopag. The significance of co-administration of eltrombopag with moderate or strong inhibitors of CYP 1A2 (eg, ciprofloxacin, fluvoxamine) and CYP 2C8 (eg, gemfibrozil, trimethoprim) on the systemic exposure of eltrombopag has not been established in clinical studies. Monitor patients for signs and symptoms of excessive eltrombopag exposure when eltrombopag is administered concomitantly with these moderate or strong inhibitors of CYP1A2 or CYP2C8).
No products indexed under this heading.

Ranitidine Hydrochloride (*In vitro* studies demonstrate that CYP1A2 and CYP2C8 are involved in the oxidative metabolism of eltrombopag. The significance of co-administration of eltrombopag with moderate or strong inhibitors of CYP 1A2 (eg, ciprofloxacin, fluvoxamine) and CYP 2C8 (eg, gemfibrozil, trimethoprim) on the systemic exposure of eltrombopag has not been established in clinical studies. Monitor patients for signs and symptoms of excessive eltrombopag exposure when eltrombopag is administered concomitantly with these moderate or strong inhibitors of CYP1A2 or CYP2C8). Products include:
Zantac 1737
Zantac Injection 1732
Zantac Pharmacy 1735

Remifentanil Hydrochloride (Studies demonstrate that eltrombopag is an inhibitor of UGT1A1, UGT1A3, UGT1A4, UGT1A6, UGT1A9, UGT2B7, and UGT2B15, enzymes involved in the metabolism of multiple drugs, such as acetaminophen, narcotics, and nonsteroidal anti-inflammatory drugs (NSAIDs). Monitor patients closely for signs of symptoms of excessive exposure to these drugs when concomitantly administered with eltrombopag).
No products indexed under this heading.

Repaglinide (*In vitro* studies demonstrate that eltrombopag is an inhibitor of the organic anion transporting polypeptide OATP1B1 and can increase the systemic exposure of other drugs that are substrates of this transporter (eg, benzylpenicillin, atorvastatin, fluvastatin, pravastatin, rosuvastatin, methotrexate, nateglinide, repaglinide, rifampin). Monitor patients closely for signs and symptoms of excessive exposure to the drugs that are substrates of OATP1B1 and consider reduction of the dose of these drugs).
No products indexed under this heading.

Rifabutin (*In vitro* studies demonstrate that CYP1A2 and CYP2C8 are involved in the oxidative metabolism of eltrombopag. The significance of co-administration of eltrombopag with inducers of CYP 1A2 (eg, tobacco, omeprazole) and CYP 2C8 (eg, rifampin) on the systemic exposure of eltrombopag has not been established in clinical studies. Monitor patients for signs and symptoms of excessive eltrombopag exposure when eltrombopag is administered concomitantly with these drugs).
No products indexed under this heading.

Rifampicin (*In vitro* studies demonstrate that CYP1A2 and CYP2C8 are involved in the oxidative metabolism of eltrombopag. The significance of co-administration of eltrombopag with inducers of CYP 1A2 (eg, tobacco, omeprazole) and CYP 2C8 (eg, rifampin) on the systemic exposure of eltrombopag has not been established in clinical studies. Monitor patients for signs and symptoms of excessive eltrombopag exposure when eltrombopag is administered concomitantly with these drugs).
No products indexed under this heading.

Rifampin (*In vitro* studies demonstrate that eltrombopag is an inhibitor of the organic anion transporting polypeptide OATP1B1 and can increase the systemic exposure of other drugs that are substrates of this transporter (eg, benzylpenicillin, atorvastatin, fluvastatin, pravastatin, rosuvastatin, methotrexate, nateglinide, repaglinide, rifampin). Monitor patients closely for signs and symptoms of excessive exposure to the drugs that are substrates of OATP1B1 and consider reduction of the dose of these drugs).
No products indexed under this heading.

Riluzole (*In vitro* studies demonstrate that CYP1A2 and CYP2C8 are involved in the oxidative metabolism of eltrombopag. The significance of co-administration of eltrombopag with other substrates of these CYP enzymes on the systemic exposure of eltrombopag has not been established in clinical studies. Monitor patients for signs and symptoms of excessive eltrombopag exposure when eltrombopag is administered concomitantly with these drugs). Products include:
Rilutek 3032

Ritonavir (*In vitro* studies demonstrate that CYP1A2 and CYP2C8 are involved in the oxidative metabolism of eltrombopag. The significance of co-administration of eltrombopag with moderate or strong inhibitors of CYP 1A2 (eg, ciprofloxacin, fluvoxamine) and CYP 2C8 (eg, gemfibrozil, trimethoprim) on the systemic exposure of eltrombopag has not been established in clinical studies. Monitor patients for signs and symptoms of excessive eltrombopag exposure when eltrombopag is administered concomitantly with these moderate or strong inhibitors of CYP1A2 or CYP2C8). Products include:
Kaletra 458
Norvir 509

Rofecoxib (Studies demonstrate that eltrombopag is an inhibitor of UGT1A1, UGT1A3, UGT1A4, UGT1A6, UGT1A9, UGT2B7, and UGT2B15, enzymes involved in the metabolism of multiple drugs, such as acetaminophen, narcotics, and nonsteroidal anti-inflammatory drugs (NSAIDs). Monitor patients closely for signs of symptoms of excessive exposure to these drugs when concomitantly administered with eltrombopag).
No products indexed under this heading.

Ropinirole Hydrochloride (*In vitro* studies demonstrate that CYP1A2 and CYP2C8 are involved in the oxidative metabolism of eltrombopag. The significance of co-administration of eltrombopag with other substrates of these CYP enzymes on the systemic exposure of eltrombopag has not been established in clinical studies. Monitor patients for signs and symptoms of excessive eltrombopag exposure when eltrombopag is administered concomitantly with these drugs). Products include:
Requip 1620
Requip XL 1628

Ropivacaine Hydrochloride (*In vitro* studies demonstrate that CYP1A2 and CYP2C8 are involved in the oxidative metabolism of eltrombopag. The significance of co-administration of eltrombopag with other substrates of these CYP enzymes on the systemic exposure of eltrombopag has not been established in clinical studies. Monitor patients for signs and symptoms of excessive eltrombopag exposure when eltrombopag is administered concomitantly with these drugs).
No products indexed under this heading.

Rosiglitazone Maleate (*In vitro* studies demonstrate that CYP1A2 and CYP2C8 are involved in the oxidative metabolism of eltrombopag. The significance of co-administration of eltrombopag with other substrates of these CYP enzymes on the systemic exposure of eltrombopag has not been established in clinical studies. Monitor patients for signs and symptoms of excessive eltrombopag exposure when eltrombopag is administered concomitantly with these drugs). Products include:
Avandamet 1345
Avandaryl 1356
Avandia 1366

Rosiglitazone/Metformin (*In vitro* studies demonstrate that CYP1A2 and CYP2C8 are involved in the oxidative metabolism of eltrombopag. The significance of co-administration of eltrombopag with other substrates of these CYP enzymes on the systemic exposure of eltrombopag has not been established in clinical studies. Monitor patients for signs and symptoms of excessive eltrombopag exposure when eltrombopag is administered concomitantly with these drugs).
No products indexed under this heading.

Rosuvastatin Calcium (In a clinical study of healthy adult subjects, administration of a single dose of rosuvastatin following repeated daily eltrombopag dosing increased plasma rosuvastatin AUC by 55% and C_{max} by 103%; a dose reduction of rosuvastatin by 50% was recommended for co-administration with eltrombopag. Use caution when concomitantly administering eltrombopag and drugs that are substrates of OATP1B1. Monitor patients closely for signs and symptoms of excessive exposure to the drugs that are substrates of OATP1B1 and consider reduction of the dose of these drugs). Products include:
Crestor 736

Selenium (Eltrombopag chelates polyvalent cations (such as iron, calcium, aluminum, magnesium, selenium, and zinc) in foods, mineral supplements, and antacids. In a clinical study, administration of eltrombopag with a polyvalent cation-containing antacid (1,524 mg aluminum hydroxide, 1,425 mg magnesium carbonate, and sodium alginate) decreased plasma eltrombopag systemic exposure by approximately 70%. Eltrombopag must not be taken within 4 hours of any medications or products containing polyvalent cations such as antacids, dairy products, and mineral supplements to avoid significant reduction in eltrombopag absorption due to chelation). Products include:
Cardio Basics 3455
Chelated Mineral 3476

Selenium Sulfide (Eltrombopag chelates polyvalent cations (such as iron, calcium, aluminum, magnesium, selenium, and zinc) in foods, mineral supplements, and antacids. In a clinical study, administration of eltrombopag with a polyvalent cation-containing antacid (1,524 mg aluminum hydroxide, 1,425 mg magnesium carbonate, and sodium alginate) decreased plasma eltrombopag systemic exposure by approximately 70%. Eltrombopag must not be taken within 4 hours of any medications or products containing polyvalent cations such as antacids, dairy products, and mineral supplements to avoid significant reduction in eltrombopag absorption due to chelation).
No products indexed under this heading.

Sildenafil Citrate (*In vitro* studies demonstrate that CYP1A2 and CYP2C8 are involved in the oxidative metabolism of eltrombopag. The significance of co-administration of eltrombopag with moderate or strong inhibitors of CYP 1A2 (eg, ciprofloxacin, fluvoxamine) and CYP 2C8 (eg, gemfibrozil, trimethoprim) on the systemic exposure of eltrombopag has not been established in clinical studies. Monitor patients for signs and symptoms of excessive eltrombopag exposure when eltrombopag is administered concomitantly with these moderate or strong inhibitors of CYP1A2 or CYP2C8).
No products indexed under this heading.

Sodium Bicarbonate (Eltrombopag chelates polyvalent cations (such as iron, calcium, aluminum, magnesium, selenium, and zinc) in foods, mineral supplements, and antacids. In a clinical study, administration of eltrombopag with a polyvalent cation-containing antacid (1,524 mg aluminum hydroxide, 1,425 mg magnesium carbonate, and sodium alginate) decreased plasma eltrombopag systemic exposure by approximately 70%. Eltrombopag must not be taken within 4 hours of any medications or products containing polyvalent cations such as antacids, dairy products, and mineral supplements to avoid significant reduction in eltrombopag absorption due to chelation).
No products indexed under this heading.

Sparfloxacin (*In vitro* studies demonstrate that CYP1A2 and CYP2C8 are involved in the oxidative metabolism of eltrombopag. The significance of co-administration of eltrombopag with moderate or strong inhibitors of CYP 1A2 (eg, ciprofloxacin, fluvoxamine) and CYP 2C8 (eg, gemfibrozil, trimethoprim) on the systemic exposure of eltrombopag has not been established in clinical studies. Monitor patients for signs and symptoms of excessive eltrombopag exposure when eltrombopag is administered concomitantly with these moderate or strong inhibitors of CYP1A2 or CYP2C8).
No products indexed under this heading.

Sufentanil Citrate (Studies demonstrate that eltrombopag is an inhibitor of UGT1A1, UGT1A3, UGT1A4, UGT1A6, UGT1A9, UGT2B7, and UGT2B15, enzymes involved in the metabolism of multiple drugs, such as acetaminophen, narcotics, and nonsteroidal anti-inflammatory drugs (NSAIDs). Monitor patients closely for signs of symptoms of excessive exposure to these drugs when concomitantly administered with eltrombopag).
No products indexed under this heading.

Sulfaphenazole (*In vitro* studies demonstrate that CYP1A2 and CYP2C8 are

involved in the oxidative metabolism of eltrombopag. The significance of co-administration of eltrombopag with moderate or strong inhibitors of CYP 1A2 (eg, ciprofloxacin, fluvoxamine) and CYP 2C8 (eg, gemfibrozil, trimethoprim) on the systemic exposure of eltrombopag has not been established in clinical studies. Monitor patients for signs and symptoms of excessive eltrombopag exposure when eltrombopag is administered concomitantly with these moderate or strong inhibitors of CYP1A2 or CYP2C8).

No products indexed under this heading.

Sulfinpyrazone (*In vitro* studies demonstrate that CYP1A2 and CYP2C8 are involved in the oxidative metabolism of eltrombopag. The significance of co-administration of eltrombopag with moderate or strong inhibitors of CYP 1A2 (eg, ciprofloxacin, fluvoxamine) and CYP 2C8 (eg, gemfibrozil, trimethoprim) on the systemic exposure of eltrombopag has not been established in clinical studies. Monitor patients for signs and symptoms of excessive eltrombopag exposure when eltrombopag is administered concomitantly with these moderate or strong inhibitors of CYP1A2 or CYP2C8).

No products indexed under this heading.

Sulindac (Studies demonstrate that eltrombopag is an inhibitor of UGT1A1, UGT1A3, UGT1A4, UGT1A6, UGT1A9, UGT2B7, and UGT2B15, enzymes involved in the metabolism of multiple drugs, such as acetaminophen, narcotics, and nonsteroidal anti-inflammatory drugs (NSAIDs). Monitor patients closely for signs of symptoms of excessive exposure to these drugs when concomitantly administered with eltrombopag). Products include:

Clinoril 2098

Tacrine Hydrochloride (*In vitro* studies demonstrate that CYP1A2 and CYP2C8 are involved in the oxidative metabolism of eltrombopag. The significance of co-administration of eltrombopag with moderate or strong inhibitors of CYP 1A2 (eg, ciprofloxacin, fluvoxamine) and CYP 2C8 (eg, gemfibrozil, trimethoprim) on the systemic exposure of eltrombopag has not been established in clinical studies. Monitor patients for signs and symptoms of excessive eltrombopag exposure when eltrombopag is administered concomitantly with these moderate or strong inhibitors of CYP1A2 or CYP2C8).

No products indexed under this heading.

Tamoxifen Citrate (*In vitro* studies demonstrate that CYP1A2 and CYP2C8 are involved in the oxidative metabolism of eltrombopag. The significance of co-administration of eltrombopag with other substrates of these CYP enzymes on the systemic exposure of eltrombopag has not been established in clinical studies. Monitor patients for signs and symptoms of excessive eltrombopag exposure when eltrombopag is administered concomitantly with these drugs).

No products indexed under this heading.

Telmisartan (*In vitro* studies demonstrate that eltrombopag is an inhibitor of UGT1A1, UGT1A3, UGT1A4, UGT1A6, UGT1A9, UGT2B7, and UGT2B15, enzymes involved in the metabolism of multiple drugs, such as acetaminophen, narcotics, and nonsteroidal anti-inflammatory drugs (NSAIDs). The significance of this inhibition on the potential for increased systemic exposure of drugs that are substrates of these UGTs following co-administration with eltrombopag has not been evaluated in clinical studies. Monitor patients closely for signs or symptoms of exces-

sive exposure to these drugs when concomitantly administered with eltrombopag). Products include:

Micardis **887**
Micardis HCT **889**

Theobromine (*In vitro* studies demonstrate that CYP1A2 and CYP2C8 are involved in the oxidative metabolism of eltrombopag. The significance of co-administration of eltrombopag with other substrates of these CYP enzymes on the systemic exposure of eltrombopag has not been established in clinical studies. Monitor patients for signs and symptoms of excessive eltrombopag exposure when eltrombopag is administered concomitantly with these drugs).

No products indexed under this heading.

Theophylline (*In vitro* studies demonstrate that CYP1A2 and CYP2C8 are involved in the oxidative metabolism of eltrombopag. The significance of co-administration of eltrombopag with other substrates of these CYP enzymes on the systemic exposure of eltrombopag has not been established in clinical studies. Monitor patients for signs and symptoms of excessive eltrombopag exposure when eltrombopag is administered concomitantly with these drugs).

No products indexed under this heading.

Theophylline Anhydrous (*In vitro* studies demonstrate that CYP1A2 and CYP2C8 are involved in the oxidative metabolism of eltrombopag. The significance of co-administration of eltrombopag with other substrates of these CYP enzymes on the systemic exposure of eltrombopag has not been established in clinical studies. Monitor patients for signs and symptoms of excessive eltrombopag exposure when eltrombopag is administered concomitantly with these drugs). Products include:

Uniphyl 2817

Theophylline Calcium Salicylate (*In vitro* studies demonstrate that CYP1A2 and CYP2C8 are involved in the oxidative metabolism of eltrombopag. The significance of co-administration of eltrombopag with other substrates of these CYP enzymes on the systemic exposure of eltrombopag has not been established in clinical studies. Monitor patients for signs and symptoms of excessive eltrombopag exposure when eltrombopag is administered concomitantly with these drugs).

No products indexed under this heading.

Theophylline Dihydroxypropyl (Glyceryl) (*In vitro* studies demonstrate that CYP1A2 and CYP2C8 are involved in the oxidative metabolism of eltrombopag. The significance of co-administration of eltrombopag with other substrates of these CYP enzymes on the systemic exposure of eltrombopag has not been established in clinical studies. Monitor patients for signs and symptoms of excessive eltrombopag exposure when eltrombopag is administered concomitantly with these drugs).

No products indexed under this heading.

Theophylline Ethylenediamine (*In vitro* studies demonstrate that CYP1A2 and CYP2C8 are involved in the oxidative metabolism of eltrombopag. The significance of co-administration of eltrombopag with other substrates of these CYP enzymes on the systemic exposure of eltrombopag has not been established in clinical studies. Monitor patients for signs and symptoms of excessive eltrombopag exposure when eltrombopag is administered concomitantly with these drugs).

No products indexed under this heading.

Theophylline Sodium Glycinate (*In vitro* studies demonstrate that CYP1A2 and CYP2C8 are involved in the oxidative metabolism of eltrombopag. The significance of co-administration of

eltrombopag with other substrates of these CYP enzymes on the systemic exposure of eltrombopag has not been established in clinical studies. Monitor patients for signs and symptoms of excessive eltrombopag exposure when eltrombopag is administered concomitantly with these drugs).

No products indexed under this heading.

Ticlopidine Hydrochloride (*In vitro* studies demonstrate that CYP1A2 and CYP2C8 are involved in the oxidative metabolism of eltrombopag. The significance of co-administration of eltrombopag with moderate or strong inhibitors of CYP 1A2 (eg, ciprofloxacin, fluvoxamine) and CYP 2C8 (eg, gemfibrozil, trimethoprim) on the systemic exposure of eltrombopag has not been established in clinical studies. Monitor patients for signs and symptoms of excessive eltrombopag exposure when eltrombopag is administered concomitantly with these moderate or strong inhibitors of CYP1A2 or CYP2C8).

No products indexed under this heading.

Tizanidine (*In vitro* studies demonstrate that CYP1A2 and CYP2C8 are involved in the oxidative metabolism of eltrombopag. The significance of co-administration of eltrombopag with other substrates of these CYP enzymes on the systemic exposure of eltrombopag has not been established in clinical studies. Monitor patients for signs and symptoms of excessive eltrombopag exposure when eltrombopag is administered concomitantly with these drugs).

No products indexed under this heading.

Tizanidine Hydrochloride (*In vitro* studies demonstrate that CYP1A2 and CYP2C8 are involved in the oxidative metabolism of eltrombopag. The significance of co-administration of eltrombopag with other substrates of these CYP enzymes on the systemic exposure of eltrombopag has not been established in clinical studies. Monitor patients for signs and symptoms of excessive eltrombopag exposure when eltrombopag is administered concomitantly with these drugs).

No products indexed under this heading.

Tobacco (*In vitro* studies demonstrate that CYP1A2 and CYP2C8 are involved in the oxidative metabolism of eltrombopag. The significance of co-administration of eltrombopag with inducers of CYP 1A2 (eg, tobacco, omeprazole) and CYP 2C8 (eg, rifampin) on the systemic exposure of eltrombopag has not been established in clinical studies. Monitor patients for signs and symptoms of excessive eltrombopag exposure when eltrombopag is administered concomitantly with these drugs).

No products indexed under this heading.

Tolbutamide (*In vitro* studies demonstrate that CYP1A2 and CYP2C8 are involved in the oxidative metabolism of eltrombopag. The significance of co-administration of eltrombopag with other substrates of these CYP enzymes on the systemic exposure of eltrombopag has not been established in clinical studies. Monitor patients for signs and symptoms of excessive eltrombopag exposure when eltrombopag is administered concomitantly with these drugs).

No products indexed under this heading.

Tolbutamide Sodium (*In vitro* studies demonstrate that CYP1A2 and CYP2C8 are involved in the oxidative metabolism of eltrombopag. The significance of co-administration of eltrombopag with other substrates of these CYP enzymes on the systemic exposure of eltrombopag has not been established in clinical studies. Monitor patients for signs and symptoms of excessive eltrom-

bopag exposure when eltrombopag is administered concomitantly with these drugs).

No products indexed under this heading.

Tolmetin Sodium (Studies demonstrate that eltrombopag is an inhibitor of UGT1A1, UGT1A3, UGT1A4, UGT1A6, UGT1A9, UGT2B7, and UGT2B15, enzymes involved in the metabolism of multiple drugs, such as acetaminophen, narcotics, and nonsteroidal anti-inflammatory drugs (NSAIDs). Monitor patients closely for signs of symptoms of excessive exposure to these drugs when concomitantly administered with eltrombopag).

No products indexed under this heading.

Tretinoin (*In vitro* studies demonstrate that CYP1A2 and CYP2C8 are involved in the oxidative metabolism of eltrombopag. The significance of co-administration of eltrombopag with other substrates of these CYP enzymes on the systemic exposure of eltrombopag has not been established in clinical studies. Monitor patients for signs and symptoms of excessive eltrombopag exposure when eltrombopag is administered concomitantly with these drugs).

No products indexed under this heading.

Trimethaphan Camsylate (*In vitro* studies demonstrate that CYP1A2 and CYP2C8 are involved in the oxidative metabolism of eltrombopag. The significance of co-administration of eltrombopag with other substrates of these CYP enzymes on the systemic exposure of eltrombopag has not been established in clinical studies. Monitor patients for signs and symptoms of excessive eltrombopag exposure when eltrombopag is administered concomitantly with these drugs).

No products indexed under this heading.

Trimethoprim (*In vitro* studies demonstrate that CYP1A2 and CYP2C8 are involved in the oxidative metabolism of eltrombopag. The significance of co-administration of eltrombopag with moderate or strong inhibitors of CYP 1A2 (eg, ciprofloxacin, fluvoxamine) and CYP 2C8 (eg, gemfibrozil, trimethoprim) on the systemic exposure of eltrombopag has not been established in clinical studies. Monitor patients for signs and symptoms of excessive eltrombopag exposure when eltrombopag is administered concomitantly with these moderate or strong inhibitors of CYP1A2 or CYP2C8).

No products indexed under this heading.

Trimethoprim Hydrochloride (*In vitro* studies demonstrate that CYP1A2 and CYP2C8 are involved in the oxidative metabolism of eltrombopag. The significance of co-administration of eltrombopag with moderate or strong inhibitors of CYP 1A2 (eg, ciprofloxacin, fluvoxamine) and CYP 2C8 (eg, gemfibrozil, trimethoprim) on the systemic exposure of eltrombopag has not been established in clinical studies. Monitor patients for signs and symptoms of excessive eltrombopag exposure when eltrombopag is administered concomitantly with these moderate or strong inhibitors of CYP1A2 or CYP2C8).

No products indexed under this heading.

Trimethoprim Sulfate (*In vitro* studies demonstrate that CYP1A2 and CYP2C8 are involved in the oxidative metabolism of eltrombopag. The significance of co-administration of eltrombopag with moderate or strong inhibitors of CYP 1A2 (eg, ciprofloxacin, fluvoxamine) and CYP 2C8 (eg, gemfibrozil, trimethoprim) on the systemic exposure of eltrombopag has not been established in clinical studies. Monitor patients for signs and symptoms of excessive eltrombopag exposure when

eltrombopag is administered concomitantly with these moderate or strong inhibitors of CYP1A2 or CYP2C8).

No products indexed under this heading.

Trimipramine Maleate (*In vitro* studies demonstrate that CYP1A2 and CYP2C8 are involved in the oxidative metabolism of eltrombopag. The significance of co-administration of eltrombopag with other substrates of these CYP enzymes on the systemic exposure of eltrombopag has not been established in clinical studies. Monitor patients for signs and symptoms of excessive eltrombopag exposure when eltrombopag is administered concomitantly with these drugs).

No products indexed under this heading.

Troleandomycin (*In vitro* studies demonstrate that CYP1A2 and CYP2C8 are involved in the oxidative metabolism of eltrombopag. The significance of co-administration of eltrombopag with moderate or strong inhibitors of CYP 1A2 (eg, ciprofloxacin, fluvoxamine) and CYP 2C8 (eg, gemfibrozil, trimethoprim) on the systemic exposure of eltrombopag has not been established in clinical studies. Monitor patients for signs and symptoms of excessive eltrombopag exposure when eltrombopag is administered concomitantly with these moderate or strong inhibitors of CYP1A2 or CYP2C8).

No products indexed under this heading.

Trovafloxacin Mesylate (*In vitro* studies demonstrate that CYP1A2 and CYP2C8 are involved in the oxidative metabolism of eltrombopag. The significance of co-administration of eltrombopag with moderate or strong inhibitors of CYP 1A2 (eg, ciprofloxacin, fluvoxamine) and CYP 2C8 (eg, gemfibrozil, trimethoprim) on the systemic exposure of eltrombopag has not been established in clinical studies. Monitor patients for signs and symptoms of excessive eltrombopag exposure when eltrombopag is administered concomitantly with these moderate or strong inhibitors of CYP1A2 or CYP2C8).

No products indexed under this heading.

Valdecoxib (Studies demonstrate that eltrombopag is an inhibitor of UGT1A1, UGT1A3, UGT1A4, UGT1A6, UGT1A9, UGT2B7, and UGT2B15, enzymes involved in the metabolism of multiple drugs, such as acetaminophen, narcotics, and nonsteroidal anti-inflammatory drugs (NSAIDs). Monitor patients closely for signs of symptoms of excessive exposure to these drugs when concomitantly administered with eltrombopag).

No products indexed under this heading.

Vardenafil Hydrochloride (*In vitro* studies demonstrate that CYP1A2 and CYP2C8 are involved in the oxidative metabolism of eltrombopag. The significance of co-administration of eltrombopag with moderate or strong inhibitors of CYP 1A2 (eg, ciprofloxacin, fluvoxamine) and CYP 2C8 (eg, gemfibrozil, trimethoprim) on the systemic exposure of eltrombopag has not been established in clinical studies. Monitor patients for signs and symptoms of excessive eltrombopag exposure when eltrombopag is administered concomitantly with these moderate or strong inhibitors of CYP1A2 or CYP2C8).
Products include:
Levitra 3157

Verapamil Hydrochloride (*In vitro* studies demonstrate that CYP1A2 and CYP2C8 are involved in the oxidative metabolism of eltrombopag. The significance of co-administration of eltrombopag with other substrates of these CYP enzymes on the systemic exposure of eltrombopag has not been established in clinical studies. Monitor patients for signs and symptoms of excessive eltrombopag exposure when

eltrombopag is administered concomitantly with these drugs). Products include:
Tarka 534

Vitamin A (*In vitro* studies demonstrate that CYP1A2 and CYP2C8 are involved in the oxidative metabolism of eltrombopag. The significance of co-administration of eltrombopag with other substrates of these CYP enzymes on the systemic exposure of eltrombopag has not been established in clinical studies. Monitor patients for signs and symptoms of excessive eltrombopag exposure when eltrombopag is administered concomitantly with these drugs).
Products include:
Cardio Basics 3455
Heplive 607
Norwegian Cod Liver Oil 919

Vitamin A Acetate (*In vitro* studies demonstrate that CYP1A2 and CYP2C8 are involved in the oxidative metabolism of eltrombopag. The significance of co-administration of eltrombopag with other substrates of these CYP enzymes on the systemic exposure of eltrombopag has not been established in clinical studies. Monitor patients for signs and symptoms of excessive eltrombopag exposure when eltrombopag is administered concomitantly with these drugs).

No products indexed under this heading.

Warfarin Sodium (*In vitro* studies demonstrate that CYP1A2 and CYP2C8 are involved in the oxidative metabolism of eltrombopag. The significance of co-administration of eltrombopag with other substrates of these CYP enzymes on the systemic exposure of eltrombopag has not been established in clinical studies. Monitor patients for signs and symptoms of excessive eltrombopag exposure when eltrombopag is administered concomitantly with these drugs).

No products indexed under this heading.

Zileuton (*In vitro* studies demonstrate that CYP1A2 and CYP2C8 are involved in the oxidative metabolism of eltrombopag. The significance of co-administration of eltrombopag with moderate or strong inhibitors of CYP 1A2 (eg, ciprofloxacin, fluvoxamine) and CYP 2C8 (eg, gemfibrozil, trimethoprim) on the systemic exposure of eltrombopag has not been established in clinical studies. Monitor patients for signs and symptoms of excessive eltrombopag exposure when eltrombopag is administered concomitantly with these moderate or strong inhibitors of CYP1A2 or CYP2C8).

No products indexed under this heading.

Zinc (Eltrombopag chelates polyvalent cations (such as iron, calcium, aluminum, magnesium, selenium, and zinc) in foods, mineral supplements, and antacids. In a clinical study, administration of eltrombopag with a polyvalent cation-containing antacid (1,524 mg aluminum hydroxide, 1,425 mg magnesium carbonate, and sodium alginate) decreased plasma eltrombopag systemic exposure by approximately 70%. Eltrombopag must not be taken within 4 hours of any medications or products containing polyvalent cations such as antacids, dairy products, and mineral supplements to avoid significant reduction in eltrombopag absorption due to chelation). Products include:
BoneMate Plus 3454
Cardio Basics 3455
Chelated Mineral 3476
CitraNatal 90 DHA Capsules 2332
CitraNatal Assure 2332
Heplive 607
Visutein 3456

Zinc Acetate (Eltrombopag chelates polyvalent cations (such as iron, calcium, aluminum, magnesium, selenium,

and zinc) in foods, mineral supplements, and antacids. In a clinical study, administration of eltrombopag with a polyvalent cation-containing antacid (1,524 mg aluminum hydroxide, 1,425 mg magnesium carbonate, and sodium alginate) decreased plasma eltrombopag systemic exposure by approximately 70%. Eltrombopag must not be taken within 4 hours of any medications or products containing polyvalent cations such as antacids, dairy products, and mineral supplements to avoid significant reduction in eltrombopag absorption due to chelation).

No products indexed under this heading.

Zinc Bisglycinate (Eltrombopag chelates polyvalent cations (such as iron, calcium, aluminum, magnesium, selenium, and zinc) in foods, mineral supplements, and antacids. In a clinical study, administration of eltrombopag with a polyvalent cation-containing antacid (1,524 mg aluminum hydroxide, 1,425 mg magnesium carbonate, and sodium alginate) decreased plasma eltrombopag systemic exposure by approximately 70%. Eltrombopag must not be taken within 4 hours of any medications or products containing polyvalent cations such as antacids, dairy products, and mineral supplements to avoid significant reduction in eltrombopag absorption due to chelation).

No products indexed under this heading.

Zinc Chloride (Eltrombopag chelates polyvalent cations (such as iron, calcium, aluminum, magnesium, selenium, and zinc) in foods, mineral supplements, and antacids. In a clinical study, administration of eltrombopag with a polyvalent cation-containing antacid (1,524 mg aluminum hydroxide, 1,425 mg magnesium carbonate, and sodium alginate) decreased plasma eltrombopag systemic exposure by approximately 70%. Eltrombopag must not be taken within 4 hours of any medications or products containing polyvalent cations such as antacids, dairy products, and mineral supplements to avoid significant reduction in eltrombopag absorption due to chelation).

No products indexed under this heading.

Zinc Citrate (Eltrombopag chelates polyvalent cations (such as iron, calcium, aluminum, magnesium, selenium, and zinc) in foods, mineral supplements, and antacids. In a clinical study, administration of eltrombopag with a polyvalent cation-containing antacid (1,524 mg aluminum hydroxide, 1,425 mg magnesium carbonate, and sodium alginate) decreased plasma eltrombopag systemic exposure by approximately 70%. Eltrombopag must not be taken within 4 hours of any medications or products containing polyvalent cations such as antacids, dairy products, and mineral supplements to avoid significant reduction in eltrombopag absorption due to chelation).
Products include:
Chelated Mineral 3476

Zinc-Containing Multivitamins (Eltrombopag chelates polyvalent cations (such as iron, calcium, aluminum, magnesium, selenium, and zinc) in foods, mineral supplements, and antacids. In a clinical study, administration of eltrombopag with a polyvalent cation-containing antacid (1,524 mg aluminum hydroxide, 1,425 mg magnesium carbonate, and sodium alginate) decreased plasma eltrombopag systemic exposure by approximately 70%. Eltrombopag must not be taken within 4 hours of any medications or products containing polyvalent cations such as antacids, dairy products, and mineral supple-

ments to avoid significant reduction in eltrombopag absorption due to chelation).

No products indexed under this heading.

Zinc Gluconate (Eltrombopag chelates polyvalent cations (such as iron, calcium, aluminum, magnesium, selenium, and zinc) in foods, mineral supplements, and antacids. In a clinical study, administration of eltrombopag with a polyvalent cation-containing antacid (1,524 mg aluminum hydroxide, 1,425 mg magnesium carbonate, and sodium alginate) decreased plasma eltrombopag systemic exposure by approximately 70%. Eltrombopag must not be taken within 4 hours of any medications or products containing polyvalent cations such as antacids, dairy products, and mineral supplements to avoid significant reduction in eltrombopag absorption due to chelation).

No products indexed under this heading.

Zinc Oxide (Eltrombopag chelates polyvalent cations (such as iron, calcium, aluminum, magnesium, selenium, and zinc) in foods, mineral supplements, and antacids. In a clinical study, administration of eltrombopag with a polyvalent cation-containing antacid (1,524 mg aluminum hydroxide, 1,425 mg magnesium carbonate, and sodium alginate) decreased plasma eltrombopag systemic exposure by approximately 70%. Eltrombopag must not be taken within 4 hours of any medications or products containing polyvalent cations such as antacids, dairy products, and mineral supplements to avoid significant reduction in eltrombopag absorption due to chelation).
Products include:
Bausch & Lomb Ocuvite Adult
50+ .... ⊙238
CitraNatal Rx 2332
Vusion Ointment 3335

Zinc Phenosulfonate (Eltrombopag chelates polyvalent cations (such as iron, calcium, aluminum, magnesium, selenium, and zinc) in foods, mineral supplements, and antacids. In a clinical study, administration of eltrombopag with a polyvalent cation-containing antacid (1,524 mg aluminum hydroxide, 1,425 mg magnesium carbonate, and sodium alginate) decreased plasma eltrombopag systemic exposure by approximately 70%. Eltrombopag must not be taken within 4 hours of any medications or products containing polyvalent cations such as antacids, dairy products, and mineral supplements to avoid significant reduction in eltrombopag absorption due to chelation).

No products indexed under this heading.

Zinc Sulfate (Eltrombopag chelates polyvalent cations (such as iron, calcium, aluminum, magnesium, selenium, and zinc) in foods, mineral supplements, and antacids. In a clinical study, administration of eltrombopag with a polyvalent cation-containing antacid (1,524 mg aluminum hydroxide, 1,425 mg magnesium carbonate, and sodium alginate) decreased plasma eltrombopag systemic exposure by approximately 70%. Eltrombopag must not be taken within 4 hours of any medications or products containing polyvalent cations such as antacids, dairy products, and mineral supplements to avoid significant reduction in eltrombopag absorption due to chelation).
Products include:
Heplive 607
Zinc-220 606

Zolmitriptan (*In vitro* studies demonstrate that CYP1A2 and CYP2C8 are involved in the oxidative metabolism of eltrombopag. The significance of co-administration of eltrombopag with other substrates of these CYP enzymes on the systemic exposure of eltrombopag

has not been established in clinical studies. Monitor patients for signs and symptoms of excessive eltrombopag exposure when eltrombopag is administered concomitantly with these drugs). Products include:
Zomig Tablets 773
Zomig Nasal Spray 768
Zomig-ZMT Tablets 773

Zopiclone (*In vitro* studies demonstrate that CYP1A2 and CYP2C8 are involved in the oxidative metabolism of eltrombopag. The significance of co-administration of eltrombopag with other substrates of these CYP enzymes on the systemic exposure of eltrombopag has not been established in clinical studies. Monitor patients for signs and symptoms of excessive eltrombopag exposure when eltrombopag is administered concomitantly with these drugs).
No products indexed under this heading.

Food Interactions

Broccoli (*In vitro* studies demonstrate that CYP1A2 and CYP2C8 are involved in the oxidative metabolism of eltrombopag. The significance of co-administration of eltrombopag with inducers of CYP 1A2 (eg, tobacco, omeprazole) and CYP 2C8 (eg, rifampin) on the systemic exposure of eltrombopag has not been established in clinical studies. Monitor patients for signs and symptoms of excessive eltrombopag exposure when eltrombopag is administered concomitantly with these drugs).

Brussel Sprouts (*In vitro* studies demonstrate that CYP1A2 and CYP2C8 are involved in the oxidative metabolism of eltrombopag. The significance of co-administration of eltrombopag with inducers of CYP 1A2 (eg, tobacco, omeprazole) and CYP 2C8 (eg, rifampin) on the systemic exposure of eltrombopag has not been established in clinical studies. Monitor patients for signs and symptoms of excessive eltrombopag exposure when eltrombopag is administered concomitantly with these drugs).

Charbroiled Food (*In vitro* studies demonstrate that CYP1A2 and CYP2C8 are involved in the oxidative metabolism of eltrombopag. The significance of co-administration of eltrombopag with inducers of CYP 1A2 (eg, tobacco, omeprazole) and CYP 2C8 (eg, rifampin) on the systemic exposure of eltrombopag has not been established in clinical studies. Monitor patients for signs and symptoms of excessive eltrombopag exposure when eltrombopag is administered concomitantly with these drugs).

Dairy products (Eltrombopag chelates polyvalent cations (such as iron, calcium, aluminum, magnesium, selenium, and zinc) in foods, mineral supplements, and antacids. In a clinical study, administration of eltrombopag with a polyvalent cation-containing antacid (1,524 mg aluminum hydroxide, 1,425 mg magnesium carbonate, and sodium alginate) decreased plasma eltrombopag systemic exposure by approximately 70%. Eltrombopag must not be taken within 4 hours of any medications or products containing polyvalent cations such as antacids, dairy products, and mineral supplements to avoid significant reduction in eltrombopag absorption due to chelation).

Food, caffeine-containing (*In vitro* studies demonstrate that CYP1A2 and CYP2C8 are involved in the oxidative metabolism of eltrombopag. The significance of co-administration of eltrombopag with other substrates of these CYP enzymes on the systemic exposure of eltrombopag has not been established in clinical studies. Monitor patients for signs and symptoms of excessive eltrombopag exposure when eltrombopag is administered concomitantly with these drugs).

Food, unspecified (Eltrombopag chelates polyvalent cations (such as iron, calcium, aluminum, magnesium, selenium, and zinc) in foods, mineral supplements, and antacids. In a clinical study, administration of eltrombopag with a polyvalent cation-containing antacid (1,524 mg aluminum hydroxide, 1,425 mg magnesium carbonate, and sodium alginate) decreased plasma eltrombopag systemic exposure by approximately 70%. Eltrombopag must not be taken within 4 hours of any medications or products containing polyvalent cations such as antacids, dairy products, and mineral supplements to avoid significant reduction in eltrombopag absorption due to chelation).

Grapefruit (*In vitro* studies demonstrate that CYP1A2 and CYP2C8 are involved in the oxidative metabolism of eltrombopag. The significance of co-administration of eltrombopag with moderate or strong inhibitors of CYP 1A2 (eg, ciprofloxacin, fluvoxamine) and CYP 2C8 (eg, gemfibrozil, trimethoprim) on the systemic exposure of eltrombopag has not been established in clinical studies. Monitor patients for signs and symptoms of excessive eltrombopag exposure when eltrombopag is administered concomitantly with these moderate or strong inhibitors of CYP1A2 or CYP2C8).

Grapefruit Juice (*In vitro* studies demonstrate that CYP1A2 and CYP2C8 are involved in the oxidative metabolism of eltrombopag. The significance of co-administration of eltrombopag with moderate or strong inhibitors of CYP 1A2 (eg, ciprofloxacin, fluvoxamine) and CYP 2C8 (eg, gemfibrozil, trimethoprim) on the systemic exposure of eltrombopag has not been established in clinical studies. Monitor patients for signs and symptoms of excessive eltrombopag exposure when eltrombopag is administered concomitantly with these moderate or strong inhibitors of CYP1A2 or CYP2C8).

Iron Amino Acid Chelate (Eltrombopag chelates polyvalent cations (such as iron, calcium, aluminum, magnesium, selenium, and zinc) in foods, mineral supplements, and antacids. In a clinical study, administration of eltrombopag with a polyvalent cation-containing antacid (1,524 mg aluminum hydroxide, 1,425 mg magnesium carbonate, and sodium alginate) decreased plasma eltrombopag systemic exposure by approximately 70%. Eltrombopag must not be taken within 4 hours of any medications or products containing polyvalent cations such as antacids, dairy products, and mineral supplements to avoid significant reduction in eltrombopag absorption due to chelation).

Meal, unspecified (Eltrombopag chelates polyvalent cations (such as iron, calcium, aluminum, magnesium, selenium, and zinc) in foods, mineral supplements, and antacids. In a clinical study, administration of eltrombopag with a polyvalent cation-containing antacid (1,524 mg aluminum hydroxide, 1,425 mg magnesium carbonate, and sodium alginate) decreased plasma eltrombopag systemic exposure by approximately 70%. Eltrombopag must not be taken within 4 hours of any medications or products containing polyvalent cations such as antacids, dairy products, and mineral supplements to avoid significant reduction in eltrombopag absorption due to chelation).

PROMETRIUM CAPSULES (100 MG, 200 MG)

(Progesterone) 3307
May interact with cytochrome p450 3a4 inhibitors (selected), estrogens, and certain other agents. Compounds in these categories include:

Acetazolamide (The metabolism of progesterone by human liver microsomes was inhibited by ketoconazole. Ketoconazole is a known inhibitor of cytochrome P450 3A4, hence these data suggest that ketoconazole or other known inhibitors of this enzyme may increase the bioavailability of progesterone. The clinical relevance of the *in vitro* findings is unknown).
No products indexed under this heading.

Acetazolamide Sodium (The metabolism of progesterone by human liver microsomes was inhibited by ketoconazole. Ketoconazole is a known inhibitor of cytochrome P450 3A4, hence these data suggest that ketoconazole or other known inhibitors of this enzyme may increase the bioavailability of progesterone. The clinical relevance of the *in vitro* findings is unknown).
No products indexed under this heading.

Amiodarone Hydrochloride (The metabolism of progesterone by human liver microsomes was inhibited by ketoconazole. Ketoconazole is a known inhibitor of cytochrome P450 3A4, hence these data suggest that ketoconazole or other known inhibitors of this enzyme may increase the bioavailability of progesterone. The clinical relevance of the *in vitro* findings is unknown).
No products indexed under this heading.

Amprenavir (The metabolism of progesterone by human liver microsomes was inhibited by ketoconazole. Ketoconazole is a known inhibitor of cytochrome P450 3A4, hence these data suggest that ketoconazole or other known inhibitors of this enzyme may increase the bioavailability of progesterone. The clinical relevance of the *in vitro* findings is unknown).
No products indexed under this heading.

Anastrozole (The metabolism of progesterone by human liver microsomes was inhibited by ketoconazole. Ketoconazole is a known inhibitor of cytochrome P450 3A4, hence these data suggest that ketoconazole or other known inhibitors of this enzyme may increase the bioavailability of progesterone. The clinical relevance of the *in vitro* findings is unknown).
No products indexed under this heading.

Aprepitant (The metabolism of progesterone by human liver microsomes was inhibited by ketoconazole. Ketoconazole is a known inhibitor of cytochrome P450 3A4, hence these data suggest that ketoconazole or other known inhibitors of this enzyme may increase the bioavailability of progesterone. The clinical relevance of the *in vitro* findings is unknown). Products include:
Emend 2124

Atazanavir (The metabolism of progesterone by human liver microsomes was inhibited by ketoconazole. Ketoconazole is a known inhibitor of cytochrome P450 3A4, hence these data suggest that ketoconazole or other known inhibitors of this enzyme may increase the bioavailability of progesterone. The clinical relevance of the *in vitro* findings is unknown).
No products indexed under this heading.

Atazanavir Sulfate (The metabolism of progesterone by human liver microsomes was inhibited by ketoconazole. Ketoconazole is a known inhibitor of cytochrome P450 3A4, hence these data suggest that ketoconazole or other known inhibitors of this enzyme may increase the bioavailability of progesterone. The clinical relevance of the *in vitro* findings is unknown).
No products indexed under this heading.

Chlorotrianisene (Co-administration of conjugated estrogens and progesterone to 29 post-menopausal women over a 12-day period resulted in an increase in total estrone concentrations (C_{max} 3.68 ng/mL to 4.93 ng/mL) and total equilin concentrations (C_{max} 2.27 ng/mL to 3.22 ng/mL) and a decrease in circulating 17β estradiol concentrations (C_{max} 0.037 ng/mL to 0.030 ng/mL). An increased risk of pulmonary embolism, DVT, stroke and MI has been reported with combined therapy. Discontinue immediately if any of these were to occur).
No products indexed under this heading.

Cimetidine (The metabolism of progesterone by human liver microsomes was inhibited by ketoconazole. Ketoconazole is a known inhibitor of cytochrome P450 3A4, hence these data suggest that ketoconazole or other known inhibitors of this enzyme may increase the bioavailability of progesterone. The clinical relevance of the *in vitro* findings is unknown).
No products indexed under this heading.

Cimetidine Hydrochloride (The metabolism of progesterone by human liver microsomes was inhibited by ketoconazole. Ketoconazole is a known inhibitor of cytochrome P450 3A4, hence these data suggest that ketoconazole or other known inhibitors of this enzyme may increase the bioavailability of progesterone. The clinical relevance of the *in vitro* findings is unknown).
No products indexed under this heading.

Ciprofloxacin (The metabolism of progesterone by human liver microsomes was inhibited by ketoconazole. Ketoconazole is a known inhibitor of cytochrome P450 3A4, hence these data suggest that ketoconazole or other known inhibitors of this enzyme may increase the bioavailability of progesterone. The clinical relevance of the *in vitro* findings is unknown). Products include:
Cipro I.V. 3082
Cipro 3073
Cipro XR 3091
Ciprodex 583

Clarithromycin (The metabolism of progesterone by human liver microsomes was inhibited by ketoconazole. Ketoconazole is a known inhibitor of cytochrome P450 3A4, hence these data suggest that ketoconazole or other known inhibitors of this enzyme may increase the bioavailability of progesterone. The clinical relevance of the *in vitro* findings is unknown). Products include:
Biaxin/Biaxin XL 412

Clotrimazole (The metabolism of progesterone by human liver microsomes was inhibited by ketoconazole. Ketoconazole is a known inhibitor of cytochrome P450 3A4, hence these data suggest that ketoconazole or other known inhibitors of this enzyme may increase the bioavailability of progesterone. The clinical relevance of the *in vitro* findings is unknown). Products include:
Lotrisone 3163

Conivaptan Hydrochloride (The metabolism of progesterone by human liver microsomes was inhibited by ketoconazole. Ketoconazole is a known inhibitor of cytochrome P450 3A4, hence these data suggest that keto-

conazole or other known inhibitors of this enzyme may increase the bioavailability of progesterone. The clinical relevance of the *in vitro* findings is unknown). Products include:

Cyclosporine (The metabolism of progesterone by human liver microsomes was inhibited by ketoconazole. Ketoconazole is a known inhibitor of cytochrome P450 3A4, hence these data suggest that ketoconazole or other known inhibitors of this enzyme may increase the bioavailability of progesterone. The clinical relevance of the *in vitro* findings is unknown). Products include:

Dalfopristin (The metabolism of progesterone by human liver microsomes was inhibited by ketoconazole. Ketoconazole is a known inhibitor of cytochrome P450 3A4, hence these data suggest that ketoconazole or other known inhibitors of this enzyme may increase the bioavailability of progesterone. The clinical relevance of the *in vitro* findings is unknown).

No products indexed under this heading.

Danazol (The metabolism of progesterone by human liver microsomes was inhibited by ketoconazole. Ketoconazole is a known inhibitor of cytochrome P450 3A4, hence these data suggest that ketoconazole or other known inhibitors of this enzyme may increase the bioavailability of progesterone. The clinical relevance of the *in vitro* findings is unknown).

No products indexed under this heading.

Darunavir (The metabolism of progesterone by human liver microsomes was inhibited by ketoconazole. Ketoconazole is a known inhibitor of cytochrome P450 3A4, hence these data suggest that ketoconazole or other known inhibitors of this enzyme may increase the bioavailability of progesterone. The clinical relevance of the *in vitro* findings is unknown).

No products indexed under this heading.

Dasatinib (The metabolism of progesterone by human liver microsomes was inhibited by ketoconazole. Ketoconazole is a known inhibitor of cytochrome P450 3A4, hence these data suggest that ketoconazole or other known inhibitors of this enzyme may increase the bioavailability of progesterone. The clinical relevance of the *in vitro* findings is unknown).

No products indexed under this heading.

Delavirdine Mesylate (The metabolism of progesterone by human liver microsomes was inhibited by ketoconazole. Ketoconazole is a known inhibitor of cytochrome P450 3A4, hence these data suggest that ketoconazole or other known inhibitors of this enzyme may increase the bioavailability of progesterone. The clinical relevance of the *in vitro* findings is unknown).

No products indexed under this heading.

Delavirine (The metabolism of progesterone by human liver microsomes was inhibited by ketoconazole. Ketoconazole is a known inhibitor of cytochrome P450 3A4, hence these data suggest that ketoconazole or other known inhibitors of this enzyme may increase the bioavailability of progesterone. The clinical relevance of the *in vitro* findings is unknown).

No products indexed under this heading.

Desloratadine (The metabolism of progesterone by human liver microsomes was inhibited by ketoconazole. Ketoconazole is a known inhibitor of cytochrome P450 3A4, hence these data suggest that ketoconazole or oth-

---

er known inhibitors of this enzyme may increase the bioavailability of progesterone. The clinical relevance of the *in vitro* findings is unknown). Products include:

Dienestrol (Co-administration of conjugated estrogens and progesterone to 29 post-menopausal women over a 12-day period resulted in an increase in total estrone concentrations (C_{max} 3.68 ng/mL to 4.93 ng/mL) and total equilin concentrations (C_{max} 2.27 ng/mL to 3.22 ng/mL) and a decrease in circulating 17β estradiol concentrations (C_{max} 0.037 ng/mL to 0.030 ng/mL). An increased risk of pulmonary embolism, DVT, stroke and MI has been reported with combined therapy. Discontinue immediately if any of these were to occur).

No products indexed under this heading.

Diethylstilbestrol (Co-administration of conjugated estrogens and progesterone to 29 post-menopausal women over a 12-day period resulted in an increase in total estrone concentrations (C_{max} 3.68 ng/mL to 4.93 ng/mL) and total equilin concentrations (C_{max} 2.27 ng/mL to 3.22 ng/mL) and a decrease in circulating 17β estradiol concentrations (C_{max} 0.037 ng/mL to 0.030 ng/mL). An increased risk of pulmonary embolism, DVT, stroke and MI has been reported with combined therapy. Discontinue immediately if any of these were to occur).

No products indexed under this heading.

Diltiazem Hydrochloride (The metabolism of progesterone by human liver microsomes was inhibited by ketoconazole. Ketoconazole is a known inhibitor of cytochrome P450 3A4, hence these data suggest that ketoconazole or other known inhibitors of this enzyme may increase the bioavailability of progesterone. The clinical relevance of the *in vitro* findings is unknown). Products include:

Diltiazem Maleate (The metabolism of progesterone by human liver microsomes was inhibited by ketoconazole. Ketoconazole is a known inhibitor of cytochrome P450 3A4, hence these data suggest that ketoconazole or other known inhibitors of this enzyme may increase the bioavailability of progesterone. The clinical relevance of the *in vitro* findings is unknown).

No products indexed under this heading.

Efavirenz (The metabolism of progesterone by human liver microsomes was inhibited by ketoconazole. Ketoconazole is a known inhibitor of cytochrome P450 3A4, hence these data suggest that ketoconazole or other known inhibitors of this enzyme may increase the bioavailability of progesterone. The clinical relevance of the *in vitro* findings is unknown). Products include:

Erythromycin (The metabolism of progesterone by human liver microsomes was inhibited by ketoconazole. Ketoconazole is a known inhibitor of cytochrome P450 3A4, hence these data suggest that ketoconazole or other known inhibitors of this enzyme may increase the bioavailability of progesterone. The clinical relevance of the *in vitro* findings is unknown).

No products indexed under this heading.

Erythromycin Estolate (The metabolism of progesterone by human liver microsomes was inhibited by ketoconazole. Ketoconazole is a known inhibitor of cytochrome P450 3A4, hence these data suggest that ketoconazole or other known inhibitors of this enzyme may increase the bioavailability of progesterone. The clinical relevance of the *in vitro* findings is unknown).

No products indexed under this heading.

Erythromycin Ethylsuccinate (The metabolism of progesterone by human liver microsomes was inhibited by ketoconazole. Ketoconazole is a known inhibitor of cytochrome P450 3A4, hence these data suggest that ketoconazole or other known inhibitors of this enzyme may increase the bioavailability of progesterone. The clinical relevance of the *in vitro* findings is unknown). Products include:

Erythromycin Gluceptate (The metabolism of progesterone by human liver microsomes was inhibited by ketoconazole. Ketoconazole is a known inhibitor of cytochrome P450 3A4, hence these data suggest that ketoconazole or other known inhibitors of this enzyme may increase the bioavailability of progesterone. The clinical relevance of the *in vitro* findings is unknown).

No products indexed under this heading.

Erythromycin Lactobionate (The metabolism of progesterone by human liver microsomes was inhibited by ketoconazole. Ketoconazole is a known inhibitor of cytochrome P450 3A4, hence these data suggest that ketoconazole or other known inhibitors of this enzyme may increase the bioavailability of progesterone. The clinical relevance of the *in vitro* findings is unknown).

No products indexed under this heading.

Erythromycin Stearate (The metabolism of progesterone by human liver microsomes was inhibited by ketoconazole. Ketoconazole is a known inhibitor of cytochrome P450 3A4, hence these data suggest that ketoconazole or other known inhibitors of this enzyme may increase the bioavailability of progesterone. The clinical relevance of the *in vitro* findings is unknown).

No products indexed under this heading.

Esomeprazole Magnesium (The metabolism of progesterone by human liver microsomes was inhibited by ketoconazole. Ketoconazole is a known inhibitor of cytochrome P450 3A4, hence these data suggest that ketoconazole or other known inhibitors of this enzyme may increase the bioavailability of progesterone. The clinical relevance of the *in vitro* findings is unknown). Products include:

Esomeprazole Sodium (The metabolism of progesterone by human liver microsomes was inhibited by ketoconazole. Ketoconazole is a known inhibitor of cytochrome P450 3A4, hence these data suggest that ketoconazole or other known inhibitors of this enzyme may increase the bioavailability of progesterone. The clinical relevance of the *in vitro* findings is unknown). Products include:

Estradiol (Co-administration of conjugated estrogens and progesterone to 29 post-menopausal women over a 12-day period resulted in an increase in total estrone concentrations (C_{max} 3.68 ng/mL to 4.93 ng/mL) and total equilin concentrations (C_{max} 2.27 ng/mL to 3.22 ng/mL) and a decrease in circulating 17β estradiol concentrations

---

(C_{max} 0.037 ng/mL to 0.030 ng/mL). An increased risk of pulmonary embolism, DVT, stroke and MI has been reported with combined therapy. Discontinue immediately if any of these were to occur). Products include:

Estrogens, Conjugated (Co-administration of conjugated estrogens and progesterone to 29 post-menopausal women over a 12-day period resulted in an increase in total estrone concentrations (C_{max} 3.68 ng/mL to 4.93 ng/mL) and total equilin concentrations (C_{max} 2.27 ng/mL to 3.22 ng/mL) and a decrease in circulating 17β estradiol concentrations (C_{max} 0.037 ng/mL to 0.03 ng/mL)). Products include:

Estrogens, Esterified (Co-administration of conjugated estrogens and progesterone to 29 post-menopausal women over a 12-day period resulted in an increase in total estrone concentrations (C_{max} 3.68 ng/mL to 4.93 ng/mL) and total equilin concentrations (C_{max} 2.27 ng/mL to 3.22 ng/mL) and a decrease in circulating 17β estradiol concentrations (C_{max} 0.037 ng/mL to 0.030 ng/mL). An increased risk of pulmonary embolism, DVT, stroke and MI has been reported with combined therapy. Discontinue immediately if any of these were to occur).

No products indexed under this heading.

Estropipate (Co-administration of conjugated estrogens and progesterone to 29 post-menopausal women over a 12-day period resulted in an increase in total estrone concentrations (C_{max} 3.68 ng/mL to 4.93 ng/mL) and total equilin concentrations (C_{max} 2.27 ng/mL to 3.22 ng/mL) and a decrease in circulating 17β estradiol concentrations (C_{max} 0.037 ng/mL to 0.030 ng/mL). An increased risk of pulmonary embolism, DVT, stroke and MI has been reported with combined therapy. Discontinue immediately if any of these were to occur).

No products indexed under this heading.

Ethinyl Estradiol (Co-administration of conjugated estrogens and progesterone to 29 post-menopausal women over a 12-day period resulted in an increase in total estrone concentrations (C_{max} 3.68 ng/mL to 4.93 ng/mL) and total equilin concentrations (C_{max} 2.27 ng/mL to 3.22 ng/mL) and a decrease in circulating 17β estradiol concentrations (C_{max} 0.037 ng/mL to 0.030 ng/mL). An increased risk of pulmonary embolism, DVT, stroke and MI has been reported with combined therapy. Discontinue immediately if any of these were to occur). Products include:

Fluconazole (The metabolism of progesterone by human liver microsomes was inhibited by ketoconazole. Ketoconazole is a known inhibitor of cytochrome P450 3A4, hence these data suggest that ketoconazole or other known inhibitors of this enzyme may increase the bioavailability of progesterone. The clinical relevance of the *in vitro* findings is unknown).
No products indexed under this heading.

Fluoxetine (The metabolism of progesterone by human liver microsomes was inhibited by ketoconazole. Ketoconazole is a known inhibitor of cytochrome P450 3A4, hence these data suggest that ketoconazole or other known inhibitors of this enzyme may increase the bioavailability of progesterone. The clinical relevance of the *in vitro* findings is unknown).
No products indexed under this heading.

Fluoxetine Hydrochloride (The metabolism of progesterone by human liver microsomes was inhibited by ketoconazole. Ketoconazole is a known inhibitor of cytochrome P450 3A4, hence these data suggest that ketoconazole or other known inhibitors of this enzyme may increase the bioavailability of progesterone. The clinical relevance of the *in vitro* findings is unknown). Products include:
Prozac Weekly 1941
Prozac Pulvules 1941
Symbyax 1965

Fluvoxamine Maleate (The metabolism of progesterone by human liver microsomes was inhibited by ketoconazole. Ketoconazole is a known inhibitor of cytochrome P450 3A4, hence these data suggest that ketoconazole or other known inhibitors of this enzyme may increase the bioavailability of progesterone. The clinical relevance of the *in vitro* findings is unknown).
No products indexed under this heading.

Fosamprenavir Calcium (The metabolism of progesterone by human liver microsomes was inhibited by ketoconazole. Ketoconazole is a known inhibitor of cytochrome P450 3A4, hence these data suggest that ketoconazole or other known inhibitors of this enzyme may increase the bioavailability of progesterone. The clinical relevance of the *in vitro* findings is unknown). Products include:
Lexiva Oral Suspension 1558
Lexiva 1558

Imatinib Mesylate (The metabolism of progesterone by human liver microsomes was inhibited by ketoconazole. Ketoconazole is a known inhibitor of cytochrome P450 3A4, hence these data suggest that ketoconazole or other known inhibitors of this enzyme may increase the bioavailability of progesterone. The clinical relevance of the *in vitro* findings is unknown). Products include:
Gleevec 2477

Indinavir Sulfate (The metabolism of progesterone by human liver microsomes was inhibited by ketoconazole. Ketoconazole is a known inhibitor of cytochrome P450 3A4, hence these data suggest that ketoconazole or other known inhibitors of this enzyme may increase the bioavailability of progesterone. The clinical relevance of the *in vitro* findings is unknown). Products include:
Crixivan 2113

Isoniazid (The metabolism of progesterone by human liver microsomes was inhibited by ketoconazole. Ketoconazole is a known inhibitor of cytochrome P450 3A4, hence these data suggest that ketoconazole or other known inhibitors of this enzyme may increase the bioavailability of progesterone. The clinical relevance of the *in vitro* findings is unknown).
No products indexed under this heading.

Itraconazole (The metabolism of progesterone by human liver microsomes was inhibited by ketoconazole. Ketoconazole is a known inhibitor of cytochrome P450 3A4, hence these data suggest that ketoconazole or other known inhibitors of this enzyme may increase the bioavailability of progesterone. The clinical relevance of the *in vitro* findings is unknown).
No products indexed under this heading.

Ketoconazole (The metabolism of progesterone by human liver microsomes was inhibited by ketoconazole. Ketoconazole is a known inhibitor of cytochrome P450 3A4, hence these data suggest that ketoconazole or other known inhibitors of this enzyme may increase the bioavailability of progesterone. The clinical relevance of the *in vitro* findings is unknown). Products include:
Extina 3319
Xolegel 3337

Lapatinib (The metabolism of progesterone by human liver microsomes was inhibited by ketoconazole. Ketoconazole is a known inhibitor of cytochrome P450 3A4, hence these data suggest that ketoconazole or other known inhibitors of this enzyme may increase the bioavailability of progesterone. The clinical relevance of the *in vitro* findings is unknown). Products include:
Tykerb 1698

Lopinavir (The metabolism of progesterone by human liver microsomes was inhibited by ketoconazole. Ketoconazole is a known inhibitor of cytochrome P450 3A4, hence these data suggest that ketoconazole or other known inhibitors of this enzyme may increase the bioavailability of progesterone. The clinical relevance of the *in vitro* findings is unknown). Products include:
Kaletra 458

Loratadine (The metabolism of progesterone by human liver microsomes was inhibited by ketoconazole. Ketoconazole is a known inhibitor of cytochrome P450 3A4, hence these data suggest that ketoconazole or other known inhibitors of this enzyme may increase the bioavailability of progesterone. The clinical relevance of the *in vitro* findings is unknown).
No products indexed under this heading.

Metronidazole (The metabolism of progesterone by human liver microsomes was inhibited by ketoconazole. Ketoconazole is a known inhibitor of cytochrome P450 3A4, hence these data suggest that ketoconazole or other known inhibitors of this enzyme may increase the bioavailability of progesterone. The clinical relevance of the *in vitro* findings is unknown). Products include:
Pylera 793

Metronidazole Benzoate (The metabolism of progesterone by human liver microsomes was inhibited by ketoconazole. Ketoconazole is a known inhibitor of cytochrome P450 3A4, hence these data suggest that ketoconazole or other known inhibitors of this enzyme may increase the bioavailability of progesterone. The clinical relevance of the *in vitro* findings is unknown).
No products indexed under this heading.

Metronidazole Hydrochloride (The metabolism of progesterone by human liver microsomes was inhibited by ketoconazole. Ketoconazole is a known inhibitor of cytochrome P450 3A4, hence these data suggest that ketoconazole or other known inhibitors of this enzyme may increase the bioavailability of progesterone. The clinical relevance of the *in vitro* findings is unknown).
No products indexed under this heading.

Metronidazole Sodium (The metabolism of progesterone by human liver microsomes was inhibited by ketoconazole. Ketoconazole is a known inhibitor of cytochrome P450 3A4, hence these data suggest that ketoconazole or other known inhibitors of this enzyme may increase the bioavailability of progesterone. The clinical relevance of the *in vitro* findings is unknown).
No products indexed under this heading.

Miconazole (The metabolism of progesterone by human liver microsomes was inhibited by ketoconazole. Ketoconazole is a known inhibitor of cytochrome P450 3A4, hence these data suggest that ketoconazole or other known inhibitors of this enzyme may increase the bioavailability of progesterone. The clinical relevance of the *in vitro* findings is unknown).
No products indexed under this heading.

Miconazole Nitrate (The metabolism of progesterone by human liver microsomes was inhibited by ketoconazole. Ketoconazole is a known inhibitor of cytochrome P450 3A4, hence these data suggest that ketoconazole or other known inhibitors of this enzyme may increase the bioavailability of progesterone. The clinical relevance of the *in vitro* findings is unknown). Products include:
Vusion Ointment 3335

Mifepristone (The metabolism of progesterone by human liver microsomes was inhibited by ketoconazole. Ketoconazole is a known inhibitor of cytochrome P450 3A4, hence these data suggest that ketoconazole or other known inhibitors of this enzyme may increase the bioavailability of progesterone. The clinical relevance of the *in vitro* findings is unknown).
No products indexed under this heading.

Nefazodone Hydrochloride (The metabolism of progesterone by human liver microsomes was inhibited by ketoconazole. Ketoconazole is a known inhibitor of cytochrome P450 3A4, hence these data suggest that ketoconazole or other known inhibitors of this enzyme may increase the bioavailability of progesterone. The clinical relevance of the *in vitro* findings is unknown).
No products indexed under this heading.

Nelfinavir Mesylate (The metabolism of progesterone by human liver microsomes was inhibited by ketoconazole. Ketoconazole is a known inhibitor of cytochrome P450 3A4, hence these data suggest that ketoconazole or other known inhibitors of this enzyme may increase the bioavailability of progesterone. The clinical relevance of the *in vitro* findings is unknown).
No products indexed under this heading.

Nevirapine (The metabolism of progesterone by human liver microsomes was inhibited by ketoconazole. Ketoconazole is a known inhibitor of cytochrome P450 3A4, hence these data suggest that ketoconazole or other known inhibitors of this enzyme may increase the bioavailability of progesterone. The clinical relevance of the *in vitro* findings is unknown). Products include:
Viramune Oral Suspension 897
Viramune Tablets 897

Niacin (The metabolism of progesterone by human liver microsomes was inhibited by ketoconazole. Ketoconazole is a known inhibitor of cytochrome P450 3A4, hence these data suggest that ketoconazole or other known inhibitors of this enzyme may increase the bioavailability of progesterone. The clinical relevance of the *in vitro* findings is unknown). Products include:
Advicor 402
Cardio Basics 3455
Niaspan 497
Simcor 524

Niacinamide (The metabolism of progesterone by human liver microsomes was inhibited by ketoconazole. Ketoconazole is a known inhibitor of cytochrome P450 3A4, hence these data suggest that ketoconazole or other known inhibitors of this enzyme may increase the bioavailability of progesterone. The clinical relevance of the *in vitro* findings is unknown). Products include:
CitraNatal 90 DHA Capsules 2332
CitraNatal Assure 2332
CitraNatal Rx 2332
Heplive 607

Niacinamide Hydroiodide (The metabolism of progesterone by human liver microsomes was inhibited by ketoconazole. Ketoconazole is a known inhibitor of cytochrome P450 3A4, hence these data suggest that ketoconazole or other known inhibitors of this enzyme may increase the bioavailability of progesterone. The clinical relevance of the *in vitro* findings is unknown).
No products indexed under this heading.

Nicotinamide (The metabolism of progesterone by human liver microsomes was inhibited by ketoconazole. Ketoconazole is a known inhibitor of cytochrome P450 3A4, hence these data suggest that ketoconazole or other known inhibitors of this enzyme may increase the bioavailability of progesterone. The clinical relevance of the *in vitro* findings is unknown).
No products indexed under this heading.

Nifedipine (The metabolism of progesterone by human liver microsomes was inhibited by ketoconazole. Ketoconazole is a known inhibitor of cytochrome P450 3A4, hence these data suggest that ketoconazole or other known inhibitors of this enzyme may increase the bioavailability of progesterone. The clinical relevance of the *in vitro* findings is unknown).
No products indexed under this heading.

Norfloxacin (The metabolism of progesterone by human liver microsomes was inhibited by ketoconazole. Ketoconazole is a known inhibitor of cytochrome P450 3A4, hence these data suggest that ketoconazole or other known inhibitors of this enzyme may increase the bioavailability of progesterone. The clinical relevance of the *in vitro* findings is unknown). Products include:
Noroxin 2220

Omeprazole (The metabolism of progesterone by human liver microsomes was inhibited by ketoconazole. Ketoconazole is a known inhibitor of cytochrome P450 3A4, hence these data suggest that ketoconazole or other known inhibitors of this enzyme may increase the bioavailability of progesterone. The clinical relevance of the *in vitro* findings is unknown).
No products indexed under this heading.

Paroxetine Hydrochloride (The metabolism of progesterone by human liver microsomes was inhibited by ketoconazole. Ketoconazole is a known inhibitor of cytochrome P450 3A4, hence these data suggest that ketoconazole or other known inhibitors of this enzyme may increase the bioavailability of progesterone. The clinical relevance of the *in vitro* findings is unknown). Products include:
Paroxetine CR 2361
Paroxetine ER 2371
Paxil 1586
Paxil CR 1596

Polyestradiol Phosphate (Co-administration of conjugated estrogens and progesterone to 29 postmenopausal women over a 12-day period resulted in an increase in total estrone concentrations (C_{max} 3.68 ng/

mL to 4.93 ng/mL) and total equilin concentrations (C_{max} 2.27 ng/mL to 3.22 ng/mL) and a decrease in circulating 17β estradiol concentrations (C_{max} 0.037 ng/mL to 0.030 ng/mL). An increased risk of pulmonary embolism, DVT, stroke and MI has been reported with combined therapy. Discontinue immediately if any of these were to occur).

No products indexed under this heading.

Posaconazole (The metabolism of progesterone by human liver microsomes was inhibited by ketoconazole. Ketoconazole is a known inhibitor of cytochrome P450 3A4, hence these data suggest that ketoconazole or other known inhibitors of this enzyme may increase the bioavailability of progesterone. The clinical relevance of the *in vitro* findings is unknown). Products include:
Noxafil 3172

Propoxyphene Hydrochloride (The metabolism of progesterone by human liver microsomes was inhibited by ketoconazole. Ketoconazole is a known inhibitor of cytochrome P450 3A4, hence these data suggest that ketoconazole or other known inhibitors of this enzyme may increase the bioavailability of progesterone. The clinical relevance of the *in vitro* findings is unknown).

No products indexed under this heading.

Propoxyphene Napsylate (The metabolism of progesterone by human liver microsomes was inhibited by ketoconazole. Ketoconazole is a known inhibitor of cytochrome P450 3A4, hence these data suggest that ketoconazole or other known inhibitors of this enzyme may increase the bioavailability of progesterone. The clinical relevance of the *in vitro* findings is unknown).

No products indexed under this heading.

Quinestrol (Co-administration of conjugated estrogens and progesterone to 29 post-menopausal women over a 12-day period resulted in an increase in total estrone concentrations (C_{max} 3.68 ng/mL to 4.93 ng/mL) and total equilin concentrations (C_{max} 2.27 ng/mL to 3.22 ng/mL) and a decrease in circulating 17β estradiol concentrations (C_{max} 0.037 ng/mL to 0.030 ng/mL). An increased risk of pulmonary embolism, DVT, stroke and MI has been reported with combined therapy. Discontinue immediately if any of these were to occur).

No products indexed under this heading.

Quinidine (The metabolism of progesterone by human liver microsomes was inhibited by ketoconazole. Ketoconazole is a known inhibitor of cytochrome P450 3A4, hence these data suggest that ketoconazole or other known inhibitors of this enzyme may increase the bioavailability of progesterone. The clinical relevance of the *in vitro* findings is unknown).

No products indexed under this heading.

Quinidine Hydrochloride (The metabolism of progesterone by human liver microsomes was inhibited by ketoconazole. Ketoconazole is a known inhibitor of cytochrome P450 3A4, hence these data suggest that ketoconazole or other known inhibitors of this enzyme may increase the bioavailability of progesterone. The clinical relevance of the *in vitro* findings is unknown).

No products indexed under this heading.

Quinidine Polygalacturonate (The metabolism of progesterone by human liver microsomes was inhibited by ketoconazole. Ketoconazole is a known inhibitor of cytochrome P450 3A4, hence these data suggest that ketoconazole or other known inhibitors of

this enzyme may increase the bioavailability of progesterone. The clinical relevance of the *in vitro* findings is unknown).

No products indexed under this heading.

Quinidine Sulfate (The metabolism of progesterone by human liver microsomes was inhibited by ketoconazole. Ketoconazole is a known inhibitor of cytochrome P450 3A4, hence these data suggest that ketoconazole or other known inhibitors of this enzyme may increase the bioavailability of progesterone. The clinical relevance of the *in vitro* findings is unknown).

No products indexed under this heading.

Quinine (The metabolism of progesterone by human liver microsomes was inhibited by ketoconazole. Ketoconazole is a known inhibitor of cytochrome P450 3A4, hence these data suggest that ketoconazole or other known inhibitors of this enzyme may increase the bioavailability of progesterone. The clinical relevance of the *in vitro* findings is unknown). Products include:
Hyland's Leg Cramps PM with Quinine 3315

Quinine Sulfate (The metabolism of progesterone by human liver microsomes was inhibited by ketoconazole. Ketoconazole is a known inhibitor of cytochrome P450 3A4, hence these data suggest that ketoconazole or other known inhibitors of this enzyme may increase the bioavailability of progesterone. The clinical relevance of the *in vitro* findings is unknown).

No products indexed under this heading.

Quinupristin (The metabolism of progesterone by human liver microsomes was inhibited by ketoconazole. Ketoconazole is a known inhibitor of cytochrome P450 3A4, hence these data suggest that ketoconazole or other known inhibitors of this enzyme may increase the bioavailability of progesterone. The clinical relevance of the *in vitro* findings is unknown).

No products indexed under this heading.

Ranitidine Bismuth Citrate (The metabolism of progesterone by human liver microsomes was inhibited by ketoconazole. Ketoconazole is a known inhibitor of cytochrome P450 3A4, hence these data suggest that ketoconazole or other known inhibitors of this enzyme may increase the bioavailability of progesterone. The clinical relevance of the *in vitro* findings is unknown).

No products indexed under this heading.

Ranitidine Hydrochloride (The metabolism of progesterone by human liver microsomes was inhibited by ketoconazole. Ketoconazole is a known inhibitor of cytochrome P450 3A4, hence these data suggest that ketoconazole or other known inhibitors of this enzyme may increase the bioavailability of progesterone. The clinical relevance of the *in vitro* findings is unknown). Products include:
Zantac 1737
Zantac Injection 1732
Zantac Pharmacy 1735

Ritonavir (The metabolism of progesterone by human liver microsomes was inhibited by ketoconazole. Ketoconazole is a known inhibitor of cytochrome P450 3A4, hence these data suggest that ketoconazole or other known inhibitors of this enzyme may increase the bioavailability of progesterone. The clinical relevance of the *in vitro* findings is unknown). Products include:
Kaletra 458
Norvir 509

Saquinavir (The metabolism of progesterone by human liver microsomes was inhibited by ketoconazole. Ketoconazole is a known inhibitor of cytochrome P450 3A4, hence these data suggest that ketoconazole or other known inhibitors of this enzyme may increase the bioavailability of progesterone. The clinical relevance of the *in vitro* findings is unknown).

No products indexed under this heading.

Saquinavir Mesylate (The metabolism of progesterone by human liver microsomes was inhibited by ketoconazole. Ketoconazole is a known inhibitor of cytochrome P450 3A4, hence these data suggest that ketoconazole or other known inhibitors of this enzyme may increase the bioavailability of progesterone. The clinical relevance of the *in vitro* findings is unknown).

No products indexed under this heading.

Sertraline Hydrochloride (The metabolism of progesterone by human liver microsomes was inhibited by ketoconazole. Ketoconazole is a known inhibitor of cytochrome P450 3A4, hence these data suggest that ketoconazole or other known inhibitors of this enzyme may increase the bioavailability of progesterone. The clinical relevance of the *in vitro* findings is unknown).

No products indexed under this heading.

Sildenafil Citrate (The metabolism of progesterone by human liver microsomes was inhibited by ketoconazole. Ketoconazole is a known inhibitor of cytochrome P450 3A4, hence these data suggest that ketoconazole or other known inhibitors of this enzyme may increase the bioavailability of progesterone. The clinical relevance of the *in vitro* findings is unknown).

No products indexed under this heading.

Telithromycin (The metabolism of progesterone by human liver microsomes was inhibited by ketoconazole. Ketoconazole is a known inhibitor of cytochrome P450 3A4, hence these data suggest that ketoconazole or other known inhibitors of this enzyme may increase the bioavailability of progesterone. The clinical relevance of the *in vitro* findings is unknown). Products include:
Ketek 2991

Troglitazone (The metabolism of progesterone by human liver microsomes was inhibited by ketoconazole. Ketoconazole is a known inhibitor of cytochrome P450 3A4, hence these data suggest that ketoconazole or other known inhibitors of this enzyme may increase the bioavailability of progesterone. The clinical relevance of the *in vitro* findings is unknown).

No products indexed under this heading.

Troleandomycin (The metabolism of progesterone by human liver microsomes was inhibited by ketoconazole. Ketoconazole is a known inhibitor of cytochrome P450 3A4, hence these data suggest that ketoconazole or other known inhibitors of this enzyme may increase the bioavailability of progesterone. The clinical relevance of the *in vitro* findings is unknown).

No products indexed under this heading.

Valproate Sodium (The metabolism of progesterone by human liver microsomes was inhibited by ketoconazole. Ketoconazole is a known inhibitor of cytochrome P450 3A4, hence these data suggest that ketoconazole or other known inhibitors of this enzyme may increase the bioavailability of progesterone. The clinical relevance of the *in vitro* findings is unknown).

No products indexed under this heading.

Vardenafil Hydrochloride (The metabolism of progesterone by human liver microsomes was inhibited by keto-

conazole. Ketoconazole is a known inhibitor of cytochrome P450 3A4, hence these data suggest that ketoconazole or other known inhibitors of this enzyme may increase the bioavailability of progesterone. The clinical relevance of the *in vitro* findings is unknown). Products include:
Levitra 3157

Verapamil Hydrochloride (The metabolism of progesterone by human liver microsomes was inhibited by ketoconazole. Ketoconazole is a known inhibitor of cytochrome P450 3A4, hence these data suggest that ketoconazole or other known inhibitors of this enzyme may increase the bioavailability of progesterone. The clinical relevance of the *in vitro* findings is unknown). Products include:
Tarka 534

Voriconazole (The metabolism of progesterone by human liver microsomes was inhibited by ketoconazole. Ketoconazole is a known inhibitor of cytochrome P450 3A4, hence these data suggest that ketoconazole or other known inhibitors of this enzyme may increase the bioavailability of progesterone. The clinical relevance of the *in vitro* findings is unknown).

No products indexed under this heading.

Zafirlukast (The metabolism of progesterone by human liver microsomes was inhibited by ketoconazole. Ketoconazole is a known inhibitor of cytochrome P450 3A4, hence these data suggest that ketoconazole or other known inhibitors of this enzyme may increase the bioavailability of progesterone. The clinical relevance of the *in vitro* findings is unknown). Products include:
Accolate 3612

Zileuton (The metabolism of progesterone by human liver microsomes was inhibited by ketoconazole. Ketoconazole is a known inhibitor of cytochrome P450 3A4, hence these data suggest that ketoconazole or other known inhibitors of this enzyme may increase the bioavailability of progesterone. The clinical relevance of the *in vitro* findings is unknown).

No products indexed under this heading.

Food Interactions

Food, unspecified (Concomitant food ingestion increased the bioavailability of progesterone relative to a fasting state when administered to post-menopausal women at a dose of 200 mg).

Grapefruit (The metabolism of progesterone by human liver microsomes was inhibited by ketoconazole. Ketoconazole is a known inhibitor of cytochrome P450 3A4, hence these data suggest that ketoconazole or other known inhibitors of this enzyme may increase the bioavailability of progesterone. The clinical relevance of the *in vitro* findings is unknown).

Grapefruit Juice (The metabolism of progesterone by human liver microsomes was inhibited by ketoconazole. Ketoconazole is a known inhibitor of cytochrome P450 3A4, hence these data suggest that ketoconazole or other known inhibitors of this enzyme may increase the bioavailability of progesterone. The clinical relevance of the *in vitro* findings is unknown).

Meal, unspecified (Concomitant food ingestion increased the bioavailability of progesterone relative to a fasting state when administered to post-menopausal women at a dose of 200 mg).

PROPECIA TABLETS
(Finasteride) 2250
None cited in PDR database.

IMPORTANT NOTE: Always consult each drug listing in the patient's regimen for possible interactions.

ProQuad Interactions Index 1520

PROQUAD
(Measles, Mumps, Rubella and Varicella Virus Vaccine Live, Measles, Mumps & Rubella Virus Vaccine, Live).... 2254
May interact with corticosteroids, immunosuppressive agents, salicylates, and certain other agents. Compounds in these categories include:

Alclometasone Dipropionate (Measles, Mumps, Rubella, and Varicella Virus Vaccine, Live may be used in individuals who are receiving topical corticosteroids or low-dose corticosteroids for asthma prophylaxis or replacement therapy, (eg, for Addison's disease). Measles, Mumps, Rubella, and Varicella Virus Vaccine, Live should not be given to individuals receiving immunosuppressive doses of corticosteroids or other immunosuppressive drugs).
No products indexed under this heading.

Aspirin (Reye's syndrome has been reported following the use of salicylates during wild-type varicella infection. Vaccine recipients should avoid use of salicylates for 6 weeks after vaccination with Measles, Mumps, Rubella, and Varicella Virus Vaccine, Live). Products include:
Aggrenox 880
Bayer Aspirin 829
Percodan 1124
St. Joseph Aspirin 2045

Aspirin, Enteric Coated (Reye's syndrome has been reported following the use of salicylates during wild-type varicella infection. Vaccine recipients should avoid use of salicylates for 6 weeks after vaccination with Measles, Mumps, Rubella, and Varicella Virus Vaccine, Live).
No products indexed under this heading.

Aspirin Buffered (Reye's syndrome has been reported following the use of salicylates during wild-type varicella infection. Vaccine recipients should avoid use of salicylates for 6 weeks after vaccination with Measles, Mumps, Rubella, and Varicella Virus Vaccine, Live).
No products indexed under this heading.

Azathioprine (Measles, Mumps, Rubella, and Varicella Virus Vaccine, Live may be used in individuals who are receiving topical corticosteroids or low-dose corticosteroids for asthma prophylaxis or replacement therapy, (eg, for Addison's disease). Measles, Mumps, Rubella, and Varicella Virus Vaccine, Live should not be given to individuals receiving immunosuppressive doses of corticosteroids or other immunosuppressive drugs).
No products indexed under this heading.

Basiliximab (Measles, Mumps, Rubella, and Varicella Virus Vaccine, Live may be used in individuals who are receiving topical corticosteroids or low-dose corticosteroids for asthma prophylaxis or replacement therapy, (eg, for Addison's disease). Measles, Mumps, Rubella, and Varicella Virus Vaccine, Live should not be given to individuals receiving immunosuppressive doses of corticosteroids or other immunosuppressive drugs). Products include:
Simulect 2524

Beclomethasone Dipropionate (Measles, Mumps, Rubella, and Varicella Virus Vaccine, Live may be used in individuals who are receiving topical corticosteroids or low-dose corticosteroids for asthma prophylaxis or replacement therapy, (eg, for Addison's disease). Measles, Mumps, Rubella, and Varicella Virus Vaccine, Live should not be given to individuals receiving immunosuppressive doses of corticosteroids or other immunosuppressive drugs). Products include:
Qvar 3398

Beclomethasone Dipropionate Monohydrate (Measles, Mumps, Rubella, and Varicella Virus Vaccine, Live may be used in individuals who are receiving topical corticosteroids or low-dose corticosteroids for asthma prophylaxis or replacement therapy, (eg, for Addison's disease). Measles, Mumps, Rubella, and Varicella Virus Vaccine, Live should not be given to individuals receiving immunosuppressive doses of corticosteroids or other immunosuppressive drugs). Products include:
Beconase AQ 1386

Betamethasone (Measles, Mumps, Rubella, and Varicella Virus Vaccine, Live may be used in individuals who are receiving topical corticosteroids or low-dose corticosteroids for asthma prophylaxis or replacement therapy, (eg, for Addison's disease). Measles, Mumps, Rubella, and Varicella Virus Vaccine, Live should not be given to individuals receiving immunosuppressive doses of corticosteroids or other immunosuppressive drugs).
No products indexed under this heading.

Betamethasone Acetate (Measles, Mumps, Rubella, and Varicella Virus Vaccine, Live may be used in individuals who are receiving topical corticosteroids or low-dose corticosteroids for asthma prophylaxis or replacement therapy, (eg, for Addison's disease). Measles, Mumps, Rubella, and Varicella Virus Vaccine, Live should not be given to individuals receiving immunosuppressive doses of corticosteroids or other immunosuppressive drugs).
No products indexed under this heading.

Betamethasone Benzoate (Measles, Mumps, Rubella, and Varicella Virus Vaccine, Live may be used in individuals who are receiving topical corticosteroids or low-dose corticosteroids for asthma prophylaxis or replacement therapy, (eg, for Addison's disease). Measles, Mumps, Rubella, and Varicella Virus Vaccine, Live should not be given to individuals receiving immunosuppressive doses of corticosteroids or other immunosuppressive drugs).
No products indexed under this heading.

Betamethasone Dipropionate (Measles, Mumps, Rubella, and Varicella Virus Vaccine, Live may be used in individuals who are receiving topical corticosteroids or low-dose corticosteroids for asthma prophylaxis or replacement therapy, (eg, for Addison's disease). Measles, Mumps, Rubella, and Varicella Virus Vaccine, Live should not be given to individuals receiving immunosuppressive doses of corticosteroids or other immunosuppressive drugs). Products include:
Diprolene Lotion 0.05% 3108
Diprolene Ointment 0.05% 3109
Diprolene AF Cream 0.05% 3107
Lotrisone 3163

Betamethasone Sodium Phosphate (Measles, Mumps, Rubella, and Varicella Virus Vaccine, Live may be used in individuals who are receiving topical corticosteroids or low-dose corticosteroids for asthma prophylaxis or replacement therapy, (eg, for Addison's disease). Measles, Mumps, Rubella, and Varicella Virus Vaccine, Live should not be given to individuals receiving immunosuppressive doses of corticosteroids or other immunosuppressive drugs).
No products indexed under this heading.

Betamethasone Valerate (Measles, Mumps, Rubella, and Varicella Virus Vaccine, Live may be used in individuals who are receiving topical corticosteroids or low-dose corticosteroids for asthma prophylaxis or replacement therapy, (eg, for Addison's disease). Measles, Mumps, Rubella, and Varicella Virus Vaccine, Live should not be given to individuals receiving immunosuppressive doses of corticosteroids or other immunosuppressive drugs). Products include:
Luxiq 3321

Budesonide (Measles, Mumps, Rubella, and Varicella Virus Vaccine, Live may be used in individuals who are receiving topical corticosteroids or low-dose corticosteroids for asthma prophylaxis or replacement therapy, (eg, for Addison's disease). Measles, Mumps, Rubella, and Varicella Virus Vaccine, Live should not be given to individuals receiving immunosuppressive doses of corticosteroids or other immunosuppressive drugs). Products include:
Pulmicort Flexhaler 714
Symbicort 80/4.5 720
Symbicort 160/4.5 720

Choline Magnesium Trisalicylate (Reye's syndrome has been reported following the use of salicylates during wild-type varicella infection. Vaccine recipients should avoid use of salicylates for 6 weeks after vaccination with Measles, Mumps, Rubella, and Varicella Virus Vaccine, Live).
No products indexed under this heading.

Ciclesonide (Measles, Mumps, Rubella, and Varicella Virus Vaccine, Live may be used in individuals who are receiving topical corticosteroids or low-dose corticosteroids for asthma prophylaxis or replacement therapy, (eg, for Addison's disease). Measles, Mumps, Rubella, and Varicella Virus Vaccine, Live should not be given to individuals receiving immunosuppressive doses of corticosteroids or other immunosuppressive drugs).
No products indexed under this heading.

Cortisone Acetate (Measles, Mumps, Rubella, and Varicella Virus Vaccine, Live may be used in individuals who are receiving topical corticosteroids or low-dose corticosteroids for asthma prophylaxis or replacement therapy, (eg, for Addison's disease). Measles, Mumps, Rubella, and Varicella Virus Vaccine, Live should not be given to individuals receiving immunosuppressive doses of corticosteroids or other immunosuppressive drugs).
No products indexed under this heading.

Cyclosporine (Measles, Mumps, Rubella, and Varicella Virus Vaccine, Live may be used in individuals who are receiving topical corticosteroids or low-dose corticosteroids for asthma prophylaxis or replacement therapy, (eg, for Addison's disease). Measles, Mumps, Rubella, and Varicella Virus Vaccine, Live should not be given to individuals receiving immunosuppressive doses of corticosteroids or other immunosuppressive drugs). Products include:
Gengraf 440
Neoral Oral Solution 2496
Neoral Capsules 2496
Restasis 605

Desoximetasone (Measles, Mumps, Rubella, and Varicella Virus Vaccine, Live may be used in individuals who are receiving topical corticosteroids or low-dose corticosteroids for asthma prophylaxis or replacement therapy, (eg, for Addison's disease). Measles, Mumps, Rubella, and Varicella Virus Vaccine, Live should not be given to individuals receiving immunosuppressive doses of corticosteroids or other immunosuppressive drugs).
No products indexed under this heading.

Dexamethasone (Measles, Mumps, Rubella, and Varicella Virus Vaccine, Live may be used in individuals who are receiving topical corticosteroids or low-dose corticosteroids for asthma prophylaxis or replacement therapy, (eg, for Addison's disease). Measles, Mumps, Rubella, and Varicella Virus Vaccine, Live should not be given to individuals receiving immunosuppressive doses of corticosteroids or other immunosuppressive drugs). Products include:
Ciprodex 583
Ozurdex .... ⊙223
Tobramycin and Dexamethasone Ophthalmic Suspension .... ⊙251

Dexamethasone Acetate (Measles, Mumps, Rubella, and Varicella Virus Vaccine, Live may be used in individuals who are receiving topical corticosteroids or low-dose corticosteroids for asthma prophylaxis or replacement therapy, (eg, for Addison's disease). Measles, Mumps, Rubella, and Varicella Virus Vaccine, Live should not be given to individuals receiving immunosuppressive doses of corticosteroids or other immunosuppressive drugs).
No products indexed under this heading.

Dexamethasone Phosphate (Measles, Mumps, Rubella, and Varicella Virus Vaccine, Live may be used in individuals who are receiving topical corticosteroids or low-dose corticosteroids for asthma prophylaxis or replacement therapy, (eg, for Addison's disease). Measles, Mumps, Rubella, and Varicella Virus Vaccine, Live should not be given to individuals receiving immunosuppressive doses of corticosteroids or other immunosuppressive drugs).
No products indexed under this heading.

Dexamethasone Sodium (Measles, Mumps, Rubella, and Varicella Virus Vaccine, Live may be used in individuals who are receiving topical corticosteroids or low-dose corticosteroids for asthma prophylaxis or replacement therapy, (eg, for Addison's disease). Measles, Mumps, Rubella, and Varicella Virus Vaccine, Live should not be given to individuals receiving immunosuppressive doses of corticosteroids or other immunosuppressive drugs).
No products indexed under this heading.

Dexamethasone Sodium Phosphate (Measles, Mumps, Rubella, and Varicella Virus Vaccine, Live may be used in individuals who are receiving topical corticosteroids or low-dose corticosteroids for asthma prophylaxis or replacement therapy, (eg, for Addison's disease). Measles, Mumps, Rubella, and Varicella Virus Vaccine, Live should not be given to individuals receiving immunosuppressive doses of corticosteroids or other immunosuppressive drugs).
No products indexed under this heading.

Dexamethasone Sodium Phosphate Injection (Measles, Mumps, Rubella, and Varicella Virus Vaccine, Live may be used in individuals who are receiving topical corticosteroids or low-dose corticosteroids for asthma prophylaxis or replacement therapy, (eg, for Addison's disease). Measles, Mumps, Rubella, and Varicella Virus Vaccine, Live should not be given to individuals receiving immunosuppressive doses of corticosteroids or other immunosuppressive drugs).
No products indexed under this heading.

Diflorasone Diacetate (Measles, Mumps, Rubella, and Varicella Virus Vaccine, Live may be used in individuals who are receiving topical corticosteroids or low-dose corticosteroids for asthma prophylaxis or replacement therapy, (eg, for Addison's disease). Measles, Mumps, Rubella, and Varicella Virus Vaccine, Live should not be given to individuals receiving immunosuppressive doses of corticosteroids or other immunosuppressive drugs).
No products indexed under this heading.

1521 Interactions Index ProQuad

Diflunisal (Reye's syndrome has been reported following the use of salicylates during wild-type varicella infection. Vaccine recipients should avoid use of salicylates for 6 weeks after vaccination with Measles, Mumps, Rubella, and Varicella Virus Vaccine, Live).
No products indexed under this heading.

Fludrocortisone Acetate (Measles, Mumps, Rubella, and Varicella Virus Vaccine, Live may be used in individuals who are receiving topical corticosteroids or low-dose corticosteroids for asthma prophylaxis or replacement therapy, (eg, for Addison's disease). Measles, Mumps, Rubella, and Varicella Virus Vaccine, Live should not be given to individuals receiving immunosuppressive doses of corticosteroids or other immunosuppressive drugs).
No products indexed under this heading.

Flumethasone Pivalate (Measles, Mumps, Rubella, and Varicella Virus Vaccine, Live may be used in individuals who are receiving topical corticosteroids or low-dose corticosteroids for asthma prophylaxis or replacement therapy, (eg, for Addison's disease). Measles, Mumps, Rubella, and Varicella Virus Vaccine, Live should not be given to individuals receiving immunosuppressive doses of corticosteroids or other immunosuppressive drugs).
No products indexed under this heading.

Flunisolide Hemihydrate (Measles, Mumps, Rubella, and Varicella Virus Vaccine, Live may be used in individuals who are receiving topical corticosteroids or low-dose corticosteroids for asthma prophylaxis or replacement therapy, (eg, for Addison's disease). Measles, Mumps, Rubella, and Varicella Virus Vaccine, Live should not be given to individuals receiving immunosuppressive doses of corticosteroids or other immunosuppressive drugs).
No products indexed under this heading.

Fluticasone Furoate (Measles, Mumps, Rubella, and Varicella Virus Vaccine, Live may be used in individuals who are receiving topical corticosteroids or low-dose corticosteroids for asthma prophylaxis or replacement therapy, (eg, for Addison's disease). Measles, Mumps, Rubella, and Varicella Virus Vaccine, Live should not be given to individuals receiving immunosuppressive doses of corticosteroids or other immunosuppressive drugs). Products include:
Veramyst **1713**

Fluticasone Propionate (Measles, Mumps, Rubella, and Varicella Virus Vaccine, Live may be used in individuals who are receiving topical corticosteroids or low-dose corticosteroids for asthma prophylaxis or replacement therapy, (eg, for Addison's disease). Measles, Mumps, Rubella, and Varicella Virus Vaccine, Live should not be given to individuals receiving immunosuppressive doses of corticosteroids or other immunosuppressive drugs). Products include:
Advair 100/50 .... **1275**
Advair 250/50 .... **1275**
Advair 500/50 .... **1275**
Advair HFA 45/21 .... **1288**
Advair HFA 115/21 .... **1288**
Advair HFA 230/21 .... **1288**
Flonase **1459**
Flovent Diskus **1463**
Flovent HFA **1470**

Globulin, Immune (Human) (Immune globulins administered concomitantly with Measles, Mumps, Rubella, and Varicella Virus Vaccine, Live may interfere with the expected immune response. Vaccination should be deferred for at least 3 months following blood plasma transfusions, or administration of immune globulins (IG)). Products include:

Hydrocortisone (Measles, Mumps, Rubella, and Varicella Virus Vaccine, Live may be used in individuals who are receiving topical corticosteroids or low-dose corticosteroids for asthma prophylaxis or replacement therapy, (eg, for Addison's disease). Measles, Mumps, Rubella, and Varicella Virus Vaccine, Live should not be given to individuals receiving immunosuppressive doses of corticosteroids or other immunosuppressive drugs).
No products indexed under this heading.

Hydrocortisone (Alcohol) (Measles, Mumps, Rubella, and Varicella Virus Vaccine, Live may be used in individuals who are receiving topical corticosteroids or low-dose corticosteroids for asthma prophylaxis or replacement therapy, (eg, for Addison's disease). Measles, Mumps, Rubella, and Varicella Virus Vaccine, Live should not be given to individuals receiving immunosuppressive doses of corticosteroids or other immunosuppressive drugs).
No products indexed under this heading.

Hydrocortisone Acetate (Measles, Mumps, Rubella, and Varicella Virus Vaccine, Live may be used in individuals who are receiving topical corticosteroids or low-dose corticosteroids for asthma prophylaxis or replacement therapy, (eg, for Addison's disease). Measles, Mumps, Rubella, and Varicella Virus Vaccine, Live should not be given to individuals receiving immunosuppressive doses of corticosteroids or other immunosuppressive drugs).
No products indexed under this heading.

Hydrocortisone Butyrate (Measles, Mumps, Rubella, and Varicella Virus Vaccine, Live may be used in individuals who are receiving topical corticosteroids or low-dose corticosteroids for asthma prophylaxis or replacement therapy, (eg, for Addison's disease). Measles, Mumps, Rubella, and Varicella Virus Vaccine, Live should not be given to individuals receiving immunosuppressive doses of corticosteroids or other immunosuppressive drugs).
No products indexed under this heading.

Hydrocortisone Cypionate (Measles, Mumps, Rubella, and Varicella Virus Vaccine, Live may be used in individuals who are receiving topical corticosteroids or low-dose corticosteroids for asthma prophylaxis or replacement therapy, (eg, for Addison's disease). Measles, Mumps, Rubella, and Varicella Virus Vaccine, Live should not be given to individuals receiving immunosuppressive doses of corticosteroids or other immunosuppressive drugs).
No products indexed under this heading.

Hydrocortisone Hemisuccinate (Measles, Mumps, Rubella, and Varicella Virus Vaccine, Live may be used in individuals who are receiving topical corticosteroids or low-dose corticosteroids for asthma prophylaxis or replacement therapy, (eg, for Addison's disease). Measles, Mumps, Rubella, and Varicella Virus Vaccine, Live should not be given to individuals receiving immunosuppressive doses of corticosteroids or other immunosuppressive drugs).
No products indexed under this heading.

Hydrocortisone Probutate (Measles, Mumps, Rubella, and Varicella Virus Vaccine, Live may be used in individuals who are receiving topical corticosteroids or low-dose corticosteroids for asthma prophylaxis or replacement therapy, (eg, for Addison's disease). Measles, Mumps, Rubella, and Varicella Virus Vaccine, Live should not be given to individuals receiving immunosuppressive doses of corticosteroids or other immunosuppressive drugs).
No products indexed under this heading.

Hydrocortisone Sodium Phosphate (Measles, Mumps, Rubella, and Varicella Virus Vaccine, Live may be used in individuals who are receiving topical corticosteroids or low-dose corticosteroids for asthma prophylaxis or replacement therapy, (eg, for Addison's disease). Measles, Mumps, Rubella, and Varicella Virus Vaccine, Live should not be given to individuals receiving immunosuppressive doses of corticosteroids or other immunosuppressive drugs).
No products indexed under this heading.

Hydrocortisone Sodium Succinate (Measles, Mumps, Rubella, and Varicella Virus Vaccine, Live may be used in individuals who are receiving topical corticosteroids or low-dose corticosteroids for asthma prophylaxis or replacement therapy, (eg, for Addison's disease). Measles, Mumps, Rubella, and Varicella Virus Vaccine, Live should not be given to individuals receiving immunosuppressive doses of corticosteroids or other immunosuppressive drugs).
No products indexed under this heading.

Hydrocortisone Valerate (Measles, Mumps, Rubella, and Varicella Virus Vaccine, Live may be used in individuals who are receiving topical corticosteroids or low-dose corticosteroids for asthma prophylaxis or replacement therapy, (eg, for Addison's disease). Measles, Mumps, Rubella, and Varicella Virus Vaccine, Live should not be given to individuals receiving immunosuppressive doses of corticosteroids or other immunosuppressive drugs).
No products indexed under this heading.

Magnesium Salicylate (Reye's syndrome has been reported following the use of salicylates during wild-type varicella infection. Vaccine recipients should avoid use of salicylates for 6 weeks after vaccination with Measles, Mumps, Rubella, and Varicella Virus Vaccine, Live).
No products indexed under this heading.

Methylprednisolone (Measles, Mumps, Rubella, and Varicella Virus Vaccine, Live may be used in individuals who are receiving topical corticosteroids or low-dose corticosteroids for asthma prophylaxis or replacement therapy, (eg, for Addison's disease). Measles, Mumps, Rubella, and Varicella Virus Vaccine, Live should not be given to individuals receiving immunosuppressive doses of corticosteroids or other immunosuppressive drugs).
No products indexed under this heading.

Methylprednisolone Acetate (Measles, Mumps, Rubella, and Varicella Virus Vaccine, Live may be used in individuals who are receiving topical corticosteroids or low-dose corticosteroids for asthma prophylaxis or replacement therapy, (eg, for Addison's disease). Measles, Mumps, Rubella, and Varicella Virus Vaccine, Live should not be given to individuals receiving immunosuppressive doses of corticosteroids or other immunosuppressive drugs).
No products indexed under this heading.

Methylprednisolone Sodium Succinate (Measles, Mumps, Rubella, and Varicella Virus Vaccine, Live may be used in individuals who are receiving topical corticosteroids or low-dose corticosteroids for asthma prophylaxis or replacement therapy, (eg, for Addison's disease). Measles, Mumps, Rubella, and Varicella Virus Vaccine, Live should not be given to individuals receiving immunosuppressive doses of corticosteroids or other immunosuppressive drugs).
No products indexed under this heading.

Mometasone Furoate (Measles, Mumps, Rubella, and Varicella Virus Vaccine, Live may be used in individuals who are receiving topical corticosteroids or low-dose corticosteroids for asthma prophylaxis or replacement therapy, (eg, for Addison's disease). Measles, Mumps, Rubella, and Varicella Virus Vaccine, Live should not be given to individuals receiving immunosuppressive doses of corticosteroids or other immunosuppressive drugs). Products include:
Asmanex **3058**
Elocon Cream **3111**
Elocon Lotion **3112**
Elocon Ointment **3114**

Mometasone Furoate Monohydrate (Measles, Mumps, Rubella, and Varicella Virus Vaccine, Live may be used in individuals who are receiving topical corticosteroids or low-dose corticosteroids for asthma prophylaxis or replacement therapy, (eg, for Addison's disease). Measles, Mumps, Rubella, and Varicella Virus Vaccine, Live should not be given to individuals receiving immunosuppressive doses of corticosteroids or other immunosuppressive drugs). Products include:
Nasonex **3166**

Muromonab-CD3 (Measles, Mumps, Rubella, and Varicella Virus Vaccine, Live may be used in individuals who are receiving topical corticosteroids or low-dose corticosteroids for asthma prophylaxis or replacement therapy, (eg, for Addison's disease). Measles, Mumps, Rubella, and Varicella Virus Vaccine, Live should not be given to individuals receiving immunosuppressive doses of corticosteroids or other immunosuppressive drugs). Products include:
Orthoclone OKT3 .... **949**

Mycophenolate Mofetil (Measles, Mumps, Rubella, and Varicella Virus Vaccine, Live may be used in individuals who are receiving topical corticosteroids or low-dose corticosteroids for asthma prophylaxis or replacement therapy, (eg, for Addison's disease). Measles, Mumps, Rubella, and Varicella Virus Vaccine, Live should not be given to individuals receiving immunosuppressive doses of corticosteroids or other immunosuppressive drugs).
No products indexed under this heading.

Prednisolone (Measles, Mumps, Rubella, and Varicella Virus Vaccine, Live may be used in individuals who are receiving topical corticosteroids or low-dose corticosteroids for asthma prophylaxis or replacement therapy, (eg, for Addison's disease). Measles, Mumps, Rubella, and Varicella Virus Vaccine, Live should not be given to individuals receiving immunosuppressive doses of corticosteroids or other immunosuppressive drugs).
No products indexed under this heading.

Prednisolone Acetate (Measles, Mumps, Rubella, and Varicella Virus Vaccine, Live may be used in individuals who are receiving topical corticosteroids or low-dose corticosteroids for asthma prophylaxis or replacement therapy, (eg, for Addison's disease). Measles, Mumps, Rubella, and Varicella Virus Vaccine, Live should not be given to individuals receiving immunosuppressive doses of corticosteroids or other immunosuppressive drugs). Products include:
Blephamide .... ⊙ **212**, ⊙ **214**
Pred Forte .... ⊙ **225**
Pred Mild .... ⊙ **230**
Pred-G .... ⊙ **226**, ⊙ **227**

Prednisolone Sodium Phosphate (Measles, Mumps, Rubella, and Varicella Virus Vaccine, Live may be used in individuals who are receiving topical corticosteroids or low-dose corticosteroids

ProQuad Interactions Index 1522

for asthma prophylaxis or replacement therapy, (eg, for Addison's disease). Measles, Mumps, Rubella, and Varicella Virus Vaccine, Live should not be given to individuals receiving immunosuppressive doses of corticosteroids or other immunosuppressive drugs).
No products indexed under this heading.

Prednisolone Tebutate (Measles, Mumps, Rubella, and Varicella Virus Vaccine, Live may be used in individuals who are receiving topical corticosteroids or low-dose corticosteroids for asthma prophylaxis or replacement therapy, (eg, for Addison's disease). Measles, Mumps, Rubella, and Varicella Virus Vaccine, Live should not be given to individuals receiving immunosuppressive doses of corticosteroids or other immunosuppressive drugs).
No products indexed under this heading.

Prednisone (Measles, Mumps, Rubella, and Varicella Virus Vaccine, Live may be used in individuals who are receiving topical corticosteroids or low-dose corticosteroids for asthma prophylaxis or replacement therapy, (eg, for Addison's disease). Measles, Mumps, Rubella, and Varicella Virus Vaccine, Live should not be given to individuals receiving immunosuppressive doses of corticosteroids or other immunosuppressive drugs).
No products indexed under this heading.

Prednisone sodium phosphate (Measles, Mumps, Rubella, and Varicella Virus Vaccine, Live may be used in individuals who are receiving topical corticosteroids or low-dose corticosteroids for asthma prophylaxis or replacement therapy, (eg, for Addison's disease). Measles, Mumps, Rubella, and Varicella Virus Vaccine, Live should not be given to individuals receiving immunosuppressive doses of corticosteroids or other immunosuppressive drugs).
No products indexed under this heading.

Rapamycin (Measles, Mumps, Rubella, and Varicella Virus Vaccine, Live may be used in individuals who are receiving topical corticosteroids or low-dose corticosteroids for asthma prophylaxis or replacement therapy, (eg, for Addison's disease). Measles, Mumps, Rubella, and Varicella Virus Vaccine, Live should not be given to individuals receiving immunosuppressive doses of corticosteroids or other immunosuppressive drugs).
No products indexed under this heading.

Salsalate (Reye's syndrome has been reported following the use of salicylates during wild-type varicella infection. Vaccine recipients should avoid use of salicylates for 6 weeks after vaccination with Measles, Mumps, Rubella, and Varicella Virus Vaccine, Live).
No products indexed under this heading.

Sirolimus (Measles, Mumps, Rubella, and Varicella Virus Vaccine, Live may be used in individuals who are receiving topical corticosteroids or low-dose corticosteroids for asthma prophylaxis or replacement therapy, (eg, for Addison's disease). Measles, Mumps, Rubella, and Varicella Virus Vaccine, Live should not be given to individuals receiving immunosuppressive doses of corticosteroids or other immunosuppressive drugs). Products include:
Rapamune 3579

Tacrolimus (Measles, Mumps, Rubella, and Varicella Virus Vaccine, Live may be used in individuals who are receiving topical corticosteroids or low-dose corticosteroids for asthma prophylaxis or replacement therapy, (eg, for Addison's disease). Measles, Mumps, Rubella, and Varicella Virus Vaccine, Live should not be given to individuals receiving immunosuppressive doses of corticosteroids or other immunosuppressive drugs). Products include:
Prograf Capsules 677
Prograf Injection 677
Protopic 685

Triamcinolone (Measles, Mumps, Rubella, and Varicella Virus Vaccine, Live may be used in individuals who are receiving topical corticosteroids or low-dose corticosteroids for asthma prophylaxis or replacement therapy, (eg, for Addison's disease). Measles, Mumps, Rubella, and Varicella Virus Vaccine, Live should not be given to individuals receiving immunosuppressive doses of corticosteroids or other immunosuppressive drugs).
No products indexed under this heading.

Triamcinolone Acetonide (Measles, Mumps, Rubella, and Varicella Virus Vaccine, Live may be used in individuals who are receiving topical corticosteroids or low-dose corticosteroids for asthma prophylaxis or replacement therapy, (eg, for Addison's disease). Measles, Mumps, Rubella, and Varicella Virus Vaccine, Live should not be given to individuals receiving immunosuppressive doses of corticosteroids or other immunosuppressive drugs). Products include:
Azmacort 408
Nasacort AQ 3019

Triamcinolone Diacetate (Measles, Mumps, Rubella, and Varicella Virus Vaccine, Live may be used in individuals who are receiving topical corticosteroids or low-dose corticosteroids for asthma prophylaxis or replacement therapy, (eg, for Addison's disease). Measles, Mumps, Rubella, and Varicella Virus Vaccine, Live should not be given to individuals receiving immunosuppressive doses of corticosteroids or other immunosuppressive drugs).
No products indexed under this heading.

Triamcinolone Hexacetonide (Measles, Mumps, Rubella, and Varicella Virus Vaccine, Live may be used in individuals who are receiving topical corticosteroids or low-dose corticosteroids for asthma prophylaxis or replacement therapy, (eg, for Addison's disease). Measles, Mumps, Rubella, and Varicella Virus Vaccine, Live should not be given to individuals receiving immunosuppressive doses of corticosteroids or other immunosuppressive drugs).
No products indexed under this heading.

PROSCAR TABLETS

(Finasteride) 2257
None cited in PDR database.

PROTONIX DELAYED-RELEASE TABLETS

(Pantoprazole Sodium) 3571
May interact with iron containing oral preparations, and certain other agents. Compounds in these categories include:

Atazanavir (Concomitant administration of pantoprazole may reduce the plasma levels of atazanavir. Concomitant use of atazanavir and proton pump inhibitors is not recommended. Concomitant use may substantially decrease atazanavir concentration and thereby reduce its therapeutic effect).
No products indexed under this heading.

Atazanavir Sulfate (Concomitant administration of pantoprazole may reduce the plasma levels of atazanavir. Concomitant use of atazanavir and proton pump inhibitors is not recommended. Concomitant use may substantially decrease atazanavir concentration and thereby reduce its therapeutic effect).
No products indexed under this heading.

Bacampicillin Hydrochloride (Pantoprazole produces sustained inhibition of gastric acid secretion; pantoprazole may interfere with the absorption of certain drugs, such as ampicillin esters, where gastric pH is an important determinant of the bioavailability).
No products indexed under this heading.

Ferrous Fumarate (Pantoprazole produces sustained inhibition of gastric acid secretion; pantoprazole may interfere with the absorption of certain drugs, such as iron salts, where gastric pH is an important determinant of the bioavailability). Products include:
PreNexa 3473

Ferrous Gluconate (Pantoprazole produces sustained inhibition of gastric acid secretion; pantoprazole may interfere with the absorption of certain drugs, such as iron salts, where gastric pH is an important determinant of the bioavailability). Products include:
CitraNatal Assure 2332
CitraNatal Rx 2332

Ferrous Sulfate (Pantoprazole produces sustained inhibition of gastric acid secretion; pantoprazole may interfere with the absorption of certain drugs, such as iron salts, where gastric pH is an important determinant of the bioavailability).
No products indexed under this heading.

Iron (Pantoprazole produces sustained inhibition of gastric acid secretion; pantoprazole may interfere with the absorption of certain drugs, such as iron salts, where gastric pH is an important determinant of the bioavailability).
No products indexed under this heading.

Ketoconazole (Pantoprazole produces sustained inhibition of gastric acid secretion; pantoprazole may interfere with the absorption of certain drugs, such as ketoconazole, where gastric pH is an important determinant of the bioavailability). Products include:
Extina 3319
Xolegel 3337

Polysaccharide Iron Complex (Pantoprazole produces sustained inhibition of gastric acid secretion; pantoprazole may interfere with the absorption of certain drugs, such as iron salts, where gastric pH is an important determinant of the bioavailability). Products include:
Nu-Iron 150 2321

Warfarin Sodium (There have been reports of increased INR and prothrombin time in patients receiving proton pump inhibitors, including pantoprazole and warfarin concomitantly. Patients treated with proton pump inhibitors and warfarin concomitantly should be monitored for increases in INR and prothrombin time).
No products indexed under this heading.

PROTONIX I.V.

(Pantoprazole Sodium) 3575
See Protonix Delayed-Release Tablets

PROTOPIC OINTMENT

(Tacrolimus) 685
May interact with calcium channel blockers, erythromycin, and certain other agents. Compounds in these categories include:

Amlodipine Besylate (Co-administration of known CYP3A4 inhibitors, such as calcium channel blockers, in patients with widespread and/or erythrodermic disease should be done with caution; based on its minimal extent of absorption, interactions of Protopic Ointment with systemically administered drugs are unlikely to occur but cannot be ruled out). Products include:
Azor 1010
Exforge 2443
Exforge HCT 2449

Bepridil Hydrochloride (Co-administration of known CYP3A4 inhibitors, such as calcium channel blockers, in patients with widespread and/or erythrodermic disease should be done with caution; based on its minimal extent of absorption, interactions of Protopic Ointment with systemically administered drugs are unlikely to occur but cannot be ruled out).
No products indexed under this heading.

Cimetidine (Co-administration of known CYP3A4 inhibitors, such as cimetidine, in patients with widespread and/or erythrodermic disease should be done with caution; based on its minimal extent of absorption, interactions of Protopic Ointment with systemically administered drugs are unlikely to occur but cannot be ruled out).
No products indexed under this heading.

Cimetidine Hydrochloride (Co-administration of known CYP3A4 inhibitors, such as cimetidine, in patients with widespread and/or erythrodermic disease should be done with caution; based on its minimal extent of absorption, interactions of Protopic Ointment with systemically administered drugs are unlikely to occur but cannot be ruled out).
No products indexed under this heading.

Diltiazem Hydrochloride (Co-administration of known CYP3A4 inhibitors, such as calcium channel blockers, in patients with widespread and/or erythrodermic disease should be done with caution; based on its minimal extent of absorption, interactions of Protopic Ointment with systemically administered drugs are unlikely to occur but cannot be ruled out). Products include:
Cardizem LA 423

Erythromycin (Co-administration of known CYP3A4 inhibitors, such as erythromycin, in patients with widespread and/or erythrodermic disease should be done with caution; based on its minimal extent of absorption, interactions of Protopic Ointment with systemically administered drugs are unlikely to occur but cannot be ruled out).
No products indexed under this heading.

Erythromycin, Topical (Co-administration of known CYP3A4 inhibitors, such as erythromycin, in patients with widespread and/or erythrodermic disease should be done with caution; based on its minimal extent of absorption, interactions of Protopic Ointment with systemically administered drugs are unlikely to occur but cannot be ruled out).
No products indexed under this heading.

Erythromycin Estolate (Co-administration of known CYP3A4 inhibitors, such as erythromycin, in patients with widespread and/or erythrodermic disease should be done with caution; based on its minimal extent of absorption, interactions of Protopic Ointment with systemically administered drugs are unlikely to occur but cannot be ruled out).
No products indexed under this heading.

Erythromycin Ethylsuccinate (Co-administration of known CYP3A4 inhibitors, such as erythromycin, in patients with widespread and/or erythrodermic disease should be done with caution; based on its minimal extent of absorption, interactions of Protopic Ointment with systemically administered drugs are unlikely to occur but cannot be ruled out). Products include:
E.E.S. 437
EryPed 435

(⊙ Described in PDR® for Ophthalmic Medicines)

Erythromycin Gluceptate (Co-administration of known CYP3A4 inhibitors, such as erythromycin, in patients with widespread and/or erythrodermic disease should be done with caution; based on its minimal extent of absorption, interactions of Protopic Ointment with systemically administered drugs are unlikely to occur but cannot be ruled out).
No products indexed under this heading.

Erythromycin Lactobionate (Co-administration of known CYP3A4 inhibitors, such as erythromycin, in patients with widespread and/or erythrodermic disease should be done with caution; based on its minimal extent of absorption, interactions of Protopic Ointment with systemically administered drugs are unlikely to occur but cannot be ruled out).
No products indexed under this heading.

Erythromycin Stearate (Co-administration of known CYP3A4 inhibitors, such as erythromycin, in patients with widespread and/or erythrodermic disease should be done with caution; based on its minimal extent of absorption, interactions of Protopic Ointment with systemically administered drugs are unlikely to occur but cannot be ruled out).
No products indexed under this heading.

Felodipine (Co-administration of known CYP3A4 inhibitors, such as calcium channel blockers, in patients with widespread and/or erythrodermic disease should be done with caution; based on its minimal extent of absorption, interactions of Protopic Ointment with systemically administered drugs are unlikely to occur but cannot be ruled out).
No products indexed under this heading.

Fluconazole (Co-administration of known CYP3A4 inhibitors, such as fluconazole, in patients with widespread and/or erythrodermic disease should be done with caution; based on its minimal extent of absorption, interactions of Protopic Ointment with systemically administered drugs are unlikely to occur but cannot be ruled out).
No products indexed under this heading.

Isradipine (Co-administration of known CYP3A4 inhibitors, such as calcium channel blockers, in patients with widespread and/or erythrodermic disease should be done with caution; based on its minimal extent of absorption, interactions of Protopic Ointment with systemically administered drugs are unlikely to occur but cannot be ruled out).
Products include:

Itraconazole (Co-administration of known CYP3A4 inhibitors, such as itraconazole, in patients with widespread and/or erythrodermic disease should be done with caution; based on its minimal extent of absorption, interactions of Protopic Ointment with systemically administered drugs are unlikely to occur but cannot be ruled out).
No products indexed under this heading.

Ketoconazole (Co-administration of known CYP3A4 inhibitors, such as ketoconazole, in patients with widespread and/or erythrodermic disease should be done with caution; based on its minimal extent of absorption, interactions of Protopic Ointment with systemically administered drugs are unlikely to occur but cannot be ruled out). Products include:

Mibefradil Dihydrochloride (Co-administration of known CYP3A4 inhibitors, such as calcium channel blockers, in patients with widespread and/or erythrodermic disease should be done with caution; based on its minimal extent of absorption, interactions of Protopic Ointment with systemically administered drugs are unlikely to occur but cannot be ruled out).
No products indexed under this heading.

Nicardipine (Co-administration of known CYP3A4 inhibitors, such as calcium channel blockers, in patients with widespread and/or erythrodermic disease should be done with caution; based on its minimal extent of absorption, interactions of Protopic Ointment with systemically administered drugs are unlikely to occur but cannot be ruled out).
No products indexed under this heading.

Nicardipine Hydrochloride (Co-administration of known CYP3A4 inhibitors, such as calcium channel blockers, in patients with widespread and/or erythrodermic disease should be done with caution; based on its minimal extent of absorption, interactions of Protopic Ointment with systemically administered drugs are unlikely to occur but cannot be ruled out).
No products indexed under this heading.

Nifedipine (Co-administration of known CYP3A4 inhibitors, such as calcium channel blockers, in patients with widespread and/or erythrodermic disease should be done with caution; based on its minimal extent of absorption, interactions of Protopic Ointment with systemically administered drugs are unlikely to occur but cannot be ruled out).
No products indexed under this heading.

Nimodipine (Co-administration of known CYP3A4 inhibitors, such as calcium channel blockers, in patients with widespread and/or erythrodermic disease should be done with caution; based on its minimal extent of absorption, interactions of Protopic Ointment with systemically administered drugs are unlikely to occur but cannot be ruled out).
No products indexed under this heading.

Nisoldipine (Co-administration of known CYP3A4 inhibitors, such as calcium channel blockers, in patients with widespread and/or erythrodermic disease should be done with caution; based on its minimal extent of absorption, interactions of Protopic Ointment with systemically administered drugs are unlikely to occur but cannot be ruled out).
No products indexed under this heading.

Verapamil Hydrochloride (Co-administration of known CYP3A4 inhibitors, such as calcium channel blockers, in patients with widespread and/or erythrodermic disease should be done with caution; based on its minimal extent of absorption, interactions of Protopic Ointment with systemically administered drugs are unlikely to occur but cannot be ruled out). Products include:

PROVENTIL HFA INHALATION AEROSOL

May interact with beta-blockers, loop diuretics, monoamine oxidase inhibitors, nonpotassium-sparing diuretics, thiazides, tricyclic antidepressants, and certain other agents. Compounds in these categories include:

Acebutolol Hydrochloride (Co-administration with beta adrenergic blocking agent blocks the pulmonary effect of beta agonists and may produce severe bronchospasm in asthmatic patients; co-administer with caution).
No products indexed under this heading.

Amitriptyline Hydrochloride (Action of albuterol on the cardiovascular system may be potentiated by tricyclic antidepressants; co-administer with caution).
No products indexed under this heading.

Amoxapine (Action of albuterol on the cardiovascular system may be potentiated by tricyclic antidepressants; co-administer with caution).
No products indexed under this heading.

Atenolol (Co-administration with beta adrenergic blocking agent blocks the pulmonary effect of beta agonists and may produce severe bronchospasm in asthmatic patients; co-administer with caution).
No products indexed under this heading.

Bendroflumethiazide (The ECG changes and hypokalemia which may result from administration of nonpotassium-sparing diuretics can be acutely worsened by beta agonists. Caution is advised in the co-administration of beta agonists with nonpotassium-sparing diuretics).
No products indexed under this heading.

Betaxolol Hydrochloride (Co-administration with beta adrenergic blocking agent blocks the pulmonary effect of beta agonists and may produce severe bronchospasm in asthmatic patients; co-administer with caution).
No products indexed under this heading.

Bisoprolol Fumarate (Co-administration with beta adrenergic blocking agent blocks the pulmonary effect of beta agonists and may produce severe bronchospasm in asthmatic patients; co-administer with caution).
No products indexed under this heading.

Bumetanide (The ECG changes and hypokalemia which may result from administration of nonpotassium-sparing diuretics can be acutely worsened by beta agonists. Caution is advised in the co-administration of beta agonists with nonpotassium-sparing diuretics).
No products indexed under this heading.

Carteolol Hydrochloride (Co-administration with beta adrenergic blocking agent blocks the pulmonary effect of beta agonists and may produce severe bronchospasm in asthmatic patients; co-administer with caution).
No products indexed under this heading.

Carvedilol (Co-administration with beta adrenergic blocking agent blocks the pulmonary effect of beta agonists and may produce severe bronchospasm in asthmatic patients; co-administer with caution). Products include:

Carvedilol Phosphate (Co-administration with beta adrenergic blocking agent blocks the pulmonary effect of beta agonists and may produce severe bronchospasm in asthmatic patients; co-administer with caution). Products include:

Chlorothiazide (The ECG changes and hypokalemia which may result from administration of nonpotassium-sparing diuretics can be acutely worsened by beta agonists. Caution is advised in the co-administration of beta agonists with nonpotassium-sparing diuretics).
No products indexed under this heading.

Chlorothiazide Sodium (The ECG changes and hypokalemia which may result from administration of nonpotassium-sparing diuretics can be

acutely worsened by beta agonists. Caution is advised in the co-administration of beta agonists with nonpotassium-sparing diuretics).
Products include:

Clomipramine Hydrochloride (Action of albuterol on the cardiovascular system may be potentiated by tricyclic antidepressants; co-administer with caution).
No products indexed under this heading.

Desipramine Hydrochloride (Action of albuterol on the cardiovascular system may be potentiated by tricyclic antidepressants; co-administer with caution).
No products indexed under this heading.

Digoxin (Mean decreases in serum digoxin levels have been demonstrated with intravenous and oral albuterol).
Products include:

Doxepin Hydrochloride (Action of albuterol on the cardiovascular system may be potentiated by tricyclic antidepressants; co-administer with caution).
No products indexed under this heading.

Esmolol Hydrochloride (Co-administration with beta adrenergic blocking agent blocks the pulmonary effect of beta agonists and may produce severe bronchospasm in asthmatic patients; co-administer with caution).
No products indexed under this heading.

Ethacrynic Acid (The ECG changes and hypokalemia which may result from administration of nonpotassium-sparing diuretics can be acutely worsened by beta agonists. Caution is advised in the co-administration of beta agonists with nonpotassium-sparing diuretics).
No products indexed under this heading.

Furosemide (The ECG changes and hypokalemia which may result from administration of nonpotassium-sparing diuretics can be acutely worsened by beta agonists. Caution is advised in the co-administration of beta agonists with nonpotassium-sparing diuretics).
Products include:

Hydrochlorothiazide (The ECG changes and hypokalemia which may result from administration of nonpotassium-sparing diuretics can be acutely worsened by beta agonists. Caution is advised in the co-administration of beta agonists with nonpotassium-sparing diuretics).
Products include:

Hydroflumethiazide (The ECG changes and hypokalemia which may result from administration of nonpotassium-sparing diuretics can be acutely worsened by beta agonists. Caution is advised in the co-administration of beta agonists with nonpotassium-sparing diuretics).
No products indexed under this heading.

Imipramine Hydrochloride (Action of albuterol on the cardiovascular system may be potentiated by tricyclic antidepressants; co-administer with caution).
No products indexed under this heading.

IMPORTANT NOTE: Always consult each drug listing in the patient's regimen for possible interactions.

Imipramine Pamoate (Action of albuterol on the cardiovascular system may be potentiated by tricyclic antidepressants; co-administer with caution).
No products indexed under this heading.

Isocarboxazid (Action of albuterol on the cardiovascular system may be potentiated by MAO inhibitors; co-administer with caution). Products include:
Marplan **3481**

Labetalol Hydrochloride (Co-administration with beta adrenergic blocking agent blocks the pulmonary effect of beta agonists and may produce severe bronchospasm in asthmatic patients; co-administer with caution).
No products indexed under this heading.

Levobunolol Hydrochloride (Co-administration with beta adrenergic blocking agent blocks the pulmonary effect of beta agonists and may produce severe bronchospasm in asthmatic patients; co-administer with caution).
No products indexed under this heading.

Maprotiline Hydrochloride (Action of albuterol on the cardiovascular system may be potentiated by tricyclic antidepressants; co-administer with caution).
No products indexed under this heading.

Methyclothiazide (The ECG changes and hypokalemia which may result from administration of nonpotassium-sparing diuretics can be acutely worsened by beta agonists. Caution is advised in the co-administration of beta agonists with nonpotassium-sparing diuretics).
No products indexed under this heading.

Metipranolol Hydrochloride (Co-administration with beta adrenergic blocking agent blocks the pulmonary effect of beta agonists and may produce severe bronchospasm in asthmatic patients; co-administer with caution).
No products indexed under this heading.

Metoprolol Succinate (Co-administration with beta adrenergic blocking agent blocks the pulmonary effect of beta agonists and may produce severe bronchospasm in asthmatic patients; co-administer with caution). Products include:
Toprol XL **732**

Metoprolol Tartrate (Co-administration with beta adrenergic blocking agent blocks the pulmonary effect of beta agonists and may produce severe bronchospasm in asthmatic patients; co-administer with caution).
No products indexed under this heading.

Moclobemide (Action of albuterol on the cardiovascular system may be potentiated by MAO inhibitors; co-administer with caution).
No products indexed under this heading.

Nadolol (Co-administration with beta adrenergic blocking agent blocks the pulmonary effect of beta agonists and may produce severe bronchospasm in asthmatic patients; co-administer with caution). Products include:
Nadolol **2359**

Nebivolol (Co-administration with beta adrenergic blocking agent blocks the pulmonary effect of beta agonists and may produce severe bronchospasm in asthmatic patients; co-administer with caution). Products include:
Bystolic **1147**

Nortriptyline Hydrochloride (Action of albuterol on the cardiovascular system may be potentiated by tricyclic antidepressants; co-administer with caution).
No products indexed under this heading.

Pargyline Hydrochloride (Action of albuterol on the cardiovascular system may be potentiated by MAO inhibitors; co-administer with caution).
No products indexed under this heading.

Penbutolol Sulfate (Co-administration with beta adrenergic blocking agent blocks the pulmonary effect of beta agonists and may produce severe bronchospasm in asthmatic patients; co-administer with caution).
No products indexed under this heading.

Phenelzine Sulfate (Action of albuterol on the cardiovascular system may be potentiated by MAO inhibitors; co-administer with caution).
No products indexed under this heading.

Pindolol (Co-administration with beta adrenergic blocking agent blocks the pulmonary effect of beta agonists and may produce severe bronchospasm in asthmatic patients; co-administer with caution).
No products indexed under this heading.

Polythiazide (The ECG changes and hypokalemia which may result from administration of nonpotassium-sparing diuretics can be acutely worsened by beta agonists. Caution is advised in the co-administration of beta agonists with nonpotassium-sparing diuretics).
No products indexed under this heading.

Procarbazine Hydrochloride (Action of albuterol on the cardiovascular system may be potentiated by MAO inhibitors; co-administer with caution).
No products indexed under this heading.

Propranolol Hydrochloride (Co-administration with beta adrenergic blocking agent blocks the pulmonary effect of beta agonists and may produce severe bronchospasm in asthmatic patients; co-administer with caution). Products include:
InnoPran XL **1517**

Protriptyline Hydrochloride (Action of albuterol on the cardiovascular system may be potentiated by tricyclic antidepressants; co-administer with caution).
No products indexed under this heading.

Rasagiline Mesylate (Action of albuterol on the cardiovascular system may be potentiated by MAO inhibitors; co-administer with caution). Products include:
Azilect **3383**

Selegiline (Action of albuterol on the cardiovascular system may be potentiated by MAO inhibitors; co-administer with caution). Products include:
Emsam **3623**

Selegiline Hydrochloride (Action of albuterol on the cardiovascular system may be potentiated by MAO inhibitors; co-administer with caution). Products include:
Eldepryl **3312**

Sotalol Hydrochloride (Co-administration with beta adrenergic blocking agent blocks the pulmonary effect of beta agonists and may produce severe bronchospasm in asthmatic patients; co-administer with caution).
No products indexed under this heading.

Timolol Hemihydrate (Co-administration with beta adrenergic blocking agent blocks the pulmonary effect of beta agonists and may produce severe bronchospasm in asthmatic patients; co-administer with caution). Products include:
Betimol **3490**

Timolol Maleate (Co-administration with beta adrenergic blocking agent blocks the pulmonary effect of beta agonists and may produce severe bronchospasm in asthmatic patients; co-administer with caution). Products include:
Combigan **601**
Dorzolamide
Hydrochloride/Timolol Maleate
Ophthalmic Solution...................... ⊙**243**
Timoptic in Ocudose .... ⊙**231**

Torsemide (The ECG changes and hypokalemia which may result from administration of nonpotassium-sparing diuretics can be acutely worsened by beta agonists. Caution is advised in the co-administration of beta agonists with nonpotassium-sparing diuretics).
No products indexed under this heading.

Tranylcypromine Sulfate (Action of albuterol on the cardiovascular system may be potentiated by MAO inhibitors; co-administer with caution). Products include:
Parnate **1584**

Trimipramine Maleate (Action of albuterol on the cardiovascular system may be potentiated by tricyclic antidepressants; co-administer with caution).
No products indexed under this heading.

PROVIGIL TABLETS

(Modafinil) **983**
May interact with alcohols, cytochrome p450 2c9 substrates (selected), cytochrome p450 3a4 inducers (selected), cytochrome p450 3a4 inhibitors (selected), cytochrome p450 3a4 substrates (selected), monoamine oxidase inhibitors, oral contraceptives, phenytoin, selective serotonin reuptake inhibitors, tricyclic antidepressants, xanthines, and certain other agents. Compounds in these categories include:

Acarbose (An apparent concentration-related suppression of CYP2C9 activity was observed in human hepatocytes after exposure to modafinil *in vitro* suggesting that there is a potential for a metabolic interaction between modafinil and substrates of CYP2C9).
No products indexed under this heading.

Acetazolamide (Co-administration of potent inhibitors of CYP3A4 could alter the plasma levels of modafinil).
No products indexed under this heading.

Acetazolamide Sodium (Co-administration of potent inhibitors of CYP3A4 could alter the plasma levels of modafinil).
No products indexed under this heading.

Alfentanil Hydrochloride (Chronic administration of modafinil can increase the elimination of substrates of CYP3A4. Dose adjustments may be necessary for patients being treated with these and similar medications).
No products indexed under this heading.

Allium sativum (Co-administration of potent inducers of CYP3A4 could alter the plasma levels of modafinil).
No products indexed under this heading.

Alprazolam (Chronic administration of modafinil can increase the elimination of substrates of CYP3A4. Dose adjustments may be necessary for patients being treated with these and similar medications).
No products indexed under this heading.

Aminoglutethimide (Co-administration of potent inducers of CYP3A4 could alter the plasma levels of modafinil).
No products indexed under this heading.

Aminophylline (Chronic administration of modafinil may cause modest induction of CYP3A4, thus reducing the levels, to a lesser degree, of co-administered substrate for that enzyme system, such as theophylline).
No products indexed under this heading.

Amiodarone Hydrochloride (Chronic administration of modafinil can increase the elimination of substrates of CYP3A4. Dose adjustments may be necessary for patients being treated with these and similar medications).
No products indexed under this heading.

Amitriptyline Hydrochloride (CYP2C19 provides an ancillary pathway for the metabolism of certain tricyclic antidepressants that are primarily metabolized by CYP2D6. In tricyclic-treated patients deficient in CYP2D6, the amount of metabolism by CYP2C19 may be substantially increased. Modafinil may cause elevation of the levels of these tricyclics in this subset of patients. A reduction in the dose of tricyclic agents might be needed in these patients).
No products indexed under this heading.

Amlodipine Besylate (Chronic administration of modafinil can increase the elimination of substrates of CYP3A4. Dose adjustments may be necessary for patients being treated with these and similar medications). Products include:
Azor **1010**
Exforge **2443**
Exforge HCT **2449**

Amoxapine (CYP2C19 provides an ancillary pathway for the metabolism of certain tricyclic antidepressants that are primarily metabolized by CYP2D6. In tricyclic-treated patients deficient in CYP2D6, the amount of metabolism by CYP2C19 may be substantially increased. Modafinil may cause elevation of the levels of these tricyclics in this subset of patients. A reduction in the dose of tricyclic agents might be needed in these patients).
No products indexed under this heading.

Amprenavir (Co-administration of potent inhibitors of CYP3A4 could alter the plasma levels of modafinil).
No products indexed under this heading.

Anastrozole (Co-administration of potent inhibitors of CYP3A4 could alter the plasma levels of modafinil).
No products indexed under this heading.

Aprepitant (Chronic administration of modafinil can increase the elimination of substrates of CYP3A4. Dose adjustments may be necessary for patients being treated with these and similar medications). Products include:
Emend **2124**

Astemizole (Chronic administration of modafinil can increase the elimination of substrates of CYP3A4. Dose adjustments may be necessary for patients being treated with these and similar medications).
No products indexed under this heading.

Atazanavir (Co-administration of potent inhibitors of CYP3A4 could alter the plasma levels of modafinil).
No products indexed under this heading.

Atazanavir Sulfate (Co-administration of potent inhibitors of CYP3A4 could alter the plasma levels of modafinil).
No products indexed under this heading.

Atorvastatin Calcium (Chronic administration of modafinil can increase the elimination of substrates of CYP3A4. Dose adjustments may be necessary for patients being treated with these and similar medications). Products include:
Lipitor **2703**

Belladonna Ergotamine (Chronic administration of modafinil can increase the elimination of substrates of CYP3A4. Dose adjustments may be necessary for patients being treated with these and similar medications).
No products indexed under this heading.

Betamethasone (Co-administration of potent inducers of CYP3A4 could alter the plasma levels of modafinil).
No products indexed under this heading.

Betamethasone Acetate (Co-administration of potent inducers of CYP3A4 could alter the plasma levels of modafinil).
No products indexed under this heading.

(⊙ Described in PDR® for Ophthalmic Medicines)

Betamethasone Benzoate (Co-administration of potent inducers of CYP3A4 could alter the plasma levels of modafinil).
No products indexed under this heading.

Betamethasone Dipropionate (Co-administration of potent inducers of CYP3A4 could alter the plasma levels of modafinil). Products include:
Diprolene Lotion 0.05% **3108**
Diprolene Ointment 0.05% **3109**
Diprolene AF Cream 0.05% **3107**
Lotrisone **3163**

Betamethasone Sodium Phosphate (Co-administration of potent inducers of CYP3A4 could alter the plasma levels of modafinil).
No products indexed under this heading.

Betamethasone Valerate (Co-administration of potent inducers of CYP3A4 could alter the plasma levels of modafinil). Products include:
Luxíq **3321**

Bosentan (Co-administration of potent inducers of CYP3A4 could alter the plasma levels of modafinil). Products include:
Tracleer **573**

Buspirone Hydrochloride (Chronic administration of modafinil can increase the elimination of substrates of CYP3A4. Dose adjustments may be necessary for patients being treated with these and similar medications).
No products indexed under this heading.

Busulfan (Chronic administration of modafinil can increase the elimination of substrates of CYP3A4. Dose adjustments may be necessary for patients being treated with these and similar medications). Products include:
Myleran **1581**

Candesartan Cilexetil (An apparent concentration-related suppression of CYP2C9 activity was observed in human hepatocytes after exposure to modafinil *in vitro* suggesting that there is a potential for a metabolic interaction between modafinil and substrates of CYP2C9). Products include:
Atacand **697**
Atacand HCT **700**

Carbamazepine (Chronic administration of modafinil may cause induction of its metabolism; co-administration of potent inducers of CYP3A4, such as carbamazepine, could alter the levels of modafinil due to the partial involvement of that enzyme in the metabolic elimination of the compound). Products include:
Carbatrol **3280**
Equetro **3477**

Carvedilol (An apparent concentration-related suppression of CYP2C9 activity was observed in human hepatocytes after exposure to modafinil *in vitro* suggesting that there is a potential for a metabolic interaction between modafinil and substrates of CYP2C9). Products include:
Coreg **1409**

Celecoxib (An apparent concentration-related suppression of CYP2C9 activity was observed in human hepatocytes after exposure to modafinil *in vitro* suggesting that there is a potential for a metabolic interaction between modafinil and substrates of CYP2C9). Products include:
Celebrex **3272**

Cerivastatin Sodium (Chronic administration of modafinil can increase the elimination of substrates of CYP3A4. Dose adjustments may be necessary for patients being treated with these and similar medications).
No products indexed under this heading.

Chlorpheniramine (Chronic administration of modafinil can increase the elimination of substrates of CYP3A4. Dose adjustments may be necessary for patients being treated with these and similar medications).
No products indexed under this heading.

Chlorpheniramine Maleate (Chronic administration of modafinil can increase the elimination of substrates of CYP3A4. Dose adjustments may be necessary for patients being treated with these and similar medications).
No products indexed under this heading.

Chlorpheniramine Polistirex (Chronic administration of modafinil can increase the elimination of substrates of CYP3A4. Dose adjustments may be necessary for patients being treated with these and similar medications). Products include:
Tussionex **3443**

Chlorpheniramine Tannate (Chronic administration of modafinil can increase the elimination of substrates of CYP3A4. Dose adjustments may be necessary for patients being treated with these and similar medications).
No products indexed under this heading.

Chlorpropamide (An apparent concentration-related suppression of CYP2C9 activity was observed in human hepatocytes after exposure to modafinil *in vitro* suggesting that there is a potential for a metabolic interaction between modafinil and substrates of CYP2C9).
No products indexed under this heading.

Cimetidine (Co-administration of potent inhibitors of CYP3A4 could alter the plasma levels of modafinil).
No products indexed under this heading.

Cimetidine Hydrochloride (Co-administration of potent inhibitors of CYP3A4 could alter the plasma levels of modafinil).
No products indexed under this heading.

Ciprofloxacin (Co-administration of potent inducers of CYP3A4 could alter the plasma levels of modafinil). Products include:
Cipro I.V. **3082**
Cipro **3073**
Cipro XR **3091**
Ciprodex **583**

Ciprofloxacin Hydrochloride (Co-administration of potent inducers of CYP3A4 could alter the plasma levels of modafinil). Products include:
Cipro **3073**

Cisapride (Chronic administration of modafinil can increase the elimination of substrates of CYP3A4. Dose adjustments may be necessary for patients being treated with these and similar medications).
No products indexed under this heading.

Cisplatin (Co-administration of potent inducers of CYP3A4 could alter the plasma levels of modafinil).
No products indexed under this heading.

Citalopram Hydrobromide (Modafinil is a reversible inhibitor of the CYP2C19; the levels of CYP2D6 substrates, such as selective serotonin reuptake inhibitors, which have ancillary routes of elimination through CYP2D6, may be increased by co-administration of modafinil). Products include:
Celexa **1153**

Clarithromycin (Chronic administration of modafinil can increase the elimination of substrates of CYP3A4. Dose adjustments may be necessary for patients being treated with these and similar medications). Products include:
Biaxin/Biaxin XL **412**

Clomipramine Hydrochloride (Co-administration has resulted in one incident of increased levels of clomipramine and its active metabolite desmethylclomipramine).
No products indexed under this heading.

Clotrimazole (Co-administration of potent inhibitors of CYP3A4 could alter the plasma levels of modafinil). Products include:
Lotrisone **3163**

Conivaptan Hydrochloride (Co-administration of potent inhibitors of CYP3A4 could alter the plasma levels of modafinil). Products include:
Vaprisol **689**

Cortisone Acetate (Co-administration of potent inducers of CYP3A4 could alter the plasma levels of modafinil).
No products indexed under this heading.

Cyclosporine (The blood levels of cyclosporine may be reduced when used with modafinil. Monitoring of circulating cyclosporine concentrations and appropriate dosage adjustment for cyclosporine should be considered when these drugs are used concomitantly). Products include:
Gengraf **440**
Neoral Oral Solution **2496**
Neoral Capsules **2496**
Restasis **605**

Dalfopristin (Co-administration of potent inhibitors of CYP3A4 could alter the plasma levels of modafinil).
No products indexed under this heading.

Danazol (Co-administration of potent inhibitors of CYP3A4 could alter the plasma levels of modafinil).
No products indexed under this heading.

Darunavir (Co-administration of potent inhibitors of CYP3A4 could alter the plasma levels of modafinil).
No products indexed under this heading.

Dasatinib (Co-administration of potent inhibitors of CYP3A4 could alter the plasma levels of modafinil).
No products indexed under this heading.

Delavirdine Mesylate (Co-administration of potent inhibitors of CYP3A4 could alter the plasma levels of modafinil).
No products indexed under this heading.

Delavirine (Co-administration of potent inhibitors of CYP3A4 could alter the plasma levels of modafinil).
No products indexed under this heading.

Desipramine Hydrochloride (CYP2C19 provides an ancillary pathway for the metabolism of certain tricyclic antidepressants that are primarily metabolized by CYP2D6. In tricyclic-treated patients deficient in CYP2D6, the amount of metabolism by CYP2C19 may be substantially increased. Modafinil may cause elevation of the levels of these tricyclics in this subset of patients. A reduction in the dose of tricyclic agents might be needed in these patients).
No products indexed under this heading.

Desloratadine (Co-administration of potent inhibitors of CYP3A4 could alter the plasma levels of modafinil). Products include:
Clarinex Syrup **3098**
Clarinex **3098**
Clarinex Reditabs **3098**
Clarinex-D 12-Hour **3101**
Clarinex-D **3104**

Desogestrel (The effectiveness of steroidal contraceptives may be reduced when used with modafinil tablets and for one month after discontinuation of therapy. Alternative or concomitant methods of contraception are recommended for patients treated with modafinil tablets and for one month after discontinuation of modafinil).
No products indexed under this heading.

Dexamethasone (Co-administration of potent inducers of CYP3A4 could alter the plasma levels of modafinil). Products include:
Ciprodex **583**
Ozurdex .... **⊙223**
Tobramycin and Dexamethasone Ophthalmic Suspension .... **⊙251**

Dexamethasone Acetate (Co-administration of potent inducers of CYP3A4 could alter the plasma levels of modafinil).
No products indexed under this heading.

Dexamethasone Phosphate (Co-administration of potent inducers of CYP3A4 could alter the plasma levels of modafinil).
No products indexed under this heading.

Dexamethasone Sodium (Co-administration of potent inducers of CYP3A4 could alter the plasma levels of modafinil).
No products indexed under this heading.

Dexamethasone Sodium Phosphate (Co-administration of potent inducers of CYP3A4 could alter the plasma levels of modafinil).
No products indexed under this heading.

Dexamethasone Sodium Phosphate Injection (Co-administration of potent inducers of CYP3A4 could alter the plasma levels of modafinil).
No products indexed under this heading.

Dextroamphetamine (Absorption of modafinil may be delayed by approximately one hour when co-administered with dextroamphetamine).
No products indexed under this heading.

Dextroamphetamine Saccharate (Absorption of modafinil may be delayed by approximately one hour when co-administered with dextroamphetamine).
No products indexed under this heading.

Dextroamphetamine Sulfate (Absorption of modafinil may be delayed by approximately one hour when co-administered with dextroamphetamine). Products include:
Dexedrine **1425**

Dextromethorphan (An apparent concentration-related suppression of CYP2C9 activity was observed in human hepatocytes after exposure to modafinil *in vitro* suggesting that there is a potential for a metabolic interaction between modafinil and substrates of CYP2C9).
No products indexed under this heading.

Diazepam (Modafinil is a reversible inhibitor of the CYP2C19; co-administration with drugs that are largely eliminated via this pathway, such as diazepam, may increase the circulating levels of diazepam). Products include:
Valium Tablets **2880**

Diclofenac Potassium (An apparent concentration-related suppression of CYP2C9 activity was observed in human hepatocytes after exposure to modafinil *in vitro* suggesting that there is a potential for a metabolic interaction between modafinil and substrates of CYP2C9).
No products indexed under this heading.

Diclofenac Sodium (An apparent concentration-related suppression of CYP2C9 activity was observed in human hepatocytes after exposure to modafinil *in vitro* suggesting that there is a potential for a metabolic interaction between modafinil and substrates of CYP2C9).
No products indexed under this heading.

Dihydroergotamine Mesylate (Chronic administration of modafinil can increase the elimination of substrates of CYP3A4. Dose adjustments may be necessary for patients being treated with these and similar medications).
No products indexed under this heading.

IMPORTANT NOTE: Always consult each drug listing in the patient's regimen for possible interactions.

(⊙ Described in PDR® for Ophthalmic Medicines)

1527 Interactions Index Provigil

Fluvoxamine (Modafinil is a reversible inhibitor of the CYP2C19; the levels of CYP2D6 substrates, such as selective serotonin reuptake inhibitors, which have ancillary routes of elimination through CYP2D6, may be increased by co-administration of modafinil).
No products indexed under this heading.

Fluvoxamine Maleate (Modafinil is a reversible inhibitor of the CYP2C19; the levels of CYP2D6 substrates, such as selective serotonin reuptake inhibitors, which have ancillary routes of elimination through CYP2D6, may be increased by co-administration of modafinil).
No products indexed under this heading.

Fosamprenavir Calcium (Co-administration of potent inhibitors of CYP3A4 could alter the plasma levels of modafinil). Products include:
Lexiva Oral Suspension 1558
Lexiva 1558

Fosphenytoin (Modafinil is a reversible inhibitor of the CYP2C19; co-administration with drugs that are largely eliminated via this pathway, such as phenytoin, may increase the circulating levels of phenytoin).
No products indexed under this heading.

Fosphenytoin Sodium (Modafinil is a reversible inhibitor of the CYP2C19; co-administration with drugs that are largely eliminated via this pathway, such as phenytoin, may increase the circulating levels of phenytoin).
No products indexed under this heading.

Garlic Extract (Co-administration of potent inducers of CYP3A4 could alter the plasma levels of modafinil).
No products indexed under this heading.

Garlic Oil (Co-administration of potent inducers of CYP3A4 could alter the plasma levels of modafinil).
No products indexed under this heading.

Glimepiride (An apparent concentration-related suppression of CYP2C9 activity was observed in human hepatocytes after exposure to modafinil *in vitro* suggesting that there is a potential for a metabolic interaction between modafinil and substrates of CYP2C9). Products include:
Avandaryl 1356
Duetact 3354

Glipizide (An apparent concentration-related suppression of CYP2C9 activity was observed in human hepatocytes after exposure to modafinil *in vitro* suggesting that there is a potential for a metabolic interaction between modafinil and substrates of CYP2C9).
No products indexed under this heading.

Haloperidol (Chronic administration of modafinil can increase the elimination of substrates of CYP3A4. Dose adjustments may be necessary for patients being treated with these and similar medications).
No products indexed under this heading.

Haloperidol Decanoate (Chronic administration of modafinil can increase the elimination of substrates of CYP3A4. Dose adjustments may be necessary for patients being treated with these and similar medications).
No products indexed under this heading.

Haloperidol Lactate (Chronic administration of modafinil can increase the elimination of substrates of CYP3A4. Dose adjustments may be necessary for patients being treated with these and similar medications).
No products indexed under this heading.

Hydrocortisone (Co-administration of potent inducers of CYP3A4 could alter the plasma levels of modafinil).
No products indexed under this heading.

Hydrocortisone (Alcohol) (Co-administration of potent inducers of CYP3A4 could alter the plasma levels of modafinil).
No products indexed under this heading.

Hydrocortisone Acetate (Co-administration of potent inducers of CYP3A4 could alter the plasma levels of modafinil).
No products indexed under this heading.

Hydrocortisone Butyrate (Co-administration of potent inducers of CYP3A4 could alter the plasma levels of modafinil).
No products indexed under this heading.

Hydrocortisone Cypionate (Co-administration of potent inducers of CYP3A4 could alter the plasma levels of modafinil).
No products indexed under this heading.

Hydrocortisone Hemisuccinate (Co-administration of potent inducers of CYP3A4 could alter the plasma levels of modafinil).
No products indexed under this heading.

Hydrocortisone Probutate (Co-administration of potent inducers of CYP3A4 could alter the plasma levels of modafinil).
No products indexed under this heading.

Hydrocortisone Sodium Phosphate (Co-administration of potent inducers of CYP3A4 could alter the plasma levels of modafinil).
No products indexed under this heading.

Hydrocortisone Sodium Succinate (Co-administration of potent inducers of CYP3A4 could alter the plasma levels of modafinil).
No products indexed under this heading.

Hydrocortisone Valerate (Co-administration of potent inducers of CYP3A4 could alter the plasma levels of modafinil).
No products indexed under this heading.

Hypericum (Co-administration of potent inducers of CYP3A4 could alter the plasma levels of modafinil).
No products indexed under this heading.

Hypericum Perforatum (Co-administration of potent inducers of CYP3A4 could alter the plasma levels of modafinil). Products include:
Traumeel 1800

Ibuprofen (An apparent concentration-related suppression of CYP2C9 activity was observed in human hepatocytes after exposure to modafinil *in vitro* suggesting that there is a potential for a metabolic interaction between modafinil and substrates of CYP2C9). Products include:
Motrin IB 2043
Children's Motrin 2044
Children's Motrin Non-Staining Dye-Free 2044
Infants' Motrin 2044
Infants' Motrin Dye-Free 2044
Junior Strength Motrin 2044
Vicoprofen 564

Imatinib Mesylate (Co-administration of potent inhibitors of CYP3A4 could alter the plasma levels of modafinil). Products include:
Gleevec 2477

Imipramine Hydrochloride (CYP2C19 provides an ancillary pathway for the metabolism of certain tricyclic antidepressants that are primarily metabolized by CYP2D6. In tricyclic-treated patients deficient in CYP2D6, the amount of metabolism by CYP2C19 may be substantially increased. Modafinil may cause elevation of the levels of these tricyclics in this subset of patients. A reduction in the dose of tricyclic agents might be needed in these patients).
No products indexed under this heading.

Imipramine Pamoate (CYP2C19 provides an ancillary pathway for the metabolism of certain tricyclic antidepressants that are primarily metabolized by CYP2D6. In tricyclic-treated patients deficient in CYP2D6, the amount of metabolism by CYP2C19 may be substantially increased. Modafinil may cause elevation of the levels of these tricyclics in this subset of patients. A reduction in the dose of tricyclic agents might be needed in these patients).
No products indexed under this heading.

Indinavir Sulfate (Chronic administration of modafinil can increase the elimination of substrates of CYP3A4. Dose adjustments may be necessary for patients being treated with these and similar medications). Products include:
Crixivan 2113

Indomethacin (An apparent concentration-related suppression of CYP2C9 activity was observed in human hepatocytes after exposure to modafinil *in vitro* suggesting that there is a potential for a metabolic interaction between modafinil and substrates of CYP2C9). Products include:
Indocin 2167

Indomethacin Sodium Trihydrate (An apparent concentration-related suppression of CYP2C9 activity was observed in human hepatocytes after exposure to modafinil *in vitro* suggesting that there is a potential for a metabolic interaction between modafinil and substrates of CYP2C9). Products include:
Indocin I.V. 2007

Irbesartan (An apparent concentration-related suppression of CYP2C9 activity was observed in human hepatocytes after exposure to modafinil *in vitro* suggesting that there is a potential for a metabolic interaction between modafinil and substrates of CYP2C9). Products include:
Avalide 2956
Avapro 2962

Isocarboxazid (Co-administration requires caution; no interaction studies have been performed). Products include:
Marplan 3481

Isoniazid (Co-administration of potent inhibitors of CYP3A4 could alter the plasma levels of modafinil).
No products indexed under this heading.

Isradipine (Chronic administration of modafinil can increase the elimination of substrates of CYP3A4. Dose adjustments may be necessary for patients being treated with these and similar medications). Products include:
DynaCirc CR 1432

Itraconazole (Chronic administration of modafinil may cause induction of its metabolism; co-administration of potent inhibitors of CYP3A4, such as itraconazole, could alter the levels of modafinil due to the partial involvement of that enzyme in the metabolic elimination of the compound).
No products indexed under this heading.

Ixabepilone (Chronic administration of modafinil can increase the elimination of substrates of CYP3A4. Dose adjustments may be necessary for patients being treated with these and similar medications).
No products indexed under this heading.

Ketoconazole (Chronic administration of modafinil may cause induction of its metabolism; co-administration of potent inhibitors of CYP3A4, such as ketoconazole, could alter the levels of modafinil due to the partial involvement of that enzyme in the metabolic elimination of the compound). Products include:
Extina 3319
Xolegel 3337

Ketoprofen (An apparent concentration-related suppression of CYP2C9 activity was observed in human hepatocytes after exposure to modafinil *in vitro* suggesting that there is a potential for a metabolic interaction between modafinil and substrates of CYP2C9).
No products indexed under this heading.

Ketorolac Tromethamine (An apparent concentration-related suppression of CYP2C9 activity was observed in human hepatocytes after exposure to modafinil *in vitro* suggesting that there is a potential for a metabolic interaction between modafinil and substrates of CYP2C9). Products include:
Acuvail .... ⊙209

Lansoprazole (An apparent concentration-related suppression of CYP2C9 activity was observed in human hepatocytes after exposure to modafinil *in vitro* suggesting that there is a potential for a metabolic interaction between modafinil and substrates of CYP2C9).
No products indexed under this heading.

Lapatinib (Co-administration of potent inhibitors of CYP3A4 could alter the plasma levels of modafinil). Products include:
Tykerb 1698

Levonorgestrel (The effectiveness of steroidal contraceptives may be reduced when used with modafinil tablets and for one month after discontinuation of therapy. Alternative or concomitant methods of contraception are recommended for patients treated with modafinil tablets and for one month after discontinuation of modafinil). Products include:
Climara Pro 847
LoSeasonique 3407
Lybrel 3514
Mirena 854
Plan B 3416
Seasonique 3418

Lidocaine (Chronic administration of modafinil can increase the elimination of substrates of CYP3A4. Dose adjustments may be necessary for patients being treated with these and similar medications). Products include:
Lidoderm 1107

Lidocaine Hydrochloride (Chronic administration of modafinil can increase the elimination of substrates of CYP3A4. Dose adjustments may be necessary for patients being treated with these and similar medications).
No products indexed under this heading.

Lopinavir (Co-administration of potent inhibitors of CYP3A4 could alter the plasma levels of modafinil). Products include:
Kaletra 458

Loratadine (Co-administration of potent inhibitors of CYP3A4 could alter the plasma levels of modafinil).
No products indexed under this heading.

Losartan Potassium (An apparent concentration-related suppression of CYP2C9 activity was observed in human hepatocytes after exposure to modafinil *in vitro* suggesting that there is a potential for a metabolic interaction between modafinil and substrates of CYP2C9). Products include:
Cozaar 2106
Hyzaar 2162
Hyzaar 100-12.5 2162

Lovastatin (Chronic administration of modafinil can increase the elimination of substrates of CYP3A4. Dose adjustments may be necessary for patients being treated with these and similar medications). Products include:
Advicor 402
Mevacor 2212

IMPORTANT NOTE: Always consult each drug listing in the patient's regimen for possible interactions.

Maprotiline Hydrochloride (CYP2C19 provides an ancillary pathway for the metabolism of certain tricyclic antidepressants that are primarily metabolized by CYP2D6. In tricyclic-treated patients deficient in CYP2D6, the amount of metabolism by CYP2C19 may be substantially increased. Modafinil may cause elevation of the levels of these tricyclics in this subset of patients. A reduction in the dose of tricyclic agents might be needed in these patients).
No products indexed under this heading.

Meclofenamate Sodium (An apparent concentration-related suppression of CYP2C9 activity was observed in human hepatocytes after exposure to modafinil *in vitro* suggesting that there is a potential for a metabolic interaction between modafinil and substrates of CYP2C9).
No products indexed under this heading.

Mefenamic Acid (An apparent concentration-related suppression of CYP2C9 activity was observed in human hepatocytes after exposure to modafinil *in vitro* suggesting that there is a potential for a metabolic interaction between modafinil and substrates of CYP2C9).
No products indexed under this heading.

Meloxicam (An apparent concentration-related suppression of CYP2C9 activity was observed in human hepatocytes after exposure to modafinil *in vitro* suggesting that there is a potential for a metabolic interaction between modafinil and substrates of CYP2C9).
No products indexed under this heading.

Mephenytoin (Co-administration of potent inducers of CYP3A4 could alter the plasma levels of modafinil).
No products indexed under this heading.

Mestranol (The effectiveness of steroidal contraceptives may be reduced when used with modafinil tablets and for one month after discontinuation of therapy. Alternative or concomitant methods of contraception are recommended for patients treated with modafinil tablets and for one month after discontinuation of modafinil).
No products indexed under this heading.

Metformin Hydrochloride (An apparent concentration-related suppression of CYP2C9 activity was observed in human hepatocytes after exposure to modafinil *in vitro* suggesting that there is a potential for a metabolic interaction between modafinil and substrates of CYP2C9). Products include:
ActoPlus 3338
Avandamet 1345
Janumet 2188

Methadone Hydrochloride (Chronic administration of modafinil can increase the elimination of substrates of CYP3A4. Dose adjustments may be necessary for patients being treated with these and similar medications).
No products indexed under this heading.

Methsuximide (Co-administration of potent inducers of CYP3A4 could alter the plasma levels of modafinil).
No products indexed under this heading.

Methylphenidate Hydrochloride (May delay absorption of modafinil by approximately one hour; no significant alterations in pharmacokinetics of either drug). Products include:
Concerta 2598
Metadate CD 3439

Methylprednisolone (Co-administration of potent inducers of CYP3A4 could alter the plasma levels of modafinil).
No products indexed under this heading.

Methylprednisolone Acetate (Co-administration of potent inducers of CYP3A4 could alter the plasma levels of modafinil).
No products indexed under this heading.

Methylprednisolone Sodium Succinate (Co-administration of potent inducers of CYP3A4 could alter the plasma levels of modafinil).
No products indexed under this heading.

Metronidazole (Co-administration of potent inhibitors of CYP3A4 could alter the plasma levels of modafinil). Products include:
Pylera 793

Metronidazole Benzoate (Co-administration of potent inhibitors of CYP3A4 could alter the plasma levels of modafinil).
No products indexed under this heading.

Metronidazole Hydrochloride (Co-administration of potent inhibitors of CYP3A4 could alter the plasma levels of modafinil).
No products indexed under this heading.

Metronidazole Sodium (Co-administration of potent inhibitors of CYP3A4 could alter the plasma levels of modafinil).
No products indexed under this heading.

Miconazole (Co-administration of potent inhibitors of CYP3A4 could alter the plasma levels of modafinil).
No products indexed under this heading.

Miconazole Nitrate (Co-administration of potent inhibitors of CYP3A4 could alter the plasma levels of modafinil). Products include:
Vusion Ointment 3335

Midazolam Hydrochloride (Chronic administration of modafinil can increase the elimination of substrates of CYP3A4. Dose adjustments may be necessary for patients being treated with these and similar medications).
No products indexed under this heading.

Mifepristone (Co-administration of potent inhibitors of CYP3A4 could alter the plasma levels of modafinil).
No products indexed under this heading.

Miglitol (An apparent concentration-related suppression of CYP2C9 activity was observed in human hepatocytes after exposure to modafinil *in vitro* suggesting that there is a potential for a metabolic interaction between modafinil and substrates of CYP2C9).
No products indexed under this heading.

Mirtazapine (An apparent concentration-related suppression of CYP2C9 activity was observed in human hepatocytes after exposure to modafinil *in vitro* suggesting that there is a potential for a metabolic interaction between modafinil and substrates of CYP2C9). Products include:
Remeron Tablets 3214
RemeronSolTab Tablets 3219

Moclobemide (Co-administration requires caution; no interaction studies have been performed).
No products indexed under this heading.

Montelukast Sodium (An apparent concentration-related suppression of CYP2C9 activity was observed in human hepatocytes after exposure to modafinil *in vitro* suggesting that there is a potential for a metabolic interaction between modafinil and substrates of CYP2C9). Products include:
Singulair 2270

Nabumetone (An apparent concentration-related suppression of CYP2C9 activity was observed in human hepatocytes after exposure to modafinil *in vitro* suggesting that there is a potential for a metabolic interaction between modafinil and substrates of CYP2C9).
No products indexed under this heading.

Nafcillin Sodium (Co-administration of potent inducers of CYP3A4 could alter the plasma levels of modafinil).
No products indexed under this heading.

Naproxen (An apparent concentration-related suppression of CYP2C9 activity was observed in human hepatocytes after exposure to modafinil *in vitro* suggesting that there is a potential for a metabolic interaction between modafinil and substrates of CYP2C9). Products include:
EC-Naprosyn 2850
Naprosyn 2850
Anaprox/Naprosyn 2850

Naproxen Sodium (An apparent concentration-related suppression of CYP2C9 activity was observed in human hepatocytes after exposure to modafinil *in vitro* suggesting that there is a potential for a metabolic interaction between modafinil and substrates of CYP2C9). Products include:
Anaprox 2850
Anaprox DS 2850
Treximet 1681

Nateglinide (An apparent concentration-related suppression of CYP2C9 activity was observed in human hepatocytes after exposure to modafinil *in vitro* suggesting that there is a potential for a metabolic interaction between modafinil and substrates of CYP2C9).
No products indexed under this heading.

Nefazodone Hydrochloride (Chronic administration of modafinil can increase the elimination of substrates of CYP3A4. Dose adjustments may be necessary for patients being treated with these and similar medications).
No products indexed under this heading.

Nelfinavir Mesylate (Chronic administration of modafinil can increase the elimination of substrates of CYP3A4. Dose adjustments may be necessary for patients being treated with these and similar medications).
No products indexed under this heading.

Nevirapine (Co-administration of potent inducers of CYP3A4 could alter the plasma levels of modafinil). Products include:
Viramune Oral Suspension 897
Viramune Tablets 897

Niacin (Co-administration of potent inhibitors of CYP3A4 could alter the plasma levels of modafinil). Products include:
Advicor 402
Cardio Basics 3455
Niaspan 497
Simcor 524

Niacinamide (Co-administration of potent inhibitors of CYP3A4 could alter the plasma levels of modafinil). Products include:
CitraNatal 90 DHA Capsules 2332
CitraNatal Assure 2332
CitraNatal Rx 2332
Heplive 607

Niacinamide Hydroiodide (Co-administration of potent inhibitors of CYP3A4 could alter the plasma levels of modafinil).
No products indexed under this heading.

Nicardipine (Chronic administration of modafinil can increase the elimination of substrates of CYP3A4. Dose adjustments may be necessary for patients being treated with these and similar medications).
No products indexed under this heading.

Nicardipine Hydrochloride (Chronic administration of modafinil can increase the elimination of substrates of CYP3A4. Dose adjustments may be necessary for patients being treated with these and similar medications).
No products indexed under this heading.

Nicotinamide (Co-administration of potent inhibitors of CYP3A4 could alter the plasma levels of modafinil).
No products indexed under this heading.

Nifedipine (Chronic administration of modafinil can increase the elimination of substrates of CYP3A4. Dose adjustments may be necessary for patients being treated with these and similar medications).
No products indexed under this heading.

Nimodipine (Chronic administration of modafinil can increase the elimination of substrates of CYP3A4. Dose adjustments may be necessary for patients being treated with these and similar medications).
No products indexed under this heading.

Nisoldipine (Chronic administration of modafinil can increase the elimination of substrates of CYP3A4. Dose adjustments may be necessary for patients being treated with these and similar medications).
No products indexed under this heading.

Nitrendipine (Chronic administration of modafinil can increase the elimination of substrates of CYP3A4. Dose adjustments may be necessary for patients being treated with these and similar medications).
No products indexed under this heading.

Norethindrone (The effectiveness of steroidal contraceptives may be reduced when used with modafinil tablets and for one month after discontinuation of therapy. Alternative or concomitant methods of contraception are recommended for patients treated with modafinil tablets and for one month after discontinuation of modafinil). Products include:
Ortho Micronor 2660

Norethindrone Acetate (Chronic administration of modafinil can increase the elimination of substrates of CYP3A4. Dose adjustments may be necessary for patients being treated with these and similar medications). Products include:
Activella 2561

Norethynodrel (The effectiveness of steroidal contraceptives may be reduced when used with modafinil tablets and for one month after discontinuation of therapy. Alternative or concomitant methods of contraception are recommended for patients treated with modafinil tablets and for one month after discontinuation of modafinil).
No products indexed under this heading.

Norfloxacin (Co-administration of potent inhibitors of CYP3A4 could alter the plasma levels of modafinil). Products include:
Noroxin 2220

Norgestimate (The effectiveness of steroidal contraceptives may be reduced when used with modafinil tablets and for one month after discontinuation of therapy. Alternative or concomitant methods of contraception are recommended for patients treated with modafinil tablets and for one month after discontinuation of modafinil). Products include:
Ortho-Cyclen/Ortho Tri-Cyclen 2663
Ortho Tri-Cyclen Lo Tablets 2673

Norgestrel (The effectiveness of steroidal contraceptives may be reduced when used with modafinil tablets and for one month after discontinuation of therapy. Alternative or concomitant methods of contraception are recommended for patients treated with modafinil tablets and for one month after discontinuation of modafinil).
No products indexed under this heading.

Nortriptyline Hydrochloride (CYP2C19 provides an ancillary pathway for the metabolism of certain tricy-

(☉ Described in PDR® for Ophthalmic Medicines)

1529 **Interactions Index** **Provigil**

clic antidepressants that are primarily metabolized by CYP2D6. In tricyclic-treated patients deficient in CYP2D6, the amount of metabolism by CYP2C19 may be substantially increased. Modafinil may cause elevation of the levels of these tricyclics in this subset of patients. A reduction in the dose of tricyclic agents might be needed in these patients).
No products indexed under this heading.

Omeprazole (An apparent concentration-related suppression of CYP2C9 activity was observed in human hepatocytes after exposure to modafinil *in vitro* suggesting that there is a potential for a metabolic interaction between modafinil and substrates of CYP2C9).
No products indexed under this heading.

Ondansetron (Chronic administration of modafinil can increase the elimination of substrates of CYP3A4. Dose adjustments may be necessary for patients being treated with these and similar medications).
No products indexed under this heading.

Ondansetron Hydrochloride (Chronic administration of modafinil can increase the elimination of substrates of CYP3A4. Dose adjustments may be necessary for patients being treated with these and similar medications). Products include:
Zofran Injection **1750**
Zofran **1756**
Zofran ODT **1756**

Oxaprozin (An apparent concentration-related suppression of CYP2C9 activity was observed in human hepatocytes after exposure to modafinil *in vitro* suggesting that there is a potential for a metabolic interaction between modafinil and substrates of CYP2C9).
No products indexed under this heading.

Oxcarbazepine (Co-administration of potent inducers of CYP3A4 could alter the plasma levels of modafinil).
No products indexed under this heading.

Paclitaxel (Chronic administration of modafinil can increase the elimination of substrates of CYP3A4. Dose adjustments may be necessary for patients being treated with these and similar medications).
No products indexed under this heading.

Pargyline Hydrochloride (Co-administration requires caution; no interaction studies have been performed).
No products indexed under this heading.

Paroxetine (Modafinil is a reversible inhibitor of the CYP2C19; the levels of CYP2D6 substrates, such as selective serotonin reuptake inhibitors, which have ancillary routes of elimination through CYP2D6, may be increased by co-administration of modafinil).
No products indexed under this heading.

Paroxetine Hydrochloride (Modafinil is a reversible inhibitor of the CYP2C19; the levels of CYP2D6 substrates, such as selective serotonin reuptake inhibitors, which have ancillary routes of elimination through CYP2D6, may be increased by co-administration of modafinil). Products include:
Paroxetine CR **2361**
Paroxetine ER **2371**
Paxil **1586**
Paxil CR **1596**

Paroxetine Mesylate (Modafinil is a reversible inhibitor of the CYP2C19; the levels of CYP2D6 substrates, such as selective serotonin reuptake inhibitors, which have ancillary routes of elimination through CYP2D6, may be increased by co-administration of modafinil).
No products indexed under this heading.

Phenelzine Sulfate (Co-administration requires caution; no interaction studies have been performed).
No products indexed under this heading.

Phenobarbital (Chronic administration of modafinil may cause induction of its metabolism; co-administration of potent inducers of CYP3A4, such as phenobarbital, could alter the levels of modafinil due to the partial involvement of that enzyme in the metabolic elimination of the compound). Products include:
Donnatal **2711**

Phenobarbital Sodium (Co-administration of potent inducers of CYP3A4 could alter the plasma levels of modafinil).
No products indexed under this heading.

Phenylbutazone (An apparent concentration-related suppression of CYP2C9 activity was observed in human hepatocytes after exposure to modafinil *in vitro* suggesting that there is a potential for a metabolic interaction between modafinil and substrates of CYP2C9).
No products indexed under this heading.

Phenytoin (Modafinil is a reversible inhibitor of the CYP2C19; co-administration with drugs that are largely eliminated via this pathway, such as phenytoin, may increase the circulating levels of phenytoin).
No products indexed under this heading.

Phenytoin Sodium (Modafinil is a reversible inhibitor of the CYP2C19; co-administration with drugs that are largely eliminated via this pathway, such as phenytoin, may increase the circulating levels of phenytoin). Products include:
Phenytek Capsules **2380**

Pimozide (Chronic administration of modafinil can increase the elimination of substrates of CYP3A4. Dose adjustments may be necessary for patients being treated with these and similar medications).
No products indexed under this heading.

Pioglitazone Hydrochloride (An apparent concentration-related suppression of CYP2C9 activity was observed in human hepatocytes after exposure to modafinil *in vitro* suggesting that there is a potential for a metabolic interaction between modafinil and substrates of CYP2C9). Products include:
ActoPlus **3338**
Actos **3345**
Duetact **3354**

Piroxicam (An apparent concentration-related suppression of CYP2C9 activity was observed in human hepatocytes after exposure to modafinil *in vitro* suggesting that there is a potential for a metabolic interaction between modafinil and substrates of CYP2C9).
No products indexed under this heading.

Polyestradiol Phosphate (Chronic administration of modafinil can increase the elimination of substrates of CYP3A4. Dose adjustments may be necessary for patients being treated with these and similar medications).
No products indexed under this heading.

Posaconazole (Co-administration of potent inhibitors of CYP3A4 could alter the plasma levels of modafinil). Products include:
Noxafil **3172**

Prednisolone (Co-administration of potent inducers of CYP3A4 could alter the plasma levels of modafinil).
No products indexed under this heading.

Prednisolone Acetate (Co-administration of potent inducers of CYP3A4 could alter the plasma levels of modafinil). Products include:
Blephamide .... ⊙**212**, ⊙**214**
Pred Forte .... ⊙**225**
Pred Mild .... ⊙**230**
Pred-G .... ⊙**226**, ⊙**227**

Prednisolone Sodium Phosphate (Co-administration of potent inducers of CYP3A4 could alter the plasma levels of modafinil).
No products indexed under this heading.

Prednisolone Tebutate (Co-administration of potent inducers of CYP3A4 could alter the plasma levels of modafinil).
No products indexed under this heading.

Prednisone (Co-administration of potent inducers of CYP3A4 could alter the plasma levels of modafinil).
No products indexed under this heading.

Prednisone sodium phosphate (Co-administration of potent inducers of CYP3A4 could alter the plasma levels of modafinil).
No products indexed under this heading.

Primidone (Co-administration of potent inducers of CYP3A4 could alter the plasma levels of modafinil).
No products indexed under this heading.

Procarbazine Hydrochloride (Co-administration requires caution; no interaction studies have been performed).
No products indexed under this heading.

Propoxyphene Hydrochloride (Co-administration of potent inhibitors of CYP3A4 could alter the plasma levels of modafinil).
No products indexed under this heading.

Propoxyphene Napsylate (Co-administration of potent inhibitors of CYP3A4 could alter the plasma levels of modafinil).
No products indexed under this heading.

Propranolol Hydrochloride (Modafinil is a reversible inhibitor of the CYP2C19; co-administration with drugs that are largely eliminated via this pathway, such as propranolol, may increase the circulating levels of propranolol). Products include:
InnoPran XL **1517**

Protriptyline Hydrochloride (CYP2C19 provides an ancillary pathway for the metabolism of certain tricyclic antidepressants that are primarily metabolized by CYP2D6. In tricyclic-treated patients deficient in CYP2D6, the amount of metabolism by CYP2C19 may be substantially increased. Modafinil may cause elevation of the levels of these tricyclics in this subset of patients. A reduction in the dose of tricyclic agents might be needed in these patients).
No products indexed under this heading.

Quinidine (Co-administration of potent inhibitors of CYP3A4 could alter the plasma levels of modafinil).
No products indexed under this heading.

Quinidine Gluconate (Chronic administration of modafinil can increase the elimination of substrates of CYP3A4. Dose adjustments may be necessary for patients being treated with these and similar medications).
No products indexed under this heading.

Quinidine Hydrochloride (Co-administration of potent inhibitors of CYP3A4 could alter the plasma levels of modafinil).
No products indexed under this heading.

Quinidine Polygalacturonate (Chronic administration of modafinil can increase the elimination of substrates of CYP3A4. Dose adjustments may be necessary for patients being treated with these and similar medications).
No products indexed under this heading.

Quinidine Sulfate (Chronic administration of modafinil can increase the elimination of substrates of CYP3A4. Dose adjustments may be necessary for patients being treated with these and similar medications).
No products indexed under this heading.

Quinine (Co-administration of potent inhibitors of CYP3A4 could alter the plasma levels of modafinil). Products include:
Hyland's Leg Cramps PM with Quinine **3315**

Quinine Sulfate (Co-administration of potent inhibitors of CYP3A4 could alter the plasma levels of modafinil).
No products indexed under this heading.

Quinupristin (Co-administration of potent inhibitors of CYP3A4 could alter the plasma levels of modafinil).
No products indexed under this heading.

Ranitidine Bismuth Citrate (Co-administration of potent inhibitors of CYP3A4 could alter the plasma levels of modafinil).
No products indexed under this heading.

Ranitidine Hydrochloride (Co-administration of potent inhibitors of CYP3A4 could alter the plasma levels of modafinil). Products include:
Zantac **1737**
Zantac Injection **1732**
Zantac Pharmacy **1735**

Rasagiline Mesylate (Co-administration requires caution; no interaction studies have been performed). Products include:
Azilect **3383**

Repaglinide (An apparent concentration-related suppression of CYP2C9 activity was observed in human hepatocytes after exposure to modafinil *in vitro* suggesting that there is a potential for a metabolic interaction between modafinil and substrates of CYP2C9).
No products indexed under this heading.

Rifabutin (Chronic administration of modafinil can increase the elimination of substrates of CYP3A4. Dose adjustments may be necessary for patients being treated with these and similar medications).
No products indexed under this heading.

Rifampicin (Co-administration of potent inducers of CYP3A4 could alter the plasma levels of modafinil).
No products indexed under this heading.

Rifampin (Chronic administration of modafinil may cause induction of its metabolism; co-administration of potent inducers of CYP3A4, such as rifampin, could alter the levels of modafinil due to the partial involvement of that enzyme in the metabolic elimination of the compound).
No products indexed under this heading.

Rifapentine (Co-administration of potent inducers of CYP3A4 could alter the plasma levels of modafinil).
No products indexed under this heading.

Ritonavir (Chronic administration of modafinil can increase the elimination of substrates of CYP3A4. Dose adjustments may be necessary for patients being treated with these and similar medications). Products include:
Kaletra **458**
Norvir **509**

Rofecoxib (An apparent concentration-related suppression of CYP2C9 activity was observed in human hepatocytes after exposure to modafinil *in vitro* suggesting that there is a potential for a metabolic interaction between modafinil and substrates of CYP2C9).
No products indexed under this heading.

Rosiglitazone Maleate (An apparent concentration-related suppression of CYP2C9 activity was observed in

IMPORTANT NOTE: Always consult each drug listing in the patient's regimen for possible interactions.

(⊙ Described in PDR® for Ophthalmic Medicines)

1531 Interactions Index Prozac

Verapamil Hydrochloride (Chronic administration of modafinil can increase the elimination of substrates of CYP3A4. Dose adjustments may be necessary for patients being treated with these and similar medications). Products include:
Tarka 534

Vinblastine Sulfate (Chronic administration of modafinil can increase the elimination of substrates of CYP3A4. Dose adjustments may be necessary for patients being treated with these and similar medications).
No products indexed under this heading.

Vincristine Sulfate (Chronic administration of modafinil can increase the elimination of substrates of CYP3A4. Dose adjustments may be necessary for patients being treated with these and similar medications).
No products indexed under this heading.

Voriconazole (An apparent concentration-related suppression of CYP2C9 activity was observed in human hepatocytes after exposure to modafinil *in vitro* suggesting that there is a potential for a metabolic interaction between modafinil and substrates of CYP2C9).
No products indexed under this heading.

Warfarin Sodium (There were no significant changes in the pharmacokinetic profile of warfarin in healthy subjects given a single dose of warfarin following chronic administration of modafinil relative to the profiles in subjects given placebo. However, more frequent monitoring of prothrombin times/INR is advisable whenever modafinil is co-administered with warfarin).
No products indexed under this heading.

Zafirlukast (An apparent concentration-related suppression of CYP2C9 activity was observed in human hepatocytes after exposure to modafinil *in vitro* suggesting that there is a potential for a metabolic interaction between modafinil and substrates of CYP2C9). Products include:
Accolate 3612

Zileuton (An apparent concentration-related suppression of CYP2C9 activity was observed in human hepatocytes after exposure to modafinil *in vitro* suggesting that there is a potential for a metabolic interaction between modafinil and substrates of CYP2C9).
No products indexed under this heading.

Food Interactions

Alcohol (The use of modafinil in combination with alcohol has not been studied. It is advisable to avoid alcohol while taking modafinil).

Beer, reduced-alcohol (The use of modafinil in combination with alcohol has not been studied. It is advisable to avoid alcohol while taking modafinil).

Beer, unspecified (The use of modafinil in combination with alcohol has not been studied. It is advisable to avoid alcohol while taking modafinil).

Food, unspecified (Delays the absorption (t_{max}) by approximately one hour; no effect on overall bioavailability).

Grapefruit (Co-administration of potent inhibitors of CYP3A4 could alter the plasma levels of modafinil).

Grapefruit Juice (Co-administration of potent inhibitors of CYP3A4 could alter the plasma levels of modafinil).

Wine, Chianti (The use of modafinil in combination with alcohol has not been studied. It is advisable to avoid alcohol while taking modafinil).

Wine, Red (The use of modafinil in combination with alcohol has not been studied. It is advisable to avoid alcohol while taking modafinil).

Wine, unspecified (The use of modafinil in combination with alcohol has not been studied. It is advisable to avoid alcohol while taking modafinil).

Wine products (The use of modafinil in combination with alcohol has not been studied. It is advisable to avoid alcohol while taking modafinil).

PROZAC WEEKLY CAPSULES

(Fluoxetine Hydrochloride) 1941

May interact with alcohols, antiarrhythmics, anticoagulants, antidepressant drugs, antipsychotic agents, aspirin-acetylsalicylic acid, atypical antipsychotics, centrally-acting drugs, cytochrome p450 2d6 substrates (selected), dopamine antagonists, highly protein bound drugs (selected), insulin, lithium preparations, monoamine oxidase inhibitors, non-steroidal anti-inflammatory agents, oral hypoglycemic agents, phenothiazines, phenytoin, selective serotonin reuptake inhibitors, serotonin and norepinephrine reuptake inhibitors, serotoninergic agents, tricyclic antidepressants, triptans, and certain other agents. Compounds in these categories include:

Acarbose (In patients with diabetes, fluoxetine may alter glycemic control. Hypoglycemia has occurred during therapy with fluoxetine, and hyperglycemia has developed following discontinuation of the drug. As is true with many other types of medication when taken concurrently by patients with diabetes, oral hypoglycemic dosage may need to be adjusted when therapy with fluoxetine is instituted or discontinued).
No products indexed under this heading.

Acebutolol Hydrochloride (Co-administration of fluoxetine with other drugs that are metabolized by CYP2D6, including antiarrhythmics (eg, propafenone, flecainide, and others) should be approached with caution. Therapy with medications that are predominantly metabolized by the CYP2D6 system and that have a relatively narrow therapeutic index should be initiated at the low end of the dose range if a patient is receiving fluoxetine concurrently or has taken it in the previous 5 weeks. If fluoxetine is added to the treatment regimen of a patient already receiving a drug metabolized by CYP2D6, the need for decreased dose of the original medication should be considered).
No products indexed under this heading.

Adenosine (Co-administration of fluoxetine with other drugs that are metabolized by CYP2D6, including antiarrhythmics (eg, propafenone, flecainide, and others) should be approached with caution. Therapy with medications that are predominantly metabolized by the CYP2D6 system and that have a relatively narrow therapeutic index should be initiated at the low end of the dose range if a patient is receiving fluoxetine concurrently or has taken it in the previous 5 weeks. If fluoxetine is added to the treatment regimen of a patient already receiving a drug metabolized by CYP2D6, the need for decreased dose of the original medication should be considered). Products include:
Adenocard 656
Adenoscan 657

Alfentanil Hydrochloride (Caution is advised if the concomitant administration of fluoxetine and CNS-acting drugs is required. In evaluating individual cases, consideration should be given to using lower initial doses of the concomitantly administered drugs, using conservative titration schedules, and monitoring of clinical status).
No products indexed under this heading.

Almotriptan Malate (Based on the mechanism of action of SNRIs and SSRIs, including fluoxetine, and the potential for serotonin syndrome, caution is advised when fluoxetine is co-administered with other drugs that may affect the serotonergic neurotransmitter systems, such as triptans. There have been rare postmarketing reports of serotonin syndrome with use of an SSRI and a triptan. If concomitant treatment of fluoxetine with a triptan is clinically warranted, careful observation of the patient is advised, particularly during treatment initiation and dose increases). Products include:
Axert 2593

Alprazolam (Co-administration of alprazolam and fluoxetine has resulted in increased alprazolam plasma concentrations and in further psychomotor performance decrement due to increased alprazolam levels).
No products indexed under this heading.

Amiodarone Hydrochloride (Because fluoxetine is tightly bound to plasma protein, adverse effects may result from displacement of protein-bound fluoxetine by other tightly-bound drugs).
No products indexed under this heading.

Amitriptyline Hydrochloride (Because fluoxetine is tightly bound to plasma protein, adverse effects may result from displacement of protein-bound fluoxetine by other tightly-bound drugs).
No products indexed under this heading.

Amoxapine (Co-administration of fluoxetine with other drugs that are metabolized by CYP2D6, including certain antidepressants (eg, TCAs), should be approached with caution. Therapy with medications that are predominantly metabolized by the CYP2D6 system and that have a relatively narrow therapeutic index should be initiated at the low end of the dose range if a patient is receiving fluoxetine concurrently or has taken it in the previous 5 weeks. The dose of TCAs may need to be reduced and plasma TCA concentrations may need to be monitored temporarily when fluoxetine is co-administered or has been recently discontinued).
No products indexed under this heading.

Amphetamine Aspartate (Co-administration of fluoxetine with other drugs that are metabolized by CYP2D6, including certain antidepressants (eg, TCAs), antipsychotics (eg, phenothiazines and most atypicals), and antiarrhythmics (eg, propafenone, flecainide, and others) should be approached with caution. Therapy with medications that are predominantly metabolized by the CYP2D6 system and that have a relatively narrow therapeutic index should be initiated at the low end of the dose range if a patient is receiving fluoxetine concurrently or has taken it in the previous 5 weeks. Thus, his/her dosing requirements resemble those of poor metabolizers. If fluoxetine is added to the treatment regimen of a patient already receiving a drug metabolized by CYP2D6, the need for decreased dose of the original medication should be considered).
No products indexed under this heading.

Amphetamine Aspartate Monohydrate (Co-administration of fluoxetine with other drugs that are metabolized by CYP2D6, including certain antidepressants (eg, TCAs), antipsychotics (eg, phenothiazines and most atypicals), and antiarrhythmics (eg, propafenone, flecainide, and others) should be approached with caution. Therapy with medications that are predominantly metabolized by the CYP2D6 system and that have a relatively narrow therapeutic index should be initiated at the low end of the dose range if a patient is receiving fluoxetine concurrently or has taken it in the previous 5 weeks. Thus, his/her dosing requirements resemble those of poor metabolizers. If fluoxetine is added to the treatment regimen of a patient already receiving a drug metabolized by CYP2D6, the need for decreased dose of the original medication should be considered).
No products indexed under this heading.

Amphetamine Resins (Caution is advised if the concomitant administration of fluoxetine and CNS-acting drugs is required. In evaluating individual cases, consideration should be given to using lower initial doses of the concomitantly administered drugs, using conservative titration schedules, and monitoring of clinical status).
No products indexed under this heading.

Amphetamine Sulfate (Co-administration of fluoxetine with other drugs that are metabolized by CYP2D6, including certain antidepressants (eg, TCAs), antipsychotics (eg, phenothiazines and most atypicals), and antiarrhythmics (eg, propafenone, flecainide, and others) should be approached with caution. Therapy with medications that are predominantly metabolized by the CYP2D6 system and that have a relatively narrow therapeutic index should be initiated at the low end of the dose range if a patient is receiving fluoxetine concurrently or has taken it in the previous 5 weeks. Thus, his/her dosing requirements resemble those of poor metabolizers. If fluoxetine is added to the treatment regimen of a patient already receiving a drug metabolized by CYP2D6, the need for decreased dose of the original medication should be considered).
No products indexed under this heading.

Anisindione (SNRIs and SSRIs, including fluoxetine, may increase the risk of bleeding reactions. Concomitant use of anticoagulants may add to this risk. Case reports and epidemiological studies (case-control and cohort design) have demonstrated an association between use of drugs that interfere with serotonin reuptake and the occurrence of gastrointestinal bleeding. Bleeding reactions related to SNRIs and SSRIs use have ranged from ecchymoses, hematomas, epistaxis, and petechiae to life-threatening hemorrhages. Patients should be cautioned about the risk of bleeding associated with the concomitant use of fluoxetine and other drugs that affect coagulation).
No products indexed under this heading.

Aprobarbital (Caution is advised if the concomitant administration of fluoxetine and CNS-acting drugs is required. In evaluating individual cases, consideration should be given to using lower initial doses of the concomitantly administered drugs, using conservative titration schedules, and monitoring of clinical status).
No products indexed under this heading.

Ardeparin Sodium (SNRIs and SSRIs, including fluoxetine, may increase the risk of bleeding reactions. Concomitant use of anticoagulants may add to this risk. Case reports and epidemiological studies (case-control and cohort design) have demonstrated an association between use of drugs that interfere with serotonin reuptake and the occurrence of gastrointestinal bleeding. Bleeding reactions related to SNRIs and SSRIs use have ranged from ecchymoses, hematomas, epistaxis, and petechiae to life-threatening hemorrhages. Patients should be cautioned about the risk of bleeding associated with the concomitant use of fluoxetine and other drugs that affect coagulation).
No products indexed under this heading.

Aripiprazole (Co-administration of fluoxetine with other drugs that are metabolized by CYP2D6, including

IMPORTANT NOTE: Always consult each drug listing in the patient's regimen for possible interactions.

Prozac Interactions Index 1532

antipsychotics (eg, phenothiazines and most atypicals), should be approached with caution. Therapy with medications that are predominantly metabolized by the CYP2D6 system and that have a relatively narrow therapeutic index should be initiated at the low end of the dose range if a patient is receiving fluoxetine concurrently or has taken it in the previous 5 weeks. If fluoxetine is added to the treatment regimen of a patient already receiving a drug metabolized by CYP2D6, the need for decreased dose of the original medication should be considered).
No products indexed under this heading.

Aspirin (Epidemiological studies of the case-control and cohort design that have demonstrated an association between use of psychotropic drugs that interfere with serotonin reuptake and the occurrence of upper gastrointestinal bleeding have also shown that concurrent use of aspirin may potentiate this risk of bleeding). Products include:
Aggrenox 880
Bayer Aspirin 829
Percodan 1124
St. Joseph Aspirin 2045

Aspirin, Enteric Coated (Epidemiological studies of the case-control and cohort design that have demonstrated an association between use of psychotropic drugs that interfere with serotonin reuptake and the occurrence of upper gastrointestinal bleeding have also shown that concurrent use of aspirin may potentiate this risk of bleeding).
No products indexed under this heading.

Aspirin Buffered (Epidemiological studies of the case-control and cohort design that have demonstrated an association between use of psychotropic drugs that interfere with serotonin reuptake and the occurrence of upper gastrointestinal bleeding have also shown that concurrent use of aspirin may potentiate this risk of bleeding).
No products indexed under this heading.

Atomoxetine Hydrochloride (Co-administration of fluoxetine with other drugs that are metabolized by CYP2D6, including certain antidepressants (eg, TCAs), antipsychotics (eg, phenothiazines and most atypicals), and antiarrhythmics (eg, propafenone, flecainide, and others) should be approached with caution. Therapy with medications that are predominantly metabolized by the CYP2D6 system and that have a relatively narrow therapeutic index should be initiated at the low end of the dose range if a patient is receiving fluoxetine concurrently or has taken it in the previous 5 weeks. Thus, his/her dosing requirements resemble those of poor metabolizers. If fluoxetine is added to the treatment regimen of a patient already receiving a drug metabolized by CYP2D6, the need for decreased dose of the original medication should be considered). Products include:
Strattera 1957

Atovaquone (Because fluoxetine is tightly bound to plasma protein, adverse effects may result from displacement of protein-bound fluoxetine by other tightly-bound drugs). Products include:
Malarone Pediatric Tablets 1572
Malarone 1572
Mepron Suspension 1576

Bisoprolol Fumarate (Co-administration of fluoxetine with other drugs that are metabolized by CYP2D6, including certain antidepressants (eg, TCAs), antipsychotics (eg, phenothiazines and most atypicals), and antiarrhythmics (eg, propafenone, flecainide, and others) should be approached with caution. Therapy with medications that are predominantly metabolized by the CYP2D6 system and that have a relatively narrow therapeutic index should be initiated at the low end of the dose range if a patient is receiving fluoxetine concurrently or has taken it in the previous 5 weeks. Thus, his/her dosing requirements resemble those of poor metabolizers. If fluoxetine is added to the treatment regimen of a patient already receiving a drug metabolized by CYP2D6, the need for decreased dose of the original medication should be considered).
No products indexed under this heading.

Bretylium Tosylate (Co-administration of fluoxetine with other drugs that are metabolized by CYP2D6, including antiarrhythmics (eg, propafenone, flecainide, and others) should be approached with caution. Therapy with medications that are predominantly metabolized by the CYP2D6 system and that have a relatively narrow therapeutic index should be initiated at the low end of the dose range if a patient is receiving fluoxetine concurrently or has taken it in the previous 5 weeks. If fluoxetine is added to the treatment regimen of a patient already receiving a drug metabolized by CYP2D6, the need for decreased dose of the original medication should be considered).
No products indexed under this heading.

Buprenorphine Hydrochloride (Caution is advised if the concomitant administration of fluoxetine and CNS-acting drugs is required. In evaluating individual cases, consideration should be given to using lower initial doses of the concomitantly administered drugs, using conservative titration schedules, and monitoring of clinical status).
No products indexed under this heading.

Bupropion Hydrochloride (Co-administration of fluoxetine with other drugs that are metabolized by CYP2D6, including certain antidepressants (eg, TCAs), should be approached with caution. Therapy with medications that are predominantly metabolized by the CYP2D6 system and that have a relatively narrow therapeutic index should be initiated at the low end of the dose range if a patient is receiving fluoxetine concurrently or has taken it in the previous 5 weeks. If fluoxetine is added to the treatment regimen of a patient already receiving a drug metabolized by CYP2D6, the need for decreased dose of the original medication should be considered). Products include:
Aplenzin 2948
Wellbutrin 1719
Wellbutrin SR 1725
Zyban 1762

Buspirone Hydrochloride (Caution is advised if the concomitant administration of fluoxetine and CNS-acting drugs is required. In evaluating individual cases, consideration should be given to using lower initial doses of the concomitantly administered drugs, using conservative titration schedules, and monitoring of clinical status).
No products indexed under this heading.

Butabarbital (Caution is advised if the concomitant administration of fluoxetine and CNS-acting drugs is required. In evaluating individual cases, consideration should be given to using lower initial doses of the concomitantly administered drugs, using conservative titration schedules, and monitoring of clinical status).
No products indexed under this heading.

Butalbital (Caution is advised if the concomitant administration of fluoxetine and CNS-acting drugs is required. In evaluating individual cases, consideration should be given to using lower initial doses of the concomitantly administered drugs, using conservative titration schedules, and monitoring of clinical status).
No products indexed under this heading.

Captopril (Co-administration of fluoxetine with other drugs that are metabolized by CYP2D6, including certain antidepressants (eg, TCAs), antipsychotics (eg, phenothiazines and most atypicals), and antiarrhythmics (eg, propafenone, flecainide, and others) should be approached with caution. Therapy with medications that are predominantly metabolized by the CYP2D6 system and that have a relatively narrow therapeutic index should be initiated at the low end of the dose range if a patient is receiving fluoxetine concurrently or has taken it in the previous 5 weeks. Thus, his/her dosing requirements resemble those of poor metabolizers. If fluoxetine is added to the treatment regimen of a patient already receiving a drug metabolized by CYP2D6, the need for decreased dose of the original medication should be considered). Products include:
Captopril 2341

Carbamazepine (Patients on stable doses of carbamazepine have developed elevated plasma anticonvulsant concentrations and clinical anticonvulsant toxicity following initiation of concomitant fluoxetine treatment). Products include:
Carbatrol 3280
Equetro 3477

Carvedilol (Co-administration of fluoxetine with other drugs that are metabolized by CYP2D6, including certain antidepressants (eg, TCAs), antipsychotics (eg, phenothiazines and most atypicals), and antiarrhythmics (eg, propafenone, flecainide, and others) should be approached with caution. Therapy with medications that are predominantly metabolized by the CYP2D6 system and that have a relatively narrow therapeutic index should be initiated at the low end of the dose range if a patient is receiving fluoxetine concurrently or has taken it in the previous 5 weeks. Thus, his/her dosing requirements resemble those of poor metabolizers. If fluoxetine is added to the treatment regimen of a patient already receiving a drug metabolized by CYP2D6, the need for decreased dose of the original medication should be considered). Products include:
Coreg 1409

Cefonicid Sodium (Because fluoxetine is tightly bound to plasma protein, adverse effects may result from displacement of protein-bound fluoxetine by other tightly-bound drugs).
No products indexed under this heading.

Celecoxib (Epidemiological studies of the case-control and cohort design that have demonstrated an association between use of psychotropic drugs that interfere with serotonin reuptake and the occurrence of upper gastrointestinal bleeding have also shown that concurrent use of an NSAID may potentiate this risk of bleeding). Products include:
Celebrex 3272

Cevimeline Hydrochloride (Co-administration of fluoxetine with other drugs that are metabolized by CYP2D6, including certain antidepressants (eg, TCAs), antipsychotics (eg, phenothiazines and most atypicals), and antiarrhythmics (eg, propafenone, flecainide, and others) should be approached with caution. Therapy with medications that are predominantly metabolized by the CYP2D6 system and that have a relatively narrow therapeutic index should be initiated at the low end of the dose range if a patient is receiving fluoxetine concurrently or has taken it in the previous 5 weeks. Thus, his/her dosing requirements resemble those of poor metabolizers. If fluoxetine is added to the treatment regimen of a patient already receiving a drug metabolized by CYP2D6, the need for decreased dose of the original medication should be considered). Products include:
Evoxac 1027

Chlordiazepoxide (Because fluoxetine is tightly bound to plasma protein, adverse effects may result from displacement of protein-bound fluoxetine by other tightly-bound drugs).
No products indexed under this heading.

Chlordiazepoxide Hydrochloride (Because fluoxetine is tightly bound to plasma protein, adverse effects may result from displacement of protein-bound fluoxetine by other tightly-bound drugs).
No products indexed under this heading.

Chlorpromazine (Because fluoxetine is tightly bound to plasma protein, adverse effects may result from displacement of protein-bound fluoxetine by other tightly-bound drugs).
No products indexed under this heading.

Chlorpromazine Hydrochloride (Because fluoxetine is tightly bound to plasma protein, adverse effects may result from displacement of protein-bound fluoxetine by other tightly-bound drugs).
No products indexed under this heading.

Chlorpropamide (In patients with diabetes, fluoxetine may alter glycemic control. Hypoglycemia has occurred during therapy with fluoxetine, and hyperglycemia has developed following discontinuation of the drug. As is true with many other types of medication when taken concurrently by patients with diabetes, oral hypoglycemic dosage may need to be adjusted when therapy with fluoxetine is instituted or discontinued).
No products indexed under this heading.

Chlorprothixene (Co-administration of fluoxetine with other drugs that are metabolized by CYP2D6, including antipsychotics (eg, phenothiazines and most atypicals), should be approached with caution. Therapy with medications that are predominantly metabolized by the CYP2D6 system and that have a relatively narrow therapeutic index should be initiated at the low end of the dose range if a patient is receiving fluoxetine concurrently or has taken it in the previous 5 weeks. If fluoxetine is added to the treatment regimen of a patient already receiving a drug metabolized by CYP2D6, the need for decreased dose of the original medication should be considered).
No products indexed under this heading.

Chlorprothixene Hydrochloride (Co-administration of fluoxetine with other drugs that are metabolized by CYP2D6, including antipsychotics (eg, phenothiazines and most atypicals), should be approached with caution. Therapy with medications that are predominantly metabolized by the CYP2D6 system and that have a relatively narrow therapeutic index should be initiated at the low end of the dose range if a patient is receiving fluoxetine concurrently or has taken it in the previous 5 weeks. If fluoxetine is added to the treatment regimen of a patient already receiving a drug metabolized by CYP2D6, the need for decreased dose of the original medication should be considered).
No products indexed under this heading.

1533 **Interactions Index** **Prozac**

Chlorprothixene Lactate (Co-administration of fluoxetine with other drugs that are metabolized by CYP2D6, including antipsychotics (eg, phenothiazines and most atypicals), should be approached with caution. Therapy with medications that are predominantly metabolized by the CYP2D6 system and that have a relatively narrow therapeutic index should be initiated at the low end of the dose range if a patient is receiving fluoxetine concurrently or has taken it in the previous 5 weeks. If fluoxetine is added to the treatment regimen of a patient already receiving a drug metabolized by CYP2D6, the need for decreased dose of the original medication should be considered).
No products indexed under this heading.

Citalopram Hydrobromide (Based on the mechanism of action of SSRIs, including fluoxetine, and the potential for serotonin syndrome, caution is advised when fluoxetine is co-administered with other drugs that may affect the serotonergic neurotransmitter systems, such as triptans, linezolid (an antibiotic which is a reversible non-selective MAOI), lithium, tramadol, or St. John's wort. The concomitant use of fluoxetine with SSRIs is not recommended). Products include:
Celexa **1153**

Clomipramine Hydrochloride (Because fluoxetine is tightly bound to plasma protein, adverse effects may result from displacement of protein-bound fluoxetine by other tightly-bound drugs).
No products indexed under this heading.

Clorazepate Dipotassium (Caution is advised if the concomitant administration of fluoxetine and CNS-acting drugs is required. In evaluating individual cases, consideration should be given to using lower initial doses of the concomitantly administered drugs, using conservative titration schedules, and monitoring of clinical status).
No products indexed under this heading.

Clozapine (Some clinical data suggests a possible pharmacodynamic and/or pharmacokinetic interaction between SSRIs and antipsychotics. Elevation of blood levels of clozapine has been observed in patients receiving concomitant fluoxetine).
No products indexed under this heading.

Codeine Phosphate (Co-administration of fluoxetine with other drugs that are metabolized by CYP2D6, including certain antidepressants (eg, TCAs), antipsychotics (eg, phenothiazines and most atypicals), and antiarrhythmics (eg, propafenone, flecainide, and others) should be approached with caution. Therapy with medications that are predominantly metabolized by the CYP2D6 system and that have a relatively narrow therapeutic index should be initiated at the low end of the dose range if a patient is receiving fluoxetine concurrently or has taken it in the previous 5 weeks. Thus, his/her dosing requirements resemble those of poor metabolizers. If fluoxetine is added to the treatment regimen of a patient already receiving a drug metabolized by CYP2D6, the need for decreased dose of the original medication should be considered). Products include:
Tylenol with Codeine **2691**

Codeine Sulfate (Co-administration of fluoxetine with other drugs that are metabolized by CYP2D6, including certain antidepressants (eg, TCAs), antipsychotics (eg, phenothiazines and most atypicals), and antiarrhythmics (eg, propafenone, flecainide, and others) should be approached with caution. Therapy with medications that are predominantly metabolized by the CYP2D6 system and that have a relatively narrow therapeutic index should be initiated at the low end of the dose range if a patient is receiving fluoxetine concurrently or has taken it in the previous 5 weeks. Thus, his/her dosing requirements resemble those of poor metabolizers. If fluoxetine is added to the treatment regimen of a patient already receiving a drug metabolized by CYP2D6, the need for decreased dose of the original medication should be considered).
No products indexed under this heading.

Cyclobenzaprine Hydrochloride (Co-administration of fluoxetine with other drugs that are metabolized by CYP2D6, including certain antidepressants (eg, TCAs), antipsychotics (eg, phenothiazines and most atypicals), and antiarrhythmics (eg, propafenone, flecainide, and others) should be approached with caution. Therapy with medications that are predominantly metabolized by the CYP2D6 system and that have a relatively narrow therapeutic index should be initiated at the low end of the dose range if a patient is receiving fluoxetine concurrently or has taken it in the previous 5 weeks. Thus, his/her dosing requirements resemble those of poor metabolizers. If fluoxetine is added to the treatment regimen of a patient already receiving a drug metabolized by CYP2D6, the need for decreased dose of the original medication should be considered). Products include:
Amrix **964**

Cyclosporine (Because fluoxetine is tightly bound to plasma protein, adverse effects may result from displacement of protein-bound fluoxetine by other tightly-bound drugs). Products include:
Gengraf **440**
Neoral Oral Solution **2496**
Neoral Capsules **2496**
Restasis **605**

Dalteparin Sodium (SNRIs and SSRIs, including fluoxetine, may increase the risk of bleeding reactions. Concomitant use of anticoagulants may add to this risk. Case reports and epidemiological studies (case-control and cohort design) have demonstrated an association between use of drugs that interfere with serotonin reuptake and the occurrence of gastrointestinal bleeding. Bleeding reactions related to SNRIs and SSRIs use have ranged from ecchymoses, hematomas, epistaxis, and petechiae to life-threatening hemorrhages. Patients should be cautioned about the risk of bleeding associated with the concomitant use of fluoxetine and other drugs that affect coagulation). Products include:
Fragmin **1058**

Danaparoid Sodium (SNRIs and SSRIs, including fluoxetine, may increase the risk of bleeding reactions. Concomitant use of anticoagulants may add to this risk. Case reports and epidemiological studies (case-control and cohort design) have demonstrated an association between use of drugs that interfere with serotonin reuptake and the occurrence of gastrointestinal bleeding. Bleeding reactions related to SNRIs and SSRIs use have ranged from ecchymoses, hematomas, epistaxis, and petechiae to life-threatening hemorrhages. Patients should be cautioned about the risk of bleeding associated with the concomitant use of fluoxetine and other drugs that affect coagulation).
No products indexed under this heading.

Debrisoquine (Co-administration of fluoxetine with other drugs that are metabolized by CYP2D6, including certain antidepressants (eg, TCAs), antipsychotics (eg, phenothiazines and most atypicals), and antiarrhythmics (eg, propafenone, flecainide, and others) should be approached with caution. Therapy with medications that are predominantly metabolized by the CYP2D6 system and that have a relatively narrow therapeutic index should be initiated at the low end of the dose range if a patient is receiving fluoxetine concurrently or has taken it in the previous 5 weeks. Thus, his/her dosing requirements resemble those of poor metabolizers. If fluoxetine is added to the treatment regimen of a patient already receiving a drug metabolized by CYP2D6, the need for decreased dose of the original medication should be considered).
No products indexed under this heading.

Desflurane (Caution is advised if the concomitant administration of fluoxetine and CNS-acting drugs is required. In evaluating individual cases, consideration should be given to using lower initial doses of the concomitantly administered drugs, using conservative titration schedules, and monitoring of clinical status).
No products indexed under this heading.

Desipramine Hydrochloride (In 2 studies, previously stable plasma levels of desipramine have increased greater than 2- to 10-fold when fluoxetine has been administered in combination. This influence may persist for 3 weeks or longer after fluoxetineis discontinued. Thus, the dose of TCAs may need to be monitored temporarily when fluoxetine is co-administered or has been recently discontinued).
No products indexed under this heading.

Desvenlafaxine Succinate (Based on the mechanism of action of SNRIs including fluoxetine, and the potential for serotonin syndrome, caution is advised when fluoxetine is co-administered with other drugs that may affect the serotonergic neurotransmitter systems, such as triptans, linezolid (an antibiotic which is a reversible non-selective MAOI), lithium, tramadol, or St. John's wort. The concomitant use of fluoxetine with SNRIs is not recommended). Products include:
Pristiq **3564**

Dexfenfluramine Hydrochloride (Co-administration of fluoxetine with other drugs that are metabolized by CYP2D6, including certain antidepressants (eg, TCAs), antipsychotics (eg, phenothiazines and most atypicals), and antiarrhythmics (eg, propafenone, flecainide, and others) should be approached with caution. Therapy with medications that are predominantly metabolized by the CYP2D6 system and that have a relatively narrow therapeutic index should be initiated at the low end of the dose range if a patient is receiving fluoxetine concurrently or has taken it in the previous 5 weeks. Thus, his/her dosing requirements resemble those of poor metabolizers. If fluoxetine is added to the treatment regimen of a patient already receiving a drug metabolized by CYP2D6, the need for decreased dose of the original medication should be considered).
No products indexed under this heading.

Dexmethylphenidate Hydrochloride (Caution is advised if the concomitant administration of fluoxetine and CNS-acting drugs is required. In evaluating individual cases, consideration should be given to using lower initial doses of the concomitantly administered drugs, using conservative titration schedules, and monitoring of clinical status). Products include:
Focalin XR **2472**

Dextroamphetamine (Caution is advised if the concomitant administration of fluoxetine and CNS-acting drugs is required. In evaluating individual cases, consideration should be given to using lower initial doses of the concomitantly administered drugs, using conservative titration schedules, and monitoring of clinical status).
No products indexed under this heading.

Dextroamphetamine Saccharate (Caution is advised if the concomitant administration of fluoxetine and CNS-acting drugs is required. In evaluating individual cases, consideration should be given to using lower initial doses of the concomitantly administered drugs, using conservative titration schedules, and monitoring of clinical status).
No products indexed under this heading.

Dextroamphetamine Sulfate (Caution is advised if the concomitant administration of fluoxetine and CNS-acting drugs is required. In evaluating individual cases, consideration should be given to using lower initial doses of the concomitantly administered drugs, using conservative titration schedules, and monitoring of clinical status). Products include:
Dexedrine **1425**

Dextromethorphan Hydrobromide (Co-administration of fluoxetine with other drugs that are metabolized by CYP2D6, including certain antidepressants (eg, TCAs), antipsychotics (eg, phenothiazines and most atypicals), and antiarrhythmics (eg, propafenone, flecainide, and others) should be approached with caution. Therapy with medications that are predominantly metabolized by the CYP2D6 system and that have a relatively narrow therapeutic index should be initiated at the low end of the dose range if a patient is receiving fluoxetine concurrently or has taken it in the previous 5 weeks. Thus, his/her dosing requirements resemble those of poor metabolizers. If fluoxetine is added to the treatment regimen of a patient already receiving a drug metabolized by CYP2D6, the need for decreased dose of the original medication should be considered).
No products indexed under this heading.

Dextromethorphan Polistirex (Co-administration of fluoxetine with other drugs that are metabolized by CYP2D6, including certain antidepressants (eg, TCAs), antipsychotics (eg, phenothiazines and most atypicals), and antiarrhythmics (eg, propafenone, flecainide, and others) should be approached with caution. Therapy with medications that are predominantly metabolized by the CYP2D6 system and that have a relatively narrow therapeutic index should be initiated at the low end of the dose range if a patient is receiving fluoxetine concurrently or has taken it in the previous 5 weeks. Thus, his/her dosing requirements resemble those of poor metabolizers. If fluoxetine is added to the treatment regimen of a patient already receiving a drug metabolized by CYP2D6, the need for decreased dose of the original medication should be considered).
No products indexed under this heading.

Dezocine (Caution is advised if the concomitant administration of fluoxetine and CNS-acting drugs is required. In evaluating individual cases, consideration should be given to using lower initial doses of the concomitantly administered drugs, using conservative titration schedules, and monitoring of clinical status).
No products indexed under this heading.

Diazepam (The half-life of concurrently administered diazepam may be prolonged in some patients). Products include:

IMPORTANT NOTE: Always consult each drug listing in the patient's regimen for possible interactions.

Prozac Interactions Index 1534

Valium Tablets 2880

Diclofenac Epolamine (Epidemiological studies of the case-control and cohort design that have demonstrated an association between use of psychotropic drugs that interfere with serotonin reuptake and the occurrence of upper gastrointestinal bleeding have also shown that concurrent use of an NSAID may potentiate this risk of bleeding). Products include:

Flector 1839

Diclofenac Potassium (Epidemiological studies of the case-control and cohort design that have demonstrated an association between use of psychotropic drugs that interfere with serotonin reuptake and the occurrence of upper gastrointestinal bleeding have also shown that concurrent use of an NSAID may potentiate this risk of bleeding).

No products indexed under this heading.

Diclofenac Sodium (Epidemiological studies of the case-control and cohort design that have demonstrated an association between use of psychotropic drugs that interfere with serotonin reuptake and the occurrence of upper gastrointestinal bleeding have also shown that concurrent use of an NSAID may potentiate this risk of bleeding).

No products indexed under this heading.

Dicumarol (SNRIs and SSRIs, including fluoxetine, may increase the risk of bleeding reactions. Concomitant use of anticoagulants may add to this risk. Case reports and epidemiological studies (case-control and cohort design) have demonstrated an association between use of drugs that interfere with serotonin reuptake and the occurrence of gastrointestinal bleeding. Bleeding reactions related to SNRIs and SSRIs use have ranged from ecchymoses, hematomas, epistaxis, and petechiae to life-threatening hemorrhages. Patients should be cautioned about the risk of bleeding associated with the concomitant use of fluoxetine and other drugs that affect coagulation).

No products indexed under this heading.

Digitalis Glycoside Preparations (Because fluoxetine is tightly bound to plasma protein, adverse effects may result from displacement of protein-bound fluoxetine by other tightly-bound drugs).

No products indexed under this heading.

Digitalis Lanata (Because fluoxetine is tightly bound to plasma protein, adverse effects may result from displacement of protein-bound fluoxetine by other tightly-bound drugs).

No products indexed under this heading.

Digitalis Purpurea (Because fluoxetine is tightly bound to plasma protein, adverse effects may result from displacement of protein-bound fluoxetine by other tightly-bound drugs).

No products indexed under this heading.

Dipyridamole (Because fluoxetine is tightly bound to plasma protein, adverse effects may result from displacement of protein-bound fluoxetine by other tightly-bound drugs). Products include:

Aggrenox 880

Disopyramide Phosphate (Co-administration of fluoxetine with other drugs that are metabolized by CYP2D6, including antiarrhythmics (eg, propafenone, flecainide, and others) should be approached with caution. Therapy with medications that are predominantly metabolized by the CYP2D6 system and that have a relatively narrow therapeutic index should be initiated at the low end of the dose range if a patient is receiving fluoxetine concurrently or has taken it in the previous 5 weeks. If fluoxetine is added to the treatment regimen of a patient already receiving a drug metabolized by CYP2D6, the need for decreased dose of the original medication should be considered).

No products indexed under this heading.

Dofetilide (Co-administration of fluoxetine with other drugs that are metabolized by CYP2D6, including antiarrhythmics (eg, propafenone, flecainide, and others) should be approached with caution. Therapy with medications that are predominantly metabolized by the CYP2D6 system and that have a relatively narrow therapeutic index should be initiated at the low end of the dose range if a patient is receiving fluoxetine concurrently or has taken it in the previous 5 weeks. If fluoxetine is added to the treatment regimen of a patient already receiving a drug metabolized by CYP2D6, the need for decreased dose of the original medication should be considered).

No products indexed under this heading.

Dolasetron Mesylate (Co-administration of fluoxetine with other drugs that are metabolized by CYP2D6, including certain antidepressants (eg, TCAs), antipsychotics (eg, phenothiazines and most atypicals), and antiarrhythmics (eg, propafenone, flecainide, and others) should be approached with caution. Therapy with medications that are predominantly metabolized by the CYP2D6 system and that have a relatively narrow therapeutic index should be initiated at the low end of the dose range if a patient is receiving fluoxetine concurrently or has taken it in the previous 5 weeks. Thus, his/her dosing requirements resemble those of poor metabolizers. If fluoxetine is added to the treatment regimen of a patient already receiving a drug metabolized by CYP2D6, the need for decreased dose of the original medication should be considered). Products include:

Anzemet Injection 2931
Anzemet Tablets 2934

Donepezil Hydrochloride (Co-administration of fluoxetine with other drugs that are metabolized by CYP2D6, including certain antidepressants (eg, TCAs), antipsychotics (eg, phenothiazines and most atypicals), and antiarrhythmics (eg, propafenone, flecainide, and others) should be approached with caution. Therapy with medications that are predominantly metabolized by the CYP2D6 system and that have a relatively narrow therapeutic index should be initiated at the low end of the dose range if a patient is receiving fluoxetine concurrently or has taken it in the previous 5 weeks. Thus, his/her dosing requirements resemble those of poor metabolizers. If fluoxetine is added to the treatment regimen of a patient already receiving a drug metabolized by CYP2D6, the need for decreased dose of the original medication should be considered). Products include:

Aricept 1045
Aricept ODT 1045

Doxepin Hydrochloride (Co-administration of fluoxetine with other drugs that are metabolized by CYP2D6, including certain antidepressants (eg, TCAs), should be approached with caution. Therapy with medications that are predominantly metabolized by the CYP2D6 system and that have a relatively narrow therapeutic index should be initiated at the low end of the dose range if a patient is receiving fluoxetine concurrently or has taken it in the previous 5 weeks. The dose of TCAs may need to be reduced and plasma TCA concentrations may need to be monitored temporarily when fluoxetine is co-administered or has been recently discontinued).

No products indexed under this heading.

Droperidol (Caution is advised if the concomitant administration of fluoxetine and CNS-acting drugs is required. In evaluating individual cases, consideration should be given to using lower initial doses of the concomitantly administered drugs, using conservative titration schedules, and monitoring of clinical status).

No products indexed under this heading.

Drugs, unspecified (Patients should be advised to inform their physician if they are taking, or plan to take, any prescription medication, including Symbyax, Sarafem, or over-the-counter drugs. Patients should also be advised to inform their physicians if they plan to discontinue any medications they are taking while on fluoxetine).

No products indexed under this heading.

Duloxetine Hydrochloride (Based on the mechanism of action of SNRIs including fluoxetine, and the potential for serotonin syndrome, caution is advised when fluoxetine is co-administered with other drugs that may affect the serotonergic neurotransmitter systems, such as triptans, linezolid (an antibiotic which is a reversible non-selective MAOI), lithium, tramadol, or St. John's wort. The concomitant use of fluoxetine with SNRIs is not recommended). Products include:

Cymbalta 1871

Eletriptan Hydrobromide (Based on the mechanism of action of SNRIs and SSRIs, including fluoxetine, and the potential for serotonin syndrome, caution is advised when fluoxetine is co-administered with other drugs that may affect the serotonergic neurotransmitter systems, such as triptans. There have been rare postmarketing reports of serotonin syndrome with use of an SSRI and a triptan. If concomitant treatment of fluoxetine with a triptan is clinically warranted, careful observation of the patient is advised, particularly during treatment initiation and dose increases).

No products indexed under this heading.

Encainide Hydrochloride (Co-administration of fluoxetine with other drugs that are metabolized by CYP2D6, including certain antidepressants (eg, TCAs), antipsychotics (eg, phenothiazines and most atypicals), and antiarrhythmics (eg, propafenone, flecainide, and others) should be approached with caution. Therapy with medications that are predominantly metabolized by the CYP2D6 system and that have a relatively narrow therapeutic index should be initiated at the low end of the dose range if a patient is receiving fluoxetine concurrently or has taken it in the previous 5 weeks. Thus, his/her dosing requirements resemble those of poor metabolizers. If fluoxetine is added to the treatment regimen of a patient already receiving a drug metabolized by CYP2D6, the need for decreased dose of the original medication should be considered).

No products indexed under this heading.

Enflurane (Caution is advised if the concomitant administration of fluoxetine and CNS-acting drugs is required. In evaluating individual cases, consideration should be given to using lower initial doses of the concomitantly administered drugs, using conservative titration schedules, and monitoring of clinical status).

No products indexed under this heading.

Enoxaparin Sodium (SNRIs and SSRIs, including fluoxetine, may increase the risk of bleeding reactions. Concomitant use of anticoagulants may add to this risk. Case reports and epidemiological studies (case-control and cohort design) have demonstrated an association between use of drugs that interfere with serotonin reuptake and the occurrence of gastrointestinal bleeding. Bleeding reactions related to SNRIs and SSRIs use have ranged from ecchymoses, hematomas, epistaxis, and petechiae to life-threatening hemorrhages. Patients should be cautioned about the risk of bleeding associated with the concomitant use of fluoxetine and other drugs that affect coagulation). Products include:

Lovenox 3005

Escitalopram Oxalate (Based on the mechanism of action of SSRIs, including fluoxetine, and the potential for serotonin syndrome, caution is advised when fluoxetine is co-administered with other drugs that may affect the serotonergic neurotransmitter systems, such as triptans, linezolid (an antibiotic which is a reversible non-selective MAOI), lithium, tramadol, or St. John's wort. The concomitant use of fluoxetine with SSRIs is not recommended). Products include:

Lexapro Oral Suspension 1160
Lexapro Tablets 1160

Estazolam (Caution is advised if the concomitant administration of fluoxetine and CNS-acting drugs is required. In evaluating individual cases, consideration should be given to using lower initial doses of the concomitantly administered drugs, using conservative titration schedules, and monitoring of clinical status).

No products indexed under this heading.

Ethanol (Caution is advised if the concomitant administration of fluoxetine and CNS-acting drugs is required. In evaluating individual cases, consideration should be given to using lower initial doses of the concomitantly administered drugs, using conservative titration schedules, and monitoring of clinical status).

No products indexed under this heading.

Ethchlorvynol (Caution is advised if the concomitant administration of fluoxetine and CNS-acting drugs is required. In evaluating individual cases, consideration should be given to using lower initial doses of the concomitantly administered drugs, using conservative titration schedules, and monitoring of clinical status).

No products indexed under this heading.

Ethinamate (Caution is advised if the concomitant administration of fluoxetine and CNS-acting drugs is required. In evaluating individual cases, consideration should be given to using lower initial doses of the concomitantly administered drugs, using conservative titration schedules, and monitoring of clinical status).

No products indexed under this heading.

Ethyl Alcohol (Caution is advised if the concomitant administration of fluoxetine and CNS-acting drugs is required. In evaluating individual cases, consideration should be given to using lower initial doses of the concomitantly administered drugs, using conservative titration schedules, and monitoring of clinical status).

No products indexed under this heading.

Etodolac (Epidemiological studies of the case-control and cohort design that have demonstrated an association between use of psychotropic drugs that interfere with serotonin reuptake and the occurrence of upper gastrointestinal bleeding have also shown that concurrent use of an NSAID may potentiate this risk of bleeding).

No products indexed under this heading.

1535 Interactions Index Prozac

Fenoprofen Calcium (Epidemiological studies of the case-control and cohort design that have demonstrated an association between use of psychotropic drugs that interfere with serotonin reuptake and the occurrence of upper gastrointestinal bleeding have also shown that concurrent use of an NSAID may potentiate this risk of bleeding).
No products indexed under this heading.

Fentanyl (Co-administration of fluoxetine with other drugs that are metabolized by CYP2D6, including certain antidepressants (eg, TCAs), antipsychotics (eg, phenothiazines and most atypicals), and antiarrhythmics (eg, propafenone, flecainide, and others) should be approached with caution. Therapy with medications that are predominantly metabolized by the CYP2D6 system and that have a relatively narrow therapeutic index should be initiated at the low end of the dose range if a patient is receiving fluoxetine concurrently or has taken it in the previous 5 weeks. Thus, his/her dosing requirements resemble those of poor metabolizers. If fluoxetine is added to the treatment regimen of a patient already receiving a drug metabolized by CYP2D6, the need for decreased dose of the original medication should be considered). Products include:
Duragesic 2604
Fentanyl Transdermal System 2346
Onsolis 2054

Fentanyl Citrate (Co-administration of fluoxetine with other drugs that are metabolized by CYP2D6, including certain antidepressants (eg, TCAs), antipsychotics (eg, phenothiazines and most atypicals), and antiarrhythmics (eg, propafenone, flecainide, and others) should be approached with caution. Therapy with medications that are predominantly metabolized by the CYP2D6 system and that have a relatively narrow therapeutic index should be initiated at the low end of the dose range if a patient is receiving fluoxetine concurrently or has taken it in the previous 5 weeks. Thus, his/her dosing requirements resemble those of poor metabolizers. If fluoxetine is added to the treatment regimen of a patient already receiving a drug metabolized by CYP2D6, the need for decreased dose of the original medication should be considered). Products include:
Fentora 966

Flecainide Acetate (Co-administration of fluoxetine with other drugs that are metabolized by CYP2D6, including antiarrhythmics (eg, propafenone, flecainide, and others) should be approached with caution. Therapy with medications that are predominantly metabolized by the CYP2D6 system and that have a relatively narrow therapeutic index should be initiated at the low end of the dose range if a patient is receiving fluoxetine concurrently or has taken it in the previous 5 weeks. If fluoxetine is added to the treatment regimen of a patient already receiving a drug metabolized by CYP2D6, the need for decreased dose of the original medication should be considered).
No products indexed under this heading.

Fluoxetine (Based on the mechanism of action of SSRIs, including fluoxetine, and the potential for serotonin syndrome, caution is advised when fluoxetine is co-administered with other drugs that may affect the serotonergic neurotransmitter systems, such as triptans, linezolid (an antibiotic which is a reversible non-selective MAOI), lithium, tramadol, or St. John's wort. The concomitant use of fluoxetine with SSRIs is not recommended).
No products indexed under this heading.

Fluphenazine Decanoate (Co-administration of fluoxetine with other drugs that are metabolized by CYP2D6, including antipsychotics (eg, phenothiazines and most atypicals) should be approached with caution. Therapy with medications that are predominantly metabolized by the CYP2D6 system and that have a relatively narrow therapeutic index should be initiated at the low end of the dose range if a patient is receiving fluoxetine concurrently or has taken it in the previous 5 weeks. If fluoxetine is added to the treatment regimen of a patient already receiving a drug metabolized by CYP2D6, the need for decreased dose of the original medication should be considered).
No products indexed under this heading.

Fluphenazine Enanthate (Co-administration of fluoxetine with other drugs that are metabolized by CYP2D6, including antipsychotics (eg, phenothiazines and most atypicals) should be approached with caution. Therapy with medications that are predominantly metabolized by the CYP2D6 system and that have a relatively narrow therapeutic index should be initiated at the low end of the dose range if a patient is receiving fluoxetine concurrently or has taken it in the previous 5 weeks. If fluoxetine is added to the treatment regimen of a patient already receiving a drug metabolized by CYP2D6, the need for decreased dose of the original medication should be considered).
No products indexed under this heading.

Fluphenazine Hydrochloride (Co-administration of fluoxetine with other drugs that are metabolized by CYP2D6, including antipsychotics (eg, phenothiazines and most atypicals) should be approached with caution. Therapy with medications that are predominantly metabolized by the CYP2D6 system and that have a relatively narrow therapeutic index should be initiated at the low end of the dose range if a patient is receiving fluoxetine concurrently or has taken it in the previous 5 weeks. If fluoxetine is added to the treatment regimen of a patient already receiving a drug metabolized by CYP2D6, the need for decreased dose of the original medication should be considered).
No products indexed under this heading.

Flurazepam Hydrochloride (Because fluoxetine is tightly bound to plasma protein, adverse effects may result from displacement of protein-bound fluoxetine by other tightly-bound drugs).
No products indexed under this heading.

Flurbiprofen (Epidemiological studies of the case-control and cohort design that have demonstrated an association between use of psychotropic drugs that interfere with serotonin reuptake and the occurrence of upper gastrointestinal bleeding have also shown that concurrent use of an NSAID may potentiate this risk of bleeding).
No products indexed under this heading.

Fluvoxamine (Based on the mechanism of action of SSRIs, including fluoxetine, and the potential for serotonin syndrome, caution is advised when fluoxetine is co-administered with other drugs that may affect the serotonergic neurotransmitter systems, such as triptans, linezolid (an antibiotic which is a reversible non-selective MAOI), lithium, tramadol, or St. John's wort. The concomitant use of fluoxetine with SSRIs is not recommended).
No products indexed under this heading.

Fluvoxamine Maleate (Based on the mechanism of action of SSRIs, including fluoxetine, and the potential for serotonin syndrome, caution is advised when fluoxetine is co-administered with other drugs that may affect the serotonergic neurotransmitter systems, such as triptans, linezolid (an antibiotic which is a reversible non-selective MAOI), lithium, tramadol, or St. John's wort. The concomitant use of fluoxetine with SSRIs is not recommended).
No products indexed under this heading.

Fondaparinux Sodium (SNRIs and SSRIs, including fluoxetine, may increase the risk of bleeding reactions. Concomitant use of anticoagulants may add to this risk. Case reports and epidemiological studies (case-control and cohort design) have demonstrated an association between use of drugs that interfere with serotonin reuptake and the occurrence of gastrointestinal bleeding. Bleeding reactions related to SNRIs and SSRIs use have ranged from ecchymoses, hematomas, epistaxis, and petechiae to life-threatening hemorrhages. Patients should be cautioned about the risk of bleeding associated with the concomitant use of fluoxetine and other drugs that affect coagulation). Products include:
Arixtra 1320

Formoterol Fumarate (Co-administration of fluoxetine with other drugs that are metabolized by CYP2D6, including certain antidepressants (eg, TCAs), antipsychotics (eg, phenothiazines and most atypicals), and antiarrhythmics (eg, propafenone, flecainide, and others) should be approached with caution. Therapy with medications that are predominantly metabolized by the CYP2D6 system and that have a relatively narrow therapeutic index should be initiated at the low end of the dose range if a patient is receiving fluoxetine concurrently or has taken it in the previous 5 weeks. Thus, his/her dosing requirements resemble those of poor metabolizers. If fluoxetine is added to the treatment regimen of a patient already receiving a drug metabolized by CYP2D6, the need for decreased dose of the original medication should be considered). Products include:
Foradil 3121
Perforomist 3634

Fosphenytoin (Patients on stable doses of phenytoin have developed elevated plasma phenytoin concentrations and clinical anticonvulsant toxicity following initiation of concomitant fluoxetine therapy).
No products indexed under this heading.

Fosphenytoin Sodium (Patients on stable doses of phenytoin have developed elevated plasma phenytoin concentrations and clinical anticonvulsant toxicity following initiation of concomitant fluoxetine therapy).
No products indexed under this heading.

Frovatriptan Succinate (Based on the mechanism of action of SNRIs and SSRIs, including fluoxetine, and the potential for serotonin syndrome, caution is advised when fluoxetine is co-administered with other drugs that may affect the serotonergic neurotransmitter systems, such as triptans. There have been rare postmarketing reports of serotonin syndrome with use of an SSRI and a triptan. If concomitant treatment of fluoxetine with a triptan is clinically warranted, careful observation of the patient is advised, particularly during treatment initiation and dose increases). Products include:
Frova 1103

Galantamine Hydrobromide (Co-administration of fluoxetine with other drugs that are metabolized by CYP2D6, including certain antidepressants (eg, TCAs), antipsychotics (eg, phenothiazines and most atypicals), and antiarrhythmics (eg, propafenone, flecainide, and others) should be approached with caution. Therapy with medications that are predominantly metabolized by the CYP2D6 system and that have a relatively narrow therapeutic index should be initiated at the low end of the dose range if a patient is receiving fluoxetine concurrently or has taken it in the previous 5 weeks. Thus, his/her dosing requirements resemble those of poor metabolizers. If fluoxetine is added to the treatment regimen of a patient already receiving a drug metabolized by CYP2D6, the need for decreased dose of the original medication should be considered).
No products indexed under this heading.

Glibenclamide (In patients with diabetes, fluoxetine may alter glycemic control. Hypoglycemia has occurred during therapy with fluoxetine, and hyperglycemia has developed following discontinuation of the drug. As is true with many other types of medication when taken concurrently by patients with diabetes, oral hypoglycemic dosage may need to be adjusted when therapy with fluoxetine is instituted or discontinued).
No products indexed under this heading.

Glimepiride (In patients with diabetes, fluoxetine may alter glycemic control. Hypoglycemia has occurred during therapy with fluoxetine, and hyperglycemia has developed following discontinuation of the drug. As is true with many other types of medication when taken concurrently by patients with diabetes, oral hypoglycemic dosage may need to be adjusted when therapy with fluoxetine is instituted or discontinued). Products include:
Avandaryl 1356
Duetact 3354

Glipizide (In patients with diabetes, fluoxetine may alter glycemic control. Hypoglycemia has occurred during therapy with fluoxetine, and hyperglycemia has developed following discontinuation of the drug. As is true with many other types of medication when taken concurrently by patients with diabetes, oral hypoglycemic dosage may need to be adjusted when therapy with fluoxetine is instituted or discontinued).
No products indexed under this heading.

Glutethimide (Caution is advised if the concomitant administration of fluoxetine and CNS-acting drugs is required. In evaluating individual cases, consideration should be given to using lower initial doses of the concomitantly administered drugs, using conservative titration schedules, and monitoring of clinical status).
No products indexed under this heading.

Glyburide (In patients with diabetes, fluoxetine may alter glycemic control. Hypoglycemia has occurred during therapy with fluoxetine, and hyperglycemia has developed following discontinuation of the drug. As is true with many other types of medication when taken concurrently by patients with diabetes, oral hypoglycemic dosage may need to be adjusted when therapy with fluoxetine is instituted or discontinued).
No products indexed under this heading.

Haloperidol (Some clinical data suggests a possible pharmacodynamic and/or pharmacokinetic interaction between SSRIs and antipsychotics. Elevation of blood levels of haloperidol has been observed in patients receiving concomitant fluoxetine).
No products indexed under this heading.

Haloperidol Decanoate (Some clinical data suggests a possible pharmacodynamic and/or pharmacokinetic interaction between SSRIs and antipsychotics. Elevation of blood levels of haloperidol has been observed in patients receiving concomitant fluoxetine).
No products indexed under this heading.

IMPORTANT NOTE: Always consult each drug listing in the patient's regimen for possible interactions.

Prozac Interactions Index 1536

Haloperidol Lactate (Some clinical data suggests a possible pharmacodynamic and/or pharmacokinetic interaction between SSRIs and antipsychotics. Elevation of blood levels of haloperidol has been observed in patients receiving concomitant fluoxetine).
No products indexed under this heading.

Heparin Calcium (SNRIs and SSRIs, including fluoxetine, may increase the risk of bleeding reactions. Concomitant use of anticoagulants may add to this risk. Case reports and epidemiological studies (case-control and cohort design) have demonstrated an association between use of drugs that interfere with serotonin reuptake and the occurrence of gastrointestinal bleeding. Bleeding reactions related to SNRIs and SSRIs use have ranged from ecchymoses, hematomas, epistaxis, and petechiae to life-threatening hemorrhages. Patients should be cautioned about the risk of bleeding associated with the concomitant use of fluoxetine and other drugs that affect coagulation).
No products indexed under this heading.

Heparin Sodium (SNRIs and SSRIs, including fluoxetine, may increase the risk of bleeding reactions. Concomitant use of anticoagulants may add to this risk. Case reports and epidemiological studies (case-control and cohort design) have demonstrated an association between use of drugs that interfere with serotonin reuptake and the occurrence of gastrointestinal bleeding. Bleeding reactions related to SNRIs and SSRIs use have ranged from ecchymoses, hematomas, epistaxis, and petechiae to life-threatening hemorrhages. Patients should be cautioned about the risk of bleeding associated with the concomitant use of fluoxetine and other drugs that affect coagulation).
No products indexed under this heading.

Herbal Medicines, unspecified (Patients should be advised to inform their physician if they are taking, or plan to take, any prescription medication, including herbal supplements. Patients should also be advised to inform their physicians if they plan to discontinue any medications they are taking while on fluoxetine).
No products indexed under this heading.

Hydrocodone Bitartrate (Co-administration of fluoxetine with other drugs that are metabolized by CYP2D6, including certain antidepressants (eg, TCAs), antipsychotics (eg, phenothiazines and most atypicals), and antiarrhythmics (eg, propafenone, flecainide, and others) should be approached with caution. Therapy with medications that are predominantly metabolized by the CYP2D6 system and that have a relatively narrow therapeutic index should be initiated at the low end of the dose range if a patient is receiving fluoxetine concurrently or has taken it in the previous 5 weeks. Thus, his/her dosing requirements resemble those of poor metabolizers. If fluoxetine is added to the treatment regimen of a patient already receiving a drug metabolized by CYP2D6, the need for decreased dose of the original medication should be considered). Products include:
Vicodin ... 560
Vicodin ES ... 561
Vicodin HP ... 563
Vicoprofen ... 564
Zydone ... 1138

Hydrocodone Polistirex (Caution is advised if the concomitant administration of fluoxetine and CNS-acting drugs is required. In evaluating individual cases, consideration should be given to using lower initial doses of the concomitantly administered drugs, using conservative titration schedules, and monitoring of clinical status). Products include:
Tussionex ... 3443

Hydromorphone Hydrochloride (Caution is advised if the concomitant administration of fluoxetine and CNS-acting drugs is required. In evaluating individual cases, consideration should be given to using lower initial doses of the concomitantly administered drugs, using conservative titration schedules, and monitoring of clinical status). Products include:
Dilaudid Injection ... 2800
Dilaudid Oral ... 2797
Dilaudid Tablets ... 2797
Dilaudid-HP ... 2800

Hydroxyamphetamine Hydrobromide (Caution is advised if the concomitant administration of fluoxetine and CNS-acting drugs is required. In evaluating individual cases, consideration should be given to using lower initial doses of the concomitantly administered drugs, using conservative titration schedules, and monitoring of clinical status).
No products indexed under this heading.

Hydroxyzine Hydrochloride (Caution is advised if the concomitant administration of fluoxetine and CNS-acting drugs is required. In evaluating individual cases, consideration should be given to using lower initial doses of the concomitantly administered drugs, using conservative titration schedules, and monitoring of clinical status).
No products indexed under this heading.

Hypericum (Based on the mechanism of action of SNRIs and SSRIs and the potential for serotonin syndrome, caution is advised when fluoxetine is co-administered with other drugs that may effect the serotonergic neurotransmitter systems, such as St. John's wort).
No products indexed under this heading.

Hypericum Perforatum (Based on the mechanism of action of SNRIs and SSRIs and the potential for serotonin syndrome, caution is advised when fluoxetine is co-administered with other drugs that may effect the serotonergic neurotransmitter systems, such as St. John's wort). Products include:
Traumeel ... 1800

Ibuprofen (Epidemiological studies of the case-control and cohort design that have demonstrated an association between use of psychotropic drugs that interfere with serotonin reuptake and the occurrence of upper gastrointestinal bleeding have also shown that concurrent use of an NSAID may potentiate this risk of bleeding). Products include:
Motrin IB ... 2043
Children's Motrin ... 2044
Children's Motrin Non-Staining Dye-Free ... 2044
Infants' Motrin ... 2044
Infants' Motrin Dye-Free ... 2044
Junior Strength Motrin ... 2044
Vicoprofen ... 564

Imipramine Hydrochloride (In 2 studies, previously stable plasma levels of imipramine have increased greater than 2- to 10-fold when fluoxetine has been administered in combination. This influence may persist for 3 weeks or longer after fluoxetineis discontinued. Thus, the dose of TCAs may need to be monitored temporarily when fluoxetine is co-administered or has been recently discontinued).
No products indexed under this heading.

Imipramine Pamoate (In 2 studies, previously stable plasma levels of imipramine have increased greater than 2- to 10-fold when fluoxetine has been administered in combination. This influence may persist for 3 weeks or longer after fluoxetineis discontinued. Thus, the dose of TCAs may need to be monitored temporarily when fluoxetine is co-administered or has been recently discontinued).
No products indexed under this heading.

Indomethacin (Epidemiological studies of the case-control and cohort design that have demonstrated an association between use of psychotropic drugs that interfere with serotonin reuptake and the occurrence of upper gastrointestinal bleeding have also shown that concurrent use of an NSAID may potentiate this risk of bleeding). Products include:
Indocin ... 2167

Indomethacin Sodium Trihydrate (Epidemiological studies of the case-control and cohort design that have demonstrated an association between use of psychotropic drugs that interfere with serotonin reuptake and the occurrence of upper gastrointestinal bleeding have also shown that concurrent use of an NSAID may potentiate this risk of bleeding). Products include:
Indocin I.V. ... 2007

Indoramin Hydrochloride (Co-administration of fluoxetine with other drugs that are metabolized by CYP2D6, including certain antidepressants (eg, TCAs), antipsychotics (eg, phenothiazines and most atypicals), and antiarrhythmics (eg, propafenone, flecainide, and others) should be approached with caution. Therapy with medications that are predominantly metabolized by the CYP2D6 system and that have a relatively narrow therapeutic index should be initiated at the low end of the dose range if a patient is receiving fluoxetine concurrently or has taken it in the previous 5 weeks. Thus, his/her dosing requirements resemble those of poor metabolizers. If fluoxetine is added to the treatment regimen of a patient already receiving a drug metabolized by CYP2D6, the need for decreased dose of the original medication should be considered).
No products indexed under this heading.

Insulin (In patients with diabetes, fluoxetine may alter glycemic control. Hypoglycemia has occurred during therapy with fluoxetine, and hyperglycemia has developed following discontinuation of the drug. As is true with many other types of medication when taken concurrently by patients with diabetes, insulin dosage may need to be adjusted when therapy with fluoxetine is instituted or discontinued).
No products indexed under this heading.

Insulin, Human, Zinc Suspension (In patients with diabetes, fluoxetine may alter glycemic control. Hypoglycemia has occurred during therapy with fluoxetine, and hyperglycemia has developed following discontinuation of the drug. As is true with many other types of medication when taken concurrently by patients with diabetes, insulin dosage may need to be adjusted when therapy with fluoxetine is instituted or discontinued).
No products indexed under this heading.

Insulin, Human (rDNA origin) (In patients with diabetes, fluoxetine may alter glycemic control. Hypoglycemia has occurred during therapy with fluoxetine, and hyperglycemia has developed following discontinuation of the drug. As is true with many other types of medication when taken concurrently by patients with diabetes, insulin dosage may need to be adjusted when therapy with fluoxetine is instituted or discontinued). Products include:
Exubera ... 2717

Insulin, Human NPH (In patients with diabetes, fluoxetine may alter glycemic control. Hypoglycemia has occurred during therapy with fluoxetine, and hyperglycemia has developed following discontinuation of the drug. As is true with many other types of medication when taken concurrently by patients with diabetes, insulin dosage may need to be adjusted when therapy with fluoxetine is instituted or discontinued). Products include:
Humulin N Vial ... 1934

Insulin, Human Regular (In patients with diabetes, fluoxetine may alter glycemic control. Hypoglycemia has occurred during therapy with fluoxetine, and hyperglycemia has developed following discontinuation of the drug. As is true with many other types of medication when taken concurrently by patients with diabetes, insulin dosage may need to be adjusted when therapy with fluoxetine is instituted or discontinued). Products include:
Humulin R ... 1937
Humulin R (U-500) ... 1939

Insulin, Human Regular and Human NPH Mixture (In patients with diabetes, fluoxetine may alter glycemic control. Hypoglycemia has occurred during therapy with fluoxetine, and hyperglycemia has developed following discontinuation of the drug. As is true with many other types of medication when taken concurrently by patients with diabetes, insulin dosage may need to be adjusted when therapy with fluoxetine is instituted or discontinued). Products include:
Humulin 50/50 ... 1930
Humulin 70/30 Vial ... 1931

Insulin, NPH (In patients with diabetes, fluoxetine may alter glycemic control. Hypoglycemia has occurred during therapy with fluoxetine, and hyperglycemia has developed following discontinuation of the drug. As is true with many other types of medication when taken concurrently by patients with diabetes, insulin dosage may need to be adjusted when therapy with fluoxetine is instituted or discontinued).
No products indexed under this heading.

Insulin, Regular (In patients with diabetes, fluoxetine may alter glycemic control. Hypoglycemia has occurred during therapy with fluoxetine, and hyperglycemia has developed following discontinuation of the drug. As is true with many other types of medication when taken concurrently by patients with diabetes, insulin dosage may need to be adjusted when therapy with fluoxetine is instituted or discontinued).
No products indexed under this heading.

Insulin, Regular and NPH mixture (In patients with diabetes, fluoxetine may alter glycemic control. Hypoglycemia has occurred during therapy with fluoxetine, and hyperglycemia has developed following discontinuation of the drug. As is true with many other types of medication when taken concurrently by patients with diabetes, insulin dosage may need to be adjusted when therapy with fluoxetine is instituted or discontinued).
No products indexed under this heading.

Insulin, Zinc Crystals (In patients with diabetes, fluoxetine may alter glycemic control. Hypoglycemia has occurred during therapy with fluoxetine, and hyperglycemia has developed following discontinuation of the drug. As is true with many other types of medication when taken concurrently by patients with diabetes, insulin dosage

(⊙ Described in PDR® for Ophthalmic Medicines)

may need to be adjusted when therapy with fluoxetine is instituted or discontinued).

No products indexed under this heading.

Insulin, Zinc Suspension (In patients with diabetes, fluoxetine may alter glycemic control. Hypoglycemia has occurred during therapy with fluoxetine, and hyperglycemia has developed following discontinuation of the drug. As is true with many other types of medication when taken concurrently by patients with diabetes, insulin dosage may need to be adjusted when therapy with fluoxetine is instituted or discontinued).

No products indexed under this heading.

Insulin Aspart (In patients with diabetes, fluoxetine may alter glycemic control. Hypoglycemia has occurred during therapy with fluoxetine, and hyperglycemia has developed following discontinuation of the drug. As is true with many other types of medication when taken concurrently by patients with diabetes, insulin dosage may need to be adjusted when therapy with fluoxetine is instituted or discontinued).

No products indexed under this heading.

Insulin Aspart, Human (In patients with diabetes, fluoxetine may alter glycemic control. Hypoglycemia has occurred during therapy with fluoxetine, and hyperglycemia has developed following discontinuation of the drug. As is true with many other types of medication when taken concurrently by patients with diabetes, insulin dosage may need to be adjusted when therapy with fluoxetine is instituted or discontinued). Products include:

NovoLog Mix 70/30 2581

Insulin Aspart, Human Regular (In patients with diabetes, fluoxetine may alter glycemic control. Hypoglycemia has occurred during therapy with fluoxetine, and hyperglycemia has developed following discontinuation of the drug. As is true with many other types of medication when taken concurrently by patients with diabetes, insulin dosage may need to be adjusted when therapy with fluoxetine is instituted or discontinued). Products include:

NovoLog 2575

Insulin Aspart Protamine, Human (In patients with diabetes, fluoxetine may alter glycemic control. Hypoglycemia has occurred during therapy with fluoxetine, and hyperglycemia has developed following discontinuation of the drug. As is true with many other types of medication when taken concurrently by patients with diabetes, insulin dosage may need to be adjusted when therapy with fluoxetine is instituted or discontinued). Products include:

NovoLog Mix 70/30 2581

Insulin Detemir (rDNA Origin) (In patients with diabetes, fluoxetine may alter glycemic control. Hypoglycemia has occurred during therapy with fluoxetine, and hyperglycemia has developed following discontinuation of the drug. As is true with many other types of medication when taken concurrently by patients with diabetes, insulin dosage may need to be adjusted when therapy with fluoxetine is instituted or discontinued). Products include:

Levemir 2566

Insulin Glargine (In patients with diabetes, fluoxetine may alter glycemic control. Hypoglycemia has occurred during therapy with fluoxetine, and hyperglycemia has developed following discontinuation of the drug. As is true with many other types of medication when taken concurrently by patients with diabetes, insulin dosage may need to be adjusted when therapy with fluoxetine is instituted or discontinued). Products include:

Lantus 2996

Insulin Glulisine (In patients with diabetes, fluoxetine may alter glycemic control. Hypoglycemia has occurred during therapy with fluoxetine, and hyperglycemia has developed following discontinuation of the drug. As is true with many other types of medication when taken concurrently by patients with diabetes, insulin dosage may need to be adjusted when therapy with fluoxetine is instituted or discontinued). Products include:

Apidra 2937
Apidra SoloStar 2937

Insulin Lispro, Human (In patients with diabetes, fluoxetine may alter glycemic control. Hypoglycemia has occurred during therapy with fluoxetine, and hyperglycemia has developed following discontinuation of the drug. As is true with many other types of medication when taken concurrently by patients with diabetes, insulin dosage may need to be adjusted when therapy with fluoxetine is instituted or discontinued). Products include:

Humalog 1910
Humalog Mix 1914
Humalog Mix75/25 1917

Insulin Lispro Protamine, Human (In patients with diabetes, fluoxetine may alter glycemic control. Hypoglycemia has occurred during therapy with fluoxetine, and hyperglycemia has developed following discontinuation of the drug. As is true with many other types of medication when taken concurrently by patients with diabetes, insulin dosage may need to be adjusted when therapy with fluoxetine is instituted or discontinued). Products include:

Humalog Mix 1914
Humalog Mix75/25 1917

Isocarboxazid (Fluoxetine is contraindicated for use with monoamine oxidase inhibitors (MAOIs). There have been reports of serious, sometimes fatal, reactions (including hyperthermia, rigidity, myoclonus, autonomic instability with possible rapid fluctuations of vital signs, and mental status changes that include extreme agitation progressing to delirium and coma) in patients receiving fluoxetine in combination with MAOI, and in patients who have recently discontinued fluoxetine and are then started on an MAOI. Some cases presented with features resembling neuroleptic malignant syndrome. Therefore, fluoxetine should not be used in combination with an MAOI, or within a minimum of 14 days of discontinuing therapy with an MAOI. Since fluoxetine and its major metabolite have very long elimination half-lives, at least 5 weeks perhaps longer, especially if fluoxetine has been prescribed chronically and/or at higher doses, should be allowed after stopping fluoxetine before starting an MAOI). Products include:

Marplan 3481

Isoflurane (Caution is advised if the concomitant administration of fluoxetine and CNS-acting drugs is required. In evaluating individual cases, consideration should be given to using lower initial doses of the concomitantly administered drugs, using conservative titration schedules, and monitoring of clinical status).

No products indexed under this heading.

Ketamine Hydrochloride (Caution is advised if the concomitant administration of fluoxetine and CNS-acting drugs is required. In evaluating individual cases, consideration should be given to using lower initial doses of the concomitantly administered drugs, using conservative titration schedules, and monitoring of clinical status).

No products indexed under this heading.

Ketoprofen (Epidemiological studies of the case-control and cohort design that have demonstrated an association between use of psychotropic drugs that interfere with serotonin reuptake and the occurrence of upper gastrointestinal bleeding have also shown that concurrent use of an NSAID may potentiate this risk of bleeding).

No products indexed under this heading.

Ketorolac Tromethamine (Epidemiological studies of the case-control and cohort design that have demonstrated an association between use of psychotropic drugs that interfere with serotonin reuptake and the occurrence of upper gastrointestinal bleeding have also shown that concurrent use of an NSAID may potentiate this risk of bleeding). Products include:

Acuvail .... ⊙ 209

Labetalol Hydrochloride (Co-administration of fluoxetine with other drugs that are metabolized by CYP2D6, including certain antidepressants (eg, TCAs), antipsychotics (eg, phenothiazines and most atypicals), and antiarrhythmics (eg, propafenone, flecainide, and others) should be approached with caution. Therapy with medications that are predominantly metabolized by the CYP2D6 system and that have a relatively narrow therapeutic index should be initiated at the low end of the dose range if a patient is receiving fluoxetine concurrently or has taken it in the previous 5 weeks. Thus, his/her dosing requirements resemble those of poor metabolizers. If fluoxetine is added to the treatment regimen of a patient already receiving a drug metabolized by CYP2D6, the need for decreased dose of the original medication should be considered).

No products indexed under this heading.

Levomethadyl Acetate Hydrochloride (Caution is advised if the concomitant administration of fluoxetine and CNS-acting drugs is required. In evaluating individual cases, consideration should be given to using lower initial doses of the concomitantly administered drugs, using conservative titration schedules, and monitoring of clinical status).

No products indexed under this heading.

Levorphanol Tartrate (Caution is advised if the concomitant administration of fluoxetine and CNS-acting drugs is required. In evaluating individual cases, consideration should be given to using lower initial doses of the concomitantly administered drugs, using conservative titration schedules, and monitoring of clinical status).

No products indexed under this heading.

Lidocaine (Co-administration of fluoxetine with other drugs that are metabolized by CYP2D6, including certain antidepressants (eg, TCAs), antipsychotics (eg, phenothiazines and most atypicals), and antiarrhythmics (eg, propafenone, flecainide, and others) should be approached with caution. Therapy with medications that are predominantly metabolized by the CYP2D6 system and that have a relatively narrow therapeutic index should be initiated at the low end of the dose range if a patient is receiving fluoxetine concurrently or has taken it in the previous 5 weeks. Thus, his/her dosing requirements resemble those of poor metabolizers. If fluoxetine is added to the treatment regimen of a patient already receiving a drug metabolized by CYP2D6, the need for decreased dose of the original medication should be considered). Products include:

Lidoderm 1107

Lidocaine Hydrochloride (Co-administration of fluoxetine with other drugs that are metabolized by CYP2D6,

---

including antiarrhythmics (eg, propafenone, flecainide, and others) should be approached with caution. Therapy with medications that are predominantly metabolized by the CYP2D6 system and that have a relatively narrow therapeutic index should be initiated at the low end of the dose range if a patient is receiving fluoxetine concurrently or has taken it in the previous 5 weeks. If fluoxetine is added to the treatment regimen of a patient already receiving a drug metabolized by CYP2D6, the need for decreased dose of the original medication should be considered).

No products indexed under this heading.

Linezolid (Based on the mechanism of action of SNRIs and SSRIs, including fluoxetine, and the potential for serotonin syndrome, caution is advised when fluoxetine is co-administered with other drugs that may affect the serotonergic neurotransmitter systems, such as linezolid (an antibiotic which is a reversible non-selective MAOI)). Products include:

Zyvox 2769

Lisdexamfetamine Dimesylate (Caution is advised if the concomitant administration of fluoxetine and CNS-acting drugs is required. In evaluating individual cases, consideration should be given to using lower initial doses of the concomitantly administered drugs, using conservative titration schedules, and monitoring of clinical status). Products include:

Vyvanse 3298

Lithium (Based on the mechanism of action of SNRIs and SSRIs, including fluoxetine, and the potential for serotonin syndrome, caution is advised when fluoxetine is co-administered with other drugs that may affect the serotonergic neurotransmitter systems, such as lithium. There have been reports of both increased and decreased lithium levels when lithium was used concomitantly with fluoxetine. Cases of lithium toxicity and increased serotonergic effects have been reported. Lithium levels should be monitored when these drugs are administered concomitantly).

No products indexed under this heading.

Lithium Carbonate (Based on the mechanism of action of SNRIs and SSRIs, including fluoxetine, and the potential for serotonin syndrome, caution is advised when fluoxetine is co-administered with other drugs that may affect the serotonergic neurotransmitter systems, such as lithium. There have been reports of both increased and decreased lithium levels when lithium was used concomitantly with fluoxetine. Cases of lithium toxicity and increased serotonergic effects have been reported. Lithium levels should be monitored when these drugs are administered concomitantly).

No products indexed under this heading.

Lithium Citrate (Based on the mechanism of action of SNRIs and SSRIs, including fluoxetine, and the potential for serotonin syndrome, caution is advised when fluoxetine is co-administered with other drugs that may affect the serotonergic neurotransmitter systems, such as lithium. There have been reports of both increased and decreased lithium levels when lithium was used concomitantly with fluoxetine. Cases of lithium toxicity and increased serotonergic effects have been reported. Lithium levels should be monitored when these drugs are administered concomitantly).

No products indexed under this heading.

IMPORTANT NOTE: Always consult each drug listing in the patient's regimen for possible interactions.

Prozac Interactions Index 1538

Lorazepam (Caution is advised if the concomitant administration of fluoxetine and CNS-acting drugs is required. In evaluating individual cases, consideration should be given to using lower initial doses of the concomitantly administered drugs, using conservative titration schedules, and monitoring of clinical status).
No products indexed under this heading.

Low Molecular Weight Heparins (SNRIs and SSRIs, including fluoxetine, may increase the risk of bleeding reactions. Concomitant use of anticoagulants may add to this risk. Case reports and epidemiological studies (case-control and cohort design) have demonstrated an association between use of drugs that interfere with serotonin reuptake and the occurrence of gastrointestinal bleeding. Bleeding reactions related to SNRIs and SSRIs use have ranged from ecchymoses, hematomas, epistaxis, and petechiae to life-threatening hemorrhages. Patients should be cautioned about the risk of bleeding associated with the concomitant use of fluoxetine and other drugs that affect coagulation).
No products indexed under this heading.

Loxapine Hydrochloride (Co-administration of fluoxetine with other drugs that are metabolized by CYP2D6, including antipsychotics (eg, phenothiazines and most atypicals), should be approached with caution. Therapy with medications that are predominantly metabolized by the CYP2D6 system and that have a relatively narrow therapeutic index should be initiated at the low end of the dose range if a patient is receiving fluoxetine concurrently or has taken it in the previous 5 weeks. If fluoxetine is added to the treatment regimen of a patient already receiving a drug metabolized by CYP2D6, the need for decreased dose of the original medication should be considered).
No products indexed under this heading.

Loxapine Succinate (Co-administration of fluoxetine with other drugs that are metabolized by CYP2D6, including antipsychotics (eg, phenothiazines and most atypicals), should be approached with caution. Therapy with medications that are predominantly metabolized by the CYP2D6 system and that have a relatively narrow therapeutic index should be initiated at the low end of the dose range if a patient is receiving fluoxetine concurrently or has taken it in the previous 5 weeks. If fluoxetine is added to the treatment regimen of a patient already receiving a drug metabolized by CYP2D6, the need for decreased dose of the original medication should be considered).
No products indexed under this heading.

Maprotiline Hydrochloride (Co-administration of fluoxetine with other drugs that are metabolized by CYP2D6, including certain antidepressants (eg, TCAs), should be approached with caution. Therapy with medications that are predominantly metabolized by the CYP2D6 system and that have a relatively narrow therapeutic index should be initiated at the low end of the dose range if a patient is receiving fluoxetine concurrently or has taken it in the previous 5 weeks. The dose of TCAs may need to be reduced and plasma TCA concentrations may need to be monitored temporarily when fluoxetine is co-administered or has been recently discontinued).
No products indexed under this heading.

Meclofenamate Sodium (Epidemiological studies of the case-control and cohort design that have demonstrated an association between use of psychotropic drugs that interfere with serotonin reuptake and the occurrence of upper gastrointestinal bleeding have also shown that concurrent use of an NSAID may potentiate this risk of bleeding).
No products indexed under this heading.

Mefenamic Acid (Epidemiological studies of the case-control and cohort design that have demonstrated an association between use of psychotropic drugs that interfere with serotonin reuptake and the occurrence of upper gastrointestinal bleeding have also shown that concurrent use of an NSAID may potentiate this risk of bleeding).
No products indexed under this heading.

Meloxicam (Epidemiological studies of the case-control and cohort design that have demonstrated an association between use of psychotropic drugs that interfere with serotonin reuptake and the occurrence of upper gastrointestinal bleeding have also shown that concurrent use of an NSAID may potentiate this risk of bleeding).
No products indexed under this heading.

Meperidine Hydrochloride (Co-administration of fluoxetine with other drugs that are metabolized by CYP2D6, including certain antidepressants (eg, TCAs), antipsychotics (eg, phenothiazines and most atypicals), and antiarrhythmics (eg, propafenone, flecainide, and others) should be approached with caution. Therapy with medications that are predominantly metabolized by the CYP2D6 system and that have a relatively narrow therapeutic index should be initiated at the low end of the dose range if a patient is receiving fluoxetine concurrently or has taken it in the previous 5 weeks. Thus, his/her dosing requirements resemble those of poor metabolizers. If fluoxetine is added to the treatment regimen of a patient already receiving a drug metabolized by CYP2D6, the need for decreased dose of the original medication should be considered).
No products indexed under this heading.

Mephobarbital (Caution is advised if the concomitant administration of fluoxetine and CNS-acting drugs is required. In evaluating individual cases, consideration should be given to using lower initial doses of the concomitantly administered drugs, using conservative titration schedules, and monitoring of clinical status).
No products indexed under this heading.

Meprobamate (Caution is advised if the concomitant administration of fluoxetine and CNS-acting drugs is required. In evaluating individual cases, consideration should be given to using lower initial doses of the concomitantly administered drugs, using conservative titration schedules, and monitoring of clinical status).
No products indexed under this heading.

Mesoridazine Besylate (Co-administration of fluoxetine with other drugs that are metabolized by CYP2D6, including antipsychotics (eg, phenothiazines and most atypicals) should be approached with caution. Therapy with medications that are predominantly metabolized by the CYP2D6 system and that have a relatively narrow therapeutic index should be initiated at the low end of the dose range if a patient is receiving fluoxetine concurrently or has taken it in the previous 5 weeks. If fluoxetine is added to the treatment regimen of a patient already receiving a drug metabolized by CYP2D6, the need for decreased dose of the original medication should be considered).
No products indexed under this heading.

Metformin Hydrochloride (In patients with diabetes, fluoxetine may alter glycemic control. Hypoglycemia has occurred during therapy with fluoxetine, and hyperglycemia has developed following discontinuation of the drug. As is true with many other types of medication when taken concurrently by patients with diabetes, oral hypoglycemic dosage may need to be adjusted when therapy with fluoxetine is instituted or discontinued). Products include:
ActoPlus **3338**
Avandamet **1345**
Janumet **2188**

Methadone Hydrochloride (Co-administration of fluoxetine with other drugs that are metabolized by CYP2D6, including certain antidepressants (eg, TCAs), antipsychotics (eg, phenothiazines and most atypicals), and antiarrhythmics (eg, propafenone, flecainide, and others) should be approached with caution. Therapy with medications that are predominantly metabolized by the CYP2D6 system and that have a relatively narrow therapeutic index should be initiated at the low end of the dose range if a patient is receiving fluoxetine concurrently or has taken it in the previous 5 weeks. Thus, his/her dosing requirements resemble those of poor metabolizers. If fluoxetine is added to the treatment regimen of a patient already receiving a drug metabolized by CYP2D6, the need for decreased dose of the original medication should be considered).
No products indexed under this heading.

Methamphetamine Hydrochloride (Co-administration of fluoxetine with other drugs that are metabolized by CYP2D6, including certain antidepressants (eg, TCAs), antipsychotics (eg, phenothiazines and most atypicals), and antiarrhythmics (eg, propafenone, flecainide, and others) should be approached with caution. Therapy with medications that are predominantly metabolized by the CYP2D6 system and that have a relatively narrow therapeutic index should be initiated at the low end of the dose range if a patient is receiving fluoxetine concurrently or has taken it in the previous 5 weeks. Thus, his/her dosing requirements resemble those of poor metabolizers. If fluoxetine is added to the treatment regimen of a patient already receiving a drug metabolized by CYP2D6, the need for decreased dose of the original medication should be considered).
No products indexed under this heading.

Methohexital Sodium (Caution is advised if the concomitant administration of fluoxetine and CNS-acting drugs is required. In evaluating individual cases, consideration should be given to using lower initial doses of the concomitantly administered drugs, using conservative titration schedules, and monitoring of clinical status).
No products indexed under this heading.

Methotrimeprazine (Co-administration of fluoxetine with other drugs that are metabolized by CYP2D6, including antipsychotics (eg, phenothiazines and most atypicals) should be approached with caution. Therapy with medications that are predominantly metabolized by the CYP2D6 system and that have a relatively narrow therapeutic index should be initiated at the low end of the dose range if a patient is receiving fluoxetine concurrently or has taken it in the previous 5 weeks. If fluoxetine is added to the treatment regimen of a patient already receiving a drug metabolized by CYP2D6, the need for decreased dose of the original medication should be considered).
No products indexed under this heading.

Methoxyflurane (Caution is advised if the concomitant administration of fluoxetine and CNS-acting drugs is required. In evaluating individual cases, consideration should be given to using lower initial doses of the concomitantly administered drugs, using conservative titration schedules, and monitoring of clinical status).
No products indexed under this heading.

Methoxyphenamine (Co-administration of fluoxetine with other drugs that are metabolized by CYP2D6, including certain antidepressants (eg, TCAs), antipsychotics (eg, phenothiazines and most atypicals), and antiarrhythmics (eg, propafenone, flecainide, and others) should be approached with caution. Therapy with medications that are predominantly metabolized by the CYP2D6 system and that have a relatively narrow therapeutic index should be initiated at the low end of the dose range if a patient is receiving fluoxetine concurrently or has taken it in the previous 5 weeks. Thus, his/her dosing requirements resemble those of poor metabolizers. If fluoxetine is added to the treatment regimen of a patient already receiving a drug metabolized by CYP2D6, the need for decreased dose of the original medication should be considered).
No products indexed under this heading.

Methylphenidate (Caution is advised if the concomitant administration of fluoxetine and CNS-acting drugs is required. In evaluating individual cases, consideration should be given to using lower initial doses of the concomitantly administered drugs, using conservative titration schedules, and monitoring of clinical status). Products include:
Daytrana **3283**

Methylphenidate Hydrochloride (Caution is advised if the concomitant administration of fluoxetine and CNS-acting drugs is required. In evaluating individual cases, consideration should be given to using lower initial doses of the concomitantly administered drugs, using conservative titration schedules, and monitoring of clinical status). Products include:
Concerta **2598**
Metadate CD **3439**

Metoclopramide Hydrochloride (The development of a potentially life-threatening serotonin syndrome or neuroleptic malignant syndrome (NMS)-like reactions have been reported with SNRIs and SSRIs alone, including fluoxetine treatment, but particularly with concomitant use of dopamine antagonists). Products include:
Metozolv ODT **2901**

Metoprolol Succinate (Co-administration of fluoxetine with other drugs that are metabolized by CYP2D6, including certain antidepressants (eg, TCAs), antipsychotics (eg, phenothiazines and most atypicals), and antiarrhythmics (eg, propafenone, flecainide, and others) should be approached with caution. Therapy with medications that are predominantly metabolized by the CYP2D6 system and that have a relatively narrow therapeutic index should be initiated at the low end of the dose range if a patient is receiving fluoxetine concurrently or has taken it in the previous 5 weeks. Thus, his/her dosing requirements resemble those of poor metabolizers. If fluoxetine is added to the treatment regimen of a patient already receiving a drug metabolized by CYP2D6, the need for decreased dose of the original medication should be considered). Products include:

1539 **Interactions Index** **Prozac**

Toprol XL 732

Metoprolol Tartrate (Co-administration of fluoxetine with other drugs that are metabolized by CYP2D6, including certain antidepressants (eg, TCAs), antipsychotics (eg, phenothiazines and most atypicals), and antiarrhythmics (eg, propafenone, flecainide, and others) should be approached with caution. Therapy with medications that are predominantly metabolized by the CYP2D6 system and that have a relatively narrow therapeutic index should be initiated at the low end of the dose range if a patient is receiving fluoxetine concurrently or has taken it in the previous 5 weeks. Thus, his/her dosing requirements resemble those of poor metabolizers. If fluoxetine is added to the treatment regimen of a patient already receiving a drug metabolized by CYP2D6, the need for decreased dose of the original medication should be considered).

No products indexed under this heading.

Mexiletine Hydrochloride (Co-administration of fluoxetine with other drugs that are metabolized by CYP2D6, including antiarrhythmics (eg, propafenone, flecainide, and others) should be approached with caution. Therapy with medications that are predominantly metabolized by the CYP2D6 system and that have a relatively narrow therapeutic index should be initiated at the low end of the dose range if a patient is receiving fluoxetine concurrently or has taken it in the previous 5 weeks. If fluoxetine is added to the treatment regimen of a patient already receiving a drug metabolized by CYP2D6, the need for decreased dose of the original medication should be considered).

No products indexed under this heading.

Midazolam Hydrochloride (Because fluoxetine is tightly bound to plasma protein, adverse effects may result from displacement of protein-bound fluoxetine by other tightly-bound drugs).

No products indexed under this heading.

Miglitol (In patients with diabetes, fluoxetine may alter glycemic control. Hypoglycemia has occurred during therapy with fluoxetine, and hyperglycemia has developed following discontinuation of the drug. As is true with many other types of medication when taken concurrently by patients with diabetes, oral hypoglycemic dosage may need to be adjusted when therapy with fluoxetine is instituted or discontinued).

No products indexed under this heading.

Mirtazapine (Co-administration of fluoxetine with other drugs that are metabolized by CYP2D6, including certain antidepressants (eg, TCAs), should be approached with caution. Therapy with medications that are predominantly metabolized by the CYP2D6 system and that have a relatively narrow therapeutic index should be initiated at the low end of the dose range if a patient is receiving fluoxetine concurrently or has taken it in the previous 5 weeks. If fluoxetine is added to the treatment regimen of a patient already receiving a drug metabolized by CYP2D6, the need for decreased dose of the original medication should be considered). Products include:

Remeron Tablets 3214
RemeronSolTab Tablets 3219

Moclobemide (Fluoxetine is contraindicated for use with monoamine oxidase inhibitors (MAOIs). There have been reports of serious, sometimes fatal, reactions (including hyperthermia, rigidity, myoclonus, autonomic instability with possible rapid fluctuations of vital signs, and mental status changes that include extreme agitation progressing to delirium and coma) in patients receiving fluoxetine in combination with MAOI, and in patients who have recently discontinued fluoxetine and are then started on an MAOI. Some cases presented with features resembling neuroleptic malignant syndrome. Therefore, fluoxetine should not be used in combination with an MAOI, or within a minimum of 14 days of discontinuing therapy with an MAOI. Since fluoxetine and its major metabolite have very long elimination half-lives, at least 5 weeks perhaps longer, especially if fluoxetine has been prescribed chronically and/or at higher doses, should be allowed after stopping fluoxetine before starting an MAOI).

No products indexed under this heading.

Molindone Hydrochloride (Co-administration of fluoxetine with other drugs that are metabolized by CYP2D6, including antipsychotics (eg, phenothiazines and most atypicals), should be approached with caution. Therapy with medications that are predominantly metabolized by the CYP2D6 system and that have a relatively narrow therapeutic index should be initiated at the low end of the dose range if a patient is receiving fluoxetine concurrently or has taken it in the previous 5 weeks. If fluoxetine is added to the treatment regimen of a patient already receiving a drug metabolized by CYP2D6, the need for decreased dose of the original medication should be considered). Products include:

Moban 1108

Moricizine Hydrochloride (Co-administration of fluoxetine with other drugs that are metabolized by CYP2D6, including antiarrhythmics (eg, propafenone, flecainide, and others) should be approached with caution. Therapy with medications that are predominantly metabolized by the CYP2D6 system and that have a relatively narrow therapeutic index should be initiated at the low end of the dose range if a patient is receiving fluoxetine concurrently or has taken it in the previous 5 weeks. If fluoxetine is added to the treatment regimen of a patient already receiving a drug metabolized by CYP2D6, the need for decreased dose of the original medication should be considered).

No products indexed under this heading.

Morphine Sulfate (Co-administration of fluoxetine with other drugs that are metabolized by CYP2D6, including certain antidepressants (eg, TCAs), antipsychotics (eg, phenothiazines and most atypicals), and antiarrhythmics (eg, propafenone, flecainide, and others) should be approached with caution. Therapy with medications that are predominantly metabolized by the CYP2D6 system and that have a relatively narrow therapeutic index should be initiated at the low end of the dose range if a patient is receiving fluoxetine concurrently or has taken it in the previous 5 weeks. Thus, his/her dosing requirements resemble those of poor metabolizers. If fluoxetine is added to the treatment regimen of a patient already receiving a drug metabolized by CYP2D6, the need for decreased dose of the original medication should be considered). Products include:

Avinza 1822
Embeda 1831
MS Contin 2803

Nabumetone (Epidemiological studies of the case-control and cohort design that have demonstrated an association between use of psychotropic drugs that interfere with serotonin reuptake and the occurrence of upper gastrointestinal bleeding have also shown that concurrent use of an NSAID may potentiate this risk of bleeding).

No products indexed under this heading.

Naproxen (Epidemiological studies of the case-control and cohort design that have demonstrated an association between use of psychotropic drugs that interfere with serotonin reuptake and the occurrence of upper gastrointestinal bleeding have also shown that concurrent use of an NSAID may potentiate this risk of bleeding). Products include:

EC-Naprosyn 2850
Naprosyn 2850
Anaprox/Naprosyn 2850

Naproxen Sodium (Epidemiological studies of the case-control and cohort design that have demonstrated an association between use of psychotropic drugs that interfere with serotonin reuptake and the occurrence of upper gastrointestinal bleeding have also shown that concurrent use of an NSAID may potentiate this risk of bleeding). Products include:

Anaprox 2850
Anaprox DS 2850
Treximet 1681

Naratriptan Hydrochloride (Based on the mechanism of action of SNRIs and SSRIs, including fluoxetine, and the potential for serotonin syndrome, caution is advised when fluoxetine is co-administered with other drugs that may affect the serotonergic neurotransmitter systems, such as triptans. There have been rare postmarketing reports of serotonin syndrome with use of an SSRI and a triptan. If concomitant treatment of fluoxetine with a triptan is clinically warranted, careful observation of the patient is advised, particularly during treatment initiation and dose increases). Products include:

Amerge 1306

Nateglinide (In patients with diabetes, fluoxetine may alter glycemic control. Hypoglycemia has occurred during therapy with fluoxetine, and hyperglycemia has developed following discontinuation of the drug. As is true with many other types of medication when taken concurrently by patients with diabetes, oral hypoglycemic dosage may need to be adjusted when therapy with fluoxetine is instituted or discontinued).

No products indexed under this heading.

Nefazodone Hydrochloride (Based on the mechanism of action of SNRIs including fluoxetine, and the potential for serotonin syndrome, caution is advised when fluoxetine is co-administered with other drugs that may affect the serotonergic neurotransmitter systems, such as triptans, linezolid (an antibiotic which is a reversible non-selective MAOI), lithium, tramadol, or St. John's wort. The concomitant use of fluoxetine with SNRIs is not recommended).

No products indexed under this heading.

Nelfinavir Mesylate (Co-administration of fluoxetine with other drugs that are metabolized by CYP2D6, including certain antidepressants (eg, TCAs), antipsychotics (eg, phenothiazines and most atypicals), and antiarrhythmics (eg, propafenone, flecainide, and others) should be approached with caution. Therapy with medications that are predominantly metabolized by the CYP2D6 system and that have a relatively narrow therapeutic index should be initiated at the low end of the dose range if a patient is receiving fluoxetine concurrently or has taken it in the previous 5 weeks. Thus, his/her dosing requirements resemble those of poor metabolizers. If fluoxetine is added to the treatment regimen of a patient already receiving a drug metabolized by CYP2D6, the need for decreased dose of the original medication should be considered).

No products indexed under this heading.

Nortriptyline Hydrochloride (Because fluoxetine is tightly bound to plasma protein, adverse effects may result from displacement of protein-bound fluoxetine by other tightly-bound drugs).

No products indexed under this heading.

Olanzapine (Fluoxetine (60 mg single dose or 60 mg daily dose for 8 days) causes a small (mean 16%) increase in the maximum concentration of olanzapine and a small (mean 16%) decrease in olanzapine clearance. The magnitude of the impact of this factor is small in comparison to the overall variability between individuals, and, therefore, dose modification is not routinely recommended). Products include:

Symbyax 1965
Zyprexa 1984
Zyprexa IntraMuscular 1984
Zyprexa ZYDIS 1984

Omeprazole (Co-administration of fluoxetine with other drugs that are metabolized by CYP2D6, including certain antidepressants (eg, TCAs), antipsychotics (eg, phenothiazines and most atypicals), and antiarrhythmics (eg, propafenone, flecainide, and others) should be approached with caution. Therapy with medications that are predominantly metabolized by the CYP2D6 system and that have a relatively narrow therapeutic index should be initiated at the low end of the dose range if a patient is receiving fluoxetine concurrently or has taken it in the previous 5 weeks. Thus, his/her dosing requirements resemble those of poor metabolizers. If fluoxetine is added to the treatment regimen of a patient already receiving a drug metabolized by CYP2D6, the need for decreased dose of the original medication should be considered).

No products indexed under this heading.

Ondansetron (Co-administration of fluoxetine with other drugs that are metabolized by CYP2D6, including certain antidepressants (eg, TCAs), antipsychotics (eg, phenothiazines and most atypicals), and antiarrhythmics (eg, propafenone, flecainide, and others) should be approached with caution. Therapy with medications that are predominantly metabolized by the CYP2D6 system and that have a relatively narrow therapeutic index should be initiated at the low end of the dose range if a patient is receiving fluoxetine concurrently or has taken it in the previous 5 weeks. Thus, his/her dosing requirements resemble those of poor metabolizers. If fluoxetine is added to the treatment regimen of a patient already receiving a drug metabolized by CYP2D6, the need for decreased dose of the original medication should be considered).

No products indexed under this heading.

Ondansetron Hydrochloride (Co-administration of fluoxetine with other drugs that are metabolized by CYP2D6, including certain antidepressants (eg, TCAs), antipsychotics (eg, phenothiazines and most atypicals), and antiarrhythmics (eg, propafenone, flecainide, and others) should be approached with caution. Therapy with medications that are predominantly metabolized by the CYP2D6 system and that have a relatively narrow therapeutic index should be initiated at the low end of the dose range if a patient is receiving fluoxetine concurrently or has taken it in the previous 5 weeks. Thus, his/her dosing requirements resemble those of poor metabolizers. If fluoxetine is added to the treatment regimen of a patient already receiving a drug metabolized by CYP2D6, the need for decreased dose of the original medication should be considered). Products include:

Zofran Injection 1750
Zofran 1756

IMPORTANT NOTE: Always consult each drug listing in the patient's regimen for possible interactions.

Prozac Interactions Index 1540

Zofran ODT 1756

Oxaprozin (Epidemiological studies of the case-control and cohort design that have demonstrated an association between use of psychotropic drugs that interfere with serotonin reuptake and the occurrence of upper gastrointestinal bleeding have also shown that concurrent use of an NSAID may potentiate this risk of bleeding).
No products indexed under this heading.

Oxazepam (Because fluoxetine is tightly bound to plasma protein, adverse effects may result from displacement of protein-bound fluoxetine by other tightly-bound drugs).
No products indexed under this heading.

Oxycodone Hydrochloride (Co-administration of fluoxetine with other drugs that are metabolized by CYP2D6, including certain antidepressants (eg, TCAs), antipsychotics (eg, phenothiazines and most atypicals), and antiarrhythmics (eg, propafenone, flecainide, and others) should be approached with caution. Therapy with medications that are predominantly metabolized by the CYP2D6 system and that have a relatively narrow therapeutic index should be initiated at the low end of the dose range if a patient is receiving fluoxetine concurrently or has taken it in the previous 5 weeks. Thus, his/her dosing requirements resemble those of poor metabolizers. If fluoxetine is added to the treatment regimen of a patient already receiving a drug metabolized by CYP2D6, the need for decreased dose of the original medication should be considered). Products include:
OxyContin 2807
Percocet 1121
Percodan 1124

Paclitaxel (Co-administration of fluoxetine with other drugs that are metabolized by CYP2D6, including certain antidepressants (eg, TCAs), antipsychotics (eg, phenothiazines and most atypicals), and antiarrhythmics (eg, propafenone, flecainide, and others) should be approached with caution. Therapy with medications that are predominantly metabolized by the CYP2D6 system and that have a relatively narrow therapeutic index should be initiated at the low end of the dose range if a patient is receiving fluoxetine concurrently or has taken it in the previous 5 weeks. Thus, his/her dosing requirements resemble those of poor metabolizers. If fluoxetine is added to the treatment regimen of a patient already receiving a drug metabolized by CYP2D6, the need for decreased dose of the original medication should be considered).
No products indexed under this heading.

Paliperidone (Co-administration of fluoxetine with other drugs that are metabolized by CYP2D6, including antipsychotics (eg, phenothiazines and most atypicals), should be approached with caution. Therapy with medications that are predominantly metabolized by the CYP2D6 system and that have a relatively narrow therapeutic index should be initiated at the low end of the dose range if a patient is receiving fluoxetine concurrently or has taken it in the previous 5 weeks. If fluoxetine is added to the treatment regimen of a patient already receiving a drug metabolized by CYP2D6, the need for decreased dose of the original medication should be considered). Products include:
Invega 2613
Invega Sustenna 2621

Pargyline Hydrochloride (Fluoxetine is contraindicated for use with monoamine oxidase inhibitors (MAOIs). There have been reports of serious, sometimes fatal, reactions (including hyperthermia, rigidity, myoclonus, autonomic instability with possible rapid fluctuations of vital signs, and mental status changes that include extreme agitation progressing to delirium and coma) in patients receiving fluoxetine in combination with MAOI, and in patients who have recently discontinued fluoxetine and are then started on an MAOI. Some cases presented with features resembling neuroleptic malignant syndrome. Therefore, fluoxetine should not be used in combination with an MAOI, or within a minimum of 14 days of discontinuing therapy with an MAOI. Since fluoxetine and its major metabolite have very long elimination half-lives, at least 5 weeks perhaps longer, especially if fluoxetine has been prescribed chronically and/or at higher doses, should be allowed after stopping fluoxetine before starting an MAOI).
No products indexed under this heading.

Paroxetine (Based on the mechanism of action of SSRIs, including fluoxetine, and the potential for serotonin syndrome, caution is advised when fluoxetine is co-administered with other drugs that may affect the serotonergic neurotransmitter systems, such as triptans, linezolid (an antibiotic which is a reversible non-selective MAOI), lithium, tramadol, or St. John's wort. The concomitant use of fluoxetine with SSRIs is not recommended).
No products indexed under this heading.

Paroxetine Hydrochloride (Based on the mechanism of action of SSRIs, including fluoxetine, and the potential for serotonin syndrome, caution is advised when fluoxetine is co-administered with other drugs that may affect the serotonergic neurotransmitter systems, such as triptans, linezolid (an antibiotic which is a reversible non-selective MAOI), lithium, tramadol, or St. John's wort. The concomitant use of fluoxetine with SSRIs is not recommended). Products include:
Paroxetine CR 2361
Paroxetine ER 2371
Paxil 1586
Paxil CR 1596

Paroxetine Mesylate (Based on the mechanism of action of SSRIs, including fluoxetine, and the potential for serotonin syndrome, caution is advised when fluoxetine is co-administered with other drugs that may affect the serotonergic neurotransmitter systems, such as triptans, linezolid (an antibiotic which is a reversible non-selective MAOI), lithium, tramadol, or St. John's wort. The concomitant use of fluoxetine with SSRIs is not recommended).
No products indexed under this heading.

Pemoline (Caution is advised if the concomitant administration of fluoxetine and CNS-acting drugs is required. In evaluating individual cases, consideration should be given to using lower initial doses of the concomitantly administered drugs, using conservative titration schedules, and monitoring of clinical status).
No products indexed under this heading.

Pentobarbital Sodium (Caution is advised if the concomitant administration of fluoxetine and CNS-acting drugs is required. In evaluating individual cases, consideration should be given to using lower initial doses of the concomitantly administered drugs, using conservative titration schedules, and monitoring of clinical status). Products include:
Nembutal 2012

Perphenazine (Co-administration of fluoxetine with other drugs that are metabolized by CYP2D6, including antipsychotics (eg, phenothiazines and most atypicals) should be approached with caution. Therapy with medications that are predominantly metabolized by the CYP2D6 system and that have a relatively narrow therapeutic index should be initiated at the low end of the dose range if a patient is receiving fluoxetine concurrently or has taken it in the previous 5 weeks. If fluoxetine is added to the treatment regimen of a patient already receiving a drug metabolized by CYP2D6, the need for decreased dose of the original medication should be considered).
No products indexed under this heading.

Phenelzine Sulfate (Fluoxetine is contraindicated for use with monoamine oxidase inhibitors (MAOIs). There have been reports of serious, sometimes fatal, reactions (including hyperthermia, rigidity, myoclonus, autonomic instability with possible rapid fluctuations of vital signs, and mental status changes that include extreme agitation progressing to delirium and coma) in patients receiving fluoxetine in combination with MAOI, and in patients who have recently discontinued fluoxetine and are then started on an MAOI. Some cases presented with features resembling neuroleptic malignant syndrome. Therefore, fluoxetine should not be used in combination with an MAOI, or within a minimum of 14 days of discontinuing therapy with an MAOI. Since fluoxetine and its major metabolite have very long elimination half-lives, at least 5 weeks perhaps longer, especially if fluoxetine has been prescribed chronically and/or at higher doses, should be allowed after stopping fluoxetine before starting an MAOI).
No products indexed under this heading.

Phenobarbital (Caution is advised if the concomitant administration of fluoxetine and CNS-acting drugs is required. In evaluating individual cases, consideration should be given to using lower initial doses of the concomitantly administered drugs, using conservative titration schedules, and monitoring of clinical status). Products include:
Donnatal 2711

Phenobarbital Sodium (Caution is advised if the concomitant administration of fluoxetine and CNS-acting drugs is required. In evaluating individual cases, consideration should be given to using lower initial doses of the concomitantly administered drugs, using conservative titration schedules, and monitoring of clinical status).
No products indexed under this heading.

Phenothiazine Derivatives (Co-administration of fluoxetine with other drugs that are metabolized by CYP2D6, including antipsychotics (eg, phenothiazines and most atypicals) should be approached with caution. Therapy with medications that are predominantly metabolized by the CYP2D6 system and that have a relatively narrow therapeutic index should be initiated at the low end of the dose range if a patient is receiving fluoxetine concurrently or has taken it in the previous 5 weeks. If fluoxetine is added to the treatment regimen of a patient already receiving a drug metabolized by CYP2D6, the need for decreased dose of the original medication should be considered).
No products indexed under this heading.

Phenothiazines (Co-administration of fluoxetine with other drugs that are metabolized by CYP2D6, including antipsychotics (eg, phenothiazines and most atypicals) should be approached with caution. Therapy with medications that are predominantly metabolized by the CYP2D6 system and that have a relatively narrow therapeutic index should be initiated at the low end of the dose range if a patient is receiving fluoxetine concurrently or has taken it in the previous 5 weeks. If fluoxetine is added to the treatment regimen of a patient already receiving a drug metabolized by CYP2D6, the need for decreased dose of the original medication should be considered).
No products indexed under this heading.

Phenylbutazone (Epidemiological studies of the case-control and cohort design that have demonstrated an association between use of psychotropic drugs that interfere with serotonin reuptake and the occurrence of upper gastrointestinal bleeding have also shown that concurrent use of an NSAID may potentiate this risk of bleeding).
No products indexed under this heading.

Phenytoin (Patients on stable doses of phenytoin have developed elevated plasma phenytoin concentrations and clinical anticonvulsant toxicity following initiation of concomitant fluoxetine therapy).
No products indexed under this heading.

Phenytoin Sodium (Patients on stable doses of phenytoin have developed elevated plasma phenytoin concentrations and clinical anticonvulsant toxicity following initiation of concomitant fluoxetine therapy). Products include:
Phenytek Capsules 2380

Pimozide (Concomitant use in patients taking pimozide is contraindicated. Clinical studies of pimozide with other antidepressants demonstrate an increase in drug interaction or QT_c prolongation. While a specific study with pimozide and fluoxetine has not been conducted, the potential for drug interactions or QT_c prolongation warrants restricting the concurrent use of pimozide and fluoxetine).
No products indexed under this heading.

Pindolol (Co-administration of fluoxetine with other drugs that are metabolized by CYP2D6, including certain antidepressants (eg, TCAs), antipsychotics (eg, phenothiazines and most atypicals), and antiarrhythmics (eg, propafenone, flecainide, and others) should be approached with caution. Therapy with medications that are predominantly metabolized by the CYP2D6 system and that have a relatively narrow therapeutic index should be initiated at the low end of the dose range if a patient is receiving fluoxetine concurrently or has taken it in the previous 5 weeks. Thus, his/her dosing requirements resemble those of poor metabolizers. If fluoxetine is added to the treatment regimen of a patient already receiving a drug metabolized by CYP2D6, the need for decreased dose of the original medication should be considered).
No products indexed under this heading.

Pioglitazone Hydrochloride (In patients with diabetes, fluoxetine may alter glycemic control. Hypoglycemia has occurred during therapy with fluoxetine, and hyperglycemia has developed following discontinuation of the drug. As is true with many other types of medication when taken concurrently by patients with diabetes, oral hypoglycemic dosage may need to be adjusted when therapy with fluoxetine is instituted or discontinued). Products include:
ActoPlus 3338
Actos 3345
Duetact 3354

Piroxicam (Epidemiological studies of the case-control and cohort design that have demonstrated an association between use of psychotropic drugs that interfere with serotonin reuptake and the occurrence of upper gastrointestinal bleeding have also shown that concurrent use of an NSAID may potentiate this risk of bleeding).
No products indexed under this heading.

1541 **Interactions Index** **Prozac**

Prazepam (Caution is advised if the concomitant administration of fluoxetine and CNS-acting drugs is required. In evaluating individual cases, consideration should be given to using lower initial doses of the concomitantly administered drugs, using conservative titration schedules, and monitoring of clinical status).
No products indexed under this heading.

Procainamide Hydrochloride (Co-administration of fluoxetine with other drugs that are metabolized by CYP2D6, including antiarrhythmics (eg, propafenone, flecainide, and others) should be approached with caution. Therapy with medications that are predominantly metabolized by the CYP2D6 system and that have a relatively narrow therapeutic index should be initiated at the low end of the dose range if a patient is receiving fluoxetine concurrently or has taken it in the previous 5 weeks. If fluoxetine is added to the treatment regimen of a patient already receiving a drug metabolized by CYP2D6, the need for decreased dose of the original medication should be considered).
No products indexed under this heading.

Procarbazine Hydrochloride (Fluoxetine is contraindicated for use with monoamine oxidase inhibitors (MAOIs). There have been reports of serious, sometimes fatal, reactions (including hyperthermia, rigidity, myoclonus, autonomic instability with possible rapid fluctuations of vital signs, and mental status changes that include extreme agitation progressing to delirium and coma) in patients receiving fluoxetine in combination with MAOI, and in patients who have recently discontinued fluoxetine and are then started on an MAOI. Some cases presented with features resembling neuroleptic malignant syndrome. Therefore, fluoxetine should not be used in combination with an MAOI, or within a minimum of 14 days of discontinuing therapy with an MAOI. Since fluoxetine and its major metabolite have very long elimination half-lives, at least 5 weeks perhaps longer, especially if fluoxetine has been prescribed chronically and/or at higher doses, should be allowed after stopping fluoxetine before starting an MAOI).
No products indexed under this heading.

Prochlorperazine (Co-administration of fluoxetine with other drugs that are metabolized by CYP2D6, including antipsychotics (eg, phenothiazines and most atypicals) should be approached with caution. Therapy with medications that are predominantly metabolized by the CYP2D6 system and that have a relatively narrow therapeutic index should be initiated at the low end of the dose range if a patient is receiving fluoxetine concurrently or has taken it in the previous 5 weeks. If fluoxetine is added to the treatment regimen of a patient already receiving a drug metabolized by CYP2D6, the need for decreased dose of the original medication should be considered).
No products indexed under this heading.

Prochlorperazine Edisylate (Co-administration of fluoxetine with other drugs that are metabolized by CYP2D6, including antipsychotics (eg, phenothiazines and most atypicals) should be approached with caution. Therapy with medications that are predominantly metabolized by the CYP2D6 system and that have a relatively narrow therapeutic index should be initiated at the low end of the dose range if a patient is receiving fluoxetine concurrently or has taken it in the previous 5 weeks. If fluoxetine is added to the treatment regimen of a patient already receiving a drug metabolized by CYP2D6, the need for decreased dose of the original medication should be considered).
No products indexed under this heading.

Prochlorperazine Maleate (Co-administration of fluoxetine with other drugs that are metabolized by CYP2D6, including antipsychotics (eg, phenothiazines and most atypicals) should be approached with caution. Therapy with medications that are predominantly metabolized by the CYP2D6 system and that have a relatively narrow therapeutic index should be initiated at the low end of the dose range if a patient is receiving fluoxetine concurrently or has taken it in the previous 5 weeks. If fluoxetine is added to the treatment regimen of a patient already receiving a drug metabolized by CYP2D6, the need for decreased dose of the original medication should be considered).
No products indexed under this heading.

Promethazine (Co-administration of fluoxetine with other drugs that are metabolized by CYP2D6, including antipsychotics (eg, phenothiazines and most atypicals) should be approached with caution. Therapy with medications that are predominantly metabolized by the CYP2D6 system and that have a relatively narrow therapeutic index should be initiated at the low end of the dose range if a patient is receiving fluoxetine concurrently or has taken it in the previous 5 weeks. If fluoxetine is added to the treatment regimen of a patient already receiving a drug metabolized by CYP2D6, the need for decreased dose of the original medication should be considered).
No products indexed under this heading.

Promethazine Hydrochloride (Co-administration of fluoxetine with other drugs that are metabolized by CYP2D6, including antipsychotics (eg, phenothiazines and most atypicals) should be approached with caution. Therapy with medications that are predominantly metabolized by the CYP2D6 system and that have a relatively narrow therapeutic index should be initiated at the low end of the dose range if a patient is receiving fluoxetine concurrently or has taken it in the previous 5 weeks. If fluoxetine is added to the treatment regimen of a patient already receiving a drug metabolized by CYP2D6, the need for decreased dose of the original medication should be considered).
No products indexed under this heading.

Propafenone Hydrochloride (Co-administration of fluoxetine with other drugs that are metabolized by CYP2D6, including antiarrhythmics (eg, propafenone, flecainide, and others) should be approached with caution. Therapy with medications that are predominantly metabolized by the CYP2D6 system and that have a relatively narrow therapeutic index should be initiated at the low end of the dose range if a patient is receiving fluoxetine concurrently or has taken it in the previous 5 weeks. If fluoxetine is added to the treatment regimen of a patient already receiving a drug metabolized by CYP2D6, the need for decreased dose of the original medication should be considered). Products include:
Rythmol **1648**
Rythmol SR **1652**

Propofol (Caution is advised if the concomitant administration of fluoxetine and CNS-acting drugs is required. In evaluating individual cases, consideration should be given to using lower initial doses of the concomitantly administered drugs, using conservative titration schedules, and monitoring of clinical status).
No products indexed under this heading.

Propoxyphene Hydrochloride (Co-administration of fluoxetine with other drugs that are metabolized by CYP2D6, including certain antidepressants (eg, TCAs), antipsychotics (eg, phenothiazines and most atypicals), and antiarrhythmics (eg, propafenone, flecainide, and others) should be approached with caution. Therapy with medications that are predominantly metabolized by the CYP2D6 system and that have a relatively narrow therapeutic index should be initiated at the low end of the dose range if a patient is receiving fluoxetine concurrently or has taken it in the previous 5 weeks. Thus, his/her dosing requirements resemble those of poor metabolizers. If fluoxetine is added to the treatment regimen of a patient already receiving a drug metabolized by CYP2D6, the need for decreased dose of the original medication should be considered).
No products indexed under this heading.

Propoxyphene Napsylate (Co-administration of fluoxetine with other drugs that are metabolized by CYP2D6, including certain antidepressants (eg, TCAs), antipsychotics (eg, phenothiazines and most atypicals), and antiarrhythmics (eg, propafenone, flecainide, and others) should be approached with caution. Therapy with medications that are predominantly metabolized by the CYP2D6 system and that have a relatively narrow therapeutic index should be initiated at the low end of the dose range if a patient is receiving fluoxetine concurrently or has taken it in the previous 5 weeks. Thus, his/her dosing requirements resemble those of poor metabolizers. If fluoxetine is added to the treatment regimen of a patient already receiving a drug metabolized by CYP2D6, the need for decreased dose of the original medication should be considered).
No products indexed under this heading.

Propranolol Hydrochloride (Because fluoxetine is tightly bound to plasma protein, adverse effects may result from displacement of protein-bound fluoxetine by other tightly-bound drugs). Products include:
InnoPran XL **1517**

Protriptyline Hydrochloride (Co-administration of fluoxetine with other drugs that are metabolized by CYP2D6, including certain antidepressants (eg, TCAs), should be approached with caution. Therapy with medications that are predominantly metabolized by the CYP2D6 system and that have a relatively narrow therapeutic index should be initiated at the low end of the dose range if a patient is receiving fluoxetine concurrently or has taken it in the previous 5 weeks. The dose of TCAs may need to be reduced and plasma TCA concentrations may need to be monitored temporarily when fluoxetine is co-administered or has been recently discontinued).
No products indexed under this heading.

Quazepam (Caution is advised if the concomitant administration of fluoxetine and CNS-acting drugs is required. In evaluating individual cases, consideration should be given to using lower initial doses of the concomitantly administered drugs, using conservative titration schedules, and monitoring of clinical status).
No products indexed under this heading.

Quetiapine Fumarate (Co-administration of fluoxetine with other drugs that are metabolized by CYP2D6, including antipsychotics (eg, phenothiazines and most atypicals), should be approached with caution. Therapy with medications that are predominantly metabolized by the CYP2D6 system and that have a relatively narrow therapeutic index should be initiated at the low end of the dose range if a patient is receiving fluoxetine concurrently or has taken it in the previous 5 weeks. If fluoxetine is added to the treatment regimen of a patient already receiving a drug metabolized by CYP2D6, the need for decreased dose of the original medication should be considered). Products include:
Seroquel **750**
Seroquel XR **759**

Quinidine Gluconate (Co-administration of fluoxetine with other drugs that are metabolized by CYP2D6, including antiarrhythmics (eg, propafenone, flecainide, and others) should be approached with caution. Therapy with medications that are predominantly metabolized by the CYP2D6 system and that have a relatively narrow therapeutic index should be initiated at the low end of the dose range if a patient is receiving fluoxetine concurrently or has taken it in the previous 5 weeks. If fluoxetine is added to the treatment regimen of a patient already receiving a drug metabolized by CYP2D6, the need for decreased dose of the original medication should be considered).
No products indexed under this heading.

Quinidine Hydrochloride (Co-administration of fluoxetine with other drugs that are metabolized by CYP2D6, including certain antidepressants (eg, TCAs), antipsychotics (eg, phenothiazines and most atypicals), and antiarrhythmics (eg, propafenone, flecainide, and others) should be approached with caution. Therapy with medications that are predominantly metabolized by the CYP2D6 system and that have a relatively narrow therapeutic index should be initiated at the low end of the dose range if a patient is receiving fluoxetine concurrently or has taken it in the previous 5 weeks. Thus, his/her dosing requirements resemble those of poor metabolizers. If fluoxetine is added to the treatment regimen of a patient already receiving a drug metabolized by CYP2D6, the need for decreased dose of the original medication should be considered).
No products indexed under this heading.

Quinidine Polygalacturonate (Co-administration of fluoxetine with other drugs that are metabolized by CYP2D6, including antiarrhythmics (eg, propafenone, flecainide, and others) should be approached with caution. Therapy with medications that are predominantly metabolized by the CYP2D6 system and that have a relatively narrow therapeutic index should be initiated at the low end of the dose range if a patient is receiving fluoxetine concurrently or has taken it in the previous 5 weeks. If fluoxetine is added to the treatment regimen of a patient already receiving a drug metabolized by CYP2D6, the need for decreased dose of the original medication should be considered).
No products indexed under this heading.

Quinidine Sulfate (Co-administration of fluoxetine with other drugs that are metabolized by CYP2D6, including antiarrhythmics (eg, propafenone, flecainide, and others) should be approached with caution. Therapy with medications that are predominantly metabolized by the CYP2D6 system and that have a relatively narrow therapeutic index should be initiated at the low end of the dose range if a patient is receiving fluoxetine concurrently or has taken it in the previous 5 weeks. If fluoxetine is added to the treatment regimen of a patient already receiving a drug metabolized by CYP2D6, the need for decreased dose of the original medication should be considered).
No products indexed under this heading.

IMPORTANT NOTE: Always consult each drug listing in the patient's regimen for possible interactions.

Rasagiline Mesylate (Fluoxetine is contraindicated for use with monoamine oxidase inhibitors (MAOIs). There have been reports of serious, sometimes fatal, reactions (including hyperthermia, rigidity, myoclonus, autonomic instability with possible rapid fluctuations of vital signs, and mental status changes that include extreme agitation progressing to delirium and coma) in patients receiving fluoxetine in combination with MAOI, and in patients who have recently discontinued fluoxetine and are then started on an MAOI. Some cases presented with features resembling neuroleptic malignant syndrome. Therefore, fluoxetine should not be used in combination with an MAOI, or within a minimum of 14 days of discontinuing therapy with an MAOI. Since fluoxetine and its major metabolite have very long elimination half-lives, at least 5 weeks perhaps longer, especially if fluoxetine has been prescribed chronically and/or at higher doses, should be allowed after stopping fluoxetine before starting an MAOI). Products include:

Azilect 3383

Remifentanil Hydrochloride (Caution is advised if the concomitant administration of fluoxetine and CNS-acting drugs is required. In evaluating individual cases, consideration should be given to using lower initial doses of the concomitantly administered drugs, using conservative titration schedules, and monitoring of clinical status).

No products indexed under this heading.

Repaglinide (In patients with diabetes, fluoxetine may alter glycemic control. Hypoglycemia has occurred during therapy with fluoxetine, and hyperglycemia has developed following discontinuation of the drug. As is true with many other types of medication when taken concurrently by patients with diabetes, oral hypoglycemic dosage may need to be adjusted when therapy with fluoxetine is instituted or discontinued).

No products indexed under this heading.

Risperidone (Co-administration of fluoxetine with other drugs that are metabolized by CYP2D6, including antipsychotics (eg, phenothiazines and most atypicals), should be approached with caution. Therapy with medications that are predominantly metabolized by the CYP2D6 system and that have a relatively narrow therapeutic index should be initiated at the low end of the dose range if a patient is receiving fluoxetine concurrently or has taken it in the previous 5 weeks. If fluoxetine is added to the treatment regimen of a patient already receiving a drug metabolized by CYP2D6, the need for decreased dose of the original medication should be considered). Products include:

Risperdal Consta 2682

Ritonavir (Co-administration of fluoxetine with other drugs that are metabolized by CYP2D6, including certain antidepressants (eg, TCAs), antipsychotics (eg, phenothiazines and most atypicals), and antiarrhythmics (eg, propafenone, flecainide, and others) should be approached with caution. Therapy with medications that are predominantly metabolized by the CYP2D6 system and that have a relatively narrow therapeutic index should be initiated at the low end of the dose range if a patient is receiving fluoxetine concurrently or has taken it in the previous 5 weeks. Thus, his/her dosing requirements resemble those of poor metabolizers. If fluoxetine is added to the treatment regimen of a patient already receiving a drug metabolized by CYP2D6, the need for decreased dose of the original medication should be considered). Products include:

Kaletra 458

Norvir 509

Rizatriptan Benzoate (Based on the mechanism of action of SNRIs and SSRIs, including fluoxetine, and the potential for serotonin syndrome, caution is advised when fluoxetine is co-administered with other drugs that may affect the serotonergic neurotransmitter systems, such as triptans. There have been rare postmarketing reports of serotonin syndrome with use of an SSRI and a triptan. If concomitant treatment of fluoxetine with a triptan is clinically warranted, careful observation of the patient is advised, particularly during treatment initiation and dose increases). Products include:

Maxalt 2206
Maxalt-MLT 2206

Rofecoxib (Epidemiological studies of the case-control and cohort design that have demonstrated an association between use of psychotropic drugs that interfere with serotonin reuptake and the occurrence of upper gastrointestinal bleeding have also shown that concurrent use of an NSAID may potentiate this risk of bleeding).

No products indexed under this heading.

Rosiglitazone Maleate (In patients with diabetes, fluoxetine may alter glycemic control. Hypoglycemia has occurred during therapy with fluoxetine, and hyperglycemia has developed following discontinuation of the drug. As is true with many other types of medication when taken concurrently by patients with diabetes, oral hypoglycemic dosage may need to be adjusted when therapy with fluoxetine is instituted or discontinued). Products include:

Avandamet 1345
Avandaryl 1356
Avandia 1366

Secobarbital Sodium (Caution is advised if the concomitant administration of fluoxetine and CNS-acting drugs is required. In evaluating individual cases, consideration should be given to using lower initial doses of the concomitantly administered drugs, using conservative titration schedules, and monitoring of clinical status).

No products indexed under this heading.

Selegiline (Fluoxetine is contraindicated for use with monoamine oxidase inhibitors (MAOIs). There have been reports of serious, sometimes fatal, reactions (including hyperthermia, rigidity, myoclonus, autonomic instability with possible rapid fluctuations of vital signs, and mental status changes that include extreme agitation progressing to delirium and coma) in patients receiving fluoxetine in combination with MAOI, and in patients who have recently discontinued fluoxetine and are then started on an MAOI. Some cases presented with features resembling neuroleptic malignant syndrome. Therefore, fluoxetine should not be used in combination with an MAOI, or within a minimum of 14 days of discontinuing therapy with an MAOI. Since fluoxetine and its major metabolite have very long elimination half-lives, at least 5 weeks perhaps longer, especially if fluoxetine has been prescribed chronically and/or at higher doses, should be allowed after stopping fluoxetine before starting an MAOI). Products include:

Emsam 3623

Selegiline Hydrochloride (Fluoxetine is contraindicated for use with monoamine oxidase inhibitors (MAOIs). There have been reports of serious, sometimes fatal, reactions (including hyperthermia, rigidity, myoclonus, autonomic instability with possible rapid fluctuations of vital signs, and mental status changes that include extreme agitation progressing to delirium and coma) in patients receiving fluoxetine in combination with MAOI, and in patients who have recently discontinued fluoxetine and are then started on an MAOI. Some cases presented with features resembling neuroleptic malignant syndrome. Therefore, fluoxetine should not be used in combination with an MAOI, or within a minimum of 14 days of discontinuing therapy with an MAOI. Since fluoxetine and its major metabolite have very long elimination half-lives, at least 5 weeks perhaps longer, especially if fluoxetine has been prescribed chronically and/or at higher doses, should be allowed after stopping fluoxetine before starting an MAOI). Products include:

Eldepryl 3312

Sertraline Hydrochloride (Based on the mechanism of action of SSRIs, including fluoxetine, and the potential for serotonin syndrome, caution is advised when fluoxetine is co-administered with other drugs that may affect the serotonergic neurotransmitter systems, such as triptans, linezolid (an antibiotic which is a reversible nonselective MAOI), lithium, tramadol, or St. John's wort. The concomitant use of fluoxetine with SSRIs is not recommended).

No products indexed under this heading.

Sevoflurane (Caution is advised if the concomitant administration of fluoxetine and CNS-acting drugs is required. In evaluating individual cases, consideration should be given to using lower initial doses of the concomitantly administered drugs, using conservative titration schedules, and monitoring of clinical status). Products include:

Ultane 554

Sitagliptin Phosphate (In patients with diabetes, fluoxetine may alter glycemic control. Hypoglycemia has occurred during therapy with fluoxetine, and hyperglycemia has developed following discontinuation of the drug. As is true with many other types of medication when taken concurrently by patients with diabetes, oral hypoglycemic dosage may need to be adjusted when therapy with fluoxetine is instituted or discontinued). Products include:

Janumet 2188
Januvia 2196

Sodium Oxybate (Caution is advised if the concomitant administration of fluoxetine and CNS-acting drugs is required. In evaluating individual cases, consideration should be given to using lower initial doses of the concomitantly administered drugs, using conservative titration schedules, and monitoring of clinical status).

No products indexed under this heading.

Sotalol Hydrochloride (Co-administration of fluoxetine with other drugs that are metabolized by CYP2D6, including antiarrhythmics (eg, propafenone, flecainide, and others) should be approached with caution. Therapy with medications that are predominantly metabolized by the CYP2D6 system and that have a relatively narrow therapeutic index should be initiated at the low end of the dose range if a patient is receiving fluoxetine concurrently or has taken it in the previous 5 weeks. If fluoxetine is added to the treatment regimen of a patient already receiving a drug metabolized by CYP2D6, the need for decreased dose of the original medication should be considered).

No products indexed under this heading.

Sufentanil Citrate (Caution is advised if the concomitant administration of fluoxetine and CNS-acting drugs is required. In evaluating individual cases, consideration should be given to using lower initial doses of the concomitantly administered drugs, using conservative titration schedules, and monitoring of clinical status).

No products indexed under this heading.

Sulindac (Epidemiological studies of the case-control and cohort design that have demonstrated an association between use of psychotropic drugs that interfere with serotonin reuptake and the occurrence of upper gastrointestinal bleeding have also shown that concurrent use of an NSAID may potentiate this risk of bleeding). Products include:

Clinoril 2098

Sumatriptan (Based on the mechanism of action of SNRIs and SSRIs, including fluoxetine, and the potential for serotonin syndrome, caution is advised when fluoxetine is co-administered with other drugs that may affect the serotonergic neurotransmitter systems, such as triptans. There have been rare postmarketing reports of serotonin syndrome with use of an SSRI and a triptan. If concomitant treatment of fluoxetine with a triptan is clinically warranted, careful observation of the patient is advised, particularly during treatment initiation and dose increases). Products include:

Imitrex Nasal 1503

Sumatriptan Succinate (Based on the mechanism of action of SNRIs and SSRIs, including fluoxetine, and the potential for serotonin syndrome, caution is advised when fluoxetine is co-administered with other drugs that may affect the serotonergic neurotransmitter systems, such as triptans. There have been rare postmarketing reports of serotonin syndrome with use of an SSRI and a triptan. If concomitant treatment of fluoxetine with a triptan is clinically warranted, careful observation of the patient is advised, particularly during treatment initiation and dose increases). Products include:

Imitrex 1497
Imitrex Tablets 1508
Treximet 1681

Tamoxifen Citrate (Co-administration of fluoxetine with other drugs that are metabolized by CYP2D6, including certain antidepressants (eg, TCAs), antipsychotics (eg, phenothiazines and most atypicals), and antiarrhythmics (eg, propafenone, flecainide, and others) should be approached with caution. Therapy with medications that are predominantly metabolized by the CYP2D6 system and that have a relatively narrow therapeutic index should be initiated at the low end of the dose range if a patient is receiving fluoxetine concurrently or has taken it in the previous 5 weeks. Thus, his/her dosing requirements resemble those of poor metabolizers. If fluoxetine is added to the treatment regimen of a patient already receiving a drug metabolized by CYP2D6, the need for decreased dose of the original medication should be considered).

No products indexed under this heading.

Temazepam (Because fluoxetine is tightly bound to plasma protein, adverse effects may result from displacement of protein-bound fluoxetine by other tightly-bound drugs).

No products indexed under this heading.

Teniposide (Co-administration of fluoxetine with other drugs that are metabolized by CYP2D6, including certain antidepressants (eg, TCAs), antipsychotics (eg, phenothiazines and most atypicals), and antiarrhythmics (eg, propafenone, flecainide, and others) should be approached with caution. Therapy

with medications that are predominantly metabolized by the CYP2D6 system and that have a relatively narrow therapeutic index should be initiated at the low end of the dose range if a patient is receiving fluoxetine concurrently or has taken it in the previous 5 weeks. Thus, his/her dosing requirements resemble those of poor metabolizers. If fluoxetine is added to the treatment regimen of a patient already receiving a drug metabolized by CYP2D6, the need for decreased dose of the original medication should be considered).

No products indexed under this heading.

Testosterone (Co-administration of fluoxetine with other drugs that are metabolized by CYP2D6, including certain antidepressants (eg, TCAs), antipsychotics (eg, phenothiazines and most atypicals), and antiarrhythmics (eg, propafenone, flecainide, and others) should be approached with caution. Therapy with medications that are predominantly metabolized by the CYP2D6 system and that have a relatively narrow therapeutic index should be initiated at the low end of the dose range if a patient is receiving fluoxetine concurrently or has taken it in the previous 5 weeks. Thus, his/her dosing requirements resemble those of poor metabolizers. If fluoxetine is added to the treatment regimen of a patient already receiving a drug metabolized by CYP2D6, the need for decreased dose of the original medication should be considered). Products include:

AndroGel 3456

Testosterone Cypionate (Co-administration of fluoxetine with other drugs that are metabolized by CYP2D6, including certain antidepressants (eg, TCAs), antipsychotics (eg, phenothiazines and most atypicals), and antiarrhythmics (eg, propafenone, flecainide, and others) should be approached with caution. Therapy with medications that are predominantly metabolized by the CYP2D6 system and that have a relatively narrow therapeutic index should be initiated at the low end of the dose range if a patient is receiving fluoxetine concurrently or has taken it in the previous 5 weeks. Thus, his/her dosing requirements resemble those of poor metabolizers. If fluoxetine is added to the treatment regimen of a patient already receiving a drug metabolized by CYP2D6, the need for decreased dose of the original medication should be considered).

No products indexed under this heading.

Testosterone Enanthate (Co-administration of fluoxetine with other drugs that are metabolized by CYP2D6, including certain antidepressants (eg, TCAs), antipsychotics (eg, phenothiazines and most atypicals), and antiarrhythmics (eg, propafenone, flecainide, and others) should be approached with caution. Therapy with medications that are predominantly metabolized by the CYP2D6 system and that have a relatively narrow therapeutic index should be initiated at the low end of the dose range if a patient is receiving fluoxetine concurrently or has taken it in the previous 5 weeks. Thus, his/her dosing requirements resemble those of poor metabolizers. If fluoxetine is added to the treatment regimen of a patient already receiving a drug metabolized by CYP2D6, the need for decreased dose of the original medication should be considered). Products include:

Delatestryl 1102

Testosterone Propionate (Co-administration of fluoxetine with other drugs that are metabolized by CYP2D6, including certain antidepressants (eg, TCAs), antipsychotics (eg, phenothiazines and most atypicals), and antiar-

rhythmics (eg, propafenone, flecainide, and others) should be approached with caution. Therapy with medications that are predominantly metabolized by the CYP2D6 system and that have a relatively narrow therapeutic index should be initiated at the low end of the dose range if a patient is receiving fluoxetine concurrently or has taken it in the previous 5 weeks. Thus, his/her dosing requirements resemble those of poor metabolizers. If fluoxetine is added to the treatment regimen of a patient already receiving a drug metabolized by CYP2D6, the need for decreased dose of the original medication should be considered).

No products indexed under this heading.

Thiamylal Sodium (Caution is advised if the concomitant administration of fluoxetine and CNS-acting drugs is required. In evaluating individual cases, consideration should be given to using lower initial doses of the concomitantly administered drugs, using conservative titration schedules, and monitoring of clinical status).

No products indexed under this heading.

Thioridazine (Fluoxetine is contraindicated for use with thioridazine due to QT$_c$ interval prolongation and potential for elevated thioridazine plasma levels. Do not use thioridazine within 5 weeks of discontinuing fluoxetine. Thioridazine administration produces a dose-related prolongation of the QT$_c$ interval, which is associated with serious ventricular arrhythmias, such as torsades de pointes-type arrhythmias, and sudden death. This risk is expected to increase with fluoxetine-induced inhibition of thioridazine metabolism).

No products indexed under this heading.

Thioridazine Hydrochloride (Fluoxetine is contraindicated for use with thioridazine due to QT$_c$ interval prolongation and potential for elevated thioridazine plasma levels. Do not use thioridazine within 5 weeks of discontinuing fluoxetine. Thioridazine administration produces a dose-related prolongation of the QT$_c$ interval, which is associated with serious ventricular arrhythmias, such as torsades de pointes-type arrhythmias, and sudden death. This risk is expected to increase with fluoxetine-induced inhibition of thioridazine metabolism). Products include:

Thioridazine Hydrochloride 2384

Thiothixene (Co-administration of fluoxetine with other drugs that are metabolized by CYP2D6, including antipsychotics (eg, phenothiazines and most atypicals), should be approached with caution. Therapy with medications that are predominantly metabolized by the CYP2D6 system and that have a relatively narrow therapeutic index should be initiated at the low end of the dose range if a patient is receiving fluoxetine concurrently or has taken it in the previous 5 weeks. If fluoxetine is added to the treatment regimen of a patient already receiving a drug metabolized by CYP2D6, the need for decreased dose of the original medication should be considered). Products include:

Thiothixene 2386

Timolol Maleate (Co-administration of fluoxetine with other drugs that are metabolized by CYP2D6, including certain antidepressants (eg, TCAs), antipsychotics (eg, phenothiazines and most atypicals), and antiarrhythmics (eg, propafenone, flecainide, and others) should be approached with caution. Therapy with medications that are predominantly metabolized by the CYP2D6 system and that have a relatively narrow therapeutic index should be initiated at the low end of the dose range if a patient is receiving fluoxetine concurrently or has taken it in the previous 5 weeks. Thus,

his/her dosing requirements resemble those of poor metabolizers. If fluoxetine is added to the treatment regimen of a patient already receiving a drug metabolized by CYP2D6, the need for decreased dose of the original medication should be considered). Products include:

Combigan 601
Dorzolamide
Hydrochloride/Timolol Maleate
Ophthalmic Solution....................⊙243
Timoptic in Ocudose ....⊙231

Tinzaparin Sodium (SNRIs and SSRIs, including fluoxetine, may increase the risk of bleeding reactions. Concomitant use of anticoagulants may add to this risk. Case reports and epidemiological studies (case-control and cohort design) have demonstrated an association between use of drugs that interfere with serotonin reuptake and the occurrence of gastrointestinal bleeding. Bleeding reactions related to SNRIs and SSRIs use have ranged from ecchymoses, hematomas, epistaxis, and petechiae to life-threatening hemorrhages. Patients should be cautioned about the risk of bleeding associated with the concomitant use of fluoxetine and other drugs that affect coagulation).

No products indexed under this heading.

Tocainide Hydrochloride (Co-administration of fluoxetine with other drugs that are metabolized by CYP2D6, including antiarrhythmics (eg, propafenone, flecainide, and others) should be approached with caution. Therapy with medications that are predominantly metabolized by the CYP2D6 system and that have a relatively narrow therapeutic index should be initiated at the low end of the dose range if a patient is receiving fluoxetine concurrently or has taken it in the previous 5 weeks. If fluoxetine is added to the treatment regimen of a patient already receiving a drug metabolized by CYP2D6, the need for decreased dose of the original medication should be considered).

No products indexed under this heading.

Tolazamide (In patients with diabetes, fluoxetine may alter glycemic control. Hypoglycemia has occurred during therapy with fluoxetine, and hyperglycemia has developed following discontinuation of the drug. As is true with many other types of medication when taken concurrently by patients with diabetes, oral hypoglycemic dosage may need to be adjusted when therapy with fluoxetine is instituted or discontinued).

No products indexed under this heading.

Tolbutamide (In patients with diabetes, fluoxetine may alter glycemic control. Hypoglycemia has occurred during therapy with fluoxetine, and hyperglycemia has developed following discontinuation of the drug. As is true with many other types of medication when taken concurrently by patients with diabetes, oral hypoglycemic dosage may need to be adjusted when therapy with fluoxetine is instituted or discontinued).

No products indexed under this heading.

Tolmetin Sodium (Epidemiological studies of the case-control and cohort design that have demonstrated an association between use of psychotropic drugs that interfere with serotonin reuptake and the occurrence of upper gastrointestinal bleeding have also shown that concurrent use of an NSAID may potentiate this risk of bleeding).

No products indexed under this heading.

Tolterodine Tartrate (Co-administration of fluoxetine with other drugs that are metabolized by CYP2D6, including certain antidepressants (eg, TCAs), antipsychotics (eg, phenothiazines and most atypicals), and antiarrhythmics (eg, propafenone, flecainide,

and others) should be approached with caution. Therapy with medications that are predominantly metabolized by the CYP2D6 system and that have a relatively narrow therapeutic index should be initiated at the low end of the dose range if a patient is receiving fluoxetine concurrently or has taken it in the previous 5 weeks. Thus, his/her dosing requirements resemble those of poor metabolizers. If fluoxetine is added to the treatment regimen of a patient already receiving a drug metabolized by CYP2D6, the need for decreased dose of the original medication should be considered).

No products indexed under this heading.

Tramadol Hydrochloride (Based on the mechanism of action of SNRIs and SSRIs and the potential for serotonin syndrome, caution is advised when fluoxetine is co-administered with other drugs that may effect the serotonergic neurotransmitter systems, such as tramadol). Products include:

Ryzolt 2813
Ultram ER 2693

Tranylcypromine Sulfate (Fluoxetine is contraindicated for use with monoamine oxidase inhibitors (MAOIs). There have been reports of serious, sometimes fatal, reactions (including hyperthermia, rigidity, myoclonus, autonomic instability with possible rapid fluctuations of vital signs, and mental status changes that include extreme agitation progressing to delirium and coma) in patients receiving fluoxetine in combination with MAOI, and in patients who have recently discontinued fluoxetine and are then started on an MAOI. Some cases presented with features resembling neuroleptic malignant syndrome. Therefore, fluoxetine should not be used in combination with an MAOI, or within a minimum of 14 days of discontinuing therapy with an MAOI. Since fluoxetine and its major metabolite have very long elimination half-lives, at least 5 weeks perhaps longer, especially if fluoxetine has been prescribed chronically and/or at higher doses, should be allowed after stopping fluoxetine before starting an MAOI). Products include:

Parnate 1584

Trazodone Hydrochloride (Co-administration of fluoxetine with other drugs that are metabolized by CYP2D6, including certain antidepressants (eg, TCAs), should be approached with caution. Therapy with medications that are predominantly metabolized by the CYP2D6 system and that have a relatively narrow therapeutic index should be initiated at the low end of the dose range if a patient is receiving fluoxetine concurrently or has taken it in the previous 5 weeks. If fluoxetine is added to the treatment regimen of a patient already receiving a drug metabolized by CYP2D6, the need for decreased dose of the original medication should be considered).

No products indexed under this heading.

Triazolam (Co-administration of fluoxetine with other drugs that are metabolized by CYP2D6, including certain antidepressants (eg, TCAs), antipsychotics (eg, phenothiazines and most atypicals), and antiarrhythmics (eg, propafenone, flecainide, and others) should be approached with caution. Therapy with medications that are predominantly metabolized by the CYP2D6 system and that have a relatively narrow therapeutic index should be initiated at the low end of the dose range if a patient is receiving fluoxetine concurrently or has taken it in the previous 5 weeks. Thus, his/her dosing requirements resemble those of poor metabolizers. If fluoxetine is added to the treatment regimen of a patient already receiving a drug metab-

Prozac Interactions Index 1544

olized by CYP2D6, the need for decreased dose of the original medication should be considered).
No products indexed under this heading.

Trifluoperazine Hydrochloride (Co-administration of fluoxetine with other drugs that are metabolized by CYP2D6, including antipsychotics (eg, phenothiazines and most atypicals) should be approached with caution. Therapy with medications that are predominantly metabolized by the CYP2D6 system and that have a relatively narrow therapeutic index should be initiated at the low end of the dose range if a patient is receiving fluoxetine concurrently or has taken it in the previous 5 weeks. If fluoxetine is added to the treatment regimen of a patient already receiving a drug metabolized by CYP2D6, the need for decreased dose of the original medication should be considered).
No products indexed under this heading.

Trimipramine Maleate (Because fluoxetine is tightly bound to plasma protein, adverse effects may result from displacement of protein-bound fluoxetine by other tightly-bound drugs).
No products indexed under this heading.

Troglitazone (In patients with diabetes, fluoxetine may alter glycemic control. Hypoglycemia has occurred during therapy with fluoxetine, and hyperglycemia has developed following discontinuation of the drug. As is true with many other types of medication when taken concurrently by patients with diabetes, oral hypoglycemic dosage may need to be adjusted when therapy with fluoxetine is instituted or discontinued).
No products indexed under this heading.

Tryptophan (Patients receiving fluoxetine in combination with tryptophan experienced adverse reactions, including agitation, restlessness, and gastrointestinal distress. The concomitant use with tryptophan is not recommended).
No products indexed under this heading.

Valdecoxib (Epidemiological studies of the case-control and cohort design that have demonstrated an association between use of psychotropic drugs that interfere with serotonin reuptake and the occurrence of upper gastrointestinal bleeding have also shown that concurrent use of an NSAID may potentiate this risk of bleeding).
No products indexed under this heading.

Venlafaxine Hydrochloride (Based on the mechanism of action of SNRIs including fluoxetine, and the potential for serotonin syndrome, caution is advised when fluoxetine is co-administered with other drugs that may affect the serotonergic neurotransmitter systems, such as triptans, linezolid (an antibiotic which is a reversible non-selective MAOI), lithium, tramadol, or St. John's wort. The concomitant use of fluoxetine with SNRIs is not recommended). Products include:
Effexor XR 3504
Venlafaxine Hydrochloride Tablets ... 2388

Verapamil Hydrochloride (Co-administration of fluoxetine with other drugs that are metabolized by CYP2D6, including antiarrhythmics (eg, propafenone, flecainide, and others) should be approached with caution. Therapy with medications that are predominantly metabolized by the CYP2D6 system and that have a relatively narrow therapeutic index should be initiated at the low end of the dose range if a patient is receiving fluoxetine concurrently or has taken it in the previous 5 weeks. If fluoxetine is added to the treatment regimen of a patient already receiving a drug metabolized by CYP2D6, the need for decreased dose of the original medication should be considered). Products include:
Tarka 534

Vinblastine Sulfate (Co-administration of fluoxetine with other drugs that are metabolized by CYP2D6, including certain antidepressants (eg, TCAs), antipsychotics (eg, phenothiazines and most atypicals), and antiarrhythmics (eg, propafenone, flecainide, and others) should be approached with caution. Therapy with medications that are predominantly metabolized by the CYP2D6 system and that have a relatively narrow therapeutic index should be initiated at the low end of the dose range if a patient is receiving fluoxetine concurrently or has taken it in the previous 5 weeks. Thus, his/her dosing requirements resemble those of poor metabolizers. If fluoxetine is added to the treatment regimen of a patient already receiving a drug metabolized by CYP2D6, the need for decreased dose of the original medication should be considered).
No products indexed under this heading.

Warfarin Sodium (Altered anticoagulant effects, including increased bleeding, have been reported when SNRIs or SSRIs are co-administered with warfarin. Patients receiving warfarin therapy should be carefully monitored when fluoxetine is initiated or discontinued. The administration of fluoxetine to a patient taking another drug that is tightly bound to protein (eg, warfarin) may cause a shift in plasma concentrations potentially resulting in an adverse effect).
No products indexed under this heading.

Zaleplon (Caution is advised if the concomitant administration of fluoxetine and CNS-acting drugs is required. In evaluating individual cases, consideration should be given to using lower initial doses of the concomitantly administered drugs, using conservative titration schedules, and monitoring of clinical status).
No products indexed under this heading.

Ziprasidone Hydrochloride (Co-administration of fluoxetine with other drugs that are metabolized by CYP2D6, including antipsychotics (eg, phenothiazines and most atypicals), should be approached with caution. Therapy with medications that are predominantly metabolized by the CYP2D6 system and that have a relatively narrow therapeutic index should be initiated at the low end of the dose range if a patient is receiving fluoxetine concurrently or has taken it in the previous 5 weeks. If fluoxetine is added to the treatment regimen of a patient already receiving a drug metabolized by CYP2D6, the need for decreased dose of the original medication should be considered). Products include:
Geodon 2723

Ziprasidone Mesylate (Co-administration of fluoxetine with other drugs that are metabolized by CYP2D6, including antipsychotics (eg, phenothiazines and most atypicals), should be approached with caution. Therapy with medications that are predominantly metabolized by the CYP2D6 system and that have a relatively narrow therapeutic index should be initiated at the low end of the dose range if a patient is receiving fluoxetine concurrently or has taken it in the previous 5 weeks. If fluoxetine is added to the treatment regimen of a patient already receiving a drug metabolized by CYP2D6, the need for decreased dose of the original medication should be considered). Products include:
Geodon 2723

Zolmitriptan (Based on the mechanism of action of SNRIs and SSRIs, including fluoxetine, and the potential for serotonin syndrome, caution is advised when fluoxetine is co-administered with other drugs that may affect the serotonergic neurotransmitter systems, such as triptans. There have been rare postmarketing reports of serotonin syndrome with use of an SSRI and a triptan. If concomitant treatment of fluoxetine with a triptan is clinically warranted, careful observation of the patient is advised, particularly during treatment initiation and dose increases). Products include:
Zomig Tablets 773
Zomig Nasal Spray 768
Zomig-ZMT Tablets 773

Zolpidem Tartrate (Caution is advised if the concomitant administration of fluoxetine and CNS-acting drugs is required. In evaluating individual cases, consideration should be given to using lower initial doses of the concomitantly administered drugs, using conservative titration schedules, and monitoring of clinical status). Products include:
Ambien 2920
Ambien CR 2925

Zonisamide (Co-administration of fluoxetine with other drugs that are metabolized by CYP2D6, including certain antidepressants (eg, TCAs), antipsychotics (eg, phenothiazines and most atypicals), and antiarrhythmics (eg, propafenone, flecainide, and others) should be approached with caution. Therapy with medications that are predominantly metabolized by the CYP2D6 system and that have a relatively narrow therapeutic index should be initiated at the low end of the dose range if a patient is receiving fluoxetine concurrently or has taken it in the previous 5 weeks. Thus, his/her dosing requirements resemble those of poor metabolizers. If fluoxetine is added to the treatment regimen of a patient already receiving a drug metabolized by CYP2D6, the need for decreased dose of the original medication should be considered). Products include:
Zonegran 1081

Food Interactions

Alcohol (Caution is advised if the concomitant administration of fluoxetine and CNS-acting drugs is required. In evaluating individual cases, consideration should be given to using lower initial doses of the concomitantly administered drugs, using conservative titration schedules, and monitoring of clinical status).

Beer, reduced-alcohol (Concurrent use with alcohol requires caution).

Beer, unspecified (Concurrent use with alcohol requires caution).

Wine, Chianti (Concurrent use with alcohol requires caution).

Wine, Red (Concurrent use with alcohol requires caution).

Wine, unspecified (Concurrent use with alcohol requires caution).

Wine products (Concurrent use with alcohol requires caution).

PROZAC PULVULES

(Fluoxetine Hydrochloride) 1941
See Prozac Weekly Capsules

PULMICORT FLEXHALER

(Budesonide) 714
May interact with cytochrome p450 3a4 inhibitors (selected), and certain other agents. Compounds in these categories include:

Acetazolamide (Concomitant administration of budesonide with known inhibitors of CYP3A4 may inhibit the metabolism of, and increase the systemic exposure to, budesonide; care should be exercised).
No products indexed under this heading.

Acetazolamide Sodium (Concomitant administration of budesonide with known inhibitors of CYP3A4 may inhibit the metabolism of, and increase the systemic exposure to, budesonide; care should be exercised).
No products indexed under this heading.

Amiodarone Hydrochloride (Concomitant administration of budesonide with known inhibitors of CYP3A4 may inhibit the metabolism of, and increase the systemic exposure to, budesonide; care should be exercised).
No products indexed under this heading.

Amprenavir (Concomitant administration of budesonide with known inhibitors of CYP3A4 may inhibit the metabolism of, and increase the systemic exposure to, budesonide; care should be exercised).
No products indexed under this heading.

Anastrozole (Concomitant administration of budesonide with known inhibitors of CYP3A4 may inhibit the metabolism of, and increase the systemic exposure to, budesonide; care should be exercised).
No products indexed under this heading.

Aprepitant (Concomitant administration of budesonide with known inhibitors of CYP3A4 may inhibit the metabolism of, and increase the systemic exposure to, budesonide; care should be exercised). Products include:
Emend 2124

Atazanavir (Concomitant administration of budesonide with known inhibitors of CYP3A4 may inhibit the metabolism of, and increase the systemic exposure to, budesonide; care should be exercised).
No products indexed under this heading.

Atazanavir Sulfate (Concomitant administration of budesonide with known inhibitors of CYP3A4 may inhibit the metabolism of, and increase the systemic exposure to, budesonide; care should be exercised).
No products indexed under this heading.

Cimetidine (Co-administration of budesonide with cimetidine caused a slight decrease in budesonide clearance and a corresponding increase in its oral bioavailability).
No products indexed under this heading.

Cimetidine Hydrochloride (Concomitant administration of budesonide with known inhibitors of CYP3A4 may inhibit the metabolism of, and increase the systemic exposure to, budesonide; care should be exercised).
No products indexed under this heading.

Ciprofloxacin (Concomitant administration of budesonide with known inhibitors of CYP3A4 may inhibit the metabolism of, and increase the systemic exposure to, budesonide; care should be exercised). Products include:
Cipro I.V. 3082
Cipro 3073
Cipro XR 3091
Ciprodex 583

Clarithromycin (Concomitant administration of budesonide with known inhibitors of CYP3A4 may inhibit the metabolism of, and increase the systemic exposure to, budesonide; care should be exercised). Products include:
Biaxin/Biaxin XL 412

Clotrimazole (Concomitant administration of budesonide with known inhibitors of CYP3A4 may inhibit the metabolism of, and increase the systemic exposure to, budesonide; care should be exercised). Products include:
Lotrisone 3163

Conivaptan Hydrochloride (Concomitant administration of budesonide with known inhibitors of CYP3A4 may inhibit the metabolism of, and increase

1545 Interactions Index Pulmicort

the systemic exposure to, budesonide; care should be exercised). Products include:
Vaprisol 689

Cyclosporine (Concomitant administration of budesonide with known inhibitors of CYP3A4 may inhibit the metabolism of, and increase the systemic exposure to, budesonide; care should be exercised). Products include:
Gengraf 440
Neoral Oral Solution 2496
Neoral Capsules 2496
Restasis 605

Dalfopristin (Concomitant administration of budesonide with known inhibitors of CYP3A4 may inhibit the metabolism of, and increase the systemic exposure to, budesonide; care should be exercised).
No products indexed under this heading.

Danazol (Concomitant administration of budesonide with known inhibitors of CYP3A4 may inhibit the metabolism of, and increase the systemic exposure to, budesonide; care should be exercised).
No products indexed under this heading.

Darunavir (Concomitant administration of budesonide with known inhibitors of CYP3A4 may inhibit the metabolism of, and increase the systemic exposure to, budesonide; care should be exercised).
No products indexed under this heading.

Dasatinib (Concomitant administration of budesonide with known inhibitors of CYP3A4 may inhibit the metabolism of, and increase the systemic exposure to, budesonide; care should be exercised).
No products indexed under this heading.

Delavirdine Mesylate (Concomitant administration of budesonide with known inhibitors of CYP3A4 may inhibit the metabolism of, and increase the systemic exposure to, budesonide; care should be exercised).
No products indexed under this heading.

Delavirine (Concomitant administration of budesonide with known inhibitors of CYP3A4 may inhibit the metabolism of, and increase the systemic exposure to, budesonide; care should be exercised).
No products indexed under this heading.

Desloratadine (Concomitant administration of budesonide with known inhibitors of CYP3A4 may inhibit the metabolism of, and increase the systemic exposure to, budesonide; care should be exercised). Products include:
Clarinex Syrup 3098
Clarinex 3098
Clarinex Reditabs 3098
Clarinex-D 12-Hour 3101
Clarinex-D 3104

Diltiazem Hydrochloride (Concomitant administration of budesonide with known inhibitors of CYP3A4 may inhibit the metabolism of, and increase the systemic exposure to, budesonide; care should be exercised). Products include:
Cardizem LA 423

Diltiazem Maleate (Concomitant administration of budesonide with known inhibitors of CYP3A4 may inhibit the metabolism of, and increase the systemic exposure to, budesonide; care should be exercised).
No products indexed under this heading.

Efavirenz (Concomitant administration of budesonide with known inhibitors of CYP3A4 may inhibit the metabolism of, and increase the systemic exposure to, budesonide; care should be exercised). Products include:
Atripla 906

Erythromycin (Concomitant administration of budesonide with known inhibitors of CYP3A4 may inhibit the metabolism of, and increase the systemic exposure to, budesonide; care should be exercised).
No products indexed under this heading.

Erythromycin Estolate (Concomitant administration of budesonide with known inhibitors of CYP3A4 may inhibit the metabolism of, and increase the systemic exposure to, budesonide; care should be exercised).
No products indexed under this heading.

Erythromycin Ethylsuccinate (Concomitant administration of budesonide with known inhibitors of CYP3A4 may inhibit the metabolism of, and increase the systemic exposure to, budesonide; care should be exercised). Products include:
E.E.S. 437
EryPed 435

Erythromycin Gluceptate (Concomitant administration of budesonide with known inhibitors of CYP3A4 may inhibit the metabolism of, and increase the systemic exposure to, budesonide; care should be exercised).
No products indexed under this heading.

Erythromycin Lactobionate (Concomitant administration of budesonide with known inhibitors of CYP3A4 may inhibit the metabolism of, and increase the systemic exposure to, budesonide; care should be exercised).
No products indexed under this heading.

Erythromycin Stearate (Concomitant administration of budesonide with known inhibitors of CYP3A4 may inhibit the metabolism of, and increase the systemic exposure to, budesonide; care should be exercised).
No products indexed under this heading.

Esomeprazole Magnesium (Concomitant administration of budesonide with known inhibitors of CYP3A4 may inhibit the metabolism of, and increase the systemic exposure to, budesonide; care should be exercised). Products include:
Nexium Capsules 704
Nexium Oral Suspension 704

Esomeprazole Sodium (Concomitant administration of budesonide with known inhibitors of CYP3A4 may inhibit the metabolism of, and increase the systemic exposure to, budesonide; care should be exercised). Products include:
Nexium I.V. 712

Fluconazole (Concomitant administration of budesonide with known inhibitors of CYP3A4 may inhibit the metabolism of, and increase the systemic exposure to, budesonide; care should be exercised).
No products indexed under this heading.

Fluoxetine (Concomitant administration of budesonide with known inhibitors of CYP3A4 may inhibit the metabolism of, and increase the systemic exposure to, budesonide; care should be exercised).
No products indexed under this heading.

Fluoxetine Hydrochloride (Concomitant administration of budesonide with known inhibitors of CYP3A4 may inhibit the metabolism of, and increase the systemic exposure to, budesonide; care should be exercised). Products include:
Prozac Weekly 1941
Prozac Pulvules 1941
Symbyax 1965

Fluvoxamine Maleate (Concomitant administration of budesonide with known inhibitors of CYP3A4 may inhibit the metabolism of, and increase the systemic exposure to, budesonide; care should be exercised).
No products indexed under this heading.

Fosamprenavir Calcium (Concomitant administration of budesonide with known inhibitors of CYP3A4 may inhibit the metabolism of, and increase the systemic exposure to, budesonide; care should be exercised). Products include:
Lexiva Oral Suspension 1558
Lexiva 1558

Imatinib Mesylate (Concomitant administration of budesonide with known inhibitors of CYP3A4 may inhibit the metabolism of, and increase the systemic exposure to, budesonide; care should be exercised). Products include:
Gleevec 2477

Indinavir Sulfate (Concomitant administration of budesonide with known inhibitors of CYP3A4 may inhibit the metabolism of, and increase the systemic exposure to, budesonide; care should be exercised). Products include:
Crixivan 2113

Isoniazid (Concomitant administration of budesonide with known inhibitors of CYP3A4 may inhibit the metabolism of, and increase the systemic exposure to, budesonide; care should be exercised).
No products indexed under this heading.

Itraconazole (Concomitant administration of budesonide with known inhibitors of CYP3A4 may inhibit the metabolism of, and increase the systemic exposure to, budesonide; care should be exercised).
No products indexed under this heading.

Ketoconazole (Concomitant administration of budesonide with known inhibitors of CYP3A4 may inhibit the metabolism of, and increase the systemic exposure to, budesonide; care should be exercised). Products include:
Extina 3319
Xolegel 3337

Lapatinib (Concomitant administration of budesonide with known inhibitors of CYP3A4 may inhibit the metabolism of, and increase the systemic exposure to, budesonide; care should be exercised). Products include:
Tykerb 1698

Lopinavir (Concomitant administration of budesonide with known inhibitors of CYP3A4 may inhibit the metabolism of, and increase the systemic exposure to, budesonide; care should be exercised). Products include:
Kaletra 458

Loratadine (Concomitant administration of budesonide with known inhibitors of CYP3A4 may inhibit the metabolism of, and increase the systemic exposure to, budesonide; care should be exercised).
No products indexed under this heading.

Metronidazole (Concomitant administration of budesonide with known inhibitors of CYP3A4 may inhibit the metabolism of, and increase the systemic exposure to, budesonide; care should be exercised). Products include:
Pylera 793

Metronidazole Benzoate (Concomitant administration of budesonide with known inhibitors of CYP3A4 may inhibit the metabolism of, and increase the systemic exposure to, budesonide; care should be exercised).
No products indexed under this heading.

Metronidazole Hydrochloride (Concomitant administration of budesonide with known inhibitors of CYP3A4 may inhibit the metabolism of, and increase the systemic exposure to, budesonide; care should be exercised).
No products indexed under this heading.

Metronidazole Sodium (Concomitant administration of budesonide with known inhibitors of CYP3A4 may inhibit the metabolism of, and increase the systemic exposure to, budesonide; care should be exercised).
No products indexed under this heading.

Miconazole (Concomitant administration of budesonide with known inhibitors of CYP3A4 may inhibit the metabolism of, and increase the systemic exposure to, budesonide; care should be exercised).
No products indexed under this heading.

Miconazole Nitrate (Concomitant administration of budesonide with known inhibitors of CYP3A4 may inhibit the metabolism of, and increase the systemic exposure to, budesonide; care should be exercised). Products include:
Vusion Ointment 3335

Mifepristone (Concomitant administration of budesonide with known inhibitors of CYP3A4 may inhibit the metabolism of, and increase the systemic exposure to, budesonide; care should be exercised).
No products indexed under this heading.

Nefazodone Hydrochloride (Concomitant administration of budesonide with known inhibitors of CYP3A4 may inhibit the metabolism of, and increase the systemic exposure to, budesonide; care should be exercised).
No products indexed under this heading.

Nelfinavir Mesylate (Concomitant administration of budesonide with known inhibitors of CYP3A4 may inhibit the metabolism of, and increase the systemic exposure to, budesonide; care should be exercised).
No products indexed under this heading.

Nevirapine (Concomitant administration of budesonide with known inhibitors of CYP3A4 may inhibit the metabolism of, and increase the systemic exposure to, budesonide; care should be exercised). Products include:
Viramune Oral Suspension 897
Viramune Tablets 897

Niacin (Concomitant administration of budesonide with known inhibitors of CYP3A4 may inhibit the metabolism of, and increase the systemic exposure to, budesonide; care should be exercised). Products include:
Advicor 402
Cardio Basics 3455
Niaspan 497
Simcor 524

Niacinamide (Concomitant administration of budesonide with known inhibitors of CYP3A4 may inhibit the metabolism of, and increase the systemic exposure to, budesonide; care should be exercised). Products include:
CitraNatal 90 DHA Capsules 2332
CitraNatal Assure 2332
CitraNatal Rx 2332
Heplive 607

Niacinamide Hydroiodide (Concomitant administration of budesonide with known inhibitors of CYP3A4 may inhibit the metabolism of, and increase the systemic exposure to, budesonide; care should be exercised).
No products indexed under this heading.

Nicotinamide (Concomitant administration of budesonide with known inhibitors of CYP3A4 may inhibit the metabolism of, and increase the systemic exposure to, budesonide; care should be exercised).
No products indexed under this heading.

Nifedipine (Concomitant administration of budesonide with known inhibitors of CYP3A4 may inhibit the metabolism of, and increase the systemic exposure to, budesonide; care should be exercised).
No products indexed under this heading.

Norfloxacin (Concomitant administration of budesonide with known inhibitors of CYP3A4 may inhibit the metabolism of, and increase the systemic exposure to, budesonide; care should be exercised). Products include:
Noroxin 2220

IMPORTANT NOTE: Always consult each drug listing in the patient's regimen for possible interactions.

Omeprazole (Concomitant administration of budesonide with known inhibitors of CYP3A4 may inhibit the metabolism of, and increase the systemic exposure to, budesonide; care should be exercised).

No products indexed under this heading.

Paroxetine Hydrochloride (Concomitant administration of budesonide with known inhibitors of CYP3A4 may inhibit the metabolism of, and increase the systemic exposure to, budesonide; care should be exercised). Products include:

Paroxetine CR 2361
Paroxetine ER 2371
Paxil 1586
Paxil CR 1596

Posaconazole (Concomitant administration of budesonide with known inhibitors of CYP3A4 may inhibit the metabolism of, and increase the systemic exposure to, budesonide; care should be exercised). Products include:

Noxafil 3172

Propoxyphene Hydrochloride (Concomitant administration of budesonide with known inhibitors of CYP3A4 may inhibit the metabolism of, and increase the systemic exposure to, budesonide; care should be exercised).

No products indexed under this heading.

Propoxyphene Napsylate (Concomitant administration of budesonide with known inhibitors of CYP3A4 may inhibit the metabolism of, and increase the systemic exposure to, budesonide; care should be exercised).

No products indexed under this heading.

Quinidine (Concomitant administration of budesonide with known inhibitors of CYP3A4 may inhibit the metabolism of, and increase the systemic exposure to, budesonide; care should be exercised).

No products indexed under this heading.

Quinidine Hydrochloride (Concomitant administration of budesonide with known inhibitors of CYP3A4 may inhibit the metabolism of, and increase the systemic exposure to, budesonide; care should be exercised).

No products indexed under this heading.

Quinidine Polygalacturonate (Concomitant administration of budesonide with known inhibitors of CYP3A4 may inhibit the metabolism of, and increase the systemic exposure to, budesonide; care should be exercised).

No products indexed under this heading.

Quinidine Sulfate (Concomitant administration of budesonide with known inhibitors of CYP3A4 may inhibit the metabolism of, and increase the systemic exposure to, budesonide; care should be exercised).

No products indexed under this heading.

Quinine (Concomitant administration of budesonide with known inhibitors of CYP3A4 may inhibit the metabolism of, and increase the systemic exposure to, budesonide; care should be exercised). Products include:

Hyland's Leg Cramps PM with Quinine 3315

Quinine Sulfate (Concomitant administration of budesonide with known inhibitors of CYP3A4 may inhibit the metabolism of, and increase the systemic exposure to, budesonide; care should be exercised).

No products indexed under this heading.

Quinupristin (Concomitant administration of budesonide with known inhibitors of CYP3A4 may inhibit the metabolism of, and increase the systemic exposure to, budesonide; care should be exercised).

No products indexed under this heading.

Ranitidine Bismuth Citrate (Concomitant administration of budesonide with known inhibitors of CYP3A4 may inhibit the metabolism of, and increase the systemic exposure to, budesonide; care should be exercised).

No products indexed under this heading.

Ranitidine Hydrochloride (Concomitant administration of budesonide with known inhibitors of CYP3A4 may inhibit the metabolism of, and increase the systemic exposure to, budesonide; care should be exercised). Products include:

Zantac 1737
Zantac Injection 1732
Zantac Pharmacy 1735

Ritonavir (Concomitant administration of budesonide with known inhibitors of CYP3A4 may inhibit the metabolism of, and increase the systemic exposure to, budesonide; care should be exercised). Products include:

Kaletra 458
Norvir 509

Saquinavir (Concomitant administration of budesonide with known inhibitors of CYP3A4 may inhibit the metabolism of, and increase the systemic exposure to, budesonide; care should be exercised).

No products indexed under this heading.

Saquinavir Mesylate (Concomitant administration of budesonide with known inhibitors of CYP3A4 may inhibit the metabolism of, and increase the systemic exposure to, budesonide; care should be exercised).

No products indexed under this heading.

Sertraline Hydrochloride (Concomitant administration of budesonide with known inhibitors of CYP3A4 may inhibit the metabolism of, and increase the systemic exposure to, budesonide; care should be exercised).

No products indexed under this heading.

Sildenafil Citrate (Concomitant administration of budesonide with known inhibitors of CYP3A4 may inhibit the metabolism of, and increase the systemic exposure to, budesonide; care should be exercised).

No products indexed under this heading.

Telithromycin (Concomitant administration of budesonide with known inhibitors of CYP3A4 may inhibit the metabolism of, and increase the systemic exposure to, budesonide; care should be exercised). Products include:

Ketek 2991

Troglitazone (Concomitant administration of budesonide with known inhibitors of CYP3A4 may inhibit the metabolism of, and increase the systemic exposure to, budesonide; care should be exercised).

No products indexed under this heading.

Troleandomycin (Concomitant administration of budesonide with known inhibitors of CYP3A4 may inhibit the metabolism of, and increase the systemic exposure to, budesonide; care should be exercised).

No products indexed under this heading.

Valproate Sodium (Concomitant administration of budesonide with known inhibitors of CYP3A4 may inhibit the metabolism of, and increase the systemic exposure to, budesonide; care should be exercised).

No products indexed under this heading.

Vardenafil Hydrochloride (Concomitant administration of budesonide with known inhibitors of CYP3A4 may inhibit the metabolism of, and increase the systemic exposure to, budesonide; care should be exercised). Products include:

Levitra 3157

Verapamil Hydrochloride (Concomitant administration of budesonide with known inhibitors of CYP3A4 may inhibit the metabolism of, and increase the

systemic exposure to, budesonide; care should be exercised). Products include:

Tarka 534

Voriconazole (Concomitant administration of budesonide with known inhibitors of CYP3A4 may inhibit the metabolism of, and increase the systemic exposure to, budesonide; care should be exercised).

No products indexed under this heading.

Zafirlukast (Concomitant administration of budesonide with known inhibitors of CYP3A4 may inhibit the metabolism of, and increase the systemic exposure to, budesonide; care should be exercised). Products include:

Accolate 3612

Zileuton (Concomitant administration of budesonide with known inhibitors of CYP3A4 may inhibit the metabolism of, and increase the systemic exposure to, budesonide; care should be exercised).

No products indexed under this heading.

Food Interactions

Grapefruit (Concomitant administration of budesonide with known inhibitors of CYP3A4 may inhibit the metabolism of, and increase the systemic exposure to, budesonide; care should be exercised).

Grapefruit Juice (Concomitant administration of budesonide with known inhibitors of CYP3A4 may inhibit the metabolism of, and increase the systemic exposure to, budesonide; care should be exercised).

PULMOZYME INHALATION SOLUTION

(Dornase Alfa) 1214
None cited in PDR database.

PYLERA CAPSULES

(Bismuth Subcitrate Potassium, Metronidazole, Tetracycline Hydrochloride) 793
May interact with alcohols, antacids, anticoagulants, lithium preparations, oral contraceptives, penicillins, phenytoin, and certain other agents. Compounds in these categories include:

Aluminum Carbonate (Absorption of Pylera is impaired by antacids containing aluminum, calcium, or magnesium).

No products indexed under this heading.

Aluminum Hydroxide (Absorption of Pylera is impaired by antacids containing aluminum, calcium, or magnesium).

No products indexed under this heading.

Amoxicillin (Since bacteriostatic drugs, such as Pylera class of antibiotics, may interfere with the bactericidal action of penicillin, it is not advisable to administer these drugs concomitantly). Products include:

Amoxil Capsules 1311
Amoxil Chewable Tablets 1311
Amoxil 1311
Amoxil Powder 1311
Augmentin 1331
Augmentin Tablets 1335
Augmentin ES-600 1338
Augmentin XR 1342
Moxatag 2321

Amoxicillin Trihydrate (Since bacteriostatic drugs, such as Pylera class of antibiotics, may interfere with the bactericidal action of penicillin, it is not advisable to administer these drugs concomitantly).

No products indexed under this heading.

Ampicillin (Since bacteriostatic drugs, such as Pylera class of antibiotics, may interfere with the bactericidal action of penicillin, it is not advisable to administer these drugs concomitantly).

No products indexed under this heading.

Ampicillin Sodium (Since bacteriostatic drugs, such as Pylera class of antibiotics, may interfere with the bactericidal action of penicillin, it is not advisable to administer these drugs concomitantly).

No products indexed under this heading.

Ampicillin Trihydrate (Since bacteriostatic drugs, such as Pylera class of antibiotics, may interfere with the bactericidal action of penicillin, it is not advisable to administer these drugs concomitantly).

No products indexed under this heading.

Anisindione (Pylera has been reported to potentiate the anticoagulant effect of warfarin and other oral coumarin anticoagulant, resulting in a prolongation of prothrombin time. Therefore, frequent monitoring therapy with appropriate adjustment of the anticoagulant dosage is warranted with initiation of Pylera).

No products indexed under this heading.

Ardeparin Sodium (Pylera has been reported to potentiate the anticoagulant effect of warfarin and other oral coumarin anticoagulant, resulting in a prolongation of prothrombin time. Therefore, frequent monitoring therapy with appropriate adjustment of the anticoagulant dosage is warranted with initiation of Pylera).

No products indexed under this heading.

Azlocillin Sodium (Since bacteriostatic drugs, such as Pylera class of antibiotics, may interfere with the bactericidal action of penicillin, it is not advisable to administer these drugs concomitantly).

No products indexed under this heading.

Bacampicillin Hydrochloride (Since bacteriostatic drugs, such as Pylera class of antibiotics, may interfere with the bactericidal action of penicillin, it is not advisable to administer these drugs concomitantly).

No products indexed under this heading.

Calcium Carbonate (Absorption of Pylera is impaired by antacids containing aluminum, calcium, or magnesium). Products include:

Chelated Mineral 3476
Pepcid Complete 1822
Extra Strength Rolaids Softchews Vanilla Creme 2045

Carbenicillin Disodium (Since bacteriostatic drugs, such as Pylera class of antibiotics, may interfere with the bactericidal action of penicillin, it is not advisable to administer these drugs concomitantly).

No products indexed under this heading.

Carbenicillin Indanyl Sodium (Since bacteriostatic drugs, such as Pylera class of antibiotics, may interfere with the bactericidal action of penicillin, it is not advisable to administer these drugs concomitantly).

No products indexed under this heading.

Cimetidine (The simultaneous administration of drugs that decrease microsomal liver enzyme activity, such as cimetidine, may prolong the half-life and decrease plasma clearance of pylera).

No products indexed under this heading.

Cloxacillin (Since bacteriostatic drugs, such as Pylera class of antibiotics, may interfere with the bactericidal action of penicillin, it is not advisable to administer these drugs concomitantly).

No products indexed under this heading.

Cloxacillin Sodium (Since bacteriostatic drugs, such as Pylera class of antibiotics, may interfere with the bactericidal action of penicillin, it is not advisable to administer these drugs concomitantly).

No products indexed under this heading.

Cloxacillin Sodium Monohydrate
(Since bacteriostatic drugs, such as Pylera class of antibiotics, may interfere with the bactericidal action of penicillin, it is not advisable to administer these drugs concomitantly).
No products indexed under this heading.

Dalteparin Sodium (Pylera has been reported to potentiate the anticoagulant effect of warfarin and other oral coumarin anticoagulant, resulting in a prolongation of prothrombin time. Therefore, frequent monitoring therapy with appropriate adjustment of the anticoagulant dosage is warranted with initiation of Pylera). Products include:

Danaparoid Sodium (Pylera has been reported to potentiate the anticoagulant effect of warfarin and other oral coumarin anticoagulant, resulting in a prolongation of prothrombin time. Therefore, frequent monitoring therapy with appropriate adjustment of the anticoagulant dosage is warranted with initiation of Pylera).
No products indexed under this heading.

Desogestrel (Concurrent use of Pylera may render oral contraceptives less effective. Patients should be advised to use a different or additional form of contraceptives).
No products indexed under this heading.

Dicloxacillin (Since bacteriostatic drugs, such as Pylera class of antibiotics, may interfere with the bactericidal action of penicillin, it is not advisable to administer these drugs concomitantly).
No products indexed under this heading.

Dicloxacillin Sodium (Since bacteriostatic drugs, such as Pylera class of antibiotics, may interfere with the bactericidal action of penicillin, it is not advisable to administer these drugs concomitantly).
No products indexed under this heading.

Dicumarol (Pylera has been reported to potentiate the anticoagulant effect of warfarin and other oral coumarin anticoagulant, resulting in a prolongation of prothrombin time. Therefore, frequent monitoring therapy with appropriate adjustment of the anticoagulant dosage is warranted with initiation of Pylera).
No products indexed under this heading.

Disodium Carbenicillin (Since bacteriostatic drugs, such as Pylera class of antibiotics, may interfere with the bactericidal action of penicillin, it is not advisable to administer these drugs concomitantly).
No products indexed under this heading.

Enoxaparin Sodium (Pylera has been reported to potentiate the anticoagulant effect of warfarin and other oral coumarin anticoagulant, resulting in a prolongation of prothrombin time. Therefore, frequent monitoring therapy with appropriate adjustment of the anticoagulant dosage is warranted with initiation of Pylera). Products include:

Ethanol (Alcoholic beverages should not be consumed during Pylera therapy and for at least 1 day afterward. Psychotic reactions have been reported in alcoholic patients who are using Pylera and disulfiram concurrently. Pylera should not be given to patients who have taken disulfiram within the last 2 weeks).
No products indexed under this heading.

Ethinyl Estradiol (Concurrent use of Pylera may render oral contraceptives less effective. Patients should be advised to use a different or additional form of contraceptives). Products include:

Ethyl Alcohol (Alcoholic beverages should not be consumed during Pylera therapy and for at least 1 day afterward. Psychotic reactions have been reported in alcoholic patients who are using Pylera and disulfiram concurrently. Pylera should not be given to patients who have taken disulfiram within the last 2 weeks).
No products indexed under this heading.

Ethynodiol Diacetate (Concurrent use of Pylera may render oral contraceptives less effective. Patients should be advised to use a different or additional form of contraceptives).
No products indexed under this heading.

Fondaparinux Sodium (Pylera has been reported to potentiate the anticoagulant effect of warfarin and other oral coumarin anticoagulant, resulting in a prolongation of prothrombin time. Therefore, frequent monitoring therapy with appropriate adjustment of the anticoagulant dosage is warranted with initiation of Pylera). Products include:

Fosphenytoin (The simultaneous administration of drugs that induce microsomal liver enzymes, such as phenytoin, may accelerate the elimination of Pylera, resulting in reduced plasma levels. Impaired clearance of phenytoin has also been reported in this situation).
No products indexed under this heading.

Fosphenytoin Sodium (The simultaneous administration of drugs that induce microsomal liver enzymes, such as phenytoin, may accelerate the elimination of Pylera, resulting in reduced plasma levels. Impaired clearance of phenytoin has also been reported in this situation).
No products indexed under this heading.

Heparin Calcium (Pylera has been reported to potentiate the anticoagulant effect of warfarin and other oral coumarin anticoagulant, resulting in a prolongation of prothrombin time. Therefore, frequent monitoring therapy with appropriate adjustment of the anticoagulant dosage is warranted with initiation of Pylera).
No products indexed under this heading.

Heparin Sodium (Pylera has been reported to potentiate the anticoagulant effect of warfarin and other oral coumarin anticoagulant, resulting in a prolongation of prothrombin time. Therefore, frequent monitoring therapy with appropriate adjustment of the anticoagulant dosage is warranted with initiation of Pylera).
No products indexed under this heading.

Levonorgestrel (Concurrent use of Pylera may render oral contraceptives less effective. Patients should be advised to use a different or additional form of contraceptives). Products include:

Lithium (In patients stabilized on relatively high doses of lithium, short-term Pylera therapy has been associated with elevation of serum lithium and, in a few cases, signs of lithium toxicity).
No products indexed under this heading.

Lithium Carbonate (In patients stabilized on relatively high doses of lithium, short-term Pylera therapy has been associated with elevation of serum lithium and, in a few cases, signs of lithium toxicity).
No products indexed under this heading.

Lithium Citrate (In patients stabilized on relatively high doses of lithium, short-term Pylera therapy has been associated with elevation of serum lithium and, in a few cases, signs of lithium toxicity).
No products indexed under this heading.

Low Molecular Weight Heparins (Pylera has been reported to potentiate the anticoagulant effect of warfarin and other oral coumarin anticoagulant, resulting in a prolongation of prothrombin time. Therefore, frequent monitoring therapy with appropriate adjustment of the anticoagulant dosage is warranted with initiation of Pylera).
No products indexed under this heading.

Magaldrate (Absorption of Pylera is impaired by antacids containing aluminum, calcium, or magnesium).
No products indexed under this heading.

Magnesium Carbonate (Absorption of Pylera is impaired by antacids containing aluminum, calcium, or magnesium).
No products indexed under this heading.

Magnesium Hydroxide (Absorption of Pylera is impaired by antacids containing aluminum, calcium, or magnesium). Products include:

Magnesium Oxide (Absorption of Pylera is impaired by antacids containing aluminum, calcium, or magnesium). Products include:

Magnesium Trisilicate (Absorption of Pylera is impaired by antacids containing aluminum, calcium, or magnesium).
No products indexed under this heading.

Mestranol (Concurrent use of Pylera may render oral contraceptives less effective. Patients should be advised to use a different or additional form of contraceptives).
No products indexed under this heading.

Methicillin Sodium (Since bacteriostatic drugs, such as Pylera class of antibiotics, may interfere with the bactericidal action of penicillin, it is not advisable to administer these drugs concomitantly).
No products indexed under this heading.

Methoxyflurane (The concurrent use of tetracycline and methoxyflurane has been reported to result in fatal renal toxicity).
No products indexed under this heading.

Mezlocillin Sodium (Since bacteriostatic drugs, such as Pylera class of antibiotics, may interfere with the bactericidal action of penicillin, it is not advisable to administer these drugs concomitantly).
No products indexed under this heading.

Nafcillin Sodium (Since bacteriostatic drugs, such as Pylera class of antibiotics, may interfere with the bactericidal action of penicillin, it is not advisable to administer these drugs concomitantly).
No products indexed under this heading.

Norethindrone (Concurrent use of Pylera may render oral contraceptives less effective. Patients should be advised to use a different or additional form of contraceptives). Products include:

Norethynodrel (Concurrent use of Pylera may render oral contraceptives less effective. Patients should be advised to use a different or additional form of contraceptives).
No products indexed under this heading.

Norgestimate (Concurrent use of Pylera may render oral contraceptives less effective. Patients should be advised to use a different or additional form of contraceptives). Products include:

Norgestrel (Concurrent use of Pylera may render oral contraceptives less effective. Patients should be advised to use a different or additional form of contraceptives).
No products indexed under this heading.

Oxacillin (Since bacteriostatic drugs, such as Pylera class of antibiotics, may interfere with the bactericidal action of penicillin, it is not advisable to administer these drugs concomitantly).
No products indexed under this heading.

Oxacillin Sodium (Since bacteriostatic drugs, such as Pylera class of antibiotics, may interfere with the bactericidal action of penicillin, it is not advisable to administer these drugs concomitantly).
No products indexed under this heading.

Penicillin, Potassium Phenoxymethyl (Since bacteriostatic drugs, such as Pylera class of antibiotics, may interfere with the bactericidal action of penicillin, it is not advisable to administer these drugs concomitantly).
No products indexed under this heading.

Penicillin G Benzathine (Since bacteriostatic drugs, such as Pylera class of antibiotics, may interfere with the bactericidal action of penicillin, it is not advisable to administer these drugs concomitantly). Products include:

Penicillin G Dibenzylethyenediamine (Since bacteriostatic drugs, such as Pylera class of antibiotics, may interfere with the bactericidal action of penicillin, it is not advisable to administer these drugs concomitantly).
No products indexed under this heading.

Penicillin G Potassium (Since bacteriostatic drugs, such as Pylera class of antibiotics, may interfere with the bactericidal action of penicillin, it is not advisable to administer these drugs concomitantly).
No products indexed under this heading.

Penicillin G Procaine (Since bacteriostatic drugs, such as Pylera class of antibiotics, may interfere with the bactericidal action of penicillin, it is not advisable to administer these drugs concomitantly). Products include:

Penicillin G Sodium (Since bacteriostatic drugs, such as Pylera class of antibiotics, may interfere with the bactericidal action of penicillin, it is not advisable to administer these drugs concomitantly).
No products indexed under this heading.

Penicillin V (Since bacteriostatic drugs, such as Pylera class of antibiotics, may interfere with the bactericidal action of penicillin, it is not advisable to administer these drugs concomitantly).
No products indexed under this heading.

Penicillin V Potassium (Since bacteriostatic drugs, such as Pylera class of antibiotics, may interfere with the bactericidal action of penicillin, it is not advisable to administer these drugs concomitantly).
No products indexed under this heading.

Penicillins (Since bacteriostatic drugs, such as Pylera class of antibiotics, may interfere with the bactericidal action of penicillin, it is not advisable to administer these drugs concomitantly).
No products indexed under this heading.

Phenobarbital (The simultaneous administration of drugs that induce microsomal liver enzymes, such as phenobarbital, may accelerate the elimination of pylera, resulting in reduced plasma levels. Impaired clearance of phenobarbital has also been reported in this situation). Products include:
Donnatal 2711

Phenytoin (The simultaneous administration of drugs that induce microsomal liver enzymes, such as phenytoin, may accelerate the elimination of Pylera, resulting in reduced plasma levels. Impaired clearance of phenytoin has also been reported in this situation).
No products indexed under this heading.

Phenytoin Sodium (The simultaneous administration of drugs that induce microsomal liver enzymes, such as phenytoin, may accelerate the elimination of Pylera, resulting in reduced plasma levels. Impaired clearance of phenytoin has also been reported in this situation). Products include:
Phenytek Capsules 2380

Piperacillin Sodium (Since bacteriostatic drugs, such as Pylera class of antibiotics, may interfere with the bactericidal action of penicillin, it is not advisable to administer these drugs concomitantly). Products include:
Zosyn 3607

Sodium Bicarbonate (Absorption of Pylera is impaired by antacids containing aluminum, calcium, or magnesium).
No products indexed under this heading.

Sodium Cloxacillin Monohydrate (Since bacteriostatic drugs, such as Pylera class of antibiotics, may interfere with the bactericidal action of penicillin, it is not advisable to administer these drugs concomitantly).
No products indexed under this heading.

Ticarcillin Disodium (Since bacteriostatic drugs, such as Pylera class of antibiotics, may interfere with the bactericidal action of penicillin, it is not advisable to administer these drugs concomitantly). Products include:
Timentin ADD-Vantage 1670
Timentin Galaxy 1674
Timentin 1666
Timentin Pharmacy 1678

Tinzaparin Sodium (Pylera has been reported to potentiate the anticoagulant effect of warfarin and other oral coumarin anticoagulant, resulting in a prolongation of prothrombin time. Therefore, frequent monitoring therapy with appropriate adjustment of the anticoagulant dosage is warranted with initiation of Pylera).
No products indexed under this heading.

Vitamins, Multiple (Absorption of Pylera is impaired by preparations containing iron, zinc, or sodium bicarbonate). Products include:
Mega Antioxidant 3476

Warfarin Sodium (Pylera has been reported to potentiate the anticoagulant effect of warfarin and other oral coumarin anticoagulant, resulting in a prolongation of prothrombin time. Therefore, frequent monitoring therapy with appropriate adjustment of the anticoagulant dosage is warranted with initiation of Pylera).
No products indexed under this heading.

Food Interactions

Alcohol (Alcoholic beverages should not be consumed during Pylera therapy and for at least 1 day afterward. Psychotic reactions have been reported in alcohol-

ic patients who are using Pylera and disulfiram concurrently. Pylera should not be given to patients who have taken disulfiram within the last 2 weeks).

Beer, reduced-alcohol (Alcoholic beverages should not be consumed during Pylera therapy and for at least 1 day afterward. Psychotic reactions have been reported in alcoholic patients who are using Pylera and disulfiram concurrently. Pylera should not be given to patients who have taken disulfiram within the last 2 weeks).

Beer, unspecified (Alcoholic beverages should not be consumed during Pylera therapy and for at least 1 day afterward. Psychotic reactions have been reported in alcoholic patients who are using Pylera and disulfiram concurrently. Pylera should not be given to patients who have taken disulfiram within the last 2 weeks).

Dairy products (Absorption of Pylera is impaired by milk or dairy products).

Wine, Chianti (Alcoholic beverages should not be consumed during Pylera therapy and for at least 1 day afterward. Psychotic reactions have been reported in alcoholic patients who are using Pylera and disulfiram concurrently. Pylera should not be given to patients who have taken disulfiram within the last 2 weeks).

Wine, Red (Alcoholic beverages should not be consumed during Pylera therapy and for at least 1 day afterward. Psychotic reactions have been reported in alcoholic patients who are using Pylera and disulfiram concurrently. Pylera should not be given to patients who have taken disulfiram within the last 2 weeks).

Wine, unspecified (Alcoholic beverages should not be consumed during Pylera therapy and for at least 1 day afterward. Psychotic reactions have been reported in alcoholic patients who are using Pylera and disulfiram concurrently. Pylera should not be given to patients who have taken disulfiram within the last 2 weeks).

Wine products (Alcoholic beverages should not be consumed during Pylera therapy and for at least 1 day afterward. Psychotic reactions have been reported in alcoholic patients who are using Pylera and disulfiram concurrently. Pylera should not be given to patients who have taken disulfiram within the last 2 weeks).

QUIXIN OPHTHALMIC SOLUTION

(Levofloxacin) 3493
May interact with xanthines, and certain other agents. Compounds in these categories include:

Aminophylline (Systemic administration of some quinolones has been shown to elevate plasma concentrations of theophylline).
No products indexed under this heading.

Caffeine (Systemic administration of some quinolones has been shown to interfere with the metabolism of caffeine).
No products indexed under this heading.

Caffeine Citrate (Systemic administration of some quinolones has been shown to interfere with the metabolism of caffeine).
No products indexed under this heading.

Cyclosporine (Systemic administration of some quinolones has been associated with transient elevations of serum creatinine in patients receiving systemic cyclosporine concomitantly). Products include:

Gengraf 440
Neoral Oral Solution 2496
Neoral Capsules 2496
Restasis 605

Dyphylline (Systemic administration of some quinolones has been shown to elevate plasma concentrations of theophylline).
No products indexed under this heading.

Theophylline (Systemic administration of some quinolones has been shown to elevate plasma concentrations of theophylline).
No products indexed under this heading.

Theophylline Anhydrous (Systemic administration of some quinolones has been shown to elevate plasma concentrations of theophylline). Products include:
Uniphyl 2817

Theophylline Calcium Salicylate (Systemic administration of some quinolones has been shown to elevate plasma concentrations of theophylline).
No products indexed under this heading.

Theophylline Dihydroxypropyl (Glyceryl) (Systemic administration of some quinolones has been shown to elevate plasma concentrations of theophylline).
No products indexed under this heading.

Theophylline Ethylenediamine (Systemic administration of some quinolones has been shown to elevate plasma concentrations of theophylline).
No products indexed under this heading.

Theophylline Sodium Glycinate (Systemic administration of some quinolones has been shown to elevate plasma concentrations of theophylline).
No products indexed under this heading.

Warfarin Sodium (Systemic administration of some quinolones has been shown to enhance the effects of the oral anticoagulant warfarin).
No products indexed under this heading.

QVAR INHALATION AEROSOL

(Beclomethasone Dipropionate) 3398
None cited in PDR database.

RANEXA EXTENDED-RELEASE TABLETS

(Ranolazine) 1255
May interact with antipsychotic agents, class 1A antiarrhythmics, class III antiarrhythmics, cytochrome p450 2d6 inhibitors (selected), cytochrome p450 2d6 substrates (selected), cytochrome p450 3a inducers (selected), cytochrome p450 3a inhibitors (selected), cytochrome p450 3a substrates (selected), P-glycoprotein inducers, P-glycoprotein inhibitors, phenytoin, tricyclic antidepressants, and certain other agents. Compounds in these categories include:

Alfentanil Hydrochloride (The plasma levels of simvastatin, a CYP3A substrate, and its active metabolite are each increased about 2-fold in healthy subjects receiving simvastatin (80 mg once daily) and ranolazine (1000 mg twice daily). Dose adjustments of simvastatin are not required when ranolazine is co-administered with simvastatin).
No products indexed under this heading.

Allium sativum (Avoid co-administration of ranolazine and CYP3A inducers, such as rifampin, rifabutin, rifapentin, phenobarbital, phenytoin, carbamazepine, and St. John's wort. Rifampin (600 mg once daily) decreases the plasma concentration of ranolazine (1000 mg twice daily) by approximately 95% by induction of CYP3A and, probably, P-gp).
No products indexed under this heading.

Alprazolam (The plasma levels of simvastatin, a CYP3A substrate, and its active metabolite are each increased about 2-fold in healthy subjects receiving simvastatin (80 mg once daily) and ranolazine (1000 mg twice daily). Dose adjustments of simvastatin are not required when ranolazine is co-administered with simvastatin).
No products indexed under this heading.

Aminophylline (The plasma levels of simvastatin, a CYP3A substrate, and its active metabolite are each increased about 2-fold in healthy subjects receiving simvastatin (80 mg once daily) and ranolazine (1000 mg twice daily). Dose adjustments of simvastatin are not required when ranolazine is co-administered with simvastatin).
No products indexed under this heading.

Amiodarone Hydrochloride (Because of possible additive effects on the QT interval, ranolazine should be avoided in patients receiving drugs that prolong the QTc interval, such as Class IA (eg, quinidine) and Class III (eg, dofetilide, sotalol) antiarrhythmics, and antipsychotics (eg, thioridazine, ziprasidone)).
No products indexed under this heading.

Amitriptyline Hydrochloride (The potent CYP2D6 inhibitor, paroxetine (20 mg once daily), increases ranolazine concentrations 1.2-fold. No dose adjustment of ranolazine is required in patients treated with CYP2D6 inhibitors).
No products indexed under this heading.

Amlodipine Besylate (Down-titrate ranozaline based on clinical response in patients concomitantly treated with P-gp inhibitors, such as cyclosporine). Products include:
Azor 1010
Exforge 2443
Exforge HCT 2449

Amoxapine (The potent CYP2D6 inhibitor, paroxetine (20 mg once daily), increases ranolazine concentrations 1.2-fold. No dose adjustment of ranolazine is required in patients treated with CYP2D6 inhibitors).
No products indexed under this heading.

Amphetamine Aspartate (Ranolazine or its metabolites partially inhibit CYP2D6. There are no studies of concomitant use of ranolazine with other drugs metabolized by CYP2D6, such as tricyclic antidepressants and antipsychotics, but lower doses of CYP2D6 substrates may be required).
No products indexed under this heading.

Amphetamine Aspartate Monohydrate (Ranolazine or its metabolites partially inhibit CYP2D6. There are no studies of concomitant use of ranolazine with other drugs metabolized by CYP2D6, such as tricyclic antidepressants and antipsychotics, but lower doses of CYP2D6 substrates may be required).
No products indexed under this heading.

Amphetamine Sulfate (Ranolazine or its metabolites partially inhibit CYP2D6. There are no studies of concomitant use of ranolazine with other drugs metabolized by CYP2D6, such as tricyclic antidepressants and antipsychotics, but lower doses of CYP2D6 substrates may be required).
No products indexed under this heading.

Amprenavir (Concurrent administration of ranolazine and CYP3A inhibitors is contraindicated. Do not use ranolazine with strong CYP3A inhibitors, including ketoconazole, itraconazole, clarithromycin, nefazodone, nelfinavir, ritonavir, indinavir, and saquinavir. Limit the dose of ranolazine to 500 mg twice daily in patients on moderate CYP3A inhibitors, including diltiazem, verapamil, aprepitant, erythromycin, flucona-

zole, and grapefruit juice or grapefruit-containing products. Weak CYP3A inhibitors such as simvastatin (20 mg once daily) and cimetidine (400 mg three times daily) do not increase the exposure to ranolazine in healthy volunteers).

No products indexed under this heading.

Aprepitant (Concurrent administration of ranolazine and CYP3A inhibitors is contraindicated. Do not use ranolazine with strong CYP3A inhibitors, including ketoconazole, itraconazole, clarithromycin, nefazodone, nelfinavir, ritonavir, indinavir, and saquinavir. Limit the dose of ranolazine to 500 mg twice daily in patients on moderate CYP3A inhibitors, including diltiazem, verapamil, aprepitant, erythromycin, fluconazole, and grapefruit juice or grapefruit-containing products. Weak CYP3A inhibitors such as simvastatin (20 mg once daily) and cimetidine (400 mg three times daily) do not increase the exposure to ranolazine in healthy volunteers). Products include:

Aripiprazole (Ranolazine can inhibit the activity of CYP2D6 and thus, the metabolism of drugs that are mainly metabolized by this enzyme (eg, some antipsychotics) may be impaired and exposure to these drugs increased. The dose of such drugs may have to be reduced when ranolazine is co-administered).

No products indexed under this heading.

Astemizole (The plasma levels of simvastatin, a CYP3A substrate, and its active metabolite are each increased about 2-fold in healthy subjects receiving simvastatin (80 mg once daily) and ranolazine (1000 mg twice daily). Dose adjustments of simvastatin are not required when ranolazine is co-administered with simvastatin).

No products indexed under this heading.

Atenolol (Down-titrate ranozaline based on clinical response in patients concomitantly treated with P-gp inhibitors, such as cyclosporine).

No products indexed under this heading.

Atomoxetine Hydrochloride (Ranolazine or its metabolites partially inhibit CYP2D6. There are no studies of concomitant use of ranolazine with other drugs metabolized by CYP2D6, such as tricyclic antidepressants and antipsychotics, but lower doses of CYP2D6 substrates may be required). Products include:

Atorvastatin Calcium (Down-titrate ranozaline based on clinical response in patients concomitantly treated with P-gp inhibitors, such as cyclosporine). Products include:

Azithromycin Dihydrate (Down-titrate ranozaline based on clinical response in patients concomitantly treated with P-gp inhibitors, such as cyclosporine).

No products indexed under this heading.

Bisoprolol Fumarate (Ranolazine or its metabolites partially inhibit CYP2D6. There are no studies of concomitant use of ranolazine with other drugs metabolized by CYP2D6, such as tricyclic antidepressants and antipsychotics, but lower doses of CYP2D6 substrates may be required).

No products indexed under this heading.

Bretylium Tosylate (Because of possible additive effects on the QT interval, ranolazine should be avoided in patients receiving drugs that prolong the QTc interval, such as Class IA (eg, quinidine) and Class III (eg, dofetilide, sotalol) antiarrhythmics, and antipsychotics (eg, thioridazine, ziprasidone)).

No products indexed under this heading.

Bromocriptine Mesylate (The plasma levels of simvastatin, a CYP3A substrate, and its active metabolite are each increased about 2-fold in healthy subjects receiving simvastatin (80 mg once daily) and ranolazine (1000 mg twice daily). Dose adjustments of simvastatin are not required when ranolazine is co-administered with simvastatin).

No products indexed under this heading.

Bupropion Hydrochloride (The potent CYP2D6 inhibitor, paroxetine (20 mg once daily), increases ranolazine concentrations 1.2-fold. No dose adjustment of ranolazine is required in patients treated with CYP2D6 inhibitors). Products include:

Buspirone Hydrochloride (The plasma levels of simvastatin, a CYP3A substrate, and its active metabolite are each increased about 2-fold in healthy subjects receiving simvastatin (80 mg once daily) and ranolazine (1000 mg twice daily). Dose adjustments of simvastatin are not required when ranolazine is co-administered with simvastatin).

No products indexed under this heading.

Busulfan (The plasma levels of simvastatin, a CYP3A substrate, and its active metabolite are each increased about 2-fold in healthy subjects receiving simvastatin (80 mg once daily) and ranolazine (1000 mg twice daily). Dose adjustments of simvastatin are not required when ranolazine is co-administered with simvastatin). Products include:

Captopril (Ranolazine or its metabolites partially inhibit CYP2D6. There are no studies of concomitant use of ranolazine with other drugs metabolized by CYP2D6, such as tricyclic antidepressants and antipsychotics, but lower doses of CYP2D6 substrates may be required). Products include:

Carbamazepine (Avoid co-administration of ranolazine and CYP3A inducers, such as rifampin, rifabutin, rifapentin, phenobarbital, phenytoin, carbamazepine, and St. John's wort. Rifampin (600 mg once daily) decreases the plasma concentration of ranolazine (1000 mg twice daily) by approximately 95% by induction of CYP3A and, probably, P-gp). Products include:

Carvedilol (Ranolazine or its metabolites partially inhibit CYP2D6. There are no studies of concomitant use of ranolazine with other drugs metabolized by CYP2D6, such as tricyclic antidepressants and antipsychotics, but lower doses of CYP2D6 substrates may be required). Products include:

Carvedilol Phosphate (Down-titrate ranozaline based on clinical response in patients concomitantly treated with P-gp inhibitors, such as cyclosporine). Products include:

Celecoxib (The potent CYP2D6 inhibitor, paroxetine (20 mg once daily), increases ranolazine concentrations 1.2-fold. No dose adjustment of ranolazine is required in patients treated with CYP2D6 inhibitors). Products include:

Cerivastatin Sodium (The plasma levels of simvastatin, a CYP3A substrate, and its active metabolite are each increased about 2-fold in healthy subjects receiving simvastatin (80 mg once daily) and ranolazine (1000 mg twice daily). Dose adjustments of simvastatin are not required when ranolazine is co-administered with simvastatin).

No products indexed under this heading.

Cevimeline Hydrochloride (Ranolazine or its metabolites partially inhibit CYP2D6. There are no studies of concomitant use of ranolazine with other drugs metabolized by CYP2D6, such as tricyclic antidepressants and antipsychotics, but lower doses of CYP2D6 substrates may be required). Products include:

Chloroquine (The potent CYP2D6 inhibitor, paroxetine (20 mg once daily), increases ranolazine concentrations 1.2-fold. No dose adjustment of ranolazine is required in patients treated with CYP2D6 inhibitors).

No products indexed under this heading.

Chloroquine Hydrochloride (The potent CYP2D6 inhibitor, paroxetine (20 mg once daily), increases ranolazine concentrations 1.2-fold. No dose adjustment of ranolazine is required in patients treated with CYP2D6 inhibitors).

No products indexed under this heading.

Chloroquine Phosphate (The potent CYP2D6 inhibitor, paroxetine (20 mg once daily), increases ranolazine concentrations 1.2-fold. No dose adjustment of ranolazine is required in patients treated with CYP2D6 inhibitors).

No products indexed under this heading.

Chlorpheniramine (The potent CYP2D6 inhibitor, paroxetine (20 mg once daily), increases ranolazine concentrations 1.2-fold. No dose adjustment of ranolazine is required in patients treated with CYP2D6 inhibitors).

No products indexed under this heading.

Chlorpheniramine Maleate (The potent CYP2D6 inhibitor, paroxetine (20 mg once daily), increases ranolazine concentrations 1.2-fold. No dose adjustment of ranolazine is required in patients treated with CYP2D6 inhibitors).

No products indexed under this heading.

Chlorpheniramine Polistirex (The potent CYP2D6 inhibitor, paroxetine (20 mg once daily), increases ranolazine concentrations 1.2-fold. No dose adjustment of ranolazine is required in patients treated with CYP2D6 inhibitors). Products include:

Chlorpheniramine Tannate (The potent CYP2D6 inhibitor, paroxetine (20 mg once daily), increases ranolazine concentrations 1.2-fold. No dose adjustment of ranolazine is required in patients treated with CYP2D6 inhibitors).

No products indexed under this heading.

Chlorpromazine (Ranolazine can inhibit the activity of CYP2D6 and thus, the metabolism of drugs that are mainly metabolized by this enzyme (eg, some antipsychotics) may be impaired and exposure to these drugs increased. The dose of such drugs may have to be reduced when ranolazine is co-administered).

No products indexed under this heading.

Chlorpromazine Hydrochloride (Ranolazine can inhibit the activity of CYP2D6 and thus, the metabolism of drugs that are mainly metabolized by this enzyme (eg, some antipsychotics) may be impaired and exposure to these drugs increased. The dose of such drugs may have to be reduced when ranolazine is co-administered).

No products indexed under this heading.

Chlorpropamide (Ranolazine or its metabolites partially inhibit CYP2D6. There are no studies of concomitant use of ranolazine with other drugs metabolized by CYP2D6, such as tricyclic antidepressants and antipsychotics, but lower doses of CYP2D6 substrates may be required).

No products indexed under this heading.

Chlorprothixene (Ranolazine can inhibit the activity of CYP2D6 and thus, the metabolism of drugs that are mainly metabolized by this enzyme (eg, some antipsychotics) may be impaired and exposure to these drugs increased. The dose of such drugs may have to be reduced when ranolazine is co-administered).

No products indexed under this heading.

Chlorprothixene Hydrochloride (Ranolazine can inhibit the activity of CYP2D6 and thus, the metabolism of drugs that are mainly metabolized by this enzyme (eg, some antipsychotics) may be impaired and exposure to these drugs increased. The dose of such drugs may have to be reduced when ranolazine is co-administered).

No products indexed under this heading.

Chlorprothixene Lactate (Ranolazine can inhibit the activity of CYP2D6 and thus, the metabolism of drugs that are mainly metabolized by this enzyme (eg, some antipsychotics) may be impaired and exposure to these drugs increased. The dose of such drugs may have to be reduced when ranolazine is co-administered).

No products indexed under this heading.

Cilostazol (The plasma levels of simvastatin, a CYP3A substrate, and its active metabolite are each increased about 2-fold in healthy subjects receiving simvastatin (80 mg once daily) and ranolazine (1000 mg twice daily). Dose adjustments of simvastatin are not required when ranolazine is co-administered with simvastatin).

No products indexed under this heading.

Cimetidine (Concurrent administration of ranolazine and CYP3A inhibitors is contraindicated. Do not use ranolazine with strong CYP3A inhibitors, including ketoconazole, itraconazole, clarithromycin, nefazodone, nelfinavir, ritonavir, indinavir, and saquinavir. Limit the dose of ranolazine to 500 mg twice daily in patients on moderate CYP3A inhibitors, including diltiazem, verapamil, aprepitant, erythromycin, fluconazole, and grapefruit juice or grapefruit-containing products. Weak CYP3A inhibitors such as simvastatin (20 mg once daily) and cimetidine (400 mg three times daily) do not increase the exposure to ranolazine in healthy volunteers).

No products indexed under this heading.

Cimetidine Hydrochloride (Concurrent administration of ranolazine and CYP3A inhibitors is contraindicated. Do not use ranolazine with strong CYP3A inhibitors, including ketoconazole, itraconazole, clarithromycin, nefazodone, nelfinavir, ritonavir, indinavir, and saquinavir. Limit the dose of ranolazine to 500 mg twice daily in patients on moderate CYP3A inhibitors, including diltiazem, verapamil, aprepitant, erythromycin, fluconazole, and grapefruit juice or grapefruit-containing products. Weak CYP3A inhibitors such as simvastatin (20 mg once daily) and cimetidine

---

IMPORTANT NOTE: Always consult each drug listing in the patient's regimen for possible interactions.

(400 mg three times daily) do not increase the exposure to ranolazine in healthy volunteers).
No products indexed under this heading.

Ciprofloxacin (Concurrent administration of ranolazine and CYP3A inhibitors is contraindicated. Do not use ranolazine with strong CYP3A inhibitors, including ketoconazole, itraconazole, clarithromycin, nefazodone, nelfinavir, ritonavir, indinavir, and saquinavir. Limit the dose of ranolazine to 500 mg twice daily in patients on moderate CYP3A inhibitors, including diltiazem, verapamil, aprepitant, erythromycin, fluconazole, and grapefruit juice or grapefruit-containing products. Weak CYP3A inhibitors such as simvastatin (20 mg once daily) and cimetidine (400 mg three times daily) do not increase the exposure to ranolazine in healthy volunteers). Products include:
Cipro I.V. 3082
Cipro 3073
Cipro XR 3091
Ciprodex 583

Ciprofloxacin Hydrochloride (Concurrent administration of ranolazine and CYP3A inhibitors is contraindicated. Do not use ranolazine with strong CYP3A inhibitors, including ketoconazole, itraconazole, clarithromycin, nefazodone, nelfinavir, ritonavir, indinavir, and saquinavir. Limit the dose of ranolazine to 500 mg twice daily in patients on moderate CYP3A inhibitors, including diltiazem, verapamil, aprepitant, erythromycin, fluconazole, and grapefruit juice or grapefruit-containing products. Weak CYP3A inhibitors such as simvastatin (20 mg once daily) and cimetidine (400 mg three times daily) do not increase the exposure to ranolazine in healthy volunteers). Products include:
Cipro 3073

Cisapride (The plasma levels of simvastatin, a CYP3A substrate, and its active metabolite are each increased about 2-fold in healthy subjects receiving simvastatin (80 mg once daily) and ranolazine (1000 mg twice daily). Dose adjustments of simvastatin are not required when ranolazine is co-administered with simvastatin).
No products indexed under this heading.

Citalopram Hydrobromide (The potent CYP2D6 inhibitor, paroxetine (20 mg once daily), increases ranolazine concentrations 1.2-fold. No dose adjustment of ranolazine is required in patients treated with CYP2D6 inhibitors). Products include:
Celexa 1153

Clarithromycin (Concurrent administration of ranolazine and CYP3A inhibitors is contraindicated. Do not use ranolazine with strong CYP3A inhibitors, including ketoconazole, itraconazole, clarithromycin, nefazodone, nelfinavir, ritonavir, indinavir, and saquinavir. Limit the dose of ranolazine to 500 mg twice daily in patients on moderate CYP3A inhibitors, including diltiazem, verapamil, aprepitant, erythromycin, fluconazole, and grapefruit juice or grapefruit-containing products. Weak CYP3A inhibitors such as simvastatin (20 mg once daily) and cimetidine (400 mg three times daily) do not increase the exposure to ranolazine in healthy volunteers). Products include:
Biaxin/Biaxin XL 412

Clomipramine Hydrochloride (The potent CYP2D6 inhibitor, paroxetine (20 mg once daily), increases ranolazine concentrations 1.2-fold. No dose adjustment of ranolazine is required in patients treated with CYP2D6 inhibitors).
No products indexed under this heading.

Clotrimazole (Avoid co-administration of ranolazine and CYP3A inducers, such as rifampin, rifabutin, rifapentin, phenobarbital, phenytoin, carbamazepine, and St. John's wort. Rifampin (600 mg once daily) decreases the plasma concentration of ranolazine (1000 mg twice daily) by approximately 95% by induction of CYP3A and, probably, P-gp). Products include:
Lotrisone 3163

Clotrimazole, Topical (Avoid co-administration of ranolazine and CYP3A inducers, such as rifampin, rifabutin, rifapentin, phenobarbital, phenytoin, carbamazepine, and St. John's wort. Rifampin (600 mg once daily) decreases the plasma concentration of ranolazine (1000 mg twice daily) by approximately 95% by induction of CYP3A and, probably, P-gp).
No products indexed under this heading.

Clozapine (Ranolazine can inhibit the activity of CYP2D6 and thus, the metabolism of drugs that are mainly metabolized by this enzyme (eg, some antipsychotics) may be impaired and exposure to these drugs increased. The dose of such drugs may have to be reduced when ranolazine is co-administered).
No products indexed under this heading.

Cocaine Hydrochloride (The potent CYP2D6 inhibitor, paroxetine (20 mg once daily), increases ranolazine concentrations 1.2-fold. No dose adjustment of ranolazine is required in patients treated with CYP2D6 inhibitors).
No products indexed under this heading.

Codeine Phosphate (Ranolazine or its metabolites partially inhibit CYP2D6. There are no studies of concomitant use of ranolazine with other drugs metabolized by CYP2D6, such as tricyclic antidepressants and antipsychotics, but lower doses of CYP2D6 substrates may be required). Products include:
Tylenol with Codeine 2691

Codeine Sulfate (Ranolazine or its metabolites partially inhibit CYP2D6. There are no studies of concomitant use of ranolazine with other drugs metabolized by CYP2D6, such as tricyclic antidepressants and antipsychotics, but lower doses of CYP2D6 substrates may be required).
No products indexed under this heading.

Cyclobenzaprine Hydrochloride (Ranolazine or its metabolites partially inhibit CYP2D6. There are no studies of concomitant use of ranolazine with other drugs metabolized by CYP2D6, such as tricyclic antidepressants and antipsychotics, but lower doses of CYP2D6 substrates may be required). Products include:
Amrix 964

Cyclosporine (Down-titrate ranolazine based on clinical response in patients concomitantly treated with P-gp inhibitors, such as cyclosporine). Products include:
Gengraf 440
Neoral Oral Solution 2496
Neoral Capsules 2496
Restasis 605

Debrisoquine (Ranolazine or its metabolites partially inhibit CYP2D6. There are no studies of concomitant use of ranolazine with other drugs metabolized by CYP2D6, such as tricyclic antidepressants and antipsychotics, but lower doses of CYP2D6 substrates may be required).
No products indexed under this heading.

Delavirdine Mesylate (Concurrent administration of ranolazine and CYP3A inhibitors is contraindicated. Do not use ranolazine with strong CYP3A inhibitors, including ketoconazole, itraconazole, clarithromycin, nefazodone, nelfinavir, ritonavir, indinavir, and saquinavir. Limit the dose of ranolazine to 500 mg twice daily in patients on moderate CYP3A inhibitors, including diltiazem, verapamil, aprepitant, erythromycin, fluconazole, and grapefruit juice or grapefruit-containing products. Weak CYP3A inhibitors such as simvastatin (20 mg once daily) and cimetidine (400 mg three times daily) do not increase the exposure to ranolazine in healthy volunteers).
No products indexed under this heading.

Desipramine Hydrochloride (The potent CYP2D6 inhibitor, paroxetine (20 mg once daily), increases ranolazine concentrations 1.2-fold. No dose adjustment of ranolazine is required in patients treated with CYP2D6 inhibitors).
No products indexed under this heading.

Desogestrel (The plasma levels of simvastatin, a CYP3A substrate, and its active metabolite are each increased about 2-fold in healthy subjects receiving simvastatin (80 mg once daily) and ranolazine (1000 mg twice daily). Dose adjustments of simvastatin are not required when ranolazine is co-administered with simvastatin).
No products indexed under this heading.

Dexamethasone (Avoid co-administration of ranolazine and CYP3A inducers, such as rifampin, rifabutin, rifapentin, phenobarbital, phenytoin, carbamazepine, and St. John's wort. Rifampin (600 mg once daily) decreases the plasma concentration of ranolazine (1000 mg twice daily) by approximately 95% by induction of CYP3A and, probably, P-gp). Products include:
Ciprodex 583
Ozurdex .... ⊙ 223
Tobramycin and Dexamethasone Ophthalmic Suspension .... ⊙ 251

Dexamethasone Acetate (The plasma levels of simvastatin, a CYP3A substrate, and its active metabolite are each increased about 2-fold in healthy subjects receiving simvastatin (80 mg once daily) and ranolazine (1000 mg twice daily). Dose adjustments of simvastatin are not required when ranolazine is co-administered with simvastatin).
No products indexed under this heading.

Dexamethasone Phosphate (The plasma levels of simvastatin, a CYP3A substrate, and its active metabolite are each increased about 2-fold in healthy subjects receiving simvastatin (80 mg once daily) and ranolazine (1000 mg twice daily). Dose adjustments of simvastatin are not required when ranolazine is co-administered with simvastatin).
No products indexed under this heading.

Dexamethasone Sodium (The plasma levels of simvastatin, a CYP3A substrate, and its active metabolite are each increased about 2-fold in healthy subjects receiving simvastatin (80 mg once daily) and ranolazine (1000 mg twice daily). Dose adjustments of simvastatin are not required when ranolazine is co-administered with simvastatin).
No products indexed under this heading.

Dexamethasone Sodium Phosphate (The plasma levels of simvastatin, a CYP3A substrate, and its active metabolite are each increased about 2-fold in healthy subjects receiving simvastatin (80 mg once daily) and ranolazine (1000 mg twice daily). Dose adjustments of simvastatin are not required when ranolazine is co-administered with simvastatin).
No products indexed under this heading.

Dexfenfluramine Hydrochloride (Ranolazine or its metabolites partially inhibit CYP2D6. There are no studies of concomitant use of ranolazine with other drugs metabolized by CYP2D6, such as tricyclic antidepressants and antipsychotics, but lower doses of CYP2D6 substrates may be required).
No products indexed under this heading.

Dextromethorphan Hydrobromide (Ranolazine or its metabolites partially inhibit CYP2D6. There are no studies of concomitant use of ranolazine with other drugs metabolized by CYP2D6, such as tricyclic antidepressants and antipsychotics, but lower doses of CYP2D6 substrates may be required).
No products indexed under this heading.

Dextromethorphan Polistirex (Ranolazine or its metabolites partially inhibit CYP2D6. There are no studies of concomitant use of ranolazine with other drugs metabolized by CYP2D6, such as tricyclic antidepressants and antipsychotics, but lower doses of CYP2D6 substrates may be required).
No products indexed under this heading.

Diazepam (The plasma levels of simvastatin, a CYP3A substrate, and its active metabolite are each increased about 2-fold in healthy subjects receiving simvastatin (80 mg once daily) and ranolazine (1000 mg twice daily). Dose adjustments of simvastatin are not required when ranolazine is co-administered with simvastatin). Products include:
Valium Tablets 2880

Digoxin (Co-administration of ranolazine and digoxin causes 1.5-fold elevation of digoxin plasma concentrations. The dose of digoxin may have to be adjusted when ranolazine is co-administered with digoxin). Products include:
Lanoxin Injection 1546
Lanoxin Injection Pediatric 1549
Lanoxin Tablets 1553

Dihydroergotamine Mesylate (The plasma levels of simvastatin, a CYP3A substrate, and its active metabolite are each increased about 2-fold in healthy subjects receiving simvastatin (80 mg once daily) and ranolazine (1000 mg twice daily). Dose adjustments of simvastatin are not required when ranolazine is co-administered with simvastatin).
No products indexed under this heading.

Diltiazem Hydrochloride (Concurrent administration of ranolazine and CYP3A inhibitors is contraindicated. Do not use ranolazine with strong CYP3A inhibitors, including ketoconazole, itraconazole, clarithromycin, nefazodone, nelfinavir, ritonavir, indinavir, and saquinavir. Limit the dose of ranolazine to 500 mg twice daily in patients on moderate CYP3A inhibitors, including diltiazem, verapamil, aprepitant, erythromycin, fluconazole, and grapefruit juice or grapefruit-containing products. Weak CYP3A inhibitors such as simvastatin (20 mg once daily) and cimetidine (400 mg three times daily) do not increase the exposure to ranolazine in healthy volunteers). Products include:
Cardizem LA 423

Diltiazem Maleate (Concurrent administration of ranolazine and CYP3A inhibitors is contraindicated. Do not use ranolazine with strong CYP3A inhibitors, including ketoconazole, itraconazole, clarithromycin, nefazodone, nelfinavir, ritonavir, indinavir, and saquinavir. Limit the dose of ranolazine to 500 mg twice daily in patients on moderate CYP3A inhibitors, including diltiazem, verapamil, aprepitant, erythromycin, fluconazole, and grapefruit juice or grapefruit-containing products. Weak CYP3A inhibitors such as simvastatin (20 mg once daily) and cimetidine (400 mg three times daily) do not increase the exposure to ranolazine in healthy volunteers).
No products indexed under this heading.

(⊙ Described in PDR® for Ophthalmic Medicines)

1551 Interactions Index Ranexa

Diphenhydramine (The potent CYP2D6 inhibitor, paroxetine (20 mg once daily), increases ranolazine concentrations 1.2-fold. No dose adjustment of ranolazine is required in patients treated with CYP2D6 inhibitors).
No products indexed under this heading.

Diphenhydramine Hydrochloride (The potent CYP2D6 inhibitor, paroxetine (20 mg once daily), increases ranolazine concentrations 1.2-fold. No dose adjustment of ranolazine is required in patients treated with CYP2D6 inhibitors). Products include:
Benadryl Allergy Ultratab 2042
Children's Benadryl Allergy Liquid 2042

Dirithromycin (Down-titrate ranozaline based on clinical response in patients concomitantly treated with P-gp inhibitors, such as cyclosporine).
No products indexed under this heading.

Disopyramide (Because of possible additive effects on the QT interval, ranolazine should be avoided in patients receiving drugs that prolong the QTc interval, such as Class IA (eg, quinidine) and Class III (eg, dofetilide, sotalol) antiarrhythmics, and antipsychotics (eg, thioridazine, ziprasidone)).
No products indexed under this heading.

Disopyramide Phosphate (Because of possible additive effects on the QT interval, ranolazine should be avoided in patients receiving drugs that prolong the QTc interval, such as Class IA (eg, quinidine) and Class III (eg, dofetilide, sotalol) antiarrhythmics, and antipsychotics (eg, thioridazine, ziprasidone)).
No products indexed under this heading.

Dolasetron Mesylate (Ranolazine or its metabolites partially inhibit CYP2D6. There are no studies of concomitant use of ranolazine with other drugs metabolized by CYP2D6, such as tricyclic antidepressants and antipsychotics, but lower doses of CYP2D6 substrates may be required). Products include:
Anzemet Injection 2931
Anzemet Tablets 2934

Donepezil Hydrochloride (Ranolazine or its metabolites partially inhibit CYP2D6. There are no studies of concomitant use of ranolazine with other drugs metabolized by CYP2D6, such as tricyclic antidepressants and antipsychotics, but lower doses of CYP2D6 substrates may be required). Products include:
Aricept 1045
Aricept ODT 1045

Doxepin Hydrochloride (The potent CYP2D6 inhibitor, paroxetine (20 mg once daily), increases ranolazine concentrations 1.2-fold. No dose adjustment of ranolazine is required in patients treated with CYP2D6 inhibitors).
No products indexed under this heading.

Doxorubicin Hydrochloride (The plasma levels of simvastatin, a CYP3A substrate, and its active metabolite are each increased about 2-fold in healthy subjects receiving simvastatin (80 mg once daily) and ranolazine (1000 mg twice daily). Dose adjustments of simvastatin are not required when ranolazine is co-administered with simvastatin).
No products indexed under this heading.

Dronabinol (The plasma levels of simvastatin, a CYP3A substrate, and its active metabolite are each increased about 2-fold in healthy subjects receiving simvastatin (80 mg once daily) and ranolazine (1000 mg twice daily). Dose adjustments of simvastatin are not required when ranolazine is co-administered with simvastatin).
No products indexed under this heading.

Dyphylline (The plasma levels of simvastatin, a CYP3A substrate, and its active metabolite are each increased about 2-fold in healthy subjects receiving simvastatin (80 mg once daily) and ranolazine (1000 mg twice daily). Dose adjustments of simvastatin are not required when ranolazine is co-administered with simvastatin).
No products indexed under this heading.

Efavirenz (Concurrent administration of ranolazine and CYP3A inhibitors is contraindicated. Do not use ranolazine with strong CYP3A inhibitors, including ketoconazole, itraconazole, clarithromycin, nefazodone, nelfinavir, ritonavir, indinavir, and saquinavir. Limit the dose of ranolazine to 500 mg twice daily in patients on moderate CYP3A inhibitors, including diltiazem, verapamil, aprepitant, erythromycin, fluconazole, and grapefruit juice or grapefruit-containing products. Weak CYP3A inhibitors such as simvastatin (20 mg once daily) and cimetidine (400 mg three times daily) do not increase the exposure to ranolazine in healthy volunteers). Products include:
Atripla 906

Elacridar (Down-titrate ranozaline based on clinical response in patients concomitantly treated with P-gp inhibitors, such as cyclosporine).
No products indexed under this heading.

Encainide Hydrochloride (Ranolazine or its metabolites partially inhibit CYP2D6. There are no studies of concomitant use of ranolazine with other drugs metabolized by CYP2D6, such as tricyclic antidepressants and antipsychotics, but lower doses of CYP2D6 substrates may be required).
No products indexed under this heading.

Ergotamine Tartrate (The plasma levels of simvastatin, a CYP3A substrate, and its active metabolite are each increased about 2-fold in healthy subjects receiving simvastatin (80 mg once daily) and ranolazine (1000 mg twice daily). Dose adjustments of simvastatin are not required when ranolazine is co-administered with simvastatin).
No products indexed under this heading.

Erythromycin (Concurrent administration of ranolazine and CYP3A inhibitors is contraindicated. Do not use ranolazine with strong CYP3A inhibitors, including ketoconazole, itraconazole, clarithromycin, nefazodone, nelfinavir, ritonavir, indinavir, and saquinavir. Limit the dose of ranolazine to 500 mg twice daily in patients on moderate CYP3A inhibitors, including diltiazem, verapamil, aprepitant, erythromycin, fluconazole, and grapefruit juice or grapefruit-containing products. Weak CYP3A inhibitors such as simvastatin (20 mg once daily) and cimetidine (400 mg three times daily) do not increase the exposure to ranolazine in healthy volunteers).
No products indexed under this heading.

Erythromycin, Topical (Down-titrate ranozaline based on clinical response in patients concomitantly treated with P-gp inhibitors, such as cyclosporine).
No products indexed under this heading.

Erythromycin Estolate (Down-titrate ranozaline based on clinical response in patients concomitantly treated with P-gp inhibitors, such as cyclosporine).
No products indexed under this heading.

Erythromycin Ethylsuccinate (Down-titrate ranozaline based on clinical response in patients concomitantly treated with P-gp inhibitors, such as cyclosporine). Products include:
E.E.S. 437
EryPed 435

Erythromycin Gluceptate (Down-titrate ranozaline based on clinical response in patients concomitantly treated with P-gp inhibitors, such as cyclosporine).
No products indexed under this heading.

Erythromycin Lactobionate (Down-titrate ranozaline based on clinical response in patients concomitantly treated with P-gp inhibitors, such as cyclosporine).
No products indexed under this heading.

Erythromycin Stearate (Down-titrate ranozaline based on clinical response in patients concomitantly treated with P-gp inhibitors, such as cyclosporine).
No products indexed under this heading.

Escitalopram Oxalate (The potent CYP2D6 inhibitor, paroxetine (20 mg once daily), increases ranolazine concentrations 1.2-fold. No dose adjustment of ranolazine is required in patients treated with CYP2D6 inhibitors). Products include:
Lexapro Oral Suspension 1160
Lexapro Tablets 1160

Estrogen (The plasma levels of simvastatin, a CYP3A substrate, and its active metabolite are each increased about 2-fold in healthy subjects receiving simvastatin (80 mg once daily) and ranolazine (1000 mg twice daily). Dose adjustments of simvastatin are not required when ranolazine is co-administered with simvastatin).
No products indexed under this heading.

Estrogens, Conjugated (The plasma levels of simvastatin, a CYP3A substrate, and its active metabolite are each increased about 2-fold in healthy subjects receiving simvastatin (80 mg once daily) and ranolazine (1000 mg twice daily). Dose adjustments of simvastatin are not required when ranolazine is co-administered with simvastatin). Products include:
Premarin Intravenous 3528
Premarin Tablets 3533
Premarin Vaginal Cream 3540
Premphase 3549
Prempro 3549

Estrogens, Conjugated, Synthetic A (The plasma levels of simvastatin, a CYP3A substrate, and its active metabolite are each increased about 2-fold in healthy subjects receiving simvastatin (80 mg once daily) and ranolazine (1000 mg twice daily). Dose adjustments of simvastatin are not required when ranolazine is co-administered with simvastatin).
No products indexed under this heading.

Estrogens, Esterified (The plasma levels of simvastatin, a CYP3A substrate, and its active metabolite are each increased about 2-fold in healthy subjects receiving simvastatin (80 mg once daily) and ranolazine (1000 mg twice daily). Dose adjustments of simvastatin are not required when ranolazine is co-administered with simvastatin).
No products indexed under this heading.

Ethinyl Estradiol (The plasma levels of simvastatin, a CYP3A substrate, and its active metabolite are each increased about 2-fold in healthy subjects receiving simvastatin (80 mg once daily) and ranolazine (1000 mg twice daily). Dose adjustments of simvastatin are not required when ranolazine is co-administered with simvastatin). Products include:
LoSeasonique 3407
Lybrel 3514
NuvaRing 3181
Ortho Evra 2648
Ortho-Cyclen/Ortho Tri-Cyclen 2663
Ortho Tri-Cyclen Lo Tablets 2673
Seasonique 3418
Yaz 864

Ethosuximide (Avoid co-administration of ranolazine and CYP3A inducers, such as rifampin, rifabutin, rifapentin, phenobarbital, phenytoin, carbamazepine, and St. John's wort. Rifampin (600 mg once daily) decreases the plasma concentration of ranolazine (1000 mg twice daily) by approximately 95% by induction of CYP3A and, probably, P-gp).
No products indexed under this heading.

Ethynodiol Diacetate (The plasma levels of simvastatin, a CYP3A substrate, and its active metabolite are each increased about 2-fold in healthy subjects receiving simvastatin (80 mg once daily) and ranolazine (1000 mg twice daily). Dose adjustments of simvastatin are not required when ranolazine is co-administered with simvastatin).
No products indexed under this heading.

Etoposide (The plasma levels of simvastatin, a CYP3A substrate, and its active metabolite are each increased about 2-fold in healthy subjects receiving simvastatin (80 mg once daily) and ranolazine (1000 mg twice daily). Dose adjustments of simvastatin are not required when ranolazine is co-administered with simvastatin).
No products indexed under this heading.

Etoposide Phosphate (The plasma levels of simvastatin, a CYP3A substrate, and its active metabolite are each increased about 2-fold in healthy subjects receiving simvastatin (80 mg once daily) and ranolazine (1000 mg twice daily). Dose adjustments of simvastatin are not required when ranolazine is co-administered with simvastatin).
No products indexed under this heading.

Felodipine (The plasma levels of simvastatin, a CYP3A substrate, and its active metabolite are each increased about 2-fold in healthy subjects receiving simvastatin (80 mg once daily) and ranolazine (1000 mg twice daily). Dose adjustments of simvastatin are not required when ranolazine is co-administered with simvastatin).
No products indexed under this heading.

Fentanyl (Ranolazine or its metabolites partially inhibit CYP2D6. There are no studies of concomitant use of ranolazine with other drugs metabolized by CYP2D6, such as tricyclic antidepressants and antipsychotics, but lower doses of CYP2D6 substrates may be required). Products include:
Duragesic 2604
Fentanyl Transdermal System 2346
Onsolis 2054

Fentanyl Citrate (Ranolazine or its metabolites partially inhibit CYP2D6. There are no studies of concomitant use of ranolazine with other drugs metabolized by CYP2D6, such as tricyclic antidepressants and antipsychotics, but lower doses of CYP2D6 substrates may be required). Products include:
Fentora 966

Flecainide Acetate (Ranolazine or its metabolites partially inhibit CYP2D6. There are no studies of concomitant use of ranolazine with other drugs metabolized by CYP2D6, such as tricyclic antidepressants and antipsychotics, but lower doses of CYP2D6 substrates may be required).
No products indexed under this heading.

Fluconazole (Concurrent administration of ranolazine and CYP3A inhibitors is contraindicated. Do not use ranolazine with strong CYP3A inhibitors, including ketoconazole, itraconazole, clarithromycin, nefazodone, nelfinavir, ritonavir, indinavir, and saquinavir. Limit the dose of ranolazine to 500 mg twice daily in patients on moderate CYP3A inhibitors, including diltiazem, verapamil, aprepitant, erythromycin, fluconazole, and grapefruit juice or grapefruit-

containing products. Weak CYP3A inhibitors such as simvastatin (20 mg once daily) and cimetidine (400 mg three times daily) do not increase the exposure to ranolazine in healthy volunteers).
No products indexed under this heading.

Fluoxetine (Concurrent administration of ranolazine and CYP3A inhibitors is contraindicated. Do not use ranolazine with strong CYP3A inhibitors, including ketoconazole, itraconazole, clarithromycin, nefazodone, nelfinavir, ritonavir, indinavir, and saquinavir. Limit the dose of ranolazine to 500 mg twice daily in patients on moderate CYP3A inhibitors, including diltiazem, verapamil, aprepitant, erythromycin, fluconazole, and grapefruit juice or grapefruit-containing products. Weak CYP3A inhibitors such as simvastatin (20 mg once daily) and cimetidine (400 mg three times daily) do not increase the exposure to ranolazine in healthy volunteers).
No products indexed under this heading.

Fluoxetine Hydrochloride (Concurrent administration of ranolazine and CYP3A inhibitors is contraindicated. Do not use ranolazine with strong CYP3A inhibitors, including ketoconazole, itraconazole, clarithromycin, nefazodone, nelfinavir, ritonavir, indinavir, and saquinavir. Limit the dose of ranolazine to 500 mg twice daily in patients on moderate CYP3A inhibitors, including diltiazem, verapamil, aprepitant, erythromycin, fluconazole, and grapefruit juice or grapefruit-containing products. Weak CYP3A inhibitors such as simvastatin (20 mg once daily) and cimetidine (400 mg three times daily) do not increase the exposure to ranolazine in healthy volunteers). Products include:
Prozac Weekly 1941
Prozac Pulvules 1941
Symbyax 1965

Fluphenazine Decanoate (Ranolazine can inhibit the activity of CYP2D6 and thus, the metabolism of drugs that are mainly metabolized by this enzyme (eg, some antipsychotics) may be impaired and exposure to these drugs increased. The dose of such drugs may have to be reduced when ranolazine is co-administered).
No products indexed under this heading.

Fluphenazine Enanthate (Ranolazine can inhibit the activity of CYP2D6 and thus, the metabolism of drugs that are mainly metabolized by this enzyme (eg, some antipsychotics) may be impaired and exposure to these drugs increased. The dose of such drugs may have to be reduced when ranolazine is co-administered).
No products indexed under this heading.

Fluphenazine Hydrochloride (Ranolazine can inhibit the activity of CYP2D6 and thus, the metabolism of drugs that are mainly metabolized by this enzyme (eg, some antipsychotics) may be impaired and exposure to these drugs increased. The dose of such drugs may have to be reduced when ranolazine is co-administered).
No products indexed under this heading.

Fluvoxamine Maleate (Concurrent administration of ranolazine and CYP3A inhibitors is contraindicated. Do not use ranolazine with strong CYP3A inhibitors, including ketoconazole, itraconazole, clarithromycin, nefazodone, nelfinavir, ritonavir, indinavir, and saquinavir. Limit the dose of ranolazine to 500 mg twice daily in patients on moderate CYP3A inhibitors, including diltiazem, verapamil, aprepitant, erythromycin, fluconazole, and grapefruit juice or grapefruit-containing products. Weak CYP3A inhibitors such as simvastatin (20 mg once daily) and cimetidine (400 mg three times daily) do not increase the exposure to ranolazine in healthy volunteers).
No products indexed under this heading.

Formoterol Fumarate (Ranolazine or its metabolites partially inhibit CYP2D6. There are no studies of concomitant use of ranolazine with other drugs metabolized by CYP2D6, such as tricyclic antidepressants and antipsychotics, but lower doses of CYP2D6 substrates may be required). Products include:
Foradil 3121
Perforomist 3634

Fosamprenavir Calcium (Avoid co-administration of ranolazine and CYP3A inducers, such as rifampin, rifabutin, rifapentin, phenobarbital, phenytoin, carbamazepine, and St. John's wort. Rifampin (600 mg once daily) decreases the plasma concentration of ranolazine (1000 mg twice daily) by approximately 95% by induction of CYP3A and, probably, P-gp). Products include:
Lexiva Oral Suspension 1558
Lexiva 1558

Fosphenytoin (Co-administration of ranolazine and an inducer of P-gp (eg, phenytoin) should be avoided).
No products indexed under this heading.

Fosphenytoin Sodium (Co-administration of ranolazine and an inducer of P-gp (eg, phenytoin) should be avoided).
No products indexed under this heading.

Galantamine Hydrobromide (Ranolazine or its metabolites partially inhibit CYP2D6. There are no studies of concomitant use of ranolazine with other drugs metabolized by CYP2D6, such as tricyclic antidepressants and antipsychotics, but lower doses of CYP2D6 substrates may be required).
No products indexed under this heading.

Glyburide (The plasma levels of simvastatin, a CYP3A substrate, and its active metabolite are each increased about 2-fold in healthy subjects receiving simvastatin (80 mg once daily) and ranolazine (1000 mg twice daily). Dose adjustments of simvastatin are not required when ranolazine is co-administered with simvastatin).
No products indexed under this heading.

Halofantrine Hydrochloride (The potent CYP2D6 inhibitor, paroxetine (20 mg once daily), increases ranolazine concentrations 1.2-fold. No dose adjustment of ranolazine is required in patients treated with CYP2D6 inhibitors).
No products indexed under this heading.

Haloperidol (Ranolazine can inhibit the activity of CYP2D6 and thus, the metabolism of drugs that are mainly metabolized by this enzyme (eg, some antipsychotics) may be impaired and exposure to these drugs increased. The dose of such drugs may have to be reduced when ranolazine is co-administered).
No products indexed under this heading.

Haloperidol Decanoate (Ranolazine can inhibit the activity of CYP2D6 and thus, the metabolism of drugs that are mainly metabolized by this enzyme (eg, some antipsychotics) may be impaired and exposure to these drugs increased. The dose of such drugs may have to be reduced when ranolazine is co-administered).
No products indexed under this heading.

Haloperidol Lactate (Ranolazine can inhibit the activity of CYP2D6 and thus, the metabolism of drugs that are mainly metabolized by this enzyme (eg, some antipsychotics) may be impaired and exposure to these drugs increased. The dose of such drugs may have to be reduced when ranolazine is co-administered).
No products indexed under this heading.

Hydrocodone Bitartrate (Ranolazine or its metabolites partially inhibit CYP2D6. There are no studies of concomitant use of ranolazine with other drugs metabolized by CYP2D6, such as tricyclic antidepressants and antipsychotics, but lower doses of CYP2D6 substrates may be required). Products include:
Vicodin 560
Vicodin ES 561
Vicodin HP 563
Vicoprofen 564
Zydone 1138

Hydroxychloroquine Sulfate (The potent CYP2D6 inhibitor, paroxetine (20 mg once daily), increases ranolazine concentrations 1.2-fold. No dose adjustment of ranolazine is required in patients treated with CYP2D6 inhibitors).
No products indexed under this heading.

Hypericum (Avoid co-administration of ranolazine and CYP3A inducers, such as rifampin, rifabutin, rifapentin, phenobarbital, phenytoin, carbamazepine, and St. John's wort. Rifampin (600 mg once daily) decreases the plasma concentration of ranolazine (1000 mg twice daily) by approximately 95% by induction of CYP3A and, probably, P-gp).
No products indexed under this heading.

Hypericum Perforatum (Avoid co-administration of ranolazine and CYP3A inducers, such as rifampin, rifabutin, rifapentin, phenobarbital, phenytoin, carbamazepine, and St. John's wort. Rifampin (600 mg once daily) decreases the plasma concentration of ranolazine (1000 mg twice daily) by approximately 95% by induction of CYP3A and, probably, P-gp). Products include:
Traumeel 1800

Imatinib Mesylate (The potent CYP2D6 inhibitor, paroxetine (20 mg once daily), increases ranolazine concentrations 1.2-fold. No dose adjustment of ranolazine is required in patients treated with CYP2D6 inhibitors). Products include:
Gleevec 2477

Imipramine Hydrochloride (The potent CYP2D6 inhibitor, paroxetine (20 mg once daily), increases ranolazine concentrations 1.2-fold. No dose adjustment of ranolazine is required in patients treated with CYP2D6 inhibitors).
No products indexed under this heading.

Imipramine Pamoate (The potent CYP2D6 inhibitor, paroxetine (20 mg once daily), increases ranolazine concentrations 1.2-fold. No dose adjustment of ranolazine is required in patients treated with CYP2D6 inhibitors).
No products indexed under this heading.

Indinavir Sulfate (Concurrent administration of ranolazine and CYP3A inhibitors is contraindicated. Do not use ranolazine with strong CYP3A inhibitors, including ketoconazole, itraconazole, clarithromycin, nefazodone, nelfinavir, ritonavir, indinavir, and saquinavir. Limit the dose of ranolazine to 500 mg twice daily in patients on moderate CYP3A inhibitors, including diltiazem, verapamil, aprepitant, erythromycin, fluconazole, and grapefruit juice or grapefruit-containing products. Weak CYP3A inhibitors such as simvastatin (20 mg once daily) and cimetidine (400 mg three times daily) do not increase the exposure to ranolazine in healthy volunteers). Products include:
Crixivan 2113

Indoramin Hydrochloride (Ranolazine or its metabolites partially inhibit CYP2D6. There are no studies of concomitant use of ranolazine with other drugs metabolized by CYP2D6, such as tricyclic antidepressants and antipsychotics, but lower doses of CYP2D6 substrates may be required).
No products indexed under this heading.

Isoniazid (Concurrent administration of ranolazine and CYP3A inhibitors is contraindicated. Do not use ranolazine with strong CYP3A inhibitors, including ketoconazole, itraconazole, clarithromycin, nefazodone, nelfinavir, ritonavir, indinavir, and saquinavir. Limit the dose of ranolazine to 500 mg twice daily in patients on moderate CYP3A inhibitors, including diltiazem, verapamil, aprepitant, erythromycin, fluconazole, and grapefruit juice or grapefruit-containing products. Weak CYP3A inhibitors such as simvastatin (20 mg once daily) and cimetidine (400 mg three times daily) do not increase the exposure to ranolazine in healthy volunteers).
No products indexed under this heading.

Isradipine (The plasma levels of simvastatin, a CYP3A substrate, and its active metabolite are each increased about 2-fold in healthy subjects receiving simvastatin (80 mg once daily) and ranolazine (1000 mg twice daily). Dose adjustments of simvastatin are not required when ranolazine is co-administered with simvastatin). Products include:
DynaCirc CR 1432

Itraconazole (Concurrent administration of ranolazine and CYP3A inhibitors is contraindicated. Do not use ranolazine with strong CYP3A inhibitors, including ketoconazole, itraconazole, clarithromycin, nefazodone, nelfinavir, ritonavir, indinavir, and saquinavir. Limit the dose of ranolazine to 500 mg twice daily in patients on moderate CYP3A inhibitors, including diltiazem, verapamil, aprepitant, erythromycin, fluconazole, and grapefruit juice or grapefruit-containing products. Weak CYP3A inhibitors such as simvastatin (20 mg once daily) and cimetidine (400 mg three times daily) do not increase the exposure to ranolazine in healthy volunteers).
No products indexed under this heading.

Ketoconazole (Concomitant use of ranolazine with ketoconazole is contraindicated. As a potent inhibitor of CYP3A, ketoconazole (200 mg b.i.d.) increases average steady-state plasma concentrations of ranolazine 3.2-fold. Ranolazine should not be used during treatment with ketoconazole. Ranolazine is primarily metabolized by CYP3A. Use of ranolazine with potent or moderately potent inhibitors of CYP3A should be avoided because concomitant administration will increase ranolazine plasma levels and QTc prolongation). Products include:
Extina 3319
Xolegel 3337

Labetalol Hydrochloride (Ranolazine or its metabolites partially inhibit CYP2D6. There are no studies of concomitant use of ranolazine with other drugs metabolized by CYP2D6, such as tricyclic antidepressants and antipsychotics, but lower doses of CYP2D6 substrates may be required).
No products indexed under this heading.

Levonorgestrel (The plasma levels of simvastatin, a CYP3A substrate, and its active metabolite are each increased about 2-fold in healthy subjects receiving simvastatin (80 mg once daily) and ranolazine (1000 mg twice daily). Dose adjustments of simvastatin are not required when ranolazine is co-administered with simvastatin). Products include:

Climara Pro 847
LoSeasonique 3407
Lybrel 3514
Mirena 854
Plan B 3416
Seasonique 3418

Lidocaine (Ranolazine or its metabolites partially inhibit CYP2D6. There are no studies of concomitant use of ranolazine with other drugs metabolized by CYP2D6, such as tricyclic antidepressants and antipsychotics, but lower doses of CYP2D6 substrates may be required). Products include:
Lidoderm 1107

Lidocaine Hydrochloride (Ranolazine or its metabolites partially inhibit CYP2D6. There are no studies of concomitant use of ranolazine with other drugs metabolized by CYP2D6, such as tricyclic antidepressants and antipsychotics, but lower doses of CYP2D6 substrates may be required).
No products indexed under this heading.

Lithium (Ranolazine can inhibit the activity of CYP2D6 and thus, the metabolism of drugs that are mainly metabolized by this enzyme (eg, some antipsychotics) may be impaired and exposure to these drugs increased. The dose of such drugs may have to be reduced when ranolazine is co-administered).
No products indexed under this heading.

Lithium Carbonate (Ranolazine can inhibit the activity of CYP2D6 and thus, the metabolism of drugs that are mainly metabolized by this enzyme (eg, some antipsychotics) may be impaired and exposure to these drugs increased. The dose of such drugs may have to be reduced when ranolazine is co-administered).
No products indexed under this heading.

Lithium Citrate (Ranolazine can inhibit the activity of CYP2D6 and thus, the metabolism of drugs that are mainly metabolized by this enzyme (eg, some antipsychotics) may be impaired and exposure to these drugs increased. The dose of such drugs may have to be reduced when ranolazine is co-administered).
No products indexed under this heading.

Lopinavir (Concurrent administration of ranolazine and CYP3A inhibitors is contraindicated. Do not use ranolazine with strong CYP3A inhibitors, including ketoconazole, itraconazole, clarithromycin, nefazodone, nelfinavir, ritonavir, indinavir, and saquinavir. Limit the dose of ranolazine to 500 mg twice daily in patients on moderate CYP3A inhibitors, including diltiazem, verapamil, aprepitant, erythromycin, fluconazole, and grapefruit juice or grapefruit-containing products. Weak CYP3A inhibitors such as simvastatin (20 mg once daily) and cimetidine (400 mg three times daily) do not increase the exposure to ranolazine in healthy volunteers). Products include:
Kaletra 458

Lovastatin (The plasma levels of simvastatin, a CYP3A substrate, and its active metabolite are each increased about 2-fold in healthy subjects receiving simvastatin (80 mg once daily) and ranolazine (1000 mg twice daily). Dose adjustments of simvastatin are not required when ranolazine is co-administered with simvastatin).
Products include:
Advicor 402
Mevacor 2212

Loxapine Hydrochloride (Ranolazine can inhibit the activity of CYP2D6 and thus, the metabolism of drugs that are mainly metabolized by this enzyme (eg, some antipsychotics) may be impaired and exposure to these drugs increased. The dose of such drugs may have to be reduced when ranolazine is co-administered).
No products indexed under this heading.

Loxapine Succinate (Ranolazine can inhibit the activity of CYP2D6 and thus, the metabolism of drugs that are mainly metabolized by this enzyme (eg, some antipsychotics) may be impaired and exposure to these drugs increased. The dose of such drugs may have to be reduced when ranolazine is co-administered).
No products indexed under this heading.

Maprotiline Hydrochloride (The potent CYP2D6 inhibitor, paroxetine (20 mg once daily), increases ranolazine concentrations 1.2-fold. No dose adjustment of ranolazine is required in patients treated with CYP2D6 inhibitors).
No products indexed under this heading.

Meperidine Hydrochloride (Ranolazine or its metabolites partially inhibit CYP2D6. There are no studies of concomitant use of ranolazine with other drugs metabolized by CYP2D6, such as tricyclic antidepressants and antipsychotics, but lower doses of CYP2D6 substrates may be required).
No products indexed under this heading.

Mesoridazine Besylate (Ranolazine can inhibit the activity of CYP2D6 and thus, the metabolism of drugs that are mainly metabolized by this enzyme (eg, some antipsychotics) may be impaired and exposure to these drugs increased. The dose of such drugs may have to be reduced when ranolazine is co-administered).
No products indexed under this heading.

Mestranol (The plasma levels of simvastatin, a CYP3A substrate, and its active metabolite are each increased about 2-fold in healthy subjects receiving simvastatin (80 mg once daily) and ranolazine (1000 mg twice daily). Dose adjustments of simvastatin are not required when ranolazine is co-administered with simvastatin).
No products indexed under this heading.

Methadone Hydrochloride (The potent CYP2D6 inhibitor, paroxetine (20 mg once daily), increases ranolazine concentrations 1.2-fold. No dose adjustment of ranolazine is required in patients treated with CYP2D6 inhibitors).
No products indexed under this heading.

Methamphetamine Hydrochloride (Ranolazine or its metabolites partially inhibit CYP2D6. There are no studies of concomitant use of ranolazine with other drugs metabolized by CYP2D6, such as tricyclic antidepressants and antipsychotics, but lower doses of CYP2D6 substrates may be required).
No products indexed under this heading.

Methotrimeprazine (Ranolazine can inhibit the activity of CYP2D6 and thus, the metabolism of drugs that are mainly metabolized by this enzyme (eg, some antipsychotics) may be impaired and exposure to these drugs increased. The dose of such drugs may have to be reduced when ranolazine is co-administered).
No products indexed under this heading.

Methoxyphenamine (Ranolazine or its metabolites partially inhibit CYP2D6. There are no studies of concomitant use of ranolazine with other drugs metabolized by CYP2D6, such as tricyclic antidepressants and antipsychotics, but lower doses of CYP2D6 substrates may be required).
No products indexed under this heading.

Methylprednisolone (The plasma levels of simvastatin, a CYP3A substrate, and its active metabolite are each increased about 2-fold in healthy subjects receiving simvastatin (80 mg once daily) and ranolazine (1000 mg twice daily). Dose adjustments of simvastatin are not required when ranolazine is co-administered with simvastatin).
No products indexed under this heading.

Methylprednisolone Acetate (The plasma levels of simvastatin, a CYP3A substrate, and its active metabolite are each increased about 2-fold in healthy subjects receiving simvastatin (80 mg once daily) and ranolazine (1000 mg twice daily). Dose adjustments of simvastatin are not required when ranolazine is co-administered with simvastatin).
No products indexed under this heading.

Methylprednisolone Sodium Succinate (The plasma levels of simvastatin, a CYP3A substrate, and its active metabolite are each increased about 2-fold in healthy subjects receiving simvastatin (80 mg once daily) and ranolazine (1000 mg twice daily). Dose adjustments of simvastatin are not required when ranolazine is co-administered with simvastatin).
No products indexed under this heading.

Metoprolol Succinate (Ranolazine or its metabolites partially inhibit CYP2D6. There are no studies of concomitant use of ranolazine with other drugs metabolized by CYP2D6, such as tricyclic antidepressants and antipsychotics, but lower doses of CYP2D6 substrates may be required). Products include:
Toprol XL 732

Metoprolol Tartrate (Ranolazine or its metabolites partially inhibit CYP2D6. There are no studies of concomitant use of ranolazine with other drugs metabolized by CYP2D6, such as tricyclic antidepressants and antipsychotics, but lower doses of CYP2D6 substrates may be required).
No products indexed under this heading.

Metronidazole (Concurrent administration of ranolazine and CYP3A inhibitors is contraindicated. Do not use ranolazine with strong CYP3A inhibitors, including ketoconazole, itraconazole, clarithromycin, nefazodone, nelfinavir, ritonavir, indinavir, and saquinavir. Limit the dose of ranolazine to 500 mg twice daily in patients on moderate CYP3A inhibitors, including diltiazem, verapamil, aprepitant, erythromycin, fluconazole, and grapefruit juice or grapefruit-containing products. Weak CYP3A inhibitors such as simvastatin (20 mg once daily) and cimetidine (400 mg three times daily) do not increase the exposure to ranolazine in healthy volunteers). Products include:
Pylera 793

Metronidazole Benzoate (Concurrent administration of ranolazine and CYP3A inhibitors is contraindicated. Do not use ranolazine with strong CYP3A inhibitors, including ketoconazole, itraconazole, clarithromycin, nefazodone, nelfinavir, ritonavir, indinavir, and saquinavir. Limit the dose of ranolazine to 500 mg twice daily in patients on moderate CYP3A inhibitors, including diltiazem, verapamil, aprepitant, erythromycin, fluconazole, and grapefruit juice or grapefruit-containing products. Weak CYP3A inhibitors such as simvastatin (20 mg once daily) and cimetidine (400 mg three times daily) do not increase the exposure to ranolazine in healthy volunteers).
No products indexed under this heading.

Metronidazole Hydrochloride (Concurrent administration of ranolazine and CYP3A inhibitors is contraindicated. Do not use ranolazine with strong CYP3A inhibitors, including ketoconazole, itraconazole, clarithromycin, nefazodone, nelfinavir, ritonavir, indinavir, and saquinavir. Limit the dose of ranolazine to 500 mg twice daily in patients on moderate CYP3A inhibitors, including diltiazem, verapamil, aprepitant, erythromycin, fluconazole, and grapefruit juice or grapefruit-containing products. Weak CYP3A inhibitors such as simvastatin (20 mg once daily) and cimetidine (400 mg three times daily) do not increase the exposure to ranolazine in healthy volunteers).
No products indexed under this heading.

Mexiletine Hydrochloride (Ranolazine or its metabolites partially inhibit CYP2D6. There are no studies of concomitant use of ranolazine with other drugs metabolized by CYP2D6, such as tricyclic antidepressants and antipsychotics, but lower doses of CYP2D6 substrates may be required).
No products indexed under this heading.

Mibefradil Dihydrochloride (The potent CYP2D6 inhibitor, paroxetine (20 mg once daily), increases ranolazine concentrations 1.2-fold. No dose adjustment of ranolazine is required in patients treated with CYP2D6 inhibitors).
No products indexed under this heading.

Miconazole (Concurrent administration of ranolazine and CYP3A inhibitors is contraindicated. Do not use ranolazine with strong CYP3A inhibitors, including ketoconazole, itraconazole, clarithromycin, nefazodone, nelfinavir, ritonavir, indinavir, and saquinavir. Limit the dose of ranolazine to 500 mg twice daily in patients on moderate CYP3A inhibitors, including diltiazem, verapamil, aprepitant, erythromycin, fluconazole, and grapefruit juice or grapefruit-containing products. Weak CYP3A inhibitors such as simvastatin (20 mg once daily) and cimetidine (400 mg three times daily) do not increase the exposure to ranolazine in healthy volunteers).
No products indexed under this heading.

Midazolam Hydrochloride (The plasma levels of simvastatin, a CYP3A substrate, and its active metabolite are each increased about 2-fold in healthy subjects receiving simvastatin (80 mg once daily) and ranolazine (1000 mg twice daily). Dose adjustments of simvastatin are not required when ranolazine is co-administered with simvastatin).
No products indexed under this heading.

Mirtazapine (Ranolazine or its metabolites partially inhibit CYP2D6. There are no studies of concomitant use of ranolazine with other drugs metabolized by CYP2D6, such as tricyclic antidepressants and antipsychotics, but lower doses of CYP2D6 substrates may be required). Products include:
Remeron Tablets 3214
RemeronSolTab Tablets 3219

Moclobemide (The potent CYP2D6 inhibitor, paroxetine (20 mg once daily), increases ranolazine concentrations 1.2-fold. No dose adjustment of ranolazine is required in patients treated with CYP2D6 inhibitors).
No products indexed under this heading.

Modafinil (Avoid co-administration of ranolazine and CYP3A inducers, such as rifampin, rifabutin, rifapentin, phenobarbital, phenytoin, carbamazepine, and St. John's wort. Rifampin (600 mg once daily) decreases the plasma concentra-

tion of ranolazine (1000 mg twice daily) by approximately 95% by induction of CYP3A and, probably, P-gp). Products include:

Provigil 983

Molindone Hydrochloride (Ranolazine can inhibit the activity of CYP2D6 and thus, the metabolism of drugs that are mainly metabolized by this enzyme (eg, some antipsychotics) may be impaired and exposure to these drugs increased. The dose of such drugs may have to be reduced when ranolazine is co-administered). Products include:

Moban 1108

Moricizine Hydrochloride (Because of possible additive effects on the QT interval, ranolazine should be avoided in patients receiving drugs that prolong the QTc interval, such as Class IA (eg, quinidine) and Class III (eg, dofetilide, sotalol) antiarrhythmics, and antipsychotics (eg, thioridazine, ziprasidone)).

No products indexed under this heading.

Morphine Sulfate (Ranolazine or its metabolites partially inhibit CYP2D6. There are no studies of concomitant use of ranolazine with other drugs metabolized by CYP2D6, such as tricyclic antidepressants and antipsychotics, but lower doses of CYP2D6 substrates may be required). Products include:

Avinza 1822
Embeda 1831
MS Contin 2803

Nefazodone Hydrochloride (Concurrent administration of ranolazine and CYP3A inhibitors is contraindicated. Do not use ranolazine with strong CYP3A inhibitors, including ketoconazole, itraconazole, clarithromycin, nefazodone, nelfinavir, ritonavir, indinavir, and saquinavir. Limit the dose of ranolazine to 500 mg twice daily in patients on moderate CYP3A inhibitors, including diltiazem, verapamil, aprepitant, erythromycin, fluconazole, and grapefruit juice or grapefruit-containing products. Weak CYP3A inhibitors such as simvastatin (20 mg once daily) and cimetidine (400 mg three times daily) do not increase the exposure to ranolazine in healthy volunteers).

No products indexed under this heading.

Nelfinavir Mesylate (Concurrent administration of ranolazine and CYP3A inhibitors is contraindicated. Do not use ranolazine with strong CYP3A inhibitors, including ketoconazole, itraconazole, clarithromycin, nefazodone, nelfinavir, ritonavir, indinavir, and saquinavir. Limit the dose of ranolazine to 500 mg twice daily in patients on moderate CYP3A inhibitors, including diltiazem, verapamil, aprepitant, erythromycin, fluconazole, and grapefruit juice or grapefruit-containing products. Weak CYP3A inhibitors such as simvastatin (20 mg once daily) and cimetidine (400 mg three times daily) do not increase the exposure to ranolazine in healthy volunteers).

No products indexed under this heading.

Nevirapine (Avoid co-administration of ranolazine and CYP3A inducers, such as rifampin, rifabutin, rifapentin, phenobarbital, phenytoin, carbamazepine, and St. John's wort. Rifampin (600 mg once daily) decreases the plasma concentration of ranolazine (1000 mg twice daily) by approximately 95% by induction of CYP3A and, probably, P-gp). Products include:

Viramune Oral Suspension 897
Viramune Tablets 897

Nicardipine (The plasma levels of simvastatin, a CYP3A substrate, and its active metabolite are each increased about 2-fold in healthy subjects receiving simvastatin (80 mg once daily) and ranolazine (1000 mg twice daily). Dose adjustments of simvastatin are not required when ranolazine is co-administered with simvastatin).

No products indexed under this heading.

Nicardipine Hydrochloride (The plasma levels of simvastatin, a CYP3A substrate, and its active metabolite are each increased about 2-fold in healthy subjects receiving simvastatin (80 mg once daily) and ranolazine (1000 mg twice daily). Dose adjustments of simvastatin are not required when ranolazine is co-administered with simvastatin).

No products indexed under this heading.

Nifedipine (Concurrent administration of ranolazine and CYP3A inhibitors is contraindicated. Do not use ranolazine with strong CYP3A inhibitors, including ketoconazole, itraconazole, clarithromycin, nefazodone, nelfinavir, ritonavir, indinavir, and saquinavir. Limit the dose of ranolazine to 500 mg twice daily in patients on moderate CYP3A inhibitors, including diltiazem, verapamil, aprepitant, erythromycin, fluconazole, and grapefruit juice or grapefruit-containing products. Weak CYP3A inhibitors such as simvastatin (20 mg once daily) and cimetidine (400 mg three times daily) do not increase the exposure to ranolazine in healthy volunteers).

No products indexed under this heading.

Nimodipine (The plasma levels of simvastatin, a CYP3A substrate, and its active metabolite are each increased about 2-fold in healthy subjects receiving simvastatin (80 mg once daily) and ranolazine (1000 mg twice daily). Dose adjustments of simvastatin are not required when ranolazine is co-administered with simvastatin).

No products indexed under this heading.

Nisoldipine (The plasma levels of simvastatin, a CYP3A substrate, and its active metabolite are each increased about 2-fold in healthy subjects receiving simvastatin (80 mg once daily) and ranolazine (1000 mg twice daily). Dose adjustments of simvastatin are not required when ranolazine is co-administered with simvastatin).

No products indexed under this heading.

Norethindrone (The plasma levels of simvastatin, a CYP3A substrate, and its active metabolite are each increased about 2-fold in healthy subjects receiving simvastatin (80 mg once daily) and ranolazine (1000 mg twice daily). Dose adjustments of simvastatin are not required when ranolazine is co-administered with simvastatin). Products include:

Ortho Micronor 2660

Norfloxacin (Concurrent administration of ranolazine and CYP3A inhibitors is contraindicated. Do not use ranolazine with strong CYP3A inhibitors, including ketoconazole, itraconazole, clarithromycin, nefazodone, nelfinavir, ritonavir, indinavir, and saquinavir. Limit the dose of ranolazine to 500 mg twice daily in patients on moderate CYP3A inhibitors, including diltiazem, verapamil, aprepitant, erythromycin, fluconazole, and grapefruit juice or grapefruit-containing products. Weak CYP3A inhibitors such as simvastatin (20 mg once daily) and cimetidine (400 mg three times daily) do not increase the exposure to ranolazine in healthy volunteers). Products include:

Noroxin 2220

Norgestrel (The plasma levels of simvastatin, a CYP3A substrate, and its active metabolite are each increased about 2-fold in healthy subjects receiving simvastatin (80 mg once daily) and ranolazine (1000 mg twice daily). Dose adjustments of simvastatin are not required when ranolazine is co-administered with simvastatin).

No products indexed under this heading.

Nortriptyline Hydrochloride (The potent CYP2D6 inhibitor, paroxetine (20 mg once daily), increases ranolazine concentrations 1.2-fold. No dose adjustment of ranolazine is required in patients treated with CYP2D6 inhibitors).

No products indexed under this heading.

Olanzapine (Ranolazine can inhibit the activity of CYP2D6 and thus, the metabolism of drugs that are mainly metabolized by this enzyme (eg, some antipsychotics) may be impaired and exposure to these drugs increased. The dose of such drugs may have to be reduced when ranolazine is co-administered). Products include:

Symbyax 1965
Zyprexa 1984
Zyprexa IntraMuscular 1984
Zyprexa ZYDIS 1984

Omeprazole (Ranolazine or its metabolites partially inhibit CYP2D6. There are no studies of concomitant use of ranolazine with other drugs metabolized by CYP2D6, such as tricyclic antidepressants and antipsychotics, but lower doses of CYP2D6 substrates may be required).

No products indexed under this heading.

Ondansetron (Ranolazine or its metabolites partially inhibit CYP2D6. There are no studies of concomitant use of ranolazine with other drugs metabolized by CYP2D6, such as tricyclic antidepressants and antipsychotics, but lower doses of CYP2D6 substrates may be required).

No products indexed under this heading.

Ondansetron Hydrochloride (Ranolazine or its metabolites partially inhibit CYP2D6. There are no studies of concomitant use of ranolazine with other drugs metabolized by CYP2D6, such as tricyclic antidepressants and antipsychotics, but lower doses of CYP2D6 substrates may be required). Products include:

Zofran Injection 1750
Zofran 1756
Zofran ODT 1756

Oxycodone Hydrochloride (Ranolazine or its metabolites partially inhibit CYP2D6. There are no studies of concomitant use of ranolazine with other drugs metabolized by CYP2D6, such as tricyclic antidepressants and antipsychotics, but lower doses of CYP2D6 substrates may be required). Products include:

OxyContin 2807
Percocet 1121
Percodan 1124

Paclitaxel (Ranolazine or its metabolites partially inhibit CYP2D6. There are no studies of concomitant use of ranolazine with other drugs metabolized by CYP2D6, such as tricyclic antidepressants and antipsychotics, but lower doses of CYP2D6 substrates may be required).

No products indexed under this heading.

Paliperidone (Ranolazine can inhibit the activity of CYP2D6 and thus, the metabolism of drugs that are mainly metabolized by this enzyme (eg, some antipsychotics) may be impaired and exposure to these drugs increased. The dose of such drugs may have to be reduced when ranolazine is co-administered). Products include:

Invega 2613
Invega Sustenna 2621

Paroxetine (Paroxetine, a potent inhibitor of CYP2D6, increased average steady-state plasma concentrations of ranolazine 1.2-fold. No dose adjustment of ranolazine is required in patients treated with paroxetine).

No products indexed under this heading.

Paroxetine Hydrochloride (Paroxetine, a potent inhibitor of CYP2D6, increased average steady-state plasma concentrations of ranolazine 1.2-fold. No dose adjustment of ranolazine is required in patients treated with paroxetine). Products include:

Paroxetine CR 2361
Paroxetine ER 2371
Paxil 1586
Paxil CR 1596

Paroxetine Mesylate (Paroxetine, a potent inhibitor of CYP2D6, increased average steady-state plasma concentrations of ranolazine 1.2-fold. No dose adjustment of ranolazine is required in patients treated with paroxetine).

No products indexed under this heading.

Perphenazine (Ranolazine can inhibit the activity of CYP2D6 and thus, the metabolism of drugs that are mainly metabolized by this enzyme (eg, some antipsychotics) may be impaired and exposure to these drugs increased. The dose of such drugs may have to be reduced when ranolazine is co-administered).

No products indexed under this heading.

Phenobarbital (Avoid co-administration of ranolazine and CYP3A inducers, such as rifampin, rifabutin, rifapentin, phenobarbital, phenytoin, carbamazepine, and St. John's wort. Rifampin (600 mg once daily) decreases the plasma concentration of ranolazine (1000 mg twice daily) by approximately 95% by induction of CYP3A and, probably, P-gp). Products include:

Donnatal 2711

Phenobarbital Sodium (Avoid co-administration of ranolazine and CYP3A inducers, such as rifampin, rifabutin, rifapentin, phenobarbital, phenytoin, carbamazepine, and St. John's wort. Rifampin (600 mg once daily) decreases the plasma concentration of ranolazine (1000 mg twice daily) by approximately 95% by induction of CYP3A and, probably, P-gp).

No products indexed under this heading.

Phenothiazine Derivatives (Avoid co-administration of ranolazine and CYP3A inducers, such as rifampin, rifabutin, rifapentin, phenobarbital, phenytoin, carbamazepine, and St. John's wort. Rifampin (600 mg once daily) decreases the plasma concentration of ranolazine (1000 mg twice daily) by approximately 95% by induction of CYP3A and, probably, P-gp).

No products indexed under this heading.

Phenothiazines (Avoid co-administration of ranolazine and CYP3A inducers, such as rifampin, rifabutin, rifapentin, phenobarbital, phenytoin, carbamazepine, and St. John's wort. Rifampin (600 mg once daily) decreases the plasma concentration of ranolazine (1000 mg twice daily) by approximately 95% by induction of CYP3A and, probably, P-gp).

No products indexed under this heading.

Phenytoin (Avoid co-administration of ranolazine and CYP3A inducers, such as rifampin, rifabutin, rifapentin, phenobarbital, phenytoin, carbamazepine, and St. John's wort. Rifampin (600 mg once daily) decreases the plasma concentration of ranolazine (1000 mg twice daily) by approximately 95% by induction of CYP3A and, probably, P-gp).

No products indexed under this heading.

1555 Interactions Index Ranexa

Phenytoin Sodium (Avoid co-administration of ranolazine and CYP3A inducers, such as rifampin, rifabutin, rifapentin, phenobarbital, phenytoin, carbamazepine, and St. John's wort. Rifampin (600 mg once daily) decreases the plasma concentration of ranolazine (1000 mg twice daily) by approximately 95% by induction of CYP3A and, probably, P-gp). Products include:
Phenytek Capsules 2380

Pimozide (Ranolazine can inhibit the activity of CYP2D6 and thus, the metabolism of drugs that are mainly metabolized by this enzyme (eg, some antipsychotics) may be impaired and exposure to these drugs increased. The dose of such drugs may have to be reduced when ranolazine is co-administered).
No products indexed under this heading.

Pindolol (Ranolazine or its metabolites partially inhibit CYP2D6. There are no studies of concomitant use of ranolazine with other drugs metabolized by CYP2D6, such as tricyclic antidepressants and antipsychotics, but lower doses of CYP2D6 substrates may be required).
No products indexed under this heading.

Procainamide (Because of possible additive effects on the QT interval, ranolazine should be avoided in patients receiving drugs that prolong the QTc interval, such as Class IA (eg, quinidine) and Class III (eg, dofetilide, sotalol) antiarrhythmics, and antipsychotics (eg, thioridazine, ziprasidone)).
No products indexed under this heading.

Prochlorperazine (Ranolazine can inhibit the activity of CYP2D6 and thus, the metabolism of drugs that are mainly metabolized by this enzyme (eg, some antipsychotics) may be impaired and exposure to these drugs increased. The dose of such drugs may have to be reduced when ranolazine is co-administered).
No products indexed under this heading.

Prochlorperazine Edisylate (Avoid co-administration of ranolazine and CYP3A inducers, such as rifampin, rifabutin, rifapentin, phenobarbital, phenytoin, carbamazepine, and St. John's wort. Rifampin (600 mg once daily) decreases the plasma concentration of ranolazine (1000 mg twice daily) by approximately 95% by induction of CYP3A and, probably, P-gp).
No products indexed under this heading.

Prochlorperazine Maleate (Avoid co-administration of ranolazine and CYP3A inducers, such as rifampin, rifabutin, rifapentin, phenobarbital, phenytoin, carbamazepine, and St. John's wort. Rifampin (600 mg once daily) decreases the plasma concentration of ranolazine (1000 mg twice daily) by approximately 95% by induction of CYP3A and, probably, P-gp).
No products indexed under this heading.

Promethazine (Avoid co-administration of ranolazine and CYP3A inducers, such as rifampin, rifabutin, rifapentin, phenobarbital, phenytoin, carbamazepine, and St. John's wort. Rifampin (600 mg once daily) decreases the plasma concentration of ranolazine (1000 mg twice daily) by approximately 95% by induction of CYP3A and, probably, P-gp).
No products indexed under this heading.

Promethazine Hydrochloride (Avoid co-administration of ranolazine and CYP3A inducers, such as rifampin, rifabutin, rifapentin, phenobarbital, phenytoin, carbamazepine, and St. John's wort. Rifampin (600 mg once daily) decreases the plasma concentration of ranolazine (1000 mg twice daily) by approximately 95% by induction of CYP3A and, probably, P-gp).
No products indexed under this heading.

Propafenone Hydrochloride (The potent CYP2D6 inhibitor, paroxetine (20 mg once daily), increases ranolazine concentrations 1.2-fold. No dose adjustment of ranolazine is required in patients treated with CYP2D6 inhibitors). Products include:
Rythmol 1648
Rythmol SR 1652

Propoxyphene Hydrochloride (The potent CYP2D6 inhibitor, paroxetine (20 mg once daily), increases ranolazine concentrations 1.2-fold. No dose adjustment of ranolazine is required in patients treated with CYP2D6 inhibitors).
No products indexed under this heading.

Propoxyphene Napsylate (The potent CYP2D6 inhibitor, paroxetine (20 mg once daily), increases ranolazine concentrations 1.2-fold. No dose adjustment of ranolazine is required in patients treated with CYP2D6 inhibitors).
No products indexed under this heading.

Propranolol Hydrochloride (Ranolazine or its metabolites partially inhibit CYP2D6. There are no studies of concomitant use of ranolazine with other drugs metabolized by CYP2D6, such as tricyclic antidepressants and antipsychotics, but lower doses of CYP2D6 substrates may be required). Products include:
InnoPran XL 1517

Protriptyline Hydrochloride (The potent CYP2D6 inhibitor, paroxetine (20 mg once daily), increases ranolazine concentrations 1.2-fold. No dose adjustment of ranolazine is required in patients treated with CYP2D6 inhibitors).
No products indexed under this heading.

Quetiapine Fumarate (Ranolazine can inhibit the activity of CYP2D6 and thus, the metabolism of drugs that are mainly metabolized by this enzyme (eg, some antipsychotics) may be impaired and exposure to these drugs increased. The dose of such drugs may have to be reduced when ranolazine is co-administered). Products include:
Seroquel 750
Seroquel XR 759

Quinacrine Hydrochloride (The potent CYP2D6 inhibitor, paroxetine (20 mg once daily), increases ranolazine concentrations 1.2-fold. No dose adjustment of ranolazine is required in patients treated with CYP2D6 inhibitors).
No products indexed under this heading.

Quinidine (Because of possible additive effects on the QT interval, ranolazine should be avoided in patients receiving drugs that prolong the QTc interval, such as Class IA (eg, quinidine) and Class III (eg, dofetilide, sotalol) antiarrhythmics, and antipsychotics (eg, thioridazine, ziprasidone)).
No products indexed under this heading.

Quinidine Gluconate (Because of possible additive effects on the QT interval, ranolazine should be avoided in patients receiving drugs that prolong the QTc interval, such as Class IA (eg, quinidine) and Class III (eg, dofetilide, sotalol) antiarrhythmics, and antipsychotics (eg, thioridazine, ziprasidone)).
No products indexed under this heading.

Quinidine Hydrochloride (Because of possible additive effects on the QT interval, ranolazine should be avoided in patients receiving drugs that prolong the QTc interval, such as Class IA (eg, quinidine) and Class III (eg, dofetilide, sotalol) antiarrhythmics, and antipsychotics (eg, thioridazine, ziprasidone)).
No products indexed under this heading.

Quinidine Polygalacturonate (Because of possible additive effects on the QT interval, ranolazine should be avoided in patients receiving drugs that prolong the QTc interval, such as Class IA (eg, quinidine) and Class III (eg, dofetilide, sotalol) antiarrhythmics, and antipsychotics (eg, thioridazine, ziprasidone)).
No products indexed under this heading.

Quinidine Sulfate (Because of possible additive effects on the QT interval, ranolazine should be avoided in patients receiving drugs that prolong the QTc interval, such as Class IA (eg, quinidine) and Class III (eg, dofetilide, sotalol) antiarrhythmics, and antipsychotics (eg, thioridazine, ziprasidone)).
No products indexed under this heading.

Quinine (Concurrent administration of ranolazine and CYP3A inhibitors is contraindicated. Do not use ranolazine with strong CYP3A inhibitors, including ketoconazole, itraconazole, clarithromycin, nefazodone, nelfinavir, ritonavir, indinavir, and saquinavir. Limit the dose of ranolazine to 500 mg twice daily in patients on moderate CYP3A inhibitors, including diltiazem, verapamil, aprepitant, erythromycin, fluconazole, and grapefruit juice or grapefruit-containing products. Weak CYP3A inhibitors such as simvastatin (20 mg once daily) and cimetidine (400 mg three times daily) do not increase the exposure to ranolazine in healthy volunteers). Products include:
Hyland's Leg Cramps PM with Quinine 3315

Quinine Sulfate (Concurrent administration of ranolazine and CYP3A inhibitors is contraindicated. Do not use ranolazine with strong CYP3A inhibitors, including ketoconazole, itraconazole, clarithromycin, nefazodone, nelfinavir, ritonavir, indinavir, and saquinavir. Limit the dose of ranolazine to 500 mg twice daily in patients on moderate CYP3A inhibitors, including diltiazem, verapamil, aprepitant, erythromycin, fluconazole, and grapefruit juice or grapefruit-containing products. Weak CYP3A inhibitors such as simvastatin (20 mg once daily) and cimetidine (400 mg three times daily) do not increase the exposure to ranolazine in healthy volunteers).
No products indexed under this heading.

Ranitidine Bismuth Citrate (The potent CYP2D6 inhibitor, paroxetine (20 mg once daily), increases ranolazine concentrations 1.2-fold. No dose adjustment of ranolazine is required in patients treated with CYP2D6 inhibitors).
No products indexed under this heading.

Ranitidine Hydrochloride (The potent CYP2D6 inhibitor, paroxetine (20 mg once daily), increases ranolazine concentrations 1.2-fold. No dose adjustment of ranolazine is required in patients treated with CYP2D6 inhibitors). Products include:
Zantac 1737
Zantac Injection 1732
Zantac Pharmacy 1735

Rifabutin (Avoid co-administration of ranolazine and CYP3A inducers, such as rifampin, rifabutin, rifapentin, phenobarbital, phenytoin, carbamazepine, and St. John's wort. Rifampin (600 mg once daily) decreases the plasma concentration of ranolazine (1000 mg twice daily) by approximately 95% by induction of CYP3A and, probably, P-gp).
No products indexed under this heading.

Rifampicin (Avoid co-administration of ranolazine and CYP3A inducers, such as rifampin, rifabutin, rifapentin, phenobarbital, phenytoin, carbamazepine, and St. John's wort. Rifampin (600 mg once daily) decreases the plasma concentration of ranolazine (1000 mg twice daily) by approximately 95% by induction of CYP3A and, probably, P-gp).
No products indexed under this heading.

Rifampin (Co-administration of ranolazine and CYP3A inducers (eg, rifampin) should be avoided. Rifampin (600 mg once daily) decreases the plasma concentration of ranolazine (1000 mg twice daily) by approximately 95% by induction of CYP3A and, probably, P-gp).
No products indexed under this heading.

Rifapentine (Avoid co-administration of ranolazine and CYP3A inducers, such as rifampin, rifabutin, rifapentin, phenobarbital, phenytoin, carbamazepine, and St. John's wort. Rifampin (600 mg once daily) decreases the plasma concentration of ranolazine (1000 mg twice daily) by approximately 95% by induction of CYP3A and, probably, P-gp).
No products indexed under this heading.

Risperidone (Ranolazine can inhibit the activity of CYP2D6 and thus, the metabolism of drugs that are mainly metabolized by this enzyme (eg, some antipsychotics) may be impaired and exposure to these drugs increased. The dose of such drugs may have to be reduced when ranolazine is co-administered). Products include:
Risperdal Consta 2682

Ritonavir (Concurrent administration of ranolazine and CYP3A inhibitors is contraindicated. Do not use ranolazine with strong CYP3A inhibitors, including ketoconazole, itraconazole, clarithromycin, nefazodone, nelfinavir, ritonavir, indinavir, and saquinavir. Limit the dose of ranolazine to 500 mg twice daily in patients on moderate CYP3A inhibitors, including diltiazem, verapamil, aprepitant, erythromycin, fluconazole, and grapefruit juice or grapefruit-containing products. Weak CYP3A inhibitors such as simvastatin (20 mg once daily) and cimetidine (400 mg three times daily) do not increase the exposure to ranolazine in healthy volunteers). Products include:
Kaletra 458
Norvir 509

Saquinavir (Concurrent administration of ranolazine and CYP3A inhibitors is contraindicated. Do not use ranolazine with strong CYP3A inhibitors, including ketoconazole, itraconazole, clarithromycin, nefazodone, nelfinavir, ritonavir, indinavir, and saquinavir. Limit the dose of ranolazine to 500 mg twice daily in patients on moderate CYP3A inhibitors, including diltiazem, verapamil, aprepitant, erythromycin, fluconazole, and grapefruit juice or grapefruit-containing products. Weak CYP3A inhibitors such as simvastatin (20 mg once daily) and cimetidine (400 mg three times daily) do not increase the exposure to ranolazine in healthy volunteers).
No products indexed under this heading.

Saquinavir Mesylate (Concurrent administration of ranolazine and CYP3A inhibitors is contraindicated. Do not use ranolazine with strong CYP3A inhibitors, including ketoconazole, itraconazole, clarithromycin, nefazodone, nelfinavir,

IMPORTANT NOTE: Always consult each drug listing in the patient's regimen for possible interactions.

ritonavir, indinavir, and saquinavir. Limit the dose of ranolazine to 500 mg twice daily in patients on moderate CYP3A inhibitors, including diltiazem, verapamil, aprepitant, erythromycin, fluconazole, and grapefruit juice or grapefruit-containing products. Weak CYP3A inhibitors such as simvastatin (20 mg once daily) and cimetidine (400 mg three times daily) do not increase the exposure to ranolazine in healthy volunteers).
No products indexed under this heading.

Sertraline Hydrochloride (Concurrent administration of ranolazine and CYP3A inhibitors is contraindicated. Do not use ranolazine with strong CYP3A inhibitors, including ketoconazole, itraconazole, clarithromycin, nefazodone, nelfinavir, ritonavir, indinavir, and saquinavir. Limit the dose of ranolazine to 500 mg twice daily in patients on moderate CYP3A inhibitors, including diltiazem, verapamil, aprepitant, erythromycin, fluconazole, and grapefruit juice or grapefruit-containing products. Weak CYP3A inhibitors such as simvastatin (20 mg once daily) and cimetidine (400 mg three times daily) do not increase the exposure to ranolazine in healthy volunteers).
No products indexed under this heading.

Sildenafil Citrate (The potent CYP2D6 inhibitor, paroxetine (20 mg once daily), increases ranolazine concentrations 1.2-fold. No dose adjustment of ranolazine is required in patients treated with CYP2D6 inhibitors).
No products indexed under this heading.

Simvastatin (The plasma levels of simvastatin, a CYP3A substrate, and its active metabolite are each increased about 2-fold in healthy subjects receiving simvastatin (80 mg once daily) and ranolazine (1000 mg twice daily). Dose adjustments of simvastatin are not required when ranolazine is co-administered with simvastatin).
Products include:
Simcor **524**
Vytorin 10/10 .... **2303, 3240**
Vytorin 10/20 .... **2303, 3240**
Vytorin 10/40 .... **2303, 3240**
Vytorin 10/80 .... **2303, 3240**
Zocor **2289**

Sirolimus (The plasma levels of simvastatin, a CYP3A substrate, and its active metabolite are each increased about 2-fold in healthy subjects receiving simvastatin (80 mg once daily) and ranolazine (1000 mg twice daily). Dose adjustments of simvastatin are not required when ranolazine is co-administered with simvastatin).
Products include:
Rapamune **3579**

Sotalol Hydrochloride (Because of possible additive effects on the QT interval, ranolazine should be avoided in patients receiving drugs that prolong the QTc interval, such as Class IA (eg, quinidine) and Class III (eg, dofetilide, sotalol) antiarrhythmics, and antipsychotics (eg, thioridazine, ziprasidone)).
No products indexed under this heading.

Tacrolimus (The plasma levels of simvastatin, a CYP3A substrate, and its active metabolite are each increased about 2-fold in healthy subjects receiving simvastatin (80 mg once daily) and ranolazine (1000 mg twice daily). Dose adjustments of simvastatin are not required when ranolazine is co-administered with simvastatin).
Products include:
Prograf Capsules **677**
Prograf Injection **677**
Protopic **685**

Tamoxifen Citrate (Ranolazine or its metabolites partially inhibit CYP2D6. There are no studies of concomitant use of ranolazine with other drugs metabolized by CYP2D6, such as tricyclic antidepressants and antipsychotics, but lower doses of CYP2D6 substrates may be required).
No products indexed under this heading.

Teniposide (Ranolazine or its metabolites partially inhibit CYP2D6. There are no studies of concomitant use of ranolazine with other drugs metabolized by CYP2D6, such as tricyclic antidepressants and antipsychotics, but lower doses of CYP2D6 substrates may be required).
No products indexed under this heading.

Terbinafine Hydrochloride (The potent CYP2D6 inhibitor, paroxetine (20 mg once daily), increases ranolazine concentrations 1.2-fold. No dose adjustment of ranolazine is required in patients treated with CYP2D6 inhibitors).
No products indexed under this heading.

Terfenadine (The plasma levels of simvastatin, a CYP3A substrate, and its active metabolite are each increased about 2-fold in healthy subjects receiving simvastatin (80 mg once daily) and ranolazine (1000 mg twice daily). Dose adjustments of simvastatin are not required when ranolazine is co-administered with simvastatin).
No products indexed under this heading.

Testosterone (Ranolazine or its metabolites partially inhibit CYP2D6. There are no studies of concomitant use of ranolazine with other drugs metabolized by CYP2D6, such as tricyclic antidepressants and antipsychotics, but lower doses of CYP2D6 substrates may be required). Products include:
AndroGel **3456**

Testosterone Cypionate (Ranolazine or its metabolites partially inhibit CYP2D6. There are no studies of concomitant use of ranolazine with other drugs metabolized by CYP2D6, such as tricyclic antidepressants and antipsychotics, but lower doses of CYP2D6 substrates may be required).
No products indexed under this heading.

Testosterone Enanthate (Ranolazine or its metabolites partially inhibit CYP2D6. There are no studies of concomitant use of ranolazine with other drugs metabolized by CYP2D6, such as tricyclic antidepressants and antipsychotics, but lower doses of CYP2D6 substrates may be required). Products include:
Delatestryl **1102**

Testosterone Propionate (Ranolazine or its metabolites partially inhibit CYP2D6. There are no studies of concomitant use of ranolazine with other drugs metabolized by CYP2D6, such as tricyclic antidepressants and antipsychotics, but lower doses of CYP2D6 substrates may be required).
No products indexed under this heading.

Theophylline (The plasma levels of simvastatin, a CYP3A substrate, and its active metabolite are each increased about 2-fold in healthy subjects receiving simvastatin (80 mg once daily) and ranolazine (1000 mg twice daily). Dose adjustments of simvastatin are not required when ranolazine is co-administered with simvastatin).
No products indexed under this heading.

Theophylline Anhydrous (The plasma levels of simvastatin, a CYP3A substrate, and its active metabolite are each increased about 2-fold in healthy subjects receiving simvastatin (80 mg once daily) and ranolazine (1000 mg twice daily). Dose adjustments of simvastatin are not required when ranolazine is co-administered with simvastatin). Products include:
Uniphyl **2817**

Theophylline Calcium Salicylate (The plasma levels of simvastatin, a CYP3A substrate, and its active metabolite are each increased about 2-fold in healthy subjects receiving simvastatin (80 mg once daily) and ranolazine (1000 mg twice daily). Dose adjustments of simvastatin are not required when ranolazine is co-administered with simvastatin).
No products indexed under this heading.

Theophylline Sodium Glycinate (The plasma levels of simvastatin, a CYP3A substrate, and its active metabolite are each increased about 2-fold in healthy subjects receiving simvastatin (80 mg once daily) and ranolazine (1000 mg twice daily). Dose adjustments of simvastatin are not required when ranolazine is co-administered with simvastatin).
No products indexed under this heading.

Thioridazine (Ranolazine or its metabolites partially inhibit CYP2D6. There are no studies of concomitant use of ranolazine with other drugs metabolized by CYP2D6, such as tricyclic antidepressants and antipsychotics, but lower doses of CYP2D6 substrates may be required).
No products indexed under this heading.

Thioridazine Hydrochloride (Ranolazine can inhibit the activity of CYP2D6 and thus, the metabolism of drugs that are mainly metabolized by this enzyme (eg, some antipsychotics) may be impaired and exposure to these drugs increased. The dose of such drugs may have to be reduced when ranolazine is co-administered). Products include:
Thioridazine Hydrochloride **2384**

Thiothixene (Ranolazine can inhibit the activity of CYP2D6 and thus, the metabolism of drugs that are mainly metabolized by this enzyme (eg, some antipsychotics) may be impaired and exposure to these drugs increased. The dose of such drugs may have to be reduced when ranolazine is co-administered).
Products include:
Thiothixene **2386**

Tiagabine Hydrochloride (The plasma levels of simvastatin, a CYP3A substrate, and its active metabolite are each increased about 2-fold in healthy subjects receiving simvastatin (80 mg once daily) and ranolazine (1000 mg twice daily). Dose adjustments of simvastatin are not required when ranolazine is co-administered with simvastatin).
Products include:
Gabitril **972**

Timolol Maleate (Ranolazine or its metabolites partially inhibit CYP2D6. There are no studies of concomitant use of ranolazine with other drugs metabolized by CYP2D6, such as tricyclic antidepressants and antipsychotics, but lower doses of CYP2D6 substrates may be required). Products include:
Combigan **601**
Dorzolamide Hydrochloride/Timolol Maleate Ophthalmic Solution .... ⊙**243**
Timoptic in Ocudose .... ⊙**231**

Tolterodine Tartrate (Ranolazine or its metabolites partially inhibit CYP2D6. There are no studies of concomitant use of ranolazine with other drugs metabolized by CYP2D6, such as tricyclic antidepressants and antipsychotics, but lower doses of CYP2D6 substrates may be required).
No products indexed under this heading.

Tramadol Hydrochloride (Ranolazine or its metabolites partially inhibit CYP2D6. There are no studies of concomitant use of ranolazine with other drugs metabolized by CYP2D6, such as tricyclic antidepressants and antipsychotics, but lower doses of CYP2D6 substrates may be required). Products include:
Ryzolt **2813**
Ultram ER **2693**

Trazodone Hydrochloride (Ranolazine or its metabolites partially inhibit CYP2D6. There are no studies of concomitant use of ranolazine with other drugs metabolized by CYP2D6, such as tricyclic antidepressants and antipsychotics, but lower doses of CYP2D6 substrates may be required).
No products indexed under this heading.

Triazolam (Ranolazine or its metabolites partially inhibit CYP2D6. There are no studies of concomitant use of ranolazine with other drugs metabolized by CYP2D6, such as tricyclic antidepressants and antipsychotics, but lower doses of CYP2D6 substrates may be required).
No products indexed under this heading.

Trifluoperazine Hydrochloride (Ranolazine can inhibit the activity of CYP2D6 and thus, the metabolism of drugs that are mainly metabolized by this enzyme (eg, some antipsychotics) may be impaired and exposure to these drugs increased. The dose of such drugs may have to be reduced when ranolazine is co-administered).
No products indexed under this heading.

Trimipramine Maleate (The potent CYP2D6 inhibitor, paroxetine (20 mg once daily), increases ranolazine concentrations 1.2-fold. No dose adjustment of ranolazine is required in patients treated with CYP2D6 inhibitors).
No products indexed under this heading.

Troleandomycin (Concurrent administration of ranolazine and CYP3A inhibitors is contraindicated. Do not use ranolazine with strong CYP3A inhibitors, including ketoconazole, itraconazole, clarithromycin, nefazodone, nelfinavir, ritonavir, indinavir, and saquinavir. Limit the dose of ranolazine to 500 mg twice daily in patients on moderate CYP3A inhibitors, including diltiazem, verapamil, aprepitant, erythromycin, fluconazole, and grapefruit juice or grapefruit-containing products. Weak CYP3A inhibitors such as simvastatin (20 mg once daily) and cimetidine (400 mg three times daily) do not increase the exposure to ranolazine in healthy volunteers).
No products indexed under this heading.

Vardenafil Hydrochloride (The potent CYP2D6 inhibitor, paroxetine (20 mg once daily), increases ranolazine concentrations 1.2-fold. No dose adjustment of ranolazine is required in patients treated with CYP2D6 inhibitors). Products include:
Levitra **3157**

Venlafaxine Hydrochloride (Concurrent administration of ranolazine and CYP3A inhibitors is contraindicated. Do not use ranolazine with strong CYP3A inhibitors, including ketoconazole, itraconazole, clarithromycin, nefazodone, nelfinavir, ritonavir, indinavir, and saquinavir. Limit the dose of ranolazine to 500 mg twice daily in patients on moderate CYP3A inhibitors, including diltiazem, verapamil, aprepitant, erythromycin, fluconazole, and grapefruit juice or grapefruit-containing products. Weak CYP3A inhibitors such as simvastatin (20 mg once daily) and cimetidine (400 mg three times daily) do not increase the exposure to ranolazine in healthy volunteers). Products include:
Effexor XR **3504**
Venlafaxine Hydrochloride Tablets **2388**

Verapamil Hydrochloride (Concomitant use is contraindicated. Ranolazine

is primarily metabolized by CYP3A. Use of ranolazine with potent or moderately potent inhibitors of CYP3A should be avoided because concomitant administration will increase ranolazine plasma levels and QTc prolongation. Verapamil 120 mg t.i.d. increases ranolazine steady-state plasma concentrations about 2-fold). Products include:

Tarka 534

Vinblastine Sulfate (Ranolazine or its metabolites partially inhibit CYP2D6. There are no studies of concomitant use of ranolazine with other drugs metabolized by CYP2D6, such as tricyclic antidepressants and antipsychotics, but lower doses of CYP2D6 substrates may be required).

No products indexed under this heading.

Vincristine Sulfate (The plasma levels of simvastatin, a CYP3A substrate, and its active metabolite are each increased about 2-fold in healthy subjects receiving simvastatin (80 mg once daily) and ranolazine (1000 mg twice daily). Dose adjustments of simvastatin are not required when ranolazine is co-administered with simvastatin).

No products indexed under this heading.

Voriconazole (Concurrent administration of ranolazine and CYP3A inhibitors is contraindicated. Do not use ranolazine with strong CYP3A inhibitors, including ketoconazole, itraconazole, clarithromycin, nefazodone, nelfinavir, ritonavir, indinavir, and saquinavir. Limit the dose of ranolazine to 500 mg twice daily in patients on moderate CYP3A inhibitors, including diltiazem, verapamil, aprepitant, erythromycin, fluconazole, and grapefruit juice or grapefruit-containing products. Weak CYP3A inhibitors such as simvastatin (20 mg once daily) and cimetidine (400 mg three times daily) do not increase the exposure to ranolazine in healthy volunteers).

No products indexed under this heading.

Warfarin Sodium (The plasma levels of simvastatin, a CYP3A substrate, and its active metabolite are each increased about 2-fold in healthy subjects receiving simvastatin (80 mg once daily) and ranolazine (1000 mg twice daily). Dose adjustments of simvastatin are not required when ranolazine is co-administered with simvastatin).

No products indexed under this heading.

Zafirlukast (Concurrent administration of ranolazine and CYP3A inhibitors is contraindicated. Do not use ranolazine with strong CYP3A inhibitors, including ketoconazole, itraconazole, clarithromycin, nefazodone, nelfinavir, ritonavir, indinavir, and saquinavir. Limit the dose of ranolazine to 500 mg twice daily in patients on moderate CYP3A inhibitors, including diltiazem, verapamil, aprepitant, erythromycin, fluconazole, and grapefruit juice or grapefruit-containing products. Weak CYP3A inhibitors such as simvastatin (20 mg once daily) and cimetidine (400 mg three times daily) do not increase the exposure to ranolazine in healthy volunteers). Products include:

Accolate 3612

Zileuton (Concurrent administration of ranolazine and CYP3A inhibitors is contraindicated. Do not use ranolazine with strong CYP3A inhibitors, including ketoconazole, itraconazole, clarithromycin, nefazodone, nelfinavir, ritonavir, indinavir, and saquinavir. Limit the dose of ranolazine to 500 mg twice daily in patients on moderate CYP3A inhibitors, including diltiazem, verapamil, aprepitant, erythromycin, fluconazole, and grapefruit juice or grapefruit-containing products. Weak CYP3A inhibitors such as simvastatin (20 mg once daily) and

cimetidine (400 mg three times daily) do not increase the exposure to ranolazine in healthy volunteers).

No products indexed under this heading.

Ziprasidone Hydrochloride (Ranolazine can inhibit the activity of CYP2D6 and thus, the metabolism of drugs that are mainly metabolized by this enzyme (eg, some antipsychotics) may be impaired and exposure to these drugs increased. The dose of such drugs may have to be reduced when ranolazine is co-administered). Products include:

Geodon 2723

Zonisamide (Ranolazine or its metabolites partially inhibit CYP2D6. There are no studies of concomitant use of ranolazine with other drugs metabolized by CYP2D6, such as tricyclic antidepressants and antipsychotics, but lower doses of CYP2D6 substrates may be required). Products include:

Zonegran 1081

Food Interactions

Grapefruit (Concomitant use is contraindicated. Ranolazine is primarily metabolized by CYP3A. Use of ranolazine with potent or moderately potent inhibitors of CYP3A should be avoided because concomitant administration will increase ranolazine plasma levels and QTc prolongation).

Grapefruit Juice (Concomitant use is contraindicated. Ranolazine is primarily metabolized by CYP3A. Use of ranolazine with potent or moderately potent inhibitors of CYP3A should be avoided because concomitant administration will increase ranolazine plasma levels and QTc prolongation).

RAPAMUNE ORAL SOLUTION
(Sirolimus) 3579
See Rapamune Tablets

RAPAMUNE TABLETS
(Sirolimus) 3579

May interact with ACE inhibitors, corticosteroids, cytochrome p450 3a4 inducers (selected), cytochrome p450 3a4 inhibitors (selected), cytochrome p450 3a4 inhibitors, potent (selected), cytochrome p450 3a4 substrates (selected), erythromycin, fibrates, HMG-CoA reductase inhibitors, P-glycoprotein inhibitors, phenytoin, protease inhibitors, vaccines, live, and certain other agents. Compounds in these categories include:

Acetazolamide (Caution when using sirolimus with CYP3A4 inhibitors. The dosage of sirolimus and/or co-administered CYP3A4 inhibitors may need to be adjusted).

No products indexed under this heading.

Acetazolamide Sodium (Caution when using sirolimus with CYP3A4 inhibitors. The dosage of sirolimus and/or co-administered CYP3A4 inhibitors may need to be adjusted).

No products indexed under this heading.

Alclometasone Dipropionate (Safety and efficacy information from a controlled clinical trial in pediatric and adolescent (<18 years of age) renal transplant patients judged to be at high-immunologic risk, defined as a history of one or more acute rejection episodes and/or the presence of chronic allograft nephropathy, do not support the chronic use of sirolimus in combination with calcineurin inhibitors and corticosteroids, due to the higher incidence of lipid abnormalities and deterioration of renal function associated with these immunosuppressive regimens compared to calcineurin inhibitors, without increased benefit with respect to acute rejection, graft survival, or patient survival).

No products indexed under this heading.

Alfentanil Hydrochloride (Care should be exercised when drugs or other substances that are substrates of CYP3A4 are administered concomitantly with sirolimus).

No products indexed under this heading.

Allium sativum (Sirolimus is known to be a substrate for cytochrome P-450 3A4 (CYP3A4). Inducers of CYP3A4 may decrease sirolimus concentrations. Co-administration of sirolimus with strong inducers of CYP3A4 is not recommended).

No products indexed under this heading.

Alprazolam (Care should be exercised when drugs or other substances that are substrates of CYP3A4 are administered concomitantly with sirolimus).

No products indexed under this heading.

Aminoglutethimide (Sirolimus is known to be a substrate for cytochrome P-450 3A4 (CYP3A4). Inducers of CYP3A4 may decrease sirolimus concentrations. Co-administration of sirolimus with strong inducers of CYP3A4 is not recommended).

No products indexed under this heading.

Amiodarone Hydrochloride (Sirolimus is known to be a substrate for p-glycoprotein (P-gp). Inhibitors of P-gp may increase sirolimus concentrations. Co-administration of sirolimus with strong inhibitors of P-gp is not recommended).

No products indexed under this heading.

Amitriptyline Hydrochloride (Care should be exercised when drugs or other substances that are substrates of CYP3A4 are administered concomitantly with sirolimus).

No products indexed under this heading.

Amlodipine Besylate (Sirolimus is known to be a substrate for p-glycoprotein (P-gp). Inhibitors of P-gp may increase sirolimus concentrations. Co-administration of sirolimus with strong inhibitors of P-gp is not recommended). Products include:

Azor 1010
Exforge 2443
Exforge HCT 2449

Amprenavir (Exercise caution when using sirolimus with drugs or agents that are modulators of CYP3A4. Co-administration of sirolimus with HIV protease inhibitors may increase sirolimus blood concentrations. The dosage of sirolimus and/or the HIV protease inhibitor may need to be adjusted).

No products indexed under this heading.

Anastrozole (Caution when using sirolimus with CYP3A4 inhibitors. The dosage of sirolimus and/or co-administered CYP3A4 inhibitors may need to be adjusted).

No products indexed under this heading.

Aprepitant (Care should be exercised when drugs or other substances that are substrates of CYP3A4 are administered concomitantly with sirolimus). Products include:

Emend 2124

Astemizole (Care should be exercised when drugs or other substances that are substrates of CYP3A4 are administered concomitantly with sirolimus).

No products indexed under this heading.

Atazanavir (Exercise caution when using sirolimus with drugs or agents that are modulators of CYP3A4. Co-administration of sirolimus with HIV protease inhibitors may increase sirolimus blood concentrations. The dosage of sirolimus and/or the HIV protease inhibitor may need to be adjusted).

No products indexed under this heading.

Atazanavir Sulfate (Exercise caution when using sirolimus with drugs or agents that are modulators of CYP3A4. Co-administration of sirolimus with HIV protease inhibitors may increase sirolimus blood concentrations. The dosage of sirolimus and/or the HIV protease inhibitor may need to be adjusted).

No products indexed under this heading.

Atenolol (Sirolimus is known to be a substrate for p-glycoprotein (P-gp). Inhibitors of P-gp may increase sirolimus concentrations. Co-administration of sirolimus with strong inhibitors of P-gp is not recommended).

No products indexed under this heading.

Atorvastatin Calcium (Sirolimus is known to be a substrate for p-glycoprotein (P-gp). Inhibitors of P-gp may increase sirolimus concentrations. Co-administration of sirolimus with strong inhibitors of P-gp is not recommended). Products include:

Lipitor 2703

Azithromycin Dihydrate (Sirolimus is known to be a substrate for p-glycoprotein (P-gp). Inhibitors of P-gp may increase sirolimus concentrations. Co-administration of sirolimus with strong inhibitors of P-gp is not recommended).

No products indexed under this heading.

BCG Vaccine (Immunosuppressants may affect response to vaccination. Therefore, during treatment with sirolimus, vaccination may be less effective. The use of live vaccines should be avoided).

No products indexed under this heading.

Beclomethasone Dipropionate (Safety and efficacy information from a controlled clinical trial in pediatric and adolescent (<18 years of age) renal transplant patients judged to be at high-immunologic risk, defined as a history of one or more acute rejection episodes and/or the presence of chronic allograft nephropathy, do not support the chronic use of sirolimus in combination with calcineurin inhibitors and corticosteroids, due to the higher incidence of lipid abnormalities and deterioration of renal function associated with these immunosuppressive regimens compared to calcineurin inhibitors, without increased benefit with respect to acute rejection, graft survival, or patient survival). Products include:

Qvar 3398

Beclomethasone Dipropionate Monohydrate (Safety and efficacy information from a controlled clinical trial in pediatric and adolescent (<18 years of age) renal transplant patients judged to be at high-immunologic risk, defined as a history of one or more acute rejection episodes and/or the presence of chronic allograft nephropathy, do not support the chronic use of sirolimus in combination with calcineurin inhibitors and corticosteroids, due to the higher incidence of lipid abnormalities and deterioration of renal function associated with these immunosuppressive regimens compared to calcineurin inhibitors, without increased benefit with respect to acute rejection, graft survival, or patient survival). Products include:

Beconase AQ 1386

Belladonna Ergotamine (Care should be exercised when drugs or other substances that are substrates of CYP3A4 are administered concomitantly with sirolimus).

No products indexed under this heading.

Benazepril Hydrochloride (Sirolimus has been associated with the development of angioedema. The concomitant use of sirolimus with other drugs known to cause angioedema, such as ACE-inhibitors, may increase the risk of developing angioedema).
No products indexed under this heading.

Betamethasone (Sirolimus is known to be a substrate for cytochrome P-450 3A4 (CYP3A4). Inducers of CYP3A4 may decrease sirolimus concentrations. Co-administration of sirolimus with strong inducers of CYP3A4 is not recommended).
No products indexed under this heading.

Betamethasone Acetate (Sirolimus is known to be a substrate for cytochrome P-450 3A4 (CYP3A4). Inducers of CYP3A4 may decrease sirolimus concentrations. Co-administration of sirolimus with strong inducers of CYP3A4 is not recommended).
No products indexed under this heading.

Betamethasone Benzoate (Sirolimus is known to be a substrate for cytochrome P-450 3A4 (CYP3A4). Inducers of CYP3A4 may decrease sirolimus concentrations. Co-administration of sirolimus with strong inducers of CYP3A4 is not recommended).
No products indexed under this heading.

Betamethasone Dipropionate (Sirolimus is known to be a substrate for cytochrome P-450 3A4 (CYP3A4). Inducers of CYP3A4 may decrease sirolimus concentrations. Co-administration of sirolimus with strong inducers of CYP3A4 is not recommended). Products include:

Betamethasone Sodium Phosphate (Sirolimus is known to be a substrate for cytochrome P-450 3A4 (CYP3A4). Inducers of CYP3A4 may decrease sirolimus concentrations. Co-administration of sirolimus with strong inducers of CYP3A4 is not recommended).
No products indexed under this heading.

Betamethasone Valerate (Sirolimus is known to be a substrate for cytochrome P-450 3A4 (CYP3A4). Inducers of CYP3A4 may decrease sirolimus concentrations. Co-administration of sirolimus with strong inducers of CYP3A4 is not recommended). Products include:

Bosentan (Sirolimus is known to be a substrate for cytochrome P-450 3A4 (CYP3A4). Inducers of CYP3A4 may decrease sirolimus concentrations. Co-administration of sirolimus with strong inducers of CYP3A4 is not recommended). Products include:

Bromocriptine Mesylate (Exercise caution when using sirolimus with drugs or agents that are modulators of CYP3A4. Co-administration of sirolimus with bromocriptine may increase sirolimus blood concentrations. The dosage of sirolimus and/or bromocriptine may need to be adjusted).
No products indexed under this heading.

Budesonide (Safety and efficacy information from a controlled clinical trial in pediatric and adolescent (<18 years of age) renal transplant patients judged to be at high-immunologic risk, defined as a history of one or more acute rejection episodes and/or the presence of chronic allograft nephropathy, do not support the chronic use of sirolimus in combination with calcineurin inhibitors and corticosteroids, due to the higher incidence of lipid abnormalities and deterioration of renal function associated with these immunosuppressive regimens compared to calcineurin inhibitors, without increased benefit with respect to acute rejection, graft survival, or patient survival). Products include:

Buspirone Hydrochloride (Care should be exercised when drugs or other substances that are substrates of CYP3A4 are administered concomitantly with sirolimus).
No products indexed under this heading.

Busulfan (Care should be exercised when drugs or other substances that are substrates of CYP3A4 are administered concomitantly with sirolimus). Products include:

Captopril (Sirolimus has been associated with the development of angioedema. The concomitant use of sirolimus with other drugs known to cause angioedema, such as ACE-inhibitors, may increase the risk of developing angioedema). Products include:

Carbamazepine (Exercise caution when using sirolimus with drugs or agents that are modulators of CYP3A4. Co-administration of sirolimus with carbamazepine may decrease sirolimus blood concentrations. The dosage of sirolimus and/or carbamazepine may need to be adjusted). Products include:

Carvedilol (Sirolimus is known to be a substrate for p-glycoprotein (P-gp). Inhibitors of P-gp may increase sirolimus concentrations. Co-administration of sirolimus with strong inhibitors of P-gp is not recommended). Products include:

Carvedilol Phosphate (Sirolimus is known to be a substrate for p-glycoprotein (P-gp). Inhibitors of P-gp may increase sirolimus concentrations. Co-administration of sirolimus with strong inhibitors of P-gp is not recommended). Products include:

Cerivastatin Sodium (During sirolimus therapy with cyclosporine, patients administered an HMG-CoA reductase inhibitor and/or fibrate should be monitored for the possible development of rhabdomyolysis and other adverse effects. In clinical trials, the concomitant administration of sirolimus and HMG-CoA reductase inhibitors appeared to be well-tolerated).
No products indexed under this heading.

Chlorpheniramine (Care should be exercised when drugs or other substances that are substrates of CYP3A4 are administered concomitantly with sirolimus).
No products indexed under this heading.

Chlorpheniramine Maleate (Care should be exercised when drugs or other substances that are substrates of CYP3A4 are administered concomitantly with sirolimus).
No products indexed under this heading.

Chlorpheniramine Polistirex (Care should be exercised when drugs or other substances that are substrates of CYP3A4 are administered concomitantly with sirolimus). Products include:

Chlorpheniramine Tannate (Care should be exercised when drugs or other substances that are substrates of CYP3A4 are administered concomitantly with sirolimus).
No products indexed under this heading.

Ciclesonide (Safety and efficacy information from a controlled clinical trial in pediatric and adolescent (<18 years of age) renal transplant patients judged to be at high-immunologic risk, defined as a history of one or more acute rejection episodes and/or the presence of chronic allograft nephropathy, do not support the chronic use of sirolimus in combination with calcineurin inhibitors and corticosteroids, due to the higher incidence of lipid abnormalities and deterioration of renal function associated with these immunosuppressive regimens compared to calcineurin inhibitors, without increased benefit with respect to acute rejection, graft survival, or patient survival).
No products indexed under this heading.

Cimetidine (Exercise caution when using sirolimus with drugs or agents that are modulators of CYP3A4. Co-administration of sirolimus with cimetidine may increase sirolimus blood concentrations. The dosage of sirolimus and/or cimetidine may need to be adjusted).
No products indexed under this heading.

Cimetidine Hydrochloride (Exercise caution when using sirolimus with drugs or agents that are modulators of CYP3A4. Co-administration of sirolimus with cimetidine may increase sirolimus blood concentrations. The dosage of sirolimus and/or cimetidine may need to be adjusted).
No products indexed under this heading.

Ciprofloxacin (Sirolimus is known to be a substrate for cytochrome P-450 3A4 (CYP3A4). Inducers of CYP3A4 may decrease sirolimus concentrations. Co-administration of sirolimus with strong inducers of CYP3A4 is not recommended). Products include:

Ciprofloxacin Hydrochloride (Sirolimus is known to be a substrate for cytochrome P-450 3A4 (CYP3A4). Inducers of CYP3A4 may decrease sirolimus concentrations. Co-administration of sirolimus with strong inducers of CYP3A4 is not recommended). Products include:

Cisapride (Exercise caution when using sirolimus with drugs or agents that are modulators of CYP3A4. Co-administration of sirolimus with cisapride may increase sirolimus blood concentrations. The dosage of sirolimus and/or cisapride may need to be adjusted).
No products indexed under this heading.

Cisplatin (Sirolimus is known to be a substrate for cytochrome P-450 3A4 (CYP3A4). Inducers of CYP3A4 may decrease sirolimus concentrations. Co-administration of sirolimus with strong inducers of CYP3A4 is not recommended).
No products indexed under this heading.

Clarithromycin (Sirolimus is known to be a substrate for cytochrome P-450 3A4 (CYP3A4). Co-administration of sirolimus with strong inhibitors of CYP3A4 such as clarithromycin is not recommended). Products include:

Clofibrate (During sirolimus therapy with cyclosporine, patients administered a fibrate should be monitored for the possible development of rhabdomyolysis and other adverse effects. In clinical trials, the concomitant administration of sirolimus and fibrates appeared to be well-tolerated).
No products indexed under this heading.

Clotrimazole (Exercise caution when using sirolimus with drugs or agents that are modulators of CYP3A4. Co-administration of sirolimus with clotrimazole may increase sirolimus blood concentrations. The dosage of sirolimus and/or clotrimazole may need to be adjusted). Products include:

Conivaptan Hydrochloride (Caution when using sirolimus with CYP3A4 inhibitors. The dosage of sirolimus and/or co-administered CYP3A4 inhibitors may need to be adjusted). Products include:

Cortisone Acetate (Sirolimus is known to be a substrate for cytochrome P-450 3A4 (CYP3A4). Inducers of CYP3A4 may decrease sirolimus concentrations. Co-administration of sirolimus with strong inducers of CYP3A4 is not recommended).
No products indexed under this heading.

Cyclosporine (Cyclosporine, a substrate and inhibitor of CYP3A4 and P-gp, was shown to increase sirolimus concentrations when co-administered with sirolimus. To reduce this, it is recommended that sirolimus be taken 4 hours after administration of cyclosporine oral solution, modified and/or cyclosporine capsules, modified. If cyclosporine is withdrawn from combination therapy with sirolimus, higher doses of sirolimus are needed to maintain recommended sirolimus trough concentration ranges. In studies of de novo livertransplant patients, the use of sirolimus in combination with cyclosporine, was associated with an increase in HAT (Hepatic Artery Thrombosis), (7% in combination vs. 2% in the control arm). Use of sirolimus in liver transplant patients is not recommended). Products include:

Dalfopristin (Caution when using sirolimus with CYP3A4 inhibitors. The dosage of sirolimus and/or co-administered CYP3A4 inhibitors may need to be adjusted).
No products indexed under this heading.

Danazol (Exercise caution when using sirolimus with drugs or agents that are modulators of CYP3A4. Co-administration of sirolimus with danazol may increase sirolimus blood concentrations. The dosage of sirolimus and/or danazol may need to be adjusted).
No products indexed under this heading.

Darunavir (Exercise caution when using sirolimus with drugs or agents that are modulators of CYP3A4. Co-administration of sirolimus with HIV protease inhibitors may increase sirolimus blood concentrations. The dosage of sirolimus and/or the HIV protease inhibitor may need to be adjusted).
No products indexed under this heading.

Dasatinib (Caution when using sirolimus with CYP3A4 inhibitors. The dosage of sirolimus and/or co-administered CYP3A4 inhibitors may need to be adjusted).
No products indexed under this heading.

Delavirdine Mesylate (Sirolimus is known to be a substrate for cytochrome P-450 3A4 (CYP3A4). Inhibitors of CYP3A4 may increase sirolimus concentrations. Co-administration of sirolimus with strong inhibitors of CYP3A4 is not recommended).
No products indexed under this heading.

Delavirine (Sirolimus is known to be a substrate for cytochrome P-450 3A4 (CYP3A4). Inhibitors of CYP3A4 may increase sirolimus concentrations. Co-administration of sirolimus with strong inhibitors of CYP3A4 is not recommended).
No products indexed under this heading.

Desloratadine (Caution when using sirolimus with CYP3A4 inhibitors. The dosage of sirolimus and/or co-administered CYP3A4 inhibitors may need to be adjusted). Products include:
- Clarinex Syrup **3098**
- Clarinex **3098**
- Clarinex Reditabs **3098**
- Clarinex-D 12-Hour **3101**
- Clarinex-D **3104**

Desogestrel (Care should be exercised when drugs or other substances that are substrates of CYP3A4 are administered concomitantly with sirolimus).
No products indexed under this heading.

Desoximetasone (Safety and efficacy information from a controlled clinical trial in pediatric and adolescent (<18 years of age) renal transplant patients judged to be at high-immunologic risk, defined as a history of one or more acute rejection episodes and/or the presence of chronic allograft nephropathy, do not support the chronic use of sirolimus in combination with calcineurin inhibitors and corticosteroids, due to the higher incidence of lipid abnormalities and deterioration of renal function associated with these immunosuppressive regimens compared to calcineurin inhibitors, without increased benefit with respect to acute rejection, graft survival, or patient survival).
No products indexed under this heading.

Dexamethasone (Sirolimus is known to be a substrate for cytochrome P-450 3A4 (CYP3A4). Inducers of CYP3A4 may decrease sirolimus concentrations. Co-administration of sirolimus with strong inducers of CYP3A4 is not recommended). Products include:
- Ciprodex **583**
- Ozurdex .... ⊙**223**
- Tobramycin and Dexamethasone Ophthalmic Suspension .... ⊙**251**

Dexamethasone Acetate (Sirolimus is known to be a substrate for cytochrome P-450 3A4 (CYP3A4). Inducers of CYP3A4 may decrease sirolimus concentrations. Co-administration of sirolimus with strong inducers of CYP3A4 is not recommended).
No products indexed under this heading.

Dexamethasone Phosphate (Sirolimus is known to be a substrate for cytochrome P-450 3A4 (CYP3A4). Inducers of CYP3A4 may decrease sirolimus concentrations. Co-administration of sirolimus with strong inducers of CYP3A4 is not recommended).
No products indexed under this heading.

Dexamethasone Sodium (Sirolimus is known to be a substrate for cytochrome P-450 3A4 (CYP3A4). Inducers of CYP3A4 may decrease sirolimus concentrations. Co-administration of sirolimus with strong inducers of CYP3A4 is not recommended).
No products indexed under this heading.

Dexamethasone Sodium Phosphate (Sirolimus is known to be a substrate for cytochrome P-450 3A4 (CYP3A4). Inducers of CYP3A4 may decrease sirolimus concentrations. Co-administration of sirolimus with strong inducers of CYP3A4 is not recommended).
No products indexed under this heading.

Dexamethasone Sodium Phosphate Injection (Sirolimus is known to be a substrate for cytochrome P-450 3A4 (CYP3A4). Inducers of CYP3A4 may decrease sirolimus concentrations. Co-administration of sirolimus with strong inducers of CYP3A4 is not recommended).
No products indexed under this heading.

Diazepam (Care should be exercised when drugs or other substances that are substrates of CYP3A4 are administered concomitantly with sirolimus). Products include:
- Valium Tablets **2880**

Diflorasone Diacetate (Safety and efficacy information from a controlled clinical trial in pediatric and adolescent (<18 years of age) renal transplant patients judged to be at high-immunologic risk, defined as a history of one or more acute rejection episodes and/or the presence of chronic allograft nephropathy, do not support the chronic use of sirolimus in combination with calcineurin inhibitors and corticosteroids, due to the higher incidence of lipid abnormalities and deterioration of renal function associated with these immunosuppressive regimens compared to calcineurin inhibitors, without increased benefit with respect to acute rejection, graft survival, or patient survival).
No products indexed under this heading.

Digoxin (Sirolimus is known to be a substrate for p-glycoprotein (P-gp). Inhibitors of P-gp may increase sirolimus concentrations. Co-administration of sirolimus with strong inhibitors of P-gp is not recommended). Products include:
- Lanoxin Injection **1546**
- Lanoxin Injection Pediatric **1549**
- Lanoxin Tablets **1553**

Dihydroergotamine Mesylate (Care should be exercised when drugs or other substances that are substrates of CYP3A4 are administered concomitantly with sirolimus).
No products indexed under this heading.

Diltiazem Hydrochloride (Diltiazem is a substrate and inhibitor of CYP3A4 and P-gp; sirolimus concentrations should be monitored and a dose adjustment may be necessary. The simultaneous oral administration of 10 mg of sirolimus oral solution and 120 mg of diltiazem to 18 healthy volunteers significantly affected the bioavailability of sirolimus. Sirolimus C_{max}, t_{max}, and AUC were increased 1.4-, 1.3-, and 1.6-fold, respectively. Sirolimus did not affect the pharmacokinetics of either diltiazem or its metabolites desacetyldiltiazem and desmethyldiltiazem). Products include:
- Cardizem LA **423**

Diltiazem Maleate (Diltiazem is a substrate and inhibitor of CYP3A4 and P-gp; sirolimus concentrations should be monitored and a dose adjustment may be necessary. The simultaneous oral administration of 10 mg of sirolimus oral solution and 120 mg of diltiazem to 18 healthy volunteers significantly affected the bioavailability of sirolimus. Sirolimus C_{max}, t_{max}, and AUC were increased 1.4-, 1.3-, and 1.6-fold, respectively. Sirolimus did not affect the pharmacokinetics of either diltiazem or its metabolites desacetyldiltiazem and desmethyldiltiazem).
No products indexed under this heading.

Dirithromycin (Sirolimus is known to be a substrate for p-glycoprotein (P-gp). Inhibitors of P-gp may increase sirolimus concentrations. Co-administration of sirolimus with strong inhibitors of P-gp is not recommended).
No products indexed under this heading.

Disopyramide (Care should be exercised when drugs or other substances that are substrates of CYP3A4 are administered concomitantly with sirolimus).
No products indexed under this heading.

Disopyramide Phosphate (Care should be exercised when drugs or other substances that are substrates of CYP3A4 are administered concomitantly with sirolimus).
No products indexed under this heading.

Disulfiram (Care should be exercised when drugs or other substances that are substrates of CYP3A4 are administered concomitantly with sirolimus).
No products indexed under this heading.

Doxorubicin Hydrochloride (Care should be exercised when drugs or other substances that are substrates of CYP3A4 are administered concomitantly with sirolimus).
No products indexed under this heading.

Dronabinol (Care should be exercised when drugs or other substances that are substrates of CYP3A4 are administered concomitantly with sirolimus).
No products indexed under this heading.

Efavirenz (Sirolimus is known to be a substrate for cytochrome P-450 3A4 (CYP3A4). Inducers of CYP3A4 may decrease sirolimus concentrations. Co-administration of sirolimus with strong inducers of CYP3A4 is not recommended). Products include:
- Atripla **906**

Elacridar (Sirolimus is known to be a substrate for p-glycoprotein (P-gp). Inhibitors of P-gp may increase sirolimus concentrations. Co-administration of sirolimus with strong inhibitors of P-gp is not recommended).
No products indexed under this heading.

Enalapril Maleate (Sirolimus has been associated with the development of angioedema. The concomitant use of sirolimus with other drugs known to cause angioedema, such as ACE-inhibitors, may increase the risk of developing angioedema).
No products indexed under this heading.

Enalaprilat (Sirolimus has been associated with the development of angioedema. The concomitant use of sirolimus with other drugs known to cause angioedema, such as ACE-inhibitors, may increase the risk of developing angioedema).
No products indexed under this heading.

Ergotamine Tartrate (Care should be exercised when drugs or other substances that are substrates of CYP3A4 are administered concomitantly with sirolimus).
No products indexed under this heading.

Erythromycin (Erythromycin is a substrate and inhibitor of CYP3A4 and P-gp; co-administration of sirolimus oral solution or tablets and erythromycin is not recommended. The simultaneous oral administration of 2 mg daily of sirolimus oral solution and 800 mg q 8h of erythromycin as erythromycin ethylsuccinate tablets at steady state to 24 healthy volunteers significantly affected the bioavailability of sirolimus and erythromycin. Sirolimus C_{max} and AUC were increased 4.4- and 4.2-fold, respectively, and t_{max} was increased by 0.4 hour. Erythromycin C_{max} and AUC were increased 1.6- and 1.7-fold, respectively, and t_{max} was increased by 0.3 hour).
No products indexed under this heading.

Erythromycin, Topical (Erythromycin is a substrate and inhibitor of CYP3A4 and P-gp; co-administration of sirolimus oral solution or tablets and erythromycin is not recommended. The simultaneous oral administration of 2 mg daily of sirolimus oral solution and 800 mg q 8h of erythromycin as erythromycin ethylsuccinate tablets at steady state to 24 healthy volunteers significantly affected the bioavailability of sirolimus and erythromycin. Sirolimus C_{max} and AUC were increased 4.4- and 4.2-fold, respectively, and t_{max} was increased by 0.4 hour. Erythromycin C_{max} and AUC were increased 1.6- and 1.7-fold, respectively, and t_{max} was increased by 0.3 hour).
No products indexed under this heading.

Erythromycin Estolate (Erythromycin is a substrate and inhibitor of CYP3A4 and P-gp; co-administration of sirolimus oral solution or tablets and erythromycin is not recommended. The simultaneous oral administration of 2 mg daily of sirolimus oral solution and 800 mg q 8h of erythromycin as erythromycin ethylsuccinate tablets at steady state to 24 healthy volunteers significantly affected the bioavailability of sirolimus and erythromycin. Sirolimus C_{max} and AUC were increased 4.4- and 4.2-fold, respectively, and t_{max} was increased by 0.4 hour. Erythromycin C_{max} and AUC were increased 1.6- and 1.7-fold, respectively, and t_{max} was increased by 0.3 hour).
No products indexed under this heading.

Erythromycin Ethylsuccinate (Erythromycin is a substrate and inhibitor of CYP3A4 and P-gp; co-administration of sirolimus oral solution or tablets and erythromycin is not recommended. The simultaneous oral administration of 2 mg daily of sirolimus oral solution and 800 mg q 8h of erythromycin as erythromycin ethylsuccinate tablets at steady state to 24 healthy volunteers significantly affected the bioavailability of sirolimus and erythromycin. Sirolimus C_{max} and AUC were increased 4.4- and 4.2-fold, respectively, and t_{max} was increased by 0.4 hour. Erythromycin C_{max} and AUC were increased 1.6- and 1.7-fold, respectively, and t_{max} was increased by 0.3 hour). Products include:
- E.E.S. **437**
- EryPed **435**

Erythromycin Gluceptate (Erythromycin is a substrate and inhibitor of CYP3A4 and P-gp; co-administration of sirolimus oral solution or tablets and erythromycin is not recommended. The simultaneous oral administration of 2 mg daily of sirolimus oral solution and 800 mg q 8h of erythromycin as erythromycin ethylsuccinate tablets at steady state to 24 healthy volunteers significantly affected the bioavailability of sirolimus and erythromycin. Sirolimus C_{max} and AUC were increased 4.4- and 4.2-fold, respectively, and t_{max} was increased by 0.4 hour. Erythromycin C_{max} and AUC were increased 1.6- and 1.7-fold, respectively, and t_{max} was increased by 0.3 hour).
No products indexed under this heading.

Erythromycin Lactobionate (Erythromycin is a substrate and inhibitor of CYP3A4 and P-gp; co-administration of sirolimus oral solution or tablets and erythromycin is not recommended. The simultaneous oral administration of 2 mg daily of sirolimus oral solution and 800 mg q 8h of erythromycin as erythromycin ethylsuccinate tablets at steady state to 24 healthy volunteers significantly affected the bioavailability of sirolimus and erythromycin. Sirolimus C_{max} and AUC were increased 4.4- and 4.2-fold, respectively, and t_{max} was increased by 0.4 hour. Erythromycin C_{max} and AUC were increased 1.6- and 1.7-fold, respectively, and t_{max} was increased by 0.3 hour).
No products indexed under this heading.

Erythromycin Stearate (Erythromycin is a substrate and inhibitor of CYP3A4 and P-gp; co-administration of sirolimus oral solution or tablets and erythromycin is not recommended. The simultaneous oral administration of 2 mg daily of sirolimus oral solution and 800 mg q 8h of erythromycin as erythromycin ethylsuccinate tablets at steady state to 24 healthy volunteers significantly affected the bioavailability of sirolimus and erythromycin. Sirolimus C_{max} and AUC were increased 4.4- and 4.2-fold, respectively, and t_{max} was increased by 0.4 hour. Erythromycin

C_{max} and AUC were increased 1.6- and 1.7-fold, respectively, and t_{max} was increased by 0.3 hour).
No products indexed under this heading.

Esomeprazole Magnesium (Caution when using sirolimus with CYP3A4 inhibitors. The dosage of sirolimus and/or co-administered CYP3A4 inhibitors may need to be adjusted). Products include:

Esomeprazole Sodium (Caution when using sirolimus with CYP3A4 inhibitors. The dosage of sirolimus and/or co-administered CYP3A4 inhibitors may need to be adjusted). Products include:

Estradiol (Care should be exercised when drugs or other substances that are substrates of CYP3A4 are administered concomitantly with sirolimus). Products include:

Estradiol Benzoate (Care should be exercised when drugs or other substances that are substrates of CYP3A4 are administered concomitantly with sirolimus).
No products indexed under this heading.

Estradiol Cypionate (Care should be exercised when drugs or other substances that are substrates of CYP3A4 are administered concomitantly with sirolimus).
No products indexed under this heading.

Estradiol Valerate (Care should be exercised when drugs or other substances that are substrates of CYP3A4 are administered concomitantly with sirolimus).
No products indexed under this heading.

Ethinyl Estradiol (Care should be exercised when drugs or other substances that are substrates of CYP3A4 are administered concomitantly with sirolimus). Products include:

Ethosuximide (Care should be exercised when drugs or other substances that are substrates of CYP3A4 are administered concomitantly with sirolimus).
No products indexed under this heading.

Ethynodiol Diacetate (Care should be exercised when drugs or other substances that are substrates of CYP3A4 are administered concomitantly with sirolimus).
No products indexed under this heading.

Etoposide (Care should be exercised when drugs or other substances that are substrates of CYP3A4 are administered concomitantly with sirolimus).
No products indexed under this heading.

Etoposide Phosphate (Care should be exercised when drugs or other substances that are substrates of CYP3A4 are administered concomitantly with sirolimus).
No products indexed under this heading.

Felbamate (Sirolimus is known to be a substrate for cytochrome P-450 3A4 (CYP3A4). Inducers of CYP3A4 may decrease sirolimus concentrations. Co-administration of sirolimus with strong inducers of CYP3A4 is not recommended).
No products indexed under this heading.

Felodipine (Care should be exercised when drugs or other substances that are substrates of CYP3A4 are administered concomitantly with sirolimus).
No products indexed under this heading.

Fenofibrate (During sirolimus therapy with cyclosporine, patients administered a fibrate should be monitored for the possible development of rhabdomyolysis and other adverse effects. In clinical trials, the concomitant administration of sirolimus and fibrates appeared to be well-tolerated). Products include:

Fentanyl (Care should be exercised when drugs or other substances that are substrates of CYP3A4 are administered concomitantly with sirolimus). Products include:

Fentanyl Citrate (Care should be exercised when drugs or other substances that are substrates of CYP3A4 are administered concomitantly with sirolimus). Products include:

Fluconazole (Exercise caution when using sirolimus with drugs or agents that are modulators of CYP3A4. Co-administration of sirolimus with fluconazole may increase sirolimus blood concentrations. The dosage of sirolimus and/or fluconazole may need to be adjusted).
No products indexed under this heading.

Fludrocortisone Acetate (Sirolimus is known to be a substrate for cytochrome P-450 3A4 (CYP3A4). Inducers of CYP3A4 may decrease sirolimus concentrations. Co-administration of sirolimus with strong inducers of CYP3A4 is not recommended).
No products indexed under this heading.

Flumethasone Pivalate (Safety and efficacy information from a controlled clinical trial in pediatric and adolescent (<18 years of age) renal transplant patients judged to be at high-immunologic risk, defined as a history of one or more acute rejection episodes and/or the presence of chronic allograft nephropathy, do not support the chronic use of sirolimus in combination with calcineurin inhibitors and corticosteroids, due to the higher incidence of lipid abnormalities and deterioration of renal function associated with these immunosuppressive regimens compared to calcineurin inhibitors, without increased benefit with respect to acute rejection, graft survival, or patient survival).
No products indexed under this heading.

Flunisolide Hemihydrate (Safety and efficacy information from a controlled clinical trial in pediatric and adolescent (<18 years of age) renal transplant patients judged to be at high-immunologic risk, defined as a history of one or more acute rejection episodes and/or the presence of chronic allograft nephropathy, do not support the chronic use of sirolimus in combination with calcineurin inhibitors and corticosteroids, due to the higher incidence of lipid abnormalities and deterioration of renal function associated with these immunosuppressive regimens compared to calcineurin inhibitors, without

increased benefit with respect to acute rejection, graft survival, or patient survival).
No products indexed under this heading.

Fluoxetine (Caution when using sirolimus with CYP3A4 inhibitors. The dosage of sirolimus and/or co-administered CYP3A4 inhibitors may need to be adjusted).
No products indexed under this heading.

Fluoxetine Hydrochloride (Caution when using sirolimus with CYP3A4 inhibitors. The dosage of sirolimus and/or co-administered CYP3A4 inhibitors may need to be adjusted). Products include:

Fluticasone Furoate (Safety and efficacy information from a controlled clinical trial in pediatric and adolescent (<18 years of age) renal transplant patients judged to be at high-immunologic risk, defined as a history of one or more acute rejection episodes and/or the presence of chronic allograft nephropathy, do not support the chronic use of sirolimus in combination with calcineurin inhibitors and corticosteroids, due to the higher incidence of lipid abnormalities and deterioration of renal function associated with these immunosuppressive regimens compared to calcineurin inhibitors, without increased benefit with respect to acute rejection, graft survival, or patient survival). Products include:

Fluticasone Propionate (Safety and efficacy information from a controlled clinical trial in pediatric and adolescent (<18 years of age) renal transplant patients judged to be at high-immunologic risk, defined as a history of one or more acute rejection episodes and/or the presence of chronic allograft nephropathy, do not support the chronic use of sirolimus in combination with calcineurin inhibitors and corticosteroids, due to the higher incidence of lipid abnormalities and deterioration of renal function associated with these immunosuppressive regimens compared to calcineurin inhibitors, without increased benefit with respect to acute rejection, graft survival, or patient survival). Products include:

Fluvastatin Sodium (During sirolimus therapy with cyclosporine, patients administered an HMG-CoA reductase inhibitor and/or fibrate should be monitored for the possible development of rhabdomyolysis and other adverse effects. In clinical trials, the concomitant administration of sirolimus and HMG-CoA reductase inhibitors appeared to be well-tolerated).
No products indexed under this heading.

Fluvoxamine Maleate (Caution when using sirolimus with CYP3A4 inhibitors. The dosage of sirolimus and/or co-administered CYP3A4 inhibitors may need to be adjusted).
No products indexed under this heading.

Fosamprenavir Calcium (Exercise caution when using sirolimus with drugs or agents that are modulators of CYP3A4. Co-administration of sirolimus with HIV protease inhibitors may increase sirolimus blood concentrations. The dosage of sirolimus and/or the HIV protease inhibitor may need to be adjusted). Products include:

Fosinopril Sodium (Sirolimus has been associated with the development of angioedema. The concomitant use of sirolimus with other drugs known to cause angioedema, such as ACE-inhibitors, may increase the risk of developing angioedema).
No products indexed under this heading.

Fosphenytoin (Exercise caution when using sirolimus with drugs or agents that are modulators of CYP3A4. Co-administration of sirolimus with phenytoin may decrease sirolimus blood concentrations. The dosage of sirolimus and/or phenytoin may need to be adjusted).
No products indexed under this heading.

Fosphenytoin Sodium (Exercise caution when using sirolimus with drugs or agents that are modulators of CYP3A4. Co-administration of sirolimus with phenytoin may decrease sirolimus blood concentrations. The dosage of sirolimus and/or phenytoin may need to be adjusted).
No products indexed under this heading.

Garlic Extract (Sirolimus is known to be a substrate for cytochrome P-450 3A4 (CYP3A4). Inducers of CYP3A4 may decrease sirolimus concentrations. Co-administration of sirolimus with strong inducers of CYP3A4 is not recommended).
No products indexed under this heading.

Garlic Oil (Sirolimus is known to be a substrate for cytochrome P-450 3A4 (CYP3A4). Inducers of CYP3A4 may decrease sirolimus concentrations. Co-administration of sirolimus with strong inducers of CYP3A4 is not recommended).
No products indexed under this heading.

Gemfibrozil (During sirolimus therapy with cyclosporine, patients administered a fibrate should be monitored for the possible development of rhabdomyolysis and other adverse effects. In clinical trials, the concomitant administration of sirolimus and fibrates appeared to be well-tolerated).
No products indexed under this heading.

Haloperidol (Care should be exercised when drugs or other substances that are substrates of CYP3A4 are administered concomitantly with sirolimus).
No products indexed under this heading.

Haloperidol Decanoate (Care should be exercised when drugs or other substances that are substrates of CYP3A4 are administered concomitantly with sirolimus).
No products indexed under this heading.

Haloperidol Lactate (Care should be exercised when drugs or other substances that are substrates of CYP3A4 are administered concomitantly with sirolimus).
No products indexed under this heading.

Hydrocortisone (Sirolimus is known to be a substrate for cytochrome P-450 3A4 (CYP3A4). Inducers of CYP3A4 may decrease sirolimus concentrations. Co-administration of sirolimus with strong inducers of CYP3A4 is not recommended).
No products indexed under this heading.

Hydrocortisone (Alcohol) (Sirolimus is known to be a substrate for cytochrome P-450 3A4 (CYP3A4). Inducers of CYP3A4 may decrease sirolimus concentrations. Co-administration of sirolimus with strong inducers of CYP3A4 is not recommended).

1561 Interactions Index Rapamune

Hydrocortisone Acetate (Sirolimus is known to be a substrate for cytochrome P-450 3A4 (CYP3A4). Inducers of CYP3A4 may decrease sirolimus concentrations. Co-administration of sirolimus with strong inducers of CYP3A4 is not recommended).
No products indexed under this heading.

Hydrocortisone Butyrate (Sirolimus is known to be a substrate for cytochrome P-450 3A4 (CYP3A4). Inducers of CYP3A4 may decrease sirolimus concentrations. Co-administration of sirolimus with strong inducers of CYP3A4 is not recommended).
No products indexed under this heading.

Hydrocortisone Cypionate (Sirolimus is known to be a substrate for cytochrome P-450 3A4 (CYP3A4). Inducers of CYP3A4 may decrease sirolimus concentrations. Co-administration of sirolimus with strong inducers of CYP3A4 is not recommended).
No products indexed under this heading.

Hydrocortisone Hemisuccinate (Sirolimus is known to be a substrate for cytochrome P-450 3A4 (CYP3A4). Inducers of CYP3A4 may decrease sirolimus concentrations. Co-administration of sirolimus with strong inducers of CYP3A4 is not recommended).
No products indexed under this heading.

Hydrocortisone Probutate (Sirolimus is known to be a substrate for cytochrome P-450 3A4 (CYP3A4). Inducers of CYP3A4 may decrease sirolimus concentrations. Co-administration of sirolimus with strong inducers of CYP3A4 is not recommended).
No products indexed under this heading.

Hydrocortisone Sodium Phosphate (Sirolimus is known to be a substrate for cytochrome P-450 3A4 (CYP3A4). Inducers of CYP3A4 may decrease sirolimus concentrations. Co-administration of sirolimus with strong inducers of CYP3A4 is not recommended).
No products indexed under this heading.

Hydrocortisone Sodium Succinate (Sirolimus is known to be a substrate for cytochrome P-450 3A4 (CYP3A4). Inducers of CYP3A4 may decrease sirolimus concentrations. Co-administration of sirolimus with strong inducers of CYP3A4 is not recommended).
No products indexed under this heading.

Hydrocortisone Valerate (Sirolimus is known to be a substrate for cytochrome P-450 3A4 (CYP3A4). Inducers of CYP3A4 may decrease sirolimus concentrations. Co-administration of sirolimus with strong inducers of CYP3A4 is not recommended).
No products indexed under this heading.

Hypericum (St. John's wort (hypericum perforatum) induces CYP3A4 and P-gp. Since sirolimus is a substrate for both cytochrome CYP3A4 and P-gp, there is the potential that the use of St. John's wort in patients receiving sirolimus could result in reduced sirolimus concentrations).
No products indexed under this heading.

Hypericum Perforatum (Sirolimus is known to be a substrate for cytochrome P-450 3A4 (CYP3A4). Inducers of CYP3A4 may decrease sirolimus concentrations. Co-administration of sirolimus with strong inducers of CYP3A4 is not recommended). Products include:
Traumeel 1800

Imatinib Mesylate (Caution when using sirolimus with CYP3A4 inhibitors. The dosage of sirolimus and/or co-administered CYP3A4 inhibitors may need to be adjusted). Products include:
Gleevec 2477

Indinavir Sulfate (Exercise caution when using sirolimus with drugs or agents that are modulators of CYP3A4. Co-administration of sirolimus with indinavir may increase sirolimus blood concentrations. The dosage of sirolimus and/or indinavir may need to be adjusted). Products include:
Crixivan 2113

Influenza Vaccine, Live Attenuated (Immunosuppressants may affect response to vaccination. Therefore, during treatment with sirolimus, vaccination may be less effective. The use of live vaccines should be avoided).
No products indexed under this heading.

Influenza Virus Vaccine Live, Intranasal (Immunosuppressants may affect response to vaccination. Therefore, during treatment with sirolimus, vaccination may be less effective. The use of live vaccines should be avoided). Products include:
FluMist 2078

Isoniazid (Caution when using sirolimus with CYP3A4 inhibitors. The dosage of sirolimus and/or co-administered CYP3A4 inhibitors may need to be adjusted).
No products indexed under this heading.

Isradipine (Care should be exercised when drugs or other substances that are substrates of CYP3A4 are administered concomitantly with sirolimus). Products include:
DynaCirc CR 1432

Itraconazole (Sirolimus is known to be a substrate for cytochrome P-450 3A4 (CYP3A4). Co-administration of sirolimus with strong inhibitors of CYP3A4 such as itraconazole is not recommended).
No products indexed under this heading.

Ixabepilone (Care should be exercised when drugs or other substances that are substrates of CYP3A4 are administered concomitantly with sirolimus).
No products indexed under this heading.

Ketoconazole (Ketoconazole is a strong inhibitor of CYP3A4 and P-gp; co-administration of sirolimus oral solution or tablets and ketoconazole is not recommended. Multiple-dose ketoconazole administration significantly affected the rate and extent of absorption and sirolimus exposure after administration of sirolimus oral solution, as reflected by increases in sirolimus C_{max}, t_{max}, and AUC of 4.3-fold, 38%, and 10.9-fold, respectively. However, the terminal t1/2 of sirolimus was not changed. Single-dose sirolimus did not affect steady-state 12-hour plasma ketoconazole concentrations). Products include:
Extina 3319
Xolegel 3337

Lapatinib (Caution when using sirolimus with CYP3A4 inhibitors. The dosage of sirolimus and/or co-administered CYP3A4 inhibitors may need to be adjusted). Products include:
Tykerb 1698

Levonorgestrel (Care should be exercised when drugs or other substances that are substrates of CYP3A4 are administered concomitantly with sirolimus). Products include:
Climara Pro 847
LoSeasonique 3407
Lybrel 3514
Mirena 854
Plan B 3416
Seasonique 3418

Lidocaine (Care should be exercised when drugs or other substances that are substrates of CYP3A4 are administered concomitantly with sirolimus). Products include:
Lidoderm 1107

Lidocaine Hydrochloride (Care should be exercised when drugs or other substances that are substrates of CYP3A4 are administered concomitantly with sirolimus).
No products indexed under this heading.

Lisinopril (Sirolimus has been associated with the development of angioedema. The concomitant use of sirolimus with other drugs known to cause angioedema, such as ACE-inhibitors, may increase the risk of developing angioedema). Products include:
Prinivil 2241
Prinzide 2246

Lopinavir (Exercise caution when using sirolimus with drugs or agents that are modulators of CYP3A4. Co-administration of sirolimus with HIV protease inhibitors may increase sirolimus blood concentrations. The dosage of sirolimus and/or the HIV protease inhibitor may need to be adjusted). Products include:
Kaletra 458

Loratadine (Caution when using sirolimus with CYP3A4 inhibitors. The dosage of sirolimus and/or co-administered CYP3A4 inhibitors may need to be adjusted).
No products indexed under this heading.

Lovastatin (During sirolimus therapy with cyclosporine, patients administered an HMG-CoA reductase inhibitor and/or fibrate should be monitored for the possible development of rhabdomyolysis and other adverse effects. In clinical trials, the concomitant administration of sirolimus and HMG-CoA reductase inhibitors appeared to be well-tolerated). Products include:
Advicor 402
Mevacor 2212

Measles, Mumps, Rubella and Varicella Virus Vaccine Live (Immunosuppressants may affect response to vaccination. Therefore, during treatment with sirolimus, vaccination may be less effective. The use of live vaccines should be avoided). Products include:
ProQuad 2254

Measles, Mumps & Rubella Virus Vaccine, Live (Immunosuppressants may affect response to vaccination. Therefore, during treatment with sirolimus, vaccination may be less effective. The use of live vaccines should be avoided). Products include:
M-M-R II 2203
ProQuad 2254

Measles & Rubella Virus Vaccine Live (Immunosuppressants may affect response to vaccination. Therefore, during treatment with sirolimus, vaccination may be less effective. The use of live vaccines should be avoided).
No products indexed under this heading.

Measles Virus Vaccine Live (Immunosuppressants may affect response to vaccination. Therefore, during treatment with sirolimus, vaccination may be less effective. The use of live vaccines should be avoided). Products include:
Attenuvax 2086

Mephenytoin (Sirolimus is known to be a substrate for cytochrome P-450 3A4 (CYP3A4). Inducers of CYP3A4 may decrease sirolimus concentrations. Co-administration of sirolimus with strong inducers of CYP3A4 is not recommended).
No products indexed under this heading.

Mestranol (Care should be exercised when drugs or other substances that are substrates of CYP3A4 are administered concomitantly with sirolimus).
No products indexed under this heading.

Methadone Hydrochloride (Care should be exercised when drugs or other substances that are substrates of CYP3A4 are administered concomitantly with sirolimus).
No products indexed under this heading.

Methsuximide (Sirolimus is known to be a substrate for cytochrome P-450 3A4 (CYP3A4). Inducers of CYP3A4 may decrease sirolimus concentrations. Co-administration of sirolimus with strong inducers of CYP3A4 is not recommended).
No products indexed under this heading.

Methylprednisolone (Sirolimus is known to be a substrate for cytochrome P-450 3A4 (CYP3A4). Inducers of CYP3A4 may decrease sirolimus concentrations. Co-administration of sirolimus with strong inducers of CYP3A4 is not recommended).
No products indexed under this heading.

Methylprednisolone Acetate (Sirolimus is known to be a substrate for cytochrome P-450 3A4 (CYP3A4). Inducers of CYP3A4 may decrease sirolimus concentrations. Co-administration of sirolimus with strong inducers of CYP3A4 is not recommended).
No products indexed under this heading.

Methylprednisolone Sodium Succinate (Sirolimus is known to be a substrate for cytochrome P-450 3A4 (CYP3A4). Inducers of CYP3A4 may decrease sirolimus concentrations. Co-administration of sirolimus with strong inducers of CYP3A4 is not recommended).
No products indexed under this heading.

Metoclopramide Hydrochloride (Exercise caution when using sirolimus with drugs or agents that are modulators of CYP3A4. Co-administration of sirolimus with metoclopramide may increase sirolimus blood concentrations. The dosage of sirolimus and/or metoclopramide may need to be adjusted). Products include:
Metozolv ODT 2901

Metronidazole (Caution when using sirolimus with CYP3A4 inhibitors. The dosage of sirolimus and/or co-administered CYP3A4 inhibitors may need to be adjusted). Products include:
Pylera 793

Metronidazole Benzoate (Caution when using sirolimus with CYP3A4 inhibitors. The dosage of sirolimus and/or co-administered CYP3A4 inhibitors may need to be adjusted).
No products indexed under this heading.

Metronidazole Hydrochloride (Caution when using sirolimus with CYP3A4 inhibitors. The dosage of sirolimus and/or co-administered CYP3A4 inhibitors may need to be adjusted).
No products indexed under this heading.

Metronidazole Sodium (Caution when using sirolimus with CYP3A4 inhibitors. The dosage of sirolimus and/or co-administered CYP3A4 inhibitors may need to be adjusted).
No products indexed under this heading.

Mibefradil Dihydrochloride (Sirolimus is known to be a substrate for p-glycoprotein (P-gp). Inhibitors of P-gp may increase sirolimus concentrations. Co-administration of sirolimus with strong inhibitors of P-gp is not recommended).
No products indexed under this heading.

Miconazole (Caution when using sirolimus with CYP3A4 inhibitors. The dosage of sirolimus and/or co-administered CYP3A4 inhibitors may need to be adjusted).
No products indexed under this heading.

Miconazole Nitrate (Caution when using sirolimus with CYP3A4 inhibitors.

IMPORTANT NOTE: Always consult each drug listing in the patient's regimen for possible interactions.

Rapamune Interactions Index 1562

The dosage of sirolimus and/or co-administered CYP3A4 inhibitors may need to be adjusted). Products include:
Vusion Ointment 3335

Midazolam Hydrochloride (Care should be exercised when drugs or other substances that are substrates of CYP3A4 are administered concomitantly with sirolimus).
No products indexed under this heading.

Mifepristone (Caution when using sirolimus with CYP3A4 inhibitors. The dosage of sirolimus and/or co-administered CYP3A4 inhibitors may need to be adjusted).
No products indexed under this heading.

Modafinil (Sirolimus is known to be a substrate for cytochrome P-450 3A4 (CYP3A4). Inducers of CYP3A4 may decrease sirolimus concentrations. Co-administration of sirolimus with strong inducers of CYP3A4 is not recommended). Products include:
Provigil 983

Moexipril Hydrochloride (Sirolimus has been associated with the development of angioedema. The concomitant use of sirolimus with other drugs known to cause angioedema, such as ACE-inhibitors, may increase the risk of developing angioedema).
No products indexed under this heading.

Mometasone Furoate (Safety and efficacy information from a controlled clinical trial in pediatric and adolescent (<18 years of age) renal transplant patients judged to be at high-immunologic risk, defined as a history of one or more acute rejection episodes and/or the presence of chronic allograft nephropathy, do not support the chronic use of sirolimus in combination with calcineurin inhibitors and corticosteroids, due to the higher incidence of lipid abnormalities and deterioration of renal function associated with these immunosuppressive regimens compared to calcineurin inhibitors, without increased benefit with respect to acute rejection, graft survival, or patient survival). Products include:
Asmanex 3058
Elocon Cream 3111
Elocon Lotion 3112
Elocon Ointment 3114

Mometasone Furoate Monohydrate (Safety and efficacy information from a controlled clinical trial in pediatric and adolescent (<18 years of age) renal transplant patients judged to be at high-immunologic risk, defined as a history of one or more acute rejection episodes and/or the presence of chronic allograft nephropathy, do not support the chronic use of sirolimus in combination with calcineurin inhibitors and corticosteroids, due to the higher incidence of lipid abnormalities and deterioration of renal function associated with these immunosuppressive regimens compared to calcineurin inhibitors, without increased benefit with respect to acute rejection, graft survival, or patient survival). Products include:
Nasonex 3166

Mumps Virus Vaccine, Live (Immunosuppressants may affect response to vaccination. Therefore, during treatment with sirolimus, vaccination may be less effective. The use of live vaccines should be avoided). Products include:
Mumpsvax 2218

Nafcillin Sodium (Sirolimus is known to be a substrate for cytochrome P-450 3A4 (CYP3A4). Inducers of CYP3A4 may decrease sirolimus concentrations. Co-administration of sirolimus with strong inducers of CYP3A4 is not recommended).
No products indexed under this heading.

Nefazodone Hydrochloride (Care should be exercised when drugs or other substances that are substrates of CYP3A4 are administered concomitantly with sirolimus).
No products indexed under this heading.

Nelfinavir Mesylate (Exercise caution when using sirolimus with drugs or agents that are modulators of CYP3A4. Co-administration of sirolimus with HIV protease inhibitors may increase sirolimus blood concentrations. The dosage of sirolimus and/or the HIV protease inhibitor may need to be adjusted).
No products indexed under this heading.

Nevirapine (Sirolimus is known to be a substrate for cytochrome P-450 3A4 (CYP3A4). Inducers of CYP3A4 may decrease sirolimus concentrations. Co-administration of sirolimus with strong inducers of CYP3A4 is not recommended). Products include:
Viramune Oral Suspension 897
Viramune Tablets 897

Niacin (Caution when using sirolimus with CYP3A4 inhibitors. The dosage of sirolimus and/or co-administered CYP3A4 inhibitors may need to be adjusted). Products include:
Advicor 402
Cardio Basics 3455
Niaspan 497
Simcor 524

Niacinamide (Caution when using sirolimus with CYP3A4 inhibitors. The dosage of sirolimus and/or co-administered CYP3A4 inhibitors may need to be adjusted). Products include:
CitraNatal 90 DHA Capsules 2332
CitraNatal Assure 2332
CitraNatal Rx 2332
Heplive 607

Niacinamide Hydroiodide (Caution when using sirolimus with CYP3A4 inhibitors. The dosage of sirolimus and/or co-administered CYP3A4 inhibitors may need to be adjusted).
No products indexed under this heading.

Nicardipine (Exercise caution when using sirolimus with drugs or agents that are modulators of CYP3A4. Co-administration of sirolimus with nicardipine may increase sirolimus blood concentrations. The dosage of sirolimus and/or nicardipine may need to be adjusted).
No products indexed under this heading.

Nicardipine Hydrochloride (Exercise caution when using sirolimus with drugs or agents that are modulators of CYP3A4. Co-administration of sirolimus with nicardipine may increase sirolimus blood concentrations. The dosage of sirolimus and/or nicardipine may need to be adjusted).
No products indexed under this heading.

Nicotinamide (Caution when using sirolimus with CYP3A4 inhibitors. The dosage of sirolimus and/or co-administered CYP3A4 inhibitors may need to be adjusted).
No products indexed under this heading.

Nifedipine (Care should be exercised when drugs or other substances that are substrates of CYP3A4 are administered concomitantly with sirolimus).
No products indexed under this heading.

Nimodipine (Care should be exercised when drugs or other substances that are substrates of CYP3A4 are administered concomitantly with sirolimus).
No products indexed under this heading.

Nisoldipine (Care should be exercised when drugs or other substances that are substrates of CYP3A4 are administered concomitantly with sirolimus).
No products indexed under this heading.

Nitrendipine (Care should be exercised when drugs or other substances that are substrates of CYP3A4 are administered concomitantly with sirolimus).
No products indexed under this heading.

Norethindrone (Care should be exercised when drugs or other substances that are substrates of CYP3A4 are administered concomitantly with sirolimus). Products include:
Ortho Micronor 2660

Norethindrone Acetate (Care should be exercised when drugs or other substances that are substrates of CYP3A4 are administered concomitantly with sirolimus). Products include:
Activella 2561

Norfloxacin (Caution when using sirolimus with CYP3A4 inhibitors. The dosage of sirolimus and/or co-administered CYP3A4 inhibitors may need to be adjusted). Products include:
Noroxin 2220

Norgestrel (Care should be exercised when drugs or other substances that are substrates of CYP3A4 are administered concomitantly with sirolimus).
No products indexed under this heading.

Omeprazole (Caution when using sirolimus with CYP3A4 inhibitors. The dosage of sirolimus and/or co-administered CYP3A4 inhibitors may need to be adjusted).
No products indexed under this heading.

Ondansetron (Care should be exercised when drugs or other substances that are substrates of CYP3A4 are administered concomitantly with sirolimus).
No products indexed under this heading.

Ondansetron Hydrochloride (Care should be exercised when drugs or other substances that are substrates of CYP3A4 are administered concomitantly with sirolimus). Products include:
Zofran Injection 1750
Zofran 1756
Zofran ODT 1756

Oxcarbazepine (Sirolimus is known to be a substrate for cytochrome P-450 3A4 (CYP3A4). Inducers of CYP3A4 may decrease sirolimus concentrations. Co-administration of sirolimus with strong inducers of CYP3A4 is not recommended).
No products indexed under this heading.

Paclitaxel (Care should be exercised when drugs or other substances that are substrates of CYP3A4 are administered concomitantly with sirolimus).
No products indexed under this heading.

Paroxetine Hydrochloride (Caution when using sirolimus with CYP3A4 inhibitors. The dosage of sirolimus and/or co-administered CYP3A4 inhibitors may need to be adjusted). Products include:
Paroxetine CR 2361
Paroxetine ER 2371
Paxil 1586
Paxil CR 1596

Perindopril Erbumine (Sirolimus has been associated with the development of angioedema. The concomitant use of sirolimus with other drugs known to cause angioedema, such as ACE-inhibitors, may increase the risk of developing angioedema).
No products indexed under this heading.

Phenobarbital (Exercise caution when using sirolimus with drugs or agents that are modulators of CYP3A4. Co-administration of sirolimus with phenobarbital may decrease sirolimus blood concentrations. The dosage of sirolimus and/or phenobarbital may need to be adjusted). Products include:
Donnatal 2711

Phenobarbital Sodium (Exercise caution when using sirolimus with drugs or agents that are modulators of CYP3A4. Co-administration of sirolimus with phenobarbital may decrease sirolimus blood concentrations. The dosage of sirolimus and/or phenobarbital may need to be adjusted).
No products indexed under this heading.

Phenytoin (Exercise caution when using sirolimus with drugs or agents that are modulators of CYP3A4. Co-administration of sirolimus with phenytoin may decrease sirolimus blood concentrations. The dosage of sirolimus and/or phenytoin may need to be adjusted).
No products indexed under this heading.

Phenytoin Sodium (Exercise caution when using sirolimus with drugs or agents that are modulators of CYP3A4. Co-administration of sirolimus with phenytoin may decrease sirolimus blood concentrations. The dosage of sirolimus and/or phenytoin may need to be adjusted). Products include:
Phenytek Capsules 2380

Pimozide (Care should be exercised when drugs or other substances that are substrates of CYP3A4 are administered concomitantly with sirolimus).
No products indexed under this heading.

Poliovirus Vaccine, Live, Oral, Trivalent, Types 1,2,3 (Sabin) (Immunosuppressants may affect response to vaccination. Therefore, during treatment with sirolimus, vaccination may be less effective. The use of live vaccines should be avoided).
No products indexed under this heading.

Polyestradiol Phosphate (Care should be exercised when drugs or other substances that are substrates of CYP3A4 are administered concomitantly with sirolimus).
No products indexed under this heading.

Posaconazole (Caution when using sirolimus with CYP3A4 inhibitors. The dosage of sirolimus and/or co-administered CYP3A4 inhibitors may need to be adjusted). Products include:
Noxafil 3172

Pravastatin Sodium (During sirolimus therapy with cyclosporine, patients administered an HMG-CoA reductase inhibitor and/or fibrate should be monitored for the possible development of rhabdomyolysis and other adverse effects. In clinical trials, the concomitant administration of sirolimus and HMG-CoA reductase inhibitors appeared to be well-tolerated).
No products indexed under this heading.

Prednisolone (Sirolimus is known to be a substrate for cytochrome P-450 3A4 (CYP3A4). Inducers of CYP3A4 may decrease sirolimus concentrations. Co-administration of sirolimus with strong inducers of CYP3A4 is not recommended).
No products indexed under this heading.

Prednisolone Acetate (Sirolimus is known to be a substrate for cytochrome P-450 3A4 (CYP3A4). Inducers of CYP3A4 may decrease sirolimus concentrations. Co-administration of sirolimus with strong inducers of CYP3A4 is not recommended). Products include:
Blephamide .... ⊙212, ⊙214
Pred Forte .... ⊙225
Pred Mild .... ⊙230
Pred-G .... ⊙226, ⊙227

Prednisolone Sodium Phosphate (Sirolimus is known to be a substrate for cytochrome P-450 3A4 (CYP3A4). Inducers of CYP3A4 may decrease sirolimus concentrations. Co-administration of sirolimus with strong inducers of CYP3A4 is not recommended).
No products indexed under this heading.

Prednisolone Tebutate (Sirolimus is known to be a substrate for cytochrome P-450 3A4 (CYP3A4). Inducers of CYP3A4 may decrease sirolimus concentrations. Co-administration of sirolimus with strong inducers of CYP3A4 is not recommended).
No products indexed under this heading.

Prednisone (Sirolimus is known to be a substrate for cytochrome P-450 3A4 (CYP3A4). Inducers of CYP3A4 may decrease sirolimus concentrations. Co-administration of sirolimus with strong inducers of CYP3A4 is not recommended).
No products indexed under this heading.

Prednisone sodium phosphate (Sirolimus is known to be a substrate for cytochrome P-450 3A4 (CYP3A4). Inducers of CYP3A4 may decrease sirolimus concentrations. Co-administration of sirolimus with strong inducers of CYP3A4 is not recommended).
No products indexed under this heading.

Primidone (Sirolimus is known to be a substrate for cytochrome P-450 3A4 (CYP3A4). Inducers of CYP3A4 may decrease sirolimus concentrations. Co-administration of sirolimus with strong inducers of CYP3A4 is not recommended).
No products indexed under this heading.

Propoxyphene Hydrochloride (Caution when using sirolimus with CYP3A4 inhibitors. The dosage of sirolimus and/or co-administered CYP3A4 inhibitors may need to be adjusted).
No products indexed under this heading.

Propoxyphene Napsylate (Caution when using sirolimus with CYP3A4 inhibitors. The dosage of sirolimus and/or co-administered CYP3A4 inhibitors may need to be adjusted).
No products indexed under this heading.

Quinapril Hydrochloride (Sirolimus has been associated with the development of angioedema. The concomitant use of sirolimus with other drugs known to cause angioedema, such as ACE-inhibitors, may increase the risk of developing angioedema).
No products indexed under this heading.

Quinidine (Sirolimus is known to be a substrate for p-glycoprotein (P-gp). Inhibitors of P-gp may increase sirolimus concentrations. Co-administration of sirolimus with strong inhibitors of P-gp is not recommended).
No products indexed under this heading.

Quinidine Gluconate (Sirolimus is known to be a substrate for p-glycoprotein (P-gp). Inhibitors of P-gp may increase sirolimus concentrations. Co-administration of sirolimus with strong inhibitors of P-gp is not recommended).
No products indexed under this heading.

Quinidine Hydrochloride (Sirolimus is known to be a substrate for p-glycoprotein (P-gp). Inhibitors of P-gp may increase sirolimus concentrations. Co-administration of sirolimus with strong inhibitors of P-gp is not recommended).
No products indexed under this heading.

Quinidine Polygalacturonate (Sirolimus is known to be a substrate for p-glycoprotein (P-gp). Inhibitors of P-gp may increase sirolimus concentrations. Co-administration of sirolimus with strong inhibitors of P-gp is not recommended).
No products indexed under this heading.

Quinidine Sulfate (Sirolimus is known to be a substrate for p-glycoprotein (P-gp). Inhibitors of P-gp may increase sirolimus concentrations. Co-administration of sirolimus with strong inhibitors of P-gp is not recommended).
No products indexed under this heading.

Quinine (Caution when using sirolimus with CYP3A4 inhibitors. The dosage of sirolimus and/or co-administered CYP3A4 inhibitors may need to be adjusted). Products include:
Hyland's Leg Cramps PM with Quinine...................................... **3315**

Quinine Sulfate (Caution when using sirolimus with CYP3A4 inhibitors. The dosage of sirolimus and/or co-administered CYP3A4 inhibitors may need to be adjusted).
No products indexed under this heading.

Quinupristin (Caution when using sirolimus with CYP3A4 inhibitors. The dosage of sirolimus and/or co-administered CYP3A4 inhibitors may need to be adjusted).
No products indexed under this heading.

Ramipril (Sirolimus has been associated with the development of angioedema. The concomitant use of sirolimus with other drugs known to cause angioedema, such as ACE-inhibitors, may increase the risk of developing angioedema).
No products indexed under this heading.

Ranitidine Bismuth Citrate (Caution when using sirolimus with CYP3A4 inhibitors. The dosage of sirolimus and/or co-administered CYP3A4 inhibitors may need to be adjusted).
No products indexed under this heading.

Ranitidine Hydrochloride (Caution when using sirolimus with CYP3A4 inhibitors. The dosage of sirolimus and/or co-administered CYP3A4 inhibitors may need to be adjusted). Products include:
Zantac **1737**
Zantac Injection **1732**
Zantac Pharmacy **1735**

Rifabutin (Sirolimus is known to be a substrate for cytochrome P-450 3A4 (CYP3A4). Co-administration of sirolimus with strong inducers of CYP3A4 such as rifabutin is not recommended).
No products indexed under this heading.

Rifampicin (Sirolimus is known to be a substrate for cytochrome P-450 3A4 (CYP3A4). Inducers of CYP3A4 may decrease sirolimus concentrations. Co-administration of sirolimus with strong inducers of CYP3A4 is not recommended).
No products indexed under this heading.

Rifampin (Rifampin is a strong inducer of CYP3A4 and P-gp; co-administration of sirolimus oral solution or tablets and rifampin is not recommended. In patients where rifampin is indicated, alternative therapeutic agents with less enzyme induction potential should be considered. Pretreatment of 14 healthy volunteers with multiple doses of rifampin, 600 mg daily for 14 days, followed by a single 20-mg dose of sirolimus oral solution, greatly decreased sirolimus AUC and C_{max} by about 82% and 71%, respectively).
No products indexed under this heading.

Rifapentine (Exercise caution when using sirolimus with drugs or agents that are modulators of CYP3A4. Co-administration of sirolimus with rifapentine may decrease sirolimus blood concentrations. The dosage of sirolimus and/or rifapentine may need to be adjusted).
No products indexed under this heading.

Ritonavir (Exercise caution when using sirolimus with drugs or agents that are modulators of CYP3A4. Co-administration of sirolimus with ritonavir may increase sirolimus blood concentrations. The dosage of sirolimus and/or ritonavir may need to be adjusted). Products include:
Kaletra **458**
Norvir **509**

Rosuvastatin Calcium (During sirolimus therapy with cyclosporine, patients administered an HMG-CoA reductase inhibitor and/or fibrate should be monitored for the possible development of rhabdomyolysis and other adverse effects. In clinical trials, the concomitant administration of sirolimus and HMG-CoA reductase inhibitors appeared to be well-tolerated). Products include:
Crestor **736**

Rotavirus Vaccine, Live, Oral, Tetravalent (Immunosuppressants may affect response to vaccination. Therefore, during treatment with sirolimus, vaccination may be less effective. The use of live vaccines should be avoided).
No products indexed under this heading.

Rubella & Mumps Virus Vaccine Live (Immunosuppressants may affect response to vaccination. Therefore, during treatment with sirolimus, vaccination may be less effective. The use of live vaccines should be avoided).
No products indexed under this heading.

Rubella Virus Vaccine Live (Immunosuppressants may affect response to vaccination. Therefore, during treatment with sirolimus, vaccination may be less effective. The use of live vaccines should be avoided). Products include:
Meruvax II **2210**

Saquinavir (Exercise caution when using sirolimus with drugs or agents that are modulators of CYP3A4. Co-administration of sirolimus with HIV protease inhibitors may increase sirolimus blood concentrations. The dosage of sirolimus and/or the HIV protease inhibitor may need to be adjusted).
No products indexed under this heading.

Saquinavir Mesylate (Exercise caution when using sirolimus with drugs or agents that are modulators of CYP3A4. Co-administration of sirolimus with HIV protease inhibitors may increase sirolimus blood concentrations. The dosage of sirolimus and/or the HIV protease inhibitor may need to be adjusted).
No products indexed under this heading.

Sertraline Hydrochloride (Care should be exercised when drugs or other substances that are substrates of CYP3A4 are administered concomitantly with sirolimus).
No products indexed under this heading.

Sildenafil Citrate (Care should be exercised when drugs or other substances that are substrates of CYP3A4 are administered concomitantly with sirolimus).
No products indexed under this heading.

Simvastatin (During sirolimus therapy with cyclosporine, patients administered an HMG-CoA reductase inhibitor and/or fibrate should be monitored for the possible development of rhabdomyolysis and other adverse effects. In clinical trials, the concomitant administration of sirolimus and HMG-CoA reductase inhibitors appeared to be well-tolerated). Products include:
Simcor **524**
Vytorin 10/10 .... **2303, 3240**
Vytorin 10/20 .... **2303, 3240**
Vytorin 10/40 .... **2303, 3240**
Vytorin 10/80 .... **2303, 3240**
Zocor **2289**

Smallpox Vaccine (Immunosuppressants may affect response to vaccination. Therefore, during treatment with sirolimus, vaccination may be less effective. The use of live vaccines should be avoided).
No products indexed under this heading.

Spirapril Hydrochloride (Sirolimus has been associated with the development of angioedema. The concomitant use of sirolimus with other drugs known to cause angioedema, such as ACE-inhibitors, may increase the risk of developing angioedema).
No products indexed under this heading.

Sulfinpyrazone (Sirolimus is known to be a substrate for cytochrome P-450 3A4 (CYP3A4). Inducers of CYP3A4 may decrease sirolimus concentrations. Co-administration of sirolimus with strong inducers of CYP3A4 is not recommended).
No products indexed under this heading.

Tacrolimus (The use of sirolimus in combination with tacrolimus was associated with excess mortality and graft loss in a study in de novo liver transplant patients (22% in combination versus 9% on tacrolimus alone). Many of these patients had evidence of infection at or near the time of death. In this and another study in de novo liver transplant patients, the use of sirolimus in combination with tacrolimus was associated with an increase in hepatic artery thrombosis (HAT) (7% in combination versus 2% in the control arm); most cases of HAT occurred within 30 days post-transplantation, and most led to graft loss or death. The safety and efficacy of sirolimus in liver transplant patients has not been established and is, therefore, not recommended). Products include:
Prograf Capsules **677**
Prograf Injection **677**
Protopic **685**

Tadalafil (Care should be exercised when drugs or other substances that are substrates of CYP3A4 are administered concomitantly with sirolimus). Products include:
Adcirca **3461**
Cialis **1861**

Tamoxifen Citrate (Sirolimus is known to be a substrate for p-glycoprotein (P-gp). Inhibitors of P-gp may increase sirolimus concentrations. Co-administration of sirolimus with strong inhibitors of P-gp is not recommended).
No products indexed under this heading.

Telithromycin (Sirolimus is known to be a substrate for cytochrome P-450 3A4 (CYP3A4). Co-administration of sirolimus with strong inhibitors of CYP3A4 such as telithromycin is not recommended). Products include:
Ketek **2991**

Terfenadine (Care should be exercised when drugs or other substances that are substrates of CYP3A4 are administered concomitantly with sirolimus).
No products indexed under this heading.

Theophyllinate (Sirolimus is known to be a substrate for cytochrome P-450 3A4 (CYP3A4). Inducers of CYP3A4 may decrease sirolimus concentrations. Co-administration of sirolimus with strong inducers of CYP3A4 is not recommended).
No products indexed under this heading.

Theophylline (Care should be exercised when drugs or other substances that are substrates of CYP3A4 are administered concomitantly with sirolimus).
No products indexed under this heading.

Theophylline Anhydrous (Care should be exercised when drugs or other substances that are substrates of CYP3A4 are administered concomitantly with sirolimus). Products include:
Uniphyl **2817**

Theophylline Calcium Salicylate (Care should be exercised when drugs or other substances that are substrates of CYP3A4 are administered concomitantly with sirolimus).
 No products indexed under this heading.

Theophylline Dihydroxypropyl (Glyceryl) (Care should be exercised when drugs or other substances that are substrates of CYP3A4 are administered concomitantly with sirolimus).
 No products indexed under this heading.

Theophylline Ethylenediamine (Care should be exercised when drugs or other substances that are substrates of CYP3A4 are administered concomitantly with sirolimus).
 No products indexed under this heading.

Theophylline Sodium Glycinate (Care should be exercised when drugs or other substances that are substrates of CYP3A4 are administered concomitantly with sirolimus).
 No products indexed under this heading.

Tiagabine Hydrochloride (Care should be exercised when drugs or other substances that are substrates of CYP3A4 are administered concomitantly with sirolimus). Products include:
 Gabitril 972

Tipranavir (Exercise caution when using sirolimus with drugs or agents that are modulators of CYP3A4. Co-administration of sirolimus with HIV protease inhibitors may increase sirolimus blood concentrations. The dosage of sirolimus and/or the HIV protease inhibitor may need to be adjusted).
 No products indexed under this heading.

Tolterodine Tartrate (Care should be exercised when drugs or other substances that are substrates of CYP3A4 are administered concomitantly with sirolimus).
 No products indexed under this heading.

Trandolapril (Sirolimus has been associated with the development of angioedema. The concomitant use of sirolimus with other drugs known to cause angioedema, such as ACE-inhibitors, may increase the risk of developing angioedema). Products include:
 Mavik 489
 Tarka 534

Trazodone Hydrochloride (Care should be exercised when drugs or other substances that are substrates of CYP3A4 are administered concomitantly with sirolimus).
 No products indexed under this heading.

Triamcinolone (Sirolimus is known to be a substrate for cytochrome P-450 3A4 (CYP3A4). Inducers of CYP3A4 may decrease sirolimus concentrations. Co-administration of sirolimus with strong inducers of CYP3A4 is not recommended).
 No products indexed under this heading.

Triamcinolone Acetonide (Sirolimus is known to be a substrate for cytochrome P-450 3A4 (CYP3A4). Inducers of CYP3A4 may decrease sirolimus concentrations. Co-administration of sirolimus with strong inducers of CYP3A4 is not recommended). Products include:
 Azmacort 408
 Nasacort AQ 3019

Triamcinolone Diacetate (Sirolimus is known to be a substrate for cytochrome P-450 3A4 (CYP3A4). Inducers of CYP3A4 may decrease sirolimus concentrations. Co-administration of sirolimus with strong inducers of CYP3A4 is not recommended).
 No products indexed under this heading.

Triamcinolone Hexacetonide (Sirolimus is known to be a substrate for cytochrome P-450 3A4 (CYP3A4). Inducers of CYP3A4 may decrease sirolimus concentrations. Co-administration of sirolimus with strong inducers of CYP3A4 is not recommended).
 No products indexed under this heading.

Triazolam (Care should be exercised when drugs or other substances that are substrates of CYP3A4 are administered concomitantly with sirolimus).
 No products indexed under this heading.

Troglitazone (Sirolimus is known to be a substrate for cytochrome P-450 3A4 (CYP3A4). Inducers of CYP3A4 may decrease sirolimus concentrations. Co-administration of sirolimus with strong inducers of CYP3A4 is not recommended).
 No products indexed under this heading.

Troleandomycin (Exercise caution when using sirolimus with drugs or agents that are modulators of CYP3A4. Co-administration of sirolimus with troleandomycin may increase sirolimus blood concentrations. The dosage of sirolimus and/or troleandomycin may need to be adjusted).
 No products indexed under this heading.

Typhoid Vaccine (Immunosuppressants may affect response to vaccination. Therefore, during treatment with sirolimus, vaccination may be less effective. The use of live vaccines should be avoided).
 No products indexed under this heading.

Valproate Sodium (Caution when using sirolimus with CYP3A4 inhibitors. The dosage of sirolimus and/or co-administered CYP3A4 inhibitors may need to be adjusted).
 No products indexed under this heading.

Vardenafil Hydrochloride (Care should be exercised when drugs or other substances that are substrates of CYP3A4 are administered concomitantly with sirolimus). Products include:
 Levitra 3157

Varicella Virus Vaccine, Live (Immunosuppressants may affect response to vaccination. Therefore, during treatment with sirolimus, vaccination may be less effective. The use of live vaccines should be avoided). Products include:
 Varivax 2285

Verapamil Hydrochloride (Verapamil is a substrate and inhibitor of CYP3A4 and P-gp; sirolimus concentrations should be monitored and a dose adjustment may be necessary. The simultaneous oral administration of 2 mg daily of sirolimus oral solution and 180 mg q 12h of verapamil at steady state to 26 healthy volunteers significantly affected the bioavailability of sirolimus and verapamil. Sirolimus C_{max} and AUC were increased 2.3- and 2.2-fold, respectively, without substantial change in t_{max}. The C_{max} and AUC of the pharmacologically active S(-) enantiomer of verapamil were both increased 1.5-fold and t_{max} was decreased by 1.2 hour). Products include:
 Tarka 534

Vinblastine Sulfate (Care should be exercised when drugs or other substances that are substrates of CYP3A4 are administered concomitantly with sirolimus).
 No products indexed under this heading.

Vincristine Sulfate (Care should be exercised when drugs or other substances that are substrates of CYP3A4 are administered concomitantly with sirolimus).
 No products indexed under this heading.

Voriconazole (Sirolimus is known to be a substrate for cytochrome P-450 3A4 (CYP3A4). Co-administration of sirolimus with strong inhibitors of CYP3A4 such as voriconazole is not recommended).
 No products indexed under this heading.

Warfarin Sodium (Care should be exercised when drugs or other substances that are substrates of CYP3A4 are administered concomitantly with sirolimus).
 No products indexed under this heading.

Yellow Fever Vaccine (Immunosuppressants may affect response to vaccination. Therefore, during treatment with sirolimus, vaccination may be less effective. The use of live vaccines should be avoided).
 No products indexed under this heading.

Zafirlukast (Caution when using sirolimus with CYP3A4 inhibitors. The dosage of sirolimus and/or co-administered CYP3A4 inhibitors may need to be adjusted). Products include:
 Accolate 3612

Zileuton (Caution when using sirolimus with CYP3A4 inhibitors. The dosage of sirolimus and/or co-administered CYP3A4 inhibitors may need to be adjusted).
 No products indexed under this heading.

Zoster Vaccine Live (Immunosuppressants may affect response to vaccination. Therefore, during treatment with sirolimus, vaccination may be less effective. The use of live vaccines should be avoided). Products include:
 Zostavax 2299

Food Interactions

Food, unspecified (In healthy subjects, a high-fat meal (861.8 kcal, 54.9% kcal from fat) increased the mean total exposure (AUC) of sirolimus by 23% to 35% compared with fasting. The effect of food on the mean sirolimus C_{max} was inconsistent depending on the sirolimus dosage form evaluated).

Grapefruit (Caution when using sirolimus with CYP3A4 inhibitors. The dosage of sirolimus and/or co-administered CYP3A4 inhibitors may need to be adjusted).

Grapefruit Juice (Because grapefruit juice inhibits the CYP3A4-mediated metabolism of sirolimus, it must not be taken with or be used for dilution of sirolimus).

REBETOL CAPSULES

(Ribavirin) 3207
May interact with antacids. Compounds in these categories include:

Aluminum Carbonate (Co-administration of ribavirin capsules with an antacid containing magnesium, aluminum and simethicone resulted in a 14% decrease in mean ribavirin AUC. The clinical relevance of results from this study is unknown).
 No products indexed under this heading.

Aluminum Hydroxide (Co-administration of ribavirin capsules with an antacid containing magnesium, aluminum and simethicone resulted in a 14% decrease in mean ribavirin AUC. The clinical relevance of results from this study is unknown).
 No products indexed under this heading.

Calcium Carbonate (Co-administration of ribavirin capsules with an antacid containing magnesium, aluminum and simethicone resulted in a 14% decrease in mean ribavirin AUC. The clinical relevance of results from this study is unknown). Products include:
 Chelated Mineral 3476

 Pepcid Complete 1822
 Extra Strength Rolaids Softchews Vanilla Creme 2045

Didanosine (Co-administration of ribavirin and didanosine is not recommended due to reports of fatal hepatic failure, peripheral neuropathy, pancreatitis, and symptomatic hyperlactactemia/lactic acidosis in clinical trials).
 No products indexed under this heading.

Magaldrate (Co-administration of ribavirin capsules with an antacid containing magnesium, aluminum and simethicone resulted in a 14% decrease in mean ribavirin AUC. The clinical relevance of results from this study is unknown).
 No products indexed under this heading.

Magnesium Carbonate (Co-administration of ribavirin capsules with an antacid containing magnesium, aluminum and simethicone resulted in a 14% decrease in mean ribavirin AUC. The clinical relevance of results from this study is unknown).
 No products indexed under this heading.

Magnesium Hydroxide (Co-administration of ribavirin capsules with an antacid containing magnesium, aluminum and simethicone resulted in a 14% decrease in mean ribavirin AUC. The clinical relevance of results from this study is unknown). Products include:
 Fleet Pedia-Lax Chewable Tablets 1144
 Pepcid Complete 1822

Magnesium Oxide (Co-administration of ribavirin capsules with an antacid containing magnesium, aluminum and simethicone resulted in a 14% decrease in mean ribavirin AUC. The clinical relevance of results from this study is unknown). Products include:
 Beelith 873

Magnesium Trisilicate (Co-administration of ribavirin capsules with an antacid containing magnesium, aluminum and simethicone resulted in a 14% decrease in mean ribavirin AUC. The clinical relevance of results from this study is unknown).
 No products indexed under this heading.

Sodium Bicarbonate (Co-administration of ribavirin capsules with an antacid containing magnesium, aluminum and simethicone resulted in a 14% decrease in mean ribavirin AUC. The clinical relevance of results from this study is unknown).
 No products indexed under this heading.

Stavudine (Ribavirin may antagonize the in vitro anti-viral activity of stavudine against HIV; concomitant use of ribavirin with stavudine should be used with caution).
 No products indexed under this heading.

Zidovudine (Ribavirin may antagonize the in vitro anti-viral activity of zidovudine against HIV; concomitant use of ribavirin with zidovudine should be used with caution). Products include:
 Combivir 1404
 Retrovir 1634
 Retrovir IV 1640
 Trizivir 1688

REBETOL ORAL SOLUTION

(Ribavirin) 3207
See Rebetol Capsules

REBIF PREFILLED SYRINGE FOR INJECTION

(Interferon Beta-1a) 1096
May interact with agents associated with myelosuppression, hepatotoxic drugs, killed/inactivated vaccines, vaccines, live. Compounds in these categories include:

Altretamine (Due to its potential to cause neutropenia and lymphopenia,

proper monitoring of patients is required if interferon β-1a is given in combination with myelosuppressive agents). Products include:

Hexalen **1066**

Amiodarone Hydrochloride (The potential risk of interferon β-1a used in combination with known hepatotoxic products should be considered prior to administration or when adding new agents to the regimen of patients on therapy. Reduction of interferon β-1 dose should be considered if SGPT rises above 5 times the upper limit of normal. The dose may be gradually re-escalated when enzyme levels have normalized).

No products indexed under this heading.

Amitriptyline Hydrochloride (The potential risk of interferon β-1a used in combination with known hepatotoxic products should be considered prior to administration or when adding new agents to the regimen of patients on therapy. Reduction of interferon β-1 dose should be considered if SGPT rises above 5 times the upper limit of normal. The dose may be gradually re-escalated when enzyme levels have normalized).

No products indexed under this heading.

Amoxapine (The potential risk of interferon β-1a used in combination with known hepatotoxic products should be considered prior to administration or when adding new agents to the regimen of patients on therapy. Reduction of interferon β-1 dose should be considered if SGPT rises above 5 times the upper limit of normal. The dose may be gradually re-escalated when enzyme levels have normalized).

No products indexed under this heading.

Amoxicillin (The potential risk of interferon β-1a used in combination with known hepatotoxic products should be considered prior to administration or when adding new agents to the regimen of patients on therapy. Reduction of interferon β-1 dose should be considered if SGPT rises above 5 times the upper limit of normal. The dose may be gradually re-escalated when enzyme levels have normalized). Products include:

Amoxil Capsules **1311**
Amoxil Chewable Tablets **1311**
Amoxil **1311**
Amoxil Powder **1311**
Augmentin **1331**
Augmentin Tablets **1335**
Augmentin ES-600 .... **1338**
Augmentin XR **1342**
Moxatag **2321**

Amoxicillin Trihydrate (The potential risk of interferon β-1a used in combination with known hepatotoxic products should be considered prior to administration or when adding new agents to the regimen of patients on therapy. Reduction of interferon β-1 dose should be considered if SGPT rises above 5 times the upper limit of normal. The dose may be gradually re-escalated when enzyme levels have normalized).

No products indexed under this heading.

Ampicillin (The potential risk of interferon β-1a used in combination with known hepatotoxic products should be considered prior to administration or when adding new agents to the regimen of patients on therapy. Reduction of interferon β-1 dose should be considered if SGPT rises above 5 times the upper limit of normal. The dose may be gradually re-escalated when enzyme levels have normalized).

No products indexed under this heading.

Ampicillin Sodium (The potential risk of interferon β-1a used in combination with known hepatotoxic products should be considered prior to administration or when adding new agents to the regimen of patients on therapy. Reduction of interferon β-1 dose should be considered if SGPT rises above 5 times the upper limit of normal. The dose may be gradually re-escalated when enzyme levels have normalized).

No products indexed under this heading.

Ampicillin Trihydrate (The potential risk of interferon β-1a used in combination with known hepatotoxic products should be considered prior to administration or when adding new agents to the regimen of patients on therapy. Reduction of interferon β-1 dose should be considered if SGPT rises above 5 times the upper limit of normal. The dose may be gradually re-escalated when enzyme levels have normalized).

No products indexed under this heading.

Amprenavir (The potential risk of interferon β-1a used in combination with known hepatotoxic products should be considered prior to administration or when adding new agents to the regimen of patients on therapy. Reduction of interferon β-1 dose should be considered if SGPT rises above 5 times the upper limit of normal. The dose may be gradually re-escalated when enzyme levels have normalized).

No products indexed under this heading.

Atazanavir (The potential risk of interferon β-1a used in combination with known hepatotoxic products should be considered prior to administration or when adding new agents to the regimen of patients on therapy. Reduction of interferon β-1 dose should be considered if SGPT rises above 5 times the upper limit of normal. The dose may be gradually re-escalated when enzyme levels have normalized).

No products indexed under this heading.

Atazanavir Sulfate (The potential risk of interferon β-1a used in combination with known hepatotoxic products should be considered prior to administration or when adding new agents to the regimen of patients on therapy. Reduction of interferon β-1 dose should be considered if SGPT rises above 5 times the upper limit of normal. The dose may be gradually re-escalated when enzyme levels have normalized).

No products indexed under this heading.

Atorvastatin Calcium (The potential risk of interferon β-1a used in combination with known hepatotoxic products should be considered prior to administration or when adding new agents to the regimen of patients on therapy. Reduction of interferon β-1 dose should be considered if SGPT rises above 5 times the upper limit of normal. The dose may be gradually re-escalated when enzyme levels have normalized). Products include:

Lipitor **2703**

Azathioprine (The potential risk of interferon β-1a used in combination with known hepatotoxic products should be considered prior to administration or when adding new agents to the regimen of patients on therapy. Reduction of interferon β-1 dose should be considered if SGPT rises above 5 times the upper limit of normal. The dose may be gradually re-escalated when enzyme levels have normalized).

No products indexed under this heading.

Azathioprine Sodium (The potential risk of interferon β-1a used in combination with known hepatotoxic products should be considered prior to administration or when adding new agents to the regimen of patients on therapy. Reduction of interferon β-1 dose should be considered if SGPT rises above 5 times the upper limit of normal. The dose may be gradually re-escalated when enzyme levels have normalized).

No products indexed under this heading.

Azlocillin Sodium (The potential risk of interferon β-1a used in combination with known hepatotoxic products should be considered prior to administration or when adding new agents to the regimen of patients on therapy. Reduction of interferon β-1 dose should be considered if SGPT rises above 5 times the upper limit of normal. The dose may be gradually re-escalated when enzyme levels have normalized).

No products indexed under this heading.

Bacampicillin Hydrochloride (The potential risk of interferon β-1a used in combination with known hepatotoxic products should be considered prior to administration or when adding new agents to the regimen of patients on therapy. Reduction of interferon β-1 dose should be considered if SGPT rises above 5 times the upper limit of normal. The dose may be gradually re-escalated when enzyme levels have normalized).

No products indexed under this heading.

BCG Vaccine (Patients receiving interferon β-1a may receive concomitant vaccination, the overall effectiveness of such vaccination is unknown).

No products indexed under this heading.

Bendroflumethiazide (The potential risk of interferon β-1a used in combination with known hepatotoxic products should be considered prior to administration or when adding new agents to the regimen of patients on therapy. Reduction of interferon β-1 dose should be considered if SGPT rises above 5 times the upper limit of normal. The dose may be gradually re-escalated when enzyme levels have normalized).

No products indexed under this heading.

Bupropion (The potential risk of interferon β-1a used in combination with known hepatotoxic products should be considered prior to administration or when adding new agents to the regimen of patients on therapy. Reduction of interferon β-1 dose should be considered if SGPT rises above 5 times the upper limit of normal. The dose may be gradually re-escalated when enzyme levels have normalized).

No products indexed under this heading.

Bupropion Hydrochloride (The potential risk of interferon β-1a used in combination with known hepatotoxic products should be considered prior to administration or when adding new agents to the regimen of patients on therapy. Reduction of interferon β-1 dose should be considered if SGPT rises above 5 times the upper limit of normal. The dose may be gradually re-escalated when enzyme levels have normalized). Products include:

Aplenzin **2948**
Wellbutrin **1719**
Wellbutrin SR **1725**
Zyban **1762**

Busulfan (Due to its potential to cause neutropenia and lymphopenia, proper monitoring of patients is required if interferon β-1a is given in combination with myelosuppressive agents). Products include:

Myleran **1581**

Carbamazepine (The potential risk of interferon β-1a used in combination with known hepatotoxic products should be considered prior to administration or when adding new agents to the regimen of patients on therapy. Reduction of interferon β-1 dose should be considered if SGPT rises above 5 times the upper limit of normal. The dose may be gradually re-escalated when enzyme levels have normalized). Products include:

Carbatrol **3280**
Equetro **3477**

Carbenicillin Disodium (The potential risk of interferon β-1a used in combination with known hepatotoxic products should be considered prior to administration or when adding new agents to the regimen of patients on therapy. Reduction of interferon β-1 dose should be considered if SGPT rises above 5 times the upper limit of normal. The dose may be gradually re-escalated when enzyme levels have normalized).

No products indexed under this heading.

Carbenicillin Indanyl Sodium (The potential risk of interferon β-1a used in combination with known hepatotoxic products should be considered prior to administration or when adding new agents to the regimen of patients on therapy. Reduction of interferon β-1 dose should be considered if SGPT rises above 5 times the upper limit of normal. The dose may be gradually re-escalated when enzyme levels have normalized).

No products indexed under this heading.

Celecoxib (The potential risk of interferon β-1a used in combination with known hepatotoxic products should be considered prior to administration or when adding new agents to the regimen of patients on therapy. Reduction of interferon β-1 dose should be considered if SGPT rises above 5 times the upper limit of normal. The dose may be gradually re-escalated when enzyme levels have normalized). Products include:

Celebrex **3272**

Cerivastatin Sodium (The potential risk of interferon β-1a used in combination with known hepatotoxic products should be considered prior to administration or when adding new agents to the regimen of patients on therapy. Reduction of interferon β-1 dose should be considered if SGPT rises above 5 times the upper limit of normal. The dose may be gradually re-escalated when enzyme levels have normalized).

No products indexed under this heading.

Chlorambucil (Due to its potential to cause neutropenia and lymphopenia, proper monitoring of patients is required if interferon β-1a is given in combination with myelosuppressive agents). Products include:

Leukeran **1557**

Chloramphenicol (Due to its potential to cause neutropenia and lymphopenia, proper monitoring of patients is required if interferon β-1a is given in combination with myelosuppressive agents).

No products indexed under this heading.

Chloramphenicol Palmitate (Due to its potential to cause neutropenia and lymphopenia, proper monitoring of patients is required if interferon β-1a is given in combination with myelosuppressive agents).

No products indexed under this heading.

Chloramphenicol Sodium Succinate (Due to its potential to cause neutropenia and lymphopenia, proper monitoring of patients is required if interferon β-1a is given in combination with myelosuppressive agents).

No products indexed under this heading.

Chlorothiazide (The potential risk of interferon β-1a used in combination with known hepatotoxic products should be considered prior to administration or when adding new agents to the regimen of patients on therapy. Reduction of interferon β-1 dose should be considered if SGPT rises above 5 times the upper limit of normal. The dose may be gradually re-escalated when enzyme levels have normalized).

No products indexed under this heading.

Rebif Interactions Index 1566

Chlorothiazide Sodium (The potential risk of interferon β-1a used in combination with known hepatotoxic products should be considered prior to administration or when adding new agents to the regimen of patients on therapy. Reduction of interferon β-1 dose should be considered if SGPT rises above 5 times the upper limit of normal. The dose may be gradually re-escalated when enzyme levels have normalized). Products include:
Diuril Intravenous 2009

Chlorpromazine (The potential risk of interferon β-1a used in combination with known hepatotoxic products should be considered prior to administration or when adding new agents to the regimen of patients on therapy. Reduction of interferon β-1 dose should be considered if SGPT rises above 5 times the upper limit of normal. The dose may be gradually re-escalated when enzyme levels have normalized).
No products indexed under this heading.

Chlorpromazine Hydrochloride (The potential risk of interferon β-1a used in combination with known hepatotoxic products should be considered prior to administration or when adding new agents to the regimen of patients on therapy. Reduction of interferon β-1 dose should be considered if SGPT rises above 5 times the upper limit of normal. The dose may be gradually re-escalated when enzyme levels have normalized).
No products indexed under this heading.

Chlorpropamide (The potential risk of interferon β-1a used in combination with known hepatotoxic products should be considered prior to administration or when adding new agents to the regimen of patients on therapy. Reduction of interferon β-1 dose should be considered if SGPT rises above 5 times the upper limit of normal. The dose may be gradually re-escalated when enzyme levels have normalized).
No products indexed under this heading.

Cladribine (Due to its potential to cause neutropenia and lymphopenia, proper monitoring of patients is required if interferon β-1a is given in combination with myelosuppressive agents). Products include:
Leustatin 946

Clomipramine Hydrochloride (The potential risk of interferon β-1a used in combination with known hepatotoxic products should be considered prior to administration or when adding new agents to the regimen of patients on therapy. Reduction of interferon β-1 dose should be considered if SGPT rises above 5 times the upper limit of normal. The dose may be gradually re-escalated when enzyme levels have normalized).
No products indexed under this heading.

Cloxacillin (The potential risk of interferon β-1a used in combination with known hepatotoxic products should be considered prior to administration or when adding new agents to the regimen of patients on therapy. Reduction of interferon β-1 dose should be considered if SGPT rises above 5 times the upper limit of normal. The dose may be gradually re-escalated when enzyme levels have normalized).
No products indexed under this heading.

Cloxacillin Sodium (The potential risk of interferon β-1a used in combination with known hepatotoxic products should be considered prior to administration or when adding new agents to the regimen of patients on therapy. Reduction of interferon β-1 dose should be considered if SGPT rises above 5 times the upper limit of normal. The dose may be gradually re-escalated when enzyme levels have normalized).
No products indexed under this heading.

Cloxacillin Sodium Monohydrate (The potential risk of interferon β-1a used in combination with known hepatotoxic products should be considered prior to administration or when adding new agents to the regimen of patients on therapy. Reduction of interferon β-1 dose should be considered if SGPT rises above 5 times the upper limit of normal. The dose may be gradually re-escalated when enzyme levels have normalized).
No products indexed under this heading.

Cyclosporine (The potential risk of interferon β-1a used in combination with known hepatotoxic products should be considered prior to administration or when adding new agents to the regimen of patients on therapy. Reduction of interferon β-1 dose should be considered if SGPT rises above 5 times the upper limit of normal. The dose may be gradually re-escalated when enzyme levels have normalized). Products include:
Gengraf 440
Neoral Oral Solution 2496
Neoral Capsules 2496
Restasis 605

Darunavir (The potential risk of interferon β-1a used in combination with known hepatotoxic products should be considered prior to administration or when adding new agents to the regimen of patients on therapy. Reduction of interferon β-1 dose should be considered if SGPT rises above 5 times the upper limit of normal. The dose may be gradually re-escalated when enzyme levels have normalized).
No products indexed under this heading.

Daunorubicin Citrate Liposome (Due to its potential to cause neutropenia and lymphopenia, proper monitoring of patients is required if interferon β-1a is given in combination with myelosuppressive agents).
No products indexed under this heading.

Daunorubicin Hydrochloride (Due to its potential to cause neutropenia and lymphopenia, proper monitoring of patients is required if interferon β-1a is given in combination with myelosuppressive agents).
No products indexed under this heading.

Demeclocycline Hydrochloride (The potential risk of interferon β-1a used in combination with known hepatotoxic products should be considered prior to administration or when adding new agents to the regimen of patients on therapy. Reduction of interferon β-1 dose should be considered if SGPT rises above 5 times the upper limit of normal. The dose may be gradually re-escalated when enzyme levels have normalized).
No products indexed under this heading.

Desipramine Hydrochloride (The potential risk of interferon β-1a used in combination with known hepatotoxic products should be considered prior to administration or when adding new agents to the regimen of patients on therapy. Reduction of interferon β-1 dose should be considered if SGPT rises above 5 times the upper limit of normal. The dose may be gradually re-escalated when enzyme levels have normalized).
No products indexed under this heading.

Dexrazoxane (Due to its potential to cause neutropenia and lymphopenia, proper monitoring of patients is required if interferon β-1a is given in combination with myelosuppressive agents).
No products indexed under this heading.

Diclofenac Epolamine (The potential risk of interferon β-1a used in combination with known hepatotoxic products should be considered prior to administration or when adding new agents to the regimen of patients on therapy. Reduction of interferon β-1 dose should be considered if SGPT rises above 5 times the upper limit of normal. The dose may be gradually re-escalated when enzyme levels have normalized). Products include:
Flector 1839

Diclofenac Potassium (The potential risk of interferon β-1a used in combination with known hepatotoxic products should be considered prior to administration or when adding new agents to the regimen of patients on therapy. Reduction of interferon β-1 dose should be considered if SGPT rises above 5 times the upper limit of normal. The dose may be gradually re-escalated when enzyme levels have normalized).
No products indexed under this heading.

Diclofenac Sodium (The potential risk of interferon β-1a used in combination with known hepatotoxic products should be considered prior to administration or when adding new agents to the regimen of patients on therapy. Reduction of interferon β-1 dose should be considered if SGPT rises above 5 times the upper limit of normal. The dose may be gradually re-escalated when enzyme levels have normalized).
No products indexed under this heading.

Dicloxacillin (The potential risk of interferon β-1a used in combination with known hepatotoxic products should be considered prior to administration or when adding new agents to the regimen of patients on therapy. Reduction of interferon β-1 dose should be considered if SGPT rises above 5 times the upper limit of normal. The dose may be gradually re-escalated when enzyme levels have normalized).
No products indexed under this heading.

Dicloxacillin Sodium (The potential risk of interferon β-1a used in combination with known hepatotoxic products should be considered prior to administration or when adding new agents to the regimen of patients on therapy. Reduction of interferon β-1 dose should be considered if SGPT rises above 5 times the upper limit of normal. The dose may be gradually re-escalated when enzyme levels have normalized).
No products indexed under this heading.

Diphtheria & Tetanus Toxoids and Acellular Pertussis Vaccine Adsorbed, Hepatitis B (recombinant) and Inactivated Poliovirus Vaccine Combined (Patients receiving interferon β-1a may receive concomitant vaccination, the overall effectiveness of such vaccination is unknown).
No products indexed under this heading.

Disodium Carbenicillin (The potential risk of interferon β-1a used in combination with known hepatotoxic products should be considered prior to administration or when adding new agents to the regimen of patients on therapy. Reduction of interferon β-1 dose should be considered if SGPT rises above 5 times the upper limit of normal. The dose may be gradually re-escalated when enzyme levels have normalized).
No products indexed under this heading.

Divalproex Sodium (The potential risk of interferon β-1a used in combination with known hepatotoxic products should be considered prior to administration or when adding new agents to the regimen of patients on therapy. Reduction of interferon β-1 dose should be considered if SGPT rises above 5 times the upper limit of normal. The dose may be gradually re-escalated when enzyme levels have normalized). Products include:
Depakote ER 426

Doxepin Hydrochloride (The potential risk of interferon β-1a used in combination with known hepatotoxic products should be considered prior to administration or when adding new agents to the regimen of patients on therapy. Reduction of interferon β-1 dose should be considered if SGPT rises above 5 times the upper limit of normal. The dose may be gradually re-escalated when enzyme levels have normalized).
No products indexed under this heading.

Doxorubicin Hydrochloride (Due to its potential to cause neutropenia and lymphopenia, proper monitoring of patients is required if interferon β-1a is given in combination with myelosuppressive agents).
No products indexed under this heading.

Doxorubicin Hydrochloride Liposome (Due to its potential to cause neutropenia and lymphopenia, proper monitoring of patients is required if interferon β-1a is given in combination with myelosuppressive agents). Products include:
Doxil 939

Doxycycline (The potential risk of interferon β-1a used in combination with known hepatotoxic products should be considered prior to administration or when adding new agents to the regimen of patients on therapy. Reduction of interferon β-1 dose should be considered if SGPT rises above 5 times the upper limit of normal. The dose may be gradually re-escalated when enzyme levels have normalized).
No products indexed under this heading.

Doxycycline Calcium (The potential risk of interferon β-1a used in combination with known hepatotoxic products should be considered prior to administration or when adding new agents to the regimen of patients on therapy. Reduction of interferon β-1 dose should be considered if SGPT rises above 5 times the upper limit of normal. The dose may be gradually re-escalated when enzyme levels have normalized).
No products indexed under this heading.

Doxycycline Hyclate (The potential risk of interferon β-1a used in combination with known hepatotoxic products should be considered prior to administration or when adding new agents to the regimen of patients on therapy. Reduction of interferon β-1 dose should be considered if SGPT rises above 5 times the upper limit of normal. The dose may be gradually re-escalated when enzyme levels have normalized).
No products indexed under this heading.

Doxycycline Monohydrate (The potential risk of interferon β-1a used in combination with known hepatotoxic products should be considered prior to administration or when adding new agents to the regimen of patients on therapy. Reduction of interferon β-1 dose should be considered if SGPT rises above 5 times the upper limit of normal. The dose may be gradually re-escalated when enzyme levels have normalized).
No products indexed under this heading.

Duloxetine Hydrochloride (The potential risk of interferon β-1a used in combination with known hepatotoxic products should be considered prior to administration or when adding new agents to the regimen of patients on therapy. Reduction of interferon β-1 dose should be considered if SGPT rises above 5 times the upper limit of

normal. The dose may be gradually re-escalated when enzyme levels have normalized). Products include:

Cymbalta 1871

Erythromycin (The potential risk of interferon β-1a used in combination with known hepatotoxic products should be considered prior to administration or when adding new agents to the regimen of patients on therapy. Reduction of interferon β-1 dose should be considered if SGPT rises above 5 times the upper limit of normal. The dose may be gradually re-escalated when enzyme levels have normalized).

No products indexed under this heading.

Erythromycin, Topical (The potential risk of interferon β-1a used in combination with known hepatotoxic products should be considered prior to administration or when adding new agents to the regimen of patients on therapy. Reduction of interferon β-1 dose should be considered if SGPT rises above 5 times the upper limit of normal. The dose may be gradually re-escalated when enzyme levels have normalized).

No products indexed under this heading.

Erythromycin Estolate (The potential risk of interferon β-1a used in combination with known hepatotoxic products should be considered prior to administration or when adding new agents to the regimen of patients on therapy. Reduction of interferon β-1 dose should be considered if SGPT rises above 5 times the upper limit of normal. The dose may be gradually re-escalated when enzyme levels have normalized).

No products indexed under this heading.

Erythromycin Ethylsuccinate (The potential risk of interferon β-1a used in combination with known hepatotoxic products should be considered prior to administration or when adding new agents to the regimen of patients on therapy. Reduction of interferon β-1 dose should be considered if SGPT rises above 5 times the upper limit of normal. The dose may be gradually re-escalated when enzyme levels have normalized). Products include:

E.E.S. 437
EryPed 435

Erythromycin Gluceptate (The potential risk of interferon β-1a used in combination with known hepatotoxic products should be considered prior to administration or when adding new agents to the regimen of patients on therapy. Reduction of interferon β-1 dose should be considered if SGPT rises above 5 times the upper limit of normal. The dose may be gradually re-escalated when enzyme levels have normalized).

No products indexed under this heading.

Erythromycin Lactobionate (The potential risk of interferon β-1a used in combination with known hepatotoxic products should be considered prior to administration or when adding new agents to the regimen of patients on therapy. Reduction of interferon β-1 dose should be considered if SGPT rises above 5 times the upper limit of normal. The dose may be gradually re-escalated when enzyme levels have normalized).

No products indexed under this heading.

Erythromycin Stearate (The potential risk of interferon β-1a used in combination with known hepatotoxic products should be considered prior to administration or when adding new agents to the regimen of patients on therapy. Reduction of interferon β-1 dose should be considered if SGPT rises above 5 times the upper limit of normal. The dose may be gradually re-escalated when enzyme levels have normalized).

No products indexed under this heading.

Etodolac (The potential risk of interferon β-1a used in combination with known hepatotoxic products should be considered prior to administration or when adding new agents to the regimen of patients on therapy. Reduction of interferon β-1 dose should be considered if SGPT rises above 5 times the upper limit of normal. The dose may be gradually re-escalated when enzyme levels have normalized).

No products indexed under this heading.

Felbamate (The potential risk of interferon β-1a used in combination with known hepatotoxic products should be considered prior to administration or when adding new agents to the regimen of patients on therapy. Reduction of interferon β-1 dose should be considered if SGPT rises above 5 times the upper limit of normal. The dose may be gradually re-escalated when enzyme levels have normalized).

No products indexed under this heading.

Fenofibrate (The potential risk of interferon β-1a used in combination with known hepatotoxic products should be considered prior to administration or when adding new agents to the regimen of patients on therapy. Reduction of interferon β-1 dose should be considered if SGPT rises above 5 times the upper limit of normal. The dose may be gradually re-escalated when enzyme levels have normalized). Products include:

Fenoglide 3263
Tricor 544
Trilipix 548

Fenoprofen Calcium (The potential risk of interferon β-1a used in combination with known hepatotoxic products should be considered prior to administration or when adding new agents to the regimen of patients on therapy. Reduction of interferon β-1 dose should be considered if SGPT rises above 5 times the upper limit of normal. The dose may be gradually re-escalated when enzyme levels have normalized).

No products indexed under this heading.

Fluconazole (The potential risk of interferon β-1a used in combination with known hepatotoxic products should be considered prior to administration or when adding new agents to the regimen of patients on therapy. Reduction of interferon β-1 dose should be considered if SGPT rises above 5 times the upper limit of normal. The dose may be gradually re-escalated when enzyme levels have normalized).

No products indexed under this heading.

Fludarabine Phosphate (Due to its potential to cause neutropenia and lymphopenia, proper monitoring of patients is required if interferon β-1a is given in combination with myelosuppressive agents). Products include:

Oforta 3023

Flurbiprofen (The potential risk of interferon β-1a used in combination with known hepatotoxic products should be considered prior to administration or when adding new agents to the regimen of patients on therapy. Reduction of interferon β-1 dose should be considered if SGPT rises above 5 times the upper limit of normal. The dose may be gradually re-escalated when enzyme levels have normalized).

No products indexed under this heading.

Flurbiprofen Sodium (The potential risk of interferon β-1a used in combination with known hepatotoxic products should be considered prior to administration or when adding new agents to the regimen of patients on therapy. Reduction of interferon β-1 dose should be considered if SGPT rises above 5 times the upper limit of normal. The dose may be gradually re-escalated when enzyme levels have normalized).

No products indexed under this heading.

Fluvastatin Sodium (The potential risk of interferon β-1a used in combination with known hepatotoxic products should be considered prior to administration or when adding new agents to the regimen of patients on therapy. Reduction of interferon β-1 dose should be considered if SGPT rises above 5 times the upper limit of normal. The dose may be gradually re-escalated when enzyme levels have normalized).

No products indexed under this heading.

Fosamprenavir Calcium (The potential risk of interferon β-1a used in combination with known hepatotoxic products should be considered prior to administration or when adding new agents to the regimen of patients on therapy. Reduction of interferon β-1 dose should be considered if SGPT rises above 5 times the upper limit of normal. The dose may be gradually re-escalated when enzyme levels have normalized). Products include:

Lexiva Oral Suspension 1558
Lexiva 1558

Fosphenytoin (The potential risk of interferon β-1a used in combination with known hepatotoxic products should be considered prior to administration or when adding new agents to the regimen of patients on therapy. Reduction of interferon β-1 dose should be considered if SGPT rises above 5 times the upper limit of normal. The dose may be gradually re-escalated when enzyme levels have normalized).

No products indexed under this heading.

Fosphenytoin Sodium (The potential risk of interferon β-1a used in combination with known hepatotoxic products should be considered prior to administration or when adding new agents to the regimen of patients on therapy. Reduction of interferon β-1 dose should be considered if SGPT rises above 5 times the upper limit of normal. The dose may be gradually re-escalated when enzyme levels have normalized).

No products indexed under this heading.

Gemcitabine Hydrochloride (Due to its potential to cause neutropenia and lymphopenia, proper monitoring of patients is required if interferon β-1a is given in combination with myelosuppressive agents). Products include:

Gemzar 1900

Gemfibrozil (The potential risk of interferon β-1a used in combination with known hepatotoxic products should be considered prior to administration or when adding new agents to the regimen of patients on therapy. Reduction of interferon β-1 dose should be considered if SGPT rises above 5 times the upper limit of normal. The dose may be gradually re-escalated when enzyme levels have normalized).

No products indexed under this heading.

Gemtuzumab Ozogamicin (Due to its potential to cause neutropenia and lymphopenia, proper monitoring of patients is required if interferon β-1a is given in combination with myelosuppressive agents). Products include:

Mylotarg 3524

Glimepiride (The potential risk of interferon β-1a used in combination with known hepatotoxic products should be considered prior to administration or when adding new agents to the regimen of patients on therapy. Reduction of interferon β-1 dose should be considered if SGPT rises above 5 times the upper limit of normal. The dose may be gradually re-escalated when enzyme levels have normalized). Products include:

Avandaryl 1356
Duetact 3354

Glipizide (The potential risk of interferon β-1a used in combination with known hepatotoxic products should be considered prior to administration or when adding new agents to the regimen of patients on therapy. Reduction of interferon β-1 dose should be considered if SGPT rises above 5 times the upper limit of normal. The dose may be gradually re-escalated when enzyme levels have normalized).

No products indexed under this heading.

Glyburide (The potential risk of interferon β-1a used in combination with known hepatotoxic products should be considered prior to administration or when adding new agents to the regimen of patients on therapy. Reduction of interferon β-1 dose should be considered if SGPT rises above 5 times the upper limit of normal. The dose may be gradually re-escalated when enzyme levels have normalized).

No products indexed under this heading.

Griseofulvin (The potential risk of interferon β-1a used in combination with known hepatotoxic products should be considered prior to administration or when adding new agents to the regimen of patients on therapy. Reduction of interferon β-1 dose should be considered if SGPT rises above 5 times the upper limit of normal. The dose may be gradually re-escalated when enzyme levels have normalized).

No products indexed under this heading.

Halothane (The potential risk of interferon β-1a used in combination with known hepatotoxic products should be considered prior to administration or when adding new agents to the regimen of patients on therapy. Reduction of interferon β-1 dose should be considered if SGPT rises above 5 times the upper limit of normal. The dose may be gradually re-escalated when enzyme levels have normalized).

No products indexed under this heading.

Heparin (The potential risk of interferon β-1a used in combination with known hepatotoxic products should be considered prior to administration or when adding new agents to the regimen of patients on therapy. Reduction of interferon β-1 dose should be considered if SGPT rises above 5 times the upper limit of normal. The dose may be gradually re-escalated when enzyme levels have normalized).

No products indexed under this heading.

Heparin Calcium (The potential risk of interferon β-1a used in combination with known hepatotoxic products should be considered prior to administration or when adding new agents to the regimen of patients on therapy. Reduction of interferon β-1 dose should be considered if SGPT rises above 5 times the upper limit of normal. The dose may be gradually re-escalated when enzyme levels have normalized).

No products indexed under this heading.

Heparin Sodium (The potential risk of interferon β-1a used in combination with known hepatotoxic products should be considered prior to administration or when adding new agents to the regimen of patients on therapy. Reduction of interferon β-1 dose should be considered if SGPT rises above 5 times the upper limit of normal. The dose may be gradually re-escalated when enzyme levels have normalized).

No products indexed under this heading.

Hepatitis A Vaccine, Inactivated (Patients receiving interferon β-1a may receive concomitant vaccination, the overall effectiveness of such vaccination is unknown). Products include:

Havrix 1485

IMPORTANT NOTE: Always consult each drug listing in the patient's regimen for possible interactions.

Hydralazine (The potential risk of interferon β-1a used in combination with known hepatotoxic products should be considered prior to administration or when adding new agents to the regimen of patients on therapy. Reduction of interferon β-1 dose should be considered if SGPT rises above 5 times the upper limit of normal. The dose may be gradually re-escalated when enzyme levels have normalized).

No products indexed under this heading.

Hydralazine Hydrochloride (The potential risk of interferon β-1a used in combination with known hepatotoxic products should be considered prior to administration or when adding new agents to the regimen of patients on therapy. Reduction of interferon β-1 dose should be considered if SGPT rises above 5 times the upper limit of normal. The dose may be gradually re-escalated when enzyme levels have normalized).

No products indexed under this heading.

Hydrochlorothiazide (The potential risk of interferon β-1a used in combination with known hepatotoxic products should be considered prior to administration or when adding new agents to the regimen of patients on therapy. Reduction of interferon β-1 dose should be considered if SGPT rises above 5 times the upper limit of normal. The dose may be gradually re-escalated when enzyme levels have normalized). Products include:

Hydrochlorothiazide Hydrochloride (The potential risk of interferon β-1a used in combination with known hepatotoxic products should be considered prior to administration or when adding new agents to the regimen of patients on therapy. Reduction of interferon β-1 dose should be considered if SGPT rises above 5 times the upper limit of normal. The dose may be gradually re-escalated when enzyme levels have normalized).

No products indexed under this heading.

Hydroflumethiazide (The potential risk of interferon β-1a used in combination with known hepatotoxic products should be considered prior to administration or when adding new agents to the regimen of patients on therapy. Reduction of interferon β-1 dose should be considered if SGPT rises above 5 times the upper limit of normal. The dose may be gradually re-escalated when enzyme levels have normalized).

No products indexed under this heading.

Ibuprofen (The potential risk of interferon β-1a used in combination with known hepatotoxic products should be considered prior to administration or when adding new agents to the regimen of patients on therapy. Reduction of interferon β-1 dose should be considered if SGPT rises above 5 times the upper limit of normal. The dose may be gradually re-escalated when enzyme levels have normalized). Products include:

Idarubicin Hydrochloride (Due to its potential to cause neutropenia and lymphopenia, proper monitoring of patients is required if interferon β-1a is given in combination with myelosuppressive agents).

No products indexed under this heading.

Imatinib Mesylate (The potential risk of interferon β-1a used in combination with known hepatotoxic products should be considered prior to administration or when adding new agents to the regimen of patients on therapy. Reduction of interferon β-1 dose should be considered if SGPT rises above 5 times the upper limit of normal. The dose may be gradually re-escalated when enzyme levels have normalized). Products include:

Imipramine Hydrochloride (The potential risk of interferon β-1a used in combination with known hepatotoxic products should be considered prior to administration or when adding new agents to the regimen of patients on therapy. Reduction of interferon β-1 dose should be considered if SGPT rises above 5 times the upper limit of normal. The dose may be gradually re-escalated when enzyme levels have normalized).

No products indexed under this heading.

Imipramine Pamoate (The potential risk of interferon β-1a used in combination with known hepatotoxic products should be considered prior to administration or when adding new agents to the regimen of patients on therapy. Reduction of interferon β-1 dose should be considered if SGPT rises above 5 times the upper limit of normal. The dose may be gradually re-escalated when enzyme levels have normalized).

No products indexed under this heading.

Indinavir Sulfate (The potential risk of interferon β-1a used in combination with known hepatotoxic products should be considered prior to administration or when adding new agents to the regimen of patients on therapy. Reduction of interferon β-1 dose should be considered if SGPT rises above 5 times the upper limit of normal. The dose may be gradually re-escalated when enzyme levels have normalized). Products include:

Indomethacin (The potential risk of interferon β-1a used in combination with known hepatotoxic products should be considered prior to administration or when adding new agents to the regimen of patients on therapy. Reduction of interferon β-1 dose should be considered if SGPT rises above 5 times the upper limit of normal. The dose may be gradually re-escalated when enzyme levels have normalized). Products include:

Indomethacin Sodium Trihydrate (The potential risk of interferon β-1a used in combination with known hepatotoxic products should be considered prior to administration or when adding new agents to the regimen of patients on therapy. Reduction of interferon β-1 dose should be considered if SGPT rises above 5 times the upper limit of normal. The dose may be gradually re-escalated when enzyme levels have normalized). Products include:

Influenza Vaccine, Live Attenuated (Patients receiving interferon β-1a may receive concomitant vaccination, the overall effectiveness of such vaccination is unknown).

No products indexed under this heading.

Influenza Virus Vaccine (Patients receiving interferon β-1a may receive concomitant vaccination, the overall effectiveness of such vaccination is unknown). Products include:

Influenza Virus Vaccine Live, Intranasal (Patients receiving interferon β-1a may receive concomitant vaccination, the overall effectiveness of such vaccination is unknown). Products include:

Interferon alfa-2a, Recombinant (Due to its potential to cause neutropenia and lymphopenia, proper monitoring of patients is required if interferon β-1a is given in combination with myelosuppressive agents).

No products indexed under this heading.

Irinotecan Hydrochloride (Due to its potential to cause neutropenia and lymphopenia, proper monitoring of patients is required if interferon β-1a is given in combination with myelosuppressive agents).

No products indexed under this heading.

Isoniazid (The potential risk of interferon β-1a used in combination with known hepatotoxic products should be considered prior to administration or when adding new agents to the regimen of patients on therapy. Reduction of interferon β-1 dose should be considered if SGPT rises above 5 times the upper limit of normal. The dose may be gradually re-escalated when enzyme levels have normalized).

No products indexed under this heading.

Isotretinoin (The potential risk of interferon β-1a used in combination with known hepatotoxic products should be considered prior to administration or when adding new agents to the regimen of patients on therapy. Reduction of interferon β-1 dose should be considered if SGPT rises above 5 times the upper limit of normal. The dose may be gradually re-escalated when enzyme levels have normalized). Products include:

Itraconazole (The potential risk of interferon β-1a used in combination with known hepatotoxic products should be considered prior to administration or when adding new agents to the regimen of patients on therapy. Reduction of interferon β-1 dose should be considered if SGPT rises above 5 times the upper limit of normal. The dose may be gradually re-escalated when enzyme levels have normalized).

No products indexed under this heading.

Japanese Encephalitis Vaccine Inactivated (Patients receiving interferon β-1a may receive concomitant vaccination, the overall effectiveness of such vaccination is unknown).

No products indexed under this heading.

Ketoconazole (The potential risk of interferon β-1a used in combination with known hepatotoxic products should be considered prior to administration or when adding new agents to the regimen of patients on therapy. Reduction of interferon β-1 dose should be considered if SGPT rises above 5 times the upper limit of normal. The dose may be gradually re-escalated when enzyme levels have normalized). Products include:

Ketoprofen (The potential risk of interferon β-1a used in combination with known hepatotoxic products should be considered prior to administration or when adding new agents to the regimen of patients on therapy. Reduction of interferon β-1 dose should be considered if SGPT rises above 5 times the upper limit of normal. The dose may be gradually re-escalated when enzyme levels have normalized).

No products indexed under this heading.

Ketorolac Tromethamine (The potential risk of interferon β-1a used in combination with known hepatotoxic products should be considered prior to administration or when adding new agents to the regimen of patients on therapy. Reduction of interferon β-1 dose should be considered if SGPT rises above 5 times the upper limit of normal. The dose may be gradually re-escalated when enzyme levels have normalized). Products include:

Labetalol Hydrochloride (The potential risk of interferon β-1a used in combination with known hepatotoxic products should be considered prior to administration or when adding new agents to the regimen of patients on therapy. Reduction of interferon β-1 dose should be considered if SGPT rises above 5 times the upper limit of normal. The dose may be gradually re-escalated when enzyme levels have normalized).

No products indexed under this heading.

Leflunomide (The potential risk of interferon β-1a used in combination with known hepatotoxic products should be considered prior to administration or when adding new agents to the regimen of patients on therapy. Reduction of interferon β-1 dose should be considered if SGPT rises above 5 times the upper limit of normal. The dose may be gradually re-escalated when enzyme levels have normalized).

No products indexed under this heading.

Lopinavir (The potential risk of interferon β-1a used in combination with known hepatotoxic products should be considered prior to administration or when adding new agents to the regimen of patients on therapy. Reduction of interferon β-1 dose should be considered if SGPT rises above 5 times the upper limit of normal. The dose may be gradually re-escalated when enzyme levels have normalized). Products include:

Lovastatin (The potential risk of interferon β-1a used in combination with known hepatotoxic products should be considered prior to administration or when adding new agents to the regimen of patients on therapy. Reduction of interferon β-1 dose should be considered if SGPT rises above 5 times the upper limit of normal. The dose may be gradually re-escalated when enzyme levels have normalized). Products include:

Maprotiline Hydrochloride (The potential risk of interferon β-1a used in combination with known hepatotoxic products should be considered prior to administration or when adding new agents to the regimen of patients on therapy. Reduction of interferon β-1 dose should be considered if SGPT rises above 5 times the upper limit of normal. The dose may be gradually re-escalated when enzyme levels have normalized).

No products indexed under this heading.

Maraviroc (The potential risk of interferon β-1a used in combination with known hepatotoxic products should be

1569 Interactions Index Rebif

considered prior to administration or when adding new agents to the regimen of patients on therapy. Reduction of interferon β-1 dose should be considered if SGPT rises above 5 times the upper limit of normal. The dose may be gradually re-escalated when enzyme levels have normalized). Products include:
Selzentry 2740

Measles, Mumps, Rubella and Varicella Virus Vaccine Live (Patients receiving interferon β-1a may receive concomitant vaccination, the overall effectiveness of such vaccination is unknown). Products include:
ProQuad 2254

Measles, Mumps & Rubella Virus Vaccine, Live (Patients receiving interferon β-1a may receive concomitant vaccination, the overall effectiveness of such vaccination is unknown). Products include:
M-M-R II 2203
ProQuad 2254

Measles & Rubella Virus Vaccine Live (Patients receiving interferon β-1a may receive concomitant vaccination, the overall effectiveness of such vaccination is unknown).
No products indexed under this heading.

Measles Virus Vaccine Live (Patients receiving interferon β-1a may receive concomitant vaccination, the overall effectiveness of such vaccination is unknown). Products include:
Attenuvax 2086

Meclofenamate Sodium (The potential risk of interferon β-1a used in combination with known hepatotoxic products should be considered prior to administration or when adding new agents to the regimen of patients on therapy. Reduction of interferon β-1 dose should be considered if SGPT rises above 5 times the upper limit of normal. The dose may be gradually re-escalated when enzyme levels have normalized).
No products indexed under this heading.

Mefenamic Acid (The potential risk of interferon β-1a used in combination with known hepatotoxic products should be considered prior to administration or when adding new agents to the regimen of patients on therapy. Reduction of interferon β-1 dose should be considered if SGPT rises above 5 times the upper limit of normal. The dose may be gradually re-escalated when enzyme levels have normalized).
No products indexed under this heading.

Meloxicam (The potential risk of interferon β-1a used in combination with known hepatotoxic products should be considered prior to administration or when adding new agents to the regimen of patients on therapy. Reduction of interferon β-1 dose should be considered if SGPT rises above 5 times the upper limit of normal. The dose may be gradually re-escalated when enzyme levels have normalized).
No products indexed under this heading.

Melphalan Hydrochloride (Due to its potential to cause neutropenia and lymphopenia, proper monitoring of patients is required if interferon β-1a is given in combination with myelosuppressive agents). Products include:
Alkeran for Injection 1300

Mephenytoin (The potential risk of interferon β-1a used in combination with known hepatotoxic products should be considered prior to administration or when adding new agents to the regimen of patients on therapy. Reduction of interferon β-1 dose should be considered if SGPT rises above 5 times the upper limit of normal. The dose may be gradually re-escalated when enzyme levels have normalized).
No products indexed under this heading.

Mercaptopurine (Due to its potential to cause neutropenia and lymphopenia, proper monitoring of patients is required if interferon β-1a is given in combination with myelosuppressive agents).
No products indexed under this heading.

Methacycline Hydrochloride (The potential risk of interferon β-1a used in combination with known hepatotoxic products should be considered prior to administration or when adding new agents to the regimen of patients on therapy. Reduction of interferon β-1 dose should be considered if SGPT rises above 5 times the upper limit of normal. The dose may be gradually re-escalated when enzyme levels have normalized).
No products indexed under this heading.

Methicillin Sodium (The potential risk of interferon β-1a used in combination with known hepatotoxic products should be considered prior to administration or when adding new agents to the regimen of patients on therapy. Reduction of interferon β-1 dose should be considered if SGPT rises above 5 times the upper limit of normal. The dose may be gradually re-escalated when enzyme levels have normalized).
No products indexed under this heading.

Methimazole (The potential risk of interferon β-1a used in combination with known hepatotoxic products should be considered prior to administration or when adding new agents to the regimen of patients on therapy. Reduction of interferon β-1 dose should be considered if SGPT rises above 5 times the upper limit of normal. The dose may be gradually re-escalated when enzyme levels have normalized).
No products indexed under this heading.

Methotrexate (The potential risk of interferon β-1a used in combination with known hepatotoxic products should be considered prior to administration or when adding new agents to the regimen of patients on therapy. Reduction of interferon β-1 dose should be considered if SGPT rises above 5 times the upper limit of normal. The dose may be gradually re-escalated when enzyme levels have normalized).
No products indexed under this heading.

Methotrexate Sodium (The potential risk of interferon β-1a used in combination with known hepatotoxic products should be considered prior to administration or when adding new agents to the regimen of patients on therapy. Reduction of interferon β-1 dose should be considered if SGPT rises above 5 times the upper limit of normal. The dose may be gradually re-escalated when enzyme levels have normalized).
No products indexed under this heading.

Methyclothiazide (The potential risk of interferon β-1a used in combination with known hepatotoxic products should be considered prior to administration or when adding new agents to the regimen of patients on therapy. Reduction of interferon β-1 dose should be considered if SGPT rises above 5 times the upper limit of normal. The dose may be gradually re-escalated when enzyme levels have normalized).
No products indexed under this heading.

Mezlocillin Sodium (The potential risk of interferon β-1a used in combination with known hepatotoxic products should be considered prior to administration or when adding new agents to the regimen of patients on therapy. Reduction of interferon β-1 dose should be considered if SGPT rises above 5 times the upper limit of normal. The dose may be gradually re-escalated when enzyme levels have normalized).
No products indexed under this heading.

Minocycline Hydrochloride (The potential risk of interferon β-1a used in combination with known hepatotoxic products should be considered prior to administration or when adding new agents to the regimen of patients on therapy. Reduction of interferon β-1 dose should be considered if SGPT rises above 5 times the upper limit of normal. The dose may be gradually re-escalated when enzyme levels have normalized). Products include:
Solodyn 2073

Mitoxantrone Hydrochloride (Due to its potential to cause neutropenia and lymphopenia, proper monitoring of patients is required if interferon β-1a is given in combination with myelosuppressive agents). Products include:
Novantrone 1088

Mumps Virus Vaccine, Live (Patients receiving interferon β-1a may receive concomitant vaccination, the overall effectiveness of such vaccination is unknown). Products include:
Mumpsvax 2218

Nabumetone (The potential risk of interferon β-1a used in combination with known hepatotoxic products should be considered prior to administration or when adding new agents to the regimen of patients on therapy. Reduction of interferon β-1 dose should be considered if SGPT rises above 5 times the upper limit of normal. The dose may be gradually re-escalated when enzyme levels have normalized).
No products indexed under this heading.

Nafcillin Sodium (The potential risk of interferon β-1a used in combination with known hepatotoxic products should be considered prior to administration or when adding new agents to the regimen of patients on therapy. Reduction of interferon β-1 dose should be considered if SGPT rises above 5 times the upper limit of normal. The dose may be gradually re-escalated when enzyme levels have normalized).
No products indexed under this heading.

Naproxen (The potential risk of interferon β-1a used in combination with known hepatotoxic products should be considered prior to administration or when adding new agents to the regimen of patients on therapy. Reduction of interferon β-1 dose should be considered if SGPT rises above 5 times the upper limit of normal. The dose may be gradually re-escalated when enzyme levels have normalized). Products include:
EC-Naprosyn 2850
Naprosyn 2850
Anaprox/Naprosyn 2850

Naproxen Sodium (The potential risk of interferon β-1a used in combination with known hepatotoxic products should be considered prior to administration or when adding new agents to the regimen of patients on therapy. Reduction of interferon β-1 dose should be considered if SGPT rises above 5 times the upper limit of normal. The dose may be gradually re-escalated when enzyme levels have normalized). Products include:
Anaprox 2850
Anaprox DS 2850
Treximet 1681

Nefazodone Hydrochloride (The potential risk of interferon β-1a used in combination with known hepatotoxic products should be considered prior to administration or when adding new agents to the regimen of patients on therapy. Reduction of interferon β-1 dose should be considered if SGPT rises above 5 times the upper limit of normal. The dose may be gradually re-escalated when enzyme levels have normalized).
No products indexed under this heading.

Nelfinavir Mesylate (The potential risk of interferon β-1a used in combination with known hepatotoxic products should be considered prior to administration or when adding new agents to the regimen of patients on therapy. Reduction of interferon β-1 dose should be considered if SGPT rises above 5 times the upper limit of normal. The dose may be gradually re-escalated when enzyme levels have normalized).
No products indexed under this heading.

Nevirapine (The potential risk of interferon β-1a used in combination with known hepatotoxic products should be considered prior to administration or when adding new agents to the regimen of patients on therapy. Reduction of interferon β-1 dose should be considered if SGPT rises above 5 times the upper limit of normal. The dose may be gradually re-escalated when enzyme levels have normalized). Products include:
Viramune Oral Suspension 897
Viramune Tablets 897

Niacin (The potential risk of interferon β-1a used in combination with known hepatotoxic products should be considered prior to administration or when adding new agents to the regimen of patients on therapy. Reduction of interferon β-1 dose should be considered if SGPT rises above 5 times the upper limit of normal. The dose may be gradually re-escalated when enzyme levels have normalized). Products include:
Advicor 402
Cardio Basics 3455
Niaspan 497
Simcor 524

Niacinamide (The potential risk of interferon β-1a used in combination with known hepatotoxic products should be considered prior to administration or when adding new agents to the regimen of patients on therapy. Reduction of interferon β-1 dose should be considered if SGPT rises above 5 times the upper limit of normal. The dose may be gradually re-escalated when enzyme levels have normalized). Products include:
CitraNatal 90 DHA Capsules 2332
CitraNatal Assure 2332
CitraNatal Rx 2332
Heplive 607

Niacinamide Hydroiodide (The potential risk of interferon β-1a used in combination with known hepatotoxic products should be considered prior to administration or when adding new agents to the regimen of patients on therapy. Reduction of interferon β-1 dose should be considered if SGPT rises above 5 times the upper limit of normal. The dose may be gradually re-escalated when enzyme levels have normalized).
No products indexed under this heading.

Nicotinic Acid (The potential risk of interferon β-1a used in combination with known hepatotoxic products should be considered prior to administration or when adding new agents to the regimen of patients on therapy. Reduction of interferon β-1 dose should be considered if SGPT rises above 5 times the upper limit of normal. The dose may be gradually re-escalated when enzyme levels have normalized).
No products indexed under this heading.

Nitrofurantoin (The potential risk of interferon β-1a used in combination with known hepatotoxic products should be considered prior to administration or when adding new agents to the regimen of patients on therapy. Reduction of

interferon β-1 dose should be considered if SGPT rises above 5 times the upper limit of normal. The dose may be gradually re-escalated when enzyme levels have normalized).
No products indexed under this heading.

Nitrofurantoin Macrocrystals (The potential risk of interferon β-1a used in combination with known hepatotoxic products should be considered prior to administration or when adding new agents to the regimen of patients on therapy. Reduction of interferon β-1 dose should be considered if SGPT rises above 5 times the upper limit of normal. The dose may be gradually re-escalated when enzyme levels have normalized).
No products indexed under this heading.

Nitrofurantoin Monohydrate (The potential risk of interferon β-1a used in combination with known hepatotoxic products should be considered prior to administration or when adding new agents to the regimen of patients on therapy. Reduction of interferon β-1 dose should be considered if SGPT rises above 5 times the upper limit of normal. The dose may be gradually re-escalated when enzyme levels have normalized).
No products indexed under this heading.

Nitrofurantoin Sodium (The potential risk of interferon β-1a used in combination with known hepatotoxic products should be considered prior to administration or when adding new agents to the regimen of patients on therapy. Reduction of interferon β-1 dose should be considered if SGPT rises above 5 times the upper limit of normal. The dose may be gradually re-escalated when enzyme levels have normalized).
No products indexed under this heading.

Nortriptyline Hydrochloride (The potential risk of interferon β-1a used in combination with known hepatotoxic products should be considered prior to administration or when adding new agents to the regimen of patients on therapy. Reduction of interferon β-1 dose should be considered if SGPT rises above 5 times the upper limit of normal. The dose may be gradually re-escalated when enzyme levels have normalized).
No products indexed under this heading.

Oxacillin (The potential risk of interferon β-1a used in combination with known hepatotoxic products should be considered prior to administration or when adding new agents to the regimen of patients on therapy. Reduction of interferon β-1 dose should be considered if SGPT rises above 5 times the upper limit of normal. The dose may be gradually re-escalated when enzyme levels have normalized).
No products indexed under this heading.

Oxacillin Sodium (The potential risk of interferon β-1a used in combination with known hepatotoxic products should be considered prior to administration or when adding new agents to the regimen of patients on therapy. Reduction of interferon β-1 dose should be considered if SGPT rises above 5 times the upper limit of normal. The dose may be gradually re-escalated when enzyme levels have normalized).
No products indexed under this heading.

Oxaprozin (The potential risk of interferon β-1a used in combination with known hepatotoxic products should be considered prior to administration or when adding new agents to the regimen of patients on therapy. Reduction of interferon β-1 dose should be considered if SGPT rises above 5 times the upper limit of normal. The dose may be gradually re-escalated when enzyme levels have normalized).
No products indexed under this heading.

Oxymetholone (The potential risk of interferon β-1a used in combination with known hepatotoxic products should be considered prior to administration or when adding new agents to the regimen of patients on therapy. Reduction of interferon β-1 dose should be considered if SGPT rises above 5 times the upper limit of normal. The dose may be gradually re-escalated when enzyme levels have normalized).
No products indexed under this heading.

Oxytetracycline (The potential risk of interferon β-1a used in combination with known hepatotoxic products should be considered prior to administration or when adding new agents to the regimen of patients on therapy. Reduction of interferon β-1 dose should be considered if SGPT rises above 5 times the upper limit of normal. The dose may be gradually re-escalated when enzyme levels have normalized).
No products indexed under this heading.

Oxytetracycline Hydrochloride (The potential risk of interferon β-1a used in combination with known hepatotoxic products should be considered prior to administration or when adding new agents to the regimen of patients on therapy. Reduction of interferon β-1 dose should be considered if SGPT rises above 5 times the upper limit of normal. The dose may be gradually re-escalated when enzyme levels have normalized).
No products indexed under this heading.

Penicillin, Potassium Phenoxymethyl (The potential risk of interferon β-1a used in combination with known hepatotoxic products should be considered prior to administration or when adding new agents to the regimen of patients on therapy. Reduction of interferon β-1 dose should be considered if SGPT rises above 5 times the upper limit of normal. The dose may be gradually re-escalated when enzyme levels have normalized).
No products indexed under this heading.

Penicillin G Benzathine (The potential risk of interferon β-1a used in combination with known hepatotoxic products should be considered prior to administration or when adding new agents to the regimen of patients on therapy. Reduction of interferon β-1 dose should be considered if SGPT rises above 5 times the upper limit of normal. The dose may be gradually re-escalated when enzyme levels have normalized). Products include:
Bicillin C-R Injectable Suspension **1826**
Bicillin L-A **1828**

Penicillin G Dibenzylethyenediamine (The potential risk of interferon β-1a used in combination with known hepatotoxic products should be considered prior to administration or when adding new agents to the regimen of patients on therapy. Reduction of interferon β-1 dose should be considered if SGPT rises above 5 times the upper limit of normal. The dose may be gradually re-escalated when enzyme levels have normalized).
No products indexed under this heading.

Penicillin G Potassium (The potential risk of interferon β-1a used in combination with known hepatotoxic products should be considered prior to administration or when adding new agents to the regimen of patients on therapy. Reduction of interferon β-1 dose should be considered if SGPT rises above 5 times the upper limit of normal. The dose may be gradually re-escalated when enzyme levels have normalized).
No products indexed under this heading.

Penicillin G Procaine (The potential risk of interferon β-1a used in combination with known hepatotoxic products should be considered prior to administration or when adding new agents to the regimen of patients on therapy. Reduction of interferon β-1 dose should be considered if SGPT rises above 5 times the upper limit of normal. The dose may be gradually re-escalated when enzyme levels have normalized). Products include:
Bicillin C-R Injectable Suspension **1826**
Bicillin L-A **1828**

Penicillin G Sodium (The potential risk of interferon β-1a used in combination with known hepatotoxic products should be considered prior to administration or when adding new agents to the regimen of patients on therapy. Reduction of interferon β-1 dose should be considered if SGPT rises above 5 times the upper limit of normal. The dose may be gradually re-escalated when enzyme levels have normalized).
No products indexed under this heading.

Penicillin V (The potential risk of interferon β-1a used in combination with known hepatotoxic products should be considered prior to administration or when adding new agents to the regimen of patients on therapy. Reduction of interferon β-1 dose should be considered if SGPT rises above 5 times the upper limit of normal. The dose may be gradually re-escalated when enzyme levels have normalized).
No products indexed under this heading.

Penicillin V Potassium (The potential risk of interferon β-1a used in combination with known hepatotoxic products should be considered prior to administration or when adding new agents to the regimen of patients on therapy. Reduction of interferon β-1 dose should be considered if SGPT rises above 5 times the upper limit of normal. The dose may be gradually re-escalated when enzyme levels have normalized).
No products indexed under this heading.

Penicillins (The potential risk of interferon β-1a used in combination with known hepatotoxic products should be considered prior to administration or when adding new agents to the regimen of patients on therapy. Reduction of interferon β-1 dose should be considered if SGPT rises above 5 times the upper limit of normal. The dose may be gradually re-escalated when enzyme levels have normalized).
No products indexed under this heading.

Phenylbutazone (The potential risk of interferon β-1a used in combination with known hepatotoxic products should be considered prior to administration or when adding new agents to the regimen of patients on therapy. Reduction of interferon β-1 dose should be considered if SGPT rises above 5 times the upper limit of normal. The dose may be gradually re-escalated when enzyme levels have normalized).
No products indexed under this heading.

Phenytoin (The potential risk of interferon β-1a used in combination with known hepatotoxic products should be considered prior to administration or when adding new agents to the regimen of patients on therapy. Reduction of interferon β-1 dose should be considered if SGPT rises above 5 times the upper limit of normal. The dose may be gradually re-escalated when enzyme levels have normalized).
No products indexed under this heading.

Phenytoin Sodium (The potential risk of interferon β-1a used in combination with known hepatotoxic products should be considered prior to administration or when adding new agents to the regimen of patients on therapy. Reduction of interferon β-1 dose should be considered if SGPT rises above 5 times the upper limit of normal. The dose may be gradually re-escalated when enzyme levels have normalized). Products include:
Phenytek Capsules **2380**

Pioglitazone Hydrochloride (The potential risk of interferon β-1a used in combination with known hepatotoxic products should be considered prior to administration or when adding new agents to the regimen of patients on therapy. Reduction of interferon β-1 dose should be considered if SGPT rises above 5 times the upper limit of normal. The dose may be gradually re-escalated when enzyme levels have normalized). Products include:
ActoPlus **3338**
Actos **3345**
Duetact **3354**

Piperacillin Sodium (The potential risk of interferon β-1a used in combination with known hepatotoxic products should be considered prior to administration or when adding new agents to the regimen of patients on therapy. Reduction of interferon β-1 dose should be considered if SGPT rises above 5 times the upper limit of normal. The dose may be gradually re-escalated when enzyme levels have normalized). Products include:
Zosyn **3607**

Piroxicam (The potential risk of interferon β-1a used in combination with known hepatotoxic products should be considered prior to administration or when adding new agents to the regimen of patients on therapy. Reduction of interferon β-1 dose should be considered if SGPT rises above 5 times the upper limit of normal. The dose may be gradually re-escalated when enzyme levels have normalized).
No products indexed under this heading.

Pneumococcal vaccine, diphtheria conjugate (Patients receiving interferon β-1a may receive concomitant vaccination, the overall effectiveness of such vaccination is unknown). Products include:
Prevnar **3557**

Pneumococcal Vaccine, Polyvalent (Patients receiving interferon β-1a may receive concomitant vaccination, the overall effectiveness of such vaccination is unknown). Products include:
Pneumovax 23 .... **2230**

Poliovirus Vaccine, Live, Oral, Trivalent, Types 1,2,3 (Sabin) (Patients receiving interferon β-1a may receive concomitant vaccination, the overall effectiveness of such vaccination is unknown).
No products indexed under this heading.

Poliovirus Vaccine Inactivated (Patients receiving interferon β-1a may receive concomitant vaccination, the overall effectiveness of such vaccination is unknown). Products include:
Pediarix **1606**

Polythiazide (The potential risk of interferon β-1a used in combination with known hepatotoxic products should be considered prior to administration or when adding new agents to the regimen of patients on therapy. Reduction of interferon β-1 dose should be considered if SGPT rises above 5 times the upper limit of normal. The dose may be gradually re-escalated when enzyme levels have normalized).
No products indexed under this heading.

Pravastatin Sodium (The potential risk of interferon β-1a used in combination with known hepatotoxic products should be considered prior to administration or when adding new agents to the regimen of patients on therapy. Reduction of interferon β-1 dose should be considered if SGPT rises above 5 times the upper limit of normal. The

1571 Interactions Index Rebif

dose may be gradually re-escalated when enzyme levels have normalized).
No products indexed under this heading.

Procainamide (The potential risk of interferon β-1a used in combination with known hepatotoxic products should be considered prior to administration or when adding new agents to the regimen of patients on therapy. Reduction of interferon β-1 dose should be considered if SGPT rises above 5 times the upper limit of normal. The dose may be gradually re-escalated when enzyme levels have normalized).
No products indexed under this heading.

Procainamide Hydrochloride (The potential risk of interferon β-1a used in combination with known hepatotoxic products should be considered prior to administration or when adding new agents to the regimen of patients on therapy. Reduction of interferon β-1 dose should be considered if SGPT rises above 5 times the upper limit of normal. The dose may be gradually re-escalated when enzyme levels have normalized).
No products indexed under this heading.

Propylthiouracil (The potential risk of interferon β-1a used in combination with known hepatotoxic products should be considered prior to administration or when adding new agents to the regimen of patients on therapy. Reduction of interferon β-1 dose should be considered if SGPT rises above 5 times the upper limit of normal. The dose may be gradually re-escalated when enzyme levels have normalized).
No products indexed under this heading.

Protriptyline Hydrochloride (The potential risk of interferon β-1a used in combination with known hepatotoxic products should be considered prior to administration or when adding new agents to the regimen of patients on therapy. Reduction of interferon β-1 dose should be considered if SGPT rises above 5 times the upper limit of normal. The dose may be gradually re-escalated when enzyme levels have normalized).
No products indexed under this heading.

Rifampin (The potential risk of interferon β-1a used in combination with known hepatotoxic products should be considered prior to administration or when adding new agents to the regimen of patients on therapy. Reduction of interferon β-1 dose should be considered if SGPT rises above 5 times the upper limit of normal. The dose may be gradually re-escalated when enzyme levels have normalized).
No products indexed under this heading.

Ritonavir (The potential risk of interferon β-1a used in combination with known hepatotoxic products should be considered prior to administration or when adding new agents to the regimen of patients on therapy. Reduction of interferon β-1 dose should be considered if SGPT rises above 5 times the upper limit of normal. The dose may be gradually re-escalated when enzyme levels have normalized). Products include:
Kaletra 458
Norvir 509

Rofecoxib (The potential risk of interferon β-1a used in combination with known hepatotoxic products should be considered prior to administration or when adding new agents to the regimen of patients on therapy. Reduction of interferon β-1 dose should be considered if SGPT rises above 5 times the upper limit of normal. The dose may be gradually re-escalated when enzyme levels have normalized).
No products indexed under this heading.

Rosuvastatin Calcium (The potential risk of interferon β-1a used in combination with known hepatotoxic products should be considered prior to administration or when adding new agents to the regimen of patients on therapy. Reduction of interferon β-1 dose should be considered if SGPT rises above 5 times the upper limit of normal. The dose may be gradually re-escalated when enzyme levels have normalized). Products include:
Crestor 736

Rotavirus Vaccine, Live, Oral, Tetravalent (Patients receiving interferon β-1a may receive concomitant vaccination, the overall effectiveness of such vaccination is unknown).
No products indexed under this heading.

Rubella & Mumps Virus Vaccine Live (Patients receiving interferon β-1a may receive concomitant vaccination, the overall effectiveness of such vaccination is unknown).
No products indexed under this heading.

Rubella Virus Vaccine Live (Patients receiving interferon β-1a may receive concomitant vaccination, the overall effectiveness of such vaccination is unknown). Products include:
Meruvax II 2210

Saquinavir (The potential risk of interferon β-1a used in combination with known hepatotoxic products should be considered prior to administration or when adding new agents to the regimen of patients on therapy. Reduction of interferon β-1 dose should be considered if SGPT rises above 5 times the upper limit of normal. The dose may be gradually re-escalated when enzyme levels have normalized).
No products indexed under this heading.

Saquinavir Mesylate (The potential risk of interferon β-1a used in combination with known hepatotoxic products should be considered prior to administration or when adding new agents to the regimen of patients on therapy. Reduction of interferon β-1 dose should be considered if SGPT rises above 5 times the upper limit of normal. The dose may be gradually re-escalated when enzyme levels have normalized).
No products indexed under this heading.

Simvastatin (The potential risk of interferon β-1a used in combination with known hepatotoxic products should be considered prior to administration or when adding new agents to the regimen of patients on therapy. Reduction of interferon β-1 dose should be considered if SGPT rises above 5 times the upper limit of normal. The dose may be gradually re-escalated when enzyme levels have normalized). Products include:
Simcor 524
Vytorin 10/10 ..... 2303, 3240
Vytorin 10/20 ..... 2303, 3240
Vytorin 10/40 ..... 2303, 3240
Vytorin 10/80 ..... 2303, 3240
Zocor 2289

Smallpox Vaccine (Patients receiving interferon β-1a may receive concomitant vaccination, the overall effectiveness of such vaccination is unknown).
No products indexed under this heading.

Sodium Cloxacillin Monohydrate (The potential risk of interferon β-1a used in combination with known hepatotoxic products should be considered prior to administration or when adding new agents to the regimen of patients on therapy. Reduction of interferon β-1 dose should be considered if SGPT rises above 5 times the upper limit of normal. The dose may be gradually re-escalated when enzyme levels have normalized).
No products indexed under this heading.

Statins (The potential risk of interferon β-1a used in combination with known hepatotoxic products should be considered prior to administration or when adding new agents to the regimen of patients on therapy. Reduction of interferon β-1 dose should be considered if SGPT rises above 5 times the upper limit of normal. The dose may be gradually re-escalated when enzyme levels have normalized).
No products indexed under this heading.

Sulfacytine (The potential risk of interferon β-1a used in combination with known hepatotoxic products should be considered prior to administration or when adding new agents to the regimen of patients on therapy. Reduction of interferon β-1 dose should be considered if SGPT rises above 5 times the upper limit of normal. The dose may be gradually re-escalated when enzyme levels have normalized).
No products indexed under this heading.

Sulfamethizole (The potential risk of interferon β-1a used in combination with known hepatotoxic products should be considered prior to administration or when adding new agents to the regimen of patients on therapy. Reduction of interferon β-1 dose should be considered if SGPT rises above 5 times the upper limit of normal. The dose may be gradually re-escalated when enzyme levels have normalized).
No products indexed under this heading.

Sulfamethoxazole (The potential risk of interferon β-1a used in combination with known hepatotoxic products should be considered prior to administration or when adding new agents to the regimen of patients on therapy. Reduction of interferon β-1 dose should be considered if SGPT rises above 5 times the upper limit of normal. The dose may be gradually re-escalated when enzyme levels have normalized).
No products indexed under this heading.

Sulfasalazine (The potential risk of interferon β-1a used in combination with known hepatotoxic products should be considered prior to administration or when adding new agents to the regimen of patients on therapy. Reduction of interferon β-1 dose should be considered if SGPT rises above 5 times the upper limit of normal. The dose may be gradually re-escalated when enzyme levels have normalized).
No products indexed under this heading.

Sulfinpyrazone (The potential risk of interferon β-1a used in combination with known hepatotoxic products should be considered prior to administration or when adding new agents to the regimen of patients on therapy. Reduction of interferon β-1 dose should be considered if SGPT rises above 5 times the upper limit of normal. The dose may be gradually re-escalated when enzyme levels have normalized).
No products indexed under this heading.

Sulfisoxazole Acetyl (The potential risk of interferon β-1a used in combination with known hepatotoxic products should be considered prior to administration or when adding new agents to the regimen of patients on therapy. Reduction of interferon β-1 dose should be considered if SGPT rises above 5 times the upper limit of normal. The dose may be gradually re-escalated when enzyme levels have normalized).
No products indexed under this heading.

Sulfisoxazole Diolamine (The potential risk of interferon β-1a used in combination with known hepatotoxic products should be considered prior to administration or when adding new agents to the regimen of patients on therapy. Reduction of interferon β-1 dose should be considered if SGPT rises above 5 times the upper limit of normal. The dose may be gradually re-escalated when enzyme levels have normalized).
No products indexed under this heading.

Sulindac (The potential risk of interferon β-1a used in combination with known hepatotoxic products should be considered prior to administration or when adding new agents to the regimen of patients on therapy. Reduction of interferon β-1 dose should be considered if SGPT rises above 5 times the upper limit of normal. The dose may be gradually re-escalated when enzyme levels have normalized). Products include:
Clinoril 2098

Tacrine Hydrochloride (The potential risk of interferon β-1a used in combination with known hepatotoxic products should be considered prior to administration or when adding new agents to the regimen of patients on therapy. Reduction of interferon β-1 dose should be considered if SGPT rises above 5 times the upper limit of normal. The dose may be gradually re-escalated when enzyme levels have normalized).
No products indexed under this heading.

Tamoxifen Citrate (The potential risk of interferon β-1a used in combination with known hepatotoxic products should be considered prior to administration or when adding new agents to the regimen of patients on therapy. Reduction of interferon β-1 dose should be considered if SGPT rises above 5 times the upper limit of normal. The dose may be gradually re-escalated when enzyme levels have normalized).
No products indexed under this heading.

Telithromycin (The potential risk of interferon β-1a used in combination with known hepatotoxic products should be considered prior to administration or when adding new agents to the regimen of patients on therapy. Reduction of interferon β-1 dose should be considered if SGPT rises above 5 times the upper limit of normal. The dose may be gradually re-escalated when enzyme levels have normalized). Products include:
Ketek 2991

Temozolomide (Due to its potential to cause neutropenia and lymphopenia, proper monitoring of patients is required if interferon β-1a is given in combination with myelosuppressive agents). Products include:
Temodar 3230
Temodar Injection 3230

Tetracycline Hydrochloride (The potential risk of interferon β-1a used in combination with known hepatotoxic products should be considered prior to administration or when adding new agents to the regimen of patients on therapy. Reduction of interferon β-1 dose should be considered if SGPT rises above 5 times the upper limit of normal. The dose may be gradually re-escalated when enzyme levels have normalized). Products include:
Pylera 793

Tetracycline Phosphate Complex (The potential risk of interferon β-1a used in combination with known hepatotoxic products should be considered prior to administration or when adding new agents to the regimen of patients on therapy. Reduction of interferon β-1 dose should be considered if SGPT rises above 5 times the upper limit of normal. The dose may be gradually re-escalated when enzyme levels have normalized).
No products indexed under this heading.

Thiazide Diuretics (The potential risk of interferon β-1a used in combination with known hepatotoxic products should be considered prior to administration or when adding new agents to the regimen

Rebif Interactions Index 1572

of patients on therapy. Reduction of interferon β-1 dose should be considered if SGPT rises above 5 times the upper limit of normal. The dose may be gradually re-escalated when enzyme levels have normalized).
No products indexed under this heading.

Thiazides (The potential risk of interferon β-1a used in combination with known hepatotoxic products should be considered prior to administration or when adding new agents to the regimen of patients on therapy. Reduction of interferon β-1 dose should be considered if SGPT rises above 5 times the upper limit of normal. The dose may be gradually re-escalated when enzyme levels have normalized).
No products indexed under this heading.

Thioguanine (Due to its potential to cause neutropenia and lymphopenia, proper monitoring of patients is required if interferon β-1a is given in combination with myelosuppressive agents). Products include:
Tabloid 1664

Ticarcillin Disodium (The potential risk of interferon β-1a used in combination with known hepatotoxic products should be considered prior to administration or when adding new agents to the regimen of patients on therapy. Reduction of interferon β-1 dose should be considered if SGPT rises above 5 times the upper limit of normal. The dose may be gradually re-escalated when enzyme levels have normalized). Products include:
Timentin ADD-Vantage 1670
Timentin Galaxy 1674
Timentin 1666
Timentin Pharmacy 1678

Tipranavir (The potential risk of interferon β-1a used in combination with known hepatotoxic products should be considered prior to administration or when adding new agents to the regimen of patients on therapy. Reduction of interferon β-1 dose should be considered if SGPT rises above 5 times the upper limit of normal. The dose may be gradually re-escalated when enzyme levels have normalized).
No products indexed under this heading.

Tolazamide (The potential risk of interferon β-1a used in combination with known hepatotoxic products should be considered prior to administration or when adding new agents to the regimen of patients on therapy. Reduction of interferon β-1 dose should be considered if SGPT rises above 5 times the upper limit of normal. The dose may be gradually re-escalated when enzyme levels have normalized).
No products indexed under this heading.

Tolbutamide (The potential risk of interferon β-1a used in combination with known hepatotoxic products should be considered prior to administration or when adding new agents to the regimen of patients on therapy. Reduction of interferon β-1 dose should be considered if SGPT rises above 5 times the upper limit of normal. The dose may be gradually re-escalated when enzyme levels have normalized).
No products indexed under this heading.

Tolbutamide Sodium (The potential risk of interferon β-1a used in combination with known hepatotoxic products should be considered prior to administration or when adding new agents to the regimen of patients on therapy. Reduction of interferon β-1 dose should be considered if SGPT rises above 5 times the upper limit of normal. The dose may be gradually re-escalated when enzyme levels have normalized).
No products indexed under this heading.

Tolmetin Sodium (The potential risk of interferon β-1a used in combination with known hepatotoxic products should be considered prior to administration or when adding new agents to the regimen of patients on therapy. Reduction of interferon β-1 dose should be considered if SGPT rises above 5 times the upper limit of normal. The dose may be gradually re-escalated when enzyme levels have normalized).
No products indexed under this heading.

Trimethoprim (The potential risk of interferon β-1a used in combination with known hepatotoxic products should be considered prior to administration or when adding new agents to the regimen of patients on therapy. Reduction of interferon β-1 dose should be considered if SGPT rises above 5 times the upper limit of normal. The dose may be gradually re-escalated when enzyme levels have normalized).
No products indexed under this heading.

Trimethoprim Hydrochloride (The potential risk of interferon β-1a used in combination with known hepatotoxic products should be considered prior to administration or when adding new agents to the regimen of patients on therapy. Reduction of interferon β-1 dose should be considered if SGPT rises above 5 times the upper limit of normal. The dose may be gradually re-escalated when enzyme levels have normalized).
No products indexed under this heading.

Trimethoprim Sulfate (The potential risk of interferon β-1a used in combination with known hepatotoxic products should be considered prior to administration or when adding new agents to the regimen of patients on therapy. Reduction of interferon β-1 dose should be considered if SGPT rises above 5 times the upper limit of normal. The dose may be gradually re-escalated when enzyme levels have normalized).
No products indexed under this heading.

Trimipramine Maleate (The potential risk of interferon β-1a used in combination with known hepatotoxic products should be considered prior to administration or when adding new agents to the regimen of patients on therapy. Reduction of interferon β-1 dose should be considered if SGPT rises above 5 times the upper limit of normal. The dose may be gradually re-escalated when enzyme levels have normalized).
No products indexed under this heading.

Typhoid Vaccine (Patients receiving interferon β-1a may receive concomitant vaccination, the overall effectiveness of such vaccination is unknown).
No products indexed under this heading.

Valdecoxib (The potential risk of interferon β-1a used in combination with known hepatotoxic products should be considered prior to administration or when adding new agents to the regimen of patients on therapy. Reduction of interferon β-1 dose should be considered if SGPT rises above 5 times the upper limit of normal. The dose may be gradually re-escalated when enzyme levels have normalized).
No products indexed under this heading.

Valproate Sodium (The potential risk of interferon β-1a used in combination with known hepatotoxic products should be considered prior to administration or when adding new agents to the regimen of patients on therapy. Reduction of interferon β-1 dose should be considered if SGPT rises above 5 times the upper limit of normal. The dose may be gradually re-escalated when enzyme levels have normalized).
No products indexed under this heading.

Valproic Acid (The potential risk of interferon β-1a used in combination with known hepatotoxic products should be considered prior to administration or when adding new agents to the regimen of patients on therapy. Reduction of interferon β-1 dose should be considered if SGPT rises above 5 times the upper limit of normal. The dose may be gradually re-escalated when enzyme levels have normalized).
No products indexed under this heading.

Varicella Virus Vaccine, Live (Patients receiving interferon β-1a may receive concomitant vaccination, the overall effectiveness of such vaccination is unknown). Products include:
Varivax 2285

Vinorelbine Tartrate (Due to its potential to cause neutropenia and lymphopenia, proper monitoring of patients is required if interferon β-1a is given in combination with myelosuppressive agents).
No products indexed under this heading.

Voriconazole (The potential risk of interferon β-1a used in combination with known hepatotoxic products should be considered prior to administration or when adding new agents to the regimen of patients on therapy. Reduction of interferon β-1 dose should be considered if SGPT rises above 5 times the upper limit of normal. The dose may be gradually re-escalated when enzyme levels have normalized).
No products indexed under this heading.

Yellow Fever Vaccine (Patients receiving interferon β-1a may receive concomitant vaccination, the overall effectiveness of such vaccination is unknown).
No products indexed under this heading.

Zoster Vaccine Live (Patients receiving interferon β-1a may receive concomitant vaccination, the overall effectiveness of such vaccination is unknown). Products include:
Zostavax 2299

RECLAST INJECTION

(Zoledronic Acid) 2509
May interact with aminoglycosides, antineoplastics, cationic drugs that are eliminated by renal tubular, corticosteroids, diuretics, loop diuretics, nephrotoxic agents, non-steroidal anti-inflammatory agents, and certain other agents. Compounds in these categories include:

Abacavir Sulfate (Caution is indicated when zoledronic acid is used with other potentially nephrotoxic drugs such as nonsteroidal anti-inflammatory drugs. Renal impairment has been observed following the administration of zoledronic acid, especially in patients with pre-existing renal compromise or other risk factors including concomitant nephrotoxic medications). Products include:
Epzicom 1448
Trizivir 1688
Ziagen 1740

Acyclovir (Caution is indicated when zoledronic acid is used with other potentially nephrotoxic drugs such as nonsteroidal anti-inflammatory drugs. Renal impairment has been observed following the administration of zoledronic acid, especially in patients with pre-existing renal compromise or other risk factors including concomitant nephrotoxic medications). Products include:
Zovirax 1760

Acyclovir Sodium (Caution is indicated when zoledronic acid is used with other potentially nephrotoxic drugs such as nonsteroidal anti-inflammatory drugs. Renal impairment has been observed following the administration of zoledronic acid, especially in patients with pre-existing renal compromise or other risk factors including concomitant nephrotoxic medications).
No products indexed under this heading.

Alatrofloxacin Mesylate (Caution is indicated when zoledronic acid is used with other potentially nephrotoxic drugs such as nonsteroidal anti-inflammatory drugs. Renal impairment has been observed following the administration of zoledronic acid, especially in patients with pre-existing renal compromise or other risk factors including concomitant nephrotoxic medications).
No products indexed under this heading.

Alclometasone Dipropionate (Osteonecrosis of the jaw (ONJ) has been reported in patients treated with bisphosphonates, including zoledronic acid. A dental examination with appropriate preventive dentistry should be considered prior to treatment with bisphosphonates in patients with a history of concomitant risk factors for ONJ (eg, corticosteroids). While on treatment, patients with concomitant risk factors should avoid invasive dental procedures if possible).
No products indexed under this heading.

Aldesleukin (Caution is indicated when zoledronic acid is used with other potentially nephrotoxic drugs such as nonsteroidal anti-inflammatory drugs. Renal impairment has been observed following the administration of zoledronic acid, especially in patients with pre-existing renal compromise or other risk factors including concomitant nephrotoxic medications). Products include:
Proleukin 2504

Altretamine (Osteonecrosis of the jaw (ONJ) has been reported in patients treated with bisphosphonates, including zoledronic acid. A dental examination with appropriate preventive dentistry should be considered prior to treatment with bisphosphonates in patients with a history of concomitant risk factors for ONJ (eg, chemotherapy). While on treatment, patients with concomitant risk factors should avoid invasive dental procedures if possible). Products include:
Hexalen 1066

Amikacin Sulfate (Caution is advised when bisphosphonates, including zoledronic acid, are administered with aminoglycosides, since these agents may have an additive effect to lower serum calcium level for prolonged periods).
No products indexed under this heading.

Amiloride Hydrochloride (Renal impairment has been observed following the administration of zoledronic acid, especially in patients with pre-existing renal compromise or other risk factors including concomitant diuretic therapy).
No products indexed under this heading.

Amoxicillin (Caution is indicated when zoledronic acid is used with other potentially nephrotoxic drugs such as nonsteroidal anti-inflammatory drugs. Renal impairment has been observed following the administration of zoledronic acid, especially in patients with pre-existing renal compromise or other risk factors including concomitant nephrotoxic medications). Products include:
Amoxil Capsules 1311
Amoxil Chewable Tablets 1311
Amoxil 1311
Amoxil Powder 1311
Augmentin 1331
Augmentin Tablets 1335
Augmentin ES-600 1338
Augmentin XR 1342
Moxatag 2321

1573 Interactions Index Reclast

Amoxicillin Trihydrate (Caution is indicated when zoledronic acid is used with other potentially nephrotoxic drugs such as nonsteroidal anti-inflammatory drugs. Renal impairment has been observed following the administration of zoledronic acid, especially in patients with pre-existing renal compromise or other risk factors including concomitant nephrotoxic medications).
No products indexed under this heading.

Amphotericin B (Caution is indicated when zoledronic acid is used with other potentially nephrotoxic drugs such as nonsteroidal anti-inflammatory drugs. Renal impairment has been observed following the administration of zoledronic acid, especially in patients with pre-existing renal compromise or other risk factors including concomitant nephrotoxic medications).
No products indexed under this heading.

Amphotericin B, liposomal (Caution is indicated when zoledronic acid is used with other potentially nephrotoxic drugs such as nonsteroidal anti-inflammatory drugs. Renal impairment has been observed following the administration of zoledronic acid, especially in patients with pre-existing renal compromise or other risk factors including concomitant nephrotoxic medications). Products include:
AmBisome 659

Amphotericin B Cholesteryl Sulfate (Caution is indicated when zoledronic acid is used with other potentially nephrotoxic drugs such as nonsteroidal anti-inflammatory drugs. Renal impairment has been observed following the administration of zoledronic acid, especially in patients with pre-existing renal compromise or other risk factors including concomitant nephrotoxic medications).
No products indexed under this heading.

Amphotericin B Lipid Complex (Caution is indicated when zoledronic acid is used with other potentially nephrotoxic drugs such as nonsteroidal anti-inflammatory drugs. Renal impairment has been observed following the administration of zoledronic acid, especially in patients with pre-existing renal compromise or other risk factors including concomitant nephrotoxic medications).
No products indexed under this heading.

Ampicillin (Caution is indicated when zoledronic acid is used with other potentially nephrotoxic drugs such as nonsteroidal anti-inflammatory drugs. Renal impairment has been observed following the administration of zoledronic acid, especially in patients with pre-existing renal compromise or other risk factors including concomitant nephrotoxic medications).
No products indexed under this heading.

Ampicillin Sodium (Caution is indicated when zoledronic acid is used with other potentially nephrotoxic drugs such as nonsteroidal anti-inflammatory drugs. Renal impairment has been observed following the administration of zoledronic acid, especially in patients with pre-existing renal compromise or other risk factors including concomitant nephrotoxic medications).
No products indexed under this heading.

Ampicillin Trihydrate (Caution is indicated when zoledronic acid is used with other potentially nephrotoxic drugs such as nonsteroidal anti-inflammatory drugs. Renal impairment has been observed following the administration of zoledronic acid, especially in patients with pre-existing renal compromise or other risk factors including concomitant nephrotoxic medications).
No products indexed under this heading.

Amprenavir (Caution is indicated when zoledronic acid is used with other potentially nephrotoxic drugs such as nonsteroidal anti-inflammatory drugs. Renal impairment has been observed following the administration of zoledronic acid, especially in patients with pre-existing renal compromise or other risk factors including concomitant nephrotoxic medications).
No products indexed under this heading.

Anastrozole (Osteonecrosis of the jaw (ONJ) has been reported in patients treated with bisphosphonates, including zoledronic acid. A dental examination with appropriate preventive dentistry should be considered prior to treatment with bisphosphonates in patients with a history of concomitant risk factors for ONJ (eg, chemotherapy). While on treatment, patients with concomitant risk factors should avoid invasive dental procedures if possible).
No products indexed under this heading.

Asparaginase (Osteonecrosis of the jaw (ONJ) has been reported in patients treated with bisphosphonates, including zoledronic acid. A dental examination with appropriate preventive dentistry should be considered prior to treatment with bisphosphonates in patients with a history of concomitant risk factors for ONJ (eg, chemotherapy). While on treatment, patients with concomitant risk factors should avoid invasive dental procedures if possible). Products include:
Elspar 2005, 2122

Aspirin (Caution is indicated when zoledronic acid is used with other potentially nephrotoxic drugs such as nonsteroidal anti-inflammatory drugs. Renal impairment has been observed following the administration of zoledronic acid, especially in patients with pre-existing renal compromise or other risk factors including concomitant nephrotoxic medications). Products include:
Aggrenox 880
Bayer Aspirin 829
Percodan 1124
St. Joseph Aspirin 2045

Atazanavir (Caution is indicated when zoledronic acid is used with other potentially nephrotoxic drugs such as nonsteroidal anti-inflammatory drugs. Renal impairment has been observed following the administration of zoledronic acid, especially in patients with pre-existing renal compromise or other risk factors including concomitant nephrotoxic medications).
No products indexed under this heading.

Atorvastatin Calcium (Caution is indicated when zoledronic acid is used with other potentially nephrotoxic drugs such as nonsteroidal anti-inflammatory drugs. Renal impairment has been observed following the administration of zoledronic acid, especially in patients with pre-existing renal compromise or other risk factors including concomitant nephrotoxic medications). Products include:
Lipitor 2703

Azithromycin Dihydrate (Caution is indicated when zoledronic acid is used with other potentially nephrotoxic drugs such as nonsteroidal anti-inflammatory drugs. Renal impairment has been observed following the administration of zoledronic acid, especially in patients with pre-existing renal compromise or other risk factors including concomitant nephrotoxic medications).
No products indexed under this heading.

Azlocillin Sodium (Caution is indicated when zoledronic acid is used with other potentially nephrotoxic drugs such as nonsteroidal anti-inflammatory drugs. Renal impairment has been observed following the administration of zoledronic acid, especially in patients with pre-existing renal compromise or other risk factors including concomitant nephrotoxic medications).
No products indexed under this heading.

Aztreonam (Caution is indicated when zoledronic acid is used with other potentially nephrotoxic drugs such as nonsteroidal anti-inflammatory drugs. Renal impairment has been observed following the administration of zoledronic acid, especially in patients with pre-existing renal compromise or other risk factors including concomitant nephrotoxic medications).
No products indexed under this heading.

Bacampicillin Hydrochloride (Caution is indicated when zoledronic acid is used with other potentially nephrotoxic drugs such as nonsteroidal anti-inflammatory drugs. Renal impairment has been observed following the administration of zoledronic acid, especially in patients with pre-existing renal compromise or other risk factors including concomitant nephrotoxic medications).
No products indexed under this heading.

Bacitracin (Caution is indicated when zoledronic acid is used with other potentially nephrotoxic drugs such as nonsteroidal anti-inflammatory drugs. Renal impairment has been observed following the administration of zoledronic acid, especially in patients with pre-existing renal compromise or other risk factors including concomitant nephrotoxic medications).
No products indexed under this heading.

Bacitracin Zinc (Caution is indicated when zoledronic acid is used with other potentially nephrotoxic drugs such as nonsteroidal anti-inflammatory drugs. Renal impairment has been observed following the administration of zoledronic acid, especially in patients with pre-existing renal compromise or other risk factors including concomitant nephrotoxic medications).
No products indexed under this heading.

Balsalazide Disodium (Caution is indicated when zoledronic acid is used with other potentially nephrotoxic drugs such as nonsteroidal anti-inflammatory drugs. Renal impairment has been observed following the administration of zoledronic acid, especially in patients with pre-existing renal compromise or other risk factors including concomitant nephrotoxic medications).
No products indexed under this heading.

Beclomethasone Dipropionate (Osteonecrosis of the jaw (ONJ) has been reported in patients treated with bisphosphonates, including zoledronic acid. A dental examination with appropriate preventive dentistry should be considered prior to treatment with bisphosphonates in patients with a history of concomitant risk factors for ONJ (eg, corticosteroids). While on treatment, patients with concomitant risk factors should avoid invasive dental procedures if possible). Products include:
Qvar 3398

Beclomethasone Dipropionate Monohydrate (Osteonecrosis of the jaw (ONJ) has been reported in patients treated with bisphosphonates, including zoledronic acid. A dental examination with appropriate preventive dentistry should be considered prior to treatment with bisphosphonates in patients with a history of concomitant risk factors for ONJ (eg, corticosteroids). While on treatment, patients with concomitant risk factors should avoid invasive dental procedures if possible). Products include:
Beconase AQ 1386

Benazepril Hydrochloride (Caution is indicated when zoledronic acid is used with other potentially nephrotoxic drugs such as nonsteroidal anti-inflammatory drugs. Renal impairment has been observed following the administration of zoledronic acid, especially in patients with pre-existing renal compromise or other risk factors including concomitant nephrotoxic medications).
No products indexed under this heading.

Bendroflumethiazide (Renal impairment has been observed following the administration of zoledronic acid, especially in patients with pre-existing renal compromise or other risk factors including concomitant diuretic therapy).
No products indexed under this heading.

Betamethasone (Osteonecrosis of the jaw (ONJ) has been reported in patients treated with bisphosphonates, including zoledronic acid. A dental examination with appropriate preventive dentistry should be considered prior to treatment with bisphosphonates in patients with a history of concomitant risk factors for ONJ (eg, corticosteroids). While on treatment, patients with concomitant risk factors should avoid invasive dental procedures if possible).
No products indexed under this heading.

Betamethasone Acetate (Osteonecrosis of the jaw (ONJ) has been reported in patients treated with bisphosphonates, including zoledronic acid. A dental examination with appropriate preventive dentistry should be considered prior to treatment with bisphosphonates in patients with a history of concomitant risk factors for ONJ (eg, corticosteroids). While on treatment, patients with concomitant risk factors should avoid invasive dental procedures if possible).
No products indexed under this heading.

Betamethasone Benzoate (Osteonecrosis of the jaw (ONJ) has been reported in patients treated with bisphosphonates, including zoledronic acid. A dental examination with appropriate preventive dentistry should be considered prior to treatment with bisphosphonates in patients with a history of concomitant risk factors for ONJ (eg, corticosteroids). While on treatment, patients with concomitant risk factors should avoid invasive dental procedures if possible).
No products indexed under this heading.

Betamethasone Dipropionate (Osteonecrosis of the jaw (ONJ) has been reported in patients treated with bisphosphonates, including zoledronic acid. A dental examination with appropriate preventive dentistry should be considered prior to treatment with bisphosphonates in patients with a history of concomitant risk factors for ONJ (eg, corticosteroids). While on treatment, patients with concomitant risk factors should avoid invasive dental procedures if possible). Products include:
Diprolene Lotion 0.05% 3108
Diprolene Ointment 0.05% 3109
Diprolene AF Cream 0.05% 3107
Lotrisone 3163

Betamethasone Sodium Phosphate (Osteonecrosis of the jaw (ONJ) has been reported in patients treated with bisphosphonates, including zoledronic acid. A dental examination with appropriate preventive dentistry should be considered prior to treatment with bisphosphonates in patients with a history of concomitant risk factors for ONJ (eg, corticosteroids). While on

IMPORTANT NOTE: Always consult each drug listing in the patient's regimen for possible interactions.

treatment, patients with concomitant risk factors should avoid invasive dental procedures if possible).

No products indexed under this heading.

Betamethasone Valerate (Osteonecrosis of the jaw (ONJ) has been reported in patients treated with bisphosphonates, including zoledronic acid. A dental examination with appropriate preventive dentistry should be considered prior to treatment with bisphosphonates in patients with a history of concomitant risk factors for ONJ (eg, corticosteroids). While on treatment, patients with concomitant risk factors should avoid invasive dental procedures if possible). Products include:

Luxíq 3321

Bicalutamide (Osteonecrosis of the jaw (ONJ) has been reported in patients treated with bisphosphonates, including zoledronic acid. A dental examination with appropriate preventive dentistry should be considered prior to treatment with bisphosphonates in patients with a history of concomitant risk factors for ONJ (eg, chemotherapy). While on treatment, patients with concomitant risk factors should avoid invasive dental procedures if possible).

No products indexed under this heading.

Bleomycin Sulfate (Osteonecrosis of the jaw (ONJ) has been reported in patients treated with bisphosphonates, including zoledronic acid. A dental examination with appropriate preventive dentistry should be considered prior to treatment with bisphosphonates in patients with a history of concomitant risk factors for ONJ (eg, chemotherapy). While on treatment, patients with concomitant risk factors should avoid invasive dental procedures if possible).

No products indexed under this heading.

Budesonide (Osteonecrosis of the jaw (ONJ) has been reported in patients treated with bisphosphonates, including zoledronic acid. A dental examination with appropriate preventive dentistry should be considered prior to treatment with bisphosphonates in patients with a history of concomitant risk factors for ONJ (eg, corticosteroids). While on treatment, patients with concomitant risk factors should avoid invasive dental procedures if possible). Products include:

Pulmicort Flexhaler 714
Symbicort 80/4.5 720
Symbicort 160/4.5 720

Bumetanide (Caution should be exercised when zoledronic acid is used in combination with loop diuretics due to an increased risk of hypocalcemia).

No products indexed under this heading.

Busulfan (Osteonecrosis of the jaw (ONJ) has been reported in patients treated with bisphosphonates, including zoledronic acid. A dental examination with appropriate preventive dentistry should be considered prior to treatment with bisphosphonates in patients with a history of concomitant risk factors for ONJ (eg, chemotherapy). While on treatment, patients with concomitant risk factors should avoid invasive dental procedures if possible). Products include:

Myleran 1581

Caffeine (Caution is indicated when zoledronic acid is used with other potentially nephrotoxic drugs such as nonsteroidal anti-inflammatory drugs. Renal impairment has been observed following the administration of zoledronic acid, especially in patients with pre-existing renal compromise or other risk factors including concomitant nephrotoxic medications).

No products indexed under this heading.

Captopril (Caution is indicated when zoledronic acid is used with other

potentially nephrotoxic drugs such as nonsteroidal anti-inflammatory drugs. Renal impairment has been observed following the administration of zoledronic acid, especially in patients with pre-existing renal compromise or other risk factors including concomitant nephrotoxic medications). Products include:

Captopril 2341

Carbenicillin Disodium (Caution is indicated when zoledronic acid is used with other potentially nephrotoxic drugs such as nonsteroidal anti-inflammatory drugs. Renal impairment has been observed following the administration of zoledronic acid, especially in patients with pre-existing renal compromise or other risk factors including concomitant nephrotoxic medications).

No products indexed under this heading.

Carbenicillin Indanyl Sodium (Caution is indicated when zoledronic acid is used with other potentially nephrotoxic drugs such as nonsteroidal anti-inflammatory drugs. Renal impairment has been observed following the administration of zoledronic acid, especially in patients with pre-existing renal compromise or other risk factors including concomitant nephrotoxic medications).

No products indexed under this heading.

Carboplatin (Caution is indicated when zoledronic acid is used with other potentially nephrotoxic drugs such as nonsteroidal anti-inflammatory drugs. Renal impairment has been observed following the administration of zoledronic acid, especially in patients with pre-existing renal compromise or other risk factors including concomitant nephrotoxic medications).

No products indexed under this heading.

Carmustine (BCNU) (Caution is indicated when zoledronic acid is used with other potentially nephrotoxic drugs such as nonsteroidal anti-inflammatory drugs. Renal impairment has been observed following the administration of zoledronic acid, especially in patients with pre-existing renal compromise or other risk factors including concomitant nephrotoxic medications).

No products indexed under this heading.

Cefaclor (Caution is indicated when zoledronic acid is used with other potentially nephrotoxic drugs such as nonsteroidal anti-inflammatory drugs. Renal impairment has been observed following the administration of zoledronic acid, especially in patients with pre-existing renal compromise or other risk factors including concomitant nephrotoxic medications).

No products indexed under this heading.

Cefadroxil (Caution is indicated when zoledronic acid is used with other potentially nephrotoxic drugs such as nonsteroidal anti-inflammatory drugs. Renal impairment has been observed following the administration of zoledronic acid, especially in patients with pre-existing renal compromise or other risk factors including concomitant nephrotoxic medications).

No products indexed under this heading.

Cefamandole Nafate (Caution is indicated when zoledronic acid is used with other potentially nephrotoxic drugs such as nonsteroidal anti-inflammatory drugs. Renal impairment has been observed following the administration of zoledronic acid, especially in patients with pre-existing renal compromise or other risk factors including concomitant nephrotoxic medications).

No products indexed under this heading.

Cefazolin Sodium (Caution is indicated when zoledronic acid is used with other potentially nephrotoxic drugs such as nonsteroidal anti-inflammatory drugs. Renal impairment has been observed following the administration of zoledronic acid, especially in patients with pre-existing renal compromise or other risk factors including concomitant nephrotoxic medications).

No products indexed under this heading.

Cefdinir (Caution is indicated when zoledronic acid is used with other potentially nephrotoxic drugs such as nonsteroidal anti-inflammatory drugs. Renal impairment has been observed following the administration of zoledronic acid, especially in patients with pre-existing renal compromise or other risk factors including concomitant nephrotoxic medications). Products include:

Omnicef Capsules 518
Omnicef Oral Suspension 518

Cefepime Hydrochloride (Caution is indicated when zoledronic acid is used with other potentially nephrotoxic drugs such as nonsteroidal anti-inflammatory drugs. Renal impairment has been observed following the administration of zoledronic acid, especially in patients with pre-existing renal compromise or other risk factors including concomitant nephrotoxic medications).

No products indexed under this heading.

Cefixime (Caution is indicated when zoledronic acid is used with other potentially nephrotoxic drugs such as nonsteroidal anti-inflammatory drugs. Renal impairment has been observed following the administration of zoledronic acid, especially in patients with pre-existing renal compromise or other risk factors including concomitant nephrotoxic medications). Products include:

Suprax for Oral Suspension 2038
Suprax Tablets 2038

Cefmetazole Sodium (Caution is indicated when zoledronic acid is used with other potentially nephrotoxic drugs such as nonsteroidal anti-inflammatory drugs. Renal impairment has been observed following the administration of zoledronic acid, especially in patients with pre-existing renal compromise or other risk factors including concomitant nephrotoxic medications).

No products indexed under this heading.

Cefonicid Sodium (Caution is indicated when zoledronic acid is used with other potentially nephrotoxic drugs such as nonsteroidal anti-inflammatory drugs. Renal impairment has been observed following the administration of zoledronic acid, especially in patients with pre-existing renal compromise or other risk factors including concomitant nephrotoxic medications).

No products indexed under this heading.

Cefoperazone Sodium (Caution is indicated when zoledronic acid is used with other potentially nephrotoxic drugs such as nonsteroidal anti-inflammatory drugs. Renal impairment has been observed following the administration of zoledronic acid, especially in patients with pre-existing renal compromise or other risk factors including concomitant nephrotoxic medications).

No products indexed under this heading.

Ceforanide (Caution is indicated when zoledronic acid is used with other potentially nephrotoxic drugs such as nonsteroidal anti-inflammatory drugs. Renal impairment has been observed following the administration of zoledronic acid, especially in patients with pre-existing renal compromise or other risk factors including concomitant nephrotoxic medications).

No products indexed under this heading.

Cefotaxime Sodium (Caution is indicated when zoledronic acid is used with other potentially nephrotoxic drugs such as nonsteroidal anti-inflammatory drugs. Renal impairment has been observed following the administration of zoledronic acid, especially in patients with pre-existing renal compromise or other risk factors including concomitant nephrotoxic medications).

No products indexed under this heading.

Cefotetan (Caution is indicated when zoledronic acid is used with other potentially nephrotoxic drugs such as nonsteroidal anti-inflammatory drugs. Renal impairment has been observed following the administration of zoledronic acid, especially in patients with pre-existing renal compromise or other risk factors including concomitant nephrotoxic medications).

No products indexed under this heading.

Cefoxitin Sodium (Caution is indicated when zoledronic acid is used with other potentially nephrotoxic drugs such as nonsteroidal anti-inflammatory drugs. Renal impairment has been observed following the administration of zoledronic acid, especially in patients with pre-existing renal compromise or other risk factors including concomitant nephrotoxic medications).

No products indexed under this heading.

Cefpodoxime Proxetil (Caution is indicated when zoledronic acid is used with other potentially nephrotoxic drugs such as nonsteroidal anti-inflammatory drugs. Renal impairment has been observed following the administration of zoledronic acid, especially in patients with pre-existing renal compromise or other risk factors including concomitant nephrotoxic medications).

No products indexed under this heading.

Cefprozil (Caution is indicated when zoledronic acid is used with other potentially nephrotoxic drugs such as nonsteroidal anti-inflammatory drugs. Renal impairment has been observed following the administration of zoledronic acid, especially in patients with pre-existing renal compromise or other risk factors including concomitant nephrotoxic medications).

No products indexed under this heading.

Ceftazidime (Caution is indicated when zoledronic acid is used with other potentially nephrotoxic drugs such as nonsteroidal anti-inflammatory drugs. Renal impairment has been observed following the administration of zoledronic acid, especially in patients with pre-existing renal compromise or other risk factors including concomitant nephrotoxic medications). Products include:

Fortaz 1481

Ceftizoxime Sodium (Caution is indicated when zoledronic acid is used with other potentially nephrotoxic drugs such as nonsteroidal anti-inflammatory drugs. Renal impairment has been observed following the administration of zoledronic acid, especially in patients with pre-existing renal compromise or other risk factors including concomitant nephrotoxic medications).

No products indexed under this heading.

Ceftriaxone Sodium (Caution is indicated when zoledronic acid is used with other potentially nephrotoxic drugs such as nonsteroidal anti-inflammatory drugs. Renal impairment has been observed following the administration of zoledronic acid, especially in patients with pre-existing renal compromise or other risk factors including concomitant nephrotoxic medications). Products include:

Rocephin 2859

Cefuroxime Axetil (Caution is indicated when zoledronic acid is used with

other potentially nephrotoxic drugs such as nonsteroidal anti-inflammatory drugs. Renal impairment has been observed following the administration of zoledronic acid, especially in patients with pre-existing renal compromise or other risk factors including concomitant nephrotoxic medications). Products include:

Ceftin 1399

Cefuroxime Sodium (Caution is indicated when zoledronic acid is used with other potentially nephrotoxic drugs such as nonsteroidal anti-inflammatory drugs. Renal impairment has been observed following the administration of zoledronic acid, especially in patients with pre-existing renal compromise or other risk factors including concomitant nephrotoxic medications).

No products indexed under this heading.

Celecoxib (Caution is indicated when zoledronic acid is used with other potentially nephrotoxic drugs such as nonsteroidal anti-inflammatory drugs. Renal impairment has been observed following the administration of zoledronic acid, especially in patients with pre-existing renal compromise or other risk factors including concomitant nephrotoxic medications). Products include:

Celebrex 3272

Cephalexin (Caution is indicated when zoledronic acid is used with other potentially nephrotoxic drugs such as nonsteroidal anti-inflammatory drugs. Renal impairment has been observed following the administration of zoledronic acid, especially in patients with pre-existing renal compromise or other risk factors including concomitant nephrotoxic medications).

No products indexed under this heading.

Cephalothin Sodium (Caution is indicated when zoledronic acid is used with other potentially nephrotoxic drugs such as nonsteroidal anti-inflammatory drugs. Renal impairment has been observed following the administration of zoledronic acid, especially in patients with pre-existing renal compromise or other risk factors including concomitant nephrotoxic medications).

No products indexed under this heading.

Cephapirin Sodium (Caution is indicated when zoledronic acid is used with other potentially nephrotoxic drugs such as nonsteroidal anti-inflammatory drugs. Renal impairment has been observed following the administration of zoledronic acid, especially in patients with pre-existing renal compromise or other risk factors including concomitant nephrotoxic medications).

No products indexed under this heading.

Cephradine (Caution is indicated when zoledronic acid is used with other potentially nephrotoxic drugs such as nonsteroidal anti-inflammatory drugs. Renal impairment has been observed following the administration of zoledronic acid, especially in patients with pre-existing renal compromise or other risk factors including concomitant nephrotoxic medications).

No products indexed under this heading.

Cerivastatin Sodium (Caution is indicated when zoledronic acid is used with other potentially nephrotoxic drugs such as nonsteroidal anti-inflammatory drugs. Renal impairment has been observed following the administration of zoledronic acid, especially in patients with pre-existing renal compromise or other risk factors including concomitant nephrotoxic medications).

No products indexed under this heading.

Chlorambucil (Osteonecrosis of the jaw (ONJ) has been reported in patients treated with bisphosphonates, including zoledronic acid. A dental examination

with appropriate preventive dentistry should be considered prior to treatment with bisphosphonates in patients with a history of concomitant risk factors for ONJ (eg, chemotherapy). While on treatment, patients with concomitant risk factors should avoid invasive dental procedures if possible). Products include:

Leukeran 1557

Chlorothiazide (Renal impairment has been observed following the administration of zoledronic acid, especially in patients with pre-existing renal compromise or other risk factors including concomitant diuretic therapy).

No products indexed under this heading.

Chlorothiazide Sodium (Renal impairment has been observed following the administration of zoledronic acid, especially in patients with pre-existing renal compromise or other risk factors including concomitant diuretic therapy). Products include:

Diuril Intravenous 2009

Chlorpropamide (Caution is indicated when zoledronic acid is used with other potentially nephrotoxic drugs such as nonsteroidal anti-inflammatory drugs. Renal impairment has been observed following the administration of zoledronic acid, especially in patients with pre-existing renal compromise or other risk factors including concomitant nephrotoxic medications).

No products indexed under this heading.

Chlorthalidone (Renal impairment has been observed following the administration of zoledronic acid, especially in patients with pre-existing renal compromise or other risk factors including concomitant diuretic therapy). Products include:

Clorpres 2344

Ciclesonide (Osteonecrosis of the jaw (ONJ) has been reported in patients treated with bisphosphonates, including zoledronic acid. A dental examination with appropriate preventive dentistry should be considered prior to treatment with bisphosphonates in patients with a history of concomitant risk factors for ONJ (eg, corticosteroids). While on treatment, patients with concomitant risk factors should avoid invasive dental procedures if possible).

No products indexed under this heading.

Cidofovir (Caution is indicated when zoledronic acid is used with other potentially nephrotoxic drugs such as nonsteroidal anti-inflammatory drugs. Renal impairment has been observed following the administration of zoledronic acid, especially in patients with pre-existing renal compromise or other risk factors including concomitant nephrotoxic medications).

No products indexed under this heading.

Cilastatin Sodium (Caution is indicated when zoledronic acid is used with other potentially nephrotoxic drugs such as nonsteroidal anti-inflammatory drugs. Renal impairment has been observed following the administration of zoledronic acid, especially in patients with pre-existing renal compromise or other risk factors including concomitant nephrotoxic medications). Products include:

Primaxin I.M. 2232
Primaxin I.V. 2235

Cimetidine (Caution is indicated when zoledronic acid is used with other potentially nephrotoxic drugs such as nonsteroidal anti-inflammatory drugs. Renal impairment has been observed following the administration of zoledronic acid, especially in patients with pre-existing renal compromise or other risk factors including concomitant nephrotoxic medications).

No products indexed under this heading.

Cimetidine Hydrochloride (Caution is indicated when zoledronic acid is used with other potentially nephrotoxic drugs such as nonsteroidal anti-inflammatory drugs. Renal impairment has been observed following the administration of zoledronic acid, especially in patients with pre-existing renal compromise or other risk factors including concomitant nephrotoxic medications).

No products indexed under this heading.

Cisplatin (Caution is indicated when zoledronic acid is used with other potentially nephrotoxic drugs such as nonsteroidal anti-inflammatory drugs. Renal impairment has been observed following the administration of zoledronic acid, especially in patients with pre-existing renal compromise or other risk factors including concomitant nephrotoxic medications).

No products indexed under this heading.

Cladribine (Caution is indicated when zoledronic acid is used with other potentially nephrotoxic drugs such as nonsteroidal anti-inflammatory drugs. Renal impairment has been observed following the administration of zoledronic acid, especially in patients with pre-existing renal compromise or other risk factors including concomitant nephrotoxic medications). Products include:

Leustatin 946

Clozapine (Caution is indicated when zoledronic acid is used with other potentially nephrotoxic drugs such as nonsteroidal anti-inflammatory drugs. Renal impairment has been observed following the administration of zoledronic acid, especially in patients with pre-existing renal compromise or other risk factors including concomitant nephrotoxic medications).

No products indexed under this heading.

Colistimethate Sodium (Caution is indicated when zoledronic acid is used with other potentially nephrotoxic drugs such as nonsteroidal anti-inflammatory drugs. Renal impairment has been observed following the administration of zoledronic acid, especially in patients with pre-existing renal compromise or other risk factors including concomitant nephrotoxic medications).

No products indexed under this heading.

Colistin Sulfate (Caution is indicated when zoledronic acid is used with other potentially nephrotoxic drugs such as nonsteroidal anti-inflammatory drugs. Renal impairment has been observed following the administration of zoledronic acid, especially in patients with pre-existing renal compromise or other risk factors including concomitant nephrotoxic medications).

No products indexed under this heading.

Cortisone Acetate (Osteonecrosis of the jaw (ONJ) has been reported in patients treated with bisphosphonates, including zoledronic acid. A dental examination with appropriate preventive dentistry should be considered prior to treatment with bisphosphonates in patients with a history of concomitant risk factors for ONJ (eg, corticosteroids). While on treatment, patients with concomitant risk factors should avoid invasive dental procedures if possible).

No products indexed under this heading.

Cyclophosphamide (Caution is indicated when zoledronic acid is used with other potentially nephrotoxic drugs such as nonsteroidal anti-inflammatory drugs. Renal impairment has been observed following the administration of zoledronic acid, especially in patients with pre-existing renal compromise or other risk factors including concomitant nephrotoxic medications).

No products indexed under this heading.

Cyclosporine (Caution is indicated when zoledronic acid is used with other potentially nephrotoxic drugs such as nonsteroidal anti-inflammatory drugs. Renal impairment has been observed following the administration of zoledronic acid, especially in patients with pre-existing renal compromise or other risk factors including concomitant nephrotoxic medications). Products include:

Gengraf 440
Neoral Oral Solution 2496
Neoral Capsules 2496
Restasis 605

Cytarabine (Caution is indicated when zoledronic acid is used with other potentially nephrotoxic drugs such as nonsteroidal anti-inflammatory drugs. Renal impairment has been observed following the administration of zoledronic acid, especially in patients with pre-existing renal compromise or other risk factors including concomitant nephrotoxic medications).

No products indexed under this heading.

Cytarabine Liposome (Caution is indicated when zoledronic acid is used with other potentially nephrotoxic drugs such as nonsteroidal anti-inflammatory drugs. Renal impairment has been observed following the administration of zoledronic acid, especially in patients with pre-existing renal compromise or other risk factors including concomitant nephrotoxic medications).

No products indexed under this heading.

Dacarbazine (Osteonecrosis of the jaw (ONJ) has been reported in patients treated with bisphosphonates, including zoledronic acid. A dental examination with appropriate preventive dentistry should be considered prior to treatment with bisphosphonates in patients with a history of concomitant risk factors for ONJ (eg, chemotherapy). While on treatment, patients with concomitant risk factors should avoid invasive dental procedures if possible).

No products indexed under this heading.

Daunorubicin Citrate (Osteonecrosis of the jaw (ONJ) has been reported in patients treated with bisphosphonates, including zoledronic acid. A dental examination with appropriate preventive dentistry should be considered prior to treatment with bisphosphonates in patients with a history of concomitant risk factors for ONJ (eg, chemotherapy). While on treatment, patients with concomitant risk factors should avoid invasive dental procedures if possible).

No products indexed under this heading.

Daunorubicin Hydrochloride (Osteonecrosis of the jaw (ONJ) has been reported in patients treated with bisphosphonates, including zoledronic acid. A dental examination with appropriate preventive dentistry should be considered prior to treatment with bisphosphonates in patients with a history of concomitant risk factors for ONJ (eg, chemotherapy). While on treatment, patients with concomitant risk factors should avoid invasive dental procedures if possible).

No products indexed under this heading.

Delavirdine Mesylate (Caution is indicated when zoledronic acid is used with other potentially nephrotoxic drugs such as nonsteroidal anti-inflammatory drugs. Renal impairment has been observed following the administration of zoledronic acid, especially in patients with pre-existing renal compromise or other risk factors including concomitant nephrotoxic medications).

No products indexed under this heading.

Denileukin Diftitox (Osteonecrosis of the jaw (ONJ) has been reported in patients treated with bisphosphonates, including zoledronic acid. A dental

examination with appropriate preventive dentistry should be considered prior to treatment with bisphosphonates in patients with a history of concomitant risk factors for ONJ (eg, chemotherapy). While on treatment, patients with concomitant risk factors should avoid invasive dental procedures if possible). Products include:

Ontak 1068

Desoximetasone (Osteonecrosis of the jaw (ONJ) has been reported in patients treated with bisphosphonates, including zoledronic acid. A dental examination with appropriate preventive dentistry should be considered prior to treatment with bisphosphonates in patients with a history of concomitant risk factors for ONJ (eg, corticosteroids). While on treatment, patients with concomitant risk factors should avoid invasive dental procedures if possible).

No products indexed under this heading.

Dexamethasone (Osteonecrosis of the jaw (ONJ) has been reported in patients treated with bisphosphonates, including zoledronic acid. A dental examination with appropriate preventive dentistry should be considered prior to treatment with bisphosphonates in patients with a history of concomitant risk factors for ONJ (eg, corticosteroids). While on treatment, patients with concomitant risk factors should avoid invasive dental procedures if possible). Products include:

Ciprodex 583
Ozurdex .... ⊙ 223
Tobramycin and Dexamethasone
Ophthalmic Suspension .... ⊙ 251

Dexamethasone Acetate (Osteonecrosis of the jaw (ONJ) has been reported in patients treated with bisphosphonates, including zoledronic acid. A dental examination with appropriate preventive dentistry should be considered prior to treatment with bisphosphonates in patients with a history of concomitant risk factors for ONJ (eg, corticosteroids). While on treatment, patients with concomitant risk factors should avoid invasive dental procedures if possible).

No products indexed under this heading.

Dexamethasone Phosphate (Osteonecrosis of the jaw (ONJ) has been reported in patients treated with bisphosphonates, including zoledronic acid. A dental examination with appropriate preventive dentistry should be considered prior to treatment with bisphosphonates in patients with a history of concomitant risk factors for ONJ (eg, corticosteroids). While on treatment, patients with concomitant risk factors should avoid invasive dental procedures if possible).

No products indexed under this heading.

Dexamethasone Sodium (Osteonecrosis of the jaw (ONJ) has been reported in patients treated with bisphosphonates, including zoledronic acid. A dental examination with appropriate preventive dentistry should be considered prior to treatment with bisphosphonates in patients with a history of concomitant risk factors for ONJ (eg, corticosteroids). While on treatment, patients with concomitant risk factors should avoid invasive dental procedures if possible).

No products indexed under this heading.

Dexamethasone Sodium Phosphate (Osteonecrosis of the jaw (ONJ) has been reported in patients treated with bisphosphonates, including zoledronic acid. A dental examination with appropriate preventive dentistry should be considered prior to treatment with bisphosphonates in patients with a history of concomitant risk factors for ONJ (eg, corticosteroids). While on

treatment, patients with concomitant risk factors should avoid invasive dental procedures if possible).

No products indexed under this heading.

Dexamethasone Sodium Phosphate Injection (Osteonecrosis of the jaw (ONJ) has been reported in patients treated with bisphosphonates, including zoledronic acid. A dental examination with appropriate preventive dentistry should be considered prior to treatment with bisphosphonates in patients with a history of concomitant risk factors for ONJ (eg, corticosteroids). While on treatment, patients with concomitant risk factors should avoid invasive dental procedures if possible).

No products indexed under this heading.

Diatrizoate Meglumine (Caution is indicated when zoledronic acid is used with other potentially nephrotoxic drugs such as nonsteroidal anti-inflammatory drugs. Renal impairment has been observed following the administration of zoledronic acid, especially in patients with pre-existing renal compromise or other risk factors including concomitant nephrotoxic medications).

No products indexed under this heading.

Diatrizoate Sodium (Caution is indicated when zoledronic acid is used with other potentially nephrotoxic drugs such as nonsteroidal anti-inflammatory drugs. Renal impairment has been observed following the administration of zoledronic acid, especially in patients with pre-existing renal compromise or other risk factors including concomitant nephrotoxic medications).

No products indexed under this heading.

Diclofenac Epolamine (Caution is indicated when zoledronic acid is used with other potentially nephrotoxic drugs such as nonsteroidal anti-inflammatory drugs. Renal impairment has been observed following the administration of zoledronic acid, especially in patients with pre-existing renal compromise or other risk factors including concomitant nephrotoxic medications). Products include:

Flector 1839

Diclofenac Potassium (Caution is indicated when zoledronic acid is used with other potentially nephrotoxic drugs such as nonsteroidal anti-inflammatory drugs. Renal impairment has been observed following the administration of zoledronic acid, especially in patients with pre-existing renal compromise or other risk factors including concomitant nephrotoxic medications).

No products indexed under this heading.

Diclofenac Sodium (Caution is indicated when zoledronic acid is used with other potentially nephrotoxic drugs such as nonsteroidal anti-inflammatory drugs. Renal impairment has been observed following the administration of zoledronic acid, especially in patients with pre-existing renal compromise or other risk factors including concomitant nephrotoxic medications).

No products indexed under this heading.

Dicloxacillin Sodium (Caution is indicated when zoledronic acid is used with other potentially nephrotoxic drugs such as nonsteroidal anti-inflammatory drugs. Renal impairment has been observed following the administration of zoledronic acid, especially in patients with pre-existing renal compromise or other risk factors including concomitant nephrotoxic medications).

No products indexed under this heading.

Didanosine (Caution is indicated when zoledronic acid is used with other potentially nephrotoxic drugs such as nonsteroidal anti-inflammatory drugs. Renal impairment has been observed following the administration of zoledronic acid, especially in patients with pre-existing renal compromise or other risk factors including concomitant nephrotoxic medications).

No products indexed under this heading.

Diflorasone Diacetate (Osteonecrosis of the jaw (ONJ) has been reported in patients treated with bisphosphonates, including zoledronic acid. A dental examination with appropriate preventive dentistry should be considered prior to treatment with bisphosphonates in patients with a history of concomitant risk factors for ONJ (eg, corticosteroids). While on treatment, patients with concomitant risk factors should avoid invasive dental procedures if possible).

No products indexed under this heading.

Digoxin (Renal impairment has been observed following the administration of zoledronic acid in patients with pre-existing renal compromise or other risk factors. In patients with renal impairment, the exposure to concomitant medications that are primarily renally excreted (eg, digoxin) may increase. Consider monitoring serum creatinine in patients at risk for renal impairment who are taking concomitant medications that are primarily excreted by the kidney). Products include:

Lanoxin Injection 1546
Lanoxin Injection Pediatric 1549
Lanoxin Tablets 1553

Dihydrostreptomycin (Caution is advised when bisphosphonates, including zoledronic acid, are administered with aminoglycosides, since these agents may have an additive effect to lower serum calcium level for prolonged periods).

No products indexed under this heading.

Docetaxel (Osteonecrosis of the jaw (ONJ) has been reported in patients treated with bisphosphonates, including zoledronic acid. A dental examination with appropriate preventive dentistry should be considered prior to treatment with bisphosphonates in patients with a history of concomitant risk factors for ONJ (eg, chemotherapy). While on treatment, patients with concomitant risk factors should avoid invasive dental procedures if possible). Products include:

Taxotere 3035

Doxorubicin Hydrochloride (Osteonecrosis of the jaw (ONJ) has been reported in patients treated with bisphosphonates, including zoledronic acid. A dental examination with appropriate preventive dentistry should be considered prior to treatment with bisphosphonates in patients with a history of concomitant risk factors for ONJ (eg, chemotherapy). While on treatment, patients with concomitant risk factors should avoid invasive dental procedures if possible).

No products indexed under this heading.

Efavirenz (Caution is indicated when zoledronic acid is used with other potentially nephrotoxic drugs such as nonsteroidal anti-inflammatory drugs. Renal impairment has been observed following the administration of zoledronic acid, especially in patients with pre-existing renal compromise or other risk factors including concomitant nephrotoxic medications). Products include:

Atripla 906

Emtricitabine (Caution is indicated when zoledronic acid is used with other potentially nephrotoxic drugs such as nonsteroidal anti-inflammatory drugs.

Renal impairment has been observed following the administration of zoledronic acid, especially in patients with pre-existing renal compromise or other risk factors including concomitant nephrotoxic medications). Products include:

Atripla 906
Emtriva 1238
Emtriva Oral Solution 1238
Truvada 1258

Enalapril Maleate (Caution is indicated when zoledronic acid is used with other potentially nephrotoxic drugs such as nonsteroidal anti-inflammatory drugs. Renal impairment has been observed following the administration of zoledronic acid, especially in patients with pre-existing renal compromise or other risk factors including concomitant nephrotoxic medications).

No products indexed under this heading.

Enalaprilat (Caution is indicated when zoledronic acid is used with other potentially nephrotoxic drugs such as nonsteroidal anti-inflammatory drugs. Renal impairment has been observed following the administration of zoledronic acid, especially in patients with pre-existing renal compromise or other risk factors including concomitant nephrotoxic medications).

No products indexed under this heading.

Enfuvirtide (Caution is indicated when zoledronic acid is used with other potentially nephrotoxic drugs such as nonsteroidal anti-inflammatory drugs. Renal impairment has been observed following the administration of zoledronic acid, especially in patients with pre-existing renal compromise or other risk factors including concomitant nephrotoxic medications).

No products indexed under this heading.

Epirubicin Hydrochloride (Osteonecrosis of the jaw (ONJ) has been reported in patients treated with bisphosphonates, including zoledronic acid. A dental examination with appropriate preventive dentistry should be considered prior to treatment with bisphosphonates in patients with a history of concomitant risk factors for ONJ (eg, chemotherapy). While on treatment, patients with concomitant risk factors should avoid invasive dental procedures if possible).

No products indexed under this heading.

Estramustine Phosphate Sodium (Osteonecrosis of the jaw (ONJ) has been reported in patients treated with bisphosphonates, including zoledronic acid. A dental examination with appropriate preventive dentistry should be considered prior to treatment with bisphosphonates in patients with a history of concomitant risk factors for ONJ (eg, chemotherapy). While on treatment, patients with concomitant risk factors should avoid invasive dental procedures if possible).

No products indexed under this heading.

Ethacrynic Acid (Caution should be exercised when zoledronic acid is used in combination with loop diuretics due to an increased risk of hypocalcemia).

No products indexed under this heading.

Ethiodized Oil (Caution is indicated when zoledronic acid is used with other potentially nephrotoxic drugs such as nonsteroidal anti-inflammatory drugs. Renal impairment has been observed following the administration of zoledronic acid, especially in patients with pre-existing renal compromise or other risk factors including concomitant nephrotoxic medications).

No products indexed under this heading.

Etodolac (Caution is indicated when zoledronic acid is used with other potentially nephrotoxic drugs such as nonsteroidal anti-inflammatory drugs. Renal impairment has been observed following the administration of zoledronic acid, especially in patients with pre-existing renal compromise or other risk factors including concomitant nephrotoxic medications).
No products indexed under this heading.

Etoposide (Osteonecrosis of the jaw (ONJ) has been reported in patients treated with bisphosphonates, including zoledronic acid. A dental examination with appropriate preventive dentistry should be considered prior to treatment with bisphosphonates in patients with a history of concomitant risk factors for ONJ (eg, chemotherapy). While on treatment, patients with concomitant risk factors should avoid invasive dental procedures if possible).
No products indexed under this heading.

Exemestane (Osteonecrosis of the jaw (ONJ) has been reported in patients treated with bisphosphonates, including zoledronic acid. A dental examination with appropriate preventive dentistry should be considered prior to treatment with bisphosphonates in patients with a history of concomitant risk factors for ONJ (eg, chemotherapy). While on treatment, patients with concomitant risk factors should avoid invasive dental procedures if possible). Products include:
Aromasin **2758**

Fenoprofen Calcium (Caution is indicated when zoledronic acid is used with other potentially nephrotoxic drugs such as nonsteroidal anti-inflammatory drugs. Renal impairment has been observed following the administration of zoledronic acid, especially in patients with pre-existing renal compromise or other risk factors including concomitant nephrotoxic medications).
No products indexed under this heading.

Filgrastim (Caution is indicated when zoledronic acid is used with other potentially nephrotoxic drugs such as nonsteroidal anti-inflammatory drugs. Renal impairment has been observed following the administration of zoledronic acid, especially in patients with pre-existing renal compromise or other risk factors including concomitant nephrotoxic medications). Products include:
Neupogen **631**

Floxuridine (Osteonecrosis of the jaw (ONJ) has been reported in patients treated with bisphosphonates, including zoledronic acid. A dental examination with appropriate preventive dentistry should be considered prior to treatment with bisphosphonates in patients with a history of concomitant risk factors for ONJ (eg, chemotherapy). While on treatment, patients with concomitant risk factors should avoid invasive dental procedures if possible).
No products indexed under this heading.

Fludrocortisone Acetate (Osteonecrosis of the jaw (ONJ) has been reported in patients treated with bisphosphonates, including zoledronic acid. A dental examination with appropriate preventive dentistry should be considered prior to treatment with bisphosphonates in patients with a history of concomitant risk factors for ONJ (eg, corticosteroids). While on treatment, patients with concomitant risk factors should avoid invasive dental procedures if possible).
No products indexed under this heading.

Flumethasone Pivalate (Osteonecrosis of the jaw (ONJ) has been reported in patients treated with bisphosphonates, including zoledronic acid. A dental examination with appropriate preven-

tive dentistry should be considered prior to treatment with bisphosphonates in patients with a history of concomitant risk factors for ONJ (eg, corticosteroids). While on treatment, patients with concomitant risk factors should avoid invasive dental procedures if possible).
No products indexed under this heading.

Flunisolide Hemihydrate (Osteonecrosis of the jaw (ONJ) has been reported in patients treated with bisphosphonates, including zoledronic acid. A dental examination with appropriate preventive dentistry should be considered prior to treatment with bisphosphonates in patients with a history of concomitant risk factors for ONJ (eg, corticosteroids). While on treatment, patients with concomitant risk factors should avoid invasive dental procedures if possible).
No products indexed under this heading.

Fluorouracil (Caution is indicated when zoledronic acid is used with other potentially nephrotoxic drugs such as nonsteroidal anti-inflammatory drugs. Renal impairment has been observed following the administration of zoledronic acid, especially in patients with pre-existing renal compromise or other risk factors including concomitant nephrotoxic medications). Products include:
Carac **2966**

Flurbiprofen (Caution is indicated when zoledronic acid is used with other potentially nephrotoxic drugs such as nonsteroidal anti-inflammatory drugs. Renal impairment has been observed following the administration of zoledronic acid, especially in patients with pre-existing renal compromise or other risk factors including concomitant nephrotoxic medications).
No products indexed under this heading.

Flutamide (Osteonecrosis of the jaw (ONJ) has been reported in patients treated with bisphosphonates, including zoledronic acid. A dental examination with appropriate preventive dentistry should be considered prior to treatment with bisphosphonates in patients with a history of concomitant risk factors for ONJ (eg, chemotherapy). While on treatment, patients with concomitant risk factors should avoid invasive dental procedures if possible).
No products indexed under this heading.

Fluticasone Furoate (Osteonecrosis of the jaw (ONJ) has been reported in patients treated with bisphosphonates, including zoledronic acid. A dental examination with appropriate preventive dentistry should be considered prior to treatment with bisphosphonates in patients with a history of concomitant risk factors for ONJ (eg, corticosteroids). While on treatment, patients with concomitant risk factors should avoid invasive dental procedures if possible). Products include:
Veramyst **1713**

Fluticasone Propionate (Osteonecrosis of the jaw (ONJ) has been reported in patients treated with bisphosphonates, including zoledronic acid. A dental examination with appropriate preventive dentistry should be considered prior to treatment with bisphosphonates in patients with a history of concomitant risk factors for ONJ (eg, corticosteroids). While on treatment, patients with concomitant risk factors should avoid invasive dental procedures if possible). Products include:
Advair 100/50 .... **1275**
Advair 250/50 .... **1275**
Advair 500/50 .... **1275**
Advair HFA 45/21 .... **1288**
Advair HFA 115/21 .... **1288**
Advair HFA 230/21 .... **1288**
Flonase **1459**

Flovent Diskus **1463**
Flovent HFA **1470**

Fluvastatin Sodium (Caution is indicated when zoledronic acid is used with other potentially nephrotoxic drugs such as nonsteroidal anti-inflammatory drugs. Renal impairment has been observed following the administration of zoledronic acid, especially in patients with pre-existing renal compromise or other risk factors including concomitant nephrotoxic medications).
No products indexed under this heading.

Foscarnet Sodium (Caution is indicated when zoledronic acid is used with other potentially nephrotoxic drugs such as nonsteroidal anti-inflammatory drugs. Renal impairment has been observed following the administration of zoledronic acid, especially in patients with pre-existing renal compromise or other risk factors including concomitant nephrotoxic medications).
No products indexed under this heading.

Fosinopril Sodium (Caution is indicated when zoledronic acid is used with other potentially nephrotoxic drugs such as nonsteroidal anti-inflammatory drugs. Renal impairment has been observed following the administration of zoledronic acid, especially in patients with pre-existing renal compromise or other risk factors including concomitant nephrotoxic medications).
No products indexed under this heading.

Furosemide (Caution should be exercised when zoledronic acid is used in combination with loop diuretics due to an increased risk of hypocalcemia).
Products include:
Furosemide **2354**

Gadopentetate Dimeglumine (Caution is indicated when zoledronic acid is used with other potentially nephrotoxic drugs such as nonsteroidal anti-inflammatory drugs. Renal impairment has been observed following the administration of zoledronic acid, especially in patients with pre-existing renal compromise or other risk factors including concomitant nephrotoxic medications).
No products indexed under this heading.

Gemcitabine Hydrochloride (Osteonecrosis of the jaw (ONJ) has been reported in patients treated with bisphosphonates, including zoledronic acid. A dental examination with appropriate preventive dentistry should be considered prior to treatment with bisphosphonates in patients with a history of concomitant risk factors for ONJ (eg, chemotherapy). While on treatment, patients with concomitant risk factors should avoid invasive dental procedures if possible). Products include:
Gemzar **1900**

Gentamicin (Caution is advised when bisphosphonates, including zoledronic acid, are administered with aminoglycosides, since these agents may have an additive effect to lower serum calcium level for prolonged periods).
No products indexed under this heading.

Gentamicin Sulfate (Caution is advised when bisphosphonates, including zoledronic acid, are administered with aminoglycosides, since these agents may have an additive effect to lower serum calcium level for prolonged periods). Products include:
Pred-G .... ⊙**226**, ⊙**227**

Glipizide (Caution is indicated when zoledronic acid is used with other potentially nephrotoxic drugs such as nonsteroidal anti-inflammatory drugs. Renal impairment has been observed following the administration of zoledronic acid, especially in patients with pre-existing renal compromise or other risk factors including concomitant nephrotoxic medications).
No products indexed under this heading.

Globulin, Immune (Human) (Caution is indicated when zoledronic acid is used with other potentially nephrotoxic drugs such as nonsteroidal anti-inflammatory drugs. Renal impairment has been observed following the administration of zoledronic acid, especially in patients with pre-existing renal compromise or other risk factors including concomitant nephrotoxic medications). Products include:

Glyburide (Caution is indicated when zoledronic acid is used with other potentially nephrotoxic drugs such as nonsteroidal anti-inflammatory drugs. Renal impairment has been observed following the administration of zoledronic acid, especially in patients with pre-existing renal compromise or other risk factors including concomitant nephrotoxic medications).
No products indexed under this heading.

Gold Therapy (Caution is indicated when zoledronic acid is used with other potentially nephrotoxic drugs such as nonsteroidal anti-inflammatory drugs. Renal impairment has been observed following the administration of zoledronic acid, especially in patients with pre-existing renal compromise or other risk factors including concomitant nephrotoxic medications).
No products indexed under this heading.

HMG-CoA Reductase Inhibitors (Caution is indicated when zoledronic acid is used with other potentially nephrotoxic drugs such as nonsteroidal anti-inflammatory drugs. Renal impairment has been observed following the administration of zoledronic acid, especially in patients with pre-existing renal compromise or other risk factors including concomitant nephrotoxic medications).
No products indexed under this heading.

Hydrochlorothiazide (Renal impairment has been observed following the administration of zoledronic acid, especially in patients with pre-existing renal compromise or other risk factors including concomitant diuretic therapy).
Products include:
Atacand HCT **700**
Avalide **2956**
Benicar HCT **1017**
Diovan HCT **2419**
Dyazide **1429**
Exforge HCT **2449**
Hyzaar **2162**
Hyzaar 100-12.5 .... **2162**
Micardis HCT **889**
Prinzide **2246**
Tekturna HCT **2541**
Teveten HCT **541**

Hydrocortisone (Osteonecrosis of the jaw (ONJ) has been reported in patients treated with bisphosphonates, including zoledronic acid. A dental examination with appropriate preventive dentistry should be considered prior to treatment with bisphosphonates in patients with a history of concomitant risk factors for ONJ (eg, corticosteroids). While on treatment, patients with concomitant risk factors should avoid invasive dental procedures if possible).
No products indexed under this heading.

Hydrocortisone (Alcohol) (Osteonecrosis of the jaw (ONJ) has been reported in patients treated with bisphosphonates, including zoledronic acid. A dental examination with appropriate preventive dentistry should be considered prior to treatment with bisphosphonates in patients with a history of concomitant risk factors for ONJ (eg, corticosteroids). While on treatment, patients with concomitant risk factors should avoid invasive dental procedures if possible).
No products indexed under this heading.

Hydrocortisone Acetate (Osteonecrosis of the jaw (ONJ) has been report-

ed in patients treated with bisphosphonates, including zoledronic acid. A dental examination with appropriate preventive dentistry should be considered prior to treatment with bisphosphonates in patients with a history of concomitant risk factors for ONJ (eg, corticosteroids). While on treatment, patients with concomitant risk factors should avoid invasive dental procedures if possible).
No products indexed under this heading.

Hydrocortisone Butyrate (Osteonecrosis of the jaw (ONJ) has been reported in patients treated with bisphosphonates, including zoledronic acid. A dental examination with appropriate preventive dentistry should be considered prior to treatment with bisphosphonates in patients with a history of concomitant risk factors for ONJ (eg, corticosteroids). While on treatment, patients with concomitant risk factors should avoid invasive dental procedures if possible).
No products indexed under this heading.

Hydrocortisone Cypionate (Osteonecrosis of the jaw (ONJ) has been reported in patients treated with bisphosphonates, including zoledronic acid. A dental examination with appropriate preventive dentistry should be considered prior to treatment with bisphosphonates in patients with a history of concomitant risk factors for ONJ (eg, corticosteroids). While on treatment, patients with concomitant risk factors should avoid invasive dental procedures if possible).
No products indexed under this heading.

Hydrocortisone Hemisuccinate (Osteonecrosis of the jaw (ONJ) has been reported in patients treated with bisphosphonates, including zoledronic acid. A dental examination with appropriate preventive dentistry should be considered prior to treatment with bisphosphonates in patients with a history of concomitant risk factors for ONJ (eg, corticosteroids). While on treatment, patients with concomitant risk factors should avoid invasive dental procedures if possible).
No products indexed under this heading.

Hydrocortisone Probutate (Osteonecrosis of the jaw (ONJ) has been reported in patients treated with bisphosphonates, including zoledronic acid. A dental examination with appropriate preventive dentistry should be considered prior to treatment with bisphosphonates in patients with a history of concomitant risk factors for ONJ (eg, corticosteroids). While on treatment, patients with concomitant risk factors should avoid invasive dental procedures if possible).
No products indexed under this heading.

Hydrocortisone Sodium Phosphate (Osteonecrosis of the jaw (ONJ) has been reported in patients treated with bisphosphonates, including zoledronic acid. A dental examination with appropriate preventive dentistry should be considered prior to treatment with bisphosphonates in patients with a history of concomitant risk factors for ONJ (eg, corticosteroids). While on treatment, patients with concomitant risk factors should avoid invasive dental procedures if possible).
No products indexed under this heading.

Hydrocortisone Sodium Succinate (Osteonecrosis of the jaw (ONJ) has been reported in patients treated with bisphosphonates, including zoledronic acid. A dental examination with appropriate preventive dentistry should be considered prior to treatment with bisphosphonates in patients with a history of concomitant risk factors for ONJ (eg, corticosteroids). While on treatment, patients with concomitant risk factors should avoid invasive dental procedures if possible).
No products indexed under this heading.

Hydrocortisone Valerate (Osteonecrosis of the jaw (ONJ) has been reported in patients treated with bisphosphonates, including zoledronic acid. A dental examination with appropriate preventive dentistry should be considered prior to treatment with bisphosphonates in patients with a history of concomitant risk factors for ONJ (eg, corticosteroids). While on treatment, patients with concomitant risk factors should avoid invasive dental procedures if possible).
No products indexed under this heading.

Hydroflumethiazide (Renal impairment has been observed following the administration of zoledronic acid, especially in patients with pre-existing renal compromise or other risk factors including concomitant diuretic therapy).
No products indexed under this heading.

Hydroxyurea (Osteonecrosis of the jaw (ONJ) has been reported in patients treated with bisphosphonates, including zoledronic acid. A dental examination with appropriate preventive dentistry should be considered prior to treatment with bisphosphonates in patients with a history of concomitant risk factors for ONJ (eg, chemotherapy). While on treatment, patients with concomitant risk factors should avoid invasive dental procedures if possible).
No products indexed under this heading.

Ibuprofen (Caution is indicated when zoledronic acid is used with other potentially nephrotoxic drugs such as nonsteroidal anti-inflammatory drugs. Renal impairment has been observed following the administration of zoledronic acid, especially in patients with pre-existing renal compromise or other risk factors including concomitant nephrotoxic medications). Products include:

- Motrin IB 2043
- Children's Motrin 2044
- Children's Motrin Non-Staining Dye-Free 2044
- Infants' Motrin 2044
- Infants' Motrin Dye-Free 2044
- Junior Strength Motrin 2044
- Vicoprofen 564

Idarubicin Hydrochloride (Caution is indicated when zoledronic acid is used with other potentially nephrotoxic drugs such as nonsteroidal anti-inflammatory drugs. Renal impairment has been observed following the administration of zoledronic acid, especially in patients with pre-existing renal compromise or other risk factors including concomitant nephrotoxic medications).
No products indexed under this heading.

Ifosfamide (Caution is indicated when zoledronic acid is used with other potentially nephrotoxic drugs such as nonsteroidal anti-inflammatory drugs. Renal impairment has been observed following the administration of zoledronic acid, especially in patients with pre-existing renal compromise or other risk factors including concomitant nephrotoxic medications).
No products indexed under this heading.

Imipenem (Caution is indicated when zoledronic acid is used with other potentially nephrotoxic drugs such as nonsteroidal anti-inflammatory drugs. Renal impairment has been observed following the administration of zoledronic acid, especially in patients with pre-existing renal compromise or other risk factors including concomitant nephrotoxic medications). Products include:

- Primaxin I.M. 2232
- Primaxin I.V. 2235

Immune Globulin Intravenous (Human) (Caution is indicated when zoledronic acid is used with other potentially nephrotoxic drugs such as nonsteroidal anti-inflammatory drugs. Renal impairment has been observed following the administration of zoledronic acid, especially in patients with pre-existing renal compromise or other risk factors including concomitant nephrotoxic medications). Products include:

- Flebogamma 5% DIF 1794
- Gammagard 812, 815
- Gamunex 3374

Indapamide (Renal impairment has been observed following the administration of zoledronic acid, especially in patients with pre-existing renal compromise or other risk factors including concomitant diuretic therapy). Products include:

- Indapamide 2356

Indinavir Sulfate (Caution is indicated when zoledronic acid is used with other potentially nephrotoxic drugs such as nonsteroidal anti-inflammatory drugs. Renal impairment has been observed following the administration of zoledronic acid, especially in patients with pre-existing renal compromise or other risk factors including concomitant nephrotoxic medications). Products include:

- Crixivan 2113

Indomethacin (Caution is indicated when zoledronic acid is used with other potentially nephrotoxic drugs such as nonsteroidal anti-inflammatory drugs. Renal impairment has been observed following the administration of zoledronic acid, especially in patients with pre-existing renal compromise or other risk factors including concomitant nephrotoxic medications). Products include:

- Indocin 2167

Indomethacin Sodium Trihydrate (Caution is indicated when zoledronic acid is used with other potentially nephrotoxic drugs such as nonsteroidal anti-inflammatory drugs. Renal impairment has been observed following the administration of zoledronic acid, especially in patients with pre-existing renal compromise or other risk factors including concomitant nephrotoxic medications). Products include:

- Indocin I.V. 2007

Interferon alfa-2a, Recombinant (Osteonecrosis of the jaw (ONJ) has been reported in patients treated with bisphosphonates, including zoledronic acid. A dental examination with appropriate preventive dentistry should be considered prior to treatment with bisphosphonates in patients with a history of concomitant risk factors for ONJ (eg, chemotherapy). While on treatment, patients with concomitant risk factors should avoid invasive dental procedures if possible).
No products indexed under this heading.

Interferon alfa-2b, Recombinant (Osteonecrosis of the jaw (ONJ) has been reported in patients treated with bisphosphonates, including zoledronic acid. A dental examination with appropriate preventive dentistry should be considered prior to treatment with bisphosphonates in patients with a history of concomitant risk factors for ONJ (eg, chemotherapy). While on treatment, patients with concomitant risk factors should avoid invasive dental procedures if possible). Products include:

- Intron A 3140

Interferon Beta-1b (Caution is indicated when zoledronic acid is used with other potentially nephrotoxic drugs such as nonsteroidal anti-inflammatory drugs. Renal impairment has been observed following the administration of zoledronic acid, especially in patients with pre-existing renal compromise or other risk factors including concomitant nephrotoxic medications). Products include:

- Betaseron 836
- Extavia 2459

Interleuken-2 (Caution is indicated when zoledronic acid is used with other potentially nephrotoxic drugs such as nonsteroidal anti-inflammatory drugs. Renal impairment has been observed following the administration of zoledronic acid, especially in patients with pre-existing renal compromise or other risk factors including concomitant nephrotoxic medications).
No products indexed under this heading.

Iodamide Meglumine (Caution is indicated when zoledronic acid is used with other potentially nephrotoxic drugs such as nonsteroidal anti-inflammatory drugs. Renal impairment has been observed following the administration of zoledronic acid, especially in patients with pre-existing renal compromise or other risk factors including concomitant nephrotoxic medications).
No products indexed under this heading.

Iohexol (Caution is indicated when zoledronic acid is used with other potentially nephrotoxic drugs such as nonsteroidal anti-inflammatory drugs. Renal impairment has been observed following the administration of zoledronic acid, especially in patients with pre-existing renal compromise or other risk factors including concomitant nephrotoxic medications).
No products indexed under this heading.

Iopamidol (Caution is indicated when zoledronic acid is used with other potentially nephrotoxic drugs such as nonsteroidal anti-inflammatory drugs. Renal impairment has been observed following the administration of zoledronic acid, especially in patients with pre-existing renal compromise or other risk factors including concomitant nephrotoxic medications).
No products indexed under this heading.

Iopanoic Acid (Caution is indicated when zoledronic acid is used with other potentially nephrotoxic drugs such as nonsteroidal anti-inflammatory drugs. Renal impairment has been observed following the administration of zoledronic acid, especially in patients with pre-existing renal compromise or other risk factors including concomitant nephrotoxic medications).
No products indexed under this heading.

Iothalamate Meglumine (Caution is indicated when zoledronic acid is used with other potentially nephrotoxic drugs such as nonsteroidal anti-inflammatory drugs. Renal impairment has been observed following the administration of zoledronic acid, especially in patients with pre-existing renal compromise or other risk factors including concomitant nephrotoxic medications).
No products indexed under this heading.

Ioxaglate Meglumine (Caution is indicated when zoledronic acid is used with other potentially nephrotoxic drugs such as nonsteroidal anti-inflammatory drugs. Renal impairment has been observed following the administration of zoledronic acid, especially in patients with pre-existing renal compromise or other risk factors including concomitant nephrotoxic medications).
No products indexed under this heading.

1579 **Interactions Index** **Reclast**

Ioxaglate Sodium (Caution is indicated when zoledronic acid is used with other potentially nephrotoxic drugs such as nonsteroidal anti-inflammatory drugs. Renal impairment has been observed following the administration of zoledronic acid, especially in patients with pre-existing renal compromise or other risk factors including concomitant nephrotoxic medications).
No products indexed under this heading.

Irinotecan Hydrochloride (Osteonecrosis of the jaw (ONJ) has been reported in patients treated with bisphosphonates, including zoledronic acid. A dental examination with appropriate preventive dentistry should be considered prior to treatment with bisphosphonates in patients with a history of concomitant risk factors for ONJ (eg, chemotherapy). While on treatment, patients with concomitant risk factors should avoid invasive dental procedures if possible).
No products indexed under this heading.

Kanamycin Sulfate (Caution is advised when bisphosphonates, including zoledronic acid, are administered with aminoglycosides, since these agents may have an additive effect to lower serum calcium level for prolonged periods).
No products indexed under this heading.

Ketoprofen (Caution is indicated when zoledronic acid is used with other potentially nephrotoxic drugs such as nonsteroidal anti-inflammatory drugs. Renal impairment has been observed following the administration of zoledronic acid, especially in patients with pre-existing renal compromise or other risk factors including concomitant nephrotoxic medications).
No products indexed under this heading.

Ketorolac Tromethamine (Caution is indicated when zoledronic acid is used with other potentially nephrotoxic drugs such as nonsteroidal anti-inflammatory drugs. Renal impairment has been observed following the administration of zoledronic acid, especially in patients with pre-existing renal compromise or other risk factors including concomitant nephrotoxic medications). Products include:
Acuvail .... ⊙ 209

Lamium album (Caution is indicated when zoledronic acid is used with other potentially nephrotoxic drugs such as nonsteroidal anti-inflammatory drugs. Renal impairment has been observed following the administration of zoledronic acid, especially in patients with pre-existing renal compromise or other risk factors including concomitant nephrotoxic medications).
No products indexed under this heading.

Levamisole Hydrochloride (Osteonecrosis of the jaw (ONJ) has been reported in patients treated with bisphosphonates, including zoledronic acid. A dental examination with appropriate preventive dentistry should be considered prior to treatment with bisphosphonates in patients with a history of concomitant risk factors for ONJ (eg, chemotherapy). While on treatment, patients with concomitant risk factors should avoid invasive dental procedures if possible).
No products indexed under this heading.

Lisinopril (Caution is indicated when zoledronic acid is used with other potentially nephrotoxic drugs such as nonsteroidal anti-inflammatory drugs. Renal impairment has been observed following the administration of zoledronic acid, especially in patients with pre-existing renal compromise or other risk factors including concomitant nephrotoxic medications). Products include:
Prinivil 2241
Prinzide 2246

Lithium (Caution is indicated when zoledronic acid is used with other potentially nephrotoxic drugs such as nonsteroidal anti-inflammatory drugs. Renal impairment has been observed following the administration of zoledronic acid, especially in patients with pre-existing renal compromise or other risk factors including concomitant nephrotoxic medications).
No products indexed under this heading.

Lithium Carbonate (Caution is indicated when zoledronic acid is used with other potentially nephrotoxic drugs such as nonsteroidal anti-inflammatory drugs. Renal impairment has been observed following the administration of zoledronic acid, especially in patients with pre-existing renal compromise or other risk factors including concomitant nephrotoxic medications).
No products indexed under this heading.

Lithium Citrate (Caution is indicated when zoledronic acid is used with other potentially nephrotoxic drugs such as nonsteroidal anti-inflammatory drugs. Renal impairment has been observed following the administration of zoledronic acid, especially in patients with pre-existing renal compromise or other risk factors including concomitant nephrotoxic medications).
No products indexed under this heading.

Lomustine (CCNU) (Osteonecrosis of the jaw (ONJ) has been reported in patients treated with bisphosphonates, including zoledronic acid. A dental examination with appropriate preventive dentistry should be considered prior to treatment with bisphosphonates in patients with a history of concomitant risk factors for ONJ (eg, chemotherapy). While on treatment, patients with concomitant risk factors should avoid invasive dental procedures if possible).
No products indexed under this heading.

Lopinavir (Caution is indicated when zoledronic acid is used with other potentially nephrotoxic drugs such as nonsteroidal anti-inflammatory drugs. Renal impairment has been observed following the administration of zoledronic acid, especially in patients with pre-existing renal compromise or other risk factors including concomitant nephrotoxic medications). Products include:
Kaletra 458

Loracarbef (Caution is indicated when zoledronic acid is used with other potentially nephrotoxic drugs such as nonsteroidal anti-inflammatory drugs. Renal impairment has been observed following the administration of zoledronic acid, especially in patients with pre-existing renal compromise or other risk factors including concomitant nephrotoxic medications).
No products indexed under this heading.

Lovastatin (Caution is indicated when zoledronic acid is used with other potentially nephrotoxic drugs such as nonsteroidal anti-inflammatory drugs. Renal impairment has been observed following the administration of zoledronic acid, especially in patients with pre-existing renal compromise or other risk factors including concomitant nephrotoxic medications). Products include:
Advicor 402
Mevacor 2212

Mechlorethamine Hydrochloride (Osteonecrosis of the jaw (ONJ) has been reported in patients treated with bisphosphonates, including zoledronic acid. A dental examination with appropriate preventive dentistry should be considered prior to treatment with bisphosphonates in patients with a history of concomitant risk factors for ONJ (eg, chemotherapy). While on treatment, patients with concomitant risk factors should avoid invasive dental procedures if possible). Products include:
Mustargen 2010

Meclofenamate Sodium (Caution is indicated when zoledronic acid is used with other potentially nephrotoxic drugs such as nonsteroidal anti-inflammatory drugs. Renal impairment has been observed following the administration of zoledronic acid, especially in patients with pre-existing renal compromise or other risk factors including concomitant nephrotoxic medications).
No products indexed under this heading.

Mefenamic Acid (Caution is indicated when zoledronic acid is used with other potentially nephrotoxic drugs such as nonsteroidal anti-inflammatory drugs. Renal impairment has been observed following the administration of zoledronic acid, especially in patients with pre-existing renal compromise or other risk factors including concomitant nephrotoxic medications).
No products indexed under this heading.

Megestrol Acetate (Osteonecrosis of the jaw (ONJ) has been reported in patients treated with bisphosphonates, including zoledronic acid. A dental examination with appropriate preventive dentistry should be considered prior to treatment with bisphosphonates in patients with a history of concomitant risk factors for ONJ (eg, chemotherapy). While on treatment, patients with concomitant risk factors should avoid invasive dental procedures if possible). Products include:
Megace ES 2698

Meloxicam (Caution is indicated when zoledronic acid is used with other potentially nephrotoxic drugs such as nonsteroidal anti-inflammatory drugs. Renal impairment has been observed following the administration of zoledronic acid, especially in patients with pre-existing renal compromise or other risk factors including concomitant nephrotoxic medications).
No products indexed under this heading.

Melphalan (Osteonecrosis of the jaw (ONJ) has been reported in patients treated with bisphosphonates, including zoledronic acid. A dental examination with appropriate preventive dentistry should be considered prior to treatment with bisphosphonates in patients with a history of concomitant risk factors for ONJ (eg, chemotherapy). While on treatment, patients with concomitant risk factors should avoid invasive dental procedures if possible). Products include:
Alkeran 1302

Melphalan Hydrochloride (Caution is indicated when zoledronic acid is used with other potentially nephrotoxic drugs such as nonsteroidal anti-inflammatory drugs. Renal impairment has been observed following the administration of zoledronic acid, especially in patients with pre-existing renal compromise or other risk factors including concomitant nephrotoxic medications). Products include:
Alkeran for Injection 1300

Mercaptopurine (Osteonecrosis of the jaw (ONJ) has been reported in patients treated with bisphosphonates, including zoledronic acid. A dental examination with appropriate preventive dentistry should be considered prior to treatment with bisphosphonates in patients with a history of concomitant risk factors for ONJ (eg, chemotherapy). While on treatment, patients with concomitant risk factors should avoid invasive dental procedures if possible).
No products indexed under this heading.

Mesalamine (Caution is indicated when zoledronic acid is used with other potentially nephrotoxic drugs such as nonsteroidal anti-inflammatory drugs. Renal impairment has been observed following the administration of zoledronic acid, especially in patients with pre-existing renal compromise or other risk factors including concomitant nephrotoxic medications). Products include:
Apriso 2899
Asacol 2786
Asacol HD 2787
Canasa 782
Lialda 3295
Pentasa 3297

Methimazole (Caution is indicated when zoledronic acid is used with other potentially nephrotoxic drugs such as nonsteroidal anti-inflammatory drugs. Renal impairment has been observed following the administration of zoledronic acid, especially in patients with pre-existing renal compromise or other risk factors including concomitant nephrotoxic medications).
No products indexed under this heading.

Methotrexate (Caution is indicated when zoledronic acid is used with other potentially nephrotoxic drugs such as nonsteroidal anti-inflammatory drugs. Renal impairment has been observed following the administration of zoledronic acid, especially in patients with pre-existing renal compromise or other risk factors including concomitant nephrotoxic medications).
No products indexed under this heading.

Methotrexate Sodium (Caution is indicated when zoledronic acid is used with other potentially nephrotoxic drugs such as nonsteroidal anti-inflammatory drugs. Renal impairment has been observed following the administration of zoledronic acid, especially in patients with pre-existing renal compromise or other risk factors including concomitant nephrotoxic medications).
No products indexed under this heading.

Methyclothiazide (Renal impairment has been observed following the administration of zoledronic acid, especially in patients with pre-existing renal compromise or other risk factors including concomitant diuretic therapy).
No products indexed under this heading.

Methylprednisolone (Osteonecrosis of the jaw (ONJ) has been reported in patients treated with bisphosphonates, including zoledronic acid. A dental examination with appropriate preventive dentistry should be considered prior to treatment with bisphosphonates in patients with a history of concomitant risk factors for ONJ (eg, corticosteroids). While on treatment, patients with concomitant risk factors should avoid invasive dental procedures if possible).
No products indexed under this heading.

Methylprednisolone Acetate (Osteonecrosis of the jaw (ONJ) has been reported in patients treated with bisphosphonates, including zoledronic acid. A dental examination with appropriate preventive dentistry should be considered prior to treatment with bisphosphonates in patients with a history of concomitant risk factors for ONJ (eg, corticosteroids). While on treatment, patients with concomitant risk factors should avoid invasive dental procedures if possible).
No products indexed under this heading.

Methylprednisolone Sodium Succinate (Osteonecrosis of the jaw (ONJ) has been reported in patients treated with bisphosphonates, including zoledronic acid. A dental examination with appropriate preventive dentistry should be considered prior to treatment with bisphosphonates in patients with a

IMPORTANT NOTE: Always consult each drug listing in the patient's regimen for possible interactions.

history of concomitant risk factors for ONJ (eg, corticosteroids). While on treatment, patients with concomitant risk factors should avoid invasive dental procedures if possible).
No products indexed under this heading.

Metolazone (Renal impairment has been observed following the administration of zoledronic acid, especially in patients with pre-existing renal compromise or other risk factors including concomitant diuretic therapy).
No products indexed under this heading.

Mezlocillin Sodium (Caution is indicated when zoledronic acid is used with other potentially nephrotoxic drugs such as nonsteroidal anti-inflammatory drugs. Renal impairment has been observed following the administration of zoledronic acid, especially in patients with pre-existing renal compromise or other risk factors including concomitant nephrotoxic medications).
No products indexed under this heading.

Minocycline Hydrochloride (Caution is indicated when zoledronic acid is used with other potentially nephrotoxic drugs such as nonsteroidal anti-inflammatory drugs. Renal impairment has been observed following the administration of zoledronic acid, especially in patients with pre-existing renal compromise or other risk factors including concomitant nephrotoxic medications). Products include:
Solodyn 2073

Mitomycin (Mitomycin-C) (Caution is indicated when zoledronic acid is used with other potentially nephrotoxic drugs such as nonsteroidal anti-inflammatory drugs. Renal impairment has been observed following the administration of zoledronic acid, especially in patients with pre-existing renal compromise or other risk factors including concomitant nephrotoxic medications).
No products indexed under this heading.

Mitotane (Osteonecrosis of the jaw (ONJ) has been reported in patients treated with bisphosphonates, including zoledronic acid. A dental examination with appropriate preventive dentistry should be considered prior to treatment with bisphosphonates in patients with a history of concomitant risk factors for ONJ (eg, chemotherapy). While on treatment, patients with concomitant risk factors should avoid invasive dental procedures if possible).
No products indexed under this heading.

Mitoxantrone Hydrochloride (Osteonecrosis of the jaw (ONJ) has been reported in patients treated with bisphosphonates, including zoledronic acid. A dental examination with appropriate preventive dentistry should be considered prior to treatment with bisphosphonates in patients with a history of concomitant risk factors for ONJ (eg, chemotherapy). While on treatment, patients with concomitant risk factors should avoid invasive dental procedures if possible). Products include:
Novantrone 1088

Moexipril Hydrochloride (Caution is indicated when zoledronic acid is used with other potentially nephrotoxic drugs such as nonsteroidal anti-inflammatory drugs. Renal impairment has been observed following the administration of zoledronic acid, especially in patients with pre-existing renal compromise or other risk factors including concomitant nephrotoxic medications).
No products indexed under this heading.

Mometasone Furoate (Osteonecrosis of the jaw (ONJ) has been reported in patients treated with bisphosphonates, including zoledronic acid. A dental examination with appropriate preventive dentistry should be considered prior to treatment with bisphosphonates in patients with a history of concomitant risk factors for ONJ (eg, corticosteroids). While on treatment, patients with concomitant risk factors should avoid invasive dental procedures if possible). Products include:
Asmanex 3058
Elocon Cream 3111
Elocon Lotion 3112
Elocon Ointment 3114

Mometasone Furoate Monohydrate (Osteonecrosis of the jaw (ONJ) has been reported in patients treated with bisphosphonates, including zoledronic acid. A dental examination with appropriate preventive dentistry should be considered prior to treatment with bisphosphonates in patients with a history of concomitant risk factors for ONJ (eg, corticosteroids). While on treatment, patients with concomitant risk factors should avoid invasive dental procedures if possible). Products include:
Nasonex 3166

Morphine Sulfate (Renal impairment has been observed following the administration of zoledronic acid in patients with pre-existing renal compromise or other risk factors. In patients with renal impairment, the exposure to concomitant medications that are primarily renally excreted (eg, digoxin) may increase. Consider monitoring serum creatinine in patients at risk for renal impairment who are taking concomitant medications that are primarily excreted by the kidney). Products include:
Avinza 1822
Embeda 1831
MS Contin 2803

Muromonab-CD3 (Caution is indicated when zoledronic acid is used with other potentially nephrotoxic drugs such as nonsteroidal anti-inflammatory drugs. Renal impairment has been observed following the administration of zoledronic acid, especially in patients with pre-existing renal compromise or other risk factors including concomitant nephrotoxic medications). Products include:
Orthoclone OKT3 949

Nabumetone (Caution is indicated when zoledronic acid is used with other potentially nephrotoxic drugs such as nonsteroidal anti-inflammatory drugs. Renal impairment has been observed following the administration of zoledronic acid, especially in patients with pre-existing renal compromise or other risk factors including concomitant nephrotoxic medications).
No products indexed under this heading.

Nafcillin Sodium (Caution is indicated when zoledronic acid is used with other potentially nephrotoxic drugs such as nonsteroidal anti-inflammatory drugs. Renal impairment has been observed following the administration of zoledronic acid, especially in patients with pre-existing renal compromise or other risk factors including concomitant nephrotoxic medications).
No products indexed under this heading.

Naproxen (Caution is indicated when zoledronic acid is used with other potentially nephrotoxic drugs such as nonsteroidal anti-inflammatory drugs. Renal impairment has been observed following the administration of zoledronic acid, especially in patients with pre-existing renal compromise or other risk factors including concomitant nephrotoxic medications). Products include:
EC-Naprosyn 2850
Naprosyn 2850
Anaprox/Naprosyn 2850

Naproxen Sodium (Caution is indicated when zoledronic acid is used with other potentially nephrotoxic drugs such as nonsteroidal anti-inflammatory drugs. Renal impairment has been observed following the administration of zoledronic acid, especially in patients with pre-existing renal compromise or other risk factors including concomitant nephrotoxic medications). Products include:
Anaprox 2850
Anaprox DS 2850
Treximet 1681

Nelfinavir Mesylate (Caution is indicated when zoledronic acid is used with other potentially nephrotoxic drugs such as nonsteroidal anti-inflammatory drugs. Renal impairment has been observed following the administration of zoledronic acid, especially in patients with pre-existing renal compromise or other risk factors including concomitant nephrotoxic medications).
No products indexed under this heading.

Neomycin (Caution is advised when bisphosphonates, including zoledronic acid, are administered with aminoglycosides, since these agents may have an additive effect to lower serum calcium level for prolonged periods).
No products indexed under this heading.

Neomycin, oral (Caution is advised when bisphosphonates, including zoledronic acid, are administered with aminoglycosides, since these agents may have an additive effect to lower serum calcium level for prolonged periods).
No products indexed under this heading.

Neomycin Sulfate (Caution is advised when bisphosphonates, including zoledronic acid, are administered with aminoglycosides, since these agents may have an additive effect to lower serum calcium level for prolonged periods).
No products indexed under this heading.

Nevirapine (Caution is indicated when zoledronic acid is used with other potentially nephrotoxic drugs such as nonsteroidal anti-inflammatory drugs. Renal impairment has been observed following the administration of zoledronic acid, especially in patients with pre-existing renal compromise or other risk factors including concomitant nephrotoxic medications). Products include:
Viramune Oral Suspension 897
Viramune Tablets 897

Norfloxacin (Caution is indicated when zoledronic acid is used with other potentially nephrotoxic drugs such as nonsteroidal anti-inflammatory drugs. Renal impairment has been observed following the administration of zoledronic acid, especially in patients with pre-existing renal compromise or other risk factors including concomitant nephrotoxic medications). Products include:
Noroxin 2220

Olsalazine Sodium (Caution is indicated when zoledronic acid is used with other potentially nephrotoxic drugs such as nonsteroidal anti-inflammatory drugs. Renal impairment has been observed following the administration of zoledronic acid, especially in patients with pre-existing renal compromise or other risk factors including concomitant nephrotoxic medications).
No products indexed under this heading.

Omeprazole (Caution is indicated when zoledronic acid is used with other potentially nephrotoxic drugs such as nonsteroidal anti-inflammatory drugs. Renal impairment has been observed following the administration of zoledronic acid, especially in patients with pre-existing renal compromise or other risk factors including concomitant nephrotoxic medications).
No products indexed under this heading.

Oxaliplatin (Osteonecrosis of the jaw (ONJ) has been reported in patients treated with bisphosphonates, including zoledronic acid. A dental examination with appropriate preventive dentistry should be considered prior to treatment with bisphosphonates in patients with a history of concomitant risk factors for ONJ (eg, chemotherapy). While on treatment, patients with concomitant risk factors should avoid invasive dental procedures if possible). Products include:
Eloxatin 2975

Oxaprozin (Caution is indicated when zoledronic acid is used with other potentially nephrotoxic drugs such as nonsteroidal anti-inflammatory drugs. Renal impairment has been observed following the administration of zoledronic acid, especially in patients with pre-existing renal compromise or other risk factors including concomitant nephrotoxic medications).
No products indexed under this heading.

Paclitaxel (Osteonecrosis of the jaw (ONJ) has been reported in patients treated with bisphosphonates, including zoledronic acid. A dental examination with appropriate preventive dentistry should be considered prior to treatment with bisphosphonates in patients with a history of concomitant risk factors for ONJ (eg, chemotherapy). While on treatment, patients with concomitant risk factors should avoid invasive dental procedures if possible).
No products indexed under this heading.

Pamidronate Disodium (Caution is indicated when zoledronic acid is used with other potentially nephrotoxic drugs such as nonsteroidal anti-inflammatory drugs. Renal impairment has been observed following the administration of zoledronic acid, especially in patients with pre-existing renal compromise or other risk factors including concomitant nephrotoxic medications).
No products indexed under this heading.

Paroxetine Hydrochloride (Caution is indicated when zoledronic acid is used with other potentially nephrotoxic drugs such as nonsteroidal anti-inflammatory drugs. Renal impairment has been observed following the administration of zoledronic acid, especially in patients with pre-existing renal compromise or other risk factors including concomitant nephrotoxic medications). Products include:
Paroxetine CR 2361
Paroxetine ER 2371
Paxil 1586
Paxil CR 1596

Penicillamine (Caution is indicated when zoledronic acid is used with other potentially nephrotoxic drugs such as nonsteroidal anti-inflammatory drugs. Renal impairment has been observed following the administration of zoledronic acid, especially in patients with pre-existing renal compromise or other risk factors including concomitant nephrotoxic medications).
No products indexed under this heading.

Penicillin G Benzathine (Caution is indicated when zoledronic acid is used with other potentially nephrotoxic drugs such as nonsteroidal anti-inflammatory drugs. Renal impairment has been observed following the administration of zoledronic acid, especially in patients with pre-existing renal compromise or other risk factors including concomitant nephrotoxic medications). Products include:
Bicillin C-R Injectable Suspension 1826
Bicillin L-A 1828

Penicillin G Potassium (Caution is indicated when zoledronic acid is used with other potentially nephrotoxic drugs such as nonsteroidal anti-inflammatory drugs. Renal impairment has been observed following the administration of zoledronic acid, especially in patients with pre-existing renal compromise or other risk factors including concomitant nephrotoxic medications).
No products indexed under this heading.

Penicillin G Procaine (Caution is indicated when zoledronic acid is used with other potentially nephrotoxic drugs such as nonsteroidal anti-inflammatory drugs. Renal impairment has been observed following the administration of zoledronic acid, especially in patients with pre-existing renal compromise or other risk factors including concomitant nephrotoxic medications). Products include:
Bicillin C-R Injectable Suspension 1826
Bicillin L-A 1828

Penicillin G Sodium (Caution is indicated when zoledronic acid is used with other potentially nephrotoxic drugs such as nonsteroidal anti-inflammatory drugs. Renal impairment has been observed following the administration of zoledronic acid, especially in patients with pre-existing renal compromise or other risk factors including concomitant nephrotoxic medications).
No products indexed under this heading.

Penicillin V Potassium (Caution is indicated when zoledronic acid is used with other potentially nephrotoxic drugs such as nonsteroidal anti-inflammatory drugs. Renal impairment has been observed following the administration of zoledronic acid, especially in patients with pre-existing renal compromise or other risk factors including concomitant nephrotoxic medications).
No products indexed under this heading.

Pentamidine Isethionate (Caution is indicated when zoledronic acid is used with other potentially nephrotoxic drugs such as nonsteroidal anti-inflammatory drugs. Renal impairment has been observed following the administration of zoledronic acid, especially in patients with pre-existing renal compromise or other risk factors including concomitant nephrotoxic medications).
No products indexed under this heading.

Perindopril Erbumine (Caution is indicated when zoledronic acid is used with other potentially nephrotoxic drugs such as nonsteroidal anti-inflammatory drugs. Renal impairment has been observed following the administration of zoledronic acid, especially in patients with pre-existing renal compromise or other risk factors including concomitant nephrotoxic medications).
No products indexed under this heading.

Phenylbutazone (Caution is indicated when zoledronic acid is used with other potentially nephrotoxic drugs such as nonsteroidal anti-inflammatory drugs. Renal impairment has been observed following the administration of zoledronic acid, especially in patients with pre-existing renal compromise or other risk factors including concomitant nephrotoxic medications).
No products indexed under this heading.

Piroxicam (Caution is indicated when zoledronic acid is used with other potentially nephrotoxic drugs such as nonsteroidal anti-inflammatory drugs. Renal impairment has been observed following the administration of zoledronic acid, especially in patients with pre-existing renal compromise or other risk factors including concomitant nephrotoxic medications).
No products indexed under this heading.

Plicamycin (Caution is indicated when zoledronic acid is used with other potentially nephrotoxic drugs such as nonsteroidal anti-inflammatory drugs. Renal impairment has been observed following the administration of zoledronic acid, especially in patients with pre-existing renal compromise or other risk factors including concomitant nephrotoxic medications).
No products indexed under this heading.

Polymyxin (Caution is indicated when zoledronic acid is used with other potentially nephrotoxic drugs such as nonsteroidal anti-inflammatory drugs. Renal impairment has been observed following the administration of zoledronic acid, especially in patients with pre-existing renal compromise or other risk factors including concomitant nephrotoxic medications).
No products indexed under this heading.

Polymyxin B Sulfate (Caution is indicated when zoledronic acid is used with other potentially nephrotoxic drugs such as nonsteroidal anti-inflammatory drugs. Renal impairment has been observed following the administration of zoledronic acid, especially in patients with pre-existing renal compromise or other risk factors including concomitant nephrotoxic medications).
No products indexed under this heading.

Polythiazide (Renal impairment has been observed following the administration of zoledronic acid, especially in patients with pre-existing renal compromise or other risk factors including concomitant diuretic therapy).
No products indexed under this heading.

Pravastatin Sodium (Caution is indicated when zoledronic acid is used with other potentially nephrotoxic drugs such as nonsteroidal anti-inflammatory drugs. Renal impairment has been observed following the administration of zoledronic acid, especially in patients with pre-existing renal compromise or other risk factors including concomitant nephrotoxic medications).
No products indexed under this heading.

Prednisolone (Osteonecrosis of the jaw (ONJ) has been reported in patients treated with bisphosphonates, including zoledronic acid. A dental examination with appropriate preventive dentistry should be considered prior to treatment with bisphosphonates in patients with a history of concomitant risk factors for ONJ (eg, corticosteroids). While on treatment, patients with concomitant risk factors should avoid invasive dental procedures if possible).
No products indexed under this heading.

Prednisolone Acetate (Osteonecrosis of the jaw (ONJ) has been reported in patients treated with bisphosphonates, including zoledronic acid. A dental examination with appropriate preventive dentistry should be considered prior to treatment with bisphosphonates in patients with a history of concomitant risk factors for ONJ (eg, corticosteroids). While on treatment, patients with concomitant risk factors should avoid invasive dental procedures if possible).
Products include:
Blephamide .... ⊙**212,** ⊙**214**
Pred Forte .... ⊙**225**
Pred Mild .... ⊙**230**
Pred-G .... ⊙**226,** ⊙**227**

Prednisolone Sodium Phosphate (Osteonecrosis of the jaw (ONJ) has been reported in patients treated with bisphosphonates, including zoledronic acid. A dental examination with appropriate preventive dentistry should be considered prior to treatment with bisphosphonates in patients with a history of concomitant risk factors for ONJ (eg, corticosteroids). While on treatment,

patients with concomitant risk factors should avoid invasive dental procedures if possible).
No products indexed under this heading.

Prednisolone Tebutate (Osteonecrosis of the jaw (ONJ) has been reported in patients treated with bisphosphonates, including zoledronic acid. A dental examination with appropriate preventive dentistry should be considered prior to treatment with bisphosphonates in patients with a history of concomitant risk factors for ONJ (eg, corticosteroids). While on treatment, patients with concomitant risk factors should avoid invasive dental procedures if possible).
No products indexed under this heading.

Prednisone (Osteonecrosis of the jaw (ONJ) has been reported in patients treated with bisphosphonates, including zoledronic acid. A dental examination with appropriate preventive dentistry should be considered prior to treatment with bisphosphonates in patients with a history of concomitant risk factors for ONJ (eg, corticosteroids). While on treatment, patients with concomitant risk factors should avoid invasive dental procedures if possible).
No products indexed under this heading.

Prednisone sodium phosphate (Osteonecrosis of the jaw (ONJ) has been reported in patients treated with bisphosphonates, including zoledronic acid. A dental examination with appropriate preventive dentistry should be considered prior to treatment with bisphosphonates in patients with a history of concomitant risk factors for ONJ (eg, corticosteroids). While on treatment, patients with concomitant risk factors should avoid invasive dental procedures if possible).
No products indexed under this heading.

Procainamide Hydrochloride (Renal impairment has been observed following the administration of zoledronic acid in patients with pre-existing renal compromise or other risk factors. In patients with renal impairment, the exposure to concomitant medications that are primarily renally excreted (eg, digoxin) may increase. Consider monitoring serum creatinine in patients at risk for renal impairment who are taking concomitant medications that are primarily excreted by the kidney).
No products indexed under this heading.

Procarbazine Hydrochloride (Osteonecrosis of the jaw (ONJ) has been reported in patients treated with bisphosphonates, including zoledronic acid. A dental examination with appropriate preventive dentistry should be considered prior to treatment with bisphosphonates in patients with a history of concomitant risk factors for ONJ (eg, chemotherapy). While on treatment, patients with concomitant risk factors should avoid invasive dental procedures if possible).
No products indexed under this heading.

Quinapril Hydrochloride (Caution is indicated when zoledronic acid is used with other potentially nephrotoxic drugs such as nonsteroidal anti-inflammatory drugs. Renal impairment has been observed following the administration of zoledronic acid, especially in patients with pre-existing renal compromise or other risk factors including concomitant nephrotoxic medications).
No products indexed under this heading.

Quinidine Gluconate (Renal impairment has been observed following the administration of zoledronic acid in patients with pre-existing renal compromise or other risk factors. In patients with renal impairment, the exposure to concomitant medications that are primarily renally excreted (eg, digoxin)

may increase. Consider monitoring serum creatinine in patients at risk for renal impairment who are taking concomitant medications that are primarily excreted by the kidney).
No products indexed under this heading.

Quinidine Polygalacturonate (Renal impairment has been observed following the administration of zoledronic acid in patients with pre-existing renal compromise or other risk factors. In patients with renal impairment, the exposure to concomitant medications that are primarily renally excreted (eg, digoxin) may increase. Consider monitoring serum creatinine in patients at risk for renal impairment who are taking concomitant medications that are primarily excreted by the kidney).
No products indexed under this heading.

Quinidine Sulfate (Renal impairment has been observed following the administration of zoledronic acid in patients with pre-existing renal compromise or other risk factors. In patients with renal impairment, the exposure to concomitant medications that are primarily renally excreted (eg, digoxin) may increase. Consider monitoring serum creatinine in patients at risk for renal impairment who are taking concomitant medications that are primarily excreted by the kidney).
No products indexed under this heading.

Quinine Sulfate (Renal impairment has been observed following the administration of zoledronic acid in patients with pre-existing renal compromise or other risk factors. In patients with renal impairment, the exposure to concomitant medications that are primarily renally excreted (eg, digoxin) may increase. Consider monitoring serum creatinine in patients at risk for renal impairment who are taking concomitant medications that are primarily excreted by the kidney).
No products indexed under this heading.

Rabeprazole Sodium (Caution is indicated when zoledronic acid is used with other potentially nephrotoxic drugs such as nonsteroidal anti-inflammatory drugs. Renal impairment has been observed following the administration of zoledronic acid, especially in patients with pre-existing renal compromise or other risk factors including concomitant nephrotoxic medications). Products include:
Aciphex 1035

Radiation (Osteonecrosis of the jaw (ONJ) has been reported in patients treated with bisphosphonates, including zoledronic acid. A dental examination with appropriate preventive dentistry should be considered prior to treatment with bisphosphonates in patients with a history of concomitant risk factors for ONJ (eg, radiotherapy). While on treatment, patients with concomitant risk factors should avoid invasive dental procedures if possible).
No products indexed under this heading.

Ramipril (Caution is indicated when zoledronic acid is used with other potentially nephrotoxic drugs such as nonsteroidal anti-inflammatory drugs. Renal impairment has been observed following the administration of zoledronic acid, especially in patients with pre-existing renal compromise or other risk factors including concomitant nephrotoxic medications).
No products indexed under this heading.

Ranitidine Hydrochloride (Renal impairment has been observed following the administration of zoledronic acid in patients with pre-existing renal compromise or other risk factors. In patients with renal impairment, the exposure to concomitant medications that are primarily renally excreted (eg,

---

IMPORTANT NOTE: Always consult each drug listing in the patient's regimen for possible interactions.

digoxin) may increase. Consider monitoring serum creatinine in patients at risk for renal impairment who are taking concomitant medications that are primarily excreted by the kidney). Products include:

Rifampin (Caution is indicated when zoledronic acid is used with other potentially nephrotoxic drugs such as nonsteroidal anti-inflammatory drugs. Renal impairment has been observed following the administration of zoledronic acid, especially in patients with pre-existing renal compromise or other risk factors including concomitant nephrotoxic medications).
No products indexed under this heading.

Riluzole (Caution is indicated when zoledronic acid is used with other potentially nephrotoxic drugs such as nonsteroidal anti-inflammatory drugs. Renal impairment has been observed following the administration of zoledronic acid, especially in patients with pre-existing renal compromise or other risk factors including concomitant nephrotoxic medications). Products include:

Ritonavir (Caution is indicated when zoledronic acid is used with other potentially nephrotoxic drugs such as nonsteroidal anti-inflammatory drugs. Renal impairment has been observed following the administration of zoledronic acid, especially in patients with pre-existing renal compromise or other risk factors including concomitant nephrotoxic medications). Products include:

Rofecoxib (Caution is indicated when zoledronic acid is used with other potentially nephrotoxic drugs such as nonsteroidal anti-inflammatory drugs. Renal impairment has been observed following the administration of zoledronic acid, especially in patients with pre-existing renal compromise or other risk factors including concomitant nephrotoxic medications).
No products indexed under this heading.

Saquinavir (Caution is indicated when zoledronic acid is used with other potentially nephrotoxic drugs such as nonsteroidal anti-inflammatory drugs. Renal impairment has been observed following the administration of zoledronic acid, especially in patients with pre-existing renal compromise or other risk factors including concomitant nephrotoxic medications).
No products indexed under this heading.

Sibutramine Hydrochloride Monohydrate (Caution is indicated when zoledronic acid is used with other potentially nephrotoxic drugs such as nonsteroidal anti-inflammatory drugs. Renal impairment has been observed following the administration of zoledronic acid, especially in patients with pre-existing renal compromise or other risk factors including concomitant nephrotoxic medications). Products include:

Simvastatin (Caution is indicated when zoledronic acid is used with other potentially nephrotoxic drugs such as nonsteroidal anti-inflammatory drugs. Renal impairment has been observed following the administration of zoledronic acid, especially in patients with pre-existing renal compromise or other risk factors including concomitant nephrotoxic medications). Products include:

Spirapril Hydrochloride (Caution is indicated when zoledronic acid is used with other potentially nephrotoxic drugs such as nonsteroidal anti-inflammatory drugs. Renal impairment has been observed following the administration of zoledronic acid, especially in patients with pre-existing renal compromise or other risk factors including concomitant nephrotoxic medications).
No products indexed under this heading.

Spironolactone (Renal impairment has been observed following the administration of zoledronic acid, especially in patients with pre-existing renal compromise or other risk factors including concomitant diuretic therapy).
No products indexed under this heading.

Stavudine (Caution is indicated when zoledronic acid is used with other potentially nephrotoxic drugs such as nonsteroidal anti-inflammatory drugs. Renal impairment has been observed following the administration of zoledronic acid, especially in patients with pre-existing renal compromise or other risk factors including concomitant nephrotoxic medications).
No products indexed under this heading.

Streptomycin Sulfate (Caution is advised when bisphosphonates, including zoledronic acid, are administered with aminoglycosides, since these agents may have an additive effect to lower serum calcium level for prolonged periods).
No products indexed under this heading.

Streptozocin (Caution is indicated when zoledronic acid is used with other potentially nephrotoxic drugs such as nonsteroidal anti-inflammatory drugs. Renal impairment has been observed following the administration of zoledronic acid, especially in patients with pre-existing renal compromise or other risk factors including concomitant nephrotoxic medications).
No products indexed under this heading.

Sulfacytine (Caution is indicated when zoledronic acid is used with other potentially nephrotoxic drugs such as nonsteroidal anti-inflammatory drugs. Renal impairment has been observed following the administration of zoledronic acid, especially in patients with pre-existing renal compromise or other risk factors including concomitant nephrotoxic medications).
No products indexed under this heading.

Sulfamethizole (Caution is indicated when zoledronic acid is used with other potentially nephrotoxic drugs such as nonsteroidal anti-inflammatory drugs. Renal impairment has been observed following the administration of zoledronic acid, especially in patients with pre-existing renal compromise or other risk factors including concomitant nephrotoxic medications).
No products indexed under this heading.

Sulfamethoxazole (Caution is indicated when zoledronic acid is used with other potentially nephrotoxic drugs such as nonsteroidal anti-inflammatory drugs. Renal impairment has been observed following the administration of zoledronic acid, especially in patients with pre-existing renal compromise or other risk factors including concomitant nephrotoxic medications).
No products indexed under this heading.

Sulfasalazine (Caution is indicated when zoledronic acid is used with other potentially nephrotoxic drugs such as nonsteroidal anti-inflammatory drugs. Renal impairment has been observed following the administration of zoledronic acid, especially in patients with pre-existing renal compromise or other risk factors including concomitant nephrotoxic medications).
No products indexed under this heading.

Sulfinpyrazone (Caution is indicated when zoledronic acid is used with other potentially nephrotoxic drugs such as nonsteroidal anti-inflammatory drugs. Renal impairment has been observed following the administration of zoledronic acid, especially in patients with pre-existing renal compromise or other risk factors including concomitant nephrotoxic medications).
No products indexed under this heading.

Sulfisoxazole Acetyl (Caution is indicated when zoledronic acid is used with other potentially nephrotoxic drugs such as nonsteroidal anti-inflammatory drugs. Renal impairment has been observed following the administration of zoledronic acid, especially in patients with pre-existing renal compromise or other risk factors including concomitant nephrotoxic medications).
No products indexed under this heading.

Sulfisoxazole Diolamine (Caution is indicated when zoledronic acid is used with other potentially nephrotoxic drugs such as nonsteroidal anti-inflammatory drugs. Renal impairment has been observed following the administration of zoledronic acid, especially in patients with pre-existing renal compromise or other risk factors including concomitant nephrotoxic medications).
No products indexed under this heading.

Sulindac (Caution is indicated when zoledronic acid is used with other potentially nephrotoxic drugs such as nonsteroidal anti-inflammatory drugs. Renal impairment has been observed following the administration of zoledronic acid, especially in patients with pre-existing renal compromise or other risk factors including concomitant nephrotoxic medications). Products include:

Tacrolimus (Caution is indicated when zoledronic acid is used with other potentially nephrotoxic drugs such as nonsteroidal anti-inflammatory drugs. Renal impairment has been observed following the administration of zoledronic acid, especially in patients with pre-existing renal compromise or other risk factors including concomitant nephrotoxic medications). Products include:

Tamoxifen Citrate (Osteonecrosis of the jaw (ONJ) has been reported in patients treated with bisphosphonates, including zoledronic acid. A dental examination with appropriate preventive dentistry should be considered prior to treatment with bisphosphonates in patients with a history of concomitant risk factors for ONJ (eg, chemotherapy). While on treatment, patients with concomitant risk factors should avoid invasive dental procedures if possible).
No products indexed under this heading.

Teniposide (Osteonecrosis of the jaw (ONJ) has been reported in patients treated with bisphosphonates, including zoledronic acid. A dental examination with appropriate preventive dentistry should be considered prior to treatment with bisphosphonates in patients with a history of concomitant risk factors for ONJ (eg, chemotherapy). While on treat-

ment, patients with concomitant risk factors should avoid invasive dental procedures if possible).
No products indexed under this heading.

Tenofovir Disoproxil Fumarate (Caution is indicated when zoledronic acid is used with other potentially nephrotoxic drugs such as nonsteroidal anti-inflammatory drugs. Renal impairment has been observed following the administration of zoledronic acid, especially in patients with pre-existing renal compromise or other risk factors including concomitant nephrotoxic medications). Products include:

Thioguanine (Caution is indicated when zoledronic acid is used with other potentially nephrotoxic drugs such as nonsteroidal anti-inflammatory drugs. Renal impairment has been observed following the administration of zoledronic acid, especially in patients with pre-existing renal compromise or other risk factors including concomitant nephrotoxic medications). Products include:

Thiotepa (Osteonecrosis of the jaw (ONJ) has been reported in patients treated with bisphosphonates, including zoledronic acid. A dental examination with appropriate preventive dentistry should be considered prior to treatment with bisphosphonates in patients with a history of concomitant risk factors for ONJ (eg, chemotherapy). While on treatment, patients with concomitant risk factors should avoid invasive dental procedures if possible).
No products indexed under this heading.

Ticarcillin Disodium (Caution is indicated when zoledronic acid is used with other potentially nephrotoxic drugs such as nonsteroidal anti-inflammatory drugs. Renal impairment has been observed following the administration of zoledronic acid, especially in patients with pre-existing renal compromise or other risk factors including concomitant nephrotoxic medications). Products include:

Tobramycin (Caution is advised when bisphosphonates, including zoledronic acid, are administered with aminoglycosides, since these agents may have an additive effect to lower serum calcium level for prolonged periods). Products include:

Tobramycin Sulfate (Caution is advised when bisphosphonates, including zoledronic acid, are administered with aminoglycosides, since these agents may have an additive effect to lower serum calcium level for prolonged periods).
No products indexed under this heading.

Tolazamide (Caution is indicated when zoledronic acid is used with other potentially nephrotoxic drugs such as nonsteroidal anti-inflammatory drugs. Renal impairment has been observed following the administration of zoledronic acid, especially in patients with pre-existing renal compromise or other risk factors including concomitant nephrotoxic medications).
No products indexed under this heading.

1583 Interactions Index Refludan

Tolbutamide (Caution is indicated when zoledronic acid is used with other potentially nephrotoxic drugs such as nonsteroidal anti-inflammatory drugs. Renal impairment has been observed following the administration of zoledronic acid, especially in patients with pre-existing renal compromise or other risk factors including concomitant nephrotoxic medications).
No products indexed under this heading.

Tolmetin Sodium (Caution is indicated when zoledronic acid is used with other potentially nephrotoxic drugs such as nonsteroidal anti-inflammatory drugs. Renal impairment has been observed following the administration of zoledronic acid, especially in patients with pre-existing renal compromise or other risk factors including concomitant nephrotoxic medications).
No products indexed under this heading.

Topotecan Hydrochloride (Osteonecrosis of the jaw (ONJ) has been reported in patients treated with bisphosphonates, including zoledronic acid. A dental examination with appropriate preventive dentistry should be considered prior to treatment with bisphosphonates in patients with a history of concomitant risk factors for ONJ (eg, chemotherapy). While on treatment, patients with concomitant risk factors should avoid invasive dental procedures if possible). Products include:
Hycamtin **1491**
Hycamtin Capsules **1488**

Toremifene Citrate (Osteonecrosis of the jaw (ONJ) has been reported in patients treated with bisphosphonates, including zoledronic acid. A dental examination with appropriate preventive dentistry should be considered prior to treatment with bisphosphonates in patients with a history of concomitant risk factors for ONJ (eg, chemotherapy). While on treatment, patients with concomitant risk factors should avoid invasive dental procedures if possible).
No products indexed under this heading.

Torsemide (Caution should be exercised when zoledronic acid is used in combination with loop diuretics due to an increased risk of hypocalcemia).
No products indexed under this heading.

Trandolapril (Caution is indicated when zoledronic acid is used with other potentially nephrotoxic drugs such as nonsteroidal anti-inflammatory drugs. Renal impairment has been observed following the administration of zoledronic acid, especially in patients with pre-existing renal compromise or other risk factors including concomitant nephrotoxic medications). Products include:
Mavik **489**
Tarka **534**

Triamcinolone (Osteonecrosis of the jaw (ONJ) has been reported in patients treated with bisphosphonates, including zoledronic acid. A dental examination with appropriate preventive dentistry should be considered prior to treatment with bisphosphonates in patients with a history of concomitant risk factors for ONJ (eg, corticosteroids). While on treatment, patients with concomitant risk factors should avoid invasive dental procedures if possible).
No products indexed under this heading.

Triamcinolone Acetonide (Osteonecrosis of the jaw (ONJ) has been reported in patients treated with bisphosphonates, including zoledronic acid. A dental examination with appropriate preventive dentistry should be considered prior to treatment with bisphosphonates in patients with a history of concomitant risk factors for ONJ (eg, corticosteroids). While on treatment, patients with concomitant risk factors should avoid invasive dental procedures if possible). Products include:
Azmacort **408**
Nasacort AQ **3019**

Triamcinolone Diacetate (Osteonecrosis of the jaw (ONJ) has been reported in patients treated with bisphosphonates, including zoledronic acid. A dental examination with appropriate preventive dentistry should be considered prior to treatment with bisphosphonates in patients with a history of concomitant risk factors for ONJ (eg, corticosteroids). While on treatment, patients with concomitant risk factors should avoid invasive dental procedures if possible).
No products indexed under this heading.

Triamcinolone Hexacetonide (Osteonecrosis of the jaw (ONJ) has been reported in patients treated with bisphosphonates, including zoledronic acid. A dental examination with appropriate preventive dentistry should be considered prior to treatment with bisphosphonates in patients with a history of concomitant risk factors for ONJ (eg, corticosteroids). While on treatment, patients with concomitant risk factors should avoid invasive dental procedures if possible).
No products indexed under this heading.

Triamterene (Renal impairment has been observed following the administration of zoledronic acid, especially in patients with pre-existing renal compromise or other risk factors including concomitant diuretic therapy). Products include:
Dyazide **1429**
Dyrenium **3495**

Trimethadione (Caution is indicated when zoledronic acid is used with other potentially nephrotoxic drugs such as nonsteroidal anti-inflammatory drugs. Renal impairment has been observed following the administration of zoledronic acid, especially in patients with pre-existing renal compromise or other risk factors including concomitant nephrotoxic medications).
No products indexed under this heading.

Trimethoprim (Renal impairment has been observed following the administration of zoledronic acid in patients with pre-existing renal compromise or other risk factors. In patients with renal impairment, the exposure to concomitant medications that are primarily renally excreted (eg, digoxin) may increase. Consider monitoring serum creatinine in patients at risk for renal impairment who are taking concomitant medications that are primarily excreted by the kidney).
No products indexed under this heading.

Trimethoprim Sulfate (Renal impairment has been observed following the administration of zoledronic acid in patients with pre-existing renal compromise or other risk factors. In patients with renal impairment, the exposure to concomitant medications that are primarily renally excreted (eg, digoxin) may increase. Consider monitoring serum creatinine in patients at risk for renal impairment who are taking concomitant medications that are primarily excreted by the kidney).
No products indexed under this heading.

Trovafloxacin Mesylate (Caution is indicated when zoledronic acid is used with other potentially nephrotoxic drugs such as nonsteroidal anti-inflammatory drugs. Renal impairment has been observed following the administration of zoledronic acid, especially in patients with pre-existing renal compromise or other risk factors including concomitant nephrotoxic medications).
No products indexed under this heading.

Tyropanoate Sodium (Caution is indicated when zoledronic acid is used with other potentially nephrotoxic drugs such as nonsteroidal anti-inflammatory drugs. Renal impairment has been observed following the administration of zoledronic acid, especially in patients with pre-existing renal compromise or other risk factors including concomitant nephrotoxic medications).
No products indexed under this heading.

Valacyclovir Hydrochloride (Caution is indicated when zoledronic acid is used with other potentially nephrotoxic drugs such as nonsteroidal anti-inflammatory drugs. Renal impairment has been observed following the administration of zoledronic acid, especially in patients with pre-existing renal compromise or other risk factors including concomitant nephrotoxic medications). Products include:
Valtrex **1702**

Valdecoxib (Caution is indicated when zoledronic acid is used with other potentially nephrotoxic drugs such as nonsteroidal anti-inflammatory drugs. Renal impairment has been observed following the administration of zoledronic acid, especially in patients with pre-existing renal compromise or other risk factors including concomitant nephrotoxic medications).
No products indexed under this heading.

Valrubicin (Osteonecrosis of the jaw (ONJ) has been reported in patients treated with bisphosphonates, including zoledronic acid. A dental examination with appropriate preventive dentistry should be considered prior to treatment with bisphosphonates in patients with a history of concomitant risk factors for ONJ (eg, chemotherapy). While on treatment, patients with concomitant risk factors should avoid invasive dental procedures if possible). Products include:
Valstar **1131**

Vancomycin Hydrochloride (Renal impairment has been observed following the administration of zoledronic acid in patients with pre-existing renal compromise or other risk factors. In patients with renal impairment, the exposure to concomitant medications that are primarily renally excreted (eg, digoxin) may increase. Consider monitoring serum creatinine in patients at risk for renal impairment who are taking concomitant medications that are primarily excreted by the kidney).
No products indexed under this heading.

Vincristine Sulfate (Osteonecrosis of the jaw (ONJ) has been reported in patients treated with bisphosphonates, including zoledronic acid. A dental examination with appropriate preventive dentistry should be considered prior to treatment with bisphosphonates in patients with a history of concomitant risk factors for ONJ (eg, chemotherapy). While on treatment, patients with concomitant risk factors should avoid invasive dental procedures if possible).
No products indexed under this heading.

Vinorelbine Tartrate (Osteonecrosis of the jaw (ONJ) has been reported in patients treated with bisphosphonates, including zoledronic acid. A dental examination with appropriate preventive dentistry should be considered prior to treatment with bisphosphonates in patients with a history of concomitant risk factors for ONJ (eg, chemotherapy). While on treatment, patients with concomitant risk factors should avoid invasive dental procedures if possible).
No products indexed under this heading.

Voriconazole (Caution is indicated when zoledronic acid is used with other potentially nephrotoxic drugs such as nonsteroidal anti-inflammatory drugs. Renal impairment has been observed following the administration of zoledronic acid, especially in patients with pre-existing renal compromise or other risk factors including concomitant nephrotoxic medications).
No products indexed under this heading.

Zalcitabine (Caution is indicated when zoledronic acid is used with other potentially nephrotoxic drugs such as nonsteroidal anti-inflammatory drugs. Renal impairment has been observed following the administration of zoledronic acid, especially in patients with pre-existing renal compromise or other risk factors including concomitant nephrotoxic medications).
No products indexed under this heading.

Zidovudine (Caution is indicated when zoledronic acid is used with other potentially nephrotoxic drugs such as nonsteroidal anti-inflammatory drugs. Renal impairment has been observed following the administration of zoledronic acid, especially in patients with pre-existing renal compromise or other risk factors including concomitant nephrotoxic medications). Products include:
Combivir **1404**
Retrovir **1634**
Retrovir IV **1640**
Trizivir **1688**

RECOMBINATE

(Antihemophilic Factor (Recombinant)) **821**
None cited in PDR database.

RECOMBIVAX HB

(Hepatitis B Vaccine, Recombinant) **2262**
None cited in PDR database.

REFACTO VIALS

(Antihemophilic Factor (Recombinant)) **3589**
None cited in PDR database.

REFLUDAN FOR INJECTION

(Lepirudin) **860**
May interact with non-steroidal anti-inflammatory agents, oral anticoagulants, thrombolytics, and certain other agents. Compounds in these categories include:

Alteplase (Concomitant therapy with thrombolytics may increase the risk of bleeding complications and considerably enhance the effect of Refludan on aPTT prolongation). Products include:
Activase **1183**
Cathflo **1192**

Anisindione (Concomitant therapy with oral anticoagulants may increase the risk of bleeding).
No products indexed under this heading.

Anistreplase (Concomitant therapy with thrombolytics may increase the risk of bleeding complications and considerably enhance the effect of Refludan on aPTT prolongation).
No products indexed under this heading.

Aspirin (Concomitant therapy with drugs that affect platelet function, such as aspirin, may increase the risk of bleeding). Products include:
Aggrenox **880**
Bayer Aspirin **829**
Percodan **1124**
St. Joseph Aspirin **2045**

Bivalirudin (Concomitant therapy with thrombolytics may increase the risk of bleeding complications and considerably enhance the effect of Refludan on aPTT prolongation). Products include:

IMPORTANT NOTE: Always consult each drug listing in the patient's regimen for possible interactions.

(⊙ Described in PDR® for Ophthalmic Medicines)

REMERON TABLETS

(Mirtazapine) 3214
May interact with alcohols, antihypertensives, drugs affecting hepatic drug metabolizing enzyme systems, monoamine oxidase inhibitors, and certain other agents. Compounds in these categories include:

Acebutolol Hydrochloride (Mirtazapine should be used with caution in patients with known cardiovascular or cerebrovascular disease that could be exacerbated by hypotension (history of myocardial infarction, angina, or ischemic stroke) and conditions that would predispose patients to hypotension (dehydration, hypovolemia, and treatment with antihypertensive medication)).
No products indexed under this heading.

Aliskiren (Mirtazapine should be used with caution in patients with known cardiovascular or cerebrovascular disease that could be exacerbated by hypotension (history of myocardial infarction, angina, or ischemic stroke) and conditions that would predispose patients to hypotension (dehydration, hypovolemia, and treatment with antihypertensive medication)). Products include:
Tekturna 2538
Tekturna HCT 2541
Valturna 3637

Amlodipine Besylate (Mirtazapine should be used with caution in patients with known cardiovascular or cerebrovascular disease that could be exacerbated by hypotension (history of myocardial infarction, angina, or ischemic stroke) and conditions that would predispose patients to hypotension (dehy-

Remeron Interactions Index 1586

dration, hypovolemia, and treatment with antihypertensive medication)). Products include:

Azor ... 1010
Exforge ... 2443
Exforge HCT ... 2449

Atenolol (Mirtazapine should be used with caution in patients with known cardiovascular or cerebrovascular disease that could be exacerbated by hypotension (history of myocardial infarction, angina, or ischemic stroke) and conditions that would predispose patients to hypotension (dehydration, hypovolemia, and treatment with antihypertensive medication)).
No products indexed under this heading.

Benazepril Hydrochloride (Mirtazapine should be used with caution in patients with known cardiovascular or cerebrovascular disease that could be exacerbated by hypotension (history of myocardial infarction, angina, or ischemic stroke) and conditions that would predispose patients to hypotension (dehydration, hypovolemia, and treatment with antihypertensive medication)).
No products indexed under this heading.

Bendroflumethiazide (Mirtazapine should be used with caution in patients with known cardiovascular or cerebrovascular disease that could be exacerbated by hypotension (history of myocardial infarction, angina, or ischemic stroke) and conditions that would predispose patients to hypotension (dehydration, hypovolemia, and treatment with antihypertensive medication)).
No products indexed under this heading.

Betaxolol Hydrochloride (Mirtazapine should be used with caution in patients with known cardiovascular or cerebrovascular disease that could be exacerbated by hypotension (history of myocardial infarction, angina, or ischemic stroke) and conditions that would predispose patients to hypotension (dehydration, hypovolemia, and treatment with antihypertensive medication)).
No products indexed under this heading.

Bisoprolol Fumarate (Mirtazapine should be used with caution in patients with known cardiovascular or cerebrovascular disease that could be exacerbated by hypotension (history of myocardial infarction, angina, or ischemic stroke) and conditions that would predispose patients to hypotension (dehydration, hypovolemia, and treatment with antihypertensive medication)).
No products indexed under this heading.

Candesartan Cilexetil (Mirtazapine should be used with caution in patients with known cardiovascular or cerebrovascular disease that could be exacerbated by hypotension (history of myocardial infarction, angina, or ischemic stroke) and conditions that would predispose patients to hypotension (dehydration, hypovolemia, and treatment with antihypertensive medication)). Products include:

Atacand ... 697
Atacand HCT ... 700

Captopril (Mirtazapine should be used with caution in patients with known cardiovascular or cerebrovascular disease that could be exacerbated by hypotension (history of myocardial infarction, angina, or ischemic stroke) and conditions that would predispose patients to hypotension (dehydration, hypovolemia, and treatment with antihypertensive medication)). Products include:

Captopril ... 2341

Carbamazepine (The metabolism and pharmacokinetics of mirtazapine may be affected by the induction or inhibition of drug-metabolizing enzymes). Products include:

Carbatrol ... 3280
Equetro ... 3477

Carteolol Hydrochloride (Mirtazapine should be used with caution in patients with known cardiovascular or cerebrovascular disease that could be exacerbated by hypotension (history of myocardial infarction, angina, or ischemic stroke) and conditions that would predispose patients to hypotension (dehydration, hypovolemia, and treatment with antihypertensive medication)).
No products indexed under this heading.

Carvedilol (Mirtazapine should be used with caution in patients with known cardiovascular or cerebrovascular disease that could be exacerbated by hypotension (history of myocardial infarction, angina, or ischemic stroke) and conditions that would predispose patients to hypotension (dehydration, hypovolemia, and treatment with antihypertensive medication)). Products include:

Coreg ... 1409

Carvedilol Phosphate (Mirtazapine should be used with caution in patients with known cardiovascular or cerebrovascular disease that could be exacerbated by hypotension (history of myocardial infarction, angina, or ischemic stroke) and conditions that would predispose patients to hypotension (dehydration, hypovolemia, and treatment with antihypertensive medication)). Products include:

Coreg CR ... 1416

Chlorothiazide (Mirtazapine should be used with caution in patients with known cardiovascular or cerebrovascular disease that could be exacerbated by hypotension (history of myocardial infarction, angina, or ischemic stroke) and conditions that would predispose patients to hypotension (dehydration, hypovolemia, and treatment with antihypertensive medication)).
No products indexed under this heading.

Chlorothiazide Sodium (Mirtazapine should be used with caution in patients with known cardiovascular or cerebrovascular disease that could be exacerbated by hypotension (history of myocardial infarction, angina, or ischemic stroke) and conditions that would predispose patients to hypotension (dehydration, hypovolemia, and treatment with antihypertensive medication)). Products include:

Diuril Intravenous ... 2009

Chlorthalidone (Mirtazapine should be used with caution in patients with known cardiovascular or cerebrovascular disease that could be exacerbated by hypotension (history of myocardial infarction, angina, or ischemic stroke) and conditions that would predispose patients to hypotension (dehydration, hypovolemia, and treatment with antihypertensive medication)). Products include:

Clorpres ... 2344

Cimetidine (The metabolism and pharmacokinetics of mirtazapine may be affected by the induction or inhibition of drug-metabolizing enzymes).
No products indexed under this heading.

Cimetidine Hydrochloride (The metabolism and pharmacokinetics of mirtazapine may be affected by the induction or inhibition of drug-metabolizing enzymes).
No products indexed under this heading.

Clonidine (Mirtazapine should be used with caution in patients with known cardiovascular or cerebrovascular disease that could be exacerbated by hypotension (history of myocardial infarction, angina, or ischemic stroke) and conditions that would predispose patients to hypotension (dehydration, hypovolemia, and treatment with antihypertensive medication)). Products include:

Catapres-TTS ... 884

Clonidine Hydrochloride (Mirtazapine should be used with caution in patients with known cardiovascular or cerebrovascular disease that could be exacerbated by hypotension (history of myocardial infarction, angina, or ischemic stroke) and conditions that would predispose patients to hypotension (dehydration, hypovolemia, and treatment with antihypertensive medication)). Products include:

Clorpres ... 2344

Deserpidine (Mirtazapine should be used with caution in patients with known cardiovascular or cerebrovascular disease that could be exacerbated by hypotension (history of myocardial infarction, angina, or ischemic stroke) and conditions that would predispose patients to hypotension (dehydration, hypovolemia, and treatment with antihypertensive medication)).
No products indexed under this heading.

Diazepam (Concomitant administration of diazepam (15 mg) had a minimal effect on plasma levels of mirtazapine (15 mg) in 6 healthy male subjects. However, the impairment of motor skills produced by mirtazapine has been shown to be additive with those caused by diazepam. Accordingly, patients should be advised to avoid diazepam and other similar drugs while taking mirtazapine). Products include:

Valium Tablets ... 2880

Diazoxide (Mirtazapine should be used with caution in patients with known cardiovascular or cerebrovascular disease that could be exacerbated by hypotension (history of myocardial infarction, angina, or ischemic stroke) and conditions that would predispose patients to hypotension (dehydration, hypovolemia, and treatment with antihypertensive medication)). Products include:

Proglycem ... 1179
Proglycem Suspension ... 1179

Diltiazem Hydrochloride (Mirtazapine should be used with caution in patients with known cardiovascular or cerebrovascular disease that could be exacerbated by hypotension (history of myocardial infarction, angina, or ischemic stroke) and conditions that would predispose patients to hypotension (dehydration, hypovolemia, and treatment with antihypertensive medication)). Products include:

Cardizem LA ... 423

Diltiazem Maleate (Mirtazapine should be used with caution in patients with known cardiovascular or cerebrovascular disease that could be exacerbated by hypotension (history of myocardial infarction, angina, or ischemic stroke) and conditions that would predispose patients to hypotension (dehydration, hypovolemia, and treatment with antihypertensive medication)).
No products indexed under this heading.

Doxazosin Mesylate (Mirtazapine should be used with caution in patients with known cardiovascular or cerebrovascular disease that could be exacerbated by hypotension (history of myocardial infarction, angina, or ischemic stroke) and conditions that would predispose patients to hypotension (dehydration, hypovolemia, and treatment with antihypertensive medication)).
No products indexed under this heading.

Drugs, unspecified (Patients should be advised to inform their physician if they are taking, on intend to take, any prescription or over-the-counter drugs, since there is a potential for mirtazapine to interact with other drugs).
No products indexed under this heading.

Enalapril Maleate (Mirtazapine should be used with caution in patients with known cardiovascular or cerebrovascular disease that could be exacerbated by hypotension (history of myocardial infarction, angina, or ischemic stroke) and conditions that would predispose patients to hypotension (dehydration, hypovolemia, and treatment with antihypertensive medication)).
No products indexed under this heading.

Enalaprilat (Mirtazapine should be used with caution in patients with known cardiovascular or cerebrovascular disease that could be exacerbated by hypotension (history of myocardial infarction, angina, or ischemic stroke) and conditions that would predispose patients to hypotension (dehydration, hypovolemia, and treatment with antihypertensive medication)).
No products indexed under this heading.

Eprosartan Mesylate (Mirtazapine should be used with caution in patients with known cardiovascular or cerebrovascular disease that could be exacerbated by hypotension (history of myocardial infarction, angina, or ischemic stroke) and conditions that would predispose patients to hypotension (dehydration, hypovolemia, and treatment with antihypertensive medication)). Products include:

Teveten ... 538
Teveten HCT ... 541

Erythromycin (The metabolism and pharmacokinetics of mirtazapine may be affected by the induction or inhibition of drug-metabolizing enzymes).
No products indexed under this heading.

Erythromycin Estolate (The metabolism and pharmacokinetics of mirtazapine may be affected by the induction or inhibition of drug-metabolizing enzymes).
No products indexed under this heading.

Erythromycin Ethylsuccinate (The metabolism and pharmacokinetics of mirtazapine may be affected by the induction or inhibition of drug-metabolizing enzymes). Products include:

E.E.S. ... 437
EryPed ... 435

Erythromycin Gluceptate (The metabolism and pharmacokinetics of mirtazapine may be affected by the induction or inhibition of drug-metabolizing enzymes).
No products indexed under this heading.

Erythromycin Lactobionate (The metabolism and pharmacokinetics of mirtazapine may be affected by the induction or inhibition of drug-metabolizing enzymes).
No products indexed under this heading.

Erythromycin Stearate (The metabolism and pharmacokinetics of mirtazapine may be affected by the induction or inhibition of drug-metabolizing enzymes).
No products indexed under this heading.

Esmolol Hydrochloride (Mirtazapine should be used with caution in patients with known cardiovascular or cerebrovascular disease that could be exacerbated by hypotension (history of myocardial infarction, angina, or ischemic stroke) and conditions that would predispose patients to hypotension (dehydration, hypovolemia, and treatment with antihypertensive medication)).
No products indexed under this heading.

1587 Interactions Index Remeron

Ethanol (Concomitant administration of alcohol (equivalent to 60 g) had a minimal effect on plasma levels of mirtazapine (15 mg) in healthy male subjects. However, the impairment of cognitive and motor skills produced by mirtazapine were shown to be additive with those produced by alcohol. Accordingly, patients should be advised to avoid alcohol while taking mirtazapine).
No products indexed under this heading.

Ethyl Alcohol (Concomitant administration of alcohol (equivalent to 60 g) had a minimal effect on plasma levels of mirtazapine (15 mg) in healthy male subjects. However, the impairment of cognitive and motor skills produced by mirtazapine were shown to be additive with those produced by alcohol. Accordingly, patients should be advised to avoid alcohol while taking mirtazapine).
No products indexed under this heading.

Felodipine (Mirtazapine should be used with caution in patients with known cardiovascular or cerebrovascular disease that could be exacerbated by hypotension (history of myocardial infarction, angina, or ischemic stroke) and conditions that would predispose patients to hypotension (dehydration, hypovolemia, and treatment with antihypertensive medication)).
No products indexed under this heading.

Fosinopril Sodium (Mirtazapine should be used with caution in patients with known cardiovascular or cerebrovascular disease that could be exacerbated by hypotension (history of myocardial infarction, angina, or ischemic stroke) and conditions that would predispose patients to hypotension (dehydration, hypovolemia, and treatment with antihypertensive medication)).
No products indexed under this heading.

Fosphenytoin Sodium (The metabolism and pharmacokinetics of mirtazapine may be affected by the induction or inhibition of drug-metabolizing enzymes).
No products indexed under this heading.

Furosemide (Mirtazapine should be used with caution in patients with known cardiovascular or cerebrovascular disease that could be exacerbated by hypotension (history of myocardial infarction, angina, or ischemic stroke) and conditions that would predispose patients to hypotension (dehydration, hypovolemia, and treatment with antihypertensive medication)). Products include:
Furosemide 2354

Guanabenz Acetate (Mirtazapine should be used with caution in patients with known cardiovascular or cerebrovascular disease that could be exacerbated by hypotension (history of myocardial infarction, angina, or ischemic stroke) and conditions that would predispose patients to hypotension (dehydration, hypovolemia, and treatment with antihypertensive medication)).
No products indexed under this heading.

Guanethidine (Mirtazapine should be used with caution in patients with known cardiovascular or cerebrovascular disease that could be exacerbated by hypotension (history of myocardial infarction, angina, or ischemic stroke) and conditions that would predispose patients to hypotension (dehydration, hypovolemia, and treatment with antihypertensive medication)).
No products indexed under this heading.

Guanethidine Monosulfate (Mirtazapine should be used with caution in patients with known cardiovascular or cerebrovascular disease that could be exacerbated by hypotension (history of myocardial infarction, angina, or ischemic stroke) and conditions that would predispose patients to hypotension (dehydration, hypovolemia, and treatment with antihypertensive medication)).
No products indexed under this heading.

Guanethidine Sulfate (Mirtazapine should be used with caution in patients with known cardiovascular or cerebrovascular disease that could be exacerbated by hypotension (history of myocardial infarction, angina, or ischemic stroke) and conditions that would predispose patients to hypotension (dehydration, hypovolemia, and treatment with antihypertensive medication)).
No products indexed under this heading.

Hydralazine Hydrochloride (Mirtazapine should be used with caution in patients with known cardiovascular or cerebrovascular disease that could be exacerbated by hypotension (history of myocardial infarction, angina, or ischemic stroke) and conditions that would predispose patients to hypotension (dehydration, hypovolemia, and treatment with antihypertensive medication)).
No products indexed under this heading.

Hydrochlorothiazide (Mirtazapine should be used with caution in patients with known cardiovascular or cerebrovascular disease that could be exacerbated by hypotension (history of myocardial infarction, angina, or ischemic stroke) and conditions that would predispose patients to hypotension (dehydration, hypovolemia, and treatment with antihypertensive medication)). Products include:
Atacand HCT 700
Avalide 2956
Benicar HCT 1017
Diovan HCT 2419
Dyazide 1429
Exforge HCT 2449
Hyzaar 2162
Hyzaar 100-12.5 2162
Micardis HCT 889
Prinzide 2246
Tekturna HCT 2541
Teveten HCT 541

Hydroflumethiazide (Mirtazapine should be used with caution in patients with known cardiovascular or cerebrovascular disease that could be exacerbated by hypotension (history of myocardial infarction, angina, or ischemic stroke) and conditions that would predispose patients to hypotension (dehydration, hypovolemia, and treatment with antihypertensive medication)).
No products indexed under this heading.

Indapamide (Mirtazapine should be used with caution in patients with known cardiovascular or cerebrovascular disease that could be exacerbated by hypotension (history of myocardial infarction, angina, or ischemic stroke) and conditions that would predispose patients to hypotension (dehydration, hypovolemia, and treatment with antihypertensive medication)). Products include:
Indapamide 2356

Irbesartan (Mirtazapine should be used with caution in patients with known cardiovascular or cerebrovascular disease that could be exacerbated by hypotension (history of myocardial infarction, angina, or ischemic stroke) and conditions that would predispose patients to hypotension (dehydration, hypovolemia, and treatment with antihypertensive medication)). Products include:
Avalide 2956
Avapro 2962

Isocarboxazid (In patients receiving other drugs for major depressive disorder in combination with a monoamine oxidase inhibitor (MAOI) and in patients who have recently discontinued a drug for major depressive disorder and then are started on an MAOI, there have been reports of serious and sometimes fatal reactions, including nausea, vomiting, flushing, dizziness, tremor, myoclonus, rigidity, diaphoresis, hyperthermia, autonomic instability with rapid fluctuations of vital signs, seizures, and mental status changes ranging from agitation to coma. Although there are no human data pertinent to such an interaction with mirtazapine tablets, it is recommended that mirtazapine not be used in combination with an MAOI, or within 14 days of initiating or discontinuing therapy with an MAOI). Products include:
Marplan 3481

Isradipine (Mirtazapine should be used with caution in patients with known cardiovascular or cerebrovascular disease that could be exacerbated by hypotension (history of myocardial infarction, angina, or ischemic stroke) and conditions that would predispose patients to hypotension (dehydration, hypovolemia, and treatment with antihypertensive medication)). Products include:
DynaCirc CR 1432

Labetalol Hydrochloride (Mirtazapine should be used with caution in patients with known cardiovascular or cerebrovascular disease that could be exacerbated by hypotension (history of myocardial infarction, angina, or ischemic stroke) and conditions that would predispose patients to hypotension (dehydration, hypovolemia, and treatment with antihypertensive medication)).
No products indexed under this heading.

Lisinopril (Mirtazapine should be used with caution in patients with known cardiovascular or cerebrovascular disease that could be exacerbated by hypotension (history of myocardial infarction, angina, or ischemic stroke) and conditions that would predispose patients to hypotension (dehydration, hypovolemia, and treatment with antihypertensive medication)). Products include:
Prinivil 2241
Prinzide 2246

Losartan Potassium (Mirtazapine should be used with caution in patients with known cardiovascular or cerebrovascular disease that could be exacerbated by hypotension (history of myocardial infarction, angina, or ischemic stroke) and conditions that would predispose patients to hypotension (dehydration, hypovolemia, and treatment with antihypertensive medication)). Products include:
Cozaar 2106
Hyzaar 2162
Hyzaar 100-12.5 2162

Mecamylamine Hydrochloride (Mirtazapine should be used with caution in patients with known cardiovascular or cerebrovascular disease that could be exacerbated by hypotension (history of myocardial infarction, angina, or ischemic stroke) and conditions that would predispose patients to hypotension (dehydration, hypovolemia, and treatment with antihypertensive medication)).
No products indexed under this heading.

Methyclothiazide (Mirtazapine should be used with caution in patients with known cardiovascular or cerebrovascular disease that could be exacerbated by hypotension (history of myocardial infarction, angina, or ischemic stroke) and conditions that would predispose patients to hypotension (dehydration, hypovolemia, and treatment with antihypertensive medication)).
No products indexed under this heading.

Methyldopa (Mirtazapine should be used with caution in patients with known cardiovascular or cerebrovascular disease that could be exacerbated by hypotension (history of myocardial infarction, angina, or ischemic stroke) and conditions that would predispose patients to hypotension (dehydration, hypovolemia, and treatment with antihypertensive medication)).
No products indexed under this heading.

Methyldopate Hydrochloride (Mirtazapine should be used with caution in patients with known cardiovascular or cerebrovascular disease that could be exacerbated by hypotension (history of myocardial infarction, angina, or ischemic stroke) and conditions that would predispose patients to hypotension (dehydration, hypovolemia, and treatment with antihypertensive medication)).
No products indexed under this heading.

Metolazone (Mirtazapine should be used with caution in patients with known cardiovascular or cerebrovascular disease that could be exacerbated by hypotension (history of myocardial infarction, angina, or ischemic stroke) and conditions that would predispose patients to hypotension (dehydration, hypovolemia, and treatment with antihypertensive medication)).
No products indexed under this heading.

Metoprolol Succinate (Mirtazapine should be used with caution in patients with known cardiovascular or cerebrovascular disease that could be exacerbated by hypotension (history of myocardial infarction, angina, or ischemic stroke) and conditions that would predispose patients to hypotension (dehydration, hypovolemia, and treatment with antihypertensive medication)). Products include:
Toprol XL 732

Metoprolol Tartrate (Mirtazapine should be used with caution in patients with known cardiovascular or cerebrovascular disease that could be exacerbated by hypotension (history of myocardial infarction, angina, or ischemic stroke) and conditions that would predispose patients to hypotension (dehydration, hypovolemia, and treatment with antihypertensive medication)).
No products indexed under this heading.

Metyrosine (Mirtazapine should be used with caution in patients with known cardiovascular or cerebrovascular disease that could be exacerbated by hypotension (history of myocardial infarction, angina, or ischemic stroke) and conditions that would predispose patients to hypotension (dehydration, hypovolemia, and treatment with antihypertensive medication)).
No products indexed under this heading.

Mibefradil Dihydrochloride (Mirtazapine should be used with caution in patients with known cardiovascular or cerebrovascular disease that could be exacerbated by hypotension (history of myocardial infarction, angina, or ischemic stroke) and conditions that would predispose patients to hypotension (dehydration, hypovolemia, and treatment with antihypertensive medication)).
No products indexed under this heading.

Remeron Interactions Index 1588

Minoxidil (Mirtazapine should be used with caution in patients with known cardiovascular or cerebrovascular disease that could be exacerbated by hypotension (history of myocardial infarction, angina, or ischemic stroke) and conditions that would predispose patients to hypotension (dehydration, hypovolemia, and treatment with antihypertensive medication)).
No products indexed under this heading.

Moclobemide (In patients receiving other drugs for major depressive disorder in combination with a monoamine oxidase inhibitor (MAOI) and in patients who have recently discontinued a drug for major depressive disorder and then are started on an MAOI, there have been reports of serious and sometimes fatal reactions, including nausea, vomiting, flushing, dizziness, tremor, myoclonus, rigidity, diaphoresis, hyperthermia, autonomic instability with rapid fluctuations of vital signs, seizures, and mental status changes ranging from agitation to coma. Although there are no human data pertinent to such an interaction with mirtazapine tablets, it is recommended that mirtazapine not be used in combination with an MAOI, or within 14 days of initiating or discontinuing therapy with an MAOI).
No products indexed under this heading.

Moexipril Hydrochloride (Mirtazapine should be used with caution in patients with known cardiovascular or cerebrovascular disease that could be exacerbated by hypotension (history of myocardial infarction, angina, or ischemic stroke) and conditions that would predispose patients to hypotension (dehydration, hypovolemia, and treatment with antihypertensive medication)).
No products indexed under this heading.

Nadolol (Mirtazapine should be used with caution in patients with known cardiovascular or cerebrovascular disease that could be exacerbated by hypotension (history of myocardial infarction, angina, or ischemic stroke) and conditions that would predispose patients to hypotension (dehydration, hypovolemia, and treatment with antihypertensive medication)). Products include:
Nadolol 2359

Nebivolol (Mirtazapine should be used with caution in patients with known cardiovascular or cerebrovascular disease that could be exacerbated by hypotension (history of myocardial infarction, angina, or ischemic stroke) and conditions that would predispose patients to hypotension (dehydration, hypovolemia, and treatment with antihypertensive medication)). Products include:
Bystolic 1147

Nicardipine Hydrochloride (Mirtazapine should be used with caution in patients with known cardiovascular or cerebrovascular disease that could be exacerbated by hypotension (history of myocardial infarction, angina, or ischemic stroke) and conditions that would predispose patients to hypotension (dehydration, hypovolemia, and treatment with antihypertensive medication)).
No products indexed under this heading.

Nifedipine (Mirtazapine should be used with caution in patients with known cardiovascular or cerebrovascular disease that could be exacerbated by hypotension (history of myocardial infarction, angina, or ischemic stroke) and conditions that would predispose patients to hypotension (dehydration, hypovolemia, and treatment with antihypertensive medication)).
No products indexed under this heading.

Nisoldipine (Mirtazapine should be used with caution in patients with known cardiovascular or cerebrovascular disease that could be exacerbated by hypotension (history of myocardial infarction, angina, or ischemic stroke) and conditions that would predispose patients to hypotension (dehydration, hypovolemia, and treatment with antihypertensive medication)).
No products indexed under this heading.

Nitroglycerin (Mirtazapine should be used with caution in patients with known cardiovascular or cerebrovascular disease that could be exacerbated by hypotension (history of myocardial infarction, angina, or ischemic stroke) and conditions that would predispose patients to hypotension (dehydration, hypovolemia, and treatment with antihypertensive medication)). Products include:
Nitro-Dur 3170
Nitrolingual 3266

Pargyline Hydrochloride (In patients receiving other drugs for major depressive disorder in combination with a monoamine oxidase inhibitor (MAOI) and in patients who have recently discontinued a drug for major depressive disorder and then are started on an MAOI, there have been reports of serious and sometimes fatal reactions, including nausea, vomiting, flushing, dizziness, tremor, myoclonus, rigidity, diaphoresis, hyperthermia, autonomic instability with rapid fluctuations of vital signs, seizures, and mental status changes ranging from agitation to coma. Although there are no human data pertinent to such an interaction with mirtazapine tablets, it is recommended that mirtazapine not be used in combination with an MAOI, or within 14 days of initiating or discontinuing therapy with an MAOI).
No products indexed under this heading.

Penbutolol Sulfate (Mirtazapine should be used with caution in patients with known cardiovascular or cerebrovascular disease that could be exacerbated by hypotension (history of myocardial infarction, angina, or ischemic stroke) and conditions that would predispose patients to hypotension (dehydration, hypovolemia, and treatment with antihypertensive medication)).
No products indexed under this heading.

Perindopril Erbumine (Mirtazapine should be used with caution in patients with known cardiovascular or cerebrovascular disease that could be exacerbated by hypotension (history of myocardial infarction, angina, or ischemic stroke) and conditions that would predispose patients to hypotension (dehydration, hypovolemia, and treatment with antihypertensive medication)).
No products indexed under this heading.

Phenelzine Sulfate (In patients receiving other drugs for major depressive disorder in combination with a monoamine oxidase inhibitor (MAOI) and in patients who have recently discontinued a drug for major depressive disorder and then are started on an MAOI, there have been reports of serious and sometimes fatal reactions, including nausea, vomiting, flushing, dizziness, tremor, myoclonus, rigidity, diaphoresis, hyperthermia, autonomic instability with rapid fluctuations of vital signs, seizures, and mental status changes ranging from agitation to coma. Although there are no human data pertinent to such an interaction with mirtazapine tablets, it is recommended that mirtazapine not be used in combination with an MAOI, or within 14 days of initiating or discontinuing therapy with an MAOI).
No products indexed under this heading.

Phenobarbital (The metabolism and pharmacokinetics of mirtazapine may be affected by the induction or inhibition of drug-metabolizing enzymes). Products include:
Donnatal 2711

Phenoxybenzamine Hydrochloride (Mirtazapine should be used with caution in patients with known cardiovascular or cerebrovascular disease that could be exacerbated by hypotension (history of myocardial infarction, angina, or ischemic stroke) and conditions that would predispose patients to hypotension (dehydration, hypovolemia, and treatment with antihypertensive medication)). Products include:
Dibenzyline 3495

Phentolamine Mesylate (Mirtazapine should be used with caution in patients with known cardiovascular or cerebrovascular disease that could be exacerbated by hypotension (history of myocardial infarction, angina, or ischemic stroke) and conditions that would predispose patients to hypotension (dehydration, hypovolemia, and treatment with antihypertensive medication)).
No products indexed under this heading.

Phenytoin (The metabolism and pharmacokinetics of mirtazapine may be affected by the induction or inhibition of drug-metabolizing enzymes).
No products indexed under this heading.

Phenytoin Sodium (The metabolism and pharmacokinetics of mirtazapine may be affected by the induction or inhibition of drug-metabolizing enzymes). Products include:
Phenytek Capsules 2380

Pindolol (Mirtazapine should be used with caution in patients with known cardiovascular or cerebrovascular disease that could be exacerbated by hypotension (history of myocardial infarction, angina, or ischemic stroke) and conditions that would predispose patients to hypotension (dehydration, hypovolemia, and treatment with antihypertensive medication)).
No products indexed under this heading.

Polythiazide (Mirtazapine should be used with caution in patients with known cardiovascular or cerebrovascular disease that could be exacerbated by hypotension (history of myocardial infarction, angina, or ischemic stroke) and conditions that would predispose patients to hypotension (dehydration, hypovolemia, and treatment with antihypertensive medication)).
No products indexed under this heading.

Prazosin Hydrochloride (Mirtazapine should be used with caution in patients with known cardiovascular or cerebrovascular disease that could be exacerbated by hypotension (history of myocardial infarction, angina, or ischemic stroke) and conditions that would predispose patients to hypotension (dehydration, hypovolemia, and treatment with antihypertensive medication)).
No products indexed under this heading.

Prescription Drugs, unspecified (Patients should be advised to inform their physician if they are taking, on intend to take, any prescription or over-the-counter drugs, since there is a potential for mirtazapine to interact with other drugs).
No products indexed under this heading.

Procarbazine Hydrochloride (In patients receiving other drugs for major depressive disorder in combination with a monoamine oxidase inhibitor (MAOI) and in patients who have recently discontinued a drug for major depressive disorder and then are started on an MAOI, there have been reports of serious and sometimes fatal reactions, including nausea, vomiting, flushing, dizziness, tremor, myoclonus, rigidity, diaphoresis, hyperthermia, autonomic instability with rapid fluctuations of vital signs, seizures, and mental status changes ranging from agitation to coma. Although there are no human data pertinent to such an interaction with mirtazapine tablets, it is recommended that mirtazapine not be used in combination with an MAOI, or within 14 days of initiating or discontinuing therapy with an MAOI).
No products indexed under this heading.

Propranolol Hydrochloride (Mirtazapine should be used with caution in patients with known cardiovascular or cerebrovascular disease that could be exacerbated by hypotension (history of myocardial infarction, angina, or ischemic stroke) and conditions that would predispose patients to hypotension (dehydration, hypovolemia, and treatment with antihypertensive medication)). Products include:
InnoPran XL 1517

Quinapril Hydrochloride (Mirtazapine should be used with caution in patients with known cardiovascular or cerebrovascular disease that could be exacerbated by hypotension (history of myocardial infarction, angina, or ischemic stroke) and conditions that would predispose patients to hypotension (dehydration, hypovolemia, and treatment with antihypertensive medication)).
No products indexed under this heading.

Ramipril (Mirtazapine should be used with caution in patients with known cardiovascular or cerebrovascular disease that could be exacerbated by hypotension (history of myocardial infarction, angina, or ischemic stroke) and conditions that would predispose patients to hypotension (dehydration, hypovolemia, and treatment with antihypertensive medication)).
No products indexed under this heading.

Rasagiline Mesylate (In patients receiving other drugs for major depressive disorder in combination with a monoamine oxidase inhibitor (MAOI) and in patients who have recently discontinued a drug for major depressive disorder and then are started on an MAOI, there have been reports of serious and sometimes fatal reactions, including nausea, vomiting, flushing, dizziness, tremor, myoclonus, rigidity, diaphoresis, hyperthermia, autonomic instability with rapid fluctuations of vital signs, seizures, and mental status changes ranging from agitation to coma. Although there are no human data pertinent to such an interaction with mirtazapine tablets, it is recommended that mirtazapine not be used in combination with an MAOI, or within 14 days of initiating or discontinuing therapy with an MAOI). Products include:
Azilect 3383

Rauwolfia Serpentina (Mirtazapine should be used with caution in patients with known cardiovascular or cerebrovascular disease that could be exacerbated by hypotension (history of myocardial infarction, angina, or ischemic stroke) and conditions that would predispose patients to hypotension (dehydration, hypovolemia, and treatment with antihypertensive medication)).
No products indexed under this heading.

(⊙ Described in PDR® for Ophthalmic Medicines)

Rescinnamine (Mirtazapine should be used with caution in patients with known cardiovascular or cerebrovascular disease that could be exacerbated by hypotension (history of myocardial infarction, angina, or ischemic stroke) and conditions that would predispose patients to hypotension (dehydration, hypovolemia, and treatment with antihypertensive medication)).
No products indexed under this heading.

Reserpine (Mirtazapine should be used with caution in patients with known cardiovascular or cerebrovascular disease that could be exacerbated by hypotension (history of myocardial infarction, angina, or ischemic stroke) and conditions that would predispose patients to hypotension (dehydration, hypovolemia, and treatment with antihypertensive medication)).
No products indexed under this heading.

Selegiline (In patients receiving other drugs for major depressive disorder in combination with a monoamine oxidase inhibitor (MAOI) and in patients who have recently discontinued a drug for major depressive disorder and then are started on an MAOI, there have been reports of serious and sometimes fatal reactions, including nausea, vomiting, flushing, dizziness, tremor, myoclonus, rigidity, diaphoresis, hyperthermia, autonomic instability with rapid fluctuations of vital signs, seizures, and mental status changes ranging from agitation to coma. Although there are no human data pertinent to such an interaction with mirtazapine tablets, it is recommended that mirtazapine not be used in combination with an MAOI, or within 14 days of initiating or discontinuing therapy with an MAOI). Products include:
Emsam 3623

Selegiline Hydrochloride (In patients receiving other drugs for major depressive disorder in combination with a monoamine oxidase inhibitor (MAOI) and in patients who have recently discontinued a drug for major depressive disorder and then are started on an MAOI, there have been reports of serious and sometimes fatal reactions, including nausea, vomiting, flushing, dizziness, tremor, myoclonus, rigidity, diaphoresis, hyperthermia, autonomic instability with rapid fluctuations of vital signs, seizures, and mental status changes ranging from agitation to coma. Although there are no human data pertinent to such an interaction with mirtazapine tablets, it is recommended that mirtazapine not be used in combination with an MAOI, or within 14 days of initiating or discontinuing therapy with an MAOI). Products include:
Eldepryl 3312

Sodium Nitroprusside (Mirtazapine should be used with caution in patients with known cardiovascular or cerebrovascular disease that could be exacerbated by hypotension (history of myocardial infarction, angina, or ischemic stroke) and conditions that would predispose patients to hypotension (dehydration, hypovolemia, and treatment with antihypertensive medication)).
No products indexed under this heading.

Sotalol Hydrochloride (Mirtazapine should be used with caution in patients with known cardiovascular or cerebrovascular disease that could be exacerbated by hypotension (history of myocardial infarction, angina, or ischemic stroke) and conditions that would predispose patients to hypotension (dehydration, hypovolemia, and treatment with antihypertensive medication)).
No products indexed under this heading.

Spirapril Hydrochloride (Mirtazapine should be used with caution in patients with known cardiovascular or cerebrovascular disease that could be exacerbated by hypotension (history of myocardial infarction, angina, or ischemic stroke) and conditions that would predispose patients to hypotension (dehydration, hypovolemia, and treatment with antihypertensive medication)).
No products indexed under this heading.

Telmisartan (Mirtazapine should be used with caution in patients with known cardiovascular or cerebrovascular disease that could be exacerbated by hypotension (history of myocardial infarction, angina, or ischemic stroke) and conditions that would predispose patients to hypotension (dehydration, hypovolemia, and treatment with antihypertensive medication)). Products include:
Micardis 887
Micardis HCT 889

Terazosin Hydrochloride (Mirtazapine should be used with caution in patients with known cardiovascular or cerebrovascular disease that could be exacerbated by hypotension (history of myocardial infarction, angina, or ischemic stroke) and conditions that would predispose patients to hypotension (dehydration, hypovolemia, and treatment with antihypertensive medication)).
No products indexed under this heading.

Theophyllinate (The metabolism and pharmacokinetics of mirtazapine may be affected by the induction or inhibition of drug-metabolizing enzymes).
No products indexed under this heading.

Theophylline (The metabolism and pharmacokinetics of mirtazapine may be affected by the induction or inhibition of drug-metabolizing enzymes).
No products indexed under this heading.

Theophylline Anhydrous (The metabolism and pharmacokinetics of mirtazapine may be affected by the induction or inhibition of drug-metabolizing enzymes). Products include:
Uniphyl 2817

Theophylline Calcium Salicylate (The metabolism and pharmacokinetics of mirtazapine may be affected by the induction or inhibition of drug-metabolizing enzymes).
No products indexed under this heading.

Theophylline Dihydroxypropyl (Glyceryl) (The metabolism and pharmacokinetics of mirtazapine may be affected by the induction or inhibition of drug-metabolizing enzymes).
No products indexed under this heading.

Theophylline Ethylenediamine (The metabolism and pharmacokinetics of mirtazapine may be affected by the induction or inhibition of drug-metabolizing enzymes).
No products indexed under this heading.

Theophylline Sodium Glycinate (The metabolism and pharmacokinetics of mirtazapine may be affected by the induction or inhibition of drug-metabolizing enzymes).
No products indexed under this heading.

Timolol Maleate (Mirtazapine should be used with caution in patients with known cardiovascular or cerebrovascular disease that could be exacerbated by hypotension (history of myocardial infarction, angina, or ischemic stroke) and conditions that would predispose patients to hypotension (dehydration, hypovolemia, and treatment with antihypertensive medication)). Products include:
Combigan 601
Dorzolamide Hydrochloride/Timolol Maleate Ophthalmic Solution .... ⊙243
Timoptic in Ocudose .... ⊙231

Torsemide (Mirtazapine should be used with caution in patients with known cardiovascular or cerebrovascular disease that could be exacerbated by hypotension (history of myocardial infarction, angina, or ischemic stroke) and conditions that would predispose patients to hypotension (dehydration, hypovolemia, and treatment with antihypertensive medication)).
No products indexed under this heading.

Trandolapril (Mirtazapine should be used with caution in patients with known cardiovascular or cerebrovascular disease that could be exacerbated by hypotension (history of myocardial infarction, angina, or ischemic stroke) and conditions that would predispose patients to hypotension (dehydration, hypovolemia, and treatment with antihypertensive medication)). Products include:
Mavik 489
Tarka 534

Tranylcypromine Sulfate (In patients receiving other drugs for major depressive disorder in combination with a monoamine oxidase inhibitor (MAOI) and in patients who have recently discontinued a drug for major depressive disorder and then are started on an MAOI, there have been reports of serious and sometimes fatal reactions, including nausea, vomiting, flushing, dizziness, tremor, myoclonus, rigidity, diaphoresis, hyperthermia, autonomic instability with rapid fluctuations of vital signs, seizures, and mental status changes ranging from agitation to coma. Although there are no human data pertinent to such an interaction with mirtazapine tablets, it is recommended that mirtazapine not be used in combination with an MAOI, or within 14 days of initiating or discontinuing therapy with an MAOI). Products include:
Parnate 1584

Trimethaphan Camsylate (Mirtazapine should be used with caution in patients with known cardiovascular or cerebrovascular disease that could be exacerbated by hypotension (history of myocardial infarction, angina, or ischemic stroke) and conditions that would predispose patients to hypotension (dehydration, hypovolemia, and treatment with antihypertensive medication)).
No products indexed under this heading.

Valsartan (Mirtazapine should be used with caution in patients with known cardiovascular or cerebrovascular disease that could be exacerbated by hypotension (history of myocardial infarction, angina, or ischemic stroke) and conditions that would predispose patients to hypotension (dehydration, hypovolemia, and treatment with antihypertensive medication)). Products include:
Diovan 2413
Diovan HCT 2419
Exforge 2443
Exforge HCT 2449
Valturna 3637

Verapamil Hydrochloride (Mirtazapine should be used with caution in patients with known cardiovascular or cerebrovascular disease that could be exacerbated by hypotension (history of myocardial infarction, angina, or ischemic stroke) and conditions that would predispose patients to hypotension (dehydration, hypovolemia, and treatment with antihypertensive medication)). Products include:
Tarka 534

Food Interactions

Alcohol (Concomitant administration of alcohol (equivalent to 60 g) had a minimal effect on plasma levels of mirtazapine (15 mg) in healthy male subjects. However, the impairment of cognitive and motor skills produced by mirtazapine were shown to be additive with those produced by alcohol. Accordingly, patients should be advised to avoid alcohol while taking mirtazapine).

Beer, reduced-alcohol (Concomitant administration of alcohol (equivalent to 60 g) had a minimal effect on plasma levels of mirtazapine (15 mg) in healthy male subjects. However, the impairment of cognitive and motor skills produced by mirtazapine were shown to be additive with those produced by alcohol. Accordingly, patients should be advised to avoid alcohol while taking mirtazapine).

Beer, unspecified (Concomitant administration of alcohol (equivalent to 60 g) had a minimal effect on plasma levels of mirtazapine (15 mg) in healthy male subjects. However, the impairment of cognitive and motor skills produced by mirtazapine were shown to be additive with those produced by alcohol. Accordingly, patients should be advised to avoid alcohol while taking mirtazapine).

Wine, Chianti (Concomitant administration of alcohol (equivalent to 60 g) had a minimal effect on plasma levels of mirtazapine (15 mg) in healthy male subjects. However, the impairment of cognitive and motor skills produced by mirtazapine were shown to be additive with those produced by alcohol. Accordingly, patients should be advised to avoid alcohol while taking mirtazapine).

Wine, Red (Concomitant administration of alcohol (equivalent to 60 g) had a minimal effect on plasma levels of mirtazapine (15 mg) in healthy male subjects. However, the impairment of cognitive and motor skills produced by mirtazapine were shown to be additive with those produced by alcohol. Accordingly, patients should be advised to avoid alcohol while taking mirtazapine).

Wine, unspecified (Concomitant administration of alcohol (equivalent to 60 g) had a minimal effect on plasma levels of mirtazapine (15 mg) in healthy male subjects. However, the impairment of cognitive and motor skills produced by mirtazapine were shown to be additive with those produced by alcohol. Accordingly, patients should be advised to avoid alcohol while taking mirtazapine).

Wine products (Concomitant administration of alcohol (equivalent to 60 g) had a minimal effect on plasma levels of mirtazapine (15 mg) in healthy male subjects. However, the impairment of cognitive and motor skills produced by mirtazapine were shown to be additive with those produced by alcohol. Accordingly, patients should be advised to avoid alcohol while taking mirtazapine).

REMERONSOLTAB TABLETS

(Mirtazapine) 3219
See Remeron Tablets

REMICADE FOR IV INJECTION

(Infliximab) 919
May interact with vaccines, live, and certain other agents. Compounds in these categories include:

IMPORTANT NOTE: Always consult each drug listing in the patient's regimen for possible interactions.

2-Amino-6-Mercaptopurine (Rare post-marketing cases of hepatosplenic T-cell lymphoma have been reported in adolescent and young adult patients with Crohns's disease treated with infliximab; all of these hepatosplenic T-cell lymphomas with infliximab have occurred in patients on concomitant treatment with 6-mercaptopurine).
No products indexed under this heading.

Anakinra (Concurrent administration of etanercept (another TNFα-blocking agent) and anakinra (an interleukin-1 receptor antagonist) has been associated with an increased risk of serious infections, and increased risk of neutropenia and no additional benefit compared to these medical products alone. Other TNFα-blocking agents (infliximab) used in combination with anakinra may also result in similar toxicites. Therefore, the combination of infliximab and anakinra is not recommended).
Products include:
Kineret 877

Azathioprine (Rare post-marketing cases of hepatosplenic T-cell lymphoma have been reported in adolescent and young adult patients with Crohns's disease treated with infliximab; all of these hepatosplenic T-cell lymphomas with infliximab have occurred in patients on concomitant treatment with azathioprine).
No products indexed under this heading.

Azathioprine Sodium (Rare post-marketing cases of hepatosplenic T-cell lymphoma have been reported in adolescent and young adult patients with Crohns's disease treated with infliximab; all of these hepatosplenic T-cell lymphomas with infliximab have occurred in patients on concomitant treatment with azathioprine).
No products indexed under this heading.

BCG Vaccine (No data vailable on the response to vaccination with live vaccines or on the secondary transmission of infection by live vaccines in patients receiving anti-TNF therapy. It is recommended that live vaccines not be given concomitantly with infliximab. All pediatric Crohn's disease patients should be brought up to date with all vaccinations prior to initiating infliximab therapy).
No products indexed under this heading.

Influenza Vaccine, Live Attenuated (No data vailable on the response to vaccination with live vaccines or on the secondary transmission of infection by live vaccines in patients receiving anti-TNF therapy. It is recommended that live vaccines not be given concomitantly with infliximab. All pediatric Crohn's disease patients should be brought up to date with all vaccinations prior to initiating infliximab therapy).
No products indexed under this heading.

Influenza Virus Vaccine Live, Intranasal (No data vailable on the response to vaccination with live vaccines or on the secondary transmission of infection by live vaccines in patients receiving anti-TNF therapy. It is recommended that live vaccines not be given concomitantly with infliximab. All pediatric Crohn's disease patients should be brought up to date with all vaccinations prior to initiating infliximab therapy).
Products include:
FluMist 2078

Measles, Mumps, Rubella and Varicella Virus Vaccine Live (No data vailable on the response to vaccination with live vaccines or on the secondary transmission of infection by live vaccines in patients receiving anti-TNF therapy. It is recommended that live vaccines not be given concomitantly with infliximab. All pediatric Crohn's disease patients should be brought up to

date with all vaccinations prior to initiating infliximab therapy). Products include:
ProQuad 2254

Measles, Mumps & Rubella Virus Vaccine, Live (No data vailable on the response to vaccination with live vaccines or on the secondary transmission of infection by live vaccines in patients receiving anti-TNF therapy. It is recommended that live vaccines not be given concomitantly with infliximab. All pediatric Crohn's disease patients should be brought up to date with all vaccinations prior to initiating infliximab therapy).
Products include:
M-M-R II 2203
ProQuad 2254

Measles & Rubella Virus Vaccine Live (No data vailable on the response to vaccination with live vaccines or on the secondary transmission of infection by live vaccines in patients receiving anti-TNF therapy. It is recommended that live vaccines not be given concomitantly with infliximab. All pediatric Crohn's disease patients should be brought up to date with all vaccinations prior to initiating infliximab therapy).
No products indexed under this heading.

Measles Virus Vaccine Live (No data vailable on the response to vaccination with live vaccines or on the secondary transmission of infection by live vaccines in patients receiving anti-TNF therapy. It is recommended that live vaccines not be given concomitantly with infliximab. All pediatric Crohn's disease patients should be brought up to date with all vaccinations prior to initiating infliximab therapy). Products include:
Attenuvax 2086

Mercaptopurine (Rare post-marketing cases of hepatosplenic T-cell lymphoma have been reported in adolescent and young adult patients with Crohns's disease treated with infliximab; all of these hepatosplenic T-cell lymphomas with infliximab have occurred in patients on concomitant treatment with 6-mercaptopurine).
No products indexed under this heading.

Mumps Virus Vaccine, Live (No data vailable on the response to vaccination with live vaccines or on the secondary transmission of infection by live vaccines in patients receiving anti-TNF therapy. It is recommended that live vaccines not be given concomitantly with infliximab. All pediatric Crohn's disease patients should be brought up to date with all vaccinations prior to initiating infliximab therapy). Products include:
Mumpsvax 2218

Poliovirus Vaccine, Live, Oral, Trivalent, Types 1,2,3 (Sabin) (No data vailable on the response to vaccination with live vaccines or on the secondary transmission of infection by live vaccines in patients receiving anti-TNF therapy. It is recommended that live vaccines not be given concomitantly with infliximab. All pediatric Crohn's disease patients should be brought up to date with all vaccinations prior to initiating infliximab therapy).
No products indexed under this heading.

Rotavirus Vaccine, Live, Oral, Tetravalent (No data vailable on the response to vaccination with live vaccines or on the secondary transmission of infection by live vaccines in patients receiving anti-TNF therapy. It is recommended that live vaccines not be given concomitantly with infliximab. All pediatric Crohn's disease patients should be brought up to date with all vaccinations prior to initiating infliximab therapy).
No products indexed under this heading.

Rubella & Mumps Virus Vaccine Live (No data vailable on the response to vaccination with live vaccines or on the secondary transmission of infection by live vaccines in patients receiving anti-TNF therapy. It is recommended that live vaccines not be given concomitantly with infliximab. All pediatric Crohn's disease patients should be brought up to date with all vaccinations prior to initiating infliximab therapy).
No products indexed under this heading.

Rubella Virus Vaccine Live (No data vailable on the response to vaccination with live vaccines or on the secondary transmission of infection by live vaccines in patients receiving anti-TNF therapy. It is recommended that live vaccines not be given concomitantly with infliximab. All pediatric Crohn's disease patients should be brought up to date with all vaccinations prior to initiating infliximab therapy). Products include:
Meruvax II 2210

Smallpox Vaccine (No data vailable on the response to vaccination with live vaccines or on the secondary transmission of infection by live vaccines in patients receiving anti-TNF therapy. It is recommended that live vaccines not be given concomitantly with infliximab. All pediatric Crohn's disease patients should be brought up to date with all vaccinations prior to initiating infliximab therapy).
No products indexed under this heading.

Typhoid Vaccine (No data vailable on the response to vaccination with live vaccines or on the secondary transmission of infection by live vaccines in patients receiving anti-TNF therapy. It is recommended that live vaccines not be given concomitantly with infliximab. All pediatric Crohn's disease patients should be brought up to date with all vaccinations prior to initiating infliximab therapy).
No products indexed under this heading.

Varicella Virus Vaccine, Live (No data vailable on the response to vaccination with live vaccines or on the secondary transmission of infection by live vaccines in patients receiving anti-TNF therapy. It is recommended that live vaccines not be given concomitantly with infliximab. All pediatric Crohn's disease patients should be brought up to date with all vaccinations prior to initiating infliximab therapy). Products include:
Varivax 2285

Yellow Fever Vaccine (No data vailable on the response to vaccination with live vaccines or on the secondary transmission of infection by live vaccines in patients receiving anti-TNF therapy. It is recommended that live vaccines not be given concomitantly with infliximab. All pediatric Crohn's disease patients should be brought up to date with all vaccinations prior to initiating infliximab therapy).
No products indexed under this heading.

Zoster Vaccine Live (No data vailable on the response to vaccination with live vaccines or on the secondary transmission of infection by live vaccines in patients receiving anti-TNF therapy. It is recommended that live vaccines not be given concomitantly with infliximab. All pediatric Crohn's disease patients should be brought up to date with all vaccinations prior to initiating infliximab therapy). Products include:
Zostavax 2299

REOPRO VIALS
(Abciximab) 1952
May interact with anticoagulants, non-steroidal anti-inflammatory agents, oral anticoagulants, thrombolytics, and certain other agents. Compounds in these categories include:

Alteplase (Co-administration with thrombolytics may be associated with an increase in bleeding). Products include:
Activase 1183
Cathflo 1192

Anisindione (Co-administration of oral anticoagulants within seven days is contraindicated unless prothrombin time is less than or equal to 1.2 times control; concurrent use with other anticoagulant agents may be associated with an increase in bleeding).
No products indexed under this heading.

Anistreplase (Co-administration with thrombolytics may be associated with an increase in bleeding).
No products indexed under this heading.

Ardeparin Sodium (Co-administration with other anticoagulant agents may be associated with an increase in bleeding).
No products indexed under this heading.

Aspirin (Co-administration with antiplatelet agents, such as aspirin, may be associated with an increase in bleeding). Products include:
Aggrenox 880
Bayer Aspirin 829
Percodan 1124
St. Joseph Aspirin 2045

Bivalirudin (Co-administration with thrombolytics may be associated with an increase in bleeding). Products include:
Angiomax for Injection 2061

Celecoxib (Co-administration with antiplatelet agents, such as non-steroidal anti-inflammatory agents, may be associated with an increase in bleeding). Products include:
Celebrex 3272

Clopidogrel Bisulfate (Co-administration with antiplatelet agents, such as clopidogrel, may be associated with an increase in bleeding). Products include:
Plavix 3027

Dalteparin Sodium (Co-administration with other anticoagulant agents may be associated with an increase in bleeding). Products include:
Fragmin 1058

Danaparoid Sodium (Co-administration with other anticoagulant agents may be associated with an increase in bleeding).
No products indexed under this heading.

Dextran (Co-administration with intravenous dextran before percutaneous coronary intervention, or intent to use it during an intervention is contraindicated).
No products indexed under this heading.

Diclofenac Epolamine (Co-administration with antiplatelet agents, such as non-steroidal anti-inflammatory agents, may be associated with an increase in bleeding). Products include:
Flector 1839

Diclofenac Potassium (Co-administration with antiplatelet agents, such as non-steroidal anti-inflammatory agents, may be associated with an increase in bleeding).
No products indexed under this heading.

Diclofenac Sodium (Co-administration with antiplatelet agents, such as non-steroidal anti-inflammatory agents, may be associated with an increase in bleeding).
No products indexed under this heading.

Dicumarol (Co-administration of oral anticoagulants within seven days is contraindicated unless prothrombin time is less than or equal to 1.2 times control; concurrent use with other anticoagulant agents may be associated with an increase in bleeding).
No products indexed under this heading.

1591 **Interactions Index** **Requip**

Dipyridamole (Co-administration with antiplatelet agents, such as dipyridamole, may be associated with an increase in bleeding). Products include:
Aggrenox 880

Enoxaparin Sodium (Co-administration with other anticoagulant agents may be associated with an increase in bleeding). Products include:
Lovenox 3005

Etodolac (Co-administration with antiplatelet agents, such as non-steroidal anti-inflammatory agents, may be associated with an increase in bleeding).
No products indexed under this heading.

Fenoprofen Calcium (Co-administration with antiplatelet agents, such as non-steroidal anti-inflammatory agents, may be associated with an increase in bleeding).
No products indexed under this heading.

Flurbiprofen (Co-administration with antiplatelet agents, such as non-steroidal anti-inflammatory agents, may be associated with an increase in bleeding).
No products indexed under this heading.

Fondaparinux Sodium (Co-administration with other anticoagulant agents may be associated with an increase in bleeding). Products include:
Arixtra 1320

Heparin Calcium (Co-administration with other anticoagulant agents may be associated with an increase in bleeding).
No products indexed under this heading.

Heparin Sodium (Co-administration with other anticoagulant agents may be associated with an increase in bleeding).
No products indexed under this heading.

Ibuprofen (Co-administration with antiplatelet agents, such as non-steroidal anti-inflammatory agents, may be associated with an increase in bleeding). Products include:
Motrin IB 2043
Children's Motrin 2044
Children's Motrin Non-Staining Dye-Free 2044
Infants' Motrin 2044
Infants' Motrin Dye-Free 2044
Junior Strength Motrin 2044
Vicoprofen 564

Indomethacin (Co-administration with antiplatelet agents, such as non-steroidal anti-inflammatory agents, may be associated with an increase in bleeding). Products include:
Indocin 2167

Indomethacin Sodium Trihydrate (Co-administration with antiplatelet agents, such as non-steroidal anti-inflammatory agents, may be associated with an increase in bleeding). Products include:
Indocin I.V. 2007

Ketoprofen (Co-administration with antiplatelet agents, such as non-steroidal anti-inflammatory agents, may be associated with an increase in bleeding).
No products indexed under this heading.

Ketorolac Tromethamine (Co-administration with antiplatelet agents, such as non-steroidal anti-inflammatory agents, may be associated with an increase in bleeding). Products include:
Acuvail .... ⊙209

Low Molecular Weight Heparins (Co-administration with other anticoagulant agents may be associated with an increase in bleeding).
No products indexed under this heading.

Meclofenamate Sodium (Co-administration with antiplatelet agents, such as non-steroidal anti-inflammatory agents, may be associated with an increase in bleeding).
No products indexed under this heading.

Mefenamic Acid (Co-administration with antiplatelet agents, such as non-steroidal anti-inflammatory agents, may be associated with an increase in bleeding).
No products indexed under this heading.

Meloxicam (Co-administration with antiplatelet agents, such as non-steroidal anti-inflammatory agents, may be associated with an increase in bleeding).
No products indexed under this heading.

Nabumetone (Co-administration with antiplatelet agents, such as non-steroidal anti-inflammatory agents, may be associated with an increase in bleeding).
No products indexed under this heading.

Naproxen (Co-administration with antiplatelet agents, such as non-steroidal anti-inflammatory agents, may be associated with an increase in bleeding). Products include:
EC-Naprosyn 2850
Naprosyn 2850
Anaprox/Naprosyn 2850

Naproxen Sodium (Co-administration with antiplatelet agents, such as non-steroidal anti-inflammatory agents, may be associated with an increase in bleeding). Products include:
Anaprox 2850
Anaprox DS 2850
Treximet 1681

Oxaprozin (Co-administration with antiplatelet agents, such as non-steroidal anti-inflammatory agents, may be associated with an increase in bleeding).
No products indexed under this heading.

Phenylbutazone (Co-administration with antiplatelet agents, such as non-steroidal anti-inflammatory agents, may be associated with an increase in bleeding).
No products indexed under this heading.

Piroxicam (Co-administration with antiplatelet agents, such as non-steroidal anti-inflammatory agents, may be associated with an increase in bleeding).
No products indexed under this heading.

Reteplase (Co-administration with thrombolytics may be associated with an increase in bleeding).
No products indexed under this heading.

Rofecoxib (Co-administration with antiplatelet agents, such as non-steroidal anti-inflammatory agents, may be associated with an increase in bleeding).
No products indexed under this heading.

Streptokinase (Co-administration with thrombolytics may be associated with an increase in bleeding).
No products indexed under this heading.

Sulindac (Co-administration with antiplatelet agents, such as non-steroidal anti-inflammatory agents, may be associated with an increase in bleeding). Products include:
Clinoril 2098

Ticlopidine Hydrochloride (Co-administration with antiplatelet agents, such as ticlopidine, may be associated with an increase in bleeding).
No products indexed under this heading.

Tinzaparin Sodium (Co-administration with other anticoagulant agents may be associated with an increase in bleeding).
No products indexed under this heading.

Tolmetin Sodium (Co-administration with antiplatelet agents, such as non-steroidal anti-inflammatory agents, may be associated with an increase in bleeding).
No products indexed under this heading.

Urokinase (Co-administration with thrombolytics may be associated with an increase in bleeding).
No products indexed under this heading.

Valdecoxib (Co-administration with antiplatelet agents, such as non-steroidal anti-inflammatory agents, may be associated with an increase in bleeding).
No products indexed under this heading.

Warfarin Sodium (Co-administration of oral anticoagulants within seven days is contraindicated unless prothrombin time is less than or equal to 1.2 times control; concurrent use with other anticoagulant agents may be associated with an increase in bleeding).
No products indexed under this heading.

REQUIP TABLETS

(Ropinirole Hydrochloride) 1620
May interact with alcohols, antidepressant drugs, antipsychotic agents, benzodiazepines, butyrophenones, central nervous system depressants, cytochrome p450 1a2 inducers (selected), cytochrome p450 1a2 inhibitors (selected), cytochrome p450 1a2 substrates (selected), dopamine antagonists, estrogens, highly metabolized sedatives and hypnotics, hypnotics and sedatives, phenothiazines, sedating antihistamines, and certain other agents. Compounds in these categories include:

Acetaminophen (*In vitro* metabolism studies showed that CYP1A2 is the major enzyme responsible for the metabolism of ropinirole. There is thus the potential for inducers or inhibitors of this enzyme to alter the clearance of ropinirole. Therefore, if therapy with a drug known to be a potent inducer or inhibitor of CYP1A2 is stopped or started during treatment with ropinirole, adjustment of the dose of ropinirole may be required). Products include:
Percocet 1121
Tylenol 2049
Tylenol 8 Hour 2049
Extra Strength Tylenol Caplets, Cool Caplets, and EZ Tabs 2049
Extra Strength Tylenol Adult Rapid Blast Liquid 2049
Extra Strength Tylenol Rapid Release 2049
Tylenol with Codeine 2691
Tylenol Arthritis Pain Extended Release Geltabs/Caplets 2049
Children's Tylenol Suspension Liquid 2048
Children's Tylenol Meltaways 2048
Tylenol, Infants' Drops 2048
Junior Tylenol 2048
Vicodin 560
Vicodin ES 561
Vicodin HP 563
Zydone 1138

Acrivastine (Before initiating treatment patients should be advised of the potential to develop drowsiness and specifically asked about factors that may increase the risk such as concomitant sedating medications. If a patient develops significant daytime sleepiness or episodes of falling asleep during activities that require active participation (eg, conversations, eating, etc.), therapy should ordinarily be discontinued. If a decision is made to continue, patients should be advised to not drive and to avoid other potentially dangerous activities).
No products indexed under this heading.

Alatrofloxacin Mesylate (*In vitro* metabolism studies showed that CYP1A2 is the major enzyme responsible for the metabolism of ropinirole. There is thus the potential for inducers or inhibitors of this enzyme to alter the clearance of ropinirole. Therefore, if therapy with a drug known to be a potent inducer or inhibitor of CYP1A2 is stopped or started during treatment with ropinirole, adjustment of the dose of ropinirole may be required).
No products indexed under this heading.

Alfentanil Hydrochloride (Sedating medications (such as alcohol or CNS depressants), may increase the risk of somnolence or falling asleep while engaged in activities of daily living. Because of possible additive effects, caution should be advised when patients are taking other sedating medications, alcohol, or other CNS depressants (eg, benzodiazepines, antipsychotics, antidepressants) in combination with ropinirole).
No products indexed under this heading.

Alprazolam (Sedating medications (such as alcohol or CNS depressants), may increase the risk of somnolence or falling asleep while engaged in activities of daily living. Because of possible additive effects, caution should be advised when patients are taking other sedating medications, alcohol, or other CNS depressants (eg, benzodiazepines, antipsychotics, antidepressants) in combination with ropinirole).
No products indexed under this heading.

Aminophylline (*In vitro* metabolism studies showed that CYP1A2 is the major enzyme responsible for the metabolism of ropinirole. There is thus the potential for inducers or inhibitors of this enzyme to alter the clearance of ropinirole. Therefore, if therapy with a drug known to be a potent inducer or inhibitor of CYP1A2 is stopped or started during treatment with ropinirole, adjustment of the dose of ropinirole may be required).
No products indexed under this heading.

Amiodarone Hydrochloride (*In vitro* metabolism studies showed that CYP1A2 is the major enzyme responsible for the metabolism of ropinirole. There is thus the potential for inducers or inhibitors of this enzyme to alter the clearance of ropinirole. Therefore, if therapy with a drug known to be a potent inducer or inhibitor of CYP1A2 is stopped or started during treatment with ropinirole, adjustment of the dose of ropinirole may be required).
No products indexed under this heading.

Amitriptyline Hydrochloride (Because of possible additive effects, caution should be advised when patients are taking other sedating medications, alcohol, or other CNS depressants (eg, benzodiazepines, antipsychotics, antidepressants) in combination with ropinirole).
No products indexed under this heading.

Amobarbital (Sedating medications (such as alcohol or CNS depressants), may increase the risk of somnolence or falling asleep while engaged in activities of daily living. Because of possible additive effects, caution should be advised when patients are taking other sedating medications, alcohol, or other CNS depressants (eg, benzodiazepines, antipsychotics, antidepressants) in combination with ropinirole).
No products indexed under this heading.

Amobarbital Sodium (Sedating medications (such as alcohol or CNS depressants), may increase the risk of somnolence or falling asleep while engaged in activities of daily living. Because of possible additive effects, caution should be advised when patients are taking other sedating medications, alcohol, or other CNS depressants (eg, benzodiazepines, antipsychotics, antidepressants) in combination with ropinirole).
No products indexed under this heading.

IMPORTANT NOTE: Always consult each drug listing in the patient's regimen for possible interactions.

Amoxapine (Because of possible additive effects, caution should be advised when patients are taking other sedating medications, alcohol, or other CNS depressants (eg, benzodiazepines, antipsychotics, antidepressants) in combination with ropinirole).
No products indexed under this heading.

Anagrelide Hydrochloride (In vitro metabolism studies showed that CYP1A2 is the major enzyme responsible for the metabolism of ropinirole. There is thus the potential for inducers or inhibitors of this enzyme to alter the clearance of ropinirole. Therefore, if therapy with a drug known to be a potent inducer or inhibitor of CYP1A2 is stopped or started during treatment with ropinirole, adjustment of the dose of ropinirole may be required).
No products indexed under this heading.

Anastrozole (In vitro metabolism studies showed that CYP1A2 is the major enzyme responsible for the metabolism of ropinirole. There is thus the potential for inducers or inhibitors of this enzyme to alter the clearance of ropinirole. Therefore, if therapy with a drug known to be a potent inducer or inhibitor of CYP1A2 is stopped or started during treatment with ropinirole, adjustment of the dose of ropinirole may be required).
No products indexed under this heading.

Aprobarbital (Sedating medications (such as alcohol or CNS depressants), may increase the risk of somnolence or falling asleep while engaged in activities of daily living. Because of possible additive effects, caution should be advised when patients are taking other sedating medications, alcohol, or other CNS depressants (eg, benzodiazepines, antipsychotics, antidepressants) in combination with ropinirole).
No products indexed under this heading.

Aripiprazole (Because of possible additive effects, caution should be advised when patients are taking other sedating medications, alcohol, or other CNS depressants (eg, antipsychotics) in combination with ropinirole).
No products indexed under this heading.

Azatadine Maleate (Before initiating treatment patients should be advised of the potential to develop drowsiness and specifically asked about factors that may increase the risk such as concomitant sedating medications. If a patient develops significant daytime sleepiness or episodes of falling asleep during activities that require active participation (eg, conversations, eating, etc.), therapy should ordinarily be discontinued. If a decision is made to continue, patients should be advised to not drive and to avoid other potentially dangerous activities).
No products indexed under this heading.

Bromodiphenhydramine Hydrochloride (Before initiating treatment patients should be advised of the potential to develop drowsiness and specifically asked about factors that may increase the risk such as concomitant sedating medications. If a patient develops significant daytime sleepiness or episodes of falling asleep during activities that require active participation (eg, conversations, eating, etc.), therapy should ordinarily be discontinued. If a decision is made to continue, patients should be advised to not drive and to avoid other potentially dangerous activities).
No products indexed under this heading.

Brompheniramine Maleate (Before initiating treatment patients should be advised of the potential to develop drowsiness and specifically asked about factors that may increase the risk such as concomitant sedating medications. If a patient develops significant daytime

sleepiness or episodes of falling asleep during activities that require active participation (eg, conversations, eating, etc.), therapy should ordinarily be discontinued. If a decision is made to continue, patients should be advised to not drive and to avoid other potentially dangerous activities).
No products indexed under this heading.

Buprenorphine Hydrochloride (Sedating medications (such as alcohol or CNS depressants), may increase the risk of somnolence or falling asleep while engaged in activities of daily living. Because of possible additive effects, caution should be advised when patients are taking other sedating medications, alcohol, or other CNS depressants (eg, benzodiazepines, antipsychotics, antidepressants) in combination with ropinirole).
No products indexed under this heading.

Bupropion Hydrochloride (Because of possible additive effects, caution should be advised when patients are taking other sedating medications, alcohol, or other CNS depressants (eg, benzodiazepines, antipsychotics, antidepressants) in combination with ropinirole). Products include:
Aplenzin **2948**
Wellbutrin **1719**
Wellbutrin SR **1725**
Zyban **1762**

Buspirone Hydrochloride (Sedating medications (such as alcohol or CNS depressants), may increase the risk of somnolence or falling asleep while engaged in activities of daily living. Because of possible additive effects, caution should be advised when patients are taking other sedating medications, alcohol, or other CNS depressants (eg, benzodiazepines, antipsychotics, antidepressants) in combination with ropinirole).
No products indexed under this heading.

Butabarbital (Sedating medications (such as alcohol or CNS depressants), may increase the risk of somnolence or falling asleep while engaged in activities of daily living. Because of possible additive effects, caution should be advised when patients are taking other sedating medications, alcohol, or other CNS depressants (eg, benzodiazepines, antipsychotics, antidepressants) in combination with ropinirole).
No products indexed under this heading.

Butabarbital Sodium (Sedating medications (such as alcohol or CNS depressants), may increase the risk of somnolence or falling asleep while engaged in activities of daily living. Because of possible additive effects, caution should be advised when patients are taking other sedating medications, alcohol, or other CNS depressants (eg, benzodiazepines, antipsychotics, antidepressants) in combination with ropinirole).
No products indexed under this heading.

Butalbital (Sedating medications (such as alcohol or CNS depressants), may increase the risk of somnolence or falling asleep while engaged in activities of daily living. Because of possible additive effects, caution should be advised when patients are taking other sedating medications, alcohol, or other CNS depressants (eg, benzodiazepines, antipsychotics, antidepressants) in combination with ropinirole).
No products indexed under this heading.

Caffeine (In vitro metabolism studies showed that CYP1A2 is the major enzyme responsible for the metabolism of ropinirole. There is thus the potential for inducers or inhibitors of this enzyme to alter the clearance of ropinirole. Therefore, if therapy with a drug known to be a potent inducer or inhibitor of CYP1A2 is stopped or started during

treatment with ropinirole, adjustment of the dose of ropinirole may be required).
No products indexed under this heading.

Caffeine Anhydrous (In vitro metabolism studies showed that CYP1A2 is the major enzyme responsible for the metabolism of ropinirole. There is thus the potential for inducers or inhibitors of this enzyme to alter the clearance of ropinirole. Therefore, if therapy with a drug known to be a potent inducer or inhibitor of CYP1A2 is stopped or started during treatment with ropinirole, adjustment of the dose of ropinirole may be required).
No products indexed under this heading.

Caffeine Citrate (In vitro metabolism studies showed that CYP1A2 is the major enzyme responsible for the metabolism of ropinirole. There is thus the potential for inducers or inhibitors of this enzyme to alter the clearance of ropinirole. Therefore, if therapy with a drug known to be a potent inducer or inhibitor of CYP1A2 is stopped or started during treatment with ropinirole, adjustment of the dose of ropinirole may be required).
No products indexed under this heading.

Caffeine-containing medications (In vitro metabolism studies showed that CYP1A2 is the major enzyme responsible for the metabolism of ropinirole. There is thus the potential for inducers or inhibitors of this enzyme to alter the clearance of ropinirole. Therefore, if therapy with a drug known to be a potent inducer or inhibitor of CYP1A2 is stopped or started during treatment with ropinirole, adjustment of the dose of ropinirole may be required).
No products indexed under this heading.

Caffeine Sodium Benzoate (In vitro metabolism studies showed that CYP1A2 is the major enzyme responsible for the metabolism of ropinirole. There is thus the potential for inducers or inhibitors of this enzyme to alter the clearance of ropinirole. Therefore, if therapy with a drug known to be a potent inducer or inhibitor of CYP1A2 is stopped or started during treatment with ropinirole, adjustment of the dose of ropinirole may be required).
No products indexed under this heading.

Carbamazepine (In vitro metabolism studies showed that CYP1A2 is the major enzyme responsible for the metabolism of ropinirole. There is thus the potential for inducers or inhibitors of this enzyme to alter the clearance of ropinirole. Therefore, if therapy with a drug known to be a potent inducer or inhibitor of CYP1A2 is stopped or started during treatment with ropinirole, adjustment of the dose of ropinirole may be required). Products include:
Carbatrol **3280**
Equetro **3477**

Chloral Hydrate (Before initiating treatment patients should be advised of the potential to develop drowsiness and specifically asked about factors that may increase the risk such as concomitant sedating medications. If a patient develops significant daytime sleepiness or episodes of falling asleep during activities that require active participation (eg, conversations, eating, etc.), therapy should ordinarily be discontinued. If a decision is made to continue, patients should be advised to not drive and to avoid other potentially dangerous activities).
No products indexed under this heading.

Chlordiazepoxide (Sedating medications (such as alcohol or CNS depressants), may increase the risk of somnolence or falling asleep while engaged in activities of daily living. Because of possible additive effects, caution should be advised when patients are taking other

sedating medications, alcohol, or other CNS depressants (eg, benzodiazepines, antipsychotics, antidepressants) in combination with ropinirole).
No products indexed under this heading.

Chlordiazepoxide Hydrochloride (Sedating medications (such as alcohol or CNS depressants), may increase the risk of somnolence or falling asleep while engaged in activities of daily living. Because of possible additive effects, caution should be advised when patients are taking other sedating medications, alcohol, or other CNS depressants (eg, benzodiazepines, antipsychotics, antidepressants) in combination with ropinirole).
No products indexed under this heading.

Chlorotrianisene (Population pharmacokinetic analysis revealed that estrogens (mainly ethinylestradiol: intake 0.6 to 3 mg over 4-month to 23-year period) reduced the oral clearance of ropinirole by 36% in 16 patients. Dosage adjustment is not needed for initiating ropinirole in patients on estrogen therapy because patients are individually titrated with ropinirole to tolerance or adequate effect. If estrogen therapy is stopped or started during treatment with ropinirole, then adjustment of the dose of ropinirole may be required).
No products indexed under this heading.

Chlorpheniramine Maleate (Before initiating treatment patients should be advised of the potential to develop drowsiness and specifically asked about factors that may increase the risk such as concomitant sedating medications. If a patient develops significant daytime sleepiness or episodes of falling asleep during activities that require active participation (eg, conversations, eating, etc.), therapy should ordinarily be discontinued. If a decision is made to continue, patients should be advised to not drive and to avoid other potentially dangerous activities).
No products indexed under this heading.

Chlorpheniramine Polistirex (Before initiating treatment patients should be advised of the potential to develop drowsiness and specifically asked about factors that may increase the risk such as concomitant sedating medications. If a patient develops significant daytime sleepiness or episodes of falling asleep during activities that require active participation (eg, conversations, eating, etc.), therapy should ordinarily be discontinued. If a decision is made to continue, patients should be advised to not drive and to avoid other potentially dangerous activities). Products include:
Tussionex **3443**

Chlorpheniramine Tannate (Before initiating treatment patients should be advised of the potential to develop drowsiness and specifically asked about factors that may increase the risk such as concomitant sedating medications. If a patient develops significant daytime sleepiness or episodes of falling asleep during activities that require active participation (eg, conversations, eating, etc.), therapy should ordinarily be discontinued. If a decision is made to continue, patients should be advised to not drive and to avoid other potentially dangerous activities).
No products indexed under this heading.

Chlorpromazine (Sedating medications (such as alcohol or CNS depressants), may increase the risk of somnolence or falling asleep while engaged in activities of daily living. Because of possible additive effects, caution should be advised when patients are taking other sedating medications, alcohol, or other

1593 **Interactions Index** **Requip**

CNS depressants (eg, benzodiazepines, antipsychotics, antidepressants) in combination with ropinirole).
No products indexed under this heading.

Chlorpromazine Hydrochloride (Sedating medications (such as alcohol or CNS depressants), may increase the risk of somnolence or falling asleep while engaged in activities of daily living. Because of possible additive effects, caution should be advised when patients are taking other sedating medications, alcohol, or other CNS depressants (eg, benzodiazepines, antipsychotics, antidepressants) in combination with ropinirole).
No products indexed under this heading.

Chlorprothixene (Sedating medications (such as alcohol or CNS depressants), may increase the risk of somnolence or falling asleep while engaged in activities of daily living. Because of possible additive effects, caution should be advised when patients are taking other sedating medications, alcohol, or other CNS depressants (eg, benzodiazepines, antipsychotics, antidepressants) in combination with ropinirole).
No products indexed under this heading.

Chlorprothixene Hydrochloride (Sedating medications (such as alcohol or CNS depressants), may increase the risk of somnolence or falling asleep while engaged in activities of daily living. Because of possible additive effects, caution should be advised when patients are taking other sedating medications, alcohol, or other CNS depressants (eg, benzodiazepines, antipsychotics, antidepressants) in combination with ropinirole).
No products indexed under this heading.

Chlorprothixene Lactate (Sedating medications (such as alcohol or CNS depressants), may increase the risk of somnolence or falling asleep while engaged in activities of daily living. Because of possible additive effects, caution should be advised when patients are taking other sedating medications, alcohol, or other CNS depressants (eg, benzodiazepines, antipsychotics, antidepressants) in combination with ropinirole).
No products indexed under this heading.

Cimetidine (*In vitro* metabolism studies showed that CYP1A2 is the major enzyme responsible for the metabolism of ropinirole. There is thus the potential for inducers or inhibitors of this enzyme to alter the clearance of ropinirole. Therefore, if therapy with a drug known to be a potent inducer or inhibitor of CYP1A2 is stopped or started during treatment with ropinirole, adjustment of the dose of ropinirole may be required).
No products indexed under this heading.

Cimetidine Hydrochloride (*In vitro* metabolism studies showed that CYP1A2 is the major enzyme responsible for the metabolism of ropinirole. There is thus the potential for inducers or inhibitors of this enzyme to alter the clearance of ropinirole. Therefore, if therapy with a drug known to be a potent inducer or inhibitor of CYP1A2 is stopped or started during treatment with ropinirole, adjustment of the dose of ropinirole may be required).
No products indexed under this heading.

Ciprofloxacin (*In vitro* metabolism studies showed that CYP1A2 is the major enzyme responsible for the metabolism of ropinirole. There is thus the potential for inducers or inhibitors of this enzyme to alter the clearance of ropinirole. Therefore, if therapy with a drug known to be a potent inducer or inhibitor of CYP1A2 is stopped or started during treatment with ropinirole, adjustment of the dose of ropinirole may be required. Co-administration of ciprofloxacin (500 mg bid), an inhibitor of CYP1A2, with immediate-release ropinirole increased the AUC of ropinirole by 84% on average and C_{max} by 60%). Products include:
Cipro I.V. **3082**
Cipro **3073**
Cipro XR **3091**
Ciprodex **583**

Ciprofloxacin Hydrochloride (*In vitro* metabolism studies showed that CYP1A2 is the major enzyme responsible for the metabolism of ropinirole. There is thus the potential for inducers or inhibitors of this enzyme to alter the clearance of ropinirole. Therefore, if therapy with a drug known to be a potent inducer or inhibitor of CYP1A2 is stopped or started during treatment with ropinirole, adjustment of the dose of ropinirole may be required. Co-administration of ciprofloxacin (500 mg bid), an inhibitor of CYP1A2, with immediate-release ropinirole increased the AUC of ropinirole by 84% on average and C_{max} by 60%). Products include:
Cipro **3073**

Citalopram Hydrobromide (Because of possible additive effects, caution should be advised when patients are taking other sedating medications, alcohol, or other CNS depressants (eg, benzodiazepines, antipsychotics, antidepressants) in combination with ropinirole). Products include:
Celexa **1153**

Clarithromycin (*In vitro* metabolism studies showed that CYP1A2 is the major enzyme responsible for the metabolism of ropinirole. There is thus the potential for inducers or inhibitors of this enzyme to alter the clearance of ropinirole. Therefore, if therapy with a drug known to be a potent inducer or inhibitor of CYP1A2 is stopped or started during treatment with ropinirole, adjustment of the dose of ropinirole may be required). Products include:
Biaxin/Biaxin XL **412**

Clemastine Fumarate (Before initiating treatment patients should be advised of the potential to develop drowsiness and specifically asked about factors that may increase the risk such as concomitant sedating medications. If a patient develops significant daytime sleepiness or episodes of falling asleep during activities that require active participation (eg, conversations, eating, etc.), therapy should ordinarily be discontinued. If a decision is made to continue, patients should be advised to not drive and to avoid other potentially dangerous activities).
No products indexed under this heading.

Clomipramine Hydrochloride (*In vitro* metabolism studies showed that CYP1A2 is the major enzyme responsible for the metabolism of ropinirole. There is thus the potential for inducers or inhibitors of this enzyme to alter the clearance of ropinirole. Therefore, if therapy with a drug known to be a potent inducer or inhibitor of CYP1A2 is stopped or started during treatment with ropinirole, adjustment of the dose of ropinirole may be required).
No products indexed under this heading.

Clonazepam (Sedating medications (such as alcohol or CNS depressants), may increase the risk of somnolence or falling asleep while engaged in activities of daily living. Because of possible additive effects, caution should be advised when patients are taking other sedating medications, alcohol, or other CNS depressants (eg, benzodiazepines, antipsychotics, antidepressants) in combination with ropinirole). Products include:
Klonopin **2855**

Clopidogrel Bisulfate (*In vitro* metabolism studies showed that CYP1A2 is the major enzyme responsible for the metabolism of ropinirole. There is thus the potential for inducers or inhibitors of this enzyme to alter the clearance of ropinirole. Therefore, if therapy with a drug known to be a potent inducer or inhibitor of CYP1A2 is stopped or started during treatment with ropinirole, adjustment of the dose of ropinirole may be required). Products include:
Plavix **3027**

Clorazepate Dipotassium (Sedating medications (such as alcohol or CNS depressants), may increase the risk of somnolence or falling asleep while engaged in activities of daily living. Because of possible additive effects, caution should be advised when patients are taking other sedating medications, alcohol, or other CNS depressants (eg, benzodiazepines, antipsychotics, antidepressants) in combination with ropinirole).
No products indexed under this heading.

Clozapine (Sedating medications (such as alcohol or CNS depressants), may increase the risk of somnolence or falling asleep while engaged in activities of daily living. Because of possible additive effects, caution should be advised when patients are taking other sedating medications, alcohol, or other CNS depressants (eg, benzodiazepines, antipsychotics, antidepressants) in combination with ropinirole).
No products indexed under this heading.

Codeine Phosphate (Sedating medications (such as alcohol or CNS depressants), may increase the risk of somnolence or falling asleep while engaged in activities of daily living. Because of possible additive effects, caution should be advised when patients are taking other sedating medications, alcohol, or other CNS depressants (eg, benzodiazepines, antipsychotics, antidepressants) in combination with ropinirole). Products include:
Tylenol with Codeine **2691**

Codeine Sulfate (Sedating medications (such as alcohol or CNS depressants), may increase the risk of somnolence or falling asleep while engaged in activities of daily living. Because of possible additive effects, caution should be advised when patients are taking other sedating medications, alcohol, or other CNS depressants (eg, benzodiazepines, antipsychotics, antidepressants) in combination with ropinirole).
No products indexed under this heading.

Cyclobenzaprine (*In vitro* metabolism studies showed that CYP1A2 is the major enzyme responsible for the metabolism of ropinirole. There is thus the potential for inducers or inhibitors of this enzyme to alter the clearance of ropinirole. Therefore, if therapy with a drug known to be a potent inducer or inhibitor of CYP1A2 is stopped or started during treatment with ropinirole, adjustment of the dose of ropinirole may be required).
No products indexed under this heading.

Cyclobenzaprine Hydrochloride (*In vitro* metabolism studies showed that CYP1A2 is the major enzyme responsible for the metabolism of ropinirole. There is thus the potential for inducers or inhibitors of this enzyme to alter the clearance of ropinirole. Therefore, if therapy with a drug known to be a potent inducer or inhibitor of CYP1A2 is stopped or started during treatment with ropinirole, adjustment of the dose of ropinirole may be required). Products include:
Amrix **964**

Cyproheptadine Hydrochloride (Before initiating treatment patients should be advised of the potential to develop drowsiness and specifically asked about factors that may increase the risk such as concomitant sedating medications. If a patient develops significant daytime sleepiness or episodes of falling asleep during activities that require active participation (eg, conversations, eating, etc.), therapy should ordinarily be discontinued. If a decision is made to continue, patients should be advised to not drive and to avoid other potentially dangerous activities).
No products indexed under this heading.

Desflurane (Sedating medications (such as alcohol or CNS depressants), may increase the risk of somnolence or falling asleep while engaged in activities of daily living. Because of possible additive effects, caution should be advised when patients are taking other sedating medications, alcohol, or other CNS depressants (eg, benzodiazepines, antipsychotics, antidepressants) in combination with ropinirole).
No products indexed under this heading.

Desipramine Hydrochloride (Because of possible additive effects, caution should be advised when patients are taking other sedating medications, alcohol, or other CNS depressants (eg, benzodiazepines, antipsychotics, antidepressants) in combination with ropinirole).
No products indexed under this heading.

Desogestrel (*In vitro* metabolism studies showed that CYP1A2 is the major enzyme responsible for the metabolism of ropinirole. There is thus the potential for inducers or inhibitors of this enzyme to alter the clearance of ropinirole. Therefore, if therapy with a drug known to be a potent inducer or inhibitor of CYP1A2 is stopped or started during treatment with ropinirole, adjustment of the dose of ropinirole may be required).
No products indexed under this heading.

Dexchlorpheniramine Maleate (Before initiating treatment patients should be advised of the potential to develop drowsiness and specifically asked about factors that may increase the risk such as concomitant sedating medications. If a patient develops significant daytime sleepiness or episodes of falling asleep during activities that require active participation (eg, conversations, eating, etc.), therapy should ordinarily be discontinued. If a decision is made to continue, patients should be advised to not drive and to avoid other potentially dangerous activities).
No products indexed under this heading.

Dezocine (Sedating medications (such as alcohol or CNS depressants), may increase the risk of somnolence or falling asleep while engaged in activities of daily living. Because of possible additive effects, caution should be advised when patients are taking other sedating medications, alcohol, or other CNS depressants (eg, benzodiazepines, antipsychotics, antidepressants) in combination with ropinirole).
No products indexed under this heading.

Diazepam (Sedating medications (such as alcohol or CNS depressants), may increase the risk of somnolence or falling asleep while engaged in activities of daily living. Because of possible additive effects, caution should be advised when patients are taking other sedating medications, alcohol, or other CNS depressants (eg, benzodiazepines, antipsychotics, antidepressants) in combination with ropinirole). Products include:
Valium Tablets **2880**

Dienestrol (Population pharmacokinetic analysis revealed that estrogens (mainly ethinylestradiol: intake 0.6 to 3 mg over 4-month to 23-year period) reduced the oral clearance of ropinirole

Requip Interactions Index 1594

by 36% in 16 patients. Dosage adjustment is not needed for initiating ropinirole in patients on estrogen therapy because patients are individually titrated with ropinirole to tolerance or adequate effect. If estrogen therapy is stopped or started during treatment with ropinirole, then adjustment of the dose of ropinirole may be required).

No products indexed under this heading.

Diethylstilbestrol (Population pharmacokinetic analysis revealed that estrogens (mainly ethinylestradiol: intake 0.6 to 3 mg over 4-month to 23-year period) reduced the oral clearance of ropinirole by 36% in 16 patients. Dosage adjustment is not needed for initiating ropinirole in patients on estrogen therapy because patients are individually titrated with ropinirole to tolerance or adequate effect. If estrogen therapy is stopped or started during treatment with ropinirole, then adjustment of the dose of ropinirole may be required).

No products indexed under this heading.

Diltiazem Hydrochloride (*In vitro* metabolism studies showed that CYP1A2 is the major enzyme responsible for the metabolism of ropinirole. There is thus the potential for inducers or inhibitors of this enzyme to alter the clearance of ropinirole. Therefore, if therapy with a drug known to be a potent inducer or inhibitor of CYP1A2 is stopped or started during treatment with ropinirole, adjustment of the dose of ropinirole may be required). Products include:

Cardizem LA 423

Diltiazem Maleate (*In vitro* metabolism studies showed that CYP1A2 is the major enzyme responsible for the metabolism of ropinirole. There is thus the potential for inducers or inhibitors of this enzyme to alter the clearance of ropinirole. Therefore, if therapy with a drug known to be a potent inducer or inhibitor of CYP1A2 is stopped or started during treatment with ropinirole, adjustment of the dose of ropinirole may be required).

No products indexed under this heading.

Diphenhydramine Hydrochloride (Before initiating treatment patients should be advised of the potential to develop drowsiness and specifically asked about factors that may increase the risk such as concomitant sedating medications. If a patient develops significant daytime sleepiness or episodes of falling asleep during activities that require active participation (eg, conversations, eating, etc.), therapy should ordinarily be discontinued. If a decision is made to continue, patients should be advised to not drive and to avoid other potentially dangerous activities). Products include:

Benadryl Allergy Ultratab 2042

Children's Benadryl Allergy Liquid 2042

Diphenylpyraline Hydrochloride (Before initiating treatment patients should be advised of the potential to develop drowsiness and specifically asked about factors that may increase the risk such as concomitant sedating medications. If a patient develops significant daytime sleepiness or episodes of falling asleep during activities that require active participation (eg, conversations, eating, etc.), therapy should ordinarily be discontinued. If a decision is made to continue, patients should be advised to not drive and to avoid other potentially dangerous activities).

No products indexed under this heading.

Doxepin Hydrochloride (Because of possible additive effects, caution should be advised when patients are taking other sedating medications, alcohol, or other CNS depressants (eg, benzodiazepines, antipsychotics, antidepressants) in combination with ropinirole).

No products indexed under this heading.

Droperidol (Sedating medications (such as alcohol or CNS depressants), may increase the risk of somnolence or falling asleep while engaged in activities of daily living. Because of possible additive effects, caution should be advised when patients are taking other sedating medications, alcohol, or other CNS depressants (eg, benzodiazepines, antipsychotics, antidepressants) in combination with ropinirole).

No products indexed under this heading.

Enflurane (Sedating medications (such as alcohol or CNS depressants), may increase the risk of somnolence or falling asleep while engaged in activities of daily living. Because of possible additive effects, caution should be advised when patients are taking other sedating medications, alcohol, or other CNS depressants (eg, benzodiazepines, antipsychotics, antidepressants) in combination with ropinirole).

No products indexed under this heading.

Enoxacin (*In vitro* metabolism studies showed that CYP1A2 is the major enzyme responsible for the metabolism of ropinirole. There is thus the potential for inducers or inhibitors of this enzyme to alter the clearance of ropinirole. Therefore, if therapy with a drug known to be a potent inducer or inhibitor of CYP1A2 is stopped or started during treatment with ropinirole, adjustment of the dose of ropinirole may be required).

No products indexed under this heading.

Erythromycin (*In vitro* metabolism studies showed that CYP1A2 is the major enzyme responsible for the metabolism of ropinirole. There is thus the potential for inducers or inhibitors of this enzyme to alter the clearance of ropinirole. Therefore, if therapy with a drug known to be a potent inducer or inhibitor of CYP1A2 is stopped or started during treatment with ropinirole, adjustment of the dose of ropinirole may be required).

No products indexed under this heading.

Erythromycin, Topical (*In vitro* metabolism studies showed that CYP1A2 is the major enzyme responsible for the metabolism of ropinirole. There is thus the potential for inducers or inhibitors of this enzyme to alter the clearance of ropinirole. Therefore, if therapy with a drug known to be a potent inducer or inhibitor of CYP1A2 is stopped or started during treatment with ropinirole, adjustment of the dose of ropinirole may be required).

No products indexed under this heading.

Erythromycin Estolate (*In vitro* metabolism studies showed that CYP1A2 is the major enzyme responsible for the metabolism of ropinirole. There is thus the potential for inducers or inhibitors of this enzyme to alter the clearance of ropinirole. Therefore, if therapy with a drug known to be a potent inducer or inhibitor of CYP1A2 is stopped or started during treatment with ropinirole, adjustment of the dose of ropinirole may be required).

No products indexed under this heading.

Erythromycin Ethylsuccinate (*In vitro* metabolism studies showed that CYP1A2 is the major enzyme responsible for the metabolism of ropinirole. There is thus the potential for inducers or inhibitors of this enzyme to alter the clearance of ropinirole. Therefore, if therapy with a drug known to be a potent inducer or inhibitor of CYP1A2 is stopped or started during treatment with ropinirole, adjustment of the dose of ropinirole may be required). Products include:

E.E.S. 437

EryPed 435

Erythromycin Gluceptate (*In vitro* metabolism studies showed that CYP1A2 is the major enzyme responsible for the metabolism of ropinirole. There is thus the potential for inducers or inhibitors of this enzyme to alter the clearance of ropinirole. Therefore, if therapy with a drug known to be a potent inducer or inhibitor of CYP1A2 is stopped or started during treatment with ropinirole, adjustment of the dose of ropinirole may be required).

No products indexed under this heading.

Erythromycin Lactobionate (*In vitro* metabolism studies showed that CYP1A2 is the major enzyme responsible for the metabolism of ropinirole. There is thus the potential for inducers or inhibitors of this enzyme to alter the clearance of ropinirole. Therefore, if therapy with a drug known to be a potent inducer or inhibitor of CYP1A2 is stopped or started during treatment with ropinirole, adjustment of the dose of ropinirole may be required).

No products indexed under this heading.

Erythromycin Stearate (*In vitro* metabolism studies showed that CYP1A2 is the major enzyme responsible for the metabolism of ropinirole. There is thus the potential for inducers or inhibitors of this enzyme to alter the clearance of ropinirole. Therefore, if therapy with a drug known to be a potent inducer or inhibitor of CYP1A2 is stopped or started during treatment with ropinirole, adjustment of the dose of ropinirole may be required).

No products indexed under this heading.

Escitalopram Oxalate (Because of possible additive effects, caution should be advised when patients are taking other sedating medications, alcohol, or other CNS depressants (eg, benzodiazepines, antipsychotics, antidepressants) in combination with ropinirole). Products include:

Lexapro Oral Suspension 1160

Lexapro Tablets 1160

Esomeprazole Magnesium (*In vitro* metabolism studies showed that CYP1A2 is the major enzyme responsible for the metabolism of ropinirole. There is thus the potential for inducers or inhibitors of this enzyme to alter the clearance of ropinirole. Therefore, if therapy with a drug known to be a potent inducer or inhibitor of CYP1A2 is stopped or started during treatment with ropinirole, adjustment of the dose of ropinirole may be required). Products include:

Nexium Capsules 704

Nexium Oral Suspension 704

Esomeprazole Sodium (*In vitro* metabolism studies showed that CYP1A2 is the major enzyme responsible for the metabolism of ropinirole. There is thus the potential for inducers or inhibitors of this enzyme to alter the clearance of ropinirole. Therefore, if therapy with a drug known to be a potent inducer or inhibitor of CYP1A2 is stopped or started during treatment with ropinirole, adjustment of the dose of ropinirole may be required). Products include:

Nexium I.V. 712

Estazolam (Sedating medications (such as alcohol or CNS depressants), may increase the risk of somnolence or falling asleep while engaged in activities of daily living. Because of possible additive effects, caution should be advised when patients are taking other sedating medications, alcohol, or other CNS depressants (eg, benzodiazepines, antipsychotics, antidepressants) in combination with ropinirole).

No products indexed under this heading.

Estradiol (Population pharmacokinetic analysis revealed that estrogens (mainly ethinylestradiol: intake 0.6 to 3 mg over 4-month to 23-year period) reduced the oral clearance of ropinirole by 36% in 16 patients. Dosage adjustment is not needed for initiating ropinirole in patients on estrogen therapy because patients are individually titrated with ropinirole to tolerance or adequate effect. If estrogen therapy is stopped or started during treatment with ropinirole, then adjustment of the dose of ropinirole may be required). Products include:

Activella 2561

Angeliq 831

Climara 841

Climara Pro 847

Divigel 3467

Estrasorb 1777

Vagifem 2589

Estradiol Benzoate (*In vitro* metabolism studies showed that CYP1A2 is the major enzyme responsible for the metabolism of ropinirole. There is thus the potential for inducers or inhibitors of this enzyme to alter the clearance of ropinirole. Therefore, if therapy with a drug known to be a potent inducer or inhibitor of CYP1A2 is stopped or started during treatment with ropinirole, adjustment of the dose of ropinirole may be required).

No products indexed under this heading.

Estradiol Cypionate (*In vitro* metabolism studies showed that CYP1A2 is the major enzyme responsible for the metabolism of ropinirole. There is thus the potential for inducers or inhibitors of this enzyme to alter the clearance of ropinirole. Therefore, if therapy with a drug known to be a potent inducer or inhibitor of CYP1A2 is stopped or started during treatment with ropinirole, adjustment of the dose of ropinirole may be required).

No products indexed under this heading.

Estrogens, Conjugated (Population pharmacokinetic analysis revealed that estrogens (mainly ethinylestradiol: intake 0.6 to 3 mg over 4-month to 23-year period) reduced the oral clearance of ropinirole by 36% in 16 patients. Dosage adjustment is not needed for initiating ropinirole in patients on estrogen therapy because patients are individually titrated with ropinirole to tolerance or adequate effect. If estrogen therapy is stopped or started during treatment with ropinirole, then adjustment of the dose of ropinirole may be required). Products include:

Premarin Intravenous 3528

Premarin Tablets 3533

Premarin Vaginal Cream 3540

Premphase 3549

Prempro 3549

Estrogens, Esterified (Population pharmacokinetic analysis revealed that estrogens (mainly ethinylestradiol: intake 0.6 to 3 mg over 4-month to 23-year period) reduced the oral clearance of ropinirole by 36% in 16 patients. Dosage adjustment is not needed for initiating ropinirole in patients on estrogen therapy because patients are individually titrated with ropinirole to tolerance or adequate effect. If estrogen therapy is stopped or started during treatment with ropinirole, then adjustment of the dose of ropinirole may be required).

No products indexed under this heading.

Estropipate (Population pharmacokinetic analysis revealed that estrogens (mainly ethinylestradiol: intake 0.6 to 3 mg over 4-month to 23-year period)

reduced the oral clearance of ropinirole by 36% in 16 patients. Dosage adjustment is not needed for initiating ropinirole in patients on estrogen therapy because patients are individually titrated with ropinirole to tolerance or adequate effect. If estrogen therapy is stopped or started during treatment with ropinirole, then adjustment of the dose of ropinirole may be required).
No products indexed under this heading.

Ethanol (Sedating medications (such as alcohol or CNS depressants), may increase the risk of somnolence or falling asleep while engaged in activities of daily living. Because of possible additive effects, caution should be advised when patients are taking other sedating medications, alcohol, or other CNS depressants (eg, benzodiazepines, antipsychotics, antidepressants) in combination with ropinirole).
No products indexed under this heading.

Ethchlorvynol (Sedating medications (such as alcohol or CNS depressants), may increase the risk of somnolence or falling asleep while engaged in activities of daily living. Because of possible additive effects, caution should be advised when patients are taking other sedating medications, alcohol, or other CNS depressants (eg, benzodiazepines, antipsychotics, antidepressants) in combination with ropinirole).
No products indexed under this heading.

Ethinamate (Sedating medications (such as alcohol or CNS depressants), may increase the risk of somnolence or falling asleep while engaged in activities of daily living. Because of possible additive effects, caution should be advised when patients are taking other sedating medications, alcohol, or other CNS depressants (eg, benzodiazepines, antipsychotics, antidepressants) in combination with ropinirole).
No products indexed under this heading.

Ethinyl Estradiol (Population pharmacokinetic analysis revealed that estrogens (mainly ethinylestradiol: intake 0.6 to 3 mg over 4-month to 23-year period) reduced the oral clearance of ropinirole by 36% in 16 patients. Dosage adjustment is not needed for initiating ropinirole in patients on estrogen therapy because patients are individually titrated with ropinirole to tolerance or adequate effect. If estrogen therapy is stopped or started during treatment with ropinirole, then adjustment of the dose of ropinirole may be required). Products include:
- LoSeasonique **3407**
- Lybrel **3514**
- NuvaRing **3181**
- Ortho Evra **2648**
- Ortho-Cyclen/Ortho Tri-Cyclen **2663**
- Ortho Tri-Cyclen Lo Tablets **2673**
- Seasonique **3418**
- Yaz **864**

Ethyl Alcohol (Sedating medications (such as alcohol or CNS depressants), may increase the risk of somnolence or falling asleep while engaged in activities of daily living. Because of possible additive effects, caution should be advised when patients are taking other sedating medications, alcohol, or other CNS depressants (eg, benzodiazepines, antipsychotics, antidepressants) in combination with ropinirole).
No products indexed under this heading.

Fentanyl (Sedating medications (such as alcohol or CNS depressants), may increase the risk of somnolence or falling asleep while engaged in activities of daily living. Because of possible additive effects, caution should be advised when patients are taking other sedating medications, alcohol, or other CNS depressants (eg, benzodiazepines, antipsychotics, antidepressants) in combination with ropinirole). Products include:
- Duragesic **2604**
- Fentanyl Transdermal System **2346**
- Onsolis **2054**

Fentanyl Citrate (Sedating medications (such as alcohol or CNS depressants), may increase the risk of somnolence or falling asleep while engaged in activities of daily living. Because of possible additive effects, caution should be advised when patients are taking other sedating medications, alcohol, or other CNS depressants (eg, benzodiazepines, antipsychotics, antidepressants) in combination with ropinirole). Products include:
- Fentora **966**

Fluoxetine Hydrochloride (Because of possible additive effects, caution should be advised when patients are taking other sedating medications, alcohol, or other CNS depressants (eg, benzodiazepines, antipsychotics, antidepressants) in combination with ropinirole). Products include:
- Prozac Weekly **1941**
- Prozac Pulvules **1941**
- Symbyax **1965**

Fluphenazine Decanoate (Sedating medications (such as alcohol or CNS depressants), may increase the risk of somnolence or falling asleep while engaged in activities of daily living. Because of possible additive effects, caution should be advised when patients are taking other sedating medications, alcohol, or other CNS depressants (eg, benzodiazepines, antipsychotics, antidepressants) in combination with ropinirole).
No products indexed under this heading.

Fluphenazine Enanthate (Sedating medications (such as alcohol or CNS depressants), may increase the risk of somnolence or falling asleep while engaged in activities of daily living. Because of possible additive effects, caution should be advised when patients are taking other sedating medications, alcohol, or other CNS depressants (eg, benzodiazepines, antipsychotics, antidepressants) in combination with ropinirole).
No products indexed under this heading.

Fluphenazine Hydrochloride (Sedating medications (such as alcohol or CNS depressants), may increase the risk of somnolence or falling asleep while engaged in activities of daily living. Because of possible additive effects, caution should be advised when patients are taking other sedating medications, alcohol, or other CNS depressants (eg, benzodiazepines, antipsychotics, antidepressants) in combination with ropinirole).
No products indexed under this heading.

Flurazepam Hydrochloride (Sedating medications (such as alcohol or CNS depressants), may increase the risk of somnolence or falling asleep while engaged in activities of daily living. Because of possible additive effects, caution should be advised when patients are taking other sedating medications, alcohol, or other CNS depressants (eg, benzodiazepines, antipsychotics, antidepressants) in combination with ropinirole).
No products indexed under this heading.

Flutamide (*In vitro* metabolism studies showed that CYP1A2 is the major enzyme responsible for the metabolism of ropinirole. There is thus the potential for inducers or inhibitors of this enzyme to alter the clearance of ropinirole. Therefore, if therapy with a drug known to be a potent inducer or inhibitor of CYP1A2 is stopped or started during treatment with ropinirole, adjustment of the dose of ropinirole may be required).
No products indexed under this heading.

Fluticasone Propionate (*In vitro* metabolism studies showed that CYP1A2 is the major enzyme responsible for the metabolism of ropinirole. There is thus the potential for inducers or inhibitors of this enzyme to alter the clearance of ropinirole. Therefore, if therapy with a drug known to be a potent inducer or inhibitor of CYP1A2 is stopped or started during treatment with ropinirole, adjustment of the dose of ropinirole may be required). Products include:
- Advair 100/50 .... **1275**
- Advair 250/50 .... **1275**
- Advair 500/50 .... **1275**
- Advair HFA 45/21 .... **1288**
- Advair HFA 115/21 .... **1288**
- Advair HFA 230/21 .... **1288**
- Flonase **1459**
- Flovent Diskus **1463**
- Flovent HFA **1470**

Fluvoxamine (Because of possible additive effects, caution should be advised when patients are taking other sedating medications, alcohol, or other CNS depressants (eg, benzodiazepines, antipsychotics, antidepressants) in combination with ropinirole).
No products indexed under this heading.

Fluvoxamine Maleate (Because of possible additive effects, caution should be advised when patients are taking other sedating medications, alcohol, or other CNS depressants (eg, benzodiazepines, antipsychotics, antidepressants) in combination with ropinirole).
No products indexed under this heading.

Gatifloxacin (*In vitro* metabolism studies showed that CYP1A2 is the major enzyme responsible for the metabolism of ropinirole. There is thus the potential for inducers or inhibitors of this enzyme to alter the clearance of ropinirole. Therefore, if therapy with a drug known to be a potent inducer or inhibitor of CYP1A2 is stopped or started during treatment with ropinirole, adjustment of the dose of ropinirole may be required).
No products indexed under this heading.

Gemifloxacin Mesylate (*In vitro* metabolism studies showed that CYP1A2 is the major enzyme responsible for the metabolism of ropinirole. There is thus the potential for inducers or inhibitors of this enzyme to alter the clearance of ropinirole. Therefore, if therapy with a drug known to be a potent inducer or inhibitor of CYP1A2 is stopped or started during treatment with ropinirole, adjustment of the dose of ropinirole may be required).
No products indexed under this heading.

Glutethimide (Sedating medications (such as alcohol or CNS depressants), may increase the risk of somnolence or falling asleep while engaged in activities of daily living. Because of possible additive effects, caution should be advised when patients are taking other sedating medications, alcohol, or other CNS depressants (eg, benzodiazepines, antipsychotics, antidepressants) in combination with ropinirole).
No products indexed under this heading.

Grepafloxacin Hydrochloride (*In vitro* metabolism studies showed that CYP1A2 is the major enzyme responsible for the metabolism of ropinirole. There is thus the potential for inducers or inhibitors of this enzyme to alter the clearance of ropinirole. Therefore, if therapy with a drug known to be a potent inducer or inhibitor of CYP1A2 is stopped or started during treatment with ropinirole, adjustment of the dose of ropinirole may be required).
No products indexed under this heading.

Halazepam (Sedating medications (such as alcohol or CNS depressants), may increase the risk of somnolence or falling asleep while engaged in activities of daily living. Because of possible additive effects, caution should be advised when patients are taking other sedating medications, alcohol, or other CNS depressants (eg, benzodiazepines, antipsychotics, antidepressants) in combination with ropinirole).
No products indexed under this heading.

Haloperidol (Sedating medications (such as alcohol or CNS depressants), may increase the risk of somnolence or falling asleep while engaged in activities of daily living. Because of possible additive effects, caution should be advised when patients are taking other sedating medications, alcohol, or other CNS depressants (eg, benzodiazepines, antipsychotics, antidepressants) in combination with ropinirole).
No products indexed under this heading.

Haloperidol Decanoate (Sedating medications (such as alcohol or CNS depressants), may increase the risk of somnolence or falling asleep while engaged in activities of daily living. Because of possible additive effects, caution should be advised when patients are taking other sedating medications, alcohol, or other CNS depressants (eg, benzodiazepines, antipsychotics, antidepressants) in combination with ropinirole).
No products indexed under this heading.

Haloperidol Lactate (Sedating medications (such as alcohol or CNS depressants), may increase the risk of somnolence or falling asleep while engaged in activities of daily living. Because of possible additive effects, caution should be advised when patients are taking other sedating medications, alcohol, or other CNS depressants (eg, benzodiazepines, antipsychotics, antidepressants) in combination with ropinirole).
No products indexed under this heading.

Hexobarbital (Sedating medications (such as alcohol or CNS depressants), may increase the risk of somnolence or falling asleep while engaged in activities of daily living. Because of possible additive effects, caution should be advised when patients are taking other sedating medications, alcohol, or other CNS depressants (eg, benzodiazepines, antipsychotics, antidepressants) in combination with ropinirole).
No products indexed under this heading.

Hydrocodone Bitartrate (Sedating medications (such as alcohol or CNS depressants), may increase the risk of somnolence or falling asleep while engaged in activities of daily living. Because of possible additive effects, caution should be advised when patients are taking other sedating medications, alcohol, or other CNS depressants (eg, benzodiazepines, antipsychotics, antidepressants) in combination with ropinirole). Products include:
- Vicodin **560**
- Vicodin ES **561**
- Vicodin HP **563**
- Vicoprofen **564**
- Zydone **1138**

Hydrocodone Polistirex (Sedating medications (such as alcohol or CNS depressants), may increase the risk of somnolence or falling asleep while engaged in activities of daily living. Because of possible additive effects, caution should be advised when patients are taking other sedating medications, alcohol, or other CNS depressants (eg, benzodiazepines, antipsychotics, antidepressants) in combination with ropinirole). Products include:

Requip Interactions Index 1596

Tussionex 3443

Hydromorphone (Sedating medications (such as alcohol or CNS depressants), may increase the risk of somnolence or falling asleep while engaged in activities of daily living. Because of possible additive effects, caution should be advised when patients are taking other sedating medications, alcohol, or other CNS depressants (eg, benzodiazepines, antipsychotics, antidepressants) in combination with ropinirole).
No products indexed under this heading.

Hydromorphone Hydrochloride (Sedating medications (such as alcohol or CNS depressants), may increase the risk of somnolence or falling asleep while engaged in activities of daily living. Because of possible additive effects, caution should be advised when patients are taking other sedating medications, alcohol, or other CNS depressants (eg, benzodiazepines, antipsychotics, antidepressants) in combination with ropinirole). Products include:
Dilaudid Injection 2800
Dilaudid Oral 2797
Dilaudid Tablets 2797
Dilaudid-HP 2800

Hydroxyzine Hydrochloride (Sedating medications (such as alcohol or CNS depressants), may increase the risk of somnolence or falling asleep while engaged in activities of daily living. Because of possible additive effects, caution should be advised when patients are taking other sedating medications, alcohol, or other CNS depressants (eg, benzodiazepines, antipsychotics, antidepressants) in combination with ropinirole).
No products indexed under this heading.

Hypericum (*In vitro* metabolism studies showed that CYP1A2 is the major enzyme responsible for the metabolism of ropinirole. There is thus the potential for inducers or inhibitors of this enzyme to alter the clearance of ropinirole. Therefore, if therapy with a drug known to be a potent inducer or inhibitor of CYP1A2 is stopped or started during treatment with ropinirole, adjustment of the dose of ropinirole may be required).
No products indexed under this heading.

Hypericum Perforatum (*In vitro* metabolism studies showed that CYP1A2 is the major enzyme responsible for the metabolism of ropinirole. There is thus the potential for inducers or inhibitors of this enzyme to alter the clearance of ropinirole. Therefore, if therapy with a drug known to be a potent inducer or inhibitor of CYP1A2 is stopped or started during treatment with ropinirole, adjustment of the dose of ropinirole may be required). Products include:
Traumeel 1800

Imipramine Hydrochloride (Because of possible additive effects, caution should be advised when patients are taking other sedating medications, alcohol, or other CNS depressants (eg, benzodiazepines, antipsychotics, antidepressants) in combination with ropinirole).
No products indexed under this heading.

Imipramine Pamoate (Because of possible additive effects, caution should be advised when patients are taking other sedating medications, alcohol, or other CNS depressants (eg, benzodiazepines, antipsychotics, antidepressants) in combination with ropinirole).
No products indexed under this heading.

Insulin (*In vitro* metabolism studies showed that CYP1A2 is the major enzyme responsible for the metabolism of ropinirole. There is thus the potential for inducers or inhibitors of this enzyme to alter the clearance of ropinirole. Therefore, if therapy with a drug known to be a potent inducer or inhibitor of CYP1A2 is stopped or started during treatment with ropinirole, adjustment of the dose of ropinirole may be required).
No products indexed under this heading.

Insulin, Human, Zinc Suspension (*In vitro* metabolism studies showed that CYP1A2 is the major enzyme responsible for the metabolism of ropinirole. There is thus the potential for inducers or inhibitors of this enzyme to alter the clearance of ropinirole. Therefore, if therapy with a drug known to be a potent inducer or inhibitor of CYP1A2 is stopped or started during treatment with ropinirole, adjustment of the dose of ropinirole may be required).
No products indexed under this heading.

Insulin, Human (rDNA origin) (*In vitro* metabolism studies showed that CYP1A2 is the major enzyme responsible for the metabolism of ropinirole. There is thus the potential for inducers or inhibitors of this enzyme to alter the clearance of ropinirole. Therefore, if therapy with a drug known to be a potent inducer or inhibitor of CYP1A2 is stopped or started during treatment with ropinirole, adjustment of the dose of ropinirole may be required). Products include:
Exubera 2717

Insulin, Human NPH (*In vitro* metabolism studies showed that CYP1A2 is the major enzyme responsible for the metabolism of ropinirole. There is thus the potential for inducers or inhibitors of this enzyme to alter the clearance of ropinirole. Therefore, if therapy with a drug known to be a potent inducer or inhibitor of CYP1A2 is stopped or started during treatment with ropinirole, adjustment of the dose of ropinirole may be required). Products include:
Humulin N Vial 1934

Insulin, Human Regular (*In vitro* metabolism studies showed that CYP1A2 is the major enzyme responsible for the metabolism of ropinirole. There is thus the potential for inducers or inhibitors of this enzyme to alter the clearance of ropinirole. Therefore, if therapy with a drug known to be a potent inducer or inhibitor of CYP1A2 is stopped or started during treatment with ropinirole, adjustment of the dose of ropinirole may be required). Products include:
Humulin R 1937
Humulin R (U-500) 1939

Insulin, Human Regular and Human NPH Mixture (*In vitro* metabolism studies showed that CYP1A2 is the major enzyme responsible for the metabolism of ropinirole. There is thus the potential for inducers or inhibitors of this enzyme to alter the clearance of ropinirole. Therefore, if therapy with a drug known to be a potent inducer or inhibitor of CYP1A2 is stopped or started during treatment with ropinirole, adjustment of the dose of ropinirole may be required). Products include:
Humulin 50/50 1930
Humulin 70/30 Vial 1931

Insulin, NPH (*In vitro* metabolism studies showed that CYP1A2 is the major enzyme responsible for the metabolism of ropinirole. There is thus the potential for inducers or inhibitors of this enzyme to alter the clearance of ropinirole. Therefore, if therapy with a drug known to be a potent inducer or inhibitor of CYP1A2 is stopped or started during treatment with ropinirole, adjustment of the dose of ropinirole may be required).
No products indexed under this heading.

Insulin, Regular (*In vitro* metabolism studies showed that CYP1A2 is the major enzyme responsible for the metabolism of ropinirole. There is thus the potential for inducers or inhibitors of this enzyme to alter the clearance of ropinirole. Therefore, if therapy with a drug known to be a potent inducer or inhibitor of CYP1A2 is stopped or started during treatment with ropinirole, adjustment of the dose of ropinirole may be required).
No products indexed under this heading.

Insulin, Regular and NPH mixture (*In vitro* metabolism studies showed that CYP1A2 is the major enzyme responsible for the metabolism of ropinirole. There is thus the potential for inducers or inhibitors of this enzyme to alter the clearance of ropinirole. Therefore, if therapy with a drug known to be a potent inducer or inhibitor of CYP1A2 is stopped or started during treatment with ropinirole, adjustment of the dose of ropinirole may be required).
No products indexed under this heading.

Insulin, Zinc Crystals (*In vitro* metabolism studies showed that CYP1A2 is the major enzyme responsible for the metabolism of ropinirole. There is thus the potential for inducers or inhibitors of this enzyme to alter the clearance of ropinirole. Therefore, if therapy with a drug known to be a potent inducer or inhibitor of CYP1A2 is stopped or started during treatment with ropinirole, adjustment of the dose of ropinirole may be required).
No products indexed under this heading.

Insulin, Zinc Suspension (*In vitro* metabolism studies showed that CYP1A2 is the major enzyme responsible for the metabolism of ropinirole. There is thus the potential for inducers or inhibitors of this enzyme to alter the clearance of ropinirole. Therefore, if therapy with a drug known to be a potent inducer or inhibitor of CYP1A2 is stopped or started during treatment with ropinirole, adjustment of the dose of ropinirole may be required).
No products indexed under this heading.

Insulin Aspart (*In vitro* metabolism studies showed that CYP1A2 is the major enzyme responsible for the metabolism of ropinirole. There is thus the potential for inducers or inhibitors of this enzyme to alter the clearance of ropinirole. Therefore, if therapy with a drug known to be a potent inducer or inhibitor of CYP1A2 is stopped or started during treatment with ropinirole, adjustment of the dose of ropinirole may be required).
No products indexed under this heading.

Insulin Aspart, Human (*In vitro* metabolism studies showed that CYP1A2 is the major enzyme responsible for the metabolism of ropinirole. There is thus the potential for inducers or inhibitors of this enzyme to alter the clearance of ropinirole. Therefore, if therapy with a drug known to be a potent inducer or inhibitor of CYP1A2 is stopped or started during treatment with ropinirole, adjustment of the dose of ropinirole may be required). Products include:
NovoLog Mix 70/30 2581

Insulin Aspart, Human Regular (*In vitro* metabolism studies showed that CYP1A2 is the major enzyme responsible for the metabolism of ropinirole. There is thus the potential for inducers or inhibitors of this enzyme to alter the clearance of ropinirole. Therefore, if therapy with a drug known to be a potent inducer or inhibitor of CYP1A2 is stopped or started during treatment with ropinirole, adjustment of the dose of ropinirole may be required). Products include:
NovoLog 2575

Insulin Aspart Protamine, Human (*In vitro* metabolism studies showed that CYP1A2 is the major enzyme responsible for the metabolism of ropinirole. There is thus the potential for inducers or inhibitors of this enzyme to alter the clearance of ropinirole. Therefore, if therapy with a drug known to be a potent inducer or inhibitor of CYP1A2 is stopped or started during treatment with ropinirole, adjustment of the dose of ropinirole may be required). Products include:
NovoLog Mix 70/30 2581

Insulin Detemir (rDNA Origin) (*In vitro* metabolism studies showed that CYP1A2 is the major enzyme responsible for the metabolism of ropinirole. There is thus the potential for inducers or inhibitors of this enzyme to alter the clearance of ropinirole. Therefore, if therapy with a drug known to be a potent inducer or inhibitor of CYP1A2 is stopped or started during treatment with ropinirole, adjustment of the dose of ropinirole may be required). Products include:
Levemir 2566

Insulin Glargine (*In vitro* metabolism studies showed that CYP1A2 is the major enzyme responsible for the metabolism of ropinirole. There is thus the potential for inducers or inhibitors of this enzyme to alter the clearance of ropinirole. Therefore, if therapy with a drug known to be a potent inducer or inhibitor of CYP1A2 is stopped or started during treatment with ropinirole, adjustment of the dose of ropinirole may be required). Products include:
Lantus 2996

Insulin Glulisine (*In vitro* metabolism studies showed that CYP1A2 is the major enzyme responsible for the metabolism of ropinirole. There is thus the potential for inducers or inhibitors of this enzyme to alter the clearance of ropinirole. Therefore, if therapy with a drug known to be a potent inducer or inhibitor of CYP1A2 is stopped or started during treatment with ropinirole, adjustment of the dose of ropinirole may be required). Products include:
Apidra 2937
Apidra SoloStar 2937

Insulin Lispro, Human (*In vitro* metabolism studies showed that CYP1A2 is the major enzyme responsible for the metabolism of ropinirole. There is thus the potential for inducers or inhibitors of this enzyme to alter the clearance of ropinirole. Therefore, if therapy with a drug known to be a potent inducer or inhibitor of CYP1A2 is stopped or started during treatment with ropinirole, adjustment of the dose of ropinirole may be required). Products include:
Humalog 1910
Humalog Mix 1914
Humalog Mix75/25 1917

Insulin Lispro Protamine, Human (*In vitro* metabolism studies showed that CYP1A2 is the major enzyme responsible for the metabolism of ropinirole. There is thus the potential for inducers or inhibitors of this enzyme to alter the clearance of ropinirole. Therefore, if therapy with a drug known to be a potent inducer or inhibitor of CYP1A2 is stopped or started during treatment with ropinirole, adjustment of the dose of ropinirole may be required). Products include:
Humalog Mix 1914
Humalog Mix75/25 1917

Isocarboxazid (Because of possible additive effects, caution should be advised when patients are taking other sedating medications, alcohol, or other CNS depressants (eg, benzodiazepines, antipsychotics, antidepressants) in combination with ropinirole). Products include:
Marplan 3481

Isoflurane (Sedating medications (such as alcohol or CNS depressants),

may increase the risk of somnolence or falling asleep while engaged in activities of daily living. Because of possible additive effects, caution should be advised when patients are taking other sedating medications, alcohol, or other CNS depressants (eg, benzodiazepines, antipsychotics, antidepressants) in combination with ropinirole.
No products indexed under this heading.

Isoniazid (*In vitro* metabolism studies showed that CYP1A2 is the major enzyme responsible for the metabolism of ropinirole. There is thus the potential for inducers or inhibitors of this enzyme to alter the clearance of ropinirole. Therefore, if therapy with a drug known to be a potent inducer or inhibitor of CYP1A2 is stopped or started during treatment with ropinirole, adjustment of the dose of ropinirole may be required).
No products indexed under this heading.

Ketamine Hydrochloride (Sedating medications (such as alcohol or CNS depressants), may increase the risk of somnolence or falling asleep while engaged in activities of daily living. Because of possible additive effects, caution should be advised when patients are taking other sedating medications, alcohol, or other CNS depressants (eg, benzodiazepines, antipsychotics, antidepressants) in combination with ropinirole).
No products indexed under this heading.

Ketoconazole (*In vitro* metabolism studies showed that CYP1A2 is the major enzyme responsible for the metabolism of ropinirole. There is thus the potential for inducers or inhibitors of this enzyme to alter the clearance of ropinirole. Therefore, if therapy with a drug known to be a potent inducer or inhibitor of CYP1A2 is stopped or started during treatment with ropinirole, adjustment of the dose of ropinirole may be required). Products include:

Lansoprazole (*In vitro* metabolism studies showed that CYP1A2 is the major enzyme responsible for the metabolism of ropinirole. There is thus the potential for inducers or inhibitors of this enzyme to alter the clearance of ropinirole. Therefore, if therapy with a drug known to be a potent inducer or inhibitor of CYP1A2 is stopped or started during treatment with ropinirole, adjustment of the dose of ropinirole may be required).
No products indexed under this heading.

Levobupivacaine Hydrochloride (*In vitro* metabolism studies showed that CYP1A2 is the major enzyme responsible for the metabolism of ropinirole. There is thus the potential for inducers or inhibitors of this enzyme to alter the clearance of ropinirole. Therefore, if therapy with a drug known to be a potent inducer or inhibitor of CYP1A2 is stopped or started during treatment with ropinirole, adjustment of the dose of ropinirole may be required).
No products indexed under this heading.

Levodopa (Co-administration of carbidopa+L-dopa (Sinemet) with ropinirole (2 mg tid) had no effect on the steady-state pharmacokinetics of ropinirole. Oral administration of ropinirole (2 mg tid) increased mean steady-state C_{max} of L-dopa by 20%, but its AUC was unaffected. Of 208 patients being treated with both L-dopa and ropinirole in placebo-controlled advanced Parkinson's disease trials, there were reports of syncope in 6 (2.9%) compared to 2 of 120 (1.7%) of placebo/L-dopa patients. In patients treated with ropinirole and L-dopa for advanced Parkinson's disease, 10.1% (21 of 208) were reported to experience hallucinations, compared to 4.2% (5 of 120) of

patients treated with placebo and L-dopa. Hallucinations were of sufficient severity to cause discontinuation of treatment in 1.9% of the advanced Parkinson's disease patients, compared to 1.7% of placebo patients. Ropinirole may potentiate the dopaminergic side effects of L-dopa and may cause and/or exacerbate pre-existing dyskinesia in patients treated with L-dopa for Parkinson's disease. Decreasing the dose of L-dopa may ameliorate this side effect). Products include:

Levofloxacin (*In vitro* metabolism studies showed that CYP1A2 is the major enzyme responsible for the metabolism of ropinirole. There is thus the potential for inducers or inhibitors of this enzyme to alter the clearance of ropinirole. Therefore, if therapy with a drug known to be a potent inducer or inhibitor of CYP1A2 is stopped or started during treatment with ropinirole, adjustment of the dose of ropinirole may be required). Products include:

Levomethadyl Acetate Hydrochloride (Sedating medications (such as alcohol or CNS depressants), may increase the risk of somnolence or falling asleep while engaged in activities of daily living. Because of possible additive effects, caution should be advised when patients are taking other sedating medications, alcohol, or other CNS depressants (eg, benzodiazepines, antipsychotics, antidepressants) in combination with ropinirole).
No products indexed under this heading.

Levonorgestrel (*In vitro* metabolism studies showed that CYP1A2 is the major enzyme responsible for the metabolism of ropinirole. There is thus the potential for inducers or inhibitors of this enzyme to alter the clearance of ropinirole. Therefore, if therapy with a drug known to be a potent inducer or inhibitor of CYP1A2 is stopped or started during treatment with ropinirole, adjustment of the dose of ropinirole may be required). Products include:

Levorphanol Tartrate (Sedating medications (such as alcohol or CNS depressants), may increase the risk of somnolence or falling asleep while engaged in activities of daily living. Because of possible additive effects, caution should be advised when patients are taking other sedating medications, alcohol, or other CNS depressants (eg, benzodiazepines, antipsychotics, antidepressants) in combination with ropinirole).
No products indexed under this heading.

Lithium (Because of possible additive effects, caution should be advised when patients are taking other sedating medications, alcohol, or other CNS depressants (eg, antipsychotics) in combination with ropinirole).
No products indexed under this heading.

Lithium Carbonate (Because of possible additive effects, caution should be advised when patients are taking other sedating medications, alcohol, or other CNS depressants (eg, antipsychotics) in combination with ropinirole).
No products indexed under this heading.

Lithium Citrate (Because of possible additive effects, caution should be advised when patients are taking other sedating medications, alcohol, or other CNS depressants (eg, antipsychotics) in combination with ropinirole).
No products indexed under this heading.

Lomefloxacin Hydrochloride (*In vitro* metabolism studies showed that CYP1A2 is the major enzyme responsible for the metabolism of ropinirole. There is thus the potential for inducers or inhibitors of this enzyme to alter the clearance of ropinirole. Therefore, if therapy with a drug known to be a potent inducer or inhibitor of CYP1A2 is stopped or started during treatment with ropinirole, adjustment of the dose of ropinirole may be required).
No products indexed under this heading.

Lorazepam (Sedating medications (such as alcohol or CNS depressants), may increase the risk of somnolence or falling asleep while engaged in activities of daily living. Because of possible additive effects, caution should be advised when patients are taking other sedating medications, alcohol, or other CNS depressants (eg, benzodiazepines, antipsychotics, antidepressants) in combination with ropinirole).
No products indexed under this heading.

Loxapine Hydrochloride (Sedating medications (such as alcohol or CNS depressants), may increase the risk of somnolence or falling asleep while engaged in activities of daily living. Because of possible additive effects, caution should be advised when patients are taking other sedating medications, alcohol, or other CNS depressants (eg, benzodiazepines, antipsychotics, antidepressants) in combination with ropinirole).
No products indexed under this heading.

Loxapine Succinate (Sedating medications (such as alcohol or CNS depressants), may increase the risk of somnolence or falling asleep while engaged in activities of daily living. Because of possible additive effects, caution should be advised when patients are taking other sedating medications, alcohol, or other CNS depressants (eg, benzodiazepines, antipsychotics, antidepressants) in combination with ropinirole).
No products indexed under this heading.

Maprotiline Hydrochloride (Because of possible additive effects, caution should be advised when patients are taking other sedating medications, alcohol, or other CNS depressants (eg, benzodiazepines, antipsychotics, antidepressants) in combination with ropinirole).
No products indexed under this heading.

Meperidine Hydrochloride (Sedating medications (such as alcohol or CNS depressants), may increase the risk of somnolence or falling asleep while engaged in activities of daily living. Because of possible additive effects, caution should be advised when patients are taking other sedating medications, alcohol, or other CNS depressants (eg, benzodiazepines, antipsychotics, antidepressants) in combination with ropinirole).
No products indexed under this heading.

Mephobarbital (Sedating medications (such as alcohol or CNS depressants), may increase the risk of somnolence or falling asleep while engaged in activities of daily living. Because of possible additive effects, caution should be advised when patients are taking other sedating medications, alcohol, or other CNS depressants (eg, benzodiazepines, antipsychotics, antidepressants) in combination with ropinirole).
No products indexed under this heading.

Meprobamate (Sedating medications (such as alcohol or CNS depressants), may increase the risk of somnolence or falling asleep while engaged in activities of daily living. Because of possible additive effects, caution should be advised when patients are taking other sedating medications, alcohol, or other CNS depressants (eg, benzodiazepines, antipsychotics, antidepressants) in combination with ropinirole).
No products indexed under this heading.

Mesoridazine Besylate (Sedating medications (such as alcohol or CNS depressants), may increase the risk of somnolence or falling asleep while engaged in activities of daily living. Because of possible additive effects, caution should be advised when patients are taking other sedating medications, alcohol, or other CNS depressants (eg, benzodiazepines, antipsychotics, antidepressants) in combination with ropinirole).
No products indexed under this heading.

Mestranol (*In vitro* metabolism studies showed that CYP1A2 is the major enzyme responsible for the metabolism of ropinirole. There is thus the potential for inducers or inhibitors of this enzyme to alter the clearance of ropinirole. Therefore, if therapy with a drug known to be a potent inducer or inhibitor of CYP1A2 is stopped or started during treatment with ropinirole, adjustment of the dose of ropinirole may be required).
No products indexed under this heading.

Methadone Hydrochloride (Sedating medications (such as alcohol or CNS depressants), may increase the risk of somnolence or falling asleep while engaged in activities of daily living. Because of possible additive effects, caution should be advised when patients are taking other sedating medications, alcohol, or other CNS depressants (eg, benzodiazepines, antipsychotics, antidepressants) in combination with ropinirole).
No products indexed under this heading.

Methdilazine Hydrochloride (Before initiating treatment patients should be advised of the potential to develop drowsiness and specifically asked about factors that may increase the risk such as concomitant sedating medications. If a patient develops significant daytime sleepiness or episodes of falling asleep during activities that require active participation (eg, conversations, eating, etc.), therapy should ordinarily be discontinued. If a decision is made to continue, patients should be advised to not drive and to avoid other potentially dangerous activities).
No products indexed under this heading.

Methohexital Sodium (Sedating medications (such as alcohol or CNS depressants), may increase the risk of somnolence or falling asleep while engaged in activities of daily living. Because of possible additive effects, caution should be advised when patients are taking other sedating medications, alcohol, or other CNS depressants (eg, benzodiazepines, antipsychotics, antidepressants) in combination with ropinirole).
No products indexed under this heading.

Methotrimeprazine (Sedating medications (such as alcohol or CNS depressants), may increase the risk of somnolence or falling asleep while engaged in activities of daily living. Because of possible additive effects, caution should be advised when patients are taking other sedating medications, alcohol, or other CNS depressants (eg, benzodiazepines, antipsychotics, antidepressants) in combination with ropinirole).
No products indexed under this heading.

Methoxsalen (*In vitro* metabolism studies showed that CYP1A2 is the

Requip Interactions Index 1598

major enzyme responsible for the metabolism of ropinirole. There is thus the potential for inducers or inhibitors of this enzyme to alter the clearance of ropinirole. Therefore, if therapy with a drug known to be a potent inducer or inhibitor of CYP1A2 is stopped or started during treatment with ropinirole, adjustment of the dose of ropinirole may be required).
No products indexed under this heading.

Methoxyflurane (Sedating medications (such as alcohol or CNS depressants), may increase the risk of somnolence or falling asleep while engaged in activities of daily living. Because of possible additive effects, caution should be advised when patients are taking other sedating medications, alcohol, or other CNS depressants (eg, benzodiazepines, antipsychotics, antidepressants) in combination with ropinirole).
No products indexed under this heading.

Metoclopramide Hydrochloride (Since ropinirole is a dopamine agonist, it is possible that dopamine antagonists such as neuroleptics (eg, phenothiazines, butyrophenones, thioxanthenes) or metoclopramide hydrochloride may diminish the effectiveness of ropinirole. Patients with a history or presence of major psychotic disorders should be treated with dopamine agonists only if the potential benefits outweigh the risks). Products include:
Metozolv ODT 2901

Mexiletine Hydrochloride (*In vitro* metabolism studies showed that CYP1A2 is the major enzyme responsible for the metabolism of ropinirole. There is thus the potential for inducers or inhibitors of this enzyme to alter the clearance of ropinirole. Therefore, if therapy with a drug known to be a potent inducer or inhibitor of CYP1A2 is stopped or started during treatment with ropinirole, adjustment of the dose of ropinirole may be required).
No products indexed under this heading.

Mibefradil Dihydrochloride (*In vitro* metabolism studies showed that CYP1A2 is the major enzyme responsible for the metabolism of ropinirole. There is thus the potential for inducers or inhibitors of this enzyme to alter the clearance of ropinirole. Therefore, if therapy with a drug known to be a potent inducer or inhibitor of CYP1A2 is stopped or started during treatment with ropinirole, adjustment of the dose of ropinirole may be required).
No products indexed under this heading.

Midazolam Hydrochloride (Sedating medications (such as alcohol or CNS depressants), may increase the risk of somnolence or falling asleep while engaged in activities of daily living. Because of possible additive effects, caution should be advised when patients are taking other sedating medications, alcohol, or other CNS depressants (eg, benzodiazepines, antipsychotics, antidepressants) in combination with ropinirole).
No products indexed under this heading.

Mirtazapine (Because of possible additive effects, caution should be advised when patients are taking other sedating medications, alcohol, or other CNS depressants (eg, benzodiazepines, antipsychotics, antidepressants) in combination with ropinirole). Products include:
Remeron Tablets 3214
RemeronSolTab Tablets 3219

Molindone Hydrochloride (Sedating medications (such as alcohol or CNS depressants), may increase the risk of somnolence or falling asleep while engaged in activities of daily living. Because of possible additive effects, caution should be advised when patients are taking other sedating medications, alcohol, or other CNS depressants (eg, benzodiazepines, antipsychotics, antidepressants) in combination with ropinirole). Products include:
Moban 1108

Morphine Sulfate (Sedating medications (such as alcohol or CNS depressants), may increase the risk of somnolence or falling asleep while engaged in activities of daily living. Because of possible additive effects, caution should be advised when patients are taking other sedating medications, alcohol, or other CNS depressants (eg, benzodiazepines, antipsychotics, antidepressants) in combination with ropinirole). Products include:
Avinza 1822
Embeda 1831
MS Contin 2803

Morphine Sulfate, Liposomal (Sedating medications (such as alcohol or CNS depressants), may increase the risk of somnolence or falling asleep while engaged in activities of daily living. Because of possible additive effects, caution should be advised when patients are taking other sedating medications, alcohol, or other CNS depressants (eg, benzodiazepines, antipsychotics, antidepressants) in combination with ropinirole).
No products indexed under this heading.

Moxifloxacin Hydrochloride (*In vitro* metabolism studies showed that CYP1A2 is the major enzyme responsible for the metabolism of ropinirole. There is thus the potential for inducers or inhibitors of this enzyme to alter the clearance of ropinirole. Therefore, if therapy with a drug known to be a potent inducer or inhibitor of CYP1A2 is stopped or started during treatment with ropinirole, adjustment of the dose of ropinirole may be required). Products include:
Avelox 3064
Vigamox 589

Nafcillin Sodium (*In vitro* metabolism studies showed that CYP1A2 is the major enzyme responsible for the metabolism of ropinirole. There is thus the potential for inducers or inhibitors of this enzyme to alter the clearance of ropinirole. Therefore, if therapy with a drug known to be a potent inducer or inhibitor of CYP1A2 is stopped or started during treatment with ropinirole, adjustment of the dose of ropinirole may be required).
No products indexed under this heading.

Nalidixic Acid (*In vitro* metabolism studies showed that CYP1A2 is the major enzyme responsible for the metabolism of ropinirole. There is thus the potential for inducers or inhibitors of this enzyme to alter the clearance of ropinirole. Therefore, if therapy with a drug known to be a potent inducer or inhibitor of CYP1A2 is stopped or started during treatment with ropinirole, adjustment of the dose of ropinirole may be required).
No products indexed under this heading.

Naproxen (*In vitro* metabolism studies showed that CYP1A2 is the major enzyme responsible for the metabolism of ropinirole. There is thus the potential for inducers or inhibitors of this enzyme to alter the clearance of ropinirole. Therefore, if therapy with a drug known to be a potent inducer or inhibitor of CYP1A2 is stopped or started during treatment with ropinirole, adjustment of the dose of ropinirole may be required). Products include:
EC-Naprosyn 2850
Naprosyn 2850
Anaprox/Naprosyn 2850

Naproxen Sodium (*In vitro* metabolism studies showed that CYP1A2 is the major enzyme responsible for the metabolism of ropinirole. There is thus the potential for inducers or inhibitors of this enzyme to alter the clearance of ropinirole. Therefore, if therapy with a drug known to be a potent inducer or inhibitor of CYP1A2 is stopped or started during treatment with ropinirole, adjustment of the dose of ropinirole may be required). Products include:
Anaprox 2850
Anaprox DS 2850
Treximet 1681

Nefazodone Hydrochloride (Because of possible additive effects, caution should be advised when patients are taking other sedating medications, alcohol, or other CNS depressants (eg, benzodiazepines, antipsychotics, antidepressants) in combination with ropinirole).
No products indexed under this heading.

Nicotine (*In vitro* metabolism studies showed that CYP1A2 is the major enzyme responsible for the metabolism of ropinirole. There is thus the potential for inducers or inhibitors of this enzyme to alter the clearance of ropinirole. Therefore, if therapy with a drug known to be a potent inducer or inhibitor of CYP1A2 is stopped or started during treatment with ropinirole, adjustment of the dose of ropinirole may be required).
No products indexed under this heading.

Nicotine Polacrilex (*In vitro* metabolism studies showed that CYP1A2 is the major enzyme responsible for the metabolism of ropinirole. There is thus the potential for inducers or inhibitors of this enzyme to alter the clearance of ropinirole. Therefore, if therapy with a drug known to be a potent inducer or inhibitor of CYP1A2 is stopped or started during treatment with ropinirole, adjustment of the dose of ropinirole may be required).
No products indexed under this heading.

Nicotine Salicylate (*In vitro* metabolism studies showed that CYP1A2 is the major enzyme responsible for the metabolism of ropinirole. There is thus the potential for inducers or inhibitors of this enzyme to alter the clearance of ropinirole. Therefore, if therapy with a drug known to be a potent inducer or inhibitor of CYP1A2 is stopped or started during treatment with ropinirole, adjustment of the dose of ropinirole may be required).
No products indexed under this heading.

Nicotine Sulfate (*In vitro* metabolism studies showed that CYP1A2 is the major enzyme responsible for the metabolism of ropinirole. There is thus the potential for inducers or inhibitors of this enzyme to alter the clearance of ropinirole. Therefore, if therapy with a drug known to be a potent inducer or inhibitor of CYP1A2 is stopped or started during treatment with ropinirole, adjustment of the dose of ropinirole may be required).
No products indexed under this heading.

Norethindrone (*In vitro* metabolism studies showed that CYP1A2 is the major enzyme responsible for the metabolism of ropinirole. There is thus the potential for inducers or inhibitors of this enzyme to alter the clearance of ropinirole. Therefore, if therapy with a drug known to be a potent inducer or inhibitor of CYP1A2 is stopped or started during treatment with ropinirole, adjustment of the dose of ropinirole may be required). Products include:
Ortho Micronor 2660

Norethindrone Acetate (*In vitro* metabolism studies showed that CYP1A2 is the major enzyme responsible for the metabolism of ropinirole. There is thus the potential for inducers or inhibitors of this enzyme to alter the clearance of ropinirole. Therefore, if therapy with a drug known to be a potent inducer or inhibitor of CYP1A2 is stopped or started during treatment with ropinirole, adjustment of the dose of ropinirole may be required). Products include:
Activella 2561

Norfloxacin (*In vitro* metabolism studies showed that CYP1A2 is the major enzyme responsible for the metabolism of ropinirole. There is thus the potential for inducers or inhibitors of this enzyme to alter the clearance of ropinirole. Therefore, if therapy with a drug known to be a potent inducer or inhibitor of CYP1A2 is stopped or started during treatment with ropinirole, adjustment of the dose of ropinirole may be required). Products include:
Noroxin 2220

Norgestrel (*In vitro* metabolism studies showed that CYP1A2 is the major enzyme responsible for the metabolism of ropinirole. There is thus the potential for inducers or inhibitors of this enzyme to alter the clearance of ropinirole. Therefore, if therapy with a drug known to be a potent inducer or inhibitor of CYP1A2 is stopped or started during treatment with ropinirole, adjustment of the dose of ropinirole may be required).
No products indexed under this heading.

Nortriptyline Hydrochloride (Because of possible additive effects, caution should be advised when patients are taking other sedating medications, alcohol, or other CNS depressants (eg, benzodiazepines, antipsychotics, antidepressants) in combination with ropinirole).
No products indexed under this heading.

Ofloxacin (*In vitro* metabolism studies showed that CYP1A2 is the major enzyme responsible for the metabolism of ropinirole. There is thus the potential for inducers or inhibitors of this enzyme to alter the clearance of ropinirole. Therefore, if therapy with a drug known to be a potent inducer or inhibitor of CYP1A2 is stopped or started during treatment with ropinirole, adjustment of the dose of ropinirole may be required).
No products indexed under this heading.

Olanzapine (Sedating medications (such as alcohol or CNS depressants), may increase the risk of somnolence or falling asleep while engaged in activities of daily living. Because of possible additive effects, caution should be advised when patients are taking other sedating medications, alcohol, or other CNS depressants (eg, benzodiazepines, antipsychotics, antidepressants) in combination with ropinirole). Products include:
Symbyax 1965
Zyprexa 1984
Zyprexa IntraMuscular 1984
Zyprexa ZYDIS 1984

Omeprazole (*In vitro* metabolism studies showed that CYP1A2 is the major enzyme responsible for the metabolism of ropinirole. There is thus the potential for inducers or inhibitors of this enzyme to alter the clearance of ropinirole. Therefore, if therapy with a drug known to be a potent inducer or inhibitor of CYP1A2 is stopped or started during treatment with ropinirole, adjustment of the dose of ropinirole may be required).
No products indexed under this heading.

Omeprazole Magnesium (*In vitro* metabolism studies showed that CYP1A2 is the major enzyme responsible for the metabolism of ropinirole. There is thus the potential for inducers or inhibitors of this enzyme to alter the clearance of ropinirole. Therefore, if therapy with a drug known to be a potent inducer or inhibitor of CYP1A2 is

1599 Interactions Index Requip

stopped or started during treatment with ropinirole, adjustment of the dose of ropinirole may be required).
No products indexed under this heading.

Ondansetron (*In vitro* metabolism studies showed that CYP1A2 is the major enzyme responsible for the metabolism of ropinirole. There is thus the potential for inducers or inhibitors of this enzyme to alter the clearance of ropinirole. Therefore, if therapy with a drug known to be a potent inducer or inhibitor of CYP1A2 is stopped or started during treatment with ropinirole, adjustment of the dose of ropinirole may be required).
No products indexed under this heading.

Ondansetron Hydrochloride (*In vitro* metabolism studies showed that CYP1A2 is the major enzyme responsible for the metabolism of ropinirole. There is thus the potential for inducers or inhibitors of this enzyme to alter the clearance of ropinirole. Therefore, if therapy with a drug known to be a potent inducer or inhibitor of CYP1A2 is stopped or started during treatment with ropinirole, adjustment of the dose of ropinirole may be required). Products include:
Zofran Injection 1750
Zofran 1756
Zofran ODT 1756

Oxazepam (Sedating medications (such as alcohol or CNS depressants), may increase the risk of somnolence or falling asleep while engaged in activities of daily living. Because of possible additive effects, caution should be advised when patients are taking other sedating medications, alcohol, or other CNS depressants (eg, benzodiazepines, antipsychotics, antidepressants) in combination with ropinirole).
No products indexed under this heading.

Oxycodone Hydrochloride (Sedating medications (such as alcohol or CNS depressants), may increase the risk of somnolence or falling asleep while engaged in activities of daily living. Because of possible additive effects, caution should be advised when patients are taking other sedating medications, alcohol, or other CNS depressants (eg, benzodiazepines, antipsychotics, antidepressants) in combination with ropinirole). Products include:
OxyContin 2807
Percocet 1121
Percodan 1124

Oxycodone Terephthalate (Sedating medications (such as alcohol or CNS depressants), may increase the risk of somnolence or falling asleep while engaged in activities of daily living. Because of possible additive effects, caution should be advised when patients are taking other sedating medications, alcohol, or other CNS depressants (eg, benzodiazepines, antipsychotics, antidepressants) in combination with ropinirole).
No products indexed under this heading.

Oxymorphone Hydrochloride (Sedating medications (such as alcohol or CNS depressants), may increase the risk of somnolence or falling asleep while engaged in activities of daily living. Because of possible additive effects, caution should be advised when patients are taking other sedating medications, alcohol, or other CNS depressants (eg, benzodiazepines, antipsychotics, antidepressants) in combination with ropinirole). Products include:
Opana 1110
Opana ER 1114

Paliperidone (Because of possible additive effects, caution should be advised when patients are taking other sedating medications, alcohol, or other CNS depressants (eg, antipsychotics) in combination with ropinirole). Products include:
Invega 2613
Invega Sustenna 2621

Paroxetine (Because of possible additive effects, caution should be advised when patients are taking other sedating medications, alcohol, or other CNS depressants (eg, benzodiazepines, antipsychotics, antidepressants) in combination with ropinirole).
No products indexed under this heading.

Paroxetine Hydrochloride (Because of possible additive effects, caution should be advised when patients are taking other sedating medications, alcohol, or other CNS depressants (eg, benzodiazepines, antipsychotics, antidepressants) in combination with ropinirole). Products include:
Paroxetine CR 2361
Paroxetine ER 2371
Paxil 1586
Paxil CR 1596

Paroxetine Mesylate (Because of possible additive effects, caution should be advised when patients are taking other sedating medications, alcohol, or other CNS depressants (eg, benzodiazepines, antipsychotics, antidepressants) in combination with ropinirole).
No products indexed under this heading.

Pentobarbital (Sedating medications (such as alcohol or CNS depressants), may increase the risk of somnolence or falling asleep while engaged in activities of daily living. Because of possible additive effects, caution should be advised when patients are taking other sedating medications, alcohol, or other CNS depressants (eg, benzodiazepines, antipsychotics, antidepressants) in combination with ropinirole).
No products indexed under this heading.

Pentobarbital Sodium (Sedating medications (such as alcohol or CNS depressants), may increase the risk of somnolence or falling asleep while engaged in activities of daily living. Because of possible additive effects, caution should be advised when patients are taking other sedating medications, alcohol, or other CNS depressants (eg, benzodiazepines, antipsychotics, antidepressants) in combination with ropinirole). Products include:
Nembutal 2012

Perphenazine (Sedating medications (such as alcohol or CNS depressants), may increase the risk of somnolence or falling asleep while engaged in activities of daily living. Because of possible additive effects, caution should be advised when patients are taking other sedating medications, alcohol, or other CNS depressants (eg, benzodiazepines, antipsychotics, antidepressants) in combination with ropinirole).
No products indexed under this heading.

Phenelzine Sulfate (Because of possible additive effects, caution should be advised when patients are taking other sedating medications, alcohol, or other CNS depressants (eg, benzodiazepines, antipsychotics, antidepressants) in combination with ropinirole).
No products indexed under this heading.

Phenobarbital (Sedating medications (such as alcohol or CNS depressants), may increase the risk of somnolence or falling asleep while engaged in activities of daily living. Because of possible additive effects, caution should be advised when patients are taking other sedating medications, alcohol, or other CNS depressants (eg, benzodiazepines, antipsychotics, antidepressants) in combination with ropinirole). Products include:
Donnatal 2711

Phenobarbital Sodium (Sedating medications (such as alcohol or CNS depressants), may increase the risk of somnolence or falling asleep while engaged in activities of daily living. Because of possible additive effects, caution should be advised when patients are taking other sedating medications, alcohol, or other CNS depressants (eg, benzodiazepines, antipsychotics, antidepressants) in combination with ropinirole).
No products indexed under this heading.

Phenothiazine Derivatives (Since ropinirole is a dopamine agonist, it is possible that dopamine antagonists such as neuroleptics (eg, phenothiazines, butyrophenones, thioxanthenes) or metoclopramide may diminish the effectiveness of ropinirole. Patients with a history or presence of major psychotic disorders should be treated with dopamine agonists only if the potential benefits outweigh the risks).
No products indexed under this heading.

Phenothiazines (Since ropinirole is a dopamine agonist, it is possible that dopamine antagonists such as neuroleptics (eg, phenothiazines, butyrophenones, thioxanthenes) or metoclopramide may diminish the effectiveness of ropinirole. Patients with a history or presence of major psychotic disorders should be treated with dopamine agonists only if the potential benefits outweigh the risks).
No products indexed under this heading.

Phenytoin (*In vitro* metabolism studies showed that CYP1A2 is the major enzyme responsible for the metabolism of ropinirole. There is thus the potential for inducers or inhibitors of this enzyme to alter the clearance of ropinirole. Therefore, if therapy with a drug known to be a potent inducer or inhibitor of CYP1A2 is stopped or started during treatment with ropinirole, adjustment of the dose of ropinirole may be required).
No products indexed under this heading.

Phenytoin Sodium (*In vitro* metabolism studies showed that CYP1A2 is the major enzyme responsible for the metabolism of ropinirole. There is thus the potential for inducers or inhibitors of this enzyme to alter the clearance of ropinirole. Therefore, if therapy with a drug known to be a potent inducer or inhibitor of CYP1A2 is stopped or started during treatment with ropinirole, adjustment of the dose of ropinirole may be required). Products include:
Phenytek Capsules 2380

Pimozide (Because of possible additive effects, caution should be advised when patients are taking other sedating medications, alcohol, or other CNS depressants (eg, antipsychotics) in combination with ropinirole).
No products indexed under this heading.

Polyestradiol Phosphate (Population pharmacokinetic analysis revealed that estrogens (mainly ethinylestradiol: intake 0.6 to 3 mg over 4-month to 23-year period) reduced the oral clearance of ropinirole by 36% in 16 patients. Dosage adjustment is not needed for initiating ropinirole in patients on estrogen therapy because patients are individually titrated with ropinirole to tolerance or adequate effect. If estrogen therapy is stopped or started during treatment with ropinirole, then adjustment of the dose of ropinirole may be required).
No products indexed under this heading.

Prazepam (Sedating medications (such as alcohol or CNS depressants), may increase the risk of somnolence or falling asleep while engaged in activities of daily living. Because of possible additive effects, caution should be advised when patients are taking other sedating medications, alcohol, or other CNS depressants (eg, benzodiazepines, antipsychotics, antidepressants) in combination with ropinirole).
No products indexed under this heading.

Primidone (*In vitro* metabolism studies showed that CYP1A2 is the major enzyme responsible for the metabolism of ropinirole. There is thus the potential for inducers or inhibitors of this enzyme to alter the clearance of ropinirole. Therefore, if therapy with a drug known to be a potent inducer or inhibitor of CYP1A2 is stopped or started during treatment with ropinirole, adjustment of the dose of ropinirole may be required).
No products indexed under this heading.

Prochlorperazine (Sedating medications (such as alcohol or CNS depressants), may increase the risk of somnolence or falling asleep while engaged in activities of daily living. Because of possible additive effects, caution should be advised when patients are taking other sedating medications, alcohol, or other CNS depressants (eg, benzodiazepines, antipsychotics, antidepressants) in combination with ropinirole).
No products indexed under this heading.

Prochlorperazine Edisylate (Sedating medications (such as alcohol or CNS depressants), may increase the risk of somnolence or falling asleep while engaged in activities of daily living. Because of possible additive effects, caution should be advised when patients are taking other sedating medications, alcohol, or other CNS depressants (eg, benzodiazepines, antipsychotics, antidepressants) in combination with ropinirole).
No products indexed under this heading.

Prochlorperazine Maleate (Sedating medications (such as alcohol or CNS depressants), may increase the risk of somnolence or falling asleep while engaged in activities of daily living. Because of possible additive effects, caution should be advised when patients are taking other sedating medications, alcohol, or other CNS depressants (eg, benzodiazepines, antipsychotics, antidepressants) in combination with ropinirole).
No products indexed under this heading.

Promethazine (Sedating medications (such as alcohol or CNS depressants), may increase the risk of somnolence or falling asleep while engaged in activities of daily living. Because of possible additive effects, caution should be advised when patients are taking other sedating medications, alcohol, or other CNS depressants (eg, benzodiazepines, antipsychotics, antidepressants) in combination with ropinirole).
No products indexed under this heading.

Promethazine Hydrochloride (Sedating medications (such as alcohol or CNS depressants), may increase the risk of somnolence or falling asleep while engaged in activities of daily living. Because of possible additive effects, caution should be advised when patients are taking other sedating medications, alcohol, or other CNS depressants (eg, benzodiazepines, antipsychotics, antidepressants) in combination with ropinirole).
No products indexed under this heading.

Propafenone Hydrochloride (*In vitro* metabolism studies showed that CYP1A2 is the major enzyme responsible for the metabolism of ropinirole. There is thus the potential for inducers or inhibitors of this enzyme to alter the clearance of ropinirole. Therefore, if therapy with a drug known to be a potent inducer or inhibitor of CYP1A2 is stopped or started during treatment

with ropinirole, adjustment of the dose of ropinirole may be required). Products include:

Propofol (Sedating medications (such as alcohol or CNS depressants), may increase the risk of somnolence or falling asleep while engaged in activities of daily living. Because of possible additive effects, caution should be advised when patients are taking other sedating medications, alcohol, or other CNS depressants (eg, benzodiazepines, antipsychotics, antidepressants) in combination with ropinirole).
No products indexed under this heading.

Propoxyphene Hydrochloride (Sedating medications (such as alcohol or CNS depressants), may increase the risk of somnolence or falling asleep while engaged in activities of daily living. Because of possible additive effects, caution should be advised when patients are taking other sedating medications, alcohol, or other CNS depressants (eg, benzodiazepines, antipsychotics, antidepressants) in combination with ropinirole).
No products indexed under this heading.

Propoxyphene Napsylate (Sedating medications (such as alcohol or CNS depressants), may increase the risk of somnolence or falling asleep while engaged in activities of daily living. Because of possible additive effects, caution should be advised when patients are taking other sedating medications, alcohol, or other CNS depressants (eg, benzodiazepines, antipsychotics, antidepressants) in combination with ropinirole).
No products indexed under this heading.

Propranolol Hydrochloride (In vitro metabolism studies showed that CYP1A2 is the major enzyme responsible for the metabolism of ropinirole. There is thus the potential for inducers or inhibitors of this enzyme to alter the clearance of ropinirole. Therefore, if therapy with a drug known to be a potent inducer or inhibitor of CYP1A2 is stopped or started during treatment with ropinirole, adjustment of the dose of ropinirole may be required). Products include:

Protriptyline Hydrochloride (Because of possible additive effects, caution should be advised when patients are taking other sedating medications, alcohol, or other CNS depressants (eg, benzodiazepines, antipsychotics, antidepressants) in combination with ropinirole).
No products indexed under this heading.

Pyrilamine Maleate (Before initiating treatment patients should be advised of the potential to develop drowsiness and specifically asked about factors that may increase the risk such as concomitant sedating medications. If a patient develops significant daytime sleepiness or episodes of falling asleep during activities that require active participation (eg, conversations, eating, etc.), therapy should ordinarily be discontinued. If a decision is made to continue, patients should be advised to not drive and to avoid other potentially dangerous activities).
No products indexed under this heading.

Pyrilamine Tannate (Before initiating treatment patients should be advised of the potential to develop drowsiness and specifically asked about factors that may increase the risk such as concomitant sedating medications. If a patient develops significant daytime sleepiness or episodes of falling asleep during activities that require active participation (eg, conversations, eating, etc.), therapy should ordinarily be discontin-

ued. If a decision is made to continue, patients should be advised to not drive and to avoid other potentially dangerous activities).
No products indexed under this heading.

Quazepam (Sedating medications (such as alcohol or CNS depressants), may increase the risk of somnolence or falling asleep while engaged in activities of daily living. Because of possible additive effects, caution should be advised when patients are taking other sedating medications, alcohol, or other CNS depressants (eg, benzodiazepines, antipsychotics, antidepressants) in combination with ropinirole).
No products indexed under this heading.

Quetiapine Fumarate (Sedating medications (such as alcohol or CNS depressants), may increase the risk of somnolence or falling asleep while engaged in activities of daily living. Because of possible additive effects, caution should be advised when patients are taking other sedating medications, alcohol, or other CNS depressants (eg, benzodiazepines, antipsychotics, antidepressants) in combination with ropinirole). Products include:

Quinestrol (Population pharmacokinetic analysis revealed that estrogens (mainly ethinylestradiol: intake 0.6 to 3 mg over 4-month to 23-year period) reduced the oral clearance of ropinirole by 36% in 16 patients. Dosage adjustment is not needed for initiating ropinirole in patients on estrogen therapy because patients are individually titrated with ropinirole to tolerance or adequate effect. If estrogen therapy is stopped or started during treatment with ropinirole, then adjustment of the dose of ropinirole may be required).
No products indexed under this heading.

Ramelteon (Before initiating treatment patients should be advised of the potential to develop drowsiness and specifically asked about factors that may increase the risk such as concomitant sedating medications. If a patient develops significant daytime sleepiness or episodes of falling asleep during activities that require active participation (eg, conversations, eating, etc.), therapy should ordinarily be discontinued. If a decision is made to continue, patients should be advised to not drive and to avoid other potentially dangerous activities). Products include:

Ranitidine Bismuth Citrate (In vitro metabolism studies showed that CYP1A2 is the major enzyme responsible for the metabolism of ropinirole. There is thus the potential for inducers or inhibitors of this enzyme to alter the clearance of ropinirole. Therefore, if therapy with a drug known to be a potent inducer or inhibitor of CYP1A2 is stopped or started during treatment with ropinirole, adjustment of the dose of ropinirole may be required).
No products indexed under this heading.

Ranitidine Hydrochloride (In vitro metabolism studies showed that CYP1A2 is the major enzyme responsible for the metabolism of ropinirole. There is thus the potential for inducers or inhibitors of this enzyme to alter the clearance of ropinirole. Therefore, if therapy with a drug known to be a potent inducer or inhibitor of CYP1A2 is stopped or started during treatment with ropinirole, adjustment of the dose of ropinirole may be required). Products include:

Remifentanil Hydrochloride (Sedating medications (such as alcohol or CNS depressants), may increase the risk of somnolence or falling asleep while engaged in activities of daily living. Because of possible additive effects, caution should be advised when patients are taking other sedating medications, alcohol, or other CNS depressants (eg, benzodiazepines, antipsychotics, antidepressants) in combination with ropinirole).
No products indexed under this heading.

Rifampicin (In vitro metabolism studies showed that CYP1A2 is the major enzyme responsible for the metabolism of ropinirole. There is thus the potential for inducers or inhibitors of this enzyme to alter the clearance of ropinirole. Therefore, if therapy with a drug known to be a potent inducer or inhibitor of CYP1A2 is stopped or started during treatment with ropinirole, adjustment of the dose of ropinirole may be required).
No products indexed under this heading.

Rifampin (In vitro metabolism studies showed that CYP1A2 is the major enzyme responsible for the metabolism of ropinirole. There is thus the potential for inducers or inhibitors of this enzyme to alter the clearance of ropinirole. Therefore, if therapy with a drug known to be a potent inducer or inhibitor of CYP1A2 is stopped or started during treatment with ropinirole, adjustment of the dose of ropinirole may be required).
No products indexed under this heading.

Riluzole (In vitro metabolism studies showed that CYP1A2 is the major enzyme responsible for the metabolism of ropinirole. There is thus the potential for inducers or inhibitors of this enzyme to alter the clearance of ropinirole. Therefore, if therapy with a drug known to be a potent inducer or inhibitor of CYP1A2 is stopped or started during treatment with ropinirole, adjustment of the dose of ropinirole may be required). Products include:

Risperidone (Sedating medications (such as alcohol or CNS depressants), may increase the risk of somnolence or falling asleep while engaged in activities of daily living. Because of possible additive effects, caution should be advised when patients are taking other sedating medications, alcohol, or other CNS depressants (eg, benzodiazepines, antipsychotics, antidepressants) in combination with ropinirole). Products include:

Ritonavir (In vitro metabolism studies showed that CYP1A2 is the major enzyme responsible for the metabolism of ropinirole. There is thus the potential for inducers or inhibitors of this enzyme to alter the clearance of ropinirole. Therefore, if therapy with a drug known to be a potent inducer or inhibitor of CYP1A2 is stopped or started during treatment with ropinirole, adjustment of the dose of ropinirole may be required). Products include:

Ropivacaine Hydrochloride (In vitro metabolism studies showed that CYP1A2 is the major enzyme responsible for the metabolism of ropinirole. There is thus the potential for inducers or inhibitors of this enzyme to alter the clearance of ropinirole. Therefore, if therapy with a drug known to be a potent inducer or inhibitor of CYP1A2 is stopped or started during treatment with ropinirole, adjustment of the dose of ropinirole may be required).
No products indexed under this heading.

Secobarbital Sodium (Sedating medications (such as alcohol or CNS depressants), may increase the risk of

somnolence or falling asleep while engaged in activities of daily living. Because of possible additive effects, caution should be advised when patients are taking other sedating medications, alcohol, or other CNS depressants (eg, benzodiazepines, antipsychotics, antidepressants) in combination with ropinirole).
No products indexed under this heading.

Selegiline (Because of possible additive effects, caution should be advised when patients are taking other sedating medications, alcohol, or other CNS depressants (eg, benzodiazepines, antipsychotics, antidepressants) in combination with ropinirole). Products include:

Selegiline Hydrochloride (Because of possible additive effects, caution should be advised when patients are taking other sedating medications, alcohol, or other CNS depressants (eg, benzodiazepines, antipsychotics, antidepressants) in combination with ropinirole). Products include:

Sertraline Hydrochloride (Because of possible additive effects, caution should be advised when patients are taking other sedating medications, alcohol, or other CNS depressants (eg, benzodiazepines, antipsychotics, antidepressants) in combination with ropinirole).
No products indexed under this heading.

Sevoflurane (Sedating medications (such as alcohol or CNS depressants), may increase the risk of somnolence or falling asleep while engaged in activities of daily living. Because of possible additive effects, caution should be advised when patients are taking other sedating medications, alcohol, or other CNS depressants (eg, benzodiazepines, antipsychotics, antidepressants) in combination with ropinirole). Products include:

Sildenafil Citrate (In vitro metabolism studies showed that CYP1A2 is the major enzyme responsible for the metabolism of ropinirole. There is thus the potential for inducers or inhibitors of this enzyme to alter the clearance of ropinirole. Therefore, if therapy with a drug known to be a potent inducer or inhibitor of CYP1A2 is stopped or started during treatment with ropinirole, adjustment of the dose of ropinirole may be required).
No products indexed under this heading.

Sodium Butabarbital (Sedating medications (such as alcohol or CNS depressants), may increase the risk of somnolence or falling asleep while engaged in activities of daily living. Because of possible additive effects, caution should be advised when patients are taking other sedating medications, alcohol, or other CNS depressants (eg, benzodiazepines, antipsychotics, antidepressants) in combination with ropinirole).
No products indexed under this heading.

Sodium Oxybate (Sedating medications (such as alcohol or CNS depressants), may increase the risk of somnolence or falling asleep while engaged in activities of daily living. Because of possible additive effects, caution should be advised when patients are taking other sedating medications, alcohol, or other CNS depressants (eg, benzodiazepines, antipsychotics, antidepressants) in combination with ropinirole).
No products indexed under this heading.

Sodium Pentobarbital (Sedating medications (such as alcohol or CNS depressants), may increase the risk of somnolence or falling asleep while engaged in activities of daily living.

1601 Interactions Index Requip

Because of possible additive effects, caution should be advised when patients are taking other sedating medications, alcohol, or other CNS depressants (eg, benzodiazepines, antipsychotics, antidepressants) in combination with ropinirole).
No products indexed under this heading.

Sparfloxacin (*In vitro* metabolism studies showed that CYP1A2 is the major enzyme responsible for the metabolism of ropinirole. There is thus the potential for inducers or inhibitors of this enzyme to alter the clearance of ropinirole. Therefore, if therapy with a drug known to be a potent inducer or inhibitor of CYP1A2 is stopped or started during treatment with ropinirole, adjustment of the dose of ropinirole may be required).
No products indexed under this heading.

Sufentanil Citrate (Sedating medications (such as alcohol or CNS depressants), may increase the risk of somnolence or falling asleep while engaged in activities of daily living. Because of possible additive effects, caution should be advised when patients are taking other sedating medications, alcohol, or other CNS depressants (eg, benzodiazepines, antipsychotics, antidepressants) in combination with ropinirole).
No products indexed under this heading.

Tacrine Hydrochloride (*In vitro* metabolism studies showed that CYP1A2 is the major enzyme responsible for the metabolism of ropinirole. There is thus the potential for inducers or inhibitors of this enzyme to alter the clearance of ropinirole. Therefore, if therapy with a drug known to be a potent inducer or inhibitor of CYP1A2 is stopped or started during treatment with ropinirole, adjustment of the dose of ropinirole may be required).
No products indexed under this heading.

Talbutal (Sedating medications (such as alcohol or CNS depressants), may increase the risk of somnolence or falling asleep while engaged in activities of daily living. Because of possible additive effects, caution should be advised when patients are taking other sedating medications, alcohol, or other CNS depressants (eg, benzodiazepines, antipsychotics, antidepressants) in combination with ropinirole).
No products indexed under this heading.

Tamoxifen Citrate (*In vitro* metabolism studies showed that CYP1A2 is the major enzyme responsible for the metabolism of ropinirole. There is thus the potential for inducers or inhibitors of this enzyme to alter the clearance of ropinirole. Therefore, if therapy with a drug known to be a potent inducer or inhibitor of CYP1A2 is stopped or started during treatment with ropinirole, adjustment of the dose of ropinirole may be required).
No products indexed under this heading.

Temazepam (Sedating medications (such as alcohol or CNS depressants), may increase the risk of somnolence or falling asleep while engaged in activities of daily living. Because of possible additive effects, caution should be advised when patients are taking other sedating medications, alcohol, or other CNS depressants (eg, benzodiazepines, antipsychotics, antidepressants) in combination with ropinirole).
No products indexed under this heading.

Theobromine (*In vitro* metabolism studies showed that CYP1A2 is the major enzyme responsible for the metabolism of ropinirole. There is thus the potential for inducers or inhibitors of this enzyme to alter the clearance of ropinirole. Therefore, if therapy with a drug known to be a potent inducer or inhibitor of CYP1A2 is stopped or started during treatment with ropinirole, adjustment of the dose of ropinirole may be required).
No products indexed under this heading.

Theophylline (*In vitro* metabolism studies showed that CYP1A2 is the major enzyme responsible for the metabolism of ropinirole. There is thus the potential for inducers or inhibitors of this enzyme to alter the clearance of ropinirole. Therefore, if therapy with a drug known to be a potent inducer or inhibitor of CYP1A2 is stopped or started during treatment with ropinirole, adjustment of the dose of ropinirole may be required).
No products indexed under this heading.

Theophylline Anhydrous (*In vitro* metabolism studies showed that CYP1A2 is the major enzyme responsible for the metabolism of ropinirole. There is thus the potential for inducers or inhibitors of this enzyme to alter the clearance of ropinirole. Therefore, if therapy with a drug known to be a potent inducer or inhibitor of CYP1A2 is stopped or started during treatment with ropinirole, adjustment of the dose of ropinirole may be required). Products include:
Uniphyl 2817

Theophylline Calcium Salicylate (*In vitro* metabolism studies showed that CYP1A2 is the major enzyme responsible for the metabolism of ropinirole. There is thus the potential for inducers or inhibitors of this enzyme to alter the clearance of ropinirole. Therefore, if therapy with a drug known to be a potent inducer or inhibitor of CYP1A2 is stopped or started during treatment with ropinirole, adjustment of the dose of ropinirole may be required).
No products indexed under this heading.

Theophylline Dihydroxypropyl (Glyceryl) (*In vitro* metabolism studies showed that CYP1A2 is the major enzyme responsible for the metabolism of ropinirole. There is thus the potential for inducers or inhibitors of this enzyme to alter the clearance of ropinirole. Therefore, if therapy with a drug known to be a potent inducer or inhibitor of CYP1A2 is stopped or started during treatment with ropinirole, adjustment of the dose of ropinirole may be required).
No products indexed under this heading.

Theophylline Ethylenediamine (*In vitro* metabolism studies showed that CYP1A2 is the major enzyme responsible for the metabolism of ropinirole. There is thus the potential for inducers or inhibitors of this enzyme to alter the clearance of ropinirole. Therefore, if therapy with a drug known to be a potent inducer or inhibitor of CYP1A2 is stopped or started during treatment with ropinirole, adjustment of the dose of ropinirole may be required).
No products indexed under this heading.

Theophylline Sodium Glycinate (*In vitro* metabolism studies showed that CYP1A2 is the major enzyme responsible for the metabolism of ropinirole. There is thus the potential for inducers or inhibitors of this enzyme to alter the clearance of ropinirole. Therefore, if therapy with a drug known to be a potent inducer or inhibitor of CYP1A2 is stopped or started during treatment with ropinirole, adjustment of the dose of ropinirole may be required).
No products indexed under this heading.

Thiamylal Sodium (Sedating medications (such as alcohol or CNS depressants), may increase the risk of somnolence or falling asleep while engaged in activities of daily living. Because of possible additive effects, caution should be advised when patients are taking other sedating medications, alcohol, or other CNS depressants (eg, benzodiazepines, antipsychotics, antidepressants) in combination with ropinirole).
No products indexed under this heading.

Thioridazine (Sedating medications (such as alcohol or CNS depressants), may increase the risk of somnolence or falling asleep while engaged in activities of daily living. Because of possible additive effects, caution should be advised when patients are taking other sedating medications, alcohol, or other CNS depressants (eg, benzodiazepines, antipsychotics, antidepressants) in combination with ropinirole).
No products indexed under this heading.

Thioridazine Hydrochloride (Sedating medications (such as alcohol or CNS depressants), may increase the risk of somnolence or falling asleep while engaged in activities of daily living. Because of possible additive effects, caution should be advised when patients are taking other sedating medications, alcohol, or other CNS depressants (eg, benzodiazepines, antipsychotics, antidepressants) in combination with ropinirole). Products include:
Thioridazine Hydrochloride 2384

Thiothixene (Sedating medications (such as alcohol or CNS depressants), may increase the risk of somnolence or falling asleep while engaged in activities of daily living. Because of possible additive effects, caution should be advised when patients are taking other sedating medications, alcohol, or other CNS depressants (eg, benzodiazepines, antipsychotics, antidepressants) in combination with ropinirole). Products include:
Thiothixene 2386

Thiothixene Hydrochloride (Sedating medications (such as alcohol or CNS depressants), may increase the risk of somnolence or falling asleep while engaged in activities of daily living. Because of possible additive effects, caution should be advised when patients are taking other sedating medications, alcohol, or other CNS depressants (eg, benzodiazepines, antipsychotics, antidepressants) in combination with ropinirole).
No products indexed under this heading.

Ticlopidine Hydrochloride (*In vitro* metabolism studies showed that CYP1A2 is the major enzyme responsible for the metabolism of ropinirole. There is thus the potential for inducers or inhibitors of this enzyme to alter the clearance of ropinirole. Therefore, if therapy with a drug known to be a potent inducer or inhibitor of CYP1A2 is stopped or started during treatment with ropinirole, adjustment of the dose of ropinirole may be required).
No products indexed under this heading.

Tizanidine (*In vitro* metabolism studies showed that CYP1A2 is the major enzyme responsible for the metabolism of ropinirole. There is thus the potential for inducers or inhibitors of this enzyme to alter the clearance of ropinirole. Therefore, if therapy with a drug known to be a potent inducer or inhibitor of CYP1A2 is stopped or started during treatment with ropinirole, adjustment of the dose of ropinirole may be required).
No products indexed under this heading.

Tizanidine Hydrochloride (*In vitro* metabolism studies showed that CYP1A2 is the major enzyme responsible for the metabolism of ropinirole. There is thus the potential for inducers or inhibitors of this enzyme to alter the clearance of ropinirole. Therefore, if therapy with a drug known to be a potent inducer or inhibitor of CYP1A2 is stopped or started during treatment with ropinirole, adjustment of the dose of ropinirole may be required).
No products indexed under this heading.

Tobacco (Cigarette smoking is expected to increase the clearance of ropinirole since CYP1A2 is known to be induced by smoking. In one study in patients with restless legs syndrome, cigarette smokers had an approximate 30% lower C_{max} and a 38% lower AUC than nonsmokers, when those parameters were normalized for dose).
No products indexed under this heading.

Tranylcypromine Sulfate (Because of possible additive effects, caution should be advised when patients are taking other sedating medications, alcohol, or other CNS depressants (eg, benzodiazepines, antipsychotics, antidepressants) in combination with ropinirole). Products include:
Parnate 1584

Trazodone Hydrochloride (Because of possible additive effects, caution should be advised when patients are taking other sedating medications, alcohol, or other CNS depressants (eg, benzodiazepines, antipsychotics, antidepressants) in combination with ropinirole).
No products indexed under this heading.

Triazolam (Sedating medications (such as alcohol or CNS depressants), may increase the risk of somnolence or falling asleep while engaged in activities of daily living. Because of possible additive effects, caution should be advised when patients are taking other sedating medications, alcohol, or other CNS depressants (eg, benzodiazepines, antipsychotics, antidepressants) in combination with ropinirole).
No products indexed under this heading.

Trifluoperazine Hydrochloride (Sedating medications (such as alcohol or CNS depressants), may increase the risk of somnolence or falling asleep while engaged in activities of daily living. Because of possible additive effects, caution should be advised when patients are taking other sedating medications, alcohol, or other CNS depressants (eg, benzodiazepines, antipsychotics, antidepressants) in combination with ropinirole).
No products indexed under this heading.

Trimeprazine Tartrate (Before initiating treatment patients should be advised of the potential to develop drowsiness and specifically asked about factors that may increase the risk such as concomitant sedating medications. If a patient develops significant daytime sleepiness or episodes of falling asleep during activities that require active participation (eg, conversations, eating, etc.), therapy should ordinarily be discontinued. If a decision is made to continue, patients should be advised to not drive and to avoid other potentially dangerous activities).
No products indexed under this heading.

Trimethaphan Camsylate (*In vitro* metabolism studies showed that CYP1A2 is the major enzyme responsible for the metabolism of ropinirole. There is thus the potential for inducers or inhibitors of this enzyme to alter the clearance of ropinirole. Therefore, if therapy with a drug known to be a potent inducer or inhibitor of CYP1A2 is stopped or started during treatment with ropinirole, adjustment of the dose of ropinirole may be required).
No products indexed under this heading.

IMPORTANT NOTE: Always consult each drug listing in the patient's regimen for possible interactions.

Trimipramine Maleate (Because of possible additive effects, caution should be advised when patients are taking other sedating medications, alcohol, or other CNS depressants (eg, benzodiazepines, antipsychotics, antidepressants) in combination with ropinirole).

No products indexed under this heading.

Tripelennamine Hydrochloride (Before initiating treatment patients should be advised of the potential to develop drowsiness and specifically asked about factors that may increase the risk such as concomitant sedating medications. If a patient develops significant daytime sleepiness or episodes of falling asleep during activities that require active participation (eg, conversations, eating, etc.), therapy should ordinarily be discontinued. If a decision is made to continue, patients should be advised to not drive and to avoid other potentially dangerous activities).

No products indexed under this heading.

Triprolidine Hydrochloride (Before initiating treatment patients should be advised of the potential to develop drowsiness and specifically asked about factors that may increase the risk such as concomitant sedating medications. If a patient develops significant daytime sleepiness or episodes of falling asleep during activities that require active participation (eg, conversations, eating, etc.), therapy should ordinarily be discontinued. If a decision is made to continue, patients should be advised to not drive and to avoid other potentially dangerous activities).

No products indexed under this heading.

Troleandomycin (In vitro metabolism studies showed that CYP1A2 is the major enzyme responsible for the metabolism of ropinirole. There is thus the potential for inducers or inhibitors of this enzyme to alter the clearance of ropinirole. Therefore, if therapy with a drug known to be a potent inducer or inhibitor of CYP1A2 is stopped or started during treatment with ropinirole, adjustment of the dose of ropinirole may be required).

No products indexed under this heading.

Trovafloxacin Mesylate (In vitro metabolism studies showed that CYP1A2 is the major enzyme responsible for the metabolism of ropinirole. There is thus the potential for inducers or inhibitors of this enzyme to alter the clearance of ropinirole. Therefore, if therapy with a drug known to be a potent inducer or inhibitor of CYP1A2 is stopped or started during treatment with ropinirole, adjustment of the dose of ropinirole may be required).

No products indexed under this heading.

Vardenafil Hydrochloride (In vitro metabolism studies showed that CYP1A2 is the major enzyme responsible for the metabolism of ropinirole. There is thus the potential for inducers or inhibitors of this enzyme to alter the clearance of ropinirole. Therefore, if therapy with a drug known to be a potent inducer or inhibitor of CYP1A2 is stopped or started during treatment with ropinirole, adjustment of the dose of ropinirole may be required). Products include:

Venlafaxine Hydrochloride (Because of possible additive effects, caution should be advised when patients are taking other sedating medications, alcohol, or other CNS depressants (eg, benzodiazepines, antipsychotics, antidepressants) in combination with ropinirole). Products include:

Verapamil Hydrochloride (In vitro metabolism studies showed that CYP1A2 is the major enzyme responsible for the metabolism of ropinirole. There is thus the potential for inducers or inhibitors of this enzyme to alter the clearance of ropinirole. Therefore, if therapy with a drug known to be a potent inducer or inhibitor of CYP1A2 is stopped or started during treatment with ropinirole, adjustment of the dose of ropinirole may be required). Products include:

Warfarin Sodium (In vitro metabolism studies showed that CYP1A2 is the major enzyme responsible for the metabolism of ropinirole. There is thus the potential for inducers or inhibitors of this enzyme to alter the clearance of ropinirole. Therefore, if therapy with a drug known to be a potent inducer or inhibitor of CYP1A2 is stopped or started during treatment with ropinirole, adjustment of the dose of ropinirole may be required).

No products indexed under this heading.

Zaleplon (Sedating medications (such as alcohol or CNS depressants), may increase the risk of somnolence or falling asleep while engaged in activities of daily living. Because of possible additive effects, caution should be advised when patients are taking other sedating medications, alcohol, or other CNS depressants (eg, benzodiazepines, antipsychotics, antidepressants) in combination with ropinirole).

No products indexed under this heading.

Zileuton (In vitro metabolism studies showed that CYP1A2 is the major enzyme responsible for the metabolism of ropinirole. There is thus the potential for inducers or inhibitors of this enzyme to alter the clearance of ropinirole. Therefore, if therapy with a drug known to be a potent inducer or inhibitor of CYP1A2 is stopped or started during treatment with ropinirole, adjustment of the dose of ropinirole may be required).

No products indexed under this heading.

Ziprasidone Hydrochloride (Sedating medications (such as alcohol or CNS depressants), may increase the risk of somnolence or falling asleep while engaged in activities of daily living. Because of possible additive effects, caution should be advised when patients are taking other sedating medications, alcohol, or other CNS depressants (eg, benzodiazepines, antipsychotics, antidepressants) in combination with ropinirole). Products include:

Zolmitriptan (In vitro metabolism studies showed that CYP1A2 is the major enzyme responsible for the metabolism of ropinirole. There is thus the potential for inducers or inhibitors of this enzyme to alter the clearance of ropinirole. Therefore, if therapy with a drug known to be a potent inducer or inhibitor of CYP1A2 is stopped or started during treatment with ropinirole, adjustment of the dose of ropinirole may be required). Products include:

Zolpidem Tartrate (Sedating medications (such as alcohol or CNS depressants), may increase the risk of somnolence or falling asleep while engaged in activities of daily living. Because of possible additive effects, caution should be advised when patients are taking other sedating medications, alcohol, or other CNS depressants (eg, benzodiazepines, antipsychotics, antidepressants) in combination with ropinirole). Products include:

Food Interactions

Alcohol (Sedating medications (such as alcohol or CNS depressants), the presence of sleeping disorders, or other medications that increase plasma levels of ropinirole, may increase the risk of somnolence or falling asleep while engaged in activities of daily living. Because of possible additive effects, caution should be advised when patients are taking other sedating medications, alcohol, or other CNS depressants (eg, benzodiazepines, antipsychotics, antidepressants) in combination with ropinirole).

Beer, reduced-alcohol (Sedating medications (such as alcohol or CNS depressants), may increase the risk of somnolence or falling asleep while engaged in activities of daily living. Because of possible additive effects, caution should be advised when patients are taking other sedating medications, alcohol, or other CNS depressants in combination with ropinirole).

Beer, unspecified (Sedating medications (such as alcohol or CNS depressants), may increase the risk of somnolence or falling asleep while engaged in activities of daily living. Because of possible additive effects, caution should be advised when patients are taking other sedating medications, alcohol, or other CNS depressants in combination with ropinirole).

Broccoli (In vitro metabolism studies showed that CYP1A2 is the major enzyme responsible for the metabolism of ropinirole. There is thus the potential for inducers or inhibitors of this enzyme to alter the clearance of ropinirole. Therefore, if therapy with a drug known to be a potent inducer or inhibitor of CYP1A2 is stopped or started during treatment with ropinirole, adjustment of the dose of ropinirole may be required).

Brussel Sprouts (In vitro metabolism studies showed that CYP1A2 is the major enzyme responsible for the metabolism of ropinirole. There is thus the potential for inducers or inhibitors of this enzyme to alter the clearance of ropinirole. Therefore, if therapy with a drug known to be a potent inducer or inhibitor of CYP1A2 is stopped or started during treatment with ropinirole, adjustment of the dose of ropinirole may be required).

Charbroiled Food (In vitro metabolism studies showed that CYP1A2 is the major enzyme responsible for the metabolism of ropinirole. There is thus the potential for inducers or inhibitors of this enzyme to alter the clearance of ropinirole. Therefore, if therapy with a drug known to be a potent inducer or inhibitor of CYP1A2 is stopped or started during treatment with ropinirole, adjustment of the dose of ropinirole may be required).

Food, caffeine-containing (In vitro metabolism studies showed that CYP1A2 is the major enzyme responsible for the metabolism of ropinirole. There is thus the potential for inducers or inhibitors of this enzyme to alter the clearance of ropinirole. Therefore, if therapy with a drug known to be a potent inducer or inhibitor of CYP1A2 is stopped or started during treatment with ropinirole, adjustment of the dose of ropinirole may be required).

Food, unspecified (Food does not affect the extent of absorption of ropinirole, although its T_{max} is increased by 2.5 hours and its C_{max} is decreased by approximately 25% when the drug is taken with a high-fat meal).

Grapefruit (In vitro metabolism studies showed that CYP1A2 is the major enzyme responsible for the metabolism of ropinirole. There is thus the potential for inducers or inhibitors of this enzyme to alter the clearance of ropinirole. Therefore, if therapy with a drug known to be a potent inducer or inhibitor of CYP1A2 is stopped or started during treatment with ropinirole, adjustment of the dose of ropinirole may be required).

Grapefruit Juice (In vitro metabolism studies showed that CYP1A2 is the major enzyme responsible for the metabolism of ropinirole. There is thus the potential for inducers or inhibitors of this enzyme to alter the clearance of ropinirole. Therefore, if therapy with a drug known to be a potent inducer or inhibitor of CYP1A2 is stopped or started during treatment with ropinirole, adjustment of the dose of ropinirole may be required).

Meal, unspecified (Food does not affect the extent of absorption of ropinirole, although its T_{max} is increased by 2.5 hours and its C_{max} is decreased by approximately 25% when the drug is taken with a high-fat meal).

Wine, Chianti (Sedating medications (such as alcohol or CNS depressants), may increase the risk of somnolence or falling asleep while engaged in activities of daily living. Because of possible additive effects, caution should be advised when patients are taking other sedating medications, alcohol, or other CNS depressants in combination with ropinirole).

Wine, Red (Sedating medications (such as alcohol or CNS depressants), may increase the risk of somnolence or falling asleep while engaged in activities of daily living. Because of possible additive effects, caution should be advised when patients are taking other sedating medications, alcohol, or other CNS depressants in combination with ropinirole).

Wine, unspecified (Sedating medications (such as alcohol or CNS depressants), may increase the risk of somnolence or falling asleep while engaged in activities of daily living. Because of possible additive effects, caution should be advised when patients are taking other sedating medications, alcohol, or other CNS depressants in combination with ropinirole).

Wine products (Sedating medications (such as alcohol or CNS depressants), may increase the risk of somnolence or falling asleep while engaged in activities of daily living. Because of possible additive effects, caution should be advised when patients are taking other sedating medications, alcohol, or other CNS depressants in combination with ropinirole).

REQUIP XL TABLETS

(Ropinirole Hydrochloride) 1628

May interact with alcohols, antidepressant drugs, antipsychotic agents, benzodiazepines, butyrophenones, central nervous system depressants, cytochrome p450 1a2 inducers (selected), cytochrome p450 1a2 inhibitors (selected), cytochrome p450 1a2 substrates (selected), dopamine antagonists, estrogens, highly metabolized sedatives and hypnotics, hypnotics and sedatives, phenothiazines, sedating antihistamines, and certain other agents. Compounds in these categories include:

(⊙ Described in PDR® for Ophthalmic Medicines)

Acetaminophen (*In vitro* metabolism studies showed that CYP1A2 is the major enzyme responsible for the metabolism of ropinirole. There is thus the potential for inducers or inhibitors of this enzyme to alter the clearance of ropinirole. Therefore, if therapy with a drug known to be a potent inducer or inhibitor of CYP1A2 is stopped or started during treatment with ropinirole, adjustment of the dose of ropinirole may be required). Products include:

Acrivastine (Before initiating treatment patients should be advised of the potential to develop drowsiness and specifically asked about factors that may increase the risk such as concomitant sedating medications. If a patient develops significant daytime sleepiness or episodes of falling asleep during activities that require active participation (eg, conversations, eating, etc.), therapy should ordinarily be discontinued. If a decision is made to continue, patients should be advised to not drive and to avoid other potentially dangerous activities).

No products indexed under this heading.

Alatrofloxacin Mesylate (*In vitro* metabolism studies showed that CYP1A2 is the major enzyme responsible for the metabolism of ropinirole. There is thus the potential for inducers or inhibitors of this enzyme to alter the clearance of ropinirole. Therefore, if therapy with a drug known to be a potent inducer or inhibitor of CYP1A2 is stopped or started during treatment with ropinirole, adjustment of the dose of ropinirole may be required).

No products indexed under this heading.

Alfentanil Hydrochloride (Sedating medications (such as alcohol or CNS depressants), may increase the risk of somnlence or falling asleep while engaged in activities of daily living. Because of possible additive effects, caution should be advised when patients are taking other sedating medications, alcohol, or other CNS depressants (eg, benzodiazepines, antipsychotics, antidepressants) in combination with ropinirole).

No products indexed under this heading.

Alprazolam (Sedating medications (such as alcohol or CNS depressants), may increase the risk of somnlence or falling asleep while engaged in activities of daily living. Because of possible additive effects, caution should be advised when patients are taking other sedating medications, alcohol, or other CNS depressants (eg, benzodiazepines, antipsychotics, antidepressants) in combination with ropinirole).

No products indexed under this heading.

Aminophylline (*In vitro* metabolism studies showed that CYP1A2 is the major enzyme responsible for the metabolism of ropinirole. There is thus the potential for inducers or inhibitors of this enzyme to alter the clearance of

ropinirole. Therefore, if therapy with a drug known to be a potent inducer or inhibitor of CYP1A2 is stopped or started during treatment with ropinirole, adjustment of the dose of ropinirole may be required).

No products indexed under this heading.

Amiodarone Hydrochloride (*In vitro* metabolism studies showed that CYP1A2 is the major enzyme responsible for the metabolism of ropinirole. There is thus the potential for inducers or inhibitors of this enzyme to alter the clearance of ropinirole. Therefore, if therapy with a drug known to be a potent inducer or inhibitor of CYP1A2 is stopped or started during treatment with ropinirole, adjustment of the dose of ropinirole may be required).

No products indexed under this heading.

Amitriptyline Hydrochloride (Because of possible additive effects, caution should be advised when patients are taking other sedating medications, alcohol, or other CNS depressants (eg, benzodiazepines, antipsychotics, antidepressants) in combination with ropinirole).

No products indexed under this heading.

Amobarbital (Sedating medications (such as alcohol or CNS depressants), may increase the risk of somnlence or falling asleep while engaged in activities of daily living. Because of possible additive effects, caution should be advised when patients are taking other sedating medications, alcohol, or other CNS depressants (eg, benzodiazepines, antipsychotics, antidepressants) in combination with ropinirole).

No products indexed under this heading.

Amobarbital Sodium (Sedating medications (such as alcohol or CNS depressants), may increase the risk of somnlence or falling asleep while engaged in activities of daily living. Because of possible additive effects, caution should be advised when patients are taking other sedating medications, alcohol, or other CNS depressants (eg, benzodiazepines, antipsychotics, antidepressants) in combination with ropinirole).

No products indexed under this heading.

Amoxapine (Because of possible additive effects, caution should be advised when patients are taking other sedating medications, alcohol, or other CNS depressants (eg, benzodiazepines, antipsychotics, antidepressants) in combination with ropinirole).

No products indexed under this heading.

Anagrelide Hydrochloride (*In vitro* metabolism studies showed that CYP1A2 is the major enzyme responsible for the metabolism of ropinirole. There is thus the potential for inducers or inhibitors of this enzyme to alter the clearance of ropinirole. Therefore, if therapy with a drug known to be a potent inducer or inhibitor of CYP1A2 is stopped or started during treatment with ropinirole, adjustment of the dose of ropinirole may be required).

No products indexed under this heading.

Anastrozole (*In vitro* metabolism studies showed that CYP1A2 is the major enzyme responsible for the metabolism of ropinirole. There is thus the potential for inducers or inhibitors of this enzyme to alter the clearance of ropinirole. Therefore, if therapy with a drug known to be a potent inducer or inhibitor of CYP1A2 is stopped or started during treatment with ropinirole, adjustment of the dose of ropinirole may be required).

No products indexed under this heading.

Aprobarbital (Sedating medications (such as alcohol or CNS depressants), may increase the risk of somnlence or falling asleep while engaged in activities of daily living. Because of possible addi-

tive effects, caution should be advised when patients are taking other sedating medications, alcohol, or other CNS depressants (eg, benzodiazepines, antipsychotics, antidepressants) in combination with ropinirole).

No products indexed under this heading.

Aripiprazole (Because of possible additive effects, caution should be advised when patients are taking other sedating medications, alcohol, or other CNS depressants (eg, antipsychotics) in combination with ropinirole).

No products indexed under this heading.

Azatadine Maleate (Before initiating treatment patients should be advised of the potential to develop drowsiness and specifically asked about factors that may increase the risk such as concomitant sedating medications. If a patient develops significant daytime sleepiness or episodes of falling asleep during activities that require active participation (eg, conversations, eating, etc.), therapy should ordinarily be discontinued. If a decision is made to continue, patients should be advised to not drive and to avoid other potentially dangerous activities).

No products indexed under this heading.

Bromodiphenhydramine Hydrochloride (Before initiating treatment patients should be advised of the potential to develop drowsiness and specifically asked about factors that may increase the risk such as concomitant sedating medications. If a patient develops significant daytime sleepiness or episodes of falling asleep during activities that require active participation (eg, conversations, eating, etc.), therapy should ordinarily be discontinued. If a decision is made to continue, patients should be advised to not drive and to avoid other potentially dangerous activities).

No products indexed under this heading.

Brompheniramine Maleate (Before initiating treatment patients should be advised of the potential to develop drowsiness and specifically asked about factors that may increase the risk such as concomitant sedating medications. If a patient develops significant daytime sleepiness or episodes of falling asleep during activities that require active participation (eg, conversations, eating, etc.), therapy should ordinarily be discontinued. If a decision is made to continue, patients should be advised to not drive and to avoid other potentially dangerous activities).

No products indexed under this heading.

Buprenorphine Hydrochloride (Sedating medications (such as alcohol or CNS depressants), may increase the risk of somnlence or falling asleep while engaged in activities of daily living. Because of possible additive effects, caution should be advised when patients are taking other sedating medications, alcohol, or other CNS depressants (eg, benzodiazepines, antipsychotics, antidepressants) in combination with ropinirole).

No products indexed under this heading.

Bupropion Hydrochloride (Because of possible additive effects, caution should be advised when patients are taking other sedating medications, alcohol, or other CNS depressants (eg, benzodiazepines, antipsychotics, antidepressants) in combination with ropinirole). Products include:

Buspirone Hydrochloride (Sedating medications (such as alcohol or CNS depressants), may increase the risk of somnlence or falling asleep while

engaged in activities of daily living. Because of possible additive effects, caution should be advised when patients are taking other sedating medications, alcohol, or other CNS depressants (eg, benzodiazepines, antipsychotics, antidepressants) in combination with ropinirole).

No products indexed under this heading.

Butabarbital (Sedating medications (such as alcohol or CNS depressants), may increase the risk of somnlence or falling asleep while engaged in activities of daily living. Because of possible additive effects, caution should be advised when patients are taking other sedating medications, alcohol, or other CNS depressants (eg, benzodiazepines, antipsychotics, antidepressants) in combination with ropinirole).

No products indexed under this heading.

Butabarbital Sodium (Sedating medications (such as alcohol or CNS depressants), may increase the risk of somnlence or falling asleep while engaged in activities of daily living. Because of possible additive effects, caution should be advised when patients are taking other sedating medications, alcohol, or other CNS depressants (eg, benzodiazepines, antipsychotics, antidepressants) in combination with ropinirole).

No products indexed under this heading.

Butalbital (Sedating medications (such as alcohol or CNS depressants), may increase the risk of somnlence or falling asleep while engaged in activities of daily living. Because of possible additive effects, caution should be advised when patients are taking other sedating medications, alcohol, or other CNS depressants (eg, benzodiazepines, antipsychotics, antidepressants) in combination with ropinirole).

No products indexed under this heading.

Caffeine (*In vitro* metabolism studies showed that CYP1A2 is the major enzyme responsible for the metabolism of ropinirole. There is thus the potential for inducers or inhibitors of this enzyme to alter the clearance of ropinirole. Therefore, if therapy with a drug known to be a potent inducer or inhibitor of CYP1A2 is stopped or started during treatment with ropinirole, adjustment of the dose of ropinirole may be required).

No products indexed under this heading.

Caffeine Anhydrous (*In vitro* metabolism studies showed that CYP1A2 is the major enzyme responsible for the metabolism of ropinirole. There is thus the potential for inducers or inhibitors of this enzyme to alter the clearance of ropinirole. Therefore, if therapy with a drug known to be a potent inducer or inhibitor of CYP1A2 is stopped or started during treatment with ropinirole, adjustment of the dose of ropinirole may be required).

No products indexed under this heading.

Caffeine Citrate (*In vitro* metabolism studies showed that CYP1A2 is the major enzyme responsible for the metabolism of ropinirole. There is thus the potential for inducers or inhibitors of this enzyme to alter the clearance of ropinirole. Therefore, if therapy with a drug known to be a potent inducer or inhibitor of CYP1A2 is stopped or started during treatment with ropinirole, adjustment of the dose of ropinirole may be required).

No products indexed under this heading.

Caffeine-containing medications (*In vitro* metabolism studies showed that CYP1A2 is the major enzyme responsible for the metabolism of ropinirole. There is thus the potential for inducers or inhibitors of this enzyme to alter the clearance of ropinirole. Therefore, if therapy with a drug known to be a potent inducer or inhibitor of CYP1A2

Requip XL Interactions Index 1604

is stopped or started during treatment with ropinirole, adjustment of the dose of ropinirole may be required).
No products indexed under this heading.

Caffeine Sodium Benzoate (*In vitro* metabolism studies showed that CYP1A2 is the major enzyme responsible for the metabolism of ropinirole. There is thus the potential for inducers or inhibitors of this enzyme to alter the clearance of ropinirole. Therefore, if therapy with a drug known to be a potent inducer or inhibitor of CYP1A2 is stopped or started during treatment with ropinirole, adjustment of the dose of ropinirole may be required).
No products indexed under this heading.

Carbamazepine (*In vitro* metabolism studies showed that CYP1A2 is the major enzyme responsible for the metabolism of ropinirole. There is thus the potential for inducers or inhibitors of this enzyme to alter the clearance of ropinirole. Therefore, if therapy with a drug known to be a potent inducer or inhibitor of CYP1A2 is stopped or started during treatment with ropinirole, adjustment of the dose of ropinirole may be required). Products include:
Carbatrol 3280
Equetro 3477

Chloral Hydrate (Before initiating treatment patients should be advised of the potential to develop drowsiness and specifically asked about factors that may increase the risk such as concomitant sedating medications. If a patient develops significant daytime sleepiness or episodes of falling asleep during activities that require active participation (eg, conversations, eating, etc.), therapy should ordinarily be discontinued. If a decision is made to continue, patients should be advised to not drive and to avoid other potentially dangerous activities).
No products indexed under this heading.

Chlordiazepoxide (Sedating medications (such as alcohol or CNS depressants), may increase the risk of somnlence or falling asleep while engaged in activities of daily living. Because of possible additive effects, caution should be advised when patients are taking other sedating medications, alcohol, or other CNS depressants (eg, benzodiazepines, antipsychotics, antidepressants) in combination with ropinirole).
No products indexed under this heading.

Chlordiazepoxide Hydrochloride (Sedating medications (such as alcohol or CNS depressants), may increase the risk of somnlence or falling asleep while engaged in activities of daily living. Because of possible additive effects, caution should be advised when patients are taking other sedating medications, alcohol, or other CNS depressants (eg, benzodiazepines, antipsychotics, antidepressants) in combination with ropinirole).
No products indexed under this heading.

Chlorotrianisene (Population pharmacokinetic analysis revealed that higher doses of estrogens (usually associated with hormone replacement therapy) reduced the oral clearance of ropinirole by approximately 35%. Dosage adjustment is not needed for initiating ropinirole in patients on estrogen therapy because patients are individually titrated with ropinirole to tolerance or adequate effect. If estrogen therapy is stopped or started during treatment with ropinirole, then adjustment of the dose of ropinirole may be required).
No products indexed under this heading.

Chlorpheniramine Maleate (Before initiating treatment patients should be advised of the potential to develop drowsiness and specifically asked about factors that may increase the risk such as concomitant sedating medications. If a patient develops significant daytime sleepiness or episodes of falling asleep during activities that require active participation (eg, conversations, eating, etc.), therapy should ordinarily be discontinued. If a decision is made to continue, patients should be advised to not drive and to avoid other potentially dangerous activities).
No products indexed under this heading.

Chlorpheniramine Polistirex (Before initiating treatment patients should be advised of the potential to develop drowsiness and specifically asked about factors that may increase the risk such as concomitant sedating medications. If a patient develops significant daytime sleepiness or episodes of falling asleep during activities that require active participation (eg, conversations, eating, etc.), therapy should ordinarily be discontinued. If a decision is made to continue, patients should be advised to not drive and to avoid other potentially dangerous activities). Products include:
Tussionex 3443

Chlorpheniramine Tannate (Before initiating treatment patients should be advised of the potential to develop drowsiness and specifically asked about factors that may increase the risk such as concomitant sedating medications. If a patient develops significant daytime sleepiness or episodes of falling asleep during activities that require active participation (eg, conversations, eating, etc.), therapy should ordinarily be discontinued. If a decision is made to continue, patients should be advised to not drive and to avoid other potentially dangerous activities).
No products indexed under this heading.

Chlorpromazine (Sedating medications (such as alcohol or CNS depressants), may increase the risk of somnlence or falling asleep while engaged in activities of daily living. Because of possible additive effects, caution should be advised when patients are taking other sedating medications, alcohol, or other CNS depressants (eg, benzodiazepines, antipsychotics, antidepressants) in combination with ropinirole).
No products indexed under this heading.

Chlorpromazine Hydrochloride (Sedating medications (such as alcohol or CNS depressants), may increase the risk of somnlence or falling asleep while engaged in activities of daily living. Because of possible additive effects, caution should be advised when patients are taking other sedating medications, alcohol, or other CNS depressants (eg, benzodiazepines, antipsychotics, antidepressants) in combination with ropinirole).
No products indexed under this heading.

Chlorprothixene (Sedating medications (such as alcohol or CNS depressants), may increase the risk of somnlence or falling asleep while engaged in activities of daily living. Because of possible additive effects, caution should be advised when patients are taking other sedating medications, alcohol, or other CNS depressants (eg, benzodiazepines, antipsychotics, antidepressants) in combination with ropinirole).
No products indexed under this heading.

Chlorprothixene Hydrochloride (Sedating medications (such as alcohol or CNS depressants), may increase the risk of somnlence or falling asleep while engaged in activities of daily living. Because of possible additive effects, caution should be advised when patients are taking other sedating medications, alcohol, or other CNS depressants (eg, benzodiazepines, antipsychotics, antidepressants) in combination with ropinirole).
No products indexed under this heading.

Chlorprothixene Lactate (Sedating medications (such as alcohol or CNS depressants), may increase the risk of somnlence or falling asleep while engaged in activities of daily living. Because of possible additive effects, caution should be advised when patients are taking other sedating medications, alcohol, or other CNS depressants (eg, benzodiazepines, antipsychotics, antidepressants) in combination with ropinirole).
No products indexed under this heading.

Cimetidine (*In vitro* metabolism studies showed that CYP1A2 is the major enzyme responsible for the metabolism of ropinirole. There is thus the potential for inducers or inhibitors of this enzyme to alter the clearance of ropinirole. Therefore, if therapy with a drug known to be a potent inducer or inhibitor of CYP1A2 is stopped or started during treatment with ropinirole, adjustment of the dose of ropinirole may be required).
No products indexed under this heading.

Cimetidine Hydrochloride (*In vitro* metabolism studies showed that CYP1A2 is the major enzyme responsible for the metabolism of ropinirole. There is thus the potential for inducers or inhibitors of this enzyme to alter the clearance of ropinirole. Therefore, if therapy with a drug known to be a potent inducer or inhibitor of CYP1A2 is stopped or started during treatment with ropinirole, adjustment of the dose of ropinirole may be required).
No products indexed under this heading.

Ciprofloxacin (*In vitro* metabolism studies showed that CYP1A2 is the major enzyme responsible for the metabolism of ropinirole. There is thus the potential for inducers or inhibitors of this enzyme to alter the clearance of ropinirole. Therefore, if therapy with a drug known to be a potent inducer or inhibitor of CYP1A2 is stopped or started during treatment with ropinirole, adjustment of the dose of ropinirole may be required. Co-administration of ciprofloxacin, an inhibitor of CYP1A2, with immediate-release ropinirole increased the AUC of ropinirole by 84% on average and C_{max} by 60%). Products include:
Cipro I.V. 3082
Cipro 3073
Cipro XR 3091
Ciprodex 583

Ciprofloxacin Hydrochloride (*In vitro* metabolism studies showed that CYP1A2 is the major enzyme responsible for the metabolism of ropinirole. There is thus the potential for inducers or inhibitors of this enzyme to alter the clearance of ropinirole. Therefore, if therapy with a drug known to be a potent inducer or inhibitor of CYP1A2 is stopped or started during treatment with ropinirole, adjustment of the dose of ropinirole may be required. Co-administration of ciprofloxacin, an inhibitor of CYP1A2, with immediate-release ropinirole increased the AUC of ropinirole by 84% on average and C_{max} by 60%). Products include:
Cipro 3073

Citalopram Hydrobromide (Because of possible additive effects, caution should be advised when patients are taking other sedating medications, alcohol, or other CNS depressants (eg, benzodiazepines, antipsychotics, antidepressants) in combination with ropinirole). Products include:
Celexa 1153

Clarithromycin (*In vitro* metabolism studies showed that CYP1A2 is the major enzyme responsible for the metabolism of ropinirole. There is thus the potential for inducers or inhibitors of this enzyme to alter the clearance of ropinirole. Therefore, if therapy with a drug known to be a potent inducer or inhibitor of CYP1A2 is stopped or started during treatment with ropinirole, adjustment of the dose of ropinirole may be required). Products include:
Biaxin/Biaxin XL 412

Clemastine Fumarate (Before initiating treatment patients should be advised of the potential to develop drowsiness and specifically asked about factors that may increase the risk such as concomitant sedating medications. If a patient develops significant daytime sleepiness or episodes of falling asleep during activities that require active participation (eg, conversations, eating, etc.), therapy should ordinarily be discontinued. If a decision is made to continue, patients should be advised to not drive and to avoid other potentially dangerous activities).
No products indexed under this heading.

Clomipramine Hydrochloride (*In vitro* metabolism studies showed that CYP1A2 is the major enzyme responsible for the metabolism of ropinirole. There is thus the potential for inducers or inhibitors of this enzyme to alter the clearance of ropinirole. Therefore, if therapy with a drug known to be a potent inducer or inhibitor of CYP1A2 is stopped or started during treatment with ropinirole, adjustment of the dose of ropinirole may be required).
No products indexed under this heading.

Clonazepam (Sedating medications (such as alcohol or CNS depressants), may increase the risk of somnlence or falling asleep while engaged in activities of daily living. Because of possible additive effects, caution should be advised when patients are taking other sedating medications, alcohol, or other CNS depressants (eg, benzodiazepines, antipsychotics, antidepressants) in combination with ropinirole). Products include:
Klonopin 2855

Clopidogrel Bisulfate (*In vitro* metabolism studies showed that CYP1A2 is the major enzyme responsible for the metabolism of ropinirole. There is thus the potential for inducers or inhibitors of this enzyme to alter the clearance of ropinirole. Therefore, if therapy with a drug known to be a potent inducer or inhibitor of CYP1A2 is stopped or started during treatment with ropinirole, adjustment of the dose of ropinirole may be required). Products include:
Plavix 3027

Clorazepate Dipotassium (Sedating medications (such as alcohol or CNS depressants), may increase the risk of somnlence or falling asleep while engaged in activities of daily living. Because of possible additive effects, caution should be advised when patients are taking other sedating medications, alcohol, or other CNS depressants (eg, benzodiazepines, antipsychotics, antidepressants) in combination with ropinirole).
No products indexed under this heading.

Clozapine (Sedating medications (such as alcohol or CNS depressants), may increase the risk of somnlence or falling asleep while engaged in activities of daily living. Because of possible additive effects, caution should be advised when patients are taking other sedating medications, alcohol, or other CNS depressants (eg, benzodiazepines, antipsychotics, antidepressants) in combination with ropinirole).
No products indexed under this heading.

1605 Interactions Index Requip XL

Codeine Phosphate (Sedating medications (such as alcohol or CNS depressants), may increase the risk of somnlence or falling asleep while engaged in activities of daily living. Because of possible additive effects, caution should be advised when patients are taking other sedating medications, alcohol, or other CNS depressants (eg, benzodiazepines, antipsychotics, antidepressants) in combination with ropinirole). Products include:
Tylenol with Codeine 2691

Codeine Sulfate (Sedating medications (such as alcohol or CNS depressants), may increase the risk of somnlence or falling asleep while engaged in activities of daily living. Because of possible additive effects, caution should be advised when patients are taking other sedating medications, alcohol, or other CNS depressants (eg, benzodiazepines, antipsychotics, antidepressants) in combination with ropinirole).
No products indexed under this heading.

Cyclobenzaprine (*In vitro* metabolism studies showed that CYP1A2 is the major enzyme responsible for the metabolism of ropinirole. There is thus the potential for inducers or inhibitors of this enzyme to alter the clearance of ropinirole. Therefore, if therapy with a drug known to be a potent inducer or inhibitor of CYP1A2 is stopped or started during treatment with ropinirole, adjustment of the dose of ropinirole may be required).
No products indexed under this heading.

Cyclobenzaprine Hydrochloride (*In vitro* metabolism studies showed that CYP1A2 is the major enzyme responsible for the metabolism of ropinirole. There is thus the potential for inducers or inhibitors of this enzyme to alter the clearance of ropinirole. Therefore, if therapy with a drug known to be a potent inducer or inhibitor of CYP1A2 is stopped or started during treatment with ropinirole, adjustment of the dose of ropinirole may be required). Products include:
Amrix 964

Cyproheptadine Hydrochloride (Before initiating treatment patients should be advised of the potential to develop drowsiness and specifically asked about factors that may increase the risk such as concomitant sedating medications. If a patient develops significant daytime sleepiness or episodes of falling asleep during activities that require active participation (eg, conversations, eating, etc.), therapy should ordinarily be discontinued. If a decision is made to continue, patients should be advised to not drive and to avoid other potentially dangerous activities).
No products indexed under this heading.

Desflurane (Sedating medications (such as alcohol or CNS depressants), may increase the risk of somnlence or falling asleep while engaged in activities of daily living. Because of possible additive effects, caution should be advised when patients are taking other sedating medications, alcohol, or other CNS depressants (eg, benzodiazepines, antipsychotics, antidepressants) in combination with ropinirole).
No products indexed under this heading.

Desipramine Hydrochloride (Because of possible additive effects, caution should be advised when patients are taking other sedating medications, alcohol, or other CNS depressants (eg, benzodiazepines, antipsychotics, antidepressants) in combination with ropinirole).
No products indexed under this heading.

Desogestrel (*In vitro* metabolism studies showed that CYP1A2 is the major enzyme responsible for the metabolism of ropinirole. There is thus the potential for inducers or inhibitors of this enzyme to alter the clearance of ropinirole. Therefore, if therapy with a drug known to be a potent inducer or inhibitor of CYP1A2 is stopped or started during treatment with ropinirole, adjustment of the dose of ropinirole may be required).
No products indexed under this heading.

Dexchlorpheniramine Maleate (Before initiating treatment patients should be advised of the potential to develop drowsiness and specifically asked about factors that may increase the risk such as concomitant sedating medications. If a patient develops significant daytime sleepiness or episodes of falling asleep during activities that require active participation (eg, conversations, eating, etc.), therapy should ordinarily be discontinued. If a decision is made to continue, patients should be advised to not drive and to avoid other potentially dangerous activities).
No products indexed under this heading.

Dezocine (Sedating medications (such as alcohol or CNS depressants), may increase the risk of somnlence or falling asleep while engaged in activities of daily living. Because of possible additive effects, caution should be advised when patients are taking other sedating medications, alcohol, or other CNS depressants (eg, benzodiazepines, antipsychotics, antidepressants) in combination with ropinirole).
No products indexed under this heading.

Diazepam (Sedating medications (such as alcohol or CNS depressants), may increase the risk of somnlence or falling asleep while engaged in activities of daily living. Because of possible additive effects, caution should be advised when patients are taking other sedating medications, alcohol, or other CNS depressants (eg, benzodiazepines, antipsychotics, antidepressants) in combination with ropinirole). Products include:
Valium Tablets 2880

Dienestrol (Population pharmacokinetic analysis revealed that higher doses of estrogens (usually associated with hormone replacement therapy) reduced the oral clearance of ropinirole by approximately 35%. Dosage adjustment is not needed for initiating ropinirole in patients on estrogen therapy because patients are individually titrated with ropinirole to tolerance or adequate effect. If estrogen therapy is stopped or started during treatment with ropinirole, then adjustment of the dose of ropinirole may be required).
No products indexed under this heading.

Diethylstilbestrol (Population pharmacokinetic analysis revealed that higher doses of estrogens (usually associated with hormone replacement therapy) reduced the oral clearance of ropinirole by approximately 35%. Dosage adjustment is not needed for initiating ropinirole in patients on estrogen therapy because patients are individually titrated with ropinirole to tolerance or adequate effect. If estrogen therapy is stopped or started during treatment with ropinirole, then adjustment of the dose of ropinirole may be required).
No products indexed under this heading.

Diltiazem Hydrochloride (*In vitro* metabolism studies showed that CYP1A2 is the major enzyme responsible for the metabolism of ropinirole. There is thus the potential for inducers or inhibitors of this enzyme to alter the clearance of ropinirole. Therefore, if therapy with a drug known to be a potent inducer or inhibitor of CYP1A2 is stopped or started during treatment with ropinirole, adjustment of the dose of ropinirole may be required). Products include:
Cardizem LA 423

Diltiazem Maleate (*In vitro* metabolism studies showed that CYP1A2 is the major enzyme responsible for the metabolism of ropinirole. There is thus the potential for inducers or inhibitors of this enzyme to alter the clearance of ropinirole. Therefore, if therapy with a drug known to be a potent inducer or inhibitor of CYP1A2 is stopped or started during treatment with ropinirole, adjustment of the dose of ropinirole may be required).
No products indexed under this heading.

Diphenhydramine Hydrochloride (Before initiating treatment patients should be advised of the potential to develop drowsiness and specifically asked about factors that may increase the risk such as concomitant sedating medications. If a patient develops significant daytime sleepiness or episodes of falling asleep during activities that require active participation (eg, conversations, eating, etc.), therapy should ordinarily be discontinued. If a decision is made to continue, patients should be advised to not drive and to avoid other potentially dangerous activities). Products include:
Benadryl Allergy Ultratab 2042
Children's Benadryl Allergy Liquid 2042

Diphenylpyraline Hydrochloride (Before initiating treatment patients should be advised of the potential to develop drowsiness and specifically asked about factors that may increase the risk such as concomitant sedating medications. If a patient develops significant daytime sleepiness or episodes of falling asleep during activities that require active participation (eg, conversations, eating, etc.), therapy should ordinarily be discontinued. If a decision is made to continue, patients should be advised to not drive and to avoid other potentially dangerous activities).
No products indexed under this heading.

Doxepin Hydrochloride (Because of possible additive effects, caution should be advised when patients are taking other sedating medications, alcohol, or other CNS depressants (eg, benzodiazepines, antipsychotics, antidepressants) in combination with ropinirole).
No products indexed under this heading.

Droperidol (Sedating medications (such as alcohol or CNS depressants), may increase the risk of somnlence or falling asleep while engaged in activities of daily living. Because of possible additive effects, caution should be advised when patients are taking other sedating medications, alcohol, or other CNS depressants (eg, benzodiazepines, antipsychotics, antidepressants) in combination with ropinirole).
No products indexed under this heading.

Enflurane (Sedating medications (such as alcohol or CNS depressants), may increase the risk of somnlence or falling asleep while engaged in activities of daily living. Because of possible additive effects, caution should be advised when patients are taking other sedating medications, alcohol, or other CNS depressants (eg, benzodiazepines, antipsychotics, antidepressants) in combination with ropinirole).
No products indexed under this heading.

Enoxacin (*In vitro* metabolism studies showed that CYP1A2 is the major enzyme responsible for the metabolism of ropinirole. There is thus the potential for inducers or inhibitors of this enzyme to alter the clearance of ropinirole. Therefore, if therapy with a drug known to be a potent inducer or inhibitor of CYP1A2 is stopped or started during treatment with ropinirole, adjustment of the dose of ropinirole may be required).
No products indexed under this heading.

Entacapone (The incidence of hallucination is increased in patients over age 65. Co-administration of entacapone and L-dopa with ropinirole may also increase the risk of hallucination. In a placebo-controlled clinical trial, hallucination occured in 0 of 43 patients taking entacapone plus L-dopa, in 9 of 155 patients taking ropinirole plus L-dopa (6%), and in 7 of 47 patients taking entacapone with ropinirole plus L-dopa (15%)). Products include:
Comtan 2409
Stalevo 2526

Erythromycin (*In vitro* metabolism studies showed that CYP1A2 is the major enzyme responsible for the metabolism of ropinirole. There is thus the potential for inducers or inhibitors of this enzyme to alter the clearance of ropinirole. Therefore, if therapy with a drug known to be a potent inducer or inhibitor of CYP1A2 is stopped or started during treatment with ropinirole, adjustment of the dose of ropinirole may be required).
No products indexed under this heading.

Erythromycin, Topical (*In vitro* metabolism studies showed that CYP1A2 is the major enzyme responsible for the metabolism of ropinirole. There is thus the potential for inducers or inhibitors of this enzyme to alter the clearance of ropinirole. Therefore, if therapy with a drug known to be a potent inducer or inhibitor of CYP1A2 is stopped or started during treatment with ropinirole, adjustment of the dose of ropinirole may be required).
No products indexed under this heading.

Erythromycin Estolate (*In vitro* metabolism studies showed that CYP1A2 is the major enzyme responsible for the metabolism of ropinirole. There is thus the potential for inducers or inhibitors of this enzyme to alter the clearance of ropinirole. Therefore, if therapy with a drug known to be a potent inducer or inhibitor of CYP1A2 is stopped or started during treatment with ropinirole, adjustment of the dose of ropinirole may be required).
No products indexed under this heading.

Erythromycin Ethylsuccinate (*In vitro* metabolism studies showed that CYP1A2 is the major enzyme responsible for the metabolism of ropinirole. There is thus the potential for inducers or inhibitors of this enzyme to alter the clearance of ropinirole. Therefore, if therapy with a drug known to be a potent inducer or inhibitor of CYP1A2 is stopped or started during treatment with ropinirole, adjustment of the dose of ropinirole may be required). Products include:
E.E.S. 437
EryPed 435

Erythromycin Gluceptate (*In vitro* metabolism studies showed that CYP1A2 is the major enzyme responsible for the metabolism of ropinirole. There is thus the potential for inducers or inhibitors of this enzyme to alter the clearance of ropinirole. Therefore, if therapy with a drug known to be a potent inducer or inhibitor of CYP1A2 is stopped or started during treatment with ropinirole, adjustment of the dose of ropinirole may be required).
No products indexed under this heading.

Erythromycin Lactobionate (*In vitro* metabolism studies showed that CYP1A2 is the major enzyme responsible for the metabolism of ropinirole. There is thus the potential for inducers or inhibitors of this enzyme to alter the clearance of ropinirole. Therefore, if therapy with a drug known to be a potent inducer or inhibitor of CYP1A2 is

stopped or started during treatment with ropinirole, adjustment of the dose of ropinirole may be required).
No products indexed under this heading.

Erythromycin Stearate (*In vitro* metabolism studies showed that CYP1A2 is the major enzyme responsible for the metabolism of ropinirole. There is thus the potential for inducers or inhibitors of this enzyme to alter the clearance of ropinirole. Therefore, if therapy with a drug known to be a potent inducer or inhibitor of CYP1A2 is stopped or started during treatment with ropinirole, adjustment of the dose of ropinirole may be required).
No products indexed under this heading.

Escitalopram Oxalate (Because of possible additive effects, caution should be advised when patients are taking other sedating medications, alcohol, or other CNS depressants (eg, benzodiazepines, antipsychotics, antidepressants) in combination with ropinirole). Products include:

Esomeprazole Magnesium (*In vitro* metabolism studies showed that CYP1A2 is the major enzyme responsible for the metabolism of ropinirole. There is thus the potential for inducers or inhibitors of this enzyme to alter the clearance of ropinirole. Therefore, if therapy with a drug known to be a potent inducer or inhibitor of CYP1A2 is stopped or started during treatment with ropinirole, adjustment of the dose of ropinirole may be required). Products include:

Esomeprazole Sodium (*In vitro* metabolism studies showed that CYP1A2 is the major enzyme responsible for the metabolism of ropinirole. There is thus the potential for inducers or inhibitors of this enzyme to alter the clearance of ropinirole. Therefore, if therapy with a drug known to be a potent inducer or inhibitor of CYP1A2 is stopped or started during treatment with ropinirole, adjustment of the dose of ropinirole may be required). Products include:

Estazolam (Sedating medications (such as alcohol or CNS depressants), may increase the risk of somnlence or falling asleep while engaged in activities of daily living. Because of possible additive effects, caution should be advised when patients are taking other sedating medications, alcohol, or other CNS depressants (eg, benzodiazepines, antipsychotics, antidepressants) in combination with ropinirole).
No products indexed under this heading.

Estradiol (Population pharmacokinetic analysis revealed that higher doses of estrogens (usually associated with hormone replacement therapy) reduced the oral clearance of ropinirole by approximately 35%. Dosage adjustment is not needed for initiating ropinirole in patients on estrogen therapy because patients are individually titrated with ropinirole to tolerance or adequate effect. If estrogen therapy is stopped or started during treatment with ropinirole, then adjustment of the dose of ropinirole may be required) Products include:

Estradiol Benzoate (*In vitro* metabolism studies showed that CYP1A2 is the

major enzyme responsible for the metabolism of ropinirole. There is thus the potential for inducers or inhibitors of this enzyme to alter the clearance of ropinirole. Therefore, if therapy with a drug known to be a potent inducer or inhibitor of CYP1A2 is stopped or started during treatment with ropinirole, adjustment of the dose of ropinirole may be required).
No products indexed under this heading.

Estradiol Cypionate (*In vitro* metabolism studies showed that CYP1A2 is the major enzyme responsible for the metabolism of ropinirole. There is thus the potential for inducers or inhibitors of this enzyme to alter the clearance of ropinirole. Therefore, if therapy with a drug known to be a potent inducer or inhibitor of CYP1A2 is stopped or started during treatment with ropinirole, adjustment of the dose of ropinirole may be required).
No products indexed under this heading.

Estrogens, Conjugated (Population pharmacokinetic analysis revealed that higher doses of estrogens (usually associated with hormone replacement therapy) reduced the oral clearance of ropinirole by approximately 35%. Dosage adjustment is not needed for initiating ropinirole in patients on estrogen therapy because patients are individually titrated with ropinirole to tolerance or adequate effect. If estrogen therapy is stopped or started during treatment with ropinirole, then adjustment of the dose of ropinirole may be required). Products include:

Estrogens, Esterified (Population pharmacokinetic analysis revealed that higher doses of estrogens (usually associated with hormone replacement therapy) reduced the oral clearance of ropinirole by approximately 35%. Dosage adjustment is not needed for initiating ropinirole in patients on estrogen therapy because patients are individually titrated with ropinirole to tolerance or adequate effect. If estrogen therapy is stopped or started during treatment with ropinirole, then adjustment of the dose of ropinirole may be required).
No products indexed under this heading.

Estropipate (Population pharmacokinetic analysis revealed that higher doses of estrogens (usually associated with hormone replacement therapy) reduced the oral clearance of ropinirole by approximately 35%. Dosage adjustment is not needed for initiating ropinirole in patients on estrogen therapy because patients are individually titrated with ropinirole to tolerance or adequate effect. If estrogen therapy is stopped or started during treatment with ropinirole, then adjustment of the dose of ropinirole may be required).
No products indexed under this heading.

Ethanol (Sedating medications (such as alcohol or CNS depressants), may increase the risk of somnlence or falling asleep while engaged in activities of daily living. Because of possible additive effects, caution should be advised when patients are taking other sedating medications, alcohol, or other CNS depressants (eg, benzodiazepines, antipsychotics, antidepressants) in combination with ropinirole).
No products indexed under this heading.

Ethchlorvynol (Sedating medications (such as alcohol or CNS depressants), may increase the risk of somnlence or falling asleep while engaged in activities of daily living. Because of possible additive effects, caution should be advised when patients are taking other sedating

medications, alcohol, or other CNS depressants (eg, benzodiazepines, antipsychotics, antidepressants) in combination with ropinirole).
No products indexed under this heading.

Ethinamate (Sedating medications (such as alcohol or CNS depressants), may increase the risk of somnlence or falling asleep while engaged in activities of daily living. Because of possible additive effects, caution should be advised when patients are taking other sedating medications, alcohol, or other CNS depressants (eg, benzodiazepines, antipsychotics, antidepressants) in combination with ropinirole).
No products indexed under this heading.

Ethinyl Estradiol (Population pharmacokinetic analysis revealed that higher doses of estrogens (usually associated with hormone replacement therapy) reduced the oral clearance of ropinirole by approximately 35%. Dosage adjustment is not needed for initiating ropinirole in patients on estrogen therapy because patients are individually titrated with ropinirole to tolerance or adequate effect. If estrogen therapy is stopped or started during treatment with ropinirole, then adjustment of the dose of ropinirole may be required). Products include:

Ethyl Alcohol (Sedating medications (such as alcohol or CNS depressants), may increase the risk of somnlence or falling asleep while engaged in activities of daily living. Because of possible additive effects, caution should be advised when patients are taking other sedating medications, alcohol, or other CNS depressants (eg, benzodiazepines, antipsychotics, antidepressants) in combination with ropinirole).
No products indexed under this heading.

Fentanyl (Sedating medications (such as alcohol or CNS depressants), may increase the risk of somnlence or falling asleep while engaged in activities of daily living. Because of possible additive effects, caution should be advised when patients are taking other sedating medications, alcohol, or other CNS depressants (eg, benzodiazepines, antipsychotics, antidepressants) in combination with ropinirole). Products include:

Fentanyl Citrate (Sedating medications (such as alcohol or CNS depressants), may increase the risk of somnlence or falling asleep while engaged in activities of daily living. Because of possible additive effects, caution should be advised when patients are taking other sedating medications, alcohol, or other CNS depressants (eg, benzodiazepines, antipsychotics, antidepressants) in combination with ropinirole). Products include:

Fluoxetine Hydrochloride (Because of possible additive effects, caution should be advised when patients are taking other sedating medications, alcohol, or other CNS depressants (eg, benzodiazepines, antipsychotics, antidepressants) in combination with ropinirole). Products include:

Fluphenazine Decanoate (Sedating medications (such as alcohol or CNS depressants), may increase the risk of somnlence or falling asleep while engaged in activities of daily living. Because of possible additive effects, caution should be advised when patients are taking other sedating medications, alcohol, or other CNS depressants (eg, benzodiazepines, antipsychotics, antidepressants) in combination with ropinirole).
No products indexed under this heading.

Fluphenazine Enanthate (Sedating medications (such as alcohol or CNS depressants), may increase the risk of somnlence or falling asleep while engaged in activities of daily living. Because of possible additive effects, caution should be advised when patients are taking other sedating medications, alcohol, or other CNS depressants (eg, benzodiazepines, antipsychotics, antidepressants) in combination with ropinirole).
No products indexed under this heading.

Fluphenazine Hydrochloride (Sedating medications (such as alcohol or CNS depressants), may increase the risk of somnlence or falling asleep while engaged in activities of daily living. Because of possible additive effects, caution should be advised when patients are taking other sedating medications, alcohol, or other CNS depressants (eg, benzodiazepines, antipsychotics, antidepressants) in combination with ropinirole).
No products indexed under this heading.

Flurazepam Hydrochloride (Sedating medications (such as alcohol or CNS depressants), may increase the risk of somnlence or falling asleep while engaged in activities of daily living. Because of possible additive effects, caution should be advised when patients are taking other sedating medications, alcohol, or other CNS depressants (eg, benzodiazepines, antipsychotics, antidepressants) in combination with ropinirole).
No products indexed under this heading.

Flutamide (*In vitro* metabolism studies showed that CYP1A2 is the major enzyme responsible for the metabolism of ropinirole. There is thus the potential for inducers or inhibitors of this enzyme to alter the clearance of ropinirole. Therefore, if therapy with a drug known to be a potent inducer or inhibitor of CYP1A2 is stopped or started during treatment with ropinirole, adjustment of the dose of ropinirole may be required).
No products indexed under this heading.

Fluticasone Propionate (*In vitro* metabolism studies showed that CYP1A2 is the major enzyme responsible for the metabolism of ropinirole. There is thus the potential for inducers or inhibitors of this enzyme to alter the clearance of ropinirole. Therefore, if therapy with a drug known to be a potent inducer or inhibitor of CYP1A2 is stopped or started during treatment with ropinirole, adjustment of the dose of ropinirole may be required). Products include:

Fluvoxamine (Because of possible additive effects, caution should be advised when patients are taking other sedating medications, alcohol, or other CNS depressants (eg, benzodiazepines, antipsychotics, antidepressants) in combination with ropinirole).
No products indexed under this heading.

Fluvoxamine Maleate (Because of possible additive effects, caution should be advised when patients are taking other sedating medications, alcohol, or other CNS depressants (eg, benzodiazepines, antipsychotics, antidepressants) in combination with ropinirole).
No products indexed under this heading.

Gatifloxacin (In vitro metabolism studies showed that CYP1A2 is the major enzyme responsible for the metabolism of ropinirole. There is thus the potential for inducers or inhibitors of this enzyme to alter the clearance of ropinirole. Therefore, if therapy with a drug known to be a potent inducer or inhibitor of CYP1A2 is stopped or started during treatment with ropinirole, adjustment of the dose of ropinirole may be required).
No products indexed under this heading.

Gemifloxacin Mesylate (In vitro metabolism studies showed that CYP1A2 is the major enzyme responsible for the metabolism of ropinirole. There is thus the potential for inducers or inhibitors of this enzyme to alter the clearance of ropinirole. Therefore, if therapy with a drug known to be a potent inducer or inhibitor of CYP1A2 is stopped or started during treatment with ropinirole, adjustment of the dose of ropinirole may be required).
No products indexed under this heading.

Glutethimide (Sedating medications (such as alcohol or CNS depressants), may increase the risk of somnlence or falling asleep while engaged in activities of daily living. Because of possible additive effects, caution should be advised when patients are taking other sedating medications, alcohol, or other CNS depressants (eg, benzodiazepines, antipsychotics, antidepressants) in combination with ropinirole).
No products indexed under this heading.

Grepafloxacin Hydrochloride (In vitro metabolism studies showed that CYP1A2 is the major enzyme responsible for the metabolism of ropinirole. There is thus the potential for inducers or inhibitors of this enzyme to alter the clearance of ropinirole. Therefore, if therapy with a drug known to be a potent inducer or inhibitor of CYP1A2 is stopped or started during treatment with ropinirole, adjustment of the dose of ropinirole may be required).
No products indexed under this heading.

Halazepam (Sedating medications (such as alcohol or CNS depressants), may increase the risk of somnlence or falling asleep while engaged in activities of daily living. Because of possible additive effects, caution should be advised when patients are taking other sedating medications, alcohol, or other CNS depressants (eg, benzodiazepines, antipsychotics, antidepressants) in combination with ropinirole).
No products indexed under this heading.

Haloperidol (Sedating medications (such as alcohol or CNS depressants), may increase the risk of somnlence or falling asleep while engaged in activities of daily living. Because of possible additive effects, caution should be advised when patients are taking other sedating medications, alcohol, or other CNS depressants (eg, benzodiazepines, antipsychotics, antidepressants) in combination with ropinirole).
No products indexed under this heading.

Haloperidol Decanoate (Sedating medications (such as alcohol or CNS

depressants), may increase the risk of somnlence or falling asleep while engaged in activities of daily living. Because of possible additive effects, caution should be advised when patients are taking other sedating medications, alcohol, or other CNS depressants (eg, benzodiazepines, antipsychotics, antidepressants) in combination with ropinirole).
No products indexed under this heading.

Haloperidol Lactate (Sedating medications (such as alcohol or CNS depressants), may increase the risk of somnlence or falling asleep while engaged in activities of daily living. Because of possible additive effects, caution should be advised when patients are taking other sedating medications, alcohol, or other CNS depressants (eg, benzodiazepines, antipsychotics, antidepressants) in combination with ropinirole).
No products indexed under this heading.

Hexobarbital (Sedating medications (such as alcohol or CNS depressants), may increase the risk of somnlence or falling asleep while engaged in activities of daily living. Because of possible additive effects, caution should be advised when patients are taking other sedating medications, alcohol, or other CNS depressants (eg, benzodiazepines, antipsychotics, antidepressants) in combination with ropinirole).
No products indexed under this heading.

Hydrocodone Bitartrate (Sedating medications (such as alcohol or CNS depressants), may increase the risk of somnlence or falling asleep while engaged in activities of daily living. Because of possible additive effects, caution should be advised when patients are taking other sedating medications, alcohol, or other CNS depressants (eg, benzodiazepines, antipsychotics, antidepressants) in combination with ropinirole). Products include:

Hydrocodone Polistirex (Sedating medications (such as alcohol or CNS depressants), may increase the risk of somnlence or falling asleep while engaged in activities of daily living. Because of possible additive effects, caution should be advised when patients are taking other sedating medications, alcohol, or other CNS depressants (eg, benzodiazepines, antipsychotics, antidepressants) in combination with ropinirole). Products include:

Hydromorphone (Sedating medications (such as alcohol or CNS depressants), may increase the risk of somnlence or falling asleep while engaged in activities of daily living. Because of possible additive effects, caution should be advised when patients are taking other sedating medications, alcohol, or other CNS depressants (eg, benzodiazepines, antipsychotics, antidepressants) in combination with ropinirole).
No products indexed under this heading.

Hydromorphone Hydrochloride (Sedating medications (such as alcohol or CNS depressants), may increase the risk of somnlence or falling asleep while engaged in activities of daily living. Because of possible additive effects, caution should be advised when patients are taking other sedating medications, alcohol, or other CNS depressants (eg, benzodiazepines, antipsychotics, antidepressants) in combination with ropinirole). Products include:

Hydroxyzine Hydrochloride (Sedating medications (such as alcohol or CNS depressants), may increase the risk of somnlence or falling asleep while engaged in activities of daily living. Because of possible additive effects, caution should be advised when patients are taking other sedating medications, alcohol, or other CNS depressants (eg, benzodiazepines, antipsychotics, antidepressants) in combination with ropinirole).
No products indexed under this heading.

Hypericum (In vitro metabolism studies showed that CYP1A2 is the major enzyme responsible for the metabolism of ropinirole. There is thus the potential for inducers or inhibitors of this enzyme to alter the clearance of ropinirole. Therefore, if therapy with a drug known to be a potent inducer or inhibitor of CYP1A2 is stopped or started during treatment with ropinirole, adjustment of the dose of ropinirole may be required).
No products indexed under this heading.

Hypericum Perforatum (In vitro metabolism studies showed that CYP1A2 is the major enzyme responsible for the metabolism of ropinirole. There is thus the potential for inducers or inhibitors of this enzyme to alter the clearance of ropinirole. Therefore, if therapy with a drug known to be a potent inducer or inhibitor of CYP1A2 is stopped or started during treatment with ropinirole, adjustment of the dose of ropinirole may be required). Products include:

Imipramine Hydrochloride (Because of possible additive effects, caution should be advised when patients are taking other sedating medications, alcohol, or other CNS depressants (eg, benzodiazepines, antipsychotics, antidepressants) in combination with ropinirole).
No products indexed under this heading.

Imipramine Pamoate (Because of possible additive effects, caution should be advised when patients are taking other sedating medications, alcohol, or other CNS depressants (eg, benzodiazepines, antipsychotics, antidepressants) in combination with ropinirole).
No products indexed under this heading.

Insulin (In vitro metabolism studies showed that CYP1A2 is the major enzyme responsible for the metabolism of ropinirole. There is thus the potential for inducers or inhibitors of this enzyme to alter the clearance of ropinirole. Therefore, if therapy with a drug known to be a potent inducer or inhibitor of CYP1A2 is stopped or started during treatment with ropinirole, adjustment of the dose of ropinirole may be required).
No products indexed under this heading.

Insulin, Human, Zinc Suspension (In vitro metabolism studies showed that CYP1A2 is the major enzyme responsible for the metabolism of ropinirole. There is thus the potential for inducers or inhibitors of this enzyme to alter the clearance of ropinirole. Therefore, if therapy with a drug known to be a potent inducer or inhibitor of CYP1A2 is stopped or started during treatment with ropinirole, adjustment of the dose of ropinirole may be required).
No products indexed under this heading.

Insulin, Human (rDNA origin) (In vitro metabolism studies showed that CYP1A2 is the major enzyme responsible for the metabolism of ropinirole. There is thus the potential for inducers or inhibitors of this enzyme to alter the clearance of ropinirole. Therefore, if

therapy with a drug known to be a potent inducer or inhibitor of CYP1A2 is stopped or started during treatment with ropinirole, adjustment of the dose of ropinirole may be required). Products include:

Insulin, Human NPH (In vitro metabolism studies showed that CYP1A2 is the major enzyme responsible for the metabolism of ropinirole. There is thus the potential for inducers or inhibitors of this enzyme to alter the clearance of ropinirole. Therefore, if therapy with a drug known to be a potent inducer or inhibitor of CYP1A2 is stopped or started during treatment with ropinirole, adjustment of the dose of ropinirole may be required). Products include:

Insulin, Human Regular (In vitro metabolism studies showed that CYP1A2 is the major enzyme responsible for the metabolism of ropinirole. There is thus the potential for inducers or inhibitors of this enzyme to alter the clearance of ropinirole. Therefore, if therapy with a drug known to be a potent inducer or inhibitor of CYP1A2 is stopped or started during treatment with ropinirole, adjustment of the dose of ropinirole may be required). Products include:

Insulin, Human Regular and Human NPH Mixture (In vitro metabolism studies showed that CYP1A2 is the major enzyme responsible for the metabolism of ropinirole. There is thus the potential for inducers or inhibitors of this enzyme to alter the clearance of ropinirole. Therefore, if therapy with a drug known to be a potent inducer or inhibitor of CYP1A2 is stopped or started during treatment with ropinirole, adjustment of the dose of ropinirole may be required). Products include:

Insulin, NPH (In vitro metabolism studies showed that CYP1A2 is the major enzyme responsible for the metabolism of ropinirole. There is thus the potential for inducers or inhibitors of this enzyme to alter the clearance of ropinirole. Therefore, if therapy with a drug known to be a potent inducer or inhibitor of CYP1A2 is stopped or started during treatment with ropinirole, adjustment of the dose of ropinirole may be required).
No products indexed under this heading.

Insulin, Regular (In vitro metabolism studies showed that CYP1A2 is the major enzyme responsible for the metabolism of ropinirole. There is thus the potential for inducers or inhibitors of this enzyme to alter the clearance of ropinirole. Therefore, if therapy with a drug known to be a potent inducer or inhibitor of CYP1A2 is stopped or started during treatment with ropinirole, adjustment of the dose of ropinirole may be required).
No products indexed under this heading.

Insulin, Regular and NPH mixture (In vitro metabolism studies showed that CYP1A2 is the major enzyme responsible for the metabolism of ropinirole. There is thus the potential for inducers or inhibitors of this enzyme to alter the clearance of ropinirole. Therefore, if therapy with a drug known to be a potent inducer or inhibitor of CYP1A2 is stopped or started during treatment with ropinirole, adjustment of the dose of ropinirole may be required).
No products indexed under this heading.

Insulin, Zinc Crystals (In vitro metabolism studies showed that CYP1A2 is the major enzyme responsible for the metabolism of ropinirole. There is thus the potential for inducers or inhibitors of

IMPORTANT NOTE: Always consult each drug listing in the patient's regimen for possible interactions.

this enzyme to alter the clearance of ropinirole. Therefore, if therapy with a drug known to be a potent inducer or inhibitor of CYP1A2 is stopped or started during treatment with ropinirole, adjustment of the dose of ropinirole may be required).

No products indexed under this heading.

Insulin, Zinc Suspension (In vitro metabolism studies showed that CYP1A2 is the major enzyme responsible for the metabolism of ropinirole. There is thus the potential for inducers or inhibitors of this enzyme to alter the clearance of ropinirole. Therefore, if therapy with a drug known to be a potent inducer or inhibitor of CYP1A2 is stopped or started during treatment with ropinirole, adjustment of the dose of ropinirole may be required).

No products indexed under this heading.

Insulin Aspart (In vitro metabolism studies showed that CYP1A2 is the major enzyme responsible for the metabolism of ropinirole. There is thus the potential for inducers or inhibitors of this enzyme to alter the clearance of ropinirole. Therefore, if therapy with a drug known to be a potent inducer or inhibitor of CYP1A2 is stopped or started during treatment with ropinirole, adjustment of the dose of ropinirole may be required).

No products indexed under this heading.

Insulin Aspart, Human (In vitro metabolism studies showed that CYP1A2 is the major enzyme responsible for the metabolism of ropinirole. There is thus the potential for inducers or inhibitors of this enzyme to alter the clearance of ropinirole. Therefore, if therapy with a drug known to be a potent inducer or inhibitor of CYP1A2 is stopped or started during treatment with ropinirole, adjustment of the dose of ropinirole may be required). Products include:

NovoLog Mix 70/30 2581

Insulin Aspart, Human Regular (In vitro metabolism studies showed that CYP1A2 is the major enzyme responsible for the metabolism of ropinirole. There is thus the potential for inducers or inhibitors of this enzyme to alter the clearance of ropinirole. Therefore, if therapy with a drug known to be a potent inducer or inhibitor of CYP1A2 is stopped or started during treatment with ropinirole, adjustment of the dose of ropinirole may be required). Products include:

NovoLog 2575

Insulin Aspart Protamine, Human (In vitro metabolism studies showed that CYP1A2 is the major enzyme responsible for the metabolism of ropinirole. There is thus the potential for inducers or inhibitors of this enzyme to alter the clearance of ropinirole. Therefore, if therapy with a drug known to be a potent inducer or inhibitor of CYP1A2 is stopped or started during treatment with ropinirole, adjustment of the dose of ropinirole may be required). Products include:

NovoLog Mix 70/30 2581

Insulin Detemir (rDNA Origin) (In vitro metabolism studies showed that CYP1A2 is the major enzyme responsible for the metabolism of ropinirole. There is thus the potential for inducers or inhibitors of this enzyme to alter the clearance of ropinirole. Therefore, if therapy with a drug known to be a potent inducer or inhibitor of CYP1A2 is stopped or started during treatment with ropinirole, adjustment of the dose of ropinirole may be required). Products include:

Levemir 2566

Insulin Glargine (In vitro metabolism studies showed that CYP1A2 is the major enzyme responsible for the

metabolism of ropinirole. There is thus the potential for inducers or inhibitors of this enzyme to alter the clearance of ropinirole. Therefore, if therapy with a drug known to be a potent inducer or inhibitor of CYP1A2 is stopped or started during treatment with ropinirole, adjustment of the dose of ropinirole may be required). Products include:

Lantus 2996

Insulin Glulisine (In vitro metabolism studies showed that CYP1A2 is the major enzyme responsible for the metabolism of ropinirole. There is thus the potential for inducers or inhibitors of this enzyme to alter the clearance of ropinirole. Therefore, if therapy with a drug known to be a potent inducer or inhibitor of CYP1A2 is stopped or started during treatment with ropinirole, adjustment of the dose of ropinirole may be required). Products include:

Apidra 2937
Apidra SoloStar 2937

Insulin Lispro, Human (In vitro metabolism studies showed that CYP1A2 is the major enzyme responsible for the metabolism of ropinirole. There is thus the potential for inducers or inhibitors of this enzyme to alter the clearance of ropinirole. Therefore, if therapy with a drug known to be a potent inducer or inhibitor of CYP1A2 is stopped or started during treatment with ropinirole, adjustment of the dose of ropinirole may be required). Products include:

Humalog 1910
Humalog Mix 1914
Humalog Mix75/25 1917

Insulin Lispro Protamine, Human (In vitro metabolism studies showed that CYP1A2 is the major enzyme responsible for the metabolism of ropinirole. There is thus the potential for inducers or inhibitors of this enzyme to alter the clearance of ropinirole. Therefore, if therapy with a drug known to be a potent inducer or inhibitor of CYP1A2 is stopped or started during treatment with ropinirole, adjustment of the dose of ropinirole may be required). Products include:

Humalog Mix 1914
Humalog Mix75/25 1917

Isocarboxazid (Because of possible additive effects, caution should be advised when patients are taking other sedating medications, alcohol, or other CNS depressants (eg, benzodiazepines, antipsychotics, antidepressants) in combination with ropinirole). Products include:

Marplan 3481

Isoflurane (Sedating medications (such as alcohol or CNS depressants), may increase the risk of somnlence or falling asleep while engaged in activities of daily living. Because of possible additive effects, caution should be advised when patients are taking other sedating medications, alcohol, or other CNS depressants (eg, benzodiazepines, antipsychotics, antidepressants) in combination with ropinirole).

No products indexed under this heading.

Isoniazid (In vitro metabolism studies showed that CYP1A2 is the major enzyme responsible for the metabolism of ropinirole. There is thus the potential for inducers or inhibitors of this enzyme to alter the clearance of ropinirole. Therefore, if therapy with a drug known to be a potent inducer or inhibitor of CYP1A2 is stopped or started during treatment with ropinirole, adjustment of the dose of ropinirole may be required).

No products indexed under this heading.

Ketamine Hydrochloride (Sedating medications (such as alcohol or CNS depressants), may increase the risk of somnlence or falling asleep while engaged in activities of daily living.

Because of possible additive effects, caution should be advised when patients are taking other sedating medications, alcohol, or other CNS depressants (eg, benzodiazepines, antipsychotics, antidepressants) in combination with ropinirole).

No products indexed under this heading.

Ketoconazole (In vitro metabolism studies showed that CYP1A2 is the major enzyme responsible for the metabolism of ropinirole. There is thus the potential for inducers or inhibitors of this enzyme to alter the clearance of ropinirole. Therefore, if therapy with a drug known to be a potent inducer or inhibitor of CYP1A2 is stopped or started during treatment with ropinirole, adjustment of the dose of ropinirole may be required). Products include:

Extina 3319
Xolegel 3337

Lansoprazole (In vitro metabolism studies showed that CYP1A2 is the major enzyme responsible for the metabolism of ropinirole. There is thus the potential for inducers or inhibitors of this enzyme to alter the clearance of ropinirole. Therefore, if therapy with a drug known to be a potent inducer or inhibitor of CYP1A2 is stopped or started during treatment with ropinirole, adjustment of the dose of ropinirole may be required).

No products indexed under this heading.

Levobupivacaine Hydrochloride (In vitro metabolism studies showed that CYP1A2 is the major enzyme responsible for the metabolism of ropinirole. There is thus the potential for inducers or inhibitors of this enzyme to alter the clearance of ropinirole. Therefore, if therapy with a drug known to be a potent inducer or inhibitor of CYP1A2 is stopped or started during treatment with ropinirole, adjustment of the dose of ropinirole may be required).

No products indexed under this heading.

Levodopa (Co-administration of carbidopa+L-dopa (Sinemet) with immediate-release ropinirole had no effect on the steady-state pharmacokinetics of ropinirole. Oral administration of immediate-release ropinirole increased mean steady-state C_{max} of L-dopa by 20%, but its AUC was unaffected. The incidence of hallucination is increased in patients over age 65. Co-administration of entacapone and L-dopa with ropinirole may also increase the risk of hallucination. In a placebo-controlled clinical trial, hallucination occured in 0 of 43 patients taking entacapone plus L-dopa, in 9 of 155 patients taking ropinirole plus L-dopa (6%), and in 7 of 47 patients taking entacapone with ropinirole plus L-dopa (15%). Ropinirole may potentiate the dopaminergic side effects of L-dopa and may cause and/or exacerbate pre-existing dyskinesia in patients treated with L-dopa for Parkinson's disease. Decreasing the dose of a dopaminergic drug may ameliorate this side effect). Products include:

Stalevo 2526

Levofloxacin (In vitro metabolism studies showed that CYP1A2 is the major enzyme responsible for the metabolism of ropinirole. There is thus the potential for inducers or inhibitors of this enzyme to alter the clearance of ropinirole. Therefore, if therapy with a drug known to be a potent inducer or inhibitor of CYP1A2 is stopped or started during treatment with ropinirole, adjustment of the dose of ropinirole may be required). Products include:

Iquix 3492
Levaquin 2629
Levaquin in 5% Dextrose 2629
Quixin 3493

Levomethadyl Acetate Hydrochloride (Sedating medications (such as alcohol or CNS depressants), may increase the risk of somnlence or falling asleep while engaged in activities of daily living. Because of possible additive effects, caution should be advised when patients are taking other sedating medications, alcohol, or other CNS depressants (eg, benzodiazepines, antipsychotics, antidepressants) in combination with ropinirole).

No products indexed under this heading.

Levonorgestrel (In vitro metabolism studies showed that CYP1A2 is the major enzyme responsible for the metabolism of ropinirole. There is thus the potential for inducers or inhibitors of this enzyme to alter the clearance of ropinirole. Therefore, if therapy with a drug known to be a potent inducer or inhibitor of CYP1A2 is stopped or started during treatment with ropinirole, adjustment of the dose of ropinirole may be required). Products include:

Climara Pro 847
LoSeasonique 3407
Lybrel 3514
Mirena 854
Plan B 3416
Seasonique 3418

Levorphanol Tartrate (Sedating medications (such as alcohol or CNS depressants), may increase the risk of somnlence or falling asleep while engaged in activities of daily living. Because of possible additive effects, caution should be advised when patients are taking other sedating medications, alcohol, or other CNS depressants (eg, benzodiazepines, antipsychotics, antidepressants) in combination with ropinirole).

No products indexed under this heading.

Lithium (Because of possible additive effects, caution should be advised when patients are taking other sedating medications, alcohol, or other CNS depressants (eg, antipsychotics) in combination with ropinirole).

No products indexed under this heading.

Lithium Carbonate (Because of possible additive effects, caution should be advised when patients are taking other sedating medications, alcohol, or other CNS depressants (eg, antipsychotics) in combination with ropinirole).

No products indexed under this heading.

Lithium Citrate (Because of possible additive effects, caution should be advised when patients are taking other sedating medications, alcohol, or other CNS depressants (eg, antipsychotics) in combination with ropinirole).

No products indexed under this heading.

Lomefloxacin Hydrochloride (In vitro metabolism studies showed that CYP1A2 is the major enzyme responsible for the metabolism of ropinirole. There is thus the potential for inducers or inhibitors of this enzyme to alter the clearance of ropinirole. Therefore, if therapy with a drug known to be a potent inducer or inhibitor of CYP1A2 is stopped or started during treatment with ropinirole, adjustment of the dose of ropinirole may be required).

No products indexed under this heading.

Lorazepam (Sedating medications (such as alcohol or CNS depressants), may increase the risk of somnlence or falling asleep while engaged in activities of daily living. Because of possible additive effects, caution should be advised when patients are taking other sedating medications, alcohol, or other CNS depressants (eg, benzodiazepines, antipsychotics, antidepressants) in combination with ropinirole).

No products indexed under this heading.

Loxapine Hydrochloride (Sedating medications (such as alcohol or CNS

depressants), may increase the risk of somnlence or falling asleep while engaged in activities of daily living. Because of possible additive effects, caution should be advised when patients are taking other sedating medications, alcohol, or other CNS depressants (eg, benzodiazepines, antipsychotics, antidepressants) in combination with ropinirole).

No products indexed under this heading.

Loxapine Succinate (Sedating medications (such as alcohol or CNS depressants), may increase the risk of somnlence or falling asleep while engaged in activities of daily living. Because of possible additive effects, caution should be advised when patients are taking other sedating medications, alcohol, or other CNS depressants (eg, benzodiazepines, antipsychotics, antidepressants) in combination with ropinirole).

No products indexed under this heading.

Maprotiline Hydrochloride (Because of possible additive effects, caution should be advised when patients are taking other sedating medications, alcohol, or other CNS depressants (eg, benzodiazepines, antipsychotics, antidepressants) in combination with ropinirole).

No products indexed under this heading.

Meperidine Hydrochloride (Sedating medications (such as alcohol or CNS depressants), may increase the risk of somnlence or falling asleep while engaged in activities of daily living. Because of possible additive effects, caution should be advised when patients are taking other sedating medications, alcohol, or other CNS depressants (eg, benzodiazepines, antipsychotics, antidepressants) in combination with ropinirole).

No products indexed under this heading.

Mephobarbital (Sedating medications (such as alcohol or CNS depressants), may increase the risk of somnlence or falling asleep while engaged in activities of daily living. Because of possible additive effects, caution should be advised when patients are taking other sedating medications, alcohol, or other CNS depressants (eg, benzodiazepines, antipsychotics, antidepressants) in combination with ropinirole).

No products indexed under this heading.

Meprobamate (Sedating medications (such as alcohol or CNS depressants), may increase the risk of somnlence or falling asleep while engaged in activities of daily living. Because of possible additive effects, caution should be advised when patients are taking other sedating medications, alcohol, or other CNS depressants (eg, benzodiazepines, antipsychotics, antidepressants) in combination with ropinirole).

No products indexed under this heading.

Mesoridazine Besylate (Sedating medications (such as alcohol or CNS depressants), may increase the risk of somnlence or falling asleep while engaged in activities of daily living. Because of possible additive effects, caution should be advised when patients are taking other sedating medications, alcohol, or other CNS depressants (eg, benzodiazepines, antipsychotics, antidepressants) in combination with ropinirole).

No products indexed under this heading.

Mestranol (In vitro metabolism studies showed that CYP1A2 is the major enzyme responsible for the metabolism of ropinirole. There is thus the potential for inducers or inhibitors of this enzyme to alter the clearance of ropinirole. Therefore, if therapy with a drug known to be a potent inducer or inhibitor of CYP1A2 is stopped or started during

treatment with ropinirole, adjustment of the dose of ropinirole may be required).

No products indexed under this heading.

Methadone Hydrochloride (Sedating medications (such as alcohol or CNS depressants), may increase the risk of somnlence or falling asleep while engaged in activities of daily living. Because of possible additive effects, caution should be advised when patients are taking other sedating medications, alcohol, or other CNS depressants (eg, benzodiazepines, antipsychotics, antidepressants) in combination with ropinirole).

No products indexed under this heading.

Methdilazine Hydrochloride (Before initiating treatment patients should be advised of the potential to develop drowsiness and specifically asked about factors that may increase the risk such as concomitant sedating medications. If a patient develops significant daytime sleepiness or episodes of falling asleep during activities that require active participation (eg, conversations, eating, etc.), therapy should ordinarily be discontinued. If a decision is made to continue, patients should be advised to not drive and to avoid other potentially dangerous activities).

No products indexed under this heading.

Methohexital Sodium (Sedating medications (such as alcohol or CNS depressants), may increase the risk of somnlence or falling asleep while engaged in activities of daily living. Because of possible additive effects, caution should be advised when patients are taking other sedating medications, alcohol, or other CNS depressants (eg, benzodiazepines, antipsychotics, antidepressants) in combination with ropinirole).

No products indexed under this heading.

Methotrimeprazine (Sedating medications (such as alcohol or CNS depressants), may increase the risk of somnlence or falling asleep while engaged in activities of daily living. Because of possible additive effects, caution should be advised when patients are taking other sedating medications, alcohol, or other CNS depressants (eg, benzodiazepines, antipsychotics, antidepressants) in combination with ropinirole).

No products indexed under this heading.

Methoxsalen (In vitro metabolism studies showed that CYP1A2 is the major enzyme responsible for the metabolism of ropinirole. There is thus the potential for inducers or inhibitors of this enzyme to alter the clearance of ropinirole. Therefore, if therapy with a drug known to be a potent inducer or inhibitor of CYP1A2 is stopped or started during treatment with ropinirole, adjustment of the dose of ropinirole may be required).

No products indexed under this heading.

Methoxyflurane (Sedating medications (such as alcohol or CNS depressants), may increase the risk of somnlence or falling asleep while engaged in activities of daily living. Because of possible additive effects, caution should be advised when patients are taking other sedating medications, alcohol, or other CNS depressants (eg, benzodiazepines, antipsychotics, antidepressants) in combination with ropinirole).

No products indexed under this heading.

Metoclopramide Hydrochloride (Since ropinirole is a dopamine agonist, it is possible that dopamine antagonists such as neuroleptics (eg, phenothiazines, butyrophenones, thioxanthenes) or metoclopramide hydrochloride may diminish the effectiveness of ropinirole. Patients with a history or presence of major psychotic disorders should be

treated with dopamine agonists only if the potential benefits outweigh the risks). Products include:
Metozolv ODT 2901

Mexiletine Hydrochloride (In vitro metabolism studies showed that CYP1A2 is the major enzyme responsible for the metabolism of ropinirole. There is thus the potential for inducers or inhibitors of this enzyme to alter the clearance of ropinirole. Therefore, if therapy with a drug known to be a potent inducer or inhibitor of CYP1A2 is stopped or started during treatment with ropinirole, adjustment of the dose of ropinirole may be required).

No products indexed under this heading.

Mibefradil Dihydrochloride (In vitro metabolism studies showed that CYP1A2 is the major enzyme responsible for the metabolism of ropinirole. There is thus the potential for inducers or inhibitors of this enzyme to alter the clearance of ropinirole. Therefore, if therapy with a drug known to be a potent inducer or inhibitor of CYP1A2 is stopped or started during treatment with ropinirole, adjustment of the dose of ropinirole may be required).

No products indexed under this heading.

Midazolam Hydrochloride (Sedating medications (such as alcohol or CNS depressants), may increase the risk of somnlence or falling asleep while engaged in activities of daily living. Because of possible additive effects, caution should be advised when patients are taking other sedating medications, alcohol, or other CNS depressants (eg, benzodiazepines, antipsychotics, antidepressants) in combination with ropinirole).

No products indexed under this heading.

Mirtazapine (Because of possible additive effects, caution should be advised when patients are taking other sedating medications, alcohol, or other CNS depressants (eg, benzodiazepines, antipsychotics, antidepressants) in combination with ropinirole). Products include:
Remeron Tablets 3214
RemeronSolTab Tablets 3219

Molindone Hydrochloride (Sedating medications (such as alcohol or CNS depressants), may increase the risk of somnlence or falling asleep while engaged in activities of daily living. Because of possible additive effects, caution should be advised when patients are taking other sedating medications, alcohol, or other CNS depressants (eg, benzodiazepines, antipsychotics, antidepressants) in combination with ropinirole). Products include:
Moban 1108

Morphine Sulfate (Sedating medications (such as alcohol or CNS depressants), may increase the risk of somnlence or falling asleep while engaged in activities of daily living. Because of possible additive effects, caution should be advised when patients are taking other sedating medications, alcohol, or other CNS depressants (eg, benzodiazepines, antipsychotics, antidepressants) in combination with ropinirole). Products include:
Avinza 1822
Embeda 1831
MS Contin 2803

Morphine Sulfate, Liposomal (Sedating medications (such as alcohol or CNS depressants), may increase the risk of somnlence or falling asleep while engaged in activities of daily living. Because of possible additive effects, caution should be advised when patients are taking other sedating medications, alcohol, or other CNS depres-

sants (eg, benzodiazepines, antipsychotics, antidepressants) in combination with ropinirole).

No products indexed under this heading.

Moxifloxacin Hydrochloride (In vitro metabolism studies showed that CYP1A2 is the major enzyme responsible for the metabolism of ropinirole. There is thus the potential for inducers or inhibitors of this enzyme to alter the clearance of ropinirole. Therefore, if therapy with a drug known to be a potent inducer or inhibitor of CYP1A2 is stopped or started during treatment with ropinirole, adjustment of the dose of ropinirole may be required). Products include:
Avelox 3064
Vigamox 589

Nafcillin Sodium (In vitro metabolism studies showed that CYP1A2 is the major enzyme responsible for the metabolism of ropinirole. There is thus the potential for inducers or inhibitors of this enzyme to alter the clearance of ropinirole. Therefore, if therapy with a drug known to be a potent inducer or inhibitor of CYP1A2 is stopped or started during treatment with ropinirole, adjustment of the dose of ropinirole may be required).

No products indexed under this heading.

Nalidixic Acid (In vitro metabolism studies showed that CYP1A2 is the major enzyme responsible for the metabolism of ropinirole. There is thus the potential for inducers or inhibitors of this enzyme to alter the clearance of ropinirole. Therefore, if therapy with a drug known to be a potent inducer or inhibitor of CYP1A2 is stopped or started during treatment with ropinirole, adjustment of the dose of ropinirole may be required).

No products indexed under this heading.

Naproxen (In vitro metabolism studies showed that CYP1A2 is the major enzyme responsible for the metabolism of ropinirole. There is thus the potential for inducers or inhibitors of this enzyme to alter the clearance of ropinirole. Therefore, if therapy with a drug known to be a potent inducer or inhibitor of CYP1A2 is stopped or started during treatment with ropinirole, adjustment of the dose of ropinirole may be required). Products include:
EC-Naprosyn 2850
Naprosyn 2850
Anaprox/Naprosyn 2850

Naproxen Sodium (In vitro metabolism studies showed that CYP1A2 is the major enzyme responsible for the metabolism of ropinirole. There is thus the potential for inducers or inhibitors of this enzyme to alter the clearance of ropinirole. Therefore, if therapy with a drug known to be a potent inducer or inhibitor of CYP1A2 is stopped or started during treatment with ropinirole, adjustment of the dose of ropinirole may be required). Products include:
Anaprox 2850
Anaprox DS 2850
Treximet 1681

Nefazodone Hydrochloride (Because of possible additive effects, caution should be advised when patients are taking other sedating medications, alcohol, or other CNS depressants (eg, benzodiazepines, antipsychotics, antidepressants) in combination with ropinirole).

No products indexed under this heading.

Nicotine (In vitro metabolism studies showed that CYP1A2 is the major enzyme responsible for the metabolism of ropinirole. There is thus the potential for inducers or inhibitors of this enzyme to alter the clearance of ropinirole. Therefore, if therapy with a drug known to be a potent inducer or inhibitor of CYP1A2 is stopped or started during

treatment with ropinirole, adjustment of the dose of ropinirole may be required).
No products indexed under this heading.

Nicotine Polacrilex (*In vitro* metabolism studies showed that CYP1A2 is the major enzyme responsible for the metabolism of ropinirole. There is thus the potential for inducers or inhibitors of this enzyme to alter the clearance of ropinirole. Therefore, if therapy with a drug known to be a potent inducer or inhibitor of CYP1A2 is stopped or started during treatment with ropinirole, adjustment of the dose of ropinirole may be required).
No products indexed under this heading.

Nicotine Salicylate (*In vitro* metabolism studies showed that CYP1A2 is the major enzyme responsible for the metabolism of ropinirole. There is thus the potential for inducers or inhibitors of this enzyme to alter the clearance of ropinirole. Therefore, if therapy with a drug known to be a potent inducer or inhibitor of CYP1A2 is stopped or started during treatment with ropinirole, adjustment of the dose of ropinirole may be required).
No products indexed under this heading.

Nicotine Sulfate (*In vitro* metabolism studies showed that CYP1A2 is the major enzyme responsible for the metabolism of ropinirole. There is thus the potential for inducers or inhibitors of this enzyme to alter the clearance of ropinirole. Therefore, if therapy with a drug known to be a potent inducer or inhibitor of CYP1A2 is stopped or started during treatment with ropinirole, adjustment of the dose of ropinirole may be required).
No products indexed under this heading.

Norethindrone (*In vitro* metabolism studies showed that CYP1A2 is the major enzyme responsible for the metabolism of ropinirole. There is thus the potential for inducers or inhibitors of this enzyme to alter the clearance of ropinirole. Therefore, if therapy with a drug known to be a potent inducer or inhibitor of CYP1A2 is stopped or started during treatment with ropinirole, adjustment of the dose of ropinirole may be required). Products include:

Norethindrone Acetate (*In vitro* metabolism studies showed that CYP1A2 is the major enzyme responsible for the metabolism of ropinirole. There is thus the potential for inducers or inhibitors of this enzyme to alter the clearance of ropinirole. Therefore, if therapy with a drug known to be a potent inducer or inhibitor of CYP1A2 is stopped or started during treatment with ropinirole, adjustment of the dose of ropinirole may be required). Products include:

Norfloxacin (*In vitro* metabolism studies showed that CYP1A2 is the major enzyme responsible for the metabolism of ropinirole. There is thus the potential for inducers or inhibitors of this enzyme to alter the clearance of ropinirole. Therefore, if therapy with a drug known to be a potent inducer or inhibitor of CYP1A2 is stopped or started during treatment with ropinirole, adjustment of the dose of ropinirole may be required). Products include:

Norgestrel (*In vitro* metabolism studies showed that CYP1A2 is the major enzyme responsible for the metabolism of ropinirole. There is thus the potential for inducers or inhibitors of this enzyme to alter the clearance of ropinirole. Therefore, if therapy with a drug known to be a potent inducer or inhibitor of CYP1A2 is stopped or started during

treatment with ropinirole, adjustment of the dose of ropinirole may be required).
No products indexed under this heading.

Nortriptyline Hydrochloride (Because of possible additive effects, caution should be advised when patients are taking other sedating medications, alcohol, or other CNS depressants (eg, benzodiazepines, antipsychotics, antidepressants) in combination with ropinirole).
No products indexed under this heading.

Ofloxacin (*In vitro* metabolism studies showed that CYP1A2 is the major enzyme responsible for the metabolism of ropinirole. There is thus the potential for inducers or inhibitors of this enzyme to alter the clearance of ropinirole. Therefore, if therapy with a drug known to be a potent inducer or inhibitor of CYP1A2 is stopped or started during treatment with ropinirole, adjustment of the dose of ropinirole may be required).
No products indexed under this heading.

Olanzapine (Sedating medications (such as alcohol or CNS depressants), may increase the risk of somnlence or falling asleep while engaged in activities of daily living. Because of possible additive effects, caution should be advised when patients are taking other sedating medications, alcohol, or other CNS depressants (eg, benzodiazepines, antipsychotics, antidepressants) in combination with ropinirole). Products include:

Omeprazole (*In vitro* metabolism studies showed that CYP1A2 is the major enzyme responsible for the metabolism of ropinirole. There is thus the potential for inducers or inhibitors of this enzyme to alter the clearance of ropinirole. Therefore, if therapy with a drug known to be a potent inducer or inhibitor of CYP1A2 is stopped or started during treatment with ropinirole, adjustment of the dose of ropinirole may be required).
No products indexed under this heading.

Omeprazole Magnesium (*In vitro* metabolism studies showed that CYP1A2 is the major enzyme responsible for the metabolism of ropinirole. There is thus the potential for inducers or inhibitors of this enzyme to alter the clearance of ropinirole. Therefore, if therapy with a drug known to be a potent inducer or inhibitor of CYP1A2 is stopped or started during treatment with ropinirole, adjustment of the dose of ropinirole may be required).
No products indexed under this heading.

Ondansetron (*In vitro* metabolism studies showed that CYP1A2 is the major enzyme responsible for the metabolism of ropinirole. There is thus the potential for inducers or inhibitors of this enzyme to alter the clearance of ropinirole. Therefore, if therapy with a drug known to be a potent inducer or inhibitor of CYP1A2 is stopped or started during treatment with ropinirole, adjustment of the dose of ropinirole may be required).
No products indexed under this heading.

Ondansetron Hydrochloride (*In vitro* metabolism studies showed that CYP1A2 is the major enzyme responsible for the metabolism of ropinirole. There is thus the potential for inducers or inhibitors of this enzyme to alter the clearance of ropinirole. Therefore, if therapy with a drug known to be a potent inducer or inhibitor of CYP1A2 is stopped or started during treatment with ropinirole, adjustment of the dose of ropinirole may be required). Products include:

Oxazepam (Sedating medications (such as alcohol or CNS depressants), may increase the risk of somnlence or falling asleep while engaged in activities of daily living. Because of possible additive effects, caution should be advised when patients are taking other sedating medications, alcohol, or other CNS depressants (eg, benzodiazepines, antipsychotics, antidepressants) in combination with ropinirole).
No products indexed under this heading.

Oxycodone Hydrochloride (Sedating medications (such as alcohol or CNS depressants), may increase the risk of somnlence or falling asleep while engaged in activities of daily living. Because of possible additive effects, caution should be advised when patients are taking other sedating medications, alcohol, or other CNS depressants (eg, benzodiazepines, antipsychotics, antidepressants) in combination with ropinirole). Products include:

Oxycodone Terephthalate (Sedating medications (such as alcohol or CNS depressants), may increase the risk of somnlence or falling asleep while engaged in activities of daily living. Because of possible additive effects, caution should be advised when patients are taking other sedating medications, alcohol, or other CNS depressants (eg, benzodiazepines, antipsychotics, antidepressants) in combination with ropinirole).
No products indexed under this heading.

Oxymorphone Hydrochloride (Sedating medications (such as alcohol or CNS depressants), may increase the risk of somnlence or falling asleep while engaged in activities of daily living. Because of possible additive effects, caution should be advised when patients are taking other sedating medications, alcohol, or other CNS depressants (eg, benzodiazepines, antipsychotics, antidepressants) in combination with ropinirole). Products include:

Paliperidone (Because of possible additive effects, caution should be advised when patients are taking other sedating medications, alcohol, or other CNS depressants (eg, antipsychotics) in combination with ropinirole). Products include:

Paroxetine (Because of possible additive effects, caution should be advised when patients are taking other sedating medications, alcohol, or other CNS depressants (eg, benzodiazepines, antipsychotics, antidepressants) in combination with ropinirole).
No products indexed under this heading.

Paroxetine Hydrochloride (Because of possible additive effects, caution should be advised when patients are taking other sedating medications, alcohol, or other CNS depressants (eg, benzodiazepines, antipsychotics, antidepressants) in combination with ropinirole). Products include:

Paroxetine Mesylate (Because of possible additive effects, caution should be advised when patients are taking other sedating medications, alcohol, or other CNS depressants (eg, benzodiazepines, antipsychotics, antidepressants) in combination with ropinirole).
No products indexed under this heading.

Pentobarbital (Sedating medications (such as alcohol or CNS depressants), may increase the risk of somnlence or falling asleep while engaged in activities of daily living. Because of possible additive effects, caution should be advised when patients are taking other sedating medications, alcohol, or other CNS depressants (eg, benzodiazepines, antipsychotics, antidepressants) in combination with ropinirole).
No products indexed under this heading.

Pentobarbital Sodium (Sedating medications (such as alcohol or CNS depressants), may increase the risk of somnlence or falling asleep while engaged in activities of daily living. Because of possible additive effects, caution should be advised when patients are taking other sedating medications, alcohol, or other CNS depressants (eg, benzodiazepines, antipsychotics, antidepressants) in combination with ropinirole). Products include:

Perphenazine (Sedating medications (such as alcohol or CNS depressants), may increase the risk of somnlence or falling asleep while engaged in activities of daily living. Because of possible additive effects, caution should be advised when patients are taking other sedating medications, alcohol, or other CNS depressants (eg, benzodiazepines, antipsychotics, antidepressants) in combination with ropinirole).
No products indexed under this heading.

Phenelzine Sulfate (Because of possible additive effects, caution should be advised when patients are taking other sedating medications, alcohol, or other CNS depressants (eg, benzodiazepines, antipsychotics, antidepressants) in combination with ropinirole).
No products indexed under this heading.

Phenobarbital (Sedating medications (such as alcohol or CNS depressants), may increase the risk of somnlence or falling asleep while engaged in activities of daily living. Because of possible additive effects, caution should be advised when patients are taking other sedating medications, alcohol, or other CNS depressants (eg, benzodiazepines, antipsychotics, antidepressants) in combination with ropinirole). Products include:

Phenobarbital Sodium (Sedating medications (such as alcohol or CNS depressants), may increase the risk of somnlence or falling asleep while engaged in activities of daily living. Because of possible additive effects, caution should be advised when patients are taking other sedating medications, alcohol, or other CNS depressants (eg, benzodiazepines, antipsychotics, antidepressants) in combination with ropinirole).
No products indexed under this heading.

Phenothiazine Derivatives (Since ropinirole is a dopamine agonist, it is possible that dopamine antagonists such as neuroleptics (eg, phenothiazines, butyrophenones, thioxanthenes) or metoclopramide may diminish the effectiveness of ropinirole. Patients with a history or presence of major psychotic disorders should be treated with dopamine agonists only if the potential benefits outweigh the risks).
No products indexed under this heading.

(⊙ Described in PDR® for Ophthalmic Medicines)

1611 Interactions Index Requip XL

Phenothiazines (Since ropinirole is a dopamine agonist, it is possible that dopamine antagonists such as neuroleptics (eg, phenothiazines, butyrophenones, thioxanthenes) or metoclopramide may diminish the effectiveness of ropinirole. Patients with a history or presence of major psychotic disorders should be treated with dopamine agonists only if the potential benefits outweigh the risks).
No products indexed under this heading.

Phenytoin (*In vitro* metabolism studies showed that CYP1A2 is the major enzyme responsible for the metabolism of ropinirole. There is thus the potential for inducers or inhibitors of this enzyme to alter the clearance of ropinirole. Therefore, if therapy with a drug known to be a potent inducer or inhibitor of CYP1A2 is stopped or started during treatment with ropinirole, adjustment of the dose of ropinirole may be required).
No products indexed under this heading.

Phenytoin Sodium (*In vitro* metabolism studies showed that CYP1A2 is the major enzyme responsible for the metabolism of ropinirole. There is thus the potential for inducers or inhibitors of this enzyme to alter the clearance of ropinirole. Therefore, if therapy with a drug known to be a potent inducer or inhibitor of CYP1A2 is stopped or started during treatment with ropinirole, adjustment of the dose of ropinirole may be required). Products include:
Phenytek Capsules **2380**

Pimozide (Because of possible additive effects, caution should be advised when patients are taking other sedating medications, alcohol, or other CNS depressants (eg, antipsychotics) in combination with ropinirole).
No products indexed under this heading.

Polyestradiol Phosphate (Population pharmacokinetic analysis revealed that higher doses of estrogens (usually associated with hormone replacement therapy) reduced the oral clearance of ropinirole by approximately 35%. Dosage adjustment is not needed for initiating ropinirole in patients on estrogen therapy because patients are individually titrated with ropinirole to tolerance or adequate effect. If estrogen therapy is stopped or started during treatment with ropinirole, then adjustment of the dose of ropinirole may be required).
No products indexed under this heading.

Prazepam (Sedating medications (such as alcohol or CNS depressants), may increase the risk of somnlence or falling asleep while engaged in activities of daily living. Because of possible additive effects, caution should be advised when patients are taking other sedating medications, alcohol, or other CNS depressants (eg, benzodiazepines, antipsychotics, antidepressants) in combination with ropinirole).
No products indexed under this heading.

Primidone (*In vitro* metabolism studies showed that CYP1A2 is the major enzyme responsible for the metabolism of ropinirole. There is thus the potential for inducers or inhibitors of this enzyme to alter the clearance of ropinirole. Therefore, if therapy with a drug known to be a potent inducer or inhibitor of CYP1A2 is stopped or started during treatment with ropinirole, adjustment of the dose of ropinirole may be required).
No products indexed under this heading.

Prochlorperazine (Sedating medications (such as alcohol or CNS depressants), may increase the risk of somnlence or falling asleep while engaged in activities of daily living. Because of possible additive effects, caution should be advised when patients are taking other sedating medications, alcohol, or other CNS depressants (eg, benzodiazepines, antipsychotics, antidepressants) in combination with ropinirole).
No products indexed under this heading.

Prochlorperazine Edisylate (Sedating medications (such as alcohol or CNS depressants), may increase the risk of somnlence or falling asleep while engaged in activities of daily living. Because of possible additive effects, caution should be advised when patients are taking other sedating medications, alcohol, or other CNS depressants (eg, benzodiazepines, antipsychotics, antidepressants) in combination with ropinirole).
No products indexed under this heading.

Prochlorperazine Maleate (Sedating medications (such as alcohol or CNS depressants), may increase the risk of somnlence or falling asleep while engaged in activities of daily living. Because of possible additive effects, caution should be advised when patients are taking other sedating medications, alcohol, or other CNS depressants (eg, benzodiazepines, antipsychotics, antidepressants) in combination with ropinirole).
No products indexed under this heading.

Promethazine (Sedating medications (such as alcohol or CNS depressants), may increase the risk of somnlence or falling asleep while engaged in activities of daily living. Because of possible additive effects, caution should be advised when patients are taking other sedating medications, alcohol, or other CNS depressants (eg, benzodiazepines, antipsychotics, antidepressants) in combination with ropinirole).
No products indexed under this heading.

Promethazine Hydrochloride (Sedating medications (such as alcohol or CNS depressants), may increase the risk of somnlence or falling asleep while engaged in activities of daily living. Because of possible additive effects, caution should be advised when patients are taking other sedating medications, alcohol, or other CNS depressants (eg, benzodiazepines, antipsychotics, antidepressants) in combination with ropinirole).
No products indexed under this heading.

Propafenone Hydrochloride (*In vitro* metabolism studies showed that CYP1A2 is the major enzyme responsible for the metabolism of ropinirole. There is thus the potential for inducers or inhibitors of this enzyme to alter the clearance of ropinirole. Therefore, if therapy with a drug known to be a potent inducer or inhibitor of CYP1A2 is stopped or started during treatment with ropinirole, adjustment of the dose of ropinirole may be required). Products include:
Rythmol **1648**
Rythmol SR **1652**

Propofol (Sedating medications (such as alcohol or CNS depressants), may increase the risk of somnlence or falling asleep while engaged in activities of daily living. Because of possible additive effects, caution should be advised when patients are taking other sedating medications, alcohol, or other CNS depressants (eg, benzodiazepines, antipsychotics, antidepressants) in combination with ropinirole).
No products indexed under this heading.

Propoxyphene Hydrochloride (Sedating medications (such as alcohol or CNS depressants), may increase the risk of somnlence or falling asleep while engaged in activities of daily living. Because of possible additive effects, caution should be advised when patients are taking other sedating medications, alcohol, or other CNS depressants (eg, benzodiazepines, antipsychotics, antidepressants) in combination with ropinirole).
No products indexed under this heading.

Propoxyphene Napsylate (Sedating medications (such as alcohol or CNS depressants), may increase the risk of somnlence or falling asleep while engaged in activities of daily living. Because of possible additive effects, caution should be advised when patients are taking other sedating medications, alcohol, or other CNS depressants (eg, benzodiazepines, antipsychotics, antidepressants) in combination with ropinirole).
No products indexed under this heading.

Propranolol Hydrochloride (*In vitro* metabolism studies showed that CYP1A2 is the major enzyme responsible for the metabolism of ropinirole. There is thus the potential for inducers or inhibitors of this enzyme to alter the clearance of ropinirole. Therefore, if therapy with a drug known to be a potent inducer or inhibitor of CYP1A2 is stopped or started during treatment with ropinirole, adjustment of the dose of ropinirole may be required). Products include:
InnoPran XL **1517**

Protriptyline Hydrochloride (Because of possible additive effects, caution should be advised when patients are taking other sedating medications, alcohol, or other CNS depressants (eg, benzodiazepines, antipsychotics, antidepressants) in combination with ropinirole).
No products indexed under this heading.

Pyrilamine Maleate (Before initiating treatment patients should be advised of the potential to develop drowsiness and specifically asked about factors that may increase the risk such as concomitant sedating medications. If a patient develops significant daytime sleepiness or episodes of falling asleep during activities that require active participation (eg, conversations, eating, etc.), therapy should ordinarily be discontinued. If a decision is made to continue, patients should be advised to not drive and to avoid other potentially dangerous activities).
No products indexed under this heading.

Pyrilamine Tannate (Before initiating treatment patients should be advised of the potential to develop drowsiness and specifically asked about factors that may increase the risk such as concomitant sedating medications. If a patient develops significant daytime sleepiness or episodes of falling asleep during activities that require active participation (eg, conversations, eating, etc.), therapy should ordinarily be discontinued. If a decision is made to continue, patients should be advised to not drive and to avoid other potentially dangerous activities).
No products indexed under this heading.

Quazepam (Sedating medications (such as alcohol or CNS depressants), may increase the risk of somnlence or falling asleep while engaged in activities of daily living. Because of possible additive effects, caution should be advised when patients are taking other sedating medications, alcohol, or other CNS depressants (eg, benzodiazepines, antipsychotics, antidepressants) in combination with ropinirole).
No products indexed under this heading.

Quetiapine Fumarate (Sedating medications (such as alcohol or CNS depressants), may increase the risk of somnlence or falling asleep while engaged in activities of daily living. Because of possible additive effects, caution should be advised when patients are taking other sedating medications, alcohol, or other CNS depressants (eg, benzodiazepines, antipsychotics, antidepressants) in combination with ropinirole). Products include:
Seroquel **750**
Seroquel XR **759**

Quinestrol (Population pharmacokinetic analysis revealed that higher doses of estrogens (usually associated with hormone replacement therapy) reduced the oral clearance of ropinirole by approximately 35%. Dosage adjustment is not needed for initiating ropinirole in patients on estrogen therapy because patients are individually titrated with ropinirole to tolerance or adequate effect. If estrogen therapy is stopped or started during treatment with ropinirole, then adjustment of the dose of ropinirole may be required).
No products indexed under this heading.

Ramelteon (Before initiating treatment patients should be advised of the potential to develop drowsiness and specifically asked about factors that may increase the risk such as concomitant sedating medications. If a patient develops significant daytime sleepiness or episodes of falling asleep during activities that require active participation (eg, conversations, eating, etc.), therapy should ordinarily be discontinued. If a decision is made to continue, patients should be advised to not drive and to avoid other potentially dangerous activities). Products include:
Rozerem **3366**

Ranitidine Bismuth Citrate (*In vitro* metabolism studies showed that CYP1A2 is the major enzyme responsible for the metabolism of ropinirole. There is thus the potential for inducers or inhibitors of this enzyme to alter the clearance of ropinirole. Therefore, if therapy with a drug known to be a potent inducer or inhibitor of CYP1A2 is stopped or started during treatment with ropinirole, adjustment of the dose of ropinirole may be required).
No products indexed under this heading.

Ranitidine Hydrochloride (*In vitro* metabolism studies showed that CYP1A2 is the major enzyme responsible for the metabolism of ropinirole. There is thus the potential for inducers or inhibitors of this enzyme to alter the clearance of ropinirole. Therefore, if therapy with a drug known to be a potent inducer or inhibitor of CYP1A2 is stopped or started during treatment with ropinirole, adjustment of the dose of ropinirole may be required). Products include:
Zantac **1737**
Zantac Injection **1732**
Zantac Pharmacy **1735**

Remifentanil Hydrochloride (Sedating medications (such as alcohol or CNS depressants), may increase the risk of somnlence or falling asleep while engaged in activities of daily living. Because of possible additive effects, caution should be advised when patients are taking other sedating medications, alcohol, or other CNS depressants (eg, benzodiazepines, antipsychotics, antidepressants) in combination with ropinirole).
No products indexed under this heading.

Rifampicin (*In vitro* metabolism studies showed that CYP1A2 is the major enzyme responsible for the metabolism of ropinirole. There is thus the potential for inducers or inhibitors of this enzyme to alter the clearance of ropinirole. Therefore, if therapy with a drug known to be a potent inducer or inhibitor of CYP1A2 is stopped or started during treatment with ropinirole, adjustment of the dose of ropinirole may be required).
No products indexed under this heading.

Requip XL Interactions Index 1612

Rifampin (*In vitro* metabolism studies showed that CYP1A2 is the major enzyme responsible for the metabolism of ropinirole. There is thus the potential for inducers or inhibitors of this enzyme to alter the clearance of ropinirole. Therefore, if therapy with a drug known to be a potent inducer or inhibitor of CYP1A2 is stopped or started during treatment with ropinirole, adjustment of the dose of ropinirole may be required).
No products indexed under this heading.

Riluzole (*In vitro* metabolism studies showed that CYP1A2 is the major enzyme responsible for the metabolism of ropinirole. There is thus the potential for inducers or inhibitors of this enzyme to alter the clearance of ropinirole. Therefore, if therapy with a drug known to be a potent inducer or inhibitor of CYP1A2 is stopped or started during treatment with ropinirole, adjustment of the dose of ropinirole may be required). Products include:
Rilutek 3032

Risperidone (Sedating medications (such as alcohol or CNS depressants), may increase the risk of somnlence or falling asleep while engaged in activities of daily living. Because of possible additive effects, caution should be advised when patients are taking other sedating medications, alcohol, or other CNS depressants (eg, benzodiazepines, antipsychotics, antidepressants) in combination with ropinirole). Products include:
Risperdal Consta 2682

Ritonavir (*In vitro* metabolism studies showed that CYP1A2 is the major enzyme responsible for the metabolism of ropinirole. There is thus the potential for inducers or inhibitors of this enzyme to alter the clearance of ropinirole. Therefore, if therapy with a drug known to be a potent inducer or inhibitor of CYP1A2 is stopped or started during treatment with ropinirole, adjustment of the dose of ropinirole may be required). Products include:
Kaletra 458
Norvir 509

Ropivacaine Hydrochloride (*In vitro* metabolism studies showed that CYP1A2 is the major enzyme responsible for the metabolism of ropinirole. There is thus the potential for inducers or inhibitors of this enzyme to alter the clearance of ropinirole. Therefore, if therapy with a drug known to be a potent inducer or inhibitor of CYP1A2 is stopped or started during treatment with ropinirole, adjustment of the dose of ropinirole may be required).
No products indexed under this heading.

Secobarbital Sodium (Sedating medications (such as alcohol or CNS depressants), may increase the risk of somnlence or falling asleep while engaged in activities of daily living. Because of possible additive effects, caution should be advised when patients are taking other sedating medications, alcohol, or other CNS depressants (eg, benzodiazepines, antipsychotics, antidepressants) in combination with ropinirole).
No products indexed under this heading.

Selegiline (Because of possible additive effects, caution should be advised when patients are taking other sedating medications, alcohol, or other CNS depressants (eg, benzodiazepines, antipsychotics, antidepressants) in combination with ropinirole). Products include:
Emsam 3623

Selegiline Hydrochloride (Because of possible additive effects, caution should be advised when patients are taking other sedating medications, alcohol, or other CNS depressants (eg, benzodiazepines, antipsychotics, antidepressants) in combination with ropinirole). Products include:
Eldepryl 3312

Sertraline Hydrochloride (Because of possible additive effects, caution should be advised when patients are taking other sedating medications, alcohol, or other CNS depressants (eg, benzodiazepines, antipsychotics, antidepressants) in combination with ropinirole).
No products indexed under this heading.

Sevoflurane (Sedating medications (such as alcohol or CNS depressants), may increase the risk of somnlence or falling asleep while engaged in activities of daily living. Because of possible additive effects, caution should be advised when patients are taking other sedating medications, alcohol, or other CNS depressants (eg, benzodiazepines, antipsychotics, antidepressants) in combination with ropinirole). Products include:
Ultane 554

Sildenafil Citrate (*In vitro* metabolism studies showed that CYP1A2 is the major enzyme responsible for the metabolism of ropinirole. There is thus the potential for inducers or inhibitors of this enzyme to alter the clearance of ropinirole. Therefore, if therapy with a drug known to be a potent inducer or inhibitor of CYP1A2 is stopped or started during treatment with ropinirole, adjustment of the dose of ropinirole may be required).
No products indexed under this heading.

Sodium Butabarbital (Sedating medications (such as alcohol or CNS depressants), may increase the risk of somnlence or falling asleep while engaged in activities of daily living. Because of possible additive effects, caution should be advised when patients are taking other sedating medications, alcohol, or other CNS depressants (eg, benzodiazepines, antipsychotics, antidepressants) in combination with ropinirole).
No products indexed under this heading.

Sodium Oxybate (Sedating medications (such as alcohol or CNS depressants), may increase the risk of somnlence or falling asleep while engaged in activities of daily living. Because of possible additive effects, caution should be advised when patients are taking other sedating medications, alcohol, or other CNS depressants (eg, benzodiazepines, antipsychotics, antidepressants) in combination with ropinirole).
No products indexed under this heading.

Sodium Pentobarbital (Sedating medications (such as alcohol or CNS depressants), may increase the risk of somnlence or falling asleep while engaged in activities of daily living. Because of possible additive effects, caution should be advised when patients are taking other sedating medications, alcohol, or other CNS depressants (eg, benzodiazepines, antipsychotics, antidepressants) in combination with ropinirole).
No products indexed under this heading.

Sparfloxacin (*In vitro* metabolism studies showed that CYP1A2 is the major enzyme responsible for the metabolism of ropinirole. There is thus the potential for inducers or inhibitors of this enzyme to alter the clearance of ropinirole. Therefore, if therapy with a drug known to be a potent inducer or inhibitor of CYP1A2 is stopped or started during treatment with ropinirole, adjustment of the dose of ropinirole may be required).
No products indexed under this heading.

Sufentanil Citrate (Sedating medications (such as alcohol or CNS depressants), may increase the risk of somnlence or falling asleep while engaged in activities of daily living. Because of possible additive effects, caution should be advised when patients are taking other sedating medications, alcohol, or other CNS depressants (eg, benzodiazepines, antipsychotics, antidepressants) in combination with ropinirole).
No products indexed under this heading.

Tacrine Hydrochloride (*In vitro* metabolism studies showed that CYP1A2 is the major enzyme responsible for the metabolism of ropinirole. There is thus the potential for inducers or inhibitors of this enzyme to alter the clearance of ropinirole. Therefore, if therapy with a drug known to be a potent inducer or inhibitor of CYP1A2 is stopped or started during treatment with ropinirole, adjustment of the dose of ropinirole may be required).
No products indexed under this heading.

Talbutal (Sedating medications (such as alcohol or CNS depressants), may increase the risk of somnlence or falling asleep while engaged in activities of daily living. Because of possible additive effects, caution should be advised when patients are taking other sedating medications, alcohol, or other CNS depressants (eg, benzodiazepines, antipsychotics, antidepressants) in combination with ropinirole).
No products indexed under this heading.

Tamoxifen Citrate (*In vitro* metabolism studies showed that CYP1A2 is the major enzyme responsible for the metabolism of ropinirole. There is thus the potential for inducers or inhibitors of this enzyme to alter the clearance of ropinirole. Therefore, if therapy with a drug known to be a potent inducer or inhibitor of CYP1A2 is stopped or started during treatment with ropinirole, adjustment of the dose of ropinirole may be required).
No products indexed under this heading.

Temazepam (Sedating medications (such as alcohol or CNS depressants), may increase the risk of somnlence or falling asleep while engaged in activities of daily living. Because of possible additive effects, caution should be advised when patients are taking other sedating medications, alcohol, or other CNS depressants (eg, benzodiazepines, antipsychotics, antidepressants) in combination with ropinirole).
No products indexed under this heading.

Theobromine (*In vitro* metabolism studies showed that CYP1A2 is the major enzyme responsible for the metabolism of ropinirole. There is thus the potential for inducers or inhibitors of this enzyme to alter the clearance of ropinirole. Therefore, if therapy with a drug known to be a potent inducer or inhibitor of CYP1A2 is stopped or started during treatment with ropinirole, adjustment of the dose of ropinirole may be required).
No products indexed under this heading.

Theophylline (*In vitro* metabolism studies showed that CYP1A2 is the major enzyme responsible for the metabolism of ropinirole. There is thus the potential for inducers or inhibitors of this enzyme to alter the clearance of ropinirole. Therefore, if therapy with a drug known to be a potent inducer or inhibitor of CYP1A2 is stopped or started during treatment with ropinirole, adjustment of the dose of ropinirole may be required).
No products indexed under this heading.

Theophylline Anhydrous (*In vitro* metabolism studies showed that CYP1A2 is the major enzyme responsible for the metabolism of ropinirole. There is thus the potential for inducers or inhibitors of this enzyme to alter the clearance of ropinirole. Therefore, if therapy with a drug known to be a potent inducer or inhibitor of CYP1A2 is stopped or started during treatment with ropinirole, adjustment of the dose of ropinirole may be required). Products include:
Uniphyl 2817

Theophylline Calcium Salicylate (*In vitro* metabolism studies showed that CYP1A2 is the major enzyme responsible for the metabolism of ropinirole. There is thus the potential for inducers or inhibitors of this enzyme to alter the clearance of ropinirole. Therefore, if therapy with a drug known to be a potent inducer or inhibitor of CYP1A2 is stopped or started during treatment with ropinirole, adjustment of the dose of ropinirole may be required).
No products indexed under this heading.

Theophylline Dihydroxypropyl (Glyceryl) (*In vitro* metabolism studies showed that CYP1A2 is the major enzyme responsible for the metabolism of ropinirole. There is thus the potential for inducers or inhibitors of this enzyme to alter the clearance of ropinirole. Therefore, if therapy with a drug known to be a potent inducer or inhibitor of CYP1A2 is stopped or started during treatment with ropinirole, adjustment of the dose of ropinirole may be required).
No products indexed under this heading.

Theophylline Ethylenediamine (*In vitro* metabolism studies showed that CYP1A2 is the major enzyme responsible for the metabolism of ropinirole. There is thus the potential for inducers or inhibitors of this enzyme to alter the clearance of ropinirole. Therefore, if therapy with a drug known to be a potent inducer or inhibitor of CYP1A2 is stopped or started during treatment with ropinirole, adjustment of the dose of ropinirole may be required).
No products indexed under this heading.

Theophylline Sodium Glycinate (*In vitro* metabolism studies showed that CYP1A2 is the major enzyme responsible for the metabolism of ropinirole. There is thus the potential for inducers or inhibitors of this enzyme to alter the clearance of ropinirole. Therefore, if therapy with a drug known to be a potent inducer or inhibitor of CYP1A2 is stopped or started during treatment with ropinirole, adjustment of the dose of ropinirole may be required).
No products indexed under this heading.

Thiamylal Sodium (Sedating medications (such as alcohol or CNS depressants), may increase the risk of somnlence or falling asleep while engaged in activities of daily living. Because of possible additive effects, caution should be advised when patients are taking other sedating medications, alcohol, or other CNS depressants (eg, benzodiazepines, antipsychotics, antidepressants) in combination with ropinirole).
No products indexed under this heading.

Thioridazine (Sedating medications (such as alcohol or CNS depressants), may increase the risk of somnlence or falling asleep while engaged in activities of daily living. Because of possible additive effects, caution should be advised when patients are taking other sedating medications, alcohol, or other CNS depressants (eg, benzodiazepines, antipsychotics, antidepressants) in combination with ropinirole).
No products indexed under this heading.

Thioridazine Hydrochloride (Sedating medications (such as alcohol or CNS depressants), may increase the risk of somnlence or falling asleep while engaged in activities of daily living. Because of possible additive effects, caution should be advised when patients are taking other sedating medications, alcohol, or other CNS depres-

sants (eg, benzodiazepines, antipsychotics, antidepressants) in combination with ropinirole). Products include:
Thioridazine Hydrochloride 2384

Thiothixene (Sedating medications (such as alcohol or CNS depressants), may increase the risk of somnlence or falling asleep while engaged in activities of daily living. Because of possible additive effects, caution should be advised when patients are taking other sedating medications, alcohol, or other CNS depressants (eg, benzodiazepines, antipsychotics, antidepressants) in combination with ropinirole). Products include:
Thiothixene 2386

Thiothixene Hydrochloride (Sedating medications (such as alcohol or CNS depressants), may increase the risk of somnlence or falling asleep while engaged in activities of daily living. Because of possible additive effects, caution should be advised when patients are taking other sedating medications, alcohol, or other CNS depressants (eg, benzodiazepines, antipsychotics, antidepressants) in combination with ropinirole).
No products indexed under this heading.

Ticlopidine Hydrochloride (*In vitro* metabolism studies showed that CYP1A2 is the major enzyme responsible for the metabolism of ropinirole. There is thus the potential for inducers or inhibitors of this enzyme to alter the clearance of ropinirole. Therefore, if therapy with a drug known to be a potent inducer or inhibitor of CYP1A2 is stopped or started during treatment with ropinirole, adjustment of the dose of ropinirole may be required).
No products indexed under this heading.

Tizanidine (*In vitro* metabolism studies showed that CYP1A2 is the major enzyme responsible for the metabolism of ropinirole. There is thus the potential for inducers or inhibitors of this enzyme to alter the clearance of ropinirole. Therefore, if therapy with a drug known to be a potent inducer or inhibitor of CYP1A2 is stopped or started during treatment with ropinirole, adjustment of the dose of ropinirole may be required).
No products indexed under this heading.

Tizanidine Hydrochloride (*In vitro* metabolism studies showed that CYP1A2 is the major enzyme responsible for the metabolism of ropinirole. There is thus the potential for inducers or inhibitors of this enzyme to alter the clearance of ropinirole. Therefore, if therapy with a drug known to be a potent inducer or inhibitor of CYP1A2 is stopped or started during treatment with ropinirole, adjustment of the dose of ropinirole may be required).
No products indexed under this heading.

Tobacco (Cigarette smoking is expected to increase the clearance of ropinirole since CYP1A2 is known to be induced by smoking. In one study in patients with restless legs syndrome, cigarette smokers had an approximate 30% lower C_{max} and a 38% lower AUC than nonsmokers, when those parameters were normalized for dose).
No products indexed under this heading.

Tranylcypromine Sulfate (Because of possible additive effects, caution should be advised when patients are taking other sedating medications, alcohol, or other CNS depressants (eg, benzodiazepines, antipsychotics, antidepressants) in combination with ropinirole). Products include:
Parnate 1584

Trazodone Hydrochloride (Because of possible additive effects, caution should be advised when patients are taking other sedating medications, alcohol, or other CNS depressants (eg, benzodiazepines, antipsychotics, antidepressants) in combination with ropinirole).
No products indexed under this heading.

Triazolam (Sedating medications (such as alcohol or CNS depressants), may increase the risk of somnlence or falling asleep while engaged in activities of daily living. Because of possible additive effects, caution should be advised when patients are taking other sedating medications, alcohol, or other CNS depressants (eg, benzodiazepines, antipsychotics, antidepressants) in combination with ropinirole).
No products indexed under this heading.

Trifluoperazine Hydrochloride (Sedating medications (such as alcohol or CNS depressants), may increase the risk of somnlence or falling asleep while engaged in activities of daily living. Because of possible additive effects, caution should be advised when patients are taking other sedating medications, alcohol, or other CNS depressants (eg, benzodiazepines, antipsychotics, antidepressants) in combination with ropinirole).
No products indexed under this heading.

Trimeprazine Tartrate (Before initiating treatment patients should be advised of the potential to develop drowsiness and specifically asked about factors that may increase the risk such as concomitant sedating medications. If a patient develops significant daytime sleepiness or episodes of falling asleep during activities that require active participation (eg, conversations, eating, etc.), therapy should ordinarily be discontinued. If a decision is made to continue, patients should be advised to not drive and to avoid other potentially dangerous activities).
No products indexed under this heading.

Trimethaphan Camsylate (*In vitro* metabolism studies showed that CYP1A2 is the major enzyme responsible for the metabolism of ropinirole. There is thus the potential for inducers or inhibitors of this enzyme to alter the clearance of ropinirole. Therefore, if therapy with a drug known to be a potent inducer or inhibitor of CYP1A2 is stopped or started during treatment with ropinirole, adjustment of the dose of ropinirole may be required).
No products indexed under this heading.

Trimipramine Maleate (Because of possible additive effects, caution should be advised when patients are taking other sedating medications, alcohol, or other CNS depressants (eg, benzodiazepines, antipsychotics, antidepressants) in combination with ropinirole).
No products indexed under this heading.

Tripelennamine Hydrochloride (Before initiating treatment patients should be advised of the potential to develop drowsiness and specifically asked about factors that may increase the risk such as concomitant sedating medications. If a patient develops significant daytime sleepiness or episodes of falling asleep during activities that require active participation (eg, conversations, eating, etc.), therapy should ordinarily be discontinued. If a decision is made to continue, patients should be advised to not drive and to avoid other potentially dangerous activities).
No products indexed under this heading.

Triprolidine Hydrochloride (Before initiating treatment patients should be advised of the potential to develop drowsiness and specifically asked about factors that may increase the risk such as concomitant sedating medications. If a patient develops significant daytime sleepiness or episodes of falling asleep during activities that require active participation (eg, conversations, eating, etc.), therapy should ordinarily be discontinued. If a decision is made to continue, patients should be advised to not drive and to avoid other potentially dangerous activities).
No products indexed under this heading.

Troleandomycin (*In vitro* metabolism studies showed that CYP1A2 is the major enzyme responsible for the metabolism of ropinirole. There is thus the potential for inducers or inhibitors of this enzyme to alter the clearance of ropinirole. Therefore, if therapy with a drug known to be a potent inducer or inhibitor of CYP1A2 is stopped or started during treatment with ropinirole, adjustment of the dose of ropinirole may be required).
No products indexed under this heading.

Trovafloxacin Mesylate (*In vitro* metabolism studies showed that CYP1A2 is the major enzyme responsible for the metabolism of ropinirole. There is thus the potential for inducers or inhibitors of this enzyme to alter the clearance of ropinirole. Therefore, if therapy with a drug known to be a potent inducer or inhibitor of CYP1A2 is stopped or started during treatment with ropinirole, adjustment of the dose of ropinirole may be required).
No products indexed under this heading.

Vardenafil Hydrochloride (*In vitro* metabolism studies showed that CYP1A2 is the major enzyme responsible for the metabolism of ropinirole. There is thus the potential for inducers or inhibitors of this enzyme to alter the clearance of ropinirole. Therefore, if therapy with a drug known to be a potent inducer or inhibitor of CYP1A2 is stopped or started during treatment with ropinirole, adjustment of the dose of ropinirole may be required). Products include:
Levitra 3157

Venlafaxine Hydrochloride (Because of possible additive effects, caution should be advised when patients are taking other sedating medications, alcohol, or other CNS depressants (eg, benzodiazepines, antipsychotics, antidepressants) in combination with ropinirole). Products include:
Effexor XR 3504
Venlafaxine Hydrochloride Tablets ... 2388

Verapamil Hydrochloride (*In vitro* metabolism studies showed that CYP1A2 is the major enzyme responsible for the metabolism of ropinirole. There is thus the potential for inducers or inhibitors of this enzyme to alter the clearance of ropinirole. Therefore, if therapy with a drug known to be a potent inducer or inhibitor of CYP1A2 is stopped or started during treatment with ropinirole, adjustment of the dose of ropinirole may be required). Products include:
Tarka 534

Warfarin Sodium (*In vitro* metabolism studies showed that CYP1A2 is the major enzyme responsible for the metabolism of ropinirole. There is thus the potential for inducers or inhibitors of this enzyme to alter the clearance of ropinirole. Therefore, if therapy with a drug known to be a potent inducer or inhibitor of CYP1A2 is stopped or started during treatment with ropinirole, adjustment of the dose of ropinirole may be required).
No products indexed under this heading.

Zaleplon (Sedating medications (such as alcohol or CNS depressants), may increase the risk of somnlence or falling asleep while engaged in activities of daily living. Because of possible additive effects, caution should be advised when patients are taking other sedating medications, alcohol, or other CNS depressants (eg, benzodiazepines, antipsychotics, antidepressants) in combination with ropinirole).
No products indexed under this heading.

Zileuton (*In vitro* metabolism studies showed that CYP1A2 is the major enzyme responsible for the metabolism of ropinirole. There is thus the potential for inducers or inhibitors of this enzyme to alter the clearance of ropinirole. Therefore, if therapy with a drug known to be a potent inducer or inhibitor of CYP1A2 is stopped or started during treatment with ropinirole, adjustment of the dose of ropinirole may be required).
No products indexed under this heading.

Ziprasidone Hydrochloride (Sedating medications (such as alcohol or CNS depressants), may increase the risk of somnlence or falling asleep while engaged in activities of daily living. Because of possible additive effects, caution should be advised when patients are taking other sedating medications, alcohol, or other CNS depressants (eg, benzodiazepines, antipsychotics, antidepressants) in combination with ropinirole). Products include:
Geodon 2723

Zolmitriptan (*In vitro* metabolism studies showed that CYP1A2 is the major enzyme responsible for the metabolism of ropinirole. There is thus the potential for inducers or inhibitors of this enzyme to alter the clearance of ropinirole. Therefore, if therapy with a drug known to be a potent inducer or inhibitor of CYP1A2 is stopped or started during treatment with ropinirole, adjustment of the dose of ropinirole may be required). Products include:
Zomig Tablets 773
Zomig Nasal Spray 768
Zomig-ZMT Tablets 773

Zolpidem Tartrate (Sedating medications (such as alcohol or CNS depressants), may increase the risk of somnlence or falling asleep while engaged in activities of daily living. Because of possible additive effects, caution should be advised when patients are taking other sedating medications, alcohol, or other CNS depressants (eg, benzodiazepines, antipsychotics, antidepressants) in combination with ropinirole). Products include:
Ambien 2920
Ambien CR 2925

Food Interactions

Alcohol (Sedating medications (such as alcohol or CNS depressants), the presence of sleeping disorders, or other medications that increase plasma levels of ropinirole, may increase the risk of somnolence or falling asleep while engaged in activities of daily living. Because of possible additive effects, caution should be advised when patients are taking other sedating medications, alcohol, or other CNS depressants (eg, benzodiazepines, antipsychotics, antidepressants) in combination with ropinirole).

Beer, reduced-alcohol (Sedating medications (such as alcohol or CNS depressants), may increase the risk of somnolence or falling asleep while engaged in activities of daily living. Because of possible additive effects, caution should be advised when patients are taking other sedating medications, alcohol, or other CNS depressants in combination with ropinirole).

IMPORTANT NOTE: Always consult each drug listing in the patient's regimen for possible interactions.

Beer, unspecified (Sedating medications (such as alcohol or CNS depressants), may increase the risk of somnolence or falling asleep while engaged in activities of daily living. Because of possible additive effects, caution should be advised when patients are taking other sedating medications, alcohol, or other CNS depressants in combination with ropinirole).

Broccoli (*In vitro* metabolism studies showed that CYP1A2 is the major enzyme responsible for the metabolism of ropinirole. There is thus the potential for inducers or inhibitors of this enzyme to alter the clearance of ropinirole. Therefore, if therapy with a drug known to be a potent inducer or inhibitor of CYP1A2 is stopped or started during treatment with ropinirole, adjustment of the dose of ropinirole may be required).

Brussel Sprouts (*In vitro* metabolism studies showed that CYP1A2 is the major enzyme responsible for the metabolism of ropinirole. There is thus the potential for inducers or inhibitors of this enzyme to alter the clearance of ropinirole. Therefore, if therapy with a drug known to be a potent inducer or inhibitor of CYP1A2 is stopped or started during treatment with ropinirole, adjustment of the dose of ropinirole may be required).

Charbroiled Food (*In vitro* metabolism studies showed that CYP1A2 is the major enzyme responsible for the metabolism of ropinirole. There is thus the potential for inducers or inhibitors of this enzyme to alter the clearance of ropinirole. Therefore, if therapy with a drug known to be a potent inducer or inhibitor of CYP1A2 is stopped or started during treatment with ropinirole, adjustment of the dose of ropinirole may be required).

Food, caffeine-containing (*In vitro* metabolism studies showed that CYP1A2 is the major enzyme responsible for the metabolism of ropinirole. There is thus the potential for inducers or inhibitors of this enzyme to alter the clearance of ropinirole. Therefore, if therapy with a drug known to be a potent inducer or inhibitor of CYP1A2 is stopped or started during treatment with ropinirole, adjustment of the dose of ropinirole may be required).

Food, unspecified (In a single-dose study, administration of ropinirole to healthy volunteers with food (eg, high-fat meal) increased AUC by approximately 30% and C_{max} by approximately 44%, compared with dosing under fasted conditions. In a repeat-dose study in patients with Parkinson's disease, food (eg, high-fat meal) increased AUC by approximately 20% and C_{max} by approximately 44%; T_{max} was prolonged by 3 hours (median prolongation) compared with dosing under fasted conditions).

Grapefruit (*In vitro* metabolism studies showed that CYP1A2 is the major enzyme responsible for the metabolism of ropinirole. There is thus the potential for inducers or inhibitors of this enzyme to alter the clearance of ropinirole. Therefore, if therapy with a drug known to be a potent inducer or inhibitor of CYP1A2 is stopped or started during treatment with ropinirole, adjustment of the dose of ropinirole may be required).

Grapefruit Juice (*In vitro* metabolism studies showed that CYP1A2 is the major enzyme responsible for the metabolism of ropinirole. There is thus the potential for inducers or inhibitors of this enzyme to alter the clearance of ropinirole. Therefore, if therapy with a drug known to be a potent inducer or inhibitor of CYP1A2 is stopped or started during treatment with ropinirole, adjustment of the dose of ropinirole may be required).

Meal, unspecified (In a single-dose study, administration of ropinirole to healthy volunteers with food (eg, high-fat meal) increased AUC by approximately 30% and C_{max} by approximately 44%, compared with dosing under fasted conditions. In a repeat-dose study in patients with Parkinson's disease, food (eg, high-fat meal) increased AUC by approximately 20% and C_{max} by approximately 44%; T_{max} was prolonged by 3 hours (median prolongation) compared with dosing under fasted conditions).

Wine, Chianti (Sedating medications (such as alcohol or CNS depressants), may increase the risk of somnolence or falling asleep while engaged in activities of daily living. Because of possible additive effects, caution should be advised when patients are taking other sedating medications, alcohol, or other CNS depressants in combination with ropinirole).

Wine, Red (Sedating medications (such as alcohol or CNS depressants), may increase the risk of somnolence or falling asleep while engaged in activities of daily living. Because of possible additive effects, caution should be advised when patients are taking other sedating medications, alcohol, or other CNS depressants in combination with ropinirole).

Wine, unspecified (Sedating medications (such as alcohol or CNS depressants), may increase the risk of somnolence or falling asleep while engaged in activities of daily living. Because of possible additive effects, caution should be advised when patients are taking other sedating medications, alcohol, or other CNS depressants in combination with ropinirole).

Wine products (Sedating medications (such as alcohol or CNS depressants), may increase the risk of somnolence or falling asleep while engaged in activities of daily living. Because of possible additive effects, caution should be advised when patients are taking other sedating medications, alcohol, or other CNS depressants in combination with ropinirole).

RESTASIS OPHTHALMIC EMULSION

(Cyclosporine) 605
None cited in PDR database.

RETROVIR CAPSULES

(Zidovudine) 1634
See Retrovir Tablets

RETROVIR IV INFUSION

(Zidovudine) 1640
See Retrovir Tablets

RETROVIR SYRUP

(Zidovudine) 1634
See Retrovir Tablets

RETROVIR TABLETS

(Zidovudine) 1634
May interact with agents associated with myelosuppression, cytotoxic drugs, interferon alpha, nucleoside analogues, nucleoside/nucleotide analogue reverse transcriptase inhibitors, phenytoin, valproate, and certain other agents. Compounds in these categories include:

Abacavir Sulfate (Some nucleoside analogues affecting DNA replication antagonize the *in vitro* antiviral activity of zidovudine against HIV-1; concomitant use of such drugs should be avoided). Products include:
Epzicom 1448
Trizivir 1688
Ziagen 1740

Acyclovir (Some nucleoside analogues affecting DNA replication antagonize the *in vitro* antiviral activity of zidovudine against HIV-1; concomitant use of such drugs should be avoided). Products include:
Zovirax 1760

Acyclovir Sodium (Some nucleoside analogues affecting DNA replication antagonize the *in vitro* antiviral activity of zidovudine against HIV-1; concomitant use of such drugs should be avoided).
No products indexed under this heading.

Adefovir dipivoxil (Some nucleoside analogues affecting DNA replication antagonize the *in vitro* antiviral activity of zidovudine against HIV-1; concomitant use of such drugs should be avoided). Products include:
Hepsera 1244

Altretamine (Co-administration with bone marrow suppressive agents may increase the hematological toxicity of zidovudine). Products include:
Hexalen 1066

Atovaquone (Co-administration results in an increased AUC of zidovudine by 31%. Routine dose modification of zidovudine is not warranted). Products include:
Malarone Pediatric Tablets 1572
Malarone 1572
Mepron Suspension 1576

Bleomycin Sulfate (Co-administration with cytotoxic agents may increase the hematologic toxicity of zidovudine).
No products indexed under this heading.

Busulfan (Co-administration with bone marrow suppressive agents may increase the hematological toxicity of zidovudine). Products include:
Myleran 1581

Chlorambucil (Co-administration with bone marrow suppressive agents may increase the hematological toxicity of zidovudine). Products include:
Leukeran 1557

Chloramphenicol (Co-administration with bone marrow suppressive agents may increase the hematological toxicity of zidovudine).
No products indexed under this heading.

Chloramphenicol Palmitate (Co-administration with bone marrow suppressive agents may increase the hematological toxicity of zidovudine).
No products indexed under this heading.

Chloramphenicol Sodium Succinate (Co-administration with bone marrow suppressive agents may increase the hematological toxicity of zidovudine).
No products indexed under this heading.

Cladribine (Co-administration with bone marrow suppressive agents may increase the hematological toxicity of zidovudine). Products include:
Leustatin 946

Cyclophosphamide (Co-administration with cytotoxic agents may increase the hematologic toxicity of zidovudine).
No products indexed under this heading.

Daunorubicin Citrate Liposome (Co-administration with bone marrow suppressive agents may increase the hematological toxicity of zidovudine).
No products indexed under this heading.

Daunorubicin Hydrochloride (Co-administration with cytotoxic agents may increase the hematologic toxicity of zidovudine).
No products indexed under this heading.

Dexrazoxane (Co-administration with bone marrow suppressive agents may increase the hematological toxicity of zidovudine).
No products indexed under this heading.

Didanosine (Some nucleoside analogues affecting DNA replication antagonize the *in vitro* antiviral activity of zidovudine against HIV-1; concomitant use of such drugs should be avoided).
No products indexed under this heading.

Divalproex Sodium (Co-administration of valproic acid results in an increased AUC of zidovudine by 80%. Routine dose modification of zidovudine is not warranted). Products include:
Depakote ER 426

Doxorubicin Hydrochloride (Concomitant use of zidovudine with doxorubicin should be avoided since an antagonistic relationship has been demonstrated *in vitro*).
No products indexed under this heading.

Doxorubicin Hydrochloride Liposome (Concomitant use of zidovudine with doxorubicin should be avoided since an antagonistic relationship has been demonstrated *in vitro*). Products include:
Doxil 939

Emtricitabine (Some nucleoside analogues affecting DNA replication antagonize the *in vitro* antiviral activity of zidovudine against HIV-1; concomitant use of such drugs should be avoided). Products include:
Atripla 906
Emtriva 1238
Emtriva Oral Solution 1238
Truvada 1258

Epirubicin Hydrochloride (Co-administration with cytotoxic agents may increase the hematologic toxicity of zidovudine).
No products indexed under this heading.

Fluconazole (Co-administration results in an increased AUC of zidovudine by 74%. Routine dose modification of zidovudine is not warranted).
No products indexed under this heading.

Fludarabine Phosphate (Co-administration with bone marrow suppressive agents may increase the hematological toxicity of zidovudine). Products include:
Oforta 3023

Fluorouracil (Co-administration with cytotoxic agents may increase the hematologic toxicity of zidovudine). Products include:
Carac 2966

Fosphenytoin (Co-administration has resulted in low phenytoin levels in some patients and a high level in one case; a 30% decrease in oral zidovudine clearance was observed with phenytoin).
No products indexed under this heading.

Fosphenytoin Sodium (Co-administration has resulted in low phenytoin levels in some patients and a high level in one case; a 30% decrease in oral zidovudine clearance was observed with phenytoin).
No products indexed under this heading.

Ganciclovir Sodium (Co-administration with ganciclovir may increase the hematologic toxicity of zidovudine).
No products indexed under this heading.

Gemcitabine Hydrochloride (Co-administration with bone marrow suppressive agents may increase the hematological toxicity of zidovudine). Products include:

IMPORTANT NOTE: Always consult each drug listing in the patient's regimen for possible interactions.

Anagrelide Hydrochloride (CYP 1A2 is the principal isoenzyme involved in the initial oxidative metabolism of riluzole; potential interactions may occur when riluzole is given concurrently with other agents which are also metabolized primarily by CYP 1A2 (eg, theophylline, caffeine, and tacrine)).
No products indexed under this heading.

Anastrozole (Potential inhibitors of CYP 1A2 (eg, caffeine, phenacetin, theophylline, amitriptyline, and quinolones) could decrease the rate of riluzole elimination).
No products indexed under this heading.

Atazanavir (Caution should be exercised if the practitioner chooses to prescribe riluzole in combination with potentially hepatotoxic drugs (eg, allopurinol, methyldopa, sulfasalazine)).
No products indexed under this heading.

Atazanavir Sulfate (Caution should be exercised if the practitioner chooses to prescribe riluzole in combination with potentially hepatotoxic drugs (eg, allopurinol, methyldopa, sulfasalazine)).
No products indexed under this heading.

Atorvastatin Calcium (Caution should be exercised if the practitioner chooses to prescribe riluzole in combination with potentially hepatotoxic drugs (eg, allopurinol, methyldopa, sulfasalazine)). Products include:
Lipitor 2703

Azathioprine (Caution should be exercised if the practitioner chooses to prescribe riluzole in combination with potentially hepatotoxic drugs (eg, allopurinol, methyldopa, sulfasalazine)).
No products indexed under this heading.

Azathioprine Sodium (Caution should be exercised if the practitioner chooses to prescribe riluzole in combination with potentially hepatotoxic drugs (eg, allopurinol, methyldopa, sulfasalazine)).
No products indexed under this heading.

Azlocillin Sodium (Caution should be exercised if the practitioner chooses to prescribe riluzole in combination with potentially hepatotoxic drugs (eg, allopurinol, methyldopa, sulfasalazine)).
No products indexed under this heading.

Bacampicillin Hydrochloride (Caution should be exercised if the practitioner chooses to prescribe riluzole in combination with potentially hepatotoxic drugs (eg, allopurinol, methyldopa, sulfasalazine)).
No products indexed under this heading.

Bendroflumethiazide (Caution should be exercised if the practitioner chooses to prescribe riluzole in combination with potentially hepatotoxic drugs (eg, allopurinol, methyldopa, sulfasalazine)).
No products indexed under this heading.

Bupropion (Caution should be exercised if the practitioner chooses to prescribe riluzole in combination with potentially hepatotoxic drugs (eg, allopurinol, methyldopa, sulfasalazine)).
No products indexed under this heading.

Bupropion Hydrochloride (Caution should be exercised if the practitioner chooses to prescribe riluzole in combination with potentially hepatotoxic drugs (eg, allopurinol, methyldopa, sulfasalazine)). Products include:
Aplenzin 2948
Wellbutrin 1719
Wellbutrin SR 1725
Zyban 1762

Caffeine (Potential inhibitors of CYP1A2, such as caffeine, could decrease the rate of riluzole elimination. CYP1A2 is the principal isoenzyme involved in the initial oxidative metabolism of riluzole; potential interactions may occur when riluzole is given concurrently with other agents which are also metabolized primarily by CYP1A2 (eg, caffeine)).
No products indexed under this heading.

Caffeine Anhydrous (Potential inhibitors of CYP1A2, such as caffeine, could decrease the rate of riluzole elimination. CYP1A2 is the principal isoenzyme involved in the initial oxidative metabolism of riluzole; potential interactions may occur when riluzole is given concurrently with other agents which are also metabolized primarily by CYP1A2 (eg, caffeine)).
No products indexed under this heading.

Caffeine Citrate (Potential inhibitors of CYP1A2, such as caffeine, could decrease the rate of riluzole elimination. CYP1A2 is the principal isoenzyme involved in the initial oxidative metabolism of riluzole; potential interactions may occur when riluzole is given concurrently with other agents which are also metabolized primarily by CYP1A2 (eg, caffeine)).
No products indexed under this heading.

Caffeine-containing medications (Potential inhibitors of CYP1A2, such as caffeine, could decrease the rate of riluzole elimination. CYP1A2 is the principal isoenzyme involved in the initial oxidative metabolism of riluzole; potential interactions may occur when riluzole is given concurrently with other agents which are also metabolized primarily by CYP1A2 (eg, caffeine)).
No products indexed under this heading.

Caffeine Sodium Benzoate (Potential inhibitors of CYP1A2, such as caffeine, could decrease the rate of riluzole elimination. CYP1A2 is the principal isoenzyme involved in the initial oxidative metabolism of riluzole; potential interactions may occur when riluzole is given concurrently with other agents which are also metabolized primarily by CYP1A2 (eg, caffeine)).
No products indexed under this heading.

Carbamazepine (Caution should be exercised if the practitioner chooses to prescribe riluzole in combination with potentially hepatotoxic drugs (eg, allopurinol, methyldopa, sulfasalazine)). Products include:
Carbatrol 3280
Equetro 3477

Carbenicillin Disodium (Caution should be exercised if the practitioner chooses to prescribe riluzole in combination with potentially hepatotoxic drugs (eg, allopurinol, methyldopa, sulfasalazine)).
No products indexed under this heading.

Carbenicillin Indanyl Sodium (Caution should be exercised if the practitioner chooses to prescribe riluzole in combination with potentially hepatotoxic drugs (eg, allopurinol, methyldopa, sulfasalazine)).
No products indexed under this heading.

Celecoxib (Caution should be exercised if the practitioner chooses to prescribe riluzole in combination with potentially hepatotoxic drugs (eg, allopurinol, methyldopa, sulfasalazine)). Products include:
Celebrex 3272

Cerivastatin Sodium (Caution should be exercised if the practitioner chooses to prescribe riluzole in combination with potentially hepatotoxic drugs (eg, allopurinol, methyldopa, sulfasalazine)).
No products indexed under this heading.

Chlordiazepoxide (CYP 1A2 is the principal isoenzyme involved in the initial oxidative metabolism of riluzole; potential interactions may occur when riluzole is given concurrently with other agents which are also metabolized primarily by CYP 1A2 (eg, theophylline, caffeine, and tacrine)).
No products indexed under this heading.

Chlordiazepoxide Hydrochloride (CYP 1A2 is the principal isoenzyme involved in the initial oxidative metabolism of riluzole; potential interactions may occur when riluzole is given concurrently with other agents which are also metabolized primarily by CYP 1A2 (eg, theophylline, caffeine, and tacrine)).
No products indexed under this heading.

Chlorothiazide (Caution should be exercised if the practitioner chooses to prescribe riluzole in combination with potentially hepatotoxic drugs (eg, allopurinol, methyldopa, sulfasalazine)).
No products indexed under this heading.

Chlorothiazide Sodium (Caution should be exercised if the practitioner chooses to prescribe riluzole in combination with potentially hepatotoxic drugs (eg, allopurinol, methyldopa, sulfasalazine)). Products include:
Diuril Intravenous 2009

Chlorpromazine (Caution should be exercised if the practitioner chooses to prescribe riluzole in combination with potentially hepatotoxic drugs (eg, allopurinol, methyldopa, sulfasalazine)).
No products indexed under this heading.

Chlorpromazine Hydrochloride (Caution should be exercised if the practitioner chooses to prescribe riluzole in combination with potentially hepatotoxic drugs (eg, allopurinol, methyldopa, sulfasalazine)).
No products indexed under this heading.

Chlorpropamide (Caution should be exercised if the practitioner chooses to prescribe riluzole in combination with potentially hepatotoxic drugs (eg, allopurinol, methyldopa, sulfasalazine)).
No products indexed under this heading.

Cimetidine (Potential inhibitors of CYP 1A2 (eg, caffeine, phenacetin, theophylline, amitriptyline, and quinolones) could decrease the rate of riluzole elimination).
No products indexed under this heading.

Cimetidine Hydrochloride (Potential inhibitors of CYP 1A2 (eg, caffeine, phenacetin, theophylline, amitriptyline, and quinolones) could decrease the rate of riluzole elimination).
No products indexed under this heading.

Ciprofloxacin (Potential inhibitors of CYP 1A2 (eg, caffeine, phenacetin, theophylline, amitriptyline, and quinolones) could decrease the rate of riluzole elimination). Products include:
Cipro I.V. 3082
Cipro 3073
Cipro XR 3091
Ciprodex 583

Ciprofloxacin Hydrochloride (Potential inhibitors of CYP 1A2 (eg, caffeine, phenacetin, theophylline, amitriptyline, and quinolones) could decrease the rate of riluzole elimination). Products include:
Cipro 3073

Citalopram Hydrobromide (Potential inducers of CYP 1A2 (eg, cigarette smoke, charcoal-broiled food, rifampicin, and omeprazole) could increase the rate of riluzole elimination). Products include:
Celexa 1153

Clarithromycin (Potential inhibitors of CYP 1A2 (eg, caffeine, phenacetin, theophylline, amitriptyline, and quinolones) could decrease the rate of riluzole elimination). Products include:
Biaxin/Biaxin XL 412

Clomipramine Hydrochloride (Caution should be exercised if the practitioner chooses to prescribe riluzole in combination with potentially hepatotoxic drugs (eg, allopurinol, methyldopa, sulfasalazine)).
No products indexed under this heading.

Clopidogrel Bisulfate (CYP 1A2 is the principal isoenzyme involved in the initial oxidative metabolism of riluzole; potential interactions may occur when riluzole is given concurrently with other agents which are also metabolized primarily by CYP 1A2 (eg, theophylline, caffeine, and tacrine)). Products include:
Plavix 3027

Cloxacillin (Caution should be exercised if the practitioner chooses to prescribe riluzole in combination with potentially hepatotoxic drugs (eg, allopurinol, methyldopa, sulfasalazine)).
No products indexed under this heading.

Cloxacillin Sodium (Caution should be exercised if the practitioner chooses to prescribe riluzole in combination with potentially hepatotoxic drugs (eg, allopurinol, methyldopa, sulfasalazine)).
No products indexed under this heading.

Cloxacillin Sodium Monohydrate (Caution should be exercised if the practitioner chooses to prescribe riluzole in combination with potentially hepatotoxic drugs (eg, allopurinol, methyldopa, sulfasalazine)).
No products indexed under this heading.

Clozapine (CYP 1A2 is the principal isoenzyme involved in the initial oxidative metabolism of riluzole; potential interactions may occur when riluzole is given concurrently with other agents which are also metabolized primarily by CYP 1A2 (eg, theophylline, caffeine, and tacrine)).
No products indexed under this heading.

Cyclobenzaprine (CYP 1A2 is the principal isoenzyme involved in the initial oxidative metabolism of riluzole; potential interactions may occur when riluzole is given concurrently with other agents which are also metabolized primarily by CYP 1A2 (eg, theophylline, caffeine, and tacrine)).
No products indexed under this heading.

Cyclobenzaprine Hydrochloride (CYP 1A2 is the principal isoenzyme involved in the initial oxidative metabolism of riluzole; potential interactions may occur when riluzole is given concurrently with other agents which are also metabolized primarily by CYP 1A2 (eg, theophylline, caffeine, and tacrine)). Products include:
Amrix 964

Cyclosporine (Caution should be exercised if the practitioner chooses to prescribe riluzole in combination with potentially hepatotoxic drugs (eg, allopurinol, methyldopa, sulfasalazine)). Products include:
Gengraf 440
Neoral Oral Solution 2496
Neoral Capsules 2496
Restasis 605

Darunavir (Caution should be exercised if the practitioner chooses to prescribe riluzole in combination with potentially hepatotoxic drugs (eg, allopurinol, methyldopa, sulfasalazine)).
No products indexed under this heading.

Demeclocycline Hydrochloride (Caution should be exercised if the practitioner chooses to prescribe riluzole in combination with potentially hepatotoxic drugs (eg, allopurinol, methyldopa, sulfasalazine)).
No products indexed under this heading.

IMPORTANT NOTE: Always consult each drug listing in the patient's regimen for possible interactions.

IMPORTANT NOTE: Always consult each drug listing in the patient's regimen for possible interactions.

Rilutek Interactions Index 1620

Nicotine (Potential inducers of CYP 1A2 (eg, cigarette smoke, charcoal-broiled food, rifampicin, and omeprazole) could increase the rate of riluzole elimination).
No products indexed under this heading.

Nicotine Polacrilex (Potential inducers of CYP 1A2 (eg, cigarette smoke, charcoal-broiled food, rifampicin, and omeprazole) could increase the rate of riluzole elimination).
No products indexed under this heading.

Nicotine Salicylate (Potential inducers of CYP 1A2 (eg, cigarette smoke, charcoal-broiled food, rifampicin, and omeprazole) could increase the rate of riluzole elimination).
No products indexed under this heading.

Nicotine Sulfate (Potential inducers of CYP 1A2 (eg, cigarette smoke, charcoal-broiled food, rifampicin, and omeprazole) could increase the rate of riluzole elimination).
No products indexed under this heading.

Nicotinic Acid (Caution should be exercised if the practitioner chooses to prescribe riluzole in combination with potentially hepatotoxic drugs (eg, allopurinol, methyldopa, sulfasalazine)).
No products indexed under this heading.

Nitrofurantoin (Caution should be exercised if the practitioner chooses to prescribe riluzole in combination with potentially hepatotoxic drugs (eg, allopurinol, methyldopa, sulfasalazine)).
No products indexed under this heading.

Nitrofurantoin Macrocrystals (Caution should be exercised if the practitioner chooses to prescribe riluzole in combination with potentially hepatotoxic drugs (eg, allopurinol, methyldopa, sulfasalazine)).
No products indexed under this heading.

Nitrofurantoin Monohydrate (Caution should be exercised if the practitioner chooses to prescribe riluzole in combination with potentially hepatotoxic drugs (eg, allopurinol, methyldopa, sulfasalazine)).
No products indexed under this heading.

Nitrofurantoin Sodium (Caution should be exercised if the practitioner chooses to prescribe riluzole in combination with potentially hepatotoxic drugs (eg, allopurinol, methyldopa, sulfasalazine)).
No products indexed under this heading.

Norethindrone (Potential inhibitors of CYP 1A2 (eg, caffeine, phenacetin, theophylline, amitriptyline, and quinolones) could decrease the rate of riluzole elimination). Products include:
Ortho Micronor **2660**

Norethindrone Acetate (Potential inhibitors of CYP 1A2 (eg, caffeine, phenacetin, theophylline, amitriptyline, and quinolones) could decrease the rate of riluzole elimination). Products include:
Activella **2561**

Norfloxacin (Potential inhibitors of CYP 1A2 (eg, caffeine, phenacetin, theophylline, amitriptyline, and quinolones) could decrease the rate of riluzole elimination). Products include:
Noroxin **2220**

Norgestrel (Potential inhibitors of CYP 1A2 (eg, caffeine, phenacetin, theophylline, amitriptyline, and quinolones) could decrease the rate of riluzole elimination).
No products indexed under this heading.

Nortriptyline Hydrochloride (Caution should be exercised if the practitioner chooses to prescribe riluzole in combination with potentially hepatotoxic drugs (eg, allopurinol, methyldopa, sulfasalazine)).
No products indexed under this heading.

Ofloxacin (Potential inhibitors of CYP 1A2 (eg, caffeine, phenacetin, theophylline, amitriptyline, and quinolones) could decrease the rate of riluzole elimination).
No products indexed under this heading.

Olanzapine (CYP 1A2 is the principal isoenzyme involved in the initial oxidative metabolism of riluzole; potential interactions may occur when riluzole is given concurrently with other agents which are also metabolized primarily by CYP 1A2 (eg, theophylline, caffeine, and tacrine)). Products include:
Symbyax **1965**
Zyprexa **1984**
Zyprexa IntraMuscular **1984**
Zyprexa ZYDIS **1984**

Omeprazole (Potential inducers of CYP1A2, such as omeprazole, could increase the rate of riluzole elimination).
No products indexed under this heading.

Omeprazole Magnesium (Potential inhibitors of CYP 1A2 (eg, caffeine, phenacetin, theophylline, amitriptyline, and quinolones) could decrease the rate of riluzole elimination).
No products indexed under this heading.

Ondansetron (CYP 1A2 is the principal isoenzyme involved in the initial oxidative metabolism of riluzole; potential interactions may occur when riluzole is given concurrently with other agents which are also metabolized primarily by CYP 1A2 (eg, theophylline, caffeine, and tacrine)).
No products indexed under this heading.

Ondansetron Hydrochloride (CYP 1A2 is the principal isoenzyme involved in the initial oxidative metabolism of riluzole; potential interactions may occur when riluzole is given concurrently with other agents which are also metabolized primarily by CYP 1A2 (eg, theophylline, caffeine, and tacrine)). Products include:
Zofran Injection **1750**
Zofran **1756**
Zofran ODT **1756**

Oxacillin (Caution should be exercised if the practitioner chooses to prescribe riluzole in combination with potentially hepatotoxic drugs (eg, allopurinol, methyldopa, sulfasalazine)).
No products indexed under this heading.

Oxacillin Sodium (Caution should be exercised if the practitioner chooses to prescribe riluzole in combination with potentially hepatotoxic drugs (eg, allopurinol, methyldopa, sulfasalazine)).
No products indexed under this heading.

Oxaprozin (Caution should be exercised if the practitioner chooses to prescribe riluzole in combination with potentially hepatotoxic drugs (eg, allopurinol, methyldopa, sulfasalazine)).
No products indexed under this heading.

Oxymetholone (Caution should be exercised if the practitioner chooses to prescribe riluzole in combination with potentially hepatotoxic drugs (eg, allopurinol, methyldopa, sulfasalazine)).
No products indexed under this heading.

Oxytetracycline (Caution should be exercised if the practitioner chooses to prescribe riluzole in combination with potentially hepatotoxic drugs (eg, allopurinol, methyldopa, sulfasalazine)).
No products indexed under this heading.

Oxytetracycline Hydrochloride (Caution should be exercised if the practitioner chooses to prescribe riluzole in combination with potentially hepatotoxic drugs (eg, allopurinol, methyldopa, sulfasalazine)).
No products indexed under this heading.

Paroxetine (Potential inhibitors of CYP 1A2 (eg, caffeine, phenacetin, theophylline, amitriptyline, and quinolones) could decrease the rate of riluzole elimination).
No products indexed under this heading.

Paroxetine Hydrochloride (Potential inhibitors of CYP 1A2 (eg, caffeine, phenacetin, theophylline, amitriptyline, and quinolones) could decrease the rate of riluzole elimination). Products include:
Paroxetine CR **2361**
Paroxetine ER **2371**
Paxil **1586**
Paxil CR **1596**

Paroxetine Mesylate (Potential inhibitors of CYP 1A2 (eg, caffeine, phenacetin, theophylline, amitriptyline, and quinolones) could decrease the rate of riluzole elimination).
No products indexed under this heading.

Penicillin, Potassium Phenoxymethyl (Caution should be exercised if the practitioner chooses to prescribe riluzole in combination with potentially hepatotoxic drugs (eg, allopurinol, methyldopa, sulfasalazine)).
No products indexed under this heading.

Penicillin G Benzathine (Caution should be exercised if the practitioner chooses to prescribe riluzole in combination with potentially hepatotoxic drugs (eg, allopurinol, methyldopa, sulfasalazine)). Products include:
Bicillin C-R Injectable Suspension **1826**
Bicillin L-A **1828**

Penicillin G Dibenzylethyenediamine (Caution should be exercised if the practitioner chooses to prescribe riluzole in combination with potentially hepatotoxic drugs (eg, allopurinol, methyldopa, sulfasalazine)).
No products indexed under this heading.

Penicillin G Potassium (Caution should be exercised if the practitioner chooses to prescribe riluzole in combination with potentially hepatotoxic drugs (eg, allopurinol, methyldopa, sulfasalazine)).
No products indexed under this heading.

Penicillin G Procaine (Caution should be exercised if the practitioner chooses to prescribe riluzole in combination with potentially hepatotoxic drugs (eg, allopurinol, methyldopa, sulfasalazine)). Products include:
Bicillin C-R Injectable Suspension **1826**
Bicillin L-A **1828**

Penicillin G Sodium (Caution should be exercised if the practitioner chooses to prescribe riluzole in combination with potentially hepatotoxic drugs (eg, allopurinol, methyldopa, sulfasalazine)).
No products indexed under this heading.

Penicillin V (Caution should be exercised if the practitioner chooses to prescribe riluzole in combination with potentially hepatotoxic drugs (eg, allopurinol, methyldopa, sulfasalazine)).
No products indexed under this heading.

Penicillin V Potassium (Caution should be exercised if the practitioner chooses to prescribe riluzole in combination with potentially hepatotoxic drugs (eg, allopurinol, methyldopa, sulfasalazine)).
No products indexed under this heading.

Penicillins (Caution should be exercised if the practitioner chooses to prescribe riluzole in combination with potentially hepatotoxic drugs (eg, allopurinol, methyldopa, sulfasalazine)).
No products indexed under this heading.

Phenacetin (Potential inhibitors of CYP1A2, such as phenacetin, could decrease the rate of riluzole elimination).
No products indexed under this heading.

Phenobarbital (Potential inducers of CYP 1A2 (eg, cigarette smoke, charcoal-broiled food, rifampicin, and omeprazole) could increase the rate of riluzole elimination). Products include:
Donnatal **2711**

Phenobarbital Sodium (Potential inducers of CYP 1A2 (eg, cigarette smoke, charcoal-broiled food, rifampicin, and omeprazole) could increase the rate of riluzole elimination).
No products indexed under this heading.

Phenylbutazone (Caution should be exercised if the practitioner chooses to prescribe riluzole in combination with potentially hepatotoxic drugs (eg, allopurinol, methyldopa, sulfasalazine)).
No products indexed under this heading.

Phenytoin (Caution should be exercised if the practitioner chooses to prescribe riluzole in combination with potentially hepatotoxic drugs (eg, allopurinol, methyldopa, sulfasalazine)).
No products indexed under this heading.

Phenytoin Sodium (Caution should be exercised if the practitioner chooses to prescribe riluzole in combination with potentially hepatotoxic drugs (eg, allopurinol, methyldopa, sulfasalazine)). Products include:
Phenytek Capsules **2380**

Pioglitazone Hydrochloride (Caution should be exercised if the practitioner chooses to prescribe riluzole in combination with potentially hepatotoxic drugs (eg, allopurinol, methyldopa, sulfasalazine)). Products include:
ActoPlus **3338**
Actos **3345**
Duetact **3354**

Piperacillin Sodium (Caution should be exercised if the practitioner chooses to prescribe riluzole in combination with potentially hepatotoxic drugs (eg, allopurinol, methyldopa, sulfasalazine)). Products include:
Zosyn **3607**

Piroxicam (Caution should be exercised if the practitioner chooses to prescribe riluzole in combination with potentially hepatotoxic drugs (eg, allopurinol, methyldopa, sulfasalazine)).
No products indexed under this heading.

Polythiazide (Caution should be exercised if the practitioner chooses to prescribe riluzole in combination with potentially hepatotoxic drugs (eg, allopurinol, methyldopa, sulfasalazine)).
No products indexed under this heading.

Pravastatin Sodium (Caution should be exercised if the practitioner chooses to prescribe riluzole in combination with potentially hepatotoxic drugs (eg, allopurinol, methyldopa, sulfasalazine)).
No products indexed under this heading.

Primidone (Potential inducers of CYP 1A2 (eg, cigarette smoke, charcoal-broiled food, rifampicin, and omeprazole) could increase the rate of riluzole elimination).
No products indexed under this heading.

Procainamide (Caution should be exercised if the practitioner chooses to prescribe riluzole in combination with potentially hepatotoxic drugs (eg, allopurinol, methyldopa, sulfasalazine)).
No products indexed under this heading.

Procainamide Hydrochloride (Caution should be exercised if the practitioner chooses to prescribe riluzole in combination with potentially hepatotoxic drugs (eg, allopurinol, methyldopa, sulfasalazine)).
No products indexed under this heading.

Propafenone Hydrochloride (CYP 1A2 is the principal isoenzyme involved in the initial oxidative metabolism of riluzole; potential interactions may occur when riluzole is given concurrently with other agents which are also metabolized primarily by CYP 1A2 (eg, theophylline, caffeine, and tacrine)). Products include:

1621 **Interactions Index** **Rilutek**

Rythmol 1648
Rythmol SR 1652

Propranolol Hydrochloride (CYP 1A2 is the principal isoenzyme involved in the initial oxidative metabolism of riluzole; potential interactions may occur when riluzole is given concurrently with other agents which are also metabolized primarily by CYP 1A2 (eg, theophylline, caffeine, and tacrine)). Products include:
InnoPran XL 1517

Propylthiouracil (Caution should be exercised if the practitioner chooses to prescribe riluzole in combination with potentially hepatotoxic drugs (eg, allopurinol, methyldopa, sulfasalazine)).
No products indexed under this heading.

Protriptyline Hydrochloride (Caution should be exercised if the practitioner chooses to prescribe riluzole in combination with potentially hepatotoxic drugs (eg, allopurinol, methyldopa, sulfasalazine)).
No products indexed under this heading.

Ranitidine Bismuth Citrate (Potential inhibitors of CYP 1A2 (eg, caffeine, phenacetin, theophylline, amitriptyline, and quinolones) could decrease the rate of riluzole elimination).
No products indexed under this heading.

Ranitidine Hydrochloride (Potential inhibitors of CYP 1A2 (eg, caffeine, phenacetin, theophylline, amitriptyline, and quinolones) could decrease the rate of riluzole elimination). Products include:
Zantac 1737
Zantac Injection 1732
Zantac Pharmacy 1735

Rifampicin (Potential inducers of CYP1A2, such as rifampicin, could increase the rate of riluzole elimination).
No products indexed under this heading.

Rifampin (Caution should be exercised if the practitioner chooses to prescribe riluzole in combination with potentially hepatotoxic drugs (eg, allopurinol, methyldopa, sulfasalazine)).
No products indexed under this heading.

Ritonavir (Caution should be exercised if the practitioner chooses to prescribe riluzole in combination with potentially hepatotoxic drugs (eg, allopurinol, methyldopa, sulfasalazine)). Products include:
Kaletra 458
Norvir 509

Rofecoxib (Caution should be exercised if the practitioner chooses to prescribe riluzole in combination with potentially hepatotoxic drugs (eg, allopurinol, methyldopa, sulfasalazine)).
No products indexed under this heading.

Ropinirole Hydrochloride (CYP 1A2 is the principal isoenzyme involved in the initial oxidative metabolism of riluzole; potential interactions may occur when riluzole is given concurrently with other agents which are also metabolized primarily by CYP 1A2 (eg, theophylline, caffeine, and tacrine)). Products include:
Requip 1620
Requip XL 1628

Ropivacaine Hydrochloride (CYP 1A2 is the principal isoenzyme involved in the initial oxidative metabolism of riluzole; potential interactions may occur when riluzole is given concurrently with other agents which are also metabolized primarily by CYP 1A2 (eg, theophylline, caffeine, and tacrine)).
No products indexed under this heading.

Rosuvastatin Calcium (Caution should be exercised if the practitioner chooses to prescribe riluzole in combination with potentially hepatotoxic drugs (eg, allopurinol, methyldopa, sulfasalazine)). Products include:
Crestor 736

Saquinavir (Caution should be exercised if the practitioner chooses to prescribe riluzole in combination with potentially hepatotoxic drugs (eg, allopurinol, methyldopa, sulfasalazine)).
No products indexed under this heading.

Saquinavir Mesylate (Caution should be exercised if the practitioner chooses to prescribe riluzole in combination with potentially hepatotoxic drugs (eg, allopurinol, methyldopa, sulfasalazine)).
No products indexed under this heading.

Sildenafil Citrate (Potential inhibitors of CYP 1A2 (eg, caffeine, phenacetin, theophylline, amitriptyline, and quinolones) could decrease the rate of riluzole elimination).
No products indexed under this heading.

Simvastatin (Caution should be exercised if the practitioner chooses to prescribe riluzole in combination with potentially hepatotoxic drugs (eg, allopurinol, methyldopa, sulfasalazine)). Products include:
Simcor 524
Vytorin 10/10 .... 2303, 3240
Vytorin 10/20 .... 2303, 3240
Vytorin 10/40 .... 2303, 3240
Vytorin 10/80 .... 2303, 3240
Zocor 2289

Sodium Cloxacillin Monohydrate (Caution should be exercised if the practitioner chooses to prescribe riluzole in combination with potentially hepatotoxic drugs (eg, allopurinol, methyldopa, sulfasalazine)).
No products indexed under this heading.

Sparfloxacin (Potential inhibitors of CYP 1A2 (eg, caffeine, phenacetin, theophylline, amitriptyline, and quinolones) could decrease the rate of riluzole elimination).
No products indexed under this heading.

Statins (Caution should be exercised if the practitioner chooses to prescribe riluzole in combination with potentially hepatotoxic drugs (eg, allopurinol, methyldopa, sulfasalazine)).
No products indexed under this heading.

Sulfacytine (Caution should be exercised if the practitioner chooses to prescribe riluzole in combination with potentially hepatotoxic drugs (eg, allopurinol, methyldopa, sulfasalazine)).
No products indexed under this heading.

Sulfamethizole (Caution should be exercised if the practitioner chooses to prescribe riluzole in combination with potentially hepatotoxic drugs (eg, allopurinol, methyldopa, sulfasalazine)).
No products indexed under this heading.

Sulfamethoxazole (Caution should be exercised if the practitioner chooses to prescribe riluzole in combination with potentially hepatotoxic drugs (eg, allopurinol, methyldopa, sulfasalazine)).
No products indexed under this heading.

Sulfasalazine (Caution should be exercised if the practitioner chooses to prescribe riluzole in combination with potentially hepatotoxic drugs (eg, sulfasalazine)).
No products indexed under this heading.

Sulfinpyrazone (Caution should be exercised if the practitioner chooses to prescribe riluzole in combination with potentially hepatotoxic drugs (eg, allopurinol, methyldopa, sulfasalazine)).
No products indexed under this heading.

Sulfisoxazole Acetyl (Caution should be exercised if the practitioner chooses to prescribe riluzole in combination with potentially hepatotoxic drugs (eg, allopurinol, methyldopa, sulfasalazine)).
No products indexed under this heading.

Sulfisoxazole Diolamine (Caution should be exercised if the practitioner chooses to prescribe riluzole in combination with potentially hepatotoxic drugs (eg, allopurinol, methyldopa, sulfasalazine)).
No products indexed under this heading.

Sulindac (Caution should be exercised if the practitioner chooses to prescribe riluzole in combination with potentially hepatotoxic drugs (eg, allopurinol, methyldopa, sulfasalazine)). Products include:
Clinoril 2098

Tacrine Hydrochloride (CYP1A2 is the principal isoenzyme involved in the initial oxidative metabolism of riluzole; potential interaction may occur when co-administered with other agents, such as tacrine, which are also metabolized primarily by CYP1A2).
No products indexed under this heading.

Tamoxifen Citrate (Caution should be exercised if the practitioner chooses to prescribe riluzole in combination with potentially hepatotoxic drugs (eg, allopurinol, methyldopa, sulfasalazine)).
No products indexed under this heading.

Telithromycin (Caution should be exercised if the practitioner chooses to prescribe riluzole in combination with potentially hepatotoxic drugs (eg, allopurinol, methyldopa, sulfasalazine)). Products include:
Ketek 2991

Tetracycline Hydrochloride (Caution should be exercised if the practitioner chooses to prescribe riluzole in combination with potentially hepatotoxic drugs (eg, allopurinol, methyldopa, sulfasalazine)). Products include:
Pylera 793

Tetracycline Phosphate Complex (Caution should be exercised if the practitioner chooses to prescribe riluzole in combination with potentially hepatotoxic drugs (eg, allopurinol, methyldopa, sulfasalazine)).
No products indexed under this heading.

Theobromine (CYP 1A2 is the principal isoenzyme involved in the initial oxidative metabolism of riluzole; potential interactions may occur when riluzole is given concurrently with other agents which are also metabolized primarily by CYP 1A2 (eg, theophylline, caffeine, and tacrine)).
No products indexed under this heading.

Theophylline (Potential inhibitors of CYP1A2, such as theophylline, could decrease the rate of riluzole elimination. CYP1A2 is the principal isoenzyme involved in the initial oxidative metabolism of riluzole; potential interactions may occur when riluzole is given concurrently with other agents which are also metabolized primarily by CYP1A2 (eg, theophylline)).
No products indexed under this heading.

Theophylline Anhydrous (Potential inhibitors of CYP1A2, such as theophylline, could decrease the rate of riluzole elimination. CYP1A2 is the principal isoenzyme involved in the initial oxidative metabolism of riluzole; potential interactions may occur when riluzole is given concurrently with other agents which are also metabolized primarily by CYP1A2 (eg, theophylline)). Products include:
Uniphyl 2817

Theophylline Calcium Salicylate (Potential inhibitors of CYP1A2, such as theophylline, could decrease the rate of riluzole elimination. CYP1A2 is the principal isoenzyme involved in the initial oxidative metabolism of riluzole; potential interactions may occur when riluzole is given concurrently with other agents which are also metabolized primarily by CYP1A2 (eg, theophylline)).
No products indexed under this heading.

Theophylline Dihydroxypropyl (Glyceryl) (Potential inhibitors of CYP1A2, such as theophylline, could decrease the rate of riluzole elimination. CYP1A2 is the principal isoenzyme involved in the initial oxidative metabolism of riluzole; potential interactions may occur when riluzole is given concurrently with other agents which are also metabolized primarily by CYP1A2 (eg, theophylline)).
No products indexed under this heading.

Theophylline Ethylenediamine (Potential inhibitors of CYP1A2, such as theophylline, could decrease the rate of riluzole elimination. CYP1A2 is the principal isoenzyme involved in the initial oxidative metabolism of riluzole; potential interactions may occur when riluzole is given concurrently with other agents which are also metabolized primarily by CYP1A2 (eg, theophylline)).
No products indexed under this heading.

Theophylline Sodium Glycinate (Potential inhibitors of CYP1A2, such as theophylline, could decrease the rate of riluzole elimination. CYP1A2 is the principal isoenzyme involved in the initial oxidative metabolism of riluzole; potential interactions may occur when riluzole is given concurrently with other agents which are also metabolized primarily by CYP1A2 (eg, theophylline)).
No products indexed under this heading.

Thiazide Diuretics (Caution should be exercised if the practitioner chooses to prescribe riluzole in combination with potentially hepatotoxic drugs (eg, allopurinol, methyldopa, sulfasalazine)).
No products indexed under this heading.

Thiazides (Caution should be exercised if the practitioner chooses to prescribe riluzole in combination with potentially hepatotoxic drugs (eg, allopurinol, methyldopa, sulfasalazine)).
No products indexed under this heading.

Ticarcillin Disodium (Caution should be exercised if the practitioner chooses to prescribe riluzole in combination with potentially hepatotoxic drugs (eg, allopurinol, methyldopa, sulfasalazine)). Products include:
Timentin ADD-Vantage 1670
Timentin Galaxy 1674
Timentin 1666
Timentin Pharmacy 1678

Ticlopidine Hydrochloride (Potential inhibitors of CYP 1A2 (eg, caffeine, phenacetin, theophylline, amitriptyline, and quinolones) could decrease the rate of riluzole elimination).
No products indexed under this heading.

Tipranavir (Caution should be exercised if the practitioner chooses to prescribe riluzole in combination with potentially hepatotoxic drugs (eg, allopurinol, methyldopa, sulfasalazine)).
No products indexed under this heading.

Tizanidine (CYP 1A2 is the principal isoenzyme involved in the initial oxidative metabolism of riluzole; potential interactions may occur when riluzole is given concurrently with other agents which are also metabolized primarily by CYP 1A2 (eg, theophylline, caffeine, and tacrine)).
No products indexed under this heading.

Tizanidine Hydrochloride (CYP 1A2 is the principal isoenzyme involved in the initial oxidative metabolism of riluzole; potential interactions may occur when riluzole is given concurrently with other agents which are also metabolized primarily by CYP 1A2 (eg, theophylline, caffeine, and tacrine)).
No products indexed under this heading.

Tobacco (Potential inducers of CYP1A2, such as cigarette smoke, could increase the rate of riluzole elimination).
No products indexed under this heading.

Tolazamide (Caution should be exercised if the practitioner chooses to prescribe riluzole in combination with potentially hepatotoxic drugs (eg, allopurinol, methyldopa, sulfasalazine)).
No products indexed under this heading.

Tolbutamide (Caution should be exercised if the practitioner chooses to prescribe riluzole in combination with potentially hepatotoxic drugs (eg, allopurinol, methyldopa, sulfasalazine)).
No products indexed under this heading.

Tolbutamide Sodium (Caution should be exercised if the practitioner chooses to prescribe riluzole in combination with potentially hepatotoxic drugs (eg, allopurinol, methyldopa, sulfasalazine)).
No products indexed under this heading.

Tolmetin Sodium (Caution should be exercised if the practitioner chooses to prescribe riluzole in combination with potentially hepatotoxic drugs (eg, allopurinol, methyldopa, sulfasalazine)).
No products indexed under this heading.

Trimethaphan Camsylate (CYP 1A2 is the principal isoenzyme involved in the initial oxidative metabolism of riluzole; potential interactions may occur when riluzole is given concurrently with other agents which are also metabolized primarily by CYP 1A2 (eg, theophylline, caffeine, and tacrine)).
No products indexed under this heading.

Trimethoprim (Caution should be exercised if the practitioner chooses to prescribe riluzole in combination with potentially hepatotoxic drugs (eg, allopurinol, methyldopa, sulfasalazine)).
No products indexed under this heading.

Trimethoprim Hydrochloride (Caution should be exercised if the practitioner chooses to prescribe riluzole in combination with potentially hepatotoxic drugs (eg, allopurinol, methyldopa, sulfasalazine)).
No products indexed under this heading.

Trimethoprim Sulfate (Caution should be exercised if the practitioner chooses to prescribe riluzole in combination with potentially hepatotoxic drugs (eg, allopurinol, methyldopa, sulfasalazine)).
No products indexed under this heading.

Trimipramine Maleate (Caution should be exercised if the practitioner chooses to prescribe riluzole in combination with potentially hepatotoxic drugs (eg, allopurinol, methyldopa, sulfasalazine)).
No products indexed under this heading.

Troleandomycin (Potential inhibitors of CYP 1A2 (eg, caffeine, phenacetin, theophylline, amitriptyline, and quinolones) could decrease the rate of riluzole elimination).
No products indexed under this heading.

Trovafloxacin Mesylate (Potential inhibitors of CYP 1A2 (eg, caffeine, phenacetin, theophylline, amitriptyline, and quinolones) could decrease the rate of riluzole elimination).
No products indexed under this heading.

Valdecoxib (Caution should be exercised if the practitioner chooses to prescribe riluzole in combination with potentially hepatotoxic drugs (eg, allopurinol, methyldopa, sulfasalazine)).
No products indexed under this heading.

Valproate Sodium (Caution should be exercised if the practitioner chooses to prescribe riluzole in combination with potentially hepatotoxic drugs (eg, allopurinol, methyldopa, sulfasalazine)).
No products indexed under this heading.

Valproic Acid (Caution should be exercised if the practitioner chooses to prescribe riluzole in combination with potentially hepatotoxic drugs (eg, allopurinol, methyldopa, sulfasalazine)).
No products indexed under this heading.

Vardenafil Hydrochloride (Potential inhibitors of CYP 1A2 (eg, caffeine, phenacetin, theophylline, amitriptyline, and quinolones) could decrease the rate of riluzole elimination). Products include:
Levitra 3157

Verapamil Hydrochloride (CYP 1A2 is the principal isoenzyme involved in the initial oxidative metabolism of riluzole; potential interactions may occur when riluzole is given concurrently with other agents which are also metabolized primarily by CYP 1A2 (eg, theophylline, caffeine, and tacrine)). Products include:
Tarka 534

Voriconazole (Caution should be exercised if the practitioner chooses to prescribe riluzole in combination with potentially hepatotoxic drugs (eg, allopurinol, methyldopa, sulfasalazine)).
No products indexed under this heading.

Warfarin Sodium (CYP 1A2 is the principal isoenzyme involved in the initial oxidative metabolism of riluzole; potential interactions may occur when riluzole is given concurrently with other agents which are also metabolized primarily by CYP 1A2 (eg, theophylline, caffeine, and tacrine)).
No products indexed under this heading.

Zileuton (Potential inhibitors of CYP 1A2 (eg, caffeine, phenacetin, theophylline, amitriptyline, and quinolones) could decrease the rate of riluzole elimination).
No products indexed under this heading.

Zolmitriptan (CYP 1A2 is the principal isoenzyme involved in the initial oxidative metabolism of riluzole; potential interactions may occur when riluzole is given concurrently with other agents which are also metabolized primarily by CYP 1A2 (eg, theophylline, caffeine, and tacrine)). Products include:
Zomig Tablets 773
Zomig Nasal Spray 768
Zomig-ZMT Tablets 773

Food Interactions

Alcohol (Whether alcohol increases the risk of serious hepatotoxicity with riluzole is unknown; therefore, patients being treated with riluzole should be discouraged from drinking excessive amounts of alcohol).

Beer, reduced-alcohol (Whether alcohol increases the risk of serious hepatotoxicity with riluzole is unknown; therefore, patients being treated with riluzole should be discouraged from drinking excessive amounts of alcohol).

Beer, unspecified (Whether alcohol increases the risk of serious hepatotoxicity with riluzole is unknown; therefore, patients being treated with riluzole should be discouraged from drinking excessive amounts of alcohol).

Beverages, caffeine-containing (Potential inhibitors of CYP1A2, such as caffeine, could decrease the rate of riluzole elimination. CYP1A2 is the principal isoenzyme involved in the initial oxidative metabolism of riluzole; potential interactions may occur when riluzole is given concurrently with other agents which are also metabolized primarily by CYP1A2 (eg, caffeine)).

Broccoli (Potential inducers of CYP 1A2 (eg, cigarette smoke, charcoal-broiled food, rifampicin, and omeprazole) could increase the rate of riluzole elimination).

Brussel Sprouts (Potential inducers of CYP 1A2 (eg, cigarette smoke, charcoal-broiled food, rifampicin, and omeprazole) could increase the rate of riluzole elimination).

Charbroiled Food (Potential inducers of CYP 1A2 (eg, cigarette smoke, charcoal-broiled food, rifampicin, and omeprazole) could increase the rate of riluzole elimination).

Diet, high-lipid (Co-administration with high-fat meal decreases absorption, reduces AUC by about 20% and peak blood levels by about 45%).

Food, caffeine-containing (Potential inhibitors of CYP1A2, such as caffeine, could decrease the rate of riluzole elimination. CYP1A2 is the principal isoenzyme involved in the initial oxidative metabolism of riluzole; potential interactions may occur when riluzole is given concurrently with other agents which are also metabolized primarily by CYP1A2 (eg, caffeine)).

Food, charcoal-broiled (Potential inducers of CYP1A2, such as charcoal-broiled food, could increase the rate of riluzole elimination).

Grapefruit (Potential inhibitors of CYP 1A2 (eg, caffeine, phenacetin, theophylline, amitriptyline, and quinolones) could decrease the rate of riluzole elimination).

Grapefruit Juice (Potential inhibitors of CYP 1A2 (eg, caffeine, phenacetin, theophylline, amitriptyline, and quinolones) could decrease the rate of riluzole elimination).

Wine, Chianti (Whether alcohol increases the risk of serious hepatotoxicity with riluzole is unknown; therefore, patients being treated with riluzole should be discouraged from drinking excessive amounts of alcohol).

Wine, Red (Whether alcohol increases the risk of serious hepatotoxicity with riluzole is unknown; therefore, patients being treated with riluzole should be discouraged from drinking excessive amounts of alcohol).

Wine, unspecified (Whether alcohol increases the risk of serious hepatotoxicity with riluzole is unknown; therefore, patients being treated with riluzole should be discouraged from drinking excessive amounts of alcohol).

Wine products (Whether alcohol increases the risk of serious hepatotoxicity with riluzole is unknown; therefore, patients being treated with riluzole should be discouraged from drinking excessive amounts of alcohol).

RISPERDAL CONSTA LONG-ACTING INJECTION

(Risperidone) 2682

May interact with alcohols, antihypertensives, centrally-acting drugs, cytochrome p450 1a2 substrates (selected), cytochrome p450 2c19 substrates (selected), cytochrome p450 2c9 substrates (selected), cytochrome p450 2d6 inhibitors (selected), cytochrome p450 3a4 inducers (selected), cytochrome p450 3a4 substrates (selected), dopamine agonists, phenytoin, valproate, and certain other agents. Compounds in these categories include:

Acarbose (*In vitro* studies showed that drugs metabolized by other CYP isozymes, including 1A1, 1A2, 2C9, 2C19, and 3A4, are only weak inhibitors of risperidone metabolism).
No products indexed under this heading.

Acebutolol Hydrochloride (Because of its potential for inducing hypotension, risperidone may enhance the hypotensive effects of other therapeutic agents with this potential).
No products indexed under this heading.

Acetaminophen (*In vitro* studies showed that drugs metabolized by other CYP isozymes, including 1A1, 1A2, 2C9, 2C19, and 3A4, are only weak inhibitors of risperidone metabolism). Products include:
Percocet 1121
Tylenol 2049
Tylenol 8 Hour 2049
Extra Strength Tylenol Caplets, Cool Caplets, and EZ Tabs 2049
Extra Strength Tylenol Adult Rapid Blast Liquid 2049
Extra Strength Tylenol Rapid Release 2049
Tylenol with Codeine 2691
Tylenol Arthritis Pain Extended Release Geltabs/Caplets 2049
Children's Tylenol Suspension Liquid 2048
Children's Tylenol Meltaways 2048
Tylenol, Infants' Drops 2048
Junior Tylenol 2048
Vicodin 560
Vicodin ES 561
Vicodin HP 563
Zydone 1138

Alatrofloxacin Mesylate (*In vitro* studies showed that drugs metabolized by other CYP isozymes, including 1A1, 1A2, 2C9, 2C19, and 3A4, are only weak inhibitors of risperidone metabolism).
No products indexed under this heading.

Alfentanil Hydrochloride (Given the primary CNS effects of risperidone, caution should be used if taken in combination with other centrally-acting drugs).
No products indexed under this heading.

Aliskiren (Because of its potential for inducing hypotension, risperidone may enhance the hypotensive effects of other therapeutic agents with this potential). Products include:
Tekturna 2538
Tekturna HCT 2541
Valturna 3637

Allium sativum (Co-administration of known CYP3A4 enzyme inducers with risperidone may cause decreases in the combined plasma concentrations of ripseridone and 9-hydroxyrisperidone, which could lead to decreased efficacy of risperidone treatment. At the initiation of therapy with known hepatic enzyme inducers, patients should be closely monitored during the first 4–8 weeks, since the dose of risperidone may need to be adjusted. A dose increase, or additional oral risperidone, may need to be considered. On discontinuation of CYP3A4 hepatic enzyme inducers, the dosage of risperidone should be re-evaluated and, if necessary, decreased).
No products indexed under this heading.

Alprazolam (Given the primary CNS effects of risperidone, caution should be used if taken in combination with other centrally-acting drugs).
No products indexed under this heading.

Aminoglutethimide (Co-administration of known CYP3A4 enzyme inducers with risperidone may cause decreases in the combined plasma concentrations of ripseridone and 9-hydroxyrisperidone, which could lead to decreased efficacy of risperidone treatment. At the initiation of therapy with known hepatic enzyme inducers, patients should be closely monitored during the first 4–8 weeks, since the dose of risperidone may need to be adjusted. A dose increase, or additional oral risperidone, may need to be considered. On discontinuation of CYP3A4 hepatic enzyme inducers, the dosage of risperidone should be re-evaluated and, if necessary, decreased).
No products indexed under this heading.

Aminophylline (*In vitro* studies showed that drugs metabolized by other CYP isozymes, including 1A1, 1A2, 2C9, 2C19, and 3A4, are only weak inhibitors of risperidone metabolism).
No products indexed under this heading.

Amiodarone Hydrochloride (*In vitro* studies showed that drugs metabolized by other CYP isozymes, including 1A1, 1A2, 2C9, 2C19, and 3A4, are only weak inhibitors of risperidone metabolism).
No products indexed under this heading.

Amitriptyline Hydrochloride (*In vitro* studies showed that drugs metabolized by other CYP isozymes, including 1A1, 1A2, 2C9, 2C19, and 3A4, are only weak inhibitors of risperidone metabolism).
No products indexed under this heading.

Amlodipine Besylate (Because of its potential for inducing hypotension, risperidone may enhance the hypotensive effects of other therapeutic agents with this potential). Products include:
Azor **1010**
Exforge **2443**
Exforge HCT **2449**

Amoxapine (*In vitro* studies showed that drugs metabolized by other CYP isozymes, including 1A1, 1A2, 2C9, 2C19, and 3A4, are only weak inhibitors of risperidone metabolism).
No products indexed under this heading.

Amphetamine Aspartate (Given the primary CNS effects of risperidone, caution should be used if taken in combination with other centrally-acting drugs).
No products indexed under this heading.

Amphetamine Aspartate Monohydrate (Given the primary CNS effects of risperidone, caution should be used if taken in combination with other centrally-acting drugs).
No products indexed under this heading.

Amphetamine Resins (Given the primary CNS effects of risperidone, caution should be used if taken in combination with other centrally-acting drugs).
No products indexed under this heading.

Amphetamine Sulfate (Given the primary CNS effects of risperidone, caution should be used if taken in combination with other centrally-acting drugs).
No products indexed under this heading.

Anagrelide Hydrochloride (*In vitro* studies showed that drugs metabolized by other CYP isozymes, including 1A1, 1A2, 2C9, 2C19, and 3A4, are only weak inhibitors of risperidone metabolism).
No products indexed under this heading.

Aprepitant (Co-administration of known CYP3A4 enzyme inducers with risperidone may cause decreases in the combined plasma concentrations of ripseridone and 9-hydroxyrisperidone, which could lead to decreased efficacy of risperidone treatment. At the initiation of therapy with known hepatic enzyme inducers, patients should be closely monitored during the first 4–8 weeks, since the dose of risperidone may need to be adjusted. A dose increase, or additional oral risperidone, may need to be considered. On discontinuation of CYP3A4 hepatic enzyme inducers, the dosage of risperidone should be re-evaluated and, if necessary, decreased). Products include:
Emend **2124**

Aprobarbital (Given the primary CNS effects of risperidone, caution should be used if taken in combination with other centrally-acting drugs).
No products indexed under this heading.

Astemizole (*In vitro* studies showed that drugs metabolized by other CYP isozymes, including 1A1, 1A2, 2C9, 2C19, and 3A4, are only weak inhibitors of risperidone metabolism).
No products indexed under this heading.

Atenolol (Because of its potential for inducing hypotension, risperidone may enhance the hypotensive effects of other therapeutic agents with this potential).
No products indexed under this heading.

Atorvastatin Calcium (*In vitro* studies showed that drugs metabolized by other CYP isozymes, including 1A1, 1A2, 2C9, 2C19, and 3A4, are only weak inhibitors of risperidone metabolism). Products include:
Lipitor **2703**

Belladonna Ergotamine (*In vitro* studies showed that drugs metabolized by other CYP isozymes, including 1A1, 1A2, 2C9, 2C19, and 3A4, are only weak inhibitors of risperidone metabolism).
No products indexed under this heading.

Benazepril Hydrochloride (Because of its potential for inducing hypotension, risperidone may enhance the hypotensive effects of other therapeutic agents with this potential).
No products indexed under this heading.

Bendroflumethiazide (Because of its potential for inducing hypotension, risperidone may enhance the hypotensive effects of other therapeutic agents with this potential).
No products indexed under this heading.

Betamethasone (Co-administration of known CYP3A4 enzyme inducers with risperidone may cause decreases in the combined plasma concentrations of ripseridone and 9-hydroxyrisperidone, which could lead to decreased efficacy of risperidone treatment. At the initiation of therapy with known hepatic enzyme inducers, patients should be closely monitored during the first 4–8 weeks, since the dose of risperidone may need to be adjusted. A dose increase, or additional oral risperidone, may need to be considered. On discontinuation of CYP3A4 hepatic enzyme inducers, the dosage of risperidone should be re-evaluated and, if necessary, decreased).
No products indexed under this heading.

Betamethasone Acetate (Co-administration of known CYP3A4 enzyme inducers with risperidone may cause decreases in the combined plasma concentrations of ripseridone and 9-hydroxyrisperidone, which could lead to decreased efficacy of risperidone treatment. At the initiation of therapy with known hepatic enzyme inducers, patients should be closely monitored during the first 4–8 weeks, since the dose of risperidone may need to be adjusted. A dose increase, or additional oral risperidone, may need to be considered. On discontinuation of CYP3A4 hepatic enzyme inducers, the dosage of risperidone should be re-evaluated and, if necessary, decreased).
No products indexed under this heading.

Betamethasone Benzoate (Co-administration of known CYP3A4 enzyme inducers with risperidone may cause decreases in the combined plasma concentrations of ripseridone and 9-hydroxyrisperidone, which could lead to decreased efficacy of risperidone treatment. At the initiation of therapy with known hepatic enzyme inducers, patients should be closely monitored during the first 4–8 weeks, since the dose of risperidone may need to be adjusted. A dose increase, or additional oral risperidone, may need to be considered. On discontinuation of CYP3A4 hepatic enzyme inducers, the dosage of risperidone should be re-evaluated and, if necessary, decreased).
No products indexed under this heading.

Betamethasone Dipropionate (Co-administration of known CYP3A4 enzyme inducers with risperidone may cause decreases in the combined plasma concentrations of ripseridone and 9-hydroxyrisperidone, which could lead to decreased efficacy of risperidone treatment. At the initiation of therapy with known hepatic enzyme inducers, patients should be closely monitored during the first 4–8 weeks, since the dose of risperidone may need to be adjusted. A dose increase, or additional oral risperidone, may need to be considered. On discontinuation of CYP3A4 hepatic enzyme inducers, the dosage of risperidone should be re-evaluated and, if necessary, decreased). Products include:
Diprolene Lotion 0.05% **3108**
Diprolene Ointment 0.05% **3109**
Diprolene AF Cream 0.05% **3107**
Lotrisone **3163**

Betamethasone Sodium Phosphate (Co-administration of known CYP3A4 enzyme inducers with risperidone may cause decreases in the combined plasma concentrations of ripseridone and 9-hydroxyrisperidone, which could lead to decreased efficacy of risperidone treatment. At the initiation of therapy with known hepatic enzyme inducers, patients should be closely monitored during the first 4–8 weeks, since the dose of risperidone may need to be adjusted. A dose increase, or additional oral risperidone, may need to be considered. On discontinuation of CYP3A4 hepatic enzyme inducers, the dosage of risperidone should be re-evaluated and, if necessary, decreased).
No products indexed under this heading.

Betamethasone Valerate (Co-administration of known CYP3A4 enzyme inducers with risperidone may cause decreases in the combined plasma concentrations of ripseridone and 9-hydroxyrisperidone, which could lead to decreased efficacy of risperidone treatment. At the initiation of therapy with known hepatic enzyme inducers, patients should be closely monitored during the first 4–8 weeks, since the dose of risperidone may need to be adjusted. A dose increase, or additional oral risperidone, may need to be considered. On discontinuation of CYP3A4 hepatic enzyme inducers, the dosage of risperidone should be re-evaluated and, if necessary, decreased). Products include:
Luxiq **3321**

Betaxolol Hydrochloride (Because of its potential for inducing hypotension, risperidone may enhance the hypotensive effects of other therapeutic agents with this potential).
No products indexed under this heading.

Bisoprolol Fumarate (Because of its potential for inducing hypotension, risperidone may enhance the hypotensive effects of other therapeutic agents with this potential).
No products indexed under this heading.

Bosentan (Co-administration of known CYP3A4 enzyme inducers with risperidone may cause decreases in the combined plasma concentrations of ripseridone and 9-hydroxyrisperidone, which could lead to decreased efficacy of risperidone treatment. At the initiation of therapy with known hepatic enzyme inducers, patients should be closely monitored during the first 4–8 weeks, since the dose of risperidone may need to be adjusted. A dose increase, or additional oral risperidone, may need to be considered. On discontinuation of CYP3A4 hepatic enzyme inducers, the dosage of risperidone should be re-evaluated and, if necessary, decreased). Products include:
Tracleer **573**

Bromocriptine Mesylate (Risperidone may antagonize the effect of dopamine agonists).
No products indexed under this heading.

Buprenorphine Hydrochloride (Given the primary CNS effects of risperidone, caution should be used if taken in combination with other centrally-acting drugs).
No products indexed under this heading.

Bupropion Hydrochloride (Risperidone is metabolized to 9-hydroxyrisperidone by CYP2D6. Drug interactions that reduce the metabolism of risperidone to 9-hydroxyrisperidone would increase the plasma concentrations of risperidone and lower the concentrations of 9-hydroxyrisperidone). Products include:
Aplenzin **2948**
Wellbutrin **1719**
Wellbutrin SR **1725**
Zyban **1762**

Buspirone Hydrochloride (Given the primary CNS effects of risperidone, caution should be used if taken in combination with other centrally-acting drugs).
No products indexed under this heading.

Busulfan (*In vitro* studies showed that drugs metabolized by other CYP isozymes, including 1A1, 1A2, 2C9, 2C19, and 3A4, are only weak inhibitors of risperidone metabolism). Products include:
Myleran **1581**

Butabarbital (Given the primary CNS effects of risperidone, caution should be used if taken in combination with other centrally-acting drugs).
No products indexed under this heading.

Butalbital (Given the primary CNS effects of risperidone, caution should be used if taken in combination with other centrally-acting drugs).
No products indexed under this heading.

Caffeine (*In vitro* studies showed that drugs metabolized by other CYP isozymes, including 1A1, 1A2, 2C9, 2C19, and 3A4, are only weak inhibitors of risperidone metabolism).
No products indexed under this heading.

Caffeine Anhydrous (*In vitro* studies showed that drugs metabolized by other CYP isozymes, including 1A1, 1A2, 2C9, 2C19, and 3A4, are only weak inhibitors of risperidone metabolism).
No products indexed under this heading.

Caffeine Citrate (*In vitro* studies showed that drugs metabolized by other CYP isozymes, including 1A1, 1A2, 2C9, 2C19, and 3A4, are only weak inhibitors of risperidone metabolism).
No products indexed under this heading.

Caffeine-containing medications (*In vitro* studies showed that drugs metabolized by other CYP isozymes, including 1A1, 1A2, 2C9, 2C19, and 3A4, are only weak inhibitors of risperidone metabolism).
No products indexed under this heading.

Caffeine Sodium Benzoate (*In vitro* studies showed that drugs metabolized by other CYP isozymes, including 1A1, 1A2, 2C9, 2C19, and 3A4, are only weak inhibitors of risperidone metabolism).
No products indexed under this heading.

Candesartan Cilexetil (Because of its potential for inducing hypotension, risperidone may enhance the hypotensive effects of other therapeutic agents with this potential). Products include:
Atacand **697**
Atacand HCT **700**

Captopril (Because of its potential for inducing hypotension, risperidone may enhance the hypotensive effects of other therapeutic agents with this potential). Products include:

Carbamazepine (Carbamazepine co-administration with oral risperidone decreased the steady state plasma concentrations of risperidone and 9-hydroxyrisperidone by about 50%. Plasma concentrations of carbamazepine did not appear to be affected. At initiation of therapy with carbamazepine, patients should be closely monitored during the first 4-8 weeks, since the dose of resperidone may need to be adjusted. A dose increase, or additional oral risperidone, may be considered. On discontinuation of carbamazepine, the dosage of risperidone should be re-evaluated and, if necessary, decreased). Products include:

Carisoprodol (In vitro studies showed that drugs metabolized by other CYP isozymes, including 1A1, 1A2, 2C9, 2C19, and 3A4, are only weak inhibitors of risperidone metabolism).
No products indexed under this heading.

Carteolol Hydrochloride (Because of its potential for inducing hypotension, risperidone may enhance the hypotensive effects of other therapeutic agents with this potential).
No products indexed under this heading.

Carvedilol (Because of its potential for inducing hypotension, risperidone may enhance the hypotensive effects of other therapeutic agents with this potential). Products include:

Carvedilol Phosphate (Because of its potential for inducing hypotension, risperidone may enhance the hypotensive effects of other therapeutic agents with this potential). Products include:

Celecoxib (Risperidone is metabolized to 9-hydroxyrisperidone by CYP2D6. Drug interactions that reduce the metabolism of risperidone to 9-hydroxyrisperidone would increase the plasma concentrations of risperidone and lower the concentrations of 9-hydroxyrisperidone). Products include:

Cerivastatin Sodium (In vitro studies showed that drugs metabolized by other CYP isozymes, including 1A1, 1A2, 2C9, 2C19, and 3A4, are only weak inhibitors of risperidone metabolism).
No products indexed under this heading.

Chlordiazepoxide (Given the primary CNS effects of risperidone, caution should be used if taken in combination with other centrally-acting drugs).
No products indexed under this heading.

Chlordiazepoxide Hydrochloride (Given the primary CNS effects of risperidone, caution should be used if taken in combination with other centrally-acting drugs).
No products indexed under this heading.

Chloroquine (Risperidone is metabolized to 9-hydroxyrisperidone by CYP2D6. Drug interactions that reduce the metabolism of risperidone to 9-hydroxyrisperidone would increase the plasma concentrations of risperidone and lower the concentrations of 9-hydroxyrisperidone).
No products indexed under this heading.

Chloroquine Hydrochloride (Risperidone is metabolized to 9-hydroxyrisperidone by CYP2D6. Drug interactions that reduce the metabolism of risperidone to 9-hydroxyrisperidone would increase the plasma concentrations of risperidone and lower the concentrations of 9-hydroxyrisperidone).
No products indexed under this heading.

Chloroquine Phosphate (Risperidone is metabolized to 9-hydroxyrisperidone by CYP2D6. Drug interactions that reduce the metabolism of risperidone to 9-hydroxyrisperidone would increase the plasma concentrations of risperidone and lower the concentrations of 9-hydroxyrisperidone).
No products indexed under this heading.

Chlorothiazide (Because of its potential for inducing hypotension, risperidone may enhance the hypotensive effects of other therapeutic agents with this potential).
No products indexed under this heading.

Chlorothiazide Sodium (Because of its potential for inducing hypotension, risperidone may enhance the hypotensive effects of other therapeutic agents with this potential). Products include:

Chlorpheniramine (Risperidone is metabolized to 9-hydroxyrisperidone by CYP2D6. Drug interactions that reduce the metabolism of risperidone to 9-hydroxyrisperidone would increase the plasma concentrations of risperidone and lower the concentrations of 9-hydroxyrisperidone).
No products indexed under this heading.

Chlorpheniramine Maleate (Risperidone is metabolized to 9-hydroxyrisperidone by CYP2D6. Drug interactions that reduce the metabolism of risperidone to 9-hydroxyrisperidone would increase the plasma concentrations of risperidone and lower the concentrations of 9-hydroxyrisperidone).
No products indexed under this heading.

Chlorpheniramine Polistirex (Risperidone is metabolized to 9-hydroxyrisperidone by CYP2D6. Drug interactions that reduce the metabolism of risperidone to 9-hydroxyrisperidone would increase the plasma concentrations of risperidone and lower the concentrations of 9-hydroxyrisperidone). Products include:

Chlorpheniramine Tannate (Risperidone is metabolized to 9-hydroxyrisperidone by CYP2D6. Drug interactions that reduce the metabolism of risperidone to 9-hydroxyrisperidone would increase the plasma concentrations of risperidone and lower the concentrations of 9-hydroxyrisperidone).
No products indexed under this heading.

Chlorpromazine (Given the primary CNS effects of risperidone, caution should be used if taken in combination with other centrally-acting drugs).
No products indexed under this heading.

Chlorpromazine Hydrochloride (Given the primary CNS effects of risperidone, caution should be used if taken in combination with other centrally-acting drugs).
No products indexed under this heading.

Chlorpropamide (In vitro studies showed that drugs metabolized by other CYP isozymes, including 1A1, 1A2, 2C9, 2C19, and 3A4, are only weak inhibitors of risperidone metabolism).
No products indexed under this heading.

Chlorprothixene (Given the primary CNS effects of risperidone, caution should be used if taken in combination with other centrally-acting drugs).
No products indexed under this heading.

Chlorprothixene Hydrochloride (Given the primary CNS effects of risperidone, caution should be used if taken in combination with other centrally-acting drugs).
No products indexed under this heading.

Chlorprothixene Lactate (Given the primary CNS effects of risperidone, caution should be used if taken in combination with other centrally-acting drugs).
No products indexed under this heading.

Chlorthalidone (Because of its potential for inducing hypotension, risperidone may enhance the hypotensive effects of other therapeutic agents with this potential). Products include:

Cilostazol (In vitro studies showed that drugs metabolized by other CYP isozymes, including 1A1, 1A2, 2C9, 2C19, and 3A4, are only weak inhibitors of risperidone metabolism).
No products indexed under this heading.

Cimetidine (Cimetidine increased the bioavailability of oral risperidone by 64%. However, cimetidine did not affect the AUC of risperidone and 9-hydroxyrisperidone combined).
No products indexed under this heading.

Cimetidine Hydrochloride (Cimetidine increased the bioavailability of oral risperidone by 64%. However, cimetidine did not affect the AUC of risperidone and 9-hydroxyrisperidone combined).
No products indexed under this heading.

Ciprofloxacin (In vitro studies showed that drugs metabolized by other CYP isozymes, including 1A1, 1A2, 2C9, 2C19, and 3A4, are only weak inhibitors of risperidone metabolism). Products include:

Ciprofloxacin Hydrochloride (In vitro studies showed that drugs metabolized by other CYP isozymes, including 1A1, 1A2, 2C9, 2C19, and 3A4, are only weak inhibitors of risperidone metabolism). Products include:

Cisapride (In vitro studies showed that drugs metabolized by other CYP isozymes, including 1A1, 1A2, 2C9, 2C19, and 3A4, are only weak inhibitors of risperidone metabolism).
No products indexed under this heading.

Cisplatin (Co-administration of known CYP3A4 enzyme inducers with risperidone may cause decreases in the combined plasma concentrations of risperidone and 9-hydroxyrisperidone, which could lead to decreased efficacy of risperidone treatment. At the initiation of therapy with known hepatic enzyme inducers, patients should be closely monitored during the first 4–8 weeks, since the dose of risperidone may need to be adjusted. A dose increase, or additional oral risperidone, may need to be considered. On discontinuation of CYP3A4 hepatic enzyme inducers, the dosage of risperidone should be re-evaluated and, if necessary, decreased).
No products indexed under this heading.

Citalopram Hydrobromide (Risperidone is metabolized to 9-hydroxyrisperidone by CYP2D6. Drug interactions that reduce the metabolism of risperidone to 9-hydroxyrisperidone would increase the plasma concentrations of risperidone and lower the concentrations of 9-hydroxyrisperidone). Products include:

Clarithromycin (In vitro studies showed that drugs metabolized by other CYP isozymes, including 1A1, 1A2, 2C9, 2C19, and 3A4, are only weak inhibitors of risperidone metabolism). Products include:

Clomipramine Hydrochloride (In vitro studies showed that drugs metabolized by other CYP isozymes, including 1A1, 1A2, 2C9, 2C19, and 3A4, are only weak inhibitors of risperidone metabolism).
No products indexed under this heading.

Clonidine (Because of its potential for inducing hypotension, risperidone may enhance the hypotensive effects of other therapeutic agents with this potential). Products include:

Clonidine Hydrochloride (Because of its potential for inducing hypotension, risperidone may enhance the hypotensive effects of other therapeutic agents with this potential). Products include:

Clopidogrel Bisulfate (In vitro studies showed that drugs metabolized by other CYP isozymes, including 1A1, 1A2, 2C9, 2C19, and 3A4, are only weak inhibitors of risperidone metabolism). Products include:

Clorazepate Dipotassium (Given the primary CNS effects of risperidone, caution should be used if taken in combination with other centrally-acting drugs).
No products indexed under this heading.

Clozapine (Chronic administration of clozapine with risperidone may decrease the clearance of risperidone).
No products indexed under this heading.

Cocaine Hydrochloride (Risperidone is metabolized to 9-hydroxyrisperidone by CYP2D6. Drug interactions that reduce the metabolism of risperidone to 9-hydroxyrisperidone would increase the plasma concentrations of risperidone and lower the concentrations of 9-hydroxyrisperidone).
No products indexed under this heading.

Codeine Phosphate (Given the primary CNS effects of risperidone, caution should be used if taken in combination with other centrally-acting drugs). Products include:

Codeine Sulfate (Given the primary CNS effects of risperidone, caution should be used if taken in combination with other centrally-acting drugs).
No products indexed under this heading.

Cortisone Acetate (Co-administration of known CYP3A4 enzyme inducers with risperidone may cause decreases in the combined plasma concentrations of risperidone and 9-hydroxyrisperidone, which could lead to decreased efficacy of risperidone treatment. At the initiation of therapy with known hepatic enzyme inducers, patients should be closely monitored during the first 4–8 weeks, since the dose of risperidone may need to be adjusted. A dose increase, or additional oral risperidone, may need to be considered. On discontinuation of CYP3A4 hepatic enzyme inducers, the dosage of risperidone should be re-evaluated and, if necessary, decreased).
No products indexed under this heading.

Cyclobenzaprine (In vitro studies showed that drugs metabolized by other CYP isozymes, including 1A1, 1A2, 2C9, 2C19, and 3A4, are only weak inhibitors of risperidone metabolism).
No products indexed under this heading.

Cyclobenzaprine Hydrochloride (In vitro studies showed that drugs metabolized by other CYP isozymes, including

1A1, 1A2, 2C9, 2C19, and 3A4, are only weak inhibitors of risperidone metabolism). Products include:

Amrix **964**

Cyclophosphamide (*In vitro* studies showed that drugs metabolized by other CYP isozymes, including 1A1, 1A2, 2C9, 2C19, and 3A4, are only weak inhibitors of risperidone metabolism).

No products indexed under this heading.

Cyclosporine (*In vitro* studies showed that drugs metabolized by other CYP isozymes, including 1A1, 1A2, 2C9, 2C19, and 3A4, are only weak inhibitors of risperidone metabolism). Products include:

Gengraf **440**
Neoral Oral Solution **2496**
Neoral Capsules **2496**
Restasis **605**

Deserpidine (Because of its potential for inducing hypotension, risperidone may enhance the hypotensive effects of other therapeutic agents with this potential).

No products indexed under this heading.

Desflurane (Given the primary CNS effects of risperidone, caution should be used if taken in combination with other centrally-acting drugs).

No products indexed under this heading.

Desipramine Hydrochloride (*In vitro* studies showed that drugs metabolized by other CYP isozymes, including 1A1, 1A2, 2C9, 2C19, and 3A4, are only weak inhibitors of risperidone metabolism).

No products indexed under this heading.

Desogestrel (*In vitro* studies showed that drugs metabolized by other CYP isozymes, including 1A1, 1A2, 2C9, 2C19, and 3A4, are only weak inhibitors of risperidone metabolism).

No products indexed under this heading.

Dexamethasone (Co-administration of known CYP3A4 enzyme inducers with risperidone may cause decreases in the combined plasma concentrations of ripseridone and 9-hydroxyrisperidone, which could lead to decreased efficacy of risperidone treatment. At the initiation of therapy with known hepatic enzyme inducers, patients should be closely monitored during the first 4–8 weeks, since the dose of risperidone may need to be adjusted. A dose increase, or additional oral risperidone, may need to be considered. On discontinuation of CYP3A4 hepatic enzyme inducers, the dosage of risperidone should be re-evaluated and, if necessary, decreased). Products include:

Ciprodex **583**
Ozurdex ....⊙**223**
Tobramycin and Dexamethasone Ophthalmic Suspension ....⊙**251**

Dexamethasone Acetate (Co-administration of known CYP3A4 enzyme inducers with risperidone may cause decreases in the combined plasma concentrations of ripseridone and 9-hydroxyrisperidone, which could lead to decreased efficacy of risperidone treatment. At the initiation of therapy with known hepatic enzyme inducers, patients should be closely monitored during the first 4–8 weeks, since the dose of risperidone may need to be adjusted. A dose increase, or additional oral risperidone, may need to be considered. On discontinuation of CYP3A4 hepatic enzyme inducers, the dosage of risperidone should be re-evaluated and, if necessary, decreased).

No products indexed under this heading.

Dexamethasone Phosphate (Co-administration of known CYP3A4 enzyme inducers with risperidone may cause decreases in the combined plasma concentrations of ripseridone and 9-hydroxyrisperidone, which could lead to decreased efficacy of risperidone

treatment. At the initiation of therapy with known hepatic enzyme inducers, patients should be closely monitored during the first 4–8 weeks, since the dose of risperidone may need to be adjusted. A dose increase, or additional oral risperidone, may need to be considered. On discontinuation of CYP3A4 hepatic enzyme inducers, the dosage of risperidone should be re-evaluated and, if necessary, decreased).

No products indexed under this heading.

Dexamethasone Sodium (Co-administration of known CYP3A4 enzyme inducers with risperidone may cause decreases in the combined plasma concentrations of ripseridone and 9-hydroxyrisperidone, which could lead to decreased efficacy of risperidone treatment. At the initiation of therapy with known hepatic enzyme inducers, patients should be closely monitored during the first 4–8 weeks, since the dose of risperidone may need to be adjusted. A dose increase, or additional oral risperidone, may need to be considered. On discontinuation of CYP3A4 hepatic enzyme inducers, the dosage of risperidone should be re-evaluated and, if necessary, decreased).

No products indexed under this heading.

Dexamethasone Sodium Phosphate (Co-administration of known CYP3A4 enzyme inducers with risperidone may cause decreases in the combined plasma concentrations of ripseridone and 9-hydroxyrisperidone, which could lead to decreased efficacy of risperidone treatment. At the initiation of therapy with known hepatic enzyme inducers, patients should be closely monitored during the first 4–8 weeks, since the dose of risperidone may need to be adjusted. A dose increase, or additional oral risperidone, may need to be considered. On discontinuation of CYP3A4 hepatic enzyme inducers, the dosage of risperidone should be re-evaluated and, if necessary, decreased).

No products indexed under this heading.

Dexamethasone Sodium Phosphate Injection (Co-administration of known CYP3A4 enzyme inducers with risperidone may cause decreases in the combined plasma concentrations of ripseridone and 9-hydroxyrisperidone, which could lead to decreased efficacy of risperidone treatment. At the initiation of therapy with known hepatic enzyme inducers, patients should be closely monitored during the first 4–8 weeks, since the dose of risperidone may need to be adjusted. A dose increase, or additional oral risperidone, may need to be considered. On discontinuation of CYP3A4 hepatic enzyme inducers, the dosage of risperidone should be re-evaluated and, if necessary, decreased).

No products indexed under this heading.

Dexmethylphenidate Hydrochloride (Given the primary CNS effects of risperidone, caution should be used if taken in combination with other centrally-acting drugs). Products include:

Focalin XR **2472**

Dextroamphetamine (Given the primary CNS effects of risperidone, caution should be used if taken in combination with other centrally-acting drugs).

No products indexed under this heading.

Dextroamphetamine Saccharate (Given the primary CNS effects of risperidone, caution should be used if taken in combination with other centrally-acting drugs).

No products indexed under this heading.

Dextroamphetamine Sulfate (Given the primary CNS effects of risperidone,

caution should be used if taken in combination with other centrally-acting drugs). Products include:

Dexedrine **1425**

Dextromethorphan (*In vitro* studies showed that drugs metabolized by other CYP isozymes, including 1A1, 1A2, 2C9, 2C19, and 3A4, are only weak inhibitors of risperidone metabolism).

No products indexed under this heading.

Dextromethorphan Hydrobromide (*In vitro* studies showed that drugs metabolized by other CYP isozymes, including 1A1, 1A2, 2C9, 2C19, and 3A4, are only weak inhibitors of risperidone metabolism).

No products indexed under this heading.

Dezocine (Given the primary CNS effects of risperidone, caution should be used if taken in combination with other centrally-acting drugs).

No products indexed under this heading.

Diazepam (Given the primary CNS effects of risperidone, caution should be used if taken in combination with other centrally-acting drugs). Products include:

Valium Tablets **2880**

Diazoxide (Because of its potential for inducing hypotension, risperidone may enhance the hypotensive effects of other therapeutic agents with this potential). Products include:

Proglycem **1179**
Proglycem Suspension **1179**

Diclofenac Potassium (*In vitro* studies showed that drugs metabolized by other CYP isozymes, including 1A1, 1A2, 2C9, 2C19, and 3A4, are only weak inhibitors of risperidone metabolism).

No products indexed under this heading.

Diclofenac Sodium (*In vitro* studies showed that drugs metabolized by other CYP isozymes, including 1A1, 1A2, 2C9, 2C19, and 3A4, are only weak inhibitors of risperidone metabolism).

No products indexed under this heading.

Dihydroergotamine Mesylate (*In vitro* studies showed that drugs metabolized by other CYP isozymes, including 1A1, 1A2, 2C9, 2C19, and 3A4, are only weak inhibitors of risperidone metabolism).

No products indexed under this heading.

Diltiazem Hydrochloride (*In vitro* studies showed that drugs metabolized by other CYP isozymes, including 1A1, 1A2, 2C9, 2C19, and 3A4, are only weak inhibitors of risperidone metabolism). Products include:

Cardizem LA **423**

Diltiazem Maleate (*In vitro* studies showed that drugs metabolized by other CYP isozymes, including 1A1, 1A2, 2C9, 2C19, and 3A4, are only weak inhibitors of risperidone metabolism).

No products indexed under this heading.

Diphenhydramine (Risperidone is metabolized to 9-hydroxyrisperidone by CYP2D6. Drug interactions that reduce the metabolism of risperidone to 9-hydroxyrisperidone would increase the plasma concentrations of risperidone and lower the concentrations of 9-hydroxyrisperidone).

No products indexed under this heading.

Diphenhydramine Hydrochloride (Risperidone is metabolized to 9-hydroxyrisperidone by CYP2D6. Drug interactions that reduce the metabolism of risperidone to 9-hydroxyrisperidone would increase the plasma concentrations of risperidone and lower the concentrations of 9-hydroxyrisperidone). Products include:

Benadryl Allergy Ultratab **2042**
Children's Benadryl Allergy Liquid **2042**

Disopyramide (*In vitro* studies showed that drugs metabolized by other CYP isozymes, including 1A1, 1A2, 2C9, 2C19, and 3A4, are only weak inhibitors of risperidone metabolism).

No products indexed under this heading.

Disopyramide Phosphate (*In vitro* studies showed that drugs metabolized by other CYP isozymes, including 1A1, 1A2, 2C9, 2C19, and 3A4, are only weak inhibitors of risperidone metabolism).

No products indexed under this heading.

Disulfiram (*In vitro* studies showed that drugs metabolized by other CYP isozymes, including 1A1, 1A2, 2C9, 2C19, and 3A4, are only weak inhibitors of risperidone metabolism).

No products indexed under this heading.

Divalproex Sodium (Repeated oral doses of risperidone (4 mg qd) did not affect the pre-dose or average plasma concentrations exposure (AUC) of valproate (1000 mg/day in three divided doses) compared to placebo (n=21). However, there was a 20% increase of valproate peak plasma concentration (C$_{max}$) after concomitant administration of oral risperidone). Products include:

Depakote ER **426**

Dopamine Hydrochloride (Risperidone may antagonize the effect of dopamine agonists).

No products indexed under this heading.

Doxazosin Mesylate (Because of its potential for inducing hypotension, risperidone may enhance the hypotensive effects of other therapeutic agents with this potential).

No products indexed under this heading.

Doxepin Hydrochloride (*In vitro* studies showed that drugs metabolized by other CYP isozymes, including 1A1, 1A2, 2C9, 2C19, and 3A4, are only weak inhibitors of risperidone metabolism).

No products indexed under this heading.

Doxorubicin Hydrochloride (Co-administration of known CYP3A4 enzyme inducers with risperidone may cause decreases in the combined plasma concentrations of ripseridone and 9-hydroxyrisperidone, which could lead to decreased efficacy of risperidone treatment. At the initiation of therapy with known hepatic enzyme inducers, patients should be closely monitored during the first 4–8 weeks, since the dose of risperidone may need to be adjusted. A dose increase, or additional oral risperidone, may need to be considered. On discontinuation of CYP3A4 hepatic enzyme inducers, the dosage of risperidone should be re-evaluated and, if necessary, decreased).

No products indexed under this heading.

Dronabinol (*In vitro* studies showed that drugs metabolized by other CYP isozymes, including 1A1, 1A2, 2C9, 2C19, and 3A4, are only weak inhibitors of risperidone metabolism).

No products indexed under this heading.

Droperidol (Given the primary CNS effects of risperidone, caution should be used if taken in combination with other centrally-acting drugs).

No products indexed under this heading.

Efavirenz (Co-administration of known CYP3A4 enzyme inducers with risperidone may cause decreases in the combined plasma concentrations of ripseridone and 9-hydroxyrisperidone, which could lead to decreased efficacy of risperidone treatment. At the initiation of therapy with known hepatic enzyme inducers, patients should be closely monitored during the first 4–8 weeks, since the dose of risperidone may need to be adjusted. A dose increase, or additional oral risperidone, may need to be considered. On discontinuation of

---

IMPORTANT NOTE: Always consult each drug listing in the patient's regimen for possible interactions.

Flurbiprofen (In vitro studies showed that drugs metabolized by other CYP isozymes, including 1A1, 1A2, 2C9, 2C19, and 3A4, are only weak inhibitors of risperidone metabolism).
No products indexed under this heading.

Flurbiprofen Sodium (In vitro studies showed that drugs metabolized by other CYP isozymes, including 1A1, 1A2, 2C9, 2C19, and 3A4, are only weak inhibitors of risperidone metabolism).
No products indexed under this heading.

Flutamide (In vitro studies showed that drugs metabolized by other CYP isozymes, including 1A1, 1A2, 2C9, 2C19, and 3A4, are only weak inhibitors of risperidone metabolism).
No products indexed under this heading.

Fluticasone Propionate (In vitro studies showed that drugs metabolized by other CYP isozymes, including 1A1, 1A2, 2C9, 2C19, and 3A4, are only weak inhibitors of risperidone metabolism). Products include:

Fluvastatin Sodium (In vitro studies showed that drugs metabolized by other CYP isozymes, including 1A1, 1A2, 2C9, 2C19, and 3A4, are only weak inhibitors of risperidone metabolism).
No products indexed under this heading.

Fluvoxamine Maleate (In vitro studies showed that drugs metabolized by other CYP isozymes, including 1A1, 1A2, 2C9, 2C19, and 3A4, are only weak inhibitors of risperidone metabolism).
No products indexed under this heading.

Formoterol Fumarate (In vitro studies showed that drugs metabolized by other CYP isozymes, including 1A1, 1A2, 2C9, 2C19, and 3A4, are only weak inhibitors of risperidone metabolism). Products include:

Fosinopril Sodium (Because of its potential for inducing hypotension, risperidone may enhance the hypotensive effects of other therapeutic agents with this potential).
No products indexed under this heading.

Fosphenytoin (Co-administration of known CYP3A4 enzyme inducers (eg, phenytoin) with risperidone may cause decreases in the combined plasma concentrations of risperidone and 9-hydroxyrisperidone, which could lead to decreased efficacy of risperidone treatment. At the initiation of therapy with known hepatic enzyme inducers, patients should be closely monitored during the first 4–8 weeks, since the dose of risperidone may need to be adjusted. A dose increase, or additional oral risperidone, may need to be considered. On discontinuation of CYP3A4 hepatic enzyme inducers, the dosage of risperidone should be re-evaluated and, if necessary, decreased).
No products indexed under this heading.

Fosphenytoin Sodium (Co-administration of known CYP3A4 enzyme inducers (eg, phenytoin) with risperidone may cause decreases in the combined plasma concentrations of risperidone and 9-hydroxyrisperidone, which could lead to decreased efficacy of risperidone treatment. At the initiation of therapy with known hepatic enzyme inducers, patients should be closely monitored during the first 4–8 weeks, since the dose of risperidone may need to be adjusted. A dose

increase, or additional oral risperidone, may need to be considered. On discontinuation of CYP3A4 hepatic enzyme inducers, the dosage of risperidone should be re-evaluated and, if necessary, decreased).
No products indexed under this heading.

Furosemide (In 2 of 4 placebo-controlled trials in elderly patients with dementia-related psychosis, a higher incidence of mortality was observed in patients treated with furosemide plus oral risperidone when compared to patients treated with oral risperidone alone or with oral placebo plus furosemide. No pathological mechanism has been identified to explain this finding, and no consistent pattern for cause of death was observed. An increase of mortality in elderly patients with dementia-related psychosis was seen with the use of oral risperidone regardless of concomitant use with furosemide). Products include:

Gabapentin (In vitro studies showed that drugs metabolized by other CYP isozymes, including 1A1, 1A2, 2C9, 2C19, and 3A4, are only weak inhibitors of risperidone metabolism).
No products indexed under this heading.

Garlic Extract (Co-administration of known CYP3A4 enzyme inducers with risperidone may cause decreases in the combined plasma concentrations of risperidone and 9-hydroxyrisperidone, which could lead to decreased efficacy of risperidone treatment. At the initiation of therapy with known hepatic enzyme inducers, patients should be closely monitored during the first 4–8 weeks, since the dose of risperidone may need to be adjusted. A dose increase, or additional oral risperidone, may need to be considered. On discontinuation of CYP3A4 hepatic enzyme inducers, the dosage of risperidone should be re-evaluated and, if necessary, decreased).
No products indexed under this heading.

Garlic Oil (Co-administration of known CYP3A4 enzyme inducers with risperidone may cause decreases in the combined plasma concentrations of risperidone and 9-hydroxyrisperidone, which could lead to decreased efficacy of risperidone treatment. At the initiation of therapy with known hepatic enzyme inducers, patients should be closely monitored during the first 4–8 weeks, since the dose of risperidone may need to be adjusted. A dose increase, or additional oral risperidone, may need to be considered. On discontinuation of CYP3A4 hepatic enzyme inducers, the dosage of risperidone should be re-evaluated and, if necessary, decreased).
No products indexed under this heading.

Glimepiride (In vitro studies showed that drugs metabolized by other CYP isozymes, including 1A1, 1A2, 2C9, 2C19, and 3A4, are only weak inhibitors of risperidone metabolism). Products include:

Glipizide (In vitro studies showed that drugs metabolized by other CYP isozymes, including 1A1, 1A2, 2C9, 2C19, and 3A4, are only weak inhibitors of risperidone metabolism).
No products indexed under this heading.

Glutethimide (Given the primary CNS effects of risperidone, caution should be used if taken in combination with other centrally-acting drugs).
No products indexed under this heading.

Grepafloxacin Hydrochloride (In vitro studies showed that drugs metabolized by other CYP isozymes, including 1A1, 1A2, 2C9, 2C19, and 3A4, are only weak inhibitors of risperidone metabolism).
No products indexed under this heading.

Guanabenz Acetate (Because of its potential for inducing hypotension, risperidone may enhance the hypotensive effects of other therapeutic agents with this potential).
No products indexed under this heading.

Guanethidine (Because of its potential for inducing hypotension, risperidone may enhance the hypotensive effects of other therapeutic agents with this potential).
No products indexed under this heading.

Guanethidine Monosulfate (Because of its potential for inducing hypotension, risperidone may enhance the hypotensive effects of other therapeutic agents with this potential).
No products indexed under this heading.

Guanethidine Sulfate (Because of its potential for inducing hypotension, risperidone may enhance the hypotensive effects of other therapeutic agents with this potential).
No products indexed under this heading.

Halofantrine Hydrochloride (Risperidone is metabolized to 9-hydroxyrisperidone by CYP2D6. Drug interactions that reduce the metabolism of risperidone to 9-hydroxyrisperidone would increase the plasma concentrations of risperidone and lower the concentrations of 9-hydroxyrisperidone).
No products indexed under this heading.

Haloperidol (Given the primary CNS effects of risperidone, caution should be used if taken in combination with other centrally-acting drugs).
No products indexed under this heading.

Haloperidol Decanoate (Given the primary CNS effects of risperidone, caution should be used if taken in combination with other centrally-acting drugs).
No products indexed under this heading.

Haloperidol Lactate (In vitro studies showed that drugs metabolized by other CYP isozymes, including 1A1, 1A2, 2C9, 2C19, and 3A4, are only weak inhibitors of risperidone metabolism).
No products indexed under this heading.

Hydralazine Hydrochloride (Because of its potential for inducing hypotension, risperidone may enhance the hypotensive effects of other therapeutic agents with this potential).
No products indexed under this heading.

Hydrochlorothiazide (Because of its potential for inducing hypotension, risperidone may enhance the hypotensive effects of other therapeutic agents with this potential). Products include:

Hydrocodone Bitartrate (Given the primary CNS effects of risperidone, caution should be used if taken in combination with other centrally-acting drugs). Products include:

Hydrocodone Polistirex (Given the primary CNS effects of risperidone, caution should be used if taken in combination with other centrally-acting drugs). Products include:

Hydrocortisone (Co-administration of known CYP3A4 enzyme inducers with risperidone may cause decreases in the combined plasma concentrations of risperidone and 9-hydroxyrisperidone, which could lead to decreased efficacy of risperidone treatment. At the initiation of therapy with known hepatic enzyme inducers, patients should be closely monitored during the first 4–8 weeks, since the dose of risperidone may need to be adjusted. A dose increase, or additional oral risperidone, may need to be considered. On discontinuation of CYP3A4 hepatic enzyme inducers, the dosage of risperidone should be re-evaluated and, if necessary, decreased).
No products indexed under this heading.

Hydrocortisone (Alcohol) (Co-administration of known CYP3A4 enzyme inducers with risperidone may cause decreases in the combined plasma concentrations of risperidone and 9-hydroxyrisperidone, which could lead to decreased efficacy of risperidone treatment. At the initiation of therapy with known hepatic enzyme inducers, patients should be closely monitored during the first 4–8 weeks, since the dose of risperidone may need to be adjusted. A dose increase, or additional oral risperidone, may need to be considered. On discontinuation of CYP3A4 hepatic enzyme inducers, the dosage of risperidone should be re-evaluated and, if necessary, decreased).
No products indexed under this heading.

Hydrocortisone Acetate (Co-administration of known CYP3A4 enzyme inducers with risperidone may cause decreases in the combined plasma concentrations of risperidone and 9-hydroxyrisperidone, which could lead to decreased efficacy of risperidone treatment. At the initiation of therapy with known hepatic enzyme inducers, patients should be closely monitored during the first 4–8 weeks, since the dose of risperidone may need to be adjusted. A dose increase, or additional oral risperidone, may need to be considered. On discontinuation of CYP3A4 hepatic enzyme inducers, the dosage of risperidone should be re-evaluated and, if necessary, decreased).
No products indexed under this heading.

Hydrocortisone Butyrate (Co-administration of known CYP3A4 enzyme inducers with risperidone may cause decreases in the combined plasma concentrations of risperidone and 9-hydroxyrisperidone, which could lead to decreased efficacy of risperidone treatment. At the initiation of therapy with known hepatic enzyme inducers, patients should be closely monitored during the first 4–8 weeks, since the dose of risperidone may need to be adjusted. A dose increase, or additional oral risperidone, may need to be considered. On discontinuation of CYP3A4 hepatic enzyme inducers, the dosage of risperidone should be re-evaluated and, if necessary, decreased).
No products indexed under this heading.

Hydrocortisone Cypionate (Co-administration of known CYP3A4 enzyme inducers with risperidone may cause decreases in the combined plasma concentrations of risperidone and 9-hydroxyrisperidone, which could lead to decreased efficacy of risperidone treatment. At the initiation of therapy with known hepatic enzyme inducers, patients should be closely monitored during the first 4–8 weeks, since the

isozymes, including 1A1, 1A2, 2C9, 2C19, and 3A4, are only weak inhibitors of risperidone metabolism). Products include:
Lidoderm 1107

Lidocaine Hydrochloride (*In vitro* studies showed that drugs metabolized by other CYP isozymes, including 1A1, 1A2, 2C9, 2C19, and 3A4, are only weak inhibitors of risperidone metabolism).
No products indexed under this heading.

Lisdexamfetamine Dimesylate (Given the primary CNS effects of risperidone, caution should be used if taken in combination with other centrally-acting drugs). Products include:
Vyvanse 3298

Lisinopril (Because of its potential for inducing hypotension, risperidone may enhance the hypotensive effects of other therapeutic agents with this potential). Products include:
Prinivil 2241
Prinzide 2246

Lomefloxacin Hydrochloride (*In vitro* studies showed that drugs metabolized by other CYP isozymes, including 1A1, 1A2, 2C9, 2C19, and 3A4, are only weak inhibitors of risperidone metabolism).
No products indexed under this heading.

Lorazepam (Given the primary CNS effects of risperidone, caution should be used if taken in combination with other centrally-acting drugs).
No products indexed under this heading.

Losartan Potassium (Because of its potential for inducing hypotension, risperidone may enhance the hypotensive effects of other therapeutic agents with this potential). Products include:
Cozaar 2106
Hyzaar 2162
Hyzaar 100-12.5 2162

Lovastatin (*In vitro* studies showed that drugs metabolized by other CYP isozymes, including 1A1, 1A2, 2C9, 2C19, and 3A4, are only weak inhibitors of risperidone metabolism). Products include:
Advicor 402
Mevacor 2212

Loxapine Hydrochloride (Given the primary CNS effects of risperidone, caution should be used if taken in combination with other centrally-acting drugs).
No products indexed under this heading.

Loxapine Succinate (Given the primary CNS effects of risperidone, caution should be used if taken in combination with other centrally-acting drugs).
No products indexed under this heading.

Maprotiline Hydrochloride (*In vitro* studies showed that drugs metabolized by other CYP isozymes, including 1A1, 1A2, 2C9, 2C19, and 3A4, are only weak inhibitors of risperidone metabolism).
No products indexed under this heading.

Mecamylamine Hydrochloride (Because of its potential for inducing hypotension, risperidone may enhance the hypotensive effects of other therapeutic agents with this potential).
No products indexed under this heading.

Meclofenamate Sodium (*In vitro* studies showed that drugs metabolized by other CYP isozymes, including 1A1, 1A2, 2C9, 2C19, and 3A4, are only weak inhibitors of risperidone metabolism).
No products indexed under this heading.

Mefenamic Acid (*In vitro* studies showed that drugs metabolized by other CYP isozymes, including 1A1, 1A2, 2C9, 2C19, and 3A4, are only weak inhibitors of risperidone metabolism).
No products indexed under this heading.

Meloxicam (*In vitro* studies showed that drugs metabolized by other CYP isozymes, including 1A1, 1A2, 2C9, 2C19, and 3A4, are only weak inhibitors of risperidone metabolism).
No products indexed under this heading.

Meperidine Hydrochloride (Given the primary CNS effects of risperidone, caution should be used if taken in combination with other centrally-acting drugs).
No products indexed under this heading.

Mephenytoin (Co-administration of known CYP3A4 enzyme inducers with risperidone may cause decreases in the combined plasma concentrations of ripseridone and 9-hydroxyrisperidone, which could lead to decreased efficacy of risperidone treatment. At the initiation of therapy with known hepatic enzyme inducers, patients should be closely monitored during the first 4–8 weeks, since the dose of risperidone may need to be adjusted. A dose increase, or additional oral risperidone, may need to be considered. On discontinuation of CYP3A4 hepatic enzyme inducers, the dosage of risperidone should be re-evaluated and, if necessary, decreased).
No products indexed under this heading.

Mephobarbital (Given the primary CNS effects of risperidone, caution should be used if taken in combination with other centrally-acting drugs).
No products indexed under this heading.

Meprobamate (Given the primary CNS effects of risperidone, caution should be used if taken in combination with other centrally-acting drugs).
No products indexed under this heading.

Mesoridazine Besylate (Given the primary CNS effects of risperidone, caution should be used if taken in combination with other centrally-acting drugs).
No products indexed under this heading.

Mestranol (*In vitro* studies showed that drugs metabolized by other CYP isozymes, including 1A1, 1A2, 2C9, 2C19, and 3A4, are only weak inhibitors of risperidone metabolism).
No products indexed under this heading.

Metformin Hydrochloride (*In vitro* studies showed that drugs metabolized by other CYP isozymes, including 1A1, 1A2, 2C9, 2C19, and 3A4, are only weak inhibitors of risperidone metabolism). Products include:
ActoPlus 3338
Avandamet 1345
Janumet 2188

Methadone Hydrochloride (Given the primary CNS effects of risperidone, caution should be used if taken in combination with other centrally-acting drugs).
No products indexed under this heading.

Methamphetamine Hydrochloride (Given the primary CNS effects of risperidone, caution should be used if taken in combination with other centrally-acting drugs).
No products indexed under this heading.

Methohexital Sodium (Given the primary CNS effects of risperidone, caution should be used if taken in combination with other centrally-acting drugs).
No products indexed under this heading.

Methotrimeprazine (Given the primary CNS effects of risperidone, caution should be used if taken in combination with other centrally-acting drugs).
No products indexed under this heading.

Methoxyflurane (Given the primary CNS effects of risperidone, caution should be used if taken in combination with other centrally-acting drugs).
No products indexed under this heading.

Methsuximide (Co-administration of known CYP3A4 enzyme inducers with risperidone may cause decreases in the combined plasma concentrations of ripseridone and 9-hydroxyrisperidone, which could lead to decreased efficacy of risperidone treatment. At the initiation of therapy with known hepatic enzyme inducers, patients should be closely monitored during the first 4–8 weeks, since the dose of risperidone may need to be adjusted. A dose increase, or additional oral risperidone, may need to be considered. On discontinuation of CYP3A4 hepatic enzyme inducers, the dosage of risperidone should be re-evaluated and, if necessary, decreased).
No products indexed under this heading.

Methyclothiazide (Because of its potential for inducing hypotension, risperidone may enhance the hypotensive effects of other therapeutic agents with this potential).
No products indexed under this heading.

Methyldopa (Because of its potential for inducing hypotension, risperidone may enhance the hypotensive effects of other therapeutic agents with this potential).
No products indexed under this heading.

Methyldopate Hydrochloride (Because of its potential for inducing hypotension, risperidone may enhance the hypotensive effects of other therapeutic agents with this potential).
No products indexed under this heading.

Methylphenidate (Given the primary CNS effects of risperidone, caution should be used if taken in combination with other centrally-acting drugs). Products include:
Daytrana 3283

Methylphenidate Hydrochloride (Given the primary CNS effects of risperidone, caution should be used if taken in combination with other centrally-acting drugs). Products include:
Concerta 2598
Metadate CD 3439

Methylprednisolone (Co-administration of known CYP3A4 enzyme inducers with risperidone may cause decreases in the combined plasma concentrations of ripseridone and 9-hydroxyrisperidone, which could lead to decreased efficacy of risperidone treatment. At the initiation of therapy with known hepatic enzyme inducers, patients should be closely monitored during the first 4–8 weeks, since the dose of risperidone may need to be adjusted. A dose increase, or additional oral risperidone, may need to be considered. On discontinuation of CYP3A4 hepatic enzyme inducers, the dosage of risperidone should be re-evaluated and, if necessary, decreased).
No products indexed under this heading.

Methylprednisolone Acetate (Co-administration of known CYP3A4 enzyme inducers with risperidone may cause decreases in the combined plasma concentrations of ripseridone and 9-hydroxyrisperidone, which could lead to decreased efficacy of risperidone treatment. At the initiation of therapy with known hepatic enzyme inducers, patients should be closely monitored during the first 4–8 weeks, since the dose of risperidone may need to be adjusted. A dose increase, or additional oral risperidone, may need to be considered. On discontinuation of CYP3A4 hepatic enzyme inducers, the dosage of risperidone should be re-evaluated and, if necessary, decreased).
No products indexed under this heading.

Methylprednisolone Sodium Succinate (Co-administration of known CYP3A4 enzyme inducers with risperidone may cause decreases in the combined plasma concentrations of ripseridone and 9-hydroxyrisperidone, which could lead to decreased efficacy of risperidone treatment. At the initiation of therapy with known hepatic enzyme inducers, patients should be closely monitored during the first 4–8 weeks, since the dose of risperidone may need to be adjusted. A dose increase, or additional oral risperidone, may need to be considered. On discontinuation of CYP3A4 hepatic enzyme inducers, the dosage of risperidone should be re-evaluated and, if necessary, decreased).
No products indexed under this heading.

Metolazone (Because of its potential for inducing hypotension, risperidone may enhance the hypotensive effects of other therapeutic agents with this potential).
No products indexed under this heading.

Metoprolol Succinate (Because of its potential for inducing hypotension, risperidone may enhance the hypotensive effects of other therapeutic agents with this potential). Products include:
Toprol XL 732

Metoprolol Tartrate (Because of its potential for inducing hypotension, risperidone may enhance the hypotensive effects of other therapeutic agents with this potential).
No products indexed under this heading.

Metyrosine (Because of its potential for inducing hypotension, risperidone may enhance the hypotensive effects of other therapeutic agents with this potential).
No products indexed under this heading.

Mexiletine Hydrochloride (*In vitro* studies showed that drugs metabolized by other CYP isozymes, including 1A1, 1A2, 2C9, 2C19, and 3A4, are only weak inhibitors of risperidone metabolism).
No products indexed under this heading.

Mibefradil Dihydrochloride (Because of its potential for inducing hypotension, risperidone may enhance the hypotensive effects of other therapeutic agents with this potential).
No products indexed under this heading.

Midazolam Hydrochloride (Given the primary CNS effects of risperidone, caution should be used if taken in combination with other centrally-acting drugs).
No products indexed under this heading.

Miglitol (*In vitro* studies showed that drugs metabolized by other CYP isozymes, including 1A1, 1A2, 2C9, 2C19, and 3A4, are only weak inhibitors of risperidone metabolism).
No products indexed under this heading.

Minoxidil (Because of its potential for inducing hypotension, risperidone may enhance the hypotensive effects of other therapeutic agents with this potential).
No products indexed under this heading.

Mirtazapine (*In vitro* studies showed that drugs metabolized by other CYP isozymes, including 1A1, 1A2, 2C9, 2C19, and 3A4, are only weak inhibitors of risperidone metabolism). Products include:
Remeron Tablets 3214
RemeronSolTab Tablets 3219

Moclobemide (Risperidone is metabolized to 9-hydroxyrisperidone by CYP2D6. Drug interactions that reduce the metabolism of risperidone to 9-hydroxyrisperidone would increase the plasma concentrations of risperidone and lower the concentrations of 9-hydroxyrisperidone).
No products indexed under this heading.

Modafinil (Co-administration of known CYP3A4 enzyme inducers with risperidone may cause decreases in the combined plasma concentrations of ripseri-

done and 9-hydroxyrisperidone, which could lead to decreased efficacy of risperidone treatment. At the initiation of therapy with known hepatic enzyme inducers, patients should be closely monitored during the first 4–8 weeks, since the dose of risperidone may need to be adjusted. A dose increase, or additional oral risperidone, may need to be considered. On discontinuation of CYP3A4 hepatic enzyme inducers, the dosage of risperidone should be re-evaluated and, if necessary, decreased). Products include:

Moexipril Hydrochloride (Because of its potential for inducing hypotension, risperidone may enhance the hypotensive effects of other therapeutic agents with this potential).
No products indexed under this heading.

Molindone Hydrochloride (Given the primary CNS effects of risperidone, caution should be used if taken in combination with other centrally-acting drugs). Products include:

Montelukast Sodium (In vitro studies showed that drugs metabolized by other CYP isozymes, including 1A1, 1A2, 2C9, 2C19, and 3A4, are only weak inhibitors of risperidone metabolism). Products include:

Morphine Sulfate (Given the primary CNS effects of risperidone, caution should be used if taken in combination with other centrally-acting drugs). Products include:

Moxifloxacin Hydrochloride (In vitro studies showed that drugs metabolized by other CYP isozymes, including 1A1, 1A2, 2C9, 2C19, and 3A4, are only weak inhibitors of risperidone metabolism). Products include:

Nabumetone (In vitro studies showed that drugs metabolized by other CYP isozymes, including 1A1, 1A2, 2C9, 2C19, and 3A4, are only weak inhibitors of risperidone metabolism).
No products indexed under this heading.

Nadolol (Because of its potential for inducing hypotension, risperidone may enhance the hypotensive effects of other therapeutic agents with this potential). Products include:

Nafcillin Sodium (In vitro studies showed that drugs metabolized by other CYP isozymes, including 1A1, 1A2, 2C9, 2C19, and 3A4, are only weak inhibitors of risperidone metabolism).
No products indexed under this heading.

Naproxen (In vitro studies showed that drugs metabolized by other CYP isozymes, including 1A1, 1A2, 2C9, 2C19, and 3A4, are only weak inhibitors of risperidone metabolism). Products include:

Naproxen Sodium (In vitro studies showed that drugs metabolized by other CYP isozymes, including 1A1, 1A2, 2C9, 2C19, and 3A4, are only weak inhibitors of risperidone metabolism). Products include:

Nateglinide (In vitro studies showed that drugs metabolized by other CYP isozymes, including 1A1, 1A2, 2C9, 2C19, and 3A4, are only weak inhibitors of risperidone metabolism).
No products indexed under this heading.

Nebivolol (Because of its potential for inducing hypotension, risperidone may enhance the hypotensive effects of other therapeutic agents with this potential). Products include:

Nefazodone Hydrochloride (In vitro studies showed that drugs metabolized by other CYP isozymes, including 1A1, 1A2, 2C9, 2C19, and 3A4, are only weak inhibitors of risperidone metabolism).
No products indexed under this heading.

Nelfinavir Mesylate (In vitro studies showed that drugs metabolized by other CYP isozymes, including 1A1, 1A2, 2C9, 2C19, and 3A4, are only weak inhibitors of risperidone metabolism).
No products indexed under this heading.

Nevirapine (Co-administration of known CYP3A4 enzyme inducers with risperidone may cause decreases in the combined plasma concentrations of ripseridone and 9-hydroxyrisperidone, which could lead to decreased efficacy of risperidone treatment. At the initiation of therapy with known hepatic enzyme inducers, patients should be closely monitored during the first 4–8 weeks, since the dose of risperidone may need to be adjusted. A dose increase, or additional oral risperidone, may need to be considered. On discontinuation of CYP3A4 hepatic enzyme inducers, the dosage of risperidone should be re-evaluated and, if necessary, decreased). Products include:

Nicardipine (In vitro studies showed that drugs metabolized by other CYP isozymes, including 1A1, 1A2, 2C9, 2C19, and 3A4, are only weak inhibitors of risperidone metabolism).
No products indexed under this heading.

Nicardipine Hydrochloride (Because of its potential for inducing hypotension, risperidone may enhance the hypotensive effects of other therapeutic agents with this potential).
No products indexed under this heading.

Nicotine Polacrilex (In vitro studies showed that drugs metabolized by other CYP isozymes, including 1A1, 1A2, 2C9, 2C19, and 3A4, are only weak inhibitors of risperidone metabolism).
No products indexed under this heading.

Nicotine Salicylate (In vitro studies showed that drugs metabolized by other CYP isozymes, including 1A1, 1A2, 2C9, 2C19, and 3A4, are only weak inhibitors of risperidone metabolism).
No products indexed under this heading.

Nicotine Sulfate (In vitro studies showed that drugs metabolized by other CYP isozymes, including 1A1, 1A2, 2C9, 2C19, and 3A4, are only weak inhibitors of risperidone metabolism).
No products indexed under this heading.

Nifedipine (Because of its potential for inducing hypotension, risperidone may enhance the hypotensive effects of other therapeutic agents with this potential).
No products indexed under this heading.

Nilutamide (In vitro studies showed that drugs metabolized by other CYP isozymes, including 1A1, 1A2, 2C9, 2C19, and 3A4, are only weak inhibitors of risperidone metabolism).
No products indexed under this heading.

Nimodipine (In vitro studies showed that drugs metabolized by other CYP isozymes, including 1A1, 1A2, 2C9, 2C19, and 3A4, are only weak inhibitors of risperidone metabolism).
No products indexed under this heading.

Nisoldipine (Because of its potential for inducing hypotension, risperidone may enhance the hypotensive effects of other therapeutic agents with this potential).
No products indexed under this heading.

Nitrendipine (In vitro studies showed that drugs metabolized by other CYP isozymes, including 1A1, 1A2, 2C9, 2C19, and 3A4, are only weak inhibitors of risperidone metabolism).
No products indexed under this heading.

Nitroglycerin (Because of its potential for inducing hypotension, risperidone may enhance the hypotensive effects of other therapeutic agents with this potential). Products include:

Norethindrone (In vitro studies showed that drugs metabolized by other CYP isozymes, including 1A1, 1A2, 2C9, 2C19, and 3A4, are only weak inhibitors of risperidone metabolism). Products include:

Norethindrone Acetate (In vitro studies showed that drugs metabolized by other CYP isozymes, including 1A1, 1A2, 2C9, 2C19, and 3A4, are only weak inhibitors of risperidone metabolism). Products include:

Norfloxacin (In vitro studies showed that drugs metabolized by other CYP isozymes, including 1A1, 1A2, 2C9, 2C19, and 3A4, are only weak inhibitors of risperidone metabolism). Products include:

Norgestrel (In vitro studies showed that drugs metabolized by other CYP isozymes, including 1A1, 1A2, 2C9, 2C19, and 3A4, are only weak inhibitors of risperidone metabolism).
No products indexed under this heading.

Nortriptyline Hydrochloride (In vitro studies showed that drugs metabolized by other CYP isozymes, including 1A1, 1A2, 2C9, 2C19, and 3A4, are only weak inhibitors of risperidone metabolism).
No products indexed under this heading.

Ofloxacin (In vitro studies showed that drugs metabolized by other CYP isozymes, including 1A1, 1A2, 2C9, 2C19, and 3A4, are only weak inhibitors of risperidone metabolism).
No products indexed under this heading.

Olanzapine (Given the primary CNS effects of risperidone, caution should be used if taken in combination with other centrally-acting drugs). Products include:

Omeprazole (In vitro studies showed that drugs metabolized by other CYP isozymes, including 1A1, 1A2, 2C9, 2C19, and 3A4, are only weak inhibitors of risperidone metabolism).
No products indexed under this heading.

Omeprazole Magnesium (In vitro studies showed that drugs metabolized by other CYP isozymes, including 1A1, 1A2, 2C9, 2C19, and 3A4, are only weak inhibitors of risperidone metabolism).
No products indexed under this heading.

Ondansetron (In vitro studies showed that drugs metabolized by other CYP isozymes, including 1A1, 1A2, 2C9, 2C19, and 3A4, are only weak inhibitors of risperidone metabolism).
No products indexed under this heading.

Ondansetron Hydrochloride (In vitro studies showed that drugs metabolized by other CYP isozymes, including 1A1, 1A2, 2C9, 2C19, and 3A4, are only weak inhibitors of risperidone metabolism). Products include:

Oxaprozin (In vitro studies showed that drugs metabolized by other CYP isozymes, including 1A1, 1A2, 2C9, 2C19, and 3A4, are only weak inhibitors of risperidone metabolism).
No products indexed under this heading.

Oxazepam (Given the primary CNS effects of risperidone, caution should be used if taken in combination with other centrally-acting drugs).
No products indexed under this heading.

Oxcarbazepine (Co-administration of known CYP3A4 enzyme inducers with risperidone may cause decreases in the combined plasma concentrations of ripseridone and 9-hydroxyrisperidone, which could lead to decreased efficacy of risperidone treatment. At the initiation of therapy with known hepatic enzyme inducers, patients should be closely monitored during the first 4–8 weeks, since the dose of risperidone may need to be adjusted. A dose increase, or additional oral risperidone, may need to be considered. On discontinuation of CYP3A4 hepatic enzyme inducers, the dosage of risperidone should be re-evaluated and, if necessary, decreased).
No products indexed under this heading.

Oxycodone Hydrochloride (Given the primary CNS effects of risperidone, caution should be used if taken in combination with other centrally-acting drugs). Products include:

Paclitaxel (In vitro studies showed that drugs metabolized by other CYP isozymes, including 1A1, 1A2, 2C9, 2C19, and 3A4, are only weak inhibitors of risperidone metabolism).
No products indexed under this heading.

Pantoprazole Sodium (In vitro studies showed that drugs metabolized by other CYP isozymes, including 1A1, 1A2, 2C9, 2C19, and 3A4, are only weak inhibitors of risperidone metabolism). Products include:

Paramethadione (In vitro studies showed that drugs metabolized by other CYP isozymes, including 1A1, 1A2, 2C9, 2C19, and 3A4, are only weak inhibitors of risperidone metabolism).
No products indexed under this heading.

Paroxetine (Paroxetine (20 mg qd), a CYP2D6 inhibitor, has been shown to increase the plasma concentration of risperidone 3-9 fold. Paroxetine lowered the concentration of 9-hydroxyrisperidone by about 10%. When concomitant paroxetine is initiated or discontinued, the dose of risperidone should be re-evaluated. When initiation of paroxetine is considered, patients may be placed on a lower dose of risperidone between 2-4 weeks before the planned start of paroxetine therapy to adjust for the expected increase in plasma concentrations of risperidone).
No products indexed under this heading.

Paroxetine Hydrochloride (Paroxetine (20 mg qd), a CYP2D6 inhibitor, has

been shown to increase the plasma concentration of risperidone 3-9 fold. Paroxetine lowered the concentration of 9-hydroxyrisperidone by about 10%. When concomitant paroxetine is initiated or discontinued, the dose of risperidone should be re-evaluated. When initiation of paroxetine is considered, patients may be placed on a lower dose of risperidone between 2-4 weeks before the planned start of paroxetine therapy to adjust for the expected increase in plasma concentrations of risperidone). Products include:

Paroxetine CR 2361
Paroxetine ER 2371
Paxil 1586
Paxil CR 1596

Paroxetine Mesylate (Paroxetine (20 mg qd), a CYP2D6 inhibitor, has been shown to increase the plasma concentration of risperidone 3-9 fold. Paroxetine lowered the concentration of 9-hydroxyrisperidone by about 10%. When concomitant paroxetine is initiated or discontinued, the dose of risperidone should be re-evaluated. When initiation of paroxetine is considered, patients may be placed on a lower dose of risperidone between 2-4 weeks before the planned start of paroxetine therapy to adjust for the expected increase in plasma concentrations of risperidone).
No products indexed under this heading.

Pemoline (Given the primary CNS effects of risperidone, caution should be used if taken in combination with other centrally-acting drugs).
No products indexed under this heading.

Penbutolol Sulfate (Because of its potential for inducing hypotension, risperidone may enhance the hypotensive effects of other therapeutic agents with this potential).
No products indexed under this heading.

Pentamidine Isethionate (*In vitro* studies showed that drugs metabolized by other CYP isozymes, including 1A1, 1A2, 2C9, 2C19, and 3A4, are only weak inhibitors of risperidone metabolism).
No products indexed under this heading.

Pentobarbital Sodium (Given the primary CNS effects of risperidone, caution should be used if taken in combination with other centrally-acting drugs). Products include:

Nembutal 2012

Pergolide Mesylate (Risperidone may antagonize the effect of dopamine agonists).
No products indexed under this heading.

Perindopril Erbumine (Because of its potential for inducing hypotension, risperidone may enhance the hypotensive effects of other therapeutic agents with this potential).
No products indexed under this heading.

Perphenazine (Given the primary CNS effects of risperidone, caution should be used if taken in combination with other centrally-acting drugs).
No products indexed under this heading.

Phenacemide (*In vitro* studies showed that drugs metabolized by other CYP isozymes, including 1A1, 1A2, 2C9, 2C19, and 3A4, are only weak inhibitors of risperidone metabolism).
No products indexed under this heading.

Phenobarbital (Co-administration of known CYP3A4 enzyme inducers (eg, phenobarbital) with risperidone may cause decreases in the combined plasma concentrations of ripseridone and 9-hydroxyrisperidone, which could lead to decreased efficacy of risperidone treatment. At the initiation of therapy with known hepatic enzyme inducers, patients should be closely monitored during the first 4–8 weeks, since the dose of risperidone may need to be adjusted. A dose increase, or additional oral risperidone, may need to be considered. On discontinuation of CYP3A4 hepatic enzyme inducers, the dosage of risperidone should be re-evaluated and, if necessary, decreased). Products include:

Donnatal 2711

Phenobarbital Sodium (Co-administration of known CYP3A4 enzyme inducers (eg, phenobarbital) with risperidone may cause decreases in the combined plasma concentrations of ripseridone and 9-hydroxyrisperidone, which could lead to decreased efficacy of risperidone treatment. At the initiation of therapy with known hepatic enzyme inducers, patients should be closely monitored during the first 4–8 weeks, since the dose of risperidone may need to be adjusted. A dose increase, or additional oral risperidone, may need to be considered. On discontinuation of CYP3A4 hepatic enzyme inducers, the dosage of risperidone should be re-evaluated and, if necessary, decreased).
No products indexed under this heading.

Phenoxybenzamine Hydrochloride (Because of its potential for inducing hypotension, risperidone may enhance the hypotensive effects of other therapeutic agents with this potential). Products include:

Dibenzyline 3495

Phensuximide (*In vitro* studies showed that drugs metabolized by other CYP isozymes, including 1A1, 1A2, 2C9, 2C19, and 3A4, are only weak inhibitors of risperidone metabolism).
No products indexed under this heading.

Phentolamine Mesylate (Because of its potential for inducing hypotension, risperidone may enhance the hypotensive effects of other therapeutic agents with this potential).
No products indexed under this heading.

Phenylbutazone (*In vitro* studies showed that drugs metabolized by other CYP isozymes, including 1A1, 1A2, 2C9, 2C19, and 3A4, are only weak inhibitors of risperidone metabolism).
No products indexed under this heading.

Phenytoin (Co-administration of known CYP3A4 enzyme inducers (eg, phenytoin) with risperidone may cause decreases in the combined plasma concentrations of ripseridone and 9-hydroxyrisperidone, which could lead to decreased efficacy of risperidone treatment. At the initiation of therapy with known hepatic enzyme inducers, patients should be closely monitored during the first 4–8 weeks, since the dose of risperidone may need to be adjusted. A dose increase, or additional oral risperidone, may need to be considered. On discontinuation of CYP3A4 hepatic enzyme inducers, the dosage of risperidone should be re-evaluated and, if necessary, decreased).
No products indexed under this heading.

Phenytoin Sodium (Co-administration of known CYP3A4 enzyme inducers (eg, phenytoin) with risperidone may cause decreases in the combined plasma concentrations of ripseridone and 9-hydroxyrisperidone, which could lead to decreased efficacy of risperidone treatment. At the initiation of therapy with known hepatic enzyme inducers, patients should be closely monitored during the first 4–8 weeks, since the dose of risperidone may need to be adjusted. A dose increase, or additional oral risperidone, may need to be considered. On discontinuation of CYP3A4 hepatic enzyme inducers, the dosage of risperidone should be re-evaluated and, if necessary, decreased). Products include:

Phenytek Capsules 2380

Pimozide (*In vitro* studies showed that drugs metabolized by other CYP isozymes, including 1A1, 1A2, 2C9, 2C19, and 3A4, are only weak inhibitors of risperidone metabolism).
No products indexed under this heading.

Pindolol (Because of its potential for inducing hypotension, risperidone may enhance the hypotensive effects of other therapeutic agents with this potential).
No products indexed under this heading.

Pioglitazone Hydrochloride (*In vitro* studies showed that drugs metabolized by other CYP isozymes, including 1A1, 1A2, 2C9, 2C19, and 3A4, are only weak inhibitors of risperidone metabolism). Products include:

ActoPlus 3338
Actos 3345
Duetact 3354

Piroxicam (*In vitro* studies showed that drugs metabolized by other CYP isozymes, including 1A1, 1A2, 2C9, 2C19, and 3A4, are only weak inhibitors of risperidone metabolism).
No products indexed under this heading.

Polyestradiol Phosphate (*In vitro* studies showed that drugs metabolized by other CYP isozymes, including 1A1, 1A2, 2C9, 2C19, and 3A4, are only weak inhibitors of risperidone metabolism).
No products indexed under this heading.

Polythiazide (Because of its potential for inducing hypotension, risperidone may enhance the hypotensive effects of other therapeutic agents with this potential).
No products indexed under this heading.

Pramipexole Dihydrochloride (Risperidone may antagonize the effect of dopamine agonists).
No products indexed under this heading.

Prazepam (Given the primary CNS effects of risperidone, caution should be used if taken in combination with other centrally-acting drugs).
No products indexed under this heading.

Prazosin Hydrochloride (Because of its potential for inducing hypotension, risperidone may enhance the hypotensive effects of other therapeutic agents with this potential).
No products indexed under this heading.

Prednisolone (Co-administration of known CYP3A4 enzyme inducers with risperidone may cause decreases in the combined plasma concentrations of ripseridone and 9-hydroxyrisperidone, which could lead to decreased efficacy of risperidone treatment. At the initiation of therapy with known hepatic enzyme inducers, patients should be closely monitored during the first 4–8 weeks, since the dose of risperidone may need to be adjusted. A dose increase, or additional oral risperidone, may need to be considered. On discontinuation of CYP3A4 hepatic enzyme inducers, the dosage of risperidone should be re-evaluated and, if necessary, decreased).
No products indexed under this heading.

Prednisolone Acetate (Co-administration of known CYP3A4 enzyme inducers with risperidone may cause decreases in the combined plasma concentrations of ripseridone and 9-hydroxyrisperidone, which could lead to decreased efficacy of risperidone treatment. At the initiation of therapy with known hepatic enzyme inducers, patients should be closely monitored during the first 4–8 weeks, since the dose of risperidone may need to be adjusted. A dose increase, or additional oral risperidone, may need to be considered. On discontinuation of CYP3A4 hepatic enzyme inducers, the dosage of risperidone should be re-evaluated and, if necessary, decreased). Products include:

Blephamide .... ⊙212, ⊙214
Pred Forte .... ⊙225
Pred Mild .... ⊙230
Pred-G .... ⊙226, ⊙227

Prednisolone Sodium Phosphate (Co-administration of known CYP3A4 enzyme inducers with risperidone may cause decreases in the combined plasma concentrations of ripseridone and 9-hydroxyrisperidone, which could lead to decreased efficacy of risperidone treatment. At the initiation of therapy with known hepatic enzyme inducers, patients should be closely monitored during the first 4–8 weeks, since the dose of risperidone may need to be adjusted. A dose increase, or additional oral risperidone, may need to be considered. On discontinuation of CYP3A4 hepatic enzyme inducers, the dosage of risperidone should be re-evaluated and, if necessary, decreased).
No products indexed under this heading.

Prednisolone Tebutate (Co-administration of known CYP3A4 enzyme inducers with risperidone may cause decreases in the combined plasma concentrations of ripseridone and 9-hydroxyrisperidone, which could lead to decreased efficacy of risperidone treatment. At the initiation of therapy with known hepatic enzyme inducers, patients should be closely monitored during the first 4–8 weeks, since the dose of risperidone may need to be adjusted. A dose increase, or additional oral risperidone, may need to be considered. On discontinuation of CYP3A4 hepatic enzyme inducers, the dosage of risperidone should be re-evaluated and, if necessary, decreased).
No products indexed under this heading.

Prednisone (Co-administration of known CYP3A4 enzyme inducers with risperidone may cause decreases in the combined plasma concentrations of ripseridone and 9-hydroxyrisperidone, which could lead to decreased efficacy of risperidone treatment. At the initiation of therapy with known hepatic enzyme inducers, patients should be closely monitored during the first 4–8 weeks, since the dose of risperidone may need to be adjusted. A dose increase, or additional oral risperidone, may need to be considered. On discontinuation of CYP3A4 hepatic enzyme inducers, the dosage of risperidone should be re-evaluated and, if necessary, decreased).
No products indexed under this heading.

Prednisone sodium phosphate (Co-administration of known CYP3A4 enzyme inducers with risperidone may cause decreases in the combined plasma concentrations of ripseridone and 9-hydroxyrisperidone, which could lead to decreased efficacy of risperidone treatment. At the initiation of therapy with known hepatic enzyme inducers, patients should be closely monitored during the first 4–8 weeks, since the dose of risperidone may need to be adjusted. A dose increase, or additional oral risperidone, may need to be considered. On discontinuation of CYP3A4 hepatic enzyme inducers, the dosage of risperidone should be re-evaluated and, if necessary, decreased).
No products indexed under this heading.

Primidone (Co-administration of known CYP3A4 enzyme inducers with risperidone may cause decreases in the combined plasma concentrations of ripseridone and 9-hydroxyrisperidone, which could lead to decreased efficacy of risperidone treatment. At the initiation of therapy with known hepatic enzyme inducers, patients should be closely monitored during the first 4–8

weeks, since the dose of risperidone may need to be adjusted. A dose increase, or additional oral risperidone, may need to be considered. On discontinuation of CYP3A4 hepatic enzyme inducers, the dosage of risperidone should be re-evaluated and, if necessary, decreased).
No products indexed under this heading.

Prochlorperazine (Given the primary CNS effects of risperidone, caution should be used if taken in combination with other centrally-acting drugs).
No products indexed under this heading.

Progesterone (In vitro studies showed that drugs metabolized by other CYP isozymes, including 1A1, 1A2, 2C9, 2C19, and 3A4, are only weak inhibitors of risperidone metabolism). Products include:

Proguanil Hydrochloride (In vitro studies showed that drugs metabolized by other CYP isozymes, including 1A1, 1A2, 2C9, 2C19, and 3A4, are only weak inhibitors of risperidone metabolism). Products include:

Promethazine Hydrochloride (Given the primary CNS effects of risperidone, caution should be used if taken in combination with other centrally-acting drugs).
No products indexed under this heading.

Propafenone Hydrochloride (In vitro studies showed that drugs metabolized by other CYP isozymes, including 1A1, 1A2, 2C9, 2C19, and 3A4, are only weak inhibitors of risperidone metabolism). Products include:

Propofol (Given the primary CNS effects of risperidone, caution should be used if taken in combination with other centrally-acting drugs).
No products indexed under this heading.

Propoxyphene Hydrochloride (Given the primary CNS effects of risperidone, caution should be used if taken in combination with other centrally-acting drugs).
No products indexed under this heading.

Propoxyphene Napsylate (Given the primary CNS effects of risperidone, caution should be used if taken in combination with other centrally-acting drugs).
No products indexed under this heading.

Propranolol Hydrochloride (In vitro studies showed that drugs metabolized by other CYP isozymes, including 1A1, 1A2, 2C9, 2C19, and 3A4, are only weak inhibitors of risperidone metabolism). Products include:

Protriptyline Hydrochloride (In vitro studies showed that drugs metabolized by other CYP isozymes, including 1A1, 1A2, 2C9, 2C19, and 3A4, are only weak inhibitors of risperidone metabolism).
No products indexed under this heading.

Quazepam (Given the primary CNS effects of risperidone, caution should be used if taken in combination with other centrally-acting drugs).
No products indexed under this heading.

Quetiapine Fumarate (Given the primary CNS effects of risperidone, caution should be used if taken in combination with other centrally-acting drugs). Products include:

Quinacrine Hydrochloride (Risperidone is metabolized to 9-hydroxyrisperidone by CYP2D6. Drug interactions that reduce the metabolism of risperidone to 9-hydroxyrisperidone would increase the plasma concentrations of risperidone and lower the concentrations of 9-hydroxyrisperidone).
No products indexed under this heading.

Quinapril Hydrochloride (Because of its potential for inducing hypotension, risperidone may enhance the hypotensive effects of other therapeutic agents with this potential).
No products indexed under this heading.

Quinidine (Risperidone is metabolized to 9-hydroxyrisperidone by CYP2D6. Drug interactions that reduce the metabolism of risperidone to 9-hydroxyrisperidone would increase the plasma concentrations of risperidone and lower the concentrations of 9-hydroxyrisperidone).
No products indexed under this heading.

Quinidine Gluconate (Risperidone is metabolized to 9-hydroxyrisperidone by CYP2D6. Drug interactions that reduce the metabolism of risperidone to 9-hydroxyrisperidone would increase the plasma concentrations of risperidone and lower the concentrations of 9-hydroxyrisperidone).
No products indexed under this heading.

Quinidine Hydrochloride (Risperidone is metabolized to 9-hydroxyrisperidone by CYP2D6. Drug interactions that reduce the metabolism of risperidone to 9-hydroxyrisperidone would increase the plasma concentrations of risperidone and lower the concentrations of 9-hydroxyrisperidone).
No products indexed under this heading.

Quinidine Polygalacturonate (Risperidone is metabolized to 9-hydroxyrisperidone by CYP2D6. Drug interactions that reduce the metabolism of risperidone to 9-hydroxyrisperidone would increase the plasma concentrations of risperidone and lower the concentrations of 9-hydroxyrisperidone).
No products indexed under this heading.

Quinidine Sulfate (Risperidone is metabolized to 9-hydroxyrisperidone by CYP2D6. Drug interactions that reduce the metabolism of risperidone to 9-hydroxyrisperidone would increase the plasma concentrations of risperidone and lower the concentrations of 9-hydroxyrisperidone).
No products indexed under this heading.

Rabeprazole Sodium (In vitro studies showed that drugs metabolized by other CYP isozymes, including 1A1, 1A2, 2C9, 2C19, and 3A4, are only weak inhibitors of risperidone metabolism). Products include:

Ramipril (Because of its potential for inducing hypotension, risperidone may enhance the hypotensive effects of other therapeutic agents with this potential).
No products indexed under this heading.

Ranitidine Bismuth Citrate (Ranitidine increased the bioavailability of oral risperidone by 26%. Ranitidine increased the AUC of risperidone and 9-hydroxyrisperidone combined by 20%).
No products indexed under this heading.

Ranitidine Hydrochloride (Ranitidine increased the bioavailability of oral risperidone by 26%. Ranitidine increased the AUC of risperidone and 9-hydroxyrisperidone combined by 20%). Products include:

Rauwolfia Serpentina (Because of its potential for inducing hypotension, risperidone may enhance the hypotensive effects of other therapeutic agents with this potential).
No products indexed under this heading.

Remifentanil Hydrochloride (Given the primary CNS effects of risperidone, caution should be used if taken in combination with other centrally-acting drugs).
No products indexed under this heading.

Repaglinide (In vitro studies showed that drugs metabolized by other CYP isozymes, including 1A1, 1A2, 2C9, 2C19, and 3A4, are only weak inhibitors of risperidone metabolism).
No products indexed under this heading.

Rescinnamine (Because of its potential for inducing hypotension, risperidone may enhance the hypotensive effects of other therapeutic agents with this potential).
No products indexed under this heading.

Reserpine (Because of its potential for inducing hypotension, risperidone may enhance the hypotensive effects of other therapeutic agents with this potential).
No products indexed under this heading.

Rifabutin (Co-administration of known CYP3A4 enzyme inducers with risperidone may cause decreases in the combined plasma concentrations of ripseridone and 9-hydroxyrisperidone, which could lead to decreased efficacy of risperidone treatment. At the initiation of therapy with known hepatic enzyme inducers, patients should be closely monitored during the first 4–8 weeks, since the dose of risperidone may need to be adjusted. A dose increase, or additional oral risperidone, may need to be considered. On discontinuation of CYP3A4 hepatic enzyme inducers, the dosage of risperidone should be re-evaluated and, if necessary, decreased).
No products indexed under this heading.

Rifampicin (Co-administration of known CYP3A4 enzyme inducers with risperidone may cause decreases in the combined plasma concentrations of ripseridone and 9-hydroxyrisperidone, which could lead to decreased efficacy of risperidone treatment. At the initiation of therapy with known hepatic enzyme inducers, patients should be closely monitored during the first 4–8 weeks, since the dose of risperidone may need to be adjusted. A dose increase, or additional oral risperidone, may need to be considered. On discontinuation of CYP3A4 hepatic enzyme inducers, the dosage of risperidone should be re-evaluated and, if necessary, decreased).
No products indexed under this heading.

Rifampin (Co-administration of known CYP3A4 enzyme inducers (eg, rifampin) with risperidone may cause decreases in the combined plasma concentrations of ripseridone and 9-hydroxyrisperidone, which could lead to decreased efficacy of risperidone treatment. At the initiation of therapy with known hepatic enzyme inducers, patients should be closely monitored during the first 4–8 weeks, since the dose of risperidone may need to be adjusted. A dose increase, or additional oral risperidone, may need to be considered. On discontinuation of CYP3A4 hepatic enzyme inducers, the dosage of risperidone should be re-evaluated and, if necessary, decreased).
No products indexed under this heading.

Rifapentine (Co-administration of known CYP3A4 enzyme inducers with risperidone may cause decreases in the combined plasma concentrations of ripseridone and 9-hydroxyrisperidone, which could lead to decreased efficacy of risperidone treatment. At the initiation of therapy with known hepatic enzyme inducers, patients should be closely monitored during the first 4–8 weeks, since the dose of risperidone may need to be adjusted. A dose increase, or additional oral risperidone, may need to be considered. On discontinuation of CYP3A4 hepatic enzyme inducers, the dosage of risperidone should be re-evaluated and, if necessary, decreased).
No products indexed under this heading.

Riluzole (In vitro studies showed that drugs metabolized by other CYP isozymes, including 1A1, 1A2, 2C9, 2C19, and 3A4, are only weak inhibitors of risperidone metabolism). Products include:

Ritonavir (In vitro studies showed that drugs metabolized by other CYP isozymes, including 1A1, 1A2, 2C9, 2C19, and 3A4, are only weak inhibitors of risperidone metabolism). Products include:

Rofecoxib (In vitro studies showed that drugs metabolized by other CYP isozymes, including 1A1, 1A2, 2C9, 2C19, and 3A4, are only weak inhibitors of risperidone metabolism).
No products indexed under this heading.

Ropinirole Hydrochloride (Risperidone may antagonize the effect of dopamine agonists). Products include:

Ropivacaine Hydrochloride (In vitro studies showed that drugs metabolized by other CYP isozymes, including 1A1, 1A2, 2C9, 2C19, and 3A4, are only weak inhibitors of risperidone metabolism).
No products indexed under this heading.

Rosiglitazone Maleate (In vitro studies showed that drugs metabolized by other CYP isozymes, including 1A1, 1A2, 2C9, 2C19, and 3A4, are only weak inhibitors of risperidone metabolism). Products include:

Saquinavir (In vitro studies showed that drugs metabolized by other CYP isozymes, including 1A1, 1A2, 2C9, 2C19, and 3A4, are only weak inhibitors of risperidone metabolism).
No products indexed under this heading.

Saquinavir Mesylate (In vitro studies showed that drugs metabolized by other CYP isozymes, including 1A1, 1A2, 2C9, 2C19, and 3A4, are only weak inhibitors of risperidone metabolism).
No products indexed under this heading.

Secobarbital Sodium (Given the primary CNS effects of risperidone, caution should be used if taken in combination with other centrally-acting drugs).
No products indexed under this heading.

Sertraline Hydrochloride (Risperidone is metabolized to 9-hydroxyrisperidone by CYP2D6. Drug interactions that reduce the metabolism of risperidone to 9-hydroxyrisperidone would increase the plasma concentrations of risperidone and lower the concentrations of 9-hydroxyrisperidone).
No products indexed under this heading.

Sevoflurane (Given the primary CNS effects of risperidone, caution should be used if taken in combination with other centrally-acting drugs). Products include:

Sildenafil Citrate (Risperidone is metabolized to 9-hydroxyrisperidone by CYP2D6. Drug interactions that reduce the metabolism of risperidone to 9-hydroxyrisperidone would increase the plasma concentrations of risperidone and lower the concentrations of 9-hydroxyrisperidone).
No products indexed under this heading.

Simvastatin (*In vitro* studies showed that drugs metabolized by other CYP isozymes, including 1A1, 1A2, 2C9, 2C19, and 3A4, are only weak inhibitors of risperidone metabolism). Products include:
Simcor **524**
Vytorin 10/10 .... **2303, 3240**
Vytorin 10/20 .... **2303, 3240**
Vytorin 10/40 .... **2303, 3240**
Vytorin 10/80 .... **2303, 3240**
Zocor **2289**

Sirolimus (*In vitro* studies showed that drugs metabolized by other CYP isozymes, including 1A1, 1A2, 2C9, 2C19, and 3A4, are only weak inhibitors of risperidone metabolism). Products include:
Rapamune **3579**

Sodium Nitroprusside (Because of its potential for inducing hypotension, risperidone may enhance the hypotensive effects of other therapeutic agents with this potential).
No products indexed under this heading.

Sodium Oxybate (Given the primary CNS effects of risperidone, caution should be used if taken in combination with other centrally-acting drugs).
No products indexed under this heading.

Sotalol Hydrochloride (Because of its potential for inducing hypotension, risperidone may enhance the hypotensive effects of other therapeutic agents with this potential).
No products indexed under this heading.

Spirapril Hydrochloride (Because of its potential for inducing hypotension, risperidone may enhance the hypotensive effects of other therapeutic agents with this potential).
No products indexed under this heading.

Sufentanil Citrate (Given the primary CNS effects of risperidone, caution should be used if taken in combination with other centrally-acting drugs).
No products indexed under this heading.

Sulfamethoxazole (*In vitro* studies showed that drugs metabolized by other CYP isozymes, including 1A1, 1A2, 2C9, 2C19, and 3A4, are only weak inhibitors of risperidone metabolism).
No products indexed under this heading.

Sulfinpyrazone (Co-administration of known CYP3A4 enzyme inducers with risperidone may cause decreases in the combined plasma concentrations of ripseridone and 9-hydroxyrisperidone, which could lead to decreased efficacy of risperidone treatment. At the initiation of therapy with known hepatic enzyme inducers, patients should be closely monitored during the first 4–8 weeks, since the dose of risperidone may need to be adjusted. A dose increase, or additional oral risperidone, may need to be considered. On discontinuation of CYP3A4 hepatic enzyme inducers, the dosage of risperidone should be re-evaluated and, if necessary, decreased).
No products indexed under this heading.

Sulindac (*In vitro* studies showed that drugs metabolized by other CYP isozymes, including 1A1, 1A2, 2C9, 2C19, and 3A4, are only weak inhibitors of risperidone metabolism). Products include:
Clinoril **2098**

Suprofen (*In vitro* studies showed that drugs metabolized by other CYP isozymes, including 1A1, 1A2, 2C9, 2C19, and 3A4, are only weak inhibitors of risperidone metabolism).
No products indexed under this heading.

Tacrine Hydrochloride (*In vitro* studies showed that drugs metabolized by other CYP isozymes, including 1A1, 1A2, 2C9, 2C19, and 3A4, are only weak inhibitors of risperidone metabolism).
No products indexed under this heading.

Tacrolimus (*In vitro* studies showed that drugs metabolized by other CYP isozymes, including 1A1, 1A2, 2C9, 2C19, and 3A4, are only weak inhibitors of risperidone metabolism). Products include:
Prograf Capsules **677**
Prograf Injection **677**
Protopic **685**

Tadalafil (*In vitro* studies showed that drugs metabolized by other CYP isozymes, including 1A1, 1A2, 2C9, 2C19, and 3A4, are only weak inhibitors of risperidone metabolism). Products include:
Adcirca **3461**
Cialis **1861**

Tamoxifen Citrate (*In vitro* studies showed that drugs metabolized by other CYP isozymes, including 1A1, 1A2, 2C9, 2C19, and 3A4, are only weak inhibitors of risperidone metabolism).
No products indexed under this heading.

Telmisartan (Because of its potential for inducing hypotension, risperidone may enhance the hypotensive effects of other therapeutic agents with this potential). Products include:
Micardis **887**
Micardis HCT **889**

Temazepam (Given the primary CNS effects of risperidone, caution should be used if taken in combination with other centrally-acting drugs).
No products indexed under this heading.

Teniposide (*In vitro* studies showed that drugs metabolized by other CYP isozymes, including 1A1, 1A2, 2C9, 2C19, and 3A4, are only weak inhibitors of risperidone metabolism).
No products indexed under this heading.

Terazosin Hydrochloride (Because of its potential for inducing hypotension, risperidone may enhance the hypotensive effects of other therapeutic agents with this potential).
No products indexed under this heading.

Terbinafine Hydrochloride (Risperidone is metabolized to 9-hydroxyrisperidone by CYP2D6. Drug interactions that reduce the metabolism of risperidone to 9-hydroxyrisperidone would increase the plasma concentrations of risperidone and lower the concentrations of 9-hydroxyrisperidone).
No products indexed under this heading.

Terfenadine (*In vitro* studies showed that drugs metabolized by other CYP isozymes, including 1A1, 1A2, 2C9, 2C19, and 3A4, are only weak inhibitors of risperidone metabolism).
No products indexed under this heading.

Theobromine (*In vitro* studies showed that drugs metabolized by other CYP isozymes, including 1A1, 1A2, 2C9, 2C19, and 3A4, are only weak inhibitors of risperidone metabolism).
No products indexed under this heading.

Theophyllinate (Co-administration of known CYP3A4 enzyme inducers with risperidone may cause decreases in the combined plasma concentrations of ripseridone and 9-hydroxyrisperidone, which could lead to decreased efficacy of risperidone treatment. At the initiation of therapy with known hepatic enzyme inducers, patients should be closely monitored during the first 4–8 weeks, since the dose of risperidone may need to be adjusted. A dose increase, or additional oral risperidone, may need to be considered. On discontinuation of CYP3A4 hepatic enzyme inducers, the dosage of risperidone should be re-evaluated and, if necessary, decreased).
No products indexed under this heading.

Theophylline (*In vitro* studies showed that drugs metabolized by other CYP isozymes, including 1A1, 1A2, 2C9, 2C19, and 3A4, are only weak inhibitors of risperidone metabolism).
No products indexed under this heading.

Theophylline Anhydrous (*In vitro* studies showed that drugs metabolized by other CYP isozymes, including 1A1, 1A2, 2C9, 2C19, and 3A4, are only weak inhibitors of risperidone metabolism). Products include:
Uniphyl **2817**

Theophylline Calcium Salicylate (*In vitro* studies showed that drugs metabolized by other CYP isozymes, including 1A1, 1A2, 2C9, 2C19, and 3A4, are only weak inhibitors of risperidone metabolism).
No products indexed under this heading.

Theophylline Dihydroxypropyl (Glyceryl) (*In vitro* studies showed that drugs metabolized by other CYP isozymes, including 1A1, 1A2, 2C9, 2C19, and 3A4, are only weak inhibitors of risperidone metabolism).
No products indexed under this heading.

Theophylline Ethylenediamine (*In vitro* studies showed that drugs metabolized by other CYP isozymes, including 1A1, 1A2, 2C9, 2C19, and 3A4, are only weak inhibitors of risperidone metabolism).
No products indexed under this heading.

Theophylline Sodium Glycinate (*In vitro* studies showed that drugs metabolized by other CYP isozymes, including 1A1, 1A2, 2C9, 2C19, and 3A4, are only weak inhibitors of risperidone metabolism).
No products indexed under this heading.

Thiamylal Sodium (Given the primary CNS effects of risperidone, caution should be used if taken in combination with other centrally-acting drugs).
No products indexed under this heading.

Thioridazine (*In vitro* studies showed that drugs metabolized by other CYP isozymes, including 1A1, 1A2, 2C9, 2C19, and 3A4, are only weak inhibitors of risperidone metabolism).
No products indexed under this heading.

Thioridazine Hydrochloride (Given the primary CNS effects of risperidone, caution should be used if taken in combination with other centrally-acting drugs). Products include:
Thioridazine Hydrochloride **2384**

Thiothixene (Given the primary CNS effects of risperidone, caution should be used if taken in combination with other centrally-acting drugs). Products include:
Thiothixene **2386**

Tiagabine Hydrochloride (*In vitro* studies showed that drugs metabolized by other CYP isozymes, including 1A1, 1A2, 2C9, 2C19, and 3A4, are only weak inhibitors of risperidone metabolism). Products include:
Gabitril **972**

Timolol Maleate (Because of its potential for inducing hypotension, risperidone may enhance the hypotensive effects of other therapeutic agents with this potential). Products include:
Combigan **601**
Dorzolamide Hydrochloride/Timolol Maleate Ophthalmic Solution .... ⊙**243**
Timoptic in Ocudose .... ⊙**231**

Tizanidine (*In vitro* studies showed that drugs metabolized by other CYP isozymes, including 1A1, 1A2, 2C9, 2C19, and 3A4, are only weak inhibitors of risperidone metabolism).
No products indexed under this heading.

Tizanidine Hydrochloride (*In vitro* studies showed that drugs metabolized by other CYP isozymes, including 1A1, 1A2, 2C9, 2C19, and 3A4, are only weak inhibitors of risperidone metabolism).
No products indexed under this heading.

Tolazamide (*In vitro* studies showed that drugs metabolized by other CYP isozymes, including 1A1, 1A2, 2C9, 2C19, and 3A4, are only weak inhibitors of risperidone metabolism).
No products indexed under this heading.

Tolbutamide (*In vitro* studies showed that drugs metabolized by other CYP isozymes, including 1A1, 1A2, 2C9, 2C19, and 3A4, are only weak inhibitors of risperidone metabolism).
No products indexed under this heading.

Tolbutamide Sodium (*In vitro* studies showed that drugs metabolized by other CYP isozymes, including 1A1, 1A2, 2C9, 2C19, and 3A4, are only weak inhibitors of risperidone metabolism).
No products indexed under this heading.

Tolmetin Sodium (*In vitro* studies showed that drugs metabolized by other CYP isozymes, including 1A1, 1A2, 2C9, 2C19, and 3A4, are only weak inhibitors of risperidone metabolism).
No products indexed under this heading.

Tolterodine Tartrate (*In vitro* studies showed that drugs metabolized by other CYP isozymes, including 1A1, 1A2, 2C9, 2C19, and 3A4, are only weak inhibitors of risperidone metabolism).
No products indexed under this heading.

Topiramate (Oral risperidone administered at doses from 1-6 mg/day concomitantly with topiramate 400 mg/day resulted in a 23% decrease in risperidone C_{max} and a 33% decrease in risperidone $AUC_{0\text{-}12\ hour}$ at steady state. Minimal reductions in the exposure to risperidone and 9-hydroxyrisperidone combined, and no change for 9-hydroxyrisperidone were observed. This interaction is unlikely to be of clinical significance).
No products indexed under this heading.

Torsemide (Because of its potential for inducing hypotension, risperidone may enhance the hypotensive effects of other therapeutic agents with this potential).
No products indexed under this heading.

Trandolapril (Because of its potential for inducing hypotension, risperidone may enhance the hypotensive effects of other therapeutic agents with this potential). Products include:
Mavik **489**
Tarka **534**

Trazodone Hydrochloride (*In vitro* studies showed that drugs metabolized by other CYP isozymes, including 1A1, 1A2, 2C9, 2C19, and 3A4, are only weak inhibitors of risperidone metabolism).
No products indexed under this heading.

Triamcinolone (Co-administration of known CYP3A4 enzyme inducers with risperidone may cause decreases in the combined plasma concentrations of ripseridone and 9-hydroxyrisperidone, which could lead to decreased efficacy of risperidone treatment. At the initiation of therapy with known hepatic enzyme inducers, patients should be closely monitored during the first 4–8 weeks, since the dose of risperidone may need to be adjusted. A dose increase, or additional oral risperidone, may need to be considered. On discon-

IMPORTANT NOTE: Always consult each drug listing in the patient's regimen for possible interactions.

tinuation of CYP3A4 hepatic enzyme inducers, the dosage of risperidone should be re-evaluated and, if necessary, decreased.

No products indexed under this heading.

Triamcinolone Acetonide (Co-administration of known CYP3A4 enzyme inducers with risperidone may cause decreases in the combined plasma concentrations of ripseridone and 9-hydroxyrisperidone, which could lead to decreased efficacy of risperidone treatment. At the initiation of therapy with known hepatic enzyme inducers, patients should be closely monitored during the first 4–8 weeks, since the dose of risperidone may need to be adjusted. A dose increase, or additional oral risperidone, may need to be considered. On discontinuation of CYP3A4 hepatic enzyme inducers, the dosage of risperidone should be re-evaluated and, if necessary, decreased). Products include:

Triamcinolone Diacetate (Co-administration of known CYP3A4 enzyme inducers with risperidone may cause decreases in the combined plasma concentrations of ripseridone and 9-hydroxyrisperidone, which could lead to decreased efficacy of risperidone treatment. At the initiation of therapy with known hepatic enzyme inducers, patients should be closely monitored during the first 4–8 weeks, since the dose of risperidone may need to be adjusted. A dose increase, or additional oral risperidone, may need to be considered. On discontinuation of CYP3A4 hepatic enzyme inducers, the dosage of risperidone should be re-evaluated and, if necessary, decreased).

No products indexed under this heading.

Triamcinolone Hexacetonide (Co-administration of known CYP3A4 enzyme inducers with risperidone may cause decreases in the combined plasma concentrations of ripseridone and 9-hydroxyrisperidone, which could lead to decreased efficacy of risperidone treatment. At the initiation of therapy with known hepatic enzyme inducers, patients should be closely monitored during the first 4–8 weeks, since the dose of risperidone may need to be adjusted. A dose increase, or additional oral risperidone, may need to be considered. On discontinuation of CYP3A4 hepatic enzyme inducers, the dosage of risperidone should be re-evaluated and, if necessary, decreased).

No products indexed under this heading.

Triazolam (Given the primary CNS effects of risperidone, caution should be used if taken in combination with other centrally-acting drugs).

No products indexed under this heading.

Trifluoperazine Hydrochloride (Given the primary CNS effects of risperidone, caution should be used if taken in combination with other centrally-acting drugs).

No products indexed under this heading.

Trimethadione (In vitro studies showed that drugs metabolized by other CYP isozymes, including 1A1, 1A2, 2C9, 2C19, and 3A4, are only weak inhibitors of risperidone metabolism).

No products indexed under this heading.

Trimethaphan Camsylate (In vitro studies showed that drugs metabolized by other CYP isozymes, including 1A1, 1A2, 2C9, 2C19, and 3A4, are only weak inhibitors of risperidone metabolism).

No products indexed under this heading.

Trimipramine Maleate (In vitro studies showed that drugs metabolized by other CYP isozymes, including 1A1, 1A2, 2C9, 2C19, and 3A4, are only weak inhibitors of risperidone metabolism).

No products indexed under this heading.

Troglitazone (Co-administration of known CYP3A4 enzyme inducers with risperidone may cause decreases in the combined plasma concentrations of ripseridone and 9-hydroxyrisperidone, which could lead to decreased efficacy of risperidone treatment. At the initiation of therapy with known hepatic enzyme inducers, patients should be closely monitored during the first 4–8 weeks, since the dose of risperidone may need to be adjusted. A dose increase, or additional oral risperidone, may need to be considered. On discontinuation of CYP3A4 hepatic enzyme inducers, the dosage of risperidone should be re-evaluated and, if necessary, decreased).

No products indexed under this heading.

Trovafloxacin Mesylate (In vitro studies showed that drugs metabolized by other CYP isozymes, including 1A1, 1A2, 2C9, 2C19, and 3A4, are only weak inhibitors of risperidone metabolism).

No products indexed under this heading.

Valdecoxib (In vitro studies showed that drugs metabolized by other CYP isozymes, including 1A1, 1A2, 2C9, 2C19, and 3A4, are only weak inhibitors of risperidone metabolism).

No products indexed under this heading.

Valproate Sodium (Repeated oral doses of risperidone (4 mg qd) did not affect the pre-dose or average plasma concentrations exposure (AUC) of valproate (1000 mg/day in three divided doses) compared to placebo (n=21). However, there was a 20% increase of valproate peak plasma concentration (C_{max}) after concomitant administration of oral risperidone).

No products indexed under this heading.

Valproic Acid (Repeated oral doses of risperidone (4 mg qd) did not affect the pre-dose or average plasma concentrations exposure (AUC) of valproate (1000 mg/day in three divided doses) compared to placebo (n=21). However, there was a 20% increase of valproate peak plasma concentration (C_{max}) after concomitant administration of oral risperidone).

No products indexed under this heading.

Valsartan (Because of its potential for inducing hypotension, risperidone may enhance the hypotensive effects of other therapeutic agents with this potential). Products include:

Vardenafil Hydrochloride (Risperidone is metabolized to 9-hydroxyrisperidone by CYP2D6. Drug interactions that reduce the metabolism of risperidone to 9-hydroxyrisperidone would increase the plasma concentrations of risperidone and lower the concentrations of 9-hydroxyrisperidone). Products include:

Verapamil Hydrochloride (In vitro studies showed that drugs metabolized by other CYP isozymes, including 1A1, 1A2, 2C9, 2C19, and 3A4, are only weak inhibitors of risperidone metabolism). Products include:

Vinblastine Sulfate (In vitro studies showed that drugs metabolized by other CYP isozymes, including 1A1, 1A2, 2C9, 2C19, and 3A4, are only weak inhibitors of risperidone metabolism).

No products indexed under this heading.

Vincristine Sulfate (In vitro studies showed that drugs metabolized by other CYP isozymes, including 1A1, 1A2, 2C9, 2C19, and 3A4, are only weak inhibitors of risperidone metabolism).

No products indexed under this heading.

Voriconazole (In vitro studies showed that drugs metabolized by other CYP isozymes, including 1A1, 1A2, 2C9, 2C19, and 3A4, are only weak inhibitors of risperidone metabolism).

No products indexed under this heading.

Warfarin Sodium (In vitro studies showed that drugs metabolized by other CYP isozymes, including 1A1, 1A2, 2C9, 2C19, and 3A4, are only weak inhibitors of risperidone metabolism).

No products indexed under this heading.

Zafirlukast (In vitro studies showed that drugs metabolized by other CYP isozymes, including 1A1, 1A2, 2C9, 2C19, and 3A4, are only weak inhibitors of risperidone metabolism). Products include:

Zaleplon (Given the primary CNS effects of risperidone, caution should be used if taken in combination with other centrally-acting drugs).

No products indexed under this heading.

Zileuton (In vitro studies showed that drugs metabolized by other CYP isozymes, including 1A1, 1A2, 2C9, 2C19, and 3A4, are only weak inhibitors of risperidone metabolism).

No products indexed under this heading.

Ziprasidone Hydrochloride (Given the primary CNS effects of risperidone, caution should be used if taken in combination with other centrally-acting drugs). Products include:

Zolmitriptan (In vitro studies showed that drugs metabolized by other CYP isozymes, including 1A1, 1A2, 2C9, 2C19, and 3A4, are only weak inhibitors of risperidone metabolism). Products include:

Zolpidem Tartrate (Given the primary CNS effects of risperidone, caution should be used if taken in combination with other centrally-acting drugs). Products include:

Zonisamide (In vitro studies showed that drugs metabolized by other CYP isozymes, including 1A1, 1A2, 2C9, 2C19, and 3A4, are only weak inhibitors of risperidone metabolism). Products include:

Food Interactions

Alcohol (Given the primary CNS effects of risperidone, caution should be used if taken in combination with alcohol).

Beer, reduced-alcohol (Given the primary CNS effects of risperidone, caution should be used if taken in combination with alcohol).

Beer, unspecified (Given the primary CNS effects of risperidone, caution should be used if taken in combination with alcohol).

Food, caffeine-containing (In vitro studies showed that drugs metabolized by other CYP isozymes, including 1A1, 1A2, 2C9, 2C19, and 3A4, are only weak inhibitors of risperidone metabolism).

Wine, Chianti (Given the primary CNS effects of risperidone, caution should be used if taken in combination with alcohol).

Wine, Red (Given the primary CNS effects of risperidone, caution should be used if taken in combination with alcohol).

Wine, unspecified (Given the primary CNS effects of risperidone, caution should be used if taken in combination with alcohol).

Wine products (Given the primary CNS effects of risperidone, caution should be used if taken in combination with alcohol).

RITUXAN I.V.

May interact with disease-modifying antirheumatic drugs, vaccines, live, and certain other agents. Compounds in these categories include:

Abatacept (Limited data are available on the safety of the use of biologic agents or DMARDs other than methotrexate in patients exhibiting peripheral B-cell depletion following treatment with rituximab. Observe patients closely for signs of infection if biologic agents and/or DMARDs are used concomitantly).

No products indexed under this heading.

Adalimumab (Limited data are available on the safety of the use of biologic agents or DMARDs other than methotrexate in patients exhibiting peripheral B-cell depletion following treatment with rituximab. Observe patients closely for signs of infection if biologic agents and/or DMARDs are used concomitantly). Products include:

Anakinra (Limited data are available on the safety of the use of biologic agents or DMARDs other than methotrexate in patients exhibiting peripheral B-cell depletion following treatment with rituximab. Observe patients closely for signs of infection if biologic agents and/or DMARDs are used concomitantly). Products include:

Auranofin (Limited data are available on the safety of the use of biologic agents or DMARDs other than methotrexate in patients exhibiting peripheral B-cell depletion following treatment with rituximab. Observe patients closely for signs of infection if biologic agents and/or DMARDs are used concomitantly).

No products indexed under this heading.

Azathioprine (Limited data are available on the safety of the use of biologic agents or DMARDs other than methotrexate in patients exhibiting peripheral B-cell depletion following treatment with rituximab. Observe patients closely for signs of infection if biologic agents and/or DMARDs are used concomitantly).

No products indexed under this heading.

Azathioprine Sodium (Limited data are available on the safety of the use of biologic agents or DMARDs other than methotrexate in patients exhibiting peripheral B-cell depletion following treatment with rituximab. Observe patients closely for signs of infection if biologic agents and/or DMARDs are used concomitantly).

No products indexed under this heading.

1635 Interactions Index Rocephin

BCG Vaccine (The safety of immunization with live viral vaccines following rituximab therapy has not been studied and vaccination with live virus vaccines is not recommended. For Non-Hodgkin's Lymphoma (NHL) patients, the benefits of primary or booster vaccinations should be weighed against the risks of delay in initiation of rituximab therapy).
No products indexed under this heading.

Cisplatin (Renal toxicity has occured in patients with Non-Hodgkin's Lymphoma (NHL) administered concomitant cisplatin therapy. The combination of cisplatin and rituximab is not an approved treatment regimen. Use extreme caution if this combination is used in clinical trials and monitor closely for signs of renal failure).
No products indexed under this heading.

Cyclophosphamide (Limited data are available on the safety of the use of biologic agents or DMARDs other than methotrexate in patients exhibiting peripheral B-cell depletion following treatment with rituximab. Observe patients closely for signs of infection if biologic agents and/or DMARDs are used concomitantly).
No products indexed under this heading.

Cyclosporine (Limited data are available on the safety of the use of biologic agents or DMARDs other than methotrexate in patients exhibiting peripheral B-cell depletion following treatment with rituximab. Observe patients closely for signs of infection if biologic agents and/or DMARDs are used concomitantly). Products include:
Gengraf 440
Neoral Oral Solution 2496
Neoral Capsules 2496
Restasis 605

Etanercept (Limited data are available on the safety of the use of biologic agents or DMARDs other than methotrexate in patients exhibiting peripheral B-cell depletion following treatment with rituximab. Observe patients closely for signs of infection if biologic agents and/or DMARDs are used concomitantly). Products include:
Enbrel 613

Gold Sodium Thiomalate (Limited data are available on the safety of the use of biologic agents or DMARDs other than methotrexate in patients exhibiting peripheral B-cell depletion following treatment with rituximab. Observe patients closely for signs of infection if biologic agents and/or DMARDs are used concomitantly).
No products indexed under this heading.

Gold Therapy (Limited data are available on the safety of the use of biologic agents or DMARDs other than methotrexate in patients exhibiting peripheral B-cell depletion following treatment with rituximab. Observe patients closely for signs of infection if biologic agents and/or DMARDs are used concomitantly).
No products indexed under this heading.

Hydroxychloroquine Sulfate (Limited data are available on the safety of the use of biologic agents or DMARDs other than methotrexate in patients exhibiting peripheral B-cell depletion following treatment with rituximab. Observe patients closely for signs of infection if biologic agents and/or DMARDs are used concomitantly).
No products indexed under this heading.

Infliximab (Limited data are available on the safety of the use of biologic agents or DMARDs other than methotrexate in patients exhibiting peripheral B-cell depletion following treatment with rituximab. Observe patients closely for signs of infection if biologic agents and/or DMARDs are used concomitantly). Products include:
Remicade 919

Influenza Vaccine, Live Attenuated (The safety of immunization with live viral vaccines following rituximab therapy has not been studied and vaccination with live virus vaccines is not recommended. For Non-Hodgkin's Lymphoma (NHL) patients, the benefits of primary or booster vaccinations should be weighed against the risks of delay in initiation of rituximab therapy).
No products indexed under this heading.

Influenza Virus Vaccine Live, Intranasal (The safety of immunization with live viral vaccines following rituximab therapy has not been studied and vaccination with live virus vaccines is not recommended. For Non-Hodgkin's Lymphoma (NHL) patients, the benefits of primary or booster vaccinations should be weighed against the risks of delay in initiation of rituximab therapy). Products include:
FluMist 2078

Leflunomide (Limited data are available on the safety of the use of biologic agents or DMARDs other than methotrexate in patients exhibiting peripheral B-cell depletion following treatment with rituximab. Observe patients closely for signs of infection if biologic agents and/or DMARDs are used concomitantly).
No products indexed under this heading.

Measles, Mumps, Rubella and Varicella Virus Vaccine Live (The safety of immunization with live viral vaccines following rituximab therapy has not been studied and vaccination with live virus vaccines is not recommended. For Non-Hodgkin's Lymphoma (NHL) patients, the benefits of primary or booster vaccinations should be weighed against the risks of delay in initiation of rituximab therapy). Products include:
ProQuad 2254

Measles, Mumps & Rubella Virus Vaccine, Live (The safety of immunization with live viral vaccines following rituximab therapy has not been studied and vaccination with live virus vaccines is not recommended. For Non-Hodgkin's Lymphoma (NHL) patients, the benefits of primary or booster vaccinations should be weighed against the risks of delay in initiation of rituximab therapy). Products include:
M-M-R II 2203
ProQuad 2254

Measles & Rubella Virus Vaccine Live (The safety of immunization with live viral vaccines following rituximab therapy has not been studied and vaccination with live virus vaccines is not recommended. For Non-Hodgkin's Lymphoma (NHL) patients, the benefits of primary or booster vaccinations should be weighed against the risks of delay in initiation of rituximab therapy).
No products indexed under this heading.

Measles Virus Vaccine Live (The safety of immunization with live viral vaccines following rituximab therapy has not been studied and vaccination with live virus vaccines is not recommended. For Non-Hodgkin's Lymphoma (NHL) patients, the benefits of primary or booster vaccinations should be weighed against the risks of delay in initiation of rituximab therapy). Products include:
Attenuvax 2086

Methotrexate (Limited data are available on the safety of the use of biologic agents or DMARDs other than methotrexate in patients exhibiting peripheral B-cell depletion following treatment with rituximab. Observe patients closely for signs of infection if biologic agents and/or DMARDs are used concomitantly).
No products indexed under this heading.

Methotrexate Sodium (Limited data are available on the safety of the use of biologic agents or DMARDs other than methotrexate in patients exhibiting peripheral B-cell depletion following treatment with rituximab. Observe patients closely for signs of infection if biologic agents and/or DMARDs are used concomitantly).
No products indexed under this heading.

Minocycline Hydrochloride (Limited data are available on the safety of the use of biologic agents or DMARDs other than methotrexate in patients exhibiting peripheral B-cell depletion following treatment with rituximab. Observe patients closely for signs of infection if biologic agents and/or DMARDs are used concomitantly). Products include:
Solodyn 2073

Mumps Virus Vaccine, Live (The safety of immunization with live viral vaccines following rituximab therapy has not been studied and vaccination with live virus vaccines is not recommended. For Non-Hodgkin's Lymphoma (NHL) patients, the benefits of primary or booster vaccinations should be weighed against the risks of delay in initiation of rituximab therapy). Products include:
Mumpsvax 2218

Penicillamine (Limited data are available on the safety of the use of biologic agents or DMARDs other than methotrexate in patients exhibiting peripheral B-cell depletion following treatment with rituximab. Observe patients closely for signs of infection if biologic agents and/or DMARDs are used concomitantly).
No products indexed under this heading.

Poliovirus Vaccine, Live, Oral, Trivalent, Types 1,2,3 (Sabin) (The safety of immunization with live viral vaccines following rituximab therapy has not been studied and vaccination with live virus vaccines is not recommended. For Non-Hodgkin's Lymphoma (NHL) patients, the benefits of primary or booster vaccinations should be weighed against the risks of delay in initiation of rituximab therapy).
No products indexed under this heading.

Rotavirus Vaccine, Live, Oral, Tetravalent (The safety of immunization with live viral vaccines following rituximab therapy has not been studied and vaccination with live virus vaccines is not recommended. For Non-Hodgkin's Lymphoma (NHL) patients, the benefits of primary or booster vaccinations should be weighed against the risks of delay in initiation of rituximab therapy).
No products indexed under this heading.

Rubella & Mumps Virus Vaccine Live (The safety of immunization with live viral vaccines following rituximab therapy has not been studied and vaccination with live virus vaccines is not recommended. For Non-Hodgkin's Lymphoma (NHL) patients, the benefits of primary or booster vaccinations should be weighed against the risks of delay in initiation of rituximab therapy).
No products indexed under this heading.

Rubella Virus Vaccine Live (The safety of immunization with live viral vaccines following rituximab therapy has not been studied and vaccination with live virus vaccines is not recommended. For Non-Hodgkin's Lymphoma (NHL) patients, the benefits of primary or booster vaccinations should be weighed against the risks of delay in initiation of rituximab therapy). Products include:
Meruvax II 2210

Smallpox Vaccine (The safety of immunization with live viral vaccines following rituximab therapy has not been studied and vaccination with live virus vaccines is not recommended. For Non-Hodgkin's Lymphoma (NHL) patients, the benefits of primary or booster vaccinations should be weighed against the risks of delay in initiation of rituximab therapy).
No products indexed under this heading.

Sulfasalazine (Limited data are available on the safety of the use of biologic agents or DMARDs other than methotrexate in patients exhibiting peripheral B-cell depletion following treatment with rituximab. Observe patients closely for signs of infection if biologic agents and/or DMARDs are used concomitantly).
No products indexed under this heading.

Typhoid Vaccine (The safety of immunization with live viral vaccines following rituximab therapy has not been studied and vaccination with live virus vaccines is not recommended. For Non-Hodgkin's Lymphoma (NHL) patients, the benefits of primary or booster vaccinations should be weighed against the risks of delay in initiation of rituximab therapy).
No products indexed under this heading.

Varicella Virus Vaccine, Live (The safety of immunization with live viral vaccines following rituximab therapy has not been studied and vaccination with live virus vaccines is not recommended. For Non-Hodgkin's Lymphoma (NHL) patients, the benefits of primary or booster vaccinations should be weighed against the risks of delay in initiation of rituximab therapy). Products include:
Varivax 2285

Yellow Fever Vaccine (The safety of immunization with live viral vaccines following rituximab therapy has not been studied and vaccination with live virus vaccines is not recommended. For Non-Hodgkin's Lymphoma (NHL) patients, the benefits of primary or booster vaccinations should be weighed against the risks of delay in initiation of rituximab therapy).
No products indexed under this heading.

Zoster Vaccine Live (The safety of immunization with live viral vaccines following rituximab therapy has not been studied and vaccination with live virus vaccines is not recommended. For Non-Hodgkin's Lymphoma (NHL) patients, the benefits of primary or booster vaccinations should be weighed against the risks of delay in initiation of rituximab therapy). Products include:
Zostavax 2299

ROCEPHIN INJECTABLE VIALS

(Ceftriaxone Sodium) 2859
May interact with calcium preparations, and certain other agents. Compounds in these categories include:

Calcium Carbonate (Do not use diluents containing calcium to reconstitute ceftriaxone or to further dilute a reconstituted vial for IV administration because a precipitate can form. Precipitation of ceftriaxone-calcium can also occur when ceftriaxone is mixed with calcium-containing solutions in the same IV administration line. Ceftriaxone must not be administered simultaneously with calcium-containing IV solutions, including continuous calcium-containing infusions, such as parenteral nutrition via a Y-site. However, in patients other than neonates, ceftriaxone and calcium-containing solutions may be administered sequentially of one another if the infusion lines are thoroughly flushed between infusions with a compatible fluid. *In vitro* studies using adult and

IMPORTANT NOTE: Always consult each drug listing in the patient's regimen for possible interactions.

neonatal plasma from umbilical cord blood demonstrated that neonates have an increased risk of precipitation of ceftriaxone-calcium). Products include:

Calcium Chloride (Do not use diluents containing calcium to reconstitute ceftriaxone or to further dilute a reconstituted vial for IV administration because a precipitate can form. Precipitation of ceftriaxone-calcium can also occur when ceftriaxone is mixed with calcium-containing solutions in the same IV administration line. Ceftriaxone must not be administered simultaneously with calcium-containing IV solutions, including continuous calcium-containing infusions, such as parenteral nutrition via a Y-site. However, in patients other than neonates, ceftriaxone and calcium-containing solutions may be administered sequentially of one another if the infusion lines are thoroughly flushed between infusions with a compatible fluid. *In vitro* studies using adult and neonatal plasma from umbilical cord blood demonstrated that neonates have an increased risk of precipitation of ceftriaxone-calcium).

No products indexed under this heading.

Calcium Citrate (Do not use diluents containing calcium to reconstitute ceftriaxone or to further dilute a reconstituted vial for IV administration because a precipitate can form. Precipitation of ceftriaxone-calcium can also occur when ceftriaxone is mixed with calcium-containing solutions in the same IV administration line. Ceftriaxone must not be administered simultaneously with calcium-containing IV solutions, including continuous calcium-containing infusions, such as parenteral nutrition via a Y-site. However, in patients other than neonates, ceftriaxone and calcium-containing solutions may be administered sequentially of one another if the infusion lines are thoroughly flushed between infusions with a compatible fluid. *In vitro* studies using adult and neonatal plasma from umbilical cord blood demonstrated that neonates have an increased risk of precipitation of ceftriaxone-calcium). Products include:

Calcium Glubionate (Do not use diluents containing calcium to reconstitute ceftriaxone or to further dilute a reconstituted vial for IV administration because a precipitate can form. Precipitation of ceftriaxone-calcium can also occur when ceftriaxone is mixed with calcium-containing solutions in the same IV administration line. Ceftriaxone must not be administered simultaneously with calcium-containing IV solutions, including continuous calcium-containing infusions, such as parenteral nutrition via a Y-site. However, in patients other than neonates, ceftriaxone and calcium-containing solutions may be administered sequentially of one another if the infusion lines are thoroughly flushed between infusions with a compatible fluid. *In vitro* studies using adult and neonatal plasma from umbilical cord blood demonstrated that neonates have an increased risk of precipitation of ceftriaxone-calcium).

No products indexed under this heading.

Diluent, Calcium-Containing (Do not use diluents containing calcium to reconstitute ceftriaxone or to further dilute a reconstituted vial for IV administration because a precipitate can form. Precipitation of ceftriaxone-calcium can

also occur when ceftriaxone is mixed with calcium-containing solutions in the same IV administration line. Ceftriaxone must not be administered simultaneously with calcium-containing IV solutions, including continuous calcium-containing infusions, such as parenteral nutrition via a Y-site. However, in patients other than neonates, ceftriaxone and calcium-containing solutions may be administered sequentially of one another if the infusion lines are thoroughly flushed between infusions with a compatible fluid. *In vitro* studies using adult and neonatal plasma from umbilical cord blood demonstrated that neonates have an increased risk of precipitation of ceftriaxone-calcium).

No products indexed under this heading.

EXTRA STRENGTH ROLAIDS SOFTCHEWS VANILLA CREME

Drugs, Oral, unspecified (Antacids may interact with certain prescription drugs).

No products indexed under this heading.

ROMAZICON INJECTION

May interact with antidepressant drugs, neuromuscular blocking agents, and certain other agents. Compounds in these categories include:

Amitriptyline Hydrochloride (Toxic effects of cyclic antidepressant may emerge with the reversal of the benzodiazepine effect).

No products indexed under this heading.

Amoxapine (Toxic effects of cyclic antidepressants may emerge with the reversal of the benzodiazepine effect).

No products indexed under this heading.

Atracurium Besylate (Romazicon should not be used until the effects of neuromuscular blockade have been fully reversed).

No products indexed under this heading.

Bupropion Hydrochloride (Toxic effects of cyclic antidepressants may emerge with the reversal of the benzodiazepine effect). Products include:

Cisatracurium Besylate (Romazicon should not be used until the effects of neuromuscular blockade have been fully reversed). Products include:

Citalopram Hydrobromide (Toxic effects of cyclic antidepressants may emerge with the reversal of the benzodiazepine effect). Products include:

Decamethonium (Romazicon should not be used until the effects of neuromuscular blockade have been fully reversed).

No products indexed under this heading.

Desipramine Hydrochloride (Toxic effects of cyclic antidepressants may emerge with the reversal of the benzodiazepine effect).

No products indexed under this heading.

Doxacurium Chloride (Romazicon should not be used until the effects of neuromuscular blockade have been fully reversed).

No products indexed under this heading.

Doxepin Hydrochloride (Toxic effects of cyclic antidepressants may emerge with the reversal of the benzodiazepine effect).

No products indexed under this heading.

d-Tubocurarine (Romazicon should not be used until the effects of neuromuscular blockade have been fully reversed).

No products indexed under this heading.

Escitalopram Oxalate (Toxic effects of cyclic antidepressants may emerge with the reversal of the benzodiazepine effect). Products include:

Fluoxetine Hydrochloride (Toxic effects of cyclic antidepressants may emerge with the reversal of the benzodiazepine effect). Products include:

Fluvoxamine (Toxic effects of cyclic antidepressants may emerge with the reversal of the benzodiazepine effect).

No products indexed under this heading.

Fluvoxamine Maleate (Toxic effects of cyclic antidepressants may emerge with the reversal of the benzodiazepine effect).

No products indexed under this heading.

Gallamine (Romazicon should not be used until the effects of neuromuscular blockade have been fully reversed).

No products indexed under this heading.

Gallamine Triethiodide (Romazicon should not be used until the effects of neuromuscular blockade have been fully reversed).

No products indexed under this heading.

Imipramine Hydrochloride (Toxic effects of cyclic antidepressants may emerge with the reversal of the benzodiazepine effect).

No products indexed under this heading.

Imipramine Pamoate (Toxic effects of cyclic antidepressants may emerge with the reversal of the benzodiazepine effect).

No products indexed under this heading.

Isocarboxazid (Toxic effects of cyclic antidepressants may emerge with the reversal of the benzodiazepine effect). Products include:

Maprotiline Hydrochloride (Toxic effects of cyclic antidepressants may emerge with the reversal of the benzodiazepine effect).

No products indexed under this heading.

Metocurine Iodide (Romazicon should not be used until the effects of neuromuscular blockade have been fully reversed).

No products indexed under this heading.

Mirtazapine (Toxic effects of cyclic antidepressants may emerge with the reversal of the benzodiazepine effect). Products include:

Mivacurium Chloride (Romazicon should not be used until the effects of neuromuscular blockade have been fully reversed).

No products indexed under this heading.

Nefazodone Hydrochloride (Toxic effects of cyclic antidepressants may emerge with the reversal of the benzodiazepine effect).

No products indexed under this heading.

Nortriptyline Hydrochloride (Toxic effects of cyclic antidepressants may emerge with the reversal of the benzodiazepine effect).

No products indexed under this heading.

Pancuronium Bromide (Romazicon should not be used until the effects of neuromuscular blockade have been fully reversed).

No products indexed under this heading.

Paroxetine (Toxic effects of cyclic antidepressants may emerge with the reversal of the benzodiazepine effect).

No products indexed under this heading.

Paroxetine Hydrochloride (Toxic effects of cyclic antidepressants may emerge with the reversal of the benzodiazepine effect). Products include:

Paroxetine Mesylate (Toxic effects of cyclic antidepressants may emerge with the reversal of the benzodiazepine effect).

No products indexed under this heading.

Phenelzine Sulfate (Toxic effects of cyclic antidepressants may emerge with the reversal of the benzodiazepine effect).

No products indexed under this heading.

Protriptyline Hydrochloride (Toxic effects of cyclic antidepressants may emerge with the reversal of the benzodiazepine effect).

No products indexed under this heading.

Rapacuronium Bromide (Romazicon should not be used until the effects of neuromuscular blockade have been fully reversed).

No products indexed under this heading.

Rocuronium Bromide (Romazicon should not be used until the effects of neuromuscular blockade have been fully reversed). Products include:

Selegiline (Toxic effects of cyclic antidepressants may emerge with the reversal of the benzodiazepine effect). Products include:

Selegiline Hydrochloride (Toxic effects of cyclic antidepressants may emerge with the reversal of the benzodiazepine effect). Products include:

Sertraline Hydrochloride (Toxic effects of cyclic antidepressants may emerge with the reversal of the benzodiazepine effect).

No products indexed under this heading.

Succinylcholine Chloride (Romazicon should not be used until the effects of neuromuscular blockade have been fully reversed).

No products indexed under this heading.

Tranylcypromine Sulfate (Toxic effects of cyclic antidepressants may emerge with the reversal of the benzodiazepine effect). Products include:

Trazodone Hydrochloride (Toxic effects of cyclic antidepressants may emerge with the reversal of the benzodiazepine effect).

No products indexed under this heading.

Trimipramine Maleate (Toxic effects of cyclic antidepressants may emerge with the reversal of the benzodiazepine effect).

No products indexed under this heading.

Tubocurarine Chloride (Romazicon should not be used until the effects of neuromuscular blockade have been fully reversed).

No products indexed under this heading.

Vecuronium Bromide (Romazicon should not be used until the effects of neuromuscular blockade have been fully reversed).

No products indexed under this heading.

Venlafaxine Hydrochloride (Toxic effects of cyclic antidepressants may emerge with the reversal of the benzodiazepine effect). Products include:

(⊙ Described in PDR® for Ophthalmic Medicines)

Food Interactions

Food, unspecified (Ingestion of food during an IV infusion results in a 50% increase in clearance).

ROSAC WASH

(Sodium Sulfacetamide) 3326
None cited in PDR database.

ROTARIX ORAL SUSPENSION

(Rotavirus Vaccine, Live, Oral) 1644
May interact with alkylating agents, antimetabolites, corticosteroids, cytotoxic drugs, immunosuppressive agents, and certain other agents. Compounds in these categories include:

Alclometasone Dipropionate (Immunosuppressive therapies, including corticosteroids (used in greater than physiologic doses) may reduce the immune response to rotavirus vaccine).
　　No products indexed under this heading.

Azathioprine (Immunosuppressive therapies may reduce the immune response to rotavirus vaccine).
　　No products indexed under this heading.

Basiliximab (Immunosuppressive therapies may reduce the immune response to rotavirus vaccine). Products include:
　　Simulect 2524

Beclomethasone Dipropionate (Immunosuppressive therapies, including corticosteroids (used in greater than physiologic doses) may reduce the immune response to rotavirus vaccine). Products include:
　　Qvar 3398

Beclomethasone Dipropionate Monohydrate (Immunosuppressive therapies, including corticosteroids (used in greater than physiologic doses) may reduce the immune response to rotavirus vaccine). Products include:
　　Beconase AQ 1386

Betamethasone (Immunosuppressive therapies, including corticosteroids (used in greater than physiologic doses) may reduce the immune response to rotavirus vaccine).
　　No products indexed under this heading.

Betamethasone Acetate (Immunosuppressive therapies, including corticosteroids (used in greater than physiologic doses) may reduce the immune response to rotavirus vaccine).
　　No products indexed under this heading.

Betamethasone Benzoate (Immunosuppressive therapies, including corticosteroids (used in greater than physiologic doses) may reduce the immune response to rotavirus vaccine).
　　No products indexed under this heading.

Betamethasone Dipropionate (Immunosuppressive therapies, including corticosteroids (used in greater than physiologic doses) may reduce the immune response to rotavirus vaccine). Products include:
　　Diprolene Lotion 0.05% 3108
　　Diprolene Ointment 0.05% 3109
　　Diprolene AF Cream 0.05% 3107
　　Lotrisone 3163

Betamethasone Sodium Phosphate (Immunosuppressive therapies, including corticosteroids (used in greater than physiologic doses) may reduce the immune response to rotavirus vaccine).
　　No products indexed under this heading.

Betamethasone Valerate (Immunosuppressive therapies, including corticosteroids (used in greater than physiologic doses) may reduce the immune response to rotavirus vaccine). Products include:
　　Luxiq 3321

Bleomycin Sulfate (Immunosuppressive therapies, including cytotoxic drugs, may reduce the immune response to rotavirus vaccine).
　　No products indexed under this heading.

Budesonide (Immunosuppressive therapies, including corticosteroids (used in greater than physiologic doses) may reduce the immune response to rotavirus vaccine). Products include:
　　Pulmicort Flexhaler 714
　　Symbicort 80/4.5 720
　　Symbicort 160/4.5 720

Busulfan (Immunosuppressive therapies, including alkylating agents, may reduce the immune response to rotavirus vaccine). Products include:
　　Myleran 1581

Capecitabine (Immunosuppressive therapies, including antimetabolites, may reduce the immune response to rotavirus vaccine). Products include:
　　Xeloda 2882

Carmustine (BCNU) (Immunosuppressive therapies, including alkylating agents, may reduce the immune response to rotavirus vaccine).
　　No products indexed under this heading.

Chlorambucil (Immunosuppressive therapies, including alkylating agents, may reduce the immune response to rotavirus vaccine). Products include:
　　Leukeran 1557

Ciclesonide (Immunosuppressive therapies, including corticosteroids (used in greater than physiologic doses) may reduce the immune response to rotavirus vaccine).
　　No products indexed under this heading.

Cladribine (Immunosuppressive therapies, including antimetabolites, may reduce the immune response to rotavirus vaccine). Products include:
　　Leustatin 946

Cortisone Acetate (Immunosuppressive therapies, including corticosteroids (used in greater than physiologic doses) may reduce the immune response to rotavirus vaccine).
　　No products indexed under this heading.

Cyclophosphamide (Immunosuppressive therapies, including alkylating agents, may reduce the immune response to rotavirus vaccine).
　　No products indexed under this heading.

Cyclosporine (Immunosuppressive therapies may reduce the immune response to rotavirus vaccine). Products include:
　　Gengraf 440
　　Neoral Oral Solution 2496
　　Neoral Capsules 2496
　　Restasis 605

Cytarabine (Immunosuppressive therapies, including antimetabolites, may reduce the immune response to rotavirus vaccine).
　　No products indexed under this heading.

Dacarbazine (Immunosuppressive therapies, including alkylating agents, may reduce the immune response to rotavirus vaccine).
　　No products indexed under this heading.

Daunorubicin Hydrochloride (Immunosuppressive therapies, including cytotoxic drugs, may reduce the immune response to rotavirus vaccine).
　　No products indexed under this heading.

Desoximetasone (Immunosuppressive therapies, including corticosteroids (used in greater than physiologic doses) may reduce the immune response to rotavirus vaccine).
　　No products indexed under this heading.

Dexamethasone (Immunosuppressive therapies, including corticosteroids (used in greater than physiologic doses) may reduce the immune response to rotavirus vaccine). Products include:

Ciprodex 583
Ozurdex .... ⊙223
Tobramycin and Dexamethasone Ophthalmic Suspension .... ⊙251

Dexamethasone Acetate (Immunosuppressive therapies, including corticosteroids (used in greater than physiologic doses) may reduce the immune response to rotavirus vaccine).
　　No products indexed under this heading.

Dexamethasone Phosphate (Immunosuppressive therapies, including corticosteroids (used in greater than physiologic doses) may reduce the immune response to rotavirus vaccine).
　　No products indexed under this heading.

Dexamethasone Sodium (Immunosuppressive therapies, including corticosteroids (used in greater than physiologic doses) may reduce the immune response to rotavirus vaccine).
　　No products indexed under this heading.

Dexamethasone Sodium Phosphate (Immunosuppressive therapies, including corticosteroids (used in greater than physiologic doses) may reduce the immune response to rotavirus vaccine).
　　No products indexed under this heading.

Dexamethasone Sodium Phosphate Injection (Immunosuppressive therapies, including corticosteroids (used in greater than physiologic doses) may reduce the immune response to rotavirus vaccine).
　　No products indexed under this heading.

Diflorasone Diacetate (Immunosuppressive therapies, including corticosteroids (used in greater than physiologic doses) may reduce the immune response to rotavirus vaccine).
　　No products indexed under this heading.

Doxorubicin Hydrochloride (Immunosuppressive therapies, including cytotoxic drugs, may reduce the immune response to rotavirus vaccine).
　　No products indexed under this heading.

Epirubicin Hydrochloride (Immunosuppressive therapies, including cytotoxic drugs, may reduce the immune response to rotavirus vaccine).
　　No products indexed under this heading.

Floxuridine (Immunosuppressive therapies, including antimetabolites, may reduce the immune response to rotavirus vaccine).
　　No products indexed under this heading.

Fludarabine Phosphate (Immunosuppressive therapies, including antimetabolites, may reduce the immune response to rotavirus vaccine). Products include:
　　Oforta 3023

Fludrocortisone Acetate (Immunosuppressive therapies, including corticosteroids (used in greater than physiologic doses) may reduce the immune response to rotavirus vaccine).
　　No products indexed under this heading.

Flumethasone Pivalate (Immunosuppressive therapies, including corticosteroids (used in greater than physiologic doses) may reduce the immune response to rotavirus vaccine).
　　No products indexed under this heading.

Flunisolide Hemihydrate (Immunosuppressive therapies, including corticosteroids (used in greater than physiologic doses) may reduce the immune response to rotavirus vaccine).
　　No products indexed under this heading.

Fluorouracil (Immunosuppressive therapies, including antimetabolites, may reduce the immune response to rotavirus vaccine). Products include:
　　Carac 2966

Fluticasone Furoate (Immunosuppressive therapies, including corticosteroids (used in greater than physiologic

doses) may reduce the immune response to rotavirus vaccine). Products include:
　　Veramyst 1713

Fluticasone Propionate (Immunosuppressive therapies, including corticosteroids (used in greater than physiologic doses) may reduce the immune response to rotavirus vaccine). Products include:
　　Advair 100/50 1275
　　Advair 250/50 1275
　　Advair 500/50 1275
　　Advair HFA 45/21 1288
　　Advair HFA 115/21 1288
　　Advair HFA 230/21 1288
　　Flonase 1459
　　Flovent Diskus 1463
　　Flovent HFA 1470

Gemcitabine Hydrochloride (Immunosuppressive therapies, including antimetabolites, may reduce the immune response to rotavirus vaccine). Products include:
　　Gemzar 1900

Hydrocortisone (Immunosuppressive therapies, including corticosteroids (used in greater than physiologic doses) may reduce the immune response to rotavirus vaccine).
　　No products indexed under this heading.

Hydrocortisone (Alcohol) (Immunosuppressive therapies, including corticosteroids (used in greater than physiologic doses) may reduce the immune response to rotavirus vaccine).
　　No products indexed under this heading.

Hydrocortisone Acetate (Immunosuppressive therapies, including corticosteroids (used in greater than physiologic doses) may reduce the immune response to rotavirus vaccine).
　　No products indexed under this heading.

Hydrocortisone Butyrate (Immunosuppressive therapies, including corticosteroids (used in greater than physiologic doses) may reduce the immune response to rotavirus vaccine).
　　No products indexed under this heading.

Hydrocortisone Cypionate (Immunosuppressive therapies, including corticosteroids (used in greater than physiologic doses) may reduce the immune response to rotavirus vaccine).
　　No products indexed under this heading.

Hydrocortisone Hemisuccinate (Immunosuppressive therapies, including corticosteroids (used in greater than physiologic doses) may reduce the immune response to rotavirus vaccine).
　　No products indexed under this heading.

Hydrocortisone Probutate (Immunosuppressive therapies, including corticosteroids (used in greater than physiologic doses) may reduce the immune response to rotavirus vaccine).
　　No products indexed under this heading.

Hydrocortisone Sodium Phosphate (Immunosuppressive therapies, including corticosteroids (used in greater than physiologic doses) may reduce the immune response to rotavirus vaccine).
　　No products indexed under this heading.

Hydrocortisone Sodium Succinate (Immunosuppressive therapies, including corticosteroids (used in greater than physiologic doses) may reduce the immune response to rotavirus vaccine).
　　No products indexed under this heading.

Hydrocortisone Valerate (Immunosuppressive therapies, including corticosteroids (used in greater than physiologic doses) may reduce the immune response to rotavirus vaccine).
　　No products indexed under this heading.

Hydroxyurea (Immunosuppressive therapies, including cytotoxic drugs, may reduce the immune response to rotavirus vaccine).
　　No products indexed under this heading.

IMPORTANT NOTE: Always consult each drug listing in the patient's regimen for possible interactions.

(⊙ Described in PDR® for Ophthalmic Medicines)

1639 Interactions Index RotaTeq

Cyclosporine (Immunosuppressive therapies including irradiation, antimetabolites, alkylating agents, cytotoxic drugs and corticosteroids (used in greater than physiologic doses) may reduce the immune response to vaccines). Products include:
Gengraf 440
Neoral Oral Solution 2496
Neoral Capsules 2496
Restasis 605

Cytarabine (Immunosuppresive therapies including antimetabolites may reduce the immune response to vaccines).
No products indexed under this heading.

Dacarbazine (Immunosuppressive therapies including alkylating agents may reduce the immune response to vaccines).
No products indexed under this heading.

Daunorubicin Hydrochloride (Immunosuppressive therapies including cytotoxic drugs may reduce the immune response to vaccines).
No products indexed under this heading.

Desoximetasone (Immunosuppressive therapies including corticosteroids (used in greater than physiologic doses) may reduce the immune response to vaccines).
No products indexed under this heading.

Dexamethasone (Immunosuppressive therapies including corticosteroids (used in greater than physiologic doses) may reduce the immune response to vaccines). Products include:
Ciprodex 583
Ozurdex .... ⊙223
Tobramycin and Dexamethasone Ophthalmic Suspension .... ⊙251

Dexamethasone Acetate (Immunosuppressive therapies including corticosteroids (used in greater than physiologic doses) may reduce the immune response to vaccines).
No products indexed under this heading.

Dexamethasone Phosphate (Immunosuppressive therapies including corticosteroids (used in greater than physiologic doses) may reduce the immune response to vaccines).
No products indexed under this heading.

Dexamethasone Sodium (Immunosuppressive therapies including corticosteroids (used in greater than physiologic doses) may reduce the immune response to vaccines).
No products indexed under this heading.

Dexamethasone Sodium Phosphate (Immunosuppressive therapies including corticosteroids (used in greater than physiologic doses) may reduce the immune response to vaccines).
No products indexed under this heading.

Dexamethasone Sodium Phosphate Injection (Immunosuppressive therapies including corticosteroids (used in greater than physiologic doses) may reduce the immune response to vaccines).
No products indexed under this heading.

Diflorasone Diacetate (Immunosuppressive therapies including corticosteroids (used in greater than physiologic doses) may reduce the immune response to vaccines).
No products indexed under this heading.

Doxorubicin Hydrochloride (Immunosuppressive therapies including cytotoxic drugs may reduce the immune response to vaccines).
No products indexed under this heading.

Epirubicin Hydrochloride (Immunosuppressive therapies including cytotoxic drugs may reduce the immune response to vaccines).
No products indexed under this heading.

Floxuridine (Immunosuppresive therapies including antimetabolites may reduce the immune response to vaccines).
No products indexed under this heading.

Fludarabine Phosphate (Immunosuppresive therapies including antimetabolites may reduce the immune response to vaccines). Products include:
Oforta 3023

Fludrocortisone Acetate (Immunosuppressive therapies including corticosteroids (used in greater than physiologic doses) may reduce the immune response to vaccines).
No products indexed under this heading.

Flumethasone Pivalate (Immunosuppressive therapies including corticosteroids (used in greater than physiologic doses) may reduce the immune response to vaccines).
No products indexed under this heading.

Flunisolide Hemihydrate (Immunosuppressive therapies including corticosteroids (used in greater than physiologic doses) may reduce the immune response to vaccines).
No products indexed under this heading.

Fluorouracil (Immunosuppresive therapies including antimetabolites may reduce the immune response to vaccines). Products include:
Carac 2966

Fluticasone Furoate (Immunosuppressive therapies including corticosteroids (used in greater than physiologic doses) may reduce the immune response to vaccines). Products include:
Veramyst 1713

Fluticasone Propionate (Immunosuppressive therapies including corticosteroids (used in greater than physiologic doses) may reduce the immune response to vaccines). Products include:
Advair 100/50 1275
Advair 250/50 1275
Advair 500/50 1275
Advair HFA 45/21 1288
Advair HFA 115/21 1288
Advair HFA 230/21 1288
Flonase 1459
Flovent Diskus 1463
Flovent HFA 1470

Gemcitabine Hydrochloride (Immunosuppresive therapies including antimetabolites may reduce the immune response to vaccines). Products include:
Gemzar 1900

Hydrocortisone (Immunosuppressive therapies including corticosteroids (used in greater than physiologic doses) may reduce the immune response to vaccines).
No products indexed under this heading.

Hydrocortisone (Alcohol) (Immunosuppressive therapies including corticosteroids (used in greater than physiologic doses) may reduce the immune response to vaccines).
No products indexed under this heading.

Hydrocortisone Acetate (Immunosuppressive therapies including corticosteroids (used in greater than physiologic doses) may reduce the immune response to vaccines).
No products indexed under this heading.

Hydrocortisone Butyrate (Immunosuppressive therapies including corticosteroids (used in greater than physiologic doses) may reduce the immune response to vaccines).
No products indexed under this heading.

Hydrocortisone Cypionate (Immunosuppressive therapies including corticosteroids (used in greater than physiologic doses) may reduce the immune response to vaccines).
No products indexed under this heading.

Hydrocortisone Hemisuccinate (Immunosuppressive therapies including corticosteroids (used in greater than physiologic doses) may reduce the immune response to vaccines).
No products indexed under this heading.

Hydrocortisone Probutate (Immunosuppressive therapies including corticosteroids (used in greater than physiologic doses) may reduce the immune response to vaccines).
No products indexed under this heading.

Hydrocortisone Sodium Phosphate (Immunosuppressive therapies including corticosteroids (used in greater than physiologic doses) may reduce the immune response to vaccines).
No products indexed under this heading.

Hydrocortisone Sodium Succinate (Immunosuppressive therapies including corticosteroids (used in greater than physiologic doses) may reduce the immune response to vaccines).
No products indexed under this heading.

Hydrocortisone Valerate (Immunosuppressive therapies including corticosteroids (used in greater than physiologic doses) may reduce the immune response to vaccines).
No products indexed under this heading.

Hydroxyurea (Immunosuppressive therapies including cytotoxic drugs may reduce the immune response to vaccines).
No products indexed under this heading.

Lomustine (CCNU) (Immunosuppressive therapies including alkylating agents may reduce the immune response to vaccines).
No products indexed under this heading.

Mechlorethamine Hydrochloride (Immunosuppressive therapies including alkylating agents may reduce the immune response to vaccines). Products include:
Mustargen 2010

Melphalan (Immunosuppressive therapies including alkylating agents may reduce the immune response to vaccines). Products include:
Alkeran 1302

Mercaptopurine (Immunosuppresive therapies including antimetabolites may reduce the immune response to vaccines).
No products indexed under this heading.

Methotrexate (Immunosuppresive therapies including antimetabolites may reduce the immune response to vaccines).
No products indexed under this heading.

Methotrexate Sodium (Immunosuppresive therapies including antimetabolites may reduce the immune response to vaccines).
No products indexed under this heading.

Methylprednisolone (Immunosuppressive therapies including corticosteroids (used in greater than physiologic doses) may reduce the immune response to vaccines).
No products indexed under this heading.

Methylprednisolone Acetate (Immunosuppressive therapies including corticosteroids (used in greater than physiologic doses) may reduce the immune response to vaccines).
No products indexed under this heading.

Methylprednisolone Sodium Succinate (Immunosuppressive therapies including corticosteroids (used in greater than physiologic doses) may reduce the immune response to vaccines).
No products indexed under this heading.

Mitotane (Immunosuppressive therapies including cytotoxic drugs may reduce the immune response to vaccines).
No products indexed under this heading.

Mitoxantrone Hydrochloride (Immunosuppressive therapies including cytotoxic drugs may reduce the immune response to vaccines). Products include:
Novantrone 1088

Mometasone Furoate (Immunosuppressive therapies including corticosteroids (used in greater than physiologic doses) may reduce the immune response to vaccines). Products include:
Asmanex 3058
Elocon Cream 3111
Elocon Lotion 3112
Elocon Ointment 3114

Mometasone Furoate Monohydrate (Immunosuppressive therapies including corticosteroids (used in greater than physiologic doses) may reduce the immune response to vaccines). Products include:
Nasonex 3166

Muromonab-CD3 (Immunosuppressive therapies including irradiation, antimetabolites, alkylating agents, cytotoxic drugs and corticosteroids (used in greater than physiologic doses) may reduce the immune response to vaccines). Products include:
Orthoclone OKT3 949

Mycophenolate Mofetil (Immunosuppressive therapies including irradiation, antimetabolites, alkylating agents, cytotoxic drugs and corticosteroids (used in greater than physiologic doses) may reduce the immune response to vaccines).
No products indexed under this heading.

Pentostatin (Immunosuppresive therapies including antimetabolites may reduce the immune response to vaccines).
No products indexed under this heading.

Prednisolone (Immunosuppressive therapies including corticosteroids (used in greater than physiologic doses) may reduce the immune response to vaccines).
No products indexed under this heading.

Prednisolone Acetate (Immunosuppressive therapies including corticosteroids (used in greater than physiologic doses) may reduce the immune response to vaccines). Products include:
Blephamide .... ⊙212, ⊙214
Pred Forte .... ⊙225
Pred Mild .... ⊙230
Pred-G .... ⊙226, ⊙227

Prednisolone Sodium Phosphate (Immunosuppressive therapies including corticosteroids (used in greater than physiologic doses) may reduce the immune response to vaccines).
No products indexed under this heading.

Prednisolone Tebutate (Immunosuppressive therapies including corticosteroids (used in greater than physiologic doses) may reduce the immune response to vaccines).
No products indexed under this heading.

Prednisone (Immunosuppressive therapies including corticosteroids (used in greater than physiologic doses) may reduce the immune response to vaccines).
No products indexed under this heading.

Prednisone sodium phosphate (Immunosuppressive therapies including corticosteroids (used in greater than physiologic doses) may reduce the immune response to vaccines).
No products indexed under this heading.

IMPORTANT NOTE: Always consult each drug listing in the patient's regimen for possible interactions.

Procarbazine Hydrochloride (Immunosuppressive therapies including cytotoxic drugs may reduce the immune response to vaccines).
No products indexed under this heading.

Radiation (Immunosuppressive therapies including irradiation (used in greater than physiologic doses) may reduce the immune response to vaccines).
No products indexed under this heading.

Rapamycin (Immunosuppressive therapies including irradiation, antimetabolites, alkylating agents, cytotoxic drugs and corticosteroids (used in greater than physiologic doses) may reduce the immune response to vaccines).
No products indexed under this heading.

Sirolimus (Immunosuppressive therapies including irradiation, antimetabolites, alkylating agents, cytotoxic drugs and corticosteroids (used in greater than physiologic doses) may reduce the immune response to vaccines).
Products include:

Tacrolimus (Immunosuppressive therapies including irradiation, antimetabolites, alkylating agents, cytotoxic drugs and corticosteroids (used in greater than physiologic doses) may reduce the immune response to vaccines).
Products include:

Tamoxifen Citrate (Immunosuppressive therapies including cytotoxic drugs may reduce the immune response to vaccines).
No products indexed under this heading.

Thioguanine (Immunosuppressive therapies including antimetabolites may reduce the immune response to vaccines). Products include:

Thiotepa (Immunosuppressive therapies including alkylating agents may reduce the immune response to vaccines).
No products indexed under this heading.

Triamcinolone (Immunosuppressive therapies including corticosteroids (used in greater than physiologic doses) may reduce the immune response to vaccines).
No products indexed under this heading.

Triamcinolone Acetonide (Immunosuppressive therapies including corticosteroids (used in greater than physiologic doses) may reduce the immune response to vaccines). Products include:

Triamcinolone Diacetate (Immunosuppressive therapies including corticosteroids (used in greater than physiologic doses) may reduce the immune response to vaccines).
No products indexed under this heading.

Triamcinolone Hexacetonide (Immunosuppressive therapies including corticosteroids (used in greater than physiologic doses) may reduce the immune response to vaccines).
No products indexed under this heading.

Vinblastine Sulfate (Immunosuppressive therapies including cytotoxic drugs may reduce the immune response to vaccines).
No products indexed under this heading.

Vincristine Sulfate (Immunosuppressive therapies including cytotoxic drugs may reduce the immune response to vaccines).
No products indexed under this heading.

Vinorelbine Tartrate (Immunosuppressive therapies including cytotoxic drugs may reduce the immune response to vaccines).
No products indexed under this heading.

ROZEREM TABLETS
May interact with alcohols, central nervous system depressants, cytochrome p450 1a2 inhibitors (selected), cytochrome p450 2c9 inhibitors (selected), cytochrome p450 3a4 inhibitors, potent (selected), cytochrome p450 inducers (selected), and certain other agents. Compounds in these categories include:

Alatrofloxacin Mesylate (Ramelteon should be administered with caution to patients taking less strong CYP1A2 inhibitors).
No products indexed under this heading.

Alfentanil Hydrochloride (Complex behaviors, such as "sleep driving" (eg, driving while not fully awake after ingestion of hypnotic) and other complex behaviors (eg, preparing and eating food, making phone calls, or having sex), with amnesia for the event, have been reported in association with hypnotic use. The use of alcohol and other CNS depressants may increase the risk of such behaviors).
No products indexed under this heading.

Allium cepa (Efficacy may be reduced when ramelteon is used in combination with strong CYP enzyme inducers). Products include:

Allium sativum (Efficacy may be reduced when ramelteon is used in combination with strong CYP enzyme inducers).
No products indexed under this heading.

Allium schoenoprasum (Efficacy may be reduced when ramelteon is used in combination with strong CYP enzyme inducers).
No products indexed under this heading.

Allium ursinum (Efficacy may be reduced when ramelteon is used in combination with strong CYP enzyme inducers).
No products indexed under this heading.

Alprazolam (Complex behaviors, such as "sleep driving" (eg, driving while not fully awake after ingestion of hypnotic) and other complex behaviors (eg, preparing and eating food, making phone calls, or having sex), with amnesia for the event, have been reported in association with hypnotic use. The use of alcohol and other CNS depressants may increase the risk of such behaviors).
No products indexed under this heading.

Aminoglutethimide (Efficacy may be reduced when ramelteon is used in combination with strong CYP enzyme inducers).
No products indexed under this heading.

Amiodarone Hydrochloride (Ramelteon should be administered with caution to patients taking less strong CYP1A2 inhibitors).
No products indexed under this heading.

Amobarbital (Complex behaviors, such as "sleep driving" (eg, driving while not fully awake after ingestion of hypnotic) and other complex behaviors (eg, preparing and eating food, making phone calls, or having sex), with amnesia for the event, have been reported in association with hypnotic use. The use of alcohol and other CNS depressants may increase the risk of such behaviors).
No products indexed under this heading.

Amobarbital Sodium (Complex behaviors, such as "sleep driving" (eg,

driving while not fully awake after ingestion of hypnotic) and other complex behaviors (eg, preparing and eating food, making phone calls, or having sex), with amnesia for the event, have been reported in association with hypnotic use. The use of alcohol and other CNS depressants may increase the risk of such behaviors).
No products indexed under this heading.

Amprenavir (Ramelteon should be administered with caution in subjects taking strong CYP3A4 inhibitors).
No products indexed under this heading.

Anastrozole (Ramelteon should be administered to patients taking less strong CYP1A2 inhibitors).
No products indexed under this heading.

Aprepitant (Efficacy may be reduced when ramelteon is used in combination with strong CYP enzyme inducers). Products include:

Aprobarbital (Complex behaviors, such as "sleep driving" (eg, driving while not fully awake after ingestion of hypnotic) and other complex behaviors (eg, preparing and eating food, making phone calls, or having sex), with amnesia for the event, have been reported in association with hypnotic use. The use of alcohol and other CNS depressants may increase the risk of such behaviors).
No products indexed under this heading.

Atazanavir (Ramelteon should be administered with caution in subjects taking strong CYP3A4 inhibitors).
No products indexed under this heading.

Atazanavir Sulfate (Ramelteon should be administered with caution in subjects taking strong CYP3A4 inhibitors).
No products indexed under this heading.

Bendroflumethiazide (Ramelteon should be administered with caution in subjects taking strong CYP2C9 inhibitors).
No products indexed under this heading.

Betamethasone (Efficacy may be reduced when ramelteon is used in combination with strong CYP enzyme inducers).
No products indexed under this heading.

Betamethasone Acetate (Efficacy may be reduced when ramelteon is used in combination with strong CYP enzyme inducers).
No products indexed under this heading.

Betamethasone Benzoate (Efficacy may be reduced when ramelteon is used in combination with strong CYP enzyme inducers).
No products indexed under this heading.

Betamethasone Dipropionate (Efficacy may be reduced when ramelteon is used in combination with strong CYP enzyme inducers). Products include:

Betamethasone Sodium Phosphate (Efficacy may be reduced when ramelteon is used in combination with strong CYP enzyme inducers).
No products indexed under this heading.

Betamethasone Valerate (Efficacy may be reduced when ramelteon is used in combination with strong CYP enzyme inducers). Products include:

Bosentan (Efficacy may be reduced when ramelteon is used in combination with strong CYP enzyme inducers). Products include:

Buprenorphine Hydrochloride (Complex behaviors, such as "sleep

driving" (eg, driving while not fully awake after ingestion of hypnotic) and other complex behaviors (eg, preparing and eating food, making phone calls, or having sex), with amnesia for the event, have been reported in association with hypnotic use. The use of alcohol and other CNS depressants may increase the risk of such behaviors).
No products indexed under this heading.

Buspirone Hydrochloride (Complex behaviors, such as "sleep driving" (eg, driving while not fully awake after ingestion of hypnotic) and other complex behaviors (eg, preparing and eating food, making phone calls, or having sex), with amnesia for the event, have been reported in association with hypnotic use. The use of alcohol and other CNS depressants may increase the risk of such behaviors).
No products indexed under this heading.

Butabarbital (Complex behaviors, such as "sleep driving" (eg, driving while not fully awake after ingestion of hypnotic) and other complex behaviors (eg, preparing and eating food, making phone calls, or having sex), with amnesia for the event, have been reported in association with hypnotic use. The use of alcohol and other CNS depressants may increase the risk of such behaviors).
No products indexed under this heading.

Butabarbital Sodium (Complex behaviors, such as "sleep driving" (eg, driving while not fully awake after ingestion of hypnotic) and other complex behaviors (eg, preparing and eating food, making phone calls, or having sex), with amnesia for the event, have been reported in association with hypnotic use. The use of alcohol and other CNS depressants may increase the risk of such behaviors).
No products indexed under this heading.

Butalbital (Complex behaviors, such as "sleep driving" (eg, driving while not fully awake after ingestion of hypnotic) and other complex behaviors (eg, preparing and eating food, making phone calls, or having sex), with amnesia for the event, have been reported in association with hypnotic use. The use of alcohol and other CNS depressants may increase the risk of such behaviors).
No products indexed under this heading.

Carbamazepine (Efficacy may be reduced when ramelteon is used in combination with strong CYP enzyme inducers). Products include:

Chloramphenicol (Ramelteon should be administered with caution in subjects taking strong CYP2C9 inhibitors).
No products indexed under this heading.

Chloramphenicol Palmitate (Ramelteon should be administered with caution in subjects taking strong CYP2C9 inhibitors).
No products indexed under this heading.

Chloramphenicol Sodium Succinate (Ramelteon should be administered with caution in subjects taking strong CYP2C9 inhibitors).
No products indexed under this heading.

Chlordiazepoxide (Complex behaviors, such as "sleep driving" (eg, driving while not fully awake after ingestion of hypnotic) and other complex behaviors (eg, preparing and eating food, making phone calls, or having sex), with amnesia for the event, have been reported in association with hypnotic use. The use of alcohol and other CNS depressants may increase the risk of such behaviors).
No products indexed under this heading.

Chlordiazepoxide Hydrochloride (Complex behaviors, such as "sleep

1641 Interactions Index Rozerem

driving" (eg, driving while not fully awake after ingestion of hypnotic) and other complex behaviors (eg, preparing and eating food, making phone calls, or having sex), with amnesia for the event, have been reported in association with hypnotic use. The use of alcohol and other CNS depressants may increase the risk of such behaviors).
No products indexed under this heading.

Chlorothiazide (Ramelteon should be administered with caution in subjects taking strong CYP2C9 inhibitors).
No products indexed under this heading.

Chlorothiazide Sodium (Ramelteon should be administered with caution in subjects taking strong CYP2C9 inhibitors). Products include:
Diuril Intravenous 2009

Chlorpromazine (Complex behaviors, such as "sleep driving" (eg, driving while not fully awake after ingestion of hypnotic) and other complex behaviors (eg, preparing and eating food, making phone calls, or having sex), with amnesia for the event, have been reported in association with hypnotic use. The use of alcohol and other CNS depressants may increase the risk of such behaviors).
No products indexed under this heading.

Chlorpromazine Hydrochloride (Complex behaviors, such as "sleep driving" (eg, driving while not fully awake after ingestion of hypnotic) and other complex behaviors (eg, preparing and eating food, making phone calls, or having sex), with amnesia for the event, have been reported in association with hypnotic use. The use of alcohol and other CNS depressants may increase the risk of such behaviors).
No products indexed under this heading.

Chlorpropamide (Ramelteon should be administered with caution in subjects taking strong CYP2C9 inhibitors).
No products indexed under this heading.

Chlorprothixene (Complex behaviors, such as "sleep driving" (eg, driving while not fully awake after ingestion of hypnotic) and other complex behaviors (eg, preparing and eating food, making phone calls, or having sex), with amnesia for the event, have been reported in association with hypnotic use. The use of alcohol and other CNS depressants may increase the risk of such behaviors).
No products indexed under this heading.

Chlorprothixene Hydrochloride (Complex behaviors, such as "sleep driving" (eg, driving while not fully awake after ingestion of hypnotic) and other complex behaviors (eg, preparing and eating food, making phone calls, or having sex), with amnesia for the event, have been reported in association with hypnotic use. The use of alcohol and other CNS depressants may increase the risk of such behaviors).
No products indexed under this heading.

Chlorprothixene Lactate (Complex behaviors, such as "sleep driving" (eg, driving while not fully awake after ingestion of hypnotic) and other complex behaviors (eg, preparing and eating food, making phone calls, or having sex), with amnesia for the event, have been reported in association with hypnotic use. The use of alcohol and other CNS depressants may increase the risk of such behaviors).
No products indexed under this heading.

Cimetidine (Ramelteon should be administered with caution to patients taking less strong CYP1A2 inhibitors).
No products indexed under this heading.

Cimetidine Hydrochloride (Ramelteon should be administered with caution to patients taking less strong CYP1A2 inhibitors).
No products indexed under this heading.

Ciprofloxacin (Ramelteon should be administered with caution to patients taking less strong CYP1A2 inhibitors). Products include:
Cipro I.V. 3082
Cipro 3073
Cipro XR 3091
Ciprodex 583

Ciprofloxacin Hydrochloride (Ramelteon should be administered with caution to patients taking less strong CYP1A2 inhibitors). Products include:
Cipro 3073

Cisplatin (Efficacy may be reduced when ramelteon is used in combination with strong CYP enzyme inducers).
No products indexed under this heading.

Citalopram Hydrobromide (Efficacy may be reduced when ramelteon is used in combination with strong CYP enzyme inducers). Products include:
Celexa 1153

Clarithromycin (Ramelteon should be administered with caution in subjects taking strong CYP3A4 inhibitors). Products include:
Biaxin/Biaxin XL 412

Clonazepam (Complex behaviors, such as "sleep driving" (eg, driving while not fully awake after ingestion of hypnotic) and other complex behaviors (eg, preparing and eating food, making phone calls, or having sex), with amnesia for the event, have been reported in association with hypnotic use. The use of alcohol and other CNS depressants may increase the risk of such behaviors). Products include:
Klonopin 2855

Clopidogrel Bisulfate (Ramelteon should be administered with caution in subjects taking strong CYP2C9 inhibitors). Products include:
Plavix 3027

Clopidogrel Hydrogen Sulfate (Ramelteon should be administered with caution in subjects taking strong CYP2C9 inhibitors).
No products indexed under this heading.

Clorazepate Dipotassium (Complex behaviors, such as "sleep driving" (eg, driving while not fully awake after ingestion of hypnotic) and other complex behaviors (eg, preparing and eating food, making phone calls, or having sex), with amnesia for the event, have been reported in association with hypnotic use. The use of alcohol and other CNS depressants may increase the risk of such behaviors).
No products indexed under this heading.

Clotrimazole (Ramelteon should be administered with caution in subjects taking strong CYP2C9 inhibitors). Products include:
Lotrisone 3163

Clozapine (Complex behaviors, such as "sleep driving" (eg, driving while not fully awake after ingestion of hypnotic) and other complex behaviors (eg, preparing and eating food, making phone calls, or having sex), with amnesia for the event, have been reported in association with hypnotic use. The use of alcohol and other CNS depressants may increase the risk of such behaviors).
No products indexed under this heading.

Codeine Phosphate (Complex behaviors, such as "sleep driving" (eg, driving while not fully awake after ingestion of hypnotic) and other complex behaviors (eg, preparing and eating food, making phone calls, or having sex), with amnesia for the event, have been reported in association with hypnotic use. The use of alcohol and other CNS depressants may increase the risk of such behaviors). Products include:
Tylenol with Codeine 2691

Codeine Sulfate (Complex behaviors, such as "sleep driving" (eg, driving while not fully awake after ingestion of hypnotic) and other complex behaviors (eg, preparing and eating food, making phone calls, or having sex), with amnesia for the event, have been reported in association with hypnotic use. The use of alcohol and other CNS depressants may increase the risk of such behaviors).
No products indexed under this heading.

Cortisone Acetate (Efficacy may be reduced when ramelteon is used in combination with strong CYP enzyme inducers).
No products indexed under this heading.

Delavirdine Mesylate (Ramelteon should be administered with caution in subjects taking strong CYP3A4 inhibitors).
No products indexed under this heading.

Delavirine (Ramelteon should be administered with caution in subjects taking strong CYP3A4 inhibitors).
No products indexed under this heading.

Desflurane (Complex behaviors, such as "sleep driving" (eg, driving while not fully awake after ingestion of hypnotic) and other complex behaviors (eg, preparing and eating food, making phone calls, or having sex), with amnesia for the event, have been reported in association with hypnotic use. The use of alcohol and other CNS depressants may increase the risk of such behaviors).
No products indexed under this heading.

Desogestrel (Ramelteon should be administered with caution to patients taking less strong CYP1A2 inhibitors).
No products indexed under this heading.

Dexamethasone (Efficacy may be reduced when ramelteon is used in combination with strong CYP enzyme inducers). Products include:
Ciprodex 583
Ozurdex ..... ⊙ 223
Tobramycin and Dexamethasone Ophthalmic Suspension ..... ⊙ 251

Dexamethasone Acetate (Efficacy may be reduced when ramelteon is used in combination with strong CYP enzyme inducers).
No products indexed under this heading.

Dexamethasone Phosphate (Efficacy may be reduced when ramelteon is used in combination with strong CYP enzyme inducers).
No products indexed under this heading.

Dexamethasone Sodium (Efficacy may be reduced when ramelteon is used in combination with strong CYP enzyme inducers).
No products indexed under this heading.

Dexamethasone Sodium Phosphate (Efficacy may be reduced when ramelteon is used in combination with strong CYP enzyme inducers).
No products indexed under this heading.

Dexamethasone Sodium Phosphate Injection (Efficacy may be reduced when ramelteon is used in combination with strong CYP enzyme inducers).
No products indexed under this heading.

Dezocine (Complex behaviors, such as "sleep driving" (eg, driving while not fully awake after ingestion of hypnotic) and other complex behaviors (eg, preparing and eating food, making phone calls, or having sex), with amnesia for the event, have been reported in association with hypnotic use. The use of alcohol and other CNS depressants may increase the risk of such behaviors).
No products indexed under this heading.

Diazepam (Complex behaviors, such as "sleep driving" (eg, driving while not fully awake after ingestion of hypnotic) and other complex behaviors (eg, preparing and eating food, making phone calls, or having sex), with amnesia for the event, have been reported in association with hypnotic use. The use of alcohol and other CNS depressants may increase the risk of such behaviors). Products include:
Valium Tablets 2880

Diclofenac Epolamine (Ramelteon should be administered with caution in subjects taking strong CYP2C9 inhibitors). Products include:
Flector 1839

Diclofenac Potassium (Ramelteon should be administered with caution in subjects taking strong CYP2C9 inhibitors).
No products indexed under this heading.

Diclofenac Sodium (Ramelteon should be administered with caution in subjects taking strong CYP2C9 inhibitors).
No products indexed under this heading.

Diltiazem Hydrochloride (Efficacy may be reduced when ramelteon is used in combination with strong CYP enzyme inducers). Products include:
Cardizem LA 423

Diltiazem Maleate (Efficacy may be reduced when ramelteon is used in combination with strong CYP enzyme inducers).
No products indexed under this heading.

Disulfiram (Ramelteon should be administered with caution in subjects taking strong CYP2C9 inhibitors).
No products indexed under this heading.

Doxorubicin Hydrochloride (Efficacy may be reduced when ramelteon is used in combination with strong CYP enzyme inducers).
No products indexed under this heading.

Droperidol (Complex behaviors, such as "sleep driving" (eg, driving while not fully awake after ingestion of hypnotic) and other complex behaviors (eg, preparing and eating food, making phone calls, or having sex), with amnesia for the event, have been reported in association with hypnotic use. The use of alcohol and other CNS depressants may increase the risk of such behaviors).
No products indexed under this heading.

Efavirenz (Ramelteon should be administered with caution in subjects taking strong CYP2C9 inhibitors). Products include:
Atripla 906

Enflurane (Complex behaviors, such as "sleep driving" (eg, driving while not fully awake after ingestion of hypnotic) and other complex behaviors (eg, preparing and eating food, making phone calls, or having sex), with amnesia for the event, have been reported in association with hypnotic use. The use of alcohol and other CNS depressants may increase the risk of such behaviors).
No products indexed under this heading.

Enoxacin (Ramelteon should be administered with caution to patients taking less strong CYP1A2 inhibitors).
No products indexed under this heading.

Erythromycin (Efficacy may be reduced when ramelteon is used in combination with strong CYP enzyme inducers).
No products indexed under this heading.

Erythromycin, Topical (Efficacy may be reduced when ramelteon is used in combination with strong CYP enzyme inducers).
No products indexed under this heading.

Erythromycin Estolate (Efficacy may be reduced when ramelteon is used in combination with strong CYP enzyme inducers).
No products indexed under this heading.

Erythromycin Ethylsuccinate (Efficacy may be reduced when ramelteon is used in combination with strong CYP enzyme inducers). Products include:

IMPORTANT NOTE: Always consult each drug listing in the patient's regimen for possible interactions.

Erythromycin Gluceptate (Efficacy may be reduced when ramelteon is used in combination with strong CYP enzyme inducers).
No products indexed under this heading.

Erythromycin Lactobionate (Efficacy may be reduced when ramelteon is used in combination with strong CYP enzyme inducers).
No products indexed under this heading.

Erythromycin Stearate (Efficacy may be reduced when ramelteon is used in combination with strong CYP enzyme inducers).
No products indexed under this heading.

Escitalopram Oxalate (Efficacy may be reduced when ramelteon is used in combination with strong CYP enzyme inducers). Products include:

Esomeprazole Magnesium (Ramelteon should be administered with caution to patients taking less strong CYP1A2 inhibitors). Products include:

Esomeprazole Sodium (Ramelteon should be administered with caution to patients taking less strong CYP1A2 inhibitors). Products include:

Estazolam (Complex behaviors, such as "sleep driving" (eg, driving while not fully awake after ingestion of hypnotic) and other complex behaviors (eg, preparing and eating food, making phone calls, or having sex), with amnesia for the event, have been reported in association with hypnotic use. The use of alcohol and other CNS depressants may increase the risk of such behaviors).
No products indexed under this heading.

Ethanol (Efficacy may be reduced when ramelteon is used in combination with strong CYP enzyme inducers).
No products indexed under this heading.

Ethchlorvynol (Complex behaviors, such as "sleep driving" (eg, driving while not fully awake after ingestion of hypnotic) and other complex behaviors (eg, preparing and eating food, making phone calls, or having sex), with amnesia for the event, have been reported in association with hypnotic use. The use of alcohol and other CNS depressants may increase the risk of such behaviors).
No products indexed under this heading.

Ethinamate (Complex behaviors, such as "sleep driving" (eg, driving while not fully awake after ingestion of hypnotic) and other complex behaviors (eg, preparing and eating food, making phone calls, or having sex), with amnesia for the event, have been reported in association with hypnotic use. The use of alcohol and other CNS depressants may increase the risk of such behaviors).
No products indexed under this heading.

Ethinyl Estradiol (Ramelteon should be administered with caution to patients taking less strong CYP1A2 inhibitors). Products include:

Ethosuximide (Efficacy may be reduced when ramelteon is used in combination with strong CYP enzyme inducers).
No products indexed under this heading.

Ethyl Alcohol (Complex behaviors, such as "sleep driving" (eg, driving while

not fully awake after ingestion of hypnotic) and other complex behaviors (eg, preparing and eating food, making phone calls, or having sex), with amnesia for the event, have been reported in association with hypnotic use. The use of alcohol and other CNS depressants may increase the risk of such behaviors).
No products indexed under this heading.

Fat (When administered with a high-fat meal, the AUC_{0-inf} for a single 16 mg dose of ramelteon was 31% higher and the C_{max} was 22% lower than when given in a fasted state. Median T_{max} was delayed by approximately 45 minutes when ramelteon was administered with food. Effects of food on the AUC values for M-II were similar. It is, therefore, recommended that ramelteon not be taken with or immediately after a high-fat meal).
No products indexed under this heading.

Felbamate (Efficacy may be reduced when ramelteon is used in combination with strong CYP enzyme inducers).
No products indexed under this heading.

Fenofibrate (Ramelteon should be administered with caution in subjects taking strong CYP2C9 inhibitors). Products include:

Fentanyl (Complex behaviors, such as "sleep driving" (eg, driving while not fully awake after ingestion of hypnotic) and other complex behaviors (eg, preparing and eating food, making phone calls, or having sex), with amnesia for the event, have been reported in association with hypnotic use. The use of alcohol and other CNS depressants may increase the risk of such behaviors). Products include:

Fentanyl Citrate (Complex behaviors, such as "sleep driving" (eg, driving while not fully awake after ingestion of hypnotic) and other complex behaviors (eg, preparing and eating food, making phone calls, or having sex), with amnesia for the event, have been reported in association with hypnotic use. The use of alcohol and other CNS depressants may increase the risk of such behaviors). Products include:

Fluconazole (The total and peak systemic exposure (AUC_{0-inf} and C_{max}) of ramelteon after a single 16 mg dose of ramelteon was increased by approximately 150% when administered with fluconazole. Similar increases were also seen in M-II exposure. Ramelteon should be administered with caution in subjects taking strong CYP2C9 inhibitors, such as fluconazole).
No products indexed under this heading.

Fludrocortisone Acetate (Efficacy may be reduced when ramelteon is used in combination with strong CYP enzyme inducers).
No products indexed under this heading.

Fluorouracil (Ramelteon should be administered with caution in subjects taking strong CYP2C9 inhibitors). Products include:

Fluoxetine Hydrochloride (Ramelteon should be administered with caution in subjects taking strong CYP2C9 inhibitors). Products include:

Fluphenazine Decanoate (Complex behaviors, such as "sleep driving" (eg, driving while not fully awake after inges-

tion of hypnotic) and other complex behaviors (eg, preparing and eating food, making phone calls, or having sex), with amnesia for the event, have been reported in association with hypnotic use. The use of alcohol and other CNS depressants may increase the risk of such behaviors).
No products indexed under this heading.

Fluphenazine Enanthate (Complex behaviors, such as "sleep driving" (eg, driving while not fully awake after ingestion of hypnotic) and other complex behaviors (eg, preparing and eating food, making phone calls, or having sex), with amnesia for the event, have been reported in association with hypnotic use. The use of alcohol and other CNS depressants may increase the risk of such behaviors).
No products indexed under this heading.

Fluphenazine Hydrochloride (Complex behaviors, such as "sleep driving" (eg, driving while not fully awake after ingestion of hypnotic) and other complex behaviors (eg, preparing and eating food, making phone calls, or having sex), with amnesia for the event, have been reported in association with hypnotic use. The use of alcohol and other CNS depressants may increase the risk of such behaviors).
No products indexed under this heading.

Flurazepam Hydrochloride (Complex behaviors, such as "sleep driving" (eg, driving while not fully awake after ingestion of hypnotic) and other complex behaviors (eg, preparing and eating food, making phone calls, or having sex), with amnesia for the event, have been reported in association with hypnotic use. The use of alcohol and other CNS depressants may increase the risk of such behaviors).
No products indexed under this heading.

Flurbiprofen (Ramelteon should be administered with caution in subjects taking strong CYP2C9 inhibitors).
No products indexed under this heading.

Flurbiprofen Sodium (Ramelteon should be administered with caution in subjects taking strong CYP2C9 inhibitors).
No products indexed under this heading.

Fluvastatin Sodium (Ramelteon should be administered with caution in subjects taking strong CYP2C9 inhibitors).
No products indexed under this heading.

Fluvoxamine (Co-administration of ramelteon and fluvoxamine is contraindicated. When fluvoxamine 100 mg twice daily was administered for 3 days prior to single-dose co-administration of ramelteon 16 mg and fluvoxamine, the AUC_{0-inf} for ramelteon increased approximately 190-fold, and the C_{max} increased approximately 70-fold, compared to ramelteon administered alone. Ramelteon should not be used in combination with fluvoxamine. Other less potent CYP1A2 inhibitors have not been adequately studied. Ramelteon should be administered with caution to patients taking less strong CYP1A2 inhibitors).
No products indexed under this heading.

Fluvoxamine Maleate (Ramelteon should be administered with caution to patients taking less strong CYP1A2 inhibitors).
No products indexed under this heading.

Fosamprenavir Calcium (Ramelteon should be administered with caution in subjects taking strong CYP3A4 inhibitors). Products include:

Fosphenytoin (Efficacy may be reduced when ramelteon is used in combination with strong CYP enzyme inducers).
No products indexed under this heading.

Fosphenytoin Sodium (Efficacy may be reduced when ramelteon is used in combination with strong CYP enzyme inducers).
No products indexed under this heading.

Garlic Extract (Efficacy may be reduced when ramelteon is used in combination with strong CYP enzyme inducers).
No products indexed under this heading.

Garlic Oil (Efficacy may be reduced when ramelteon is used in combination with strong CYP enzyme inducers).
No products indexed under this heading.

Gatifloxacin (Ramelteon should be administered with caution to patients taking less strong CYP1A2 inhibitors).
No products indexed under this heading.

Gemfibrozil (Ramelteon should be administered with caution in subjects taking strong CYP2C9 inhibitors).
No products indexed under this heading.

Gemifloxacin Mesylate (Ramelteon should be administered with caution to patients taking less strong CYP1A2 inhibitors).
No products indexed under this heading.

Glipizide (Ramelteon should be administered with caution in subjects taking strong CYP2C9 inhibitors).
No products indexed under this heading.

Glutethimide (Complex behaviors, such as "sleep driving" (eg, driving while not fully awake after ingestion of hypnotic) and other complex behaviors (eg, preparing and eating food, making phone calls, or having sex), with amnesia for the event, have been reported in association with hypnotic use. The use of alcohol and other CNS depressants may increase the risk of such behaviors).
No products indexed under this heading.

Glyburide (Ramelteon should be administered with caution in subjects taking strong CYP2C9 inhibitors).
No products indexed under this heading.

Grepafloxacin Hydrochloride (Ramelteon should be administered with caution to patients taking less strong CYP1A2 inhibitors).
No products indexed under this heading.

Halazepam (Complex behaviors, such as "sleep driving" (eg, driving while not fully awake after ingestion of hypnotic) and other complex behaviors (eg, preparing and eating food, making phone calls, or having sex), with amnesia for the event, have been reported in association with hypnotic use. The use of alcohol and other CNS depressants may increase the risk of such behaviors).
No products indexed under this heading.

Haloperidol (Complex behaviors, such as "sleep driving" (eg, driving while not fully awake after ingestion of hypnotic) and other complex behaviors (eg, preparing and eating food, making phone calls, or having sex), with amnesia for the event, have been reported in association with hypnotic use. The use of alcohol and other CNS depressants may increase the risk of such behaviors).
No products indexed under this heading.

Haloperidol Decanoate (Complex behaviors, such as "sleep driving" (eg, driving while not fully awake after ingestion of hypnotic) and other complex behaviors (eg, preparing and eating food, making phone calls, or having sex), with amnesia for the event, have been reported in association with hypnotic use. The use of alcohol and other CNS depressants may increase the risk of such behaviors).
No products indexed under this heading.

IMPORTANT NOTE: Always consult each drug listing in the patient's regimen for possible interactions.

Levofloxacin (Ramelteon should be administered with caution to patients taking less strong CYP1A2 inhibitors).
Products include:
Iquix 3492
Levaquin 2629
Levaquin in 5% Dextrose 2629
Quixin 3493

Levomethadyl Acetate Hydrochloride (Complex behaviors, such as "sleep driving" (eg, driving while not fully awake after ingestion of hypnotic) and other complex behaviors (eg, preparing and eating food, making phone calls, or having sex), with amnesia for the event, have been reported in association with hypnotic use. The use of alcohol and other CNS depressants may increase the risk of such behaviors).
No products indexed under this heading.

Levonorgestrel (Ramelteon should be administered with caution to patients taking less strong CYP1A2 inhibitors).
Products include:
Climara Pro 847
LoSeasonique 3407
Lybrel 3514
Mirena 854
Plan B 3416
Seasonique 3418

Levorphanol Tartrate (Complex behaviors, such as "sleep driving" (eg, driving while not fully awake after ingestion of hypnotic) and other complex behaviors (eg, preparing and eating food, making phone calls, or having sex), with amnesia for the event, have been reported in association with hypnotic use. The use of alcohol and other CNS depressants may increase the risk of such behaviors).
No products indexed under this heading.

Lomefloxacin Hydrochloride (Ramelteon should be administered with caution to patients taking less strong CYP1A2 inhibitors).
No products indexed under this heading.

Lopinavir (Ramelteon should be administered with caution in subjects taking strong CYP3A4 inhibitors).
Products include:
Kaletra 458

Lorazepam (Complex behaviors, such as "sleep driving" (eg, driving while not fully awake after ingestion of hypnotic) and other complex behaviors (eg, preparing and eating food, making phone calls, or having sex), with amnesia for the event, have been reported in association with hypnotic use. The use of alcohol and other CNS depressants may increase the risk of such behaviors).
No products indexed under this heading.

Lovastatin (Ramelteon should be administered with caution in subjects taking strong CYP2C9 inhibitors).
Products include:
Advicor 402
Mevacor 2212

Loxapine Hydrochloride (Complex behaviors, such as "sleep driving" (eg, driving while not fully awake after ingestion of hypnotic) and other complex behaviors (eg, preparing and eating food, making phone calls, or having sex), with amnesia for the event, have been reported in association with hypnotic use. The use of alcohol and other CNS depressants may increase the risk of such behaviors).
No products indexed under this heading.

Loxapine Succinate (Complex behaviors, such as "sleep driving" (eg, driving while not fully awake after ingestion of hypnotic) and other complex behaviors (eg, preparing and eating food, making phone calls, or having sex), with amnesia for the event, have been reported in association with hypnotic use. The use of alcohol and other CNS depressants may increase the risk of such behaviors).
No products indexed under this heading.

Meperidine Hydrochloride (Complex behaviors, such as "sleep driving" (eg, driving while not fully awake after ingestion of hypnotic) and other complex behaviors (eg, preparing and eating food, making phone calls, or having sex), with amnesia for the event, have been reported in association with hypnotic use. The use of alcohol and other CNS depressants may increase the risk of such behaviors).
No products indexed under this heading.

Mephenytoin (Efficacy may be reduced when ramelteon is used in combination with strong CYP enzyme inducers).
No products indexed under this heading.

Mephobarbital (Complex behaviors, such as "sleep driving" (eg, driving while not fully awake after ingestion of hypnotic) and other complex behaviors (eg, preparing and eating food, making phone calls, or having sex), with amnesia for the event, have been reported in association with hypnotic use. The use of alcohol and other CNS depressants may increase the risk of such behaviors).
No products indexed under this heading.

Meprobamate (Complex behaviors, such as "sleep driving" (eg, driving while not fully awake after ingestion of hypnotic) and other complex behaviors (eg, preparing and eating food, making phone calls, or having sex), with amnesia for the event, have been reported in association with hypnotic use. The use of alcohol and other CNS depressants may increase the risk of such behaviors).
No products indexed under this heading.

Mesoridazine Besylate (Complex behaviors, such as "sleep driving" (eg, driving while not fully awake after ingestion of hypnotic) and other complex behaviors (eg, preparing and eating food, making phone calls, or having sex), with amnesia for the event, have been reported in association with hypnotic use. The use of alcohol and other CNS depressants may increase the risk of such behaviors).
No products indexed under this heading.

Mestranol (Ramelteon should be administered with caution to patients taking less strong CYP1A2 inhibitors).
No products indexed under this heading.

Methadone Hydrochloride (Complex behaviors, such as "sleep driving" (eg, driving while not fully awake after ingestion of hypnotic) and other complex behaviors (eg, preparing and eating food, making phone calls, or having sex), with amnesia for the event, have been reported in association with hypnotic use. The use of alcohol and other CNS depressants may increase the risk of such behaviors).
No products indexed under this heading.

Methohexital Sodium (Complex behaviors, such as "sleep driving" (eg, driving while not fully awake after ingestion of hypnotic) and other complex behaviors (eg, preparing and eating food, making phone calls, or having sex), with amnesia for the event, have been reported in association with hypnotic use. The use of alcohol and other CNS depressants may increase the risk of such behaviors).
No products indexed under this heading.

Methotrimeprazine (Complex behaviors, such as "sleep driving" (eg, driving while not fully awake after ingestion of hypnotic) and other complex behaviors (eg, preparing and eating food, making phone calls, or having sex), with amnesia for the event, have been reported in association with hypnotic use. The use of alcohol and other CNS depressants may increase the risk of such behaviors).
No products indexed under this heading.

Methoxsalen (Ramelteon should be administered with caution to patients taking less strong CYP1A2 inhibitors).
No products indexed under this heading.

Methoxyflurane (Complex behaviors, such as "sleep driving" (eg, driving while not fully awake after ingestion of hypnotic) and other complex behaviors (eg, preparing and eating food, making phone calls, or having sex), with amnesia for the event, have been reported in association with hypnotic use. The use of alcohol and other CNS depressants may increase the risk of such behaviors).
No products indexed under this heading.

Methsuximide (Efficacy may be reduced when ramelteon is used in combination with strong CYP enzyme inducers).
No products indexed under this heading.

Methyclothiazide (Ramelteon should be administered with caution in subjects taking strong CYP2C9 inhibitors).
No products indexed under this heading.

Methylprednisolone (Efficacy may be reduced when ramelteon is used in combination with strong CYP enzyme inducers).
No products indexed under this heading.

Methylprednisolone Acetate (Efficacy may be reduced when ramelteon is used in combination with strong CYP enzyme inducers).
No products indexed under this heading.

Methylprednisolone Sodium Succinate (Efficacy may be reduced when ramelteon is used in combination with strong CYP enzyme inducers).
No products indexed under this heading.

Metronidazole (Ramelteon should be administered with caution in subjects taking strong CYP2C9 inhibitors).
Products include:
Pylera 793

Metronidazole Benzoate (Ramelteon should be administered with caution in subjects taking strong CYP2C9 inhibitors).
No products indexed under this heading.

Metronidazole Hydrochloride (Ramelteon should be administered with caution in subjects taking strong CYP2C9 inhibitors).
No products indexed under this heading.

Metronidazole Sodium (Ramelteon should be administered with caution in subjects taking strong CYP2C9 inhibitors).
No products indexed under this heading.

Mexiletine Hydrochloride (Ramelteon should be administered with caution to patients taking less strong CYP1A2 inhibitors).
No products indexed under this heading.

Mibefradil Dihydrochloride (Ramelteon should be administered with caution to patients taking less strong CYP1A2 inhibitors).
No products indexed under this heading.

Miconazole (Ramelteon should be administered with caution in subjects taking strong CYP2C9 inhibitors).
No products indexed under this heading.

Miconazole Nitrate (Ramelteon should be administered with caution in subjects taking strong CYP2C9 inhibitors). Products include:
Vusion Ointment 3335

Midazolam Hydrochloride (Complex behaviors, such as "sleep driving" (eg, driving while not fully awake after ingestion of hypnotic) and other complex behaviors (eg, preparing and eating food, making phone calls, or having sex), with amnesia for the event, have been reported in association with hypnotic use. The use of alcohol and other CNS depressants may increase the risk of such behaviors).
No products indexed under this heading.

Modafinil (Ramelteon should be administered with caution in subjects taking strong CYP2C9 inhibitors).
Products include:
Provigil 983

Molindone Hydrochloride (Complex behaviors, such as "sleep driving" (eg, driving while not fully awake after ingestion of hypnotic) and other complex behaviors (eg, preparing and eating food, making phone calls, or having sex), with amnesia for the event, have been reported in association with hypnotic use. The use of alcohol and other CNS depressants may increase the risk of such behaviors). Products include:
Moban 1108

Morphine Sulfate (Complex behaviors, such as "sleep driving" (eg, driving while not fully awake after ingestion of hypnotic) and other complex behaviors (eg, preparing and eating food, making phone calls, or having sex), with amnesia for the event, have been reported in association with hypnotic use. The use of alcohol and other CNS depressants may increase the risk of such behaviors). Products include:
Avinza 1822
Embeda 1831
MS Contin 2803

Morphine Sulfate, Liposomal (Complex behaviors, such as "sleep driving" (eg, driving while not fully awake after ingestion of hypnotic) and other complex behaviors (eg, preparing and eating food, making phone calls, or having sex), with amnesia for the event, have been reported in association with hypnotic use. The use of alcohol and other CNS depressants may increase the risk of such behaviors).
No products indexed under this heading.

Moxifloxacin Hydrochloride (Ramelteon should be administered with caution to patients taking less strong CYP1A2 inhibitors). Products include:
Avelox 3064
Vigamox 589

Nafcillin Sodium (Efficacy may be reduced when ramelteon is used in combination with strong CYP enzyme inducers).
No products indexed under this heading.

Nalidixic Acid (Ramelteon should be administered with caution to patients taking less strong CYP1A2 inhibitors).
No products indexed under this heading.

Nefazodone Hydrochloride (Ramelteon should be administered with caution in subjects taking strong CYP3A4 inhibitors).
No products indexed under this heading.

Nelfinavir Mesylate (Ramelteon should be administered with caution in subjects taking strong CYP3A4 inhibitors).
No products indexed under this heading.

Nevirapine (Efficacy may be reduced when ramelteon is used in combination with strong CYP enzyme inducers).
Products include:
Viramune Oral Suspension 897
Viramune Tablets 897

Nicotine (Efficacy may be reduced when ramelteon is used in combination with strong CYP enzyme inducers).
No products indexed under this heading.

Nicotine Polacrilex (Efficacy may be reduced when ramelteon is used in combination with strong CYP enzyme inducers).
No products indexed under this heading.

IMPORTANT NOTE: Always consult each drug listing in the patient's regimen for possible interactions.

sex), with amnesia for the event, have been reported in association with hypnotic use. The use of alcohol and other CNS depressants may increase the risk of such behaviors). Products include:

Seroquel 750
Seroquel XR 759

Ranitidine Bismuth Citrate (Ramelteon should be administered with caution to patients taking less strong CYP1A2 inhibitors).
No products indexed under this heading.

Ranitidine Hydrochloride (Ramelteon should be administered with caution to patients taking less strong CYP1A2 inhibitors). Products include:

Zantac 1737
Zantac Injection 1732
Zantac Pharmacy 1735

Remifentanil Hydrochloride (Complex behaviors, such as "sleep driving" (eg, driving while not fully awake after ingestion of hypnotic) and other complex behaviors (eg, preparing and eating food, making phone calls, or having sex), with amnesia for the event, have been reported in association with hypnotic use. The use of alcohol and other CNS depressants may increase the risk of such behaviors).
No products indexed under this heading.

Rifabutin (Efficacy may be reduced when ramelteon is used in combination with strong CYP enzyme inducers).
No products indexed under this heading.

Rifampicin (Efficacy may be reduced when ramelteon is used in combination with strong CYP enzyme inducers).
No products indexed under this heading.

Rifampin (Administration of rifampin 600 mg once daily for 11 days resulted in a mean decrease of approximately 80% (40% to 90%) in total exposure to ramelteon and metabolite M-II, (both $AUC_{0\text{-}inf}$ and C_{max}), after a single 32 mg dose of ramelteon. Efficacy may be reduced when ramelteon is used in combination with strong CYP enzyme inducers, such as rifampin).
No products indexed under this heading.

Rifapentine (Efficacy may be reduced when ramelteon is used in combination with strong CYP enzyme inducers).
No products indexed under this heading.

Risperidone (Complex behaviors, such as "sleep driving" (eg, driving while not fully awake after ingestion of hypnotic) and other complex behaviors (eg, preparing and eating food, making phone calls, or having sex), with amnesia for the event, have been reported in association with hypnotic use. The use of alcohol and other CNS depressants may increase the risk of such behaviors). Products include:

Risperdal Consta 2682

Ritonavir (Ramelteon should be administered with caution in subjects taking strong CYP3A4 inhibitors). Products include:

Kaletra 458
Norvir 509

Saquinavir (Ramelteon should be administered with caution in subjects taking strong CYP3A4 inhibitors).
No products indexed under this heading.

Saquinavir Mesylate (Ramelteon should be administered with caution in subjects taking strong CYP3A4 inhibitors).
No products indexed under this heading.

Secobarbital Sodium (Efficacy may be reduced when ramelteon is used in combination with strong CYP enzyme inducers).
No products indexed under this heading.

Sertraline Hydrochloride (Ramelteon should be administered with caution in subjects taking strong CYP2C9 inhibitors).
No products indexed under this heading.

Sevoflurane (Complex behaviors, such as "sleep driving" (eg, driving while not fully awake after ingestion of hypnotic) and other complex behaviors (eg, preparing and eating food, making phone calls, or having sex), with amnesia for the event, have been reported in association with hypnotic use. The use of alcohol and other CNS depressants may increase the risk of such behaviors). Products include:

Ultane 554

Sildenafil Citrate (Ramelteon should be administered with caution to patients taking less strong CYP1A2 inhibitors).
No products indexed under this heading.

Sodium Butabarbital (Complex behaviors, such as "sleep driving" (eg, driving while not fully awake after ingestion of hypnotic) and other complex behaviors (eg, preparing and eating food, making phone calls, or having sex), with amnesia for the event, have been reported in association with hypnotic use. The use of alcohol and other CNS depressants may increase the risk of such behaviors).
No products indexed under this heading.

Sodium Oxybate (Complex behaviors, such as "sleep driving" (eg, driving while not fully awake after ingestion of hypnotic) and other complex behaviors (eg, preparing and eating food, making phone calls, or having sex), with amnesia for the event, have been reported in association with hypnotic use. The use of alcohol and other CNS depressants may increase the risk of such behaviors).
No products indexed under this heading.

Sodium Pentobarbital (Complex behaviors, such as "sleep driving" (eg, driving while not fully awake after ingestion of hypnotic) and other complex behaviors (eg, preparing and eating food, making phone calls, or having sex), with amnesia for the event, have been reported in association with hypnotic use. The use of alcohol and other CNS depressants may increase the risk of such behaviors).
No products indexed under this heading.

Sparfloxacin (Ramelteon should be administered with caution to patients taking less strong CYP1A2 inhibitors).
No products indexed under this heading.

Sufentanil Citrate (Complex behaviors, such as "sleep driving" (eg, driving while not fully awake after ingestion of hypnotic) and other complex behaviors (eg, preparing and eating food, making phone calls, or having sex), with amnesia for the event, have been reported in association with hypnotic use. The use of alcohol and other CNS depressants may increase the risk of such behaviors).
No products indexed under this heading.

Sulfacytine (Ramelteon should be administered with caution in subjects taking strong CYP2C9 inhibitors).
No products indexed under this heading.

Sulfamethizole (Ramelteon should be administered with caution in subjects taking strong CYP2C9 inhibitors).
No products indexed under this heading.

Sulfamethoxazole (Ramelteon should be administered with caution in subjects taking strong CYP2C9 inhibitors).
No products indexed under this heading.

Sulfasalazine (Ramelteon should be administered with caution in subjects taking strong CYP2C9 inhibitors).
No products indexed under this heading.

Sulfinpyrazone (Ramelteon should be administered with caution in subjects taking strong CYP2C9 inhibitors).
No products indexed under this heading.

Sulfisoxazole Acetyl (Ramelteon should be administered with caution in subjects taking strong CYP2C9 inhibitors).
No products indexed under this heading.

Sulfisoxazole Diolamine (Ramelteon should be administered with caution in subjects taking strong CYP2C9 inhibitors).
No products indexed under this heading.

Tacrine Hydrochloride (Ramelteon should be administered with caution to patients taking less strong CYP1A2 inhibitors).
No products indexed under this heading.

Talbutal (Complex behaviors, such as "sleep driving" (eg, driving while not fully awake after ingestion of hypnotic) and other complex behaviors (eg, preparing and eating food, making phone calls, or having sex), with amnesia for the event, have been reported in association with hypnotic use. The use of alcohol and other CNS depressants may increase the risk of such behaviors).
No products indexed under this heading.

Telithromycin (Ramelteon should be administered with caution in subjects taking strong CYP3A4 inhibitors). Products include:

Ketek 2991

Temazepam (Complex behaviors, such as "sleep driving" (eg, driving while not fully awake after ingestion of hypnotic) and other complex behaviors (eg, preparing and eating food, making phone calls, or having sex), with amnesia for the event, have been reported in association with hypnotic use. The use of alcohol and other CNS depressants may increase the risk of such behaviors).
No products indexed under this heading.

Terconazole (Ramelteon should be administered with caution in subjects taking strong CYP2C9 inhibitors).
No products indexed under this heading.

Theophyllinate (Efficacy may be reduced when ramelteon is used in combination with strong CYP enzyme inducers).
No products indexed under this heading.

Theophylline (Efficacy may be reduced when ramelteon is used in combination with strong CYP enzyme inducers).
No products indexed under this heading.

Theophylline Anhydrous (Efficacy may be reduced when ramelteon is used in combination with strong CYP enzyme inducers). Products include:

Uniphyl 2817

Theophylline Calcium Salicylate (Efficacy may be reduced when ramelteon is used in combination with strong CYP enzyme inducers).
No products indexed under this heading.

Theophylline Dihydroxypropyl (Glyceryl) (Efficacy may be reduced when ramelteon is used in combination with strong CYP enzyme inducers).
No products indexed under this heading.

Theophylline Ethylenediamine (Efficacy may be reduced when ramelteon is used in combination with strong CYP enzyme inducers).
No products indexed under this heading.

Theophylline Sodium Glycinate (Efficacy may be reduced when ramelteon is used in combination with strong CYP enzyme inducers).
No products indexed under this heading.

Thiamylal Sodium (Complex behaviors, such as "sleep driving" (eg, driving while not fully awake after ingestion of hypnotic) and other complex behaviors (eg, preparing and eating food, making phone calls, or having sex), with amnesia for the event, have been reported in association with hypnotic use. The use of alcohol and other CNS depressants may increase the risk of such behaviors).
No products indexed under this heading.

Thioridazine (Complex behaviors, such as "sleep driving" (eg, driving while not fully awake after ingestion of hypnotic) and other complex behaviors (eg, preparing and eating food, making phone calls, or having sex), with amnesia for the event, have been reported in association with hypnotic use. The use of alcohol and other CNS depressants may increase the risk of such behaviors).
No products indexed under this heading.

Thioridazine Hydrochloride (Complex behaviors, such as "sleep driving" (eg, driving while not fully awake after ingestion of hypnotic) and other complex behaviors (eg, preparing and eating food, making phone calls, or having sex), with amnesia for the event, have been reported in association with hypnotic use. The use of alcohol and other CNS depressants may increase the risk of such behaviors). Products include:

Thioridazine Hydrochloride 2384

Thiothixene (Complex behaviors, such as "sleep driving" (eg, driving while not fully awake after ingestion of hypnotic) and other complex behaviors (eg, preparing and eating food, making phone calls, or having sex), with amnesia for the event, have been reported in association with hypnotic use. The use of alcohol and other CNS depressants may increase the risk of such behaviors). Products include:

Thiothixene 2386

Thiothixene Hydrochloride (Complex behaviors, such as "sleep driving" (eg, driving while not fully awake after ingestion of hypnotic) and other complex behaviors (eg, preparing and eating food, making phone calls, or having sex), with amnesia for the event, have been reported in association with hypnotic use. The use of alcohol and other CNS depressants may increase the risk of such behaviors).
No products indexed under this heading.

Ticlopidine Hydrochloride (Ramelteon should be administered with caution to patients taking less strong CYP1A2 inhibitors).
No products indexed under this heading.

Tobacco (Efficacy may be reduced when ramelteon is used in combination with strong CYP enzyme inducers).
No products indexed under this heading.

Tolazamide (Ramelteon should be administered with caution in subjects taking strong CYP2C9 inhibitors).
No products indexed under this heading.

Tolbutamide (Ramelteon should be administered with caution in subjects taking strong CYP2C9 inhibitors).
No products indexed under this heading.

Tolbutamide Sodium (Ramelteon should be administered with caution in subjects taking strong CYP2C9 inhibitors).
No products indexed under this heading.

Triamcinolone (Efficacy may be reduced when ramelteon is used in combination with strong CYP enzyme inducers).
No products indexed under this heading.

Triamcinolone Acetonide (Efficacy may be reduced when ramelteon is used in combination with strong CYP enzyme inducers). Products include:

Azmacort 408
Nasacort AQ 3019

Triamcinolone Diacetate (Efficacy may be reduced when ramelteon is used in combination with strong CYP enzyme inducers).
No products indexed under this heading.

Triamcinolone Hexacetonide (Efficacy may be reduced when ramelteon is used in combination with strong CYP enzyme inducers).
No products indexed under this heading.

Triazolam (Complex behaviors, such as "sleep driving" (eg, driving while not fully awake after ingestion of hypnotic) and other complex behaviors (eg, preparing and eating food, making phone calls, or having sex), with amnesia for the event, have been reported in association with hypnotic use. The use of alcohol and other CNS depressants may increase the risk of such behaviors).
No products indexed under this heading.

Trifluoperazine Hydrochloride (Complex behaviors, such as "sleep driving" (eg, driving while not fully awake after ingestion of hypnotic) and other complex behaviors (eg, preparing and eating food, making phone calls, or having sex), with amnesia for the event, have been reported in association with hypnotic use. The use of alcohol and other CNS depressants may increase the risk of such behaviors).
No products indexed under this heading.

Troglitazone (Ramelteon should be administered with caution in subjects taking strong CYP2C9 inhibitors).
No products indexed under this heading.

Troleandomycin (Ramelteon should be administered with caution in subjects taking strong CYP3A4 inhibitors).
No products indexed under this heading.

Trovafloxacin Mesylate (Ramelteon should be administered with caution to patients taking less strong CYP1A2 inhibitors).
No products indexed under this heading.

Vardenafil Hydrochloride (Ramelteon should be administered with caution to patients taking less strong CYP1A2 inhibitors). Products include:
Levitra **3157**

Voriconazole (Ramelteon should be administered with caution in subjects taking strong CYP3A4 inhibitors).
No products indexed under this heading.

Zafirlukast (Ramelteon should be administered with caution in subjects taking strong CYP2C9 inhibitors). Products include:
Accolate **3612**

Zaleplon (Complex behaviors, such as "sleep driving" (eg, driving while not fully awake after ingestion of hypnotic) and other complex behaviors (eg, preparing and eating food, making phone calls, or having sex), with amnesia for the event, have been reported in association with hypnotic use. The use of alcohol and other CNS depressants may increase the risk of such behaviors).
No products indexed under this heading.

Zileuton (Ramelteon should be administered with caution to patients taking less strong CYP1A2 inhibitors).
No products indexed under this heading.

Ziprasidone Hydrochloride (Complex behaviors, such as "sleep driving" (eg, driving while not fully awake after ingestion of hypnotic) and other complex behaviors (eg, preparing and eating food, making phone calls, or having sex), with amnesia for the event, have been reported in association with hypnotic use. The use of alcohol and other CNS depressants may increase the risk of such behaviors). Products include:
Geodon **2723**

Zolpidem Tartrate (Complex behaviors, such as "sleep driving" (eg, driving while not fully awake after ingestion of hypnotic) and other complex behaviors (eg, preparing and eating food, making phone calls, or having sex), with amnesia for the event, have been reported in association with hypnotic use. The use of alcohol and other CNS depressants may increase the risk of such behaviors). Products include:
Ambien **2920**
Ambien CR **2925**

Food Interactions

Alcohol (Complex behaviors, such as "sleep driving" (eg, driving while not fully awake after ingestion of hypnotic) and other complex behaviors (eg, preparing and eating food, making phone calls, or having sex), with amnesia for the event, have been reported in association with hypnotic use. The use of alcohol and other CNS depressants may increase the risk of such behaviors).

Beer, reduced-alcohol (Complex behaviors, such as "sleep driving" (eg, driving while not fully awake after ingestion of hypnotic) and other complex behaviors (eg, preparing and eating food, making phone calls, or having sex), with amnesia for the event, have been reported in association with hypnotic use. The use of alcohol and other CNS depressants may increase the risk of such behaviors).

Beer, unspecified (Complex behaviors, such as "sleep driving" (eg, driving while not fully awake after ingestion of hypnotic) and other complex behaviors (eg, preparing and eating food, making phone calls, or having sex), with amnesia for the event, have been reported in association with hypnotic use. The use of alcohol and other CNS depressants may increase the risk of such behaviors).

Broccoli (Efficacy may be reduced when ramelteon is used in combination with strong CYP enzyme inducers).

Brussel Sprouts (Efficacy may be reduced when ramelteon is used in combination with strong CYP enzyme inducers).

Charbroiled Food (Efficacy may be reduced when ramelteon is used in combination with strong CYP enzyme inducers).

Food, unspecified (When administered with a high-fat meal, the $AUC_{0\text{-inf}}$ for a single 16 mg dose of ramelteon was 31% higher and the C_{max} was 22% lower than when given in a fasted state. Median T_{max} was delayed by approximately 45 minutes when ramelteon was administered with food. Effects of food on the AUC values for M-II were similar. It is, therefore, recommended that ramelteon not be taken with or immediately after a high-fat meal).

Grapefruit (Ramelteon should be administered with caution to patients taking less strong CYP1A2 inhibitors).

Grapefruit Juice (Ramelteon should be administered with caution to patients taking less strong CYP1A2 inhibitors).

Meal, unspecified (When administered with a high-fat meal, the $AUC_{0\text{-inf}}$ for a single 16 mg dose of ramelteon was 31% higher and the C_{max} was 22% lower than when given in a fasted state. Median T_{max} was delayed by approximately 45 minutes when ramelteon was administered with food. Effects of food on the AUC values for M-II were similar. It is, therefore, recommended that ramelteon not be taken with or immediately after a high-fat meal).

Wine, Chianti (Complex behaviors, such as "sleep driving" (eg, driving while not fully awake after ingestion of hypnotic) and other complex behaviors (eg, preparing and eating food, making phone calls, or having sex), with amnesia for the event, have been reported in association with hypnotic use. The use of alcohol and other CNS depressants may increase the risk of such behaviors).

Wine, Red (Complex behaviors, such as "sleep driving" (eg, driving while not fully awake after ingestion of hypnotic) and other complex behaviors (eg, preparing and eating food, making phone calls, or having sex), with amnesia for the event, have been reported in association with hypnotic use. The use of alcohol and other CNS depressants may increase the risk of such behaviors).

Wine, unspecified (Complex behaviors, such as "sleep driving" (eg, driving while not fully awake after ingestion of hypnotic) and other complex behaviors (eg, preparing and eating food, making phone calls, or having sex), with amnesia for the event, have been reported in association with hypnotic use. The use of alcohol and other CNS depressants may increase the risk of such behaviors).

Wine products (Complex behaviors, such as "sleep driving" (eg, driving while not fully awake after ingestion of hypnotic) and other complex behaviors (eg, preparing and eating food, making phone calls, or having sex), with amnesia for the event, have been reported in association with hypnotic use. The use of alcohol and other CNS depressants may increase the risk of such behaviors).

RYTHMOL TABLETS

(Propafenone Hydrochloride) **1648**
May interact with beta-blockers, cytochrome p450 1a2 inhibitors (selected), cytochrome p450 2d6 inhibitors (selected), cytochrome p450 2d6 substrates (selected), cytochrome p450 3a4 inhibitors (selected), erythromycin, haloperidols, quinidine, and certain other agents. Compounds in these categories include:

Acebutolol Hydrochloride (Concomitant use of propafenone and propranolol in healthy subjects increased propranolol plasma concentrations at steady state by 113%. In 4 patients, administration of metoprolol with propafenone increased the metoprolol plasma concentrations at steady state by 100% to 400%. The pharmacokinetics of propafenone was not affected by the co-administration of either propranolol or metoprolol. In clinical trials using propafenone immediate release tablets, patients who were receiving β-blockers concurrently did not experience an increased incidence of side effects).
No products indexed under this heading.

Acetazolamide (Propafenone is metabolized by CYP3A4. Drugs that inhibit CYP3A4 can be expected to cause increased plasma levels of propafenone. Appropriate monitoring is recommended when propafenone is used together with such drugs).
No products indexed under this heading.

Acetazolamide Sodium (Propafenone is metabolized by CYP3A4. Drugs that inhibit CYP3A4 can be expected to cause increased plasma levels of propafenone. Appropriate monitoring is recommended when propafenone is used together with such drugs).
No products indexed under this heading.

Alatrofloxacin Mesylate (Propafenone is metabolized by CYP1A2. Drugs that inhibit CYP1A2 can be expected to cause increased plasma levels of propafenone. Appropriate monitoring is recommended when propafenone is used together with such drugs).
No products indexed under this heading.

Amiodarone Hydrochloride (Concomitant administration of propafenone and amiodarone can affect conduction and repolarization and is not recommended).
No products indexed under this heading.

Amitriptyline Hydrochloride (Propafenone is metabolized by CYP2D6 (major pathway). Drugs that inhibit CYP2D6 can be expected to cause increased plasma levels of propafenone. Appropriate monitoring is recommended when propafenone is used together with such drugs).
No products indexed under this heading.

Amoxapine (Propafenone is metabolized by CYP2D6 (major pathway). Drugs that inhibit CYP2D6 can be expected to cause increased plasma levels of propafenone. Appropriate monitoring is recommended when propafenone is used together with such drugs).
No products indexed under this heading.

Amphetamine Aspartate (Propafenone is an inhibitor of CYP2D6. Co-administration of propafenone with drugs metabolized by CYP2D6 might lead to increased plasma concentrations of these drugs).
No products indexed under this heading.

Amphetamine Aspartate Monohydrate (Propafenone is an inhibitor of CYP2D6. Co-administration of propafenone with drugs metabolized by CYP2D6 might lead to increased plasma concentrations of these drugs).
No products indexed under this heading.

Amphetamine Sulfate (Propafenone is an inhibitor of CYP2D6. Co-administration of propafenone with drugs metabolized by CYP2D6 might lead to increased plasma concentrations of these drugs).
No products indexed under this heading.

Amprenavir (Propafenone is metabolized by CYP3A4. Drugs that inhibit CYP3A4 can be expected to cause increased plasma levels of propafenone. Appropriate monitoring is recommended when propafenone is used together with such drugs).
No products indexed under this heading.

Anastrozole (Propafenone is metabolized by CYP1A2. Drugs that inhibit CYP1A2 can be expected to cause increased plasma levels of propafenone. Appropriate monitoring is recommended when propafenone is used together with such drugs).
No products indexed under this heading.

Aprepitant (Propafenone is metabolized by CYP3A4. Drugs that inhibit CYP3A4 can be expected to cause increased plasma levels of propafenone. Appropriate monitoring is recommended when propafenone is used together with such drugs). Products include:
Emend **2124**

Atazanavir (Propafenone is metabolized by CYP3A4. Drugs that inhibit CYP3A4 can be expected to cause increased plasma levels of propafenone. Appropriate monitoring is recommended when propafenone is used together with such drugs).
No products indexed under this heading.

Atazanavir Sulfate (Propafenone is metabolized by CYP3A4. Drugs that inhibit CYP3A4 can be expected to cause increased plasma levels of propafenone. Appropriate monitoring is recommended when propafenone is used together with such drugs).
No products indexed under this heading.

Atenolol (Concomitant use of propafenone and propranolol in healthy subjects increased propranolol plasma concentrations at steady state by 113%. In 4 patients, administration of

metoprolol with propafenone increased the metoprolol plasma concentrations at steady state by 100% to 400%. The pharmacokinetics of propafenone was not affected by the co-administration of either propranolol or metoprolol. In clinical trials using propafenone immediate release tablets, patients who were receiving β-blockers concurrently did not experience an increased incidence of side effects).

No products indexed under this heading.

Atomoxetine Hydrochloride (Propafenone is an inhibitor of CYP2D6. Co-administration of propafenone with drugs metabolized by CYP2D6 might lead to increased plasma concentrations of these drugs). Products include:
Strattera 1957

Betaxolol Hydrochloride (Concomitant use of propafenone and propranolol in healthy subjects increased propranolol plasma concentrations at steady state by 113%. In 4 patients, administration of metoprolol with propafenone increased the metoprolol plasma concentrations at steady state by 100% to 400%. The pharmacokinetics of propafenone was not affected by the co-administration of either propranolol or metoprolol. In clinical trials using propafenone immediate release tablets, patients who were receiving β-blockers concurrently did not experience an increased incidence of side effects).

No products indexed under this heading.

Bisoprolol Fumarate (Concomitant use of propafenone and propranolol in healthy subjects increased propranolol plasma concentrations at steady state by 113%. In 4 patients, administration of metoprolol with propafenone increased the metoprolol plasma concentrations at steady state by 100% to 400%. The pharmacokinetics of propafenone was not affected by the co-administration of either propranolol or metoprolol. In clinical trials using propafenone immediate release tablets, patients who were receiving β-blockers concurrently did not experience an increased incidence of side effects).

No products indexed under this heading.

Bupropion Hydrochloride (Propafenone is metabolized by CYP2D6 (major pathway). Drugs that inhibit CYP2D6 can be expected to cause increased plasma levels of propafenone. Appropriate monitoring is recommended when propafenone is used together with such drugs).
Products include:
Aplenzin 2948
Wellbutrin 1719
Wellbutrin SR 1725
Zyban 1762

Captopril (Propafenone is an inhibitor of CYP2D6. Co-administration of propafenone with drugs metabolized by CYP2D6 might lead to increased plasma concentrations of these drugs). Products include:
Captopril 2341

Carteolol Hydrochloride (Concomitant use of propafenone and propranolol in healthy subjects increased propranolol plasma concentrations at steady state by 113%. In 4 patients, administration of metoprolol with propafenone increased the metoprolol plasma concentrations at steady state by 100% to 400%. The pharmacokinetics of propafenone was not affected by the co-administration of either propranolol or metoprolol. In clinical trials using propafenone immediate release tablets, patients who were receiving β-blockers concurrently did not experience an increased incidence of side effects).

No products indexed under this heading.

Carvedilol (Concomitant use of propafenone and propranolol in healthy subjects increased propranolol plasma

concentrations at steady state by 113%. In 4 patients, administration of metoprolol with propafenone increased the metoprolol plasma concentrations at steady state by 100% to 400%. The pharmacokinetics of propafenone was not affected by the co-administration of either propranolol or metoprolol. In clinical trials using propafenone immediate release tablets, patients who were receiving β-blockers concurrently did not experience an increased incidence of side effects). Products include:
Coreg 1409

Carvedilol Phosphate (Concomitant use of propafenone and propranolol in healthy subjects increased propranolol plasma concentrations at steady state by 113%. In 4 patients, administration of metoprolol with propafenone increased the metoprolol plasma concentrations at steady state by 100% to 400%. The pharmacokinetics of propafenone was not affected by the co-administration of either propranolol or metoprolol. In clinical trials using propafenone immediate release tablets, patients who were receiving β-blockers concurrently did not experience an increased incidence of side effects). Products include:
Coreg CR 1416

Celecoxib (Propafenone is metabolized by CYP2D6 (major pathway). Drugs that inhibit CYP2D6 can be expected to cause increased plasma levels of propafenone. Appropriate monitoring is recommended when propafenone is used together with such drugs). Products include:
Celebrex 3272

Cevimeline Hydrochloride (Propafenone is an inhibitor of CYP2D6. Co-administration of propafenone with drugs metabolized by CYP2D6 might lead to increased plasma concentrations of these drugs). Products include:
Evoxac 1027

Chloroquine (Propafenone is metabolized by CYP2D6 (major pathway). Drugs that inhibit CYP2D6 can be expected to cause increased plasma levels of propafenone. Appropriate monitoring is recommended when propafenone is used together with such drugs).

No products indexed under this heading.

Chloroquine Hydrochloride (Propafenone is metabolized by CYP2D6 (major pathway). Drugs that inhibit CYP2D6 can be expected to cause increased plasma levels of propafenone. Appropriate monitoring is recommended when propafenone is used together with such drugs).

No products indexed under this heading.

Chloroquine Phosphate (Propafenone is metabolized by CYP2D6 (major pathway). Drugs that inhibit CYP2D6 can be expected to cause increased plasma levels of propafenone. Appropriate monitoring is recommended when propafenone is used together with such drugs).

No products indexed under this heading.

Chlorpheniramine (Propafenone is metabolized by CYP2D6 (major pathway). Drugs that inhibit CYP2D6 can be expected to cause increased plasma levels of propafenone. Appropriate monitoring is recommended when propafenone is used together with such drugs).

No products indexed under this heading.

Chlorpheniramine Maleate (Propafenone is metabolized by CYP2D6 (major pathway). Drugs that inhibit CYP2D6 can be expected to cause increased plasma levels of propafenone. Appropriate monitoring is recommended when propafenone is used together with such drugs).

No products indexed under this heading.

Chlorpheniramine Polistirex (Propafenone is metabolized by CYP2D6 (major pathway). Drugs that inhibit CYP2D6 can be expected to cause increased plasma levels of propafenone. Appropriate monitoring is recommended when propafenone is used together with such drugs). Products include:
Tussionex 3443

Chlorpheniramine Tannate (Propafenone is metabolized by CYP2D6 (major pathway). Drugs that inhibit CYP2D6 can be expected to cause increased plasma levels of propafenone. Appropriate monitoring is recommended when propafenone is used together with such drugs).

No products indexed under this heading.

Chlorpromazine (Propafenone is an inhibitor of CYP2D6. Co-administration of propafenone with drugs metabolized by CYP2D6 might lead to increased plasma concentrations of these drugs).

No products indexed under this heading.

Chlorpromazine Hydrochloride (Propafenone is an inhibitor of CYP2D6. Co-administration of propafenone with drugs metabolized by CYP2D6 might lead to increased plasma concentrations of these drugs).

No products indexed under this heading.

Chlorpropamide (Propafenone is an inhibitor of CYP2D6. Co-administration of propafenone with drugs metabolized by CYP2D6 might lead to increased plasma concentrations of these drugs).

No products indexed under this heading.

Cimetidine (Concomitant administration of propafenone immediate release tablets and cimetidine in 12 healthy subjects resulted in a 20% increase in steady-state plasma concentrations of propafenone).

No products indexed under this heading.

Cimetidine Hydrochloride (Concomitant administration of propafenone immediate release tablets and cimetidine in 12 healthy subjects resulted in a 20% increase in steady-state plasma concentrations of propafenone).

No products indexed under this heading.

Ciprofloxacin (Propafenone is metabolized by CYP1A2. Drugs that inhibit CYP1A2 can be expected to cause increased plasma levels of propafenone. Appropriate monitoring is recommended when propafenone is used together with such drugs). Products include:
Cipro I.V. 3082
Cipro 3073
Cipro XR 3091
Ciprodex 583

Ciprofloxacin Hydrochloride (Propafenone is metabolized by CYP1A2. Drugs that inhibit CYP1A2 can be expected to cause increased plasma levels of propafenone. Appropriate monitoring is recommended when propafenone is used together with such drugs). Products include:
Cipro 3073

Citalopram Hydrobromide (Propafenone is metabolized by CYP2D6 (major pathway). Drugs that inhibit CYP2D6 can be expected to cause increased plasma levels of propafenone. Appropriate monitoring is recommended when propafenone is used together with such drugs). Products include:
Celexa 1153

Clarithromycin (Propafenone is metabolized by CYP1A2. Drugs that inhibit CYP1A2 can be expected to cause increased plasma levels of propafenone. Appropriate monitoring is recommended when propafenone is used together with such drugs). Products include:

Biaxin/Biaxin XL 412

Clomipramine Hydrochloride (Propafenone is metabolized by CYP2D6 (major pathway). Drugs that inhibit CYP2D6 can be expected to cause increased plasma levels of propafenone. Appropriate monitoring is recommended when propafenone is used together with such drugs).

No products indexed under this heading.

Clotrimazole (Propafenone is metabolized by CYP3A4. Drugs that inhibit CYP3A4 can be expected to cause increased plasma levels of propafenone. Appropriate monitoring is recommended when propafenone is used together with such drugs). Products include:
Lotrisone 3163

Clozapine (Propafenone is an inhibitor of CYP2D6. Co-administration of propafenone with drugs metabolized by CYP2D6 might lead to increased plasma concentrations of these drugs).

No products indexed under this heading.

Cocaine Hydrochloride (Propafenone is metabolized by CYP2D6 (major pathway). Drugs that inhibit CYP2D6 can be expected to cause increased plasma levels of propafenone. Appropriate monitoring is recommended when propafenone is used together with such drugs).

No products indexed under this heading.

Codeine Phosphate (Propafenone is an inhibitor of CYP2D6. Co-administration of propafenone with drugs metabolized by CYP2D6 might lead to increased plasma concentrations of these drugs). Products include:
Tylenol with Codeine 2691

Codeine Sulfate (Propafenone is an inhibitor of CYP2D6. Co-administration of propafenone with drugs metabolized by CYP2D6 might lead to increased plasma concentrations of these drugs).

No products indexed under this heading.

Conivaptan Hydrochloride (Propafenone is metabolized by CYP3A4. Drugs that inhibit CYP3A4 can be expected to cause increased plasma levels of propafenone. Appropriate monitoring is recommended when propafenone is used together with such drugs). Products include:
Vaprisol 689

Cyclobenzaprine Hydrochloride (Propafenone is an inhibitor of CYP2D6. Co-administration of propafenone with drugs metabolized by CYP2D6 might lead to increased plasma concentrations of these drugs). Products include:
Amrix 964

Cyclosporine (Propafenone is metabolized by CYP3A4. Drugs that inhibit CYP3A4 can be expected to cause increased plasma levels of propafenone. Appropriate monitoring is recommended when propafenone is used together with such drugs). Products include:
Gengraf 440
Neoral Oral Solution 2496
Neoral Capsules 2496
Restasis 605

Dalfopristin (Propafenone is metabolized by CYP3A4. Drugs that inhibit CYP3A4 can be expected to cause increased plasma levels of propafenone. Appropriate monitoring is recommended when propafenone is used together with such drugs).

No products indexed under this heading.

Danazol (Propafenone is metabolized by CYP3A4. Drugs that inhibit CYP3A4 can be expected to cause increased plasma levels of propafenone. Appropriate monitoring is recommended when propafenone is used together with such drugs).

No products indexed under this heading.

Darunavir (Propafenone is metabolized by CYP3A4. Drugs that inhibit CYP3A4 can be expected to cause increased plasma levels of propafenone. Appropriate monitoring is recommended when propafenone is used together with such drugs).
No products indexed under this heading.

Dasatinib (Propafenone is metabolized by CYP3A4. Drugs that inhibit CYP3A4 can be expected to cause increased plasma levels of propafenone. Appropriate monitoring is recommended when propafenone is used together with such drugs).
No products indexed under this heading.

Debrisoquine (Propafenone is an inhibitor of CYP2D6. Co-administration of propafenone with drugs metabolized by CYP2D6 might lead to increased plasma concentrations of these drugs).
No products indexed under this heading.

Delavirdine Mesylate (Propafenone is metabolized by CYP3A4. Drugs that inhibit CYP3A4 can be expected to cause increased plasma levels of propafenone. Appropriate monitoring is recommended when propafenone is used together with such drugs).
No products indexed under this heading.

Delavirine (Propafenone is metabolized by CYP3A4. Drugs that inhibit CYP3A4 can be expected to cause increased plasma levels of propafenone. Appropriate monitoring is recommended when propafenone is used together with such drugs).
No products indexed under this heading.

Desipramine Hydrochloride (Co-administration of drugs which are metabolized and inhibited by CYP2D6, such as desipramine, may lead to increased levels of propafenone and desipramine. Appropriate monitoring is recommended when propafenone is used together with desipramine).
No products indexed under this heading.

Desloratadine (Propafenone is metabolized by CYP3A4. Drugs that inhibit CYP3A4 can be expected to cause increased plasma levels of propafenone. Appropriate monitoring is recommended when propafenone is used together with such drugs).
Products include:

Desogestrel (Propafenone is metabolized by CYP1A2. Drugs that inhibit CYP1A2 can be expected to cause increased plasma levels of propafenone. Appropriate monitoring is recommended when propafenone is used together with such drugs).
No products indexed under this heading.

Dexfenfluramine Hydrochloride (Propafenone is an inhibitor of CYP2D6. Co-administration of propafenone with drugs metabolized by CYP2D6 might lead to increased plasma concentrations of these drugs).
No products indexed under this heading.

Dextromethorphan Hydrobromide (Propafenone is an inhibitor of CYP2D6. Co-administration of propafenone with drugs metabolized by CYP2D6 might lead to increased plasma concentrations of these drugs).
No products indexed under this heading.

Dextromethorphan Polistirex (Propafenone is an inhibitor of CYP2D6. Co-administration of propafenone with drugs metabolized by CYP2D6 might lead to increased plasma concentrations of these drugs).
No products indexed under this heading.

Digoxin (Concomitant use of propafenone and digoxin increased steady-state serum digoxin exposure (AUC) in patients by 60% to 270%, and decreased the clearance of digoxin by 31% to 67%. Plasma digoxin levels of patients receiving propafenone should be monitored and digoxin dosage adjusted as needed). Products include:

Diltiazem Hydrochloride (Propafenone is metabolized by CYP3A4. Drugs that inhibit CYP3A4 can be expected to cause increased plasma levels of propafenone. Appropriate monitoring is recommended when propafenone is used together with such drugs). Products include:

Diltiazem Maleate (Propafenone is metabolized by CYP3A4. Drugs that inhibit CYP3A4 can be expected to cause increased plasma levels of propafenone. Appropriate monitoring is recommended when propafenone is used together with such drugs).
No products indexed under this heading.

Diphenhydramine (Propafenone is metabolized by CYP2D6 (major pathway). Drugs that inhibit CYP2D6 can be expected to cause increased plasma levels of propafenone. Appropriate monitoring is recommended when propafenone is used together with such drugs).
No products indexed under this heading.

Diphenhydramine Hydrochloride (Propafenone is metabolized by CYP2D6 (major pathway). Drugs that inhibit CYP2D6 can be expected to cause increased plasma levels of propafenone. Appropriate monitoring is recommended when propafenone is used together with such drugs).
Products include:

Dolasetron Mesylate (Propafenone is an inhibitor of CYP2D6. Co-administration of propafenone with drugs metabolized by CYP2D6 might lead to increased plasma concentrations of these drugs). Products include:

Donepezil Hydrochloride (Propafenone is an inhibitor of CYP2D6. Co-administration of propafenone with drugs metabolized by CYP2D6 might lead to increased plasma concentrations of these drugs). Products include:

Doxepin Hydrochloride (Propafenone is metabolized by CYP2D6 (major pathway). Drugs that inhibit CYP2D6 can be expected to cause increased plasma levels of propafenone. Appropriate monitoring is recommended when propafenone is used together with such drugs).
No products indexed under this heading.

Efavirenz (Propafenone is metabolized by CYP3A4. Drugs that inhibit CYP3A4 can be expected to cause increased plasma levels of propafenone. Appropriate monitoring is recommended when propafenone is used together with such drugs). Products include:

Encainide Hydrochloride (Propafenone is an inhibitor of CYP2D6. Co-administration of propafenone with drugs metabolized by CYP2D6 might lead to increased plasma concentrations of these drugs).
No products indexed under this heading.

Enoxacin (Propafenone is metabolized by CYP1A2. Drugs that inhibit CYP1A2 can be expected to cause increased plasma levels of propafenone. Appropriate monitoring is recommended when propafenone is used together with such drugs).
No products indexed under this heading.

Erythromycin (Propafenone is metabolized by CYP3A4. Drugs that inhibit CYP3A4 (such as erythromycin) can be expected to cause increased plasma levels of propafenone. Appropriate monitoring is recommended when propafenone is used together with such drugs).
No products indexed under this heading.

Erythromycin, Topical (Propafenone is metabolized by CYP3A4. Drugs that inhibit CYP3A4 (such as erythromycin) can be expected to cause increased plasma levels of propafenone. Appropriate monitoring is recommended when propafenone is used together with such drugs).
No products indexed under this heading.

Erythromycin Estolate (Propafenone is metabolized by CYP3A4. Drugs that inhibit CYP3A4 (such as erythromycin) can be expected to cause increased plasma levels of propafenone. Appropriate monitoring is recommended when propafenone is used together with such drugs).
No products indexed under this heading.

Erythromycin Ethylsuccinate (Propafenone is metabolized by CYP3A4. Drugs that inhibit CYP3A4 (such as erythromycin) can be expected to cause increased plasma levels of propafenone. Appropriate monitoring is recommended when propafenone is used together with such drugs).
Products include:

Erythromycin Gluceptate (Propafenone is metabolized by CYP3A4. Drugs that inhibit CYP3A4 (such as erythromycin) can be expected to cause increased plasma levels of propafenone. Appropriate monitoring is recommended when propafenone is used together with such drugs).
No products indexed under this heading.

Erythromycin Lactobionate (Propafenone is metabolized by CYP3A4. Drugs that inhibit CYP3A4 (such as erythromycin) can be expected to cause increased plasma levels of propafenone. Appropriate monitoring is recommended when propafenone is used together with such drugs).
No products indexed under this heading.

Erythromycin Stearate (Propafenone is metabolized by CYP3A4. Drugs that inhibit CYP3A4 (such as erythromycin) can be expected to cause increased plasma levels of propafenone. Appropriate monitoring is recommended when propafenone is used together with such drugs).
No products indexed under this heading.

Escitalopram Oxalate (Propafenone is metabolized by CYP2D6 (major pathway). Drugs that inhibit CYP2D6 can be expected to cause increased plasma levels of propafenone. Appropriate monitoring is recommended when propafenone is used together with such drugs). Products include:

Esmolol Hydrochloride (Concomitant use of propafenone and propranolol in healthy subjects increased propranolol plasma concentrations at steady state by 113%. In 4 patients, administration of metoprolol with propafenone increased the metoprolol plasma concentrations at steady state by 100% to 400%. The pharmacokinetics of propafenone was not affected by the co-administration of either propranolol or metoprolol. In clinical trials using propafenone immediate release tablets, patients who were receiving β-blockers concurrently did not experience an increased incidence of side effects).
No products indexed under this heading.

Esomeprazole Magnesium (Propafenone is metabolized by CYP1A2. Drugs that inhibit CYP1A2 can be expected to cause increased plasma levels of propafenone. Appropriate monitoring is recommended when propafenone is used together with such drugs). Products include:

Esomeprazole Sodium (Propafenone is metabolized by CYP1A2. Drugs that inhibit CYP1A2 can be expected to cause increased plasma levels of propafenone. Appropriate monitoring is recommended when propafenone is used together with such drugs). Products include:

Ethinyl Estradiol (Propafenone is metabolized by CYP1A2. Drugs that inhibit CYP1A2 can be expected to cause increased plasma levels of propafenone. Appropriate monitoring is recommended when propafenone is used together with such drugs).
Products include:

Fentanyl (Propafenone is an inhibitor of CYP2D6. Co-administration of propafenone with drugs metabolized by CYP2D6 might lead to increased plasma concentrations of these drugs).
Products include:

Fentanyl Citrate (Propafenone is an inhibitor of CYP2D6. Co-administration of propafenone with drugs metabolized by CYP2D6 might lead to increased plasma concentrations of these drugs). Products include:

Flecainide Acetate (Propafenone is an inhibitor of CYP2D6. Co-administration of propafenone with drugs metabolized by CYP2D6 might lead to increased plasma concentrations of these drugs).
No products indexed under this heading.

Fluconazole (Propafenone is metabolized by CYP3A4. Drugs that inhibit CYP3A4 can be expected to cause increased plasma levels of propafenone. Appropriate monitoring is recommended when propafenone is used together with such drugs).
No products indexed under this heading.

Fluoxetine (Concomitant administration of propafenone and fluoxetine in extensive metabolizers increased the S propafenone C_{max} and AUC by 39% and 50%, respectively, and the R propafenone C_{max} and AUC by 71% and 50%, respectively).
No products indexed under this heading.

Fluoxetine Hydrochloride (Concomitant administration of propafenone and fluoxetine in extensive metabolizers increased the S propafenone C_{max} and AUC by 39% and 50%, respectively, and the R propafenone C_{max} and AUC by 71% and 50%, respectively). Products include:

IMPORTANT NOTE: Always consult each drug listing in the patient's regimen for possible interactions.

Symbyax 1965

Fluphenazine Decanoate (Propafenone is metabolized by CYP2D6 (major pathway). Drugs that inhibit CYP2D6 can be expected to cause increased plasma levels of propafenone. Appropriate monitoring is recommended when propafenone is used together with such drugs).
No products indexed under this heading.

Fluphenazine Enanthate (Propafenone is metabolized by CYP2D6 (major pathway). Drugs that inhibit CYP2D6 can be expected to cause increased plasma levels of propafenone. Appropriate monitoring is recommended when propafenone is used together with such drugs).
No products indexed under this heading.

Fluphenazine Hydrochloride (Propafenone is metabolized by CYP2D6 (major pathway). Drugs that inhibit CYP2D6 can be expected to cause increased plasma levels of propafenone. Appropriate monitoring is recommended when propafenone is used together with such drugs).
No products indexed under this heading.

Fluvoxamine (Propafenone is metabolized by CYP1A2. Drugs that inhibit CYP1A2 can be expected to cause increased plasma levels of propafenone. Appropriate monitoring is recommended when propafenone is used together with such drugs).
No products indexed under this heading.

Fluvoxamine Maleate (Propafenone is metabolized by CYP2D6 (major pathway). Drugs that inhibit CYP2D6 can be expected to cause increased plasma levels of propafenone. Appropriate monitoring is recommended when propafenone is used together with such drugs).
No products indexed under this heading.

Formoterol Fumarate (Propafenone is an inhibitor of CYP2D6. Co-administration of propafenone with drugs metabolized by CYP2D6 might lead to increased plasma concentrations of these drugs). Products include:
Foradil 3121
Perforomist 3634

Fosamprenavir Calcium (Propafenone is metabolized by CYP3A4. Drugs that inhibit CYP3A4 can be expected to cause increased plasma levels of propafenone. Appropriate monitoring is recommended when propafenone is used together with such drugs). Products include:
Lexiva Oral Suspension 1558
Lexiva 1558

Galantamine Hydrobromide (Propafenone is an inhibitor of CYP2D6. Co-administration of propafenone with drugs metabolized by CYP2D6 might lead to increased plasma concentrations of these drugs).
No products indexed under this heading.

Gatifloxacin (Propafenone is metabolized by CYP1A2. Drugs that inhibit CYP1A2 can be expected to cause increased plasma levels of propafenone. Appropriate monitoring is recommended when propafenone is used together with such drugs).
No products indexed under this heading.

Gemifloxacin Mesylate (Propafenone is metabolized by CYP1A2. Drugs that inhibit CYP1A2 can be expected to cause increased plasma levels of propafenone. Appropriate monitoring is recommended when propafenone is used together with such drugs).
No products indexed under this heading.

Grepafloxacin Hydrochloride (Propafenone is metabolized by CYP1A2. Drugs that inhibit CYP1A2 can be expected to cause increased plasma levels of propafenone. Appropriate monitoring is recommended when propafenone is used together with such drugs).
No products indexed under this heading.

Halofantrine Hydrochloride (Propafenone is metabolized by CYP2D6 (major pathway). Drugs that inhibit CYP2D6 can be expected to cause increased plasma levels of propafenone. Appropriate monitoring is recommended when propafenone is used together with such drugs).
No products indexed under this heading.

Haloperidol (Propafenone is metabolized by CYP2D6 (major pathway). Drugs that inhibit CYP2D6 can be expected to cause increased plasma levels of propafenone. Appropriate monitoring is recommended when propafenone is used together with such drugs).
No products indexed under this heading.

Haloperidol Decanoate (Propafenone is metabolized by CYP2D6 (major pathway). Drugs that inhibit CYP2D6 can be expected to cause increased plasma levels of propafenone. Appropriate monitoring is recommended when propafenone is used together with such drugs).
No products indexed under this heading.

Haloperidol Lactate (Propafenone is metabolized by CYP2D6 (major pathway). Drugs that inhibit CYP2D6 can be expected to cause increased plasma levels of propafenone. Appropriate monitoring is recommended when propafenone is used together with such drugs).
No products indexed under this heading.

Hydrocodone Bitartrate (Propafenone is an inhibitor of CYP2D6. Co-administration of propafenone with drugs metabolized by CYP2D6 might lead to increased plasma concentrations of these drugs). Products include:
Vicodin 560
Vicodin ES 561
Vicodin HP 563
Vicoprofen 564
Zydone 1138

Hydroxychloroquine Sulfate (Propafenone is metabolized by CYP2D6 (major pathway). Drugs that inhibit CYP2D6 can be expected to cause increased plasma levels of propafenone. Appropriate monitoring is recommended when propafenone is used together with such drugs).
No products indexed under this heading.

Imatinib Mesylate (Propafenone is metabolized by CYP2D6 (major pathway). Drugs that inhibit CYP2D6 can be expected to cause increased plasma levels of propafenone. Appropriate monitoring is recommended when propafenone is used together with such drugs). Products include:
Gleevec 2477

Imipramine Hydrochloride (Propafenone is metabolized by CYP2D6. Co-administration of propafenone with drugs metabolized by CYP2D6 (such as imipramine) might lead to increased plasma concentrations of imipramine).
No products indexed under this heading.

Imipramine Pamoate (Propafenone is metabolized by CYP2D6. Co-administration of propafenone with drugs metabolized by CYP2D6 (such as imipramine) might lead to increased plasma concentrations of imipramine).
No products indexed under this heading.

Indinavir Sulfate (Propafenone is metabolized by CYP3A4. Drugs that inhibit CYP3A4 can be expected to cause increased plasma levels of propafenone. Appropriate monitoring is recommended when propafenone is used together with such drugs).
Products include:
Crixivan 2113

Indoramin Hydrochloride (Propafenone is an inhibitor of CYP2D6. Co-administration of propafenone with drugs metabolized by CYP2D6 might lead to increased plasma concentrations of these drugs).
No products indexed under this heading.

Isoniazid (Propafenone is metabolized by CYP1A2. Drugs that inhibit CYP1A2 can be expected to cause increased plasma levels of propafenone. Appropriate monitoring is recommended when propafenone is used together with such drugs).
No products indexed under this heading.

Itraconazole (Propafenone is metabolized by CYP3A4. Drugs that inhibit CYP3A4 can be expected to cause increased plasma levels of propafenone. Appropriate monitoring is recommended when propafenone is used together with such drugs).
No products indexed under this heading.

Ketoconazole (Propafenone is metabolized by CYP3A4. Drugs that inhibit CYP3A4 (such as ketoconazole) can be expected to cause increased plasma levels of propafenone. Appropriate monitoring is recommended when propafenone is used together with such drugs). Products include:
Extina 3319
Xolegel 3337

Labetalol Hydrochloride (Concomitant use of propafenone and propranolol in healthy subjects increased propranolol plasma concentrations at steady state by 113%. In 4 patients, administration of metoprolol with propafenone increased the metoprolol plasma concentrations at steady state by 100% to 400%. The pharmacokinetics of propafenone was not affected by the co-administration of either propranolol or metoprolol. In clinical trials using propafenone immediate release tablets, patients who were receiving β-blockers concurrently did not experience an increased incidence of side effects).
No products indexed under this heading.

Lapatinib (Propafenone is metabolized by CYP3A4. Drugs that inhibit CYP3A4 can be expected to cause increased plasma levels of propafenone. Appropriate monitoring is recommended when propafenone is used together with such drugs). Products include:
Tykerb 1698

Levobunolol Hydrochloride (Concomitant use of propafenone and propranolol in healthy subjects increased propranolol plasma concentrations at steady state by 113%. In 4 patients, administration of metoprolol with propafenone increased the metoprolol plasma concentrations at steady state by 100% to 400%. The pharmacokinetics of propafenone was not affected by the co-administration of either propranolol or metoprolol. In clinical trials using propafenone immediate release tablets, patients who were receiving β-blockers concurrently did not experience an increased incidence of side effects).
No products indexed under this heading.

Levofloxacin (Propafenone is metabolized by CYP1A2. Drugs that inhibit CYP1A2 can be expected to cause increased plasma levels of propafenone. Appropriate monitoring is recommended when propafenone is used together with such drugs). Products include:
Iquix 3492
Levaquin 2629
Levaquin in 5% Dextrose 2629

Quixin 3493

Levonorgestrel (Propafenone is metabolized by CYP1A2. Drugs that inhibit CYP1A2 can be expected to cause increased plasma levels of propafenone. Appropriate monitoring is recommended when propafenone is used together with such drugs). Products include:
Climara Pro 847
LoSeasonique 3407
Lybrel 3514
Mirena 854
Plan B 3416
Seasonique 3418

Lidocaine (No significant effects on the pharmacokinetics of propafenone or lidocaine have been seen following their concomitant use in patients. However, concomitant use of propafenone and lidocaine have been reported to increase the risks of central nervous system side effects of lidocaine). Products include:
Lidoderm 1107

Lidocaine Base (No significant effects on the pharmacokinetics of propafenone or lidocaine have been seen following their concomitant use in patients. However, concomitant use of propafenone and lidocaine have been reported to increase the risks of central nervous system side effects of lidocaine).
No products indexed under this heading.

Lidocaine Hydrochloride (No significant effects on the pharmacokinetics of propafenone or lidocaine have been seen following their concomitant use in patients. However, concomitant use of propafenone and lidocaine have been reported to increase the risks of central nervous system side effects of lidocaine).
No products indexed under this heading.

Lomefloxacin Hydrochloride (Propafenone is metabolized by CYP1A2. Drugs that inhibit CYP1A2 can be expected to cause increased plasma levels of propafenone. Appropriate monitoring is recommended when propafenone is used together with such drugs).
No products indexed under this heading.

Lopinavir (Propafenone is metabolized by CYP3A4. Drugs that inhibit CYP3A4 can be expected to cause increased plasma levels of propafenone. Appropriate monitoring is recommended when propafenone is used together with such drugs). Products include:
Kaletra 458

Loratadine (Propafenone is metabolized by CYP3A4. Drugs that inhibit CYP3A4 can be expected to cause increased plasma levels of propafenone. Appropriate monitoring is recommended when propafenone is used together with such drugs).
No products indexed under this heading.

Maprotiline Hydrochloride (Propafenone is metabolized by CYP2D6 (major pathway). Drugs that inhibit CYP2D6 can be expected to cause increased plasma levels of propafenone. Appropriate monitoring is recommended when propafenone is used together with such drugs).
No products indexed under this heading.

Meperidine Hydrochloride (Propafenone is an inhibitor of CYP2D6. Co-administration of propafenone with drugs metabolized by CYP2D6 might lead to increased plasma concentrations of these drugs).
No products indexed under this heading.

Mestranol (Propafenone is metabolized by CYP1A2. Drugs that inhibit CYP1A2 can be expected to cause increased plasma levels of propafenone. Appropriate monitoring is recommended when propafenone is used together with such drugs).
No products indexed under this heading.

Methadone Hydrochloride (Propafenone is metabolized by CYP2D6 (major pathway). Drugs that inhibit CYP2D6 can be expected to cause increased plasma levels of propafenone. Appropriate monitoring is recommended when propafenone is used together with such drugs).
No products indexed under this heading.

Methamphetamine Hydrochloride (Propafenone is an inhibitor of CYP2D6. Co-administration of propafenone with drugs metabolized by CYP2D6 might lead to increased plasma concentrations of these drugs).
No products indexed under this heading.

Methoxsalen (Propafenone is metabolized by CYP1A2. Drugs that inhibit CYP1A2 can be expected to cause increased plasma levels of propafenone. Appropriate monitoring is recommended when propafenone is used together with such drugs).
No products indexed under this heading.

Methoxyphenamine (Propafenone is an inhibitor of CYP2D6. Co-administration of propafenone with drugs metabolized by CYP2D6 might lead to increased plasma concentrations of these drugs).
No products indexed under this heading.

Metipranolol Hydrochloride (Concomitant use of propafenone and propranolol in healthy subjects increased propranolol plasma concentrations at steady state by 113%. In 4 patients, administration of metoprolol with propafenone increased the metoprolol plasma concentrations at steady state by 100% to 400%. The pharmacokinetics of propafenone was not affected by the co-administration of either propranolol or metoprolol. In clinical trials using propafenone immediate release tablets, patients who were receiving β-blockers concurrently did not experience an increased incidence of side effects).
No products indexed under this heading.

Metoprolol Succinate (In 4 patients, administration of metoprolol with propafenone increased the metoprolol plasma concentrations at steady state by 100% to 400%. The pharmacokinetics of propafenone was not affected by the co-administration of metoprolol. In clinical trials using propafenone immediate release tablets, patients who were receiving β-blockers concurrently did not experience an increased incidence of side effects). Products include:
Toprol XL 732

Metoprolol Tartrate (In 4 patients, administration of metoprolol with propafenone increased the metoprolol plasma concentrations at steady state by 100% to 400%. The pharmacokinetics of propafenone was not affected by the co-administration of metoprolol. In clinical trials using propafenone immediate release tablets, patients who were receiving β-blockers concurrently did not experience an increased incidence of side effects).
No products indexed under this heading.

Metronidazole (Propafenone is metabolized by CYP3A4. Drugs that inhibit CYP3A4 can be expected to cause increased plasma levels of propafenone. Appropriate monitoring is recommended when propafenone is used together with such drugs). Products include:
Pylera 793

Metronidazole Benzoate (Propafenone is metabolized by CYP3A4. Drugs that inhibit CYP3A4 can be expected to cause increased plasma levels of propafenone. Appropriate monitoring is recommended when propafenone is used together with such drugs).
No products indexed under this heading.

Metronidazole Hydrochloride (Propafenone is metabolized by CYP3A4. Drugs that inhibit CYP3A4 can be expected to cause increased plasma levels of propafenone. Appropriate monitoring is recommended when propafenone is used together with such drugs).
No products indexed under this heading.

Metronidazole Sodium (Propafenone is metabolized by CYP3A4. Drugs that inhibit CYP3A4 can be expected to cause increased plasma levels of propafenone. Appropriate monitoring is recommended when propafenone is used together with such drugs).
No products indexed under this heading.

Mexiletine Hydrochloride (Propafenone is metabolized by CYP1A2. Drugs that inhibit CYP1A2 can be expected to cause increased plasma levels of propafenone. Appropriate monitoring is recommended when propafenone is used together with such drugs).
No products indexed under this heading.

Mibefradil Dihydrochloride (Propafenone is metabolized by CYP2D6 (major pathway). Drugs that inhibit CYP2D6 can be expected to cause increased plasma levels of propafenone. Appropriate monitoring is recommended when propafenone is used together with such drugs).
No products indexed under this heading.

Miconazole (Propafenone is metabolized by CYP3A4. Drugs that inhibit CYP3A4 can be expected to cause increased plasma levels of propafenone. Appropriate monitoring is recommended when propafenone is used together with such drugs).
No products indexed under this heading.

Miconazole Nitrate (Propafenone is metabolized by CYP3A4. Drugs that inhibit CYP3A4 can be expected to cause increased plasma levels of propafenone. Appropriate monitoring is recommended when propafenone is used together with such drugs).
Products include:
Vusion Ointment 3335

Mifepristone (Propafenone is metabolized by CYP3A4. Drugs that inhibit CYP3A4 can be expected to cause increased plasma levels of propafenone. Appropriate monitoring is recommended when propafenone is used together with such drugs).
No products indexed under this heading.

Mirtazapine (Propafenone is an inhibitor of CYP2D6. Co-administration of propafenone with drugs metabolized by CYP2D6 might lead to increased plasma concentrations of these drugs).
Products include:
Remeron Tablets 3214
RemeronSolTab Tablets 3219

Moclobemide (Propafenone is metabolized by CYP2D6 (major pathway). Drugs that inhibit CYP2D6 can be expected to cause increased plasma levels of propafenone. Appropriate monitoring is recommended when propafenone is used together with such drugs).
No products indexed under this heading.

Morphine Sulfate (Propafenone is an inhibitor of CYP2D6. Co-administration of propafenone with drugs metabolized

by CYP2D6 might lead to increased plasma concentrations of these drugs). Products include:
Avinza 1822
Embeda 1831
MS Contin 2803

Moxifloxacin Hydrochloride (Propafenone is metabolized by CYP1A2. Drugs that inhibit CYP1A2 can be expected to cause increased plasma levels of propafenone. Appropriate monitoring is recommended when propafenone is used together with such drugs). Products include:
Avelox 3064
Vigamox 589

Nadolol (Concomitant use of propafenone and propranolol in healthy subjects increased propranolol plasma concentrations at steady state by 113%. In 4 patients, administration of metoprolol with propafenone increased the metoprolol plasma concentrations at steady state by 100% to 400%. The pharmacokinetics of propafenone was not affected by the co-administration of either propranolol or metoprolol. In clinical trials using propafenone immediate release tablets, patients who were receiving β-blockers concurrently did not experience an increased incidence of side effects. Products include:
Nadolol 2359

Nalidixic Acid (Propafenone is metabolized by CYP1A2. Drugs that inhibit CYP1A2 can be expected to cause increased plasma levels of propafenone. Appropriate monitoring is recommended when propafenone is used together with such drugs).
No products indexed under this heading.

Nebivolol (Concomitant use of propafenone and propranolol in healthy subjects increased propranolol plasma concentrations at steady state by 113%. In 4 patients, administration of metoprolol with propafenone increased the metoprolol plasma concentrations at steady state by 100% to 400%. The pharmacokinetics of propafenone was not affected by the co-administration of either propranolol or metoprolol. In clinical trials using propafenone immediate release tablets, patients who were receiving β-blockers concurrently did not experience an increased incidence of side effects). Products include:
Bystolic 1147

Nefazodone Hydrochloride (Propafenone is metabolized by CYP3A4. Drugs that inhibit CYP3A4 can be expected to cause increased plasma levels of propafenone. Appropriate monitoring is recommended when propafenone is used together with such drugs).
No products indexed under this heading.

Nelfinavir Mesylate (Propafenone is metabolized by CYP3A4. Drugs that inhibit CYP3A4 can be expected to cause increased plasma levels of propafenone. Appropriate monitoring is recommended when propafenone is used together with such drugs).
No products indexed under this heading.

Nevirapine (Propafenone is metabolized by CYP3A4. Drugs that inhibit CYP3A4 can be expected to cause increased plasma levels of propafenone. Appropriate monitoring is recommended when propafenone is used together with such drugs).
Products include:
Viramune Oral Suspension 897
Viramune Tablets 897

Niacin (Propafenone is metabolized by CYP3A4. Drugs that inhibit CYP3A4 can be expected to cause increased plasma levels of propafenone. Appropriate monitoring is recommended when propafenone is used together with such drugs). Products include:

Advicor 402
Cardio Basics 3455
Niaspan 497
Simcor 524

Niacinamide (Propafenone is metabolized by CYP3A4. Drugs that inhibit CYP3A4 can be expected to cause increased plasma levels of propafenone. Appropriate monitoring is recommended when propafenone is used together with such drugs).
Products include:
CitraNatal 90 DHA Capsules 2332
CitraNatal Assure 2332
CitraNatal Rx 2332
Heplive 607

Niacinamide Hydroiodide (Propafenone is metabolized by CYP3A4. Drugs that inhibit CYP3A4 can be expected to cause increased plasma levels of propafenone. Appropriate monitoring is recommended when propafenone is used together with such drugs).
No products indexed under this heading.

Nicotinamide (Propafenone is metabolized by CYP3A4. Drugs that inhibit CYP3A4 can be expected to cause increased plasma levels of propafenone. Appropriate monitoring is recommended when propafenone is used together with such drugs).
No products indexed under this heading.

Nifedipine (Propafenone is metabolized by CYP3A4. Drugs that inhibit CYP3A4 can be expected to cause increased plasma levels of propafenone. Appropriate monitoring is recommended when propafenone is used together with such drugs).
No products indexed under this heading.

Norethindrone (Propafenone is metabolized by CYP1A2. Drugs that inhibit CYP1A2 can be expected to cause increased plasma levels of propafenone. Appropriate monitoring is recommended when propafenone is used together with such drugs).
Products include:
Ortho Micronor 2660

Norethindrone Acetate (Propafenone is metabolized by CYP1A2. Drugs that inhibit CYP1A2 can be expected to cause increased plasma levels of propafenone. Appropriate monitoring is recommended when propafenone is used together with such drugs). Products include:
Activella 2561

Norfloxacin (Propafenone is metabolized by CYP1A2. Drugs that inhibit CYP1A2 can be expected to cause increased plasma levels of propafenone. Appropriate monitoring is recommended when propafenone is used together with such drugs).
Products include:
Noroxin 2220

Norgestrel (Propafenone is metabolized by CYP1A2. Drugs that inhibit CYP1A2 can be expected to cause increased plasma levels of propafenone. Appropriate monitoring is recommended when propafenone is used together with such drugs).
No products indexed under this heading.

Nortriptyline Hydrochloride (Propafenone is metabolized by CYP2D6 (major pathway). Drugs that inhibit CYP2D6 can be expected to cause increased plasma levels of propafenone. Appropriate monitoring is recommended when propafenone is used together with such drugs).
No products indexed under this heading.

Rythmol Interactions Index 1652

Ofloxacin (Propafenone is metabolized by CYP1A2. Drugs that inhibit CYP1A2 can be expected to cause increased plasma levels of propafenone. Appropriate monitoring is recommended when propafenone is used together with such drugs).
No products indexed under this heading.

Olanzapine (Propafenone is an inhibitor of CYP2D6. Co-administration of propafenone with drugs metabolized by CYP2D6 might lead to increased plasma concentrations of these drugs). Products include:
Symbyax 1965
Zyprexa 1984
Zyprexa IntraMuscular 1984
Zyprexa ZYDIS 1984

Omeprazole (Propafenone is metabolized by CYP1A2. Drugs that inhibit CYP1A2 can be expected to cause increased plasma levels of propafenone. Appropriate monitoring is recommended when propafenone is used together with such drugs).
No products indexed under this heading.

Omeprazole Magnesium (Propafenone is metabolized by CYP1A2. Drugs that inhibit CYP1A2 can be expected to cause increased plasma levels of propafenone. Appropriate monitoring is recommended when propafenone is used together with such drugs).
No products indexed under this heading.

Ondansetron (Propafenone is an inhibitor of CYP2D6. Co-administration of propafenone with drugs metabolized by CYP2D6 might lead to increased plasma concentrations of these drugs).
No products indexed under this heading.

Ondansetron Hydrochloride (Propafenone is an inhibitor of CYP2D6. Co-administration of propafenone with drugs metabolized by CYP2D6 might lead to increased plasma concentrations of these drugs). Products include:
Zofran Injection 1750
Zofran 1756
Zofran ODT 1756

Orlistat (Orlistat may limit the fraction of propafenone available for absorption. In post-marketing reports, abrupt cessation of orlistat in patients stabilized on propafenone has resulted in severe adverse events including convulsions, atrioventricular block and acute circulatory failure). Products include:
Xenical 2893

Oxycodone Hydrochloride (Propafenone is an inhibitor of CYP2D6. Co-administration of propafenone with drugs metabolized by CYP2D6 might lead to increased plasma concentrations of these drugs). Products include:
OxyContin 2807
Percocet 1121
Percodan 1124

Paclitaxel (Propafenone is an inhibitor of CYP2D6. Co-administration of propafenone with drugs metabolized by CYP2D6 might lead to increased plasma concentrations of these drugs).
No products indexed under this heading.

Paroxetine (Propafenone is metabolized by CYP2D6 (major pathway). Drugs that inhibit CYP2D6 (such as paroxetine), can be expected to cause increased plasma levels of propafenone. Appropriate monitoring is recommended when propafenone is used together with such drugs).
No products indexed under this heading.

Paroxetine Hydrochloride (Propafenone is metabolized by CYP2D6 (major pathway). Drugs that inhibit CYP2D6 (such as paroxetine), can be expected to cause increased plasma levels of propafenone. Appropriate monitoring is recommended when propafenone is used together with such drugs). Products include:
Paroxetine CR 2361
Paroxetine ER 2371
Paxil 1586
Paxil CR 1596

Paroxetine Mesylate (Propafenone is metabolized by CYP2D6 (major pathway). Drugs that inhibit CYP2D6 (such as paroxetine), can be expected to cause increased plasma levels of propafenone. Appropriate monitoring is recommended when propafenone is used together with such drugs).
No products indexed under this heading.

Penbutolol Sulfate (Concomitant use of propafenone and propranolol in healthy subjects increased propranolol plasma concentrations at steady state by 113%. In 4 patients, administration of metoprolol with propafenone increased the metoprolol plasma concentrations at steady state by 100% to 400%. The pharmacokinetics of propafenone was not affected by the co-administration of either propranolol or metoprolol. In clinical trials using propafenone immediate release tablets, patients who were receiving β-blockers concurrently did not experience an increased incidence of side effects).
No products indexed under this heading.

Perphenazine (Propafenone is metabolized by CYP2D6 (major pathway). Drugs that inhibit CYP2D6 can be expected to cause increased plasma levels of propafenone. Appropriate monitoring is recommended when propafenone is used together with such drugs).
No products indexed under this heading.

Pindolol (Concomitant use of propafenone and propranolol in healthy subjects increased propranolol plasma concentrations at steady state by 113%. In 4 patients, administration of metoprolol with propafenone increased the metoprolol plasma concentrations at steady state by 100% to 400%. The pharmacokinetics of propafenone was not affected by the co-administration of either propranolol or metoprolol. In clinical trials using propafenone immediate release tablets, patients who were receiving β-blockers concurrently did not experience an increased incidence of side effects).
No products indexed under this heading.

Posaconazole (Propafenone is metabolized by CYP3A4. Drugs that inhibit CYP3A4 can be expected to cause increased plasma levels of propafenone. Appropriate monitoring is recommended when propafenone is used together with such drugs). Products include:
Noxafil 3172

Propoxyphene Hydrochloride (Propafenone is metabolized by CYP2D6 (major pathway). Drugs that inhibit CYP2D6 can be expected to cause increased plasma levels of propafenone. Appropriate monitoring is recommended when propafenone is used together with such drugs).
No products indexed under this heading.

Propoxyphene Napsylate (Propafenone is metabolized by CYP2D6 (major pathway). Drugs that inhibit CYP2D6 can be expected to cause increased plasma levels of propafenone. Appropriate monitoring is recommended when propafenone is used together with such drugs).
No products indexed under this heading.

Propranolol (Concomitant use of propafenone and propranolol in healthy subjects increased propranolol plasma concentrations at steady state by 113%. The pharmacokinetics of propafenone was not affected by the co-administration of propranolol. In clinical trials using propafenone immediate release tablets, patients who were receiving β-blockers concurrently did not experience an increased incidence of side effects).
No products indexed under this heading.

Propranolol Hydrochloride (Concomitant use of propafenone and propranolol in healthy subjects increased propranolol plasma concentrations at steady state by 113%. The pharmacokinetics of propafenone was not affected by the co-administration of propranolol. In clinical trials using propafenone immediate release tablets, patients who were receiving β-blockers concurrently did not experience an increased incidence of side effects). Products include:
InnoPran XL 1517

Protriptyline Hydrochloride (Propafenone is metabolized by CYP2D6 (major pathway). Drugs that inhibit CYP2D6 can be expected to cause increased plasma levels of propafenone. Appropriate monitoring is recommended when propafenone is used together with such drugs).
No products indexed under this heading.

Quetiapine Fumarate (Propafenone is an inhibitor of CYP2D6. Co-administration of propafenone with drugs metabolized by CYP2D6 might lead to increased plasma concentrations of these drugs). Products include:
Seroquel 750
Seroquel XR 759

Quinacrine Hydrochloride (Propafenone is metabolized by CYP2D6 (major pathway). Drugs that inhibit CYP2D6 can be expected to cause increased plasma levels of propafenone. Appropriate monitoring is recommended when propafenone is used together with such drugs).
No products indexed under this heading.

Quinidine (Small doses of quinidine completely inhibit the CYP2D6 hydroxylation metabolic pathways, making all patients, in effect, slow metabolizers. Concomitant administration of quinidine (50 mg TID) with 150 mg immediate release propafenone TID decreased the clearance of propafenone by 60% in extensive metabolizers (EM), making them poor metabolizers (PM). Steady-state plasma concentrations increased by more than 2-fold for propafenone, and decreased 50% for 5-OH-propafenone. A 100 mg dose of quinidine increased steady-state concentrations of propafenone 3-fold. Concomitant use of propafenone and quinidine is not recommended).
No products indexed under this heading.

Quinidine Gluconate (Small doses of quinidine completely inhibit the CYP2D6 hydroxylation metabolic pathways, making all patients, in effect, slow metabolizers. Concomitant administration of quinidine (50 mg TID) with 150 mg immediate release propafenone TID decreased the clearance of propafenone by 60% in extensive metabolizers (EM), making them poor metabolizers (PM). Steady-state plasma concentrations increased by more than 2-fold for propafenone, and decreased 50% for 5-OH-propafenone. A 100 mg dose of quinidine increased steady-state concentrations of propafenone 3-fold. Concomitant use of propafenone and quinidine is not recommended).
No products indexed under this heading.

Quinidine Hydrochloride (Small doses of quinidine completely inhibit the CYP2D6 hydroxylation metabolic pathways, making all patients, in effect, slow metabolizers. Concomitant administration of quinidine (50 mg TID) with 150 mg immediate release propafenone TID decreased the clearance of propafenone by 60% in extensive metabolizers (EM), making them poor metabolizers (PM). Steady-state plasma concentrations increased by more than 2-fold for propafenone, and decreased 50% for 5-OH-propafenone. A 100 mg dose of quinidine increased steady-state concentrations of propafenone 3-fold. Concomitant use of propafenone and quinidine is not recommended).
No products indexed under this heading.

Quinidine Polygalacturonate (Small doses of quinidine completely inhibit the CYP2D6 hydroxylation metabolic pathways, making all patients, in effect, slow metabolizers. Concomitant administration of quinidine (50 mg TID) with 150 mg immediate release propafenone TID decreased the clearance of propafenone by 60% in extensive metabolizers (EM), making them poor metabolizers (PM). Steady-state plasma concentrations increased by more than 2-fold for propafenone, and decreased 50% for 5-OH-propafenone. A 100 mg dose of quinidine increased steady-state concentrations of propafenone 3-fold. Concomitant use of propafenone and quinidine is not recommended).
No products indexed under this heading.

Quinidine Sulfate (Small doses of quinidine completely inhibit the CYP2D6 hydroxylation metabolic pathways, making all patients, in effect, slow metabolizers. Concomitant administration of quinidine (50 mg TID) with 150 mg immediate release propafenone TID decreased the clearance of propafenone by 60% in extensive metabolizers (EM), making them poor metabolizers (PM). Steady-state plasma concentrations increased by more than 2-fold for propafenone, and decreased 50% for 5-OH-propafenone. A 100 mg dose of quinidine increased steady-state concentrations of propafenone 3-fold. Concomitant use of propafenone and quinidine is not recommended).
No products indexed under this heading.

Quinine (Propafenone is metabolized by CYP3A4. Drugs that inhibit CYP3A4 can be expected to cause increased plasma levels of propafenone. Appropriate monitoring is recommended when propafenone is used together with such drugs). Products include:
Hyland's Leg Cramps PM with Quinine 3315

Quinine Sulfate (Propafenone is metabolized by CYP3A4. Drugs that inhibit CYP3A4 can be expected to cause increased plasma levels of propafenone. Appropriate monitoring is recommended when propafenone is used together with such drugs).
No products indexed under this heading.

Quinupristin (Propafenone is metabolized by CYP3A4. Drugs that inhibit CYP3A4 can be expected to cause increased plasma levels of propafenone. Appropriate monitoring is recommended when propafenone is used together with such drugs).
No products indexed under this heading.

Ranitidine Bismuth Citrate (Propafenone is metabolized by CYP2D6 (major pathway). Drugs that inhibit CYP2D6 can be expected to cause increased plasma levels of propafenone. Appropriate monitoring is recommended when propafenone is used together with such drugs).
No products indexed under this heading.

Ranitidine Hydrochloride (Propafenone is metabolized by CYP2D6 (major pathway). Drugs that inhibit CYP2D6 can be expected to cause increased plasma levels of propafenone. Appropriate monitoring is recommended when propafenone is used together with such drugs). Products include:
Zantac 1737
Zantac Injection 1732
Zantac Pharmacy 1735

Rifampin (Concomitant administration of rifampin and propafenone in extensive metabolizers decreased the plasma concentrations of propafenone by 67% with a corresponding decrease of 5OH-propafenone by 65%. The concentrations of norpropafenone increased by 30%. In poor metabolizers, there was a 50% decrease in propafenone plasma concentrations and an increase in the AUC and C_{max} of norpropafenone by 74% and 20%, respectively. Urinary excretion of propafenone and its metabolites decreased significantly. Similar results were noted in elderly patients: both the AUC and C_{max} of propafenone decreased by 84%, with a corresponding decrease in AUC and C_{max} of 5OH-propafenone by 69% and 57%).
No products indexed under this heading.

Risperidone (Propafenone is an inhibitor of CYP2D6. Co-administration of propafenone with drugs metabolized by CYP2D6 might lead to increased plasma concentrations of these drugs). Products include:
Risperdal Consta 2682

Ritonavir (Propafenone is metabolized by CYP2D6 (major pathway) and CYP3A4. Drugs that inhibit CYP2D6 and CYP3A4 (such as ritonavir) can be expected to cause increased plasma levels of propafenone. Appropriate monitoring is recommended when propafenone is used together with such drugs). Products include:
Kaletra 458
Norvir 509

Saquinavir (Propafenone is metabolized by CYP3A4. Drugs that inhibit CYP3A4 (such as saquinavir) can be expected to cause increased plasma levels of propafenone. Appropriate monitoring is recommended when propafenone is used together with such drugs).
No products indexed under this heading.

Saquinavir Mesylate (Propafenone is metabolized by CYP3A4. Drugs that inhibit CYP3A4 (such as saquinavir) can be expected to cause increased plasma levels of propafenone. Appropriate monitoring is recommended when propafenone is used together with such drugs).
No products indexed under this heading.

Sertraline Hydrochloride (Propafenone is metabolized by CYP2D6 (major pathway). Drugs that inhibit CYP2D6 (such as sertaline) can be expected to cause increased plasma levels of propafenone. Appropriate monitoring is recommended when propafenone is used together with such drugs).
No products indexed under this heading.

Sildenafil Citrate (Propafenone is metabolized by CYP2D6 (major pathway). Drugs that inhibit CYP2D6 can be expected to cause increased plasma levels of propafenone. Appropriate monitoring is recommended when propafenone is used together with such drugs).
No products indexed under this heading.

Sotalol Hydrochloride (Concomitant use of propafenone and propranolol in healthy subjects increased propranolol plasma concentrations at steady state by 113%. In 4 patients, administration of metoprolol with propafenone increased the metoprolol plasma concentrations at steady state by 100% to 400%. The pharmacokinetics of propafenone was not affected by the co-administration of either propranolol or metoprolol. In clinical trials using propafenone immediate release tablets, patients who were receiving β-blockers concurrently did not experience an increased incidence of side effects).
No products indexed under this heading.

Sparfloxacin (Propafenone is metabolized by CYP1A2. Drugs that inhibit CYP1A2 can be expected to cause increased plasma levels of propafenone. Appropriate monitoring is recommended when propafenone is used together with such drugs).
No products indexed under this heading.

Tacrine Hydrochloride (Propafenone is metabolized by CYP1A2. Drugs that inhibit CYP1A2 can be expected to cause increased plasma levels of propafenone. Appropriate monitoring is recommended when propafenone is used together with such drugs).
No products indexed under this heading.

Tamoxifen Citrate (Propafenone is an inhibitor of CYP2D6. Co-administration of propafenone with drugs metabolized by CYP2D6 might lead to increased plasma concentrations of these drugs).
No products indexed under this heading.

Telithromycin (Propafenone is metabolized by CYP3A4. Drugs that inhibit CYP3A4 can be expected to cause increased plasma levels of propafenone. Appropriate monitoring is recommended when propafenone is used together with such drugs). Products include:
Ketek 2991

Teniposide (Propafenone is an inhibitor of CYP2D6. Co-administration of propafenone with drugs metabolized by CYP2D6 might lead to increased plasma concentrations of these drugs).
No products indexed under this heading.

Terbinafine Hydrochloride (Propafenone is metabolized by CYP2D6 (major pathway). Drugs that inhibit CYP2D6 can be expected to cause increased plasma levels of propafenone. Appropriate monitoring is recommended when propafenone is used together with such drugs).
No products indexed under this heading.

Testosterone (Propafenone is an inhibitor of CYP2D6. Co-administration of propafenone with drugs metabolized by CYP2D6 might lead to increased plasma concentrations of these drugs). Products include:
AndroGel 3456

Testosterone Cypionate (Propafenone is an inhibitor of CYP2D6. Co-administration of propafenone with drugs metabolized by CYP2D6 might lead to increased plasma concentrations of these drugs).
No products indexed under this heading.

Testosterone Enanthate (Propafenone is an inhibitor of CYP2D6. Co-administration of propafenone with drugs metabolized by CYP2D6 might lead to increased plasma concentrations of these drugs). Products include:
Delatestryl 1102

Testosterone Propionate (Propafenone is an inhibitor of CYP2D6. Co-administration of propafenone with drugs metabolized by CYP2D6 might lead to increased plasma concentrations of these drugs).
No products indexed under this heading.

Thioridazine (Propafenone is an inhibitor of CYP2D6. Co-administration of propafenone with drugs metabolized by CYP2D6 might lead to increased plasma concentrations of these drugs).
No products indexed under this heading.

Thioridazine Hydrochloride (Propafenone is metabolized by CYP2D6 (major pathway). Drugs that inhibit CYP2D6 can be expected to cause increased plasma levels of propafenone. Appropriate monitoring is recommended when propafenone is used together with such drugs). Products include:
Thioridazine Hydrochloride 2384

Ticlopidine Hydrochloride (Propafenone is metabolized by CYP1A2. Drugs that inhibit CYP1A2 can be expected to cause increased plasma levels of propafenone. Appropriate monitoring is recommended when propafenone is used together with such drugs).
No products indexed under this heading.

Timolol Hemihydrate (Concomitant use of propafenone and propranolol in healthy subjects increased propranolol plasma concentrations at steady state by 113%. In 4 patients, administration of metoprolol with propafenone increased the metoprolol plasma concentrations at steady state by 100% to 400%. The pharmacokinetics of propafenone was not affected by the co-administration of either propranolol or metoprolol. In clinical trials using propafenone immediate release tablets, patients who were receiving β-blockers concurrently did not experience an increased incidence of side effects). Products include:
Betimol 3490

Timolol Maleate (Concomitant use of propafenone and propranolol in healthy subjects increased propranolol plasma concentrations at steady state by 113%. In 4 patients, administration of metoprolol with propafenone increased the metoprolol plasma concentrations at steady state by 100% to 400%. The pharmacokinetics of propafenone was not affected by the co-administration of either propranolol or metoprolol. In clinical trials using propafenone immediate release tablets, patients who were receiving β-blockers concurrently did not experience an increased incidence of side effects). Products include:
Combigan 601
Dorzolamide Hydrochloride/Timolol Maleate Ophthalmic Solution .... ⊙ 243
Timoptic in Ocudose .... ⊙ 231

Tolterodine Tartrate (Propafenone is an inhibitor of CYP2D6. Co-administration of propafenone with drugs metabolized by CYP2D6 might lead to increased plasma concentrations of these drugs).
No products indexed under this heading.

Tramadol Hydrochloride (Propafenone is an inhibitor of CYP2D6. Co-administration of propafenone with drugs metabolized by CYP2D6 might lead to increased plasma concentrations of these drugs). Products include:
Ryzolt 2813
Ultram ER 2693

Trazodone Hydrochloride (Propafenone is an inhibitor of CYP2D6. Co-administration of propafenone with drugs metabolized by CYP2D6 might lead to increased plasma concentrations of these drugs).
No products indexed under this heading.

Triazolam (Propafenone is an inhibitor of CYP2D6. Co-administration of propafenone with drugs metabolized by CYP2D6 might lead to increased plasma concentrations of these drugs).
No products indexed under this heading.

Trimipramine Maleate (Propafenone is metabolized by CYP2D6 (major pathway). Drugs that inhibit CYP2D6 can be expected to cause increased plasma levels of propafenone. Appropriate monitoring is recommended when propafenone is used together with such drugs).
No products indexed under this heading.

Troglitazone (Propafenone is metabolized by CYP3A4. Drugs that inhibit CYP3A4 can be expected to cause increased plasma levels of propafenone. Appropriate monitoring is recommended when propafenone is used together with such drugs).
No products indexed under this heading.

Troleandomycin (Propafenone is metabolized by CYP1A2. Drugs that inhibit CYP1A2 can be expected to cause increased plasma levels of propafenone. Appropriate monitoring is recommended when propafenone is used together with such drugs).
No products indexed under this heading.

Trovafloxacin Mesylate (Propafenone is metabolized by CYP1A2. Drugs that inhibit CYP1A2 can be expected to cause increased plasma levels of propafenone. Appropriate monitoring is recommended when propafenone is used together with such drugs).
No products indexed under this heading.

Valproate Sodium (Propafenone is metabolized by CYP3A4. Drugs that inhibit CYP3A4 can be expected to cause increased plasma levels of propafenone. Appropriate monitoring is recommended when propafenone is used together with such drugs).
No products indexed under this heading.

Vardenafil Hydrochloride (Propafenone is metabolized by CYP2D6 (major pathway). Drugs that inhibit CYP2D6 can be expected to cause increased plasma levels of propafenone. Appropriate monitoring is recommended when propafenone is used together with such drugs). Products include:
Levitra 3157

Venlafaxine Hydrochloride (Propafenone is an inhibitor of CYP2D6. Co-administration of propafenone with drugs metabolized by CYP2D6 (such as venlafaxine) might lead to increased plasma levels of venlafaxine). Products include:
Effexor XR 3504
Venlafaxine Hydrochloride Tablets ... 2388

Verapamil Hydrochloride (Propafenone is metabolized by CYP3A4. Drugs that inhibit CYP3A4 can be expected to cause increased plasma levels of propafenone. Appropriate monitoring is recommended when propafenone is used together with such drugs). Products include:
Tarka 534

Vinblastine Sulfate (Propafenone is an inhibitor of CYP2D6. Co-administration of propafenone with drugs metabolized by CYP2D6 might lead to increased plasma concentrations of these drugs).
No products indexed under this heading.

Voriconazole (Propafenone is metabolized by CYP3A4. Drugs that inhibit CYP3A4 can be expected to cause increased plasma levels of propafenone. Appropriate monitoring is recommended when propafenone is used together with such drugs).
No products indexed under this heading.

Warfarin Sodium (The concomitant administration of propafenone and warfarin increased warfarin plasma concentrations at steady state by 39% in healthy volunteers and prolonged the prothrombin time in patients taking warfarin. Adjustment of the warfarin dose should be guided by monitoring prothrombin time).
No products indexed under this heading.

Zafirlukast (Propafenone is metabolized by CYP3A4. Drugs that inhibit CYP3A4 can be expected to cause increased plasma levels of propafenone. Appropriate monitoring is recommended when propafenone is used together with such drugs). Products include:
Accolate 3612

IMPORTANT NOTE: Always consult each drug listing in the patient's regimen for possible interactions.

Rythmol Interactions Index 1654

Zileuton (Propafenone is metabolized by CYP1A2. Drugs that inhibit CYP1A2 can be expected to cause increased plasma levels of propafenone. Appropriate monitoring is recommended when propafenone is used together with such drugs).
No products indexed under this heading.

Zonisamide (Propafenone is an inhibitor of CYP2D6. Co-administration of propafenone with drugs metabolized by CYP2D6 might lead to increased plasma concentrations of these drugs). Products include:
Zonegran 1081

Food Interactions

Grapefruit (Propafenone is metabolized by CYP1A2. Drugs that inhibit CYP1A2 can be expected to cause increased plasma levels of propafenone. Appropriate monitoring is recommended when propafenone is used together with such drugs).

Grapefruit Juice (Propafenone is metabolized by CYP3A4. Agents that inhibit CYP3A4 (such as grapefruit juice), can be expected to cause increased plasma levels of propafenone. Appropriate monitoring is recommended when propafenone is used together with such agents).

RYTHMOL SR EXTENDED RELEASE CAPSULES
(Propafenone Hydrochloride) 1652
May interact with cardiac glycosides, class 1A antiarrhythmics, class III antiarrhythmics, cytochrome p450 1a2 inhibitors (selected), cytochrome p450 2d6 inhibitors (selected), cytochrome p450 3a4 inhibitors (selected), drugs that prolong the QT interval, local anesthetics, macrolide antibiotics, phenothiazines, quinidine, tricyclic antidepressants, and certain other agents. Compounds in these categories include:

Acetazolamide (Drugs that inhibit CYP3A4 might lead to increased plasma levels of propafenone; patients should be closely monitored and the propafenone dose adjusted accordingly).
No products indexed under this heading.

Acetazolamide Sodium (Drugs that inhibit CYP3A4 might lead to increased plasma levels of propafenone; patients should be closely monitored and the propafenone dose adjusted accordingly).
No products indexed under this heading.

Alatrofloxacin Mesylate (Drugs that inhibit CYP1A2 might lead to increased plasma levels of propafenone; patients should be closely monitored and the propafenone dose adjusted accordingly).
No products indexed under this heading.

Alprazolam (The use of propafenone in conjunction with other drugs that prolong the QT interval has not been extensively studied and is not recommended).
No products indexed under this heading.

Amiodarone Hydrochloride (The use of propafenone in conjunction with other drugs that prolong the QT interval has not been extensively studied and is not recommended).
No products indexed under this heading.

Amitriptyline Hydrochloride (The use of propafenone in conjunction with other drugs that prolong the QT interval has not been extensively studied and is not recommended).
No products indexed under this heading.

Amoxapine (The use of propafenone in conjunction with other drugs that prolong the QT interval has not been extensively studied and is not recommended).
No products indexed under this heading.

Amprenavir (Drugs that inhibit CYP3A4 might lead to increased plasma levels of propafenone; patients should be closely monitored and the propafenone dose adjusted accordingly).
No products indexed under this heading.

Anastrozole (Drugs that inhibit CYP1A2 might lead to increased plasma levels of propafenone; patients should be closely monitored and the propafenone dose adjusted accordingly).
No products indexed under this heading.

Aprepitant (Drugs that inhibit CYP3A4 might lead to increased plasma levels of propafenone; patients should be closely monitored and the propafenone dose adjusted accordingly). Products include:
Emend 2124

Articaine Hydrochloride (Concomitant use of local anesthetics may increase the risk of CNS side effects).
No products indexed under this heading.

Astemizole (The use of propafenone in conjunction with other drugs that prolong the QT interval has not been extensively studied and is not recommended).
No products indexed under this heading.

Atazanavir (Drugs that inhibit CYP3A4 might lead to increased plasma levels of propafenone; patients should be closely monitored and the propafenone dose adjusted accordingly).
No products indexed under this heading.

Atazanavir Sulfate (Drugs that inhibit CYP3A4 might lead to increased plasma levels of propafenone; patients should be closely monitored and the propafenone dose adjusted accordingly).
No products indexed under this heading.

Azithromycin Dihydrate (The use of propafenone in conjunction with other drugs that prolong the QT interval has not been extensively studied and is not recommended).
No products indexed under this heading.

Bepridil Hydrochloride (The use of propafenone in conjunction with other drugs that prolong the QT interval has not been extensively studied and is not recommended).
No products indexed under this heading.

Bretylium Tosylate (The use of propafenone in conjunction with other drugs that prolong the QT interval has not been extensively studied and is not recommended).
No products indexed under this heading.

Bupivacaine Hydrochloride (Concomitant use of local anesthetics may increase the risk of CNS side effects).
No products indexed under this heading.

Bupropion Hydrochloride (Drugs that inhibit CYP2D6 might lead to increased plasma levels of propafenone; patients should be closely monitored and the propafenone dose adjusted accordingly). Products include:
Aplenzin 2948
Wellbutrin 1719
Wellbutrin SR 1725
Zyban 1762

Buspirone Hydrochloride (The use of propafenone in conjunction with other drugs that prolong the QT interval has not been extensively studied and is not recommended).
No products indexed under this heading.

Celecoxib (Drugs that inhibit CYP2D6 might lead to increased plasma levels of propafenone; patients should be closely monitored and the propafenone dose adjusted accordingly). Products include:
Celebrex 3272

Chlordiazepoxide (The use of propafenone in conjunction with other drugs that prolong the QT interval has not been extensively studied and is not recommended).
No products indexed under this heading.

Chlordiazepoxide Hydrochloride (The use of propafenone in conjunction with other drugs that prolong the QT interval has not been extensively studied and is not recommended).
No products indexed under this heading.

Chloroprocaine Hydrochloride (Concomitant use of local anesthetics may increase the risk of CNS side effects).
No products indexed under this heading.

Chloroquine (Drugs that inhibit CYP2D6 might lead to increased plasma levels of propafenone; patients should be closely monitored and the propafenone dose adjusted accordingly).
No products indexed under this heading.

Chloroquine Hydrochloride (Drugs that inhibit CYP2D6 might lead to increased plasma levels of propafenone; patients should be closely monitored and the propafenone dose adjusted accordingly).
No products indexed under this heading.

Chloroquine Phosphate (Drugs that inhibit CYP2D6 might lead to increased plasma levels of propafenone; patients should be closely monitored and the propafenone dose adjusted accordingly).
No products indexed under this heading.

Chlorpheniramine (Drugs that inhibit CYP2D6 might lead to increased plasma levels of propafenone; patients should be closely monitored and the propafenone dose adjusted accordingly).
No products indexed under this heading.

Chlorpheniramine Maleate (Drugs that inhibit CYP2D6 might lead to increased plasma levels of propafenone; patients should be closely monitored and the propafenone dose adjusted accordingly).
No products indexed under this heading.

Chlorpheniramine Polistirex (Drugs that inhibit CYP2D6 might lead to increased plasma levels of propafenone; patients should be closely monitored and the propafenone dose adjusted accordingly). Products include:
Tussionex 3443

Chlorpheniramine Tannate (Drugs that inhibit CYP2D6 might lead to increased plasma levels of propafenone; patients should be closely monitored and the propafenone dose adjusted accordingly).
No products indexed under this heading.

Chlorpromazine (The use of propafenone in conjunction with other drugs that prolong the QT interval has not been extensively studied and is not recommended).
No products indexed under this heading.

Chlorpromazine Hydrochloride (The use of propafenone in conjunction with other drugs that prolong the QT interval has not been extensively studied and is not recommended).
No products indexed under this heading.

Chlorprothixene (The use of propafenone in conjunction with other drugs that prolong the QT interval has not been extensively studied and is not recommended).
No products indexed under this heading.

Chlorprothixene Hydrochloride (The use of propafenone in conjunction with other drugs that prolong the QT interval has not been extensively studied and is not recommended).
No products indexed under this heading.

Cimetidine (Increases steady-state plasma concentrations with no detectable changes in electrocardiographic parameters).
No products indexed under this heading.

Cimetidine Hydrochloride (Increases steady-state plasma concentrations with no detectable changes in electrocardiographic parameters).
No products indexed under this heading.

Ciprofloxacin (Drugs that inhibit CYP1A2 might lead to increased plasma levels of propafenone; patients should be closely monitored and the propafenone dose adjusted accordingly). Products include:
Cipro I.V. 3082
Cipro 3073
Cipro XR 3091
Ciprodex 583

Ciprofloxacin Hydrochloride (Drugs that inhibit CYP1A2 might lead to increased plasma levels of propafenone; patients should be closely monitored and the propafenone dose adjusted accordingly). Products include:
Cipro 3073

Cisapride (The use of propafenone in conjunction with other drugs that prolong the QT interval has not been extensively studied and is not recommended).
No products indexed under this heading.

Citalopram Hydrobromide (Drugs that inhibit CYP2D6 might lead to increased plasma levels of propafenone; patients should be closely monitored and the propafenone dose adjusted accordingly). Products include:
Celexa 1153

Clarithromycin (The use of propafenone in conjunction with other drugs that prolong the QT interval has not been extensively studied and is not recommended). Products include:
Biaxin/Biaxin XL 412

Clomipramine Hydrochloride (The use of propafenone in conjunction with other drugs that prolong the QT interval has not been extensively studied and is not recommended).
No products indexed under this heading.

Clorazepate Dipotassium (The use of propafenone in conjunction with other drugs that prolong the QT interval has not been extensively studied and is not recommended).
No products indexed under this heading.

Clotrimazole (Drugs that inhibit CYP3A4 might lead to increased plasma levels of propafenone; patients should be closely monitored and the propafenone dose adjusted accordingly). Products include:
Lotrisone 3163

Clozapine (The use of propafenone in conjunction with other drugs that prolong the QT interval has not been extensively studied and is not recommended).
No products indexed under this heading.

Cocaine Hydrochloride (Concomitant use of local anesthetics may increase the risk of CNS side effects).
No products indexed under this heading.

Conivaptan Hydrochloride (Drugs that inhibit CYP3A4 might lead to increased plasma levels of propafenone; patients should be closely monitored and the propafenone dose adjusted accordingly). Products include:
Vaprisol 689

Cyclosporine (Drugs that inhibit CYP3A4 might lead to increased plas-

ma levels of propafenone; patients should be closely monitored and the propafenone dose adjusted accordingly). Products include:

Gengraf	440
Neoral Oral Solution	2496
Neoral Capsules	2496
Restasis	605

Dalfopristin (Drugs that inhibit CYP3A4 might lead to increased plasma levels of propafenone; patients should be closely monitored and the propafenone dose adjusted accordingly).

No products indexed under this heading.

Danazol (Drugs that inhibit CYP3A4 might lead to increased plasma levels of propafenone; patients should be closely monitored and the propafenone dose adjusted accordingly).

No products indexed under this heading.

Darunavir (Drugs that inhibit CYP3A4 might lead to increased plasma levels of propafenone; patients should be closely monitored and the propafenone dose adjusted accordingly).

No products indexed under this heading.

Dasatinib (Drugs that inhibit CYP3A4 might lead to increased plasma levels of propafenone; patients should be closely monitored and the propafenone dose adjusted accordingly).

No products indexed under this heading.

Delavirdine Mesylate (Drugs that inhibit CYP3A4 might lead to increased plasma levels of propafenone; patients should be closely monitored and the propafenone dose adjusted accordingly).

No products indexed under this heading.

Delavirine (Drugs that inhibit CYP3A4 might lead to increased plasma levels of propafenone; patients should be closely monitored and the propafenone dose adjusted accordingly).

No products indexed under this heading.

Desipramine Hydrochloride (Co-administration may result in elevated serum desipramine levels).

No products indexed under this heading.

Deslanoside (Potential for elevated digoxin levels; dosage reduction of digitalis may be necessary).

No products indexed under this heading.

Desloratadine (Drugs that inhibit CYP3A4 might lead to increased plasma levels of propafenone; patients should be closely monitored and the propafenone dose adjusted accordingly). Products include:

Clarinex Syrup	3098
Clarinex	3098
Clarinex Reditabs	3098
Clarinex-D 12-Hour	3101
Clarinex-D	3104

Desogestrel (Drugs that inhibit CYP1A2 might lead to increased plasma levels of propafenone; patients should be closely monitored and the propafenone dose adjusted accordingly).

No products indexed under this heading.

Diazepam (The use of propafenone in conjunction with other drugs that prolong the QT interval has not been extensively studied and is not recommended). Products include:

Valium Tablets	2880

Digitalis Glycoside Preparations (Potential for elevated digoxin levels; dosage reduction of digitalis may be necessary).

No products indexed under this heading.

Digitalis Lanata (Potential for elevated digoxin levels; dosage reduction of digitalis may be necessary).

No products indexed under this heading.

Digitalis Purpurea (Potential for elevated digoxin levels; dosage reduction of digitalis may be necessary).

No products indexed under this heading.

Digitoxin (Potential for elevated digoxin levels; dosage reduction of digitalis may be necessary).

No products indexed under this heading.

Digoxin (Potential for elevated digoxin levels; dosage reduction of digitalis may be necessary). Products include:

Lanoxin Injection	1546
Lanoxin Injection Pediatric	1549
Lanoxin Tablets	1553

Diltiazem Hydrochloride (Drugs that inhibit CYP3A4 might lead to increased plasma levels of propafenone; patients should be closely monitored and the propafenone dose adjusted accordingly). Products include:

Cardizem LA	423

Diltiazem Maleate (Drugs that inhibit CYP3A4 might lead to increased plasma levels of propafenone; patients should be closely monitored and the propafenone dose adjusted accordingly).

No products indexed under this heading.

Diphenhydramine (Drugs that inhibit CYP2D6 might lead to increased plasma levels of propafenone; patients should be closely monitored and the propafenone dose adjusted accordingly).

No products indexed under this heading.

Diphenhydramine Hydrochloride (Drugs that inhibit CYP2D6 might lead to increased plasma levels of propafenone; patients should be closely monitored and the propafenone dose adjusted accordingly). Products include:

Benadryl Allergy Ultratab	2042
Children's Benadryl Allergy Liquid	2042

Dirithromycin (The use of propafenone in conjunction with other drugs that prolong the QT interval has not been extensively studied and is not recommended).

No products indexed under this heading.

Disopyramide (The use of propafenone in conjunction with other drugs that prolong the QT interval has not been extensively studied and is not recommended).

No products indexed under this heading.

Disopyramide Phosphate (The use of propafenone in conjunction with other drugs that prolong the QT interval has not been extensively studied and is not recommended).

No products indexed under this heading.

Dofetilide (The use of propafenone in conjunction with other drugs that prolong the QT interval has not been extensively studied and is not recommended).

No products indexed under this heading.

Doxepin Hydrochloride (The use of propafenone in conjunction with other drugs that prolong the QT interval has not been extensively studied and is not recommended).

No products indexed under this heading.

Droperidol (The use of propafenone in conjunction with other drugs that prolong the QT interval has not been extensively studied and is not recommended).

No products indexed under this heading.

Efavirenz (Drugs that inhibit CYP3A4 might lead to increased plasma levels of propafenone; patients should be closely monitored and the propafenone dose adjusted accordingly). Products include:

Atripla	906

Enoxacin (Drugs that inhibit CYP1A2 might lead to increased plasma levels of propafenone; patients should be closely monitored and the propafenone dose adjusted accordingly).

No products indexed under this heading.

Erythromycin (The use of propafenone in conjunction with other drugs that prolong the QT interval has not been extensively studied and is not recommended).

No products indexed under this heading.

Erythromycin Estolate (The use of propafenone in conjunction with other drugs that prolong the QT interval has not been extensively studied and is not recommended).

No products indexed under this heading.

Erythromycin Ethylsuccinate (The use of propafenone in conjunction with other drugs that prolong the QT interval has not been extensively studied and is not recommended). Products include:

E.E.S.	437
EryPed	435

Erythromycin Gluceptate (The use of propafenone in conjunction with other drugs that prolong the QT interval has not been extensively studied and is not recommended).

No products indexed under this heading.

Erythromycin Lactobionate (The use of propafenone in conjunction with other drugs that prolong the QT interval has not been extensively studied and is not recommended).

No products indexed under this heading.

Erythromycin Stearate (The use of propafenone in conjunction with other drugs that prolong the QT interval has not been extensively studied and is not recommended).

No products indexed under this heading.

Escitalopram Oxalate (Drugs that inhibit CYP2D6 might lead to increased plasma levels of propafenone; patients should be closely monitored and the propafenone dose adjusted accordingly). Products include:

Lexapro Oral Suspension	1160
Lexapro Tablets	1160

Esomeprazole Magnesium (Drugs that inhibit CYP1A2 might lead to increased plasma levels of propafenone; patients should be closely monitored and the propafenone dose adjusted accordingly). Products include:

Nexium Capsules	704
Nexium Oral Suspension	704

Esomeprazole Sodium (Drugs that inhibit CYP1A2 might lead to increased plasma levels of propafenone; patients should be closely monitored and the propafenone dose adjusted accordingly). Products include:

Nexium I.V.	712

Ethinyl Estradiol (Drugs that inhibit CYP1A2 might lead to increased plasma levels of propafenone; patients should be closely monitored and the propafenone dose adjusted accordingly). Products include:

LoSeasonique	3407
Lybrel	3514
NuvaRing	3181
Ortho Evra	2648
Ortho-Cyclen/Ortho Tri-Cyclen	2663
Ortho Tri-Cyclen Lo Tablets	2673
Seasonique	3418
Yaz	864

Etidocaine Hydrochloride (Concomitant use of local anesthetics may increase the risk of CNS side effects).

No products indexed under this heading.

Flecainide Acetate (The use of propafenone in conjunction with other drugs that prolong the QT interval has not been extensively studied and is not recommended).

No products indexed under this heading.

Fluconazole (Drugs that inhibit CYP3A4 might lead to increased plasma levels of propafenone; patients should be closely monitored and the propafenone dose adjusted accordingly).

No products indexed under this heading.

Fluoxetine (Drugs that inhibit CYP2D6 might lead to increased plasma levels of propafenone; patients should be closely monitored and the propafenone dose adjusted accordingly).

No products indexed under this heading.

Fluoxetine Hydrochloride (Drugs that inhibit CYP2D6 might lead to increased plasma levels of propafenone; patients should be closely monitored and the propafenone dose adjusted accordingly). Products include:

Prozac Weekly	1941
Prozac Pulvules	1941
Symbyax	1965

Fluphenazine Decanoate (The use of propafenone in conjunction with other drugs that prolong the QT interval has not been extensively studied and is not recommended).

No products indexed under this heading.

Fluphenazine Enanthate (The use of propafenone in conjunction with other drugs that prolong the QT interval has not been extensively studied and is not recommended).

No products indexed under this heading.

Fluphenazine Hydrochloride (The use of propafenone in conjunction with other drugs that prolong the QT interval has not been extensively studied and is not recommended).

No products indexed under this heading.

Fluvoxamine (Drugs that inhibit CYP1A2 might lead to increased plasma levels of propafenone; patients should be closely monitored and the propafenone dose adjusted accordingly).

No products indexed under this heading.

Fluvoxamine Maleate (Drugs that inhibit CYP2D6 might lead to increased plasma levels of propafenone; patients should be closely monitored and the propafenone dose adjusted accordingly).

No products indexed under this heading.

Fosamprenavir Calcium (Drugs that inhibit CYP3A4 might lead to increased plasma levels of propafenone; patients should be closely monitored and the propafenone dose adjusted accordingly). Products include:

Lexiva Oral Suspension	1558
Lexiva	1558

Gatifloxacin (Drugs that inhibit CYP1A2 might lead to increased plasma levels of propafenone; patients should be closely monitored and the propafenone dose adjusted accordingly).

No products indexed under this heading.

Gemifloxacin Mesylate (Drugs that inhibit CYP1A2 might lead to increased plasma levels of propafenone; patients should be closely monitored and the propafenone dose adjusted accordingly).

No products indexed under this heading.

Grepafloxacin Hydrochloride (Drugs that inhibit CYP1A2 might lead to increased plasma levels of propafenone; patients should be closely monitored and the propafenone dose adjusted accordingly).

No products indexed under this heading.

Halofantrine Hydrochloride (Drugs that inhibit CYP2D6 might lead to increased plasma levels of propafenone; patients should be closely monitored and the propafenone dose adjusted accordingly).

No products indexed under this heading.

IMPORTANT NOTE: Always consult each drug listing in the patient's regimen for possible interactions.

Rythmol SR Interactions Index 1656

Haloperidol (The use of propafenone in conjunction with other drugs that prolong the QT interval has not been extensively studied and is not recommended).
No products indexed under this heading.

Haloperidol Decanoate (The use of propafenone in conjunction with other drugs that prolong the QT interval has not been extensively studied and is not recommended).
No products indexed under this heading.

Haloperidol Lactate (The use of propafenone in conjunction with other drugs that prolong the QT interval has not been extensively studied and is not recommended).
No products indexed under this heading.

Hydroxychloroquine Sulfate (Drugs that inhibit CYP2D6 might lead to increased plasma levels of propafenone; patients should be closely monitored and the propafenone dose adjusted accordingly).
No products indexed under this heading.

Hydroxyzine Hydrochloride (The use of propafenone in conjunction with other drugs that prolong the QT interval has not been extensively studied and is not recommended).
No products indexed under this heading.

Imatinib Mesylate (Drugs that inhibit CYP2D6 might lead to increased plasma levels of propafenone; patients should be closely monitored and the propafenone dose adjusted accordingly). Products include:
Gleevec 2477

Imipramine Hydrochloride (The use of propafenone in conjunction with other drugs that prolong the QT interval has not been extensively studied and is not recommended).
No products indexed under this heading.

Imipramine Pamoate (The use of propafenone in conjunction with other drugs that prolong the QT interval has not been extensively studied and is not recommended).
No products indexed under this heading.

Indinavir Sulfate (Drugs that inhibit CYP3A4 might lead to increased plasma levels of propafenone; patients should be closely monitored and the propafenone dose adjusted accordingly). Products include:
Crixivan 2113

Isocarboxazid (The use of propafenone in conjunction with other drugs that prolong the QT interval has not been extensively studied and is not recommended). Products include:
Marplan 3481

Isoniazid (Drugs that inhibit CYP1A2 might lead to increased plasma levels of propafenone; patients should be closely monitored and the propafenone dose adjusted accordingly).
No products indexed under this heading.

Itraconazole (Drugs that inhibit CYP3A4 might lead to increased plasma levels of propafenone; patients should be closely monitored and the propafenone dose adjusted accordingly).
No products indexed under this heading.

Ketoconazole (Drugs that inhibit CYP1A2 might lead to increased plasma levels of propafenone; patients should be closely monitored and the propafenone dose adjusted accordingly). Products include:
Extina 3319
Xolegel 3337

Lapatinib (Drugs that inhibit CYP3A4 might lead to increased plasma levels of propafenone; patients should be closely monitored and the propafenone dose adjusted accordingly). Products include:
Tykerb 1698

Levobupivacaine Hydrochloride (Concomitant use of local anesthetics may increase the risk of CNS side effects).
No products indexed under this heading.

Levofloxacin (Drugs that inhibit CYP1A2 might lead to increased plasma levels of propafenone; patients should be closely monitored and the propafenone dose adjusted accordingly). Products include:
Iquix 3492
Levaquin 2629
Levaquin in 5% Dextrose 2629
Quixin 3493

Levonorgestrel (Drugs that inhibit CYP1A2 might lead to increased plasma levels of propafenone; patients should be closely monitored and the propafenone dose adjusted accordingly). Products include:
Climara Pro 847
LoSeasonique 3407
Lybrel 3514
Mirena 854
Plan B 3416
Seasonique 3418

Lidocaine (The use of propafenone in conjunction with other drugs that prolong the QT interval has not been extensively studied and is not recommended). Products include:
Lidoderm 1107

Lidocaine Hydrochloride (The use of propafenone in conjunction with other drugs that prolong the QT interval has not been extensively studied and is not recommended).
No products indexed under this heading.

Lithium Carbonate (The use of propafenone in conjunction with other drugs that prolong the QT interval has not been extensively studied and is not recommended).
No products indexed under this heading.

Lithium Citrate (The use of propafenone in conjunction with other drugs that prolong the QT interval has not been extensively studied and is not recommended).
No products indexed under this heading.

Lomefloxacin Hydrochloride (Drugs that inhibit CYP1A2 might lead to increased plasma levels of propafenone; patients should be closely monitored and the propafenone dose adjusted accordingly).
No products indexed under this heading.

Lopinavir (Drugs that inhibit CYP3A4 might lead to increased plasma levels of propafenone; patients should be closely monitored and the propafenone dose adjusted accordingly). Products include:
Kaletra 458

Loratadine (Drugs that inhibit CYP3A4 might lead to increased plasma levels of propafenone; patients should be closely monitored and the propafenone dose adjusted accordingly).
No products indexed under this heading.

Lorazepam (The use of propafenone in conjunction with other drugs that prolong the QT interval has not been extensively studied and is not recommended).
No products indexed under this heading.

Loxapine Hydrochloride (The use of propafenone in conjunction with other drugs that prolong the QT interval has not been extensively studied and is not recommended).
No products indexed under this heading.

Loxapine Succinate (The use of propafenone in conjunction with other drugs that prolong the QT interval has not been extensively studied and is not recommended).
No products indexed under this heading.

Maprotiline Hydrochloride (The use of propafenone in conjunction with other drugs that prolong the QT interval has not been extensively studied and is not recommended).
No products indexed under this heading.

Mepivacaine Hydrochloride (Concomitant use of local anesthetics may increase the risk of CNS side effects).
No products indexed under this heading.

Meprobamate (The use of propafenone in conjunction with other drugs that prolong the QT interval has not been extensively studied and is not recommended).
No products indexed under this heading.

Mesoridazine Besylate (The use of propafenone in conjunction with other drugs that prolong the QT interval has not been extensively studied and is not recommended).
No products indexed under this heading.

Mestranol (Drugs that inhibit CYP1A2 might lead to increased plasma levels of propafenone; patients should be closely monitored and the propafenone dose adjusted accordingly).
No products indexed under this heading.

Methadone Hydrochloride (Drugs that inhibit CYP2D6 might lead to increased plasma levels of propafenone; patients should be closely monitored and the propafenone dose adjusted accordingly).
No products indexed under this heading.

Methotrimeprazine (The use of propafenone in conjunction with other drugs that prolong the QT interval has not been extensively studied and is not recommended).
No products indexed under this heading.

Methoxsalen (Drugs that inhibit CYP1A2 might lead to increased plasma levels of propafenone; patients should be closely monitored and the propafenone dose adjusted accordingly).
No products indexed under this heading.

Metoprolol Succinate (Coadministration can result in substantial increases in metoprolol concentration and elimination half-life; increased plasma levels of metoprolol could overcome its cardioselectivity). Products include:
Toprol XL 732

Metoprolol Tartrate (Coadministration can result in substantial increases in metoprolol concentration and elimination half-life; increased plasma levels of metoprolol could overcome its cardioselectivity).
No products indexed under this heading.

Metronidazole (Drugs that inhibit CYP3A4 might lead to increased plasma levels of propafenone; patients should be closely monitored and the propafenone dose adjusted accordingly). Products include:
Pylera 793

Metronidazole Benzoate (Drugs that inhibit CYP3A4 might lead to increased plasma levels of propafenone; patients should be closely monitored and the propafenone dose adjusted accordingly).
No products indexed under this heading.

Metronidazole Hydrochloride (Drugs that inhibit CYP3A4 might lead to increased plasma levels of propafenone; patients should be closely monitored and the propafenone dose adjusted accordingly).
No products indexed under this heading.

Metronidazole Sodium (Drugs that inhibit CYP3A4 might lead to increased plasma levels of propafenone; patients should be closely monitored and the propafenone dose adjusted accordingly).
No products indexed under this heading.

Mexiletine Hydrochloride (The use of propafenone in conjunction with other drugs that prolong the QT interval has not been extensively studied and is not recommended).
No products indexed under this heading.

Mibefradil Dihydrochloride (Drugs that inhibit CYP2D6 might lead to increased plasma levels of propafenone; patients should be closely monitored and the propafenone dose adjusted accordingly).
No products indexed under this heading.

Miconazole (Drugs that inhibit CYP3A4 might lead to increased plasma levels of propafenone; patients should be closely monitored and the propafenone dose adjusted accordingly).
No products indexed under this heading.

Miconazole Nitrate (Drugs that inhibit CYP3A4 might lead to increased plasma levels of propafenone; patients should be closely monitored and the propafenone dose adjusted accordingly). Products include:
Vusion Ointment 3335

Midazolam Hydrochloride (The use of propafenone in conjunction with other drugs that prolong the QT interval has not been extensively studied and is not recommended).
No products indexed under this heading.

Mifepristone (Drugs that inhibit CYP3A4 might lead to increased plasma levels of propafenone; patients should be closely monitored and the propafenone dose adjusted accordingly).
No products indexed under this heading.

Moclobemide (Drugs that inhibit CYP2D6 might lead to increased plasma levels of propafenone; patients should be closely monitored and the propafenone dose adjusted accordingly).
No products indexed under this heading.

Molindone Hydrochloride (The use of propafenone in conjunction with other drugs that prolong the QT interval has not been extensively studied and is not recommended). Products include:
Moban 1108

Moricizine Hydrochloride (Class Ia antiarrythmic agents should be withheld for at least five half-lives prior to dosing with extended release propafenone. The use of propafenone with Class Ia antiarrythmic agents is not recommended).
No products indexed under this heading.

Moxifloxacin Hydrochloride (Drugs that inhibit CYP1A2 might lead to increased plasma levels of propafenone; patients should be closely monitored and the propafenone dose adjusted accordingly). Products include:
Avelox 3064
Vigamox 589

Nalidixic Acid (Drugs that inhibit CYP1A2 might lead to increased plasma levels of propafenone; patients should be closely monitored and the propafenone dose adjusted accordingly).
No products indexed under this heading.

Nefazodone Hydrochloride (Drugs that inhibit CYP3A4 might lead to increased plasma levels of propafenone; patients should be closely monitored and the propafenone dose adjusted accordingly).
No products indexed under this heading.

Nelfinavir Mesylate (Drugs that inhibit CYP3A4 might lead to increased plasma levels of propafenone; patients should be closely monitored and the propafenone dose adjusted accordingly).
No products indexed under this heading.

Nevirapine (Drugs that inhibit CYP3A4 might lead to increased plasma levels

IMPORTANT NOTE: Always consult each drug listing in the patient's regimen for possible interactions.

Saquinavir (Drugs that inhibit CYP3A4 might lead to increased plasma levels of propafenone; patients should be closely monitored and the propafenone dose adjusted accordingly).

No products indexed under this heading.

Saquinavir Mesylate (Drugs that inhibit CYP3A4 might lead to increased plasma levels of propafenone; patients should be closely monitored and the propafenone dose adjusted accordingly).

No products indexed under this heading.

Sertraline Hydrochloride (Drugs that inhibit CYP2D6 might lead to increased plasma levels of propafenone; patients should be closely monitored and the propafenone dose adjusted accordingly).

No products indexed under this heading.

Sildenafil Citrate (Drugs that inhibit CYP2D6 might lead to increased plasma levels of propafenone; patients should be closely monitored and the propafenone dose adjusted accordingly).

No products indexed under this heading.

Sotalol Hydrochloride (Class III antiarrythmic agents should be withheld for at least five half-lives prior to dosing with extended release propafenone. The use of propafenone with Class III antiarrythmic agents is not recommended).

No products indexed under this heading.

Sparfloxacin (Drugs that inhibit CYP1A2 might lead to increased plasma levels of propafenone; patients should be closely monitored and the propafenone dose adjusted accordingly).

No products indexed under this heading.

Tacrine Hydrochloride (Drugs that inhibit CYP1A2 might lead to increased plasma levels of propafenone; patients should be closely monitored and the propafenone dose adjusted accordingly).

No products indexed under this heading.

Telithromycin (Drugs that inhibit CYP3A4 might lead to increased plasma levels of propafenone; patients should be closely monitored and the propafenone dose adjusted accordingly). Products include:
Ketek 2991

Terbinafine Hydrochloride (Drugs that inhibit CYP2D6 might lead to increased plasma levels of propafenone; patients should be closely monitored and the propafenone dose adjusted accordingly).

No products indexed under this heading.

Tetracaine Hydrochloride (Concomitant use of local anesthetics may increase the risk of CNS side effects).

No products indexed under this heading.

Thioridazine (The use of propafenone in conjunction with other drugs that prolong the QT interval has not been extensively studied and is not recommended).

No products indexed under this heading.

Thioridazine Hydrochloride (The use of propafenone in conjunction with other drugs that prolong the QT interval has not been extensively studied and is not recommended). Products include:
Thioridazine Hydrochloride 2384

Thiothixene (The use of propafenone in conjunction with other drugs that prolong the QT interval has not been extensively studied and is not recommended). Products include:
Thiothixene 2386

Ticlopidine Hydrochloride (Drugs that inhibit CYP1A2 might lead to increased plasma levels of propafenone; patients should be closely monitored and the propafenone dose adjusted accordingly).

No products indexed under this heading.

Tocainide Hydrochloride (The use of propafenone in conjunction with other drugs that prolong the QT interval has not been extensively studied and is not recommended).

No products indexed under this heading.

Tranylcypromine Sulfate (The use of propafenone in conjunction with other drugs that prolong the QT interval has not been extensively studied and is not recommended). Products include:
Parnate 1584

Trifluoperazine Hydrochloride (The use of propafenone in conjunction with other drugs that prolong the QT interval has not been extensively studied and is not recommended).

No products indexed under this heading.

Trimipramine Maleate (The use of propafenone in conjunction with other drugs that prolong the QT interval has not been extensively studied and is not recommended).

No products indexed under this heading.

Troglitazone (Drugs that inhibit CYP3A4 might lead to increased plasma levels of propafenone; patients should be closely monitored and the propafenone dose adjusted accordingly).

No products indexed under this heading.

Troleandomycin (The use of propafenone in conjunction with other drugs that prolong the QT interval has not been extensively studied and is not recommended).

No products indexed under this heading.

Trovafloxacin Mesylate (Drugs that inhibit CYP1A2 might lead to increased plasma levels of propafenone; patients should be closely monitored and the propafenone dose adjusted accordingly).

No products indexed under this heading.

Valproate Sodium (Drugs that inhibit CYP3A4 might lead to increased plasma levels of propafenone; patients should be closely monitored and the propafenone dose adjusted accordingly).

No products indexed under this heading.

Vardenafil Hydrochloride (Drugs that inhibit CYP2D6 might lead to increased plasma levels of propafenone; patients should be closely monitored and the propafenone dose adjusted accordingly). Products include:
Levitra 3157

Verapamil Hydrochloride (Drugs that inhibit CYP3A4 might lead to increased plasma levels of propafenone; patients should be closely monitored and the propafenone dose adjusted accordingly). Products include:
Tarka 534

Voriconazole (Drugs that inhibit CYP3A4 might lead to increased plasma levels of propafenone; patients should be closely monitored and the propafenone dose adjusted accordingly).

No products indexed under this heading.

Warfarin Sodium (Increase in mean steady-state plasma levels of warfarin resulting in increased prothrombin time).

No products indexed under this heading.

Zafirlukast (Drugs that inhibit CYP3A4 might lead to increased plasma levels of propafenone; patients should be closely monitored and the propafenone dose adjusted accordingly). Products include:
Accolate 3612

Zileuton (Drugs that inhibit CYP1A2 might lead to increased plasma levels of propafenone; patients should be closely monitored and the propafenone dose adjusted accordingly).

No products indexed under this heading.

Ziprasidone Hydrochloride (The use of propafenone in conjunction with other drugs that prolong the QT interval has not been extensively studied and is not recommended). Products include:
Geodon 2723

Food Interactions

Food, unspecified (Increased peak blood level and bioavailability in a single dose study).

Grapefruit (Drugs that inhibit CYP1A2 might lead to increased plasma levels of propafenone; patients should be closely monitored and the propafenone dose adjusted accordingly).

Grapefruit Juice (Drugs that inhibit CYP1A2 might lead to increased plasma levels of propafenone; patients should be closely monitored and the propafenone dose adjusted accordingly).

RYZOLT
EXTENDED-RELEASE
TABLETS
(Tramadol Hydrochloride) 2813
May interact with alcohols, alpha adrenergic blockers, anesthetics, antidepressant drugs, central nervous system depressants, cytochrome p450 2d6 inhibitors (selected), cytochrome p450 3a4 inducers (selected), cytochrome p450 3a4 inhibitors (selected), drugs which lower seizure threshold, erythromycin, hypnotics and sedatives, lithium preparations, monoamine oxidase inhibitors, narcotic analgesics, phenothiazines, quinidine, selective serotonin reuptake inhibitors, serotonin and norepinephrine reuptake inhibitors, skeletal muscle relaxants, tranquilizers, tricyclic antidepressants, triptans, and certain other agents. Compounds in these categories include:

Acetazolamide (Concomitant administration of CYP3A4 inhibitors, such as ketoconazole and erythromycin, may reduce metabolic clearance of tramadol increasing the risk for serious adverse events including seizures and serotonin syndrome).

No products indexed under this heading.

Acetazolamide Sodium (Concomitant administration of CYP3A4 inhibitors, such as ketoconazole and erythromycin, may reduce metabolic clearance of tramadol increasing the risk for serious adverse events including seizures and serotonin syndrome).

No products indexed under this heading.

Alfentanil Hydrochloride (Concomitant use of tramadol hydrochloride increases the seizure risk in patients taking other opioids. Tramadol should be used with caution and in reduced dosages when administered to patients receiving CNS depressants such as opioids or narcotics. Tramadol increases the risk of CNS and respiratory depression in these patients).

No products indexed under this heading.

Alfuzosin Hydrochloride (There have been postmarketing reports of serotonin syndrome with use of tramadol and alpha2-adrenergic blockers). Products include:
Uroxatral 3050

Allium sativum (Administration of CYP3A4 inducers, such as rifampin or St. John's Wort, with tramadol hydrochloride may effect the metabolism of tramadol leading to altered tramadol exposure).

No products indexed under this heading.

Almotriptan Malate (Caution is advised when tramadol is co-administered with other drugs that may affect the serotonergic neurotransmitter systems, such as triptans. If concomitant treatment of tramadol with a drug affecting the serotonergic neurotransmitter system is clinically warranted,

careful observation of the patient is advised, particularly during treatment initiation and dose increases). Products include:
Axert 2593

Alprazolam (Administration of tramadol may increase the seizure risk in patients taking neuroleptics or other drugs that reduce the seizure threshold).

No products indexed under this heading.

Aminoglutethimide (Administration of CYP3A4 inducers, such as rifampin or St. John's Wort, with tramadol hydrochloride may effect the metabolism of tramadol leading to altered tramadol exposure).

No products indexed under this heading.

Amiodarone Hydrochloride (Concomitant administration of CYP2D6 inhibitors such as quinidine, fluoxetine, paroxetine and amitriptyline may reduce metabolic clearance of tramadol increasing the risk for serious adverse events including seizures and serotonin syndrome. *In vitro* drug interaction studies in human liver microsomes indicate that inhibitors of CYP2D6 inhibit the metabolism of tramadol to various degrees, suggesting that concomitant administration of these compounds could result in increases in tramadol concentrations and decreased concentrations of M1. The full pharmacological impact of these alterations in terms of either efficacy or safety is unknown).

No products indexed under this heading.

Amitriptyline Hydrochloride (Administration of tramadol may increase the seizure risk in patients taking neuroleptics or other drugs that reduce the seizure threshold).

No products indexed under this heading.

Amobarbital (Tramadol hydrochloride should be used with caution and in reduced dosages when administered to patients receiving CNS depressants, such as alcohol, opioids, anesthetic agents, narcotics, phenothiazines, tranquilizers, or sedative hypnotics. Tramadol hydrochloride increases the risk of CNS and respiratory depression).

No products indexed under this heading.

Amobarbital Sodium (Tramadol hydrochloride should be used with caution and in reduced dosages when administered to patients receiving CNS depressants, such as alcohol, opioids, anesthetic agents, narcotics, phenothiazines, tranquilizers, or sedative hypnotics. Tramadol hydrochloride increases the risk of CNS and respiratory depression).

No products indexed under this heading.

Amoxapine (Administration of tramadol may increase the seizure risk in patients taking neuroleptics or other drugs that reduce the seizure threshold).

No products indexed under this heading.

Amprenavir (Concomitant administration of CYP3A4 inhibitors, such as ketoconazole and erythromycin, may reduce metabolic clearance of tramadol increasing the risk for serious adverse events including seizures and serotonin syndrome).

No products indexed under this heading.

Anastrozole (Concomitant administration of CYP3A4 inhibitors, such as ketoconazole and erythromycin, may reduce metabolic clearance of tramadol increasing the risk for serious adverse events including seizures and serotonin syndrome).

No products indexed under this heading.

(⊙ Described in PDR® for Ophthalmic Medicines)

Apomorphine (Concomitant use of tramadol hydrochloride increases the seizure risk in patients taking other opioids. Tramadol should be used with caution and in reduced dosages when administered to patients receiving CNS depressants such as opioids or narcotics. Tramadol increases the risk of CNS and respiratory depression in these patients).
No products indexed under this heading.

Apomorphine Hydrochloride (Concomitant use of tramadol hydrochloride increases the seizure risk in patients taking other opioids. Tramadol should be used with caution and in reduced dosages when administered to patients receiving CNS depressants such as opioids or narcotics. Tramadol increases the risk of CNS and respiratory depression in these patients).
No products indexed under this heading.

Apraclonidine Hydrochloride (There have been postmarketing reports of serotonin syndrome with use of tramadol and alpha2-adrenergic blockers).
No products indexed under this heading.

Aprepitant (Concomitant administration of CYP3A4 inhibitors, such as ketoconazole and erythromycin, may reduce metabolic clearance of tramadol increasing the risk for serious adverse events including seizures and serotonin syndrome). Products include:
Emend 2124

Aprobarbital (Tramadol hydrochloride should be used with caution and in reduced dosages when administered to patients receiving CNS depressants, such as alcohol, opioids, anesthetic agents, narcotics, phenothiazines, tranquilizers, or sedative hypnotics. Tramadol hydrochloride increases the risk of CNS and respiratory depression).
No products indexed under this heading.

Articaine Hydrochloride (Tramadol hydrochloride should be used with caution and in reduced dosages when administered to patients receiving CNS depressants, such as anesthetic agents. Tramadol hydrochloride increases the risk of CNS and respiratory depression).
No products indexed under this heading.

Atazanavir (Concomitant administration of CYP3A4 inhibitors, such as ketoconazole and erythromycin, may reduce metabolic clearance of tramadol increasing the risk for serious adverse events including seizures and serotonin syndrome).
No products indexed under this heading.

Atazanavir Sulfate (Concomitant administration of CYP3A4 inhibitors, such as ketoconazole and erythromycin, may reduce metabolic clearance of tramadol increasing the risk for serious adverse events including seizures and serotonin syndrome).
No products indexed under this heading.

Atracurium Besylate (Because of its added depressant effects, tramadol should be prescribed with caution for those patients whose medical condition requires the concomitant administration of muscle relaxants, or other CNS-depressant drugs. Patients should be advised of the additive depressant effects of these combinations).
No products indexed under this heading.

Baclofen (Because of its added depressant effects, tramadol should be prescribed with caution for those patients whose medical condition requires the concomitant administration of muscle relaxants, or other CNS-depressant drugs. Patients should be advised of the additive depressant effects of these combinations).
No products indexed under this heading.

Benzocaine (Tramadol hydrochloride should be used with caution and in reduced dosages when administered to patients receiving CNS depressants, such as anesthetic agents. Tramadol hydrochloride increases the risk of CNS and respiratory depression).
No products indexed under this heading.

Betamethasone (Administration of CYP3A4 inducers, such as rifampin or St. John's Wort, with tramadol hydrochloride may effect the metabolism of tramadol leading to altered tramadol exposure).
No products indexed under this heading.

Betamethasone Acetate (Administration of CYP3A4 inducers, such as rifampin or St. John's Wort, with tramadol hydrochloride may effect the metabolism of tramadol leading to altered tramadol exposure).
No products indexed under this heading.

Betamethasone Benzoate (Administration of CYP3A4 inducers, such as rifampin or St. John's Wort, with tramadol hydrochloride may effect the metabolism of tramadol leading to altered tramadol exposure).
No products indexed under this heading.

Betamethasone Dipropionate (Administration of CYP3A4 inducers, such as rifampin or St. John's Wort, with tramadol hydrochloride may effect the metabolism of tramadol leading to altered tramadol exposure). Products include:
Diprolene Lotion 0.05% 3108
Diprolene Ointment 0.05% 3109
Diprolene AF Cream 0.05% 3107
Lotrisone 3163

Betamethasone Sodium Phosphate (Administration of CYP3A4 inducers, such as rifampin or St. John's Wort, with tramadol hydrochloride may effect the metabolism of tramadol leading to altered tramadol exposure).
No products indexed under this heading.

Betamethasone Valerate (Administration of CYP3A4 inducers, such as rifampin or St. John's Wort, with tramadol hydrochloride may effect the metabolism of tramadol leading to altered tramadol exposure). Products include:
Luxiq 3321

Bosentan (Administration of CYP3A4 inducers, such as rifampin or St. John's Wort, with tramadol hydrochloride may effect the metabolism of tramadol leading to altered tramadol exposure). Products include:
Tracleer 573

Bupivacaine Hydrochloride (Tramadol hydrochloride should be used with caution and in reduced dosages when administered to patients receiving CNS depressants, such as anesthetic agents. Tramadol hydrochloride increases the risk of CNS and respiratory depression).
No products indexed under this heading.

Buprenorphine Hydrochloride (Concomitant use of tramadol hydrochloride increases the seizure risk in patients taking other opioids. Tramadol should be used with caution and in reduced dosages when administered to patients receiving CNS depressants such as opioids or narcotics. Tramadol increases the risk of CNS and respiratory depression in these patients).
No products indexed under this heading.

Bupropion Hydrochloride (Concomitant administration of CYP2D6 inhibitors such as quinidine, fluoxetine, paroxetine and amitriptyline may reduce metabolic clearance of tramadol increasing the risk for serious adverse events including seizures and serotonin syndrome. *In vitro* drug interaction studies in human liver microsomes indicate that inhibitors of CYP2D6 inhibit the metabolism of tramadol to various degrees, suggesting that concomitant administration of these compounds could result in increases in tramadol concentrations and decreased concentrations of M1. The full pharmacological impact of these alterations in terms of either efficacy or safety is unknown). Products include:
Aplenzin 2948
Wellbutrin 1719
Wellbutrin SR 1725
Zyban 1762

Buspirone Hydrochloride (Tramadol hydrochloride should be used with caution and in reduced dosages when administered to patients receiving CNS depressants, such as alcohol, opioids, anesthetic agents, narcotics, phenothiazines, tranquilizers, or sedative hypnotics. Tramadol hydrochloride increases the risk of CNS and respiratory depression).
No products indexed under this heading.

Butabarbital (Tramadol hydrochloride should be used with caution and in reduced dosages when administered to patients receiving CNS depressants, such as sedative hypnotics. Tramadol hydrochloride increases the risk of CNS and respiratory depression).
No products indexed under this heading.

Butabarbital Sodium (Tramadol hydrochloride should be used with caution and in reduced dosages when administered to patients receiving CNS depressants, such as sedative hypnotics. Tramadol hydrochloride increases the risk of CNS and respiratory depression).
No products indexed under this heading.

Butalbital (Tramadol hydrochloride should be used with caution and in reduced dosages when administered to patients receiving CNS depressants, such as sedative hypnotics. Tramadol hydrochloride increases the risk of CNS and respiratory depression).
No products indexed under this heading.

Carbamazepine (Patients taking carbamazepine, a CYP3A4 inducer, may have a significantly reduced analgesic effect of tramadol. Because carbamazepine increases tramadol metabolism and because of the seizure risk associated with tramadol, concomitant administration of tramadol hydrochloride and carbamazepine is not recommended). Products include:
Carbatrol 3280
Equetro 3477

Carisoprodol (Because of its added depressant effects, tramadol should be prescribed with caution for those patients whose medical condition requires the concomitant administration of muscle relaxants, or other CNS-depressant drugs. Patients should be advised of the additive depressant effects of these combinations).
No products indexed under this heading.

Celecoxib (Concomitant administration of CYP2D6 inhibitors such as quinidine, fluoxetine, paroxetine and amitriptyline may reduce metabolic clearance of tramadol increasing the risk for serious adverse events including seizures and serotonin syndrome. *In vitro* drug interaction studies in human liver microsomes indicate that inhibitors of CYP2D6 inhibit the metabolism of tramadol to various degrees, suggesting that concomitant administration of these compounds could result in increases in tramadol concentrations and decreased concentrations of M1. The full pharmacological impact of these alterations in terms of either efficacy or safety is unknown). Products include:
Celebrex 3272

Chloral Hydrate (Tramadol hydrochloride should be used with caution and in reduced dosages when administered to patients receiving CNS depressants, such as sedative hypnotics. Tramadol hydrochloride increases the risk of CNS and respiratory depression).
No products indexed under this heading.

Chlordiazepoxide (Administration of tramadol may increase the seizure risk in patients taking neuroleptics or other drugs that reduce the seizure threshold).
No products indexed under this heading.

Chlordiazepoxide Hydrochloride (Administration of tramadol may increase the seizure risk in patients taking neuroleptics or other drugs that reduce the seizure threshold).
No products indexed under this heading.

Chloroprocaine Hydrochloride (Tramadol hydrochloride should be used with caution and in reduced dosages when administered to patients receiving CNS depressants, such as anesthetic agents. Tramadol hydrochloride increases the risk of CNS and respiratory depression).
No products indexed under this heading.

Chloroquine (Concomitant administration of CYP2D6 inhibitors such as quinidine, fluoxetine, paroxetine and amitriptyline may reduce metabolic clearance of tramadol increasing the risk for serious adverse events including seizures and serotonin syndrome. *In vitro* drug interaction studies in human liver microsomes indicate that inhibitors of CYP2D6 inhibit the metabolism of tramadol to various degrees, suggesting that concomitant administration of these compounds could result in increases in tramadol concentrations and decreased concentrations of M1. The full pharmacological impact of these alterations in terms of either efficacy or safety is unknown).
No products indexed under this heading.

Chloroquine Hydrochloride (Concomitant administration of CYP2D6 inhibitors such as quinidine, fluoxetine, paroxetine and amitriptyline may reduce metabolic clearance of tramadol increasing the risk for serious adverse events including seizures and serotonin syndrome. *In vitro* drug interaction studies in human liver microsomes indicate that inhibitors of CYP2D6 inhibit the metabolism of tramadol to various degrees, suggesting that concomitant administration of these compounds could result in increases in tramadol concentrations and decreased concentrations of M1. The full pharmacological impact of these alterations in terms of either efficacy or safety is unknown).
No products indexed under this heading.

Chloroquine Phosphate (Concomitant administration of CYP2D6 inhibitors such as quinidine, fluoxetine, paroxetine and amitriptyline may reduce metabolic clearance of tramadol increasing the risk for serious adverse events including seizures and serotonin syndrome. *In vitro* drug interaction studies in human liver microsomes indicate that inhibitors of CYP2D6 inhibit the metabolism of tramadol to various degrees, suggesting that concomitant administration of these compounds could result in increases in tramadol concentrations and decreased concentrations of M1. The full pharmacological impact of these alterations in terms of either efficacy or safety is unknown).
No products indexed under this heading.

Chlorpheniramine (Concomitant administration of CYP2D6 inhibitors such as quinidine, fluoxetine, paroxetine and amitriptyline may reduce metabolic clearance of tramadol increasing the risk for serious adverse events includ-

Ryzolt **Interactions Index** 1660

ing seizures and serotonin syndrome. *In vitro* drug interaction studies in human liver microsomes indicate that inhibitors of CYP2D6 inhibit the metabolism of tramadol to various degrees, suggesting that concomitant administration of these compounds could result in increases in tramadol concentrations and decreased concentrations of M1. The full pharmacological impact of these alterations in terms of either efficacy or safety is unknown).
No products indexed under this heading.

Chlorpheniramine Maleate (Concomitant administration of CYP2D6 inhibitors such as quinidine, fluoxetine, paroxetine and amitriptyline may reduce metabolic clearance of tramadol increasing the risk for serious adverse events including seizures and serotonin syndrome. *In vitro* drug interaction studies in human liver microsomes indicate that inhibitors of CYP2D6 inhibit the metabolism of tramadol to various degrees, suggesting that concomitant administration of these compounds could result in increases in tramadol concentrations and decreased concentrations of M1. The full pharmacological impact of these alterations in terms of either efficacy or safety is unknown).
No products indexed under this heading.

Chlorpheniramine Polistirex (Concomitant administration of CYP2D6 inhibitors such as quinidine, fluoxetine, paroxetine and amitriptyline may reduce metabolic clearance of tramadol increasing the risk for serious adverse events including seizures and serotonin syndrome. *In vitro* drug interaction studies in human liver microsomes indicate that inhibitors of CYP2D6 inhibit the metabolism of tramadol to various degrees, suggesting that concomitant administration of these compounds could result in increases in tramadol concentrations and decreased concentrations of M1. The full pharmacological impact of these alterations in terms of either efficacy or safety is unknown). Products include:
Tussionex 3443

Chlorpheniramine Tannate (Concomitant administration of CYP2D6 inhibitors such as quinidine, fluoxetine, paroxetine and amitriptyline may reduce metabolic clearance of tramadol increasing the risk for serious adverse events including seizures and serotonin syndrome. *In vitro* drug interaction studies in human liver microsomes indicate that inhibitors of CYP2D6 inhibit the metabolism of tramadol to various degrees, suggesting that concomitant administration of these compounds could result in increases in tramadol concentrations and decreased concentrations of M1. The full pharmacological impact of these alterations in terms of either efficacy or safety is unknown).
No products indexed under this heading.

Chlorpromazine (Administration of tramadol may increase the seizure risk in patients taking neuroleptics or other drugs that reduce the seizure threshold).
No products indexed under this heading.

Chlorpromazine Hydrochloride (Administration of tramadol may increase the seizure risk in patients taking neuroleptics or other drugs that reduce the seizure threshold).
No products indexed under this heading.

Chlorprothixene (Tramadol hydrochloride should be used with caution and in reduced dosages when administered to patients receiving CNS depressants, such as alcohol, opioids, anesthetic agents, narcotics, phenothiazines, tranquilizers, or sedative hypnotics. Tramadol hydrochloride increases the risk of CNS and respiratory depression).
No products indexed under this heading.

Chlorprothixene Hydrochloride (Tramadol hydrochloride should be used with caution and in reduced dosages when administered to patients receiving CNS depressants, such as alcohol, opioids, anesthetic agents, narcotics, phenothiazines, tranquilizers, or sedative hypnotics. Tramadol hydrochloride increases the risk of CNS and respiratory depression).
No products indexed under this heading.

Chlorprothixene Lactate (Tramadol hydrochloride should be used with caution and in reduced dosages when administered to patients receiving CNS depressants, such as alcohol, opioids, anesthetic agents, narcotics, phenothiazines, tranquilizers, or sedative hypnotics. Tramadol hydrochloride increases the risk of CNS and respiratory depression).
No products indexed under this heading.

Chlorzoxazone (Because of its added depressant effects, tramadol should be prescribed with caution for those patients whose medical condition requires the concomitant administration of muscle relaxants, or other CNS-depressant drugs. Patients should be advised of the additive depressant effects of these combinations).
No products indexed under this heading.

Cimetidine (Concomitant administration of CYP2D6 inhibitors such as quinidine, fluoxetine, paroxetine and amitriptyline may reduce metabolic clearance of tramadol increasing the risk for serious adverse events including seizures and serotonin syndrome. *In vitro* drug interaction studies in human liver microsomes indicate that inhibitors of CYP2D6 inhibit the metabolism of tramadol to various degrees, suggesting that concomitant administration of these compounds could result in increases in tramadol concentrations and decreased concentrations of M1. The full pharmacological impact of these alterations in terms of either efficacy or safety is unknown).
No products indexed under this heading.

Cimetidine Hydrochloride (Concomitant administration of CYP2D6 inhibitors such as quinidine, fluoxetine, paroxetine and amitriptyline may reduce metabolic clearance of tramadol increasing the risk for serious adverse events including seizures and serotonin syndrome. *In vitro* drug interaction studies in human liver microsomes indicate that inhibitors of CYP2D6 inhibit the metabolism of tramadol to various degrees, suggesting that concomitant administration of these compounds could result in increases in tramadol concentrations and decreased concentrations of M1. The full pharmacological impact of these alterations in terms of either efficacy or safety is unknown).
No products indexed under this heading.

Ciprofloxacin (Concomitant administration of CYP3A4 inhibitors, such as ketoconazole and erythromycin, may reduce metabolic clearance of tramadol increasing the risk for serious adverse events including seizures and serotonin syndrome). Products include:
Cipro I.V. 3082
Cipro 3073
Cipro XR 3091
Ciprodex 583

Ciprofloxacin Hydrochloride (Administration of CYP3A4 inducers, such as rifampin or St. John's Wort, with tramadol hydrochloride may effect the metabolism of tramadol leading to altered tramadol exposure). Products include:
Cipro 3073

Cisatracurium Besylate (Because of its added depressant effects, tramadol should be prescribed with caution for those patients whose medical condition requires the concomitant administration of muscle relaxants, or other CNS-depressant drugs. Patients should be advised of the additive depressant effects of these combinations). Products include:
Nimbex 503

Cisplatin (Administration of CYP3A4 inducers, such as rifampin or St. John's Wort, with tramadol hydrochloride may effect the metabolism of tramadol leading to altered tramadol exposure).
No products indexed under this heading.

Citalopram Hydrobromide (Concomitant use of tramadol hydrochloride increases the seizure risk in patients taking selective serotonin reuptake inhibitors (SSRI antidepressants or anorectics). There have been postmarketing reports of serotonin syndrome with use of tramadol and SSRIs/SNRIs. Caution is advised when tramadol is co-administered with other drugs that may affect the serotonergic neurotransmitter systems, such as SSRIs. If concomitant treatment of tramadol with a drug affecting the serotonergic neurotransmitter system is clinically warranted, careful observation of the patient is advised, particularly during treatment initiation and dose increases). Products include:
Celexa 1153

Clarithromycin (Concomitant administration of CYP3A4 inhibitors, such as ketoconazole and erythromycin, may reduce metabolic clearance of tramadol increasing the risk for serious adverse events including seizures and serotonin syndrome). Products include:
Biaxin/Biaxin XL 412

Clomipramine Hydrochloride (Administration of tramadol may increase the seizure risk in patients taking neuroleptics or other drugs that reduce the seizure threshold).
No products indexed under this heading.

Clonazepam (Tramadol hydrochloride should be used with caution and in reduced dosages when administered to patients receiving CNS depressants, such as alcohol, opioids, anesthetic agents, narcotics, phenothiazines, tranquilizers, or sedative hypnotics. Tramadol hydrochloride increases the risk of CNS and respiratory depression). Products include:
Klonopin 2855

Clonidine (There have been postmarketing reports of serotonin syndrome with use of tramadol and alpha2-adrenergic blockers). Products include:
Catapres-TTS 884

Clonidine Hydrochloride (There have been postmarketing reports of serotonin syndrome with use of tramadol and alpha2-adrenergic blockers). Products include:
Clorpres 2344

Clorazepate Dipotassium (Tramadol hydrochloride should be used with caution and in reduced dosages when administered to patients receiving CNS depressants, such as alcohol, opioids, anesthetic agents, narcotics, phenothiazines, tranquilizers, or sedative hypnotics. Tramadol hydrochloride increases the risk of CNS and respiratory depression).
No products indexed under this heading.

Clotrimazole (Concomitant administration of CYP3A4 inhibitors, such as ketoconazole and erythromycin, may reduce metabolic clearance of tramadol increasing the risk for serious adverse events including seizures and serotonin syndrome). Products include:
Lotrisone 3163

Clozapine (Tramadol hydrochloride should be used with caution and in reduced dosages when administered to patients receiving CNS depressants, such as alcohol, opioids, anesthetic agents, narcotics, phenothiazines, tranquilizers, or sedative hypnotics. Tramadol hydrochloride increases the risk of CNS and respiratory depression).
No products indexed under this heading.

Cocaine Hydrochloride (Tramadol hydrochloride should be used with caution and in reduced dosages when administered to patients receiving CNS depressants, such as anesthetic agents. Tramadol hydrochloride increases the risk of CNS and respiratory depression).
No products indexed under this heading.

Codeine Phosphate (Concomitant use of tramadol hydrochloride increases the seizure risk in patients taking other opioids. Tramadol should be used with caution and in reduced dosages when administered to patients receiving CNS depressants such as opioids or narcotics. Tramadol increases the risk of CNS and respiratory depression in these patients). Products include:
Tylenol with Codeine 2691

Codeine Sulfate (Concomitant use of tramadol hydrochloride increases the seizure risk in patients taking other opioids. Tramadol should be used with caution and in reduced dosages when administered to patients receiving CNS depressants such as opioids or narcotics. Tramadol increases the risk of CNS and respiratory depression in these patients).
No products indexed under this heading.

Conivaptan Hydrochloride (Concomitant administration of CYP3A4 inhibitors, such as ketoconazole and erythromycin, may reduce metabolic clearance of tramadol increasing the risk for serious adverse events including seizures and serotonin syndrome). Products include:
Vaprisol 689

Cortisone Acetate (Administration of CYP3A4 inducers, such as rifampin or St. John's Wort, with tramadol hydrochloride may effect the metabolism of tramadol leading to altered tramadol exposure).
No products indexed under this heading.

Cyclobenzaprine (Concomitant use of tramadol hydrochloride increases the seizure risk in patients taking tricyclic compounds, such as cyclobenzaprine).
No products indexed under this heading.

Cyclobenzaprine Hydrochloride (Concomitant use of tramadol hydrochloride increases the seizure risk in patients taking tricyclic compounds, such as cyclobenzaprine). Products include:
Amrix 964

Cyclosporine (Concomitant administration of CYP3A4 inhibitors, such as ketoconazole and erythromycin, may reduce metabolic clearance of tramadol increasing the risk for serious adverse events including seizures and serotonin syndrome). Products include:
Gengraf 440
Neoral Oral Solution 2496
Neoral Capsules 2496
Restasis 605

Dalfopristin (Concomitant administration of CYP3A4 inhibitors, such as ketoconazole and erythromycin, may reduce metabolic clearance of tramadol increasing the risk for serious adverse events including seizures and serotonin syndrome).
No products indexed under this heading.

Danazol (Concomitant administration of CYP3A4 inhibitors, such as ketoconazole and erythromycin, may reduce metabolic clearance of tramadol increasing the risk for serious adverse events including seizures and serotonin syndrome).
No products indexed under this heading.

Dantrolene Sodium (Because of its added depressant effects, tramadol should be prescribed with caution for those patients whose medical condition requires the concomitant administration of muscle relaxants, or other CNS-depressant drugs. Patients should be advised of the additive depressant effects of these combinations).
No products indexed under this heading.

Darunavir (Concomitant administration of CYP3A4 inhibitors, such as ketoconazole and erythromycin, may reduce metabolic clearance of tramadol increasing the risk for serious adverse events including seizures and serotonin syndrome).
No products indexed under this heading.

Dasatinib (Concomitant administration of CYP3A4 inhibitors, such as ketoconazole and erythromycin, may reduce metabolic clearance of tramadol increasing the risk for serious adverse events including seizures and serotonin syndrome).
No products indexed under this heading.

Delavirdine Mesylate (Concomitant administration of CYP3A4 inhibitors, such as ketoconazole and erythromycin, may reduce metabolic clearance of tramadol increasing the risk for serious adverse events including seizures and serotonin syndrome).
No products indexed under this heading.

Delavirine (Concomitant administration of CYP3A4 inhibitors, such as ketoconazole and erythromycin, may reduce metabolic clearance of tramadol increasing the risk for serious adverse events including seizures and serotonin syndrome).
No products indexed under this heading.

Desflurane (Tramadol hydrochloride should be used with caution and in reduced dosages when administered to patients receiving CNS depressants, such as alcohol, opioids, anesthetic agents, narcotics, phenothiazines, tranquilizers, or sedative hypnotics. Tramadol hydrochloride increases the risk of CNS and respiratory depression).
No products indexed under this heading.

Desipramine Hydrochloride (Administration of tramadol may increase the seizure risk in patients taking neuroleptics or other drugs that reduce the seizure threshold).
No products indexed under this heading.

Desloratadine (Concomitant administration of CYP3A4 inhibitors, such as ketoconazole and erythromycin, may reduce metabolic clearance of tramadol increasing the risk for serious adverse events including seizures and serotonin syndrome). Products include:
Clarinex Syrup 3098
Clarinex 3098
Clarinex Reditabs 3098
Clarinex-D 12-Hour 3101
Clarinex-D 3104

Desvenlafaxine Succinate (There have been postmarketing reports of serotonin syndrome with use of tramadol and SSRIs/SNRIs. Caution is advised when tramadol is co-

administered with other drugs that may affect the serotonergic neurotransmitter systems, such as SSRIs. If concomitant treatment of tramadol with a drug affecting the serotonergic neurotransmitter system is clinically warranted, careful observation of the patient is advised, particularly during treatment initiation and dose increases). Products include:
Pristiq 3564

Dexamethasone (Administration of CYP3A4 inducers, such as rifampin or St. John's Wort, with tramadol hydrochloride may effect the metabolism of tramadol leading to altered tramadol exposure). Products include:
Ciprodex 583
Ozurdex .... ⊙223
Tobramycin and Dexamethasone
  Ophthalmic Suspension .... ⊙251

Dexamethasone Acetate (Administration of CYP3A4 inducers, such as rifampin or St. John's Wort, with tramadol hydrochloride may effect the metabolism of tramadol leading to altered tramadol exposure).
No products indexed under this heading.

Dexamethasone Phosphate (Administration of CYP3A4 inducers, such as rifampin or St. John's Wort, with tramadol hydrochloride may effect the metabolism of tramadol leading to altered tramadol exposure).
No products indexed under this heading.

Dexamethasone Sodium (Administration of CYP3A4 inducers, such as rifampin or St. John's Wort, with tramadol hydrochloride may effect the metabolism of tramadol leading to altered tramadol exposure).
No products indexed under this heading.

Dexamethasone Sodium Phosphate (Administration of CYP3A4 inducers, such as rifampin or St. John's Wort, with tramadol hydrochloride may effect the metabolism of tramadol leading to altered tramadol exposure).
No products indexed under this heading.

Dexamethasone Sodium Phosphate Injection (Administration of CYP3A4 inducers, such as rifampin or St. John's Wort, with tramadol hydrochloride may effect the metabolism of tramadol leading to altered tramadol exposure).
No products indexed under this heading.

Dezocine (Concomitant use of tramadol hydrochloride increases the seizure risk in patients taking other opioids. Tramadol should be used with caution and in reduced dosages when administered to patients receiving CNS depressants such as opioids or narcotics. Tramadol increases the risk of CNS and respiratory depression in these patients).
No products indexed under this heading.

Diazepam (Administration of tramadol may increase the seizure risk in patients taking neuroleptics or other drugs that reduce the seizure threshold). Products include:
Valium Tablets 2880

Dibucaine (Tramadol hydrochloride should be used with caution and in reduced dosages when administered to patients receiving CNS depressants, such as anesthetic agents. Tramadol hydrochloride increases the risk of CNS and respiratory depression).
No products indexed under this heading.

Dibucaine Hydrochloride (Tramadol hydrochloride should be used with caution and in reduced dosages when administered to patients receiving CNS depressants, such as anesthetic agents. Tramadol hydrochloride increases the risk of CNS and respiratory depression).
No products indexed under this heading.

Digoxin (Post-marketing surveillance of tramadol has revealed rare reports of digoxin toxicity). Products include:
Lanoxin Injection 1546
Lanoxin Injection Pediatric 1549
Lanoxin Tablets 1553

Dihydrocodeine Bitartrate (Concomitant use of tramadol hydrochloride increases the seizure risk in patients taking other opioids. Tramadol should be used with caution and in reduced dosages when administered to patients receiving CNS depressants such as opioids or narcotics. Tramadol increases the risk of CNS and respiratory depression in these patients).
No products indexed under this heading.

Dihydrocodeinone Bitartrate (Concomitant use of tramadol hydrochloride increases the seizure risk in patients taking other opioids. Tramadol should be used with caution and in reduced dosages when administered to patients receiving CNS depressants such as opioids or narcotics. Tramadol increases the risk of CNS and respiratory depression in these patients).
No products indexed under this heading.

Diltiazem Hydrochloride (Concomitant administration of CYP3A4 inhibitors, such as ketoconazole and erythromycin, may reduce metabolic clearance of tramadol increasing the risk for serious adverse events including seizures and serotonin syndrome). Products include:
Cardizem LA 423

Diltiazem Maleate (Concomitant administration of CYP3A4 inhibitors, such as ketoconazole and erythromycin, may reduce metabolic clearance of tramadol increasing the risk for serious adverse events including seizures and serotonin syndrome).
No products indexed under this heading.

Diphenhydramine (Concomitant administration of CYP2D6 inhibitors such as quinidine, fluoxetine, paroxetine and amitriptyline may reduce metabolic clearance of tramadol increasing the risk for serious adverse events including seizures and serotonin syndrome. *In vitro* drug interaction studies in human liver microsomes indicate that inhibitors of CYP2D6 inhibit the metabolism of tramadol to various degrees, suggesting that concomitant administration of these compounds could result in increases in tramadol concentrations and decreased concentrations of M1. The full pharmacological impact of these alterations in terms of either efficacy or safety is unknown).
No products indexed under this heading.

Diphenhydramine Hydrochloride (Concomitant administration of CYP2D6 inhibitors such as quinidine, fluoxetine, paroxetine and amitriptyline may reduce metabolic clearance of tramadol increasing the risk for serious adverse events including seizures and serotonin syndrome. *In vitro* drug interaction studies in human liver microsomes indicate that inhibitors of CYP2D6 inhibit the metabolism of tramadol to various degrees, suggesting that concomitant administration of these compounds could result in increases in tramadol concentrations and decreased concentrations of M1. The full pharmacological impact of these alterations in terms of either efficacy or safety is unknown).
Products include:
Benadryl Allergy Ultratab 2042
Children's Benadryl Allergy Liquid 2042

Doxacurium Chloride (Because of its added depressant effects, tramadol should be prescribed with caution for those patients whose medical condition requires the concomitant administration of muscle relaxants, or other CNS-depressant drugs. Patients should be advised of the additive depressant effects of these combinations).
No products indexed under this heading.

Doxazosin Mesylate (There have been postmarketing reports of serotonin syndrome with use of tramadol and alpha2-adrenergic blockers).
No products indexed under this heading.

Doxepin Hydrochloride (Administration of tramadol may increase the seizure risk in patients taking neuroleptics or other drugs that reduce the seizure threshold).
No products indexed under this heading.

Doxorubicin Hydrochloride (Administration of CYP3A4 inducers, such as rifampin or St. John's Wort, with tramadol hydrochloride may effect the metabolism of tramadol leading to altered tramadol exposure).
No products indexed under this heading.

Droperidol (Tramadol hydrochloride should be used with caution and in reduced dosages when administered to patients receiving CNS depressants, such as alcohol, opioids, anesthetic agents, narcotics, phenothiazines, tranquilizers, or sedative hypnotics. Tramadol hydrochloride increases the risk of CNS and respiratory depression).
No products indexed under this heading.

d-Tubocurarine (Because of its added depressant effects, tramadol should be prescribed with caution for those patients whose medical condition requires the concomitant administration of muscle relaxants, or other CNS-depressant drugs. Patients should be advised of the additive depressant effects of these combinations).
No products indexed under this heading.

Duloxetine Hydrochloride (There have been postmarketing reports of serotonin syndrome with use of tramadol and SSRIs/SNRIs. Caution is advised when tramadol is co-administered with other drugs that may affect the serotonergic neurotransmitter systems, such as SSRIs. If concomitant treatment of tramadol with a drug affecting the serotonergic neurotransmitter system is clinically warranted, careful observation of the patient is advised, particularly during treatment initiation and dose increases). Products include:
Cymbalta 1871

Efavirenz (Concomitant administration of CYP3A4 inhibitors, such as ketoconazole and erythromycin, may reduce metabolic clearance of tramadol increasing the risk for serious adverse events including seizures and serotonin syndrome). Products include:
Atripla 906

Eletriptan Hydrobromide (Caution is advised when tramadol is co-administered with other drugs that may affect the serotonergic neurotransmitter systems, such as triptans. If concomitant treatment of tramadol with a drug affecting the serotonergic neurotransmitter system is clinically warranted, careful observation of the patient is advised, particularly during treatment initiation and dose increases).
No products indexed under this heading.

IMPORTANT NOTE: Always consult each drug listing in the patient's regimen for possible interactions.

Enflurane (Tramadol hydrochloride should be used with caution and in reduced dosages when administered to patients receiving CNS depressants, such as alcohol, opioids, anesthetic agents, narcotics, phenothiazines, tranquilizers, or sedative hypnotics. Tramadol hydrochloride increases the risk of CNS and respiratory depression).
No products indexed under this heading.

Erythromycin (Concomitant administration of CYP3A4 inhibitors, such as ketoconazole and erythromycin, may reduce metabolic clearance of tramadol increasing the risk for serious adverse events including seizures and serotonin syndrome).
No products indexed under this heading.

Erythromycin, Topical (Concomitant administration of CYP3A4 inhibitors, such as ketoconazole and erythromycin, may reduce metabolic clearance of tramadol increasing the risk for serious adverse events including seizures and serotonin syndrome).
No products indexed under this heading.

Erythromycin Estolate (Concomitant administration of CYP3A4 inhibitors, such as ketoconazole and erythromycin, may reduce metabolic clearance of tramadol increasing the risk for serious adverse events including seizures and serotonin syndrome).
No products indexed under this heading.

Erythromycin Ethylsuccinate (Concomitant administration of CYP3A4 inhibitors, such as ketoconazole and erythromycin, may reduce metabolic clearance of tramadol increasing the risk for serious adverse events including seizures and serotonin syndrome). Products include:
E.E.S. 437
EryPed 435

Erythromycin Gluceptate (Concomitant administration of CYP3A4 inhibitors, such as ketoconazole and erythromycin, may reduce metabolic clearance of tramadol increasing the risk for serious adverse events including seizures and serotonin syndrome).
No products indexed under this heading.

Erythromycin Lactobionate (Concomitant administration of CYP3A4 inhibitors, such as ketoconazole and erythromycin, may reduce metabolic clearance of tramadol increasing the risk for serious adverse events including seizures and serotonin syndrome).
No products indexed under this heading.

Erythromycin Stearate (Concomitant administration of CYP3A4 inhibitors, such as ketoconazole and erythromycin, may reduce metabolic clearance of tramadol increasing the risk for serious adverse events including seizures and serotonin syndrome).
No products indexed under this heading.

Escitalopram Oxalate (Concomitant use of tramadol hydrochloride increases the seizure risk in patients taking selective serotonin reuptake inhibitors (SSRI antidepressants or anorectics). There have been postmarketing reports of serotonin syndrome with use of tramadol and SSRIs/SNRIs. Caution is advised when tramadol is co-administered with other drugs that may affect the serotonergic neurotransmitter systems, such as SSRIs. If concomitant treatment of tramadol with a drug affecting the serotonergic neurotransmitter system is clinically warranted, careful observation of the patient is advised, particularly during treatment initiation and dose increases). Products include:
Lexapro Oral Suspension 1160
Lexapro Tablets 1160

Esomeprazole Magnesium (Concomitant administration of CYP3A4 inhibitors, such as ketoconazole and erythromycin, may reduce metabolic clearance of tramadol increasing the risk for serious adverse events including seizures and serotonin syndrome). Products include:
Nexium Capsules 704
Nexium Oral Suspension 704

Esomeprazole Sodium (Concomitant administration of CYP3A4 inhibitors, such as ketoconazole and erythromycin, may reduce metabolic clearance of tramadol increasing the risk for serious adverse events including seizures and serotonin syndrome). Products include:
Nexium I.V. 712

Estazolam (Tramadol hydrochloride should be used with caution and in reduced dosages when administered to patients receiving CNS depressants, such as sedative hypnotics. Tramadol hydrochloride increases the risk of CNS and respiratory depression).
No products indexed under this heading.

Ethanol (Tramadol hydrochloride should be used with caution and in reduced dosages when administered to patients receiving CNS depressants, such as alcohol, opioids, anesthetic agents, narcotics, phenothiazines, tranquilizers, or sedative hypnotics. Tramadol hydrochloride increases the risk of CNS and respiratory depression).
No products indexed under this heading.

Ethchlorvynol (Tramadol hydrochloride should be used with caution and in reduced dosages when administered to patients receiving CNS depressants, such as sedative hypnotics. Tramadol hydrochloride increases the risk of CNS and respiratory depression).
No products indexed under this heading.

Ethinamate (Tramadol hydrochloride should be used with caution and in reduced dosages when administered to patients receiving CNS depressants, such as sedative hypnotics. Tramadol hydrochloride increases the risk of CNS and respiratory depression).
No products indexed under this heading.

Ethosuximide (Administration of CYP3A4 inducers, such as rifampin or St. John's Wort, with tramadol hydrochloride may effect the metabolism of tramadol leading to altered tramadol exposure).
No products indexed under this heading.

Ethyl Alcohol (Tramadol hydrochloride should be used with caution and in reduced dosages when administered to patients receiving CNS depressants, such as alcohol, opioids, anesthetic agents, narcotics, phenothiazines, tranquilizers, or sedative hypnotics. Tramadol hydrochloride increases the risk of CNS and respiratory depression).
No products indexed under this heading.

Etidocaine Hydrochloride (Tramadol hydrochloride should be used with caution and in reduced dosages when administered to patients receiving CNS depressants, such as anesthetic agents. Tramadol hydrochloride increases the risk of CNS and respiratory depression).
No products indexed under this heading.

Fat (Co-administration with a high fat meal did not significantly affect AUC (overall exposure to tramadol); however, C_{max} (peak plasma concentration) increased 67% following a single 300 mg tablet administration and 54% following a single 200 mg tablet administration. Tramadol hydrochloride was administered without regard to food in all clinical trials).
No products indexed under this heading.

Felbamate (Administration of CYP3A4 inducers, such as rifampin or St. John's Wort, with tramadol hydrochloride may effect the metabolism of tramadol leading to altered tramadol exposure).
No products indexed under this heading.

Fentanyl (Concomitant use of tramadol hydrochloride increases the seizure risk in patients taking other opioids. Tramadol should be used with caution and in reduced dosages when administered to patients receiving CNS depressants such as opioids or narcotics. Tramadol increases the risk of CNS and respiratory depression in these patients). Products include:
Duragesic 2604
Fentanyl Transdermal System 2346
Onsolis 2054

Fentanyl Citrate (Concomitant use of tramadol hydrochloride increases the seizure risk in patients taking other opioids. Tramadol should be used with caution and in reduced dosages when administered to patients receiving CNS depressants such as opioids or narcotics. Tramadol increases the risk of CNS and respiratory depression in these patients). Products include:
Fentora 966

Fluconazole (Concomitant administration of CYP3A4 inhibitors, such as ketoconazole and erythromycin, may reduce metabolic clearance of tramadol increasing the risk for serious adverse events including seizures and serotonin syndrome).
No products indexed under this heading.

Fludrocortisone Acetate (Administration of CYP3A4 inducers, such as rifampin or St. John's Wort, with tramadol hydrochloride may effect the metabolism of tramadol leading to altered tramadol exposure).
No products indexed under this heading.

Fluoxetine (Concomitant use of tramadol hydrochloride increases the seizure risk in patients taking selective serotonin reuptake inhibitors (SSRI antidepressants or anorectics). There have been postmarketing reports of serotonin syndrome with use of tramadol and SSRIs/SNRIs. Caution is advised when tramadol is co-administered with other drugs that may affect the serotonergic neurotransmitter systems, such as SSRIs. If concomitant treatment of tramadol with a drug affecting the serotonergic neurotransmitter system is clinically warranted, careful observation of the patient is advised, particularly during treatment initiation and dose increases).
No products indexed under this heading.

Fluoxetine Hydrochloride (Administration of tramadol may increase the seizure risk in patients taking neuroleptics or other drugs that reduce the seizure threshold). Products include:
Prozac Weekly 1941
Prozac Pulvules 1941
Symbyax 1965

Fluphenazine Decanoate (Administration of tramadol may increase the seizure risk in patients taking neuroleptics or other drugs that reduce the seizure threshold).
No products indexed under this heading.

Fluphenazine Enanthate (Administration of tramadol may increase the seizure risk in patients taking neuroleptics or other drugs that reduce the seizure threshold).
No products indexed under this heading.

Fluphenazine Hydrochloride (Administration of tramadol may increase the seizure risk in patients taking neuroleptics or other drugs that reduce the seizure threshold).
No products indexed under this heading.

Flurazepam Hydrochloride (Tramadol hydrochloride should be used with caution and in reduced dosages when administered to patients receiving CNS depressants, such as sedative hypnotics. Tramadol hydrochloride increases the risk of CNS and respiratory depression).
No products indexed under this heading.

Fluvoxamine (Concomitant use of tramadol hydrochloride increases the seizure risk in patients taking selective serotonin reuptake inhibitors (SSRI antidepressants or anorectics). There have been postmarketing reports of serotonin syndrome with use of tramadol and SSRIs/SNRIs. Caution is advised when tramadol is co-administered with other drugs that may affect the serotonergic neurotransmitter systems, such as SSRIs. If concomitant treatment of tramadol with a drug affecting the serotonergic neurotransmitter system is clinically warranted, careful observation of the patient is advised, particularly during treatment initiation and dose increases).
No products indexed under this heading.

Fluvoxamine Maleate (Concomitant use of tramadol hydrochloride increases the seizure risk in patients taking selective serotonin reuptake inhibitors (SSRI antidepressants or anorectics). There have been postmarketing reports of serotonin syndrome with use of tramadol and SSRIs/SNRIs. Caution is advised when tramadol is co-administered with other drugs that may affect the serotonergic neurotransmitter systems, such as SSRIs. If concomitant treatment of tramadol with a drug affecting the serotonergic neurotransmitter system is clinically warranted, careful observation of the patient is advised, particularly during treatment initiation and dose increases).
No products indexed under this heading.

Fosamprenavir Calcium (Concomitant administration of CYP3A4 inhibitors, such as ketoconazole and erythromycin, may reduce metabolic clearance of tramadol increasing the risk for serious adverse events including seizures and serotonin syndrome). Products include:
Lexiva Oral Suspension 1558
Lexiva 1558

Fosphenytoin Sodium (Administration of CYP3A4 inducers, such as rifampin or St. John's Wort, with tramadol hydrochloride may effect the metabolism of tramadol leading to altered tramadol exposure).
No products indexed under this heading.

Frovatriptan Succinate (Caution is advised when tramadol is co-administered with other drugs that may affect the serotonergic neurotransmitter systems, such as triptans. If concomitant treatment of tramadol with a drug affecting the serotonergic neurotransmitter system is clinically warranted, careful observation of the patient is advised, particularly during treatment initiation and dose increases). Products include:
Frova 1103

Gallamine (Because of its added depressant effects, tramadol should be prescribed with caution for those patients whose medical condition requires the concomitant administration of muscle relaxants, or other CNS-depressant drugs. Patients should be advised of the additive depressant effects of these combinations).
No products indexed under this heading.

Gallamine Triethiodide (Because of its added depressant effects, tramadol should be prescribed with caution for those patients whose medical condition requires the concomitant administration of muscle relaxants, or other CNS-depressant drugs. Patients should be advised of the additive depressant effects of these combinations).
No products indexed under this heading.

Garlic Extract (Administration of CYP3A4 inducers, such as rifampin or St. John's Wort, with tramadol hydrochloride may effect the metabolism of tramadol leading to altered tramadol exposure).
No products indexed under this heading.

Garlic Oil (Administration of CYP3A4 inducers, such as rifampin or St. John's Wort, with tramadol hydrochloride may effect the metabolism of tramadol leading to altered tramadol exposure).
No products indexed under this heading.

Glutethimide (Tramadol hydrochloride should be used with caution and in reduced dosages when administered to patients receiving CNS depressants, such as sedative hypnotics. Tramadol hydrochloride increases the risk of CNS and respiratory depression).
No products indexed under this heading.

Halazepam (Tramadol hydrochloride should be used with caution and in reduced dosages when administered to patients receiving CNS depressants, such as alcohol, opioids, anesthetic agents, narcotics, phenothiazines, tranquilizers, or sedative hypnotics. Tramadol hydrochloride increases the risk of CNS and respiratory depression).
No products indexed under this heading.

Halofantrine Hydrochloride (Concomitant administration of CYP2D6 inhibitors such as quinidine, fluoxetine, paroxetine and amitriptyline may reduce metabolic clearance of tramadol increasing the risk for serious adverse events including seizures and serotonin syndrome. In vitro drug interaction studies in human liver microsomes indicate that inhibitors of CYP2D6 inhibit the metabolism of tramadol to various degrees, suggesting that concomitant administration of these compounds could result in increases in tramadol concentrations and decreased concentrations of M1. The full pharmacological impact of these alterations in terms of either efficacy or safety is unknown).
No products indexed under this heading.

Haloperidol (Administration of tramadol may increase the seizure risk in patients taking neuroleptics or other drugs that reduce the seizure threshold).
No products indexed under this heading.

Haloperidol Decanoate (Administration of tramadol may increase the seizure risk in patients taking neuroleptics or other drugs that reduce the seizure threshold).
No products indexed under this heading.

Haloperidol Lactate (Tramadol hydrochloride should be used with caution and in reduced dosages when administered to patients receiving CNS depressants, such as alcohol, opioids, anesthetic agents, narcotics, phenothiazines, tranquilizers, or sedative hypnotics. Tramadol hydrochloride increases the risk of CNS and respiratory depression).
No products indexed under this heading.

Halothane (Tramadol hydrochloride should be used with caution and in reduced dosages when administered to patients receiving CNS depressants, such as anesthetic agents. Tramadol hydrochloride increases the risk of CNS and respiratory depression).
No products indexed under this heading.

Hexobarbital (Tramadol hydrochloride should be used with caution and in reduced dosages when administered to patients receiving CNS depressants, such as alcohol, opioids, anesthetic agents, narcotics, phenothiazines, tranquilizers, or sedative hypnotics. Tramadol hydrochloride increases the risk of CNS and respiratory depression).
No products indexed under this heading.

Hydrocodone Bitartrate (Concomitant use of tramadol hydrochloride increases the seizure risk in patients taking other opioids. Tramadol should be used with caution and in reduced dosages when administered to patients receiving CNS depressants such as opioids or narcotics. Tramadol increases the risk of CNS and respiratory depression in these patients).
Products include:
Vicodin 560
Vicodin ES 561
Vicodin HP 563
Vicoprofen 564
Zydone 1138

Hydrocodone Polistirex (Concomitant use of tramadol hydrochloride increases the seizure risk in patients taking other opioids. Tramadol should be used with caution and in reduced dosages when administered to patients receiving CNS depressants such as opioids or narcotics. Tramadol increases the risk of CNS and respiratory depression in these patients).
Products include:
Tussionex 3443

Hydrocortisone (Administration of CYP3A4 inducers, such as rifampin or St. John's Wort, with tramadol hydrochloride may effect the metabolism of tramadol leading to altered tramadol exposure).
No products indexed under this heading.

Hydrocortisone (Alcohol) (Administration of CYP3A4 inducers, such as rifampin or St. John's Wort, with tramadol hydrochloride may effect the metabolism of tramadol leading to altered tramadol exposure).
No products indexed under this heading.

Hydrocortisone Acetate (Administration of CYP3A4 inducers, such as rifampin or St. John's Wort, with tramadol hydrochloride may effect the metabolism of tramadol leading to altered tramadol exposure).
No products indexed under this heading.

Hydrocortisone Butyrate (Administration of CYP3A4 inducers, such as rifampin or St. John's Wort, with tramadol hydrochloride may effect the metabolism of tramadol leading to altered tramadol exposure).
No products indexed under this heading.

Hydrocortisone Cypionate (Administration of CYP3A4 inducers, such as rifampin or St. John's Wort, with tramadol hydrochloride may effect the metabolism of tramadol leading to altered tramadol exposure).
No products indexed under this heading.

Hydrocortisone Hemisuccinate (Administration of CYP3A4 inducers, such as rifampin or St. John's Wort, with tramadol hydrochloride may effect the metabolism of tramadol leading to altered tramadol exposure).
No products indexed under this heading.

Hydrocortisone Probutate (Administration of CYP3A4 inducers, such as rifampin or St. John's Wort, with tramadol hydrochloride may effect the metabolism of tramadol leading to altered tramadol exposure).
No products indexed under this heading.

Hydrocortisone Sodium Phosphate (Administration of CYP3A4 inducers, such as rifampin or St. John's Wort, with tramadol hydrochloride may effect the metabolism of tramadol leading to altered tramadol exposure).
No products indexed under this heading.

Hydrocortisone Sodium Succinate (Administration of CYP3A4 inducers, such as rifampin or St. John's Wort, with tramadol hydrochloride may effect the metabolism of tramadol leading to altered tramadol exposure).
No products indexed under this heading.

Hydrocortisone Valerate (Administration of CYP3A4 inducers, such as rifampin or St. John's Wort, with tramadol hydrochloride may effect the metabolism of tramadol leading to altered tramadol exposure).
No products indexed under this heading.

Hydromorphone (Concomitant use of tramadol hydrochloride increases the seizure risk in patients taking other opioids. Tramadol should be used with caution and in reduced dosages when administered to patients receiving CNS depressants such as opioids or narcotics. Tramadol increases the risk of CNS and respiratory depression in these patients).
No products indexed under this heading.

Hydromorphone Hydrochloride (Concomitant use of tramadol hydrochloride increases the seizure risk in patients taking other opioids. Tramadol should be used with caution and in reduced dosages when administered to patients receiving CNS depressants such as opioids or narcotics. Tramadol increases the risk of CNS and respiratory depression in these patients).
Products include:
Dilaudid Injection 2800
Dilaudid Oral 2797
Dilaudid Tablets 2797
Dilaudid-HP 2800

Hydroxychloroquine Sulfate (Concomitant administration of CYP2D6 inhibitors such as quinidine, fluoxetine, paroxetine and amitriptyline may reduce metabolic clearance of tramadol increasing the risk for serious adverse events including seizures and serotonin syndrome. In vitro drug interaction studies in human liver microsomes indicate that inhibitors of CYP2D6 inhibit the metabolism of tramadol to various degrees, suggesting that concomitant administration of these compounds could result in increases in tramadol concentrations and decreased concentrations of M1. The full pharmacological impact of these alterations in terms of either efficacy or safety is unknown).
No products indexed under this heading.

Hydroxyzine Hydrochloride (Tramadol hydrochloride should be used with caution and in reduced dosages when administered to patients receiving CNS depressants, such as alcohol, opioids, anesthetic agents, narcotics, phenothiazines, tranquilizers, or sedative hypnotics. Tramadol hydrochloride increases the risk of CNS and respiratory depression).
No products indexed under this heading.

Hypericum (Administration of CYP3A4 inducers, such as rifampin or St. John's Wort, with tramadol hydrochloride may effect the metabolism of tramadol leading to altered tramadol exposure).
No products indexed under this heading.

Hypericum Perforatum (Caution is advised when tramadol is co-administered with other drugs that may affect the serotonergic neurotransmitter systems, such as St. John's Wort. If concomitant treatment of tramadol with a drug affecting the serotonergic neurotransmitter system is clinically warranted, careful observation of the

patient is advised, particularly during treatment initiation and dose increases).
Products include:
Traumeel 1800

Imatinib Mesylate (Concomitant administration of CYP2D6 inhibitors such as quinidine, fluoxetine, paroxetine and amitriptyline may reduce metabolic clearance of tramadol increasing the risk for serious adverse events including seizures and serotonin syndrome. In vitro drug interaction studies in human liver microsomes indicate that inhibitors of CYP2D6 inhibit the metabolism of tramadol to various degrees, suggesting that concomitant administration of these compounds could result in increases in tramadol concentrations and decreased concentrations of M1. The full pharmacological impact of these alterations in terms of either efficacy or safety is unknown). Products include:
Gleevec 2477

Imipramine Hydrochloride (Administration of tramadol may increase the seizure risk in patients taking neuroleptics or other drugs that reduce the seizure threshold).
No products indexed under this heading.

Imipramine Pamoate (Administration of tramadol may increase the seizure risk in patients taking neuroleptics or other drugs that reduce the seizure threshold).
No products indexed under this heading.

Indinavir Sulfate (Concomitant administration of CYP3A4 inhibitors, such as ketoconazole and erythromycin, may reduce metabolic clearance of tramadol increasing the risk for serious adverse events including seizures and serotonin syndrome). Products include:
Crixivan 2113

Isocarboxazid (Administration of tramadol may enhance the seizure risk in patients taking monoamine oxidase (MAO) inhibitors. There have been post-marketing reports of serotonin syndrome with use of tramadol and monoamine oxidase inhibitors. Caution is advised when tramadol is co-administered with other drugs that may affect the serotonergic neurotransmitter systems, such as MAOIs. If concomitant treatment of tramadol with a drug affecting the serotonergic neurotransmitter system is clinically warranted, careful observation of the patient is advised, particularly during treatment initiation and dose increases). Products include:
Marplan 3481

Isoflurane (Tramadol hydrochloride should be used with caution and in reduced dosages when administered to patients receiving CNS depressants, such as alcohol, opioids, anesthetic agents, narcotics, phenothiazines, tranquilizers, or sedative hypnotics. Tramadol hydrochloride increases the risk of CNS and respiratory depression).
No products indexed under this heading.

Isoniazid (Concomitant administration of CYP3A4 inhibitors, such as ketoconazole and erythromycin, may reduce metabolic clearance of tramadol increasing the risk for serious adverse events including seizures and serotonin syndrome).
No products indexed under this heading.

Itraconazole (Concomitant administration of CYP3A4 inhibitors, such as ketoconazole and erythromycin, may reduce metabolic clearance of tramadol increasing the risk for serious adverse events including seizures and serotonin syndrome).
No products indexed under this heading.

IMPORTANT NOTE: Always consult each drug listing in the patient's regimen for possible interactions.

Ketamine Hydrochloride (Tramadol hydrochloride should be used with caution and in reduced dosages when administered to patients receiving CNS depressants, such as alcohol, opioids, anesthetic agents, narcotics, phenothiazines, tranquilizers, or sedative hypnotics. Tramadol hydrochloride increases the risk of CNS and respiratory depression).
No products indexed under this heading.

Ketoconazole (Concomitant administration of CYP3A4 inhibitors, such as ketoconazole and erythromycin, may reduce metabolic clearance of tramadol increasing the risk for serious adverse events including seizures and serotonin syndrome). Products include:
Extina 3319
Xolegel 3337

Lapatinib (Concomitant administration of CYP3A4 inhibitors, such as ketoconazole and erythromycin, may reduce metabolic clearance of tramadol increasing the risk for serious adverse events including seizures and serotonin syndrome). Products include:
Tykerb 1698

Levobupivacaine Hydrochloride (Tramadol hydrochloride should be used with caution and in reduced dosages when administered to patients receiving CNS depressants, such as anesthetic agents. Tramadol hydrochloride increases the risk of CNS and respiratory depression).
No products indexed under this heading.

Levomethadyl Acetate Hydrochloride (Tramadol hydrochloride should be used with caution and in reduced dosages when administered to patients receiving CNS depressants, such as alcohol, opioids, anesthetic agents, narcotics, phenothiazines, tranquilizers, or sedative hypnotics. Tramadol hydrochloride increases the risk of CNS and respiratory depression).
No products indexed under this heading.

Levorphanol Tartrate (Concomitant use of tramadol hydrochloride increases the seizure risk in patients taking other opioids. Tramadol should be used with caution and in reduced dosages when administered to patients receiving CNS depressants such as opioids or narcotics. Tramadol increases the risk of CNS and respiratory depression in these patients).
No products indexed under this heading.

Lidocaine (Tramadol hydrochloride should be used with caution and in reduced dosages when administered to patients receiving CNS depressants, such as anesthetic agents. Tramadol hydrochloride increases the risk of CNS and respiratory depression). Products include:
Lidoderm 1107

Lidocaine Base (Tramadol hydrochloride should be used with caution and in reduced dosages when administered to patients receiving CNS depressants, such as anesthetic agents. Tramadol hydrochloride increases the risk of CNS and respiratory depression).
No products indexed under this heading.

Lidocaine Hydrochloride (Tramadol hydrochloride should be used with caution and in reduced dosages when administered to patients receiving CNS depressants, such as anesthetic agents. Tramadol hydrochloride increases the risk of CNS and respiratory depression).
No products indexed under this heading.

Lithium (Caution is advised when tramadol is co-administered with other drugs that may affect the serotonergic neurotransmitter systems, such as lithium. If concomitant treatment of tramadol with a drug affecting the serotonergic neurotransmitter system is clinically warranted, careful observation of the patient is advised, particularly during treatment initiation and dose increases).
No products indexed under this heading.

Lithium Carbonate (Caution is advised when tramadol is co-administered with other drugs that may affect the serotonergic neurotransmitter systems, such as lithium. If concomitant treatment of tramadol with a drug affecting the serotonergic neurotransmitter system is clinically warranted, careful observation of the patient is advised, particularly during treatment initiation and dose increases).
No products indexed under this heading.

Lithium Citrate (Caution is advised when tramadol is co-administered with other drugs that may affect the serotonergic neurotransmitter systems, such as lithium. If concomitant treatment of tramadol with a drug affecting the serotonergic neurotransmitter system is clinically warranted, careful observation of the patient is advised, particularly during treatment initiation and dose increases).
No products indexed under this heading.

Lopinavir (Concomitant administration of CYP3A4 inhibitors, such as ketoconazole and erythromycin, may reduce metabolic clearance of tramadol increasing the risk for serious adverse events including seizures and serotonin syndrome). Products include:
Kaletra 458

Loratadine (Concomitant administration of CYP3A4 inhibitors, such as ketoconazole and erythromycin, may reduce metabolic clearance of tramadol increasing the risk for serious adverse events including seizures and serotonin syndrome).
No products indexed under this heading.

Lorazepam (Tramadol hydrochloride should be used with caution and in reduced dosages when administered to patients receiving CNS depressants, such as sedative hypnotics. Tramadol hydrochloride increases the risk of CNS and respiratory depression).
No products indexed under this heading.

Loxapine Hydrochloride (Tramadol hydrochloride should be used with caution and in reduced dosages when administered to patients receiving CNS depressants, such as alcohol, opioids, anesthetic agents, narcotics, phenothiazines, tranquilizers, or sedative hypnotics. Tramadol hydrochloride increases the risk of CNS and respiratory depression).
No products indexed under this heading.

Loxapine Succinate (Tramadol hydrochloride should be used with caution and in reduced dosages when administered to patients receiving CNS depressants, such as alcohol, opioids, anesthetic agents, narcotics, phenothiazines, tranquilizers, or sedative hypnotics. Tramadol hydrochloride increases the risk of CNS and respiratory depression).
No products indexed under this heading.

Maprotiline Hydrochloride (Administration of tramadol may increase the seizure risk in patients taking neuroleptics or other drugs that reduce the seizure threshold).
No products indexed under this heading.

Meperidine Hydrochloride (Concomitant use of tramadol hydrochloride increases the seizure risk in patients taking other opioids. Tramadol should be used with caution and in reduced dosages when administered to patients receiving CNS depressants such as opioids or narcotics. Tramadol increases the risk of CNS and respiratory depression in these patients).
No products indexed under this heading.

Mephenytoin (Administration of CYP3A4 inducers, such as rifampin or St. John's Wort, with tramadol hydrochloride may effect the metabolism of tramadol leading to altered tramadol exposure).
No products indexed under this heading.

Mephobarbital (Tramadol hydrochloride should be used with caution and in reduced dosages when administered to patients receiving CNS depressants, such as alcohol, opioids, anesthetic agents, narcotics, phenothiazines, tranquilizers, or sedative hypnotics. Tramadol hydrochloride increases the risk of CNS and respiratory depression).
No products indexed under this heading.

Mepivacaine Hydrochloride (Tramadol hydrochloride should be used with caution and in reduced dosages when administered to patients receiving CNS depressants, such as anesthetic agents. Tramadol hydrochloride increases the risk of CNS and respiratory depression).
No products indexed under this heading.

Meprobamate (Tramadol hydrochloride should be used with caution and in reduced dosages when administered to patients receiving CNS depressants, such as alcohol, opioids, anesthetic agents, narcotics, phenothiazines, tranquilizers, or sedative hypnotics. Tramadol hydrochloride increases the risk of CNS and respiratory depression).
No products indexed under this heading.

Mesoridazine Besylate (Administration of tramadol may increase the seizure risk in patients taking neuroleptics or other drugs that reduce the seizure threshold).
No products indexed under this heading.

Metaxalone (Because of its added depressant effects, tramadol should be prescribed with caution for those patients whose medical condition requires the concomitant administration of muscle relaxants, or other CNS-depressant drugs. Patients should be advised of the additive depressant effects of these combinations).
Products include:
Skelaxin 1848

Methadone Hydrochloride (Concomitant use of tramadol hydrochloride increases the seizure risk in patients taking other opioids. Tramadol should be used with caution and in reduced dosages when administered to patients receiving CNS depressants such as opioids or narcotics. Tramadol increases the risk of CNS and respiratory depression in these patients).
No products indexed under this heading.

Methocarbamol (Because of its added depressant effects, tramadol should be prescribed with caution for those patients whose medical condition requires the concomitant administration of muscle relaxants, or other CNS-depressant drugs. Patients should be advised of the additive depressant effects of these combinations).
No products indexed under this heading.

Methohexital Sodium (Tramadol hydrochloride should be used with caution and in reduced dosages when administered to patients receiving CNS depressants, such as alcohol, opioids, anesthetic agents, narcotics, phenothiazines, tranquilizers, or sedative hypnotics. Tramadol hydrochloride increases the risk of CNS and respiratory depression).
No products indexed under this heading.

Methotrimeprazine (Tramadol hydrochloride should be used with caution and in reduced dosages when administered to patients receiving CNS depressants, such as alcohol, opioids, anesthetic agents, narcotics, phenothiazines, tranquilizers, or sedative hypnotics. Tramadol hydrochloride increases the risk of CNS and respiratory depression).
No products indexed under this heading.

Methoxyflurane (Tramadol hydrochloride should be used with caution and in reduced dosages when administered to patients receiving CNS depressants, such as alcohol, opioids, anesthetic agents, narcotics, phenothiazines, tranquilizers, or sedative hypnotics. Tramadol hydrochloride increases the risk of CNS and respiratory depression).
No products indexed under this heading.

Methsuximide (Administration of CYP3A4 inducers, such as rifampin or St. John's Wort, with tramadol hydrochloride may effect the metabolism of tramadol leading to altered tramadol exposure).
No products indexed under this heading.

Methylprednisolone (Administration of CYP3A4 inducers, such as rifampin or St. John's Wort, with tramadol hydrochloride may effect the metabolism of tramadol leading to altered tramadol exposure).
No products indexed under this heading.

Methylprednisolone Acetate (Administration of CYP3A4 inducers, such as rifampin or St. John's Wort, with tramadol hydrochloride may effect the metabolism of tramadol leading to altered tramadol exposure).
No products indexed under this heading.

Methylprednisolone Sodium Succinate (Administration of CYP3A4 inducers, such as rifampin or St. John's Wort, with tramadol hydrochloride may effect the metabolism of tramadol leading to altered tramadol exposure).
No products indexed under this heading.

Metocurine Iodide (Because of its added depressant effects, tramadol should be prescribed with caution for those patients whose medical condition requires the concomitant administration of muscle relaxants, or other CNS-depressant drugs. Patients should be advised of the additive depressant effects of these combinations).
No products indexed under this heading.

Metronidazole (Concomitant administration of CYP3A4 inhibitors, such as ketoconazole and erythromycin, may reduce metabolic clearance of tramadol increasing the risk for serious adverse events including seizures and serotonin syndrome). Products include:
Pylera 793

Metronidazole Benzoate (Concomitant administration of CYP3A4 inhibitors, such as ketoconazole and erythromycin, may reduce metabolic clearance of tramadol increasing the risk for serious adverse events including seizures and serotonin syndrome).
No products indexed under this heading.

1665 **Interactions Index** **Ryzolt**

Metronidazole Hydrochloride (Concomitant administration of CYP3A4 inhibitors, such as ketoconazole and erythromycin, may reduce metabolic clearance of tramadol increasing the risk for serious adverse events including seizures and serotonin syndrome).
No products indexed under this heading.

Metronidazole Sodium (Concomitant administration of CYP3A4 inhibitors, such as ketoconazole and erythromycin, may reduce metabolic clearance of tramadol increasing the risk for serious adverse events including seizures and serotonin syndrome).
No products indexed under this heading.

Mibefradil Dihydrochloride (Concomitant administration of CYP2D6 inhibitors such as quinidine, fluoxetine, paroxetine and amitriptyline may reduce metabolic clearance of tramadol increasing the risk for serious adverse events including seizures and serotonin syndrome. *In vitro* drug interaction studies in human liver microsomes indicate that inhibitors of CYP2D6 inhibit the metabolism of tramadol to various degrees, suggesting that concomitant administration of these compounds could result in increases in tramadol concentrations and decreased concentrations of M1. The full pharmacological impact of these alterations in terms of either efficacy or safety is unknown).
No products indexed under this heading.

Miconazole (Concomitant administration of CYP3A4 inhibitors, such as ketoconazole and erythromycin, may reduce metabolic clearance of tramadol increasing the risk for serious adverse events including seizures and serotonin syndrome).
No products indexed under this heading.

Miconazole Nitrate (Concomitant administration of CYP3A4 inhibitors, such as ketoconazole and erythromycin, may reduce metabolic clearance of tramadol increasing the risk for serious adverse events including seizures and serotonin syndrome). Products include:
Vusion Ointment 3335

Midazolam Hydrochloride (Tramadol hydrochloride should be used with caution and in reduced dosages when administered to patients receiving CNS depressants, such as sedative hypnotics. Tramadol hydrochloride increases the risk of CNS and respiratory depression).
No products indexed under this heading.

Mifepristone (Concomitant administration of CYP3A4 inhibitors, such as ketoconazole and erythromycin, may reduce metabolic clearance of tramadol increasing the risk for serious adverse events including seizures and serotonin syndrome).
No products indexed under this heading.

Mirtazapine (Prescribe tramadol with caution for patients taking antidepressant drugs. Serious potential consequences of overdosage with tramadol are central nervous system depression, respiratory depression and death. In treating an overdose, primary attention should be given to maintaining adequate ventilation along with general supportive treatment). Products include:
Remeron Tablets 3214
RemeronSolTab Tablets 3219

Mivacurium Chloride (Because of its added depressant effects, tramadol should be prescribed with caution for those patients whose medical condition requires the concomitant administration of muscle relaxants, or other CNS-depressant drugs. Patients should be advised of the additive depressant effects of these combinations).
No products indexed under this heading.

Moclobemide (Administration of tramadol may enhance the seizure risk in patients taking monoamine oxidase (MAO) inhibitors. There have been postmarketing reports of serotonin syndrome with use of tramadol and monoamine oxidase inhibitors. Caution is advised when tramadol is coadministered with other drugs that may affect the serotonergic neurotransmitter systems, such as MAOIs. If concomitant treatment of tramadol with a drug affecting the serotonergic neurotransmitter system is clinically warranted, careful observation of the patient is advised, particularly during treatment initiation and dose increases).
No products indexed under this heading.

Modafinil (Administration of CYP3A4 inducers, such as rifampin or St. John's Wort, with tramadol hydrochloride may effect the metabolism of tramadol leading to altered tramadol exposure). Products include:
Provigil 983

Molindone Hydrochloride (Tramadol hydrochloride should be used with caution and in reduced dosages when administered to patients receiving CNS depressants, such as alcohol, opioids, anesthetic agents, narcotics, phenothiazines, tranquilizers, or sedative hypnotics. Tramadol hydrochloride increases the risk of CNS and respiratory depression). Products include:
Moban 1108

Morphine Sulfate (Concomitant use of tramadol hydrochloride increases the seizure risk in patients taking other opioids. Tramadol should be used with caution and in reduced dosages when administered to patients receiving CNS depressants such as opioids or narcotics. Tramadol increases the risk of CNS and respiratory depression in these patients). Products include:
Avinza 1822
Embeda 1831
MS Contin 2803

Morphine Sulfate, Liposomal (Concomitant use of tramadol hydrochloride increases the seizure risk in patients taking other opioids. Tramadol should be used with caution and in reduced dosages when administered to patients receiving CNS depressants such as opioids or narcotics. Tramadol increases the risk of CNS and respiratory depression in these patients).
No products indexed under this heading.

Nafcillin Sodium (Administration of CYP3A4 inducers, such as rifampin or St. John's Wort, with tramadol hydrochloride may effect the metabolism of tramadol leading to altered tramadol exposure).
No products indexed under this heading.

Naloxone Hydrochloride (In tramadol overdose, naloxone administration may increase the risk of seizures).
No products indexed under this heading.

Naratriptan Hydrochloride (Caution is advised when tramadol is coadministered with other drugs that may affect the serotonergic neurotransmitter systems, such as triptans. If concomitant treatment of tramadol with a drug affecting the serotonergic neurotransmitter system is clinically warranted, careful observation of the patient is advised, particularly during treatment initiation and dose increases). Products include:
Amerge 1306

Nefazodone Hydrochloride (Concomitant administration of CYP3A4 inhibitors, such as ketoconazole and erythromycin, may reduce metabolic clearance of tramadol increasing the risk for serious adverse events including seizures and serotonin syndrome).
No products indexed under this heading.

Nelfinavir Mesylate (Concomitant administration of CYP3A4 inhibitors, such as ketoconazole and erythromycin, may reduce metabolic clearance of tramadol increasing the risk for serious adverse events including seizures and serotonin syndrome).
No products indexed under this heading.

Nevirapine (Concomitant administration of CYP3A4 inhibitors, such as ketoconazole and erythromycin, may reduce metabolic clearance of tramadol increasing the risk for serious adverse events including seizures and serotonin syndrome). Products include:
Viramune Oral Suspension 897
Viramune Tablets 897

Niacin (Concomitant administration of CYP3A4 inhibitors, such as ketoconazole and erythromycin, may reduce metabolic clearance of tramadol increasing the risk for serious adverse events including seizures and serotonin syndrome). Products include:
Advicor 402
Cardio Basics 3455
Niaspan 497
Simcor 524

Niacinamide (Concomitant administration of CYP3A4 inhibitors, such as ketoconazole and erythromycin, may reduce metabolic clearance of tramadol increasing the risk for serious adverse events including seizures and serotonin syndrome). Products include:
CitraNatal 90 DHA Capsules 2332
CitraNatal Assure 2332
CitraNatal Rx 2332
Heplive 607

Niacinamide Hydroiodide (Concomitant administration of CYP3A4 inhibitors, such as ketoconazole and erythromycin, may reduce metabolic clearance of tramadol increasing the risk for serious adverse events including seizures and serotonin syndrome).
No products indexed under this heading.

Nicotinamide (Concomitant administration of CYP3A4 inhibitors, such as ketoconazole and erythromycin, may reduce metabolic clearance of tramadol increasing the risk for serious adverse events including seizures and serotonin syndrome).
No products indexed under this heading.

Nifedipine (Concomitant administration of CYP3A4 inhibitors, such as ketoconazole and erythromycin, may reduce metabolic clearance of tramadol increasing the risk for serious adverse events including seizures and serotonin syndrome).
No products indexed under this heading.

Norepinephrine Bitartrate (Tramadol has been shown to inhibit reuptake of norepinephrine and serotonin *in vitro*, as have some other opioid analgesics. These mechanisms may contribute independently to the overall analgesic profile of tramadol).
No products indexed under this heading.

Norepinephrine Hydrochloride (Tramadol has been shown to inhibit reuptake of norepinephrine and serotonin *in vitro*, as have some other opioid analgesics. These mechanisms may contribute independently to the overall analgesic profile of tramadol).
No products indexed under this heading.

Norfloxacin (Concomitant administration of CYP3A4 inhibitors, such as ketoconazole and erythromycin, may reduce metabolic clearance of tramadol increasing the risk for serious adverse events including seizures and serotonin syndrome). Products include:
Noroxin 2220

Nortriptyline Hydrochloride (Administration of tramadol may increase the seizure risk in patients taking neuroleptics or other drugs that reduce the seizure threshold).
No products indexed under this heading.

Olanzapine (Tramadol hydrochloride should be used with caution and in reduced dosages when administered to patients receiving CNS depressants, such as alcohol, opioids, anesthetic agents, narcotics, phenothiazines, tranquilizers, or sedative hypnotics. Tramadol hydrochloride increases the risk of CNS and respiratory depression). Products include:
Symbyax 1965
Zyprexa 1984
Zyprexa IntraMuscular 1984
Zyprexa ZYDIS 1984

Omeprazole (Concomitant administration of CYP3A4 inhibitors, such as ketoconazole and erythromycin, may reduce metabolic clearance of tramadol increasing the risk for serious adverse events including seizures and serotonin syndrome).
No products indexed under this heading.

Orphenadrine Citrate (Because of its added depressant effects, tramadol should be prescribed with caution for those patients whose medical condition requires the concomitant administration of muscle relaxants, or other CNS-depressant drugs. Patients should be advised of the additive depressant effects of these combinations).
No products indexed under this heading.

Oxazepam (Administration of tramadol may increase the seizure risk in patients taking neuroleptics or other drugs that reduce the seizure threshold).
No products indexed under this heading.

Oxcarbazepine (Administration of CYP3A4 inducers, such as rifampin or St. John's Wort, with tramadol hydrochloride may effect the metabolism of tramadol leading to altered tramadol exposure).
No products indexed under this heading.

Oxycodone Hydrochloride (Concomitant use of tramadol hydrochloride increases the seizure risk in patients taking other opioids. Tramadol should be used with caution and in reduced dosages when administered to patients receiving CNS depressants such as opioids or narcotics. Tramadol increases the risk of CNS and respiratory depression in these patients). Products include:
OxyContin 2807
Percocet 1121
Percodan 1124

Oxycodone Terephthalate (Concomitant use of tramadol hydrochloride increases the seizure risk in patients taking other opioids. Tramadol should be used with caution and in reduced dosages when administered to patients receiving CNS depressants such as opioids or narcotics. Tramadol increases the risk of CNS and respiratory depression in these patients).
No products indexed under this heading.

Oxymorphone Hydrochloride (Concomitant use of tramadol hydrochloride increases the seizure risk in patients taking other opioids. Tramadol should be used with caution and in reduced dosages when administered to patients receiving CNS depressants such as opioids or narcotics. Tramadol increases the risk of CNS and respiratory depression in these patients). Products include:
Opana 1110
Opana ER 1114

IMPORTANT NOTE: Always consult each drug listing in the patient's regimen for possible interactions.

Pancuronium Bromide (Because of its added depressant effects, tramadol should be prescribed with caution for those patients whose medical condition requires the concomitant administration of muscle relaxants, or other CNS-depressant drugs. Patients should be advised of the additive depressant effects of these combinations).
No products indexed under this heading.

Pargyline Hydrochloride (Administration of tramadol may enhance the seizure risk in patients taking monoamine oxidase (MAO) inhibitors. There have been post-marketing reports of serotonin syndrome with use of tramadol and monoamine oxidase inhibitors. Caution is advised when tramadol is co-administered with other drugs that may affect the serotonergic neurotransmitter systems, such as MAOIs. If concomitant treatment of tramadol with a drug affecting the serotonergic neurotransmitter system is clinically warranted, careful observation of the patient is advised, particularly during treatment initiation and dose increases).
No products indexed under this heading.

Paroxetine (Concomitant use of tramadol hydrochloride increases the seizure risk in patients taking selective serotonin reuptake inhibitors (SSRI antidepressants or anorectics). There have been postmarketing reports of serotonin syndrome with use of tramadol and SSRIs/SNRIs. Caution is advised when tramadol is co-administered with other drugs that may affect the serotonergic neurotransmitter systems, such as SSRIs. If concomitant treatment of tramadol with a drug affecting the serotonergic neurotransmitter system is clinically warranted, careful observation of the patient is advised, particularly during treatment initiation and dose increases).
No products indexed under this heading.

Paroxetine Hydrochloride (Concomitant use of tramadol hydrochloride increases the seizure risk in patients taking selective serotonin reuptake inhibitors (SSRI antidepressants or anorectics). There have been postmarketing reports of serotonin syndrome with use of tramadol and SSRIs/SNRIs. Caution is advised when tramadol is co-administered with other drugs that may affect the serotonergic neurotransmitter systems, such as SSRIs. If concomitant treatment of tramadol with a drug affecting the serotonergic neurotransmitter system is clinically warranted, careful observation of the patient is advised, particularly during treatment initiation and dose increases). Products include:

Paroxetine CR 2361
Paroxetine ER 2371
Paxil 1586
Paxil CR 1596

Paroxetine Mesylate (Concomitant use of tramadol hydrochloride increases the seizure risk in patients taking selective serotonin reuptake inhibitors (SSRI antidepressants or anorectics). There have been postmarketing reports of serotonin syndrome with use of tramadol and SSRIs/SNRIs. Caution is advised when tramadol is co-administered with other drugs that may affect the serotonergic neurotransmitter systems, such as SSRIs. If concomitant treatment of tramadol with a drug affecting the serotonergic neurotransmitter system is clinically warranted, careful observation of the patient is advised, particularly during treatment initiation and dose increases).
No products indexed under this heading.

Pentobarbital (Tramadol hydrochloride should be used with caution and in reduced dosages when administered to patients receiving CNS depressants, such as alcohol, opioids, anesthetic agents, narcotics, phenothiazines, tranquilizers, or sedative hypnotics. Tramadol hydrochloride increases the risk of CNS and respiratory depression).
No products indexed under this heading.

Pentobarbital Sodium (Tramadol hydrochloride should be used with caution and in reduced dosages when administered to patients receiving CNS depressants, such as alcohol, opioids, anesthetic agents, narcotics, phenothiazines, tranquilizers, or sedative hypnotics. Tramadol hydrochloride increases the risk of CNS and respiratory depression). Products include:

Nembutal 2012

Perphenazine (Administration of tramadol may increase the seizure risk in patients taking neuroleptics or other drugs that reduce the seizure threshold).
No products indexed under this heading.

Phenelzine Sulfate (Administration of tramadol may enhance the seizure risk in patients taking monoamine oxidase (MAO) inhibitors. There have been post-marketing reports of serotonin syndrome with use of tramadol and monoamine oxidase inhibitors. Caution is advised when tramadol is co-administered with other drugs that may affect the serotonergic neurotransmitter systems, such as MAOIs. If concomitant treatment of tramadol with a drug affecting the serotonergic neurotransmitter system is clinically warranted, careful observation of the patient is advised, particularly during treatment initiation and dose increases).
No products indexed under this heading.

Phenobarbital (Tramadol hydrochloride should be used with caution and in reduced dosages when administered to patients receiving CNS depressants, such as alcohol, opioids, anesthetic agents, narcotics, phenothiazines, tranquilizers, or sedative hypnotics. Tramadol hydrochloride increases the risk of CNS and respiratory depression). Products include:

Donnatal 2711

Phenobarbital Sodium (Tramadol hydrochloride should be used with caution and in reduced dosages when administered to patients receiving CNS depressants, such as alcohol, opioids, anesthetic agents, narcotics, phenothiazines, tranquilizers, or sedative hypnotics. Tramadol hydrochloride increases the risk of CNS and respiratory depression).
No products indexed under this heading.

Phenothiazine Derivatives (Tramadol hydrochloride should be used with caution and in reduced dosages when administered to patients receiving CNS depressants, such as phenothiazines. Tramadol hydrochloride increases the risk of CNS and respiratory depression).
No products indexed under this heading.

Phenothiazines (Tramadol hydrochloride should be used with caution and in reduced dosages when administered to patients receiving CNS depressants, such as phenothiazines. Tramadol hydrochloride increases the risk of CNS and respiratory depression).
No products indexed under this heading.

Phenytoin (Administration of CYP3A4 inducers, such as rifampin or St. John's Wort, with tramadol hydrochloride may effect the metabolism of tramadol leading to altered tramadol exposure).
No products indexed under this heading.

Phenytoin Sodium (Administration of CYP3A4 inducers, such as rifampin or St. John's Wort, with tramadol hydro-

chloride may effect the metabolism of tramadol leading to altered tramadol exposure). Products include:

Phenytek Capsules 2380

Pipecuronium Bromide (Because of its added depressant effects, tramadol should be prescribed with caution for those patients whose medical condition requires the concomitant administration of muscle relaxants, or other CNS-depressant drugs. Patients should be advised of the additive depressant effects of these combinations).
No products indexed under this heading.

Posaconazole (Concomitant administration of CYP3A4 inhibitors, such as ketoconazole and erythromycin, may reduce metabolic clearance of tramadol increasing the risk for serious adverse events including seizures and serotonin syndrome). Products include:

Noxafil 3172

Prazepam (Administration of tramadol may increase the seizure risk in patients taking neuroleptics or other drugs that reduce the seizure threshold).
No products indexed under this heading.

Prazosin Hydrochloride (There have been postmarketing reports of serotonin syndrome with use of tramadol and alpha2-adrenergic blockers).
No products indexed under this heading.

Prednisolone (Administration of CYP3A4 inducers, such as rifampin or St. John's Wort, with tramadol hydrochloride may effect the metabolism of tramadol leading to altered tramadol exposure).
No products indexed under this heading.

Prednisolone Acetate (Administration of CYP3A4 inducers, such as rifampin or St. John's Wort, with tramadol hydrochloride may effect the metabolism of tramadol leading to altered tramadol exposure). Products include:

Blephamide .... ☉212, ☉214
Pred Forte .... ☉225
Pred Mild .... ☉230
Pred-G .... ☉226, ☉227

Prednisolone Sodium Phosphate (Administration of CYP3A4 inducers, such as rifampin or St. John's Wort, with tramadol hydrochloride may effect the metabolism of tramadol leading to altered tramadol exposure).
No products indexed under this heading.

Prednisolone Tebutate (Administration of CYP3A4 inducers, such as rifampin or St. John's Wort, with tramadol hydrochloride may effect the metabolism of tramadol leading to altered tramadol exposure).
No products indexed under this heading.

Prednisone (Administration of CYP3A4 inducers, such as rifampin or St. John's Wort, with tramadol hydrochloride may effect the metabolism of tramadol leading to altered tramadol exposure).
No products indexed under this heading.

Prednisone sodium phosphate (Administration of CYP3A4 inducers, such as rifampin or St. John's Wort, with tramadol hydrochloride may effect the metabolism of tramadol leading to altered tramadol exposure).
No products indexed under this heading.

Prilocaine (Tramadol hydrochloride should be used with caution and in reduced dosages when administered to patients receiving CNS depressants, such as anesthetic agents. Tramadol hydrochloride increases the risk of CNS and respiratory depression).
No products indexed under this heading.

Prilocaine Hydrochloride (Tramadol hydrochloride should be used with caution and in reduced dosages when administered to patients receiving CNS depressants, such as anesthetic agents. Tramadol hydrochloride increases the risk of CNS and respiratory depression).
No products indexed under this heading.

Primidone (Administration of CYP3A4 inducers, such as rifampin or St. John's Wort, with tramadol hydrochloride may effect the metabolism of tramadol leading to altered tramadol exposure).
No products indexed under this heading.

Procaine (Tramadol hydrochloride should be used with caution and in reduced dosages when administered to patients receiving CNS depressants, such as anesthetic agents. Tramadol hydrochloride increases the risk of CNS and respiratory depression).
No products indexed under this heading.

Procaine Hydrochloride (Tramadol hydrochloride should be used with caution and in reduced dosages when administered to patients receiving CNS depressants, such as anesthetic agents. Tramadol hydrochloride increases the risk of CNS and respiratory depression).
No products indexed under this heading.

Procarbazine Hydrochloride (Administration of tramadol may enhance the seizure risk in patients taking monoamine oxidase (MAO) inhibitors. There have been post-marketing reports of serotonin syndrome with use of tramadol and monoamine oxidase inhibitors. Caution is advised when tramadol is co-administered with other drugs that may affect the serotonergic neurotransmitter systems, such as MAOIs. If concomitant treatment of tramadol with a drug affecting the serotonergic neurotransmitter system is clinically warranted, careful observation of the patient is advised, particularly during treatment initiation and dose increases).
No products indexed under this heading.

Prochlorperazine (Administration of tramadol may increase the seizure risk in patients taking neuroleptics or other drugs that reduce the seizure threshold).
No products indexed under this heading.

Prochlorperazine Edisylate (Tramadol hydrochloride should be used with caution and in reduced dosages when administered to patients receiving CNS depressants, such as alcohol, opioids, anesthetic agents, narcotics, phenothiazines, tranquilizers, or sedative hypnotics. Tramadol hydrochloride increases the risk of CNS and respiratory depression).
No products indexed under this heading.

Prochlorperazine Maleate (Tramadol hydrochloride should be used with caution and in reduced dosages when administered to patients receiving CNS depressants, such as alcohol, opioids, anesthetic agents, narcotics, phenothiazines, tranquilizers, or sedative hypnotics. Tramadol hydrochloride increases the risk of CNS and respiratory depression).
No products indexed under this heading.

Promethazine (Concomitant use of tramadol increases the seizure risk in patients taking tricyclic compounds, such as promethazine).
No products indexed under this heading.

Promethazine Hydrochloride (Concomitant use of tramadol increases the seizure risk in patients taking tricyclic compounds, such as promethazine).
No products indexed under this heading.

Propafenone Hydrochloride (Concomitant administration of CYP2D6

1667 Interactions Index Ryzolt

inhibitors such as quinidine, fluoxetine, paroxetine and amitriptyline may reduce metabolic clearance of tramadol increasing the risk for serious adverse events including seizures and serotonin syndrome. *In vitro* drug interaction studies in human liver microsomes indicate that inhibitors of CYP2D6 inhibit the metabolism of tramadol to various degrees, suggesting that concomitant administration of these compounds could result in increases in tramadol concentrations and decreased concentrations of M1. The full pharmacological impact of these alterations in terms of either efficacy or safety is unknown). Products include:

Rythmol 1648
Rythmol SR 1652

Proparacaine Hydrochloride (Tramadol hydrochloride should be used with caution and in reduced dosages when administered to patients receiving CNS depressants, such as anesthetic agents. Tramadol hydrochloride increases the risk of CNS and respiratory depression).
No products indexed under this heading.

Propofol (Tramadol hydrochloride should be used with caution and in reduced dosages when administered to patients receiving CNS depressants, such as sedative hypnotics. Tramadol hydrochloride increases the risk of CNS and respiratory depression).
No products indexed under this heading.

Propoxyphene Hydrochloride (Concomitant use of tramadol hydrochloride increases the seizure risk in patients taking other opioids. Tramadol should be used with caution and in reduced dosages when administered to patients receiving CNS depressants such as opioids or narcotics. Tramadol increases the risk of CNS and respiratory depression in these patients).
No products indexed under this heading.

Propoxyphene Napsylate (Concomitant use of tramadol hydrochloride increases the seizure risk in patients taking other opioids. Tramadol should be used with caution and in reduced dosages when administered to patients receiving CNS depressants such as opioids or narcotics. Tramadol increases the risk of CNS and respiratory depression in these patients).
No products indexed under this heading.

Protriptyline Hydrochloride (Administration of tramadol may increase the seizure risk in patients taking neuroleptics or other drugs that reduce the seizure threshold).
No products indexed under this heading.

Quazepam (Tramadol hydrochloride should be used with caution and in reduced dosages when administered to patients receiving CNS depressants, such as sedative hypnotics. Tramadol hydrochloride increases the risk of CNS and respiratory depression).
No products indexed under this heading.

Quetiapine Fumarate (Tramadol hydrochloride should be used with caution and in reduced dosages when administered to patients receiving CNS depressants, such as alcohol, opioids, anesthetic agents, narcotics, phenothiazines, tranquilizers, or sedative hypnotics. Tramadol hydrochloride increases the risk of CNS and respiratory depression). Products include:

Seroquel 750
Seroquel XR 759

Quinacrine Hydrochloride (Concomitant administration of CYP2D6 inhibitors such as quinidine, fluoxetine, paroxetine and amitriptyline may reduce metabolic clearance of tramadol increasing the risk for serious adverse events including seizures and serotonin syndrome. *In vitro* drug interaction studies in human liver microsomes indicate that inhibitors of CYP2D6 inhibit the metabolism of tramadol to various degrees, suggesting that concomitant administration of these compounds could result in increases in tramadol concentrations and decreased concentrations of M1. The full pharmacological impact of these alterations in terms of either efficacy or safety is unknown).
No products indexed under this heading.

Quinidine (Concomitant administration of CYP2D6 inhibitors such as quinidine, fluoxetine, paroxetine and amitriptyline may reduce metabolic clearance of tramadol increasing the risk for serious adverse events including seizures and serotonin syndrome. *In vitro* drug interaction studies in human liver microsomes indicate that inhibitors of CYP2D6 inhibit the metabolism of tramadol to various degrees, suggesting that concomitant administration of these compounds could result in increases in tramadol concentrations and decreased concentrations of M1. The full pharmacological impact of these alterations in terms of either efficacy or safety is unknown).
No products indexed under this heading.

Quinidine Gluconate (Concomitant administration of CYP2D6 inhibitors such as quinidine, fluoxetine, paroxetine and amitriptyline may reduce metabolic clearance of tramadol increasing the risk for serious adverse events including seizures and serotonin syndrome. *In vitro* drug interaction studies in human liver microsomes indicate that inhibitors of CYP2D6 inhibit the metabolism of tramadol to various degrees, suggesting that concomitant administration of these compounds could result in increases in tramadol concentrations and decreased concentrations of M1. The full pharmacological impact of these alterations in terms of either efficacy or safety is unknown).
No products indexed under this heading.

Quinidine Hydrochloride (Concomitant administration of CYP2D6 inhibitors such as quinidine, fluoxetine, paroxetine and amitriptyline may reduce metabolic clearance of tramadol increasing the risk for serious adverse events including seizures and serotonin syndrome. *In vitro* drug interaction studies in human liver microsomes indicate that inhibitors of CYP2D6 inhibit the metabolism of tramadol to various degrees, suggesting that concomitant administration of these compounds could result in increases in tramadol concentrations and decreased concentrations of M1. The full pharmacological impact of these alterations in terms of either efficacy or safety is unknown).
No products indexed under this heading.

Quinidine Polygalacturonate (Concomitant administration of CYP2D6 inhibitors such as quinidine, fluoxetine, paroxetine and amitriptyline may reduce metabolic clearance of tramadol increasing the risk for serious adverse events including seizures and serotonin syndrome. *In vitro* drug interaction studies in human liver microsomes indicate that inhibitors of CYP2D6 inhibit the metabolism of tramadol to various degrees, suggesting that concomitant administration of these compounds could result in increases in tramadol concentrations and decreased concentrations of M1. The full pharmacological impact of these alterations in terms of either efficacy or safety is unknown).
No products indexed under this heading.

Quinidine Sulfate (Concomitant administration of CYP2D6 inhibitors such as quinidine, fluoxetine, paroxetine and amitriptyline may reduce metabolic clearance of tramadol increasing the risk for serious adverse events including seizures and serotonin syndrome. *In vitro* drug interaction studies in human liver microsomes indicate that inhibitors of CYP2D6 inhibit the metabolism of tramadol to various degrees, suggesting that concomitant administration of these compounds could result in increases in tramadol concentrations and decreased concentrations of M1. The full pharmacological impact of these alterations in terms of either efficacy or safety is unknown).
No products indexed under this heading.

Quinine (Concomitant administration of CYP3A4 inhibitors, such as ketoconazole and erythromycin, may reduce metabolic clearance of tramadol increasing the risk for serious adverse events including seizures and serotonin syndrome). Products include:

Hyland's Leg Cramps PM with Quinine 3315

Quinine Sulfate (Concomitant administration of CYP3A4 inhibitors, such as ketoconazole and erythromycin, may reduce metabolic clearance of tramadol increasing the risk for serious adverse events including seizures and serotonin syndrome).
No products indexed under this heading.

Quinupristin (Concomitant administration of CYP3A4 inhibitors, such as ketoconazole and erythromycin, may reduce metabolic clearance of tramadol increasing the risk for serious adverse events including seizures and serotonin syndrome).
No products indexed under this heading.

Ramelteon (Tramadol hydrochloride should be used with caution and in reduced dosages when administered to patients receiving CNS depressants, such as sedative hypnotics. Tramadol hydrochloride increases the risk of CNS and respiratory depression). Products include:

Rozerem 3366

Ranitidine Bismuth Citrate (Concomitant administration of CYP2D6 inhibitors such as quinidine, fluoxetine, paroxetine and amitriptyline may reduce metabolic clearance of tramadol increasing the risk for serious adverse events including seizures and serotonin syndrome. *In vitro* drug interaction studies in human liver microsomes indicate that inhibitors of CYP2D6 inhibit the metabolism of tramadol to various degrees, suggesting that concomitant administration of these compounds could result in increases in tramadol concentrations and decreased concentrations of M1. The full pharmacological impact of these alterations in terms of either efficacy or safety is unknown).
No products indexed under this heading.

Ranitidine Hydrochloride (Concomitant administration of CYP2D6 inhibitors such as quinidine, fluoxetine, paroxetine and amitriptyline may reduce metabolic clearance of tramadol increasing the risk for serious adverse events including seizures and serotonin syndrome. *In vitro* drug interaction studies in human liver microsomes indicate that inhibitors of CYP2D6 inhibit the metabolism of tramadol to various degrees, suggesting that concomitant administration of these compounds could result in increases in tramadol concentrations and decreased concentrations of M1. The full pharmacological impact of these alterations in terms of either efficacy or safety is unknown). Products include:

Zantac 1737
Zantac Injection 1732
Zantac Pharmacy 1735

Rapacuronium Bromide (Because of its added depressant effects, tramadol should be prescribed with caution for those patients whose medical condition requires the concomitant administration of muscle relaxants, or other CNS-depressant drugs. Patients should be advised of the additive depressant effects of these combinations).
No products indexed under this heading.

Rasagiline Mesylate (Administration of tramadol may enhance the seizure risk in patients taking monoamine oxidase (MAO) inhibitors. There have been post-marketing reports of serotonin syndrome with use of tramadol and monoamine oxidase inhibitors. Caution is advised when tramadol is co-administered with other drugs that may affect the serotonergic neurotransmitter systems, such as MAOIs. If concomitant treatment of tramadol with a drug affecting the serotonergic neurotransmitter system is clinically warranted, careful observation of the patient is advised, particularly during treatment initiation and dose increases). Products include:

Azilect 3383

Remifentanil Hydrochloride (Concomitant use of tramadol hydrochloride increases the seizure risk in patients taking other opioids. Tramadol should be used with caution and in reduced dosages when administered to patients receiving CNS depressants such as opioids or narcotics. Tramadol increases the risk of CNS and respiratory depression in these patients).
No products indexed under this heading.

Rifabutin (Administration of CYP3A4 inducers, such as rifampin or St. John's Wort, with tramadol hydrochloride may effect the metabolism of tramadol leading to altered tramadol exposure).
No products indexed under this heading.

Rifampicin (Administration of CYP3A4 inducers, such as rifampin or St. John's Wort, with tramadol hydrochloride may effect the metabolism of tramadol leading to altered tramadol exposure).
No products indexed under this heading.

Rifampin (Administration of CYP3A4 inducers, such as rifampin or St. John's Wort, with tramadol hydrochloride may effect the metabolism of tramadol leading to altered tramadol exposure).
No products indexed under this heading.

Rifapentine (Administration of CYP3A4 inducers, such as rifampin or St. John's Wort, with tramadol hydrochloride may effect the metabolism of tramadol leading to altered tramadol exposure).
No products indexed under this heading.

Risperidone (Tramadol hydrochloride should be used with caution and in reduced dosages when administered to patients receiving CNS depressants, such as alcohol, opioids, anesthetic agents, narcotics, phenothiazines, tranquilizers, or sedative hypnotics. Tramadol hydrochloride increases the risk of CNS and respiratory depression). Products include:

Risperdal Consta 2682

Ritonavir (Concomitant administration of CYP2D6 inhibitors such as quinidine, fluoxetine, paroxetine and amitriptyline may reduce metabolic clearance of tramadol increasing the risk for serious adverse events including seizures and serotonin syndrome. *In vitro* drug interaction studies in human liver microsomes indicate that inhibitors of CYP2D6 inhibit the metabolism of tramadol to various degrees, suggesting that concomitant administration of these compounds could result in increases in tramadol concentrations and decreased concentrations of M1. The full pharmacological impact of

Ryzolt | Interactions Index | 1668

these alterations in terms of either efficacy or safety is unknown). Products include:
Kaletra 458
Norvir 509

Rizatriptan Benzoate (Caution is advised when tramadol is co-administered with other drugs that may affect the serotonergic neurotransmitter systems, such as triptans. If concomitant treatment of tramadol with a drug affecting the serotonergic neurotransmitter system is clinically warranted, careful observation of the patient is advised, particularly during treatment initiation and dose increases). Products include:
Maxalt 2206
Maxalt-MLT 2206

Rocuronium Bromide (Because of its added depressant effects, tramadol should be prescribed with caution for those patients whose medical condition requires the concomitant administration of muscle relaxants, or other CNS-depressant drugs. Patients should be advised of the additive depressant effects of these combinations). Products include:
Zemuron 3249

Ropivacaine Hydrochloride (Tramadol hydrochloride should be used with caution and in reduced dosages when administered to patients receiving CNS depressants, such as anesthetic agents. Tramadol hydrochloride increases the risk of CNS and respiratory depression).
No products indexed under this heading.

Saquinavir (Concomitant administration of CYP3A4 inhibitors, such as ketoconazole and erythromycin, may reduce metabolic clearance of tramadol increasing the risk for serious adverse events including seizures and serotonin syndrome).
No products indexed under this heading.

Saquinavir Mesylate (Concomitant administration of CYP3A4 inhibitors, such as ketoconazole and erythromycin, may reduce metabolic clearance of tramadol increasing the risk for serious adverse events including seizures and serotonin syndrome).
No products indexed under this heading.

Secobarbital Sodium (Tramadol hydrochloride should be used with caution and in reduced dosages when administered to patients receiving CNS depressants, such as sedative hypnotics. Tramadol hydrochloride increases the risk of CNS and respiratory depression).
No products indexed under this heading.

Selegiline (Administration of tramadol may enhance the seizure risk in patients taking monoamine oxidase (MAO) inhibitors. There have been post-marketing reports of serotonin syndrome with use of tramadol and monoamine oxidase inhibitors. Caution is advised when tramadol is co-administered with other drugs that may affect the serotonergic neurotransmitter systems, such as MAOIs. If concomitant treatment of tramadol with a drug affecting the serotonergic neurotransmitter system is clinically warranted, careful observation of the patient is advised, particularly during treatment initiation and dose increases). Products include:
Emsam 3623

Selegiline Hydrochloride (Administration of tramadol may enhance the seizure risk in patients taking monoamine oxidase (MAO) inhibitors. There have been post-marketing reports of serotonin syndrome with use of tramadol and monoamine oxidase inhibitors. Caution is advised when tramadol is co-administered with other drugs that may affect the serotonergic neurotransmitter systems, such as MAOIs. If concomitant treatment of tramadol with a drug affecting the serotonergic neurotransmitter system is clinically warranted, careful observation of the patient is advised, particularly during treatment initiation and dose increases). Products include:
Eldepryl 3312

Sertraline Hydrochloride (Concomitant use of tramadol hydrochloride increases the seizure risk in patients taking selective serotonin reuptake inhibitors (SSRI antidepressants or anorectics). There have been postmarketing reports of serotonin syndrome with use of tramadol and SSRIs/SNRIs. Caution is advised when tramadol is co-administered with other drugs that may affect the serotonergic neurotransmitter systems, such as SSRIs. If concomitant treatment of tramadol with a drug affecting the serotonergic neurotransmitter system is clinically warranted, careful observation of the patient is advised, particularly during treatment initiation and dose increases).
No products indexed under this heading.

Sevoflurane (Tramadol hydrochloride should be used with caution and in reduced dosages when administered to patients receiving CNS depressants, such as alcohol, opioids, anesthetic agents, narcotics, phenothiazines, tranquilizers, or sedative hypnotics. Tramadol hydrochloride increases the risk of CNS and respiratory depression). Products include:
Ultane 554

Sildenafil Citrate (Concomitant administration of CYP2D6 inhibitors such as quinidine, fluoxetine, paroxetine and amitriptyline may reduce metabolic clearance of tramadol increasing the risk for serious adverse events including seizures and serotonin syndrome. *In vitro* drug interaction studies in human liver microsomes indicate that inhibitors of CYP2D6 inhibit the metabolism of tramadol to various degrees, suggesting that concomitant administration of these compounds could result in increases in tramadol concentrations and decreased concentrations of M1. The full pharmacological impact of these alterations in terms of either efficacy or safety is unknown).
No products indexed under this heading.

Sodium Butabarbital (Tramadol hydrochloride should be used with caution and in reduced dosages when administered to patients receiving CNS depressants, such as sedative hypnotics. Tramadol hydrochloride increases the risk of CNS and respiratory depression).
No products indexed under this heading.

Sodium Oxybate (Tramadol hydrochloride should be used with caution and in reduced dosages when administered to patients receiving CNS depressants, such as alcohol, opioids, anesthetic agents, narcotics, phenothiazines, tranquilizers, or sedative hypnotics. Tramadol hydrochloride increases the risk of CNS and respiratory depression).
No products indexed under this heading.

Sodium Pentobarbital (Tramadol hydrochloride should be used with caution and in reduced dosages when administered to patients receiving CNS depressants, such as alcohol, opioids, anesthetic agents, narcotics, phenothiazines, tranquilizers, or sedative hypnotics. Tramadol hydrochloride increases the risk of CNS and respiratory depression).
No products indexed under this heading.

Succinylcholine Chloride (Because of its added depressant effects, tramadol should be prescribed with caution for those patients whose medical condition requires the concomitant administration of muscle relaxants, or other CNS-depressant drugs. Patients should be advised of the additive depressant effects of these combinations).
No products indexed under this heading.

Sufentanil Citrate (Concomitant use of tramadol hydrochloride increases the seizure risk in patients taking other opioids. Tramadol should be used with caution and in reduced dosages when administered to patients receiving CNS depressants such as opioids or narcotics. Tramadol increases the risk of CNS and respiratory depression in these patients).
No products indexed under this heading.

Sulfinpyrazone (Administration of CYP3A4 inducers, such as rifampin or St. John's Wort, with tramadol hydrochloride may effect the metabolism of tramadol leading to altered tramadol exposure).
No products indexed under this heading.

Sumatriptan (Caution is advised when tramadol is co-administered with other drugs that may affect the serotonergic neurotransmitter systems, such as triptans. If concomitant treatment of tramadol with a drug affecting the serotonergic neurotransmitter system is clinically warranted, careful observation of the patient is advised, particularly during treatment initiation and dose increases). Products include:
Imitrex Nasal 1503

Sumatriptan Succinate (Caution is advised when tramadol is co-administered with other drugs that may affect the serotonergic neurotransmitter systems, such as triptans. If concomitant treatment of tramadol with a drug affecting the serotonergic neurotransmitter system is clinically warranted, careful observation of the patient is advised, particularly during treatment initiation and dose increases). Products include:
Imitrex 1497
Imitrex Tablets 1508
Treximet 1681

Talbutal (Tramadol hydrochloride should be used with caution and in reduced dosages when administered to patients receiving CNS depressants, such as alcohol, opioids, anesthetic agents, narcotics, phenothiazines, tranquilizers, or sedative hypnotics. Tramadol hydrochloride increases the risk of CNS and respiratory depression).
No products indexed under this heading.

Tamsulosin Hydrochloride (There have been postmarketing reports of serotonin syndrome with use of tramadol and alpha2-adrenergic blockers).
No products indexed under this heading.

Telithromycin (Concomitant administration of CYP3A4 inhibitors, such as ketoconazole and erythromycin, may reduce metabolic clearance of tramadol increasing the risk for serious adverse events including seizures and serotonin syndrome). Products include:
Ketek 2991

Temazepam (Tramadol hydrochloride should be used with caution and in reduced dosages when administered to patients receiving CNS depressants, such as sedative hypnotics. Tramadol hydrochloride increases the risk of CNS and respiratory depression).
No products indexed under this heading.

Terazosin Hydrochloride (There have been postmarketing reports of serotonin syndrome with use of tramadol and alpha2-adrenergic blockers).
No products indexed under this heading.

Terbinafine Hydrochloride (Concomitant administration of CYP2D6 inhibitors such as quinidine, fluoxetine, paroxetine and amitriptyline may reduce metabolic clearance of tramadol increasing the risk for serious adverse events including seizures and serotonin syndrome. *In vitro* drug interaction studies in human liver microsomes indicate that inhibitors of CYP2D6 inhibit the metabolism of tramadol to various degrees, suggesting that concomitant administration of these compounds could result in increases in tramadol concentrations and decreased concentrations of M1. The full pharmacological impact of these alterations in terms of either efficacy or safety is unknown).
No products indexed under this heading.

Tetracaine (Tramadol hydrochloride should be used with caution and in reduced dosages when administered to patients receiving CNS depressants, such as anesthetic agents. Tramadol hydrochloride increases the risk of CNS and respiratory depression).
No products indexed under this heading.

Tetracaine Hydrochloride (Tramadol hydrochloride should be used with caution and in reduced dosages when administered to patients receiving CNS depressants, such as anesthetic agents. Tramadol hydrochloride increases the risk of CNS and respiratory depression).
No products indexed under this heading.

Theophyllinate (Administration of CYP3A4 inducers, such as rifampin or St. John's Wort, with tramadol hydrochloride may effect the metabolism of tramadol leading to altered tramadol exposure).
No products indexed under this heading.

Theophylline (Administration of CYP3A4 inducers, such as rifampin or St. John's Wort, with tramadol hydrochloride may effect the metabolism of tramadol leading to altered tramadol exposure).
No products indexed under this heading.

Theophylline Anhydrous (Administration of CYP3A4 inducers, such as rifampin or St. John's Wort, with tramadol hydrochloride may effect the metabolism of tramadol leading to altered tramadol exposure). Products include:
Uniphyl 2817

Theophylline Calcium Salicylate (Administration of CYP3A4 inducers, such as rifampin or St. John's Wort, with tramadol hydrochloride may effect the metabolism of tramadol leading to altered tramadol exposure).
No products indexed under this heading.

Theophylline Dihydroxypropyl (Glyceryl) (Administration of CYP3A4 inducers, such as rifampin or St. John's Wort, with tramadol hydrochloride may effect the metabolism of tramadol leading to altered tramadol exposure).
No products indexed under this heading.

Theophylline Ethylenediamine (Administration of CYP3A4 inducers, such as rifampin or St. John's Wort, with tramadol hydrochloride may effect the metabolism of tramadol leading to altered tramadol exposure).
No products indexed under this heading.

Theophylline Sodium Glycinate (Administration of CYP3A4 inducers, such as rifampin or St. John's Wort, with tramadol hydrochloride may effect the metabolism of tramadol leading to altered tramadol exposure).
No products indexed under this heading.

Thiamylal Sodium (Tramadol hydrochloride should be used with caution and in reduced dosages when administered to patients receiving CNS depressants, such as alcohol, opioids, anesthetic agents, narcotics, phenothiazines, tranquilizers, or sedative hypnotics. Tramadol hydrochloride increases the risk of CNS and respiratory depression).
No products indexed under this heading.

Thioridazine (Tramadol hydrochloride should be used with caution and in reduced dosages when administered to patients receiving CNS depressants, such as alcohol, opioids, anesthetic agents, narcotics, phenothiazines, tranquilizers, or sedative hypnotics. Tramadol hydrochloride increases the risk of CNS and respiratory depression).
No products indexed under this heading.

Thioridazine Hydrochloride (Administration of tramadol may increase the seizure risk in patients taking neuroleptics or other drugs that reduce the seizure threshold). Products include:
Thioridazine Hydrochloride 2384

Thiothixene (Tramadol hydrochloride should be used with caution and in reduced dosages when administered to patients receiving CNS depressants, such as alcohol, opioids, anesthetic agents, narcotics, phenothiazines, tranquilizers, or sedative hypnotics. Tramadol hydrochloride increases the risk of CNS and respiratory depression).
Products include:
Thiothixene 2386

Thiothixene Hydrochloride (Tramadol hydrochloride should be used with caution and in reduced dosages when administered to patients receiving CNS depressants, such as alcohol, opioids, anesthetic agents, narcotics, phenothiazines, tranquilizers, or sedative hypnotics. Tramadol hydrochloride increases the risk of CNS and respiratory depression).
No products indexed under this heading.

Tizanidine (Because of its added depressant effects, tramadol should be prescribed with caution for those patients whose medical condition requires the concomitant administration of muscle relaxants, or other CNS-depressant drugs. Patients should be advised of the additive depressant effects of these combinations).
No products indexed under this heading.

Tizanidine Hydrochloride (Because of its added depressant effects, tramadol should be prescribed with caution for those patients whose medical condition requires the concomitant administration of muscle relaxants, or other CNS-depressant drugs. Patients should be advised of the additive depressant effects of these combinations).
No products indexed under this heading.

Tranylcypromine Sulfate (Administration of tramadol may enhance the seizure risk in patients taking monoamine oxidase (MAO) inhibitors. There have been post-marketing reports of serotonin syndrome with use of tramadol and monoamine oxidase inhibitors. Caution is advised when tramadol is co-administered with other drugs that may affect the serotonergic neurotransmitter systems, such as MAOIs. If concomitant treatment of tramadol with a drug affecting the serotonergic neurotransmitter system is clinically warranted, careful observation of the patient is advised, particularly during treatment initiation and dose increases). Products include:
Parnate 1584

Trazodone Hydrochloride (Administration of tramadol may increase the seizure risk in patients taking neuroleptics or other drugs that reduce the seizure threshold).
No products indexed under this heading.

Triamcinolone (Administration of CYP3A4 inducers, such as rifampin or St. John's Wort, with tramadol hydrochloride may effect the metabolism of tramadol leading to altered tramadol exposure).
No products indexed under this heading.

Triamcinolone Acetonide (Administration of CYP3A4 inducers, such as rifampin or St. John's Wort, with tramadol hydrochloride may effect the metabolism of tramadol leading to altered tramadol exposure). Products include:
Azmacort **408**
Nasacort AQ **3019**

Triamcinolone Diacetate (Administration of CYP3A4 inducers, such as rifampin or St. John's Wort, with tramadol hydrochloride may effect the metabolism of tramadol leading to altered tramadol exposure).
No products indexed under this heading.

Triamcinolone Hexacetonide (Administration of CYP3A4 inducers, such as rifampin or St. John's Wort, with tramadol hydrochloride may effect the metabolism of tramadol leading to altered tramadol exposure).
No products indexed under this heading.

Triazolam (Tramadol hydrochloride should be used with caution and in reduced dosages when administered to patients receiving CNS depressants, such as sedative hypnotics. Tramadol hydrochloride increases the risk of CNS and respiratory depression).
No products indexed under this heading.

Trifluoperazine Hydrochloride (Administration of tramadol may increase the seizure risk in patients taking neuroleptics or other drugs that reduce the seizure threshold).
No products indexed under this heading.

Trimipramine Maleate (Administration of tramadol may increase the seizure risk in patients taking neuroleptics or other drugs that reduce the seizure threshold).
No products indexed under this heading.

Troglitazone (Concomitant administration of CYP3A4 inhibitors, such as ketoconazole and erythromycin, may reduce metabolic clearance of tramadol increasing the risk for serious adverse events including seizures and serotonin syndrome).
No products indexed under this heading.

Troleandomycin (Concomitant administration of CYP3A4 inhibitors, such as ketoconazole and erythromycin, may reduce metabolic clearance of tramadol increasing the risk for serious adverse events including seizures and serotonin syndrome).
No products indexed under this heading.

Tubocurarine Chloride (Because of its added depressant effects, tramadol should be prescribed with caution for those patients whose medical condition requires the concomitant administration of muscle relaxants, or other CNS-depressant drugs. Patients should be advised of the additive depressant effects of these combinations).
No products indexed under this heading.

Valproate Sodium (Concomitant administration of CYP3A4 inhibitors, such as ketoconazole and erythromycin, may reduce metabolic clearance of tramadol increasing the risk for serious adverse events including seizures and serotonin syndrome).
No products indexed under this heading.

Vardenafil Hydrochloride (Concomitant administration of CYP2D6 inhibitors

such as quinidine, fluoxetine, paroxetine and amitriptyline may reduce metabolic clearance of tramadol increasing the risk for serious adverse events including seizures and serotonin syndrome. *In vitro* drug interaction studies in human liver microsomes indicate that inhibitors of CYP2D6 inhibit the metabolism of tramadol to various degrees, suggesting that concomitant administration of these compounds could result in increases in tramadol concentrations and decreased concentrations of M1. The full pharmacological impact of these alterations in terms of either efficacy or safety is unknown). Products include:
Levitra **3157**

Vecuronium Bromide (Because of its added depressant effects, tramadol should be prescribed with caution for those patients whose medical condition requires the concomitant administration of muscle relaxants, or other CNS-depressant drugs. Patients should be advised of the additive depressant effects of these combinations).
No products indexed under this heading.

Venlafaxine Hydrochloride (Prescribe tramadol with caution for patients taking antidepressant drugs. Serious potential consequences of overdosage with tramadol are central nervous system depression, respiratory depression and death. In treating an overdose, primary attention should be given to maintaining adequate ventilation along with general supportive treatment). Products include:
Effexor XR **3504**
Venlafaxine Hydrochloride Tablets ... **2388**

Verapamil Hydrochloride (Concomitant administration of CYP3A4 inhibitors, such as ketoconazole and erythromycin, may reduce metabolic clearance of tramadol increasing the risk for serious adverse events including seizures and serotonin syndrome). Products include:
Tarka **534**

Voriconazole (Concomitant administration of CYP3A4 inhibitors, such as ketoconazole and erythromycin, may reduce metabolic clearance of tramadol increasing the risk for serious adverse events including seizures and serotonin syndrome).
No products indexed under this heading.

Warfarin Sodium (Post-marketing surveillance of tramadol has revealed rare reports of alteration of warfarin effect, including elevation of prothrombin times).
No products indexed under this heading.

Zafirlukast (Concomitant administration of CYP3A4 inhibitors, such as ketoconazole and erythromycin, may reduce metabolic clearance of tramadol increasing the risk for serious adverse events including seizures and serotonin syndrome). Products include:
Accolate **3612**

Zaleplon (Tramadol hydrochloride should be used with caution and in reduced dosages when administered to patients receiving CNS depressants, such as sedative hypnotics. Tramadol hydrochloride increases the risk of CNS and respiratory depression).
No products indexed under this heading.

Zileuton (Concomitant administration of CYP3A4 inhibitors, such as ketoconazole and erythromycin, may reduce metabolic clearance of tramadol increasing the risk for serious adverse events including seizures and serotonin syndrome).
No products indexed under this heading.

Ziprasidone Hydrochloride (Tramadol hydrochloride should be used with caution and in reduced dosages when administered to patients receiving CNS

depressants, such as alcohol, opioids, anesthetic agents, narcotics, phenothiazines, tranquilizers, or sedative hypnotics. Tramadol hydrochloride increases the risk of CNS and respiratory depression). Products include:
Geodon **2723**

Zolmitriptan (Caution is advised when tramadol is co-administered with other drugs that may affect the serotonergic neurotransmitter systems, such as triptans. If concomitant treatment of tramadol with a drug affecting the serotonergic neurotransmitter system is clinically warranted, careful observation of the patient is advised, particularly during treatment initiation and dose increases). Products include:
Zomig Tablets **773**
Zomig Nasal Spray **768**
Zomig-ZMT Tablets **773**

Zolpidem Tartrate (Tramadol hydrochloride should be used with caution and in reduced dosages when administered to patients receiving CNS depressants, such as sedative hypnotics. Tramadol hydrochloride increases the risk of CNS and respiratory depression). Products include:
Ambien **2920**
Ambien CR **2925**

Food Interactions

Alcohol (Tramadol hydrochloride should be used with caution and in reduced dosages when administered to patients receiving CNS depressants, such as alcohol, opioids, anesthetic agents, narcotics, phenothiazines, tranquilizers, or sedative hypnotics. Tramadol hydrochloride increases the risk of CNS and respiratory depression).

Beer, reduced-alcohol (Patients should be cautioned about the concomitant use of tramadol products and alcohol because of potentially serious CNS-additive effects of these agents. When large doses of tramadol are administered with alcohol, respiratory depression may result. Prescribe tramadol with caution for patients who use alcohol in excess).

Beer, unspecified (Patients should be cautioned about the concomitant use of tramadol products and alcohol because of potentially serious CNS-additive effects of these agents. When large doses of tramadol are administered with alcohol, respiratory depression may result. Prescribe tramadol with caution for patients who use alcohol in excess).

Food, unspecified (Co-administration with a high fat meal did not significantly affect AUC (overall exposure to tramadol); however, C_{max} (peak plasma concentration) increased 67% following a single 300 mg tablet administration and 54% following a single 200 mg tablet administration. Tramadol hydrochloride was administered without regard to food in all clinical trials).

Grapefruit (Concomitant administration of CYP3A4 inhibitors, such as ketoconazole and erythromycin, may reduce metabolic clearance of tramadol increasing the risk for serious adverse events including seizures and serotonin syndrome).

Grapefruit Juice (Concomitant administration of CYP3A4 inhibitors, such as ketoconazole and erythromycin, may reduce metabolic clearance of tramadol increasing the risk for serious adverse events including seizures and serotonin syndrome).

Meal, unspecified (Co-administration with a high fat meal did not significantly affect AUC (overall exposure to tramadol); however, C_{max} (peak plasma con-

centration) increased 67% following a single 300 mg tablet administration and 54% following a single 200 mg tablet administration. Tramadol hydrochloride was administered without regard to food in all clinical trials).

Wine, Chianti (Patients should be cautioned about the concomitant use of tramadol products and alcohol because of potentially serious CNS-additive effects of these agents. When large doses of tramadol are administered with alcohol, respiratory depression may result. Prescribe tramadol with caution for patients who use alcohol in excess).

Wine, Red (Patients should be cautioned about the concomitant use of tramadol products and alcohol because of potentially serious CNS-additive effects of these agents. When large doses of tramadol are administered with alcohol, respiratory depression may result. Prescribe tramadol with caution for patients who use alcohol in excess).

Wine, unspecified (Patients should be cautioned about the concomitant use of tramadol products and alcohol because of potentially serious CNS-additive effects of these agents. When large doses of tramadol are administered with alcohol, respiratory depression may result. Prescribe tramadol with caution for patients who use alcohol in excess).

Wine products (Patients should be cautioned about the concomitant use of tramadol products and alcohol because of potentially serious CNS-additive effects of these agents. When large doses of tramadol are administered with alcohol, respiratory depression may result. Prescribe tramadol with caution for patients who use alcohol in excess).

SABRIL FOR ORAL SOLUTION

(Vigabatrin) 2017
May interact with phenytoin, valproate, and certain other agents. Compounds in these categories include:

Clonazepam (In a study of 12 healthy volunteers, clonazepam (0.5 mg) co-administration had no effect on vigabatrin (1.5 g twice daily) concentrations. Vigabatrin increases the mean C_{max} of clonazepam by 30% and decreases the mean t_{max} by 45%). Products include:
Klonopin 2855

Divalproex Sodium (When co-administered with vigabatrin, sodium valproate plasma concentrations were reduced by an average of 8%). Products include:
Depakote ER 426

Drugs, unspecified (Vigabatrin should not be used with other drugs associated with serious adverse ophthalmic effects such as retinopathy or glaucoma unless the benefits clearly outweigh the risks).
No products indexed under this heading.

Fosphenytoin (A 16% to 20% average reduction in total phenytoin plasma levels was reported in controlled clinical studies).
No products indexed under this heading.

Fosphenytoin Sodium (A 16% to 20% average reduction in total phenytoin plasma levels was reported in controlled clinical studies).
No products indexed under this heading.

Phenobarbital (When co-administered with vigabatrin, phenobarbital concentration (from phenobarbital or primidone) was reduced by an average of 8% to 16%). Products include:
Donnatal 2711

Phenobarbital Sodium (When co-administered with vigabatrin, phenobarbital concentration (from phenobarbital or primidone) was reduced by an average of 8% to 16%).
No products indexed under this heading.

Phenytoin (A 16% to 20% average reduction in total phenytoin plasma levels was reported in controlled clinical studies).
No products indexed under this heading.

Phenytoin Sodium (A 16% to 20% average reduction in total phenytoin plasma levels was reported in controlled clinical studies). Products include:
Phenytek Capsules 2380

Primidone (When co-administered with vigabatrin, phenobarbital concentration (from phenobarbital or primidone) was reduced by an average of 8% to 16%).
No products indexed under this heading.

Valproate Sodium (When co-administered with vigabatrin, sodium valproate plasma concentrations were reduced by an average of 8%).
No products indexed under this heading.

Valproic Acid (When co-administered with vigabatrin, sodium valproate plasma concentrations were reduced by an average of 8%).
No products indexed under this heading.

SABRIL TABLETS

(Vigabatrin) 2025
See Sabril Oral Solution

ST. JOSEPH 81 MG ASPIRIN CHEWABLE AND ENTERIC COATED TABLETS

(Aspirin) 2045
May interact with ACE inhibitors, alcohols, anticoagulants, beta-blockers, diuretics, non-steroidal anti-inflammatory agents, oral hypoglycemic agents, phenytoin, valproate, and certain other agents. Compounds in these categories include:

Acarbose (Moderate doses of aspirin may increase the effectiveness of oral hypoglycemic agents leading to hypoglycemia).
No products indexed under this heading.

Acebutolol Hydrochloride (Decreased hypotensive effects of beta-blockers).
No products indexed under this heading.

Acetazolamide (Co-administration can lead to high serum concentrations of acetazolamide and its toxicity).
No products indexed under this heading.

Acetazolamide Sodium (Co-administration can lead to high serum concentrations of acetazolamide and its toxicity).
No products indexed under this heading.

Amiloride Hydrochloride (Diminished effectiveness of diuretics in patients with underlying renal or cardiovascular disease).
No products indexed under this heading.

Anisindione (Patients on anticoagulant therapy are at increased risk of bleeding).
No products indexed under this heading.

Ardeparin Sodium (Patients on anticoagulant therapy are at increased risk of bleeding).
No products indexed under this heading.

Atenolol (Decreased hypotensive effects of beta-blockers).
No products indexed under this heading.

Benazepril Hydrochloride (Co-administration may result in diminished hyponatremic and hypotensive effects of ACE inhibitors).
No products indexed under this heading.

Bendroflumethiazide (Diminished effectiveness of diuretics in patients with underlying renal or cardiovascular disease).
No products indexed under this heading.

Betaxolol Hydrochloride (Decreased hypotensive effects of beta-blockers).
No products indexed under this heading.

Bisoprolol Fumarate (Decreased hypotensive effects of beta-blockers).
No products indexed under this heading.

Bumetanide (Diminished effectiveness of diuretics in patients with underlying renal or cardiovascular disease).
No products indexed under this heading.

Captopril (Co-administration may result in diminished hyponatremic and hypotensive effects of ACE inhibitors). Products include:
Captopril 2341

Carteolol Hydrochloride (Decreased hypotensive effects of beta-blockers).
No products indexed under this heading.

Carvedilol (Decreased hypotensive effects of beta-blockers). Products include:
Coreg 1409

Carvedilol Phosphate (Decreased hypotensive effects of beta-blockers). Products include:
Coreg CR 1416

Celecoxib (Co-administration may increase bleeding or lead to decreased renal function). Products include:
Celebrex 3272

Chlorothiazide (Diminished effectiveness of diuretics in patients with underlying renal or cardiovascular disease).
No products indexed under this heading.

Chlorothiazide Sodium (Diminished effectiveness of diuretics in patients with underlying renal or cardiovascular disease). Products include:
Diuril Intravenous 2009

Chlorpropamide (Moderate doses of aspirin may increase the effectiveness of oral hypoglycemic agents leading to hypoglycemia).
No products indexed under this heading.

Chlorthalidone (Diminished effectiveness of diuretics in patients with underlying renal or cardiovascular disease). Products include:
Clorpres 2344

Dalteparin Sodium (Patients on anticoagulant therapy are at increased risk of bleeding). Products include:
Fragmin 1058

Danaparoid Sodium (Patients on anticoagulant therapy are at increased risk of bleeding).
No products indexed under this heading.

Diclofenac Epolamine (Co-administration may increase bleeding or lead to decreased renal function). Products include:
Flector 1839

Diclofenac Potassium (Co-administration may increase bleeding or lead to decreased renal function).
No products indexed under this heading.

Diclofenac Sodium (Co-administration may increase bleeding or lead to decreased renal function).
No products indexed under this heading.

Dicumarol (Patients on anticoagulant therapy are at increased risk of bleeding).
No products indexed under this heading.

Divalproex Sodium (Salicylate can displace protein-bound valproic acid leading to an increase in serum valproic acid levels). Products include:
Depakote ER 426

Enalapril Maleate (Co-administration may result in diminished hyponatremic and hypotensive effects of ACE inhibitors).
No products indexed under this heading.

Enalaprilat (Co-administration may result in diminished hyponatremic and hypotensive effects of ACE inhibitors).
No products indexed under this heading.

Enoxaparin Sodium (Patients on anticoagulant therapy are at increased risk of bleeding). Products include:
Lovenox 3005

Esmolol Hydrochloride (Decreased hypotensive effects of beta-blockers).
No products indexed under this heading.

Ethacrynic Acid (Diminished effectiveness of diuretics in patients with underlying renal or cardiovascular disease).
No products indexed under this heading.

Ethanol (Chronic heavy alcohol users, 3 or more drinks per day, in combination with analgesic/antipyretic drug products containing aspirin increases the risk of adverse GI events, including stomach bleeding).
No products indexed under this heading.

Ethyl Alcohol (Chronic heavy alcohol users, 3 or more drinks per day, in combination with analgesic/antipyretic drug products containing aspirin increases the risk of adverse GI events, including stomach bleeding).
No products indexed under this heading.

Etodolac (Co-administration may increase bleeding or lead to decreased renal function).
No products indexed under this heading.

Fenoprofen Calcium (Co-administration may increase bleeding or lead to decreased renal function).
No products indexed under this heading.

Flurbiprofen (Co-administration may increase bleeding or lead to decreased renal function).
No products indexed under this heading.

Fondaparinux Sodium (Patients on anticoagulant therapy are at increased risk of bleeding). Products include:
Arixtra 1320

Fosinopril Sodium (Co-administration may result in diminished hyponatremic and hypotensive effects of ACE inhibitors).
No products indexed under this heading.

Fosphenytoin (Salicylate can displace protein-bound phenytoin leading to a decrease in the total concentration of phenytoin).
No products indexed under this heading.

Fosphenytoin Sodium (Salicylate can displace protein-bound phenytoin leading to a decrease in the total concentration of phenytoin).
No products indexed under this heading.

Furosemide (Diminished effectiveness of diuretics in patients with underlying renal or cardiovascular disease). Products include:
Furosemide 2354

Glibenclamide (Moderate doses of aspirin may increase the effectiveness of oral hypoglycemic agents leading to hypoglycemia).
No products indexed under this heading.

Glimepiride (Moderate doses of aspirin may increase the effectiveness of oral hypoglycemic agents leading to hypoglycemia). Products include:
Avandaryl 1356
Duetact 3354

Glipizide (Moderate doses of aspirin may increase the effectiveness of oral hypoglycemic agents leading to hypoglycemia).
No products indexed under this heading.

Glyburide (Moderate doses of aspirin may increase the effectiveness of oral hypoglycemic agents leading to hypoglycemia).
No products indexed under this heading.

Heparin Calcium (Patients on anticoagulant therapy are at increased risk of bleeding).
No products indexed under this heading.

Heparin Sodium (Aspirin can increase the anticoagulant activity of heparin increasing bleeding risk).
No products indexed under this heading.

Hydrochlorothiazide (Diminished effectiveness of diuretics in patients with underlying renal or cardiovascular disease). Products include:

Atacand HCT	700
Avalide	2956
Benicar HCT	1017
Diovan HCT	2419
Dyazide	1429
Exforge HCT	2449
Hyzaar	2162
Hyzaar 100-12.5	2162
Micardis HCT	889
Prinzide	2246
Tekturna HCT	2541
Teveten HCT	541

Hydroflumethiazide (Diminished effectiveness of diuretics in patients with underlying renal or cardiovascular disease).
No products indexed under this heading.

Ibuprofen (Co-administration may increase bleeding or lead to decreased renal function). Products include:

Motrin IB	2043
Children's Motrin	2044
Children's Motrin Non-Staining Dye-Free	2044
Infants' Motrin	2044
Infants' Motrin Dye-Free	2044
Junior Strength Motrin	2044
Vicoprofen	564

Indapamide (Diminished effectiveness of diuretics in patients with underlying renal or cardiovascular disease). Products include:

Indapamide	2356

Indomethacin (Co-administration may increase bleeding or lead to decreased renal function). Products include:

Indocin	2167

Indomethacin Sodium Trihydrate (Co-administration may increase bleeding or lead to decreased renal function). Products include:

Indocin I.V.	2007

Ketoprofen (Co-administration may increase bleeding or lead to decreased renal function).
No products indexed under this heading.

Ketorolac Tromethamine (Co-administration may increase bleeding or lead to decreased renal function). Products include:

Acuvail	⊙209

Labetalol Hydrochloride (Decreased hypotensive effects of beta-blockers).
No products indexed under this heading.

Levobunolol Hydrochloride (Decreased hypotensive effects of beta-blockers).
No products indexed under this heading.

Lisinopril (Co-administration may result in diminished hyponatremic and hypotensive effects of ACE inhibitors). Products include:

Prinivil	2241
Prinzide	2246

Low Molecular Weight Heparins (Patients on anticoagulant therapy are at increased risk of bleeding).
No products indexed under this heading.

Meclofenamate Sodium (Co-administration may increase bleeding or lead to decreased renal function).
No products indexed under this heading.

Mefenamic Acid (Co-administration may increase bleeding or lead to decreased renal function).
No products indexed under this heading.

Meloxicam (Co-administration may increase bleeding or lead to decreased renal function).
No products indexed under this heading.

Metformin Hydrochloride (Moderate doses of aspirin may increase the effectiveness of oral hypoglycemic agents leading to hypoglycemia). Products include:

ActoPlus	3338
Avandamet	1345
Janumet	2188

Methotrexate Sodium (Salicylate can inhibit renal clearance of methotrexate leading to bone marrow toxicity, especially in the elderly or renal impaired).
No products indexed under this heading.

Methyclothiazide (Diminished effectiveness of diuretics in patients with underlying renal or cardiovascular disease).
No products indexed under this heading.

Metipranolol Hydrochloride (Decreased hypotensive effects of beta-blockers).
No products indexed under this heading.

Metolazone (Diminished effectiveness of diuretics in patients with underlying renal or cardiovascular disease).
No products indexed under this heading.

Metoprolol Succinate (Decreased hypotensive effects of beta-blockers). Products include:

Toprol XL	732

Metoprolol Tartrate (Decreased hypotensive effects of beta-blockers).
No products indexed under this heading.

Miglitol (Moderate doses of aspirin may increase the effectiveness of oral hypoglycemic agents leading to hypoglycemia).
No products indexed under this heading.

Moexipril Hydrochloride (Co-administration may result in diminished hyponatremic and hypotensive effects of ACE inhibitors).
No products indexed under this heading.

Nabumetone (Co-administration may increase bleeding or lead to decreased renal function).
No products indexed under this heading.

Nadolol (Decreased hypotensive effects of beta-blockers). Products include:

Nadolol	2359

Naproxen (Co-administration may increase bleeding or lead to decreased renal function). Products include:

EC-Naprosyn	2850
Naprosyn	2850
Anaprox/Naprosyn	2850

Naproxen Sodium (Co-administration may increase bleeding or lead to decreased renal function). Products include:

Anaprox	2850
Anaprox DS	2850
Treximet	1681

Nateglinide (Moderate doses of aspirin may increase the effectiveness of oral hypoglycemic agents leading to hypoglycemia).
No products indexed under this heading.

Nebivolol (Decreased hypotensive effects of beta-blockers). Products include:

Bystolic	1147

Oxaprozin (Co-administration may increase bleeding or lead to decreased renal function).
No products indexed under this heading.

Penbutolol Sulfate (Decreased hypotensive effects of beta-blockers).
No products indexed under this heading.

Perindopril Erbumine (Co-administration may result in diminished hyponatremic and hypotensive effects of ACE inhibitors).
No products indexed under this heading.

Phenylbutazone (Co-administration may increase bleeding or lead to decreased renal function).
No products indexed under this heading.

Phenytoin (Salicylate can displace protein-bound phenytoin leading to a decrease in the total concentration of phenytoin).
No products indexed under this heading.

Phenytoin Sodium (Salicylate can displace protein-bound phenytoin leading to a decrease in the total concentration of phenytoin). Products include:

Phenytek Capsules	2380

Pindolol (Decreased hypotensive effects of beta-blockers).
No products indexed under this heading.

Pioglitazone Hydrochloride (Moderate doses of aspirin may increase the effectiveness of oral hypoglycemic agents leading to hypoglycemia). Products include:

ActoPlus	3338
Actos	3345
Duetact	3354

Piroxicam (Co-administration may increase bleeding or lead to decreased renal function).
No products indexed under this heading.

Polythiazide (Diminished effectiveness of diuretics in patients with underlying renal or cardiovascular disease).
No products indexed under this heading.

Probenecid (Salicylate antagonizes the uricosuric action of probenecid).
No products indexed under this heading.

Propranolol Hydrochloride (Decreased hypotensive effects of beta-blockers). Products include:

InnoPran XL	1517

Quinapril Hydrochloride (Co-administration may result in diminished hyponatremic and hypotensive effects of ACE inhibitors).
No products indexed under this heading.

Ramipril (Co-administration may result in diminished hyponatremic and hypotensive effects of ACE inhibitors).
No products indexed under this heading.

Repaglinide (Moderate doses of aspirin may increase the effectiveness of oral hypoglycemic agents leading to hypoglycemia).
No products indexed under this heading.

Rofecoxib (Co-administration may increase bleeding or lead to decreased renal function).
No products indexed under this heading.

Rosiglitazone Maleate (Moderate doses of aspirin may increase the effectiveness of oral hypoglycemic agents leading to hypoglycemia). Products include:

Avandamet	1345
Avandaryl	1356
Avandia	1366

Sitagliptin Phosphate (Moderate doses of aspirin may increase the effectiveness of oral hypoglycemic agents leading to hypoglycemia). Products include:

Janumet	2188
Januvia	2196

Sotalol Hydrochloride (Decreased hypotensive effects of beta-blockers).
No products indexed under this heading.

Spirapril Hydrochloride (Co-administration may result in diminished hyponatremic and hypotensive effects of ACE inhibitors).
No products indexed under this heading.

Spironolactone (Diminished effectiveness of diuretics in patients with underlying renal or cardiovascular disease).
No products indexed under this heading.

Sulfinpyrazone (Salicylate antagonizes the uricosuric action of sulfinpyrazone).
No products indexed under this heading.

Sulindac (Co-administration may increase bleeding or lead to decreased renal function). Products include:

Clinoril	2098

Timolol Hemihydrate (Decreased hypotensive effects of beta-blockers). Products include:

Betimol	3490

Timolol Maleate (Decreased hypotensive effects of beta-blockers). Products include:

Combigan	601
Dorzolamide Hydrochloride/Timolol Maleate Ophthalmic Solution	⊙243
Timoptic in Ocudose	⊙231

Tinzaparin Sodium (Patients on anticoagulant therapy are at increased risk of bleeding).
No products indexed under this heading.

Tolazamide (Moderate doses of aspirin may increase the effectiveness of oral hypoglycemic agents leading to hypoglycemia).
No products indexed under this heading.

Tolbutamide (Moderate doses of aspirin may increase the effectiveness of oral hypoglycemic agents leading to hypoglycemia).
No products indexed under this heading.

Tolmetin Sodium (Co-administration may increase bleeding or lead to decreased renal function).
No products indexed under this heading.

Torsemide (Diminished effectiveness of diuretics in patients with underlying renal or cardiovascular disease).
No products indexed under this heading.

Trandolapril (Co-administration may result in diminished hyponatremic and hypotensive effects of ACE inhibitors). Products include:

Mavik	489
Tarka	534

Triamterene (Diminished effectiveness of diuretics in patients with underlying renal or cardiovascular disease). Products include:

Dyazide	1429
Dyrenium	3495

Troglitazone (Moderate doses of aspirin may increase the effectiveness of oral hypoglycemic agents leading to hypoglycemia).
No products indexed under this heading.

Valdecoxib (Co-administration may increase bleeding or lead to decreased renal function).
No products indexed under this heading.

Valproate Sodium (Salicylate can displace protein-bound valproic acid leading to an increase in serum valproic acid levels).
No products indexed under this heading.

Valproic Acid (Salicylate can displace protein-bound valproic acid leading to an increase in serum valproic acid levels).
No products indexed under this heading.

Warfarin Sodium (Aspirin can displace Warfarin from protein binding sites leading to prolongation of both the prothrombin time and the bleeding time).
No products indexed under this heading.

Food Interactions

Alcohol (Chronic heavy alcohol users, 3 or more drinks per day, in combination with analgesic/antipyretic drug products containing aspirin increases the risk of

---

IMPORTANT NOTE: Always consult each drug listing in the patient's regimen for possible interactions.

St. Joseph Interactions Index 1672

adverse GI events, including stomach bleeding).

Beer, reduced-alcohol (Chronic heavy alcohol users, 3 or more drinks per day, in combination with analgesic/antipyretic drug products containing aspirin increases the risk of adverse GI events, including stomach bleeding).

Beer, unspecified (Chronic heavy alcohol users, 3 or more drinks per day, in combination with analgesic/antipyretic drug products containing aspirin increases the risk of adverse GI events, including stomach bleeding).

Wine, Chianti (Chronic heavy alcohol users, 3 or more drinks per day, in combination with analgesic/antipyretic drug products containing aspirin increases the risk of adverse GI events, including stomach bleeding).

Wine, Red (Chronic heavy alcohol users, 3 or more drinks per day, in combination with analgesic/antipyretic drug products containing aspirin increases the risk of adverse GI events, including stomach bleeding).

Wine, unspecified (Chronic heavy alcohol users, 3 or more drinks per day, in combination with analgesic/antipyretic drug products containing aspirin increases the risk of adverse GI events, including stomach bleeding).

Wine products (Chronic heavy alcohol users, 3 or more drinks per day, in combination with analgesic/antipyretic drug products containing aspirin increases the risk of adverse GI events, including stomach bleeding).

SALAGEN TABLETS

(Pilocarpine Hydrochloride) 1072

May interact with anticholinergics, beta-blockers, parasympathomimetics. Compounds in these categories include:

Acebutolol Hydrochloride (Pilocarpine should be administered with caution in patients taking beta adrenergic antagonists because of the possibility of conduction disturbances).
No products indexed under this heading.

Atenolol (Pilocarpine should be administered with caution in patients taking beta adrenergic antagonists because of the possibility of conduction disturbances).
No products indexed under this heading.

Atropine Sulfate (Pilocarpine might antagonize the anticholinergic effects of drugs used concomitantly. These effects should be considered when anticholinergic properties may be contributing to the therapeutic effect of concomitant medication). Products include:
Donnatal 2711

Belladonna Alkaloids (Pilocarpine might antagonize the anticholinergic effects of drugs used concomitantly. These effects should be considered when anticholinergic properties may be contributing to the therapeutic effect of concomitant medication). Products include:
Hyland's Teething Tablets 3316

Benztropine Mesylate (Pilocarpine might antagonize the anticholinergic effects of drugs used concomitantly. These effects should be considered when anticholinergic properties may be contributing to the therapeutic effect of concomitant medication).
No products indexed under this heading.

Betaxolol Hydrochloride (Pilocarpine should be administered with caution in patients taking beta adrenergic antagonists because of the possibility of conduction disturbances).
No products indexed under this heading.

Biperiden Hydrochloride (Pilocarpine might antagonize the anticholinergic effects of drugs used concomitantly. These effects should be considered when anticholinergic properties may be contributing to the therapeutic effect of concomitant medication).
No products indexed under this heading.

Bisoprolol Fumarate (Pilocarpine should be administered with caution in patients taking beta adrenergic antagonists because of the possibility of conduction disturbances).
No products indexed under this heading.

Carteolol Hydrochloride (Pilocarpine should be administered with caution in patients taking beta adrenergic antagonists because of the possibility of conduction disturbances).
No products indexed under this heading.

Carvedilol (Pilocarpine should be administered with caution in patients taking beta adrenergic antagonists because of the possibility of conduction disturbances). Products include:
Coreg 1409

Carvedilol Phosphate (Pilocarpine should be administered with caution in patients taking beta adrenergic antagonists because of the possibility of conduction disturbances). Products include:
Coreg CR 1416

Cevimeline Hydrochloride (Drugs with parasympathomimetic effects administered concurrently with pilocarpine would be expected to result in additive pharmacologic effects). Products include:
Evoxac 1027

Clidinium Bromide (Pilocarpine might antagonize the anticholinergic effects of drugs used concomitantly. These effects should be considered when anticholinergic properties may be contributing to the therapeutic effect of concomitant medication).
No products indexed under this heading.

Dicyclomine Hydrochloride (Pilocarpine might antagonize the anticholinergic effects of drugs used concomitantly. These effects should be considered when anticholinergic properties may be contributing to the therapeutic effect of concomitant medication). Products include:
Bentyl Capsules 780
Bentyl Injection 780
Bentyl Syrup 780
Bentyl Tablets 780

Edrophonium Chloride (Drugs with parasympathomimetic effects administered concurrently with pilocarpine would be expected to result in additive pharmacologic effects).
No products indexed under this heading.

Esmolol Hydrochloride (Pilocarpine should be administered with caution in patients taking beta adrenergic antagonists because of the possibility of conduction disturbances).
No products indexed under this heading.

Glycopyrrolate (Pilocarpine might antagonize the anticholinergic effects of drugs used concomitantly. These effects should be considered when anticholinergic properties may be contributing to the therapeutic effect of concomitant medication).
No products indexed under this heading.

Hyoscyamine (Pilocarpine might antagonize the anticholinergic effects of drugs used concomitantly. These effects should be considered when anticholinergic properties may be contributing to the therapeutic effect of concomitant medication).
No products indexed under this heading.

Hyoscyamine Sulfate (Pilocarpine might antagonize the anticholinergic effects of drugs used concomitantly. These effects should be considered when anticholinergic properties may be contributing to the therapeutic effect of concomitant medication). Products include:
Donnatal 2711

Ipratropium Bromide (Pilocarpine might antagonize the anticholinergic effects of drugs used concomitantly. These effects should be considered when anticholinergic properties may be contributing to the therapeutic effect of concomitant medication).
No products indexed under this heading.

Labetalol Hydrochloride (Pilocarpine should be administered with caution in patients taking beta adrenergic antagonists because of the possibility of conduction disturbances).
No products indexed under this heading.

Levobunolol Hydrochloride (Pilocarpine should be administered with caution in patients taking beta adrenergic antagonists because of the possibility of conduction disturbances).
No products indexed under this heading.

Mepenzolate Bromide (Pilocarpine might antagonize the anticholinergic effects of drugs used concomitantly. These effects should be considered when anticholinergic properties may be contributing to the therapeutic effect of concomitant medication).
No products indexed under this heading.

Metipranolol Hydrochloride (Pilocarpine should be administered with caution in patients taking beta adrenergic antagonists because of the possibility of conduction disturbances).
No products indexed under this heading.

Metoprolol Succinate (Pilocarpine should be administered with caution in patients taking beta adrenergic antagonists because of the possibility of conduction disturbances). Products include:
Toprol XL 732

Metoprolol Tartrate (Pilocarpine should be administered with caution in patients taking beta adrenergic antagonists because of the possibility of conduction disturbances).
No products indexed under this heading.

Nadolol (Pilocarpine should be administered with caution in patients taking beta adrenergic antagonists because of the possibility of conduction disturbances). Products include:
Nadolol 2359

Nebivolol (Pilocarpine should be administered with caution in patients taking beta adrenergic antagonists because of the possibility of conduction disturbances). Products include:
Bystolic 1147

Neostigmine Bromide (Drugs with parasympathomimetic effects administered concurrently with pilocarpine would be expected to result in additive pharmacologic effects).
No products indexed under this heading.

Neostigmine Methylsulfate (Drugs with parasympathomimetic effects administered concurrently with pilocarpine would be expected to result in additive pharmacologic effects).
No products indexed under this heading.

Oxybutynin Chloride (Pilocarpine might antagonize the anticholinergic effects of drugs used concomitantly. These effects should be considered when anticholinergic properties may be contributing to the therapeutic effect of concomitant medication).
No products indexed under this heading.

Penbutolol Sulfate (Pilocarpine should be administered with caution in patients taking beta adrenergic antagonists because of the possibility of conduction disturbances).
No products indexed under this heading.

Pindolol (Pilocarpine should be administered with caution in patients taking beta adrenergic antagonists because of the possibility of conduction disturbances).
No products indexed under this heading.

Procyclidine Hydrochloride (Pilocarpine might antagonize the anticholinergic effects of drugs used concomitantly. These effects should be considered when anticholinergic properties may be contributing to the therapeutic effect of concomitant medication).
No products indexed under this heading.

Propantheline Bromide (Pilocarpine might antagonize the anticholinergic effects of drugs used concomitantly. These effects should be considered when anticholinergic properties may be contributing to the therapeutic effect of concomitant medication).
No products indexed under this heading.

Propranolol Hydrochloride (Pilocarpine should be administered with caution in patients taking beta adrenergic antagonists because of the possibility of conduction disturbances). Products include:
InnoPran XL 1517

Pyridostigmine Bromide (Drugs with parasympathomimetic effects administered concurrently with pilocarpine would be expected to result in additive pharmacologic effects).
No products indexed under this heading.

Scopolamine (Pilocarpine might antagonize the anticholinergic effects of drugs used concomitantly. These effects should be considered when anticholinergic properties may be contributing to the therapeutic effect of concomitant medication). Products include:
Transderm Scōp 2397

Scopolamine Hydrobromide (Pilocarpine might antagonize the anticholinergic effects of drugs used concomitantly. These effects should be considered when anticholinergic properties may be contributing to the therapeutic effect of concomitant medication). Products include:
Donnatal 2711

Sotalol Hydrochloride (Pilocarpine should be administered with caution in patients taking beta adrenergic antagonists because of the possibility of conduction disturbances).
No products indexed under this heading.

Timolol Hemihydrate (Pilocarpine should be administered with caution in patients taking beta adrenergic antagonists because of the possibility of conduction disturbances). Products include:
Betimol 3490

Timolol Maleate (Pilocarpine should be administered with caution in patients taking beta adrenergic antagonists because of the possibility of conduction disturbances). Products include:
Combigan 601
Dorzolamide Hydrochloride/Timolol Maleate Ophthalmic Solution .... ⊙243
Timoptic in Ocudose .... ⊙231

Tolterodine Tartrate (Pilocarpine might antagonize the anticholinergic effects of drugs used concomitantly. These effects should be considered when anticholinergic properties may be contributing to the therapeutic effect of concomitant medication).
No products indexed under this heading.

Tridihexethyl Chloride (Pilocarpine might antagonize the anticholinergic effects of drugs used concomitantly. These effects should be considered when anticholinergic properties may be contributing to the therapeutic effect of concomitant medication).
No products indexed under this heading.

(⊙ Described in PDR® for Ophthalmic Medicines)

Trihexyphenidyl Hydrochloride
(Pilocarpine might antagonize the anticholinergic effects of drugs used concomitantly. These effects should be considered when anticholinergic properties may be contributing to the therapeutic effect of concomitant medication).
No products indexed under this heading.

SALONPAS ARTHRITIS PAIN

(Menthol, Methyl Salicylate) **1805**
May interact with alcohols, anticoagulants, corticosteroids, non-steroidal anti-inflammatory agents. Compounds in these categories include:

Alclometasone Dipropionate (Taking a steroid may increase the chance of stomach bleeding).
No products indexed under this heading.

Anisindione (Taking a blood thinning agent (eg, anticoagulants) may increase the chance of stomach bleeding).
No products indexed under this heading.

Ardeparin Sodium (Taking a blood thinning agent (eg, anticoagulants) may increase the chance of stomach bleeding).
No products indexed under this heading.

Beclomethasone Dipropionate
(Taking a steroid may increase the chance of stomach bleeding). Products include:
Qvar **3398**

Beclomethasone Dipropionate Monohydrate (Taking a steroid may increase the chance of stomach bleeding). Products include:
Beconase AQ **1386**

Betamethasone (Taking a steroid may increase the chance of stomach bleeding).
No products indexed under this heading.

Betamethasone Acetate (Taking a steroid may increase the chance of stomach bleeding).
No products indexed under this heading.

Betamethasone Benzoate (Taking a steroid may increase the chance of stomach bleeding).
No products indexed under this heading.

Betamethasone Dipropionate (Taking a steroid may increase the chance of stomach bleeding). Products include:
Diprolene Lotion 0.05% **3108**
Diprolene Ointment 0.05% **3109**
Diprolene AF Cream 0.05% **3107**
Lotrisone **3163**

Betamethasone Sodium Phosphate (Taking a steroid may increase the chance of stomach bleeding).
No products indexed under this heading.

Betamethasone Valerate (Taking a steroid may increase the chance of stomach bleeding). Products include:
Luxíq **3321**

Budesonide (Taking a steroid may increase the chance of stomach bleeding). Products include:
Pulmicort Flexhaler **714**
Symbicort 80/4.5 .... **720**
Symbicort 160/4.5 .... **720**

Celecoxib (Taking other drugs containing an NSAID (eg, aspirin, ibuprofen, naproxen, or others) may increase the chance of stomach bleeding). Products include:
Celebrex **3272**

Ciclesonide (Taking a steroid may increase the chance of stomach bleeding).
No products indexed under this heading.

Cortisone Acetate (Taking a steroid may increase the chance of stomach bleeding).
No products indexed under this heading.

Dalteparin Sodium (Taking a blood thinning agent (eg, anticoagulants) may increase the chance of stomach bleeding). Products include:
Fragmin **1058**

Danaparoid Sodium (Taking a blood thinning agent (eg, anticoagulants) may increase the chance of stomach bleeding).
No products indexed under this heading.

Desoximetasone (Taking a steroid may increase the chance of stomach bleeding).
No products indexed under this heading.

Dexamethasone (Taking a steroid may increase the chance of stomach bleeding). Products include:
Ciprodex **583**
Ozurdex .... ⊙**223**
Tobramycin and Dexamethasone
Ophthalmic Suspension............... ⊙**251**

Dexamethasone Acetate (Taking a steroid may increase the chance of stomach bleeding).
No products indexed under this heading.

Dexamethasone Phosphate (Taking a steroid may increase the chance of stomach bleeding).
No products indexed under this heading.

Dexamethasone Sodium (Taking a steroid may increase the chance of stomach bleeding).
No products indexed under this heading.

Dexamethasone Sodium Phosphate (Taking a steroid may increase the chance of stomach bleeding).
No products indexed under this heading.

Dexamethasone Sodium Phosphate Injection (Taking a steroid may increase the chance of stomach bleeding).
No products indexed under this heading.

Diclofenac Epolamine (Taking other drugs containing an NSAID (eg, aspirin, ibuprofen, naproxen, or others) may increase the chance of stomach bleeding). Products include:
Flector **1839**

Diclofenac Potassium (Taking other drugs containing an NSAID (eg, aspirin, ibuprofen, naproxen, or others) may increase the chance of stomach bleeding).
No products indexed under this heading.

Diclofenac Sodium (Taking other drugs containing an NSAID (eg, aspirin, ibuprofen, naproxen, or others) may increase the chance of stomach bleeding).
No products indexed under this heading.

Dicumarol (Taking a blood thinning agent (eg, anticoagulants) may increase the chance of stomach bleeding).
No products indexed under this heading.

Diflorasone Diacetate (Taking a steroid may increase the chance of stomach bleeding).
No products indexed under this heading.

Enoxaparin Sodium (Taking a blood thinning agent (eg, anticoagulants) may increase the chance of stomach bleeding). Products include:
Lovenox **3005**

Ethanol (Having 3 or more alcoholic drinks everyday may increase the chance of stomach bleeding).
No products indexed under this heading.

Ethyl Alcohol (Having 3 or more alcoholic drinks everyday may increase the chance of stomach bleeding).
No products indexed under this heading.

Etodolac (Taking other drugs containing an NSAID (eg, aspirin, ibuprofen, naproxen, or others) may increase the chance of stomach bleeding).
No products indexed under this heading.

Fenoprofen Calcium (Taking other drugs containing an NSAID (eg, aspirin, ibuprofen, naproxen, or others) may increase the chance of stomach bleeding).
No products indexed under this heading.

Fludrocortisone Acetate (Taking a steroid may increase the chance of stomach bleeding).
No products indexed under this heading.

Flumethasone Pivalate (Taking a steroid may increase the chance of stomach bleeding).
No products indexed under this heading.

Flunisolide Hemihydrate (Taking a steroid may increase the chance of stomach bleeding).
No products indexed under this heading.

Flurbiprofen (Taking other drugs containing an NSAID (eg, aspirin, ibuprofen, naproxen, or others) may increase the chance of stomach bleeding).
No products indexed under this heading.

Fluticasone Furoate (Taking a steroid may increase the chance of stomach bleeding). Products include:
Veramyst **1713**

Fluticasone Propionate (Taking a steroid may increase the chance of stomach bleeding). Products include:
Advair 100/50 .... **1275**
Advair 250/50 .... **1275**
Advair 500/50 .... **1275**
Advair HFA 45/21 .... **1288**
Advair HFA 115/21 .... **1288**
Advair HFA 230/21 .... **1288**
Flonase **1459**
Flovent Diskus **1463**
Flovent HFA **1470**

Fondaparinux Sodium (Taking a blood thinning agent (eg, anticoagulants) may increase the chance of stomach bleeding). Products include:
Arixtra **1320**

Heparin Calcium (Taking a blood thinning agent (eg, anticoagulants) may increase the chance of stomach bleeding).
No products indexed under this heading.

Heparin Sodium (Taking a blood thinning agent (eg, anticoagulants) may increase the chance of stomach bleeding).
No products indexed under this heading.

Hydrocortisone (Taking a steroid may increase the chance of stomach bleeding).
No products indexed under this heading.

Hydrocortisone (Alcohol) (Taking a steroid may increase the chance of stomach bleeding).
No products indexed under this heading.

Hydrocortisone Acetate (Taking a steroid may increase the chance of stomach bleeding).
No products indexed under this heading.

Hydrocortisone Butyrate (Taking a steroid may increase the chance of stomach bleeding).
No products indexed under this heading.

Hydrocortisone Cypionate (Taking a steroid may increase the chance of stomach bleeding).
No products indexed under this heading.

Hydrocortisone Hemisuccinate (Taking a steroid may increase the chance of stomach bleeding).
No products indexed under this heading.

Hydrocortisone Probutate (Taking a steroid may increase the chance of stomach bleeding).
No products indexed under this heading.

Hydrocortisone Sodium Phosphate (Taking a steroid may increase the chance of stomach bleeding).
No products indexed under this heading.

Hydrocortisone Sodium Succinate
(Taking a steroid may increase the chance of stomach bleeding).
No products indexed under this heading.

Hydrocortisone Valerate (Taking a steroid may increase the chance of stomach bleeding).
No products indexed under this heading.

Ibuprofen (Taking other drugs containing an NSAID (eg, aspirin, ibuprofen, naproxen, or others) may increase the chance of stomach bleeding). Products include:
Motrin IB **2043**
Children's Motrin **2044**
Children's Motrin Non-Staining
Dye-Free.................................... **2044**
Infants' Motrin **2044**
Infants' Motrin Dye-Free **2044**
Junior Strength Motrin **2044**
Vicoprofen **564**

Indomethacin (Taking other drugs containing an NSAID (eg, aspirin, ibuprofen, naproxen, or others) may increase the chance of stomach bleeding). Products include:
Indocin **2167**

Indomethacin Sodium Trihydrate (Taking other drugs containing an NSAID (eg, aspirin, ibuprofen, naproxen, or others) may increase the chance of stomach bleeding). Products include:
Indocin I.V. **2007**

Ketoprofen (Taking other drugs containing an NSAID (eg, aspirin, ibuprofen, naproxen, or others) may increase the chance of stomach bleeding).
No products indexed under this heading.

Ketorolac Tromethamine (Taking other drugs containing an NSAID (eg, aspirin, ibuprofen, naproxen, or others) may increase the chance of stomach bleeding). Products include:
Acuvail .... ⊙**209**

Low Molecular Weight Heparins (Taking a blood thinning agent (eg, anticoagulants) may increase the chance of stomach bleeding).
No products indexed under this heading.

Meclofenamate Sodium (Taking other drugs containing an NSAID (eg, aspirin, ibuprofen, naproxen, or others) may increase the chance of stomach bleeding).
No products indexed under this heading.

Mefenamic Acid (Taking other drugs containing an NSAID (eg, aspirin, ibuprofen, naproxen, or others) may increase the chance of stomach bleeding).
No products indexed under this heading.

Meloxicam (Taking other drugs containing an NSAID (eg, aspirin, ibuprofen, naproxen, or others) may increase the chance of stomach bleeding).
No products indexed under this heading.

Methylprednisolone (Taking a steroid may increase the chance of stomach bleeding).
No products indexed under this heading.

Methylprednisolone Acetate (Taking a steroid may increase the chance of stomach bleeding).
No products indexed under this heading.

Methylprednisolone Sodium Succinate (Taking a steroid may increase the chance of stomach bleeding).
No products indexed under this heading.

Mometasone Furoate (Taking a steroid may increase the chance of stomach bleeding). Products include:
Asmanex **3058**
Elocon Cream **3111**
Elocon Lotion **3112**
Elocon Ointment **3114**

Mometasone Furoate Monohydrate (Taking a steroid may increase the chance of stomach bleeding). Products include:
Nasonex **3166**

Nabumetone (Taking other drugs containing an NSAID (eg, aspirin, ibuprofen, naproxen, or others) may increase the chance of stomach bleeding).
No products indexed under this heading.

Naproxen (Taking other drugs containing an NSAID (eg, aspirin, ibuprofen, naproxen, or others) may increase the chance of stomach bleeding). Products include:
EC-Naprosyn 2850
Naprosyn 2850
Anaprox/Naprosyn 2850

Naproxen Sodium (Taking other drugs containing an NSAID (eg, aspirin, ibuprofen, naproxen, or others) may increase the chance of stomach bleeding). Products include:
Anaprox 2850
Anaprox DS 2850
Treximet 1681

Oxaprozin (Taking other drugs containing an NSAID (eg, aspirin, ibuprofen, naproxen, or others) may increase the chance of stomach bleeding).
No products indexed under this heading.

Phenylbutazone (Taking other drugs containing an NSAID (eg, aspirin, ibuprofen, naproxen, or others) may increase the chance of stomach bleeding).
No products indexed under this heading.

Piroxicam (Taking other drugs containing an NSAID (eg, aspirin, ibuprofen, naproxen, or others) may increase the chance of stomach bleeding).
No products indexed under this heading.

Prednisolone (Taking a steroid may increase the chance of stomach bleeding).
No products indexed under this heading.

Prednisolone Acetate (Taking a steroid may increase the chance of stomach bleeding). Products include:
Blephamide .... ⊙212, ⊙214
Pred Forte .... ⊙225
Pred Mild .... ⊙230
Pred-G .... ⊙226, ⊙227

Prednisolone Sodium Phosphate (Taking a steroid may increase the chance of stomach bleeding).
No products indexed under this heading.

Prednisolone Tebutate (Taking a steroid may increase the chance of stomach bleeding).
No products indexed under this heading.

Prednisone (Taking a steroid may increase the chance of stomach bleeding).
No products indexed under this heading.

Prednisone sodium phosphate (Taking a steroid may increase the chance of stomach bleeding).
No products indexed under this heading.

Rofecoxib (Taking other drugs containing an NSAID (eg, aspirin, ibuprofen, naproxen, or others) may increase the chance of stomach bleeding).
No products indexed under this heading.

Sulindac (Taking other drugs containing an NSAID (eg, aspirin, ibuprofen, naproxen, or others) may increase the chance of stomach bleeding). Products include:
Clinoril 2098

Tinzaparin Sodium (Taking a blood thinning agent (eg, anticoagulants) may increase the chance of stomach bleeding).
No products indexed under this heading.

Tolmetin Sodium (Taking other drugs containing an NSAID (eg, aspirin, ibuprofen, naproxen, or others) may increase the chance of stomach bleeding).
No products indexed under this heading.

Triamcinolone (Taking a steroid may increase the chance of stomach bleeding).
No products indexed under this heading.

Triamcinolone Acetonide (Taking a steroid may increase the chance of stomach bleeding). Products include:
Azmacort 408
Nasacort AQ 3019

Triamcinolone Diacetate (Taking a steroid may increase the chance of stomach bleeding).
No products indexed under this heading.

Triamcinolone Hexacetonide (Taking a steroid may increase the chance of stomach bleeding).
No products indexed under this heading.

Valdecoxib (Taking other drugs containing an NSAID (eg, aspirin, ibuprofen, naproxen, or others) may increase the chance of stomach bleeding).
No products indexed under this heading.

Warfarin Sodium (Taking a blood thinning agent (eg, anticoagulants) may increase the chance of stomach bleeding).
No products indexed under this heading.

Food Interactions

Alcohol (Having 3 or more alcoholic drinks everyday may increase the chance of stomach bleeding).

Beer, reduced-alcohol (Having 3 or more alcoholic drinks everyday may increase the chance of stomach bleeding).

Beer, unspecified (Having 3 or more alcoholic drinks everyday may increase the chance of stomach bleeding).

Wine, Chianti (Having 3 or more alcoholic drinks everyday may increase the chance of stomach bleeding).

Wine, Red (Having 3 or more alcoholic drinks everyday may increase the chance of stomach bleeding).

Wine, unspecified (Having 3 or more alcoholic drinks everyday may increase the chance of stomach bleeding).

Wine products (Having 3 or more alcoholic drinks everyday may increase the chance of stomach bleeding).

SALONPAS PAIN RELIEF PATCH

(Menthol, Methyl Salicylate) 1805
May interact with alcohols, anticoagulants, corticosteroids, non-steroidal anti-inflammatory agents. Compounds in these categories include:

Alclometasone Dipropionate (Taking a steroid may increase the chance of stomach bleeding).
No products indexed under this heading.

Anisindione (Taking a blood thinning agent (eg, anticoagulants) may increase the chance of stomach bleeding).
No products indexed under this heading.

Ardeparin Sodium (Taking a blood thinning agent (eg, anticoagulants) may increase the chance of stomach bleeding).
No products indexed under this heading.

Beclomethasone Dipropionate (Taking a steroid may increase the chance of stomach bleeding). Products include:
Qvar 3398

Beclomethasone Dipropionate Monohydrate (Taking a steroid may increase the chance of stomach bleeding). Products include:
Beconase AQ 1386

Betamethasone (Taking a steroid may increase the chance of stomach bleeding).
No products indexed under this heading.

Betamethasone Acetate (Taking a steroid may increase the chance of stomach bleeding).
No products indexed under this heading.

Betamethasone Benzoate (Taking a steroid may increase the chance of stomach bleeding).
No products indexed under this heading.

Betamethasone Dipropionate (Taking a steroid may increase the chance of stomach bleeding). Products include:
Diprolene Lotion 0.05% 3108
Diprolene Ointment 0.05% 3109
Diprolene AF Cream 0.05% 3107
Lotrisone 3163

Betamethasone Sodium Phosphate (Taking a steroid may increase the chance of stomach bleeding).
No products indexed under this heading.

Betamethasone Valerate (Taking a steroid may increase the chance of stomach bleeding). Products include:
Luxíq 3321

Budesonide (Taking a steroid may increase the chance of stomach bleeding). Products include:
Pulmicort Flexhaler 714
Symbicort 80/4.5 720
Symbicort 160/4.5 720

Celecoxib (Taking other drugs containing an NSAID (eg, aspirin, ibuprofen, naproxen, or others) may increase the chance of stomach bleeding). Products include:
Celebrex 3272

Ciclesonide (Taking a steroid may increase the chance of stomach bleeding).
No products indexed under this heading.

Cortisone Acetate (Taking a steroid may increase the chance of stomach bleeding).
No products indexed under this heading.

Dalteparin Sodium (Taking a blood thinning agent (eg, anticoagulants) may increase the chance of stomach bleeding). Products include:
Fragmin 1058

Danaparoid Sodium (Taking a blood thinning agent (eg, anticoagulants) may increase the chance of stomach bleeding).
No products indexed under this heading.

Desoximetasone (Taking a steroid may increase the chance of stomach bleeding).
No products indexed under this heading.

Dexamethasone (Taking a steroid may increase the chance of stomach bleeding). Products include:
Ciprodex 583
Ozurdex .... ⊙223
Tobramycin and Dexamethasone
Ophthalmic Suspension .... ⊙251

Dexamethasone Acetate (Taking a steroid may increase the chance of stomach bleeding).
No products indexed under this heading.

Dexamethasone Phosphate (Taking a steroid may increase the chance of stomach bleeding).
No products indexed under this heading.

Dexamethasone Sodium (Taking a steroid may increase the chance of stomach bleeding).
No products indexed under this heading.

Dexamethasone Sodium Phosphate (Taking a steroid may increase the chance of stomach bleeding).
No products indexed under this heading.

Dexamethasone Sodium Phosphate Injection (Taking a steroid may increase the chance of stomach bleeding).
No products indexed under this heading.

Diclofenac Epolamine (Taking other drugs containing an NSAID (eg, aspirin, ibuprofen, naproxen, or others) may increase the chance of stomach bleeding). Products include:
Flector 1839

Diclofenac Potassium (Taking other drugs containing an NSAID (eg, aspirin, ibuprofen, naproxen, or others) may increase the chance of stomach bleeding).
No products indexed under this heading.

Diclofenac Sodium (Taking other drugs containing an NSAID (eg, aspirin, ibuprofen, naproxen, or others) may increase the chance of stomach bleeding).
No products indexed under this heading.

Dicumarol (Taking a blood thinning agent (eg, anticoagulants) may increase the chance of stomach bleeding).
No products indexed under this heading.

Diflorasone Diacetate (Taking a steroid may increase the chance of stomach bleeding).
No products indexed under this heading.

Enoxaparin Sodium (Taking a blood thinning agent (eg, anticoagulants) may increase the chance of stomach bleeding). Products include:
Lovenox 3005

Ethanol (Having 3 or more alcoholic drinks everyday may increase the chance of stomach bleeding).
No products indexed under this heading.

Ethyl Alcohol (Having 3 or more alcoholic drinks everyday may increase the chance of stomach bleeding).
No products indexed under this heading.

Etodolac (Taking other drugs containing an NSAID (eg, aspirin, ibuprofen, naproxen, or others) may increase the chance of stomach bleeding).
No products indexed under this heading.

Fenoprofen Calcium (Taking other drugs containing an NSAID (eg, aspirin, ibuprofen, naproxen, or others) may increase the chance of stomach bleeding).
No products indexed under this heading.

Fludrocortisone Acetate (Taking a steroid may increase the chance of stomach bleeding).
No products indexed under this heading.

Flumethasone Pivalate (Taking a steroid may increase the chance of stomach bleeding).
No products indexed under this heading.

Flunisolide Hemihydrate (Taking a steroid may increase the chance of stomach bleeding).
No products indexed under this heading.

Flurbiprofen (Taking other drugs containing an NSAID (eg, aspirin, ibuprofen, naproxen, or others) may increase the chance of stomach bleeding).
No products indexed under this heading.

Fluticasone Furoate (Taking a steroid may increase the chance of stomach bleeding). Products include:
Veramyst 1713

Fluticasone Propionate (Taking a steroid may increase the chance of stomach bleeding). Products include:
Advair 100/50 1275
Advair 250/50 1275
Advair 500/50 1275
Advair HFA 45/21 1288
Advair HFA 115/21 1288
Advair HFA 230/21 1288
Flonase 1459
Flovent Diskus 1463
Flovent HFA 1470

Fondaparinux Sodium (Taking a blood thinning agent (eg, anticoagulants) may increase the chance of stomach bleeding). Products include:
Arixtra 1320

Heparin Calcium (Taking a blood thinning agent (eg, anticoagulants) may increase the chance of stomach bleeding).
No products indexed under this heading.

(⊙ Described in PDR® for Ophthalmic Medicines)

Heparin Sodium (Taking a blood thinning agent (eg, anticoagulants) may increase the chance of stomach bleeding).
No products indexed under this heading.

Hydrocortisone (Taking a steroid may increase the chance of stomach bleeding).
No products indexed under this heading.

Hydrocortisone (Alcohol) (Taking a steroid may increase the chance of stomach bleeding).
No products indexed under this heading.

Hydrocortisone Acetate (Taking a steroid may increase the chance of stomach bleeding).
No products indexed under this heading.

Hydrocortisone Butyrate (Taking a steroid may increase the chance of stomach bleeding).
No products indexed under this heading.

Hydrocortisone Cypionate (Taking a steroid may increase the chance of stomach bleeding).
No products indexed under this heading.

Hydrocortisone Hemisuccinate (Taking a steroid may increase the chance of stomach bleeding).
No products indexed under this heading.

Hydrocortisone Probutate (Taking a steroid may increase the chance of stomach bleeding).
No products indexed under this heading.

Hydrocortisone Sodium Phosphate (Taking a steroid may increase the chance of stomach bleeding).
No products indexed under this heading.

Hydrocortisone Sodium Succinate (Taking a steroid may increase the chance of stomach bleeding).
No products indexed under this heading.

Hydrocortisone Valerate (Taking a steroid may increase the chance of stomach bleeding).
No products indexed under this heading.

Ibuprofen (Taking other drugs containing an NSAID (eg, aspirin, ibuprofen, naproxen, or others) may increase the chance of stomach bleeding). Products include:
Motrin IB 2043
Children's Motrin 2044
Children's Motrin Non-Staining Dye-Free 2044
Infants' Motrin 2044
Infants' Motrin Dye-Free 2044
Junior Strength Motrin 2044
Vicoprofen 564

Indomethacin (Taking other drugs containing an NSAID (eg, aspirin, ibuprofen, naproxen, or others) may increase the chance of stomach bleeding). Products include:
Indocin 2167

Indomethacin Sodium Trihydrate (Taking other drugs containing an NSAID (eg, aspirin, ibuprofen, naproxen, or others) may increase the chance of stomach bleeding). Products include:
Indocin I.V. 2007

Ketoprofen (Taking other drugs containing an NSAID (eg, aspirin, ibuprofen, naproxen, or others) may increase the chance of stomach bleeding).
No products indexed under this heading.

Ketorolac Tromethamine (Taking other drugs containing an NSAID (eg, aspirin, ibuprofen, naproxen, or others) may increase the chance of stomach bleeding). Products include:
Acuvail .... ⊙209

Low Molecular Weight Heparins (Taking a blood thinning agent (eg, anticoagulants) may increase the chance of stomach bleeding).
No products indexed under this heading.

Meclofenamate Sodium (Taking other drugs containing an NSAID (eg, aspirin, ibuprofen, naproxen, or others) may increase the chance of stomach bleeding).
No products indexed under this heading.

Mefenamic Acid (Taking other drugs containing an NSAID (eg, aspirin, ibuprofen, naproxen, or others) may increase the chance of stomach bleeding).
No products indexed under this heading.

Meloxicam (Taking other drugs containing an NSAID (eg, aspirin, ibuprofen, naproxen, or others) may increase the chance of stomach bleeding).
No products indexed under this heading.

Methylprednisolone (Taking a steroid may increase the chance of stomach bleeding).
No products indexed under this heading.

Methylprednisolone Acetate (Taking a steroid may increase the chance of stomach bleeding).
No products indexed under this heading.

Methylprednisolone Sodium Succinate (Taking a steroid may increase the chance of stomach bleeding).
No products indexed under this heading.

Mometasone Furoate (Taking a steroid may increase the chance of stomach bleeding). Products include:
Asmanex 3058
Elocon Cream 3111
Elocon Lotion 3112
Elocon Ointment 3114

Mometasone Furoate Monohydrate (Taking a steroid may increase the chance of stomach bleeding). Products include:
Nasonex 3166

Nabumetone (Taking other drugs containing an NSAID (eg, aspirin, ibuprofen, naproxen, or others) may increase the chance of stomach bleeding).
No products indexed under this heading.

Naproxen (Taking other drugs containing an NSAID (eg, aspirin, ibuprofen, naproxen, or others) may increase the chance of stomach bleeding). Products include:
EC-Naprosyn 2850
Naprosyn 2850
Anaprox/Naprosyn 2850

Naproxen Sodium (Taking other drugs containing an NSAID (eg, aspirin, ibuprofen, naproxen, or others) may increase the chance of stomach bleeding). Products include:
Anaprox 2850
Anaprox DS 2850
Treximet 1681

Oxaprozin (Taking other drugs containing an NSAID (eg, aspirin, ibuprofen, naproxen, or others) may increase the chance of stomach bleeding).
No products indexed under this heading.

Phenylbutazone (Taking other drugs containing an NSAID (eg, aspirin, ibuprofen, naproxen, or others) may increase the chance of stomach bleeding).
No products indexed under this heading.

Piroxicam (Taking other drugs containing an NSAID (eg, aspirin, ibuprofen, naproxen, or others) may increase the chance of stomach bleeding).
No products indexed under this heading.

Prednisolone (Taking a steroid may increase the chance of stomach bleeding).
No products indexed under this heading.

Prednisolone Acetate (Taking a steroid may increase the chance of stomach bleeding). Products include:
Blephamide .... ⊙212, ⊙214
Pred Forte .... ⊙225
Pred Mild .... ⊙230
Pred-G .... ⊙226, ⊙227

Prednisolone Sodium Phosphate (Taking a steroid may increase the chance of stomach bleeding).
No products indexed under this heading.

Prednisolone Tebutate (Taking a steroid may increase the chance of stomach bleeding).
No products indexed under this heading.

Prednisone (Taking a steroid may increase the chance of stomach bleeding).
No products indexed under this heading.

Prednisone sodium phosphate (Taking a steroid may increase the chance of stomach bleeding).
No products indexed under this heading.

Rofecoxib (Taking other drugs containing an NSAID (eg, aspirin, ibuprofen, naproxen, or others) may increase the chance of stomach bleeding).
No products indexed under this heading.

Sulindac (Taking other drugs containing an NSAID (eg, aspirin, ibuprofen, naproxen, or others) may increase the chance of stomach bleeding). Products include:
Clinoril 2098

Tinzaparin Sodium (Taking a blood thinning agent (eg, anticoagulants) may increase the chance of stomach bleeding).
No products indexed under this heading.

Tolmetin Sodium (Taking other drugs containing an NSAID (eg, aspirin, ibuprofen, naproxen, or others) may increase the chance of stomach bleeding).
No products indexed under this heading.

Triamcinolone (Taking a steroid may increase the chance of stomach bleeding).
No products indexed under this heading.

Triamcinolone Acetonide (Taking a steroid may increase the chance of stomach bleeding). Products include:
Azmacort 408
Nasacort AQ 3019

Triamcinolone Diacetate (Taking a steroid may increase the chance of stomach bleeding).
No products indexed under this heading.

Triamcinolone Hexacetonide (Taking a steroid may increase the chance of stomach bleeding).
No products indexed under this heading.

Valdecoxib (Taking other drugs containing an NSAID (eg, aspirin, ibuprofen, naproxen, or others) may increase the chance of stomach bleeding).
No products indexed under this heading.

Warfarin Sodium (Taking a blood thinning agent (eg, anticoagulants) may increase the chance of stomach bleeding).
No products indexed under this heading.

Food Interactions

Alcohol (Having 3 or more alcoholic drinks everyday may increase the chance of stomach bleeding).

Beer, reduced-alcohol (Having 3 or more alcoholic drinks everyday may increase the chance of stomach bleeding).

Beer, unspecified (Having 3 or more alcoholic drinks everyday may increase the chance of stomach bleeding).

Wine, Chianti (Having 3 or more alcoholic drinks everyday may increase the chance of stomach bleeding).

Wine, Red (Having 3 or more alcoholic drinks everyday may increase the chance of stomach bleeding).

Wine, unspecified (Having 3 or more alcoholic drinks everyday may increase the chance of stomach bleeding).

Wine products (Having 3 or more alcoholic drinks everyday may increase the chance of stomach bleeding).

SANDOSTATIN INJECTION

(Octreotide Acetate) 2517
See Sandostatin LAR Depot

SANDOSTATIN LAR DEPOT

(Octreotide Acetate) 2519
May interact with beta-blockers, cytochrome p450 3a4 substrates (selected), drugs which undergo biotransformation by cytochrome p-450 mixed function oxidase, insulin, oral hypoglycemic agents, quinidine, and certain other agents. Compounds in these categories include:

Acarbose (Octreotide inhibits the secretion of insulin and glucagon. Therefore, blood glucose levels should be monitored when octreotide is initiated or when the dose is altered and antidiabetic treatment should be adjusted accordingly).
No products indexed under this heading.

Acebutolol Hydrochloride (Concomitant administration of bradycardia inducing drugs (eg, beta blockers) may have an additive effect on the reduction of heart rate associated with octreotide. Dose adjustment of concomitant medication may be necessary).
No products indexed under this heading.

Acetaminophen (Limited published data indicate that somatostatin analogs may decrease the metabolic clearance of compounds known to be metabolized by cytochrome P450 enzymes, which may be due to the suppression of growth hormone). Products include:
Percocet 1121
Tylenol 2049
Tylenol 8 Hour 2049
Extra Strength Tylenol Caplets, Cool Caplets, and EZ Tabs 2049
Extra Strength Tylenol Adult Rapid Blast Liquid 2049
Extra Strength Tylenol Rapid Release 2049
Tylenol with Codeine 2691
Tylenol Arthritis Pain Extended Release Geltabs/Caplets 2049
Children's Tylenol Suspension Liquid 2048
Children's Tylenol Meltaways 2048
Tylenol, Infants' Drops 2048
Junior Tylenol 2048
Vicodin 560
Vicodin ES 561
Vicodin HP 563
Zydone 1138

Alatrofloxacin Mesylate (Limited published data indicate that somatostatin analogs may decrease the metabolic clearance of compounds known to be metabolized by cytochrome P450 enzymes, which may be due to the suppression of growth hormone).
No products indexed under this heading.

Alfentanil Hydrochloride (Limited published data indicate that somatostatin analogs may decrease the metabolic clearance of compounds known to be metabolized by cytochrome P450 enzymes, which may be due to the suppression of growth hormone. Since it cannot be excluded that octreotide may have this effect, other drugs mainly metabolized by CYP3A4 and which have a low therapeutic index (eg, quinidine, terfenadine) should therefore be used with caution).
No products indexed under this heading.

Alprazolam (Limited published data indicate that somatostatin analogs may decrease the metabolic clearance of compounds known to be metabolized by cytochrome P450 enzymes, which may be due to the suppression of growth hormone. Since it cannot be excluded that octreotide may have this effect, other drugs mainly metabolized by CYP3A4 and which have a low thera-

Sandostatin LAR Interactions Index 1676

peutic index (eg, quinidine, terfenadine) should therefore be used with caution).
No products indexed under this heading.

Aminophylline (Limited published data indicate that somatostatin analogs may decrease the metabolic clearance of compounds known to be metabolized by cytochrome P450 enzymes, which may be due to the suppression of growth hormone).
No products indexed under this heading.

Amiodarone Hydrochloride (Limited published data indicate that somatostatin analogs may decrease the metabolic clearance of compounds known to be metabolized by cytochrome P450 enzymes, which may be due to the suppression of growth hormone. Since it cannot be excluded that octreotide may have this effect, other drugs mainly metabolized by CYP3A4 and which have a low therapeutic index (eg, quinidine, terfenadine) should therefore be used with caution).
No products indexed under this heading.

Amitriptyline Hydrochloride (Limited published data indicate that somatostatin analogs may decrease the metabolic clearance of compounds known to be metabolized by cytochrome P450 enzymes, which may be due to the suppression of growth hormone. Since it cannot be excluded that octreotide may have this effect, other drugs mainly metabolized by CYP3A4 and which have a low therapeutic index (eg, quinidine, terfenadine) should therefore be used with caution).
No products indexed under this heading.

Amlodipine Besylate (Limited published data indicate that somatostatin analogs may decrease the metabolic clearance of compounds known to be metabolized by cytochrome P450 enzymes, which may be due to the suppression of growth hormone. Since it cannot be excluded that octreotide may have this effect, other drugs mainly metabolized by CYP3A4 and which have a low therapeutic index (eg, quinidine, terfenadine) should therefore be used with caution). Products include:
Azor 1010
Exforge 2443
Exforge HCT 2449

Amoxapine (Limited published data indicate that somatostatin analogs may decrease the metabolic clearance of compounds known to be metabolized by cytochrome P450 enzymes, which may be due to the suppression of growth hormone).
No products indexed under this heading.

Amphetamine Aspartate (Limited published data indicate that somatostatin analogs may decrease the metabolic clearance of compounds known to be metabolized by cytochrome P450 enzymes, which may be due to the suppression of growth hormone).
No products indexed under this heading.

Amphetamine Aspartate Monohydrate (Limited published data indicate that somatostatin analogs may decrease the metabolic clearance of compounds known to be metabolized by cytochrome P450 enzymes, which may be due to the suppression of growth hormone).
No products indexed under this heading.

Amphetamine Sulfate (Limited published data indicate that somatostatin analogs may decrease the metabolic clearance of compounds known to be metabolized by cytochrome P450 enzymes, which may be due to the suppression of growth hormone).
No products indexed under this heading.

Anagrelide Hydrochloride (Limited published data indicate that somatostatin analogs may decrease the metabolic clearance of compounds known to be metabolized by cytochrome P450 enzymes, which may be due to the suppression of growth hormone).
No products indexed under this heading.

Aprepitant (Limited published data indicate that somatostatin analogs may decrease the metabolic clearance of compounds known to be metabolized by cytochrome P450 enzymes, which may be due to the suppression of growth hormone. Since it cannot be excluded that octreotide may have this effect, other drugs mainly metabolized by CYP3A4 and which have a low therapeutic index (eg, quinidine, terfenadine) should therefore be used with caution). Products include:
Emend 2124

Astemizole (Limited published data indicate that somatostatin analogs may decrease the metabolic clearance of compounds known to be metabolized by cytochrome P450 enzymes, which may be due to the suppression of growth hormone. Since it cannot be excluded that octreotide may have this effect, other drugs mainly metabolized by CYP3A4 and which have a low therapeutic index (eg, quinidine, terfenadine) should therefore be used with caution).
No products indexed under this heading.

Atenolol (Concomitant administration of bradycardia inducing drugs (eg, beta blockers) may have an additive effect on the reduction of heart rate associated with octreotide. Dose adjustment of concomitant medication may be necessary).
No products indexed under this heading.

Atomoxetine Hydrochloride (Limited published data indicate that somatostatin analogs may decrease the metabolic clearance of compounds known to be metabolized by cytochrome P450 enzymes, which may be due to the suppression of growth hormone). Products include:
Strattera 1957

Atorvastatin Calcium (Limited published data indicate that somatostatin analogs may decrease the metabolic clearance of compounds known to be metabolized by cytochrome P450 enzymes, which may be due to the suppression of growth hormone. Since it cannot be excluded that octreotide may have this effect, other drugs mainly metabolized by CYP3A4 and which have a low therapeutic index (eg, quinidine, terfenadine) should therefore be used with caution). Products include:
Lipitor 2703

Belladonna Ergotamine (Limited published data indicate that somatostatin analogs may decrease the metabolic clearance of compounds known to be metabolized by cytochrome P450 enzymes, which may be due to the suppression of growth hormone. Since it cannot be excluded that octreotide may have this effect, other drugs mainly metabolized by CYP3A4 and which have a low therapeutic index (eg, quinidine, terfenadine) should therefore be used with caution).
No products indexed under this heading.

Benzphetamine Hydrochloride (Limited published data indicate that somatostatin analogs may decrease the metabolic clearance of compounds known to be metabolized by cytochrome P450 enzymes, which may be due to the suppression of growth hormone).
No products indexed under this heading.

Betaxolol Hydrochloride (Concomitant administration of bradycardia inducing drugs (eg, beta blockers) may have an additive effect on the reduction of heart rate associated with octreotide. Dose adjustment of concomitant medication may be necessary).
No products indexed under this heading.

Bisoprolol Fumarate (Concomitant administration of bradycardia inducing drugs (eg, beta blockers) may have an additive effect on the reduction of heart rate associated with octreotide. Dose adjustment of concomitant medication may be necessary).
No products indexed under this heading.

Bromocriptine Mesylate (Concomitant administration of octreotide and bromocriptine increases the availability of bromocriptine).
No products indexed under this heading.

Buspirone Hydrochloride (Limited published data indicate that somatostatin analogs may decrease the metabolic clearance of compounds known to be metabolized by cytochrome P450 enzymes, which may be due to the suppression of growth hormone. Since it cannot be excluded that octreotide may have this effect, other drugs mainly metabolized by CYP3A4 and which have a low therapeutic index (eg, quinidine, terfenadine) should therefore be used with caution).
No products indexed under this heading.

Busulfan (Limited published data indicate that somatostatin analogs may decrease the metabolic clearance of compounds known to be metabolized by cytochrome P450 enzymes, which may be due to the suppression of growth hormone. Since it cannot be excluded that octreotide may have this effect, other drugs mainly metabolized by CYP3A4 and which have a low therapeutic index (eg, quinidine, terfenadine) should therefore be used with caution). Products include:
Myleran 1581

Caffeine (Limited published data indicate that somatostatin analogs may decrease the metabolic clearance of compounds known to be metabolized by cytochrome P450 enzymes, which may be due to the suppression of growth hormone).
No products indexed under this heading.

Caffeine Anhydrous (Limited published data indicate that somatostatin analogs may decrease the metabolic clearance of compounds known to be metabolized by cytochrome P450 enzymes, which may be due to the suppression of growth hormone).
No products indexed under this heading.

Caffeine Citrate (Limited published data indicate that somatostatin analogs may decrease the metabolic clearance of compounds known to be metabolized by cytochrome P450 enzymes, which may be due to the suppression of growth hormone).
No products indexed under this heading.

Caffeine-containing medications (Limited published data indicate that somatostatin analogs may decrease the metabolic clearance of compounds known to be metabolized by cytochrome P450 enzymes, which may be due to the suppression of growth hormone).
No products indexed under this heading.

Caffeine Sodium Benzoate (Limited published data indicate that somatostatin analogs may decrease the metabolic clearance of compounds known to be metabolized by cytochrome P450 enzymes, which may be due to the suppression of growth hormone).
No products indexed under this heading.

Candesartan Cilexetil (Limited published data indicate that somatostatin analogs may decrease the metabolic clearance of compounds known to be metabolized by cytochrome P450 enzymes, which may be due to the suppression of growth hormone). Products include:
Atacand 697
Atacand HCT 700

Captopril (Limited published data indicate that somatostatin analogs may decrease the metabolic clearance of compounds known to be metabolized by cytochrome P450 enzymes, which may be due to the suppression of growth hormone). Products include:
Captopril 2341

Carbamazepine (Limited published data indicate that somatostatin analogs may decrease the metabolic clearance of compounds known to be metabolized by cytochrome P450 enzymes, which may be due to the suppression of growth hormone. Since it cannot be excluded that octreotide may have this effect, other drugs mainly metabolized by CYP3A4 and which have a low therapeutic index (eg, quinidine, terfenadine) should therefore be used with caution). Products include:
Carbatrol 3280
Equetro 3477

Carisoprodol (Limited published data indicate that somatostatin analogs may decrease the metabolic clearance of compounds known to be metabolized by cytochrome P450 enzymes, which may be due to the suppression of growth hormone).
No products indexed under this heading.

Carteolol Hydrochloride (Concomitant administration of bradycardia inducing drugs (eg, beta blockers) may have an additive effect on the reduction of heart rate associated with octreotide. Dose adjustment of concomitant medication may be necessary).
No products indexed under this heading.

Carvedilol (Concomitant administration of bradycardia inducing drugs (eg, beta blockers) may have an additive effect on the reduction of heart rate associated with octreotide. Dose adjustment of concomitant medication may be necessary). Products include:
Coreg 1409

Carvedilol Phosphate (Concomitant administration of bradycardia inducing drugs (eg, beta blockers) may have an additive effect on the reduction of heart rate associated with octreotide. Dose adjustment of concomitant medication may be necessary). Products include:
Coreg CR 1416

Celecoxib (Limited published data indicate that somatostatin analogs may decrease the metabolic clearance of compounds known to be metabolized by cytochrome P450 enzymes, which may be due to the suppression of growth hormone). Products include:
Celebrex 3272

Cerivastatin Sodium (Limited published data indicate that somatostatin analogs may decrease the metabolic clearance of compounds known to be metabolized by cytochrome P450 enzymes, which may be due to the suppression of growth hormone. Since it cannot be excluded that octreotide may have this effect, other drugs mainly metabolized by CYP3A4 and which have a low therapeutic index (eg, quinidine, terfenadine) should therefore be used with caution).
No products indexed under this heading.

Cevimeline Hydrochloride (Limited published data indicate that somatostatin analogs may decrease the metabolic clearance of compounds known to be metabolized by cytochrome P450

enzymes, which may be due to the suppression of growth hormone). Products include:

Evoxac 1027

Chlordiazepoxide (Limited published data indicate that somatostatin analogs may decrease the metabolic clearance of compounds known to be metabolized by cytochrome P450 enzymes, which may be due to the suppression of growth hormone).

No products indexed under this heading.

Chlordiazepoxide Hydrochloride (Limited published data indicate that somatostatin analogs may decrease the metabolic clearance of compounds known to be metabolized by cytochrome P450 enzymes, which may be due to the suppression of growth hormone).

No products indexed under this heading.

Chlorpheniramine (Limited published data indicate that somatostatin analogs may decrease the metabolic clearance of compounds known to be metabolized by cytochrome P450 enzymes, which may be due to the suppression of growth hormone. Since it cannot be excluded that octreotide may have this effect, other drugs mainly metabolized by CYP3A4 and which have a low therapeutic index (eg, quinidine, terfenadine) should therefore be used with caution).

No products indexed under this heading.

Chlorpheniramine Maleate (Limited published data indicate that somatostatin analogs may decrease the metabolic clearance of compounds known to be metabolized by cytochrome P450 enzymes, which may be due to the suppression of growth hormone. Since it cannot be excluded that octreotide may have this effect, other drugs mainly metabolized by CYP3A4 and which have a low therapeutic index (eg, quinidine, terfenadine) should therefore be used with caution).

No products indexed under this heading.

Chlorpheniramine Polistirex (Limited published data indicate that somatostatin analogs may decrease the metabolic clearance of compounds known to be metabolized by cytochrome P450 enzymes, which may be due to the suppression of growth hormone. Since it cannot be excluded that octreotide may have this effect, other drugs mainly metabolized by CYP3A4 and which have a low therapeutic index (eg, quinidine, terfenadine) should therefore be used with caution). Products include:

Tussionex 3443

Chlorpheniramine Tannate (Limited published data indicate that somatostatin analogs may decrease the metabolic clearance of compounds known to be metabolized by cytochrome P450 enzymes, which may be due to the suppression of growth hormone. Since it cannot be excluded that octreotide may have this effect, other drugs mainly metabolized by CYP3A4 and which have a low therapeutic index (eg, quinidine, terfenadine) should therefore be used with caution).

No products indexed under this heading.

Chlorpromazine (Limited published data indicate that somatostatin analogs may decrease the metabolic clearance of compounds known to be metabolized by cytochrome P450 enzymes, which may be due to the suppression of growth hormone).

No products indexed under this heading.

Chlorpromazine Hydrochloride (Limited published data indicate that somatostatin analogs may decrease the metabolic clearance of compounds known to be metabolized by cytochrome P450 enzymes, which may be due to the suppression of growth hormone).

No products indexed under this heading.

Chlorpropamide (Octreotide inhibits the secretion of insulin and glucagon. Therefore, blood glucose levels should be monitored when octreotide is initiated or when the dose is altered and antidiabetic treatment should be adjusted accordingly).

No products indexed under this heading.

Cilostazol (Limited published data indicate that somatostatin analogs may decrease the metabolic clearance of compounds known to be metabolized by cytochrome P450 enzymes, which may be due to the suppression of growth hormone).

No products indexed under this heading.

Cimetidine Hydrochloride (Limited published data indicate that somatostatin analogs may decrease the metabolic clearance of compounds known to be metabolized by cytochrome P450 enzymes, which may be due to the suppression of growth hormone).

No products indexed under this heading.

Ciprofloxacin (Limited published data indicate that somatostatin analogs may decrease the metabolic clearance of compounds known to be metabolized by cytochrome P450 enzymes, which may be due to the suppression of growth hormone). Products include:

Cipro I.V. 3082
Cipro 3073
Cipro XR 3091
Ciprodex 583

Ciprofloxacin Hydrochloride (Limited published data indicate that somatostatin analogs may decrease the metabolic clearance of compounds known to be metabolized by cytochrome P450 enzymes, which may be due to the suppression of growth hormone). Products include:

Cipro 3073

Cisapride (Limited published data indicate that somatostatin analogs may decrease the metabolic clearance of compounds known to be metabolized by cytochrome P450 enzymes, which may be due to the suppression of growth hormone. Since it cannot be excluded that octreotide may have this effect, other drugs mainly metabolized by CYP3A4 and which have a low therapeutic index (eg, quinidine, terfenadine) should therefore be used with caution).

No products indexed under this heading.

Citalopram Hydrobromide (Limited published data indicate that somatostatin analogs may decrease the metabolic clearance of compounds known to be metabolized by cytochrome P450 enzymes, which may be due to the suppression of growth hormone). Products include:

Celexa 1153

Clarithromycin (Limited published data indicate that somatostatin analogs may decrease the metabolic clearance of compounds known to be metabolized by cytochrome P450 enzymes, which may be due to the suppression of growth hormone. Since it cannot be excluded that octreotide may have this effect, other drugs mainly metabolized by CYP3A4 and which have a low therapeutic index (eg, quinidine, terfenadine) should therefore be used with caution). Products include:

Biaxin/Biaxin XL 412

Clomipramine Hydrochloride (Limited published data indicate that somatostatin analogs may decrease the metabolic clearance of compounds known to be metabolized by cytochrome P450 enzymes, which may be due to the suppression of growth hormone).

No products indexed under this heading.

Clopidogrel Bisulfate (Limited published data indicate that somatostatin analogs may decrease the metabolic clearance of compounds known to be metabolized by cytochrome P450 enzymes, which may be due to the suppression of growth hormone). Products include:

Plavix 3027

Clopidogrel Hydrogen Sulfate (Limited published data indicate that somatostatin analogs may decrease the metabolic clearance of compounds known to be metabolized by cytochrome P450 enzymes, which may be due to the suppression of growth hormone).

No products indexed under this heading.

Clozapine (Limited published data indicate that somatostatin analogs may decrease the metabolic clearance of compounds known to be metabolized by cytochrome P450 enzymes, which may be due to the suppression of growth hormone).

No products indexed under this heading.

Codeine Phosphate (Limited published data indicate that somatostatin analogs may decrease the metabolic clearance of compounds known to be metabolized by cytochrome P450 enzymes, which may be due to the suppression of growth hormone). Products include:

Tylenol with Codeine 2691

Codeine Sulfate (Limited published data indicate that somatostatin analogs may decrease the metabolic clearance of compounds known to be metabolized by cytochrome P450 enzymes, which may be due to the suppression of growth hormone).

No products indexed under this heading.

Cyclobenzaprine (Limited published data indicate that somatostatin analogs may decrease the metabolic clearance of compounds known to be metabolized by cytochrome P450 enzymes, which may be due to the suppression of growth hormone).

No products indexed under this heading.

Cyclobenzaprine Hydrochloride (Limited published data indicate that somatostatin analogs may decrease the metabolic clearance of compounds known to be metabolized by cytochrome P450 enzymes, which may be due to the suppression of growth hormone). Products include:

Amrix 964

Cyclophosphamide (Limited published data indicate that somatostatin analogs may decrease the metabolic clearance of compounds known to be metabolized by cytochrome P450 enzymes, which may be due to the suppression of growth hormone).

No products indexed under this heading.

Cyclosporine (Concomitant administration of octreotide injection with cyclosporine may decrease blood levels of cyclosporine and result in transplant rejection). Products include:

Gengraf 440
Neoral Oral Solution 2496
Neoral Capsules 2496
Restasis 605

Desipramine Hydrochloride (Limited published data indicate that somatostatin analogs may decrease the metabolic clearance of compounds known to be metabolized by cytochrome P450 enzymes, which may be due to the suppression of growth hormone).

No products indexed under this heading.

Desogestrel (Limited published data indicate that somatostatin analogs may decrease the metabolic clearance of compounds known to be metabolized by cytochrome P450 enzymes, which may be due to the suppression of growth hormone. Since it cannot be excluded that octreotide may have this effect, other drugs mainly metabolized by CYP3A4 and which have a low therapeutic index (eg, quinidine, terfenadine) should therefore be used with caution).

No products indexed under this heading.

Dexamethasone (Limited published data indicate that somatostatin analogs may decrease the metabolic clearance of compounds known to be metabolized by cytochrome P450 enzymes, which may be due to the suppression of growth hormone). Products include:

Ciprodex .... ˙583
Ozurdex .... ⊙223
Tobramycin and Dexamethasone Ophthalmic Suspension .... ⊙251

Dexamethasone Acetate (Limited published data indicate that somatostatin analogs may decrease the metabolic clearance of compounds known to be metabolized by cytochrome P450 enzymes, which may be due to the suppression of growth hormone).

No products indexed under this heading.

Dexamethasone Phosphate (Limited published data indicate that somatostatin analogs may decrease the metabolic clearance of compounds known to be metabolized by cytochrome P450 enzymes, which may be due to the suppression of growth hormone).

No products indexed under this heading.

Dexamethasone Sodium (Limited published data indicate that somatostatin analogs may decrease the metabolic clearance of compounds known to be metabolized by cytochrome P450 enzymes, which may be due to the suppression of growth hormone).

No products indexed under this heading.

Dexamethasone Sodium Phosphate (Limited published data indicate that somatostatin analogs may decrease the metabolic clearance of compounds known to be metabolized by cytochrome P450 enzymes, which may be due to the suppression of growth hormone).

No products indexed under this heading.

Dexfenfluramine Hydrochloride (Limited published data indicate that somatostatin analogs may decrease the metabolic clearance of compounds known to be metabolized by cytochrome P450 enzymes, which may be due to the suppression of growth hormone).

No products indexed under this heading.

Dextromethorphan (Limited published data indicate that somatostatin analogs may decrease the metabolic clearance of compounds known to be metabolized by cytochrome P450 enzymes, which may be due to the suppression of growth hormone).

No products indexed under this heading.

Dextromethorphan Hydrobromide (Limited published data indicate that somatostatin analogs may decrease the metabolic clearance of compounds known to be metabolized by cytochrome P450 enzymes, which may be due to the suppression of growth hormone).

No products indexed under this heading.

IMPORTANT NOTE: Always consult each drug listing in the patient's regimen for possible interactions.

Sandostatin LAR | Interactions Index | 1678

Dextromethorphan Polistirex (Limited published data indicate that somatostatin analogs may decrease the metabolic clearance of compounds known to be metabolized by cytochrome P450 enzymes, which may be due to the suppression of growth hormone).
No products indexed under this heading.

Diazepam (Limited published data indicate that somatostatin analogs may decrease the metabolic clearance of compounds known to be metabolized by cytochrome P450 enzymes, which may be due to the suppression of growth hormone. Since it cannot be excluded that octreotide may have this effect, other drugs mainly metabolized by CYP3A4 and which have a low therapeutic index (eg, quinidine, terfenadine) should therefore be used with caution). Products include:
Valium Tablets 2880

Diclofenac Potassium (Limited published data indicate that somatostatin analogs may decrease the metabolic clearance of compounds known to be metabolized by cytochrome P450 enzymes, which may be due to the suppression of growth hormone).
No products indexed under this heading.

Diclofenac Sodium (Limited published data indicate that somatostatin analogs may decrease the metabolic clearance of compounds known to be metabolized by cytochrome P450 enzymes, which may be due to the suppression of growth hormone).
No products indexed under this heading.

Dihydroergotamine Mesylate (Limited published data indicate that somatostatin analogs may decrease the metabolic clearance of compounds known to be metabolized by cytochrome P450 enzymes, which may be due to the suppression of growth hormone. Since it cannot be excluded that octreotide may have this effect, other drugs mainly metabolized by CYP3A4 and which have a low therapeutic index (eg, quinidine, terfenadine) should therefore be used with caution).
No products indexed under this heading.

Diltiazem Hydrochloride (Limited published data indicate that somatostatin analogs may decrease the metabolic clearance of compounds known to be metabolized by cytochrome P450 enzymes, which may be due to the suppression of growth hormone. Since it cannot be excluded that octreotide may have this effect, other drugs mainly metabolized by CYP3A4 and which have a low therapeutic index (eg, quinidine, terfenadine) should therefore be used with caution). Products include:
Cardizem LA 423

Diltiazem Maleate (Limited published data indicate that somatostatin analogs may decrease the metabolic clearance of compounds known to be metabolized by cytochrome P450 enzymes, which may be due to the suppression of growth hormone. Since it cannot be excluded that octreotide may have this effect, other drugs mainly metabolized by CYP3A4 and which have a low therapeutic index (eg, quinidine, terfenadine) should therefore be used with caution).
No products indexed under this heading.

Disopyramide (Limited published data indicate that somatostatin analogs may decrease the metabolic clearance of compounds known to be metabolized by cytochrome P450 enzymes, which may be due to the suppression of growth hormone. Since it cannot be excluded that octreotide may have this effect, other drugs mainly metabolized by CYP3A4 and which have a low therapeutic index (eg, quinidine, terfenadine) should therefore be used with caution).
No products indexed under this heading.

Disopyramide Phosphate (Limited published data indicate that somatostatin analogs may decrease the metabolic clearance of compounds known to be metabolized by cytochrome P450 enzymes, which may be due to the suppression of growth hormone. Since it cannot be excluded that octreotide may have this effect, other drugs mainly metabolized by CYP3A4 and which have a low therapeutic index (eg, quinidine, terfenadine) should therefore be used with caution).
No products indexed under this heading.

Disulfiram (Limited published data indicate that somatostatin analogs may decrease the metabolic clearance of compounds known to be metabolized by cytochrome P450 enzymes, which may be due to the suppression of growth hormone. Since it cannot be excluded that octreotide may have this effect, other drugs mainly metabolized by CYP3A4 and which have a low therapeutic index (eg, quinidine, terfenadine) should therefore be used with caution).
No products indexed under this heading.

Divalproex Sodium (Limited published data indicate that somatostatin analogs may decrease the metabolic clearance of compounds known to be metabolized by cytochrome P450 enzymes, which may be due to the suppression of growth hormone). Products include:
Depakote ER 426

Docetaxel (Limited published data indicate that somatostatin analogs may decrease the metabolic clearance of compounds known to be metabolized by cytochrome P450 enzymes, which may be due to the suppression of growth hormone). Products include:
Taxotere 3035

Dolasetron Mesylate (Limited published data indicate that somatostatin analogs may decrease the metabolic clearance of compounds known to be metabolized by cytochrome P450 enzymes, which may be due to the suppression of growth hormone). Products include:
Anzemet Injection 2931
Anzemet Tablets 2934

Donepezil Hydrochloride (Limited published data indicate that somatostatin analogs may decrease the metabolic clearance of compounds known to be metabolized by cytochrome P450 enzymes, which may be due to the suppression of growth hormone). Products include:
Aricept 1045
Aricept ODT 1045

Doxepin Hydrochloride (Limited published data indicate that somatostatin analogs may decrease the metabolic clearance of compounds known to be metabolized by cytochrome P450 enzymes, which may be due to the suppression of growth hormone).
No products indexed under this heading.

Doxorubicin Hydrochloride (Limited published data indicate that somatostatin analogs may decrease the metabolic clearance of compounds known to be metabolized by cytochrome P450 enzymes, which may be due to the suppression of growth hormone. Since it cannot be excluded that octreotide may have this effect, other drugs mainly metabolized by CYP3A4 and which have a low therapeutic index (eg, quinidine, terfenadine) should therefore be used with caution).
No products indexed under this heading.

Dronabinol (Limited published data indicate that somatostatin analogs may decrease the metabolic clearance of compounds known to be metabolized by cytochrome P450 enzymes, which may be due to the suppression of growth hormone. Since it cannot be excluded that octreotide may have this effect, other drugs mainly metabolized by CYP3A4 and which have a low therapeutic index (eg, quinidine, terfenadine) should therefore be used with caution).
No products indexed under this heading.

Drugs, Oral, unspecified (Octreotide has been associated with alterations in nutrient absorption, so it may have an effect on absorption of orally administered drugs).
No products indexed under this heading.

Drugs that Undergo Biotransformation by Cytochrome P-450 Mixed Function Oxidase (Limited published data indicate that somatostatin analogs may decrease the metabolic clearance of compounds known to be metabolized by cytochrome P450 enzymes, which may be due to the suppression of growth hormone).
No products indexed under this heading.

Dyphylline (Limited published data indicate that somatostatin analogs may decrease the metabolic clearance of compounds known to be metabolized by cytochrome P450 enzymes, which may be due to the suppression of growth hormone).
No products indexed under this heading.

Encainide Hydrochloride (Limited published data indicate that somatostatin analogs may decrease the metabolic clearance of compounds known to be metabolized by cytochrome P450 enzymes, which may be due to the suppression of growth hormone).
No products indexed under this heading.

Enoxacin (Limited published data indicate that somatostatin analogs may decrease the metabolic clearance of compounds known to be metabolized by cytochrome P450 enzymes, which may be due to the suppression of growth hormone).
No products indexed under this heading.

Eprosartan Mesylate (Limited published data indicate that somatostatin analogs may decrease the metabolic clearance of compounds known to be metabolized by cytochrome P450 enzymes, which may be due to the suppression of growth hormone). Products include:
Teveten 538
Teveten HCT 541

Ergotamine Tartrate (Limited published data indicate that somatostatin analogs may decrease the metabolic clearance of compounds known to be metabolized by cytochrome P450 enzymes, which may be due to the suppression of growth hormone. Since it cannot be excluded that octreotide may have this effect, other drugs mainly metabolized by CYP3A4 and which have a low therapeutic index (eg, quinidine, terfenadine) should therefore be used with caution).
No products indexed under this heading.

Erythromycin (Limited published data indicate that somatostatin analogs may decrease the metabolic clearance of compounds known to be metabolized by cytochrome P450 enzymes, which may be due to the suppression of growth hormone. Since it cannot be excluded that octreotide may have this effect, other drugs mainly metabolized by CYP3A4 and which have a low therapeutic index (eg, quinidine, terfenadine) should therefore be used with caution).
No products indexed under this heading.

Erythromycin Estolate (Limited published data indicate that somatostatin analogs may decrease the metabolic clearance of compounds known to be metabolized by cytochrome P450 enzymes, which may be due to the suppression of growth hormone. Since it cannot be excluded that octreotide may have this effect, other drugs mainly metabolized by CYP3A4 and which have a low therapeutic index (eg, quinidine, terfenadine) should therefore be used with caution).
No products indexed under this heading.

Erythromycin Ethylsuccinate (Limited published data indicate that somatostatin analogs may decrease the metabolic clearance of compounds known to be metabolized by cytochrome P450 enzymes, which may be due to the suppression of growth hormone. Since it cannot be excluded that octreotide may have this effect, other drugs mainly metabolized by CYP3A4 and which have a low therapeutic index (eg, quinidine, terfenadine) should therefore be used with caution). Products include:
E.E.S. 437
EryPed 435

Erythromycin Gluceptate (Limited published data indicate that somatostatin analogs may decrease the metabolic clearance of compounds known to be metabolized by cytochrome P450 enzymes, which may be due to the suppression of growth hormone. Since it cannot be excluded that octreotide may have this effect, other drugs mainly metabolized by CYP3A4 and which have a low therapeutic index (eg, quinidine, terfenadine) should therefore be used with caution).
No products indexed under this heading.

Erythromycin Lactobionate (Limited published data indicate that somatostatin analogs may decrease the metabolic clearance of compounds known to be metabolized by cytochrome P450 enzymes, which may be due to the suppression of growth hormone. Since it cannot be excluded that octreotide may have this effect, other drugs mainly metabolized by CYP3A4 and which have a low therapeutic index (eg, quinidine, terfenadine) should therefore be used with caution).
No products indexed under this heading.

Erythromycin Stearate (Limited published data indicate that somatostatin analogs may decrease the metabolic clearance of compounds known to be metabolized by cytochrome P450 enzymes, which may be due to the suppression of growth hormone. Since it cannot be excluded that octreotide may have this effect, other drugs mainly metabolized by CYP3A4 and which have a low therapeutic index (eg, quinidine, terfenadine) should therefore be used with caution).
No products indexed under this heading.

Esmolol Hydrochloride (Concomitant administration of bradycardia inducing drugs (eg, beta blockers) may have an additive effect on the reduction of heart rate associated with octreotide. Dose adjustment of concomitant medication may be necessary).
No products indexed under this heading.

Esomeprazole Magnesium (Limited published data indicate that somatostatin analogs may decrease the metabolic clearance of compounds known to be metabolized by cytochrome P450 enzymes, which may be due to the suppression of growth hormone). Products include:
Nexium Capsules 704
Nexium Oral Suspension 704

Esomeprazole Sodium (Limited published data indicate that somatostatin analogs may decrease the metabolic clearance of compounds known to be metabolized by cytochrome P450 enzymes, which may be due to the suppression of growth hormone). Products include:
Nexium I.V. 712

Estradiol (Limited published data indicate that somatostatin analogs may

decrease the metabolic clearance of compounds known to be metabolized by cytochrome P450 enzymes, which may be due to the suppression of growth hormone. Since it cannot be excluded that octreotide may have this effect, other drugs mainly metabolized by CYP3A4 and which have a low therapeutic index (eg, quinidine, terfenadine) should therefore be used with caution). Products include:

Estradiol Benzoate (Limited published data indicate that somatostatin analogs may decrease the metabolic clearance of compounds known to be metabolized by cytochrome P450 enzymes, which may be due to the suppression of growth hormone. Since it cannot be excluded that octreotide may have this effect, other drugs mainly metabolized by CYP3A4 and which have a low therapeutic index (eg, quinidine, terfenadine) should therefore be used with caution).
No products indexed under this heading.

Estradiol Cypionate (Limited published data indicate that somatostatin analogs may decrease the metabolic clearance of compounds known to be metabolized by cytochrome P450 enzymes, which may be due to the suppression of growth hormone. Since it cannot be excluded that octreotide may have this effect, other drugs mainly metabolized by CYP3A4 and which have a low therapeutic index (eg, quinidine, terfenadine) should therefore be used with caution).
No products indexed under this heading.

Estradiol Valerate (Limited published data indicate that somatostatin analogs may decrease the metabolic clearance of compounds known to be metabolized by cytochrome P450 enzymes, which may be due to the suppression of growth hormone. Since it cannot be excluded that octreotide may have this effect, other drugs mainly metabolized by CYP3A4 and which have a low therapeutic index (eg, quinidine, terfenadine) should therefore be used with caution).
No products indexed under this heading.

Estrogen (Limited published data indicate that somatostatin analogs may decrease the metabolic clearance of compounds known to be metabolized by cytochrome P450 enzymes, which may be due to the suppression of growth hormone).
No products indexed under this heading.

Estrogens, Conjugated (Limited published data indicate that somatostatin analogs may decrease the metabolic clearance of compounds known to be metabolized by cytochrome P450 enzymes, which may be due to the suppression of growth hormone). Products include:

Estrogens, Conjugated, Synthetic A (Limited published data indicate that somatostatin analogs may decrease the metabolic clearance of compounds known to be metabolized by cytochrome P450 enzymes, which may be due to the suppression of growth hormone).
No products indexed under this heading.

Estrogens, Esterified (Limited published data indicate that somatostatin analogs may decrease the metabolic clearance of compounds known to be metabolized by cytochrome P450 enzymes, which may be due to the suppression of growth hormone).
No products indexed under this heading.

Ethinyl Estradiol (Limited published data indicate that somatostatin analogs may decrease the metabolic clearance of compounds known to be metabolized by cytochrome P450 enzymes, which may be due to the suppression of growth hormone. Since it cannot be excluded that octreotide may have this effect, other drugs mainly metabolized by CYP3A4 and which have a low therapeutic index (eg, quinidine, terfenadine) should therefore be used with caution). Products include:

Ethosuximide (Limited published data indicate that somatostatin analogs may decrease the metabolic clearance of compounds known to be metabolized by cytochrome P450 enzymes, which may be due to the suppression of growth hormone. Since it cannot be excluded that octreotide may have this effect, other drugs mainly metabolized by CYP3A4 and which have a low therapeutic index (eg, quinidine, terfenadine) should therefore be used with caution).
No products indexed under this heading.

Ethotoin (Limited published data indicate that somatostatin analogs may decrease the metabolic clearance of compounds known to be metabolized by cytochrome P450 enzymes, which may be due to the suppression of growth hormone).
No products indexed under this heading.

Ethynodiol Diacetate (Limited published data indicate that somatostatin analogs may decrease the metabolic clearance of compounds known to be metabolized by cytochrome P450 enzymes, which may be due to the suppression of growth hormone. Since it cannot be excluded that octreotide may have this effect, other drugs mainly metabolized by CYP3A4 and which have a low therapeutic index (eg, quinidine, terfenadine) should therefore be used with caution).
No products indexed under this heading.

Etodolac (Limited published data indicate that somatostatin analogs may decrease the metabolic clearance of compounds known to be metabolized by cytochrome P450 enzymes, which may be due to the suppression of growth hormone).
No products indexed under this heading.

Etoposide (Limited published data indicate that somatostatin analogs may decrease the metabolic clearance of compounds known to be metabolized by cytochrome P450 enzymes, which may be due to the suppression of growth hormone. Since it cannot be excluded that octreotide may have this effect, other drugs mainly metabolized by CYP3A4 and which have a low therapeutic index (eg, quinidine, terfenadine) should therefore be used with caution).
No products indexed under this heading.

Etoposide Phosphate (Limited published data indicate that somatostatin analogs may decrease the metabolic clearance of compounds known to be metabolized by cytochrome P450 enzymes, which may be due to the suppression of growth hormone. Since it

cannot be excluded that octreotide may have this effect, other drugs mainly metabolized by CYP3A4 and which have a low therapeutic index (eg, quinidine, terfenadine) should therefore be used with caution).
No products indexed under this heading.

Felbamate (Limited published data indicate that somatostatin analogs may decrease the metabolic clearance of compounds known to be metabolized by cytochrome P450 enzymes, which may be due to the suppression of growth hormone).
No products indexed under this heading.

Felodipine (Limited published data indicate that somatostatin analogs may decrease the metabolic clearance of compounds known to be metabolized by cytochrome P450 enzymes, which may be due to the suppression of growth hormone. Since it cannot be excluded that octreotide may have this effect, other drugs mainly metabolized by CYP3A4 and which have a low therapeutic index (eg, quinidine, terfenadine) should therefore be used with caution).
No products indexed under this heading.

Fenoprofen Calcium (Limited published data indicate that somatostatin analogs may decrease the metabolic clearance of compounds known to be metabolized by cytochrome P450 enzymes, which may be due to the suppression of growth hormone).
No products indexed under this heading.

Fentanyl (Limited published data indicate that somatostatin analogs may decrease the metabolic clearance of compounds known to be metabolized by cytochrome P450 enzymes, which may be due to the suppression of growth hormone. Since it cannot be excluded that octreotide may have this effect, other drugs mainly metabolized by CYP3A4 and which have a low therapeutic index (eg, quinidine, terfenadine) should therefore be used with caution). Products include:

Fentanyl Citrate (Limited published data indicate that somatostatin analogs may decrease the metabolic clearance of compounds known to be metabolized by cytochrome P450 enzymes, which may be due to the suppression of growth hormone. Since it cannot be excluded that octreotide may have this effect, other drugs mainly metabolized by CYP3A4 and which have a low therapeutic index (eg, quinidine, terfenadine) should therefore be used with caution). Products include:

Flecainide Acetate (Limited published data indicate that somatostatin analogs may decrease the metabolic clearance of compounds known to be metabolized by cytochrome P450 enzymes, which may be due to the suppression of growth hormone).
No products indexed under this heading.

Fluoxetine (Limited published data indicate that somatostatin analogs may decrease the metabolic clearance of compounds known to be metabolized by cytochrome P450 enzymes, which may be due to the suppression of growth hormone).
No products indexed under this heading.

Fluoxetine Hydrochloride (Limited published data indicate that somatostatin analogs may decrease the metabolic clearance of compounds known to be metabolized by cytochrome P450 enzymes, which may be due to the suppression of growth hormone). Products include:

Fluphenazine Decanoate (Limited published data indicate that somatostatin analogs may decrease the metabolic clearance of compounds known to be metabolized by cytochrome P450 enzymes, which may be due to the suppression of growth hormone).
No products indexed under this heading.

Fluphenazine Enanthate (Limited published data indicate that somatostatin analogs may decrease the metabolic clearance of compounds known to be metabolized by cytochrome P450 enzymes, which may be due to the suppression of growth hormone).
No products indexed under this heading.

Fluphenazine Hydrochloride (Limited published data indicate that somatostatin analogs may decrease the metabolic clearance of compounds known to be metabolized by cytochrome P450 enzymes, which may be due to the suppression of growth hormone).
No products indexed under this heading.

Flurbiprofen (Limited published data indicate that somatostatin analogs may decrease the metabolic clearance of compounds known to be metabolized by cytochrome P450 enzymes, which may be due to the suppression of growth hormone).
No products indexed under this heading.

Flurbiprofen Sodium (Limited published data indicate that somatostatin analogs may decrease the metabolic clearance of compounds known to be metabolized by cytochrome P450 enzymes, which may be due to the suppression of growth hormone).
No products indexed under this heading.

Flutamide (Limited published data indicate that somatostatin analogs may decrease the metabolic clearance of compounds known to be metabolized by cytochrome P450 enzymes, which may be due to the suppression of growth hormone).
No products indexed under this heading.

Fluticasone Propionate (Limited published data indicate that somatostatin analogs may decrease the metabolic clearance of compounds known to be metabolized by cytochrome P450 enzymes, which may be due to the suppression of growth hormone). Products include:

Fluvastatin Sodium (Limited published data indicate that somatostatin analogs may decrease the metabolic clearance of compounds known to be metabolized by cytochrome P450 enzymes, which may be due to the suppression of growth hormone).
No products indexed under this heading.

Fluvoxamine Maleate (Limited published data indicate that somatostatin analogs may decrease the metabolic clearance of compounds known to be metabolized by cytochrome P450 enzymes, which may be due to the suppression of growth hormone).
No products indexed under this heading.

Formoterol Fumarate (Limited published data indicate that somatostatin analogs may decrease the metabolic clearance of compounds known to be metabolized by cytochrome P450 enzymes, which may be due to the suppression of growth hormone). Products include:

IMPORTANT NOTE: Always consult each drug listing in the patient's regimen for possible interactions.

Insulin Lispro Protamine, Human (Octreotide inhibits the secretion of insulin and glucagon. Therefore, blood glucose levels should be monitored when octreotide is initiated or when the dose is altered and antidiabetic treatment should be adjusted accordingly. Products include:

Irbesartan (Limited published data indicate that somatostatin analogs may decrease the metabolic clearance of compounds known to be metabolized by cytochrome P450 enzymes, which may be due to the suppression of growth hormone). Products include:

Isotretinoin (Limited published data indicate that somatostatin analogs may decrease the metabolic clearance of compounds known to be metabolized by cytochrome P450 enzymes, which may be due to the suppression of growth hormone). Products include:

Isradipine (Limited published data indicate that somatostatin analogs may decrease the metabolic clearance of compounds known to be metabolized by cytochrome P450 enzymes, which may be due to the suppression of growth hormone. Since it cannot be excluded that octreotide may have this effect, other drugs mainly metabolized by CYP3A4 and which have a low therapeutic index (eg, quinidine, terfenadine) should therefore be used with caution). Products include:

Itraconazole (Limited published data indicate that somatostatin analogs may decrease the metabolic clearance of compounds known to be metabolized by cytochrome P450 enzymes, which may be due to the suppression of growth hormone. Since it cannot be excluded that octreotide may have this effect, other drugs mainly metabolized by CYP3A4 and which have a low therapeutic index (eg, quinidine, terfenadine) should therefore be used with caution).
No products indexed under this heading.

Ixabepilone (Limited published data indicate that somatostatin analogs may decrease the metabolic clearance of compounds known to be metabolized by cytochrome P450 enzymes, which may be due to the suppression of growth hormone. Since it cannot be excluded that octreotide may have this effect, other drugs mainly metabolized by CYP3A4 and which have a low therapeutic index (eg, quinidine, terfenadine) should therefore be used with caution).
No products indexed under this heading.

Ketoconazole (Limited published data indicate that somatostatin analogs may decrease the metabolic clearance of compounds known to be metabolized by cytochrome P450 enzymes, which may be due to the suppression of growth hormone. Since it cannot be excluded that octreotide may have this effect, other drugs mainly metabolized by CYP3A4 and which have a low therapeutic index (eg, quinidine, terfenadine) should therefore be used with caution). Products include:

Ketoprofen (Limited published data indicate that somatostatin analogs may decrease the metabolic clearance of compounds known to be metabolized by cytochrome P450 enzymes, which may be due to the suppression of growth hormone).
No products indexed under this heading.

Ketorolac Tromethamine (Limited published data indicate that somatostatin analogs may decrease the metabolic clearance of compounds known to be metabolized by cytochrome P450 enzymes, which may be due to the suppression of growth hormone). Products include:

Labetalol Hydrochloride (Concomitant administration of bradycardia inducing drugs (eg, beta blockers) may have an additive effect on the reduction of heart rate associated with octreotide. Dose adjustment of concomitant medication may be necessary).
No products indexed under this heading.

Lamotrigine (Limited published data indicate that somatostatin analogs may decrease the metabolic clearance of compounds known to be metabolized by cytochrome P450 enzymes, which may be due to the suppression of growth hormone). Products include:

Lansoprazole (Limited published data indicate that somatostatin analogs may decrease the metabolic clearance of compounds known to be metabolized by cytochrome P450 enzymes, which may be due to the suppression of growth hormone).
No products indexed under this heading.

Levetiracetam (Limited published data indicate that somatostatin analogs may decrease the metabolic clearance of compounds known to be metabolized by cytochrome P450 enzymes, which may be due to the suppression of growth hormone). Products include:

Levobunolol Hydrochloride (Concomitant administration of bradycardia inducing drugs (eg, beta blockers) may have an additive effect on the reduction of heart rate associated with octreotide. Dose adjustment of concomitant medication may be necessary).
No products indexed under this heading.

Levobupivacaine Hydrochloride (Limited published data indicate that somatostatin analogs may decrease the metabolic clearance of compounds known to be metabolized by cytochrome P450 enzymes, which may be due to the suppression of growth hormone).
No products indexed under this heading.

Levonorgestrel (Limited published data indicate that somatostatin analogs may decrease the metabolic clearance of compounds known to be metabolized by cytochrome P450 enzymes, which may be due to the suppression of growth hormone. Since it cannot be excluded that octreotide may have this effect, other drugs mainly metabolized by CYP3A4 and which have a low therapeutic index (eg, quinidine, terfenadine) should therefore be used with caution). Products include:

Lidocaine (Limited published data indicate that somatostatin analogs may decrease the metabolic clearance of compounds known to be metabolized by cytochrome P450 enzymes, which may be due to the suppression of growth hormone. Since it cannot be excluded that octreotide may have this effect, other drugs mainly metabolized by CYP3A4 and which have a low therapeutic index (eg, quinidine, terfenadine) should therefore be used with caution). Products include:

Lidocaine Base (Limited published data indicate that somatostatin analogs may decrease the metabolic clearance of compounds known to be metabolized by cytochrome P450 enzymes, which may be due to the suppression of growth hormone).
No products indexed under this heading.

Lidocaine Hydrochloride (Limited published data indicate that somatostatin analogs may decrease the metabolic clearance of compounds known to be metabolized by cytochrome P450 enzymes, which may be due to the suppression of growth hormone. Since it cannot be excluded that octreotide may have this effect, other drugs mainly metabolized by CYP3A4 and which have a low therapeutic index (eg, quinidine, terfenadine) should therefore be used with caution).
No products indexed under this heading.

Lomefloxacin Hydrochloride (Limited published data indicate that somatostatin analogs may decrease the metabolic clearance of compounds known to be metabolized by cytochrome P450 enzymes, which may be due to the suppression of growth hormone).
No products indexed under this heading.

Losartan Potassium (Limited published data indicate that somatostatin analogs may decrease the metabolic clearance of compounds known to be metabolized by cytochrome P450 enzymes, which may be due to the suppression of growth hormone). Products include:

Lovastatin (Limited published data indicate that somatostatin analogs may decrease the metabolic clearance of compounds known to be metabolized by cytochrome P450 enzymes, which may be due to the suppression of growth hormone. Since it cannot be excluded that octreotide may have this effect, other drugs mainly metabolized by CYP3A4 and which have a low therapeutic index (eg, quinidine, terfenadine) should therefore be used with caution). Products include:

Maprotiline Hydrochloride (Limited published data indicate that somatostatin analogs may decrease the metabolic clearance of compounds known to be metabolized by cytochrome P450 enzymes, which may be due to the suppression of growth hormone).
No products indexed under this heading.

Meclofenamate Sodium (Limited published data indicate that somatostatin analogs may decrease the metabolic clearance of compounds known to be metabolized by cytochrome P450 enzymes, which may be due to the suppression of growth hormone).
No products indexed under this heading.

Mefenamic Acid (Limited published data indicate that somatostatin analogs may decrease the metabolic clearance of compounds known to be metabolized by cytochrome P450 enzymes, which may be due to the suppression of growth hormone).
No products indexed under this heading.

Meloxicam (Limited published data indicate that somatostatin analogs may decrease the metabolic clearance of compounds known to be metabolized by cytochrome P450 enzymes, which may be due to the suppression of growth hormone).
No products indexed under this heading.

Meperidine Hydrochloride (Limited published data indicate that somatostatin analogs may decrease the metabolic clearance of compounds known to be metabolized by cytochrome P450 enzymes, which may be due to the suppression of growth hormone).
No products indexed under this heading.

Mephenytoin (Limited published data indicate that somatostatin analogs may decrease the metabolic clearance of compounds known to be metabolized by cytochrome P450 enzymes, which may be due to the suppression of growth hormone).
No products indexed under this heading.

Mephobarbital (Limited published data indicate that somatostatin analogs may decrease the metabolic clearance of compounds known to be metabolized by cytochrome P450 enzymes, which may be due to the suppression of growth hormone).
No products indexed under this heading.

Meprobamate (Limited published data indicate that somatostatin analogs may decrease the metabolic clearance of compounds known to be metabolized by cytochrome P450 enzymes, which may be due to the suppression of growth hormone).
No products indexed under this heading.

Mestranol (Limited published data indicate that somatostatin analogs may decrease the metabolic clearance of compounds known to be metabolized by cytochrome P450 enzymes, which may be due to the suppression of growth hormone. Since it cannot be excluded that octreotide may have this effect, other drugs mainly metabolized by CYP3A4 and which have a low therapeutic index (eg, quinidine, terfenadine) should therefore be used with caution).
No products indexed under this heading.

Metformin Hydrochloride (Octreotide inhibits the secretion of insulin and glucagon. Therefore, blood glucose levels should be monitored when octreotide is initiated or when the dose is altered and antidiabetic treatment should be adjusted accordingly. Products include:

Methadone Hydrochloride (Limited published data indicate that somatostatin analogs may decrease the metabolic clearance of compounds known to be metabolized by cytochrome P450 enzymes, which may be due to the suppression of growth hormone. Since it cannot be excluded that octreotide may have this effect, other drugs mainly metabolized by CYP3A4 and which have a low therapeutic index (eg, quinidine, terfenadine) should therefore be used with caution).
No products indexed under this heading.

Methamphetamine Hydrochloride (Limited published data indicate that somatostatin analogs may decrease the metabolic clearance of compounds known to be metabolized by cytochrome P450 enzymes, which may be due to the suppression of growth hormone).
No products indexed under this heading.

Methsuximide (Limited published data indicate that somatostatin analogs may decrease the metabolic clearance of compounds known to be metabolized by cytochrome P450 enzymes, which may be due to the suppression of growth hormone).
No products indexed under this heading.

Sandostatin LAR Interactions Index 1682

Metipranolol Hydrochloride (Concomitant administration of bradycardia inducing drugs (eg, beta blockers) may have an additive effect on the reduction of heart rate associated with octreotide. Dose adjustment of concomitant medication may be necessary).
No products indexed under this heading.

Metoprolol Succinate (Concomitant administration of bradycardia inducing drugs (eg, beta blockers) may have an additive effect on the reduction of heart rate associated with octreotide. Dose adjustment of concomitant medication may be necessary). Products include:
Toprol XL 732

Metoprolol Tartrate (Concomitant administration of bradycardia inducing drugs (eg, beta blockers) may have an additive effect on the reduction of heart rate associated with octreotide. Dose adjustment of concomitant medication may be necessary).
No products indexed under this heading.

Mexiletine Hydrochloride (Limited published data indicate that somatostatin analogs may decrease the metabolic clearance of compounds known to be metabolized by cytochrome P450 enzymes, which may be due to the suppression of growth hormone).
No products indexed under this heading.

Midazolam Hydrochloride (Limited published data indicate that somatostatin analogs may decrease the metabolic clearance of compounds known to be metabolized by cytochrome P450 enzymes, which may be due to the suppression of growth hormone. Since it cannot be excluded that octreotide may have this effect, other drugs mainly metabolized by CYP3A4 and which have a low therapeutic index (eg, quinidine, terfenadine) should therefore be used with caution).
No products indexed under this heading.

Miglitol (Octreotide inhibits the secretion of insulin and glucagon. Therefore, blood glucose levels should be monitored when octreotide is initiated or when the dose is altered and antidiabetic treatment should be adjusted accordingly).
No products indexed under this heading.

Mirtazapine (Limited published data indicate that somatostatin analogs may decrease the metabolic clearance of compounds known to be metabolized by cytochrome P450 enzymes, which may be due to the suppression of growth hormone). Products include:
Remeron Tablets 3214
RemeronSolTab Tablets 3219

Montelukast Sodium (Limited published data indicate that somatostatin analogs may decrease the metabolic clearance of compounds known to be metabolized by cytochrome P450 enzymes, which may be due to the suppression of growth hormone). Products include:
Singulair 2270

Morphine Sulfate (Limited published data indicate that somatostatin analogs may decrease the metabolic clearance of compounds known to be metabolized by cytochrome P450 enzymes, which may be due to the suppression of growth hormone). Products include:
Avinza 1822
Embeda 1831
MS Contin 2803

Moxifloxacin Hydrochloride (Limited published data indicate that somatostatin analogs may decrease the metabolic clearance of compounds known to be metabolized by cytochrome P450 enzymes, which may be due to the suppression of growth hormone). Products include:
Avelox 3064
Vigamox 589

Nabumetone (Limited published data indicate that somatostatin analogs may decrease the metabolic clearance of compounds known to be metabolized by cytochrome P450 enzymes, which may be due to the suppression of growth hormone).
No products indexed under this heading.

Nadolol (Concomitant administration of bradycardia inducing drugs (eg, beta blockers) may have an additive effect on the reduction of heart rate associated with octreotide. Dose adjustment of concomitant medication may be necessary). Products include:
Nadolol 2359

Nafcillin Sodium (Limited published data indicate that somatostatin analogs may decrease the metabolic clearance of compounds known to be metabolized by cytochrome P450 enzymes, which may be due to the suppression of growth hormone).
No products indexed under this heading.

Naproxen (Limited published data indicate that somatostatin analogs may decrease the metabolic clearance of compounds known to be metabolized by cytochrome P450 enzymes, which may be due to the suppression of growth hormone). Products include:
EC-Naprosyn 2850
Naprosyn 2850
Anaprox/Naprosyn 2850

Naproxen Sodium (Limited published data indicate that somatostatin analogs may decrease the metabolic clearance of compounds known to be metabolized by cytochrome P450 enzymes, which may be due to the suppression of growth hormone). Products include:
Anaprox 2850
Anaprox DS 2850
Treximet 1681

Nateglinide (Octreotide inhibits the secretion of insulin and glucagon. Therefore, blood glucose levels should be monitored when octreotide is initiated or when the dose is altered and antidiabetic treatment should be adjusted accordingly).
No products indexed under this heading.

Nebivolol (Concomitant administration of bradycardia inducing drugs (eg, beta blockers) may have an additive effect on the reduction of heart rate associated with octreotide. Dose adjustment of concomitant medication may be necessary). Products include:
Bystolic 1147

Nefazodone Hydrochloride (Limited published data indicate that somatostatin analogs may decrease the metabolic clearance of compounds known to be metabolized by cytochrome P450 enzymes, which may be due to the suppression of growth hormone. Since it cannot be excluded that octreotide may have this effect, other drugs mainly metabolized by CYP3A4 and which have a low therapeutic index (eg, quinidine, terfenadine) should therefore be used with caution).
No products indexed under this heading.

Nelfinavir Mesylate (Limited published data indicate that somatostatin analogs may decrease the metabolic clearance of compounds known to be metabolized by cytochrome P450 enzymes, which may be due to the suppression of growth hormone. Since it cannot be excluded that octreotide may have this effect, other drugs mainly metabolized by CYP3A4 and which have a low therapeutic index (eg, quinidine, terfenadine) should therefore be used with caution).
No products indexed under this heading.

Nicardipine (Limited published data indicate that somatostatin analogs may decrease the metabolic clearance of compounds known to be metabolized by cytochrome P450 enzymes, which may be due to the suppression of growth hormone. Since it cannot be excluded that octreotide may have this effect, other drugs mainly metabolized by CYP3A4 and which have a low therapeutic index (eg, quinidine, terfenadine) should therefore be used with caution).
No products indexed under this heading.

Nicardipine Hydrochloride (Limited published data indicate that somatostatin analogs may decrease the metabolic clearance of compounds known to be metabolized by cytochrome P450 enzymes, which may be due to the suppression of growth hormone. Since it cannot be excluded that octreotide may have this effect, other drugs mainly metabolized by CYP3A4 and which have a low therapeutic index (eg, quinidine, terfenadine) should therefore be used with caution).
No products indexed under this heading.

Nicotine Polacrilex (Limited published data indicate that somatostatin analogs may decrease the metabolic clearance of compounds known to be metabolized by cytochrome P450 enzymes, which may be due to the suppression of growth hormone).
No products indexed under this heading.

Nicotine Salicylate (Limited published data indicate that somatostatin analogs may decrease the metabolic clearance of compounds known to be metabolized by cytochrome P450 enzymes, which may be due to the suppression of growth hormone).
No products indexed under this heading.

Nicotine Sulfate (Limited published data indicate that somatostatin analogs may decrease the metabolic clearance of compounds known to be metabolized by cytochrome P450 enzymes, which may be due to the suppression of growth hormone).
No products indexed under this heading.

Nifedipine (Limited published data indicate that somatostatin analogs may decrease the metabolic clearance of compounds known to be metabolized by cytochrome P450 enzymes, which may be due to the suppression of growth hormone. Since it cannot be excluded that octreotide may have this effect, other drugs mainly metabolized by CYP3A4 and which have a low therapeutic index (eg, quinidine, terfenadine) should therefore be used with caution).
No products indexed under this heading.

Nilutamide (Limited published data indicate that somatostatin analogs may decrease the metabolic clearance of compounds known to be metabolized by cytochrome P450 enzymes, which may be due to the suppression of growth hormone).
No products indexed under this heading.

Nimodipine (Limited published data indicate that somatostatin analogs may decrease the metabolic clearance of compounds known to be metabolized by cytochrome P450 enzymes, which may be due to the suppression of growth hormone. Since it cannot be excluded that octreotide may have this effect, other drugs mainly metabolized by CYP3A4 and which have a low therapeutic index (eg, quinidine, terfenadine) should therefore be used with caution).
No products indexed under this heading.

Nisoldipine (Limited published data indicate that somatostatin analogs may decrease the metabolic clearance of compounds known to be metabolized by cytochrome P450 enzymes, which may be due to the suppression of growth hormone. Since it cannot be excluded that octreotide may have this effect, other drugs mainly metabolized by CYP3A4 and which have a low therapeutic index (eg, quinidine, terfenadine) should therefore be used with caution).
No products indexed under this heading.

Nitrendipine (Limited published data indicate that somatostatin analogs may decrease the metabolic clearance of compounds known to be metabolized by cytochrome P450 enzymes, which may be due to the suppression of growth hormone. Since it cannot be excluded that octreotide may have this effect, other drugs mainly metabolized by CYP3A4 and which have a low therapeutic index (eg, quinidine, terfenadine) should therefore be used with caution).
No products indexed under this heading.

Norethindrone (Limited published data indicate that somatostatin analogs may decrease the metabolic clearance of compounds known to be metabolized by cytochrome P450 enzymes, which may be due to the suppression of growth hormone. Since it cannot be excluded that octreotide may have this effect, other drugs mainly metabolized by CYP3A4 and which have a low therapeutic index (eg, quinidine, terfenadine) should therefore be used with caution). Products include:
Ortho Micronor 2660

Norethindrone Acetate (Limited published data indicate that somatostatin analogs may decrease the metabolic clearance of compounds known to be metabolized by cytochrome P450 enzymes, which may be due to the suppression of growth hormone. Since it cannot be excluded that octreotide may have this effect, other drugs mainly metabolized by CYP3A4 and which have a low therapeutic index (eg, quinidine, terfenadine) should therefore be used with caution). Products include:
Activella 2561

Norfloxacin (Limited published data indicate that somatostatin analogs may decrease the metabolic clearance of compounds known to be metabolized by cytochrome P450 enzymes, which may be due to the suppression of growth hormone). Products include:
Noroxin 2220

Norgestrel (Limited published data indicate that somatostatin analogs may decrease the metabolic clearance of compounds known to be metabolized by cytochrome P450 enzymes, which may be due to the suppression of growth hormone. Since it cannot be excluded that octreotide may have this effect, other drugs mainly metabolized by CYP3A4 and which have a low therapeutic index (eg, quinidine, terfenadine) should therefore be used with caution).
No products indexed under this heading.

Nortriptyline Hydrochloride (Limited published data indicate that somatostatin analogs may decrease the metabolic clearance of compounds known to be metabolized by cytochrome P450 enzymes, which may be due to the suppression of growth hormone).
No products indexed under this heading.

Ofloxacin (Limited published data indicate that somatostatin analogs may decrease the metabolic clearance of compounds known to be metabolized by cytochrome P450 enzymes, which may be due to the suppression of growth hormone).
No products indexed under this heading.

Olanzapine (Limited published data indicate that somatostatin analogs may decrease the metabolic clearance of compounds known to be metabolized by cytochrome P450 enzymes, which may be due to the suppression of growth hormone). Products include:
Symbyax 1965
Zyprexa 1984
Zyprexa IntraMuscular 1984
Zyprexa ZYDIS 1984

Omeprazole (Limited published data indicate that somatostatin analogs may decrease the metabolic clearance of compounds known to be metabolized by cytochrome P450 enzymes, which may be due to the suppression of growth hormone).
No products indexed under this heading.

Omeprazole Magnesium (Limited published data indicate that somatostatin analogs may decrease the metabolic clearance of compounds known to be metabolized by cytochrome P450 enzymes, which may be due to the suppression of growth hormone).
No products indexed under this heading.

Ondansetron (Limited published data indicate that somatostatin analogs may decrease the metabolic clearance of compounds known to be metabolized by cytochrome P450 enzymes, which may be due to the suppression of growth hormone. Since it cannot be excluded that octreotide may have this effect, other drugs mainly metabolized by CYP3A4 and which have a low therapeutic index (eg, quinidine, terfenadine) should therefore be used with caution).
No products indexed under this heading.

Ondansetron Hydrochloride (Limited published data indicate that somatostatin analogs may decrease the metabolic clearance of compounds known to be metabolized by cytochrome P450 enzymes, which may be due to the suppression of growth hormone. Since it cannot be excluded that octreotide may have this effect, other drugs mainly metabolized by CYP3A4 and which have a low therapeutic index (eg, quinidine, terfenadine) should therefore be used with caution). Products include:
Zofran Injection 1750
Zofran 1756
Zofran ODT 1756

Oxaprozin (Limited published data indicate that somatostatin analogs may decrease the metabolic clearance of compounds known to be metabolized by cytochrome P450 enzymes, which may be due to the suppression of growth hormone).
No products indexed under this heading.

Oxcarbazepine (Limited published data indicate that somatostatin analogs may decrease the metabolic clearance of compounds known to be metabolized by cytochrome P450 enzymes, which may be due to the suppression of growth hormone).
No products indexed under this heading.

Oxycodone Hydrochloride (Limited published data indicate that somatostatin analogs may decrease the metabolic clearance of compounds known to be metabolized by cytochrome P450 enzymes, which may be due to the suppression of growth hormone). Products include:
OxyContin 2807
Percocet 1121
Percodan 1124

Paclitaxel (Limited published data indicate that somatostatin analogs may decrease the metabolic clearance of compounds known to be metabolized by cytochrome P450 enzymes, which may be due to the suppression of growth hormone. Since it cannot be excluded that octreotide may have this effect, other drugs mainly metabolized by CYP3A4 and which have a low therapeutic index (eg, quinidine, terfenadine) should therefore be used with caution).
No products indexed under this heading.

Pantoprazole Sodium (Limited published data indicate that somatostatin analogs may decrease the metabolic clearance of compounds known to be metabolized by cytochrome P450

enzymes, which may be due to the suppression of growth hormone). Products include:
Protonix Tablets 3571
Protonix 3575

Paramethadione (Limited published data indicate that somatostatin analogs may decrease the metabolic clearance of compounds known to be metabolized by cytochrome P450 enzymes, which may be due to the suppression of growth hormone).
No products indexed under this heading.

Paroxetine Hydrochloride (Limited published data indicate that somatostatin analogs may decrease the metabolic clearance of compounds known to be metabolized by cytochrome P450 enzymes, which may be due to the suppression of growth hormone). Products include:
Paroxetine CR 2361
Paroxetine ER 2371
Paxil 1586
Paxil CR 1596

Penbutolol Sulfate (Concomitant administration of bradycardia inducing drugs (eg, beta blockers) may have an additive effect on the reduction of heart rate associated with octreotide. Dose adjustment of concomitant medication may be necessary).
No products indexed under this heading.

Pentamidine Isethionate (Limited published data indicate that somatostatin analogs may decrease the metabolic clearance of compounds known to be metabolized by cytochrome P450 enzymes, which may be due to the suppression of growth hormone).
No products indexed under this heading.

Phenacemide (Limited published data indicate that somatostatin analogs may decrease the metabolic clearance of compounds known to be metabolized by cytochrome P450 enzymes, which may be due to the suppression of growth hormone).
No products indexed under this heading.

Phenobarbital (Limited published data indicate that somatostatin analogs may decrease the metabolic clearance of compounds known to be metabolized by cytochrome P450 enzymes, which may be due to the suppression of growth hormone). Products include:
Donnatal 2711

Phenobarbital Sodium (Limited published data indicate that somatostatin analogs may decrease the metabolic clearance of compounds known to be metabolized by cytochrome P450 enzymes, which may be due to the suppression of growth hormone).
No products indexed under this heading.

Phensuximide (Limited published data indicate that somatostatin analogs may decrease the metabolic clearance of compounds known to be metabolized by cytochrome P450 enzymes, which may be due to the suppression of growth hormone).
No products indexed under this heading.

Phenylbutazone (Limited published data indicate that somatostatin analogs may decrease the metabolic clearance of compounds known to be metabolized by cytochrome P450 enzymes, which may be due to the suppression of growth hormone).
No products indexed under this heading.

Phenytoin (Limited published data indicate that somatostatin analogs may decrease the metabolic clearance of compounds known to be metabolized by cytochrome P450 enzymes, which may be due to the suppression of growth hormone).
No products indexed under this heading.

Phenytoin Sodium (Limited published data indicate that somatostatin analogs

may decrease the metabolic clearance of compounds known to be metabolized by cytochrome P450 enzymes, which may be due to the suppression of growth hormone). Products include:
Phenytek Capsules 2380

Pimozide (Limited published data indicate that somatostatin analogs may decrease the metabolic clearance of compounds known to be metabolized by cytochrome P450 enzymes, which may be due to the suppression of growth hormone. Since it cannot be excluded that octreotide may have this effect, other drugs mainly metabolized by CYP3A4 and which have a low therapeutic index (eg, quinidine, terfenadine) should therefore be used with caution).
No products indexed under this heading.

Pindolol (Concomitant administration of bradycardia inducing drugs (eg, beta blockers) may have an additive effect on the reduction of heart rate associated with octreotide. Dose adjustment of concomitant medication may be necessary).
No products indexed under this heading.

Pioglitazone Hydrochloride (Octreotide inhibits the secretion of insulin and glucagon. Therefore, blood glucose levels should be monitored when octreotide is initiated or when the dose is altered and antidiabetic treatment should be adjusted accordingly). Products include:
ActoPlus 3338
Actos 3345
Duetact 3354

Piroxicam (Limited published data indicate that somatostatin analogs may decrease the metabolic clearance of compounds known to be metabolized by cytochrome P450 enzymes, which may be due to the suppression of growth hormone).
No products indexed under this heading.

Polyestradiol Phosphate (Limited published data indicate that somatostatin analogs may decrease the metabolic clearance of compounds known to be metabolized by cytochrome P450 enzymes, which may be due to the suppression of growth hormone. Since it cannot be excluded that octreotide may have this effect, other drugs mainly metabolized by CYP3A4 and which have a low therapeutic index (eg, quinidine, terfenadine) should therefore be used with caution).
No products indexed under this heading.

Primidone (Limited published data indicate that somatostatin analogs may decrease the metabolic clearance of compounds known to be metabolized by cytochrome P450 enzymes, which may be due to the suppression of growth hormone).
No products indexed under this heading.

Progesterone (Limited published data indicate that somatostatin analogs may decrease the metabolic clearance of compounds known to be metabolized by cytochrome P450 enzymes, which may be due to the suppression of growth hormone). Products include:
Crinone 4% 996
Crinone 8% 996
Prometrium 3307

Proguanil Hydrochloride (Limited published data indicate that somatostatin analogs may decrease the metabolic clearance of compounds known to be metabolized by cytochrome P450 enzymes, which may be due to the suppression of growth hormone). Products include:
Malarone Pediatric Tablets 1572
Malarone 1572

Propafenone Hydrochloride (Limited published data indicate that somatostatin analogs may decrease the metabolic clearance of compounds known

to be metabolized by cytochrome P450 enzymes, which may be due to the suppression of growth hormone). Products include:
Rythmol 1648
Rythmol SR 1652

Propoxyphene Hydrochloride (Limited published data indicate that somatostatin analogs may decrease the metabolic clearance of compounds known to be metabolized by cytochrome P450 enzymes, which may be due to the suppression of growth hormone).
No products indexed under this heading.

Propoxyphene Napsylate (Limited published data indicate that somatostatin analogs may decrease the metabolic clearance of compounds known to be metabolized by cytochrome P450 enzymes, which may be due to the suppression of growth hormone).
No products indexed under this heading.

Propranolol Hydrochloride (Concomitant administration of bradycardia inducing drugs (eg, beta blockers) may have an additive effect on the reduction of heart rate associated with octreotide. Dose adjustment of concomitant medication may be necessary). Products include:
InnoPran XL 1517

Protriptyline Hydrochloride (Limited published data indicate that somatostatin analogs may decrease the metabolic clearance of compounds known to be metabolized by cytochrome P450 enzymes, which may be due to the suppression of growth hormone).
No products indexed under this heading.

Quetiapine Fumarate (Limited published data indicate that somatostatin analogs may decrease the metabolic clearance of compounds known to be metabolized by cytochrome P450 enzymes, which may be due to the suppression of growth hormone). Products include:
Seroquel 750
Seroquel XR 759

Quinidine (Limited published data indicate that somatostatin analogs may decrease the metabolic clearance of compounds known to be metabolized by cytochrome P450 enzymes, which may be due to the suppression of growth hormone. Since it cannot be excluded that octreotide may have this effect, other drugs mainly metabolized by CYP3A4 and which have a low therapeutic index such as quinidine, should therefore be used with caution).
No products indexed under this heading.

Quinidine Gluconate (Limited published data indicate that somatostatin analogs may decrease the metabolic clearance of compounds known to be metabolized by cytochrome P450 enzymes, which may be due to the suppression of growth hormone. Since it cannot be excluded that octreotide may have this effect, other drugs mainly metabolized by CYP3A4 and which have a low therapeutic index such as quinidine, should therefore be used with caution).
No products indexed under this heading.

Quinidine Hydrochloride (Limited published data indicate that somatostatin analogs may decrease the metabolic clearance of compounds known to be metabolized by cytochrome P450 enzymes, which may be due to the suppression of growth hormone. Since it cannot be excluded that octreotide may have this effect, other drugs mainly metabolized by CYP3A4 and which have a low therapeutic index such as quinidine, should therefore be used with caution).
No products indexed under this heading.

Quinidine Polygalacturonate (Limited published data indicate that soma-

tostatin analogs may decrease the metabolic clearance of compounds known to be metabolized by cytochrome P450 enzymes, which may be due to the suppression of growth hormone. Since it cannot be excluded that octreotide may have this effect, other drugs mainly metabolized by CYP3A4 and which have a low therapeutic index such as quinidine, should therefore be used with caution).

No products indexed under this heading.

Quinidine Sulfate (Limited published data indicate that somatostatin analogs may decrease the metabolic clearance of compounds known to be metabolized by cytochrome P450 enzymes, which may be due to the suppression of growth hormone. Since it cannot be excluded that octreotide may have this effect, other drugs mainly metabolized by CYP3A4 and which have a low therapeutic index such as quinidine, should therefore be used with caution).

No products indexed under this heading.

Quinine (Limited published data indicate that somatostatin analogs may decrease the metabolic clearance of compounds known to be metabolized by cytochrome P450 enzymes, which may be due to the suppression of growth hormone). Products include:
Hyland's Leg Cramps PM with
Quinine 3315

Quinine Sulfate (Limited published data indicate that somatostatin analogs may decrease the metabolic clearance of compounds known to be metabolized by cytochrome P450 enzymes, which may be due to the suppression of growth hormone).

No products indexed under this heading.

Rabeprazole Sodium (Limited published data indicate that somatostatin analogs may decrease the metabolic clearance of compounds known to be metabolized by cytochrome P450 enzymes, which may be due to the suppression of growth hormone). Products include:
Aciphex 1035

Repaglinide (Octreotide inhibits the secretion of insulin and glucagon. Therefore, blood glucose levels should be monitored when octreotide is initiated or when the dose is altered and antidiabetic treatment should be adjusted accordingly).

No products indexed under this heading.

Rifabutin (Limited published data indicate that somatostatin analogs may decrease the metabolic clearance of compounds known to be metabolized by cytochrome P450 enzymes, which may be due to the suppression of growth hormone. Since it cannot be excluded that octreotide may have this effect, other drugs mainly metabolized by CYP3A4 and which have a low therapeutic index (eg, quinidine, terfenadine) should therefore be used with caution).

No products indexed under this heading.

Riluzole (Limited published data indicate that somatostatin analogs may decrease the metabolic clearance of compounds known to be metabolized by cytochrome P450 enzymes, which may be due to the suppression of growth hormone). Products include:
Rilutek 3032

Risperidone (Limited published data indicate that somatostatin analogs may decrease the metabolic clearance of compounds known to be metabolized by cytochrome P450 enzymes, which may be due to the suppression of growth hormone). Products include:
Risperdal Consta 2682

Ritonavir (Limited published data indicate that somatostatin analogs may decrease the metabolic clearance of compounds known to be metabolized

by cytochrome P450 enzymes, which may be due to the suppression of growth hormone. Since it cannot be excluded that octreotide may have this effect, other drugs mainly metabolized by CYP3A4 and which have a low therapeutic index (eg, quinidine, terfenadine) should therefore be used with caution). Products include:
Kaletra 458
Norvir 509

Rofecoxib (Limited published data indicate that somatostatin analogs may decrease the metabolic clearance of compounds known to be metabolized by cytochrome P450 enzymes, which may be due to the suppression of growth hormone).

No products indexed under this heading.

Ropinirole Hydrochloride (Limited published data indicate that somatostatin analogs may decrease the metabolic clearance of compounds known to be metabolized by cytochrome P450 enzymes, which may be due to the suppression of growth hormone). Products include:
Requip 1620
Requip XL 1628

Ropivacaine Hydrochloride (Limited published data indicate that somatostatin analogs may decrease the metabolic clearance of compounds known to be metabolized by cytochrome P450 enzymes, which may be due to the suppression of growth hormone).

No products indexed under this heading.

Rosiglitazone (Limited published data indicate that somatostatin analogs may decrease the metabolic clearance of compounds known to be metabolized by cytochrome P450 enzymes, which may be due to the suppression of growth hormone).

No products indexed under this heading.

Rosiglitazone Maleate (Octreotide inhibits the secretion of insulin and glucagon. Therefore, blood glucose levels should be monitored when octreotide is initiated or when the dose is altered and antidiabetic treatment should be adjusted accordingly). Products include:
Avandamet 1345
Avandaryl 1356
Avandia 1366

Rosiglitazone/Metformin (Limited published data indicate that somatostatin analogs may decrease the metabolic clearance of compounds known to be metabolized by cytochrome P450 enzymes, which may be due to the suppression of growth hormone).

No products indexed under this heading.

Saquinavir (Limited published data indicate that somatostatin analogs may decrease the metabolic clearance of compounds known to be metabolized by cytochrome P450 enzymes, which may be due to the suppression of growth hormone. Since it cannot be excluded that octreotide may have this effect, other drugs mainly metabolized by CYP3A4 and which have a low therapeutic index (eg, quinidine, terfenadine) should therefore be used with caution).

No products indexed under this heading.

Saquinavir Mesylate (Limited published data indicate that somatostatin analogs may decrease the metabolic clearance of compounds known to be metabolized by cytochrome P450 enzymes, which may be due to the suppression of growth hormone. Since it cannot be excluded that octreotide may have this effect, other drugs mainly metabolized by CYP3A4 and which have a low therapeutic index (eg, quinidine, terfenadine) should therefore be used with caution).

No products indexed under this heading.

Sertraline Hydrochloride (Limited published data indicate that somatostatin analogs may decrease the metabolic clearance of compounds known to be metabolized by cytochrome P450 enzymes, which may be due to the suppression of growth hormone. Since it cannot be excluded that octreotide may have this effect, other drugs mainly metabolized by CYP3A4 and which have a low therapeutic index (eg, quinidine, terfenadine) should therefore be used with caution).

No products indexed under this heading.

Sildenafil Citrate (Limited published data indicate that somatostatin analogs may decrease the metabolic clearance of compounds known to be metabolized by cytochrome P450 enzymes, which may be due to the suppression of growth hormone. Since it cannot be excluded that octreotide may have this effect, other drugs mainly metabolized by CYP3A4 and which have a low therapeutic index (eg, quinidine, terfenadine) should therefore be used with caution).

No products indexed under this heading.

Simvastatin (Limited published data indicate that somatostatin analogs may decrease the metabolic clearance of compounds known to be metabolized by cytochrome P450 enzymes, which may be due to the suppression of growth hormone. Since it cannot be excluded that octreotide may have this effect, other drugs mainly metabolized by CYP3A4 and which have a low therapeutic index (eg, quinidine, terfenadine) should therefore be used with caution). Products include:
Simcor 524
Vytorin 10/10 .... 2303, 3240
Vytorin 10/20 .... 2303, 3240
Vytorin 10/40 .... 2303, 3240
Vytorin 10/80 .... 2303, 3240
Zocor 2289

Sirolimus (Limited published data indicate that somatostatin analogs may decrease the metabolic clearance of compounds known to be metabolized by cytochrome P450 enzymes, which may be due to the suppression of growth hormone. Since it cannot be excluded that octreotide may have this effect, other drugs mainly metabolized by CYP3A4 and which have a low therapeutic index (eg, quinidine, terfenadine) should therefore be used with caution). Products include:
Rapamune 3579

Sitagliptin Phosphate (Octreotide inhibits the secretion of insulin and glucagon. Therefore, blood glucose levels should be monitored when octreotide is initiated or when the dose is altered and antidiabetic treatment should be adjusted accordingly). Products include:
Janumet 2188
Januvia 2196

Sotalol Hydrochloride (Concomitant administration of bradycardia inducing drugs (eg, beta blockers) may have an additive effect on the reduction of heart rate associated with octreotide. Dose adjustment of concomitant medication may be necessary).

No products indexed under this heading.

Sulfamethoxazole (Limited published data indicate that somatostatin analogs may decrease the metabolic clearance of compounds known to be metabolized by cytochrome P450 enzymes, which may be due to the suppression of growth hormone).

No products indexed under this heading.

Sulindac (Limited published data indicate that somatostatin analogs may decrease the metabolic clearance of compounds known to be metabolized by cytochrome P450 enzymes, which may be due to the suppression of growth hormone). Products include:
Clinoril 2098

Suprofen (Limited published data indicate that somatostatin analogs may decrease the metabolic clearance of compounds known to be metabolized by cytochrome P450 enzymes, which may be due to the suppression of growth hormone).

No products indexed under this heading.

Tacrine Hydrochloride (Limited published data indicate that somatostatin analogs may decrease the metabolic clearance of compounds known to be metabolized by cytochrome P450 enzymes, which may be due to the suppression of growth hormone).

No products indexed under this heading.

Tacrolimus (Limited published data indicate that somatostatin analogs may decrease the metabolic clearance of compounds known to be metabolized by cytochrome P450 enzymes, which may be due to the suppression of growth hormone. Since it cannot be excluded that octreotide may have this effect, other drugs mainly metabolized by CYP3A4 and which have a low therapeutic index (eg, quinidine, terfenadine) should therefore be used with caution). Products include:
Prograf Capsules 677
Prograf Injection 677
Protopic 685

Tadalafil (Limited published data indicate that somatostatin analogs may decrease the metabolic clearance of compounds known to be metabolized by cytochrome P450 enzymes, which may be due to the suppression of growth hormone. Since it cannot be excluded that octreotide may have this effect, other drugs mainly metabolized by CYP3A4 and which have a low therapeutic index (eg, quinidine, terfenadine) should therefore be used with caution). Products include:
Adcirca 3461
Cialis 1861

Tamoxifen Citrate (Limited published data indicate that somatostatin analogs may decrease the metabolic clearance of compounds known to be metabolized by cytochrome P450 enzymes, which may be due to the suppression of growth hormone. Since it cannot be excluded that octreotide may have this effect, other drugs mainly metabolized by CYP3A4 and which have a low therapeutic index (eg, quinidine, terfenadine) should therefore be used with caution).

No products indexed under this heading.

Telmisartan (Limited published data indicate that somatostatin analogs may decrease the metabolic clearance of compounds known to be metabolized by cytochrome P450 enzymes, which may be due to the suppression of growth hormone). Products include:
Micardis 887
Micardis HCT 889

Teniposide (Limited published data indicate that somatostatin analogs may decrease the metabolic clearance of compounds known to be metabolized by cytochrome P450 enzymes, which may be due to the suppression of growth hormone).

No products indexed under this heading.

Terfenadine (Limited published data indicate that somatostatin analogs may decrease the metabolic clearance of compounds known to be metabolized by cytochrome P450 enzymes, which may be due to the suppression of growth hormone. Since it cannot be excluded that octreotide may have this effect, other drugs mainly metabolized by CYP3A4 and which have a low therapeutic index such as terfenadine, should therefore be used with caution).

No products indexed under this heading.

Testosterone (Limited published data indicate that somatostatin analogs may

decrease the metabolic clearance of compounds known to be metabolized by cytochrome P450 enzymes, which may be due to the suppression of growth hormone). Products include:

AndroGel **3456**

Testosterone Cypionate (Limited published data indicate that somatostatin analogs may decrease the metabolic clearance of compounds known to be metabolized by cytochrome P450 enzymes, which may be due to the suppression of growth hormone).

No products indexed under this heading.

Testosterone Enanthate (Limited published data indicate that somatostatin analogs may decrease the metabolic clearance of compounds known to be metabolized by cytochrome P450 enzymes, which may be due to the suppression of growth hormone). Products include:

Delatestryl **1102**

Testosterone Propionate (Limited published data indicate that somatostatin analogs may decrease the metabolic clearance of compounds known to be metabolized by cytochrome P450 enzymes, which may be due to the suppression of growth hormone).

No products indexed under this heading.

Theophylline (Limited published data indicate that somatostatin analogs may decrease the metabolic clearance of compounds known to be metabolized by cytochrome P450 enzymes, which may be due to the suppression of growth hormone. Since it cannot be excluded that octreotide may have this effect, other drugs mainly metabolized by CYP3A4 and which have a low therapeutic index (eg, quinidine, terfenadine) should therefore be used with caution).

No products indexed under this heading.

Theophylline Anhydrous (Limited published data indicate that somatostatin analogs may decrease the metabolic clearance of compounds known to be metabolized by cytochrome P450 enzymes, which may be due to the suppression of growth hormone. Since it cannot be excluded that octreotide may have this effect, other drugs mainly metabolized by CYP3A4 and which have a low therapeutic index (eg, quinidine, terfenadine) should therefore be used with caution). Products include:

Uniphyl **2817**

Theophylline Calcium Salicylate (Limited published data indicate that somatostatin analogs may decrease the metabolic clearance of compounds known to be metabolized by cytochrome P450 enzymes, which may be due to the suppression of growth hormone. Since it cannot be excluded that octreotide may have this effect, other drugs mainly metabolized by CYP3A4 and which have a low therapeutic index (eg, quinidine, terfenadine) should therefore be used with caution).

No products indexed under this heading.

Theophylline Dihydroxypropyl (Glyceryl) (Limited published data indicate that somatostatin analogs may decrease the metabolic clearance of compounds known to be metabolized by cytochrome P450 enzymes, which may be due to the suppression of growth hormone. Since it cannot be excluded that octreotide may have this effect, other drugs mainly metabolized by CYP3A4 and which have a low therapeutic index (eg, quinidine, terfenadine) should therefore be used with caution).

No products indexed under this heading.

Theophylline Ethylenediamine (Limited published data indicate that somatostatin analogs may decrease the metabolic clearance of compounds known to be metabolized by cytochrome P450 enzymes, which may be

due to the suppression of growth hormone. Since it cannot be excluded that octreotide may have this effect, other drugs mainly metabolized by CYP3A4 and which have a low therapeutic index (eg, quinidine, terfenadine) should therefore be used with caution).

No products indexed under this heading.

Theophylline Sodium Glycinate (Limited published data indicate that somatostatin analogs may decrease the metabolic clearance of compounds known to be metabolized by cytochrome P450 enzymes, which may be due to the suppression of growth hormone. Since it cannot be excluded that octreotide may have this effect, other drugs mainly metabolized by CYP3A4 and which have a low therapeutic index (eg, quinidine, terfenadine) should therefore be used with caution).

No products indexed under this heading.

Thioridazine (Limited published data indicate that somatostatin analogs may decrease the metabolic clearance of compounds known to be metabolized by cytochrome P450 enzymes, which may be due to the suppression of growth hormone).

No products indexed under this heading.

Thioridazine Hydrochloride (Limited published data indicate that somatostatin analogs may decrease the metabolic clearance of compounds known to be metabolized by cytochrome P450 enzymes, which may be due to the suppression of growth hormone). Products include:

Thioridazine Hydrochloride **2384**

Tiagabine Hydrochloride (Limited published data indicate that somatostatin analogs may decrease the metabolic clearance of compounds known to be metabolized by cytochrome P450 enzymes, which may be due to the suppression of growth hormone. Since it cannot be excluded that octreotide may have this effect, other drugs mainly metabolized by CYP3A4 and which have a low therapeutic index (eg, quinidine, terfenadine) should therefore be used with caution). Products include:

Gabitril **972**

Timolol Hemihydrate (Concomitant administration of bradycardia inducing drugs (eg, beta blockers) may have an additive effect on the reduction of heart rate associated with octreotide. Dose adjustment of concomitant medication may be necessary). Products include:

Betimol **3490**

Timolol Maleate (Concomitant administration of bradycardia inducing drugs (eg, beta blockers) may have an additive effect on the reduction of heart rate associated with octreotide. Dose adjustment of concomitant medication may be necessary). Products include:

Combigan **601**
Dorzolamide
    Hydrochloride/Timolol Maleate
    Ophthalmic Solution ....⊙**243**
Timoptic in Ocudose ....⊙**231**

Tolazamide (Octreotide inhibits the secretion of insulin and glucagon. Therefore, blood glucose levels should be monitored when octreotide is initiated or when the dose is altered and antidiabetic treatment should be adjusted accordingly).

No products indexed under this heading.

Tolbutamide (Octreotide inhibits the secretion of insulin and glucagon. Therefore, blood glucose levels should be monitored when octreotide is initiated or when the dose is altered and antidiabetic treatment should be adjusted accordingly).

No products indexed under this heading.

Tolbutamide Sodium (Limited published data indicate that somatostatin analogs may decrease the metabolic clearance of compounds known to be metabolized by cytochrome P450 enzymes, which may be due to the suppression of growth hormone).

No products indexed under this heading.

Tolmetin Sodium (Limited published data indicate that somatostatin analogs may decrease the metabolic clearance of compounds known to be metabolized by cytochrome P450 enzymes, which may be due to the suppression of growth hormone).

No products indexed under this heading.

Tolterodine Tartrate (Limited published data indicate that somatostatin analogs may decrease the metabolic clearance of compounds known to be metabolized by cytochrome P450 enzymes, which may be due to the suppression of growth hormone. Since it cannot be excluded that octreotide may have this effect, other drugs mainly metabolized by CYP3A4 and which have a low therapeutic index (eg, quinidine, terfenadine) should therefore be used with caution).

No products indexed under this heading.

Topiramate (Limited published data indicate that somatostatin analogs may decrease the metabolic clearance of compounds known to be metabolized by cytochrome P450 enzymes, which may be due to the suppression of growth hormone).

No products indexed under this heading.

Torsemide (Limited published data indicate that somatostatin analogs may decrease the metabolic clearance of compounds known to be metabolized by cytochrome P450 enzymes, which may be due to the suppression of growth hormone).

No products indexed under this heading.

Tramadol Hydrochloride (Limited published data indicate that somatostatin analogs may decrease the metabolic clearance of compounds known to be metabolized by cytochrome P450 enzymes, which may be due to the suppression of growth hormone). Products include:

Ryzolt **2813**
Ultram ER **2693**

Trazodone Hydrochloride (Limited published data indicate that somatostatin analogs may decrease the metabolic clearance of compounds known to be metabolized by cytochrome P450 enzymes, which may be due to the suppression of growth hormone. Since it cannot be excluded that octreotide may have this effect, other drugs mainly metabolized by CYP3A4 and which have a low therapeutic index (eg, quinidine, terfenadine) should therefore be used with caution).

No products indexed under this heading.

Tretinoin (Limited published data indicate that somatostatin analogs may decrease the metabolic clearance of compounds known to be metabolized by cytochrome P450 enzymes, which may be due to the suppression of growth hormone).

No products indexed under this heading.

Triazolam (Limited published data indicate that somatostatin analogs may decrease the metabolic clearance of compounds known to be metabolized by cytochrome P450 enzymes, which may be due to the suppression of growth hormone. Since it cannot be excluded that octreotide may have this effect, other drugs mainly metabolized by CYP3A4 and which have a low therapeutic index (eg, quinidine, terfenadine) should therefore be used with caution).

No products indexed under this heading.

Trimethadione (Limited published data indicate that somatostatin analogs may decrease the metabolic clearance of compounds known to be metabolized by cytochrome P450 enzymes, which may be due to the suppression of growth hormone).

No products indexed under this heading.

Trimethaphan Camsylate (Limited published data indicate that somatostatin analogs may decrease the metabolic clearance of compounds known to be metabolized by cytochrome P450 enzymes, which may be due to the suppression of growth hormone).

No products indexed under this heading.

Trimipramine Maleate (Limited published data indicate that somatostatin analogs may decrease the metabolic clearance of compounds known to be metabolized by cytochrome P450 enzymes, which may be due to the suppression of growth hormone).

No products indexed under this heading.

Troglitazone (Octreotide inhibits the secretion of insulin and glucagon. Therefore, blood glucose levels should be monitored when octreotide is initiated or when the dose is altered and antidiabetic treatment should be adjusted accordingly).

No products indexed under this heading.

Trovafloxacin Mesylate (Limited published data indicate that somatostatin analogs may decrease the metabolic clearance of compounds known to be metabolized by cytochrome P450 enzymes, which may be due to the suppression of growth hormone).

No products indexed under this heading.

Valdecoxib (Limited published data indicate that somatostatin analogs may decrease the metabolic clearance of compounds known to be metabolized by cytochrome P450 enzymes, which may be due to the suppression of growth hormone).

No products indexed under this heading.

Valproate Sodium (Limited published data indicate that somatostatin analogs may decrease the metabolic clearance of compounds known to be metabolized by cytochrome P450 enzymes, which may be due to the suppression of growth hormone).

No products indexed under this heading.

Valproic Acid (Limited published data indicate that somatostatin analogs may decrease the metabolic clearance of compounds known to be metabolized by cytochrome P450 enzymes, which may be due to the suppression of growth hormone).

No products indexed under this heading.

Valsartan (Limited published data indicate that somatostatin analogs may decrease the metabolic clearance of compounds known to be metabolized by cytochrome P450 enzymes, which may be due to the suppression of growth hormone). Products include:

Diovan **2413**
Diovan HCT **2419**
Exforge **2443**
Exforge HCT **2449**
Valturna **3637**

Vardenafil Hydrochloride (Limited published data indicate that somatostatin analogs may decrease the metabolic clearance of compounds known to be metabolized by cytochrome P450 enzymes, which may be due to the suppression of growth hormone. Since it cannot be excluded that octreotide may have this effect, other drugs mainly metabolized by CYP3A4 and which have a low therapeutic index (eg, quinidine, terfenadine) should therefore be used with caution). Products include:

Levitra **3157**

IMPORTANT NOTE: Always consult each drug listing in the patient's regimen for possible interactions.

Venlafaxine Hydrochloride (Limited published data indicate that somatostatin analogs may decrease the metabolic clearance of compounds known to be metabolized by cytochrome P450 enzymes, which may be due to the suppression of growth hormone). Products include:

Verapamil Hydrochloride (Limited published data indicate that somatostatin analogs may decrease the metabolic clearance of compounds known to be metabolized by cytochrome P450 enzymes, which may be due to the suppression of growth hormone. Since it cannot be excluded that octreotide may have this effect, other drugs mainly metabolized by CYP3A4 and which have a low therapeutic index (eg, quinidine, terfenadine) should therefore be used with caution). Products include:

Vinblastine Sulfate (Limited published data indicate that somatostatin analogs may decrease the metabolic clearance of compounds known to be metabolized by cytochrome P450 enzymes, which may be due to the suppression of growth hormone. Since it cannot be excluded that octreotide may have this effect, other drugs mainly metabolized by CYP3A4 and which have a low therapeutic index (eg, quinidine, terfenadine) should therefore be used with caution).
No products indexed under this heading.

Vincristine Sulfate (Limited published data indicate that somatostatin analogs may decrease the metabolic clearance of compounds known to be metabolized by cytochrome P450 enzymes, which may be due to the suppression of growth hormone. Since it cannot be excluded that octreotide may have this effect, other drugs mainly metabolized by CYP3A4 and which have a low therapeutic index (eg, quinidine, terfenadine) should therefore be used with caution).
No products indexed under this heading.

Vitamin A (Limited published data indicate that somatostatin analogs may decrease the metabolic clearance of compounds known to be metabolized by cytochrome P450 enzymes, which may be due to the suppression of growth hormone). Products include:

Vitamin A Acetate (Limited published data indicate that somatostatin analogs may decrease the metabolic clearance of compounds known to be metabolized by cytochrome P450 enzymes, which may be due to the suppression of growth hormone).
No products indexed under this heading.

Voriconazole (Limited published data indicate that somatostatin analogs may decrease the metabolic clearance of compounds known to be metabolized by cytochrome P450 enzymes, which may be due to the suppression of growth hormone).
No products indexed under this heading.

Warfarin Sodium (Limited published data indicate that somatostatin analogs may decrease the metabolic clearance of compounds known to be metabolized by cytochrome P450 enzymes, which may be due to the suppression of growth hormone. Since it cannot be excluded that octreotide may have this effect, other drugs mainly metabolized by CYP3A4 and which have a low therapeutic index (eg, quinidine, terfenadine) should therefore be used with caution).
No products indexed under this heading.

Zafirlukast (Limited published data indicate that somatostatin analogs may

decrease the metabolic clearance of compounds known to be metabolized by cytochrome P450 enzymes, which may be due to the suppression of growth hormone). Products include:

Zileuton (Limited published data indicate that somatostatin analogs may decrease the metabolic clearance of compounds known to be metabolized by cytochrome P450 enzymes, which may be due to the suppression of growth hormone).
No products indexed under this heading.

Zolmitriptan (Limited published data indicate that somatostatin analogs may decrease the metabolic clearance of compounds known to be metabolized by cytochrome P450 enzymes, which may be due to the suppression of growth hormone). Products include:

Zonisamide (Limited published data indicate that somatostatin analogs may decrease the metabolic clearance of compounds known to be metabolized by cytochrome P450 enzymes, which may be due to the suppression of growth hormone). Products include:

Zopiclone (Limited published data indicate that somatostatin analogs may decrease the metabolic clearance of compounds known to be metabolized by cytochrome P450 enzymes, which may be due to the suppression of growth hormone).
No products indexed under this heading.

Food Interactions
Beverages, caffeine-containing (Limited published data indicate that somatostatin analogs may decrease the metabolic clearance of compounds known to be metabolized by cytochrome P450 enzymes, which may be due to the suppression of growth hormone).

Food, caffeine-containing (Limited published data indicate that somatostatin analogs may decrease the metabolic clearance of compounds known to be metabolized by cytochrome P450 enzymes, which may be due to the suppression of growth hormone).

SANTYL COLLAGENASE OINTMENT
(Collagenase) 1799

Antiseptics (The enzymatic activity of collagenase is adversely affected by heavy metal ions which are in some antiseptics. When use of such agents is suspected, the site should be cleaned by repeated washing with normal saline before applying collagenase).
No products indexed under this heading.

Cortisone Acetate (Chronic concurrent use may result in systemic manifestations of hypersensitivity to collagenase).
No products indexed under this heading.

Soap (The enzymatic activity of collagenase is adversely affected by certain detergents. When use of such agents is suspected, the site should be cleaned by repeated washing with normal saline before applying collagenase).
No products indexed under this heading.

SAPHRIS TABLETS
(Asenapine) 3223
May interact with alcohols, antibiotics, anticholinergics, antihypertensives, antipsychotic agents, centrally-acting drugs, class 1A antiarrhythmics, class III antiarrhythmics, cytochrome p450 2d6 inhibitors (selected), cytochrome p450 2d6 substrates (selected), drugs that prolong the QT interval, quinidine, valproate, and certain other agents. Compounds in these categories include:

Acebutolol Hydrochloride (Because of its α1-adrenergic antagonism with potential for inducing hypotension, asenapine may enhance the effects of certain antihypertensive agents).
No products indexed under this heading.

Alatrofloxacin Mesylate (The use of asenapine should be avoided in combination with other drugs known to prolong the QTc interval, including antibiotics (eg, gatifloxacin, moxifloxacin)).
No products indexed under this heading.

Alfentanil Hydrochloride (Given the primary CNS effects of asenapine, caution should be used when it is taken in combination with other centrally-acting drugs or alcohol).
No products indexed under this heading.

Aliskiren (Because of its α1-adrenergic antagonism with potential for inducing hypotension, asenapine may enhance the effects of certain antihypertensive agents). Products include:

Alprazolam (The use of asenapine should be avoided in combination with other drugs known to prolong the QTc interval).
No products indexed under this heading.

Amikacin Sulfate (The use of asenapine should be avoided in combination with other drugs known to prolong the QTc interval, including antibiotics (eg, gatifloxacin, moxifloxacin)).
No products indexed under this heading.

Amiodarone Hydrochloride (The use of asenapine should be avoided in combination with other drugs known to prolong the QTc interval, including Class 3 antiarrhythmics (eg, amiodarone)).
No products indexed under this heading.

Amitriptyline Hydrochloride (The use of asenapine should be avoided in combination with other drugs known to prolong the QTc interval).
No products indexed under this heading.

Amlodipine Besylate (Because of its α1-adrenergic antagonism with potential for inducing hypotension, asenapine may enhance the effects of certain antihypertensive agents). Products include:

Amoxapine (The use of asenapine should be avoided in combination with other drugs known to prolong the QTc interval).
No products indexed under this heading.

Amoxicillin (The use of asenapine should be avoided in combination with other drugs known to prolong the QTc interval, including antibiotics (eg, gatifloxacin, moxifloxacin)). Products include:

Amoxicillin Trihydrate (The use of asenapine should be avoided in combination with other drugs known to prolong the QTc interval, including antibiotics (eg, gatifloxacin, moxifloxacin)).
No products indexed under this heading.

Amphetamine Aspartate (Given the primary CNS effects of asenapine, caution should be used when it is taken in combination with other centrally-acting drugs or alcohol).
No products indexed under this heading.

Amphetamine Aspartate Monohydrate (Given the primary CNS effects of asenapine, caution should be used when it is taken in combination with other centrally-acting drugs or alcohol).
No products indexed under this heading.

Amphetamine Resins (Given the primary CNS effects of asenapine, caution should be used when it is taken in combination with other centrally-acting drugs or alcohol).
No products indexed under this heading.

Amphetamine Sulfate (Given the primary CNS effects of asenapine, caution should be used when it is taken in combination with other centrally-acting drugs or alcohol).
No products indexed under this heading.

Ampicillin (The use of asenapine should be avoided in combination with other drugs known to prolong the QTc interval, including antibiotics (eg, gatifloxacin, moxifloxacin)).
No products indexed under this heading.

Ampicillin Sodium (The use of asenapine should be avoided in combination with other drugs known to prolong the QTc interval, including antibiotics (eg, gatifloxacin, moxifloxacin)).
No products indexed under this heading.

Ampicillin Trihydrate (The use of asenapine should be avoided in combination with other drugs known to prolong the QTc interval, including antibiotics (eg, gatifloxacin, moxifloxacin)).
No products indexed under this heading.

Antibiotics, non-penicillin, unspecified (The use of asenapine should be avoided in combination with other drugs known to prolong the QTc interval, including antibiotics (eg, gatifloxacin, moxifloxacin)).
No products indexed under this heading.

Aprobarbital (Given the primary CNS effects of asenapine, caution should be used when it is taken in combination with other centrally-acting drugs or alcohol).
No products indexed under this heading.

Aripiprazole (The use of asenapine should be avoided in combination with other drugs known to prolong the QTc interval, including antipsychotic medications (eg, ziprasidone, chlorpromazine, thioridazine)).
No products indexed under this heading.

Astemizole (The use of asenapine should be avoided in combination with other drugs known to prolong the QTc interval).
No products indexed under this heading.

Atenolol (Because of its α1-adrenergic antagonism with potential for inducing hypotension, asenapine may enhance the effects of certain antihypertensive agents).
No products indexed under this heading.

Atomoxetine Hydrochloride (Asenapine should be co-administered cautiously with drugs that are both substrates and inhibitors for CYP2D6). Products include:

Atropine Sulfate (Appropriate care is advised when prescribing asenapine for patients receiving concomitant medication with anticholinergic activity). Products include:

Azithromycin Dihydrate (The use of asenapine should be avoided in combination with other drugs known to prolong the QTc interval, including antibiotics (eg, gatifloxacin, moxifloxacin)).
No products indexed under this heading.

1687 **Interactions Index** **Saphris**

Azlocillin Sodium (The use of asenapine should be avoided in combination with other drugs known to prolong the QTc interval, including antibiotics (eg, gatifloxacin, moxifloxacin)).
No products indexed under this heading.

Aztreonam (The use of asenapine should be avoided in combination with other drugs known to prolong the QTc interval, including antibiotics (eg, gatifloxacin, moxifloxacin)).
No products indexed under this heading.

Bacampicillin Hydrochloride (The use of asenapine should be avoided in combination with other drugs known to prolong the QTc interval, including antibiotics (eg, gatifloxacin, moxifloxacin)).
No products indexed under this heading.

Belladonna Alkaloids (Appropriate care is advised when prescribing asenapine for patients receiving concomitant medication with anticholinergic activity). Products include:
Hyland's Teething Tablets **3316**

Benazepril Hydrochloride (Because of its α1-adrenergic antagonism with potential for inducing hypotension, asenapine may enhance the effects of certain antihypertensive agents).
No products indexed under this heading.

Bendroflumethiazide (Because of its α1-adrenergic antagonism with potential for inducing hypotension, asenapine may enhance the effects of certain antihypertensive agents).
No products indexed under this heading.

Benztropine Mesylate (Appropriate care is advised when prescribing asenapine for patients receiving concomitant medication with anticholinergic activity).
No products indexed under this heading.

Betaxolol Hydrochloride (Because of its α1-adrenergic antagonism with potential for inducing hypotension, asenapine may enhance the effects of certain antihypertensive agents).
No products indexed under this heading.

Biperiden Hydrochloride (Appropriate care is advised when prescribing asenapine for patients receiving concomitant medication with anticholinergic activity).
No products indexed under this heading.

Bisoprolol Fumarate (Because of its α1-adrenergic antagonism with potential for inducing hypotension, asenapine may enhance the effects of certain antihypertensive agents).
No products indexed under this heading.

Bretylium Tosylate (The use of asenapine should be avoided in combination with other drugs known to prolong the QTc interval).
No products indexed under this heading.

Buprenorphine Hydrochloride (Given the primary CNS effects of asenapine, caution should be used when it is taken in combination with other centrally-acting drugs or alcohol).
No products indexed under this heading.

Bupropion Hydrochloride (Asenapine should be co-administered cautiously with drugs that are both substrates and inhibitors for CYP2D6). Products include:
Aplenzin **2948**
Wellbutrin **1719**
Wellbutrin SR **1725**
Zyban **1762**

Buspirone Hydrochloride (The use of asenapine should be avoided in combination with other drugs known to prolong the QTc interval).
No products indexed under this heading.

Butabarbital (Given the primary CNS effects of asenapine, caution should be used when it is taken in combination with other centrally-acting drugs or alcohol).
No products indexed under this heading.

Butalbital (Given the primary CNS effects of asenapine, caution should be used when it is taken in combination with other centrally-acting drugs or alcohol).
No products indexed under this heading.

Candesartan Cilexetil (Because of its α1-adrenergic antagonism with potential for inducing hypotension, asenapine may enhance the effects of certain antihypertensive agents). Products include:
Atacand **697**
Atacand HCT **700**

Captopril (Because of its α1-adrenergic antagonism with potential for inducing hypotension, asenapine may enhance the effects of certain antihypertensive agents). Products include:
Captopril **2341**

Carbamazepine (Asenapine is cleared primarily through direct glucuronidation by UGT1A4 and oxidative metabolism by cytochrome P450 isoenzymes (predominantly CYP1A2). Co-administration of carbamazepine, a CYP3A4 inducer (400 mg bid daily for 15 days), with asenapine (5 mg single dose) decreased the C_{max} of asenapine by 16% and decreased the AUC of asenapine by 16%. No dosage adjustment of asenapine is required). Products include:
Carbatrol **3280**
Equetro **3477**

Carbenicillin Disodium (The use of asenapine should be avoided in combination with other drugs known to prolong the QTc interval, including antibiotics (eg, gatifloxacin, moxifloxacin)).
No products indexed under this heading.

Carbenicillin Indanyl Sodium (The use of asenapine should be avoided in combination with other drugs known to prolong the QTc interval, including antibiotics (eg, gatifloxacin, moxifloxacin)).
No products indexed under this heading.

Carteolol Hydrochloride (Because of its α1-adrenergic antagonism with potential for inducing hypotension, asenapine may enhance the effects of certain antihypertensive agents).
No products indexed under this heading.

Carvedilol (Because of its α1-adrenergic antagonism with potential for inducing hypotension, asenapine may enhance the effects of certain antihypertensive agents). Products include:
Coreg **1409**

Carvedilol Phosphate (Because of its α1-adrenergic antagonism with potential for inducing hypotension, asenapine may enhance the effects of certain antihypertensive agents). Products include:
Coreg CR **1416**

Cefaclor (The use of asenapine should be avoided in combination with other drugs known to prolong the QTc interval, including antibiotics (eg, gatifloxacin, moxifloxacin)).
No products indexed under this heading.

Cefadroxil (The use of asenapine should be avoided in combination with other drugs known to prolong the QTc interval, including antibiotics (eg, gatifloxacin, moxifloxacin)).
No products indexed under this heading.

Cefamandole Nafate (The use of asenapine should be avoided in combination with other drugs known to prolong the QTc interval, including antibiotics (eg, gatifloxacin, moxifloxacin)).
No products indexed under this heading.

Cefazolin Sodium (The use of asenapine should be avoided in combination with other drugs known to prolong the QTc interval, including antibiotics (eg, gatifloxacin, moxifloxacin)).
No products indexed under this heading.

Cefixime (The use of asenapine should be avoided in combination with other drugs known to prolong the QTc interval, including antibiotics (eg, gatifloxacin, moxifloxacin)). Products include:
Suprax for Oral Suspension **2038**
Suprax Tablets **2038**

Cefmetazole Sodium (The use of asenapine should be avoided in combination with other drugs known to prolong the QTc interval, including antibiotics (eg, gatifloxacin, moxifloxacin)).
No products indexed under this heading.

Cefonicid Sodium (The use of asenapine should be avoided in combination with other drugs known to prolong the QTc interval, including antibiotics (eg, gatifloxacin, moxifloxacin)).
No products indexed under this heading.

Cefoperazone Sodium (The use of asenapine should be avoided in combination with other drugs known to prolong the QTc interval, including antibiotics (eg, gatifloxacin, moxifloxacin)).
No products indexed under this heading.

Ceforanide (The use of asenapine should be avoided in combination with other drugs known to prolong the QTc interval, including antibiotics (eg, gatifloxacin, moxifloxacin)).
No products indexed under this heading.

Cefotaxime Sodium (The use of asenapine should be avoided in combination with other drugs known to prolong the QTc interval, including antibiotics (eg, gatifloxacin, moxifloxacin)).
No products indexed under this heading.

Cefotetan (The use of asenapine should be avoided in combination with other drugs known to prolong the QTc interval, including antibiotics (eg, gatifloxacin, moxifloxacin)).
No products indexed under this heading.

Cefoxitin Sodium (The use of asenapine should be avoided in combination with other drugs known to prolong the QTc interval, including antibiotics (eg, gatifloxacin, moxifloxacin)).
No products indexed under this heading.

Cefpodoxime Proxetil (The use of asenapine should be avoided in combination with other drugs known to prolong the QTc interval, including antibiotics (eg, gatifloxacin, moxifloxacin)).
No products indexed under this heading.

Cefprozil (The use of asenapine should be avoided in combination with other drugs known to prolong the QTc interval, including antibiotics (eg, gatifloxacin, moxifloxacin)).
No products indexed under this heading.

Ceftazidime (The use of asenapine should be avoided in combination with other drugs known to prolong the QTc interval, including antibiotics (eg, gatifloxacin, moxifloxacin)). Products include:
Fortaz **1481**

Ceftizoxime Sodium (The use of asenapine should be avoided in combination with other drugs known to prolong the QTc interval, including antibiotics (eg, gatifloxacin, moxifloxacin)).
No products indexed under this heading.

Ceftriaxone Sodium (The use of asenapine should be avoided in combination with other drugs known to prolong the QTc interval, including antibiotics (eg, gatifloxacin, moxifloxacin)). Products include:
Rocephin **2859**

Cefuroxime Axetil (The use of asenapine should be avoided in combination with other drugs known to prolong the QTc interval, including antibiotics (eg, gatifloxacin, moxifloxacin)). Products include:
Ceftin **1399**

Cefuroxime Sodium (The use of asenapine should be avoided in combination with other drugs known to prolong the QTc interval, including antibiotics (eg, gatifloxacin, moxifloxacin)).
No products indexed under this heading.

Celecoxib (Asenapine should be co-administered cautiously with drugs that are both substrates and inhibitors for CYP2D6). Products include:
Celebrex **3272**

Cephalexin (The use of asenapine should be avoided in combination with other drugs known to prolong the QTc interval, including antibiotics (eg, gatifloxacin, moxifloxacin)).
No products indexed under this heading.

Cephalothin Sodium (The use of asenapine should be avoided in combination with other drugs known to prolong the QTc interval, including antibiotics (eg, gatifloxacin, moxifloxacin)).
No products indexed under this heading.

Cephapirin Sodium (The use of asenapine should be avoided in combination with other drugs known to prolong the QTc interval, including antibiotics (eg, gatifloxacin, moxifloxacin)).
No products indexed under this heading.

Cephradine (The use of asenapine should be avoided in combination with other drugs known to prolong the QTc interval, including antibiotics (eg, gatifloxacin, moxifloxacin)).
No products indexed under this heading.

Cevimeline Hydrochloride (Asenapine should be co-administered cautiously with drugs that are both substrates and inhibitors for CYP2D6). Products include:
Evoxac **1027**

Chloramphenicol (The use of asenapine should be avoided in combination with other drugs known to prolong the QTc interval, including antibiotics (eg, gatifloxacin, moxifloxacin)).
No products indexed under this heading.

Chloramphenicol Palmitate (The use of asenapine should be avoided in combination with other drugs known to prolong the QTc interval, including antibiotics (eg, gatifloxacin, moxifloxacin)).
No products indexed under this heading.

Chloramphenicol Sodium Succinate (The use of asenapine should be avoided in combination with other drugs known to prolong the QTc interval, including antibiotics (eg, gatifloxacin, moxifloxacin)).
No products indexed under this heading.

Chlordiazepoxide (The use of asenapine should be avoided in combination with other drugs known to prolong the QTc interval).
No products indexed under this heading.

Chlordiazepoxide Hydrochloride (The use of asenapine should be avoided in combination with other drugs known to prolong the QTc interval).
No products indexed under this heading.

Chloroquine (Asenapine should be co-administered cautiously with drugs that are both substrates and inhibitors for CYP2D6).
No products indexed under this heading.

Chloroquine Hydrochloride (Asenapine should be co-administered cautiously with drugs that are both substrates and inhibitors for CYP2D6).
No products indexed under this heading.

Chloroquine Phosphate (Asenapine should be co-administered cautiously with drugs that are both substrates and inhibitors for CYP2D6).
No products indexed under this heading.

IMPORTANT NOTE: Always consult each drug listing in the patient's regimen for possible interactions.

Saphris Interactions Index 1688

Chlorothiazide (Because of its α1-adrenergic antagonism with potential for inducing hypotension, asenapine may enhance the effects of certain antihypertensive agents).
No products indexed under this heading.

Chlorothiazide Sodium (Because of its α1-adrenergic antagonism with potential for inducing hypotension, asenapine may enhance the effects of certain antihypertensive agents). Products include:
Diuril Intravenous 2009

Chlorpheniramine (Asenapine should be co-administered cautiously with drugs that are both substrates and inhibitors for CYP2D6).
No products indexed under this heading.

Chlorpheniramine Maleate (Asenapine should be co-administered cautiously with drugs that are both substrates and inhibitors for CYP2D6).
No products indexed under this heading.

Chlorpheniramine Polistirex (Asenapine should be co-administered cautiously with drugs that are both substrates and inhibitors for CYP2D6). Products include:
Tussionex 3443

Chlorpheniramine Tannate (Asenapine should be co-administered cautiously with drugs that are both substrates and inhibitors for CYP2D6).
No products indexed under this heading.

Chlorpromazine (The use of asenapine should be avoided in combination with other drugs known to prolong QTc, including antipsychotic medications (eg, chlorpromazine)).
No products indexed under this heading.

Chlorpromazine Hydrochloride (The use of asenapine should be avoided in combination with other drugs known to prolong QTc, including antipsychotic medications (eg, chlorpromazine)).
No products indexed under this heading.

Chlorpropamide (Asenapine should be co-administered cautiously with drugs that are both substrates and inhibitors for CYP2D6).
No products indexed under this heading.

Chlorprothixene (The use of asenapine should be avoided in combination with other drugs known to prolong the QTc interval, including antipsychotic medications (eg, ziprasidone, chlorpromazine, thioridazine)).
No products indexed under this heading.

Chlorprothixene Hydrochloride (The use of asenapine should be avoided in combination with other drugs known to prolong the QTc interval, including antipsychotic medications (eg, ziprasidone, chlorpromazine, thioridazine)).
No products indexed under this heading.

Chlorprothixene Lactate (The use of asenapine should be avoided in combination with other drugs known to prolong the QTc interval, including antipsychotic medications (eg, ziprasidone, chlorpromazine, thioridazine)).
No products indexed under this heading.

Chlorthalidone (Because of its α1-adrenergic antagonism with potential for inducing hypotension, asenapine may enhance the effects of certain antihypertensive agents). Products include:
Clorpres 2344

Cilastatin Sodium (The use of asenapine should be avoided in combination with other drugs known to prolong the QTc interval, including antibiotics (eg, gatifloxacin, moxifloxacin)). Products include:
Primaxin I.M. 2232
Primaxin I.V. 2235

Cimetidine (Asenapine is cleared primarily through direct glucuronidation by UGT1A4 and oxidative metabolism by cytochrome P450 isoenzymes (predominantly CYP1A2). Co-administration of cimetidine, a CYP3A4/2D6/1A2 inhibitor (800 mg bid for 8 days), with asenapine (5 mg single dose) decreased the C_{max} of asenapine by 13% and increased the AUC of asenapine by 1%. No dosage adjustment of asenapine is necessary).
No products indexed under this heading.

Cimetidine Hydrochloride (Asenapine is cleared primarily through direct glucuronidation by UGT1A4 and oxidative metabolism by cytochrome P450 isoenzymes (predominantly CYP1A2). Co-administration of cimetidine, a CYP3A4/2D6/1A2 inhibitor (800 mg bid for 8 days), with asenapine (5 mg single dose) decreased the C_{max} of asenapine by 13% and increased the AUC of asenapine by 1%. No dosage adjustment of asenapine is necessary).
No products indexed under this heading.

Ciprofloxacin (The use of asenapine should be avoided in combination with other drugs known to prolong the QTc interval, including antibiotics (eg, gatifloxacin, moxifloxacin)). Products include:
Cipro I.V. 3082
Cipro 3073
Cipro XR 3091
Ciprodex 583

Ciprofloxacin Hydrochloride (The use of asenapine should be avoided in combination with other drugs known to prolong the QTc interval, including antibiotics (eg, gatifloxacin, moxifloxacin)). Products include:
Cipro 3073

Citalopram Hydrobromide (Asenapine should be co-administered cautiously with drugs that are both substrates and inhibitors for CYP2D6). Products include:
Celexa 1153

Clarithromycin (The use of asenapine should be avoided in combination with other drugs known to prolong the QTc interval, including antibiotics (eg, gatifloxacin, moxifloxacin)). Products include:
Biaxin/Biaxin XL 412

Clidinium Bromide (Appropriate care is advised when prescribing asenapine for patients receiving concomitant medication with anticholinergic activity).
No products indexed under this heading.

Clomipramine Hydrochloride (The use of asenapine should be avoided in combination with other drugs known to prolong the QTc interval).
No products indexed under this heading.

Clonidine (Because of its α1-adrenergic antagonism with potential for inducing hypotension, asenapine may enhance the effects of certain antihypertensive agents). Products include:
Catapres-TTS 884

Clonidine Hydrochloride (Because of its α1-adrenergic antagonism with potential for inducing hypotension, asenapine may enhance the effects of certain antihypertensive agents). Products include:
Clorpres 2344

Clorazepate Dipotassium (The use of asenapine should be avoided in combination with other drugs known to prolong the QTc interval).
No products indexed under this heading.

Clotrimazole (The use of asenapine should be avoided in combination with other drugs known to prolong the QTc interval, including antibiotics (eg, gatifloxacin, moxifloxacin)). Products include:
Lotrisone 3163

Cloxacillin (The use of asenapine should be avoided in combination with other drugs known to prolong the QTc interval, including antibiotics (eg, gatifloxacin, moxifloxacin)).
No products indexed under this heading.

Cloxacillin Sodium (The use of asenapine should be avoided in combination with other drugs known to prolong the QTc interval, including antibiotics (eg, gatifloxacin, moxifloxacin)).
No products indexed under this heading.

Cloxacillin Sodium Monohydrate (The use of asenapine should be avoided in combination with other drugs known to prolong the QTc interval, including antibiotics (eg, gatifloxacin, moxifloxacin)).
No products indexed under this heading.

Clozapine (The use of asenapine should be avoided in combination with other drugs known to prolong the QTc interval, including antipsychotic medications (eg, ziprasidone, chlorpromazine, thioridazine)).
No products indexed under this heading.

Cocaine Hydrochloride (Asenapine should be co-administered cautiously with drugs that are both substrates and inhibitors for CYP2D6).
No products indexed under this heading.

Codeine Phosphate (Given the primary CNS effects of asenapine, caution should be used when it is taken in combination with other centrally-acting drugs or alcohol). Products include:
Tylenol with Codeine 2691

Codeine Sulfate (Given the primary CNS effects of asenapine, caution should be used when it is taken in combination with other centrally-acting drugs or alcohol).
No products indexed under this heading.

Cyclobenzaprine Hydrochloride (Asenapine should be co-administered cautiously with drugs that are both substrates and inhibitors for CYP2D6). Products include:
Amrix 964

Daunorubicin Hydrochloride (The use of asenapine should be avoided in combination with other drugs known to prolong the QTc interval, including antibiotics (eg, gatifloxacin, moxifloxacin)).
No products indexed under this heading.

Debrisoquine (Asenapine should be co-administered cautiously with drugs that are both substrates and inhibitors for CYP2D6).
No products indexed under this heading.

Demeclocycline Hydrochloride (The use of asenapine should be avoided in combination with other drugs known to prolong the QTc interval, including antibiotics (eg, gatifloxacin, moxifloxacin)).
No products indexed under this heading.

Deserpidine (Because of its α1-adrenergic antagonism with potential for inducing hypotension, asenapine may enhance the effects of certain antihypertensive agents).
No products indexed under this heading.

Desflurane (Given the primary CNS effects of asenapine, caution should be used when it is taken in combination with other centrally-acting drugs or alcohol).
No products indexed under this heading.

Desipramine Hydrochloride (The use of asenapine should be avoided in combination with other drugs known to prolong the QTc interval).
No products indexed under this heading.

Dexfenfluramine Hydrochloride (Asenapine should be co-administered cautiously with drugs that are both substrates and inhibitors for CYP2D6).
No products indexed under this heading.

Dexmethylphenidate Hydrochloride (Given the primary CNS effects of asenapine, caution should be used when it is taken in combination with other centrally-acting drugs or alcohol). Products include:
Focalin XR 2472

Dextroamphetamine (Given the primary CNS effects of asenapine, caution should be used when it is taken in combination with other centrally-acting drugs or alcohol).
No products indexed under this heading.

Dextroamphetamine Saccharate (Given the primary CNS effects of asenapine, caution should be used when it is taken in combination with other centrally-acting drugs or alcohol).
No products indexed under this heading.

Dextroamphetamine Sulfate (Given the primary CNS effects of asenapine, caution should be used when it is taken in combination with other centrally-acting drugs or alcohol). Products include:
Dexedrine 1425

Dextromethorphan (*In vitro* studies indicate that asenapine weakly inhibits CYP2D6. Following co-administration of dextromethorphan and asenapine in healthy subjects, the ratio of dextrorphan/dextromethorphan (DX/DM) as a marker of CYP2D6 activity was measured. Indicative of CYP2D6 inhibition, treatment with asenapine 5 mg twice daily decreased the DX/DM ratio to 0.43).
No products indexed under this heading.

Dextromethorphan Hydrobromide (*In vitro* studies indicate that asenapine weakly inhibits CYP2D6. Following co-administration of dextromethorphan and asenapine in healthy subjects, the ratio of dextrorphan/dextromethorphan (DX/DM) as a marker of CYP2D6 activity was measured. Indicative of CYP2D6 inhibition, treatment with asenapine 5 mg twice daily decreased the DX/DM ratio to 0.43).
No products indexed under this heading.

Dextromethorphan Polistirex (*In vitro* studies indicate that asenapine weakly inhibits CYP2D6. Following co-administration of dextromethorphan and asenapine in healthy subjects, the ratio of dextrorphan/dextromethorphan (DX/DM) as a marker of CYP2D6 activity was measured. Indicative of CYP2D6 inhibition, treatment with asenapine 5 mg twice daily decreased the DX/DM ratio to 0.43).
No products indexed under this heading.

Dextromethorphan Tannate (*In vitro* studies indicate that asenapine weakly inhibits CYP2D6. Following co-administration of dextromethorphan and asenapine in healthy subjects, the ratio of dextrorphan/dextromethorphan (DX/DM) as a marker of CYP2D6 activity was measured. Indicative of CYP2D6 inhibition, treatment with asenapine 5 mg twice daily decreased the DX/DM ratio to 0.43).
No products indexed under this heading.

Dezocine (Given the primary CNS effects of asenapine, caution should be used when it is taken in combination with other centrally-acting drugs or alcohol).
No products indexed under this heading.

Diazepam (The use of asenapine should be avoided in combination with other drugs known to prolong the QTc interval). Products include:
Valium Tablets 2880

Diazoxide (Because of its α1-adrenergic antagonism with potential for inducing hypotension, asenapine may enhance the effects of certain antihypertensive agents). Products include:
Proglycem 1179

IMPORTANT NOTE: Always consult each drug listing in the patient's regimen for possible interactions.

Saphris Interactions Index 1690

therapeutic dose of fluvoxamine was administered, a greater increase in asenapine plasma concentrations would be expected. Co-administration of fluvoxamine with asenapine should be done with caution).
No products indexed under this heading.

Formoterol Fumarate (Asenapine should be co-administered cautiously with drugs that are both substrates and inhibitors for CYP2D6). Products include:
Foradil 3121
Perforomist 3634

Fosinopril Sodium (Because of its α1-adrenergic antagonism with potential for inducing hypotension, asenapine may enhance the effects of certain antihypertensive agents).
No products indexed under this heading.

Furosemide (Because of its α1-adrenergic antagonism with potential for inducing hypotension, asenapine may enhance the effects of certain antihypertensive agents). Products include:
Furosemide 2354

Galantamine Hydrobromide (Asenapine should be co-administered cautiously with drugs that are both substrates and inhibitors for CYP2D6).
No products indexed under this heading.

Gatifloxacin (The use of asenapine should be avoided in combination with other drugs known to prolong the QTc interval, including antibiotics (eg, gatifloxacin)).
No products indexed under this heading.

Gemifloxacin Mesylate (The use of asenapine should be avoided in combination with other drugs known to prolong the QTc interval, including antibiotics (eg, gatifloxacin, moxifloxacin)).
No products indexed under this heading.

Gentamicin Sulfate (The use of asenapine should be avoided in combination with other drugs known to prolong the QTc interval, including antibiotics (eg, gatifloxacin, moxifloxacin)). Products include:
Pred-G .... ⊙226, ⊙227

Glutethimide (Given the primary CNS effects of asenapine, caution should be used when it is taken in combination with other centrally-acting drugs or alcohol).
No products indexed under this heading.

Glycopyrrolate (Appropriate care is advised when prescribing asenapine for patients receiving concomitant medication with anticholinergic activity).
No products indexed under this heading.

Grepafloxacin Hydrochloride (The use of asenapine should be avoided in combination with other drugs known to prolong the QTc interval, including antibiotics (eg, gatifloxacin, moxifloxacin)).
No products indexed under this heading.

Griseofulvin (The use of asenapine should be avoided in combination with other drugs known to prolong the QTc interval, including antibiotics (eg, gatifloxacin, moxifloxacin)).
No products indexed under this heading.

Guanabenz Acetate (Because of its α1-adrenergic antagonism with potential for inducing hypotension, asenapine may enhance the effects of certain antihypertensive agents).
No products indexed under this heading.

Guanethidine (Because of its α1-adrenergic antagonism with potential for inducing hypotension, asenapine may enhance the effects of certain antihypertensive agents).
No products indexed under this heading.

Guanethidine Monosulfate (Because of its α1-adrenergic antagonism with potential for inducing hypotension, asenapine may enhance the effects of certain antihypertensive agents).
No products indexed under this heading.

Guanethidine Sulfate (Because of its α1-adrenergic antagonism with potential for inducing hypotension, asenapine may enhance the effects of certain antihypertensive agents).
No products indexed under this heading.

Halofantrine Hydrochloride (Asenapine should be co-administered cautiously with drugs that are both substrates and inhibitors for CYP2D6).
No products indexed under this heading.

Haloperidol (The use of asenapine should be avoided in combination with other drugs known to prolong the QTc interval, including antipsychotic medications (eg, ziprasidone, chlorpromazine, thioridazine)).
No products indexed under this heading.

Haloperidol Decanoate (The use of asenapine should be avoided in combination with other drugs known to prolong the QTc interval, including antipsychotic medications (eg, ziprasidone, chlorpromazine, thioridazine)).
No products indexed under this heading.

Haloperidol Lactate (The use of asenapine should be avoided in combination with other drugs known to prolong the QTc interval, including antipsychotic medications (eg, ziprasidone, chlorpromazine, thioridazine)).
No products indexed under this heading.

Hydralazine Hydrochloride (Because of its α1-adrenergic antagonism with potential for inducing hypotension, asenapine may enhance the effects of certain antihypertensive agents).
No products indexed under this heading.

Hydrochlorothiazide (Because of its α1-adrenergic antagonism with potential for inducing hypotension, asenapine may enhance the effects of certain antihypertensive agents). Products include:
Atacand HCT 700
Avalide 2956
Benicar HCT 1017
Diovan HCT 2419
Dyazide 1429
Exforge HCT 2449
Hyzaar 2162
Hyzaar 100-12.5 2162
Micardis HCT 889
Prinzide 2246
Tekturna HCT 2541
Teveten HCT 541

Hydrocodone Bitartrate (Given the primary CNS effects of asenapine, caution should be used when it is taken in combination with other centrally-acting drugs or alcohol). Products include:
Vicodin 560
Vicodin ES 561
Vicodin HP 563
Vicoprofen 564
Zydone 1138

Hydrocodone Polistirex (Given the primary CNS effects of asenapine, caution should be used when it is taken in combination with other centrally-acting drugs or alcohol). Products include:
Tussionex 3443

Hydroflumethiazide (Because of its α1-adrenergic antagonism with potential for inducing hypotension, asenapine may enhance the effects of certain antihypertensive agents).
No products indexed under this heading.

Hydromorphone Hydrochloride (Given the primary CNS effects of asenapine, caution should be used when it is taken in combination with other centrally-acting drugs or alcohol). Products include:
Dilaudid Injection 2800
Dilaudid Oral 2797
Dilaudid Tablets 2797
Dilaudid-HP 2800

Hydroxyamphetamine Hydrobromide (Given the primary CNS effects of asenapine, caution should be used when it is taken in combination with other centrally-acting drugs or alcohol).
No products indexed under this heading.

Hydroxychloroquine Sulfate (Asenapine should be co-administered cautiously with drugs that are both substrates and inhibitors for CYP2D6).
No products indexed under this heading.

Hydroxyzine Hydrochloride (The use of asenapine should be avoided in combination with other drugs known to prolong the QTc interval).
No products indexed under this heading.

Hyoscyamine (Appropriate care is advised when prescribing asenapine for patients receiving concomitant medication with anticholinergic activity).
No products indexed under this heading.

Hyoscyamine Sulfate (Appropriate care is advised when prescribing asenapine for patients receiving concomitant medication with anticholinergic activity). Products include:
Donnatal 2711

Idarubicin Hydrochloride (The use of asenapine should be avoided in combination with other drugs known to prolong the QTc interval, including antibiotics (eg, gatifloxacin, moxifloxacin)).
No products indexed under this heading.

Imatinib Mesylate (Asenapine should be co-administered cautiously with drugs that are both substrates and inhibitors for CYP2D6). Products include:
Gleevec 2477

Imipenem (The use of asenapine should be avoided in combination with other drugs known to prolong the QTc interval, including antibiotics (eg, gatifloxacin, moxifloxacin)). Products include:
Primaxin I.M. 2232
Primaxin I.V. 2235

Imipramine Hydrochloride (Asenapine is cleared primarily through direct glucuronidation by UGT1A4 and oxidative metabolism by cytochrome P450 isoenzymes (predominantly CYP1A2). Co-administration of imipramine, a CYP1A2/2C19/3A4 inhibitor (75 mg single dose), with asenapine (5 mg single dose) increased the C_{max} of asenapine by 17% and the AUC of asenapine by 10%. No dosage adjustment of asenapine is necessary).
No products indexed under this heading.

Imipramine Pamoate (Asenapine is cleared primarily through direct glucuronidation by UGT1A4 and oxidative metabolism by cytochrome P450 isoenzymes (predominantly CYP1A2). Co-administration of imipramine, a CYP1A2/2C19/3A4 inhibitor (75 mg single dose), with asenapine (5 mg single dose) increased the C_{max} of asenapine by 17% and the AUC of asenapine by 10%. No dosage adjustment of asenapine is necessary).
No products indexed under this heading.

Indapamide (Because of its α1-adrenergic antagonism with potential for inducing hypotension, asenapine may enhance the effects of certain antihypertensive agents). Products include:
Indapamide 2356

Indoramin Hydrochloride (Asenapine should be co-administered cautiously with drugs that are both substrates and inhibitors for CYP2D6).
No products indexed under this heading.

Ipratropium Bromide (Appropriate care is advised when prescribing asenapine for patients receiving concomitant medication with anticholinergic activity).
No products indexed under this heading.

Irbesartan (Because of its α1-adrenergic antagonism with potential for inducing hypotension, asenapine may enhance the effects of certain antihypertensive agents). Products include:
Avalide 2956
Avapro 2962

Isocarboxazid (The use of asenapine should be avoided in combination with other drugs known to prolong the QTc interval). Products include:
Marplan 3481

Isoflurane (Given the primary CNS effects of asenapine, caution should be used when it is taken in combination with other centrally-acting drugs or alcohol).
No products indexed under this heading.

Isradipine (Because of its α1-adrenergic antagonism with potential for inducing hypotension, asenapine may enhance the effects of certain antihypertensive agents). Products include:
DynaCirc CR 1432

Kanamycin Sulfate (The use of asenapine should be avoided in combination with other drugs known to prolong the QTc interval, including antibiotics (eg, gatifloxacin, moxifloxacin)).
No products indexed under this heading.

Ketamine Hydrochloride (Given the primary CNS effects of asenapine, caution should be used when it is taken in combination with other centrally-acting drugs or alcohol).
No products indexed under this heading.

Labetalol Hydrochloride (Because of its α1-adrenergic antagonism with potential for inducing hypotension, asenapine may enhance the effects of certain antihypertensive agents).
No products indexed under this heading.

Levofloxacin (The use of asenapine should be avoided in combination with other drugs known to prolong the QTc interval, including antibiotics (eg, gatifloxacin, moxifloxacin)). Products include:
Iquix 3492
Levaquin 2629
Levaquin in 5% Dextrose 2629
Quixin 3493

Levomethadyl Acetate Hydrochloride (Given the primary CNS effects of asenapine, caution should be used when it is taken in combination with other centrally-acting drugs or alcohol).
No products indexed under this heading.

Levorphanol Tartrate (Given the primary CNS effects of asenapine, caution should be used when it is taken in combination with other centrally-acting drugs or alcohol).
No products indexed under this heading.

Lidocaine (The use of asenapine should be avoided in combination with other drugs known to prolong the QTc interval). Products include:
Lidoderm 1107

Lidocaine Hydrochloride (The use of asenapine should be avoided in combination with other drugs known to prolong the QTc interval).
No products indexed under this heading.

Lisdexamfetamine Dimesylate (Given the primary CNS effects of asenapine, caution should be used when it is taken in combination with other centrally-acting drugs or alcohol). Products include:
Vyvanse 3298

Lisinopril (Because of its α1-adrenergic antagonism with potential for inducing hypotension, asenapine

(⊙ Described in PDR® for Ophthalmic Medicines)

may enhance the effects of certain anti-hypertensive agents). Products include:

Lithium (The use of asenapine should be avoided in combination with other drugs known to prolong the QTc interval, including antipsychotic medications (eg, ziprasidone, chlorpromazine, thioridazine)).

No products indexed under this heading.

Lithium Carbonate (The use of asenapine should be avoided in combination with other drugs known to prolong the QTc interval, including antipsychotic medications (eg, ziprasidone, chlorpromazine, thioridazine)).

No products indexed under this heading.

Lithium Citrate (The use of asenapine should be avoided in combination with other drugs known to prolong the QTc interval, including antipsychotic medications (eg, ziprasidone, chlorpromazine, thioridazine)).

No products indexed under this heading.

Lomefloxacin Hydrochloride (The use of asenapine should be avoided in combination with other drugs known to prolong the QTc interval, including antibiotics (eg, gatifloxacin, moxifloxacin)).

No products indexed under this heading.

Loracarbef (The use of asenapine should be avoided in combination with other drugs known to prolong the QTc interval, including antibiotics (eg, gatifloxacin, moxifloxacin)).

No products indexed under this heading.

Lorazepam (The use of asenapine should be avoided in combination with other drugs known to prolong the QTc interval).

No products indexed under this heading.

Losartan Potassium (Because of its α1-adrenergic antagonism with potential for inducing hypotension, asenapine may enhance the effects of certain antihypertensive agents). Products include:

Loxapine Hydrochloride (The use of asenapine should be avoided in combination with other drugs known to prolong the QTc interval, including antipsychotic medications (eg, ziprasidone, chlorpromazine, thioridazine)).

No products indexed under this heading.

Loxapine Succinate (The use of asenapine should be avoided in combination with other drugs known to prolong the QTc interval, including antipsychotic medications (eg, ziprasidone, chlorpromazine, thioridazine)).

No products indexed under this heading.

Maprotiline Hydrochloride (The use of asenapine should be avoided in combination with other drugs known to prolong the QTc interval).

No products indexed under this heading.

Mecamylamine Hydrochloride (Because of its α1-adrenergic antagonism with potential for inducing hypotension, asenapine may enhance the effects of certain antihypertensive agents).

No products indexed under this heading.

Mepenzolate Bromide (Appropriate care is advised when prescribing asenapine for patients receiving concomitant medication with anticholinergic activity).

No products indexed under this heading.

Meperidine Hydrochloride (Given the primary CNS effects of asenapine, caution should be used when it is taken in combination with other centrally-acting drugs or alcohol).

No products indexed under this heading.

Mephobarbital (Given the primary CNS effects of asenapine, caution should be used when it is taken in combination with other centrally-acting drugs or alcohol).

No products indexed under this heading.

Meprobamate (The use of asenapine should be avoided in combination with other drugs known to prolong the QTc interval).

No products indexed under this heading.

Mesoridazine Besylate (The use of asenapine should be avoided in combination with other drugs known to prolong the QTc interval, including antipsychotic medications (eg, ziprasidone, chlorpromazine, thioridazine)).

No products indexed under this heading.

Methacycline Hydrochloride (The use of asenapine should be avoided in combination with other drugs known to prolong the QTc interval, including antibiotics (eg, gatifloxacin, moxifloxacin)).

No products indexed under this heading.

Methadone Hydrochloride (Given the primary CNS effects of asenapine, caution should be used when it is taken in combination with other centrally-acting drugs or alcohol).

No products indexed under this heading.

Methamphetamine Hydrochloride (Given the primary CNS effects of asenapine, caution should be used when it is taken in combination with other centrally-acting drugs or alcohol).

No products indexed under this heading.

Methicillin Sodium (The use of asenapine should be avoided in combination with other drugs known to prolong the QTc interval, including antibiotics (eg, gatifloxacin, moxifloxacin)).

No products indexed under this heading.

Methohexital Sodium (Given the primary CNS effects of asenapine, caution should be used when it is taken in combination with other centrally-acting drugs or alcohol).

No products indexed under this heading.

Methotrimeprazine (The use of asenapine should be avoided in combination with other drugs known to prolong the QTc interval, including antipsychotic medications (eg, ziprasidone, chlorpromazine, thioridazine)).

No products indexed under this heading.

Methoxyflurane (Given the primary CNS effects of asenapine, caution should be used when it is taken in combination with other centrally-acting drugs or alcohol).

No products indexed under this heading.

Methoxyphenamine (Asenapine should be co-administered cautiously with drugs that are both substrates and inhibitors for CYP2D6).

No products indexed under this heading.

Methyclothiazide (Because of its α1-adrenergic antagonism with potential for inducing hypotension, asenapine may enhance the effects of certain antihypertensive agents).

No products indexed under this heading.

Methyldopa (Because of its α1-adrenergic antagonism with potential for inducing hypotension, asenapine may enhance the effects of certain antihypertensive agents).

No products indexed under this heading.

Methyldopate Hydrochloride (Because of its α1-adrenergic antagonism with potential for inducing hypotension, asenapine may enhance the effects of certain antihypertensive agents).

No products indexed under this heading.

Methylphenidate (Given the primary CNS effects of asenapine, caution should be used when it is taken in combination with other centrally-acting drugs or alcohol). Products include:

Methylphenidate Hydrochloride (Given the primary CNS effects of asenapine, caution should be used when it is taken in combination with other centrally-acting drugs or alcohol). Products include:

Metolazone (Because of its α1-adrenergic antagonism with potential for inducing hypotension, asenapine may enhance the effects of certain antihypertensive agents).

No products indexed under this heading.

Metoprolol Succinate (Because of its α1-adrenergic antagonism with potential for inducing hypotension, asenapine may enhance the effects of certain antihypertensive agents). Products include:

Metoprolol Tartrate (Because of its α1-adrenergic antagonism with potential for inducing hypotension, asenapine may enhance the effects of certain antihypertensive agents).

No products indexed under this heading.

Metyrosine (Because of its α1-adrenergic antagonism with potential for inducing hypotension, asenapine may enhance the effects of certain antihypertensive agents).

No products indexed under this heading.

Mexiletine Hydrochloride (The use of asenapine should be avoided in combination with other drugs known to prolong the QTc interval).

No products indexed under this heading.

Mezlocillin Sodium (The use of asenapine should be avoided in combination with other drugs known to prolong the QTc interval, including antibiotics (eg, gatifloxacin, moxifloxacin)).

No products indexed under this heading.

Mibefradil Dihydrochloride (Because of its α1-adrenergic antagonism with potential for inducing hypotension, asenapine may enhance the effects of certain antihypertensive agents).

No products indexed under this heading.

Midazolam Hydrochloride (The use of asenapine should be avoided in combination with other drugs known to prolong the QTc interval).

No products indexed under this heading.

Minocycline Hydrochloride (The use of asenapine should be avoided in combination with other drugs known to prolong the QTc interval, including antibiotics (eg, gatifloxacin, moxifloxacin)). Products include:

Minoxidil (Because of its α1-adrenergic antagonism with potential for inducing hypotension, asenapine may enhance the effects of certain antihypertensive agents).

No products indexed under this heading.

Mirtazapine (Asenapine should be co-administered cautiously with drugs that are both substrates and inhibitors for CYP2D6). Products include:

Moclobemide (Asenapine should be co-administered cautiously with drugs that are both substrates and inhibitors for CYP2D6).

No products indexed under this heading.

Moexipril Hydrochloride (Because of its α1-adrenergic antagonism with potential for inducing hypotension, asenapine may enhance the effects of certain antihypertensive agents).

No products indexed under this heading.

Molindone Hydrochloride (The use of asenapine should be avoided in combination with other drugs known to pro-

long the QTc interval, including antipsychotic medications (eg, ziprasidone, chlorpromazine, thioridazine)). Products include:

Moricizine Hydrochloride (The use of asenapine should be avoided in combination with other drugs known to prolong the QTc interval, including Class 1A antiarrhythmics (eg, quinidine, procainamide)).

No products indexed under this heading.

Morphine Sulfate (Given the primary CNS effects of asenapine, caution should be used when it is taken in combination with other centrally-acting drugs or alcohol). Products include:

Moxifloxacin Hydrochloride (The use of asenapine should be avoided in combination with other drugs known to prolong the QTc interval, including antibiotics (eg, moxifloxacin)). Products include:

Nadolol (Because of its α1-adrenergic antagonism with potential for inducing hypotension, asenapine may enhance the effects of certain antihypertensive agents). Products include:

Nafcillin Sodium (The use of asenapine should be avoided in combination with other drugs known to prolong the QTc interval, including antibiotics (eg, gatifloxacin, moxifloxacin)).

No products indexed under this heading.

Nebivolol (Because of its α1-adrenergic antagonism with potential for inducing hypotension, asenapine may enhance the effects of certain antihypertensive agents). Products include:

Nelfinavir Mesylate (Asenapine should be co-administered cautiously with drugs that are both substrates and inhibitors for CYP2D6).

No products indexed under this heading.

Nicardipine Hydrochloride (Because of its α1-adrenergic antagonism with potential for inducing hypotension, asenapine may enhance the effects of certain antihypertensive agents).

No products indexed under this heading.

Nifedipine (Because of its α1-adrenergic antagonism with potential for inducing hypotension, asenapine may enhance the effects of certain antihypertensive agents).

No products indexed under this heading.

Nisoldipine (Because of its α1-adrenergic antagonism with potential for inducing hypotension, asenapine may enhance the effects of certain antihypertensive agents).

No products indexed under this heading.

Nitroglycerin (Because of its α1-adrenergic antagonism with potential for inducing hypotension, asenapine may enhance the effects of certain antihypertensive agents). Products include:

Norfloxacin (The use of asenapine should be avoided in combination with other drugs known to prolong the QTc interval, including antibiotics (eg, gatifloxacin, moxifloxacin)). Products include:

Nortriptyline Hydrochloride (The use of asenapine should be avoided in combination with other drugs known to prolong the QTc interval).

No products indexed under this heading.

IMPORTANT NOTE: Always consult each drug listing in the patient's regimen for possible interactions.

Ofloxacin (The use of asenapine should be avoided in combination with other drugs known to prolong the QTc interval, including antibiotics (eg, gatifloxacin, moxifloxacin)).

No products indexed under this heading.

Olanzapine (The use of asenapine should be avoided in combination with other drugs known to prolong the QTc interval, including antipsychotic medications (eg, ziprasidone, chlorpromazine, thioridazine)). Products include:

Omeprazole (Asenapine should be co-administered cautiously with drugs that are both substrates and inhibitors for CYP2D6).

No products indexed under this heading.

Ondansetron (Asenapine should be co-administered cautiously with drugs that are both substrates and inhibitors for CYP2D6).

No products indexed under this heading.

Ondansetron Hydrochloride (Asenapine should be co-administered cautiously with drugs that are both substrates and inhibitors for CYP2D6). Products include:

Oxacillin (The use of asenapine should be avoided in combination with other drugs known to prolong the QTc interval, including antibiotics (eg, gatifloxacin, moxifloxacin)).

No products indexed under this heading.

Oxacillin Sodium (The use of asenapine should be avoided in combination with other drugs known to prolong the QTc interval, including antibiotics (eg, gatifloxacin, moxifloxacin)).

No products indexed under this heading.

Oxazepam (The use of asenapine should be avoided in combination with other drugs known to prolong the QTc interval).

No products indexed under this heading.

Oxybutynin Chloride (Appropriate care is advised when prescribing asenapine for patients receiving concomitant medication with anticholinergic activity).

No products indexed under this heading.

Oxycodone Hydrochloride (Given the primary CNS effects of asenapine, caution should be used when it is taken in combination with other centrally-acting drugs or alcohol). Products include:

Oxytetracycline Hydrochloride (The use of asenapine should be avoided in combination with other drugs known to prolong the QTc interval, including antibiotics (eg, gatifloxacin, moxifloxacin)).

No products indexed under this heading.

Paclitaxel (Asenapine should be co-administered cautiously with drugs that are both substrates and inhibitors for CYP2D6).

No products indexed under this heading.

Paliperidone (The use of asenapine should be avoided in combination with other drugs known to prolong the QTc interval, including antipsychotic medications (eg, ziprasidone, chlorpromazine, thioridazine)). Products include:

Paroxetine (Asenapine is cleared primarily through direct glucuronidation by UGT1A4 and oxidative metabolism by cytochrome P450 isoenzymes (predom-

inantly CYP1A2). Co-administration with paroxetine, a CYP2D6 inhibitor and substrate, (20 mg qd for 9 days) with asenapine (5 mg single dose) decreased the C_{max} of asenapine by 13% and the AUC of asenapine by 9%. No dosage adjustment is necessary. In addition, *in vitro* studies indicate that asenapine weakly inhibits CYP2D6. Co-administration of a single 20 mg dose of paroxetine during treatment with 5 mg asenapine twice daily in 15 healthy male subjects resulted in an almost 2-fold increase in paroxetine exposure. Asenapine may enhance the inhibitory effects of paroxetine on its own metabolism).

No products indexed under this heading.

Paroxetine Hydrochloride (Asenapine is cleared primarily through direct glucuronidation by UGT1A4 and oxidative metabolism by cytochrome P450 isoenzymes (predominantly CYP1A2). Co-administration with paroxetine, a CYP2D6 inhibitor and substrate, (20 mg qd for 9 days) with asenapine (5 mg single dose) decreased the C_{max} of asenapine by 13% and the AUC of asenapine by 9%. No dosage adjustment is necessary. In addition, *in vitro* studies indicate that asenapine weakly inhibits CYP2D6. Co-administration of a single 20 mg dose of paroxetine during treatment with 5 mg asenapine twice daily in 15 healthy male subjects resulted in an almost 2-fold increase in paroxetine exposure. Asenapine may enhance the inhibitory effects of paroxetine on its own metabolism). Products include:

Paroxetine Mesylate (Asenapine is cleared primarily through direct glucuronidation by UGT1A4 and oxidative metabolism by cytochrome P450 isoenzymes (predominantly CYP1A2). Co-administration with paroxetine, a CYP2D6 inhibitor and substrate, (20 mg qd for 9 days) with asenapine (5 mg single dose) decreased the C_{max} of asenapine by 13% and the AUC of asenapine by 9%. No dosage adjustment is necessary. In addition, *in vitro* studies indicate that asenapine weakly inhibits CYP2D6. Co-administration of a single 20 mg dose of paroxetine during treatment with 5 mg asenapine twice daily in 15 healthy male subjects resulted in an almost 2-fold increase in paroxetine exposure. Asenapine may enhance the inhibitory effects of paroxetine on its own metabolism).

No products indexed under this heading.

Pemoline (Given the primary CNS effects of asenapine, caution should be used when it is taken in combination with other centrally-acting drugs or alcohol).

No products indexed under this heading.

Penbutolol Sulfate (Because of its α1-adrenergic antagonism with potential for inducing hypotension, asenapine may enhance the effects of certain antihypertensive agents).

No products indexed under this heading.

Penicillin, Potassium Phenoxymethyl (The use of asenapine should be avoided in combination with other drugs known to prolong the QTc interval, including antibiotics (eg, gatifloxacin, moxifloxacin)).

No products indexed under this heading.

Penicillin G Benzathine (The use of asenapine should be avoided in combination with other drugs known to prolong the QTc interval, including antibiotics (eg, gatifloxacin, moxifloxacin)). Products include:

Penicillin G Dibenzylethenediamine (The use of asenapine should be avoided in combination with other drugs known to prolong the QTc interval, including antibiotics (eg, gatifloxacin, moxifloxacin)).

No products indexed under this heading.

Penicillin G Potassium (The use of asenapine should be avoided in combination with other drugs known to prolong the QTc interval, including antibiotics (eg, gatifloxacin, moxifloxacin)).

No products indexed under this heading.

Penicillin G Procaine (The use of asenapine should be avoided in combination with other drugs known to prolong the QTc interval, including antibiotics (eg, gatifloxacin, moxifloxacin)). Products include:

Penicillin G Sodium (The use of asenapine should be avoided in combination with other drugs known to prolong the QTc interval, including antibiotics (eg, gatifloxacin, moxifloxacin)).

No products indexed under this heading.

Penicillin V (The use of asenapine should be avoided in combination with other drugs known to prolong the QTc interval, including antibiotics (eg, gatifloxacin, moxifloxacin)).

No products indexed under this heading.

Penicillin V Potassium (The use of asenapine should be avoided in combination with other drugs known to prolong the QTc interval, including antibiotics (eg, gatifloxacin, moxifloxacin)).

No products indexed under this heading.

Penicillins (The use of asenapine should be avoided in combination with other drugs known to prolong the QTc interval, including antibiotics (eg, gatifloxacin, moxifloxacin)).

No products indexed under this heading.

Pentobarbital Sodium (Given the primary CNS effects of asenapine, caution should be used when it is taken in combination with other centrally-acting drugs or alcohol). Products include:

Perindopril Erbumine (Because of its α1-adrenergic antagonism with potential for inducing hypotension, asenapine may enhance the effects of certain antihypertensive agents).

No products indexed under this heading.

Perphenazine (The use of asenapine should be avoided in combination with other drugs known to prolong the QTc interval, including antipsychotic medications (eg, ziprasidone, chlorpromazine, thioridazine)).

No products indexed under this heading.

Phenelzine Sulfate (The use of asenapine should be avoided in combination with other drugs known to prolong the QTc interval).

No products indexed under this heading.

Phenobarbital (Given the primary CNS effects of asenapine, caution should be used when it is taken in combination with other centrally-acting drugs or alcohol). Products include:

Phenobarbital Sodium (Given the primary CNS effects of asenapine, caution should be used when it is taken in combination with other centrally-acting drugs or alcohol).

No products indexed under this heading.

Phenoxybenzamine Hydrochloride (Because of its α1-adrenergic antagonism with potential for inducing hypotension, asenapine may enhance the effects of certain antihypertensive agents). Products include:

Phentolamine Mesylate (Because of its α1-adrenergic antagonism with potential for inducing hypotension, asenapine may enhance the effects of certain antihypertensive agents).

No products indexed under this heading.

Pimozide (The use of asenapine should be avoided in combination with other drugs known to prolong the QTc interval, including antipsychotic medications (eg, ziprasidone, chlorpromazine, thioridazine)).

No products indexed under this heading.

Pindolol (Because of its α1-adrenergic antagonism with potential for inducing hypotension, asenapine may enhance the effects of certain antihypertensive agents).

No products indexed under this heading.

Piperacillin Sodium (The use of asenapine should be avoided in combination with other drugs known to prolong the QTc interval, including antibiotics (eg, gatifloxacin, moxifloxacin)). Products include:

Polythiazide (Because of its α1-adrenergic antagonism with potential for inducing hypotension, asenapine may enhance the effects of certain antihypertensive agents).

No products indexed under this heading.

Prazepam (The use of asenapine should be avoided in combination with other drugs known to prolong the QTc interval).

No products indexed under this heading.

Prazosin Hydrochloride (Because of its α1-adrenergic antagonism with potential for inducing hypotension, asenapine may enhance the effects of certain antihypertensive agents).

No products indexed under this heading.

Procainamide (The use of asenapine should be avoided in combination with other drugs known to prolong the QTc interval, including Class 1A antiarrhythmics (eg, procainamide)).

No products indexed under this heading.

Procainamide Hydrochloride (The use of asenapine should be avoided in combination with other drugs known to prolong the QTc interval, including Class 1A antiarrhythmics (eg, procainamide)).

No products indexed under this heading.

Prochlorperazine (The use of asenapine should be avoided in combination with other drugs known to prolong the QTc interval, including antipsychotic medications (eg, ziprasidone, chlorpromazine, thioridazine)).

No products indexed under this heading.

Procyclidine Hydrochloride (Appropriate care is advised when prescribing asenapine for patients receiving concomitant medication with anticholinergic activity).

No products indexed under this heading.

Promethazine Hydrochloride (The use of asenapine should be avoided in combination with other drugs known to prolong the QTc interval).

No products indexed under this heading.

Propafenone Hydrochloride (The use of asenapine should be avoided in combination with other drugs known to prolong the QTc interval). Products include:

Propantheline Bromide (Appropriate care is advised when prescribing asenapine for patients receiving concomitant medication with anticholinergic activity).

No products indexed under this heading.

Propofol (Given the primary CNS effects of asenapine, caution should be used when it is taken in combination with other centrally-acting drugs or alcohol).
No products indexed under this heading.

Propoxyphene Hydrochloride (Given the primary CNS effects of asenapine, caution should be used when it is taken in combination with other centrally-acting drugs or alcohol).
No products indexed under this heading.

Propoxyphene Napsylate (Given the primary CNS effects of asenapine, caution should be used when it is taken in combination with other centrally-acting drugs or alcohol).
No products indexed under this heading.

Propranolol Hydrochloride (Because of its α1-adrenergic antagonism with potential for inducing hypotension, asenapine may enhance the effects of certain antihypertensive agents). Products include:

Protriptyline Hydrochloride (The use of asenapine should be avoided in combination with other drugs known to prolong the QTc interval).
No products indexed under this heading.

Quazepam (Given the primary CNS effects of asenapine, caution should be used when it is taken in combination with other centrally-acting drugs or alcohol).
No products indexed under this heading.

Quetiapine Fumarate (The use of asenapine should be avoided in combination with other drugs known to prolong the QTc interval, including antipsychotic medications (eg, ziprasidone, chlorpromazine, thioridazine)). Products include:

Quinacrine Hydrochloride (Asenapine should be co-administered cautiously with drugs that are both substrates and inhibitors for CYP2D6).
No products indexed under this heading.

Quinapril Hydrochloride (Because of its α1-adrenergic antagonism with potential for inducing hypotension, asenapine may enhance the effects of certain antihypertensive agents).
No products indexed under this heading.

Quinidine (The use of asenapine should be avoided in combination with other drugs known to prolong the QTc interval including Class 1A antiarrhythmics (eg, quinidine)).
No products indexed under this heading.

Quinidine Gluconate (The use of asenapine should be avoided in combination with other drugs known to prolong the QTc interval including Class 1A antiarrhythmics (eg, quinidine)).
No products indexed under this heading.

Quinidine Hydrochloride (The use of asenapine should be avoided in combination with other drugs known to prolong the QTc interval including Class 1A antiarrhythmics (eg, quinidine)).
No products indexed under this heading.

Quinidine Polygalacturonate (The use of asenapine should be avoided in combination with other drugs known to prolong the QTc interval including Class 1A antiarrhythmics (eg, quinidine)).
No products indexed under this heading.

Quinidine Sulfate (The use of asenapine should be avoided in combination with other drugs known to prolong the QTc interval including Class 1A antiarrhythmics (eg, quinidine)).
No products indexed under this heading.

Ramipril (Because of its α1-adrenergic antagonism with potential for inducing hypotension, asenapine may enhance the effects of certain antihypertensive agents).
No products indexed under this heading.

Ranitidine Bismuth Citrate (Asenapine should be co-administered cautiously with drugs that are both substrates and inhibitors for CYP2D6).
No products indexed under this heading.

Ranitidine Hydrochloride (Asenapine should be co-administered cautiously with drugs that are both substrates and inhibitors for CYP2D6). Products include:

Rauwolfia Serpentina (Because of its α1-adrenergic antagonism with potential for inducing hypotension, asenapine may enhance the effects of certain antihypertensive agents).
No products indexed under this heading.

Remifentanil Hydrochloride (Given the primary CNS effects of asenapine, caution should be used when it is taken in combination with other centrally-acting drugs or alcohol).
No products indexed under this heading.

Rescinnamine (Because of its α1-adrenergic antagonism with potential for inducing hypotension, asenapine may enhance the effects of certain antihypertensive agents).
No products indexed under this heading.

Reserpine (Because of its α1-adrenergic antagonism with potential for inducing hypotension, asenapine may enhance the effects of certain antihypertensive agents).
No products indexed under this heading.

Risperidone (The use of asenapine should be avoided in combination with other drugs known to prolong the QTc interval, including antipsychotic medications (eg, ziprasidone, chlorpromazine, thioridazine)). Products include:

Ritonavir (Asenapine should be co-administered cautiously with drugs that are both substrates and inhibitors for CYP2D6). Products include:

Scopolamine (Appropriate care is advised when prescribing asenapine for patients receiving concomitant medication with anticholinergic activity). Products include:

Scopolamine Hydrobromide (Appropriate care is advised when prescribing asenapine for patients receiving concomitant medication with anticholinergic activity). Products include:

Secobarbital Sodium (Given the primary CNS effects of asenapine, caution should be used when it is taken in combination with other centrally-acting drugs or alcohol).
No products indexed under this heading.

Sertraline Hydrochloride (Asenapine should be co-administered cautiously with drugs that are both substrates and inhibitors for CYP2D6).
No products indexed under this heading.

Sevoflurane (Given the primary CNS effects of asenapine, caution should be used when it is taken in combination with other centrally-acting drugs or alcohol). Products include:

Sildenafil Citrate (Asenapine should be co-administered cautiously with drugs that are both substrates and inhibitors for CYP2D6).
No products indexed under this heading.

Sodium Cloxacillin Monohydrate (The use of asenapine should be avoided in combination with other drugs known to prolong the QTc interval, including antibiotics (eg, gatifloxacin, moxifloxacin)).
No products indexed under this heading.

Sodium Nitroprusside (Because of its α1-adrenergic antagonism with potential for inducing hypotension, asenapine may enhance the effects of certain antihypertensive agents).
No products indexed under this heading.

Sodium Oxybate (Given the primary CNS effects of asenapine, caution should be used when it is taken in combination with other centrally-acting drugs or alcohol).
No products indexed under this heading.

Sotalol Hydrochloride (The use of asenapine should be avoided in combination with other drugs known to prolong the QTc interval, including Class 3 antiarrhythmics (eg, sotalol)).
No products indexed under this heading.

Sparfloxacin (The use of asenapine should be avoided in combination with other drugs known to prolong the QTc interval, including antibiotics (eg, gatifloxacin, moxifloxacin)).
No products indexed under this heading.

Spirapril Hydrochloride (Because of its α1-adrenergic antagonism with potential for inducing hypotension, asenapine may enhance the effects of certain antihypertensive agents).
No products indexed under this heading.

Streptomycin Sulfate (The use of asenapine should be avoided in combination with other drugs known to prolong the QTc interval, including antibiotics (eg, gatifloxacin, moxifloxacin)).
No products indexed under this heading.

Sufentanil Citrate (Given the primary CNS effects of asenapine, caution should be used when it is taken in combination with other centrally-acting drugs or alcohol).
No products indexed under this heading.

Sulfamethizole (The use of asenapine should be avoided in combination with other drugs known to prolong the QTc interval, including antibiotics (eg, gatifloxacin, moxifloxacin)).
No products indexed under this heading.

Sulfamethoxazole (The use of asenapine should be avoided in combination with other drugs known to prolong the QTc interval, including antibiotics (eg, gatifloxacin, moxifloxacin)).
No products indexed under this heading.

Sulfisoxazole Acetyl (The use of asenapine should be avoided in combination with other drugs known to prolong the QTc interval, including antibiotics (eg, gatifloxacin, moxifloxacin)).
No products indexed under this heading.

Sulfisoxazole Diolamine (The use of asenapine should be avoided in combination with other drugs known to prolong the QTc interval, including antibiotics (eg, gatifloxacin, moxifloxacin)).
No products indexed under this heading.

Tamoxifen Citrate (Asenapine should be co-administered cautiously with drugs that are both substrates and inhibitors for CYP2D6).
No products indexed under this heading.

Telmisartan (Because of its α1-adrenergic antagonism with potential for inducing hypotension, asenapine may enhance the effects of certain antihypertensive agents). Products include:

Temazepam (Given the primary CNS effects of asenapine, caution should be used when it is taken in combination with other centrally-acting drugs or alcohol).
No products indexed under this heading.

Teniposide (Asenapine should be co-administered cautiously with drugs that are both substrates and inhibitors for CYP2D6).
No products indexed under this heading.

Terazosin Hydrochloride (Because of its α1-adrenergic antagonism with potential for inducing hypotension, asenapine may enhance the effects of certain antihypertensive agents).
No products indexed under this heading.

Terbinafine Hydrochloride (Asenapine should be co-administered cautiously with drugs that are both substrates and inhibitors for CYP2D6).
No products indexed under this heading.

Testosterone (Asenapine should be co-administered cautiously with drugs that are both substrates and inhibitors for CYP2D6). Products include:

Testosterone Cypionate (Asenapine should be co-administered cautiously with drugs that are both substrates and inhibitors for CYP2D6).
No products indexed under this heading.

Testosterone Enanthate (Asenapine should be co-administered cautiously with drugs that are both substrates and inhibitors for CYP2D6). Products include:

Testosterone Propionate (Asenapine should be co-administered cautiously with drugs that are both substrates and inhibitors for CYP2D6).
No products indexed under this heading.

Tetracycline Hydrochloride (The use of asenapine should be avoided in combination with other drugs known to prolong the QTc interval, including antibiotics (eg, gatifloxacin, moxifloxacin)). Products include:

Thiamylal Sodium (Given the primary CNS effects of asenapine, caution should be used when it is taken in combination with other centrally-acting drugs or alcohol).
No products indexed under this heading.

Thioridazine (The use of asenapine should be avoided in combination with other drugs known to prolong the QTc interval, including antipsychotic medications (eg, thioridazine)).
No products indexed under this heading.

Thioridazine Hydrochloride (The use of asenapine should be avoided in combination with other drugs known to prolong the QTc interval, including antipsychotic medications (eg, thioridazine)). Products include:

Thiothixene (The use of asenapine should be avoided in combination with other drugs known to prolong the QTc interval, including antipsychotic medications (eg, ziprasidone, chlorpromazine, thioridazine)). Products include:

Ticarcillin Disodium (The use of asenapine should be avoided in combination with other drugs known to prolong the QTc interval, including antibiotics (eg, gatifloxacin, moxifloxacin)). Products include:

Timolol Maleate (Because of its α1-adrenergic antagonism with potential for inducing hypotension, asenapine

IMPORTANT NOTE: Always consult each drug listing in the patient's regimen for possible interactions.

may enhance the effects of certain antihypertensive agents). Products include:

Tobramycin (The use of asenapine should be avoided in combination with other drugs known to prolong the QTc interval, including antibiotics (eg, gatifloxacin, moxifloxacin)). Products include:

Tobramycin Sulfate (The use of asenapine should be avoided in combination with other drugs known to prolong the QTc interval, including antibiotics (eg, gatifloxacin, moxifloxacin)).
No products indexed under this heading.

Tocainide Hydrochloride (The use of asenapine should be avoided in combination with other drugs known to prolong the QTc interval).
No products indexed under this heading.

Tolterodine Tartrate (Appropriate care is advised when prescribing asenapine for patients receiving concomitant medication with anticholinergic activity).
No products indexed under this heading.

Torsemide (Because of its α1-adrenergic antagonism with potential for inducing hypotension, asenapine may enhance the effects of certain antihypertensive agents).
No products indexed under this heading.

Tramadol Hydrochloride (Asenapine should be co-administered cautiously with drugs that are both substrates and inhibitors for CYP2D6). Products include:

Trandolapril (Because of its α1-adrenergic antagonism with potential for inducing hypotension, asenapine may enhance the effects of certain antihypertensive agents). Products include:

Tranylcypromine Sulfate (The use of asenapine should be avoided in combination with other drugs known to prolong the QTc interval). Products include:

Trazodone Hydrochloride (Asenapine should be co-administered cautiously with drugs that are both substrates and inhibitors for CYP2D6).
No products indexed under this heading.

Triazolam (Given the primary CNS effects of asenapine, caution should be used when it is taken in combination with other centrally-acting drugs or alcohol).
No products indexed under this heading.

Tridihexethyl Chloride (Appropriate care is advised when prescribing asenapine for patients receiving concomitant medication with anticholinergic activity).
No products indexed under this heading.

Trifluoperazine Hydrochloride (The use of asenapine should be avoided in combination with other drugs known to prolong the QTc interval, including antipsychotic medications (eg, ziprasidone, chlorpromazine, thioridazine)).
No products indexed under this heading.

Trihexyphenidyl Hydrochloride (Appropriate care is advised when prescribing asenapine for patients receiving concomitant medication with anticholinergic activity).
No products indexed under this heading.

Trimethaphan Camsylate (Because of its α1-adrenergic antagonism with potential for inducing hypotension, asenapine may enhance the effects of certain antihypertensive agents).
No products indexed under this heading.

Trimipramine Maleate (The use of asenapine should be avoided in combination with other drugs known to prolong the QTc interval.
No products indexed under this heading.

Troleandomycin (The use of asenapine should be avoided in combination with other drugs known to prolong the QTc interval, including antibiotics (eg, gatifloxacin, moxifloxacin)).
No products indexed under this heading.

Trovafloxacin Mesylate (The use of asenapine should be avoided in combination with other drugs known to prolong the QTc interval, including antibiotics (eg, gatifloxacin, moxifloxacin)).
No products indexed under this heading.

Valproate Sodium (Asenapine is cleared primarily through direct glucuronidation by UGT1A4 and oxidative metabolism by cytochrome P450 isoenzymes (predominantly CYP1A2). Co-administration of valproate (500 mg bid for 9 days), a UGT1A4 inhibitor, with asenapine (5 mg single dose) increased the C_{max} of asenapine by 2% and decreased the AUC of asenapine by 1%. No asenapine dose adjustment is required).
No products indexed under this heading.

Valproic Acid (Asenapine is cleared primarily through direct glucuronidation by UGT1A4 and oxidative metabolism by cytochrome P450 isoenzymes (predominantly CYP1A2). Co-administration of valproate (500 mg bid for 9 days), a UGT1A4 inhibitor, with asenapine (5 mg single dose) increased the C_{max} of asenapine by 2% and decreased the AUC of asenapine by 1%. No asenapine dose adjustment is required).
No products indexed under this heading.

Valsartan (Because of its α1-adrenergic antagonism with potential for inducing hypotension, asenapine may enhance the effects of certain antihypertensive agents). Products include:

Vardenafil Hydrochloride (Asenapine should be co-administered cautiously with drugs that are both substrates and inhibitors for CYP2D6). Products include:

Venlafaxine Hydrochloride (Asenapine should be co-administered cautiously with drugs that are both substrates and inhibitors for CYP2D6). Products include:

Verapamil Hydrochloride (Because of its α1-adrenergic antagonism with potential for inducing hypotension, asenapine may enhance the effects of certain antihypertensive agents). Products include:

Vinblastine Sulfate (Asenapine should be co-administered cautiously with drugs that are both substrates and inhibitors for CYP2D6).
No products indexed under this heading.

Water, Sterile (In clinical trials establishing the efficacy and safety of asenapine, patients were instructed to avoid drinking for 10 minutes following sublingual dosing. The effect of water administration following 10 mg sublingual asenapine dosing was studied at different time points of 2, 5, 10, and 30

minutes in 15 healthy male subjects. The exposure of asenapine following administration of water 10 minutes after sublingual dosing was equivalent to that which water was administered 30 minutes after dosing. Reduced exposure to asenapine was observed following water administration at 2 minutes (19% decrease) and 5 minutes (10% decrease). Patients should be instructed to not eat or drink for 10 minutes after administration).
No products indexed under this heading.

Zaleplon (Given the primary CNS effects of asenapine, caution should be used when it is taken in combination with other centrally-acting drugs or alcohol).
No products indexed under this heading.

Ziprasidone Hydrochloride (The use of asenapine should be avoided in combination with other drugs known to prolong the QTc interval, including antipsychotic medications (eg, ziprasidone)). Products include:

Ziprasidone Mesylate (The use of asenapine should be avoided in combination with other drugs known to prolong the QTc interval, including antipsychotic medications (eg, ziprasidone)). Products include:

Zolpidem Tartrate (Given the primary CNS effects of asenapine, caution should be used when it is taken in combination with other centrally-acting drugs or alcohol). Products include:

Zonisamide (Asenapine should be co-administered cautiously with drugs that are both substrates and inhibitors for CYP2D6). Products include:

Food Interactions

Alcohol (Given the primary CNS effects of asenapine, caution should be used when it is taken in combination with other centrally-acting drugs or alcohol).

Beer, reduced-alcohol (Given the primary CNS effects of asenapine, caution should be used when it is taken in combination with other centrally-acting drugs or alcohol).

Beer, unspecified (Given the primary CNS effects of asenapine, caution should be used when it is taken in combination with other centrally-acting drugs or alcohol).

Food, unspecified (A crossover study in 26 healthy male subjects was performed to evaluate the effect of food on the pharmacokinetics of a single 5 mg dose of asenapine. Consumption of food immediately prior to sublingual administration decreased asenapine exposure by 20%; consumption of food 4 hours after sublingual administration decreased asenapine exposure by about 10%. These effects are probably due to increased hepatic blood flow. Patients should be instructed to not eat or drink for 10 minutes after administration of asenapine).

Meal, unspecified (A crossover study in 26 healthy male subjects was performed to evaluate the effect of food on the pharmacokinetics of a single 5 mg dose of asenapine. Consumption of food immediately prior to sublingual administration decreased asenapine exposure by 20%; consumption of food 4 hours after sublingual administration decreased asenapine exposure by about 10%. These effects are probably due to increased hepatic blood flow. Patients should be instructed to not eat or drink

for 10 minutes after administration of asenapine).

Wine, Chianti (Given the primary CNS effects of asenapine, caution should be used when it is taken in combination with other centrally-acting drugs or alcohol).

Wine, Red (Given the primary CNS effects of asenapine, caution should be used when it is taken in combination with other centrally-acting drugs or alcohol).

Wine, unspecified (Given the primary CNS effects of asenapine, caution should be used when it is taken in combination with other centrally-acting drugs or alcohol).

Wine products (Given the primary CNS effects of asenapine, caution should be used when it is taken in combination with other centrally-acting drugs or alcohol).

SARAPIN VIALS

None cited in PDR database.

SAVELLA TABLETS

May interact with 5HT1-receptor agonists, alcohols, anticoagulants, antipsychotic agents, aspirin-acetylsalicylic acid, centrally-acting drugs, diuretics, dopamine antagonists, epinephrine-containing products, lithium preparations, monoamine oxidase inhibitors, non-steroidal anti-inflammatory agents, selective serotonin reuptake inhibitors, serotoninergic agents, triptans, and certain other agents. Compounds in these categories include:

Alfentanil Hydrochloride (Given the primary central nervous system effects of milnacipran hydrochloride, caution should be used when it is taken in combination with other centrally acting drugs, including those with a similar mechanism of action).
No products indexed under this heading.

Almotriptan Malate (The development of a potentially life-threatening serotonin syndrome or Neuroleptic Malignant Syndrome (NMS)-like reactions have been reported with SNRIs and SSRIs alone, including milnacipran hydrochloride, but particularly with concomitant use of serotonergic drugs (including triptans)). Products include:

Alprazolam (Given the primary central nervous system effects of milnacipran hydrochloride, caution should be used when it is taken in combination with other centrally acting drugs, including those with a similar mechanism of action).
No products indexed under this heading.

Amiloride Hydrochloride (Hyponatremia may occur as a result of treatment with SSRIs and SNRIs, including milnacipran. Elderly patients may be at greater risk of developing hyponatremia with SNRIs, SSRIs, or milnacipran. Also, patients taking diuretics or who are otherwise volume-depleted may be at greater risk. Discontinuation of milnacipran should be considered in patients with symptomatic hyponatremia).
No products indexed under this heading.

Amphetamine Aspartate (Given the primary central nervous system effects of milnacipran hydrochloride, caution should be used when it is taken in combination with other centrally acting drugs, including those with a similar mechanism of action).
No products indexed under this heading.

1695 Interactions Index Savella

Amphetamine Aspartate Monohydrate (Given the primary central nervous system effects of milnacipran hydrochloride, caution should be used when it is taken in combination with other centrally acting drugs, including those with a similar mechanism of action).
No products indexed under this heading.

Amphetamine Resins (Given the primary central nervous system effects of milnacipran hydrochloride, caution should be used when it is taken in combination with other centrally acting drugs, including those with a similar mechanism of action).
No products indexed under this heading.

Amphetamine Sulfate (Given the primary central nervous system effects of milnacipran hydrochloride, caution should be used when it is taken in combination with other centrally acting drugs, including those with a similar mechanism of action).
No products indexed under this heading.

Anisindione (Concomitant use of other anticoagulants with milnacipran hydrochloride may add to the risk of bleeding events of SSRIs and SNRIs).
No products indexed under this heading.

Aprobarbital (Given the primary central nervous system effects of milnacipran hydrochloride, caution should be used when it is taken in combination with other centrally acting drugs, including those with a similar mechanism of action).
No products indexed under this heading.

Ardeparin Sodium (Concomitant use of other anticoagulants with milnacipran hydrochloride may add to the risk of bleeding events of SSRIs and SNRIs).
No products indexed under this heading.

Aripiprazole (The development of a potentially life-threatening serotonin syndrome or Neuroleptic Malignant Syndrome (NMS)-like reactions have been reported with SNRIs and SSRIs alone, including milnacipran hydrochloride, particularly with concomitant use of antipsychotics).
No products indexed under this heading.

Aspirin (Concomitant use of aspirin with milnacipran hydrochloride may add to the risk of bleeding events of SSRIs and SNRIs). Products include:
Aggrenox 880
Bayer Aspirin 829
Percodan 1124
St. Joseph Aspirin 2045

Aspirin, Enteric Coated (Concomitant use of aspirin with milnacipran hydrochloride may add to the risk of bleeding events of SSRIs and SNRIs).
No products indexed under this heading.

Aspirin Buffered (Concomitant use of aspirin with milnacipran hydrochloride may add to the risk of bleeding events of SSRIs and SNRIs).
No products indexed under this heading.

Bendroflumethiazide (Hyponatremia may occur as a result of treatment with SSRIs and SNRIs, including milnacipran. Elderly patients may be at greater risk of developing hyponatremia with SNRIs, SSRIs, or milnacipran. Also, patients taking diuretics or who are otherwise volume-depleted may be at greater risk. Discontinuation of milnacipran should be considered in patients with symptomatic hyponatremia).
No products indexed under this heading.

Bumetanide (Hyponatremia may occur as a result of treatment with SSRIs and SNRIs, including milnacipran. Elderly patients may be at greater risk of developing hyponatremia with SNRIs, SSRIs, or milnacipran. Also, patients taking diuretics or who are otherwise volume-depleted may be at greater risk. Discontinuation of milnacipran should be considered in patients with symptomatic hyponatremia).
No products indexed under this heading.

Buprenorphine Hydrochloride (Given the primary central nervous system effects of milnacipran hydrochloride, caution should be used when it is taken in combination with other centrally acting drugs, including those with a similar mechanism of action).
No products indexed under this heading.

Buspirone Hydrochloride (Given the primary central nervous system effects of milnacipran hydrochloride, caution should be used when it is taken in combination with other centrally acting drugs, including those with a similar mechanism of action).
No products indexed under this heading.

Butabarbital (Given the primary central nervous system effects of milnacipran hydrochloride, caution should be used when it is taken in combination with other centrally acting drugs, including those with a similar mechanism of action).
No products indexed under this heading.

Butalbital (Given the primary central nervous system effects of milnacipran hydrochloride, caution should be used when it is taken in combination with other centrally acting drugs, including those with a similar mechanism of action).
No products indexed under this heading.

Celecoxib (Concomitant use of nonsteroidal anti-inflammatory drugs with milnacipran hydrochloride may add to the risk of bleeding events of SSRIs and SNRIs). Products include:
Celebrex 3272

Chlordiazepoxide (Given the primary central nervous system effects of milnacipran hydrochloride, caution should be used when it is taken in combination with other centrally acting drugs, including those with a similar mechanism of action).
No products indexed under this heading.

Chlordiazepoxide Hydrochloride (Given the primary central nervous system effects of milnacipran hydrochloride, caution should be used when it is taken in combination with other centrally acting drugs, including those with a similar mechanism of action).
No products indexed under this heading.

Chlorothiazide (Hyponatremia may occur as a result of treatment with SSRIs and SNRIs, including milnacipran. Elderly patients may be at greater risk of developing hyponatremia with SNRIs, SSRIs, or milnacipran. Also, patients taking diuretics or who are otherwise volume-depleted may be at greater risk. Discontinuation of milnacipran should be considered in patients with symptomatic hyponatremia).
No products indexed under this heading.

Chlorothiazide Sodium (Hyponatremia may occur as a result of treatment with SSRIs and SNRIs, including milnacipran. Elderly patients may be at greater risk of developing hyponatremia with SNRIs, SSRIs, or milnacipran. Also, patients taking diuretics or who are otherwise volume-depleted may be at greater risk. Discontinuation of milnacipran should be considered in patients with symptomatic hyponatremia). Products include:
Diuril Intravenous 2009

Chlorpromazine (The development of a potentially life-threatening serotonin syndrome or Neuroleptic Malignant Syndrome (NMS)-like reactions have been reported with SNRIs and SSRIs alone, including milnacipran hydrochloride, particularly with concomitant use of antipsychotics).
No products indexed under this heading.

Chlorpromazine Hydrochloride (The development of a potentially life-threatening serotonin syndrome or Neuroleptic Malignant Syndrome (NMS)-like reactions have been reported with SNRIs and SSRIs alone, including milnacipran hydrochloride, particularly with concomitant use of antipsychotics).
No products indexed under this heading.

Chlorprothixene (The development of a potentially life-threatening serotonin syndrome or Neuroleptic Malignant Syndrome (NMS)-like reactions have been reported with SNRIs and SSRIs alone, including milnacipran hydrochloride, particularly with concomitant use of antipsychotics).
No products indexed under this heading.

Chlorprothixene Hydrochloride (The development of a potentially life-threatening serotonin syndrome or Neuroleptic Malignant Syndrome (NMS)-like reactions have been reported with SNRIs and SSRIs alone, including milnacipran hydrochloride, particularly with concomitant use of antipsychotics).
No products indexed under this heading.

Chlorprothixene Lactate (The development of a potentially life-threatening serotonin syndrome or Neuroleptic Malignant Syndrome (NMS)-like reactions have been reported with SNRIs and SSRIs alone, including milnacipran hydrochloride, particularly with concomitant use of antipsychotics).
No products indexed under this heading.

Chlorthalidone (Hyponatremia may occur as a result of treatment with SSRIs and SNRIs, including milnacipran. Elderly patients may be at greater risk of developing hyponatremia with SNRIs, SSRIs, or milnacipran. Also, patients taking diuretics or who are otherwise volume-depleted may be at greater risk. Discontinuation of milnacipran should be considered in patients with symptomatic hyponatremia). Products include:
Clorpres 2344

Citalopram Hydrobromide (The development of a potentially life-threatening serotonin syndrome or Neuroleptic Malignant Syndrome (NMS)-like reactions have been reported with SNRIs and SSRIs alone, including milnacipran hydrochloride, but particularly with concomitant use of serotonergic drugs (including triptans)). Products include:
Celexa 1153

Clomipramine Hydrochloride (An increase in euphoria and postural hypotension was observed in patients who switched from clomipramine to milnacipran hydrochloride. Switching from clomipramine (75 mg once a day) to milnacipran hydrochloride (100 mg/day) without a washout period did not lead to clinically significant changes in the pharmacokinetics of milnacipran hydrochloride. Monitoring of patients during treatment switch is recommended).
No products indexed under this heading.

Clonidine (Co-administration of clonidine with milnacipran hydrochloride may inhibit clonidine's anti-hypertensive effect). Products include:
Catapres-TTS 884

Clonidine Hydrochloride (Co-administration of clonidine with milnacipran hydrochloride may inhibit clonidine's anti-hypertensive effect). Products include:
Clorpres 2344

Clorazepate Dipotassium (Given the primary central nervous system effects of milnacipran hydrochloride, caution should be used when it is taken in combination with other centrally acting drugs, including those with a similar mechanism of action).
No products indexed under this heading.

Clozapine (The development of a potentially life-threatening serotonin syndrome or Neuroleptic Malignant Syndrome (NMS)-like reactions have been reported with SNRIs and SSRIs alone, including milnacipran hydrochloride, particularly with concomitant use of antipsychotics).
No products indexed under this heading.

Codeine Phosphate (Given the primary central nervous system effects of milnacipran hydrochloride, caution should be used when it is taken in combination with other centrally acting drugs, including those with a similar mechanism of action). Products include:
Tylenol with Codeine 2691

Codeine Sulfate (Given the primary central nervous system effects of milnacipran hydrochloride, caution should be used when it is taken in combination with other centrally acting drugs, including those with a similar mechanism of action).
No products indexed under this heading.

Dalteparin Sodium (Concomitant use of other anticoagulants with milnacipran hydrochloride may add to the risk of bleeding events of SSRIs and SNRIs). Products include:
Fragmin 1058

Danaparoid Sodium (Concomitant use of other anticoagulants with milnacipran hydrochloride may add to the risk of bleeding events of SSRIs and SNRIs).
No products indexed under this heading.

Desflurane (Given the primary central nervous system effects of milnacipran hydrochloride, caution should be used when it is taken in combination with other centrally acting drugs, including those with a similar mechanism of action).
No products indexed under this heading.

Dexmethylphenidate Hydrochloride (Given the primary central nervous system effects of milnacipran hydrochloride, caution should be used when it is taken in combination with other centrally acting drugs, including those with a similar mechanism of action). Products include:
Focalin XR 2472

Dextroamphetamine (Given the primary central nervous system effects of milnacipran hydrochloride, caution should be used when it is taken in combination with other centrally acting drugs, including those with a similar mechanism of action).
No products indexed under this heading.

Dextroamphetamine Saccharate (Given the primary central nervous system effects of milnacipran hydrochloride, caution should be used when it is taken in combination with other centrally acting drugs, including those with a similar mechanism of action).
No products indexed under this heading.

Dextroamphetamine Sulfate (Given the primary central nervous system effects of milnacipran hydrochloride, caution should be used when it is taken in combination with other centrally acting drugs, including those with a similar mechanism of action). Products include:
Dexedrine 1425

IMPORTANT NOTE: Always consult each drug listing in the patient's regimen for possible interactions.

Savella Interactions Index 1696

Dezocine (Given the primary central nervous system effects of milnacipran hydrochloride, caution should be used when it is taken in combination with other centrally acting drugs, including those with a similar mechanism of action).
No products indexed under this heading.

Diazepam (Given the primary central nervous system effects of milnacipran hydrochloride, caution should be used when it is taken in combination with other centrally acting drugs, including those with a similar mechanism of action). Products include:
Valium Tablets ... 2880

Diclofenac Epolamine (Concomitant use of nonsteroidal anti-inflammatory drugs with milnacipran hydrochloride may add to the risk of bleeding events of SSRIs and SNRIs). Products include:
Flector ... 1839

Diclofenac Potassium (Concomitant use of nonsteroidal anti-inflammatory drugs with milnacipran hydrochloride may add to the risk of bleeding events of SSRIs and SNRIs).
No products indexed under this heading.

Diclofenac Sodium (Concomitant use of nonsteroidal anti-inflammatory drugs with milnacipran hydrochloride may add to the risk of bleeding events of SSRIs and SNRIs).
No products indexed under this heading.

Dicumarol (Concomitant use of other anticoagulants with milnacipran hydrochloride may add to the risk of bleeding events of SSRIs and SNRIs).
No products indexed under this heading.

Digoxin (Use of milnacipran hydrochloride concomitantly with digoxin may be associated with potentiation of adverse hemodynamic effects. Postural hypotension and tachycardia have been reported in combination therapy with intravenously administered digoxin (1 mg). Co-administration of milnacipran hydrochloride and intravenous digoxin should be avoided). Products include:
Lanoxin Injection ... 1546
Lanoxin Injection Pediatric ... 1549
Lanoxin Tablets ... 1553

Droperidol (Given the primary central nervous system effects of milnacipran hydrochloride, caution should be used when it is taken in combination with other centrally acting drugs, including those with a similar mechanism of action).
No products indexed under this heading.

Eletriptan Hydrobromide (The development of a potentially life-threatening serotonin syndrome or Neuroleptic Malignant Syndrome (NMS)-like reactions have been reported with SNRIs and SSRIs alone, including milnacipran hydrochloride, but particularly with concomitant use of serotonergic drugs (including triptans)).
No products indexed under this heading.

Enflurane (Given the primary central nervous system effects of milnacipran hydrochloride, caution should be used when it is taken in combination with other centrally acting drugs, including those with a similar mechanism of action).
No products indexed under this heading.

Enoxaparin Sodium (Concomitant use of other anticoagulants with milnacipran hydrochloride may add to the risk of bleeding events of SSRIs and SNRIs). Products include:
Lovenox ... 3005

Epinephrine (Milnacipran hydrochloride inhibits the reuptake of norepinephrine. Therefore, concomitant use of milnacipran hydrochloride with epinephrine and norepinephrine may be associated with paroxysmal hypertension and possible arrhythmia). Products include:
EpiPen ... 3631
Twinject ... 3268

Epinephrine, Racemic (Milnacipran hydrochloride inhibits the reuptake of norepinephrine. Therefore, concomitant use of milnacipran hydrochloride with epinephrine and norepinephrine may be associated with paroxysmal hypertension and possible arrhythmia).
No products indexed under this heading.

Epinephrine Bitartrate (Milnacipran hydrochloride inhibits the reuptake of norepinephrine. Therefore, concomitant use of milnacipran hydrochloride with epinephrine and norepinephrine may be associated with paroxysmal hypertension and possible arrhythmia).
No products indexed under this heading.

Epinephrine Hydrochloride (Milnacipran hydrochloride inhibits the reuptake of norepinephrine. Therefore, concomitant use of milnacipran hydrochloride with epinephrine and norepinephrine may be associated with paroxysmal hypertension and possible arrhythmia).
No products indexed under this heading.

Escitalopram Oxalate (The development of a potentially life-threatening serotonin syndrome or Neuroleptic Malignant Syndrome (NMS)-like reactions have been reported with SNRIs and SSRIs alone, including milnacipran hydrochloride, but particularly with concomitant use of serotonergic drugs (including triptans)). Products include:
Lexapro Oral Suspension ... 1160
Lexapro Tablets ... 1160

Estazolam (Given the primary central nervous system effects of milnacipran hydrochloride, caution should be used when it is taken in combination with other centrally acting drugs, including those with a similar mechanism of action).
No products indexed under this heading.

Ethacrynic Acid (Hyponatremia may occur as a result of treatment with SSRIs and SNRIs, including milnacipran. Elderly patients may be at greater risk of developing hyponatremia with SNRIs, SSRIs, or milnacipran. Also, patients taking diuretics or who are otherwise volume-depleted may be at greater risk. Discontinuation of milnacipran should be considered in patients with symptomatic hyponatremia).
No products indexed under this heading.

Ethanol (Milnacipran hydrochloride should not be prescribed to patients with substantial alcohol use or evidence of chronic liver disease because it is possible that milnacipran hydrochloride may aggravate pre-existing liver disease).
No products indexed under this heading.

Ethchlorvynol (Given the primary central nervous system effects of milnacipran hydrochloride, caution should be used when it is taken in combination with other centrally acting drugs, including those with a similar mechanism of action).
No products indexed under this heading.

Ethinamate (Given the primary central nervous system effects of milnacipran hydrochloride, caution should be used when it is taken in combination with other centrally acting drugs, including those with a similar mechanism of action).
No products indexed under this heading.

Ethyl Alcohol (Milnacipran hydrochloride should not be prescribed to patients with substantial alcohol use or evidence of chronic liver disease because it is possible that milnacipran hydrochloride may aggravate pre-existing liver disease).
No products indexed under this heading.

Etodolac (Concomitant use of nonsteroidal anti-inflammatory drugs with milnacipran hydrochloride may add to the risk of bleeding events of SSRIs and SNRIs).
No products indexed under this heading.

Fenoprofen Calcium (Concomitant use of nonsteroidal anti-inflammatory drugs with milnacipran hydrochloride may add to the risk of bleeding events of SSRIs and SNRIs).
No products indexed under this heading.

Fentanyl (Given the primary central nervous system effects of milnacipran hydrochloride, caution should be used when it is taken in combination with other centrally acting drugs, including those with a similar mechanism of action). Products include:
Duragesic ... 2604
Fentanyl Transdermal System ... 2346
Onsolis ... 2054

Fentanyl Citrate (Given the primary central nervous system effects of milnacipran hydrochloride, caution should be used when it is taken in combination with other centrally acting drugs, including those with a similar mechanism of action). Products include:
Fentora ... 966

Fluoxetine (Co-administration of milnacipran hydrochloride with other inhibitors of serotonin reuptake may result in hypertension and coronary artery vasoconstriction, through additive serotonergic effects).
No products indexed under this heading.

Fluoxetine Hydrochloride (The development of a potentially life-threatening serotonin syndrome or Neuroleptic Malignant Syndrome (NMS)-like reactions have been reported with SNRIs and SSRIs alone, including milnacipran hydrochloride, but particularly with concomitant use of serotonergic drugs (including triptans)). Products include:
Prozac Weekly ... 1941
Prozac Pulvules ... 1941
Symbyax ... 1965

Fluphenazine Decanoate (The development of a potentially life-threatening serotonin syndrome or Neuroleptic Malignant Syndrome (NMS)-like reactions have been reported with SNRIs and SSRIs alone, including milnacipran hydrochloride, particularly with concomitant use of antipsychotics).
No products indexed under this heading.

Fluphenazine Enanthate (The development of a potentially life-threatening serotonin syndrome or Neuroleptic Malignant Syndrome (NMS)-like reactions have been reported with SNRIs and SSRIs alone, including milnacipran hydrochloride, particularly with concomitant use of antipsychotics).
No products indexed under this heading.

Fluphenazine Hydrochloride (The development of a potentially life-threatening serotonin syndrome or Neuroleptic Malignant Syndrome (NMS)-like reactions have been reported with SNRIs and SSRIs alone, including milnacipran hydrochloride, particularly with concomitant use of antipsychotics).
No products indexed under this heading.

Flurazepam Hydrochloride (Given the primary central nervous system effects of milnacipran hydrochloride, caution should be used when it is taken in combination with other centrally acting drugs, including those with a similar mechanism of action).
No products indexed under this heading.

Flurbiprofen (Concomitant use of nonsteroidal anti-inflammatory drugs with milnacipran hydrochloride may add to the risk of bleeding events of SSRIs and SNRIs).
No products indexed under this heading.

Fluvoxamine (Co-administration of milnacipran hydrochloride with other inhibitors of serotonin reuptake may result in hypertension and coronary artery vasoconstriction, through additive serotonergic effects).
No products indexed under this heading.

Fluvoxamine Maleate (The development of a potentially life-threatening serotonin syndrome or Neuroleptic Malignant Syndrome (NMS)-like reactions have been reported with SNRIs and SSRIs alone, including milnacipran hydrochloride, but particularly with concomitant use of serotonergic drugs (including triptans)).
No products indexed under this heading.

Fondaparinux Sodium (Concomitant use of other anticoagulants with milnacipran hydrochloride may add to the risk of bleeding events of SSRIs and SNRIs). Products include:
Arixtra ... 1320

Frovatriptan Succinate (The development of a potentially life-threatening serotonin syndrome or Neuroleptic Malignant Syndrome (NMS)-like reactions have been reported with SNRIs and SSRIs alone, including milnacipran hydrochloride, but particularly with concomitant use of serotonergic drugs (including triptans)). Products include:
Frova ... 1103

Furosemide (Hyponatremia may occur as a result of treatment with SSRIs and SNRIs, including milnacipran. Elderly patients may be at greater risk of developing hyponatremia with SNRIs, SSRIs, or milnacipran. Also, patients taking diuretics or who are otherwise volume-depleted may be at greater risk. Discontinuation of milnacipran should be considered in patients with symptomatic hyponatremia). Products include:
Furosemide ... 2354

Glutethimide (Given the primary central nervous system effects of milnacipran hydrochloride, caution should be used when it is taken in combination with other centrally acting drugs, including those with a similar mechanism of action).
No products indexed under this heading.

Haloperidol (The development of a potentially life-threatening serotonin syndrome or Neuroleptic Malignant Syndrome (NMS)-like reactions have been reported with SNRIs and SSRIs alone, including milnacipran hydrochloride, particularly with concomitant use of antipsychotics).
No products indexed under this heading.

Haloperidol Decanoate (The development of a potentially life-threatening serotonin syndrome or Neuroleptic Malignant Syndrome (NMS)-like reactions have been reported with SNRIs and SSRIs alone, including milnacipran hydrochloride, particularly with concomitant use of antipsychotics).
No products indexed under this heading.

Haloperidol Lactate (The development of a potentially life-threatening serotonin syndrome or Neuroleptic Malignant Syndrome (NMS)-like reactions have been reported with SNRIs and SSRIs alone, including milnacipran hydrochloride, particularly with concomitant use of antipsychotics).
No products indexed under this heading.

Heparin Calcium (Concomitant use of other anticoagulants with milnacipran hydrochloride may add to the risk of bleeding events of SSRIs and SNRIs).
No products indexed under this heading.

Heparin Sodium (Concomitant use of other anticoagulants with milnacipran hydrochloride may add to the risk of bleeding events of SSRIs and SNRIs).
No products indexed under this heading.

(⊙ Described in PDR® for Ophthalmic Medicines)

Hydrochlorothiazide (Hyponatremia may occur as a result of treatment with SSRIs and SNRIs, including milnacipran. Elderly patients may be at greater risk of developing hyponatremia with SNRIs, SSRIs, or milnacipran. Also, patients taking diuretics or who are otherwise volume-depleted may be at greater risk. Discontinuation of milnacipran should be considered in patients with symptomatic hyponatremia). Products include:

Hydrocodone Bitartrate (Given the primary central nervous system effects of milnacipran hydrochloride, caution should be used when it is taken in combination with other centrally acting drugs, including those with a similar mechanism of action). Products include:

Hydrocodone Polistirex (Given the primary central nervous system effects of milnacipran hydrochloride, caution should be used when it is taken in combination with other centrally acting drugs, including those with a similar mechanism of action). Products include:

Hydroflumethiazide (Hyponatremia may occur as a result of treatment with SSRIs and SNRIs, including milnacipran. Elderly patients may be at greater risk of developing hyponatremia with SNRIs, SSRIs, or milnacipran. Also, patients taking diuretics or who are otherwise volume-depleted may be at greater risk. Discontinuation of milnacipran should be considered in patients with symptomatic hyponatremia).
No products indexed under this heading.

Hydromorphone Hydrochloride (Given the primary central nervous system effects of milnacipran hydrochloride, caution should be used when it is taken in combination with other centrally acting drugs, including those with a similar mechanism of action). Products include:

Hydroxyamphetamine Hydrobromide (Given the primary central nervous system effects of milnacipran hydrochloride, caution should be used when it is taken in combination with other centrally acting drugs, including those with a similar mechanism of action).
No products indexed under this heading.

Hydroxyzine Hydrochloride (Given the primary central nervous system effects of milnacipran hydrochloride, caution should be used when it is taken in combination with other centrally acting drugs, including those with a similar mechanism of action).
No products indexed under this heading.

Ibuprofen (Concomitant use of nonsteroidal anti-inflammatory drugs with milnacipran hydrochloride may add to the risk of bleeding events of SSRIs and SNRIs). Products include:

Indapamide (Hyponatremia may occur as a result of treatment with SSRIs and SNRIs, including milnacipran. Elderly patients may be at greater risk of developing hyponatremia with SNRIs, SSRIs, or milnacipran. Also, patients taking diuretics or who are otherwise volume-depleted may be at greater risk. Discontinuation of milnacipran should be considered in patients with symptomatic hyponatremia). Products include:

Indomethacin (Concomitant use of nonsteroidal anti-inflammatory drugs with milnacipran hydrochloride may add to the risk of bleeding events of SSRIs and SNRIs). Products include:

Indomethacin Sodium Trihydrate (Concomitant use of nonsteroidal anti-inflammatory drugs with milnacipran hydrochloride may add to the risk of bleeding events of SSRIs and SNRIs). Products include:

Isocarboxazid (Concomitant use of milnacipran hydrochloride in patients taking monoamine oxidase inhibitors (MAOIs) is contraindicated. In patients receiving a serotonin reuptake inhibitor in combination with a monoamine oxidase inhibitor (MAOI), there have been reports of serious, sometimes fatal, reactions including hyperthermia, rigidity, myoclonus, autonomic instability with possible rapid fluctuations of vital signs, and mental status changes that include extreme agitation progressing to delirium and coma. It is recommended that milnacipran should not be used in combination with a MAOI, or within 14 days of discontinuing treatment with a MAOI. At least 5 days should be allowed after stopping milnacipran before starting a MAOI). Products include:

Isoflurane (Given the primary central nervous system effects of milnacipran hydrochloride, caution should be used when it is taken in combination with other centrally acting drugs, including those with a similar mechanism of action).
No products indexed under this heading.

Ketamine Hydrochloride (Given the primary central nervous system effects of milnacipran hydrochloride, caution should be used when it is taken in combination with other centrally acting drugs, including those with a similar mechanism of action).
No products indexed under this heading.

Ketoprofen (Concomitant use of nonsteroidal anti-inflammatory drugs with milnacipran hydrochloride may add to the risk of bleeding events of SSRIs and SNRIs).
No products indexed under this heading.

Ketorolac Tromethamine (Concomitant use of nonsteroidal anti-inflammatory drugs with milnacipran hydrochloride may add to the risk of bleeding events of SSRIs and SNRIs). Products include:

Levomethadyl Acetate Hydrochloride (Given the primary central nervous system effects of milnacipran hydrochloride, caution should be used when it is taken in combination with other centrally acting drugs, including those with a similar mechanism of action).
No products indexed under this heading.

Levorphanol Tartrate (Given the primary central nervous system effects of milnacipran hydrochloride, caution should be used when it is taken in combination with other centrally acting drugs, including those with a similar mechanism of action).
No products indexed under this heading.

Lisdexamfetamine Dimesylate (Given the primary central nervous system effects of milnacipran hydrochloride, caution should be used when it is taken in combination with other centrally acting drugs, including those with a similar mechanism of action). Products include:

Lithium (The development of a potentially life-threatening serotonin syndrome or Neuroleptic Malignant Syndrome (NMS)-like reactions have been reported with SNRIs and SSRIs alone, including milnacipran hydrochloride, particularly with concomitant use of antipsychotics).
No products indexed under this heading.

Lithium Carbonate (The development of a potentially life-threatening serotonin syndrome or Neuroleptic Malignant Syndrome (NMS)-like reactions have been reported with SNRIs and SSRIs alone, including milnacipran hydrochloride, particularly with concomitant use of antipsychotics).
No products indexed under this heading.

Lithium Citrate (The development of a potentially life-threatening serotonin syndrome or Neuroleptic Malignant Syndrome (NMS)-like reactions have been reported with SNRIs and SSRIs alone, including milnacipran hydrochloride, particularly with concomitant use of antipsychotics).
No products indexed under this heading.

Lorazepam (Given the primary central nervous system effects of milnacipran hydrochloride, caution should be used when it is taken in combination with other centrally acting drugs, including those with a similar mechanism of action).
No products indexed under this heading.

Low Molecular Weight Heparins (Concomitant use of other anticoagulants with milnacipran hydrochloride may add to the risk of bleeding events of SSRIs and SNRIs).
No products indexed under this heading.

Loxapine Hydrochloride (The development of a potentially life-threatening serotonin syndrome or Neuroleptic Malignant Syndrome (NMS)-like reactions have been reported with SNRIs and SSRIs alone, including milnacipran hydrochloride, particularly with concomitant use of antipsychotics).
No products indexed under this heading.

Loxapine Succinate (The development of a potentially life-threatening serotonin syndrome or Neuroleptic Malignant Syndrome (NMS)-like reactions have been reported with SNRIs and SSRIs alone, including milnacipran hydrochloride, particularly with concomitant use of antipsychotics).
No products indexed under this heading.

Meclofenamate Sodium (Concomitant use of nonsteroidal anti-inflammatory drugs with milnacipran hydrochloride may add to the risk of bleeding events of SSRIs and SNRIs).
No products indexed under this heading.

Mefenamic Acid (Concomitant use of nonsteroidal anti-inflammatory drugs with milnacipran hydrochloride may add to the risk of bleeding events of SSRIs and SNRIs).
No products indexed under this heading.

Meloxicam (Concomitant use of nonsteroidal anti-inflammatory drugs with milnacipran hydrochloride may add to the risk of bleeding events of SSRIs and SNRIs).
No products indexed under this heading.

Meperidine Hydrochloride (Given the primary central nervous system effects of milnacipran hydrochloride, caution should be used when it is taken in combination with other centrally acting drugs, including those with a similar mechanism of action).
No products indexed under this heading.

Mephobarbital (Given the primary central nervous system effects of milnacipran hydrochloride, caution should be used when it is taken in combination with other centrally acting drugs, including those with a similar mechanism of action).
No products indexed under this heading.

Meprobamate (Given the primary central nervous system effects of milnacipran hydrochloride, caution should be used when it is taken in combination with other centrally acting drugs, including those with a similar mechanism of action).
No products indexed under this heading.

Mesoridazine Besylate (The development of a potentially life-threatening serotonin syndrome or Neuroleptic Malignant Syndrome (NMS)-like reactions have been reported with SNRIs and SSRIs alone, including milnacipran hydrochloride, particularly with concomitant use of antipsychotics).
No products indexed under this heading.

Methadone Hydrochloride (Given the primary central nervous system effects of milnacipran hydrochloride, caution should be used when it is taken in combination with other centrally acting drugs, including those with a similar mechanism of action).
No products indexed under this heading.

Methamphetamine Hydrochloride (Given the primary central nervous system effects of milnacipran hydrochloride, caution should be used when it is taken in combination with other centrally acting drugs, including those with a similar mechanism of action).
No products indexed under this heading.

Methohexital Sodium (Given the primary central nervous system effects of milnacipran hydrochloride, caution should be used when it is taken in combination with other centrally acting drugs, including those with a similar mechanism of action).
No products indexed under this heading.

Methotrimeprazine (The development of a potentially life-threatening serotonin syndrome or Neuroleptic Malignant Syndrome (NMS)-like reactions have been reported with SNRIs and SSRIs alone, including milnacipran hydrochloride, particularly with concomitant use of antipsychotics).
No products indexed under this heading.

Methoxyflurane (Given the primary central nervous system effects of milnacipran hydrochloride, caution should be used when it is taken in combination with other centrally acting drugs, including those with a similar mechanism of action).
No products indexed under this heading.

Methyclothiazide (Hyponatremia may occur as a result of treatment with SSRIs and SNRIs, including milnacipran. Elderly patients may be at greater risk of developing hyponatremia with SNRIs, SSRIs, or milnacipran. Also, patients taking diuretics or who are otherwise volume-depleted may be at greater risk. Discontinuation of milnacipran should be considered in patients with symptomatic hyponatremia).
No products indexed under this heading.

IMPORTANT NOTE: Always consult each drug listing in the patient's regimen for possible interactions.

Savella Interactions Index 1698

Methylphenidate (Given the primary central nervous system effects of milnacipran hydrochloride, caution should be used when it is taken in combination with other centrally acting drugs, including those with a similar mechanism of action). Products include:
Daytrana 3283

Methylphenidate Hydrochloride (Given the primary central nervous system effects of milnacipran hydrochloride, caution should be used when it is taken in combination with other centrally acting drugs, including those with a similar mechanism of action). Products include:
Concerta 2598
Metadate CD 3439

Metoclopramide Hydrochloride (The development of a potentially life-threatening serotonin syndrome or Neuroleptic Malignant Syndrome (NMS)-like reactions have been reported with SNRIs and SSRIs alone, including milnacipran hydrochloride, but particularly with concomitant use of other dopamine antagonists). Products include:
Metozolv ODT 2901

Metolazone (Hyponatremia may occur as a result of treatment with SSRIs and SNRIs, including milnacipran. Elderly patients may be at greater risk of developing hyponatremia with SNRIs, SSRIs, or milnacipran. Also, patients taking diuretics or who are otherwise volume-depleted may be at greater risk. Discontinuation of milnacipran should be considered in patients with symptomatic hyponatremia).
No products indexed under this heading.

Midazolam Hydrochloride (Given the primary central nervous system effects of milnacipran hydrochloride, caution should be used when it is taken in combination with other centrally acting drugs, including those with a similar mechanism of action).
No products indexed under this heading.

Moclobemide (Concomitant use of milnacipran hydrochloride in patients taking monoamine oxidase inhibitors (MAOIs) is contraindicated. In patients receiving a serotonin reuptake inhibitor in combination with a monoamine oxidase inhibitor (MAOI), there have been reports of serious, sometimes fatal, reactions including hyperthermia, rigidity, myoclonus, autonomic instability with possible rapid fluctuations of vital signs, and mental status changes that include extreme agitation progressing to delirium and coma. It is recommended that milnacipran should not be used in combination with a MAOI, or within 14 days of discontinuing treatment with a MAOI. At least 5 days should be allowed after stopping milnacipran before starting a MAOI).
No products indexed under this heading.

Molindone Hydrochloride (The development of a potentially life-threatening serotonin syndrome or Neuroleptic Malignant Syndrome (NMS)-like reactions have been reported with SNRIs and SSRIs alone, including milnacipran hydrochloride, particularly with concomitant use of antipsychotics). Products include:
Moban 1108

Morphine Sulfate (Given the primary central nervous system effects of milnacipran hydrochloride, caution should be used when it is taken in combination with other centrally acting drugs, including those with a similar mechanism of action). Products include:
Avinza 1822
Embeda 1831
MS Contin 2803

Nabumetone (Concomitant use of nonsteroidal anti-inflammatory drugs with milnacipran hydrochloride may add to the risk of bleeding events of SSRIs and SNRIs).
No products indexed under this heading.

Naproxen (Concomitant use of nonsteroidal anti-inflammatory drugs with milnacipran hydrochloride may add to the risk of bleeding events of SSRIs and SNRIs). Products include:
EC-Naprosyn 2850
Naprosyn 2850
Anaprox/Naprosyn 2850

Naproxen Sodium (Concomitant use of nonsteroidal anti-inflammatory drugs with milnacipran hydrochloride may add to the risk of bleeding events of SSRIs and SNRIs). Products include:
Anaprox 2850
Anaprox DS 2850
Treximet 1681

Naratriptan Hydrochloride (The development of a potentially life-threatening serotonin syndrome or Neuroleptic Malignant Syndrome (NMS)-like reactions have been reported with SNRIs and SSRIs alone, including milnacipran hydrochloride, but particularly with concomitant use of serotonergic drugs (including triptans)). Products include:
Amerge 1306

Norepinephrine Bitartrate (Milnacipran hydrochloride inhibits the reuptake of norepinephrine. Therefore, concomitant use of milnacipran hydrochloride with epinephrine and norepinephrine may be associated with paroxysmal hypertension and possible arrhythmia).
No products indexed under this heading.

Norepinephrine Hydrochloride (Milnacipran hydrochloride inhibits the reuptake of norepinephrine. Therefore, concomitant use of milnacipran hydrochloride with epinephrine and norepinephrine may be associated with paroxysmal hypertension and possible arrhythmia).
No products indexed under this heading.

Olanzapine (The development of a potentially life-threatening serotonin syndrome or Neuroleptic Malignant Syndrome (NMS)-like reactions have been reported with SNRIs and SSRIs alone, including milnacipran hydrochloride, particularly with concomitant use of antipsychotics). Products include:
Symbyax 1965
Zyprexa 1984
Zyprexa IntraMuscular 1984
Zyprexa ZYDIS 1984

Oxaprozin (Concomitant use of nonsteroidal anti-inflammatory drugs with milnacipran hydrochloride may add to the risk of bleeding events of SSRIs and SNRIs).
No products indexed under this heading.

Oxazepam (Given the primary central nervous system effects of milnacipran hydrochloride, caution should be used when it is taken in combination with other centrally acting drugs, including those with a similar mechanism of action).
No products indexed under this heading.

Oxycodone Hydrochloride (Given the primary central nervous system effects of milnacipran hydrochloride, caution should be used when it is taken in combination with other centrally acting drugs, including those with a similar mechanism of action). Products include:
OxyContin 2807
Percocet 1121
Percodan 1124

Paliperidone (The development of a potentially life-threatening serotonin syndrome or Neuroleptic Malignant Syndrome (NMS)-like reactions have been reported with SNRIs and SSRIs alone, including milnacipran hydrochloride, particularly with concomitant use of antipsychotics). Products include:
Invega 2613
Invega Sustenna 2621

Pargyline Hydrochloride (Concomitant use of milnacipran hydrochloride in patients taking monoamine oxidase inhibitors (MAOIs) is contraindicated. In patients receiving a serotonin reuptake inhibitor in combination with a monoamine oxidase inhibitor (MAOI), there have been reports of serious, sometimes fatal, reactions including hyperthermia, rigidity, myoclonus, autonomic instability with possible rapid fluctuations of vital signs, and mental status changes that include extreme agitation progressing to delirium and coma. It is recommended that milnacipran should not be used in combination with a MAOI, or within 14 days of discontinuing treatment with a MAOI. At least 5 days should be allowed after stopping milnacipran before starting a MAOI).
No products indexed under this heading.

Paroxetine (Co-administration of milnacipran hydrochloride with other inhibitors of serotonin reuptake may result in hypertension and coronary artery vasoconstriction, through additive serotonergic effects).
No products indexed under this heading.

Paroxetine Hydrochloride (The development of a potentially life-threatening serotonin syndrome or Neuroleptic Malignant Syndrome (NMS)-like reactions have been reported with SNRIs and SSRIs alone, including milnacipran hydrochloride, but particularly with concomitant use of serotonergic drugs (including triptans)). Products include:
Paroxetine CR 2361
Paroxetine ER 2371
Paxil 1586
Paxil CR 1596

Paroxetine Mesylate (Co-administration of milnacipran hydrochloride with other inhibitors of serotonin reuptake may result in hypertension and coronary artery vasoconstriction, through additive serotonergic effects).
No products indexed under this heading.

Pemoline (Given the primary central nervous system effects of milnacipran hydrochloride, caution should be used when it is taken in combination with other centrally acting drugs, including those with a similar mechanism of action).
No products indexed under this heading.

Pentobarbital Sodium (Given the primary central nervous system effects of milnacipran hydrochloride, caution should be used when it is taken in combination with other centrally acting drugs, including those with a similar mechanism of action). Products include:
Nembutal 2012

Perphenazine (The development of a potentially life-threatening serotonin syndrome or Neuroleptic Malignant Syndrome (NMS)-like reactions have been reported with SNRIs and SSRIs alone, including milnacipran hydrochloride, particularly with concomitant use of antipsychotics).
No products indexed under this heading.

Phenelzine Sulfate (Concomitant use of milnacipran hydrochloride in patients taking monoamine oxidase inhibitors (MAOIs) is contraindicated. In patients receiving a serotonin reuptake inhibitor in combination with a monoamine oxidase inhibitor (MAOI), there have been reports of serious, sometimes fatal, reactions including hyperthermia, rigidity, myoclonus, autonomic instability with possible rapid fluctuations of vital signs, and mental status changes that include extreme agitation progressing to delirium and coma. It is recommended that milnacipran should not be used in combination with a MAOI, or within 14 days of discontinuing treatment with a MAOI. At least 5 days should be allowed after stopping milnacipran before starting a MAOI).
No products indexed under this heading.

Phenobarbital (Given the primary central nervous system effects of milnacipran hydrochloride, caution should be used when it is taken in combination with other centrally acting drugs, including those with a similar mechanism of action). Products include:
Donnatal 2711

Phenobarbital Sodium (Given the primary central nervous system effects of milnacipran hydrochloride, caution should be used when it is taken in combination with other centrally acting drugs, including those with a similar mechanism of action).
No products indexed under this heading.

Phenylbutazone (Concomitant use of nonsteroidal anti-inflammatory drugs with milnacipran hydrochloride may add to the risk of bleeding events of SSRIs and SNRIs).
No products indexed under this heading.

Pimozide (The development of a potentially life-threatening serotonin syndrome or Neuroleptic Malignant Syndrome (NMS)-like reactions have been reported with SNRIs and SSRIs alone, including milnacipran hydrochloride, particularly with concomitant use of antipsychotics).
No products indexed under this heading.

Piroxicam (Concomitant use of nonsteroidal anti-inflammatory drugs with milnacipran hydrochloride may add to the risk of bleeding events of SSRIs and SNRIs).
No products indexed under this heading.

Polythiazide (Hyponatremia may occur as a result of treatment with SSRIs and SNRIs, including milnacipran. Elderly patients may be at greater risk of developing hyponatremia with SNRIs, SSRIs, or milnacipran. Also, patients taking diuretics or who are otherwise volume-depleted may be at greater risk. Discontinuation of milnacipran should be considered in patients with symptomatic hyponatremia).
No products indexed under this heading.

Prazepam (Given the primary central nervous system effects of milnacipran hydrochloride, caution should be used when it is taken in combination with other centrally acting drugs, including those with a similar mechanism of action).
No products indexed under this heading.

Procarbazine Hydrochloride (Concomitant use of milnacipran hydrochloride in patients taking monoamine oxidase inhibitors (MAOIs) is contraindicated. In patients receiving a serotonin reuptake inhibitor in combination with a monoamine oxidase inhibitor (MAOI), there have been reports of serious, sometimes fatal, reactions including hyperthermia, rigidity, myoclonus, autonomic instability with possible rapid fluctuations of vital signs, and mental status changes that include extreme agitation progressing to delirium and coma. It is recommended that milnacipran should not be used in combination with a MAOI, or within 14 days of discontinuing treatment with a MAOI. At least 5 days should be allowed after stopping milnacipran before starting a MAOI).
No products indexed under this heading.

(⊙ Described in PDR® for Ophthalmic Medicines)

1699 Interactions Index Savella

Prochlorperazine (The development of a potentially life-threatening serotonin syndrome or Neuroleptic Malignant Syndrome (NMS)-like reactions have been reported with SNRIs and SSRIs alone, including milnacipran hydrochloride, particularly with concomitant use of antipsychotics).
No products indexed under this heading.

Promethazine (The development of a potentially life-threatening serotonin syndrome or Neuroleptic Malignant Syndrome (NMS)-like reactions have been reported with SNRIs and SSRIs alone, including milnacipran hydrochloride, but particularly with concomitant use of other dopamine antagonists).
No products indexed under this heading.

Promethazine Hydrochloride (The development of a potentially life-threatening serotonin syndrome or Neuroleptic Malignant Syndrome (NMS)-like reactions have been reported with SNRIs and SSRIs alone, including milnacipran hydrochloride, but particularly with concomitant use of other dopamine antagonists).
No products indexed under this heading.

Propofol (Given the primary central nervous system effects of milnacipran hydrochloride, caution should be used when it is taken in combination with other centrally acting drugs, including those with a similar mechanism of action).
No products indexed under this heading.

Propoxyphene Hydrochloride (Given the primary central nervous system effects of milnacipran hydrochloride, caution should be used when it is taken in combination with other centrally acting drugs, including those with a similar mechanism of action).
No products indexed under this heading.

Propoxyphene Napsylate (Given the primary central nervous system effects of milnacipran hydrochloride, caution should be used when it is taken in combination with other centrally acting drugs, including those with a similar mechanism of action).
No products indexed under this heading.

Quazepam (Given the primary central nervous system effects of milnacipran hydrochloride, caution should be used when it is taken in combination with other centrally acting drugs, including those with a similar mechanism of action).
No products indexed under this heading.

Quetiapine Fumarate (The development of a potentially life-threatening serotonin syndrome or Neuroleptic Malignant Syndrome (NMS)-like reactions have been reported with SNRIs and SSRIs alone, including milnacipran hydrochloride, particularly with concomitant use of antipsychotics). Products include:
Seroquel 750
Seroquel XR 759

Rasagiline Mesylate (Concomitant use of milnacipran hydrochloride in patients taking monoamine oxidase inhibitors (MAOIs) is contraindicated. In patients receiving a serotonin reuptake inhibitor in combination with a monoamine oxidase inhibitor (MAOI), there have been reports of serious, sometimes fatal, reactions including hyperthermia, rigidity, myoclonus, autonomic instability with possible rapid fluctuations of vital signs, and mental status changes that include extreme agitation progressing to delirium and coma. It is recommended that milnacipran should not be used in combination with a MAOI, or within 14 days of discontinuing treatment with a MAOI. At least 5 days should be allowed after stopping milnacipran before starting a MAOI). Products include:
Azilect 3383

Remifentanil Hydrochloride (Given the primary central nervous system effects of milnacipran hydrochloride, caution should be used when it is taken in combination with other centrally acting drugs, including those with a similar mechanism of action).
No products indexed under this heading.

Risperidone (The development of a potentially life-threatening serotonin syndrome or Neuroleptic Malignant Syndrome (NMS)-like reactions have been reported with SNRIs and SSRIs alone, including milnacipran hydrochloride, particularly with concomitant use of antipsychotics). Products include:
Risperdal Consta 2682

Rizatriptan Benzoate (The development of a potentially life-threatening serotonin syndrome or Neuroleptic Malignant Syndrome (NMS)-like reactions have been reported with SNRIs and SSRIs alone, including milnacipran hydrochloride, but particularly with concomitant use of serotonergic drugs (including triptans)). Products include:
Maxalt 2206
Maxalt-MLT 2206

Rofecoxib (Concomitant use of nonsteroidal anti-inflammatory drugs with milnacipran hydrochloride may add to the risk of bleeding events of SSRIs and SNRIs).
No products indexed under this heading.

Secobarbital Sodium (Given the primary central nervous system effects of milnacipran hydrochloride, caution should be used when it is taken in combination with other centrally acting drugs, including those with a similar mechanism of action).
No products indexed under this heading.

Selegiline (Concomitant use of milnacipran hydrochloride in patients taking monoamine oxidase inhibitors (MAOIs) is contraindicated. In patients receiving a serotonin reuptake inhibitor in combination with a monoamine oxidase inhibitor (MAOI), there have been reports of serious, sometimes fatal, reactions including hyperthermia, rigidity, myoclonus, autonomic instability with possible rapid fluctuations of vital signs, and mental status changes that include extreme agitation progressing to delirium and coma. It is recommended that milnacipran should not be used in combination with a MAOI, or within 14 days of discontinuing treatment with a MAOI. At least 5 days should be allowed after stopping milnacipran before starting a MAOI). Products include:
Emsam 3623

Selegiline Hydrochloride (Concomitant use of milnacipran hydrochloride in patients taking monoamine oxidase inhibitors (MAOIs) is contraindicated. In patients receiving a serotonin reuptake inhibitor in combination with a monoamine oxidase inhibitor (MAOI), there have been reports of serious, sometimes fatal, reactions including hyperthermia, rigidity, myoclonus, autonomic instability with possible rapid fluctuations of vital signs, and mental status changes that include extreme agitation progressing to delirium and coma. It is recommended that milnacipran should not be used in combination with a MAOI, or within 14 days of discontinuing treatment with a MAOI. At least 5 days should be allowed after stopping milnacipran before starting a MAOI). Products include:
Eldepryl 3312

Sertraline Hydrochloride (The development of a potentially life-threatening serotonin syndrome or Neuroleptic Malignant Syndrome (NMS)-like reactions have been reported with SNRIs and SSRIs alone, including milnacipran hydrochloride, but particularly with concomitant use of serotonergic drugs (including triptans)).
No products indexed under this heading.

Sevoflurane (Given the primary central nervous system effects of milnacipran hydrochloride, caution should be used when it is taken in combination with other centrally acting drugs, including those with a similar mechanism of action). Products include:
Ultane 554

Sodium Oxybate (Given the primary central nervous system effects of milnacipran hydrochloride, caution should be used when it is taken in combination with other centrally acting drugs, including those with a similar mechanism of action).
No products indexed under this heading.

Spironolactone (Hyponatremia may occur as a result of treatment with SSRIs and SNRIs, including milnacipran. Elderly patients may be at greater risk of developing hyponatremia with SNRIs, SSRIs, or milnacipran. Also, patients taking diuretics or who are otherwise volume-depleted may be at greater risk. Discontinuation of milnacipran should be considered in patients with symptomatic hyponatremia).
No products indexed under this heading.

Sufentanil Citrate (Given the primary central nervous system effects of milnacipran hydrochloride, caution should be used when it is taken in combination with other centrally acting drugs, including those with a similar mechanism of action).
No products indexed under this heading.

Sulindac (Concomitant use of nonsteroidal anti-inflammatory drugs with milnacipran hydrochloride may add to the risk of bleeding events of SSRIs and SNRIs). Products include:
Clinoril 2098

Sumatriptan (The development of a potentially life-threatening serotonin syndrome or Neuroleptic Malignant Syndrome (NMS)-like reactions have been reported with SNRIs and SSRIs alone, including milnacipran hydrochloride, but particularly with concomitant use of serotonergic drugs (including triptans)). Products include:
Imitrex Nasal 1503

Sumatriptan Succinate (The development of a potentially life-threatening serotonin syndrome or Neuroleptic Malignant Syndrome (NMS)-like reactions have been reported with SNRIs and SSRIs alone, including milnacipran hydrochloride, but particularly with concomitant use of serotonergic drugs (including triptans)). Products include:
Imitrex 1497
Imitrex Tablets 1508
Treximet 1681

Temazepam (Given the primary central nervous system effects of milnacipran hydrochloride, caution should be used when it is taken in combination with other centrally acting drugs, including those with a similar mechanism of action).
No products indexed under this heading.

Thiamylal Sodium (Given the primary central nervous system effects of milnacipran hydrochloride, caution should be used when it is taken in combination with other centrally acting drugs, including those with a similar mechanism of action).
No products indexed under this heading.

Thioridazine Hydrochloride (The development of a potentially life-threatening serotonin syndrome or Neuroleptic Malignant Syndrome (NMS)-like reactions have been reported with SNRIs and SSRIs alone, including milnacipran hydrochloride, particularly with concomitant use of antipsychotics). Products include:
Thioridazine Hydrochloride 2384

Thiothixene (The development of a potentially life-threatening serotonin syndrome or Neuroleptic Malignant Syndrome (NMS)-like reactions have been reported with SNRIs and SSRIs alone, including milnacipran hydrochloride, particularly with concomitant use of antipsychotics). Products include:
Thiothixene 2386

Tinzaparin Sodium (Concomitant use of other anticoagulants with milnacipran hydrochloride may add to the risk of bleeding events of SSRIs and SNRIs).
No products indexed under this heading.

Tolmetin Sodium (Concomitant use of nonsteroidal anti-inflammatory drugs with milnacipran hydrochloride may add to the risk of bleeding events of SSRIs and SNRIs).
No products indexed under this heading.

Torsemide (Hyponatremia may occur as a result of treatment with SSRIs and SNRIs, including milnacipran. Elderly patients may be at greater risk of developing hyponatremia with SNRIs, SSRIs, or milnacipran. Also, patients taking diuretics or who are otherwise volume-depleted may be at greater risk. Discontinuation of milnacipran should be considered in patients with symptomatic hyponatremia).
No products indexed under this heading.

Tramadol Hydrochloride (Patients should be cautioned about the risk of serotonin syndrome with concomitant use of milnacipran hydrochloride and tramadol). Products include:
Ryzolt 2813
Ultram ER 2693

Tranylcypromine Sulfate (Concomitant use of milnacipran hydrochloride in patients taking monoamine oxidase inhibitors (MAOIs) is contraindicated. In patients receiving a serotonin reuptake inhibitor in combination with a monoamine oxidase inhibitor (MAOI), there have been reports of serious, sometimes fatal, reactions including hyperthermia, rigidity, myoclonus, autonomic instability with possible rapid fluctuations of vital signs, and mental status changes that include extreme agitation progressing to delirium and coma. It is recommended that milnacipran should not be used in combination with a MAOI, or within 14 days of discontinuing treatment with a MAOI. At least 5 days should be allowed after stopping milnacipran before starting a MAOI). Products include:
Parnate 1584

Triamterene (Hyponatremia may occur as a result of treatment with SSRIs and SNRIs, including milnacipran. Elderly patients may be at greater risk of developing hyponatremia with SNRIs, SSRIs, or milnacipran. Also, patients taking diuretics or who are otherwise volume-depleted may be at greater risk. Discontinuation of milnacipran should be considered in patients with symptomatic hyponatremia). Products include:
Dyazide 1429
Dyrenium 3495

Triazolam (Given the primary central nervous system effects of milnacipran hydrochloride, caution should be used when it is taken in combination with other centrally acting drugs, including those with a similar mechanism of action).
No products indexed under this heading.

IMPORTANT NOTE: Always consult each drug listing in the patient's regimen for possible interactions.

Trifluoperazine Hydrochloride (The development of a potentially life-threatening serotonin syndrome or Neuroleptic Malignant Syndrome (NMS)-like reactions have been reported with SNRIs and SSRIs alone, including milnacipran hydrochloride, particularly with concomitant use of antipsychotics).
No products indexed under this heading.

Tryptophan (The concomitant use of milnacipran hydrochloride with serotonin precursors (such as tryptophan) is not recommended).
No products indexed under this heading.

Valdecoxib (Concomitant use of nonsteroidal anti-inflammatory drugs with milnacipran hydrochloride may add to the risk of bleeding events of SSRIs and SNRIs).
No products indexed under this heading.

Venlafaxine Hydrochloride (The development of a potentially life-threatening serotonin syndrome or Neuroleptic Malignant Syndrome (NMS)-like reactions have been reported with SNRIs and SSRIs alone, including milnacipran hydrochloride, but particularly with concomitant use of serotonergic drugs (including triptans)). Products include:
Effexor XR 3504
Venlafaxine Hydrochloride Tablets ... 2388

Warfarin Sodium (Concomitant use of warfarin with milnacipran hydrochloride may add to the risk of bleeding events of SSRIs and SNRIs).
No products indexed under this heading.

Zaleplon (Given the primary central nervous system effects of milnacipran hydrochloride, caution should be used when it is taken in combination with other centrally acting drugs, including those with a similar mechanism of action).
No products indexed under this heading.

Ziprasidone Hydrochloride (The development of a potentially life-threatening serotonin syndrome or Neuroleptic Malignant Syndrome (NMS)-like reactions have been reported with SNRIs and SSRIs alone, including milnacipran hydrochloride, particularly with concomitant use of antipsychotics).
Products include:
Geodon 2723

Zolmitriptan (The development of a potentially life-threatening serotonin syndrome or Neuroleptic Malignant Syndrome (NMS)-like reactions have been reported with SNRIs and SSRIs alone, including milnacipran hydrochloride, but particularly with concomitant use of serotonergic drugs (including triptans)).
Products include:
Zomig Tablets 773
Zomig Nasal Spray 768
Zomig-ZMT Tablets 773

Zolpidem Tartrate (Given the primary central nervous system effects of milnacipran hydrochloride, caution should be used when it is taken in combination with other centrally acting drugs, including those with a similar mechanism of action). Products include:
Ambien 2920
Ambien CR 2925

Food Interactions

Alcohol (Milnacipran hydrochloride should not be prescribed to patients with substantial alcohol use or evidence of chronic liver disease because it is possible that milnacipran hydrochloride may aggravate pre-existing liver disease).

Beer, reduced-alcohol (Milnacipran hydrochloride should not be prescribed to patients with substantial alcohol use or evidence of chronic liver disease because it is possible that milnacipran hydrochloride may aggravate pre-existing liver disease).

Beer, unspecified (Milnacipran hydrochloride should not be prescribed to patients with substantial alcohol use or evidence of chronic liver disease because it is possible that milnacipran hydrochloride may aggravate pre-existing liver disease).

Wine, Chianti (Milnacipran hydrochloride should not be prescribed to patients with substantial alcohol use or evidence of chronic liver disease because it is possible that milnacipran hydrochloride may aggravate pre-existing liver disease).

Wine, Red (Milnacipran hydrochloride should not be prescribed to patients with substantial alcohol use or evidence of chronic liver disease because it is possible that milnacipran hydrochloride may aggravate pre-existing liver disease).

Wine, unspecified (Milnacipran hydrochloride should not be prescribed to patients with substantial alcohol use or evidence of chronic liver disease because it is possible that milnacipran hydrochloride may aggravate pre-existing liver disease).

Wine products (Milnacipran hydrochloride should not be prescribed to patients with substantial alcohol use or evidence of chronic liver disease because it is possible that milnacipran hydrochloride may aggravate pre-existing liver disease).

SEASONIQUE TABLETS

(Ethinyl Estradiol, Levonorgestrel) 3418
May interact with ampicillins, antibiotics, anticonvulsants, barbiturates, cytochrome p450 3a4 inhibitors (selected), phenytoin, prednisolone, protease inhibitors, salicylates, tetracyclines, theophyllines, and certain other agents. Compounds in these categories include:

Acetaminophen (Acetaminophen may increase plasma ethinyl estradiol levels, possibly by inhibition of conjugation. Decreased plasma concentrations of acetaminophen have been noted when co-administered with combination oral contraceptives). Products include:
Percocet 1121
Tylenol 2049
Tylenol 8 Hour 2049
Extra Strength Tylenol Caplets, Cool Caplets, and EZ Tabs 2049
Extra Strength Tylenol Adult Rapid Blast Liquid 2049
Extra Strength Tylenol Rapid Release 2049
Tylenol with Codeine 2691
Tylenol Arthritis Pain Extended Release Geltabs/Caplets 2049
Children's Tylenol Suspension Liquid 2048
Chlidren's Tylenol Meltaways 2048
Tylenol, Infants' Drops 2048
Junior Tylenol 2048
Vicodin 560
Vicodin ES 561
Vicodin HP 563
Zydone 1138

Acetaminophen-containing products (Acetaminophen may increase plasma ethinyl estradiol levels, possibly by inhibition of conjugation. Decreased plasma concentrations of acetaminophen have been noted when co-administered with combination oral contraceptives).
No products indexed under this heading.

Acetazolamide (CYP3A4 inhibitors may increase plasma ethinyl estradiol levels).
No products indexed under this heading.

Acetazolamide Sodium (CYP3A4 inhibitors may increase plasma ethinyl estradiol levels).
No products indexed under this heading.

Alatrofloxacin Mesylate (Contraceptive effectiveness may be reduced when hormonal contraceptives are co-administered with antibiotics and other drugs that increase metabolism of contraceptive steroids. This could result in unintended pregnancy or breakthrough bleeding).
No products indexed under this heading.

Amikacin Sulfate (Contraceptive effectiveness may be reduced when hormonal contraceptives are co-administered with antibiotics and other drugs that increase metabolism of contraceptive steroids. This could result in unintended pregnancy or breakthrough bleeding).
No products indexed under this heading.

Amiodarone Hydrochloride (CYP3A4 inhibitors may increase plasma ethinyl estradiol levels).
No products indexed under this heading.

Amobarbital (Contraceptive effectivness may be reduced when hormonal contraceptives are co-administered with drugs that increase the metabolism of contraceptive steroids, such as barbiturates).
No products indexed under this heading.

Amobarbital Sodium (Contraceptive effectivness may be reduced when hormonal contraceptives are co-administered with drugs that increase the metabolism of contraceptive steroids, such as barbiturates).
No products indexed under this heading.

Amoxicillin (Contraceptive effectiveness may be reduced when hormonal contraceptives are co-administered with antibiotics and other drugs that increase metabolism of contraceptive steroids. This could result in unintended pregnancy or breakthrough bleeding).
Products include:
Amoxil Capsules 1311
Amoxil Chewable Tablets 1311
Amoxil 1311
Amoxil Powder 1311
Augmentin 1331
Augmentin Tablets 1335
Augmentin ES-600 1338
Augmentin XR 1342
Moxatag 2321

Amoxicillin Trihydrate (Contraceptive effectiveness may be reduced when hormonal contraceptives are co-administered with antibiotics and other drugs that increase metabolism of contraceptive steroids. This could result in unintended pregnancy or breakthrough bleeding).
No products indexed under this heading.

Ampicillin (Contraceptive effectiveness may be reduced when hormonal contraceptives are co-administered with antibiotics and other drugs that increase metabolism of contraceptive steroids. This could result in unintended pregnancy or breakthrough bleeding).
No products indexed under this heading.

Ampicillin Sodium (Contraceptive effectiveness may be reduced when hormonal contraceptives are co-administered with antibiotics and other drugs that increase metabolism of contraceptive steroids. This could result in unintended pregnancy or breakthrough bleeding).
No products indexed under this heading.

Ampicillin Trihydrate (Contraceptive effectiveness may be reduced when hormonal contraceptives are co-administered with antibiotics and other drugs that increase metabolism of contraceptive steroids. This could result in unintended pregnancy or breakthrough bleeding).
No products indexed under this heading.

Amprenavir (Several protease inhibitors have been studied with co-administration of oral combination hormonal contraceptives with significant changes (increase and decrease) in the plasma levels of the estrogen and progestin being noted in some cases. The safety and efficacy of combination oral contraceptive products may be affected with co-administration of anti-HIV protease inhibitors).
No products indexed under this heading.

Anastrozole (CYP3A4 inhibitors may increase plasma ethinyl estradiol levels).
No products indexed under this heading.

Antibiotics, non-penicillin, unspecified (Contraceptive effectiveness may be reduced when hormonal contraceptives are co-administered with antibiotics and other drugs that increase metabolism of contraceptive steroids. This could result in unintended pregnancy or breakthrough bleeding).
No products indexed under this heading.

Aprepitant (CYP3A4 inhibitors may increase plasma ethinyl estradiol levels). Products include:
Emend 2124

Aprobarbital (Contraceptive effectivness may be reduced when hormonal contraceptives are co-administered with drugs that increase the metabolism of contraceptive steroids, such as barbiturates).
No products indexed under this heading.

Ascorbic Acid (Ascorbic acid may increase plasma ethinyl estradiol levels, possibly by inhibition of conjugation).
No products indexed under this heading.

Aspirin (Increased clearance of salicylic acid due to induction of conjugation has been noted when co-administered with combination oral contraceptives).
Products include:
Aggrenox 880
Bayer Aspirin 829
Percodan 1124
St. Joseph Aspirin 2045

Aspirin, Enteric Coated (Increased clearance of salicylic acid due to induction of conjugation has been noted when co-administered with combination oral contraceptives).
No products indexed under this heading.

Aspirin Buffered (Increased clearance of salicylic acid due to induction of conjugation has been noted when co-administered with combination oral contraceptives).
No products indexed under this heading.

Atazanavir (Several protease inhibitors have been studied with co-administration of oral combination hormonal contraceptives with significant changes (increase and decrease) in the plasma levels of the estrogen and progestin being noted in some cases. The safety and efficacy of combination oral contraceptive products may be affected with co-administration of anti-HIV protease inhibitors).
No products indexed under this heading.

Atazanavir Sulfate (Several protease inhibitors have been studied with co-administration of oral combination hormonal contraceptives with significant changes (increase and decrease) in the plasma levels of the estrogen and progestin being noted in some cases. The safety and efficacy of combination oral contraceptive products may be affected with co-administration of anti-HIV protease inhibitors).
No products indexed under this heading.

Atorvastatin Calcium (Co-administration of atorvastatin and certain combination oral contraceptives containing ethinyl estradiol increase AUC values for ethinyl estradiol by approximately 20%). Products include:
Lipitor 2703

1701 Interactions Index Seasonique

Azithromycin Dihydrate (Contraceptive effectiveness may be reduced when hormonal contraceptives are co-administered with antibiotics and other drugs that increase metabolism of contraceptive steroids. This could result in unintended pregnancy or breakthrough bleeding).
No products indexed under this heading.

Azlocillin Sodium (Contraceptive effectiveness may be reduced when hormonal contraceptives are co-administered with antibiotics and other drugs that increase metabolism of contraceptive steroids. This could result in unintended pregnancy or breakthrough bleeding).
No products indexed under this heading.

Aztreonam (Contraceptive effectiveness may be reduced when hormonal contraceptives are co-administered with antibiotics and other drugs that increase metabolism of contraceptive steroids. This could result in unintended pregnancy or breakthrough bleeding).
No products indexed under this heading.

Bacampicillin Hydrochloride (Contraceptive effectiveness may be reduced when hormonal contraceptives are co-administered with antibiotics and other drugs that increase metabolism of contraceptive steroids. This could result in unintended pregnancy or breakthrough bleeding).
No products indexed under this heading.

Butabarbital (Contraceptive effectivness may be reduced when hormonal contraceptives are co-administered with drugs that increase the metabolism of contraceptive steroids, such as barbiturates).
No products indexed under this heading.

Butabarbital Sodium (Contraceptive effectivness may be reduced when hormonal contraceptives are co-administered with drugs that increase the metabolism of contraceptive steroids, such as barbiturates).
No products indexed under this heading.

Butalbital (Contraceptive effectivness may be reduced when hormonal contraceptives are co-administered with drugs that increase the metabolism of contraceptive steroids, such as barbiturates).
No products indexed under this heading.

Carbamazepine (Contraceptive effectiveness may be reduced when hormonal contraceptives are co-administered with drugs that increase the metabolism of contraceptive steroids, such as carbamazepine).
Products include:
Carbatrol 3280
Equetro 3477

Carbenicillin Disodium (Contraceptive effectiveness may be reduced when hormonal contraceptives are co-administered with antibiotics and other drugs that increase metabolism of contraceptive steroids. This could result in unintended pregnancy or breakthrough bleeding).
No products indexed under this heading.

Carbenicillin Indanyl Sodium (Contraceptive effectiveness may be reduced when hormonal contraceptives are co-administered with antibiotics and other drugs that increase metabolism of contraceptive steroids. This could result in unintended pregnancy or breakthrough bleeding).
No products indexed under this heading.

Cefaclor (Contraceptive effectiveness may be reduced when hormonal contraceptives are co-administered with antibiotics and other drugs that increase metabolism of contraceptive steroids. This could result in unintended pregnancy or breakthrough bleeding).
No products indexed under this heading.

Cefadroxil (Contraceptive effectiveness may be reduced when hormonal contraceptives are co-administered with antibiotics and other drugs that increase metabolism of contraceptive steroids. This could result in unintended pregnancy or breakthrough bleeding).
No products indexed under this heading.

Cefamandole Nafate (Contraceptive effectiveness may be reduced when hormonal contraceptives are co-administered with antibiotics and other drugs that increase metabolism of contraceptive steroids. This could result in unintended pregnancy or breakthrough bleeding).
No products indexed under this heading.

Cefazolin Sodium (Contraceptive effectiveness may be reduced when hormonal contraceptives are co-administered with antibiotics and other drugs that increase metabolism of contraceptive steroids. This could result in unintended pregnancy or breakthrough bleeding).
No products indexed under this heading.

Cefixime (Contraceptive effectiveness may be reduced when hormonal contraceptives are co-administered with antibiotics and other drugs that increase metabolism of contraceptive steroids. This could result in unintended pregnancy or breakthrough bleeding). Products include:
Suprax for Oral Suspension 2038
Suprax Tablets 2038

Cefmetazole Sodium (Contraceptive effectiveness may be reduced when hormonal contraceptives are co-administered with antibiotics and other drugs that increase metabolism of contraceptive steroids. This could result in unintended pregnancy or breakthrough bleeding).
No products indexed under this heading.

Cefonicid Sodium (Contraceptive effectiveness may be reduced when hormonal contraceptives are co-administered with antibiotics and other drugs that increase metabolism of contraceptive steroids. This could result in unintended pregnancy or breakthrough bleeding).
No products indexed under this heading.

Cefoperazone Sodium (Contraceptive effectiveness may be reduced when hormonal contraceptives are co-administered with antibiotics and other drugs that increase metabolism of contraceptive steroids. This could result in unintended pregnancy or breakthrough bleeding).
No products indexed under this heading.

Ceforanide (Contraceptive effectiveness may be reduced when hormonal contraceptives are co-administered with antibiotics and other drugs that increase metabolism of contraceptive steroids. This could result in unintended pregnancy or breakthrough bleeding).
No products indexed under this heading.

Cefotaxime Sodium (Contraceptive effectiveness may be reduced when hormonal contraceptives are co-administered with antibiotics and other drugs that increase metabolism of contraceptive steroids. This could result in unintended pregnancy or breakthrough bleeding).
No products indexed under this heading.

Cefotetan (Contraceptive effectiveness may be reduced when hormonal contraceptives are co-administered with antibiotics and other drugs that increase metabolism of contraceptive steroids. This could result in unintended pregnancy or breakthrough bleeding).
No products indexed under this heading.

Cefoxitin Sodium (Contraceptive effectiveness may be reduced when hormonal contraceptives are co-administered with antibiotics and other drugs that increase metabolism of contraceptive steroids. This could result in unintended pregnancy or breakthrough bleeding).
No products indexed under this heading.

Cefpodoxime Proxetil (Contraceptive effectiveness may be reduced when hormonal contraceptives are co-administered with antibiotics and other drugs that increase metabolism of contraceptive steroids. This could result in unintended pregnancy or breakthrough bleeding).
No products indexed under this heading.

Cefprozil (Contraceptive effectiveness may be reduced when hormonal contraceptives are co-administered with antibiotics and other drugs that increase metabolism of contraceptive steroids. This could result in unintended pregnancy or breakthrough bleeding).
No products indexed under this heading.

Ceftazidime (Contraceptive effectiveness may be reduced when hormonal contraceptives are co-administered with antibiotics and other drugs that increase metabolism of contraceptive steroids. This could result in unintended pregnancy or breakthrough bleeding).
Products include:
Fortaz 1481

Ceftizoxime Sodium (Contraceptive effectiveness may be reduced when hormonal contraceptives are co-administered with antibiotics and other drugs that increase metabolism of contraceptive steroids. This could result in unintended pregnancy or breakthrough bleeding).
No products indexed under this heading.

Ceftriaxone Sodium (Contraceptive effectiveness may be reduced when hormonal contraceptives are co-administered with antibiotics and other drugs that increase metabolism of contraceptive steroids. This could result in unintended pregnancy or breakthrough bleeding). Products include:
Rocephin 2859

Cefuroxime Axetil (Contraceptive effectiveness may be reduced when hormonal contraceptives are co-administered with antibiotics and other drugs that increase metabolism of contraceptive steroids. This could result in unintended pregnancy or breakthrough bleeding). Products include:
Ceftin 1399

Cefuroxime Sodium (Contraceptive effectiveness may be reduced when hormonal contraceptives are co-administered with antibiotics and other drugs that increase metabolism of contraceptive steroids. This could result in unintended pregnancy or breakthrough bleeding).
No products indexed under this heading.

Cephalexin (Contraceptive effectiveness may be reduced when hormonal contraceptives are co-administered with antibiotics and other drugs that increase metabolism of contraceptive steroids. This could result in unintended pregnancy or breakthrough bleeding).
No products indexed under this heading.

Cephalothin Sodium (Contraceptive effectiveness may be reduced when hormonal contraceptives are co-administered with antibiotics and other drugs that increase metabolism of contraceptive steroids. This could result in unintended pregnancy or breakthrough bleeding).
No products indexed under this heading.

Cephapirin Sodium (Contraceptive effectiveness may be reduced when hormonal contraceptives are co-administered with antibiotics and other drugs that increase metabolism of contraceptive steroids. This could result in unintended pregnancy or breakthrough bleeding).
No products indexed under this heading.

Cephradine (Contraceptive effectiveness may be reduced when hormonal contraceptives are co-administered with antibiotics and other drugs that increase metabolism of contraceptive steroids. This could result in unintended pregnancy or breakthrough bleeding).
No products indexed under this heading.

Chloramphenicol (Contraceptive effectiveness may be reduced when hormonal contraceptives are co-administered with antibiotics and other drugs that increase metabolism of contraceptive steroids. This could result in unintended pregnancy or breakthrough bleeding).
No products indexed under this heading.

Chloramphenicol Palmitate (Contraceptive effectiveness may be reduced when hormonal contraceptives are co-administered with antibiotics and other drugs that increase metabolism of contraceptive steroids. This could result in unintended pregnancy or breakthrough bleeding).
No products indexed under this heading.

Chloramphenicol Sodium Succinate (Contraceptive effectiveness may be reduced when hormonal contraceptives are co-administered with antibiotics and other drugs that increase metabolism of contraceptive steroids. This could result in unintended pregnancy or breakthrough bleeding).
No products indexed under this heading.

Choline Magnesium Trisalicylate (Increased clearance of salicylic acid due to induction of conjugation has been noted when co-administered with combination oral contraceptives).
No products indexed under this heading.

Cilastatin Sodium (Contraceptive effectiveness may be reduced when hormonal contraceptives are co-administered with antibiotics and other drugs that increase metabolism of contraceptive steroids. This could result in unintended pregnancy or breakthrough bleeding). Products include:
Primaxin I.M. 2232
Primaxin I.V. 2235

Cimetidine (CYP3A4 inhibitors may increase plasma ethinyl estradiol levels).
No products indexed under this heading.

Cimetidine Hydrochloride (CYP3A4 inhibitors may increase plasma ethinyl estradiol levels).
No products indexed under this heading.

Ciprofloxacin (CYP3A4 inhibitors may increase plasma ethinyl estradiol levels). Products include:
Cipro I.V. 3082
Cipro 3073
Cipro XR 3091
Ciprodex 583

Ciprofloxacin Hydrochloride (Contraceptive effectiveness may be reduced when hormonal contraceptives are co-administered with antibiotics and other drugs that increase metabolism of contraceptive steroids. This could result in unintended pregnancy or breakthrough bleeding). Products include:
Cipro 3073

Clarithromycin (CYP3A4 inhibitors may increase plasma ethinyl estradiol levels). Products include:
Biaxin/Biaxin XL 412

IMPORTANT NOTE: Always consult each drug listing in the patient's regimen for possible interactions.

Gatifloxacin (Contraceptive effectiveness may be reduced when hormonal contraceptives are co-administered with antibiotics and other drugs that increase metabolism of contraceptive steroids. This could result in unintended pregnancy or breakthrough bleeding).
No products indexed under this heading.

Gemifloxacin Mesylate (Contraceptive effectiveness may be reduced when hormonal contraceptives are co-administered with antibiotics and other drugs that increase metabolism of contraceptive steroids. This could result in unintended pregnancy or breakthrough bleeding).
No products indexed under this heading.

Gentamicin Sulfate (Contraceptive effectiveness may be reduced when hormonal contraceptives are co-administered with antibiotics and other drugs that increase metabolism of contraceptive steroids. This could result in unintended pregnancy or breakthrough bleeding). Products include:
Pred-G .... ⊙ **226**, ⊙ **227**

Grepafloxacin Hydrochloride (Contraceptive effectiveness may be reduced when hormonal contraceptives are co-administered with antibiotics and other drugs that increase metabolism of contraceptive steroids. This could result in unintended pregnancy or breakthrough bleeding).
No products indexed under this heading.

Griseofulvin (Contraceptive effectiveness may be reduced when hormonal contraceptives are co-administered with drugs that increase the metabolism of contraceptive steroids, such as griseofulvin).
No products indexed under this heading.

Hexobarbital (Contraceptive effectivness may be reduced when hormonal contraceptives are co-administered with drugs that increase the metabolism of contraceptive steroids, such as barbiturates).
No products indexed under this heading.

Hypericum (Herbal products containing St. John's Wort (hypericum perforatum) may induce hepatic enzymes (cytochrome p450) and p-glycoprotein transporter and may reduce the effectiveness of contraceptive steroids. This may also result in breakthrough bleeding).
No products indexed under this heading.

Hypericum Perforatum (Herbal products containing St. John's Wort (hypericum perforatum) may induce hepatic enzymes (cytochrome p450) and p-glycoprotein transporter and may reduce the effectiveness of contraceptive steroids. This may also result in breakthrough bleeding). Products include:
Traumeel **1800**

Idarubicin Hydrochloride (Contraceptive effectiveness may be reduced when hormonal contraceptives are co-administered with antibiotics and other drugs that increase metabolism of contraceptive steroids. This could result in unintended pregnancy or breakthrough bleeding).
No products indexed under this heading.

Imatinib Mesylate (CYP3A4 inhibitors may increase plasma ethinyl estradiol levels). Products include:
Gleevec **2477**

Imipenem (Contraceptive effectiveness may be reduced when hormonal contraceptives are co-administered with antibiotics and other drugs that increase metabolism of contraceptive steroids. This could result in unintended pregnancy or breakthrough bleeding). Products include:
Primaxin I.M. **2232**
Primaxin I.V. **2235**

Indinavir Sulfate (Several protease inhibitors have been studied with co-administration of oral combination hormonal contraceptives with significant changes (increase and decrease) in the plasma levels of the estrogen and progestin being noted in some cases. The safety and efficacy of combination oral contraceptive products may be affected with co-administration of anti-HIV protease inhibitors). Products include:
Crixivan **2113**

Isoniazid (CYP3A4 inhibitors may increase plasma ethinyl estradiol levels).
No products indexed under this heading.

Itraconazole (CYP3A4 inhibitors may increase plasma ethinyl estradiol levels).
No products indexed under this heading.

Kanamycin Sulfate (Contraceptive effectiveness may be reduced when hormonal contraceptives are co-administered with antibiotics and other drugs that increase metabolism of contraceptive steroids. This could result in unintended pregnancy or breakthrough bleeding).
No products indexed under this heading.

Ketoconazole (CYP3A4 inhibitors may increase plasma ethinyl estradiol levels). Products include:
Extina **3319**
Xolegel **3337**

Lamotrigine (Combination oral contraceptives have been shown to significantly decrease plasma concentrations of lamotrigine likely due to induction of lamotrigine glucuronidation. This may reduce seizure control; therefore, dosage adjustments of lamotrigine may be necessary). Products include:
Lamictal **1522**
Lamictal ODT **1522**
Lamictal XR **1536**

Lapatinib (CYP3A4 inhibitors may increase plasma ethinyl estradiol levels). Products include:
Tykerb **1698**

Levetiracetam (Contraceptive effectiveness may be reduced when hormonal contraceptives are co-administered with anticonvulsants and other drugs that increase metabolism of contraceptive steroids. This could result in unintended pregnancy or breakthrough bleeding). Products include:
Keppra XR **3434**

Levofloxacin (Contraceptive effectiveness may be reduced when hormonal contraceptives are co-administered with antibiotics and other drugs that increase metabolism of contraceptive steroids. This could result in unintended pregnancy or breakthrough bleeding). Products include:
Iquix **3492**
Levaquin **2629**
Levaquin in 5% Dextrose **2629**
Quixin **3493**

Lomefloxacin Hydrochloride (Contraceptive effectiveness may be reduced when hormonal contraceptives are co-administered with antibiotics and other drugs that increase metabolism of contraceptive steroids. This could result in unintended pregnancy or breakthrough bleeding).
No products indexed under this heading.

Lopinavir (Several protease inhibitors have been studied with co-administration of oral combination hormonal contraceptives with significant changes (increase and decrease) in the plasma levels of the estrogen and progestin being noted in some cases. The safety and efficacy of combination oral contraceptive products may be affected with co-administration of anti-HIV protease inhibitors). Products include:
Kaletra **458**

Loracarbef (Contraceptive effectiveness may be reduced when hormonal contraceptives are co-administered with antibiotics and other drugs that increase metabolism of contraceptive steroids. This could result in unintended pregnancy or breakthrough bleeding).
No products indexed under this heading.

Loratadine (CYP3A4 inhibitors may increase plasma ethinyl estradiol levels).
No products indexed under this heading.

Magnesium Salicylate (Increased clearance of salicylic acid due to induction of conjugation has been noted when co-administered with combination oral contraceptives).
No products indexed under this heading.

Mephenytoin (Contraceptive effectiveness may be reduced when hormonal contraceptives are co-administered with anticonvulsants and other drugs that increase metabolism of contraceptive steroids. This could result in unintended pregnancy or breakthrough bleeding).
No products indexed under this heading.

Mephobarbital (Contraceptive effectivness may be reduced when hormonal contraceptives are co-administered with drugs that increase the metabolism of contraceptive steroids, such as barbiturates).
No products indexed under this heading.

Methacycline Hydrochloride (Several cases of contraceptive failure and breakthrough bleeding have been reported in the literature concomitant administration of antibiotics, such as tetracyclines; however, clinical pharmacology studies investigating drug interactions between combined oral contraceptives and these antibiotics have reported inconsistent results).
No products indexed under this heading.

Methicillin Sodium (Contraceptive effectiveness may be reduced when hormonal contraceptives are co-administered with antibiotics and other drugs that increase metabolism of contraceptive steroids. This could result in unintended pregnancy or breakthrough bleeding).
No products indexed under this heading.

Methsuximide (Contraceptive effectiveness may be reduced when hormonal contraceptives are co-administered with anticonvulsants and other drugs that increase metabolism of contraceptive steroids. This could result in unintended pregnancy or breakthrough bleeding).
No products indexed under this heading.

Metronidazole (CYP3A4 inhibitors may increase plasma ethinyl estradiol levels). Products include:
Pylera **793**

Metronidazole Benzoate (CYP3A4 inhibitors may increase plasma ethinyl estradiol levels).
No products indexed under this heading.

Metronidazole Hydrochloride (CYP3A4 inhibitors may increase plasma ethinyl estradiol levels).
No products indexed under this heading.

Metronidazole Sodium (CYP3A4 inhibitors may increase plasma ethinyl estradiol levels).
No products indexed under this heading.

Mezlocillin Sodium (Contraceptive effectiveness may be reduced when hormonal contraceptives are co-administered with antibiotics and other drugs that increase metabolism of contraceptive steroids. This could result in unintended pregnancy or breakthrough bleeding).
No products indexed under this heading.

Miconazole (CYP3A4 inhibitors may increase plasma ethinyl estradiol levels).
No products indexed under this heading.

Miconazole Nitrate (CYP3A4 inhibitors may increase plasma ethinyl estradiol levels). Products include:
Vusion Ointment **3335**

Mifepristone (CYP3A4 inhibitors may increase plasma ethinyl estradiol levels).
No products indexed under this heading.

Minocycline Hydrochloride (Several cases of contraceptive failure and breakthrough bleeding have been reported in the literature concomitant administration of antibiotics, such as tetracyclines; however, clinical pharmacology studies investigating drug interactions between combined oral contraceptives and these antibiotics have reported inconsistent results). Products include:
Solodyn **2073**

Morphine Sulfate (Increased clearance of morphine due to induction of conjugation has been noted when co-administered with combination oral contraceptives). Products include:
Avinza **1822**
Embeda **1831**
MS Contin **2803**

Moxifloxacin Hydrochloride (Contraceptive effectiveness may be reduced when hormonal contraceptives are co-administered with antibiotics and other drugs that increase metabolism of contraceptive steroids. This could result in unintended pregnancy or breakthrough bleeding). Products include:
Avelox **3064**
Vigamox **589**

Nafcillin Sodium (Contraceptive effectiveness may be reduced when hormonal contraceptives are co-administered with antibiotics and other drugs that increase metabolism of contraceptive steroids. This could result in unintended pregnancy or breakthrough bleeding).
No products indexed under this heading.

Nefazodone Hydrochloride (CYP3A4 inhibitors may increase plasma ethinyl estradiol levels).
No products indexed under this heading.

Nelfinavir Mesylate (Several protease inhibitors have been studied with co-administration of oral combination hormonal contraceptives with significant changes (increase and decrease) in the plasma levels of the estrogen and progestin being noted in some cases. The safety and efficacy of combination oral contraceptive products may be affected with co-administration of anti-HIV protease inhibitors).
No products indexed under this heading.

Nevirapine (CYP3A4 inhibitors may increase plasma ethinyl estradiol levels). Products include:
Viramune Oral Suspension **897**
Viramune Tablets **897**

Niacin (CYP3A4 inhibitors may increase plasma ethinyl estradiol levels). Products include:
Advicor **402**
Cardio Basics **3455**
Niaspan **497**
Simcor **524**

Niacinamide (CYP3A4 inhibitors may increase plasma ethinyl estradiol levels). Products include:
CitraNatal 90 DHA Capsules **2332**
CitraNatal Assure **2332**
CitraNatal Rx **2332**
Heplive **607**

Niacinamide Hydroiodide (CYP3A4 inhibitors may increase plasma ethinyl estradiol levels).
No products indexed under this heading.

IMPORTANT NOTE: Always consult each drug listing in the patient's regimen for possible interactions.

Nicotinamide (CYP3A4 inhibitors may increase plasma ethinyl estradiol levels).
No products indexed under this heading.

Nifedipine (CYP3A4 inhibitors may increase plasma ethinyl estradiol levels).
No products indexed under this heading.

Norfloxacin (CYP3A4 inhibitors may increase plasma ethinyl estradiol levels). Products include:
Noroxin **2220**

Ofloxacin (Contraceptive effectiveness may be reduced when hormonal contraceptives are co-administered with antibiotics and other drugs that increase metabolism of contraceptive steroids. This could result in unintended pregnancy or breakthrough bleeding).
No products indexed under this heading.

Omeprazole (CYP3A4 inhibitors may increase plasma ethinyl estradiol levels).
No products indexed under this heading.

Oxacillin (Contraceptive effectiveness may be reduced when hormonal contraceptives are co-administered with antibiotics and other drugs that increase metabolism of contraceptive steroids. This could result in unintended pregnancy or breakthrough bleeding).
No products indexed under this heading.

Oxacillin Sodium (Contraceptive effectiveness may be reduced when hormonal contraceptives are co-administered with antibiotics and other drugs that increase metabolism of contraceptive steroids. This could result in unintended pregnancy or breakthrough bleeding).
No products indexed under this heading.

Oxcarbazepine (Contraceptive effectiveness may be reduced when hormonal contraceptives are co-administered with drugs that increase the metabolism of contraceptive steroids, such as oxcarbazepine).
No products indexed under this heading.

Oxytetracycline (Several cases of contraceptive failure and breakthrough bleeding have been reported in the literature concomitant administration of antibiotics, such as tetracyclines; however, clinical pharmacology studies investigating drug interactions between combined oral contraceptives and these antibiotics have reported inconsistent results).
No products indexed under this heading.

Oxytetracycline Hydrochloride (Several cases of contraceptive failure and breakthrough bleeding have been reported in the literature concomitant administration of antibiotics, such as tetracyclines; however, clinical pharmacology studies investigating drug interactions between combined oral contraceptives and these antibiotics have reported inconsistent results).
No products indexed under this heading.

Paramethadione (Contraceptive effectiveness may be reduced when hormonal contraceptives are co-administered with anticonvulsants and other drugs that increase metabolism of contraceptive steroids. This could result in unintended pregnancy or breakthrough bleeding).
No products indexed under this heading.

Paroxetine Hydrochloride (CYP3A4 inhibitors may increase plasma ethinyl estradiol levels). Products include:
Paroxetine CR **2361**
Paroxetine ER **2371**
Paxil **1586**
Paxil CR **1596**

Penicillin, Potassium Phenoxymethyl (Contraceptive effectiveness may be reduced when hormonal contraceptives are co-administered with antibiotics and other drugs that increase metabolism of contraceptive steroids. This could result in unintended pregnancy or breakthrough bleeding).
No products indexed under this heading.

Penicillin G Benzathine (Contraceptive effectiveness may be reduced when hormonal contraceptives are co-administered with antibiotics and other drugs that increase metabolism of contraceptive steroids. This could result in unintended pregnancy or breakthrough bleeding). Products include:
Bicillin C-R Injectable Suspension **1826**
Bicillin L-A **1828**

Penicillin G Dibenzylethyenediamine (Contraceptive effectiveness may be reduced when hormonal contraceptives are co-administered with antibiotics and other drugs that increase metabolism of contraceptive steroids. This could result in unintended pregnancy or breakthrough bleeding).
No products indexed under this heading.

Penicillin G Potassium (Contraceptive effectiveness may be reduced when hormonal contraceptives are co-administered with antibiotics and other drugs that increase metabolism of contraceptive steroids. This could result in unintended pregnancy or breakthrough bleeding).
No products indexed under this heading.

Penicillin G Procaine (Contraceptive effectiveness may be reduced when hormonal contraceptives are co-administered with antibiotics and other drugs that increase metabolism of contraceptive steroids. This could result in unintended pregnancy or breakthrough bleeding). Products include:
Bicillin C-R Injectable Suspension **1826**
Bicillin L-A **1828**

Penicillin G Sodium (Contraceptive effectiveness may be reduced when hormonal contraceptives are co-administered with antibiotics and other drugs that increase metabolism of contraceptive steroids. This could result in unintended pregnancy or breakthrough bleeding).
No products indexed under this heading.

Penicillin V (Contraceptive effectiveness may be reduced when hormonal contraceptives are co-administered with antibiotics and other drugs that increase metabolism of contraceptive steroids. This could result in unintended pregnancy or breakthrough bleeding).
No products indexed under this heading.

Penicillin V Potassium (Contraceptive effectiveness may be reduced when hormonal contraceptives are co-administered with antibiotics and other drugs that increase metabolism of contraceptive steroids. This could result in unintended pregnancy or breakthrough bleeding).
No products indexed under this heading.

Penicillins (Contraceptive effectiveness may be reduced when hormonal contraceptives are co-administered with antibiotics and other drugs that increase metabolism of contraceptive steroids. This could result in unintended pregnancy or breakthrough bleeding).
No products indexed under this heading.

Pentobarbital (Contraceptive effectivness may be reduced when hormonal contraceptives are co-administered with drugs that increase the metabolism of contraceptive steroids, such as barbiturates).
No products indexed under this heading.

Pentobarbital Sodium (Contraceptive effectivness may be reduced when hormonal contraceptives are co-administered with drugs that increase the metabolism of contraceptive steroids, such as barbiturates). Products include:
Nembutal **2012**

Phenacemide (Contraceptive effectiveness may be reduced when hormonal contraceptives are co-administered with anticonvulsants and other drugs that increase metabolism of contraceptive steroids. This could result in unintended pregnancy or breakthrough bleeding).
No products indexed under this heading.

Phenobarbital (Contraceptive effectivness may be reduced when hormonal contraceptives are co-administered with drugs that increase the metabolism of contraceptive steroids, such as barbiturates). Products include:
Donnatal **2711**

Phenobarbital Sodium (Contraceptive effectivness may be reduced when hormonal contraceptives are co-administered with drugs that increase the metabolism of contraceptive steroids, such as barbiturates).
No products indexed under this heading.

Phensuximide (Contraceptive effectiveness may be reduced when hormonal contraceptives are co-administered with anticonvulsants and other drugs that increase metabolism of contraceptive steroids. This could result in unintended pregnancy or breakthrough bleeding).
No products indexed under this heading.

Phenylbutazone (Contraceptive effectiveness may be reduced when hormonal contraceptives are co-administered with drugs that increase the metabolism of contraceptive steroids, such as phenylbutazone).
No products indexed under this heading.

Phenytoin (Contraceptive effectivness may be reduced when hormonal contraceptives are co-administered with drugs that increase the metabolism of contraceptive steroids, such as phenytoin).
No products indexed under this heading.

Phenytoin Sodium (Contraceptive effectivness may be reduced when hormonal contraceptives are co-administered with drugs that increase the metabolism of contraceptive steroids, such as phenytoin). Products include:
Phenytek Capsules **2380**

Piperacillin Sodium (Contraceptive effectiveness may be reduced when hormonal contraceptives are co-administered with antibiotics and other drugs that increase metabolism of contraceptive steroids. This could result in unintended pregnancy or breakthrough bleeding). Products include:
Zosyn **3607**

Posaconazole (CYP3A4 inhibitors may increase plasma ethinyl estradiol levels). Products include:
Noxafil **3172**

Prednisolone (Combination hormonal contraceptives containing some synthetic estrogens (eg, ethinyl estradiol) may inhibit the metabolism of other compounds. Increased plasma concentrations of prednisolone have been reported with concomitant administration of combination oral contraceptives).
No products indexed under this heading.

Prednisolone Acetate (Combination hormonal contraceptives containing some synthetic estrogens (eg, ethinyl estradiol) may inhibit the metabolism of other compounds. Increased plasma concentrations of prednisolone have been reported with concomitant administration of combination oral contraceptives). Products include:
Blephamide .... ⊙**212**, ⊙**214**
Pred Forte .... ⊙**225**
Pred Mild .... ⊙**230**
Pred-G .... ⊙**226**, ⊙**227**

Prednisolone Sodium Phosphate (Combination hormonal contraceptives containing some synthetic estrogens (eg, ethinyl estradiol) may inhibit the metabolism of other compounds. Increased plasma concentrations of prednisolone have been reported with concomitant administration of combination oral contraceptives).
No products indexed under this heading.

Prednisolone Tebutate (Combination hormonal contraceptives containing some synthetic estrogens (eg, ethinyl estradiol) may inhibit the metabolism of other compounds. Increased plasma concentrations of prednisolone have been reported with concomitant administration of combination oral contraceptives).
No products indexed under this heading.

Primidone (Contraceptive effectiveness may be reduced when hormonal contraceptives are co-administered with anticonvulsants and other drugs that increase metabolism of contraceptive steroids. This could result in unintended pregnancy or breakthrough bleeding).
No products indexed under this heading.

Propoxyphene Hydrochloride (CYP3A4 inhibitors may increase plasma ethinyl estradiol levels).
No products indexed under this heading.

Propoxyphene Napsylate (CYP3A4 inhibitors may increase plasma ethinyl estradiol levels).
No products indexed under this heading.

Quinidine (CYP3A4 inhibitors may increase plasma ethinyl estradiol levels).
No products indexed under this heading.

Quinidine Hydrochloride (CYP3A4 inhibitors may increase plasma ethinyl estradiol levels).
No products indexed under this heading.

Quinidine Polygalacturonate (CYP3A4 inhibitors may increase plasma ethinyl estradiol levels).
No products indexed under this heading.

Quinidine Sulfate (CYP3A4 inhibitors may increase plasma ethinyl estradiol levels).
No products indexed under this heading.

Quinine (CYP3A4 inhibitors may increase plasma ethinyl estradiol levels). Products include:
Hyland's Leg Cramps PM with Quinine **3315**

Quinine Sulfate (CYP3A4 inhibitors may increase plasma ethinyl estradiol levels).
No products indexed under this heading.

Quinupristin (CYP3A4 inhibitors may increase plasma ethinyl estradiol levels).
No products indexed under this heading.

Ranitidine Bismuth Citrate (CYP3A4 inhibitors may increase plasma ethinyl estradiol levels).
No products indexed under this heading.

Ranitidine Hydrochloride (CYP3A4 inhibitors may increase plasma ethinyl estradiol levels). Products include:
Zantac **1737**
Zantac Injection **1732**
Zantac Pharmacy **1735**

Rifampin (Contraceptive effectiveness may be reduced when hormonal contraceptives are co-administered with drugs that increase the metabolism of contraceptive steroids, such as rifampin).
No products indexed under this heading.

Ritonavir (Several protease inhibitors have been studied with co-administration of oral combination hormonal contraceptives with significant changes (increase and decrease) in the

plasma levels of the estrogen and progestin being noted in some cases. The safety and efficacy of combination oral contraceptive products may be affected with co-administration of anti-HIV protease inhibitors). Products include:

Rufinamide (Contraceptive effectiveness may be reduced when hormonal contraceptives are co-administered with anticonvulsants and other drugs that increase metabolism of contraceptive steroids. This could result in unintended pregnancy or breakthrough bleeding). Products include:

Salsalate (Increased clearance of salicylic acid due to induction of conjugation has been noted when co-administered with combination oral contraceptives).
No products indexed under this heading.

Saquinavir (Several protease inhibitors have been studied with co-administration of oral combination hormonal contraceptives with significant changes (increase and decrease) in the plasma levels of the estrogen and progestin being noted in some cases. The safety and efficacy of combination oral contraceptive products may be affected with co-administration of anti-HIV protease inhibitors).
No products indexed under this heading.

Saquinavir Mesylate (Several protease inhibitors have been studied with co-administration of oral combination hormonal contraceptives with significant changes (increase and decrease) in the plasma levels of the estrogen and progestin being noted in some cases. The safety and efficacy of combination oral contraceptive products may be affected with co-administration of anti-HIV protease inhibitors).
No products indexed under this heading.

Secobarbital Sodium (Contraceptive effectivness may be reduced when hormonal contraceptives are co-administered with drugs that increase the metabolism of contraceptive steroids, such as barbiturates).
No products indexed under this heading.

Sertraline Hydrochloride (CYP3A4 inhibitors may increase plasma ethinyl estradiol levels).
No products indexed under this heading.

Sildenafil Citrate (CYP3A4 inhibitors may increase plasma ethinyl estradiol levels).
No products indexed under this heading.

Sodium Butabarbital (Contraceptive effectivness may be reduced when hormonal contraceptives are co-administered with drugs that increase the metabolism of contraceptive steroids, such as barbiturates).
No products indexed under this heading.

Sodium Cloxacillin Monohydrate (Contraceptive effectiveness may be reduced when hormonal contraceptives are co-administered with antibiotics and other drugs that increase metabolism of contraceptive steroids. This could result in unintended pregnancy or breakthrough bleeding).
No products indexed under this heading.

Sodium Pentobarbital (Contraceptive effectivness may be reduced when hormonal contraceptives are co-administered with drugs that increase the metabolism of contraceptive steroids, such as barbiturates).

Sparfloxacin (Contraceptive effectiveness may be reduced when hormonal contraceptives are co-administered with antibiotics and other drugs that increase metabolism of contraceptive steroids. This could result in unintended pregnancy or breakthrough bleeding).
No products indexed under this heading.

Streptomycin Sulfate (Contraceptive effectiveness may be reduced when hormonal contraceptives are co-administered with antibiotics and other drugs that increase metabolism of contraceptive steroids. This could result in unintended pregnancy or breakthrough bleeding).
No products indexed under this heading.

Sulfamethizole (Contraceptive effectiveness may be reduced when hormonal contraceptives are co-administered with antibiotics and other drugs that increase metabolism of contraceptive steroids. This could result in unintended pregnancy or breakthrough bleeding).
No products indexed under this heading.

Sulfamethoxazole (Contraceptive effectiveness may be reduced when hormonal contraceptives are co-administered with antibiotics and other drugs that increase metabolism of contraceptive steroids. This could result in unintended pregnancy or breakthrough bleeding).
No products indexed under this heading.

Sulfisoxazole Acetyl (Contraceptive effectiveness may be reduced when hormonal contraceptives are co-administered with antibiotics and other drugs that increase metabolism of contraceptive steroids. This could result in unintended pregnancy or breakthrough bleeding).
No products indexed under this heading.

Sulfisoxazole Diolamine (Contraceptive effectiveness may be reduced when hormonal contraceptives are co-administered with antibiotics and other drugs that increase metabolism of contraceptive steroids. This could result in unintended pregnancy or breakthrough bleeding).
No products indexed under this heading.

Telithromycin (CYP3A4 inhibitors may increase plasma ethinyl estradiol levels). Products include:

Temazepam (Increased clearance of temazepam due to induction of conjugation has been noted when co-administered with combination oral contraceptives).
No products indexed under this heading.

Tetracycline Hydrochloride (Several cases of contraceptive failure and breakthrough bleeding have been reported in the literature concomitant administration of antibiotics, such as tetracyclines; however, clinical pharmacology studies investigating drug interactions between combined oral contraceptives and these antibiotics have reported inconsistent results). Products include:

Tetracycline Phosphate Complex (Several cases of contraceptive failure and breakthrough bleeding have been reported in the literature concomitant administration of antibiotics, such as tetracyclines; however, clinical pharmacology studies investigating drug interactions between combined oral contraceptives and these antibiotics have reported inconsistent results).
No products indexed under this heading.

Theophylline (Combination hormonal contraceptives containing some synthetic estrogens (eg, ethinyl estradiol) may inhibit the metabolism of other compounds. Increased plasma concentrations of theophylline have been reported with concomitant administration of combination oral contraceptives).
No products indexed under this heading.

Theophylline Anhydrous (Combination hormonal contraceptives containing some synthetic estrogens (eg, ethinyl estradiol) may inhibit the metabolism of other compounds. Increased plasma concentrations of theophylline have been reported with concomitant administration of combination oral contraceptives). Products include:

Theophylline Calcium Salicylate (Combination hormonal contraceptives containing some synthetic estrogens (eg, ethinyl estradiol) may inhibit the metabolism of other compounds. Increased plasma concentrations of theophylline have been reported with concomitant administration of combination oral contraceptives).
No products indexed under this heading.

Theophylline Dihydroxypropyl (Glyceryl) (Combination hormonal contraceptives containing some synthetic estrogens (eg, ethinyl estradiol) may inhibit the metabolism of other compounds. Increased plasma concentrations of theophylline have been reported with concomitant administration of combination oral contraceptives).
No products indexed under this heading.

Theophylline Ethylenediamine (Combination hormonal contraceptives containing some synthetic estrogens (eg, ethinyl estradiol) may inhibit the metabolism of other compounds. Increased plasma concentrations of theophylline have been reported with concomitant administration of combination oral contraceptives).
No products indexed under this heading.

Theophylline Sodium Glycinate (Combination hormonal contraceptives containing some synthetic estrogens (eg, ethinyl estradiol) may inhibit the metabolism of other compounds. Increased plasma concentrations of theophylline have been reported with concomitant administration of combination oral contraceptives).
No products indexed under this heading.

Thiamylal Sodium (Contraceptive effectivness may be reduced when hormonal contraceptives are co-administered with drugs that increase the metabolism of contraceptive steroids, such as barbiturates).
No products indexed under this heading.

Tiagabine Hydrochloride (Contraceptive effectiveness may be reduced when hormonal contraceptives are co-administered with anticonvulsants and other drugs that increase metabolism of contraceptive steroids. This could result in unintended pregnancy or breakthrough bleeding). Products include:

Ticarcillin Disodium (Contraceptive effectiveness may be reduced when hormonal contraceptives are co-administered with antibiotics and other drugs that increase metabolism of contraceptive steroids. This could result in unintended pregnancy or breakthrough bleeding). Products include:

Tipranavir (Several protease inhibitors have been studied with co-administration of oral combination hormonal contraceptives with significant changes (increase and decrease) in the plasma levels of the estrogen and progestin being noted in some cases. The safety and efficacy of combination oral contraceptive products may be affected with co-administration of anti-HIV protease inhibitors).
No products indexed under this heading.

Tobacco (Cigarette smoking increases the risk of serious cardiovascular side effects from oral contraceptive use. This risk increases with age and with heavy smoking (15 or more cigarettes per day) and is quite marked in women over 35 years of age. Women who use oral contraceptives should be strongly advised not to smoke).
No products indexed under this heading.

Tobramycin (Contraceptive effectiveness may be reduced when hormonal contraceptives are co-administered with antibiotics and other drugs that increase metabolism of contraceptive steroids. This could result in unintended pregnancy or breakthrough bleeding). Products include:

Tobramycin Sulfate (Contraceptive effectiveness may be reduced when hormonal contraceptives are co-administered with antibiotics and other drugs that increase metabolism of contraceptive steroids. This could result in unintended pregnancy or breakthrough bleeding).
No products indexed under this heading.

Topiramate (Contraceptive effectiveness may be reduced when hormonal contraceptives are co-administered with drugs that increase the metabolism of contraceptive steroids, such as topiramate).
No products indexed under this heading.

Trimethadione (Contraceptive effectiveness may be reduced when hormonal contraceptives are co-administered with anticonvulsants and other drugs that increase metabolism of contraceptive steroids. This could result in unintended pregnancy or breakthrough bleeding).
No products indexed under this heading.

Troglitazone (CYP3A4 inhibitors may increase plasma ethinyl estradiol levels).
No products indexed under this heading.

Troleandomycin (CYP3A4 inhibitors may increase plasma ethinyl estradiol levels).
No products indexed under this heading.

Trovafloxacin Mesylate (Contraceptive effectiveness may be reduced when hormonal contraceptives are co-administered with antibiotics and other drugs that increase metabolism of contraceptive steroids. This could result in unintended pregnancy or breakthrough bleeding).
No products indexed under this heading.

Valproate Sodium (CYP3A4 inhibitors may increase plasma ethinyl estradiol levels).
No products indexed under this heading.

Valproic Acid (Contraceptive effectiveness may be reduced when hormonal contraceptives are co-administered with anticonvulsants and other drugs that increase metabolism of contraceptive steroids. This could result in unintended pregnancy or breakthrough bleeding).
No products indexed under this heading.

Vardenafil Hydrochloride (CYP3A4 inhibitors may increase plasma ethinyl estradiol levels). Products include:

Verapamil Hydrochloride (CYP3A4 inhibitors may increase plasma ethinyl estradiol levels). Products include:

Tarka 534

Vitamin C (Ascorbic acid may increase plasma ethinyl estradiol levels, possibly by inhibition of conjugation). Products include:

Bausch & Lomb Ocuvite Adult
50+ .... ☉238
Bio-C 3454
BoneMate Plus 3454
Cardio Basics 3455
CitraNatal 90 DHA Capsules 2332
CitraNatal Assure 2332
CitraNatal Rx 2332
Ferralet 2333
Heplive 607
Meili Clear 607
MoviPrep Oral Solution 2905
PreNexa 3473
Proflavanol 90 3476

Voriconazole (CYP3A4 inhibitors may increase plasma ethinyl estradiol levels).

No products indexed under this heading.

Zafirlukast (CYP3A4 inhibitors may increase plasma ethinyl estradiol levels). Products include:

Accolate 3612

Zileuton (CYP3A4 inhibitors may increase plasma ethinyl estradiol levels).

No products indexed under this heading.

Zonisamide (Contraceptive effectiveness may be reduced when hormonal contraceptives are co-administered with anticonvulsants and other drugs that increase metabolism of contraceptive steroids. This could result in unintended pregnancy or breakthrough bleeding). Products include:

Zonegran 1081

Food Interactions

Grapefruit (CYP3A4 inhibitors may increase plasma ethinyl estradiol levels).

Grapefruit Juice (CYP3A4 inhibitors may increase plasma ethinyl estradiol levels).

SELZENTRY TABLETS

(Maraviroc) 2740

May interact with antihypertensives, cytochrome p450 2d6 substrates (selected), cytochrome p450 3a inducers (selected), cytochrome p450 3a inhibitors (selected), P-glycoprotein inducers, P-glycoprotein inhibitors, and certain other agents. Compounds in these categories include:

Acebutolol Hydrochloride (Caution should be used when administering maraviroc in patients with a history of postural hypotension or on concomitant medication known to lower blood pressure).

No products indexed under this heading.

Aliskiren (Caution should be used when administering maraviroc in patients with a history of postural hypotension or on concomitant medication known to lower blood pressure). Products include:

Tekturna 2538
Tekturna HCT 2541
Valturna 3637

Allium sativum (Maraviroc is a substrate of CYP3A and Pgp and hence its pharmacokinetics are likely to be modulated by inhibitors and inducers of these enzymes/transporters. The CYP3A inducers rifampin and efavirenz decreased the C$_{max}$ and AUC of maraviroc).

No products indexed under this heading.

Amiodarone Hydrochloride (Maraviroc is a substrate of CYP3A and Pgp and hence its pharmacokinetics are likely to be modulated by inhibitors and inducers of these enzymes/transporters. The CYP3A/Pgp inhibitors ketoconazole, lopinavir/ritonavir, ritonavir, saquinavir and atazanavir all increased the C$_{max}$ and AUC of maraviroc).

No products indexed under this heading.

Amitriptyline Hydrochloride (Maraviroc had no effect on the debrisoquine metabolic ratio (MR) at 300 mg twice or less in vivo and did not cause inhibition of CYP2D6 in vitro until concentrations> 100 µM. However, there was 234% increase in debrisoquine MR on treatment compared to baseline at 600 mg once daily, suggesting potential inhibition of CYP2D6 at higher dose).

No products indexed under this heading.

Amlodipine Besylate (Caution should be used when administering maraviroc in patients with a history of postural hypotension or on concomitant medication known to lower blood pressure). Products include:

Azor 1010
Exforge 2443
Exforge HCT 2449

Amphetamine Aspartate (Maraviroc had no effect on the debrisoquine metabolic ratio (MR) at 300 mg twice or less in vivo and did not cause inhibition of CYP2D6 in vitro until concentrations> 100 µM. However, there was 234% increase in debrisoquine MR on treatment compared to baseline at 600 mg once daily, suggesting potential inhibition of CYP2D6 at higher dose).

No products indexed under this heading.

Amphetamine Aspartate Monohydrate (Maraviroc had no effect on the debrisoquine metabolic ratio (MR) at 300 mg twice or less in vivo and did not cause inhibition of CYP2D6 in vitro until concentrations> 100 µM. However, there was 234% increase in debrisoquine MR on treatment compared to baseline at 600 mg once daily, suggesting potential inhibition of CYP2D6 at higher dose).

No products indexed under this heading.

Amphetamine Sulfate (Maraviroc had no effect on the debrisoquine metabolic ratio (MR) at 300 mg twice or less in vivo and did not cause inhibition of CYP2D6 in vitro until concentrations> 100 µM. However, there was 234% increase in debrisoquine MR on treatment compared to baseline at 600 mg once daily, suggesting potential inhibition of CYP2D6 at higher dose).

No products indexed under this heading.

Amprenavir (Maraviroc is a substrate of CYP3A and Pgp and hence its pharmacokinetics are likely to be modulated by inhibitors and inducers of these enzymes/transporters. The CYP3A/Pgp inhibitors ketoconazole, lopinavir/ritonavir, ritonavir, saquinavir and atazanavir all increased the C$_{max}$ and AUC of maraviroc).

No products indexed under this heading.

Aprepitant (Maraviroc is a substrate of CYP3A and Pgp and hence its pharmacokinetics are likely to be modulated by inhibitors and inducers of these enzymes/transporters. The CYP3A/Pgp inhibitors ketoconazole, lopinavir/ritonavir, ritonavir, saquinavir and atazanavir all increased the C$_{max}$ and AUC of maraviroc). Products include:

Emend 2124

Atazanavir (The CYP3A/Pgp inhibitor atazanavir increased the C$_{max}$ and AUC of maraviroc).

No products indexed under this heading.

Atazanavir Sulfate (The CYP3A/Pgp inhibitor atazanavir increased the C$_{max}$ and AUC of maraviroc).

No products indexed under this heading.

Atenolol (Caution should be used when administering maraviroc in patients with a history of postural hypotension or on concomitant medication known to lower blood pressure).

No products indexed under this heading.

Atomoxetine Hydrochloride (Maraviroc had no effect on the debrisoquine metabolic ratio (MR) at 300 mg twice or less in vivo and did not cause inhibition of CYP2D6 in vitro until concentrations> 100 µM. However, there was 234% increase in debrisoquine MR on treatment compared to baseline at 600 mg once daily, suggesting potential inhibition of CYP2D6 at higher dose). Products include:

Strattera 1957

Atorvastatin Calcium (Maraviroc is a substrate of CYP3A and Pgp and hence its pharmacokinetics are likely to be modulated by inhibitors and inducers of these enzymes/transporters. The CYP3A/Pgp inhibitors ketoconazole, lopinavir/ritonavir, ritonavir, saquinavir and atazanavir all increased the C$_{max}$ and AUC of maraviroc). Products include:

Lipitor 2703

Azithromycin Dihydrate (Maraviroc is a substrate of CYP3A and Pgp and hence its pharmacokinetics are likely to be modulated by inhibitors and inducers of these enzymes/transporters. The CYP3A/Pgp inhibitors ketoconazole, lopinavir/ritonavir, ritonavir, saquinavir and atazanavir all increased the C$_{max}$ and AUC of maraviroc).

No products indexed under this heading.

Benazepril Hydrochloride (Caution should be used when administering maraviroc in patients with a history of postural hypotension or on concomitant medication known to lower blood pressure).

No products indexed under this heading.

Bendroflumethiazide (Caution should be used when administering maraviroc in patients with a history of postural hypotension or on concomitant medication known to lower blood pressure).

No products indexed under this heading.

Betaxolol Hydrochloride (Caution should be used when administering maraviroc in patients with a history of postural hypotension or on concomitant medication known to lower blood pressure).

No products indexed under this heading.

Bisoprolol Fumarate (Caution should be used when administering maraviroc in patients with a history of postural hypotension or on concomitant medication known to lower blood pressure).

No products indexed under this heading.

Candesartan Cilexetil (Caution should be used when administering maraviroc in patients with a history of postural hypotension or on concomitant medication known to lower blood pressure). Products include:

Atacand 697
Atacand HCT 700

Captopril (Caution should be used when administering maraviroc in patients with a history of postural hypotension or on concomitant medication known to lower blood pressure). Products include:

Captopril 2341

Carbamazepine (Maraviroc is a substrate of CYP3A and Pgp and hence its pharmacokinetics are likely to be modulated by inhibitors and inducers of these enzymes/transporters. The CYP3A

inducers rifampin and efavirenz decreased the C$_{max}$ and AUC of maraviroc). Products include:

Carbatrol 3280
Equetro 3477

Carteolol Hydrochloride (Caution should be used when administering maraviroc in patients with a history of postural hypotension or on concomitant medication known to lower blood pressure).

No products indexed under this heading.

Carvedilol (Caution should be used when administering maraviroc in patients with a history of postural hypotension or on concomitant medication known to lower blood pressure). Products include:

Coreg 1409

Carvedilol Phosphate (Caution should be used when administering maraviroc in patients with a history of postural hypotension or on concomitant medication known to lower blood pressure). Products include:

Coreg CR 1416

Cevimeline Hydrochloride (Maraviroc had no effect on the debrisoquine metabolic ratio (MR) at 300 mg twice or less in vivo and did not cause inhibition of CYP2D6 in vitro until concentrations> 100 µM. However, there was 234% increase in debrisoquine MR on treatment compared to baseline at 600 mg once daily, suggesting potential inhibition of CYP2D6 at higher dose). Products include:

Evoxac 1027

Chlorothiazide (Caution should be used when administering maraviroc in patients with a history of postural hypotension or on concomitant medication known to lower blood pressure).

No products indexed under this heading.

Chlorothiazide Sodium (Caution should be used when administering maraviroc in patients with a history of postural hypotension or on concomitant medication known to lower blood pressure). Products include:

Diuril Intravenous 2009

Chlorpromazine (Maraviroc is a substrate of CYP3A and Pgp and hence its pharmacokinetics are likely to be modulated by inhibitors and inducers of these enzymes/transporters. The CYP3A/Pgp inhibitors ketoconazole, lopinavir/ritonavir, ritonavir, saquinavir and atazanavir all increased the C$_{max}$ and AUC of maraviroc).

No products indexed under this heading.

Chlorpromazine Hydrochloride (Maraviroc is a substrate of CYP3A and Pgp and hence its pharmacokinetics are likely to be modulated by inhibitors and inducers of these enzymes/transporters. The CYP3A/Pgp inhibitors ketoconazole, lopinavir/ritonavir, ritonavir, saquinavir and atazanavir all increased the C$_{max}$ and AUC of maraviroc).

No products indexed under this heading.

Chlorpropamide (Maraviroc had no effect on the debrisoquine metabolic ratio (MR) at 300 mg twice or less in vivo and did not cause inhibition of CYP2D6 in vitro until concentrations> 100 µM. However, there was 234% increase in debrisoquine MR on treatment compared to baseline at 600 mg once daily, suggesting potential inhibition of CYP2D6 at higher dose).

No products indexed under this heading.

Chlorthalidone (Caution should be used when administering maraviroc in patients with a history of postural hypotension or on concomitant medication known to lower blood pressure). Products include:

Clorpres 2344

Cimetidine (Maraviroc is a substrate of CYP3A and Pgp and hence its pharmacokinetics are likely to be modulated by inhibitors and inducers of these enzymes/transporters. The CYP3A/Pgp inhibitors ketoconazole, lopinavir/ritonavir, ritonavir, saquinavir and atazanavir all increased the C_{max} and AUC of maraviroc).
No products indexed under this heading.

Cimetidine Hydrochloride (Maraviroc is a substrate of CYP3A and Pgp and hence its pharmacokinetics are likely to be modulated by inhibitors and inducers of these enzymes/transporters. The CYP3A/Pgp inhibitors ketoconazole, lopinavir/ritonavir, ritonavir, saquinavir and atazanavir all increased the C_{max} and AUC of maraviroc).
No products indexed under this heading.

Ciprofloxacin (Maraviroc is a substrate of CYP3A and Pgp and hence its pharmacokinetics are likely to be modulated by inhibitors and inducers of these enzymes/transporters. The CYP3A/Pgp inhibitors ketoconazole, lopinavir/ritonavir, ritonavir, saquinavir and atazanavir all increased the C_{max} and AUC of maraviroc). Products include:
Cipro I.V. 3082
Cipro 3073
Cipro XR 3091
Ciprodex 583

Ciprofloxacin Hydrochloride (Maraviroc is a substrate of CYP3A and Pgp and hence its pharmacokinetics are likely to be modulated by inhibitors and inducers of these enzymes/transporters. The CYP3A/Pgp inhibitors ketoconazole, lopinavir/ritonavir, ritonavir, saquinavir and atazanavir all increased the C_{max} and AUC of maraviroc). Products include:
Cipro 3073

Clarithromycin (Maraviroc is a substrate of CYP3A and Pgp and hence its pharmacokinetics are likely to be modulated by inhibitors and inducers of these enzymes/transporters. The CYP3A/Pgp inhibitors ketoconazole, lopinavir/ritonavir, ritonavir, saquinavir and atazanavir all increased the C_{max} and AUC of maraviroc). Products include:
Biaxin/Biaxin XL 412

Clomipramine Hydrochloride (Maraviroc had no effect on the debrisoquine metabolic ratio (MR) at 300 mg twice or less in vivo and did not cause inhibition of CYP2D6 in vitro until concentrations> 100 µM. However, there was 234% increase in debrisoquine MR on treatment compared to baseline at 600 mg once daily, suggesting potential inhibition of CYP2D6 at higher dose).
No products indexed under this heading.

Clonidine (Caution should be used when administering maraviroc in patients with a history of postural hypotension or on concomitant medication known to lower blood pressure). Products include:
Catapres-TTS 884

Clonidine Hydrochloride (Caution should be used when administering maraviroc in patients with a history of postural hypotension or on concomitant medication known to lower blood pressure). Products include:
Clorpres 2344

Clotrimazole (Maraviroc is a substrate of CYP3A and Pgp and hence its pharmacokinetics are likely to be modulated by inhibitors and inducers of these enzymes/transporters. The CYP3A/Pgp inhibitors ketoconazole, lopinavir/ritonavir, ritonavir, saquinavir and atazanavir all increased the C_{max} and AUC of maraviroc). Products include:
Lotrisone 3163

Clotrimazole, Topical (Maraviroc is a substrate of CYP3A and Pgp and hence its pharmacokinetics are likely to be modulated by inhibitors and inducers of these enzymes/transporters. The CYP3A/Pgp inhibitors ketoconazole, lopinavir/ritonavir, ritonavir, saquinavir and atazanavir all increased the C_{max} and AUC of maraviroc).
No products indexed under this heading.

Clozapine (Maraviroc had no effect on the debrisoquine metabolic ratio (MR) at 300 mg twice or less in vivo and did not cause inhibition of CYP2D6 in vitro until concentrations> 100 µM. However, there was 234% increase in debrisoquine MR on treatment compared to baseline at 600 mg once daily, suggesting potential inhibition of CYP2D6 at higher dose).
No products indexed under this heading.

Codeine Phosphate (Maraviroc had no effect on the debrisoquine metabolic ratio (MR) at 300 mg twice or less in vivo and did not cause inhibition of CYP2D6 in vitro until concentrations> 100 µM. However, there was 234% increase in debrisoquine MR on treatment compared to baseline at 600 mg once daily, suggesting potential inhibition of CYP2D6 at higher dose). Products include:
Tylenol with Codeine 2691

Codeine Sulfate (Maraviroc had no effect on the debrisoquine metabolic ratio (MR) at 300 mg twice or less in vivo and did not cause inhibition of CYP2D6 in vitro until concentrations> 100 µM. However, there was 234% increase in debrisoquine MR on treatment compared to baseline at 600 mg once daily, suggesting potential inhibition of CYP2D6 at higher dose).
No products indexed under this heading.

Cyclobenzaprine Hydrochloride (Maraviroc had no effect on the debrisoquine metabolic ratio (MR) at 300 mg twice or less in vivo and did not cause inhibition of CYP2D6 in vitro until concentrations> 100 µM. However, there was 234% increase in debrisoquine MR on treatment compared to baseline at 600 mg once daily, suggesting potential inhibition of CYP2D6 at higher dose). Products include:
Amrix 964

Cyclosporine (Maraviroc is a substrate of CYP3A and Pgp and hence its pharmacokinetics are likely to be modulated by inhibitors and inducers of these enzymes/transporters. The CYP3A/Pgp inhibitors ketoconazole, lopinavir/ritonavir, ritonavir, saquinavir and atazanavir all increased the C_{max} and AUC of maraviroc). Products include:
Gengraf 440
Neoral Oral Solution 2496
Neoral Capsules 2496
Restasis 605

Debrisoquine (Maraviroc had no effect on the debrisoquine metabolic ratio (MR) at 300 mg twice or less in vivo and did not cause inhibition of CYP2D6 in vitro until concentrations> 100 µM. However, there was 234% increase in debrisoquine MR on treatment compared to baseline at 600 mg once daily, suggesting potential inhibition of CYP2D6 at higher dose).
No products indexed under this heading.

Delavirdine Mesylate (Maraviroc is a substrate of CYP3A and Pgp and hence its pharmacokinetics are likely to be modulated by inhibitors and inducers of these enzymes/transporters. The CYP3A/Pgp inhibitors ketoconazole, lopinavir/ritonavir, ritonavir, saquinavir and atazanavir all increased the C_{max} and AUC of maraviroc).
No products indexed under this heading.

Deserpidine (Caution should be used when administering maraviroc in patients with a history of postural hypotension or on concomitant medication known to lower blood pressure).
No products indexed under this heading.

Desipramine Hydrochloride (Maraviroc had no effect on the debrisoquine metabolic ratio (MR) at 300 mg twice or less in vivo and did not cause inhibition of CYP2D6 in vitro until concentrations> 100 µM. However, there was 234% increase in debrisoquine MR on treatment compared to baseline at 600 mg once daily, suggesting potential inhibition of CYP2D6 at higher dose).
No products indexed under this heading.

Dexamethasone (Maraviroc is a substrate of CYP3A and Pgp and hence its pharmacokinetics are likely to be modulated by inhibitors and inducers of these enzymes/transporters. The CYP3A inducers rifampin and efavirenz decreased the C_{max} and AUC of maraviroc). Products include:
Ciprodex 583
Ozurdex ....⊙223
Tobramycin and Dexamethasone
Ophthalmic Suspension ....⊙251

Dexfenfluramine Hydrochloride (Maraviroc had no effect on the debrisoquine metabolic ratio (MR) at 300 mg twice or less in vivo and did not cause inhibition of CYP2D6 in vitro until concentrations> 100 µM. However, there was 234% increase in debrisoquine MR on treatment compared to baseline at 600 mg once daily, suggesting potential inhibition of CYP2D6 at higher dose).
No products indexed under this heading.

Dextromethorphan Hydrobromide (Maraviroc had no effect on the debrisoquine metabolic ratio (MR) at 300 mg twice or less in vivo and did not cause inhibition of CYP2D6 in vitro until concentrations> 100 µM. However, there was 234% increase in debrisoquine MR on treatment compared to baseline at 600 mg once daily, suggesting potential inhibition of CYP2D6 at higher dose).
No products indexed under this heading.

Dextromethorphan Polistirex (Maraviroc had no effect on the debrisoquine metabolic ratio (MR) at 300 mg twice or less in vivo and did not cause inhibition of CYP2D6 in vitro until concentrations> 100 µM. However, there was 234% increase in debrisoquine MR on treatment compared to baseline at 600 mg once daily, suggesting potential inhibition of CYP2D6 at higher dose).
No products indexed under this heading.

Diazoxide (Caution should be used when administering maraviroc in patients with a history of postural hypotension or on concomitant medication known to lower blood pressure). Products include:
Proglycem 1179
Proglycem Suspension 1179

Digoxin (Maraviroc is a substrate of CYP3A and Pgp and hence its pharmacokinetics are likely to be modulated by inhibitors and inducers of these enzymes/transporters. The CYP3A/Pgp inhibitors ketoconazole, lopinavir/ritonavir, ritonavir, saquinavir and atazanavir all increased the C_{max} and AUC of maraviroc). Products include:
Lanoxin Injection 1546
Lanoxin Injection Pediatric 1549
Lanoxin Tablets 1553

Diltiazem Hydrochloride (Caution should be used when administering maraviroc in patients with a history of postural hypotension or on concomitant medication known to lower blood pressure). Products include:

Cardizem LA 423

Diltiazem Maleate (Caution should be used when administering maraviroc in patients with a history of postural hypotension or on concomitant medication known to lower blood pressure).
No products indexed under this heading.

Dirithromycin (Maraviroc is a substrate of CYP3A and Pgp and hence its pharmacokinetics are likely to be modulated by inhibitors and inducers of these enzymes/transporters. The CYP3A/Pgp inhibitors ketoconazole, lopinavir/ritonavir, ritonavir, saquinavir and atazanavir all increased the C_{max} and AUC of maraviroc).
No products indexed under this heading.

Dolasetron Mesylate (Maraviroc had no effect on the debrisoquine metabolic ratio (MR) at 300 mg twice or less in vivo and did not cause inhibition of CYP2D6 in vitro until concentrations> 100 µM. However, there was 234% increase in debrisoquine MR on treatment compared to baseline at 600 mg once daily, suggesting potential inhibition of CYP2D6 at higher dose). Products include:
Anzemet Injection 2931
Anzemet Tablets 2934

Donepezil Hydrochloride (Maraviroc had no effect on the debrisoquine metabolic ratio (MR) at 300 mg twice or less in vivo and did not cause inhibition of CYP2D6 in vitro until concentrations> 100 µM. However, there was 234% increase in debrisoquine MR on treatment compared to baseline at 600 mg once daily, suggesting potential inhibition of CYP2D6 at higher dose). Products include:
Aricept 1045
Aricept ODT 1045

Doxazosin Mesylate (Caution should be used when administering maraviroc in patients with a history of postural hypotension or on concomitant medication known to lower blood pressure).
No products indexed under this heading.

Doxepin Hydrochloride (Maraviroc had no effect on the debrisoquine metabolic ratio (MR) at 300 mg twice or less in vivo and did not cause inhibition of CYP2D6 in vitro until concentrations> 100 µM. However, there was 234% increase in debrisoquine MR on treatment compared to baseline at 600 mg once daily, suggesting potential inhibition of CYP2D6 at higher dose).
No products indexed under this heading.

Efavirenz (The CYP3A inducer efavirenz decreased the C_{max} and AUC of maraviroc). Products include:
Atripla 906

Elacridar (Maraviroc is a substrate of CYP3A and Pgp and hence its pharmacokinetics are likely to be modulated by inhibitors and inducers of these enzymes/transporters. The CYP3A/Pgp inhibitors ketoconazole, lopinavir/ritonavir, ritonavir, saquinavir and atazanavir all increased the C_{max} and AUC of maraviroc).
No products indexed under this heading.

Enalapril Maleate (Caution should be used when administering maraviroc in patients with a history of postural hypotension or on concomitant medication known to lower blood pressure).
No products indexed under this heading.

Enalaprilat (Caution should be used when administering maraviroc in patients with a history of postural hypotension or on concomitant medication known to lower blood pressure).
No products indexed under this heading.

Encainide Hydrochloride (Maraviroc had no effect on the debrisoquine metabolic ratio (MR) at 300 mg twice or less in vivo and did not cause inhibition of CYP2D6 in vitro until concentrations>

IMPORTANT NOTE: Always consult each drug listing in the patient's regimen for possible interactions.

100 μM. However, there was 234% increase in debrisoquine MR on treatment compared to baseline at 600 mg once daily, suggesting potential inhibition of CYP2D6 at higher dose).
No products indexed under this heading.

Enfuvirtide (Maraviroc was additive/synergistic with the HIV fusion inhibitor enfuvirtide).
No products indexed under this heading.

Eprosartan Mesylate (Caution should be used when administering maraviroc in patients with a history of postural hypotension or on concomitant medication known to lower blood pressure). Products include:

Erythromycin (Maraviroc is a substrate of CYP3A and Pgp and hence its pharmacokinetics are likely to be modulated by inhibitors and inducers of these enzymes/transporters. The CYP3A/Pgp inhibitors ketoconazole, lopinavir/ritonavir, ritonavir, saquinavir and atazanavir all increased the C_{max} and AUC of maraviroc).
No products indexed under this heading.

Erythromycin, Topical (Maraviroc is a substrate of CYP3A and Pgp and hence its pharmacokinetics are likely to be modulated by inhibitors and inducers of these enzymes/transporters. The CYP3A/Pgp inhibitors ketoconazole, lopinavir/ritonavir, ritonavir, saquinavir and atazanavir all increased the C_{max} and AUC of maraviroc).
No products indexed under this heading.

Erythromycin Estolate (Maraviroc is a substrate of CYP3A and Pgp and hence its pharmacokinetics are likely to be modulated by inhibitors and inducers of these enzymes/transporters. The CYP3A/Pgp inhibitors ketoconazole, lopinavir/ritonavir, ritonavir, saquinavir and atazanavir all increased the C_{max} and AUC of maraviroc).
No products indexed under this heading.

Erythromycin Ethylsuccinate (Maraviroc is a substrate of CYP3A and Pgp and hence its pharmacokinetics are likely to be modulated by inhibitors and inducers of these enzymes/transporters. The CYP3A/Pgp inhibitors ketoconazole, lopinavir/ritonavir, ritonavir, saquinavir and atazanavir all increased the C_{max} and AUC of maraviroc). Products include:

Erythromycin Gluceptate (Maraviroc is a substrate of CYP3A and Pgp and hence its pharmacokinetics are likely to be modulated by inhibitors and inducers of these enzymes/transporters. The CYP3A/Pgp inhibitors ketoconazole, lopinavir/ritonavir, ritonavir, saquinavir and atazanavir all increased the C_{max} and AUC of maraviroc).
No products indexed under this heading.

Erythromycin Lactobionate (Maraviroc is a substrate of CYP3A and Pgp and hence its pharmacokinetics are likely to be modulated by inhibitors and inducers of these enzymes/transporters. The CYP3A/Pgp inhibitors ketoconazole, lopinavir/ritonavir, ritonavir, saquinavir and atazanavir all increased the C_{max} and AUC of maraviroc).
No products indexed under this heading.

Erythromycin Stearate (Maraviroc is a substrate of CYP3A and Pgp and hence its pharmacokinetics are likely to be modulated by inhibitors and inducers of these enzymes/transporters. The CYP3A/Pgp inhibitors ketoconazole, lopinavir/ritonavir, ritonavir, saquinavir and atazanavir all increased the C_{max} and AUC of maraviroc).
No products indexed under this heading.

Esmolol Hydrochloride (Caution should be used when administering maraviroc in patients with a history of postural hypotension or on concomitant medication known to lower blood pressure).
No products indexed under this heading.

Ethosuximide (Maraviroc is a substrate of CYP3A and Pgp and hence its pharmacokinetics are likely to be modulated by inhibitors and inducers of these enzymes/transporters. The CYP3A inducers rifampin and efavirenz decreased the C_{max} and AUC of maraviroc).
No products indexed under this heading.

Fat (Co-administration of a 300 mg tablet with a high fat breakfast reduced maraviroc C_{max} and AUC by 33% in healthy volunteers. There were no food restrictions in the studies that demonstrated the efficacy and safety of maraviroc. Therefore, maraviroc can be taken with or without food at the recommended dose).
No products indexed under this heading.

Felodipine (Caution should be used when administering maraviroc in patients with a history of postural hypotension or on concomitant medication known to lower blood pressure).
No products indexed under this heading.

Fentanyl (Maraviroc had no effect on the debrisoquine metabolic ratio (MR) at 300 mg twice or less in vivo and did not cause inhibition of CYP2D6 in vitro until concentrations> 100 μM. However, there was 234% increase in debrisoquine MR on treatment compared to baseline at 600 mg once daily, suggesting potential inhibition of CYP2D6 at higher dose). Products include:

Fentanyl Citrate (Maraviroc had no effect on the debrisoquine metabolic ratio (MR) at 300 mg twice or less in vivo and did not cause inhibition of CYP2D6 in vitro until concentrations> 100 μM. However, there was 234% increase in debrisoquine MR on treatment compared to baseline at 600 mg once daily, suggesting potential inhibition of CYP2D6 at higher dose). Products include:

Flecainide Acetate (Maraviroc had no effect on the debrisoquine metabolic ratio (MR) at 300 mg twice or less in vivo and did not cause inhibition of CYP2D6 in vitro until concentrations> 100 μM. However, there was 234% increase in debrisoquine MR on treatment compared to baseline at 600 mg once daily, suggesting potential inhibition of CYP2D6 at higher dose).
No products indexed under this heading.

Fluconazole (Maraviroc is a substrate of CYP3A and Pgp and hence its pharmacokinetics are likely to be modulated by inhibitors and inducers of these enzymes/transporters. The CYP3A/Pgp inhibitors ketoconazole, lopinavir/ritonavir, ritonavir, saquinavir and atazanavir all increased the C_{max} and AUC of maraviroc).
No products indexed under this heading.

Fluoxetine (Maraviroc is a substrate of CYP3A and Pgp and hence its pharmacokinetics are likely to be modulated by inhibitors and inducers of these enzymes/transporters. The CYP3A/Pgp inhibitors ketoconazole, lopinavir/ritonavir, ritonavir, saquinavir and atazanavir all increased the C_{max} and AUC of maraviroc).
No products indexed under this heading.

Fluoxetine Hydrochloride (Maraviroc is a substrate of CYP3A and Pgp and hence its pharmacokinetics are likely to be modulated by inhibitors and

inducers of these enzymes/transporters. The CYP3A/Pgp inhibitors ketoconazole, lopinavir/ritonavir, ritonavir, saquinavir and atazanavir all increased the C_{max} and AUC of maraviroc). Products include:

Fluphenazine Decanoate (Maraviroc is a substrate of CYP3A and Pgp and hence its pharmacokinetics are likely to be modulated by inhibitors and inducers of these enzymes/transporters. The CYP3A/Pgp inhibitors ketoconazole, lopinavir/ritonavir, ritonavir, saquinavir and atazanavir all increased the C_{max} and AUC of maraviroc).
No products indexed under this heading.

Fluphenazine Enanthate (Maraviroc is a substrate of CYP3A and Pgp and hence its pharmacokinetics are likely to be modulated by inhibitors and inducers of these enzymes/transporters. The CYP3A/Pgp inhibitors ketoconazole, lopinavir/ritonavir, ritonavir, saquinavir and atazanavir all increased the C_{max} and AUC of maraviroc).
No products indexed under this heading.

Fluphenazine Hydrochloride (Maraviroc is a substrate of CYP3A and Pgp and hence its pharmacokinetics are likely to be modulated by inhibitors and inducers of these enzymes/transporters. The CYP3A/Pgp inhibitors ketoconazole, lopinavir/ritonavir, ritonavir, saquinavir and atazanavir all increased the C_{max} and AUC of maraviroc).
No products indexed under this heading.

Fluvoxamine Maleate (Maraviroc is a substrate of CYP3A and Pgp and hence its pharmacokinetics are likely to be modulated by inhibitors and inducers of these enzymes/transporters. The CYP3A/Pgp inhibitors ketoconazole, lopinavir/ritonavir, ritonavir, saquinavir and atazanavir all increased the C_{max} and AUC of maraviroc).
No products indexed under this heading.

Formoterol Fumarate (Maraviroc had no effect on the debrisoquine metabolic ratio (MR) at 300 mg twice or less in vivo and did not cause inhibition of CYP2D6 in vitro until concentrations> 100 μM. However, there was 234% increase in debrisoquine MR on treatment compared to baseline at 600 mg once daily, suggesting potential inhibition of CYP2D6 at higher dose). Products include:

Fosamprenavir Calcium (Maraviroc is a substrate of CYP3A and Pgp and hence its pharmacokinetics are likely to be modulated by inhibitors and inducers of these enzymes/transporters. The CYP3A/Pgp inhibitors ketoconazole, lopinavir/ritonavir, ritonavir, saquinavir and atazanavir all increased the C_{max} and AUC of maraviroc). Products include:

Fosinopril Sodium (Caution should be used when administering maraviroc in patients with a history of postural hypotension or on concomitant medication known to lower blood pressure).
No products indexed under this heading.

Furosemide (Caution should be used when administering maraviroc in patients with a history of postural hypotension or on concomitant medication known to lower blood pressure). Products include:

Galantamine Hydrobromide (Maraviroc had no effect on the debrisoquine metabolic ratio (MR) at 300 mg twice or less in vivo and did not cause

inhibition of CYP2D6 in vitro until concentrations> 100 μM. However, there was 234% increase in debrisoquine MR on treatment compared to baseline at 600 mg once daily, suggesting potential inhibition of CYP2D6 at higher dose).
No products indexed under this heading.

Guanabenz Acetate (Caution should be used when administering maraviroc in patients with a history of postural hypotension or on concomitant medication known to lower blood pressure).
No products indexed under this heading.

Guanethidine (Caution should be used when administering maraviroc in patients with a history of postural hypotension or on concomitant medication known to lower blood pressure).
No products indexed under this heading.

Guanethidine Monosulfate (Caution should be used when administering maraviroc in patients with a history of postural hypotension or on concomitant medication known to lower blood pressure).
No products indexed under this heading.

Guanethidine Sulfate (Caution should be used when administering maraviroc in patients with a history of postural hypotension or on concomitant medication known to lower blood pressure).
No products indexed under this heading.

Haloperidol (Maraviroc had no effect on the debrisoquine metabolic ratio (MR) at 300 mg twice or less in vivo and did not cause inhibition of CYP2D6 in vitro until concentrations> 100 μM. However, there was 234% increase in debrisoquine MR on treatment compared to baseline at 600 mg once daily, suggesting potential inhibition of CYP2D6 at higher dose).
No products indexed under this heading.

Haloperidol Decanoate (Maraviroc had no effect on the debrisoquine metabolic ratio (MR) at 300 mg twice or less in vivo and did not cause inhibition of CYP2D6 in vitro until concentrations> 100 μM. However, there was 234% increase in debrisoquine MR on treatment compared to baseline at 600 mg once daily, suggesting potential inhibition of CYP2D6 at higher dose).
No products indexed under this heading.

Hydralazine Hydrochloride (Caution should be used when administering maraviroc in patients with a history of postural hypotension or on concomitant medication known to lower blood pressure).
No products indexed under this heading.

Hydrochlorothiazide (Caution should be used when administering maraviroc in patients with a history of postural hypotension or on concomitant medication known to lower blood pressure). Products include:

Hydrocodone Bitartrate (Maraviroc had no effect on the debrisoquine metabolic ratio (MR) at 300 mg twice or less in vivo and did not cause inhibition of CYP2D6 in vitro until concentrations> 100 μM. However, there was 234% increase in debrisoquine MR on treatment compared to baseline at 600 mg

once daily, suggesting potential inhibition of CYP2D6 at higher dose).
Products include:
Vicodin 560
Vicodin ES 561
Vicodin HP 563
Vicoprofen 564
Zydone 1138

Hydroflumethiazide (Caution should be used when administering maraviroc in patients with a history of postural hypotension or on concomitant medication known to lower blood pressure).
No products indexed under this heading.

Hypericum (Maraviroc is a substrate of CYP3A and Pgp and hence its pharmacokinetics are likely to be modulated by inhibitors and inducers of these enzymes/transporters. The CYP3A/Pgp inhibitors ketoconazole, lopinavir/ritonavir, ritonavir, saquinavir and atazanavir all increased the C_{max} and AUC of maraviroc).
No products indexed under this heading.

Hypericum Perforatum (Concomitant use of maraviroc and St. John's Wort (hypericum perforatum) or products containing St. John's Wort is not recommended. Co-administration of maraviroc with St. John's Wort is expected to substantially decrease maraviroc concentrations and may result in suboptimal levels of maraviroc and lead to loss of virologic response and possible resistance to maraviroc).
Products include:
Traumeel 1800

Imipramine Hydrochloride (Maraviroc had no effect on the debrisoquine metabolic ratio (MR) at 300 mg twice or less in vivo and did not cause inhibition of CYP2D6 in vitro until concentrations> 100 µM. However, there was 234% increase in debrisoquine MR on treatment compared to baseline at 600 mg once daily, suggesting potential inhibition of CYP2D6 at higher dose).
No products indexed under this heading.

Imipramine Pamoate (Maraviroc had no effect on the debrisoquine metabolic ratio (MR) at 300 mg twice or less in vivo and did not cause inhibition of CYP2D6 in vitro until concentrations> 100 µM. However, there was 234% increase in debrisoquine MR on treatment compared to baseline at 600 mg once daily, suggesting potential inhibition of CYP2D6 at higher dose).
No products indexed under this heading.

Indapamide (Caution should be used when administering maraviroc in patients with a history of postural hypotension or on concomitant medication known to lower blood pressure).
Products include:
Indapamide 2356

Indinavir Sulfate (Maraviroc is a substrate of CYP3A and Pgp and hence its pharmacokinetics are likely to be modulated by inhibitors and inducers of these enzymes/transporters. The CYP3A/Pgp inhibitors ketoconazole, lopinavir/ritonavir, ritonavir, saquinavir and atazanavir all increased the C_{max} and AUC of maraviroc). Products include:
Crixivan 2113

Indoramin Hydrochloride (Maraviroc had no effect on the debrisoquine metabolic ratio (MR) at 300 mg twice or less in vivo and did not cause inhibition of CYP2D6 in vitro until concentrations> 100 µM. However, there was 234% increase in debrisoquine MR on treatment compared to baseline at 600 mg once daily, suggesting potential inhibition of CYP2D6 at higher dose).
No products indexed under this heading.

Irbesartan (Caution should be used when administering maraviroc in patients with a history of postural hypo-

tension or on concomitant medication known to lower blood pressure).
Products include:
Avalide 2956
Avapro 2962

Isoniazid (Maraviroc is a substrate of CYP3A and Pgp and hence its pharmacokinetics are likely to be modulated by inhibitors and inducers of these enzymes/transporters. The CYP3A/Pgp inhibitors ketoconazole, lopinavir/ritonavir, ritonavir, saquinavir and atazanavir all increased the C_{max} and AUC of maraviroc).
No products indexed under this heading.

Isradipine (Caution should be used when administering maraviroc in patients with a history of postural hypotension or on concomitant medication known to lower blood pressure).
Products include:
DynaCirc CR 1432

Itraconazole (Maraviroc is a substrate of CYP3A and Pgp and hence its pharmacokinetics are likely to be modulated by inhibitors and inducers of these enzymes/transporters. The CYP3A/Pgp inhibitors ketoconazole, lopinavir/ritonavir, ritonavir, saquinavir and atazanavir all increased the C_{max} and AUC of maraviroc).
No products indexed under this heading.

Ketoconazole (The CYP3A/Pgp inhibitor ketoconazole increased the C_{max} and AUC of maraviroc). Products include:
Extina 3319
Xolegel 3337

Labetalol Hydrochloride (Caution should be used when administering maraviroc in patients with a history of postural hypotension or on concomitant medication known to lower blood pressure).
No products indexed under this heading.

Lidocaine (Maraviroc had no effect on the debrisoquine metabolic ratio (MR) at 300 mg twice or less in vivo and did not cause inhibition of CYP2D6 in vitro until concentrations> 100 µM. However, there was 234% increase in debrisoquine MR on treatment compared to baseline at 600 mg once daily, suggesting potential inhibition of CYP2D6 at higher dose). Products include:
Lidoderm 1107

Lidocaine Hydrochloride (Maraviroc had no effect on the debrisoquine metabolic ratio (MR) at 300 mg twice or less in vivo and did not cause inhibition of CYP2D6 in vitro until concentrations> 100 µM. However, there was 234% increase in debrisoquine MR on treatment compared to baseline at 600 mg once daily, suggesting potential inhibition of CYP2D6 at higher dose).
No products indexed under this heading.

Lisinopril (Caution should be used when administering maraviroc in patients with a history of postural hypotension or on concomitant medication known to lower blood pressure).
Products include:
Prinivil 2241
Prinzide 2246

Lopinavir (The CYP3A/Pgp inhibitor lopinavir increased the C_{max} and AUC of maraviroc). Products include:
Kaletra 458

Losartan Potassium (Caution should be used when administering maraviroc in patients with a history of postural hypotension or on concomitant medication known to lower blood pressure).
Products include:
Cozaar 2106
Hyzaar 2162
Hyzaar 100-12.5 2162

Maprotiline Hydrochloride (Maraviroc had no effect on the debrisoquine metabolic ratio (MR) at 300 mg twice or

less in vivo and did not cause inhibition of CYP2D6 in vitro until concentrations> 100 µM. However, there was 234% increase in debrisoquine MR on treatment compared to baseline at 600 mg once daily, suggesting potential inhibition of CYP2D6 at higher dose).
No products indexed under this heading.

Mecamylamine Hydrochloride (Caution should be used when administering maraviroc in patients with a history of postural hypotension or on concomitant medication known to lower blood pressure).
No products indexed under this heading.

Meperidine Hydrochloride (Maraviroc had no effect on the debrisoquine metabolic ratio (MR) at 300 mg twice or less in vivo and did not cause inhibition of CYP2D6 in vitro until concentrations> 100 µM. However, there was 234% increase in debrisoquine MR on treatment compared to baseline at 600 mg once daily, suggesting potential inhibition of CYP2D6 at higher dose).
No products indexed under this heading.

Mesoridazine Besylate (Maraviroc is a substrate of CYP3A and Pgp and hence its pharmacokinetics are likely to be modulated by inhibitors and inducers of these enzymes/transporters. The CYP3A/Pgp inhibitors ketoconazole, lopinavir/ritonavir, ritonavir, saquinavir and atazanavir all increased the C_{max} and AUC of maraviroc).
No products indexed under this heading.

Methadone Hydrochloride (Maraviroc had no effect on the debrisoquine metabolic ratio (MR) at 300 mg twice or less in vivo and did not cause inhibition of CYP2D6 in vitro until concentrations> 100 µM. However, there was 234% increase in debrisoquine MR on treatment compared to baseline at 600 mg once daily, suggesting potential inhibition of CYP2D6 at higher dose).
No products indexed under this heading.

Methamphetamine Hydrochloride (Maraviroc had no effect on the debrisoquine metabolic ratio (MR) at 300 mg twice or less in vivo and did not cause inhibition of CYP2D6 in vitro until concentrations> 100 µM. However, there was 234% increase in debrisoquine MR on treatment compared to baseline at 600 mg once daily, suggesting potential inhibition of CYP2D6 at higher dose).
No products indexed under this heading.

Methoxyphenamine (Maraviroc had no effect on the debrisoquine metabolic ratio (MR) at 300 mg twice or less in vivo and did not cause inhibition of CYP2D6 in vitro until concentrations> 100 µM. However, there was 234% increase in debrisoquine MR on treatment compared to baseline at 600 mg once daily, suggesting potential inhibition of CYP2D6 at higher dose).
No products indexed under this heading.

Methyclothiazide (Caution should be used when administering maraviroc in patients with a history of postural hypotension or on concomitant medication known to lower blood pressure).
No products indexed under this heading.

Methyldopa (Caution should be used when administering maraviroc in patients with a history of postural hypotension or on concomitant medication known to lower blood pressure).
No products indexed under this heading.

Methyldopate Hydrochloride (Caution should be used when administering maraviroc in patients with a history of postural hypotension or on concomitant medication known to lower blood pressure).
No products indexed under this heading.

Metolazone (Caution should be used when administering maraviroc in patients with a history of postural hypotension or on concomitant medication known to lower blood pressure).
No products indexed under this heading.

Metoprolol Succinate (Caution should be used when administering maraviroc in patients with a history of postural hypotension or on concomitant medication known to lower blood pressure). Products include:
Toprol XL 732

Metoprolol Tartrate (Caution should be used when administering maraviroc in patients with a history of postural hypotension or on concomitant medication known to lower blood pressure).
No products indexed under this heading.

Metronidazole (Maraviroc is a substrate of CYP3A and Pgp and hence its pharmacokinetics are likely to be modulated by inhibitors and inducers of these enzymes/transporters. The CYP3A/Pgp inhibitors ketoconazole, lopinavir/ritonavir, ritonavir, saquinavir and atazanavir all increased the C_{max} and AUC of maraviroc). Products include:
Pylera 793

Metronidazole Benzoate (Maraviroc is a substrate of CYP3A and Pgp and hence its pharmacokinetics are likely to be modulated by inhibitors and inducers of these enzymes/transporters. The CYP3A/Pgp inhibitors ketoconazole, lopinavir/ritonavir, ritonavir, saquinavir and atazanavir all increased the C_{max} and AUC of maraviroc).
No products indexed under this heading.

Metronidazole Hydrochloride (Maraviroc is a substrate of CYP3A and Pgp and hence its pharmacokinetics are likely to be modulated by inhibitors and inducers of these enzymes/transporters. The CYP3A/Pgp inhibitors ketoconazole, lopinavir/ritonavir, ritonavir, saquinavir and atazanavir all increased the C_{max} and AUC of maraviroc).
No products indexed under this heading.

Metyrosine (Caution should be used when administering maraviroc in patients with a history of postural hypotension or on concomitant medication known to lower blood pressure).
No products indexed under this heading.

Mexiletine Hydrochloride (Maraviroc had no effect on the debrisoquine metabolic ratio (MR) at 300 mg twice or less in vivo and did not cause inhibition of CYP2D6 in vitro until concentrations> 100 µM. However, there was 234% increase in debrisoquine MR on treatment compared to baseline at 600 mg once daily, suggesting potential inhibition of CYP2D6 at higher dose).
No products indexed under this heading.

Mibefradil Dihydrochloride (Caution should be used when administering maraviroc in patients with a history of postural hypotension or on concomitant medication known to lower blood pressure).
No products indexed under this heading.

Miconazole (Maraviroc is a substrate of CYP3A and Pgp and hence its pharmacokinetics are likely to be modulated by inhibitors and inducers of these enzymes/transporters. The CYP3A/Pgp inhibitors ketoconazole, lopinavir/ritonavir, ritonavir, saquinavir and atazanavir all increased the C_{max} and AUC of maraviroc).
No products indexed under this heading.

Minoxidil (Caution should be used when administering maraviroc in patients with a history of postural hypotension or on concomitant medication known to lower blood pressure).
No products indexed under this heading.

Mirtazapine (Maraviroc had no effect on the debrisoquine metabolic ratio

(MR) at 300 mg twice or less *in vivo* and did not cause inhibition of CYP2D6 *in vitro* until concentrations> 100 μM. However, there was 234% increase in debrisoquine MR on treatment compared to baseline at 600 mg once daily, suggesting potential inhibition of CYP2D6 at higher dose). Products include:

Modafinil (Maraviroc is a substrate of CYP3A and Pgp and hence its pharmacokinetics are likely to be modulated by inhibitors and inducers of these enzymes/transporters. The CYP3A inducers rifampin and efavirenz decreased the C_{max} and AUC of maraviroc). Products include:

Moexipril Hydrochloride (Caution should be used when administering maraviroc in patients with a history of postural hypotension or on concomitant medication known to lower blood pressure).

No products indexed under this heading.

Morphine Sulfate (Maraviroc had no effect on the debrisoquine metabolic ratio (MR) at 300 mg twice or less *in vivo* and did not cause inhibition of CYP2D6 *in vitro* until concentrations> 100 μM. However, there was 234% increase in debrisoquine MR on treatment compared to baseline at 600 mg once daily, suggesting potential inhibition of CYP2D6 at higher dose). Products include:

Nadolol (Caution should be used when administering maraviroc in patients with a history of postural hypotension or on concomitant medication known to lower blood pressure). Products include:

Nebivolol (Caution should be used when administering maraviroc in patients with a history of postural hypotension or on concomitant medication known to lower blood pressure). Products include:

Nefazodone Hydrochloride (Maraviroc is a substrate of CYP3A and Pgp and hence its pharmacokinetics are likely to be modulated by inhibitors and inducers of these enzymes/transporters. The CYP3A/Pgp inhibitors ketoconazole, lopinavir/ritonavir, ritonavir, saquinavir and atazanavir all increased the C_{max} and AUC of maraviroc).

No products indexed under this heading.

Nelfinavir Mesylate (Maraviroc is a substrate of CYP3A and Pgp and hence its pharmacokinetics are likely to be modulated by inhibitors and inducers of these enzymes/transporters. The CYP3A/Pgp inhibitors ketoconazole, lopinavir/ritonavir, ritonavir, saquinavir and atazanavir all increased the C_{max} and AUC of maraviroc).

No products indexed under this heading.

Nevirapine (Maraviroc is a substrate of CYP3A and Pgp and hence its pharmacokinetics are likely to be modulated by inhibitors and inducers of these enzymes/transporters. The CYP3A inducers rifampin and efavirenz decreased the C_{max} and AUC of maraviroc). Products include:

Nicardipine Hydrochloride (Caution should be used when administering maraviroc in patients with a history of postural hypotension or on concomitant medication known to lower blood pressure).

No products indexed under this heading.

Nifedipine (Caution should be used when administering maraviroc in patients with a history of postural hypotension or on concomitant medication known to lower blood pressure).

No products indexed under this heading.

Nisoldipine (Caution should be used when administering maraviroc in patients with a history of postural hypotension or on concomitant medication known to lower blood pressure).

No products indexed under this heading.

Nitroglycerin (Caution should be used when administering maraviroc in patients with a history of postural hypotension or on concomitant medication known to lower blood pressure). Products include:

Norfloxacin (Maraviroc is a substrate of CYP3A and Pgp and hence its pharmacokinetics are likely to be modulated by inhibitors and inducers of these enzymes/transporters. The CYP3A/Pgp inhibitors ketoconazole, lopinavir/ritonavir, ritonavir, saquinavir and atazanavir all increased the C_{max} and AUC of maraviroc). Products include:

Nortriptyline Hydrochloride (Maraviroc had no effect on the debrisoquine metabolic ratio (MR) at 300 mg twice or less *in vivo* and did not cause inhibition of CYP2D6 *in vitro* until concentrations> 100 μM. However, there was 234% increase in debrisoquine MR on treatment compared to baseline at 600 mg once daily, suggesting potential inhibition of CYP2D6 at higher dose).

No products indexed under this heading.

Olanzapine (Maraviroc had no effect on the debrisoquine metabolic ratio (MR) at 300 mg twice or less *in vivo* and did not cause inhibition of CYP2D6 *in vitro* until concentrations> 100 μM. However, there was 234% increase in debrisoquine MR on treatment compared to baseline at 600 mg once daily, suggesting potential inhibition of CYP2D6 at higher dose). Products include:

Omeprazole (Maraviroc had no effect on the debrisoquine metabolic ratio (MR) at 300 mg twice or less *in vivo* and did not cause inhibition of CYP2D6 *in vitro* until concentrations> 100 μM. However, there was 234% increase in debrisoquine MR on treatment compared to baseline at 600 mg once daily, suggesting potential inhibition of CYP2D6 at higher dose).

No products indexed under this heading.

Ondansetron (Maraviroc had no effect on the debrisoquine metabolic ratio (MR) at 300 mg twice or less *in vivo* and did not cause inhibition of CYP2D6 *in vitro* until concentrations> 100 μM. However, there was 234% increase in debrisoquine MR on treatment compared to baseline at 600 mg once daily, suggesting potential inhibition of CYP2D6 at higher dose).

No products indexed under this heading.

Ondansetron Hydrochloride (Maraviroc had no effect on the debrisoquine metabolic ratio (MR) at 300 mg twice or less *in vivo* and did not cause inhibition of CYP2D6 *in vitro* until concentrations> 100 μM. However, there was 234% increase in debrisoquine MR on treatment compared to baseline at 600 mg once daily, suggesting potential inhibition of CYP2D6 at higher dose). Products include:

Oxycodone Hydrochloride (Maraviroc had no effect on the debrisoquine metabolic ratio (MR) at 300 mg twice or less *in vivo* and did not cause inhibition of CYP2D6 *in vitro* until concentrations> 100 μM. However, there was 234% increase in debrisoquine MR on treatment compared to baseline at 600 mg once daily, suggesting potential inhibition of CYP2D6 at higher dose). Products include:

Paclitaxel (Maraviroc had no effect on the debrisoquine metabolic ratio (MR) at 300 mg twice or less *in vivo* and did not cause inhibition of CYP2D6 *in vitro* until concentrations> 100 μM. However, there was 234% increase in debrisoquine MR on treatment compared to baseline at 600 mg once daily, suggesting potential inhibition of CYP2D6 at higher dose).

No products indexed under this heading.

Paroxetine Hydrochloride (Maraviroc is a substrate of CYP3A and Pgp and hence its pharmacokinetics are likely to be modulated by inhibitors and inducers of these enzymes/transporters. The CYP3A/Pgp inhibitors ketoconazole, lopinavir/ritonavir, ritonavir, saquinavir and atazanavir all increased the C_{max} and AUC of maraviroc). Products include:

Penbutolol Sulfate (Caution should be used when administering maraviroc in patients with a history of postural hypotension or on concomitant medication known to lower blood pressure).

No products indexed under this heading.

Perindopril Erbumine (Caution should be used when administering maraviroc in patients with a history of postural hypotension or on concomitant medication known to lower blood pressure).

No products indexed under this heading.

Perphenazine (Maraviroc is a substrate of CYP3A and Pgp and hence its pharmacokinetics are likely to be modulated by inhibitors and inducers of these enzymes/transporters. The CYP3A/Pgp inhibitors ketoconazole, lopinavir/ritonavir, ritonavir, saquinavir and atazanavir all increased the C_{max} and AUC of maraviroc).

No products indexed under this heading.

Phenobarbital (Maraviroc is a substrate of CYP3A and Pgp and hence its pharmacokinetics are likely to be modulated by inhibitors and inducers of these enzymes/transporters. The CYP3A inducers rifampin and efavirenz decreased the C_{max} and AUC of maraviroc). Products include:

Phenobarbital Sodium (Maraviroc is a substrate of CYP3A and Pgp and hence its pharmacokinetics are likely to be modulated by inhibitors and inducers of these enzymes/transporters. The CYP3A inducers rifampin and efavirenz decreased the C_{max} and AUC of maraviroc).

No products indexed under this heading.

Phenothiazine Derivatives (Maraviroc is a substrate of CYP3A and Pgp and hence its pharmacokinetics are likely to be modulated by inhibitors and inducers of these enzymes/transporters. The CYP3A/Pgp inhibitors ketoconazole, lopinavir/ritonavir, ritonavir, saquinavir and atazanavir all increased the C_{max} and AUC of maraviroc).

No products indexed under this heading.

Phenothiazines (Maraviroc is a substrate of CYP3A and Pgp and hence its pharmacokinetics are likely to be modulated by inhibitors and inducers of these enzymes/transporters. The CYP3A/Pgp inhibitors ketoconazole, lopinavir/ritonavir, ritonavir, saquinavir and atazanavir all increased the C_{max} and AUC of maraviroc).

No products indexed under this heading.

Phenoxybenzamine Hydrochloride (Caution should be used when administering maraviroc in patients with a history of postural hypotension or on concomitant medication known to lower blood pressure). Products include:

Phentolamine Mesylate (Caution should be used when administering maraviroc in patients with a history of postural hypotension or on concomitant medication known to lower blood pressure).

No products indexed under this heading.

Phenytoin (Maraviroc is a substrate of CYP3A and Pgp and hence its pharmacokinetics are likely to be modulated by inhibitors and inducers of these enzymes/transporters. The CYP3A inducers rifampin and efavirenz decreased the C_{max} and AUC of maraviroc).

No products indexed under this heading.

Phenytoin Sodium (Maraviroc is a substrate of CYP3A and Pgp and hence its pharmacokinetics are likely to be modulated by inhibitors and inducers of these enzymes/transporters. The CYP3A inducers rifampin and efavirenz decreased the C_{max} and AUC of maraviroc). Products include:

Pindolol (Caution should be used when administering maraviroc in patients with a history of postural hypotension or on concomitant medication known to lower blood pressure).

No products indexed under this heading.

Polythiazide (Caution should be used when administering maraviroc in patients with a history of postural hypotension or on concomitant medication known to lower blood pressure).

No products indexed under this heading.

Prazosin Hydrochloride (Caution should be used when administering maraviroc in patients with a history of postural hypotension or on concomitant medication known to lower blood pressure).

No products indexed under this heading.

Prochlorperazine (Maraviroc is a substrate of CYP3A and Pgp and hence its pharmacokinetics are likely to be modulated by inhibitors and inducers of these enzymes/transporters. The CYP3A/Pgp inhibitors ketoconazole, lopinavir/ritonavir, ritonavir, saquinavir and atazanavir all increased the C_{max} and AUC of maraviroc).

No products indexed under this heading.

Prochlorperazine Edisylate (Maraviroc is a substrate of CYP3A and Pgp and hence its pharmacokinetics are likely to be modulated by inhibitors and inducers of these enzymes/transporters. The CYP3A/Pgp inhibitors ketoconazole, lopinavir/ritonavir, ritonavir, saquinavir and atazanavir all increased the C_{max} and AUC of maraviroc).

No products indexed under this heading.

Prochlorperazine Maleate (Maraviroc is a substrate of CYP3A and Pgp and hence its pharmacokinetics are likely to be modulated by inhibitors and inducers of these enzymes/transporters. The CYP3A/Pgp inhibitors ketoconazole, lopinavir/ritonavir, ritonavir, saquinavir and atazanavir all increased the C_{max} and AUC of maraviroc).
No products indexed under this heading.

Promethazine (Maraviroc is a substrate of CYP3A and Pgp and hence its pharmacokinetics are likely to be modulated by inhibitors and inducers of these enzymes/transporters. The CYP3A/Pgp inhibitors ketoconazole, lopinavir/ritonavir, ritonavir, saquinavir and atazanavir all increased the C_{max} and AUC of maraviroc).
No products indexed under this heading.

Promethazine Hydrochloride (Maraviroc is a substrate of CYP3A and Pgp and hence its pharmacokinetics are likely to be modulated by inhibitors and inducers of these enzymes/transporters. The CYP3A/Pgp inhibitors ketoconazole, lopinavir/ritonavir, ritonavir, saquinavir and atazanavir all increased the C_{max} and AUC of maraviroc).
No products indexed under this heading.

Propafenone Hydrochloride (Maraviroc had no effect on the debrisoquine metabolic ratio (MR) at 300 mg twice or less *in vivo* and did not cause inhibition of CYP2D6 *in vitro* until concentrations> 100 μM. However, there was 234% increase in debrisoquine MR on treatment compared to baseline at 600 mg once daily, suggesting potential inhibition of CYP2D6 at higher dose). Products include:
Rythmol 1648
Rythmol SR 1652

Propoxyphene Hydrochloride (Maraviroc had no effect on the debrisoquine metabolic ratio (MR) at 300 mg twice or less *in vivo* and did not cause inhibition of CYP2D6 *in vitro* until concentrations> 100 μM. However, there was 234% increase in debrisoquine MR on treatment compared to baseline at 600 mg once daily, suggesting potential inhibition of CYP2D6 at higher dose).
No products indexed under this heading.

Propoxyphene Napsylate (Maraviroc had no effect on the debrisoquine metabolic ratio (MR) at 300 mg twice or less *in vivo* and did not cause inhibition of CYP2D6 *in vitro* until concentrations> 100 μM. However, there was 234% increase in debrisoquine MR on treatment compared to baseline at 600 mg once daily, suggesting potential inhibition of CYP2D6 at higher dose).
No products indexed under this heading.

Propranolol Hydrochloride (Caution should be used when administering maraviroc in patients with a history of postural hypotension or on concomitant medication known to lower blood pressure). Products include:
InnoPran XL 1517

Quetiapine Fumarate (Maraviroc had no effect on the debrisoquine metabolic ratio (MR) at 300 mg twice or less *in vivo* and did not cause inhibition of CYP2D6 *in vitro* until concentrations> 100 μM. However, there was 234% increase in debrisoquine MR on treatment compared to baseline at 600 mg once daily, suggesting potential inhibition of CYP2D6 at higher dose). Products include:
Seroquel 750
Seroquel XR 759

Quinapril Hydrochloride (Caution should be used when administering maraviroc in patients with a history of postural hypotension or on concomitant medication known to lower blood pressure).
No products indexed under this heading.

Quinidine (Maraviroc is a substrate of CYP3A and Pgp and hence its pharmacokinetics are likely to be modulated by inhibitors and inducers of these enzymes/transporters. The CYP3A/Pgp inhibitors ketoconazole, lopinavir/ritonavir, ritonavir, saquinavir and atazanavir all increased the C_{max} and AUC of maraviroc).
No products indexed under this heading.

Quinidine Gluconate (Maraviroc is a substrate of CYP3A and Pgp and hence its pharmacokinetics are likely to be modulated by inhibitors and inducers of these enzymes/transporters. The CYP3A/Pgp inhibitors ketoconazole, lopinavir/ritonavir, ritonavir, saquinavir and atazanavir all increased the C_{max} and AUC of maraviroc).
No products indexed under this heading.

Quinidine Hydrochloride (Maraviroc is a substrate of CYP3A and Pgp and hence its pharmacokinetics are likely to be modulated by inhibitors and inducers of these enzymes/transporters. The CYP3A/Pgp inhibitors ketoconazole, lopinavir/ritonavir, ritonavir, saquinavir and atazanavir all increased the C_{max} and AUC of maraviroc).
No products indexed under this heading.

Quinidine Polygalacturonate (Maraviroc is a substrate of CYP3A and Pgp and hence its pharmacokinetics are likely to be modulated by inhibitors and inducers of these enzymes/transporters. The CYP3A/Pgp inhibitors ketoconazole, lopinavir/ritonavir, ritonavir, saquinavir and atazanavir all increased the C_{max} and AUC of maraviroc).
No products indexed under this heading.

Quinidine Sulfate (Maraviroc is a substrate of CYP3A and Pgp and hence its pharmacokinetics are likely to be modulated by inhibitors and inducers of these enzymes/transporters. The CYP3A/Pgp inhibitors ketoconazole, lopinavir/ritonavir, ritonavir, saquinavir and atazanavir all increased the C_{max} and AUC of maraviroc).
No products indexed under this heading.

Quinine (Maraviroc is a substrate of CYP3A and Pgp and hence its pharmacokinetics are likely to be modulated by inhibitors and inducers of these enzymes/transporters. The CYP3A/Pgp inhibitors ketoconazole, lopinavir/ritonavir, ritonavir, saquinavir and atazanavir all increased the C_{max} and AUC of maraviroc). Products include:
Hyland's Leg Cramps PM with Quinine 3315

Quinine Sulfate (Maraviroc is a substrate of CYP3A and Pgp and hence its pharmacokinetics are likely to be modulated by inhibitors and inducers of these enzymes/transporters. The CYP3A/Pgp inhibitors ketoconazole, lopinavir/ritonavir, ritonavir, saquinavir and atazanavir all increased the C_{max} and AUC of maraviroc).
No products indexed under this heading.

Ramipril (Caution should be used when administering maraviroc in patients with a history of postural hypotension or on concomitant medication known to lower blood pressure).
No products indexed under this heading.

Rauwolfia Serpentina (Caution should be used when administering maraviroc in patients with a history of postural hypotension or on concomitant medication known to lower blood pressure).
No products indexed under this heading.

Rescinnamine (Caution should be used when administering maraviroc in patients with a history of postural hypotension or on concomitant medication known to lower blood pressure).
No products indexed under this heading.

Reserpine (Caution should be used when administering maraviroc in patients with a history of postural hypotension or on concomitant medication known to lower blood pressure).
No products indexed under this heading.

Rifabutin (Maraviroc is a substrate of CYP3A and Pgp and hence its pharmacokinetics are likely to be modulated by inhibitors and inducers of these enzymes/transporters. The CYP3A inducers rifampin and efavirenz decreased the C_{max} and AUC of maraviroc).
No products indexed under this heading.

Rifampicin (Maraviroc is a substrate of CYP3A and Pgp and hence its pharmacokinetics are likely to be modulated by inhibitors and inducers of these enzymes/transporters. The CYP3A inducers rifampin and efavirenz decreased the C_{max} and AUC of maraviroc).
No products indexed under this heading.

Rifampin (The CYP3A inducer rifampin decreased the C_{max} and AUC of maraviroc).
No products indexed under this heading.

Rifapentine (Maraviroc is a substrate of CYP3A and Pgp and hence its pharmacokinetics are likely to be modulated by inhibitors and inducers of these enzymes/transporters. The CYP3A inducers rifampin and efavirenz decreased the C_{max} and AUC of maraviroc).
No products indexed under this heading.

Risperidone (Maraviroc had no effect on the debrisoquine metabolic ratio (MR) at 300 mg twice or less *in vivo* and did not cause inhibition of CYP2D6 *in vitro* until concentrations> 100 μM. However, there was 234% increase in debrisoquine MR on treatment compared to baseline at 600 mg once daily, suggesting potential inhibition of CYP2D6 at higher dose). Products include:
Risperdal Consta 2682

Ritonavir (The CYP3A/Pgp inhibitor ritonavir increased the C_{max} and AUC of maraviroc). Products include:
Kaletra 458
Norvir 509

Saquinavir (The CYP3A/Pgp inhibitor saquinavir increased the C_{max} and AUC of maraviroc).
No products indexed under this heading.

Saquinavir Mesylate (The CYP3A/Pgp inhibitor saquinavir increased the C_{max} and AUC of maraviroc).
No products indexed under this heading.

Sertraline Hydrochloride (Maraviroc is a substrate of CYP3A and Pgp and hence its pharmacokinetics are likely to be modulated by inhibitors and inducers of these enzymes/transporters. The CYP3A/Pgp inhibitors ketoconazole, lopinavir/ritonavir, ritonavir, saquinavir and atazanavir all increased the C_{max} and AUC of maraviroc).
No products indexed under this heading.

Sodium Nitroprusside (Caution should be used when administering maraviroc in patients with a history of postural hypotension or on concomitant medication known to lower blood pressure).
No products indexed under this heading.

Sotalol Hydrochloride (Caution should be used when administering maraviroc in patients with a history of postural hypotension or on concomitant medication known to lower blood pressure).
No products indexed under this heading.

Spirapril Hydrochloride (Caution should be used when administering maraviroc in patients with a history of postural hypotension or on concomitant medication known to lower blood pressure).
No products indexed under this heading.

Tamoxifen Citrate (Maraviroc is a substrate of CYP3A and Pgp and hence its pharmacokinetics are likely to be modulated by inhibitors and inducers of these enzymes/transporters. The CYP3A/Pgp inhibitors ketoconazole, lopinavir/ritonavir, ritonavir, saquinavir and atazanavir all increased the C_{max} and AUC of maraviroc).
No products indexed under this heading.

Telmisartan (Caution should be used when administering maraviroc in patients with a history of postural hypotension or on concomitant medication known to lower blood pressure).
Products include:
Micardis 887
Micardis HCT 889

Teniposide (Maraviroc had no effect on the debrisoquine metabolic ratio (MR) at 300 mg twice or less *in vivo* and did not cause inhibition of CYP2D6 *in vitro* until concentrations> 100 μM. However, there was 234% increase in debrisoquine MR on treatment compared to baseline at 600 mg once daily, suggesting potential inhibition of CYP2D6 at higher dose).
No products indexed under this heading.

Terazosin Hydrochloride (Caution should be used when administering maraviroc in patients with a history of postural hypotension or on concomitant medication known to lower blood pressure).
No products indexed under this heading.

Testosterone (Maraviroc had no effect on the debrisoquine metabolic ratio (MR) at 300 mg twice or less *in vivo* and did not cause inhibition of CYP2D6 *in vitro* until concentrations> 100 μM. However, there was 234% increase in debrisoquine MR on treatment compared to baseline at 600 mg once daily, suggesting potential inhibition of CYP2D6 at higher dose). Products include:
AndroGel 3456

Testosterone Cypionate (Maraviroc had no effect on the debrisoquine metabolic ratio (MR) at 300 mg twice or less *in vivo* and did not cause inhibition of CYP2D6 *in vitro* until concentrations> 100 μM. However, there was 234% increase in debrisoquine MR on treatment compared to baseline at 600 mg once daily, suggesting potential inhibition of CYP2D6 at higher dose).
No products indexed under this heading.

Testosterone Enanthate (Maraviroc had no effect on the debrisoquine metabolic ratio (MR) at 300 mg twice or less *in vivo* and did not cause inhibition of CYP2D6 *in vitro* until concentrations> 100 μM. However, there was 234% increase in debrisoquine MR on treatment compared to baseline at 600 mg once daily, suggesting potential inhibition of CYP2D6 at higher dose).
Products include:
Delatestryl 1102

Testosterone Propionate (Maraviroc had no effect on the debrisoquine metabolic ratio (MR) at 300 mg twice or less *in vivo* and did not cause inhibition of CYP2D6 *in vitro* until concentrations> 100 μM. However, there was 234% increase in debrisoquine MR on treat-

Selzentry Interactions Index 1712

ment compared to baseline at 600 mg once daily, suggesting potential inhibition of CYP2D6 at higher dose).
No products indexed under this heading.

Thioridazine (Maraviroc is a substrate of CYP3A and Pgp and hence its pharmacokinetics are likely to be modulated by inhibitors and inducers of these enzymes/transporters. The CYP3A/Pgp inhibitors ketoconazole, lopinavir/ritonavir, ritonavir, saquinavir and atazanavir all increased the C_{max} and AUC of maraviroc).
No products indexed under this heading.

Thioridazine Hydrochloride (Maraviroc is a substrate of CYP3A and Pgp and hence its pharmacokinetics are likely to be modulated by inhibitors and inducers of these enzymes/transporters. The CYP3A/Pgp inhibitors ketoconazole, lopinavir/ritonavir, ritonavir, saquinavir and atazanavir all increased the C_{max} and AUC of maraviroc). Products include:
Thioridazine Hydrochloride 2384

Timolol Maleate (Caution should be used when administering maraviroc in patients with a history of postural hypotension or on concomitant medication known to lower blood pressure).
Products include:
Combigan 601
Dorzolamide Hydrochloride/Timolol Maleate Ophthalmic Solution .... ⊙243
Timoptic in Ocudose .... ⊙231

Tolterodine Tartrate (Maraviroc had no effect on the debrisoquine metabolic ratio (MR) at 300 mg twice or less *in vivo* and did not cause inhibition of CYP2D6 *in vitro* until concentrations> 100 µM. However, there was 234% increase in debrisoquine MR on treatment compared to baseline at 600 mg once daily, suggesting potential inhibition of CYP2D6 at higher dose).
No products indexed under this heading.

Torsemide (Caution should be used when administering maraviroc in patients with a history of postural hypotension or on concomitant medication known to lower blood pressure).
No products indexed under this heading.

Tramadol Hydrochloride (Maraviroc had no effect on the debrisoquine metabolic ratio (MR) at 300 mg twice or less *in vivo* and did not cause inhibition of CYP2D6 *in vitro* until concentrations> 100 µM. However, there was 234% increase in debrisoquine MR on treatment compared to baseline at 600 mg once daily, suggesting potential inhibition of CYP2D6 at higher dose).
Products include:
Ryzolt 2813
Ultram ER 2693

Trandolapril (Caution should be used when administering maraviroc in patients with a history of postural hypotension or on concomitant medication known to lower blood pressure).
Products include:
Mavik 489
Tarka 534

Trazodone Hydrochloride (Maraviroc had no effect on the debrisoquine metabolic ratio (MR) at 300 mg twice or less *in vivo* and did not cause inhibition of CYP2D6 *in vitro* until concentrations> 100 µM. However, there was 234% increase in debrisoquine MR on treatment compared to baseline at 600 mg once daily, suggesting potential inhibition of CYP2D6 at higher dose).
No products indexed under this heading.

Triazolam (Maraviroc had no effect on the debrisoquine metabolic ratio (MR) at 300 mg twice or less *in vivo* and did not cause inhibition of CYP2D6 *in vitro* until concentrations> 100 µM. However, there was 234% increase in debrisoquine MR on treatment compared to baseline at 600 mg once daily, suggesting potential inhibition of CYP2D6 at higher dose).
No products indexed under this heading.

Trifluoperazine Hydrochloride (Maraviroc is a substrate of CYP3A and Pgp and hence its pharmacokinetics are likely to be modulated by inhibitors and inducers of these enzymes/transporters. The CYP3A/Pgp inhibitors ketoconazole, lopinavir/ritonavir, ritonavir, saquinavir and atazanavir all increased the C_{max} and AUC of maraviroc).
No products indexed under this heading.

Trimethaphan Camsylate (Caution should be used when administering maraviroc in patients with a history of postural hypotension or on concomitant medication known to lower blood pressure).
No products indexed under this heading.

Trimipramine Maleate (Maraviroc had no effect on the debrisoquine metabolic ratio (MR) at 300 mg twice or less *in vivo* and did not cause inhibition of CYP2D6 *in vitro* until concentrations> 100 µM. However, there was 234% increase in debrisoquine MR on treatment compared to baseline at 600 mg once daily, suggesting potential inhibition of CYP2D6 at higher dose).
No products indexed under this heading.

Troleandomycin (Maraviroc is a substrate of CYP3A and Pgp and hence its pharmacokinetics are likely to be modulated by inhibitors and inducers of these enzymes/transporters. The CYP3A/Pgp inhibitors ketoconazole, lopinavir/ritonavir, ritonavir, saquinavir and atazanavir all increased the C_{max} and AUC of maraviroc).
No products indexed under this heading.

Valsartan (Caution should be used when administering maraviroc in patients with a history of postural hypotension or on concomitant medication known to lower blood pressure).
Products include:
Diovan 2413
Diovan HCT 2419
Exforge 2443
Exforge HCT 2449
Valturna 3637

Venlafaxine Hydrochloride (Maraviroc is a substrate of CYP3A and Pgp and hence its pharmacokinetics are likely to be modulated by inhibitors and inducers of these enzymes/transporters. The CYP3A/Pgp inhibitors ketoconazole, lopinavir/ritonavir, ritonavir, saquinavir and atazanavir all increased the C_{max} and AUC of maraviroc). Products include:
Effexor XR 3504
Venlafaxine Hydrochloride Tablets ... 2388

Verapamil Hydrochloride (Caution should be used when administering maraviroc in patients with a history of postural hypotension or on concomitant medication known to lower blood pressure). Products include:
Tarka 534

Vinblastine Sulfate (Maraviroc had no effect on the debrisoquine metabolic ratio (MR) at 300 mg twice or less *in vivo* and did not cause inhibition of CYP2D6 *in vitro* until concentrations> 100 µM. However, there was 234% increase in debrisoquine MR on treatment compared to baseline at 600 mg once daily, suggesting potential inhibition of CYP2D6 at higher dose).
No products indexed under this heading.

Voriconazole (Maraviroc is a substrate of CYP3A and Pgp and hence its pharmacokinetics are likely to be modulated by inhibitors and inducers of these enzymes/transporters. The CYP3A/Pgp inhibitors ketoconazole, lopinavir/ritonavir, ritonavir, saquinavir and atazanavir all increased the C_{max} and AUC of maraviroc).
No products indexed under this heading.

Zafirlukast (Maraviroc is a substrate of CYP3A and Pgp and hence its pharmacokinetics are likely to be modulated by inhibitors and inducers of these enzymes/transporters. The CYP3A/Pgp inhibitors ketoconazole, lopinavir/ritonavir, ritonavir, saquinavir and atazanavir all increased the C_{max} and AUC of maraviroc). Products include:
Accolate 3612

Zileuton (Maraviroc is a substrate of CYP3A and Pgp and hence its pharmacokinetics are likely to be modulated by inhibitors and inducers of these enzymes/transporters. The CYP3A/Pgp inhibitors ketoconazole, lopinavir/ritonavir, ritonavir, saquinavir and atazanavir all increased the C_{max} and AUC of maraviroc).
No products indexed under this heading.

Zonisamide (Maraviroc had no effect on the debrisoquine metabolic ratio (MR) at 300 mg twice or less *in vivo* and did not cause inhibition of CYP2D6 *in vitro* until concentrations> 100 µM. However, there was 234% increase in debrisoquine MR on treatment compared to baseline at 600 mg once daily, suggesting potential inhibition of CYP2D6 at higher dose). Products include:
Zonegran 1081

Food Interactions

Food, unspecified (Co-administration of a 300 mg tablet with a high fat breakfast reduced maraviroc C_{max} and AUC by 33% in healthy volunteers. There were no food restrictions in the studies that demonstrated the efficacy and safety of maraviroc. Therefore, maraviroc can be taken with or without food at the recommended dose).

Grapefruit (Maraviroc is a substrate of CYP3A and Pgp and hence its pharmacokinetics are likely to be modulated by inhibitors and inducers of these enzymes/transporters. The CYP3A/Pgp inhibitors ketoconazole, lopinavir/ritonavir, ritonavir, saquinavir and atazanavir all increased the C_{max} and AUC of maraviroc).

Grapefruit Juice (Maraviroc is a substrate of CYP3A and Pgp and hence its pharmacokinetics are likely to be modulated by inhibitors and inducers of these enzymes/transporters. The CYP3A/Pgp inhibitors ketoconazole, lopinavir/ritonavir, ritonavir, saquinavir and atazanavir all increased the C_{max} and AUC of maraviroc).

Meal, unspecified (Co-administration of a 300 mg tablet with a high fat breakfast reduced maraviroc C_{max} and AUC by 33% in healthy volunteers. There were no food restrictions in the studies that demonstrated the efficacy and safety of maraviroc. Therefore, maraviroc can be taken with or without food at the recommended dose).

SEN-SEI-RO LIQUID GOLD

(Dietary Supplement) 1849
None cited in PDR database.

SEN-SEI-RO LIQUID ROYAL

(Dietary Supplement) 1849
None cited in PDR database.

SEN-SEI-RO POWDER GOLD

(Dietary Supplement) 1849
None cited in PDR database.

SENSIPAR TABLETS

(Cinacalcet Hydrochloride) 640
May interact with cytochrome p450 2d6 substrates (selected), cytochrome p450 3a4 inhibitors (selected), cytochrome p450 3a4 inhibitors, potent (selected), erythromycin, tricyclic antidepressants, and certain other agents. Compounds in these categories include:

Acetazolamide (Co-administration of ketoconazole, a strong inhibitor of CYP3A4, increased cinacalcet exposure following a single 90 mg dose of cinacalcet by 2.3-fold. Dose adjustment of cinacalcet may be required and PTH and serum calcium concentrations should be closely monitored if a patient initiates or discontinues therapy with a strong CYP3A4 inhibitor (eg, ketoconazole, erythromycin, itraconazole)).
No products indexed under this heading.

Acetazolamide Sodium (Co-administration of ketoconazole, a strong inhibitor of CYP3A4, increased cinacalcet exposure following a single 90 mg dose of cinacalcet by 2.3-fold. Dose adjustment of cinacalcet may be required and PTH and serum calcium concentrations should be closely monitored if a patient initiates or discontinues therapy with a strong CYP3A4 inhibitor (eg, ketoconazole, erythromycin, itraconazole)).
No products indexed under this heading.

Amiodarone Hydrochloride (Co-administration of ketoconazole, a strong inhibitor of CYP3A4, increased cinacalcet exposure following a single 90 mg dose of cinacalcet by 2.3-fold. Dose adjustment of cinacalcet may be required and PTH and serum calcium concentrations should be closely monitored if a patient initiates or discontinues therapy with a strong CYP3A4 inhibitor (eg, ketoconazole, erythromycin, itraconazole)).
No products indexed under this heading.

Amitriptyline Hydrochloride (Cinacalcet is a strong *in vitro*, as well as *in vivo*, inhibitor of CYP2D6. Therefore, dose adjustments of concomitant medications that are predominantly metabolized by CYP2D6 and particularly those with a narrow therapeutic index may be required. Concurrent administration of 25 mg or 100 mg cinacalcet with 50 mg amitriptyline increased amitriptyline exposure and nortriptyline (active metabolite) exposure by approximately 20% in CYP2D6 extensive metabolizers).
No products indexed under this heading.

Amoxapine (Cinacalcet is a strong *in vitro*, as well as *in vivo*, inhibitor of CYP2D6. Therefore, dose adjustments of concomitant medications that are predominantly metabolized by CYP2D6 (eg, metoprolol and carvedilol) and particularly those with a narrow therapeutic index (eg, flecainide, vinblastine, thioridazine and most tricyclic antidepressants) may be required).
No products indexed under this heading.

Amphetamine Aspartate (Cinacalcet is a strong *in vitro*, as well as *in vivo*, inhibitor of CYP2D6. Therefore, dose adjustments of concomitant medications that are predominantly metabolized by CYP2D6 (eg, metoprolol and carvedilol) and particularly those with a narrow therapeutic index (eg, flecainide, vinblastine, thioridazine and most tricyclic antidepressants) may be required).
No products indexed under this heading.

Amphetamine Aspartate Monohydrate (Cinacalcet is a strong *in vitro*,

(⊙ Described in PDR® for Ophthalmic Medicines)

as well as *in vivo*, inhibitor of CYP2D6. Therefore, dose adjustments of concomitant medications that are predominantly metabolized by CYP2D6 (eg, metoprolol and carvedilol) and particularly those with a narrow therapeutic index (eg, flecainide, vinblastine, thioridazine and most tricyclic antidepressants) may be required).
No products indexed under this heading.

Amphetamine Sulfate (Cinacalcet is a strong *in vitro*, as well as *in vivo*, inhibitor of CYP2D6. Therefore, dose adjustments of concomitant medications that are predominantly metabolized by CYP2D6 (eg, metoprolol and carvedilol) and particularly those with a narrow therapeutic index (eg, flecainide, vinblastine, thioridazine and most tricyclic antidepressants) may be required).
No products indexed under this heading.

Amprenavir (Co-administration of ketoconazole, a strong inhibitor of CYP3A4, increased cinacalcet exposure following a single 90 mg dose of cinacalcet by 2.3-fold. Dose adjustment of cinacalcet may be required and PTH and serum calcium concentrations should be closely monitored if a patient initiates or discontinues therapy with a strong CYP3A4 inhibitor (eg, ketoconazole, erythromycin, itraconazole)).
No products indexed under this heading.

Anastrozole (Co-administration of ketoconazole, a strong inhibitor of CYP3A4, increased cinacalcet exposure following a single 90 mg dose of cinacalcet by 2.3-fold. Dose adjustment of cinacalcet may be required and PTH and serum calcium concentrations should be closely monitored if a patient initiates or discontinues therapy with a strong CYP3A4 inhibitor (eg, ketoconazole, erythromycin, itraconazole)).
No products indexed under this heading.

Aprepitant (Co-administration of ketoconazole, a strong inhibitor of CYP3A4, increased cinacalcet exposure following a single 90 mg dose of cinacalcet by 2.3-fold. Dose adjustment of cinacalcet may be required and PTH and serum calcium concentrations should be closely monitored if a patient initiates or discontinues therapy with a strong CYP3A4 inhibitor (eg, ketoconazole, erythromycin, itraconazole)). Products include:
Emend 2124

Atazanavir (Co-administration of ketoconazole, a strong inhibitor of CYP3A4, increased cinacalcet exposure following a single 90 mg dose of cinacalcet by 2.3-fold. Dose adjustment of cinacalcet may be required and PTH and serum calcium concentrations should be closely monitored if a patient initiates or discontinues therapy with a strong CYP3A4 inhibitor (eg, ketoconazole, erythromycin, itraconazole)).
No products indexed under this heading.

Atazanavir Sulfate (Co-administration of ketoconazole, a strong inhibitor of CYP3A4, increased cinacalcet exposure following a single 90 mg dose of cinacalcet by 2.3-fold. Dose adjustment of cinacalcet may be required and PTH and serum calcium concentrations should be closely monitored if a patient initiates or discontinues therapy with a strong CYP3A4 inhibitor (eg, ketoconazole, erythromycin, itraconazole)).
No products indexed under this heading.

Atomoxetine Hydrochloride (Cinacalcet is a strong *in vitro*, as well as *in vivo*, inhibitor of CYP2D6. Therefore, dose adjustments of concomitant medications that are predominantly metabolized by CYP2D6 (eg, metoprolol and carvedilol) and particularly those with a narrow therapeutic index (eg, flecainide, vinblastine, thioridazine and most tricyclic antidepressants) may be required). Products include:
Strattera 1957

Bisoprolol Fumarate (Cinacalcet is a strong *in vitro*, as well as *in vivo*, inhibitor of CYP2D6. Therefore, dose adjustments of concomitant medications that are predominantly metabolized by CYP2D6 (eg, metoprolol and carvedilol) and particularly those with a narrow therapeutic index (eg, flecainide, vinblastine, thioridazine and most tricyclic antidepressants) may be required).
No products indexed under this heading.

Captopril (Cinacalcet is a strong *in vitro*, as well as *in vivo*, inhibitor of CYP2D6. Therefore, dose adjustments of concomitant medications that are predominantly metabolized by CYP2D6 (eg, metoprolol and carvedilol) and particularly those with a narrow therapeutic index (eg, flecainide, vinblastine, thioridazine and most tricyclic antidepressants) may be required). Products include:
Captopril 2341

Carvedilol (Cinacalcet is a strong *in vitro*, as well as *in vivo*, inhibitor of CYP2D6. Therefore, dose adjustments of concomitant medications that are predominantly metabolized by CYP2D6 (eg, metoprolol and carvedilol) and particularly those with a narrow therapeutic index (eg, flecainide, vinblastine, thioridazine and most tricyclic antidepressants) may be required). Products include:
Coreg 1409

Carvedilol Phosphate (Cinacalcet is a strong *in vitro*, as well as *in vivo*, inhibitor of CYP2D6. Therefore, dose adjustments of concomitant medications that are predominantly metabolized by CYP2D6 (eg, metoprolol and carvedilol) and particularly those with a narrow therapeutic index (eg, flecainide, vinblastine, thioridazine and most tricyclic antidepressants) may be required). Products include:
Coreg CR 1416

Cevimeline Hydrochloride (Cinacalcet is a strong *in vitro*, as well as *in vivo*, inhibitor of CYP2D6. Therefore, dose adjustments of concomitant medications that are predominantly metabolized by CYP2D6 (eg, metoprolol and carvedilol) and particularly those with a narrow therapeutic index (eg, flecainide, vinblastine, thioridazine and most tricyclic antidepressants) may be required). Products include:
Evoxac 1027

Chlorpromazine (Cinacalcet is a strong *in vitro*, as well as *in vivo*, inhibitor of CYP2D6. Therefore, dose adjustments of concomitant medications that are predominantly metabolized by CYP2D6 (eg, metoprolol and carvedilol) and particularly those with a narrow therapeutic index (eg, flecainide, vinblastine, thioridazine and most tricyclic antidepressants) may be required).
No products indexed under this heading.

Chlorpromazine Hydrochloride (Cinacalcet is a strong *in vitro*, as well as *in vivo*, inhibitor of CYP2D6. Therefore, dose adjustments of concomitant medications that are predominantly metabolized by CYP2D6 (eg, metoprolol and carvedilol) and particularly those with a narrow therapeutic index (eg, flecainide, vinblastine, thioridazine and most tricyclic antidepressants) may be required).
No products indexed under this heading.

Chlorpropamide (Cinacalcet is a strong *in vitro*, as well as *in vivo*, inhibitor of CYP2D6. Therefore, dose adjustments of concomitant medications that are predominantly metabolized by CYP2D6 (eg, metoprolol and carvedilol) and particularly those with a narrow therapeutic index (eg, flecainide, vinblastine, thioridazine and most tricyclic antidepressants) may be required).
No products indexed under this heading.

Cimetidine (Co-administration of ketoconazole, a strong inhibitor of CYP3A4, increased cinacalcet exposure following a single 90 mg dose of cinacalcet by 2.3-fold. Dose adjustment of cinacalcet may be required and PTH and serum calcium concentrations should be closely monitored if a patient initiates or discontinues therapy with a strong CYP3A4 inhibitor (eg, ketoconazole, erythromycin, itraconazole)).
No products indexed under this heading.

Cimetidine Hydrochloride (Co-administration of ketoconazole, a strong inhibitor of CYP3A4, increased cinacalcet exposure following a single 90 mg dose of cinacalcet by 2.3-fold. Dose adjustment of cinacalcet may be required and PTH and serum calcium concentrations should be closely monitored if a patient initiates or discontinues therapy with a strong CYP3A4 inhibitor (eg, ketoconazole, erythromycin, itraconazole)).
No products indexed under this heading.

Ciprofloxacin (Co-administration of ketoconazole, a strong inhibitor of CYP3A4, increased cinacalcet exposure following a single 90 mg dose of cinacalcet by 2.3-fold. Dose adjustment of cinacalcet may be required and PTH and serum calcium concentrations should be closely monitored if a patient initiates or discontinues therapy with a strong CYP3A4 inhibitor (eg, ketoconazole, erythromycin, itraconazole)). Products include:
Cipro I.V. 3082
Cipro 3073
Cipro XR 3091
Ciprodex 583

Clarithromycin (Co-administration of ketoconazole, a strong inhibitor of CYP3A4, increased cinacalcet exposure following a single 90 mg dose of cinacalcet by 2.3-fold. Dose adjustment of cinacalcet may be required and PTH and serum calcium concentrations should be closely monitored if a patient initiates or discontinues therapy with a strong CYP3A4 inhibitor (eg, ketoconazole, erythromycin, itraconazole)). Products include:
Biaxin/Biaxin XL 412

Clomipramine Hydrochloride (Cinacalcet is a strong *in vitro*, as well as *in vivo*, inhibitor of CYP2D6. Therefore, dose adjustments of concomitant medications that are predominantly metabolized by CYP2D6 (eg, metoprolol and carvedilol) and particularly those with a narrow therapeutic index (eg, flecainide, vinblastine, thioridazine and most tricyclic antidepressants) may be required).
No products indexed under this heading.

Clotrimazole (Co-administration of ketoconazole, a strong inhibitor of CYP3A4, increased cinacalcet exposure following a single 90 mg dose of cinacalcet by 2.3-fold. Dose adjustment of cinacalcet may be required and PTH and serum calcium concentrations should be closely monitored if a patient initiates or discontinues therapy with a strong CYP3A4 inhibitor (eg, ketoconazole, erythromycin, itraconazole)). Products include:
Lotrisone 3163

Clozapine (Cinacalcet is a strong *in vitro*, as well as *in vivo*, inhibitor of CYP2D6. Therefore, dose adjustments of concomitant medications that are predominantly metabolized by CYP2D6 (eg, metoprolol and carvedilol) and particularly those with a narrow therapeutic index (eg, flecainide, vinblastine, thioridazine and most tricyclic antidepressants) may be required).
No products indexed under this heading.

Codeine Phosphate (Cinacalcet is a strong *in vitro*, as well as *in vivo*, inhibitor of CYP2D6. Therefore, dose adjustments of concomitant medications that are predominantly metabolized by CYP2D6 (eg, metoprolol and carvedilol) and particularly those with a narrow therapeutic index (eg, flecainide, vinblastine, thioridazine and most tricyclic antidepressants) may be required). Products include:
Tylenol with Codeine 2691

Codeine Sulfate (Cinacalcet is a strong *in vitro*, as well as *in vivo*, inhibitor of CYP2D6. Therefore, dose adjustments of concomitant medications that are predominantly metabolized by CYP2D6 (eg, metoprolol and carvedilol) and particularly those with a narrow therapeutic index (eg, flecainide, vinblastine, thioridazine and most tricyclic antidepressants) may be required).
No products indexed under this heading.

Conivaptan Hydrochloride (Co-administration of ketoconazole, a strong inhibitor of CYP3A4, increased cinacalcet exposure following a single 90 mg dose of cinacalcet by 2.3-fold. Dose adjustment of cinacalcet may be required and PTH and serum calcium concentrations should be closely monitored if a patient initiates or discontinues therapy with a strong CYP3A4 inhibitor (eg, ketoconazole, erythromycin, itraconazole)). Products include:
Vaprisol 689

Cyclobenzaprine Hydrochloride (Cinacalcet is a strong *in vitro*, as well as *in vivo*, inhibitor of CYP2D6. Therefore, dose adjustments of concomitant medications that are predominantly metabolized by CYP2D6 (eg, metoprolol and carvedilol) and particularly those with a narrow therapeutic index (eg, flecainide, vinblastine, thioridazine and most tricyclic antidepressants) may be required). Products include:
Amrix 964

Cyclosporine (Co-administration of ketoconazole, a strong inhibitor of CYP3A4, increased cinacalcet exposure following a single 90 mg dose of cinacalcet by 2.3-fold. Dose adjustment of cinacalcet may be required and PTH and serum calcium concentrations should be closely monitored if a patient initiates or discontinues therapy with a strong CYP3A4 inhibitor (eg, ketoconazole, erythromycin, itraconazole)). Products include:
Gengraf 440
Neoral Oral Solution 2496
Neoral Capsules 2496
Restasis 605

Dalfopristin (Co-administration of ketoconazole, a strong inhibitor of CYP3A4, increased cinacalcet exposure following a single 90 mg dose of cinacalcet by 2.3-fold. Dose adjustment of cinacalcet may be required and PTH and serum calcium concentrations should be closely monitored if a patient initiates or discontinues therapy with a strong CYP3A4 inhibitor (eg, ketoconazole, erythromycin, itraconazole)).
No products indexed under this heading.

Danazol (Co-administration of ketoconazole, a strong inhibitor of CYP3A4, increased cinacalcet exposure following a single 90 mg dose of cinacalcet by 2.3-fold. Dose adjustment of cinacalcet may be required and PTH and serum calcium concentrations should be closely monitored if a patient initiates or discontinues therapy with a strong CYP3A4 inhibitor (eg, ketoconazole, erythromycin, itraconazole)).
No products indexed under this heading.

Darunavir (Co-administration of keto-conazole, a strong inhibitor of CYP3A4, increased cinacalcet exposure following a single 90 mg dose of cinacalcet by 2.3-fold. Dose adjustment of cinacalcet may be required and PTH and serum calcium concentrations should be close-ly monitored if a patient initiates or dis-continues therapy with a strong CYP3A4 inhibitor (eg, ketoconazole, erythromycin, itraconazole)).
No products indexed under this heading.

Dasatinib (Co-administration of keto-conazole, a strong inhibitor of CYP3A4, increased cinacalcet exposure following a single 90 mg dose of cinacalcet by 2.3-fold. Dose adjustment of cinacalcet may be required and PTH and serum calcium concentrations should be close-ly monitored if a patient initiates or dis-continues therapy with a strong CYP3A4 inhibitor (eg, ketoconazole, erythromycin, itraconazole)).
No products indexed under this heading.

Debrisoquine (Cinacalcet is a strong *in vitro*, as well as *in vivo*, inhibitor of CYP2D6. Therefore, dose adjustments of concomitant medications that are predominantly metabolized by CYP2D6 (eg, metoprolol and carvedilol) and par-ticularly those with a narrow therapeutic index (eg, flecainide, vinblastine, thiorid-azine and most tricyclic antidepres-sants) may be required).
No products indexed under this heading.

Delavirdine Mesylate (Co-administration of ketoconazole, a strong inhibitor of CYP3A4, increased cinacalcet exposure following a single 90 mg dose of cinacalcet by 2.3-fold. Dose adjustment of cinacalcet may be required and PTH and serum calcium concentrations should be closely moni-tored if a patient initiates or discontin-ues therapy with a strong CYP3A4 inhib-itor (eg, ketoconazole, erythromycin, itraconazole)).
No products indexed under this heading.

Delavirine (Co-administration of keto-conazole, a strong inhibitor of CYP3A4, increased cinacalcet exposure following a single 90 mg dose of cinacalcet by 2.3-fold. Dose adjustment of cinacalcet may be required and PTH and serum calcium concentrations should be close-ly monitored if a patient initiates or dis-continues therapy with a strong CYP3A4 inhibitor (eg, ketoconazole, erythromycin, itraconazole)).
No products indexed under this heading.

Desipramine Hydrochloride (Cinac-alcet is a strong *in vitro*, as well as *in vivo*, inhibitor of CYP2D6. Therefore, dose adjustments of concomitant medi-cations that are predominantly metabo-lized by CYP2D6 and particularly those with a narrow therapeutic index may be required. Concurrent administration of cinacalcet (90 mg) with desipramine (50 mg) increased the exposure of desi-pramine by 3.6-fold in CYP2D6 exten-sive metabolizers).
No products indexed under this heading.

Desloratadine (Co-administration of ketoconazole, a strong inhibitor of CYP3A4, increased cinacalcet exposure following a single 90 mg dose of cina-calcet by 2.3-fold. Dose adjustment of cinacalcet may be required and PTH and serum calcium concentrations should be closely monitored if a patient initiates or discontinues therapy with a strong CYP3A4 inhibitor (eg, ketocona-zole, erythromycin, itraconazole)). Products include:
Clarinex Syrup 3098
Clarinex 3098
Clarinex Reditabs 3098
Clarinex-D 12-Hour 3101
Clarinex-D 3104

Dexfenfluramine Hydrochloride (Cinacalcet is a strong *in vitro*, as well

as *in vivo*, inhibitor of CYP2D6. There-fore, dose adjustments of concomitant medications that are predominantly metabolized by CYP2D6 (eg, metoprolol and carvedilol) and particularly those with a narrow therapeutic index (eg, flecainide, vinblastine, thioridazine and most tricyclic antidepressants) may be required).
No products indexed under this heading.

Dextromethorphan Hydrobromide (Cinacalcet is a strong *in vitro*, as well as *in vivo*, inhibitor of CYP2D6. There-fore, dose adjustments of concomitant medications that are predominantly metabolized by CYP2D6 (eg, metoprolol and carvedilol) and particularly those with a narrow therapeutic index (eg, flecainide, vinblastine, thioridazine and most tricyclic antidepressants) may be required).
No products indexed under this heading.

Dextromethorphan Polistirex (Cina-calcet is a strong *in vitro*, as well as *in vivo*, inhibitor of CYP2D6. Therefore, dose adjustments of concomitant medi-cations that are predominantly metabo-lized by CYP2D6 (eg, metoprolol and carvedilol) and particularly those with a narrow therapeutic index (eg, flecainide, vinblastine, thioridazine and most tricy-clic antidepressants) may be required).
No products indexed under this heading.

Diltiazem Hydrochloride (Co-administration of ketoconazole, a strong inhibitor of CYP3A4, increased cinacalcet exposure following a single 90 mg dose of cinacalcet by 2.3-fold. Dose adjustment of cinacalcet may be required and PTH and serum calcium concentrations should be closely moni-tored if a patient initiates or discontin-ues therapy with a strong CYP3A4 inhib-itor (eg, ketoconazole, erythromycin, itraconazole)). Products include:
Cardizem LA 423

Diltiazem Maleate (Co-administration of ketoconazole, a strong inhibitor of CYP3A4, increased cinacalcet exposure following a single 90 mg dose of cina-calcet by 2.3-fold. Dose adjustment of cinacalcet may be required and PTH and serum calcium concentrations should be closely monitored if a patient initiates or discontinues therapy with a strong CYP3A4 inhibitor (eg, ketocona-zole, erythromycin, itraconazole)).
No products indexed under this heading.

Dolasetron Mesylate (Cinacalcet is a strong *in vitro*, as well as *in vivo*, inhibi-tor of CYP2D6. Therefore, dose adjust-ments of concomitant medications that are predominantly metabolized by CYP2D6 (eg, metoprolol and carvedilol) and particularly those with a narrow therapeutic index (eg, flecainide, vin-blastine, thioridazine and most tricyclic antidepressants) may be required). Products include:
Anzemet Injection 2931
Anzemet Tablets 2934

Donepezil Hydrochloride (Cinacal-cet is a strong *in vitro*, as well as *in vivo*, inhibitor of CYP2D6. Therefore, dose adjustments of concomitant medi-cations that are predominantly metabo-lized by CYP2D6 (eg, metoprolol and carvedilol) and particularly those with a narrow therapeutic index (eg, flecainide, vinblastine, thioridazine and most tricy-clic antidepressants) may be required). Products include:
Aricept 1045
Aricept ODT 1045

Doxepin Hydrochloride (Cinacalcet is a strong *in vitro*, as well as *in vivo*, inhibitor of CYP2D6. Therefore, dose adjustments of concomitant medica-tions that are predominantly metabo-lized by CYP2D6 (eg, metoprolol and carvedilol) and particularly those with a narrow therapeutic index (eg, flecainide,

vinblastine, thioridazine and most tricy-clic antidepressants) may be required).
No products indexed under this heading.

Efavirenz (Co-administration of keto-conazole, a strong inhibitor of CYP3A4, increased cinacalcet exposure following a single 90 mg dose of cinacalcet by 2.3-fold. Dose adjustment of cinacalcet may be required and PTH and serum calcium concentrations should be close-ly monitored if a patient initiates or dis-continues therapy with a strong CYP3A4 inhibitor (eg, ketoconazole, erythromycin, itraconazole)). Products include:
Atripla 906

Encainide Hydrochloride (Cinacal-cet is a strong *in vitro*, as well as *in vivo*, inhibitor of CYP2D6. Therefore, dose adjustments of concomitant medi-cations that are predominantly metabo-lized by CYP2D6 (eg, metoprolol and carvedilol) and particularly those with a narrow therapeutic index (eg, flecainide, vinblastine, thioridazine and most tricy-clic antidepressants) may be required).
No products indexed under this heading.

Erythromycin (Co-administration of ketoconazole, a strong inhibitor of CYP3A4, increased cinacalcet exposure following a single 90 mg dose of cina-calcet by 2.3-fold. Dose adjustment of cinacalcet may be required and PTH and serum calcium concentrations should be closely monitored if a patient initiates or discontinues therapy with a strong CYP3A4 inhibitor (eg, ketocona-zole, erythromycin, itraconazole)).
No products indexed under this heading.

Erythromycin, Topical (Co-administration of ketoconazole, a strong inhibitor of CYP3A4, increased cinacalcet exposure following a single 90 mg dose of cinacalcet by 2.3-fold. Dose adjustment of cinacalcet may be required and PTH and serum calcium concentrations should be closely moni-tored if a patient initiates or discontin-ues therapy with a strong CYP3A4 inhib-itor (eg, ketoconazole, erythromycin, itraconazole)).
No products indexed under this heading.

Erythromycin Estolate (Co-administration of ketoconazole, a strong inhibitor of CYP3A4, increased cinacalcet exposure following a single 90 mg dose of cinacalcet by 2.3-fold. Dose adjustment of cinacalcet may be required and PTH and serum calcium concentrations should be closely moni-tored if a patient initiates or discontin-ues therapy with a strong CYP3A4 inhib-itor (eg, ketoconazole, erythromycin, itraconazole)).
No products indexed under this heading.

Erythromycin Ethylsuccinate (Co-administration of ketoconazole, a strong inhibitor of CYP3A4, increased cinacalcet exposure following a single 90 mg dose of cinacalcet by 2.3-fold. Dose adjustment of cinacalcet may be required and PTH and serum calcium concentrations should be closely moni-tored if a patient initiates or discontin-ues therapy with a strong CYP3A4 inhib-itor (eg, ketoconazole, erythromycin, itraconazole)). Products include:
E.E.S. 437
EryPed 435

Erythromycin Gluceptate (Co-administration of ketoconazole, a strong inhibitor of CYP3A4, increased cinacalcet exposure following a single 90 mg dose of cinacalcet by 2.3-fold. Dose adjustment of cinacalcet may be required and PTH and serum calcium concentrations should be closely moni-tored if a patient initiates or discontin-ues therapy with a strong CYP3A4 inhib-itor (eg, ketoconazole, erythromycin, itraconazole)).
No products indexed under this heading.

Erythromycin Lactobionate (Co-administration of ketoconazole, a strong inhibitor of CYP3A4, increased cinacalcet exposure following a single 90 mg dose of cinacalcet by 2.3-fold. Dose adjustment of cinacalcet may be required and PTH and serum calcium concentrations should be closely moni-tored if a patient initiates or discontin-ues therapy with a strong CYP3A4 inhib-itor (eg, ketoconazole, erythromycin, itraconazole)).
No products indexed under this heading.

Erythromycin Stearate (Co-administration of ketoconazole, a strong inhibitor of CYP3A4, increased cinacalcet exposure following a single 90 mg dose of cinacalcet by 2.3-fold. Dose adjustment of cinacalcet may be required and PTH and serum calcium concentrations should be closely moni-tored if a patient initiates or discontin-ues therapy with a strong CYP3A4 inhib-itor (eg, ketoconazole, erythromycin, itraconazole)).
No products indexed under this heading.

Esomeprazole Magnesium (Co-administration of ketoconazole, a strong inhibitor of CYP3A4, increased cinacalcet exposure following a single 90 mg dose of cinacalcet by 2.3-fold. Dose adjustment of cinacalcet may be required and PTH and serum calcium concentrations should be closely moni-tored if a patient initiates or discontin-ues therapy with a strong CYP3A4 inhib-itor (eg, ketoconazole, erythromycin, itraconazole)). Products include:
Nexium Capsules 704
Nexium Oral Suspension 704

Esomeprazole Sodium (Co-administration of ketoconazole, a strong inhibitor of CYP3A4, increased cinacalcet exposure following a single 90 mg dose of cinacalcet by 2.3-fold. Dose adjustment of cinacalcet may be required and PTH and serum calcium concentrations should be closely moni-tored if a patient initiates or discontin-ues therapy with a strong CYP3A4 inhib-itor (eg, ketoconazole, erythromycin, itraconazole)). Products include:
Nexium I.V. 712

Fat (A food-effect study in healthy vol-unteers indicated that the C_{max} and area under the curve (AUC$_{(0-inf)}$) were increased 82% and 68%, respectively, when cinacalcet was administered with a high-fat meal compared to fasting. C_{max} and AUC$_{(0-inf)}$ of cinacalcet were increased 65% and 50%, respectively, when cinacalcet was administered with a low-fat meal compared to fasting).
No products indexed under this heading.

Fentanyl (Cinacalcet is a strong *in vitro*, as well as *in vivo*, inhibitor of CYP2D6. Therefore, dose adjustments of concomitant medications that are predominantly metabolized by CYP2D6 (eg, metoprolol and carvedilol) and par-ticularly those with a narrow therapeutic index (eg, flecainide, vinblastine, thiorid-azine and most tricyclic antidepres-sants) may be required). Products include:
Duragesic 2604
Fentanyl Transdermal System 2346
Onsolis 2054

Fentanyl Citrate (Cinacalcet is a strong *in vitro*, as well as *in vivo*, inhibi-tor of CYP2D6. Therefore, dose adjust-ments of concomitant medications that are predominantly metabolized by CYP2D6 (eg, metoprolol and carvedilol) and particularly those with a narrow therapeutic index (eg, flecainide, vin-blastine, thioridazine and most tricyclic antidepressants) may be required). Products include:
Fentora 966

Flecainide Acetate (Cinacalcet is a strong *in vitro*, as well as *in vivo*, inhibi-

tor of CYP2D6. Therefore, dose adjustments of concomitant medications that are predominantly metabolized by CYP2D6 (eg, metoprolol and carvedilol) and particularly those with a narrow therapeutic index (eg, flecainide, vinblastine, thioridazine and most tricyclic antidepressants) may be required).
No products indexed under this heading.

Fluconazole (Co-administration of ketoconazole, a strong inhibitor of CYP3A4, increased cinacalcet exposure following a single 90 mg dose of cinacalcet by 2.3-fold. Dose adjustment of cinacalcet may be required and PTH and serum calcium concentrations should be closely monitored if a patient initiates or discontinues therapy with a strong CYP3A4 inhibitor (eg, ketoconazole, erythromycin, itraconazole)).
No products indexed under this heading.

Fluoxetine (Co-administration of ketoconazole, a strong inhibitor of CYP3A4, increased cinacalcet exposure following a single 90 mg dose of cinacalcet by 2.3-fold. Dose adjustment of cinacalcet may be required and PTH and serum calcium concentrations should be closely monitored if a patient initiates or discontinues therapy with a strong CYP3A4 inhibitor (eg, ketoconazole, erythromycin, itraconazole)).
No products indexed under this heading.

Fluoxetine Hydrochloride (Co-administration of ketoconazole, a strong inhibitor of CYP3A4, increased cinacalcet exposure following a single 90 mg dose of cinacalcet by 2.3-fold. Dose adjustment of cinacalcet may be required and PTH and serum calcium concentrations should be closely monitored if a patient initiates or discontinues therapy with a strong CYP3A4 inhibitor (eg, ketoconazole, erythromycin, itraconazole)). Products include:
Prozac Weekly 1941
Prozac Pulvules 1941
Symbyax 1965

Fluphenazine Decanoate (Cinacalcet is a strong *in vitro*, as well as *in vivo*, inhibitor of CYP2D6. Therefore, dose adjustments of concomitant medications that are predominantly metabolized by CYP2D6 (eg, metoprolol and carvedilol) and particularly those with a narrow therapeutic index (eg, flecainide, vinblastine, thioridazine and most tricyclic antidepressants) may be required).
No products indexed under this heading.

Fluphenazine Enanthate (Cinacalcet is a strong *in vitro*, as well as *in vivo*, inhibitor of CYP2D6. Therefore, dose adjustments of concomitant medications that are predominantly metabolized by CYP2D6 (eg, metoprolol and carvedilol) and particularly those with a narrow therapeutic index (eg, flecainide, vinblastine, thioridazine and most tricyclic antidepressants) may be required).
No products indexed under this heading.

Fluphenazine Hydrochloride (Cinacalcet is a strong *in vitro*, as well as *in vivo*, inhibitor of CYP2D6. Therefore, dose adjustments of concomitant medications that are predominantly metabolized by CYP2D6 (eg, metoprolol and carvedilol) and particularly those with a narrow therapeutic index (eg, flecainide, vinblastine, thioridazine and most tricyclic antidepressants) may be required).
No products indexed under this heading.

Fluvoxamine Maleate (Co-administration of ketoconazole, a strong inhibitor of CYP3A4, increased cinacalcet exposure following a single 90 mg dose of cinacalcet by 2.3-fold. Dose adjustment of cinacalcet may be required and PTH and serum calcium concentrations should be closely monitored if a patient initiates or discontinues therapy with a strong CYP3A4 inhibitor (eg, ketoconazole, erythromycin, itraconazole)).
No products indexed under this heading.

Formoterol Fumarate (Cinacalcet is a strong *in vitro*, as well as *in vivo*, inhibitor of CYP2D6. Therefore, dose adjustments of concomitant medications that are predominantly metabolized by CYP2D6 (eg, metoprolol and carvedilol) and particularly those with a narrow therapeutic index (eg, flecainide, vinblastine, thioridazine and most tricyclic antidepressants) may be required). Products include:
Foradil 3121
Perforomist 3634

Fosamprenavir Calcium (Co-administration of ketoconazole, a strong inhibitor of CYP3A4, increased cinacalcet exposure following a single 90 mg dose of cinacalcet by 2.3-fold. Dose adjustment of cinacalcet may be required and PTH and serum calcium concentrations should be closely monitored if a patient initiates or discontinues therapy with a strong CYP3A4 inhibitor (eg, ketoconazole, erythromycin, itraconazole)). Products include:
Lexiva Oral Suspension 1558
Lexiva 1558

Galantamine Hydrobromide (Cinacalcet is a strong *in vitro*, as well as *in vivo*, inhibitor of CYP2D6. Therefore, dose adjustments of concomitant medications that are predominantly metabolized by CYP2D6 (eg, metoprolol and carvedilol) and particularly those with a narrow therapeutic index (eg, flecainide, vinblastine, thioridazine and most tricyclic antidepressants) may be required).
No products indexed under this heading.

Haloperidol (Cinacalcet is a strong *in vitro*, as well as *in vivo*, inhibitor of CYP2D6. Therefore, dose adjustments of concomitant medications that are predominantly metabolized by CYP2D6 (eg, metoprolol and carvedilol) and particularly those with a narrow therapeutic index (eg, flecainide, vinblastine, thioridazine and most tricyclic antidepressants) may be required).
No products indexed under this heading.

Haloperidol Decanoate (Cinacalcet is a strong *in vitro*, as well as *in vivo*, inhibitor of CYP2D6. Therefore, dose adjustments of concomitant medications that are predominantly metabolized by CYP2D6 (eg, metoprolol and carvedilol) and particularly those with a narrow therapeutic index (eg, flecainide, vinblastine, thioridazine and most tricyclic antidepressants) may be required).
No products indexed under this heading.

Hydrocodone Bitartrate (Cinacalcet is a strong *in vitro*, as well as *in vivo*, inhibitor of CYP2D6. Therefore, dose adjustments of concomitant medications that are predominantly metabolized by CYP2D6 (eg, metoprolol and carvedilol) and particularly those with a narrow therapeutic index (eg, flecainide, vinblastine, thioridazine and most tricyclic antidepressants) may be required). Products include:
Vicodin 560
Vicodin ES 561
Vicodin HP 563
Vicoprofen 564
Zydone 1138

Imatinib Mesylate (Co-administration of ketoconazole, a strong inhibitor of CYP3A4, increased cinacalcet exposure following a single 90 mg dose of cinacalcet by 2.3-fold. Dose adjustment of cinacalcet may be required and PTH and serum calcium concentrations should be closely monitored if a patient initiates or discontinues therapy with a strong CYP3A4 inhibitor (eg, ketoconazole, erythromycin, itraconazole)). Products include:
Gleevec 2477

Imipramine Hydrochloride (Cinacalcet is a strong *in vitro*, as well as *in vivo*, inhibitor of CYP2D6. Therefore, dose adjustments of concomitant medications that are predominantly metabolized by CYP2D6 (eg, metoprolol and carvedilol) and particularly those with a narrow therapeutic index (eg, flecainide, vinblastine, thioridazine and most tricyclic antidepressants) may be required).
No products indexed under this heading.

Imipramine Pamoate (Cinacalcet is a strong *in vitro*, as well as *in vivo*, inhibitor of CYP2D6. Therefore, dose adjustments of concomitant medications that are predominantly metabolized by CYP2D6 (eg, metoprolol and carvedilol) and particularly those with a narrow therapeutic index (eg, flecainide, vinblastine, thioridazine and most tricyclic antidepressants) may be required).
No products indexed under this heading.

Indinavir Sulfate (Co-administration of ketoconazole, a strong inhibitor of CYP3A4, increased cinacalcet exposure following a single 90 mg dose of cinacalcet by 2.3-fold. Dose adjustment of cinacalcet may be required and PTH and serum calcium concentrations should be closely monitored if a patient initiates or discontinues therapy with a strong CYP3A4 inhibitor (eg, ketoconazole, erythromycin, itraconazole)). Products include:
Crixivan 2113

Indoramin Hydrochloride (Cinacalcet is a strong *in vitro*, as well as *in vivo*, inhibitor of CYP2D6. Therefore, dose adjustments of concomitant medications that are predominantly metabolized by CYP2D6 (eg, metoprolol and carvedilol) and particularly those with a narrow therapeutic index (eg, flecainide, vinblastine, thioridazine and most tricyclic antidepressants) may be required).
No products indexed under this heading.

Isoniazid (Co-administration of ketoconazole, a strong inhibitor of CYP3A4, increased cinacalcet exposure following a single 90 mg dose of cinacalcet by 2.3-fold. Dose adjustment of cinacalcet may be required and PTH and serum calcium concentrations should be closely monitored if a patient initiates or discontinues therapy with a strong CYP3A4 inhibitor (eg, ketoconazole, erythromycin, itraconazole)).
No products indexed under this heading.

Itraconazole (Co-administration of ketoconazole, a strong inhibitor of CYP3A4, increased cinacalcet exposure following a single 90 mg dose of cinacalcet by 2.3-fold. Dose adjustment of cinacalcet may be required and PTH and serum calcium concentrations should be closely monitored if a patient initiates or discontinues therapy with a strong CYP3A4 inhibitor (eg, ketoconazole, erythromycin, itraconazole)).
No products indexed under this heading.

Ketoconazole (Co-administration of ketoconazole, a strong inhibitor of CYP3A4, increased cinacalcet exposure following a single 90 mg dose of cinacalcet by 2.3-fold. Dose adjustment of cinacalcet may be required and PTH and serum calcium concentrations should be closely monitored if a patient initiates or discontinues therapy with a strong CYP3A4 inhibitor (eg, ketoconazole, erythromycin, itraconazole)). Products include:
Extina 3319
Xolegel 3337

Labetalol Hydrochloride (Cinacalcet is a strong *in vitro*, as well as *in vivo*, inhibitor of CYP2D6. Therefore, dose adjustments of concomitant medications that are predominantly metabolized by CYP2D6 (eg, metoprolol and carvedilol) and particularly those with a narrow therapeutic index (eg, flecainide, vinblastine, thioridazine and most tricyclic antidepressants) may be required).
No products indexed under this heading.

Lapatinib (Co-administration of ketoconazole, a strong inhibitor of CYP3A4, increased cinacalcet exposure following a single 90 mg dose of cinacalcet by 2.3-fold. Dose adjustment of cinacalcet may be required and PTH and serum calcium concentrations should be closely monitored if a patient initiates or discontinues therapy with a strong CYP3A4 inhibitor (eg, ketoconazole, erythromycin, itraconazole)). Products include:
Tykerb 1698

Lidocaine (Cinacalcet is a strong *in vitro*, as well as *in vivo*, inhibitor of CYP2D6. Therefore, dose adjustments of concomitant medications that are predominantly metabolized by CYP2D6 (eg, metoprolol and carvedilol) and particularly those with a narrow therapeutic index (eg, flecainide, vinblastine, thioridazine and most tricyclic antidepressants) may be required). Products include:
Lidoderm 1107

Lidocaine Hydrochloride (Cinacalcet is a strong *in vitro*, as well as *in vivo*, inhibitor of CYP2D6. Therefore, dose adjustments of concomitant medications that are predominantly metabolized by CYP2D6 (eg, metoprolol and carvedilol) and particularly those with a narrow therapeutic index (eg, flecainide, vinblastine, thioridazine and most tricyclic antidepressants) may be required).
No products indexed under this heading.

Lopinavir (Co-administration of ketoconazole, a strong inhibitor of CYP3A4, increased cinacalcet exposure following a single 90 mg dose of cinacalcet by 2.3-fold. Dose adjustment of cinacalcet may be required and PTH and serum calcium concentrations should be closely monitored if a patient initiates or discontinues therapy with a strong CYP3A4 inhibitor (eg, ketoconazole, erythromycin, itraconazole)). Products include:
Kaletra 458

Loratadine (Co-administration of ketoconazole, a strong inhibitor of CYP3A4, increased cinacalcet exposure following a single 90 mg dose of cinacalcet by 2.3-fold. Dose adjustment of cinacalcet may be required and PTH and serum calcium concentrations should be closely monitored if a patient initiates or discontinues therapy with a strong CYP3A4 inhibitor (eg, ketoconazole, erythromycin, itraconazole)).
No products indexed under this heading.

Maprotiline Hydrochloride (Cinacalcet is a strong *in vitro*, as well as *in vivo*, inhibitor of CYP2D6. Therefore, dose adjustments of concomitant medications that are predominantly metabolized by CYP2D6 (eg, metoprolol and carvedilol) and particularly those with a narrow therapeutic index (eg, flecainide, vinblastine, thioridazine and most tricyclic antidepressants) may be required).
No products indexed under this heading.

Meperidine Hydrochloride (Cinacalcet is a strong *in vitro*, as well as *in vivo*, inhibitor of CYP2D6. Therefore, dose adjustments of concomitant medications that are predominantly metabolized by CYP2D6 (eg, metoprolol and carvedilol) and particularly those with a narrow therapeutic index (eg, flecainide, vinblastine, thioridazine and most tricyclic antidepressants) may be required).
No products indexed under this heading.

Methadone Hydrochloride (Cinacalcet is a strong *in vitro*, as well as *in vivo*, inhibitor of CYP2D6. Therefore, dose adjustments of concomitant medications that are predominantly metabo-

IMPORTANT NOTE: Always consult each drug listing in the patient's regimen for possible interactions.

lized by CYP2D6 (eg, metoprolol and carvedilol) and particularly those with a narrow therapeutic index (eg, flecainide, vinblastine, thioridazine and most tricyclic antidepressants) may be required).
No products indexed under this heading.

Methamphetamine Hydrochloride (Cinacalcet is a strong in vitro, as well as in vivo, inhibitor of CYP2D6. Therefore, dose adjustments of concomitant medications that are predominantly metabolized by CYP2D6 (eg, metoprolol and carvedilol) and particularly those with a narrow therapeutic index (eg, flecainide, vinblastine, thioridazine and most tricyclic antidepressants) may be required).
No products indexed under this heading.

Methoxyphenamine (Cinacalcet is a strong in vitro, as well as in vivo, inhibitor of CYP2D6. Therefore, dose adjustments of concomitant medications that are predominantly metabolized by CYP2D6 (eg, metoprolol and carvedilol) and particularly those with a narrow therapeutic index (eg, flecainide, vinblastine, thioridazine and most tricyclic antidepressants) may be required).
No products indexed under this heading.

Metoprolol Succinate (Cinacalcet is a strong in vitro, as well as in vivo, inhibitor of CYP2D6. Therefore, dose adjustments of concomitant medications that are predominantly metabolized by CYP2D6 (eg, metoprolol and carvedilol) and particularly those with a narrow therapeutic index (eg, flecainide, vinblastine, thioridazine and most tricyclic antidepressants) may be required). Products include:
Toprol XL 732

Metoprolol Tartrate (Cinacalcet is a strong in vitro, as well as in vivo, inhibitor of CYP2D6. Therefore, dose adjustments of concomitant medications that are predominantly metabolized by CYP2D6 (eg, metoprolol and carvedilol) and particularly those with a narrow therapeutic index (eg, flecainide, vinblastine, thioridazine and most tricyclic antidepressants) may be required).
No products indexed under this heading.

Metronidazole (Co-administration of ketoconazole, a strong inhibitor of CYP3A4, increased cinacalcet exposure following a single 90 mg dose of cinacalcet by 2.3-fold. Dose adjustment of cinacalcet may be required and PTH and serum calcium concentrations should be closely monitored if a patient initiates or discontinues therapy with a strong CYP3A4 inhibitor (eg, ketoconazole, erythromycin, itraconazole)). Products include:
Pylera 793

Metronidazole Benzoate (Co-administration of ketoconazole, a strong inhibitor of CYP3A4, increased cinacalcet exposure following a single 90 mg dose of cinacalcet by 2.3-fold. Dose adjustment of cinacalcet may be required and PTH and serum calcium concentrations should be closely monitored if a patient initiates or discontinues therapy with a strong CYP3A4 inhibitor (eg, ketoconazole, erythromycin, itraconazole)).
No products indexed under this heading.

Metronidazole Hydrochloride (Co-administration of ketoconazole, a strong inhibitor of CYP3A4, increased cinacalcet exposure following a single 90 mg dose of cinacalcet by 2.3-fold. Dose adjustment of cinacalcet may be required and PTH and serum calcium concentrations should be closely monitored if a patient initiates or discontinues therapy with a strong CYP3A4 inhibitor (eg, ketoconazole, erythromycin, itraconazole)).
No products indexed under this heading.

Metronidazole Sodium (Co-administration of ketoconazole, a strong inhibitor of CYP3A4, increased cinacalcet exposure following a single 90 mg dose of cinacalcet by 2.3-fold. Dose adjustment of cinacalcet may be required and PTH and serum calcium concentrations should be closely monitored if a patient initiates or discontinues therapy with a strong CYP3A4 inhibitor (eg, ketoconazole, erythromycin, itraconazole)).
No products indexed under this heading.

Mexiletine Hydrochloride (Cinacalcet is a strong in vitro, as well as in vivo, inhibitor of CYP2D6. Therefore, dose adjustments of concomitant medications that are predominantly metabolized by CYP2D6 (eg, metoprolol and carvedilol) and particularly those with a narrow therapeutic index (eg, flecainide, vinblastine, thioridazine and most tricyclic antidepressants) may be required).
No products indexed under this heading.

Miconazole (Co-administration of ketoconazole, a strong inhibitor of CYP3A4, increased cinacalcet exposure following a single 90 mg dose of cinacalcet by 2.3-fold. Dose adjustment of cinacalcet may be required and PTH and serum calcium concentrations should be closely monitored if a patient initiates or discontinues therapy with a strong CYP3A4 inhibitor (eg, ketoconazole, erythromycin, itraconazole)).
No products indexed under this heading.

Miconazole Nitrate (Co-administration of ketoconazole, a strong inhibitor of CYP3A4, increased cinacalcet exposure following a single 90 mg dose of cinacalcet by 2.3-fold. Dose adjustment of cinacalcet may be required and PTH and serum calcium concentrations should be closely monitored if a patient initiates or discontinues therapy with a strong CYP3A4 inhibitor (eg, ketoconazole, erythromycin, itraconazole)). Products include:
Vusion Ointment 3335

Mifepristone (Co-administration of ketoconazole, a strong inhibitor of CYP3A4, increased cinacalcet exposure following a single 90 mg dose of cinacalcet by 2.3-fold. Dose adjustment of cinacalcet may be required and PTH and serum calcium concentrations should be closely monitored if a patient initiates or discontinues therapy with a strong CYP3A4 inhibitor (eg, ketoconazole, erythromycin, itraconazole)).
No products indexed under this heading.

Mirtazapine (Cinacalcet is a strong in vitro, as well as in vivo, inhibitor of CYP2D6. Therefore, dose adjustments of concomitant medications that are predominantly metabolized by CYP2D6 (eg, metoprolol and carvedilol) and particularly those with a narrow therapeutic index (eg, flecainide, vinblastine, thioridazine and most tricyclic antidepressants) may be required). Products include:
Remeron Tablets 3214
RemeronSolTab Tablets 3219

Morphine Sulfate (Cinacalcet is a strong in vitro, as well as in vivo, inhibitor of CYP2D6. Therefore, dose adjustments of concomitant medications that are predominantly metabolized by CYP2D6 (eg, metoprolol and carvedilol) and particularly those with a narrow therapeutic index (eg, flecainide, vinblastine, thioridazine and most tricyclic antidepressants) may be required). Products include:
Avinza 1822
Embeda 1831
MS Contin 2803

Nefazodone Hydrochloride (Co-administration of ketoconazole, a strong inhibitor of CYP3A4, increased cinacalcet exposure following a single

90 mg dose of cinacalcet by 2.3-fold. Dose adjustment of cinacalcet may be required and PTH and serum calcium concentrations should be closely monitored if a patient initiates or discontinues therapy with a strong CYP3A4 inhibitor (eg, ketoconazole, erythromycin, itraconazole)).
No products indexed under this heading.

Nelfinavir Mesylate (Co-administration of ketoconazole, a strong inhibitor of CYP3A4, increased cinacalcet exposure following a single 90 mg dose of cinacalcet by 2.3-fold. Dose adjustment of cinacalcet may be required and PTH and serum calcium concentrations should be closely monitored if a patient initiates or discontinues therapy with a strong CYP3A4 inhibitor (eg, ketoconazole, erythromycin, itraconazole)).
No products indexed under this heading.

Nevirapine (Co-administration of ketoconazole, a strong inhibitor of CYP3A4, increased cinacalcet exposure following a single 90 mg dose of cinacalcet by 2.3-fold. Dose adjustment of cinacalcet may be required and PTH and serum calcium concentrations should be closely monitored if a patient initiates or discontinues therapy with a strong CYP3A4 inhibitor (eg, ketoconazole, erythromycin, itraconazole)). Products include:
Viramune Oral Suspension 897
Viramune Tablets 897

Niacin (Co-administration of ketoconazole, a strong inhibitor of CYP3A4, increased cinacalcet exposure following a single 90 mg dose of cinacalcet by 2.3-fold. Dose adjustment of cinacalcet may be required and PTH and serum calcium concentrations should be closely monitored if a patient initiates or discontinues therapy with a strong CYP3A4 inhibitor (eg, ketoconazole, erythromycin, itraconazole)). Products include:
Advicor 402
Cardio Basics 3455
Niaspan 497
Simcor 524

Niacinamide (Co-administration of ketoconazole, a strong inhibitor of CYP3A4, increased cinacalcet exposure following a single 90 mg dose of cinacalcet by 2.3-fold. Dose adjustment of cinacalcet may be required and PTH and serum calcium concentrations should be closely monitored if a patient initiates or discontinues therapy with a strong CYP3A4 inhibitor (eg, ketoconazole, erythromycin, itraconazole)). Products include:
CitraNatal 90 DHA Capsules 2332
CitraNatal Assure 2332
CitraNatal Rx 2332
Heplive 607

Niacinamide Hydroiodide (Co-administration of ketoconazole, a strong inhibitor of CYP3A4, increased cinacalcet exposure following a single 90 mg dose of cinacalcet by 2.3-fold. Dose adjustment of cinacalcet may be required and PTH and serum calcium concentrations should be closely monitored if a patient initiates or discontinues therapy with a strong CYP3A4 inhibitor (eg, ketoconazole, erythromycin, itraconazole)).
No products indexed under this heading.

Nicotinamide (Co-administration of ketoconazole, a strong inhibitor of CYP3A4, increased cinacalcet exposure following a single 90 mg dose of cinacalcet by 2.3-fold. Dose adjustment of cinacalcet may be required and PTH and serum calcium concentrations should be closely monitored if a patient initiates or discontinues therapy with a strong CYP3A4 inhibitor (eg, ketoconazole, erythromycin, itraconazole)).
No products indexed under this heading.

Nifedipine (Co-administration of ketoconazole, a strong inhibitor of CYP3A4, increased cinacalcet exposure following a single 90 mg dose of cinacalcet by 2.3-fold. Dose adjustment of cinacalcet may be required and PTH and serum calcium concentrations should be closely monitored if a patient initiates or discontinues therapy with a strong CYP3A4 inhibitor (eg, ketoconazole, erythromycin, itraconazole)).
No products indexed under this heading.

Norfloxacin (Co-administration of ketoconazole, a strong inhibitor of CYP3A4, increased cinacalcet exposure following a single 90 mg dose of cinacalcet by 2.3-fold. Dose adjustment of cinacalcet may be required and PTH and serum calcium concentrations should be closely monitored if a patient initiates or discontinues therapy with a strong CYP3A4 inhibitor (eg, ketoconazole, erythromycin, itraconazole)). Products include:
Noroxin 2220

Nortriptyline Hydrochloride (Cinacalcet is a strong in vitro, as well as in vivo, inhibitor of CYP2D6. Therefore, dose adjustments of concomitant medications that are predominantly metabolized by CYP2D6 (eg, metoprolol and carvedilol) and particularly those with a narrow therapeutic index (eg, flecainide, vinblastine, thioridazine and most tricyclic antidepressants) may be required).
No products indexed under this heading.

Olanzapine (Cinacalcet is a strong in vitro, as well as in vivo, inhibitor of CYP2D6. Therefore, dose adjustments of concomitant medications that are predominantly metabolized by CYP2D6 (eg, metoprolol and carvedilol) and particularly those with a narrow therapeutic index (eg, flecainide, vinblastine, thioridazine and most tricyclic antidepressants) may be required). Products include:
Symbyax 1965
Zyprexa 1984
Zyprexa IntraMuscular 1984
Zyprexa ZYDIS 1984

Omeprazole (Co-administration of ketoconazole, a strong inhibitor of CYP3A4, increased cinacalcet exposure following a single 90 mg dose of cinacalcet by 2.3-fold. Dose adjustment of cinacalcet may be required and PTH and serum calcium concentrations should be closely monitored if a patient initiates or discontinues therapy with a strong CYP3A4 inhibitor (eg, ketoconazole, erythromycin, itraconazole)).
No products indexed under this heading.

Ondansetron (Cinacalcet is a strong in vitro, as well as in vivo, inhibitor of CYP2D6. Therefore, dose adjustments of concomitant medications that are predominantly metabolized by CYP2D6 (eg, metoprolol and carvedilol) and particularly those with a narrow therapeutic index (eg, flecainide, vinblastine, thioridazine and most tricyclic antidepressants) may be required).
No products indexed under this heading.

Ondansetron Hydrochloride (Cinacalcet is a strong in vitro, as well as in vivo, inhibitor of CYP2D6. Therefore, dose adjustments of concomitant medications that are predominantly metabolized by CYP2D6 (eg, metoprolol and carvedilol) and particularly those with a narrow therapeutic index (eg, flecainide, vinblastine, thioridazine and most tricyclic antidepressants) may be required). Products include:
Zofran Injection 1750
Zofran 1756
Zofran ODT 1756

Oxycodone Hydrochloride (Cinacalcet is a strong in vitro, as well as in vivo, inhibitor of CYP2D6. Therefore, dose adjustments of concomitant medi-

cations that are predominantly metabolized by CYP2D6 (eg, metoprolol and carvedilol) and particularly those with a narrow therapeutic index (eg, flecainide, vinblastine, thioridazine and most tricyclic antidepressants) may be required). Products include:

OxyContin **2807**
Percocet **1121**
Percodan **1124**

Paclitaxel (Cinacalcet is a strong *in vitro*, as well as *in vivo*, inhibitor of CYP2D6. Therefore, dose adjustments of concomitant medications that are predominantly metabolized by CYP2D6 (eg, metoprolol and carvedilol) and particularly those with a narrow therapeutic index (eg, flecainide, vinblastine, thioridazine and most tricyclic antidepressants) may be required).
No products indexed under this heading.

Paroxetine Hydrochloride (Co-administration of ketoconazole, a strong inhibitor of CYP3A4, increased cinacalcet exposure following a single 90 mg dose of cinacalcet by 2.3-fold. Dose adjustment of cinacalcet may be required and PTH and serum calcium concentrations should be closely monitored if a patient initiates or discontinues therapy with a strong CYP3A4 inhibitor (eg, ketoconazole, erythromycin, itraconazole)). Products include:

Paroxetine CR **2361**
Paroxetine ER **2371**
Paxil **1586**
Paxil CR **1596**

Pindolol (Cinacalcet is a strong *in vitro*, as well as *in vivo*, inhibitor of CYP2D6. Therefore, dose adjustments of concomitant medications that are predominantly metabolized by CYP2D6 (eg, metoprolol and carvedilol) and particularly those with a narrow therapeutic index (eg, flecainide, vinblastine, thioridazine and most tricyclic antidepressants) may be required).
No products indexed under this heading.

Posaconazole (Co-administration of ketoconazole, a strong inhibitor of CYP3A4, increased cinacalcet exposure following a single 90 mg dose of cinacalcet by 2.3-fold. Dose adjustment of cinacalcet may be required and PTH and serum calcium concentrations should be closely monitored if a patient initiates or discontinues therapy with a strong CYP3A4 inhibitor (eg, ketoconazole, erythromycin, itraconazole)). Products include:

Noxafil **3172**

Propafenone Hydrochloride (Cinacalcet is a strong *in vitro*, as well as *in vivo*, inhibitor of CYP2D6. Therefore, dose adjustments of concomitant medications that are predominantly metabolized by CYP2D6 (eg, metoprolol and carvedilol) and particularly those with a narrow therapeutic index (eg, flecainide, vinblastine, thioridazine and most tricyclic antidepressants) may be required). Products include:

Rythmol **1648**
Rythmol SR **1652**

Propoxyphene Hydrochloride (Co-administration of ketoconazole, a strong inhibitor of CYP3A4, increased cinacalcet exposure following a single 90 mg dose of cinacalcet by 2.3-fold. Dose adjustment of cinacalcet may be required and PTH and serum calcium concentrations should be closely monitored if a patient initiates or discontinues therapy with a strong CYP3A4 inhibitor (eg, ketoconazole, erythromycin, itraconazole)).
No products indexed under this heading.

Propoxyphene Napsylate (Co-administration of ketoconazole, a strong inhibitor of CYP3A4, increased cinacalcet exposure following a single 90 mg dose of cinacalcet by 2.3-fold. Dose adjustment of cinacalcet may be required and PTH and serum calcium concentrations should be closely monitored if a patient initiates or discontinues therapy with a strong CYP3A4 inhibitor (eg, ketoconazole, erythromycin, itraconazole)).
No products indexed under this heading.

Propranolol Hydrochloride (Cinacalcet is a strong *in vitro*, as well as *in vivo*, inhibitor of CYP2D6. Therefore, dose adjustments of concomitant medications that are predominantly metabolized by CYP2D6 (eg, metoprolol and carvedilol) and particularly those with a narrow therapeutic index (eg, flecainide, vinblastine, thioridazine and most tricyclic antidepressants) may be required). Products include:

InnoPran XL **1517**

Protriptyline Hydrochloride (Cinacalcet is a strong *in vitro*, as well as *in vivo*, inhibitor of CYP2D6. Therefore, dose adjustments of concomitant medications that are predominantly metabolized by CYP2D6 (eg, metoprolol and carvedilol) and particularly those with a narrow therapeutic index (eg, flecainide, vinblastine, thioridazine and most tricyclic antidepressants) may be required).
No products indexed under this heading.

Quetiapine Fumarate (Cinacalcet is a strong *in vitro*, as well as *in vivo*, inhibitor of CYP2D6. Therefore, dose adjustments of concomitant medications that are predominantly metabolized by CYP2D6 (eg, metoprolol and carvedilol) and particularly those with a narrow therapeutic index (eg, flecainide, vinblastine, thioridazine and most tricyclic antidepressants) may be required). Products include:

Seroquel **750**
Seroquel XR **759**

Quinidine (Co-administration of ketoconazole, a strong inhibitor of CYP3A4, increased cinacalcet exposure following a single 90 mg dose of cinacalcet by 2.3-fold. Dose adjustment of cinacalcet may be required and PTH and serum calcium concentrations should be closely monitored if a patient initiates or discontinues therapy with a strong CYP3A4 inhibitor (eg, ketoconazole, erythromycin, itraconazole)).
No products indexed under this heading.

Quinidine Gluconate (Cinacalcet is a strong *in vitro*, as well as *in vivo*, inhibitor of CYP2D6. Therefore, dose adjustments of concomitant medications that are predominantly metabolized by CYP2D6 (eg, metoprolol and carvedilol) and particularly those with a narrow therapeutic index (eg, flecainide, vinblastine, thioridazine and most tricyclic antidepressants) may be required).
No products indexed under this heading.

Quinidine Hydrochloride (Co-administration of ketoconazole, a strong inhibitor of CYP3A4, increased cinacalcet exposure following a single 90 mg dose of cinacalcet by 2.3-fold. Dose adjustment of cinacalcet may be required and PTH and serum calcium concentrations should be closely monitored if a patient initiates or discontinues therapy with a strong CYP3A4 inhibitor (eg, ketoconazole, erythromycin, itraconazole)).
No products indexed under this heading.

Quinidine Polygalacturonate (Co-administration of ketoconazole, a strong inhibitor of CYP3A4, increased cinacalcet exposure following a single 90 mg dose of cinacalcet by 2.3-fold. Dose adjustment of cinacalcet may be required and PTH and serum calcium concentrations should be closely monitored if a patient initiates or discontinues therapy with a strong CYP3A4 inhibitor (eg, ketoconazole, erythromycin, itraconazole)).
No products indexed under this heading.

Quinidine Sulfate (Co-administration of ketoconazole, a strong inhibitor of CYP3A4, increased cinacalcet exposure following a single 90 mg dose of cinacalcet by 2.3-fold. Dose adjustment of cinacalcet may be required and PTH and serum calcium concentrations should be closely monitored if a patient initiates or discontinues therapy with a strong CYP3A4 inhibitor (eg, ketoconazole, erythromycin, itraconazole)).
No products indexed under this heading.

Quinine (Co-administration of ketoconazole, a strong inhibitor of CYP3A4, increased cinacalcet exposure following a single 90 mg dose of cinacalcet by 2.3-fold. Dose adjustment of cinacalcet may be required and PTH and serum calcium concentrations should be closely monitored if a patient initiates or discontinues therapy with a strong CYP3A4 inhibitor (eg, ketoconazole, erythromycin, itraconazole)). Products include:

Hyland's Leg Cramps PM with Quinine **3315**

Quinine Sulfate (Co-administration of ketoconazole, a strong inhibitor of CYP3A4, increased cinacalcet exposure following a single 90 mg dose of cinacalcet by 2.3-fold. Dose adjustment of cinacalcet may be required and PTH and serum calcium concentrations should be closely monitored if a patient initiates or discontinues therapy with a strong CYP3A4 inhibitor (eg, ketoconazole, erythromycin, itraconazole)).
No products indexed under this heading.

Quinupristin (Co-administration of ketoconazole, a strong inhibitor of CYP3A4, increased cinacalcet exposure following a single 90 mg dose of cinacalcet by 2.3-fold. Dose adjustment of cinacalcet may be required and PTH and serum calcium concentrations should be closely monitored if a patient initiates or discontinues therapy with a strong CYP3A4 inhibitor (eg, ketoconazole, erythromycin, itraconazole)).
No products indexed under this heading.

Ranitidine Bismuth Citrate (Co-administration of ketoconazole, a strong inhibitor of CYP3A4, increased cinacalcet exposure following a single 90 mg dose of cinacalcet by 2.3-fold. Dose adjustment of cinacalcet may be required and PTH and serum calcium concentrations should be closely monitored if a patient initiates or discontinues therapy with a strong CYP3A4 inhibitor (eg, ketoconazole, erythromycin, itraconazole)).
No products indexed under this heading.

Ranitidine Hydrochloride (Co-administration of ketoconazole, a strong inhibitor of CYP3A4, increased cinacalcet exposure following a single 90 mg dose of cinacalcet by 2.3-fold. Dose adjustment of cinacalcet may be required and PTH and serum calcium concentrations should be closely monitored if a patient initiates or discontinues therapy with a strong CYP3A4 inhibitor (eg, ketoconazole, erythromycin, itraconazole)). Products include:

Zantac **1737**
Zantac Injection **1732**
Zantac Pharmacy **1735**

Risperidone (Cinacalcet is a strong *in vitro*, as well as *in vivo*, inhibitor of CYP2D6. Therefore, dose adjustments of concomitant medications that are predominantly metabolized by CYP2D6 (eg, metoprolol and carvedilol) and particularly those with a narrow therapeutic index (eg, flecainide, vinblastine, thioridazine and most tricyclic antidepressants) may be required). Products include:

Risperdal Consta **2682**

Ritonavir (Co-administration of ketoconazole, a strong inhibitor of CYP3A4, increased cinacalcet exposure following a single 90 mg dose of cinacalcet by 2.3-fold. Dose adjustment of cinacalcet may be required and PTH and serum calcium concentrations should be closely monitored if a patient initiates or discontinues therapy with a strong CYP3A4 inhibitor (eg, ketoconazole, erythromycin, itraconazole)). Products include:

Kaletra **458**
Norvir **509**

Saquinavir (Co-administration of ketoconazole, a strong inhibitor of CYP3A4, increased cinacalcet exposure following a single 90 mg dose of cinacalcet by 2.3-fold. Dose adjustment of cinacalcet may be required and PTH and serum calcium concentrations should be closely monitored if a patient initiates or discontinues therapy with a strong CYP3A4 inhibitor (eg, ketoconazole, erythromycin, itraconazole)).
No products indexed under this heading.

Saquinavir Mesylate (Co-administration of ketoconazole, a strong inhibitor of CYP3A4, increased cinacalcet exposure following a single 90 mg dose of cinacalcet by 2.3-fold. Dose adjustment of cinacalcet may be required and PTH and serum calcium concentrations should be closely monitored if a patient initiates or discontinues therapy with a strong CYP3A4 inhibitor (eg, ketoconazole, erythromycin, itraconazole)).
No products indexed under this heading.

Sertraline Hydrochloride (Co-administration of ketoconazole, a strong inhibitor of CYP3A4, increased cinacalcet exposure following a single 90 mg dose of cinacalcet by 2.3-fold. Dose adjustment of cinacalcet may be required and PTH and serum calcium concentrations should be closely monitored if a patient initiates or discontinues therapy with a strong CYP3A4 inhibitor (eg, ketoconazole, erythromycin, itraconazole)).
No products indexed under this heading.

Sildenafil Citrate (Co-administration of ketoconazole, a strong inhibitor of CYP3A4, increased cinacalcet exposure following a single 90 mg dose of cinacalcet by 2.3-fold. Dose adjustment of cinacalcet may be required and PTH and serum calcium concentrations should be closely monitored if a patient initiates or discontinues therapy with a strong CYP3A4 inhibitor (eg, ketoconazole, erythromycin, itraconazole)).
No products indexed under this heading.

Tamoxifen Citrate (Cinacalcet is a strong *in vitro*, as well as *in vivo*, inhibitor of CYP2D6. Therefore, dose adjustments of concomitant medications that are predominantly metabolized by CYP2D6 (eg, metoprolol and carvedilol) and particularly those with a narrow therapeutic index (eg, flecainide, vinblastine, thioridazine and most tricyclic antidepressants) may be required).
No products indexed under this heading.

Telithromycin (Co-administration of ketoconazole, a strong inhibitor of CYP3A4, increased cinacalcet exposure following a single 90 mg dose of cinacalcet by 2.3-fold. Dose adjustment of cinacalcet may be required and PTH and serum calcium concentrations should be closely monitored if a patient initiates or discontinues therapy with a strong CYP3A4 inhibitor (eg, ketoconazole, erythromycin, itraconazole)). Products include:

Ketek **2991**

Teniposide (Cinacalcet is a strong *in vitro*, as well as *in vivo*, inhibitor of CYP2D6. Therefore, dose adjustments of concomitant medications that are predominantly metabolized by CYP2D6 (eg, metoprolol and carvedilol) and particularly those with a narrow therapeutic

index (eg, flecainide, vinblastine, thioridazine and most tricyclic antidepressants) may be required).
No products indexed under this heading.

Testosterone (Cinacalcet is a strong in vitro, as well as in vivo, inhibitor of CYP2D6. Therefore, dose adjustments of concomitant medications that are predominantly metabolized by CYP2D6 (eg, metoprolol and carvedilol) and particularly those with a narrow therapeutic index (eg, flecainide, vinblastine, thioridazine and most tricyclic antidepressants) may be required). Products include:
AndroGel 3456

Testosterone Cypionate (Cinacalcet is a strong in vitro, as well as in vivo, inhibitor of CYP2D6. Therefore, dose adjustments of concomitant medications that are predominantly metabolized by CYP2D6 (eg, metoprolol and carvedilol) and particularly those with a narrow therapeutic index (eg, flecainide, vinblastine, thioridazine and most tricyclic antidepressants) may be required).
No products indexed under this heading.

Testosterone Enanthate (Cinacalcet is a strong in vitro, as well as in vivo, inhibitor of CYP2D6. Therefore, dose adjustments of concomitant medications that are predominantly metabolized by CYP2D6 (eg, metoprolol and carvedilol) and particularly those with a narrow therapeutic index (eg, flecainide, vinblastine, thioridazine and most tricyclic antidepressants) may be required). Products include:
Delatestryl 1102

Testosterone Propionate (Cinacalcet is a strong in vitro, as well as in vivo, inhibitor of CYP2D6. Therefore, dose adjustments of concomitant medications that are predominantly metabolized by CYP2D6 (eg, metoprolol and carvedilol) and particularly those with a narrow therapeutic index (eg, flecainide, vinblastine, thioridazine and most tricyclic antidepressants) may be required).
No products indexed under this heading.

Thioridazine (Cinacalcet is a strong in vitro, as well as in vivo, inhibitor of CYP2D6. Therefore, dose adjustments of concomitant medications that are predominantly metabolized by CYP2D6 (eg, metoprolol and carvedilol) and particularly those with a narrow therapeutic index (eg, flecainide, vinblastine, thioridazine and most tricyclic antidepressants) may be required).
No products indexed under this heading.

Thioridazine Hydrochloride (Cinacalcet is a strong in vitro, as well as in vivo, inhibitor of CYP2D6. Therefore, dose adjustments of concomitant medications that are predominantly metabolized by CYP2D6 (eg, metoprolol and carvedilol) and particularly those with a narrow therapeutic index (eg, flecainide, vinblastine, thioridazine and most tricyclic antidepressants) may be required). Products include:
Thioridazine Hydrochloride 2384

Timolol Maleate (Cinacalcet is a strong in vitro, as well as in vivo, inhibitor of CYP2D6. Therefore, dose adjustments of concomitant medications that are predominantly metabolized by CYP2D6 (eg, metoprolol and carvedilol) and particularly those with a narrow therapeutic index (eg, flecainide, vinblastine, thioridazine and most tricyclic antidepressants) may be required). Products include:
Combigan 601
Dorzolamide Hydrochloride/Timolol Maleate Ophthalmic Solution .... ⊙243
Timoptic in Ocudose .... ⊙231

Tolterodine Tartrate (Cinacalcet is a strong in vitro, as well as in vivo, inhibitor of CYP2D6. Therefore, dose adjust-

ments of concomitant medications that are predominantly metabolized by CYP2D6 (eg, metoprolol and carvedilol) and particularly those with a narrow therapeutic index (eg, flecainide, vinblastine, thioridazine and most tricyclic antidepressants) may be required).
No products indexed under this heading.

Tramadol Hydrochloride (Cinacalcet is a strong in vitro, as well as in vivo, inhibitor of CYP2D6. Therefore, dose adjustments of concomitant medications that are predominantly metabolized by CYP2D6 (eg, metoprolol and carvedilol) and particularly those with a narrow therapeutic index (eg, flecainide, vinblastine, thioridazine and most tricyclic antidepressants) may be required). Products include:
Ryzolt 2813
Ultram ER 2693

Trazodone Hydrochloride (Cinacalcet is a strong in vitro, as well as in vivo, inhibitor of CYP2D6. Therefore, dose adjustments of concomitant medications that are predominantly metabolized by CYP2D6 (eg, metoprolol and carvedilol) and particularly those with a narrow therapeutic index (eg, flecainide, vinblastine, thioridazine and most tricyclic antidepressants) may be required).
No products indexed under this heading.

Triazolam (Cinacalcet is a strong in vitro, as well as in vivo, inhibitor of CYP2D6. Therefore, dose adjustments of concomitant medications that are predominantly metabolized by CYP2D6 (eg, metoprolol and carvedilol) and particularly those with a narrow therapeutic index (eg, flecainide, vinblastine, thioridazine and most tricyclic antidepressants) may be required).
No products indexed under this heading.

Trimipramine Maleate (Cinacalcet is a strong in vitro, as well as in vivo, inhibitor of CYP2D6. Therefore, dose adjustments of concomitant medications that are predominantly metabolized by CYP2D6 (eg, metoprolol and carvedilol) and particularly those with a narrow therapeutic index (eg, flecainide, vinblastine, thioridazine and most tricyclic antidepressants) may be required).
No products indexed under this heading.

Troglitazone (Co-administration of ketoconazole, a strong inhibitor of CYP3A4, increased cinacalcet exposure following a single 90 mg dose of cinacalcet by 2.3-fold. Dose adjustment of cinacalcet may be required and PTH and serum calcium concentrations should be closely monitored if a patient initiates or discontinues therapy with a strong CYP3A4 inhibitor (eg, ketoconazole, erythromycin, itraconazole)).
No products indexed under this heading.

Troleandomycin (Co-administration of ketoconazole, a strong inhibitor of CYP3A4, increased cinacalcet exposure following a single 90 mg dose of cinacalcet by 2.3-fold. Dose adjustment of cinacalcet may be required and PTH and serum calcium concentrations should be closely monitored if a patient initiates or discontinues therapy with a strong CYP3A4 inhibitor (eg, ketoconazole, erythromycin, itraconazole)).
No products indexed under this heading.

Valproate Sodium (Co-administration of ketoconazole, a strong inhibitor of CYP3A4, increased cinacalcet exposure following a single 90 mg dose of cinacalcet by 2.3-fold. Dose adjustment of cinacalcet may be required and PTH and serum calcium concentrations should be closely monitored if a patient initiates or discontinues therapy with a strong CYP3A4 inhibitor (eg, ketoconazole, erythromycin, itraconazole)).
No products indexed under this heading.

Vardenafil Hydrochloride (Co-administration of ketoconazole, a

strong inhibitor of CYP3A4, increased cinacalcet exposure following a single 90 mg dose of cinacalcet by 2.3-fold. Dose adjustment of cinacalcet may be required and PTH and serum calcium concentrations should be closely monitored if a patient initiates or discontinues therapy with a strong CYP3A4 inhibitor (eg, ketoconazole, erythromycin, itraconazole)). Products include:
Levitra 3157

Venlafaxine Hydrochloride (Cinacalcet is a strong in vitro, as well as in vivo, inhibitor of CYP2D6. Therefore, dose adjustments of concomitant medications that are predominantly metabolized by CYP2D6 (eg, metoprolol and carvedilol) and particularly those with a narrow therapeutic index (eg, flecainide, vinblastine, thioridazine and most tricyclic antidepressants) may be required). Products include:
Effexor XR 3504
Venlafaxine Hydrochloride Tablets ... 2388

Verapamil Hydrochloride (Co-administration of ketoconazole, a strong inhibitor of CYP3A4, increased cinacalcet exposure following a single 90 mg dose of cinacalcet by 2.3-fold. Dose adjustment of cinacalcet may be required and PTH and serum calcium concentrations should be closely monitored if a patient initiates or discontinues therapy with a strong CYP3A4 inhibitor (eg, ketoconazole, erythromycin, itraconazole)). Products include:
Tarka 534

Vinblastine Sulfate (Cinacalcet is a strong in vitro, as well as in vivo, inhibitor of CYP2D6. Therefore, dose adjustments of concomitant medications that are predominantly metabolized by CYP2D6 (eg, metoprolol and carvedilol) and particularly those with a narrow therapeutic index (eg, flecainide, vinblastine, thioridazine and most tricyclic antidepressants) may be required).
No products indexed under this heading.

Voriconazole (Co-administration of ketoconazole, a strong inhibitor of CYP3A4, increased cinacalcet exposure following a single 90 mg dose of cinacalcet by 2.3-fold. Dose adjustment of cinacalcet may be required and PTH and serum calcium concentrations should be closely monitored if a patient initiates or discontinues therapy with a strong CYP3A4 inhibitor (eg, ketoconazole, erythromycin, itraconazole)).
No products indexed under this heading.

Zafirlukast (Co-administration of ketoconazole, a strong inhibitor of CYP3A4, increased cinacalcet exposure following a single 90 mg dose of cinacalcet by 2.3-fold. Dose adjustment of cinacalcet may be required and PTH and serum calcium concentrations should be closely monitored if a patient initiates or discontinues therapy with a strong CYP3A4 inhibitor (eg, ketoconazole, erythromycin, itraconazole)). Products include:
Accolate 3612

Zileuton (Co-administration of ketoconazole, a strong inhibitor of CYP3A4, increased cinacalcet exposure following a single 90 mg dose of cinacalcet by 2.3-fold. Dose adjustment of cinacalcet may be required and PTH and serum calcium concentrations should be closely monitored if a patient initiates or discontinues therapy with a strong CYP3A4 inhibitor (eg, ketoconazole, erythromycin, itraconazole)).
No products indexed under this heading.

Zonisamide (Cinacalcet is a strong in vitro, as well as in vivo, inhibitor of CYP2D6. Therefore, dose adjustments of concomitant medications that are predominantly metabolized by CYP2D6 (eg, metoprolol and carvedilol) and particularly those with a narrow therapeutic index (eg, flecainide, vinblastine, thiorid-

azine and most tricyclic antidepressants) may be required). Products include:
Zonegran 1081

Food Interactions

Food, unspecified (A food-effect study in healthy volunteers indicated that the C_{max} and area under the curve ($AUC_{(0-inf)}$) were increased 82% and 68%, respectively, when cinacalcet was administered with a high-fat meal compared to fasting. C_{max} and $AUC_{(0-inf)}$ of cinacalcet were increased 65% and 50%, respectively, when cinacalcet was administered with a low-fat meal compared to fasting).

Grapefruit (Co-administration of ketoconazole, a strong inhibitor of CYP3A4, increased cinacalcet exposure following a single 90 mg dose of cinacalcet by 2.3-fold. Dose adjustment of cinacalcet may be required and PTH and serum calcium concentrations should be closely monitored if a patient initiates or discontinues therapy with a strong CYP3A4 inhibitor (eg, ketoconazole, erythromycin, itraconazole)).

Grapefruit Juice (Co-administration of ketoconazole, a strong inhibitor of CYP3A4, increased cinacalcet exposure following a single 90 mg dose of cinacalcet by 2.3-fold. Dose adjustment of cinacalcet may be required and PTH and serum calcium concentrations should be closely monitored if a patient initiates or discontinues therapy with a strong CYP3A4 inhibitor (eg, ketoconazole, erythromycin, itraconazole)).

Meal, unspecified (A food-effect study in healthy volunteers indicated that the C_{max} and area under the curve ($AUC_{(0-inf)}$) were increased 82% and 68%, respectively, when cinacalcet was administered with a high-fat meal compared to fasting. C_{max} and $AUC_{(0-inf)}$ of cinacalcet were increased 65% and 50%, respectively, when cinacalcet was administered with a low-fat meal compared to fasting).

SEREVENT DISKUS

(Salmeterol Xinafoate) 1656
May interact with beta-blockers, cytochrome p450 3a4 inhibitors (selected), monoamine oxidase inhibitors, nonpotassium-sparing diuretics, tricyclic antidepressants. Compounds in these categories include:

Acebutolol Hydrochloride (Beta-adrenergic blockers may produce severe bronchospasm in asthmatic patients, however, beta blockers do not block the pulmonary effect of beta-agonists).
No products indexed under this heading.

Acetazolamide (Co-administration of salmeterol and a strong CYP3A4 inhibitor ketoconazole resulted in a significant increase in plasma salmeterol exposure as determined by a 16-fold increase in AUC mainly due to increased bioavailability of swallowed portion of the dose. Although there was no statistical effect on the mean QTc, co-administration of salmeterol and ketoconazole was associated with more frequent increases in QTc duration compared with salmeterol and placebo administration. Due to the potential increased risk of cardiovascular adverse events, the concomitant use of salmeterol with strong CYP3A4 inhibitors, (eg, ketoconazole, ritonavir, atazanavir, clarithromycin, indinavir, itraconazole, nefazodone, nelfinavir, saquinavir, telithromycin) is not recommended).
No products indexed under this heading.

Acetazolamide Sodium (Co-administration of salmeterol and a strong CYP3A4 inhibitor ketoconazole resulted in a significant increase in plasma salmeterol exposure as determined

by a 16-fold increase in AUC mainly due to increased bioavailability of swallowed portion of the dose. Although there was no statistical effect on the mean QTc, co-administration of salmeterol and ketoconazole was associated with more frequent increases in QTc duration compared with salmeterol and placebo administration. Due to the potential increased risk of cardiovascular adverse events, the concomitant use of salmeterol with strong CYP3A4 inhibitors, (eg, ketoconazole, ritonavir, atazanavir, clarithromycin, indinavir, itraconazole, nefazodone, nelfinavir, saquinavir, telithromycin) is not recommended).
No products indexed under this heading.

Amiodarone Hydrochloride (Co-administration of salmeterol and a strong CYP3A4 inhibitor ketoconazole resulted in a significant increase in plasma salmeterol exposure as determined by a 16-fold increase in AUC mainly due to increased bioavailability of swallowed portion of the dose. Although there was no statistical effect on the mean QTc, co-administration of salmeterol and ketoconazole was associated with more frequent increases in QTc duration compared with salmeterol and placebo administration. Due to the potential increased risk of cardiovascular adverse events, the concomitant use of salmeterol with strong CYP3A4 inhibitors, (eg, ketoconazole, ritonavir, atazanavir, clarithromycin, indinavir, itraconazole, nefazodone, nelfinavir, saquinavir, telithromycin) is not recommended).
No products indexed under this heading.

Amitriptyline Hydrochloride (The action of salmeterol on the vascular system may be potentiated by tricyclic antidepressant).
No products indexed under this heading.

Amoxapine (The action of salmeterol on the vascular system may be potentiated by tricyclic antidepressant).
No products indexed under this heading.

Amprenavir (Co-administration of salmeterol and a strong CYP3A4 inhibitor ketoconazole resulted in a significant increase in plasma salmeterol exposure as determined by a 16-fold increase in AUC mainly due to increased bioavailability of swallowed portion of the dose. Although there was no statistical effect on the mean QTc, co-administration of salmeterol and ketoconazole was associated with more frequent increases in QTc duration compared with salmeterol and placebo administration. Due to the potential increased risk of cardiovascular adverse events, the concomitant use of salmeterol with strong CYP3A4 inhibitors, (eg, ketoconazole, ritonavir, atazanavir, clarithromycin, indinavir, itraconazole, nefazodone, nelfinavir, saquinavir, telithromycin) is not recommended).
No products indexed under this heading.

Anastrozole (Co-administration of salmeterol and a strong CYP3A4 inhibitor ketoconazole resulted in a significant increase in plasma salmeterol exposure as determined by a 16-fold increase in AUC mainly due to increased bioavailability of swallowed portion of the dose. Although there was no statistical effect on the mean QTc, co-administration of salmeterol and ketoconazole was associated with more frequent increases in QTc duration compared with salmeterol and placebo administration. Due to the potential increased risk of cardiovascular adverse events, the concomitant use of salmeterol with strong CYP3A4 inhibitors, (eg, ketoconazole, ritonavir, atazanavir, clarithromycin, indinavir, itraconazole, nefazodone, nelfinavir, saquinavir, telithromycin) is not recommended).
No products indexed under this heading.

Aprepitant (Co-administration of salmeterol and a strong CYP3A4 inhibitor ketoconazole resulted in a significant increase in plasma salmeterol exposure as determined by a 16-fold increase in AUC mainly due to increased bioavailability of swallowed portion of the dose. Although there was no statistical effect on the mean QTc, co-administration of salmeterol and ketoconazole was associated with more frequent increases in QTc duration compared with salmeterol and placebo administration. Due to the potential increased risk of cardiovascular adverse events, the concomitant use of salmeterol with strong CYP3A4 inhibitors, (eg, ketoconazole, ritonavir, atazanavir, clarithromycin, indinavir, itraconazole, nefazodone, nelfinavir, saquinavir, telithromycin) is not recommended). Products include:
Emend **2124**

Atazanavir (Co-administration of salmeterol and a strong CYP3A4 inhibitor ketoconazole resulted in a significant increase in plasma salmeterol exposure as determined by a 16-fold increase in AUC mainly due to increased bioavailability of swallowed portion of the dose. Although there was no statistical effect on the mean QTc, co-administration of salmeterol and ketoconazole was associated with more frequent increases in QTc duration compared with salmeterol and placebo administration. Due to the potential increased risk of cardiovascular adverse events, the concomitant use of salmeterol with strong CYP3A4 inhibitors, (eg, ketoconazole, ritonavir, atazanavir, clarithromycin, indinavir, itraconazole, nefazodone, nelfinavir, saquinavir, telithromycin) is not recommended).
No products indexed under this heading.

Atazanavir Sulfate (Co-administration of salmeterol and a strong CYP3A4 inhibitor ketoconazole resulted in a significant increase in plasma salmeterol exposure as determined by a 16-fold increase in AUC mainly due to increased bioavailability of swallowed portion of the dose. Although there was no statistical effect on the mean QTc, co-administration of salmeterol and ketoconazole was associated with more frequent increases in QTc duration compared with salmeterol and placebo administration. Due to the potential increased risk of cardiovascular adverse events, the concomitant use of salmeterol with strong CYP3A4 inhibitors, (eg, ketoconazole, ritonavir, atazanavir, clarithromycin, indinavir, itraconazole, nefazodone, nelfinavir, saquinavir, telithromycin) is not recommended).
No products indexed under this heading.

Atenolol (Beta-adrenergic blockers may produce severe bronchospasm in asthmatic patients, however, beta blockers do not block the pulmonary effect of beta-agonists).
No products indexed under this heading.

Bendroflumethiazide (The ECG changes and/or hypokalemia that may result from the administration of nonpotassium-sparing diuretics can be acutely worsened by beta-agonists, especially when the recommended dose of beta-agonist is exceeded).
No products indexed under this heading.

Betaxolol Hydrochloride (Beta-adrenergic blockers may produce severe bronchospasm in asthmatic patients, however, beta blockers do not block the pulmonary effect of beta-agonists).
No products indexed under this heading.

Bisoprolol Fumarate (Beta-adrenergic blockers may produce severe bronchospasm in asthmatic patients, however, beta blockers do not block the pulmonary effect of beta-agonists).
No products indexed under this heading.

Bumetanide (The ECG changes and/or hypokalemia that may result from the administration of nonpotassium-sparing diuretics can be acutely worsened by beta-agonists, especially when the recommended dose of beta-agonist is exceeded).
No products indexed under this heading.

Carteolol Hydrochloride (Beta-adrenergic blockers may produce severe bronchospasm in asthmatic patients, however, beta blockers do not block the pulmonary effect of beta-agonists).
No products indexed under this heading.

Carvedilol (Beta-adrenergic blockers may produce severe bronchospasm in asthmatic patients, however, beta blockers do not block the pulmonary effect of beta-agonists). Products include:
Coreg **1409**

Carvedilol Phosphate (Beta-adrenergic blockers may produce severe bronchospasm in asthmatic patients, however, beta blockers do not block the pulmonary effect of beta-agonists). Products include:
Coreg CR **1416**

Chlorothiazide (The ECG changes and/or hypokalemia that may result from the administration of nonpotassium-sparing diuretics can be acutely worsened by beta-agonists, especially when the recommended dose of beta-agonist is exceeded).
No products indexed under this heading.

Chlorothiazide Sodium (The ECG changes and/or hypokalemia that may result from the administration of nonpotassium-sparing diuretics can be acutely worsened by beta-agonists, especially when the recommended dose of beta-agonist is exceeded). Products include:
Diuril Intravenous **2009**

Cimetidine (Co-administration of salmeterol and a strong CYP3A4 inhibitor ketoconazole resulted in a significant increase in plasma salmeterol exposure as determined by a 16-fold increase in AUC mainly due to increased bioavailability of swallowed portion of the dose. Although there was no statistical effect on the mean QTc, co-administration of salmeterol and ketoconazole was associated with more frequent increases in QTc duration compared with salmeterol and placebo administration. Due to the potential increased risk of cardiovascular adverse events, the concomitant use of salmeterol with strong CYP3A4 inhibitors, (eg, ketoconazole, ritonavir, atazanavir, clarithromycin, indinavir, itraconazole, nefazodone, nelfinavir, saquinavir, telithromycin) is not recommended).
No products indexed under this heading.

Cimetidine Hydrochloride (Co-administration of salmeterol and a strong CYP3A4 inhibitor ketoconazole resulted in a significant increase in plasma salmeterol exposure as determined by a 16-fold increase in AUC mainly due to increased bioavailability of swallowed portion of the dose. Although there was no statistical effect on the mean QTc, co-administration of salmeterol and ketoconazole was associated with more frequent increases in QTc duration compared with salmeterol and placebo administration. Due to the potential increased risk of cardiovascular adverse events, the concomitant use of salmeterol with strong CYP3A4 inhibitors, (eg, ketoconazole, ritonavir, atazanavir, clarithromycin, indinavir, itraconazole, nefazodone, nelfinavir, saquinavir, telithromycin) is not recommended).
No products indexed under this heading.

Ciprofloxacin (Co-administration of salmeterol and a strong CYP3A4 inhibitor ketoconazole resulted in a significant increase in plasma salmeterol exposure as determined by a 16-fold increase in AUC mainly due to increased bioavailability of swallowed portion of the dose. Although there was no statistical effect on the mean QTc, co-administration of salmeterol and ketoconazole was associated with more frequent increases in QTc duration compared with salmeterol and placebo administration. Due to the potential increased risk of cardiovascular adverse events, the concomitant use of salmeterol with strong CYP3A4 inhibitors, (eg, ketoconazole, ritonavir, atazanavir, clarithromycin, indinavir, itraconazole, nefazodone, nelfinavir, saquinavir, telithromycin) is not recommended). Products include:
Cipro I.V. **3082**
Cipro **3073**
Cipro XR **3091**
Ciprodex **583**

Clarithromycin (Co-administration of salmeterol and a strong CYP3A4 inhibitor ketoconazole resulted in a significant increase in plasma salmeterol exposure as determined by a 16-fold increase in AUC mainly due to increased bioavailability of swallowed portion of the dose. Although there was no statistical effect on the mean QTc, co-administration of salmeterol and ketoconazole was associated with more frequent increases in QTc duration compared with salmeterol and placebo administration. Due to the potential increased risk of cardiovascular adverse events, the concomitant use of salmeterol with strong CYP3A4 inhibitors, (eg, ketoconazole, ritonavir, atazanavir, clarithromycin, indinavir, itraconazole, nefazodone, nelfinavir, saquinavir, telithromycin) is not recommended). Products include:
Biaxin/Biaxin XL **412**

Clomipramine Hydrochloride (The action of salmeterol on the vascular system may be potentiated by tricyclic antidepressant).
No products indexed under this heading.

Clotrimazole (Co-administration of salmeterol and a strong CYP3A4 inhibitor ketoconazole resulted in a significant increase in plasma salmeterol exposure as determined by a 16-fold increase in AUC mainly due to increased bioavailability of swallowed portion of the dose. Although there was no statistical effect on the mean QTc, co-administration of salmeterol and ketoconazole was associated with more frequent increases in QTc duration compared with salmeterol and placebo administration. Due to the potential increased risk of cardiovascular adverse events, the concomitant use of salmeterol with strong CYP3A4 inhibitors, (eg, ketoconazole, ritonavir, atazanavir, clarithromycin, indinavir, itraconazole, nefazodone, nelfinavir, saquinavir, telithromycin) is not recommended). Products include:
Lotrisone **3163**

Conivaptan Hydrochloride (Co-administration of salmeterol and a strong CYP3A4 inhibitor ketoconazole resulted in a significant increase in plasma salmeterol exposure as determined by a 16-fold increase in AUC mainly due to increased bioavailability of swallowed portion of the dose. Although there was no statistical effect on the mean QTc, co-administration of salmeterol and ketoconazole was associated with more frequent increases in QTc duration compared with salmeterol and placebo administration. Due to the potential increased risk of cardiovascular adverse events, the concomitant use of salmeterol with strong CYP3A4 inhibitors, (eg, ketoconazole, ritonavir, atazanavir, clarithromycin, indinavir, itraconazole,

zole, nefazodone, nelfinavir, saquinavir, telithromycin) is not recommended).
Products include:
Vaprisol **689**

Cyclosporine (Co-administration of salmeterol and a strong CYP3A4 inhibitor ketoconazole resulted in a significant increase in plasma salmeterol exposure as determined by a 16-fold increase in AUC mainly due to increased bioavailability of swallowed portion of the dose. Although there was no statistical effect on the mean QTc, co-administration of salmeterol and ketoconazole was associated with more frequent increases in QTc duration compared with salmeterol and placebo administration. Due to the potential increased risk of cardiovascular adverse events, the concomitant use of salmeterol with strong CYP3A4 inhibitors, (eg, ketoconazole, ritonavir, atazanavir, clarithromycin, indinavir, itraconazole, nefazodone, nelfinavir, saquinavir, telithromycin) is not recommended).
Products include:
Gengraf **440**
Neoral Oral Solution **2496**
Neoral Capsules **2496**
Restasis **605**

Dalfopristin (Co-administration of salmeterol and a strong CYP3A4 inhibitor ketoconazole resulted in a significant increase in plasma salmeterol exposure as determined by a 16-fold increase in AUC mainly due to increased bioavailability of swallowed portion of the dose. Although there was no statistical effect on the mean QTc, co-administration of salmeterol and ketoconazole was associated with more frequent increases in QTc duration compared with salmeterol and placebo administration. Due to the potential increased risk of cardiovascular adverse events, the concomitant use of salmeterol with strong CYP3A4 inhibitors, (eg, ketoconazole, ritonavir, atazanavir, clarithromycin, indinavir, itraconazole, nefazodone, nelfinavir, saquinavir, telithromycin) is not recommended).
No products indexed under this heading.

Danazol (Co-administration of salmeterol and a strong CYP3A4 inhibitor ketoconazole resulted in a significant increase in plasma salmeterol exposure as determined by a 16-fold increase in AUC mainly due to increased bioavailability of swallowed portion of the dose. Although there was no statistical effect on the mean QTc, co-administration of salmeterol and ketoconazole was associated with more frequent increases in QTc duration compared with salmeterol and placebo administration. Due to the potential increased risk of cardiovascular adverse events, the concomitant use of salmeterol with strong CYP3A4 inhibitors, (eg, ketoconazole, ritonavir, atazanavir, clarithromycin, indinavir, itraconazole, nefazodone, nelfinavir, saquinavir, telithromycin) is not recommended).
No products indexed under this heading.

Darunavir (Co-administration of salmeterol and a strong CYP3A4 inhibitor ketoconazole resulted in a significant increase in plasma salmeterol exposure as determined by a 16-fold increase in AUC mainly due to increased bioavailability of swallowed portion of the dose. Although there was no statistical effect on the mean QTc, co-administration of salmeterol and ketoconazole was associated with more frequent increases in QTc duration compared with salmeterol and placebo administration. Due to the potential increased risk of cardiovascular adverse events, the concomitant use of salmeterol with strong CYP3A4 inhibitors, (eg, ketoconazole, ritonavir, atazanavir, clarithromycin, indinavir, itraconazole, nefazodone, nelfinavir, saquinavir, telithromycin) is not recommended).
No products indexed under this heading.

Dasatinib (Co-administration of salmeterol and a strong CYP3A4 inhibitor ketoconazole resulted in a significant increase in plasma salmeterol exposure as determined by a 16-fold increase in AUC mainly due to increased bioavailability of swallowed portion of the dose. Although there was no statistical effect on the mean QTc, co-administration of salmeterol and ketoconazole was associated with more frequent increases in QTc duration compared with salmeterol and placebo administration. Due to the potential increased risk of cardiovascular adverse events, the concomitant use of salmeterol with strong CYP3A4 inhibitors, (eg, ketoconazole, ritonavir, atazanavir, clarithromycin, indinavir, itraconazole, nefazodone, nelfinavir, saquinavir, telithromycin) is not recommended).
No products indexed under this heading.

Delavirdine Mesylate (Co-administration of salmeterol and a strong CYP3A4 inhibitor ketoconazole resulted in a significant increase in plasma salmeterol exposure as determined by a 16-fold increase in AUC mainly due to increased bioavailability of swallowed portion of the dose. Although there was no statistical effect on the mean QTc, co-administration of salmeterol and ketoconazole was associated with more frequent increases in QTc duration compared with salmeterol and placebo administration. Due to the potential increased risk of cardiovascular adverse events, the concomitant use of salmeterol with strong CYP3A4 inhibitors, (eg, ketoconazole, ritonavir, atazanavir, clarithromycin, indinavir, itraconazole, nefazodone, nelfinavir, saquinavir, telithromycin) is not recommended).
No products indexed under this heading.

Delavirine (Co-administration of salmeterol and a strong CYP3A4 inhibitor ketoconazole resulted in a significant increase in plasma salmeterol exposure as determined by a 16-fold increase in AUC mainly due to increased bioavailability of swallowed portion of the dose. Although there was no statistical effect on the mean QTc, co-administration of salmeterol and ketoconazole was associated with more frequent increases in QTc duration compared with salmeterol and placebo administration. Due to the potential increased risk of cardiovascular adverse events, the concomitant use of salmeterol with strong CYP3A4 inhibitors, (eg, ketoconazole, ritonavir, atazanavir, clarithromycin, indinavir, itraconazole, nefazodone, nelfinavir, saquinavir, telithromycin) is not recommended).
No products indexed under this heading.

Desipramine Hydrochloride (The action of salmeterol on the vascular system may be potentiated by tricyclic antidepressant).
No products indexed under this heading.

Desloratadine (Co-administration of salmeterol and a strong CYP3A4 inhibitor ketoconazole resulted in a significant increase in plasma salmeterol exposure as determined by a 16-fold increase in AUC mainly due to increased bioavailability of swallowed portion of the dose. Although there was no statistical effect on the mean QTc, co-administration of salmeterol and ketoconazole was associated with more frequent increases in QTc duration compared with salmeterol and placebo administration. Due to the potential increased risk of cardiovascular adverse events, the concomitant use of salmeterol with strong CYP3A4 inhibitors, (eg, ketoconazole, ritonavir, atazanavir, clarithromycin, indinavir, itraconazole, nefazodone, nelfinavir, saquinavir, telithromycin) is not recommended).
Products include:
Clarinex Syrup **3098**
Clarinex **3098**
Clarinex Reditabs **3098**
Clarinex-D 12-Hour **3101**
Clarinex-D **3104**

Diltiazem Hydrochloride (Co-administration of salmeterol and a strong CYP3A4 inhibitor ketoconazole resulted in a significant increase in plasma salmeterol exposure as determined by a 16-fold increase in AUC mainly due to increased bioavailability of swallowed portion of the dose. Although there was no statistical effect on the mean QTc, co-administration of salmeterol and ketoconazole was associated with more frequent increases in QTc duration compared with salmeterol and placebo administration. Due to the potential increased risk of cardiovascular adverse events, the concomitant use of salmeterol with strong CYP3A4 inhibitors, (eg, ketoconazole, ritonavir, atazanavir, clarithromycin, indinavir, itraconazole, nefazodone, nelfinavir, saquinavir, telithromycin) is not recommended).
Products include:
Cardizem LA **423**

Diltiazem Maleate (Co-administration of salmeterol and a strong CYP3A4 inhibitor ketoconazole resulted in a significant increase in plasma salmeterol exposure as determined by a 16-fold increase in AUC mainly due to increased bioavailability of swallowed portion of the dose. Although there was no statistical effect on the mean QTc, co-administration of salmeterol and ketoconazole was associated with more frequent increases in QTc duration compared with salmeterol and placebo administration. Due to the potential increased risk of cardiovascular adverse events, the concomitant use of salmeterol with strong CYP3A4 inhibitors, (eg, ketoconazole, ritonavir, atazanavir, clarithromycin, indinavir, itraconazole, nefazodone, nelfinavir, saquinavir, telithromycin) is not recommended).
No products indexed under this heading.

Doxepin Hydrochloride (The action of salmeterol on the vascular system may be potentiated by tricyclic antidepressant).
No products indexed under this heading.

Efavirenz (Co-administration of salmeterol and a strong CYP3A4 inhibitor ketoconazole resulted in a significant increase in plasma salmeterol exposure as determined by a 16-fold increase in AUC mainly due to increased bioavailability of swallowed portion of the dose. Although there was no statistical effect on the mean QTc, co-administration of salmeterol and ketoconazole was associated with more frequent increases in QTc duration compared with salmeterol and placebo administration. Due to the potential increased risk of cardiovascular adverse events, the concomitant use of salmeterol with strong CYP3A4 inhibitors, (eg, ketoconazole, ritonavir, atazanavir, clarithromycin, indinavir, itraconazole, nefazodone, nelfinavir, saquinavir, telithromycin) is not recommended).
Products include:
Atripla **906**

Erythromycin (Co-administration of salmeterol and a strong CYP3A4 inhibitor ketoconazole resulted in a significant increase in plasma salmeterol exposure as determined by a 16-fold increase in AUC mainly due to increased bioavailability of swallowed portion of the dose. Although there was no statistical effect on the mean QTc, co-administration of salmeterol and ketoconazole was associated with more frequent increases in QTc duration compared with salmeterol and placebo administration. Due to the potential increased risk of cardiovascular adverse events, the concomitant use of salmeterol with strong CYP3A4 inhibitors, (eg, ketoconazole, ritonavir, ataza-

navir, clarithromycin, indinavir, itraconazole, nefazodone, nelfinavir, saquinavir, telithromycin) is not recommended).
No products indexed under this heading.

Erythromycin Estolate (Co-administration of salmeterol and a strong CYP3A4 inhibitor ketoconazole resulted in a significant increase in plasma salmeterol exposure as determined by a 16-fold increase in AUC mainly due to increased bioavailability of swallowed portion of the dose. Although there was no statistical effect on the mean QTc, co-administration of salmeterol and ketoconazole was associated with more frequent increases in QTc duration compared with salmeterol and placebo administration. Due to the potential increased risk of cardiovascular adverse events, the concomitant use of salmeterol with strong CYP3A4 inhibitors, (eg, ketoconazole, ritonavir, atazanavir, clarithromycin, indinavir, itraconazole, nefazodone, nelfinavir, saquinavir, telithromycin) is not recommended).
No products indexed under this heading.

Erythromycin Ethylsuccinate (Co-administration of salmeterol and a strong CYP3A4 inhibitor ketoconazole resulted in a significant increase in plasma salmeterol exposure as determined by a 16-fold increase in AUC mainly due to increased bioavailability of swallowed portion of the dose. Although there was no statistical effect on the mean QTc, co-administration of salmeterol and ketoconazole was associated with more frequent increases in QTc duration compared with salmeterol and placebo administration. Due to the potential increased risk of cardiovascular adverse events, the concomitant use of salmeterol with strong CYP3A4 inhibitors, (eg, ketoconazole, ritonavir, atazanavir, clarithromycin, indinavir, itraconazole, nefazodone, nelfinavir, saquinavir, telithromycin) is not recommended).
Products include:
E.E.S. **437**
EryPed **435**

Erythromycin Gluceptate (Co-administration of salmeterol and a strong CYP3A4 inhibitor ketoconazole resulted in a significant increase in plasma salmeterol exposure as determined by a 16-fold increase in AUC mainly due to increased bioavailability of swallowed portion of the dose. Although there was no statistical effect on the mean QTc, co-administration of salmeterol and ketoconazole was associated with more frequent increases in QTc duration compared with salmeterol and placebo administration. Due to the potential increased risk of cardiovascular adverse events, the concomitant use of salmeterol with strong CYP3A4 inhibitors, (eg, ketoconazole, ritonavir, atazanavir, clarithromycin, indinavir, itraconazole, nefazodone, nelfinavir, saquinavir, telithromycin) is not recommended).
No products indexed under this heading.

Erythromycin Lactobionate (Co-administration of salmeterol and a strong CYP3A4 inhibitor ketoconazole resulted in a significant increase in plasma salmeterol exposure as determined by a 16-fold increase in AUC mainly due to increased bioavailability of swallowed portion of the dose. Although there was no statistical effect on the mean QTc, co-administration of salmeterol and ketoconazole was associated with more frequent increases in QTc duration compared with salmeterol and placebo administration. Due to the potential increased risk of cardiovascular adverse events, the concomitant use of salmeterol with strong CYP3A4 inhibitors, (eg, ketoconazole, ritonavir, ataza-

1721 Interactions Index Serevent

navir, clarithromycin, indinavir, itraconazole, nefazodone, nelfinavir, saquinavir, telithromycin) is not recommended).
No products indexed under this heading.

Erythromycin Stearate (Co-administration of salmeterol and a strong CYP3A4 inhibitor ketoconazole resulted in a significant increase in plasma salmeterol exposure as determined by a 16-fold increase in AUC mainly due to increased bioavailability of swallowed portion of the dose. Although there was no statistical effect on the mean QTc, co-administration of salmeterol and ketoconazole was associated with more frequent increases in QTc duration compared with salmeterol and placebo administration. Due to the potential increased risk of cardiovascular adverse events, the concomitant use of salmeterol with strong CYP3A4 inhibitors, (eg, ketoconazole, ritonavir, atazanavir, clarithromycin, indinavir, itraconazole, nefazodone, nelfinavir, saquinavir, telithromycin) is not recommended).
No products indexed under this heading.

Esmolol Hydrochloride (Beta-adrenergic blockers may produce severe bronchospasm in asthmatic patients, however, beta blockers do not block the pulmonary effect of beta-agonists).
No products indexed under this heading.

Esomeprazole Magnesium (Co-administration of salmeterol and a strong CYP3A4 inhibitor ketoconazole resulted in a significant increase in plasma salmeterol exposure as determined by a 16-fold increase in AUC mainly due to increased bioavailability of swallowed portion of the dose. Although there was no statistical effect on the mean QTc, co-administration of salmeterol and ketoconazole was associated with more frequent increases in QTc duration compared with salmeterol and placebo administration. Due to the potential increased risk of cardiovascular adverse events, the concomitant use of salmeterol with strong CYP3A4 inhibitors, (eg, ketoconazole, ritonavir, atazanavir, clarithromycin, indinavir, itraconazole, nefazodone, nelfinavir, saquinavir, telithromycin) is not recommended).
Products include:
Nexium Capsules 704
Nexium Oral Suspension 704

Esomeprazole Sodium (Co-administration of salmeterol and a strong CYP3A4 inhibitor ketoconazole resulted in a significant increase in plasma salmeterol exposure as determined by a 16-fold increase in AUC mainly due to increased bioavailability of swallowed portion of the dose. Although there was no statistical effect on the mean QTc, co-administration of salmeterol and ketoconazole was associated with more frequent increases in QTc duration compared with salmeterol and placebo administration. Due to the potential increased risk of cardiovascular adverse events, the concomitant use of salmeterol with strong CYP3A4 inhibitors, (eg, ketoconazole, ritonavir, atazanavir, clarithromycin, indinavir, itraconazole, nefazodone, nelfinavir, saquinavir, telithromycin) is not recommended).
Products include:
Nexium I.V. 712

Ethacrynic Acid (The ECG changes and/or hypokalemia that may result from the administration of nonpotassium-sparing diuretics can be acutely worsened by beta-agonists, especially when the recommended dose of beta-agonist is exceeded).
No products indexed under this heading.

Fluconazole (Co-administration of salmeterol and a strong CYP3A4 inhibitor ketoconazole resulted in a significant increase in plasma salmeterol exposure as determined by a 16-fold increase in AUC mainly due to increased bioavailability of swallowed portion of the dose. Although there was no statistical effect on the mean QTc, co-administration of salmeterol and ketoconazole was associated with more frequent increases in QTc duration compared with salmeterol and placebo administration. Due to the potential increased risk of cardiovascular adverse events, the concomitant use of salmeterol with strong CYP3A4 inhibitors, (eg, ketoconazole, ritonavir, atazanavir, clarithromycin, indinavir, itraconazole, nefazodone, nelfinavir, saquinavir, telithromycin) is not recommended).
No products indexed under this heading.

Fluoxetine (Co-administration of salmeterol and a strong CYP3A4 inhibitor ketoconazole resulted in a significant increase in plasma salmeterol exposure as determined by a 16-fold increase in AUC mainly due to increased bioavailability of swallowed portion of the dose. Although there was no statistical effect on the mean QTc, co-administration of salmeterol and ketoconazole was associated with more frequent increases in QTc duration compared with salmeterol and placebo administration. Due to the potential increased risk of cardiovascular adverse events, the concomitant use of salmeterol with strong CYP3A4 inhibitors, (eg, ketoconazole, ritonavir, atazanavir, clarithromycin, indinavir, itraconazole, nefazodone, nelfinavir, saquinavir, telithromycin) is not recommended).
No products indexed under this heading.

Fluoxetine Hydrochloride (Co-administration of salmeterol and a strong CYP3A4 inhibitor ketoconazole resulted in a significant increase in plasma salmeterol exposure as determined by a 16-fold increase in AUC mainly due to increased bioavailability of swallowed portion of the dose. Although there was no statistical effect on the mean QTc, co-administration of salmeterol and ketoconazole was associated with more frequent increases in QTc duration compared with salmeterol and placebo administration. Due to the potential increased risk of cardiovascular adverse events, the concomitant use of salmeterol with strong CYP3A4 inhibitors, (eg, ketoconazole, ritonavir, atazanavir, clarithromycin, indinavir, itraconazole, nefazodone, nelfinavir, saquinavir, telithromycin) is not recommended).
Products include:
Prozac Weekly 1941
Prozac Pulvules 1941
Symbyax 1965

Fluvoxamine Maleate (Co-administration of salmeterol and a strong CYP3A4 inhibitor ketoconazole resulted in a significant increase in plasma salmeterol exposure as determined by a 16-fold increase in AUC mainly due to increased bioavailability of swallowed portion of the dose. Although there was no statistical effect on the mean QTc, co-administration of salmeterol and ketoconazole was associated with more frequent increases in QTc duration compared with salmeterol and placebo administration. Due to the potential increased risk of cardiovascular adverse events, the concomitant use of salmeterol with strong CYP3A4 inhibitors, (eg, ketoconazole, ritonavir, atazanavir, clarithromycin, indinavir, itraconazole, nefazodone, nelfinavir, saquinavir, telithromycin) is not recommended).
No products indexed under this heading.

Fosamprenavir Calcium (Co-administration of salmeterol and a strong CYP3A4 inhibitor ketoconazole resulted in a significant increase in plasma salmeterol exposure as determined by a 16-fold increase in AUC mainly due to increased bioavailability of swallowed portion of the dose. Although there was no statistical effect on the mean QTc, co-administration of salmeterol and ketoconazole was associated with more frequent increases in QTc duration compared with salmeterol and placebo administration. Due to the potential increased risk of cardiovascular adverse events, the concomitant use of salmeterol with strong CYP3A4 inhibitors, (eg, ketoconazole, ritonavir, atazanavir, clarithromycin, indinavir, itraconazole, nefazodone, nelfinavir, saquinavir, telithromycin) is not recommended).
Products include:
Lexiva Oral Suspension 1558
Lexiva 1558

Furosemide (The ECG changes and/or hypokalemia that may result from the administration of nonpotassium-sparing diuretics can be acutely worsened by beta-agonists, especially when the recommended dose of beta-agonist is exceeded). Products include:
Furosemide 2354

Hydrochlorothiazide (The ECG changes and/or hypokalemia that may result from the administration of nonpotassium-sparing diuretics can be acutely worsened by beta-agonists, especially when the recommended dose of beta-agonist is exceeded).
Products include:
Atacand HCT 700
Avalide 2956
Benicar HCT 1017
Diovan HCT 2419
Dyazide 1429
Exforge HCT 2449
Hyzaar 2162
Hyzaar 100-12.5 2162
Micardis HCT 889
Prinzide 2246
Tekturna HCT 2541
Teveten HCT 541

Hydroflumethiazide (The ECG changes and/or hypokalemia that may result from the administration of nonpotassium-sparing diuretics can be acutely worsened by beta-agonists, especially when the recommended dose of beta-agonist is exceeded).
No products indexed under this heading.

Imatinib Mesylate (Co-administration of salmeterol and a strong CYP3A4 inhibitor ketoconazole resulted in a significant increase in plasma salmeterol exposure as determined by a 16-fold increase in AUC mainly due to increased bioavailability of swallowed portion of the dose. Although there was no statistical effect on the mean QTc, co-administration of salmeterol and ketoconazole was associated with more frequent increases in QTc duration compared with salmeterol and placebo administration. Due to the potential increased risk of cardiovascular adverse events, the concomitant use of salmeterol with strong CYP3A4 inhibitors, (eg, ketoconazole, ritonavir, atazanavir, clarithromycin, indinavir, itraconazole, nefazodone, nelfinavir, saquinavir, telithromycin) is not recommended).
Products include:
Gleevec 2477

Imipramine Hydrochloride (The action of salmeterol on the vascular system may be potentiated by tricyclic antidepressant).
No products indexed under this heading.

Imipramine Pamoate (The action of salmeterol on the vascular system may be potentiated by tricyclic antidepressant).
No products indexed under this heading.

Indinavir Sulfate (Co-administration of salmeterol and a strong CYP3A4 inhibitor ketoconazole resulted in a significant increase in plasma salmeterol exposure as determined by a 16-fold increase in AUC mainly due to increased bioavailability of swallowed portion of the dose. Although there was no statistical effect on the mean QTc, co-administration of salmeterol and ketoconazole was associated with more frequent increases in QTc duration compared with salmeterol and placebo administration. Due to the potential increased risk of cardiovascular adverse events, the concomitant use of salmeterol with strong CYP3A4 inhibitors, (eg, ketoconazole, ritonavir, atazanavir, clarithromycin, indinavir, itraconazole, nefazodone, nelfinavir, saquinavir, telithromycin) is not recommended).
Products include:
Crixivan 2113

Isocarboxazid (The action of salmeterol on the vascular system may be potentiated by a MAO inhibitor).
Products include:
Marplan 3481

Isoniazid (Co-administration of salmeterol and a strong CYP3A4 inhibitor ketoconazole resulted in a significant increase in plasma salmeterol exposure as determined by a 16-fold increase in AUC mainly due to increased bioavailability of swallowed portion of the dose. Although there was no statistical effect on the mean QTc, co-administration of salmeterol and ketoconazole was associated with more frequent increases in QTc duration compared with salmeterol and placebo administration. Due to the potential increased risk of cardiovascular adverse events, the concomitant use of salmeterol with strong CYP3A4 inhibitors, (eg, ketoconazole, ritonavir, atazanavir, clarithromycin, indinavir, itraconazole, nefazodone, nelfinavir, saquinavir, telithromycin) is not recommended).
No products indexed under this heading.

Itraconazole (Co-administration of salmeterol and a strong CYP3A4 inhibitor ketoconazole resulted in a significant increase in plasma salmeterol exposure as determined by a 16-fold increase in AUC mainly due to increased bioavailability of swallowed portion of the dose. Although there was no statistical effect on the mean QTc, co-administration of salmeterol and ketoconazole was associated with more frequent increases in QTc duration compared with salmeterol and placebo administration. Due to the potential increased risk of cardiovascular adverse events, the concomitant use of salmeterol with strong CYP3A4 inhibitors, (eg, ketoconazole, ritonavir, atazanavir, clarithromycin, indinavir, itraconazole, nefazodone, nelfinavir, saquinavir, telithromycin) is not recommended).
No products indexed under this heading.

Ketoconazole (Co-administration of salmeterol and a strong CYP3A4 inhibitor ketoconazole resulted in a significant increase in plasma salmeterol exposure as determined by a 16-fold increase in AUC mainly due to increased bioavailability of swallowed portion of the dose. Although there was no statistical effect on the mean QTc, co-administration of salmeterol and ketoconazole was associated with more frequent increases in QTc duration compared with salmeterol and placebo administration. Due to the potential increased risk of cardiovascular adverse events, the concomitant use of salmeterol with strong CYP3A4 inhibitors, (eg, ketoconazole) is not recommended). Products include:
Extina 3319
Xolegel 3337

Labetalol Hydrochloride (Beta-adrenergic blockers may produce severe bronchospasm in asthmatic patients, however, beta blockers do not block the pulmonary effect of beta-agonists).
No products indexed under this heading.

Lapatinib (Co-administration of salmeterol and a strong CYP3A4 inhibitor ketoconazole resulted in a significant increase in plasma salmeterol exposure as determined by a 16-fold increase in

AUC mainly due to increased bioavailability of swallowed portion of the dose. Although there was no statistical effect on the mean QTc, co-administration of salmeterol and ketoconazole was associated with more frequent increases in QTc duration compared with salmeterol and placebo administration. Due to the potential increased risk of cardiovascular adverse events, the concomitant use of salmeterol with strong CYP3A4 inhibitors, (eg, ketoconazole, ritonavir, atazanavir, clarithromycin, indinavir, itraconazole, nefazodone, nelfinavir, saquinavir, telithromycin) is not recommended). Products include:

Tykerb 1698

Levobunolol Hydrochloride (Beta-adrenergic blockers may produce severe bronchospasm in asthmatic patients, however, beta blockers do not block the pulmonary effect of beta-agonists).

No products indexed under this heading.

Lopinavir (Co-administration of salmeterol and a strong CYP3A4 inhibitor ketoconazole resulted in a significant increase in plasma salmeterol exposure as determined by a 16-fold increase in AUC mainly due to increased bioavailability of swallowed portion of the dose. Although there was no statistical effect on the mean QTc, co-administration of salmeterol and ketoconazole was associated with more frequent increases in QTc duration compared with salmeterol and placebo administration. Due to the potential increased risk of cardiovascular adverse events, the concomitant use of salmeterol with strong CYP3A4 inhibitors, (eg, ketoconazole, ritonavir, atazanavir, clarithromycin, indinavir, itraconazole, nefazodone, nelfinavir, saquinavir, telithromycin) is not recommended). Products include:

Kaletra 458

Loratadine (Co-administration of salmeterol and a strong CYP3A4 inhibitor ketoconazole resulted in a significant increase in plasma salmeterol exposure as determined by a 16-fold increase in AUC mainly due to increased bioavailability of swallowed portion of the dose. Although there was no statistical effect on the mean QTc, co-administration of salmeterol and ketoconazole was associated with more frequent increases in QTc duration compared with salmeterol and placebo administration. Due to the potential increased risk of cardiovascular adverse events, the concomitant use of salmeterol with strong CYP3A4 inhibitors, (eg, ketoconazole, ritonavir, atazanavir, clarithromycin, indinavir, itraconazole, nefazodone, nelfinavir, saquinavir, telithromycin) is not recommended).

No products indexed under this heading.

Maprotiline Hydrochloride (The action of salmeterol on the vascular system may be potentiated by tricyclic antidepressant).

No products indexed under this heading.

Methyclothiazide (The ECG changes and/or hypokalemia that may result from the administration of nonpotassium-sparing diuretics can be acutely worsened by beta-agonists, especially when the recommended dose of beta-agonist is exceeded).

No products indexed under this heading.

Metipranolol Hydrochloride (Beta-adrenergic blockers may produce severe bronchospasm in asthmatic patients, however, beta blockers do not block the pulmonary effect of beta-agonists).

No products indexed under this heading.

Metoprolol Succinate (Beta-adrenergic blockers may produce severe bronchospasm in asthmatic patients, however, beta blockers do not block the pulmonary effect of beta-agonists). Products include:

Toprol XL 732

Metoprolol Tartrate (Beta-adrenergic blockers may produce severe bronchospasm in asthmatic patients, however, beta blockers do not block the pulmonary effect of beta-agonists).

No products indexed under this heading.

Metronidazole (Co-administration of salmeterol and a strong CYP3A4 inhibitor ketoconazole resulted in a significant increase in plasma salmeterol exposure as determined by a 16-fold increase in AUC mainly due to increased bioavailability of swallowed portion of the dose. Although there was no statistical effect on the mean QTc, co-administration of salmeterol and ketoconazole was associated with more frequent increases in QTc duration compared with salmeterol and placebo administration. Due to the potential increased risk of cardiovascular adverse events, the concomitant use of salmeterol with strong CYP3A4 inhibitors, (eg, ketoconazole, ritonavir, atazanavir, clarithromycin, indinavir, itraconazole, nefazodone, nelfinavir, saquinavir, telithromycin) is not recommended). Products include:

Pylera 793

Metronidazole Benzoate (Co-administration of salmeterol and a strong CYP3A4 inhibitor ketoconazole resulted in a significant increase in plasma salmeterol exposure as determined by a 16-fold increase in AUC mainly due to increased bioavailability of swallowed portion of the dose. Although there was no statistical effect on the mean QTc, co-administration of salmeterol and ketoconazole was associated with more frequent increases in QTc duration compared with salmeterol and placebo administration. Due to the potential increased risk of cardiovascular adverse events, the concomitant use of salmeterol with strong CYP3A4 inhibitors, (eg, ketoconazole, ritonavir, atazanavir, clarithromycin, indinavir, itraconazole, nefazodone, nelfinavir, saquinavir, telithromycin) is not recommended).

No products indexed under this heading.

Metronidazole Hydrochloride (Co-administration of salmeterol and a strong CYP3A4 inhibitor ketoconazole resulted in a significant increase in plasma salmeterol exposure as determined by a 16-fold increase in AUC mainly due to increased bioavailability of swallowed portion of the dose. Although there was no statistical effect on the mean QTc, co-administration of salmeterol and ketoconazole was associated with more frequent increases in QTc duration compared with salmeterol and placebo administration. Due to the potential increased risk of cardiovascular adverse events, the concomitant use of salmeterol with strong CYP3A4 inhibitors, (eg, ketoconazole, ritonavir, atazanavir, clarithromycin, indinavir, itraconazole, nefazodone, nelfinavir, saquinavir, telithromycin) is not recommended).

No products indexed under this heading.

Metronidazole Sodium (Co-administration of salmeterol and a strong CYP3A4 inhibitor ketoconazole resulted in a significant increase in plasma salmeterol exposure as determined by a 16-fold increase in AUC mainly due to increased bioavailability of swallowed portion of the dose. Although there was no statistical effect on the mean QTc, co-administration of salmeterol and ketoconazole was associated with more frequent increases in QTc duration compared with salmeterol and placebo administration. Due to the potential increased risk of cardiovascular adverse events, the concomitant use of salmeterol with strong CYP3A4 inhibitors, (eg, ketoconazole, ritonavir, atazanavir, clarithromycin, indinavir, itraconazole, nefazodone, nelfinavir, saquinavir, telithromycin) is not recommended).

No products indexed under this heading.

Miconazole (Co-administration of salmeterol and a strong CYP3A4 inhibitor ketoconazole resulted in a significant increase in plasma salmeterol exposure as determined by a 16-fold increase in AUC mainly due to increased bioavailability of swallowed portion of the dose. Although there was no statistical effect on the mean QTc, co-administration of salmeterol and ketoconazole was associated with more frequent increases in QTc duration compared with salmeterol and placebo administration. Due to the potential increased risk of cardiovascular adverse events, the concomitant use of salmeterol with strong CYP3A4 inhibitors, (eg, ketoconazole, ritonavir, atazanavir, clarithromycin, indinavir, itraconazole, nefazodone, nelfinavir, saquinavir, telithromycin) is not recommended).

No products indexed under this heading.

Miconazole Nitrate (Co-administration of salmeterol and a strong CYP3A4 inhibitor ketoconazole resulted in a significant increase in plasma salmeterol exposure as determined by a 16-fold increase in AUC mainly due to increased bioavailability of swallowed portion of the dose. Although there was no statistical effect on the mean QTc, co-administration of salmeterol and ketoconazole was associated with more frequent increases in QTc duration compared with salmeterol and placebo administration. Due to the potential increased risk of cardiovascular adverse events, the concomitant use of salmeterol with strong CYP3A4 inhibitors, (eg, ketoconazole, ritonavir, atazanavir, clarithromycin, indinavir, itraconazole, nefazodone, nelfinavir, saquinavir, telithromycin) is not recommended). Products include:

Vusion Ointment 3335

Mifepristone (Co-administration of salmeterol and a strong CYP3A4 inhibitor ketoconazole resulted in a significant increase in plasma salmeterol exposure as determined by a 16-fold increase in AUC mainly due to increased bioavailability of swallowed portion of the dose. Although there was no statistical effect on the mean QTc, co-administration of salmeterol and ketoconazole was associated with more frequent increases in QTc duration compared with salmeterol and placebo administration. Due to the potential increased risk of cardiovascular adverse events, the concomitant use of salmeterol with strong CYP3A4 inhibitors, (eg, ketoconazole, ritonavir, atazanavir, clarithromycin, indinavir, itraconazole, nefazodone, nelfinavir, saquinavir, telithromycin) is not recommended).

No products indexed under this heading.

Moclobemide (The action of salmeterol on the vascular system may be potentiated by a MAO inhibitor).

No products indexed under this heading.

Nadolol (Beta-adrenergic blockers may produce severe bronchospasm in asthmatic patients, however, beta blockers do not block the pulmonary effect of beta-agonists). Products include:

Nadolol 2359

Nebivolol (Beta-adrenergic blockers may produce severe bronchospasm in asthmatic patients, however, beta blockers do not block the pulmonary effect of beta-agonists). Products include:

Bystolic 1147

Nefazodone Hydrochloride (Co-administration of salmeterol and a strong CYP3A4 inhibitor ketoconazole resulted in a significant increase in plasma salmeterol exposure as determined by a 16-fold increase in AUC mainly due to increased bioavailability of swallowed portion of the dose. Although there was no statistical effect on the mean QTc, co-administration of salmeterol and ketoconazole was associated with more frequent increases in QTc duration compared with salmeterol and placebo administration. Due to the potential increased risk of cardiovascular adverse events, the concomitant use of salmeterol with strong CYP3A4 inhibitors, (eg, ketoconazole, ritonavir, atazanavir, clarithromycin, indinavir, itraconazole, nefazodone, nelfinavir, saquinavir, telithromycin) is not recommended).

No products indexed under this heading.

Nelfinavir Mesylate (Co-administration of salmeterol and a strong CYP3A4 inhibitor ketoconazole resulted in a significant increase in plasma salmeterol exposure as determined by a 16-fold increase in AUC mainly due to increased bioavailability of swallowed portion of the dose. Although there was no statistical effect on the mean QTc, co-administration of salmeterol and ketoconazole was associated with more frequent increases in QTc duration compared with salmeterol and placebo administration. Due to the potential increased risk of cardiovascular adverse events, the concomitant use of salmeterol with strong CYP3A4 inhibitors, (eg, ketoconazole, ritonavir, atazanavir, clarithromycin, indinavir, itraconazole, nefazodone, nelfinavir, saquinavir, telithromycin) is not recommended).

No products indexed under this heading.

Nevirapine (Co-administration of salmeterol and a strong CYP3A4 inhibitor ketoconazole resulted in a significant increase in plasma salmeterol exposure as determined by a 16-fold increase in AUC mainly due to increased bioavailability of swallowed portion of the dose. Although there was no statistical effect on the mean QTc, co-administration of salmeterol and ketoconazole was associated with more frequent increases in QTc duration compared with salmeterol and placebo administration. Due to the potential increased risk of cardiovascular adverse events, the concomitant use of salmeterol with strong CYP3A4 inhibitors, (eg, ketoconazole, ritonavir, atazanavir, clarithromycin, indinavir, itraconazole, nefazodone, nelfinavir, saquinavir, telithromycin) is not recommended). Products include:

Viramune Oral Suspension 897
Viramune Tablets 897

Niacin (Co-administration of salmeterol and a strong CYP3A4 inhibitor ketoconazole resulted in a significant increase in plasma salmeterol exposure as determined by a 16-fold increase in AUC mainly due to increased bioavailability of swallowed portion of the dose. Although there was no statistical effect on the mean QTc, co-administration of salmeterol and ketoconazole was associated with more frequent increases in QTc duration compared with salmeterol and placebo administration. Due to the potential increased risk of cardiovascular adverse events, the concomitant use of salmeterol with strong CYP3A4 inhibitors, (eg, ketoconazole, ritonavir, atazanavir, clarithromycin, indinavir, itraconazole, nefazodone, nelfinavir, saquinavir, telithromycin) is not recommended). Products include:

Advicor 402
Cardio Basics 3455
Niaspan 497
Simcor 524

Niacinamide (Co-administration of salmeterol and a strong CYP3A4 inhibitor ketoconazole resulted in a significant increase in plasma salmeterol exposure as determined by a 16-fold increase in AUC mainly due to increased bioavailability of swallowed portion of

1723 **Interactions Index** **Serevent**

the dose. Although there was no statistical effect on the mean QTc, co-administration of salmeterol and ketoconazole was associated with more frequent increases in QTc duration compared with salmeterol and placebo administration. Due to the potential increased risk of cardiovascular adverse events, the concomitant use of salmeterol with strong CYP3A4 inhibitors, (eg, ketoconazole, ritonavir, atazanavir, clarithromycin, indinavir, itraconazole, nefazodone, nelfinavir, saquinavir, telithromycin) is not recommended).
Products include:
CitraNatal 90 DHA Capsules 2332
CitraNatal Assure 2332
CitraNatal Rx 2332
Heplive 607

Niacinamide Hydroiodide (Co-administration of salmeterol and a strong CYP3A4 inhibitor ketoconazole resulted in a significant increase in plasma salmeterol exposure as determined by a 16-fold increase in AUC mainly due to increased bioavailability of swallowed portion of the dose. Although there was no statistical effect on the mean QTc, co-administration of salmeterol and ketoconazole was associated with more frequent increases in QTc duration compared with salmeterol and placebo administration. Due to the potential increased risk of cardiovascular adverse events, the concomitant use of salmeterol with strong CYP3A4 inhibitors, (eg, ketoconazole, ritonavir, atazanavir, clarithromycin, indinavir, itraconazole, nefazodone, nelfinavir, saquinavir, telithromycin) is not recommended).
No products indexed under this heading.

Nicotinamide (Co-administration of salmeterol and a strong CYP3A4 inhibitor ketoconazole resulted in a significant increase in plasma salmeterol exposure as determined by a 16-fold increase in AUC mainly due to increased bioavailability of swallowed portion of the dose. Although there was no statistical effect on the mean QTc, co-administration of salmeterol and ketoconazole was associated with more frequent increases in QTc duration compared with salmeterol and placebo administration. Due to the potential increased risk of cardiovascular adverse events, the concomitant use of salmeterol with strong CYP3A4 inhibitors, (eg, ketoconazole, ritonavir, atazanavir, clarithromycin, indinavir, itraconazole, nefazodone, nelfinavir, saquinavir, telithromycin) is not recommended).
No products indexed under this heading.

Nifedipine (Co-administration of salmeterol and a strong CYP3A4 inhibitor ketoconazole resulted in a significant increase in plasma salmeterol exposure as determined by a 16-fold increase in AUC mainly due to increased bioavailability of swallowed portion of the dose. Although there was no statistical effect on the mean QTc, co-administration of salmeterol and ketoconazole was associated with more frequent increases in QTc duration compared with salmeterol and placebo administration. Due to the potential increased risk of cardiovascular adverse events, the concomitant use of salmeterol with strong CYP3A4 inhibitors, (eg, ketoconazole, ritonavir, atazanavir, clarithromycin, indinavir, itraconazole, nefazodone, nelfinavir, saquinavir, telithromycin) is not recommended).
No products indexed under this heading.

Norfloxacin (Co-administration of salmeterol and a strong CYP3A4 inhibitor ketoconazole resulted in a significant increase in plasma salmeterol exposure as determined by a 16-fold increase in AUC mainly due to increased bioavailability of swallowed portion of the dose. Although there was no statistical effect on the mean QTc, co-administration of salmeterol and ketoconazole was associated with more frequent increases in QTc duration compared with salmeterol and placebo administration. Due to the potential increased risk of cardiovascular adverse events, the concomitant use of salmeterol with strong CYP3A4 inhibitors, (eg, ketoconazole, ritonavir, atazanavir, clarithromycin, indinavir, itraconazole, nefazodone, nelfinavir, saquinavir, telithromycin) is not recommended).
Products include:
Noroxin 2220

Nortriptyline Hydrochloride (The action of salmeterol on the vascular system may be potentiated by tricyclic antidepressant).
No products indexed under this heading.

Omeprazole (Co-administration of salmeterol and a strong CYP3A4 inhibitor ketoconazole resulted in a significant increase in plasma salmeterol exposure as determined by a 16-fold increase in AUC mainly due to increased bioavailability of swallowed portion of the dose. Although there was no statistical effect on the mean QTc, co-administration of salmeterol and ketoconazole was associated with more frequent increases in QTc duration compared with salmeterol and placebo administration. Due to the potential increased risk of cardiovascular adverse events, the concomitant use of salmeterol with strong CYP3A4 inhibitors, (eg, ketoconazole, ritonavir, atazanavir, clarithromycin, indinavir, itraconazole, nefazodone, nelfinavir, saquinavir, telithromycin) is not recommended).
No products indexed under this heading.

Pargyline Hydrochloride (The action of salmeterol on the vascular system may be potentiated by a MAO inhibitor).
No products indexed under this heading.

Paroxetine Hydrochloride (Co-administration of salmeterol and a strong CYP3A4 inhibitor ketoconazole resulted in a significant increase in plasma salmeterol exposure as determined by a 16-fold increase in AUC mainly due to increased bioavailability of swallowed portion of the dose. Although there was no statistical effect on the mean QTc, co-administration of salmeterol and ketoconazole was associated with more frequent increases in QTc duration compared with salmeterol and placebo administration. Due to the potential increased risk of cardiovascular adverse events, the concomitant use of salmeterol with strong CYP3A4 inhibitors, (eg, ketoconazole, ritonavir, atazanavir, clarithromycin, indinavir, itraconazole, nefazodone, nelfinavir, saquinavir, telithromycin) is not recommended).
Products include:
Paroxetine CR 2361
Paroxetine ER 2371
Paxil 1586
Paxil CR 1596

Penbutolol Sulfate (Beta-adrenergic blockers may produce severe bronchospasm in asthmatic patients, however, beta blockers do not block the pulmonary effect of beta-agonists).
No products indexed under this heading.

Phenelzine Sulfate (The action of salmeterol on the vascular system may be potentiated by a MAO inhibitor).
No products indexed under this heading.

Pindolol (Beta-adrenergic blockers may produce severe bronchospasm in asthmatic patients, however, beta blockers do not block the pulmonary effect of beta-agonists).
No products indexed under this heading.

Polythiazide (The ECG changes and/or hypokalemia that may result from the administration of nonpotassium-sparing diuretics can be acutely worsened by beta-agonists, especially when the recommended dose of beta-agonist is exceeded).
No products indexed under this heading.

Posaconazole (Co-administration of salmeterol and a strong CYP3A4 inhibitor ketoconazole resulted in a significant increase in plasma salmeterol exposure as determined by a 16-fold increase in AUC mainly due to increased bioavailability of swallowed portion of the dose. Although there was no statistical effect on the mean QTc, co-administration of salmeterol and ketoconazole was associated with more frequent increases in QTc duration compared with salmeterol and placebo administration. Due to the potential increased risk of cardiovascular adverse events, the concomitant use of salmeterol with strong CYP3A4 inhibitors, (eg, ketoconazole, ritonavir, atazanavir, clarithromycin, indinavir, itraconazole, nefazodone, nelfinavir, saquinavir, telithromycin) is not recommended).
Products include:
Noxafil 3172

Procarbazine Hydrochloride (The action of salmeterol on the vascular system may be potentiated by a MAO inhibitor).
No products indexed under this heading.

Propoxyphene Hydrochloride (Co-administration of salmeterol and a strong CYP3A4 inhibitor ketoconazole resulted in a significant increase in plasma salmeterol exposure as determined by a 16-fold increase in AUC mainly due to increased bioavailability of swallowed portion of the dose. Although there was no statistical effect on the mean QTc, co-administration of salmeterol and ketoconazole was associated with more frequent increases in QTc duration compared with salmeterol and placebo administration. Due to the potential increased risk of cardiovascular adverse events, the concomitant use of salmeterol with strong CYP3A4 inhibitors, (eg, ketoconazole, ritonavir, atazanavir, clarithromycin, indinavir, itraconazole, nefazodone, nelfinavir, saquinavir, telithromycin) is not recommended).
No products indexed under this heading.

Propoxyphene Napsylate (Co-administration of salmeterol and a strong CYP3A4 inhibitor ketoconazole resulted in a significant increase in plasma salmeterol exposure as determined by a 16-fold increase in AUC mainly due to increased bioavailability of swallowed portion of the dose. Although there was no statistical effect on the mean QTc, co-administration of salmeterol and ketoconazole was associated with more frequent increases in QTc duration compared with salmeterol and placebo administration. Due to the potential increased risk of cardiovascular adverse events, the concomitant use of salmeterol with strong CYP3A4 inhibitors, (eg, ketoconazole, ritonavir, atazanavir, clarithromycin, indinavir, itraconazole, nefazodone, nelfinavir, saquinavir, telithromycin) is not recommended).
No products indexed under this heading.

Propranolol Hydrochloride (Beta-adrenergic blockers may produce severe bronchospasm in asthmatic patients, however, beta blockers do not block the pulmonary effect of beta-agonists). Products include:
InnoPran XL 1517

Protriptyline Hydrochloride (The action of salmeterol on the vascular system may be potentiated by tricyclic antidepressant).
No products indexed under this heading.

Quinidine (Co-administration of salmeterol and a strong CYP3A4 inhibitor ketoconazole resulted in a significant increase in plasma salmeterol exposure as determined by a 16-fold increase in AUC mainly due to increased bioavailability of swallowed portion of the dose. Although there was no statistical effect on the mean QTc, co-administration of salmeterol and ketoconazole was associated with more frequent increases in QTc duration compared with salmeterol and placebo administration. Due to the potential increased risk of cardiovascular adverse events, the concomitant use of salmeterol with strong CYP3A4 inhibitors, (eg, ketoconazole, ritonavir, atazanavir, clarithromycin, indinavir, itraconazole, nefazodone, nelfinavir, saquinavir, telithromycin) is not recommended).
No products indexed under this heading.

Quinidine Hydrochloride (Co-administration of salmeterol and a strong CYP3A4 inhibitor ketoconazole resulted in a significant increase in plasma salmeterol exposure as determined by a 16-fold increase in AUC mainly due to increased bioavailability of swallowed portion of the dose. Although there was no statistical effect on the mean QTc, co-administration of salmeterol and ketoconazole was associated with more frequent increases in QTc duration compared with salmeterol and placebo administration. Due to the potential increased risk of cardiovascular adverse events, the concomitant use of salmeterol with strong CYP3A4 inhibitors, (eg, ketoconazole, ritonavir, atazanavir, clarithromycin, indinavir, itraconazole, nefazodone, nelfinavir, saquinavir, telithromycin) is not recommended).
No products indexed under this heading.

Quinidine Polygalacturonate (Co-administration of salmeterol and a strong CYP3A4 inhibitor ketoconazole resulted in a significant increase in plasma salmeterol exposure as determined by a 16-fold increase in AUC mainly due to increased bioavailability of swallowed portion of the dose. Although there was no statistical effect on the mean QTc, co-administration of salmeterol and ketoconazole was associated with more frequent increases in QTc duration compared with salmeterol and placebo administration. Due to the potential increased risk of cardiovascular adverse events, the concomitant use of salmeterol with strong CYP3A4 inhibitors, (eg, ketoconazole, ritonavir, atazanavir, clarithromycin, indinavir, itraconazole, nefazodone, nelfinavir, saquinavir, telithromycin) is not recommended).
No products indexed under this heading.

Quinidine Sulfate (Co-administration of salmeterol and a strong CYP3A4 inhibitor ketoconazole resulted in a significant increase in plasma salmeterol exposure as determined by a 16-fold increase in AUC mainly due to increased bioavailability of swallowed portion of the dose. Although there was no statistical effect on the mean QTc, co-administration of salmeterol and ketoconazole was associated with more frequent increases in QTc duration compared with salmeterol and placebo administration. Due to the potential increased risk of cardiovascular adverse events, the concomitant use of salmeterol with strong CYP3A4 inhibitors, (eg, ketoconazole, ritonavir, atazanavir, clarithromycin, indinavir, itraconazole, nefazodone, nelfinavir, saquinavir, telithromycin) is not recommended).
No products indexed under this heading.

Quinine (Co-administration of salmeterol and a strong CYP3A4 inhibitor ketoconazole resulted in a significant increase in plasma salmeterol exposure as determined by a 16-fold increase in AUC mainly due to increased bioavail-

ability of swallowed portion of the dose. Although there was no statistical effect on the mean QTc, co-administration of salmeterol and ketoconazole was associated with more frequent increases in QTc duration compared with salmeterol and placebo administration. Due to the potential increased risk of cardiovascular adverse events, the concomitant use of salmeterol with strong CYP3A4 inhibitors, (eg, ketoconazole, ritonavir, atazanavir, clarithromycin, indinavir, itraconazole, nefazodone, nelfinavir, saquinavir, telithromycin) is not recommended). Products include:

Hyland's Leg Cramps PM with Quinine 3315

Quinine Sulfate (Co-administration of salmeterol and a strong CYP3A4 inhibitor ketoconazole resulted in a significant increase in plasma salmeterol exposure as determined by a 16-fold increase in AUC mainly due to increased bioavailability of swallowed portion of the dose. Although there was no statistical effect on the mean QTc, co-administration of salmeterol and ketoconazole was associated with more frequent increases in QTc duration compared with salmeterol and placebo administration. Due to the potential increased risk of cardiovascular adverse events, the concomitant use of salmeterol with strong CYP3A4 inhibitors, (eg, ketoconazole, ritonavir, atazanavir, clarithromycin, indinavir, itraconazole, nefazodone, nelfinavir, saquinavir, telithromycin) is not recommended).

No products indexed under this heading.

Quinupristin (Co-administration of salmeterol and a strong CYP3A4 inhibitor ketoconazole resulted in a significant increase in plasma salmeterol exposure as determined by a 16-fold increase in AUC mainly due to increased bioavailability of swallowed portion of the dose. Although there was no statistical effect on the mean QTc, co-administration of salmeterol and ketoconazole was associated with more frequent increases in QTc duration compared with salmeterol and placebo administration. Due to the potential increased risk of cardiovascular adverse events, the concomitant use of salmeterol with strong CYP3A4 inhibitors, (eg, ketoconazole, ritonavir, atazanavir, clarithromycin, indinavir, itraconazole, nefazodone, nelfinavir, saquinavir, telithromycin) is not recommended).

No products indexed under this heading.

Ranitidine Bismuth Citrate (Co-administration of salmeterol and a strong CYP3A4 inhibitor ketoconazole resulted in a significant increase in plasma salmeterol exposure as determined by a 16-fold increase in AUC mainly due to increased bioavailability of swallowed portion of the dose. Although there was no statistical effect on the mean QTc, co-administration of salmeterol and ketoconazole was associated with more frequent increases in QTc duration compared with salmeterol and placebo administration. Due to the potential increased risk of cardiovascular adverse events, the concomitant use of salmeterol with strong CYP3A4 inhibitors, (eg, ketoconazole, ritonavir, atazanavir, clarithromycin, indinavir, itraconazole, nefazodone, nelfinavir, saquinavir, telithromycin) is not recommended).

No products indexed under this heading.

Ranitidine Hydrochloride (Co-administration of salmeterol and a strong CYP3A4 inhibitor ketoconazole resulted in a significant increase in plasma salmeterol exposure as determined by a 16-fold increase in AUC mainly due to increased bioavailability of swallowed portion of the dose. Although there was no statistical effect on the mean QTc, co-administration of salmeterol and ketoconazole was associated with more frequent increases in QTc duration compared with salmeterol and placebo administration. Due to the potential increased risk of cardiovascular adverse events, the concomitant use of salmeterol with strong CYP3A4 inhibitors, (eg, ketoconazole, ritonavir, atazanavir, clarithromycin, indinavir, itraconazole, nefazodone, nelfinavir, saquinavir, telithromycin) is not recommended). Products include:

Zantac 1737
Zantac Injection 1732
Zantac Pharmacy 1735

Rasagiline Mesylate (The action of salmeterol on the vascular system may be potentiated by a MAO inhibitor). Products include:

Azilect 3383

Ritonavir (Co-administration of salmeterol and a strong CYP3A4 inhibitor ketoconazole resulted in a significant increase in plasma salmeterol exposure as determined by a 16-fold increase in AUC mainly due to increased bioavailability of swallowed portion of the dose. Although there was no statistical effect on the mean QTc, co-administration of salmeterol and ketoconazole was associated with more frequent increases in QTc duration compared with salmeterol and placebo administration. Due to the potential increased risk of cardiovascular adverse events, the concomitant use of salmeterol with strong CYP3A4 inhibitors, (eg, ketoconazole, ritonavir, atazanavir, clarithromycin, indinavir, itraconazole, nefazodone, nelfinavir, saquinavir, telithromycin) is not recommended). Products include:

Kaletra 458
Norvir 509

Saquinavir (Co-administration of salmeterol and a strong CYP3A4 inhibitor ketoconazole resulted in a significant increase in plasma salmeterol exposure as determined by a 16-fold increase in AUC mainly due to increased bioavailability of swallowed portion of the dose. Although there was no statistical effect on the mean QTc, co-administration of salmeterol and ketoconazole was associated with more frequent increases in QTc duration compared with salmeterol and placebo administration. Due to the potential increased risk of cardiovascular adverse events, the concomitant use of salmeterol with strong CYP3A4 inhibitors, (eg, ketoconazole, ritonavir, atazanavir, clarithromycin, indinavir, itraconazole, nefazodone, nelfinavir, saquinavir, telithromycin) is not recommended).

No products indexed under this heading.

Saquinavir Mesylate (Co-administration of salmeterol and a strong CYP3A4 inhibitor ketoconazole resulted in a significant increase in plasma salmeterol exposure as determined by a 16-fold increase in AUC mainly due to increased bioavailability of swallowed portion of the dose. Although there was no statistical effect on the mean QTc, co-administration of salmeterol and ketoconazole was associated with more frequent increases in QTc duration compared with salmeterol and placebo administration. Due to the potential increased risk of cardiovascular adverse events, the concomitant use of salmeterol with strong CYP3A4 inhibitors, (eg, ketoconazole, ritonavir, atazanavir, clarithromycin, indinavir, itraconazole, nefazodone, nelfinavir, saquinavir, telithromycin) is not recommended).

No products indexed under this heading.

Selegiline (The action of salmeterol on the vascular system may be potentiated by a MAO inhibitor). Products include:

Emsam 3623

Selegiline Hydrochloride (The action of salmeterol on the vascular system may be potentiated by a MAO inhibitor). Products include:

Eldepryl 3312

Sertraline Hydrochloride (Co-administration of salmeterol and a strong CYP3A4 inhibitor ketoconazole resulted in a significant increase in plasma salmeterol exposure as determined by a 16-fold increase in AUC mainly due to increased bioavailability of swallowed portion of the dose. Although there was no statistical effect on the mean QTc, co-administration of salmeterol and ketoconazole was associated with more frequent increases in QTc duration compared with salmeterol and placebo administration. Due to the potential increased risk of cardiovascular adverse events, the concomitant use of salmeterol with strong CYP3A4 inhibitors, (eg, ketoconazole, ritonavir, atazanavir, clarithromycin, indinavir, itraconazole, nefazodone, nelfinavir, saquinavir, telithromycin) is not recommended).

No products indexed under this heading.

Sildenafil Citrate (Co-administration of salmeterol and a strong CYP3A4 inhibitor ketoconazole resulted in a significant increase in plasma salmeterol exposure as determined by a 16-fold increase in AUC mainly due to increased bioavailability of swallowed portion of the dose. Although there was no statistical effect on the mean QTc, co-administration of salmeterol and ketoconazole was associated with more frequent increases in QTc duration compared with salmeterol and placebo administration. Due to the potential increased risk of cardiovascular adverse events, the concomitant use of salmeterol with strong CYP3A4 inhibitors, (eg, ketoconazole, ritonavir, atazanavir, clarithromycin, indinavir, itraconazole, nefazodone, nelfinavir, saquinavir, telithromycin) is not recommended).

No products indexed under this heading.

Sotalol Hydrochloride (Beta-adrenergic blockers may produce severe bronchospasm in asthmatic patients, however, beta blockers do not block the pulmonary effect of beta-agonists).

No products indexed under this heading.

Telithromycin (Co-administration of salmeterol and a strong CYP3A4 inhibitor ketoconazole resulted in a significant increase in plasma salmeterol exposure as determined by a 16-fold increase in AUC mainly due to increased bioavailability of swallowed portion of the dose. Although there was no statistical effect on the mean QTc, co-administration of salmeterol and ketoconazole was associated with more frequent increases in QTc duration compared with salmeterol and placebo administration. Due to the potential increased risk of cardiovascular adverse events, the concomitant use of salmeterol with strong CYP3A4 inhibitors, (eg, ketoconazole, ritonavir, atazanavir, clarithromycin, indinavir, itraconazole, nefazodone, nelfinavir, saquinavir, telithromycin) is not recommended). Products include:

Ketek 2991

Timolol Hemihydrate (Beta-adrenergic blockers may produce severe bronchospasm in asthmatic patients, however, beta blockers do not block the pulmonary effect of beta-agonists). Products include:

Betimol 3490

Timolol Maleate (Beta-adrenergic blockers may produce severe bronchospasm in asthmatic patients, however, beta blockers do not block the pulmonary effect of beta-agonists). Products include:

Combigan 601
Dorzolamide Hydrochloride/Timolol Maleate Ophthalmic Solution .... ⊙243
Timoptic in Ocudose .... ⊙231

Torsemide (The ECG changes and/or hypokalemia that may result from the administration of nonpotassium-sparing diuretics can be acutely worsened by beta-agonists, especially when the recommended dose of beta-agonist is exceeded).

No products indexed under this heading.

Tranylcypromine Sulfate (The action of salmeterol on the vascular system may be potentiated by a MAO inhibitor). Products include:

Parnate 1584

Trimipramine Maleate (The action of salmeterol on the vascular system may be potentiated by tricyclic antidepressant).

No products indexed under this heading.

Troglitazone (Co-administration of salmeterol and a strong CYP3A4 inhibitor ketoconazole resulted in a significant increase in plasma salmeterol exposure as determined by a 16-fold increase in AUC mainly due to increased bioavailability of swallowed portion of the dose. Although there was no statistical effect on the mean QTc, co-administration of salmeterol and ketoconazole was associated with more frequent increases in QTc duration compared with salmeterol and placebo administration. Due to the potential increased risk of cardiovascular adverse events, the concomitant use of salmeterol with strong CYP3A4 inhibitors, (eg, ketoconazole, ritonavir, atazanavir, clarithromycin, indinavir, itraconazole, nefazodone, nelfinavir, saquinavir, telithromycin) is not recommended).

No products indexed under this heading.

Troleandomycin (Co-administration of salmeterol and a strong CYP3A4 inhibitor ketoconazole resulted in a significant increase in plasma salmeterol exposure as determined by a 16-fold increase in AUC mainly due to increased bioavailability of swallowed portion of the dose. Although there was no statistical effect on the mean QTc, co-administration of salmeterol and ketoconazole was associated with more frequent increases in QTc duration compared with salmeterol and placebo administration. Due to the potential increased risk of cardiovascular adverse events, the concomitant use of salmeterol with strong CYP3A4 inhibitors, (eg, ketoconazole, ritonavir, atazanavir, clarithromycin, indinavir, itraconazole, nefazodone, nelfinavir, saquinavir, telithromycin) is not recommended).

No products indexed under this heading.

Valproate Sodium (Co-administration of salmeterol and a strong CYP3A4 inhibitor ketoconazole resulted in a significant increase in plasma salmeterol exposure as determined by a 16-fold increase in AUC mainly due to increased bioavailability of swallowed portion of the dose. Although there was no statistical effect on the mean QTc, co-administration of salmeterol and ketoconazole was associated with more frequent increases in QTc duration compared with salmeterol and placebo administration. Due to the potential increased risk of cardiovascular adverse events, the concomitant use of salmeterol with strong CYP3A4 inhibitors, (eg, ketoconazole, ritonavir, atazanavir, clarithromycin, indinavir, itraconazole, nefazodone, nelfinavir, saquinavir, telithromycin) is not recommended).

No products indexed under this heading.

Vardenafil Hydrochloride (Co-administration of salmeterol and a strong CYP3A4 inhibitor ketoconazole resulted in a significant increase in plasma salmeterol exposure as determined by a 16-fold increase in AUC mainly due to increased bioavailability of swallowed portion of the dose. Although there was no statistical effect on the mean QTc, co-administration of salmeterol and

1725 Interactions Index Seroquel

ketoconazole was associated with more frequent increases in QTc duration compared with salmeterol and placebo administration. Due to the potential increased risk of cardiovascular adverse events, the concomitant use of salmeterol with strong CYP3A4 inhibitors, (eg, ketoconazole, ritonavir, atazanavir, clarithromycin, indinavir, itraconazole, nefazodone, nelfinavir, saquinavir, telithromycin) is not recommended).
Products include:
Levitra 3157

Verapamil Hydrochloride (Co-administration of salmeterol and a strong CYP3A4 inhibitor ketoconazole resulted in a significant increase in plasma salmeterol exposure as determined by a 16-fold increase in AUC mainly due to increased bioavailability of swallowed portion of the dose. Although there was no statistical effect on the mean QTc, co-administration of salmeterol and ketoconazole was associated with more frequent increases in QTc duration compared with salmeterol and placebo administration. Due to the potential increased risk of cardiovascular adverse events, the concomitant use of salmeterol with strong CYP3A4 inhibitors, (eg, ketoconazole, ritonavir, atazanavir, clarithromycin, indinavir, itraconazole, nefazodone, nelfinavir, saquinavir, telithromycin) is not recommended).
Products include:
Tarka 534

Voriconazole (Co-administration of salmeterol and a strong CYP3A4 inhibitor ketoconazole resulted in a significant increase in plasma salmeterol exposure as determined by a 16-fold increase in AUC mainly due to increased bioavailability of swallowed portion of the dose. Although there was no statistical effect on the mean QTc, co-administration of salmeterol and ketoconazole was associated with more frequent increases in QTc duration compared with salmeterol and placebo administration. Due to the potential increased risk of cardiovascular adverse events, the concomitant use of salmeterol with strong CYP3A4 inhibitors, (eg, ketoconazole, ritonavir, atazanavir, clarithromycin, indinavir, itraconazole, nefazodone, nelfinavir, saquinavir, telithromycin) is not recommended).
No products indexed under this heading.

Zafirlukast (Co-administration of salmeterol and a strong CYP3A4 inhibitor ketoconazole resulted in a significant increase in plasma salmeterol exposure as determined by a 16-fold increase in AUC mainly due to increased bioavailability of swallowed portion of the dose. Although there was no statistical effect on the mean QTc, co-administration of salmeterol and ketoconazole was associated with more frequent increases in QTc duration compared with salmeterol and placebo administration. Due to the potential increased risk of cardiovascular adverse events, the concomitant use of salmeterol with strong CYP3A4 inhibitors, (eg, ketoconazole, ritonavir, atazanavir, clarithromycin, indinavir, itraconazole, nefazodone, nelfinavir, saquinavir, telithromycin) is not recommended).
Products include:
Accolate 3612

Zileuton (Co-administration of salmeterol and a strong CYP3A4 inhibitor ketoconazole resulted in a significant increase in plasma salmeterol exposure as determined by a 16-fold increase in AUC mainly due to increased bioavailability of swallowed portion of the dose. Although there was no statistical effect on the mean QTc, co-administration of salmeterol and ketoconazole was associated with more frequent increases in QTc duration compared with salmeterol and placebo administration. Due to the potential increased risk of cardiovascular adverse events, the concomitant use of salmeterol with strong CYP3A4 inhibitors, (eg, ketoconazole, ritonavir, atazanavir, clarithromycin, indinavir, itraconazole, nefazodone, nelfinavir, saquinavir, telithromycin) is not recommended).
No products indexed under this heading.

Food Interactions

Grapefruit (Co-administration of salmeterol and a strong CYP3A4 inhibitor ketoconazole resulted in a significant increase in plasma salmeterol exposure as determined by a 16-fold increase in AUC mainly due to increased bioavailability of swallowed portion of the dose. Although there was no statistical effect on the mean QTc, co-administration of salmeterol and ketoconazole was associated with more frequent increases in QTc duration compared with salmeterol and placebo administration. Due to the potential increased risk of cardiovascular adverse events, the concomitant use of salmeterol with strong CYP3A4 inhibitors, (eg, ketoconazole, ritonavir, atazanavir, clarithromycin, indinavir, itraconazole, nefazodone, nelfinavir, saquinavir, telithromycin) is not recommended).

Grapefruit Juice (Co-administration of salmeterol and a strong CYP3A4 inhibitor ketoconazole resulted in a significant increase in plasma salmeterol exposure as determined by a 16-fold increase in AUC mainly due to increased bioavailability of swallowed portion of the dose. Although there was no statistical effect on the mean QTc, co-administration of salmeterol and ketoconazole was associated with more frequent increases in QTc duration compared with salmeterol and placebo administration. Due to the potential increased risk of cardiovascular adverse events, the concomitant use of salmeterol with strong CYP3A4 inhibitors, (eg, ketoconazole, ritonavir, atazanavir, clarithromycin, indinavir, itraconazole, nefazodone, nelfinavir, saquinavir, telithromycin) is not recommended).

SEROMYCIN CAPSULES

(Cycloserine) 1956
May interact with alcohols, antituberculosis drugs, and certain other agents. Compounds in these categories include:

Aminosalicylic Acid (Co-administration has been associated with a few instances of vitamin B12 and/or folic acid deficiency, megaloblastic anemia, and sideroblastic anemia).
Products include:
Paser 1820

p-Aminosalicylic Acid (Co-administration has been associated with a few instances of vitamin B12 and/or folic acid deficiency, megaloblastic anemia, and sideroblastic anemia).
No products indexed under this heading.

Ethambutol Hydrochloride (Co-administration has been associated with a few instances of vitamin B12 and/or folic acid deficiency, megaloblastic anemia, and sideroblastic anemia).
No products indexed under this heading.

Ethanol (Concurrent use increases the possibility and risk of epileptic episodes).
No products indexed under this heading.

Ethionamide (Co-administration has been reported to potentiate neurotoxic side effects).
No products indexed under this heading.

Ethyl Alcohol (Concurrent use increases the possibility and risk of epileptic episodes).
No products indexed under this heading.

Isoniazid (Co-administration may result in increased incidence of CNS effects, such as dizziness or drowsiness).
No products indexed under this heading.

Pyrazinamide (Co-administration has been associated with a few instances of vitamin B12 and/or folic acid deficiency, megaloblastic anemia, and sideroblastic anemia).
No products indexed under this heading.

Rifampin (Co-administration has been associated with a few instances of vitamin B12 and/or folic acid deficiency, megaloblastic anemia, and sideroblastic anemia).
No products indexed under this heading.

Rifapentine (Co-administration has been associated with a few instances of vitamin B12 and/or folic acid deficiency, megaloblastic anemia, and sideroblastic anemia).
No products indexed under this heading.

Food Interactions

Alcohol (Concurrent use increases the possibility and risk of epileptic episodes).

Beer, reduced-alcohol (Concurrent use increases the possibility and risk of epileptic episodes).

Beer, unspecified (Concurrent use increases the possibility and risk of epileptic episodes).

Wine, Chianti (Concurrent use increases the possibility and risk of epileptic episodes).

Wine, Red (Concurrent use increases the possibility and risk of epileptic episodes).

Wine, unspecified (Concurrent use increases the possibility and risk of epileptic episodes).

Wine products (Concurrent use increases the possibility and risk of epileptic episodes).

SEROQUEL TABLETS

(Quetiapine Fumarate) 750
May interact with alcohols, antihypertensives, barbiturates, central nervous system depressants, central nervous system stimulants, cytochrome p450 3a4 inducers (selected), cytochrome p450 3a4 inhibitors (selected), dopamine agonists, glucocorticoids, phenytoin, and certain other agents. Compounds in these categories include:

Acebutolol Hydrochloride (Enhanced effects of certain anti-hypertensive agents).
No products indexed under this heading.

Acetazolamide (Co-administration with an inhibitor of CYP4503A may reduce oral clearance of quetiapine, resulting in an increase in maximum plasma concentration of quetiapine; dose adjustment of quetiapine will be necessary).
No products indexed under this heading.

Acetazolamide Sodium (Co-administration with an inhibitor of CYP4503A may reduce oral clearance of quetiapine, resulting in an increase in maximum plasma concentration of quetiapine; dose adjustment of quetiapine will be necessary).
No products indexed under this heading.

Alfentanil Hydrochloride (Caution should be used when quetiapine is taken in combination with other centrally acting drugs).
No products indexed under this heading.

Aliskiren (Enhanced effects of certain anti-hypertensive agents). Products include:
Tekturna 2538
Tekturna HCT 2541
Valturna 3637

Allium sativum (Co-administration of quetiapine and CYP450 3A4 inducer increased the mean oral clearance of quetiapine by 5-fold. Increased doses of quetiapine may be required to maintain control of symptoms of schizophrenia in patients receiving quetiapine and phenytoin, or other hepatic enzyme inducers (eg, carbamazepine, barbiturates, rifampin and glucocorticoids)).
No products indexed under this heading.

Alprazolam (Caution should be used when quetiapine is taken in combination with other centrally acting drugs).
No products indexed under this heading.

Aminoglutethimide (Co-administration of quetiapine and CYP450 3A4 inducer increased the mean oral clearance of quetiapine by 5-fold. Increased doses of quetiapine may be required to maintain control of symptoms of schizophrenia in patients receiving quetiapine and phenytoin, or other hepatic enzyme inducers (eg, carbamazepine, barbiturates, rifampin and glucocorticoids)).
No products indexed under this heading.

Amiodarone Hydrochloride (Co-administration with an inhibitor of CYP4503A may reduce oral clearance of quetiapine, resulting in an increase in maximum plasma concentration of quetiapine; dose adjustment of quetiapine will be necessary).
No products indexed under this heading.

Amlodipine Besylate (Enhanced effects of certain anti-hypertensive agents). Products include:
Azor 1010
Exforge 2443
Exforge HCT 2449

Amobarbital (Co-administration with hepatic enzyme inducers, such as barbiturates, may increase oral clearance).
No products indexed under this heading.

Amobarbital Sodium (Co-administration with hepatic enzyme inducers, such as barbiturates, may increase oral clearance).
No products indexed under this heading.

Amphetamine Aspartate (Caution should be used when quetiapine is taken in combination with other centrally acting drugs).
No products indexed under this heading.

Amphetamine Aspartate Monohydrate (Caution should be used when quetiapine is taken in combination with other centrally acting drugs).
No products indexed under this heading.

Amphetamine Resins (Caution should be used when quetiapine is taken in combination with other centrally acting drugs).
No products indexed under this heading.

Amphetamine Sulfate (Caution should be used when quetiapine is taken in combination with other centrally acting drugs).
No products indexed under this heading.

Amprenavir (Co-administration with an inhibitor of CYP4503A may reduce oral clearance of quetiapine, resulting in an increase in maximum plasma concentration of quetiapine; dose adjustment of quetiapine will be necessary).
No products indexed under this heading.

Anastrozole (Co-administration with an inhibitor of CYP4503A may reduce oral clearance of quetiapine, resulting in an increase in maximum plasma concentration of quetiapine; dose adjustment of quetiapine will be necessary).
No products indexed under this heading.

Aprepitant (Co-administration with an inhibitor of CYP4503A may reduce oral clearance of quetiapine, resulting in an increase in maximum plasma concentration of quetiapine; dose adjustment of quetiapine will be necessary). Products include:

IMPORTANT NOTE: Always consult each drug listing in the patient's regimen for possible interactions.

Emend 2124

Aprobarbital (Co-administration with hepatic enzyme inducers, such as barbiturates, may increase oral clearance).
No products indexed under this heading.

Atazanavir (Co-administration with an inhibitor of CYP4503A may reduce oral clearance of quetiapine, resulting in an increase in maximum plasma concentration of quetiapine; dose adjustment of quetiapine will be necessary).
No products indexed under this heading.

Atazanavir Sulfate (Co-administration with an inhibitor of CYP4503A may reduce oral clearance of quetiapine, resulting in an increase in maximum plasma concentration of quetiapine; dose adjustment of quetiapine will be necessary).
No products indexed under this heading.

Atenolol (Enhanced effects of certain anti-hypertensive agents).
No products indexed under this heading.

Benazepril Hydrochloride (Enhanced effects of certain anti-hypertensive agents).
No products indexed under this heading.

Bendroflumethiazide (Enhanced effects of certain anti-hypertensive agents).
No products indexed under this heading.

Betamethasone (Co-administration of quetiapine and CYP450 3A4 inducer increased the mean oral clearance of quetiapine by 5-fold. Increased doses of quetiapine may be required to maintain control of symptoms of schizophrenia in patients receiving quetiapine and phenytoin, or other hepatic enzyme inducers (eg, carbamazepine, barbiturates, rifampin and glucocorticoids)).
No products indexed under this heading.

Betamethasone Acetate (Co-administration with hepatic enzyme inducers, such as glucocorticosteroids, may increase oral clearance).
No products indexed under this heading.

Betamethasone Benzoate (Co-administration of quetiapine and CYP450 3A4 inducer increased the mean oral clearance of quetiapine by 5-fold. Increased doses of quetiapine may be required to maintain control of symptoms of schizophrenia in patients receiving quetiapine and phenytoin, or other hepatic enzyme inducers (eg, carbamazepine, barbiturates, rifampin and glucocorticoids)).
No products indexed under this heading.

Betamethasone Dipropionate (Co-administration of quetiapine and CYP450 3A4 inducer increased the mean oral clearance of quetiapine by 5-fold. Increased doses of quetiapine may be required to maintain control of symptoms of schizophrenia in patients receiving quetiapine and phenytoin, or other hepatic enzyme inducers (eg, carbamazepine, barbiturates, rifampin and glucocorticoids)). Products include:
Diprolene Lotion 0.05% 3108
Diprolene Ointment 0.05% 3109
Diprolene AF Cream 0.05% 3107
Lotrisone 3163

Betamethasone Sodium Phosphate (Co-administration with hepatic enzyme inducers, such as glucocorticosteroids, may increase oral clearance).
No products indexed under this heading.

Betamethasone Valerate (Co-administration of quetiapine and CYP450 3A4 inducer increased the mean oral clearance of quetiapine by 5-fold. Increased doses of quetiapine may be required to maintain control of symptoms of schizophrenia in patients receiving quetiapine and phenytoin, or other hepatic enzyme inducers (eg, carbamazepine, barbiturates, rifampin and glucocorticoids)). Products include:

Luxiq 3321

Betaxolol Hydrochloride (Enhanced effects of certain anti-hypertensive agents).
No products indexed under this heading.

Bisoprolol Fumarate (Enhanced effects of certain anti-hypertensive agents).
No products indexed under this heading.

Bosentan (Co-administration of quetiapine and CYP450 3A4 inducer increased the mean oral clearance of quetiapine by 5-fold. Increased doses of quetiapine may be required to maintain control of symptoms of schizophrenia in patients receiving quetiapine and phenytoin, or other hepatic enzyme inducers (eg, carbamazepine, barbiturates, rifampin and glucocorticoids)). Products include:
Tracleer 573

Bromocriptine Mesylate (Quetiapine may antagonize the effects of dopamine agonists).
No products indexed under this heading.

Budesonide (Co-administration with hepatic enzyme inducers, such as glucocorticosteroids, may increase oral clearance). Products include:
Pulmicort Flexhaler 714
Symbicort 80/4.5 720
Symbicort 160/4.5 720

Buprenorphine Hydrochloride (Caution should be used when quetiapine is taken in combination with other centrally acting drugs).
No products indexed under this heading.

Buspirone Hydrochloride (Caution should be used when quetiapine is taken in combination with other centrally acting drugs).
No products indexed under this heading.

Butabarbital (Co-administration with hepatic enzyme inducers, such as barbiturates, may increase oral clearance).
No products indexed under this heading.

Butabarbital Sodium (Co-administration with hepatic enzyme inducers, such as barbiturates, may increase oral clearance).
No products indexed under this heading.

Butalbital (Co-administration with hepatic enzyme inducers, such as barbiturates, may increase oral clearance).
No products indexed under this heading.

Candesartan Cilexetil (Enhanced effects of certain anti-hypertensive agents). Products include:
Atacand 697
Atacand HCT 700

Captopril (Enhanced effects of certain anti-hypertensive agents). Products include:
Captopril 2341

Carbamazepine (Co-administration with hepatic enzyme inducers, such as carbamazepine, may increase oral clearance). Products include:
Carbatrol 3280
Equetro 3477

Carteolol Hydrochloride (Enhanced effects of certain anti-hypertensive agents).
No products indexed under this heading.

Carvedilol (Enhanced effects of certain anti-hypertensive agents). Products include:
Coreg 1409

Carvedilol Phosphate (Enhanced effects of certain anti-hypertensive agents). Products include:
Coreg CR 1416

Chlordiazepoxide (Caution should be used when quetiapine is taken in combination with other centrally acting drugs).
No products indexed under this heading.

Chlordiazepoxide Hydrochloride (Caution should be used when quetiapine is taken in combination with other centrally acting drugs).
No products indexed under this heading.

Chlorothiazide (Enhanced effects of certain anti-hypertensive agents).
No products indexed under this heading.

Chlorothiazide Sodium (Enhanced effects of certain anti-hypertensive agents). Products include:
Diuril Intravenous 2009

Chlorpromazine (Caution should be used when quetiapine is taken in combination with other centrally acting drugs).
No products indexed under this heading.

Chlorpromazine Hydrochloride (Caution should be used when quetiapine is taken in combination with other centrally acting drugs).
No products indexed under this heading.

Chlorprothixene (Caution should be used when quetiapine is taken in combination with other centrally acting drugs).
No products indexed under this heading.

Chlorprothixene Hydrochloride (Caution should be used when quetiapine is taken in combination with other centrally acting drugs).
No products indexed under this heading.

Chlorprothixene Lactate (Caution should be used when quetiapine is taken in combination with other centrally acting drugs).
No products indexed under this heading.

Chlorthalidone (Enhanced effects of certain anti-hypertensive agents). Products include:
Clorpres 2344

Cimetidine (Co-administration with an inhibitor of CYP4503A may reduce oral clearance of quetiapine, resulting in an increase in maximum plasma concentration of quetiapine; dose adjustment of quetiapine will be necessary).
No products indexed under this heading.

Cimetidine Hydrochloride (Co-administration with an inhibitor of CYP4503A may reduce oral clearance of quetiapine, resulting in an increase in maximum plasma concentration of quetiapine; dose adjustment of quetiapine will be necessary).
No products indexed under this heading.

Ciprofloxacin (Co-administration with an inhibitor of CYP4503A may reduce oral clearance of quetiapine, resulting in an increase in maximum plasma concentration of quetiapine; dose adjustment of quetiapine will be necessary). Products include:
Cipro I.V. 3082
Cipro 3073
Cipro XR 3091
Ciprodex 583

Ciprofloxacin Hydrochloride (Co-administration of quetiapine and CYP450 3A4 inducer increased the mean oral clearance of quetiapine by 5-fold. Increased doses of quetiapine may be required to maintain control of symptoms of schizophrenia in patients receiving quetiapine and phenytoin, or other hepatic enzyme inducers (eg, carbamazepine, barbiturates, rifampin and glucocorticoids)). Products include:
Cipro 3073

Cisplatin (Co-administration of quetiapine and CYP450 3A4 inducer increased the mean oral clearance of quetiapine by 5-fold. Increased doses of quetiapine may be required to maintain control of symptoms of schizophrenia in patients receiving quetiapine and phenytoin, or other hepatic enzyme inducers (eg, carbamazepine, barbiturates, rifampin and glucocorticoids)).
No products indexed under this heading.

Clarithromycin (Co-administration with an inhibitor of CYP4503A may reduce oral clearance of quetiapine, resulting in an increase in maximum plasma concentration of quetiapine; dose adjustment of quetiapine will be necessary). Products include:
Biaxin/Biaxin XL 412

Clonazepam (Caution should be used when quetiapine is taken in combination with other centrally acting drugs). Products include:
Klonopin 2855

Clonidine (Enhanced effects of certain anti-hypertensive agents). Products include:
Catapres-TTS 884

Clonidine Hydrochloride (Enhanced effects of certain anti-hypertensive agents). Products include:
Clorpres 2344

Clorazepate Dipotassium (Caution should be used when quetiapine is taken in combination with other centrally acting drugs).
No products indexed under this heading.

Clotrimazole (Co-administration with an inhibitor of CYP4503A may reduce oral clearance of quetiapine, resulting in an increase in maximum plasma concentration of quetiapine; dose adjustment of quetiapine will be necessary). Products include:
Lotrisone 3163

Clozapine (Caution should be used when quetiapine is taken in combination with other centrally acting drugs).
No products indexed under this heading.

Codeine Phosphate (Caution should be used when quetiapine is taken in combination with other centrally acting drugs). Products include:
Tylenol with Codeine 2691

Codeine Sulfate (Caution should be used when quetiapine is taken in combination with other centrally acting drugs).
No products indexed under this heading.

Conivaptan Hydrochloride (Co-administration with an inhibitor of CYP4503A may reduce oral clearance of quetiapine, resulting in an increase in maximum plasma concentration of quetiapine; dose adjustment of quetiapine will be necessary). Products include:
Vaprisol 689

Cortisone Acetate (Co-administration with hepatic enzyme inducers, such as glucocorticosteroids, may increase oral clearance).
No products indexed under this heading.

Cyclosporine (Co-administration with an inhibitor of CYP4503A may reduce oral clearance of quetiapine, resulting in an increase in maximum plasma concentration of quetiapine; dose adjustment of quetiapine will be necessary). Products include:
Gengraf 440
Neoral Oral Solution 2496
Neoral Capsules 2496
Restasis 605

Dalfopristin (Co-administration with an inhibitor of CYP4503A may reduce oral clearance of quetiapine, resulting in an increase in maximum plasma concentration of quetiapine; dose adjustment of quetiapine will be necessary).
No products indexed under this heading.

Danazol (Co-administration with an inhibitor of CYP4503A may reduce oral clearance of quetiapine, resulting in an increase in maximum plasma concentration of quetiapine; dose adjustment of quetiapine will be necessary).
No products indexed under this heading.

Darunavir (Co-administration with an inhibitor of CYP4503A may reduce oral clearance of quetiapine, resulting in an increase in maximum plasma concentration of quetiapine; dose adjustment of quetiapine will be necessary).
No products indexed under this heading.

Dasatinib (Co-administration with an inhibitor of CYP4503A may reduce oral clearance of quetiapine, resulting in an increase in maximum plasma concentration of quetiapine; dose adjustment of quetiapine will be necessary).
No products indexed under this heading.

Delavirdine Mesylate (Co-administration with an inhibitor of CYP4503A may reduce oral clearance of quetiapine, resulting in an increase in maximum plasma concentration of quetiapine; dose adjustment of quetiapine will be necessary).
No products indexed under this heading.

Delavirine (Co-administration with an inhibitor of CYP4503A may reduce oral clearance of quetiapine, resulting in an increase in maximum plasma concentration of quetiapine; dose adjustment of quetiapine will be necessary).
No products indexed under this heading.

Deserpidine (Enhanced effects of certain anti-hypertensive agents).
No products indexed under this heading.

Desflurane (Caution should be used when quetiapine is taken in combination with other centrally acting drugs).
No products indexed under this heading.

Desloratadine (Co-administration with an inhibitor of CYP4503A may reduce oral clearance of quetiapine, resulting in an increase in maximum plasma concentration of quetiapine; dose adjustment of quetiapine will be necessary).
Products include:
Clarinex Syrup 3098
Clarinex 3098
Clarinex Reditabs 3098
Clarinex-D 12-Hour 3101
Clarinex-D 3104

Dexamethasone (Co-administration with hepatic enzyme inducers, such as glucocorticosteroids, may increase oral clearance). Products include:
Ciprodex 583
Ozurdex .... ⊙223
Tobramycin and Dexamethasone Ophthalmic Suspension .... ⊙251

Dexamethasone Acetate (Co-administration with hepatic enzyme inducers, such as glucocorticosteroids, may increase oral clearance).
No products indexed under this heading.

Dexamethasone Phosphate (Co-administration of quetiapine and CYP450 3A4 inducer increased the mean oral clearance of quetiapine by 5-fold. Increased doses of quetiapine may be required to maintain control of symptoms of schizophrenia in patients receiving quetiapine and phenytoin, or other hepatic enzyme inducers (eg, carbamazepine, barbiturates, rifampin and glucocorticoids)).
No products indexed under this heading.

Dexamethasone Sodium (Co-administration of quetiapine and CYP450 3A4 inducer increased the mean oral clearance of quetiapine by 5-fold. Increased doses of quetiapine may be required to maintain control of symptoms of schizophrenia in patients receiving quetiapine and phenytoin, or other hepatic enzyme inducers (eg, carbamazepine, barbiturates, rifampin and glucocorticoids)).
No products indexed under this heading.

Dexamethasone Sodium Phosphate (Co-administration with hepatic enzyme inducers, such as glucocorticosteroids, may increase oral clearance).
No products indexed under this heading.

Dexamethasone Sodium Phosphate Injection (Co-administration of quetiapine and CYP450 3A4 inducer increased the mean oral clearance of quetiapine by 5-fold. Increased doses of quetiapine may be required to maintain control of symptoms of schizophrenia in patients receiving quetiapine and phenytoin, or other hepatic enzyme inducers (eg, carbamazepine, barbiturates, rifampin and glucocorticoids)).
No products indexed under this heading.

Dexmethylphenidate Hydrochloride (Caution should be used when quetiapine is taken in combination with other centrally acting drugs). Products include:
Focalin XR 2472

Dextroamphetamine (Caution should be used when quetiapine is taken in combination with other centrally acting drugs).
No products indexed under this heading.

Dextroamphetamine Saccharate (Caution should be used when quetiapine is taken in combination with other centrally acting drugs).
No products indexed under this heading.

Dextroamphetamine Sulfate (Caution should be used when quetiapine is taken in combination with other centrally acting drugs). Products include:
Dexedrine 1425

Dezocine (Caution should be used when quetiapine is taken in combination with other centrally acting drugs).
No products indexed under this heading.

Diazepam (Caution should be used when quetiapine is taken in combination with other centrally acting drugs). Products include:
Valium Tablets 2880

Diazoxide (Enhanced effects of certain anti-hypertensive agents). Products include:
Proglycem 1179
Proglycem Suspension 1179

Diltiazem Hydrochloride (Enhanced effects of certain anti-hypertensive agents). Products include:
Cardizem LA 423

Diltiazem Maleate (Enhanced effects of certain anti-hypertensive agents).
No products indexed under this heading.

Divalproex Sodium (Co-administration of quetiapine (150 mg bid) and divalproex (500 mg bid) increased the mean maximum plasma concentration of quetiapine at steady state by 17% without affecting the extent of absorption or mean oral clearance. Co-administration also decreased the mean maximum concentration and extent of absorption of total and free valproic acid at steady state by 10% to 12% and increased mean oral clearance of total valproic acid by 11%). Products include:
Depakote ER 426

Dopamine Hydrochloride (Quetiapine may antagonize the effects of dopamine agonists).
No products indexed under this heading.

Doxazosin Mesylate (Enhanced effects of certain anti-hypertensive agents).
No products indexed under this heading.

Doxorubicin Hydrochloride (Co-administration of quetiapine and CYP450 3A4 inducer increased the mean oral clearance of quetiapine by 5-fold. Increased doses of quetiapine may be required to maintain control of symptoms of schizophrenia in patients receiving quetiapine and phenytoin, or other hepatic enzyme inducers (eg, carbamazepine, barbiturates, rifampin and glucocorticoids)).
No products indexed under this heading.

Droperidol (Caution should be used when quetiapine is taken in combination with other centrally acting drugs).
No products indexed under this heading.

Efavirenz (Co-administration with an inhibitor of CYP4503A may reduce oral clearance of quetiapine, resulting in an increase in maximum plasma concentration of quetiapine; dose adjustment of quetiapine will be necessary). Products include:
Atripla 906

Enalapril Maleate (Enhanced effects of certain anti-hypertensive agents).
No products indexed under this heading.

Enalaprilat (Enhanced effects of certain anti-hypertensive agents).
No products indexed under this heading.

Enflurane (Caution should be used when quetiapine is taken in combination with other centrally acting drugs).
No products indexed under this heading.

Eprosartan Mesylate (Enhanced effects of certain anti-hypertensive agents). Products include:
Teveten 538
Teveten HCT 541

Erythromycin (Co-administration with an inhibitor of CYP4503A may reduce oral clearance of quetiapine, resulting in an increase in maximum plasma concentration of quetiapine; dose adjustment of quetiapine will be necessary).
No products indexed under this heading.

Erythromycin Estolate (Co-administration with an inhibitor of CYP4503A may reduce oral clearance of quetiapine, resulting in an increase in maximum plasma concentration of quetiapine; dose adjustment of quetiapine will be necessary).
No products indexed under this heading.

Erythromycin Ethylsuccinate (Co-administration with an inhibitor of CYP4503A may reduce oral clearance of quetiapine, resulting in an increase in maximum plasma concentration of quetiapine; dose adjustment of quetiapine will be necessary). Products include:
E.E.S. 437
EryPed 435

Erythromycin Gluceptate (Co-administration with an inhibitor of CYP4503A may reduce oral clearance of quetiapine, resulting in an increase in maximum plasma concentration of quetiapine; dose adjustment of quetiapine will be necessary).
No products indexed under this heading.

Erythromycin Lactobionate (Co-administration with an inhibitor of CYP4503A may reduce oral clearance of quetiapine, resulting in an increase in maximum plasma concentration of quetiapine; dose adjustment of quetiapine will be necessary).
No products indexed under this heading.

Erythromycin Stearate (Co-administration with an inhibitor of CYP4503A may reduce oral clearance of quetiapine, resulting in an increase in maximum plasma concentration of quetiapine; dose adjustment of quetiapine will be necessary).
No products indexed under this heading.

Esmolol Hydrochloride (Enhanced effects of certain anti-hypertensive agents).
No products indexed under this heading.

Esomeprazole Magnesium (Co-administration with an inhibitor of CYP4503A may reduce oral clearance of quetiapine, resulting in an increase in maximum plasma concentration of quetiapine; dose adjustment of quetiapine will be necessary). Products include:
Nexium Capsules 704
Nexium Oral Suspension 704

Esomeprazole Sodium (Co-administration with an inhibitor of

CYP4503A may reduce oral clearance of quetiapine, resulting in an increase in maximum plasma concentration of quetiapine; dose adjustment of quetiapine will be necessary). Products include:
Nexium I.V. 712

Estazolam (Caution should be used when quetiapine is taken in combination with other centrally acting drugs).
No products indexed under this heading.

Ethanol (Quetiapine potentiated the cognitive and motor effects of alcohol in a clinical trial in subjects with selected psychotic disorders. Alcoholic beverages should be avoided while taking quetiapine).
No products indexed under this heading.

Ethchlorvynol (Caution should be used when quetiapine is taken in combination with other centrally acting drugs).
No products indexed under this heading.

Ethinamate (Caution should be used when quetiapine is taken in combination with other centrally acting drugs).
No products indexed under this heading.

Ethosuximide (Co-administration of quetiapine and CYP450 3A4 inducer increased the mean oral clearance of quetiapine by 5-fold. Increased doses of quetiapine may be required to maintain control of symptoms of schizophrenia in patients receiving quetiapine and phenytoin, or other hepatic enzyme inducers (eg, carbamazepine, barbiturates, rifampin and glucocorticoids)).
No products indexed under this heading.

Ethyl Alcohol (Quetiapine potentiated the cognitive and motor effects of alcohol in a clinical trial in subjects with selected psychotic disorders. Alcoholic beverages should be avoided while taking quetiapine).
No products indexed under this heading.

Felbamate (Co-administration of quetiapine and CYP450 3A4 inducer increased the mean oral clearance of quetiapine by 5-fold. Increased doses of quetiapine may be required to maintain control of symptoms of schizophrenia in patients receiving quetiapine and phenytoin, or other hepatic enzyme inducers (eg, carbamazepine, barbiturates, rifampin and glucocorticoids)).
No products indexed under this heading.

Felodipine (Enhanced effects of certain anti-hypertensive agents).
No products indexed under this heading.

Fentanyl (Caution should be used when quetiapine is taken in combination with other centrally acting drugs). Products include:
Duragesic 2604
Fentanyl Transdermal System 2346
Onsolis 2054

Fentanyl Citrate (Caution should be used when quetiapine is taken in combination with other centrally acting drugs). Products include:
Fentora 966

Fluconazole (Co-administration with an inhibitor of CYP4503A may reduce oral clearance of quetiapine, resulting in an increase in maximum plasma concentration of quetiapine; dose adjustment of quetiapine will be necessary).
No products indexed under this heading.

Fludrocortisone Acetate (Co-administration with hepatic enzyme inducers, such as glucocorticosteroids, may increase oral clearance).
No products indexed under this heading.

Fluoxetine (Co-administration with an inhibitor of CYP4503A may reduce oral clearance of quetiapine, resulting in an increase in maximum plasma concentration of quetiapine; dose adjustment of quetiapine will be necessary).
No products indexed under this heading.

Itraconazole (Co-administration with an inhibitor of CYP4503A may reduce oral clearance of quetiapine, resulting in an increase in maximum plasma concentration of quetiapine; dose adjustment of quetiapine will be necessary).
No products indexed under this heading.

Ketamine Hydrochloride (Caution should be used when quetiapine is taken in combination with other centrally acting drugs).
No products indexed under this heading.

Ketoconazole (Co-administration of ketoconazole, a potent inhibitor of CYP4503A, reduced oral clearance of quetiapine by 84%, resulting in a 335% increase in maximum plasma concentration of quetiapine; dose adjustment of quetiapine will be necessary if it is used with ketoconazole). Products include:

Labetalol Hydrochloride (Enhanced effects of certain anti-hypertensive agents).
No products indexed under this heading.

Lapatinib (Co-administration with an inhibitor of CYP4503A may reduce oral clearance of quetiapine, resulting in an increase in maximum plasma concentration of quetiapine; dose adjustment of quetiapine will be necessary). Products include:

Levodopa (Quetiapine may antagonize the effects of levodopa). Products include:

Levomethadyl Acetate Hydrochloride (Caution should be used when quetiapine is taken in combination with other centrally acting drugs).
No products indexed under this heading.

Levorphanol Tartrate (Caution should be used when quetiapine is taken in combination with other centrally acting drugs).
No products indexed under this heading.

Lisdexamfetamine Dimesylate (Caution should be used when quetiapine is taken in combination with other centrally acting drugs). Products include:

Lisinopril (Enhanced effects of certain anti-hypertensive agents). Products include:

Lopinavir (Co-administration with an inhibitor of CYP4503A may reduce oral clearance of quetiapine, resulting in an increase in maximum plasma concentration of quetiapine; dose adjustment of quetiapine will be necessary). Products include:

Loratadine (Co-administration with an inhibitor of CYP4503A may reduce oral clearance of quetiapine, resulting in an increase in maximum plasma concentration of quetiapine; dose adjustment of quetiapine will be necessary).
No products indexed under this heading.

Lorazepam (Co-administration has resulted in reduced (20%) mean oral clearance of lorazepam).
No products indexed under this heading.

Losartan Potassium (Enhanced effects of certain anti-hypertensive agents). Products include:

Loxapine Hydrochloride (Caution should be used when quetiapine is taken in combination with other centrally acting drugs).
No products indexed under this heading.

Loxapine Succinate (Caution should be used when quetiapine is taken in combination with other centrally acting drugs).
No products indexed under this heading.

Mecamylamine Hydrochloride (Enhanced effects of certain anti-hypertensive agents).
No products indexed under this heading.

Meperidine Hydrochloride (Caution should be used when quetiapine is taken in combination with other centrally acting drugs).
No products indexed under this heading.

Mephenytoin (Co-administration of quetiapine and CYP450 3A4 inducer increased the mean oral clearance of quetiapine by 5-fold. Increased doses of quetiapine may be required to maintain control of symptoms of schizophrenia in patients receiving quetiapine and phenytoin, or other hepatic enzyme inducers (eg, carbamazepine, barbiturates, rifampin and glucocorticoids)).
No products indexed under this heading.

Mephobarbital (Co-administration with hepatic enzyme inducers, such as barbiturates, may increase oral clearance).
No products indexed under this heading.

Meprobamate (Caution should be used when quetiapine is taken in combination with other centrally acting drugs).
No products indexed under this heading.

Mesoridazine Besylate (Caution should be used when quetiapine is taken in combination with other centrally acting drugs).
No products indexed under this heading.

Methadone Hydrochloride (Caution should be used when quetiapine is taken in combination with other centrally acting drugs).
No products indexed under this heading.

Methamphetamine Hydrochloride (Caution should be used when quetiapine is taken in combination with other centrally acting drugs).
No products indexed under this heading.

Methohexital Sodium (Caution should be used when quetiapine is taken in combination with other centrally acting drugs).
No products indexed under this heading.

Methotrimeprazine (Caution should be used when quetiapine is taken in combination with other centrally acting drugs).
No products indexed under this heading.

Methoxyflurane (Caution should be used when quetiapine is taken in combination with other centrally acting drugs).
No products indexed under this heading.

Methsuximide (Co-administration of quetiapine and CYP450 3A4 inducer increased the mean oral clearance of quetiapine by 5-fold. Increased doses of quetiapine may be required to maintain control of symptoms of schizophrenia in patients receiving quetiapine and phenytoin, or other hepatic enzyme inducers (eg, carbamazepine, barbiturates, rifampin and glucocorticoids)).
No products indexed under this heading.

Methyclothiazide (Enhanced effects of certain anti-hypertensive agents).
No products indexed under this heading.

Methyldopa (Enhanced effects of certain anti-hypertensive agents).
No products indexed under this heading.

Methyldopate Hydrochloride (Enhanced effects of certain anti-hypertensive agents).
No products indexed under this heading.

Methylphenidate (Caution should be used when quetiapine is taken in combination with other centrally acting drugs). Products include:

Methylphenidate Hydrochloride (Caution should be used when quetiapine is taken in combination with other centrally acting drugs). Products include:

Methylprednisolone (Co-administration of quetiapine and CYP450 3A4 inducer increased the mean oral clearance of quetiapine by 5-fold. Increased doses of quetiapine may be required to maintain control of symptoms of schizophrenia in patients receiving quetiapine and phenytoin, or other hepatic enzyme inducers (eg, carbamazepine, barbiturates, rifampin and glucocorticoids)).
No products indexed under this heading.

Methylprednisolone Acetate (Co-administration with hepatic enzyme inducers, such as glucocorticosteroids, may increase oral clearance).
No products indexed under this heading.

Methylprednisolone Sodium Succinate (Co-administration with hepatic enzyme inducers, such as glucocorticosteroids, may increase oral clearance).
No products indexed under this heading.

Metolazone (Enhanced effects of certain anti-hypertensive agents).
No products indexed under this heading.

Metoprolol Succinate (Enhanced effects of certain anti-hypertensive agents). Products include:

Metoprolol Tartrate (Enhanced effects of certain anti-hypertensive agents).
No products indexed under this heading.

Metronidazole (Co-administration with an inhibitor of CYP4503A may reduce oral clearance of quetiapine, resulting in an increase in maximum plasma concentration of quetiapine; dose adjustment of quetiapine will be necessary). Products include:

Metronidazole Benzoate (Co-administration with an inhibitor of CYP4503A may reduce oral clearance of quetiapine, resulting in an increase in maximum plasma concentration of quetiapine; dose adjustment of quetiapine will be necessary).
No products indexed under this heading.

Metronidazole Hydrochloride (Co-administration with an inhibitor of CYP4503A may reduce oral clearance of quetiapine, resulting in an increase in maximum plasma concentration of quetiapine; dose adjustment of quetiapine will be necessary).
No products indexed under this heading.

Metronidazole Sodium (Co-administration with an inhibitor of CYP4503A may reduce oral clearance of quetiapine, resulting in an increase in maximum plasma concentration of quetiapine; dose adjustment of quetiapine will be necessary).
No products indexed under this heading.

Metyrosine (Enhanced effects of certain anti-hypertensive agents).
No products indexed under this heading.

Mibefradil Dihydrochloride (Enhanced effects of certain anti-hypertensive agents).
No products indexed under this heading.

Miconazole (Co-administration with an inhibitor of CYP4503A may reduce oral clearance of quetiapine, resulting in an increase in maximum plasma concentration of quetiapine; dose adjustment of quetiapine will be necessary).
No products indexed under this heading.

Miconazole Nitrate (Co-administration with an inhibitor of

CYP4503A may reduce oral clearance of quetiapine, resulting in an increase in maximum plasma concentration of quetiapine; dose adjustment of quetiapine will be necessary). Products include:

Midazolam Hydrochloride (Caution should be used when quetiapine is taken in combination with other centrally acting drugs).
No products indexed under this heading.

Mifepristone (Co-administration with an inhibitor of CYP4503A may reduce oral clearance of quetiapine, resulting in an increase in maximum plasma concentration of quetiapine; dose adjustment of quetiapine will be necessary).
No products indexed under this heading.

Minoxidil (Enhanced effects of certain anti-hypertensive agents).
No products indexed under this heading.

Modafinil (Co-administration of quetiapine and CYP450 3A4 inducer increased the mean oral clearance of quetiapine by 5-fold. Increased doses of quetiapine may be required to maintain control of symptoms of schizophrenia in patients receiving quetiapine and phenytoin, or other hepatic enzyme inducers (eg, carbamazepine, barbiturates, rifampin and glucocorticoids)). Products include:

Moexipril Hydrochloride (Enhanced effects of certain anti-hypertensive agents).
No products indexed under this heading.

Molindone Hydrochloride (Caution should be used when quetiapine is taken in combination with other centrally acting drugs). Products include:

Morphine Sulfate (Caution should be used when quetiapine is taken in combination with other centrally acting drugs). Products include:

Morphine Sulfate, Liposomal (Caution should be used when quetiapine is taken in combination with other centrally acting drugs).
No products indexed under this heading.

Nadolol (Enhanced effects of certain anti-hypertensive agents). Products include:

Nafcillin Sodium (Co-administration of quetiapine and CYP450 3A4 inducer increased the mean oral clearance of quetiapine by 5-fold. Increased doses of quetiapine may be required to maintain control of symptoms of schizophrenia in patients receiving quetiapine and phenytoin, or other hepatic enzyme inducers (eg, carbamazepine, barbiturates, rifampin and glucocorticoids)).
No products indexed under this heading.

Nebivolol (Enhanced effects of certain anti-hypertensive agents). Products include:

Nefazodone Hydrochloride (Co-administration with an inhibitor of CYP4503A may reduce oral clearance of quetiapine, resulting in an increase in maximum plasma concentration of quetiapine; dose adjustment of quetiapine will be necessary).
No products indexed under this heading.

Nelfinavir Mesylate (Co-administration with an inhibitor of CYP4503A may reduce oral clearance of quetiapine, resulting in an increase in maximum plasma concentration of quetiapine; dose adjustment of quetiapine will be necessary).
No products indexed under this heading.

Nevirapine (Co-administration with an inhibitor of CYP4503A may reduce oral

clearance of quetiapine, resulting in an increase in maximum plasma concentration of quetiapine; dose adjustment of quetiapine will be necessary). Products include:

Niacin (Co-administration with an inhibitor of CYP4503A may reduce oral clearance of quetiapine, resulting in an increase in maximum plasma concentration of quetiapine; dose adjustment of quetiapine will be necessary). Products include:

Niacinamide (Co-administration with an inhibitor of CYP4503A may reduce oral clearance of quetiapine, resulting in an increase in maximum plasma concentration of quetiapine; dose adjustment of quetiapine will be necessary). Products include:

Niacinamide Hydroiodide (Co-administration with an inhibitor of CYP4503A may reduce oral clearance of quetiapine, resulting in an increase in maximum plasma concentration of quetiapine; dose adjustment of quetiapine will be necessary).
No products indexed under this heading.

Nicardipine Hydrochloride (Enhanced effects of certain anti-hypertensive agents).
No products indexed under this heading.

Nicotinamide (Co-administration with an inhibitor of CYP4503A may reduce oral clearance of quetiapine, resulting in an increase in maximum plasma concentration of quetiapine; dose adjustment of quetiapine will be necessary).
No products indexed under this heading.

Nifedipine (Enhanced effects of certain anti-hypertensive agents).
No products indexed under this heading.

Nisoldipine (Enhanced effects of certain anti-hypertensive agents).
No products indexed under this heading.

Nitroglycerin (Enhanced effects of certain anti-hypertensive agents). Products include:

Norfloxacin (Co-administration with an inhibitor of CYP4503A may reduce oral clearance of quetiapine, resulting in an increase in maximum plasma concentration of quetiapine; dose adjustment of quetiapine will be necessary). Products include:

Olanzapine (Caution should be used when quetiapine is taken in combination with other centrally acting drugs). Products include:

Omeprazole (Co-administration with an inhibitor of CYP4503A may reduce oral clearance of quetiapine, resulting in an increase in maximum plasma concentration of quetiapine; dose adjustment of quetiapine will be necessary).
No products indexed under this heading.

Oxazepam (Caution should be used when quetiapine is taken in combination with other centrally acting drugs).
No products indexed under this heading.

Oxcarbazepine (Co-administration of quetiapine and CYP450 3A4 inducer increased the mean oral clearance of quetiapine by 5-fold. Increased doses of quetiapine may be required to maintain control of symptoms of schizophrenia in patients receiving quetiapine and phenytoin, or other hepatic enzyme inducers (eg, carbamazepine, barbiturates, rifampin and glucocorticoids)).
No products indexed under this heading.

Oxycodone Hydrochloride (Caution should be used when quetiapine is taken in combination with other centrally acting drugs). Products include:

Oxycodone Terephthalate (Caution should be used when quetiapine is taken in combination with other centrally acting drugs).
No products indexed under this heading.

Oxymorphone Hydrochloride (Caution should be used when quetiapine is taken in combination with other centrally acting drugs). Products include:

Paroxetine Hydrochloride (Co-administration with an inhibitor of CYP4503A may reduce oral clearance of quetiapine, resulting in an increase in maximum plasma concentration of quetiapine; dose adjustment of quetiapine will be necessary). Products include:

Pemoline (Caution should be used when quetiapine is taken in combination with other centrally acting drugs).
No products indexed under this heading.

Penbutolol Sulfate (Enhanced effects of certain anti-hypertensive agents).
No products indexed under this heading.

Pentobarbital (Co-administration with hepatic enzyme inducers, such as barbiturates, may increase oral clearance).
No products indexed under this heading.

Pentobarbital Sodium (Co-administration with hepatic enzyme inducers, such as barbiturates, may increase oral clearance). Products include:

Pergolide Mesylate (Quetiapine may antagonize the effects of dopamine agonists).
No products indexed under this heading.

Perindopril Erbumine (Enhanced effects of certain anti-hypertensive agents).
No products indexed under this heading.

Perphenazine (Caution should be used when quetiapine is taken in combination with other centrally acting drugs).
No products indexed under this heading.

Phenobarbital (Co-administration with hepatic enzyme inducers, such as barbiturates, may increase oral clearance). Products include:

Phenobarbital Sodium (Co-administration with hepatic enzyme inducers, such as barbiturates, may increase oral clearance).
No products indexed under this heading.

Phenoxybenzamine Hydrochloride (Enhanced effects of certain anti-hypertensive agents). Products include:

Phentolamine Mesylate (Enhanced effects of certain anti-hypertensive agents).
No products indexed under this heading.

Phenytoin (Co-administration has resulted in increased mean oral clearance of quetiapine by 5-fold; increased dose of quetiapine may be required).
No products indexed under this heading.

Phenytoin Sodium (Co-administration has resulted in increased mean oral clearance of quetiapine by 5-fold; increased dose of quetiapine may be required). Products include:

Pindolol (Enhanced effects of certain anti-hypertensive agents).
No products indexed under this heading.

Polythiazide (Enhanced effects of certain anti-hypertensive agents).
No products indexed under this heading.

Posaconazole (Co-administration with an inhibitor of CYP4503A may reduce oral clearance of quetiapine, resulting in an increase in maximum plasma concentration of quetiapine; dose adjustment of quetiapine will be necessary). Products include:

Pramipexole Dihydrochloride (Quetiapine may antagonize the effects of dopamine agonists).
No products indexed under this heading.

Prazepam (Caution should be used when quetiapine is taken in combination with other centrally acting drugs).
No products indexed under this heading.

Prazosin Hydrochloride (Enhanced effects of certain anti-hypertensive agents).
No products indexed under this heading.

Prednisolone (Co-administration of quetiapine and CYP450 3A4 inducer increased the mean oral clearance of quetiapine by 5-fold. Increased doses of quetiapine may be required to maintain control of symptoms of schizophrenia in patients receiving quetiapine and phenytoin, or other hepatic enzyme inducers (eg, carbamazepine, barbiturates, rifampin and glucocorticoids)).
No products indexed under this heading.

Prednisolone Acetate (Co-administration with hepatic enzyme inducers, such as glucocorticosteroids, may increase oral clearance). Products include:

Prednisolone Sodium Phosphate (Co-administration with hepatic enzyme inducers, such as glucocorticosteroids, may increase oral clearance).
No products indexed under this heading.

Prednisolone Tebutate (Co-administration with hepatic enzyme inducers, such as glucocorticosteroids, may increase oral clearance).
No products indexed under this heading.

Prednisone (Co-administration with hepatic enzyme inducers, such as glucocorticosteroids, may increase oral clearance).
No products indexed under this heading.

Prednisone sodium phosphate (Co-administration of quetiapine and CYP450 3A4 inducer increased the mean oral clearance of quetiapine by 5-fold. Increased doses of quetiapine may be required to maintain control of symptoms of schizophrenia in patients receiving quetiapine and phenytoin, or other hepatic enzyme inducers (eg, carbamazepine, barbiturates, rifampin and glucocorticoids)).
No products indexed under this heading.

Primidone (Co-administration of quetiapine and CYP450 3A4 inducer increased the mean oral clearance of quetiapine by 5-fold. Increased doses of quetiapine may be required to maintain control of symptoms of schizophrenia in patients receiving quetiapine and phenytoin, or other hepatic enzyme inducers (eg, carbamazepine, barbiturates, rifampin and glucocorticoids)).
No products indexed under this heading.

Prochlorperazine (Caution should be used when quetiapine is taken in combination with other centrally acting drugs).
No products indexed under this heading.

Prochlorperazine Edisylate (Caution should be used when quetiapine is taken in combination with other centrally acting drugs).
No products indexed under this heading.

Prochlorperazine Maleate (Caution should be used when quetiapine is taken in combination with other centrally acting drugs).
No products indexed under this heading.

Promethazine (Caution should be used when quetiapine is taken in combination with other centrally acting drugs).
No products indexed under this heading.

Promethazine Hydrochloride (Caution should be used when quetiapine is taken in combination with other centrally acting drugs).
No products indexed under this heading.

Propofol (Caution should be used when quetiapine is taken in combination with other centrally acting drugs).
No products indexed under this heading.

Propoxyphene Hydrochloride (Caution should be used when quetiapine is taken in combination with other centrally acting drugs).
No products indexed under this heading.

Propoxyphene Napsylate (Caution should be used when quetiapine is taken in combination with other centrally acting drugs).
No products indexed under this heading.

Propranolol Hydrochloride (Enhanced effects of certain anti-hypertensive agents). Products include:

Quazepam (Caution should be used when quetiapine is taken in combination with other centrally acting drugs).
No products indexed under this heading.

Quinapril Hydrochloride (Enhanced effects of certain anti-hypertensive agents).
No products indexed under this heading.

Quinidine (Co-administration with an inhibitor of CYP4503A may reduce oral clearance of quetiapine, resulting in an increase in maximum plasma concentration of quetiapine; dose adjustment of quetiapine will be necessary).
No products indexed under this heading.

Quinidine Hydrochloride (Co-administration with an inhibitor of CYP4503A may reduce oral clearance of quetiapine, resulting in an increase in maximum plasma concentration of quetiapine; dose adjustment of quetiapine will be necessary).
No products indexed under this heading.

Quinidine Polygalacturonate (Co-administration with an inhibitor of CYP4503A may reduce oral clearance of quetiapine, resulting in an increase in maximum plasma concentration of quetiapine; dose adjustment of quetiapine will be necessary).
No products indexed under this heading.

1731 **Interactions Index** **Seroquel**

Quinidine Sulfate (Co-administration with an inhibitor of CYP4503A may reduce oral clearance of quetiapine, resulting in an increase in maximum plasma concentration of quetiapine; dose adjustment of quetiapine will be necessary).
No products indexed under this heading.

Quinine (Co-administration with an inhibitor of CYP4503A may reduce oral clearance of quetiapine, resulting in an increase in maximum plasma concentration of quetiapine; dose adjustment of quetiapine will be necessary). Products include:
Hyland's Leg Cramps PM with Quinine 3315

Quinine Sulfate (Co-administration with an inhibitor of CYP4503A may reduce oral clearance of quetiapine, resulting in an increase in maximum plasma concentration of quetiapine; dose adjustment of quetiapine will be necessary).
No products indexed under this heading.

Quinupristin (Co-administration with an inhibitor of CYP4503A may reduce oral clearance of quetiapine, resulting in an increase in maximum plasma concentration of quetiapine; dose adjustment of quetiapine will be necessary).
No products indexed under this heading.

Ramipril (Enhanced effects of certain anti-hypertensive agents).
No products indexed under this heading.

Ranitidine Bismuth Citrate (Co-administration with an inhibitor of CYP4503A may reduce oral clearance of quetiapine, resulting in an increase in maximum plasma concentration of quetiapine; dose adjustment of quetiapine will be necessary).
No products indexed under this heading.

Ranitidine Hydrochloride (Co-administration with an inhibitor of CYP4503A may reduce oral clearance of quetiapine, resulting in an increase in maximum plasma concentration of quetiapine; dose adjustment of quetiapine will be necessary). Products include:
Zantac 1737
Zantac Injection 1732
Zantac Pharmacy 1735

Rauwolfia Serpentina (Enhanced effects of certain anti-hypertensive agents).
No products indexed under this heading.

Remifentanil Hydrochloride (Caution should be used when quetiapine is taken in combination with other centrally acting drugs).
No products indexed under this heading.

Rescinnamine (Enhanced effects of certain anti-hypertensive agents).
No products indexed under this heading.

Reserpine (Enhanced effects of certain anti-hypertensive agents).
No products indexed under this heading.

Rifabutin (Co-administration of quetiapine and CYP450 3A4 inducer increased the mean oral clearance of quetiapine by 5-fold. Increased doses of quetiapine may be required to maintain control of symptoms of schizophrenia in patients receiving quetiapine and phenytoin, or other hepatic enzyme inducers (eg, carbamazepine, barbiturates, rifampin and glucocorticoids)).
No products indexed under this heading.

Rifampicin (Co-administration of quetiapine and CYP450 3A4 inducer increased the mean oral clearance of quetiapine by 5-fold. Increased doses of quetiapine may be required to maintain control of symptoms of schizophrenia in patients receiving quetiapine and phenytoin, or other hepatic enzyme inducers (eg, carbamazepine, barbiturates, rifampin and glucocorticoids)).
No products indexed under this heading.

Rifampin (Co-administration of quetiapine and CYP450 3A4 inducer increased the mean oral clearance of quetiapine by 5-fold. Increased doses of quetiapine may be required to maintain control of symptoms of schizophrenia in patients receiving quetiapine and phenytoin, or other hepatic enzyme inducers (eg, carbamazepine, barbiturates, rifampin and glucocorticoids)).
No products indexed under this heading.

Rifapentine (Co-administration of quetiapine and CYP450 3A4 inducer increased the mean oral clearance of quetiapine by 5-fold. Increased doses of quetiapine may be required to maintain control of symptoms of schizophrenia in patients receiving quetiapine and phenytoin, or other hepatic enzyme inducers (eg, carbamazepine, barbiturates, rifampin and glucocorticoids)).
No products indexed under this heading.

Risperidone (Caution should be used when quetiapine is taken in combination with other centrally acting drugs). Products include:
Risperdal Consta 2682

Ritonavir (Co-administration with an inhibitor of CYP4503A may reduce oral clearance of quetiapine, resulting in an increase in maximum plasma concentration of quetiapine; dose adjustment of quetiapine will be necessary). Products include:
Kaletra 458
Norvir 509

Ropinirole Hydrochloride (Quetiapine may antagonize the effects of dopamine agonists). Products include:
Requip 1620
Requip XL 1628

Saquinavir (Co-administration with an inhibitor of CYP4503A may reduce oral clearance of quetiapine, resulting in an increase in maximum plasma concentration of quetiapine; dose adjustment of quetiapine will be necessary).
No products indexed under this heading.

Saquinavir Mesylate (Co-administration with an inhibitor of CYP4503A may reduce oral clearance of quetiapine, resulting in an increase in maximum plasma concentration of quetiapine; dose adjustment of quetiapine will be necessary).
No products indexed under this heading.

Secobarbital Sodium (Co-administration with hepatic enzyme inducers, such as barbiturates, may increase oral clearance).
No products indexed under this heading.

Sertraline Hydrochloride (Co-administration with an inhibitor of CYP4503A may reduce oral clearance of quetiapine, resulting in an increase in maximum plasma concentration of quetiapine; dose adjustment of quetiapine will be necessary).
No products indexed under this heading.

Sevoflurane (Caution should be used when quetiapine is taken in combination with other centrally acting drugs). Products include:
Ultane 554

Sildenafil Citrate (Co-administration with an inhibitor of CYP4503A may reduce oral clearance of quetiapine, resulting in an increase in maximum plasma concentration of quetiapine; dose adjustment of quetiapine will be necessary).
No products indexed under this heading.

Sodium Butabarbital (Co-administration with hepatic enzyme inducers, such as barbiturates, may increase oral clearance).
No products indexed under this heading.

Sodium Nitroprusside (Enhanced effects of certain anti-hypertensive agents).
No products indexed under this heading.

Sodium Oxybate (Caution should be used when quetiapine is taken in combination with other centrally acting drugs).
No products indexed under this heading.

Sodium Pentobarbital (Co-administration with hepatic enzyme inducers, such as barbiturates, may increase oral clearance).
No products indexed under this heading.

Sotalol Hydrochloride (Enhanced effects of certain anti-hypertensive agents).
No products indexed under this heading.

Spirapril Hydrochloride (Enhanced effects of certain anti-hypertensive agents).
No products indexed under this heading.

Sufentanil Citrate (Caution should be used when quetiapine is taken in combination with other centrally acting drugs).
No products indexed under this heading.

Sulfinpyrazone (Co-administration of quetiapine and CYP450 3A4 inducer increased the mean oral clearance of quetiapine by 5-fold. Increased doses of quetiapine may be required to maintain control of symptoms of schizophrenia in patients receiving quetiapine and phenytoin, or other hepatic enzyme inducers (eg, carbamazepine, barbiturates, rifampin and glucocorticoids)).
No products indexed under this heading.

Talbutal (Caution should be used when quetiapine is taken in combination with other centrally acting drugs).
No products indexed under this heading.

Telithromycin (Co-administration with an inhibitor of CYP4503A may reduce oral clearance of quetiapine, resulting in an increase in maximum plasma concentration of quetiapine; dose adjustment of quetiapine will be necessary). Products include:
Ketek 2991

Telmisartan (Enhanced effects of certain anti-hypertensive agents). Products include:
Micardis 887
Micardis HCT 889

Temazepam (Caution should be used when quetiapine is taken in combination with other centrally acting drugs).
No products indexed under this heading.

Terazosin Hydrochloride (Enhanced effects of certain anti-hypertensive agents).
No products indexed under this heading.

Theophyllinate (Co-administration of quetiapine and CYP450 3A4 inducer increased the mean oral clearance of quetiapine by 5-fold. Increased doses of quetiapine may be required to maintain control of symptoms of schizophrenia in patients receiving quetiapine and phenytoin, or other hepatic enzyme inducers (eg, carbamazepine, barbiturates, rifampin and glucocorticoids)).
No products indexed under this heading.

Theophylline (Co-administration of quetiapine and CYP450 3A4 inducer increased the mean oral clearance of quetiapine by 5-fold. Increased doses of quetiapine may be required to maintain control of symptoms of schizophrenia in patients receiving quetiapine and phenytoin, or other hepatic enzyme inducers (eg, carbamazepine, barbiturates, rifampin and glucocorticoids)).
No products indexed under this heading.

Theophylline Anhydrous (Co-administration of quetiapine and CYP450 3A4 inducer increased the mean oral clearance of quetiapine by 5-fold. Increased doses of quetiapine may be required to maintain control of symptoms of schizophrenia in patients receiving quetiapine and phenytoin, or other hepatic enzyme inducers (eg, carbamazepine, barbiturates, rifampin and glucocorticoids)). Products include:
Uniphyl 2817

Theophylline Calcium Salicylate (Co-administration of quetiapine and CYP450 3A4 inducer increased the mean oral clearance of quetiapine by 5-fold. Increased doses of quetiapine may be required to maintain control of symptoms of schizophrenia in patients receiving quetiapine and phenytoin, or other hepatic enzyme inducers (eg, carbamazepine, barbiturates, rifampin and glucocorticoids)).
No products indexed under this heading.

Theophylline Dihydroxypropyl (Glyceryl) (Co-administration of quetiapine and CYP450 3A4 inducer increased the mean oral clearance of quetiapine by 5-fold. Increased doses of quetiapine may be required to maintain control of symptoms of schizophrenia in patients receiving quetiapine and phenytoin, or other hepatic enzyme inducers (eg, carbamazepine, barbiturates, rifampin and glucocorticoids)).
No products indexed under this heading.

Theophylline Ethylenediamine (Co-administration of quetiapine and CYP450 3A4 inducer increased the mean oral clearance of quetiapine by 5-fold. Increased doses of quetiapine may be required to maintain control of symptoms of schizophrenia in patients receiving quetiapine and phenytoin, or other hepatic enzyme inducers (eg, carbamazepine, barbiturates, rifampin and glucocorticoids)).
No products indexed under this heading.

Theophylline Sodium Glycinate (Co-administration of quetiapine and CYP450 3A4 inducer increased the mean oral clearance of quetiapine by 5-fold. Increased doses of quetiapine may be required to maintain control of symptoms of schizophrenia in patients receiving quetiapine and phenytoin, or other hepatic enzyme inducers (eg, carbamazepine, barbiturates, rifampin and glucocorticoids)).
No products indexed under this heading.

Thiamylal Sodium (Co-administration with hepatic enzyme inducers, such as barbiturates, may increase oral clearance).
No products indexed under this heading.

Thioridazine (Increases the oral clearance of quetiapine by 65%).
No products indexed under this heading.

Thioridazine Hydrochloride (Caution should be used when quetiapine is taken in combination with other centrally acting drugs). Products include:
Thioridazine Hydrochloride 2384

Thiothixene (Caution should be used when quetiapine is taken in combination with other centrally acting drugs). Products include:
Thiothixene 2386

Thiothixene Hydrochloride (Caution should be used when quetiapine is taken in combination with other centrally acting drugs).
No products indexed under this heading.

Timolol Maleate (Enhanced effects of certain anti-hypertensive agents). Products include:
Combigan 601
Dorzolamide Hydrochloride/Timolol Maleate Ophthalmic Solution .... ⊙ 243
Timoptic in Ocudose .... ⊙ 231

Torsemide (Enhanced effects of certain anti-hypertensive agents).
No products indexed under this heading.

Trandolapril (Enhanced effects of certain anti-hypertensive agents). Products include:
Mavik 489

IMPORTANT NOTE: Always consult each drug listing in the patient's regimen for possible interactions.

Seroquel Interactions Index 1732

Tarka ... 534

Triamcinolone (Co-administration with hepatic enzyme inducers, such as glucocorticosteroids, may increase oral clearance).
No products indexed under this heading.

Triamcinolone Acetonide (Co-administration with hepatic enzyme inducers, such as glucocorticosteroids, may increase oral clearance). Products include:
Azmacort ... 408
Nasacort AQ ... 3019

Triamcinolone Diacetate (Co-administration with hepatic enzyme inducers, such as glucocorticosteroids, may increase oral clearance).
No products indexed under this heading.

Triamcinolone Hexacetonide (Co-administration with hepatic enzyme inducers, such as glucocorticosteroids, may increase oral clearance).
No products indexed under this heading.

Triazolam (Caution should be used when quetiapine is taken in combination with other centrally acting drugs).
No products indexed under this heading.

Trifluoperazine Hydrochloride (Caution should be used when quetiapine is taken in combination with other centrally acting drugs).
No products indexed under this heading.

Trimethaphan Camsylate (Enhanced effects of certain anti-hypertensive agents).
No products indexed under this heading.

Troglitazone (Co-administration with an inhibitor of CYP4503A may reduce oral clearance of quetiapine, resulting in an increase in maximum plasma concentration of quetiapine; dose adjustment of quetiapine will be necessary).
No products indexed under this heading.

Troleandomycin (Co-administration with an inhibitor of CYP4503A may reduce oral clearance of quetiapine, resulting in an increase in maximum plasma concentration of quetiapine; dose adjustment of quetiapine will be necessary).
No products indexed under this heading.

Valproate Sodium (Co-administration with an inhibitor of CYP4503A may reduce oral clearance of quetiapine, resulting in an increase in maximum plasma concentration of quetiapine; dose adjustment of quetiapine will be necessary).
No products indexed under this heading.

Valsartan (Enhanced effects of certain anti-hypertensive agents). Products include:
Diovan ... 2413
Diovan HCT ... 2419
Exforge ... 2443
Exforge HCT ... 2449
Valturna ... 3637

Vardenafil Hydrochloride (Co-administration with an inhibitor of CYP4503A may reduce oral clearance of quetiapine, resulting in an increase in maximum plasma concentration of quetiapine; dose adjustment of quetiapine will be necessary). Products include:
Levitra ... 3157

Verapamil Hydrochloride (Enhanced effects of certain anti-hypertensive agents). Products include:
Tarka ... 534

Voriconazole (Co-administration with an inhibitor of CYP4503A may reduce oral clearance of quetiapine, resulting in an increase in maximum plasma concentration of quetiapine; dose adjustment of quetiapine will be necessary).
No products indexed under this heading.

Zafirlukast (Co-administration with an inhibitor of CYP4503A may reduce oral clearance of quetiapine, resulting in an increase in maximum plasma concentration of quetiapine; dose adjustment of quetiapine will be necessary). Products include:
Accolate ... 3612

Zaleplon (Caution should be used when quetiapine is taken in combination with other centrally acting drugs).
No products indexed under this heading.

Zileuton (Co-administration with an inhibitor of CYP4503A may reduce oral clearance of quetiapine, resulting in an increase in maximum plasma concentration of quetiapine; dose adjustment of quetiapine will be necessary).
No products indexed under this heading.

Ziprasidone Hydrochloride (Caution should be used when quetiapine is taken in combination with other centrally acting drugs). Products include:
Geodon ... 2723

Zolpidem Tartrate (Caution should be used when quetiapine is taken in combination with other centrally acting drugs). Products include:
Ambien ... 2920
Ambien CR ... 2925

Food Interactions

Alcohol (The cognitive and motor effect of alcohol is potentiated; alcohol use should be avoided).

Beer, reduced-alcohol (Quetiapine potentiated the cognitive and motor effects of alcohol in a clinical trial in subjects with selected psychotic disorders. Alcoholic beverages should be avoided while taking quetiapine).

Beer, unspecified (Quetiapine potentiated the cognitive and motor effects of alcohol in a clinical trial in subjects with selected psychotic disorders. Alcoholic beverages should be avoided while taking quetiapine).

Food, unspecified (The bioavailability of quetiapine is marginally affected by administration with food, with C_{max} and AUC values increased by 25% and 15%, respectively).

Grapefruit (Co-administration with an inhibitor of CYP4503A may reduce oral clearance of quetiapine, resulting in an increase in maximum plasma concentration of quetiapine; dose adjustment of quetiapine will be necessary).

Grapefruit Juice (Co-administration with an inhibitor of CYP4503A may reduce oral clearance of quetiapine, resulting in an increase in maximum plasma concentration of quetiapine; dose adjustment of quetiapine will be necessary).

Wine, Chianti (Quetiapine potentiated the cognitive and motor effects of alcohol in a clinical trial in subjects with selected psychotic disorders. Alcoholic beverages should be avoided while taking quetiapine).

Wine, Red (Quetiapine potentiated the cognitive and motor effects of alcohol in a clinical trial in subjects with selected psychotic disorders. Alcoholic beverages should be avoided while taking quetiapine).

Wine, unspecified (Quetiapine potentiated the cognitive and motor effects of alcohol in a clinical trial in subjects with selected psychotic disorders. Alcoholic beverages should be avoided while taking quetiapine).

Wine products (Quetiapine potentiated the cognitive and motor effects of alcohol in a clinical trial in subjects with selected psychotic disorders. Alcoholic beverages should be avoided while taking quetiapine).

SEROQUEL XR EXTENDED-RELEASE TABLETS

(Quetiapine Fumarate) ... 759
May interact with alcohols, anticholinergics, antihypertensives, barbiturates, centrally-acting drugs, cytochrome p450 3a4 inducers (selected), cytochrome p450 3a4 inhibitors (selected), dopamine agonists, glucocorticoids, hepatic microsomal enzyme inducers, phenytoin, and certain other agents. Compounds in these categories include:

Acebutolol Hydrochloride (Because of its potential for inducing hypotension, quetiapine may enhance the effects of certain antihypertensive agents).
No products indexed under this heading.

Acetazolamide (Co-administration of quetiapine with cytochrome P450 3A inhibitors may decrease the clearance of quetiapine. Caution (reduced dosage) of quetiapine may be necessary when co-administered with other cytochrome P450 3A inhibitors).
No products indexed under this heading.

Acetazolamide Sodium (Co-administration of quetiapine with cytochrome P450 3A inhibitors may decrease the clearance of quetiapine. Caution (reduced dosage) of quetiapine may be necessary when co-administered with other cytochrome P450 3A inhibitors).
No products indexed under this heading.

Alfentanil Hydrochloride (Given the primary CNS effects of quetiapine, caution should be used when it is taken in combination with other centrally acting drugs. Quetiapine potentiated the cognitive and motor effects of alcohol in a clinical trial in subjects with selected psychotic disorders, and alcoholic beverages should be limited while taking quetiapine).
No products indexed under this heading.

Aliskiren (Because of its potential for inducing hypotension, quetiapine may enhance the effects of certain antihypertensive agents). Products include:
Tekturna ... 2538
Tekturna HCT ... 2541
Valturna ... 3637

Allium sativum (Co-administration of quetiapine with hepatic enzyme inducers may increase the clearance of quetiapine. Higher doses of quetiapine may be required when co-administered with hepatic enzyme inducers).
No products indexed under this heading.

Alprazolam (Given the primary CNS effects of quetiapine, caution should be used when it is taken in combination with other centrally acting drugs. Quetiapine potentiated the cognitive and motor effects of alcohol in a clinical trial in subjects with selected psychotic disorders, and alcoholic beverages should be limited while taking quetiapine).
No products indexed under this heading.

Aminoglutethimide (Co-administration of quetiapine with hepatic enzyme inducers may increase the clearance of quetiapine. Higher doses of quetiapine may be required when co-administered with hepatic enzyme inducers).
No products indexed under this heading.

Amiodarone Hydrochloride (Co-administration of quetiapine with cytochrome P450 3A inhibitors may decrease the clearance of quetiapine. Caution (reduced dosage) of quetiapine may be necessary when co-administered with other cytochrome P450 3A inhibitors).
No products indexed under this heading.

Amlodipine Besylate (Because of its potential for inducing hypotension, quetiapine may enhance the effects of certain antihypertensive agents). Products include:
Azor ... 1010
Exforge ... 2443
Exforge HCT ... 2449

Amobarbital (Co-administration of quetiapine with hepatic enzyme inducers (eg, barbiturates) may increase the clearance of quetiapine. Higher doses of quetiapine may be required when co-administered with hepatic enzyme inducers).
No products indexed under this heading.

Amobarbital Sodium (Co-administration of quetiapine with hepatic enzyme inducers (eg, barbiturates) may increase the clearance of quetiapine. Higher doses of quetiapine may be required when co-administered with hepatic enzyme inducers).
No products indexed under this heading.

Amphetamine Aspartate (Given the primary CNS effects of quetiapine, caution should be used when it is taken in combination with other centrally acting drugs. Quetiapine potentiated the cognitive and motor effects of alcohol in a clinical trial in subjects with selected psychotic disorders, and alcoholic beverages should be limited while taking quetiapine).
No products indexed under this heading.

Amphetamine Aspartate Monohydrate (Given the primary CNS effects of quetiapine, caution should be used when it is taken in combination with other centrally acting drugs. Quetiapine potentiated the cognitive and motor effects of alcohol in a clinical trial in subjects with selected psychotic disorders, and alcoholic beverages should be limited while taking quetiapine).
No products indexed under this heading.

Amphetamine Resins (Given the primary CNS effects of quetiapine, caution should be used when it is taken in combination with other centrally acting drugs. Quetiapine potentiated the cognitive and motor effects of alcohol in a clinical trial in subjects with selected psychotic disorders, and alcoholic beverages should be limited while taking quetiapine).
No products indexed under this heading.

Amphetamine Sulfate (Given the primary CNS effects of quetiapine, caution should be used when it is taken in combination with other centrally acting drugs. Quetiapine potentiated the cognitive and motor effects of alcohol in a clinical trial in subjects with selected psychotic disorders, and alcoholic beverages should be limited while taking quetiapine).
No products indexed under this heading.

Amprenavir (Co-administration of quetiapine with cytochrome P450 3A inhibitors may decrease the clearance of quetiapine. Caution (reduced dosage) of quetiapine may be necessary when co-administered with other cytochrome P450 3A inhibitors).
No products indexed under this heading.

Anastrozole (Co-administration of quetiapine with cytochrome P450 3A inhibitors may decrease the clearance of quetiapine. Caution (reduced dosage) of quetiapine may be necessary when co-administered with other cytochrome P450 3A inhibitors).
No products indexed under this heading.

Aprepitant (Co-administration of quetiapine with hepatic enzyme inducers may increase the clearance of quetiapine. Higher doses of quetiapine may be required when co-administered with hepatic enzyme inducers). Products include:
Emend ... 2124

1733 Interactions Index Seroquel XR

Aprobarbital (Co-administration of quetiapine with hepatic enzyme inducers (eg, barbiturates) may increase the clearance of quetiapine. Higher doses of quetiapine may be required when co-administered with hepatic enzyme inducers).
No products indexed under this heading.

Atazanavir (Co-administration of quetiapine with cytochrome P450 3A inhibitors may decrease the clearance of quetiapine. Caution (reduced dosage) of quetiapine may be necessary when co-administered with other cytochrome P450 3A inhibitors).
No products indexed under this heading.

Atazanavir Sulfate (Co-administration of quetiapine with cytochrome P450 3A inhibitors may decrease the clearance of quetiapine. Caution (reduced dosage) of quetiapine may be necessary when co-administered with other cytochrome P450 3A inhibitors).
No products indexed under this heading.

Atenolol (Because of its potential for inducing hypotension, quetiapine may enhance the effects of certain antihypertensive agents).
No products indexed under this heading.

Atropine Sulfate (Disruption of the body's ability to reduce core body temperature has been atributed to antipsychotic agents. Appropriate care is advised when co-administering quetiapine with agents which may contribute to an elevation in core body temperature such as anticholinergics). Products include:
Donnatal 2711

Belladonna Alkaloids (Disruption of the body's ability to reduce core body temperature has been atributed to antipsychotic agents. Appropriate care is advised when co-administering quetiapine with agents which may contribute to an elevation in core body temperature such as anticholinergics). Products include:
Hyland's Teething Tablets 3316

Benazepril Hydrochloride (Because of its potential for inducing hypotension, quetiapine may enhance the effects of certain antihypertensive agents).
No products indexed under this heading.

Bendroflumethiazide (Because of its potential for inducing hypotension, quetiapine may enhance the effects of certain antihypertensive agents).
No products indexed under this heading.

Benztropine Mesylate (Disruption of the body's ability to reduce core body temperature has been atributed to antipsychotic agents. Appropriate care is advised when co-administering quetiapine with agents which may contribute to an elevation in core body temperature such as anticholinergics).
No products indexed under this heading.

Betamethasone (Co-administration of quetiapine with hepatic enzyme inducers may increase the clearance of quetiapine. Higher doses of quetiapine may be required when co-administered with hepatic enzyme inducers).
No products indexed under this heading.

Betamethasone Acetate (Co-administration of quetiapine with hepatic enzyme inducers (eg, glucocorticoids) may increase the clearance of quetiapine. Higher doses of quetiapine may be required when co-administered with hepatic enzyme inducers).
No products indexed under this heading.

Betamethasone Benzoate (Quetiapine oral clearance is increased by the prototype cytochrome P450 3A4 inducer phenytoin. Dose adjustment of quetiapine is necessary. Higher maintenance doses of quetiapine may be required when it is co-administered with other enzyme inducers such as carbamazepine and phenobarbital).
No products indexed under this heading.

Betamethasone Dipropionate (Quetiapine oral clearance is increased by the prototype cytochrome P450 3A4 inducer phenytoin. Dose adjustment of quetiapine is necessary. Higher maintenance doses of quetiapine may be required when it is co-administered with other enzyme inducers such as carbamazepine and phenobarbital). Products include:
Diprolene Lotion 0.05% 3108
Diprolene Ointment 0.05% 3109
Diprolene AF Cream 0.05% 3107
Lotrisone 3163

Betamethasone Sodium Phosphate (Co-administration of quetiapine with hepatic enzyme inducers (eg, glucocorticoids) may increase the clearance of quetiapine. Higher doses of quetiapine may be required when co-administered with hepatic enzyme inducers).
No products indexed under this heading.

Betamethasone Valerate (Quetiapine oral clearance is increased by the prototype cytochrome P450 3A4 inducer phenytoin. Dose adjustment of quetiapine is necessary. Higher maintenance doses of quetiapine may be required when it is co-administered with other enzyme inducers such as carbamazepine and phenobarbital). Products include:
Luxíq 3321

Betaxolol Hydrochloride (Because of its potential for inducing hypotension, quetiapine may enhance the effects of certain antihypertensive agents).
No products indexed under this heading.

Biperiden Hydrochloride (Disruption of the body's ability to reduce core body temperature has been atributed to antipsychotic agents. Appropriate care is advised when co-administering quetiapine with agents which may contribute to an elevation in core body temperature such as anticholinergics).
No products indexed under this heading.

Bisoprolol Fumarate (Because of its potential for inducing hypotension, quetiapine may enhance the effects of certain antihypertensive agents).
No products indexed under this heading.

Bosentan (Co-administration of quetiapine with hepatic enzyme inducers may increase the clearance of quetiapine. Higher doses of quetiapine may be required when co-administered with hepatic enzyme inducers). Products include:
Tracleer 573

Bromocriptine Mesylate (Quetiapine may antagonize the effects of dopamine agonists).
No products indexed under this heading.

Budesonide (Co-administration of quetiapine with hepatic enzyme inducers (eg, glucocorticoids) may increase the clearance of quetiapine. Higher doses of quetiapine may be required when co-administered with hepatic enzyme inducers). Products include:
Pulmicort Flexhaler 714
Symbicort 80/4.5 720
Symbicort 160/4.5 720

Buprenorphine Hydrochloride (Given the primary CNS effects of quetiapine, caution should be used when it is taken in combination with other centrally acting drugs. Quetiapine potentiated the cognitive and motor effects of alcohol in a clinical trial in subjects with selected psychotic disorders, and alcoholic beverages should be limited while taking quetiapine).
No products indexed under this heading.

Buspirone Hydrochloride (Given the primary CNS effects of quetiapine, caution should be used when it is taken in combination with other centrally acting drugs. Quetiapine potentiated the cognitive and motor effects of alcohol in a clinical trial in subjects with selected psychotic disorders, and alcoholic beverages should be limited while taking quetiapine).
No products indexed under this heading.

Butabarbital (Co-administration of quetiapine with hepatic enzyme inducers (eg, barbiturates) may increase the clearance of quetiapine. Higher doses of quetiapine may be required when co-administered with hepatic enzyme inducers).
No products indexed under this heading.

Butabarbital Sodium (Co-administration of quetiapine with hepatic enzyme inducers (eg, barbiturates) may increase the clearance of quetiapine. Higher doses of quetiapine may be required when co-administered with hepatic enzyme inducers).
No products indexed under this heading.

Butalbital (Co-administration of quetiapine with hepatic enzyme inducers (eg, barbiturates) may increase the clearance of quetiapine. Higher doses of quetiapine may be required when co-administered with hepatic enzyme inducers).
No products indexed under this heading.

Candesartan Cilexetil (Because of its potential for inducing hypotension, quetiapine may enhance the effects of certain antihypertensive agents). Products include:
Atacand 697
Atacand HCT 700

Captopril (Because of its potential for inducing hypotension, quetiapine may enhance the effects of certain antihypertensive agents). Products include:
Captopril 2341

Carbamazepine (Co-administration of quetiapine with hepatic enzyme inducers may increase the clearance of quetiapine. Higher doses of quetiapine may be required when co-administered with hepatic enzyme inducers). Products include:
Carbatrol 3280
Equetro 3477

Carteolol Hydrochloride (Because of its potential for inducing hypotension, quetiapine may enhance the effects of certain antihypertensive agents).
No products indexed under this heading.

Carvedilol (Because of its potential for inducing hypotension, quetiapine may enhance the effects of certain antihypertensive agents). Products include:
Coreg 1409

Carvedilol Phosphate (Because of its potential for inducing hypotension, quetiapine may enhance the effects of certain antihypertensive agents). Products include:
Coreg CR 1416

Chlordiazepoxide (Given the primary CNS effects of quetiapine, caution should be used when it is taken in combination with other centrally acting drugs. Quetiapine potentiated the cognitive and motor effects of alcohol in a clinical trial in subjects with selected psychotic disorders, and alcoholic beverages should be limited while taking quetiapine).
No products indexed under this heading.

Chlordiazepoxide Hydrochloride (Given the primary CNS effects of quetiapine, caution should be used when it is taken in combination with other centrally acting drugs. Quetiapine potentiated the cognitive and motor effects of alcohol in a clinical trial in subjects with selected psychotic disorders, and alcoholic beverages should be limited while taking quetiapine).
No products indexed under this heading.

Chlorothiazide (Because of its potential for inducing hypotension, quetiapine may enhance the effects of certain antihypertensive agents).
No products indexed under this heading.

Chlorothiazide Sodium (Because of its potential for inducing hypotension, quetiapine may enhance the effects of certain antihypertensive agents). Products include:
Diuril Intravenous 2009

Chlorpromazine (Given the primary CNS effects of quetiapine, caution should be used when it is taken in combination with other centrally acting drugs. Quetiapine potentiated the cognitive and motor effects of alcohol in a clinical trial in subjects with selected psychotic disorders, and alcoholic beverages should be limited while taking quetiapine).
No products indexed under this heading.

Chlorpromazine Hydrochloride (Given the primary CNS effects of quetiapine, caution should be used when it is taken in combination with other centrally acting drugs. Quetiapine potentiated the cognitive and motor effects of alcohol in a clinical trial in subjects with selected psychotic disorders, and alcoholic beverages should be limited while taking quetiapine).
No products indexed under this heading.

Chlorpropamide (Co-administration of quetiapine with hepatic enzyme inducers may increase the clearance of quetiapine. Higher doses of quetiapine may be required when co-administered with hepatic enzyme inducers).
No products indexed under this heading.

Chlorprothixene (Given the primary CNS effects of quetiapine, caution should be used when it is taken in combination with other centrally acting drugs. Quetiapine potentiated the cognitive and motor effects of alcohol in a clinical trial in subjects with selected psychotic disorders, and alcoholic beverages should be limited while taking quetiapine).
No products indexed under this heading.

Chlorprothixene Hydrochloride (Given the primary CNS effects of quetiapine, caution should be used when it is taken in combination with other centrally acting drugs. Quetiapine potentiated the cognitive and motor effects of alcohol in a clinical trial in subjects with selected psychotic disorders, and alcoholic beverages should be limited while taking quetiapine).
No products indexed under this heading.

IMPORTANT NOTE: Always consult each drug listing in the patient's regimen for possible interactions.

1735 Interactions Index Seroquel XR

Dezocine (Given the primary CNS effects of quetiapine, caution should be used when it is taken in combination with other centrally acting drugs. Quetiapine potentiated the cognitive and motor effects of alcohol in a clinical trial in subjects with selected psychotic disorders, and alcoholic beverages should be limited while taking quetiapine).
No products indexed under this heading.

Diazepam (Given the primary CNS effects of quetiapine, caution should be used when it is taken in combination with other centrally acting drugs. Quetiapine potentiated the cognitive and motor effects of alcohol in a clinical trial in subjects with selected psychotic disorders, and alcoholic beverages should be limited while taking quetiapine).
Products include:
Valium Tablets 2880

Diazoxide (Because of its potential for inducing hypotension, quetiapine may enhance the effects of certain antihypertensive agents). Products include:
Proglycem 1179
Proglycem Suspension 1179

Dicyclomine Hydrochloride (Disruption of the body's ability to reduce core body temperature has been atributed to antipsychotic agents. Appropriate care is advised when co-administering quetiapine with agents which may contribute to an elevation in core body temperature such as anticholinergics).
Products include:
Bentyl Capsules 780
Bentyl Injection 780
Bentyl Syrup 780
Bentyl Tablets 780

Diltiazem Hydrochloride (Because of its potential for inducing hypotension, quetiapine may enhance the effects of certain antihypertensive agents).
Products include:
Cardizem LA 423

Diltiazem Maleate (Because of its potential for inducing hypotension, quetiapine may enhance the effects of certain antihypertensive agents).
No products indexed under this heading.

Divalproex Sodium (Co-administration of quetiapine (150 mg twice daily) and divalproex (500 mg twice daily) increased the mean maximum plasma concentration of quetiapine at steady-state by 17% without affecting the extent of absorption or mean oral clearance while the mean maximum concentration and extent of absorption of total and free valproic acid at steady-state were decreased by 10 to 12%. The mean oral clearance of total valproic acid (administered as divalproex 500 mg twice daily) was increased by 11% in the presence of quetiapine (150 mg twice daily)).
Products include:
Depakote ER 426

Dopamine Hydrochloride (Quetiapine may antagonize the effects of dopamine agonists).
No products indexed under this heading.

Doxazosin Mesylate (Because of its potential for inducing hypotension, quetiapine may enhance the effects of certain antihypertensive agents).
No products indexed under this heading.

Doxorubicin Hydrochloride (Co-administration of quetiapine with hepatic enzyme inducers may increase the clearance of quetiapine. Higher doses of quetiapine may be required when co-administered with hepatic enzyme inducers).
No products indexed under this heading.

Droperidol (Given the primary CNS effects of quetiapine, caution should be used when it is taken in combination with other centrally acting drugs. Quetiapine potentiated the cognitive and motor effects of alcohol in a clinical trial in subjects with selected psychotic disorders, and alcoholic beverages should be limited while taking quetiapine).
No products indexed under this heading.

Efavirenz (Co-administration of quetiapine with hepatic enzyme inducers may increase the clearance of quetiapine. Higher doses of quetiapine may be required when co-administered with hepatic enzyme inducers). Products include:
Atripla 906

Enalapril Maleate (Because of its potential for inducing hypotension, quetiapine may enhance the effects of certain antihypertensive agents).
No products indexed under this heading.

Enalaprilat (Because of its potential for inducing hypotension, quetiapine may enhance the effects of certain antihypertensive agents).
No products indexed under this heading.

Enflurane (Given the primary CNS effects of quetiapine, caution should be used when it is taken in combination with other centrally acting drugs. Quetiapine potentiated the cognitive and motor effects of alcohol in a clinical trial in subjects with selected psychotic disorders, and alcoholic beverages should be limited while taking quetiapine).
No products indexed under this heading.

Eprosartan Mesylate (Because of its potential for inducing hypotension, quetiapine may enhance the effects of certain antihypertensive agents). Products include:
Teveten 538
Teveten HCT 541

Erythromycin (Co-administration of quetiapine with hepatic enzyme inducers may increase the clearance of quetiapine. Higher doses of quetiapine may be required when co-administered with hepatic enzyme inducers).
No products indexed under this heading.

Erythromycin, Topical (Co-administration of quetiapine with hepatic enzyme inducers may increase the clearance of quetiapine. Higher doses of quetiapine may be required when co-administered with hepatic enzyme inducers).
No products indexed under this heading.

Erythromycin Estolate (Co-administration of quetiapine with hepatic enzyme inducers may increase the clearance of quetiapine. Higher doses of quetiapine may be required when co-administered with hepatic enzyme inducers).
No products indexed under this heading.

Erythromycin Ethylsuccinate (Co-administration of quetiapine with hepatic enzyme inducers may increase the clearance of quetiapine. Higher doses of quetiapine may be required when co-administered with hepatic enzyme inducers). Products include:
E.E.S. 437
EryPed 435

Erythromycin Gluceptate (Co-administration of quetiapine with hepatic enzyme inducers may increase the clearance of quetiapine. Higher doses of quetiapine may be required when co-administered with hepatic enzyme inducers).
No products indexed under this heading.

Erythromycin Lactobionate (Co-administration of quetiapine with hepatic enzyme inducers may increase the clearance of quetiapine. Higher doses of quetiapine may be required when co-administered with hepatic enzyme inducers).
No products indexed under this heading.

Erythromycin Stearate (Co-administration of quetiapine with hepatic enzyme inducers may increase the clearance of quetiapine. Higher doses of quetiapine may be required when co-administered with hepatic enzyme inducers).
No products indexed under this heading.

Escitalopram Oxalate (Co-administration of quetiapine with hepatic enzyme inducers may increase the clearance of quetiapine. Higher doses of quetiapine may be required when co-administered with hepatic enzyme inducers). Products include:
Lexapro Oral Suspension 1160
Lexapro Tablets 1160

Esmolol Hydrochloride (Because of its potential for inducing hypotension, quetiapine may enhance the effects of certain antihypertensive agents).
No products indexed under this heading.

Esomeprazole Magnesium (Co-administration of quetiapine with hepatic enzyme inducers may increase the clearance of quetiapine. Higher doses of quetiapine may be required when co-administered with hepatic enzyme inducers). Products include:
Nexium Capsules 704
Nexium Oral Suspension 704

Esomeprazole Sodium (Co-administration of quetiapine with hepatic enzyme inducers may increase the clearance of quetiapine. Higher doses of quetiapine may be required when co-administered with hepatic enzyme inducers). Products include:
Nexium I.V. 712

Estazolam (Given the primary CNS effects of quetiapine, caution should be used when it is taken in combination with other centrally acting drugs. Quetiapine potentiated the cognitive and motor effects of alcohol in a clinical trial in subjects with selected psychotic disorders, and alcoholic beverages should be limited while taking quetiapine).
No products indexed under this heading.

Ethanol (Co-administration of quetiapine with hepatic enzyme inducers may increase the clearance of quetiapine. Higher doses of quetiapine may be required when co-administered with hepatic enzyme inducers).
No products indexed under this heading.

Ethchlorvynol (Given the primary CNS effects of quetiapine, caution should be used when it is taken in combination with other centrally acting drugs. Quetiapine potentiated the cognitive and motor effects of alcohol in a clinical trial in subjects with selected psychotic disorders, and alcoholic beverages should be limited while taking quetiapine).
No products indexed under this heading.

Ethinamate (Given the primary CNS effects of quetiapine, caution should be used when it is taken in combination with other centrally acting drugs. Quetiapine potentiated the cognitive and motor effects of alcohol in a clinical trial in subjects with selected psychotic disorders, and alcoholic beverages should be limited while taking quetiapine).
No products indexed under this heading.

Ethosuximide (Co-administration of quetiapine with hepatic enzyme inducers may increase the clearance of quetiapine. Higher doses of quetiapine may be required when co-administered with hepatic enzyme inducers).
No products indexed under this heading.

Ethyl Alcohol (Co-administration of quetiapine with hepatic enzyme inducers may increase the clearance of quetiapine. Higher doses of quetiapine may be required when co-administered with hepatic enzyme inducers).
No products indexed under this heading.

Fat (A high fat meal (approximately 800 to 1000 calories) was found to produce statistically significant increases in the quetiapine C_{max} and AUC of 44% to 52% and 20% to 22%, respectively, for the 50 mg and 300 mg tablets. In comparison, a light meal (approximately 300 calories) had no significant effect on the C_{max} or AUC of quetiapine. It is recommended that quetiapine be taken without food or with a light meal).
No products indexed under this heading.

Felbamate (Co-administration of quetiapine with hepatic enzyme inducers may increase the clearance of quetiapine. Higher doses of quetiapine may be required when co-administered with hepatic enzyme inducers).
No products indexed under this heading.

Felodipine (Because of its potential for inducing hypotension, quetiapine may enhance the effects of certain antihypertensive agents).
No products indexed under this heading.

Fentanyl (Given the primary CNS effects of quetiapine, caution should be used when it is taken in combination with other centrally acting drugs. Quetiapine potentiated the cognitive and motor effects of alcohol in a clinical trial in subjects with selected psychotic disorders, and alcoholic beverages should be limited while taking quetiapine).
Products include:
Duragesic 2604
Fentanyl Transdermal System 2346
Onsolis 2054

Fentanyl Citrate (Given the primary CNS effects of quetiapine, caution should be used when it is taken in combination with other centrally acting drugs. Quetiapine potentiated the cognitive and motor effects of alcohol in a clinical trial in subjects with selected psychotic disorders, and alcoholic beverages should be limited while taking quetiapine). Products include:
Fentora 966

Fluconazole (Co-administration of quetiapine with cytochrome P450 3A inhibitors may decrease the clearance of quetiapine. Caution (reduced dosage) of quetiapine may be necessary when co-administered with other cytochrome P450 3A inhibitors).
No products indexed under this heading.

Fludrocortisone Acetate (Co-administration of quetiapine with hepatic enzyme inducers (eg, glucocorticoids) may increase the clearance of quetiapine. Higher doses of quetiapine may be required when co-administered with hepatic enzyme inducers).
No products indexed under this heading.

Fluoxetine (Co-administration of quetiapine with cytochrome P450 3A inhibitors may decrease the clearance of quetiapine. Caution (reduced dosage) of quetiapine may be necessary when co-administered with other cytochrome P450 3A inhibitors).
No products indexed under this heading.

Fluoxetine Hydrochloride (Co-administration of quetiapine with cytochrome P450 3A inhibitors may decrease the clearance of quetiapine. Caution (reduced dosage) of quetiapine may be necessary when co-administered with other cytochrome P450 3A inhibitors). Products include:
Prozac Weekly 1941
Prozac Pulvules 1941
Symbyax 1965

IMPORTANT NOTE: Always consult each drug listing in the patient's regimen for possible interactions.

Fluphenazine Decanoate (Given the primary CNS effects of quetiapine, caution should be used when it is taken in combination with other centrally acting drugs. Quetiapine potentiated the cognitive and motor effects of alcohol in a clinical trial in subjects with selected psychotic disorders, and alcoholic beverages should be limited while taking quetiapine).
No products indexed under this heading.

Fluphenazine Enanthate (Given the primary CNS effects of quetiapine, caution should be used when it is taken in combination with other centrally acting drugs. Quetiapine potentiated the cognitive and motor effects of alcohol in a clinical trial in subjects with selected psychotic disorders, and alcoholic beverages should be limited while taking quetiapine).
No products indexed under this heading.

Fluphenazine Hydrochloride (Given the primary CNS effects of quetiapine, caution should be used when it is taken in combination with other centrally acting drugs. Quetiapine potentiated the cognitive and motor effects of alcohol in a clinical trial in subjects with selected psychotic disorders, and alcoholic beverages should be limited while taking quetiapine).
No products indexed under this heading.

Flurazepam Hydrochloride (Given the primary CNS effects of quetiapine, caution should be used when it is taken in combination with other centrally acting drugs. Quetiapine potentiated the cognitive and motor effects of alcohol in a clinical trial in subjects with selected psychotic disorders, and alcoholic beverages should be limited while taking quetiapine).
No products indexed under this heading.

Fluvoxamine (Co-administration of quetiapine with hepatic enzyme inducers may increase the clearance of quetiapine. Higher doses of quetiapine may be required when co-administered with hepatic enzyme inducers).
No products indexed under this heading.

Fluvoxamine Maleate (Co-administration of quetiapine with hepatic enzyme inducers may increase the clearance of quetiapine. Higher doses of quetiapine may be required when co-administered with hepatic enzyme inducers).
No products indexed under this heading.

Fosamprenavir Calcium (Co-administration of quetiapine with cytochrome P450 3A inhibitors may decrease the clearance of quetiapine. Caution (reduced dosage) of quetiapine may be necessary when co-administered with other cytochrome P450 3A inhibitors). Products include:
Lexiva Oral Suspension 1558
Lexiva 1558

Fosinopril Sodium (Because of its potential for inducing hypotension, quetiapine may enhance the effects of certain antihypertensive agents).
No products indexed under this heading.

Fosphenytoin (Co-administration of quetiapine (250 mg three times/day) and phenytoin (100 mg three times/day) increased the mean oral clearance of quetiapine by 5-fold. Increased doses of quetiapine may be required to maintain control symptoms of schizophrenia in patients receiving quetiapine and phenytoin. Caution should be taken if phenytoin is withdrawn and replaced with a non-inducer (eg, valproate)).
No products indexed under this heading.

Fosphenytoin Sodium (Co-administration of quetiapine (250 mg three times/day) and phenytoin (100 mg three times/day) increased the mean oral clearance of quetiapine by 5-fold. Increased doses of quetiapine may be required to maintain control symptoms of schizophrenia in patients receiving quetiapine and phenytoin. Caution should be taken if phenytoin is withdrawn and replaced with a non-inducer (eg, valproate)).
No products indexed under this heading.

Furosemide (Because of its potential for inducing hypotension, quetiapine may enhance the effects of certain antihypertensive agents). Products include:
Furosemide 2354

Garlic Extract (Co-administration of quetiapine with hepatic enzyme inducers may increase the clearance of quetiapine. Higher doses of quetiapine may be required when co-administered with hepatic enzyme inducers).
No products indexed under this heading.

Garlic Oil (Co-administration of quetiapine with hepatic enzyme inducers may increase the clearance of quetiapine. Higher doses of quetiapine may be required when co-administered with hepatic enzyme inducers).
No products indexed under this heading.

Glipizide (Co-administration of quetiapine with hepatic enzyme inducers may increase the clearance of quetiapine. Higher doses of quetiapine may be required when co-administered with hepatic enzyme inducers).
No products indexed under this heading.

Glutethimide (Given the primary CNS effects of quetiapine, caution should be used when it is taken in combination with other centrally acting drugs. Quetiapine potentiated the cognitive and motor effects of alcohol in a clinical trial in subjects with selected psychotic disorders, and alcoholic beverages should be limited while taking quetiapine).
No products indexed under this heading.

Glyburide (Co-administration of quetiapine with hepatic enzyme inducers may increase the clearance of quetiapine. Higher doses of quetiapine may be required when co-administered with hepatic enzyme inducers).
No products indexed under this heading.

Glycopyrrolate (Disruption of the body's ability to reduce core body temperature has been atributed to antipsychotic agents. Appropriate care is advised when co-administering quetiapine with agents which may contribute to an elevation in core body temperature such as anticholinergics).
No products indexed under this heading.

Guanabenz Acetate (Because of its potential for inducing hypotension, quetiapine may enhance the effects of certain antihypertensive agents).
No products indexed under this heading.

Guanethidine (Because of its potential for inducing hypotension, quetiapine may enhance the effects of certain antihypertensive agents).
No products indexed under this heading.

Guanethidine Monosulfate (Because of its potential for inducing hypotension, quetiapine may enhance the effects of certain antihypertensive agents).
No products indexed under this heading.

Guanethidine Sulfate (Because of its potential for inducing hypotension, quetiapine may enhance the effects of certain antihypertensive agents).
No products indexed under this heading.

Haloperidol (Given the primary CNS effects of quetiapine, caution should be used when it is taken in combination with other centrally acting drugs. Quetiapine potentiated the cognitive and motor effects of alcohol in a clinical trial in subjects with selected psychotic disorders, and alcoholic beverages should be limited while taking quetiapine).
No products indexed under this heading.

Haloperidol Decanoate (Given the primary CNS effects of quetiapine, caution should be used when it is taken in combination with other centrally acting drugs. Quetiapine potentiated the cognitive and motor effects of alcohol in a clinical trial in subjects with selected psychotic disorders, and alcoholic beverages should be limited while taking quetiapine).
No products indexed under this heading.

Hepatic Enzyme-Inducing Agents (Co-administration of quetiapine with hepatic enzyme inducers may increase the clearance of quetiapine. Higher doses of quetiapine may be required when co-administered with hepatic enzyme inducers).
No products indexed under this heading.

Hexobarbital (Co-administration of quetiapine with hepatic enzyme inducers (eg, barbiturates) may increase the clearance of quetiapine. Higher doses of quetiapine may be required when co-administered with hepatic enzyme inducers).
No products indexed under this heading.

Hydralazine Hydrochloride (Because of its potential for inducing hypotension, quetiapine may enhance the effects of certain antihypertensive agents).
No products indexed under this heading.

Hydrochlorothiazide (Because of its potential for inducing hypotension, quetiapine may enhance the effects of certain antihypertensive agents). Products include:
Atacand HCT 700
Avalide 2956
Benicar HCT 1017
Diovan HCT 2419
Dyazide 1429
Exforge HCT 2449
Hyzaar 2162
Hyzaar 100-12.5 2162
Micardis HCT 889
Prinzide 2246
Tekturna HCT 2541
Teveten HCT 541

Hydrocodone Bitartrate (Given the primary CNS effects of quetiapine, caution should be used when it is taken in combination with other centrally acting drugs. Quetiapine potentiated the cognitive and motor effects of alcohol in a clinical trial in subjects with selected psychotic disorders, and alcoholic beverages should be limited while taking quetiapine). Products include:
Vicodin 560
Vicodin ES 561
Vicodin HP 563
Vicoprofen 564
Zydone 1138

Hydrocodone Polistirex (Given the primary CNS effects of quetiapine, caution should be used when it is taken in combination with other centrally acting drugs. Quetiapine potentiated the cognitive and motor effects of alcohol in a clinical trial in subjects with selected psychotic disorders, and alcoholic beverages should be limited while taking quetiapine). Products include:
Tussionex 3443

Hydrocortisone (Co-administration of quetiapine with hepatic enzyme inducers (eg, glucocorticoids) may increase the clearance of quetiapine. Higher doses of quetiapine may be required when co-administered with hepatic enzyme inducers).
No products indexed under this heading.

Hydrocortisone (Alcohol) (Co-administration of quetiapine with hepatic enzyme inducers may increase the clearance of quetiapine. Higher doses of quetiapine may be required when co-administered with hepatic enzyme inducers).
No products indexed under this heading.

Hydrocortisone Acetate (Co-administration of quetiapine with hepatic enzyme inducers (eg, glucocorticoids) may increase the clearance of quetiapine. Higher doses of quetiapine may be required when co-administered with hepatic enzyme inducers).
No products indexed under this heading.

Hydrocortisone Butyrate (Co-administration of quetiapine with hepatic enzyme inducers may increase the clearance of quetiapine. Higher doses of quetiapine may be required when co-administered with hepatic enzyme inducers).
No products indexed under this heading.

Hydrocortisone Cypionate (Co-administration of quetiapine with hepatic enzyme inducers may increase the clearance of quetiapine. Higher doses of quetiapine may be required when co-administered with hepatic enzyme inducers).
No products indexed under this heading.

Hydrocortisone Hemisuccinate (Co-administration of quetiapine with hepatic enzyme inducers may increase the clearance of quetiapine. Higher doses of quetiapine may be required when co-administered with hepatic enzyme inducers).
No products indexed under this heading.

Hydrocortisone Probutate (Co-administration of quetiapine with hepatic enzyme inducers may increase the clearance of quetiapine. Higher doses of quetiapine may be required when co-administered with hepatic enzyme inducers).
No products indexed under this heading.

Hydrocortisone Sodium Phosphate (Co-administration of quetiapine with hepatic enzyme inducers (eg, glucocorticoids) may increase the clearance of quetiapine. Higher doses of quetiapine may be required when co-administered with hepatic enzyme inducers).
No products indexed under this heading.

Hydrocortisone Sodium Succinate (Co-administration of quetiapine with hepatic enzyme inducers (eg, glucocorticoids) may increase the clearance of quetiapine. Higher doses of quetiapine may be required when co-administered with hepatic enzyme inducers).
No products indexed under this heading.

Hydrocortisone Valerate (Co-administration of quetiapine with hepatic enzyme inducers may increase the clearance of quetiapine. Higher doses of quetiapine may be required when co-administered with hepatic enzyme inducers).
No products indexed under this heading.

Hydroflumethiazide (Because of its potential for inducing hypotension, quetiapine may enhance the effects of certain antihypertensive agents).
No products indexed under this heading.

Hydromorphone Hydrochloride (Given the primary CNS effects of quetiapine, caution should be used when it is taken in combination with other centrally acting drugs. Quetiapine potentiated the cognitive and motor effects of alcohol in a clinical trial in subjects with selected psychotic disorders, and alcoholic beverages should be limited while taking quetiapine). Products include:
Dilaudid Injection 2800
Dilaudid Oral 2797
Dilaudid Tablets 2797
Dilaudid-HP 2800

IMPORTANT NOTE: Always consult each drug listing in the patient's regimen for possible interactions.

(⊙ Described in PDR® for Ophthalmic Medicines)

Moexipril Hydrochloride (Because of its potential for inducing hypotension, quetiapine may enhance the effects of certain antihypertensive agents). No products indexed under this heading.

Molindone Hydrochloride (Given the primary CNS effects of quetiapine, caution should be used when it is taken in combination with other centrally acting drugs. Quetiapine potentiated the cognitive and motor effects of alcohol in a clinical trial in subjects with selected psychotic disorders, and alcoholic beverages should be limited while taking quetiapine). Products include:

Morphine Sulfate (Given the primary CNS effects of quetiapine, caution should be used when it is taken in combination with other centrally acting drugs. Quetiapine potentiated the cognitive and motor effects of alcohol in a clinical trial in subjects with selected psychotic disorders, and alcoholic beverages should be limited while taking quetiapine). Products include:

Nadolol (Because of its potential for inducing hypotension, quetiapine may enhance the effects of certain antihypertensive agents). Products include:

Nafcillin Sodium (Co-administration of quetiapine with hepatic enzyme inducers may increase the clearance of quetiapine. Higher doses of quetiapine may be required when co-administered with hepatic enzyme inducers). No products indexed under this heading.

Nebivolol (Because of its potential for inducing hypotension, quetiapine may enhance the effects of certain antihypertensive agents). Products include:

Nefazodone Hydrochloride (Co-administration of quetiapine with cytochrome P450 3A inhibitors may decrease the clearance of quetiapine. Caution (reduced dosage) of quetiapine may be necessary when co-administered with other cytochrome P450 3A inhibitors). No products indexed under this heading.

Nelfinavir Mesylate (Co-administration of quetiapine with cytochrome P450 3A inhibitors may decrease the clearance of quetiapine. Caution (reduced dosage) of quetiapine may be necessary when co-administered with other cytochrome P450 3A inhibitors). No products indexed under this heading.

Nevirapine (Co-administration of quetiapine with hepatic enzyme inducers may increase the clearance of quetiapine. Higher doses of quetiapine may be required when co-administered with hepatic enzyme inducers). Products include:

Niacin (Co-administration of quetiapine with cytochrome P450 3A inhibitors may decrease the clearance of quetiapine. Caution (reduced dosage) of quetiapine may be necessary when co-administered with other cytochrome P450 3A inhibitors). Products include:

Niacinamide (Co-administration of quetiapine with cytochrome P450 3A inhibitors may decrease the clearance of quetiapine. Caution (reduced dosage) of quetiapine may be necessary when co-administered with other cytochrome P450 3A inhibitors). Products include:

Niacinamide Hydroiodide (Co-administration of quetiapine with cytochrome P450 3A inhibitors may decrease the clearance of quetiapine. Caution (reduced dosage) of quetiapine may be necessary when co-administered with other cytochrome P450 3A inhibitors). No products indexed under this heading.

Nicardipine Hydrochloride (Because of its potential for inducing hypotension, quetiapine may enhance the effects of certain antihypertensive agents). No products indexed under this heading.

Nicotinamide (Co-administration of quetiapine with cytochrome P450 3A inhibitors may decrease the clearance of quetiapine. Caution (reduced dosage) of quetiapine may be necessary when co-administered with other cytochrome P450 3A inhibitors). No products indexed under this heading.

Nicotine (Co-administration of quetiapine with hepatic enzyme inducers may increase the clearance of quetiapine. Higher doses of quetiapine may be required when co-administered with hepatic enzyme inducers). No products indexed under this heading.

Nicotine Polacrilex (Co-administration of quetiapine with hepatic enzyme inducers may increase the clearance of quetiapine. Higher doses of quetiapine may be required when co-administered with hepatic enzyme inducers). No products indexed under this heading.

Nicotine Salicylate (Co-administration of quetiapine with hepatic enzyme inducers may increase the clearance of quetiapine. Higher doses of quetiapine may be required when co-administered with hepatic enzyme inducers). No products indexed under this heading.

Nicotine Sulfate (Co-administration of quetiapine with hepatic enzyme inducers may increase the clearance of quetiapine. Higher doses of quetiapine may be required when co-administered with hepatic enzyme inducers). No products indexed under this heading.

Nifedipine (Because of its potential for inducing hypotension, quetiapine may enhance the effects of certain antihypertensive agents). No products indexed under this heading.

Nisoldipine (Because of its potential for inducing hypotension, quetiapine may enhance the effects of certain antihypertensive agents). No products indexed under this heading.

Nitroglycerin (Because of its potential for inducing hypotension, quetiapine may enhance the effects of certain antihypertensive agents). Products include:

Norethindrone (Co-administration of quetiapine with hepatic enzyme inducers may increase the clearance of quetiapine. Higher doses of quetiapine may be required when co-administered with hepatic enzyme inducers). Products include:

Norethindrone Acetate (Co-administration of quetiapine with hepatic enzyme inducers may increase the clearance of quetiapine. Higher doses of quetiapine may be required when co-administered with hepatic enzyme inducers). Products include:

Norfloxacin (Co-administration of quetiapine with cytochrome P450 3A inhibi-

tors may decrease the clearance of quetiapine. Caution (reduced dosage) of quetiapine may be necessary when co-administered with other cytochrome P450 3A inhibitors). Products include:

Olanzapine (Given the primary CNS effects of quetiapine, caution should be used when it is taken in combination with other centrally acting drugs. Quetiapine potentiated the cognitive and motor effects of alcohol in a clinical trial in subjects with selected psychotic disorders, and alcoholic beverages should be limited while taking quetiapine). Products include:

Omeprazole (Co-administration of quetiapine with hepatic enzyme inducers may increase the clearance of quetiapine. Higher doses of quetiapine may be required when co-administered with hepatic enzyme inducers). No products indexed under this heading.

Omeprazole Magnesium (Co-administration of quetiapine with hepatic enzyme inducers may increase the clearance of quetiapine. Higher doses of quetiapine may be required when co-administered with hepatic enzyme inducers). No products indexed under this heading.

Oxazepam (Given the primary CNS effects of quetiapine, caution should be used when it is taken in combination with other centrally acting drugs. Quetiapine potentiated the cognitive and motor effects of alcohol in a clinical trial in subjects with selected psychotic disorders, and alcoholic beverages should be limited while taking quetiapine). No products indexed under this heading.

Oxcarbazepine (Co-administration of quetiapine with hepatic enzyme inducers may increase the clearance of quetiapine. Higher doses of quetiapine may be required when co-administered with hepatic enzyme inducers). No products indexed under this heading.

Oxybutynin Chloride (Disruption of the body's ability to reduce core body temperature has been attributed to antipsychotic agents. Appropriate care is advised when co-administering quetiapine with agents which may contribute to an elevation in core body temperature such as anticholinergics). No products indexed under this heading.

Oxycodone Hydrochloride (Given the primary CNS effects of quetiapine, caution should be used when it is taken in combination with other centrally acting drugs. Quetiapine potentiated the cognitive and motor effects of alcohol in a clinical trial in subjects with selected psychotic disorders, and alcoholic beverages should be limited while taking quetiapine). Products include:

Paroxetine Hydrochloride (Co-administration of quetiapine with cytochrome P450 3A inhibitors may decrease the clearance of quetiapine. Caution (reduced dosage) of quetiapine may be necessary when co-administered with other cytochrome P450 3A inhibitors). Products include:

Pemoline (Given the primary CNS effects of quetiapine, caution should be used when it is taken in combination with other centrally acting drugs. Quetiapine potentiated the cognitive and motor effects of alcohol in a clinical trial in subjects with selected psychotic disorders, and alcoholic beverages should be limited while taking quetiapine). No products indexed under this heading.

Penbutolol Sulfate (Because of its potential for inducing hypotension, quetiapine may enhance the effects of certain antihypertensive agents). No products indexed under this heading.

Pentobarbital (Co-administration of quetiapine with hepatic enzyme inducers (eg, barbiturates) may increase the clearance of quetiapine. Higher doses of quetiapine may be required when co-administered with hepatic enzyme inducers). No products indexed under this heading.

Pentobarbital Sodium (Co-administration of quetiapine with hepatic enzyme inducers (eg, barbiturates) may increase the clearance of quetiapine. Higher doses of quetiapine may be required when co-administered with hepatic enzyme inducers). Products include:

Pergolide Mesylate (Quetiapine may antagonize the effects of dopamine agonists). No products indexed under this heading.

Perindopril Erbumine (Because of its potential for inducing hypotension, quetiapine may enhance the effects of certain antihypertensive agents). No products indexed under this heading.

Perphenazine (Given the primary CNS effects of quetiapine, caution should be used when it is taken in combination with other centrally acting drugs. Quetiapine potentiated the cognitive and motor effects of alcohol in a clinical trial in subjects with selected psychotic disorders, and alcoholic beverages should be limited while taking quetiapine). No products indexed under this heading.

Phenobarbital (Co-administration of quetiapine with hepatic enzyme inducers (eg, barbiturates) may increase the clearance of quetiapine. Higher doses of quetiapine may be required when co-administered with hepatic enzyme inducers). Products include:

Phenobarbital Sodium (Co-administration of quetiapine with hepatic enzyme inducers (eg, barbiturates) may increase the clearance of quetiapine. Higher doses of quetiapine may be required when co-administered with hepatic enzyme inducers). No products indexed under this heading.

Phenoxybenzamine Hydrochloride (Because of its potential for inducing hypotension, quetiapine may enhance the effects of certain antihypertensive agents). Products include:

Phentolamine Mesylate (Because of its potential for inducing hypotension, quetiapine may enhance the effects of certain antihypertensive agents). No products indexed under this heading.

Phenylbutazone (Co-administration of quetiapine with hepatic enzyme inducers may increase the clearance of quetiapine. Higher doses of quetiapine may be required when co-administered with hepatic enzyme inducers). No products indexed under this heading.

Phenytoin (Co-administration of quetiapine (250 mg three times/day) and phenytoin (100 mg three times/day) increased the mean oral clearance of quetiapine by 5-fold. Increased doses of

quetiapine may be required to maintain control symptoms of schizophrenia in patients receiving quetiapine and phenytoin. Caution should be taken if phenytoin is withdrawn and replaced with a non-inducer (eg, valproate)).
No products indexed under this heading.

Phenytoin Sodium (Co-administration of quetiapine (250 mg three times/day) and phenytoin (100 mg three times/day) increased the mean oral clearance of quetiapine by 5-fold. Increased doses of quetiapine may be required to maintain control symptoms of schizophrenia in patients receiving quetiapine and phenytoin. Caution should be taken if phenytoin is withdrawn and replaced with a non-inducer (eg, valproate)). Products include:
Phenytek Capsules **2380**

Pindolol (Because of its potential for inducing hypotension, quetiapine may enhance the effects of certain antihypertensive agents).
No products indexed under this heading.

Polythiazide (Because of its potential for inducing hypotension, quetiapine may enhance the effects of certain antihypertensive agents).
No products indexed under this heading.

Posaconazole (Co-administration of quetiapine with cytochrome P450 3A inhibitors may decrease the clearance of quetiapine. Caution (reduced dosage) of quetiapine may be necessary when co-administered with other cytochrome P450 3A inhibitors). Products include:
Noxafil **3172**

Pramipexole Dihydrochloride (Quetiapine may antagonize the effects of dopamine agonists).
No products indexed under this heading.

Prazepam (Given the primary CNS effects of quetiapine, caution should be used when it is taken in combination with other centrally acting drugs. Quetiapine potentiated the cognitive and motor effects of alcohol in a clinical trial in subjects with selected psychotic disorders, and alcoholic beverages should be limited while taking quetiapine).
No products indexed under this heading.

Prazosin Hydrochloride (Because of its potential for inducing hypotension, quetiapine may enhance the effects of certain antihypertensive agents).
No products indexed under this heading.

Prednisolone (Co-administration of quetiapine with hepatic enzyme inducers may increase the clearance of quetiapine. Higher doses of quetiapine may be required when co-administered with hepatic enzyme inducers).
No products indexed under this heading.

Prednisolone Acetate (Co-administration of quetiapine with hepatic enzyme inducers (eg, glucocorticoids) may increase the clearance of quetiapine. Higher doses of quetiapine may be required when co-administered with hepatic enzyme inducers).
Products include:
Blephamide .... ⊙**212**, ⊙**214**
Pred Forte .... ⊙**225**
Pred Mild .... ⊙**230**
Pred-G .... ⊙**226**, ⊙**227**

Prednisolone Sodium Phosphate (Co-administration of quetiapine with hepatic enzyme inducers (eg, glucocorticoids) may increase the clearance of quetiapine. Higher doses of quetiapine may be required when co-administered with hepatic enzyme inducers).
No products indexed under this heading.

Prednisolone Tebutate (Co-administration of quetiapine with hepatic enzyme inducers (eg, glucocorticoids) may increase the clearance of quetiapine. Higher doses of quetiapine may be required when co-administered with hepatic enzyme inducers).
No products indexed under this heading.

Prednisone (Co-administration of quetiapine with hepatic enzyme inducers (eg, glucocorticoids) may increase the clearance of quetiapine. Higher doses of quetiapine may be required when co-administered with hepatic enzyme inducers).
No products indexed under this heading.

Prednisone sodium phosphate (Co-administration of quetiapine with hepatic enzyme inducers may increase the clearance of quetiapine. Higher doses of quetiapine may be required when co-administered with hepatic enzyme inducers).
No products indexed under this heading.

Primidone (Co-administration of quetiapine with hepatic enzyme inducers may increase the clearance of quetiapine. Higher doses of quetiapine may be required when co-administered with hepatic enzyme inducers).
No products indexed under this heading.

Prochlorperazine (Given the primary CNS effects of quetiapine, caution should be used when it is taken in combination with other centrally acting drugs. Quetiapine potentiated the cognitive and motor effects of alcohol in a clinical trial in subjects with selected psychotic disorders, and alcoholic beverages should be limited while taking quetiapine).
No products indexed under this heading.

Procyclidine Hydrochloride (Disruption of the body's ability to reduce core body temperature has been atributed to antipsychotic agents. Appropriate care is advised when co-administering quetiapine with agents which may contribute to an elevation in core body temperature such as anticholinergics).
No products indexed under this heading.

Promethazine Hydrochloride (Given the primary CNS effects of quetiapine, caution should be used when it is taken in combination with other centrally acting drugs. Quetiapine potentiated the cognitive and motor effects of alcohol in a clinical trial in subjects with selected psychotic disorders, and alcoholic beverages should be limited while taking quetiapine).
No products indexed under this heading.

Propantheline Bromide (Disruption of the body's ability to reduce core body temperature has been atributed to antipsychotic agents. Appropriate care is advised when co-administering quetiapine with agents which may contribute to an elevation in core body temperature such as anticholinergics).
No products indexed under this heading.

Propofol (Given the primary CNS effects of quetiapine, caution should be used when it is taken in combination with other centrally acting drugs. Quetiapine potentiated the cognitive and motor effects of alcohol in a clinical trial in subjects with selected psychotic disorders, and alcoholic beverages should be limited while taking quetiapine).
No products indexed under this heading.

Propoxyphene Hydrochloride (Given the primary CNS effects of quetiapine, caution should be used when it is taken in combination with other centrally acting drugs. Quetiapine potentiated the cognitive and motor effects of alcohol in a clinical trial in subjects with selected psychotic disorders, and alcoholic beverages should be limited while taking quetiapine).
No products indexed under this heading.

Propoxyphene Napsylate (Given the primary CNS effects of quetiapine, caution should be used when it is taken in combination with other centrally acting drugs. Quetiapine potentiated the cognitive and motor effects of alcohol in a clinical trial in subjects with selected psychotic disorders, and alcoholic beverages should be limited while taking quetiapine).
No products indexed under this heading.

Propranolol Hydrochloride (Because of its potential for inducing hypotension, quetiapine may enhance the effects of certain antihypertensive agents). Products include:
InnoPran XL **1517**

Quazepam (Given the primary CNS effects of quetiapine, caution should be used when it is taken in combination with other centrally acting drugs. Quetiapine potentiated the cognitive and motor effects of alcohol in a clinical trial in subjects with selected psychotic disorders, and alcoholic beverages should be limited while taking quetiapine).
No products indexed under this heading.

Quinapril Hydrochloride (Because of its potential for inducing hypotension, quetiapine may enhance the effects of certain antihypertensive agents).
No products indexed under this heading.

Quinidine (Co-administration of quetiapine with cytochrome P450 3A inhibitors may decrease the clearance of quetiapine. Caution (reduced dosage) of quetiapine may be necessary when co-administered with other cytochrome P450 3A inhibitors).
No products indexed under this heading.

Quinidine Hydrochloride (Co-administration of quetiapine with cytochrome P450 3A inhibitors may decrease the clearance of quetiapine. Caution (reduced dosage) of quetiapine may be necessary when co-administered with other cytochrome P450 3A inhibitors).
No products indexed under this heading.

Quinidine Polygalacturonate (Co-administration of quetiapine with cytochrome P450 3A inhibitors may decrease the clearance of quetiapine. Caution (reduced dosage) of quetiapine may be necessary when co-administered with other cytochrome P450 3A inhibitors).
No products indexed under this heading.

Quinidine Sulfate (Co-administration of quetiapine with cytochrome P450 3A inhibitors may decrease the clearance of quetiapine. Caution (reduced dosage) of quetiapine may be necessary when co-administered with other cytochrome P450 3A inhibitors).
No products indexed under this heading.

Quinine (Co-administration of quetiapine with cytochrome P450 3A inhibitors may decrease the clearance of quetiapine. Caution (reduced dosage) of quetiapine may be necessary when co-administered with other cytochrome P450 3A inhibitors). Products include:
Hyland's Leg Cramps PM with Quinine **3315**

Quinine Sulfate (Co-administration of quetiapine with cytochrome P450 3A inhibitors may decrease the clearance of quetiapine. Caution (reduced dosage) of quetiapine may be necessary when co-administered with other cytochrome P450 3A inhibitors).
No products indexed under this heading.

Quinupristin (Co-administration of quetiapine with cytochrome P450 3A inhibitors may decrease the clearance of quetiapine. Caution (reduced dosage) of quetiapine may be necessary when co-administered with other cytochrome P450 3A inhibitors).
No products indexed under this heading.

Ramipril (Because of its potential for inducing hypotension, quetiapine may enhance the effects of certain antihypertensive agents).
No products indexed under this heading.

Ranitidine Bismuth Citrate (Co-administration of quetiapine with cytochrome P450 3A inhibitors may decrease the clearance of quetiapine. Caution (reduced dosage) of quetiapine may be necessary when co-administered with other cytochrome P450 3A inhibitors).
No products indexed under this heading.

Ranitidine Hydrochloride (Co-administration of quetiapine with cytochrome P450 3A inhibitors may decrease the clearance of quetiapine. Caution (reduced dosage) of quetiapine may be necessary when co-administered with other cytochrome P450 3A inhibitors). Products include:
Zantac **1737**
Zantac Injection **1732**
Zantac Pharmacy **1735**

Rauwolfia Serpentina (Because of its potential for inducing hypotension, quetiapine may enhance the effects of certain antihypertensive agents).
No products indexed under this heading.

Remifentanil Hydrochloride (Given the primary CNS effects of quetiapine, caution should be used when it is taken in combination with other centrally acting drugs. Quetiapine potentiated the cognitive and motor effects of alcohol in a clinical trial in subjects with selected psychotic disorders, and alcoholic beverages should be limited while taking quetiapine).
No products indexed under this heading.

Rescinnamine (Because of its potential for inducing hypotension, quetiapine may enhance the effects of certain antihypertensive agents).
No products indexed under this heading.

Reserpine (Because of its potential for inducing hypotension, quetiapine may enhance the effects of certain antihypertensive agents).
No products indexed under this heading.

Rifabutin (Co-administration of quetiapine with hepatic enzyme inducers may increase the clearance of quetiapine. Higher doses of quetiapine may be required when co-administered with hepatic enzyme inducers).
No products indexed under this heading.

Rifampicin (Co-administration of quetiapine with hepatic enzyme inducers may increase the clearance of quetiapine. Higher doses of quetiapine may be required when co-administered with hepatic enzyme inducers).
No products indexed under this heading.

Rifampin (Co-administration of quetiapine with hepatic enzyme inducers may increase the clearance of quetiapine. Higher doses of quetiapine may be required when co-administered with hepatic enzyme inducers).
No products indexed under this heading.

Rifapentine (Co-administration of quetiapine with hepatic enzyme inducers may increase the clearance of quetiapine. Higher doses of quetiapine may be required when co-administered with hepatic enzyme inducers).
No products indexed under this heading.

Risperidone (Given the primary CNS effects of quetiapine, caution should be used when it is taken in combination with other centrally acting drugs. Quetiapine potentiated the cognitive and motor effects of alcohol in a clinical trial in subjects with selected psychotic disorders, and alcoholic beverages should be limited while taking quetiapine).
Products include:
Risperdal Consta **2682**

(⊙ Described in PDR® for Ophthalmic Medicines)

1741 Interactions Index Seroquel XR

Ritonavir (Co-administration of quetiapine with hepatic enzyme inducers may increase the clearance of quetiapine. Higher doses of quetiapine may be required when co-administered with hepatic enzyme inducers). Products include:
Kaletra 458
Norvir 509

Ropinirole Hydrochloride (Quetiapine may antagonize the effects of dopamine agonists). Products include:
Requip 1620
Requip XL 1628

Saquinavir (Co-administration of quetiapine with cytochrome P450 3A inhibitors may decrease the clearance of quetiapine. Caution (reduced dosage) of quetiapine may be necessary when co-administered with other cytochrome P450 3A inhibitors).
No products indexed under this heading.

Saquinavir Mesylate (Co-administration of quetiapine with cytochrome P450 3A inhibitors may decrease the clearance of quetiapine. Caution (reduced dosage) of quetiapine may be necessary when co-administered with other cytochrome P450 3A inhibitors).
No products indexed under this heading.

Scopolamine (Disruption of the body's ability to reduce core body temperature has been atributed to antipsychotic agents. Appropriate care is advised when co-administering quetiapine with agents which may contribute to an elevation in core body temperature such as anticholinergics). Products include:
Transderm Scōp 2397

Scopolamine Hydrobromide (Disruption of the body's ability to reduce core body temperature has been atributed to antipsychotic agents. Appropriate care is advised when co-administering quetiapine with agents which may contribute to an elevation in core body temperature such as anticholinergics). Products include:
Donnatal 2711

Secobarbital Sodium (Co-administration of quetiapine with hepatic enzyme inducers (eg, barbiturates) may increase the clearance of quetiapine. Higher doses of quetiapine may be required when co-administered with hepatic enzyme inducers).
No products indexed under this heading.

Sertraline Hydrochloride (Co-administration of quetiapine with cytochrome P450 3A inhibitors may decrease the clearance of quetiapine. Caution (reduced dosage) of quetiapine may be necessary when co-administered with other cytochrome P450 3A inhibitors).
No products indexed under this heading.

Sevoflurane (Given the primary CNS effects of quetiapine, caution should be used when it is taken in combination with other centrally acting drugs. Quetiapine potentiated the cognitive and motor effects of alcohol in a clinical trial in subjects with selected psychotic disorders, and alcoholic beverages should be limited while taking quetiapine). Products include:
Ultane 554

Sildenafil Citrate (Co-administration of quetiapine with cytochrome P450 3A inhibitors may decrease the clearance of quetiapine. Caution (reduced dosage) of quetiapine may be necessary when co-administered with other cytochrome P450 3A inhibitors).
No products indexed under this heading.

Sodium Butabarbital (Co-administration of quetiapine with hepatic enzyme inducers (eg, barbiturates) may increase the clearance of quetiapine. Higher doses of quetiapine may be required when co-administered with hepatic enzyme inducers).
No products indexed under this heading.

Sodium Nitroprusside (Because of its potential for inducing hypotension, quetiapine may enhance the effects of certain antihypertensive agents).
No products indexed under this heading.

Sodium Oxybate (Given the primary CNS effects of quetiapine, caution should be used when it is taken in combination with other centrally acting drugs. Quetiapine potentiated the cognitive and motor effects of alcohol in a clinical trial in subjects with selected psychotic disorders, and alcoholic beverages should be limited while taking quetiapine).
No products indexed under this heading.

Sodium Pentobarbital (Co-administration of quetiapine with hepatic enzyme inducers (eg, barbiturates) may increase the clearance of quetiapine. Higher doses of quetiapine may be required when co-administered with hepatic enzyme inducers).
No products indexed under this heading.

Sotalol Hydrochloride (Because of its potential for inducing hypotension, quetiapine may enhance the effects of certain antihypertensive agents).
No products indexed under this heading.

Spirapril Hydrochloride (Because of its potential for inducing hypotension, quetiapine may enhance the effects of certain antihypertensive agents).
No products indexed under this heading.

Sufentanil Citrate (Given the primary CNS effects of quetiapine, caution should be used when it is taken in combination with other centrally acting drugs. Quetiapine potentiated the cognitive and motor effects of alcohol in a clinical trial in subjects with selected psychotic disorders, and alcoholic beverages should be limited while taking quetiapine).
No products indexed under this heading.

Sulfinpyrazone (Quetiapine oral clearance is increased by the prototype cytochrome P450 3A4 inducer phenytoin. Dose adjustment of quetiapine is necessary. Higher maintenance doses of quetiapine may be required when it is co-administered with other enzyme inducers such as carbamazepine and phenobarbital).
No products indexed under this heading.

Telithromycin (Co-administration of quetiapine with cytochrome P450 3A inhibitors may decrease the clearance of quetiapine. Caution (reduced dosage) of quetiapine may be necessary when co-administered with other cytochrome P450 3A inhibitors). Products include:
Ketek 2991

Telmisartan (Because of its potential for inducing hypotension, quetiapine may enhance the effects of certain antihypertensive agents). Products include:
Micardis 887
Micardis HCT 889

Temazepam (Given the primary CNS effects of quetiapine, caution should be used when it is taken in combination with other centrally acting drugs. Quetiapine potentiated the cognitive and motor effects of alcohol in a clinical trial in subjects with selected psychotic disorders, and alcoholic beverages should be limited while taking quetiapine).
No products indexed under this heading.

Terazosin Hydrochloride (Because of its potential for inducing hypotension, quetiapine may enhance the effects of certain antihypertensive agents).
No products indexed under this heading.

Theophyllinate (Quetiapine oral clearance is increased by the prototype cytochrome P450 3A4 inducer phenytoin. Dose adjustment of quetiapine is necessary. Higher maintenance doses of quetiapine may be required when it is co-administered with other enzyme inducers such as carbamazepine and phenobarbital).
No products indexed under this heading.

Theophylline (Co-administration of quetiapine with hepatic enzyme inducers may increase the clearance of quetiapine. Higher doses of quetiapine may be required when co-administered with hepatic enzyme inducers).
No products indexed under this heading.

Theophylline Anhydrous (Co-administration of quetiapine with hepatic enzyme inducers may increase the clearance of quetiapine. Higher doses of quetiapine may be required when co-administered with hepatic enzyme inducers). Products include:
Uniphyl 2817

Theophylline Calcium Salicylate (Co-administration of quetiapine with hepatic enzyme inducers may increase the clearance of quetiapine. Higher doses of quetiapine may be required when co-administered with hepatic enzyme inducers).
No products indexed under this heading.

Theophylline Dihydroxypropyl (Glyceryl) (Co-administration of quetiapine with hepatic enzyme inducers may increase the clearance of quetiapine. Higher doses of quetiapine may be required when co-administered with hepatic enzyme inducers).
No products indexed under this heading.

Theophylline Ethylenediamine (Co-administration of quetiapine with hepatic enzyme inducers may increase the clearance of quetiapine. Higher doses of quetiapine may be required when co-administered with hepatic enzyme inducers).
No products indexed under this heading.

Theophylline Sodium Glycinate (Co-administration of quetiapine with hepatic enzyme inducers may increase the clearance of quetiapine. Higher doses of quetiapine may be required when co-administered with hepatic enzyme inducers).
No products indexed under this heading.

Thiamylal Sodium (Co-administration of quetiapine with hepatic enzyme inducers (eg, barbiturates) may increase the clearance of quetiapine. Higher doses of quetiapine may be required when co-administered with hepatic enzyme inducers).
No products indexed under this heading.

Thioridazine (Thioridazine (200 mg twice daily) increased the oral clearance of quetiapine (300 mg twice daily) by 65%).
No products indexed under this heading.

Thioridazine Hydrochloride (Thioridazine (200 mg twice daily) increased the oral clearance of quetiapine (300 mg twice daily) by 65%). Products include:
Thioridazine Hydrochloride 2384

Thiothixene (Given the primary CNS effects of quetiapine, caution should be used when it is taken in combination with other centrally acting drugs. Quetiapine potentiated the cognitive and motor effects of alcohol in a clinical trial in subjects with selected psychotic disorders, and alcoholic beverages should be limited while taking quetiapine). Products include:
Thiothixene 2386

Timolol Maleate (Because of its potential for inducing hypotension, quetiapine may enhance the effects of certain antihypertensive agents). Products include:
Combigan 601
Dorzolamide Hydrochloride/Timolol Maleate Ophthalmic Solution .... ⊙243
Timoptic in Ocudose .... ⊙231

Tobacco (Co-administration of quetiapine with hepatic enzyme inducers may increase the clearance of quetiapine. Higher doses of quetiapine may be required when co-administered with hepatic enzyme inducers).
No products indexed under this heading.

Tolazamide (Co-administration of quetiapine with hepatic enzyme inducers may increase the clearance of quetiapine. Higher doses of quetiapine may be required when co-administered with hepatic enzyme inducers).
No products indexed under this heading.

Tolbutamide (Co-administration of quetiapine with hepatic enzyme inducers may increase the clearance of quetiapine. Higher doses of quetiapine may be required when co-administered with hepatic enzyme inducers).
No products indexed under this heading.

Tolterodine Tartrate (Disruption of the body's ability to reduce core body temperature has been atributed to antipsychotic agents. Appropriate care is advised when co-administering quetiapine with agents which may contribute to an elevation in core body temperature such as anticholinergics).
No products indexed under this heading.

Torsemide (Because of its potential for inducing hypotension, quetiapine may enhance the effects of certain antihypertensive agents).
No products indexed under this heading.

Trandolapril (Because of its potential for inducing hypotension, quetiapine may enhance the effects of certain antihypertensive agents). Products include:
Mavik 489
Tarka 534

Triamcinolone (Co-administration of quetiapine with hepatic enzyme inducers (eg, glucocorticoids) may increase the clearance of quetiapine. Higher doses of quetiapine may be required when co-administered with hepatic enzyme inducers).
No products indexed under this heading.

Triamcinolone Acetonide (Co-administration of quetiapine with hepatic enzyme inducers (eg, glucocorticoids) may increase the clearance of quetiapine. Higher doses of quetiapine may be required when co-administered with hepatic enzyme inducers). Products include:
Azmacort 408
Nasacort AQ 3019

Triamcinolone Diacetate (Co-administration of quetiapine with hepatic enzyme inducers (eg, glucocorticoids) may increase the clearance of quetiapine. Higher doses of quetiapine may be required when co-administered with hepatic enzyme inducers).
No products indexed under this heading.

Triamcinolone Hexacetonide (Co-administration of quetiapine with hepatic enzyme inducers (eg, glucocorticoids) may increase the clearance of quetiapine. Higher doses of quetiapine may be required when co-administered with hepatic enzyme inducers).
No products indexed under this heading.

IMPORTANT NOTE: Always consult each drug listing in the patient's regimen for possible interactions.

Triazolam (Given the primary CNS effects of quetiapine, caution should be used when it is taken in combination with other centrally acting drugs. Quetiapine potentiated the cognitive and motor effects of alcohol in a clinical trial in subjects with selected psychotic disorders, and alcoholic beverages should be limited while taking quetiapine).
No products indexed under this heading.

Tridihexethyl Chloride (Disruption of the body's ability to reduce core body temperature has been atributed to antipsychotic agents. Appropriate care is advised when co-administering quetiapine with agents which may contribute to an elevation in core body temperature such as anticholinergics).
No products indexed under this heading.

Trifluoperazine Hydrochloride (Given the primary CNS effects of quetiapine, caution should be used when it is taken in combination with other centrally acting drugs. Quetiapine potentiated the cognitive and motor effects of alcohol in a clinical trial in subjects with selected psychotic disorders, and alcoholic beverages should be limited while taking quetiapine).
No products indexed under this heading.

Trihexyphenidyl Hydrochloride (Disruption of the body's ability to reduce core body temperature has been atributed to antipsychotic agents. Appropriate care is advised when co-administering quetiapine with agents which may contribute to an elevation in core body temperature such as anticholinergics).
No products indexed under this heading.

Trimethaphan Camsylate (Because of its potential for inducing hypotension, quetiapine may enhance the effects of certain antihypertensive agents).
No products indexed under this heading.

Troglitazone (Co-administration of quetiapine with hepatic enzyme inducers may increase the clearance of quetiapine. Higher doses of quetiapine may be required when co-administered with hepatic enzyme inducers).
No products indexed under this heading.

Troleandomycin (Co-administration of quetiapine with cytochrome P450 3A inhibitors may decrease the clearance of quetiapine. Caution (reduced dosage) of quetiapine may be necessary when co-administered with other cytochrome P450 3A inhibitors).
No products indexed under this heading.

Valproate Sodium (Co-administration of quetiapine with cytochrome P450 3A inhibitors may decrease the clearance of quetiapine. Caution (reduced dosage) of quetiapine may be necessary when co-administered with other cytochrome P450 3A inhibitors).
No products indexed under this heading.

Valproic Acid (The mean maximum concentration and extent of absorption of total and free valproic acid at steady-state were decreased by 10 to 12% when divalproex (500 mg twice daily) was administered with quetiapine (150 mg twice daily). The mean oral clearance of total valproic acid (administered as divalproex 500 mg twice daily) was increased by 11% in the presence of quetiapine (150 mg twice daily). The changes were not significant).
No products indexed under this heading.

Valsartan (Because of its potential for inducing hypotension, quetiapine may enhance the effects of certain antihypertensive agents). Products include:

Vardenafil Hydrochloride (Co-administration of quetiapine with cytochrome P450 3A inhibitors may decrease the clearance of quetiapine. Caution (reduced dosage) of quetiapine may be necessary when co-administered with other cytochrome P450 3A inhibitors). Products include:

Verapamil Hydrochloride (Because of its potential for inducing hypotension, quetiapine may enhance the effects of certain antihypertensive agents). Products include:

Voriconazole (Co-administration of quetiapine with cytochrome P450 3A inhibitors may decrease the clearance of quetiapine. Caution (reduced dosage) of quetiapine may be necessary when co-administered with other cytochrome P450 3A inhibitors).
No products indexed under this heading.

Zafirlukast (Co-administration of quetiapine with cytochrome P450 3A inhibitors may decrease the clearance of quetiapine. Caution (reduced dosage) of quetiapine may be necessary when co-administered with other cytochrome P450 3A inhibitors). Products include:

Zaleplon (Given the primary CNS effects of quetiapine, caution should be used when it is taken in combination with other centrally acting drugs. Quetiapine potentiated the cognitive and motor effects of alcohol in a clinical trial in subjects with selected psychotic disorders, and alcoholic beverages should be limited while taking quetiapine).
No products indexed under this heading.

Zileuton (Co-administration of quetiapine with cytochrome P450 3A inhibitors may decrease the clearance of quetiapine. Caution (reduced dosage) of quetiapine may be necessary when co-administered with other cytochrome P450 3A inhibitors).
No products indexed under this heading.

Ziprasidone Hydrochloride (Given the primary CNS effects of quetiapine, caution should be used when it is taken in combination with other centrally acting drugs. Quetiapine potentiated the cognitive and motor effects of alcohol in a clinical trial in subjects with selected psychotic disorders, and alcoholic beverages should be limited while taking quetiapine). Products include:

Zolpidem Tartrate (Given the primary CNS effects of quetiapine, caution should be used when it is taken in combination with other centrally acting drugs. Quetiapine potentiated the cognitive and motor effects of alcohol in a clinical trial in subjects with selected psychotic disorders, and alcoholic beverages should be limited while taking quetiapine). Products include:

Food Interactions

Alcohol (Given the primary CNS effects of quetiapine, caution should be used when it is taken in combination with other centrally acting drugs. Quetiapine potentiated the cognitive and motor effects of alcohol in a clinical trial in subjects with selected psychotic disorders, and alcoholic beverages should be limited while taking quetiapine).

Beer, reduced-alcohol (Given the primary CNS effects of quetiapine, caution should be used when it is taken in combination with other centrally acting drugs. Quetiapine potentiated the cognitive and motor effects of alcohol in a clinical trial in subjects with selected psychotic disorders, and alcoholic beverages should be limited while taking quetiapine).

Beer, unspecified (Given the primary CNS effects of quetiapine, caution should be used when it is taken in combination with other centrally acting drugs. Quetiapine potentiated the cognitive and motor effects of alcohol in a clinical trial in subjects with selected psychotic disorders, and alcoholic beverages should be limited while taking quetiapine).

Broccoli (Co-administration of quetiapine with hepatic enzyme inducers may increase the clearance of quetiapine. Higher doses of quetiapine may be required when co-administered with hepatic enzyme inducers).

Brussel Sprouts (Co-administration of quetiapine with hepatic enzyme inducers may increase the clearance of quetiapine. Higher doses of quetiapine may be required when co-administered with hepatic enzyme inducers).

Charbroiled Food (Co-administration of quetiapine with hepatic enzyme inducers may increase the clearance of quetiapine. Higher doses of quetiapine may be required when co-administered with hepatic enzyme inducers).

Food, unspecified (A high fat meal (approximately 800 to 1000 calories) was found to produce statistically significant increases in the quetiapine C_{max} and AUC of 44% to 52% and 20% to 22%, respectively, for the 50 mg and 300 mg tablets. In comparison, a light meal (approximately 300 calories) had no significant effect on the C_{max} or AUC of quetiapine. It is recommended that quetiapine be taken without food or with a light meal).

Grapefruit (Co-administration of quetiapine with cytochrome P450 3A inhibitors may decrease the clearance of quetiapine. Caution (reduced dosage) of quetiapine may be necessary when co-administered with other cytochrome P450 3A inhibitors).

Grapefruit Juice (Co-administration of quetiapine with cytochrome P450 3A inhibitors may decrease the clearance of quetiapine. Caution (reduced dosage) of quetiapine may be necessary when co-administered with other cytochrome P450 3A inhibitors).

Meal, unspecified (A high fat meal (approximately 800 to 1000 calories) was found to produce statistically significant increases in the quetiapine C_{max} and AUC of 44% to 52% and 20% to 22%, respectively, for the 50 mg and 300 mg tablets. In comparison, a light meal (approximately 300 calories) had no significant effect on the C_{max} or AUC of quetiapine. It is recommended that quetiapine be taken without food or with a light meal).

Wine, Chianti (Given the primary CNS effects of quetiapine, caution should be used when it is taken in combination with other centrally acting drugs. Quetiapine potentiated the cognitive and motor effects of alcohol in a clinical trial in subjects with selected psychotic disorders, and alcoholic beverages should be limited while taking quetiapine).

Wine, Red (Given the primary CNS effects of quetiapine, caution should be used when it is taken in combination with other centrally acting drugs. Quetiapine potentiated the cognitive and motor effects of alcohol in a clinical trial in subjects with selected psychotic disorders, and alcoholic beverages should be limited while taking quetiapine).

Wine, unspecified (Given the primary CNS effects of quetiapine, caution should be used when it is taken in combination with other centrally acting drugs.

Quetiapine potentiated the cognitive and motor effects of alcohol in a clinical trial in subjects with selected psychotic disorders, and alcoholic beverages should be limited while taking quetiapine).

Wine products (Given the primary CNS effects of quetiapine, caution should be used when it is taken in combination with other centrally acting drugs. Quetiapine potentiated the cognitive and motor effects of alcohol in a clinical trial in subjects with selected psychotic disorders, and alcoholic beverages should be limited while taking quetiapine).

SIMCOR TABLETS
(Niacin, Simvastatin) **524**
May interact with antihypertensives, aspirin-acetylsalicylic acid, bile acid sequestering agents, cytochrome p450 3a4 inhibitors (selected), fibrates, oral anticoagulants, and certain other agents. Compounds in these categories include:

Acebutolol Hydrochloride (Niacin may potentiate the effects of ganglionic blocking agents and vasoactive drugs resulting in postural hypotension).
No products indexed under this heading.

Acetazolamide (Potent inhibitors of CYP3A4 increase the risk of myopathy by reducing the elimination of simvastatin. Hence when simvastatin is used with a potent inhibitor of CYP3A4, elevated plasma levels of HMG-CoA reductase inhibitory activity can increase the risk of myopathy and rhabdomyolysis, particularly with higher doses of simvastatin. Concomitant use of drugs labeled as potent inhibitors of CYP3A4 should be avoided unless the benefits of combined therapy outweigh the increased risk. If treatment with itraconazole, ketoconazole, erythromycin, clarithromycin or telithromycin is unavoidable, therapy with Simcor should be suspended during the course of treatment).
No products indexed under this heading.

Acetazolamide Sodium (Potent inhibitors of CYP3A4 increase the risk of myopathy by reducing the elimination of simvastatin. Hence when simvastatin is used with a potent inhibitor of CYP3A4, elevated plasma levels of HMG-CoA reductase inhibitory activity can increase the risk of myopathy and rhabdomyolysis, particularly with higher doses of simvastatin. Concomitant use of drugs labeled as potent inhibitors of CYP3A4 should be avoided unless the benefits of combined therapy outweigh the increased risk. If treatment with itraconazole, ketoconazole, erythromycin, clarithromycin or telithromycin is unavoidable, therapy with Simcor should be suspended during the course of treatment).
No products indexed under this heading.

Aliskiren (Niacin may potentiate the effects of ganglionic blocking agents and vasoactive drugs resulting in postural hypotension). Products include:

Amiodarone Hydrochloride (The risk of myopathy/rhabdomyolysis is increased by concomitant administration of amiodarone or verapamil with higher doses of simvastatin. Combination with Simcor should be limited to the 20 mg once daily dose of simvastatin).
No products indexed under this heading.

Amlodipine Besylate (Niacin may potentiate the effects of ganglionic blocking agents and vasoactive drugs resulting in postural hypotension). Products include:

Amprenavir (Potent inhibitors of CYP3A4 increase the risk of myopathy by reducing the elimination of simvastatin. Hence when simvastatin is used with a potent inhibitor of CYP3A4, elevated plasma levels of HMG-CoA reductase inhibitory activity can increase the risk of myopathy and rhabdomyolysis, particularly with higher doses of simvastatin. Concomitant use of drugs labeled as potent inhibitors of CYP3A4 should be avoided unless the benefits of combined therapy outweigh the increased risk. If treatment with itraconazole, ketoconazole, erythromycin, clarithromycin or telithromycin is unavoidable, therapy with Simcor should be suspended during the course of treatment).
No products indexed under this heading.

Anastrozole (Potent inhibitors of CYP3A4 increase the risk of myopathy by reducing the elimination of simvastatin. Hence when simvastatin is used with a potent inhibitor of CYP3A4, elevated plasma levels of HMG-CoA reductase inhibitory activity can increase the risk of myopathy and rhabdomyolysis, particularly with higher doses of simvastatin. Concomitant use of drugs labeled as potent inhibitors of CYP3A4 should be avoided unless the benefits of combined therapy outweigh the increased risk. If treatment with itraconazole, ketoconazole, erythromycin, clarithromycin or telithromycin is unavoidable, therapy with Simcor should be suspended during the course of treatment).
No products indexed under this heading.

Anisindione (Co-administration prolongs INR. Achieve stable INR prior to starting Simcor. Monitor INR frequently until stable upon initiation or alteration of Simcor therapy).
No products indexed under this heading.

Aprepitant (Potent inhibitors of CYP3A4 increase the risk of myopathy by reducing the elimination of simvastatin. Hence when simvastatin is used with a potent inhibitor of CYP3A4, elevated plasma levels of HMG-CoA reductase inhibitory activity can increase the risk of myopathy and rhabdomyolysis, particularly with higher doses of simvastatin. Concomitant use of drugs labeled as potent inhibitors of CYP3A4 should be avoided unless the benefits of combined therapy outweigh the increased risk. If treatment with itraconazole, ketoconazole, erythromycin, clarithromycin or telithromycin is unavoidable, therapy with Simcor should be suspended during the course of treatment). Products include:
Emend 2124

Aspirin (Concomitant use of aspirin may decrease the metabolic clearance of niacin. The clinical relevance of this finding is unclear). Products include:
Aggrenox 880
Bayer Aspirin 829
Percodan 1124
St. Joseph Aspirin 2045

Aspirin, Enteric Coated (Concomitant use of aspirin may decrease the metabolic clearance of niacin. The clinical relevance of this finding is unclear).
No products indexed under this heading.

Aspirin Buffered (Concomitant use of aspirin may decrease the metabolic clearance of niacin. The clinical relevance of this finding is unclear).
No products indexed under this heading.

Atazanavir (Potent inhibitors of CYP3A4 increase the risk of myopathy by reducing the elimination of simvastatin. Hence when simvastatin is used with a potent inhibitor of CYP3A4, elevated plasma levels of HMG-CoA reductase inhibitory activity can increase the risk of myopathy and rhabdomyolysis, particularly with higher doses of simvastatin. Concomitant use of drugs labeled as potent inhibitors of CYP3A4 should

be avoided unless the benefits of combined therapy outweigh the increased risk. If treatment with itraconazole, ketoconazole, erythromycin, clarithromycin or telithromycin is unavoidable, therapy with Simcor should be suspended during the course of treatment).
No products indexed under this heading.

Atazanavir Sulfate (Potent inhibitors of CYP3A4 increase the risk of myopathy by reducing the elimination of simvastatin. Hence when simvastatin is used with a potent inhibitor of CYP3A4, elevated plasma levels of HMG-CoA reductase inhibitory activity can increase the risk of myopathy and rhabdomyolysis, particularly with higher doses of simvastatin. Concomitant use of drugs labeled as potent inhibitors of CYP3A4 should be avoided unless the benefits of combined therapy outweigh the increased risk. If treatment with itraconazole, ketoconazole, erythromycin, clarithromycin or telithromycin is unavoidable, therapy with Simcor should be suspended during the course of treatment).
No products indexed under this heading.

Atenolol (Niacin may potentiate the effects of ganglionic blocking agents and vasoactive drugs resulting in postural hypotension).
No products indexed under this heading.

Benazepril Hydrochloride (Niacin may potentiate the effects of ganglionic blocking agents and vasoactive drugs resulting in postural hypotension).
No products indexed under this heading.

Bendroflumethiazide (Niacin may potentiate the effects of ganglionic blocking agents and vasoactive drugs resulting in postural hypotension).
No products indexed under this heading.

Betaxolol Hydrochloride (Niacin may potentiate the effects of ganglionic blocking agents and vasoactive drugs resulting in postural hypotension).
No products indexed under this heading.

Bisoprolol Fumarate (Niacin may potentiate the effects of ganglionic blocking agents and vasoactive drugs resulting in postural hypotension).
No products indexed under this heading.

Candesartan Cilexetil (Niacin may potentiate the effects of ganglionic blocking agents and vasoactive drugs resulting in postural hypotension). Products include:
Atacand 697
Atacand HCT 700

Captopril (Niacin may potentiate the effects of ganglionic blocking agents and vasoactive drugs resulting in postural hypotension). Products include:
Captopril 2341

Carteolol Hydrochloride (Niacin may potentiate the effects of ganglionic blocking agents and vasoactive drugs resulting in postural hypotension).
No products indexed under this heading.

Carvedilol (Niacin may potentiate the effects of ganglionic blocking agents and vasoactive drugs resulting in postural hypotension). Products include:
Coreg 1409

Carvedilol Phosphate (Niacin may potentiate the effects of ganglionic blocking agents and vasoactive drugs resulting in postural hypotension). Products include:
Coreg CR 1416

Chlorothiazide (Niacin may potentiate the effects of ganglionic blocking agents and vasoactive drugs resulting in postural hypotension).
No products indexed under this heading.

Chlorothiazide Sodium (Niacin may potentiate the effects of ganglionic blocking agents and vasoactive drugs resulting in postural hypotension).
Products include:

Diuril Intravenous 2009

Chlorthalidone (Niacin may potentiate the effects of ganglionic blocking agents and vasoactive drugs resulting in postural hypotension). Products include:
Clorpres 2344

Cholestyramine (An *in vitro* study was carried out investigating the niacin-binding capacity of colestipol and cholestyramine. About 98% of available niacin was bound to colestipol, with 10% to 30% binding to cholestyramine. These results suggest that 4 to 6 hours, or as great an interval as possible, should elapse between the ingestion of bile acid-binding resins and the administration of Simcor).
No products indexed under this heading.

Cimetidine (Potent inhibitors of CYP3A4 increase the risk of myopathy by reducing the elimination of simvastatin. Hence when simvastatin is used with a potent inhibitor of CYP3A4, elevated plasma levels of HMG-CoA reductase inhibitory activity can increase the risk of myopathy and rhabdomyolysis, particularly with higher doses of simvastatin. Concomitant use of drugs labeled as potent inhibitors of CYP3A4 should be avoided unless the benefits of combined therapy outweigh the increased risk. If treatment with itraconazole, ketoconazole, erythromycin, clarithromycin or telithromycin is unavoidable, therapy with Simcor should be suspended during the course of treatment).
No products indexed under this heading.

Cimetidine Hydrochloride (Potent inhibitors of CYP3A4 increase the risk of myopathy by reducing the elimination of simvastatin. Hence when simvastatin is used with a potent inhibitor of CYP3A4, elevated plasma levels of HMG-CoA reductase inhibitory activity can increase the risk of myopathy and rhabdomyolysis, particularly with higher doses of simvastatin. Concomitant use of drugs labeled as potent inhibitors of CYP3A4 should be avoided unless the benefits of combined therapy outweigh the increased risk. If treatment with itraconazole, ketoconazole, erythromycin, clarithromycin or telithromycin is unavoidable, therapy with Simcor should be suspended during the course of treatment).
No products indexed under this heading.

Ciprofloxacin (Potent inhibitors of CYP3A4 increase the risk of myopathy by reducing the elimination of simvastatin. Hence when simvastatin is used with a potent inhibitor of CYP3A4, elevated plasma levels of HMG-CoA reductase inhibitory activity can increase the risk of myopathy and rhabdomyolysis, particularly with higher doses of simvastatin. Concomitant use of drugs labeled as potent inhibitors of CYP3A4 should be avoided unless the benefits of combined therapy outweigh the increased risk. If treatment with itraconazole, ketoconazole, erythromycin, clarithromycin or telithromycin is unavoidable, therapy with Simcor should be suspended during the course of treatment). Products include:
Cipro I.V. 3082
Cipro 3073
Cipro XR 3091
Ciprodex 583

Clarithromycin (Potent inhibitors of CYP3A4 increase the risk of myopathy by reducing the elimination of simvastatin. Hence when simvastatin is used with a potent inhibitor of CYP3A4, elevated plasma levels of HMG-CoA reductase inhibitory activity can increase the risk of myopathy and rhabdomyolysis, particularly with higher doses of simvastatin. Concomitant use of drugs labeled as potent inhibitors of CYP3A4 should be avoided unless the benefits of com-

bined therapy outweigh the increased risk. If treatment with itraconazole, ketoconazole, erythromycin, clarithromycin or telithromycin is unavoidable, therapy with Simcor should be suspended during the course of treatment). Products include:
Biaxin/Biaxin XL 412

Clofibrate (Co-administration of gemfibrozil (600 mg bid for 3 days) with simvastatin (40 mg daily) resulted in clinically significant increases in simvastatin acid AUC (185%) and peak plasma concentration (C_{max}, 112%), possibly due to inhibition of simvastatin acid glucuronidation by gemfibrozil. The increase in simvastatin exposure increases the risk of myopathy when co-administered with gemfibrozil. The combined use of Simcor with gemfibrozil should be avoided. The risk of myopathy also increases to a lesser extent when simvastatin is used in combination with other fibrates. Combination therapy with Simcor should be avoided).
No products indexed under this heading.

Clonidine (Niacin may potentiate the effects of ganglionic blocking agents and vasoactive drugs resulting in postural hypotension). Products include:
Catapres-TTS 884

Clonidine Hydrochloride (Niacin may potentiate the effects of ganglionic blocking agents and vasoactive drugs resulting in postural hypotension). Products include:
Clorpres 2344

Clotrimazole (Potent inhibitors of CYP3A4 increase the risk of myopathy by reducing the elimination of simvastatin. Hence when simvastatin is used with a potent inhibitor of CYP3A4, elevated plasma levels of HMG-CoA reductase inhibitory activity can increase the risk of myopathy and rhabdomyolysis, particularly with higher doses of simvastatin. Concomitant use of drugs labeled as potent inhibitors of CYP3A4 should be avoided unless the benefits of combined therapy outweigh the increased risk. If treatment with itraconazole, ketoconazole, erythromycin, clarithromycin or telithromycin is unavoidable, therapy with Simcor should be suspended during the course of treatment). Products include:
Lotrisone 3163

Colesevelam Hydrochloride (An *in vitro* study was carried out investigating the niacin-binding capacity of colestipol and cholestyramine. About 98% of available niacin was bound to colestipol, with 10% to 30% binding to cholestyramine. These results suggest that 4 to 6 hours, or as great an interval as possible, should elapse between the ingestion of bile acid-binding resins and the administration of Simcor). Products include:
Welchol 1029

Colestipol Hydrochloride (An *in vitro* study was carried out investigating the niacin-binding capacity of colestipol and cholestyramine. About 98% of available niacin was bound to colestipol, with 10% to 30% binding to cholestyramine. These results suggest that 4 to 6 hours, or as great an interval as possible, should elapse between the ingestion of bile acid-binding resins and the administration of Simcor).
No products indexed under this heading.

Conivaptan Hydrochloride (Potent inhibitors of CYP3A4 increase the risk of myopathy by reducing the elimination of simvastatin. Hence when simvastatin is used with a potent inhibitor of CYP3A4, elevated plasma levels of HMG-CoA reductase inhibitory activity can increase the risk of myopathy and rhabdomyolysis, particularly with higher doses of simvastatin. Concomitant use of drugs labeled as potent inhibitors of

IMPORTANT NOTE: Always consult each drug listing in the patient's regimen for possible interactions.

Simcor Interactions Index 1744

CYP3A4 should be avoided unless the benefits of combined therapy outweigh the increased risk. If treatment with itraconazole, ketoconazole, erythromycin, clarithromycin or telithromycin is unavoidable, therapy with Simcor should be suspended during the course of treatment). Products include:
Vaprisol 689

Cyclosporine (Although the mechanism is not fully understood, cyclosporine has been shown to increase the AUC of HMG-CoA reductase inhibitors. The increase in AUC for simvastatin acid is presumably due, in part, to inhibition of CYP3A4. The risk of myopathy/rhabdomyolysis is increased by concomitant administration of cyclosporine or danazol particularly with higher doses of simvastatin. Co-administration with Simcor should be avoided). Products include:
Gengraf 440
Neoral Oral Solution 2496
Neoral Capsules 2496
Restasis 605

Dalfopristin (Potent inhibitors of CYP3A4 increase the risk of myopathy by reducing the elimination of simvastatin. Hence when simvastatin is used with a potent inhibitor of CYP3A4, elevated plasma levels of HMG-CoA reductase inhibitory activity can increase the risk of myopathy and rhabdomyolysis, particularly with higher doses of simvastatin. Concomitant use of drugs labeled as potent inhibitors of CYP3A4 should be avoided unless the benefits of combined therapy outweigh the increased risk. If treatment with itraconazole, ketoconazole, erythromycin, clarithromycin or telithromycin is unavoidable, therapy with Simcor should be suspended during the course of treatment).
No products indexed under this heading.

Danazol (Although the mechanism is not fully understood, cyclosporine has been shown to increase the AUC of HMG-CoA reductase inhibitors. The increase in AUC for simvastatin acid is presumably due, in part, to inhibition of CYP3A4. The risk of myopathy/rhabdomyolysis is increased by concomitant administration of cyclosporine or danazol particularly with higher doses of simvastatin. Co-administration with Simcor should be avoided).
No products indexed under this heading.

Darunavir (Potent inhibitors of CYP3A4 increase the risk of myopathy by reducing the elimination of simvastatin. Hence when simvastatin is used with a potent inhibitor of CYP3A4, elevated plasma levels of HMG-CoA reductase inhibitory activity can increase the risk of myopathy and rhabdomyolysis, particularly with higher doses of simvastatin. Concomitant use of drugs labeled as potent inhibitors of CYP3A4 should be avoided unless the benefits of combined therapy outweigh the increased risk. If treatment with itraconazole, ketoconazole, erythromycin, clarithromycin or telithromycin is unavoidable, therapy with Simcor should be suspended during the course of treatment).
No products indexed under this heading.

Dasatinib (Potent inhibitors of CYP3A4 increase the risk of myopathy by reducing the elimination of simvastatin. Hence when simvastatin is used with a potent inhibitor of CYP3A4, elevated plasma levels of HMG-CoA reductase inhibitory activity can increase the risk of myopathy and rhabdomyolysis, particularly with higher doses of simvastatin. Concomitant use of drugs labeled as potent inhibitors of CYP3A4 should be avoided unless the benefits of combined therapy outweigh the increased risk. If treatment with itraconazole, ketoconazole, erythromycin, clarithromycin or telithromycin is unavoidable, therapy with Simcor should be suspended during the course of treatment).
No products indexed under this heading.

Delavirdine Mesylate (Potent inhibitors of CYP3A4 increase the risk of myopathy by reducing the elimination of simvastatin. Hence when simvastatin is used with a potent inhibitor of CYP3A4, elevated plasma levels of HMG-CoA reductase inhibitory activity can increase the risk of myopathy and rhabdomyolysis, particularly with higher doses of simvastatin. Concomitant use of drugs labeled as potent inhibitors of CYP3A4 should be avoided unless the benefits of combined therapy outweigh the increased risk. If treatment with itraconazole, ketoconazole, erythromycin, clarithromycin or telithromycin is unavoidable, therapy with Simcor should be suspended during the course of treatment).
No products indexed under this heading.

Delavirine (Potent inhibitors of CYP3A4 increase the risk of myopathy by reducing the elimination of simvastatin. Hence when simvastatin is used with a potent inhibitor of CYP3A4, elevated plasma levels of HMG-CoA reductase inhibitory activity can increase the risk of myopathy and rhabdomyolysis, particularly with higher doses of simvastatin. Concomitant use of drugs labeled as potent inhibitors of CYP3A4 should be avoided unless the benefits of combined therapy outweigh the increased risk. If treatment with itraconazole, ketoconazole, erythromycin, clarithromycin or telithromycin is unavoidable, therapy with Simcor should be suspended during the course of treatment).
No products indexed under this heading.

Deserpidine (Niacin may potentiate the effects of ganglionic blocking agents and vasoactive drugs resulting in postural hypotension).
No products indexed under this heading.

Desloratadine (Potent inhibitors of CYP3A4 increase the risk of myopathy by reducing the elimination of simvastatin. Hence when simvastatin is used with a potent inhibitor of CYP3A4, elevated plasma levels of HMG-CoA reductase inhibitory activity can increase the risk of myopathy and rhabdomyolysis, particularly with higher doses of simvastatin. Concomitant use of drugs labeled as potent inhibitors of CYP3A4 should be avoided unless the benefits of combined therapy outweigh the increased risk. If treatment with itraconazole, ketoconazole, erythromycin, clarithromycin or telithromycin is unavoidable, therapy with Simcor should be suspended during the course of treatment). Products include:
Clarinex Syrup 3098
Clarinex 3098
Clarinex Reditabs 3098
Clarinex-D 12-Hour 3101
Clarinex-D 3104

Diazoxide (Niacin may potentiate the effects of ganglionic blocking agents and vasoactive drugs resulting in postural hypotension). Products include:
Proglycem 1179
Proglycem Suspension 1179

Dicumarol (Co-administration prolongs INR. Achieve stable INR prior to starting Simcor. Monitor INR frequently until stable upon initiation or alteration of Simcor therapy).
No products indexed under this heading.

Digoxin (Concomitant administration of a single dose of digoxin in healthy male volunteers receiving simvastatin resulted in a slight elevation (less than 0.3 ng/mL) in digoxin concentrations in plasma (as measured by a radioimmunoassay) compared to concomitant administration of placebo and digoxin. Patients taking digoxin should be monitored appropriately when Simcor is initiated). Products include:
Lanoxin Injection 1546
Lanoxin Injection Pediatric 1549
Lanoxin Tablets 1553

Diltiazem Hydrochloride (Niacin may potentiate the effects of ganglionic blocking agents and vasoactive drugs resulting in postural hypotension). Products include:
Cardizem LA 423

Diltiazem Maleate (Niacin may potentiate the effects of ganglionic blocking agents and vasoactive drugs resulting in postural hypotension).
No products indexed under this heading.

Doxazosin Mesylate (Niacin may potentiate the effects of ganglionic blocking agents and vasoactive drugs resulting in postural hypotension).
No products indexed under this heading.

Efavirenz (Potent inhibitors of CYP3A4 increase the risk of myopathy by reducing the elimination of simvastatin. Hence when simvastatin is used with a potent inhibitor of CYP3A4, elevated plasma levels of HMG-CoA reductase inhibitory activity can increase the risk of myopathy and rhabdomyolysis, particularly with higher doses of simvastatin. Concomitant use of drugs labeled as potent inhibitors of CYP3A4 should be avoided unless the benefits of combined therapy outweigh the increased risk. If treatment with itraconazole, ketoconazole, erythromycin, clarithromycin or telithromycin is unavoidable, therapy with Simcor should be suspended during the course of treatment). Products include:
Atripla 906

Enalapril Maleate (Niacin may potentiate the effects of ganglionic blocking agents and vasoactive drugs resulting in postural hypotension).
No products indexed under this heading.

Enalaprilat (Niacin may potentiate the effects of ganglionic blocking agents and vasoactive drugs resulting in postural hypotension).
No products indexed under this heading.

Eprosartan Mesylate (Niacin may potentiate the effects of ganglionic blocking agents and vasoactive drugs resulting in postural hypotension). Products include:
Teveten 538
Teveten HCT 541

Erythromycin (Potent inhibitors of CYP3A4 increase the risk of myopathy by reducing the elimination of simvastatin. Hence when simvastatin is used with a potent inhibitor of CYP3A4, elevated plasma levels of HMG-CoA reductase inhibitory activity can increase the risk of myopathy and rhabdomyolysis, particularly with higher doses of simvastatin. Concomitant use of drugs labeled as potent inhibitors of CYP3A4 should be avoided unless the benefits of combined therapy outweigh the increased risk. If treatment with itraconazole, ketoconazole, erythromycin, clarithromycin or telithromycin is unavoidable, therapy with Simcor should be suspended during the course of treatment).
No products indexed under this heading.

Erythromycin Estolate (Potent inhibitors of CYP3A4 increase the risk of myopathy by reducing the elimination of simvastatin. Hence when simvastatin is used with a potent inhibitor of CYP3A4, elevated plasma levels of HMG-CoA reductase inhibitory activity can increase the risk of myopathy and rhabdomyolysis, particularly with higher doses of simvastatin. Concomitant use of drugs labeled as potent inhibitors of CYP3A4 should be avoided unless the benefits of combined therapy outweigh the increased risk. If treatment with itraconazole, ketoconazole, erythromycin, clarithromycin or telithromycin is unavoidable, therapy with Simcor should be suspended during the course of treatment).
No products indexed under this heading.

Erythromycin Ethylsuccinate (Potent inhibitors of CYP3A4 increase the risk of myopathy by reducing the elimination of simvastatin. Hence when simvastatin is used with a potent inhibitor of CYP3A4, elevated plasma levels of HMG-CoA reductase inhibitory activity can increase the risk of myopathy and rhabdomyolysis, particularly with higher doses of simvastatin. Concomitant use of drugs labeled as potent inhibitors of CYP3A4 should be avoided unless the benefits of combined therapy outweigh the increased risk. If treatment with itraconazole, ketoconazole, erythromycin, clarithromycin or telithromycin is unavoidable, therapy with Simcor should be suspended during the course of treatment). Products include:
E.E.S. 437
EryPed 435

Erythromycin Gluceptate (Potent inhibitors of CYP3A4 increase the risk of myopathy by reducing the elimination of simvastatin. Hence when simvastatin is used with a potent inhibitor of CYP3A4, elevated plasma levels of HMG-CoA reductase inhibitory activity can increase the risk of myopathy and rhabdomyolysis, particularly with higher doses of simvastatin. Concomitant use of drugs labeled as potent inhibitors of CYP3A4 should be avoided unless the benefits of combined therapy outweigh the increased risk. If treatment with itraconazole, ketoconazole, erythromycin, clarithromycin or telithromycin is unavoidable, therapy with Simcor should be suspended during the course of treatment).
No products indexed under this heading.

Erythromycin Lactobionate (Potent inhibitors of CYP3A4 increase the risk of myopathy by reducing the elimination of simvastatin. Hence when simvastatin is used with a potent inhibitor of CYP3A4, elevated plasma levels of HMG-CoA reductase inhibitory activity can increase the risk of myopathy and rhabdomyolysis, particularly with higher doses of simvastatin. Concomitant use of drugs labeled as potent inhibitors of CYP3A4 should be avoided unless the benefits of combined therapy outweigh the increased risk. If treatment with itraconazole, ketoconazole, erythromycin, clarithromycin or telithromycin is unavoidable, therapy with Simcor should be suspended during the course of treatment).
No products indexed under this heading.

Erythromycin Stearate (Potent inhibitors of CYP3A4 increase the risk of myopathy by reducing the elimination of simvastatin. Hence when simvastatin is used with a potent inhibitor of CYP3A4, elevated plasma levels of HMG-CoA reductase inhibitory activity can increase the risk of myopathy and rhabdomyolysis, particularly with higher doses of simvastatin. Concomitant use of drugs labeled as potent inhibitors of CYP3A4 should be avoided unless the benefits of combined therapy outweigh the increased risk. If treatment with itraconazole, ketoconazole, erythromycin, clarithromycin or telithromycin is unavoidable, therapy with Simcor should be suspended during the course of treatment).
No products indexed under this heading.

Esmolol Hydrochloride (Niacin may potentiate the effects of ganglionic blocking agents and vasoactive drugs resulting in postural hypotension).
No products indexed under this heading.

Esomeprazole Magnesium (Potent inhibitors of CYP3A4 increase the risk of myopathy by reducing the elimination of simvastatin. Hence when simvastatin is used with a potent inhibitor of CYP3A4, elevated plasma levels of HMG-CoA reductase inhibitory activity can increase the risk of myopathy and rhabdomyolysis, particularly with higher doses of simvastatin. Concomitant use of drugs labeled as potent inhibitors of CYP3A4 should be avoided unless the benefits of combined therapy outweigh the increased risk. If treatment with itraconazole, ketoconazole, erythromycin, clarithromycin or telithromycin is unavoidable, therapy with Simcor should be suspended during the course of treatment). Products include:

Nexium Capsules 704
Nexium Oral Suspension 704

Esomeprazole Sodium (Potent inhibitors of CYP3A4 increase the risk of myopathy by reducing the elimination of simvastatin. Hence when simvastatin is used with a potent inhibitor of CYP3A4, elevated plasma levels of HMG-CoA reductase inhibitory activity can increase the risk of myopathy and rhabdomyolysis, particularly with higher doses of simvastatin. Concomitant use of drugs labeled as potent inhibitors of CYP3A4 should be avoided unless the benefits of combined therapy outweigh the increased risk. If treatment with itraconazole, ketoconazole, erythromycin, clarithromycin or telithromycin is unavoidable, therapy with Simcor should be suspended during the course of treatment). Products include:

Nexium I.V. 712

Felodipine (Niacin may potentiate the effects of ganglionic blocking agents and vasoactive drugs resulting in postural hypotension).
No products indexed under this heading.

Fenofibrate (Co-administration of gemfibrozil (600 mg bid for 3 days) with simvastatin (40 mg daily) resulted in clinically significant increases in simvastatin acid AUC (185%) and peak plasma concentration (C_{max}, 112%), possibly due to inhibition of simvastatin acid glucuronidation by gemfibrozil. The increase in simvastatin exposure increases the risk of myopathy when co-administered with gemfibrozil. The combined use of Simcor with gemfibrozil should be avoided. The risk of myopathy also increases to a lesser extent when simvastatin is used in combination with other fibrates. Combination therapy with Simcor should be avoided). Products include:

Fenoglide 3263
Tricor 544
Trilipix 548

Fluconazole (Potent inhibitors of CYP3A4 increase the risk of myopathy by reducing the elimination of simvastatin. Hence when simvastatin is used with a potent inhibitor of CYP3A4, elevated plasma levels of HMG-CoA reductase inhibitory activity can increase the risk of myopathy and rhabdomyolysis, particularly with higher doses of simvastatin. Concomitant use of drugs labeled as potent inhibitors of CYP3A4 should be avoided unless the benefits of combined therapy outweigh the increased risk. If treatment with itraconazole, ketoconazole, erythromycin, clarithromycin or telithromycin is unavoidable, therapy with Simcor should be suspended during the course of treatment).
No products indexed under this heading.

Fluoxetine (Potent inhibitors of CYP3A4 increase the risk of myopathy by reducing the elimination of simvastatin. Hence when simvastatin is used with a potent inhibitor of CYP3A4, elevated plasma levels of HMG-CoA reductase inhibitory activity can increase the

risk of myopathy and rhabdomyolysis, particularly with higher doses of simvastatin. Concomitant use of drugs labeled as potent inhibitors of CYP3A4 should be avoided unless the benefits of combined therapy outweigh the increased risk. If treatment with itraconazole, ketoconazole, erythromycin, clarithromycin or telithromycin is unavoidable, therapy with Simcor should be suspended during the course of treatment).
No products indexed under this heading.

Fluoxetine Hydrochloride (Potent inhibitors of CYP3A4 increase the risk of myopathy by reducing the elimination of simvastatin. Hence when simvastatin is used with a potent inhibitor of CYP3A4, elevated plasma levels of HMG-CoA reductase inhibitory activity can increase the risk of myopathy and rhabdomyolysis, particularly with higher doses of simvastatin. Concomitant use of drugs labeled as potent inhibitors of CYP3A4 should be avoided unless the benefits of combined therapy outweigh the increased risk. If treatment with itraconazole, ketoconazole, erythromycin, clarithromycin or telithromycin is unavoidable, therapy with Simcor should be suspended during the course of treatment). Products include:

Prozac Weekly 1941
Prozac Pulvules 1941
Symbyax 1965

Fluvoxamine Maleate (Potent inhibitors of CYP3A4 increase the risk of myopathy by reducing the elimination of simvastatin. Hence when simvastatin is used with a potent inhibitor of CYP3A4, elevated plasma levels of HMG-CoA reductase inhibitory activity can increase the risk of myopathy and rhabdomyolysis, particularly with higher doses of simvastatin. Concomitant use of drugs labeled as potent inhibitors of CYP3A4 should be avoided unless the benefits of combined therapy outweigh the increased risk. If treatment with itraconazole, ketoconazole, erythromycin, clarithromycin or telithromycin is unavoidable, therapy with Simcor should be suspended during the course of treatment).
No products indexed under this heading.

Fosamprenavir Calcium (Potent inhibitors of CYP3A4 increase the risk of myopathy by reducing the elimination of simvastatin. Hence when simvastatin is used with a potent inhibitor of CYP3A4, elevated plasma levels of HMG-CoA reductase inhibitory activity can increase the risk of myopathy and rhabdomyolysis, particularly with higher doses of simvastatin. Concomitant use of drugs labeled as potent inhibitors of CYP3A4 should be avoided unless the benefits of combined therapy outweigh the increased risk. If treatment with itraconazole, ketoconazole, erythromycin, clarithromycin or telithromycin is unavoidable, therapy with Simcor should be suspended during the course of treatment). Products include:

Lexiva Oral Suspension 1558
Lexiva 1558

Fosinopril Sodium (Niacin may potentiate the effects of ganglionic blocking agents and vasoactive drugs resulting in postural hypotension).
No products indexed under this heading.

Furosemide (Niacin may potentiate the effects of ganglionic blocking agents and vasoactive drugs resulting in postural hypotension). Products include:

Furosemide 2354

Gemfibrozil (Co-administration of gemfibrozil (600 mg twice daily for 3 days) with simvastatin (40 mg daily) resulted in clinically significant increases in simvastatin acid AUC (185%) and peak plasma concentration (C, 112%), possibly due to inhibition of

simvastatin acid glucuronidation by gemfibrozil. The increase in simvastatin exposure increases the risk of myopathy when co-administered with gemfibrozil. The combined use of SIMCOR with gemfibrozil should be avoided).
No products indexed under this heading.

Guanabenz Acetate (Niacin may potentiate the effects of ganglionic blocking agents and vasoactive drugs resulting in postural hypotension).
No products indexed under this heading.

Guanethidine (Niacin may potentiate the effects of ganglionic blocking agents and vasoactive drugs resulting in postural hypotension).
No products indexed under this heading.

Guanethidine Monosulfate (Niacin may potentiate the effects of ganglionic blocking agents and vasoactive drugs resulting in postural hypotension).
No products indexed under this heading.

Guanethidine Sulfate (Niacin may potentiate the effects of ganglionic blocking agents and vasoactive drugs resulting in postural hypotension).
No products indexed under this heading.

Hydralazine Hydrochloride (Niacin may potentiate the effects of ganglionic blocking agents and vasoactive drugs resulting in postural hypotension).
No products indexed under this heading.

Hydrochlorothiazide (Niacin may potentiate the effects of ganglionic blocking agents and vasoactive drugs resulting in postural hypotension). Products include:

Atacand HCT 700
Avalide 2956
Benicar HCT 1017
Diovan HCT 2419
Dyazide 1429
Exforge HCT 2449
Hyzaar 2162
Hyzaar 100-12.5 2162
Micardis HCT 889
Prinzide 2246
Tekturna HCT 2541
Teveten HCT 541

Hydroflumethiazide (Niacin may potentiate the effects of ganglionic blocking agents and vasoactive drugs resulting in postural hypotension).
No products indexed under this heading.

Imatinib Mesylate (Potent inhibitors of CYP3A4 increase the risk of myopathy by reducing the elimination of simvastatin. Hence when simvastatin is used with a potent inhibitor of CYP3A4, elevated plasma levels of HMG-CoA reductase inhibitory activity can increase the risk of myopathy and rhabdomyolysis, particularly with higher doses of simvastatin. Concomitant use of drugs labeled as potent inhibitors of CYP3A4 should be avoided unless the benefits of combined therapy outweigh the increased risk. If treatment with itraconazole, ketoconazole, erythromycin, clarithromycin or telithromycin is unavoidable, therapy with Simcor should be suspended during the course of treatment). Products include:

Gleevec 2477

Indapamide (Niacin may potentiate the effects of ganglionic blocking agents and vasoactive drugs resulting in postural hypotension). Products include:

Indapamide 2356

Indinavir Sulfate (Potent inhibitors of CYP3A4 increase the risk of myopathy by reducing the elimination of simvastatin. Hence when simvastatin is used with a potent inhibitor of CYP3A4, elevated plasma levels of HMG-CoA reductase inhibitory activity can increase the risk of myopathy and rhabdomyolysis, particularly with higher doses of simvastatin. Concomitant use of drugs labeled as potent inhibitors of CYP3A4 should

be avoided unless the benefits of combined therapy outweigh the increased risk. If treatment with itraconazole, ketoconazole, erythromycin, clarithromycin or telithromycin is unavoidable, therapy with Simcor should be suspended during the course of treatment). Products include:

Crixivan 2113

Irbesartan (Niacin may potentiate the effects of ganglionic blocking agents and vasoactive drugs resulting in postural hypotension). Products include:

Avalide 2956
Avapro 2962

Isoniazid (Potent inhibitors of CYP3A4 increase the risk of myopathy by reducing the elimination of simvastatin. Hence when simvastatin is used with a potent inhibitor of CYP3A4, elevated plasma levels of HMG-CoA reductase inhibitory activity can increase the risk of myopathy and rhabdomyolysis, particularly with higher doses of simvastatin. Concomitant use of drugs labeled as potent inhibitors of CYP3A4 should be avoided unless the benefits of combined therapy outweigh the increased risk. If treatment with itraconazole, ketoconazole, erythromycin, clarithromycin or telithromycin is unavoidable, therapy with Simcor should be suspended during the course of treatment).
No products indexed under this heading.

Isradipine (Niacin may potentiate the effects of ganglionic blocking agents and vasoactive drugs resulting in postural hypotension). Products include:

DynaCirc CR 1432

Itraconazole (Potent inhibitors of CYP3A4 increase the risk of myopathy by reducing the elimination of simvastatin. Hence when simvastatin is used with a potent inhibitor of CYP3A4, elevated plasma levels of HMG-CoA reductase inhibitory activity can increase the risk of myopathy and rhabdomyolysis, particularly with higher doses of simvastatin. Concomitant use of drugs labeled as potent inhibitors of CYP3A4 should be avoided unless the benefits of combined therapy outweigh the increased risk. If treatment with itraconazole, ketoconazole, erythromycin, clarithromycin or telithromycin is unavoidable, therapy with Simcor should be suspended during the course of treatment).
No products indexed under this heading.

Ketoconazole (Potent inhibitors of CYP3A4 increase the risk of myopathy by reducing the elimination of simvastatin. Hence when simvastatin is used with a potent inhibitor of CYP3A4, elevated plasma levels of HMG-CoA reductase inhibitory activity can increase the risk of myopathy and rhabdomyolysis, particularly with higher doses of simvastatin. Concomitant use of drugs labeled as potent inhibitors of CYP3A4 should be avoided unless the benefits of combined therapy outweigh the increased risk. If treatment with itraconazole, ketoconazole, erythromycin, clarithromycin or telithromycin is unavoidable, therapy with Simcor should be suspended during the course of treatment). Products include:

Extina 3319
Xolegel 3337

Labetalol Hydrochloride (Niacin may potentiate the effects of ganglionic blocking agents and vasoactive drugs resulting in postural hypotension).
No products indexed under this heading.

Lapatinib (Potent inhibitors of CYP3A4 increase the risk of myopathy by reducing the elimination of simvastatin. Hence when simvastatin is used with a potent inhibitor of CYP3A4, elevated plasma levels of HMG-CoA reductase inhibitory activity can increase the risk of myopathy and rhabdomyolysis, particularly with higher doses of simvasta-

IMPORTANT NOTE: Always consult each drug listing in the patient's regimen for possible interactions.

Simcor **Interactions Index** 1746

tin. Concomitant use of drugs labeled as potent inhibitors of CYP3A4 should be avoided unless the benefits of combined therapy outweigh the increased risk. If treatment with itraconazole, ketoconazole, erythromycin, clarithromycin or telithromycin is unavoidable, therapy with Simcor should be suspended during the course of treatment). Products include:

Tykerb 1698

Lisinopril (Niacin may potentiate the effects of ganglionic blocking agents and vasoactive drugs resulting in postural hypotension). Products include:

Prinivil 2241
Prinzide 2246

Lopinavir (Potent inhibitors of CYP3A4 increase the risk of myopathy by reducing the elimination of simvastatin. Hence when simvastatin is used with a potent inhibitor of CYP3A4, elevated plasma levels of HMG-CoA reductase inhibitory activity can increase the risk of myopathy and rhabdomyolysis, particularly with higher doses of simvastatin. Concomitant use of drugs labeled as potent inhibitors of CYP3A4 should be avoided unless the benefits of combined therapy outweigh the increased risk. If treatment with itraconazole, ketoconazole, erythromycin, clarithromycin or telithromycin is unavoidable, therapy with Simcor should be suspended during the course of treatment). Products include:

Kaletra 458

Loratadine (Potent inhibitors of CYP3A4 increase the risk of myopathy by reducing the elimination of simvastatin. Hence when simvastatin is used with a potent inhibitor of CYP3A4, elevated plasma levels of HMG-CoA reductase inhibitory activity can increase the risk of myopathy and rhabdomyolysis, particularly with higher doses of simvastatin. Concomitant use of drugs labeled as potent inhibitors of CYP3A4 should be avoided unless the benefits of combined therapy outweigh the increased risk. If treatment with itraconazole, ketoconazole, erythromycin, clarithromycin or telithromycin is unavoidable, therapy with Simcor should be suspended during the course of treatment).

No products indexed under this heading.

Losartan Potassium (Niacin may potentiate the effects of ganglionic blocking agents and vasoactive drugs resulting in postural hypotension). Products include:

Cozaar 2106
Hyzaar 2162
Hyzaar 100-12.5 2162

Mecamylamine Hydrochloride (Niacin may potentiate the effects of ganglionic blocking agents and vasoactive drugs resulting in postural hypotension).

No products indexed under this heading.

Methyclothiazide (Niacin may potentiate the effects of ganglionic blocking agents and vasoactive drugs resulting in postural hypotension).

No products indexed under this heading.

Methyldopa (Niacin may potentiate the effects of ganglionic blocking agents and vasoactive drugs resulting in postural hypotension).

No products indexed under this heading.

Methyldopate Hydrochloride (Niacin may potentiate the effects of ganglionic blocking agents and vasoactive drugs resulting in postural hypotension).

No products indexed under this heading.

Metolazone (Niacin may potentiate the effects of ganglionic blocking agents and vasoactive drugs resulting in postural hypotension).

No products indexed under this heading.

Metoprolol Succinate (Niacin may potentiate the effects of ganglionic blocking agents and vasoactive drugs resulting in postural hypotension). Products include:

Toprol XL 732

Metoprolol Tartrate (Niacin may potentiate the effects of ganglionic blocking agents and vasoactive drugs resulting in postural hypotension).

No products indexed under this heading.

Metronidazole (Potent inhibitors of CYP3A4 increase the risk of myopathy by reducing the elimination of simvastatin. Hence when simvastatin is used with a potent inhibitor of CYP3A4, elevated plasma levels of HMG-CoA reductase inhibitory activity can increase the risk of myopathy and rhabdomyolysis, particularly with higher doses of simvastatin. Concomitant use of drugs labeled as potent inhibitors of CYP3A4 should be avoided unless the benefits of combined therapy outweigh the increased risk. If treatment with itraconazole, ketoconazole, erythromycin, clarithromycin or telithromycin is unavoidable, therapy with Simcor should be suspended during the course of treatment). Products include:

Pylera 793

Metronidazole Benzoate (Potent inhibitors of CYP3A4 increase the risk of myopathy by reducing the elimination of simvastatin. Hence when simvastatin is used with a potent inhibitor of CYP3A4, elevated plasma levels of HMG-CoA reductase inhibitory activity can increase the risk of myopathy and rhabdomyolysis, particularly with higher doses of simvastatin. Concomitant use of drugs labeled as potent inhibitors of CYP3A4 should be avoided unless the benefits of combined therapy outweigh the increased risk. If treatment with itraconazole, ketoconazole, erythromycin, clarithromycin or telithromycin is unavoidable, therapy with Simcor should be suspended during the course of treatment).

No products indexed under this heading.

Metronidazole Hydrochloride (Potent inhibitors of CYP3A4 increase the risk of myopathy by reducing the elimination of simvastatin. Hence when simvastatin is used with a potent inhibitor of CYP3A4, elevated plasma levels of HMG-CoA reductase inhibitory activity can increase the risk of myopathy and rhabdomyolysis, particularly with higher doses of simvastatin. Concomitant use of drugs labeled as potent inhibitors of CYP3A4 should be avoided unless the benefits of combined therapy outweigh the increased risk. If treatment with itraconazole, ketoconazole, erythromycin, clarithromycin or telithromycin is unavoidable, therapy with Simcor should be suspended during the course of treatment).

No products indexed under this heading.

Metronidazole Sodium (Potent inhibitors of CYP3A4 increase the risk of myopathy by reducing the elimination of simvastatin. Hence when simvastatin is used with a potent inhibitor of CYP3A4, elevated plasma levels of HMG-CoA reductase inhibitory activity can increase the risk of myopathy and rhabdomyolysis, particularly with higher doses of simvastatin. Concomitant use of drugs labeled as potent inhibitors of CYP3A4 should be avoided unless the benefits of combined therapy outweigh the increased risk. If treatment with itraconazole, ketoconazole, erythromycin, clarithromycin or telithromycin is unavoidable, therapy with Simcor should be suspended during the course of treatment).

No products indexed under this heading.

Metyrosine (Niacin may potentiate the effects of ganglionic blocking agents and vasoactive drugs resulting in postural hypotension).

No products indexed under this heading.

Mibefradil Dihydrochloride (Niacin may potentiate the effects of ganglionic blocking agents and vasoactive drugs resulting in postural hypotension).

No products indexed under this heading.

Miconazole (Potent inhibitors of CYP3A4 increase the risk of myopathy by reducing the elimination of simvastatin. Hence when simvastatin is used with a potent inhibitor of CYP3A4, elevated plasma levels of HMG-CoA reductase inhibitory activity can increase the risk of myopathy and rhabdomyolysis, particularly with higher doses of simvastatin. Concomitant use of drugs labeled as potent inhibitors of CYP3A4 should be avoided unless the benefits of combined therapy outweigh the increased risk. If treatment with itraconazole, ketoconazole, erythromycin, clarithromycin or telithromycin is unavoidable, therapy with Simcor should be suspended during the course of treatment).

No products indexed under this heading.

Miconazole Nitrate (Potent inhibitors of CYP3A4 increase the risk of myopathy by reducing the elimination of simvastatin. Hence when simvastatin is used with a potent inhibitor of CYP3A4, elevated plasma levels of HMG-CoA reductase inhibitory activity can increase the risk of myopathy and rhabdomyolysis, particularly with higher doses of simvastatin. Concomitant use of drugs labeled as potent inhibitors of CYP3A4 should be avoided unless the benefits of combined therapy outweigh the increased risk. If treatment with itraconazole, ketoconazole, erythromycin, clarithromycin or telithromycin is unavoidable, therapy with Simcor should be suspended during the course of treatment). Products include:

Vusion Ointment 3335

Mifepristone (Potent inhibitors of CYP3A4 increase the risk of myopathy by reducing the elimination of simvastatin. Hence when simvastatin is used with a potent inhibitor of CYP3A4, elevated plasma levels of HMG-CoA reductase inhibitory activity can increase the risk of myopathy and rhabdomyolysis, particularly with higher doses of simvastatin. Concomitant use of drugs labeled as potent inhibitors of CYP3A4 should be avoided unless the benefits of combined therapy outweigh the increased risk. If treatment with itraconazole, ketoconazole, erythromycin, clarithromycin or telithromycin is unavoidable, therapy with Simcor should be suspended during the course of treatment).

No products indexed under this heading.

Minoxidil (Niacin may potentiate the effects of ganglionic blocking agents and vasoactive drugs resulting in postural hypotension).

No products indexed under this heading.

Moexipril Hydrochloride (Niacin may potentiate the effects of ganglionic blocking agents and vasoactive drugs resulting in postural hypotension).

No products indexed under this heading.

Multivitamins with Minerals (Nutritional supplements containing large doses of niacin or related compounds may potentiate the adverse effects of Simcor). Products include:

Bios Life Slim 3454

Nadolol (Niacin may potentiate the effects of ganglionic blocking agents and vasoactive drugs resulting in postural hypotension). Products include:

Nadolol 2359

Nebivolol (Niacin may potentiate the effects of ganglionic blocking agents and vasoactive drugs resulting in postural hypotension). Products include:

Bystolic 1147

Nefazodone Hydrochloride (Potent inhibitors of CYP3A4 increase the risk of myopathy by reducing the elimination of simvastatin. Hence when simvastatin is used with a potent inhibitor of CYP3A4, elevated plasma levels of HMG-CoA reductase inhibitory activity can increase the risk of myopathy and rhabdomyolysis, particularly with higher doses of simvastatin. Concomitant use of drugs labeled as potent inhibitors of CYP3A4 should be avoided unless the benefits of combined therapy outweigh the increased risk. If treatment with itraconazole, ketoconazole, erythromycin, clarithromycin or telithromycin is unavoidable, therapy with Simcor should be suspended during the course of treatment).

No products indexed under this heading.

Nelfinavir Mesylate (Potent inhibitors of CYP3A4 increase the risk of myopathy by reducing the elimination of simvastatin. Hence when simvastatin is used with a potent inhibitor of CYP3A4, elevated plasma levels of HMG-CoA reductase inhibitory activity can increase the risk of myopathy and rhabdomyolysis, particularly with higher doses of simvastatin. Concomitant use of drugs labeled as potent inhibitors of CYP3A4 should be avoided unless the benefits of combined therapy outweigh the increased risk. If treatment with itraconazole, ketoconazole, erythromycin, clarithromycin or telithromycin is unavoidable, therapy with Simcor should be suspended during the course of treatment).

No products indexed under this heading.

Nevirapine (Potent inhibitors of CYP3A4 increase the risk of myopathy by reducing the elimination of simvastatin. Hence when simvastatin is used with a potent inhibitor of CYP3A4, elevated plasma levels of HMG-CoA reductase inhibitory activity can increase the risk of myopathy and rhabdomyolysis, particularly with higher doses of simvastatin. Concomitant use of drugs labeled as potent inhibitors of CYP3A4 should be avoided unless the benefits of combined therapy outweigh the increased risk. If treatment with itraconazole, ketoconazole, erythromycin, clarithromycin or telithromycin is unavoidable, therapy with Simcor should be suspended during the course of treatment). Products include:

Viramune Oral Suspension 897
Viramune Tablets 897

Niacinamide (Potent inhibitors of CYP3A4 increase the risk of myopathy by reducing the elimination of simvastatin. Hence when simvastatin is used with a potent inhibitor of CYP3A4, elevated plasma levels of HMG-CoA reductase inhibitory activity can increase the risk of myopathy and rhabdomyolysis, particularly with higher doses of simvastatin. Concomitant use of drugs labeled as potent inhibitors of CYP3A4 should be avoided unless the benefits of combined therapy outweigh the increased risk. If treatment with itraconazole, ketoconazole, erythromycin, clarithromycin or telithromycin is unavoidable, therapy with Simcor should be suspended during the course of treatment). Products include:

CitraNatal 90 DHA Capsules 2332
CitraNatal Assure 2332
CitraNatal Rx 2332
Heplive 607

Niacinamide Hydroiodide (Potent inhibitors of CYP3A4 increase the risk of myopathy by reducing the elimination of simvastatin. Hence when simvastatin is used with a potent inhibitor of

1747 Interactions Index Simcor

CYP3A4, elevated plasma levels of HMG-CoA reductase inhibitory activity can increase the risk of myopathy and rhabdomyolysis, particularly with higher doses of simvastatin. Concomitant use of drugs labeled as potent inhibitors of CYP3A4 should be avoided unless the benefits of combined therapy outweigh the increased risk. If treatment with itraconazole, ketoconazole, erythromycin, clarithromycin or telithromycin is unavoidable, therapy with Simcor should be suspended during the course of treatment).
No products indexed under this heading.

Nicardipine Hydrochloride (Niacin may potentiate the effects of ganglionic blocking agents and vasoactive drugs resulting in postural hypotension).
No products indexed under this heading.

Nicotinamide (Potent inhibitors of CYP3A4 increase the risk of myopathy by reducing the elimination of simvastatin. Hence when simvastatin is used with a potent inhibitor of CYP3A4, elevated plasma levels of HMG-CoA reductase inhibitory activity can increase the risk of myopathy and rhabdomyolysis, particularly with higher doses of simvastatin. Concomitant use of drugs labeled as potent inhibitors of CYP3A4 should be avoided unless the benefits of combined therapy outweigh the increased risk. If treatment with itraconazole, ketoconazole, erythromycin, clarithromycin or telithromycin is unavoidable, therapy with Simcor should be suspended during the course of treatment).
No products indexed under this heading.

Nifedipine (Niacin may potentiate the effects of ganglionic blocking agents and vasoactive drugs resulting in postural hypotension).
No products indexed under this heading.

Nisoldipine (Niacin may potentiate the effects of ganglionic blocking agents and vasoactive drugs resulting in postural hypotension).
No products indexed under this heading.

Nitroglycerin (Niacin may potentiate the effects of ganglionic blocking agents and vasoactive drugs resulting in postural hypotension). Products include:
Nitro-Dur 3170
Nitrolingual 3266

Norfloxacin (Potent inhibitors of CYP3A4 increase the risk of myopathy by reducing the elimination of simvastatin. Hence when simvastatin is used with a potent inhibitor of CYP3A4, elevated plasma levels of HMG-CoA reductase inhibitory activity can increase the risk of myopathy and rhabdomyolysis, particularly with higher doses of simvastatin. Concomitant use of drugs labeled as potent inhibitors of CYP3A4 should be avoided unless the benefits of combined therapy outweigh the increased risk. If treatment with itraconazole, ketoconazole, erythromycin, clarithromycin or telithromycin is unavoidable, therapy with Simcor should be suspended during the course of treatment). Products include:
Noroxin 2220

Nutritional Supplement (Nutritional supplements containing large doses of niacin or related compounds may potentiate the adverse effects of Simcor).
No products indexed under this heading.

Omeprazole (Potent inhibitors of CYP3A4 increase the risk of myopathy by reducing the elimination of simvastatin. Hence when simvastatin is used with a potent inhibitor of CYP3A4, elevated plasma levels of HMG-CoA reductase inhibitory activity can increase the risk of myopathy and rhabdomyolysis, particularly with higher doses of simvastatin. Concomitant use of drugs labeled as potent inhibitors of CYP3A4 should be avoided unless the benefits of combined therapy outweigh the increased risk. If treatment with itraconazole, ketoconazole, erythromycin, clarithromycin or telithromycin is unavoidable, therapy with Simcor should be suspended during the course of treatment).
No products indexed under this heading.

Paroxetine Hydrochloride (Potent inhibitors of CYP3A4 increase the risk of myopathy by reducing the elimination of simvastatin. Hence when simvastatin is used with a potent inhibitor of CYP3A4, elevated plasma levels of HMG-CoA reductase inhibitory activity can increase the risk of myopathy and rhabdomyolysis, particularly with higher doses of simvastatin. Concomitant use of drugs labeled as potent inhibitors of CYP3A4 should be avoided unless the benefits of combined therapy outweigh the increased risk. If treatment with itraconazole, ketoconazole, erythromycin, clarithromycin or telithromycin is unavoidable, therapy with Simcor should be suspended during the course of treatment). Products include:
Paroxetine CR 2361
Paroxetine ER 2371
Paxil 1586
Paxil CR 1596

Penbutolol Sulfate (Niacin may potentiate the effects of ganglionic blocking agents and vasoactive drugs resulting in postural hypotension).
No products indexed under this heading.

Perindopril Erbumine (Niacin may potentiate the effects of ganglionic blocking agents and vasoactive drugs resulting in postural hypotension).
No products indexed under this heading.

Phenoxybenzamine Hydrochloride (Niacin may potentiate the effects of ganglionic blocking agents and vasoactive drugs resulting in postural hypotension). Products include:
Dibenzyline 3495

Phentolamine Mesylate (Niacin may potentiate the effects of ganglionic blocking agents and vasoactive drugs resulting in postural hypotension).
No products indexed under this heading.

Pindolol (Niacin may potentiate the effects of ganglionic blocking agents and vasoactive drugs resulting in postural hypotension).
No products indexed under this heading.

Polythiazide (Niacin may potentiate the effects of ganglionic blocking agents and vasoactive drugs resulting in postural hypotension).
No products indexed under this heading.

Posaconazole (Potent inhibitors of CYP3A4 increase the risk of myopathy by reducing the elimination of simvastatin. Hence when simvastatin is used with a potent inhibitor of CYP3A4, elevated plasma levels of HMG-CoA reductase inhibitory activity can increase the risk of myopathy and rhabdomyolysis, particularly with higher doses of simvastatin. Concomitant use of drugs labeled as potent inhibitors of CYP3A4 should be avoided unless the benefits of combined therapy outweigh the increased risk. If treatment with itraconazole, ketoconazole, erythromycin, clarithromycin or telithromycin is unavoidable, therapy with Simcor should be suspended during the course of treatment). Products include:
Noxafil 3172

Prazosin Hydrochloride (Niacin may potentiate the effects of ganglionic blocking agents and vasoactive drugs resulting in postural hypotension).
No products indexed under this heading.

Propoxyphene Hydrochloride (Potent inhibitors of CYP3A4 increase the risk of myopathy by reducing the elimination of simvastatin. Hence when simvastatin is used with a potent inhibitor of CYP3A4, elevated plasma levels of HMG-CoA reductase inhibitory activity can increase the risk of myopathy and rhabdomyolysis, particularly with higher doses of simvastatin. Concomitant use of drugs labeled as potent inhibitors of CYP3A4 should be avoided unless the benefits of combined therapy outweigh the increased risk. If treatment with itraconazole, ketoconazole, erythromycin, clarithromycin or telithromycin is unavoidable, therapy with Simcor should be suspended during the course of treatment).
No products indexed under this heading.

Propoxyphene Napsylate (Potent inhibitors of CYP3A4 increase the risk of myopathy by reducing the elimination of simvastatin. Hence when simvastatin is used with a potent inhibitor of CYP3A4, elevated plasma levels of HMG-CoA reductase inhibitory activity can increase the risk of myopathy and rhabdomyolysis, particularly with higher doses of simvastatin. Concomitant use of drugs labeled as potent inhibitors of CYP3A4 should be avoided unless the benefits of combined therapy outweigh the increased risk. If treatment with itraconazole, ketoconazole, erythromycin, clarithromycin or telithromycin is unavoidable, therapy with Simcor should be suspended during the course of treatment).
No products indexed under this heading.

Propranolol Hydrochloride (In healthy male volunteers there was a significant decrease in mean C_{max}, but no change in AUC, for simvastatin total and active inhibitors with concomitant administration of single doses of simvastatin and propranolol. The clinical relevance of this finding is unclear. The pharmacokinetics of the enantiomers of propranolol were not affected). Products include:
InnoPran XL 1517

Quinapril Hydrochloride (Niacin may potentiate the effects of ganglionic blocking agents and vasoactive drugs resulting in postural hypotension).
No products indexed under this heading.

Quinidine (Potent inhibitors of CYP3A4 increase the risk of myopathy by reducing the elimination of simvastatin. Hence when simvastatin is used with a potent inhibitor of CYP3A4, elevated plasma levels of HMG-CoA reductase inhibitory activity can increase the risk of myopathy and rhabdomyolysis, particularly with higher doses of simvastatin. Concomitant use of drugs labeled as potent inhibitors of CYP3A4 should be avoided unless the benefits of combined therapy outweigh the increased risk. If treatment with itraconazole, ketoconazole, erythromycin, clarithromycin or telithromycin is unavoidable, therapy with Simcor should be suspended during the course of treatment).
No products indexed under this heading.

Quinidine Hydrochloride (Potent inhibitors of CYP3A4 increase the risk of myopathy by reducing the elimination of simvastatin. Hence when simvastatin is used with a potent inhibitor of CYP3A4, elevated plasma levels of HMG-CoA reductase inhibitory activity can increase the risk of myopathy and rhabdomyolysis, particularly with higher doses of simvastatin. Concomitant use of drugs labeled as potent inhibitors of CYP3A4 should be avoided unless the benefits of combined therapy outweigh the increased risk. If treatment with itraconazole, ketoconazole, erythromycin, clarithromycin or telithromycin is unavoidable, therapy with Simcor should be suspended during the course of treatment).
No products indexed under this heading.

Quinidine Polygalacturonate (Potent inhibitors of CYP3A4 increase the risk of myopathy by reducing the elimination of simvastatin. Hence when simvastatin is used with a potent inhibitor of CYP3A4, elevated plasma levels of HMG-CoA reductase inhibitory activity can increase the risk of myopathy and rhabdomyolysis, particularly with higher doses of simvastatin. Concomitant use of drugs labeled as potent inhibitors of CYP3A4 should be avoided unless the benefits of combined therapy outweigh the increased risk. If treatment with itraconazole, ketoconazole, erythromycin, clarithromycin or telithromycin is unavoidable, therapy with Simcor should be suspended during the course of treatment).
No products indexed under this heading.

Quinidine Sulfate (Potent inhibitors of CYP3A4 increase the risk of myopathy by reducing the elimination of simvastatin. Hence when simvastatin is used with a potent inhibitor of CYP3A4, elevated plasma levels of HMG-CoA reductase inhibitory activity can increase the risk of myopathy and rhabdomyolysis, particularly with higher doses of simvastatin. Concomitant use of drugs labeled as potent inhibitors of CYP3A4 should be avoided unless the benefits of combined therapy outweigh the increased risk. If treatment with itraconazole, ketoconazole, erythromycin, clarithromycin or telithromycin is unavoidable, therapy with Simcor should be suspended during the course of treatment).
No products indexed under this heading.

Quinine (Potent inhibitors of CYP3A4 increase the risk of myopathy by reducing the elimination of simvastatin. Hence when simvastatin is used with a potent inhibitor of CYP3A4, elevated plasma levels of HMG-CoA reductase inhibitory activity can increase the risk of myopathy and rhabdomyolysis, particularly with higher doses of simvastatin. Concomitant use of drugs labeled as potent inhibitors of CYP3A4 should be avoided unless the benefits of combined therapy outweigh the increased risk. If treatment with itraconazole, ketoconazole, erythromycin, clarithromycin or telithromycin is unavoidable, therapy with Simcor should be suspended during the course of treatment). Products include:
Hyland's Leg Cramps PM with Quinine 3315

Quinine Sulfate (Potent inhibitors of CYP3A4 increase the risk of myopathy by reducing the elimination of simvastatin. Hence when simvastatin is used with a potent inhibitor of CYP3A4, elevated plasma levels of HMG-CoA reductase inhibitory activity can increase the risk of myopathy and rhabdomyolysis, particularly with higher doses of simvastatin. Concomitant use of drugs labeled as potent inhibitors of CYP3A4 should be avoided unless the benefits of combined therapy outweigh the increased risk. If treatment with itraconazole, ketoconazole, erythromycin, clarithromycin or telithromycin is unavoidable, therapy with Simcor should be suspended during the course of treatment).
No products indexed under this heading.

Quinupristin (Potent inhibitors of CYP3A4 increase the risk of myopathy by reducing the elimination of simvastatin. Hence when simvastatin is used with a potent inhibitor of CYP3A4, elevated plasma levels of HMG-CoA reductase inhibitory activity can increase the risk of myopathy and rhabdomyolysis, particularly with higher doses of simvastatin. Concomitant use of drugs labeled as potent inhibitors of CYP3A4 should be avoided unless the benefits of combined therapy outweigh the increased risk. If treatment with itraconazole, ketoconazole, erythromycin, clarithro-

IMPORTANT NOTE: Always consult each drug listing in the patient's regimen for possible interactions.

Simcor Interactions Index 1748

mycin or telithromycin is unavoidable, therapy with Simcor should be suspended during the course of treatment).
No products indexed under this heading.

Ramipril (Niacin may potentiate the effects of ganglionic blocking agents and vasoactive drugs resulting in postural hypotension).
No products indexed under this heading.

Ranitidine Bismuth Citrate (Potent inhibitors of CYP3A4 increase the risk of myopathy by reducing the elimination of simvastatin. Hence when simvastatin is used with a potent inhibitor of CYP3A4, elevated plasma levels of HMG-CoA reductase inhibitory activity can increase the risk of myopathy and rhabdomyolysis, particularly with higher doses of simvastatin. Concomitant use of drugs labeled as potent inhibitors of CYP3A4 should be avoided unless the benefits of combined therapy outweigh the increased risk. If treatment with itraconazole, ketoconazole, erythromycin, clarithromycin or telithromycin is unavoidable, therapy with Simcor should be suspended during the course of treatment).
No products indexed under this heading.

Ranitidine Hydrochloride (Potent inhibitors of CYP3A4 increase the risk of myopathy by reducing the elimination of simvastatin. Hence when simvastatin is used with a potent inhibitor of CYP3A4, elevated plasma levels of HMG-CoA reductase inhibitory activity can increase the risk of myopathy and rhabdomyolysis, particularly with higher doses of simvastatin. Concomitant use of drugs labeled as potent inhibitors of CYP3A4 should be avoided unless the benefits of combined therapy outweigh the increased risk. If treatment with itraconazole, ketoconazole, erythromycin, clarithromycin or telithromycin is unavoidable, therapy with Simcor should be suspended during the course of treatment). Products include:
Zantac 1737
Zantac Injection 1732
Zantac Pharmacy 1735

Rauwolfia Serpentina (Niacin may potentiate the effects of ganglionic blocking agents and vasoactive drugs resulting in postural hypotension).
No products indexed under this heading.

Rescinnamine (Niacin may potentiate the effects of ganglionic blocking agents and vasoactive drugs resulting in postural hypotension).
No products indexed under this heading.

Reserpine (Niacin may potentiate the effects of ganglionic blocking agents and vasoactive drugs resulting in postural hypotension).
No products indexed under this heading.

Ritonavir (Potent inhibitors of CYP3A4 increase the risk of myopathy by reducing the elimination of simvastatin. Hence when simvastatin is used with a potent inhibitor of CYP3A4, elevated plasma levels of HMG-CoA reductase inhibitory activity can increase the risk of myopathy and rhabdomyolysis, particularly with higher doses of simvastatin. Concomitant use of drugs labeled as potent inhibitors of CYP3A4 should be avoided unless the benefits of combined therapy outweigh the increased risk. If treatment with itraconazole, ketoconazole, erythromycin, clarithromycin or telithromycin is unavoidable, therapy with Simcor should be suspended during the course of treatment). Products include:
Kaletra 458
Norvir 509

Saquinavir (Potent inhibitors of CYP3A4 increase the risk of myopathy by reducing the elimination of simvastatin. Hence when simvastatin is used with a potent inhibitor of CYP3A4, elevated plasma levels of HMG-CoA reductase inhibitory activity can increase the risk of myopathy and rhabdomyolysis, particularly with higher doses of simvastatin. Concomitant use of drugs labeled as potent inhibitors of CYP3A4 should be avoided unless the benefits of combined therapy outweigh the increased risk. If treatment with itraconazole, ketoconazole, erythromycin, clarithromycin or telithromycin is unavoidable, therapy with Simcor should be suspended during the course of treatment).
No products indexed under this heading.

Saquinavir Mesylate (Potent inhibitors of CYP3A4 increase the risk of myopathy by reducing the elimination of simvastatin. Hence when simvastatin is used with a potent inhibitor of CYP3A4, elevated plasma levels of HMG-CoA reductase inhibitory activity can increase the risk of myopathy and rhabdomyolysis, particularly with higher doses of simvastatin. Concomitant use of drugs labeled as potent inhibitors of CYP3A4 should be avoided unless the benefits of combined therapy outweigh the increased risk. If treatment with itraconazole, ketoconazole, erythromycin, clarithromycin or telithromycin is unavoidable, therapy with Simcor should be suspended during the course of treatment).
No products indexed under this heading.

Sertraline Hydrochloride (Potent inhibitors of CYP3A4 increase the risk of myopathy by reducing the elimination of simvastatin. Hence when simvastatin is used with a potent inhibitor of CYP3A4, elevated plasma levels of HMG-CoA reductase inhibitory activity can increase the risk of myopathy and rhabdomyolysis, particularly with higher doses of simvastatin. Concomitant use of drugs labeled as potent inhibitors of CYP3A4 should be avoided unless the benefits of combined therapy outweigh the increased risk. If treatment with itraconazole, ketoconazole, erythromycin, clarithromycin or telithromycin is unavoidable, therapy with Simcor should be suspended during the course of treatment).
No products indexed under this heading.

Sildenafil Citrate (Potent inhibitors of CYP3A4 increase the risk of myopathy by reducing the elimination of simvastatin. Hence when simvastatin is used with a potent inhibitor of CYP3A4, elevated plasma levels of HMG-CoA reductase inhibitory activity can increase the risk of myopathy and rhabdomyolysis, particularly with higher doses of simvastatin. Concomitant use of drugs labeled as potent inhibitors of CYP3A4 should be avoided unless the benefits of combined therapy outweigh the increased risk. If treatment with itraconazole, ketoconazole, erythromycin, clarithromycin or telithromycin is unavoidable, therapy with Simcor should be suspended during the course of treatment).
No products indexed under this heading.

Sodium Nitroprusside (Niacin may potentiate the effects of ganglionic blocking agents and vasoactive drugs resulting in postural hypotension).
No products indexed under this heading.

Sotalol Hydrochloride (Niacin may potentiate the effects of ganglionic blocking agents and vasoactive drugs resulting in postural hypotension).
No products indexed under this heading.

Spirapril Hydrochloride (Niacin may potentiate the effects of ganglionic blocking agents and vasoactive drugs resulting in postural hypotension).
No products indexed under this heading.

Telithromycin (Potent inhibitors of CYP3A4 increase the risk of myopathy by reducing the elimination of simvastatin. Hence when simvastatin is used with a potent inhibitor of CYP3A4, elevated plasma levels of HMG-CoA reductase inhibitory activity can increase the risk of myopathy and rhabdomyolysis, particularly with higher doses of simvastatin. Concomitant use of drugs labeled as potent inhibitors of CYP3A4 should be avoided unless the benefits of combined therapy outweigh the increased risk. If treatment with itraconazole, ketoconazole, erythromycin, clarithromycin or telithromycin is unavoidable, therapy with Simcor should be suspended during the course of treatment). Products include:
Ketek 2991

Telmisartan (Niacin may potentiate the effects of ganglionic blocking agents and vasoactive drugs resulting in postural hypotension). Products include:
Micardis 887
Micardis HCT 889

Terazosin Hydrochloride (Niacin may potentiate the effects of ganglionic blocking agents and vasoactive drugs resulting in postural hypotension).
No products indexed under this heading.

Timolol Maleate (Niacin may potentiate the effects of ganglionic blocking agents and vasoactive drugs resulting in postural hypotension). Products include:
Combigan 601
Dorzolamide Hydrochloride/Timolol Maleate Ophthalmic Solution .... ⊙243
Timoptic in Ocudose .... ⊙231

Torsemide (Niacin may potentiate the effects of ganglionic blocking agents and vasoactive drugs resulting in postural hypotension).
No products indexed under this heading.

Trandolapril (Niacin may potentiate the effects of ganglionic blocking agents and vasoactive drugs resulting in postural hypotension). Products include:
Mavik 489
Tarka 534

Trimethaphan Camsylate (Niacin may potentiate the effects of ganglionic blocking agents and vasoactive drugs resulting in postural hypotension).
No products indexed under this heading.

Troglitazone (Potent inhibitors of CYP3A4 increase the risk of myopathy by reducing the elimination of simvastatin. Hence when simvastatin is used with a potent inhibitor of CYP3A4, elevated plasma levels of HMG-CoA reductase inhibitory activity can increase the risk of myopathy and rhabdomyolysis, particularly with higher doses of simvastatin. Concomitant use of drugs labeled as potent inhibitors of CYP3A4 should be avoided unless the benefits of combined therapy outweigh the increased risk. If treatment with itraconazole, ketoconazole, erythromycin, clarithromycin or telithromycin is unavoidable, therapy with Simcor should be suspended during the course of treatment).
No products indexed under this heading.

Troleandomycin (Potent inhibitors of CYP3A4 increase the risk of myopathy by reducing the elimination of simvastatin. Hence when simvastatin is used with a potent inhibitor of CYP3A4, elevated plasma levels of HMG-CoA reductase inhibitory activity can increase the risk of myopathy and rhabdomyolysis, particularly with higher doses of simvastatin. Concomitant use of drugs labeled as potent inhibitors of CYP3A4 should be avoided unless the benefits of combined therapy outweigh the increased risk. If treatment with itraconazole, ketoconazole, erythromycin, clarithromycin or telithromycin is unavoidable, therapy with Simcor should be suspended during the course of treatment).
No products indexed under this heading.

Valproate Sodium (Potent inhibitors of CYP3A4 increase the risk of myopathy by reducing the elimination of simvastatin. Hence when simvastatin is used with a potent inhibitor of CYP3A4, elevated plasma levels of HMG-CoA reductase inhibitory activity can increase the risk of myopathy and rhabdomyolysis, particularly with higher doses of simvastatin. Concomitant use of drugs labeled as potent inhibitors of CYP3A4 should be avoided unless the benefits of combined therapy outweigh the increased risk. If treatment with itraconazole, ketoconazole, erythromycin, clarithromycin or telithromycin is unavoidable, therapy with Simcor should be suspended during the course of treatment).
No products indexed under this heading.

Valsartan (Niacin may potentiate the effects of ganglionic blocking agents and vasoactive drugs resulting in postural hypotension). Products include:
Diovan 2413
Diovan HCT 2419
Exforge 2443
Exforge HCT 2449
Valturna 3637

Vardenafil Hydrochloride (Potent inhibitors of CYP3A4 increase the risk of myopathy by reducing the elimination of simvastatin. Hence when simvastatin is used with a potent inhibitor of CYP3A4, elevated plasma levels of HMG-CoA reductase inhibitory activity can increase the risk of myopathy and rhabdomyolysis, particularly with higher doses of simvastatin. Concomitant use of drugs labeled as potent inhibitors of CYP3A4 should be avoided unless the benefits of combined therapy outweigh the increased risk. If treatment with itraconazole, ketoconazole, erythromycin, clarithromycin or telithromycin is unavoidable, therapy with Simcor should be suspended during the course of treatment). Products include:
Levitra 3157

Verapamil Hydrochloride (The risk of myopathy/rhabdomyolysis is increased by concomitant administration of amiodarone or verapamil with higher doses of simvastatin. Combination with Simcor should be limited to the 20 mg once daily dose of simvastatin). Products include:
Tarka 534

Vitamin B Complex (Nutritional supplements containing large doses of niacin or related compounds may potentiate the adverse effects of simvastatin).
No products indexed under this heading.

Vitamin B Complex With Vitamin C (Nutritional supplements containing large doses of niacin or related compounds may potentiate the adverse effects of simvastatin).
No products indexed under this heading.

Vitamins, Multiple (Nutritional supplements containing large doses of niacin or related compounds may potentiate the adverse effects of Simcor). Products include:
Mega Antioxidant 3476

Voriconazole (Potent inhibitors of CYP3A4 increase the risk of myopathy by reducing the elimination of simvastatin. Hence when simvastatin is used with a potent inhibitor of CYP3A4, elevated plasma levels of HMG-CoA reductase inhibitory activity can increase the risk of myopathy and rhabdomyolysis, particularly with higher doses of simvastatin. Concomitant use of drugs labeled as potent inhibitors of CYP3A4 should be avoided unless the benefits of combined therapy outweigh the increased risk. If treatment with itraconazole, ketoconazole, erythromycin, clarithro-

(⊙ Described in PDR® for Ophthalmic Medicines)

1749 Interactions Index Simponi

mycin or telithromycin is unavoidable, therapy with Simcor should be suspended during the course of treatment).
No products indexed under this heading.

Warfarin Sodium (Co-administration prolongs INR. Achieve stable INR prior to starting Simcor. Monitor INR frequently until stable upon initiation or alteration of Simcor therapy).
No products indexed under this heading.

Zafirlukast (Potent inhibitors of CYP3A4 increase the risk of myopathy by reducing the elimination of simvastatin. Hence when simvastatin is used with a potent inhibitor of CYP3A4, elevated plasma levels of HMG-CoA reductase inhibitory activity can increase the risk of myopathy and rhabdomyolysis, particularly with higher doses of simvastatin. Concomitant use of drugs labeled as potent inhibitors of CYP3A4 should be avoided unless the benefits of combined therapy outweigh the increased risk. If treatment with itraconazole, ketoconazole, erythromycin, clarithromycin or telithromycin is unavoidable, therapy with Simcor should be suspended during the course of treatment). Products include:
Accolate 3612

Zileuton (Potent inhibitors of CYP3A4 increase the risk of myopathy by reducing the elimination of simvastatin. Hence when simvastatin is used with a potent inhibitor of CYP3A4, elevated plasma levels of HMG-CoA reductase inhibitory activity can increase the risk of myopathy and rhabdomyolysis, particularly with higher doses of simvastatin. Concomitant use of drugs labeled as potent inhibitors of CYP3A4 should be avoided unless the benefits of combined therapy outweigh the increased risk. If treatment with itraconazole, ketoconazole, erythromycin, clarithromycin or telithromycin is unavoidable, therapy with Simcor should be suspended during the course of treatment).
No products indexed under this heading.

Food Interactions

Grapefruit (Potent inhibitors of CYP3A4 increase the risk of myopathy by reducing the elimination of simvastatin. Hence when simvastatin is used with a potent inhibitor of CYP3A4, elevated plasma levels of HMG-CoA reductase inhibitory activity can increase the risk of myopathy and rhabdomyolysis, particularly with higher doses of simvastatin. Concomitant use of drugs labeled as potent inhibitors of CYP3A4 should be avoided unless the benefits of combined therapy outweigh the increased risk. If treatment with itraconazole, ketoconazole, erythromycin, clarithromycin or telithromycin is unavoidable, therapy with Simcor should be suspended during the course of treatment).

Grapefruit Juice (Potent inhibitors of CYP3A4 increase the risk of myopathy by reducing the elimination of simvastatin. Hence when simvastatin is used with a potent inhibitor of CYP3A4, elevated plasma levels of HMG-CoA reductase inhibitory activity can increase the risk of myopathy and rhabdomyolysis, particularly with higher doses of simvastatin. Concomitant use of drugs labeled as potent inhibitors of CYP3A4 should be avoided unless the benefits of combined therapy outweigh the increased risk. If treatment with itraconazole, ketoconazole, erythromycin, clarithromycin or telithromycin is unavoidable, therapy with Simcor should be suspended during the course of treatment).

SIMPONI INJECTION

(Golimumab) 930
May interact with drugs which undergo biotransformation by cytochrome p-450 mixed function oxidase, theophyllines, vaccines, live, and certain other agents. Compounds in these categories include:

Abatacept (In controlled trials, the concurrent administration of another TNF-blocker and abatacept was associated with a greater proportion of serious infections than the use of a TNF-blocker alone; and the combination therapy, compared to the use of a TNF-blocker alone, has not demonstrated improved clinical benefit in the treatment of RA. Therefore, the combination of TNF-blockers, including golimumab, and abatacept is not recommended).
No products indexed under this heading.

Acarbose (The formation of CYP450 enzymes may be suppressed by increased levels of cytokines (eg, TNFα) during chronic inflammation. Therefore, it is expected that for a molecule that antagonizes cytokine activity, such as golimumab, the formation of CYP450 enzymes could be normalized. Upon initiation or discontinuation of golimumab in patients being treated with CYP450 substrates with a narrow therapeutic index, monitoring of the effect (eg, warfarin) or drug concentration (eg, cyclosporine or theophylline) is recommended and the individual dose of the drug product may be adjusted as needed).
No products indexed under this heading.

Acetaminophen (The formation of CYP450 enzymes may be suppressed by increased levels of cytokines (eg, TNFα) during chronic inflammation. Therefore, it is expected that for a molecule that antagonizes cytokine activity, such as golimumab, the formation of CYP450 enzymes could be normalized. Upon initiation or discontinuation of golimumab in patients being treated with CYP450 substrates with a narrow therapeutic index, monitoring of the effect (eg, warfarin) or drug concentration (eg, cyclosporine or theophylline) is recommended and the individual dose of the drug product may be adjusted as needed). Products include:
Percocet 1121
Tylenol 2049
Tylenol 8 Hour 2049
Extra Strength Tylenol Caplets, Cool Caplets, and EZ Tabs 2049
Extra Strength Tylenol Adult Rapid Blast Liquid 2049
Extra Strength Tylenol Rapid Release 2049
Tylenol with Codeine 2691
Tylenol Arthritis Pain Extended Release Geltabs/Caplets 2049
Children's Tylenol Suspension Liquid 2048
Chlidren's Tylenol Meltaways 2048
Tylenol, Infants' Drops 2048
Junior Tylenol 2048
Vicodin 560
Vicodin ES 561
Vicodin HP 563
Zydone 1138

Alatrofloxacin Mesylate (The formation of CYP450 enzymes may be suppressed by increased levels of cytokines (eg, TNFα) during chronic inflammation. Therefore, it is expected that for a molecule that antagonizes cytokine activity, such as golimumab, the formation of CYP450 enzymes could be normalized. Upon initiation or discontinuation of golimumab in patients being treated with CYP450 substrates with a narrow therapeutic index, monitoring of the effect (eg, warfarin) or drug concentration (eg, cyclosporine or theophylline) is recommended and the individual dose of the drug product may be adjusted as needed).
No products indexed under this heading.

Alfentanil Hydrochloride (The formation of CYP450 enzymes may be suppressed by increased levels of cytokines (eg, TNFα) during chronic inflammation. Therefore, it is expected that for a molecule that antagonizes cytokine activity, such as golimumab, the formation of CYP450 enzymes could be normalized. Upon initiation or discontinuation of golimumab in patients being treated with CYP450 substrates with a narrow therapeutic index, monitoring of the effect (eg, warfarin) or drug concentration (eg, cyclosporine or theophylline) is recommended and the individual dose of the drug product may be adjusted as needed).
No products indexed under this heading.

Alprazolam (The formation of CYP450 enzymes may be suppressed by increased levels of cytokines (eg, TNFα) during chronic inflammation. Therefore, it is expected that for a molecule that antagonizes cytokine activity, such as golimumab, the formation of CYP450 enzymes could be normalized. Upon initiation or discontinuation of golimumab in patients being treated with CYP450 substrates with a narrow therapeutic index, monitoring of the effect (eg, warfarin) or drug concentration (eg, cyclosporine or theophylline) is recommended and the individual dose of the drug product may be adjusted as needed).
No products indexed under this heading.

Aminophylline (The formation of CYP450 enzymes may be suppressed by increased levels of cytokines (eg, TNFα) during chronic inflammation. Therefore, it is expected that for a molecule that antagonizes cytokine activity, such as golimumab, the formation of CYP450 enzymes could be normalized. Upon initiation or discontinuation of golimumab in patients being treated with CYP450 substrates with a narrow therapeutic index, monitoring of the effect (eg, warfarin) or drug concentration (eg, cyclosporine or theophylline) is recommended and the individual dose of the drug product may be adjusted as needed).
No products indexed under this heading.

Amiodarone Hydrochloride (The formation of CYP450 enzymes may be suppressed by increased levels of cytokines (eg, TNFα) during chronic inflammation. Therefore, it is expected that for a molecule that antagonizes cytokine activity, such as golimumab, the formation of CYP450 enzymes could be normalized. Upon initiation or discontinuation of golimumab in patients being treated with CYP450 substrates with a narrow therapeutic index, monitoring of the effect (eg, warfarin) or drug concentration (eg, cyclosporine or theophylline) is recommended and the individual dose of the drug product may be adjusted as needed).
No products indexed under this heading.

Amitriptyline Hydrochloride (The formation of CYP450 enzymes may be suppressed by increased levels of cytokines (eg, TNFα) during chronic inflammation. Therefore, it is expected that for a molecule that antagonizes cytokine activity, such as golimumab, the formation of CYP450 enzymes could be normalized. Upon initiation or discontinuation of golimumab in patients being treated with CYP450 substrates with a narrow therapeutic index, monitoring of the effect (eg, warfarin) or drug concentration (eg, cyclosporine or theophylline) is recommended and the individual dose of the drug product may be adjusted as needed).
No products indexed under this heading.

Amlodipine Besylate (The formation of CYP450 enzymes may be suppressed by increased levels of cytokines (eg, TNFα) during chronic inflammation. Therefore, it is expected that for a molecule that antagonizes cytokine activity, such as golimumab, the formation of CYP450 enzymes could be normalized. Upon initiation or discontinuation of golimumab in patients being treated with CYP450 substrates with a narrow therapeutic index, monitoring of the effect (eg, warfarin) or drug concentration (eg, cyclosporine or theophylline) is recommended and the individual dose of the drug product may be adjusted as needed). Products include:
Azor 1010
Exforge 2443
Exforge HCT 2449

Amoxapine (The formation of CYP450 enzymes may be suppressed by increased levels of cytokines (eg, TNFα) during chronic inflammation. Therefore, it is expected that for a molecule that antagonizes cytokine activity, such as golimumab, the formation of CYP450 enzymes could be normalized. Upon initiation or discontinuation of golimumab in patients being treated with CYP450 substrates with a narrow therapeutic index, monitoring of the effect (eg, warfarin) or drug concentration (eg, cyclosporine or theophylline) is recommended and the individual dose of the drug product may be adjusted as needed).
No products indexed under this heading.

Amphetamine Aspartate (The formation of CYP450 enzymes may be suppressed by increased levels of cytokines (eg, TNFα) during chronic inflammation. Therefore, it is expected that for a molecule that antagonizes cytokine activity, such as golimumab, the formation of CYP450 enzymes could be normalized. Upon initiation or discontinuation of golimumab in patients being treated with CYP450 substrates with a narrow therapeutic index, monitoring of the effect (eg, warfarin) or drug concentration (eg, cyclosporine or theophylline) is recommended and the individual dose of the drug product may be adjusted as needed).
No products indexed under this heading.

Amphetamine Aspartate Monohydrate (The formation of CYP450 enzymes may be suppressed by increased levels of cytokines (eg, TNFα) during chronic inflammation. Therefore, it is expected that for a molecule that antagonizes cytokine activity, such as golimumab, the formation of CYP450 enzymes could be normalized. Upon initiation or discontinuation of golimumab in patients being treated with CYP450 substrates with a narrow therapeutic index, monitoring of the effect (eg, warfarin) or drug concentration (eg, cyclosporine or theophylline) is recommended and the individual dose of the drug product may be adjusted as needed).
No products indexed under this heading.

Amphetamine Sulfate (The formation of CYP450 enzymes may be suppressed by increased levels of cytokines (eg, TNFα) during chronic inflammation. Therefore, it is expected that for a molecule that antagonizes cytokine activity, such as golimumab, the formation of CYP450 enzymes could be normalized. Upon initiation or discontinuation of golimumab in patients being treated with CYP450 substrates with a narrow therapeutic index, monitoring of the effect (eg, warfarin) or drug concentration (eg, cyclosporine or theophylline) is recom-

mended and the individual dose of the drug product may be adjusted as needed).

No products indexed under this heading.

Anagrelide Hydrochloride (The formation of CYP450 enzymes may be suppressed by increased levels of cytokines (eg, TNFα) during chronic inflammation. Therefore, it is expected that for a molecule that antagonizes cytokine activity, such as golimumab, the formation of CYP450 enzymes could be normalized. Upon initiation or discontinuation of golimumab in patients being treated with CYP450 substrates with a narrow therapeutic index, monitoring of the effect (eg, warfarin) or drug concentration (eg, cyclosporine or theophylline) is recommended and the individual dose of the drug product may be adjusted as needed).

No products indexed under this heading.

Anakinra (The concurrent administration of anakinra (an interleukin-1 antagonist) and a TNF-blocker was associated with a greater portion of serious infections and neutropenia and no additional benefits compared with the TNF-blocker alone. Therefore, the combination of anakinra with TNF-blockers, including golimumab, is not recommended). Products include:

Kineret 877

Aprepitant (The formation of CYP450 enzymes may be suppressed by increased levels of cytokines (eg, TNFα) during chronic inflammation. Therefore, it is expected that for a molecule that antagonizes cytokine activity, such as golimumab, the formation of CYP450 enzymes could be normalized. Upon initiation or discontinuation of golimumab in patients being treated with CYP450 substrates with a narrow therapeutic index, monitoring of the effect (eg, warfarin) or drug concentration (eg, cyclosporine or theophylline) is recommended and the individual dose of the drug product may be adjusted as needed). Products include:

Emend 2124

Astemizole (The formation of CYP450 enzymes may be suppressed by increased levels of cytokines (eg, TNFα) during chronic inflammation. Therefore, it is expected that for a molecule that antagonizes cytokine activity, such as golimumab, the formation of CYP450 enzymes could be normalized. Upon initiation or discontinuation of golimumab in patients being treated with CYP450 substrates with a narrow therapeutic index, monitoring of the effect (eg, warfarin) or drug concentration (eg, cyclosporine or theophylline) is recommended and the individual dose of the drug product may be adjusted as needed).

No products indexed under this heading.

Atomoxetine Hydrochloride (The formation of CYP450 enzymes may be suppressed by increased levels of cytokines (eg, TNFα) during chronic inflammation. Therefore, it is expected that for a molecule that antagonizes cytokine activity, such as golimumab, the formation of CYP450 enzymes could be normalized. Upon initiation or discontinuation of golimumab in patients being treated with CYP450 substrates with a narrow therapeutic index, monitoring of the effect (eg, warfarin) or drug concentration (eg, cyclosporine or theophylline) is recommended and the individual dose of the drug product may be adjusted as needed). Products include:

Strattera 1957

Atorvastatin Calcium (The formation of CYP450 enzymes may be suppressed by increased levels of cytokines (eg, TNFα) during chronic inflam-

mation. Therefore, it is expected that for a molecule that antagonizes cytokine activity, such as golimumab, the formation of CYP450 enzymes could be normalized. Upon initiation or discontinuation of golimumab in patients being treated with CYP450 substrates with a narrow therapeutic index, monitoring of the effect (eg, warfarin) or drug concentration (eg, cyclosporine or theophylline) is recommended and the individual dose of the drug product may be adjusted as needed). Products include:

Lipitor 2703

BCG Vaccine (Live vaccines should not be given concurrently with golimumab).

No products indexed under this heading.

Belladonna Ergotamine (The formation of CYP450 enzymes may be suppressed by increased levels of cytokines (eg, TNFα) during chronic inflammation. Therefore, it is expected that for a molecule that antagonizes cytokine activity, such as golimumab, the formation of CYP450 enzymes could be normalized. Upon initiation or discontinuation of golimumab in patients being treated with CYP450 substrates with a narrow therapeutic index, monitoring of the effect (eg, warfarin) or drug concentration (eg, cyclosporine or theophylline) is recommended and the individual dose of the drug product may be adjusted as needed).

No products indexed under this heading.

Benzphetamine Hydrochloride (The formation of CYP450 enzymes may be suppressed by increased levels of cytokines (eg, TNFα) during chronic inflammation. Therefore, it is expected that for a molecule that antagonizes cytokine activity, such as golimumab, the formation of CYP450 enzymes could be normalized. Upon initiation or discontinuation of golimumab in patients being treated with CYP450 substrates with a narrow therapeutic index, monitoring of the effect (eg, warfarin) or drug concentration (eg, cyclosporine or theophylline) is recommended and the individual dose of the drug product may be adjusted as needed).

No products indexed under this heading.

Bisoprolol Fumarate (The formation of CYP450 enzymes may be suppressed by increased levels of cytokines (eg, TNFα) during chronic inflammation. Therefore, it is expected that for a molecule that antagonizes cytokine activity, such as golimumab, the formation of CYP450 enzymes could be normalized. Upon initiation or discontinuation of golimumab in patients being treated with CYP450 substrates with a narrow therapeutic index, monitoring of the effect (eg, warfarin) or drug concentration (eg, cyclosporine or theophylline) is recommended and the individual dose of the drug product may be adjusted as needed).

No products indexed under this heading.

Bromocriptine Mesylate (The formation of CYP450 enzymes may be suppressed by increased levels of cytokines (eg, TNFα) during chronic inflammation. Therefore, it is expected that for a molecule that antagonizes cytokine activity, such as golimumab, the formation of CYP450 enzymes could be normalized. Upon initiation or discontinuation of golimumab in patients being treated with CYP450 substrates with a narrow therapeutic index, monitoring of the effect (eg, warfarin) or drug concentration (eg, cyclosporine or theophylline) is recommended and the individual dose of the drug product may be adjusted as needed).

No products indexed under this heading.

Buspirone Hydrochloride (The formation of CYP450 enzymes may be suppressed by increased levels of cytokines (eg, TNFα) during chronic inflammation. Therefore, it is expected that for a molecule that antagonizes cytokine activity, such as golimumab, the formation of CYP450 enzymes could be normalized. Upon initiation or discontinuation of golimumab in patients being treated with CYP450 substrates with a narrow therapeutic index, monitoring of the effect (eg, warfarin) or drug concentration (eg, cyclosporine or theophylline) is recommended and the individual dose of the drug product may be adjusted as needed).

No products indexed under this heading.

Busulfan (The formation of CYP450 enzymes may be suppressed by increased levels of cytokines (eg, TNFα) during chronic inflammation. Therefore, it is expected that for a molecule that antagonizes cytokine activity, such as golimumab, the formation of CYP450 enzymes could be normalized. Upon initiation or discontinuation of golimumab in patients being treated with CYP450 substrates with a narrow therapeutic index, monitoring of the effect (eg, warfarin) or drug concentration (eg, cyclosporine or theophylline) is recommended and the individual dose of the drug product may be adjusted as needed). Products include:

Myleran 1581

Caffeine (The formation of CYP450 enzymes may be suppressed by increased levels of cytokines (eg, TNFα) during chronic inflammation. Therefore, it is expected that for a molecule that antagonizes cytokine activity, such as golimumab, the formation of CYP450 enzymes could be normalized. Upon initiation or discontinuation of golimumab in patients being treated with CYP450 substrates with a narrow therapeutic index, monitoring of the effect (eg, warfarin) or drug concentration (eg, cyclosporine or theophylline) is recommended and the individual dose of the drug product may be adjusted as needed).

No products indexed under this heading.

Caffeine Anhydrous (The formation of CYP450 enzymes may be suppressed by increased levels of cytokines (eg, TNFα) during chronic inflammation. Therefore, it is expected that for a molecule that antagonizes cytokine activity, such as golimumab, the formation of CYP450 enzymes could be normalized. Upon initiation or discontinuation of golimumab in patients being treated with CYP450 substrates with a narrow therapeutic index, monitoring of the effect (eg, warfarin) or drug concentration (eg, cyclosporine or theophylline) is recommended and the individual dose of the drug product may be adjusted as needed).

No products indexed under this heading.

Caffeine Citrate (The formation of CYP450 enzymes may be suppressed by increased levels of cytokines (eg, TNFα) during chronic inflammation. Therefore, it is expected that for a molecule that antagonizes cytokine activity, such as golimumab, the formation of CYP450 enzymes could be normalized. Upon initiation or discontinuation of golimumab in patients being treated with CYP450 substrates with a narrow therapeutic index, monitoring of the effect (eg, warfarin) or drug concentration (eg, cyclosporine or theophylline) is recommended and the individual dose of the drug product may be adjusted as needed).

No products indexed under this heading.

Caffeine-containing medications (The formation of CYP450 enzymes

may be suppressed by increased levels of cytokines (eg, TNFα) during chronic inflammation. Therefore, it is expected that for a molecule that antagonizes cytokine activity, such as golimumab, the formation of CYP450 enzymes could be normalized. Upon initiation or discontinuation of golimumab in patients being treated with CYP450 substrates with a narrow therapeutic index, monitoring of the effect (eg, warfarin) or drug concentration (eg, cyclosporine or theophylline) is recommended and the individual dose of the drug product may be adjusted as needed).

No products indexed under this heading.

Caffeine Sodium Benzoate (The formation of CYP450 enzymes may be suppressed by increased levels of cytokines (eg, TNFα) during chronic inflammation. Therefore, it is expected that for a molecule that antagonizes cytokine activity, such as golimumab, the formation of CYP450 enzymes could be normalized. Upon initiation or discontinuation of golimumab in patients being treated with CYP450 substrates with a narrow therapeutic index, monitoring of the effect (eg, warfarin) or drug concentration (eg, cyclosporine or theophylline) is recommended and the individual dose of the drug product may be adjusted as needed).

No products indexed under this heading.

Candesartan Cilexetil (The formation of CYP450 enzymes may be suppressed by increased levels of cytokines (eg, TNFα) during chronic inflammation. Therefore, it is expected that for a molecule that antagonizes cytokine activity, such as golimumab, the formation of CYP450 enzymes could be normalized. Upon initiation or discontinuation of golimumab in patients being treated with CYP450 substrates with a narrow therapeutic index, monitoring of the effect (eg, warfarin) or drug concentration (eg, cyclosporine or theophylline) is recommended and the individual dose of the drug product may be adjusted as needed). Products include:

Atacand 697
Atacand HCT 700

Captopril (The formation of CYP450 enzymes may be suppressed by increased levels of cytokines (eg, TNFα) during chronic inflammation. Therefore, it is expected that for a molecule that antagonizes cytokine activity, such as golimumab, the formation of CYP450 enzymes could be normalized. Upon initiation or discontinuation of golimumab in patients being treated with CYP450 substrates with a narrow therapeutic index, monitoring of the effect (eg, warfarin) or drug concentration (eg, cyclosporine or theophylline) is recommended and the individual dose of the drug product may be adjusted as needed). Products include:

Captopril 2341

Carbamazepine (The formation of CYP450 enzymes may be suppressed by increased levels of cytokines (eg, TNFα) during chronic inflammation. Therefore, it is expected that for a molecule that antagonizes cytokine activity, such as golimumab, the formation of CYP450 enzymes could be normalized. Upon initiation or discontinuation of golimumab in patients being treated with CYP450 substrates with a narrow therapeutic index, monitoring of the effect (eg, warfarin) or drug concentration (eg, cyclosporine or theophylline) is recommended and the individual dose of the drug product may be adjusted as needed). Products include:

Carbatrol 3280
Equetro 3477

Carisoprodol (The formation of CYP450 enzymes may be suppressed by increased levels of cytokines (eg, TNFα) during chronic inflammation. Therefore, it is expected that for a molecule that antagonizes cytokine activity, such as golimumab, the formation of CYP450 enzymes could be normalized. Upon initiation or discontinuation of golimumab in patients being treated with CYP450 substrates with a narrow therapeutic index, monitoring of the effect (eg, warfarin) or drug concentration (eg, cyclosporine or theophylline) is recommended and the individual dose of the drug product may be adjusted as needed).
No products indexed under this heading.

Carvedilol (The formation of CYP450 enzymes may be suppressed by increased levels of cytokines (eg, TNFα) during chronic inflammation. Therefore, it is expected that for a molecule that antagonizes cytokine activity, such as golimumab, the formation of CYP450 enzymes could be normalized. Upon initiation or discontinuation of golimumab in patients being treated with CYP450 substrates with a narrow therapeutic index, monitoring of the effect (eg, warfarin) or drug concentration (eg, cyclosporine or theophylline) is recommended and the individual dose of the drug product may be adjusted as needed). Products include:
Coreg 1409

Celecoxib (The formation of CYP450 enzymes may be suppressed by increased levels of cytokines (eg, TNFα) during chronic inflammation. Therefore, it is expected that for a molecule that antagonizes cytokine activity, such as golimumab, the formation of CYP450 enzymes could be normalized. Upon initiation or discontinuation of golimumab in patients being treated with CYP450 substrates with a narrow therapeutic index, monitoring of the effect (eg, warfarin) or drug concentration (eg, cyclosporine or theophylline) is recommended and the individual dose of the drug product may be adjusted as needed). Products include:
Celebrex 3272

Cerivastatin Sodium (The formation of CYP450 enzymes may be suppressed by increased levels of cytokines (eg, TNFα) during chronic inflammation. Therefore, it is expected that for a molecule that antagonizes cytokine activity, such as golimumab, the formation of CYP450 enzymes could be normalized. Upon initiation or discontinuation of golimumab in patients being treated with CYP450 substrates with a narrow therapeutic index, monitoring of the effect (eg, warfarin) or drug concentration (eg, cyclosporine or theophylline) is recommended and the individual dose of the drug product may be adjusted as needed).
No products indexed under this heading.

Cevimeline Hydrochloride (The formation of CYP450 enzymes may be suppressed by increased levels of cytokines (eg, TNFα) during chronic inflammation. Therefore, it is expected that for a molecule that antagonizes cytokine activity, such as golimumab, the formation of CYP450 enzymes could be normalized. Upon initiation or discontinuation of golimumab in patients being treated with CYP450 substrates with a narrow therapeutic index, monitoring of the effect (eg, warfarin) or drug concentration (eg, cyclosporine or theophylline) is recommended and the individual dose of the drug product may be adjusted as needed). Products include:
Evoxac 1027

Chlordiazepoxide (The formation of CYP450 enzymes may be suppressed

by increased levels of cytokines (eg, TNFα) during chronic inflammation. Therefore, it is expected that for a molecule that antagonizes cytokine activity, such as golimumab, the formation of CYP450 enzymes could be normalized. Upon initiation or discontinuation of golimumab in patients being treated with CYP450 substrates with a narrow therapeutic index, monitoring of the effect (eg, warfarin) or drug concentration (eg, cyclosporine or theophylline) is recommended and the individual dose of the drug product may be adjusted as needed).
No products indexed under this heading.

Chlordiazepoxide Hydrochloride (The formation of CYP450 enzymes may be suppressed by increased levels of cytokines (eg, TNFα) during chronic inflammation. Therefore, it is expected that for a molecule that antagonizes cytokine activity, such as golimumab, the formation of CYP450 enzymes could be normalized. Upon initiation or discontinuation of golimumab in patients being treated with CYP450 substrates with a narrow therapeutic index, monitoring of the effect (eg, warfarin) or drug concentration (eg, cyclosporine or theophylline) is recommended and the individual dose of the drug product may be adjusted as needed).
No products indexed under this heading.

Chlorpheniramine (The formation of CYP450 enzymes may be suppressed by increased levels of cytokines (eg, TNFα) during chronic inflammation. Therefore, it is expected that for a molecule that antagonizes cytokine activity, such as golimumab, the formation of CYP450 enzymes could be normalized. Upon initiation or discontinuation of golimumab in patients being treated with CYP450 substrates with a narrow therapeutic index, monitoring of the effect (eg, warfarin) or drug concentration (eg, cyclosporine or theophylline) is recommended and the individual dose of the drug product may be adjusted as needed).
No products indexed under this heading.

Chlorpheniramine Maleate (The formation of CYP450 enzymes may be suppressed by increased levels of cytokines (eg, TNFα) during chronic inflammation. Therefore, it is expected that for a molecule that antagonizes cytokine activity, such as golimumab, the formation of CYP450 enzymes could be normalized. Upon initiation or discontinuation of golimumab in patients being treated with CYP450 substrates with a narrow therapeutic index, monitoring of the effect (eg, warfarin) or drug concentration (eg, cyclosporine or theophylline) is recommended and the individual dose of the drug product may be adjusted as needed).
No products indexed under this heading.

Chlorpheniramine Polistirex (The formation of CYP450 enzymes may be suppressed by increased levels of cytokines (eg, TNFα) during chronic inflammation. Therefore, it is expected that for a molecule that antagonizes cytokine activity, such as golimumab, the formation of CYP450 enzymes could be normalized. Upon initiation or discontinuation of golimumab in patients being treated with CYP450 substrates with a narrow therapeutic index, monitoring of the effect (eg, warfarin) or drug concentration (eg, cyclosporine or theophylline) is recommended and the individual dose of the drug product may be adjusted as needed). Products include:
Tussionex 3443

Chlorpheniramine Tannate (The formation of CYP450 enzymes may be

suppressed by increased levels of cytokines (eg, TNFα) during chronic inflammation. Therefore, it is expected that for a molecule that antagonizes cytokine activity, such as golimumab, the formation of CYP450 enzymes could be normalized. Upon initiation or discontinuation of golimumab in patients being treated with CYP450 substrates with a narrow therapeutic index, monitoring of the effect (eg, warfarin) or drug concentration (eg, cyclosporine or theophylline) is recommended and the individual dose of the drug product may be adjusted as needed).
No products indexed under this heading.

Chlorpromazine (The formation of CYP450 enzymes may be suppressed by increased levels of cytokines (eg, TNFα) during chronic inflammation. Therefore, it is expected that for a molecule that antagonizes cytokine activity, such as golimumab, the formation of CYP450 enzymes could be normalized. Upon initiation or discontinuation of golimumab in patients being treated with CYP450 substrates with a narrow therapeutic index, monitoring of the effect (eg, warfarin) or drug concentration (eg, cyclosporine or theophylline) is recommended and the individual dose of the drug product may be adjusted as needed).
No products indexed under this heading.

Chlorpromazine Hydrochloride (The formation of CYP450 enzymes may be suppressed by increased levels of cytokines (eg, TNFα) during chronic inflammation. Therefore, it is expected that for a molecule that antagonizes cytokine activity, such as golimumab, the formation of CYP450 enzymes could be normalized. Upon initiation or discontinuation of golimumab in patients being treated with CYP450 substrates with a narrow therapeutic index, monitoring of the effect (eg, warfarin) or drug concentration (eg, cyclosporine or theophylline) is recommended and the individual dose of the drug product may be adjusted as needed).
No products indexed under this heading.

Chlorpropamide (The formation of CYP450 enzymes may be suppressed by increased levels of cytokines (eg, TNFα) during chronic inflammation. Therefore, it is expected that for a molecule that antagonizes cytokine activity, such as golimumab, the formation of CYP450 enzymes could be normalized. Upon initiation or discontinuation of golimumab in patients being treated with CYP450 substrates with a narrow therapeutic index, monitoring of the effect (eg, warfarin) or drug concentration (eg, cyclosporine or theophylline) is recommended and the individual dose of the drug product may be adjusted as needed).
No products indexed under this heading.

Cilostazol (The formation of CYP450 enzymes may be suppressed by increased levels of cytokines (eg, TNFα) during chronic inflammation. Therefore, it is expected that for a molecule that antagonizes cytokine activity, such as golimumab, the formation of CYP450 enzymes could be normalized. Upon initiation or discontinuation of golimumab in patients being treated with CYP450 substrates with a narrow therapeutic index, monitoring of the effect (eg, warfarin) or drug concentration (eg, cyclosporine or theophylline) is recommended and the individual dose of the drug product may be adjusted as needed).
No products indexed under this heading.

Cimetidine Hydrochloride (The formation of CYP450 enzymes may be suppressed by increased levels of

cytokines (eg, TNFα) during chronic inflammation. Therefore, it is expected that for a molecule that antagonizes cytokine activity, such as golimumab, the formation of CYP450 enzymes could be normalized. Upon initiation or discontinuation of golimumab in patients being treated with CYP450 substrates with a narrow therapeutic index, monitoring of the effect (eg, warfarin) or drug concentration (eg, cyclosporine or theophylline) is recommended and the individual dose of the drug product may be adjusted as needed).
No products indexed under this heading.

Ciprofloxacin (The formation of CYP450 enzymes may be suppressed by increased levels of cytokines (eg, TNFα) during chronic inflammation. Therefore, it is expected that for a molecule that antagonizes cytokine activity, such as golimumab, the formation of CYP450 enzymes could be normalized. Upon initiation or discontinuation of golimumab in patients being treated with CYP450 substrates with a narrow therapeutic index, monitoring of the effect (eg, warfarin) or drug concentration (eg, cyclosporine or theophylline) is recommended and the individual dose of the drug product may be adjusted as needed). Products include:
Cipro I.V. 3082
Cipro 3073
Cipro XR 3091
Ciprodex 583

Ciprofloxacin Hydrochloride (The formation of CYP450 enzymes may be suppressed by increased levels of cytokines (eg, TNFα) during chronic inflammation. Therefore, it is expected that for a molecule that antagonizes cytokine activity, such as golimumab, the formation of CYP450 enzymes could be normalized. Upon initiation or discontinuation of golimumab in patients being treated with CYP450 substrates with a narrow therapeutic index, monitoring of the effect (eg, warfarin) or drug concentration (eg, cyclosporine or theophylline) is recommended and the individual dose of the drug product may be adjusted as needed). Products include:
Cipro 3073

Cisapride (The formation of CYP450 enzymes may be suppressed by increased levels of cytokines (eg, TNFα) during chronic inflammation. Therefore, it is expected that for a molecule that antagonizes cytokine activity, such as golimumab, the formation of CYP450 enzymes could be normalized. Upon initiation or discontinuation of golimumab in patients being treated with CYP450 substrates with a narrow therapeutic index, monitoring of the effect (eg, warfarin) or drug concentration (eg, cyclosporine or theophylline) is recommended and the individual dose of the drug product may be adjusted as needed).
No products indexed under this heading.

Citalopram Hydrobromide (The formation of CYP450 enzymes may be suppressed by increased levels of cytokines (eg, TNFα) during chronic inflammation. Therefore, it is expected that for a molecule that antagonizes cytokine activity, such as golimumab, the formation of CYP450 enzymes could be normalized. Upon initiation or discontinuation of golimumab in patients being treated with CYP450 substrates with a narrow therapeutic index, monitoring of the effect (eg, warfarin) or drug concentration (eg, cyclosporine or theophylline) is recommended and the individual dose of the drug product may be adjusted as needed). Products include:
Celexa 1153

IMPORTANT NOTE: Always consult each drug listing in the patient's regimen for possible interactions.

Clarithromycin (The formation of CYP450 enzymes may be suppressed by increased levels of cytokines (eg, TNFα) during chronic inflammation. Therefore, it is expected that for a molecule that antagonizes cytokine activity, such as golimumab, the formation of CYP450 enzymes could be normalized. Upon initiation or discontinuation of golimumab in patients being treated with CYP450 substrates with a narrow therapeutic index, monitoring of the effect (eg, warfarin) or drug concentration (eg, cyclosporine or theophylline) is recommended and the individual dose of the drug product may be adjusted as needed). Products include:

Biaxin/Biaxin XL **412**

Clomipramine Hydrochloride (The formation of CYP450 enzymes may be suppressed by increased levels of cytokines (eg, TNFα) during chronic inflammation. Therefore, it is expected that for a molecule that antagonizes cytokine activity, such as golimumab, the formation of CYP450 enzymes could be normalized. Upon initiation or discontinuation of golimumab in patients being treated with CYP450 substrates with a narrow therapeutic index, monitoring of the effect (eg, warfarin) or drug concentration (eg, cyclosporine or theophylline) is recommended and the individual dose of the drug product may be adjusted as needed).

No products indexed under this heading.

Clopidogrel Bisulfate (The formation of CYP450 enzymes may be suppressed by increased levels of cytokines (eg, TNFα) during chronic inflammation. Therefore, it is expected that for a molecule that antagonizes cytokine activity, such as golimumab, the formation of CYP450 enzymes could be normalized. Upon initiation or discontinuation of golimumab in patients being treated with CYP450 substrates with a narrow therapeutic index, monitoring of the effect (eg, warfarin) or drug concentration (eg, cyclosporine or theophylline) is recommended and the individual dose of the drug product may be adjusted as needed). Products include:

Plavix **3027**

Clopidogrel Hydrogen Sulfate (The formation of CYP450 enzymes may be suppressed by increased levels of cytokines (eg, TNFα) during chronic inflammation. Therefore, it is expected that for a molecule that antagonizes cytokine activity, such as golimumab, the formation of CYP450 enzymes could be normalized. Upon initiation or discontinuation of golimumab in patients being treated with CYP450 substrates with a narrow therapeutic index, monitoring of the effect (eg, warfarin) or drug concentration (eg, cyclosporine or theophylline) is recommended and the individual dose of the drug product may be adjusted as needed).

No products indexed under this heading.

Clozapine (The formation of CYP450 enzymes may be suppressed by increased levels of cytokines (eg, TNFα) during chronic inflammation. Therefore, it is expected that for a molecule that antagonizes cytokine activity, such as golimumab, the formation of CYP450 enzymes could be normalized. Upon initiation or discontinuation of golimumab in patients being treated with CYP450 substrates with a narrow therapeutic index, monitoring of the effect (eg, warfarin) or drug concentration (eg, cyclosporine or theophylline) is recommended and the individual dose of the drug product may be adjusted as needed).

No products indexed under this heading.

Codeine Phosphate (The formation of CYP450 enzymes may be suppressed by increased levels of cytokines (eg, TNFα) during chronic inflammation. Therefore, it is expected that for a molecule that antagonizes cytokine activity, such as golimumab, the formation of CYP450 enzymes could be normalized. Upon initiation or discontinuation of golimumab in patients being treated with CYP450 substrates with a narrow therapeutic index, monitoring of the effect (eg, warfarin) or drug concentration (eg, cyclosporine or theophylline) is recommended and the individual dose of the drug product may be adjusted as needed). Products include:

Tylenol with Codeine **2691**

Codeine Sulfate (The formation of CYP450 enzymes may be suppressed by increased levels of cytokines (eg, TNFα) during chronic inflammation. Therefore, it is expected that for a molecule that antagonizes cytokine activity, such as golimumab, the formation of CYP450 enzymes could be normalized. Upon initiation or discontinuation of golimumab in patients being treated with CYP450 substrates with a narrow therapeutic index, monitoring of the effect (eg, warfarin) or drug concentration (eg, cyclosporine or theophylline) is recommended and the individual dose of the drug product may be adjusted as needed).

No products indexed under this heading.

Cyclobenzaprine (The formation of CYP450 enzymes may be suppressed by increased levels of cytokines (eg, TNFα) during chronic inflammation. Therefore, it is expected that for a molecule that antagonizes cytokine activity, such as golimumab, the formation of CYP450 enzymes could be normalized. Upon initiation or discontinuation of golimumab in patients being treated with CYP450 substrates with a narrow therapeutic index, monitoring of the effect (eg, warfarin) or drug concentration (eg, cyclosporine or theophylline) is recommended and the individual dose of the drug product may be adjusted as needed).

No products indexed under this heading.

Cyclobenzaprine Hydrochloride (The formation of CYP450 enzymes may be suppressed by increased levels of cytokines (eg, TNFα) during chronic inflammation. Therefore, it is expected that for a molecule that antagonizes cytokine activity, such as golimumab, the formation of CYP450 enzymes could be normalized. Upon initiation or discontinuation of golimumab in patients being treated with CYP450 substrates with a narrow therapeutic index, monitoring of the effect (eg, warfarin) or drug concentration (eg, cyclosporine or theophylline) is recommended and the individual dose of the drug product may be adjusted as needed). Products include:

Amrix **964**

Cyclophosphamide (The formation of CYP450 enzymes may be suppressed by increased levels of cytokines (eg, TNFα) during chronic inflammation. Therefore, it is expected that for a molecule that antagonizes cytokine activity, such as golimumab, the formation of CYP450 enzymes could be normalized. Upon initiation or discontinuation of golimumab in patients being treated with CYP450 substrates with a narrow therapeutic index, monitoring of the effect (eg, warfarin) or drug concentration (eg, cyclosporine or theophylline) is recommended and the individual dose of the drug product may be adjusted as needed).

No products indexed under this heading.

Cyclosporine (The formation of CYP450 enzymes may be suppressed by increased levels of cytokines (eg, TNFα) during chronic inflammation. Therefore, it is expected that for a molecule that antagonizes cytokine activity, such as golimumab, the formation of CYP450 enzymes could be normalized. Upon initiation or discontinuation of golimumab in patients being treated with CYP450 substrates with a narrow therapeutic index, monitoring of the effect (eg, warfarin) or drug concentration (eg, cyclosporine or theophylline) is recommended and the individual dose of the drug product may be adjusted as needed). Products include:

Gengraf **440**
Neoral Oral Solution **2496**
Neoral Capsules **2496**
Restasis **605**

Desipramine Hydrochloride (The formation of CYP450 enzymes may be suppressed by increased levels of cytokines (eg, TNFα) during chronic inflammation. Therefore, it is expected that for a molecule that antagonizes cytokine activity, such as golimumab, the formation of CYP450 enzymes could be normalized. Upon initiation or discontinuation of golimumab in patients being treated with CYP450 substrates with a narrow therapeutic index, monitoring of the effect (eg, warfarin) or drug concentration (eg, cyclosporine or theophylline) is recommended and the individual dose of the drug product may be adjusted as needed).

No products indexed under this heading.

Desogestrel (The formation of CYP450 enzymes may be suppressed by increased levels of cytokines (eg, TNFα) during chronic inflammation. Therefore, it is expected that for a molecule that antagonizes cytokine activity, such as golimumab, the formation of CYP450 enzymes could be normalized. Upon initiation or discontinuation of golimumab in patients being treated with CYP450 substrates with a narrow therapeutic index, monitoring of the effect (eg, warfarin) or drug concentration (eg, cyclosporine or theophylline) is recommended and the individual dose of the drug product may be adjusted as needed).

No products indexed under this heading.

Dexamethasone (The formation of CYP450 enzymes may be suppressed by increased levels of cytokines (eg, TNFα) during chronic inflammation. Therefore, it is expected that for a molecule that antagonizes cytokine activity, such as golimumab, the formation of CYP450 enzymes could be normalized. Upon initiation or discontinuation of golimumab in patients being treated with CYP450 substrates with a narrow therapeutic index, monitoring of the effect (eg, warfarin) or drug concentration (eg, cyclosporine or theophylline) is recommended and the individual dose of the drug product may be adjusted as needed). Products include:

Ciprodex **583**
Ozurdex .... ⊙ **223**
Tobramycin and Dexamethasone Ophthalmic Suspension .... ⊙ **251**

Dexamethasone Acetate (The formation of CYP450 enzymes may be suppressed by increased levels of cytokines (eg, TNFα) during chronic inflammation. Therefore, it is expected that for a molecule that antagonizes cytokine activity, such as golimumab, the formation of CYP450 enzymes could be normalized. Upon initiation or discontinuation of golimumab in patients being treated with CYP450 substrates with a narrow therapeutic index, monitoring of the effect (eg, warfarin) or drug concentration (eg, cyclosporine or theophylline) is recommended and the individual dose of the drug product may be adjusted as needed).

No products indexed under this heading.

Dexamethasone Phosphate (The formation of CYP450 enzymes may be suppressed by increased levels of cytokines (eg, TNFα) during chronic inflammation. Therefore, it is expected that for a molecule that antagonizes cytokine activity, such as golimumab, the formation of CYP450 enzymes could be normalized. Upon initiation or discontinuation of golimumab in patients being treated with CYP450 substrates with a narrow therapeutic index, monitoring of the effect (eg, warfarin) or drug concentration (eg, cyclosporine or theophylline) is recommended and the individual dose of the drug product may be adjusted as needed).

No products indexed under this heading.

Dexamethasone Sodium (The formation of CYP450 enzymes may be suppressed by increased levels of cytokines (eg, TNFα) during chronic inflammation. Therefore, it is expected that for a molecule that antagonizes cytokine activity, such as golimumab, the formation of CYP450 enzymes could be normalized. Upon initiation or discontinuation of golimumab in patients being treated with CYP450 substrates with a narrow therapeutic index, monitoring of the effect (eg, warfarin) or drug concentration (eg, cyclosporine or theophylline) is recommended and the individual dose of the drug product may be adjusted as needed).

No products indexed under this heading.

Dexamethasone Sodium Phosphate (The formation of CYP450 enzymes may be suppressed by increased levels of cytokines (eg, TNFα) during chronic inflammation. Therefore, it is expected that for a molecule that antagonizes cytokine activity, such as golimumab, the formation of CYP450 enzymes could be normalized. Upon initiation or discontinuation of golimumab in patients being treated with CYP450 substrates with a narrow therapeutic index, monitoring of the effect (eg, warfarin) or drug concentration (eg, cyclosporine or theophylline) is recommended and the individual dose of the drug product may be adjusted as needed).

No products indexed under this heading.

Dexfenfluramine Hydrochloride (The formation of CYP450 enzymes may be suppressed by increased levels of cytokines (eg, TNFα) during chronic inflammation. Therefore, it is expected that for a molecule that antagonizes cytokine activity, such as golimumab, the formation of CYP450 enzymes could be normalized. Upon initiation or discontinuation of golimumab in patients being treated with CYP450 substrates with a narrow therapeutic index, monitoring of the effect (eg, warfarin) or drug concentration (eg, cyclosporine or theophylline) is recommended and the individual dose of the drug product may be adjusted as needed).

No products indexed under this heading.

Dextromethorphan (The formation of CYP450 enzymes may be suppressed by increased levels of cytokines (eg, TNFα) during chronic inflammation. Therefore, it is expected that for a molecule that antagonizes cytokine activity, such as golimumab, the formation of CYP450 enzymes could be normalized. Upon initiation or discontinuation of golimumab in patients being treated with CYP450 substrates with a narrow therapeutic index, monitoring of the effect (eg, warfarin) or drug concentration (eg,

cyclosporine or theophylline) is recommended and the individual dose of the drug product may be adjusted as needed).

No products indexed under this heading.

Dextromethorphan Hydrobromide (The formation of CYP450 enzymes may be suppressed by increased levels of cytokines (eg, TNFα) during chronic inflammation. Therefore, it is expected that for a molecule that antagonizes cytokine activity, such as golimumab, the formation of CYP450 enzymes could be normalized. Upon initiation or discontinuation of golimumab in patients being treated with CYP450 substrates with a narrow therapeutic index, monitoring of the effect (eg, warfarin) or drug concentration (eg, cyclosporine or theophylline) is recommended and the individual dose of the drug product may be adjusted as needed).

No products indexed under this heading.

Dextromethorphan Polistirex (The formation of CYP450 enzymes may be suppressed by increased levels of cytokines (eg, TNFα) during chronic inflammation. Therefore, it is expected that for a molecule that antagonizes cytokine activity, such as golimumab, the formation of CYP450 enzymes could be normalized. Upon initiation or discontinuation of golimumab in patients being treated with CYP450 substrates with a narrow therapeutic index, monitoring of the effect (eg, warfarin) or drug concentration (eg, cyclosporine or theophylline) is recommended and the individual dose of the drug product may be adjusted as needed).

No products indexed under this heading.

Diazepam (The formation of CYP450 enzymes may be suppressed by increased levels of cytokines (eg, TNFα) during chronic inflammation. Therefore, it is expected that for a molecule that antagonizes cytokine activity, such as golimumab, the formation of CYP450 enzymes could be normalized. Upon initiation or discontinuation of golimumab in patients being treated with CYP450 substrates with a narrow therapeutic index, monitoring of the effect (eg, warfarin) or drug concentration (eg, cyclosporine or theophylline) is recommended and the individual dose of the drug product may be adjusted as needed). Products include:

Valium Tablets 2880

Diclofenac Potassium (The formation of CYP450 enzymes may be suppressed by increased levels of cytokines (eg, TNFα) during chronic inflammation. Therefore, it is expected that for a molecule that antagonizes cytokine activity, such as golimumab, the formation of CYP450 enzymes could be normalized. Upon initiation or discontinuation of golimumab in patients being treated with CYP450 substrates with a narrow therapeutic index, monitoring of the effect (eg, warfarin) or drug concentration (eg, cyclosporine or theophylline) is recommended and the individual dose of the drug product may be adjusted as needed).

No products indexed under this heading.

Diclofenac Sodium (The formation of CYP450 enzymes may be suppressed by increased levels of cytokines (eg, TNFα) during chronic inflammation. Therefore, it is expected that for a molecule that antagonizes cytokine activity, such as golimumab, the formation of CYP450 enzymes could be normalized. Upon initiation or discontinuation of golimumab in patients being treated with CYP450 substrates with a narrow therapeutic index, monitoring of the effect (eg, warfarin) or drug concentration (eg,

cyclosporine or theophylline) is recommended and the individual dose of the drug product may be adjusted as needed).

No products indexed under this heading.

Dihydroergotamine Mesylate (The formation of CYP450 enzymes may be suppressed by increased levels of cytokines (eg, TNFα) during chronic inflammation. Therefore, it is expected that for a molecule that antagonizes cytokine activity, such as golimumab, the formation of CYP450 enzymes could be normalized. Upon initiation or discontinuation of golimumab in patients being treated with CYP450 substrates with a narrow therapeutic index, monitoring of the effect (eg, warfarin) or drug concentration (eg, cyclosporine or theophylline) is recommended and the individual dose of the drug product may be adjusted as needed).

No products indexed under this heading.

Diltiazem Hydrochloride (The formation of CYP450 enzymes may be suppressed by increased levels of cytokines (eg, TNFα) during chronic inflammation. Therefore, it is expected that for a molecule that antagonizes cytokine activity, such as golimumab, the formation of CYP450 enzymes could be normalized. Upon initiation or discontinuation of golimumab in patients being treated with CYP450 substrates with a narrow therapeutic index, monitoring of the effect (eg, warfarin) or drug concentration (eg, cyclosporine or theophylline) is recommended and the individual dose of the drug product may be adjusted as needed). Products include:

Cardizem LA 423

Diltiazem Maleate (The formation of CYP450 enzymes may be suppressed by increased levels of cytokines (eg, TNFα) during chronic inflammation. Therefore, it is expected that for a molecule that antagonizes cytokine activity, such as golimumab, the formation of CYP450 enzymes could be normalized. Upon initiation or discontinuation of golimumab in patients being treated with CYP450 substrates with a narrow therapeutic index, monitoring of the effect (eg, warfarin) or drug concentration (eg, cyclosporine or theophylline) is recommended and the individual dose of the drug product may be adjusted as needed).

No products indexed under this heading.

Disopyramide (The formation of CYP450 enzymes may be suppressed by increased levels of cytokines (eg, TNFα) during chronic inflammation. Therefore, it is expected that for a molecule that antagonizes cytokine activity, such as golimumab, the formation of CYP450 enzymes could be normalized. Upon initiation or discontinuation of golimumab in patients being treated with CYP450 substrates with a narrow therapeutic index, monitoring of the effect (eg, warfarin) or drug concentration (eg, cyclosporine or theophylline) is recommended and the individual dose of the drug product may be adjusted as needed).

No products indexed under this heading.

Disopyramide Phosphate (The formation of CYP450 enzymes may be suppressed by increased levels of cytokines (eg, TNFα) during chronic inflammation. Therefore, it is expected that for a molecule that antagonizes cytokine activity, such as golimumab, the formation of CYP450 enzymes could be normalized. Upon initiation or discontinuation of golimumab in patients being treated with CYP450 substrates with a narrow therapeutic index, monitoring of the effect (eg, warfarin) or drug concentration (eg,

cyclosporine or theophylline) is recommended and the individual dose of the drug product may be adjusted as needed).

No products indexed under this heading.

Disulfiram (The formation of CYP450 enzymes may be suppressed by increased levels of cytokines (eg, TNFα) during chronic inflammation. Therefore, it is expected that for a molecule that antagonizes cytokine activity, such as golimumab, the formation of CYP450 enzymes could be normalized. Upon initiation or discontinuation of golimumab in patients being treated with CYP450 substrates with a narrow therapeutic index, monitoring of the effect (eg, warfarin) or drug concentration (eg, cyclosporine or theophylline) is recommended and the individual dose of the drug product may be adjusted as needed).

No products indexed under this heading.

Divalproex Sodium (The formation of CYP450 enzymes may be suppressed by increased levels of cytokines (eg, TNFα) during chronic inflammation. Therefore, it is expected that for a molecule that antagonizes cytokine activity, such as golimumab, the formation of CYP450 enzymes could be normalized. Upon initiation or discontinuation of golimumab in patients being treated with CYP450 substrates with a narrow therapeutic index, monitoring of the effect (eg, warfarin) or drug concentration (eg, cyclosporine or theophylline) is recommended and the individual dose of the drug product may be adjusted as needed). Products include:

Depakote ER 426

Docetaxel (The formation of CYP450 enzymes may be suppressed by increased levels of cytokines (eg, TNFα) during chronic inflammation. Therefore, it is expected that for a molecule that antagonizes cytokine activity, such as golimumab, the formation of CYP450 enzymes could be normalized. Upon initiation or discontinuation of golimumab in patients being treated with CYP450 substrates with a narrow therapeutic index, monitoring of the effect (eg, warfarin) or drug concentration (eg, cyclosporine or theophylline) is recommended and the individual dose of the drug product may be adjusted as needed). Products include:

Taxotere 3035

Dolasetron Mesylate (The formation of CYP450 enzymes may be suppressed by increased levels of cytokines (eg, TNFα) during chronic inflammation. Therefore, it is expected that for a molecule that antagonizes cytokine activity, such as golimumab, the formation of CYP450 enzymes could be normalized. Upon initiation or discontinuation of golimumab in patients being treated with CYP450 substrates with a narrow therapeutic index, monitoring of the effect (eg, warfarin) or drug concentration (eg, cyclosporine or theophylline) is recommended and the individual dose of the drug product may be adjusted as needed). Products include:

Anzemet Injection 2931
Anzemet Tablets 2934

Donepezil Hydrochloride (The formation of CYP450 enzymes may be suppressed by increased levels of cytokines (eg, TNFα) during chronic inflammation. Therefore, it is expected that for a molecule that antagonizes cytokine activity, such as golimumab, the formation of CYP450 enzymes could be normalized. Upon initiation or discontinuation of golimumab in patients being treated with CYP450 substrates with a narrow therapeutic index, monitoring of the effect (eg, warfarin) or drug concentration (eg, cyclosporine or theophylline) is recom-

mended and the individual dose of the drug product may be adjusted as needed). Products include:

Aricept 1045
Aricept ODT 1045

Doxepin Hydrochloride (The formation of CYP450 enzymes may be suppressed by increased levels of cytokines (eg, TNFα) during chronic inflammation. Therefore, it is expected that for a molecule that antagonizes cytokine activity, such as golimumab, the formation of CYP450 enzymes could be normalized. Upon initiation or discontinuation of golimumab in patients being treated with CYP450 substrates with a narrow therapeutic index, monitoring of the effect (eg, warfarin) or drug concentration (eg, cyclosporine or theophylline) is recommended and the individual dose of the drug product may be adjusted as needed).

No products indexed under this heading.

Doxorubicin Hydrochloride (The formation of CYP450 enzymes may be suppressed by increased levels of cytokines (eg, TNFα) during chronic inflammation. Therefore, it is expected that for a molecule that antagonizes cytokine activity, such as golimumab, the formation of CYP450 enzymes could be normalized. Upon initiation or discontinuation of golimumab in patients being treated with CYP450 substrates with a narrow therapeutic index, monitoring of the effect (eg, warfarin) or drug concentration (eg, cyclosporine or theophylline) is recommended and the individual dose of the drug product may be adjusted as needed).

No products indexed under this heading.

Dronabinol (The formation of CYP450 enzymes may be suppressed by increased levels of cytokines (eg, TNFα) during chronic inflammation. Therefore, it is expected that for a molecule that antagonizes cytokine activity, such as golimumab, the formation of CYP450 enzymes could be normalized. Upon initiation or discontinuation of golimumab in patients being treated with CYP450 substrates with a narrow therapeutic index, monitoring of the effect (eg, warfarin) or drug concentration (eg, cyclosporine or theophylline) is recommended and the individual dose of the drug product may be adjusted as needed).

No products indexed under this heading.

Drugs that Undergo Biotransformation by Cytochrome P-450 Mixed Function Oxidase (The formation of CYP450 enzymes may be suppressed by increased levels of cytokines (eg, TNFα) during chronic inflammation. Therefore, it is expected that for a molecule that antagonizes cytokine activity, such as golimumab, the formation of CYP450 enzymes could be normalized. Upon initiation or discontinuation of golimumab in patients being treated with CYP450 substrates with a narrow therapeutic index, monitoring of the effect (eg, warfarin) or drug concentration (eg, cyclosporine or theophylline) is recommended and the individual dose of the drug product may be adjusted as needed).

No products indexed under this heading.

Dyphylline (The formation of CYP450 enzymes may be suppressed by increased levels of cytokines (eg, TNFα) during chronic inflammation. Therefore, it is expected that for a molecule that antagonizes cytokine activity, such as golimumab, the formation of CYP450 enzymes could be normalized. Upon initiation or discontinuation of golimumab in patients being treated with CYP450 substrates with a narrow thera-

---

IMPORTANT NOTE: Always consult each drug listing in the patient's regimen for possible interactions.

peutic index, monitoring of the effect (eg, warfarin) or drug concentration (eg, cyclosporine or theophylline) is recommended and the individual dose of the drug product may be adjusted as needed).

No products indexed under this heading.

Encainide Hydrochloride (The formation of CYP450 enzymes may be suppressed by increased levels of cytokines (eg, TNFα) during chronic inflammation. Therefore, it is expected that for a molecule that antagonizes cytokine activity, such as golimumab, the formation of CYP450 enzymes could be normalized. Upon initiation or discontinuation of golimumab in patients being treated with CYP450 substrates with a narrow therapeutic index, monitoring of the effect (eg, warfarin) or drug concentration (eg, cyclosporine or theophylline) is recommended and the individual dose of the drug product may be adjusted as needed).

No products indexed under this heading.

Enoxacin (The formation of CYP450 enzymes may be suppressed by increased levels of cytokines (eg, TNFα) during chronic inflammation. Therefore, it is expected that for a molecule that antagonizes cytokine activity, such as golimumab, the formation of CYP450 enzymes could be normalized. Upon initiation or discontinuation of golimumab in patients being treated with CYP450 substrates with a narrow therapeutic index, monitoring of the effect (eg, warfarin) or drug concentration (eg, cyclosporine or theophylline) is recommended and the individual dose of the drug product may be adjusted as needed).

No products indexed under this heading.

Eprosartan Mesylate (The formation of CYP450 enzymes may be suppressed by increased levels of cytokines (eg, TNFα) during chronic inflammation. Therefore, it is expected that for a molecule that antagonizes cytokine activity, such as golimumab, the formation of CYP450 enzymes could be normalized. Upon initiation or discontinuation of golimumab in patients being treated with CYP450 substrates with a narrow therapeutic index, monitoring of the effect (eg, warfarin) or drug concentration (eg, cyclosporine or theophylline) is recommended and the individual dose of the drug product may be adjusted as needed). Products include:

Teveten **538**
Teveten HCT **541**

Ergotamine Tartrate (The formation of CYP450 enzymes may be suppressed by increased levels of cytokines (eg, TNFα) during chronic inflammation. Therefore, it is expected that for a molecule that antagonizes cytokine activity, such as golimumab, the formation of CYP450 enzymes could be normalized. Upon initiation or discontinuation of golimumab in patients being treated with CYP450 substrates with a narrow therapeutic index, monitoring of the effect (eg, warfarin) or drug concentration (eg, cyclosporine or theophylline) is recommended and the individual dose of the drug product may be adjusted as needed).

No products indexed under this heading.

Erythromycin (The formation of CYP450 enzymes may be suppressed by increased levels of cytokines (eg, TNFα) during chronic inflammation. Therefore, it is expected that for a molecule that antagonizes cytokine activity, such as golimumab, the formation of CYP450 enzymes could be normalized. Upon initiation or discontinuation of golimumab in patients being treated with CYP450 substrates with a narrow therapeutic index, monitoring of the effect

(eg, warfarin) or drug concentration (eg, cyclosporine or theophylline) is recommended and the individual dose of the drug product may be adjusted as needed).

No products indexed under this heading.

Erythromycin Estolate (The formation of CYP450 enzymes may be suppressed by increased levels of cytokines (eg, TNFα) during chronic inflammation. Therefore, it is expected that for a molecule that antagonizes cytokine activity, such as golimumab, the formation of CYP450 enzymes could be normalized. Upon initiation or discontinuation of golimumab in patients being treated with CYP450 substrates with a narrow therapeutic index, monitoring of the effect (eg, warfarin) or drug concentration (eg, cyclosporine or theophylline) is recommended and the individual dose of the drug product may be adjusted as needed).

No products indexed under this heading.

Erythromycin Ethylsuccinate (The formation of CYP450 enzymes may be suppressed by increased levels of cytokines (eg, TNFα) during chronic inflammation. Therefore, it is expected that for a molecule that antagonizes cytokine activity, such as golimumab, the formation of CYP450 enzymes could be normalized. Upon initiation or discontinuation of golimumab in patients being treated with CYP450 substrates with a narrow therapeutic index, monitoring of the effect (eg, warfarin) or drug concentration (eg, cyclosporine or theophylline) is recommended and the individual dose of the drug product may be adjusted as needed). Products include:

E.E.S. **437**
EryPed **435**

Erythromycin Gluceptate (The formation of CYP450 enzymes may be suppressed by increased levels of cytokines (eg, TNFα) during chronic inflammation. Therefore, it is expected that for a molecule that antagonizes cytokine activity, such as golimumab, the formation of CYP450 enzymes could be normalized. Upon initiation or discontinuation of golimumab in patients being treated with CYP450 substrates with a narrow therapeutic index, monitoring of the effect (eg, warfarin) or drug concentration (eg, cyclosporine or theophylline) is recommended and the individual dose of the drug product may be adjusted as needed).

No products indexed under this heading.

Erythromycin Lactobionate (The formation of CYP450 enzymes may be suppressed by increased levels of cytokines (eg, TNFα) during chronic inflammation. Therefore, it is expected that for a molecule that antagonizes cytokine activity, such as golimumab, the formation of CYP450 enzymes could be normalized. Upon initiation or discontinuation of golimumab in patients being treated with CYP450 substrates with a narrow therapeutic index, monitoring of the effect (eg, warfarin) or drug concentration (eg, cyclosporine or theophylline) is recommended and the individual dose of the drug product may be adjusted as needed).

No products indexed under this heading.

Erythromycin Stearate (The formation of CYP450 enzymes may be suppressed by increased levels of cytokines (eg, TNFα) during chronic inflammation. Therefore, it is expected that for a molecule that antagonizes cytokine activity, such as golimumab, the formation of CYP450 enzymes could be normalized. Upon initiation or discontinuation of golimumab in

patients being treated with CYP450 substrates with a narrow therapeutic index, monitoring of the effect (eg, warfarin) or drug concentration (eg, cyclosporine or theophylline) is recommended and the individual dose of the drug product may be adjusted as needed).

No products indexed under this heading.

Esomeprazole Magnesium (The formation of CYP450 enzymes may be suppressed by increased levels of cytokines (eg, TNFα) during chronic inflammation. Therefore, it is expected that for a molecule that antagonizes cytokine activity, such as golimumab, the formation of CYP450 enzymes could be normalized. Upon initiation or discontinuation of golimumab in patients being treated with CYP450 substrates with a narrow therapeutic index, monitoring of the effect (eg, warfarin) or drug concentration (eg, cyclosporine or theophylline) is recommended and the individual dose of the drug product may be adjusted as needed). Products include:

Nexium Capsules **704**
Nexium Oral Suspension **704**

Esomeprazole Sodium (The formation of CYP450 enzymes may be suppressed by increased levels of cytokines (eg, TNFα) during chronic inflammation. Therefore, it is expected that for a molecule that antagonizes cytokine activity, such as golimumab, the formation of CYP450 enzymes could be normalized. Upon initiation or discontinuation of golimumab in patients being treated with CYP450 substrates with a narrow therapeutic index, monitoring of the effect (eg, warfarin) or drug concentration (eg, cyclosporine or theophylline) is recommended and the individual dose of the drug product may be adjusted as needed). Products include:

Nexium I.V. **712**

Estradiol (The formation of CYP450 enzymes may be suppressed by increased levels of cytokines (eg, TNFα) during chronic inflammation. Therefore, it is expected that for a molecule that antagonizes cytokine activity, such as golimumab, the formation of CYP450 enzymes could be normalized. Upon initiation or discontinuation of golimumab in patients being treated with CYP450 substrates with a narrow therapeutic index, monitoring of the effect (eg, warfarin) or drug concentration (eg, cyclosporine or theophylline) is recommended and the individual dose of the drug product may be adjusted as needed). Products include:

Activella **2561**
Angeliq **831**
Climara **841**
Climara Pro **847**
Divigel **3467**
Estrasorb **1777**
Vagifem **2589**

Estradiol Benzoate (The formation of CYP450 enzymes may be suppressed by increased levels of cytokines (eg, TNFα) during chronic inflammation. Therefore, it is expected that for a molecule that antagonizes cytokine activity, such as golimumab, the formation of CYP450 enzymes could be normalized. Upon initiation or discontinuation of golimumab in patients being treated with CYP450 substrates with a narrow therapeutic index, monitoring of the effect (eg, warfarin) or drug concentration (eg, cyclosporine or theophylline) is recommended and the individual dose of the drug product may be adjusted as needed).

No products indexed under this heading.

Estradiol Cypionate (The formation of CYP450 enzymes may be suppressed by increased levels of cytok-

ines (eg, TNFα) during chronic inflammation. Therefore, it is expected that for a molecule that antagonizes cytokine activity, such as golimumab, the formation of CYP450 enzymes could be normalized. Upon initiation or discontinuation of golimumab in patients being treated with CYP450 substrates with a narrow therapeutic index, monitoring of the effect (eg, warfarin) or drug concentration (eg, cyclosporine or theophylline) is recommended and the individual dose of the drug product may be adjusted as needed).

No products indexed under this heading.

Estradiol Valerate (The formation of CYP450 enzymes may be suppressed by increased levels of cytokines (eg, TNFα) during chronic inflammation. Therefore, it is expected that for a molecule that antagonizes cytokine activity, such as golimumab, the formation of CYP450 enzymes could be normalized. Upon initiation or discontinuation of golimumab in patients being treated with CYP450 substrates with a narrow therapeutic index, monitoring of the effect (eg, warfarin) or drug concentration (eg, cyclosporine or theophylline) is recommended and the individual dose of the drug product may be adjusted as needed).

No products indexed under this heading.

Estrogen (The formation of CYP450 enzymes may be suppressed by increased levels of cytokines (eg, TNFα) during chronic inflammation. Therefore, it is expected that for a molecule that antagonizes cytokine activity, such as golimumab, the formation of CYP450 enzymes could be normalized. Upon initiation or discontinuation of golimumab in patients being treated with CYP450 substrates with a narrow therapeutic index, monitoring of the effect (eg, warfarin) or drug concentration (eg, cyclosporine or theophylline) is recommended and the individual dose of the drug product may be adjusted as needed).

No products indexed under this heading.

Estrogens, Conjugated (The formation of CYP450 enzymes may be suppressed by increased levels of cytokines (eg, TNFα) during chronic inflammation. Therefore, it is expected that for a molecule that antagonizes cytokine activity, such as golimumab, the formation of CYP450 enzymes could be normalized. Upon initiation or discontinuation of golimumab in patients being treated with CYP450 substrates with a narrow therapeutic index, monitoring of the effect (eg, warfarin) or drug concentration (eg, cyclosporine or theophylline) is recommended and the individual dose of the drug product may be adjusted as needed). Products include:

Premarin Intravenous **3528**
Premarin Tablets **3533**
Premarin Vaginal Cream **3540**
Premphase **3549**
Prempro **3549**

Estrogens, Conjugated, Synthetic A (The formation of CYP450 enzymes may be suppressed by increased levels of cytokines (eg, TNFα) during chronic inflammation. Therefore, it is expected that for a molecule that antagonizes cytokine activity, such as golimumab, the formation of CYP450 enzymes could be normalized. Upon initiation or discontinuation of golimumab in patients being treated with CYP450 substrates with a narrow therapeutic index, monitoring of the effect (eg, warfarin) or drug concentration (eg, cyclosporine or theophylline) is recommended and the individual dose of the drug product may be adjusted as needed).

No products indexed under this heading.

Estrogens, Esterified (The formation of CYP450 enzymes may be suppressed by increased levels of cytokines (eg, TNFα) during chronic inflammation. Therefore, it is expected that for a molecule that antagonizes cytokine activity, such as golimumab, the formation of CYP450 enzymes could be normalized. Upon initiation or discontinuation of golimumab in patients being treated with CYP450 substrates with a narrow therapeutic index, monitoring of the effect (eg, warfarin) or drug concentration (eg, cyclosporine or theophylline) is recommended and the individual dose of the drug product may be adjusted as needed).
No products indexed under this heading.

Ethinyl Estradiol (The formation of CYP450 enzymes may be suppressed by increased levels of cytokines (eg, TNFα) during chronic inflammation. Therefore, it is expected that for a molecule that antagonizes cytokine activity, such as golimumab, the formation of CYP450 enzymes could be normalized. Upon initiation or discontinuation of golimumab in patients being treated with CYP450 substrates with a narrow therapeutic index, monitoring of the effect (eg, warfarin) or drug concentration (eg, cyclosporine or theophylline) is recommended and the individual dose of the drug product may be adjusted as needed). Products include:
LoSeasonique **3407**
Lybrel **3514**
NuvaRing **3181**
Ortho Evra **2648**
Ortho-Cyclen/Ortho Tri-Cyclen **2663**
Ortho Tri-Cyclen Lo Tablets **2673**
Seasonique **3418**
Yaz **864**

Ethosuximide (The formation of CYP450 enzymes may be suppressed by increased levels of cytokines (eg, TNFα) during chronic inflammation. Therefore, it is expected that for a molecule that antagonizes cytokine activity, such as golimumab, the formation of CYP450 enzymes could be normalized. Upon initiation or discontinuation of golimumab in patients being treated with CYP450 substrates with a narrow therapeutic index, monitoring of the effect (eg, warfarin) or drug concentration (eg, cyclosporine or theophylline) is recommended and the individual dose of the drug product may be adjusted as needed).
No products indexed under this heading.

Ethotoin (The formation of CYP450 enzymes may be suppressed by increased levels of cytokines (eg, TNFα) during chronic inflammation. Therefore, it is expected that for a molecule that antagonizes cytokine activity, such as golimumab, the formation of CYP450 enzymes could be normalized. Upon initiation or discontinuation of golimumab in patients being treated with CYP450 substrates with a narrow therapeutic index, monitoring of the effect (eg, warfarin) or drug concentration (eg, cyclosporine or theophylline) is recommended and the individual dose of the drug product may be adjusted as needed).
No products indexed under this heading.

Ethynodiol Diacetate (The formation of CYP450 enzymes may be suppressed by increased levels of cytokines (eg, TNFα) during chronic inflammation. Therefore, it is expected that for a molecule that antagonizes cytokine activity, such as golimumab, the formation of CYP450 enzymes could be normalized. Upon initiation or discontinuation of golimumab in patients being treated with CYP450 substrates with a narrow therapeutic index, monitoring of the effect (eg, warfarin) or drug concentration (eg, cyclosporine or theophylline) is recommended and the individual dose of the drug product may be adjusted as needed).
No products indexed under this heading.

Etodolac (The formation of CYP450 enzymes may be suppressed by increased levels of cytokines (eg, TNFα) during chronic inflammation. Therefore, it is expected that for a molecule that antagonizes cytokine activity, such as golimumab, the formation of CYP450 enzymes could be normalized. Upon initiation or discontinuation of golimumab in patients being treated with CYP450 substrates with a narrow therapeutic index, monitoring of the effect (eg, warfarin) or drug concentration (eg, cyclosporine or theophylline) is recommended and the individual dose of the drug product may be adjusted as needed).
No products indexed under this heading.

Etoposide (The formation of CYP450 enzymes may be suppressed by increased levels of cytokines (eg, TNFα) during chronic inflammation. Therefore, it is expected that for a molecule that antagonizes cytokine activity, such as golimumab, the formation of CYP450 enzymes could be normalized. Upon initiation or discontinuation of golimumab in patients being treated with CYP450 substrates with a narrow therapeutic index, monitoring of the effect (eg, warfarin) or drug concentration (eg, cyclosporine or theophylline) is recommended and the individual dose of the drug product may be adjusted as needed).
No products indexed under this heading.

Etoposide Phosphate (The formation of CYP450 enzymes may be suppressed by increased levels of cytokines (eg, TNFα) during chronic inflammation. Therefore, it is expected that for a molecule that antagonizes cytokine activity, such as golimumab, the formation of CYP450 enzymes could be normalized. Upon initiation or discontinuation of golimumab in patients being treated with CYP450 substrates with a narrow therapeutic index, monitoring of the effect (eg, warfarin) or drug concentration (eg, cyclosporine or theophylline) is recommended and the individual dose of the drug product may be adjusted as needed).
No products indexed under this heading.

Felbamate (The formation of CYP450 enzymes may be suppressed by increased levels of cytokines (eg, TNFα) during chronic inflammation. Therefore, it is expected that for a molecule that antagonizes cytokine activity, such as golimumab, the formation of CYP450 enzymes could be normalized. Upon initiation or discontinuation of golimumab in patients being treated with CYP450 substrates with a narrow therapeutic index, monitoring of the effect (eg, warfarin) or drug concentration (eg, cyclosporine or theophylline) is recommended and the individual dose of the drug product may be adjusted as needed).
No products indexed under this heading.

Felodipine (The formation of CYP450 enzymes may be suppressed by increased levels of cytokines (eg, TNFα) during chronic inflammation. Therefore, it is expected that for a molecule that antagonizes cytokine activity, such as golimumab, the formation of CYP450 enzymes could be normalized. Upon initiation or discontinuation of golimumab in patients being treated with CYP450 substrates with a narrow therapeutic index, monitoring of the effect (eg, warfarin) or drug concentration (eg, cyclosporine or theophylline) is recommended and the individual dose of the drug product may be adjusted as needed).
No products indexed under this heading.

Fenoprofen Calcium (The formation of CYP450 enzymes may be suppressed by increased levels of cytokines (eg, TNFα) during chronic inflammation. Therefore, it is expected that for a molecule that antagonizes cytokine activity, such as golimumab, the formation of CYP450 enzymes could be normalized. Upon initiation or discontinuation of golimumab in patients being treated with CYP450 substrates with a narrow therapeutic index, monitoring of the effect (eg, warfarin) or drug concentration (eg, cyclosporine or theophylline) is recommended and the individual dose of the drug product may be adjusted as needed).
No products indexed under this heading.

Fentanyl (The formation of CYP450 enzymes may be suppressed by increased levels of cytokines (eg, TNFα) during chronic inflammation. Therefore, it is expected that for a molecule that antagonizes cytokine activity, such as golimumab, the formation of CYP450 enzymes could be normalized. Upon initiation or discontinuation of golimumab in patients being treated with CYP450 substrates with a narrow therapeutic index, monitoring of the effect (eg, warfarin) or drug concentration (eg, cyclosporine or theophylline) is recommended and the individual dose of the drug product may be adjusted as needed). Products include:
Duragesic **2604**
Fentanyl Transdermal System **2346**
Onsolis **2054**

Fentanyl Citrate (The formation of CYP450 enzymes may be suppressed by increased levels of cytokines (eg, TNFα) during chronic inflammation. Therefore, it is expected that for a molecule that antagonizes cytokine activity, such as golimumab, the formation of CYP450 enzymes could be normalized. Upon initiation or discontinuation of golimumab in patients being treated with CYP450 substrates with a narrow therapeutic index, monitoring of the effect (eg, warfarin) or drug concentration (eg, cyclosporine or theophylline) is recommended and the individual dose of the drug product may be adjusted as needed). Products include:
Fentora **966**

Flecainide Acetate (The formation of CYP450 enzymes may be suppressed by increased levels of cytokines (eg, TNFα) during chronic inflammation. Therefore, it is expected that for a molecule that antagonizes cytokine activity, such as golimumab, the formation of CYP450 enzymes could be normalized. Upon initiation or discontinuation of golimumab in patients being treated with CYP450 substrates with a narrow therapeutic index, monitoring of the effect (eg, warfarin) or drug concentration (eg, cyclosporine or theophylline) is recommended and the individual dose of the drug product may be adjusted as needed).
No products indexed under this heading.

Fluoxetine (The formation of CYP450 enzymes may be suppressed by increased levels of cytokines (eg, TNFα) during chronic inflammation. Therefore, it is expected that for a molecule that antagonizes cytokine activity, such as golimumab, the formation of CYP450 enzymes could be normalized. Upon initiation or discontinuation of golimumab in patients being treated with CYP450 substrates with a narrow therapeutic index, monitoring of the effect (eg, warfarin) or drug concentration (eg, cyclosporine or theophylline) is recommended and the individual dose of the drug product may be adjusted as needed).
No products indexed under this heading.

Fluoxetine Hydrochloride (The formation of CYP450 enzymes may be suppressed by increased levels of cytokines (eg, TNFα) during chronic inflammation. Therefore, it is expected that for a molecule that antagonizes cytokine activity, such as golimumab, the formation of CYP450 enzymes could be normalized. Upon initiation or discontinuation of golimumab in patients being treated with CYP450 substrates with a narrow therapeutic index, monitoring of the effect (eg, warfarin) or drug concentration (eg, cyclosporine or theophylline) is recommended and the individual dose of the drug product may be adjusted as needed). Products include:
Prozac Weekly **1941**
Prozac Pulvules **1941**
Symbyax **1965**

Fluphenazine Decanoate (The formation of CYP450 enzymes may be suppressed by increased levels of cytokines (eg, TNFα) during chronic inflammation. Therefore, it is expected that for a molecule that antagonizes cytokine activity, such as golimumab, the formation of CYP450 enzymes could be normalized. Upon initiation or discontinuation of golimumab in patients being treated with CYP450 substrates with a narrow therapeutic index, monitoring of the effect (eg, warfarin) or drug concentration (eg, cyclosporine or theophylline) is recommended and the individual dose of the drug product may be adjusted as needed).
No products indexed under this heading.

Fluphenazine Enanthate (The formation of CYP450 enzymes may be suppressed by increased levels of cytokines (eg, TNFα) during chronic inflammation. Therefore, it is expected that for a molecule that antagonizes cytokine activity, such as golimumab, the formation of CYP450 enzymes could be normalized. Upon initiation or discontinuation of golimumab in patients being treated with CYP450 substrates with a narrow therapeutic index, monitoring of the effect (eg, warfarin) or drug concentration (eg, cyclosporine or theophylline) is recommended and the individual dose of the drug product may be adjusted as needed).
No products indexed under this heading.

Fluphenazine Hydrochloride (The formation of CYP450 enzymes may be suppressed by increased levels of cytokines (eg, TNFα) during chronic inflammation. Therefore, it is expected that for a molecule that antagonizes cytokine activity, such as golimumab, the formation of CYP450 enzymes could be normalized. Upon initiation or discontinuation of golimumab in patients being treated with CYP450 substrates with a narrow therapeutic index, monitoring of the effect (eg, warfarin) or drug concentration (eg, cyclosporine or theophylline) is recommended and the individual dose of the drug product may be adjusted as needed).
No products indexed under this heading.

Flurbiprofen (The formation of CYP450 enzymes may be suppressed by increased levels of cytokines (eg, TNFα) during chronic inflammation. Therefore, it is expected that for a molecule that antagonizes cytokine activity, such as golimumab, the formation of CYP450 enzymes could be normalized. Upon initiation or discontinuation of golimumab in patients being treated with CYP450 substrates with a narrow thera-

peutic index, monitoring of the effect (eg, warfarin) or drug concentration (eg, cyclosporine or theophylline) is recommended and the individual dose of the drug product may be adjusted as needed).
No products indexed under this heading.

Flurbiprofen Sodium (The formation of CYP450 enzymes may be suppressed by increased levels of cytokines (eg, TNFα) during chronic inflammation. Therefore, it is expected that for a molecule that antagonizes cytokine activity, such as golimumab, the formation of CYP450 enzymes could be normalized. Upon initiation or discontinuation of golimumab in patients being treated with CYP450 substrates with a narrow therapeutic index, monitoring of the effect (eg, warfarin) or drug concentration (eg, cyclosporine or theophylline) is recommended and the individual dose of the drug product may be adjusted as needed).
No products indexed under this heading.

Flutamide (The formation of CYP450 enzymes may be suppressed by increased levels of cytokines (eg, TNFα) during chronic inflammation. Therefore, it is expected that for a molecule that antagonizes cytokine activity, such as golimumab, the formation of CYP450 enzymes could be normalized. Upon initiation or discontinuation of golimumab in patients being treated with CYP450 substrates with a narrow therapeutic index, monitoring of the effect (eg, warfarin) or drug concentration (eg, cyclosporine or theophylline) is recommended and the individual dose of the drug product may be adjusted as needed).
No products indexed under this heading.

Fluticasone Propionate (The formation of CYP450 enzymes may be suppressed by increased levels of cytokines (eg, TNFα) during chronic inflammation. Therefore, it is expected that for a molecule that antagonizes cytokine activity, such as golimumab, the formation of CYP450 enzymes could be normalized. Upon initiation or discontinuation of golimumab in patients being treated with CYP450 substrates with a narrow therapeutic index, monitoring of the effect (eg, warfarin) or drug concentration (eg, cyclosporine or theophylline) is recommended and the individual dose of the drug product may be adjusted as needed). Products include:
Advair 100/50 1275
Advair 250/50 1275
Advair 500/50 1275
Advair HFA 45/21 1288
Advair HFA 115/21 1288
Advair HFA 230/21 1288
Flonase 1459
Flovent Diskus 1463
Flovent HFA 1470

Fluvastatin Sodium (The formation of CYP450 enzymes may be suppressed by increased levels of cytokines (eg, TNFα) during chronic inflammation. Therefore, it is expected that for a molecule that antagonizes cytokine activity, such as golimumab, the formation of CYP450 enzymes could be normalized. Upon initiation or discontinuation of golimumab in patients being treated with CYP450 substrates with a narrow therapeutic index, monitoring of the effect (eg, warfarin) or drug concentration (eg, cyclosporine or theophylline) is recommended and the individual dose of the drug product may be adjusted as needed).
No products indexed under this heading.

Fluvoxamine Maleate (The formation of CYP450 enzymes may be suppressed by increased levels of cytokines (eg, TNFα) during chronic inflammation. Therefore, it is expected that for a molecule that antagonizes cytokine activity, such as golimumab, the formation of CYP450 enzymes could be normalized. Upon initiation or discontinuation of golimumab in patients being treated with CYP450 substrates with a narrow therapeutic index, monitoring of the effect (eg, warfarin) or drug concentration (eg, cyclosporine or theophylline) is recommended and the individual dose of the drug product may be adjusted as needed).
No products indexed under this heading.

Formoterol Fumarate (The formation of CYP450 enzymes may be suppressed by increased levels of cytokines (eg, TNFα) during chronic inflammation. Therefore, it is expected that for a molecule that antagonizes cytokine activity, such as golimumab, the formation of CYP450 enzymes could be normalized. Upon initiation or discontinuation of golimumab in patients being treated with CYP450 substrates with a narrow therapeutic index, monitoring of the effect (eg, warfarin) or drug concentration (eg, cyclosporine or theophylline) is recommended and the individual dose of the drug product may be adjusted as needed). Products include:
Foradil 3121
Perforomist 3634

Fosphenytoin (The formation of CYP450 enzymes may be suppressed by increased levels of cytokines (eg, TNFα) during chronic inflammation. Therefore, it is expected that for a molecule that antagonizes cytokine activity, such as golimumab, the formation of CYP450 enzymes could be normalized. Upon initiation or discontinuation of golimumab in patients being treated with CYP450 substrates with a narrow therapeutic index, monitoring of the effect (eg, warfarin) or drug concentration (eg, cyclosporine or theophylline) is recommended and the individual dose of the drug product may be adjusted as needed).
No products indexed under this heading.

Fosphenytoin Sodium (The formation of CYP450 enzymes may be suppressed by increased levels of cytokines (eg, TNFα) during chronic inflammation. Therefore, it is expected that for a molecule that antagonizes cytokine activity, such as golimumab, the formation of CYP450 enzymes could be normalized. Upon initiation or discontinuation of golimumab in patients being treated with CYP450 substrates with a narrow therapeutic index, monitoring of the effect (eg, warfarin) or drug concentration (eg, cyclosporine or theophylline) is recommended and the individual dose of the drug product may be adjusted as needed).
No products indexed under this heading.

Gabapentin (The formation of CYP450 enzymes may be suppressed by increased levels of cytokines (eg, TNFα) during chronic inflammation. Therefore, it is expected that for a molecule that antagonizes cytokine activity, such as golimumab, the formation of CYP450 enzymes could be normalized. Upon initiation or discontinuation of golimumab in patients being treated with CYP450 substrates with a narrow therapeutic index, monitoring of the effect (eg, warfarin) or drug concentration (eg, cyclosporine or theophylline) is recommended and the individual dose of the drug product may be adjusted as needed).
No products indexed under this heading.

Galantamine Hydrobromide (The formation of CYP450 enzymes may be suppressed by increased levels of cytokines (eg, TNFα) during chronic inflammation. Therefore, it is expected that for a molecule that antagonizes cytokine activity, such as golimumab, the formation of CYP450 enzymes could be normalized. Upon initiation or discontinuation of golimumab in patients being treated with CYP450 substrates with a narrow therapeutic index, monitoring of the effect (eg, warfarin) or drug concentration (eg, cyclosporine or theophylline) is recommended and the individual dose of the drug product may be adjusted as needed).
No products indexed under this heading.

Glimepiride (The formation of CYP450 enzymes may be suppressed by increased levels of cytokines (eg, TNFα) during chronic inflammation. Therefore, it is expected that for a molecule that antagonizes cytokine activity, such as golimumab, the formation of CYP450 enzymes could be normalized. Upon initiation or discontinuation of golimumab in patients being treated with CYP450 substrates with a narrow therapeutic index, monitoring of the effect (eg, warfarin) or drug concentration (eg, cyclosporine or theophylline) is recommended and the individual dose of the drug product may be adjusted as needed). Products include:
Avandaryl 1356
Duetact 3354

Glipizide (The formation of CYP450 enzymes may be suppressed by increased levels of cytokines (eg, TNFα) during chronic inflammation. Therefore, it is expected that for a molecule that antagonizes cytokine activity, such as golimumab, the formation of CYP450 enzymes could be normalized. Upon initiation or discontinuation of golimumab in patients being treated with CYP450 substrates with a narrow therapeutic index, monitoring of the effect (eg, warfarin) or drug concentration (eg, cyclosporine or theophylline) is recommended and the individual dose of the drug product may be adjusted as needed).
No products indexed under this heading.

Glyburide (The formation of CYP450 enzymes may be suppressed by increased levels of cytokines (eg, TNFα) during chronic inflammation. Therefore, it is expected that for a molecule that antagonizes cytokine activity, such as golimumab, the formation of CYP450 enzymes could be normalized. Upon initiation or discontinuation of golimumab in patients being treated with CYP450 substrates with a narrow therapeutic index, monitoring of the effect (eg, warfarin) or drug concentration (eg, cyclosporine or theophylline) is recommended and the individual dose of the drug product may be adjusted as needed).
No products indexed under this heading.

Grepafloxacin Hydrochloride (The formation of CYP450 enzymes may be suppressed by increased levels of cytokines (eg, TNFα) during chronic inflammation. Therefore, it is expected that for a molecule that antagonizes cytokine activity, such as golimumab, the formation of CYP450 enzymes could be normalized. Upon initiation or discontinuation of golimumab in patients being treated with CYP450 substrates with a narrow therapeutic index, monitoring of the effect (eg, warfarin) or drug concentration (eg, cyclosporine or theophylline) is recommended and the individual dose of the drug product may be adjusted as needed).
No products indexed under this heading.

Haloperidol (The formation of CYP450 enzymes may be suppressed by increased levels of cytokines (eg, TNFα) during chronic inflammation. Therefore, it is expected that for a molecule that antagonizes cytokine activity, such as golimumab, the formation of CYP450 enzymes could be normalized. Upon initiation or discontinuation of golimumab in patients being treated with CYP450 substrates with a narrow therapeutic index, monitoring of the effect (eg, warfarin) or drug concentration (eg, cyclosporine or theophylline) is recommended and the individual dose of the drug product may be adjusted as needed).
No products indexed under this heading.

Haloperidol Decanoate (The formation of CYP450 enzymes may be suppressed by increased levels of cytokines (eg, TNFα) during chronic inflammation. Therefore, it is expected that for a molecule that antagonizes cytokine activity, such as golimumab, the formation of CYP450 enzymes could be normalized. Upon initiation or discontinuation of golimumab in patients being treated with CYP450 substrates with a narrow therapeutic index, monitoring of the effect (eg, warfarin) or drug concentration (eg, cyclosporine or theophylline) is recommended and the individual dose of the drug product may be adjusted as needed).
No products indexed under this heading.

Haloperidol Lactate (The formation of CYP450 enzymes may be suppressed by increased levels of cytokines (eg, TNFα) during chronic inflammation. Therefore, it is expected that for a molecule that antagonizes cytokine activity, such as golimumab, the formation of CYP450 enzymes could be normalized. Upon initiation or discontinuation of golimumab in patients being treated with CYP450 substrates with a narrow therapeutic index, monitoring of the effect (eg, warfarin) or drug concentration (eg, cyclosporine or theophylline) is recommended and the individual dose of the drug product may be adjusted as needed).
No products indexed under this heading.

Hexobarbital (The formation of CYP450 enzymes may be suppressed by increased levels of cytokines (eg, TNFα) during chronic inflammation. Therefore, it is expected that for a molecule that antagonizes cytokine activity, such as golimumab, the formation of CYP450 enzymes could be normalized. Upon initiation or discontinuation of golimumab in patients being treated with CYP450 substrates with a narrow therapeutic index, monitoring of the effect (eg, warfarin) or drug concentration (eg, cyclosporine or theophylline) is recommended and the individual dose of the drug product may be adjusted as needed).
No products indexed under this heading.

Hydrocodone Bitartrate (The formation of CYP450 enzymes may be suppressed by increased levels of cytokines (eg, TNFα) during chronic inflammation. Therefore, it is expected that for a molecule that antagonizes cytokine activity, such as golimumab, the formation of CYP450 enzymes could be normalized. Upon initiation or discontinuation of golimumab in patients being treated with CYP450 substrates with a narrow therapeutic index, monitoring of the effect (eg, warfarin) or drug concentration (eg, cyclosporine or theophylline) is recommended and the individual dose of the drug product may be adjusted as needed). Products include:
Vicodin 560
Vicodin ES 561
Vicodin HP 563
Vicoprofen 564
Zydone 1138

that for a molecule that antagonizes cytokine activity, such as golimumab, the formation of CYP450 enzymes could be normalized. Upon initiation or discontinuation of golimumab in patients being treated with CYP450 substrates with a narrow therapeutic index, monitoring of the effect (eg, warfarin) or drug concentration (eg, cyclosporine or theophylline) is recommended and the individual dose of the drug product may be adjusted as needed).
No products indexed under this heading.

Levonorgestrel (The formation of CYP450 enzymes may be suppressed by increased levels of cytokines (eg, TNFα) during chronic inflammation. Therefore, it is expected that for a molecule that antagonizes cytokine activity, such as golimumab, the formation of CYP450 enzymes could be normalized. Upon initiation or discontinuation of golimumab in patients being treated with CYP450 substrates with a narrow therapeutic index, monitoring of the effect (eg, warfarin) or drug concentration (eg, cyclosporine or theophylline) is recommended and the individual dose of the drug product may be adjusted as needed). Products include:
Climara Pro 847
LoSeasonique 3407
Lybrel 3514
Mirena 854
Plan B 3416
Seasonique 3418

Lidocaine (The formation of CYP450 enzymes may be suppressed by increased levels of cytokines (eg, TNFα) during chronic inflammation. Therefore, it is expected that for a molecule that antagonizes cytokine activity, such as golimumab, the formation of CYP450 enzymes could be normalized. Upon initiation or discontinuation of golimumab in patients being treated with CYP450 substrates with a narrow therapeutic index, monitoring of the effect (eg, warfarin) or drug concentration (eg, cyclosporine or theophylline) is recommended and the individual dose of the drug product may be adjusted as needed). Products include:
Lidoderm 1107

Lidocaine Base (The formation of CYP450 enzymes may be suppressed by increased levels of cytokines (eg, TNFα) during chronic inflammation. Therefore, it is expected that for a molecule that antagonizes cytokine activity, such as golimumab, the formation of CYP450 enzymes could be normalized. Upon initiation or discontinuation of golimumab in patients being treated with CYP450 substrates with a narrow therapeutic index, monitoring of the effect (eg, warfarin) or drug concentration (eg, cyclosporine or theophylline) is recommended and the individual dose of the drug product may be adjusted as needed).
No products indexed under this heading.

Lidocaine Hydrochloride (The formation of CYP450 enzymes may be suppressed by increased levels of cytokines (eg, TNFα) during chronic inflammation. Therefore, it is expected that for a molecule that antagonizes cytokine activity, such as golimumab, the formation of CYP450 enzymes could be normalized. Upon initiation or discontinuation of golimumab in patients being treated with CYP450 substrates with a narrow therapeutic index, monitoring of the effect (eg, warfarin) or drug concentration (eg, cyclosporine or theophylline) is recommended and the individual dose of the drug product may be adjusted as needed).
No products indexed under this heading.

Lomefloxacin Hydrochloride (The formation of CYP450 enzymes may be suppressed by increased levels of cytokines (eg, TNFα) during chronic inflammation. Therefore, it is expected that for a molecule that antagonizes cytokine activity, such as golimumab, the formation of CYP450 enzymes could be normalized. Upon initiation or discontinuation of golimumab in patients being treated with CYP450 substrates with a narrow therapeutic index, monitoring of the effect (eg, warfarin) or drug concentration (eg, cyclosporine or theophylline) is recommended and the individual dose of the drug product may be adjusted as needed).
No products indexed under this heading.

Losartan Potassium (The formation of CYP450 enzymes may be suppressed by increased levels of cytokines (eg, TNFα) during chronic inflammation. Therefore, it is expected that for a molecule that antagonizes cytokine activity, such as golimumab, the formation of CYP450 enzymes could be normalized. Upon initiation or discontinuation of golimumab in patients being treated with CYP450 substrates with a narrow therapeutic index, monitoring of the effect (eg, warfarin) or drug concentration (eg, cyclosporine or theophylline) is recommended and the individual dose of the drug product may be adjusted as needed). Products include:
Cozaar 2106
Hyzaar 2162
Hyzaar 100-12.5 2162

Lovastatin (The formation of CYP450 enzymes may be suppressed by increased levels of cytokines (eg, TNFα) during chronic inflammation. Therefore, it is expected that for a molecule that antagonizes cytokine activity, such as golimumab, the formation of CYP450 enzymes could be normalized. Upon initiation or discontinuation of golimumab in patients being treated with CYP450 substrates with a narrow therapeutic index, monitoring of the effect (eg, warfarin) or drug concentration (eg, cyclosporine or theophylline) is recommended and the individual dose of the drug product may be adjusted as needed). Products include:
Advicor 402
Mevacor 2212

Maprotiline Hydrochloride (The formation of CYP450 enzymes may be suppressed by increased levels of cytokines (eg, TNFα) during chronic inflammation. Therefore, it is expected that for a molecule that antagonizes cytokine activity, such as golimumab, the formation of CYP450 enzymes could be normalized. Upon initiation or discontinuation of golimumab in patients being treated with CYP450 substrates with a narrow therapeutic index, monitoring of the effect (eg, warfarin) or drug concentration (eg, cyclosporine or theophylline) is recommended and the individual dose of the drug product may be adjusted as needed).
No products indexed under this heading.

Measles, Mumps, Rubella and Varicella Virus Vaccine Live (Live vaccines should not be given concurrently with golimumab). Products include:
ProQuad 2254

Measles, Mumps & Rubella Virus Vaccine, Live (Live vaccines should not be given concurrently with golimumab). Products include:
M-M-R II 2203
ProQuad 2254

Measles & Rubella Virus Vaccine Live (Live vaccines should not be given concurrently with golimumab).
No products indexed under this heading.

Measles Virus Vaccine Live (Live vaccines should not be given concurrently with golimumab). Products include:
Attenuvax 2086

Meclofenamate Sodium (The formation of CYP450 enzymes may be suppressed by increased levels of cytokines (eg, TNFα) during chronic inflammation. Therefore, it is expected that for a molecule that antagonizes cytokine activity, such as golimumab, the formation of CYP450 enzymes could be normalized. Upon initiation or discontinuation of golimumab in patients being treated with CYP450 substrates with a narrow therapeutic index, monitoring of the effect (eg, warfarin) or drug concentration (eg, cyclosporine or theophylline) is recommended and the individual dose of the drug product may be adjusted as needed).
No products indexed under this heading.

Mefenamic Acid (The formation of CYP450 enzymes may be suppressed by increased levels of cytokines (eg, TNFα) during chronic inflammation. Therefore, it is expected that for a molecule that antagonizes cytokine activity, such as golimumab, the formation of CYP450 enzymes could be normalized. Upon initiation or discontinuation of golimumab in patients being treated with CYP450 substrates with a narrow therapeutic index, monitoring of the effect (eg, warfarin) or drug concentration (eg, cyclosporine or theophylline) is recommended and the individual dose of the drug product may be adjusted as needed).
No products indexed under this heading.

Meloxicam (The formation of CYP450 enzymes may be suppressed by increased levels of cytokines (eg, TNFα) during chronic inflammation. Therefore, it is expected that for a molecule that antagonizes cytokine activity, such as golimumab, the formation of CYP450 enzymes could be normalized. Upon initiation or discontinuation of golimumab in patients being treated with CYP450 substrates with a narrow therapeutic index, monitoring of the effect (eg, warfarin) or drug concentration (eg, cyclosporine or theophylline) is recommended and the individual dose of the drug product may be adjusted as needed).
No products indexed under this heading.

Meperidine Hydrochloride (The formation of CYP450 enzymes may be suppressed by increased levels of cytokines (eg, TNFα) during chronic inflammation. Therefore, it is expected that for a molecule that antagonizes cytokine activity, such as golimumab, the formation of CYP450 enzymes could be normalized. Upon initiation or discontinuation of golimumab in patients being treated with CYP450 substrates with a narrow therapeutic index, monitoring of the effect (eg, warfarin) or drug concentration (eg, cyclosporine or theophylline) is recommended and the individual dose of the drug product may be adjusted as needed).
No products indexed under this heading.

Mephenytoin (The formation of CYP450 enzymes may be suppressed by increased levels of cytokines (eg, TNFα) during chronic inflammation. Therefore, it is expected that for a molecule that antagonizes cytokine activity, such as golimumab, the formation of CYP450 enzymes could be normalized. Upon initiation or discontinuation of golimumab in patients being treated with CYP450 substrates with a narrow therapeutic index, monitoring of the effect (eg, warfarin) or drug concentration (eg, cyclosporine or theophylline) is recommended and the individual dose of the drug product may be adjusted as needed).
No products indexed under this heading.

Mephobarbital (The formation of CYP450 enzymes may be suppressed by increased levels of cytokines (eg, TNFα) during chronic inflammation. Therefore, it is expected that for a molecule that antagonizes cytokine activity, such as golimumab, the formation of CYP450 enzymes could be normalized. Upon initiation or discontinuation of golimumab in patients being treated with CYP450 substrates with a narrow therapeutic index, monitoring of the effect (eg, warfarin) or drug concentration (eg, cyclosporine or theophylline) is recommended and the individual dose of the drug product may be adjusted as needed).
No products indexed under this heading.

Meprobamate (The formation of CYP450 enzymes may be suppressed by increased levels of cytokines (eg, TNFα) during chronic inflammation. Therefore, it is expected that for a molecule that antagonizes cytokine activity, such as golimumab, the formation of CYP450 enzymes could be normalized. Upon initiation or discontinuation of golimumab in patients being treated with CYP450 substrates with a narrow therapeutic index, monitoring of the effect (eg, warfarin) or drug concentration (eg, cyclosporine or theophylline) is recommended and the individual dose of the drug product may be adjusted as needed).
No products indexed under this heading.

Mestranol (The formation of CYP450 enzymes may be suppressed by increased levels of cytokines (eg, TNFα) during chronic inflammation. Therefore, it is expected that for a molecule that antagonizes cytokine activity, such as golimumab, the formation of CYP450 enzymes could be normalized. Upon initiation or discontinuation of golimumab in patients being treated with CYP450 substrates with a narrow therapeutic index, monitoring of the effect (eg, warfarin) or drug concentration (eg, cyclosporine or theophylline) is recommended and the individual dose of the drug product may be adjusted as needed).
No products indexed under this heading.

Metformin Hydrochloride (The formation of CYP450 enzymes may be suppressed by increased levels of cytokines (eg, TNFα) during chronic inflammation. Therefore, it is expected that for a molecule that antagonizes cytokine activity, such as golimumab, the formation of CYP450 enzymes could be normalized. Upon initiation or discontinuation of golimumab in patients being treated with CYP450 substrates with a narrow therapeutic index, monitoring of the effect (eg, warfarin) or drug concentration (eg, cyclosporine or theophylline) is recommended and the individual dose of the drug product may be adjusted as needed). Products include:
ActoPlus 3338
Avandamet 1345
Janumet 2188

Methadone Hydrochloride (The formation of CYP450 enzymes may be suppressed by increased levels of cytokines (eg, TNFα) during chronic inflammation. Therefore, it is expected that for a molecule that antagonizes cytokine activity, such as golimumab, the formation of CYP450 enzymes could be normalized. Upon initiation or discontinuation of golimumab in patients being treated with CYP450 substrates with a narrow therapeutic index, monitoring of the effect (eg, warfarin) or drug concentration (eg,

cyclosporine or theophylline) is recommended and the individual dose of the drug product may be adjusted as needed).
No products indexed under this heading.

Methamphetamine Hydrochloride (The formation of CYP450 enzymes may be suppressed by increased levels of cytokines (eg, TNFα) during chronic inflammation. Therefore, it is expected that for a molecule that antagonizes cytokine activity, such as golimumab, the formation of CYP450 enzymes could be normalized. Upon initiation or discontinuation of golimumab in patients being treated with CYP450 substrates with a narrow therapeutic index, monitoring of the effect (eg, warfarin) or drug concentration (eg, cyclosporine or theophylline) is recommended and the individual dose of the drug product may be adjusted as needed).
No products indexed under this heading.

Methotrexate (Patients with rheumatoid arthritis (RA), psoriatic arthritis (PsA), and ankylosing spondylitis (AS) treated with golimumab 50 mg and methotrexate (MTX) had approximately 52%, 36% and 21% higher mean steady-state trough concentrations of golimumab, respectively, compared with those treated with golimumab 50 mg without MTX. The presence of MTX also decreased anti-golimumab antibody incidence from 7% to 2%. For RA, golimumab should be used with MTX. In the PsA and AS trials, the presence or absence of concomitant MTX did not appear to influence clinical efficacy and safety parameters).
No products indexed under this heading.

Methotrexate Sodium (Patients with rheumatoid arthritis (RA), psoriatic arthritis (PsA), and ankylosing spondylitis (AS) treated with golimumab 50 mg and methotrexate (MTX) had approximately 52%, 36% and 21% higher mean steady-state trough concentrations of golimumab, respectively, compared with those treated with golimumab 50 mg without MTX. The presence of MTX also decreased anti-golimumab antibody incidence from 7% to 2%. For RA, golimumab should be used with MTX. In the PsA and AS trials, the presence or absence of concomitant MTX did not appear to influence clinical efficacy and safety parameters).
No products indexed under this heading.

Methsuximide (The formation of CYP450 enzymes may be suppressed by increased levels of cytokines (eg, TNFα) during chronic inflammation. Therefore, it is expected that for a molecule that antagonizes cytokine activity, such as golimumab, the formation of CYP450 enzymes could be normalized. Upon initiation or discontinuation of golimumab in patients being treated with CYP450 substrates with a narrow therapeutic index, monitoring of the effect (eg, warfarin) or drug concentration (eg, cyclosporine or theophylline) is recommended and the individual dose of the drug product may be adjusted as needed).
No products indexed under this heading.

Metoprolol Succinate (The formation of CYP450 enzymes may be suppressed by increased levels of cytokines (eg, TNFα) during chronic inflammation. Therefore, it is expected that for a molecule that antagonizes cytokine activity, such as golimumab, the formation of CYP450 enzymes could be normalized. Upon initiation or discontinuation of golimumab in patients being treated with CYP450 substrates with a narrow therapeutic index, monitoring of the effect (eg, warfarin) or drug concentration (eg, cyclosporine or theophylline) is recommended and the individual dose of the drug product may be adjusted as needed). Products include:
Toprol XL ... 732

Metoprolol Tartrate (The formation of CYP450 enzymes may be suppressed by increased levels of cytokines (eg, TNFα) during chronic inflammation. Therefore, it is expected that for a molecule that antagonizes cytokine activity, such as golimumab, the formation of CYP450 enzymes could be normalized. Upon initiation or discontinuation of golimumab in patients being treated with CYP450 substrates with a narrow therapeutic index, monitoring of the effect (eg, warfarin) or drug concentration (eg, cyclosporine or theophylline) is recommended and the individual dose of the drug product may be adjusted as needed).
No products indexed under this heading.

Mexiletine Hydrochloride (The formation of CYP450 enzymes may be suppressed by increased levels of cytokines (eg, TNFα) during chronic inflammation. Therefore, it is expected that for a molecule that antagonizes cytokine activity, such as golimumab, the formation of CYP450 enzymes could be normalized. Upon initiation or discontinuation of golimumab in patients being treated with CYP450 substrates with a narrow therapeutic index, monitoring of the effect (eg, warfarin) or drug concentration (eg, cyclosporine or theophylline) is recommended and the individual dose of the drug product may be adjusted as needed).
No products indexed under this heading.

Midazolam Hydrochloride (The formation of CYP450 enzymes may be suppressed by increased levels of cytokines (eg, TNFα) during chronic inflammation. Therefore, it is expected that for a molecule that antagonizes cytokine activity, such as golimumab, the formation of CYP450 enzymes could be normalized. Upon initiation or discontinuation of golimumab in patients being treated with CYP450 substrates with a narrow therapeutic index, monitoring of the effect (eg, warfarin) or drug concentration (eg, cyclosporine or theophylline) is recommended and the individual dose of the drug product may be adjusted as needed).
No products indexed under this heading.

Miglitol (The formation of CYP450 enzymes may be suppressed by increased levels of cytokines (eg, TNFα) during chronic inflammation. Therefore, it is expected that for a molecule that antagonizes cytokine activity, such as golimumab, the formation of CYP450 enzymes could be normalized. Upon initiation or discontinuation of golimumab in patients being treated with CYP450 substrates with a narrow therapeutic index, monitoring of the effect (eg, warfarin) or drug concentration (eg, cyclosporine or theophylline) is recommended and the individual dose of the drug product may be adjusted as needed).
No products indexed under this heading.

Mirtazapine (The formation of CYP450 enzymes may be suppressed by increased levels of cytokines (eg, TNFα) during chronic inflammation. Therefore, it is expected that for a molecule that antagonizes cytokine activity, such as golimumab, the formation of CYP450 enzymes could be normalized. Upon initiation or discontinuation of golimumab in patients being treated with CYP450 substrates with a narrow therapeutic index, monitoring of the effect (eg, warfarin) or drug concentration (eg, cyclosporine or theophylline) is recommended and the individual dose of the drug product may be adjusted as needed). Products include:
Remeron Tablets ... 3214
RemeronSolTab Tablets ... 3219

Montelukast Sodium (The formation of CYP450 enzymes may be suppressed by increased levels of cytokines (eg, TNFα) during chronic inflammation. Therefore, it is expected that for a molecule that antagonizes cytokine activity, such as golimumab, the formation of CYP450 enzymes could be normalized. Upon initiation or discontinuation of golimumab in patients being treated with CYP450 substrates with a narrow therapeutic index, monitoring of the effect (eg, warfarin) or drug concentration (eg, cyclosporine or theophylline) is recommended and the individual dose of the drug product may be adjusted as needed). Products include:
Singulair ... 2270

Morphine Sulfate (The formation of CYP450 enzymes may be suppressed by increased levels of cytokines (eg, TNFα) during chronic inflammation. Therefore, it is expected that for a molecule that antagonizes cytokine activity, such as golimumab, the formation of CYP450 enzymes could be normalized. Upon initiation or discontinuation of golimumab in patients being treated with CYP450 substrates with a narrow therapeutic index, monitoring of the effect (eg, warfarin) or drug concentration (eg, cyclosporine or theophylline) is recommended and the individual dose of the drug product may be adjusted as needed). Products include:
Avinza ... 1822
Embeda ... 1831
MS Contin ... 2803

Moxifloxacin Hydrochloride (The formation of CYP450 enzymes may be suppressed by increased levels of cytokines (eg, TNFα) during chronic inflammation. Therefore, it is expected that for a molecule that antagonizes cytokine activity, such as golimumab, the formation of CYP450 enzymes could be normalized. Upon initiation or discontinuation of golimumab in patients being treated with CYP450 substrates with a narrow therapeutic index, monitoring of the effect (eg, warfarin) or drug concentration (eg, cyclosporine or theophylline) is recommended and the individual dose of the drug product may be adjusted as needed). Products include:
Avelox ... 3064
Vigamox ... 589

Mumps Virus Vaccine, Live (Live vaccines should not be given concurrently with golimumab). Products include:
Mumpsvax ... 2218

Nabumetone (The formation of CYP450 enzymes may be suppressed by increased levels of cytokines (eg, TNFα) during chronic inflammation. Therefore, it is expected that for a molecule that antagonizes cytokine activity, such as golimumab, the formation of CYP450 enzymes could be normalized. Upon initiation or discontinuation of golimumab in patients being treated with CYP450 substrates with a narrow therapeutic index, monitoring of the effect (eg, warfarin) or drug concentration (eg, cyclosporine or theophylline) is recommended and the individual dose of the drug product may be adjusted as needed).
No products indexed under this heading.

Nafcillin Sodium (The formation of CYP450 enzymes may be suppressed by increased levels of cytokines (eg, TNFα) during chronic inflammation. Therefore, it is expected that for a molecule that antagonizes cytokine activity, such as golimumab, the formation of CYP450 enzymes could be normalized. Upon initiation or discontinuation of golimumab in patients being treated with CYP450 substrates with a narrow therapeutic index, monitoring of the effect (eg, warfarin) or drug concentration (eg, cyclosporine or theophylline) is recommended and the individual dose of the drug product may be adjusted as needed).
No products indexed under this heading.

Naproxen (The formation of CYP450 enzymes may be suppressed by increased levels of cytokines (eg, TNFα) during chronic inflammation. Therefore, it is expected that for a molecule that antagonizes cytokine activity, such as golimumab, the formation of CYP450 enzymes could be normalized. Upon initiation or discontinuation of golimumab in patients being treated with CYP450 substrates with a narrow therapeutic index, monitoring of the effect (eg, warfarin) or drug concentration (eg, cyclosporine or theophylline) is recommended and the individual dose of the drug product may be adjusted as needed). Products include:
EC-Naprosyn ... 2850
Naprosyn ... 2850
Anaprox/Naprosyn ... 2850

Naproxen Sodium (The formation of CYP450 enzymes may be suppressed by increased levels of cytokines (eg, TNFα) during chronic inflammation. Therefore, it is expected that for a molecule that antagonizes cytokine activity, such as golimumab, the formation of CYP450 enzymes could be normalized. Upon initiation or discontinuation of golimumab in patients being treated with CYP450 substrates with a narrow therapeutic index, monitoring of the effect (eg, warfarin) or drug concentration (eg, cyclosporine or theophylline) is recommended and the individual dose of the drug product may be adjusted as needed). Products include:
Anaprox ... 2850
Anaprox DS ... 2850
Treximet ... 1681

Nateglinide (The formation of CYP450 enzymes may be suppressed by increased levels of cytokines (eg, TNFα) during chronic inflammation. Therefore, it is expected that for a molecule that antagonizes cytokine activity, such as golimumab, the formation of CYP450 enzymes could be normalized. Upon initiation or discontinuation of golimumab in patients being treated with CYP450 substrates with a narrow therapeutic index, monitoring of the effect (eg, warfarin) or drug concentration (eg, cyclosporine or theophylline) is recommended and the individual dose of the drug product may be adjusted as needed).
No products indexed under this heading.

Nefazodone Hydrochloride (The formation of CYP450 enzymes may be suppressed by increased levels of cytokines (eg, TNFα) during chronic inflammation. Therefore, it is expected that for a molecule that antagonizes cytokine activity, such as golimumab, the formation of CYP450 enzymes could be normalized. Upon initiation or discontinuation of golimumab in patients being treated with CYP450 substrates with a narrow therapeutic index, monitoring of the effect (eg, warfarin) or drug concentration (eg, cyclosporine or theophylline) is recommended and the individual dose of the drug product may be adjusted as needed).
No products indexed under this heading.

Nelfinavir Mesylate (The formation of CYP450 enzymes may be suppressed by increased levels of cytokines (eg, TNFα) during chronic inflammation. Therefore, it is expected that

for a molecule that antagonizes cytokine activity, such as golimumab, the formation of CYP450 enzymes could be normalized. Upon initiation or discontinuation of golimumab in patients being treated with CYP450 substrates with a narrow therapeutic index, monitoring of the effect (eg, warfarin) or drug concentration (eg, cyclosporine or theophylline) is recommended and the individual dose of the drug product may be adjusted as needed).

No products indexed under this heading.

Nicardipine (The formation of CYP450 enzymes may be suppressed by increased levels of cytokines (eg, TNFα) during chronic inflammation. Therefore, it is expected that for a molecule that antagonizes cytokine activity, such as golimumab, the formation of CYP450 enzymes could be normalized. Upon initiation or discontinuation of golimumab in patients being treated with CYP450 substrates with a narrow therapeutic index, monitoring of the effect (eg, warfarin) or drug concentration (eg, cyclosporine or theophylline) is recommended and the individual dose of the drug product may be adjusted as needed).

No products indexed under this heading.

Nicardipine Hydrochloride (The formation of CYP450 enzymes may be suppressed by increased levels of cytokines (eg, TNFα) during chronic inflammation. Therefore, it is expected that for a molecule that antagonizes cytokine activity, such as golimumab, the formation of CYP450 enzymes could be normalized. Upon initiation or discontinuation of golimumab in patients being treated with CYP450 substrates with a narrow therapeutic index, monitoring of the effect (eg, warfarin) or drug concentration (eg, cyclosporine or theophylline) is recommended and the individual dose of the drug product may be adjusted as needed).

No products indexed under this heading.

Nicotine Polacrilex (The formation of CYP450 enzymes may be suppressed by increased levels of cytokines (eg, TNFα) during chronic inflammation. Therefore, it is expected that for a molecule that antagonizes cytokine activity, such as golimumab, the formation of CYP450 enzymes could be normalized. Upon initiation or discontinuation of golimumab in patients being treated with CYP450 substrates with a narrow therapeutic index, monitoring of the effect (eg, warfarin) or drug concentration (eg, cyclosporine or theophylline) is recommended and the individual dose of the drug product may be adjusted as needed).

No products indexed under this heading.

Nicotine Salicylate (The formation of CYP450 enzymes may be suppressed by increased levels of cytokines (eg, TNFα) during chronic inflammation. Therefore, it is expected that for a molecule that antagonizes cytokine activity, such as golimumab, the formation of CYP450 enzymes could be normalized. Upon initiation or discontinuation of golimumab in patients being treated with CYP450 substrates with a narrow therapeutic index, monitoring of the effect (eg, warfarin) or drug concentration (eg, cyclosporine or theophylline) is recommended and the individual dose of the drug product may be adjusted as needed).

No products indexed under this heading.

Nicotine Sulfate (The formation of CYP450 enzymes may be suppressed by increased levels of cytokines (eg, TNFα) during chronic inflammation. Therefore, it is expected that for a molecule that antagonizes cytokine activity, such as golimumab, the formation of

CYP450 enzymes could be normalized. Upon initiation or discontinuation of golimumab in patients being treated with CYP450 substrates with a narrow therapeutic index, monitoring of the effect (eg, warfarin) or drug concentration (eg, cyclosporine or theophylline) is recommended and the individual dose of the drug product may be adjusted as needed).

No products indexed under this heading.

Nifedipine (The formation of CYP450 enzymes may be suppressed by increased levels of cytokines (eg, TNFα) during chronic inflammation. Therefore, it is expected that for a molecule that antagonizes cytokine activity, such as golimumab, the formation of CYP450 enzymes could be normalized. Upon initiation or discontinuation of golimumab in patients being treated with CYP450 substrates with a narrow therapeutic index, monitoring of the effect (eg, warfarin) or drug concentration (eg, cyclosporine or theophylline) is recommended and the individual dose of the drug product may be adjusted as needed).

No products indexed under this heading.

Nilutamide (The formation of CYP450 enzymes may be suppressed by increased levels of cytokines (eg, TNFα) during chronic inflammation. Therefore, it is expected that for a molecule that antagonizes cytokine activity, such as golimumab, the formation of CYP450 enzymes could be normalized. Upon initiation or discontinuation of golimumab in patients being treated with CYP450 substrates with a narrow therapeutic index, monitoring of the effect (eg, warfarin) or drug concentration (eg, cyclosporine or theophylline) is recommended and the individual dose of the drug product may be adjusted as needed).

No products indexed under this heading.

Nimodipine (The formation of CYP450 enzymes may be suppressed by increased levels of cytokines (eg, TNFα) during chronic inflammation. Therefore, it is expected that for a molecule that antagonizes cytokine activity, such as golimumab, the formation of CYP450 enzymes could be normalized. Upon initiation or discontinuation of golimumab in patients being treated with CYP450 substrates with a narrow therapeutic index, monitoring of the effect (eg, warfarin) or drug concentration (eg, cyclosporine or theophylline) is recommended and the individual dose of the drug product may be adjusted as needed).

No products indexed under this heading.

Nisoldipine (The formation of CYP450 enzymes may be suppressed by increased levels of cytokines (eg, TNFα) during chronic inflammation. Therefore, it is expected that for a molecule that antagonizes cytokine activity, such as golimumab, the formation of CYP450 enzymes could be normalized. Upon initiation or discontinuation of golimumab in patients being treated with CYP450 substrates with a narrow therapeutic index, monitoring of the effect (eg, warfarin) or drug concentration (eg, cyclosporine or theophylline) is recommended and the individual dose of the drug product may be adjusted as needed).

No products indexed under this heading.

Nitrendipine (The formation of CYP450 enzymes may be suppressed by increased levels of cytokines (eg, TNFα) during chronic inflammation. Therefore, it is expected that for a molecule that antagonizes cytokine activity, such as golimumab, the formation of CYP450 enzymes could be normalized. Upon initiation or discontinuation of golimumab in patients being treated with

CYP450 substrates with a narrow therapeutic index, monitoring of the effect (eg, warfarin) or drug concentration (eg, cyclosporine or theophylline) is recommended and the individual dose of the drug product may be adjusted as needed).

No products indexed under this heading.

Norethindrone (The formation of CYP450 enzymes may be suppressed by increased levels of cytokines (eg, TNFα) during chronic inflammation. Therefore, it is expected that for a molecule that antagonizes cytokine activity, such as golimumab, the formation of CYP450 enzymes could be normalized. Upon initiation or discontinuation of golimumab in patients being treated with CYP450 substrates with a narrow therapeutic index, monitoring of the effect (eg, warfarin) or drug concentration (eg, cyclosporine or theophylline) is recommended and the individual dose of the drug product may be adjusted as needed). Products include:
Ortho Micronor 2660

Norethindrone Acetate (The formation of CYP450 enzymes may be suppressed by increased levels of cytokines (eg, TNFα) during chronic inflammation. Therefore, it is expected that for a molecule that antagonizes cytokine activity, such as golimumab, the formation of CYP450 enzymes could be normalized. Upon initiation or discontinuation of golimumab in patients being treated with CYP450 substrates with a narrow therapeutic index, monitoring of the effect (eg, warfarin) or drug concentration (eg, cyclosporine or theophylline) is recommended and the individual dose of the drug product may be adjusted as needed). Products include:
Activella 2561

Norfloxacin (The formation of CYP450 enzymes may be suppressed by increased levels of cytokines (eg, TNFα) during chronic inflammation. Therefore, it is expected that for a molecule that antagonizes cytokine activity, such as golimumab, the formation of CYP450 enzymes could be normalized. Upon initiation or discontinuation of golimumab in patients being treated with CYP450 substrates with a narrow therapeutic index, monitoring of the effect (eg, warfarin) or drug concentration (eg, cyclosporine or theophylline) is recommended and the individual dose of the drug product may be adjusted as needed). Products include:
Noroxin 2220

Norgestrel (The formation of CYP450 enzymes may be suppressed by increased levels of cytokines (eg, TNFα) during chronic inflammation. Therefore, it is expected that for a molecule that antagonizes cytokine activity, such as golimumab, the formation of CYP450 enzymes could be normalized. Upon initiation or discontinuation of golimumab in patients being treated with CYP450 substrates with a narrow therapeutic index, monitoring of the effect (eg, warfarin) or drug concentration (eg, cyclosporine or theophylline) is recommended and the individual dose of the drug product may be adjusted as needed).

No products indexed under this heading.

Nortriptyline Hydrochloride (The formation of CYP450 enzymes may be suppressed by increased levels of cytokines (eg, TNFα) during chronic inflammation. Therefore, it is expected that for a molecule that antagonizes cytokine activity, such as golimumab, the formation of CYP450 enzymes could be normalized. Upon initiation or discontinuation of golimumab in patients being treated with CYP450 substrates with a narrow therapeutic

index, monitoring of the effect (eg, warfarin) or drug concentration (eg, cyclosporine or theophylline) is recommended and the individual dose of the drug product may be adjusted as needed).

No products indexed under this heading.

Ofloxacin (The formation of CYP450 enzymes may be suppressed by increased levels of cytokines (eg, TNFα) during chronic inflammation. Therefore, it is expected that for a molecule that antagonizes cytokine activity, such as golimumab, the formation of CYP450 enzymes could be normalized. Upon initiation or discontinuation of golimumab in patients being treated with CYP450 substrates with a narrow therapeutic index, monitoring of the effect (eg, warfarin) or drug concentration (eg, cyclosporine or theophylline) is recommended and the individual dose of the drug product may be adjusted as needed).

No products indexed under this heading.

Olanzapine (The formation of CYP450 enzymes may be suppressed by increased levels of cytokines (eg, TNFα) during chronic inflammation. Therefore, it is expected that for a molecule that antagonizes cytokine activity, such as golimumab, the formation of CYP450 enzymes could be normalized. Upon initiation or discontinuation of golimumab in patients being treated with CYP450 substrates with a narrow therapeutic index, monitoring of the effect (eg, warfarin) or drug concentration (eg, cyclosporine or theophylline) is recommended and the individual dose of the drug product may be adjusted as needed). Products include:
Symbyax 1965
Zyprexa 1984
Zyprexa IntraMuscular 1984
Zyprexa ZYDIS 1984

Omeprazole (The formation of CYP450 enzymes may be suppressed by increased levels of cytokines (eg, TNFα) during chronic inflammation. Therefore, it is expected that for a molecule that antagonizes cytokine activity, such as golimumab, the formation of CYP450 enzymes could be normalized. Upon initiation or discontinuation of golimumab in patients being treated with CYP450 substrates with a narrow therapeutic index, monitoring of the effect (eg, warfarin) or drug concentration (eg, cyclosporine or theophylline) is recommended and the individual dose of the drug product may be adjusted as needed).

No products indexed under this heading.

Omeprazole Magnesium (The formation of CYP450 enzymes may be suppressed by increased levels of cytokines (eg, TNFα) during chronic inflammation. Therefore, it is expected that for a molecule that antagonizes cytokine activity, such as golimumab, the formation of CYP450 enzymes could be normalized. Upon initiation or discontinuation of golimumab in patients being treated with CYP450 substrates with a narrow therapeutic index, monitoring of the effect (eg, warfarin) or drug concentration (eg, cyclosporine or theophylline) is recommended and the individual dose of the drug product may be adjusted as needed).

No products indexed under this heading.

Ondansetron (The formation of CYP450 enzymes may be suppressed by increased levels of cytokines (eg, TNFα) during chronic inflammation. Therefore, it is expected that for a molecule that antagonizes cytokine activity, such as golimumab, the formation of CYP450 enzymes could be normalized. Upon initiation or discontinuation of golimumab in patients being treated with

CYP450 substrates with a narrow therapeutic index, monitoring of the effect (eg, warfarin) or drug concentration (eg, cyclosporine or theophylline) is recommended and the individual dose of the drug product may be adjusted as needed).
No products indexed under this heading.

Ondansetron Hydrochloride (The formation of CYP450 enzymes may be suppressed by increased levels of cytokines (eg, TNFα) during chronic inflammation. Therefore, it is expected that for a molecule that antagonizes cytokine activity, such as golimumab, the formation of CYP450 enzymes could be normalized. Upon initiation or discontinuation of golimumab in patients being treated with CYP450 substrates with a narrow therapeutic index, monitoring of the effect (eg, warfarin) or drug concentration (eg, cyclosporine or theophylline) is recommended and the individual dose of the drug product may be adjusted as needed). Products include:
Zofran Injection 1750
Zofran 1756
Zofran ODT 1756

Oxaprozin (The formation of CYP450 enzymes may be suppressed by increased levels of cytokines (eg, TNFα) during chronic inflammation. Therefore, it is expected that for a molecule that antagonizes cytokine activity, such as golimumab, the formation of CYP450 enzymes could be normalized. Upon initiation or discontinuation of golimumab in patients being treated with CYP450 substrates with a narrow therapeutic index, monitoring of the effect (eg, warfarin) or drug concentration (eg, cyclosporine or theophylline) is recommended and the individual dose of the drug product may be adjusted as needed).
No products indexed under this heading.

Oxcarbazepine (The formation of CYP450 enzymes may be suppressed by increased levels of cytokines (eg, TNFα) during chronic inflammation. Therefore, it is expected that for a molecule that antagonizes cytokine activity, such as golimumab, the formation of CYP450 enzymes could be normalized. Upon initiation or discontinuation of golimumab in patients being treated with CYP450 substrates with a narrow therapeutic index, monitoring of the effect (eg, warfarin) or drug concentration (eg, cyclosporine or theophylline) is recommended and the individual dose of the drug product may be adjusted as needed).
No products indexed under this heading.

Oxycodone Hydrochloride (The formation of CYP450 enzymes may be suppressed by increased levels of cytokines (eg, TNFα) during chronic inflammation. Therefore, it is expected that for a molecule that antagonizes cytokine activity, such as golimumab, the formation of CYP450 enzymes could be normalized. Upon initiation or discontinuation of golimumab in patients being treated with CYP450 substrates with a narrow therapeutic index, monitoring of the effect (eg, warfarin) or drug concentration (eg, cyclosporine or theophylline) is recommended and the individual dose of the drug product may be adjusted as needed). Products include:
OxyContin 2807
Percocet 1121
Percodan 1124

Paclitaxel (The formation of CYP450 enzymes may be suppressed by increased levels of cytokines (eg, TNFα) during chronic inflammation. Therefore, it is expected that for a molecule that antagonizes cytokine activity, such as golimumab, the formation of CYP450 enzymes could be normalized. Upon initiation or discontinuation of golimumab in patients being treated with CYP450 substrates with a narrow therapeutic index, monitoring of the effect (eg, warfarin) or drug concentration (eg, cyclosporine or theophylline) is recommended and the individual dose of the drug product may be adjusted as needed).
No products indexed under this heading.

Pantoprazole Sodium (The formation of CYP450 enzymes may be suppressed by increased levels of cytokines (eg, TNFα) during chronic inflammation. Therefore, it is expected that for a molecule that antagonizes cytokine activity, such as golimumab, the formation of CYP450 enzymes could be normalized. Upon initiation or discontinuation of golimumab in patients being treated with CYP450 substrates with a narrow therapeutic index, monitoring of the effect (eg, warfarin) or drug concentration (eg, cyclosporine or theophylline) is recommended and the individual dose of the drug product may be adjusted as needed). Products include:
Protonix Tablets 3571
Protonix 3575

Paramethadione (The formation of CYP450 enzymes may be suppressed by increased levels of cytokines (eg, TNFα) during chronic inflammation. Therefore, it is expected that for a molecule that antagonizes cytokine activity, such as golimumab, the formation of CYP450 enzymes could be normalized. Upon initiation or discontinuation of golimumab in patients being treated with CYP450 substrates with a narrow therapeutic index, monitoring of the effect (eg, warfarin) or drug concentration (eg, cyclosporine or theophylline) is recommended and the individual dose of the drug product may be adjusted as needed).
No products indexed under this heading.

Paroxetine Hydrochloride (The formation of CYP450 enzymes may be suppressed by increased levels of cytokines (eg, TNFα) during chronic inflammation. Therefore, it is expected that for a molecule that antagonizes cytokine activity, such as golimumab, the formation of CYP450 enzymes could be normalized. Upon initiation or discontinuation of golimumab in patients being treated with CYP450 substrates with a narrow therapeutic index, monitoring of the effect (eg, warfarin) or drug concentration (eg, cyclosporine or theophylline) is recommended and the individual dose of the drug product may be adjusted as needed). Products include:
Paroxetine CR 2361
Paroxetine ER 2371
Paxil 1586
Paxil CR 1596

Pentamidine Isethionate (The formation of CYP450 enzymes may be suppressed by increased levels of cytokines (eg, TNFα) during chronic inflammation. Therefore, it is expected that for a molecule that antagonizes cytokine activity, such as golimumab, the formation of CYP450 enzymes could be normalized. Upon initiation or discontinuation of golimumab in patients being treated with CYP450 substrates with a narrow therapeutic index, monitoring of the effect (eg, warfarin) or drug concentration (eg, cyclosporine or theophylline) is recommended and the individual dose of the drug product may be adjusted as needed).
No products indexed under this heading.

Phenacemide (The formation of CYP450 enzymes may be suppressed by increased levels of cytokines (eg, TNFα) during chronic inflammation. Therefore, it is expected that for a molecule that antagonizes cytokine activity, such as golimumab, the formation of CYP450 enzymes could be normalized. Upon initiation or discontinuation of golimumab in patients being treated with CYP450 substrates with a narrow therapeutic index, monitoring of the effect (eg, warfarin) or drug concentration (eg, cyclosporine or theophylline) is recommended and the individual dose of the drug product may be adjusted as needed).
No products indexed under this heading.

Phenobarbital (The formation of CYP450 enzymes may be suppressed by increased levels of cytokines (eg, TNFα) during chronic inflammation. Therefore, it is expected that for a molecule that antagonizes cytokine activity, such as golimumab, the formation of CYP450 enzymes could be normalized. Upon initiation or discontinuation of golimumab in patients being treated with CYP450 substrates with a narrow therapeutic index, monitoring of the effect (eg, warfarin) or drug concentration (eg, cyclosporine or theophylline) is recommended and the individual dose of the drug product may be adjusted as needed). Products include:
Donnatal 2711

Phenobarbital Sodium (The formation of CYP450 enzymes may be suppressed by increased levels of cytokines (eg, TNFα) during chronic inflammation. Therefore, it is expected that for a molecule that antagonizes cytokine activity, such as golimumab, the formation of CYP450 enzymes could be normalized. Upon initiation or discontinuation of golimumab in patients being treated with CYP450 substrates with a narrow therapeutic index, monitoring of the effect (eg, warfarin) or drug concentration (eg, cyclosporine or theophylline) is recommended and the individual dose of the drug product may be adjusted as needed).
No products indexed under this heading.

Phensuximide (The formation of CYP450 enzymes may be suppressed by increased levels of cytokines (eg, TNFα) during chronic inflammation. Therefore, it is expected that for a molecule that antagonizes cytokine activity, such as golimumab, the formation of CYP450 enzymes could be normalized. Upon initiation or discontinuation of golimumab in patients being treated with CYP450 substrates with a narrow therapeutic index, monitoring of the effect (eg, warfarin) or drug concentration (eg, cyclosporine or theophylline) is recommended and the individual dose of the drug product may be adjusted as needed).
No products indexed under this heading.

Phenylbutazone (The formation of CYP450 enzymes may be suppressed by increased levels of cytokines (eg, TNFα) during chronic inflammation. Therefore, it is expected that for a molecule that antagonizes cytokine activity, such as golimumab, the formation of CYP450 enzymes could be normalized. Upon initiation or discontinuation of golimumab in patients being treated with CYP450 substrates with a narrow therapeutic index, monitoring of the effect (eg, warfarin) or drug concentration (eg, cyclosporine or theophylline) is recommended and the individual dose of the drug product may be adjusted as needed).
No products indexed under this heading.

Phenytoin (The formation of CYP450 enzymes may be suppressed by increased levels of cytokines (eg, TNFα) during chronic inflammation. Therefore, it is expected that for a molecule that antagonizes cytokine activity, such as golimumab, the formation of CYP450 enzymes could be normalized. Upon initiation or discontinuation of golimumab in patients being treated with CYP450 substrates with a narrow therapeutic index, monitoring of the effect (eg, warfarin) or drug concentration (eg, cyclosporine or theophylline) is recommended and the individual dose of the drug product may be adjusted as needed).
No products indexed under this heading.

Phenytoin Sodium (The formation of CYP450 enzymes may be suppressed by increased levels of cytokines (eg, TNFα) during chronic inflammation. Therefore, it is expected that for a molecule that antagonizes cytokine activity, such as golimumab, the formation of CYP450 enzymes could be normalized. Upon initiation or discontinuation of golimumab in patients being treated with CYP450 substrates with a narrow therapeutic index, monitoring of the effect (eg, warfarin) or drug concentration (eg, cyclosporine or theophylline) is recommended and the individual dose of the drug product may be adjusted as needed). Products include:
Phenytek Capsules 2380

Pimozide (The formation of CYP450 enzymes may be suppressed by increased levels of cytokines (eg, TNFα) during chronic inflammation. Therefore, it is expected that for a molecule that antagonizes cytokine activity, such as golimumab, the formation of CYP450 enzymes could be normalized. Upon initiation or discontinuation of golimumab in patients being treated with CYP450 substrates with a narrow therapeutic index, monitoring of the effect (eg, warfarin) or drug concentration (eg, cyclosporine or theophylline) is recommended and the individual dose of the drug product may be adjusted as needed).
No products indexed under this heading.

Pindolol (The formation of CYP450 enzymes may be suppressed by increased levels of cytokines (eg, TNFα) during chronic inflammation. Therefore, it is expected that for a molecule that antagonizes cytokine activity, such as golimumab, the formation of CYP450 enzymes could be normalized. Upon initiation or discontinuation of golimumab in patients being treated with CYP450 substrates with a narrow therapeutic index, monitoring of the effect (eg, warfarin) or drug concentration (eg, cyclosporine or theophylline) is recommended and the individual dose of the drug product may be adjusted as needed).
No products indexed under this heading.

Pioglitazone Hydrochloride (The formation of CYP450 enzymes may be suppressed by increased levels of cytokines (eg, TNFα) during chronic inflammation. Therefore, it is expected that for a molecule that antagonizes cytokine activity, such as golimumab, the formation of CYP450 enzymes could be normalized. Upon initiation or discontinuation of golimumab in patients being treated with CYP450 substrates with a narrow therapeutic index, monitoring of the effect (eg, warfarin) or drug concentration (eg, cyclosporine or theophylline) is recommended and the individual dose of the drug product may be adjusted as needed). Products include:
ActoPlus 3338
Actos 3345
Duetact 3354

Piroxicam (The formation of CYP450 enzymes may be suppressed by increased levels of cytokines (eg, TNFα) during chronic inflammation. Therefore, it is expected that for a molecule that

antagonizes cytokine activity, such as golimumab, the formation of CYP450 enzymes could be normalized. Upon initiation or discontinuation of golimumab in patients being treated with CYP450 substrates with a narrow therapeutic index, monitoring of the effect (eg, warfarin) or drug concentration (eg, cyclosporine or theophylline) is recommended and the individual dose of the drug product may be adjusted as needed).

No products indexed under this heading.

Poliovirus Vaccine, Live, Oral, Trivalent, Types 1,2,3 (Sabin) (Live vaccines should not be given concurrently with golimumab).

No products indexed under this heading.

Polyestradiol Phosphate (The formation of CYP450 enzymes may be suppressed by increased levels of cytokines (eg, TNFα) during chronic inflammation. Therefore, it is expected that for a molecule that antagonizes cytokine activity, such as golimumab, the formation of CYP450 enzymes could be normalized. Upon initiation or discontinuation of golimumab in patients being treated with CYP450 substrates with a narrow therapeutic index, monitoring of the effect (eg, warfarin) or drug concentration (eg, cyclosporine or theophylline) is recommended and the individual dose of the drug product may be adjusted as needed).

No products indexed under this heading.

Primidone (The formation of CYP450 enzymes may be suppressed by increased levels of cytokines (eg, TNFα) during chronic inflammation. Therefore, it is expected that for a molecule that antagonizes cytokine activity, such as golimumab, the formation of CYP450 enzymes could be normalized. Upon initiation or discontinuation of golimumab in patients being treated with CYP450 substrates with a narrow therapeutic index, monitoring of the effect (eg, warfarin) or drug concentration (eg, cyclosporine or theophylline) is recommended and the individual dose of the drug product may be adjusted as needed).

No products indexed under this heading.

Progesterone (The formation of CYP450 enzymes may be suppressed by increased levels of cytokines (eg, TNFα) during chronic inflammation. Therefore, it is expected that for a molecule that antagonizes cytokine activity, such as golimumab, the formation of CYP450 enzymes could be normalized. Upon initiation or discontinuation of golimumab in patients being treated with CYP450 substrates with a narrow therapeutic index, monitoring of the effect (eg, warfarin) or drug concentration (eg, cyclosporine or theophylline) is recommended and the individual dose of the drug product may be adjusted as needed). Products include:

Crinone 4% **996**
Crinone 8% **996**
Prometrium **3307**

Proguanil Hydrochloride (The formation of CYP450 enzymes may be suppressed by increased levels of cytokines (eg, TNFα) during chronic inflammation. Therefore, it is expected that for a molecule that antagonizes cytokine activity, such as golimumab, the formation of CYP450 enzymes could be normalized. Upon initiation or discontinuation of golimumab in patients being treated with CYP450 substrates with a narrow therapeutic index, monitoring of the effect (eg, warfarin) or drug concentration (eg, cyclosporine or theophylline) is recommended and the individual dose of the drug product may be adjusted as needed). Products include:

Malarone Pediatric Tablets **1572**
Malarone **1572**

Propafenone Hydrochloride (The formation of CYP450 enzymes may be suppressed by increased levels of cytokines (eg, TNFα) during chronic inflammation. Therefore, it is expected that for a molecule that antagonizes cytokine activity, such as golimumab, the formation of CYP450 enzymes could be normalized. Upon initiation or discontinuation of golimumab in patients being treated with CYP450 substrates with a narrow therapeutic index, monitoring of the effect (eg, warfarin) or drug concentration (eg, cyclosporine or theophylline) is recommended and the individual dose of the drug product may be adjusted as needed). Products include:

Rythmol **1648**
Rythmol SR **1652**

Propoxyphene Hydrochloride (The formation of CYP450 enzymes may be suppressed by increased levels of cytokines (eg, TNFα) during chronic inflammation. Therefore, it is expected that for a molecule that antagonizes cytokine activity, such as golimumab, the formation of CYP450 enzymes could be normalized. Upon initiation or discontinuation of golimumab in patients being treated with CYP450 substrates with a narrow therapeutic index, monitoring of the effect (eg, warfarin) or drug concentration (eg, cyclosporine or theophylline) is recommended and the individual dose of the drug product may be adjusted as needed).

No products indexed under this heading.

Propoxyphene Napsylate (The formation of CYP450 enzymes may be suppressed by increased levels of cytokines (eg, TNFα) during chronic inflammation. Therefore, it is expected that for a molecule that antagonizes cytokine activity, such as golimumab, the formation of CYP450 enzymes could be normalized. Upon initiation or discontinuation of golimumab in patients being treated with CYP450 substrates with a narrow therapeutic index, monitoring of the effect (eg, warfarin) or drug concentration (eg, cyclosporine or theophylline) is recommended and the individual dose of the drug product may be adjusted as needed).

No products indexed under this heading.

Propranolol Hydrochloride (The formation of CYP450 enzymes may be suppressed by increased levels of cytokines (eg, TNFα) during chronic inflammation. Therefore, it is expected that for a molecule that antagonizes cytokine activity, such as golimumab, the formation of CYP450 enzymes could be normalized. Upon initiation or discontinuation of golimumab in patients being treated with CYP450 substrates with a narrow therapeutic index, monitoring of the effect (eg, warfarin) or drug concentration (eg, cyclosporine or theophylline) is recommended and the individual dose of the drug product may be adjusted as needed). Products include:

InnoPran XL **1517**

Protriptyline Hydrochloride (The formation of CYP450 enzymes may be suppressed by increased levels of cytokines (eg, TNFα) during chronic inflammation. Therefore, it is expected that for a molecule that antagonizes cytokine activity, such as golimumab, the formation of CYP450 enzymes could be normalized. Upon initiation or discontinuation of golimumab in patients being treated with CYP450 substrates with a narrow therapeutic index, monitoring of the effect (eg, warfarin) or drug concentration (eg, cyclosporine or theophylline) is recommended and the individual dose of the drug product may be adjusted as needed).

No products indexed under this heading.

Quetiapine Fumarate (The formation of CYP450 enzymes may be suppressed by increased levels of cytokines (eg, TNFα) during chronic inflammation. Therefore, it is expected that for a molecule that antagonizes cytokine activity, such as golimumab, the formation of CYP450 enzymes could be normalized. Upon initiation or discontinuation of golimumab in patients being treated with CYP450 substrates with a narrow therapeutic index, monitoring of the effect (eg, warfarin) or drug concentration (eg, cyclosporine or theophylline) is recommended and the individual dose of the drug product may be adjusted as needed). Products include:

Seroquel **750**
Seroquel XR **759**

Quinidine Gluconate (The formation of CYP450 enzymes may be suppressed by increased levels of cytokines (eg, TNFα) during chronic inflammation. Therefore, it is expected that for a molecule that antagonizes cytokine activity, such as golimumab, the formation of CYP450 enzymes could be normalized. Upon initiation or discontinuation of golimumab in patients being treated with CYP450 substrates with a narrow therapeutic index, monitoring of the effect (eg, warfarin) or drug concentration (eg, cyclosporine or theophylline) is recommended and the individual dose of the drug product may be adjusted as needed).

No products indexed under this heading.

Quinidine Hydrochloride (The formation of CYP450 enzymes may be suppressed by increased levels of cytokines (eg, TNFα) during chronic inflammation. Therefore, it is expected that for a molecule that antagonizes cytokine activity, such as golimumab, the formation of CYP450 enzymes could be normalized. Upon initiation or discontinuation of golimumab in patients being treated with CYP450 substrates with a narrow therapeutic index, monitoring of the effect (eg, warfarin) or drug concentration (eg, cyclosporine or theophylline) is recommended and the individual dose of the drug product may be adjusted as needed).

No products indexed under this heading.

Quinidine Polygalacturonate (The formation of CYP450 enzymes may be suppressed by increased levels of cytokines (eg, TNFα) during chronic inflammation. Therefore, it is expected that for a molecule that antagonizes cytokine activity, such as golimumab, the formation of CYP450 enzymes could be normalized. Upon initiation or discontinuation of golimumab in patients being treated with CYP450 substrates with a narrow therapeutic index, monitoring of the effect (eg, warfarin) or drug concentration (eg, cyclosporine or theophylline) is recommended and the individual dose of the drug product may be adjusted as needed).

No products indexed under this heading.

Quinidine Sulfate (The formation of CYP450 enzymes may be suppressed by increased levels of cytokines (eg, TNFα) during chronic inflammation. Therefore, it is expected that for a molecule that antagonizes cytokine activity, such as golimumab, the formation of CYP450 enzymes could be normalized. Upon initiation or discontinuation of golimumab in patients being treated with CYP450 substrates with a narrow therapeutic index, monitoring of the effect (eg, warfarin) or drug concentration (eg, cyclosporine or theophylline) is recommended and the individual dose of the drug product may be adjusted as needed).

No products indexed under this heading.

Quinine (The formation of CYP450 enzymes may be suppressed by increased levels of cytokines (eg, TNFα) during chronic inflammation. Therefore, it is expected that for a molecule that antagonizes cytokine activity, such as golimumab, the formation of CYP450 enzymes could be normalized. Upon initiation or discontinuation of golimumab in patients being treated with CYP450 substrates with a narrow therapeutic index, monitoring of the effect (eg, warfarin) or drug concentration (eg, cyclosporine or theophylline) is recommended and the individual dose of the drug product may be adjusted as needed). Products include:

Hyland's Leg Cramps PM with Quinine **3315**

Quinine Sulfate (The formation of CYP450 enzymes may be suppressed by increased levels of cytokines (eg, TNFα) during chronic inflammation. Therefore, it is expected that for a molecule that antagonizes cytokine activity, such as golimumab, the formation of CYP450 enzymes could be normalized. Upon initiation or discontinuation of golimumab in patients being treated with CYP450 substrates with a narrow therapeutic index, monitoring of the effect (eg, warfarin) or drug concentration (eg, cyclosporine or theophylline) is recommended and the individual dose of the drug product may be adjusted as needed).

No products indexed under this heading.

Rabeprazole Sodium (The formation of CYP450 enzymes may be suppressed by increased levels of cytokines (eg, TNFα) during chronic inflammation. Therefore, it is expected that for a molecule that antagonizes cytokine activity, such as golimumab, the formation of CYP450 enzymes could be normalized. Upon initiation or discontinuation of golimumab in patients being treated with CYP450 substrates with a narrow therapeutic index, monitoring of the effect (eg, warfarin) or drug concentration (eg, cyclosporine or theophylline) is recommended and the individual dose of the drug product may be adjusted as needed). Products include:

Aciphex **1035**

Repaglinide (The formation of CYP450 enzymes may be suppressed by increased levels of cytokines (eg, TNFα) during chronic inflammation. Therefore, it is expected that for a molecule that antagonizes cytokine activity, such as golimumab, the formation of CYP450 enzymes could be normalized. Upon initiation or discontinuation of golimumab in patients being treated with CYP450 substrates with a narrow therapeutic index, monitoring of the effect (eg, warfarin) or drug concentration (eg, cyclosporine or theophylline) is recommended and the individual dose of the drug product may be adjusted as needed).

No products indexed under this heading.

Rifabutin (The formation of CYP450 enzymes may be suppressed by increased levels of cytokines (eg, TNFα) during chronic inflammation. Therefore, it is expected that for a molecule that antagonizes cytokine activity, such as golimumab, the formation of CYP450 enzymes could be normalized. Upon initiation or discontinuation of golimumab in patients being treated with CYP450 substrates with a narrow therapeutic index, monitoring of the effect (eg, warfarin) or drug concentration (eg, cyclosporine or theophylline) is recom-

1763 Interactions Index Simponi

mended and the individual dose of the drug product may be adjusted as needed).
No products indexed under this heading.

Riluzole (The formation of CYP450 enzymes may be suppressed by increased levels of cytokines (eg, TNFα) during chronic inflammation. Therefore, it is expected that for a molecule that antagonizes cytokine activity, such as golimumab, the formation of CYP450 enzymes could be normalized. Upon initiation or discontinuation of golimumab in patients being treated with CYP450 substrates with a narrow therapeutic index, monitoring of the effect (eg, warfarin) or drug concentration (eg, cyclosporine or theophylline) is recommended and the individual dose of the drug product may be adjusted as needed). Products include:
Rilutek 3032

Risperidone (The formation of CYP450 enzymes may be suppressed by increased levels of cytokines (eg, TNFα) during chronic inflammation. Therefore, it is expected that for a molecule that antagonizes cytokine activity, such as golimumab, the formation of CYP450 enzymes could be normalized. Upon initiation or discontinuation of golimumab in patients being treated with CYP450 substrates with a narrow therapeutic index, monitoring of the effect (eg, warfarin) or drug concentration (eg, cyclosporine or theophylline) is recommended and the individual dose of the drug product may be adjusted as needed). Products include:
Risperdal Consta 2682

Ritonavir (The formation of CYP450 enzymes may be suppressed by increased levels of cytokines (eg, TNFα) during chronic inflammation. Therefore, it is expected that for a molecule that antagonizes cytokine activity, such as golimumab, the formation of CYP450 enzymes could be normalized. Upon initiation or discontinuation of golimumab in patients being treated with CYP450 substrates with a narrow therapeutic index, monitoring of the effect (eg, warfarin) or drug concentration (eg, cyclosporine or theophylline) is recommended and the individual dose of the drug product may be adjusted as needed). Products include:
Kaletra 458
Norvir 509

Rituximab (A higher rate of serious infections has been observed in rheumatoid arthritis patients treated with rituximab who received subsequent treatment with a TNF-blocker). Products include:
Rituxan 1216

Rofecoxib (The formation of CYP450 enzymes may be suppressed by increased levels of cytokines (eg, TNFα) during chronic inflammation. Therefore, it is expected that for a molecule that antagonizes cytokine activity, such as golimumab, the formation of CYP450 enzymes could be normalized. Upon initiation or discontinuation of golimumab in patients being treated with CYP450 substrates with a narrow therapeutic index, monitoring of the effect (eg, warfarin) or drug concentration (eg, cyclosporine or theophylline) is recommended and the individual dose of the drug product may be adjusted as needed).
No products indexed under this heading.

Ropinirole Hydrochloride (The formation of CYP450 enzymes may be suppressed by increased levels of cytokines (eg, TNFα) during chronic inflammation. Therefore, it is expected that for a molecule that antagonizes cytokine activity, such as golimumab, the formation of CYP450 enzymes could be normalized. Upon initiation or discontinuation of golimumab in patients being treated with CYP450 substrates with a narrow therapeutic index, monitoring of the effect (eg, warfarin) or drug concentration (eg, cyclosporine or theophylline) is recommended and the individual dose of the drug product may be adjusted as needed). Products include:
Requip 1620
Requip XL 1628

Ropivacaine Hydrochloride (The formation of CYP450 enzymes may be suppressed by increased levels of cytokines (eg, TNFα) during chronic inflammation. Therefore, it is expected that for a molecule that antagonizes cytokine activity, such as golimumab, the formation of CYP450 enzymes could be normalized. Upon initiation or discontinuation of golimumab in patients being treated with CYP450 substrates with a narrow therapeutic index, monitoring of the effect (eg, warfarin) or drug concentration (eg, cyclosporine or theophylline) is recommended and the individual dose of the drug product may be adjusted as needed).
No products indexed under this heading.

Rosiglitazone (The formation of CYP450 enzymes may be suppressed by increased levels of cytokines (eg, TNFα) during chronic inflammation. Therefore, it is expected that for a molecule that antagonizes cytokine activity, such as golimumab, the formation of CYP450 enzymes could be normalized. Upon initiation or discontinuation of golimumab in patients being treated with CYP450 substrates with a narrow therapeutic index, monitoring of the effect (eg, warfarin) or drug concentration (eg, cyclosporine or theophylline) is recommended and the individual dose of the drug product may be adjusted as needed).
No products indexed under this heading.

Rosiglitazone Maleate (The formation of CYP450 enzymes may be suppressed by increased levels of cytokines (eg, TNFα) during chronic inflammation. Therefore, it is expected that for a molecule that antagonizes cytokine activity, such as golimumab, the formation of CYP450 enzymes could be normalized. Upon initiation or discontinuation of golimumab in patients being treated with CYP450 substrates with a narrow therapeutic index, monitoring of the effect (eg, warfarin) or drug concentration (eg, cyclosporine or theophylline) is recommended and the individual dose of the drug product may be adjusted as needed). Products include:
Avandamet 1345
Avandaryl 1356
Avandia 1366

Rosiglitazone/Metformin (The formation of CYP450 enzymes may be suppressed by increased levels of cytokines (eg, TNFα) during chronic inflammation. Therefore, it is expected that for a molecule that antagonizes cytokine activity, such as golimumab, the formation of CYP450 enzymes could be normalized. Upon initiation or discontinuation of golimumab in patients being treated with CYP450 substrates with a narrow therapeutic index, monitoring of the effect (eg, warfarin) or drug concentration (eg, cyclosporine or theophylline) is recommended and the individual dose of the drug product may be adjusted as needed).
No products indexed under this heading.

Rotavirus Vaccine, Live, Oral, Tetravalent (Live vaccines should not be given concurrently with golimumab).
No products indexed under this heading.

Rubella & Mumps Virus Vaccine Live (Live vaccines should not be given concurrently with golimumab).
No products indexed under this heading.

Rubella Virus Vaccine Live (Live vaccines should not be given concurrently with golimumab). Products include:
Meruvax II 2210

Saquinavir (The formation of CYP450 enzymes may be suppressed by increased levels of cytokines (eg, TNFα) during chronic inflammation. Therefore, it is expected that for a molecule that antagonizes cytokine activity, such as golimumab, the formation of CYP450 enzymes could be normalized. Upon initiation or discontinuation of golimumab in patients being treated with CYP450 substrates with a narrow therapeutic index, monitoring of the effect (eg, warfarin) or drug concentration (eg, cyclosporine or theophylline) is recommended and the individual dose of the drug product may be adjusted as needed).
No products indexed under this heading.

Saquinavir Mesylate (The formation of CYP450 enzymes may be suppressed by increased levels of cytokines (eg, TNFα) during chronic inflammation. Therefore, it is expected that for a molecule that antagonizes cytokine activity, such as golimumab, the formation of CYP450 enzymes could be normalized. Upon initiation or discontinuation of golimumab in patients being treated with CYP450 substrates with a narrow therapeutic index, monitoring of the effect (eg, warfarin) or drug concentration (eg, cyclosporine or theophylline) is recommended and the individual dose of the drug product may be adjusted as needed).
No products indexed under this heading.

Sertraline Hydrochloride (The formation of CYP450 enzymes may be suppressed by increased levels of cytokines (eg, TNFα) during chronic inflammation. Therefore, it is expected that for a molecule that antagonizes cytokine activity, such as golimumab, the formation of CYP450 enzymes could be normalized. Upon initiation or discontinuation of golimumab in patients being treated with CYP450 substrates with a narrow therapeutic index, monitoring of the effect (eg, warfarin) or drug concentration (eg, cyclosporine or theophylline) is recommended and the individual dose of the drug product may be adjusted as needed).
No products indexed under this heading.

Sildenafil Citrate (The formation of CYP450 enzymes may be suppressed by increased levels of cytokines (eg, TNFα) during chronic inflammation. Therefore, it is expected that for a molecule that antagonizes cytokine activity, such as golimumab, the formation of CYP450 enzymes could be normalized. Upon initiation or discontinuation of golimumab in patients being treated with CYP450 substrates with a narrow therapeutic index, monitoring of the effect (eg, warfarin) or drug concentration (eg, cyclosporine or theophylline) is recommended and the individual dose of the drug product may be adjusted as needed).
No products indexed under this heading.

Simvastatin (The formation of CYP450 enzymes may be suppressed by increased levels of cytokines (eg, TNFα) during chronic inflammation. Therefore, it is expected that for a molecule that antagonizes cytokine activity, such as golimumab, the formation of CYP450 enzymes could be normalized. Upon initiation or discontinuation of golimumab in patients being treated with CYP450 substrates with a narrow therapeutic index, monitoring of the effect (eg, warfarin) or drug concentration (eg, cyclosporine or theophylline) is recommended and the individual dose of the drug product may be adjusted as needed). Products include:
Simcor 524
Vytorin 10/10 .... 2303, 3240
Vytorin 10/20 .... 2303, 3240
Vytorin 10/40 .... 2303, 3240
Vytorin 10/80 .... 2303, 3240
Zocor 2289

Sirolimus (The formation of CYP450 enzymes may be suppressed by increased levels of cytokines (eg, TNFα) during chronic inflammation. Therefore, it is expected that for a molecule that antagonizes cytokine activity, such as golimumab, the formation of CYP450 enzymes could be normalized. Upon initiation or discontinuation of golimumab in patients being treated with CYP450 substrates with a narrow therapeutic index, monitoring of the effect (eg, warfarin) or drug concentration (eg, cyclosporine or theophylline) is recommended and the individual dose of the drug product may be adjusted as needed). Products include:
Rapamune 3579

Smallpox Vaccine (Live vaccines should not be given concurrently with golimumab).
No products indexed under this heading.

Sulfamethoxazole (The formation of CYP450 enzymes may be suppressed by increased levels of cytokines (eg, TNFα) during chronic inflammation. Therefore, it is expected that for a molecule that antagonizes cytokine activity, such as golimumab, the formation of CYP450 enzymes could be normalized. Upon initiation or discontinuation of golimumab in patients being treated with CYP450 substrates with a narrow therapeutic index, monitoring of the effect (eg, warfarin) or drug concentration (eg, cyclosporine or theophylline) is recommended and the individual dose of the drug product may be adjusted as needed).
No products indexed under this heading.

Sulindac (The formation of CYP450 enzymes may be suppressed by increased levels of cytokines (eg, TNFα) during chronic inflammation. Therefore, it is expected that for a molecule that antagonizes cytokine activity, such as golimumab, the formation of CYP450 enzymes could be normalized. Upon initiation or discontinuation of golimumab in patients being treated with CYP450 substrates with a narrow therapeutic index, monitoring of the effect (eg, warfarin) or drug concentration (eg, cyclosporine or theophylline) is recommended and the individual dose of the drug product may be adjusted as needed). Products include:
Clinoril 2098

Suprofen (The formation of CYP450 enzymes may be suppressed by increased levels of cytokines (eg, TNFα) during chronic inflammation. Therefore, it is expected that for a molecule that antagonizes cytokine activity, such as golimumab, the formation of CYP450 enzymes could be normalized. Upon initiation or discontinuation of golimumab in patients being treated with CYP450 substrates with a narrow therapeutic index, monitoring of the effect (eg, warfarin) or drug concentration (eg, cyclosporine or theophylline) is recommended and the individual dose of the drug product may be adjusted as needed).
No products indexed under this heading.

Tacrine Hydrochloride (The formation of CYP450 enzymes may be suppressed by increased levels of cytokines (eg, TNFα) during chronic inflammation. Therefore, it is expected

IMPORTANT NOTE: Always consult each drug listing in the patient's regimen for possible interactions.

that for a molecule that antagonizes cytokine activity, such as golimumab, the formation of CYP450 enzymes could be normalized. Upon initiation or discontinuation of golimumab in patients being treated with CYP450 substrates with a narrow therapeutic index, monitoring of the effect (eg, warfarin) or drug concentration (eg, cyclosporine or theophylline) is recommended and the individual dose of the drug product may be adjusted as needed).

No products indexed under this heading.

Tacrolimus (The formation of CYP450 enzymes may be suppressed by increased levels of cytokines (eg, TNFα) during chronic inflammation. Therefore, it is expected that for a molecule that antagonizes cytokine activity, such as golimumab, the formation of CYP450 enzymes could be normalized. Upon initiation or discontinuation of golimumab in patients being treated with CYP450 substrates with a narrow therapeutic index, monitoring of the effect (eg, warfarin) or drug concentration (eg, cyclosporine or theophylline) is recommended and the individual dose of the drug product may be adjusted as needed). Products include:

Prograf Capsules 677
Prograf Injection 677
Protopic 685

Tadalafil (The formation of CYP450 enzymes may be suppressed by increased levels of cytokines (eg, TNFα) during chronic inflammation. Therefore, it is expected that for a molecule that antagonizes cytokine activity, such as golimumab, the formation of CYP450 enzymes could be normalized. Upon initiation or discontinuation of golimumab in patients being treated with CYP450 substrates with a narrow therapeutic index, monitoring of the effect (eg, warfarin) or drug concentration (eg, cyclosporine or theophylline) is recommended and the individual dose of the drug product may be adjusted as needed). Products include:

Adcirca 3461
Cialis 1861

Tamoxifen Citrate (The formation of CYP450 enzymes may be suppressed by increased levels of cytokines (eg, TNFα) during chronic inflammation. Therefore, it is expected that for a molecule that antagonizes cytokine activity, such as golimumab, the formation of CYP450 enzymes could be normalized. Upon initiation or discontinuation of golimumab in patients being treated with CYP450 substrates with a narrow therapeutic index, monitoring of the effect (eg, warfarin) or drug concentration (eg, cyclosporine or theophylline) is recommended and the individual dose of the drug product may be adjusted as needed).

No products indexed under this heading.

Telmisartan (The formation of CYP450 enzymes may be suppressed by increased levels of cytokines (eg, TNFα) during chronic inflammation. Therefore, it is expected that for a molecule that antagonizes cytokine activity, such as golimumab, the formation of CYP450 enzymes could be normalized. Upon initiation or discontinuation of golimumab in patients being treated with CYP450 substrates with a narrow therapeutic index, monitoring of the effect (eg, warfarin) or drug concentration (eg, cyclosporine or theophylline) is recommended and the individual dose of the drug product may be adjusted as needed). Products include:

Micardis 887
Micardis HCT 889

Teniposide (The formation of CYP450 enzymes may be suppressed by increased levels of cytokines (eg, TNFα) during chronic inflammation. Therefore, it is expected that for a molecule that antagonizes cytokine activity, such as golimumab, the formation of CYP450 enzymes could be normalized. Upon initiation or discontinuation of golimumab in patients being treated with CYP450 substrates with a narrow therapeutic index, monitoring of the effect (eg, warfarin) or drug concentration (eg, cyclosporine or theophylline) is recommended and the individual dose of the drug product may be adjusted as needed).

No products indexed under this heading.

Terfenadine (The formation of CYP450 enzymes may be suppressed by increased levels of cytokines (eg, TNFα) during chronic inflammation. Therefore, it is expected that for a molecule that antagonizes cytokine activity, such as golimumab, the formation of CYP450 enzymes could be normalized. Upon initiation or discontinuation of golimumab in patients being treated with CYP450 substrates with a narrow therapeutic index, monitoring of the effect (eg, warfarin) or drug concentration (eg, cyclosporine or theophylline) is recommended and the individual dose of the drug product may be adjusted as needed).

No products indexed under this heading.

Testosterone (The formation of CYP450 enzymes may be suppressed by increased levels of cytokines (eg, TNFα) during chronic inflammation. Therefore, it is expected that for a molecule that antagonizes cytokine activity, such as golimumab, the formation of CYP450 enzymes could be normalized. Upon initiation or discontinuation of golimumab in patients being treated with CYP450 substrates with a narrow therapeutic index, monitoring of the effect (eg, warfarin) or drug concentration (eg, cyclosporine or theophylline) is recommended and the individual dose of the drug product may be adjusted as needed). Products include:

AndroGel 3456

Testosterone Cypionate (The formation of CYP450 enzymes may be suppressed by increased levels of cytokines (eg, TNFα) during chronic inflammation. Therefore, it is expected that for a molecule that antagonizes cytokine activity, such as golimumab, the formation of CYP450 enzymes could be normalized. Upon initiation or discontinuation of golimumab in patients being treated with CYP450 substrates with a narrow therapeutic index, monitoring of the effect (eg, warfarin) or drug concentration (eg, cyclosporine or theophylline) is recommended and the individual dose of the drug product may be adjusted as needed).

No products indexed under this heading.

Testosterone Enanthate (The formation of CYP450 enzymes may be suppressed by increased levels of cytokines (eg, TNFα) during chronic inflammation. Therefore, it is expected that for a molecule that antagonizes cytokine activity, such as golimumab, the formation of CYP450 enzymes could be normalized. Upon initiation or discontinuation of golimumab in patients being treated with CYP450 substrates with a narrow therapeutic index, monitoring of the effect (eg, warfarin) or drug concentration (eg, cyclosporine or theophylline) is recommended and the individual dose of the drug product may be adjusted as needed). Products include:

Delatestryl 1102

Testosterone Propionate (The formation of CYP450 enzymes may be suppressed by increased levels of cytokines (eg, TNFα) during chronic inflammation. Therefore, it is expected that for a molecule that antagonizes cytokine activity, such as golimumab, the formation of CYP450 enzymes could be normalized. Upon initiation or discontinuation of golimumab in patients being treated with CYP450 substrates with a narrow therapeutic index, monitoring of the effect (eg, warfarin) or drug concentration (eg, cyclosporine or theophylline) is recommended and the individual dose of the drug product may be adjusted as needed).

No products indexed under this heading.

Theophylline (The formation of CYP450 enzymes may be suppressed by increased levels of cytokines (eg, TNFα) during chronic inflammation. Therefore, it is expected that for a molecule that antagonizes cytokine activity, such as golimumab, the formation of CYP450 enzymes could be normalized. Upon initiation or discontinuation of golimumab in patients being treated with CYP450 substrates with a narrow therapeutic index, monitoring of the effect (eg, warfarin) or drug concentration (eg, cyclosporine or theophylline) is recommended and the individual dose of the drug product may be adjusted as needed).

No products indexed under this heading.

Theophylline Anhydrous (The formation of CYP450 enzymes may be suppressed by increased levels of cytokines (eg, TNFα) during chronic inflammation. Therefore, it is expected that for a molecule that antagonizes cytokine activity, such as golimumab, the formation of CYP450 enzymes could be normalized. Upon initiation or discontinuation of golimumab in patients being treated with CYP450 substrates with a narrow therapeutic index, monitoring of the effect (eg, warfarin) or drug concentration (eg, cyclosporine or theophylline) is recommended and the individual dose of the drug product may be adjusted as needed). Products include:

Uniphyl 2817

Theophylline Calcium Salicylate (The formation of CYP450 enzymes may be suppressed by increased levels of cytokines (eg, TNFα) during chronic inflammation. Therefore, it is expected that for a molecule that antagonizes cytokine activity, such as golimumab, the formation of CYP450 enzymes could be normalized. Upon initiation or discontinuation of golimumab in patients being treated with CYP450 substrates with a narrow therapeutic index, monitoring of the effect (eg, warfarin) or drug concentration (eg, cyclosporine or theophylline) is recommended and the individual dose of the drug product may be adjusted as needed).

No products indexed under this heading.

Theophylline Dihydroxypropyl (Glyceryl) (The formation of CYP450 enzymes may be suppressed by increased levels of cytokines (eg, TNFα) during chronic inflammation. Therefore, it is expected that for a molecule that antagonizes cytokine activity, such as golimumab, the formation of CYP450 enzymes could be normalized. Upon initiation or discontinuation of golimumab in patients being treated with CYP450 substrates with a narrow therapeutic index, monitoring of the effect (eg, warfarin) or drug concentration (eg, cyclosporine or theophylline) is recommended and the individual dose of the drug product may be adjusted as needed).

No products indexed under this heading.

Theophylline Ethylenediamine (The formation of CYP450 enzymes may be suppressed by increased levels of cytokines (eg, TNFα) during chronic inflammation. Therefore, it is expected that for a molecule that antagonizes cytokine activity, such as golimumab, the formation of CYP450 enzymes could be normalized. Upon initiation or discontinuation of golimumab in patients being treated with CYP450 substrates with a narrow therapeutic index, monitoring of the effect (eg, warfarin) or drug concentration (eg, cyclosporine or theophylline) is recommended and the individual dose of the drug product may be adjusted as needed).

No products indexed under this heading.

Theophylline Sodium Glycinate (The formation of CYP450 enzymes may be suppressed by increased levels of cytokines (eg, TNFα) during chronic inflammation. Therefore, it is expected that for a molecule that antagonizes cytokine activity, such as golimumab, the formation of CYP450 enzymes could be normalized. Upon initiation or discontinuation of golimumab in patients being treated with CYP450 substrates with a narrow therapeutic index, monitoring of the effect (eg, warfarin) or drug concentration (eg, cyclosporine or theophylline) is recommended and the individual dose of the drug product may be adjusted as needed).

No products indexed under this heading.

Thioridazine (The formation of CYP450 enzymes may be suppressed by increased levels of cytokines (eg, TNFα) during chronic inflammation. Therefore, it is expected that for a molecule that antagonizes cytokine activity, such as golimumab, the formation of CYP450 enzymes could be normalized. Upon initiation or discontinuation of golimumab in patients being treated with CYP450 substrates with a narrow therapeutic index, monitoring of the effect (eg, warfarin) or drug concentration (eg, cyclosporine or theophylline) is recommended and the individual dose of the drug product may be adjusted as needed).

No products indexed under this heading.

Thioridazine Hydrochloride (The formation of CYP450 enzymes may be suppressed by increased levels of cytokines (eg, TNFα) during chronic inflammation. Therefore, it is expected that for a molecule that antagonizes cytokine activity, such as golimumab, the formation of CYP450 enzymes could be normalized. Upon initiation or discontinuation of golimumab in patients being treated with CYP450 substrates with a narrow therapeutic index, monitoring of the effect (eg, warfarin) or drug concentration (eg, cyclosporine or theophylline) is recommended and the individual dose of the drug product may be adjusted as needed). Products include:

Thioridazine Hydrochloride 2384

Tiagabine Hydrochloride (The formation of CYP450 enzymes may be suppressed by increased levels of cytokines (eg, TNFα) during chronic inflammation. Therefore, it is expected that for a molecule that antagonizes cytokine activity, such as golimumab, the formation of CYP450 enzymes could be normalized. Upon initiation or discontinuation of golimumab in patients being treated with CYP450 substrates with a narrow therapeutic index, monitoring of the effect (eg, warfarin) or drug concentration (eg, cyclosporine or theophylline) is recommended and the individual dose of the drug product may be adjusted as needed). Products include:

Gabitril 972

Timolol Maleate (The formation of CYP450 enzymes may be suppressed

by increased levels of cytokines (eg, TNFα) during chronic inflammation. Therefore, it is expected that for a molecule that antagonizes cytokine activity, such as golimumab, the formation of CYP450 enzymes could be normalized. Upon initiation or discontinuation of golimumab in patients being treated with CYP450 substrates with a narrow therapeutic index, monitoring of the effect (eg, warfarin) or drug concentration (eg, cyclosporine or theophylline) is recommended and the individual dose of the drug product may be adjusted as needed). Products include:

Combigan **601**
Dorzolamide Hydrochloride/Timolol Maleate Ophthalmic Solution.................... ⊙**243**
Timoptic in Ocudose .... ⊙**231**

Tolazamide (The formation of CYP450 enzymes may be suppressed by increased levels of cytokines (eg, TNFα) during chronic inflammation. Therefore, it is expected that for a molecule that antagonizes cytokine activity, such as golimumab, the formation of CYP450 enzymes could be normalized. Upon initiation or discontinuation of golimumab in patients being treated with CYP450 substrates with a narrow therapeutic index, monitoring of the effect (eg, warfarin) or drug concentration (eg, cyclosporine or theophylline) is recommended and the individual dose of the drug product may be adjusted as needed).
No products indexed under this heading.

Tolbutamide (The formation of CYP450 enzymes may be suppressed by increased levels of cytokines (eg, TNFα) during chronic inflammation. Therefore, it is expected that for a molecule that antagonizes cytokine activity, such as golimumab, the formation of CYP450 enzymes could be normalized. Upon initiation or discontinuation of golimumab in patients being treated with CYP450 substrates with a narrow therapeutic index, monitoring of the effect (eg, warfarin) or drug concentration (eg, cyclosporine or theophylline) is recommended and the individual dose of the drug product may be adjusted as needed).
No products indexed under this heading.

Tolbutamide Sodium (The formation of CYP450 enzymes may be suppressed by increased levels of cytokines (eg, TNFα) during chronic inflammation. Therefore, it is expected that for a molecule that antagonizes cytokine activity, such as golimumab, the formation of CYP450 enzymes could be normalized. Upon initiation or discontinuation of golimumab in patients being treated with CYP450 substrates with a narrow therapeutic index, monitoring of the effect (eg, warfarin) or drug concentration (eg, cyclosporine or theophylline) is recommended and the individual dose of the drug product may be adjusted as needed).
No products indexed under this heading.

Tolmetin Sodium (The formation of CYP450 enzymes may be suppressed by increased levels of cytokines (eg, TNFα) during chronic inflammation. Therefore, it is expected that for a molecule that antagonizes cytokine activity, such as golimumab, the formation of CYP450 enzymes could be normalized. Upon initiation or discontinuation of golimumab in patients being treated with CYP450 substrates with a narrow therapeutic index, monitoring of the effect (eg, warfarin) or drug concentration (eg, cyclosporine or theophylline) is recommended and the individual dose of the drug product may be adjusted as needed).
No products indexed under this heading.

Tolterodine Tartrate (The formation of CYP450 enzymes may be suppressed by increased levels of cytokines (eg, TNFα) during chronic inflammation. Therefore, it is expected that for a molecule that antagonizes cytokine activity, such as golimumab, the formation of CYP450 enzymes could be normalized. Upon initiation or discontinuation of golimumab in patients being treated with CYP450 substrates with a narrow therapeutic index, monitoring of the effect (eg, warfarin) or drug concentration (eg, cyclosporine or theophylline) is recommended and the individual dose of the drug product may be adjusted as needed).
No products indexed under this heading.

Topiramate (The formation of CYP450 enzymes may be suppressed by increased levels of cytokines (eg, TNFα) during chronic inflammation. Therefore, it is expected that for a molecule that antagonizes cytokine activity, such as golimumab, the formation of CYP450 enzymes could be normalized. Upon initiation or discontinuation of golimumab in patients being treated with CYP450 substrates with a narrow therapeutic index, monitoring of the effect (eg, warfarin) or drug concentration (eg, cyclosporine or theophylline) is recommended and the individual dose of the drug product may be adjusted as needed).
No products indexed under this heading.

Torsemide (The formation of CYP450 enzymes may be suppressed by increased levels of cytokines (eg, TNFα) during chronic inflammation. Therefore, it is expected that for a molecule that antagonizes cytokine activity, such as golimumab, the formation of CYP450 enzymes could be normalized. Upon initiation or discontinuation of golimumab in patients being treated with CYP450 substrates with a narrow therapeutic index, monitoring of the effect (eg, warfarin) or drug concentration (eg, cyclosporine or theophylline) is recommended and the individual dose of the drug product may be adjusted as needed).
No products indexed under this heading.

Tramadol Hydrochloride (The formation of CYP450 enzymes may be suppressed by increased levels of cytokines (eg, TNFα) during chronic inflammation. Therefore, it is expected that for a molecule that antagonizes cytokine activity, such as golimumab, the formation of CYP450 enzymes could be normalized. Upon initiation or discontinuation of golimumab in patients being treated with CYP450 substrates with a narrow therapeutic index, monitoring of the effect (eg, warfarin) or drug concentration (eg, cyclosporine or theophylline) is recommended and the individual dose of the drug product may be adjusted as needed). Products include:

Ryzolt **2813**
Ultram ER **2693**

Trazodone Hydrochloride (The formation of CYP450 enzymes may be suppressed by increased levels of cytokines (eg, TNFα) during chronic inflammation. Therefore, it is expected that for a molecule that antagonizes cytokine activity, such as golimumab, the formation of CYP450 enzymes could be normalized. Upon initiation or discontinuation of golimumab in patients being treated with CYP450 substrates with a narrow therapeutic index, monitoring of the effect (eg, warfarin) or drug concentration (eg, cyclosporine or theophylline) is recommended and the individual dose of the drug product may be adjusted as needed).
No products indexed under this heading.

Tretinoin (The formation of CYP450 enzymes may be suppressed by increased levels of cytokines (eg, TNFα) during chronic inflammation. Therefore, it is expected that for a molecule that antagonizes cytokine activity, such as golimumab, the formation of CYP450 enzymes could be normalized. Upon initiation or discontinuation of golimumab in patients being treated with CYP450 substrates with a narrow therapeutic index, monitoring of the effect (eg, warfarin) or drug concentration (eg, cyclosporine or theophylline) is recommended and the individual dose of the drug product may be adjusted as needed).
No products indexed under this heading.

Triazolam (The formation of CYP450 enzymes may be suppressed by increased levels of cytokines (eg, TNFα) during chronic inflammation. Therefore, it is expected that for a molecule that antagonizes cytokine activity, such as golimumab, the formation of CYP450 enzymes could be normalized. Upon initiation or discontinuation of golimumab in patients being treated with CYP450 substrates with a narrow therapeutic index, monitoring of the effect (eg, warfarin) or drug concentration (eg, cyclosporine or theophylline) is recommended and the individual dose of the drug product may be adjusted as needed).
No products indexed under this heading.

Trimethadione (The formation of CYP450 enzymes may be suppressed by increased levels of cytokines (eg, TNFα) during chronic inflammation. Therefore, it is expected that for a molecule that antagonizes cytokine activity, such as golimumab, the formation of CYP450 enzymes could be normalized. Upon initiation or discontinuation of golimumab in patients being treated with CYP450 substrates with a narrow therapeutic index, monitoring of the effect (eg, warfarin) or drug concentration (eg, cyclosporine or theophylline) is recommended and the individual dose of the drug product may be adjusted as needed).
No products indexed under this heading.

Trimethaphan Camsylate (The formation of CYP450 enzymes may be suppressed by increased levels of cytokines (eg, TNFα) during chronic inflammation. Therefore, it is expected that for a molecule that antagonizes cytokine activity, such as golimumab, the formation of CYP450 enzymes could be normalized. Upon initiation or discontinuation of golimumab in patients being treated with CYP450 substrates with a narrow therapeutic index, monitoring of the effect (eg, warfarin) or drug concentration (eg, cyclosporine or theophylline) is recommended and the individual dose of the drug product may be adjusted as needed).
No products indexed under this heading.

Trimipramine Maleate (The formation of CYP450 enzymes may be suppressed by increased levels of cytokines (eg, TNFα) during chronic inflammation. Therefore, it is expected that for a molecule that antagonizes cytokine activity, such as golimumab, the formation of CYP450 enzymes could be normalized. Upon initiation or discontinuation of golimumab in patients being treated with CYP450 substrates with a narrow therapeutic index, monitoring of the effect (eg, warfarin) or drug concentration (eg, cyclosporine or theophylline) is recommended and the individual dose of the drug product may be adjusted as needed).
No products indexed under this heading.

Troglitazone (The formation of CYP450 enzymes may be suppressed by increased levels of cytokines (eg, TNFα) during chronic inflammation. Therefore, it is expected that for a molecule that antagonizes cytokine activity, such as golimumab, the formation of CYP450 enzymes could be normalized. Upon initiation or discontinuation of golimumab in patients being treated with CYP450 substrates with a narrow therapeutic index, monitoring of the effect (eg, warfarin) or drug concentration (eg, cyclosporine or theophylline) is recommended and the individual dose of the drug product may be adjusted as needed).
No products indexed under this heading.

Trovafloxacin Mesylate (The formation of CYP450 enzymes may be suppressed by increased levels of cytokines (eg, TNFα) during chronic inflammation. Therefore, it is expected that for a molecule that antagonizes cytokine activity, such as golimumab, the formation of CYP450 enzymes could be normalized. Upon initiation or discontinuation of golimumab in patients being treated with CYP450 substrates with a narrow therapeutic index, monitoring of the effect (eg, warfarin) or drug concentration (eg, cyclosporine or theophylline) is recommended and the individual dose of the drug product may be adjusted as needed).
No products indexed under this heading.

Typhoid Vaccine (Live vaccines should not be given concurrently with golimumab).
No products indexed under this heading.

Valdecoxib (The formation of CYP450 enzymes may be suppressed by increased levels of cytokines (eg, TNFα) during chronic inflammation. Therefore, it is expected that for a molecule that antagonizes cytokine activity, such as golimumab, the formation of CYP450 enzymes could be normalized. Upon initiation or discontinuation of golimumab in patients being treated with CYP450 substrates with a narrow therapeutic index, monitoring of the effect (eg, warfarin) or drug concentration (eg, cyclosporine or theophylline) is recommended and the individual dose of the drug product may be adjusted as needed).
No products indexed under this heading.

Valproate Sodium (The formation of CYP450 enzymes may be suppressed by increased levels of cytokines (eg, TNFα) during chronic inflammation. Therefore, it is expected that for a molecule that antagonizes cytokine activity, such as golimumab, the formation of CYP450 enzymes could be normalized. Upon initiation or discontinuation of golimumab in patients being treated with CYP450 substrates with a narrow therapeutic index, monitoring of the effect (eg, warfarin) or drug concentration (eg, cyclosporine or theophylline) is recommended and the individual dose of the drug product may be adjusted as needed).
No products indexed under this heading.

Valproic Acid (The formation of CYP450 enzymes may be suppressed by increased levels of cytokines (eg, TNFα) during chronic inflammation. Therefore, it is expected that for a molecule that antagonizes cytokine activity, such as golimumab, the formation of CYP450 enzymes could be normalized. Upon initiation or discontinuation of golimumab in patients being treated with CYP450 substrates with a narrow therapeutic index, monitoring of the effect (eg, warfarin) or drug concentration (eg, cyclosporine or theophylline) is recom-

mended and the individual dose of the drug product may be adjusted as needed).
No products indexed under this heading.

Valsartan (The formation of CYP450 enzymes may be suppressed by increased levels of cytokines (eg, TNFα) during chronic inflammation. Therefore, it is expected that for a molecule that antagonizes cytokine activity, such as golimumab, the formation of CYP450 enzymes could be normalized. Upon initiation or discontinuation of golimumab in patients being treated with CYP450 substrates with a narrow therapeutic index, monitoring of the effect (eg, warfarin) or drug concentration (eg, cyclosporine or theophylline) is recommended and the individual dose of the drug product may be adjusted as needed). Products include:
Diovan 2413
Diovan HCT 2419
Exforge 2443
Exforge HCT 2449
Valturna 3637

Vardenafil Hydrochloride (The formation of CYP450 enzymes may be suppressed by increased levels of cytokines (eg, TNFα) during chronic inflammation. Therefore, it is expected that for a molecule that antagonizes cytokine activity, such as golimumab, the formation of CYP450 enzymes could be normalized. Upon initiation or discontinuation of golimumab in patients being treated with CYP450 substrates with a narrow therapeutic index, monitoring of the effect (eg, warfarin) or drug concentration (eg, cyclosporine or theophylline) is recommended and the individual dose of the drug product may be adjusted as needed). Products include:
Levitra 3157

Varicella Virus Vaccine, Live (Live vaccines should not be given concurrently with golimumab). Products include:
Varivax 2285

Venlafaxine Hydrochloride (The formation of CYP450 enzymes may be suppressed by increased levels of cytokines (eg, TNFα) during chronic inflammation. Therefore, it is expected that for a molecule that antagonizes cytokine activity, such as golimumab, the formation of CYP450 enzymes could be normalized. Upon initiation or discontinuation of golimumab in patients being treated with CYP450 substrates with a narrow therapeutic index, monitoring of the effect (eg, warfarin) or drug concentration (eg, cyclosporine or theophylline) is recommended and the individual dose of the drug product may be adjusted as needed). Products include:
Effexor XR 3504
Venlafaxine Hydrochloride Tablets 2388

Verapamil Hydrochloride (The formation of CYP450 enzymes may be suppressed by increased levels of cytokines (eg, TNFα) during chronic inflammation. Therefore, it is expected that for a molecule that antagonizes cytokine activity, such as golimumab, the formation of CYP450 enzymes could be normalized. Upon initiation or discontinuation of golimumab in patients being treated with CYP450 substrates with a narrow therapeutic index, monitoring of the effect (eg, warfarin) or drug concentration (eg, cyclosporine or theophylline) is recommended and the individual dose of the drug product may be adjusted as needed). Products include:
Tarka 534

Vinblastine Sulfate (The formation of CYP450 enzymes may be suppressed by increased levels of cytokines (eg, TNFα) during chronic inflammation. Therefore, it is expected that for a molecule that antagonizes cytokine activity, such as golimumab, the formation of CYP450 enzymes could be normalized. Upon initiation or discontinuation of golimumab in patients being treated with CYP450 substrates with a narrow therapeutic index, monitoring of the effect (eg, warfarin) or drug concentration (eg, cyclosporine or theophylline) is recommended and the individual dose of the drug product may be adjusted as needed).
No products indexed under this heading.

Vincristine Sulfate (The formation of CYP450 enzymes may be suppressed by increased levels of cytokines (eg, TNFα) during chronic inflammation. Therefore, it is expected that for a molecule that antagonizes cytokine activity, such as golimumab, the formation of CYP450 enzymes could be normalized. Upon initiation or discontinuation of golimumab in patients being treated with CYP450 substrates with a narrow therapeutic index, monitoring of the effect (eg, warfarin) or drug concentration (eg, cyclosporine or theophylline) is recommended and the individual dose of the drug product may be adjusted as needed).
No products indexed under this heading.

Vitamin A (The formation of CYP450 enzymes may be suppressed by increased levels of cytokines (eg, TNFα) during chronic inflammation. Therefore, it is expected that for a molecule that antagonizes cytokine activity, such as golimumab, the formation of CYP450 enzymes could be normalized. Upon initiation or discontinuation of golimumab in patients being treated with CYP450 substrates with a narrow therapeutic index, monitoring of the effect (eg, warfarin) or drug concentration (eg, cyclosporine or theophylline) is recommended and the individual dose of the drug product may be adjusted as needed). Products include:
Cardio Basics 3455
Heplive 607
Norwegian Cod Liver Oil 919

Vitamin A Acetate (The formation of CYP450 enzymes may be suppressed by increased levels of cytokines (eg, TNFα) during chronic inflammation. Therefore, it is expected that for a molecule that antagonizes cytokine activity, such as golimumab, the formation of CYP450 enzymes could be normalized. Upon initiation or discontinuation of golimumab in patients being treated with CYP450 substrates with a narrow therapeutic index, monitoring of the effect (eg, warfarin) or drug concentration (eg, cyclosporine or theophylline) is recommended and the individual dose of the drug product may be adjusted as needed).
No products indexed under this heading.

Voriconazole (The formation of CYP450 enzymes may be suppressed by increased levels of cytokines (eg, TNFα) during chronic inflammation. Therefore, it is expected that for a molecule that antagonizes cytokine activity, such as golimumab, the formation of CYP450 enzymes could be normalized. Upon initiation or discontinuation of golimumab in patients being treated with CYP450 substrates with a narrow therapeutic index, monitoring of the effect (eg, warfarin) or drug concentration (eg, cyclosporine or theophylline) is recommended and the individual dose of the drug product may be adjusted as needed).
No products indexed under this heading.

Warfarin Sodium (The formation of CYP450 enzymes may be suppressed by increased levels of cytokines (eg, TNFα) during chronic inflammation. Therefore, it is expected that for a molecule that antagonizes cytokine activity, such as golimumab, the formation of CYP450 enzymes could be normalized. Upon initiation or discontinuation of golimumab in patients being treated with CYP450 substrates with a narrow therapeutic index, monitoring of the effect (eg, warfarin) or drug concentration (eg, cyclosporine or theophylline) is recommended and the individual dose of the drug product may be adjusted as needed).
No products indexed under this heading.

Yellow Fever Vaccine (Live vaccines should not be given concurrently with golimumab).
No products indexed under this heading.

Zafirlukast (The formation of CYP450 enzymes may be suppressed by increased levels of cytokines (eg, TNFα) during chronic inflammation. Therefore, it is expected that for a molecule that antagonizes cytokine activity, such as golimumab, the formation of CYP450 enzymes could be normalized. Upon initiation or discontinuation of golimumab in patients being treated with CYP450 substrates with a narrow therapeutic index, monitoring of the effect (eg, warfarin) or drug concentration (eg, cyclosporine or theophylline) is recommended and the individual dose of the drug product may be adjusted as needed). Products include:
Accolate 3612

Zileuton (The formation of CYP450 enzymes may be suppressed by increased levels of cytokines (eg, TNFα) during chronic inflammation. Therefore, it is expected that for a molecule that antagonizes cytokine activity, such as golimumab, the formation of CYP450 enzymes could be normalized. Upon initiation or discontinuation of golimumab in patients being treated with CYP450 substrates with a narrow therapeutic index, monitoring of the effect (eg, warfarin) or drug concentration (eg, cyclosporine or theophylline) is recommended and the individual dose of the drug product may be adjusted as needed).
No products indexed under this heading.

Zolmitriptan (The formation of CYP450 enzymes may be suppressed by increased levels of cytokines (eg, TNFα) during chronic inflammation. Therefore, it is expected that for a molecule that antagonizes cytokine activity, such as golimumab, the formation of CYP450 enzymes could be normalized. Upon initiation or discontinuation of golimumab in patients being treated with CYP450 substrates with a narrow therapeutic index, monitoring of the effect (eg, warfarin) or drug concentration (eg, cyclosporine or theophylline) is recommended and the individual dose of the drug product may be adjusted as needed). Products include:
Zomig Tablets 773
Zomig Nasal Spray 768
Zomig-ZMT Tablets 773

Zonisamide (The formation of CYP450 enzymes may be suppressed by increased levels of cytokines (eg, TNFα) during chronic inflammation. Therefore, it is expected that for a molecule that antagonizes cytokine activity, such as golimumab, the formation of CYP450 enzymes could be normalized. Upon initiation or discontinuation of golimumab in patients being treated with CYP450 substrates with a narrow therapeutic index, monitoring of the effect (eg, warfarin) or drug concentration (eg, cyclosporine or theophylline) is recommended and the individual dose of the drug product may be adjusted as needed). Products include:
Zonegran 1081

Zopiclone (The formation of CYP450 enzymes may be suppressed by increased levels of cytokines (eg, TNFα) during chronic inflammation. Therefore, it is expected that for a molecule that antagonizes cytokine activity, such as golimumab, the formation of CYP450 enzymes could be normalized. Upon initiation or discontinuation of golimumab in patients being treated with CYP450 substrates with a narrow therapeutic index, monitoring of the effect (eg, warfarin) or drug concentration (eg, cyclosporine or theophylline) is recommended and the individual dose of the drug product may be adjusted as needed).
No products indexed under this heading.

Zoster Vaccine Live (Live vaccines should not be given concurrently with golimumab). Products include:
Zostavax 2299

Food Interactions

Beverages, caffeine-containing (The formation of CYP450 enzymes may be suppressed by increased levels of cytokines (eg, TNFα) during chronic inflammation. Therefore, it is expected that for a molecule that antagonizes cytokine activity, such as golimumab, the formation of CYP450 enzymes could be normalized. Upon initiation or discontinuation of golimumab in patients being treated with CYP450 substrates with a narrow therapeutic index, monitoring of the effect (eg, warfarin) or drug concentration (eg, cyclosporine or theophylline) is recommended and the individual dose of the drug product may be adjusted as needed).

Food, caffeine-containing (The formation of CYP450 enzymes may be suppressed by increased levels of cytokines (eg, TNFα) during chronic inflammation. Therefore, it is expected that for a molecule that antagonizes cytokine activity, such as golimumab, the formation of CYP450 enzymes could be normalized. Upon initiation or discontinuation of golimumab in patients being treated with CYP450 substrates with a narrow therapeutic index, monitoring of the effect (eg, warfarin) or drug concentration (eg, cyclosporine or theophylline) is recommended and the individual dose of the drug product may be adjusted as needed).

SIMULECT FOR INJECTION

(Basiliximab) 2524
None cited in PDR database.

SINGULAIR TABLETS

(Montelukast Sodium) 2270

Phenobarbital (Phenobarbital, which induces hepatic metabolism, decreased the AUC of montelukast approximately 40% following a single 10-mg dose of montelukast. No dosage adjustment for montelukast is recommended. It is reasonable to employ appropriate clinical monitoring when potent cytochrome P450 enzyme inducers, such as phenobarbital, are co-administered with montelukast). Products include:
Donnatal 2711

Rifampin (It is reasonable to employ appropriate clinical monitoring when potent cytochrome P450 enzyme inducers, such as rifampin, are co-administered with montelukast).
No products indexed under this heading.

SINGULAIR CHEWABLE TABLETS

(Montelukast Sodium) 2270

See Singulair Tablets

1767 Interactions Index Skelaxin

SINGULAIR ORAL GRANULES
(Montelukast Sodium) 2270
See Singulair Tablets

SKELAXIN TABLETS
(Metaxalone) 1848
May interact with alcohols, benzodiazepines, central nervous system depressants, narcotic analgesics, tricyclic antidepressants, and certain other agents. Compounds in these categories include:

Alfentanil Hydrochloride (The sedative effects of metaxalone and other CNS depressants (eg, opioids) may be additive. Therefore, caution should be exercised with patients who take more than one of these CNS depressants simultaneously).
No products indexed under this heading.

Alprazolam (The sedative effects of metaxalone and other CNS depressants (eg, benzodiazepines) may be additive. Therefore, caution should be exercised with patients who take more than one of these CNS depressants simultaneously).
No products indexed under this heading.

Amitriptyline Hydrochloride (The sedative effects of metaxalone and other CNS depressants (eg, tricyclic antidepressants) may be additive. Therefore, caution should be exercised with patients who take more than one of these CNS depressants simultaneously).
No products indexed under this heading.

Amobarbital (The sedative effects of metaxalone and other CNS depressants (eg, alcohol, benzodiazepines, opioids, tricyclic antidepressants) may be additive. Therefore, caution should be exercised with patients who take more than one of these CNS depressants simultaneously).
No products indexed under this heading.

Amobarbital Sodium (The sedative effects of metaxalone and other CNS depressants (eg, alcohol, benzodiazepines, opioids, tricyclic antidepressants) may be additive. Therefore, caution should be exercised with patients who take more than one of these CNS depressants simultaneously).
No products indexed under this heading.

Amoxapine (The sedative effects of metaxalone and other CNS depressants (eg, tricyclic antidepressants) may be additive. Therefore, caution should be exercised with patients who take more than one of these CNS depressants simultaneously).
No products indexed under this heading.

Apomorphine (The sedative effects of metaxalone and other CNS depressants (eg, opioids) may be additive. Therefore, caution should be exercised with patients who take more than one of these CNS depressants simultaneously).
No products indexed under this heading.

Apomorphine Hydrochloride (The sedative effects of metaxalone and other CNS depressants (eg, opioids) may be additive. Therefore, caution should be exercised with patients who take more than one of these CNS depressants simultaneously).
No products indexed under this heading.

Aprobarbital (The sedative effects of metaxalone and other CNS depressants (eg, alcohol, benzodiazepines, opioids, tricyclic antidepressants) may be additive. Therefore, caution should be exercised with patients who take more than one of these CNS depressants simultaneously).
No products indexed under this heading.

Buprenorphine Hydrochloride (The sedative effects of metaxalone and other CNS depressants (eg, opioids) may be additive. Therefore, caution should be exercised with patients who take more than one of these CNS depressants simultaneously).
No products indexed under this heading.

Buspirone Hydrochloride (The sedative effects of metaxalone and other CNS depressants (eg, alcohol, benzodiazepines, opioids, tricyclic antidepressants) may be additive. Therefore, caution should be exercised with patients who take more than one of these CNS depressants simultaneously).
No products indexed under this heading.

Butabarbital (The sedative effects of metaxalone and other CNS depressants (eg, alcohol, benzodiazepines, opioids, tricyclic antidepressants) may be additive. Therefore, caution should be exercised with patients who take more than one of these CNS depressants simultaneously).
No products indexed under this heading.

Butabarbital Sodium (The sedative effects of metaxalone and other CNS depressants (eg, alcohol, benzodiazepines, opioids, tricyclic antidepressants) may be additive. Therefore, caution should be exercised with patients who take more than one of these CNS depressants simultaneously).
No products indexed under this heading.

Butalbital (The sedative effects of metaxalone and other CNS depressants (eg, alcohol, benzodiazepines, opioids, tricyclic antidepressants) may be additive. Therefore, caution should be exercised with patients who take more than one of these CNS depressants simultaneously).
No products indexed under this heading.

Chlordiazepoxide (The sedative effects of metaxalone and other CNS depressants (eg, benzodiazepines) may be additive. Therefore, caution should be exercised with patients who take more than one of these CNS depressants simultaneously).
No products indexed under this heading.

Chlordiazepoxide Hydrochloride (The sedative effects of metaxalone and other CNS depressants (eg, benzodiazepines) may be additive. Therefore, caution should be exercised with patients who take more than one of these CNS depressants simultaneously).
No products indexed under this heading.

Chlorpromazine (The sedative effects of metaxalone and other CNS depressants (eg, alcohol, benzodiazepines, opioids, tricyclic antidepressants) may be additive. Therefore, caution should be exercised with patients who take more than one of these CNS depressants simultaneously).
No products indexed under this heading.

Chlorpromazine Hydrochloride (The sedative effects of metaxalone and other CNS depressants (eg, alcohol, benzodiazepines, opioids, tricyclic antidepressants) may be additive. Therefore, caution should be exercised with patients who take more than one of these CNS depressants simultaneously).
No products indexed under this heading.

Chlorprothixene (The sedative effects of metaxalone and other CNS depressants (eg, alcohol, benzodiazepines, opioids, tricyclic antidepressants) may be additive. Therefore, caution should be exercised with patients who take more than one of these CNS depressants simultaneously).
No products indexed under this heading.

Chlorprothixene Hydrochloride (The sedative effects of metaxalone and other CNS depressants (eg, alcohol, benzodiazepines, opioids, tricyclic antidepressants) may be additive. Therefore, caution should be exercised with patients who take more than one of these CNS depressants simultaneously).
No products indexed under this heading.

Chlorprothixene Lactate (The sedative effects of metaxalone and other CNS depressants (eg, alcohol, benzodiazepines, opioids, tricyclic antidepressants) may be additive. Therefore, caution should be exercised with patients who take more than one of these CNS depressants simultaneously).
No products indexed under this heading.

Clomipramine Hydrochloride (The sedative effects of metaxalone and other CNS depressants (eg, tricyclic antidepressants) may be additive. Therefore, caution should be exercised with patients who take more than one of these CNS depressants simultaneously).
No products indexed under this heading.

Clonazepam (The sedative effects of metaxalone and other CNS depressants (eg, alcohol, benzodiazepines, opioids, tricyclic antidepressants) may be additive. Therefore, caution should be exercised with patients who take more than one of these CNS depressants simultaneously). Products include:
Klonopin 2855

Clorazepate Dipotassium (The sedative effects of metaxalone and other CNS depressants (eg, benzodiazepines) may be additive. Therefore, caution should be exercised with patients who take more than one of these CNS depressants simultaneously).
No products indexed under this heading.

Clozapine (The sedative effects of metaxalone and other CNS depressants (eg, alcohol, benzodiazepines, opioids, tricyclic antidepressants) may be additive. Therefore, caution should be exercised with patients who take more than one of these CNS depressants simultaneously).
No products indexed under this heading.

Codeine Phosphate (The sedative effects of metaxalone and other CNS depressants (eg, opioids) may be additive. Therefore, caution should be exercised with patients who take more than one of these CNS depressants simultaneously). Products include:
Tylenol with Codeine 2691

Codeine Sulfate (The sedative effects of metaxalone and other CNS depressants (eg, opioids) may be additive. Therefore, caution should be exercised with patients who take more than one of these CNS depressants simultaneously).
No products indexed under this heading.

Desflurane (The sedative effects of metaxalone and other CNS depressants (eg, alcohol, benzodiazepines, opioids, tricyclic antidepressants) may be additive. Therefore, caution should be exercised with patients who take more than one of these CNS depressants simultaneously).
No products indexed under this heading.

Desipramine Hydrochloride (The sedative effects of metaxalone and other CNS depressants (eg, tricyclic antidepressants) may be additive. Therefore, caution should be exercised with patients who take more than one of these CNS depressants simultaneously).
No products indexed under this heading.

Dezocine (The sedative effects of metaxalone and other CNS depressants (eg, opioids) may be additive. Therefore, caution should be exercised with patients who take more than one of these CNS depressants simultaneously).
No products indexed under this heading.

Diazepam (The sedative effects of metaxalone and other CNS depressants (eg, benzodiazepines) may be additive. Therefore, caution should be exercised with patients who take more than one of these CNS depressants simultaneously). Products include:
Valium Tablets 2880

Dihydrocodeine Bitartrate (The sedative effects of metaxalone and other CNS depressants (eg, opioids) may be additive. Therefore, caution should be exercised with patients who take more than one of these CNS depressants simultaneously).
No products indexed under this heading.

Dihydrocodeinone Bitartrate (The sedative effects of metaxalone and other CNS depressants (eg, opioids) may be additive. Therefore, caution should be exercised with patients who take more than one of these CNS depressants simultaneously).
No products indexed under this heading.

Doxepin Hydrochloride (The sedative effects of metaxalone and other CNS depressants (eg, tricyclic antidepressants) may be additive. Therefore, caution should be exercised with patients who take more than one of these CNS depressants simultaneously).
No products indexed under this heading.

Droperidol (The sedative effects of metaxalone and other CNS depressants (eg, alcohol, benzodiazepines, opioids, tricyclic antidepressants) may be additive. Therefore, caution should be exercised with patients who take more than one of these CNS depressants simultaneously).
No products indexed under this heading.

Enflurane (The sedative effects of metaxalone and other CNS depressants (eg, alcohol, benzodiazepines, opioids, tricyclic antidepressants) may be additive. Therefore, caution should be exercised with patients who take more than one of these CNS depressants simultaneously).
No products indexed under this heading.

Estazolam (The sedative effects of metaxalone and other CNS depressants (eg, benzodiazepines) may be additive. Therefore, caution should be exercised with patients who take more than one of these CNS depressants simultaneously).
No products indexed under this heading.

Ethanol (The sedative effects of metaxalone and other CNS depressants (eg, alcohol) may be additive. Therefore, caution should be exercised with patients who take more than one of these CNS depressants simultaneously).
No products indexed under this heading.

Ethchlorvynol (The sedative effects of metaxalone and other CNS depressants (eg, alcohol, benzodiazepines, opioids, tricyclic antidepressants) may be additive. Therefore, caution should be exercised with patients who take more than one of these CNS depressants simultaneously).
No products indexed under this heading.

Ethinamate (The sedative effects of metaxalone and other CNS depressants (eg, alcohol, benzodiazepines, opioids, tricyclic antidepressants) may be additive. Therefore, caution should be exercised with patients who take more than one of these CNS depressants simultaneously).
No products indexed under this heading.

Ethyl Alcohol (The sedative effects of metaxalone and other CNS depressants (eg, alcohol) may be additive. Therefore, caution should be exercised with patients who take more than one of these CNS depressants simultaneously).
No products indexed under this heading.

Fat (Taking metaxalone with food may enhance general CNS depression. The presence of a high fat meal at the time of drug administration increased C_{max} and AUC. T_{max} was also delayed and terminal half-life was decreased under fed conditions compared to fasted conditions).
No products indexed under this heading.

Fentanyl (The sedative effects of metaxalone and other CNS depressants (eg, opioids) may be additive. Therefore, caution should be exercised with patients who take more than one of these CNS depressants simultaneously). Products include:
Duragesic 2604
Fentanyl Transdermal System 2346
Onsolis 2054

Fentanyl Citrate (The sedative effects of metaxalone and other CNS depressants (eg, opioids) may be additive. Therefore, caution should be exercised with patients who take more than one of these CNS depressants simultaneously). Products include:
Fentora 966

Fluphenazine Decanoate (The sedative effects of metaxalone and other CNS depressants (eg, alcohol, benzodiazepines, opioids, tricyclic antidepressants) may be additive. Therefore, caution should be exercised with patients who take more than one of these CNS depressants simultaneously).
No products indexed under this heading.

Fluphenazine Enanthate (The sedative effects of metaxalone and other CNS depressants (eg, alcohol, benzodiazepines, opioids, tricyclic antidepressants) may be additive. Therefore, caution should be exercised with patients who take more than one of these CNS depressants simultaneously).
No products indexed under this heading.

Fluphenazine Hydrochloride (The sedative effects of metaxalone and other CNS depressants (eg, alcohol, benzodiazepines, opioids, tricyclic antidepressants) may be additive. Therefore, caution should be exercised with patients who take more than one of these CNS depressants simultaneously).
No products indexed under this heading.

Flurazepam Hydrochloride (The sedative effects of metaxalone and other CNS depressants (eg, benzodiazepines) may be additive. Therefore, caution should be exercised with patients who take more than one of these CNS depressants simultaneously).
No products indexed under this heading.

Glutethimide (The sedative effects of metaxalone and other CNS depressants (eg, alcohol, benzodiazepines, opioids, tricyclic antidepressants) may be additive. Therefore, caution should be exercised with patients who take more than one of these CNS depressants simultaneously).
No products indexed under this heading.

Halazepam (The sedative effects of metaxalone and other CNS depressants (eg, benzodiazepines) may be additive. Therefore, caution should be exercised with patients who take more than one of these CNS depressants simultaneously).
No products indexed under this heading.

Haloperidol (The sedative effects of metaxalone and other CNS depressants (eg, alcohol, benzodiazepines, opioids, tricyclic antidepressants) may be additive. Therefore, caution should be exercised with patients who take more than one of these CNS depressants simultaneously).
No products indexed under this heading.

Haloperidol Decanoate (The sedative effects of metaxalone and other CNS depressants (eg, alcohol, benzodiazepines, opioids, tricyclic antidepressants) may be additive. Therefore, caution should be exercised with patients who take more than one of these CNS depressants simultaneously).
No products indexed under this heading.

Haloperidol Lactate (The sedative effects of metaxalone and other CNS depressants (eg, alcohol, benzodiazepines, opioids, tricyclic antidepressants) may be additive. Therefore, caution should be exercised with patients who take more than one of these CNS depressants simultaneously).
No products indexed under this heading.

Hexobarbital (The sedative effects of metaxalone and other CNS depressants (eg, alcohol, benzodiazepines, opioids, tricyclic antidepressants) may be additive. Therefore, caution should be exercised with patients who take more than one of these CNS depressants simultaneously).
No products indexed under this heading.

Hydrocodone Bitartrate (The sedative effects of metaxalone and other CNS depressants (eg, opioids) may be additive. Therefore, caution should be exercised with patients who take more than one of these CNS depressants simultaneously). Products include:
Vicodin 560
Vicodin ES 561
Vicodin HP 563
Vicoprofen 564
Zydone 1138

Hydrocodone Polistirex (The sedative effects of metaxalone and other CNS depressants (eg, opioids) may be additive. Therefore, caution should be exercised with patients who take more than one of these CNS depressants simultaneously). Products include:
Tussionex 3443

Hydromorphone (The sedative effects of metaxalone and other CNS depressants (eg, opioids) may be additive. Therefore, caution should be exercised with patients who take more than one of these CNS depressants simultaneously).
No products indexed under this heading.

Hydromorphone Hydrochloride (The sedative effects of metaxalone and other CNS depressants (eg, opioids) may be additive. Therefore, caution should be exercised with patients who take more than one of these CNS depressants simultaneously). Products include:
Dilaudid Injection 2800
Dilaudid Oral 2797
Dilaudid Tablets 2797
Dilaudid-HP 2800

Hydroxyzine Hydrochloride (The sedative effects of metaxalone and other CNS depressants (eg, alcohol, benzodiazepines, opioids, tricyclic antidepressants) may be additive. Therefore, caution should be exercised with patients who take more than one of these CNS depressants simultaneously).
No products indexed under this heading.

Imipramine Hydrochloride (The sedative effects of metaxalone and other CNS depressants (eg, tricyclic antidepressants) may be additive. Therefore, caution should be exercised with patients who take more than one of these CNS depressants simultaneously).
No products indexed under this heading.

Imipramine Pamoate (The sedative effects of metaxalone and other CNS depressants (eg, tricyclic antidepressants) may be additive. Therefore, caution should be exercised with patients who take more than one of these CNS depressants simultaneously).
No products indexed under this heading.

Isoflurane (The sedative effects of metaxalone and other CNS depressants (eg, alcohol, benzodiazepines, opioids, tricyclic antidepressants) may be additive. Therefore, caution should be exercised with patients who take more than one of these CNS depressants simultaneously).
No products indexed under this heading.

Ketamine Hydrochloride (The sedative effects of metaxalone and other CNS depressants (eg, alcohol, benzodiazepines, opioids, tricyclic antidepressants) may be additive. Therefore, caution should be exercised with patients who take more than one of these CNS depressants simultaneously).
No products indexed under this heading.

Levomethadyl Acetate Hydrochloride (The sedative effects of metaxalone and other CNS depressants (eg, alcohol, benzodiazepines, opioids, tricyclic antidepressants) may be additive. Therefore, caution should be exercised with patients who take more than one of these CNS depressants simultaneously).
No products indexed under this heading.

Levorphanol Tartrate (The sedative effects of metaxalone and other CNS depressants (eg, opioids) may be additive. Therefore, caution should be exercised with patients who take more than one of these CNS depressants simultaneously).
No products indexed under this heading.

Lorazepam (The sedative effects of metaxalone and other CNS depressants (eg, benzodiazepines) may be additive. Therefore, caution should be exercised with patients who take more than one of these CNS depressants simultaneously).
No products indexed under this heading.

Loxapine Hydrochloride (The sedative effects of metaxalone and other CNS depressants (eg, alcohol, benzodiazepines, opioids, tricyclic antidepressants) may be additive. Therefore, caution should be exercised with patients who take more than one of these CNS depressants simultaneously).
No products indexed under this heading.

Loxapine Succinate (The sedative effects of metaxalone and other CNS depressants (eg, alcohol, benzodiazepines, opioids, tricyclic antidepressants) may be additive. Therefore, caution should be exercised with patients who take more than one of these CNS depressants simultaneously).
No products indexed under this heading.

Maprotiline Hydrochloride (The sedative effects of metaxalone and other CNS depressants (eg, tricyclic antidepressants) may be additive. Therefore, caution should be exercised with patients who take more than one of these CNS depressants simultaneously).
No products indexed under this heading.

Meperidine Hydrochloride (The sedative effects of metaxalone and other CNS depressants (eg, opioids) may be additive. Therefore, caution should be exercised with patients who take more than one of these CNS depressants simultaneously).
No products indexed under this heading.

Mephobarbital (The sedative effects of metaxalone and other CNS depressants (eg, alcohol, benzodiazepines, opioids, tricyclic antidepressants) may be additive. Therefore, caution should be exercised with patients who take more than one of these CNS depressants simultaneously).
No products indexed under this heading.

Meprobamate (The sedative effects of metaxalone and other CNS depressants (eg, alcohol, benzodiazepines, opioids, tricyclic antidepressants) may be additive. Therefore, caution should be exercised with patients who take more than one of these CNS depressants simultaneously).
No products indexed under this heading.

Mesoridazine Besylate (The sedative effects of metaxalone and other CNS depressants (eg, alcohol, benzodiazepines, opioids, tricyclic antidepressants) may be additive. Therefore, caution should be exercised with patients who take more than one of these CNS depressants simultaneously).
No products indexed under this heading.

Methadone Hydrochloride (The sedative effects of metaxalone and other CNS depressants (eg, opioids) may be additive. Therefore, caution should be exercised with patients who take more than one of these CNS depressants simultaneously).
No products indexed under this heading.

Methohexital Sodium (The sedative effects of metaxalone and other CNS depressants (eg, alcohol, benzodiazepines, opioids, tricyclic antidepressants) may be additive. Therefore, caution should be exercised with patients who take more than one of these CNS depressants simultaneously).
No products indexed under this heading.

Methotrimeprazine (The sedative effects of metaxalone and other CNS depressants (eg, alcohol, benzodiazepines, opioids, tricyclic antidepressants) may be additive. Therefore, caution should be exercised with patients who take more than one of these CNS depressants simultaneously).
No products indexed under this heading.

Methoxyflurane (The sedative effects of metaxalone and other CNS depressants (eg, alcohol, benzodiazepines, opioids, tricyclic antidepressants) may be additive. Therefore, caution should be exercised with patients who take more than one of these CNS depressants simultaneously).
No products indexed under this heading.

Midazolam Hydrochloride (The sedative effects of metaxalone and other CNS depressants (eg, benzodiazepines) may be additive. Therefore, caution should be exercised with patients who take more than one of these CNS depressants simultaneously).
No products indexed under this heading.

Molindone Hydrochloride (The sedative effects of metaxalone and other CNS depressants (eg, alcohol, benzodiazepines, opioids, tricyclic antidepres-

sants) may be additive. Therefore, caution should be exercised with patients who take more than one of these CNS depressants simultaneously). Products include:

Morphine Sulfate (The sedative effects of metaxalone and other CNS depressants (eg, opioids) may be additive. Therefore, caution should be exercised with patients who take more than one of these CNS depressants simultaneously). Products include:

Morphine Sulfate, Liposomal (The sedative effects of metaxalone and other CNS depressants (eg, opioids) may be additive. Therefore, caution should be exercised with patients who take more than one of these CNS depressants simultaneously).

No products indexed under this heading.

Nortriptyline Hydrochloride (The sedative effects of metaxalone and other CNS depressants (eg, tricyclic antidepressants) may be additive. Therefore, caution should be exercised with patients who take more than one of these CNS depressants simultaneously).

No products indexed under this heading.

Olanzapine (The sedative effects of metaxalone and other CNS depressants (eg, alcohol, benzodiazepines, opioids, tricyclic antidepressants) may be additive. Therefore, caution should be exercised with patients who take more than one of these CNS depressants simultaneously). Products include:

Oxazepam (The sedative effects of metaxalone and other CNS depressants (eg, benzodiazepines) may be additive. Therefore, caution should be exercised with patients who take more than one of these CNS depressants simultaneously).

No products indexed under this heading.

Oxycodone Hydrochloride (The sedative effects of metaxalone and other CNS depressants (eg, opioids) may be additive. Therefore, caution should be exercised with patients who take more than one of these CNS depressants simultaneously). Products include:

Oxycodone Terephthalate (The sedative effects of metaxalone and other CNS depressants (eg, opioids) may be additive. Therefore, caution should be exercised with patients who take more than one of these CNS depressants simultaneously).

No products indexed under this heading.

Oxymorphone Hydrochloride (The sedative effects of metaxalone and other CNS depressants (eg, opioids) may be additive. Therefore, caution should be exercised with patients who take more than one of these CNS depressants simultaneously). Products include:

Pentobarbital (The sedative effects of metaxalone and other CNS depressants (eg, alcohol, benzodiazepines, opioids, tricyclic antidepressants) may be additive. Therefore, caution should be exercised with patients who take more than one of these CNS depressants simultaneously).

No products indexed under this heading.

Pentobarbital Sodium (The sedative effects of metaxalone and other CNS depressants (eg, alcohol, benzodiaz-

epines, opioids, tricyclic antidepressants) may be additive. Therefore, caution should be exercised with patients who take more than one of these CNS depressants simultaneously). Products include:

Perphenazine (The sedative effects of metaxalone and other CNS depressants (eg, alcohol, benzodiazepines, opioids, tricyclic antidepressants) may be additive. Therefore, caution should be exercised with patients who take more than one of these CNS depressants simultaneously).

No products indexed under this heading.

Phenobarbital (The sedative effects of metaxalone and other CNS depressants (eg, alcohol, benzodiazepines, opioids, tricyclic antidepressants) may be additive. Therefore, caution should be exercised with patients who take more than one of these CNS depressants simultaneously). Products include:

Phenobarbital Sodium (The sedative effects of metaxalone and other CNS depressants (eg, alcohol, benzodiazepines, opioids, tricyclic antidepressants) may be additive. Therefore, caution should be exercised with patients who take more than one of these CNS depressants simultaneously).

No products indexed under this heading.

Prazepam (The sedative effects of metaxalone and other CNS depressants (eg, benzodiazepines) may be additive. Therefore, caution should be exercised with patients who take more than one of these CNS depressants simultaneously).

No products indexed under this heading.

Prochlorperazine (The sedative effects of metaxalone and other CNS depressants (eg, alcohol, benzodiazepines, opioids, tricyclic antidepressants) may be additive. Therefore, caution should be exercised with patients who take more than one of these CNS depressants simultaneously).

No products indexed under this heading.

Prochlorperazine Edisylate (The sedative effects of metaxalone and other CNS depressants (eg, alcohol, benzodiazepines, opioids, tricyclic antidepressants) may be additive. Therefore, caution should be exercised with patients who take more than one of these CNS depressants simultaneously).

No products indexed under this heading.

Prochlorperazine Maleate (The sedative effects of metaxalone and other CNS depressants (eg, alcohol, benzodiazepines, opioids, tricyclic antidepressants) may be additive. Therefore, caution should be exercised with patients who take more than one of these CNS depressants simultaneously).

No products indexed under this heading.

Promethazine (The sedative effects of metaxalone and other CNS depressants (eg, alcohol, benzodiazepines, opioids, tricyclic antidepressants) may be additive. Therefore, caution should be exercised with patients who take more than one of these CNS depressants simultaneously).

No products indexed under this heading.

Promethazine Hydrochloride (The sedative effects of metaxalone and other CNS depressants (eg, alcohol, benzodiazepines, opioids, tricyclic antidepressants) may be additive. Therefore, caution should be exercised with patients who take more than one of these CNS depressants simultaneously).

No products indexed under this heading.

Propofol (The sedative effects of metaxalone and other CNS depressants (eg, alcohol, benzodiazepines, opioids, tricyclic antidepressants) may be additive. Therefore, caution should be exercised with patients who take more than one of these CNS depressants simultaneously).

No products indexed under this heading.

Propoxyphene Hydrochloride (The sedative effects of metaxalone and other CNS depressants (eg, opioids) may be additive. Therefore, caution should be exercised with patients who take more than one of these CNS depressants simultaneously).

No products indexed under this heading.

Propoxyphene Napsylate (The sedative effects of metaxalone and other CNS depressants (eg, opioids) may be additive. Therefore, caution should be exercised with patients who take more than one of these CNS depressants simultaneously).

No products indexed under this heading.

Protriptyline Hydrochloride (The sedative effects of metaxalone and other CNS depressants (eg, tricyclic antidepressants) may be additive. Therefore, caution should be exercised with patients who take more than one of these CNS depressants simultaneously).

No products indexed under this heading.

Quazepam (The sedative effects of metaxalone and other CNS depressants (eg, benzodiazepines) may be additive. Therefore, caution should be exercised with patients who take more than one of these CNS depressants simultaneously).

No products indexed under this heading.

Quetiapine Fumarate (The sedative effects of metaxalone and other CNS depressants (eg, alcohol, benzodiazepines, opioids, tricyclic antidepressants) may be additive. Therefore, caution should be exercised with patients who take more than one of these CNS depressants simultaneously). Products include:

Remifentanil Hydrochloride (The sedative effects of metaxalone and other CNS depressants (eg, opioids) may be additive. Therefore, caution should be exercised with patients who take more than one of these CNS depressants simultaneously).

No products indexed under this heading.

Risperidone (The sedative effects of metaxalone and other CNS depressants (eg, alcohol, benzodiazepines, opioids, tricyclic antidepressants) may be additive. Therefore, caution should be exercised with patients who take more than one of these CNS depressants simultaneously). Products include:

Secobarbital Sodium (The sedative effects of metaxalone and other CNS depressants (eg, alcohol, benzodiazepines, opioids, tricyclic antidepressants) may be additive. Therefore, caution should be exercised with patients who take more than one of these CNS depressants simultaneously).

No products indexed under this heading.

Sevoflurane (The sedative effects of metaxalone and other CNS depressants (eg, alcohol, benzodiazepines, opioids, tricyclic antidepressants) may be additive. Therefore, caution should be exercised with patients who take more than one of these CNS depressants simultaneously). Products include:

Sodium Butabarbital (The sedative effects of metaxalone and other CNS depressants (eg, alcohol, benzodiazepines, opioids, tricyclic antidepressants) may be additive. Therefore, caution should be exercised with patients who take more than one of these CNS depressants simultaneously).

No products indexed under this heading.

Sodium Oxybate (The sedative effects of metaxalone and other CNS depressants (eg, alcohol, benzodiazepines, opioids, tricyclic antidepressants) may be additive. Therefore, caution should be exercised with patients who take more than one of these CNS depressants simultaneously).

No products indexed under this heading.

Sodium Pentobarbital (The sedative effects of metaxalone and other CNS depressants (eg, alcohol, benzodiazepines, opioids, tricyclic antidepressants) may be additive. Therefore, caution should be exercised with patients who take more than one of these CNS depressants simultaneously).

No products indexed under this heading.

Sufentanil Citrate (The sedative effects of metaxalone and other CNS depressants (eg, opioids) may be additive. Therefore, caution should be exercised with patients who take more than one of these CNS depressants simultaneously).

No products indexed under this heading.

Talbutal (The sedative effects of metaxalone and other CNS depressants (eg, alcohol, benzodiazepines, opioids, tricyclic antidepressants) may be additive. Therefore, caution should be exercised with patients who take more than one of these CNS depressants simultaneously).

No products indexed under this heading.

Temazepam (The sedative effects of metaxalone and other CNS depressants (eg, benzodiazepines) may be additive. Therefore, caution should be exercised with patients who take more than one of these CNS depressants simultaneously).

No products indexed under this heading.

Thiamylal Sodium (The sedative effects of metaxalone and other CNS depressants (eg, alcohol, benzodiazepines, opioids, tricyclic antidepressants) may be additive. Therefore, caution should be exercised with patients who take more than one of these CNS depressants simultaneously).

No products indexed under this heading.

Thioridazine (The sedative effects of metaxalone and other CNS depressants (eg, alcohol, benzodiazepines, opioids, tricyclic antidepressants) may be additive. Therefore, caution should be exercised with patients who take more than one of these CNS depressants simultaneously).

No products indexed under this heading.

Thioridazine Hydrochloride (The sedative effects of metaxalone and other CNS depressants (eg, alcohol, benzodiazepines, opioids, tricyclic antidepressants) may be additive. Therefore, caution should be exercised with patients who take more than one of these CNS depressants simultaneously). Products include:

Thiothixene (The sedative effects of metaxalone and other CNS depressants (eg, alcohol, benzodiazepines, opioids, tricyclic antidepressants) may be additive. Therefore, caution should be exercised with patients who take more than one of these CNS depressants simultaneously). Products include:

Thiothixene Hydrochloride (The sedative effects of metaxalone and other CNS depressants (eg, alcohol, benzodiazepines, opioids, tricyclic antidepressants) may be additive. Therefore, caution should be exercised with patients who take more than one of these CNS depressants simultaneously).
No products indexed under this heading.

Triazolam (The sedative effects of metaxalone and other CNS depressants (eg, benzodiazepines) may be additive. Therefore, caution should be exercised with patients who take more than one of these CNS depressants simultaneously).
No products indexed under this heading.

Trifluoperazine Hydrochloride (The sedative effects of metaxalone and other CNS depressants (eg, alcohol, benzodiazepines, opioids, tricyclic antidepressants) may be additive. Therefore, caution should be exercised with patients who take more than one of these CNS depressants simultaneously).
No products indexed under this heading.

Trimipramine Maleate (The sedative effects of metaxalone and other CNS depressants (eg, tricyclic antidepressants) may be additive. Therefore, caution should be exercised with patients who take more than one of these CNS depressants simultaneously).
No products indexed under this heading.

Zaleplon (The sedative effects of metaxalone and other CNS depressants (eg, alcohol, benzodiazepines, opioids, tricyclic antidepressants) may be additive. Therefore, caution should be exercised with patients who take more than one of these CNS depressants simultaneously).
No products indexed under this heading.

Ziprasidone Hydrochloride (The sedative effects of metaxalone and other CNS depressants (eg, alcohol, benzodiazepines, opioids, tricyclic antidepressants) may be additive. Therefore, caution should be exercised with patients who take more than one of these CNS depressants simultaneously). Products include:
Geodon 2723

Zolpidem Tartrate (The sedative effects of metaxalone and other CNS depressants (eg, alcohol, benzodiazepines, opioids, tricyclic antidepressants) may be additive. Therefore, caution should be exercised with patients who take more than one of these CNS depressants simultaneously). Products include:
Ambien 2920
Ambien CR 2925

Food Interactions

Alcohol (The sedative effects of metaxalone and other CNS depressants (eg, alcohol) may be additive. Therefore, caution should be exercised with patients who take more than one of these CNS depressants simultaneously).

Beer, reduced-alcohol (The sedative effects of metaxalone and other CNS depressants (eg, alcohol) may be additive. Therefore, caution should be exercised with patients who take more than one of these CNS depressants simultaneously).

Beer, unspecified (The sedative effects of metaxalone and other CNS depressants (eg, alcohol) may be additive. Therefore, caution should be exercised with patients who take more than one of these CNS depressants simultaneously).

Food, unspecified (Taking metaxalone with food may enhance general CNS depression. The presence of a high fat meal at the time of drug administration increased C_{max} and AUC. T_{max} was also delayed and terminal half-life was decreased under fed conditions compared to fasted conditions).

Meal, unspecified (Taking metaxalone with food may enhance general CNS depression. The presence of a high fat meal at the time of drug administration increased C_{max} and AUC. T_{max} was also delayed and terminal half-life was decreased under fed conditions compared to fasted conditions).

Wine, Chianti (The sedative effects of metaxalone and other CNS depressants (eg, alcohol) may be additive. Therefore, caution should be exercised with patients who take more than one of these CNS depressants simultaneously).

Wine, Red (The sedative effects of metaxalone and other CNS depressants (eg, alcohol) may be additive. Therefore, caution should be exercised with patients who take more than one of these CNS depressants simultaneously).

Wine, unspecified (The sedative effects of metaxalone and other CNS depressants (eg, alcohol) may be additive. Therefore, caution should be exercised with patients who take more than one of these CNS depressants simultaneously).

Wine products (The sedative effects of metaxalone and other CNS depressants (eg, alcohol) may be additive. Therefore, caution should be exercised with patients who take more than one of these CNS depressants simultaneously).

SMILE'S PRID SALVE

(Homeopathic Formulations) 3316
None cited in PDR database.

SOLIRIS CONCENTRATED SOLUTION FOR INTRAVENOUS INFUSION

(Eculizumab) 590
None cited in PDR database.

SOLODYN EXTENDED RELEASE TABLETS

(Minocycline Hydrochloride) 2073
May interact with antacids containing aluminum, calcium and magnesium, anticoagulants, estrogens, iron containing oral preparations, iron salts, oral contraceptives, penicillins, progestins, and certain other agents. Compounds in these categories include:

Aluminum Carbonate (Absorption of tetracyclines is impaired by antacids containing aluminum, calcium, or magnesium).
No products indexed under this heading.

Aluminum Hydroxide (Absorption of tetracyclines is impaired by antacids containing aluminum, calcium, or magnesium).
No products indexed under this heading.

Amoxicillin (Since bacteriostatic drugs may interfere with the bactericidal action of penicillin, it is advisable to avoid giving tetracycline-class drugs in conjunction with penicillin). Products include:
Amoxil Capsules 1311
Amoxil Chewable Tablets 1311
Amoxil 1311
Amoxil Powder 1311
Augmentin 1331
Augmentin Tablets 1335
Augmentin ES-600 1338
Augmentin XR 1342
Moxatag 2321

Amoxicillin Trihydrate (Since bacteriostatic drugs may interfere with the bactericidal action of penicillin, it is advisable to avoid giving tetracycline-class drugs in conjunction with penicillin).
No products indexed under this heading.

Ampicillin (Since bacteriostatic drugs may interfere with the bactericidal action of penicillin, it is advisable to avoid giving tetracycline-class drugs in conjunction with penicillin).
No products indexed under this heading.

Ampicillin Sodium (Since bacteriostatic drugs may interfere with the bactericidal action of penicillin, it is advisable to avoid giving tetracycline-class drugs in conjunction with penicillin).
No products indexed under this heading.

Ampicillin Trihydrate (Since bacteriostatic drugs may interfere with the bactericidal action of penicillin, it is advisable to avoid giving tetracycline-class drugs in conjunction with penicillin).
No products indexed under this heading.

Anisindione (Because tetracyclines have been shown to depress plasma prothrombin activity, patients who are on anticoagulant therapy may require downward adjustment of their anticoagulant dosage).
No products indexed under this heading.

Ardeparin Sodium (Because tetracyclines have been shown to depress plasma prothrombin activity, patients who are on anticoagulant therapy may require downward adjustment of their anticoagulant dosage).
No products indexed under this heading.

Azlocillin Sodium (Since bacteriostatic drugs may interfere with the bactericidal action of penicillin, it is advisable to avoid giving tetracycline-class drugs in conjunction with penicillin).
No products indexed under this heading.

Bacampicillin Hydrochloride (Since bacteriostatic drugs may interfere with the bactericidal action of penicillin, it is advisable to avoid giving tetracycline-class drugs in conjunction with penicillin).
No products indexed under this heading.

Calcium Carbonate (Absorption of tetracyclines is impaired by antacids containing aluminum, calcium, or magnesium). Products include:
Chelated Mineral 3476
Pepcid Complete 1822
Extra Strength Rolaids Softchews Vanilla Creme 2045

Carbenicillin Disodium (Since bacteriostatic drugs may interfere with the bactericidal action of penicillin, it is advisable to avoid giving tetracycline-class drugs in conjunction with penicillin).
No products indexed under this heading.

Carbenicillin Indanyl Sodium (Since bacteriostatic drugs may interfere with the bactericidal action of penicillin, it is advisable to avoid giving tetracycline-class drugs in conjunction with penicillin).
No products indexed under this heading.

Chlorotrianisene (In a multi-center study to evaluate the effect of minocycline on low dose oral contraceptives, hormone levels over one menstrual cycle with and without minocycline 1 mg/kg once-daily were measured. Based on the results of this trial, minocycline-related changes in estradiol, progestinic hormone, FSH and LH plasma levels, of breakthrough bleeding, or of contraceptive failure, can not be ruled out. To avoid contraceptive failure, female patients are advised to use a second form of contraceptive during treatment with minocycline).
No products indexed under this heading.

Cloxacillin (Since bacteriostatic drugs may interfere with the bactericidal action of penicillin, it is advisable to avoid giving tetracycline-class drugs in conjunction with penicillin).
No products indexed under this heading.

Cloxacillin Sodium (Since bacteriostatic drugs may interfere with the bactericidal action of penicillin, it is advisable to avoid giving tetracycline-class drugs in conjunction with penicillin).
No products indexed under this heading.

Cloxacillin Sodium Monohydrate (Since bacteriostatic drugs may interfere with the bactericidal action of penicillin, it is advisable to avoid giving tetracycline-class drugs in conjunction with penicillin).
No products indexed under this heading.

Dalteparin Sodium (Because tetracyclines have been shown to depress plasma prothrombin activity, patients who are on anticoagulant therapy may require downward adjustment of their anticoagulant dosage). Products include:
Fragmin 1058

Danaparoid Sodium (Because tetracyclines have been shown to depress plasma prothrombin activity, patients who are on anticoagulant therapy may require downward adjustment of their anticoagulant dosage).
No products indexed under this heading.

Desogestrel (In a multi-center study to evaluate the effect of minocycline on low dose oral contraceptives, hormone levels over one menstrual cycle with and without minocycline 1 mg/kg once-daily were measured. Based on the results of this trial, minocycline-related changes in estradiol, progestinic hormone, FSH and LH plasma levels, of breakthrough bleeding, or of contraceptive failure, can not be ruled out. To avoid contraceptive failure, female patients are advised to use a second form of contraceptive during treatment with minocycline).
No products indexed under this heading.

Dicloxacillin (Since bacteriostatic drugs may interfere with the bactericidal action of penicillin, it is advisable to avoid giving tetracycline-class drugs in conjunction with penicillin).
No products indexed under this heading.

Dicloxacillin Sodium (Since bacteriostatic drugs may interfere with the bactericidal action of penicillin, it is advisable to avoid giving tetracycline-class drugs in conjunction with penicillin).
No products indexed under this heading.

Dicumarol (Because tetracyclines have been shown to depress plasma prothrombin activity, patients who are on anticoagulant therapy may require downward adjustment of their anticoagulant dosage).
No products indexed under this heading.

Dienestrol (In a multi-center study to evaluate the effect of minocycline on low dose oral contraceptives, hormone levels over one menstrual cycle with and without minocycline 1 mg/kg once-daily were measured. Based on the results of this trial, minocycline-related changes in estradiol, progestinic hormone, FSH and LH plasma levels, of breakthrough bleeding, or of contraceptive failure, can not be ruled out. To avoid contraceptive failure, female patients are advised to use a second form of contraceptive during treatment with minocycline).
No products indexed under this heading.

Diethylstilbestrol (In a multi-center study to evaluate the effect of minocycline on low dose oral contraceptives, hormone levels over one menstrual cycle with and without minocycline 1 mg/kg once-daily were measured.

1771 **Interactions Index** **Solodyn**

Based on the results of this trial, minocycline-related changes in estradiol, progestinic hormone, FSH and LH plasma levels, of breakthrough bleeding, or of contraceptive failure, can not be ruled out. To avoid contraceptive failure, female patients are advised to use a second form of contraceptive during treatment with minocycline).
No products indexed under this heading.

Disodium Carbenicillin (Since bacteriostatic drugs may interfere with the bactericidal action of penicillin, it is advisable to avoid giving tetracycline-class drugs in conjunction with penicillin).
No products indexed under this heading.

Enoxaparin Sodium (Because tetracyclines have been shown to depress plasma prothrombin activity, patients who are on anticoagulant therapy may require downward adjustment of their anticoagulant dosage). Products include:
Lovenox 3005

Estradiol (In a multi-center study to evaluate the effect of minocycline on low dose oral contraceptives, hormone levels over one menstrual cycle with and without minocycline 1 mg/kg once-daily were measured. Based on the results of this trial, minocycline-related changes in estradiol, progestinic hormone, FSH and LH plasma levels, of breakthrough bleeding, or of contraceptive failure, can not be ruled out. To avoid contraceptive failure, female patients are advised to use a second form of contraceptive during treatment with minocycline). Products include:
Activella 2561
Angeliq 831
Climara 841
Climara Pro 847
Divigel 3467
Estrasorb 1777
Vagifem 2589

Estrogens, Conjugated (In a multi-center study to evaluate the effect of minocycline on low dose oral contraceptives, hormone levels over one menstrual cycle with and without minocycline 1 mg/kg once-daily were measured. Based on the results of this trial, minocycline-related changes in estradiol, progestinic hormone, FSH and LH plasma levels, of breakthrough bleeding, or of contraceptive failure, can not be ruled out. To avoid contraceptive failure, female patients are advised to use a second form of contraceptive during treatment with minocycline). Products include:
Premarin Intravenous 3528
Premarin Tablets 3533
Premarin Vaginal Cream 3540
Premphase 3549
Prempro 3549

Estrogens, Esterified (In a multi-center study to evaluate the effect of minocycline on low dose oral contraceptives, hormone levels over one menstrual cycle with and without minocycline 1 mg/kg once-daily were measured. Based on the results of this trial, minocycline-related changes in estradiol, progestinic hormone, FSH and LH plasma levels, of breakthrough bleeding, or of contraceptive failure, can not be ruled out. To avoid contraceptive failure, female patients are advised to use a second form of contraceptive during treatment with minocycline).
No products indexed under this heading.

Estropipate (In a multi-center study to evaluate the effect of minocycline on low dose oral contraceptives, hormone levels over one menstrual cycle with and without minocycline 1 mg/kg once-daily were measured. Based on the results of this trial, minocycline-related changes in estradiol, progestinic hormone, FSH and LH plasma levels, of breakthrough bleeding, or of contraceptive failure, can not be ruled out. To avoid contraceptive failure, female patients are advised to use a second form of contraceptive during treatment with minocycline).
No products indexed under this heading.

Ethinyl Estradiol (In a multi-center study to evaluate the effect of minocycline on low dose oral contraceptives, hormone levels over one menstrual cycle with and without minocycline 1 mg/kg once-daily were measured. Based on the results of this trial, minocycline-related changes in estradiol, progestinic hormone, FSH and LH plasma levels, of breakthrough bleeding, or of contraceptive failure, can not be ruled out. To avoid contraceptive failure, female patients are advised to use a second form of contraceptive during treatment with minocycline). Products include:
LoSeasonique 3407
Lybrel 3514
NuvaRing 3181
Ortho Evra 2648
Ortho-Cyclen/Ortho Tri-Cyclen 2663
Ortho Tri-Cyclen Lo Tablets 2673
Seasonique 3418
Yaz 864

Ethynodiol Diacetate (In a multi-center study to evaluate the effect of minocycline on low dose oral contraceptives, hormone levels over one menstrual cycle with and without minocycline 1 mg/kg once-daily were measured. Based on the results of this trial, minocycline-related changes in estradiol, progestinic hormone, FSH and LH plasma levels, of breakthrough bleeding, or of contraceptive failure, can not be ruled out. To avoid contraceptive failure, female patients are advised to use a second form of contraceptive during treatment with minocycline).
No products indexed under this heading.

Ferrous Fumarate (Absorption of tetracyclines is impaired by iron-containing preparations). Products include:
PreNexa 3473

Ferrous Gluconate (Absorption of tetracyclines is impaired by iron-containing preparations). Products include:
CitraNatal Assure 2332
CitraNatal Rx 2332

Ferrous Sulfate (Absorption of tetracyclines is impaired by iron-containing preparations).
No products indexed under this heading.

Fondaparinux Sodium (Because tetracyclines have been shown to depress plasma prothrombin activity, patients who are on anticoagulant therapy may require downward adjustment of their anticoagulant dosage). Products include:
Arixtra 1320

Heparin Calcium (Because tetracyclines have been shown to depress plasma prothrombin activity, patients who are on anticoagulant therapy may require downward adjustment of their anticoagulant dosage).
No products indexed under this heading.

Heparin Sodium (Because tetracyclines have been shown to depress plasma prothrombin activity, patients who are on anticoagulant therapy may require downward adjustment of their anticoagulant dosage).
No products indexed under this heading.

Iron (Absorption of tetracyclines is impaired by iron-containing preparations).
No products indexed under this heading.

Iron, Peptonized (Absorption of tetracyclines is impaired by iron-containing preparations).
No products indexed under this heading.

Iron Cacodylate (Absorption of tetracyclines is impaired by iron-containing preparations).
No products indexed under this heading.

Iron Carbonyl (Absorption of tetracyclines is impaired by iron-containing preparations). Products include:
CitraNatal 90 DHA Capsules 2332
CitraNatal Assure 2332
CitraNatal Harmony 2332
CitraNatal Rx 2332
Ferralet 2333

Iron Dextran (Absorption of tetracyclines is impaired by iron-containing preparations).
No products indexed under this heading.

Iron Polysaccharide Complex (Absorption of tetracyclines is impaired by iron-containing preparations).
No products indexed under this heading.

Iron Sucrose (Absorption of tetracyclines is impaired by iron-containing preparations).
No products indexed under this heading.

Iron Supplements (Absorption of tetracyclines is impaired by iron-containing preparations).
No products indexed under this heading.

Isotretinoin (Concomitant use of isotretinoin and minocycline should be avoided because isotretinoin, a systemic retinoid, is also known to cause pseudotumor cerebri). Products include:
Accutane 2832

Levonorgestrel (In a multi-center study to evaluate the effect of minocycline on low dose oral contraceptives, hormone levels over one menstrual cycle with and without minocycline 1 mg/kg once-daily were measured. Based on the results of this trial, minocycline-related changes in estradiol, progestinic hormone, FSH and LH plasma levels, of breakthrough bleeding, or of contraceptive failure, can not be ruled out. To avoid contraceptive failure, female patients are advised to use a second form of contraceptive during treatment with minocycline). Products include:
Climara Pro 847
LoSeasonique 3407
Lybrel 3514
Mirena 854
Plan B 3416
Seasonique 3418

Low Molecular Weight Heparins (Because tetracyclines have been shown to depress plasma prothrombin activity, patients who are on anticoagulant therapy may require downward adjustment of their anticoagulant dosage).
No products indexed under this heading.

Magaldrate (Absorption of tetracyclines is impaired by antacids containing aluminum, calcium, or magnesium).
No products indexed under this heading.

Magnesium Carbonate (Absorption of tetracyclines is impaired by antacids containing aluminum, calcium, or magnesium).
No products indexed under this heading.

Magnesium Hydroxide (Absorption of tetracyclines is impaired by antacids containing aluminum, calcium, or magnesium). Products include:
Fleet Pedia-Lax Chewable Tablets 1144
Pepcid Complete 1822

Magnesium Oxide (Absorption of tetracyclines is impaired by antacids containing aluminum, calcium, or magnesium). Products include:
Beelith 873

Magnesium Trisilicate (Absorption of tetracyclines is impaired by antacids containing aluminum, calcium, or magnesium).
No products indexed under this heading.

Medroxyprogesterone Acetate (In a multi-center study to evaluate the effect of minocycline on low dose oral contraceptives, hormone levels over one menstrual cycle with and without minocycline 1 mg/kg once-daily were measured. Based on the results of this trial, minocycline-related changes in estradiol, progestinic hormone, FSH and LH plasma levels, of breakthrough bleeding, or of contraceptive failure, can not be ruled out. To avoid contraceptive failure, female patients are advised to use a second form of contraceptive during treatment with minocycline). Products include:
Premphase 3549
Prempro 3549

Megestrol Acetate (In a multi-center study to evaluate the effect of minocycline on low dose oral contraceptives, hormone levels over one menstrual cycle with and without minocycline 1 mg/kg once-daily were measured. Based on the results of this trial, minocycline-related changes in estradiol, progestinic hormone, FSH and LH plasma levels, of breakthrough bleeding, or of contraceptive failure, can not be ruled out. To avoid contraceptive failure, female patients are advised to use a second form of contraceptive during treatment with minocycline). Products include:
Megace ES 2698

Mestranol (In a multi-center study to evaluate the effect of minocycline on low dose oral contraceptives, hormone levels over one menstrual cycle with and without minocycline 1 mg/kg once-daily were measured. Based on the results of this trial, minocycline-related changes in estradiol, progestinic hormone, FSH and LH plasma levels, of breakthrough bleeding, or of contraceptive failure, can not be ruled out. To avoid contraceptive failure, female patients are advised to use a second form of contraceptive during treatment with minocycline).
No products indexed under this heading.

Methicillin Sodium (Since bacteriostatic drugs may interfere with the bactericidal action of penicillin, it is advisable to avoid giving tetracycline-class drugs in conjunction with penicillin).
No products indexed under this heading.

Methoxyflurane (The concurrent use of tetracycline and methoxyflurane has been reported to result in fatal renal toxicity).
No products indexed under this heading.

Mezlocillin Sodium (Since bacteriostatic drugs may interfere with the bactericidal action of penicillin, it is advisable to avoid giving tetracycline-class drugs in conjunction with penicillin).
No products indexed under this heading.

Nafcillin Sodium (Since bacteriostatic drugs may interfere with the bactericidal action of penicillin, it is advisable to avoid giving tetracycline-class drugs in conjunction with penicillin).
No products indexed under this heading.

Norethindrone (In a multi-center study to evaluate the effect of minocycline on low dose oral contraceptives, hormone levels over one menstrual cycle with and without minocycline 1 mg/kg once-daily were measured. Based on the results of this trial, minocycline-related changes in estradiol, progestinic hormone, FSH and LH plasma levels, of breakthrough bleeding, or of contraceptive failure, can not be ruled out. To avoid contraceptive failure, female

IMPORTANT NOTE: Always consult each drug listing in the patient's regimen for possible interactions.

1773 Interactions Index Stalevo

Wine products (Clinical evidence has shown that etretinate can be formed with concurrent ingestion of acitretin and ethanol).

SPIRIVA HANDIHALER

(Tiotropium Bromide) 893
May interact with anticholinergics, and certain other agents. Compounds in these categories include:

Atropine Sulfate (Co-administration of tiotropium with other anticholinergic-containing drugs (eg, ipratropium) has not been studied and is, therefore, not recommended). Products include:
Donnatal 2711

Belladonna Alkaloids (Co-administration of tiotropium with other anticholinergic-containing drugs (eg, ipratropium) has not been studied and is, therefore, not recommended). Products include:
Hyland's Teething Tablets 3316

Benztropine Mesylate (Co-administration of tiotropium with other anticholinergic-containing drugs (eg, ipratropium) has not been studied and is, therefore, not recommended).
No products indexed under this heading.

Biperiden Hydrochloride (Co-administration of tiotropium with other anticholinergic-containing drugs (eg, ipratropium) has not been studied and is, therefore, not recommended).
No products indexed under this heading.

Cimetidine (Concomitant administration of cimetidine with tiotropium resulted in a 20% increase in the $AUC_{0\text{-}4h}$, a 28% increase in the renal clearance of tiotropium and no significant change in the C_{max} and amount excreted in urine over 96 hours. Therefore, no clinically significant interaction occurred between tiotropium and cimetidine).
No products indexed under this heading.

Cimetidine Hydrochloride (Concomitant administration of cimetidine with tiotropium resulted in a 20% increase in the $AUC_{0\text{-}4h}$, a 28% increase in the renal clearance of tiotropium and no significant change in the C_{max} and amount excreted in urine over 96 hours. Therefore, no clinically significant interaction occurred between tiotropium and cimetidine).
No products indexed under this heading.

Clidinium Bromide (Co-administration of tiotropium with other anticholinergic-containing drugs (eg, ipratropium) has not been studied and is, therefore, not recommended).
No products indexed under this heading.

Dicyclomine Hydrochloride (Co-administration of tiotropium with other anticholinergic-containing drugs (eg, ipratropium) has not been studied and is, therefore, not recommended).
Products include:
Bentyl Capsules 780
Bentyl Injection 780
Bentyl Syrup 780
Bentyl Tablets 780

Glycopyrrolate (Co-administration of tiotropium with other anticholinergic-containing drugs (eg, ipratropium) has not been studied and is, therefore, not recommended).
No products indexed under this heading.

Hyoscyamine (Co-administration of tiotropium with other anticholinergic-containing drugs (eg, ipratropium) has not been studied and is, therefore, not recommended).
No products indexed under this heading.

Hyoscyamine Sulfate (Co-administration of tiotropium with other anticholinergic-containing drugs (eg, ipratropium) has not been studied and is, therefore, not recommended).
Products include:
Donnatal 2711

Ipratropium Bromide (Co-administration of tiotropium with other anticholinergic-containing drugs (eg, ipratropium) has not been studied and is, therefore, not recommended).
No products indexed under this heading.

Mepenzolate Bromide (Co-administration of tiotropium with other anticholinergic-containing drugs (eg, ipratropium) has not been studied and is, therefore, not recommended).
No products indexed under this heading.

Oxybutynin Chloride (Co-administration of tiotropium with other anticholinergic-containing drugs (eg, ipratropium) has not been studied and is, therefore, not recommended).
No products indexed under this heading.

Procyclidine Hydrochloride (Co-administration of tiotropium with other anticholinergic-containing drugs (eg, ipratropium) has not been studied and is, therefore, not recommended).
No products indexed under this heading.

Propantheline Bromide (Co-administration of tiotropium with other anticholinergic-containing drugs (eg, ipratropium) has not been studied and is, therefore, not recommended).
No products indexed under this heading.

Ranitidine Bismuth Citrate (An interaction study with tiotropium (14.4 mcg intravenous infusion over 15 minutes) and ranitidine 300 mg once daily was conducted).
No products indexed under this heading.

Ranitidine Hydrochloride (An interaction study with tiotropium (14.4 mcg intravenous infusion over 15 minutes) and ranitidine 300 mg once daily was conducted). Products include:
Zantac 1737
Zantac Injection 1732
Zantac Pharmacy 1735

Scopolamine (Co-administration of tiotropium with other anticholinergic-containing drugs (eg, ipratropium) has not been studied and is, therefore, not recommended). Products include:
Transderm Scōp 2397

Scopolamine Hydrobromide (Co-administration of tiotropium with other anticholinergic-containing drugs (eg, ipratropium) has not been studied and is, therefore, not recommended).
Products include:
Donnatal 2711

Tolterodine Tartrate (Co-administration of tiotropium with other anticholinergic-containing drugs (eg, ipratropium) has not been studied and is, therefore, not recommended).
No products indexed under this heading.

Tridihexethyl Chloride (Co-administration of tiotropium with other anticholinergic-containing drugs (eg, ipratropium) has not been studied and is, therefore, not recommended).
No products indexed under this heading.

Trihexyphenidyl Hydrochloride (Co-administration of tiotropium with other anticholinergic-containing drugs (eg, ipratropium) has not been studied and is, therefore, not recommended).
No products indexed under this heading.

SPRINGCODE SPRAY

(Sheep Placenta) 607
None cited in PDR database.

STALEVO TABLETS

(Carbidopa, Entacapone, Levodopa) 2526
May interact with ampicillins, antihypertensives, chloramphenicol, dopamine D2 antagonists, drugs metabolized by catechol-O-methyltransferase, erythromycin, iron containing oral preparations, monoamine oxidase inhibitors, phenytoin, tricyclic antidepressants, and certain other agents. Compounds in these categories include:

Acebutolol Hydrochloride (Symptomatic postural hypotension has occurred when carbidopa-levodopa was added to the treatment of a patient receiving antihypertensive drugs).
No products indexed under this heading.

Aliskiren (Symptomatic postural hypotension has occurred when carbidopa-levodopa was added to the treatment of a patient receiving antihypertensive drugs). Products include:
Tekturna 2538
Tekturna HCT 2541
Valturna 3637

Amitriptyline Hydrochloride (There have been rare reports of adverse reactions, including hypertension and dyskinesia, resulting from the concomitant use of tricylic antidepressants and carbidopa-levodopa).
No products indexed under this heading.

Amlodipine Besylate (Symptomatic postural hypotension has occurred when carbidopa-levodopa was added to the treatment of a patient receiving antihypertensive drugs). Products include:
Azor 1010
Exforge 2443
Exforge HCT 2449

Amoxapine (There have been rare reports of adverse reactions, including hypertension and dyskinesia, resulting from the concomitant use of tricylic antidepressants and carbidopa-levodopa).
No products indexed under this heading.

Ampicillin (As most entacapone excretion is via the bile, caution should be exercised when drugs known to interfere with biliary excretion, glucuronidation, and intestinal β-glucuronidase are given concurrently with entacapone).
No products indexed under this heading.

Ampicillin Sodium (As most entacapone excretion is via the bile, caution should be exercised when drugs known to interfere with biliary excretion, glucuronidation, and intestinal β-glucuronidase are given concurrently with entacapone).
No products indexed under this heading.

Ampicillin Trihydrate (As most entacapone excretion is via the bile, caution should be exercised when drugs known to interfere with biliary excretion, glucuronidation, and intestinal β-glucuronidase are given concurrently with entacapone).
No products indexed under this heading.

Apomorphine (Drugs known to be metabolized by Catechol-O-methytransferase should be administered with caution in patients receiving entacapone regardless of the route of administration (including inhalation), as their interaction may result in increased heart rates, possibly arrhythmias, and excessive changes in blood pressure).
No products indexed under this heading.

Atenolol (Symptomatic postural hypotension has occurred when carbidopa-levodopa was added to the treatment of a patient receiving antihypertensive drugs).
No products indexed under this heading.

Bacampicillin Hydrochloride (As most entacapone excretion is via the bile, caution should be exercised when drugs known to interfere with biliary excretion, glucuronidation, and intestinal β-glucuronidase are given concurrently with entacapone).
No products indexed under this heading.

Benazepril Hydrochloride (Symptomatic postural hypotension has occurred when carbidopa-levodopa was added to the treatment of a patient receiving antihypertensive drugs).
No products indexed under this heading.

Bendroflumethiazide (Symptomatic postural hypotension has occurred when carbidopa-levodopa was added to the treatment of a patient receiving antihypertensive drugs).
No products indexed under this heading.

Betaxolol Hydrochloride (Symptomatic postural hypotension has occurred when carbidopa-levodopa was added to the treatment of a patient receiving antihypertensive drugs).
No products indexed under this heading.

Bisoprolol Fumarate (Symptomatic postural hypotension has occurred when carbidopa-levodopa was added to the treatment of a patient receiving antihypertensive drugs).
No products indexed under this heading.

Bitolterol Mesylate (Drugs known to be metabolized by Catechol-O-methytransferase should be administered with caution in patients receiving entacapone regardless of the route of administration (including inhalation), as their interaction may result in increased heart rates, possibly arrhythmias, and excessive changes in blood pressure).
No products indexed under this heading.

Candesartan Cilexetil (Symptomatic postural hypotension has occurred when carbidopa-levodopa was added to the treatment of a patient receiving antihypertensive drugs). Products include:
Atacand 697
Atacand HCT 700

Captopril (Symptomatic postural hypotension has occurred when carbidopa-levodopa was added to the treatment of a patient receiving antihypertensive drugs). Products include:
Captopril 2341

Carteolol Hydrochloride (Symptomatic postural hypotension has occurred when carbidopa-levodopa was added to the treatment of a patient receiving antihypertensive drugs).
No products indexed under this heading.

Carvedilol (Symptomatic postural hypotension has occurred when carbidopa-levodopa was added to the treatment of a patient receiving antihypertensive drugs). Products include:
Coreg 1409

Carvedilol Phosphate (Symptomatic postural hypotension has occurred when carbidopa-levodopa was added to the treatment of a patient receiving antihypertensive drugs). Products include:
Coreg CR 1416

Chloramphenicol (As most entacapone excretion is via the bile, caution should be exercised when drugs known to interfere with biliary excretion, glucuronidation, and intestinal β-glucuronidase are given concurrently with entacapone).
No products indexed under this heading.

Chloramphenicol Palmitate (As most entacapone excretion is via the bile, caution should be exercised when drugs known to interfere with biliary excretion, glucuronidation, and intestinal β-glucuronidase are given concurrently with entacapone).
No products indexed under this heading.

Chloramphenicol Sodium Succinate (As most entacapone excretion is via the bile, caution should be exercised when drugs known to interfere with biliary excretion, glucuronidation, and intestinal β-glucuronidase are given concurrently with entacapone).
No products indexed under this heading.

Chlorothiazide (Symptomatic postural hypotension has occurred when carbidopa-levodopa was added to the treatment of a patient receiving antihypertensive drugs).
No products indexed under this heading.

Chlorothiazide Sodium (Symptomatic postural hypotension has occurred

IMPORTANT NOTE: Always consult each drug listing in the patient's regimen for possible interactions.

Stalevo Interactions Index 1774

when carbidopa-levodopa was added to the treatment of a patient receiving antihypertensive drugs). Products include:
Diuril Intravenous 2009

Chlorpromazine (Dopamine D2 receptor antagonists may reduce the therapeutic effects of levodopa).
No products indexed under this heading.

Chlorpromazine Hydrochloride (Dopamine D2 receptor antagonists may reduce the therapeutic effects of levodopa).
No products indexed under this heading.

Chlorprothixene (Dopamine D2 receptor antagonists may reduce the therapeutic effects of levodopa).
No products indexed under this heading.

Chlorprothixene Hydrochloride (Dopamine D2 receptor antagonists may reduce the therapeutic effects of levodopa).
No products indexed under this heading.

Chlorthalidone (Symptomatic postural hypotension has occurred when carbidopa-levodopa was added to the treatment of a patient receiving antihypertensive drugs). Products include:
Clorpres 2344

Cholestyramine (As most entacapone excretion is via the bile, caution should be exercised when drugs known to interfere with biliary excretion, glucuronidation, and intestinal β-glucuronidase are given concurrently with entacapone).
No products indexed under this heading.

Clomipramine Hydrochloride (There have been rare reports of adverse reactions, including hypertension and dyskinesia, resulting from the concomitant use of tricylic antidepressants and carbidopa-levodopa).
No products indexed under this heading.

Clonidine (Symptomatic postural hypotension has occurred when carbidopa-levodopa was added to the treatment of a patient receiving antihypertensive drugs). Products include:
Catapres-TTS 884

Clonidine Hydrochloride (Symptomatic postural hypotension has occurred when carbidopa-levodopa was added to the treatment of a patient receiving antihypertensive drugs). Products include:
Clorpres 2344

Deserpidine (Symptomatic postural hypotension has occurred when carbidopa-levodopa was added to the treatment of a patient receiving antihypertensive drugs).
No products indexed under this heading.

Desipramine Hydrochloride (There have been rare reports of adverse reactions, including hypertension and dyskinesia, resulting from the concomitant use of tricyclic antidepressants and carbidopa-levodopa).
No products indexed under this heading.

Diazoxide (Symptomatic postural hypotension has occurred when carbidopa-levodopa was added to the treatment of a patient receiving antihypertensive drugs). Products include:
Proglycem 1179
Proglycem Suspension 1179

Diltiazem Hydrochloride (Symptomatic postural hypotension has occurred when carbidopa-levodopa was added to the treatment of a patient receiving antihypertensive drugs). Products include:
Cardizem LA 423

Diltiazem Maleate (Symptomatic postural hypotension has occurred when carbidopa-levodopa was added to the treatment of a patient receiving antihypertensive drugs).
No products indexed under this heading.

Dobutamine Hydrochloride (Drugs known to be metabolized by Catechol-O-methyltransferase should be administered with caution in patients receiving entacapone regardless of the route of administration (including inhalation), as their interaction may result in increased heart rates, possibly arrhythmias, and excessive changes in blood pressure).
No products indexed under this heading.

Dopamine Hydrochloride (Drugs known to be metabolized by Catechol-O-methyltransferase should be administered with caution in patients receiving entacapone regardless of the route of administration (including inhalation), as their interaction may result in increased heart rates, possibly arrhythmias, and excessive changes in blood pressure).
No products indexed under this heading.

Doxazosin Mesylate (Symptomatic postural hypotension has occurred when carbidopa-levodopa was added to the treatment of a patient receiving antihypertensive drugs).
No products indexed under this heading.

Doxepin Hydrochloride (There have been rare reports of adverse reactions, including hypertension and dyskinesia, resulting from the concomitant use of tricylic antidepressants and carbidopa-levodopa).
No products indexed under this heading.

Enalapril Maleate (Symptomatic postural hypotension has occurred when carbidopa-levodopa was added to the treatment of a patient receiving antihypertensive drugs).
No products indexed under this heading.

Enalaprilat (Symptomatic postural hypotension has occurred when carbidopa-levodopa was added to the treatment of a patient receiving antihypertensive drugs).
No products indexed under this heading.

Epinephrine (Drugs known to be metabolized by Catechol-O-methyltransferase should be administered with caution in patients receiving entacapone regardless of the route of administration (including inhalation), as their interaction may result in increased heart rates, possibly arrhythmias, and excessive changes in blood pressure). Products include:
EpiPen 3631
Twinject 3268

Epinephrine Bitartrate (Drugs known to be metabolized by Catechol-O-methyltransferase should be administered with caution in patients receiving entacapone regardless of the route of administration (including inhalation), as their interaction may result in increased heart rates, possibly arrhythmias, and excessive changes in blood pressure).
No products indexed under this heading.

Epinephrine Hydrochloride (Drugs known to be metabolized by Catechol-O-methyltransferase should be administered with caution in patients receiving entacapone regardless of the route of administration (including inhalation), as their interaction may result in increased heart rates, possibly arrhythmias, and excessive changes in blood pressure).
No products indexed under this heading.

Eprosartan Mesylate (Symptomatic postural hypotension has occurred when carbidopa-levodopa was added to the treatment of a patient receiving antihypertensive drugs). Products include:
Teveten 538
Teveten HCT 541

Erythromycin (As most entacapone excretion is via the bile, caution should be exercised when drugs known to interfere with biliary excretion, glucuronidation, and intestinal β-glucuronidase are given concurrently with entacapone).
No products indexed under this heading.

Erythromycin, Topical (As most entacapone excretion is via the bile, caution should be exercised when drugs known to interfere with biliary excretion, glucuronidation, and intestinal β-glucuronidase are given concurrently with entacapone).
No products indexed under this heading.

Erythromycin Estolate (As most entacapone excretion is via the bile, caution should be exercised when drugs known to interfere with biliary excretion, glucuronidation, and intestinal β-glucuronidase are given concurrently with entacapone).
No products indexed under this heading.

Erythromycin Ethylsuccinate (As most entacapone excretion is via the bile, caution should be exercised when drugs known to interfere with biliary excretion, glucuronidation, and intestinal β-glucuronidase are given concurrently with entacapone). Products include:
E.E.S. 437
EryPed 435

Erythromycin Gluceptate (As most entacapone excretion is via the bile, caution should be exercised when drugs known to interfere with biliary excretion, glucuronidation, and intestinal β-glucuronidase are given concurrently with entacapone).
No products indexed under this heading.

Erythromycin Lactobionate (As most entacapone excretion is via the bile, caution should be exercised when drugs known to interfere with biliary excretion, glucuronidation, and intestinal β-glucuronidase are given concurrently with entacapone).
No products indexed under this heading.

Erythromycin Stearate (As most entacapone excretion is via the bile, caution should be exercised when drugs known to interfere with biliary excretion, glucuronidation, and intestinal β-glucuronidase are given concurrently with entacapone).
No products indexed under this heading.

Esmolol Hydrochloride (Symptomatic postural hypotension has occurred when carbidopa-levodopa was added to the treatment of a patient receiving antihypertensive drugs).
No products indexed under this heading.

Ethylpapaverine Hydrochloride (The beneficial effects of levodopa in Parkinson's disease have been reported to be reversed by papaverine).
No products indexed under this heading.

Felodipine (Symptomatic postural hypotension has occurred when carbidopa-levodopa was added to the treatment of a patient receiving antihypertensive drugs).
No products indexed under this heading.

Ferrous Fumarate (Iron salts may reduce the bioavailability of levodopa, carbidopa and entacapone). Products include:
PreNexa 3473

Ferrous Gluconate (Iron salts may reduce the bioavailability of levodopa, carbidopa and entacapone). Products include:
CitraNatal Assure 2332
CitraNatal Rx 2332

Ferrous Sulfate (Iron salts may reduce the bioavailability of levodopa, carbidopa and entacapone).
No products indexed under this heading.

Fluphenazine Decanoate (Dopamine D2 receptor antagonists may reduce the therapeutic effects of levodopa).
No products indexed under this heading.

Fluphenazine Enanthate (Dopamine D2 receptor antagonists may reduce the therapeutic effects of levodopa).
No products indexed under this heading.

Fluphenazine Hydrochloride (Dopamine D2 receptor antagonists may reduce the therapeutic effects of levodopa).
No products indexed under this heading.

Fosinopril Sodium (Symptomatic postural hypotension has occurred when carbidopa-levodopa was added to the treatment of a patient receiving antihypertensive drugs).
No products indexed under this heading.

Fosphenytoin (The beneficial effects of levodopa in Parkinson's disease have been reported to be reversed by phenytoin).
No products indexed under this heading.

Fosphenytoin Sodium (The beneficial effects of levodopa in Parkinson's disease have been reported to be reversed by phenytoin).
No products indexed under this heading.

Furosemide (Symptomatic postural hypotension has occurred when carbidopa-levodopa was added to the treatment of a patient receiving antihypertensive drugs). Products include:
Furosemide 2354

Guanabenz Acetate (Symptomatic postural hypotension has occurred when carbidopa-levodopa was added to the treatment of a patient receiving antihypertensive drugs).
No products indexed under this heading.

Guanethidine (Symptomatic postural hypotension has occurred when carbidopa-levodopa was added to the treatment of a patient receiving antihypertensive drugs).
No products indexed under this heading.

Guanethidine Monosulfate (Symptomatic postural hypotension has occurred when carbidopa-levodopa was added to the treatment of a patient receiving antihypertensive drugs).
No products indexed under this heading.

Guanethidine Sulfate (Symptomatic postural hypotension has occurred when carbidopa-levodopa was added to the treatment of a patient receiving antihypertensive drugs).
No products indexed under this heading.

Haloperidol (Dopamine D2 receptor antagonists may reduce the therapeutic effects of levodopa).
No products indexed under this heading.

Haloperidol Decanoate (Dopamine D2 receptor antagonists may reduce the therapeutic effects of levodopa).
No products indexed under this heading.

Hydralazine Hydrochloride (Symptomatic postural hypotension has occurred when carbidopa-levodopa was added to the treatment of a patient receiving antihypertensive drugs).
No products indexed under this heading.

Hydrochlorothiazide (Symptomatic postural hypotension has occurred when carbidopa-levodopa was added to the treatment of a patient receiving antihypertensive drugs). Products include:
Atacand HCT 700
Avalide 2956
Benicar HCT 1017
Diovan HCT 2419
Dyazide 1429
Exforge HCT 2449
Hyzaar 2162
Hyzaar 100-12.5 2162
Micardis HCT 889
Prinzide 2246

IMPORTANT NOTE: Always consult each drug listing in the patient's regimen for possible interactions.

Stalevo Interactions Index 1776

Probenecid (As most entacapone excretion is via the bile, caution should be exercised when drugs known to interfere with biliary excretion, glucuronidation, and intestinal β-glucuronidase are given concurrently with entacapone).
No products indexed under this heading.

Procarbazine Hydrochloride (Nonselective monoamine oxidase (MAO) inhibitors are contraindicated for use with Stalevo).
No products indexed under this heading.

Prochlorperazine (Dopamine D2 receptor antagonists may reduce the therapeutic effects of levodopa).
No products indexed under this heading.

Promethazine Hydrochloride (Dopamine D2 receptor antagonists may reduce the therapeutic effects of levodopa).
No products indexed under this heading.

Propranolol Hydrochloride (Symptomatic postural hypotension has occurred when carbidopa-levodopa was added to the treatment of a patient receiving antihypertensive drugs). Products include:
InnoPran XL 1517

Protriptyline Hydrochloride (There have been rare reports of adverse reactions, including hypertension and dyskinesia, resulting from the concomitant use of tricylic antidepressants and carbidopa-levodopa).
No products indexed under this heading.

Pyridoxine (Stalevo can be given to patients receiving supplemental pyridoxine. Oral co-administration of 10-25 mg of pyridoxine hydrochloride (vitamin B6) with levodopa may reverse the effects of levodopa by increasing the rate of aromatic amino acid decarboxylation. Carbidopa inhibits this action of pyridoxine; therefore, Stalevo can be given to patients receiving supplemental pyridoxine).
No products indexed under this heading.

Pyridoxine Hydrochloride (Stalevo can be given to patients receiving supplemental pyridoxine. Oral co-administration of 10-25 mg of pyridoxine hydrochloride (vitamin B6) with levodopa may reverse the effects of levodopa by increasing the rate of aromatic amino acid decarboxylation. Carbidopa inhibits this action of pyridoxine; therefore, Stalevo can be given to patients receiving supplemental pyridoxine).
No products indexed under this heading.

Quetiapine Fumarate (Dopamine D2 receptor antagonists may reduce the therapeutic effects of levodopa). Products include:
Seroquel 750
Seroquel XR 759

Quinapril Hydrochloride (Symptomatic postural hypotension has occurred when carbidopa-levodopa was added to the treatment of a patient receiving antihypertensive drugs).
No products indexed under this heading.

Ramipril (Symptomatic postural hypotension has occurred when carbidopa-levodopa was added to the treatment of a patient receiving antihypertensive drugs).
No products indexed under this heading.

Rasagiline Mesylate (Nonselective monoamine oxidase (MAO) inhibitors are contraindicated for use with Stalevo). Products include:
Azilect 3383

Rauwolfia Serpentina (Symptomatic postural hypotension has occurred when carbidopa-levodopa was added to the treatment of a patient receiving antihypertensive drugs).
No products indexed under this heading.

Rescinnamine (Symptomatic postural hypotension has occurred when carbidopa-levodopa was added to the treatment of a patient receiving antihypertensive drugs).
No products indexed under this heading.

Reserpine (Symptomatic postural hypotension has occurred when carbidopa-levodopa was added to the treatment of a patient receiving antihypertensive drugs).
No products indexed under this heading.

Rifampicin (As most entacapone excretion is via the bile, caution should be exercised when drugs known to interfere with biliary excretion, glucuronidation, and intestinal β-glucuronidase are given concurrently with entacapone).
No products indexed under this heading.

Risperidone (Dopamine D2 receptor antagonists may reduce the therapeutic effects of levodopa). Products include:
Risperdal Consta 2682

Selegiline (Nonselective monoamine oxidase (MAO) inhibitors are contraindicated for use with Stalevo). Products include:
Emsam 3623

Selegiline Hydrochloride (Nonselective monoamine oxidase (MAO) inhibitors are contraindicated for use with Stalevo). Products include:
Eldepryl 3312

Sodium Nitroprusside (Symptomatic postural hypotension has occurred when carbidopa-levodopa was added to the treatment of a patient receiving antihypertensive drugs).
No products indexed under this heading.

Sotalol Hydrochloride (Symptomatic postural hypotension has occurred when carbidopa-levodopa was added to the treatment of a patient receiving antihypertensive drugs).
No products indexed under this heading.

Spirapril Hydrochloride (Symptomatic postural hypotension has occurred when carbidopa-levodopa was added to the treatment of a patient receiving antihypertensive drugs).
No products indexed under this heading.

Telmisartan (Symptomatic postural hypotension has occurred when carbidopa-levodopa was added to the treatment of a patient receiving antihypertensive drugs). Products include:
Micardis 887
Micardis HCT 889

Terazosin Hydrochloride (Symptomatic postural hypotension has occurred when carbidopa-levodopa was added to the treatment of a patient receiving antihypertensive drugs).
No products indexed under this heading.

Thioridazine Hydrochloride (Dopamine D2 receptor antagonists may reduce the therapeutic effects of levodopa). Products include:
Thioridazine Hydrochloride 2384

Thiothixene (Dopamine D2 receptor antagonists may reduce the therapeutic effects of levodopa). Products include:
Thiothixene 2386

Thiothixene Hydrochloride (Dopamine D2 receptor antagonists may reduce the therapeutic effects of levodopa).
No products indexed under this heading.

Thioxanthene Derivatives (Dopamine D2 receptor antagonists may reduce the therapeutic effects of levodopa).
No products indexed under this heading.

Timolol Maleate (Symptomatic postural hypotension has occurred when carbidopa-levodopa was added to the treatment of a patient receiving antihypertensive drugs). Products include:
Combigan 601
Dorzolamide Hydrochloride/Timolol Maleate Ophthalmic Solution .... ⊙243
Timoptic in Ocudose .... ⊙231

Torsemide (Symptomatic postural hypotension has occurred when carbidopa-levodopa was added to the treatment of a patient receiving antihypertensive drugs).
No products indexed under this heading.

Trandolapril (Symptomatic postural hypotension has occurred when carbidopa-levodopa was added to the treatment of a patient receiving antihypertensive drugs). Products include:
Mavik 489
Tarka 534

Tranylcypromine Sulfate (Nonselective monoamine oxidase (MAO) inhibitors are contraindicated for use with Stalevo). Products include:
Parnate 1584

Trifluoperazine Hydrochloride (Dopamine D2 receptor antagonists may reduce the therapeutic effects of levodopa).
No products indexed under this heading.

Trimethaphan Camsylate (Symptomatic postural hypotension has occurred when carbidopa-levodopa was added to the treatment of a patient receiving antihypertensive drugs).
No products indexed under this heading.

Trimipramine Maleate (There have been rare reports of adverse reactions, including hypertension and dyskinesia, resulting from the concomitant use of tricylic antidepressants and carbidopa-levodopa).
No products indexed under this heading.

Valsartan (Symptomatic postural hypotension has occurred when carbidopa-levodopa was added to the treatment of a patient receiving antihypertensive drugs). Products include:
Diovan 2413
Diovan HCT 2419
Exforge 2443
Exforge HCT 2449
Valturna 3637

Verapamil Hydrochloride (Symptomatic postural hypotension has occurred when carbidopa-levodopa was added to the treatment of a patient receiving antihypertensive drugs). Products include:
Tarka 534

STRATTERA CAPSULES

(Atomoxetine Hydrochloride) 1957
May interact with beta-adrenergic stimulating agents, cytochrome p450 2d6 inhibitors (selected), monoamine oxidase inhibitors, quinidine, vasopressors, and certain other agents. Compounds in these categories include:

Albuterol (Atomoxetine hydrochloride should be administered with caution to patients being treated with systemically-administered (oral or intravenous) albuterol (or other β_2 agonists) because the action of albuterol on the cardiovascular system can be potentiated resulting in increases in heart rate and blood pressure. Albuterol (600 mcg IV over 2 hours) increases heart rate and blood pressure. These effects were potentiated by atomoxetine (60 mg BID for 5 days) and were most marked after the initial co-administration of albuterol and atomoxetine. However, these effects on heart rate and blood pressure were not seen in another study after the co-administration with inhaled dose of albuterol (200-800 mcg) and atomoxetine (80 mg QD for 5 days) in 21 healthy Asian subjects who were excluded for poor metabolizer status).
No products indexed under this heading.

Albuterol Sulfate (Atomoxetine hydrochloride should be administered with caution to patients being treated with systemically-administered (oral or intravenous) albuterol (or other β_2 agonists) because the action of albuterol on the cardiovascular system can be potentiated resulting in increases in heart rate and blood pressure. Albuterol (600 mcg IV over 2 hours) increases heart rate and blood pressure. These effects were potentiated by atomoxetine (60 mg BID for 5 days) and were most marked after the initial co-administration of albuterol and atomoxetine. However, these effects on heart rate and blood pressure were not seen in another study after the co-administration with inhaled dose of albuterol (200-800 mcg) and atomoxetine (80 mg QD for 5 days) in 21 healthy Asian subjects who were excluded for poor metabolizer status). Products include:
ProAir HFA 3393
Proventil HFA 3204
Ventolin HFA 1708

Amiodarone Hydrochloride (In extensive metabolizers (EMs), inhibitors of CYP2D6 (eg, paroxetine, fluoxetine, and quinidine) increase atomoxetine steady–state plasma concentrations to exposures similar to those observed in poor metabolizers (PMs)).
No products indexed under this heading.

Amitriptyline Hydrochloride (In extensive metabolizers (EMs), inhibitors of CYP2D6 (eg, paroxetine, fluoxetine, and quinidine) increase atomoxetine steady–state plasma concentrations to exposures similar to those observed in poor metabolizers (PMs)).
No products indexed under this heading.

Amoxapine (In extensive metabolizers (EMs), inhibitors of CYP2D6 (eg, paroxetine, fluoxetine, and quinidine) increase atomoxetine steady–state plasma concentrations to exposures similar to those observed in poor metabolizers (PMs)).
No products indexed under this heading.

Bitolterol Mesylate (Atomoxetine hydrochloride should be administered with caution to patients being treated with systemically-administered (oral or intravenous) albuterol (or other β_2 agonists) because the action of albuterol on the cardiovascular system can be potentiated resulting in increases in heart rate and blood pressure).
No products indexed under this heading.

Bupropion Hydrochloride (In extensive metabolizers (EMs), inhibitors of CYP2D6 (eg, paroxetine, fluoxetine, and quinidine) increase atomoxetine steady–state plasma concentrations to exposures similar to those observed in poor metabolizers (PMs)). Products include:
Aplenzin 2948
Wellbutrin 1719
Wellbutrin SR 1725
Zyban 1762

Celecoxib (In extensive metabolizers (EMs), inhibitors of CYP2D6 (eg, paroxetine, fluoxetine, and quinidine) increase atomoxetine steady–state plasma concentrations to exposures similar to those observed in poor metabolizers (PMs)). Products include:
Celebrex 3272

Chloroquine (In extensive metabolizers (EMs), inhibitors of CYP2D6 (eg, paroxetine, fluoxetine, and quinidine) increase atomoxetine steady–state plasma concentrations to exposures similar to those observed in poor metabolizers (PMs)).
No products indexed under this heading.

(⊙ Described in PDR® for Ophthalmic Medicines)

Chloroquine Hydrochloride (In extensive metabolizers (EMs), inhibitors of CYP2D6 (eg, paroxetine, fluoxetine, and quinidine) increase atomoxetine steady–state plasma concentrations to exposures similar to those observed in poor metabolizers (PMs)).
No products indexed under this heading.

Chloroquine Phosphate (In extensive metabolizers (EMs), inhibitors of CYP2D6 (eg, paroxetine, fluoxetine, and quinidine) increase atomoxetine steady–state plasma concentrations to exposures similar to those observed in poor metabolizers (PMs)).
No products indexed under this heading.

Chlorpheniramine (In extensive metabolizers (EMs), inhibitors of CYP2D6 (eg, paroxetine, fluoxetine, and quinidine) increase atomoxetine steady–state plasma concentrations to exposures similar to those observed in poor metabolizers (PMs)).
No products indexed under this heading.

Chlorpheniramine Maleate (In extensive metabolizers (EMs), inhibitors of CYP2D6 (eg, paroxetine, fluoxetine, and quinidine) increase atomoxetine steady–state plasma concentrations to exposures similar to those observed in poor metabolizers (PMs)).
No products indexed under this heading.

Chlorpheniramine Polistirex (In extensive metabolizers (EMs), inhibitors of CYP2D6 (eg, paroxetine, fluoxetine, and quinidine) increase atomoxetine steady–state plasma concentrations to exposures similar to those observed in poor metabolizers (PMs)). Products include:
Tussionex 3443

Chlorpheniramine Tannate (In extensive metabolizers (EMs), inhibitors of CYP2D6 (eg, paroxetine, fluoxetine, and quinidine) increase atomoxetine steady–state plasma concentrations to exposures similar to those observed in poor metabolizers (PMs)).
No products indexed under this heading.

Cimetidine (In extensive metabolizers (EMs), inhibitors of CYP2D6 (eg, paroxetine, fluoxetine, and quinidine) increase atomoxetine steady–state plasma concentrations to exposures similar to those observed in poor metabolizers (PMs)).
No products indexed under this heading.

Cimetidine Hydrochloride (In extensive metabolizers (EMs), inhibitors of CYP2D6 (eg, paroxetine, fluoxetine, and quinidine) increase atomoxetine steady–state plasma concentrations to exposures similar to those observed in poor metabolizers (PMs)).
No products indexed under this heading.

Citalopram Hydrobromide (In extensive metabolizers (EMs), inhibitors of CYP2D6 (eg, paroxetine, fluoxetine, and quinidine) increase atomoxetine steady–state plasma concentrations to exposures similar to those observed in poor metabolizers (PMs)). Products include:
Celexa 1153

Clomipramine Hydrochloride (In extensive metabolizers (EMs), inhibitors of CYP2D6 (eg, paroxetine, fluoxetine, and quinidine) increase atomoxetine steady–state plasma concentrations to exposures similar to those observed in poor metabolizers (PMs)).
No products indexed under this heading.

Cocaine Hydrochloride (In extensive metabolizers (EMs), inhibitors of CYP2D6 (eg, paroxetine, fluoxetine, and quinidine) increase atomoxetine steady–state plasma concentrations to exposures similar to those observed in poor metabolizers (PMs)).
No products indexed under this heading.

Desipramine Hydrochloride (In extensive metabolizers (EMs), inhibitors of CYP2D6 (eg, paroxetine, fluoxetine, and quinidine) increase atomoxetine steady–state plasma concentrations to exposures similar to those observed in poor metabolizers (PMs)).
No products indexed under this heading.

Diphenhydramine (In extensive metabolizers (EMs), inhibitors of CYP2D6 (eg, paroxetine, fluoxetine, and quinidine) increase atomoxetine steady–state plasma concentrations to exposures similar to those observed in poor metabolizers (PMs)).
No products indexed under this heading.

Diphenhydramine Hydrochloride (In extensive metabolizers (EMs), inhibitors of CYP2D6 (eg, paroxetine, fluoxetine, and quinidine) increase atomoxetine steady–state plasma concentrations to exposures similar to those observed in poor metabolizers (PMs)). Products include:
Benadryl Allergy Ultratab 2042
Children's Benadryl Allergy Liquid 2042

Dobutamine (Because of possible effects on blood pressure, atomoxetine hydrochloride should be used cautiously with pressor agents (eg, dobutamine)).
No products indexed under this heading.

Dobutamine Hydrochloride (Because of possible effects on blood pressure, atomoxetine hydrochloride should be used cautiously with pressor agents (eg, dobutamine)).
No products indexed under this heading.

Dopamine Hydrochloride (Because of possible effects on blood pressure, atomoxetine hydrochloride should be used cautiously with pressor agents (eg, dopamine)).
No products indexed under this heading.

Doxepin Hydrochloride (In extensive metabolizers (EMs), inhibitors of CYP2D6 (eg, paroxetine, fluoxetine, and quinidine) increase atomoxetine steady–state plasma concentrations to exposures similar to those observed in poor metabolizers (PMs)).
No products indexed under this heading.

Ephedrine Hydrochloride (Atomoxetine hydrochloride should be administered with caution to patients being treated with systemically-administered (oral or intravenous) albuterol (or other β_2 agonists) because the action of albuterol on the cardiovascular system can be potentiated resulting in increases in heart rate and blood pressure).
No products indexed under this heading.

Ephedrine Sulfate (Atomoxetine hydrochloride should be administered with caution to patients being treated with systemically-administered (oral or intravenous) albuterol (or other β_2 agonists) because the action of albuterol on the cardiovascular system can be potentiated resulting in increases in heart rate and blood pressure).
No products indexed under this heading.

Ephedrine Tannate (Atomoxetine hydrochloride should be administered with caution to patients being treated with systemically-administered (oral or intravenous) albuterol (or other β_2 agonists) because the action of albuterol on the cardiovascular system can be potentiated resulting in increases in heart rate and blood pressure).
No products indexed under this heading.

Epinephrine (Atomoxetine hydrochloride should be administered with caution to patients being treated with systemically-administered (oral or intravenous) albuterol (or other β_2 agonists) because the action of albuterol on the cardiovascular system can be potentiated resulting in increases in heart rate and blood pressure). Products include:

EpiPen 3631
Twinject 3268

Epinephrine Bitartrate (Because of possible effects on blood pressure, atomoxetine hydrochloride should be used cautiously with pressor agents (eg, dopamine, dobutamine)).
No products indexed under this heading.

Epinephrine Hydrochloride (Atomoxetine hydrochloride should be administered with caution to patients being treated with systemically-administered (oral or intravenous) albuterol (or other β_2 agonists) because the action of albuterol on the cardiovascular system can be potentiated resulting in increases in heart rate and blood pressure).
No products indexed under this heading.

Escitalopram Oxalate (In extensive metabolizers (EMs), inhibitors of CYP2D6 (eg, paroxetine, fluoxetine, and quinidine) increase atomoxetine steady–state plasma concentrations to exposures similar to those observed in poor metabolizers (PMs)). Products include:
Lexapro Oral Suspension 1160
Lexapro Tablets 1160

Fat (Atomoxetine hydrochloride can be administered with or without food. Administration of atomoxetine with a standard high–fat meal in adults did not affect the extent of oral absorption of atomoxetine (AUC), but did decrease the rate of absorption, resulting in a 37% lower C_{max}, and delayed T_{max} by 3 hours. In clinical trials with children and adolescents, administration of atomoxetine with food resulted in a 9% lower C_{max}).
No products indexed under this heading.

Fluoxetine (In extensive metabolizers (EMs), inhibitors of CYP2D6 (eg, fluoxetine) increase atomoxetine steady–state plasma concentrations to exposures similar to those observed in poor metabolizers (PMs). In EM individuals treated with fluoxetine, the AUC of atomoxetine is approximately 6– to 8–fold and C is about 3– to 4– fold greater than atomoxetine alone).
No products indexed under this heading.

Fluoxetine Hydrochloride (In extensive metabolizers (EMs), inhibitors of CYP2D6 (eg, fluoxetine) increase atomoxetine steady–state plasma concentrations to exposures similar to those observed in poor metabolizers (PMs). In EM individuals treated with fluoxetine, the AUC of atomoxetine is approximately 6– to 8–fold and C is about 3– to 4–fold greater than atomoxetine alone). Products include:
Prozac Weekly 1941
Prozac Pulvules 1941
Symbyax 1965

Fluphenazine Decanoate (In extensive metabolizers (EMs), inhibitors of CYP2D6 (eg, paroxetine, fluoxetine, and quinidine) increase atomoxetine steady–state plasma concentrations to exposures similar to those observed in poor metabolizers (PMs)).
No products indexed under this heading.

Fluphenazine Enanthate (In extensive metabolizers (EMs), inhibitors of CYP2D6 (eg, paroxetine, fluoxetine, and quinidine) increase atomoxetine steady–state plasma concentrations to exposures similar to those observed in poor metabolizers (PMs)).
No products indexed under this heading.

Fluphenazine Hydrochloride (In extensive metabolizers (EMs), inhibitors of CYP2D6 (eg, paroxetine, fluoxetine, and quinidine) increase atomoxetine steady–state plasma concentrations to exposures similar to those observed in poor metabolizers (PMs)).
No products indexed under this heading.

Fluvoxamine Maleate (In extensive metabolizers (EMs), inhibitors of CYP2D6 (eg, paroxetine, fluoxetine, and quinidine) increase atomoxetine steady–state plasma concentrations to exposures similar to those observed in poor metabolizers (PMs)).
No products indexed under this heading.

Halofantrine Hydrochloride (In extensive metabolizers (EMs), inhibitors of CYP2D6 (eg, paroxetine, fluoxetine, and quinidine) increase atomoxetine steady–state plasma concentrations to exposures similar to those observed in poor metabolizers (PMs)).
No products indexed under this heading.

Haloperidol (In extensive metabolizers (EMs), inhibitors of CYP2D6 (eg, paroxetine, fluoxetine, and quinidine) increase atomoxetine steady–state plasma concentrations to exposures similar to those observed in poor metabolizers (PMs)).
No products indexed under this heading.

Haloperidol Decanoate (In extensive metabolizers (EMs), inhibitors of CYP2D6 (eg, paroxetine, fluoxetine, and quinidine) increase atomoxetine steady–state plasma concentrations to exposures similar to those observed in poor metabolizers (PMs)).
No products indexed under this heading.

Haloperidol Lactate (In extensive metabolizers (EMs), inhibitors of CYP2D6 (eg, paroxetine, fluoxetine, and quinidine) increase atomoxetine steady–state plasma concentrations to exposures similar to those observed in poor metabolizers (PMs)).
No products indexed under this heading.

Hydroxychloroquine Sulfate (In extensive metabolizers (EMs), inhibitors of CYP2D6 (eg, paroxetine, fluoxetine, and quinidine) increase atomoxetine steady–state plasma concentrations to exposures similar to those observed in poor metabolizers (PMs)).
No products indexed under this heading.

Imatinib Mesylate (In extensive metabolizers (EMs), inhibitors of CYP2D6 (eg, paroxetine, fluoxetine, and quinidine) increase atomoxetine steady–state plasma concentrations to exposures similar to those observed in poor metabolizers (PMs)). Products include:
Gleevec 2477

Imipramine Hydrochloride (In extensive metabolizers (EMs), inhibitors of CYP2D6 (eg, paroxetine, fluoxetine, and quinidine) increase atomoxetine steady–state plasma concentrations to exposures similar to those observed in poor metabolizers (PMs)).
No products indexed under this heading.

Imipramine Pamoate (In extensive metabolizers (EMs), inhibitors of CYP2D6 (eg, paroxetine, fluoxetine, and quinidine) increase atomoxetine steady–state plasma concentrations to exposures similar to those observed in poor metabolizers (PMs)).
No products indexed under this heading.

Isocarboxazid (Atomoxetine hydrochloride is contraindicated with an MAOI, or within 2 weeks after discontinuing an MAOI. Treatment with an MAOI should not be initiated within 2 weeks after discontinuing atomoxetine hydrochloride. With other drugs that affect brain monoamine concentrations, there have been reports of serious, sometimes fatal reactions (including hyperthermia, rigidity, myoclonus, autonomic instability with possible rapid fluctuations of vital signs, and mental status changes that include extreme agitation progressing to delirium and coma) when taken in combination with an MAOI. Some cases presented with features resembling neuroleptic malignant syndrome. Such reactions may

IMPORTANT NOTE: Always consult each drug listing in the patient's regimen for possible interactions.

occur when these drugs are given concurrently or in close proximity). Products include:

Marplan **3481**

Isoetharine (Atomoxetine hydrochloride should be administered with caution to patients being treated with systemically-administered (oral or intravenous) albuterol (or other β_2 agonists) because the action of albuterol on the cardiovascular system can be potentiated resulting in increases in heart rate and blood pressure).

No products indexed under this heading.

Isoproterenol Hydrochloride (Atomoxetine hydrochloride should be administered with caution to patients being treated with systemically-administered (oral or intravenous) albuterol (or other β_2 agonists) because the action of albuterol on the cardiovascular system can be potentiated resulting in increases in heart rate and blood pressure).

No products indexed under this heading.

Isoproterenol Sulfate (Atomoxetine hydrochloride should be administered with caution to patients being treated with systemically-administered (oral or intravenous) albuterol (or other β_2 agonists) because the action of albuterol on the cardiovascular system can be potentiated resulting in increases in heart rate and blood pressure).

No products indexed under this heading.

Levalbuterol Hydrochloride (Atomoxetine hydrochloride should be administered with caution to patients being treated with systemically-administered (oral or intravenous) albuterol (or other β_2 agonists) because the action of albuterol on the cardiovascular system can be potentiated resulting in increases in heart rate and blood pressure).

No products indexed under this heading.

Maprotiline Hydrochloride (In extensive metabolizers (EMs), inhibitors of CYP2D6 (eg, paroxetine, fluoxetine, and quinidine) increase atomoxetine steady–state plasma concentrations to exposures similar to those observed in poor metabolizers (PMs)).

No products indexed under this heading.

Mephentermine Sulfate (Because of possible effects on blood pressure, atomoxetine hydrochloride should be used cautiously with pressor agents (eg, dopamine, dobutamine)).

No products indexed under this heading.

Metaproterenol Sulfate (Atomoxetine hydrochloride should be administered with caution to patients being treated with systemically-administered (oral or intravenous) albuterol (or other β_2 agonists) because the action of albuterol on the cardiovascular system can be potentiated resulting in increases in heart rate and blood pressure).

No products indexed under this heading.

Metaraminol Bitartrate (Because of possible effects on blood pressure, atomoxetine hydrochloride should be used cautiously with pressor agents (eg, dopamine, dobutamine)).

No products indexed under this heading.

Methadone Hydrochloride (In extensive metabolizers (EMs), inhibitors of CYP2D6 (eg, paroxetine, fluoxetine, and quinidine) increase atomoxetine steady–state plasma concentrations to exposures similar to those observed in poor metabolizers (PMs)).

No products indexed under this heading.

Methoxamine Hydrochloride (Because of possible effects on blood pressure, atomoxetine hydrochloride should be used cautiously with pressor agents (eg, dopamine, dobutamine)).

No products indexed under this heading.

Mibefradil Dihydrochloride (In extensive metabolizers (EMs), inhibitors of CYP2D6 (eg, paroxetine, fluoxetine, and quinidine) increase atomoxetine steady–state plasma concentrations to exposures similar to those observed in poor metabolizers (PMs)).

No products indexed under this heading.

Midazolam Hydrochloride (Co-administration of atomoxetine hydrochloride (60 mg BID for 12 days) with midazolam, a model compound for CYP3A4 metabolized drugs (single dose of 5 mg), resulted in 15% increase in AUC of midazolam. No dose adjustment is recommended for drugs metabolized CYP3A).

No products indexed under this heading.

Moclobemide (Atomoxetine hydrochloride is contraindicated with an MAOI, or within 2 weeks after discontinuing an MAOI. Treatment with an MAOI should not be initiated within 2 weeks after discontinuing atomoxetine hydrochloride. With other drugs that affect brain monoamine concentrations, there have been reports of serious, sometimes fatal reactions (including hyperthermia, rigidity, myoclonus, autonomic instability with possible rapid fluctuations of vital signs, and mental status changes that include extreme agitation progressing to delirium and coma) when taken in combination with an MAOI. Some cases presented with features resembling neuroleptic malignant syndrome. Such reactions may occur when these drugs are given concurrently or in close proximity).

No products indexed under this heading.

Norepinephrine Bitartrate (Because of possible effects on blood pressure, atomoxetine hydrochloride should be used cautiously with pressor agents (eg, dopamine, dobutamine)).

No products indexed under this heading.

Nortriptyline Hydrochloride (In extensive metabolizers (EMs), inhibitors of CYP2D6 (eg, paroxetine, fluoxetine, and quinidine) increase atomoxetine steady–state plasma concentrations to exposures similar to those observed in poor metabolizers (PMs)).

No products indexed under this heading.

Pargyline Hydrochloride (Atomoxetine hydrochloride is contraindicated with an MAOI, or within 2 weeks after discontinuing an MAOI. Treatment with an MAOI should not be initiated within 2 weeks after discontinuing atomoxetine hydrochloride. With other drugs that affect brain monoamine concentrations, there have been reports of serious, sometimes fatal reactions (including hyperthermia, rigidity, myoclonus, autonomic instability with possible rapid fluctuations of vital signs, and mental status changes that include extreme agitation progressing to delirium and coma) when taken in combination with an MAOI. Some cases presented with features resembling neuroleptic malignant syndrome. Such reactions may occur when these drugs are given concurrently or in close proximity).

No products indexed under this heading.

Paroxetine (In extensive metabolizers (EMs), inhibitors of CYP2D6 (eg, paroxetine) increase atomoxetine steady–state plasma concentrations to exposures similar to those observed in poor metabolizers (PMs). In EM individuals treated with paroxetine, the AUC of atomoxetine is approximately 6– to 8–fold and C is about 3– to 4– fold greater than atomoxetine alone).

No products indexed under this heading.

Paroxetine Hydrochloride (In extensive metabolizers (EMs), inhibitors of CYP2D6 (eg, paroxetine) increase atomoxetine steady–state plasma concentrations to exposures similar to those observed in poor metabolizers (PMs). In EM individuals treated with paroxetine, the AUC of atomoxetine is approximately 6– to 8–fold and C is about 3– to 4– fold greater than atomoxetine alone). Products include:

Paroxetine CR **2361**
Paroxetine ER **2371**
Paxil **1586**
Paxil CR **1596**

Paroxetine Mesylate (In extensive metabolizers (EMs), inhibitors of CYP2D6 (eg, paroxetine) increase atomoxetine steady–state plasma concentrations to exposures similar to those observed in poor metabolizers (PMs). In EM individuals treated with paroxetine, the AUC of atomoxetine is approximately 6– to 8–fold and C is about 3– to 4– fold greater than atomoxetine alone).

No products indexed under this heading.

Perphenazine (In extensive metabolizers (EMs), inhibitors of CYP2D6 (eg, paroxetine, fluoxetine, and quinidine) increase atomoxetine steady–state plasma concentrations to exposures similar to those observed in poor metabolizers (PMs)).

No products indexed under this heading.

Phenelzine Sulfate (Atomoxetine hydrochloride is contraindicated with an MAOI, or within 2 weeks after discontinuing an MAOI. Treatment with an MAOI should not be initiated within 2 weeks after discontinuing atomoxetine hydrochloride. With other drugs that affect brain monoamine concentrations, there have been reports of serious, sometimes fatal reactions (including hyperthermia, rigidity, myoclonus, autonomic instability with possible rapid fluctuations of vital signs, and mental status changes that include extreme agitation progressing to delirium and coma) when taken in combination with an MAOI. Some cases presented with features resembling neuroleptic malignant syndrome. Such reactions may occur when these drugs are given concurrently or in close proximity).

No products indexed under this heading.

Phenylephrine Hydrochloride (Because of possible effects on blood pressure, atomoxetine hydrochloride should be used cautiously with pressor agents (eg, dopamine, dobutamine)). Products include:

Sudafed PE Nasal Decongestant **2048**
Children's Sudafed PE Nasal Decongestant **2047**

Pirbuterol Acetate (Atomoxetine hydrochloride should be administered with caution to patients being treated with systemically-administered (oral or intravenous) albuterol (or other β_2 agonists) because the action of albuterol on the cardiovascular system can be potentiated resulting in increases in heart rate and blood pressure). Products include:

Maxair Autohaler **1782**

Procarbazine Hydrochloride (Atomoxetine hydrochloride is contraindicated with an MAOI, or within 2 weeks after discontinuing an MAOI. Treatment with an MAOI should not be initiated within 2 weeks after discontinuing atomoxetine hydrochloride. With other drugs that affect brain monoamine concentrations, there have been reports of serious, sometimes fatal reactions (including hyperthermia, rigidity, myoclonus, autonomic instability with possible rapid fluctuations of vital signs, and mental status changes that include extreme agitation progressing to delirium and coma) when taken in combination with an MAOI. Some cases presented with features resembling neuroleptic malignant syndrome. Such reactions may occur when these drugs are given concurrently or in close proximity).

No products indexed under this heading.

Propafenone Hydrochloride (In extensive metabolizers (EMs), inhibitors of CYP2D6 (eg, paroxetine, fluoxetine, and quinidine) increase atomoxetine steady–state plasma concentrations to exposures similar to those observed in poor metabolizers (PMs)). Products include:

Rythmol **1648**
Rythmol SR **1652**

Propoxyphene Hydrochloride (In extensive metabolizers (EMs), inhibitors of CYP2D6 (eg, paroxetine, fluoxetine, and quinidine) increase atomoxetine steady–state plasma concentrations to exposures similar to those observed in poor metabolizers (PMs)).

No products indexed under this heading.

Propoxyphene Napsylate (In extensive metabolizers (EMs), inhibitors of CYP2D6 (eg, paroxetine, fluoxetine, and quinidine) increase atomoxetine steady–state plasma concentrations to exposures similar to those observed in poor metabolizers (PMs)).

No products indexed under this heading.

Protriptyline Hydrochloride (In extensive metabolizers (EMs), inhibitors of CYP2D6 (eg, paroxetine, fluoxetine, and quinidine) increase atomoxetine steady–state plasma concentrations to exposures similar to those observed in poor metabolizers (PMs)).

No products indexed under this heading.

Quinacrine Hydrochloride (In extensive metabolizers (EMs), inhibitors of CYP2D6 (eg, paroxetine, fluoxetine, and quinidine) increase atomoxetine steady–state plasma concentrations to exposures similar to those observed in poor metabolizers (PMs)).

No products indexed under this heading.

Quinidine (In extensive metabolizers (EMs), inhibitors of CYP2D6 (eg, paroxetine, fluoxetine, and quinidine) increase atomoxetine steady–state plasma concentrations to exposures similar to those observed in poor metabolizers (PMs)).

No products indexed under this heading.

Quinidine Gluconate (In extensive metabolizers (EMs), inhibitors of CYP2D6 (eg, paroxetine, fluoxetine, and quinidine) increase atomoxetine steady–state plasma concentrations to exposures similar to those observed in poor metabolizers (PMs)).

No products indexed under this heading.

Quinidine Hydrochloride (In extensive metabolizers (EMs), inhibitors of CYP2D6 (eg, paroxetine, fluoxetine, and quinidine) increase atomoxetine steady–state plasma concentrations to exposures similar to those observed in poor metabolizers (PMs)).

No products indexed under this heading.

Quinidine Polygalacturonate (In extensive metabolizers (EMs), inhibitors of CYP2D6 (eg, paroxetine, fluoxetine, and quinidine) increase atomoxetine steady–state plasma concentrations to exposures similar to those observed in poor metabolizers (PMs)).

No products indexed under this heading.

Quinidine Sulfate (In extensive metabolizers (EMs), inhibitors of CYP2D6 (eg, paroxetine, fluoxetine, and quinidine) increase atomoxetine steady–state plasma concentrations to exposures similar to those observed in poor metabolizers (PMs)).

No products indexed under this heading.

Ranitidine Bismuth Citrate (In extensive metabolizers (EMs), inhibitors of CYP2D6 (eg, paroxetine, fluoxetine, and quinidine) increase atomoxetine steady–state plasma concentrations to exposures similar to those observed in poor metabolizers (PMs)).

No products indexed under this heading.

Ranitidine Hydrochloride (In extensive metabolizers (EMs), inhibitors of

CYP2D6 (eg, paroxetine, fluoxetine, and quinidine) increase atomoxetine steady–state plasma concentrations to exposures similar to those observed in poor metabolizers (PMs)). Products include:

Rasagiline Mesylate (Atomoxetine hydrochloride is contraindicated with an MAOI, or within 2 weeks after discontinuing an MAOI. Treatment with an MAOI should not be initiated within 2 weeks after discontinuing atomoxetine hydrochloride. With other drugs that affect brain monoamine concentrations, there have been reports of serious, sometimes fatal reactions (including hyperthermia, rigidity, myoclonus, autonomic instability with possible rapid fluctuations of vital signs, and mental status changes that include extreme agitation progressing to delirium and coma) when taken in combination with an MAOI. Some cases presented with features resembling neuroleptic malignant syndrome. Such reactions may occur when these drugs are given concurrently or in close proximity). Products include:

Ritonavir (In extensive metabolizers (EMs), inhibitors of CYP2D6 (eg, paroxetine, fluoxetine, and quinidine) increase atomoxetine steady–state plasma concentrations to exposures similar to those observed in poor metabolizers (PMs)). Products include:

Salmeterol Xinafoate (Atomoxetine hydrochloride should be administered with caution to patients being treated with systemically-administered (oral or intravenous) albuterol (or other β_2 agonists) because the action of albuterol on the cardiovascular system can be potentiated resulting in increases in heart rate and blood pressure). Products include:

Selegiline (Atomoxetine hydrochloride is contraindicated with an MAOI, or within 2 weeks after discontinuing an MAOI. Treatment with an MAOI should not be initiated within 2 weeks after discontinuing atomoxetine hydrochloride. With other drugs that affect brain monoamine concentrations, there have been reports of serious, sometimes fatal reactions (including hyperthermia, rigidity, myoclonus, autonomic instability with possible rapid fluctuations of vital signs, and mental status changes that include extreme agitation progressing to delirium and coma) when taken in combination with an MAOI. Some cases presented with features resembling neuroleptic malignant syndrome. Such reactions may occur when these drugs are given concurrently or in close proximity). Products include:

Selegiline Hydrochloride (Atomoxetine hydrochloride is contraindicated with an MAOI, or within 2 weeks after discontinuing an MAOI. Treatment with an MAOI should not be initiated within 2 weeks after discontinuing atomoxetine hydrochloride. With other drugs that affect brain monoamine concentrations, there have been reports of serious, sometimes fatal reactions (including hyperthermia, rigidity, myoclonus, autonomic instability with possible rapid fluctuations of vital signs, and mental status changes that include extreme

agitation progressing to delirium and coma) when taken in combination with an MAOI. Some cases presented with features resembling neuroleptic malignant syndrome. Such reactions may occur when these drugs are given concurrently or in close proximity). Products include:

Sertraline Hydrochloride (In extensive metabolizers (EMs), inhibitors of CYP2D6 (eg, paroxetine, fluoxetine, and quinidine) increase atomoxetine steady–state plasma concentrations to exposures similar to those observed in poor metabolizers (PMs)).

No products indexed under this heading.

Sildenafil Citrate (In extensive metabolizers (EMs), inhibitors of CYP2D6 (eg, paroxetine, fluoxetine, and quinidine) increase atomoxetine steady–state plasma concentrations to exposures similar to those observed in poor metabolizers (PMs)).

No products indexed under this heading.

Terbinafine Hydrochloride (In extensive metabolizers (EMs), inhibitors of CYP2D6 (eg, paroxetine, fluoxetine, and quinidine) increase atomoxetine steady–state plasma concentrations to exposures similar to those observed in poor metabolizers (PMs)).

No products indexed under this heading.

Terbutaline Sulfate (Atomoxetine hydrochloride should be administered with caution to patients being treated with systemically-administered (oral or intravenous) albuterol (or other β_2 agonists) because the action of albuterol on the cardiovascular system can be potentiated resulting in increases in heart rate and blood pressure).

No products indexed under this heading.

Thioridazine Hydrochloride (In extensive metabolizers (EMs), inhibitors of CYP2D6 (eg, paroxetine, fluoxetine, and quinidine) increase atomoxetine steady–state plasma concentrations to exposures similar to those observed in poor metabolizers (PMs)). Products include:

Tranylcypromine Sulfate (Atomoxetine hydrochloride is contraindicated with an MAOI, or within 2 weeks after discontinuing an MAOI. Treatment with an MAOI should not be initiated within 2 weeks after discontinuing atomoxetine hydrochloride. With other drugs that affect brain monoamine concentrations, there have been reports of serious, sometimes fatal reactions (including hyperthermia, rigidity, myoclonus, autonomic instability with possible rapid fluctuations of vital signs, and mental status changes that include extreme agitation progressing to delirium and coma) when taken in combination with an MAOI. Some cases presented with features resembling neuroleptic malignant syndrome. Such reactions may occur when these drugs are given concurrently or in close proximity). Products include:

Trimipramine Maleate (In extensive metabolizers (EMs), inhibitors of CYP2D6 (eg, paroxetine, fluoxetine, and quinidine) increase atomoxetine steady–state plasma concentrations to exposures similar to those observed in poor metabolizers (PMs)).

No products indexed under this heading.

Vardenafil Hydrochloride (In extensive metabolizers (EMs), inhibitors of CYP2D6 (eg, paroxetine, fluoxetine, and quinidine) increase atomoxetine steady–state plasma concentrations to exposures similar to those observed in poor metabolizers (PMs)). Products include:

Food Interactions

Food, unspecified (Atomoxetine hydrochloride can be administered with or without food. Administration of atomoxetine with a standard high–fat meal in adults did not affect the extent of oral absorption of atomoxetine (AUC), but did decrease the rate of absorption, resulting in a 37% lower C_{max}, and delayed T_{max} by 3 hours. In clinical trials with children and adolescents, administration of atomoxetine with food resulted in a 9% lower C_{max}).

Meal, unspecified (Atomoxetine hydrochloride can be administered with or without food. Administration of atomoxetine with a standard high–fat meal in adults did not affect the extent of oral absorption of atomoxetine (AUC), but did decrease the rate of absorption, resulting in a 37% lower C_{max}, and delayed T_{max} by 3 hours. In clinical trials with children and adolescents, administration of atomoxetine with food resulted in a 9% lower C_{max}).

STROMECTOL TABLETS

Warfarin Sodium (Post-marketing reports of increased INR have been rarely reported when ivermectin was co-administered with warfarin).

No products indexed under this heading.

SUDAFED 12 HOUR NASAL DECONGESTANT NON-DROWSY CAPLETS

See Sudafed Nasal Decongestant Tablets

SUDAFED 24 HOUR NON-DROWSY NASAL DECONGESTANT TABLETS

See Sudafed Nasal Decongestant Tablets

SUDAFED NASAL DECONGESTANT TABLETS

May interact with monoamine oxidase inhibitors. Compounds in these categories include:

Isocarboxazid (Concurrent and/or sequential use with MAO inhibitors is not recommended). Products include:

Moclobemide (Concurrent and/or sequential use with MAO inhibitors is not recommended).

No products indexed under this heading.

Pargyline Hydrochloride (Concurrent and/or sequential use with MAO inhibitors is not recommended).

No products indexed under this heading.

Phenelzine Sulfate (Concurrent and/or sequential use with MAO inhibitors is not recommended).

No products indexed under this heading.

Procarbazine Hydrochloride (Concurrent and/or sequential use with MAO inhibitors is not recommended).

No products indexed under this heading.

Rasagiline Mesylate (Concurrent and/or sequential use with MAO inhibitors is not recommended). Products include:

Selegiline (Concurrent and/or sequential use with MAO inhibitors is not recommended). Products include:

Selegiline Hydrochloride (Concurrent and/or sequential use with MAO inhibitors is not recommended). Products include:

Tranylcypromine Sulfate (Concurrent and/or sequential use with MAO inhibitors is not recommended). Products include:

Eldepryl 3312

Tranylcypromine Sulfate (Concurrent and/or sequential use with MAO inhibitors is not recommended). Products include:

SUDAFED PE NASAL DECONGESTANT TABLETS

See Sudafed Nasal Decongestant Tablets

CHILDREN'S SUDAFED NASAL DECONGESTANT LIQUID

See Sudafed Nasal Decongestant Tablets

CHILDREN'S SUDAFED PE NASAL DECONGESTANT LIQUID

May interact with monoamine oxidase inhibitors. Compounds in these categories include:

Isocarboxazid (Concurrent and/or sequential use with MAO inhibitors is not recommended). Products include:

Moclobemide (Concurrent and/or sequential use with MAO inhibitors is not recommended).

No products indexed under this heading.

Pargyline Hydrochloride (Concurrent and/or sequential use with MAO inhibitors is not recommended).

No products indexed under this heading.

Phenelzine Sulfate (Concurrent and/or sequential use with MAO inhibitors is not recommended).

No products indexed under this heading.

Procarbazine Hydrochloride (Concurrent and/or sequential use with MAO inhibitors is not recommended).

No products indexed under this heading.

Rasagiline Mesylate (Concurrent and/or sequential use with MAO inhibitors is not recommended). Products include:

Selegiline (Concurrent and/or sequential use with MAO inhibitors is not recommended). Products include:

Selegiline Hydrochloride (Concurrent and/or sequential use with MAO inhibitors is not recommended). Products include:

SUDAFED OM SINUS CONGESTION MOISTURIZING NASAL SPRAY

None cited in PDR database.

SULFAMYLON CREAM

None cited in PDR database.

SULFAMYLON FOR 5% TOPICAL SOLUTION

None cited in PDR database.

SUPPRELIN LA IMPLANT

None cited in PDR database.

IMPORTANT NOTE: Always consult each drug listing in the patient's regimen for possible interactions.

Suprax | Interactions Index | 1780

SUPRAX FOR ORAL SUSPENSION
(Cefixime) 2038
May interact with anticoagulants, and certain other agents. Compounds in these categories include:

Anisindione (Increased prothrombin time, with or without clinical bleeding, has been reported when cefixime is administered concomitantly).
No products indexed under this heading.

Ardeparin Sodium (Increased prothrombin time, with or without clinical bleeding, has been reported when cefixime is administered concomitantly).
No products indexed under this heading.

Carbamazepine (Elevated carbamazepine levels have been reported in postmarketing experience when cefixime is administered concomitantly. Drug monitoring may be of assistance in detecting alterations in carbamazepine plasma concentrations). Products include:
Carbatrol 3280
Equetro 3477

Dalteparin Sodium (Increased prothrombin time, with or without clinical bleeding, has been reported when cefixime is administered concomitantly). Products include:
Fragmin 1058

Danaparoid Sodium (Increased prothrombin time, with or without clinical bleeding, has been reported when cefixime is administered concomitantly).
No products indexed under this heading.

Dicumarol (Increased prothrombin time, with or without clinical bleeding, has been reported when cefixime is administered concomitantly).
No products indexed under this heading.

Enoxaparin Sodium (Increased prothrombin time, with or without clinical bleeding, has been reported when cefixime is administered concomitantly). Products include:
Lovenox 3005

Fondaparinux Sodium (Increased prothrombin time, with or without clinical bleeding, has been reported when cefixime is administered concomitantly). Products include:
Arixtra 1320

Heparin Calcium (Increased prothrombin time, with or without clinical bleeding, has been reported when cefixime is administered concomitantly).
No products indexed under this heading.

Heparin Sodium (Increased prothrombin time, with or without clinical bleeding, has been reported when cefixime is administered concomitantly).
No products indexed under this heading.

Low Molecular Weight Heparins (Increased prothrombin time, with or without clinical bleeding, has been reported when cefixime is administered concomitantly).
No products indexed under this heading.

Tinzaparin Sodium (Increased prothrombin time, with or without clinical bleeding, has been reported when cefixime is administered concomitantly).
No products indexed under this heading.

Warfarin Sodium (Increased prothrombin time, with or without clinical bleeding, has been reported when cefixime is administered concomitantly).
No products indexed under this heading.

Food Interactions

Food, unspecified (Cefixime, given orally, is about 40% to 50% absorbed whether administered with or without food; however, time to maximal absorption is increased approximately 0.8 hours when administered with food).

SUPRAX TABLETS
(Cefixime) 2038
See Suprax for Oral Suspension

SUTENT CAPSULES
(Sunitinib Malate) 2747
May interact with antiarrhythmics, cytochrome p450 3a4 inducers (selected), cytochrome p450 3a4 inhibitors, potent (selected), and certain other agents. Compounds in these categories include:

Acebutolol Hydrochloride (Sunitinib has been shown to prolong QT interval in a dose dependent manner; caution is advised in patients taking sunitinib and antiarrhythmics concomittantly).
No products indexed under this heading.

Adenosine (Sunitinib has been shown to prolong QT interval in a dose dependent manner; caution is advised in patients taking sunitinib and antiarrhythmics concomittantly). Products include:
Adenocard 656
Adenoscan 657

Allium sativum (Concurrent administration of sunitinib with CYP3A4 inducers (eg, rifampin) may decrease plasma sunitinib concentrations. Dose increase of sunitinib to 87.5 mg daily should be considered with co-administration).
No products indexed under this heading.

Aminoglutethimide (Concurrent administration of sunitinib with CYP3A4 inducers (eg, rifampin) may decrease plasma sunitinib concentrations. Dose increase of sunitinib to 87.5 mg daily should be considered with co-administration).
No products indexed under this heading.

Amiodarone Hydrochloride (Sunitinib has been shown to prolong QT interval in a dose dependent manner; caution is advised in patients taking sunitinib and antiarrhythmics concomittantly).
No products indexed under this heading.

Amprenavir (Concurrent administration of sunitinib with strong CYP3A4 inhibitors (eg, ketoconazole) may increase sunitinib plasma concentrations. Dose reduction of sunitinib to 37.5 mg daily is recommended with co-administration).
No products indexed under this heading.

Aprepitant (Concurrent administration of sunitinib with CYP3A4 inducers (eg, rifampin) may decrease plasma sunitinib concentrations. Dose increase of sunitinib to 87.5 mg daily should be considered with co-administration). Products include:
Emend 2124

Atazanavir (Concurrent administration of sunitinib with strong CYP3A4 inhibitors (eg, ketoconazole) may increase sunitinib plasma concentrations. Dose reduction of sunitinib to 37.5 mg daily is recommended with co-administration).
No products indexed under this heading.

Atazanavir Sulfate (Concurrent administration of sunitinib with strong CYP3A4 inhibitors (eg, ketoconazole) may increase sunitinib plasma concentrations. Dose reduction of sunitinib to 37.5 mg daily is recommended with co-administration).
No products indexed under this heading.

Betamethasone (Concurrent administration of sunitinib with CYP3A4 inducers (eg, rifampin) may decrease plasma sunitinib concentrations. Dose increase of sunitinib to 87.5 mg daily should be considered with co-administration).
No products indexed under this heading.

Betamethasone Acetate (Concurrent administration of sunitinib with CYP3A4 inducers (eg, rifampin) may decrease plasma sunitinib concentrations. Dose increase of sunitinib to 87.5 mg daily should be considered with co-administration).
No products indexed under this heading.

Betamethasone Benzoate (Concurrent administration of sunitinib with CYP3A4 inducers (eg, rifampin) may decrease plasma sunitinib concentrations. Dose increase of sunitinib to 87.5 mg daily should be considered with co-administration).
No products indexed under this heading.

Betamethasone Dipropionate (Concurrent administration of sunitinib with CYP3A4 inducers (eg, rifampin) may decrease plasma sunitinib concentrations. Dose increase of sunitinib to 87.5 mg daily should be considered with co-administration). Products include:
Diprolene Lotion 0.05% 3108
Diprolene Ointment 0.05% 3109
Diprolene AF Cream 0.05% 3107
Lotrisone 3163

Betamethasone Sodium Phosphate (Concurrent administration of sunitinib with CYP3A4 inducers (eg, rifampin) may decrease plasma sunitinib concentrations. Dose increase of sunitinib to 87.5 mg daily should be considered with co-administration).
No products indexed under this heading.

Betamethasone Valerate (Concurrent administration of sunitinib with CYP3A4 inducers (eg, rifampin) may decrease plasma sunitinib concentrations. Dose increase of sunitinib to 87.5 mg daily should be considered with co-administration). Products include:
Luxíq 3321

Bosentan (Concurrent administration of sunitinib with CYP3A4 inducers (eg, rifampin) may decrease plasma sunitinib concentrations. Dose increase of sunitinib to 87.5 mg daily should be considered with co-administration). Products include:
Tracleer 573

Bretylium Tosylate (Sunitinib has been shown to prolong QT interval in a dose dependent manner; caution is advised in patients taking sunitinib and antiarrhythmics concomittantly).
No products indexed under this heading.

Carbamazepine (Concurrent administration of sunitinib with CYP3A4 inducers (eg, rifampin) may decrease plasma sunitinib concentrations. Dose increase of sunitinib to 87.5 mg daily should be considered with co-administration). Products include:
Carbatrol 3280
Equetro 3477

Ciprofloxacin (Concurrent administration of sunitinib with CYP3A4 inducers (eg, rifampin) may decrease plasma sunitinib concentrations. Dose increase of sunitinib to 87.5 mg daily should be considered with co-administration). Products include:
Cipro I.V. 3082
Cipro 3073
Cipro XR 3091
Ciprodex 583

Ciprofloxacin Hydrochloride (Concurrent administration of sunitinib with CYP3A4 inducers (eg, rifampin) may decrease plasma sunitinib concentrations. Dose increase of sunitinib to 87.5 mg daily should be considered with co-administration). Products include:
Cipro 3073

Cisplatin (Concurrent administration of sunitinib with CYP3A4 inducers (eg, rifampin) may decrease plasma sunitinib concentrations. Dose increase of sunitinib to 87.5 mg daily should be considered with co-administration).
No products indexed under this heading.

Clarithromycin (Concurrent administration of sunitinib with strong CYP3A4 inhibitors (eg, ketoconazole) may increase sunitinib plasma concentrations. Dose reduction of sunitinib to 37.5 mg daily is recommended with co-administration). Products include:
Biaxin/Biaxin XL 412

Cortisone Acetate (Concurrent administration of sunitinib with CYP3A4 inducers (eg, rifampin) may decrease plasma sunitinib concentrations. Dose increase of sunitinib to 87.5 mg daily should be considered with co-administration).
No products indexed under this heading.

Delavirdine Mesylate (Concurrent administration of sunitinib with strong CYP3A4 inhibitors (eg, ketoconazole) may increase sunitinib plasma concentrations. Dose reduction of sunitinib to 37.5 mg daily is recommended with co-administration).
No products indexed under this heading.

Delavirine (Concurrent administration of sunitinib with strong CYP3A4 inhibitors (eg, ketoconazole) may increase sunitinib plasma concentrations. Dose reduction of sunitinib to 37.5 mg daily is recommended with co-administration).
No products indexed under this heading.

Dexamethasone (Concurrent administration of sunitinib with CYP3A4 inducers (eg, rifampin) may decrease plasma sunitinib concentrations. Dose increase of sunitinib to 87.5 mg daily should be considered with co-administration). Products include:
Ciprodex 583
Ozurdex .... ⊙ 223
Tobramycin and Dexamethasone Ophthalmic Suspension .... ⊙ 251

Dexamethasone Acetate (Concurrent administration of sunitinib with CYP3A4 inducers (eg, rifampin) may decrease plasma sunitinib concentrations. Dose increase of sunitinib to 87.5 mg daily should be considered with co-administration).
No products indexed under this heading.

Dexamethasone Phosphate (Concurrent administration of sunitinib with CYP3A4 inducers (eg, rifampin) may decrease plasma sunitinib concentrations. Dose increase of sunitinib to 87.5 mg daily should be considered with co-administration).
No products indexed under this heading.

Dexamethasone Sodium (Concurrent administration of sunitinib with CYP3A4 inducers (eg, rifampin) may decrease plasma sunitinib concentrations. Dose increase of sunitinib to 87.5 mg daily should be considered with co-administration).
No products indexed under this heading.

Dexamethasone Sodium Phosphate (Concurrent administration of sunitinib with CYP3A4 inducers (eg, rifampin) may decrease plasma sunitinib concentrations. Dose increase of sunitinib to 87.5 mg daily should be considered with co-administration).
No products indexed under this heading.

Dexamethasone Sodium Phosphate Injection (Concurrent administration of sunitinib with CYP3A4 inducers (eg, rifampin) may decrease plasma sunitinib concentrations. Dose increase of sunitinib to 87.5 mg daily should be considered with co-administration).
No products indexed under this heading.

(⊙ Described in PDR® for Ophthalmic Medicines)

1781 **Interactions Index** **Sutent**

Disopyramide Phosphate (Sunitinib has been shown to prolong QT interval in a dose dependent manner; caution is advised in patients taking sunitinib and antiarrhythmics concomittantly).
No products indexed under this heading.

Dofetilide (Sunitinib has been shown to prolong QT interval in a dose dependent manner; caution is advised in patients taking sunitinib and antiarrhythmics concomittantly).
No products indexed under this heading.

Doxorubicin Hydrochloride (Concurrent administration of sunitinib with CYP3A4 inducers (eg, rifampin) may decrease plasma sunitinib concentrations. Dose increase of sunitinib to 87.5 mg daily should be considered with co-administration).
No products indexed under this heading.

Efavirenz (Concurrent administration of sunitinib with CYP3A4 inducers (eg, rifampin) may decrease plasma sunitinib concentrations. Dose increase of sunitinib to 87.5 mg daily should be considered with co-administration). Products include:
Atripla 906

Ethosuximide (Concurrent administration of sunitinib with CYP3A4 inducers (eg, rifampin) may decrease plasma sunitinib concentrations. Dose increase of sunitinib to 87.5 mg daily should be considered with co-administration).
No products indexed under this heading.

Felbamate (Concurrent administration of sunitinib with CYP3A4 inducers (eg, rifampin) may decrease plasma sunitinib concentrations. Dose increase of sunitinib to 87.5 mg daily should be considered with co-administration).
No products indexed under this heading.

Flecainide Acetate (Sunitinib has been shown to prolong QT interval in a dose dependent manner; caution is advised in patients taking sunitinib and antiarrhythmics concomittantly).
No products indexed under this heading.

Fludrocortisone Acetate (Concurrent administration of sunitinib with CYP3A4 inducers (eg, rifampin) may decrease plasma sunitinib concentrations. Dose increase of sunitinib to 87.5 mg daily should be considered with co-administration).
No products indexed under this heading.

Fosamprenavir Calcium (Concurrent administration of sunitinib with strong CYP3A4 inhibitors (eg, ketoconazole) may increase sunitinib plasma concentrations. Dose reduction of sunitinib to 37.5 mg daily is recommended with co-administration). Products include:
Lexiva Oral Suspension 1558
Lexiva 1558

Fosphenytoin Sodium (Concurrent administration of sunitinib with CYP3A4 inducers (eg, rifampin) may decrease plasma sunitinib concentrations. Dose increase of sunitinib to 87.5 mg daily should be considered with co-administration).
No products indexed under this heading.

Garlic Extract (Concurrent administration of sunitinib with CYP3A4 inducers (eg, rifampin) may decrease plasma sunitinib concentrations. Dose increase of sunitinib to 87.5 mg daily should be considered with co-administration).
No products indexed under this heading.

Garlic Oil (Concurrent administration of sunitinib with CYP3A4 inducers (eg, rifampin) may decrease plasma sunitinib concentrations. Dose increase of sunitinib to 87.5 mg daily should be considered with co-administration).
No products indexed under this heading.

Hydrocortisone (Concurrent administration of sunitinib with CYP3A4 inducers (eg, rifampin) may decrease plasma sunitinib concentrations. Dose increase of sunitinib to 87.5 mg daily should be considered with co-administration).
No products indexed under this heading.

Hydrocortisone (Alcohol) (Concurrent administration of sunitinib with CYP3A4 inducers (eg, rifampin) may decrease plasma sunitinib concentrations. Dose increase of sunitinib to 87.5 mg daily should be considered with co-administration).
No products indexed under this heading.

Hydrocortisone Acetate (Concurrent administration of sunitinib with CYP3A4 inducers (eg, rifampin) may decrease plasma sunitinib concentrations. Dose increase of sunitinib to 87.5 mg daily should be considered with co-administration).
No products indexed under this heading.

Hydrocortisone Butyrate (Concurrent administration of sunitinib with CYP3A4 inducers (eg, rifampin) may decrease plasma sunitinib concentrations. Dose increase of sunitinib to 87.5 mg daily should be considered with co-administration).
No products indexed under this heading.

Hydrocortisone Cypionate (Concurrent administration of sunitinib with CYP3A4 inducers (eg, rifampin) may decrease plasma sunitinib concentrations. Dose increase of sunitinib to 87.5 mg daily should be considered with co-administration).
No products indexed under this heading.

Hydrocortisone Hemisuccinate (Concurrent administration of sunitinib with CYP3A4 inducers (eg, rifampin) may decrease plasma sunitinib concentrations. Dose increase of sunitinib to 87.5 mg daily should be considered with co-administration).
No products indexed under this heading.

Hydrocortisone Probutate (Concurrent administration of sunitinib with CYP3A4 inducers (eg, rifampin) may decrease plasma sunitinib concentrations. Dose increase of sunitinib to 87.5 mg daily should be considered with co-administration).
No products indexed under this heading.

Hydrocortisone Sodium Phosphate (Concurrent administration of sunitinib with CYP3A4 inducers (eg, rifampin) may decrease plasma sunitinib concentrations. Dose increase of sunitinib to 87.5 mg daily should be considered with co-administration).
No products indexed under this heading.

Hydrocortisone Sodium Succinate (Concurrent administration of sunitinib with CYP3A4 inducers (eg, rifampin) may decrease plasma sunitinib concentrations. Dose increase of sunitinib to 87.5 mg daily should be considered with co-administration).
No products indexed under this heading.

Hydrocortisone Valerate (Concurrent administration of sunitinib with CYP3A4 inducers (eg, rifampin) may decrease plasma sunitinib concentrations. Dose increase of sunitinib to 87.5 mg daily should be considered with co-administration).
No products indexed under this heading.

Hypericum (Co-administration of St. John's Wort with sunitinib may decrease plasma concentrations of sunitinib unpredictably. Avoid concurrent administration of St. John's Wort with sunitinib).
No products indexed under this heading.

Hypericum Perforatum (Co-administration of St. John's Wort with sunitinib may decrease plasma concentrations of sunitinib unpredictably. Avoid concurrent administration of St. John's Wort with sunitinib). Products include:
Traumeel 1800

Indinavir Sulfate (Concurrent administration of sunitinib with strong CYP3A4 inhibitors (eg, ketoconazole) may increase sunitinib plasma concentrations. Dose reduction of sunitinib to 37.5 mg daily is recommended with co-administration). Products include:
Crixivan 2113

Itraconazole (Concurrent administration of sunitinib with strong CYP3A4 inhibitors (eg, ketoconazole) may increase sunitinib plasma concentrations. Dose reduction of sunitinib to 37.5 mg daily is recommended with co-administration).
No products indexed under this heading.

Ketoconazole (Concurrent administration of sunitinib with strong CYP3A4 inhibitors (eg, ketoconazole) may increase sunitinib plasma concentrations. Dose reduction of sunitinib to 37.5 mg daily is recommended with co-administration). Products include:
Extina 3319
Xolegel 3337

Lidocaine Hydrochloride (Sunitinib has been shown to prolong QT interval in a dose dependent manner; caution is advised in patients taking sunitinib and antiarrhythmics concomittantly).
No products indexed under this heading.

Lopinavir (Concurrent administration of sunitinib with strong CYP3A4 inhibitors (eg, ketoconazole) may increase sunitinib plasma concentrations. Dose reduction of sunitinib to 37.5 mg daily is recommended with co-administration). Products include:
Kaletra 458

Mephenytoin (Concurrent administration of sunitinib with CYP3A4 inducers (eg, rifampin) may decrease plasma sunitinib concentrations. Dose increase of sunitinib to 87.5 mg daily should be considered with co-administration).
No products indexed under this heading.

Methsuximide (Concurrent administration of sunitinib with CYP3A4 inducers (eg, rifampin) may decrease plasma sunitinib concentrations. Dose increase of sunitinib to 87.5 mg daily should be considered with co-administration).
No products indexed under this heading.

Methylprednisolone (Concurrent administration of sunitinib with CYP3A4 inducers (eg, rifampin) may decrease plasma sunitinib concentrations. Dose increase of sunitinib to 87.5 mg daily should be considered with co-administration).
No products indexed under this heading.

Methylprednisolone Acetate (Concurrent administration of sunitinib with CYP3A4 inducers (eg, rifampin) may decrease plasma sunitinib concentrations. Dose increase of sunitinib to 87.5 mg daily should be considered with co-administration).
No products indexed under this heading.

Methylprednisolone Sodium Succinate (Concurrent administration of sunitinib with CYP3A4 inducers (eg, rifampin) may decrease plasma sunitinib concentrations. Dose increase of sunitinib to 87.5 mg daily should be considered with co-administration).
No products indexed under this heading.

Mexiletine Hydrochloride (Sunitinib has been shown to prolong QT interval in a dose dependent manner; caution is advised in patients taking sunitinib and antiarrhythmics concomittantly).
No products indexed under this heading.

Modafinil (Concurrent administration of sunitinib with CYP3A4 inducers (eg, rifampin) may decrease plasma sunitinib concentrations. Dose increase of sunitinib to 87.5 mg daily should be considered with co-administration). Products include:
Provigil 983

Moricizine Hydrochloride (Sunitinib has been shown to prolong QT interval in a dose dependent manner; caution is advised in patients taking sunitinib and antiarrhythmics concomittantly).
No products indexed under this heading.

Nafcillin Sodium (Concurrent administration of sunitinib with CYP3A4 inducers (eg, rifampin) may decrease plasma sunitinib concentrations. Dose increase of sunitinib to 87.5 mg daily should be considered with co-administration).
No products indexed under this heading.

Nefazodone Hydrochloride (Concurrent administration of sunitinib with strong CYP3A4 inhibitors (eg, ketoconazole) may increase sunitinib plasma concentrations. Dose reduction of sunitinib to 37.5 mg daily is recommended with co-administration).
No products indexed under this heading.

Nelfinavir Mesylate (Concurrent administration of sunitinib with strong CYP3A4 inhibitors (eg, ketoconazole) may increase sunitinib plasma concentrations. Dose reduction of sunitinib to 37.5 mg daily is recommended with co-administration).
No products indexed under this heading.

Nevirapine (Concurrent administration of sunitinib with CYP3A4 inducers (eg, rifampin) may decrease plasma sunitinib concentrations. Dose increase of sunitinib to 87.5 mg daily should be considered with co-administration). Products include:
Viramune Oral Suspension 897
Viramune Tablets 897

Oxcarbazepine (Concurrent administration of sunitinib with CYP3A4 inducers (eg, rifampin) may decrease plasma sunitinib concentrations. Dose increase of sunitinib to 87.5 mg daily should be considered with co-administration).
No products indexed under this heading.

Phenobarbital (Concurrent administration of sunitinib with CYP3A4 inducers (eg, rifampin) may decrease plasma sunitinib concentrations. Dose increase of sunitinib to 87.5 mg daily should be considered with co-administration). Products include:
Donnatal 2711

Phenobarbital Sodium (Concurrent administration of sunitinib with CYP3A4 inducers (eg, rifampin) may decrease plasma sunitinib concentrations. Dose increase of sunitinib to 87.5 mg daily should be considered with co-administration).
No products indexed under this heading.

Phenytoin (Concurrent administration of sunitinib with CYP3A4 inducers (eg, rifampin) may decrease plasma sunitinib concentrations. Dose increase of sunitinib to 87.5 mg daily should be considered with co-administration).
No products indexed under this heading.

Phenytoin Sodium (Concurrent administration of sunitinib with CYP3A4 inducers (eg, rifampin) may decrease plasma sunitinib concentrations. Dose increase of sunitinib to 87.5 mg daily should be considered with co-administration). Products include:
Phenytek Capsules 2380

Prednisolone (Concurrent administration of sunitinib with CYP3A4 inducers (eg, rifampin) may decrease plasma sunitinib concentrations. Dose increase of sunitinib to 87.5 mg daily should be considered with co-administration).
No products indexed under this heading.

Prednisolone Acetate (Concurrent administration of sunitinib with CYP3A4 inducers (eg, rifampin) may decrease plasma sunitinib concentrations. Dose

increase of sunitinib to 87.5 mg daily should be considered with co-administration). Products include:

Blephamide .... ⊙212, ⊙214
Pred Forte .... ⊙225
Pred Mild .... ⊙230
Pred-G .... ⊙226, ⊙227

Prednisolone Sodium Phosphate (Concurrent administration of sunitinib with CYP3A4 inducers (eg, rifampin) may decrease plasma sunitinib concentrations. Dose increase of sunitinib to 87.5 mg daily should be considered with co-administration).
No products indexed under this heading.

Prednisolone Tebutate (Concurrent administration of sunitinib with CYP3A4 inducers (eg, rifampin) may decrease plasma sunitinib concentrations. Dose increase of sunitinib to 87.5 mg daily should be considered with co-administration).
No products indexed under this heading.

Prednisone (Concurrent administration of sunitinib with CYP3A4 inducers (eg, rifampin) may decrease plasma sunitinib concentrations. Dose increase of sunitinib to 87.5 mg daily should be considered with co-administration).
No products indexed under this heading.

Prednisone sodium phosphate (Concurrent administration of sunitinib with CYP3A4 inducers (eg, rifampin) may decrease plasma sunitinib concentrations. Dose increase of sunitinib to 87.5 mg daily should be considered with co-administration).
No products indexed under this heading.

Primidone (Concurrent administration of sunitinib with CYP3A4 inducers (eg, rifampin) may decrease plasma sunitinib concentrations. Dose increase of sunitinib to 87.5 mg daily should be considered with co-administration).
No products indexed under this heading.

Procainamide Hydrochloride (Sunitinib has been shown to prolong QT interval in a dose dependent manner; caution is advised in patients taking sunitinib and antiarrhythmics concomittantly).
No products indexed under this heading.

Propafenone Hydrochloride (Sunitinib has been shown to prolong QT interval in a dose dependent manner; caution is advised in patients taking sunitinib and antiarrhythmics concomittantly). Products include:

Rythmol 1648
Rythmol SR 1652

Propranolol Hydrochloride (Sunitinib has been shown to prolong QT interval in a dose dependent manner; caution is advised in patients taking sunitinib and antiarrhythmics concomittantly). Products include:

InnoPran XL 1517

Quinidine Gluconate (Sunitinib has been shown to prolong QT interval in a dose dependent manner; caution is advised in patients taking sunitinib and antiarrhythmics concomittantly).
No products indexed under this heading.

Quinidine Polygalacturonate (Sunitinib has been shown to prolong QT interval in a dose dependent manner; caution is advised in patients taking sunitinib and antiarrhythmics concomittantly).
No products indexed under this heading.

Quinidine Sulfate (Sunitinib has been shown to prolong QT interval in a dose dependent manner; caution is advised in patients taking sunitinib and antiarrhythmics concomittantly).
No products indexed under this heading.

Rifabutin (Concurrent administration of sunitinib with CYP3A4 inducers (eg, rifampin) may decrease plasma sunitinib concentrations. Dose increase of sunitinib to 87.5 mg daily should be considered with co-administration).
No products indexed under this heading.

Rifampicin (Concurrent administration of sunitinib with CYP3A4 inducers (eg, rifampin) may decrease plasma sunitinib concentrations. Dose increase of sunitinib to 87.5 mg daily should be considered with co-administration).
No products indexed under this heading.

Rifampin (Concurrent administration of sunitinib with CYP3A4 inducers (eg, rifampin) may decrease plasma sunitinib concentrations. Dose increase of sunitinib to 87.5 mg daily should be considered with co-administration).
No products indexed under this heading.

Rifapentine (Concurrent administration of sunitinib with CYP3A4 inducers (eg, rifampin) may decrease plasma sunitinib concentrations. Dose increase of sunitinib to 87.5 mg daily should be considered with co-administration).
No products indexed under this heading.

Ritonavir (Concurrent administration of sunitinib with strong CYP3A4 inhibitors (eg, ketoconazole) may increase sunitinib plasma concentrations. Dose reduction of sunitinib to 37.5 mg daily is recommended with co-administration). Products include:

Kaletra 458
Norvir 509

Saquinavir (Concurrent administration of sunitinib with strong CYP3A4 inhibitors (eg, ketoconazole) may increase sunitinib plasma concentrations. Dose reduction of sunitinib to 37.5 mg daily is recommended with co-administration).
No products indexed under this heading.

Saquinavir Mesylate (Concurrent administration of sunitinib with strong CYP3A4 inhibitors (eg, ketoconazole) may increase sunitinib plasma concentrations. Dose reduction of sunitinib to 37.5 mg daily is recommended with co-administration).
No products indexed under this heading.

Sotalol Hydrochloride (Sunitinib has been shown to prolong QT interval in a dose dependent manner; caution is advised in patients taking sunitinib and antiarrhythmics concomittantly).
No products indexed under this heading.

Sulfinpyrazone (Concurrent administration of sunitinib with CYP3A4 inducers (eg, rifampin) may decrease plasma sunitinib concentrations. Dose increase of sunitinib to 87.5 mg daily should be considered with co-administration).
No products indexed under this heading.

Telithromycin (Concurrent administration of sunitinib with strong CYP3A4 inhibitors (eg, ketoconazole) may increase sunitinib plasma concentrations. Dose reduction of sunitinib to 37.5 mg daily is recommended with co-administration). Products include:

Ketek 2991

Theophyllinate (Concurrent administration of sunitinib with CYP3A4 inducers (eg, rifampin) may decrease plasma sunitinib concentrations. Dose increase of sunitinib to 87.5 mg daily should be considered with co-administration).
No products indexed under this heading.

Theophylline (Concurrent administration of sunitinib with CYP3A4 inducers (eg, rifampin) may decrease plasma sunitinib concentrations. Dose increase of sunitinib to 87.5 mg daily should be considered with co-administration).
No products indexed under this heading.

Theophylline Anhydrous (Concurrent administration of sunitinib with CYP3A4 inducers (eg, rifampin) may decrease plasma sunitinib concentrations. Dose increase of sunitinib to 87.5 mg daily should be considered with co-administration). Products include:

Uniphyl 2817

Theophylline Calcium Salicylate (Concurrent administration of sunitinib with CYP3A4 inducers (eg, rifampin) may decrease plasma sunitinib concentrations. Dose increase of sunitinib to 87.5 mg daily should be considered with co-administration).
No products indexed under this heading.

Theophylline Dihydroxypropyl (Glyceryl) (Concurrent administration of sunitinib with CYP3A4 inducers (eg, rifampin) may decrease plasma sunitinib concentrations. Dose increase of sunitinib to 87.5 mg daily should be considered with co-administration).
No products indexed under this heading.

Theophylline Ethylenediamine (Concurrent administration of sunitinib with CYP3A4 inducers (eg, rifampin) may decrease plasma sunitinib concentrations. Dose increase of sunitinib to 87.5 mg daily should be considered with co-administration).
No products indexed under this heading.

Theophylline Sodium Glycinate (Concurrent administration of sunitinib with CYP3A4 inducers (eg, rifampin) may decrease plasma sunitinib concentrations. Dose increase of sunitinib to 87.5 mg daily should be considered with co-administration).
No products indexed under this heading.

Tocainide Hydrochloride (Sunitinib has been shown to prolong QT interval in a dose dependent manner; caution is advised in patients taking sunitinib and antiarrhythmics concomittantly).
No products indexed under this heading.

Triamcinolone (Concurrent administration of sunitinib with CYP3A4 inducers (eg, rifampin) may decrease plasma sunitinib concentrations. Dose increase of sunitinib to 87.5 mg daily should be considered with co-administration).
No products indexed under this heading.

Triamcinolone Acetonide (Concurrent administration of sunitinib with CYP3A4 inducers (eg, rifampin) may decrease plasma sunitinib concentrations. Dose increase of sunitinib to 87.5 mg daily should be considered with co-administration). Products include:

Azmacort 408
Nasacort AQ 3019

Triamcinolone Diacetate (Concurrent administration of sunitinib with CYP3A4 inducers (eg, rifampin) may decrease plasma sunitinib concentrations. Dose increase of sunitinib to 87.5 mg daily should be considered with co-administration).
No products indexed under this heading.

Triamcinolone Hexacetonide (Concurrent administration of sunitinib with CYP3A4 inducers (eg, rifampin) may decrease plasma sunitinib concentrations. Dose increase of sunitinib to 87.5 mg daily should be considered with co-administration).
No products indexed under this heading.

Troglitazone (Concurrent administration of sunitinib with CYP3A4 inducers (eg, rifampin) may decrease plasma sunitinib concentrations. Dose increase of sunitinib to 87.5 mg daily should be considered with co-administration).
No products indexed under this heading.

Troleandomycin (Concurrent administration of sunitinib with strong CYP3A4 inhibitors (eg, ketoconazole) may increase sunitinib plasma concentrations. Dose reduction of sunitinib to 37.5 mg daily is recommended with co-administration).
No products indexed under this heading.

Verapamil Hydrochloride (Sunitinib has been shown to prolong QT interval in a dose dependent manner; caution is advised in patients taking sunitinib and antiarrhythmics concomittantly). Products include:

Tarka 534

Voriconazole (Concurrent administration of sunitinib with strong CYP3A4 inhibitors (eg, ketoconazole) may increase sunitinib plasma concentrations. Dose reduction of sunitinib to 37.5 mg daily is recommended with co-administration).
No products indexed under this heading.

Food Interactions

Grapefruit (Grapefruit may increase plasma concentrations of sunitinib malate).

Grapefruit Juice (Grapefruit may increase plasma concentrations of sunitinib malate).

SYMBICORT 80/4.5 INHALATION AEROSOL

(Budesonide, Formoterol fumarate dihydrate) 720

May interact with anticonvulsants, beta-blockers, corticosteroids, cytochrome p450 3a4 inhibitors (selected), cytochrome p450 3a4 inhibitors, potent (selected), diuretics, loop diuretics, monoamine oxidase inhibitors, nonpotassium-sparing diuretics, thiazides, tricyclic antidepressants, and certain other agents. Compounds in these categories include:

Acebutolol Hydrochloride (β-blockers (including eye drops) may not only block the pulmonary effect of β-agonists, such as formoterol, a component of Symbicort, but may produce severe bronchospasm in patients with asthma. Therefore, patients with asthma should not normally be treated with β-blockers. However, under certain circumstances, there may be no acceptable alternatives to the use of β-adrenergic blocking agents in patients with asthma. In this setting, cardioselective β-blockers could be considered, although they should be administered with caution).
No products indexed under this heading.

Acetazolamide (The main route of metabolism of corticosteroids, including budesonide, a component of Symbicort, is via cytochrome P450 (CYP) isoenzyme 3A4 (CYP3A4). After oral administration of ketoconazole, a strong inhibitor of CYP3A4, the mean plasma concentration of orally administered budesonide increased. Concomitant administration of CYP3A4 inhibitors may inhibit the metabolism of, and increase the systemic exposure to, budesonide. Caution should be exercised when considering the co-administration of Symbicort with long-term ketoconazole and other known strong CYP3A4 inhibitors (eg, ritonavir, atazanavir, clarithromycin, indinavir, itraconazole, nefazodone, nelfinavir, saquinavir, telithromycin)).
No products indexed under this heading.

Acetazolamide Sodium (The main route of metabolism of corticosteroids, including budesonide, a component of Symbicort, is via cytochrome P450 (CYP) isoenzyme 3A4 (CYP3A4). After oral administration of ketoconazole, a strong inhibitor of CYP3A4, the mean plasma concentration of orally administered budesonide increased. Concomi-

1783 **Interactions Index** **Symbicort**

tant administration of CYP3A4 inhibitors may inhibit the metabolism of, and increase the systemic exposure to, budesonide. Caution should be exercised when considering the co-administration of Symbicort with long-term ketoconazole and other known strong CYP3A4 inhibitors (eg, ritonavir, atazanavir, clarithromycin, indinavir, itraconazole, nefazodone, nelfinavir, saquinavir, telithromycin)).
No products indexed under this heading.

Alclometasone Dipropionate (Decreases in bone mineral density (BMD) have been observed with long-term administration of products containing inhaled corticosteroids. Patients with major risk factors for decreased bone mineral content, such as chronic use of drugs that can reduce bone mass (eg, oral corticosteroids), should be monitored and treated with established standards of care).
No products indexed under this heading.

Amiloride Hydrochloride (The ECG changes and/or hypokalemia that may result from the administration of non-potassium-sparing diuretics (such as loop or thiazide diuretics) can be acutely worsened by beta-agonists, especially when the recommended dose of the beta-agonist is exceeded. Although the clinical significance of these effects is not known, caution is advised in the co-administration of Symbicort with non-potassium-sparing diuretics).
No products indexed under this heading.

Amiodarone Hydrochloride (The main route of metabolism of corticosteroids, including budesonide, a component of Symbicort, is via cytochrome P450 (CYP) isoenzyme 3A4 (CYP3A4). After oral administration of ketoconazole, a strong inhibitor of CYP3A4, the mean plasma concentration of orally administered budesonide increased. Concomitant administration of CYP3A4 inhibitors may inhibit the metabolism of, and increase the systemic exposure to, budesonide. Caution should be exercised when considering the co-administration of Symbicort with long-term ketoconazole and other known strong CYP3A4 inhibitors (eg, ritonavir, atazanavir, clarithromycin, indinavir, itraconazole, nefazodone, nelfinavir, saquinavir, telithromycin)).
No products indexed under this heading.

Amitriptyline Hydrochloride (Symbicort should be administered with caution to patients being treated with tricyclic antidepressants, or within 2 weeks of discontinuation of such agents, because the action of formoterol, a component of Symbicort, on the vascular system may be potentiated by these agents. In clinical trials with Symbicort, a limited number of COPD and asthma patients received tricyclic antidepressants, and, therefore, no clinically meaningful conclusions on adverse events can be made).
No products indexed under this heading.

Amoxapine (Symbicort should be administered with caution to patients being treated with tricyclic antidepressants, or within 2 weeks of discontinuation of such agents, because the action of formoterol, a component of Symbicort, on the vascular system may be potentiated by these agents. In clinical trials with Symbicort, a limited number of COPD and asthma patients received tricyclic antidepressants, and, therefore, no clinically meaningful conclusions on adverse events can be made).
No products indexed under this heading.

Amprenavir (The main route of metabolism of corticosteroids, including budesonide, a component of Symbicort, is via cytochrome P450 (CYP) isoenzyme 3A4 (CYP3A4). After oral administration of ketoconazole, a strong inhibitor of CYP3A4, the mean plasma concentration of orally administered budesonide increased. Concomitant administration of CYP3A4 inhibitors may inhibit the metabolism of, and increase the systemic exposure to, budesonide. Caution should be exercised when considering the co-administration of Symbicort with long-term ketoconazole and other known strong CYP3A4 inhibitors (eg, ritonavir, atazanavir, clarithromycin, indinavir, itraconazole, nefazodone, nelfinavir, saquinavir, telithromycin)).
No products indexed under this heading.

Anastrozole (The main route of metabolism of corticosteroids, including budesonide, a component of Symbicort, is via cytochrome P450 (CYP) isoenzyme 3A4 (CYP3A4). After oral administration of ketoconazole, a strong inhibitor of CYP3A4, the mean plasma concentration of orally administered budesonide increased. Concomitant administration of CYP3A4 inhibitors may inhibit the metabolism of, and increase the systemic exposure to, budesonide. Caution should be exercised when considering the co-administration of Symbicort with long-term ketoconazole and other known strong CYP3A4 inhibitors (eg, ritonavir, atazanavir, clarithromycin, indinavir, itraconazole, nefazodone, nelfinavir, saquinavir, telithromycin)).
No products indexed under this heading.

Aprepitant (The main route of metabolism of corticosteroids, including budesonide, a component of Symbicort, is via cytochrome P450 (CYP) isoenzyme 3A4 (CYP3A4). After oral administration of ketoconazole, a strong inhibitor of CYP3A4, the mean plasma concentration of orally administered budesonide increased. Concomitant administration of CYP3A4 inhibitors may inhibit the metabolism of, and increase the systemic exposure to, budesonide. Caution should be exercised when considering the co-administration of Symbicort with long-term ketoconazole and other known strong CYP3A4 inhibitors (eg, ritonavir, atazanavir, clarithromycin, indinavir, itraconazole, nefazodone, nelfinavir, saquinavir, telithromycin)). Products include:
Emend **2124**

Atazanavir (The main route of metabolism of corticosteroids, including budesonide, a component of Symbicort, is via cytochrome P450 (CYP) isoenzyme 3A4 (CYP3A4). After oral administration of ketoconazole, a strong inhibitor of CYP3A4, the mean plasma concentration of orally administered budesonide increased. Concomitant administration of CYP3A4 inhibitors may inhibit the metabolism of, and increase the systemic exposure to, budesonide. Caution should be exercised when considering the co-administration of Symbicort with long-term ketoconazole and other known strong CYP3A4 inhibitors (eg, ritonavir, atazanavir, clarithromycin, indinavir, itraconazole, nefazodone, nelfinavir, saquinavir, telithromycin)).
No products indexed under this heading.

Atazanavir Sulfate (The main route of metabolism of corticosteroids, including budesonide, a component of Symbicort, is via cytochrome P450 (CYP) isoenzyme 3A4 (CYP3A4). After oral administration of ketoconazole, a strong inhibitor of CYP3A4, the mean plasma concentration of orally administered budesonide increased. Concomitant administration of CYP3A4 inhibitors may inhibit the metabolism of, and increase the systemic exposure to, budesonide. Caution should be exercised when considering the co-administration of Symbicort with long-term ketoconazole and other known strong CYP3A4 inhibitors (eg, ritonavir, atazanavir, clarithromycin, indinavir, itraconazole, nefazodone, nelfinavir, saquinavir, telithromycin)).
No products indexed under this heading.

Atenolol (β-blockers (including eye drops) may not only block the pulmonary effect of β-agonists, such as formoterol, a component of Symbicort, but may produce severe bronchospasm in patients with asthma. Therefore, patients with asthma should not normally be treated with β-blockers. However, under certain circumstances, there may be no acceptable alternatives to the use of β-adrenergic blocking agents in patients with asthma. In this setting, cardioselective β-blockers could be considered, although they should be administered with caution).
No products indexed under this heading.

Beclomethasone Dipropionate (Decreases in bone mineral density (BMD) have been observed with long-term administration of products containing inhaled corticosteroids. Patients with major risk factors for decreased bone mineral content, such as chronic use of drugs that can reduce bone mass (eg, oral corticosteroids), should be monitored and treated with established standards of care). Products include:
Qvar **3398**

Beclomethasone Dipropionate Monohydrate (Decreases in bone mineral density (BMD) have been observed with long-term administration of products containing inhaled corticosteroids. Patients with major risk factors for decreased bone mineral content, such as chronic use of drugs that can reduce bone mass (eg, oral corticosteroids), should be monitored and treated with established standards of care). Products include:
Beconase AQ **1386**

Bendroflumethiazide (The ECG changes and/or hypokalemia that may result from the administration of non-potassium-sparing diuretics (such as loop or thiazide diuretics) can be acutely worsened by β-agonists, especially when the recommended dose of the β-agonist is exceeded. Although the clinical significance of these effects is not known, caution is advised in the co-administration of Symbicort with non-potassium-sparing diuretics).
No products indexed under this heading.

Betamethasone (Decreases in bone mineral density (BMD) have been observed with long-term administration of products containing inhaled corticosteroids. Patients with major risk factors for decreased bone mineral content, such as chronic use of drugs that can reduce bone mass (eg, oral corticosteroids), should be monitored and treated with established standards of care).
No products indexed under this heading.

Betamethasone Acetate (Decreases in bone mineral density (BMD) have been observed with long-term administration of products containing inhaled corticosteroids. Patients with major risk factors for decreased bone mineral content, such as chronic use of drugs that can reduce bone mass (eg, oral corticosteroids), should be monitored and treated with established standards of care).
No products indexed under this heading.

Betamethasone Benzoate (Decreases in bone mineral density (BMD) have been observed with long-term administration of products containing inhaled corticosteroids. Patients with major risk factors for decreased bone mineral content, such as chronic use of drugs that can reduce bone mass (eg, oral corticosteroids), should be monitored and treated with established standards of care).
No products indexed under this heading.

Betamethasone Dipropionate (Decreases in bone mineral density (BMD) have been observed with long-term administration of products containing inhaled corticosteroids. Patients with major risk factors for decreased bone mineral content, such as chronic use of drugs that can reduce bone mass (eg, oral corticosteroids), should be monitored and treated with established standards of care). Products include:
Diprolene Lotion 0.05% **3108**
Diprolene Ointment 0.05% **3109**
Diprolene AF Cream 0.05% **3107**
Lotrisone **3163**

Betamethasone Sodium Phosphate (Decreases in bone mineral density (BMD) have been observed with long-term administration of products containing inhaled corticosteroids. Patients with major risk factors for decreased bone mineral content, such as chronic use of drugs that can reduce bone mass (eg, oral corticosteroids), should be monitored and treated with established standards of care).
No products indexed under this heading.

Betamethasone Valerate (Decreases in bone mineral density (BMD) have been observed with long-term administration of products containing inhaled corticosteroids. Patients with major risk factors for decreased bone mineral content, such as chronic use of drugs that can reduce bone mass (eg, oral corticosteroids), should be monitored and treated with established standards of care). Products include:
Luxíq **3321**

Betaxolol Hydrochloride (β-blockers (including eye drops) may not only block the pulmonary effect of β-agonists, such as formoterol, a component of Symbicort, but may produce severe bronchospasm in patients with asthma. Therefore, patients with asthma should not normally be treated with β-blockers. However, under certain circumstances, there may be no acceptable alternatives to the use of β-adrenergic blocking agents in patients with asthma. In this setting, cardioselective β-blockers could be considered, although they should be administered with caution).
No products indexed under this heading.

Bisoprolol Fumarate (β-blockers (including eye drops) may not only block the pulmonary effect of β-agonists, such as formoterol, a component of Symbicort, but may produce severe bronchospasm in patients with asthma. Therefore, patients with asthma should not normally be treated with β-blockers. However, under certain circumstances, there may be no acceptable alternatives to the use of β-adrenergic blocking agents in patients with asthma. In this setting, cardioselective β-blockers could be considered, although they should be administered with caution).
No products indexed under this heading.

Bumetanide (The ECG changes and/or hypokalemia that may result from the administration of non-potassium-sparing diuretics (such as loop or thiazide diuretics) can be acutely worsened by β-agonists, especially when the recommended dose of the β-agonist is exceeded. Although the clinical signifi-

IMPORTANT NOTE: Always consult each drug listing in the patient's regimen for possible interactions.

cance of these effects is not known, caution is advised in the co-administration of Symbicort with non-potassium-sparing diuretics).
No products indexed under this heading.

Carbamazepine (Decreases in bone mineral density (BMD) have been observed with long-term administration of products containing inhaled corticosteroids. Patients with major risk factors for decreased bone mineral content, such as chronic use of drugs that can reduce bone mass (eg, anticonvulsants), should be monitored and treated with established standards of care). Products include:
Carbatrol 3280
Equetro 3477

Carteolol Hydrochloride (β-blockers (including eye drops) may not only block the pulmonary effect of β-agonists, such as formoterol, a component of Symbicort, but may produce severe bronchospasm in patients with asthma. Therefore, patients with asthma should not normally be treated with β-blockers. However, under certain circumstances, there may be no acceptable alternatives to the use of β-adrenergic blocking agents in patients with asthma. In this setting, cardioselective β-blockers could be considered, although they should be administered with caution).
No products indexed under this heading.

Carvedilol (β-blockers (including eye drops) may not only block the pulmonary effect of β-agonists, such as formoterol, a component of Symbicort, but may produce severe bronchospasm in patients with asthma. Therefore, patients with asthma should not normally be treated with β-blockers. However, under certain circumstances, there may be no acceptable alternatives to the use of β-adrenergic blocking agents in patients with asthma. In this setting, cardioselective β-blockers could be considered, although they should be administered with caution). Products include:
Coreg 1409

Carvedilol Phosphate (β-blockers (including eye drops) may not only block the pulmonary effect of β-agonists, such as formoterol, a component of Symbicort, but may produce severe bronchospasm in patients with asthma. Therefore, patients with asthma should not normally be treated with β-blockers. However, under certain circumstances, there may be no acceptable alternatives to the use of β-adrenergic blocking agents in patients with asthma. In this setting, cardioselective β-blockers could be considered, although they should be administered with caution). Products include:
Coreg CR 1416

Chlorothiazide (The ECG changes and/or hypokalemia that may result from the administration of non-potassium-sparing diuretics (such as loop or thiazide diuretics) can be acutely worsened by β-agonists, especially when the recommended dose of the β-agonist is exceeded. Although the clinical significance of these effects is not known, caution is advised in the co-administration of Symbicort with non-potassium-sparing diuretics).
No products indexed under this heading.

Chlorothiazide Sodium (The ECG changes and/or hypokalemia that may result from the administration of non-potassium-sparing diuretics (such as loop or thiazide diuretics) can be acutely worsened by β-agonists, especially when the recommended dose of the β-agonist is exceeded. Although the clinical significance of these effects is not known, caution is advised in the co-administration of Symbicort with non-potassium-sparing diuretics). Products include:
Diuril Intravenous 2009

Chlorthalidone (The ECG changes and/or hypokalemia that may result from the administration of non-potassium-sparing diuretics (such as loop or thiazide diuretics) can be acutely worsened by beta-agonists, especially when the recommended dose of the beta-agonist is exceeded. Although the clinical significance of these effects is not known, caution is advised in the co-administration of Symbicort with non-potassium-sparing diuretics). Products include:
Clorpres 2344

Ciclesonide (Decreases in bone mineral density (BMD) have been observed with long-term administration of products containing inhaled corticosteroids. Patients with major risk factors for decreased bone mineral content, such as chronic use of drugs that can reduce bone mass (eg, oral corticosteroids), should be monitored and treated with established standards of care).
No products indexed under this heading.

Cimetidine (At recommended doses, cimetidine, a non-specific inhibitor of CYP enzymes, had a slight but clinically insignificant effect on the pharmacokinetics of oral budesonide).
No products indexed under this heading.

Cimetidine Hydrochloride (At recommended doses, cimetidine, a non-specific inhibitor of CYP enzymes, had a slight but clinically insignificant effect on the pharmacokinetics of oral budesonide).
No products indexed under this heading.

Ciprofloxacin (The main route of metabolism of corticosteroids, including budesonide, a component of Symbicort, is via cytochrome P450 (CYP) isoenzyme 3A4 (CYP3A4). After oral administration of ketoconazole, a strong inhibitor of CYP3A4, the mean plasma concentration of orally administered budesonide increased. Concomitant administration of CYP3A4 inhibitors may inhibit the metabolism of, and increase the systemic exposure to, budesonide. Caution should be exercised when considering the co-administration of Symbicort with long-term ketoconazole and other known strong CYP3A4 inhibitors (eg, ritonavir, atazanavir, clarithromycin, indinavir, itraconazole, nefazodone, nelfinavir, saquinavir, telithromycin)). Products include:
Cipro I.V. 3082
Cipro 3073
Cipro XR 3091
Ciprodex 583

Clarithromycin (The main route of metabolism of corticosteroids, including budesonide, a component of Symbicort, is via cytochrome P450 (CYP) isoenzyme 3A4 (CYP3A4). After oral administration of ketoconazole, a strong inhibitor of CYP3A4, the mean plasma concentration of orally administered budesonide increased. Concomitant administration of CYP3A4 inhibitors may inhibit the metabolism of, and increase the systemic exposure to, budesonide. Caution should be exercised when considering the co-administration of Symbicort with long-term ketoconazole and other known strong CYP3A4 inhibitors (eg, ritonavir, atazanavir, clarithromycin, indinavir, itraconazole, nefazodone, nelfinavir, saquinavir, telithromycin)). Products include:
Biaxin/Biaxin XL 412

Clomipramine Hydrochloride (Symbicort should be administered with caution to patients being treated with tricyclic antidepressants, or within 2 weeks of discontinuation of such agents, because the action of formoterol, a component of Symbicort, on the vascular system may be potentiated by these agents. In clinical trials with Symbicort, a limited number of COPD and asthma patients received tricyclic antidepressants, and, therefore, no clinically meaningful conclusions on adverse events can be made).
No products indexed under this heading.

Clotrimazole (The main route of metabolism of corticosteroids, including budesonide, a component of Symbicort, is via cytochrome P450 (CYP) isoenzyme 3A4 (CYP3A4). After oral administration of ketoconazole, a strong inhibitor of CYP3A4, the mean plasma concentration of orally administered budesonide increased. Concomitant administration of CYP3A4 inhibitors may inhibit the metabolism of, and increase the systemic exposure to, budesonide. Caution should be exercised when considering the co-administration of Symbicort with long-term ketoconazole and other known strong CYP3A4 inhibitors (eg, ritonavir, atazanavir, clarithromycin, indinavir, itraconazole, nefazodone, nelfinavir, saquinavir, telithromycin)). Products include:
Lotrisone 3163

Conivaptan Hydrochloride (The main route of metabolism of corticosteroids, including budesonide, a component of Symbicort, is via cytochrome P450 (CYP) isoenzyme 3A4 (CYP3A4). After oral administration of ketoconazole, a strong inhibitor of CYP3A4, the mean plasma concentration of orally administered budesonide increased. Concomitant administration of CYP3A4 inhibitors may inhibit the metabolism of, and increase the systemic exposure to, budesonide. Caution should be exercised when considering the co-administration of Symbicort with long-term ketoconazole and other known strong CYP3A4 inhibitors (eg, ritonavir, atazanavir, clarithromycin, indinavir, itraconazole, nefazodone, nelfinavir, saquinavir, telithromycin)). Products include:
Vaprisol 689

Cortisone Acetate (Decreases in bone mineral density (BMD) have been observed with long-term administration of products containing inhaled corticosteroids. Patients with major risk factors for decreased bone mineral content, such as chronic use of drugs that can reduce bone mass (eg, oral corticosteroids), should be monitored and treated with established standards of care).
No products indexed under this heading.

Cyclosporine (The main route of metabolism of corticosteroids, including budesonide, a component of Symbicort, is via cytochrome P450 (CYP) isoenzyme 3A4 (CYP3A4). After oral administration of ketoconazole, a strong inhibitor of CYP3A4, the mean plasma concentration of orally administered budesonide increased. Concomitant administration of CYP3A4 inhibitors may inhibit the metabolism of, and increase the systemic exposure to, budesonide. Caution should be exercised when considering the co-administration of Symbicort with long-term ketoconazole and other known strong CYP3A4 inhibitors (eg, ritonavir, atazanavir, clarithromycin, indinavir, itraconazole, nefazodone, nelfinavir, saquinavir, telithromycin)). Products include:
Gengraf 440
Neoral Oral Solution 2496
Neoral Capsules 2496
Restasis 605

Dalfopristin (The main route of metabolism of corticosteroids, including budesonide, a component of Symbicort, is via cytochrome P450 (CYP) isoenzyme 3A4 (CYP3A4). After oral administration of ketoconazole, a strong inhibitor of CYP3A4, the mean plasma concentration of orally administered budesonide increased. Concomitant administration of CYP3A4 inhibitors may inhibit the metabolism of, and increase the systemic exposure to, budesonide. Caution should be exercised when considering the co-administration of Symbicort with long-term ketoconazole and other known strong CYP3A4 inhibitors (eg, ritonavir, atazanavir, clarithromycin, indinavir, itraconazole, nefazodone, nelfinavir, saquinavir, telithromycin)).
No products indexed under this heading.

Danazol (The main route of metabolism of corticosteroids, including budesonide, a component of Symbicort, is via cytochrome P450 (CYP) isoenzyme 3A4 (CYP3A4). After oral administration of ketoconazole, a strong inhibitor of CYP3A4, the mean plasma concentration of orally administered budesonide increased. Concomitant administration of CYP3A4 inhibitors may inhibit the metabolism of, and increase the systemic exposure to, budesonide. Caution should be exercised when considering the co-administration of Symbicort with long-term ketoconazole and other known strong CYP3A4 inhibitors (eg, ritonavir, atazanavir, clarithromycin, indinavir, itraconazole, nefazodone, nelfinavir, saquinavir, telithromycin)).
No products indexed under this heading.

Darunavir (The main route of metabolism of corticosteroids, including budesonide, a component of Symbicort, is via cytochrome P450 (CYP) isoenzyme 3A4 (CYP3A4). After oral administration of ketoconazole, a strong inhibitor of CYP3A4, the mean plasma concentration of orally administered budesonide increased. Concomitant administration of CYP3A4 inhibitors may inhibit the metabolism of, and increase the systemic exposure to, budesonide. Caution should be exercised when considering the co-administration of Symbicort with long-term ketoconazole and other known strong CYP3A4 inhibitors (eg, ritonavir, atazanavir, clarithromycin, indinavir, itraconazole, nefazodone, nelfinavir, saquinavir, telithromycin)).
No products indexed under this heading.

Dasatinib (The main route of metabolism of corticosteroids, including budesonide, a component of Symbicort, is via cytochrome P450 (CYP) isoenzyme 3A4 (CYP3A4). After oral administration of ketoconazole, a strong inhibitor of CYP3A4, the mean plasma concentration of orally administered budesonide increased. Concomitant administration of CYP3A4 inhibitors may inhibit the metabolism of, and increase the systemic exposure to, budesonide. Caution should be exercised when considering the co-administration of Symbicort with long-term ketoconazole and other known strong CYP3A4 inhibitors (eg, ritonavir, atazanavir, clarithromycin, indinavir, itraconazole, nefazodone, nelfinavir, saquinavir, telithromycin)).
No products indexed under this heading.

Delavirdine Mesylate (The main route of metabolism of corticosteroids, including budesonide, a component of Symbicort, is via cytochrome P450 (CYP) isoenzyme 3A4 (CYP3A4). After oral administration of ketoconazole, a strong inhibitor of CYP3A4, the mean plasma concentration of orally administered budesonide increased. Concomitant administration of CYP3A4 inhibitors may inhibit the metabolism of, and increase the systemic exposure to,

1785 Interactions Index Symbicort

budesonide. Caution should be exercised when considering the co-administration of Symbicort with long-term ketoconazole and other known strong CYP3A4 inhibitors (eg, ritonavir, atazanavir, clarithromycin, indinavir, itraconazole, nefazodone, nelfinavir, saquinavir, telithromycin)).
No products indexed under this heading.

Delavirine (The main route of metabolism of corticosteroids, including budesonide, a component of Symbicort, is via cytochrome P450 (CYP) isoenzyme 3A4 (CYP3A4). After oral administration of ketoconazole, a strong inhibitor of CYP3A4, the mean plasma concentration of orally administered budesonide increased. Concomitant administration of CYP3A4 inhibitors may inhibit the metabolism of, and increase the systemic exposure to, budesonide. Caution should be exercised when considering the co-administration of Symbicort with long-term ketoconazole and other known strong CYP3A4 inhibitors (eg, ritonavir, atazanavir, clarithromycin, indinavir, itraconazole, nefazodone, nelfinavir, saquinavir, telithromycin)).
No products indexed under this heading.

Desipramine Hydrochloride (Symbicort should be administered with caution to patients being treated with tricyclic antidepressants, or within 2 weeks of discontinuation of such agents, because the action of formoterol, a component of Symbicort, on the vascular system may be potentiated by these agents. In clinical trials with Symbicort, a limited number of COPD and asthma patients received tricyclic antidepressants, and, therefore, no clinically meaningful conclusions on adverse events can be made).
No products indexed under this heading.

Desloratadine (The main route of metabolism of corticosteroids, including budesonide, a component of Symbicort, is via cytochrome P450 (CYP) isoenzyme 3A4 (CYP3A4). After oral administration of ketoconazole, a strong inhibitor of CYP3A4, the mean plasma concentration of orally administered budesonide increased. Concomitant administration of CYP3A4 inhibitors may inhibit the metabolism of, and increase the systemic exposure to, budesonide. Caution should be exercised when considering the co-administration of Symbicort with long-term ketoconazole and other known strong CYP3A4 inhibitors (eg, ritonavir, atazanavir, clarithromycin, indinavir, itraconazole, nefazodone, nelfinavir, saquinavir, telithromycin)). Products include:
Clarinex Syrup ... 3098
Clarinex ... 3098
Clarinex Reditabs ... 3098
Clarinex-D 12-Hour ... 3101
Clarinex-D ... 3104

Desoximetasone (Decreases in bone mineral density (BMD) have been observed with long-term administration of products containing inhaled corticosteroids. Patients with major risk factors for decreased bone mineral content, such as chronic use of drugs that can reduce bone mass (eg, oral corticosteroids), should be monitored and treated with established standards of care).
No products indexed under this heading.

Dexamethasone (Decreases in bone mineral density (BMD) have been observed with long-term administration of products containing inhaled corticosteroids. Patients with major risk factors for decreased bone mineral content, such as chronic use of drugs that can reduce bone mass (eg, oral corticosteroids), should be monitored and treated with established standards of care). Products include:
Ciprodex ... 583
Ozurdex ... ⊙223
Tobramycin and Dexamethasone Ophthalmic Suspension ... ⊙251

Dexamethasone Acetate (Decreases in bone mineral density (BMD) have been observed with long-term administration of products containing inhaled corticosteroids. Patients with major risk factors for decreased bone mineral content, such as chronic use of drugs that can reduce bone mass (eg, oral corticosteroids), should be monitored and treated with established standards of care).
No products indexed under this heading.

Dexamethasone Phosphate (Decreases in bone mineral density (BMD) have been observed with long-term administration of products containing inhaled corticosteroids. Patients with major risk factors for decreased bone mineral content, such as chronic use of drugs that can reduce bone mass (eg, oral corticosteroids), should be monitored and treated with established standards of care).
No products indexed under this heading.

Dexamethasone Sodium (Decreases in bone mineral density (BMD) have been observed with long-term administration of products containing inhaled corticosteroids. Patients with major risk factors for decreased bone mineral content, such as chronic use of drugs that can reduce bone mass (eg, oral corticosteroids), should be monitored and treated with established standards of care).
No products indexed under this heading.

Dexamethasone Sodium Phosphate (Decreases in bone mineral density (BMD) have been observed with long-term administration of products containing inhaled corticosteroids. Patients with major risk factors for decreased bone mineral content, such as chronic use of drugs that can reduce bone mass (eg, oral corticosteroids), should be monitored and treated with established standards of care).
No products indexed under this heading.

Dexamethasone Sodium Phosphate Injection (Decreases in bone mineral density (BMD) have been observed with long-term administration of products containing inhaled corticosteroids. Patients with major risk factors for decreased bone mineral content, such as chronic use of drugs that can reduce bone mass (eg, oral corticosteroids), should be monitored and treated with established standards of care).
No products indexed under this heading.

Diflorasone Diacetate (Decreases in bone mineral density (BMD) have been observed with long-term administration of products containing inhaled corticosteroids. Patients with major risk factors for decreased bone mineral content, such as chronic use of drugs that can reduce bone mass (eg, oral corticosteroids), should be monitored and treated with established standards of care).
No products indexed under this heading.

Diltiazem Hydrochloride (The main route of metabolism of corticosteroids, including budesonide, a component of Symbicort, is via cytochrome P450 (CYP) isoenzyme 3A4 (CYP3A4). After oral administration of ketoconazole, a strong inhibitor of CYP3A4, the mean plasma concentration of orally administered budesonide increased. Concomitant administration of CYP3A4 inhibitors may inhibit the metabolism of, and increase the systemic exposure to, budesonide. Caution should be exercised when considering the co-administration of Symbicort with long-term ketoconazole and other known strong CYP3A4 inhibitors (eg, ritonavir, atazanavir, clarithromycin, indinavir, itraconazole, nefazodone, nelfinavir, saquinavir, telithromycin)). Products include:
Cardizem LA ... 423

Diltiazem Maleate (The main route of metabolism of corticosteroids, including budesonide, a component of Symbicort, is via cytochrome P450 (CYP) isoenzyme 3A4 (CYP3A4). After oral administration of ketoconazole, a strong inhibitor of CYP3A4, the mean plasma concentration of orally administered budesonide increased. Concomitant administration of CYP3A4 inhibitors may inhibit the metabolism of, and increase the systemic exposure to, budesonide. Caution should be exercised when considering the co-administration of Symbicort with long-term ketoconazole and other known strong CYP3A4 inhibitors (eg, ritonavir, atazanavir, clarithromycin, indinavir, itraconazole, nefazodone, nelfinavir, saquinavir, telithromycin)).
No products indexed under this heading.

Divalproex Sodium (Decreases in bone mineral density (BMD) have been observed with long-term administration of products containing inhaled corticosteroids. Patients with major risk factors for decreased bone mineral content, such as chronic use of drugs that can reduce bone mass (eg, anticonvulsants), should be monitored and treated with established standards of care). Products include:
Depakote ER ... 426

Doxepin Hydrochloride (Symbicort should be administered with caution to patients being treated with tricyclic antidepressants, or within 2 weeks of discontinuation of such agents, because the action of formoterol, a component of Symbicort, on the vascular system may be potentiated by these agents. In clinical trials with Symbicort, a limited number of COPD and asthma patients received tricyclic antidepressants, and, therefore, no clinically meaningful conclusions on adverse events can be made).
No products indexed under this heading.

Efavirenz (The main route of metabolism of corticosteroids, including budesonide, a component of Symbicort, is via cytochrome P450 (CYP) isoenzyme 3A4 (CYP3A4). After oral administration of ketoconazole, a strong inhibitor of CYP3A4, the mean plasma concentration of orally administered budesonide increased. Concomitant administration of CYP3A4 inhibitors may inhibit the metabolism of, and increase the systemic exposure to, budesonide. Caution should be exercised when considering the co-administration of Symbicort with long-term ketoconazole and other known strong CYP3A4 inhibitors (eg, ritonavir, atazanavir, clarithromycin, indinavir, itraconazole, nefazodone, nelfinavir, saquinavir, telithromycin)). Products include:
Atripla ... 906

Erythromycin (The main route of metabolism of corticosteroids, including budesonide, a component of Symbicort, is via cytochrome P450 (CYP) isoenzyme 3A4 (CYP3A4). After oral administration of ketoconazole, a strong inhibitor of CYP3A4, the mean plasma concentration of orally administered budesonide increased. Concomitant administration of CYP3A4 inhibitors may inhibit the metabolism of, and increase the systemic exposure to, budesonide. Caution should be exercised when considering the co-administration of Symbicort with long-term ketoconazole and other known strong CYP3A4 inhibitors (eg, ritonavir, atazanavir, clarithromycin, indinavir, itraconazole, nefazodone, nelfinavir, saquinavir, telithromycin)).
No products indexed under this heading.

Erythromycin Estolate (The main route of metabolism of corticosteroids, including budesonide, a component of Symbicort, is via cytochrome P450 (CYP) isoenzyme 3A4 (CYP3A4). After oral administration of ketoconazole, a strong inhibitor of CYP3A4, the mean plasma concentration of orally administered budesonide increased. Concomitant administration of CYP3A4 inhibitors may inhibit the metabolism of, and increase the systemic exposure to, budesonide. Caution should be exercised when considering the co-administration of Symbicort with long-term ketoconazole and other known strong CYP3A4 inhibitors (eg, ritonavir, atazanavir, clarithromycin, indinavir, itraconazole, nefazodone, nelfinavir, saquinavir, telithromycin)).
No products indexed under this heading.

Erythromycin Ethylsuccinate (The main route of metabolism of corticosteroids, including budesonide, a component of Symbicort, is via cytochrome P450 (CYP) isoenzyme 3A4 (CYP3A4). After oral administration of ketoconazole, a strong inhibitor of CYP3A4, the mean plasma concentration of orally administered budesonide increased. Concomitant administration of CYP3A4 inhibitors may inhibit the metabolism of, and increase the systemic exposure to, budesonide. Caution should be exercised when considering the co-administration of Symbicort with long-term ketoconazole and other known strong CYP3A4 inhibitors (eg, ritonavir, atazanavir, clarithromycin, indinavir, itraconazole, nefazodone, nelfinavir, saquinavir, telithromycin)). Products include:
E.E.S. ... 437
EryPed ... 435

Erythromycin Gluceptate (The main route of metabolism of corticosteroids, including budesonide, a component of Symbicort, is via cytochrome P450 (CYP) isoenzyme 3A4 (CYP3A4). After oral administration of ketoconazole, a strong inhibitor of CYP3A4, the mean plasma concentration of orally administered budesonide increased. Concomitant administration of CYP3A4 inhibitors may inhibit the metabolism of, and increase the systemic exposure to, budesonide. Caution should be exercised when considering the co-administration of Symbicort with long-term ketoconazole and other known strong CYP3A4 inhibitors (eg, ritonavir, atazanavir, clarithromycin, indinavir, itraconazole, nefazodone, nelfinavir, saquinavir, telithromycin)).
No products indexed under this heading.

Erythromycin Lactobionate (The main route of metabolism of corticosteroids, including budesonide, a component of Symbicort, is via cytochrome P450 (CYP) isoenzyme 3A4 (CYP3A4). After oral administration of ketoconazole, a strong inhibitor of CYP3A4, the mean plasma concentration of orally administered budesonide increased. Concomitant administration of CYP3A4 inhibitors may inhibit the metabolism of, and increase the systemic exposure to, budesonide. Caution should be exercised when considering the co-administration of Symbicort with long-term ketoconazole and other known strong CYP3A4 inhibitors (eg, ritonavir, atazanavir, clarithromycin, indinavir, itraconazole, nefazodone, nelfinavir, saquinavir, telithromycin)).
No products indexed under this heading.

Erythromycin Stearate (The main route of metabolism of corticosteroids, including budesonide, a component of

IMPORTANT NOTE: Always consult each drug listing in the patient's regimen for possible interactions.

Symbicort, is via cytochrome P450 (CYP) isoenzyme 3A4 (CYP3A4). After oral administration of ketoconazole, a strong inhibitor of CYP3A4, the mean plasma concentration of orally administered budesonide increased. Concomitant administration of CYP3A4 inhibitors may inhibit the metabolism of, and increase the systemic exposure to, budesonide. Caution should be exercised when considering the co-administration of Symbicort with long-term ketoconazole and other known strong CYP3A4 inhibitors (eg, ritonavir, atazanavir, clarithromycin, indinavir, itraconazole, nefazodone, nelfinavir, saquinavir, telithromycin)).
No products indexed under this heading.

Esmolol Hydrochloride (β-blockers (including eye drops) may not only block the pulmonary effect of β-agonists, such as formoterol, a component of Symbicort, but may produce severe bronchospasm in patients with asthma. Therefore, patients with asthma should not normally be treated with β-blockers. However, under certain circumstances, there may be no acceptable alternatives to the use of β-adrenergic blocking agents in patients with asthma. In this setting, cardioselective β-blockers could be considered, although they should be administered with caution).
No products indexed under this heading.

Esomeprazole Magnesium (The main route of metabolism of corticosteroids, including budesonide, a component of Symbicort, is via cytochrome P450 (CYP) isoenzyme 3A4 (CYP3A4). After oral administration of ketoconazole, a strong inhibitor of CYP3A4, the mean plasma concentration of orally administered budesonide increased. Concomitant administration of CYP3A4 inhibitors may inhibit the metabolism of, and increase the systemic exposure to, budesonide. Caution should be exercised when considering the co-administration of Symbicort with long-term ketoconazole and other known strong CYP3A4 inhibitors (eg, ritonavir, atazanavir, clarithromycin, indinavir, itraconazole, nefazodone, nelfinavir, saquinavir, telithromycin)). Products include:
Nexium Capsules 704
Nexium Oral Suspension 704

Esomeprazole Sodium (The main route of metabolism of corticosteroids, including budesonide, a component of Symbicort, is via cytochrome P450 (CYP) isoenzyme 3A4 (CYP3A4). After oral administration of ketoconazole, a strong inhibitor of CYP3A4, the mean plasma concentration of orally administered budesonide increased. Concomitant administration of CYP3A4 inhibitors may inhibit the metabolism of, and increase the systemic exposure to, budesonide. Caution should be exercised when considering the co-administration of Symbicort with long-term ketoconazole and other known strong CYP3A4 inhibitors (eg, ritonavir, atazanavir, clarithromycin, indinavir, itraconazole, nefazodone, nelfinavir, saquinavir, telithromycin)). Products include:
Nexium I.V. 712

Ethacrynic Acid (The ECG changes and/or hypokalemia that may result from the administration of non-potassium-sparing diuretics (such as loop or thiazide diuretics) can be acutely worsened by β-agonists, especially when the recommended dose of the β-agonist is exceeded. Although the clinical significance of these effects is not known, caution is advised in the co-administration of Symbicort with non-potassium-sparing diuretics).
No products indexed under this heading.

Ethosuximide (Decreases in bone mineral density (BMD) have been observed with long-term administration of products containing inhaled corticosteroids. Patients with major risk factors for decreased bone mineral content, such as chronic use of drugs that can reduce bone mass (eg, anticonvulsants), should be monitored and treated with established standards of care).
No products indexed under this heading.

Ethotoin (Decreases in bone mineral density (BMD) have been observed with long-term administration of products containing inhaled corticosteroids. Patients with major risk factors for decreased bone mineral content, such as chronic use of drugs that can reduce bone mass (eg, anticonvulsants), should be monitored and treated with established standards of care).
No products indexed under this heading.

Felbamate (Decreases in bone mineral density (BMD) have been observed with long-term administration of products containing inhaled corticosteroids. Patients with major risk factors for decreased bone mineral content, such as chronic use of drugs that can reduce bone mass (eg, anticonvulsants), should be monitored and treated with established standards of care).
No products indexed under this heading.

Fluconazole (The main route of metabolism of corticosteroids, including budesonide, a component of Symbicort, is via cytochrome P450 (CYP) isoenzyme 3A4 (CYP3A4). After oral administration of ketoconazole, a strong inhibitor of CYP3A4, the mean plasma concentration of orally administered budesonide increased. Concomitant administration of CYP3A4 inhibitors may inhibit the metabolism of, and increase the systemic exposure to, budesonide. Caution should be exercised when considering the co-administration of Symbicort with long-term ketoconazole and other known strong CYP3A4 inhibitors (eg, ritonavir, atazanavir, clarithromycin, indinavir, itraconazole, nefazodone, nelfinavir, saquinavir, telithromycin)).
No products indexed under this heading.

Fludrocortisone Acetate (Decreases in bone mineral density (BMD) have been observed with long-term administration of products containing inhaled corticosteroids. Patients with major risk factors for decreased bone mineral content, such as chronic use of drugs that can reduce bone mass (eg, oral corticosteroids), should be monitored and treated with established standards of care).
No products indexed under this heading.

Flumethasone Pivalate (Decreases in bone mineral density (BMD) have been observed with long-term administration of products containing inhaled corticosteroids. Patients with major risk factors for decreased bone mineral content, such as chronic use of drugs that can reduce bone mass (eg, oral corticosteroids), should be monitored and treated with established standards of care).
No products indexed under this heading.

Flunisolide Hemihydrate (Decreases in bone mineral density (BMD) have been observed with long-term administration of products containing inhaled corticosteroids. Patients with major risk factors for decreased bone mineral content, such as chronic use of drugs that can reduce bone mass (eg, oral corticosteroids), should be monitored and treated with established standards of care).
No products indexed under this heading.

Fluoxetine (The main route of metabolism of corticosteroids, including budesonide, a component of Symbicort, is via cytochrome P450 (CYP) isoenzyme 3A4 (CYP3A4). After oral administration of ketoconazole, a strong inhibitor of CYP3A4, the mean plasma concentration of orally administered budesonide increased. Concomitant administration of CYP3A4 inhibitors may inhibit the metabolism of, and increase the systemic exposure to, budesonide. Caution should be exercised when considering the co-administration of Symbicort with long-term ketoconazole and other known strong CYP3A4 inhibitors (eg, ritonavir, atazanavir, clarithromycin, indinavir, itraconazole, nefazodone, nelfinavir, saquinavir, telithromycin)).
No products indexed under this heading.

Fluoxetine Hydrochloride (The main route of metabolism of corticosteroids, including budesonide, a component of Symbicort, is via cytochrome P450 (CYP) isoenzyme 3A4 (CYP3A4). After oral administration of ketoconazole, a strong inhibitor of CYP3A4, the mean plasma concentration of orally administered budesonide increased. Concomitant administration of CYP3A4 inhibitors may inhibit the metabolism of, and increase the systemic exposure to, budesonide. Caution should be exercised when considering the co-administration of Symbicort with long-term ketoconazole and other known strong CYP3A4 inhibitors (eg, ritonavir, atazanavir, clarithromycin, indinavir, itraconazole, nefazodone, nelfinavir, saquinavir, telithromycin)). Products include:
Prozac Weekly 1941
Prozac Pulvules 1941
Symbyax 1965

Fluticasone Furoate (Decreases in bone mineral density (BMD) have been observed with long-term administration of products containing inhaled corticosteroids. Patients with major risk factors for decreased bone mineral content, such as chronic use of drugs that can reduce bone mass (eg, oral corticosteroids), should be monitored and treated with established standards of care). Products include:
Veramyst 1713

Fluticasone Propionate (Decreases in bone mineral density (BMD) have been observed with long-term administration of products containing inhaled corticosteroids. Patients with major risk factors for decreased bone mineral content, such as chronic use of drugs that can reduce bone mass (eg, oral corticosteroids), should be monitored and treated with established standards of care). Products include:
Advair 100/50 1275
Advair 250/50 1275
Advair 500/50 1275
Advair HFA 45/21 1288
Advair HFA 115/21 1288
Advair HFA 230/21 1288
Flonase 1459
Flovent Diskus 1463
Flovent HFA 1470

Fluvoxamine Maleate (The main route of metabolism of corticosteroids, including budesonide, a component of Symbicort, is via cytochrome P450 (CYP) isoenzyme 3A4 (CYP3A4). After oral administration of ketoconazole, a strong inhibitor of CYP3A4, the mean plasma concentration of orally administered budesonide increased. Concomitant administration of CYP3A4 inhibitors may inhibit the metabolism of, and increase the systemic exposure to, budesonide. Caution should be exercised when considering the co-administration of Symbicort with long-term ketoconazole and other known strong CYP3A4 inhibitors (eg, ritonavir, atazanavir, clarithromycin, indinavir, itraconazole, nefazodone, nelfinavir, saquinavir, telithromycin)).
No products indexed under this heading.

Fosamprenavir Calcium (The main route of metabolism of corticosteroids, including budesonide, a component of Symbicort, is via cytochrome P450 (CYP) isoenzyme 3A4 (CYP3A4). After oral administration of ketoconazole, a strong inhibitor of CYP3A4, the mean plasma concentration of orally administered budesonide increased. Concomitant administration of CYP3A4 inhibitors may inhibit the metabolism of, and increase the systemic exposure to, budesonide. Caution should be exercised when considering the co-administration of Symbicort with long-term ketoconazole and other known strong CYP3A4 inhibitors (eg, ritonavir, atazanavir, clarithromycin, indinavir, itraconazole, nefazodone, nelfinavir, saquinavir, telithromycin)). Products include:
Lexiva Oral Suspension 1558
Lexiva 1558

Fosphenytoin (Decreases in bone mineral density (BMD) have been observed with long-term administration of products containing inhaled corticosteroids. Patients with major risk factors for decreased bone mineral content, such as chronic use of drugs that can reduce bone mass (eg, anticonvulsants), should be monitored and treated with established standards of care).
No products indexed under this heading.

Fosphenytoin Sodium (Decreases in bone mineral density (BMD) have been observed with long-term administration of products containing inhaled corticosteroids. Patients with major risk factors for decreased bone mineral content, such as chronic use of drugs that can reduce bone mass (eg, anticonvulsants), should be monitored and treated with established standards of care).
No products indexed under this heading.

Furosemide (The ECG changes and/or hypokalemia that may result from the administration of non-potassium-sparing diuretics (such as loop or thiazide diuretics) can be acutely worsened by β-agonists, especially when the recommended dose of the β-agonist is exceeded. Although the clinical significance of these effects is not known, caution is advised in the co-administration of Symbicort with non-potassium-sparing diuretics). Products include:
Furosemide 2354

Gabapentin (Decreases in bone mineral density (BMD) have been observed with long-term administration of products containing inhaled corticosteroids. Patients with major risk factors for decreased bone mineral content, such as chronic use of drugs that can reduce bone mass (eg, anticonvulsants), should be monitored and treated with established standards of care).
No products indexed under this heading.

Hydrochlorothiazide (The ECG changes and/or hypokalemia that may result from the administration of non-potassium-sparing diuretics (such as loop or thiazide diuretics) can be acutely worsened by β-agonists, especially when the recommended dose of the β-agonist is exceeded. Although the clinical significance of these effects is not known, caution is advised in the co-administration of Symbicort with non-potassium-sparing diuretics). Products include:
Atacand HCT 700
Avalide 2956
Benicar HCT 1017
Diovan HCT 2419
Dyazide 1429

Exforge HCT 2449
Hyzaar 2162
Hyzaar 100-12.5 2162
Micardis HCT 889
Prinzide 2246
Tekturna HCT 2541
Teveten HCT 541

Hydrocortisone (Decreases in bone mineral density (BMD) have been observed with long-term administration of products containing inhaled corticosteroids. Patients with major risk factors for decreased bone mineral content, such as chronic use of drugs that can reduce bone mass (eg, oral corticosteroids), should be monitored and treated with established standards of care).
No products indexed under this heading.

Hydrocortisone (Alcohol) (Decreases in bone mineral density (BMD) have been observed with long-term administration of products containing inhaled corticosteroids. Patients with major risk factors for decreased bone mineral content, such as chronic use of drugs that can reduce bone mass (eg, oral corticosteroids), should be monitored and treated with established standards of care).
No products indexed under this heading.

Hydrocortisone Acetate (Decreases in bone mineral density (BMD) have been observed with long-term administration of products containing inhaled corticosteroids. Patients with major risk factors for decreased bone mineral content, such as chronic use of drugs that can reduce bone mass (eg, oral corticosteroids), should be monitored and treated with established standards of care).
No products indexed under this heading.

Hydrocortisone Butyrate (Decreases in bone mineral density (BMD) have been observed with long-term administration of products containing inhaled corticosteroids. Patients with major risk factors for decreased bone mineral content, such as chronic use of drugs that can reduce bone mass (eg, oral corticosteroids), should be monitored and treated with established standards of care).
No products indexed under this heading.

Hydrocortisone Cypionate (Decreases in bone mineral density (BMD) have been observed with long-term administration of products containing inhaled corticosteroids. Patients with major risk factors for decreased bone mineral content, such as chronic use of drugs that can reduce bone mass (eg, oral corticosteroids), should be monitored and treated with established standards of care).
No products indexed under this heading.

Hydrocortisone Hemisuccinate (Decreases in bone mineral density (BMD) have been observed with long-term administration of products containing inhaled corticosteroids. Patients with major risk factors for decreased bone mineral content, such as chronic use of drugs that can reduce bone mass (eg, oral corticosteroids), should be monitored and treated with established standards of care).
No products indexed under this heading.

Hydrocortisone Probutate (Decreases in bone mineral density (BMD) have been observed with long-term administration of products containing inhaled corticosteroids. Patients with major risk factors for decreased bone mineral content, such as chronic use of drugs that can reduce bone mass (eg, oral corticosteroids), should be monitored and treated with established standards of care).
No products indexed under this heading.

Hydrocortisone Sodium Phosphate (Decreases in bone mineral density (BMD) have been observed with long-term administration of products containing inhaled corticosteroids. Patients with major risk factors for decreased bone mineral content, such as chronic use of drugs that can reduce bone mass (eg, oral corticosteroids), should be monitored and treated with established standards of care).
No products indexed under this heading.

Hydrocortisone Sodium Succinate (Decreases in bone mineral density (BMD) have been observed with long-term administration of products containing inhaled corticosteroids. Patients with major risk factors for decreased bone mineral content, such as chronic use of drugs that can reduce bone mass (eg, oral corticosteroids), should be monitored and treated with established standards of care).
No products indexed under this heading.

Hydrocortisone Valerate (Decreases in bone mineral density (BMD) have been observed with long-term administration of products containing inhaled corticosteroids. Patients with major risk factors for decreased bone mineral content, such as chronic use of drugs that can reduce bone mass (eg, oral corticosteroids), should be monitored and treated with established standards of care).
No products indexed under this heading.

Hydroflumethiazide (The ECG changes and/or hypokalemia that may result from the administration of non-potassium-sparing diuretics (such as loop or thiazide diuretics) can be acutely worsened by β-agonists, especially when the recommended dose of the β-agonist is exceeded. Although the clinical significance of these effects is not known, caution is advised in the co-administration of Symbicort with non-potassium-sparing diuretics).
No products indexed under this heading.

Imatinib Mesylate (The main route of metabolism of corticosteroids, including budesonide, a component of Symbicort, is via cytochrome P450 (CYP) isoenzyme 3A4 (CYP3A4). After oral administration of ketoconazole, a strong inhibitor of CYP3A4, the mean plasma concentration of orally administered budesonide increased. Concomitant administration of CYP3A4 inhibitors may inhibit the metabolism of, and increase the systemic exposure to, budesonide. Caution should be exercised when considering the co-administration of Symbicort with long-term ketoconazole and other known strong CYP3A4 inhibitors (eg, ritonavir, atazanavir, clarithromycin, indinavir, itraconazole, nefazodone, nelfinavir, saquinavir, telithromycin)). Products include:

Gleevec 2477

Imipramine Hydrochloride (Symbicort should be administered with caution to patients being treated with tricyclic antidepressants, or within 2 weeks of discontinuation of such agents, because the action of formoterol, a component of Symbicort, on the vascular system may be potentiated by these agents. In clinical trials with Symbicort, a limited number of COPD and asthma patients received tricyclic antidepressants, and, therefore, no clinically meaningful conclusions on adverse events can be made).
No products indexed under this heading.

Imipramine Pamoate (Symbicort should be administered with caution to patients being treated with tricyclic antidepressants, or within 2 weeks of discontinuation of such agents, because the action of formoterol, a component of Symbicort, on the vascular system may be potentiated by these agents. In clinical trials with Symbicort, a limited number of COPD and asthma patients received tricyclic antidepressants, and, therefore, no clinically meaningful conclusions on adverse events can be made).
No products indexed under this heading.

Indapamide (The ECG changes and/or hypokalemia that may result from the administration of non-potassium-sparing diuretics (such as loop or thiazide diuretics) can be acutely worsened by beta-agonists, especially when the recommended dose of the beta-agonist is exceeded. Although the clinical significance of these effects is not known, caution is advised in the co-administration of Symbicort with non-potassium-sparing diuretics). Products include:

Indapamide 2356

Indinavir Sulfate (The main route of metabolism of corticosteroids, including budesonide, a component of Symbicort, is via cytochrome P450 (CYP) isoenzyme 3A4 (CYP3A4). After oral administration of ketoconazole, a strong inhibitor of CYP3A4, the mean plasma concentration of orally administered budesonide increased. Concomitant administration of CYP3A4 inhibitors may inhibit the metabolism of, and increase the systemic exposure to, budesonide. Caution should be exercised when considering the co-administration of Symbicort with long-term ketoconazole and other known strong CYP3A4 inhibitors (eg, ritonavir, atazanavir, clarithromycin, indinavir, itraconazole, nefazodone, nelfinavir, saquinavir, telithromycin)). Products include:

Crixivan 2113

Isocarboxazid (Symbicort should be administered with caution to patients being treated with monoamine oxidase inhibitors or within 2 weeks of discontinuation of such agents, because the action of formoterol, a component of Symbicort, on the vascular system may be potentiated by these agents). Products include:

Marplan 3481

Isoniazid (The main route of metabolism of corticosteroids, including budesonide, a component of Symbicort, is via cytochrome P450 (CYP) isoenzyme 3A4 (CYP3A4). After oral administration of ketoconazole, a strong inhibitor of CYP3A4, the mean plasma concentration of orally administered budesonide increased. Concomitant administration of CYP3A4 inhibitors may inhibit the metabolism of, and increase the systemic exposure to, budesonide. Caution should be exercised when considering the co-administration of Symbicort with long-term ketoconazole and other known strong CYP3A4 inhibitors (eg, ritonavir, atazanavir, clarithromycin, indinavir, itraconazole, nefazodone, nelfinavir, saquinavir, telithromycin)).
No products indexed under this heading.

Itraconazole (The main route of metabolism of corticosteroids, including budesonide, a component of Symbicort, is via cytochrome P450 (CYP) isoenzyme 3A4 (CYP3A4). After oral administration of ketoconazole, a strong inhibitor of CYP3A4, the mean plasma concentration of orally administered budesonide increased. Concomitant administration of CYP3A4 inhibitors may inhibit the metabolism of, and increase the systemic exposure to, budesonide. Caution should be exercised when considering the co-administration of Symbicort with long-term ketoconazole and other known strong CYP3A4 inhibitors (eg, ritonavir, atazanavir, clarithromycin, indinavir, itraconazole, nefazodone, nelfinavir, saquinavir, telithromycin)).
No products indexed under this heading.

Ketoconazole (The main route of metabolism of corticosteroids, including budesonide, a component of Symbicort, is via cytochrome P450 (CYP) isoenzyme 3A4 (CYP3A4). After oral administration of ketoconazole, a strong inhibitor of CYP3A4, the mean plasma concentration of orally administered budesonide increased. Concomitant administration of CYP3A4 may inhibit the metabolism of, and increase the systemic exposure to, budesonide. Caution should be exercised when considering the co-administration of Symbicort with long-term ketoconazole use). Products include:

Extina 3319
Xolegel 3337

Labetalol Hydrochloride (β-blockers (including eye drops) may not only block the pulmonary effect of β-agonists, such as formoterol, a component of Symbicort, but may produce severe bronchospasm in patients with asthma. Therefore, patients with asthma should not normally be treated with β-blockers. However, under certain circumstances, there may be no acceptable alternatives to the use of β-adrenergic blocking agents in patients with asthma. In this setting, cardioselective β-blockers could be considered, although they should be administered with caution).
No products indexed under this heading.

Lamotrigine (Decreases in bone mineral density (BMD) have been observed with long-term administration of products containing inhaled corticosteroids. Patients with major risk factors for decreased bone mineral content, such as chronic use of drugs that can reduce bone mass (eg, anticonvulsants), should be monitored and treated with established standards of care). Products include:

Lamictal 1522
Lamictal ODT 1522
Lamictal XR 1536

Lapatinib (The main route of metabolism of corticosteroids, including budesonide, a component of Symbicort, is via cytochrome P450 (CYP) isoenzyme 3A4 (CYP3A4). After oral administration of ketoconazole, a strong inhibitor of CYP3A4, the mean plasma concentration of orally administered budesonide increased. Concomitant administration of CYP3A4 inhibitors may inhibit the metabolism of, and increase the systemic exposure to, budesonide. Caution should be exercised when considering the co-administration of Symbicort with long-term ketoconazole and other known strong CYP3A4 inhibitors (eg, ritonavir, atazanavir, clarithromycin, indinavir, itraconazole, nefazodone, nelfinavir, saquinavir, telithromycin)). Products include:

Tykerb 1698

Levetiracetam (Decreases in bone mineral density (BMD) have been observed with long-term administration of products containing inhaled corticosteroids. Patients with major risk factors for decreased bone mineral content, such as chronic use of drugs that can reduce bone mass (eg, anticonvulsants), should be monitored and treated with established standards of care). Products include:

Keppra XR 3434

Levobunolol Hydrochloride (β-blockers (including eye drops) may not only block the pulmonary effect of β-agonists, such as formoterol, a component of Symbicort, but may produce severe bronchospasm in patients with asthma. Therefore, patients with asthma should not normally be treated with

Symbicort Interactions Index 1788

β-blockers. However, under certain circumstances, there may be no acceptable alternatives to the use of β-adrenergic blocking agents in patients with asthma. In this setting, cardioselective β-blockers could be considered, although they should be administered with caution).
No products indexed under this heading.

Lopinavir (The main route of metabolism of corticosteroids, including budesonide, a component of Symbicort, is via cytochrome P450 (CYP) isoenzyme 3A4 (CYP3A4). After oral administration of ketoconazole, a strong inhibitor of CYP3A4, the mean plasma concentration of orally administered budesonide increased. Concomitant administration of CYP3A4 inhibitors may inhibit the metabolism of, and increase the systemic exposure to, budesonide. Caution should be exercised when considering the co-administration of Symbicort with long-term ketoconazole and other known strong CYP3A4 inhibitors (eg, ritonavir, atazanavir, clarithromycin, indinavir, itraconazole, nefazodone, nelfinavir, saquinavir, telithromycin)). Products include:
Kaletra 458

Loratadine (The main route of metabolism of corticosteroids, including budesonide, a component of Symbicort, is via cytochrome P450 (CYP) isoenzyme 3A4 (CYP3A4). After oral administration of ketoconazole, a strong inhibitor of CYP3A4, the mean plasma concentration of orally administered budesonide increased. Concomitant administration of CYP3A4 inhibitors may inhibit the metabolism of, and increase the systemic exposure to, budesonide. Caution should be exercised when considering the co-administration of Symbicort with long-term ketoconazole and other known strong CYP3A4 inhibitors (eg, ritonavir, atazanavir, clarithromycin, indinavir, itraconazole, nefazodone, nelfinavir, saquinavir, telithromycin)).
No products indexed under this heading.

Maprotiline Hydrochloride (Symbicort should be administered with caution to patients being treated with tricyclic antidepressants, or within 2 weeks of discontinuation of such agents, because the action of formoterol, a component of Symbicort, on the vascular system may be potentiated by these agents. In clinical trials with Symbicort, a limited number of COPD and asthma patients received tricyclic antidepressants, and, therefore, no clinically meaningful conclusions on adverse events can be made).
No products indexed under this heading.

Mephenytoin (Decreases in bone mineral density (BMD) have been observed with long-term administration of products containing inhaled corticosteroids. Patients with major risk factors for decreased bone mineral content, such as chronic use of drugs that can reduce bone mass (eg, anticonvulsants), should be monitored and treated with established standards of care).
No products indexed under this heading.

Methsuximide (Decreases in bone mineral density (BMD) have been observed with long-term administration of products containing inhaled corticosteroids. Patients with major risk factors for decreased bone mineral content, such as chronic use of drugs that can reduce bone mass (eg, anticonvulsants), should be monitored and treated with established standards of care).
No products indexed under this heading.

Methyclothiazide (The ECG changes and/or hypokalemia that may result from the administration of non-potassium-sparing diuretics (such as loop or thiazide diuretics) can be acutely worsened by β-agonists, especially when the recommended dose of the β-agonist is exceeded. Although the clinical significance of these effects is not known, caution is advised in the co-administration of Symbicort with non-potassium-sparing diuretics).
No products indexed under this heading.

Methylprednisolone (Decreases in bone mineral density (BMD) have been observed with long-term administration of products containing inhaled corticosteroids. Patients with major risk factors for decreased bone mineral content, such as chronic use of drugs that can reduce bone mass (eg, oral corticosteroids), should be monitored and treated with established standards of care).
No products indexed under this heading.

Methylprednisolone Acetate (Decreases in bone mineral density (BMD) have been observed with long-term administration of products containing inhaled corticosteroids. Patients with major risk factors for decreased bone mineral content, such as chronic use of drugs that can reduce bone mass (eg, oral corticosteroids), should be monitored and treated with established standards of care).
No products indexed under this heading.

Methylprednisolone Sodium Succinate (Decreases in bone mineral density (BMD) have been observed with long-term administration of products containing inhaled corticosteroids. Patients with major risk factors for decreased bone mineral content, such as chronic use of drugs that can reduce bone mass (eg, oral corticosteroids), should be monitored and treated with established standards of care).
No products indexed under this heading.

Metipranolol Hydrochloride (β-blockers (including eye drops) may not only block the pulmonary effect of β-agonists, such as formoterol, a component of Symbicort, but may produce severe bronchospasm in patients with asthma. Therefore, patients with asthma should not normally be treated with β-blockers. However, under certain circumstances, there may be no acceptable alternatives to the use of β-adrenergic blocking agents in patients with asthma. In this setting, cardioselective β-blockers could be considered, although they should be administered with caution).
No products indexed under this heading.

Metolazone (The ECG changes and/or hypokalemia that may result from the administration of non-potassium-sparing diuretics (such as loop or thiazide diuretics) can be acutely worsened by beta-agonists, especially when the recommended dose of the beta-agonist is exceeded. Although the clinical significance of these effects is not known, caution is advised in the co-administration of Symbicort with non-potassium-sparing diuretics).
No products indexed under this heading.

Metoprolol Succinate (β-blockers (including eye drops) may not only block the pulmonary effect of β-agonists, such as formoterol, a component of Symbicort, but may produce severe bronchospasm in patients with asthma. Therefore, patients with asthma should not normally be treated with β-blockers. However, under certain circumstances, there may be no acceptable alternatives to the use of β-adrenergic blocking agents in patients with asthma. In this setting, cardioselective β-blockers could be considered, although they should be administered with caution). Products include:
Toprol XL 732

Metoprolol Tartrate (β-blockers (including eye drops) may not only block the pulmonary effect of β-agonists, such as formoterol, a component of Symbicort, but may produce severe bronchospasm in patients with asthma. Therefore, patients with asthma should not normally be treated with β-blockers. However, under certain circumstances, there may be no acceptable alternatives to the use of β-adrenergic blocking agents in patients with asthma. In this setting, cardioselective β-blockers could be considered, although they should be administered with caution).
No products indexed under this heading.

Metronidazole (The main route of metabolism of corticosteroids, including budesonide, a component of Symbicort, is via cytochrome P450 (CYP) isoenzyme 3A4 (CYP3A4). After oral administration of ketoconazole, a strong inhibitor of CYP3A4, the mean plasma concentration of orally administered budesonide increased. Concomitant administration of CYP3A4 inhibitors may inhibit the metabolism of, and increase the systemic exposure to, budesonide. Caution should be exercised when considering the co-administration of Symbicort with long-term ketoconazole and other known strong CYP3A4 inhibitors (eg, ritonavir, atazanavir, clarithromycin, indinavir, itraconazole, nefazodone, nelfinavir, saquinavir, telithromycin)). Products include:
Pylera 793

Metronidazole Benzoate (The main route of metabolism of corticosteroids, including budesonide, a component of Symbicort, is via cytochrome P450 (CYP) isoenzyme 3A4 (CYP3A4). After oral administration of ketoconazole, a strong inhibitor of CYP3A4, the mean plasma concentration of orally administered budesonide increased. Concomitant administration of CYP3A4 inhibitors may inhibit the metabolism of, and increase the systemic exposure to, budesonide. Caution should be exercised when considering the co-administration of Symbicort with long-term ketoconazole and other known strong CYP3A4 inhibitors (eg, ritonavir, atazanavir, clarithromycin, indinavir, itraconazole, nefazodone, nelfinavir, saquinavir, telithromycin)).
No products indexed under this heading.

Metronidazole Hydrochloride (The main route of metabolism of corticosteroids, including budesonide, a component of Symbicort, is via cytochrome P450 (CYP) isoenzyme 3A4 (CYP3A4). After oral administration of ketoconazole, a strong inhibitor of CYP3A4, the mean plasma concentration of orally administered budesonide increased. Concomitant administration of CYP3A4 inhibitors may inhibit the metabolism of, and increase the systemic exposure to, budesonide. Caution should be exercised when considering the co-administration of Symbicort with long-term ketoconazole and other known strong CYP3A4 inhibitors (eg, ritonavir, atazanavir, clarithromycin, indinavir, itraconazole, nefazodone, nelfinavir, saquinavir, telithromycin)).
No products indexed under this heading.

Metronidazole Sodium (The main route of metabolism of corticosteroids, including budesonide, a component of Symbicort, is via cytochrome P450 (CYP) isoenzyme 3A4 (CYP3A4). After oral administration of ketoconazole, a strong inhibitor of CYP3A4, the mean plasma concentration of orally administered budesonide increased. Concomitant administration of CYP3A4 inhibitors may inhibit the metabolism of, and increase the systemic exposure to, budesonide. Caution should be exercised when considering the co-administration of Symbicort with long-term ketoconazole and other known strong CYP3A4 inhibitors (eg, ritonavir, atazanavir, clarithromycin, indinavir, itraconazole, nefazodone, nelfinavir, saquinavir, telithromycin)).
No products indexed under this heading.

Miconazole (The main route of metabolism of corticosteroids, including budesonide, a component of Symbicort, is via cytochrome P450 (CYP) isoenzyme 3A4 (CYP3A4). After oral administration of ketoconazole, a strong inhibitor of CYP3A4, the mean plasma concentration of orally administered budesonide increased. Concomitant administration of CYP3A4 inhibitors may inhibit the metabolism of, and increase the systemic exposure to, budesonide. Caution should be exercised when considering the co-administration of Symbicort with long-term ketoconazole and other known strong CYP3A4 inhibitors (eg, ritonavir, atazanavir, clarithromycin, indinavir, itraconazole, nefazodone, nelfinavir, saquinavir, telithromycin)).
No products indexed under this heading.

Miconazole Nitrate (The main route of metabolism of corticosteroids, including budesonide, a component of Symbicort, is via cytochrome P450 (CYP) isoenzyme 3A4 (CYP3A4). After oral administration of ketoconazole, a strong inhibitor of CYP3A4, the mean plasma concentration of orally administered budesonide increased. Concomitant administration of CYP3A4 inhibitors may inhibit the metabolism of, and increase the systemic exposure to, budesonide. Caution should be exercised when considering the co-administration of Symbicort with long-term ketoconazole and other known strong CYP3A4 inhibitors (eg, ritonavir, atazanavir, clarithromycin, indinavir, itraconazole, nefazodone, nelfinavir, saquinavir, telithromycin)). Products include:
Vusion Ointment 3335

Mifepristone (The main route of metabolism of corticosteroids, including budesonide, a component of Symbicort, is via cytochrome P450 (CYP) isoenzyme 3A4 (CYP3A4). After oral administration of ketoconazole, a strong inhibitor of CYP3A4, the mean plasma concentration of orally administered budesonide increased. Concomitant administration of CYP3A4 inhibitors may inhibit the metabolism of, and increase the systemic exposure to, budesonide. Caution should be exercised when considering the co-administration of Symbicort with long-term ketoconazole and other known strong CYP3A4 inhibitors (eg, ritonavir, atazanavir, clarithromycin, indinavir, itraconazole, nefazodone, nelfinavir, saquinavir, telithromycin)).
No products indexed under this heading.

Moclobemide (Symbicort should be administered with caution to patients being treated with monoamine oxidase inhibitors or within 2 weeks of discontinuation of such agents, because the action of formoterol, a component of Symbicort, on the vascular system may be potentiated by these agents).
No products indexed under this heading.

Mometasone Furoate (Decreases in bone mineral density (BMD) have been observed with long-term administration of products containing inhaled corticosteroids. Patients with major risk factors for decreased bone mineral content, such as chronic use of drugs that can reduce bone mass (eg, oral corticosteroids), should be monitored and treated with established standards of care). Products include:
Asmanex 3058
Elocon Cream 3111
Elocon Lotion 3112

1789 Interactions Index Symbicort

Elocon Ointment 3114

Mometasone Furoate Monohydrate (Decreases in bone mineral density (BMD) have been observed with long-term administration of products containing inhaled corticosteroids. Patients with major risk factors for decreased bone mineral content, such as chronic use of drugs that can reduce bone mass (eg, oral corticosteroids), should be monitored and treated with established standards of care).
Products include:
Nasonex 3166

Nadolol (β-blockers (including eye drops) may not only block the pulmonary effect of β-agonists, such as formoterol, a component of Symbicort, but may produce severe bronchospasm in patients with asthma. Therefore, patients with asthma should not normally be treated with β-blockers. However, under certain circumstances, there may be no acceptable alternatives to the use of β-adrenergic blocking agents in patients with asthma. In this setting, cardioselective β-blockers could be considered, although they should be administered with caution). Products include:
Nadolol 2359

Nebivolol (β-blockers (including eye drops) may not only block the pulmonary effect of β-agonists, such as formoterol, a component of Symbicort, but may produce severe bronchospasm in patients with asthma. Therefore, patients with asthma should not normally be treated with β-blockers. However, under certain circumstances, there may be no acceptable alternatives to the use of β-adrenergic blocking agents in patients with asthma. In this setting, cardioselective β-blockers could be considered, although they should be administered with caution). Products include:
Bystolic 1147

Nefazodone Hydrochloride (The main route of metabolism of corticosteroids, including budesonide, a component of Symbicort, is via cytochrome P450 (CYP) isoenzyme 3A4 (CYP3A4). After oral administration of ketoconazole, a strong inhibitor of CYP3A4, the mean plasma concentration of orally administered budesonide increased. Concomitant administration of CYP3A4 inhibitors may inhibit the metabolism of, and increase the systemic exposure to, budesonide. Caution should be exercised when considering the co-administration of Symbicort with long-term ketoconazole and other known strong CYP3A4 inhibitors (eg, ritonavir, atazanavir, clarithromycin, indinavir, itraconazole, nefazodone, nelfinavir, saquinavir, telithromycin)).
No products indexed under this heading.

Nelfinavir Mesylate (The main route of metabolism of corticosteroids, including budesonide, a component of Symbicort, is via cytochrome P450 (CYP) isoenzyme 3A4 (CYP3A4). After oral administration of ketoconazole, a strong inhibitor of CYP3A4, the mean plasma concentration of orally administered budesonide increased. Concomitant administration of CYP3A4 inhibitors may inhibit the metabolism of, and increase the systemic exposure to, budesonide. Caution should be exercised when considering the co-administration of Symbicort with long-term ketoconazole and other known strong CYP3A4 inhibitors (eg, ritonavir, atazanavir, clarithromycin, indinavir, itraconazole, nefazodone, nelfinavir, saquinavir, telithromycin)).
No products indexed under this heading.

Nevirapine (The main route of metabolism of corticosteroids, including budesonide, a component of Symbicort, is via cytochrome P450 (CYP) isoenzyme 3A4 (CYP3A4). After oral administration of ketoconazole, a strong inhibitor of CYP3A4, the mean plasma concentration of orally administered budesonide increased. Concomitant administration of CYP3A4 inhibitors may inhibit the metabolism of, and increase the systemic exposure to, budesonide. Caution should be exercised when considering the co-administration of Symbicort with long-term ketoconazole and other known strong CYP3A4 inhibitors (eg, ritonavir, atazanavir, clarithromycin, indinavir, itraconazole, nefazodone, nelfinavir, saquinavir, telithromycin)). Products include:
Viramune Oral Suspension 897
Viramune Tablets 897

Niacin (The main route of metabolism of corticosteroids, including budesonide, a component of Symbicort, is via cytochrome P450 (CYP) isoenzyme 3A4 (CYP3A4). After oral administration of ketoconazole, a strong inhibitor of CYP3A4, the mean plasma concentration of orally administered budesonide increased. Concomitant administration of CYP3A4 inhibitors may inhibit the metabolism of, and increase the systemic exposure to, budesonide. Caution should be exercised when considering the co-administration of Symbicort with long-term ketoconazole and other known strong CYP3A4 inhibitors (eg, ritonavir, atazanavir, clarithromycin, indinavir, itraconazole, nefazodone, nelfinavir, saquinavir, telithromycin)). Products include:
Advicor 402
Cardio Basics 3455
Niaspan 497
Simcor 524

Niacinamide (The main route of metabolism of corticosteroids, including budesonide, a component of Symbicort, is via cytochrome P450 (CYP) isoenzyme 3A4 (CYP3A4). After oral administration of ketoconazole, a strong inhibitor of CYP3A4, the mean plasma concentration of orally administered budesonide increased. Concomitant administration of CYP3A4 inhibitors may inhibit the metabolism of, and increase the systemic exposure to, budesonide. Caution should be exercised when considering the co-administration of Symbicort with long-term ketoconazole and other known strong CYP3A4 inhibitors (eg, ritonavir, atazanavir, clarithromycin, indinavir, itraconazole, nefazodone, nelfinavir, saquinavir, telithromycin)). Products include:
CitraNatal 90 DHA Capsules 2332
CitraNatal Assure 2332
CitraNatal Rx 2332
Heplive 607

Niacinamide Hydroiodide (The main route of metabolism of corticosteroids, including budesonide, a component of Symbicort, is via cytochrome P450 (CYP) isoenzyme 3A4 (CYP3A4). After oral administration of ketoconazole, a strong inhibitor of CYP3A4, the mean plasma concentration of orally administered budesonide increased. Concomitant administration of CYP3A4 inhibitors may inhibit the metabolism of, and increase the systemic exposure to, budesonide. Caution should be exercised when considering the co-administration of Symbicort with long-term ketoconazole and other known strong CYP3A4 inhibitors (eg, ritonavir, atazanavir, clarithromycin, indinavir, itraconazole, nefazodone, nelfinavir, saquinavir, telithromycin)).
No products indexed under this heading.

Nicotinamide (The main route of metabolism of corticosteroids, including budesonide, a component of Symbicort, is via cytochrome P450 (CYP) isoenzyme 3A4 (CYP3A4). After oral administration of ketoconazole, a strong inhibitor of CYP3A4, the mean plasma concentration of orally administered budesonide increased. Concomitant administration of CYP3A4 inhibitors may inhibit the metabolism of, and increase the systemic exposure to, budesonide. Caution should be exercised when considering the co-administration of Symbicort with long-term ketoconazole and other known strong CYP3A4 inhibitors (eg, ritonavir, atazanavir, clarithromycin, indinavir, itraconazole, nefazodone, nelfinavir, saquinavir, telithromycin)).
No products indexed under this heading.

Nifedipine (The main route of metabolism of corticosteroids, including budesonide, a component of Symbicort, is via cytochrome P450 (CYP) isoenzyme 3A4 (CYP3A4). After oral administration of ketoconazole, a strong inhibitor of CYP3A4, the mean plasma concentration of orally administered budesonide increased. Concomitant administration of CYP3A4 inhibitors may inhibit the metabolism of, and increase the systemic exposure to, budesonide. Caution should be exercised when considering the co-administration of Symbicort with long-term ketoconazole and other known strong CYP3A4 inhibitors (eg, ritonavir, atazanavir, clarithromycin, indinavir, itraconazole, nefazodone, nelfinavir, saquinavir, telithromycin)).
No products indexed under this heading.

Norfloxacin (The main route of metabolism of corticosteroids, including budesonide, a component of Symbicort, is via cytochrome P450 (CYP) isoenzyme 3A4 (CYP3A4). After oral administration of ketoconazole, a strong inhibitor of CYP3A4, the mean plasma concentration of orally administered budesonide increased. Concomitant administration of CYP3A4 inhibitors may inhibit the metabolism of, and increase the systemic exposure to, budesonide. Caution should be exercised when considering the co-administration of Symbicort with long-term ketoconazole and other known strong CYP3A4 inhibitors (eg, ritonavir, atazanavir, clarithromycin, indinavir, itraconazole, nefazodone, nelfinavir, saquinavir, telithromycin)). Products include:
Noroxin 2220

Nortriptyline Hydrochloride (Symbicort should be administered with caution to patients being treated with tricyclic antidepressants, or within 2 weeks of discontinuation of such agents, because the action of formoterol, a component of Symbicort, on the vascular system may be potentiated by these agents. In clinical trials with Symbicort, a limited number of COPD and asthma patients received tricyclic antidepressants, and, therefore, no clinically meaningful conclusions on adverse events can be made).
No products indexed under this heading.

Omeprazole (The main route of metabolism of corticosteroids, including budesonide, a component of Symbicort, is via cytochrome P450 (CYP) isoenzyme 3A4 (CYP3A4). After oral administration of ketoconazole, a strong inhibitor of CYP3A4, the mean plasma concentration of orally administered budesonide increased. Concomitant administration of CYP3A4 inhibitors may inhibit the metabolism of, and increase the systemic exposure to, budesonide. Caution should be exercised when considering the co-administration of Symbicort with long-term ketoconazole and other known strong CYP3A4 inhibitors (eg, ritonavir, atazanavir, clarithromycin, indinavir, itraconazole, nefazodone, nelfinavir, saquinavir, telithromycin)).
No products indexed under this heading.

Oxcarbazepine (Decreases in bone mineral density (BMD) have been observed with long-term administration of products containing inhaled corticosteroids. Patients with major risk factors for decreased bone mineral content, such as chronic use of drugs that can reduce bone mass (eg, anticonvulsants), should be monitored and treated with established standards of care).
No products indexed under this heading.

Paramethadione (Decreases in bone mineral density (BMD) have been observed with long-term administration of products containing inhaled corticosteroids. Patients with major risk factors for decreased bone mineral content, such as chronic use of drugs that can reduce bone mass (eg, anticonvulsants), should be monitored and treated with established standards of care).
No products indexed under this heading.

Pargyline Hydrochloride (Symbicort should be administered with caution to patients being treated with monoamine oxidase inhibitors or within 2 weeks of discontinuation of such agents, because the action of formoterol, a component of Symbicort, on the vascular system may be potentiated by these agents).
No products indexed under this heading.

Paroxetine Hydrochloride (The main route of metabolism of corticosteroids, including budesonide, a component of Symbicort, is via cytochrome P450 (CYP) isoenzyme 3A4 (CYP3A4). After oral administration of ketoconazole, a strong inhibitor of CYP3A4, the mean plasma concentration of orally administered budesonide increased. Concomitant administration of CYP3A4 inhibitors may inhibit the metabolism of, and increase the systemic exposure to, budesonide. Caution should be exercised when considering the co-administration of Symbicort with long-term ketoconazole and other known strong CYP3A4 inhibitors (eg, ritonavir, atazanavir, clarithromycin, indinavir, itraconazole, nefazodone, nelfinavir, saquinavir, telithromycin)). Products include:
Paroxetine CR 2361
Paroxetine ER 2371
Paxil 1586
Paxil CR 1596

Penbutolol Sulfate (β-blockers (including eye drops) may not only block the pulmonary effect of β-agonists, such as formoterol, a component of Symbicort, but may produce severe bronchospasm in patients with asthma. Therefore, patients with asthma should not normally be treated with β-blockers. However, under certain circumstances, there may be no acceptable alternatives to the use of β-adrenergic blocking agents in patients with asthma. In this setting, cardioselective β-blockers could be considered, although they should be administered with caution).
No products indexed under this heading.

Phenacemide (Decreases in bone mineral density (BMD) have been observed with long-term administration of products containing inhaled corticosteroids. Patients with major risk factors for decreased bone mineral content, such as chronic use of drugs that can reduce bone mass (eg, anticonvulsants), should be monitored and treated with established standards of care).
No products indexed under this heading.

IMPORTANT NOTE: Always consult each drug listing in the patient's regimen for possible interactions.

Phenelzine Sulfate (Symbicort should be administered with caution to patients being treated with monoamine oxidase inhibitors or within 2 weeks of discontinuation of such agents, because the action of formoterol, a component of Symbicort, on the vascular system may be potentiated by these agents).

No products indexed under this heading.

Phenobarbital (Decreases in bone mineral density (BMD) have been observed with long-term administration of products containing inhaled corticosteroids. Patients with major risk factors for decreased bone mineral content, such as chronic use of drugs that can reduce bone mass (eg, anticonvulsants), should be monitored and treated with established standards of care). Products include:

Donnatal 2711

Phenobarbital Sodium (Decreases in bone mineral density (BMD) have been observed with long-term administration of products containing inhaled corticosteroids. Patients with major risk factors for decreased bone mineral content, such as chronic use of drugs that can reduce bone mass (eg, anticonvulsants), should be monitored and treated with established standards of care).

No products indexed under this heading.

Phensuximide (Decreases in bone mineral density (BMD) have been observed with long-term administration of products containing inhaled corticosteroids. Patients with major risk factors for decreased bone mineral content, such as chronic use of drugs that can reduce bone mass (eg, anticonvulsants), should be monitored and treated with established standards of care).

No products indexed under this heading.

Phenytoin (Decreases in bone mineral density (BMD) have been observed with long-term administration of products containing inhaled corticosteroids. Patients with major risk factors for decreased bone mineral content, such as chronic use of drugs that can reduce bone mass (eg, anticonvulsants), should be monitored and treated with established standards of care).

No products indexed under this heading.

Phenytoin Sodium (Decreases in bone mineral density (BMD) have been observed with long-term administration of products containing inhaled corticosteroids. Patients with major risk factors for decreased bone mineral content, such as chronic use of drugs that can reduce bone mass (eg, anticonvulsants), should be monitored and treated with established standards of care). Products include:

Phenytek Capsules 2380

Pindolol (β-blockers (including eye drops) may not only block the pulmonary effect of β-agonists, such as formoterol, a component of Symbicort, but may produce severe bronchospasm in patients with asthma. Therefore, patients with asthma should not normally be treated with β-blockers. However, under certain circumstances, there may be no acceptable alternatives to the use of β-adrenergic blocking agents in patients with asthma. In this setting, cardioselective β-blockers could be considered, although they should be administered with caution).

No products indexed under this heading.

Polythiazide (The ECG changes and/or hypokalemia that may result from the administration of non-potassium-sparing diuretics (such as loop or thiazide diuretics) can be acutely worsened by β-agonists, especially when the recommended dose of the β-agonist is exceeded. Although the clinical significance of these effects is not known,

caution is advised in the co-administration of Symbicort with non-potassium-sparing diuretics).

No products indexed under this heading.

Posaconazole (The main route of metabolism of corticosteroids, including budesonide, a component of Symbicort, is via cytochrome P450 (CYP) isoenzyme 3A4 (CYP3A4). After oral administration of ketoconazole, a strong inhibitor of CYP3A4, the mean plasma concentration of orally administered budesonide increased. Concomitant administration of CYP3A4 inhibitors may inhibit the metabolism of, and increase the systemic exposure to, budesonide. Caution should be exercised when considering the co-administration of Symbicort with long-term ketoconazole and other known strong CYP3A4 inhibitors (eg, ritonavir, atazanavir, clarithromycin, indinavir, itraconazole, nefazodone, nelfinavir, saquinavir, telithromycin)). Products include:

Noxafil 3172

Prednisolone (Decreases in bone mineral density (BMD) have been observed with long-term administration of products containing inhaled corticosteroids. Patients with major risk factors for decreased bone mineral content, such as chronic use of drugs that can reduce bone mass (eg, oral corticosteroids), should be monitored and treated with established standards of care).

No products indexed under this heading.

Prednisolone Acetate (Decreases in bone mineral density (BMD) have been observed with long-term administration of products containing inhaled corticosteroids. Patients with major risk factors for decreased bone mineral content, such as chronic use of drugs that can reduce bone mass (eg, oral corticosteroids), should be monitored and treated with established standards of care). Products include:

Blephamide .... ⊙212, ⊙214
Pred Forte .... ⊙225
Pred Mild .... ⊙230
Pred-G .... ⊙226, ⊙227

Prednisolone Sodium Phosphate (Decreases in bone mineral density (BMD) have been observed with long-term administration of products containing inhaled corticosteroids. Patients with major risk factors for decreased bone mineral content, such as chronic use of drugs that can reduce bone mass (eg, oral corticosteroids), should be monitored and treated with established standards of care).

No products indexed under this heading.

Prednisolone Tebutate (Decreases in bone mineral density (BMD) have been observed with long-term administration of products containing inhaled corticosteroids. Patients with major risk factors for decreased bone mineral content, such as chronic use of drugs that can reduce bone mass (eg, oral corticosteroids), should be monitored and treated with established standards of care).

No products indexed under this heading.

Prednisone (Decreases in bone mineral density (BMD) have been observed with long-term administration of products containing inhaled corticosteroids. Patients with major risk factors for decreased bone mineral content, such as chronic use of drugs that can reduce bone mass (eg, oral corticosteroids), should be monitored and treated with established standards of care).

No products indexed under this heading.

Prednisone sodium phosphate (Decreases in bone mineral density (BMD) have been observed with long-term administration of products containing inhaled corticosteroids. Patients with major risk factors for decreased bone mineral content, such as chronic use of drugs that can reduce bone mass (eg, oral corticosteroids), should be monitored and treated with established standards of care).

No products indexed under this heading.

Primidone (Decreases in bone mineral density (BMD) have been observed with long-term administration of products containing inhaled corticosteroids. Patients with major risk factors for decreased bone mineral content, such as chronic use of drugs that can reduce bone mass (eg, anticonvulsants), should be monitored and treated with established standards of care).

No products indexed under this heading.

Procarbazine Hydrochloride (Symbicort should be administered with caution to patients being treated with monoamine oxidase inhibitors or within 2 weeks of discontinuation of such agents, because the action of formoterol, a component of Symbicort, on the vascular system may be potentiated by these agents).

No products indexed under this heading.

Propoxyphene Hydrochloride (The main route of metabolism of corticosteroids, including budesonide, a component of Symbicort, is via cytochrome P450 (CYP) isoenzyme 3A4 (CYP3A4). After oral administration of ketoconazole, a strong inhibitor of CYP3A4, the mean plasma concentration of orally administered budesonide increased. Concomitant administration of CYP3A4 inhibitors may inhibit the metabolism of, and increase the systemic exposure to, budesonide. Caution should be exercised when considering the co-administration of Symbicort with long-term ketoconazole and other known strong CYP3A4 inhibitors (eg, ritonavir, atazanavir, clarithromycin, indinavir, itraconazole, nefazodone, nelfinavir, saquinavir, telithromycin)).

No products indexed under this heading.

Propoxyphene Napsylate (The main route of metabolism of corticosteroids, including budesonide, a component of Symbicort, is via cytochrome P450 (CYP) isoenzyme 3A4 (CYP3A4). After oral administration of ketoconazole, a strong inhibitor of CYP3A4, the mean plasma concentration of orally administered budesonide increased. Concomitant administration of CYP3A4 inhibitors may inhibit the metabolism of, and increase the systemic exposure to, budesonide. Caution should be exercised when considering the co-administration of Symbicort with long-term ketoconazole and other known strong CYP3A4 inhibitors (eg, ritonavir, atazanavir, clarithromycin, indinavir, itraconazole, nefazodone, nelfinavir, saquinavir, telithromycin)).

No products indexed under this heading.

Propranolol Hydrochloride (β-blockers (including eye drops) may not only block the pulmonary effect of β-agonists, such as formoterol, a component of Symbicort, but may produce severe bronchospasm in patients with asthma. Therefore, patients with asthma should not normally be treated with β-blockers. However, under certain circumstances, there may be no acceptable alternatives to the use of β-adrenergic blocking agents in patients with asthma. In this setting, cardioselective β-blockers could be considered, although they should be administered with caution). Products include:

InnoPran XL 1517

Protriptyline Hydrochloride (Symbicort should be administered with caution to patients being treated with tricyclic antidepressants, or within 2 weeks of discontinuation of such agents, because the action of formoterol, a component of Symbicort, on the vascular system may be potentiated by these agents. In clinical trials with Symbicort, a limited number of COPD and asthma patients received tricyclic antidepressants, and, therefore, no clinically meaningful conclusions on adverse events can be made).

No products indexed under this heading.

Quinidine (The main route of metabolism of corticosteroids, including budesonide, a component of Symbicort, is via cytochrome P450 (CYP) isoenzyme 3A4 (CYP3A4). After oral administration of ketoconazole, a strong inhibitor of CYP3A4, the mean plasma concentration of orally administered budesonide increased. Concomitant administration of CYP3A4 inhibitors may inhibit the metabolism of, and increase the systemic exposure to, budesonide. Caution should be exercised when considering the co-administration of Symbicort with long-term ketoconazole and other known strong CYP3A4 inhibitors (eg, ritonavir, atazanavir, clarithromycin, indinavir, itraconazole, nefazodone, nelfinavir, saquinavir, telithromycin)).

No products indexed under this heading.

Quinidine Hydrochloride (The main route of metabolism of corticosteroids, including budesonide, a component of Symbicort, is via cytochrome P450 (CYP) isoenzyme 3A4 (CYP3A4). After oral administration of ketoconazole, a strong inhibitor of CYP3A4, the mean plasma concentration of orally administered budesonide increased. Concomitant administration of CYP3A4 inhibitors may inhibit the metabolism of, and increase the systemic exposure to, budesonide. Caution should be exercised when considering the co-administration of Symbicort with long-term ketoconazole and other known strong CYP3A4 inhibitors (eg, ritonavir, atazanavir, clarithromycin, indinavir, itraconazole, nefazodone, nelfinavir, saquinavir, telithromycin)).

No products indexed under this heading.

Quinidine Polygalacturonate (The main route of metabolism of corticosteroids, including budesonide, a component of Symbicort, is via cytochrome P450 (CYP) isoenzyme 3A4 (CYP3A4). After oral administration of ketoconazole, a strong inhibitor of CYP3A4, the mean plasma concentration of orally administered budesonide increased. Concomitant administration of CYP3A4 inhibitors may inhibit the metabolism of, and increase the systemic exposure to, budesonide. Caution should be exercised when considering the co-administration of Symbicort with long-term ketoconazole and other known strong CYP3A4 inhibitors (eg, ritonavir, atazanavir, clarithromycin, indinavir, itraconazole, nefazodone, nelfinavir, saquinavir, telithromycin)).

No products indexed under this heading.

Quinidine Sulfate (The main route of metabolism of corticosteroids, including budesonide, a component of Symbicort, is via cytochrome P450 (CYP) isoenzyme 3A4 (CYP3A4). After oral administration of ketoconazole, a strong inhibitor of CYP3A4, the mean plasma concentration of orally administered budesonide increased. Concomitant administration of CYP3A4 inhibitors may inhibit the metabolism of, and increase the systemic exposure to, budesonide. Caution should be exercised when considering the co-administration of Symbicort with long-term ketoconazole and other known

(⊙ Described in PDR® for Ophthalmic Medicines)

1791 Interactions Index Symbicort

strong CYP3A4 inhibitors (eg, ritonavir, atazanavir, clarithromycin, indinavir, itraconazole, nefazodone, nelfinavir, saquinavir, telithromycin)).
No products indexed under this heading.

Quinine (The main route of metabolism of corticosteroids, including budesonide, a component of Symbicort, is via cytochrome P450 (CYP) isoenzyme 3A4 (CYP3A4). After oral administration of ketoconazole, a strong inhibitor of CYP3A4, the mean plasma concentration of orally administered budesonide increased. Concomitant administration of CYP3A4 inhibitors may inhibit the metabolism of, and increase the systemic exposure to, budesonide. Caution should be exercised when considering the co-administration of Symbicort with long-term ketoconazole and other known strong CYP3A4 inhibitors (eg, ritonavir, atazanavir, clarithromycin, indinavir, itraconazole, nefazodone, nelfinavir, saquinavir, telithromycin)). Products include:
Hyland's Leg Cramps PM with Quinine 3315

Quinine Sulfate (The main route of metabolism of corticosteroids, including budesonide, a component of Symbicort, is via cytochrome P450 (CYP) isoenzyme 3A4 (CYP3A4). After oral administration of ketoconazole, a strong inhibitor of CYP3A4, the mean plasma concentration of orally administered budesonide increased. Concomitant administration of CYP3A4 inhibitors may inhibit the metabolism of, and increase the systemic exposure to, budesonide. Caution should be exercised when considering the co-administration of Symbicort with long-term ketoconazole and other known strong CYP3A4 inhibitors (eg, ritonavir, atazanavir, clarithromycin, indinavir, itraconazole, nefazodone, nelfinavir, saquinavir, telithromycin)).
No products indexed under this heading.

Quinupristin (The main route of metabolism of corticosteroids, including budesonide, a component of Symbicort, is via cytochrome P450 (CYP) isoenzyme 3A4 (CYP3A4). After oral administration of ketoconazole, a strong inhibitor of CYP3A4, the mean plasma concentration of orally administered budesonide increased. Concomitant administration of CYP3A4 inhibitors may inhibit the metabolism of, and increase the systemic exposure to, budesonide. Caution should be exercised when considering the co-administration of Symbicort with long-term ketoconazole and other known strong CYP3A4 inhibitors (eg, ritonavir, atazanavir, clarithromycin, indinavir, itraconazole, nefazodone, nelfinavir, saquinavir, telithromycin)).
No products indexed under this heading.

Ranitidine Bismuth Citrate (The main route of metabolism of corticosteroids, including budesonide, a component of Symbicort, is via cytochrome P450 (CYP) isoenzyme 3A4 (CYP3A4). After oral administration of ketoconazole, a strong inhibitor of CYP3A4, the mean plasma concentration of orally administered budesonide increased. Concomitant administration of CYP3A4 inhibitors may inhibit the metabolism of, and increase the systemic exposure to, budesonide. Caution should be exercised when considering the co-administration of Symbicort with long-term ketoconazole and other known strong CYP3A4 inhibitors (eg, ritonavir, atazanavir, clarithromycin, indinavir, itraconazole, nefazodone, nelfinavir, saquinavir, telithromycin)).
No products indexed under this heading.

Ranitidine Hydrochloride (The main route of metabolism of corticosteroids, including budesonide, a component of Symbicort, is via cytochrome P450 (CYP) isoenzyme 3A4 (CYP3A4). After oral administration of ketoconazole, a strong inhibitor of CYP3A4, the mean plasma concentration of orally administered budesonide increased. Concomitant administration of CYP3A4 inhibitors may inhibit the metabolism of, and increase the systemic exposure to, budesonide. Caution should be exercised when considering the co-administration of Symbicort with long-term ketoconazole and other known strong CYP3A4 inhibitors (eg, ritonavir, atazanavir, clarithromycin, indinavir, itraconazole, nefazodone, nelfinavir, saquinavir, telithromycin)). Products include:
Zantac 1737
Zantac Injection 1732
Zantac Pharmacy 1735

Rasagiline Mesylate (Symbicort should be administered with caution to patients being treated with monoamine oxidase inhibitors or within 2 weeks of discontinuation of such agents, because the action of formoterol, a component of Symbicort, on the vascular system may be potentiated by these agents). Products include:
Azilect 3383

Ritonavir (The main route of metabolism of corticosteroids, including budesonide, a component of Symbicort, is via cytochrome P450 (CYP) isoenzyme 3A4 (CYP3A4). After oral administration of ketoconazole, a strong inhibitor of CYP3A4, the mean plasma concentration of orally administered budesonide increased. Concomitant administration of CYP3A4 inhibitors may inhibit the metabolism of, and increase the systemic exposure to, budesonide. Caution should be exercised when considering the co-administration of Symbicort with long-term ketoconazole and other known strong CYP3A4 inhibitors (eg, ritonavir, atazanavir, clarithromycin, indinavir, itraconazole, nefazodone, nelfinavir, saquinavir, telithromycin)). Products include:
Kaletra 458
Norvir 509

Rufinamide (Decreases in bone mineral density (BMD) have been observed with long-term administration of products containing inhaled corticosteroids. Patients with major risk factors for decreased bone mineral content, such as chronic use of drugs that can reduce bone mass (eg, anticonvulsants), should be monitored and treated with established standards of care). Products include:
Banzel 1050

Saquinavir (The main route of metabolism of corticosteroids, including budesonide, a component of Symbicort, is via cytochrome P450 (CYP) isoenzyme 3A4 (CYP3A4). After oral administration of ketoconazole, a strong inhibitor of CYP3A4, the mean plasma concentration of orally administered budesonide increased. Concomitant administration of CYP3A4 inhibitors may inhibit the metabolism of, and increase the systemic exposure to, budesonide. Caution should be exercised when considering the co-administration of Symbicort with long-term ketoconazole and other known strong CYP3A4 inhibitors (eg, ritonavir, atazanavir, clarithromycin, indinavir, itraconazole, nefazodone, nelfinavir, saquinavir, telithromycin)).
No products indexed under this heading.

Saquinavir Mesylate (The main route of metabolism of corticosteroids, including budesonide, a component of Symbicort, is via cytochrome P450 (CYP) isoenzyme 3A4 (CYP3A4). After oral administration of ketoconazole, a strong inhibitor of CYP3A4, the mean plasma concentration of orally administered budesonide increased. Concomitant administration of CYP3A4 inhibitors may inhibit the metabolism of, and increase the systemic exposure to, budesonide. Caution should be exercised when considering the co-administration of Symbicort with long-term ketoconazole and other known strong CYP3A4 inhibitors (eg, ritonavir, atazanavir, clarithromycin, indinavir, itraconazole, nefazodone, nelfinavir, saquinavir, telithromycin)).
No products indexed under this heading.

Selegiline (Symbicort should be administered with caution to patients being treated with monoamine oxidase inhibitors or within 2 weeks of discontinuation of such agents, because the action of formoterol, a component of Symbicort, on the vascular system may be potentiated by these agents). Products include:
Emsam 3623

Selegiline Hydrochloride (Symbicort should be administered with caution to patients being treated with monoamine oxidase inhibitors or within 2 weeks of discontinuation of such agents, because the action of formoterol, a component of Symbicort, on the vascular system may be potentiated by these agents). Products include:
Eldepryl 3312

Sertraline Hydrochloride (The main route of metabolism of corticosteroids, including budesonide, a component of Symbicort, is via cytochrome P450 (CYP) isoenzyme 3A4 (CYP3A4). After oral administration of ketoconazole, a strong inhibitor of CYP3A4, the mean plasma concentration of orally administered budesonide increased. Concomitant administration of CYP3A4 inhibitors may inhibit the metabolism of, and increase the systemic exposure to, budesonide. Caution should be exercised when considering the co-administration of Symbicort with long-term ketoconazole and other known strong CYP3A4 inhibitors (eg, ritonavir, atazanavir, clarithromycin, indinavir, itraconazole, nefazodone, nelfinavir, saquinavir, telithromycin)).
No products indexed under this heading.

Sildenafil Citrate (The main route of metabolism of corticosteroids, including budesonide, a component of Symbicort, is via cytochrome P450 (CYP) isoenzyme 3A4 (CYP3A4). After oral administration of ketoconazole, a strong inhibitor of CYP3A4, the mean plasma concentration of orally administered budesonide increased. Concomitant administration of CYP3A4 inhibitors may inhibit the metabolism of, and increase the systemic exposure to, budesonide. Caution should be exercised when considering the co-administration of Symbicort with long-term ketoconazole and other known strong CYP3A4 inhibitors (eg, ritonavir, atazanavir, clarithromycin, indinavir, itraconazole, nefazodone, nelfinavir, saquinavir, telithromycin)).
No products indexed under this heading.

Sotalol Hydrochloride (β-blockers (including eye drops) may not only block the pulmonary effect of β-agonists, such as formoterol, a component of Symbicort, but may produce severe bronchospasm in patients with asthma. Therefore, patients with asthma should not normally be treated with β-blockers. However, under certain circumstances, there may be no acceptable alternatives to the use of β-adrenergic blocking agents in patients with asthma. In this setting, cardioselective β-blockers could be considered, although they should be administered with caution).
No products indexed under this heading.

Spironolactone (The ECG changes and/or hypokalemia that may result from the administration of non-potassium-sparing diuretics (such as loop or thiazide diuretics) can be acutely worsened by beta-agonists, especially when the recommended dose of the beta-agonist is exceeded. Although the clinical significance of these effects is not known, caution is advised in the co-administration of Symbicort with non-potassium-sparing diuretics).
No products indexed under this heading.

Telithromycin (The main route of metabolism of corticosteroids, including budesonide, a component of Symbicort, is via cytochrome P450 (CYP) isoenzyme 3A4 (CYP3A4). After oral administration of ketoconazole, a strong inhibitor of CYP3A4, the mean plasma concentration of orally administered budesonide increased. Concomitant administration of CYP3A4 inhibitors may inhibit the metabolism of, and increase the systemic exposure to, budesonide. Caution should be exercised when considering the co-administration of Symbicort with long-term ketoconazole and other known strong CYP3A4 inhibitors (eg, ritonavir, atazanavir, clarithromycin, indinavir, itraconazole, nefazodone, nelfinavir, saquinavir, telithromycin)). Products include:
Ketek 2991

Tiagabine Hydrochloride (Decreases in bone mineral density (BMD) have been observed with long-term administration of products containing inhaled corticosteroids. Patients with major risk factors for decreased bone mineral content, such as chronic use of drugs that can reduce bone mass (eg, anticonvulsants), should be monitored and treated with established standards of care). Products include:
Gabitril 972

Timolol Hemihydrate (β-blockers (including eye drops) may not only block the pulmonary effect of β-agonists, such as formoterol, a component of Symbicort, but may produce severe bronchospasm in patients with asthma. Therefore, patients with asthma should not normally be treated with β-blockers. However, under certain circumstances, there may be no acceptable alternatives to the use of β-adrenergic blocking agents in patients with asthma. In this setting, cardioselective β-blockers could be considered, although they should be administered with caution). Products include:
Betimol 3490

Timolol Maleate (β-blockers (including eye drops) may not only block the pulmonary effect of β-agonists, such as formoterol, a component of Symbicort, but may produce severe bronchospasm in patients with asthma. Therefore, patients with asthma should not normally be treated with β-blockers. However, under certain circumstances, there may be no acceptable alternatives to the use of β-adrenergic blocking agents in patients with asthma. In this setting, cardioselective β-blockers could be considered, although they should be administered with caution). Products include:
Combigan 601
Dorzolamide Hydrochloride/Timolol Maleate Ophthalmic Solution .... ⊙ 243
Timoptic in Ocudose .... ⊙ 231

Tobacco (Decreases in bone mineral density (BMD) have been observed with long-term administration of products containing inhaled corticosteroids. Patients with major risk factors for decreased bone mineral content, such as tobacco use, should be monitored and treated with established standards of care).
No products indexed under this heading.

IMPORTANT NOTE: Always consult each drug listing in the patient's regimen for possible interactions.

Topiramate (Decreases in bone mineral density (BMD) have been observed with long-term administration of products containing inhaled corticosteroids. Patients with major risk factors for decreased bone mineral content, such as chronic use of drugs that can reduce bone mass (eg, anticonvulsants), should be monitored and treated with established standards of care).
No products indexed under this heading.

Torsemide (The ECG changes and/or hypokalemia that may result from the administration of non-potassium-sparing diuretics (such as loop or thiazide diuretics) can be acutely worsened by β-agonists, especially when the recommended dose of the β-agonist is exceeded. Although the clinical significance of these effects is not known, caution is advised in the co-administration of Symbicort with non-potassium-sparing diuretics).
No products indexed under this heading.

Tranylcypromine Sulfate (Symbicort should be administered with caution to patients being treated with monoamine oxidase inhibitors or within 2 weeks of discontinuation of such agents, because the action of formoterol, a component of Symbicort, on the vascular system may be potentiated by these agents). Products include:
Parnate 1584

Triamcinolone (Decreases in bone mineral density (BMD) have been observed with long-term administration of products containing inhaled corticosteroids. Patients with major risk factors for decreased bone mineral content, such as chronic use of drugs that can reduce bone mass (eg, oral corticosteroids), should be monitored and treated with established standards of care).
No products indexed under this heading.

Triamcinolone Acetonide (Decreases in bone mineral density (BMD) have been observed with long-term administration of products containing inhaled corticosteroids. Patients with major risk factors for decreased bone mineral content, such as chronic use of drugs that can reduce bone mass (eg, oral corticosteroids), should be monitored and treated with established standards of care). Products include:
Azmacort 408
Nasacort AQ 3019

Triamcinolone Diacetate (Decreases in bone mineral density (BMD) have been observed with long-term administration of products containing inhaled corticosteroids. Patients with major risk factors for decreased bone mineral content, such as chronic use of drugs that can reduce bone mass (eg, oral corticosteroids), should be monitored and treated with established standards of care).
No products indexed under this heading.

Triamcinolone Hexacetonide (Decreases in bone mineral density (BMD) have been observed with long-term administration of products containing inhaled corticosteroids. Patients with major risk factors for decreased bone mineral content, such as chronic use of drugs that can reduce bone mass (eg, oral corticosteroids), should be monitored and treated with established standards of care).
No products indexed under this heading.

Triamterene (The ECG changes and/or hypokalemia that may result from the administration of non-potassium-sparing diuretics (such as loop or thiazide diuretics) can be acutely worsened by beta-agonists, especially when the recommended dose of the beta-agonist is exceeded. Although the clinical significance of these effects is not known, caution is advised in the co-

administration of Symbicort with non-potassium-sparing diuretics). Products include:
Dyazide 1429
Dyrenium 3495

Trimethadione (Decreases in bone mineral density (BMD) have been observed with long-term administration of products containing inhaled corticosteroids. Patients with major risk factors for decreased bone mineral content, such as chronic use of drugs that can reduce bone mass (eg, anticonvulsants), should be monitored and treated with established standards of care).
No products indexed under this heading.

Trimipramine Maleate (Symbicort should be administered with caution to patients being treated with tricyclic antidepressants, or within 2 weeks of discontinuation of such agents, because the action of formoterol, a component of Symbicort, on the vascular system may be potentiated by these agents. In clinical trials with Symbicort, a limited number of COPD and asthma patients received tricyclic antidepressants, and, therefore, no clinically meaningful conclusions on adverse events can be made).
No products indexed under this heading.

Troglitazone (The main route of metabolism of corticosteroids, including budesonide, a component of Symbicort, is via cytochrome P450 (CYP) isoenzyme 3A4 (CYP3A4). After oral administration of ketoconazole, a strong inhibitor of CYP3A4, the mean plasma concentration of orally administered budesonide increased. Concomitant administration of CYP3A4 inhibitors may inhibit the metabolism of, and increase the systemic exposure to, budesonide. Caution should be exercised when considering the co-administration of Symbicort with long-term ketoconazole and other known strong CYP3A4 inhibitors (eg, ritonavir, atazanavir, clarithromycin, indinavir, itraconazole, nefazodone, nelfinavir, saquinavir, telithromycin)).
No products indexed under this heading.

Troleandomycin (The main route of metabolism of corticosteroids, including budesonide, a component of Symbicort, is via cytochrome P450 (CYP) isoenzyme 3A4 (CYP3A4). After oral administration of ketoconazole, a strong inhibitor of CYP3A4, the mean plasma concentration of orally administered budesonide increased. Concomitant administration of CYP3A4 inhibitors may inhibit the metabolism of, and increase the systemic exposure to, budesonide. Caution should be exercised when considering the co-administration of Symbicort with long-term ketoconazole and other known strong CYP3A4 inhibitors (eg, ritonavir, atazanavir, clarithromycin, indinavir, itraconazole, nefazodone, nelfinavir, saquinavir, telithromycin)).
No products indexed under this heading.

Valproate Sodium (The main route of metabolism of corticosteroids, including budesonide, a component of Symbicort, is via cytochrome P450 (CYP) isoenzyme 3A4 (CYP3A4). After oral administration of ketoconazole, a strong inhibitor of CYP3A4, the mean plasma concentration of orally administered budesonide increased. Concomitant administration of CYP3A4 inhibitors may inhibit the metabolism of, and increase the systemic exposure to, budesonide. Caution should be exercised when considering the co-administration of Symbicort with long-term ketoconazole and other known strong CYP3A4 inhibitors (eg, ritonavir,

atazanavir, clarithromycin, indinavir, itraconazole, nefazodone, nelfinavir, saquinavir, telithromycin)).
No products indexed under this heading.

Valproic Acid (Decreases in bone mineral density (BMD) have been observed with long-term administration of products containing inhaled corticosteroids. Patients with major risk factors for decreased bone mineral content, such as chronic use of drugs that can reduce bone mass (eg, anticonvulsants), should be monitored and treated with established standards of care).
No products indexed under this heading.

Vardenafil Hydrochloride (The main route of metabolism of corticosteroids, including budesonide, a component of Symbicort, is via cytochrome P450 (CYP) isoenzyme 3A4 (CYP3A4). After oral administration of ketoconazole, a strong inhibitor of CYP3A4, the mean plasma concentration of orally administered budesonide increased. Concomitant administration of CYP3A4 inhibitors may inhibit the metabolism of, and increase the systemic exposure to, budesonide. Caution should be exercised when considering the co-administration of Symbicort with long-term ketoconazole and other known strong CYP3A4 inhibitors (eg, ritonavir, atazanavir, clarithromycin, indinavir, itraconazole, nefazodone, nelfinavir, saquinavir, telithromycin)). Products include:
Levitra 3157

Verapamil Hydrochloride (The main route of metabolism of corticosteroids, including budesonide, a component of Symbicort, is via cytochrome P450 (CYP) isoenzyme 3A4 (CYP3A4). After oral administration of ketoconazole, a strong inhibitor of CYP3A4, the mean plasma concentration of orally administered budesonide increased. Concomitant administration of CYP3A4 inhibitors may inhibit the metabolism of, and increase the systemic exposure to, budesonide. Caution should be exercised when considering the co-administration of Symbicort with long-term ketoconazole and other known strong CYP3A4 inhibitors (eg, ritonavir, atazanavir, clarithromycin, indinavir, itraconazole, nefazodone, nelfinavir, saquinavir, telithromycin)). Products include:
Tarka 534

Voriconazole (The main route of metabolism of corticosteroids, including budesonide, a component of Symbicort, is via cytochrome P450 (CYP) isoenzyme 3A4 (CYP3A4). After oral administration of ketoconazole, a strong inhibitor of CYP3A4, the mean plasma concentration of orally administered budesonide increased. Concomitant administration of CYP3A4 inhibitors may inhibit the metabolism of, and increase the systemic exposure to, budesonide. Caution should be exercised when considering the co-administration of Symbicort with long-term ketoconazole and other known strong CYP3A4 inhibitors (eg, ritonavir, atazanavir, clarithromycin, indinavir, itraconazole, nefazodone, nelfinavir, saquinavir, telithromycin)).
No products indexed under this heading.

Zafirlukast (The main route of metabolism of corticosteroids, including budesonide, a component of Symbicort, is via cytochrome P450 (CYP) isoenzyme 3A4 (CYP3A4). After oral administration of ketoconazole, a strong inhibitor of CYP3A4, the mean plasma concentration of orally administered budesonide increased. Concomitant administration of CYP3A4 inhibitors may inhibit the metabolism of, and increase the systemic exposure to, budesonide. Caution should be exercised when considering

the co-administration of Symbicort with long-term ketoconazole and other known strong CYP3A4 inhibitors (eg, ritonavir, atazanavir, clarithromycin, indinavir, itraconazole, nefazodone, nelfinavir, saquinavir, telithromycin)). Products include:
Accolate 3612

Zileuton (The main route of metabolism of corticosteroids, including budesonide, a component of Symbicort, is via cytochrome P450 (CYP) isoenzyme 3A4 (CYP3A4). After oral administration of ketoconazole, a strong inhibitor of CYP3A4, the mean plasma concentration of orally administered budesonide increased. Concomitant administration of CYP3A4 inhibitors may inhibit the metabolism of, and increase the systemic exposure to, budesonide. Caution should be exercised when considering the co-administration of Symbicort with long-term ketoconazole and other known strong CYP3A4 inhibitors (eg, ritonavir, atazanavir, clarithromycin, indinavir, itraconazole, nefazodone, nelfinavir, saquinavir, telithromycin)).
No products indexed under this heading.

Zonisamide (Decreases in bone mineral density (BMD) have been observed with long-term administration of products containing inhaled corticosteroids. Patients with major risk factors for decreased bone mineral content, such as chronic use of drugs that can reduce bone mass (eg, anticonvulsants), should be monitored and treated with established standards of care). Products include:
Zonegran 1081

Food Interactions

Grapefruit (The main route of metabolism of corticosteroids, including budesonide, a component of Symbicort, is via cytochrome P450 (CYP) isoenzyme 3A4 (CYP3A4). After oral administration of ketoconazole, a strong inhibitor of CYP3A4, the mean plasma concentration of orally administered budesonide increased. Concomitant administration of CYP3A4 inhibitors may inhibit the metabolism of, and increase the systemic exposure to, budesonide. Caution should be exercised when considering the co-administration of Symbicort with long-term ketoconazole and other known strong CYP3A4 inhibitors (eg, ritonavir, atazanavir, clarithromycin, indinavir, itraconazole, nefazodone, nelfinavir, saquinavir, telithromycin)).

Grapefruit Juice (The main route of metabolism of corticosteroids, including budesonide, a component of Symbicort, is via cytochrome P450 (CYP) isoenzyme 3A4 (CYP3A4). After oral administration of ketoconazole, a strong inhibitor of CYP3A4, the mean plasma concentration of orally administered budesonide increased. Concomitant administration of CYP3A4 inhibitors may inhibit the metabolism of, and increase the systemic exposure to, budesonide. Caution should be exercised when considering the co-administration of Symbicort with long-term ketoconazole and other known strong CYP3A4 inhibitors (eg, ritonavir, atazanavir, clarithromycin, indinavir, itraconazole, nefazodone, nelfinavir, saquinavir, telithromycin)).

SYMBICORT 160/4.5 INHALATION AEROSOL
(Budesonide, Formoterol fumarate dihydrate) 720
See Symbicort 80/4.5 Inhalation Aerosol

SYMBYAX CAPSULES
(Fluoxetine Hydrochloride, Olanzapine) 1965
May interact with alcohols, antiarrhyth-

1793 **Interactions Index** **Symbyax**

mics, anticoagulants, antidepressant drugs, antihypertensives, antipsychotic agents, aspirin-acetylsalicylic acid, centrally-acting drugs, cytochrome p450 1a2 inducers (selected), cytochrome p450 2d6 substrates (selected), diuretics, dopamine agonists, dopamine antagonists, haloperidols, highly protein bound drugs (selected), lithium preparations, monoamine oxidase inhibitors, non-steroidal anti-inflammatory agents, phenothiazines, phenytoin, selective serotonin reuptake inhibitors, serotonin and norepinephrine reuptake inhibitors, serotoninergic agents, tricyclic antidepressants, triptans, and certain other agents. Compounds in these categories include:

Acebutolol Hydrochloride (Co-administration of fluoxetine with other drugs that are metabolized by CYP2D6, including antiarrhythmics (eg, propafenone, flecainide, and others) should be approached with caution. Therapy with medications that are predominantly metabolized by the CYP2D6 system and that have a relatively narrow therapeutic index should be initiated at the low end of the dose range if a patient is receiving fluoxetine concurrently or has taken it in the previous 5 weeks. If fluoxetine is added to the treatment regimen of a patient already receiving a drug metabolized by CYP2D6, the need for a decreased dose of the original medication should be considered).
No products indexed under this heading.

Adenosine (Co-administration of fluoxetine with other drugs that are metabolized by CYP2D6, including antiarrhythmics (eg, propafenone, flecainide, and others) should be approached with caution. Therapy with medications that are predominantly metabolized by the CYP2D6 system and that have a relatively narrow therapeutic index should be initiated at the low end of the dose range if a patient is receiving fluoxetine concurrently or has taken it in the previous 5 weeks. If fluoxetine is added to the treatment regimen of a patient already receiving a drug metabolized by CYP2D6, the need for a decreased dose of the original medication should be considered). Products include:
Adenocard 656
Adenoscan 657

Alfentanil Hydrochloride (Caution is advised if the concomitant administration of Symbyax and other CNS-active drugs is required. In evaluating individual cases, consideration should be given to using lower initial doses of the concomitantly administered drugs, using conservative titration schedules and monitoring of clinical status).
No products indexed under this heading.

Aliskiren (Because of the potential for olanzapine to induce hypotension, Symbyax may enhance the effects of certain antihypertensive agents). Products include:
Tekturna 2538
Tekturna HCT 2541
Valturna 3637

Almotriptan Malate (There have been rare postmarketing reports of serotonin syndrome with use of an SSRI and a triptan. If concomitant treatment of Symbyax with a triptan is clinically warranted, careful observation of the patient is advised, particularly during treatment initiation and dose increases). Products include:
Axert 2593

Alprazolam (Co-administration of alprazolam and fluoxetine may result in increased alprazolam plasma concentrations and in further psychomotor performance decrement due to increased alprazolam levels).
No products indexed under this heading.

Amiloride Hydrochloride (Hyponatremia may occur as a result of treatment with SSRIs and SNRIs, including fluoxetine and Symbyax. In many cases, this hyponatremia appears to be the result of the syndrome of inappropriate antidiuretic hormone secretion (SIADH). Cases with serum sodium lower than 110 mmol/L have been reported and appeared to be reversible when Symbyax was discontinued. Patients taking diuretics or who are otherwise volume depleted may be at greater risk. Discontinuation of Symbyax should be considered in patients with symptomatic hyponatremia and appropriate medical intervention should be instituted).
No products indexed under this heading.

Amiodarone Hydrochloride (Co-administration of fluoxetine with other drugs that are metabolized by CYP2D6, including antiarrhythmics (eg, propafenone, flecainide, and others) should be approached with caution. Therapy with medications that are predominantly metabolized by the CYP2D6 system and that have a relatively narrow therapeutic index should be initiated at the low end of the dose range if a patient is receiving fluoxetine concurrently or has taken it in the previous 5 weeks. If fluoxetine is added to the treatment regimen of a patient already receiving a drug metabolized by CYP2D6, the need for a decreased dose of the original medication should be considered).
No products indexed under this heading.

Amitriptyline Hydrochloride (In two fluoxetine studies, previously stable plasma levels of imipramine and desipramine have increased>2- to 10-fold when fluoxetine has been administered in combination. This influence may persist for three weeks or longer after fluoxetine is discontinued. Thus, the dose of TCA may need to be reduced and plasma TCA concentrations may need to be monitored temporarily when Symbyax is co-administered or has been recently discontinued. Co-administration of fluoxetine with other drugs that are metabolized by CYP2D6, including certain antidepressants (eg, TCAs), should be approached with caution).
No products indexed under this heading.

Amlodipine Besylate (Because of the potential for olanzapine to induce hypotension, Symbyax may enhance the effects of certain antihypertensive agents). Products include:
Azor 1010
Exforge 2443
Exforge HCT 2449

Amoxapine (In two fluoxetine studies, previously stable plasma levels of imipramine and desipramine have increased>2- to 10-fold when fluoxetine has been administered in combination. This influence may persist for three weeks or longer after fluoxetine is discontinued. Thus, the dose of TCA may need to be reduced and plasma TCA concentrations may need to be monitored temporarily when Symbyax is co-administered or has been recently discontinued. Co-administration of fluoxetine with other drugs that are metabolized by CYP2D6, including certain antidepressants (eg, TCAs), should be approached with caution).
No products indexed under this heading.

Amphetamine Aspartate (Caution is advised if the concomitant administration of Symbyax and other CNS-active drugs is required. In evaluating individual cases, consideration should be given to using lower initial doses of the concomitantly administered drugs, using conservative titration schedules and monitoring of clinical status).
No products indexed under this heading.

Amphetamine Aspartate Monohydrate (Caution is advised if the concomitant administration of Symbyax and other CNS-active drugs is required. In evaluating individual cases, consideration should be given to using lower initial doses of the concomitantly administered drugs, using conservative titration schedules and monitoring of clinical status).
No products indexed under this heading.

Amphetamine Resins (Caution is advised if the concomitant administration of Symbyax and other CNS-active drugs is required. In evaluating individual cases, consideration should be given to using lower initial doses of the concomitantly administered drugs, using conservative titration schedules and monitoring of clinical status).
No products indexed under this heading.

Amphetamine Sulfate (Caution is advised if the concomitant administration of Symbyax and other CNS-active drugs is required. In evaluating individual cases, consideration should be given to using lower initial doses of the concomitantly administered drugs, using conservative titration schedules and monitoring of clinical status).
No products indexed under this heading.

Anisindione (Serotonin release by platelets plays an important role in hemostasis. Epidemiological studies of the case-control and cohort design that have demonstrated an association between use of psychotropic drugs that interfere with serotonin re-uptake and the occurrence of upper gastrointestinal bleeding have also shown that concurrent use of an NSAID or aspirin may potentiate this risk of bleeding. Patients should be cautioned about the risk of bleeding associated with the concomitant use of Symbyax and NSAIDs, aspirin, or other drugs that affect coagulation).
No products indexed under this heading.

Aprobarbital (Caution is advised if the concomitant administration of Symbyax and other CNS-active drugs is required. In evaluating individual cases, consideration should be given to using lower initial doses of the concomitantly administered drugs, using conservative titration schedules and monitoring of clinical status).
No products indexed under this heading.

Ardeparin Sodium (Serotonin release by platelets plays an important role in hemostasis. Epidemiological studies of the case-control and cohort design that have demonstrated an association between use of psychotropic drugs that interfere with serotonin re-uptake and the occurrence of upper gastrointestinal bleeding have also shown that concurrent use of an NSAID or aspirin may potentiate this risk of bleeding. Patients should be cautioned about the risk of bleeding associated with the concomitant use of Symbyax and NSAIDs, aspirin, or other drugs that affect coagulation).
No products indexed under this heading.

Aripiprazole (The development of a potentially life-threatening serotonin syndrome or neuroleptic malignant syndrome (NMS)-like reactions have been reported with SNRIs and SSRIs alone and with the concomitant use of antipsychotics. Serotonin syndrome, in its most severe form can resemble neuroleptic malignant syndrome. Patients should be monitored for the emergence of serotonin syndrome or NMS-like signs and symptoms. Treatment with Symbyax and any concomitant serotonergic or antidopaminergic agents, including antipsychotics, should be discontinued immediately, if the above reactions occur, and supportive symptomatic treatment should be initiated. In addition, co-administration of fluoxetine with other drugs metabolized by CYP2D6, including antipsychotics (eg, phenothiazines and most atypicals), should be approached with caution. Therapy with medications that are predominantly metabolized by the CYP2D6 system and that have a relatively narrow therapeutic index should be initiated at the low end of the dose range if a patient is receiving fluoxetine concurrently or has taken it in the previous 5 weeks. If fluoxetine is added to the treatment regimen of a patient already receiving a drug metabolized by CYP2D6, the need for a decreased dose of the original medication should be considered).
No products indexed under this heading.

Aspirin (Serotonin release by platelets plays an important role in hemostasis. Epidemiological studies of the case-control and cohort design that have demonstrated an association between use of psychotropic drugs that interfere with serotonin re-uptake and the occurrence of upper gastrointestinal bleeding have also shown that concurrent use of an NSAID or aspirin may potentiate this risk of bleeding. Patients should be cautioned about the risk of bleeding associated with the concomitant use of Symbyax and NSAIDs, aspirin, or other drugs that affect coagulation). Products include:
Aggrenox 880
Bayer Aspirin 829
Percodan 1124
St. Joseph Aspirin 2045

Aspirin, Enteric Coated (Serotonin release by platelets plays an important role in hemostasis. Epidemiological studies of the case-control and cohort design that have demonstrated an association between use of psychotropic drugs that interfere with serotonin re-uptake and the occurrence of upper gastrointestinal bleeding have also shown that concurrent use of an NSAID or aspirin may potentiate this risk of bleeding. Patients should be cautioned about the risk of bleeding associated with the concomitant use of Symbyax and NSAIDs, aspirin, or other drugs that affect coagulation).
No products indexed under this heading.

Aspirin Buffered (Serotonin release by platelets plays an important role in hemostasis. Epidemiological studies of the case-control and cohort design that have demonstrated an association between use of psychotropic drugs that interfere with serotonin re-uptake and the occurrence of upper gastrointestinal bleeding have also shown that concurrent use of an NSAID or aspirin may potentiate this risk of bleeding. Patients should be cautioned about the risk of bleeding associated with the concomitant use of Symbyax and NSAIDs, aspirin, or other drugs that affect coagulation).
No products indexed under this heading.

Atenolol (Because of the potential for olanzapine to induce hypotension, Symbyax may enhance the effects of certain antihypertensive agents).
No products indexed under this heading.

Atomoxetine Hydrochloride (Co-administration of fluoxetine with other drugs that are metabolized by CYP2D6 should be approached with caution. Therapy with medications that are predominantly metabolized by the CYP2D6 system and that have a relatively narrow therapeutic index should be initiated at the low end of the dose range if a patient is receiving fluoxetine concurrently or has taken it in the previous 5 weeks. If fluoxetine is added to the treatment regimen of a patient already receiving a drug metabolized by

IMPORTANT NOTE: Always consult each drug listing in the patient's regimen for possible interactions.

CYP2D6, the need for a decreased dose of the original medication should be considered). Products include:

Atovaquone (Because fluoxetine is tightly bound to plasma protein, the administration of fluoxetine to a patient taking another drug that is tightly bound to protein (eg, warfarin, digitoxin) may cause a shift in plasma concentrations, potentially resulting in an adverse effect. Conversely, adverse effects may result from displacement of protein-bound fluoxetine by other tightly bound drugs). Products include:

Benazepril Hydrochloride (Because of the potential for olanzapine to induce hypotension, Symbyax may enhance the effects of certain antihypertensive agents).

No products indexed under this heading.

Bendroflumethiazide (Because of the potential for olanzapine to induce hypotension, Symbyax may enhance the effects of certain antihypertensive agents).

No products indexed under this heading.

Betaxolol Hydrochloride (Because of the potential for olanzapine to induce hypotension, Symbyax may enhance the effects of certain antihypertensive agents).

No products indexed under this heading.

Bisoprolol Fumarate (Because of the potential for olanzapine to induce hypotension, Symbyax may enhance the effects of certain antihypertensive agents).

No products indexed under this heading.

Bretylium Tosylate (Co-administration of fluoxetine with other drugs that are metabolized by CYP2D6, including antiarrhythmics (eg, propafenone, flecainide, and others) should be approached with caution. Therapy with medications that are predominantly metabolized by the CYP2D6 system and that have a relatively narrow therapeutic index should be initiated at the low end of the dose range if a patient is receiving fluoxetine concurrently or has taken it in the previous 5 weeks. If fluoxetine is added to the treatment regimen of a patient already receiving a drug metabolized by CYP2D6, the need for a decreased dose of the original medication should be considered).

No products indexed under this heading.

Bromocriptine Mesylate (The olanzapine component of Symbyax may antagonize the effects of levodopa and dopamine agonists).

No products indexed under this heading.

Bumetanide (Hyponatremia may occur as a result of treatment with SSRIs and SNRIs, including fluoxetine and Symbyax. In many cases, this hyponatremia appears to be the result of the syndrome of inappropriate antidiuretic hormone secretion (SIADH). Cases with serum sodium lower than 110 mmol/L have been reported and appeared to be reversible when Symbyax was discontinued. Patients taking diuretics or who are otherwise volume depleted may be at greater risk. Discontinuation of Symbyax should be considered in patients with symptomatic hyponatremia and appropriate medical intervention should be instituted).

No products indexed under this heading.

Buprenorphine Hydrochloride (Caution is advised if the concomitant administration of Symbyax and other CNS-active drugs is required. In evaluating individual cases, consideration should be given to using lower initial doses of the concomitantly administered drugs, using conservative titration schedules and monitoring of clinical status).

No products indexed under this heading.

Bupropion Hydrochloride (Co-administration of fluoxetine with other drugs that are metabolized by CYP2D6, including certain antidepressants (eg, TCAs) should be approached with caution. Therapy with medications that are predominantly metabolized by the CYP2D6 system and that have a relatively narrow therapeutic index should be initiated at the low end of the dose range if a patient is receiving fluoxetine concurrently or has taken it in the previous 5 weeks. If fluoxetine is added to the treatment regimen of a patient already receiving a drug metabolized by CYP2D6, the need for a decreased dose of the original medication should be considered). Products include:

Buspirone Hydrochloride (Caution is advised if the concomitant administration of Symbyax and other CNS-active drugs is required. In evaluating individual cases, consideration should be given to using lower initial doses of the concomitantly administered drugs, using conservative titration schedules and monitoring of clinical status).

No products indexed under this heading.

Butabarbital (Caution is advised if the concomitant administration of Symbyax and other CNS-active drugs is required. In evaluating individual cases, consideration should be given to using lower initial doses of the concomitantly administered drugs, using conservative titration schedules and monitoring of clinical status).

No products indexed under this heading.

Butalbital (Caution is advised if the concomitant administration of Symbyax and other CNS-active drugs is required. In evaluating individual cases, consideration should be given to using lower initial doses of the concomitantly administered drugs, using conservative titration schedules and monitoring of clinical status).

No products indexed under this heading.

Candesartan Cilexetil (Because of the potential for olanzapine to induce hypotension, Symbyax may enhance the effects of certain antihypertensive agents). Products include:

Captopril (Because of the potential for olanzapine to induce hypotension, Symbyax may enhance the effects of certain antihypertensive agents). Products include:

Carbamazepine (Carbamazepine therapy (200 mg bid) causes an approximate 50% increase in the clearance of olanzapine. This increase is likely due to the fact that carbamazepine is a potent inducer of CYP1A2 activity. Higher daily doses of carbamazepine may cause an even greater increase in olanzapine clearance. Patients on stable doses of carbamazepine have developed elevated plasma anticonvulsant concentrations and clinical anticonvulsant toxicity following initiation of concomitant fluoxetine treatment). Products include:

Carteolol Hydrochloride (Because of the potential for olanzapine to induce hypotension, Symbyax may enhance the effects of certain antihypertensive agents).

No products indexed under this heading.

Carvedilol (Because of the potential for olanzapine to induce hypotension, Symbyax may enhance the effects of certain antihypertensive agents). Products include:

Carvedilol Phosphate (Because of the potential for olanzapine to induce hypotension, Symbyax may enhance the effects of certain antihypertensive agents). Products include:

Cefonicid Sodium (Because fluoxetine is tightly bound to plasma protein, the administration of fluoxetine to a patient taking another drug that is tightly bound to protein (eg, warfarin, digitoxin) may cause a shift in plasma concentrations, potentially resulting in an adverse effect. Conversely, adverse effects may result from displacement of protein-bound fluoxetine by other tightly bound drugs).

No products indexed under this heading.

Celecoxib (Serotonin release by platelets plays an important role in hemostasis. Epidemiological studies of the case-control and cohort design that have demonstrated an association between use of psychotropic drugs that interfere with serotonin re-uptake and the occurrence of upper gastrointestinal bleeding have also shown that concurrent use of an NSAID or aspirin may potentiate this risk of bleeding. Patients should be cautioned about the risk of bleeding associated with the concomitant use of Symbyax and NSAIDs, aspirin, or other drugs that affect coagulation). Products include:

Cevimeline Hydrochloride (Co-administration of fluoxetine with other drugs that are metabolized by CYP2D6 should be approached with caution. Therapy with medications that are predominantly metabolized by the CYP2D6 system and that have a relatively narrow therapeutic index should be initiated at the low end of the dose range if a patient is receiving fluoxetine concurrently or has taken it in the previous 5 weeks. If fluoxetine is added to the treatment regimen of a patient already receiving a drug metabolized by CYP2D6, the need for a decreased dose of the original medication should be considered). Products include:

Chlordiazepoxide (Caution is advised if the concomitant administration of Symbyax and other CNS-active drugs is required. In evaluating individual cases, consideration should be given to using lower initial doses of the concomitantly administered drugs, using conservative titration schedules and monitoring of clinical status).

No products indexed under this heading.

Chlordiazepoxide Hydrochloride (Caution is advised if the concomitant administration of Symbyax and other CNS-active drugs is required. In evaluating individual cases, consideration should be given to using lower initial doses of the concomitantly administered drugs, using conservative titration schedules and monitoring of clinical status).

No products indexed under this heading.

Chlorothiazide (Because of the potential for olanzapine to induce hypotension, Symbyax may enhance the effects of certain antihypertensive agents).

No products indexed under this heading.

Chlorothiazide Sodium (Because of the potential for olanzapine to induce hypotension, Symbyax may enhance the effects of certain antihypertensive agents). Products include:

Chlorpromazine (The development of a potentially life-threatening serotonin syndrome or neuroleptic malignant syndrome (NMS)-like reactions have been reported with SNRIs and SSRIs alone and with the concomitant use of antipsychotics. Serotonin syndrome, in its most severe form can resemble neuroleptic malignant syndrome. Patients should be monitored for the emergence of serotonin syndrome or NMS-like signs and symptoms. Treatment with Symbyax and any concomitant serotonergic or antidopaminergic agents, including antipsychotics, should be discontinued immediately, if the above reactions occur, and supportive symptomatic treatment should be initiated. In addition, co-administration of fluoxetine with other drugs metabolized by CYP2D6 including antipsychotics (eg, phenothiazines and most atypicals) should be approached with caution. Therapy with medications that are predominantly metabolized by the CYP2D6 system and that have a relatively narrow therapeutic index should be initiated at the low end of the dose range if a patient is receiving fluoxetine concurrently or has taken it in the previous 5 weeks. If fluoxetine is added to the treatment regimen of a patient already receiving a drug metabolized by CYP2D6, the need for a decreased dose of the original medication should be considered).

No products indexed under this heading.

Chlorpromazine Hydrochloride (The development of a potentially life-threatening serotonin syndrome or neuroleptic malignant syndrome (NMS)-like reactions have been reported with SNRIs and SSRIs alone and with the concomitant use of antipsychotics. Serotonin syndrome, in its most severe form can resemble neuroleptic malignant syndrome. Patients should be monitored for the emergence of serotonin syndrome or NMS-like signs and symptoms. Treatment with Symbyax and any concomitant serotonergic or antidopaminergic agents, including antipsychotics, should be discontinued immediately, if the above reactions occur, and supportive symptomatic treatment should be initiated. In addition, co-administration of fluoxetine with other drugs metabolized by CYP2D6 including antipsychotics (eg, phenothiazines and most atypicals) should be approached with caution. Therapy with medications that are predominantly metabolized by the CYP2D6 system and that have a relatively narrow therapeutic index should be initiated at the low end of the dose range if a patient is receiving fluoxetine concurrently or has taken it in the previous 5 weeks. If fluoxetine is added to the treatment regimen of a patient already receiving a drug metabolized by CYP2D6, the need for a decreased dose of the original medication should be considered).

No products indexed under this heading.

Chlorpropamide (Co-administration of fluoxetine with other drugs that are metabolized by CYP2D6 should be approached with caution. Therapy with medications that are predominantly metabolized by the CYP2D6 system and that have a relatively narrow therapeutic index should be initiated at the low end of the dose range if a patient is receiving fluoxetine concurrently or has taken it in the previous 5 weeks. If fluoxetine is added to the treatment regimen of a patient already receiving a drug

metabolized by CYP2D6, the need for a decreased dose of the original medication should be considered).

No products indexed under this heading.

Chlorprothixene (The development of a potentially life-threatening serotonin syndrome or neuroleptic malignant syndrome (NMS)-like reactions have been reported with SNRIs and SSRIs alone and with the concomitant use of antipsychotics. Serotonin syndrome, in its most severe form can resemble neuroleptic malignant syndrome. Patients should be monitored for the emergence of serotonin syndrome or NMS-like signs and symptoms. Treatment with Symbyax and any concomitant serotonergic or antidopaminergic agents, including antipsychotics, should be discontinued immediately, if the above reactions occur, and supportive symptomatic treatment should be initiated. In addition, co-administration of fluoxetine with other drugs metabolized by CYP2D6, including antipsychotics (eg, phenothiazines and most atypicals), should be approached with caution. Therapy with medications that are predominantly metabolized by the CYP2D6 system and that have a relatively narrow therapeutic index should be initiated at the low end of the dose range if a patient is receiving fluoxetine concurrently or has taken it in the previous 5 weeks. If fluoxetine is added to the treatment regimen of a patient already receiving a drug metabolized by CYP2D6, the need for a decreased dose of the original medication should be considered).

No products indexed under this heading.

Chlorprothixene Hydrochloride (The development of a potentially life-threatening serotonin syndrome or neuroleptic malignant syndrome (NMS)-like reactions have been reported with SNRIs and SSRIs alone and with the concomitant use of antipsychotics. Serotonin syndrome, in its most severe form can resemble neuroleptic malignant syndrome. Patients should be monitored for the emergence of serotonin syndrome or NMS-like signs and symptoms. Treatment with Symbyax and any concomitant serotonergic or antidopaminergic agents, including antipsychotics, should be discontinued immediately, if the above reactions occur, and supportive symptomatic treatment should be initiated. In addition, co-administration of fluoxetine with other drugs metabolized by CYP2D6, including antipsychotics (eg, phenothiazines and most atypicals), should be approached with caution. Therapy with medications that are predominantly metabolized by the CYP2D6 system and that have a relatively narrow therapeutic index should be initiated at the low end of the dose range if a patient is receiving fluoxetine concurrently or has taken it in the previous 5 weeks. If fluoxetine is added to the treatment regimen of a patient already receiving a drug metabolized by CYP2D6, the need for a decreased dose of the original medication should be considered).

No products indexed under this heading.

Chlorprothixene Lactate (The development of a potentially life-threatening serotonin syndrome or neuroleptic malignant syndrome (NMS)-like reactions have been reported with SNRIs and SSRIs alone and with the concomitant use of antipsychotics. Serotonin syndrome, in its most severe form can resemble neuroleptic malignant syndrome. Patients should be monitored for the emergence of serotonin syndrome or NMS-like signs and symptoms. Treatment with Symbyax and any concomitant serotonergic or antidopaminergic agents, including antipsychotics, should be discontinued immediately, if

the above reactions occur, and supportive symptomatic treatment should be initiated. In addition, co-administration of fluoxetine with other drugs metabolized by CYP2D6, including antipsychotics (eg, phenothiazines and most atypicals), should be approached with caution. Therapy with medications that are predominantly metabolized by the CYP2D6 system and that have a relatively narrow therapeutic index should be initiated at the low end of the dose range if a patient is receiving fluoxetine concurrently or has taken it in the previous 5 weeks. If fluoxetine is added to the treatment regimen of a patient already receiving a drug metabolized by CYP2D6, the need for a decreased dose of the original medication should be considered).

No products indexed under this heading.

Chlorthalidone (Because of the potential for olanzapine to induce hypotension, Symbyax may enhance the effects of certain antihypertensive agents). Products include:
Clorpres 2344

Citalopram Hydrobromide (The concomitant use of Symbyax with selective serotonin reuptake inhibitors (SSRIs) is not recommended). Products include:
Celexa 1153

Clomipramine Hydrochloride (In two fluoxetine studies, previously stable plasma levels of imipramine and desipramine have increased>2- to 10-fold when fluoxetine has been administered in combination. This influence may persist for three weeks or longer after fluoxetine is discontinued. Thus, the dose of TCA may need to be reduced and plasma TCA concentrations may need to be monitored temporarily when Symbyax is co-administered or has been recently discontinued. Co-administration of fluoxetine with other drugs that are metabolized by CYP2D6, including certain antidepressants (eg, TCAs), should be approached with caution).

No products indexed under this heading.

Clonidine (Because of the potential for olanzapine to induce hypotension, Symbyax may enhance the effects of certain antihypertensive agents). Products include:
Catapres-TTS 884

Clonidine Hydrochloride (Because of the potential for olanzapine to induce hypotension, Symbyax may enhance the effects of certain antihypertensive agents). Products include:
Clorpres 2344

Clorazepate Dipotassium (Caution is advised if the concomitant administration of Symbyax and other CNS-active drugs is required. In evaluating individual cases, consideration should be given to using lower initial doses of the concomitantly administered drugs, using conservative titration schedules and monitoring of clinical status).

No products indexed under this heading.

Clozapine (Elevation of blood levels of clozapine has been observed in patients receiving concomitant fluoxetine).

No products indexed under this heading.

Codeine Phosphate (Caution is advised if the concomitant administration of Symbyax and other CNS-active drugs is required. In evaluating individual cases, consideration should be given to using lower initial doses of the concomitantly administered drugs, using conservative titration schedules and monitoring of clinical status). Products include:
Tylenol with Codeine 2691

Codeine Sulfate (Caution is advised if the concomitant administration of Symbyax and other CNS-active drugs is required. In evaluating individual cases, consideration should be given to using lower initial doses of the concomitantly administered drugs, using conservative titration schedules and monitoring of clinical status).

No products indexed under this heading.

Cyclobenzaprine Hydrochloride (Co-administration of fluoxetine with other drugs that are metabolized by CYP2D6 should be approached with caution. Therapy with medications that are predominantly metabolized by the CYP2D6 system and that have a relatively narrow therapeutic index should be initiated at the low end of the dose range if a patient is receiving fluoxetine concurrently or has taken it in the previous 5 weeks. If fluoxetine is added to the treatment regimen of a patient already receiving a drug metabolized by CYP2D6, the need for a decreased dose of the original medication should be considered). Products include:
Amrix 964

Cyclosporine (Because fluoxetine is tightly bound to plasma protein, the administration of fluoxetine to a patient taking another drug that is tightly bound to protein (eg, warfarin, digitoxin) may cause a shift in plasma concentrations, potentially resulting in an adverse effect. Conversely, adverse effects may result from displacement of protein-bound fluoxetine by other tightly bound drugs). Products include:
Gengraf 440
Neoral Oral Solution 2496
Neoral Capsules 2496
Restasis 605

Dalteparin Sodium (Serotonin release by platelets plays an important role in hemostasis. Epidemiological studies of the case-control and cohort design that have demonstrated an association between use of psychotropic drugs that interfere with serotonin re-uptake and the occurrence of upper gastrointestinal bleeding have also shown that concurrent use of an NSAID or aspirin may potentiate this risk of bleeding. Patients should be cautioned about the risk of bleeding associated with the concomitant use of Symbyax and NSAIDs, aspirin, or other drugs that affect coagulation). Products include:
Fragmin 1058

Danaparoid Sodium (Serotonin release by platelets plays an important role in hemostasis. Epidemiological studies of the case-control and cohort design that have demonstrated an association between use of psychotropic drugs that interfere with serotonin re-uptake and the occurrence of upper gastrointestinal bleeding have also shown that concurrent use of an NSAID or aspirin may potentiate this risk of bleeding. Patients should be cautioned about the risk of bleeding associated with the concomitant use of Symbyax and NSAIDs, aspirin, or other drugs that affect coagulation).

No products indexed under this heading.

Debrisoquine (Co-administration of fluoxetine with other drugs that are metabolized by CYP2D6 should be approached with caution. Therapy with medications that are predominantly metabolized by the CYP2D6 system and that have a relatively narrow therapeutic index should be initiated at the low end of the dose range if a patient is receiving fluoxetine concurrently or has taken it in the previous 5 weeks. If fluoxetine is added to the treatment regimen of a patient already receiving a drug

metabolized by CYP2D6, the need for a decreased dose of the original medication should be considered).

No products indexed under this heading.

Deserpidine (Because of the potential for olanzapine to induce hypotension, Symbyax may enhance the effects of certain antihypertensive agents).

No products indexed under this heading.

Desflurane (Caution is advised if the concomitant administration of Symbyax and other CNS-active drugs is required. In evaluating individual cases, consideration should be given to using lower initial doses of the concomitantly administered drugs, using conservative titration schedules and monitoring of clinical status).

No products indexed under this heading.

Desipramine Hydrochloride (In two fluoxetine studies, previously stable plasma levels of imipramine and desipramine have increased>2- to 10-fold when fluoxetine has been administered in combination. This influence may persist for three weeks or longer after fluoxetine is discontinued. Thus, the dose of TCA may need to be reduced and plasma TCA concentrations may need to be monitored temporarily when Symbyax is co-administered or has been recently discontinued. Co-administration of fluoxetine with other drugs that are metabolized by CYP2D6, including certain antidepressants (eg, TCAs), should be approached with caution).

No products indexed under this heading.

Desvenlafaxine Succinate (The concomitant use of Symbyax with serotonin and norepinephrine reuptake inhibitors (SNRIs) is not recommended). Products include:
Pristiq 3564

Dexfenfluramine Hydrochloride (Co-administration of fluoxetine with other drugs that are metabolized by CYP2D6 should be approached with caution. Therapy with medications that are predominantly metabolized by the CYP2D6 system and that have a relatively narrow therapeutic index should be initiated at the low end of the dose range if a patient is receiving fluoxetine concurrently or has taken it in the previous 5 weeks. If fluoxetine is added to the treatment regimen of a patient already receiving a drug metabolized by CYP2D6, the need for a decreased dose of the original medication should be considered).

No products indexed under this heading.

Dexmethylphenidate Hydrochloride (Caution is advised if the concomitant administration of Symbyax and other CNS-active drugs is required. In evaluating individual cases, consideration should be given to using lower initial doses of the concomitantly administered drugs, using conservative titration schedules and monitoring of clinical status). Products include:
Focalin XR 2472

Dextroamphetamine (Caution is advised if the concomitant administration of Symbyax and other CNS-active drugs is required. In evaluating individual cases, consideration should be given to using lower initial doses of the concomitantly administered drugs, using conservative titration schedules and monitoring of clinical status).

No products indexed under this heading.

Symbyax Interactions Index 1796

Dextroamphetamine Saccharate (Caution is advised if the concomitant administration of Symbyax and other CNS-active drugs is required. In evaluating individual cases, consideration should be given to using lower initial doses of the concomitantly administered drugs, using conservative titration schedules and monitoring of clinical status).
No products indexed under this heading.

Dextroamphetamine Sulfate (Caution is advised if the concomitant administration of Symbyax and other CNS-active drugs is required. In evaluating individual cases, consideration should be given to using lower initial doses of the concomitantly administered drugs, using conservative titration schedules and monitoring of clinical status). Products include:
Dexedrine 1425

Dextromethorphan Hydrobromide (Co-administration of fluoxetine with other drugs that are metabolized by CYP2D6 should be approached with caution. Therapy with medications that are predominantly metabolized by the CYP2D6 system and that have a relatively narrow therapeutic index should be initiated at the low end of the dose range if a patient is receiving fluoxetine concurrently or has taken it in the previous 5 weeks. If fluoxetine is added to the treatment regimen of a patient already receiving a drug metabolized by CYP2D6, the need for a decreased dose of the original medication should be considered).
No products indexed under this heading.

Dextromethorphan Polistirex (Co-administration of fluoxetine with other drugs that are metabolized by CYP2D6 should be approached with caution. Therapy with medications that are predominantly metabolized by the CYP2D6 system and that have a relatively narrow therapeutic index should be initiated at the low end of the dose range if a patient is receiving fluoxetine concurrently or has taken it in the previous 5 weeks. If fluoxetine is added to the treatment regimen of a patient already receiving a drug metabolized by CYP2D6, the need for a decreased dose of the original medication should be considered).
No products indexed under this heading.

Dezocine (Caution is advised if the concomitant administration of Symbyax and other CNS-active drugs is required. In evaluating individual cases, consideration should be given to using lower initial doses of the concomitantly administered drugs, using conservative titration schedules and monitoring of clinical status).
No products indexed under this heading.

Diazepam (Co-administration of diazepam with olanzapine may potentiate the orthostatic hypotension observed with olanzapine. When concurrently administered with fluoxetine, the half-life of diazepam may be prolonged in some patients). Products include:
Valium Tablets 2880

Diazoxide (Because of the potential for olanzapine to induce hypotension, Symbyax may enhance the effects of certain antihypertensive agents). Products include:
Proglycem 1179
Proglycem Suspension 1179

Diclofenac Epolamine (Serotonin release by platelets plays an important role in hemostasis. Epidemiological studies of the case-control and cohort design that have demonstrated an association between use of psychotropic drugs that interfere with serotonin re-uptake and the occurrence of upper gastrointestinal bleeding have also shown that concurrent use of an NSAID or aspirin may potentiate this risk of bleeding. Patients should be cautioned about the risk of bleeding associated with the concomitant use of Symbyax and NSAIDs, aspirin, or other drugs that affect coagulation). Products include:
Flector 1839

Diclofenac Potassium (Serotonin release by platelets plays an important role in hemostasis. Epidemiological studies of the case-control and cohort design that have demonstrated an association between use of psychotropic drugs that interfere with serotonin re-uptake and the occurrence of upper gastrointestinal bleeding have also shown that concurrent use of an NSAID or aspirin may potentiate this risk of bleeding. Patients should be cautioned about the risk of bleeding associated with the concomitant use of Symbyax and NSAIDs, aspirin, or other drugs that affect coagulation).
No products indexed under this heading.

Diclofenac Sodium (Serotonin release by platelets plays an important role in hemostasis. Epidemiological studies of the case-control and cohort design that have demonstrated an association between use of psychotropic drugs that interfere with serotonin re-uptake and the occurrence of upper gastrointestinal bleeding have also shown that concurrent use of an NSAID or aspirin may potentiate this risk of bleeding. Patients should be cautioned about the risk of bleeding associated with the concomitant use of Symbyax and NSAIDs, aspirin, or other drugs that affect coagulation).
No products indexed under this heading.

Dicumarol (Serotonin release by platelets plays an important role in hemostasis. Epidemiological studies of the case-control and cohort design that have demonstrated an association between use of psychotropic drugs that interfere with serotonin re-uptake and the occurrence of upper gastrointestinal bleeding have also shown that concurrent use of an NSAID or aspirin may potentiate this risk of bleeding. Patients should be cautioned about the risk of bleeding associated with the concomitant use of Symbyax and NSAIDs, aspirin, or other drugs that affect coagulation).
No products indexed under this heading.

Digitalis Glycoside Preparations (Because fluoxetine is tightly bound to plasma protein, the administration of fluoxetine to a patient taking another drug that is tightly bound to protein (eg, warfarin, digitoxin) may cause a shift in plasma concentrations, potentially resulting in an adverse effect. Conversely, adverse effects may result from displacement of protein-bound fluoxetine by other tightly bound drugs).
No products indexed under this heading.

Digitalis Lanata (Because fluoxetine is tightly bound to plasma protein, the administration of fluoxetine to a patient taking another drug that is tightly bound to protein (eg, warfarin, digitoxin) may cause a shift in plasma concentrations, potentially resulting in an adverse effect. Conversely, adverse effects may result from displacement of protein-bound fluoxetine by other tightly bound drugs).
No products indexed under this heading.

Digitalis Purpurea (Because fluoxetine is tightly bound to plasma protein, the administration of fluoxetine to a patient taking another drug that is tightly bound to protein (eg, warfarin, digitoxin) may cause a shift in plasma concentrations, potentially resulting in an adverse effect. Conversely, adverse effects may result from displacement of protein-bound fluoxetine by other tightly bound drugs).
No products indexed under this heading.

Digitoxin (Because fluoxetine is tightly bound to plasma protein, the administration of fluoxetine to a patient taking another drug that is tightly bound to protein (eg, warfarin, digitoxin) may cause a shift in plasma concentrations, potentially resulting in an adverse effect. Conversely, adverse effects may result from displacement of protein-bound fluoxetine by other tightly bound drugs).
No products indexed under this heading.

Diltiazem Hydrochloride (Because of the potential for olanzapine to induce hypotension, Symbyax may enhance the effects of certain antihypertensive agents). Products include:
Cardizem LA 423

Diltiazem Maleate (Because of the potential for olanzapine to induce hypotension, Symbyax may enhance the effects of certain antihypertensive agents).
No products indexed under this heading.

Dipyridamole (Because fluoxetine is tightly bound to plasma protein, the administration of fluoxetine to a patient taking another drug that is tightly bound to protein (eg, warfarin, digitoxin) may cause a shift in plasma concentrations, potentially resulting in an adverse effect. Conversely, adverse effects may result from displacement of protein-bound fluoxetine by other tightly bound drugs). Products include:
Aggrenox 880

Disopyramide Phosphate (Co-administration of fluoxetine with other drugs that are metabolized by CYP2D6, including antiarrhythmics (eg, propafenone, flecainide, and others) should be approached with caution. Therapy with medications that are predominantly metabolized by the CYP2D6 system and that have a relatively narrow therapeutic index should be initiated at the low end of the dose range if a patient is receiving fluoxetine concurrently or has taken it in the previous 5 weeks. If fluoxetine is added to the treatment regimen of a patient already receiving a drug metabolized by CYP2D6, the need for a decreased dose of the original medication should be considered).
No products indexed under this heading.

Dofetilide (Co-administration of fluoxetine with other drugs that are metabolized by CYP2D6, including antiarrhythmics (eg, propafenone, flecainide, and others) should be approached with caution. Therapy with medications that are predominantly metabolized by the CYP2D6 system and that have a relatively narrow therapeutic index should be initiated at the low end of the dose range if a patient is receiving fluoxetine concurrently or has taken it in the previous 5 weeks. If fluoxetine is added to the treatment regimen of a patient already receiving a drug metabolized by CYP2D6, the need for a decreased dose of the original medication should be considered).
No products indexed under this heading.

Dolasetron Mesylate (Co-administration of fluoxetine with other drugs that are metabolized by CYP2D6 should be approached with caution. Therapy with medications that are predominantly metabolized by the CYP2D6 system and that have a relatively narrow therapeutic index should be initiated at the low end of the dose range if a patient is receiving fluoxetine concurrently or has taken it in the previous 5 weeks. If fluoxetine is added to the treatment regimen of a patient already receiving a drug metabolized by CYP2D6, the need for a decreased dose of the original medication should be considered). Products include:
Anzemet Injection 2931
Anzemet Tablets 2934

Donepezil Hydrochloride (Co-administration of fluoxetine with other drugs that are metabolized by CYP2D6 should be approached with caution. Therapy with medications that are predominantly metabolized by the CYP2D6 system and that have a relatively narrow therapeutic index should be initiated at the low end of the dose range if a patient is receiving fluoxetine concurrently or has taken it in the previous 5 weeks. If fluoxetine is added to the treatment regimen of a patient already receiving a drug metabolized by CYP2D6, the need for a decreased dose of the original medication should be considered). Products include:
Aricept 1045
Aricept ODT 1045

Dopamine Hydrochloride (The olanzapine component of Symbyax may antagonize the effects of levodopa and dopamine agonists).
No products indexed under this heading.

Doxazosin Mesylate (Because of the potential for olanzapine to induce hypotension, Symbyax may enhance the effects of certain antihypertensive agents).
No products indexed under this heading.

Doxepin Hydrochloride (In two fluoxetine studies, previously stable plasma levels of imipramine and desipramine have increased>2- to 10-fold when fluoxetine has been administered in combination. This influence may persist for three weeks or longer after fluoxetine is discontinued. Thus, the dose of TCA may need to be reduced and plasma TCA concentrations may need to be monitored temporarily when Symbyax is co-administered or has been recently discontinued. Co-administration of fluoxetine with other drugs that are metabolized by CYP2D6, including certain antidepressants (eg, TCAs), should be approached with caution).
No products indexed under this heading.

Droperidol (Caution is advised if the concomitant administration of Symbyax and other CNS-active drugs is required. In evaluating individual cases, consideration should be given to using lower initial doses of the concomitantly administered drugs, using conservative titration schedules and monitoring of clinical status).
No products indexed under this heading.

Duloxetine Hydrochloride (The concomitant use of Symbyax with serotonin and norepinephrine reuptake inhibitors (SNRIs) is not recommended). Products include:
Cymbalta 1871

Electroshock Therapy (There are no clinical studies establishing the benefit of the combined use of electroconvulsive therapy (ECT) and fluoxetine. There have been rare reports of prolonged seizures in patients on fluoxetine receiving ECT treatment).
No products indexed under this heading.

Eletriptan Hydrobromide (There have been rare postmarketing reports of serotonin syndrome with use of an SSRI and a triptan. If concomitant treatment of Symbyax with a triptan is clinically warranted, careful observation of the patient is advised, particularly during treatment initiation and dose increases).
No products indexed under this heading.

Enalapril Maleate (Because of the potential for olanzapine to induce hypotension, Symbyax may enhance the effects of certain antihypertensive agents).
No products indexed under this heading.

1797 Interactions Index Symbyax

Enalaprilat (Because of the potential for olanzapine to induce hypotension, Symbyax may enhance the effects of certain antihypertensive agents).
No products indexed under this heading.

Encainide Hydrochloride (Co-administration of fluoxetine with other drugs that are metabolized by CYP2D6 should be approached with caution. Therapy with medications that are predominantly metabolized by the CYP2D6 system and that have a relatively narrow therapeutic index should be initiated at the low end of the dose range if a patient is receiving fluoxetine concurrently or has taken it in the previous 5 weeks. If fluoxetine is added to the treatment regimen of a patient already receiving a drug metabolized by CYP2D6, the need for a decreased dose of the original medication should be considered).
No products indexed under this heading.

Enflurane (Caution is advised if the concomitant administration of Symbyax and other CNS-active drugs is required. In evaluating individual cases, consideration should be given to using lower initial doses of the concomitantly administered drugs, using conservative titration schedules and monitoring of clinical status).
No products indexed under this heading.

Enoxaparin Sodium (Serotonin release by platelets plays an important role in hemostasis. Epidemiological studies of the case-control and cohort design that have demonstrated an association between use of psychotropic drugs that interfere with serotonin re-uptake and the occurrence of upper gastrointestinal bleeding have also shown that concurrent use of an NSAID or aspirin may potentiate this risk of bleeding. Patients should be cautioned about the risk of bleeding associated with the concomitant use of Symbyax and NSAIDs, aspirin, or other drugs that affect coagulation). Products include:
Lovenox 3005

Eprosartan Mesylate (Because of the potential for olanzapine to induce hypotension, Symbyax may enhance the effects of certain antihypertensive agents). Products include:
Teveten 538
Teveten HCT 541

Erythromycin (Agents that induce CYP1A2 or glucuronyl transferase enzymes may cause an increase in olanzapine concentration).
No products indexed under this heading.

Erythromycin, Topical (Agents that induce CYP1A2 or glucuronyl transferase enzymes may cause an increase in olanzapine concentration).
No products indexed under this heading.

Erythromycin Estolate (Agents that induce CYP1A2 or glucuronyl transferase enzymes may cause an increase in olanzapine concentration).
No products indexed under this heading.

Erythromycin Ethylsuccinate (Agents that induce CYP1A2 or glucuronyl transferase enzymes may cause an increase in olanzapine concentration). Products include:
E.E.S. 437
EryPed 435

Erythromycin Gluceptate (Agents that induce CYP1A2 or glucuronyl transferase enzymes may cause an increase in olanzapine concentration).
No products indexed under this heading.

Erythromycin Lactobionate (Agents that induce CYP1A2 or glucuronyl transferase enzymes may cause an increase in olanzapine concentration).
No products indexed under this heading.

Erythromycin Stearate (Agents that induce CYP1A2 or glucuronyl transferase enzymes may cause an increase in olanzapine concentration).
No products indexed under this heading.

Escitalopram Oxalate (The concomitant use of Symbyax with selective serotonin reuptake inhibitors (SSRIs) is not recommended). Products include:
Lexapro Oral Suspension 1160
Lexapro Tablets 1160

Esmolol Hydrochloride (Because of the potential for olanzapine to induce hypotension, Symbyax may enhance the effects of certain antihypertensive agents).
No products indexed under this heading.

Esomeprazole Magnesium (Agents that induce CYP1A2 or glucuronyl transferase enzymes may cause an increase in olanzapine concentration). Products include:
Nexium Capsules 704
Nexium Oral Suspension 704

Esomeprazole Sodium (Agents that induce CYP1A2 or glucuronyl transferase enzymes may cause an increase in olanzapine concentration). Products include:
Nexium I.V. 712

Estazolam (Caution is advised if the concomitant administration of Symbyax and other CNS-active drugs is required. In evaluating individual cases, consideration should be given to using lower initial doses of the concomitantly administered drugs, using conservative titration schedules and monitoring of clinical status).
No products indexed under this heading.

Ethacrynic Acid (Hyponatremia may occur as a result of treatment with SSRIs and SNRIs, including fluoxetine and Symbyax. In many cases, this hyponatremia appears to be the result of the syndrome of inappropriate antidiuretic hormone secretion (SIADH). Cases with serum sodium lower than 110 mmol/L have been reported and appeared to be reversible when Symbyax was discontinued. Patients taking diuretics or who are otherwise volume depleted may be at greater risk. Discontinuation of Symbyax should be considered in patients with symptomatic hyponatremia and appropriate medical intervention should be instituted).
No products indexed under this heading.

Ethanol (The co-administration of ethanol with Symbyax may potentiate sedation and orthostatic hypotension. Patients should be advised to avoid alcohol while taking Symbyax).
No products indexed under this heading.

Ethchlorvynol (Caution is advised if the concomitant administration of Symbyax and other CNS-active drugs is required. In evaluating individual cases, consideration should be given to using lower initial doses of the concomitantly administered drugs, using conservative titration schedules and monitoring of clinical status).
No products indexed under this heading.

Ethinamate (Caution is advised if the concomitant administration of Symbyax and other CNS-active drugs is required. In evaluating individual cases, consideration should be given to using lower initial doses of the concomitantly administered drugs, using conservative titration schedules and monitoring of clinical status).
No products indexed under this heading.

Ethyl Alcohol (The co-administration of ethanol with Symbyax may potentiate sedation and orthostatic hypotension. Patients should be advised to avoid alcohol while taking Symbyax).
No products indexed under this heading.

Etodolac (Serotonin release by platelets plays an important role in hemostasis. Epidemiological studies of the case-control and cohort design that have demonstrated an association between use of psychotropic drugs that interfere with serotonin re-uptake and the occurrence of upper gastrointestinal bleeding have also shown that concurrent use of an NSAID or aspirin may potentiate this risk of bleeding. Patients should be cautioned about the risk of bleeding associated with the concomitant use of Symbyax and NSAIDs, aspirin, or other drugs that affect coagulation).
No products indexed under this heading.

Felodipine (Because of the potential for olanzapine to induce hypotension, Symbyax may enhance the effects of certain antihypertensive agents).
No products indexed under this heading.

Fenoprofen Calcium (Serotonin release by platelets plays an important role in hemostasis. Epidemiological studies of the case-control and cohort design that have demonstrated an association between use of psychotropic drugs that interfere with serotonin re-uptake and the occurrence of upper gastrointestinal bleeding have also shown that concurrent use of an NSAID or aspirin may potentiate this risk of bleeding. Patients should be cautioned about the risk of bleeding associated with the concomitant use of Symbyax and NSAIDs, aspirin, or other drugs that affect coagulation).
No products indexed under this heading.

Fentanyl (Caution is advised if the concomitant administration of Symbyax and other CNS-active drugs is required. In evaluating individual cases, consideration should be given to using lower initial doses of the concomitantly administered drugs, using conservative titration schedules and monitoring of clinical status). Products include:
Duragesic 2604
Fentanyl Transdermal System 2346
Onsolis 2054

Fentanyl Citrate (Caution is advised if the concomitant administration of Symbyax and other CNS-active drugs is required. In evaluating individual cases, consideration should be given to using lower initial doses of the concomitantly administered drugs, using conservative titration schedules and monitoring of clinical status). Products include:
Fentora 966

Flecainide Acetate (Co-administration of fluoxetine with other drugs that are metabolized by CYP2D6, including antiarrhythmics (eg, propafenone, flecainide, and others) should be approached with caution. Therapy with medications that are predominantly metabolized by the CYP2D6 system and that have a relatively narrow therapeutic index should be initiated at the low end of the dose range if a patient is receiving fluoxetine concurrently or has taken it in the previous 5 weeks. If fluoxetine is added to the treatment regimen of a patient already receiving a drug metabolized by CYP2D6, the need for a decreased dose of the original medication should be considered).
No products indexed under this heading.

Fluoxetine (The concomitant use of Symbyax with selective serotonin reuptake inhibitors (SSRIs) is not recommended).
No products indexed under this heading.

Fluphenazine Decanoate (The development of a potentially life-threatening serotonin syndrome or neuroleptic malignant syndrome (NMS)-like reactions have been reported with SNRIs and SSRIs alone and with the concomitant use of antipsychotics. Serotonin syndrome, in its most severe form can resemble neuroleptic malignant syndrome. Patients should be monitored for the emergence of serotonin syndrome or NMS-like signs and symptoms. Treatment with Symbyax and any concomitant serotonergic or antidopaminergic agents, including antipsychotics, should be discontinued immediately, if the above reactions occur, and supportive symptomatic treatment should be initiated. In addition, co-administration of fluoxetine with other drugs metabolized by CYP2D6 including antipsychotics (eg, phenothiazines and most atypicals) should be approached with caution. Therapy with medications that are predominantly metabolized by the CYP2D6 system and that have a relatively narrow therapeutic index should be initiated at the low end of the dose range if a patient is receiving fluoxetine concurrently or has taken it in the previous 5 weeks. If fluoxetine is added to the treatment regimen of a patient already receiving a drug metabolized by CYP2D6, the need for a decreased dose of the original medication should be considered).
No products indexed under this heading.

Fluphenazine Enanthate (The development of a potentially life-threatening serotonin syndrome or neuroleptic malignant syndrome (NMS)-like reactions have been reported with SNRIs and SSRIs alone and with the concomitant use of antipsychotics. Serotonin syndrome, in its most severe form can resemble neuroleptic malignant syndrome. Patients should be monitored for the emergence of serotonin syndrome or NMS-like signs and symptoms. Treatment with Symbyax and any concomitant serotonergic or antidopaminergic agents, including antipsychotics, should be discontinued immediately, if the above reactions occur, and supportive symptomatic treatment should be initiated. In addition, co-administration of fluoxetine with other drugs metabolized by CYP2D6 including antipsychotics (eg, phenothiazines and most atypicals) should be approached with caution. Therapy with medications that are predominantly metabolized by the CYP2D6 system and that have a relatively narrow therapeutic index should be initiated at the low end of the dose range if a patient is receiving fluoxetine concurrently or has taken it in the previous 5 weeks. If fluoxetine is added to the treatment regimen of a patient already receiving a drug metabolized by CYP2D6, the need for a decreased dose of the original medication should be considered).
No products indexed under this heading.

Fluphenazine Hydrochloride (The development of a potentially life-threatening serotonin syndrome or neuroleptic malignant syndrome (NMS)-like reactions have been reported with SNRIs and SSRIs alone and with the concomitant use of antipsychotics. Serotonin syndrome, in its most severe form can resemble neuroleptic malignant syndrome. Patients should be monitored for the emergence of serotonin syndrome or NMS-like signs and symptoms. Treatment with Symbyax and any concomitant serotonergic or antidopaminergic agents, including antipsychotics, should be discontinued immediately, if the above reactions occur, and supportive symptomatic treatment should be initiated. In addition, co-administration of fluoxetine with other drugs metabolized by CYP2D6 including antipsychotics (eg, phenothiazines and most atypicals) should be approached with caution. Therapy with medications that are predominantly metabolized by the CYP2D6 system and that have a relatively narrow therapeutic index should be initiated at the low end of the dose range if a patient is receiving fluoxetine concurrently or has taken it in the previous 5 weeks. If fluoxetine is added to

IMPORTANT NOTE: Always consult each drug listing in the patient's regimen for possible interactions.

Symbyax Interactions Index 1798

the treatment regimen of a patient already receiving a drug metabolized by CYP2D6, the need for a decreased dose of the original medication should be considered).
No products indexed under this heading.

Flurazepam Hydrochloride (Caution is advised if the concomitant administration of Symbyax and other CNS-active drugs is required. In evaluating individual cases, consideration should be given to using lower initial doses of the concomitantly administered drugs, using conservative titration schedules and monitoring of clinical status).
No products indexed under this heading.

Flurbiprofen (Serotonin release by platelets plays an important role in hemostasis. Epidemiological studies of the case-control and cohort design that have demonstrated an association between use of psychotropic drugs that interfere with serotonin re-uptake and the occurrence of upper gastrointestinal bleeding have also shown that concurrent use of an NSAID or aspirin may potentiate this risk of bleeding. Patients should be cautioned about the risk of bleeding associated with the concomitant use of Symbyax and NSAIDs, aspirin, or other drugs that affect coagulation).
No products indexed under this heading.

Fluvoxamine (Fluvoxamine, a CYP1A2 inhibitor, decreases the clearance of olanzapine. This results in a mean increase in olanzapine C_{max} following fluvoxamine administration of 54% in female nonsmokers and 77% in male smokers. The mean increase in olanzapine AUC is 52% and 108%, respectively. Lower doses of the olanzapine component of Symbyax should be considered in patients receiving concomitant treatment with fluvoxamine).
No products indexed under this heading.

Fluvoxamine Maleate (Fluvoxamine, a CYP1A2 inhibitor, decreases the clearance of olanzapine. This results in a mean increase in olanzapine C_{max} following fluvoxamine administration of 54% in female nonsmokers and 77% in male smokers. The mean increase in olanzapine AUC is 52% and 108%, respectively. Lower doses of the olanzapine component of Symbyax should be considered in patients receiving concomitant treatment with fluvoxamine).
No products indexed under this heading.

Fondaparinux Sodium (Serotonin release by platelets plays an important role in hemostasis. Epidemiological studies of the case-control and cohort design that have demonstrated an association between use of psychotropic drugs that interfere with serotonin re-uptake and the occurrence of upper gastrointestinal bleeding have also shown that concurrent use of an NSAID or aspirin may potentiate this risk of bleeding. Patients should be cautioned about the risk of bleeding associated with the concomitant use of Symbyax and NSAIDs, aspirin, or other drugs that affect coagulation). Products include:
Arixtra 1320

Formoterol Fumarate (Co-administration of fluoxetine with other drugs that are metabolized by CYP2D6 should be approached with caution. Therapy with medications that are predominantly metabolized by the CYP2D6 system and that have a relatively narrow therapeutic index should be initiated at the low end of the dose range if a patient is receiving fluoxetine concurrently or has taken it in the previous 5 weeks. If fluoxetine is added to the treatment regimen of a patient already receiving a drug metabolized by CYP2D6, the need for a decreased dose of the original medication should be considered). Products include:
Foradil 3121
Perforomist 3634

Fosinopril Sodium (Because of the potential for olanzapine to induce hypotension, Symbyax may enhance the effects of certain antihypertensive agents).
No products indexed under this heading.

Fosphenytoin (Patients on stable doses of phenytoin have developed elevated plasma levels of phenytoin with clinical phenytoin toxicity following initiation of concomitant fluoxetine).
No products indexed under this heading.

Fosphenytoin Sodium (Patients on stable doses of phenytoin have developed elevated plasma levels of phenytoin with clinical phenytoin toxicity following initiation of concomitant fluoxetine).
No products indexed under this heading.

Frovatriptan Succinate (There have been rare postmarketing reports of serotonin syndrome with use of an SSRI and a triptan. If concomitant treatment of Symbyax with a triptan is clinically warranted, careful observation of the patient is advised, particularly during treatment initiation and dose increases). Products include:
Frova 1103

Furosemide (Because of the potential for olanzapine to induce hypotension, Symbyax may enhance the effects of certain antihypertensive agents). Products include:
Furosemide 2354

Galantamine Hydrobromide (Co-administration of fluoxetine with other drugs that are metabolized by CYP2D6 should be approached with caution. Therapy with medications that are predominantly metabolized by the CYP2D6 system and that have a relatively narrow therapeutic index should be initiated at the low end of the dose range if a patient is receiving fluoxetine concurrently or has taken it in the previous 5 weeks. If fluoxetine is added to the treatment regimen of a patient already receiving a drug metabolized by CYP2D6, the need for a decreased dose of the original medication should be considered).
No products indexed under this heading.

Glipizide (Because fluoxetine is tightly bound to plasma protein, the administration of fluoxetine to a patient taking another drug that is tightly bound to protein (eg, warfarin, digitoxin) may cause a shift in plasma concentrations, potentially resulting in an adverse effect. Conversely, adverse effects may result from displacement of protein-bound fluoxetine by other tightly bound drugs).
No products indexed under this heading.

Glutethimide (Caution is advised if the concomitant administration of Symbyax and other CNS-active drugs is required. In evaluating individual cases, consideration should be given to using lower initial doses of the concomitantly administered drugs, using conservative titration schedules and monitoring of clinical status).
No products indexed under this heading.

Guanabenz Acetate (Because of the potential for olanzapine to induce hypotension, Symbyax may enhance the effects of certain antihypertensive agents).
No products indexed under this heading.

Guanethidine (Because of the potential for olanzapine to induce hypotension, Symbyax may enhance the effects of certain antihypertensive agents).
No products indexed under this heading.

Guanethidine Monosulfate (Because of the potential for olanzapine to induce hypotension, Symbyax may enhance the effects of certain antihypertensive agents).
No products indexed under this heading.

Guanethidine Sulfate (Because of the potential for olanzapine to induce hypotension, Symbyax may enhance the effects of certain antihypertensive agents).
No products indexed under this heading.

Haloperidol (Elevation of blood levels of haloperidol has been observed in patients receiving concomitant fluoxetine).
No products indexed under this heading.

Haloperidol Decanoate (Elevation of blood levels of haloperidol has been observed in patients receiving concomitant fluoxetine).
No products indexed under this heading.

Haloperidol Lactate (Elevation of blood levels of haloperidol has been observed in patients receiving concomitant fluoxetine).
No products indexed under this heading.

Heparin Calcium (Serotonin release by platelets plays an important role in hemostasis. Epidemiological studies of the case-control and cohort design that have demonstrated an association between use of psychotropic drugs that interfere with serotonin re-uptake and the occurrence of upper gastrointestinal bleeding have also shown that concurrent use of an NSAID or aspirin may potentiate this risk of bleeding. Patients should be cautioned about the risk of bleeding associated with the concomitant use of Symbyax and NSAIDs, aspirin, or other drugs that affect coagulation).
No products indexed under this heading.

Heparin Sodium (Serotonin release by platelets plays an important role in hemostasis. Epidemiological studies of the case-control and cohort design that have demonstrated an association between use of psychotropic drugs that interfere with serotonin re-uptake and the occurrence of upper gastrointestinal bleeding have also shown that concurrent use of an NSAID or aspirin may potentiate this risk of bleeding. Patients should be cautioned about the risk of bleeding associated with the concomitant use of Symbyax and NSAIDs, aspirin, or other drugs that affect coagulation).
No products indexed under this heading.

Hydralazine Hydrochloride (Because of the potential for olanzapine to induce hypotension, Symbyax may enhance the effects of certain antihypertensive agents).
No products indexed under this heading.

Hydrochlorothiazide (Because of the potential for olanzapine to induce hypotension, Symbyax may enhance the effects of certain antihypertensive agents). Products include:
Atacand HCT 700
Avalide 2956
Benicar HCT 1017
Diovan HCT 2419
Dyazide 1429
Exforge HCT 2449
Hyzaar 2162
Hyzaar 100-12.5 2162
Micardis HCT 889
Prinzide 2246
Tekturna HCT 2541
Teveten HCT 541

Hydrocodone Bitartrate (Caution is advised if the concomitant administration of Symbyax and other CNS-active drugs is required. In evaluating individual cases, consideration should be given to using lower initial doses of the concomitantly administered drugs, using conservative titration schedules and monitoring of clinical status). Products include:
Vicodin 560
Vicodin ES 561
Vicodin HP 563
Vicoprofen 564
Zydone 1138

Hydrocodone Polistirex (Caution is advised if the concomitant administration of Symbyax and other CNS-active drugs is required. In evaluating individual cases, consideration should be given to using lower initial doses of the concomitantly administered drugs, using conservative titration schedules and monitoring of clinical status). Products include:
Tussionex 3443

Hydroflumethiazide (Because of the potential for olanzapine to induce hypotension, Symbyax may enhance the effects of certain antihypertensive agents).
No products indexed under this heading.

Hydromorphone Hydrochloride (Caution is advised if the concomitant administration of Symbyax and other CNS-active drugs is required. In evaluating individual cases, consideration should be given to using lower initial doses of the concomitantly administered drugs, using conservative titration schedules and monitoring of clinical status). Products include:
Dilaudid Injection 2800
Dilaudid Oral 2797
Dilaudid Tablets 2797
Dilaudid-HP 2800

Hydroxyamphetamine Hydrobromide (Caution is advised if the concomitant administration of Symbyax and other CNS-active drugs is required. In evaluating individual cases, consideration should be given to using lower initial doses of the concomitantly administered drugs, using conservative titration schedules and monitoring of clinical status).
No products indexed under this heading.

Hydroxyzine Hydrochloride (Caution is advised if the concomitant administration of Symbyax and other CNS-active drugs is required. In evaluating individual cases, consideration should be given to using lower initial doses of the concomitantly administered drugs, using conservative titration schedules and monitoring of clinical status).
No products indexed under this heading.

Hypericum (Based on the mechanism of action of SNRIs and SSRIs, including Symbyax, and the potential for serotonin syndrome, caution is advised when Symbyax is co-administered with other drugs that may affect the serotonergic neurotransmitter systems, such as St. John's Wort).
No products indexed under this heading.

Hypericum Perforatum (Based on the mechanism of action of SNRIs and SSRIs, including Symbyax, and the potential for serotonin syndrome, caution is advised when Symbyax is co-administered with other drugs that may affect the serotonergic neurotransmitter systems, such as St. John's Wort). Products include:
Traumeel 1800

Ibuprofen (Serotonin release by platelets plays an important role in hemostasis. Epidemiological studies of the case-control and cohort design that have demonstrated an association between use of psychotropic drugs that interfere with serotonin re-uptake and the occurrence of upper gastrointestinal bleeding have also shown that concurrent use of an NSAID or aspirin may potentiate this risk of bleeding. Patients should be cautioned about the risk of bleeding associated with the concomitant use of Symb-

yax and NSAIDs, aspirin, or other drugs that affect coagulation). Products include:

Imipramine Hydrochloride (In two fluoxetine studies, previously stable plasma levels of imipramine and desipramine have increased>2- to 10-fold when fluoxetine has been administered in combination. This influence may persist for three weeks or longer after fluoxetine is discontinued. Thus, the dose of TCA may need to be reduced and plasma TCA concentrations may need to be monitored temporarily when Symbyax is co-administered or has been recently discontinued. Co-administration of fluoxetine with other drugs that are metabolized by CYP2D6, including certain antidepressants (eg, TCAs), should be approached with caution).

No products indexed under this heading.

Imipramine Pamoate (In two fluoxetine studies, previously stable plasma levels of imipramine and desipramine have increased>2- to 10-fold when fluoxetine has been administered in combination. This influence may persist for three weeks or longer after fluoxetine is discontinued. Thus, the dose of TCA may need to be reduced and plasma TCA concentrations may need to be monitored temporarily when Symbyax is co-administered or has been recently discontinued. Co-administration of fluoxetine with other drugs that are metabolized by CYP2D6, including certain antidepressants (eg, TCAs), should be approached with caution).

No products indexed under this heading.

Indapamide (Because of the potential for olanzapine to induce hypotension, Symbyax may enhance the effects of certain antihypertensive agents). Products include:

Indomethacin (Serotonin release by platelets plays an important role in hemostasis. Epidemiological studies of the case-control and cohort design that have demonstrated an association between use of psychotropic drugs that interfere with serotonin re-uptake and the occurrence of upper gastrointestinal bleeding have also shown that concurrent use of an NSAID or aspirin may potentiate this risk of bleeding. Patients should be cautioned about the risk of bleeding associated with the concomitant use of Symbyax and NSAIDs, aspirin, or other drugs that affect coagulation). Products include:

Indomethacin Sodium Trihydrate (Serotonin release by platelets plays an important role in hemostasis. Epidemiological studies of the case-control and cohort design that have demonstrated an association between use of psychotropic drugs that interfere with serotonin re-uptake and the occurrence of upper gastrointestinal bleeding have also shown that concurrent use of an NSAID or aspirin may potentiate this risk of bleeding. Patients should be cautioned about the risk of bleeding associated with the concomitant use of Symbyax and NSAIDs, aspirin, or other drugs that affect coagulation). Products include:

Indoramin Hydrochloride (Co-administration of fluoxetine with other drugs that are metabolized by CYP2D6 should be approached with caution. Therapy with medications that are pre-

---

dominantly metabolized by the CYP2D6 system and that have a relatively narrow therapeutic index should be initiated at the low end of the dose range if a patient is receiving fluoxetine concurrently or has taken it in the previous 5 weeks. If fluoxetine is added to the treatment regimen of a patient already receiving a drug metabolized by CYP2D6, the need for a decreased dose of the original medication should be considered).

No products indexed under this heading.

Insulin (Agents that induce CYP1A2 or glucuronyl transferase enzymes may cause an increase in olanzapine concentration).

No products indexed under this heading.

Insulin, Human, Zinc Suspension (Agents that induce CYP1A2 or glucuronyl transferase enzymes may cause an increase in olanzapine concentration).

No products indexed under this heading.

Insulin, Human (rDNA origin) (Agents that induce CYP1A2 or glucuronyl transferase enzymes may cause an increase in olanzapine concentration). Products include:

Insulin, Human NPH (Agents that induce CYP1A2 or glucuronyl transferase enzymes may cause an increase in olanzapine concentration). Products include:

Insulin, Human Regular (Agents that induce CYP1A2 or glucuronyl transferase enzymes may cause an increase in olanzapine concentration). Products include:

Insulin, Human Regular and Human NPH Mixture (Agents that induce CYP1A2 or glucuronyl transferase enzymes may cause an increase in olanzapine concentration). Products include:

Insulin, NPH (Agents that induce CYP1A2 or glucuronyl transferase enzymes may cause an increase in olanzapine concentration).

No products indexed under this heading.

Insulin, Regular (Agents that induce CYP1A2 or glucuronyl transferase enzymes may cause an increase in olanzapine concentration).

No products indexed under this heading.

Insulin, Regular and NPH mixture (Agents that induce CYP1A2 or glucuronyl transferase enzymes may cause an increase in olanzapine concentration).

No products indexed under this heading.

Insulin, Zinc Crystals (Agents that induce CYP1A2 or glucuronyl transferase enzymes may cause an increase in olanzapine concentration).

No products indexed under this heading.

Insulin, Zinc Suspension (Agents that induce CYP1A2 or glucuronyl transferase enzymes may cause an increase in olanzapine concentration).

No products indexed under this heading.

Insulin Aspart (Agents that induce CYP1A2 or glucuronyl transferase enzymes may cause an increase in olanzapine concentration).

No products indexed under this heading.

Insulin Aspart, Human (Agents that induce CYP1A2 or glucuronyl transferase enzymes may cause an increase in olanzapine concentration). Products include:

Insulin Aspart, Human Regular (Agents that induce CYP1A2 or glucuro-

---

nyl transferase enzymes may cause an increase in olanzapine concentration). Products include:

Insulin Aspart Protamine, Human (Agents that induce CYP1A2 or glucuronyl transferase enzymes may cause an increase in olanzapine concentration). Products include:

Insulin Detemir (rDNA Origin) (Agents that induce CYP1A2 or glucuronyl transferase enzymes may cause an increase in olanzapine concentration). Products include:

Insulin Glargine (Agents that induce CYP1A2 or glucuronyl transferase enzymes may cause an increase in olanzapine concentration). Products include:

Insulin Glulisine (Agents that induce CYP1A2 or glucuronyl transferase enzymes may cause an increase in olanzapine concentration). Products include:

Insulin Lispro, Human (Agents that induce CYP1A2 or glucuronyl transferase enzymes may cause an increase in olanzapine concentration). Products include:

Insulin Lispro Protamine, Human (Agents that induce CYP1A2 or glucuronyl transferase enzymes may cause an increase in olanzapine concentration). Products include:

Irbesartan (Because of the potential for olanzapine to induce hypotension, Symbyax may enhance the effects of certain antihypertensive agents). Products include:

Isocarboxazid (Concomitant use in patients taking MAO inhibitors is contraindicated. Symbyax should not be used in combination with an MAOI, or within a minimum of 14 days of discontinuing therapy with an MAOI. There have been reports of serious, sometimes fatal reactions in patients receiving fluoxetine in combination with an MAOI, and in patients who have recently discontinued fluoxetine and are then started on an MAOI. Some cases presented with features resembling neuroleptic malignant syndrome. Since fluoxetine and its major metabolite have very long elimination half-lives, at least 5 weeks (perhaps longer, especially if fluoxetine has been prescribed chronically and/or at higher doses) should be allowed after stopping Symbyax before starting an MAOI). Products include:

Isoflurane (Caution is advised if the concomitant administration of Symbyax and other CNS-active drugs is required. In evaluating individual cases, consideration should be given to using lower initial doses of the concomitantly administered drugs, using conservative titration schedules and monitoring of clinical status).

No products indexed under this heading.

Isradipine (Because of the potential for olanzapine to induce hypotension, Symbyax may enhance the effects of certain antihypertensive agents). Products include:

Ketamine Hydrochloride (Caution is advised if the concomitant administration of Symbyax and other CNS-active drugs is required. In evaluating individual cases, consideration should be given to using lower initial doses of the concomitantly administered drugs, using conservative titration schedules and monitoring of clinical status).

No products indexed under this heading.

Ketoprofen (Serotonin release by platelets plays an important role in hemostasis. Epidemiological studies of the case-control and cohort design that have demonstrated an association between use of psychotropic drugs that interfere with serotonin re-uptake and the occurrence of upper gastrointestinal bleeding have also shown that concurrent use of an NSAID or aspirin may potentiate this risk of bleeding. Patients should be cautioned about the risk of bleeding associated with the concomitant use of Symbyax and NSAIDs, aspirin, or other drugs that affect coagulation).

No products indexed under this heading.

Ketorolac Tromethamine (Serotonin release by platelets plays an important role in hemostasis. Epidemiological studies of the case-control and cohort design that have demonstrated an association between use of psychotropic drugs that interfere with serotonin re-uptake and the occurrence of upper gastrointestinal bleeding have also shown that concurrent use of an NSAID or aspirin may potentiate this risk of bleeding. Patients should be cautioned about the risk of bleeding associated with the concomitant use of Symbyax and NSAIDs, aspirin, or other drugs that affect coagulation). Products include:

Labetalol Hydrochloride (Because of the potential for olanzapine to induce hypotension, Symbyax may enhance the effects of certain antihypertensive agents).

No products indexed under this heading.

Lansoprazole (Agents that induce CYP1A2 or glucuronyl transferase enzymes may cause an increase in olanzapine concentration).

No products indexed under this heading.

Levodopa (The olanzapine component of Symbyax may antagonize the effects of levodopa and dopamine agonists). Products include:

Levomethadyl Acetate Hydrochloride (Caution is advised if the concomitant administration of Symbyax and other CNS-active drugs is required. In evaluating individual cases, consideration should be given to using lower initial doses of the concomitantly administered drugs, using conservative titration schedules and monitoring of clinical status).

No products indexed under this heading.

Levorphanol Tartrate (Caution is advised if the concomitant administration of Symbyax and other CNS-active drugs is required. In evaluating individual cases, consideration should be given to using lower initial doses of the concomitantly administered drugs, using conservative titration schedules and monitoring of clinical status).

No products indexed under this heading.

Lidocaine (Co-administration of fluoxetine with other drugs that are metabolized by CYP2D6 should be approached with caution. Therapy with medications that are predominantly metabolized by the CYP2D6 system and that have a relatively narrow therapeutic index should be initiated at the low end of the dose range if a patient is receiving fluoxetine concurrently or has taken it in the previous 5 weeks. If fluoxetine is

---

Symbyax Interactions Index 1800

added to the treatment regimen of a patient already receiving a drug metabolized by CYP2D6, the need for a decreased dose of the original medication should be considered). Products include:

Lidoderm 1107

Lidocaine Hydrochloride (Co-administration of fluoxetine with other drugs that are metabolized by CYP2D6, including antiarrhythmics (eg, propafenone, flecainide, and others) should be approached with caution. Therapy with medications that are predominantly metabolized by the CYP2D6 system and that have a relatively narrow therapeutic index should be initiated at the low end of the dose range if a patient is receiving fluoxetine concurrently or has taken it in the previous 5 weeks. If fluoxetine is added to the treatment regimen of a patient already receiving a drug metabolized by CYP2D6, the need for a decreased dose of the original medication should be considered).

No products indexed under this heading.

Linezolid (Based on the mechanism of action of SNRIs and SSRIs, including fluoxetine, and the potential for serotonin syndrome, caution is advised when fluoxetine is co-administered with other drugs that may affect the serotonergic neurotransmitter systems, such as linezolid (an antibiotic which is a reversible non-selective MAOI)). Products include:

Zyvox 2769

Lisdexamfetamine Dimesylate (Caution is advised if the concomitant administration of Symbyax and other CNS-active drugs is required. In evaluating individual cases, consideration should be given to using lower initial doses of the concomitantly administered drugs, using conservative titration schedules and monitoring of clinical status). Products include:

Vyvanse 3298

Lisinopril (Because of the potential for olanzapine to induce hypotension, Symbyax may enhance the effects of certain antihypertensive agents). Products include:

Prinivil 2241

Prinzide 2246

Lithium (There have been reports of both increased and decreased lithium levels when lithium was used concomitantly with fluoxetine. Cases of lithium toxicity and increased serotonergic effects have been reported. Lithium levels should be monitored in patients taking Symbyax concomitantly with lithium).

No products indexed under this heading.

Lithium Carbonate (There have been reports of both increased and decreased lithium levels when lithium was used concomitantly with fluoxetine. Cases of lithium toxicity and increased serotonergic effects have been reported. Lithium levels should be monitored in patients taking Symbyax concomitantly with lithium).

No products indexed under this heading.

Lithium Citrate (There have been reports of both increased and decreased lithium levels when lithium was used concomitantly with fluoxetine. Cases of lithium toxicity and increased serotonergic effects have been reported. Lithium levels should be monitored in patients taking Symbyax concomitantly with lithium).

No products indexed under this heading.

Lorazepam (Caution is advised if the concomitant administration of Symbyax and other CNS-active drugs is required. In evaluating individual cases, consideration should be given to using lower initial doses of the concomitantly administered drugs, using conservative titration schedules and monitoring of clinical status).

No products indexed under this heading.

Losartan Potassium (Because of the potential for olanzapine to induce hypotension, Symbyax may enhance the effects of certain antihypertensive agents). Products include:

Cozaar 2106

Hyzaar 2162

Hyzaar 100-12.5 2162

Low Molecular Weight Heparins (Serotonin release by platelets plays an important role in hemostasis. Epidemiological studies of the case-control and cohort design that have demonstrated an association between use of psychotropic drugs that interfere with serotonin re-uptake and the occurrence of upper gastrointestinal bleeding have also shown that concurrent use of an NSAID or aspirin may potentiate this risk of bleeding. Patients should be cautioned about the risk of bleeding associated with the concomitant use of Symbyax and NSAIDs, aspirin, or other drugs that affect coagulation).

No products indexed under this heading.

Loxapine Hydrochloride (The development of a potentially life-threatening serotonin syndrome or neuroleptic malignant syndrome (NMS)-like reactions have been reported with SNRIs and SSRIs alone and with the concomitant use of antipsychotics. Serotonin syndrome, in its most severe form can resemble neuroleptic malignant syndrome. Patients should be monitored for the emergence of serotonin syndrome or NMS-like signs and symptoms. Treatment with Symbyax and any concomitant serotonergic or antidopaminergic agents, including antipsychotics, should be discontinued immediately, if the above reactions occur, and supportive symptomatic treatment should be initiated. In addition, co-administration of fluoxetine with other drugs metabolized by CYP2D6, including antipsychotics (eg, phenothiazines and most atypicals), should be approached with caution. Therapy with medications that are predominantly metabolized by the CYP2D6 system and that have a relatively narrow therapeutic index should be initiated at the low end of the dose range if a patient is receiving fluoxetine concurrently or has taken it in the previous 5 weeks. If fluoxetine is added to the treatment regimen of a patient already receiving a drug metabolized by CYP2D6, the need for a decreased dose of the original medication should be considered).

No products indexed under this heading.

Loxapine Succinate (The development of a potentially life-threatening serotonin syndrome or neuroleptic malignant syndrome (NMS)-like reactions have been reported with SNRIs and SSRIs alone and with the concomitant use of antipsychotics. Serotonin syndrome, in its most severe form can resemble neuroleptic malignant syndrome. Patients should be monitored for the emergence of serotonin syndrome or NMS-like signs and symptoms. Treatment with Symbyax and any concomitant serotonergic or antidopaminergic agents, including antipsychotics, should be discontinued immediately, if the above reactions occur, and supportive symptomatic treatment should be initiated. In addition, co-administration of fluoxetine with other drugs metabolized by CYP2D6, including antipsychotics (eg, phenothiazines and most atypicals), should be approached with caution. Therapy with medications that are predominantly metabolized by the CYP2D6 system and that have a relatively narrow therapeutic index should be initiated at the low end of the dose range if a patient is receiving fluoxetine concurrently or has taken it in the previous 5 weeks. If fluoxetine is added to the treatment regimen of a patient already receiving a drug metabolized by CYP2D6, the need for a decreased dose of the original medication should be considered).

No products indexed under this heading.

Maprotiline Hydrochloride (In two fluoxetine studies, previously stable plasma levels of imipramine and desipramine have increased>2- to 10-fold when fluoxetine has been administered in combination. This influence may persist for three weeks or longer after fluoxetine is discontinued. Thus, the dose of TCA may need to be reduced and plasma TCA concentrations may need to be monitored temporarily when Symbyax is co-administered or has been recently discontinued. Co-administration of fluoxetine with other drugs that are metabolized by CYP2D6, including certain antidepressants (eg, TCAs), should be approached with caution).

No products indexed under this heading.

Mecamylamine Hydrochloride (Because of the potential for olanzapine to induce hypotension, Symbyax may enhance the effects of certain antihypertensive agents).

No products indexed under this heading.

Meclofenamate Sodium (Serotonin release by platelets plays an important role in hemostasis. Epidemiological studies of the case-control and cohort design that have demonstrated an association between use of psychotropic drugs that interfere with serotonin re-uptake and the occurrence of upper gastrointestinal bleeding have also shown that concurrent use of an NSAID or aspirin may potentiate this risk of bleeding. Patients should be cautioned about the risk of bleeding associated with the concomitant use of Symbyax and NSAIDs, aspirin, or other drugs that affect coagulation).

No products indexed under this heading.

Mefenamic Acid (Serotonin release by platelets plays an important role in hemostasis. Epidemiological studies of the case-control and cohort design that have demonstrated an association between use of psychotropic drugs that interfere with serotonin re-uptake and the occurrence of upper gastrointestinal bleeding have also shown that concurrent use of an NSAID or aspirin may potentiate this risk of bleeding. Patients should be cautioned about the risk of bleeding associated with the concomitant use of Symbyax and NSAIDs, aspirin, or other drugs that affect coagulation).

No products indexed under this heading.

Meloxicam (Serotonin release by platelets plays an important role in hemostasis. Epidemiological studies of the case-control and cohort design that have demonstrated an association between use of psychotropic drugs that interfere with serotonin re-uptake and the occurrence of upper gastrointestinal bleeding have also shown that concurrent use of an NSAID or aspirin may potentiate this risk of bleeding. Patients should be cautioned about the risk of bleeding associated with the concomitant use of Symbyax and NSAIDs, aspirin, or other drugs that affect coagulation).

No products indexed under this heading.

Meperidine Hydrochloride (Caution is advised if the concomitant administration of Symbyax and other CNS-active drugs is required. In evaluating individual cases, consideration should be given to using lower initial doses of the concomitantly administered drugs, using conservative titration schedules and monitoring of clinical status).

No products indexed under this heading.

Mephobarbital (Caution is advised if the concomitant administration of Symbyax and other CNS-active drugs is required. In evaluating individual cases, consideration should be given to using lower initial doses of the concomitantly administered drugs, using conservative titration schedules and monitoring of clinical status).

No products indexed under this heading.

Meprobamate (Caution is advised if the concomitant administration of Symbyax and other CNS-active drugs is required. In evaluating individual cases, consideration should be given to using lower initial doses of the concomitantly administered drugs, using conservative titration schedules and monitoring of clinical status).

No products indexed under this heading.

Mesoridazine Besylate (The development of a potentially life-threatening serotonin syndrome or neuroleptic malignant syndrome (NMS)-like reactions have been reported with SNRIs and SSRIs alone and with the concomitant use of antipsychotics. Serotonin syndrome, in its most severe form can resemble neuroleptic malignant syndrome. Patients should be monitored for the emergence of serotonin syndrome or NMS-like signs and symptoms. Treatment with Symbyax and any concomitant serotonergic or antidopaminergic agents, including antipsychotics, should be discontinued immediately, if the above reactions occur, and supportive symptomatic treatment should be initiated. In addition, co-administration of fluoxetine with other drugs metabolized by CYP2D6 including antipsychotics (eg, phenothiazines and most atypicals) should be approached with caution. Therapy with medications that are predominantly metabolized by the CYP2D6 system and that have a relatively narrow therapeutic index should be initiated at the low end of the dose range if a patient is receiving fluoxetine concurrently or has taken it in the previous 5 weeks. If fluoxetine is added to the treatment regimen of a patient already receiving a drug metabolized by CYP2D6, the need for a decreased dose of the original medication should be considered).

No products indexed under this heading.

Methadone Hydrochloride (Caution is advised if the concomitant administration of Symbyax and other CNS-active drugs is required. In evaluating individual cases, consideration should be given to using lower initial doses of the concomitantly administered drugs, using conservative titration schedules and monitoring of clinical status).

No products indexed under this heading.

Methamphetamine Hydrochloride (Caution is advised if the concomitant administration of Symbyax and other CNS-active drugs is required. In evaluating individual cases, consideration should be given to using lower initial doses of the concomitantly administered drugs, using conservative titration schedules and monitoring of clinical status).

No products indexed under this heading.

1801 **Interactions Index** **Symbyax**

Methohexital Sodium (Caution is advised if the concomitant administration of Symbyax and other CNS-active drugs is required. In evaluating individual cases, consideration should be given to using lower initial doses of the concomitantly administered drugs, using conservative titration schedules and monitoring of clinical status).
No products indexed under this heading.

Methotrimeprazine (The development of a potentially life-threatening serotonin syndrome or neuroleptic malignant syndrome (NMS)-like reactions have been reported with SNRIs and SSRIs alone and with the concomitant use of antipsychotics. Serotonin syndrome, in its most severe form can resemble neuroleptic malignant syndrome. Patients should be monitored for the emergence of serotonin syndrome or NMS-like signs and symptoms. Treatment with Symbyax and any concomitant serotonergic or antidopaminergic agents, including antipsychotics, should be discontinued immediately, if the above reactions occur, and supportive symptomatic treatment should be initiated. In addition, co-administration of fluoxetine with other drugs metabolized by CYP2D6 including antipsychotics (eg, phenothiazines and most atypicals) should be approached with caution. Therapy with medications that are predominantly metabolized by the CYP2D6 system and that have a relatively narrow therapeutic index should be initiated at the low end of the dose range if a patient is receiving fluoxetine concurrently or has taken it in the previous 5 weeks. If fluoxetine is added to the treatment regimen of a patient already receiving a drug metabolized by CYP2D6, the need for a decreased dose of the original medication should be considered).
No products indexed under this heading.

Methoxyflurane (Caution is advised if the concomitant administration of Symbyax and other CNS-active drugs is required. In evaluating individual cases, consideration should be given to using lower initial doses of the concomitantly administered drugs, using conservative titration schedules and monitoring of clinical status).
No products indexed under this heading.

Methoxyphenamine (Co-administration of fluoxetine with other drugs that are metabolized by CYP2D6 should be approached with caution. Therapy with medications that are predominantly metabolized by the CYP2D6 system and that have a relatively narrow therapeutic index should be initiated at the low end of the dose range if a patient is receiving fluoxetine concurrently or has taken it in the previous 5 weeks. If fluoxetine is added to the treatment regimen of a patient already receiving a drug metabolized by CYP2D6, the need for a decreased dose of the original medication should be considered).
No products indexed under this heading.

Methyclothiazide (Because of the potential for olanzapine to induce hypotension, Symbyax may enhance the effects of certain antihypertensive agents).
No products indexed under this heading.

Methyldopa (Because of the potential for olanzapine to induce hypotension, Symbyax may enhance the effects of certain antihypertensive agents).
No products indexed under this heading.

Methyldopate Hydrochloride (Because of the potential for olanzapine to induce hypotension, Symbyax may enhance the effects of certain antihypertensive agents).
No products indexed under this heading.

Methylphenidate (Caution is advised if the concomitant administration of Symbyax and other CNS-active drugs is required. In evaluating individual cases, consideration should be given to using lower initial doses of the concomitantly administered drugs, using conservative titration schedules and monitoring of clinical status). Products include:
Daytrana **3283**

Methylphenidate Hydrochloride (Caution is advised if the concomitant administration of Symbyax and other CNS-active drugs is required. In evaluating individual cases, consideration should be given to using lower initial doses of the concomitantly administered drugs, using conservative titration schedules and monitoring of clinical status). Products include:
Concerta **2598**
Metadate CD **3439**

Metoclopramide Hydrochloride (The development of a potentially life-threatening serotonin syndrome or neuroleptic malignant syndrome (NMS)-like reactions have been reported with SNRIs and SSRIs alone but particularly with concomitant use of serotonergic drugs (including triptans) with drugs which impair metabolism of serotonin (including MAOIs), or with antipsychotics or other dopamine antagonists. Serotonin syndrome symptoms may include mental status changes, autonomic instability, neuromuscular aberrations, and/or gastrointestinal symptoms. Serotonin syndrome, in its most severe form can resemble neuroleptic malignant syndrome. Patients should be monitored for the emergence of serotonin syndrome or NMS-like signs and symptoms. Treatment with Symbyax and any concomitant serotonergic or antidopaminergic agents, including antipsychotics, should be discontinued immediately, if the above reactions occur, and supportive symptomatic treatment should be initiated). Products include:
Metozolv ODT **2901**

Metolazone (Because of the potential for olanzapine to induce hypotension, Symbyax may enhance the effects of certain antihypertensive agents).
No products indexed under this heading.

Metoprolol Succinate (Because of the potential for olanzapine to induce hypotension, Symbyax may enhance the effects of certain antihypertensive agents). Products include:
Toprol XL **732**

Metoprolol Tartrate (Because of the potential for olanzapine to induce hypotension, Symbyax may enhance the effects of certain antihypertensive agents).
No products indexed under this heading.

Metyrosine (Because of the potential for olanzapine to induce hypotension, Symbyax may enhance the effects of certain antihypertensive agents).
No products indexed under this heading.

Mexiletine Hydrochloride (Co-administration of fluoxetine with other drugs that are metabolized by CYP2D6, including antiarrhythmics (eg, propafenone, flecainide, and others) should be approached with caution. Therapy with medications that are predominantly metabolized by the CYP2D6 system and that have a relatively narrow therapeutic index should be initiated at the low end of the dose range if a patient is receiving fluoxetine concurrently or has taken it in the previous 5 weeks. If fluoxetine is added to the treatment regimen of a patient already receiving a drug metabolized by CYP2D6, the need for a decreased dose of the original medication should be considered).
No products indexed under this heading.

Mibefradil Dihydrochloride (Because of the potential for olanzapine to induce hypotension, Symbyax may enhance the effects of certain antihypertensive agents).
No products indexed under this heading.

Midazolam Hydrochloride (Caution is advised if the concomitant administration of Symbyax and other CNS-active drugs is required. In evaluating individual cases, consideration should be given to using lower initial doses of the concomitantly administered drugs, using conservative titration schedules and monitoring of clinical status).
No products indexed under this heading.

Minoxidil (Because of the potential for olanzapine to induce hypotension, Symbyax may enhance the effects of certain antihypertensive agents).
No products indexed under this heading.

Mirtazapine (Co-administration of fluoxetine with other drugs that are metabolized by CYP2D6, including certain antidepressants (eg, TCAs) should be approached with caution. Therapy with medications that are predominantly metabolized by the CYP2D6 system and that have a relatively narrow therapeutic index should be initiated at the low end of the dose range if a patient is receiving fluoxetine concurrently or has taken it in the previous 5 weeks. If fluoxetine is added to the treatment regimen of a patient already receiving a drug metabolized by CYP2D6, the need for a decreased dose of the original medication should be considered). Products include:
Remeron Tablets **3214**
RemeronSolTab Tablets **3219**

Moclobemide (Concomitant use in patients taking MAO inhibitors is contraindicated. Symbyax should not be used in combination with an MAOI, or within a minimum of 14 days of discontinuing therapy with an MAOI. There have been reports of serious, sometimes fatal reactions in patients receiving fluoxetine in combination with an MAOI, and in patients who have recently discontinued fluoxetine and are then started on an MAOI. Some cases presented with features resembling neuroleptic malignant syndrome. Since fluoxetine and its major metabolite have very long elimination half-lives, at least 5 weeks (perhaps longer, especially if fluoxetine has been prescribed chronically and/or at higher doses) should be allowed after stopping Symbyax before starting an MAOI).
No products indexed under this heading.

Moexipril Hydrochloride (Because of the potential for olanzapine to induce hypotension, Symbyax may enhance the effects of certain antihypertensive agents).
No products indexed under this heading.

Molindone Hydrochloride (The development of a potentially life-threatening serotonin syndrome or neuroleptic malignant syndrome (NMS)-like reactions have been reported with SNRIs and SSRIs alone and with the concomitant use of antipsychotics. Serotonin syndrome, in its most severe form can resemble neuroleptic malignant syndrome. Patients should be monitored for the emergence of serotonin syndrome or NMS-like signs and symptoms. Treatment with Symbyax and any concomitant serotonergic or antidopaminergic agents, including antipsychotics, should be discontinued immediately, if the above reactions occur, and supportive symptomatic treatment should be initiated. In addition, co-administration of fluoxetine with other drugs metabolized by CYP2D6, including antipsychotics (eg, phenothiazines and most atypicals), should be approached with caution. Therapy with medications that are predominantly metabolized by the CYP2D6 system and that have a relatively narrow therapeutic index should be initiated at the low end of the dose range if a patient is receiving fluoxetine concurrently or has taken it in the previous 5 weeks. If fluoxetine is added to the treatment regimen of a patient already receiving a drug metabolized by CYP2D6, the need for a decreased dose of the original medication should be considered). Products include:
Moban **1108**

Moricizine Hydrochloride (Co-administration of fluoxetine with other drugs that are metabolized by CYP2D6, including antiarrhythmics (eg, propafenone, flecainide, and others) should be approached with caution. Therapy with medications that are predominantly metabolized by the CYP2D6 system and that have a relatively narrow therapeutic index should be initiated at the low end of the dose range if a patient is receiving fluoxetine concurrently or has taken it in the previous 5 weeks. If fluoxetine is added to the treatment regimen of a patient already receiving a drug metabolized by CYP2D6, the need for a decreased dose of the original medication should be considered).
No products indexed under this heading.

Morphine Sulfate (Caution is advised if the concomitant administration of Symbyax and other CNS-active drugs is required. In evaluating individual cases, consideration should be given to using lower initial doses of the concomitantly administered drugs, using conservative titration schedules and monitoring of clinical status). Products include:
Avinza **1822**
Embeda **1831**
MS Contin **2803**

Nabumetone (Serotonin release by platelets plays an important role in hemostasis. Epidemiological studies of the case-control and cohort design that have demonstrated an association between use of psychotropic drugs that interfere with serotonin re-uptake and the occurrence of upper gastrointestinal bleeding have also shown that concurrent use of an NSAID or aspirin may potentiate this risk of bleeding. Patients should be cautioned about the risk of bleeding associated with the concomitant use of Symbyax and NSAIDs, aspirin, or other drugs that affect coagulation).
No products indexed under this heading.

Nadolol (Because of the potential for olanzapine to induce hypotension, Symbyax may enhance the effects of certain antihypertensive agents). Products include:
Nadolol **2359**

Nafcillin Sodium (Agents that induce CYP1A2 or glucuronyl transferase enzymes may cause an increase in olanzapine concentration).
No products indexed under this heading.

Naproxen (Serotonin release by platelets plays an important role in hemostasis. Epidemiological studies of the case-control and cohort design that have demonstrated an association between use of psychotropic drugs that interfere with serotonin re-uptake and the occurrence of upper gastrointestinal bleeding have also shown that concurrent use of an NSAID or aspirin may potentiate this risk of bleeding. Patients should be cautioned about the risk of bleeding associated with the concomitant use of Symbyax and NSAIDs, aspirin, or other drugs that affect coagulation). Products include:
EC-Naprosyn **2850**
Naprosyn **2850**
Anaprox/Naprosyn **2850**

Naproxen Sodium (Serotonin release by platelets plays an important role in hemostasis. Epidemiological studies of

IMPORTANT NOTE: Always consult each drug listing in the patient's regimen for possible interactions.

Symbyax Interactions Index 1802

the case-control and cohort design that have demonstrated an association between use of psychotropic drugs that interfere with serotonin re-uptake and the occurrence of upper gastrointestinal bleeding have also shown that concurrent use of an NSAID or aspirin may potentiate this risk of bleeding. Patients should be cautioned about the risk of bleeding associated with the concomitant use of Symbyax and NSAIDs, aspirin, or other drugs that affect coagulation). Products include:

Anaprox 2850
Anaprox DS 2850
Treximet 1681

Naratriptan Hydrochloride (There have been rare postmarketing reports of serotonin syndrome with use of an SSRI and a triptan. If concomitant treatment of Symbyax with a triptan is clinically warranted, careful observation of the patient is advised, particularly during treatment initiation and dose increases). Products include:

Amerge 1306

Nebivolol (Because of the potential for olanzapine to induce hypotension, Symbyax may enhance the effects of certain antihypertensive agents). Products include:

Bystolic 1147

Nefazodone Hydrochloride (The concomitant use of Symbyax with serotonin and norepinephrine reuptake inhibitors (SNRIs) is not recommended).

No products indexed under this heading.

Nelfinavir Mesylate (Co-administration of fluoxetine with other drugs that are metabolized by CYP2D6 should be approached with caution. Therapy with medications that are predominantly metabolized by the CYP2D6 system and that have a relatively narrow therapeutic index should be initiated at the low end of the dose range if a patient is receiving fluoxetine concurrently or has taken it in the previous 5 weeks. If fluoxetine is added to the treatment regimen of a patient already receiving a drug metabolized by CYP2D6, the need for a decreased dose of the original medication should be considered).

No products indexed under this heading.

Nicardipine Hydrochloride (Because of the potential for olanzapine to induce hypotension, Symbyax may enhance the effects of certain antihypertensive agents).

No products indexed under this heading.

Nicotine (Agents that induce CYP1A2 or glucuronyl transferase enzymes may cause an increase in olanzapine concentration).

No products indexed under this heading.

Nicotine Polacrilex (Agents that induce CYP1A2 or glucuronyl transferase enzymes may cause an increase in olanzapine concentration).

No products indexed under this heading.

Nicotine Salicylate (Agents that induce CYP1A2 or glucuronyl transferase enzymes may cause an increase in olanzapine concentration).

No products indexed under this heading.

Nicotine Sulfate (Agents that induce CYP1A2 or glucuronyl transferase enzymes may cause an increase in olanzapine concentration).

No products indexed under this heading.

Nifedipine (Because of the potential for olanzapine to induce hypotension, Symbyax may enhance the effects of certain antihypertensive agents).

No products indexed under this heading.

Nisoldipine (Because of the potential for olanzapine to induce hypotension, Symbyax may enhance the effects of certain antihypertensive agents).

No products indexed under this heading.

Nitroglycerin (Because of the potential for olanzapine to induce hypotension, Symbyax may enhance the effects of certain antihypertensive agents). Products include:

Nitro-Dur 3170
Nitrolingual 3266

Nortriptyline Hydrochloride (In two fluoxetine studies, previously stable plasma levels of imipramine and desipramine have increased>2- to 10-fold when fluoxetine has been administered in combination. This influence may persist for three weeks or longer after fluoxetine is discontinued. Thus, the dose of TCA may need to be reduced and plasma TCA concentrations may need to be monitored temporarily when Symbyax is co-administered or has been recently discontinued. Co-administration of fluoxetine with other drugs that are metabolized by CYP2D6, including certain antidepressants (eg, TCAs), should be approached with caution).

No products indexed under this heading.

Omeprazole (Agents that induce CYP1A2 or glucuronyl transferase enzymes, such as omeprazole, may cause an increase in olanzapine clearance).

No products indexed under this heading.

Omeprazole Magnesium (Agents that induce CYP1A2 or glucuronyl transferase enzymes, such as omeprazole, may cause an increase in olanzapine clearance).

No products indexed under this heading.

Ondansetron (Co-administration of fluoxetine with other drugs that are metabolized by CYP2D6 should be approached with caution. Therapy with medications that are predominantly metabolized by the CYP2D6 system and that have a relatively narrow therapeutic index should be initiated at the low end of the dose range if a patient is receiving fluoxetine concurrently or has taken it in the previous 5 weeks. If fluoxetine is added to the treatment regimen of a patient already receiving a drug metabolized by CYP2D6, the need for a decreased dose of the original medication should be considered).

No products indexed under this heading.

Ondansetron Hydrochloride (Co-administration of fluoxetine with other drugs that are metabolized by CYP2D6 should be approached with caution. Therapy with medications that are predominantly metabolized by the CYP2D6 system and that have a relatively narrow therapeutic index should be initiated at the low end of the dose range if a patient is receiving fluoxetine concurrently or has taken it in the previous 5 weeks. If fluoxetine is added to the treatment regimen of a patient already receiving a drug metabolized by CYP2D6, the need for a decreased dose of the original medication should be considered). Products include:

Zofran Injection 1750
Zofran 1756
Zofran ODT 1756

Oxaprozin (Serotonin release by platelets plays an important role in hemostasis. Epidemiological studies of the case-control and cohort design that have demonstrated an association between use of psychotropic drugs that interfere with serotonin re-uptake and the occurrence of upper gastrointestinal bleeding have also shown that concurrent use of an NSAID or aspirin may potentiate this risk of bleeding. Patients should be cautioned about the risk of bleeding associated with the concomitant use of Symbyax and NSAIDs, aspirin, or other drugs that affect coagulation).

No products indexed under this heading.

Oxazepam (Caution is advised if the concomitant administration of Symbyax and other CNS-active drugs is required. In evaluating individual cases, consideration should be given to using lower initial doses of the concomitantly administered drugs, using conservative titration schedules and monitoring of clinical status).

No products indexed under this heading.

Oxycodone Hydrochloride (Caution is advised if the concomitant administration of Symbyax and other CNS-active drugs is required. In evaluating individual cases, consideration should be given to using lower initial doses of the concomitantly administered drugs, using conservative titration schedules and monitoring of clinical status). Products include:

OxyContin 2807
Percocet 1121
Percodan 1124

Paclitaxel (Co-administration of fluoxetine with other drugs that are metabolized by CYP2D6 should be approached with caution. Therapy with medications that are predominantly metabolized by the CYP2D6 system and that have a relatively narrow therapeutic index should be initiated at the low end of the dose range if a patient is receiving fluoxetine concurrently or has taken it in the previous 5 weeks. If fluoxetine is added to the treatment regimen of a patient already receiving a drug metabolized by CYP2D6, the need for a decreased dose of the original medication should be considered).

No products indexed under this heading.

Paliperidone (The development of a potentially life-threatening serotonin syndrome or neuroleptic malignant syndrome (NMS)-like reactions have been reported with SNRIs and SSRIs alone and with the concomitant use of antipsychotics. Serotonin syndrome, in its most severe form can resemble neuroleptic malignant syndrome. Patients should be monitored for the emergence of serotonin syndrome or NMS-like signs and symptoms. Treatment with Symbyax and any concomitant serotonergic or antidopaminergic agents, including antipsychotics, should be discontinued immediately, if the above reactions occur, and supportive symptomatic treatment should be initiated. In addition, co-administration of fluoxetine with other drugs metabolized by CYP2D6, including antipsychotics (eg, phenothiazines and most atypicals), should be approached with caution. Therapy with medications that are predominantly metabolized by the CYP2D6 system and that have a relatively narrow therapeutic index should be initiated at the low end of the dose range if a patient is receiving fluoxetine concurrently or has taken it in the previous 5 weeks. If fluoxetine is added to the treatment regimen of a patient already receiving a drug metabolized by CYP2D6, the need for a decreased dose of the original medication should be considered). Products include:

Invega 2613
Invega Sustenna 2621

Pargyline Hydrochloride (Concomitant use in patients taking MAO inhibitors is contraindicated. Symbyax should not be used in combination with an MAOI, or within a minimum of 14 days of discontinuing therapy with an MAOI. There have been reports of serious, sometimes fatal reactions in patients receiving fluoxetine in combination with an MAOI, and in patients who have recently discontinued fluoxetine and are then started on an MAOI. Some cases presented with features resembling neuroleptic malignant syndrome. Since fluoxetine and its major metabolite have very long elimination half-lives, at least 5 weeks (perhaps longer, especially if fluoxetine has been prescribed chronically and/or at higher doses) should be allowed after stopping Symbyax before starting an MAOI).

No products indexed under this heading.

Paroxetine (The concomitant use of Symbyax with selective serotonin reuptake inhibitors (SSRIs) is not recommended).

No products indexed under this heading.

Paroxetine Hydrochloride (The concomitant use of Symbyax with selective serotonin reuptake inhibitors (SSRIs) is not recommended). Products include:

Paroxetine CR 2361
Paroxetine ER 2371
Paxil 1586
Paxil CR 1596

Paroxetine Mesylate (The concomitant use of Symbyax with selective serotonin reuptake inhibitors (SSRIs) is not recommended).

No products indexed under this heading.

Pemoline (Caution is advised if the concomitant administration of Symbyax and other CNS-active drugs is required. In evaluating individual cases, consideration should be given to using lower initial doses of the concomitantly administered drugs, using conservative titration schedules and monitoring of clinical status).

No products indexed under this heading.

Penbutolol Sulfate (Because of the potential for olanzapine to induce hypotension, Symbyax may enhance the effects of certain antihypertensive agents).

No products indexed under this heading.

Pentobarbital Sodium (Caution is advised if the concomitant administration of Symbyax and other CNS-active drugs is required. In evaluating individual cases, consideration should be given to using lower initial doses of the concomitantly administered drugs, using conservative titration schedules and monitoring of clinical status). Products include:

Nembutal 2012

Pergolide Mesylate (The olanzapine component of Symbyax may antagonize the effects of levodopa and dopamine agonists).

No products indexed under this heading.

Perindopril Erbumine (Because of the potential for olanzapine to induce hypotension, Symbyax may enhance the effects of certain antihypertensive agents).

No products indexed under this heading.

Perphenazine (The development of a potentially life-threatening serotonin syndrome or neuroleptic malignant syndrome (NMS)-like reactions have been reported with SNRIs and SSRIs alone and with the concomitant use of antipsychotics. Serotonin syndrome, in its most severe form can resemble neuroleptic malignant syndrome. Patients should be monitored for the emergence of serotonin syndrome or NMS-like signs and symptoms. Treatment with Symbyax and any concomitant serotonergic or antidopaminergic agents, including antipsychotics, should be discontinued immediately, if the above reactions occur, and supportive symptomatic treatment should be initiated. In addition, co-administration of fluoxetine with other drugs metabolized by CYP2D6 including antipsychotics (eg, phenothiazines and most atypicals) should be approached with caution. Therapy with medications that are predominantly metabolized by the CYP2D6 system and that have a relatively narrow therapeutic index should be initiated at the low end of the dose range if a patient is receiving fluoxetine concur-

1803 Interactions Index Symbyax

rently or has taken it in the previous 5 weeks. If fluoxetine is added to the treatment regimen of a patient already receiving a drug metabolized by CYP2D6, the need for a decreased dose of the original medication should be considered).
No products indexed under this heading.

Phenelzine Sulfate (Concomitant use in patients taking MAO inhibitors is contraindicated. Symbyax should not be used in combination with an MAOI, or within a minimum of 14 days of discontinuing therapy with an MAOI. There have been reports of serious, sometimes fatal reactions in patients receiving fluoxetine in combination with an MAOI, and in patients who have recently discontinued fluoxetine and are then started on an MAOI. Some cases presented with features resembling neuroleptic malignant syndrome. Since fluoxetine and its major metabolite have very long elimination half-lives, at least 5 weeks (perhaps longer, especially if fluoxetine has been prescribed chronically and/or at higher doses) should be allowed after stopping Symbyax before starting an MAOI).
No products indexed under this heading.

Phenobarbital (Caution is advised if the concomitant administration of Symbyax and other CNS-active drugs is required. In evaluating individual cases, consideration should be given to using lower initial doses of the concomitantly administered drugs, using conservative titration schedules and monitoring of clinical status). Products include:
Donnatal 2711

Phenobarbital Sodium (Caution is advised if the concomitant administration of Symbyax and other CNS-active drugs is required. In evaluating individual cases, consideration should be given to using lower initial doses of the concomitantly administered drugs, using conservative titration schedules and monitoring of clinical status).
No products indexed under this heading.

Phenothiazine Derivatives (The development of a potentially life-threatening serotonin syndrome or neuroleptic malignant syndrome (NMS)-like reactions have been reported with SNRIs and SSRIs alone and with the concomitant use of antipsychotics. Serotonin syndrome, in its most severe form can resemble neuroleptic malignant syndrome. Patients should be monitored for the emergence of serotonin syndrome or NMS-like signs and symptoms. Treatment with Symbyax and any concomitant serotonergic or antidopaminergic agents, including antipsychotics, should be discontinued immediately, if the above reactions occur, and supportive symptomatic treatment should be initiated. In addition, co-administration of fluoxetine with other drugs metabolized by CYP2D6 including antipsychotics (eg, phenothiazines and most atypicals) should be approached with caution. Therapy with medications that are predominantly metabolized by the CYP2D6 system and that have a relatively narrow therapeutic index should be initiated at the low end of the dose range if a patient is receiving fluoxetine concurrently or has taken it in the previous 5 weeks. If fluoxetine is added to the treatment regimen of a patient already receiving a drug metabolized by CYP2D6, the need for a decreased dose of the original medication should be considered).
No products indexed under this heading.

Phenothiazines (The development of a potentially life-threatening serotonin syndrome or neuroleptic malignant syndrome (NMS)-like reactions have been reported with SNRIs and SSRIs alone and with the concomitant use of antipsychotics. Serotonin syndrome, in its most severe form can resemble neuroleptic malignant syndrome. Patients should be monitored for the emergence of serotonin syndrome or NMS-like signs and symptoms. Treatment with Symbyax and any concomitant serotonergic or antidopaminergic agents, including antipsychotics, should be discontinued immediately, if the above reactions occur, and supportive symptomatic treatment should be initiated. In addition, co-administration of fluoxetine with other drugs metabolized by CYP2D6 including antipsychotics (eg, phenothiazines and most atypicals) should be approached with caution. Therapy with medications that are predominantly metabolized by the CYP2D6 system and that have a relatively narrow therapeutic index should be initiated at the low end of the dose range if a patient is receiving fluoxetine concurrently or has taken it in the previous 5 weeks. If fluoxetine is added to the treatment regimen of a patient already receiving a drug metabolized by CYP2D6, the need for a decreased dose of the original medication should be considered).
No products indexed under this heading.

Phenoxybenzamine Hydrochloride (Because of the potential for olanzapine to induce hypotension, Symbyax may enhance the effects of certain antihypertensive agents). Products include:
Dibenzyline 3495

Phentolamine Mesylate (Because of the potential for olanzapine to induce hypotension, Symbyax may enhance the effects of certain antihypertensive agents).
No products indexed under this heading.

Phenylbutazone (Serotonin release by platelets plays an important role in hemostasis. Epidemiological studies of the case-control and cohort design that have demonstrated an association between use of psychotropic drugs that interfere with serotonin re-uptake and the occurrence of upper gastrointestinal bleeding have also shown that concurrent use of an NSAID or aspirin may potentiate this risk of bleeding. Patients should be cautioned about the risk of bleeding associated with the concomitant use of Symbyax and NSAIDs, aspirin, or other drugs that affect coagulation).
No products indexed under this heading.

Phenytoin (Patients on stable doses of phenytoin have developed elevated plasma levels of phenytoin with clinical phenytoin toxicity following initiation of concomitant fluoxetine).
No products indexed under this heading.

Phenytoin Sodium (Patients on stable doses of phenytoin have developed elevated plasma levels of phenytoin with clinical phenytoin toxicity following initiation of concomitant fluoxetine). Products include:
Phenytek Capsules 2380

Pimozide (Concomitant use of fluoxetine and pimozide is contraindicated. Clinical studies of pimozide with other antidepressants demonstrate an increase in drug interaction or QTc prolongation. While a specific study with pimozide and fluoxetine has not been conducted, the potential for drug interactions or QTc prolongation warrants restricting the concurrent use of pimozide and fluoxetine).
No products indexed under this heading.

Pindolol (Because of the potential for olanzapine to induce hypotension, Symbyax may enhance the effects of certain antihypertensive agents).
No products indexed under this heading.

Piroxicam (Serotonin release by platelets plays an important role in hemostasis. Epidemiological studies of the case-control and cohort design that have demonstrated an association between use of psychotropic drugs that interfere with serotonin re-uptake and the occurrence of upper gastrointestinal bleeding have also shown that concurrent use of an NSAID or aspirin may potentiate this risk of bleeding. Patients should be cautioned about the risk of bleeding associated with the concomitant use of Symbyax and NSAIDs, aspirin, or other drugs that affect coagulation).
No products indexed under this heading.

Polythiazide (Because of the potential for olanzapine to induce hypotension, Symbyax may enhance the effects of certain antihypertensive agents).
No products indexed under this heading.

Pramipexole Dihydrochloride (The olanzapine component of Symbyax may antagonize the effects of levodopa and dopamine agonists).
No products indexed under this heading.

Prazepam (Caution is advised if the concomitant administration of Symbyax and other CNS-active drugs is required. In evaluating individual cases, consideration should be given to using lower initial doses of the concomitantly administered drugs, using conservative titration schedules and monitoring of clinical status).
No products indexed under this heading.

Prazosin Hydrochloride (Because of the potential for olanzapine to induce hypotension, Symbyax may enhance the effects of certain antihypertensive agents).
No products indexed under this heading.

Primidone (Agents that induce CYP1A2 or glucuronyl transferase enzymes may cause an increase in olanzapine concentration).
No products indexed under this heading.

Procainamide Hydrochloride (Co-administration of fluoxetine with other drugs that are metabolized by CYP2D6, including antiarrhythmics (eg, propafenone, flecainide, and others) should be approached with caution. Therapy with medications that are predominantly metabolized by the CYP2D6 system and that have a relatively narrow therapeutic index should be initiated at the low end of the dose range if a patient is receiving fluoxetine concurrently or has taken it in the previous 5 weeks. If fluoxetine is added to the treatment regimen of a patient already receiving a drug metabolized by CYP2D6, the need for a decreased dose of the original medication should be considered).
No products indexed under this heading.

Procarbazine Hydrochloride (Concomitant use in patients taking MAO inhibitors is contraindicated. Symbyax should not be used in combination with an MAOI, or within a minimum of 14 days of discontinuing therapy with an MAOI. There have been reports of serious, sometimes fatal reactions in patients receiving fluoxetine in combination with an MAOI, and in patients who have recently discontinued fluoxetine and are then started on an MAOI. Some cases presented with features resembling neuroleptic malignant syndrome. Since fluoxetine and its major metabolite have very long elimination half-lives, at least 5 weeks (perhaps longer, especially if fluoxetine has been prescribed chronically and/or at higher doses) should be allowed after stopping Symbyax before starting an MAOI).
No products indexed under this heading.

Prochlorperazine (The development of a potentially life-threatening serotonin syndrome or neuroleptic malignant syndrome (NMS)-like reactions have been reported with SNRIs and SSRIs alone and with the concomitant use of antipsychotics. Serotonin syndrome, in its most severe form can resemble neuroleptic malignant syndrome. Patients should be monitored for the emergence of serotonin syndrome or NMS-like signs and symptoms. Treatment with Symbyax and any concomitant serotonergic or antidopaminergic agents, including antipsychotics, should be discontinued immediately, if the above reactions occur, and supportive symptomatic treatment should be initiated. In addition, co-administration of fluoxetine with other drugs metabolized by CYP2D6 including antipsychotics (eg, phenothiazines and most atypicals) should be approached with caution. Therapy with medications that are predominantly metabolized by the CYP2D6 system and that have a relatively narrow therapeutic index should be initiated at the low end of the dose range if a patient is receiving fluoxetine concurrently or has taken it in the previous 5 weeks. If fluoxetine is added to the treatment regimen of a patient already receiving a drug metabolized by CYP2D6, the need for a decreased dose of the original medication should be considered).
No products indexed under this heading.

Prochlorperazine Edisylate (The development of a potentially life-threatening serotonin syndrome or neuroleptic malignant syndrome (NMS)-like reactions have been reported with SNRIs and SSRIs alone and with the concomitant use of antipsychotics. Serotonin syndrome, in its most severe form can resemble neuroleptic malignant syndrome. Patients should be monitored for the emergence of serotonin syndrome or NMS-like signs and symptoms. Treatment with Symbyax and any concomitant serotonergic or antidopaminergic agents, including antipsychotics, should be discontinued immediately, if the above reactions occur, and supportive symptomatic treatment should be initiated. In addition, co-administration of fluoxetine with other drugs metabolized by CYP2D6 including antipsychotics (eg, phenothiazines and most atypicals) should be approached with caution. Therapy with medications that are predominantly metabolized by the CYP2D6 system and that have a relatively narrow therapeutic index should be initiated at the low end of the dose range if a patient is receiving fluoxetine concurrently or has taken it in the previous 5 weeks. If fluoxetine is added to the treatment regimen of a patient already receiving a drug metabolized by CYP2D6, the need for a decreased dose of the original medication should be considered).
No products indexed under this heading.

Prochlorperazine Maleate (The development of a potentially life-threatening serotonin syndrome or neuroleptic malignant syndrome (NMS)-like reactions have been reported with SNRIs and SSRIs alone and with the concomitant use of antipsychotics. Serotonin syndrome, in its most severe form can resemble neuroleptic malignant syndrome. Patients should be monitored for the emergence of serotonin syndrome or NMS-like signs and symptoms. Treatment with Symbyax and any concomitant serotonergic or antidopaminergic agents, including antipsychotics, should be discontinued immediately, if the above reactions occur, and supportive symptomatic treatment should be initiated. In addition, co-administration of fluoxetine with other drugs metabolized by CYP2D6 including antipsychotics (eg, phenothiazines and most atypicals) should be approached with caution. Therapy with medications that are predominantly metabolized by the CYP2D6 system and that have a rela-

IMPORTANT NOTE: Always consult each drug listing in the patient's regimen for possible interactions.

Symbyax Interactions Index 1804

tively narrow therapeutic index should be initiated at the low end of the dose range if a patient is receiving fluoxetine concurrently or has taken it in the previous 5 weeks. If fluoxetine is added to the treatment regimen of a patient already receiving a drug metabolized by CYP2D6, the need for a decreased dose of the original medication should be considered).
No products indexed under this heading.

Promethazine (The development of a potentially life-threatening serotonin syndrome or neuroleptic malignant syndrome (NMS)-like reactions have been reported with SNRIs and SSRIs alone and with the concomitant use of antipsychotics. Serotonin syndrome, in its most severe form can resemble neuroleptic malignant syndrome. Patients should be monitored for the emergence of serotonin syndrome or NMS-like signs and symptoms. Treatment with Symbyax and any concomitant serotonergic or antidopaminergic agents, including antipsychotics, should be discontinued immediately, if the above reactions occur, and supportive symptomatic treatment should be initiated. In addition, co-administration of fluoxetine with other drugs metabolized by CYP2D6 including antipsychotics (eg, phenothiazines and most atypicals) should be approached with caution. Therapy with medications that are predominantly metabolized by the CYP2D6 system and that have a relatively narrow therapeutic index should be initiated at the low end of the dose range if a patient is receiving fluoxetine concurrently or has taken it in the previous 5 weeks. If fluoxetine is added to the treatment regimen of a patient already receiving a drug metabolized by CYP2D6, the need for a decreased dose of the original medication should be considered).
No products indexed under this heading.

Promethazine Hydrochloride (The development of a potentially life-threatening serotonin syndrome or neuroleptic malignant syndrome (NMS)-like reactions have been reported with SNRIs and SSRIs alone and with the concomitant use of antipsychotics. Serotonin syndrome, in its most severe form can resemble neuroleptic malignant syndrome. Patients should be monitored for the emergence of serotonin syndrome or NMS-like signs and symptoms. Treatment with Symbyax and any concomitant serotonergic or antidopaminergic agents, including antipsychotics, should be discontinued immediately, if the above reactions occur, and supportive symptomatic treatment should be initiated. In addition, co-administration of fluoxetine with other drugs metabolized by CYP2D6 including antipsychotics (eg, phenothiazines and most atypicals) should be approached with caution. Therapy with medications that are predominantly metabolized by the CYP2D6 system and that have a relatively narrow therapeutic index should be initiated at the low end of the dose range if a patient is receiving fluoxetine concurrently or has taken it in the previous 5 weeks. If fluoxetine is added to the treatment regimen of a patient already receiving a drug metabolized by CYP2D6, the need for a decreased dose of the original medication should be considered).
No products indexed under this heading.

Propafenone Hydrochloride (Co-administration of fluoxetine with other drugs that are metabolized by CYP2D6, including antiarrhythmics (eg, propafenone, flecainide, and others) should be approached with caution. Therapy with medications that are predominantly metabolized by the CYP2D6 system and that have a relatively narrow therapeutic index should be initiated at the low end of the dose range if a patient is receiving fluoxetine concurrently or has taken it in the previous 5 weeks. If fluoxetine is added to the treatment regimen of a patient already receiving a drug metabolized by CYP2D6, the need for a decreased dose of the original medication should be considered). Products include:
Rythmol 1648
Rythmol SR 1652

Propofol (Caution is advised if the concomitant administration of Symbyax and other CNS-active drugs is required. In evaluating individual cases, consideration should be given to using lower initial doses of the concomitantly administered drugs, using conservative titration schedules and monitoring of clinical status).
No products indexed under this heading.

Propoxyphene Hydrochloride (Caution is advised if the concomitant administration of Symbyax and other CNS-active drugs is required. In evaluating individual cases, consideration should be given to using lower initial doses of the concomitantly administered drugs, using conservative titration schedules and monitoring of clinical status).
No products indexed under this heading.

Propoxyphene Napsylate (Caution is advised if the concomitant administration of Symbyax and other CNS-active drugs is required. In evaluating individual cases, consideration should be given to using lower initial doses of the concomitantly administered drugs, using conservative titration schedules and monitoring of clinical status).
No products indexed under this heading.

Propranolol Hydrochloride (Co-administration of fluoxetine with other drugs that are metabolized by CYP2D6, including antiarrhythmics (eg, propafenone, flecainide, and others) should be approached with caution. Therapy with medications that are predominantly metabolized by the CYP2D6 system and that have a relatively narrow therapeutic index should be initiated at the low end of the dose range if a patient is receiving fluoxetine concurrently or has taken it in the previous 5 weeks. If fluoxetine is added to the treatment regimen of a patient already receiving a drug metabolized by CYP2D6, the need for a decreased dose of the original medication should be considered). Products include:
InnoPran XL 1517

Protriptyline Hydrochloride (In two fluoxetine studies, previously stable plasma levels of imipramine and desipramine have increased>2- to 10-fold when fluoxetine has been administered in combination. This influence may persist for three weeks or longer after fluoxetine is discontinued. Thus, the dose of TCA may need to be reduced and plasma TCA concentrations may need to be monitored temporarily when Symbyax is co-administered or has been recently discontinued. Co-administration of fluoxetine with other drugs that are metabolized by CYP2D6, including certain antidepressants (eg, TCAs), should be approached with caution).
No products indexed under this heading.

Quazepam (Caution is advised if the concomitant administration of Symbyax and other CNS-active drugs is required. In evaluating individual cases, consideration should be given to using lower initial doses of the concomitantly administered drugs, using conservative titration schedules and monitoring of clinical status).
No products indexed under this heading.

Quetiapine Fumarate (The development of a potentially life-threatening serotonin syndrome or neuroleptic malignant syndrome (NMS)-like reactions have been reported with SNRIs and SSRIs alone but particularly with concomitant use of serotonergic drugs (including triptans) with drugs which impair metabolism of serotonin (including MAOIs), or with antipsychotics or other dopamine antagonists. Serotonin syndrome symptoms may include mental status changes, autonomic instability, neuromuscular aberrations, and/or gastrointestinal symptoms. Serotonin syndrome, in its most severe form can resemble neuroleptic malignant syndrome. Patients should be monitored for the emergence of serotonin syndrome or NMS-like signs and symptoms. Treatment with Symbyax and any concomitant serotonergic or antidopaminergic agents, including antipsychotics, should be discontinued immediately, if the above reactions occur, and supportive symptomatic treatment should be initiated). Products include:
Seroquel 750
Seroquel XR 759

Quinapril Hydrochloride (Because of the potential for olanzapine to induce hypotension, Symbyax may enhance the effects of certain antihypertensive agents).
No products indexed under this heading.

Quinidine Gluconate (Co-administration of fluoxetine with other drugs that are metabolized by CYP2D6, including antiarrhythmics (eg, propafenone, flecainide, and others) should be approached with caution. Therapy with medications that are predominantly metabolized by the CYP2D6 system and that have a relatively narrow therapeutic index should be initiated at the low end of the dose range if a patient is receiving fluoxetine concurrently or has taken it in the previous 5 weeks. If fluoxetine is added to the treatment regimen of a patient already receiving a drug metabolized by CYP2D6, the need for a decreased dose of the original medication should be considered).
No products indexed under this heading.

Quinidine Hydrochloride (Co-administration of fluoxetine with other drugs that are metabolized by CYP2D6 should be approached with caution. Therapy with medications that are predominantly metabolized by the CYP2D6 system and that have a relatively narrow therapeutic index should be initiated at the low end of the dose range if a patient is receiving fluoxetine concurrently or has taken it in the previous 5 weeks. If fluoxetine is added to the treatment regimen of a patient already receiving a drug metabolized by CYP2D6, the need for a decreased dose of the original medication should be considered).
No products indexed under this heading.

Quinidine Polygalacturonate (Co-administration of fluoxetine with other drugs that are metabolized by CYP2D6, including antiarrhythmics (eg, propafenone, flecainide, and others) should be approached with caution. Therapy with medications that are predominantly metabolized by the CYP2D6 system and that have a relatively narrow therapeutic index should be initiated at the low end of the dose range if a patient is receiving fluoxetine concurrently or has taken it in the previous 5 weeks. If fluoxetine is added to the treatment regimen of a patient already receiving a drug metabolized by CYP2D6, the need for a decreased dose of the original medication should be considered).
No products indexed under this heading.

Quinidine Sulfate (Co-administration of fluoxetine with other drugs that are metabolized by CYP2D6, including antiarrhythmics (eg, propafenone, flecainide, and others) should be approached with caution. Therapy with medications that are predominantly metabolized by the CYP2D6 system and that have a relatively narrow therapeutic index should be initiated at the low end of the dose range if a patient is receiving fluoxetine concurrently or has taken it in the previous 5 weeks. If fluoxetine is added to the treatment regimen of a patient already receiving a drug metabolized by CYP2D6, the need for a decreased dose of the original medication should be considered).
No products indexed under this heading.

Ramipril (Because of the potential for olanzapine to induce hypotension, Symbyax may enhance the effects of certain antihypertensive agents).
No products indexed under this heading.

Rasagiline Mesylate (Concomitant use in patients taking MAO inhibitors is contraindicated. Symbyax should not be used in combination with an MAOI, or within a minimum of 14 days of discontinuing therapy with an MAOI. There have been reports of serious, sometimes fatal reactions in patients receiving fluoxetine in combination with an MAOI, and in patients who have recently discontinued fluoxetine and are then started on an MAOI. Some cases presented with features resembling neuroleptic malignant syndrome. Since fluoxetine and its major metabolite have very long elimination half-lives, at least 5 weeks (perhaps longer, especially if fluoxetine has been prescribed chronically and/or at higher doses) should be allowed after stopping Symbyax before starting an MAOI). Products include:
Azilect 3383

Rauwolfia Serpentina (Because of the potential for olanzapine to induce hypotension, Symbyax may enhance the effects of certain antihypertensive agents).
No products indexed under this heading.

Remifentanil Hydrochloride (Caution is advised if the concomitant administration of Symbyax and other CNS-active drugs is required. In evaluating individual cases, consideration should be given to using lower initial doses of the concomitantly administered drugs, using conservative titration schedules and monitoring of clinical status).
No products indexed under this heading.

Rescinnamine (Because of the potential for olanzapine to induce hypotension, Symbyax may enhance the effects of certain antihypertensive agents).
No products indexed under this heading.

Reserpine (Because of the potential for olanzapine to induce hypotension, Symbyax may enhance the effects of certain antihypertensive agents).
No products indexed under this heading.

Rifampicin (Agents that induce CYP1A2 or glucuronyl transferase enzymes may cause an increase in olanzapine concentration).
No products indexed under this heading.

Rifampin (Agents that induce CYP1A2 or glucuronyl transferase enzymes, such as rifampin, may cause an increase in olanzapine clearance).
No products indexed under this heading.

Risperidone (The development of a potentially life-threatening serotonin syndrome or neuroleptic malignant syndrome (NMS)-like reactions have been reported with SNRIs and SSRIs alone and with the concomitant use of antipsychotics. Serotonin syndrome, in its most severe form can resemble neuroleptic malignant syndrome. Patients should be monitored for the emergence of serotonin syndrome or NMS-like signs and symptoms. Treatment with Symbyax and any concomitant serotonergic or antidopaminergic agents,

1805 Interactions Index Symbyax

including antipsychotics, should be discontinued immediately, if the above reactions occur, and supportive symptomatic treatment should be initiated. In addition, co-administration of fluoxetine with other drugs metabolized by CYP2D6, including antipsychotics (eg, phenothiazines and most atypicals), should be approached with caution. Therapy with medications that are predominantly metabolized by the CYP2D6 system and that have a relatively narrow therapeutic index should be initiated at the low end of the dose range if a patient is receiving fluoxetine concurrently or has taken it in the previous 5 weeks. If fluoxetine is added to the treatment regimen of a patient already receiving a drug metabolized by CYP2D6, the need for a decreased dose of the original medication should be considered). Products include:

Risperdal Consta 2682

Ritonavir (Co-administration of fluoxetine with other drugs that are metabolized by CYP2D6 should be approached with caution. Therapy with medications that are predominantly metabolized by the CYP2D6 system and that have a relatively narrow therapeutic index should be initiated at the low end of the dose range if a patient is receiving fluoxetine concurrently or has taken it in the previous 5 weeks. If fluoxetine is added to the treatment regimen of a patient already receiving a drug metabolized by CYP2D6, the need for a decreased dose of the original medication should be considered). Products include:

Kaletra 458
Norvir 509

Rizatriptan Benzoate (There have been rare postmarketing reports of serotonin syndrome with use of an SSRI and a triptan. If concomitant treatment of Symbyax with a triptan is clinically warranted, careful observation of the patient is advised, particularly during treatment initiation and dose increases). Products include:

Maxalt 2206
Maxalt-MLT 2206

Rofecoxib (Serotonin release by platelets plays an important role in hemostasis. Epidemiological studies of the case-control and cohort design that have demonstrated an association between use of psychotropic drugs that interfere with serotonin re-uptake and the occurrence of upper gastrointestinal bleeding have also shown that concurrent use of an NSAID or aspirin may potentiate this risk of bleeding. Patients should be cautioned about the risk of bleeding associated with the concomitant use of Symbyax and NSAIDs, aspirin, or other drugs that affect coagulation).

No products indexed under this heading.

Ropinirole Hydrochloride (The olanzapine component of Symbyax may antagonize the effects of levodopa and dopamine agonists). Products include:

Requip 1620
Requip XL 1628

Secobarbital Sodium (Caution is advised if the concomitant administration of Symbyax and other CNS-active drugs is required. In evaluating individual cases, consideration should be given to using lower initial doses of the concomitantly administered drugs, using conservative titration schedules and monitoring of clinical status).

No products indexed under this heading.

Selegiline (Concomitant use in patients taking MAO inhibitors is contraindicated. Symbyax should not be used in combination with an MAOI, or within a minimum of 14 days of discontinuing therapy with an MAOI. There have been reports of serious, sometimes fatal reactions in patients receiving fluoxetine in combination with an MAOI, and in patients who have recently discontinued fluoxetine and are then started on an MAOI. Some cases presented with features resembling neuroleptic malignant syndrome. Since fluoxetine and its major metabolite have very long elimination half-lives, at least 5 weeks (perhaps longer, especially if fluoxetine has been prescribed chronically and/or at higher doses) should be allowed after stopping Symbyax before starting an MAOI). Products include:

Emsam 3623

Selegiline Hydrochloride (Concomitant use in patients taking MAO inhibitors is contraindicated. Symbyax should not be used in combination with an MAOI, or within a minimum of 14 days of discontinuing therapy with an MAOI. There have been reports of serious, sometimes fatal reactions in patients receiving fluoxetine in combination with an MAOI, and in patients who have recently discontinued fluoxetine and are then started on an MAOI. Some cases presented with features resembling neuroleptic malignant syndrome. Since fluoxetine and its major metabolite have very long elimination half-lives, at least 5 weeks (perhaps longer, especially if fluoxetine has been prescribed chronically and/or at higher doses) should be allowed after stopping Symbyax before starting an MAOI). Products include:

Eldepryl 3312

Sertraline Hydrochloride (The concomitant use of Symbyax with selective serotonin reuptake inhibitors (SSRIs) is not recommended).

No products indexed under this heading.

Sevoflurane (Caution is advised if the concomitant administration of Symbyax and other CNS-active drugs is required. In evaluating individual cases, consideration should be given to using lower initial doses of the concomitantly administered drugs, using conservative titration schedules and monitoring of clinical status). Products include:

Ultane 554

Sodium Nitroprusside (Because of the potential for olanzapine to induce hypotension, Symbyax may enhance the effects of certain antihypertensive agents).

No products indexed under this heading.

Sodium Oxybate (Caution is advised if the concomitant administration of Symbyax and other CNS-active drugs is required. In evaluating individual cases, consideration should be given to using lower initial doses of the concomitantly administered drugs, using conservative titration schedules and monitoring of clinical status).

No products indexed under this heading.

Sotalol Hydrochloride (Co-administration of fluoxetine with other drugs that are metabolized by CYP2D6, including antiarrhythmics (eg, propafenone, flecainide, and others) should be approached with caution. Therapy with medications that are predominantly metabolized by the CYP2D6 system and that have a relatively narrow therapeutic index should be initiated at the low end of the dose range if a patient is receiving fluoxetine concurrently or has taken it in the previous 5 weeks. If fluoxetine is added to the treatment regimen of a patient already receiving a drug metabolized by CYP2D6, the need for a decreased dose of the original medication should be considered).

No products indexed under this heading.

Spirapril Hydrochloride (Because of the potential for olanzapine to induce hypotension, Symbyax may enhance the effects of certain antihypertensive agents).

No products indexed under this heading.

Spironolactone (Hyponatremia may occur as a result of treatment with SSRIs and SNRIs, including fluoxetine and Symbyax. In many cases, this hyponatremia appears to be the result of the syndrome of inappropriate antidiuretic hormone secretion (SIADH). Cases with serum sodium lower than 110 mmol/L have been reported and appeared to be reversible when Symbyax was discontinued. Patients taking diuretics or who are otherwise volume depleted may be at greater risk. Discontinuation of Symbyax should be considered in patients with symptomatic hyponatremia and appropriate medical intervention should be instituted).

No products indexed under this heading.

Sufentanil Citrate (Caution is advised if the concomitant administration of Symbyax and other CNS-active drugs is required. In evaluating individual cases, consideration should be given to using lower initial doses of the concomitantly administered drugs, using conservative titration schedules and monitoring of clinical status).

No products indexed under this heading.

Sulindac (Serotonin release by platelets plays an important role in hemostasis. Epidemiological studies of the case-control and cohort design that have demonstrated an association between use of psychotropic drugs that interfere with serotonin re-uptake and the occurrence of upper gastrointestinal bleeding have also shown that concurrent use of an NSAID or aspirin may potentiate this risk of bleeding. Patients should be cautioned about the risk of bleeding associated with the concomitant use of Symbyax and NSAIDs, aspirin, or other drugs that affect coagulation). Products include:

Clinoril 2098

Sumatriptan (There have been rare postmarketing reports of serotonin syndrome with use of an SSRI and a triptan. If concomitant treatment of Symbyax with a triptan is clinically warranted, careful observation of the patient is advised, particularly during treatment initiation and dose increases). Products include:

Imitrex Nasal 1503

Sumatriptan Succinate (There have been rare postmarketing reports of serotonin syndrome with use of an SSRI and a triptan. If concomitant treatment of Symbyax with a triptan is clinically warranted, careful observation of the patient is advised, particularly during treatment initiation and dose increases). Products include:

Imitrex 1497
Imitrex Tablets 1508
Treximet 1681

Tamoxifen Citrate (Co-administration of fluoxetine with other drugs that are metabolized by CYP2D6 should be approached with caution. Therapy with medications that are predominantly metabolized by the CYP2D6 system and that have a relatively narrow therapeutic index should be initiated at the low end of the dose range if a patient is receiving fluoxetine concurrently or has taken it in the previous 5 weeks. If fluoxetine is added to the treatment regimen of a patient already receiving a drug metabolized by CYP2D6, the need for a decreased dose of the original medication should be considered).

No products indexed under this heading.

Telmisartan (Because of the potential for olanzapine to induce hypotension, Symbyax may enhance the effects of certain antihypertensive agents). Products include:

Micardis 887
Micardis HCT 889

Temazepam (Caution is advised if the concomitant administration of Symbyax and other CNS-active drugs is required. In evaluating individual cases, consideration should be given to using lower initial doses of the concomitantly administered drugs, using conservative titration schedules and monitoring of clinical status).

No products indexed under this heading.

Teniposide (Co-administration of fluoxetine with other drugs that are metabolized by CYP2D6 should be approached with caution. Therapy with medications that are predominantly metabolized by the CYP2D6 system and that have a relatively narrow therapeutic index should be initiated at the low end of the dose range if a patient is receiving fluoxetine concurrently or has taken it in the previous 5 weeks. If fluoxetine is added to the treatment regimen of a patient already receiving a drug metabolized by CYP2D6, the need for a decreased dose of the original medication should be considered).

No products indexed under this heading.

Terazosin Hydrochloride (Because of the potential for olanzapine to induce hypotension, Symbyax may enhance the effects of certain antihypertensive agents).

No products indexed under this heading.

Testosterone (Co-administration of fluoxetine with other drugs that are metabolized by CYP2D6 should be approached with caution. Therapy with medications that are predominantly metabolized by the CYP2D6 system and that have a relatively narrow therapeutic index should be initiated at the low end of the dose range if a patient is receiving fluoxetine concurrently or has taken it in the previous 5 weeks. If fluoxetine is added to the treatment regimen of a patient already receiving a drug metabolized by CYP2D6, the need for a decreased dose of the original medication should be considered). Products include:

AndroGel 3456

Testosterone Cypionate (Co-administration of fluoxetine with other drugs that are metabolized by CYP2D6 should be approached with caution. Therapy with medications that are predominantly metabolized by the CYP2D6 system and that have a relatively narrow therapeutic index should be initiated at the low end of the dose range if a patient is receiving fluoxetine concurrently or has taken it in the previous 5 weeks. If fluoxetine is added to the treatment regimen of a patient already receiving a drug metabolized by CYP2D6, the need for a decreased dose of the original medication should be considered).

No products indexed under this heading.

Testosterone Enanthate (Co-administration of fluoxetine with other drugs that are metabolized by CYP2D6 should be approached with caution. Therapy with medications that are predominantly metabolized by the CYP2D6 system and that have a relatively narrow therapeutic index should be initiated at the low end of the dose range if a patient is receiving fluoxetine concurrently or has taken it in the previous 5 weeks. If fluoxetine is added to the treatment regimen of a patient already receiving a drug metabolized by CYP2D6, the need for a decreased dose of the original medication should be considered). Products include:

Delatestryl 1102

Testosterone Propionate (Co-administration of fluoxetine with other drugs that are metabolized by CYP2D6 should be approached with caution. Therapy with medications that are predominantly metabolized by the CYP2D6

IMPORTANT NOTE: Always consult each drug listing in the patient's regimen for possible interactions.

Symbyax Interactions Index 1806

system and that have a relatively narrow therapeutic index should be initiated at the low end of the dose range if a patient is receiving fluoxetine concurrently or has taken it in the previous 5 weeks. If fluoxetine is added to the treatment regimen of a patient already receiving a drug metabolized by CYP2D6, the need for a decreased dose of the original medication should be considered).
No products indexed under this heading.

Thiamylal Sodium (Caution is advised if the concomitant administration of Symbyax and other CNS-active drugs is required. In evaluating individual cases, consideration should be given to using lower initial doses of the concomitantly administered drugs, using conservative titration schedules and monitoring of clinical status).
No products indexed under this heading.

Thioridazine (Concomitant use in patients taking thioridazine is contraindicated. Thioridazine administration produces a dose-related prolongation of the QT_c interval, which is associated with serious ventricular arrhythmias, such as torsades de pointes-type arrhythmias and sudden death. This risk is expected to increase with fluoxetine-induced inhibition of thioridazine metabolism. Due to the risk of serious ventricular arrhythmias and sudden death potentially associated with elevated thioridazine plasma levels, thioridazine should not be administered with fluoxetine or within a minimum of 5 weeks after fluoxetine has been discontinued).
No products indexed under this heading.

Thioridazine Hydrochloride (Concomitant use in patients taking thioridazine is contraindicated. Thioridazine administration produces a dose-related prolongation of the QT_c interval, which is associated with serious ventricular arrhythmias, such as torsades de pointes-type arrhythmias and sudden death. This risk is expected to increase with fluoxetine-induced inhibition of thioridazine metabolism. Due to the risk of serious ventricular arrhythmias and sudden death potentially associated with elevated thioridazine plasma levels, thioridazine should not be administered with fluoxetine or within a minimum of 5 weeks after fluoxetine has been discontinued). Products include:
Thioridazine Hydrochloride 2384

Thiothixene (The development of a potentially life-threatening serotonin syndrome or neuroleptic malignant syndrome (NMS)-like reactions have been reported with SNRIs and SSRIs alone and with the concomitant use of antipsychotics. Serotonin syndrome, in its most severe form can resemble neuroleptic malignant syndrome. Patients should be monitored for the emergence of serotonin syndrome or NMS-like signs and symptoms. Treatment with Symbyax and any concomitant serotonergic or antidopaminergic agents, including antipsychotics, should be discontinued immediately, if the above reactions occur, and supportive symptomatic treatment should be initiated. In addition, co-administration of fluoxetine with other drugs metabolized by CYP2D6, including antipsychotics (eg, phenothiazines and most atypicals), should be approached with caution. Therapy with medications that are predominantly metabolized by the CYP2D6 system and that have a relatively narrow therapeutic index should be initiated at the low end of the dose range if a patient is receiving fluoxetine concurrently or has taken it in the previous 5 weeks. If fluoxetine is added to the treatment regimen of a patient already receiving a drug metabolized by CYP2D6, the need for a decreased dose of the original medication should be considered). Products include:
Thiothixene 2386

Timolol Maleate (Because of the potential for olanzapine to induce hypotension, Symbyax may enhance the effects of certain antihypertensive agents). Products include:
Combigan 601
Dorzolamide Hydrochloride/Timolol Maleate Ophthalmic Solution.................... ⊙243
Timoptic in Ocudose .... ⊙231

Tinzaparin Sodium (Serotonin release by platelets plays an important role in hemostasis. Epidemiological studies of the case-control and cohort design that have demonstrated an association between use of psychotropic drugs that interfere with serotonin reuptake and the occurrence of upper gastrointestinal bleeding have also shown that concurrent use of an NSAID or aspirin may potentiate this risk of bleeding. Patients should be cautioned about the risk of bleeding associated with the concomitant use of Symbyax and NSAIDs, aspirin, or other drugs that affect coagulation).
No products indexed under this heading.

Tobacco (Agents that induce CYP1A2 or glucuronyl transferase enzymes may cause an increase in olanzapine concentration).
No products indexed under this heading.

Tocainide Hydrochloride (Co-administration of fluoxetine with other drugs that are metabolized by CYP2D6, including antiarrhythmics (eg, propafenone, flecainide, and others) should be approached with caution. Therapy with medications that are predominantly metabolized by the CYP2D6 system and that have a relatively narrow therapeutic index should be initiated at the low end of the dose range if a patient is receiving fluoxetine concurrently or has taken it in the previous 5 weeks. If fluoxetine is added to the treatment regimen of a patient already receiving a drug metabolized by CYP2D6, the need for a decreased dose of the original medication should be considered).
No products indexed under this heading.

Tolbutamide (Because fluoxetine is tightly bound to plasma protein, the administration of fluoxetine to a patient taking another drug that is tightly bound to protein (eg, warfarin, digitoxin) may cause a shift in plasma concentrations, potentially resulting in an adverse effect. Conversely, adverse effects may result from displacement of protein-bound fluoxetine by other tightly bound drugs).
No products indexed under this heading.

Tolmetin Sodium (Serotonin release by platelets plays an important role in hemostasis. Epidemiological studies of the case-control and cohort design that have demonstrated an association between use of psychotropic drugs that interfere with serotonin re-uptake and the occurrence of upper gastrointestinal bleeding have also shown that concurrent use of an NSAID or aspirin may potentiate this risk of bleeding. Patients should be cautioned about the risk of bleeding associated with the concomitant use of Symbyax and NSAIDs, aspirin, or other drugs that affect coagulation).
No products indexed under this heading.

Tolterodine Tartrate (Co-administration of fluoxetine with other drugs that are metabolized by CYP2D6 should be approached with caution. Therapy with medications that are predominantly metabolized by the CYP2D6 system and that have a relatively narrow therapeutic index should be initiated at the low end of the dose range if a patient is receiving fluoxetine concurrently or has taken it in the previous 5 weeks. If fluoxetine is added to the treatment regimen of a patient already receiving a drug metabolized by CYP2D6, the need for a decreased dose of the original medication should be considered).
No products indexed under this heading.

Torsemide (Because of the potential for olanzapine to induce hypotension, Symbyax may enhance the effects of certain antihypertensive agents).
No products indexed under this heading.

Tramadol Hydrochloride (Based on the mechanism of action of SNRIs and SSRIs, including Symbyax, and the potential for serotonin syndrome, caution is advised when Symbyax is co-administered with other drugs that may affect the serotonergic neurotransmitter systems, such as tramadol). Products include:
Ryzolt 2813
Ultram ER 2693

Trandolapril (Because of the potential for olanzapine to induce hypotension, Symbyax may enhance the effects of certain antihypertensive agents). Products include:
Mavik 489
Tarka 534

Tranylcypromine Sulfate (Concomitant use in patients taking MAO inhibitors is contraindicated. Symbyax should not be used in combination with an MAOI, or within a minimum of 14 days of discontinuing therapy with an MAOI. There have been reports of serious, sometimes fatal reactions in patients receiving fluoxetine in combination with an MAOI, and in patients who have recently discontinued fluoxetine and are then started on an MAOI. Some cases presented with features resembling neuroleptic malignant syndrome. Since fluoxetine and its major metabolite have very long elimination half-lives, at least 5 weeks (perhaps longer, especially if fluoxetine has been prescribed chronically and/or at higher doses) should be allowed after stopping Symbyax before starting an MAOI). Products include:
Parnate 1584

Trazodone Hydrochloride (Co-administration of fluoxetine with other drugs that are metabolized by CYP2D6, including certain antidepressants (eg, TCAs) should be approached with caution. Therapy with medications that are predominantly metabolized by the CYP2D6 system and that have a relatively narrow therapeutic index should be initiated at the low end of the dose range if a patient is receiving fluoxetine concurrently or has taken it in the previous 5 weeks. If fluoxetine is added to the treatment regimen of a patient already receiving a drug metabolized by CYP2D6, the need for a decreased dose of the original medication should be considered).
No products indexed under this heading.

Triamterene (Hyponatremia may occur as a result of treatment with SSRIs and SNRIs, including fluoxetine and Symbyax. In many cases, this hyponatremia appears to be the result of the syndrome of inappropriate antidiuretic hormone secretion (SIADH). Cases with serum sodium lower than 110 mmol/L have been reported and appeared to be reversible when Symbyax was discontinued. Patients taking diuretics or who are otherwise volume depleted may be at greater risk. Discontinuation of Symbyax should be considered in patients with symptomatic hyponatremia and appropriate medical intervention should be instituted). Products include:
Dyazide 1429
Dyrenium 3495

Triazolam (Caution is advised if the concomitant administration of Symbyax and other CNS-active drugs is required. In evaluating individual cases, consideration should be given to using lower initial doses of the concomitantly administered drugs, using conservative titration schedules and monitoring of clinical status).
No products indexed under this heading.

Trifluoperazine Hydrochloride (The development of a potentially life-threatening serotonin syndrome or neuroleptic malignant syndrome (NMS)-like reactions have been reported with SNRIs and SSRIs alone and with the concomitant use of antipsychotics. Serotonin syndrome, in its most severe form can resemble neuroleptic malignant syndrome. Patients should be monitored for the emergence of serotonin syndrome or NMS-like signs and symptoms. Treatment with Symbyax and any concomitant serotonergic or antidopaminergic agents, including antipsychotics, should be discontinued immediately, if the above reactions occur, and supportive symptomatic treatment should be initiated. In addition, co-administration of fluoxetine with other drugs metabolized by CYP2D6 including antipsychotics (eg, phenothiazines and most atypicals) should be approached with caution. Therapy with medications that are predominantly metabolized by the CYP2D6 system and that have a relatively narrow therapeutic index should be initiated at the low end of the dose range if a patient is receiving fluoxetine concurrently or has taken it in the previous 5 weeks. If fluoxetine is added to the treatment regimen of a patient already receiving a drug metabolized by CYP2D6, the need for a decreased dose of the original medication should be considered).
No products indexed under this heading.

Trimethaphan Camsylate (Because of the potential for olanzapine to induce hypotension, Symbyax may enhance the effects of certain antihypertensive agents).
No products indexed under this heading.

Trimipramine Maleate (In two fluoxetine studies, previously stable plasma levels of imipramine and desipramine have increased>2- to 10-fold when fluoxetine has been administered in combination. This influence may persist for three weeks or longer after fluoxetine is discontinued. Thus, the dose of TCA may need to be reduced and plasma TCA concentrations may need to be monitored temporarily when Symbyax is co-administered or has been recently discontinued. Co-administration of fluoxetine with other drugs that are metabolized by CYP2D6, including certain antidepressants (eg, TCAs), should be approached with caution).
No products indexed under this heading.

Tryptophan (Five patients receiving fluoxetine in combination with tryptophan experienced adverse reactions, including agitation, restlessness, and gastrointestinal distress. Concomitant use with tryptophan is not recommended).
No products indexed under this heading.

L-Tryptophan (Five patients receiving fluoxetine in combination with tryptophan experienced adverse reactions, including agitation, restlessness, and gastrointestinal distress. Concomitant use of Symbyax with tryptophan is not recommended).
No products indexed under this heading.

Valdecoxib (Serotonin release by platelets plays an important role in hemostasis. Epidemiological studies of the case-control and cohort design that have demonstrated an association between use of psychotropic drugs that

(⊙ Described in PDR® for Ophthalmic Medicines)

interfere with serotonin re-uptake and the occurrence of upper gastrointestinal bleeding have also shown that concurrent use of an NSAID or aspirin may potentiate this risk of bleeding. Patients should be cautioned about the risk of bleeding associated with the concomitant use of Symbyax and NSAIDs, aspirin, or other drugs that affect coagulation).

No products indexed under this heading.

Valsartan (Because of the potential for olanzapine to induce hypotension, Symbyax may enhance the effects of certain antihypertensive agents). Products include:

Diovan **2413**
Diovan HCT **2419**
Exforge **2443**
Exforge HCT **2449**
Valturna **3637**

Venlafaxine Hydrochloride (The concomitant use of Symbyax with serotonin and norepinephrine reuptake inhibitors (SNRIs) is not recommended). Products include:

Effexor XR **3504**
Venlafaxine Hydrochloride Tablets ... **2388**

Verapamil Hydrochloride (Co-administration of fluoxetine with other drugs that are metabolized by CYP2D6, including antiarrhythmics (eg, propafenone, flecainide, and others) should be approached with caution. Therapy with medications that are predominantly metabolized by the CYP2D6 system and that have a relatively narrow therapeutic index should be initiated at the low end of the dose range if a patient is receiving fluoxetine concurrently or has taken it in the previous 5 weeks. If fluoxetine is added to the treatment regimen of a patient already receiving a drug metabolized by CYP2D6, the need for a decreased dose of the original medication should be considered). Products include:

Tarka **534**

Vinblastine Sulfate (Co-administration of fluoxetine with other drugs that are metabolized by CYP2D6 should be approached with caution. Therapy with medications that are predominantly metabolized by the CYP2D6 system and that have a relatively narrow therapeutic index should be initiated at the low end of the dose range if a patient is receiving fluoxetine concurrently or has taken it in the previous 5 weeks. If fluoxetine is added to the treatment regimen of a patient already receiving a drug metabolized by CYP2D6, the need for a decreased dose of the original medication should be considered).

No products indexed under this heading.

Warfarin Sodium (Altered anticoagulant effects, including increased bleeding, have been reported when SSRIs or SNRIs are co-administered with warfarin. Patients receiving warfarin therapy should receive careful coagulation monitoring when Symbyax is initiated or discontinued. In addition, because fluoxetine is tightly bound to plasma protein, the administration of fluoxetine to a patient taking another drug that is tightly bound to protein (eg, warfarin) may cause a shift in plasma concentrations, potentially resulting in an adverse effect. Conversely, adverse effects may result from displacement of protein-bound fluoxetine by other tightly bound drugs).

No products indexed under this heading.

Zaleplon (Caution is advised if the concomitant administration of Symbyax and other CNS-active drugs is required. In evaluating individual cases, consideration should be given to using lower initial doses of the concomitantly administered drugs, using conservative titration schedules and monitoring of clinical status).

No products indexed under this heading.

Ziprasidone Hydrochloride (The development of a potentially life-threatening serotonin syndrome or neuroleptic malignant syndrome (NMS)-like reactions have been reported with SNRIs and SSRIs alone and with the concomitant use of antipsychotics. Serotonin syndrome, in its most severe form can resemble neuroleptic malignant syndrome. Patients should be monitored for the emergence of serotonin syndrome or NMS-like signs and symptoms. Treatment with Symbyax and any concomitant serotonergic or antidopaminergic agents, including antipsychotics, should be discontinued immediately, if the above reactions occur, and supportive symptomatic treatment should be initiated. In addition, co-administration of fluoxetine with other drugs metabolized by CYP2D6, including antipsychotics (eg, phenothiazines and most atypicals), should be approached with caution. Therapy with medications that are predominantly metabolized by the CYP2D6 system and that have a relatively narrow therapeutic index should be initiated at the low end of the dose range if a patient is receiving fluoxetine concurrently or has taken it in the previous 5 weeks. If fluoxetine is added to the treatment regimen of a patient already receiving a drug metabolized by CYP2D6, the need for a decreased dose of the original medication should be considered). Products include:

Geodon **2723**

Zolmitriptan (There have been rare postmarketing reports of serotonin syndrome with use of an SSRI and a triptan. If concomitant treatment of Symbyax with a triptan is clinically warranted, careful observation of the patient is advised, particularly during treatment initiation and dose increases). Products include:

Zomig Tablets **773**
Zomig Nasal Spray **768**
Zomig-ZMT Tablets **773**

Zolpidem Tartrate (Caution is advised if the concomitant administration of Symbyax and other CNS-active drugs is required. In evaluating individual cases, consideration should be given to using lower initial doses of the concomitantly administered drugs, using conservative titration schedules and monitoring of clinical status). Products include:

Ambien **2920**
Ambien CR **2925**

Zonisamide (Co-administration of fluoxetine with other drugs that are metabolized by CYP2D6 should be approached with caution. Therapy with medications that are predominantly metabolized by the CYP2D6 system and that have a relatively narrow therapeutic index should be initiated at the low end of the dose range if a patient is receiving fluoxetine concurrently or has taken it in the previous 5 weeks. If fluoxetine is added to the treatment regimen of a patient already receiving a drug metabolized by CYP2D6, the need for a decreased dose of the original medication should be considered). Products include:

Zonegran **1081**

Food Interactions

Alcohol (The co-administration of ethanol with Symbyax may potentiate sedation and orthostatic hypotension. Patients should be advised to avoid alcohol while taking Symbyax).

Beer, reduced-alcohol (The co-administration of ethanol with Symbyax may potentiate sedation and orthostatic hypotension. Patients should be advised to avoid alcohol while taking Symbyax).

Beer, unspecified (The co-administration of ethanol with Symbyax may potentiate sedation and orthostatic hypotension. Patients should be advised to avoid alcohol while taking Symbyax).

Broccoli (Agents that induce CYP1A2 or glucuronyl transferase enzymes may cause an increase in olanzapine concentration).

Brussel Sprouts (Agents that induce CYP1A2 or glucuronyl transferase enzymes may cause an increase in olanzapine concentration).

Charbroiled Food (Agents that induce CYP1A2 or glucuronyl transferase enzymes may cause an increase in olanzapine concentration).

Wine, Chianti (The co-administration of ethanol with Symbyax may potentiate sedation and orthostatic hypotension. Patients should be advised to avoid alcohol while taking Symbyax).

Wine, Red (The co-administration of ethanol with Symbyax may potentiate sedation and orthostatic hypotension. Patients should be advised to avoid alcohol while taking Symbyax).

Wine, unspecified (The co-administration of ethanol with Symbyax may potentiate sedation and orthostatic hypotension. Patients should be advised to avoid alcohol while taking Symbyax).

Wine products (The co-administration of ethanol with Symbyax may potentiate sedation and orthostatic hypotension. Patients should be advised to avoid alcohol while taking Symbyax).

SYMLIN INJECTION

(Pramlintide Acetate) **651**

May interact with ACE inhibitors, alpha-glucosidase inhibitors, anticholinergics, drugs affecting gastrointestinal motility, fibrates, insulin, mixed agonist/antagonist opioid analgesics, monoamine oxidase inhibitors, narcotic analgesics, oral hypoglycemic agents, salicylates, sulfonamides, sulfonylureas, and certain other agents. Compounds in these categories include:

Acarbose (Concomitant use with oral anti-diabetic products, may increase the blood glucose-lowering effect and susceptibility to hypoglycemia. This may necessitate further insulin dose adjustments and particularly close monitoring of blood glucose).

No products indexed under this heading.

Acetaminophen (Concomitant use of pramlintide acetate (120 mcg) with acetaminophen (1000 mg) did not significantly alter the AUC of acetaminophen. However, pramlintide acetate decreased acetaminophen C_{max} (about 29% with simultaneous co-administration) and increased the time to maximum plasma concentration or t_{max} (ranging from 48 to 72 minutes) dependent on the time of acetaminophen administration relative to pramlintide acetate injection. Acetaminophen t_{max} was significantly increased when acetaminophen was administered simultaneously with or up to 2 hours following pramlintide acetate injection). Products include:

Percocet **1121**
Tylenol **2049**
Tylenol 8 Hour **2049**
Extra Strength Tylenol Caplets, Cool Caplets, and EZ Tabs **2049**
Extra Strength Tylenol Adult Rapid Blast Liquid **2049**
Extra Strength Tylenol Rapid Release **2049**
Tylenol with Codeine **2691**
Tylenol Arthritis Pain Extended Release Geltabs/Caplets **2049**
Children's Tylenol Suspension Liquid **2048**
Children's Tylenol Meltaways **2048**
Tylenol, Infants' Drops **2048**
Junior Tylenol **2048**
Vicodin **560**
Vicodin ES **561**
Vicodin HP **563**
Zydone **1138**

Albuterol (Due to its effects on gastric emptying, pramlintide acetate should not be considered for patients taking drugs that alter gastrointestinal motility).

No products indexed under this heading.

Albuterol Sulfate (Due to its effects on gastric emptying, pramlintide acetate should not be considered for patients taking drugs that alter gastrointestinal motility). Products include:

ProAir HFA **3393**
Proventil HFA **3204**
Ventolin HFA **1708**

Alfentanil Hydrochloride (Due to its effects on gastric emptying, pramlintide acetate should not be considered for patients taking drugs that alter gastrointestinal motility).

No products indexed under this heading.

Amitriptyline Hydrochloride (Due to its effects on gastric emptying, pramlintide acetate should not be considered for patients taking drugs that alter gastrointestinal motility).

No products indexed under this heading.

Amlodipine Besylate (Due to its effects on gastric emptying, pramlintide acetate should not be considered for patients taking drugs that alter gastrointestinal motility). Products include:

Azor **1010**
Exforge **2443**
Exforge HCT **2449**

Amoxapine (Due to its effects on gastric emptying, pramlintide acetate should not be considered for patients taking drugs that alter gastrointestinal motility).

No products indexed under this heading.

Apomorphine (Due to its effects on gastric emptying, pramlintide acetate should not be considered for patients taking drugs that alter gastrointestinal motility).

No products indexed under this heading.

Apomorphine Hydrochloride (Due to its effects on gastric emptying, pramlintide acetate should not be considered for patients taking drugs that alter gastrointestinal motility).

No products indexed under this heading.

Aspirin (Concomitant use with salicylates, may increase the blood glucose-lowering effect and susceptibility to hypoglycemia. This may necessitate further insulin dose adjustments and particularly close monitoring of blood glucose). Products include:

Aggrenox **880**
Bayer Aspirin **829**
Percodan **1124**
St. Joseph Aspirin **2045**

Aspirin, Enteric Coated (Concomitant use with salicylates, may increase the blood glucose-lowering effect and susceptibility to hypoglycemia. This may necessitate further insulin dose adjustments and particularly close monitoring of blood glucose).

No products indexed under this heading.

IMPORTANT NOTE: Always consult each drug listing in the patient's regimen for possible interactions.

Aspirin Buffered (Concomitant use with salicylates, may increase the blood glucose-lowering effect and susceptibility to hypoglycemia. This may necessitate further insulin dose adjustments and particularly close monitoring of blood glucose).
    No products indexed under this heading.

Astemizole (Due to its effects on gastric emptying, pramlintide acetate should not be considered for patients taking drugs that alter gastrointestinal motility).
    No products indexed under this heading.

Atropine Sulfate (Due to its effects on gastric emptying, pramlintide acetate should not be considered for patients taking drugs that alter gastrointestinal motility). Products include:
    Donnatal 2711

Azatadine Maleate (Due to its effects on gastric emptying, pramlintide acetate should not be considered for patients taking drugs that alter gastrointestinal motility).
    No products indexed under this heading.

Belladonna Alkaloids (Due to its effects on gastric emptying, pramlintide acetate should not be considered for patients taking drugs that alter gastrointestinal motility). Products include:
    Hyland's Teething Tablets. 3316

Benazepril Hydrochloride (Concomitant use with ACE inhibitors may increase the blood glucose-lowering effect and susceptibility to hypoglycemia. This may necessitate further insulin dose adjustments and particularly close monitoring of blood glucose).
    No products indexed under this heading.

Bendroflumethiazide (Concomitant use with salicylates, may increase the blood glucose-lowering effect and susceptibility to hypoglycemia. This may necessitate further insulin dose adjustments and particularly close monitoring of blood glucose).
    No products indexed under this heading.

Benztropine Mesylate (Due to its effects on gastric emptying, pramlintide acetate should not be considered for patients taking drugs that alter gastrointestinal motility).
    No products indexed under this heading.

Bepridil Hydrochloride (Due to its effects on gastric emptying, pramlintide acetate should not be considered for patients taking drugs that alter gastrointestinal motility).
    No products indexed under this heading.

Bethanechol Chloride (Due to its effects on gastric emptying, pramlintide acetate should not be considered for patients taking drugs that alter gastrointestinal motility).
    No products indexed under this heading.

Biperiden Hydrochloride (Due to its effects on gastric emptying, pramlintide acetate should not be considered for patients taking drugs that alter gastrointestinal motility).
    No products indexed under this heading.

Bitolterol Mesylate (Due to its effects on gastric emptying, pramlintide acetate should not be considered for patients taking drugs that alter gastrointestinal motility).
    No products indexed under this heading.

Bromocriptine Mesylate (Due to its effects on gastric emptying, pramlintide acetate should not be considered for patients taking drugs that alter gastrointestinal motility).
    No products indexed under this heading.

Bromodiphenhydramine Hydrochloride (Due to its effects on gastric emptying, pramlintide acetate should not be considered for patients taking drugs that alter gastrointestinal motility).
    No products indexed under this heading.

Brompheniramine Maleate (Due to its effects on gastric emptying, pramlintide acetate should not be considered for patients taking drugs that alter gastrointestinal motility).
    No products indexed under this heading.

Buprenorphine Hydrochloride (Due to its effects on gastric emptying, pramlintide acetate should not be considered for patients taking drugs that alter gastrointestinal motility).
    No products indexed under this heading.

Butorphanol Tartrate (Pramlintide acetate has the potential to delay the absorption of concomitantly administered oral medications. When the rapid onset of a concomitant orally administered agent is a critical determinant of effectiveness (such as analgesics), the agent should be administered at least 1 hour prior to or 2 hours after pramlintide acetate injection).
    No products indexed under this heading.

Captopril (Concomitant use with ACE inhibitors may increase the blood glucose-lowering effect and susceptibility to hypoglycemia. This may necessitate further insulin dose adjustments and particularly close monitoring of blood glucose). Products include:
    Captopril 2341

Cevimeline Hydrochloride (Due to its effects on gastric emptying, pramlintide acetate should not be considered for patients taking drugs that alter gastrointestinal motility). Products include:
    Evoxac 1027

Chlorothiazide (Concomitant use with salicylates, may increase the blood glucose-lowering effect and susceptibility to hypoglycemia. This may necessitate further insulin dose adjustments and particularly close monitoring of blood glucose).
    No products indexed under this heading.

Chlorothiazide Sodium (Concomitant use with salicylates, may increase the blood glucose-lowering effect and susceptibility to hypoglycemia. This may necessitate further insulin dose adjustments and particularly close monitoring of blood glucose). Products include:
    Diuril Intravenous 2009

Chlorpheniramine Maleate (Due to its effects on gastric emptying, pramlintide acetate should not be considered for patients taking drugs that alter gastrointestinal motility).
    No products indexed under this heading.

Chlorpheniramine Polistirex (Due to its effects on gastric emptying, pramlintide acetate should not be considered for patients taking drugs that alter gastrointestinal motility). Products include:
    Tussionex 3443

Chlorpheniramine Tannate (Due to its effects on gastric emptying, pramlintide acetate should not be considered for patients taking drugs that alter gastrointestinal motility).
    No products indexed under this heading.

Chlorpropamide (Concomitant use with oral anti-diabetic products, may increase the blood glucose-lowering effect and susceptibility to hypoglycemia. This may necessitate further insulin dose adjustments and particularly close monitoring of blood glucose).
    No products indexed under this heading.

Choline Magnesium Trisalicylate (Concomitant use with salicylates, may increase the blood glucose-lowering effect and susceptibility to hypoglycemia. This may necessitate further insulin dose adjustments and particularly close monitoring of blood glucose).
    No products indexed under this heading.

Cisapride (Due to its effects on gastric emptying, pramlintide acetate should not be considered for patients taking drugs that alter gastrointestinal motility).
    No products indexed under this heading.

Clemastine Fumarate (Due to its effects on gastric emptying, pramlintide acetate should not be considered for patients taking drugs that alter gastrointestinal motility).
    No products indexed under this heading.

Clidinium Bromide (Due to its effects on gastric emptying, pramlintide acetate should not be considered for patients taking drugs that alter gastrointestinal motility).
    No products indexed under this heading.

Clofibrate (Concomitant use with fibrates may increase the blood glucose-lowering effect and susceptibility to hypoglycemia. This may necessitate further insulin dose adjustments and particularly close monitoring of blood glucose).
    No products indexed under this heading.

Clomipramine Hydrochloride (Due to its effects on gastric emptying, pramlintide acetate should not be considered for patients taking drugs that alter gastrointestinal motility).
    No products indexed under this heading.

Codeine Phosphate (Due to its effects on gastric emptying, pramlintide acetate should not be considered for patients taking drugs that alter gastrointestinal motility). Products include:
    Tylenol with Codeine 2691

Codeine Sulfate (Due to its effects on gastric emptying, pramlintide acetate should not be considered for patients taking drugs that alter gastrointestinal motility).
    No products indexed under this heading.

Cyproheptadine Hydrochloride (Due to its effects on gastric emptying, pramlintide acetate should not be considered for patients taking drugs that alter gastrointestinal motility).
    No products indexed under this heading.

Desipramine Hydrochloride (Due to its effects on gastric emptying, pramlintide acetate should not be considered for patients taking drugs that alter gastrointestinal motility).
    No products indexed under this heading.

Dexchlorpheniramine Maleate (Due to its effects on gastric emptying, pramlintide acetate should not be considered for patients taking drugs that alter gastrointestinal motility).
    No products indexed under this heading.

Dezocine (Due to its effects on gastric emptying, pramlintide acetate should not be considered for patients taking drugs that alter gastrointestinal motility).
    No products indexed under this heading.

Dicyclomine Hydrochloride (Due to its effects on gastric emptying, pramlintide acetate should not be considered for patients taking drugs that alter gastrointestinal motility). Products include:
    Bentyl Capsules 780
    Bentyl Injection 780
    Bentyl Syrup 780
    Bentyl Tablets 780

Diflunisal (Concomitant use with salicylates, may increase the blood glucose-lowering effect and susceptibility to hypoglycemia. This may necessitate further insulin dose adjustments and particularly close monitoring of blood glucose).
    No products indexed under this heading.

Dihydrocodeine Bitartrate (Due to its effects on gastric emptying, pramlintide acetate should not be considered for patients taking drugs that alter gastrointestinal motility).
    No products indexed under this heading.

Dihydrocodeinone Bitartrate (Pramlintide acetate has the potential to delay the absorption of concomitantly administered oral medications. When the rapid onset of a concomitant orally administered agent is a critical determinant of effectiveness (such as analgesics), the agent should be administered at least 1 hour prior to or 2 hours after pramlintide acetate injection).
    No products indexed under this heading.

Diltiazem Hydrochloride (Due to its effects on gastric emptying, pramlintide acetate should not be considered for patients taking drugs that alter gastrointestinal motility). Products include:
    Cardizem LA 423

Diphenhydramine Hydrochloride (Due to its effects on gastric emptying, pramlintide acetate should not be considered for patients taking drugs that alter gastrointestinal motility). Products include:
    Benadryl Allergy Ultratab 2042
    Children's Benadryl Allergy Liquid 2042

Diphenoxylate (Due to its effects on gastric emptying, pramlintide acetate should not be considered for patients taking drugs that alter gastrointestinal motility).
    No products indexed under this heading.

Diphenoxylate Hydrochloride (Due to its effects on gastric emptying, pramlintide acetate should not be considered for patients taking drugs that alter gastrointestinal motility).
    No products indexed under this heading.

Diphenylpyraline Hydrochloride (Due to its effects on gastric emptying, pramlintide acetate should not be considered for patients taking drugs that alter gastrointestinal motility).
    No products indexed under this heading.

Disopyramide (Concomitant use with disopyramide may increase the blood glucose-lowering effect and susceptibility to hypoglycemia. This may necessitate further insulin dose adjustments and particularly close monitoring of blood glucose).
    No products indexed under this heading.

Disopyramide Phosphate (Concomitant use with disopyramide may increase the blood glucose-lowering effect and susceptibility to hypoglycemia. This may necessitate further insulin dose adjustments and particularly close monitoring of blood glucose).
    No products indexed under this heading.

Dobutamine (Due to its effects on gastric emptying, pramlintide acetate should not be considered for patients taking drugs that alter gastrointestinal motility).
    No products indexed under this heading.

Dobutamine Hydrochloride (Due to its effects on gastric emptying, pramlintide acetate should not be considered for patients taking drugs that alter gastrointestinal motility).
    No products indexed under this heading.

Domperidone (Due to its effects on gastric emptying, pramlintide acetate should not be considered for patients taking drugs that alter gastrointestinal motility).
    No products indexed under this heading.

Donepezil Hydrochloride (Due to its effects on gastric emptying, pramlintide acetate should not be considered for patients taking drugs that alter gastrointestinal motility). Products include:

Dopamine Hydrochloride (Due to its effects on gastric emptying, pramlintide acetate should not be considered for patients taking drugs that alter gastrointestinal motility).
No products indexed under this heading.

Doxepin Hydrochloride (Due to its effects on gastric emptying, pramlintide acetate should not be considered for patients taking drugs that alter gastrointestinal motility).
No products indexed under this heading.

Edrophonium Chloride (Due to its effects on gastric emptying, pramlintide acetate should not be considered for patients taking drugs that alter gastrointestinal motility).
No products indexed under this heading.

Enalapril Maleate (Concomitant use with ACE inhibitors may increase the blood glucose-lowering effect and susceptibility to hypoglycemia. This may necessitate further insulin dose adjustments and particularly close monitoring of blood glucose).
No products indexed under this heading.

Enalaprilat (Concomitant use with ACE inhibitors may increase the blood glucose-lowering effect and susceptibility to hypoglycemia. This may necessitate further insulin dose adjustments and particularly close monitoring of blood glucose).
No products indexed under this heading.

Ephedrine Hydrochloride (Due to its effects on gastric emptying, pramlintide acetate should not be considered for patients taking drugs that alter gastrointestinal motility).
No products indexed under this heading.

Ephedrine Sulfate (Due to its effects on gastric emptying, pramlintide acetate should not be considered for patients taking drugs that alter gastrointestinal motility).
No products indexed under this heading.

Ephedrine Tannate (Due to its effects on gastric emptying, pramlintide acetate should not be considered for patients taking drugs that alter gastrointestinal motility).
No products indexed under this heading.

Epinephrine (Due to its effects on gastric emptying, pramlintide acetate should not be considered for patients taking drugs that alter gastrointestinal motility). Products include:

Epinephrine Hydrochloride (Due to its effects on gastric emptying, pramlintide acetate should not be considered for patients taking drugs that alter gastrointestinal motility).
No products indexed under this heading.

Erythromycin (Due to its effects on gastric emptying, pramlintide acetate should not be considered for patients taking drugs that alter gastrointestinal motility).
No products indexed under this heading.

Erythromycin Estolate (Due to its effects on gastric emptying, pramlintide acetate should not be considered for patients taking drugs that alter gastrointestinal motility).
No products indexed under this heading.

Erythromycin Ethylsuccinate (Due to its effects on gastric emptying, pramlintide acetate should not be considered for patients taking drugs that alter gastrointestinal motility). Products include:

Erythromycin Gluceptate (Due to its effects on gastric emptying, pramlintide acetate should not be considered for patients taking drugs that alter gastrointestinal motility).
No products indexed under this heading.

Erythromycin Stearate (Due to its effects on gastric emptying, pramlintide acetate should not be considered for patients taking drugs that alter gastrointestinal motility).
No products indexed under this heading.

Felodipine (Due to its effects on gastric emptying, pramlintide acetate should not be considered for patients taking drugs that alter gastrointestinal motility).
No products indexed under this heading.

Fenofibrate (Concomitant use with fibrates may increase the blood glucose-lowering effect and susceptibility to hypoglycemia. This may necessitate further insulin dose adjustments and particularly close monitoring of blood glucose). Products include:

Fentanyl (Due to its effects on gastric emptying, pramlintide acetate should not be considered for patients taking drugs that alter gastrointestinal motility). Products include:

Fentanyl Citrate (Due to its effects on gastric emptying, pramlintide acetate should not be considered for patients taking drugs that alter gastrointestinal motility). Products include:

Fluoxetine (Concomitant use with fluoxetine may increase the blood glucose-lowering effect and susceptibility to hypoglycemia. This may necessitate further insulin dose adjustments and particularly close monitoring of blood glucose).
No products indexed under this heading.

Fluoxetine Hydrochloride (Concomitant use with fluoxetine may increase the blood glucose-lowering effect and susceptibility to hypoglycemia. This may necessitate further insulin dose adjustments and particularly close monitoring of blood glucose). Products include:

Fosinopril Sodium (Concomitant use with ACE inhibitors may increase the blood glucose-lowering effect and susceptibility to hypoglycemia. This may necessitate further insulin dose adjustments and particularly close monitoring of blood glucose).
No products indexed under this heading.

Galantamine Hydrobromide (Due to its effects on gastric emptying, pramlintide acetate should not be considered for patients taking drugs that alter gastrointestinal motility).
No products indexed under this heading.

Gemfibrozil (Concomitant use with fibrates may increase the blood glucose-lowering effect and susceptibility to hypoglycemia. This may necessitate further insulin dose adjustments and particularly close monitoring of blood glucose).
No products indexed under this heading.

Glibenclamide (Concomitant use with oral anti-diabetic products, may increase the blood glucose-lowering effect and susceptibility to hypoglycemia. This may necessitate further insulin dose adjustments and particularly close monitoring of blood glucose).
No products indexed under this heading.

Glimepiride (Concomitant use with oral anti-diabetic products, may increase the blood glucose-lowering effect and susceptibility to hypoglycemia. This may necessitate further insulin dose adjustments and particularly close monitoring of blood glucose). Products include:

Glipizide (Concomitant use with oral anti-diabetic products, may increase the blood glucose-lowering effect and susceptibility to hypoglycemia. This may necessitate further insulin dose adjustments and particularly close monitoring of blood glucose).
No products indexed under this heading.

Glyburide (Concomitant use with oral anti-diabetic products, may increase the blood glucose-lowering effect and susceptibility to hypoglycemia. This may necessitate further insulin dose adjustments and particularly close monitoring of blood glucose).
No products indexed under this heading.

Glycopyrrolate (Due to its effects on gastric emptying, pramlintide acetate should not be considered for patients taking drugs that alter gastrointestinal motility).
No products indexed under this heading.

Hydrochlorothiazide (Concomitant use with salicylates, may increase the blood glucose-lowering effect and susceptibility to hypoglycemia. This may necessitate further insulin dose adjustments and particularly close monitoring of blood glucose). Products include:

Hydrocodone Bitartrate (Due to its effects on gastric emptying, pramlintide acetate should not be considered for patients taking drugs that alter gastrointestinal motility). Products include:

Hydrocodone Polistirex (Due to its effects on gastric emptying, pramlintide acetate should not be considered for patients taking drugs that alter gastrointestinal motility). Products include:

Hydroflumethiazide (Concomitant use with salicylates, may increase the blood glucose-lowering effect and susceptibility to hypoglycemia. This may necessitate further insulin dose adjustments and particularly close monitoring of blood glucose).
No products indexed under this heading.

Hydromorphone (Due to its effects on gastric emptying, pramlintide acetate should not be considered for patients taking drugs that alter gastrointestinal motility).
No products indexed under this heading.

Hydromorphone Hydrochloride (Due to its effects on gastric emptying,

pramlintide acetate should not be considered for patients taking drugs that alter gastrointestinal motility). Products include:

Hyoscyamine (Due to its effects on gastric emptying, pramlintide acetate should not be considered for patients taking drugs that alter gastrointestinal motility).
No products indexed under this heading.

Hyoscyamine Sulfate (Due to its effects on gastric emptying, pramlintide acetate should not be considered for patients taking drugs that alter gastrointestinal motility). Products include:

Imipramine Hydrochloride (Due to its effects on gastric emptying, pramlintide acetate should not be considered for patients taking drugs that alter gastrointestinal motility).
No products indexed under this heading.

Imipramine Pamoate (Due to its effects on gastric emptying, pramlintide acetate should not be considered for patients taking drugs that alter gastrointestinal motility).
No products indexed under this heading.

Insulin (The addition of any antihyperglycemic agent, such as pramlintide acetate, to an existing regimen of one or more anti-hyperglycemic agents (eg, insulin) may necessitate further insulin dose adjustments and particularly close monitoring of blood glucose. Pramlintide acetate is used with insulin and has been associated with an increased risk of insulin-induced severe hypoglycemia, particularly in patients with type 1 diabetes).
No products indexed under this heading.

Insulin, Human, Zinc Suspension (The addition of any antihyperglycemic agent, such as pramlintide acetate, to an existing regimen of one or more anti-hyperglycemic agents (eg, insulin) may necessitate further insulin dose adjustments and particularly close monitoring of blood glucose. Pramlintide acetate is used with insulin and has been associated with an increased risk of insulin-induced severe hypoglycemia, particularly in patients with type 1 diabetes).
No products indexed under this heading.

Insulin, Human (rDNA origin) (The addition of any antihyperglycemic agent, such as pramlintide acetate, to an existing regimen of one or more anti-hyperglycemic agents (eg, insulin) may necessitate further insulin dose adjustments and particularly close monitoring of blood glucose. Pramlintide acetate is used with insulin and has been associated with an increased risk of insulin-induced severe hypoglycemia, particularly in patients with type 1 diabetes). Products include:

Insulin, Human NPH (The addition of any antihyperglycemic agent, such as pramlintide acetate, to an existing regimen of one or more anti-hyperglycemic agents (eg, insulin) may necessitate further insulin dose adjustments and particularly close monitoring of blood glucose. Pramlintide acetate is used with insulin and has been associated with an increased risk of insulin-induced severe hypoglycemia, particularly in patients with type 1 diabetes). Products include:

Insulin, Human Regular (The addition of any antihyperglycemic agent, such as pramlintide acetate, to an existing regimen of one or more anti-hyperglycemic agents (eg, insulin) may necessitate further insulin dose adjust-

ments and particularly close monitoring of blood glucose. Pramlintide acetate is used with insulin and has been associated with an increased risk of insulin-induced severe hypoglycemia, particularly in patients with type 1 diabetes). Products include:

Humulin R 1937
Humulin R (U-500) 1939

Insulin, Human Regular and Human NPH Mixture (The addition of any antihyperglycemic agent, such as pramlintide acetate, to an existing regimen of one or more anti-hyperglycemic agents (eg, insulin) may necessitate further insulin dose adjustments and particularly close monitoring of blood glucose. Pramlintide acetate is used with insulin and has been associated with an increased risk of insulin-induced severe hypoglycemia, particularly in patients with type 1 diabetes). Products include:

Humulin 50/50 1930
Humulin 70/30 Vial 1931

Insulin, NPH (The addition of any antihyperglycemic agent, such as pramlintide acetate, to an existing regimen of one or more anti-hyperglycemic agents (eg, insulin) may necessitate further insulin dose adjustments and particularly close monitoring of blood glucose. Pramlintide acetate is used with insulin and has been associated with an increased risk of insulin-induced severe hypoglycemia, particularly in patients with type 1 diabetes).
No products indexed under this heading.

Insulin, Regular (The addition of any antihyperglycemic agent, such as pramlintide acetate, to an existing regimen of one or more anti-hyperglycemic agents (eg, insulin) may necessitate further insulin dose adjustments and particularly close monitoring of blood glucose. Pramlintide acetate is used with insulin and has been associated with an increased risk of insulin-induced severe hypoglycemia, particularly in patients with type 1 diabetes).
No products indexed under this heading.

Insulin, Regular and NPH mixture (The addition of any antihyperglycemic agent, such as pramlintide acetate, to an existing regimen of one or more anti-hyperglycemic agents (eg, insulin) may necessitate further insulin dose adjustments and particularly close monitoring of blood glucose. Pramlintide acetate is used with insulin and has been associated with an increased risk of insulin-induced severe hypoglycemia, particularly in patients with type 1 diabetes).
No products indexed under this heading.

Insulin, Zinc Crystals (The addition of any antihyperglycemic agent, such as pramlintide acetate, to an existing regimen of one or more anti-hyperglycemic agents (eg, insulin) may necessitate further insulin dose adjustments and particularly close monitoring of blood glucose. Pramlintide acetate is used with insulin and has been associated with an increased risk of insulin-induced severe hypoglycemia, particularly in patients with type 1 diabetes).
No products indexed under this heading.

Insulin, Zinc Suspension (The addition of any antihyperglycemic agent, such as pramlintide acetate, to an existing regimen of one or more anti-hyperglycemic agents (eg, insulin) may necessitate further insulin dose adjustments and particularly close monitoring of blood glucose. Pramlintide acetate is used with insulin and has been associated with an increased risk of insulin-induced severe hypoglycemia, particularly in patients with type 1 diabetes).
No products indexed under this heading.

Insulin Aspart (The addition of any antihyperglycemic agent, such as pramlintide acetate, to an existing regimen of one or more anti-hyperglycemic agents (eg, insulin) may necessitate further insulin dose adjustments and particularly close monitoring of blood glucose. Pramlintide acetate is used with insulin and has been associated with an increased risk of insulin-induced severe hypoglycemia, particularly in patients with type 1 diabetes).
No products indexed under this heading.

Insulin Aspart, Human (The addition of any antihyperglycemic agent, such as pramlintide acetate, to an existing regimen of one or more anti-hyperglycemic agents (eg, insulin) may necessitate further insulin dose adjustments and particularly close monitoring of blood glucose. Pramlintide acetate is used with insulin and has been associated with an increased risk of insulin-induced severe hypoglycemia, particularly in patients with type 1 diabetes). Products include:

NovoLog Mix 70/30 2581

Insulin Aspart, Human Regular (The addition of any antihyperglycemic agent, such as pramlintide acetate, to an existing regimen of one or more anti-hyperglycemic agents (eg, insulin) may necessitate further insulin dose adjustments and particularly close monitoring of blood glucose. Pramlintide acetate is used with insulin and has been associated with an increased risk of insulin-induced severe hypoglycemia, particularly in patients with type 1 diabetes). Products include:

NovoLog 2575

Insulin Aspart Protamine, Human (The addition of any antihyperglycemic agent, such as pramlintide acetate, to an existing regimen of one or more anti-hyperglycemic agents (eg, insulin) may necessitate further insulin dose adjustments and particularly close monitoring of blood glucose. Pramlintide acetate is used with insulin and has been associated with an increased risk of insulin-induced severe hypoglycemia, particularly in patients with type 1 diabetes). Products include:

NovoLog Mix 70/30 2581

Insulin Detemir (rDNA Origin) (The addition of any antihyperglycemic agent, such as pramlintide acetate, to an existing regimen of one or more anti-hyperglycemic agents (eg, insulin) may necessitate further insulin dose adjustments and particularly close monitoring of blood glucose. Pramlintide acetate is used with insulin and has been associated with an increased risk of insulin-induced severe hypoglycemia, particularly in patients with type 1 diabetes). Products include:

Levemir 2566

Insulin Glargine (The addition of any antihyperglycemic agent, such as pramlintide acetate, to an existing regimen of one or more anti-hyperglycemic agents (eg, insulin) may necessitate further insulin dose adjustments and particularly close monitoring of blood glucose. Pramlintide acetate is used with insulin and has been associated with an increased risk of insulin-induced severe hypoglycemia, particularly in patients with type 1 diabetes). Products include:

Lantus 2996

Insulin Glulisine (The addition of any antihyperglycemic agent, such as pramlintide acetate, to an existing regimen of one or more anti-hyperglycemic agents (eg, insulin) may necessitate further insulin dose adjustments and particularly close monitoring of blood glucose. Pramlintide acetate is used with insulin and has been associated with an increased risk of insulin-induced severe hypoglycemia, particularly in patients with type 1 diabetes). Products include:

Apidra 2937
Apidra SoloStar 2937

Insulin Lispro, Human (The addition of any antihyperglycemic agent, such as pramlintide acetate, to an existing regimen of one or more anti-hyperglycemic agents (eg, insulin) may necessitate further insulin dose adjustments and particularly close monitoring of blood glucose. Pramlintide acetate is used with insulin and has been associated with an increased risk of insulin-induced severe hypoglycemia, particularly in patients with type 1 diabetes). Products include:

Humalog 1910
Humalog Mix 1914
Humalog Mix75/25 1917

Insulin Lispro Protamine, Human (The addition of any antihyperglycemic agent, such as pramlintide acetate, to an existing regimen of one or more anti-hyperglycemic agents (eg, insulin) may necessitate further insulin dose adjustments and particularly close monitoring of blood glucose. Pramlintide acetate is used with insulin and has been associated with an increased risk of insulin-induced severe hypoglycemia, particularly in patients with type 1 diabetes). Products include:

Humalog Mix 1914
Humalog Mix75/25 1917

Ipratropium Bromide (Due to its effects on gastric emptying, pramlintide acetate should not be considered for patients taking drugs that alter gastrointestinal motility).
No products indexed under this heading.

Isocarboxazid (Concomitant use with MAO inhibitors, may increase the blood glucose-lowering effect and susceptibility to hypoglycemia. This may necessitate further insulin dose adjustments and particularly close monitoring of blood glucose). Products include:

Marplan 3481

Isoetharine (Due to its effects on gastric emptying, pramlintide acetate should not be considered for patients taking drugs that alter gastrointestinal motility).
No products indexed under this heading.

Isoproterenol Hydrochloride (Due to its effects on gastric emptying, pramlintide acetate should not be considered for patients taking drugs that alter gastrointestinal motility).
No products indexed under this heading.

Isoproterenol Sulfate (Due to its effects on gastric emptying, pramlintide acetate should not be considered for patients taking drugs that alter gastrointestinal motility).
No products indexed under this heading.

Isradipine (Due to its effects on gastric emptying, pramlintide acetate should not be considered for patients taking drugs that alter gastrointestinal motility). Products include:

DynaCirc CR 1432

Levalbuterol Hydrochloride (Due to its effects on gastric emptying, pramlintide acetate should not be considered for patients taking drugs that alter gastrointestinal motility).
No products indexed under this heading.

Levorphanol Tartrate (Due to its effects on gastric emptying, pramlintide acetate should not be considered for patients taking drugs that alter gastrointestinal motility).
No products indexed under this heading.

Lisinopril (Concomitant use with ACE inhibitors may increase the blood glucose-lowering effect and susceptibility to hypoglycemia. This may necessitate further insulin dose adjustments and particularly close monitoring of blood glucose). Products include:

Prinivil 2241
Prinzide 2246

Magnesium Salicylate (Concomitant use with salicylates, may increase the blood glucose-lowering effect and susceptibility to hypoglycemia. This may necessitate further insulin dose adjustments and particularly close monitoring of blood glucose).
No products indexed under this heading.

Maprotiline Hydrochloride (Due to its effects on gastric emptying, pramlintide acetate should not be considered for patients taking drugs that alter gastrointestinal motility).
No products indexed under this heading.

Mepenzolate Bromide (Due to its effects on gastric emptying, pramlintide acetate should not be considered for patients taking drugs that alter gastrointestinal motility).
No products indexed under this heading.

Meperidine Hydrochloride (Due to its effects on gastric emptying, pramlintide acetate should not be considered for patients taking drugs that alter gastrointestinal motility).
No products indexed under this heading.

Metaproterenol Sulfate (Due to its effects on gastric emptying, pramlintide acetate should not be considered for patients taking drugs that alter gastrointestinal motility).
No products indexed under this heading.

Metformin Hydrochloride (Concomitant use with oral anti-diabetic products, may increase the blood glucose-lowering effect and susceptibility to hypoglycemia. This may necessitate further insulin dose adjustments and particularly close monitoring of blood glucose). Products include:

ActoPlus 3338
Avandamet 1345
Janumet 2188

Methadone Hydrochloride (Due to its effects on gastric emptying, pramlintide acetate should not be considered for patients taking drugs that alter gastrointestinal motility).
No products indexed under this heading.

Methdilazine Hydrochloride (Due to its effects on gastric emptying, pramlintide acetate should not be considered for patients taking drugs that alter gastrointestinal motility).
No products indexed under this heading.

Methyclothiazide (Concomitant use with salicylates, may increase the blood glucose-lowering effect and susceptibility to hypoglycemia. This may necessitate further insulin dose adjustments and particularly close monitoring of blood glucose).
No products indexed under this heading.

Metoclopramide Hydrochloride (Due to its effects on gastric emptying, pramlintide acetate should not be considered for patients taking drugs that alter gastrointestinal motility). Products include:

Metozolv ODT 2901

Mibefradil Dihydrochloride (Due to its effects on gastric emptying, pramlintide acetate should not be considered for patients taking drugs that alter gastrointestinal motility).
No products indexed under this heading.

Miglitol (Concomitant use with oral anti-diabetic products, may increase the blood glucose-lowering effect and susceptibility to hypoglycemia. This may necessitate further insulin dose adjustments and particularly close monitoring of blood glucose).
No products indexed under this heading.

1811 Interactions Index Symlin

Moclobemide (Concomitant use with MAO inhibitors, may increase the blood glucose-lowering effect and susceptibility to hypoglycemia. This may necessitate further insulin dose adjustments and particularly close monitoring of blood glucose).
No products indexed under this heading.

Moexipril Hydrochloride (Concomitant use with ACE inhibitors may increase the blood glucose-lowering effect and susceptibility to hypoglycemia. This may necessitate further insulin dose adjustments and particularly close monitoring of blood glucose).
No products indexed under this heading.

Morphine Sulfate (Due to its effects on gastric emptying, pramlintide acetate should not be considered for patients taking drugs that alter gastrointestinal motility). Products include:
Avinza **1822**
Embeda **1831**
MS Contin **2803**

Morphine Sulfate, Liposomal (Due to its effects on gastric emptying, pramlintide acetate should not be considered for patients taking drugs that alter gastrointestinal motility).
No products indexed under this heading.

Nalbuphine Hydrochloride (Pramlintide acetate has the potential to delay the absorption of concomitantly administered oral medications. When the rapid onset of a concomitant orally administered agent is a critical determinant of effectiveness (such as analgesics), the agent should be administered at least 1 hour prior to or 2 hours after pramlintide acetate injection).
No products indexed under this heading.

Nateglinide (Concomitant use with oral anti-diabetic products, may increase the blood glucose-lowering effect and susceptibility to hypoglycemia. This may necessitate further insulin dose adjustments and particularly close monitoring of blood glucose).
No products indexed under this heading.

Neostigmine Bromide (Due to its effects on gastric emptying, pramlintide acetate should not be considered for patients taking drugs that alter gastrointestinal motility).
No products indexed under this heading.

Neostigmine Methylsulfate (Due to its effects on gastric emptying, pramlintide acetate should not be considered for patients taking drugs that alter gastrointestinal motility).
No products indexed under this heading.

Nicardipine Hydrochloride (Due to its effects on gastric emptying, pramlintide acetate should not be considered for patients taking drugs that alter gastrointestinal motility).
No products indexed under this heading.

Nifedipine (Due to its effects on gastric emptying, pramlintide acetate should not be considered for patients taking drugs that alter gastrointestinal motility).
No products indexed under this heading.

Nimodipine (Due to its effects on gastric emptying, pramlintide acetate should not be considered for patients taking drugs that alter gastrointestinal motility).
No products indexed under this heading.

Nisoldipine (Due to its effects on gastric emptying, pramlintide acetate should not be considered for patients taking drugs that alter gastrointestinal motility).
No products indexed under this heading.

Nortriptyline Hydrochloride (Due to its effects on gastric emptying, pramlintide acetate should not be considered for patients taking drugs that alter gastrointestinal motility).
No products indexed under this heading.

Octreotide Acetate (Due to its effects on gastric emptying, pramlintide acetate should not be considered for patients taking drugs that alter gastrointestinal motility). Products include:
Sandostatin **2517**
Sandostatin LAR **2519**

Oral Medications, unspecified (Pramlintide has the potential to delay the absorption of co-administered oral medications. When the rapid onset of a concomitant orally administered agent is a critical determinant of effectiveness (such as analgesics), the agent should be administered at least 1 hour prior to or 2 hours after pramlintide injection).
No products indexed under this heading.

Oxybutynin Chloride (Due to its effects on gastric emptying, pramlintide acetate should not be considered for patients taking drugs that alter gastrointestinal motility).
No products indexed under this heading.

Oxycodone Hydrochloride (Due to its effects on gastric emptying, pramlintide acetate should not be considered for patients taking drugs that alter gastrointestinal motility). Products include:
OxyContin **2807**
Percocet **1121**
Percodan **1124**

Oxycodone Terephthalate (Due to its effects on gastric emptying, pramlintide acetate should not be considered for patients taking drugs that alter gastrointestinal motility).
No products indexed under this heading.

Oxymorphone Hydrochloride (Due to its effects on gastric emptying, pramlintide acetate should not be considered for patients taking drugs that alter gastrointestinal motility). Products include:
Opana **1110**
Opana ER **1114**

Oxyphenonium Bromide (Due to its effects on gastric emptying, pramlintide acetate should not be considered for patients taking drugs that alter gastrointestinal motility).
No products indexed under this heading.

Pargyline Hydrochloride (Concomitant use with MAO inhibitors, may increase the blood glucose-lowering effect and susceptibility to hypoglycemia. This may necessitate further insulin dose adjustments and particularly close monitoring of blood glucose).
No products indexed under this heading.

Pentazocine Hydrochloride (Pramlintide acetate has the potential to delay the absorption of concomitantly administered oral medications. When the rapid onset of a concomitant orally administered agent is a critical determinant of effectiveness (such as analgesics), the agent should be administered at least 1 hour prior to or 2 hours after pramlintide acetate injection).
No products indexed under this heading.

Pentazocine Lactate (Pramlintide acetate has the potential to delay the absorption of concomitantly administered oral medications. When the rapid onset of a concomitant orally administered agent is a critical determinant of effectiveness (such as analgesics), the agent should be administered at least 1 hour prior to or 2 hours after pramlintide acetate injection).
No products indexed under this heading.

Pentoxifylline (Concomitant use with pentoxifylline may increase the blood glucose-lowering effect and susceptibility to hypoglycemia. This may necessitate further insulin dose adjustments and particularly close monitoring of blood glucose).
No products indexed under this heading.

Pergolide Mesylate (Due to its effects on gastric emptying, pramlintide acetate should not be considered for patients taking drugs that alter gastrointestinal motility).
No products indexed under this heading.

Perindopril Erbumine (Concomitant use with ACE inhibitors may increase the blood glucose-lowering effect and susceptibility to hypoglycemia. This may necessitate further insulin dose adjustments and particularly close monitoring of blood glucose).
No products indexed under this heading.

Phenelzine Sulfate (Concomitant use with MAO inhibitors, may increase the blood glucose-lowering effect and susceptibility to hypoglycemia. This may necessitate further insulin dose adjustments and particularly close monitoring of blood glucose).
No products indexed under this heading.

Pioglitazone Hydrochloride (Concomitant use with oral anti-diabetic products, may increase the blood glucose-lowering effect and susceptibility to hypoglycemia. This may necessitate further insulin dose adjustments and particularly close monitoring of blood glucose). Products include:
ActoPlus **3338**
Actos **3345**
Duetact **3354**

Pirbuterol Acetate (Due to its effects on gastric emptying, pramlintide acetate should not be considered for patients taking drugs that alter gastrointestinal motility). Products include:
Maxair Autohaler **1782**

Polythiazide (Concomitant use with salicylates, may increase the blood glucose-lowering effect and susceptibility to hypoglycemia. This may necessitate further insulin dose adjustments and particularly close monitoring of blood glucose).
No products indexed under this heading.

Pramipexole Dihydrochloride (Due to its effects on gastric emptying, pramlintide acetate should not be considered for patients taking drugs that alter gastrointestinal motility).
No products indexed under this heading.

Procainamide Hydrochloride (Due to its effects on gastric emptying, pramlintide acetate should not be considered for patients taking drugs that alter gastrointestinal motility).
No products indexed under this heading.

Procarbazine Hydrochloride (Concomitant use with MAO inhibitors, may increase the blood glucose-lowering effect and susceptibility to hypoglycemia. This may necessitate further insulin dose adjustments and particularly close monitoring of blood glucose).
No products indexed under this heading.

Procyclidine Hydrochloride (Due to its effects on gastric emptying, pramlintide acetate should not be considered for patients taking drugs that alter gastrointestinal motility).
No products indexed under this heading.

Promethazine Hydrochloride (Due to its effects on gastric emptying, pramlintide acetate should not be considered for patients taking drugs that alter gastrointestinal motility).
No products indexed under this heading.

Propantheline Bromide (Due to its effects on gastric emptying, pramlintide acetate should not be considered for patients taking drugs that alter gastrointestinal motility).
No products indexed under this heading.

Propoxyphene Hydrochloride (Concomitant use with propoxyphene, may increase the blood glucose-lowering effect and susceptibility to hypoglycemia. This may necessitate further insulin dose adjustments and particularly close monitoring of blood glucose).
No products indexed under this heading.

Propoxyphene Napsylate (Concomitant use with propoxyphene, may increase the blood glucose-lowering effect and susceptibility to hypoglycemia. This may necessitate further insulin dose adjustments and particularly close monitoring of blood glucose).
No products indexed under this heading.

Protriptyline Hydrochloride (Due to its effects on gastric emptying, pramlintide acetate should not be considered for patients taking drugs that alter gastrointestinal motility).
No products indexed under this heading.

Pyridostigmine Bromide (Due to its effects on gastric emptying, pramlintide acetate should not be considered for patients taking drugs that alter gastrointestinal motility).
No products indexed under this heading.

Pyrilamine Maleate (Due to its effects on gastric emptying, pramlintide acetate should not be considered for patients taking drugs that alter gastrointestinal motility).
No products indexed under this heading.

Pyrilamine Tannate (Due to its effects on gastric emptying, pramlintide acetate should not be considered for patients taking drugs that alter gastrointestinal motility).
No products indexed under this heading.

Quinapril Hydrochloride (Concomitant use with ACE inhibitors may increase the blood glucose-lowering effect and susceptibility to hypoglycemia. This may necessitate further insulin dose adjustments and particularly close monitoring of blood glucose).
No products indexed under this heading.

Quinidine Gluconate (Due to its effects on gastric emptying, pramlintide acetate should not be considered for patients taking drugs that alter gastrointestinal motility).
No products indexed under this heading.

Quinidine Polygalacturonate (Due to its effects on gastric emptying, pramlintide acetate should not be considered for patients taking drugs that alter gastrointestinal motility).
No products indexed under this heading.

Quinidine Sulfate (Due to its effects on gastric emptying, pramlintide acetate should not be considered for patients taking drugs that alter gastrointestinal motility).
No products indexed under this heading.

Ramipril (Concomitant use with ACE inhibitors may increase the blood glucose-lowering effect and susceptibility to hypoglycemia. This may necessitate further insulin dose adjustments and particularly close monitoring of blood glucose).
No products indexed under this heading.

Rasagiline Mesylate (Concomitant use with MAO inhibitors, may increase the blood glucose-lowering effect and susceptibility to hypoglycemia. This may necessitate further insulin dose adjustments and particularly close monitoring of blood glucose). Products include:
Azilect **3383**

Remifentanil Hydrochloride (Due to its effects on gastric emptying, pramlintide acetate should not be considered for patients taking drugs that alter gastrointestinal motility).
No products indexed under this heading.

IMPORTANT NOTE: Always consult each drug listing in the patient's regimen for possible interactions.

Symlin Interactions Index 1812

Repaglinide (Concomitant use with oral anti-diabetic products, may increase the blood glucose-lowering effect and susceptibility to hypoglycemia. This may necessitate further insulin dose adjustments and particularly close monitoring of blood glucose).
No products indexed under this heading.

Rivastigmine Tartrate (Due to its effects on gastric emptying, pramlintide acetate should not be considered for patients taking drugs that alter gastrointestinal motility). Products include:
Exelon 2432
Exelon Oral 2432
Exelon Patch 2437

Ropinirole Hydrochloride (Due to its effects on gastric emptying, pramlintide acetate should not be considered for patients taking drugs that alter gastrointestinal motility). Products include:
Requip 1620
Requip XL 1628

Rosiglitazone Maleate (Concomitant use with oral anti-diabetic products, may increase the blood glucose-lowering effect and susceptibility to hypoglycemia. This may necessitate further insulin dose adjustments and particularly close monitoring of blood glucose). Products include:
Avandamet 1345
Avandaryl 1356
Avandia 1366

Salmeterol Xinafoate (Due to its effects on gastric emptying, pramlintide acetate should not be considered for patients taking drugs that alter gastrointestinal motility). Products include:
Advair 100/50 1275
Advair 250/50 1275
Advair 500/50 1275
Advair HFA 45/21 1288
Advair HFA 115/21 1288
Advair HFA 230/21 1288
Serevent Diskus 1656

Salsalate (Concomitant use with salicylates, may increase the blood glucose-lowering effect and susceptibility to hypoglycemia. This may necessitate further insulin dose adjustments and particularly close monitoring of blood glucose).
No products indexed under this heading.

Scopolamine (Due to its effects on gastric emptying, pramlintide acetate should not be considered for patients taking drugs that alter gastrointestinal motility). Products include:
Transderm Scōp 2397

Scopolamine Hydrobromide (Due to its effects on gastric emptying, pramlintide acetate should not be considered for patients taking drugs that alter gastrointestinal motility). Products include:
Donnatal 2711

Selegiline (Concomitant use with MAO inhibitors, may increase the blood glucose-lowering effect and susceptibility to hypoglycemia. This may necessitate further insulin dose adjustments and particularly close monitoring of blood glucose). Products include:
Emsam 3623

Selegiline Hydrochloride (Concomitant use with MAO inhibitors, may increase the blood glucose-lowering effect and susceptibility to hypoglycemia. This may necessitate further insulin dose adjustments and particularly close monitoring of blood glucose). Products include:
Eldepryl 3312

Sitagliptin Phosphate (Concomitant use with oral anti-diabetic products, may increase the blood glucose-lowering effect and susceptibility to hypoglycemia. This may necessitate further insulin dose adjustments and particularly close monitoring of blood glucose). Products include:
Janumet 2188
Januvia 2196

Spirapril Hydrochloride (Concomitant use with ACE inhibitors may increase the blood glucose-lowering effect and susceptibility to hypoglycemia. This may necessitate further insulin dose adjustments and particularly close monitoring of blood glucose).
No products indexed under this heading.

Sucralfate (Due to its effects on gastric emptying, pramlintide acetate should not be considered for patients taking drugs that alter gastrointestinal motility). Products include:
Carafate Suspension 784
Carafate Tablets 785

Sufentanil Citrate (Due to its effects on gastric emptying, pramlintide acetate should not be considered for patients taking drugs that alter gastrointestinal motility).
No products indexed under this heading.

Sulfacytine (Concomitant use with salicylates, may increase the blood glucose-lowering effect and susceptibility to hypoglycemia. This may necessitate further insulin dose adjustments and particularly close monitoring of blood glucose).
No products indexed under this heading.

Sulfamethizole (Concomitant use with salicylates, may increase the blood glucose-lowering effect and susceptibility to hypoglycemia. This may necessitate further insulin dose adjustments and particularly close monitoring of blood glucose).
No products indexed under this heading.

Sulfamethoxazole (Concomitant use with salicylates, may increase the blood glucose-lowering effect and susceptibility to hypoglycemia. This may necessitate further insulin dose adjustments and particularly close monitoring of blood glucose).
No products indexed under this heading.

Sulfasalazine (Concomitant use with salicylates, may increase the blood glucose-lowering effect and susceptibility to hypoglycemia. This may necessitate further insulin dose adjustments and particularly close monitoring of blood glucose).
No products indexed under this heading.

Sulfinpyrazone (Concomitant use with salicylates, may increase the blood glucose-lowering effect and susceptibility to hypoglycemia. This may necessitate further insulin dose adjustments and particularly close monitoring of blood glucose).
No products indexed under this heading.

Sulfisoxazole Acetyl (Concomitant use with salicylates, may increase the blood glucose-lowering effect and susceptibility to hypoglycemia. This may necessitate further insulin dose adjustments and particularly close monitoring of blood glucose).
No products indexed under this heading.

Sulfisoxazole Diolamine (Concomitant use with salicylates, may increase the blood glucose-lowering effect and susceptibility to hypoglycemia. This may necessitate further insulin dose adjustments and particularly close monitoring of blood glucose).
No products indexed under this heading.

Tacrine Hydrochloride (Due to its effects on gastric emptying, pramlintide acetate should not be considered for patients taking drugs that alter gastrointestinal motility).
No products indexed under this heading.

Terbutaline Sulfate (Due to its effects on gastric emptying, pramlintide acetate should not be considered for patients taking drugs that alter gastrointestinal motility).
No products indexed under this heading.

Tolazamide (Concomitant use with oral anti-diabetic products, may increase the blood glucose-lowering effect and susceptibility to hypoglycemia. This may necessitate further insulin dose adjustments and particularly close monitoring of blood glucose).
No products indexed under this heading.

Tolbutamide (Concomitant use with oral anti-diabetic products, may increase the blood glucose-lowering effect and susceptibility to hypoglycemia. This may necessitate further insulin dose adjustments and particularly close monitoring of blood glucose).
No products indexed under this heading.

Tolterodine Tartrate (Due to its effects on gastric emptying, pramlintide acetate should not be considered for patients taking drugs that alter gastrointestinal motility).
No products indexed under this heading.

Trandolapril (Concomitant use with ACE inhibitors may increase the blood glucose-lowering effect and susceptibility to hypoglycemia. This may necessitate further insulin dose adjustments and particularly close monitoring of blood glucose). Products include:
Mavik 489
Tarka 534

Tranylcypromine Sulfate (Concomitant use with MAO inhibitors, may increase the blood glucose-lowering effect and susceptibility to hypoglycemia. This may necessitate further insulin dose adjustments and particularly close monitoring of blood glucose). Products include:
Parnate 1584

Tridihexethyl Chloride (Due to its effects on gastric emptying, pramlintide acetate should not be considered for patients taking drugs that alter gastrointestinal motility).
No products indexed under this heading.

Trihexyphenidyl Hydrochloride (Due to its effects on gastric emptying, pramlintide acetate should not be considered for patients taking drugs that alter gastrointestinal motility).
No products indexed under this heading.

Trimeprazine Tartrate (Due to its effects on gastric emptying, pramlintide acetate should not be considered for patients taking drugs that alter gastrointestinal motility).
No products indexed under this heading.

Trimipramine Maleate (Due to its effects on gastric emptying, pramlintide acetate should not be considered for patients taking drugs that alter gastrointestinal motility).
No products indexed under this heading.

Tripelennamine Hydrochloride (Due to its effects on gastric emptying, pramlintide acetate should not be considered for patients taking drugs that alter gastrointestinal motility).
No products indexed under this heading.

Triprolidine Hydrochloride (Due to its effects on gastric emptying, pramlintide acetate should not be considered for patients taking drugs that alter gastrointestinal motility).
No products indexed under this heading.

Troglitazone (Concomitant use with oral anti-diabetic products, may increase the blood glucose-lowering effect and susceptibility to hypoglycemia. This may necessitate further insulin dose adjustments and particularly close monitoring of blood glucose).
No products indexed under this heading.

Verapamil Hydrochloride (Due to its effects on gastric emptying, pramlintide acetate should not be considered for patients taking drugs that alter gastrointestinal motility). Products include:
Tarka 534

SYMLINPEN
(Pramlintide Acetate) 651
See Symlin Injection

SYNAGIS INTRAMUSCULAR SOLUTION
(Palivizumab) 2082
None cited in PDR database.

SYNTHROID TABLETS
(Levothyroxine Sodium) 529
May interact with androgens, antithyroid agents, beta-blockers, cardiac glycosides, cytokines, dopamine agonists, estrogens, glucocorticoids, hepatic microsomal enzyme inducers, insulin, lithium preparations, oral anticoagulants, oral hypoglycemic agents, phenytoin, radiographic iodinated contrast media, salicylates, sulfonamides, sulfonylureas, sympathomimetics, thiazides, tricyclic antidepressants, xanthines, and certain other agents. Compounds in these categories include:

Acarbose (Requirements of oral antidiabetic agents may be reduced in hypothyroid patients with diabetes and may be subsequently increased with initiation of thyroid hormone therapy).
No products indexed under this heading.

Acebutolol Hydrochloride (Alters thyroid hormone or TSH levels; actions of some beta blockers may be impaired when hypothyroid patients become euthyroid).
No products indexed under this heading.

Albuterol (Possible increased risk of coronary insufficiency in patients with coronary artery disease).
No products indexed under this heading.

Albuterol Sulfate (Possible increased risk of coronary insufficiency in patients with coronary artery disease). Products include:
ProAir HFA 3393
Proventil HFA 3204
Ventolin HFA 1708

Aldesleukin (Cytokines have been reported to induce both hyperthyroidism or hypothyroidism; dosage adjustment may be necessary). Products include:
Proleukin 2504

Allium sativum (Alters thyroid hormone or TSH levels).
No products indexed under this heading.

Aluminum Hydroxide (Binds and decreases absorption of levothyroxine sodium from the gastrointestinal tract).
No products indexed under this heading.

Aminoglutethimide (Alters thyroid hormone or TSH levels).
No products indexed under this heading.

Aminophylline (Theophylline clearance may be decreased in hypothyroid patients and return toward normal when euthyroid state is achieved).
No products indexed under this heading.

p-Aminosalicylic Acid (Alters thyroid hormone or TSH levels).
No products indexed under this heading.

Amiodarone Hydrochloride (Amiodarone therapy alone can cause hypothyroidism or hyperthyroidism).
No products indexed under this heading.

Amitriptyline Hydrochloride (Concurrent use may increase the therapeutic and toxic effects of both drugs; onset of action of tricyclics may be accelerated).
No products indexed under this heading.

Amoxapine (Concurrent use may increase the therapeutic and toxic effects of both drugs; onset of action of tricyclics may be accelerated).
No products indexed under this heading.

IMPORTANT NOTE: Always consult each drug listing in the patient's regimen for possible interactions.

1815 Interactions Index Synthroid

Iodine, radiolabeled (Uptake of radiolabeled ions may be decreased).
No products indexed under this heading.

Iohexol (Alters thyroid hormone or TSH levels).
No products indexed under this heading.

Iopamidol (Alters thyroid hormone or TSH levels).
No products indexed under this heading.

Iopanoic Acid (Alters thyroid hormone or TSH levels).
No products indexed under this heading.

Iothalamate Meglumine (Alters thyroid hormone or TSH levels).
No products indexed under this heading.

Ioxaglate Meglumine (Alters thyroid hormone or TSH levels).
No products indexed under this heading.

Ioxaglate Sodium (Alters thyroid hormone or TSH levels).
No products indexed under this heading.

Isoproterenol Hydrochloride (Possible increased risk of coronary insufficiency in patients with coronary artery disease).
No products indexed under this heading.

Isoproterenol Sulfate (Possible increased risk of coronary insufficiency in patients with coronary artery disease).
No products indexed under this heading.

Ketamine Hydrochloride (Co-administration produces marked hypertension and tachycardia).
No products indexed under this heading.

Labetalol Hydrochloride (Alters thyroid hormone or TSH levels; actions of some beta blockers may be impaired when hypothyroid patients become euthyroid).
No products indexed under this heading.

Lansoprazole (Alters thyroid hormone or TSH levels).
No products indexed under this heading.

Levalbuterol Hydrochloride (Possible increased risk of coronary insufficiency in patients with coronary artery disease).
No products indexed under this heading.

Levobunolol Hydrochloride (Alters thyroid hormone or TSH levels; actions of some beta blockers may be impaired when hypothyroid patients become euthyroid).
No products indexed under this heading.

Levodopa (Alters thyroid hormone or TSH levels). Products include:
Stalevo 2526

Lithium (Blocks the TSH-mediated release of T4 and T3; thyroid function should therefore be carefully monitored during lithium initiation, stablization, and maintenence; if hypothyroidism occurs during lithium treatment, a higher than usual Synthroid dose may be required).
No products indexed under this heading.

Lithium Carbonate (Blocks the TSH-mediated release of T4 and T3; thyroid function should therefore be carefully monitored during lithium initiation, stablization, and maintenence; if hypothyroidism occurs during lithium treatment, a higher than usual Synthroid dose may be required).
No products indexed under this heading.

Lithium Citrate (Blocks the TSH-mediated release of T4 and T3; thyroid function should therefore be carefully monitored during lithium initiation, stablization, and maintenence; if hypothyroidism occurs during lithium treatment, a higher than usual Synthroid dose may be required).
No products indexed under this heading.

Lovastatin (Alters thyroid hormone or TSH levels). Products include:
Advicor 402
Mevacor 2212

Magnesium Salicylate (May inhibit levothyroxine sodium binding to serum proteins or alter the concentrations of serum proteins).
No products indexed under this heading.

Maprotiline Hydrochloride (Risk of cardiac arrhythmias may increase).
No products indexed under this heading.

Meclofenamate Sodium (Meclofenamic acid may inhibit levothyroxine sodium binding to serum proteins or alter the concentrations of serum proteins).
No products indexed under this heading.

Mefenamic Acid (May inhibit levothyroxine sodium binding to serum proteins or alter the concentrations of serum proteins).
No products indexed under this heading.

Mephenytoin (Alters thyroid hormone or TSH levels).
No products indexed under this heading.

Mercaptopurine (Alters thyroid hormone or TSH levels).
No products indexed under this heading.

Metaproterenol Sulfate (Possible increased risk of coronary insufficiency in patients with coronary artery disease).
No products indexed under this heading.

Metaraminol Bitartrate (Possible increased risk of coronary insufficiency in patients with coronary artery disease).
No products indexed under this heading.

Metformin Hydrochloride (Requirements of oral antidiabetic agents may be reduced in hypothyroid patients with diabetes and may be subsequently increased with initiation of thyroid hormone therapy). Products include:
ActoPlus 3338
Avandamet 1345
Janumet 2188

Methadone Hydrochloride (May inhibit levothyroxine sodium binding to serum proteins or alter the concentrations of serum proteins).
No products indexed under this heading.

Methimazole (Alters thyroid hormone or TSH levels).
No products indexed under this heading.

Methoxamine Hydrochloride (Possible increased risk of coronary insufficiency in patients with coronary artery disease).
No products indexed under this heading.

Methsuximide (Alters thyroid hormone or TSH levels).
No products indexed under this heading.

Methyclothiazide (Alters thyroid hormone or TSH levels).
No products indexed under this heading.

Methylprednisolone (Alters thyroid hormone or TSH levels).
No products indexed under this heading.

Methylprednisolone Acetate (May inhibit levothyroxine sodium binding to serum proteins or alter the concentrations of serum proteins).
No products indexed under this heading.

Methylprednisolone Sodium Succinate (May inhibit levothyroxine sodium binding to serum proteins or alter the concentrations of serum proteins).
No products indexed under this heading.

Methyltestosterone (May inhibit levothyroxine sodium binding to serum proteins or alter the concentrations of serum proteins; alters TSH or thyroid hormone levels).
No products indexed under this heading.

Metipranolol Hydrochloride (Alters thyroid hormone or TSH levels; actions of some beta blockers may be impaired when hypothyroid patients become euthyroid).
No products indexed under this heading.

Metoclopramide Hydrochloride (Alters thyroid hormone or TSH levels). Products include:
Metozolv ODT 2901

Metoprolol Succinate (Alters thyroid hormone or TSH levels; actions of some beta blockers may be impaired when hypothyroid patients become euthyroid). Products include:
Toprol XL 732

Metoprolol Tartrate (Alters thyroid hormone or TSH levels; actions of some beta blockers may be impaired when hypothyroid patients become euthyroid).
No products indexed under this heading.

Miglitol (Requirements of oral antidiabetic agents may be reduced in hypothyroid patients with diabetes and may be subsequently increased with initiation of thyroid hormone therapy).
No products indexed under this heading.

Mitotane (Alters thyroid hormone or TSH levels).
No products indexed under this heading.

Modafinil (Alters thyroid hormone or TSH levels). Products include:
Provigil 983

Nadolol (Alters thyroid hormone or TSH levels; actions of some beta blockers may be impaired when hypothyroid patients become euthyroid). Products include:
Nadolol 2359

Nafcillin Sodium (Alters thyroid hormone or TSH levels).
No products indexed under this heading.

Nateglinide (Requirements of oral antidiabetic agents may be reduced in hypothyroid patients with diabetes and may be subsequently increased with initiation of thyroid hormone therapy).
No products indexed under this heading.

Nebivolol (Alters thyroid hormone or TSH levels; actions of some beta blockers may be impaired when hypothyroid patients become euthyroid). Products include:
Bystolic 1147

Nevirapine (Alters thyroid hormone or TSH levels). Products include:
Viramune Oral Suspension 897
Viramune Tablets 897

Nicotine (Alters thyroid hormone or TSH levels).
No products indexed under this heading.

Nicotine Polacrilex (Alters thyroid hormone or TSH levels).
No products indexed under this heading.

Nicotine Salicylate (Alters thyroid hormone or TSH levels).
No products indexed under this heading.

Nicotine Sulfate (Alters thyroid hormone or TSH levels).
No products indexed under this heading.

Norepinephrine Bitartrate (Possible increased risk of coronary insufficiency in patients with coronary artery disease).
No products indexed under this heading.

Norethindrone (Alters thyroid hormone or TSH levels). Products include:
Ortho Micronor 2660

Norethindrone Acetate (Alters thyroid hormone or TSH levels). Products include:
Activella 2561

Nortriptyline Hydrochloride (Concurrent use may increase the therapeutic and toxic effects of both drugs; onset of action of tricyclics may be accelerated).
No products indexed under this heading.

Octreotide Acetate (Alters thyroid hormone or TSH levels). Products include:
Sandostatin 2517
Sandostatin LAR 2519

Omeprazole (Alters thyroid hormone or TSH levels).
No products indexed under this heading.

Omeprazole Magnesium (Alters thyroid hormone or TSH levels).
No products indexed under this heading.

Orlistat (Concurrent use may reduce the efficacy of levothyroxine by binding and delaying or preventing absorption, potentially resulting in hypothyroidism. Patients treated concomitantly with orlistat and levothyroxine should be monitored for changes in thyroid function). Products include:
Xenical 2893

Oxandrolone (May inhibit levothyroxine sodium binding to serum proteins or alter the concentrations of serum proteins; alters TSH or thyroid hormone levels).
No products indexed under this heading.

Oxcarbazepine (Alters thyroid hormone or TSH levels).
No products indexed under this heading.

Oxymetholone (May inhibit levothyroxine sodium binding to serum proteins or alter the concentrations of serum proteins; alters TSH or thyroid hormone levels).
No products indexed under this heading.

Penbutolol Sulfate (Alters thyroid hormone or TSH levels; actions of some beta blockers may be impaired when hypothyroid patients become euthyroid).
No products indexed under this heading.

Pergolide Mesylate (Alters thyroid hormone or TSH levels).
No products indexed under this heading.

Perphenazine (May inhibit levothyroxine sodium binding to serum proteins or alter the concentrations of serum proteins).
No products indexed under this heading.

Phenobarbital (Alters thyroid hormone or TSH levels). Products include:
Donnatal 2711

Phenobarbital Sodium (Alters thyroid hormone or TSH levels).
No products indexed under this heading.

Phenylbutazone (May inhibit levothyroxine sodium binding to serum proteins or alter the concentrations of serum proteins; alters thyroid hormone or TSH levels).
No products indexed under this heading.

Phenylephrine Bitartrate (Possible increased risk of coronary insufficiency in patients with coronary artery disease).
No products indexed under this heading.

Phenylephrine Hydrochloride (Possible increased risk of coronary insufficiency in patients with coronary artery disease). Products include:
Sudafed PE Nasal Decongestant 2048
Children's Sudafed PE Nasal Decongestant 2047

Phenylephrine Tannate (Possible increased risk of coronary insufficiency in patients with coronary artery disease).
No products indexed under this heading.

Phenylpropanolamine Hydrochloride (Possible increased risk of coronary insufficiency in patients with coronary artery disease).
No products indexed under this heading.

Phenytoin (May inhibit levothyroxine sodium binding to serum proteins or alter the concentrations of serum proteins; alters thyroid hormone or TSH levels).
No products indexed under this heading.

IMPORTANT NOTE: Always consult each drug listing in the patient's regimen for possible interactions.

1817 Interactions Index Tabloid

SYSTANE ULTRA LUBRICANT EYE DROPS
(Polyethylene Glycol, Propylene Glycol)... 587
None cited in PDR database.

TABLOID TABLETS
(Thioguanine) 1664
May interact with agents associated with myelosuppression, antineoplastics, drugs that inhibit thiopurine methyltransferase (TPMT), vaccines, live, and certain other agents. Compounds in these categories include:

Altretamine (The most consistent, dose-related toxicity is bone marrow suppression. The dosage of thioguanine may need to be reduced when this agent is combined with other drugs whose primary toxicity is myelosuppression). Products include:
Hexalen 1066

Anastrozole (Although the primary toxicity of thioguanine is myelosuppression, other toxicities have occasionally been observed, particularly when thioguanine is used in combination with other cancer chemotherapeutic agents).
No products indexed under this heading.

Asparaginase (Although the primary toxicity of thioguanine is myelosuppression, other toxicities have occasionally been observed, particularly when thioguanine is used in combination with other cancer chemotherapeutic agents).
Products include:
Elspar 2005, 2122

BCG Vaccine (Administration of live vaccines to immunocompromised patients should be avoided).
No products indexed under this heading.

Bicalutamide (Although the primary toxicity of thioguanine is myelosuppression, other toxicities have occasionally been observed, particularly when thioguanine is used in combination with other cancer chemotherapeutic agents).
No products indexed under this heading.

Bleomycin Sulfate (Although the primary toxicity of thioguanine is myelosuppression, other toxicities have occasionally been observed, particularly when thioguanine is used in combination with other cancer chemotherapeutic agents).
No products indexed under this heading.

Busulfan (The most consistent, dose-related toxicity is bone marrow suppression. The dosage of thioguanine may need to be reduced when this agent is combined with other drugs whose primary toxicity is myelosuppression).
Products include:
Myleran 1581

Carboplatin (Although the primary toxicity of thioguanine is myelosuppression, other toxicities have occasionally been observed, particularly when thioguanine is used in combination with other cancer chemotherapeutic agents).
No products indexed under this heading.

Carmustine (BCNU) (Although the primary toxicity of thioguanine is myelosuppression, other toxicities have occasionally been observed, particularly when thioguanine is used in combination with other cancer chemotherapeutic agents).
No products indexed under this heading.

Chlorambucil (The most consistent, dose-related toxicity is bone marrow suppression. The dosage of thioguanine may need to be reduced when this agent is combined with other drugs whose primary toxicity is myelosuppression). Products include:
Leukeran 1557

Chloramphenicol (The most consistent, dose-related toxicity is bone marrow suppression. The dosage of thioguanine may need to be reduced when this agent is combined with other drugs whose primary toxicity is myelosuppression).
No products indexed under this heading.

Chloramphenicol Palmitate (The most consistent, dose-related toxicity is bone marrow suppression. The dosage of thioguanine may need to be reduced when this agent is combined with other drugs whose primary toxicity is myelosuppression).
No products indexed under this heading.

Chloramphenicol Sodium Succinate (The most consistent, dose-related toxicity is bone marrow suppression. The dosage of thioguanine may need to be reduced when this agent is combined with other drugs whose primary toxicity is myelosuppression).
No products indexed under this heading.

Cisplatin (Although the primary toxicity of thioguanine is myelosuppression, other toxicities have occasionally been observed, particularly when thioguanine is used in combination with other cancer chemotherapeutic agents).
No products indexed under this heading.

Cladribine (The most consistent, dose-related toxicity is bone marrow suppression. The dosage of thioguanine may need to be reduced when this agent is combined with other drugs whose primary toxicity is myelosuppression). Products include:
Leustatin 946

Cyclophosphamide (Although the primary toxicity of thioguanine is myelosuppression, other toxicities have occasionally been observed, particularly when thioguanine is used in combination with other cancer chemotherapeutic agents).
No products indexed under this heading.

Cytarabine (A few cases of jaundice have been reported in patients with leukemia receiving thioguanine. Six patients had received cytarabine prior to treatment with thioguanine, and some were receiving other chemotherapy in addition to thioguanine when they became symptomatic).
No products indexed under this heading.

Dacarbazine (Although the primary toxicity of thioguanine is myelosuppression, other toxicities have occasionally been observed, particularly when thioguanine is used in combination with other cancer chemotherapeutic agents).
No products indexed under this heading.

Daunorubicin Citrate (Although the primary toxicity of thioguanine is myelosuppression, other toxicities have occasionally been observed, particularly when thioguanine is used in combination with other cancer chemotherapeutic agents).
No products indexed under this heading.

Daunorubicin Citrate Liposome (The most consistent, dose-related toxicity is bone marrow suppression. The dosage of thioguanine may need to be reduced when this agent is combined with other drugs whose primary toxicity is myelosuppression).
No products indexed under this heading.

Daunorubicin Hydrochloride (The most consistent, dose-related toxicity is bone marrow suppression. The dosage of thioguanine may need to be reduced when this agent is combined with other drugs whose primary toxicity is myelosuppression).
No products indexed under this heading.

Denileukin Diftitox (Although the primary toxicity of thioguanine is myelosuppression, other toxicities have occasionally been observed, particularly when thioguanine is used in combination with other cancer chemotherapeutic agents). Products include:
Ontak 1068

Dexrazoxane (The most consistent, dose-related toxicity is bone marrow suppression. The dosage of thioguanine may need to be reduced when this agent is combined with other drugs whose primary toxicity is myelosuppression).
No products indexed under this heading.

Docetaxel (Although the primary toxicity of thioguanine is myelosuppression, other toxicities have occasionally been observed, particularly when thioguanine is used in combination with other cancer chemotherapeutic agents).
Products include:
Taxotere 3035

Doxorubicin Hydrochloride (The most consistent, dose-related toxicity is bone marrow suppression. The dosage of thioguanine may need to be reduced when this agent is combined with other drugs whose primary toxicity is myelosuppression).
No products indexed under this heading.

Doxorubicin Hydrochloride Liposome (The most consistent, dose-related toxicity is bone marrow suppression. The dosage of thioguanine may need to be reduced when this agent is combined with other drugs whose primary toxicity is myelosuppression).
Products include:
Doxil 939

Epirubicin Hydrochloride (Although the primary toxicity of thioguanine is myelosuppression, other toxicities have occasionally been observed, particularly when thioguanine is used in combination with other cancer chemotherapeutic agents).
No products indexed under this heading.

Estramustine Phosphate Sodium (Although the primary toxicity of thioguanine is myelosuppression, other toxicities have occasionally been observed, particularly when thioguanine is used in combination with other cancer chemotherapeutic agents).
No products indexed under this heading.

Etoposide (Although the primary toxicity of thioguanine is myelosuppression, other toxicities have occasionally been observed, particularly when thioguanine is used in combination with other cancer chemotherapeutic agents).
No products indexed under this heading.

Exemestane (Although the primary toxicity of thioguanine is myelosuppression, other toxicities have occasionally been observed, particularly when thioguanine is used in combination with other cancer chemotherapeutic agents).
Products include:
Aromasin 2758

Floxuridine (Although the primary toxicity of thioguanine is myelosuppression, other toxicities have occasionally been observed, particularly when thioguanine is used in combination with other cancer chemotherapeutic agents).
No products indexed under this heading.

Fludarabine Phosphate (The most consistent, dose-related toxicity is bone marrow suppression. The dosage of thioguanine may need to be reduced when this agent is combined with other drugs whose primary toxicity is myelosuppression). Products include:
Oforta 3023

Fluorouracil (Although the primary toxicity of thioguanine is myelosuppression, other toxicities have occasionally been observed, particularly when thioguanine is used in combination with other cancer chemotherapeutic agents).
Products include:
Carac 2966

Flutamide (Although the primary toxicity of thioguanine is myelosuppression, other toxicities have occasionally been observed, particularly when thioguanine is used in combination with other cancer chemotherapeutic agents).
No products indexed under this heading.

Gemcitabine Hydrochloride (The most consistent, dose-related toxicity is bone marrow suppression. The dosage of thioguanine may need to be reduced when this agent is combined with other drugs whose primary toxicity is myelosuppression). Products include:
Gemzar 1900

Gemtuzumab Ozogamicin (The most consistent, dose-related toxicity is bone marrow suppression. The dosage of thioguanine may need to be reduced when this agent is combined with other drugs whose primary toxicity is myelosuppression). Products include:
Mylotarg 3524

Hydroxyurea (Although the primary toxicity of thioguanine is myelosuppression, other toxicities have occasionally been observed, particularly when thioguanine is used in combination with other cancer chemotherapeutic agents).
No products indexed under this heading.

Idarubicin Hydrochloride (The most consistent, dose-related toxicity is bone marrow suppression. The dosage of thioguanine may need to be reduced when this agent is combined with other drugs whose primary toxicity is myelosuppression).
No products indexed under this heading.

Ifosfamide (Although the primary toxicity of thioguanine is myelosuppression, other toxicities have occasionally been observed, particularly when thioguanine is used in combination with other cancer chemotherapeutic agents).
No products indexed under this heading.

Influenza Vaccine, Live Attenuated (Administration of live vaccines to immunocompromised patients should be avoided).
No products indexed under this heading.

Influenza Virus Vaccine Live, Intranasal (Administration of live vaccines to immunocompromised patients should be avoided). Products include:
FluMist 2078

Interferon alfa-2a, Recombinant (The most consistent, dose-related toxicity is bone marrow suppression. The dosage of thioguanine may need to be reduced when this agent is combined with other drugs whose primary toxicity is myelosuppression).
No products indexed under this heading.

Interferon alfa-2b, Recombinant (Although the primary toxicity of thioguanine is myelosuppression, other toxicities have occasionally been observed, particularly when thioguanine is used in combination with other cancer chemotherapeutic agents).
Products include:
Intron A 3140

Irinotecan Hydrochloride (The most consistent, dose-related toxicity is bone marrow suppression. The dosage of thioguanine may need to be reduced when this agent is combined with other drugs whose primary toxicity is myelosuppression).
No products indexed under this heading.

Levamisole Hydrochloride (Although the primary toxicity of thioguanine is myelosuppression, other toxicities have occasionally been observed, particularly when thioguanine is used in combination with other cancer chemotherapeutic agents).
No products indexed under this heading.

IMPORTANT NOTE: Always consult each drug listing in the patient's regimen for possible interactions.

Lomustine (CCNU) (Although the primary toxicity of thioguanine is myelosuppression, other toxicities have occasionally been observed, particularly when thioguanine is used in combination with other cancer chemotherapeutic agents).
No products indexed under this heading.

Measles, Mumps, Rubella and Varicella Virus Vaccine Live (Administration of live vaccines to immunocompromised patients should be avoided). Products include:

Measles, Mumps & Rubella Virus Vaccine, Live (Administration of live vaccines to immunocompromised patients should be avoided). Products include:

Measles & Rubella Virus Vaccine Live (Administration of live vaccines to immunocompromised patients should be avoided).
No products indexed under this heading.

Measles Virus Vaccine Live (Administration of live vaccines to immunocompromised patients should be avoided). Products include:

Mechlorethamine Hydrochloride (Although the primary toxicity of thioguanine is myelosuppression, other toxicities have occasionally been observed, particularly when thioguanine is used in combination with other cancer chemotherapeutic agents). Products include:

Megestrol Acetate (Although the primary toxicity of thioguanine is myelosuppression, other toxicities have occasionally been observed, particularly when thioguanine is used in combination with other cancer chemotherapeutic agents). Products include:

Melphalan (Although the primary toxicity of thioguanine is myelosuppression, other toxicities have occasionally been observed, particularly when thioguanine is used in combination with other cancer chemotherapeutic agents). Products include:

Melphalan Hydrochloride (The most consistent, dose-related toxicity is bone marrow suppression. The dosage of thioguanine may need to be reduced when this agent is combined with other drugs whose primary toxicity is myelosuppression). Products include:

Mercaptopurine (There is usually complete cross-resistance between mercaptopurine and thioguanine).
No products indexed under this heading.

Mesalamine (Bone marrow suppression could be exacerbated by co-administration with drugs that inhibit thiopurine methyltransferase enzyme (TPMT), such as olsalazine, mesalazine, or sulphasalazine). Products include:

Mesalazine (As there is *in vitro* evidence that aminosalicylate derivatives (eg, olsalazine, mesalazine, or sulphasalazine) inhibit the thiopurine methyltransferase (TPMT) enzyme, they should be administered with caution to patients receiving concurrent thioguanine therapy. Bone marrow suppression

could be exacerbated by co-administration with drugs that inhibit TPMT).
No products indexed under this heading.

Methotrexate (Although the primary toxicity of thioguanine is myelosuppression, other toxicities have occasionally been observed, particularly when thioguanine is used in combination with other cancer chemotherapeutic agents).
No products indexed under this heading.

Methotrexate Sodium (Although the primary toxicity of thioguanine is myelosuppression, other toxicities have occasionally been observed, particularly when thioguanine is used in combination with other cancer chemotherapeutic agents).
No products indexed under this heading.

Mitomycin (Mitomycin-C) (Although the primary toxicity of thioguanine is myelosuppression, other toxicities have occasionally been observed, particularly when thioguanine is used in combination with other cancer chemotherapeutic agents).
No products indexed under this heading.

Mitotane (Although the primary toxicity of thioguanine is myelosuppression, other toxicities have occasionally been observed, particularly when thioguanine is used in combination with other cancer chemotherapeutic agents).
No products indexed under this heading.

Mitoxantrone Hydrochloride (The most consistent, dose-related toxicity is bone marrow suppression. The dosage of thioguanine may need to be reduced when this agent is combined with other drugs whose primary toxicity is myelosuppression). Products include:

Mumps Virus Vaccine, Live (Administration of live vaccines to immunocompromised patients should be avoided). Products include:

Olsalazine Sodium (As there is *in vitro* evidence that aminosalicylate derivatives (eg, olsalazine, mesalazine, or sulphasalazine) inhibit the thiopurine methyltransferase (TPMT) enzyme, they should be administered with caution to patients receiving concurrent thioguanine therapy. Bone marrow suppression could be exacerbated by co-administration with drugs that inhibit TPMT).
No products indexed under this heading.

Oxaliplatin (Although the primary toxicity of thioguanine is myelosuppression, other toxicities have occasionally been observed, particularly when thioguanine is used in combination with other cancer chemotherapeutic agents). Products include:

Paclitaxel (Although the primary toxicity of thioguanine is myelosuppression, other toxicities have occasionally been observed, particularly when thioguanine is used in combination with other cancer chemotherapeutic agents).
No products indexed under this heading.

Poliovirus Vaccine, Live, Oral, Trivalent, Types 1,2,3 (Sabin) (Administration of live vaccines to immunocompromised patients should be avoided).
No products indexed under this heading.

Procarbazine Hydrochloride (Although the primary toxicity of thioguanine is myelosuppression, other toxicities have occasionally been observed, particularly when thioguanine is used in combination with other cancer chemotherapeutic agents).
No products indexed under this heading.

Rotavirus Vaccine, Live, Oral, Tetravalent (Administration of live vaccines to immunocompromised patients should be avoided).
No products indexed under this heading.

Rubella & Mumps Virus Vaccine Live (Administration of live vaccines to immunocompromised patients should be avoided).
No products indexed under this heading.

Rubella Virus Vaccine Live (Administration of live vaccines to immunocompromised patients should be avoided). Products include:

Smallpox Vaccine (Administration of live vaccines to immunocompromised patients should be avoided).
No products indexed under this heading.

Streptozocin (Although the primary toxicity of thioguanine is myelosuppression, other toxicities have occasionally been observed, particularly when thioguanine is used in combination with other cancer chemotherapeutic agents).
No products indexed under this heading.

Sulphasalazine (As there is *in vitro* evidence that aminosalicylate derivatives (eg, olsalazine, mesalazine, or sulphasalazine) inhibit the thiopurine methyltransferase (TPMT) enzyme, they should be administered with caution to patients receiving concurrent thioguanine therapy. Bone marrow suppression could be exacerbated by co-administration with drugs that inhibit TPMT).
No products indexed under this heading.

Tamoxifen Citrate (Although the primary toxicity of thioguanine is myelosuppression, other toxicities have occasionally been observed, particularly when thioguanine is used in combination with other cancer chemotherapeutic agents).
No products indexed under this heading.

Temozolomide (The most consistent, dose-related toxicity is bone marrow suppression. The dosage of thioguanine may need to be reduced when this agent is combined with other drugs whose primary toxicity is myelosuppression). Products include:

Teniposide (Although the primary toxicity of thioguanine is myelosuppression, other toxicities have occasionally been observed, particularly when thioguanine is used in combination with other cancer chemotherapeutic agents).
No products indexed under this heading.

Thiotepa (Although the primary toxicity of thioguanine is myelosuppression, other toxicities have occasionally been observed, particularly when thioguanine is used in combination with other cancer chemotherapeutic agents).
No products indexed under this heading.

Topotecan Hydrochloride (Although the primary toxicity of thioguanine is myelosuppression, other toxicities have occasionally been observed, particularly when thioguanine is used in combination with other cancer chemotherapeutic agents). Products include:

Toremifene Citrate (Although the primary toxicity of thioguanine is myelosuppression, other toxicities have occasionally been observed, particularly when thioguanine is used in combination with other cancer chemotherapeutic agents).
No products indexed under this heading.

Typhoid Vaccine (Administration of live vaccines to immunocompromised patients should be avoided).
No products indexed under this heading.

Valrubicin (Although the primary toxicity of thioguanine is myelosuppression, other toxicities have occasionally been observed, particularly when thioguanine is used in combination with other cancer chemotherapeutic agents). Products include:

Varicella Virus Vaccine, Live (Administration of live vaccines to immunocompromised patients should be avoided). Products include:

Vincristine Sulfate (Although the primary toxicity of thioguanine is myelosuppression, other toxicities have occasionally been observed, particularly when thioguanine is used in combination with other cancer chemotherapeutic agents).
No products indexed under this heading.

Vinorelbine Tartrate (The most consistent, dose-related toxicity is bone marrow suppression. The dosage of thioguanine may need to be reduced when this agent is combined with other drugs whose primary toxicity is myelosuppression).
No products indexed under this heading.

Yellow Fever Vaccine (Administration of live vaccines to immunocompromised patients should be avoided).
No products indexed under this heading.

Zoster Vaccine Live (Administration of live vaccines to immunocompromised patients should be avoided). Products include:

TAMIFLU CAPSULES

Influenza Vaccine, Live Attenuated (The concomitant use of oseltamivir phosphate with live attenuated influenza vaccine (LAIV) intranasal has not been evaluated. However, because of the potential for interference between these products, LAIV, should not be administered within 2 weeks before or 48 hours after administration of oseltamivir phosphate, unless medically indicated. The concern about possible interferences arises from the potential for antiviral drugs to inhibit replication of live vaccine virus. Trivalent inactivated influenza vaccine can be administered at any time relative to use of oseltamivir phosphate).
No products indexed under this heading.

Probenecid (Co-administration with probenecid results in an approximate two-fold increase in exposure to oseltamivir due to a decrease in active anionic tubular secretion in the kidneys; no dose adjustments are required due to the safety margin of oseltamivir).
No products indexed under this heading.

TAMIFLU ORAL SUSPENSION

See Tamiflu Capsules

TARCEVA TABLETS

May interact with antacids, antiangiogenic drugs, antineoplastics, corticosteroids, cytochrome p450 1a2 inducers (selected), cytochrome p450 1a2 inhibitors (selected), cytochrome p450 3a4 inducers (selected), cytochrome p450 3a4 inhibitors (selected), cytochrome p450 3a4 inhibitors, potent (selected), drugs that reduce gastric acidity, non-steroidal anti-inflammatory agents, oral anticoagulants, phenytoin, proton pump inhibitor, and certain other agents. Compounds in these categories include:

Acetazolamide (Erlotinib is metabolized predominantly by CYP3A4. Inhibitors of CYP3A4 would be expected to increase exposure. Caution should be used when co-administering erlotinib with a strong CYP3A4 inhibitor; consider a dose reduction if severe adverse reactions occur).
No products indexed under this heading.

Acetazolamide Sodium (Erlotinib is metabolized predominantly by CYP3A4. Inhibitors of CYP3A4 would be expected to increase exposure. Caution should be used when co-administering erlotinib with a strong CYP3A4 inhibitor; consider a dose reduction if severe adverse reactions occur).
No products indexed under this heading.

Alatrofloxacin Mesylate (When erlotinib was co-administered with ciprofloxacin, an inhibitor of both CYP3A4 and CYP1A2, erlotinib exposure (AUC) and maximum concentration (C_{max}) increased by 39% and 17%, respectively. In patients who are taking erlotinib with an inhibitor of both CYP3A4 and CYP1A2 like ciprofloxacin, a dose reduction of erlotinib should be considered if severe adverse reactions occur).
No products indexed under this heading.

Alclometasone Dipropionate (Gastrointestinal perforation (including fatalities) has been reported in patients receiving erlotinib. Patients receiving concomitant corticosteroids are at increased risk).
No products indexed under this heading.

Allium sativum (Pre-treatment with the CYP3A4 inducer rifampicin decreased erlotinib AUC by about 2/3 to 4/5. Use of alternative treatments lacking CYP3A4 inducing activity is strongly recommended. If an alternative treatment is unavailable, an increase in the dose of erlotinib should be considered as tolerated at two week intervals while monitoring the patient's safety. If the erlotinib dose is adjusted upward, the dose will need to be reduced immediately to the indicated starting dose upon discontinuation of the CYP3A4 inducer).
No products indexed under this heading.

Altretamine (Gastrointestinal perforation (including fatalities) has been reported in patients receiving erlotinib. Patients receiving concomitant taxane-based chemotherapy are at increased risk). Products include:
Hexalen ... 1066

Aluminum Carbonate (The use of antacids may be considered in place of histamine 2 receptor blockers (H_2 blockers) or proton pump inhibitors in patients receiving erlotinib. However, no clinical study has been conducted to evaluate the effect of antacids on erlotinib pharmacokinetics. If an antacid is necessary, the antacid dose and the erlotinib dose should be separated by several hours).
No products indexed under this heading.

Aluminum Hydroxide (The use of antacids may be considered in place of histamine 2 receptor blockers (H_2 blockers) or proton pump inhibitors in patients receiving erlotinib. However, no clinical study has been conducted to evaluate the effect of antacids on erlotinib pharmacokinetics. If an antacid is necessary, the antacid dose and the erlotinib dose should be separated by several hours).
No products indexed under this heading.

Aminoglutethimide (Pre-treatment with the CYP3A4 inducer rifampicin decreased erlotinib AUC by about 2/3 to 4/5. Use of alternative treatments lacking CYP3A4 inducing activity is strongly recommended. If an alternative treatment is unavailable, an increase in the dose of erlotinib should be considered as tolerated at two week intervals while monitoring the patient's safety. If the erlotinib dose is adjusted upward, the dose will need to be reduced immediately to the indicated starting dose upon discontinuation of the CYP3A4 inducer).
No products indexed under this heading.

Amiodarone Hydrochloride (Erlotinib is metabolized predominantly by CYP3A4. Inhibitors of CYP3A4 would be expected to increase exposure. Caution should be used when co-administering erlotinib with a strong CYP3A4 inhibitor; consider a dose reduction if severe adverse reactions occur).
No products indexed under this heading.

Amprenavir (Erlotinib is metabolized predominantly by CYP3A4. Inhibitors of CYP3A4 would be expected to increase exposure. Caution should be used when co-administering erlotinib with a strong CYP3A4 inhibitor; consider a dose reduction if severe adverse reactions occur).
No products indexed under this heading.

Anastrozole (Gastrointestinal perforation (including fatalities) has been reported in patients receiving erlotinib. Patients receiving concomitant taxane-based chemotherapy are at increased risk).
No products indexed under this heading.

Anisindione (International Normalized Ratio (INR) elevations and infrequent reports of bleeding events including gastrointestinal and non-gastrointestinal bleedings have been reported in clinical studies, some associated with concomitant warfarin administration. Patients taking warfarin or other coumarin-derivative anticoagulants should be monitored regularly for changes in prothrombin time or INR).
No products indexed under this heading.

Aprepitant (Erlotinib is metabolized predominantly by CYP3A4. Inhibitors of CYP3A4 would be expected to increase exposure. Caution should be used when co-administering erlotinib with a strong CYP3A4 inhibitor; consider a dose reduction if severe adverse reactions occur). Products include:
Emend ... 2124

Asparaginase (Gastrointestinal perforation (including fatalities) has been reported in patients receiving erlotinib. Patients receiving concomitant taxane-based chemotherapy are at increased risk). Products include:
Elspar ... 2005, 2122

Atazanavir (Erlotinib is metabolized predominantly by CYP3A4. Inhibitors of CYP3A4 would be expected to increase exposure. Caution should be used when co-administering erlotinib with a strong CYP3A4 inhibitor, such as atazanavir; consider a dose reduction if severe adverse reactions occur).
No products indexed under this heading.

Atazanavir Sulfate (Erlotinib is metabolized predominantly by CYP3A4. Inhibitors of CYP3A4 would be expected to increase exposure. Caution should be used when co-administering erlotinib with a strong CYP3A4 inhibitor, such as atazanavir; consider a dose reduction if severe adverse reactions occur).
No products indexed under this heading.

Beclomethasone Dipropionate (Gastrointestinal perforation (including fatalities) has been reported in patients receiving erlotinib. Patients receiving concomitant corticosteroids are at increased risk). Products include:
Qvar ... 3398

Beclomethasone Dipropionate Monohydrate (Gastrointestinal perforation (including fatalities) has been reported in patients receiving erlotinib. Patients receiving concomitant corticosteroids are at increased risk). Products include:
Beconase AQ ... 1386

Betamethasone (Gastrointestinal perforation (including fatalities) has been reported in patients receiving erlotinib. Patients receiving concomitant corticosteroids are at increased risk).
No products indexed under this heading.

Betamethasone Acetate (Gastrointestinal perforation (including fatalities) has been reported in patients receiving erlotinib. Patients receiving concomitant corticosteroids are at increased risk).
No products indexed under this heading.

Betamethasone Benzoate (Gastrointestinal perforation (including fatalities) has been reported in patients receiving erlotinib. Patients receiving concomitant corticosteroids are at increased risk).
No products indexed under this heading.

Betamethasone Dipropionate (Gastrointestinal perforation (including fatalities) has been reported in patients receiving erlotinib. Patients receiving concomitant corticosteroids are at increased risk). Products include:
Diprolene Lotion 0.05% ... 3108
Diprolene Ointment 0.05% ... 3109
Diprolene AF Cream 0.05% ... 3107
Lotrisone ... 3163

Betamethasone Sodium Phosphate (Gastrointestinal perforation (including fatalities) has been reported in patients receiving erlotinib. Patients receiving concomitant corticosteroids are at increased risk).
No products indexed under this heading.

Betamethasone Valerate (Gastrointestinal perforation (including fatalities) has been reported in patients receiving erlotinib. Patients receiving concomitant corticosteroids are at increased risk). Products include:
Luxiq ... 3321

Bevacizumab (Gastrointestinal perforation (including fatalities) has been reported in patients receiving erlotinib. Patients receiving concomitant anti-angiogenic agents are at increased risk. Permanently discontinue erlotinib in patients who develop gastrointestinal perforation). Products include:
Avastin ... 1187

Bicalutamide (Gastrointestinal perforation (including fatalities) has been reported in patients receiving erlotinib. Patients receiving concomitant taxane-based chemotherapy are at increased risk).
No products indexed under this heading.

Bleomycin Sulfate (Gastrointestinal perforation (including fatalities) has been reported in patients receiving erlotinib. Patients receiving concomitant taxane-based chemotherapy are at increased risk).
No products indexed under this heading.

Bosentan (Pre-treatment with the CYP3A4 inducer rifampicin decreased erlotinib AUC by about 2/3 to 4/5. Use of alternative treatments lacking CYP3A4 inducing activity is strongly recommended. If an alternative treatment is unavailable, an increase in the dose of erlotinib should be considered as tolerated at two week intervals while monitoring the patient's safety. If the erlotinib dose is adjusted upward, the dose will need to be reduced immediately to the indicated starting dose upon discontinuation of the CYP3A4 inducer). Products include:
Tracleer ... 573

Budesonide (Gastrointestinal perforation (including fatalities) has been reported in patients receiving erlotinib. Patients receiving concomitant corticosteroids are at increased risk). Products include:
Pulmicort Flexhaler ... 714
Symbicort 80/4.5 ... 720
Symbicort 160/4.5 ... 720

Busulfan (Gastrointestinal perforation (including fatalities) has been reported in patients receiving erlotinib. Patients receiving concomitant taxane-based chemotherapy are at increased risk). Products include:
Myleran ... 1581

Calcium Carbonate (The use of antacids may be considered in place of histamine 2 receptor blockers (H_2 blockers) or proton pump inhibitors in patients receiving erlotinib. However, no clinical study has been conducted to evaluate the effect of antacids on erlotinib pharmacokinetics. If an antacid is necessary, the antacid dose and the erlotinib dose should be separated by several hours). Products include:
Chelated Mineral ... 3476
Pepcid Complete ... 1822
Extra Strength Rolaids Softchews Vanilla Creme ... 2045

Carbamazepine (Pre-treatment with the CYP3A4 inducer rifampicin decreased erlotinib AUC by about 2/3 to 4/5. Use of alternative treatments lacking CYP3A4 inducing activity is strongly recommended. If an alternative treatment is unavailable, an increase in the dose of erlotinib should be considered as tolerated at two week intervals while monitoring the patient's safety. If the erlotinib dose is adjusted upward, the dose will need to be reduced immediately to the indicated starting dose upon discontinuation of the CYP3A4 inducer. CYP3A4 inducers include carbamazepine). Products include:
Carbatrol ... 3280
Equetro ... 3477

Carboplatin (Gastrointestinal perforation (including fatalities) has been reported in patients receiving erlotinib. Patients receiving concomitant taxane-based chemotherapy are at increased risk).
No products indexed under this heading.

Carmustine (BCNU) (Gastrointestinal perforation (including fatalities) has been reported in patients receiving erlotinib. Patients receiving concomitant taxane-based chemotherapy are at increased risk).
No products indexed under this heading.

Celecoxib (Gastrointestinal perforation (including fatalities) has been reported in patients receiving erlotinib. Patients receiving concomitant NSAIDs are at increased risk). Products include:
Celebrex ... 3272

Cetuximab (Gastrointestinal perforation (including fatalities) has been reported in patients receiving erlotinib. Patients receiving concomitant anti-angiogenic agents are at increased risk. Permanently discontinue erlotinib in patients who develop gastrointestinal perforation).
No products indexed under this heading.

Chlorambucil (Gastrointestinal perforation (including fatalities) has been reported in patients receiving erlotinib. Patients receiving concomitant taxane-based chemotherapy are at increased risk). Products include:
Leukeran ... 1557

Ciclesonide (Gastrointestinal perforation (including fatalities) has been reported in patients receiving erlotinib. Patients receiving concomitant corticosteroids are at increased risk).
No products indexed under this heading.

Tarceva Interactions Index 1820

Cimetidine (Drugs that alter the pH of the upper GI tract may alter the solubility of erlotinib and reduce its bioavailability).
No products indexed under this heading.

Cimetidine Hydrochloride (Drugs that alter the pH of the upper GI tract may alter the solubility of erlotinib and reduce its bioavailability).
No products indexed under this heading.

Ciprofloxacin (When erlotinib was co-administered with ciprofloxacin, an inhibitor of both CYP3A4 and CYP1A2, erlotinib exposure (AUC) and maximum concentration (C_{max}) increased by 39% and 17%, respectively. In patients who are taking erlotinib with an inhibitor of both CYP3A4 and CYP1A2 like ciprofloxacin, a dose reduction of erlotinib should be considered if severe adverse reactions occur). Products include:
Cipro I.V. ... 3082
Cipro ... 3073
Cipro XR ... 3091
Ciprodex ... 583

Ciprofloxacin Hydrochloride (When erlotinib was co-administered with ciprofloxacin, an inhibitor of both CYP3A4 and CYP1A2, erlotinib exposure (AUC) and maximum concentration (C_{max}) increased by 39% and 17%, respectively. In patients who are taking erlotinib with an inhibitor of both CYP3A4 and CYP1A2 like ciprofloxacin, a dose reduction of erlotinib should be considered if severe adverse reactions occur). Products include:
Cipro ... 3073

Cisplatin (Gastrointestinal perforation (including fatalities) has been reported in patients receiving erlotinib. Patients receiving concomitant taxane-based chemotherapy are at increased risk).
No products indexed under this heading.

Citalopram Hydrobromide (CYP1A2 inducers may decrease erlotinib plasma concentrations). Products include:
Celexa ... 1153

Clarithromycin (Erlotinib is metabolized predominantly by CYP3A4. Inhibitors of CYP3A4 would be expected to increase exposure. Caution should be used when co-administering erlotinib with a strong CYP3A4 inhibitor, such as clarithromycin; consider a dose reduction if severe adverse reactions occur). Products include:
Biaxin/Biaxin XL ... 412

Clotrimazole (Erlotinib is metabolized predominantly by CYP3A4. Inhibitors of CYP3A4 would be expected to increase exposure. Caution should be used when co-administering erlotinib with a strong CYP3A4 inhibitor; consider a dose reduction if severe adverse reactions occur). Products include:
Lotrisone ... 3163

Conivaptan Hydrochloride (Erlotinib is metabolized predominantly by CYP3A4. Inhibitors of CYP3A4 would be expected to increase exposure. Caution should be used when co-administering erlotinib with a strong CYP3A4 inhibitor; consider a dose reduction if severe adverse reactions occur). Products include:
Vaprisol ... 689

Cortisone Acetate (Gastrointestinal perforation (including fatalities) has been reported in patients receiving erlotinib. Patients receiving concomitant corticosteroids are at increased risk).
No products indexed under this heading.

Cyclophosphamide (Gastrointestinal perforation (including fatalities) has been reported in patients receiving erlotinib. Patients receiving concomitant taxane-based chemotherapy are at increased risk).
No products indexed under this heading.

Cyclosporine (Erlotinib is metabolized predominantly by CYP3A4. Inhibitors of CYP3A4 would be expected to increase exposure. Caution should be used when co-administering erlotinib with a strong CYP3A4 inhibitor; consider a dose reduction if severe adverse reactions occur). Products include:
Gengraf ... 440
Neoral Oral Solution ... 2496
Neoral Capsules ... 2496
Restasis ... 605

Dacarbazine (Gastrointestinal perforation (including fatalities) has been reported in patients receiving erlotinib. Patients receiving concomitant taxane-based chemotherapy are at increased risk).
No products indexed under this heading.

Dalfopristin (Erlotinib is metabolized predominantly by CYP3A4. Inhibitors of CYP3A4 would be expected to increase exposure. Caution should be used when co-administering erlotinib with a strong CYP3A4 inhibitor; consider a dose reduction if severe adverse reactions occur).
No products indexed under this heading.

Danazol (Erlotinib is metabolized predominantly by CYP3A4. Inhibitors of CYP3A4 would be expected to increase exposure. Caution should be used when co-administering erlotinib with a strong CYP3A4 inhibitor; consider a dose reduction if severe adverse reactions occur).
No products indexed under this heading.

Darunavir (Erlotinib is metabolized predominantly by CYP3A4. Inhibitors of CYP3A4 would be expected to increase exposure. Caution should be used when co-administering erlotinib with a strong CYP3A4 inhibitor; consider a dose reduction if severe adverse reactions occur).
No products indexed under this heading.

Dasatinib (Erlotinib is metabolized predominantly by CYP3A4. Inhibitors of CYP3A4 would be expected to increase exposure. Caution should be used when co-administering erlotinib with a strong CYP3A4 inhibitor; consider a dose reduction if severe adverse reactions occur).
No products indexed under this heading.

Daunorubicin Citrate (Gastrointestinal perforation (including fatalities) has been reported in patients receiving erlotinib. Patients receiving concomitant taxane-based chemotherapy are at increased risk).
No products indexed under this heading.

Daunorubicin Hydrochloride (Gastrointestinal perforation (including fatalities) has been reported in patients receiving erlotinib. Patients receiving concomitant taxane-based chemotherapy are at increased risk).
No products indexed under this heading.

Delavirdine Mesylate (Erlotinib is metabolized predominantly by CYP3A4. Inhibitors of CYP3A4 would be expected to increase exposure. Caution should be used when co-administering erlotinib with a strong CYP3A4 inhibitor; consider a dose reduction if severe adverse reactions occur).
No products indexed under this heading.

Delavirine (Erlotinib is metabolized predominantly by CYP3A4. Inhibitors of CYP3A4 would be expected to increase exposure. Caution should be used when co-administering erlotinib with a strong CYP3A4 inhibitor; consider a dose reduction if severe adverse reactions occur).
No products indexed under this heading.

Denileukin Diftitox (Gastrointestinal perforation (including fatalities) has been reported in patients receiving erlotinib. Patients receiving concomitant taxane-based chemotherapy are at increased risk). Products include:
Ontak ... 1068

Desloratadine (Erlotinib is metabolized predominantly by CYP3A4. Inhibitors of CYP3A4 would be expected to increase exposure. Caution should be used when co-administering erlotinib with a strong CYP3A4 inhibitor; consider a dose reduction if severe adverse reactions occur). Products include:
Clarinex Syrup ... 3098
Clarinex ... 3098
Clarinex Reditabs ... 3098
Clarinex-D 12-Hour ... 3101
Clarinex-D ... 3104

Desogestrel (When erlotinib was co-administered with ciprofloxacin, an inhibitor of both CYP3A4 and CYP1A2, erlotinib exposure (AUC) and maximum concentration (C_{max}) increased by 39% and 17%, respectively. In patients who are taking erlotinib with an inhibitor of both CYP3A4 and CYP1A2 like ciprofloxacin, a dose reduction of erlotinib should be considered if severe adverse reactions occur).
No products indexed under this heading.

Desoximetasone (Gastrointestinal perforation (including fatalities) has been reported in patients receiving erlotinib. Patients receiving concomitant corticosteroids are at increased risk).
No products indexed under this heading.

Dexamethasone (Gastrointestinal perforation (including fatalities) has been reported in patients receiving erlotinib. Patients receiving concomitant corticosteroids are at increased risk). Products include:
Ciprodex ... 583
Ozurdex ... ⊙ 223
Tobramycin and Dexamethasone Ophthalmic Suspension ... ⊙ 251

Dexamethasone Acetate (Gastrointestinal perforation (including fatalities) has been reported in patients receiving erlotinib. Patients receiving concomitant corticosteroids are at increased risk).
No products indexed under this heading.

Dexamethasone Phosphate (Gastrointestinal perforation (including fatalities) has been reported in patients receiving erlotinib. Patients receiving concomitant corticosteroids are at increased risk).
No products indexed under this heading.

Dexamethasone Sodium (Gastrointestinal perforation (including fatalities) has been reported in patients receiving erlotinib. Patients receiving concomitant corticosteroids are at increased risk).
No products indexed under this heading.

Dexamethasone Sodium Phosphate (Gastrointestinal perforation (including fatalities) has been reported in patients receiving erlotinib. Patients receiving concomitant corticosteroids are at increased risk).
No products indexed under this heading.

Dexamethasone Sodium Phosphate Injection (Gastrointestinal perforation (including fatalities) has been reported in patients receiving erlotinib. Patients receiving concomitant corticosteroids are at increased risk).
No products indexed under this heading.

Dexlansoprazole (Drugs that alter the pH of the upper GI tract may alter the solubility of erlotinib and reduce its bioavailability. Co-administration of erlotinib with omeprazole, a proton pump inhibitor, decreased the erlotinib AUC by 46%. Increasing the dose of erlotinib when co-administered with such agents is not likely to compensate for the loss of exposure. Since proton pump inhibitors affect pH of the upper GI tract for an extended period, separation of doses may not eliminate the interaction. The concomitant use of proton pump inhibitors with erlotinib should be avoided if possible). Products include:
Kapidex ... 3362

Diclofenac Epolamine (Gastrointestinal perforation (including fatalities) has been reported in patients receiving erlotinib. Patients receiving concomitant NSAIDs are at increased risk). Products include:
Flector ... 1839

Diclofenac Potassium (Gastrointestinal perforation (including fatalities) has been reported in patients receiving erlotinib. Patients receiving concomitant NSAIDs are at increased risk).
No products indexed under this heading.

Diclofenac Sodium (Gastrointestinal perforation (including fatalities) has been reported in patients receiving erlotinib. Patients receiving concomitant NSAIDs are at increased risk).
No products indexed under this heading.

Dicumarol (International Normalized Ratio (INR) elevations and infrequent reports of bleeding events including gastrointestinal and non-gastrointestinal bleedings have been reported in clinical studies, some associated with concomitant warfarin administration. Patients taking warfarin or other coumarin-derivative anticoagulants should be monitored regularly for changes in prothrombin time or INR).
No products indexed under this heading.

Diflorasone Diacetate (Gastrointestinal perforation (including fatalities) has been reported in patients receiving erlotinib. Patients receiving concomitant corticosteroids are at increased risk).
No products indexed under this heading.

Diltiazem Hydrochloride (Erlotinib is metabolized predominantly by CYP3A4. Inhibitors of CYP3A4 would be expected to increase exposure. Caution should be used when co-administering erlotinib with a strong CYP3A4 inhibitor; consider a dose reduction if severe adverse reactions occur). Products include:
Cardizem LA ... 423

Diltiazem Maleate (Erlotinib is metabolized predominantly by CYP3A4. Inhibitors of CYP3A4 would be expected to increase exposure. Caution should be used when co-administering erlotinib with a strong CYP3A4 inhibitor; consider a dose reduction if severe adverse reactions occur).
No products indexed under this heading.

Docetaxel (Gastrointestinal perforation (including fatalities) has been reported in patients receiving erlotinib. Patients receiving concomitant taxane-based chemotherapy are at increased risk). Products include:
Taxotere ... 3035

Doxorubicin Hydrochloride (Gastrointestinal perforation (including fatalities) has been reported in patients receiving erlotinib. Patients receiving concomitant taxane-based chemotherapy are at increased risk).
No products indexed under this heading.

Efavirenz (Erlotinib is metabolized predominantly by CYP3A4. Inhibitors of CYP3A4 would be expected to increase exposure. Caution should be used when co-administering erlotinib with a strong CYP3A4 inhibitor; consider a dose reduction if severe adverse reactions occur). Products include:
Atripla ... 906

Enoxacin (When erlotinib was co-administered with ciprofloxacin, an inhibitor of both CYP3A4 and CYP1A2, erlotinib exposure (AUC) and maximum concentration (C_{max}) increased by 39% and 17%, respectively. In patients who are taking erlotinib with an inhibitor of both CYP3A4 and CYP1A2 like ciprofloxacin, a dose reduction of erlotinib should be considered if severe adverse reactions occur).
No products indexed under this heading.

IMPORTANT NOTE: Always consult each drug listing in the patient's regimen for possible interactions.

while monitoring the patient's safety. If the erlotinib dose is adjusted upward, the dose will need to be reduced immediately to the indicated starting dose upon discontinuation of the CYP3A4 inducer. CYP3A4 inducers include phenytoin).

No products indexed under this heading.

Garlic Extract (Pre-treatment with the CYP3A4 inducer rifampicin decreased erlotinib AUC by about 2/3 to 4/5. Use of alternative treatments lacking CYP3A4 inducing activity is strongly recommended. If an alternative treatment is unavailable, an increase in the dose of erlotinib should be considered as tolerated at two week intervals while monitoring the patient's safety. If the erlotinib dose is adjusted upward, the dose will need to be reduced immediately to the indicated starting dose upon discontinuation of the CYP3A4 inducer).

No products indexed under this heading.

Garlic Oil (Pre-treatment with the CYP3A4 inducer rifampicin decreased erlotinib AUC by about 2/3 to 4/5. Use of alternative treatments lacking CYP3A4 inducing activity is strongly recommended. If an alternative treatment is unavailable, an increase in the dose of erlotinib should be considered as tolerated at two week intervals while monitoring the patient's safety. If the erlotinib dose is adjusted upward, the dose will need to be reduced immediately to the indicated starting dose upon discontinuation of the CYP3A4 inducer).

No products indexed under this heading.

Gatifloxacin (When erlotinib was co-administered with ciprofloxacin, an inhibitor of both CYP3A4 and CYP1A2, erlotinib exposure (AUC) and maximum concentration (C_{max}) increased by 39% and 17%, respectively. In patients who are taking erlotinib with an inhibitor of both CYP3A4 and CYP1A2 like ciprofloxacin, a dose reduction of erlotinib should be considered if severe adverse reactions occur).

No products indexed under this heading.

Gemcitabine Hydrochloride (Gastrointestinal perforation (including fatalities) has been reported in patients receiving erlotinib. Patients receiving concomitant taxane-based chemotherapy are at increased risk). Products include:

Gemzar 1900

Gemifloxacin Mesylate (When erlotinib was co-administered with ciprofloxacin, an inhibitor of both CYP3A4 and CYP1A2, erlotinib exposure (AUC) and maximum concentration (C_{max}) increased by 39% and 17%, respectively. In patients who are taking erlotinib with an inhibitor of both CYP3A4 and CYP1A2 like ciprofloxacin, a dose reduction of erlotinib should be considered if severe adverse reactions occur).

No products indexed under this heading.

Grepafloxacin Hydrochloride (When erlotinib was co-administered with ciprofloxacin, an inhibitor of both CYP3A4 and CYP1A2, erlotinib exposure (AUC) and maximum concentration (C_{max}) increased by 39% and 17%, respectively. In patients who are taking erlotinib with an inhibitor of both CYP3A4 and CYP1A2 like ciprofloxacin, a dose reduction of erlotinib should be considered if severe adverse reactions occur).

No products indexed under this heading.

Hydrocortisone (Gastrointestinal perforation (including fatalities) has been reported in patients receiving erlotinib. Patients receiving concomitant corticosteroids are at increased risk).

No products indexed under this heading.

Hydrocortisone (Alcohol) (Gastrointestinal perforation (including fatalities) has been reported in patients receiving erlotinib. Patients receiving concomitant corticosteroids are at increased risk).

No products indexed under this heading.

Hydrocortisone Acetate (Gastrointestinal perforation (including fatalities) has been reported in patients receiving erlotinib. Patients receiving concomitant corticosteroids are at increased risk).

No products indexed under this heading.

Hydrocortisone Butyrate (Gastrointestinal perforation (including fatalities) has been reported in patients receiving erlotinib. Patients receiving concomitant corticosteroids are at increased risk).

No products indexed under this heading.

Hydrocortisone Cypionate (Gastrointestinal perforation (including fatalities) has been reported in patients receiving erlotinib. Patients receiving concomitant corticosteroids are at increased risk).

No products indexed under this heading.

Hydrocortisone Hemisuccinate (Gastrointestinal perforation (including fatalities) has been reported in patients receiving erlotinib. Patients receiving concomitant corticosteroids are at increased risk).

No products indexed under this heading.

Hydrocortisone Probutate (Gastrointestinal perforation (including fatalities) has been reported in patients receiving erlotinib. Patients receiving concomitant corticosteroids are at increased risk).

No products indexed under this heading.

Hydrocortisone Sodium Phosphate (Gastrointestinal perforation (including fatalities) has been reported in patients receiving erlotinib. Patients receiving concomitant corticosteroids are at increased risk).

No products indexed under this heading.

Hydrocortisone Sodium Succinate (Gastrointestinal perforation (including fatalities) has been reported in patients receiving erlotinib. Patients receiving concomitant corticosteroids are at increased risk).

No products indexed under this heading.

Hydrocortisone Valerate (Gastrointestinal perforation (including fatalities) has been reported in patients receiving erlotinib. Patients receiving concomitant corticosteroids are at increased risk).

No products indexed under this heading.

Hydroxyurea (Gastrointestinal perforation (including fatalities) has been reported in patients receiving erlotinib. Patients receiving concomitant taxane-based chemotherapy are at increased risk).

No products indexed under this heading.

Hypericum (Pre-treatment with the CYP3A4 inducer rifampicin decreased erlotinib AUC by about 2/3 to 4/5. Use of alternative treatments lacking CYP3A4 inducing activity is strongly recommended. If an alternative treatment is unavailable, an increase in the dose of erlotinib should be considered as tolerated at two week intervals while monitoring the patient's safety. If the erlotinib dose is adjusted upward, the dose will need to be reduced immediately to the indicated starting dose upon discontinuation of the CYP3A4 inducer. CYP3A4 inducers include St. John's wort).

No products indexed under this heading.

Hypericum Perforatum (Pre-treatment with the CYP3A4 inducer rifampicin decreased erlotinib AUC by about 2/3 to 4/5. Use of alternative treatments lacking CYP3A4 inducing activity is strongly recommended. If an alternative treatment is unavailable, an

increase in the dose of erlotinib should be considered as tolerated at two week intervals while monitoring the patient's safety. If the erlotinib dose is adjusted upward, the dose will need to be reduced immediately to the indicated starting dose upon discontinuation of the CYP3A4 inducer. CYP3A4 inducers include St. John's wort). Products include:

Traumeel 1800

Ibuprofen (Gastrointestinal perforation (including fatalities) has been reported in patients receiving erlotinib. Patients receiving concomitant NSAIDs are at increased risk). Products include:

Motrin IB 2043
Children's Motrin 2044
Children's Motrin Non-Staining
    Dye-Free 2044
Infants' Motrin 2044
Infants' Motrin Dye-Free 2044
Junior Strength Motrin 2044
Vicoprofen 564

Idarubicin Hydrochloride (Gastrointestinal perforation (including fatalities) has been reported in patients receiving erlotinib. Patients receiving concomitant taxane-based chemotherapy are at increased risk).

No products indexed under this heading.

Ifosfamide (Gastrointestinal perforation (including fatalities) has been reported in patients receiving erlotinib. Patients receiving concomitant taxane-based chemotherapy are at increased risk).

No products indexed under this heading.

Imatinib Mesylate (Erlotinib is metabolized predominantly by CYP3A4. Inhibitors of CYP3A4 would be expected to increase exposure. Caution should be used when co-administering erlotinib with a strong CYP3A4 inhibitor; consider a dose reduction if severe adverse reactions occur). Products include:

Gleevec 2477

Indinavir Sulfate (Erlotinib is metabolized predominantly by CYP3A4. Inhibitors of CYP3A4 would be expected to increase exposure. Caution should be used when co-administering erlotinib with a strong CYP3A4 inhibitor, such as indinavir; consider a dose reduction if severe adverse reactions occur). Products include:

Crixivan 2113

Indomethacin (Gastrointestinal perforation (including fatalities) has been reported in patients receiving erlotinib. Patients receiving concomitant NSAIDs are at increased risk). Products include:

Indocin 2167

Indomethacin Sodium Trihydrate (Gastrointestinal perforation (including fatalities) has been reported in patients receiving erlotinib. Patients receiving concomitant NSAIDs are at increased risk). Products include:

Indocin I.V. 2007

Insulin (CYP1A2 inducers may decrease erlotinib plasma concentrations).

No products indexed under this heading.

Insulin, Human, Zinc Suspension (CYP1A2 inducers may decrease erlotinib plasma concentrations).

No products indexed under this heading.

Insulin, Human (rDNA origin) (CYP1A2 inducers may decrease erlotinib plasma concentrations). Products include:

Exubera 2717

Insulin, Human NPH (CYP1A2 inducers may decrease erlotinib plasma concentrations). Products include:

Humulin N Vial 1934

Insulin, Human Regular (CYP1A2 inducers may decrease erlotinib plasma concentrations). Products include:

Humulin R 1937

Humulin R (U-500) 1939

Insulin, Human Regular and Human NPH Mixture (CYP1A2 inducers may decrease erlotinib plasma concentrations). Products include:

Humulin 50/50 1930
Humulin 70/30 Vial 1931

Insulin, NPH (CYP1A2 inducers may decrease erlotinib plasma concentrations).

No products indexed under this heading.

Insulin, Regular (CYP1A2 inducers may decrease erlotinib plasma concentrations).

No products indexed under this heading.

Insulin, Regular and NPH mixture (CYP1A2 inducers may decrease erlotinib plasma concentrations).

No products indexed under this heading.

Insulin, Zinc Crystals (CYP1A2 inducers may decrease erlotinib plasma concentrations).

No products indexed under this heading.

Insulin, Zinc Suspension (CYP1A2 inducers may decrease erlotinib plasma concentrations).

No products indexed under this heading.

Insulin Aspart (CYP1A2 inducers may decrease erlotinib plasma concentrations).

No products indexed under this heading.

Insulin Aspart, Human (CYP1A2 inducers may decrease erlotinib plasma concentrations). Products include:

NovoLog Mix 70/30 2581

Insulin Aspart, Human Regular (CYP1A2 inducers may decrease erlotinib plasma concentrations). Products include:

NovoLog 2575

Insulin Aspart Protamine, Human (CYP1A2 inducers may decrease erlotinib plasma concentrations). Products include:

NovoLog Mix 70/30 2581

Insulin Detemir (rDNA Origin) (CYP1A2 inducers may decrease erlotinib plasma concentrations). Products include:

Levemir 2566

Insulin Glargine (CYP1A2 inducers may decrease erlotinib plasma concentrations). Products include:

Lantus 2996

Insulin Glulisine (CYP1A2 inducers may decrease erlotinib plasma concentrations). Products include:

Apidra 2937
Apidra SoloStar 2937

Insulin Lispro, Human (CYP1A2 inducers may decrease erlotinib plasma concentrations). Products include:

Humalog 1910
Humalog Mix 1914
Humalog Mix 75/25 1917

Insulin Lispro Protamine, Human (CYP1A2 inducers may decrease erlotinib plasma concentrations). Products include:

Humalog Mix 1914
Humalog Mix 75/25 1917

Interferon alfa-2a, Recombinant (Gastrointestinal perforation (including fatalities) has been reported in patients receiving erlotinib. Patients receiving concomitant taxane-based chemotherapy are at increased risk).

No products indexed under this heading.

Interferon alfa-2b, Recombinant (Gastrointestinal perforation (including fatalities) has been reported in patients receiving erlotinib. Patients receiving concomitant taxane-based chemotherapy are at increased risk). Products include:

Intron A 3140

Irinotecan Hydrochloride (Gastrointestinal perforation (including fatalities) has been reported in patients receiving erlotinib. Patients receiving concomitant taxane-based chemotherapy are at increased risk).
No products indexed under this heading.

Isoniazid (Erlotinib is metabolized predominantly by CYP3A4. Inhibitors of CYP3A4 would be expected to increase exposure. Caution should be used when co-administering erlotinib with a strong CYP3A4 inhibitor; consider a dose reduction if severe adverse reactions occur).
No products indexed under this heading.

Itraconazole (Erlotinib is metabolized predominantly by CYP3A4. Inhibitors of CYP3A4 would be expected to increase exposure. Caution should be used when co-administering erlotinib with a strong CYP3A4 inhibitor, such as itraconazole; consider a dose reduction if severe adverse reactions occur).
No products indexed under this heading.

Ketoconazole (Erlotinib is metabolized predominantly by CYP3A4. Co-treatment with the potent CYP3A4 inhibitor ketoconazole increases erlotinib AUC by 2/3. Caution should be used when co-administering erlotinib with a strong CYP3A4 inhibitor, such as ketoconazole; consider a dose reduction if severe adverse reactions occur). Products include:
Extina 3319
Xolegel 3337

Ketoprofen (Gastrointestinal perforation (including fatalities) has been reported in patients receiving erlotinib. Patients receiving concomitant NSAIDs are at increased risk).
No products indexed under this heading.

Ketorolac Tromethamine (Gastrointestinal perforation (including fatalities) has been reported in patients receiving erlotinib. Patients receiving concomitant NSAIDs are at increased risk). Products include:
Acuvail .... ⊙ 209

Lansoprazole (Drugs that alter the pH of the upper GI tract may alter the solubility of erlotinib and reduce its bioavailability. Co-administration of erlotinib with omeprazole, a proton pump inhibitor, decreased the erlotinib AUC by 46%. Increasing the dose of erlotinib when co-administered with such agents is not likely to compensate for the loss of exposure. Since proton pump inhibitors affect pH of the upper GI tract for an extended period, separation of doses may not eliminate the interaction. The concomitant use of proton pump inhibitors with erlotinib should be avoided if possible).
No products indexed under this heading.

Lapatinib (Erlotinib is metabolized predominantly by CYP3A4. Inhibitors of CYP3A4 would be expected to increase exposure. Caution should be used when co-administering erlotinib with a strong CYP3A4 inhibitor; consider a dose reduction if severe adverse reactions occur). Products include:
Tykerb 1698

Lenalidomide (Gastrointestinal perforation (including fatalities) has been reported in patients receiving erlotinib. Patients receiving concomitant anti-angiogenic agents are at increased risk. Permanently discontinue erlotinib in patients who develop gastrointestinal perforation).
No products indexed under this heading.

Levamisole Hydrochloride (Gastrointestinal perforation (including fatalities) has been reported in patients receiving erlotinib. Patients receiving concomitant taxane-based chemotherapy are at increased risk).
No products indexed under this heading.

Levofloxacin (When erlotinib was co-administered with ciprofloxacin, an inhibitor of both CYP3A4 and CYP1A2, erlotinib exposure (AUC) and maximum concentration (C_{max}) increased by 39% and 17%, respectively. In patients who are taking erlotinib with an inhibitor of both CYP3A4 and CYP1A2 like ciprofloxacin, a dose reduction of erlotinib should be considered if severe adverse reactions occur). Products include:
Iquix 3492
Levaquin 2629
Levaquin in 5% Dextrose 2629
Quixin 3493

Levonorgestrel (When erlotinib was co-administered with ciprofloxacin, an inhibitor of both CYP3A4 and CYP1A2, erlotinib exposure (AUC) and maximum concentration (C_{max}) increased by 39% and 17%, respectively. In patients who are taking erlotinib with an inhibitor of both CYP3A4 and CYP1A2 like ciprofloxacin, a dose reduction of erlotinib should be considered if severe adverse reactions occur). Products include:
Climara Pro 847
LoSeasonique 3407
Lybrel 3514
Mirena 854
Plan B 3416
Seasonique 3418

Lomefloxacin Hydrochloride (When erlotinib was co-administered with ciprofloxacin, an inhibitor of both CYP3A4 and CYP1A2, erlotinib exposure (AUC) and maximum concentration (C_{max}) increased by 39% and 17%, respectively. In patients who are taking erlotinib with an inhibitor of both CYP3A4 and CYP1A2 like ciprofloxacin, a dose reduction of erlotinib should be considered if severe adverse reactions occur).
No products indexed under this heading.

Lomustine (CCNU) (Gastrointestinal perforation (including fatalities) has been reported in patients receiving erlotinib. Patients receiving concomitant taxane-based chemotherapy are at increased risk).
No products indexed under this heading.

Lopinavir (Erlotinib is metabolized predominantly by CYP3A4. Inhibitors of CYP3A4 would be expected to increase exposure. Caution should be used when co-administering erlotinib with a strong CYP3A4 inhibitor; consider a dose reduction if severe adverse reactions occur). Products include:
Kaletra 458

Loratadine (Erlotinib is metabolized predominantly by CYP3A4. Inhibitors of CYP3A4 would be expected to increase exposure. Caution should be used when co-administering erlotinib with a strong CYP3A4 inhibitor; consider a dose reduction if severe adverse reactions occur).
No products indexed under this heading.

Magaldrate (The use of antacids may be considered in place of histamine 2 receptor blockers (H_2 blockers) or proton pump inhibitors in patients receiving erlotinib. However, no clinical study has been conducted to evaluate the effect of antacids on erlotinib pharmacokinetics. If an antacid is necessary, the antacid dose and the erlotinib dose should be separated by several hours).
No products indexed under this heading.

Magnesium Carbonate (The use of antacids may be considered in place of histamine 2 receptor blockers (H_2 blockers) or proton pump inhibitors in patients receiving erlotinib. However, no clinical study has been conducted to evaluate the effect of antacids on erlotinib pharmacokinetics. If an antacid is necessary, the antacid dose and the erlotinib dose should be separated by several hours).
No products indexed under this heading.

Magnesium Hydroxide (The use of antacids may be considered in place of histamine 2 receptor blockers (H_2 blockers) or proton pump inhibitors in patients receiving erlotinib. However, no clinical study has been conducted to evaluate the effect of antacids on erlotinib pharmacokinetics. If an antacid is necessary, the antacid dose and the erlotinib dose should be separated by several hours). Products include:
Fleet Pedia-Lax Chewable Tablets 1144
Pepcid Complete 1822

Magnesium Oxide (The use of antacids may be considered in place of histamine 2 receptor blockers (H_2 blockers) or proton pump inhibitors in patients receiving erlotinib. However, no clinical study has been conducted to evaluate the effect of antacids on erlotinib pharmacokinetics. If an antacid is necessary, the antacid dose and the erlotinib dose should be separated by several hours). Products include:
Beelith 873

Magnesium Trisilicate (The use of antacids may be considered in place of histamine 2 receptor blockers (H_2 blockers) or proton pump inhibitors in patients receiving erlotinib. However, no clinical study has been conducted to evaluate the effect of antacids on erlotinib pharmacokinetics. If an antacid is necessary, the antacid dose and the erlotinib dose should be separated by several hours).
No products indexed under this heading.

Mechlorethamine Hydrochloride (Gastrointestinal perforation (including fatalities) has been reported in patients receiving erlotinib. Patients receiving concomitant taxane-based chemotherapy are at increased risk). Products include:
Mustargen 2010

Meclofenamate Sodium (Gastrointestinal perforation (including fatalities) has been reported in patients receiving erlotinib. Patients receiving concomitant NSAIDs are at increased risk).
No products indexed under this heading.

Mefenamic Acid (Gastrointestinal perforation (including fatalities) has been reported in patients receiving erlotinib. Patients receiving concomitant NSAIDs are at increased risk).
No products indexed under this heading.

Megestrol Acetate (Gastrointestinal perforation (including fatalities) has been reported in patients receiving erlotinib. Patients receiving concomitant taxane-based chemotherapy are at increased risk). Products include:
Megace ES 2698

Meloxicam (Gastrointestinal perforation (including fatalities) has been reported in patients receiving erlotinib. Patients receiving concomitant NSAIDs are at increased risk).
No products indexed under this heading.

Melphalan (Gastrointestinal perforation (including fatalities) has been reported in patients receiving erlotinib. Patients receiving concomitant taxane-based chemotherapy are at increased risk). Products include:
Alkeran 1302

Mephenytoin (Pre-treatment with the CYP3A4 inducer rifampicin decreased erlotinib AUC by about 2/3 to 4/5. Use of alternative treatments lacking CYP3A4 inducing activity is strongly recommended. If an alternative treatment is unavailable, an increase in the dose of erlotinib should be considered as tolerated at two week intervals while monitoring the patient's safety. If the erlotinib dose is adjusted upward, the dose will need to be reduced immediately to the indicated starting dose upon discontinuation of the CYP3A4 inducer).
No products indexed under this heading.

Mercaptopurine (Gastrointestinal perforation (including fatalities) has been reported in patients receiving erlotinib. Patients receiving concomitant taxane-based chemotherapy are at increased risk).
No products indexed under this heading.

Mestranol (When erlotinib was co-administered with ciprofloxacin, an inhibitor of both CYP3A4 and CYP1A2, erlotinib exposure (AUC) and maximum concentration (C_{max}) increased by 39% and 17%, respectively. In patients who are taking erlotinib with an inhibitor of both CYP3A4 and CYP1A2 like ciprofloxacin, a dose reduction of erlotinib should be considered if severe adverse reactions occur).
No products indexed under this heading.

Methotrexate (Gastrointestinal perforation (including fatalities) has been reported in patients receiving erlotinib. Patients receiving concomitant taxane-based chemotherapy are at increased risk).
No products indexed under this heading.

Methotrexate Sodium (Gastrointestinal perforation (including fatalities) has been reported in patients receiving erlotinib. Patients receiving concomitant taxane-based chemotherapy are at increased risk).
No products indexed under this heading.

Methoxsalen (When erlotinib was co-administered with ciprofloxacin, an inhibitor of both CYP3A4 and CYP1A2, erlotinib exposure (AUC) and maximum concentration (C_{max}) increased by 39% and 17%, respectively. In patients who are taking erlotinib with an inhibitor of both CYP3A4 and CYP1A2 like ciprofloxacin, a dose reduction of erlotinib should be considered if severe adverse reactions occur).
No products indexed under this heading.

Methsuximide (Pre-treatment with the CYP3A4 inducer rifampicin decreased erlotinib AUC by about 2/3 to 4/5. Use of alternative treatments lacking CYP3A4 inducing activity is strongly recommended. If an alternative treatment is unavailable, an increase in the dose of erlotinib should be considered as tolerated at two week intervals while monitoring the patient's safety. If the erlotinib dose is adjusted upward, the dose will need to be reduced immediately to the indicated starting dose upon discontinuation of the CYP3A4 inducer).
No products indexed under this heading.

Methylprednisolone (Gastrointestinal perforation (including fatalities) has been reported in patients receiving erlotinib. Patients receiving concomitant corticosteroids are at increased risk).
No products indexed under this heading.

Methylprednisolone Acetate (Gastrointestinal perforation (including fatalities) has been reported in patients receiving erlotinib. Patients receiving concomitant corticosteroids are at increased risk).
No products indexed under this heading.

Methylprednisolone Sodium Succinate (Gastrointestinal perforation (including fatalities) has been reported in patients receiving erlotinib. Patients receiving concomitant corticosteroids are at increased risk).
No products indexed under this heading.

Metronidazole (Erlotinib is metabolized predominantly by CYP3A4. Inhibitors of CYP3A4 would be expected to increase exposure. Caution should be used when co-administering erlotinib

are taking erlotinib with an inhibitor of both CYP3A4 and CYP1A2 like ciprofloxacin, a dose reduction of erlotinib should be considered if severe adverse reactions occur).
No products indexed under this heading.

Omeprazole (Drugs that alter the pH of the upper GI tract may alter the solubility of erlotinib and reduce its bioavailability. Co-administration of erlotinib with omeprazole, a proton pump inhibitor, decreased the erlotinib AUC by 46%. Increasing the dose of erlotinib when co-administered with such agents is not likely to compensate for the loss of exposure. Since proton pump inhibitors affect pH of the upper GI tract for an extended period, separation of doses may not eliminate the interaction. The concomitant use of proton pump inhibitors with erlotinib should be avoided if possible).
No products indexed under this heading.

Omeprazole Magnesium (Drugs that alter the pH of the upper GI tract may alter the solubility of erlotinib and reduce its bioavailability. Co-administration of erlotinib with omeprazole, a proton pump inhibitor, decreased the erlotinib AUC by 46%. Increasing the dose of erlotinib when co-administered with such agents is not likely to compensate for the loss of exposure. Since proton pump inhibitors affect pH of the upper GI tract for an extended period, separation of doses may not eliminate the interaction. The concomitant use of proton pump inhibitors with erlotinib should be avoided if possible).
No products indexed under this heading.

Oxaliplatin (Gastrointestinal perforation (including fatalities) has been reported in patients receiving erlotinib. Patients receiving concomitant taxane-based chemotherapy are at increased risk). Products include:
Eloxatin **2975**

Oxaprozin (Gastrointestinal perforation (including fatalities) has been reported in patients receiving erlotinib. Patients receiving concomitant NSAIDs are at increased risk).
No products indexed under this heading.

Oxcarbazepine (Pre-treatment with the CYP3A4 inducer rifampicin decreased erlotinib AUC by about 2/3 to 4/5. Use of alternative treatments lacking CYP3A4 inducing activity is strongly recommended. If an alternative treatment is unavailable, an increase in the dose of erlotinib should be considered as tolerated at two week intervals while monitoring the patient's safety. If the erlotinib dose is adjusted upward, the dose will need to be reduced immediately to the indicated starting dose upon discontinuation of the CYP3A4 inducer).
No products indexed under this heading.

Paclitaxel (Gastrointestinal perforation (including fatalities) has been reported in patients receiving erlotinib. Patients receiving concomitant taxane-based chemotherapy are at increased risk).
No products indexed under this heading.

Pantoprazole Sodium (Drugs that alter the pH of the upper GI tract may alter the solubility of erlotinib and reduce its bioavailability. Co-administration of erlotinib with omeprazole, a proton pump inhibitor, decreased the erlotinib AUC by 46%. Increasing the dose of erlotinib when co-administered with such agents is not likely to compensate for the loss of exposure. Since proton pump inhibitors affect pH of the upper GI tract for an extended period, separation of doses may not eliminate the interaction. The concomitant use of proton pump inhibitors with erlotinib should be avoided if possible). Products include:
Protonix Tablets **3571**
Protonix **3575**

Paroxetine (When erlotinib was co-administered with ciprofloxacin, an inhibitor of both CYP3A4 and CYP1A2, erlotinib exposure (AUC) and maximum concentration (C_{max}) increased by 39% and 17%, respectively. In patients who are taking erlotinib with an inhibitor of both CYP3A4 and CYP1A2 like ciprofloxacin, a dose reduction of erlotinib should be considered if severe adverse reactions occur).
No products indexed under this heading.

Paroxetine Hydrochloride (Erlotinib is metabolized predominantly by CYP3A4. Inhibitors of CYP3A4 would be expected to increase exposure. Caution should be used when co-administering erlotinib with a strong CYP3A4 inhibitor; consider a dose reduction if severe adverse reactions occur). Products include:
Paroxetine CR **2361**
Paroxetine ER **2371**
Paxil **1586**
Paxil CR **1596**

Paroxetine Mesylate (When erlotinib was co-administered with ciprofloxacin, an inhibitor of both CYP3A4 and CYP1A2, erlotinib exposure (AUC) and maximum concentration (C_{max}) increased by 39% and 17%, respectively. In patients who are taking erlotinib with an inhibitor of both CYP3A4 and CYP1A2 like ciprofloxacin, a dose reduction of erlotinib should be considered if severe adverse reactions occur).
No products indexed under this heading.

Pegaptanib sodium (Gastrointestinal perforation (including fatalities) has been reported in patients receiving erlotinib. Patients receiving concomitant anti-angiogenic agents are at increased risk. Permanently discontinue erlotinib in patients who develop gastrointestinal perforation).
No products indexed under this heading.

Phenobarbital (Pre-treatment with the CYP3A4 inducer rifampicin decreased erlotinib AUC by about 2/3 to 4/5. Use of alternative treatments lacking CYP3A4 inducing activity is strongly recommended. If an alternative treatment is unavailable, an increase in the dose of erlotinib should be considered as tolerated at two week intervals while monitoring the patient's safety. If the erlotinib dose is adjusted upward, the dose will need to be reduced immediately to the indicated starting dose upon discontinuation of the CYP3A4 inducer. CYP3A4 inducers include phenobarbital). Products include:
Donnatal **2711**

Phenobarbital Sodium (Pre-treatment with the CYP3A4 inducer rifampicin decreased erlotinib AUC by about 2/3 to 4/5. Use of alternative treatments lacking CYP3A4 inducing activity is strongly recommended. If an alternative treatment is unavailable, an increase in the dose of erlotinib should be considered as tolerated at two week intervals while monitoring the patient's safety. If the erlotinib dose is adjusted upward, the dose will need to be reduced immediately to the indicated starting dose upon discontinuation of the CYP3A4 inducer. CYP3A4 inducers include phenobarbital).
No products indexed under this heading.

Phenylbutazone (Gastrointestinal perforation (including fatalities) has been reported in patients receiving erlotinib. Patients receiving concomitant NSAIDs are at increased risk).
No products indexed under this heading.

Phenytoin (Pre-treatment with the CYP3A4 inducer rifampicin decreased erlotinib AUC by about 2/3 to 4/5. Use of alternative treatments lacking CYP3A4 inducing activity is strongly recommended. If an alternative treatment is unavailable, an increase in the dose of erlotinib should be considered as tolerated at two week intervals while monitoring the patient's safety. If the erlotinib dose is adjusted upward, the dose will need to be reduced immediately to the indicated starting dose upon discontinuation of the CYP3A4 inducer. CYP3A4 inducers include phenytoin).
No products indexed under this heading.

Phenytoin Sodium (Pre-treatment with the CYP3A4 inducer rifampicin decreased erlotinib AUC by about 2/3 to 4/5. Use of alternative treatments lacking CYP3A4 inducing activity is strongly recommended. If an alternative treatment is unavailable, an increase in the dose of erlotinib should be considered as tolerated at two week intervals while monitoring the patient's safety. If the erlotinib dose is adjusted upward, the dose will need to be reduced immediately to the indicated starting dose upon discontinuation of the CYP3A4 inducer. CYP3A4 inducers include phenytoin). Products include:
Phenytek Capsules **2380**

Piroxicam (Gastrointestinal perforation (including fatalities) has been reported in patients receiving erlotinib. Patients receiving concomitant NSAIDs are at increased risk).
No products indexed under this heading.

Posaconazole (Erlotinib is metabolized predominantly by CYP3A4. Inhibitors of CYP3A4 would be expected to increase exposure. Caution should be used when co-administering erlotinib with a strong CYP3A4 inhibitor; consider a dose reduction if severe adverse reactions occur). Products include:
Noxafil **3172**

Prednisolone (Gastrointestinal perforation (including fatalities) has been reported in patients receiving erlotinib. Patients receiving concomitant corticosteroids are at increased risk).
No products indexed under this heading.

Prednisolone Acetate (Gastrointestinal perforation (including fatalities) has been reported in patients receiving erlotinib. Patients receiving concomitant corticosteroids are at increased risk). Products include:
Blephamide .... ⊙**212**, ⊙**214**
Pred Forte .... ⊙**225**
Pred Mild .... ⊙**230**
Pred-G .... ⊙**226**, ⊙**227**

Prednisolone Sodium Phosphate (Gastrointestinal perforation (including fatalities) has been reported in patients receiving erlotinib. Patients receiving concomitant corticosteroids are at increased risk).
No products indexed under this heading.

Prednisolone Tebutate (Gastrointestinal perforation (including fatalities) has been reported in patients receiving erlotinib. Patients receiving concomitant corticosteroids are at increased risk).
No products indexed under this heading.

Prednisone (Gastrointestinal perforation (including fatalities) has been reported in patients receiving erlotinib. Patients receiving concomitant corticosteroids are at increased risk).
No products indexed under this heading.

Prednisone sodium phosphate (Gastrointestinal perforation (including fatalities) has been reported in patients receiving erlotinib. Patients receiving concomitant corticosteroids are at increased risk).
No products indexed under this heading.

Primidone (Pre-treatment with the CYP3A4 inducer rifampicin decreased erlotinib AUC by about 2/3 to 4/5. Use of alternative treatments lacking CYP3A4 inducing activity is strongly recommended. If an alternative treatment is unavailable, an increase in the dose of erlotinib should be considered as tolerated at two week intervals while monitoring the patient's safety. If the erlotinib dose is adjusted upward, the dose will need to be reduced immediately to the indicated starting dose upon discontinuation of the CYP3A4 inducer).
No products indexed under this heading.

Procarbazine Hydrochloride (Gastrointestinal perforation (including fatalities) has been reported in patients receiving erlotinib. Patients receiving concomitant taxane-based chemotherapy are at increased risk).
No products indexed under this heading.

Propoxyphene Hydrochloride (Erlotinib is metabolized predominantly by CYP3A4. Inhibitors of CYP3A4 would be expected to increase exposure. Caution should be used when co-administering erlotinib with a strong CYP3A4 inhibitor; consider a dose reduction if severe adverse reactions occur).
No products indexed under this heading.

Propoxyphene Napsylate (Erlotinib is metabolized predominantly by CYP3A4. Inhibitors of CYP3A4 would be expected to increase exposure. Caution should be used when co-administering erlotinib with a strong CYP3A4 inhibitor; consider a dose reduction if severe adverse reactions occur).
No products indexed under this heading.

Quinidine (Erlotinib is metabolized predominantly by CYP3A4. Inhibitors of CYP3A4 would be expected to increase exposure. Caution should be used when co-administering erlotinib with a strong CYP3A4 inhibitor; consider a dose reduction if severe adverse reactions occur).
No products indexed under this heading.

Quinidine Hydrochloride (Erlotinib is metabolized predominantly by CYP3A4. Inhibitors of CYP3A4 would be expected to increase exposure. Caution should be used when co-administering erlotinib with a strong CYP3A4 inhibitor; consider a dose reduction if severe adverse reactions occur).
No products indexed under this heading.

Quinidine Polygalacturonate (Erlotinib is metabolized predominantly by CYP3A4. Inhibitors of CYP3A4 would be expected to increase exposure. Caution should be used when co-administering erlotinib with a strong CYP3A4 inhibitor; consider a dose reduction if severe adverse reactions occur).
No products indexed under this heading.

Quinidine Sulfate (Erlotinib is metabolized predominantly by CYP3A4. Inhibitors of CYP3A4 would be expected to increase exposure. Caution should be used when co-administering erlotinib with a strong CYP3A4 inhibitor; consider a dose reduction if severe adverse reactions occur).
No products indexed under this heading.

Quinine (Erlotinib is metabolized predominantly by CYP3A4. Inhibitors of CYP3A4 would be expected to increase exposure. Caution should be used when co-administering erlotinib with a strong CYP3A4 inhibitor; consider a dose reduction if severe adverse reactions occur). Products include:
Hyland's Leg Cramps PM with Quinine **3315**

IMPORTANT NOTE: Always consult each drug listing in the patient's regimen for possible interactions.

Quinine Sulfate (Erlotinib is metabolized predominantly by CYP3A4. Inhibitors of CYP3A4 would be expected to increase exposure. Caution should be used when co-administering erlotinib with a strong CYP3A4 inhibitor; consider a dose reduction if severe adverse reactions occur).
No products indexed under this heading.

Quinupristin (Erlotinib is metabolized predominantly by CYP3A4. Inhibitors of CYP3A4 would be expected to increase exposure. Caution should be used when co-administering erlotinib with a strong CYP3A4 inhibitor; consider a dose reduction if severe adverse reactions occur).
No products indexed under this heading.

Rabeprazole Sodium (Drugs that alter the pH of the upper GI tract may alter the solubility of erlotinib and reduce its bioavailability. Co-administration of erlotinib with omeprazole, a proton pump inhibitor, decreased the erlotinib AUC by 46%. Increasing the dose of erlotinib when co-administered with such agents is not likely to compensate for the loss of exposure. Since proton pump inhibitors affect pH of the upper GI tract for an extended period, separation of doses may not eliminate the interaction. The concomitant use of proton pump inhibitors with erlotinib should be avoided if possible). Products include:
Aciphex 1035

Ranibizumab (Gastrointestinal perforation (including fatalities) has been reported in patients receiving erlotinib. Patients receiving concomitant anti-angiogenic agents are at increased risk. Permanently discontinue erlotinib in patients who develop gastrointestinal perforation). Products include:
Lucentis 1201

Ranitidine Bismuth Citrate (Erlotinib is metabolized predominantly by CYP3A4. Inhibitors of CYP3A4 would be expected to increase exposure. Caution should be used when co-administering erlotinib with a strong CYP3A4 inhibitor; consider a dose reduction if severe adverse reactions occur).
No products indexed under this heading.

Ranitidine Hydrochloride (Drugs that alter the pH of the upper GI tract may alter the solubility of erlotinib and reduce its bioavailability). Products include:
Zantac 1737
Zantac Injection 1732
Zantac Pharmacy 1735

Rifabutin (Pre-treatment with the CYP3A4 inducer rifampicin decreased erlotinib AUC by about 2/3 to 4/5. Use of alternative treatments lacking CYP3A4 inducing activity is strongly recommended. If an alternative treatment is unavailable, an increase in the dose of erlotinib should be considered as tolerated at two week intervals while monitoring the patient's safety. If the erlotinib dose is adjusted upward, the dose will need to be reduced immediately to the indicated starting dose upon discontinuation of the CYP3A4 inducer. CYP3A4 inducers include rifabutin).
No products indexed under this heading.

Rifampicin (Pre-treatment with the CYP3A4 inducer rifampicin for 7 days prior to erlotinib decreased erlotinib AUC by about 2/3 to 4/5, which is equivalent to a dose of about 30 to 50 mg in NSCLC patients. In a separate study, treatment with rifampicin for 11 days, with co-administration of a single 450 mg dose of erlotinib on day 8 resulted in a mean erlotinib exposure (AUC) that was 57.6% of that observed following a single 150 mg erlotinib dose in the absence of rifampicin treatment. Use of alternative treatments lacking

CYP3A4 inducing activity is strongly recommended. If an alternative treatment is unavailable, adjusting the starting dose should be considered. If the erlotinib dose is adjusted upward, the dose will need to be reduced immediately to the indicated starting dose upon discontinuation of rifampicin or other inducers).
No products indexed under this heading.

Rifampin (Pre-treatment with the CYP3A4 inducer rifampicin decreased erlotinib AUC by about 2/3 to 4/5. Use of alternative treatments lacking CYP3A4 inducing activity is strongly recommended. If an alternative treatment is unavailable, an increase in the dose of erlotinib should be considered as tolerated at two week intervals while monitoring the patient's safety. If the erlotinib dose is adjusted upward, the dose will need to be reduced immediately to the indicated starting dose upon discontinuation of the CYP3A4 inducer).
No products indexed under this heading.

Rifapentine (Pre-treatment with the CYP3A4 inducer rifampicin decreased erlotinib AUC by about 2/3 to 4/5. Use of alternative treatments lacking CYP3A4 inducing activity is strongly recommended. If an alternative treatment is unavailable, an increase in the dose of erlotinib should be considered as tolerated at two week intervals while monitoring the patient's safety. If the erlotinib dose is adjusted upward, the dose will need to be reduced immediately to the indicated starting dose upon discontinuation of the CYP3A4 inducer. CYP3A4 inducers include rifapentine).
No products indexed under this heading.

Ritonavir (Erlotinib is metabolized predominantly by CYP3A4. Inhibitors of CYP3A4 would be expected to increase exposure. Caution should be used when co-administering erlotinib with a strong CYP3A4 inhibitor such as ritonavir; consider a dose reduction if severe adverse reactions occur). Products include:
Kaletra 458
Norvir 509

Rofecoxib (Gastrointestinal perforation (including fatalities) has been reported in patients receiving erlotinib. Patients receiving concomitant NSAIDs are at increased risk).
No products indexed under this heading.

Saquinavir (Erlotinib is metabolized predominantly by CYP3A4. Inhibitors of CYP3A4 would be expected to increase exposure. Caution should be used when co-administering erlotinib with a strong CYP3A4 inhibitor, such as saquinavir; consider a dose reduction if severe adverse reactions occur).
No products indexed under this heading.

Saquinavir Mesylate (Erlotinib is metabolized predominantly by CYP3A4. Inhibitors of CYP3A4 would be expected to increase exposure. Caution should be used when co-administering erlotinib with a strong CYP3A4 inhibitor, such as saquinavir; consider a dose reduction if severe adverse reactions occur).
No products indexed under this heading.

Sertraline Hydrochloride (Erlotinib is metabolized predominantly by CYP3A4. Inhibitors of CYP3A4 would be expected to increase exposure. Caution should be used when co-administering erlotinib with a strong CYP3A4 inhibitor; consider a dose reduction if severe adverse reactions occur).
No products indexed under this heading.

Sildenafil Citrate (Erlotinib is metabolized predominantly by CYP3A4. Inhibitors of CYP3A4 would be expected to increase exposure. Caution should be used when co-administering erlotinib with a strong CYP3A4 inhibitor; consider a dose reduction if severe adverse reactions occur).
No products indexed under this heading.

Sirolimus (Gastrointestinal perforation (including fatalities) has been reported in patients receiving erlotinib. Patients receiving concomitant anti-angiogenic agents are at increased risk. Permanently discontinue erlotinib in patients who develop gastrointestinal perforation). Products include:
Rapamune 3579

Sodium Bicarbonate (The use of antacids may be considered in place of histamine 2 receptor blockers (H_2 blockers) or proton pump inhibitors in patients receiving erlotinib. However, no clinical study has been conducted to evaluate the effect of antacids on erlotinib pharmacokinetics. If an antacid is necessary, the antacid dose and the erlotinib dose should be separated by several hours).
No products indexed under this heading.

Sorafenib (Gastrointestinal perforation (including fatalities) has been reported in patients receiving erlotinib. Patients receiving concomitant anti-angiogenic agents are at increased risk. Permanently discontinue erlotinib in patients who develop gastrointestinal perforation).
No products indexed under this heading.

Sparfloxacin (When erlotinib was co-administered with ciprofloxacin, an inhibitor of both CYP3A4 and CYP1A2, erlotinib exposure (AUC) and maximum concentration (C_{max}) increased by 39% and 17%, respectively. In patients who are taking erlotinib with an inhibitor of both CYP3A4 and CYP1A2 like ciprofloxacin, a dose reduction of erlotinib should be considered if severe adverse reactions occur).
No products indexed under this heading.

Streptozocin (Gastrointestinal perforation (including fatalities) has been reported in patients receiving erlotinib. Patients receiving concomitant taxane-based chemotherapy are at increased risk).
No products indexed under this heading.

Sulfinpyrazone (Pre-treatment with the CYP3A4 inducer rifampicin decreased erlotinib AUC by about 2/3 to 4/5. Use of alternative treatments lacking CYP3A4 inducing activity is strongly recommended. If an alternative treatment is unavailable, an increase in the dose of erlotinib should be considered as tolerated at two week intervals while monitoring the patient's safety. If the erlotinib dose is adjusted upward, the dose will need to be reduced immediately to the indicated starting dose upon discontinuation of the CYP3A4 inducer).
No products indexed under this heading.

Sulindac (Gastrointestinal perforation (including fatalities) has been reported in patients receiving erlotinib. Patients receiving concomitant NSAIDs are at increased risk). Products include:
Clinoril 2098

Sunitinib (Gastrointestinal perforation (including fatalities) has been reported in patients receiving erlotinib. Patients receiving concomitant anti-angiogenic agents are at increased risk. Permanently discontinue erlotinib in patients who develop gastrointestinal perforation).
No products indexed under this heading.

Sunitinib Malate (Gastrointestinal perforation (including fatalities) has been reported in patients receiving erlo-

tinib. Patients receiving concomitant anti-angiogenic agents are at increased risk. Permanently discontinue erlotinib in patients who develop gastrointestinal perforation). Products include:
Sutent 2747

Tacrine Hydrochloride (When erlotinib was co-administered with ciprofloxacin, an inhibitor of both CYP3A4 and CYP1A2, erlotinib exposure (AUC) and maximum concentration (C_{max}) increased by 39% and 17%, respectively. In patients who are taking erlotinib with an inhibitor of both CYP3A4 and CYP1A2 like ciprofloxacin, a dose reduction of erlotinib should be considered if severe adverse reactions occur).
No products indexed under this heading.

Tamoxifen Citrate (Gastrointestinal perforation (including fatalities) has been reported in patients receiving erlotinib. Patients receiving concomitant taxane-based chemotherapy are at increased risk).
No products indexed under this heading.

Telithromycin (Erlotinib is metabolized predominantly by CYP3A4. Inhibitors of CYP3A4 would be expected to increase exposure. Caution should be used when co-administering erlotinib with a strong CYP3A4 inhibitor, such as telithromycin; consider a dose reduction if severe adverse reactions occur). Products include:
Ketek 2991

Temsirolimus (Gastrointestinal perforation (including fatalities) has been reported in patients receiving erlotinib. Patients receiving concomitant anti-angiogenic agents are at increased risk. Permanently discontinue erlotinib in patients who develop gastrointestinal perforation). Products include:
Torisel 3592

Teniposide (Gastrointestinal perforation (including fatalities) has been reported in patients receiving erlotinib. Patients receiving concomitant taxane-based chemotherapy are at increased risk).
No products indexed under this heading.

Thalidomide (Gastrointestinal perforation (including fatalities) has been reported in patients receiving erlotinib. Patients receiving concomitant anti-angiogenic agents are at increased risk. Permanently discontinue erlotinib in patients who develop gastrointestinal perforation).
No products indexed under this heading.

Theophyllinate (Pre-treatment with the CYP3A4 inducer rifampicin decreased erlotinib AUC by about 2/3 to 4/5. Use of alternative treatments lacking CYP3A4 inducing activity is strongly recommended. If an alternative treatment is unavailable, an increase in the dose of erlotinib should be considered as tolerated at two week intervals while monitoring the patient's safety. If the erlotinib dose is adjusted upward, the dose will need to be reduced immediately to the indicated starting dose upon discontinuation of the CYP3A4 inducer).
No products indexed under this heading.

Theophylline (Pre-treatment with the CYP3A4 inducer rifampicin decreased erlotinib AUC by about 2/3 to 4/5. Use of alternative treatments lacking CYP3A4 inducing activity is strongly recommended. If an alternative treatment is unavailable, an increase in the dose of erlotinib should be considered as tolerated at two week intervals while monitoring the patient's safety. If the erlotinib dose is adjusted upward, the dose will need to be reduced immediately to the indicated starting dose upon discontinuation of the CYP3A4 inducer).
No products indexed under this heading.

Theophylline Anhydrous (Pretreatment with the CYP3A4 inducer rifampicin decreased erlotinib AUC by about 2/3 to 4/5. Use of alternative treatments lacking CYP3A4 inducing activity is strongly recommended. If an alternative treatment is unavailable, an increase in the dose of erlotinib should be considered as tolerated at two week intervals while monitoring the patient's safety. If the erlotinib dose is adjusted upward, the dose will need to be reduced immediately to the indicated starting dose upon discontinuation of the CYP3A4 inducer. Products include:
Uniphyl 2817

Theophylline Calcium Salicylate (Pre-treatment with the CYP3A4 inducer rifampicin decreased erlotinib AUC by about 2/3 to 4/5. Use of alternative treatments lacking CYP3A4 inducing activity is strongly recommended. If an alternative treatment is unavailable, an increase in the dose of erlotinib should be considered as tolerated at two week intervals while monitoring the patient's safety. If the erlotinib dose is adjusted upward, the dose will need to be reduced immediately to the indicated starting dose upon discontinuation of the CYP3A4 inducer).
No products indexed under this heading.

Theophylline Dihydroxypropyl (Glyceryl) (Pre-treatment with the CYP3A4 inducer rifampicin decreased erlotinib AUC by about 2/3 to 4/5. Use of alternative treatments lacking CYP3A4 inducing activity is strongly recommended. If an alternative treatment is unavailable, an increase in the dose of erlotinib should be considered as tolerated at two week intervals while monitoring the patient's safety. If the erlotinib dose is adjusted upward, the dose will need to be reduced immediately to the indicated starting dose upon discontinuation of the CYP3A4 inducer).
No products indexed under this heading.

Theophylline Ethylenediamine (Pre-treatment with the CYP3A4 inducer rifampicin decreased erlotinib AUC by about 2/3 to 4/5. Use of alternative treatments lacking CYP3A4 inducing activity is strongly recommended. If an alternative treatment is unavailable, an increase in the dose of erlotinib should be considered as tolerated at two week intervals while monitoring the patient's safety. If the erlotinib dose is adjusted upward, the dose will need to be reduced immediately to the indicated starting dose upon discontinuation of the CYP3A4 inducer).
No products indexed under this heading.

Theophylline Sodium Glycinate (Pre-treatment with the CYP3A4 inducer rifampicin decreased erlotinib AUC by about 2/3 to 4/5. Use of alternative treatments lacking CYP3A4 inducing activity is strongly recommended. If an alternative treatment is unavailable, an increase in the dose of erlotinib should be considered as tolerated at two week intervals while monitoring the patient's safety. If the erlotinib dose is adjusted upward, the dose will need to be reduced immediately to the indicated starting dose upon discontinuation of the CYP3A4 inducer).
No products indexed under this heading.

Thioguanine (Gastrointestinal perforation (including fatalities) has been reported in patients receiving erlotinib. Patients receiving concomitant taxane-based chemotherapy are at increased risk). Products include:
Tabloid 1664

Thiotepa (Gastrointestinal perforation (including fatalities) has been reported in patients receiving erlotinib. Patients receiving concomitant taxane-based chemotherapy are at increased risk).
No products indexed under this heading.

Ticlopidine Hydrochloride (When erlotinib was co-administered with ciprofloxacin, an inhibitor of both CYP3A4 and CYP1A2, erlotinib exposure (AUC) and maximum concentration (C_{max}) increased by 39% and 17%, respectively. In patients who are taking erlotinib with an inhibitor of both CYP3A4 and CYP1A2 like ciprofloxacin, a dose reduction of erlotinib should be considered if severe adverse reactions occur).
No products indexed under this heading.

Tobacco (Cigarette smoking has been shown to reduce erlotinib AUC. Patients should be advised to stop smoking; however, if they continue to smoke, a cautious increase in the dose of erlotinib may be considered, while monitoring the patient's safety. If the erlotinib dose is adjusted upward, the dose should be reduced immediately to the indicated starting dose upon cessation of smoking).
No products indexed under this heading.

Tolmetin Sodium (Gastrointestinal perforation (including fatalities) has been reported in patients receiving erlotinib. Patients receiving concomitant NSAIDs are at increased risk).
No products indexed under this heading.

Topotecan Hydrochloride (Gastrointestinal perforation (including fatalities) has been reported in patients receiving erlotinib. Patients receiving concomitant taxane-based chemotherapy are at increased risk). Products include:
Hycamtin 1491
Hycamtin Capsules 1488

Toremifene Citrate (Gastrointestinal perforation (including fatalities) has been reported in patients receiving erlotinib. Patients receiving concomitant taxane-based chemotherapy are at increased risk).
No products indexed under this heading.

Triamcinolone (Gastrointestinal perforation (including fatalities) has been reported in patients receiving erlotinib. Patients receiving concomitant corticosteroids are at increased risk).
No products indexed under this heading.

Triamcinolone Acetonide (Gastrointestinal perforation (including fatalities) has been reported in patients receiving erlotinib. Patients receiving concomitant corticosteroids are at increased risk). Products include:
Azmacort 408
Nasacort AQ 3019

Triamcinolone Diacetate (Gastrointestinal perforation (including fatalities) has been reported in patients receiving erlotinib. Patients receiving concomitant corticosteroids are at increased risk).
No products indexed under this heading.

Triamcinolone Hexacetonide (Gastrointestinal perforation (including fatalities) has been reported in patients receiving erlotinib. Patients receiving concomitant corticosteroids are at increased risk).
No products indexed under this heading.

Troglitazone (Erlotinib is metabolized predominantly by CYP3A4. Inhibitors of CYP3A4 would be expected to increase exposure. Caution should be used when co-administering erlotinib with a strong CYP3A4 inhibitor; consider a dose reduction if severe adverse reactions occur).
No products indexed under this heading.

Troleandomycin (Erlotinib is metabolized predominantly by CYP3A4. Inhibitors of CYP3A4 would be expected to increase exposure. Caution should be used when co-administering erlotinib with a strong CYP3A4 inhibitor, such as troleandomycin (TAO); consider a dose reduction if severe adverse reactions occur).
No products indexed under this heading.

Trovafloxacin Mesylate (When erlotinib was co-administered with ciprofloxacin, an inhibitor of both CYP3A4 and CYP1A2, erlotinib exposure (AUC) and maximum concentration (C_{max}) increased by 39% and 17%, respectively. In patients who are taking erlotinib with an inhibitor of both CYP3A4 and CYP1A2 like ciprofloxacin, a dose reduction of erlotinib should be considered if severe adverse reactions occur).
No products indexed under this heading.

Valdecoxib (Gastrointestinal perforation (including fatalities) has been reported in patients receiving erlotinib. Patients receiving concomitant NSAIDs are at increased risk).
No products indexed under this heading.

Valproate Sodium (Erlotinib is metabolized predominantly by CYP3A4. Inhibitors of CYP3A4 would be expected to increase exposure. Caution should be used when co-administering erlotinib with a strong CYP3A4 inhibitor; consider a dose reduction if severe adverse reactions occur).
No products indexed under this heading.

Valrubicin (Gastrointestinal perforation (including fatalities) has been reported in patients receiving erlotinib. Patients receiving concomitant taxane-based chemotherapy are at increased risk). Products include:
Valstar 1131

Vardenafil Hydrochloride (Erlotinib is metabolized predominantly by CYP3A4. Inhibitors of CYP3A4 would be expected to increase exposure. Caution should be used when co-administering erlotinib with a strong CYP3A4 inhibitor; consider a dose reduction if severe adverse reactions occur). Products include:
Levitra 3157

Verapamil Hydrochloride (Erlotinib is metabolized predominantly by CYP3A4. Inhibitors of CYP3A4 would be expected to increase exposure. Caution should be used when co-administering erlotinib with a strong CYP3A4 inhibitor; consider a dose reduction if severe adverse reactions occur). Products include:
Tarka 534

Vincristine Sulfate (Gastrointestinal perforation (including fatalities) has been reported in patients receiving erlotinib. Patients receiving concomitant taxane-based chemotherapy are at increased risk).
No products indexed under this heading.

Vinorelbine Tartrate (Gastrointestinal perforation (including fatalities) has been reported in patients receiving erlotinib. Patients receiving concomitant taxane-based chemotherapy are at increased risk).
No products indexed under this heading.

Voriconazole (Erlotinib is metabolized predominantly by CYP3A4. Inhibitors of CYP3A4 would be expected to increase exposure. Caution should be used when co-administering erlotinib with a strong CYP3A4 inhibitor, such as voriconazole; consider a dose reduction if severe adverse reactions occur).
No products indexed under this heading.

Warfarin Sodium (International Normalized Ratio (INR) elevations and infrequent reports of bleeding events including gastrointestinal and non-gastrointestinal bleedings have been reported in clinical studies, some associated with concomitant warfarin administration. Patients taking warfarin or other coumarin-derivative anticoagulants should be monitored regularly for changes in prothrombin time or INR).
No products indexed under this heading.

Zafirlukast (Erlotinib is metabolized predominantly by CYP3A4. Inhibitors of CYP3A4 would be expected to increase exposure. Caution should be used when co-administering erlotinib with a strong CYP3A4 inhibitor; consider a dose reduction if severe adverse reactions occur). Products include:
Accolate 3612

Zileuton (Erlotinib is metabolized predominantly by CYP3A4. Inhibitors of CYP3A4 would be expected to increase exposure. Caution should be used when co-administering erlotinib with a strong CYP3A4 inhibitor; consider a dose reduction if severe adverse reactions occur).
No products indexed under this heading.

Food Interactions

Broccoli (CYP1A2 inducers may decrease erlotinib plasma concentrations).

Brussel Sprouts (CYP1A2 inducers may decrease erlotinib plasma concentrations).

Charbroiled Food (CYP1A2 inducers may decrease erlotinib plasma concentrations).

Food, unspecified (Erlotinib is about 60% absorbed after oral administration and its bioavailability is substantially increased by food to almost 100%).

Grapefruit (Erlotinib is metabolized predominantly by CYP3A4. Inhibitors of CYP3A4 would be expected to increase exposure. Caution should be used when co-administering erlotinib with a strong CYP3A4 inhibitor, such as grapefruit; consider a dose reduction if severe adverse reactions occur).

Grapefruit Juice (Erlotinib is metabolized predominantly by CYP3A4. Inhibitors of CYP3A4 would be expected to increase exposure. Caution should be used when co-administering erlotinib with a strong CYP3A4 inhibitor, such as grapefruit juice; consider a dose reduction if severe adverse reactions occur).

Meal, unspecified (Erlotinib is about 60% absorbed after oral administration and its bioavailability is substantially increased by food to almost 100%).

TARGRETIN CAPSULES
(Bexarotene) 1074
May interact with erythromycin, insulin, oral contraceptives, oral hypoglycemic agents, phenytoin, protease inhibitors, and certain other agents. Compounds in these categories include:

Acarbose (Bexarotene could enhance the action of hypoglycemic agents resulting in hypoglycemia).
No products indexed under this heading.

Amiodarone Hydrochloride (Bexarotene is metabolized by CYP4503A4; co-administration with inhibitors of CYP4503A4, such as amiodarone, would be expected to lead to an increase in plasma bexarotene concentrations).
No products indexed under this heading.

Amprenavir (Bexarotene is metabolized by CYP4503A4; co-administration with inhibitors of CYP4503A4, such as protease inhibitors, would be expected to lead to an increase in plasma bexarotene concentrations).
No products indexed under this heading.

IMPORTANT NOTE: Always consult each drug listing in the patient's regimen for possible interactions.

1829 **Interactions Index** **Targretin**

Nefazodone Hydrochloride (Bexarotene is metabolized by CYP4503A4; co-administration with inhibitors of CYP4503A4, such as nefazodone, would be expected to lead to an increase in plasma bexarotene concentrations).
No products indexed under this heading.

Nelfinavir Mesylate (Bexarotene is metabolized by CYP4503A4; co-administration with inhibitors of CYP4503A4, such as protease inhibitors, would be expected to lead to an increase in plasma bexarotene concentrations).
No products indexed under this heading.

Norethindrone (Bexarotene may theoretically increase the rate of metabolism and reduce plasma concentrations of other substrates metabolized by CYP4503A4, including hormonal contraceptives; it is strongly recommended that two reliable forms of contraception be used concurrently, one of which should be non-hormonal). Products include:
Ortho Micronor 2660

Norethynodrel (Bexarotene may theoretically increase the rate of metabolism and reduce plasma concentrations of other substrates metabolized by CYP4503A4, including hormonal contraceptives; it is strongly recommended that two reliable forms of contraception be used concurrently, one of which should be non-hormonal).
No products indexed under this heading.

Norgestimate (Bexarotene may theoretically increase the rate of metabolism and reduce plasma concentrations of other substrates metabolized by CYP4503A4, including hormonal contraceptives; it is strongly recommended that two reliable forms of contraception be used concurrently, one of which should be non-hormonal). Products include:
Ortho-Cyclen/Ortho Tri-Cyclen 2663
Ortho Tri-Cyclen Lo Tablets 2673

Norgestrel (Bexarotene may theoretically increase the rate of metabolism and reduce plasma concentrations of other substrates metabolized by CYP4503A4, including hormonal contraceptives; it is strongly recommended that two reliable forms of contraception be used concurrently, one of which should be non-hormonal).
No products indexed under this heading.

Phenobarbital (Bexarotene is metabolized by CYP4503A4; co-administration with inducers of CYP4503A4, such as phenobarbital, may cause a reduction in plasma bexarotene concentrations). Products include:
Donnatal 2711

Phenytoin (Bexarotene is metabolized by CYP4503A4; co-administration with inducers of CYP4503A4, such as phenytoin, may cause a reduction in plasma bexarotene concentrations).
No products indexed under this heading.

Phenytoin Sodium (Bexarotene is metabolized by CYP4503A4; co-administration with inducers of CYP4503A4, such as phenytoin, may cause a reduction in plasma bexarotene concentrations). Products include:
Phenytek Capsules 2380

Pioglitazone Hydrochloride (Bexarotene could enhance the action of hypoglycemic agents resulting in hypoglycemia). Products include:
ActoPlus 3338
Actos 3345
Duetact 3354

Repaglinide (Bexarotene could enhance the action of hypoglycemic agents resulting in hypoglycemia).
No products indexed under this heading.

Rifampin (Bexarotene is metabolized by CYP4503A4; co-administration with inducers of CYP4503A4, such as rifampin, may cause a reduction in plasma bexarotene concentrations).
No products indexed under this heading.

Ritonavir (Bexarotene is metabolized by CYP4503A4; co-administration with inhibitors of CYP4503A4, such as protease inhibitors, would be expected to lead to an increase in plasma bexarotene concentrations). Products include:
Kaletra 458
Norvir 509

Rosiglitazone Maleate (Bexarotene could enhance the action of hypoglycemic agents resulting in hypoglycemia). Products include:
Avandamet 1345
Avandaryl 1356
Avandia 1366

Saquinavir (Bexarotene is metabolized by CYP4503A4; co-administration with inhibitors of CYP4503A4, such as protease inhibitors, would be expected to lead to an increase in plasma bexarotene concentrations).
No products indexed under this heading.

Saquinavir Mesylate (Bexarotene is metabolized by CYP4503A4; co-administration with inhibitors of CYP4503A4, such as protease inhibitors, would be expected to lead to an increase in plasma bexarotene concentrations).
No products indexed under this heading.

Sitagliptin Phosphate (Bexarotene could enhance the action of hypoglycemic agents resulting in hypoglycemia). Products include:
Janumet 2188
Januvia 2196

Tamoxifen Citrate (Co-administration has resulted in a modest decrease in plasma concentrations of tamoxifen).
No products indexed under this heading.

Tipranavir (Bexarotene is metabolized by CYP4503A4; co-administration with inhibitors of CYP4503A4, such as protease inhibitors, would be expected to lead to an increase in plasma bexarotene concentrations).
No products indexed under this heading.

Tolazamide (Bexarotene could enhance the action of hypoglycemic agents resulting in hypoglycemia).
No products indexed under this heading.

Tolbutamide (Bexarotene could enhance the action of hypoglycemic agents resulting in hypoglycemia).
No products indexed under this heading.

Troglitazone (Bexarotene could enhance the action of hypoglycemic agents resulting in hypoglycemia).
No products indexed under this heading.

Vitamin A (Potential for additive toxic effects because of the relationship of bexarotene to vitamin A; patients should be advised to limit their vitamin A intake). Products include:
Cardio Basics 3455
Heplive 607
Norwegian Cod Liver Oil 919

Food Interactions

Food, unspecified (Co-administration with a fat-containing meal has resulted in higher plasma bexarotene AUC and C_{max} values; because safety and efficacy data are based upon administration with food, it is recommended that Targretin capsules be administered with or immediately following a meal).

Grapefruit Juice (Bexarotene is metabolized by CYP403A4; co-administration with inhibitors of CYP4503A4, such as grapefruit juice, would be expected to lead to an increase in plasma bexarotene concentrations).

TARGRETIN GEL 1%

(Bexarotene) 1079
May interact with cytochrome p450 3a4 inducers (selected), cytochrome p450 3a4 inhibitors (selected), erythromycin, oral contraceptives, and certain other agents. Compounds in these categories include:

Acetazolamide (Drugs that affect levels of activity of cytochrome P450 3A4 may potentially affect the disposition of bexarotene).
No products indexed under this heading.

Acetazolamide Sodium (Drugs that affect levels of activity of cytochrome P450 3A4 may potentially affect the disposition of bexarotene).
No products indexed under this heading.

Allium sativum (Drugs that affect levels of activity of cytochrome P450 3A4 may potentially affect the disposition of bexarotene).
No products indexed under this heading.

Aminoglutethimide (Drugs that affect levels of activity of cytochrome P450 3A4 may potentially affect the disposition of bexarotene).
No products indexed under this heading.

Amiodarone Hydrochloride (Drugs that affect levels of activity of cytochrome P450 3A4 may potentially affect the disposition of bexarotene).
No products indexed under this heading.

Amprenavir (Drugs that affect levels of activity of cytochrome P450 3A4 may potentially affect the disposition of bexarotene).
No products indexed under this heading.

Anastrozole (Drugs that affect levels of activity of cytochrome P450 3A4 may potentially affect the disposition of bexarotene).
No products indexed under this heading.

Aprepitant (Drugs that affect levels of activity of cytochrome P450 3A4 may potentially affect the disposition of bexarotene). Products include:
Emend 2124

Atazanavir (Drugs that affect levels of activity of cytochrome P450 3A4 may potentially affect the disposition of bexarotene).
No products indexed under this heading.

Atazanavir Sulfate (Drugs that affect levels of activity of cytochrome P450 3A4 may potentially affect the disposition of bexarotene).
No products indexed under this heading.

Betamethasone (Drugs that affect levels of activity of cytochrome P450 3A4 may potentially affect the disposition of bexarotene).
No products indexed under this heading.

Betamethasone Acetate (Drugs that affect levels of activity of cytochrome P450 3A4 may potentially affect the disposition of bexarotene).
No products indexed under this heading.

Betamethasone Benzoate (Drugs that affect levels of activity of cytochrome P450 3A4 may potentially affect the disposition of bexarotene).
No products indexed under this heading.

Betamethasone Dipropionate (Drugs that affect levels of activity of cytochrome P450 3A4 may potentially affect the disposition of bexarotene). Products include:
Diprolene Lotion 0.05% 3108
Diprolene Ointment 0.05% 3109
Diprolene AF Cream 0.05% 3107
Lotrisone 3163

Betamethasone Sodium Phosphate (Drugs that affect levels of activity of cytochrome P450 3A4 may potentially affect the disposition of bexarotene).
No products indexed under this heading.

Betamethasone Valerate (Drugs that affect levels of activity of cytochrome P450 3A4 may potentially affect the disposition of bexarotene). Products include:
Luxíq 3321

Bosentan (Drugs that affect levels of activity of cytochrome P450 3A4 may potentially affect the disposition of bexarotene). Products include:
Tracleer 573

Carbamazepine (Drugs that affect levels of activity of cytochrome P450 3A4 may potentially affect the disposition of bexarotene). Products include:
Carbatrol 3280
Equetro 3477

Cimetidine (Drugs that affect levels of activity of cytochrome P450 3A4 may potentially affect the disposition of bexarotene).
No products indexed under this heading.

Cimetidine Hydrochloride (Drugs that affect levels of activity of cytochrome P450 3A4 may potentially affect the disposition of bexarotene).
No products indexed under this heading.

Ciprofloxacin (Drugs that affect levels of activity of cytochrome P450 3A4 may potentially affect the disposition of bexarotene). Products include:
Cipro I.V. 3082
Cipro 3073
Cipro XR 3091
Ciprodex 583

Ciprofloxacin Hydrochloride (Drugs that affect levels of activity of cytochrome P450 3A4 may potentially affect the disposition of bexarotene). Products include:
Cipro 3073

Cisplatin (Drugs that affect levels of activity of cytochrome P450 3A4 may potentially affect the disposition of bexarotene).
No products indexed under this heading.

Clarithromycin (Drugs that affect levels of activity of cytochrome P450 3A4 may potentially affect the disposition of bexarotene). Products include:
Biaxin/Biaxin XL 412

Clotrimazole (Drugs that affect levels of activity of cytochrome P450 3A4 may potentially affect the disposition of bexarotene). Products include:
Lotrisone 3163

Conivaptan Hydrochloride (Drugs that affect levels of activity of cytochrome P450 3A4 may potentially affect the disposition of bexarotene). Products include:
Vaprisol 689

Cortisone Acetate (Drugs that affect levels of activity of cytochrome P450 3A4 may potentially affect the disposition of bexarotene).
No products indexed under this heading.

Cyclosporine (Drugs that affect levels of activity of cytochrome P450 3A4 may potentially affect the disposition of bexarotene). Products include:
Gengraf 440
Neoral Oral Solution 2496
Neoral Capsules 2496
Restasis 605

Dalfopristin (Drugs that affect levels of activity of cytochrome P450 3A4 may potentially affect the disposition of bexarotene).
No products indexed under this heading.

Danazol (Drugs that affect levels of activity of cytochrome P450 3A4 may potentially affect the disposition of bexarotene).
No products indexed under this heading.

Darunavir (Drugs that affect levels of activity of cytochrome P450 3A4 may potentially affect the disposition of bexarotene).
No products indexed under this heading.

IMPORTANT NOTE: Always consult each drug listing in the patient's regimen for possible interactions.

Dasatinib (Drugs that affect levels of activity of cytochrome P450 3A4 may potentially affect the disposition of bexarotene).

No products indexed under this heading.

Delavirdine Mesylate (Drugs that affect levels of activity of cytochrome P450 3A4 may potentially affect the disposition of bexarotene).

No products indexed under this heading.

Delavirine (Drugs that affect levels of activity of cytochrome P450 3A4 may potentially affect the disposition of bexarotene).

No products indexed under this heading.

Desloratadine (Drugs that affect levels of activity of cytochrome P450 3A4 may potentially affect the disposition of bexarotene). Products include:

Desogestrel (Effective contraception must be used for one month prior to initiation of therapy, during therapy, and for at least one month following discontinuation of therapy; it is recommended that two reliable forms of contraception be used simultaneously unless abstinence is the chosen method.

No products indexed under this heading.

Dexamethasone (Drugs that affect levels of activity of cytochrome P450 3A4 may potentially affect the disposition of bexarotene). Products include:

Dexamethasone Acetate (Drugs that affect levels of activity of cytochrome P450 3A4 may potentially affect the disposition of bexarotene).

No products indexed under this heading.

Dexamethasone Phosphate (Drugs that affect levels of activity of cytochrome P450 3A4 may potentially affect the disposition of bexarotene).

No products indexed under this heading.

Dexamethasone Sodium (Drugs that affect levels of activity of cytochrome P450 3A4 may potentially affect the disposition of bexarotene).

No products indexed under this heading.

Dexamethasone Sodium Phosphate (Drugs that affect levels of activity of cytochrome P450 3A4 may potentially affect the disposition of bexarotene).

No products indexed under this heading.

Dexamethasone Sodium Phosphate Injection (Drugs that affect levels of activity of cytochrome P450 3A4 may potentially affect the disposition of bexarotene).

No products indexed under this heading.

Diltiazem Hydrochloride (Drugs that affect levels of activity of cytochrome P450 3A4 may potentially affect the disposition of bexarotene). Products include:

Diltiazem Maleate (Drugs that affect levels of activity of cytochrome P450 3A4 may potentially affect the disposition of bexarotene).

No products indexed under this heading.

Doxorubicin Hydrochloride (Drugs that affect levels of activity of cytochrome P450 3A4 may potentially affect the disposition of bexarotene).

No products indexed under this heading.

Efavirenz (Drugs that affect levels of activity of cytochrome P450 3A4 may potentially affect the disposition of bexarotene). Products include:

Erythromycin (Bexarotene is metabolized by CYP4503A4; co-administration with inhibitors of CYP4503A4, such as erythromycin, would be expected to lead to an increase in plasma bexarotene concentrations).

No products indexed under this heading.

Erythromycin, Topical (Bexarotene is metabolized by CYP4503A4; co-administration with inhibitors of CYP4503A4, such as erythromycin, would be expected to lead to an increase in plasma bexarotene concentrations).

No products indexed under this heading.

Erythromycin Estolate (Bexarotene is metabolized by CYP4503A4; co-administration with inhibitors of CYP4503A4, such as erythromycin, would be expected to lead to an increase in plasma bexarotene concentrations).

No products indexed under this heading.

Erythromycin Ethylsuccinate (Bexarotene is metabolized by CYP4503A4; co-administration with inhibitors of CYP4503A4, such as erythromycin, would be expected to lead to an increase in plasma bexarotene concentrations). Products include:

Erythromycin Gluceptate (Bexarotene is metabolized by CYP4503A4; co-administration with inhibitors of CYP4503A4, such as erythromycin, would be expected to lead to an increase in plasma bexarotene concentrations).

No products indexed under this heading.

Erythromycin Lactobionate (Bexarotene is metabolized by CYP4503A4; co-administration with inhibitors of CYP4503A4, such as erythromycin, would be expected to lead to an increase in plasma bexarotene concentrations).

No products indexed under this heading.

Erythromycin Stearate (Bexarotene is metabolized by CYP4503A4; co-administration with inhibitors of CYP4503A4, such as erythromycin, would be expected to lead to an increase in plasma bexarotene concentrations).

No products indexed under this heading.

Esomeprazole Magnesium (Drugs that affect levels of activity of cytochrome P450 3A4 may potentially affect the disposition of bexarotene). Products include:

Esomeprazole Sodium (Drugs that affect levels of activity of cytochrome P450 3A4 may potentially affect the disposition of bexarotene). Products include:

Ethinyl Estradiol (Effective contraception must be used for one month prior to initiation of therapy, during therapy, and for at least one month following discontinuation of therapy; it is recommended that two reliable forms of contraception be used simultaneously unless abstinence is the chosen method). Products include:

Ethosuximide (Drugs that affect levels of activity of cytochrome P450 3A4 may potentially affect the disposition of bexarotene).

No products indexed under this heading.

Ethynodiol Diacetate (Effective contraception must be used for one month prior to initiation of therapy, during therapy, and for at least one month following discontinuation of therapy; it is recommended that two reliable forms of contraception be used simultaneously unless abstinence is the chosen method).

No products indexed under this heading.

Felbamate (Drugs that affect levels of activity of cytochrome P450 3A4 may potentially affect the disposition of bexarotene).

No products indexed under this heading.

Fluconazole (Drugs that affect levels of activity of cytochrome P450 3A4 may potentially affect the disposition of bexarotene).

No products indexed under this heading.

Fludrocortisone Acetate (Drugs that affect levels of activity of cytochrome P450 3A4 may potentially affect the disposition of bexarotene).

No products indexed under this heading.

Fluoxetine (Drugs that affect levels of activity of cytochrome P450 3A4 may potentially affect the disposition of bexarotene).

No products indexed under this heading.

Fluoxetine Hydrochloride (Drugs that affect levels of activity of cytochrome P450 3A4 may potentially affect the disposition of bexarotene). Products include:

Fluvoxamine Maleate (Drugs that affect levels of activity of cytochrome P450 3A4 may potentially affect the disposition of bexarotene).

No products indexed under this heading.

Fosamprenavir Calcium (Drugs that affect levels of activity of cytochrome P450 3A4 may potentially affect the disposition of bexarotene). Products include:

Fosphenytoin Sodium (Drugs that affect levels of activity of cytochrome P450 3A4 may potentially affect the disposition of bexarotene).

No products indexed under this heading.

Garlic Extract (Drugs that affect levels of activity of cytochrome P450 3A4 may potentially affect the disposition of bexarotene).

No products indexed under this heading.

Garlic Oil (Drugs that affect levels of activity of cytochrome P450 3A4 may potentially affect the disposition of bexarotene).

No products indexed under this heading.

Gemfibrozil (Concomitant gemfibrozil was associated with increased bexarotene concentrations following oral administration of bexarotene).

No products indexed under this heading.

Hydrocortisone (Drugs that affect levels of activity of cytochrome P450 3A4 may potentially affect the disposition of bexarotene).

No products indexed under this heading.

Hydrocortisone (Alcohol) (Drugs that affect levels of activity of cytochrome P450 3A4 may potentially affect the disposition of bexarotene).

No products indexed under this heading.

Hydrocortisone Acetate (Drugs that affect levels of activity of cytochrome P450 3A4 may potentially affect the disposition of bexarotene).

No products indexed under this heading.

Hydrocortisone Butyrate (Drugs that affect levels of activity of cytochrome P450 3A4 may potentially affect the disposition of bexarotene).

No products indexed under this heading.

Hydrocortisone Cypionate (Drugs that affect levels of activity of cytochrome P450 3A4 may potentially affect the disposition of bexarotene).

No products indexed under this heading.

Hydrocortisone Hemisuccinate (Drugs that affect levels of activity of cytochrome P450 3A4 may potentially affect the disposition of bexarotene).

No products indexed under this heading.

Hydrocortisone Probutate (Drugs that affect levels of activity of cytochrome P450 3A4 may potentially affect the disposition of bexarotene).

No products indexed under this heading.

Hydrocortisone Sodium Phosphate (Drugs that affect levels of activity of cytochrome P450 3A4 may potentially affect the disposition of bexarotene).

No products indexed under this heading.

Hydrocortisone Sodium Succinate (Drugs that affect levels of activity of cytochrome P450 3A4 may potentially affect the disposition of bexarotene).

No products indexed under this heading.

Hydrocortisone Valerate (Drugs that affect levels of activity of cytochrome P450 3A4 may potentially affect the disposition of bexarotene).

No products indexed under this heading.

Hypericum (Drugs that affect levels of activity of cytochrome P450 3A4 may potentially affect the disposition of bexarotene).

No products indexed under this heading.

Hypericum Perforatum (Drugs that affect levels of activity of cytochrome P450 3A4 may potentially affect the disposition of bexarotene). Products include:

Imatinib Mesylate (Drugs that affect levels of activity of cytochrome P450 3A4 may potentially affect the disposition of bexarotene). Products include:

Indinavir Sulfate (Drugs that affect levels of activity of cytochrome P450 3A4 may potentially affect the disposition of bexarotene). Products include:

Isoniazid (Drugs that affect levels of activity of cytochrome P450 3A4 may potentially affect the disposition of bexarotene).

No products indexed under this heading.

Itraconazole (Bexarotene is metabolized by CYP4503A4; co-administration with inhibitors of CYP4503A4, such as itraconazole, could lead to an increase in plasma bexarotene concentrations).

No products indexed under this heading.

Ketoconazole (Bexarotene is metabolized vy CYP4503A4; co-administration with inhibitors of CYP4503A4, such as keoconazole, could lead to an increase in plasma concentrations). Products include:

Lapatinib (Drugs that affect levels of activity of cytochrome P450 3A4 may potentially affect the disposition of bexarotene). Products include:

Levonorgestrel (Effective contraception must be used for one month prior to initiation of therapy, during therapy, and for at least one month following discontinuation of therapy; it is recommended that two reliable forms of contraception be used simultaneously unless abstinence is the chosen method). Products include:

(⊙ Described in PDR® for Ophthalmic Medicines)

IMPORTANT NOTE: Always consult each drug listing in the patient's regimen for possible interactions.

Kaletra 458
Norvir 509

Saquinavir (Drugs that affect levels of activity of cytochrome P450 3A4 may potentially affect the disposition of bexarotene).
No products indexed under this heading.

Saquinavir Mesylate (Drugs that affect levels of activity of cytochrome P450 3A4 may potentially affect the disposition of bexarotene).
No products indexed under this heading.

Sertraline Hydrochloride (Drugs that affect levels of activity of cytochrome P450 3A4 may potentially affect the disposition of bexarotene).
No products indexed under this heading.

Sildenafil Citrate (Drugs that affect levels of activity of cytochrome P450 3A4 may potentially affect the disposition of bexarotene).
No products indexed under this heading.

Sulfinpyrazone (Drugs that affect levels of activity of cytochrome P450 3A4 may potentially affect the disposition of bexarotene).
No products indexed under this heading.

Telithromycin (Drugs that affect levels of activity of cytochrome P450 3A4 may potentially affect the disposition of bexarotene). Products include:
Ketek 2991

Theophyllinate (Drugs that affect levels of activity of cytochrome P450 3A4 may potentially affect the disposition of bexarotene).
No products indexed under this heading.

Theophylline (Drugs that affect levels of activity of cytochrome P450 3A4 may potentially affect the disposition of bexarotene).
No products indexed under this heading.

Theophylline Anhydrous (Drugs that affect levels of activity of cytochrome P450 3A4 may potentially affect the disposition of bexarotene). Products include:
Uniphyl 2817

Theophylline Calcium Salicylate (Drugs that affect levels of activity of cytochrome P450 3A4 may potentially affect the disposition of bexarotene).
No products indexed under this heading.

Theophylline Dihydroxypropyl (Glyceryl) (Drugs that affect levels of activity of cytochrome P450 3A4 may potentially affect the disposition of bexarotene).
No products indexed under this heading.

Theophylline Ethylenediamine (Drugs that affect levels of activity of cytochrome P450 3A4 may potentially affect the disposition of bexarotene).
No products indexed under this heading.

Theophylline Sodium Glycinate (Drugs that affect levels of activity of cytochrome P450 3A4 may potentially affect the disposition of bexarotene).
No products indexed under this heading.

Triamcinolone (Drugs that affect levels of activity of cytochrome P450 3A4 may potentially affect the disposition of bexarotene).
No products indexed under this heading.

Triamcinolone Acetonide (Drugs that affect levels of activity of cytochrome P450 3A4 may potentially affect the disposition of bexarotene). Products include:
Azmacort 408
Nasacort AQ 3019

Triamcinolone Diacetate (Drugs that affect levels of activity of cytochrome P450 3A4 may potentially affect the disposition of bexarotene).
No products indexed under this heading.

Triamcinolone Hexacetonide (Drugs that affect levels of activity of cytochrome P450 3A4 may potentially affect the disposition of bexarotene).
No products indexed under this heading.

Troglitazone (Drugs that affect levels of activity of cytochrome P450 3A4 may potentially affect the disposition of bexarotene).
No products indexed under this heading.

Troleandomycin (Drugs that affect levels of activity of cytochrome P450 3A4 may potentially affect the disposition of bexarotene).
No products indexed under this heading.

Valproate Sodium (Drugs that affect levels of activity of cytochrome P450 3A4 may potentially affect the disposition of bexarotene).
No products indexed under this heading.

Vardenafil Hydrochloride (Drugs that affect levels of activity of cytochrome P450 3A4 may potentially affect the disposition of bexarotene). Products include:
Levitra 3157

Verapamil Hydrochloride (Drugs that affect levels of activity of cytochrome P450 3A4 may potentially affect the disposition of bexarotene). Products include:
Tarka 534

Vitamin A (Potential for additive toxic effects because of the relationship of bexarotene to vitamin A; patients should be advised to limit their vitamin A intake). Products include:
Cardio Basics 3455
Heplive 607
Norwegian Cod Liver Oil 919

Voriconazole (Drugs that affect levels of activity of cytochrome P450 3A4 may potentially affect the disposition of bexarotene).
No products indexed under this heading.

Zafirlukast (Drugs that affect levels of activity of cytochrome P450 3A4 may potentially affect the disposition of bexarotene). Products include:
Accolate 3612

Zileuton (Drugs that affect levels of activity of cytochrome P450 3A4 may potentially affect the disposition of bexarotene).
No products indexed under this heading.

Food Interactions

Grapefruit (Bexarotene is metabolized by CYP4503A4; co-administration with inhibitors of CYP4503A4, such as grapefruit juice, could lead to an increase in plasma bexarotene concentrations).

Grapefruit Juice (Bexarotene is metabolized by CYP4503A4; co-administration with inhibitors of CYP4503A4, such as grapefruit juice, could lead to an increase in plasma bexarotene concentrations).

TARKA TABLETS

(Trandolapril, Verapamil Hydrochloride) 534

May interact with anesthetics, beta-blockers, cardiac glycosides, diuretics, erythromycin, inhalant anesthetics, lithium preparations, neuromuscular blocking agents, nitrates and nitrites, potassium preparations, potassium sparing diuretics, quinidine, theophyllines, thiazides, and certain other agents. Compounds in these categories include:

Acebutolol Hydrochloride (Co-administration of β-blockers and verapamil may result in additive effects on heart rate, atrioventricular conduction, and/or cardiac contractility. The use of verapamil in combination with a β-blocker should be used only with caution, and close monitoring).
No products indexed under this heading.

Alfentanil Hydrochloride (In patients undergoing major surgery or during anesthesia with agents that produce hypotension, trandolapril will block angiotensin II formation secondary to compensatory renin release. If hypotension occurs and is considered to be due to this mechanism, it can be corrected by volume expansion).
No products indexed under this heading.

Amiloride Hydrochloride (Use of potassium-sparing diuretics (spironolactone, triamterene, or amiloride), potassium supplements, or potassium-containing salt substitutes concomitantly with ACE inhibitors can increase the risk of hyperkalemia. If concomitant use of such agents is indicated, they should be used with caution and with appropriate monitoring of serum potassium).
No products indexed under this heading.

Amyl Nitrite (Verapamil has been given concomitantly with short- and long-acting nitrates without any undesirable drug interactions. The pharmacologic profile of both drugs and the clinical experience suggest beneficial interactions).
No products indexed under this heading.

Articaine Hydrochloride (In patients undergoing major surgery or during anesthesia with agents that produce hypotension, trandolapril will block angiotensin II formation secondary to compensatory renin release. If hypotension occurs and is considered to be due to this mechanism, it can be corrected by volume expansion).
No products indexed under this heading.

Atenolol (Co-administration of β-blockers and verapamil may result in additive effects on heart rate, atrioventricular conduction, and/or cardiac contractility. The use of verapamil in combination with a β-blocker should be used only with caution, and close monitoring).
No products indexed under this heading.

Atracurium Besylate (Clinical data and studies suggest that verapamil may potentiate the activity of neuromuscular blocking agents (curare-like and depolarizing). It may be necessary to decrease the dose of verapamil and/or the dose of the neuromuscular blocking agent when the drugs are used concomitantly).
No products indexed under this heading.

Bendroflumethiazide (Trandolapril can attenuate potassium loss caused by thiazide diuretics).
No products indexed under this heading.

Benzocaine (In patients undergoing major surgery or during anesthesia with agents that produce hypotension, trandolapril will block angiotensin II formation secondary to compensatory renin release. If hypotension occurs and is considered to be due to this mechanism, it can be corrected by volume expansion).
No products indexed under this heading.

Betaxolol Hydrochloride (Co-administration of β-blockers and verapamil may result in additive effects on heart rate, atrioventricular conduction, and/or cardiac contractility. The use of verapamil in combination with a β-blocker should be used only with caution, and close monitoring).
No products indexed under this heading.

Bisoprolol Fumarate (Co-administration of β-blockers and verapamil may result in additive effects on heart rate, atrioventricular conduction, and/or cardiac contractility. The use of verapamil in combination with a β-blocker should be used only with caution, and close monitoring).
No products indexed under this heading.

Bumetanide (Patients on diuretics, especially those on recently instituted diuretic therapy, may occasionally experience an excessive reduction of blood pressure after initiation of therapy with Tarka).
No products indexed under this heading.

Bupivacaine Hydrochloride (In patients undergoing major surgery or during anesthesia with agents that produce hypotension, trandolapril will block angiotensin II formation secondary to compensatory renin release. If hypotension occurs and is considered to be due to this mechanism, it can be corrected by volume expansion).
No products indexed under this heading.

Carbamazepine (Combined therapy of verapamil and carbamazepine may increase carbamazepine concentrations, resulting in side effects such as diplopia, ataxia, and headache).
Products include:
Carbatrol 3280
Equetro 3477

Carteolol Hydrochloride (Co-administration of β-blockers and verapamil may result in additive effects on heart rate, atrioventricular conduction, and/or cardiac contractility. The use of verapamil in combination with a β-blocker should be used only with caution, and close monitoring).
No products indexed under this heading.

Carvedilol (Co-administration of β-blockers and verapamil may result in additive effects on heart rate, atrioventricular conduction, and/or cardiac contractility. The use of verapamil in combination with a β-blocker should be used only with caution, and close monitoring). Products include:
Coreg 1409

Carvedilol Phosphate (Co-administration of β-blockers and verapamil may result in additive effects on heart rate, atrioventricular conduction, and/or cardiac contractility. The use of verapamil in combination with a β-blocker should be used only with caution, and close monitoring). Products include:
Coreg CR 1416

Chloroprocaine Hydrochloride (In patients undergoing major surgery or during anesthesia with agents that produce hypotension, trandolapril will block angiotensin II formation secondary to compensatory renin release. If hypotension occurs and is considered to be due to this mechanism, it can be corrected by volume expansion).
No products indexed under this heading.

Chlorothiazide (Trandolapril can attenuate potassium loss caused by thiazide diuretics).
No products indexed under this heading.

Chlorothiazide Sodium (Trandolapril can attenuate potassium loss caused by thiazide diuretics). Products include:
Diuril Intravenous 2009

Chlorthalidone (Patients on diuretics, especially those on recently instituted diuretic therapy, may occasionally experience an excessive reduction of blood pressure after initiation of therapy with Tarka). Products include:
Clorpres 2344

Cimetidine (Variable results on clearance have been obtained in acute studies during concomitant therapy; clearance of verapamil may be reduced or unchanged).
No products indexed under this heading.

Cimetidine Hydrochloride (Variable results on clearance have been obtained in acute studies during concomitant therapy; clearance of verapamil may be reduced or unchanged).
No products indexed under this heading.

1833 Interactions Index Tarka

Cisatracurium Besylate (Clinical data and studies suggest that verapamil may potentiate the activity of neuromuscular blocking agents (curare-like and depolarizing). It may be necessary to decrease the dose of verapamil and/or the dose of the neuromuscular blocking agent when the drugs are used concomitantly). Products include:
Nimbex 503

Clarithromycin (Hypotension, bradyarrhythmias, and lactic acidosis have been observed in patients receiving concurrent clarithromycin). Products include:
Biaxin/Biaxin XL 412

Cocaine Hydrochloride (In patients undergoing major surgery or during anesthesia with agents that produce hypotension, trandolapril will block angiotensin II formation secondary to compensatory renin release. If hypotension occurs and is considered to be due to this mechanism, it can be corrected by volume expansion).
No products indexed under this heading.

Cyclosporine (Verapamil therapy may increase serum levels of cyclosporin). Products include:
Gengraf 440
Neoral Oral Solution 2496
Neoral Capsules 2496
Restasis 605

Decamethonium (Clinical data and studies suggest that verapamil may potentiate the activity of neuromuscular blocking agents (curare-like and depolarizing). It may be necessary to decrease the dose of verapamil and/or the dose of the neuromuscular blocking agent when the drugs are used concomitantly).
No products indexed under this heading.

Desflurane (Experiments have shown that inhalation anesthetics depress cardiovascular activity by decreasing the inward movement of calcium ions. When used concomitantly, inhalation anesthetics and calcium antagonists, such as verapamil, should each be titrated carefully to avoid excessive cardiovascular depression).
No products indexed under this heading.

Deslanoside (Chronic verapamil therapy can increase serum digoxin levels by 50% to 75% during the first week, and this can result in digoxin toxicity. Verapamil may reduce total body clearance and extrarenal clearance of digitoxin by 27% and 29%, respectively. Maintenance digoxin doses should be reduced when verapamil is administered, and the patient should be carefully monitored to avoid over- or under-digitalization).
No products indexed under this heading.

Dibucaine (In patients undergoing major surgery or during anesthesia with agents that produce hypotension, trandolapril will block angiotensin II formation secondary to compensatory renin release. If hypotension occurs and is considered to be due to this mechanism, it can be corrected by volume expansion).
No products indexed under this heading.

Dibucaine Hydrochloride (In patients undergoing major surgery or during anesthesia with agents that produce hypotension, trandolapril will block angiotensin II formation secondary to compensatory renin release. If hypotension occurs and is considered to be due to this mechanism, it can be corrected by volume expansion).
No products indexed under this heading.

Digitalis Glycoside Preparations (Chronic verapamil therapy can increase serum digoxin levels by 50% to 75% during the first week, and this can result in digoxin toxicity. Verapamil may reduce total body clearance and extrarenal clearance of digitoxin by 27% and 29%, respectively. Maintenance digoxin doses should be reduced when verapamil is administered, and the patient should be carefully monitored to avoid over- or under-digitalization).
No products indexed under this heading.

Digitalis Lanata (Chronic verapamil therapy can increase serum digoxin levels by 50% to 75% during the first week, and this can result in digoxin toxicity. Verapamil may reduce total body clearance and extrarenal clearance of digitoxin by 27% and 29%, respectively. Maintenance digoxin doses should be reduced when verapamil is administered, and the patient should be carefully monitored to avoid over- or under-digitalization).
No products indexed under this heading.

Digitalis Purpurea (Chronic verapamil therapy can increase serum digoxin levels by 50% to 75% during the first week, and this can result in digoxin toxicity. Verapamil may reduce total body clearance and extrarenal clearance of digitoxin by 27% and 29%, respectively. Maintenance digoxin doses should be reduced when verapamil is administered, and the patient should be carefully monitored to avoid over- or under-digitalization).
No products indexed under this heading.

Digitoxin (Chronic verapamil therapy can increase serum digoxin levels by 50% to 75% during the first week, and this can result in digoxin toxicity. Verapamil may reduce total body clearance and extrarenal clearance of digitoxin by 27% and 29%, respectively. Maintenance digoxin doses should be reduced when verapamil is administered, and the patient should be carefully monitored to avoid over- or under-digitalization).
No products indexed under this heading.

Digoxin (Chronic verapamil therapy can increase serum digoxin levels by 50% to 75% during the first week, and this can result in digoxin toxicity. Verapamil may reduce total body clearance and extrarenal clearance of digitoxin by 27% and 29%, respectively. Maintenance digoxin doses should be reduced when verapamil is administered, and the patient should be carefully monitored to avoid over- or under-digitalization). Products include:
Lanoxin Injection 1546
Lanoxin Injection Pediatric 1549
Lanoxin Tablets 1553

Disopyramide (Data on possible interactions between verapamil and disopyramide phosphate are not available. Therefore, disopyramide should not be administered within 48 hours before or 24 hours after verapamil administration).
No products indexed under this heading.

Disopyramide Phosphate (Data on possible interactions between verapamil and disopyramide phosphate are not available. Therefore, disopyramide should not be administered within 48 hours before or 24 hours after verapamil administration).
No products indexed under this heading.

Doxacurium Chloride (Clinical data and studies suggest that verapamil may potentiate the activity of neuromuscular blocking agents (curare-like and depolarizing). It may be necessary to decrease the dose of verapamil and/or the dose of the neuromuscular blocking agent when the drugs are used concomitantly).
No products indexed under this heading.

d-Tubocurarine (Clinical data and studies suggest that verapamil may potentiate the activity of neuromuscular blocking agents (curare-like and depolarizing). It may be necessary to decrease the dose of verapamil and/or the dose of the neuromuscular blocking agent when the drugs are used concomitantly).
No products indexed under this heading.

Enflurane (Experiments have shown that inhalation anesthetics depress cardiovascular activity by decreasing the inward movement of calcium ions. When used concomitantly, inhalation anesthetics and calcium antagonists, such as verapamil, should each be titrated carefully to avoid excessive cardiovascular depression).
No products indexed under this heading.

Erythrityl Tetranitrate (Verapamil has been given concomitantly with short- and long-acting nitrates without any undesirable drug interactions. The pharmacologic profile of both drugs and the clinical experience suggest beneficial interactions).
No products indexed under this heading.

Erythromycin (Hypotension, bradyarrhythmias, and lactic acidosis have been observed in patients receiving concurrent erythromycin ethylsuccinate).
No products indexed under this heading.

Erythromycin, Topical (Hypotension, bradyarrhythmias, and lactic acidosis have been observed in patients receiving concurrent erythromycin ethylsuccinate).
No products indexed under this heading.

Erythromycin Estolate (Hypotension, bradyarrhythmias, and lactic acidosis have been observed in patients receiving concurrent erythromycin ethylsuccinate).
No products indexed under this heading.

Erythromycin Ethylsuccinate (Hypotension, bradyarrhythmias, and lactic acidosis have been observed in patients receiving concurrent erythromycin ethylsuccinate). Products include:
E.E.S. 437
EryPed 435

Erythromycin Gluceptate (Hypotension, bradyarrhythmias, and lactic acidosis have been observed in patients receiving concurrent erythromycin ethylsuccinate).
No products indexed under this heading.

Erythromycin Lactobionate (Hypotension, bradyarrhythmias, and lactic acidosis have been observed in patients receiving concurrent erythromycin ethylsuccinate).
No products indexed under this heading.

Erythromycin Stearate (Hypotension, bradyarrhythmias, and lactic acidosis have been observed in patients receiving concurrent erythromycin ethylsuccinate).
No products indexed under this heading.

Esmolol Hydrochloride (Coadministration of β-blockers and verapamil may result in additive effects on heart rate, atrioventricular conduction, and/or cardiac contractility. The use of verapamil in combination with a β-blocker should be used only with caution, and close monitoring).
No products indexed under this heading.

Ethacrynic Acid (Patients on diuretics, especially those on recently instituted diuretic therapy, may occasionally experience an excessive reduction of blood pressure after initiation of therapy with Tarka).
No products indexed under this heading.

Etidocaine Hydrochloride (In patients undergoing major surgery or during anesthesia with agents that produce hypotension, trandolapril will block angiotensin II formation secondary to compensatory renin release. If hypotension occurs and is considered to be due to this mechanism, it can be corrected by volume expansion).
No products indexed under this heading.

Fentanyl Citrate (In patients undergoing major surgery or during anesthesia with agents that produce hypotension, trandolapril will block angiotensin II formation secondary to compensatory renin release. If hypotension occurs and is considered to be due to this mechanism, it can be corrected by volume expansion). Products include:
Fentora 966

Flecainide Acetate (Concomitant use may result in additive effects on myocardial contractility, AV conduction and repolarization; concurrent use of flecainide and verapamil may result in additive inotropic effect and prolongation of atrioventricular conduction).
No products indexed under this heading.

Furosemide (Patients on diuretics, especially those on recently instituted diuretic therapy, may occasionally experience an excessive reduction of blood pressure after initiation of therapy with Tarka). Products include:
Furosemide 2354

Gallamine (Clinical data and studies suggest that verapamil may potentiate the activity of neuromuscular blocking agents (curare-like and depolarizing). It may be necessary to decrease the dose of verapamil and/or the dose of the neuromuscular blocking agent when the drugs are used concomitantly).
No products indexed under this heading.

Gallamine Triethiodide (Clinical data and studies suggest that verapamil may potentiate the activity of neuromuscular blocking agents (curare-like and depolarizing). It may be necessary to decrease the dose of verapamil and/or the dose of the neuromuscular blocking agent when the drugs are used concomitantly).
No products indexed under this heading.

Glyceryl Trinitrate (Verapamil has been given concomitantly with short- and long-acting nitrates without any undesirable drug interactions. The pharmacologic profile of both drugs and the clinical experience suggest beneficial interactions).
No products indexed under this heading.

Gold Sodium Thiomalate (Nitritoid reactions (symptoms include facial flushing, nausea, vomiting and hypotension) have been reported rarely in patients on therapy with injectable gold (sodium aurothiomalate) and concomitant ACE inhibitor therapy including Tarka).
No products indexed under this heading.

Gold Therapy (Nitritoid reactions (symptoms include facial flushing, nausea, vomiting and hypotension) have been reported rarely in patients on therapy with injectable gold (sodium aurothiomalate) and concomitant ACE inhibitor therapy including Tarka).
No products indexed under this heading.

Halothane (Experiments have shown that inhalation anesthetics depress cardiovascular activity by decreasing the inward movement of calcium ions. When used concomitantly, inhalation anesthetics and calcium antagonists, such as verapamil, should each be titrated carefully to avoid excessive cardiovascular depression).
No products indexed under this heading.

Hydrochlorothiazide (Trandolapril can attenuate potassium loss caused by thiazide diuretics). Products include:

IMPORTANT NOTE: Always consult each drug listing in the patient's regimen for possible interactions.

Hydroflumethiazide (Trandolapril can attenuate potassium loss caused by thiazide diuretics).
No products indexed under this heading.

Indapamide (Patients on diuretics, especially those on recently instituted diuretic therapy, may occasionally experience an excessive reduction of blood pressure after initiation of therapy with Tarka). Products include:

Isoflurane (Experiments have shown that inhalation anesthetics depress cardiovascular activity by decreasing the inward movement of calcium ions. When used concomitantly, inhalation anesthetics and calcium antagonists, such as verapamil, should each be titrated carefully to avoid excessive cardiovascular depression).
No products indexed under this heading.

Isosorbide Dinitrate (Verapamil has been given concomitantly with short- and long-acting nitrates without any undesirable drug interactions. The pharmacologic profile of both drugs and the clinical experience suggest beneficial interactions).
No products indexed under this heading.

Isosorbide Mononitrate (Verapamil has been given concomitantly with short- and long-acting nitrates without any undesirable drug interactions. The pharmacologic profile of both drugs and the clinical experience suggest beneficial interactions).
No products indexed under this heading.

Ketamine Hydrochloride (In patients undergoing major surgery or during anesthesia with agents that produce hypotension, trandolapril will block angiotensin II formation secondary to compensatory renin release. If hypotension occurs and is considered to be due to this mechanism, it can be corrected by volume expansion).
No products indexed under this heading.

Labetalol Hydrochloride (Co-administration of β-blockers and verapamil may result in additive effects on heart rate, atrioventricular conduction, and/or cardiac contractility. The use of verapamil in combination with a β-blocker should be used only with caution, and close monitoring).
No products indexed under this heading.

Levobunolol Hydrochloride (Co-administration of β-blockers and verapamil may result in additive effects on heart rate, atrioventricular conduction, and/or cardiac contractility. The use of verapamil in combination with a β-blocker should be used only with caution, and close monitoring).
No products indexed under this heading.

Levobupivacaine Hydrochloride (In patients undergoing major surgery or during anesthesia with agents that produce hypotension, trandolapril will block angiotensin II formation secondary to compensatory renin release. If hypotension occurs and is considered to be due to this mechanism, it can be corrected by volume expansion).
No products indexed under this heading.

Lidocaine (In patients undergoing major surgery or during anesthesia with agents that produce hypotension, trandolapril will block angiotensin II formation secondary to compensatory renin release. If hypotension occurs and is considered to be due to this mechanism, it can be corrected by volume expansion). Products include:

Lidocaine Base (In patients undergoing major surgery or during anesthesia with agents that produce hypotension, trandolapril will block angiotensin II formation secondary to compensatory renin release. If hypotension occurs and is considered to be due to this mechanism, it can be corrected by volume expansion).
No products indexed under this heading.

Lidocaine Hydrochloride (In patients undergoing major surgery or during anesthesia with agents that produce hypotension, trandolapril will block angiotensin II formation secondary to compensatory renin release. If hypotension occurs and is considered to be due to this mechanism, it can be corrected by volume expansion).
No products indexed under this heading.

Lithium (Increased sensitivity to the effects of lithium (neurotoxicity) has been reported during concomitant verapamil-lithium therapy with either no change or an increase in serum lithium levels. Tarka and lithium should be co-administered with caution, and frequent monitoring of serum lithium levels is recommended).
No products indexed under this heading.

Lithium Carbonate (Increased sensitivity to the effects of lithium (neurotoxicity) has been reported during concomitant verapamil-lithium therapy with either no change or an increase in serum lithium levels. Tarka and lithium should be co-administered with caution, and frequent monitoring of serum lithium levels is recommended).
No products indexed under this heading.

Lithium Citrate (Increased sensitivity to the effects of lithium (neurotoxicity) has been reported during concomitant verapamil-lithium therapy with either no change or an increase in serum lithium levels. Tarka and lithium should be co-administered with caution, and frequent monitoring of serum lithium levels is recommended).
No products indexed under this heading.

Mepivacaine Hydrochloride (In patients undergoing major surgery or during anesthesia with agents that produce hypotension, trandolapril will block angiotensin II formation secondary to compensatory renin release. If hypotension occurs and is considered to be due to this mechanism, it can be corrected by volume expansion).
No products indexed under this heading.

Methohexital Sodium (In patients undergoing major surgery or during anesthesia with agents that produce hypotension, trandolapril will block angiotensin II formation secondary to compensatory renin release. If hypotension occurs and is considered to be due to this mechanism, it can be corrected by volume expansion).
No products indexed under this heading.

Methoxyflurane (Experiments have shown that inhalation anesthetics depress cardiovascular activity by decreasing the inward movement of calcium ions. When used concomitantly, inhalation anesthetics and calcium antagonists, such as verapamil, should each be titrated carefully to avoid excessive cardiovascular depression).
No products indexed under this heading.

Methyclothiazide (Trandolapril can attenuate potassium loss caused by thiazide diuretics).
No products indexed under this heading.

Metipranolol Hydrochloride (Co-administration of β-blockers and verapamil may result in additive effects on heart rate, atrioventricular conduction, and/or cardiac contractility. The use of verapamil in combination with a β-blocker should be used only with caution, and close monitoring).
No products indexed under this heading.

Metocurine Iodide (Clinical data and studies suggest that verapamil may potentiate the activity of neuromuscular blocking agents (curare-like and depolarizing). It may be necessary to decrease the dose of verapamil and/or the dose of the neuromuscular blocking agent when the drugs are used concomitantly).
No products indexed under this heading.

Metolazone (Patients on diuretics, especially those on recently instituted diuretic therapy, may occasionally experience an excessive reduction of blood pressure after initiation of therapy with Tarka).
No products indexed under this heading.

Metoprolol Succinate (Co-administration of β-blockers and verapamil may result in additive effects on heart rate, atrioventricular conduction, and/or cardiac contractility. The use of verapamil in combination with a β-blocker should be used only with caution, and close monitoring). Products include:

Metoprolol Tartrate (Co-administration of β-blockers and verapamil may result in additive effects on heart rate, atrioventricular conduction, and/or cardiac contractility. The use of verapamil in combination with a β-blocker should be used only with caution, and close monitoring).
No products indexed under this heading.

Midazolam Hydrochloride (In patients undergoing major surgery or during anesthesia with agents that produce hypotension, trandolapril will block angiotensin II formation secondary to compensatory renin release. If hypotension occurs and is considered to be due to this mechanism, it can be corrected by volume expansion).
No products indexed under this heading.

Mivacurium Chloride (Clinical data and studies suggest that verapamil may potentiate the activity of neuromuscular blocking agents (curare-like and depolarizing). It may be necessary to decrease the dose of verapamil and/or the dose of the neuromuscular blocking agent when the drugs are used concomitantly).
No products indexed under this heading.

Nadolol (Co-administration of β-blockers and verapamil may result in additive effects on heart rate, atrioventricular conduction, and/or cardiac contractility. The use of verapamil in combination with a β-blocker should be used only with caution, and close monitoring). Products include:

Nebivolol (Co-administration of β-blockers and verapamil may result in additive effects on heart rate, atrioventricular conduction, and/or cardiac contractility. The use of verapamil in combination with a β-blocker should be used only with caution, and close monitoring). Products include:

Nitrate & Nitrite Preparations (Verapamil has been given concomitantly with short- and long-acting nitrates without any undesirable drug interactions. The pharmacologic profile of both drugs and the clinical experience suggest beneficial interactions).
No products indexed under this heading.

Nitrates, organic (Verapamil has been given concomitantly with short- and long-acting nitrates without any undesirable drug interactions. The pharmacologic profile of both drugs and the clinical experience suggest beneficial interactions).
No products indexed under this heading.

Nitrates and Nitrites (Verapamil has been given concomitantly with short- and long-acting nitrates without any undesirable drug interactions. The pharmacologic profile of both drugs and the clinical experience suggest beneficial interactions).
No products indexed under this heading.

Nitroglycerin (Verapamil has been given concomitantly with short- and long-acting nitrates without any undesirable drug interactions. The pharmacologic profile of both drugs and the clinical experience suggest beneficial interactions). Products include:

Nitroglycerin, long-acting formulations (Verapamil has been given concomitantly with short- and long-acting nitrates without any undesirable drug interactions. The pharmacologic profile of both drugs and the clinical experience suggest beneficial interactions).
No products indexed under this heading.

Nitroglycerin Intravenous (Verapamil has been given concomitantly with short- and long-acting nitrates without any undesirable drug interactions. The pharmacologic profile of both drugs and the clinical experience suggest beneficial interactions).
No products indexed under this heading.

Pancuronium Bromide (Clinical data and studies suggest that verapamil may potentiate the activity of neuromuscular blocking agents (curare-like and depolarizing). It may be necessary to decrease the dose of verapamil and/or the dose of the neuromuscular blocking agent when the drugs are used concomitantly).
No products indexed under this heading.

Penbutolol Sulfate (Co-administration of β-blockers and verapamil may result in additive effects on heart rate, atrioventricular conduction, and/or cardiac contractility. The use of verapamil in combination with a β-blocker should be used only with caution, and close monitoring).
No products indexed under this heading.

Pentaerythritol Tetranitrate (Verapamil has been given concomitantly with short- and long-acting nitrates without any undesirable drug interactions. The pharmacologic profile of both drugs and the clinical experience suggest beneficial interactions).
No products indexed under this heading.

Phenobarbital (Phenobarbital therapy may increase verapamil clearance). Products include:

Pindolol (Co-administration of β-blockers and verapamil may result in additive effects on heart rate, atrioventricular conduction, and/or cardiac contractility. The use of verapamil in combination with a β-blocker should be used only with caution, and close monitoring).
No products indexed under this heading.

Polythiazide (Trandolapril can attenuate potassium loss caused by thiazide diuretics).
No products indexed under this heading.

Potassium Acid Phosphate (Use of potassium-sparing diuretics (spironolactone, triamterene, or amiloride), potassium supplements, or potassium-containing salt substitutes concomitantly with ACE inhibitors can

1835 Interactions Index Tarka

increase the risk of hyperkalemia. If concomitant use of such agents is indicated, they should be used with caution and with appropriate monitoring of serum potassium). Products include:
K-Phos Original 874

Potassium Bicarbonate (Use of potassium-sparing diuretics (spironolactone, triamterene, or amiloride), potassium supplements, or potassium-containing salt substitutes concomitantly with ACE inhibitors can increase the risk of hyperkalemia. If concomitant use of such agents is indicated, they should be used with caution and with appropriate monitoring of serum potassium).
No products indexed under this heading.

Potassium Chloride (Use of potassium-sparing diuretics (spironolactone, triamterene, or amiloride), potassium supplements, or potassium-containing salt substitutes concomitantly with ACE inhibitors can increase the risk of hyperkalemia. If concomitant use of such agents is indicated, they should be used with caution and with appropriate monitoring of serum potassium). Products include:
MoviPrep Oral Solution 2905

Potassium Citrate (Use of potassium-sparing diuretics (spironolactone, triamterene, or amiloride), potassium supplements, or potassium-containing salt substitutes concomitantly with ACE inhibitors can increase the risk of hyperkalemia. If concomitant use of such agents is indicated, they should be used with caution and with appropriate monitoring of serum potassium). Products include:
Urocit-K 2333

Potassium Gluconate (Use of potassium-sparing diuretics (spironolactone, triamterene, or amiloride), potassium supplements, or potassium-containing salt substitutes concomitantly with ACE inhibitors can increase the risk of hyperkalemia. If concomitant use of such agents is indicated, they should be used with caution and with appropriate monitoring of serum potassium).
No products indexed under this heading.

Potassium Phosphate (Use of potassium-sparing diuretics (spironolactone, triamterene, or amiloride), potassium supplements, or potassium-containing salt substitutes concomitantly with ACE inhibitors can increase the risk of hyperkalemia. If concomitant use of such agents is indicated, they should be used with caution and with appropriate monitoring of serum potassium). Products include:
K-Phos Neutral 873

Prilocaine (In patients undergoing major surgery or during anesthesia with agents that produce hypotension, trandolapril will block angiotensin II formation secondary to compensatory renin release. If hypotension occurs and is considered to be due to this mechanism, it can be corrected by volume expansion).
No products indexed under this heading.

Prilocaine Hydrochloride (In patients undergoing major surgery or during anesthesia with agents that produce hypotension, trandolapril will block angiotensin II formation secondary to compensatory renin release. If hypotension occurs and is considered to be due to this mechanism, it can be corrected by volume expansion).
No products indexed under this heading.

Procaine (In patients undergoing major surgery or during anesthesia with agents that produce hypotension, trandolapril will block angiotensin II formation secondary to compensatory renin release. If hypotension occurs and is considered to be due to this mechanism, it can be corrected by volume expansion).
No products indexed under this heading.

Procaine Hydrochloride (In patients undergoing major surgery or during anesthesia with agents that produce hypotension, trandolapril will block angiotensin II formation secondary to compensatory renin release. If hypotension occurs and is considered to be due to this mechanism, it can be corrected by volume expansion).
No products indexed under this heading.

Proparacaine Hydrochloride (In patients undergoing major surgery or during anesthesia with agents that produce hypotension, trandolapril will block angiotensin II formation secondary to compensatory renin release. If hypotension occurs and is considered to be due to this mechanism, it can be corrected by volume expansion).
No products indexed under this heading.

Propofol (In patients undergoing major surgery or during anesthesia with agents that produce hypotension, trandolapril will block angiotensin II formation secondary to compensatory renin release. If hypotension occurs and is considered to be due to this mechanism, it can be corrected by volume expansion).
No products indexed under this heading.

Propranolol Hydrochloride (Co-administration of β-blockers and verapamil may result in additive effects on heart rate, atrioventricular conduction, and/or cardiac contractility. The use of verapamil in combination with a β-blocker should be used only with caution, and close monitoring). Products include:
InnoPran XL 1517

Quinidine (In a small number of patients with hypertrophic cardiomyopathy (IHSS), concomitant use of verapamil and quinidine resulted in significant hypotension. Combined therapy of verapamil and quinidine in these patients should be avoided. Verapamil counteracts the effects of quinidine on AV conduction and there has been a report of increased quinidine levels during verapamil therapy).
No products indexed under this heading.

Quinidine Gluconate (In a small number of patients with hypertrophic cardiomyopathy (IHSS), concomitant use of verapamil and quinidine resulted in significant hypotension. Combined therapy of verapamil and quinidine in these patients should be avoided. Verapamil counteracts the effects of quinidine on AV conduction and there has been a report of increased quinidine levels during verapamil therapy).
No products indexed under this heading.

Quinidine Hydrochloride (In a small number of patients with hypertrophic cardiomyopathy (IHSS), concomitant use of verapamil and quinidine resulted in significant hypotension. Combined therapy of verapamil and quinidine in these patients should be avoided. Verapamil counteracts the effects of quinidine on AV conduction and there has been a report of increased quinidine levels during verapamil therapy).
No products indexed under this heading.

Quinidine Polygalacturonate (In a small number of patients with hypertrophic cardiomyopathy (IHSS), concomitant use of verapamil and quinidine resulted in significant hypotension. Combined therapy of verapamil and quinidine in these patients should be avoided. Verapamil counteracts the effects of quinidine on AV conduction and there has been a report of increased quinidine levels during verapamil therapy).
No products indexed under this heading.

Quinidine Sulfate (In a small number of patients with hypertrophic cardiomyopathy (IHSS), concomitant use of verapamil and quinidine resulted in significant hypotension. Combined therapy of verapamil and quinidine in these patients should be avoided. Verapamil counteracts the effects of quinidine on AV conduction and there has been a report of increased quinidine levels during verapamil therapy).
No products indexed under this heading.

Rapacuronium Bromide (Clinical data and studies suggest that verapamil may potentiate the activity of neuromuscular blocking agents (curare-like and depolarizing). It may be necessary to decrease the dose of verapamil and/or the dose of the neuromuscular blocking agent when the drugs are used concomitantly).
No products indexed under this heading.

Remifentanil Hydrochloride (In patients undergoing major surgery or during anesthesia with agents that produce hypotension, trandolapril will block angiotensin II formation secondary to compensatory renin release. If hypotension occurs and is considered to be due to this mechanism, it can be corrected by volume expansion).
No products indexed under this heading.

Rifampin (Therapy with rifampin may markedly reduce oral verapamil bioavailability).
No products indexed under this heading.

Rocuronium Bromide (Clinical data and studies suggest that verapamil may potentiate the activity of neuromuscular blocking agents (curare-like and depolarizing). It may be necessary to decrease the dose of verapamil and/or the dose of the neuromuscular blocking agent when the drugs are used concomitantly). Products include:
Zemuron 3249

Ropivacaine Hydrochloride (In patients undergoing major surgery or during anesthesia with agents that produce hypotension, trandolapril will block angiotensin II formation secondary to compensatory renin release. If hypotension occurs and is considered to be due to this mechanism, it can be corrected by volume expansion).
No products indexed under this heading.

Sevoflurane (Experiments have shown that inhalation anesthetics depress cardiovascular activity by decreasing the inward movement of calcium ions. When used concomitantly, inhalation anesthetics and calcium antagonists, such as verapamil, should each be titrated carefully to avoid excessive cardiovascular depression). Products include:
Ultane 554

Sotalol Hydrochloride (Co-administration of β-blockers and verapamil may result in additive effects on heart rate, atrioventricular conduction, and/or cardiac contractility. The use of verapamil in combination with a β-blocker should be used only with caution, and close monitoring).
No products indexed under this heading.

Spironolactone (Use of potassium-sparing diuretics (spironolactone, triamterene, or amiloride), potassium supplements, or potassium-containing salt substitutes concomitantly with ACE inhibitors can increase the risk of hyperkalemia. If concomitant use of such agents is indicated, they should be used with caution and with appropriate monitoring of serum potassium).
No products indexed under this heading.

Succinylcholine Chloride (Clinical data and studies suggest that verapamil may potentiate the activity of neuromuscular blocking agents (curare-like and depolarizing). It may be necessary to decrease the dose of verapamil and/or the dose of the neuromuscular blocking agent when the drugs are used concomitantly).
No products indexed under this heading.

Sufentanil Citrate (In patients undergoing major surgery or during anesthesia with agents that produce hypotension, trandolapril will block angiotensin II formation secondary to compensatory renin release. If hypotension occurs and is considered to be due to this mechanism, it can be corrected by volume expansion).
No products indexed under this heading.

Tetracaine (In patients undergoing major surgery or during anesthesia with agents that produce hypotension, trandolapril will block angiotensin II formation secondary to compensatory renin release. If hypotension occurs and is considered to be due to this mechanism, it can be corrected by volume expansion).
No products indexed under this heading.

Tetracaine Hydrochloride (In patients undergoing major surgery or during anesthesia with agents that produce hypotension, trandolapril will block angiotensin II formation secondary to compensatory renin release. If hypotension occurs and is considered to be due to this mechanism, it can be corrected by volume expansion).
No products indexed under this heading.

Theophylline (Verapamil therapy may inhibit the clearance and increase the plasma levels of theophylline).
No products indexed under this heading.

Theophylline Anhydrous (Verapamil therapy may inhibit the clearance and increase the plasma levels of theophylline). Products include:
Uniphyl 2817

Theophylline Calcium Salicylate (Verapamil therapy may inhibit the clearance and increase the plasma levels of theophylline).
No products indexed under this heading.

Theophylline Dihydroxypropyl (Glyceryl) (Verapamil therapy may inhibit the clearance and increase the plasma levels of theophylline).
No products indexed under this heading.

Theophylline Ethylenediamine (Verapamil therapy may inhibit the clearance and increase the plasma levels of theophylline).
No products indexed under this heading.

Theophylline Sodium Glycinate (Verapamil therapy may inhibit the clearance and increase the plasma levels of theophylline).
No products indexed under this heading.

Thiamylal Sodium (In patients undergoing major surgery or during anesthesia with agents that produce hypotension, trandolapril will block angiotensin II formation secondary to compensatory renin release. If hypotension occurs and is considered to be due to this mechanism, it can be corrected by volume expansion).
No products indexed under this heading.

IMPORTANT NOTE: Always consult each drug listing in the patient's regimen for possible interactions.

Tarka **Interactions Index** 1836

Timolol Hemihydrate (Concomitant therapy with β-adrenergic blockers and verapamil may result in additive negative effects on heart rate, atrioventricular conduction, and/or cardiac contractility. The use of verapamil in combination with a β-blocker should be used only with caution, and close monitoring. Asymptomatic bradycardia (36 beats/min) with a wandering atrial pacemaker has been observed in a patient receiving concomitant timolol (a β-adrenergic blocker) eyedrops and oral verapamil). Products include:

Betimol 3490

Timolol Maleate (Concomitant therapy with β-adrenergic blockers and verapamil may result in additive negative effects on heart rate, atrioventricular conduction, and/or cardiac contractility. The use of verapamil in combination with a β-blocker should be used only with caution, and close monitoring. Asymptomatic bradycardia (36 beats/min) with a wandering atrial pacemaker has been observed in a patient receiving concomitant timolol (a β-adrenergic blocker) eyedrops and oral verapamil). Products include:

Combigan 601
Dorzolamide Hydrochloride/Timolol Maleate Ophthalmic Solution .... ⊙243
Timoptic in Ocudose .... ⊙231

Torsemide (Patients on diuretics, especially those on recently instituted diuretic therapy, may occasionally experience an excessive reduction of blood pressure after initiation of therapy with Tarka).

No products indexed under this heading.

Triamterene (Use of potassium-sparing diuretics (spironolactone, triamterene, or amiloride), potassium supplements, or potassium-containing salt substitutes concomitantly with ACE inhibitors can increase the risk of hyperkalemia. If concomitant use of such agents is indicated, they should be used with caution and with appropriate monitoring of serum potassium). Products include:

Dyazide 1429
Dyrenium 3495

Tubocurarine Chloride (Clinical data and studies suggest that verapamil may potentiate the activity of neuromuscular blocking agents (curare-like and depolarizing). It may be necessary to decrease the dose of verapamil and/or the dose of the neuromuscular blocking agent when the drugs are used concomitantly).

No products indexed under this heading.

Vecuronium Bromide (Clinical data and studies suggest that verapamil may potentiate the activity of neuromuscular blocking agents (curare-like and depolarizing). It may be necessary to decrease the dose of verapamil and/or the dose of the neuromuscular blocking agent when the drugs are used concomitantly).

No products indexed under this heading.

Food Interactions

Food, unspecified (Co-administration with food decreases verapamil bioavailability and the time to peak plasma concentration is delayed; bioavailability of trandolapril is not altered; Tarka should be administered with food).

Salt Substitutes, Potassium-Containing (Use of potassium-sparing diuretics (spironolactone, triamterene, or amiloride), potassium supplements, or potassium-containing salt substitutes concomitantly with ACE inhibitors can increase the risk of hyperkalemia. If concomitant use of such agents is indicated, they should be used with caution and with appropriate monitoring of serum potassium).

TASIGNA CAPSULES

(Nilotinib) 2533

May interact with antiarrhythmics, cytochrome p450 2b6 substrates (selected), cytochrome p450 2c8 substrates (selected), cytochrome p450 2c9 substrates (selected), cytochrome p450 2d6 substrates (selected), cytochrome p450 3a4 inducers (selected), cytochrome p450 3a4 inhibitors, potent (selected), cytochrome p450 3a4 substrates (selected), dexamethasones, drugs that prolong the QT interval, haloperidols, P-glycoprotein inhibitors, P-glycoprotein substrates (selected), phenytoin, quinidine, UDP-glucuronosyltransferase (UGT) 1A1 substrates (selected), and certain other agents. Compounds in these categories include:

Acarbose (Nilotinib is a competitive inhibitor of CYP2C9 *in vitro*, potentially increasing the concentration of drugs eliminated by CYP2C9. Caution should be exercised when co-administering nilotinib with substrates for CYP2C9 that have a narrow therapeutic index. *In vitro* studies also suggest that nilotinib may induce CYP2B6, CYP2C8 and CYP2C9, and thereby has the potential to decrease the concentrations of drugs which are eliminated by these enzymes).

No products indexed under this heading.

Acebutolol Hydrochloride (The administration of nilotinib with agents that are strong CYP3A4 inhibitors or anti-arrhythmic drugs and other drugs that may prolong QT interval should be avoided. Should treatment with any of these agents be required, it is recommended that therapy with nilotinib be interrupted. If interruption of treatment with nilotinib is not possible, patients who require treatment with a drug that prolongs QT or strongly inhibits CYP3A4 should be closely monitored for prolongation of the QT interval).

No products indexed under this heading.

Acetaminophen (Nilotinib is a competitive inhibitor of UGT1A1 *in vitro*, potentially increasing the concentrations of drugs eliminated by this enzyme). Products include:

Percocet 1121
Tylenol 2049
Tylenol 8 Hour 2049
Extra Strength Tylenol Caplets, Cool Caplets, and EZ Tabs 2049
Extra Strength Tylenol Adult Rapid Blast Liquid 2049
Extra Strength Tylenol Rapid Release 2049
Tylenol with Codeine 2691
Tylenol Arthritis Pain Extended Release Geltabs/Caplets 2049
Children's Tylenol Suspension Liquid 2048
Chlidren's Tylenol Meltaways 2048
Tylenol, Infants' Drops 2048
Junior Tylenol 2048
Vicodin 560
Vicodin ES 561
Vicodin HP 563
Zydone 1138

Acetaminophen-containing products (Nilotinib is a competitive inhibitor of UGT1A1 *in vitro*, potentially increasing the concentrations of drugs eliminated by this enzyme).

No products indexed under this heading.

Adenosine (The administration of nilotinib with agents that are strong CYP3A4 inhibitors or anti-arrhythmic drugs and other drugs that may prolong QT interval should be avoided. Should treatment with any of these agents be required, it is recommended that therapy with nilotinib be interrupted. If interruption of treatment with nilotinib is not possible, patients who require treatment with a drug that prolongs QT or strongly inhibits CYP3A4 should be closely monitored for prolongation of the QT interval). Products include:

Adenocard 656
Adenoscan 657

Alfentanil Hydrochloride (Nilotinib is a competitive inhibitor of CYP3A4 *in vitro*, potentially increasing the concentration of drugs eliminated by CYP3A4. Caution should be exercised when co-administering nilotinib with substrates for CYP3A4 that have a narrow therapeutic index).

No products indexed under this heading.

Allium sativum (The concomitant use of strong CYP3A4 inducers should be avoided. If patients must be co-administered a strong CYP3A4 inducer, the dose of nilotinib may need to be increased, depending on patient tolerability. If the strong inducer is discontinued, the nilotinib dose should be reduced to the indicated dose).

No products indexed under this heading.

Alprazolam (The administration of nilotinib with agents that prolong the QT interval should be avoided. Should treatment with any of these agents be required, it is recommended that therapy with nilotinib be interrupted. If interruption of treatment with nilotinib is not possible, patients who require treatment with a drug that prolongs the QT interval should be closely monitored for prolongation of the QT interval).

No products indexed under this heading.

Ambrisentan (Nilotinib inhibits human P-glycoprotein. If nilotinib is administered with drugs that are substrates of Pgp, increased concentrations of the substrate drug are likely, and caution should be exercised). Products include:

Letairis Tablets 1250

Aminoglutethimide (The concomitant use of strong CYP3A4 inducers should be avoided. If patients must be co-administered a strong CYP3A4 inducer, the dose of nilotinib may need to be increased, depending on patient tolerability. If the strong inducer is discontinued, the nilotinib dose should be reduced to the indicated dose).

No products indexed under this heading.

Amiodarone Hydrochloride (The administration of nilotinib with agents that are strong CYP3A4 inhibitors or anti-arrhythmic drugs (eg,amiodarone) and other drugs that may prolong QT interval should be avoided. Should treatment with any of these agents be required, it is recommended that therapy with nilotinib be interrupted. If interruption of treatment with nilotinib is not possible, patients who require treatment with a drug that prolongs QT or strongly inhibits CYP3A4 should be closely monitored for prolongation of the QT interval).

No products indexed under this heading.

Amitriptyline Hydrochloride (The administration of nilotinib with agents that prolong the QT interval should be avoided. Should treatment with any of these agents be required, it is recommended that therapy with nilotinib be interrupted. If interruption of treatment with nilotinib is not possible, patients who require treatment with a drug that prolongs the QT interval should be closely monitored for prolongation of the QT interval).

No products indexed under this heading.

Amlodipine Besylate (Nilotinib is a competitive inhibitor of CYP3A4 *in vitro*, potentially increasing the concentration of drugs eliminated by CYP3A4. Caution should be exercised when co-administering nilotinib with substrates for CYP3A4 that have a narrow therapeutic index). Products include:

Azor 1010
Exforge 2443
Exforge HCT 2449

Amoxapine (The administration of nilotinib with agents that prolong the QT interval should be avoided. Should treatment with any of these agents be required, it is recommended that therapy with nilotinib be interrupted. If interruption of treatment with nilotinib is not possible, patients who require treatment with a drug that prolongs the QT interval should be closely monitored for prolongation of the QT interval).

No products indexed under this heading.

Amphetamine Aspartate (Nilotinib is a competitive inhibitor of CYP2D6 *in vitro*, potentially increasing the concentration of drugs eliminated by CYP2D6. Caution should be exercised when co-administering nilotinib with substrates for CYP2D6 that have a narrow therapeutic index).

No products indexed under this heading.

Amphetamine Aspartate Monohydrate (Nilotinib is a competitive inhibitor of CYP2D6 *in vitro*, potentially increasing the concentration of drugs eliminated by CYP2D6. Caution should be exercised when co-administering nilotinib with substrates for CYP2D6 that have a narrow therapeutic index).

No products indexed under this heading.

Amphetamine Sulfate (Nilotinib is a competitive inhibitor of CYP2D6 *in vitro*, potentially increasing the concentration of drugs eliminated by CYP2D6. Caution should be exercised when co-administering nilotinib with substrates for CYP2D6 that have a narrow therapeutic index).

No products indexed under this heading.

Amprenavir (The administration of nilotinib with agents that are strong CYP3A4 inhibitors should be avoided. Should treatment with any of these agents be required, it is recommended that therapy with nilotinib be interrupted. If patients must be co-administered a strong CYP3A4 inhibitor, based on pharmacokinetic studies, 400 mg qd is predicted to adjust the nilotinib AUC to the AUC observed without inhibitors. However, there are no clinical data with this dose adjustment in patients receiving strong CYP3A4 inhibitors. If the strong inhibitor is discontinued, a washout period should be allowed before the nilotinib dose is adjusted upward to the indicated dose. Close monitoring for prolongation of the QT interval is indicated for patients who cannot avoid strong CYP3A4 inhibitors).

No products indexed under this heading.

Aprepitant (Nilotinib is a competitive inhibitor of CYP3A4 *in vitro*, potentially increasing the concentration of drugs eliminated by CYP3A4. Caution should be exercised when co-administering nilotinib with substrates for CYP3A4 that have a narrow therapeutic index). Products include:

Emend 2124

Astemizole (The administration of nilotinib with agents that prolong the QT interval should be avoided. Should treatment with any of these agents be required, it is recommended that therapy with nilotinib be interrupted. If interruption of treatment with nilotinib is not possible, patients who require treatment with a drug that prolongs the QT interval should be closely monitored for prolongation of the QT interval).

No products indexed under this heading.

Atazanavir (The administration of nilotinib with agents that are strong CYP3A4 inhibitors such as atazanavir should be avoided. If treatment is required, it is recommended that therapy with nilotinib be interrupted. If patients must be co-administered a strong CYP3A4 inhibitor, based on pharmacokinetic studies, 400 mg qd is predicted to adjust the nilotinib AUC to the AUC observed without inhibitors. However, there are no clinical data with this

1837 Interactions Index Tasigna

dose adjustment in patients receiving strong CYP3A4 inhibitors. If the strong inhibitor is discontinued, a washout period should be allowed before the nilotinib dose is adjusted upward to the indicated dose. Close monitoring for prolongation of the QT interval is indicated for patients who cannot avoid strong CYP3A4 inhibitors).
No products indexed under this heading.

Atazanavir Sulfate (The administration of nilotinib with agents that are strong CYP3A4 inhibitors such as atazanavir should be avoided. If treatment is required, it is recommended that therapy with nilotinib be interrupted. If patients must be co-administered a strong CYP3A4 inhibitor, based on pharmacokinetic studies, 400 mg qd is predicted to adjust the nilotinib AUC to the AUC observed without inhibitors. However, there are no clinical data with this dose adjustment in patients receiving strong CYP3A4 inhibitors. If the strong inhibitor is discontinued, a washout period should be allowed before the nilotinib dose is adjusted upward to the indicated dose. Close monitoring for prolongation of the QT interval is indicated for patients who cannot avoid strong CYP3A4 inhibitors).
No products indexed under this heading.

Atenolol (Nilotinib is a substrate of the efflux transporter P-glycoprotein (Pgp, ABCB1). If nilotinib is administered with drugs that inhibit Pgp, increased concentrations of nilotinib are likely, and caution should be exercised).
No products indexed under this heading.

Atomoxetine Hydrochloride (Nilotinib is a competitive inhibitor of CYP2D6 *in vitro*, potentially increasing the concentration of drugs eliminated by CYP2D6. Caution should be exercised when co-administering nilotinib with substrates for CYP2D6 that have a narrow therapeutic index). Products include:
Strattera 1957

Atorvastatin Calcium (Nilotinib is a competitive inhibitor of CYP3A4 *in vitro*, potentially increasing the concentration of drugs eliminated by CYP3A4. Caution should be exercised when co-administering nilotinib with substrates for CYP3A4 that have a narrow therapeutic index). Products include:
Lipitor 2703

Azithromycin Dihydrate (Nilotinib is a substrate of the efflux transporter P-glycoprotein (Pgp, ABCB1). If nilotinib is administered with drugs that inhibit Pgp, increased concentrations of nilotinib are likely, and caution should be exercised).
No products indexed under this heading.

Belladonna Ergotamine (Nilotinib is a competitive inhibitor of CYP3A4 *in vitro*, potentially increasing the concentration of drugs eliminated by CYP3A4. Caution should be exercised when co-administering nilotinib with substrates for CYP3A4 that have a narrow therapeutic index).
No products indexed under this heading.

Benzphetamine Hydrochloride (Nilotinib is a competitive inhibitor of CYP2C8 *in vitro*, potentially increasing the concentration of drugs eliminated by CYP2C8. Caution should be exercised when co-administering nilotinib with substrates for CYP2C8 that have a narrow therapeutic index. *In vitro* studies also suggest that nilotinib may induce CYP2B6, CYP2C8, and CYP2C9, and thereby has the potential to decrease the concentrations of drugs which are eliminated by these enzymes).
No products indexed under this heading.

Bepridil Hydrochloride (The administration of nilotinib with agents that are strong CYP3A4 inhibitors or anti-arrhythmic drugs and other drugs that may prolong QT interval (eg, bepridil) should be avoided. Should treatment with any of these agents be required, it is recommended that therapy with nilotinib be interrupted. If interruption of treatment with nilotinib is not possible, patients who require treatment with a drug that prolongs QT or strongly inhibits CYP3A4 should be closely monitored for prolongation of the QT interval).
No products indexed under this heading.

Betamethasone (The concomitant use of strong CYP3A4 inducers should be avoided. If patients must be co-administered a strong CYP3A4 inducer, the dose of nilotinib may need to be increased, depending on patient tolerability. If the strong inducer is discontinued, the nilotinib dose should be reduced to the indicated dose).
No products indexed under this heading.

Betamethasone Acetate (The concomitant use of strong CYP3A4 inducers should be avoided. If patients must be co-administered a strong CYP3A4 inducer, the dose of nilotinib may need to be increased, depending on patient tolerability. If the strong inducer is discontinued, the nilotinib dose should be reduced to the indicated dose).
No products indexed under this heading.

Betamethasone Benzoate (The concomitant use of strong CYP3A4 inducers should be avoided. If patients must be co-administered a strong CYP3A4 inducer, the dose of nilotinib may need to be increased, depending on patient tolerability. If the strong inducer is discontinued, the nilotinib dose should be reduced to the indicated dose).
No products indexed under this heading.

Betamethasone Dipropionate (The concomitant use of strong CYP3A4 inducers should be avoided. If patients must be co-administered a strong CYP3A4 inducer, the dose of nilotinib may need to be increased, depending on patient tolerability. If the strong inducer is discontinued, the nilotinib dose should be reduced to the indicated dose). Products include:
Diprolene Lotion 0.05% 3108
Diprolene Ointment 0.05% 3109
Diprolene AF Cream 0.05% 3107
Lotrisone 3163

Betamethasone Sodium Phosphate (The concomitant use of strong CYP3A4 inducers should be avoided. If patients must be co-administered a strong CYP3A4 inducer, the dose of nilotinib may need to be increased, depending on patient tolerability. If the strong inducer is discontinued, the nilotinib dose should be reduced to the indicated dose).
No products indexed under this heading.

Betamethasone Valerate (The concomitant use of strong CYP3A4 inducers should be avoided. If patients must be co-administered a strong CYP3A4 inducer, the dose of nilotinib may need to be increased, depending on patient tolerability. If the strong inducer is discontinued, the nilotinib dose should be reduced to the indicated dose). Products include:
Luxiq 3321

Bisoprolol Fumarate (Nilotinib is a competitive inhibitor of CYP2D6 *in vitro*, potentially increasing the concentration of drugs eliminated by CYP2D6. Caution should be exercised when co-administering nilotinib with substrates for CYP2D6 that have a narrow therapeutic index).
No products indexed under this heading.

Bosentan (The concomitant use of strong CYP3A4 inducers should be avoided. If patients must be co-administered a strong CYP3A4 inducer, the dose of nilotinib may need to be increased, depending on patient tolerability. If the strong inducer is discontinued, the nilotinib dose should be reduced to the indicated dose). Products include:
Tracleer 573

Bretylium Tosylate (The administration of nilotinib with agents that prolong the QT interval should be avoided. Should treatment with any of these agents be required, it is recommended that therapy with nilotinib be interrupted. If interruption of treatment with nilotinib is not possible, patients who require treatment with a drug that prolongs the QT interval should be closely monitored for prolongation of the QT interval).
No products indexed under this heading.

Buprenorphine Hydrochloride (Nilotinib is a competitive inhibitor of UGT1A1 *in vitro*, potentially increasing the concentrations of drugs eliminated by this enzyme).
No products indexed under this heading.

Bupropion (*In vitro* studies suggest that nilotinib may induce CYP2B6, CYP2C8 and CYP2C9, and decrease the concentrations of drugs which are eliminated by these enzymes).
No products indexed under this heading.

Bupropion Hydrochloride (*In vitro* studies suggest that nilotinib may induce CYP2B6, CYP2C8 and CYP2C9, and decrease the concentrations of drugs which are eliminated by these enzymes). Products include:
Aplenzin 2948
Wellbutrin 1719
Wellbutrin SR 1725
Zyban 1762

Buspirone Hydrochloride (The administration of nilotinib with agents that prolong the QT interval should be avoided. Should treatment with any of these agents be required, it is recommended that therapy with nilotinib be interrupted. If interruption of treatment with nilotinib is not possible, patients who require treatment with a drug that prolongs the QT interval should be closely monitored for prolongation of the QT interval).
No products indexed under this heading.

Busulfan (Nilotinib is a competitive inhibitor of CYP3A4 *in vitro*, potentially increasing the concentration of drugs eliminated by CYP3A4. Caution should be exercised when co-administering nilotinib with substrates for CYP3A4 that have a narrow therapeutic index). Products include:
Myleran 1581

Candesartan Cilexetil (Nilotinib is a competitive inhibitor of CYP2C9 *in vitro*, potentially increasing the concentration of drugs eliminated by CYP2C9. Caution should be exercised when co-administering nilotinib with substrates for CYP2C9 that have a narrow therapeutic index. *In vitro* studies also suggest that nilotinib may induce CYP2B6, CYP2C8 and CYP2C9, and thereby has the potential to decrease the concentrations of drugs which are eliminated by these enzymes). Products include:
Atacand 697
Atacand HCT 700

Captopril (Nilotinib is a competitive inhibitor of CYP2D6 *in vitro*, potentially increasing the concentration of drugs eliminated by CYP2D6. Caution should be exercised when co-administering nilotinib with substrates for CYP2D6 that have a narrow therapeutic index). Products include:
Captopril 2341

Carbamazepine (The concomitant use of strong CYP3A4 inducers such as carbamazepine should be avoided. If patients must be co-administered a strong CYP3A4 inducer, the dose of nilotinib may need to be increased, depending on patient tolerability. If the strong inducer is discontinued, the nilotinib dose should be reduced to the indicated dose). Products include:
Carbatrol 3280
Equetro 3477

Carvedilol (Nilotinib is a competitive inhibitor of CYP2C9 *in vitro*, potentially increasing the concentration of drugs eliminated by CYP2C9. Caution should be exercised when co-administering nilotinib with substrates for CYP2C9 that have a narrow therapeutic index. *In vitro* studies also suggest that nilotinib may induce CYP2B6, CYP2C8 and CYP2C9, and thereby has the potential to decrease the concentrations of drugs which are eliminated by these enzymes). Products include:
Coreg 1409

Carvedilol Phosphate (Nilotinib is a substrate of the efflux transporter P-glycoprotein (Pgp, ABCB1). If nilotinib is administered with drugs that inhibit Pgp, increased concentrations of nilotinib are likely, and caution should be exercised). Products include:
Coreg CR 1416

Celecoxib (Nilotinib is a competitive inhibitor of CYP2C9 *in vitro*, potentially increasing the concentration of drugs eliminated by CYP2C9. Caution should be exercised when co-administering nilotinib with substrates for CYP2C9 that have a narrow therapeutic index. *In vitro* studies also suggest that nilotinib may induce CYP2B6, CYP2C8 and CYP2C9, and thereby has the potential to decrease the concentrations of drugs which are eliminated by these enzymes). Products include:
Celebrex 3272

Cerivastatin Sodium (Nilotinib is a competitive inhibitor of CYP3A4 *in vitro*, potentially increasing the concentration of drugs eliminated by CYP3A4. Caution should be exercised when co-administering nilotinib with substrates for CYP3A4 that have a narrow therapeutic index).
No products indexed under this heading.

Cevimeline Hydrochloride (Nilotinib is a competitive inhibitor of CYP2D6 *in vitro*, potentially increasing the concentration of drugs eliminated by CYP2D6. Caution should be exercised when co-administering nilotinib with substrates for CYP2D6 that have a narrow therapeutic index). Products include:
Evoxac 1027

Chlordiazepoxide (The administration of nilotinib with agents that prolong the QT interval should be avoided. Should treatment with any of these agents be required, it is recommended that therapy with nilotinib be interrupted. If interruption of treatment with nilotinib is not possible, patients who require treatment with a drug that prolongs the QT interval should be closely monitored for prolongation of the QT interval).
No products indexed under this heading.

Chlordiazepoxide Hydrochloride (The administration of nilotinib with agents that prolong the QT interval should be avoided. Should treatment with any of these agents be required, it is recommended that therapy with nilotinib be interrupted. If interruption of treatment with nilotinib is not possible, patients who require treatment with a drug that prolongs the QT interval should be closely monitored for prolongation of the QT interval).
No products indexed under this heading.

Chloroquine (The administration of nilotinib with agents that are strong CYP3A4 inhibitors or anti-arrhythmic drugs and other drugs that may prolong QT interval (eg, chloroquine) should be

IMPORTANT NOTE: Always consult each drug listing in the patient's regimen for possible interactions.

avoided. Should treatment with any of these agents be required, it is recommended that therapy with nilotinib be interrupted. If interruption of treatment with nilotinib is not possible, patients who require treatment with a drug that prolongs QT or strongly inhibits CYP3A4 should be closely monitored for prolongation of the QT interval).
No products indexed under this heading.

Chloroquine Hydrochloride (The administration of nilotinib with agents that are strong CYP3A4 inhibitors or anti-arrhythmic drugs and other drugs that may prolong QT interval (eg, chloroquine) should be avoided. Should treatment with any of these agents be required, it is recommended that therapy with nilotinib be interrupted. If interruption of treatment with nilotinib is not possible, patients who require treatment with a drug that prolongs QT or strongly inhibits CYP3A4 should be closely monitored for prolongation of the QT interval).
No products indexed under this heading.

Chloroquine Phosphate (The administration of nilotinib with agents that are strong CYP3A4 inhibitors or anti-arrhythmic drugs and other drugs that may prolong QT interval (eg, chloroquine) should be avoided. Should treatment with any of these agents be required, it is recommended that therapy with nilotinib be interrupted. If interruption of treatment with nilotinib is not possible, patients who require treatment with a drug that prolongs QT or strongly inhibits CYP3A4 should be closely monitored for prolongation of the QT interval).
No products indexed under this heading.

Chlorpheniramine (Nilotinib is a competitive inhibitor of CYP3A4 *in vitro*, potentially increasing the concentration of drugs eliminated by CYP3A4. Caution should be exercised when co-administering nilotinib with substrates for CYP3A4 that have a narrow therapeutic index).
No products indexed under this heading.

Chlorpheniramine Maleate (Nilotinib is a competitive inhibitor of CYP3A4 *in vitro*, potentially increasing the concentration of drugs eliminated by CYP3A4. Caution should be exercised when co-administering nilotinib with substrates for CYP3A4 that have a narrow therapeutic index).
No products indexed under this heading.

Chlorpheniramine Polistirex (Nilotinib is a competitive inhibitor of CYP3A4 *in vitro*, potentially increasing the concentration of drugs eliminated by CYP3A4. Caution should be exercised when co-administering nilotinib with substrates for CYP3A4 that have a narrow therapeutic index). Products include:
Tussionex 3443

Chlorpheniramine Tannate (Nilotinib is a competitive inhibitor of CYP3A4 *in vitro*, potentially increasing the concentration of drugs eliminated by CYP3A4. Caution should be exercised when co-administering nilotinib with substrates for CYP3A4 that have a narrow therapeutic index).
No products indexed under this heading.

Chlorpromazine (The administration of nilotinib with agents that prolong the QT interval should be avoided. Should treatment with any of these agents be required, it is recommended that therapy with nilotinib be interrupted. If interruption of treatment with nilotinib is not possible, patients who require treatment with a drug that prolongs the QT interval should be closely monitored for prolongation of the QT interval).
No products indexed under this heading.

Chlorpromazine Hydrochloride (The administration of nilotinib with agents that prolong the QT interval should be avoided. Should treatment with any of these agents be required, it is recommended that therapy with nilotinib be interrupted. If interruption of treatment with nilotinib is not possible, patients who require treatment with a drug that prolongs the QT interval should be closely monitored for prolongation of the QT interval).
No products indexed under this heading.

Chlorpropamide (Nilotinib is a competitive inhibitor of CYP2C9 *in vitro*, potentially increasing the concentration of drugs eliminated by CYP2C9. Caution should be exercised when co-administering nilotinib with substrates for CYP2C9 that have a narrow therapeutic index. *In vitro* studies also suggest that nilotinib may induce CYP2B6, CYP2C8 and CYP2C9, and thereby has the potential to decrease the concentrations of drugs which are eliminated by these enzymes).
No products indexed under this heading.

Chlorprothixene (The administration of nilotinib with agents that prolong the QT interval should be avoided. Should treatment with any of these agents be required, it is recommended that therapy with nilotinib be interrupted. If interruption of treatment with nilotinib is not possible, patients who require treatment with a drug that prolongs the QT interval should be closely monitored for prolongation of the QT interval).
No products indexed under this heading.

Chlorprothixene Hydrochloride (The administration of nilotinib with agents that prolong the QT interval should be avoided. Should treatment with any of these agents be required, it is recommended that therapy with nilotinib be interrupted. If interruption of treatment with nilotinib is not possible, patients who require treatment with a drug that prolongs the QT interval should be closely monitored for prolongation of the QT interval).
No products indexed under this heading.

Ciprofloxacin (The concomitant use of strong CYP3A4 inducers should be avoided. If patients must be co-administered a strong CYP3A4 inducer, the dose of nilotinib may need to be increased, depending on patient tolerability. If the strong inducer is discontinued, the nilotinib dose should be reduced to the indicated dose). Products include:
Cipro I.V. 3082
Cipro 3073
Cipro XR 3091
Ciprodex 583

Ciprofloxacin Hydrochloride (The concomitant use of strong CYP3A4 inducers should be avoided. If patients must be co-administered a strong CYP3A4 inducer, the dose of nilotinib may need to be increased, depending on patient tolerability. If the strong inducer is discontinued, the nilotinib dose should be reduced to the indicated dose). Products include:
Cipro 3073

Cisapride (Nilotinib is a competitive inhibitor of CYP3A4 *in vitro*, potentially increasing the concentration of drugs eliminated by CYP3A4. Caution should be exercised when co-administering nilotinib with substrates for CYP3A4 that have a narrow therapeutic index).
No products indexed under this heading.

Cisplatin (The concomitant use of strong CYP3A4 inducers should be avoided. If patients must be co-administered a strong CYP3A4 inducer, the dose of nilotinib may need to be increased, depending on patient tolerability. If the strong inducer is discontinued, the nilotinib dose should be reduced to the indicated dose).
No products indexed under this heading.

Clarithromycin (The administration of nilotinib with agents that are strong CYP3A4 inhibitors such as clarithromycin should be avoided. If treatment is required, it is recommended that therapy with nilotinib be interrupted. If patients must be co-administered a strong CYP3A4 inhibitor, based on pharmacokinetic studies, 400 mg qd is predicted to adjust the nilotinib AUC to the AUC observed without inhibitors. However, there are no clinical data with this dose adjustment in patients receiving strong CYP3A4 inhibitors. If the strong inhibitor is discontinued, a washout period should be allowed before the nilotinib dose is adjusted upward to the indicated dose. Close monitoring for prolongation of the QT interval is indicated for patients who cannot avoid strong CYP3A4 inhibitors). Products include:
Biaxin/Biaxin XL 412

Clomipramine Hydrochloride (The administration of nilotinib with agents that prolong the QT interval should be avoided. Should treatment with any of these agents be required, it is recommended that therapy with nilotinib be interrupted. If interruption of treatment with nilotinib is not possible, patients who require treatment with a drug that prolongs the QT interval should be closely monitored for prolongation of the QT interval).
No products indexed under this heading.

Clorazepate Dipotassium (The administration of nilotinib with agents that prolong the QT interval should be avoided. Should treatment with any of these agents be required, it is recommended that therapy with nilotinib be interrupted. If interruption of treatment with nilotinib is not possible, patients who require treatment with a drug that prolongs the QT interval should be closely monitored for prolongation of the QT interval).
No products indexed under this heading.

Clozapine (The administration of nilotinib with agents that prolong the QT interval should be avoided. Should treatment with any of these agents be required, it is recommended that therapy with nilotinib be interrupted. If interruption of treatment with nilotinib is not possible, patients who require treatment with a drug that prolongs the QT interval should be closely monitored for prolongation of the QT interval).
No products indexed under this heading.

Codeine Phosphate (Nilotinib is a competitive inhibitor of CYP2D6 *in vitro*, potentially increasing the concentration of drugs eliminated by CYP2D6. Caution should be exercised when co-administering nilotinib with substrates for CYP2D6 that have a narrow therapeutic index). Products include:
Tylenol with Codeine 2691

Codeine Sulfate (Nilotinib is a competitive inhibitor of CYP2D6 *in vitro*, potentially increasing the concentration of drugs eliminated by CYP2D6. Caution should be exercised when co-administering nilotinib with substrates for CYP2D6 that have a narrow therapeutic index).
No products indexed under this heading.

Cortisone Acetate (The concomitant use of strong CYP3A4 inducers should be avoided. If patients must be co-administered a strong CYP3A4 inducer, the dose of nilotinib may need to be increased, depending on patient tolerability. If the strong inducer is discontinued, the nilotinib dose should be reduced to the indicated dose).
No products indexed under this heading.

Cyclobenzaprine Hydrochloride (Nilotinib is a competitive inhibitor of CYP2D6 *in vitro*, potentially increasing the concentration of drugs eliminated by CYP2D6. Caution should be exercised when co-administering nilotinib with substrates for CYP2D6 that have a narrow therapeutic index). Products include:
Amrix 964

Cyclophosphamide (*In vitro* studies suggest that nilotinib may induce CYP2B6, CYP2C8 and CYP2C9, and decrease the concentrations of drugs which are eliminated by these enzymes).
No products indexed under this heading.

Cyclosporine (Nilotinib is a competitive inhibitor of CYP3A4 *in vitro*, potentially increasing the concentration of drugs eliminated by CYP3A4. Caution should be exercised when co-administering nilotinib with substrates for CYP3A4 that have a narrow therapeutic index). Products include:
Gengraf 440
Neoral Oral Solution 2496
Neoral Capsules 2496
Restasis 605

Debrisoquine (Nilotinib is a competitive inhibitor of CYP2D6 *in vitro*, potentially increasing the concentration of drugs eliminated by CYP2D6. Caution should be exercised when co-administering nilotinib with substrates for CYP2D6 that have a narrow therapeutic index).
No products indexed under this heading.

Delavirdine Mesylate (The administration of nilotinib with agents that are strong CYP3A4 inhibitors should be avoided. Should treatment with any of these agents be required, it is recommended that therapy with nilotinib be interrupted. If patients must be co-administered a strong CYP3A4 inhibitor, based on pharmacokinetic studies, 400 mg qd is predicted to adjust the nilotinib AUC to the AUC observed without inhibitors. However, there are no clinical data with this dose adjustment in patients receiving strong CYP3A4 inhibitors. If the strong inhibitor is discontinued, a washout period should be allowed before the nilotinib dose is adjusted upward to the indicated dose. Close monitoring for prolongation of the QT interval is indicated for patients who cannot avoid strong CYP3A4 inhibitors).
No products indexed under this heading.

Delavirine (The administration of nilotinib with agents that are strong CYP3A4 inhibitors should be avoided. Should treatment with any of these agents be required, it is recommended that therapy with nilotinib be interrupted. If patients must be co-administered a strong CYP3A4 inhibitor, based on pharmacokinetic studies, 400 mg qd is predicted to adjust the nilotinib AUC to the AUC observed without inhibitors. However, there are no clinical data with this dose adjustment in patients receiving strong CYP3A4 inhibitors. If the strong inhibitor is discontinued, a washout period should be allowed before the nilotinib dose is adjusted upward to the indicated dose. Close monitoring for prolongation of the QT interval is indicated for patients who cannot avoid strong CYP3A4 inhibitors).
No products indexed under this heading.

Desipramine Hydrochloride (The administration of nilotinib with agents that prolong the QT interval should be avoided. Should treatment with any of these agents be required, it is recommended that therapy with nilotinib be interrupted. If interruption of treatment with nilotinib is not possible, patients who require treatment with a drug that prolongs the QT interval should be closely monitored for prolongation of the QT interval).
No products indexed under this heading.

Desogestrel (Nilotinib is a competitive inhibitor of CYP3A4 *in vitro*, potentially increasing the concentration of drugs eliminated by CYP3A4. Caution should be exercised when co-administering nilotinib with substrates for CYP3A4 that have a narrow therapeutic index).
No products indexed under this heading.

Dexamethasone (The concomitant use of strong CYP3A4 inducers such as dexamethasone should be avoided. If patients must be co-administered a strong CYP3A4 inducer, the dose of nilotinib may need to be increased, depending on patient tolerability. If the strong inducer is discontinued, the nilotinib dose should be reduced to the indicated dose). Products include:
Ciprodex 583
Ozurdex .... ⊙ 223
Tobramycin and Dexamethasone Ophthalmic Suspension .... ⊙ 251

Dexamethasone Acetate (The concomitant use of strong CYP3A4 inducers such as dexamethasone should be avoided. If patients must be co-administered a strong CYP3A4 inducer, the dose of nilotinib may need to be increased, depending on patient tolerability. If the strong inducer is discontinued, the nilotinib dose should be reduced to the indicated dose).
No products indexed under this heading.

Dexamethasone Phosphate (The concomitant use of strong CYP3A4 inducers such as dexamethasone should be avoided. If patients must be co-administered a strong CYP3A4 inducer, the dose of nilotinib may need to be increased, depending on patient tolerability. If the strong inducer is discontinued, the nilotinib dose should be reduced to the indicated dose).
No products indexed under this heading.

Dexamethasone Sodium (The concomitant use of strong CYP3A4 inducers such as dexamethasone should be avoided. If patients must be co-administered a strong CYP3A4 inducer, the dose of nilotinib may need to be increased, depending on patient tolerability. If the strong inducer is discontinued, the nilotinib dose should be reduced to the indicated dose).
No products indexed under this heading.

Dexamethasone Sodium Phosphate (The concomitant use of strong CYP3A4 inducers such as dexamethasone should be avoided. If patients must be co-administered a strong CYP3A4 inducer, the dose of nilotinib may need to be increased, depending on patient tolerability. If the strong inducer is discontinued, the nilotinib dose should be reduced to the indicated dose).
No products indexed under this heading.

Dexamethasone Sodium Phosphate Injection (The concomitant use of strong CYP3A4 inducers such as dexamethasone should be avoided. If patients must be co-administered a strong CYP3A4 inducer, the dose of nilotinib may need to be increased, depending on patient tolerability. If the strong inducer is discontinued, the nilotinib dose should be reduced to the indicated dose).
No products indexed under this heading.

Dexfenfluramine Hydrochloride (Nilotinib is a competitive inhibitor of CYP2D6 *in vitro*, potentially increasing the concentration of drugs eliminated by CYP2D6. Caution should be exercised when co-administering nilotinib with substrates for CYP2D6 that have a narrow therapeutic index).
No products indexed under this heading.

Dextromethorphan (Nilotinib is a competitive inhibitor of CYP2C9 *in vitro*, potentially increasing the concentration of drugs eliminated by CYP2C9. Caution should be exercised when co-administering nilotinib with substrates for CYP2C9 that have a narrow therapeutic index. *In vitro* studies also suggest that nilotinib may induce CYP2B6, CYP2C8 and CYP2C9, and thereby has the potential to decrease the concentrations of drugs which are eliminated by these enzymes).
No products indexed under this heading.

Dextromethorphan Hydrobromide (Nilotinib is a competitive inhibitor of CYP2D6 *in vitro*, potentially increasing the concentration of drugs eliminated by CYP2D6. Caution should be exercised when co-administering nilotinib with substrates for CYP2D6 that have a narrow therapeutic index).
No products indexed under this heading.

Dextromethorphan Polistirex (Nilotinib is a competitive inhibitor of CYP2D6 *in vitro*, potentially increasing the concentration of drugs eliminated by CYP2D6. Caution should be exercised when co-administering nilotinib with substrates for CYP2D6 that have a narrow therapeutic index).
No products indexed under this heading.

Diazepam (The administration of nilotinib with agents that prolong the QT interval should be avoided. Should treatment with any of these agents be required, it is recommended that therapy with nilotinib be interrupted. If interruption of treatment with nilotinib is not possible, patients who require treatment with a drug that prolongs the QT interval should be closely monitored for prolongation of the QT interval). Products include:
Valium Tablets 2880

Diclofenac Epolamine (*In vitro* studies suggest that nilotinib may induce CYP2B6, CYP2C8 and CYP2C9, and decrease the concentrations of drugs which are eliminated by these enzymes). Products include:
Flector 1839

Diclofenac Potassium (Nilotinib is a competitive inhibitor of CYP2C8 *in vitro*, potentially increasing the concentration of drugs eliminated by CYP2C8. Caution should be exercised when co-administering nilotinib with substrates for CYP2C8 that have a narrow therapeutic index. *In vitro* studies also suggest that nilotinib may induce CYP2B6, CYP2C8, and CYP2C9, and thereby has the potential to decrease the concentrations of drugs which are eliminated by these enzymes).
No products indexed under this heading.

Diclofenac Sodium (Nilotinib is a competitive inhibitor of CYP2C8 *in vitro*, potentially increasing the concentration of drugs eliminated by CYP2C8. Caution should be exercised when co-administering nilotinib with substrates for CYP2C8 that have a narrow therapeutic index. *In vitro* studies also suggest that nilotinib may induce CYP2B6, CYP2C8, and CYP2C9, and thereby has the potential to decrease the concentrations of drugs which are eliminated by these enzymes).
No products indexed under this heading.

Digoxin (Nilotinib is a substrate of the efflux transporter P-glycoprotein (Pgp, ABCB1). If nilotinib is administered with drugs that inhibit Pgp, increased concentrations of nilotinib are likely, and caution should be exercised). Products include:
Lanoxin Injection 1546
Lanoxin Injection Pediatric 1549
Lanoxin Tablets 1553

Digoxin Immune Fab (Ovine) (Nilotinib inhibits human P-glycoprotein. If nilotinib is administered with drugs that are substrates of Pgp, increased concentrations of the substrate drug are likely, and caution should be exercised). Products include:
Digibind 1427

Dihydroergotamine Mesylate (Nilotinib is a competitive inhibitor of CYP3A4 *in vitro*, potentially increasing the concentration of drugs eliminated by CYP3A4. Caution should be exercised when co-administering nilotinib with substrates for CYP3A4 that have a narrow therapeutic index).
No products indexed under this heading.

Diltiazem Hydrochloride (Nilotinib is a competitive inhibitor of CYP3A4 *in vitro*, potentially increasing the concentration of drugs eliminated by CYP3A4. Caution should be exercised when co-administering nilotinib with substrates for CYP3A4 that have a narrow therapeutic index). Products include:
Cardizem LA 423

Diltiazem Maleate (Nilotinib is a competitive inhibitor of CYP3A4 *in vitro*, potentially increasing the concentration of drugs eliminated by CYP3A4. Caution should be exercised when co-administering nilotinib with substrates for CYP3A4 that have a narrow therapeutic index).
No products indexed under this heading.

Dirithromycin (Nilotinib is a substrate of the efflux transporter P-glycoprotein (Pgp, ABCB1). If nilotinib is administered with drugs that inhibit Pgp, increased concentrations of nilotinib are likely, and caution should be exercised).
No products indexed under this heading.

Disopyramide (The administration of nilotinib with agents that are strong CYP3A4 inhibitors or anti-arrhythmic drugs (eg, disopyramide) and other drugs that may prolong QT interval should be avoided. Should treatment with any of these agents be required, it is recommended that therapy with nilotinib be interrupted. If interruption of treatment with nilotinib is not possible, patients who require treatment with a drug that prolongs QT or strongly inhibits CYP3A4 should be closely monitored for prolongation of the QT interval).
No products indexed under this heading.

Disopyramide Phosphate (The administration of nilotinib with agents that are strong CYP3A4 inhibitors or anti-arrhythmic drugs (eg, disopyramide) and other drugs that may prolong QT interval should be avoided. Should treatment with any of these agents be required, it is recommended that therapy with nilotinib be interrupted. If interruption of treatment with nilotinib is not possible, patients who require treatment with a drug that prolongs QT or strongly inhibits CYP3A4 should be closely monitored for prolongation of the QT interval).
No products indexed under this heading.

Disulfiram (Nilotinib is a competitive inhibitor of CYP3A4 *in vitro*, potentially increasing the concentration of drugs eliminated by CYP3A4. Caution should be exercised when co-administering nilotinib with substrates for CYP3A4 that have a narrow therapeutic index).
No products indexed under this heading.

Divalproex Sodium (*In vitro* studies suggest that nilotinib may induce CYP2B6, CYP2C8 and CYP2C9, and decrease the concentrations of drugs which are eliminated by these enzymes). Products include:
Depakote ER 426

Docetaxel (Nilotinib is a competitive inhibitor of CYP2C8 *in vitro*, potentially increasing the concentration of drugs eliminated by CYP2C8. Caution should be exercised when co-administering nilotinib with substrates for CYP2C8 that have a narrow therapeutic index. *In vitro* studies also suggest that nilotinib may induce CYP2B6, CYP2C8, and CYP2C9, and thereby has the potential to decrease the concentrations of drugs which are eliminated by these enzymes). Products include:
Taxotere 3035

Dofetilide (The administration of nilotinib with agents that prolong the QT interval should be avoided. Should treatment with any of these agents be required, it is recommended that therapy with nilotinib be interrupted. If interruption of treatment with nilotinib is not possible, patients who require treatment with a drug that prolongs the QT interval should be closely monitored for prolongation of the QT interval).
No products indexed under this heading.

Dolasetron Mesylate (Nilotinib is a competitive inhibitor of CYP2D6 *in vitro*, potentially increasing the concentration of drugs eliminated by CYP2D6. Caution should be exercised when co-administering nilotinib with substrates for CYP2D6 that have a narrow therapeutic index). Products include:
Anzemet Injection 2931
Anzemet Tablets 2934

Domperidone (Nilotinib inhibits human P-glycoprotein. If nilotinib is administered with drugs that are substrates of Pgp, increased concentrations of the substrate drug are likely, and caution should be exercised).
No products indexed under this heading.

Donepezil Hydrochloride (Nilotinib is a competitive inhibitor of CYP2D6 *in vitro*, potentially increasing the concentration of drugs eliminated by CYP2D6. Caution should be exercised when co-administering nilotinib with substrates for CYP2D6 that have a narrow therapeutic index). Products include:
Aricept 1045
Aricept ODT 1045

Doxepin Hydrochloride (The administration of nilotinib with agents that prolong the QT interval should be avoided. Should treatment with any of these agents be required, it is recommended that therapy with nilotinib be interrupted. If interruption of treatment with nilotinib is not possible, patients who require treatment with a drug that prolongs the QT interval should be closely monitored for prolongation of the QT interval).
No products indexed under this heading.

Doxorubicin Hydrochloride (Nilotinib is a competitive inhibitor of CYP3A4 *in vitro*, potentially increasing the concentration of drugs eliminated by CYP3A4. Caution should be exercised when co-administering nilotinib with substrates for CYP3A4 that have a narrow therapeutic index).
No products indexed under this heading.

Doxorubicin Hydrochloride Liposome (Nilotinib inhibits human P-glycoprotein. If nilotinib is administered with drugs that are substrates of Pgp, increased concentrations of the substrate drug are likely, and caution should be exercised). Products include:
Doxil 939

IMPORTANT NOTE: Always consult each drug listing in the patient's regimen for possible interactions.

Tasigna Interactions Index 1840

Dronabinol (Nilotinib is a competitive inhibitor of CYP3A4 *in vitro*, potentially increasing the concentration of drugs eliminated by CYP3A4. Caution should be exercised when co-administering nilotinib with substrates for CYP3A4 that have a narrow therapeutic index).
No products indexed under this heading.

Droperidol (The administration of nilotinib with agents that prolong the QT interval should be avoided. Should treatment with any of these agents be required, it is recommended that therapy with nilotinib be interrupted. If interruption of treatment with nilotinib is not possible, patients who require treatment with a drug that prolongs the QT interval should be closely monitored for prolongation of the QT interval).
No products indexed under this heading.

Efavirenz (The concomitant use of strong CYP3A4 inducers should be avoided. If patients must be co-administered a strong CYP3A4 inducer, the dose of nilotinib may need to be increased, depending on patient tolerability. If the strong inducer is discontinued, the nilotinib dose should be reduced to the indicated dose). Products include:
Atripla 906

Elacridar (Nilotinib is a substrate of the efflux transporter P-glycoprotein (Pgp, ABCB1). If nilotinib is administered with drugs that inhibit Pgp, increased concentrations of nilotinib are likely, and caution should be exercised).
No products indexed under this heading.

Encainide Hydrochloride (Nilotinib is a competitive inhibitor of CYP2D6 *in vitro*, potentially increasing the concentration of drugs eliminated by CYP2D6. Caution should be exercised when co-administering nilotinib with substrates for CYP2D6 that have a narrow therapeutic index).
No products indexed under this heading.

Eprosartan Mesylate (Nilotinib is a competitive inhibitor of CYP2C9 *in vitro*, potentially increasing the concentration of drugs eliminated by CYP2C9. Caution should be exercised when co-administering nilotinib with substrates for CYP2C9 that have a narrow therapeutic index. *In vitro* studies also suggest that nilotinib may induce CYP2B6, CYP2C8 and CYP2C9, and thereby has the potential to decrease the concentrations of drugs which are eliminated by these enzymes). Products include:
Teveten 538
Teveten HCT 541

Ergotamine Tartrate (Nilotinib is a competitive inhibitor of CYP3A4 *in vitro*, potentially increasing the concentration of drugs eliminated by CYP3A4. Caution should be exercised when co-administering nilotinib with substrates for CYP3A4 that have a narrow therapeutic index).
No products indexed under this heading.

Erythromycin (The administration of nilotinib with agents that prolong the QT interval should be avoided. Should treatment with any of these agents be required, it is recommended that therapy with nilotinib be interrupted. If interruption of treatment with nilotinib is not possible, patients who require treatment with a drug that prolongs the QT interval should be closely monitored for prolongation of the QT interval).
No products indexed under this heading.

Erythromycin, Topical (*In vitro* studies suggest that nilotinib may induce CYP2B6, CYP2C8 and CYP2C9, and decrease the concentrations of drugs which are eliminated by these enzymes).
No products indexed under this heading.

Erythromycin Estolate (The administration of nilotinib with agents that prolong the QT interval should be avoided. Should treatment with any of these agents be required, it is recommended that therapy with nilotinib be interrupted. If interruption of treatment with nilotinib is not possible, patients who require treatment with a drug that prolongs the QT interval should be closely monitored for prolongation of the QT interval).
No products indexed under this heading.

Erythromycin Ethylsuccinate (The administration of nilotinib with agents that prolong the QT interval should be avoided. Should treatment with any of these agents be required, it is recommended that therapy with nilotinib be interrupted. If interruption of treatment with nilotinib is not possible, patients who require treatment with a drug that prolongs the QT interval should be closely monitored for prolongation of the QT interval). Products include:
E.E.S. 437
EryPed 435

Erythromycin Gluceptate (The administration of nilotinib with agents that prolong the QT interval should be avoided. Should treatment with any of these agents be required, it is recommended that therapy with nilotinib be interrupted. If interruption of treatment with nilotinib is not possible, patients who require treatment with a drug that prolongs the QT interval should be closely monitored for prolongation of the QT interval).
No products indexed under this heading.

Erythromycin Lactobionate (The administration of nilotinib with agents that prolong the QT interval should be avoided. Should treatment with any of these agents be required, it is recommended that therapy with nilotinib be interrupted. If interruption of treatment with nilotinib is not possible, patients who require treatment with a drug that prolongs the QT interval should be closely monitored for prolongation of the QT interval).
No products indexed under this heading.

Erythromycin Stearate (The administration of nilotinib with agents that prolong the QT interval should be avoided. Should treatment with any of these agents be required, it is recommended that therapy with nilotinib be interrupted. If interruption of treatment with nilotinib is not possible, patients who require treatment with a drug that prolongs the QT interval should be closely monitored for prolongation of the QT interval).
No products indexed under this heading.

Estradiol (Nilotinib is a competitive inhibitor of CYP3A4 *in vitro*, potentially increasing the concentration of drugs eliminated by CYP3A4. Caution should be exercised when co-administering nilotinib with substrates for CYP3A4 that have a narrow therapeutic index). Products include:
Activella 2561
Angeliq 831
Climara 841
Climara Pro 847
Divigel 3467
Estrasorb 1777
Vagifem 2589

Estradiol Acetate (*In vitro* studies suggest that nilotinib may induce CYP2B6, CYP2C8 and CYP2C9, and decrease the concentrations of drugs which are eliminated by these enzymes).
No products indexed under this heading.

Estradiol Benzoate (Nilotinib is a competitive inhibitor of CYP3A4 *in vitro*, potentially increasing the concentration of drugs eliminated by CYP3A4. Caution should be exercised when co-administering nilotinib with substrates for CYP3A4 that have a narrow therapeutic index).
No products indexed under this heading.

Estradiol Cypionate (Nilotinib is a competitive inhibitor of CYP3A4 *in vitro*, potentially increasing the concentration of drugs eliminated by CYP3A4. Caution should be exercised when co-administering nilotinib with substrates for CYP3A4 that have a narrow therapeutic index).
No products indexed under this heading.

Estradiol Valerate (Nilotinib is a competitive inhibitor of CYP3A4 *in vitro*, potentially increasing the concentration of drugs eliminated by CYP3A4. Caution should be exercised when co-administering nilotinib with substrates for CYP3A4 that have a narrow therapeutic index).
No products indexed under this heading.

Estrogen (*In vitro* studies suggest that nilotinib may induce CYP2B6, CYP2C8 and CYP2C9, and decrease the concentrations of drugs which are eliminated by these enzymes).
No products indexed under this heading.

Estrogens, Conjugated (*In vitro* studies suggest that nilotinib may induce CYP2B6, CYP2C8 and CYP2C9, and decrease the concentrations of drugs which are eliminated by these enzymes). Products include:
Premarin Intravenous 3528
Premarin Tablets 3533
Premarin Vaginal Cream 3540
Premphase 3549
Prempro 3549

Estrogens, Conjugated, Synthetic A (*In vitro* studies suggest that nilotinib may induce CYP2B6, CYP2C8 and CYP2C9, and decrease the concentrations of drugs which are eliminated by these enzymes).
No products indexed under this heading.

Estrogens, Conjugated, Synthetic B (*In vitro* studies suggest that nilotinib may induce CYP2B6, CYP2C8 and CYP2C9, and decrease the concentrations of drugs which are eliminated by these enzymes). Products include:
Enjuvia 3401

Estrogens, Esterified (*In vitro* studies suggest that nilotinib may induce CYP2B6, CYP2C8 and CYP2C9, and decrease the concentrations of drugs which are eliminated by these enzymes).
No products indexed under this heading.

Estrone (*In vitro* studies suggest that nilotinib may induce CYP2B6, CYP2C8 and CYP2C9, and decrease the concentrations of drugs which are eliminated by these enzymes).
No products indexed under this heading.

Estropipate (*In vitro* studies suggest that nilotinib may induce CYP2B6, CYP2C8 and CYP2C9, and decrease the concentrations of drugs which are eliminated by these enzymes).
No products indexed under this heading.

Ethinyl Estradiol (Nilotinib is a competitive inhibitor of CYP3A4 *in vitro*, potentially increasing the concentration of drugs eliminated by CYP3A4. Caution should be exercised when co-administering nilotinib with substrates for CYP3A4 that have a narrow therapeutic index). Products include:
LoSeasonique 3407
Lybrel 3514
NuvaRing 3181
Ortho Evra 2648
Ortho-Cyclen/Ortho Tri-Cyclen 2663
Ortho Tri-Cyclen Lo Tablets 2673
Seasonique 3418
Yaz 864

Ethosuximide (Nilotinib is a competitive inhibitor of CYP3A4 *in vitro*, potentially increasing the concentration of drugs eliminated by CYP3A4. Caution should be exercised when co-administering nilotinib with substrates for CYP3A4 that have a narrow therapeutic index).
No products indexed under this heading.

Ethynodiol Diacetate (Nilotinib is a competitive inhibitor of CYP3A4 *in vitro*, potentially increasing the concentration of drugs eliminated by CYP3A4. Caution should be exercised when co-administering nilotinib with substrates for CYP3A4 that have a narrow therapeutic index).
No products indexed under this heading.

Etodolac (Nilotinib is a competitive inhibitor of CYP2C9 *in vitro*, potentially increasing the concentration of drugs eliminated by CYP2C9. Caution should be exercised when co-administering nilotinib with substrates for CYP2C9 that have a narrow therapeutic index. *In vitro* studies also suggest that nilotinib may induce CYP2B6, CYP2C8 and CYP2C9, and thereby has the potential to decrease the concentrations of drugs which are eliminated by these enzymes).
No products indexed under this heading.

Etoposide (Nilotinib is a competitive inhibitor of CYP3A4 *in vitro*, potentially increasing the concentration of drugs eliminated by CYP3A4. Caution should be exercised when co-administering nilotinib with substrates for CYP3A4 that have a narrow therapeutic index).
No products indexed under this heading.

Etoposide Phosphate (Nilotinib is a competitive inhibitor of CYP3A4 *in vitro*, potentially increasing the concentration of drugs eliminated by CYP3A4. Caution should be exercised when co-administering nilotinib with substrates for CYP3A4 that have a narrow therapeutic index).
No products indexed under this heading.

Fat (The bioavailability of nilotinib was increased when given with a meal. Compared to the fasted state, the systemic exposure (AUC) increased by 82% when the dose was given 30 minutes after a high fat meal. Nilotinib should not be taken with food. No food should be taken at least 2 hours before and at least one hour after the dose is taken).
No products indexed under this heading.

Felbamate (The concomitant use of strong CYP3A4 inducers should be avoided. If patients must be co-administered a strong CYP3A4 inducer, the dose of nilotinib may need to be increased, depending on patient tolerability. If the strong inducer is discontinued, the nilotinib dose should be reduced to the indicated dose).
No products indexed under this heading.

Felodipine (Nilotinib is a competitive inhibitor of CYP3A4 *in vitro*, potentially increasing the concentration of drugs eliminated by CYP3A4. Caution should be exercised when co-administering nilotinib with substrates for CYP3A4 that have a narrow therapeutic index).
No products indexed under this heading.

Fenoprofen Calcium (Nilotinib is a competitive inhibitor of CYP2C9 *in vitro*, potentially increasing the concentration of drugs eliminated by CYP2C9. Caution should be exercised when co-administering nilotinib with substrates for CYP2C9 that have a narrow therapeutic index. *In vitro* studies also suggest that nilotinib may induce CYP2B6, CYP2C8 and CYP2C9, and thereby has

1841 **Interactions Index** **Tasigna**

the potential to decrease the concentrations of drugs which are eliminated by these enzymes).
No products indexed under this heading.

Fentanyl (Nilotinib is a competitive inhibitor of CYP3A4 *in vitro*, potentially increasing the concentration of drugs eliminated by CYP3A4. Caution should be exercised when co-administering nilotinib with substrates for CYP3A4 that have a narrow therapeutic index). Products include:
Duragesic 2604
Fentanyl Transdermal System 2346
Onsolis 2054

Fentanyl Citrate (Nilotinib is a competitive inhibitor of CYP3A4 *in vitro*, potentially increasing the concentration of drugs eliminated by CYP3A4. Caution should be exercised when co-administering nilotinib with substrates for CYP3A4 that have a narrow therapeutic index). Products include:
Fentora 966

Fexofenadine Hydrochloride (Nilotinib inhibits human P-glycoprotein. If nilotinib is administered with drugs that are substrates of Pgp, increased concentrations of the substrate drug are likely, and caution should be exercised). Products include:
Allegra ODT 2911
Allegra Oral Solution 2911
Allegra 2911
Allegra-D 2915
Allegra-D 24 2918

Flecainide Acetate (The administration of nilotinib with agents that prolong the QT interval should be avoided. Should treatment with any of these agents be required, it is recommended that therapy with nilotinib be interrupted. If interruption of treatment with nilotinib is not possible, patients who require treatment with a drug that prolongs the QT interval should be closely monitored for prolongation of the QT interval).
No products indexed under this heading.

Fludrocortisone Acetate (The concomitant use of strong CYP3A4 inducers should be avoided. If patients must be co-administered a strong CYP3A4 inducer, the dose of nilotinib may need to be increased, depending on patient tolerability. If the strong inducer is discontinued, the nilotinib dose should be reduced to the indicated dose).
No products indexed under this heading.

Fluoxetine (Nilotinib is a competitive inhibitor of CYP2D6 *in vitro*, potentially increasing the concentration of drugs eliminated by CYP2D6. Caution should be exercised when co-administering nilotinib with substrates for CYP2D6 that have a narrow therapeutic index).
No products indexed under this heading.

Fluoxetine Hydrochloride (Nilotinib is a competitive inhibitor of CYP2C9 *in vitro*, potentially increasing the concentration of drugs eliminated by CYP2C9. Caution should be exercised when co-administering nilotinib with substrates for CYP2C9 that have a narrow therapeutic index. *In vitro* studies also suggest that nilotinib may induce CYP2B6, CYP2C8 and CYP2C9, and thereby has the potential to decrease the concentrations of drugs which are eliminated by these enzymes). Products include:
Prozac Weekly 1941
Prozac Pulvules 1941
Symbyax 1965

Fluphenazine Decanoate (The administration of nilotinib with agents that prolong the QT interval should be avoided. Should treatment with any of these agents be required, it is recommended that therapy with nilotinib be interrupted. If interruption of treatment with nilotinib is not possible, patients who require treatment with a drug that prolongs the QT interval should be closely monitored for prolongation of the QT interval).
No products indexed under this heading.

Fluphenazine Enanthate (The administration of nilotinib with agents that prolong the QT interval should be avoided. Should treatment with any of these agents be required, it is recommended that therapy with nilotinib be interrupted. If interruption of treatment with nilotinib is not possible, patients who require treatment with a drug that prolongs the QT interval should be closely monitored for prolongation of the QT interval).
No products indexed under this heading.

Fluphenazine Hydrochloride (The administration of nilotinib with agents that prolong the QT interval should be avoided. Should treatment with any of these agents be required, it is recommended that therapy with nilotinib be interrupted. If interruption of treatment with nilotinib is not possible, patients who require treatment with a drug that prolongs the QT interval should be closely monitored for prolongation of the QT interval).
No products indexed under this heading.

Flurbiprofen (Nilotinib is a competitive inhibitor of CYP2C9 *in vitro*, potentially increasing the concentration of drugs eliminated by CYP2C9. Caution should be exercised when co-administering nilotinib with substrates for CYP2C9 that have a narrow therapeutic index. *In vitro* studies also suggest that nilotinib may induce CYP2B6, CYP2C8 and CYP2C9, and thereby has the potential to decrease the concentrations of drugs which are eliminated by these enzymes).
No products indexed under this heading.

Flurbiprofen Sodium (Nilotinib is a competitive inhibitor of CYP2C9 *in vitro*, potentially increasing the concentration of drugs eliminated by CYP2C9. Caution should be exercised when co-administering nilotinib with substrates for CYP2C9 that have a narrow therapeutic index. *In vitro* studies also suggest that nilotinib may induce CYP2B6, CYP2C8 and CYP2C9, and thereby has the potential to decrease the concentrations of drugs which are eliminated by these enzymes).
No products indexed under this heading.

Fluvastatin Sodium (Nilotinib is a competitive inhibitor of CYP2C8 *in vitro*, potentially increasing the concentration of drugs eliminated by CYP2C8. Caution should be exercised when co-administering nilotinib with substrates for CYP2C8 that have a narrow therapeutic index. *In vitro* studies also suggest that nilotinib may induce CYP2B6, CYP2C8, and CYP2C9, and thereby has the potential to decrease the concentrations of drugs which are eliminated by these enzymes).
No products indexed under this heading.

Fluvoxamine Maleate (Nilotinib is a competitive inhibitor of CYP2D6 *in vitro*, potentially increasing the concentration of drugs eliminated by CYP2D6. Caution should be exercised when co-administering nilotinib with substrates for CYP2D6 that have a narrow therapeutic index).
No products indexed under this heading.

Formoterol Fumarate (Nilotinib is a competitive inhibitor of CYP2D6 *in vitro*, potentially increasing the concentration of drugs eliminated by CYP2D6. Caution should be exercised when co-administering nilotinib with substrates for CYP2D6 that have a narrow therapeutic index). Products include:
Foradil 3121
Perforomist 3634

Fosamprenavir Calcium (The administration of nilotinib with agents that are strong CYP3A4 inhibitors should be avoided. Should treatment with any of these agents be required, it is recommended that therapy with nilotinib be interrupted. If patients must be co-administered a strong CYP3A4 inhibitor, based on pharmacokinetic studies, 400 mg qd is predicted to adjust the nilotinib AUC to the AUC observed without inhibitors. However, there are no clinical data with this dose adjustment in patients receiving strong CYP3A4 inhibitors. If the strong inhibitor is discontinued, a washout period should be allowed before the nilotinib dose is adjusted upward to the indicated dose. Close monitoring for prolongation of the QT interval is indicated for patients who cannot avoid strong CYP3A4 inhibitors). Products include:
Lexiva Oral Suspension 1558
Lexiva 1558

Fosphenytoin (The concomitant use of strong CYP3A4 inducers such as phenytoin should be avoided. If patients must be co-administered a strong CYP3A4 inducer, the dose of nilotinib may need to be increased, depending on patient tolerability. If the strong inducer is discontinued, the nilotinib dose should be reduced to the indicated dose).
No products indexed under this heading.

Fosphenytoin Sodium (The concomitant use of strong CYP3A4 inducers such as phenytoin should be avoided. If patients must be co-administered a strong CYP3A4 inducer, the dose of nilotinib may need to be increased, depending on patient tolerability. If the strong inducer is discontinued, the nilotinib dose should be reduced to the indicated dose).
No products indexed under this heading.

Galantamine Hydrobromide (Nilotinib is a competitive inhibitor of CYP2D6 *in vitro*, potentially increasing the concentration of drugs eliminated by CYP2D6. Caution should be exercised when co-administering nilotinib with substrates for CYP2D6 that have a narrow therapeutic index).
No products indexed under this heading.

Garlic Extract (The concomitant use of strong CYP3A4 inducers should be avoided. If patients must be co-administered a strong CYP3A4 inducer, the dose of nilotinib may need to be increased, depending on patient tolerability. If the strong inducer is discontinued, the nilotinib dose should be reduced to the indicated dose).
No products indexed under this heading.

Garlic Oil (The concomitant use of strong CYP3A4 inducers should be avoided. If patients must be co-administered a strong CYP3A4 inducer, the dose of nilotinib may need to be increased, depending on patient tolerability. If the strong inducer is discontinued, the nilotinib dose should be reduced to the indicated dose).
No products indexed under this heading.

Glimepiride (Nilotinib is a competitive inhibitor of CYP2C9 *in vitro*, potentially increasing the concentration of drugs eliminated by CYP2C9. Caution should be exercised when co-administering nilotinib with substrates for CYP2C9 that have a narrow therapeutic index. *In vitro* studies also suggest that nilotinib may induce CYP2B6, CYP2C8 and CYP2C9, and thereby has the potential to decrease the concentrations of drugs which are eliminated by these enzymes). Products include:
Avandaryl 1356
Duetact 3354

Glipizide (Nilotinib is a competitive inhibitor of CYP2C9 *in vitro*, potentially increasing the concentration of drugs eliminated by CYP2C9. Caution should be exercised when co-administering nilotinib with substrates for CYP2C9 that have a narrow therapeutic index. *In vitro* studies also suggest that nilotinib may induce CYP2B6, CYP2C8 and CYP2C9, and thereby has the potential to decrease the concentrations of drugs which are eliminated by these enzymes).
No products indexed under this heading.

Halofantrine (The administration of nilotinib with agents that are strong CYP3A4 inhibitors or anti-arrhythmic drugs and other drugs that may prolong QT interval (eg, halofantrine) should be avoided. Should treatment with any of these agents be required, it is recommended that therapy with nilotinib be interrupted. If interruption of treatment with nilotinib is not possible, patients who require treatment with a drug that prolongs QT or strongly inhibits CYP3A4 should be closely monitored for prolongation of the QT interval).
No products indexed under this heading.

Halofantrine Hydrochloride (The administration of nilotinib with agents that are strong CYP3A4 inhibitors or anti-arrhythmic drugs and other drugs that may prolong QT interval (eg, halofantrine) should be avoided. Should treatment with any of these agents be required, it is recommended that therapy with nilotinib be interrupted. If interruption of treatment with nilotinib is not possible, patients who require treatment with a drug that prolongs QT or strongly inhibits CYP3A4 should be closely monitored for prolongation of the QT interval).
No products indexed under this heading.

Haloperidol (The administration of nilotinib with agents that are strong CYP3A4 inhibitors or anti-arrhythmic drugs and other drugs that may prolong QT interval (eg, haloperidol) should be avoided. Should treatment with any of these agents be required, it is recommended that therapy with nilotinib be interrupted. If interruption of treatment with nilotinib is not possible, patients who require treatment with a drug that prolongs QT or strongly inhibits CYP3A4 should be closely monitored for prolongation of the QT interval).
No products indexed under this heading.

Haloperidol Decanoate (The administration of nilotinib with agents that are strong CYP3A4 inhibitors or anti-arrhythmic drugs and other drugs that may prolong QT interval (eg, haloperidol) should be avoided. Should treatment with any of these agents be required, it is recommended that therapy with nilotinib be interrupted. If interruption of treatment with nilotinib is not possible, patients who require treatment with a drug that prolongs QT or strongly inhibits CYP3A4 should be closely monitored for prolongation of the QT interval).
No products indexed under this heading.

Haloperidol Lactate (The administration of nilotinib with agents that are strong CYP3A4 inhibitors or anti-arrhythmic drugs and other drugs that may prolong QT interval (eg, haloperidol) should be avoided. Should treatment with any of these agents be required, it is recommended that therapy with nilotinib be interrupted. If interruption of treatment with nilotinib is not possible, patients who require treatment with a drug that prolongs QT or strongly inhibits CYP3A4 should be closely monitored for prolongation of the QT interval).
No products indexed under this heading.

IMPORTANT NOTE: Always consult each drug listing in the patient's regimen for possible interactions.

Tasigna Interactions Index 1842

Halothane (*In vitro* studies suggest that nilotinib may induce CYP2B6, CYP2C8 and CYP2C9, and decrease the concentrations of drugs which are eliminated by these enzymes).
No products indexed under this heading.

Hydrocodone Bitartrate (Nilotinib is a competitive inhibitor of CYP2D6 *in vitro*, potentially increasing the concentration of drugs eliminated by CYP2D6. Caution should be exercised when co-administering nilotinib with substrates for CYP2D6 that have a narrow therapeutic index). Products include:
Vicodin 560
Vicodin ES 561
Vicodin HP 563
Vicoprofen 564
Zydone 1138

Hydrocortisone (The concomitant use of strong CYP3A4 inducers should be avoided. If patients must be co-administered a strong CYP3A4 inducer, the dose of nilotinib may need to be increased, depending on patient tolerability. If the strong inducer is discontinued, the nilotinib dose should be reduced to the indicated dose).
No products indexed under this heading.

Hydrocortisone (Alcohol) (The concomitant use of strong CYP3A4 inducers should be avoided. If patients must be co-administered a strong CYP3A4 inducer, the dose of nilotinib may need to be increased, depending on patient tolerability. If the strong inducer is discontinued, the nilotinib dose should be reduced to the indicated dose).
No products indexed under this heading.

Hydrocortisone Acetate (The concomitant use of strong CYP3A4 inducers should be avoided. If patients must be co-administered a strong CYP3A4 inducer, the dose of nilotinib may need to be increased, depending on patient tolerability. If the strong inducer is discontinued, the nilotinib dose should be reduced to the indicated dose).
No products indexed under this heading.

Hydrocortisone Butyrate (The concomitant use of strong CYP3A4 inducers should be avoided. If patients must be co-administered a strong CYP3A4 inducer, the dose of nilotinib may need to be increased, depending on patient tolerability. If the strong inducer is discontinued, the nilotinib dose should be reduced to the indicated dose).
No products indexed under this heading.

Hydrocortisone Cypionate (The concomitant use of strong CYP3A4 inducers should be avoided. If patients must be co-administered a strong CYP3A4 inducer, the dose of nilotinib may need to be increased, depending on patient tolerability. If the strong inducer is discontinued, the nilotinib dose should be reduced to the indicated dose).
No products indexed under this heading.

Hydrocortisone Hemisuccinate (The concomitant use of strong CYP3A4 inducers should be avoided. If patients must be co-administered a strong CYP3A4 inducer, the dose of nilotinib may need to be increased, depending on patient tolerability. If the strong inducer is discontinued, the nilotinib dose should be reduced to the indicated dose).
No products indexed under this heading.

Hydrocortisone Probutate (The concomitant use of strong CYP3A4 inducers should be avoided. If patients must be co-administered a strong CYP3A4 inducer, the dose of nilotinib may need to be increased, depending on patient tolerability. If the strong inducer is discontinued, the nilotinib dose should be reduced to the indicated dose).
No products indexed under this heading.

Hydrocortisone Sodium Phosphate (The concomitant use of strong CYP3A4 inducers should be avoided. If patients must be co-administered a strong CYP3A4 inducer, the dose of nilotinib may need to be increased, depending on patient tolerability. If the strong inducer is discontinued, the nilotinib dose should be reduced to the indicated dose).
No products indexed under this heading.

Hydrocortisone Sodium Succinate (The concomitant use of strong CYP3A4 inducers should be avoided. If patients must be co-administered a strong CYP3A4 inducer, the dose of nilotinib may need to be increased, depending on patient tolerability. If the strong inducer is discontinued, the nilotinib dose should be reduced to the indicated dose).
No products indexed under this heading.

Hydrocortisone Valerate (The concomitant use of strong CYP3A4 inducers should be avoided. If patients must be co-administered a strong CYP3A4 inducer, the dose of nilotinib may need to be increased, depending on patient tolerability. If the strong inducer is discontinued, the nilotinib dose should be reduced to the indicated dose).
No products indexed under this heading.

Hydroxyzine Hydrochloride (The administration of nilotinib with agents that prolong the QT interval should be avoided. Should treatment with any of these agents be required, it is recommended that therapy with nilotinib be interrupted. If interruption of treatment with nilotinib is not possible, patients who require treatment with a drug that prolongs the QT interval should be closely monitored for prolongation of the QT interval).
No products indexed under this heading.

Hypericum (Concomitant use with St. John's Wort should be avoided).
No products indexed under this heading.

Hypericum Perforatum (Concomitant use with St. John's Wort should be avoided). Products include:
Traumeel 1800

Ibuprofen (Nilotinib is a competitive inhibitor of CYP2C9 *in vitro*, potentially increasing the concentration of drugs eliminated by CYP2C9. Caution should be exercised when co-administering nilotinib with substrates for CYP2C9 that have a narrow therapeutic index. *In vitro* studies also suggest that nilotinib may induce CYP2B6, CYP2C8 and CYP2C9, and thereby has the potential to decrease the concentrations of drugs which are eliminated by these enzymes). Products include:
Motrin IB 2043
Children's Motrin 2044
Children's Motrin Non-Staining Dye-Free 2044
Infants' Motrin 2044
Infants' Motrin Dye-Free 2044
Junior Strength Motrin 2044
Vicoprofen 564

Ifosfamide (*In vitro* studies suggest that nilotinib may induce CYP2B6, CYP2C8 and CYP2C9, and decrease the concentrations of drugs which are eliminated by these enzymes).
No products indexed under this heading.

Imatinib Mesylate (In a Phase 1 trial of nilotinib 400 mg twice daily in combination with imatinib 400 mg daily or 400 mg twice daily, the AUC increased 30%-50% for nilotinib and approximately 20% for imatinib). Products include:
Gleevec 2477

Imipramine Hydrochloride (The administration of nilotinib with agents that prolong the QT interval should be avoided. Should treatment with any of these agents be required, it is recommended that therapy with nilotinib be interrupted. If interruption of treatment with nilotinib is not possible, patients who require treatment with a drug that prolongs the QT interval should be closely monitored for prolongation of the QT interval).
No products indexed under this heading.

Imipramine Pamoate (The administration of nilotinib with agents that prolong the QT interval should be avoided. Should treatment with any of these agents be required, it is recommended that therapy with nilotinib be interrupted. If interruption of treatment with nilotinib is not possible, patients who require treatment with a drug that prolongs the QT interval should be closely monitored for prolongation of the QT interval).
No products indexed under this heading.

Indinavir Sulfate (The administration of nilotinib with agents that are strong CYP3A4 inhibitors such as indinavir should be avoided. If treatment is required, it is recommended that therapy with nilotinib be interrupted. If patients must be co-administered a strong CYP3A4 inhibitor, based on pharmacokinetic studies, 400 mg qd is predicted to adjust the nilotinib AUC to the AUC observed without inhibitors. However, there are no clinical data with this dose adjustment in patients receiving strong CYP3A4 inhibitors. If the strong inhibitor is discontinued, a washout period should be allowed before the nilotinib dose is adjusted upward to the indicated dose. Close monitoring for prolongation of the QT interval is indicated for patients who cannot avoid strong CYP3A4 inhibitors). Products include:
Crixivan 2113

Indomethacin (Nilotinib is a competitive inhibitor of CYP2C9 *in vitro*, potentially increasing the concentration of drugs eliminated by CYP2C9. Caution should be exercised when co-administering nilotinib with substrates for CYP2C9 that have a narrow therapeutic index. *In vitro* studies also suggest that nilotinib may induce CYP2B6, CYP2C8 and CYP2C9, and thereby has the potential to decrease the concentrations of drugs which are eliminated by these enzymes). Products include:
Indocin 2167

Indomethacin Sodium Trihydrate (Nilotinib is a competitive inhibitor of CYP2C9 *in vitro*, potentially increasing the concentration of drugs eliminated by CYP2C9. Caution should be exercised when co-administering nilotinib with substrates for CYP2C9 that have a narrow therapeutic index. *In vitro* studies also suggest that nilotinib may induce CYP2B6, CYP2C8 and CYP2C9, and thereby has the potential to decrease the concentrations of drugs which are eliminated by these enzymes). Products include:
Indocin I.V. 2007

Indoramin Hydrochloride (Nilotinib is a competitive inhibitor of CYP2D6 *in vitro*, potentially increasing the concentration of drugs eliminated by CYP2D6. Caution should be exercised when co-administering nilotinib with substrates for CYP2D6 that have a narrow therapeutic index).
No products indexed under this heading.

Irbesartan (Nilotinib is a competitive inhibitor of CYP2C9 *in vitro*, potentially increasing the concentration of drugs eliminated by CYP2C9. Caution should be exercised when co-administering nilotinib with substrates for CYP2C9 that have a narrow therapeutic index. *In vitro* studies also suggest that nilotinib may induce CYP2B6, CYP2C8 and CYP2C9, and thereby has the potential to decrease the concentrations of drugs which are eliminated by these enzymes). Products include:
Avalide 2956
Avapro 2962

Irinotecan Hydrochloride (*In vitro* studies suggest that nilotinib may induce CYP2B6, CYP2C8 and CYP2C9, and decrease the concentrations of drugs which are eliminated by these enzymes).
No products indexed under this heading.

Isocarboxazid (The administration of nilotinib with agents that prolong the QT interval should be avoided. Should treatment with any of these agents be required, it is recommended that therapy with nilotinib be interrupted. If interruption of treatment with nilotinib is not possible, patients who require treatment with a drug that prolongs the QT interval should be closely monitored for prolongation of the QT interval). Products include:
Marplan 3481

Isotretinoin (Nilotinib is a competitive inhibitor of CYP2C8 *in vitro*, potentially increasing the concentration of drugs eliminated by CYP2C8. Caution should be exercised when co-administering nilotinib with substrates for CYP2C8 that have a narrow therapeutic index. *In vitro* studies also suggest that nilotinib may induce CYP2B6, CYP2C8, and CYP2C9, and thereby has the potential to decrease the concentrations of drugs which are eliminated by these enzymes). Products include:
Accutane 2832

Isradipine (Nilotinib is a competitive inhibitor of CYP3A4 *in vitro*, potentially increasing the concentration of drugs eliminated by CYP3A4. Caution should be exercised when co-administering nilotinib with substrates for CYP3A4 that have a narrow therapeutic index). Products include:
DynaCirc CR 1432

Itraconazole (The administration of nilotinib with agents that are strong CYP3A4 inhibitors such as itraconazole should be avoided. If treatment is required, it is recommended that therapy with nilotinib be interrupted. If patients must be co-administered a strong CYP3A4 inhibitor, based on pharmacokinetic studies, 400 mg qd is predicted to adjust the nilotinib AUC to the AUC observed without inhibitors. However, there are no clinical data with this dose adjustment in patients receiving strong CYP3A4 inhibitors. If the strong inhibitor is discontinued, a washout period should be allowed before the nilotinib dose is adjusted upward to the indicated dose. Close monitoring for prolongation of the QT interval is indicated for patients who cannot avoid strong CYP3A4 inhibitors).
No products indexed under this heading.

Ivermectin (Nilotinib inhibits human P-glycoprotein. If nilotinib is administered with drugs that are substrates of Pgp, increased concentrations of the substrate drug are likely, and caution should be exercised). Products include:
Stromectol 2277

Ixabepilone (Nilotinib is a competitive inhibitor of CYP3A4 *in vitro*, potentially increasing the concentration of drugs eliminated by CYP3A4. Caution should be exercised when co-administering nilotinib with substrates for CYP3A4 that have a narrow therapeutic index).
No products indexed under this heading.

Ketamine (*In vitro* studies suggest that nilotinib may induce CYP2B6, CYP2C8 and CYP2C9, and decrease the concentrations of drugs which are eliminated by these enzymes).
No products indexed under this heading.

Ketamine Hydrochloride (*In vitro* studies suggest that nilotinib may induce CYP2B6, CYP2C8 and CYP2C9, and decrease the concentrations of drugs which are eliminated by these enzymes).
No products indexed under this heading.

Ketoconazole (The administration of nilotinib with agents that are strong CYP3A4 inhibitors such as ketoconazole should be avoided. If treatment is required, it is recommended that therapy with nilotinib be interrupted. If patients must be co-administered a strong CYP3A4 inhibitor, based on pharmacokinetic studies, 400 mg qd is predicted to adjust the nilotinib AUC to the AUC observed without inhibitors. However, there are no clinical data with this dose adjustment in patients receiving strong CYP3A4 inhibitors. If the strong inhibitor is discontinued, a washout period should be allowed before the nilotinib dose is adjusted upward to the indicated dose. Close monitoring for prolongation of the QT interval is indicated for patients who cannot avoid strong CYP3A4 inhibitors). Products include:
Extina **3319**
Xolegel **3337**

Ketoprofen (Nilotinib is a competitive inhibitor of CYP2C9 *in vitro*, potentially increasing the concentration of drugs eliminated by CYP2C9. Caution should be exercised when co-administering nilotinib with substrates for CYP2C9 that have a narrow therapeutic index. *In vitro* studies also suggest that nilotinib may induce CYP2B6, CYP2C8 and CYP2C9, and thereby has the potential to decrease the concentrations of drugs which are eliminated by these enzymes).
No products indexed under this heading.

Ketorolac Tromethamine (Nilotinib is a competitive inhibitor of CYP2C9 *in vitro*, potentially increasing the concentration of drugs eliminated by CYP2C9. Caution should be exercised when co-administering nilotinib with substrates for CYP2C9 that have a narrow therapeutic index. *In vitro* studies also suggest that nilotinib may induce CYP2B6, CYP2C8 and CYP2C9, and thereby has the potential to decrease the concentrations of drugs which are eliminated by these enzymes). Products include:
Acuvail .... ⊙ **209**

Labetalol Hydrochloride (Nilotinib is a competitive inhibitor of CYP2D6 *in vitro*, potentially increasing the concentration of drugs eliminated by CYP2D6. Caution should be exercised when co-administering nilotinib with substrates for CYP2D6 that have a narrow therapeutic index).
No products indexed under this heading.

Lansoprazole (Nilotinib is a competitive inhibitor of CYP2C9 *in vitro*, potentially increasing the concentration of drugs eliminated by CYP2C9. Caution should be exercised when co-administering nilotinib with substrates for CYP2C9 that have a narrow therapeutic index. *In vitro* studies also suggest that nilotinib may induce CYP2B6, CYP2C8 and CYP2C9, and thereby has the potential to decrease the concentrations of drugs which are eliminated by these enzymes).
No products indexed under this heading.

Lapatinib (Nilotinib inhibits human P-glycoprotein. If nilotinib is administered with drugs that are substrates of Pgp, increased concentrations of the substrate drug are likely, and caution should be exercised). Products include:
Tykerb **1698**

Levonorgestrel (Nilotinib is a competitive inhibitor of CYP3A4 *in vitro*, potentially increasing the concentration of drugs eliminated by CYP3A4. Caution should be exercised when co-administering nilotinib with substrates for CYP3A4 that have a narrow therapeutic index). Products include:
Climara Pro **847**
LoSeasonique **3407**
Lybrel **3514**
Mirena **854**
Plan B **3416**
Seasonique **3418**

Lidocaine (The administration of nilotinib with agents that prolong the QT interval should be avoided. Should treatment with any of these agents be required, it is recommended that therapy with nilotinib be interrupted. If interruption of treatment with nilotinib is not possible, patients who require treatment with a drug that prolongs the QT interval should be closely monitored for prolongation of the QT interval). Products include:
Lidoderm **1107**

Lidocaine Base (*In vitro* studies suggest that nilotinib may induce CYP2B6, CYP2C8 and CYP2C9, and decrease the concentrations of drugs which are eliminated by these enzymes).
No products indexed under this heading.

Lidocaine Hydrochloride (The administration of nilotinib with agents that prolong the QT interval should be avoided. Should treatment with any of these agents be required, it is recommended that therapy with nilotinib be interrupted. If interruption of treatment with nilotinib is not possible, patients who require treatment with a drug that prolongs the QT interval should be closely monitored for prolongation of the QT interval).
No products indexed under this heading.

Lithium Carbonate (The administration of nilotinib with agents that prolong the QT interval should be avoided. Should treatment with any of these agents be required, it is recommended that therapy with nilotinib be interrupted. If interruption of treatment with nilotinib is not possible, patients who require treatment with a drug that prolongs the QT interval should be closely monitored for prolongation of the QT interval).
No products indexed under this heading.

Lithium Citrate (The administration of nilotinib with agents that prolong the QT interval should be avoided. Should treatment with any of these agents be required, it is recommended that therapy with nilotinib be interrupted. If interruption of treatment with nilotinib is not possible, patients who require treatment with a drug that prolongs the QT interval should be closely monitored for prolongation of the QT interval).
No products indexed under this heading.

Loperamide Hydrochloride (Nilotinib inhibits human P-glycoprotein. If nilotinib is administered with drugs that are substrates of Pgp, increased concentrations of the substrate drug are likely, and caution should be exercised). Products include:
Imodium A-D **2042**
Imodium Multi-Symptom Relief **2043**

Lopinavir (The administration of nilotinib with agents that are strong CYP3A4 inhibitors should be avoided. Should treatment with any of these agents be required, it is recommended that therapy with nilotinib be interrupted. If patients must be co-administered a strong CYP3A4 inhibitor, based on pharmacokinetic studies, 400 mg qd is predicted to adjust the nilotinib AUC to the AUC observed without inhibitors. However, there are no clinical data with this dose adjustment in patients receiving strong CYP3A4 inhibitors. If the strong inhibitor is discontinued, a washout period should be allowed before the nilotinib dose is adjusted upward to the indicated dose. Close monitoring for prolongation of the QT interval is indicated for patients who cannot avoid strong CYP3A4 inhibitors). Products include:
Kaletra **458**

Lorazepam (The administration of nilotinib with agents that prolong the QT interval should be avoided. Should treatment with any of these agents be required, it is recommended that therapy with nilotinib be interrupted. If interruption of treatment with nilotinib is not possible, patients who require treatment with a drug that prolongs the QT interval should be closely monitored for prolongation of the QT interval).
No products indexed under this heading.

Losartan Potassium (Nilotinib is a competitive inhibitor of CYP2C9 *in vitro*, potentially increasing the concentration of drugs eliminated by CYP2C9. Caution should be exercised when co-administering nilotinib with substrates for CYP2C9 that have a narrow therapeutic index. *In vitro* studies also suggest that nilotinib may induce CYP2B6, CYP2C8 and CYP2C9, and thereby has the potential to decrease the concentrations of drugs which are eliminated by these enzymes). Products include:
Cozaar **2106**
Hyzaar **2162**
Hyzaar 100-12.5 .... **2162**

Lovastatin (Nilotinib is a competitive inhibitor of CYP3A4 *in vitro*, potentially increasing the concentration of drugs eliminated by CYP3A4. Caution should be exercised when co-administering nilotinib with substrates for CYP3A4 that have a narrow therapeutic index). Products include:
Advicor **402**
Mevacor **2212**

Loxapine Hydrochloride (The administration of nilotinib with agents that prolong the QT interval should be avoided. Should treatment with any of these agents be required, it is recommended that therapy with nilotinib be interrupted. If interruption of treatment with nilotinib is not possible, patients who require treatment with a drug that prolongs the QT interval should be closely monitored for prolongation of the QT interval).
No products indexed under this heading.

Loxapine Succinate (The administration of nilotinib with agents that prolong the QT interval should be avoided. Should treatment with any of these agents be required, it is recommended that therapy with nilotinib be interrupted. If interruption of treatment with nilotinib is not possible, patients who require treatment with a drug that prolongs the QT interval should be closely monitored for prolongation of the QT interval).
No products indexed under this heading.

Maprotiline Hydrochloride (The administration of nilotinib with agents that prolong the QT interval should be avoided. Should treatment with any of these agents be required, it is recommended that therapy with nilotinib be interrupted. If interruption of treatment with nilotinib is not possible, patients who require treatment with a drug that prolongs the QT interval should be closely monitored for prolongation of the QT interval).
No products indexed under this heading.

Maraviroc (Nilotinib inhibits human P-glycoprotein. If nilotinib is administered with drugs that are substrates of Pgp, increased concentrations of the substrate drug are likely, and caution should be exercised). Products include:
Selzentry **2740**

Meclofenamate Sodium (Nilotinib is a competitive inhibitor of CYP2C9 *in vitro*, potentially increasing the concentration of drugs eliminated by CYP2C9. Caution should be exercised when co-administering nilotinib with substrates for CYP2C9 that have a narrow therapeutic index. *In vitro* studies also suggest that nilotinib may induce CYP2B6, CYP2C8 and CYP2C9, and thereby has the potential to decrease the concentrations of drugs which are eliminated by these enzymes).
No products indexed under this heading.

Mefenamic Acid (Nilotinib is a competitive inhibitor of CYP2C9 *in vitro*, potentially increasing the concentration of drugs eliminated by CYP2C9. Caution should be exercised when co-administering nilotinib with substrates for CYP2C9 that have a narrow therapeutic index. *In vitro* studies also suggest that nilotinib may induce CYP2B6, CYP2C8 and CYP2C9, and thereby has the potential to decrease the concentrations of drugs which are eliminated by these enzymes).
No products indexed under this heading.

Meloxicam (Nilotinib is a competitive inhibitor of CYP2C9 *in vitro*, potentially increasing the concentration of drugs eliminated by CYP2C9. Caution should be exercised when co-administering nilotinib with substrates for CYP2C9 that have a narrow therapeutic index. *In vitro* studies also suggest that nilotinib may induce CYP2B6, CYP2C8 and CYP2C9, and thereby has the potential to decrease the concentrations of drugs which are eliminated by these enzymes).
No products indexed under this heading.

Meperidine Hydrochloride (Nilotinib is a competitive inhibitor of CYP2D6 *in vitro*, potentially increasing the concentration of drugs eliminated by CYP2D6. Caution should be exercised when co-administering nilotinib with substrates for CYP2D6 that have a narrow therapeutic index).
No products indexed under this heading.

Mephenytoin (The concomitant use of strong CYP3A4 inducers should be avoided. If patients must be co-administered a strong CYP3A4 inducer, the dose of nilotinib may need to be increased, depending on patient tolerability. If the strong inducer is discontinued, the nilotinib dose should be reduced to the indicated dose).
No products indexed under this heading.

Mephobarbital (Nilotinib is a competitive inhibitor of CYP2C8 *in vitro*, potentially increasing the concentration of drugs eliminated by CYP2C8. Caution should be exercised when co-administering nilotinib with substrates for CYP2C8 that have a narrow therapeutic index. *In vitro* studies also suggest that nilotinib may induce CYP2B6, CYP2C8, and CYP2C9, and thereby has the potential to decrease the concentrations of drugs which are eliminated by these enzymes).
No products indexed under this heading.

Meprobamate (The administration of nilotinib with agents that prolong the QT interval should be avoided. Should treatment with any of these agents be required, it is recommended that therapy with nilotinib be interrupted. If interruption of treatment with nilotinib is not possible, patients who require treatment with a drug that prolongs the QT interval should be closely monitored for prolongation of the QT interval).
No products indexed under this heading.

Mesoridazine Besylate (The administration of nilotinib with agents that prolong the QT interval should be avoided. Should treatment with any of these agents be required, it is recommended that therapy with nilotinib be interrupted. If interruption of treatment

with nilotinib is not possible, patients who require treatment with a drug that prolongs the QT interval should be closely monitored for prolongation of the QT interval).
No products indexed under this heading.

Mestranol (Nilotinib is a competitive inhibitor of CYP3A4 *in vitro*, potentially increasing the concentration of drugs eliminated by CYP3A4. Caution should be exercised when co-administering nilotinib with substrates for CYP3A4 that have a narrow therapeutic index).
No products indexed under this heading.

Metformin Hydrochloride (Nilotinib is a competitive inhibitor of CYP2C9 *in vitro*, potentially increasing the concentration of drugs eliminated by CYP2C9. Caution should be exercised when co-administering nilotinib with substrates for CYP2C9 that have a narrow therapeutic index. *In vitro* studies also suggest that nilotinib may induce CYP2B6, CYP2C8 and CYP2C9, and thereby has the potential to decrease the concentrations of drugs which are eliminated by these enzymes). Products include:
ActoPlus 3338
Avandamet 1345
Janumet 2188

Methadone Hydrochloride (The administration of nilotinib with agents that are strong CYP3A4 inhibitors or anti-arrhythmic drugs and other drugs that may prolong QT interval (eg, methadone) should be avoided. Should treatment with any of these agents be required, it is recommended that therapy with nilotinib be interrupted. If interruption of treatment with nilotinib is not possible, patients who require treatment with a drug that prolongs QT or strongly inhibits CYP3A4 should be closely monitored for prolongation of the QT interval).
No products indexed under this heading.

Methamphetamine Hydrochloride (Nilotinib is a competitive inhibitor of CYP2D6 *in vitro*, potentially increasing the concentration of drugs eliminated by CYP2D6. Caution should be exercised when co-administering nilotinib with substrates for CYP2D6 that have a narrow therapeutic index).
No products indexed under this heading.

Methoxyphenamine (Nilotinib is a competitive inhibitor of CYP2D6 *in vitro*, potentially increasing the concentration of drugs eliminated by CYP2D6. Caution should be exercised when co-administering nilotinib with substrates for CYP2D6 that have a narrow therapeutic index).
No products indexed under this heading.

Methsuximide (The concomitant use of strong CYP3A4 inducers should be avoided. If patients must be co-administered a strong CYP3A4 inducer, the dose of nilotinib may need to be increased, depending on patient tolerability. If the strong inducer is discontinued, the nilotinib dose should be reduced to the indicated dose).
No products indexed under this heading.

Methylprednisolone (The concomitant use of strong CYP3A4 inducers should be avoided. If patients must be co-administered a strong CYP3A4 inducer, the dose of nilotinib may need to be increased, depending on patient tolerability. If the strong inducer is discontinued, the nilotinib dose should be reduced to the indicated dose).
No products indexed under this heading.

Methylprednisolone Acetate (The concomitant use of strong CYP3A4 inducers should be avoided. If patients must be co-administered a strong CYP3A4 inducer, the dose of nilotinib may need to be increased, depending on patient tolerability. If the strong inducer is discontinued, the nilotinib dose should be reduced to the indicated dose).
No products indexed under this heading.

Methylprednisolone Sodium Succinate (The concomitant use of strong CYP3A4 inducers should be avoided. If patients must be co-administered a strong CYP3A4 inducer, the dose of nilotinib may need to be increased, depending on patient tolerability. If the strong inducer is discontinued, the nilotinib dose should be reduced to the indicated dose).
No products indexed under this heading.

Methyltestosterone (*In vitro* studies suggest that nilotinib may induce CYP2B6, CYP2C8 and CYP2C9, and decrease the concentrations of drugs which are eliminated by these enzymes).
No products indexed under this heading.

Metoprolol Succinate (Nilotinib is a competitive inhibitor of CYP2D6 *in vitro*, potentially increasing the concentration of drugs eliminated by CYP2D6. Caution should be exercised when co-administering nilotinib with substrates for CYP2D6 that have a narrow therapeutic index). Products include:
Toprol XL 732

Metoprolol Tartrate (Nilotinib is a competitive inhibitor of CYP2D6 *in vitro*, potentially increasing the concentration of drugs eliminated by CYP2D6. Caution should be exercised when co-administering nilotinib with substrates for CYP2D6 that have a narrow therapeutic index).
No products indexed under this heading.

Mexiletine Hydrochloride (The administration of nilotinib with agents that prolong the QT interval should be avoided. Should treatment with any of these agents be required, it is recommended that therapy with nilotinib be interrupted. If interruption of treatment with nilotinib is not possible, patients who require treatment with a drug that prolongs the QT interval should be closely monitored for prolongation of the QT interval).
No products indexed under this heading.

Mibefradil Dihydrochloride (Nilotinib is a substrate of the efflux transporter P-glycoprotein (Pgp, ABCB1). If nilotinib is administered with drugs that inhibit Pgp, increased concentrations of nilotinib are likely, and caution should be exercised).
No products indexed under this heading.

Midazolam Hydrochloride (Single-dose administration of nilotinib with midazolam (a CYP3A4 substrate) to healthy subjects increased midazolam exposure by 30%).
No products indexed under this heading.

Miglitol (Nilotinib is a competitive inhibitor of CYP2C9 *in vitro*, potentially increasing the concentration of drugs eliminated by CYP2C9. Caution should be exercised when co-administering nilotinib with substrates for CYP2C9 that have a narrow therapeutic index. *In vitro* studies also suggest that nilotinib may induce CYP2B6, CYP2C8 and CYP2C9, and thereby has the potential to decrease the concentrations of drugs which are eliminated by these enzymes).
No products indexed under this heading.

Mirtazapine (Nilotinib is a competitive inhibitor of CYP2C9 *in vitro*, potentially increasing the concentration of drugs eliminated by CYP2C9. Caution should be exercised when co-administering nilotinib with substrates for CYP2C9 that have a narrow therapeutic index. *In vitro* studies also suggest that nilotinib may induce CYP2B6, CYP2C8 and CYP2C9, and thereby has the potential to decrease the concentrations of drugs which are eliminated by these enzymes). Products include:
Remeron Tablets 3214
RemeronSolTab Tablets 3219

Modafinil (The concomitant use of strong CYP3A4 inducers should be avoided. If patients must be co-administered a strong CYP3A4 inducer, the dose of nilotinib may need to be increased, depending on patient tolerability. If the strong inducer is discontinued, the nilotinib dose should be reduced to the indicated dose). Products include:
Provigil 983

Molindone Hydrochloride (The administration of nilotinib with agents that prolong the QT interval should be avoided. Should treatment with any of these agents be required, it is recommended that therapy with nilotinib be interrupted. If interruption of treatment with nilotinib is not possible, patients who require treatment with a drug that prolongs the QT interval should be closely monitored for prolongation of the QT interval). Products include:
Moban 1108

Montelukast Sodium (Nilotinib is a competitive inhibitor of CYP2C9 *in vitro*, potentially increasing the concentration of drugs eliminated by CYP2C9. Caution should be exercised when co-administering nilotinib with substrates for CYP2C9 that have a narrow therapeutic index. *In vitro* studies also suggest that nilotinib may induce CYP2B6, CYP2C8 and CYP2C9, and thereby has the potential to decrease the concentrations of drugs which are eliminated by these enzymes). Products include:
Singulair 2270

Moricizine Hydrochloride (The administration of nilotinib with agents that are strong CYP3A4 inhibitors or anti-arrhythmic drugs and other drugs that may prolong QT interval should be avoided. Should treatment with any of these agents be required, it is recommended that therapy with nilotinib be interrupted. If interruption of treatment with nilotinib is not possible, patients who require treatment with a drug that prolongs QT or strongly inhibits CYP3A4 should be closely monitored for prolongation of the QT interval).
No products indexed under this heading.

Morphine Sulfate (Nilotinib is a competitive inhibitor of CYP2D6 *in vitro*, potentially increasing the concentration of drugs eliminated by CYP2D6. Caution should be exercised when co-administering nilotinib with substrates for CYP2D6 that have a narrow therapeutic index). Products include:
Avinza 1822
Embeda 1831
MS Contin 2803

Moxifloxacin Hydrochloride (The administration of nilotinib with agents that are strong CYP3A4 inhibitors or anti-arrhythmic drugs and other drugs that may prolong QT interval (eg, moxifloxacin) should be avoided. Should treatment with any of these agents be required, it is recommended that therapy with nilotinib be interrupted. If interruption of treatment with nilotinib is not possible, patients who require treatment with a drug that prolongs QT or strongly inhibits CYP3A4 should be closely monitored for prolongation of the QT interval). Products include:
Avelox 3064
Vigamox 589

Nabumetone (Nilotinib is a competitive inhibitor of CYP2C9 *in vitro*, potentially increasing the concentration of drugs eliminated by CYP2C9. Caution should be exercised when co-administering nilotinib with substrates for CYP2C9 that have a narrow therapeutic index. *In vitro* studies also suggest that nilotinib may induce CYP2B6, CYP2C8 and CYP2C9, and thereby has the potential to decrease the concentrations of drugs which are eliminated by these enzymes).
No products indexed under this heading.

Nafcillin Sodium (The concomitant use of strong CYP3A4 inducers should be avoided. If patients must be co-administered a strong CYP3A4 inducer, the dose of nilotinib may need to be increased, depending on patient tolerability. If the strong inducer is discontinued, the nilotinib dose should be reduced to the indicated dose).
No products indexed under this heading.

Naproxen (Nilotinib is a competitive inhibitor of CYP2C9 *in vitro*, potentially increasing the concentration of drugs eliminated by CYP2C9. Caution should be exercised when co-administering nilotinib with substrates for CYP2C9 that have a narrow therapeutic index. *In vitro* studies also suggest that nilotinib may induce CYP2B6, CYP2C8 and CYP2C9, and thereby has the potential to decrease the concentrations of drugs which are eliminated by these enzymes). Products include:
EC-Naprosyn 2850
Naprosyn 2850
Anaprox/Naprosyn 2850

Naproxen Sodium (Nilotinib is a competitive inhibitor of CYP2C9 *in vitro*, potentially increasing the concentration of drugs eliminated by CYP2C9. Caution should be exercised when co-administering nilotinib with substrates for CYP2C9 that have a narrow therapeutic index. *In vitro* studies also suggest that nilotinib may induce CYP2B6, CYP2C8 and CYP2C9, and thereby has the potential to decrease the concentrations of drugs which are eliminated by these enzymes). Products include:
Anaprox 2850
Anaprox DS 2850
Treximet 1681

Nateglinide (Nilotinib is a competitive inhibitor of CYP2C9 *in vitro*, potentially increasing the concentration of drugs eliminated by CYP2C9. Caution should be exercised when co-administering nilotinib with substrates for CYP2C9 that have a narrow therapeutic index. *In vitro* studies also suggest that nilotinib may induce CYP2B6, CYP2C8 and CYP2C9, and thereby has the potential to decrease the concentrations of drugs which are eliminated by these enzymes).
No products indexed under this heading.

Nefazodone Hydrochloride (The administration of nilotinib with agents that are strong CYP3A4 inhibitors such as nefazodone should be avoided. If treatment is required, it is recommended that therapy with nilotinib be interrupted. If patients must be co-administered a strong CYP3A4 inhibitor, based on pharmacokinetic studies, 400 mg qd is predicted to adjust the nilotinib AUC to the AUC observed without inhibitors. However, there are no clinical data with this dose adjustment in patients receiving strong CYP3A4 inhibitors. If the strong inhibitor is discontinued, a washout period should be allowed before the nilotinib dose is adjusted upward to the indicated dose. Close monitoring for prolongation of the QT interval is indicated for patients who cannot avoid strong CYP3A4 inhibitors).
No products indexed under this heading.

1845 Interactions Index Tasigna

Nelfinavir Mesylate (The administration of nilotinib with agents that are strong CYP3A4 inhibitors such as nelfinavir should be avoided. If treatment is required, it is recommended that therapy with nilotinib be interrupted. If patients must be co-administered a strong CYP3A4 inhibitor, based on pharmacokinetic studies, 400 mg qd is predicted to adjust the nilotinib AUC to the AUC observed without inhibitors. However, there are no clinical data with this dose adjustment in patients receiving strong CYP3A4 inhibitors. If the strong inhibitor is discontinued, a washout period should be allowed before the nilotinib dose is adjusted upward to the indicated dose. Close monitoring for prolongation of the QT interval is indicated for patients who cannot avoid strong CYP3A4 inhibitors).
No products indexed under this heading.

Nevirapine (The concomitant use of strong CYP3A4 inducers should be avoided. If patients must be co-administered a strong CYP3A4 inducer, the dose of nilotinib may need to be increased, depending on patient tolerability. If the strong inducer is discontinued, the nilotinib dose should be reduced to the indicated dose). Products include:
Viramune Oral Suspension 897
Viramune Tablets 897

Nicardipine (Nilotinib is a competitive inhibitor of CYP3A4 *in vitro*, potentially increasing the concentration of drugs eliminated by CYP3A4. Caution should be exercised when co-administering nilotinib with substrates for CYP3A4 that have a narrow therapeutic index).
No products indexed under this heading.

Nicardipine Hydrochloride (Nilotinib is a competitive inhibitor of CYP3A4 *in vitro*, potentially increasing the concentration of drugs eliminated by CYP3A4. Caution should be exercised when co-administering nilotinib with substrates for CYP3A4 that have a narrow therapeutic index).
No products indexed under this heading.

Nicotine (*In vitro* studies suggest that nilotinib may induce CYP2B6, CYP2C8 and CYP2C9, and decrease the concentrations of drugs which are eliminated by these enzymes).
No products indexed under this heading.

Nicotine Polacrilex (*In vitro* studies suggest that nilotinib may induce CYP2B6, CYP2C8 and CYP2C9, and decrease the concentrations of drugs which are eliminated by these enzymes).
No products indexed under this heading.

Nicotine Salicylate (*In vitro* studies suggest that nilotinib may induce CYP2B6, CYP2C8 and CYP2C9, and decrease the concentrations of drugs which are eliminated by these enzymes).
No products indexed under this heading.

Nicotine Sulfate (*In vitro* studies suggest that nilotinib may induce CYP2B6, CYP2C8 and CYP2C9, and decrease the concentrations of drugs which are eliminated by these enzymes).
No products indexed under this heading.

Nifedipine (Nilotinib is a competitive inhibitor of CYP3A4 *in vitro*, potentially increasing the concentration of drugs eliminated by CYP3A4. Caution should be exercised when co-administering nilotinib with substrates for CYP3A4 that have a narrow therapeutic index).
No products indexed under this heading.

Nimodipine (Nilotinib is a competitive inhibitor of CYP3A4 *in vitro*, potentially increasing the concentration of drugs eliminated by CYP3A4. Caution should be exercised when co-administering nilotinib with substrates for CYP3A4 that have a narrow therapeutic index).
No products indexed under this heading.

Nisoldipine (Nilotinib is a competitive inhibitor of CYP3A4 *in vitro*, potentially increasing the concentration of drugs eliminated by CYP3A4. Caution should be exercised when co-administering nilotinib with substrates for CYP3A4 that have a narrow therapeutic index).
No products indexed under this heading.

Nitrendipine (Nilotinib is a competitive inhibitor of CYP3A4 *in vitro*, potentially increasing the concentration of drugs eliminated by CYP3A4. Caution should be exercised when co-administering nilotinib with substrates for CYP3A4 that have a narrow therapeutic index).
No products indexed under this heading.

Norethindrone (Nilotinib is a competitive inhibitor of CYP3A4 *in vitro*, potentially increasing the concentration of drugs eliminated by CYP3A4. Caution should be exercised when co-administering nilotinib with substrates for CYP3A4 that have a narrow therapeutic index). Products include:
Ortho Micronor 2660

Norethindrone Acetate (Nilotinib is a competitive inhibitor of CYP3A4 *in vitro*, potentially increasing the concentration of drugs eliminated by CYP3A4. Caution should be exercised when co-administering nilotinib with substrates for CYP3A4 that have a narrow therapeutic index). Products include:
Activella 2561

Norgestrel (Nilotinib is a competitive inhibitor of CYP3A4 *in vitro*, potentially increasing the concentration of drugs eliminated by CYP3A4. Caution should be exercised when co-administering nilotinib with substrates for CYP3A4 that have a narrow therapeutic index).
No products indexed under this heading.

Nortriptyline Hydrochloride (The administration of nilotinib with agents that prolong the QT interval should be avoided. Should treatment with any of these agents be required, it is recommended that therapy with nilotinib be interrupted. If interruption of treatment with nilotinib is not possible, patients who require treatment with a drug that prolongs the QT interval should be closely monitored for prolongation of the QT interval).
No products indexed under this heading.

Olanzapine (The administration of nilotinib with agents that prolong the QT interval should be avoided. Should treatment with any of these agents be required, it is recommended that therapy with nilotinib be interrupted. If interruption of treatment with nilotinib is not possible, patients who require treatment with a drug that prolongs the QT interval should be closely monitored for prolongation of the QT interval). Products include:
Symbyax 1965
Zyprexa 1984
Zyprexa IntraMuscular 1984
Zyprexa ZYDIS 1984

Omeprazole (Nilotinib is a competitive inhibitor of CYP2C8 *in vitro*, potentially increasing the concentration of drugs eliminated by CYP2C8. Caution should be exercised when co-administering nilotinib with substrates for CYP2C8 that have a narrow therapeutic index. *In vitro* studies also suggest that nilotinib may induce CYP2B6, CYP2C8, and CYP2C9, and thereby has the potential to decrease the concentrations of drugs which are eliminated by these enzymes).
No products indexed under this heading.

Ondansetron (Nilotinib is a competitive inhibitor of CYP3A4 *in vitro*, potentially increasing the concentration of drugs eliminated by CYP3A4. Caution should be exercised when co-administering nilotinib with substrates for CYP3A4 that have a narrow therapeutic index).
No products indexed under this heading.

Ondansetron Hydrochloride (Nilotinib is a competitive inhibitor of CYP3A4 *in vitro*, potentially increasing the concentration of drugs eliminated by CYP3A4. Caution should be exercised when co-administering nilotinib with substrates for CYP3A4 that have a narrow therapeutic index). Products include:
Zofran Injection 1750
Zofran 1756
Zofran ODT 1756

Orphenadrine Citrate (*In vitro* studies suggest that nilotinib may induce CYP2B6, CYP2C8 and CYP2C9, and decrease the concentrations of drugs which are eliminated by these enzymes).
No products indexed under this heading.

Orphenadrine Hydrochloride (*In vitro* studies suggest that nilotinib may induce CYP2B6, CYP2C8 and CYP2C9, and decrease the concentrations of drugs which are eliminated by these enzymes).
No products indexed under this heading.

Oxaprozin (Nilotinib is a competitive inhibitor of CYP2C9 *in vitro*, potentially increasing the concentration of drugs eliminated by CYP2C9. Caution should be exercised when co-administering nilotinib with substrates for CYP2C9 that have a narrow therapeutic index. *In vitro* studies also suggest that nilotinib may induce CYP2B6, CYP2C8 and CYP2C9, and thereby has the potential to decrease the concentrations of drugs which are eliminated by these enzymes).
No products indexed under this heading.

Oxazepam (The administration of nilotinib with agents that prolong the QT interval should be avoided. Should treatment with any of these agents be required, it is recommended that therapy with nilotinib be interrupted. If interruption of treatment with nilotinib is not possible, patients who require treatment with a drug that prolongs the QT interval should be closely monitored for prolongation of the QT interval).
No products indexed under this heading.

Oxcarbazepine (The concomitant use of strong CYP3A4 inducers should be avoided. If patients must be co-administered a strong CYP3A4 inducer, the dose of nilotinib may need to be increased, depending on patient tolerability. If the strong inducer is discontinued, the nilotinib dose should be reduced to the indicated dose).
No products indexed under this heading.

Oxycodone Hydrochloride (Nilotinib is a competitive inhibitor of CYP2D6 *in vitro*, potentially increasing the concentration of drugs eliminated by CYP2D6. Caution should be exercised when co-administering nilotinib with substrates for CYP2D6 that have a narrow therapeutic index). Products include:
OxyContin 2807
Percocet 1121
Percodan 1124

Paclitaxel (Nilotinib is a competitive inhibitor of CYP2C8 *in vitro*, potentially increasing the concentration of drugs eliminated by CYP2C8. Caution should be exercised when co-administering nilotinib with substrates for CYP2C8 that have a narrow therapeutic index. *In vitro* studies also suggest that nilotinib may induce CYP2B6, CYP2C8, and CYP2C9, and thereby has the potential to decrease the concentrations of drugs which are eliminated by these enzymes).
No products indexed under this heading.

Paclitaxel, protein-bound (Nilotinib inhibits human P-glycoprotein. If nilotinib is administered with drugs that are substrates of Pgp, increased concentrations of the substrate drug are likely, and caution should be exercised).
No products indexed under this heading.

Paroxetine Hydrochloride (Nilotinib is a competitive inhibitor of CYP2D6 *in vitro*, potentially increasing the concentration of drugs eliminated by CYP2D6. Caution should be exercised when co-administering nilotinib with substrates for CYP2D6 that have a narrow therapeutic index). Products include:
Paroxetine CR 2361
Paroxetine ER 2371
Paxil 1586
Paxil CR 1596

Perphenazine (The administration of nilotinib with agents that prolong the QT interval should be avoided. Should treatment with any of these agents be required, it is recommended that therapy with nilotinib be interrupted. If interruption of treatment with nilotinib is not possible, patients who require treatment with a drug that prolongs the QT interval should be closely monitored for prolongation of the QT interval).
No products indexed under this heading.

Phenelzine Sulfate (The administration of nilotinib with agents that prolong the QT interval should be avoided. Should treatment with any of these agents be required, it is recommended that therapy with nilotinib be interrupted. If interruption of treatment with nilotinib is not possible, patients who require treatment with a drug that prolongs the QT interval should be closely monitored for prolongation of the QT interval).
No products indexed under this heading.

Phenobarbital (The concomitant use of strong CYP3A4 inducers such as phenobarbital should be avoided. If patients must be co-administered a strong CYP3A4 inducer, the dose of nilotinib may need to be increased, depending on patient tolerability. If the strong inducer is discontinued, the nilotinib dose should be reduced to the indicated dose). Products include:
Donnatal 2711

Phenobarbital Sodium (The concomitant use of strong CYP3A4 inducers such as phenobarbital should be avoided. If patients must be co-administered a strong CYP3A4 inducer, the dose of nilotinib may need to be increased, depending on patient tolerability. If the strong inducer is discontinued, the nilotinib dose should be reduced to the indicated dose).
No products indexed under this heading.

Phenylbutazone (Nilotinib is a competitive inhibitor of CYP2C9 *in vitro*, potentially increasing the concentration of drugs eliminated by CYP2C9. Caution should be exercised when co-administering nilotinib with substrates for CYP2C9 that have a narrow therapeutic index. *In vitro* studies also suggest that nilotinib may induce CYP2B6, CYP2C8 and CYP2C9, and thereby has the potential to decrease the concentrations of drugs which are eliminated by these enzymes).
No products indexed under this heading.

IMPORTANT NOTE: Always consult each drug listing in the patient's regimen for possible interactions.

Tasigna Interactions Index 1846

Phenytoin (The concomitant use of strong CYP3A4 inducers such as phenytoin should be avoided. If patients must be co-administered a strong CYP3A4 inducer, the dose of nilotinib may need to be increased, depending on patient tolerability. If the strong inducer is discontinued, the nilotinib dose should be reduced to the indicated dose).
No products indexed under this heading.

Phenytoin Sodium (The concomitant use of strong CYP3A4 inducers such as phenytoin should be avoided. If patients must be co-administered a strong CYP3A4 inducer, the dose of nilotinib may need to be increased, depending on patient tolerability. If the strong inducer is discontinued, the nilotinib dose should be reduced to the indicated dose). Products include:
Phenytek Capsules 2380

Pimozide (The administration of nilotinib with agents that are strong CYP3A4 inhibitors or anti-arrhythmic drugs and other drugs that may prolong QT interval (eg, pimozide) should be avoided. Should treatment with any of these agents be required, it is recommended that therapy with nilotinib be interrupted. If interruption of treatment with nilotinib is not possible, patients who require treatment with a drug that prolongs QT or strongly inhibits CYP3A4 should be closely monitored for prolongation of the QT interval).
No products indexed under this heading.

Pindolol (Nilotinib is a competitive inhibitor of CYP2D6 *in vitro*, potentially increasing the concentration of drugs eliminated by CYP2D6. Caution should be exercised when co-administering nilotinib with substrates for CYP2D6 that have a narrow therapeutic index).
No products indexed under this heading.

Pioglitazone Hydrochloride (Nilotinib is a competitive inhibitor of CYP2C8 *in vitro*, potentially increasing the concentration of drugs eliminated by CYP2C8. Caution should be exercised when co-administering nilotinib with substrates for CYP2C8 that have a narrow therapeutic index. *In vitro* studies also suggest that nilotinib may induce CYP2B6, CYP2C8, and CYP2C9, and thereby has the potential to decrease the concentrations of drugs which are eliminated by these enzymes). Products include:
ActoPlus 3338
Actos 3345
Duetact 3354

Piroxicam (Nilotinib is a competitive inhibitor of CYP2C9 *in vitro*, potentially increasing the concentration of drugs eliminated by CYP2C9. Caution should be exercised when co-administering nilotinib with substrates for CYP2C9 that have a narrow therapeutic index. *In vitro* studies also suggest that nilotinib may induce CYP2B6, CYP2C8 and CYP2C9, and thereby has the potential to decrease the concentrations of drugs which are eliminated by these enzymes).
No products indexed under this heading.

Polyestradiol Phosphate (Nilotinib is a competitive inhibitor of CYP3A4 *in vitro*, potentially increasing the concentration of drugs eliminated by CYP3A4. Caution should be exercised when co-administering nilotinib with substrates for CYP3A4 that have a narrow therapeutic index).
No products indexed under this heading.

Posaconazole (Nilotinib inhibits human P-glycoprotein. If nilotinib is administered with drugs that are substrates of Pgp, increased concentrations of the substrate drug are likely, and caution should be exercised). Products include:
Noxafil 3172

Prazepam (The administration of nilotinib with agents that prolong the QT interval should be avoided. Should treatment with any of these agents be required, it is recommended that therapy with nilotinib be interrupted. If interruption of treatment with nilotinib is not possible, patients who require treatment with a drug that prolongs the QT interval should be closely monitored for prolongation of the QT interval).
No products indexed under this heading.

Prednisolone (The concomitant use of strong CYP3A4 inducers should be avoided. If patients must be co-administered a strong CYP3A4 inducer, the dose of nilotinib may need to be increased, depending on patient tolerability. If the strong inducer is discontinued, the nilotinib dose should be reduced to the indicated dose).
No products indexed under this heading.

Prednisolone Acetate (The concomitant use of strong CYP3A4 inducers should be avoided. If patients must be co-administered a strong CYP3A4 inducer, the dose of nilotinib may need to be increased, depending on patient tolerability. If the strong inducer is discontinued, the nilotinib dose should be reduced to the indicated dose). Products include:
Blephamide .... ⊙212, ⊙214
Pred Forte .... ⊙225
Pred Mild .... ⊙230
Pred-G .... ⊙226, ⊙227

Prednisolone Sodium Phosphate (The concomitant use of strong CYP3A4 inducers should be avoided. If patients must be co-administered a strong CYP3A4 inducer, the dose of nilotinib may need to be increased, depending on patient tolerability. If the strong inducer is discontinued, the nilotinib dose should be reduced to the indicated dose).
No products indexed under this heading.

Prednisolone Tebutate (The concomitant use of strong CYP3A4 inducers should be avoided. If patients must be co-administered a strong CYP3A4 inducer, the dose of nilotinib may need to be increased, depending on patient tolerability. If the strong inducer is discontinued, the nilotinib dose should be reduced to the indicated dose).
No products indexed under this heading.

Prednisone (The concomitant use of strong CYP3A4 inducers should be avoided. If patients must be co-administered a strong CYP3A4 inducer, the dose of nilotinib may need to be increased, depending on patient tolerability. If the strong inducer is discontinued, the nilotinib dose should be reduced to the indicated dose).
No products indexed under this heading.

Prednisone sodium phosphate (The concomitant use of strong CYP3A4 inducers should be avoided. If patients must be co-administered a strong CYP3A4 inducer, the dose of nilotinib may need to be increased, depending on patient tolerability. If the strong inducer is discontinued, the nilotinib dose should be reduced to the indicated dose).
No products indexed under this heading.

Primidone (The concomitant use of strong CYP3A4 inducers should be avoided. If patients must be co-administered a strong CYP3A4 inducer, the dose of nilotinib may need to be increased, depending on patient tolerability. If the strong inducer is discontinued, the nilotinib dose should be reduced to the indicated dose).
No products indexed under this heading.

Procainamide (The administration of nilotinib with agents that are strong CYP3A4 inhibitors or anti-arrhythmic drugs (eg, procainamide) and other drugs that may prolong QT interval should be avoided. Should treatment with any of these agents be required, it is recommended that therapy with nilotinib be interrupted. If interruption of treatment with nilotinib is not possible, patients who require treatment with a drug that prolongs QT or strongly inhibits CYP3A4 should be closely monitored for prolongation of the QT interval).
No products indexed under this heading.

Procainamide Hydrochloride (The administration of nilotinib with agents that are strong CYP3A4 inhibitors or anti-arrhythmic drugs (eg, procainamide) and other drugs that may prolong QT interval should be avoided. Should treatment with any of these agents be required, it is recommended that therapy with nilotinib be interrupted. If interruption of treatment with nilotinib is not possible, patients who require treatment with a drug that prolongs QT or strongly inhibits CYP3A4 should be closely monitored for prolongation of the QT interval).
No products indexed under this heading.

Prochlorperazine (The administration of nilotinib with agents that prolong the QT interval should be avoided. Should treatment with any of these agents be required, it is recommended that therapy with nilotinib be interrupted. If interruption of treatment with nilotinib is not possible, patients who require treatment with a drug that prolongs the QT interval should be closely monitored for prolongation of the QT interval).
No products indexed under this heading.

Promethazine (*In vitro* studies suggest that nilotinib may induce CYP2B6, CYP2C8 and CYP2C9, and decrease the concentrations of drugs which are eliminated by these enzymes).
No products indexed under this heading.

Promethazine Hydrochloride (The administration of nilotinib with agents that prolong the QT interval should be avoided. Should treatment with any of these agents be required, it is recommended that therapy with nilotinib be interrupted. If interruption of treatment with nilotinib is not possible, patients who require treatment with a drug that prolongs the QT interval should be closely monitored for prolongation of the QT interval).
No products indexed under this heading.

Propafenone Hydrochloride (The administration of nilotinib with agents that prolong the QT interval should be avoided. Should treatment with any of these agents be required, it is recommended that therapy with nilotinib be interrupted. If interruption of treatment with nilotinib is not possible, patients who require treatment with a drug that prolongs the QT interval should be closely monitored for prolongation of the QT interval). Products include:
Rythmol 1648
Rythmol SR 1652

Propofol (*In vitro* studies suggest that nilotinib may induce CYP2B6, CYP2C8 and CYP2C9, and decrease the concentrations of drugs which are eliminated by these enzymes).
No products indexed under this heading.

Propoxyphene Hydrochloride (Nilotinib is a competitive inhibitor of CYP2D6 *in vitro*, potentially increasing the concentration of drugs eliminated by CYP2D6. Caution should be exercised when co-administering nilotinib with substrates for CYP2D6 that have a narrow therapeutic index).
No products indexed under this heading.

Propoxyphene Napsylate (Nilotinib is a competitive inhibitor of CYP2D6 *in vitro*, potentially increasing the concentration of drugs eliminated by CYP2D6. Caution should be exercised when co-administering nilotinib with substrates for CYP2D6 that have a narrow therapeutic index).
No products indexed under this heading.

Propranolol Hydrochloride (The administration of nilotinib with agents that are strong CYP3A4 inhibitors or anti-arrhythmic drugs and other drugs that may prolong QT interval should be avoided. Should treatment with any of these agents be required, it is recommended that therapy with nilotinib be interrupted. If interruption of treatment with nilotinib is not possible, patients who require treatment with a drug that prolongs QT or strongly inhibits CYP3A4 should be closely monitored for prolongation of the QT interval). Products include:
InnoPran XL 1517

Protriptyline Hydrochloride (The administration of nilotinib with agents that prolong the QT interval should be avoided. Should treatment with any of these agents be required, it is recommended that therapy with nilotinib be interrupted. If interruption of treatment with nilotinib is not possible, patients who require treatment with a drug that prolongs the QT interval should be closely monitored for prolongation of the QT interval).
No products indexed under this heading.

Quetiapine Fumarate (The administration of nilotinib with agents that prolong the QT interval should be avoided. Should treatment with any of these agents be required, it is recommended that therapy with nilotinib be interrupted. If interruption of treatment with nilotinib is not possible, patients who require treatment with a drug that prolongs the QT interval should be closely monitored for prolongation of the QT interval). Products include:
Seroquel 750
Seroquel XR 759

Quinidine (The administration of nilotinib with agents that are strong CYP3A4 inhibitors or anti-arrhythmic drugs (eg, quinidine) and other drugs that may prolong QT interval should be avoided. Should treatment with any of these agents be required, it is recommended that therapy with nilotinib be interrupted. If interruption of treatment with nilotinib is not possible, patients who require treatment with a drug that prolongs QT or strongly inhibits CYP3A4 should be closely monitored for prolongation of the QT interval).
No products indexed under this heading.

Quinidine Gluconate (The administration of nilotinib with agents that are strong CYP3A4 inhibitors or anti-arrhythmic drugs (eg, quinidine) and other drugs that may prolong QT interval should be avoided. Should treatment with any of these agents be required, it is recommended that therapy with nilotinib be interrupted. If interruption of treatment with nilotinib is not possible, patients who require treatment with a drug that prolongs QT or strongly inhibits CYP3A4 should be closely monitored for prolongation of the QT interval).
No products indexed under this heading.

Quinidine Hydrochloride (The administration of nilotinib with agents that are strong CYP3A4 inhibitors or anti-arrhythmic drugs (eg, quinidine) and other drugs that may prolong QT interval should be avoided. Should treatment with any of these agents be required, it is recommended that therapy with nilotinib be interrupted. If interruption of treatment with nilotinib is not possible, patients who require treatment with a

drug that prolongs QT or strongly inhibits CYP3A4 should be closely monitored for prolongation of the QT interval.

No products indexed under this heading.

Quinidine Polygalacturonate (The administration of nilotinib with agents that are strong CYP3A4 inhibitors or anti-arrhythmic drugs (eg, quinidine) and other drugs that may prolong QT interval should be avoided. Should treatment with any of these agents be required, it is recommended that therapy with nilotinib be interrupted. If interruption of treatment with nilotinib is not possible, patients who require treatment with a drug that prolongs QT or strongly inhibits CYP3A4 should be closely monitored for prolongation of the QT interval.

No products indexed under this heading.

Quinidine Sulfate (The administration of nilotinib with agents that are strong CYP3A4 inhibitors or anti-arrhythmic drugs (eg, quinidine) and other drugs that may prolong QT interval should be avoided. Should treatment with any of these agents be required, it is recommended that therapy with nilotinib be interrupted. If interruption of treatment with nilotinib is not possible, patients who require treatment with a drug that prolongs QT or strongly inhibits CYP3A4 should be closely monitored for prolongation of the QT interval.

No products indexed under this heading.

Ranolazine (Nilotinib inhibits human P-glycoprotein. If nilotinib is administered with drugs that are substrates of Pgp, increased concentrations of the substrate drug are likely, and caution should be exercised). Products include:
Ranexa 1255

Repaglinide (Nilotinib is a competitive inhibitor of CYP2C8 *in vitro*, potentially increasing the concentration of drugs eliminated by CYP2C8. Caution should be exercised when co-administering nilotinib with substrates for CYP2C8 that have a narrow therapeutic index. *In vitro* studies also suggest that nilotinib may induce CYP2B6, CYP2C8, and CYP2C9, and thereby has the potential to decrease the concentrations of drugs which are eliminated by these enzymes).

No products indexed under this heading.

Rifabutin (The concomitant use of strong CYP3A4 inducers such as rifabutin should be avoided. If patients must be co-administered a strong CYP3A4 inducer, the dose of nilotinib may need to be increased, depending on patient tolerability. If the strong inducer is discontinued, the nilotinib dose should be reduced to the indicated dose).

No products indexed under this heading.

Rifampicin (The concomitant use of strong CYP3A4 inducers should be avoided. If patients must be co-administered a strong CYP3A4 inducer, the dose of nilotinib may need to be increased, depending on patient tolerability. If the strong inducer is discontinued, the nilotinib dose should be reduced to the indicated dose. In healthy subjects receiving the CYP3A4 inducer, rifampicin, at 600 mg daily for 12 days, systemic exposure (AUC) to nilotinib was decreased by approximately 80%).

No products indexed under this heading.

Rifampin (The concomitant use of strong CYP3A4 inducers such as rifampin, should be avoided. If patients must be co-administered a strong CYP3A4 inducer, the dose of nilotinib may need to be increased, depending on patient tolerability. If the strong inducer is discontinued, the nilotinib dose should be reduced to the indicated dose).

No products indexed under this heading.

Rifapentine (The concomitant use of strong CYP3A4 inducers such as rifapentine should be avoided. If patients must be co-administered a strong CYP3A4 inducer, the dose of nilotinib may need to be increased, depending on patient tolerability. If the strong inducer is discontinued, the nilotinib dose should be reduced to the indicated dose).

No products indexed under this heading.

Risperidone (The administration of nilotinib with agents that prolong the QT interval should be avoided. Should treatment with any of these agents be required, it is recommended that therapy with nilotinib be interrupted. If interruption of treatment with nilotinib is not possible, patients who require treatment with a drug that prolongs the QT interval should be closely monitored for prolongation of the QT interval. Products include:
Risperdal Consta 2682

Ritonavir (The administration of nilotinib with agents that are strong CYP3A4 inhibitors such as ritonavir should be avoided. If treatment is required, it is recommended that therapy with nilotinib be interrupted. If patients must be co-administered a strong CYP3A4 inhibitor, based on pharmacokinetic studies, 400 mg qd is predicted to adjust the nilotinib AUC to the AUC observed without inhibitors. However, there are no clinical data with this dose adjustment in patients receiving strong CYP3A4 inhibitors. If the strong inhibitor is discontinued, a washout period should be allowed before the nilotinib dose is adjusted upward to the indicated dose. Close monitoring for prolongation of the QT interval is indicated for patients who cannot avoid strong CYP3A4 inhibitors). Products include:
Kaletra 458
Norvir 509

Rofecoxib (Nilotinib is a competitive inhibitor of CYP2C9 *in vitro*, potentially increasing the concentration of drugs eliminated by CYP2C9. Caution should be exercised when co-administering nilotinib with substrates for CYP2C9 that have a narrow therapeutic index. *In vitro* studies also suggest that nilotinib may induce CYP2B6, CYP2C8 and CYP2C9, and thereby has the potential to decrease the concentrations of drugs which are eliminated by these enzymes).

No products indexed under this heading.

Ropivacaine Hydrochloride (*In vitro* studies suggest that nilotinib may induce CYP2B6, CYP2C8 and CYP2C9, and decrease the concentrations of drugs which are eliminated by these enzymes).

No products indexed under this heading.

Rosiglitazone Maleate (Nilotinib is a competitive inhibitor of CYP2C8 *in vitro*, potentially increasing the concentration of drugs eliminated by CYP2C8. Caution should be exercised when co-administering nilotinib with substrates for CYP2C8 that have a narrow therapeutic index. *In vitro* studies also suggest that nilotinib may induce CYP2B6, CYP2C8, and CYP2C9, and thereby has the potential to decrease the concentrations of drugs which are eliminated by these enzymes). Products include:
Avandamet 1345
Avandaryl 1356
Avandia 1366

Rosiglitazone/Metformin (Nilotinib is a competitive inhibitor of CYP2C8 *in vitro*, potentially increasing the concentration of drugs eliminated by CYP2C8. Caution should be exercised when co-administering nilotinib with substrates for CYP2C8 that have a narrow therapeutic index. *In vitro* studies also suggest that nilotinib may induce CYP2B6, CYP2C8, and CYP2C9, and thereby has the potential to decrease the concentrations of drugs which are eliminated by these enzymes).

No products indexed under this heading.

Saquinavir (The administration of nilotinib with agents that are of strong CYP3A4 inhibitors such as saquinavir should be avoided. If treatment is required, it is recommended that therapy with nilotinib be interrupted. If patients must be co-administered a strong CYP3A4 inhibitor, based on pharmacokinetic studies, 400 mg qd is predicted to adjust the nilotinib AUC to the AUC observed without inhibitors. However, there are no clinical data with this dose adjustment in patients receiving strong CYP3A4 inhibitors. If the strong inhibitor is discontinued, a washout period should be allowed before the nilotinib dose is adjusted upward to the indicated dose. Close monitoring for prolongation of the QT interval is indicated for patients who cannot avoid strong CYP3A4 inhibitors).

No products indexed under this heading.

Saquinavir Mesylate (The administration of nilotinib with agents that are of strong CYP3A4 inhibitors such as saquinavir should be avoided. If treatment is required, it is recommended that therapy with nilotinib be interrupted. If patients must be co-administered a strong CYP3A4 inhibitor, based on pharmacokinetic studies, 400 mg qd is predicted to adjust the nilotinib AUC to the AUC observed without inhibitors. However, there are no clinical data with this dose adjustment in patients receiving strong CYP3A4 inhibitors. If the strong inhibitor is discontinued, a washout period should be allowed before the nilotinib dose is adjusted upward to the indicated dose. Close monitoring for prolongation of the QT interval is indicated for patients who cannot avoid strong CYP3A4 inhibitors).

No products indexed under this heading.

Selegiline (*In vitro* studies suggest that nilotinib may induce CYP2B6, CYP2C8 and CYP2C9, and decrease the concentrations of drugs which are eliminated by these enzymes). Products include:
Emsam 3623

Selegiline Hydrochloride (*In vitro* studies suggest that nilotinib may induce CYP2B6, CYP2C8 and CYP2C9, and decrease the concentrations of drugs which are eliminated by these enzymes). Products include:
Eldepryl 3312

Sertraline Hydrochloride (Nilotinib is a competitive inhibitor of CYP3A4 *in vitro*, potentially increasing the concentration of drugs eliminated by CYP3A4. Caution should be exercised when co-administering nilotinib with substrates for CYP3A4 that have a narrow therapeutic index).

No products indexed under this heading.

Sevoflurane (*In vitro* studies suggest that nilotinib may induce CYP2B6, CYP2C8 and CYP2C9, and decrease the concentrations of drugs which are eliminated by these enzymes). Products include:
Ultane 554

Sildenafil Citrate (Nilotinib is a competitive inhibitor of CYP3A4 *in vitro*, potentially increasing the concentration of drugs eliminated by CYP3A4. Caution should be exercised when co-administering nilotinib with substrates for CYP3A4 that have a narrow therapeutic index).

No products indexed under this heading.

Simvastatin (Nilotinib is a competitive inhibitor of CYP3A4 *in vitro*, potentially increasing the concentration of drugs

eliminated by CYP3A4. Caution should be exercised when co-administering nilotinib with substrates for CYP3A4 that have a narrow therapeutic index). Products include:
Simcor 524
Vytorin 10/10 .... 2303, 3240
Vytorin 10/20 .... 2303, 3240
Vytorin 10/40 .... 2303, 3240
Vytorin 10/80 .... 2303, 3240
Zocor 2289

Sirolimus (Nilotinib is a competitive inhibitor of CYP3A4 *in vitro*, potentially increasing the concentration of drugs eliminated by CYP3A4. Caution should be exercised when co-administering nilotinib with substrates for CYP3A4 that have a narrow therapeutic index). Products include:
Rapamune 3579

Sitagliptin Phosphate (Nilotinib inhibits human P-glycoprotein. If nilotinib is administered with drugs that are substrates of Pgp, increased concentrations of the substrate drug are likely, and caution should be exercised). Products include:
Janumet 2188
Januvia 2196

Sotalol Hydrochloride (The administration of nilotinib with agents that are strong CYP3A4 inhibitors or anti-arrhythmic drugs (eg, sotalol) and other drugs that may prolong QT interval should be avoided. Should treatment with any of these agents be required, it is recommended that therapy with nilotinib be interrupted. If interruption of treatment with nilotinib is not possible, patients who require treatment with a drug that prolongs QT or strongly inhibits CYP3A4 should be closely monitored for prolongation of the QT interval.

No products indexed under this heading.

Sulfamethoxazole (Nilotinib is a competitive inhibitor of CYP2C9 *in vitro*, potentially increasing the concentration of drugs eliminated by CYP2C9. Caution should be exercised when co-administering nilotinib with substrates for CYP2C9 that have a narrow therapeutic index. *In vitro* studies also suggest that nilotinib may induce CYP2B6, CYP2C8 and CYP2C9, and thereby has the potential to decrease the concentrations of drugs which are eliminated by these enzymes).

No products indexed under this heading.

Sulfinpyrazone (The concomitant use of strong CYP3A4 inducers should be avoided. If patients must be co-administered a strong CYP3A4 inducer, the dose of nilotinib may need to be increased, depending on patient tolerability. If the strong inducer is discontinued, the nilotinib dose should be reduced to the indicated dose).

No products indexed under this heading.

Sulindac (Nilotinib is a competitive inhibitor of CYP2C9 *in vitro*, potentially increasing the concentration of drugs eliminated by CYP2C9. Caution should be exercised when co-administering nilotinib with substrates for CYP2C9 that have a narrow therapeutic index. *In vitro* studies also suggest that nilotinib may induce CYP2B6, CYP2C8 and CYP2C9, and thereby has the potential to decrease the concentrations of drugs which are eliminated by these enzymes). Products include:
Clinoril 2098

Suprofen (Nilotinib is a competitive inhibitor of CYP2C9 *in vitro*, potentially increasing the concentration of drugs eliminated by CYP2C9. Caution should be exercised when co-administering nilotinib with substrates for CYP2C9 that have a narrow therapeutic index. *In vitro* studies also suggest that nilotinib may induce CYP2B6, CYP2C8 and CYP2C9, and thereby has the potential

Tasigna Interactions Index 1848

to decrease the concentrations of drugs which are eliminated by these enzymes).
No products indexed under this heading.

Tacrolimus (Nilotinib is a competitive inhibitor of CYP3A4 *in vitro*, potentially increasing the concentration of drugs eliminated by CYP3A4. Caution should be exercised when co-administering nilotinib with substrates for CYP3A4 that have a narrow therapeutic index). Products include:
Prograf Capsules 677
Prograf Injection 677
Protopic 685

Tadalafil (Nilotinib is a competitive inhibitor of CYP3A4 *in vitro*, potentially increasing the concentration of drugs eliminated by CYP3A4. Caution should be exercised when co-administering nilotinib with substrates for CYP3A4 that have a narrow therapeutic index). Products include:
Adcirca 3461
Cialis 1861

Tamoxifen Citrate (Nilotinib is a competitive inhibitor of CYP3A4 *in vitro*, potentially increasing the concentration of drugs eliminated by CYP3A4. Caution should be exercised when co-administering nilotinib with substrates for CYP3A4 that have a narrow therapeutic index).
No products indexed under this heading.

Telithromycin (The administration of nilotinib with agents that are strong CYP3A4 inhibitors such as telithromycin should be avoided. If treatment is required, it is recommended that therapy with nilotinib be interrupted. If patients must be co-administered a strong CYP3A4 inhibitor, based on pharmacokinetic studies, 400 mg qd is predicted to adjust the nilotinib AUC to the AUC observed without inhibitors. However, there are no clinical data with this dose adjustment in patients receiving strong CYP3A4 inhibitors. If the strong inhibitor is discontinued, a washout period should be allowed before the nilotinib dose is adjusted upward to the indicated dose. Close monitoring for prolongation of the QT interval is indicated for patients who cannot avoid strong CYP3A4 inhibitors). Products include:
Ketek 2991

Telmisartan (Nilotinib is a competitive inhibitor of CYP2C9 *in vitro*, potentially increasing the concentration of drugs eliminated by CYP2C9. Caution should be exercised when co-administering nilotinib with substrates for CYP2C9 that have a narrow therapeutic index. *In vitro* studies also suggest that nilotinib may induce CYP2B6, CYP2C8 and CYP2C9, and thereby has the potential to decrease the concentrations of drugs which are eliminated by these enzymes). Products include:
Micardis 887
Micardis HCT 889

Temazepam (*In vitro* studies suggest that nilotinib may induce CYP2B6, CYP2C8 and CYP2C9, and decrease the concentrations of drugs which are eliminated by these enzymes).
No products indexed under this heading.

Temsirolimus (Nilotinib inhibits human P-glycoprotein. If nilotinib is administered with drugs that are substrates of Pgp, increased concentrations of the substrate drug are likely, and caution should be exercised). Products include:
Torisel 3592

Teniposide (Nilotinib is a competitive inhibitor of CYP2D6 *in vitro*, potentially increasing the concentration of drugs eliminated by CYP2D6. Caution should be exercised when co-administering nilotinib with substrates for CYP2D6 that have a narrow therapeutic index).
No products indexed under this heading.

Terfenadine (Nilotinib is a competitive inhibitor of CYP3A4 *in vitro*, potentially increasing the concentration of drugs eliminated by CYP3A4. Caution should be exercised when co-administering nilotinib with substrates for CYP3A4 that have a narrow therapeutic index).
No products indexed under this heading.

Testosterone (Nilotinib is a competitive inhibitor of CYP2D6 *in vitro*, potentially increasing the concentration of drugs eliminated by CYP2D6. Caution should be exercised when co-administering nilotinib with substrates for CYP2D6 that have a narrow therapeutic index). Products include:
AndroGel 3456

Testosterone Cypionate (Nilotinib is a competitive inhibitor of CYP2D6 *in vitro*, potentially increasing the concentration of drugs eliminated by CYP2D6. Caution should be exercised when co-administering nilotinib with substrates for CYP2D6 that have a narrow therapeutic index).
No products indexed under this heading.

Testosterone Enanthate (Nilotinib is a competitive inhibitor of CYP2D6 *in vitro*, potentially increasing the concentration of drugs eliminated by CYP2D6. Caution should be exercised when co-administering nilotinib with substrates for CYP2D6 that have a narrow therapeutic index). Products include:
Delatestryl 1102

Testosterone Propionate (Nilotinib is a competitive inhibitor of CYP2D6 *in vitro*, potentially increasing the concentration of drugs eliminated by CYP2D6. Caution should be exercised when co-administering nilotinib with substrates for CYP2D6 that have a narrow therapeutic index).
No products indexed under this heading.

Theophyllinate (The concomitant use of strong CYP3A4 inducers should be avoided. If patients must be co-administered a strong CYP3A4 inducer, the dose of nilotinib may need to be increased, depending on patient tolerability. If the strong inducer is discontinued, the nilotinib dose should be reduced to the indicated dose).
No products indexed under this heading.

Theophylline (Nilotinib is a competitive inhibitor of CYP3A4 *in vitro*, potentially increasing the concentration of drugs eliminated by CYP3A4. Caution should be exercised when co-administering nilotinib with substrates for CYP3A4 that have a narrow therapeutic index).
No products indexed under this heading.

Theophylline Anhydrous (Nilotinib is a competitive inhibitor of CYP3A4 *in vitro*, potentially increasing the concentration of drugs eliminated by CYP3A4. Caution should be exercised when co-administering nilotinib with substrates for CYP3A4 that have a narrow therapeutic index). Products include:
Uniphyl 2817

Theophylline Calcium Salicylate (Nilotinib is a competitive inhibitor of CYP3A4 *in vitro*, potentially increasing the concentration of drugs eliminated by CYP3A4. Caution should be exercised when co-administering nilotinib with substrates for CYP3A4 that have a narrow therapeutic index).
No products indexed under this heading.

Theophylline Dihydroxypropyl (Glyceryl) (Nilotinib is a competitive inhibitor of CYP3A4 *in vitro*, potentially increasing the concentration of drugs eliminated by CYP3A4. Caution should be exercised when co-administering nilotinib with substrates for CYP3A4 that have a narrow therapeutic index).
No products indexed under this heading.

Theophylline Ethylenediamine (Nilotinib is a competitive inhibitor of CYP3A4 *in vitro*, potentially increasing the concentration of drugs eliminated by CYP3A4. Caution should be exercised when co-administering nilotinib with substrates for CYP3A4 that have a narrow therapeutic index).
No products indexed under this heading.

Theophylline Sodium Glycinate (Nilotinib is a competitive inhibitor of CYP3A4 *in vitro*, potentially increasing the concentration of drugs eliminated by CYP3A4. Caution should be exercised when co-administering nilotinib with substrates for CYP3A4 that have a narrow therapeutic index).
No products indexed under this heading.

Thioridazine (Nilotinib is a competitive inhibitor of CYP2D6 *in vitro*, potentially increasing the concentration of drugs eliminated by CYP2D6. Caution should be exercised when co-administering nilotinib with substrates for CYP2D6 that have a narrow therapeutic index).
No products indexed under this heading.

Thioridazine Hydrochloride (The administration of nilotinib with agents that prolong the QT interval should be avoided. Should treatment with any of these agents be required, it is recommended that therapy with nilotinib be interrupted. If interruption of treatment with nilotinib is not possible, patients who require treatment with a drug that prolongs the QT interval should be closely monitored for prolongation of the QT interval). Products include:
Thioridazine Hydrochloride 2384

Thiothixene (The administration of nilotinib with agents that prolong the QT interval should be avoided. Should treatment with any of these agents be required, it is recommended that therapy with nilotinib be interrupted. If interruption of treatment with nilotinib is not possible, patients who require treatment with a drug that prolongs the QT interval should be closely monitored for prolongation of the QT interval). Products include:
Thiothixene 2386

Tiagabine Hydrochloride (Nilotinib is a competitive inhibitor of CYP3A4 *in vitro*, potentially increasing the concentration of drugs eliminated by CYP3A4. Caution should be exercised when co-administering nilotinib with substrates for CYP3A4 that have a narrow therapeutic index). Products include:
Gabitril 972

Timolol Maleate (Nilotinib is a competitive inhibitor of CYP2D6 *in vitro*, potentially increasing the concentration of drugs eliminated by CYP2D6. Caution should be exercised when co-administering nilotinib with substrates for CYP2D6 that have a narrow therapeutic index). Products include:
Combigan 601
Dorzolamide Hydrochloride/Timolol Maleate Ophthalmic Solution .... ⊙243
Timoptic in Ocudose .... ⊙231

Tipranavir (Nilotinib inhibits human P-glycoprotein. If nilotinib is administered with drugs that are substrates of Pgp, increased concentrations of the substrate drug are likely, and caution should be exercised).
No products indexed under this heading.

Tocainide Hydrochloride (The administration of nilotinib with agents that prolong the QT interval should be avoided. Should treatment with any of these agents be required, it is recommended that therapy with nilotinib be interrupted. If interruption of treatment with nilotinib is not possible, patients who require treatment with a drug that prolongs the QT interval should be closely monitored for prolongation of the QT interval).
No products indexed under this heading.

Tolazamide (Nilotinib is a competitive inhibitor of CYP2C9 *in vitro*, potentially increasing the concentration of drugs eliminated by CYP2C9. Caution should be exercised when co-administering nilotinib with substrates for CYP2C9 that have a narrow therapeutic index. *In vitro* studies also suggest that nilotinib may induce CYP2B6, CYP2C8 and CYP2C9, and thereby has the potential to decrease the concentrations of drugs which are eliminated by these enzymes).
No products indexed under this heading.

Tolbutamide (Nilotinib is a competitive inhibitor of CYP2C8 *in vitro*, potentially increasing the concentration of drugs eliminated by CYP2C8. Caution should be exercised when co-administering nilotinib with substrates for CYP2C8 that have a narrow therapeutic index. *In vitro* studies also suggest that nilotinib may induce CYP2B6, CYP2C8, and CYP2C9, and thereby has the potential to decrease the concentrations of drugs which are eliminated by these enzymes).
No products indexed under this heading.

Tolbutamide Sodium (Nilotinib is a competitive inhibitor of CYP2C8 *in vitro*, potentially increasing the concentration of drugs eliminated by CYP2C8. Caution should be exercised when co-administering nilotinib with substrates for CYP2C8 that have a narrow therapeutic index. *In vitro* studies also suggest that nilotinib may induce CYP2B6, CYP2C8, and CYP2C9, and thereby has the potential to decrease the concentrations of drugs which are eliminated by these enzymes).
No products indexed under this heading.

Tolmetin Sodium (Nilotinib is a competitive inhibitor of CYP2C9 *in vitro*, potentially increasing the concentration of drugs eliminated by CYP2C9. Caution should be exercised when co-administering nilotinib with substrates for CYP2C9 that have a narrow therapeutic index. *In vitro* studies also suggest that nilotinib may induce CYP2B6, CYP2C8 and CYP2C9, and thereby has the potential to decrease the concentrations of drugs which are eliminated by these enzymes).
No products indexed under this heading.

Tolterodine Tartrate (Nilotinib is a competitive inhibitor of CYP3A4 *in vitro*, potentially increasing the concentration of drugs eliminated by CYP3A4. Caution should be exercised when co-administering nilotinib with substrates for CYP3A4 that have a narrow therapeutic index).
No products indexed under this heading.

Torsemide (Nilotinib is a competitive inhibitor of CYP2C9 *in vitro*, potentially increasing the concentration of drugs eliminated by CYP2C9. Caution should be exercised when co-administering nilotinib with substrates for CYP2C9 that have a narrow therapeutic index. *In vitro* studies also suggest that nilotinib may induce CYP2B6, CYP2C8 and CYP2C9, and thereby has the potential to decrease the concentrations of drugs which are eliminated by these enzymes).
No products indexed under this heading.

Tramadol Hydrochloride (Nilotinib is a competitive inhibitor of CYP2D6 *in*

vitro, potentially increasing the concentration of drugs eliminated by CYP2D6. Caution should be exercised when co-administering nilotinib with substrates for CYP2D6 that have a narrow therapeutic index). Products include:

Ryzolt 2813
Ultram ER 2693

Tranylcypromine Sulfate (The administration of nilotinib with agents that prolong the QT interval should be avoided. Should treatment with any of these agents be required, it is recommended that therapy with nilotinib be interrupted. If interruption of treatment with nilotinib is not possible, patients who require treatment with a drug that prolongs the QT interval should be closely monitored for prolongation of the QT interval). Products include:

Parnate 1584

Trazodone Hydrochloride (Nilotinib is a competitive inhibitor of CYP3A4 *in vitro*, potentially increasing the concentration of drugs eliminated by CYP3A4. Caution should be exercised when co-administering nilotinib with substrates for CYP3A4 that have a narrow therapeutic index).

No products indexed under this heading.

Tretinoin (Nilotinib is a competitive inhibitor of CYP2C8 *in vitro*, potentially increasing the concentration of drugs eliminated by CYP2C8. Caution should be exercised when co-administering nilotinib with substrates for CYP2C8 that have a narrow therapeutic index. *In vitro* studies also suggest that nilotinib may induce CYP2B6, CYP2C8, and CYP2C9, and thereby has the potential to decrease the concentrations of drugs which are eliminated by these enzymes).

No products indexed under this heading.

Triamcinolone (The concomitant use of strong CYP3A4 inducers should be avoided. If patients must be co-administered a strong CYP3A4 inducer, the dose of nilotinib may need to be increased, depending on patient tolerability. If the strong inducer is discontinued, the nilotinib dose should be reduced to the indicated dose).

No products indexed under this heading.

Triamcinolone Acetonide (The concomitant use of strong CYP3A4 inducers should be avoided. If patients must be co-administered a strong CYP3A4 inducer, the dose of nilotinib may need to be increased, depending on patient tolerability. If the strong inducer is discontinued, the nilotinib dose should be reduced to the indicated dose). Products include:

Azmacort 408
Nasacort AQ 3019

Triamcinolone Diacetate (The concomitant use of strong CYP3A4 inducers should be avoided. If patients must be co-administered a strong CYP3A4 inducer, the dose of nilotinib may need to be increased, depending on patient tolerability. If the strong inducer is discontinued, the nilotinib dose should be reduced to the indicated dose).

No products indexed under this heading.

Triamcinolone Hexacetonide (The concomitant use of strong CYP3A4 inducers should be avoided. If patients must be co-administered a strong CYP3A4 inducer, the dose of nilotinib may need to be increased, depending on patient tolerability. If the strong inducer is discontinued, the nilotinib dose should be reduced to the indicated dose).

No products indexed under this heading.

Triazolam (Nilotinib is a competitive inhibitor of CYP3A4 *in vitro*, potentially increasing the concentration of drugs eliminated by CYP3A4. Caution should be exercised when co-administering nilotinib with substrates for CYP3A4 that have a narrow therapeutic index).

No products indexed under this heading.

Trifluoperazine Hydrochloride (The administration of nilotinib with agents that prolong the QT interval should be avoided. Should treatment with any of these agents be required, it is recommended that therapy with nilotinib be interrupted. If interruption of treatment with nilotinib is not possible, patients who require treatment with a drug that prolongs the QT interval should be closely monitored for prolongation of the QT interval).

No products indexed under this heading.

Trimipramine Maleate (The administration of nilotinib with agents that prolong the QT interval should be avoided. Should treatment with any of these agents be required, it is recommended that therapy with nilotinib be interrupted. If interruption of treatment with nilotinib is not possible, patients who require treatment with a drug that prolongs the QT interval should be closely monitored for prolongation of the QT interval).

No products indexed under this heading.

Troglitazone (The concomitant use of strong CYP3A4 inducers should be avoided. If patients must be co-administered a strong CYP3A4 inducer, the dose of nilotinib may need to be increased, depending on patient tolerability. If the strong inducer is discontinued, the nilotinib dose should be reduced to the indicated dose).

No products indexed under this heading.

Troleandomycin (The administration of nilotinib with agents that are strong CYP3A4 inhibitors should be avoided. Should treatment with any of these agents be required, it is recommended that therapy with nilotinib be interrupted. If patients must be co-administered a strong CYP3A4 inhibitor, based on pharmacokinetic studies, 400 mg qd is predicted to adjust the nilotinib AUC to the AUC observed without inhibitors. However, there are no clinical data with this dose adjustment in patients receiving strong CYP3A4 inhibitors. If the strong inhibitor is discontinued, a wash-out period should be allowed before the nilotinib dose is adjusted upward to the indicated dose. Close monitoring for prolongation of the QT interval is indicated for patients who cannot avoid strong CYP3A4 inhibitors).

No products indexed under this heading.

Valdecoxib (Nilotinib is a competitive inhibitor of CYP2C9 *in vitro*, potentially increasing the concentration of drugs eliminated by CYP2C9. Caution should be exercised when co-administering nilotinib with substrates for CYP2C9 that have a narrow therapeutic index. *In vitro* studies also suggest that nilotinib may induce CYP2B6, CYP2C8 and CYP2C9, and thereby has the potential to decrease the concentrations of drugs which are eliminated by these enzymes).

No products indexed under this heading.

Valproate Sodium (*In vitro* studies suggest that nilotinib may induce CYP2B6, CYP2C8 and CYP2C9, and decrease the concentrations of drugs which are eliminated by these enzymes).

No products indexed under this heading.

Valproic Acid (*In vitro* studies suggest that nilotinib may induce CYP2B6, CYP2C8 and CYP2C9, and decrease the concentrations of drugs which are eliminated by these enzymes).

No products indexed under this heading.

Valsartan (Nilotinib is a competitive inhibitor of CYP2C9 *in vitro*, potentially increasing the concentration of drugs eliminated by CYP2C9. Caution should be exercised when co-administering nilotinib with substrates for CYP2C9 that have a narrow therapeutic index. *In vitro* studies also suggest that nilotinib may induce CYP2B6, CYP2C8 and CYP2C9, and thereby has the potential to decrease the concentrations of drugs which are eliminated by these enzymes). Products include:

Diovan 2413
Diovan HCT 2419
Exforge 2443
Exforge HCT 2449
Valturna 3637

Vardenafil Hydrochloride (Nilotinib is a competitive inhibitor of CYP3A4 *in vitro*, potentially increasing the concentration of drugs eliminated by CYP3A4. Caution should be exercised when co-administering nilotinib with substrates for CYP3A4 that have a narrow therapeutic index). Products include:

Levitra 3157

Venlafaxine Hydrochloride (Nilotinib is a competitive inhibitor of CYP2D6 *in vitro*, potentially increasing the concentration of drugs eliminated by CYP2D6. Caution should be exercised when co-administering nilotinib with substrates for CYP2D6 that have a narrow therapeutic index). Products include:

Effexor XR 3504
Venlafaxine Hydrochloride Tablets ... 2388

Verapamil Hydrochloride (The administration of nilotinib with agents that are strong CYP3A4 inhibitors or anti-arrhythmic drugs and other drugs that may prolong QT interval should be avoided. Should treatment with any of these agents be required, it is recommended that therapy with nilotinib be interrupted. If interruption of treatment with nilotinib is not possible, patients who require treatment with a drug that prolongs QT or strongly inhibits CYP3A4 should be closely monitored for prolongation of the QT interval). Products include:

Tarka 534

Vinblastine Sulfate (Nilotinib is a competitive inhibitor of CYP3A4 *in vitro*, potentially increasing the concentration of drugs eliminated by CYP3A4. Caution should be exercised when co-administering nilotinib with substrates for CYP3A4 that have a narrow therapeutic index).

No products indexed under this heading.

Vincristine Sulfate (Nilotinib is a competitive inhibitor of CYP3A4 *in vitro*, potentially increasing the concentration of drugs eliminated by CYP3A4. Caution should be exercised when co-administering nilotinib with substrates for CYP3A4 that have a narrow therapeutic index).

No products indexed under this heading.

Vitamin A (Nilotinib is a competitive inhibitor of CYP2C8 *in vitro*, potentially increasing the concentration of drugs eliminated by CYP2C8. Caution should be exercised when co-administering nilotinib with substrates for CYP2C8 that have a narrow therapeutic index. *In vitro* studies also suggest that nilotinib may induce CYP2B6, CYP2C8, and CYP2C9, and thereby has the potential to decrease the concentrations of drugs which are eliminated by these enzymes). Products include:

Cardio Basics 3455
Heplive 607
Norwegian Cod Liver Oil 919

Vitamin A Acetate (Nilotinib is a competitive inhibitor of CYP2C8 *in vitro*, potentially increasing the concentration of drugs eliminated by CYP2C8. Caution should be exercised when co-administering nilotinib with substrates

for CYP2C8 that have a narrow therapeutic index. *In vitro* studies also suggest that nilotinib may induce CYP2B6, CYP2C8, and CYP2C9, and thereby has the potential to decrease the concentrations of drugs which are eliminated by these enzymes).

No products indexed under this heading.

Voriconazole (The administration of nilotinib with agents that are strong CYP3A4 inhibitors such as voriconazole should be avoided. If treatment is required, it is recommended that therapy with nilotinib be interrupted. If patients must be co-administered a strong CYP3A4 inhibitor, based on pharmacokinetic studies, 400 mg qd is predicted to adjust the nilotinib AUC to the AUC observed without inhibitors. However, there are no clinical data with this dose adjustment in patients receiving strong CYP3A4 inhibitors. If the strong inhibitor is discontinued, a washout period should be allowed before the nilotinib dose is adjusted upward to the indicated dose. Close monitoring for prolongation of the QT interval is indicated for patients who cannot avoid strong CYP3A4 inhibitors).

No products indexed under this heading.

Warfarin Sodium (Single-dose administration of nilotinib to healthy subjects did not change the pharmacokinetics and pharmacodynamics of warfarin (a CYP2C9 substrate). The ability of nilotinib to induce metabolism has not been determined *in vivo*. Caution should be exercised when co-administering nilotinib with substrates for these enzymes that have a narrow therapeutic index).

No products indexed under this heading.

Zafirlukast (Nilotinib is a competitive inhibitor of CYP2C9 *in vitro*, potentially increasing the concentration of drugs eliminated by CYP2C9. Caution should be exercised when co-administering nilotinib with substrates for CYP2C9 that have a narrow therapeutic index. *In vitro* studies also suggest that nilotinib may induce CYP2B6, CYP2C8 and CYP2C9, and thereby has the potential to decrease the concentrations of drugs which are eliminated by these enzymes). Products include:

Accolate 3612

Zileuton (Nilotinib is a competitive inhibitor of CYP2C9 *in vitro*, potentially increasing the concentration of drugs eliminated by CYP2C9. Caution should be exercised when co-administering nilotinib with substrates for CYP2C9 that have a narrow therapeutic index. *In vitro* studies also suggest that nilotinib may induce CYP2B6, CYP2C8 and CYP2C9, and thereby has the potential to decrease the concentrations of drugs which are eliminated by these enzymes).

No products indexed under this heading.

Ziprasidone Hydrochloride (The administration of nilotinib with agents that prolong the QT interval should be avoided. Should treatment with any of these agents be required, it is recommended that therapy with nilotinib be interrupted. If interruption of treatment with nilotinib is not possible, patients who require treatment with a drug that prolongs the QT interval should be closely monitored for prolongation of the QT interval). Products include:

Geodon 2723

Zonisamide (Nilotinib is a competitive inhibitor of CYP2D6 *in vitro*, potentially increasing the concentration of drugs eliminated by CYP2D6. Caution should be exercised when co-administering nilotinib with substrates for CYP2D6 that have a narrow therapeutic index). Products include:

Zonegran 1081

Zopiclone (Nilotinib is a competitive inhibitor of CYP2C8 *in vitro*, potentially

increasing the concentration of drugs eliminated by CYP2C8. Caution should be exercised when co-administering nilotinib with substrates for CYP2C8 that have a narrow therapeutic index. *In vitro* studies also suggest that nilotinib may induce CYP2B6, CYP2C8, and CYP2C9, and thereby has the potential to decrease the concentrations of drugs which are eliminated by these enzymes).

No products indexed under this heading.

Food Interactions

Food, unspecified (The bioavailability of nilotinib is increased with food. Nilotinib should not be taken with food. No food should be taken at least 2 hours before and at least one hour after the dose is taken).

Grapefruit (Concomitant use with grapefruit products may increase serum concentrations of nilotinib and should be avoided).

Grapefruit Juice (Concomitant use with grapefruit products may increase serum concentrations of nilotinib and should be avoided).

Meal, unspecified (The bioavailability of nilotinib is increased with food. Nilotinib should not be taken with food. No food should be taken at least 2 hours before and at least one hour after the dose is taken).

TAXOTERE INJECTION CONCENTRATE

(Docetaxel) 3035
May interact with cytochrome p450 3a4 inducers (selected), cytochrome p450 3a4 inhibitors (selected), cytochrome p450 3a4 substrates (selected), erythromycin, and certain other agents. Compounds in these categories include:

Acetazolamide (*In vitro* studies have shown that the metabolism of docetaxel may be modified by the concomitant administration of compounds that induce, inhibit, or are metabolized by cytochrome P450 3A4, such as cyclosporine, terfenadine, ketoconazole, erythromycin, and troleandomycin. Caution should be exercised with these drugs when treating patients receiving docetaxel as there is a potential for a significant interaction).

No products indexed under this heading.

Acetazolamide Sodium (*In vitro* studies have shown that the metabolism of docetaxel may be modified by the concomitant administration of compounds that induce, inhibit, or are metabolized by cytochrome P450 3A4, such as cyclosporine, terfenadine, ketoconazole, erythromycin, and troleandomycin. Caution should be exercised with these drugs when treating patients receiving docetaxel as there is a potential for a significant interaction).

No products indexed under this heading.

Alfentanil Hydrochloride (*In vitro* studies have shown that the metabolism of docetaxel may be modified by the concomitant administration of compounds that induce, inhibit, or are metabolized by cytochrome P450 3A4, such as cyclosporine, terfenadine, ketoconazole, erythromycin, and troleandomycin. Caution should be exercised with these drugs when treating patients receiving docetaxel as there is a potential for a significant interaction).

No products indexed under this heading.

Allium sativum (*In vitro* studies have shown that the metabolism of docetaxel may be modified by the concomitant administration of compounds that induce, inhibit, or are metabolized by cytochrome P450 3A4, such as cyclosporine, terfenadine, ketocona-

zole, erythromycin, and troleandomycin. Caution should be exercised with these drugs when treating patients receiving docetaxel as there is a potential for a significant interaction).

No products indexed under this heading.

Alprazolam (*In vitro* studies have shown that the metabolism of docetaxel may be modified by the concomitant administration of compounds that induce, inhibit, or are metabolized by cytochrome P450 3A4, such as cyclosporine, terfenadine, ketoconazole, erythromycin, and troleandomycin. Caution should be exercised with these drugs when treating patients receiving docetaxel as there is a potential for a significant interaction).

No products indexed under this heading.

Aminoglutethimide (*In vitro* studies have shown that the metabolism of docetaxel may be modified by the concomitant administration of compounds that induce, inhibit, or are metabolized by cytochrome P450 3A4, such as cyclosporine, terfenadine, ketoconazole, erythromycin, and troleandomycin. Caution should be exercised with these drugs when treating patients receiving docetaxel as there is a potential for a significant interaction).

No products indexed under this heading.

Amiodarone Hydrochloride (*In vitro* studies have shown that the metabolism of docetaxel may be modified by the concomitant administration of compounds that induce, inhibit, or are metabolized by cytochrome P450 3A4, such as cyclosporine, terfenadine, ketoconazole, erythromycin, and troleandomycin. Caution should be exercised with these drugs when treating patients receiving docetaxel as there is a potential for a significant interaction).

No products indexed under this heading.

Amitriptyline Hydrochloride (*In vitro* studies have shown that the metabolism of docetaxel may be modified by the concomitant administration of compounds that induce, inhibit, or are metabolized by cytochrome P450 3A4, such as cyclosporine, terfenadine, ketoconazole, erythromycin, and troleandomycin. Caution should be exercised with these drugs when treating patients receiving docetaxel as there is a potential for a significant interaction).

No products indexed under this heading.

Amlodipine Besylate (*In vitro* studies have shown that the metabolism of docetaxel may be modified by the concomitant administration of compounds that induce, inhibit, or are metabolized by cytochrome P450 3A4, such as cyclosporine, terfenadine, ketoconazole, erythromycin, and troleandomycin. Caution should be exercised with these drugs when treating patients receiving docetaxel as there is a potential for a significant interaction). Products include:

Azor 1010
Exforge 2443
Exforge HCT 2449

Amprenavir (*In vitro* studies have shown that the metabolism of docetaxel may be modified by the concomitant administration of compounds that induce, inhibit, or are metabolized by cytochrome P450 3A4, such as cyclosporine, terfenadine, ketoconazole, erythromycin, and troleandomycin. Caution should be exercised with these drugs when treating patients receiving docetaxel as there is a potential for a significant interaction).

No products indexed under this heading.

Anastrozole (*In vitro* studies have shown that the metabolism of docetaxel may be modified by the concomitant administration of compounds that induce, inhibit, or are metabolized by

cytochrome P450 3A4, such as cyclosporine, terfenadine, ketoconazole, erythromycin, and troleandomycin. Caution should be exercised with these drugs when treating patients receiving docetaxel as there is a potential for a significant interaction).

No products indexed under this heading.

Aprepitant (*In vitro* studies have shown that the metabolism of docetaxel may be modified by the concomitant administration of compounds that induce, inhibit, or are metabolized by cytochrome P450 3A4, such as cyclosporine, terfenadine, ketoconazole, erythromycin, and troleandomycin. Caution should be exercised with these drugs when treating patients receiving docetaxel as there is a potential for a significant interaction). Products include:
Emend 2124

Astemizole (*In vitro* studies have shown that the metabolism of docetaxel may be modified by the concomitant administration of compounds that induce, inhibit, or are metabolized by cytochrome P450 3A4, such as cyclosporine, terfenadine, ketoconazole, erythromycin, and troleandomycin. Caution should be exercised with these drugs when treating patients receiving docetaxel as there is a potential for a significant interaction).

No products indexed under this heading.

Atazanavir (*In vitro* studies have shown that the metabolism of docetaxel may be modified by the concomitant administration of compounds that induce, inhibit, or are metabolized by cytochrome P450 3A4, such as cyclosporine, terfenadine, ketoconazole, erythromycin, and troleandomycin. Caution should be exercised with these drugs when treating patients receiving docetaxel as there is a potential for a significant interaction).

No products indexed under this heading.

Atazanavir Sulfate (*In vitro* studies have shown that the metabolism of docetaxel may be modified by the concomitant administration of compounds that induce, inhibit, or are metabolized by cytochrome P450 3A4, such as cyclosporine, terfenadine, ketoconazole, erythromycin, and troleandomycin. Caution should be exercised with these drugs when treating patients receiving docetaxel as there is a potential for a significant interaction).

No products indexed under this heading.

Atorvastatin Calcium (*In vitro* studies have shown that the metabolism of docetaxel may be modified by the concomitant administration of compounds that induce, inhibit, or are metabolized by cytochrome P450 3A4, such as cyclosporine, terfenadine, ketoconazole, erythromycin, and troleandomycin. Caution should be exercised with these drugs when treating patients receiving docetaxel as there is a potential for a significant interaction). Products include:
Lipitor 2703

Belladonna Ergotamine (*In vitro* studies have shown that the metabolism of docetaxel may be modified by the concomitant administration of compounds that induce, inhibit, or are metabolized by cytochrome P450 3A4, such as cyclosporine, terfenadine, ketoconazole, erythromycin, and troleandomycin. Caution should be exercised with these drugs when treating patients receiving docetaxel as there is a potential for a significant interaction).

No products indexed under this heading.

Betamethasone (*In vitro* studies have shown that the metabolism of docetaxel may be modified by the concomitant administration of compounds that

induce, inhibit, or are metabolized by cytochrome P450 3A4, such as cyclosporine, terfenadine, ketoconazole, erythromycin, and troleandomycin. Caution should be exercised with these drugs when treating patients receiving docetaxel as there is a potential for a significant interaction).

No products indexed under this heading.

Betamethasone Acetate (*In vitro* studies have shown that the metabolism of docetaxel may be modified by the concomitant administration of compounds that induce, inhibit, or are metabolized by cytochrome P450 3A4, such as cyclosporine, terfenadine, ketoconazole, erythromycin, and troleandomycin. Caution should be exercised with these drugs when treating patients receiving docetaxel as there is a potential for a significant interaction).

No products indexed under this heading.

Betamethasone Benzoate (*In vitro* studies have shown that the metabolism of docetaxel may be modified by the concomitant administration of compounds that induce, inhibit, or are metabolized by cytochrome P450 3A4, such as cyclosporine, terfenadine, ketoconazole, erythromycin, and troleandomycin. Caution should be exercised with these drugs when treating patients receiving docetaxel as there is a potential for a significant interaction).

No products indexed under this heading.

Betamethasone Dipropionate (*In vitro* studies have shown that the metabolism of docetaxel may be modified by the concomitant administration of compounds that induce, inhibit, or are metabolized by cytochrome P450 3A4, such as cyclosporine, terfenadine, ketoconazole, erythromycin, and troleandomycin. Caution should be exercised with these drugs when treating patients receiving docetaxel as there is a potential for a significant interaction). Products include:
Diprolene Lotion 0.05% 3108
Diprolene Ointment 0.05% 3109
Diprolene AF Cream 0.05% 3107
Lotrisone 3163

Betamethasone Sodium Phosphate (*In vitro* studies have shown that the metabolism of docetaxel may be modified by the concomitant administration of compounds that induce, inhibit, or are metabolized by cytochrome P450 3A4, such as cyclosporine, terfenadine, ketoconazole, erythromycin, and troleandomycin. Caution should be exercised with these drugs when treating patients receiving docetaxel as there is a potential for a significant interaction).

No products indexed under this heading.

Betamethasone Valerate (*In vitro* studies have shown that the metabolism of docetaxel may be modified by the concomitant administration of compounds that induce, inhibit, or are metabolized by cytochrome P450 3A4, such as cyclosporine, terfenadine, ketoconazole, erythromycin, and troleandomycin. Caution should be exercised with these drugs when treating patients receiving docetaxel as there is a potential for a significant interaction). Products include:
Luxiq 3321

Bosentan (*In vitro* studies have shown that the metabolism of docetaxel may be modified by the concomitant administration of compounds that induce, inhibit, or are metabolized by cytochrome P450 3A4, such as cyclosporine, terfenadine, ketoconazole, erythromycin, and troleandomycin. Caution should be exercised with these drugs when treating patients receiving docetaxel as there is a potential for a significant interaction). Products include:

Tracleer 573

Buspirone Hydrochloride (*In vitro* studies have shown that the metabolism of docetaxel may be modified by the concomitant administration of compounds that induce, inhibit, or are metabolized by cytochrome P450 3A4, such as cyclosporine, terfenadine, ketoconazole, erythromycin, and troleandomycin. Caution should be exercised with these drugs when treating patients receiving docetaxel as there is a potential for a significant interaction).
No products indexed under this heading.

Busulfan (*In vitro* studies have shown that the metabolism of docetaxel may be modified by the concomitant administration of compounds that induce, inhibit, or are metabolized by cytochrome P450 3A4, such as cyclosporine, terfenadine, ketoconazole, erythromycin, and troleandomycin. Caution should be exercised with these drugs when treating patients receiving docetaxel as there is a potential for a significant interaction). Products include:
Myleran 1581

Carbamazepine (*In vitro* studies have shown that the metabolism of docetaxel may be modified by the concomitant administration of compounds that induce, inhibit, or are metabolized by cytochrome P450 3A4, such as cyclosporine, terfenadine, ketoconazole, erythromycin, and troleandomycin. Caution should be exercised with these drugs when treating patients receiving docetaxel as there is a potential for a significant interaction). Products include:
Carbatrol 3280
Equetro 3477

Cerivastatin Sodium (*In vitro* studies have shown that the metabolism of docetaxel may be modified by the concomitant administration of compounds that induce, inhibit, or are metabolized by cytochrome P450 3A4, such as cyclosporine, terfenadine, ketoconazole, erythromycin, and troleandomycin. Caution should be exercised with these drugs when treating patients receiving docetaxel as there is a potential for a significant interaction).
No products indexed under this heading.

Chlorpheniramine (*In vitro* studies have shown that the metabolism of docetaxel may be modified by the concomitant administration of compounds that induce, inhibit, or are metabolized by cytochrome P450 3A4, such as cyclosporine, terfenadine, ketoconazole, erythromycin, and troleandomycin. Caution should be exercised with these drugs when treating patients receiving docetaxel as there is a potential for a significant interaction).
No products indexed under this heading.

Chlorpheniramine Maleate (*In vitro* studies have shown that the metabolism of docetaxel may be modified by the concomitant administration of compounds that induce, inhibit, or are metabolized by cytochrome P450 3A4, such as cyclosporine, terfenadine, ketoconazole, erythromycin, and troleandomycin. Caution should be exercised with these drugs when treating patients receiving docetaxel as there is a potential for a significant interaction).
No products indexed under this heading.

Chlorpheniramine Polistirex (*In vitro* studies have shown that the metabolism of docetaxel may be modified by the concomitant administration of compounds that induce, inhibit, or are metabolized by cytochrome P450 3A4, such as cyclosporine, terfenadine, ketoconazole, erythromycin, and troleandomycin. Caution should be exercised with these drugs when treating patients receiving docetaxel as there is a potential for a significant interaction). Products include:
Tussionex 3443

Chlorpheniramine Tannate (*In vitro* studies have shown that the metabolism of docetaxel may be modified by the concomitant administration of compounds that induce, inhibit, or are metabolized by cytochrome P450 3A4, such as cyclosporine, terfenadine, ketoconazole, erythromycin, and troleandomycin. Caution should be exercised with these drugs when treating patients receiving docetaxel as there is a potential for a significant interaction).
No products indexed under this heading.

Cimetidine (*In vitro* studies have shown that the metabolism of docetaxel may be modified by the concomitant administration of compounds that induce, inhibit, or are metabolized by cytochrome P450 3A4, such as cyclosporine, terfenadine, ketoconazole, erythromycin, and troleandomycin. Caution should be exercised with these drugs when treating patients receiving docetaxel as there is a potential for a significant interaction).
No products indexed under this heading.

Cimetidine Hydrochloride (*In vitro* studies have shown that the metabolism of docetaxel may be modified by the concomitant administration of compounds that induce, inhibit, or are metabolized by cytochrome P450 3A4, such as cyclosporine, terfenadine, ketoconazole, erythromycin, and troleandomycin. Caution should be exercised with these drugs when treating patients receiving docetaxel as there is a potential for a significant interaction).
No products indexed under this heading.

Ciprofloxacin (*In vitro* studies have shown that the metabolism of docetaxel may be modified by the concomitant administration of compounds that induce, inhibit, or are metabolized by cytochrome P450 3A4, such as cyclosporine, terfenadine, ketoconazole, erythromycin, and troleandomycin. Caution should be exercised with these drugs when treating patients receiving docetaxel as there is a potential for a significant interaction). Products include:
Cipro I.V. 3082
Cipro 3073
Cipro XR 3091
Ciprodex 583

Ciprofloxacin Hydrochloride (*In vitro* studies have shown that the metabolism of docetaxel may be modified by the concomitant administration of compounds that induce, inhibit, or are metabolized by cytochrome P450 3A4, such as cyclosporine, terfenadine, ketoconazole, erythromycin, and troleandomycin. Caution should be exercised with these drugs when treating patients receiving docetaxel as there is a potential for a significant interaction). Products include:
Cipro 3073

Cisapride (*In vitro* studies have shown that the metabolism of docetaxel may be modified by the concomitant administration of compounds that induce, inhibit, or are metabolized by cytochrome P450 3A4, such as cyclosporine, terfenadine, ketoconazole, erythromycin, and troleandomycin. Caution should be exercised with these drugs when treating patients receiving docetaxel as there is a potential for a significant interaction).
No products indexed under this heading.

Cisplatin (*In vitro* studies have shown that the metabolism of docetaxel may be modified by the concomitant administration of compounds that induce, inhibit, or are metabolized by cytochrome P450 3A4, such as cyclosporine, terfenadine, ketoconazole, erythromycin, and troleandomycin. Caution should be exercised with these drugs when treating patients receiving docetaxel as there is a potential for a significant interaction).
No products indexed under this heading.

Clarithromycin (*In vitro* studies have shown that the metabolism of docetaxel may be modified by the concomitant administration of compounds that induce, inhibit, or are metabolized by cytochrome P450 3A4, such as cyclosporine, terfenadine, ketoconazole, erythromycin, and troleandomycin. Caution should be exercised with these drugs when treating patients receiving docetaxel as there is a potential for a significant interaction). Products include:
Biaxin/Biaxin XL 412

Clotrimazole (*In vitro* studies have shown that the metabolism of docetaxel may be modified by the concomitant administration of compounds that induce, inhibit, or are metabolized by cytochrome P450 3A4, such as cyclosporine, terfenadine, ketoconazole, erythromycin, and troleandomycin. Caution should be exercised with these drugs when treating patients receiving docetaxel as there is a potential for a significant interaction). Products include:
Lotrisone 3163

Conivaptan Hydrochloride (*In vitro* studies have shown that the metabolism of docetaxel may be modified by the concomitant administration of compounds that induce, inhibit, or are metabolized by cytochrome P450 3A4, such as cyclosporine, terfenadine, ketoconazole, erythromycin, and troleandomycin. Caution should be exercised with these drugs when treating patients receiving docetaxel as there is a potential for a significant interaction). Products include:
Vaprisol 689

Cortisone Acetate (*In vitro* studies have shown that the metabolism of docetaxel may be modified by the concomitant administration of compounds that induce, inhibit, or are metabolized by cytochrome P450 3A4, such as cyclosporine, terfenadine, ketoconazole, erythromycin, and troleandomycin. Caution should be exercised with these drugs when treating patients receiving docetaxel as there is a potential for a significant interaction).
No products indexed under this heading.

Cyclosporine (*In vitro* studies have shown that the metabolism of docetaxel may be modified by the concomitant administration of compounds that induce, inhibit, or are metabolized by cytochrome P450 3A4, such as cyclosporine. Caution should be exercised with these drugs when treating patients receiving docetaxel as there is a potential for a significant interaction). Products include:
Gengraf 440
Neoral Oral Solution 2496
Neoral Capsules 2496
Restasis 605

Dalfopristin (*In vitro* studies have shown that the metabolism of docetaxel may be modified by the concomitant administration of compounds that induce, inhibit, or are metabolized by cytochrome P450 3A4, such as cyclosporine, terfenadine, ketoconazole, erythromycin, and troleandomycin. Caution should be exercised with these drugs when treating patients receiving docetaxel as there is a potential for a significant interaction).
No products indexed under this heading.

Danazol (*In vitro* studies have shown that the metabolism of docetaxel may be modified by the concomitant administration of compounds that induce, inhibit, or are metabolized by cytochrome P450 3A4, such as cyclosporine, terfenadine, ketoconazole, erythromycin, and troleandomycin. Caution should be exercised with these drugs when treating patients receiving docetaxel as there is a potential for a significant interaction).
No products indexed under this heading.

Darunavir (*In vitro* studies have shown that the metabolism of docetaxel may be modified by the concomitant administration of compounds that induce, inhibit, or are metabolized by cytochrome P450 3A4, such as cyclosporine, terfenadine, ketoconazole, erythromycin, and troleandomycin. Caution should be exercised with these drugs when treating patients receiving docetaxel as there is a potential for a significant interaction).
No products indexed under this heading.

Dasatinib (*In vitro* studies have shown that the metabolism of docetaxel may be modified by the concomitant administration of compounds that induce, inhibit, or are metabolized by cytochrome P450 3A4, such as cyclosporine, terfenadine, ketoconazole, erythromycin, and troleandomycin. Caution should be exercised with these drugs when treating patients receiving docetaxel as there is a potential for a significant interaction).
No products indexed under this heading.

Delavirdine Mesylate (*In vitro* studies have shown that the metabolism of docetaxel may be modified by the concomitant administration of compounds that induce, inhibit, or are metabolized by cytochrome P450 3A4, such as cyclosporine, terfenadine, ketoconazole, erythromycin, and troleandomycin. Caution should be exercised with these drugs when treating patients receiving docetaxel as there is a potential for a significant interaction).
No products indexed under this heading.

Delavirine (*In vitro* studies have shown that the metabolism of docetaxel may be modified by the concomitant administration of compounds that induce, inhibit, or are metabolized by cytochrome P450 3A4, such as cyclosporine, terfenadine, ketoconazole, erythromycin, and troleandomycin. Caution should be exercised with these drugs when treating patients receiving docetaxel as there is a potential for a significant interaction).
No products indexed under this heading.

Desloratadine (*In vitro* studies have shown that the metabolism of docetaxel may be modified by the concomitant administration of compounds that induce, inhibit, or are metabolized by cytochrome P450 3A4, such as cyclosporine, terfenadine, ketoconazole, erythromycin, and troleandomycin. Caution should be exercised with these drugs when treating patients receiving docetaxel as there is a potential for a significant interaction). Products include:
Clarinex Syrup 3098
Clarinex 3098
Clarinex Reditabs 3098
Clarinex-D 12-Hour 3101
Clarinex-D 3104

Desogestrel (*In vitro* studies have shown that the metabolism of docetaxel may be modified by the concomitant administration of compounds that induce, inhibit, or are metabolized by cytochrome P450 3A4, such as cyclosporine, terfenadine, ketoconazole, erythromycin, and troleandomycin. Caution should be exercised with these

Taxotere Interactions Index 1852

drugs when treating patients receiving docetaxel as there is a potential for a significant interaction).
No products indexed under this heading.

Dexamethasone (*In vitro* studies have shown that the metabolism of docetaxel may be modified by the concomitant administration of compounds that induce, inhibit, or are metabolized by cytochrome P450 3A4, such as cyclosporine, terfenadine, ketoconazole, erythromycin, and troleandomycin. Caution should be exercised with these drugs when treating patients receiving docetaxel as there is a potential for a significant interaction). Products include:
Ciprodex 583
Ozurdex .... ⊙223
Tobramycin and Dexamethasone Ophthalmic Suspension .... ⊙251

Dexamethasone Acetate (*In vitro* studies have shown that the metabolism of docetaxel may be modified by the concomitant administration of compounds that induce, inhibit, or are metabolized by cytochrome P450 3A4, such as cyclosporine, terfenadine, ketoconazole, erythromycin, and troleandomycin. Caution should be exercised with these drugs when treating patients receiving docetaxel as there is a potential for a significant interaction).
No products indexed under this heading.

Dexamethasone Phosphate (*In vitro* studies have shown that the metabolism of docetaxel may be modified by the concomitant administration of compounds that induce, inhibit, or are metabolized by cytochrome P450 3A4, such as cyclosporine, terfenadine, ketoconazole, erythromycin, and troleandomycin. Caution should be exercised with these drugs when treating patients receiving docetaxel as there is a potential for a significant interaction).
No products indexed under this heading.

Dexamethasone Sodium (*In vitro* studies have shown that the metabolism of docetaxel may be modified by the concomitant administration of compounds that induce, inhibit, or are metabolized by cytochrome P450 3A4, such as cyclosporine, terfenadine, ketoconazole, erythromycin, and troleandomycin. Caution should be exercised with these drugs when treating patients receiving docetaxel as there is a potential for a significant interaction).
No products indexed under this heading.

Dexamethasone Sodium Phosphate (*In vitro* studies have shown that the metabolism of docetaxel may be modified by the concomitant administration of compounds that induce, inhibit, or are metabolized by cytochrome P450 3A4, such as cyclosporine, terfenadine, ketoconazole, erythromycin, and troleandomycin. Caution should be exercised with these drugs when treating patients receiving docetaxel as there is a potential for a significant interaction).
No products indexed under this heading.

Dexamethasone Sodium Phosphate Injection (*In vitro* studies have shown that the metabolism of docetaxel may be modified by the concomitant administration of compounds that induce, inhibit, or are metabolized by cytochrome P450 3A4, such as cyclosporine, terfenadine, ketoconazole, erythromycin, and troleandomycin. Caution should be exercised with these drugs when treating patients receiving docetaxel as there is a potential for a significant interaction).
No products indexed under this heading.

Diazepam (*In vitro* studies have shown that the metabolism of docetaxel may be modified by the concomitant administration of compounds that induce, inhibit, or are metabolized by cytochrome P450 3A4, such as cyclosporine, terfenadine, ketoconazole, erythromycin, and troleandomycin. Caution should be exercised with these drugs when treating patients receiving docetaxel as there is a potential for a significant interaction). Products include:
Valium Tablets 2880

Dihydroergotamine Mesylate (*In vitro* studies have shown that the metabolism of docetaxel may be modified by the concomitant administration of compounds that induce, inhibit, or are metabolized by cytochrome P450 3A4, such as cyclosporine, terfenadine, ketoconazole, erythromycin, and troleandomycin. Caution should be exercised with these drugs when treating patients receiving docetaxel as there is a potential for a significant interaction).
No products indexed under this heading.

Diltiazem Hydrochloride (*In vitro* studies have shown that the metabolism of docetaxel may be modified by the concomitant administration of compounds that induce, inhibit, or are metabolized by cytochrome P450 3A4, such as cyclosporine, terfenadine, ketoconazole, erythromycin, and troleandomycin. Caution should be exercised with these drugs when treating patients receiving docetaxel as there is a potential for a significant interaction). Products include:
Cardizem LA 423

Diltiazem Maleate (*In vitro* studies have shown that the metabolism of docetaxel may be modified by the concomitant administration of compounds that induce, inhibit, or are metabolized by cytochrome P450 3A4, such as cyclosporine, terfenadine, ketoconazole, erythromycin, and troleandomycin. Caution should be exercised with these drugs when treating patients receiving docetaxel as there is a potential for a significant interaction).
No products indexed under this heading.

Disopyramide (*In vitro* studies have shown that the metabolism of docetaxel may be modified by the concomitant administration of compounds that induce, inhibit, or are metabolized by cytochrome P450 3A4, such as cyclosporine, terfenadine, ketoconazole, erythromycin, and troleandomycin. Caution should be exercised with these drugs when treating patients receiving docetaxel as there is a potential for a significant interaction).
No products indexed under this heading.

Disopyramide Phosphate (*In vitro* studies have shown that the metabolism of docetaxel may be modified by the concomitant administration of compounds that induce, inhibit, or are metabolized by cytochrome P450 3A4, such as cyclosporine, terfenadine, ketoconazole, erythromycin, and troleandomycin. Caution should be exercised with these drugs when treating patients receiving docetaxel as there is a potential for a significant interaction).
No products indexed under this heading.

Disulfiram (*In vitro* studies have shown that the metabolism of docetaxel may be modified by the concomitant administration of compounds that induce, inhibit, or are metabolized by cytochrome P450 3A4, such as cyclosporine, terfenadine, ketoconazole, erythromycin, and troleandomycin. Caution should be exercised with these drugs when treating patients receiving docetaxel as there is a potential for a significant interaction).
No products indexed under this heading.

Doxorubicin Hydrochloride (*In vitro* studies have shown that the metabolism of docetaxel may be modified by the concomitant administration of compounds that induce, inhibit, or are metabolized by cytochrome P450 3A4, such as cyclosporine, terfenadine, ketoconazole, erythromycin, and troleandomycin. Caution should be exercised with these drugs when treating patients receiving docetaxel as there is a potential for a significant interaction).
No products indexed under this heading.

Dronabinol (*In vitro* studies have shown that the metabolism of docetaxel may be modified by the concomitant administration of compounds that induce, inhibit, or are metabolized by cytochrome P450 3A4, such as cyclosporine, terfenadine, ketoconazole, erythromycin, and troleandomycin. Caution should be exercised with these drugs when treating patients receiving docetaxel as there is a potential for a significant interaction).
No products indexed under this heading.

Efavirenz (*In vitro* studies have shown that the metabolism of docetaxel may be modified by the concomitant administration of compounds that induce, inhibit, or are metabolized by cytochrome P450 3A4, such as cyclosporine, terfenadine, ketoconazole, erythromycin, and troleandomycin. Caution should be exercised with these drugs when treating patients receiving docetaxel as there is a potential for a significant interaction). Products include:
Atripla 906

Ergotamine Tartrate (*In vitro* studies have shown that the metabolism of docetaxel may be modified by the concomitant administration of compounds that induce, inhibit, or are metabolized by cytochrome P450 3A4, such as cyclosporine, terfenadine, ketoconazole, erythromycin, and troleandomycin. Caution should be exercised with these drugs when treating patients receiving docetaxel as there is a potential for a significant interaction).
No products indexed under this heading.

Erythromycin (*In vitro* studies have shown that the metabolism of docetaxel may be modified by the concomitant administration of compounds that induce, inhibit, or are metabolized by cytochrome P450 3A4, such as cyclosporine, terfenadine, ketoconazole, erythromycin, and troleandomycin. Caution should be exercised with erythromycin when treating patients receiving docetaxel as there is a potential for a significant interaction).
No products indexed under this heading.

Erythromycin, Topical (*In vitro* studies have shown that the metabolism of docetaxel may be modified by the concomitant administration of compounds that induce, inhibit, or are metabolized by cytochrome P450 3A4, such as cyclosporine, terfenadine, ketoconazole, erythromycin, and troleandomycin. Caution should be exercised with erythromycin when treating patients receiving docetaxel as there is a potential for a significant interaction).
No products indexed under this heading.

Erythromycin Estolate (*In vitro* studies have shown that the metabolism of docetaxel may be modified by the concomitant administration of compounds that induce, inhibit, or are metabolized by cytochrome P450 3A4, such as cyclosporine, terfenadine, ketoconazole, erythromycin, and troleandomycin. Caution should be exercised with erythromycin when treating patients receiving docetaxel as there is a potential for a significant interaction).
No products indexed under this heading.

Erythromycin Ethylsuccinate (*In vitro* studies have shown that the metabolism of docetaxel may be modified by the concomitant administration of compounds that induce, inhibit, or are metabolized by cytochrome P450 3A4, such as cyclosporine, terfenadine, ketoconazole, erythromycin, and troleandomycin. Caution should be exercised with erythromycin when treating patients receiving docetaxel as there is a potential for a significant interaction). Products include:
E.E.S. 437
EryPed 435

Erythromycin Gluceptate (*In vitro* studies have shown that the metabolism of docetaxel may be modified by the concomitant administration of compounds that induce, inhibit, or are metabolized by cytochrome P450 3A4, such as cyclosporine, terfenadine, ketoconazole, erythromycin, and troleandomycin. Caution should be exercised with erythromycin when treating patients receiving docetaxel as there is a potential for a significant interaction).
No products indexed under this heading.

Erythromycin Lactobionate (*In vitro* studies have shown that the metabolism of docetaxel may be modified by the concomitant administration of compounds that induce, inhibit, or are metabolized by cytochrome P450 3A4, such as cyclosporine, terfenadine, ketoconazole, erythromycin, and troleandomycin. Caution should be exercised with erythromycin when treating patients receiving docetaxel as there is a potential for a significant interaction).
No products indexed under this heading.

Erythromycin Stearate (*In vitro* studies have shown that the metabolism of docetaxel may be modified by the concomitant administration of compounds that induce, inhibit, or are metabolized by cytochrome P450 3A4, such as cyclosporine, terfenadine, ketoconazole, erythromycin, and troleandomycin. Caution should be exercised with erythromycin when treating patients receiving docetaxel as there is a potential for a significant interaction).
No products indexed under this heading.

Esomeprazole Magnesium (*In vitro* studies have shown that the metabolism of docetaxel may be modified by the concomitant administration of compounds that induce, inhibit, or are metabolized by cytochrome P450 3A4, such as cyclosporine, terfenadine, ketoconazole, erythromycin, and troleandomycin. Caution should be exercised with these drugs when treating patients receiving docetaxel as there is a potential for a significant interaction).
Products include:
Nexium Capsules 704
Nexium Oral Suspension 704

Esomeprazole Sodium (*In vitro* studies have shown that the metabolism of docetaxel may be modified by the concomitant administration of compounds that induce, inhibit, or are metabolized by cytochrome P450 3A4, such as cyclosporine, terfenadine, ketoconazole, erythromycin, and troleandomycin. Caution should be exercised with these drugs when treating patients receiving docetaxel as there is a potential for a significant interaction). Products include:
Nexium I.V. 712

Estradiol (*In vitro* studies have shown that the metabolism of docetaxel may be modified by the concomitant administration of compounds that induce, inhibit, or are metabolized by cytochrome P450 3A4, such as cyclosporine, terfenadine, ketoconazole, erythromycin, and troleandomycin. Caution should be exercised with these drugs when treating patients receiving docetaxel as there is a potential for a significant interaction). Products include:
Activella 2561
Angeliq 831

(⊙ Described in PDR® for Ophthalmic Medicines)

1853 **Interactions Index** **Taxotere**

Climara **841**
Climara Pro **847**
Divigel **3467**
Estrasorb **1777**
Vagifem **2589**

Estradiol Benzoate (*In vitro* studies have shown that the metabolism of docetaxel may be modified by the concomitant administration of compounds that induce, inhibit, or are metabolized by cytochrome P450 3A4, such as cyclosporine, terfenadine, ketoconazole, erythromycin, and troleandomycin. Caution should be exercised with these drugs when treating patients receiving docetaxel as there is a potential for a significant interaction).
No products indexed under this heading.

Estradiol Cypionate (*In vitro* studies have shown that the metabolism of docetaxel may be modified by the concomitant administration of compounds that induce, inhibit, or are metabolized by cytochrome P450 3A4, such as cyclosporine, terfenadine, ketoconazole, erythromycin, and troleandomycin. Caution should be exercised with these drugs when treating patients receiving docetaxel as there is a potential for a significant interaction).
No products indexed under this heading.

Estradiol Valerate (*In vitro* studies have shown that the metabolism of docetaxel may be modified by the concomitant administration of compounds that induce, inhibit, or are metabolized by cytochrome P450 3A4, such as cyclosporine, terfenadine, ketoconazole, erythromycin, and troleandomycin. Caution should be exercised with these drugs when treating patients receiving docetaxel as there is a potential for a significant interaction).
No products indexed under this heading.

Ethinyl Estradiol (*In vitro* studies have shown that the metabolism of docetaxel may be modified by the concomitant administration of compounds that induce, inhibit, or are metabolized by cytochrome P450 3A4, such as cyclosporine, terfenadine, ketoconazole, erythromycin, and troleandomycin. Caution should be exercised with these drugs when treating patients receiving docetaxel as there is a potential for a significant interaction). Products include:
LoSeasonique **3407**
Lybrel **3514**
NuvaRing **3181**
Ortho Evra **2648**
Ortho-Cyclen/Ortho Tri-Cyclen **2663**
Ortho Tri-Cyclen Lo Tablets **2673**
Seasonique **3418**
Yaz **864**

Ethosuximide (*In vitro* studies have shown that the metabolism of docetaxel may be modified by the concomitant administration of compounds that induce, inhibit, or are metabolized by cytochrome P450 3A4, such as cyclosporine, terfenadine, ketoconazole, erythromycin, and troleandomycin. Caution should be exercised with these drugs when treating patients receiving docetaxel as there is a potential for a significant interaction).
No products indexed under this heading.

Ethynodiol Diacetate (*In vitro* studies have shown that the metabolism of docetaxel may be modified by the concomitant administration of compounds that induce, inhibit, or are metabolized by cytochrome P450 3A4, such as cyclosporine, terfenadine, ketoconazole, erythromycin, and troleandomycin. Caution should be exercised with these drugs when treating patients receiving docetaxel as there is a potential for a significant interaction).
No products indexed under this heading.

Etoposide (*In vitro* studies have shown that the metabolism of docetaxel may be modified by the concomitant administration of compounds that induce, inhibit, or are metabolized by cytochrome P450 3A4, such as cyclosporine, terfenadine, ketoconazole, erythromycin, and troleandomycin. Caution should be exercised with these drugs when treating patients receiving docetaxel as there is a potential for a significant interaction).
No products indexed under this heading.

Etoposide Phosphate (*In vitro* studies have shown that the metabolism of docetaxel may be modified by the concomitant administration of compounds that induce, inhibit, or are metabolized by cytochrome P450 3A4, such as cyclosporine, terfenadine, ketoconazole, erythromycin, and troleandomycin. Caution should be exercised with these drugs when treating patients receiving docetaxel as there is a potential for a significant interaction).
No products indexed under this heading.

Felbamate (*In vitro* studies have shown that the metabolism of docetaxel may be modified by the concomitant administration of compounds that induce, inhibit, or are metabolized by cytochrome P450 3A4, such as cyclosporine, terfenadine, ketoconazole, erythromycin, and troleandomycin. Caution should be exercised with these drugs when treating patients receiving docetaxel as there is a potential for a significant interaction).
No products indexed under this heading.

Felodipine (*In vitro* studies have shown that the metabolism of docetaxel may be modified by the concomitant administration of compounds that induce, inhibit, or are metabolized by cytochrome P450 3A4, such as cyclosporine, terfenadine, ketoconazole, erythromycin, and troleandomycin. Caution should be exercised with these drugs when treating patients receiving docetaxel as there is a potential for a significant interaction).
No products indexed under this heading.

Fentanyl (*In vitro* studies have shown that the metabolism of docetaxel may be modified by the concomitant administration of compounds that induce, inhibit, or are metabolized by cytochrome P450 3A4, such as cyclosporine, terfenadine, ketoconazole, erythromycin, and troleandomycin. Caution should be exercised with these drugs when treating patients receiving docetaxel as there is a potential for a significant interaction). Products include:
Duragesic **2604**
Fentanyl Transdermal System **2346**
Onsolis **2054**

Fentanyl Citrate (*In vitro* studies have shown that the metabolism of docetaxel may be modified by the concomitant administration of compounds that induce, inhibit, or are metabolized by cytochrome P450 3A4, such as cyclosporine, terfenadine, ketoconazole, erythromycin, and troleandomycin. Caution should be exercised with these drugs when treating patients receiving docetaxel as there is a potential for a significant interaction). Products include:
Fentora **966**

Fluconazole (*In vitro* studies have shown that the metabolism of docetaxel may be modified by the concomitant administration of compounds that induce, inhibit, or are metabolized by cytochrome P450 3A4, such as cyclosporine, terfenadine, ketoconazole, erythromycin, and troleandomycin. Caution should be exercised with these drugs when treating patients receiving docetaxel as there is a potential for a significant interaction).
No products indexed under this heading.

Fludrocortisone Acetate (*In vitro* studies have shown that the metabolism of docetaxel may be modified by the concomitant administration of compounds that induce, inhibit, or are metabolized by cytochrome P450 3A4, such as cyclosporine, terfenadine, ketoconazole, erythromycin, and troleandomycin. Caution should be exercised with these drugs when treating patients receiving docetaxel as there is a potential for a significant interaction).
No products indexed under this heading.

Fluoxetine (*In vitro* studies have shown that the metabolism of docetaxel may be modified by the concomitant administration of compounds that induce, inhibit, or are metabolized by cytochrome P450 3A4, such as cyclosporine, terfenadine, ketoconazole, erythromycin, and troleandomycin. Caution should be exercised with these drugs when treating patients receiving docetaxel as there is a potential for a significant interaction).
No products indexed under this heading.

Fluoxetine Hydrochloride (*In vitro* studies have shown that the metabolism of docetaxel may be modified by the concomitant administration of compounds that induce, inhibit, or are metabolized by cytochrome P450 3A4, such as cyclosporine, terfenadine, ketoconazole, erythromycin, and troleandomycin. Caution should be exercised with these drugs when treating patients receiving docetaxel as there is a potential for a significant interaction).
Products include:
Prozac Weekly **1941**
Prozac Pulvules **1941**
Symbyax **1965**

Fluvoxamine Maleate (*In vitro* studies have shown that the metabolism of docetaxel may be modified by the concomitant administration of compounds that induce, inhibit, or are metabolized by cytochrome P450 3A4, such as cyclosporine, terfenadine, ketoconazole, erythromycin, and troleandomycin. Caution should be exercised with these drugs when treating patients receiving docetaxel as there is a potential for a significant interaction).
No products indexed under this heading.

Fosamprenavir Calcium (*In vitro* studies have shown that the metabolism of docetaxel may be modified by the concomitant administration of compounds that induce, inhibit, or are metabolized by cytochrome P450 3A4, such as cyclosporine, terfenadine, ketoconazole, erythromycin, and troleandomycin. Caution should be exercised with these drugs when treating patients receiving docetaxel as there is a potential for a significant interaction).
Products include:
Lexiva Oral Suspension **1558**
Lexiva **1558**

Fosphenytoin Sodium (*In vitro* studies have shown that the metabolism of docetaxel may be modified by the concomitant administration of compounds that induce, inhibit, or are metabolized by cytochrome P450 3A4, such as cyclosporine, terfenadine, ketoconazole, erythromycin, and troleandomycin. Caution should be exercised with these drugs when treating patients receiving docetaxel as there is a potential for a significant interaction).
No products indexed under this heading.

Garlic Extract (*In vitro* studies have shown that the metabolism of docetaxel may be modified by the concomitant administration of compounds that induce, inhibit, or are metabolized by cytochrome P450 3A4, such as cyclosporine, terfenadine, ketoconazole, erythromycin, and troleandomycin. Caution should be exercised with these drugs when treating patients receiving docetaxel as there is a potential for a significant interaction).
No products indexed under this heading.

Garlic Oil (*In vitro* studies have shown that the metabolism of docetaxel may be modified by the concomitant administration of compounds that induce, inhibit, or are metabolized by cytochrome P450 3A4, such as cyclosporine, terfenadine, ketoconazole, erythromycin, and troleandomycin. Caution should be exercised with these drugs when treating patients receiving docetaxel as there is a potential for a significant interaction).
No products indexed under this heading.

Haloperidol (*In vitro* studies have shown that the metabolism of docetaxel may be modified by the concomitant administration of compounds that induce, inhibit, or are metabolized by cytochrome P450 3A4, such as cyclosporine, terfenadine, ketoconazole, erythromycin, and troleandomycin. Caution should be exercised with these drugs when treating patients receiving docetaxel as there is a potential for a significant interaction).
No products indexed under this heading.

Haloperidol Decanoate (*In vitro* studies have shown that the metabolism of docetaxel may be modified by the concomitant administration of compounds that induce, inhibit, or are metabolized by cytochrome P450 3A4, such as cyclosporine, terfenadine, ketoconazole, erythromycin, and troleandomycin. Caution should be exercised with these drugs when treating patients receiving docetaxel as there is a potential for a significant interaction).
No products indexed under this heading.

Haloperidol Lactate (*In vitro* studies have shown that the metabolism of docetaxel may be modified by the concomitant administration of compounds that induce, inhibit, or are metabolized by cytochrome P450 3A4, such as cyclosporine, terfenadine, ketoconazole, erythromycin, and troleandomycin. Caution should be exercised with these drugs when treating patients receiving docetaxel as there is a potential for a significant interaction).
No products indexed under this heading.

Hydrocortisone (*In vitro* studies have shown that the metabolism of docetaxel may be modified by the concomitant administration of compounds that induce, inhibit, or are metabolized by cytochrome P450 3A4, such as cyclosporine, terfenadine, ketoconazole, erythromycin, and troleandomycin. Caution should be exercised with these drugs when treating patients receiving docetaxel as there is a potential for a significant interaction).
No products indexed under this heading.

Hydrocortisone (Alcohol) (*In vitro* studies have shown that the metabolism of docetaxel may be modified by the concomitant administration of compounds that induce, inhibit, or are metabolized by cytochrome P450 3A4, such as cyclosporine, terfenadine, ketoconazole, erythromycin, and troleandomycin. Caution should be exercised with these drugs when treating patients receiving docetaxel as there is a potential for a significant interaction).
No products indexed under this heading.

Hydrocortisone Acetate (*In vitro* studies have shown that the metabolism of docetaxel may be modified by the concomitant administration of compounds that induce, inhibit, or are metabolized by cytochrome P450 3A4, such as cyclosporine, terfenadine, ketoconazole, erythromycin, and troleandomycin. Caution should be exercised with

these drugs when treating patients receiving docetaxel as there is a potential for a significant interaction).
No products indexed under this heading.

Hydrocortisone Butyrate (*In vitro* studies have shown that the metabolism of docetaxel may be modified by the concomitant administration of compounds that induce, inhibit, or are metabolized by cytochrome P450 3A4, such as cyclosporine, terfenadine, ketoconazole, erythromycin, and troleandomycin. Caution should be exercised with these drugs when treating patients receiving docetaxel as there is a potential for a significant interaction).
No products indexed under this heading.

Hydrocortisone Cypionate (*In vitro* studies have shown that the metabolism of docetaxel may be modified by the concomitant administration of compounds that induce, inhibit, or are metabolized by cytochrome P450 3A4, such as cyclosporine, terfenadine, ketoconazole, erythromycin, and troleandomycin. Caution should be exercised with these drugs when treating patients receiving docetaxel as there is a potential for a significant interaction).
No products indexed under this heading.

Hydrocortisone Hemisuccinate (*In vitro* studies have shown that the metabolism of docetaxel may be modified by the concomitant administration of compounds that induce, inhibit, or are metabolized by cytochrome P450 3A4, such as cyclosporine, terfenadine, ketoconazole, erythromycin, and troleandomycin. Caution should be exercised with these drugs when treating patients receiving docetaxel as there is a potential for a significant interaction).
No products indexed under this heading.

Hydrocortisone Probutate (*In vitro* studies have shown that the metabolism of docetaxel may be modified by the concomitant administration of compounds that induce, inhibit, or are metabolized by cytochrome P450 3A4, such as cyclosporine, terfenadine, ketoconazole, erythromycin, and troleandomycin. Caution should be exercised with these drugs when treating patients receiving docetaxel as there is a potential for a significant interaction).
No products indexed under this heading.

Hydrocortisone Sodium Phosphate (*In vitro* studies have shown that the metabolism of docetaxel may be modified by the concomitant administration of compounds that induce, inhibit, or are metabolized by cytochrome P450 3A4, such as cyclosporine, terfenadine, ketoconazole, erythromycin, and troleandomycin. Caution should be exercised with these drugs when treating patients receiving docetaxel as there is a potential for a significant interaction).
No products indexed under this heading.

Hydrocortisone Sodium Succinate (*In vitro* studies have shown that the metabolism of docetaxel may be modified by the concomitant administration of compounds that induce, inhibit, or are metabolized by cytochrome P450 3A4, such as cyclosporine, terfenadine, ketoconazole, erythromycin, and troleandomycin. Caution should be exercised with these drugs when treating patients receiving docetaxel as there is a potential for a significant interaction).
No products indexed under this heading.

Hydrocortisone Valerate (*In vitro* studies have shown that the metabolism of docetaxel may be modified by the concomitant administration of compounds that induce, inhibit, or are metabolized by cytochrome P450 3A4, such as cyclosporine, terfenadine, ketoconazole, erythromycin, and troleandomycin. Caution should be exercised with these drugs when treating patients receiving docetaxel as there is a potential for a significant interaction).
No products indexed under this heading.

Hypericum (*In vitro* studies have shown that the metabolism of docetaxel may be modified by the concomitant administration of compounds that induce, inhibit, or are metabolized by cytochrome P450 3A4, such as cyclosporine, terfenadine, ketoconazole, erythromycin, and troleandomycin. Caution should be exercised with these drugs when treating patients receiving docetaxel as there is a potential for a significant interaction).
No products indexed under this heading.

Hypericum Perforatum (*In vitro* studies have shown that the metabolism of docetaxel may be modified by the concomitant administration of compounds that induce, inhibit, or are metabolized by cytochrome P450 3A4, such as cyclosporine, terfenadine, ketoconazole, erythromycin, and troleandomycin. Caution should be exercised with these drugs when treating patients receiving docetaxel as there is a potential for a significant interaction). Products include:
Traumeel 1800

Imatinib Mesylate (*In vitro* studies have shown that the metabolism of docetaxel may be modified by the concomitant administration of compounds that induce, inhibit, or are metabolized by cytochrome P450 3A4, such as cyclosporine, terfenadine, ketoconazole, erythromycin, and troleandomycin. Caution should be exercised with these drugs when treating patients receiving docetaxel as there is a potential for a significant interaction). Products include:
Gleevec 2477

Indinavir Sulfate (*In vitro* studies have shown that the metabolism of docetaxel may be modified by the concomitant administration of compounds that induce, inhibit, or are metabolized by cytochrome P450 3A4, such as cyclosporine, terfenadine, ketoconazole, erythromycin, and troleandomycin. Caution should be exercised with these drugs when treating patients receiving docetaxel as there is a potential for a significant interaction). Products include:
Crixivan 2113

Isoniazid (*In vitro* studies have shown that the metabolism of docetaxel may be modified by the concomitant administration of compounds that induce, inhibit, or are metabolized by cytochrome P450 3A4, such as cyclosporine, terfenadine, ketoconazole, erythromycin, and troleandomycin. Caution should be exercised with these drugs when treating patients receiving docetaxel as there is a potential for a significant interaction).
No products indexed under this heading.

Isradipine (*In vitro* studies have shown that the metabolism of docetaxel may be modified by the concomitant administration of compounds that induce, inhibit, or are metabolized by cytochrome P450 3A4, such as cyclosporine, terfenadine, ketoconazole, erythromycin, and troleandomycin. Caution should be exercised with these drugs when treating patients receiving docetaxel as there is a potential for a significant interaction). Products include:
DynaCirc CR 1432

Itraconazole (*In vitro* studies have shown that the metabolism of docetaxel may be modified by the concomitant administration of compounds that induce, inhibit, or are metabolized by cytochrome P450 3A4, such as cyclosporine, terfenadine, ketoconazole, erythromycin, and troleandomycin. Caution should be exercised with these drugs when treating patients receiving docetaxel as there is a potential for a significant interaction).
No products indexed under this heading.

Ixabepilone (*In vitro* studies have shown that the metabolism of docetaxel may be modified by the concomitant administration of compounds that induce, inhibit, or are metabolized by cytochrome P450 3A4, such as cyclosporine, terfenadine, ketoconazole, erythromycin, and troleandomycin. Caution should be exercised with these drugs when treating patients receiving docetaxel as there is a potential for a significant interaction).
No products indexed under this heading.

Ketoconazole (*In vitro* studies have shown that the metabolism of docetaxel may be modified by the concomitant administration of compounds that induce, inhibit, or are metabolized by cytochrome P450 3A4, such as cyclosporine, terfenadine, ketoconazole, erythromycin, and troleandomycin. Caution should be exercised with these drugs when treating patients receiving docetaxel as there is a potential for a significant interaction. *In vivo* investigations show that caution should be exercised when administering ketoconazole to patients as concomitant therapy since there is a potential for a significant interaction). Products include:
Extina 3319
Xolegel 3337

Lapatinib (*In vitro* studies have shown that the metabolism of docetaxel may be modified by the concomitant administration of compounds that induce, inhibit, or are metabolized by cytochrome P450 3A4, such as cyclosporine, terfenadine, ketoconazole, erythromycin, and troleandomycin. Caution should be exercised with these drugs when treating patients receiving docetaxel as there is a potential for a significant interaction). Products include:
Tykerb 1698

Levonorgestrel (*In vitro* studies have shown that the metabolism of docetaxel may be modified by the concomitant administration of compounds that induce, inhibit, or are metabolized by cytochrome P450 3A4, such as cyclosporine, terfenadine, ketoconazole, erythromycin, and troleandomycin. Caution should be exercised with these drugs when treating patients receiving docetaxel as there is a potential for a significant interaction). Products include:
Climara Pro 847
LoSeasonique 3407
Lybrel 3514
Mirena 854
Plan B 3416
Seasonique 3418

Lidocaine (*In vitro* studies have shown that the metabolism of docetaxel may be modified by the concomitant administration of compounds that induce, inhibit, or are metabolized by cytochrome P450 3A4, such as cyclosporine, terfenadine, ketoconazole, erythromycin, and troleandomycin. Caution should be exercised with these drugs when treating patients receiving docetaxel as there is a potential for a significant interaction). Products include:
Lidoderm 1107

Lidocaine Hydrochloride (*In vitro* studies have shown that the metabolism of docetaxel may be modified by the concomitant administration of compounds that induce, inhibit, or are metabolized by cytochrome P450 3A4, such as cyclosporine, terfenadine, ketoconazole, erythromycin, and troleandomycin. Caution should be exercised with these drugs when treating patients receiving docetaxel as there is a potential for a significant interaction).
No products indexed under this heading.

Lopinavir (*In vitro* studies have shown that the metabolism of docetaxel may be modified by the concomitant administration of compounds that induce, inhibit, or are metabolized by cytochrome P450 3A4, such as cyclosporine, terfenadine, ketoconazole, erythromycin, and troleandomycin. Caution should be exercised with these drugs when treating patients receiving docetaxel as there is a potential for a significant interaction). Products include:
Kaletra 458

Loratadine (*In vitro* studies have shown that the metabolism of docetaxel may be modified by the concomitant administration of compounds that induce, inhibit, or are metabolized by cytochrome P450 3A4, such as cyclosporine, terfenadine, ketoconazole, erythromycin, and troleandomycin. Caution should be exercised with these drugs when treating patients receiving docetaxel as there is a potential for a significant interaction).
No products indexed under this heading.

Lovastatin (*In vitro* studies have shown that the metabolism of docetaxel may be modified by the concomitant administration of compounds that induce, inhibit, or are metabolized by cytochrome P450 3A4, such as cyclosporine, terfenadine, ketoconazole, erythromycin, and troleandomycin. Caution should be exercised with these drugs when treating patients receiving docetaxel as there is a potential for a significant interaction). Products include:
Advicor 402
Mevacor 2212

Mephenytoin (*In vitro* studies have shown that the metabolism of docetaxel may be modified by the concomitant administration of compounds that induce, inhibit, or are metabolized by cytochrome P450 3A4, such as cyclosporine, terfenadine, ketoconazole, erythromycin, and troleandomycin. Caution should be exercised with these drugs when treating patients receiving docetaxel as there is a potential for a significant interaction).
No products indexed under this heading.

Mestranol (*In vitro* studies have shown that the metabolism of docetaxel may be modified by the concomitant administration of compounds that induce, inhibit, or are metabolized by cytochrome P450 3A4, such as cyclosporine, terfenadine, ketoconazole, erythromycin, and troleandomycin. Caution should be exercised with these drugs when treating patients receiving docetaxel as there is a potential for a significant interaction).
No products indexed under this heading.

Methadone Hydrochloride (*In vitro* studies have shown that the metabolism of docetaxel may be modified by the concomitant administration of compounds that induce, inhibit, or are metabolized by cytochrome P450 3A4, such as cyclosporine, terfenadine, ketoconazole, erythromycin, and troleandomycin. Caution should be exercised with these drugs when treating patients receiving docetaxel as there is a potential for a significant interaction).
No products indexed under this heading.

Methsuximide (*In vitro* studies have shown that the metabolism of docetaxel may be modified by the concomitant administration of compounds that induce, inhibit, or are metabolized by cytochrome P450 3A4, such as cyclosporine, terfenadine, ketoconazole, erythromycin, and troleandomycin. Caution should be exercised with these

1855 **Interactions Index** **Taxotere**

drugs when treating patients receiving docetaxel as there is a potential for a significant interaction).
No products indexed under this heading.

Methylprednisolone (*In vitro* studies have shown that the metabolism of docetaxel may be modified by the concomitant administration of compounds that induce, inhibit, or are metabolized by cytochrome P450 3A4, such as cyclosporine, terfenadine, ketoconazole, erythromycin, and troleandomycin. Caution should be exercised with these drugs when treating patients receiving docetaxel as there is a potential for a significant interaction).
No products indexed under this heading.

Methylprednisolone Acetate (*In vitro* studies have shown that the metabolism of docetaxel may be modified by the concomitant administration of compounds that induce, inhibit, or are metabolized by cytochrome P450 3A4, such as cyclosporine, terfenadine, ketoconazole, erythromycin, and troleandomycin. Caution should be exercised with these drugs when treating patients receiving docetaxel as there is a potential for a significant interaction).
No products indexed under this heading.

Methylprednisolone Sodium Succinate (*In vitro* studies have shown that the metabolism of docetaxel may be modified by the concomitant administration of compounds that induce, inhibit, or are metabolized by cytochrome P450 3A4, such as cyclosporine, terfenadine, ketoconazole, erythromycin, and troleandomycin. Caution should be exercised with these drugs when treating patients receiving docetaxel as there is a potential for a significant interaction).
No products indexed under this heading.

Metronidazole (*In vitro* studies have shown that the metabolism of docetaxel may be modified by the concomitant administration of compounds that induce, inhibit, or are metabolized by cytochrome P450 3A4, such as cyclosporine, terfenadine, ketoconazole, erythromycin, and troleandomycin. Caution should be exercised with these drugs when treating patients receiving docetaxel as there is a potential for a significant interaction). Products include:
Pylera **793**

Metronidazole Benzoate (*In vitro* studies have shown that the metabolism of docetaxel may be modified by the concomitant administration of compounds that induce, inhibit, or are metabolized by cytochrome P450 3A4, such as cyclosporine, terfenadine, ketoconazole, erythromycin, and troleandomycin. Caution should be exercised with these drugs when treating patients receiving docetaxel as there is a potential for a significant interaction).
No products indexed under this heading.

Metronidazole Hydrochloride (*In vitro* studies have shown that the metabolism of docetaxel may be modified by the concomitant administration of compounds that induce, inhibit, or are metabolized by cytochrome P450 3A4, such as cyclosporine, terfenadine, ketoconazole, erythromycin, and troleandomycin. Caution should be exercised with these drugs when treating patients receiving docetaxel as there is a potential for a significant interaction).
No products indexed under this heading.

Metronidazole Sodium (*In vitro* studies have shown that the metabolism of docetaxel may be modified by the concomitant administration of compounds that induce, inhibit, or are metabolized by cytochrome P450 3A4, such as cyclosporine, terfenadine, ketoconazole, erythromycin, and troleandomycin. Caution should be exercised with these drugs when treating patients receiving docetaxel as there is a potential for a significant interaction).
No products indexed under this heading.

Miconazole (*In vitro* studies have shown that the metabolism of docetaxel may be modified by the concomitant administration of compounds that induce, inhibit, or are metabolized by cytochrome P450 3A4, such as cyclosporine, terfenadine, ketoconazole, erythromycin, and troleandomycin. Caution should be exercised with these drugs when treating patients receiving docetaxel as there is a potential for a significant interaction).
No products indexed under this heading.

Miconazole Nitrate (*In vitro* studies have shown that the metabolism of docetaxel may be modified by the concomitant administration of compounds that induce, inhibit, or are metabolized by cytochrome P450 3A4, such as cyclosporine, terfenadine, ketoconazole, erythromycin, and troleandomycin. Caution should be exercised with these drugs when treating patients receiving docetaxel as there is a potential for a significant interaction). Products include:
Vusion Ointment **3335**

Midazolam Hydrochloride (*In vitro* studies have shown that the metabolism of docetaxel may be modified by the concomitant administration of compounds that induce, inhibit, or are metabolized by cytochrome P450 3A4, such as cyclosporine, terfenadine, ketoconazole, erythromycin, and troleandomycin. Caution should be exercised with these drugs when treating patients receiving docetaxel as there is a potential for a significant interaction).
No products indexed under this heading.

Mifepristone (*In vitro* studies have shown that the metabolism of docetaxel may be modified by the concomitant administration of compounds that induce, inhibit, or are metabolized by cytochrome P450 3A4, such as cyclosporine, terfenadine, ketoconazole, erythromycin, and troleandomycin. Caution should be exercised with these drugs when treating patients receiving docetaxel as there is a potential for a significant interaction).
No products indexed under this heading.

Modafinil (*In vitro* studies have shown that the metabolism of docetaxel may be modified by the concomitant administration of compounds that induce, inhibit, or are metabolized by cytochrome P450 3A4, such as cyclosporine, terfenadine, ketoconazole, erythromycin, and troleandomycin. Caution should be exercised with these drugs when treating patients receiving docetaxel as there is a potential for a significant interaction). Products include:
Provigil **983**

Nafcillin Sodium (*In vitro* studies have shown that the metabolism of docetaxel may be modified by the concomitant administration of compounds that induce, inhibit, or are metabolized by cytochrome P450 3A4, such as cyclosporine, terfenadine, ketoconazole, erythromycin, and troleandomycin. Caution should be exercised with these drugs when treating patients receiving docetaxel as there is a potential for a significant interaction).
No products indexed under this heading.

Nefazodone Hydrochloride (*In vitro* studies have shown that the metabolism of docetaxel may be modified by the concomitant administration of compounds that induce, inhibit, or are metabolized by cytochrome P450 3A4, such as cyclosporine, terfenadine, ketoconazole, erythromycin, and troleandomycin. Caution should be exercised with these drugs when treating patients receiving docetaxel as there is a potential for a significant interaction).
No products indexed under this heading.

Nelfinavir Mesylate (*In vitro* studies have shown that the metabolism of docetaxel may be modified by the concomitant administration of compounds that induce, inhibit, or are metabolized by cytochrome P450 3A4, such as cyclosporine, terfenadine, ketoconazole, erythromycin, and troleandomycin. Caution should be exercised with these drugs when treating patients receiving docetaxel as there is a potential for a significant interaction).
No products indexed under this heading.

Nevirapine (*In vitro* studies have shown that the metabolism of docetaxel may be modified by the concomitant administration of compounds that induce, inhibit, or are metabolized by cytochrome P450 3A4, such as cyclosporine, terfenadine, ketoconazole, erythromycin, and troleandomycin. Caution should be exercised with these drugs when treating patients receiving docetaxel as there is a potential for a significant interaction). Products include:
Viramune Oral Suspension **897**
Viramune Tablets **897**

Niacin (*In vitro* studies have shown that the metabolism of docetaxel may be modified by the concomitant administration of compounds that induce, inhibit, or are metabolized by cytochrome P450 3A4, such as cyclosporine, terfenadine, ketoconazole, erythromycin, and troleandomycin. Caution should be exercised with these drugs when treating patients receiving docetaxel as there is a potential for a significant interaction). Products include:
Advicor **402**
Cardio Basics **3455**
Niaspan **497**
Simcor **524**

Niacinamide (*In vitro* studies have shown that the metabolism of docetaxel may be modified by the concomitant administration of compounds that induce, inhibit, or are metabolized by cytochrome P450 3A4, such as cyclosporine, terfenadine, ketoconazole, erythromycin, and troleandomycin. Caution should be exercised with these drugs when treating patients receiving docetaxel as there is a potential for a significant interaction). Products include:
CitraNatal 90 DHA Capsules **2332**
CitraNatal Assure **2332**
CitraNatal Rx **2332**
Heplive **607**

Niacinamide Hydroiodide (*In vitro* studies have shown that the metabolism of docetaxel may be modified by the concomitant administration of compounds that induce, inhibit, or are metabolized by cytochrome P450 3A4, such as cyclosporine, terfenadine, ketoconazole, erythromycin, and troleandomycin. Caution should be exercised with these drugs when treating patients receiving docetaxel as there is a potential for a significant interaction).
No products indexed under this heading.

Nicardipine (*In vitro* studies have shown that the metabolism of docetaxel may be modified by the concomitant administration of compounds that induce, inhibit, or are metabolized by cytochrome P450 3A4, such as cyclosporine, terfenadine, ketoconazole, erythromycin, and troleandomycin. Caution should be exercised with these drugs when treating patients receiving docetaxel as there is a potential for a significant interaction).
No products indexed under this heading.

Nicardipine Hydrochloride (*In vitro* studies have shown that the metabolism of docetaxel may be modified by the concomitant administration of compounds that induce, inhibit, or are metabolized by cytochrome P450 3A4, such as cyclosporine, terfenadine, ketoconazole, erythromycin, and troleandomycin. Caution should be exercised with these drugs when treating patients receiving docetaxel as there is a potential for a significant interaction).
No products indexed under this heading.

Nicotinamide (*In vitro* studies have shown that the metabolism of docetaxel may be modified by the concomitant administration of compounds that induce, inhibit, or are metabolized by cytochrome P450 3A4, such as cyclosporine, terfenadine, ketoconazole, erythromycin, and troleandomycin. Caution should be exercised with these drugs when treating patients receiving docetaxel as there is a potential for a significant interaction).
No products indexed under this heading.

Nifedipine (*In vitro* drug interaction studies revealed that docetaxel is metabolized by the CYP3A4 isoenzyme, and its metabolism can be inhibited by CYP3A4 inhibitors, such as ketoconazole, erythromycin, troleandomycin, and nifedipine. Based on *in vitro* findings, it is likely that CYP3A4 inhibitors and/or substrates may lead to substantial increases in docetaxel blood concentrations).
No products indexed under this heading.

Nimodipine (*In vitro* studies have shown that the metabolism of docetaxel may be modified by the concomitant administration of compounds that induce, inhibit, or are metabolized by cytochrome P450 3A4, such as cyclosporine, terfenadine, ketoconazole, erythromycin, and troleandomycin. Caution should be exercised with these drugs when treating patients receiving docetaxel as there is a potential for a significant interaction).
No products indexed under this heading.

Nisoldipine (*In vitro* studies have shown that the metabolism of docetaxel may be modified by the concomitant administration of compounds that induce, inhibit, or are metabolized by cytochrome P450 3A4, such as cyclosporine, terfenadine, ketoconazole, erythromycin, and troleandomycin. Caution should be exercised with these drugs when treating patients receiving docetaxel as there is a potential for a significant interaction).
No products indexed under this heading.

Nitrendipine (*In vitro* studies have shown that the metabolism of docetaxel may be modified by the concomitant administration of compounds that induce, inhibit, or are metabolized by cytochrome P450 3A4, such as cyclosporine, terfenadine, ketoconazole, erythromycin, and troleandomycin. Caution should be exercised with these drugs when treating patients receiving docetaxel as there is a potential for a significant interaction).
No products indexed under this heading.

Norethindrone (*In vitro* studies have shown that the metabolism of docetaxel may be modified by the concomitant administration of compounds that induce, inhibit, or are metabolized by cytochrome P450 3A4, such as cyclosporine, terfenadine, ketoconazole, erythromycin, and troleandomycin. Caution should be exercised with these drugs when treating patients receiving docetaxel as there is a potential for a significant interaction). Products include:
Ortho Micronor **2660**

Norethindrone Acetate (*In vitro* studies have shown that the metabolism of docetaxel may be modified by the concomitant administration of compounds that induce, inhibit, or are metabolized by cytochrome P450 3A4, such as cyclosporine, terfenadine, ketoconazole, erythromycin, and troleandomycin. Caution should be exercised with these drugs when treating patients receiving docetaxel as there is a potential for a significant interaction). Products include:
Activella **2561**

Norfloxacin (*In vitro* studies have shown that the metabolism of docetaxel may be modified by the concomitant administration of compounds that induce, inhibit, or are metabolized by cytochrome P450 3A4, such as cyclosporine, terfenadine, ketoconazole, erythromycin, and troleandomycin. Caution should be exercised with these drugs when treating patients receiving docetaxel as there is a potential for a significant interaction). Products include:
Noroxin **2220**

Norgestrel (*In vitro* studies have shown that the metabolism of docetaxel may be modified by the concomitant administration of compounds that induce, inhibit, or are metabolized by cytochrome P450 3A4, such as cyclosporine, terfenadine, ketoconazole, erythromycin, and troleandomycin. Caution should be exercised with these drugs when treating patients receiving docetaxel as there is a potential for a significant interaction).
No products indexed under this heading.

Omeprazole (*In vitro* studies have shown that the metabolism of docetaxel may be modified by the concomitant administration of compounds that induce, inhibit, or are metabolized by cytochrome P450 3A4, such as cyclosporine, terfenadine, ketoconazole, erythromycin, and troleandomycin. Caution should be exercised with these drugs when treating patients receiving docetaxel as there is a potential for a significant interaction).
No products indexed under this heading.

Ondansetron (*In vitro* studies have shown that the metabolism of docetaxel may be modified by the concomitant administration of compounds that induce, inhibit, or are metabolized by cytochrome P450 3A4, such as cyclosporine, terfenadine, ketoconazole, erythromycin, and troleandomycin. Caution should be exercised with these drugs when treating patients receiving docetaxel as there is a potential for a significant interaction).
No products indexed under this heading.

Ondansetron Hydrochloride (*In vitro* studies have shown that the metabolism of docetaxel may be modified by the concomitant administration of compounds that induce, inhibit, or are metabolized by cytochrome P450 3A4, such as cyclosporine, terfenadine, ketoconazole, erythromycin, and troleandomycin. Caution should be exercised with these drugs when treating patients receiving docetaxel as there is a potential for a significant interaction). Products include:
Zofran Injection **1750**
Zofran **1756**
Zofran ODT **1756**

Oxcarbazepine (*In vitro* studies have shown that the metabolism of docetaxel may be modified by the concomitant administration of compounds that induce, inhibit, or are metabolized by cytochrome P450 3A4, such as cyclosporine, terfenadine, ketoconazole, erythromycin, and troleandomycin. Caution should be exercised with these drugs when treating patients receiving docetaxel as there is a potential for a significant interaction).
No products indexed under this heading.

Paclitaxel (*In vitro* studies have shown that the metabolism of docetaxel may be modified by the concomitant administration of compounds that induce, inhibit, or are metabolized by cytochrome P450 3A4, such as cyclosporine, terfenadine, ketoconazole, erythromycin, and troleandomycin. Caution should be exercised with these drugs when treating patients receiving docetaxel as there is a potential for a significant interaction).
No products indexed under this heading.

Paroxetine Hydrochloride (*In vitro* studies have shown that the metabolism of docetaxel may be modified by the concomitant administration of compounds that induce, inhibit, or are metabolized by cytochrome P450 3A4, such as cyclosporine, terfenadine, ketoconazole, erythromycin, and troleandomycin. Caution should be exercised with these drugs when treating patients receiving docetaxel as there is a potential for a significant interaction). Products include:
Paroxetine CR **2361**
Paroxetine ER **2371**
Paxil **1586**
Paxil CR **1596**

Phenobarbital (*In vitro* studies have shown that the metabolism of docetaxel may be modified by the concomitant administration of compounds that induce, inhibit, or are metabolized by cytochrome P450 3A4, such as cyclosporine, terfenadine, ketoconazole, erythromycin, and troleandomycin. Caution should be exercised with these drugs when treating patients receiving docetaxel as there is a potential for a significant interaction). Products include:
Donnatal **2711**

Phenobarbital Sodium (*In vitro* studies have shown that the metabolism of docetaxel may be modified by the concomitant administration of compounds that induce, inhibit, or are metabolized by cytochrome P450 3A4, such as cyclosporine, terfenadine, ketoconazole, erythromycin, and troleandomycin. Caution should be exercised with these drugs when treating patients receiving docetaxel as there is a potential for a significant interaction).
No products indexed under this heading.

Phenytoin (*In vitro* studies have shown that the metabolism of docetaxel may be modified by the concomitant administration of compounds that induce, inhibit, or are metabolized by cytochrome P450 3A4, such as cyclosporine, terfenadine, ketoconazole, erythromycin, and troleandomycin. Caution should be exercised with these drugs when treating patients receiving docetaxel as there is a potential for a significant interaction).
No products indexed under this heading.

Phenytoin Sodium (*In vitro* studies have shown that the metabolism of docetaxel may be modified by the concomitant administration of compounds that induce, inhibit, or are metabolized by cytochrome P450 3A4, such as cyclosporine, terfenadine, ketoconazole, erythromycin, and troleandomycin. Caution should be exercised with these drugs when treating patients receiving docetaxel as there is a potential for a significant interaction). Products include:
Phenytek Capsules **2380**

Pimozide (*In vitro* studies have shown that the metabolism of docetaxel may be modified by the concomitant administration of compounds that induce, inhibit, or are metabolized by cytochrome P450 3A4, such as cyclosporine, terfenadine, ketoconazole, erythromycin, and troleandomycin. Caution should be exercised with these drugs when treating patients receiving docetaxel as there is a potential for a significant interaction).
No products indexed under this heading.

Polyestradiol Phosphate (*In vitro* studies have shown that the metabolism of docetaxel may be modified by the concomitant administration of compounds that induce, inhibit, or are metabolized by cytochrome P450 3A4, such as cyclosporine, terfenadine, ketoconazole, erythromycin, and troleandomycin. Caution should be exercised with these drugs when treating patients receiving docetaxel as there is a potential for a significant interaction).
No products indexed under this heading.

Polysorbate 80 (Docetaxel is contraindicated in patients who have a history of severe hypersensitivity reactions to docetaxel or to other drugs formulated with polysorbate 80).
No products indexed under this heading.

Posaconazole (*In vitro* studies have shown that the metabolism of docetaxel may be modified by the concomitant administration of compounds that induce, inhibit, or are metabolized by cytochrome P450 3A4, such as cyclosporine, terfenadine, ketoconazole, erythromycin, and troleandomycin. Caution should be exercised with these drugs when treating patients receiving docetaxel as there is a potential for a significant interaction). Products include:
Noxafil **3172**

Prednisolone (*In vitro* studies have shown that the metabolism of docetaxel may be modified by the concomitant administration of compounds that induce, inhibit, or are metabolized by cytochrome P450 3A4, such as cyclosporine, terfenadine, ketoconazole, erythromycin, and troleandomycin. Caution should be exercised with these drugs when treating patients receiving docetaxel as there is a potential for a significant interaction).
No products indexed under this heading.

Prednisolone Acetate (*In vitro* studies have shown that the metabolism of docetaxel may be modified by the concomitant administration of compounds that induce, inhibit, or are metabolized by cytochrome P450 3A4, such as cyclosporine, terfenadine, ketoconazole, erythromycin, and troleandomycin. Caution should be exercised with these drugs when treating patients receiving docetaxel as there is a potential for a significant interaction). Products include:
Blephamide .... ⊙**212**, ⊙**214**
Pred Forte .... ⊙**225**
Pred Mild .... ⊙**230**
Pred-G .... ⊙**226**, ⊙**227**

Prednisolone Sodium Phosphate (*In vitro* studies have shown that the metabolism of docetaxel may be modified by the concomitant administration of compounds that induce, inhibit, or are metabolized by cytochrome P450 3A4, such as cyclosporine, terfenadine, ketoconazole, erythromycin, and troleandomycin. Caution should be exercised with these drugs when treating patients receiving docetaxel as there is a potential for a significant interaction).
No products indexed under this heading.

Prednisolone Tebutate (*In vitro* studies have shown that the metabolism of docetaxel may be modified by the concomitant administration of compounds that induce, inhibit, or are metabolized by cytochrome P450 3A4, such as cyclosporine, terfenadine, ketoconazole, erythromycin, and troleandomycin. Caution should be exercised with these drugs when treating patients receiving docetaxel as there is a potential for a significant interaction).
No products indexed under this heading.

Prednisone (*In vitro* studies have shown that the metabolism of docetaxel may be modified by the concomitant administration of compounds that induce, inhibit, or are metabolized by cytochrome P450 3A4, such as cyclosporine, terfenadine, ketoconazole, erythromycin, and troleandomycin. Caution should be exercised with these drugs when treating patients receiving docetaxel as there is a potential for a significant interaction).
No products indexed under this heading.

Prednisone sodium phosphate (*In vitro* studies have shown that the metabolism of docetaxel may be modified by the concomitant administration of compounds that induce, inhibit, or are metabolized by cytochrome P450 3A4, such as cyclosporine, terfenadine, ketoconazole, erythromycin, and troleandomycin. Caution should be exercised with these drugs when treating patients receiving docetaxel as there is a potential for a significant interaction).
No products indexed under this heading.

Primidone (*In vitro* studies have shown that the metabolism of docetaxel may be modified by the concomitant administration of compounds that induce, inhibit, or are metabolized by cytochrome P450 3A4, such as cyclosporine, terfenadine, ketoconazole, erythromycin, and troleandomycin. Caution should be exercised with these drugs when treating patients receiving docetaxel as there is a potential for a significant interaction).
No products indexed under this heading.

Propoxyphene Hydrochloride (*In vitro* studies have shown that the metabolism of docetaxel may be modified by the concomitant administration of compounds that induce, inhibit, or are metabolized by cytochrome P450 3A4, such as cyclosporine, terfenadine, ketoconazole, erythromycin, and troleandomycin. Caution should be exercised with these drugs when treating patients receiving docetaxel as there is a potential for a significant interaction).
No products indexed under this heading.

Propoxyphene Napsylate (*In vitro* studies have shown that the metabolism of docetaxel may be modified by the concomitant administration of compounds that induce, inhibit, or are metabolized by cytochrome P450 3A4, such as cyclosporine, terfenadine, ketoconazole, erythromycin, and troleandomycin. Caution should be exercised with these drugs when treating patients receiving docetaxel as there is a potential for a significant interaction).
No products indexed under this heading.

Quinidine (*In vitro* studies have shown that the metabolism of docetaxel may be modified by the concomitant administration of compounds that induce, inhibit, or are metabolized by cytochrome P450 3A4, such as cyclosporine, terfenadine, ketoconazole, erythromycin, and troleandomycin. Caution should be exercised with these drugs when treating patients receiving docetaxel as there is a potential for a significant interaction).
No products indexed under this heading.

Quinidine Gluconate (*In vitro* studies have shown that the metabolism of docetaxel may be modified by the concomitant administration of compounds that induce, inhibit, or are metabolized by cytochrome P450 3A4, such as cyclosporine, terfenadine, ketoconazole, erythromycin, and troleandomycin.

Caution should be exercised with these drugs when treating patients receiving docetaxel as there is a potential for a significant interaction).

No products indexed under this heading.

Quinidine Hydrochloride (*In vitro* studies have shown that the metabolism of docetaxel may be modified by the concomitant administration of compounds that induce, inhibit, or are metabolized by cytochrome P450 3A4, such as cyclosporine, terfenadine, ketoconazole, erythromycin, and troleandomycin. Caution should be exercised with these drugs when treating patients receiving docetaxel as there is a potential for a significant interaction).

No products indexed under this heading.

Quinidine Polygalacturonate (*In vitro* studies have shown that the metabolism of docetaxel may be modified by the concomitant administration of compounds that induce, inhibit, or are metabolized by cytochrome P450 3A4, such as cyclosporine, terfenadine, ketoconazole, erythromycin, and troleandomycin. Caution should be exercised with these drugs when treating patients receiving docetaxel as there is a potential for a significant interaction).

No products indexed under this heading.

Quinidine Sulfate (*In vitro* studies have shown that the metabolism of docetaxel may be modified by the concomitant administration of compounds that induce, inhibit, or are metabolized by cytochrome P450 3A4, such as cyclosporine, terfenadine, ketoconazole, erythromycin, and troleandomycin. Caution should be exercised with these drugs when treating patients receiving docetaxel as there is a potential for a significant interaction).

No products indexed under this heading.

Quinine (*In vitro* studies have shown that the metabolism of docetaxel may be modified by the concomitant administration of compounds that induce, inhibit, or are metabolized by cytochrome P450 3A4, such as cyclosporine, terfenadine, ketoconazole, erythromycin, and troleandomycin. Caution should be exercised with these drugs when treating patients receiving docetaxel as there is a potential for a significant interaction). Products include:

Hyland's Leg Cramps PM with Quinine **3315**

Quinine Sulfate (*In vitro* studies have shown that the metabolism of docetaxel may be modified by the concomitant administration of compounds that induce, inhibit, or are metabolized by cytochrome P450 3A4, such as cyclosporine, terfenadine, ketoconazole, erythromycin, and troleandomycin. Caution should be exercised with these drugs when treating patients receiving docetaxel as there is a potential for a significant interaction).

No products indexed under this heading.

Quinupristin (*In vitro* studies have shown that the metabolism of docetaxel may be modified by the concomitant administration of compounds that induce, inhibit, or are metabolized by cytochrome P450 3A4, such as cyclosporine, terfenadine, ketoconazole, erythromycin, and troleandomycin. Caution should be exercised with these drugs when treating patients receiving docetaxel as there is a potential for a significant interaction).

No products indexed under this heading.

Ranitidine Bismuth Citrate (*In vitro* studies have shown that the metabolism of docetaxel may be modified by the concomitant administration of compounds that induce, inhibit, or are metabolized by cytochrome P450 3A4, such as cyclosporine, terfenadine, ketoconazole, erythromycin, and troleandomycin. Caution should be exercised with these drugs when treating patients receiving docetaxel as there is a potential for a significant interaction).

No products indexed under this heading.

Ranitidine Hydrochloride (*In vitro* studies have shown that the metabolism of docetaxel may be modified by the concomitant administration of compounds that induce, inhibit, or are metabolized by cytochrome P450 3A4, such as cyclosporine, terfenadine, ketoconazole, erythromycin, and troleandomycin. Caution should be exercised with these drugs when treating patients receiving docetaxel as there is a potential for a significant interaction). Products include:

Zantac **1737**
Zantac Injection **1732**
Zantac Pharmacy **1735**

Rifabutin (*In vitro* studies have shown that the metabolism of docetaxel may be modified by the concomitant administration of compounds that induce, inhibit, or are metabolized by cytochrome P450 3A4, such as cyclosporine, terfenadine, ketoconazole, erythromycin, and troleandomycin. Caution should be exercised with these drugs when treating patients receiving docetaxel as there is a potential for a significant interaction).

No products indexed under this heading.

Rifampicin (*In vitro* studies have shown that the metabolism of docetaxel may be modified by the concomitant administration of compounds that induce, inhibit, or are metabolized by cytochrome P450 3A4, such as cyclosporine, terfenadine, ketoconazole, erythromycin, and troleandomycin. Caution should be exercised with these drugs when treating patients receiving docetaxel as there is a potential for a significant interaction).

No products indexed under this heading.

Rifampin (*In vitro* studies have shown that the metabolism of docetaxel may be modified by the concomitant administration of compounds that induce, inhibit, or are metabolized by cytochrome P450 3A4, such as cyclosporine, terfenadine, ketoconazole, erythromycin, and troleandomycin. Caution should be exercised with these drugs when treating patients receiving docetaxel as there is a potential for a significant interaction).

No products indexed under this heading.

Rifapentine (*In vitro* studies have shown that the metabolism of docetaxel may be modified by the concomitant administration of compounds that induce, inhibit, or are metabolized by cytochrome P450 3A4, such as cyclosporine, terfenadine, ketoconazole, erythromycin, and troleandomycin. Caution should be exercised with these drugs when treating patients receiving docetaxel as there is a potential for a significant interaction).

No products indexed under this heading.

Ritonavir (*In vitro* studies have shown that the metabolism of docetaxel may be modified by the concomitant administration of compounds that induce, inhibit, or are metabolized by cytochrome P450 3A4, such as cyclosporine, terfenadine, ketoconazole, erythromycin, and troleandomycin. Caution should be exercised with these drugs when treating patients receiving docetaxel as there is a potential for a significant interaction). Products include:

Kaletra **458**
Norvir **509**

Saquinavir (*In vitro* studies have shown that the metabolism of docetaxel may be modified by the concomitant administration of compounds that induce, inhibit, or are metabolized by cytochrome P450 3A4, such as cyclosporine, terfenadine, ketoconazole, erythromycin, and troleandomycin. Caution should be exercised with these drugs when treating patients receiving docetaxel as there is a potential for a significant interaction).

No products indexed under this heading.

Saquinavir Mesylate (*In vitro* studies have shown that the metabolism of docetaxel may be modified by the concomitant administration of compounds that induce, inhibit, or are metabolized by cytochrome P450 3A4, such as cyclosporine, terfenadine, ketoconazole, erythromycin, and troleandomycin. Caution should be exercised with these drugs when treating patients receiving docetaxel as there is a potential for a significant interaction).

No products indexed under this heading.

Sertraline Hydrochloride (*In vitro* studies have shown that the metabolism of docetaxel may be modified by the concomitant administration of compounds that induce, inhibit, or are metabolized by cytochrome P450 3A4, such as cyclosporine, terfenadine, ketoconazole, erythromycin, and troleandomycin. Caution should be exercised with these drugs when treating patients receiving docetaxel as there is a potential for a significant interaction).

No products indexed under this heading.

Sildenafil Citrate (*In vitro* studies have shown that the metabolism of docetaxel may be modified by the concomitant administration of compounds that induce, inhibit, or are metabolized by cytochrome P450 3A4, such as cyclosporine, terfenadine, ketoconazole, erythromycin, and troleandomycin. Caution should be exercised with these drugs when treating patients receiving docetaxel as there is a potential for a significant interaction).

No products indexed under this heading.

Simvastatin (*In vitro* studies have shown that the metabolism of docetaxel may be modified by the concomitant administration of compounds that induce, inhibit, or are metabolized by cytochrome P450 3A4, such as cyclosporine, terfenadine, ketoconazole, erythromycin, and troleandomycin. Caution should be exercised with these drugs when treating patients receiving docetaxel as there is a potential for a significant interaction). Products include:

Simcor **524**
Vytorin 10/10 .... **2303, 3240**
Vytorin 10/20 .... **2303, 3240**
Vytorin 10/40 .... **2303, 3240**
Vytorin 10/80 .... **2303, 3240**
Zocor **2289**

Sirolimus (*In vitro* studies have shown that the metabolism of docetaxel may be modified by the concomitant administration of compounds that induce, inhibit, or are metabolized by cytochrome P450 3A4, such as cyclosporine, terfenadine, ketoconazole, erythromycin, and troleandomycin. Caution should be exercised with these drugs when treating patients receiving docetaxel as there is a potential for a significant interaction). Products include:

Rapamune **3579**

Sulfinpyrazone (*In vitro* studies have shown that the metabolism of docetaxel may be modified by the concomitant administration of compounds that induce, inhibit, or are metabolized by cytochrome P450 3A4, such as cyclosporine, terfenadine, ketoconazole, erythromycin, and troleandomycin. Caution should be exercised with these drugs when treating patients receiving docetaxel as there is a potential for a significant interaction).

No products indexed under this heading.

Tacrolimus (*In vitro* studies have shown that the metabolism of docetaxel may be modified by the concomitant administration of compounds that induce, inhibit, or are metabolized by cytochrome P450 3A4, such as cyclosporine, terfenadine, ketoconazole, erythromycin, and troleandomycin. Caution should be exercised with these drugs when treating patients receiving docetaxel as there is a potential for a significant interaction). Products include:

Prograf Capsules **677**
Prograf Injection **677**
Protopic **685**

Tadalafil (*In vitro* studies have shown that the metabolism of docetaxel may be modified by the concomitant administration of compounds that induce, inhibit, or are metabolized by cytochrome P450 3A4, such as cyclosporine, terfenadine, ketoconazole, erythromycin, and troleandomycin. Caution should be exercised with these drugs when treating patients receiving docetaxel as there is a potential for a significant interaction). Products include:

Adcirca **3461**
Cialis **1861**

Tamoxifen Citrate (*In vitro* studies have shown that the metabolism of docetaxel may be modified by the concomitant administration of compounds that induce, inhibit, or are metabolized by cytochrome P450 3A4, such as cyclosporine, terfenadine, ketoconazole, erythromycin, and troleandomycin. Caution should be exercised with these drugs when treating patients receiving docetaxel as there is a potential for a significant interaction).

No products indexed under this heading.

Telithromycin (*In vitro* studies have shown that the metabolism of docetaxel may be modified by the concomitant administration of compounds that induce, inhibit, or are metabolized by cytochrome P450 3A4, such as cyclosporine, terfenadine, ketoconazole, erythromycin, and troleandomycin. Caution should be exercised with these drugs when treating patients receiving docetaxel as there is a potential for a significant interaction). Products include:

Ketek **2991**

Terfenadine (*In vitro* studies have shown that the metabolism of docetaxel may be modified by the concomitant administration of compounds that induce, inhibit, or are metabolized by cytochrome P450 3A4, such as cyclosporine, terfenadine, ketoconazole, erythromycin, and troleandomycin. Caution should be exercised with these drugs when treating patients receiving docetaxel as there is a potential for a significant interaction).

No products indexed under this heading.

Theophyllinate (*In vitro* studies have shown that the metabolism of docetaxel may be modified by the concomitant administration of compounds that induce, inhibit, or are metabolized by cytochrome P450 3A4, such as cyclosporine, terfenadine, ketoconazole, erythromycin, and troleandomycin. Caution should be exercised with these drugs when treating patients receiving docetaxel as there is a potential for a significant interaction).

No products indexed under this heading.

Theophylline (*In vitro* studies have shown that the metabolism of docetaxel may be modified by the concomitant administration of compounds that induce, inhibit, or are metabolized by cytochrome P450 3A4, such as cyclosporine, terfenadine, ketoconazole, erythromycin, and troleandomycin. Caution should be exercised with these

drugs when treating patients receiving docetaxel as there is a potential for a significant interaction).
No products indexed under this heading.

Theophylline Anhydrous (*In vitro* studies have shown that the metabolism of docetaxel may be modified by the concomitant administration of compounds that induce, inhibit, or are metabolized by cytochrome P450 3A4, such as cyclosporine, terfenadine, ketoconazole, erythromycin, and troleandomycin. Caution should be exercised with these drugs when treating patients receiving docetaxel as there is a potential for a significant interaction).
Products include:
Uniphyl 2817

Theophylline Calcium Salicylate (*In vitro* studies have shown that the metabolism of docetaxel may be modified by the concomitant administration of compounds that induce, inhibit, or are metabolized by cytochrome P450 3A4, such as cyclosporine, terfenadine, ketoconazole, erythromycin, and troleandomycin. Caution should be exercised with these drugs when treating patients receiving docetaxel as there is a potential for a significant interaction).
No products indexed under this heading.

Theophylline Dihydroxypropyl (Glyceryl) (*In vitro* studies have shown that the metabolism of docetaxel may be modified by the concomitant administration of compounds that induce, inhibit, or are metabolized by cytochrome P450 3A4, such as cyclosporine, terfenadine, ketoconazole, erythromycin, and troleandomycin. Caution should be exercised with these drugs when treating patients receiving docetaxel as there is a potential for a significant interaction).
No products indexed under this heading.

Theophylline Ethylenediamine (*In vitro* studies have shown that the metabolism of docetaxel may be modified by the concomitant administration of compounds that induce, inhibit, or are metabolized by cytochrome P450 3A4, such as cyclosporine, terfenadine, ketoconazole, erythromycin, and troleandomycin. Caution should be exercised with these drugs when treating patients receiving docetaxel as there is a potential for a significant interaction).
No products indexed under this heading.

Theophylline Sodium Glycinate (*In vitro* studies have shown that the metabolism of docetaxel may be modified by the concomitant administration of compounds that induce, inhibit, or are metabolized by cytochrome P450 3A4, such as cyclosporine, terfenadine, ketoconazole, erythromycin, and troleandomycin. Caution should be exercised with these drugs when treating patients receiving docetaxel as there is a potential for a significant interaction).
No products indexed under this heading.

Tiagabine Hydrochloride (*In vitro* studies have shown that the metabolism of docetaxel may be modified by the concomitant administration of compounds that induce, inhibit, or are metabolized by cytochrome P450 3A4, such as cyclosporine, terfenadine, ketoconazole, erythromycin, and troleandomycin. Caution should be exercised with these drugs when treating patients receiving docetaxel as there is a potential for a significant interaction).
Products include:
Gabitril 972

Tolterodine Tartrate (*In vitro* studies have shown that the metabolism of docetaxel may be modified by the concomitant administration of compounds that induce, inhibit, or are metabolized by cytochrome P450 3A4, such as cyclosporine, terfenadine, ketoconazole, erythromycin, and troleandomycin. Caution should be exercised with these drugs when treating patients receiving docetaxel as there is a potential for a significant interaction).
No products indexed under this heading.

Trazodone Hydrochloride (*In vitro* studies have shown that the metabolism of docetaxel may be modified by the concomitant administration of compounds that induce, inhibit, or are metabolized by cytochrome P450 3A4, such as cyclosporine, terfenadine, ketoconazole, erythromycin, and troleandomycin. Caution should be exercised with these drugs when treating patients receiving docetaxel as there is a potential for a significant interaction).
No products indexed under this heading.

Triamcinolone (*In vitro* studies have shown that the metabolism of docetaxel may be modified by the concomitant administration of compounds that induce, inhibit, or are metabolized by cytochrome P450 3A4, such as cyclosporine, terfenadine, ketoconazole, erythromycin, and troleandomycin. Caution should be exercised with these drugs when treating patients receiving docetaxel as there is a potential for a significant interaction).
No products indexed under this heading.

Triamcinolone Acetonide (*In vitro* studies have shown that the metabolism of docetaxel may be modified by the concomitant administration of compounds that induce, inhibit, or are metabolized by cytochrome P450 3A4, such as cyclosporine, terfenadine, ketoconazole, erythromycin, and troleandomycin. Caution should be exercised with these drugs when treating patients receiving docetaxel as there is a potential for a significant interaction).
Products include:
Azmacort 408
Nasacort AQ 3019

Triamcinolone Diacetate (*In vitro* studies have shown that the metabolism of docetaxel may be modified by the concomitant administration of compounds that induce, inhibit, or are metabolized by cytochrome P450 3A4, such as cyclosporine, terfenadine, ketoconazole, erythromycin, and troleandomycin. Caution should be exercised with these drugs when treating patients receiving docetaxel as there is a potential for a significant interaction).
No products indexed under this heading.

Triamcinolone Hexacetonide (*In vitro* studies have shown that the metabolism of docetaxel may be modified by the concomitant administration of compounds that induce, inhibit, or are metabolized by cytochrome P450 3A4, such as cyclosporine, terfenadine, ketoconazole, erythromycin, and troleandomycin. Caution should be exercised with these drugs when treating patients receiving docetaxel as there is a potential for a significant interaction).
No products indexed under this heading.

Triazolam (*In vitro* studies have shown that the metabolism of docetaxel may be modified by the concomitant administration of compounds that induce, inhibit, or are metabolized by cytochrome P450 3A4, such as cyclosporine, terfenadine, ketoconazole, erythromycin, and troleandomycin. Caution should be exercised with these drugs when treating patients receiving docetaxel as there is a potential for a significant interaction).
No products indexed under this heading.

Troglitazone (*In vitro* studies have shown that the metabolism of docetaxel may be modified by the concomitant administration of compounds that induce, inhibit, or are metabolized by cytochrome P450 3A4, such as cyclosporine, terfenadine, ketoconazole, erythromycin, and troleandomycin. Caution should be exercised with these drugs when treating patients receiving docetaxel as there is a potential for a significant interaction).
No products indexed under this heading.

Troleandomycin (*In vitro* studies have shown that the metabolism of docetaxel may be modified by the concomitant administration of compounds that induce, inhibit, or are metabolized by cytochrome P450 3A4, such as cyclosporine, terfenadine, ketoconazole, erythromycin, and troleandomycin. Caution should be exercised with these drugs when treating patients receiving docetaxel as there is a potential for a significant interaction).
No products indexed under this heading.

Valproate Sodium (*In vitro* studies have shown that the metabolism of docetaxel may be modified by the concomitant administration of compounds that induce, inhibit, or are metabolized by cytochrome P450 3A4, such as cyclosporine, terfenadine, ketoconazole, erythromycin, and troleandomycin. Caution should be exercised with these drugs when treating patients receiving docetaxel as there is a potential for a significant interaction).
No products indexed under this heading.

Vardenafil Hydrochloride (*In vitro* studies have shown that the metabolism of docetaxel may be modified by the concomitant administration of compounds that induce, inhibit, or are metabolized by cytochrome P450 3A4, such as cyclosporine, terfenadine, ketoconazole, erythromycin, and troleandomycin. Caution should be exercised with these drugs when treating patients receiving docetaxel as there is a potential for a significant interaction).
Products include:
Levitra 3157

Verapamil Hydrochloride (*In vitro* studies have shown that the metabolism of docetaxel may be modified by the concomitant administration of compounds that induce, inhibit, or are metabolized by cytochrome P450 3A4, such as cyclosporine, terfenadine, ketoconazole, erythromycin, and troleandomycin. Caution should be exercised with these drugs when treating patients receiving docetaxel as there is a potential for a significant interaction).
Products include:
Tarka 534

Vinblastine Sulfate (*In vitro* studies have shown that the metabolism of docetaxel may be modified by the concomitant administration of compounds that induce, inhibit, or are metabolized by cytochrome P450 3A4, such as cyclosporine, terfenadine, ketoconazole, erythromycin, and troleandomycin. Caution should be exercised with these drugs when treating patients receiving docetaxel as there is a potential for a significant interaction).
No products indexed under this heading.

Vincristine Sulfate (*In vitro* studies have shown that the metabolism of docetaxel may be modified by the concomitant administration of compounds that induce, inhibit, or are metabolized by cytochrome P450 3A4, such as cyclosporine, terfenadine, ketoconazole, erythromycin, and troleandomycin. Caution should be exercised with these drugs when treating patients receiving docetaxel as there is a potential for a significant interaction).
No products indexed under this heading.

Voriconazole (*In vitro* studies have shown that the metabolism of docetaxel may be modified by the concomitant administration of compounds that induce, inhibit, or are metabolized by cytochrome P450 3A4, such as cyclosporine, terfenadine, ketoconazole, erythromycin, and troleandomycin. Caution should be exercised with these drugs when treating patients receiving docetaxel as there is a potential for a significant interaction).
No products indexed under this heading.

Warfarin Sodium (*In vitro* studies have shown that the metabolism of docetaxel may be modified by the concomitant administration of compounds that induce, inhibit, or are metabolized by cytochrome P450 3A4, such as cyclosporine, terfenadine, ketoconazole, erythromycin, and troleandomycin. Caution should be exercised with these drugs when treating patients receiving docetaxel as there is a potential for a significant interaction).
No products indexed under this heading.

Zafirlukast (*In vitro* studies have shown that the metabolism of docetaxel may be modified by the concomitant administration of compounds that induce, inhibit, or are metabolized by cytochrome P450 3A4, such as cyclosporine, terfenadine, ketoconazole, erythromycin, and troleandomycin. Caution should be exercised with these drugs when treating patients receiving docetaxel as there is a potential for a significant interaction). Products include:
Accolate 3612

Zileuton (*In vitro* studies have shown that the metabolism of docetaxel may be modified by the concomitant administration of compounds that induce, inhibit, or are metabolized by cytochrome P450 3A4, such as cyclosporine, terfenadine, ketoconazole, erythromycin, and troleandomycin. Caution should be exercised with these drugs when treating patients receiving docetaxel as there is a potential for a significant interaction).
No products indexed under this heading.

Food Interactions

Grapefruit (*In vitro* studies have shown that the metabolism of docetaxel may be modified by the concomitant administration of compounds that induce, inhibit, or are metabolized by cytochrome P450 3A4, such as cyclosporine, terfenadine, ketoconazole, erythromycin, and troleandomycin. Caution should be exercised with these drugs when treating patients receiving docetaxel as there is a potential for a significant interaction).

Grapefruit Juice (*In vitro* studies have shown that the metabolism of docetaxel may be modified by the concomitant administration of compounds that induce, inhibit, or are metabolized by cytochrome P450 3A4, such as cyclosporine, terfenadine, ketoconazole, erythromycin, and troleandomycin. Caution should be exercised with these drugs when treating patients receiving docetaxel as there is a potential for a significant interaction).

TĒGREEN 97 CAPSULES

(Camellia sinensis) 2778
May interact with oral anticoagulants. Compounds in these categories include:

Anisindione (Concurrent use with anticoagulants requires consultation with a physician).
No products indexed under this heading.

Dicumarol (Concurrent use with anticoagulants requires consultation with a physician).
No products indexed under this heading.

Warfarin Sodium (Concurrent use with anticoagulants requires consultation with a physician).
No products indexed under this heading.

1859 Interactions Index Tekturna HCT

TEKTURNA TABLETS
(Aliskiren) 2538

Atorvastatin Calcium (Co-administration of atorvastatin, a potent Pgp inhibitor, resulted in about a 50% increase in aliskiren C_{max} and AUC after multiple dosing). Products include:
Lipitor 2703

Cyclosporine (When aliskiren was given with cyclosporine, the blood concentrations of aliskiren were significantly increased. Concomitant use of aliskiren with cyclosporine is not recommended). Products include:
Gengraf 440
Neoral Oral Solution 2496
Neoral Capsules 2496
Restasis 605

Furosemide (Concomitant use leads to a significant decrease in furosemide blood concentrations. Patients using furosemide could find its effect diminished after starting aliskiren). Products include:
Furosemide 2354

Irbesartan (Co-administration of irbesartan reduced aliskiren C_{max} up to 50% after multiple dosing). Products include:
Avalide 2956
Avapro 2962

Ketoconazole (Co-administration of 200 mg twice-daily ketoconazole, a potent Pgp inhibitor, with aliskiren resulted in an approximate 80% increase in plasma levels of aliskiren). Products include:
Extina 3319
Xolegel 3337

TEKTURNA HCT TABLETS
(Aliskiren, Hydrochlorothiazide) 2541
May interact with alcohols, antihypertensives, barbiturates, corticosteroids, insulin, lithium preparations, narcotic analgesics, non-steroidal anti-inflammatory agents, nondepolarizing neuromuscular blocking agents, oral hypoglycemic agents, P-glycoprotein inhibitors, potassium preparations, potassium sparing diuretics, and certain other agents. Compounds in these categories include:

Acarbose (Concurrent use may require dosage adjustment of the antidiabetic drug).
No products indexed under this heading.

Acebutolol Hydrochloride (Concurrent use with other antihypertensives may cause an additive effect or potentiation).
No products indexed under this heading.

ACTH (Intensified electrolyte depletion, particularly hypokalemia with concurrent use).
No products indexed under this heading.

Alclometasone Dipropionate (Intensified electrolyte depletion, particularly hypokalemia with concurrent use).
No products indexed under this heading.

Alfentanil Hydrochloride (Potentiation of orthostatic hypotension may occur with concurrent use).
No products indexed under this heading.

Amiloride Hydrochloride (Based on experience with the use of other substances that affect the renin-angiotensin system (RAS), concomitant use of Tekturna HCT with potassium-sparing diuretics may lead to increases in serum potassium. If concomitant use is considered necessary, caution should be exercised).
No products indexed under this heading.

Amiodarone Hydrochloride (Pgp (MDR1/Mdr1a/1b) was found to be the major efflux system involved in absorption and disposition of aliskiren in preclinical studies. The potential for drug interactions at the Pgp site will likely depend on the degree of inhibition of this transporter).
No products indexed under this heading.

Amlodipine Besylate (Concurrent use with other antihypertensives may cause an additive effect or potentiation). Products include:
Azor 1010
Exforge 2443
Exforge HCT 2449

Amobarbital (Potentiation of orthostatic hypotension may occur with concurrent use).
No products indexed under this heading.

Amobarbital Sodium (Potentiation of orthostatic hypotension may occur with concurrent use).
No products indexed under this heading.

Apomorphine (Potentiation of orthostatic hypotension may occur with concurrent use).
No products indexed under this heading.

Apomorphine Hydrochloride (Potentiation of orthostatic hypotension may occur with concurrent use).
No products indexed under this heading.

Aprobarbital (Potentiation of orthostatic hypotension may occur with concurrent use).
No products indexed under this heading.

Atenolol (Concurrent use with other antihypertensives may cause an additive effect or potentiation).
No products indexed under this heading.

Atorvastatin Calcium (Co-administration of atorvastatin resulted in about a 50% increase in aliskiren C_{max} and AUC after multiple dosing). Products include:
Lipitor 2703

Atracurium Besylate (Concurrent use may increase the responsiveness to the muscle relaxant).
No products indexed under this heading.

Azithromycin Dihydrate (Pgp (MDR1/Mdr1a/1b) was found to be the major efflux system involved in absorption and disposition of aliskiren in preclinical studies. The potential for drug interactions at the Pgp site will likely depend on the degree of inhibition of this transporter).
No products indexed under this heading.

Beclomethasone Dipropionate (Intensified electrolyte depletion, particularly hypokalemia with concurrent use). Products include:
Qvar 3398

Beclomethasone Dipropionate Monohydrate (Intensified electrolyte depletion, particularly hypokalemia with concurrent use). Products include:
Beconase AQ 1386

Benazepril Hydrochloride (Concurrent use with other antihypertensives may cause an additive effect or potentiation).
No products indexed under this heading.

Bendroflumethiazide (Concurrent use with other antihypertensives may cause an additive effect or potentiation).
No products indexed under this heading.

Betamethasone (Intensified electrolyte depletion, particularly hypokalemia with concurrent use).
No products indexed under this heading.

Betamethasone Acetate (Intensified electrolyte depletion, particularly hypokalemia with concurrent use).
No products indexed under this heading.

Betamethasone Benzoate (Intensified electrolyte depletion, particularly hypokalemia with concurrent use).
No products indexed under this heading.

Betamethasone Dipropionate (Intensified electrolyte depletion, particularly hypokalemia with concurrent use). Products include:
Diprolene Lotion 0.05% 3108
Diprolene Ointment 0.05% 3109
Diprolene AF Cream 0.05% 3107
Lotrisone 3163

Betamethasone Sodium Phosphate (Intensified electrolyte depletion, particularly hypokalemia with concurrent use).
No products indexed under this heading.

Betamethasone Valerate (Intensified electrolyte depletion, particularly hypokalemia with concurrent use). Products include:
Luxiq 3321

Betaxolol Hydrochloride (Concurrent use with other antihypertensives may cause an additive effect or potentiation).
No products indexed under this heading.

Bisoprolol Fumarate (Concurrent use with other antihypertensives may cause an additive effect or potentiation).
No products indexed under this heading.

Budesonide (Intensified electrolyte depletion, particularly hypokalemia with concurrent use). Products include:
Pulmicort Flexhaler 714
Symbicort 80/4.5 720
Symbicort 160/4.5 720

Buprenorphine Hydrochloride (Potentiation of orthostatic hypotension may occur with concurrent use).
No products indexed under this heading.

Butabarbital (Potentiation of orthostatic hypotension may occur with concurrent use).
No products indexed under this heading.

Butabarbital Sodium (Potentiation of orthostatic hypotension may occur with concurrent use).
No products indexed under this heading.

Butalbital (Potentiation of orthostatic hypotension may occur with concurrent use).
No products indexed under this heading.

Candesartan Cilexetil (Concurrent use with other antihypertensives may cause an additive effect or potentiation). Products include:
Atacand 697
Atacand HCT 700

Captopril (Concurrent use with other antihypertensives may cause an additive effect or potentiation). Products include:
Captopril 2341

Carteolol Hydrochloride (Concurrent use with other antihypertensives may cause an additive effect or potentiation).
No products indexed under this heading.

Carvedilol (Concurrent use with other antihypertensives may cause an additive effect or potentiation). Products include:
Coreg 1409

Carvedilol Phosphate (Concurrent use with other antihypertensives may cause an additive effect or potentiation). Products include:
Coreg CR 1416

Celecoxib (In some patients, the administration of a nonsteroidal anti-inflammatory agent can reduce the diuretic, natriuretic, and antihypertensive effects of thiazide diuretics. Therefore, when Tekturna HCT and nonsteroidal anti-inflammatory agents are used concomitantly, the patient should be observed closely to determine if the desired effect of the diuretic is obtained). Products include:
Celebrex 3272

Chlorothiazide (Concurrent use with other antihypertensives may cause an additive effect or potentiation).
No products indexed under this heading.

Chlorothiazide Sodium (Concurrent use with other antihypertensives may cause an additive effect or potentiation). Products include:
Diuril Intravenous 2009

Chlorpropamide (Concurrent use may require dosage adjustment of the antidiabetic drug).
No products indexed under this heading.

Chlorthalidone (Concurrent use with other antihypertensives may cause an additive effect or potentiation). Products include:
Clorpres 2344

Cholestyramine (Absorption of hydrochlorothiazide is impaired in the presence of anionic exchange resins. Single doses of cholestyramine bind the hydrochlorothiazide and reduce its absorption from the gastrointestinal tract by up to 85%).
No products indexed under this heading.

Ciclesonide (Intensified electrolyte depletion, particularly hypokalemia with concurrent use).
No products indexed under this heading.

Cisatracurium Besylate (Concurrent use may increase the responsiveness to the muscle relaxant). Products include:
Nimbex 503

Clarithromycin (Pgp (MDR1/Mdr1a/1b) was found to be the major efflux system involved in absorption and disposition of aliskiren in preclinical studies. The potential for drug interactions at the Pgp site will likely depend on the degree of inhibition of this transporter). Products include:
Biaxin/Biaxin XL 412

Clonidine (Concurrent use with other antihypertensives may cause an additive effect or potentiation). Products include:
Catapres-TTS 884

Clonidine Hydrochloride (Concurrent use with other antihypertensives may cause an additive effect or potentiation). Products include:
Clorpres 2344

Codeine Phosphate (Potentiation of orthostatic hypotension may occur with concurrent use). Products include:
Tylenol with Codeine 2691

Codeine Sulfate (Potentiation of orthostatic hypotension may occur with concurrent use).
No products indexed under this heading.

Colestipol (Absorption of hydrochlorothiazide is impaired in the presence of anionic exchange resins. Single doses of colestipol resins bind the hydrochlorothiazide and reduce its absorption from the gastrointestinal tract by up to 43%).
No products indexed under this heading.

Colestipol Hydrochloride (Absorption of hydrochlorothiazide is impaired in the presence of anionic exchange resins. Single doses of colestipol resins bind the hydrochlorothiazide and reduce its absorption from the gastrointestinal tract by up to 43%).
No products indexed under this heading.

Cortisone Acetate (Intensified electrolyte depletion, particularly hypokalemia with concurrent use).
No products indexed under this heading.

Cyclosporine (Co-administration of 200 mg and 600 mg cyclosporine, a potent Pgp inhibitor, with 75 mg aliskiren resulted in an approximate 2.5-fold increase in C_{max} and 5-fold

IMPORTANT NOTE: Always consult each drug listing in the patient's regimen for possible interactions.

increase in AUC of aliskiren. Concomitant use of aliskiren with cyclosporine is not recommended). Products include:

Deserpidine (Concurrent use with other antihypertensives may cause an additive effect or potentiation).
No products indexed under this heading.

Desoximetasone (Intensified electrolyte depletion, particularly hypokalemia with concurrent use).
No products indexed under this heading.

Dexamethasone (Intensified electrolyte depletion, particularly hypokalemia with concurrent use). Products include:

Dexamethasone Acetate (Intensified electrolyte depletion, particularly hypokalemia with concurrent use).
No products indexed under this heading.

Dexamethasone Phosphate (Intensified electrolyte depletion, particularly hypokalemia with concurrent use).
No products indexed under this heading.

Dexamethasone Sodium (Intensified electrolyte depletion, particularly hypokalemia with concurrent use).
No products indexed under this heading.

Dexamethasone Sodium Phosphate (Intensified electrolyte depletion, particularly hypokalemia with concurrent use).
No products indexed under this heading.

Dexamethasone Sodium Phosphate Injection (Intensified electrolyte depletion, particularly hypokalemia with concurrent use).
No products indexed under this heading.

Dezocine (Potentiation of orthostatic hypotension may occur with concurrent use).
No products indexed under this heading.

Diazoxide (Concurrent use with other antihypertensives may cause an additive effect or potentiation). Products include:

Diclofenac Epolamine (In some patients, the administration of a nonsteroidal anti-inflammatory agent can reduce the diuretic, natriuretic, and antihypertensive effects of thiazide diuretics. Therefore, when Tekturna HCT and nonsteroidal anti-inflammatory agents are used concomitantly, the patient should be observed closely to determine if the desired effect of the diuretic is obtained). Products include:

Diclofenac Potassium (In some patients, the administration of a nonsteroidal anti-inflammatory agent can reduce the diuretic, natriuretic, and antihypertensive effects of thiazide diuretics. Therefore, when Tekturna HCT and nonsteroidal anti-inflammatory agents are used concomitantly, the patient should be observed closely to determine if the desired effect of the diuretic is obtained).
No products indexed under this heading.

Diclofenac Sodium (In some patients, the administration of a nonsteroidal anti-inflammatory agent can reduce the diuretic, natriuretic, and antihypertensive effects of thiazide diuretics. Therefore, when Tekturna HCT and nonsteroidal anti-inflammatory agents are used concomitantly, the patient should be observed closely to determine if the desired effect of the diuretic is obtained).
No products indexed under this heading.

Diflorasone Diacetate (Intensified electrolyte depletion, particularly hypokalemia with concurrent use).
No products indexed under this heading.

Digoxin (Pgp (MDR1/Mdr1a/1b) was found to be the major efflux system involved in absorption and disposition of aliskiren in preclinical studies. The potential for drug interactions at the Pgp site will likely depend on the degree of inhibition of this transporter). Products include:

Dihydrocodeine Bitartrate (Potentiation of orthostatic hypotension may occur with concurrent use).
No products indexed under this heading.

Dihydrocodeinone Bitartrate (Potentiation of orthostatic hypotension may occur with concurrent use).
No products indexed under this heading.

Diltiazem Hydrochloride (Concurrent use with other antihypertensives may cause an additive effect or potentiation). Products include:

Diltiazem Maleate (Concurrent use with other antihypertensives may cause an additive effect or potentiation).
No products indexed under this heading.

Dirithromycin (Pgp (MDR1/Mdr1a/1b) was found to be the major efflux system involved in absorption and disposition of aliskiren in preclinical studies. The potential for drug interactions at the Pgp site will likely depend on the degree of inhibition of this transporter).
No products indexed under this heading.

Doxacurium Chloride (Concurrent use may increase the responsiveness to the muscle relaxant).
No products indexed under this heading.

Doxazosin Mesylate (Concurrent use with other antihypertensives may cause an additive effect or potentiation).
No products indexed under this heading.

d-Tubocurarine (Concurrent use may increase the responsiveness to the muscle relaxant).
No products indexed under this heading.

Elacridar (Pgp (MDR1/Mdr1a/1b) was found to be the major efflux system involved in absorption and disposition of aliskiren in preclinical studies. The potential for drug interactions at the Pgp site will likely depend on the degree of inhibition of this transporter).
No products indexed under this heading.

Enalapril Maleate (Concurrent use with other antihypertensives may cause an additive effect or potentiation).
No products indexed under this heading.

Enalaprilat (Concurrent use with other antihypertensives may cause an additive effect or potentiation).
No products indexed under this heading.

Eprosartan Mesylate (Concurrent use with other antihypertensives may cause an additive effect or potentiation). Products include:

Erythromycin (Pgp (MDR1/Mdr1a/1b) was found to be the major efflux system involved in absorption and disposition of aliskiren in preclinical studies. The potential for drug interactions at the Pgp site will likely depend on the degree of inhibition of this transporter).
No products indexed under this heading.

Erythromycin, Topical (Pgp (MDR1/Mdr1a/1b) was found to be the major efflux system involved in absorption and disposition of aliskiren in preclinical studies. The potential for drug interactions at the Pgp site will likely depend on the degree of inhibition of this transporter).
No products indexed under this heading.

Erythromycin Estolate (Pgp (MDR1/Mdr1a/1b) was found to be the major efflux system involved in absorption and disposition of aliskiren in preclinical studies. The potential for drug interactions at the Pgp site will likely depend on the degree of inhibition of this transporter).
No products indexed under this heading.

Erythromycin Ethylsuccinate (Pgp (MDR1/Mdr1a/1b) was found to be the major efflux system involved in absorption and disposition of aliskiren in preclinical studies. The potential for drug interactions at the Pgp site will likely depend on the degree of inhibition of this transporter). Products include:

Erythromycin Gluceptate (Pgp (MDR1/Mdr1a/1b) was found to be the major efflux system involved in absorption and disposition of aliskiren in preclinical studies. The potential for drug interactions at the Pgp site will likely depend on the degree of inhibition of this transporter).
No products indexed under this heading.

Erythromycin Lactobionate (Pgp (MDR1/Mdr1a/1b) was found to be the major efflux system involved in absorption and disposition of aliskiren in preclinical studies. The potential for drug interactions at the Pgp site will likely depend on the degree of inhibition of this transporter).
No products indexed under this heading.

Erythromycin Stearate (Pgp (MDR1/Mdr1a/1b) was found to be the major efflux system involved in absorption and disposition of aliskiren in preclinical studies. The potential for drug interactions at the Pgp site will likely depend on the degree of inhibition of this transporter).
No products indexed under this heading.

Esmolol Hydrochloride (Concurrent use with other antihypertensives may cause an additive effect or potentiation).
No products indexed under this heading.

Ethanol (Potentiation of orthostatic hypotension may occur with concurrent use).
No products indexed under this heading.

Ethyl Alcohol (Potentiation of orthostatic hypotension may occur with concurrent use).
No products indexed under this heading.

Etodolac (In some patients, the administration of a nonsteroidal anti-inflammatory agent can reduce the diuretic, natriuretic, and antihypertensive effects of thiazide diuretics. Therefore, when Tekturna HCT and nonsteroidal anti-inflammatory agents are used concomitantly, the patient should be observed closely to determine if the desired effect of the diuretic is obtained).
No products indexed under this heading.

Felodipine (Concurrent use with other antihypertensives may cause an additive effect or potentiation).
No products indexed under this heading.

Fenoprofen Calcium (In some patients, the administration of a nonsteroidal anti-inflammatory agent can reduce the diuretic, natriuretic, and antihypertensive effects of thiazide diuretics. Therefore, when Tekturna HCT and nonsteroidal anti-inflammatory agents are used concomitantly, the patient should be observed closely to determine if the desired effect of the diuretic is obtained).
No products indexed under this heading.

Fentanyl (Potentiation of orthostatic hypotension may occur with concurrent use). Products include:

Fentanyl Citrate (Potentiation of orthostatic hypotension may occur with concurrent use). Products include:

Fludrocortisone Acetate (Intensified electrolyte depletion, particularly hypokalemia with concurrent use).
No products indexed under this heading.

Flumethasone Pivalate (Intensified electrolyte depletion, particularly hypokalemia with concurrent use).
No products indexed under this heading.

Flunisolide Hemihydrate (Intensified electrolyte depletion, particularly hypokalemia with concurrent use).
No products indexed under this heading.

Flurbiprofen (In some patients, the administration of a nonsteroidal anti-inflammatory agent can reduce the diuretic, natriuretic, and antihypertensive effects of thiazide diuretics. Therefore, when Tekturna HCT and nonsteroidal anti-inflammatory agents are used concomitantly, the patient should be observed closely to determine if the desired effect of the diuretic is obtained).
No products indexed under this heading.

Fluticasone Furoate (Intensified electrolyte depletion, particularly hypokalemia with concurrent use). Products include:

Fluticasone Propionate (Intensified electrolyte depletion, particularly hypokalemia with concurrent use). Products include:

Fosinopril Sodium (Concurrent use with other antihypertensives may cause an additive effect or potentiation).
No products indexed under this heading.

Furosemide (When aliskiren was co-administered with furosemide, the AUC and C_{max} of furosemide were reduced by about 30% and 50%, respectively. Patients receiving furosemide could find its effect diminished after starting aliskiren). Products include:

Gallamine (Concurrent use may increase the responsiveness to the muscle relaxant).
No products indexed under this heading.

Gallamine Triethiodide (Concurrent use may increase the responsiveness to the muscle relaxant).
No products indexed under this heading.

Glibenclamide (Concurrent use may require dosage adjustment of the antidiabetic drug).
No products indexed under this heading.

Glimepiride (Concurrent use may require dosage adjustment of the antidiabetic drug). Products include:

IMPORTANT NOTE: Always consult each drug listing in the patient's regimen for possible interactions.

Mefenamic Acid (In some patients, the administration of a nonsteroidal anti-inflammatory agent can reduce the diuretic, natriuretic, and antihypertensive effects of thiazide diuretics. Therefore, when Tekturna HCT and nonsteroidal anti-inflammatory agents are used concomitantly, the patient should be observed closely to determine if the desired effect of the diuretic is obtained).

No products indexed under this heading.

Meloxicam (In some patients, the administration of a nonsteroidal anti-inflammatory agent can reduce the diuretic, natriuretic, and antihypertensive effects of thiazide diuretics. Therefore, when Tekturna HCT and nonsteroidal anti-inflammatory agents are used concomitantly, the patient should be observed closely to determine if the desired effect of the diuretic is obtained).

No products indexed under this heading.

Meperidine Hydrochloride (Potentiation of orthostatic hypotension may occur with concurrent use).

No products indexed under this heading.

Mephobarbital (Potentiation of orthostatic hypotension may occur with concurrent use).

No products indexed under this heading.

Metformin Hydrochloride (Concurrent use may require dosage adjustment of the antidiabetic drug). Products include:

ActoPlus 3338
Avandamet 1345
Janumet 2188

Methadone Hydrochloride (Potentiation of orthostatic hypotension may occur with concurrent use).

No products indexed under this heading.

Methyclothiazide (Concurrent use with other antihypertensives may cause an additive effect or potentiation).

No products indexed under this heading.

Methyldopa (Concurrent use with other antihypertensives may cause an additive effect or potentiation).

No products indexed under this heading.

Methyldopate Hydrochloride (Concurrent use with other antihypertensives may cause an additive effect or potentiation).

No products indexed under this heading.

Methylprednisolone (Intensified electrolyte depletion, particularly hypokalemia with concurrent use).

No products indexed under this heading.

Methylprednisolone Acetate (Intensified electrolyte depletion, particularly hypokalemia with concurrent use).

No products indexed under this heading.

Methylprednisolone Sodium Succinate (Intensified electrolyte depletion, particularly hypokalemia with concurrent use).

No products indexed under this heading.

Metocurine Iodide (Concurrent use may increase the responsiveness to the muscle relaxant).

No products indexed under this heading.

Metolazone (Concurrent use with other antihypertensives may cause an additive effect or potentiation).

No products indexed under this heading.

Metoprolol Succinate (Concurrent use with other antihypertensives may cause an additive effect or potentiation). Products include:

Toprol XL 732

Metoprolol Tartrate (Concurrent use with other antihypertensives may cause an additive effect or potentiation).

No products indexed under this heading.

Metyrosine (Concurrent use with other antihypertensives may cause an additive effect or potentiation).

No products indexed under this heading.

Mibefradil Dihydrochloride (Concurrent use with other antihypertensives may cause an additive effect or potentiation).

No products indexed under this heading.

Miglitol (Concurrent use may require dosage adjustment of the antidiabetic drug).

No products indexed under this heading.

Minoxidil (Concurrent use with other antihypertensives may cause an additive effect or potentiation).

No products indexed under this heading.

Mivacurium Chloride (Concurrent use may increase the responsiveness to the muscle relaxant).

No products indexed under this heading.

Moexipril Hydrochloride (Concurrent use with other antihypertensives may cause an additive effect or potentiation).

No products indexed under this heading.

Mometasone Furoate (Intensified electrolyte depletion, particularly hypokalemia with concurrent use). Products include:

Asmanex 3058
Elocon Cream 3111
Elocon Lotion 3112
Elocon Ointment 3114

Mometasone Furoate Monohydrate (Intensified electrolyte depletion, particularly hypokalemia with concurrent use). Products include:

Nasonex 3166

Morphine Sulfate (Potentiation of orthostatic hypotension may occur with concurrent use). Products include:

Avinza 1822
Embeda 1831
MS Contin 2803

Morphine Sulfate, Liposomal (Potentiation of orthostatic hypotension may occur with concurrent use).

No products indexed under this heading.

Nabumetone (In some patients, the administration of a nonsteroidal anti-inflammatory agent can reduce the diuretic, natriuretic, and antihypertensive effects of thiazide diuretics. Therefore, when Tekturna HCT and nonsteroidal anti-inflammatory agents are used concomitantly, the patient should be observed closely to determine if the desired effect of the diuretic is obtained).

No products indexed under this heading.

Nadolol (Concurrent use with other antihypertensives may cause an additive effect or potentiation). Products include:

Nadolol 2359

Naproxen (In some patients, the administration of a nonsteroidal anti-inflammatory agent can reduce the diuretic, natriuretic, and antihypertensive effects of thiazide diuretics. Therefore, when Tekturna HCT and nonsteroidal anti-inflammatory agents are used concomitantly, the patient should be observed closely to determine if the desired effect of the diuretic is obtained). Products include:

EC-Naprosyn 2850
Naprosyn 2850
Anaprox/Naprosyn 2850

Naproxen Sodium (In some patients, the administration of a nonsteroidal anti-inflammatory agent can reduce the diuretic, natriuretic, and antihypertensive effects of thiazide diuretics. Therefore, when Tekturna HCT and nonsteroidal anti-inflammatory agents are used concomitantly, the patient should be

observed closely to determine if the desired effect of the diuretic is obtained). Products include:

Anaprox 2850
Anaprox DS 2850
Treximet 1681

Nateglinide (Concurrent use may require dosage adjustment of the antidiabetic drug).

No products indexed under this heading.

Nebivolol (Concurrent use with other antihypertensives may cause an additive effect or potentiation). Products include:

Bystolic 1147

Nicardipine Hydrochloride (Concurrent use with other antihypertensives may cause an additive effect or potentiation).

No products indexed under this heading.

Nifedipine (Concurrent use with other antihypertensives may cause an additive effect or potentiation).

No products indexed under this heading.

Nisoldipine (Concurrent use with other antihypertensives may cause an additive effect or potentiation).

No products indexed under this heading.

Nitroglycerin (Concurrent use with other antihypertensives may cause an additive effect or potentiation). Products include:

Nitro-Dur 3170
Nitrolingual 3266

Norepinephrine Bitartrate (Possible decreased response to pressor amines, but not sufficient to preclude their use).

No products indexed under this heading.

Norepinephrine Hydrochloride (Possible decreased response to pressor amines, but not sufficient to preclude their use).

No products indexed under this heading.

Oxaprozin (In some patients, the administration of a nonsteroidal anti-inflammatory agent can reduce the diuretic, natriuretic, and antihypertensive effects of thiazide diuretics. Therefore, when Tekturna HCT and nonsteroidal anti-inflammatory agents are used concomitantly, the patient should be observed closely to determine if the desired effect of the diuretic is obtained).

No products indexed under this heading.

Oxycodone Hydrochloride (Potentiation of orthostatic hypotension may occur with concurrent use). Products include:

OxyContin 2807
Percocet 1121
Percodan 1124

Oxycodone Terephthalate (Potentiation of orthostatic hypotension may occur with concurrent use).

No products indexed under this heading.

Oxymorphone Hydrochloride (Potentiation of orthostatic hypotension may occur with concurrent use). Products include:

Opana 1110
Opana ER 1114

Pancuronium Bromide (Concurrent use may increase the responsiveness to the muscle relaxant).

No products indexed under this heading.

Penbutolol Sulfate (Concurrent use with other antihypertensives may cause an additive effect or potentiation).

No products indexed under this heading.

Pentobarbital (Potentiation of orthostatic hypotension may occur with concurrent use).

No products indexed under this heading.

Pentobarbital Sodium (Potentiation of orthostatic hypotension may occur with concurrent use). Products include:

Nembutal 2012

Perindopril Erbumine (Concurrent use with other antihypertensives may cause an additive effect or potentiation).

No products indexed under this heading.

Phenobarbital (Potentiation of orthostatic hypotension may occur with concurrent use). Products include:

Donnatal 2711

Phenobarbital Sodium (Potentiation of orthostatic hypotension may occur with concurrent use).

No products indexed under this heading.

Phenoxybenzamine Hydrochloride (Concurrent use with other antihypertensives may cause an additive effect or potentiation). Products include:

Dibenzyline 3495

Phentolamine Mesylate (Concurrent use with other antihypertensives may cause an additive effect or potentiation).

No products indexed under this heading.

Phenylbutazone (In some patients, the administration of a nonsteroidal anti-inflammatory agent can reduce the diuretic, natriuretic, and antihypertensive effects of thiazide diuretics. Therefore, when Tekturna HCT and nonsteroidal anti-inflammatory agents are used concomitantly, the patient should be observed closely to determine if the desired effect of the diuretic is obtained).

No products indexed under this heading.

Pindolol (Concurrent use with other antihypertensives may cause an additive effect or potentiation).

No products indexed under this heading.

Pioglitazone Hydrochloride (Concurrent use may require dosage adjustment of the antidiabetic drug). Products include:

ActoPlus 3338
Actos 3345
Duetact 3354

Pipecuronium Bromide (Concurrent use may increase the responsiveness to the muscle relaxant).

No products indexed under this heading.

Piroxicam (In some patients, the administration of a nonsteroidal anti-inflammatory agent can reduce the diuretic, natriuretic, and antihypertensive effects of thiazide diuretics. Therefore, when Tekturna HCT and nonsteroidal anti-inflammatory agents are used concomitantly, the patient should be observed closely to determine if the desired effect of the diuretic is obtained).

No products indexed under this heading.

Polythiazide (Concurrent use with other antihypertensives may cause an additive effect or potentiation).

No products indexed under this heading.

Potassium Acid Phosphate (Based on experience with the use of other substances that affect the renin-angiotensin system (RAS), concomitant use of Tekturna HCT with potassium supplements or salt substitutes containing potassium, or other drugs that increase potassium may lead to increases in serum potassium. If concomitant use is considered necessary, caution should be exercised). Products include:

K-Phos Original 874

Potassium Bicarbonate (Based on experience with the use of other substances that affect the renin-angiotensin system (RAS), concomitant use of Tekturna HCT with potassium supplements or salt substitutes containing potassium, or other drugs that increase potassium may lead to increases in serum potassium. If concomitant use is considered necessary, caution should be exercised).

No products indexed under this heading.

Potassium Chloride (Based on experience with the use of other substances that affect the renin-angiotensin system (RAS), concomitant use of Tekturna HCT with potassium supplements or salt substitutes containing potassium, or other drugs that increase potassium may lead to increases in serum potassium. If concomitant use is considered necessary, caution should be exercised). Products include:

Potassium Citrate (Based on experience with the use of other substances that affect the renin-angiotensin system (RAS), concomitant use of Tekturna HCT with potassium supplements or salt substitutes containing potassium, or other drugs that increase potassium may lead to increases in serum potassium. If concomitant use is considered necessary, caution should be exercised). Products include:

Potassium Gluconate (Based on experience with the use of other substances that affect the renin-angiotensin system (RAS), concomitant use of Tekturna HCT with potassium supplements or salt substitutes containing potassium, or other drugs that increase potassium may lead to increases in serum potassium. If concomitant use is considered necessary, caution should be exercised).
No products indexed under this heading.

Potassium Phosphate (Based on experience with the use of other substances that affect the renin-angiotensin system (RAS), concomitant use of Tekturna HCT with potassium supplements or salt substitutes containing potassium, or other drugs that increase potassium may lead to increases in serum potassium. If concomitant use is considered necessary, caution should be exercised). Products include:

Prazosin Hydrochloride (Concurrent use with other antihypertensives may cause an additive effect or potentiation).
No products indexed under this heading.

Prednisolone (Intensified electrolyte depletion, particularly hypokalemia with concurrent use).
No products indexed under this heading.

Prednisolone Acetate (Intensified electrolyte depletion, particularly hypokalemia with concurrent use). Products include:

Prednisolone Sodium Phosphate (Intensified electrolyte depletion, particularly hypokalemia with concurrent use).
No products indexed under this heading.

Prednisolone Tebutate (Intensified electrolyte depletion, particularly hypokalemia with concurrent use).
No products indexed under this heading.

Prednisone (Intensified electrolyte depletion, particularly hypokalemia with concurrent use).
No products indexed under this heading.

Prednisone sodium phosphate (Intensified electrolyte depletion, particularly hypokalemia with concurrent use).
No products indexed under this heading.

Propoxyphene Hydrochloride (Potentiation of orthostatic hypotension may occur with concurrent use).
No products indexed under this heading.

Propoxyphene Napsylate (Potentiation of orthostatic hypotension may occur with concurrent use).
No products indexed under this heading.

Propranolol Hydrochloride (Concurrent use with other antihypertensives may cause an additive effect or potentiation). Products include:

Quinapril Hydrochloride (Concurrent use with other antihypertensives may cause an additive effect or potentiation).
No products indexed under this heading.

Quinidine (Pgp (MDR1/Mdr1a/1b) was found to be the major efflux system involved in absorption and disposition of aliskiren in preclinical studies. The potential for drug interactions at the Pgp site will likely depend on the degree of inhibition of this transporter).
No products indexed under this heading.

Quinidine Gluconate (Pgp (MDR1/Mdr1a/1b) was found to be the major efflux system involved in absorption and disposition of aliskiren in preclinical studies. The potential for drug interactions at the Pgp site will likely depend on the degree of inhibition of this transporter).
No products indexed under this heading.

Quinidine Hydrochloride (Pgp (MDR1/Mdr1a/1b) was found to be the major efflux system involved in absorption and disposition of aliskiren in preclinical studies. The potential for drug interactions at the Pgp site will likely depend on the degree of inhibition of this transporter).
No products indexed under this heading.

Quinidine Polygalacturonate (Pgp (MDR1/Mdr1a/1b) was found to be the major efflux system involved in absorption and disposition of aliskiren in preclinical studies. The potential for drug interactions at the Pgp site will likely depend on the degree of inhibition of this transporter).
No products indexed under this heading.

Quinidine Sulfate (Pgp (MDR1/Mdr1a/1b) was found to be the major efflux system involved in absorption and disposition of aliskiren in preclinical studies. The potential for drug interactions at the Pgp site will likely depend on the degree of inhibition of this transporter).
No products indexed under this heading.

Ramipril (Concurrent use with other antihypertensives may cause an additive effect or potentiation).
No products indexed under this heading.

Rapacuronium Bromide (Concurrent use may increase the responsiveness to the muscle relaxant).
No products indexed under this heading.

Rauwolfia Serpentina (Concurrent use with other antihypertensives may cause an additive effect or potentiation).
No products indexed under this heading.

Remifentanil Hydrochloride (Potentiation of orthostatic hypotension may occur with concurrent use).
No products indexed under this heading.

Repaglinide (Concurrent use may require dosage adjustment of the antidiabetic drug).
No products indexed under this heading.

Rescinnamine (Concurrent use with other antihypertensives may cause an additive effect or potentiation).
No products indexed under this heading.

Reserpine (Concurrent use with other antihypertensives may cause an additive effect or potentiation).
No products indexed under this heading.

Ritonavir (Pgp (MDR1/Mdr1a/1b) was found to be the major efflux system involved in absorption and disposition of aliskiren in preclinical studies. The potential for drug interactions at the Pgp site will likely depend on the degree of inhibition of this transporter). Products include:

Rocuronium Bromide (Concurrent use may increase the responsiveness to the muscle relaxant). Products include:

Rofecoxib (In some patients, the administration of a nonsteroidal anti-inflammatory agent can reduce the diuretic, natriuretic, and antihypertensive effects of thiazide diuretics. Therefore, when Tekturna HCT and nonsteroidal anti-inflammatory agents are used concomitantly, the patient should be observed closely to determine if the desired effect of the diuretic is obtained).
No products indexed under this heading.

Rosiglitazone Maleate (Concurrent use may require dosage adjustment of the antidiabetic drug). Products include:

Secobarbital Sodium (Potentiation of orthostatic hypotension may occur with concurrent use).
No products indexed under this heading.

Sitagliptin Phosphate (Concurrent use may require dosage adjustment of the antidiabetic drug). Products include:

Sodium Butabarbital (Potentiation of orthostatic hypotension may occur with concurrent use).
No products indexed under this heading.

Sodium Nitroprusside (Concurrent use with other antihypertensives may cause an additive effect or potentiation).
No products indexed under this heading.

Sodium Pentobarbital (Potentiation of orthostatic hypotension may occur with concurrent use).
No products indexed under this heading.

Sotalol Hydrochloride (Concurrent use with other antihypertensives may cause an additive effect or potentiation).
No products indexed under this heading.

Spirapril Hydrochloride (Concurrent use with other antihypertensives may cause an additive effect or potentiation).
No products indexed under this heading.

Spironolactone (Based on experience with the use of other substances that affect the renin-angiotensin system (RAS), concomitant use of Tekturna HCT with potassium-sparing diuretics may lead to increases in serum potassium. If concomitant use is considered necessary, caution should be exercised).
No products indexed under this heading.

Sufentanil Citrate (Potentiation of orthostatic hypotension may occur with concurrent use).
No products indexed under this heading.

Sulindac (In some patients, the administration of a nonsteroidal anti-inflammatory agent can reduce the diuretic, natriuretic, and antihypertensive effects of thiazide diuretics. Therefore, when Tekturna HCT and nonsteroidal anti-inflammatory agents are used concomitantly, the patient should be observed closely to determine if the desired effect of the diuretic is obtained). Products include:

Tamoxifen Citrate (Pgp (MDR1/Mdr1a/1b) was found to be the major efflux system involved in absorption and disposition of aliskiren in preclinical studies. The potential for drug interactions at the Pgp site will likely depend on the degree of inhibition of this transporter).
No products indexed under this heading.

Telmisartan (Concurrent use with other antihypertensives may cause an additive effect or potentiation). Products include:

Terazosin Hydrochloride (Concurrent use with other antihypertensives may cause an additive effect or potentiation).
No products indexed under this heading.

Thiamylal Sodium (Potentiation of orthostatic hypotension may occur with concurrent use).
No products indexed under this heading.

Timolol Maleate (Concurrent use with other antihypertensives may cause an additive effect or potentiation). Products include:

Tolazamide (Concurrent use may require dosage adjustment of the antidiabetic drug).
No products indexed under this heading.

Tolbutamide (Concurrent use may require dosage adjustment of the antidiabetic drug).
No products indexed under this heading.

Tolmetin Sodium (In some patients, the administration of a nonsteroidal anti-inflammatory agent can reduce the diuretic, natriuretic, and antihypertensive effects of thiazide diuretics. Therefore, when Tekturna HCT and nonsteroidal anti-inflammatory agents are used concomitantly, the patient should be observed closely to determine if the desired effect of the diuretic is obtained).
No products indexed under this heading.

Torsemide (Concurrent use with other antihypertensives may cause an additive effect or potentiation).
No products indexed under this heading.

Trandolapril (Concurrent use with other antihypertensives may cause an additive effect or potentiation). Products include:

Triamcinolone (Intensified electrolyte depletion, particularly hypokalemia with concurrent use).
No products indexed under this heading.

Triamcinolone Acetonide (Intensified electrolyte depletion, particularly hypokalemia with concurrent use). Products include:

Triamcinolone Diacetate (Intensified electrolyte depletion, particularly hypokalemia with concurrent use).
No products indexed under this heading.

Triamcinolone Hexacetonide (Intensified electrolyte depletion, particularly hypokalemia with concurrent use).
No products indexed under this heading.

Triamterene (Based on experience with the use of other substances that affect the renin-angiotensin system (RAS), concomitant use of Tekturna HCT with potassium-sparing diuretics may lead to increases in serum potassium. If concomitant use is considered necessary, caution should be exercised). Products include:

Trimethaphan Camsylate (Concurrent use with other antihypertensives may cause an additive effect or potentiation).
No products indexed under this heading.

IMPORTANT NOTE: Always consult each drug listing in the patient's regimen for possible interactions.

Troglitazone (Concurrent use may require dosage adjustment of the antidiabetic drug).
No products indexed under this heading.

Troleandomycin (Pgp (MDR1/Mdr1a/1b) was found to be the major efflux system involved in absorption and disposition of aliskiren in preclinical studies. The potential for drug interactions at the Pgp site will likely depend on the degree of inhibition of this transporter).
No products indexed under this heading.

Tubocurarine Chloride (Concurrent use may increase the responsiveness to tubocurarine).
No products indexed under this heading.

Valdecoxib (In some patients, the administration of a nonsteroidal anti-inflammatory agent can reduce the diuretic, natriuretic, and antihypertensive effects of thiazide diuretics. Therefore, when Tekturna HCT and nonsteroidal anti-inflammatory agents are used concomitantly, the patient should be observed closely to determine if the desired effect of the diuretic is obtained).
No products indexed under this heading.

Valsartan (Concurrent use with other antihypertensives may cause an additive effect or potentiation). Products include:
Diovan ... 2413
Diovan HCT ... 2419
Exforge ... 2443
Exforge HCT ... 2449
Valturna ... 3637

Vecuronium Bromide (Concurrent use may increase the responsiveness to the muscle relaxant).
No products indexed under this heading.

Verapamil Hydrochloride (Concurrent use with other antihypertensives may cause an additive effect or potentiation). Products include:
Tarka ... 534

Food Interactions

Alcohol (Potentiation of orthostatic hypotension may occur with concurrent use).

Beer, reduced-alcohol (Potentiation of orthostatic hypotension may occur with concurrent use).

Beer, unspecified (Potentiation of orthostatic hypotension may occur with concurrent use).

Wine, Chianti (Potentiation of orthostatic hypotension may occur with concurrent use).

Wine, Red (Potentiation of orthostatic hypotension may occur with concurrent use).

Wine, unspecified (Potentiation of orthostatic hypotension may occur with concurrent use).

Wine products (Potentiation of orthostatic hypotension may occur with concurrent use).

TEMODAR CAPSULES

(Temozolomide) ... 3230
May interact with corticosteroids, phenytoin, valproate, and certain other agents. Compounds in these categories include:

Alclometasone Dipropionate (All patients receiving temozolomide, particularly patients receiving steroids, should be observed closely for the development of PCP regardless of the regimen).
No products indexed under this heading.

Beclomethasone Dipropionate (All patients receiving temozolomide, particularly patients receiving steroids, should be observed closely for the development of PCP regardless of the regimen). Products include:
Qvar ... 3398

Beclomethasone Dipropionate Monohydrate (All patients receiving temozolomide, particularly patients receiving steroids, should be observed closely for the development of PCP regardless of the regimen). Products include:
Beconase AQ ... 1386

Betamethasone (All patients receiving temozolomide, particularly patients receiving steroids, should be observed closely for the development of PCP regardless of the regimen).
No products indexed under this heading.

Betamethasone Acetate (All patients receiving temozolomide, particularly patients receiving steroids, should be observed closely for the development of PCP regardless of the regimen).
No products indexed under this heading.

Betamethasone Benzoate (All patients receiving temozolomide, particularly patients receiving steroids, should be observed closely for the development of PCP regardless of the regimen).
No products indexed under this heading.

Betamethasone Dipropionate (All patients receiving temozolomide, particularly patients receiving steroids, should be observed closely for the development of PCP regardless of the regimen). Products include:
Diprolene Lotion 0.05% ... 3108
Diprolene Ointment 0.05% ... 3109
Diprolene AF Cream 0.05% ... 3107
Lotrisone ... 3163

Betamethasone Sodium Phosphate (All patients receiving temozolomide, particularly patients receiving steroids, should be observed closely for the development of PCP regardless of the regimen).
No products indexed under this heading.

Betamethasone Valerate (All patients receiving temozolomide, particularly patients receiving steroids, should be observed closely for the development of PCP regardless of the regimen). Products include:
Luxíq ... 3321

Budesonide (All patients receiving temozolomide, particularly patients receiving steroids, should be observed closely for the development of PCP regardless of the regimen). Products include:
Pulmicort Flexhaler ... 714
Symbicort 80/4.5 ... 720
Symbicort 160/4.5 ... 720

Carbamazepine (Temozolomide may cause myelosuppression, including prolonged pancytopenia, which may result in aplastic anemia. Exposure to concomitant medications associated with aplastic anemia, including carbamazepine, complicates assessment). Products include:
Carbatrol ... 3280
Equetro ... 3477

Ciclesonide (All patients receiving temozolomide, particularly patients receiving steroids, should be observed closely for the development of PCP regardless of the regimen).
No products indexed under this heading.

Cortisone Acetate (All patients receiving temozolomide, particularly patients receiving steroids, should be observed closely for the development of PCP regardless of the regimen).
No products indexed under this heading.

Desoximetasone (All patients receiving temozolomide, particularly patients receiving steroids, should be observed closely for the development of PCP regardless of the regimen).
No products indexed under this heading.

Dexamethasone (All patients receiving temozolomide, particularly patients receiving steroids, should be observed closely for the development of PCP regardless of the regimen). Products include:
Ciprodex ... 583
Ozurdex ... ⊙223
Tobramycin and Dexamethasone Ophthalmic Suspension ... ⊙251

Dexamethasone Acetate (All patients receiving temozolomide, particularly patients receiving steroids, should be observed closely for the development of PCP regardless of the regimen).
No products indexed under this heading.

Dexamethasone Phosphate (All patients receiving temozolomide, particularly patients receiving steroids, should be observed closely for the development of PCP regardless of the regimen).
No products indexed under this heading.

Dexamethasone Sodium (All patients receiving temozolomide, particularly patients receiving steroids, should be observed closely for the development of PCP regardless of the regimen).
No products indexed under this heading.

Dexamethasone Sodium Phosphate (All patients receiving temozolomide, particularly patients receiving steroids, should be observed closely for the development of PCP regardless of the regimen).
No products indexed under this heading.

Dexamethasone Sodium Phosphate Injection (All patients receiving temozolomide, particularly patients receiving steroids, should be observed closely for the development of PCP regardless of the regimen).
No products indexed under this heading.

Diflorasone Diacetate (All patients receiving temozolomide, particularly patients receiving steroids, should be observed closely for the development of PCP regardless of the regimen).
No products indexed under this heading.

Divalproex Sodium (Co-administration of temozolomide with valproic acid may decreases oral clearance of temozolomide by about 5%. The clinical implication of this effect is not known). Products include:
Depakote ER ... 426

Fat (Temozolomide is rapidly and completely absorbed after oral administration with a peak plasma concentration (C_{max}) achieved in a median T_{max} of 1 hour. Food reduces the rate and extent of temozolomide absorption. Mean peak plasma concentration and AUC decreased by 32% and 9%, respectively, and median T_{max} increased by 2-fold (from 1 to 2.25 hours) when temozolomide was administered after a modified high-fat breakfast).
No products indexed under this heading.

Fludrocortisone Acetate (All patients receiving temozolomide, particularly patients receiving steroids, should be observed closely for the development of PCP regardless of the regimen).
No products indexed under this heading.

Flumethasone Pivalate (All patients receiving temozolomide, particularly patients receiving steroids, should be observed closely for the development of PCP regardless of the regimen).
No products indexed under this heading.

Flunisolide Hemihydrate (All patients receiving temozolomide, particularly patients receiving steroids, should be observed closely for the development of PCP regardless of the regimen).
No products indexed under this heading.

Fluticasone Furoate (All patients receiving temozolomide, particularly patients receiving steroids, should be observed closely for the development of PCP regardless of the regimen). Products include:
Veramyst ... 1713

Fluticasone Propionate (All patients receiving temozolomide, particularly patients receiving steroids, should be observed closely for the development of PCP regardless of the regimen). Products include:
Advair 100/50 ... 1275
Advair 250/50 ... 1275
Advair 500/50 ... 1275
Advair HFA 45/21 ... 1288
Advair HFA 115/21 ... 1288
Advair HFA 230/21 ... 1288
Flonase ... 1459
Flovent Diskus ... 1463
Flovent HFA ... 1470

Fosphenytoin (Temozolomide may cause myelosuppression, including prolonged pancytopenia, which may result in aplastic anemia. Exposure to concomitant medications associated with aplastic anemia, including phenytoin, complicates assessment).
No products indexed under this heading.

Fosphenytoin Sodium (Temozolomide may cause myelosuppression, including prolonged pancytopenia, which may result in aplastic anemia. Exposure to concomitant medications associated with aplastic anemia, including phenytoin, complicates assessment).
No products indexed under this heading.

Hydrocortisone (All patients receiving temozolomide, particularly patients receiving steroids, should be observed closely for the development of PCP regardless of the regimen).
No products indexed under this heading.

Hydrocortisone (Alcohol) (All patients receiving temozolomide, particularly patients receiving steroids, should be observed closely for the development of PCP regardless of the regimen).
No products indexed under this heading.

Hydrocortisone Acetate (All patients receiving temozolomide, particularly patients receiving steroids, should be observed closely for the development of PCP regardless of the regimen).
No products indexed under this heading.

Hydrocortisone Butyrate (All patients receiving temozolomide, particularly patients receiving steroids, should be observed closely for the development of PCP regardless of the regimen).
No products indexed under this heading.

Hydrocortisone Cypionate (All patients receiving temozolomide, particularly patients receiving steroids, should be observed closely for the development of PCP regardless of the regimen).
No products indexed under this heading.

Hydrocortisone Hemisuccinate (All patients receiving temozolomide, particularly patients receiving steroids, should be observed closely for the development of PCP regardless of the regimen).
No products indexed under this heading.

Hydrocortisone Probutate (All patients receiving temozolomide, particularly patients receiving steroids, should be observed closely for the development of PCP regardless of the regimen).
No products indexed under this heading.

(⊙ Described in PDR® for Ophthalmic Medicines)

Hydrocortisone Sodium Phosphate (All patients receiving temozolomide, particularly patients receiving steroids, should be observed closely for the development of PCP regardless of the regimen).
No products indexed under this heading.

Hydrocortisone Sodium Succinate (All patients receiving temozolomide, particularly patients receiving steroids, should be observed closely for the development of PCP regardless of the regimen).
No products indexed under this heading.

Hydrocortisone Valerate (All patients receiving temozolomide, particularly patients receiving steroids, should be observed closely for the development of PCP regardless of the regimen).
No products indexed under this heading.

Methylprednisolone (All patients receiving temozolomide, particularly patients receiving steroids, should be observed closely for the development of PCP regardless of the regimen).
No products indexed under this heading.

Methylprednisolone Acetate (All patients receiving temozolomide, particularly patients receiving steroids, should be observed closely for the development of PCP regardless of the regimen).
No products indexed under this heading.

Methylprednisolone Sodium Succinate (All patients receiving temozolomide, particularly patients receiving steroids, should be observed closely for the development of PCP regardless of the regimen).
No products indexed under this heading.

Mometasone Furoate (All patients receiving temozolomide, particularly patients receiving steroids, should be observed closely for the development of PCP regardless of the regimen). Products include:

Asmanex	3058
Elocon Cream	3111
Elocon Lotion	3112
Elocon Ointment	3114

Mometasone Furoate Monohydrate (All patients receiving temozolomide, particularly patients receiving steroids, should be observed closely for the development of PCP regardless of the regimen). Products include:

Nasonex	3166

Phenytoin (Temozolomide may cause myelosuppression, including prolonged pancytopenia, which may result in aplastic anemia. Exposure to concomitant medications associated with aplastic anemia, including phenytoin, complicates assessment).
No products indexed under this heading.

Phenytoin Sodium (Temozolomide may cause myelosuppression, including prolonged pancytopenia, which may result in aplastic anemia. Exposure to concomitant medications associated with aplastic anemia, including phenytoin, complicates assessment). Products include:

Phenytek Capsules	2380

Prednisolone (All patients receiving temozolomide, particularly patients receiving steroids, should be observed closely for the development of PCP regardless of the regimen).
No products indexed under this heading.

Prednisolone Acetate (All patients receiving temozolomide, particularly patients receiving steroids, should be observed closely for the development of PCP regardless of the regimen). Products include:

Blephamide	☉212, ☉214
Pred Forte	☉225
Pred Mild	☉230

Pred-G .... ☉226, ☉227

Prednisolone Sodium Phosphate (All patients receiving temozolomide, particularly patients receiving steroids, should be observed closely for the development of PCP regardless of the regimen).
No products indexed under this heading.

Prednisolone Tebutate (All patients receiving temozolomide, particularly patients receiving steroids, should be observed closely for the development of PCP regardless of the regimen).
No products indexed under this heading.

Prednisone (All patients receiving temozolomide, particularly patients receiving steroids, should be observed closely for the development of PCP regardless of the regimen).
No products indexed under this heading.

Prednisone sodium phosphate (All patients receiving temozolomide, particularly patients receiving steroids, should be observed closely for the development of PCP regardless of the regimen).
No products indexed under this heading.

Steroids, unspecified (All patients receiving temozolomide, particularly patients receiving steroids, should be observed closely for the development of PCP regardless of the regimen).
No products indexed under this heading.

Sulfamethoxazole (Temozolomide may cause myelosuppression, including prolonged pancytopenia, which may result in aplastic anemia. Exposure to concomitant medications associated with aplastic anemia, including sulfamethoxazole/trimethoprim, complicates assessment).
No products indexed under this heading.

Triamcinolone (All patients receiving temozolomide, particularly patients receiving steroids, should be observed closely for the development of PCP regardless of the regimen).
No products indexed under this heading.

Triamcinolone Acetonide (All patients receiving temozolomide, particularly patients receiving steroids, should be observed closely for the development of PCP regardless of the regimen). Products include:

Azmacort	☉408
Nasacort AQ	3019

Triamcinolone Diacetate (All patients receiving temozolomide, particularly patients receiving steroids, should be observed closely for the development of PCP regardless of the regimen).
No products indexed under this heading.

Triamcinolone Hexacetonide (All patients receiving temozolomide, particularly patients receiving steroids, should be observed closely for the development of PCP regardless of the regimen).
No products indexed under this heading.

Trimethoprim (Temozolomide may cause myelosuppression, including prolonged pancytopenia, which may result in aplastic anemia. Exposure to concomitant medications associated with aplastic anemia, including sulfamethoxazole/trimethoprim, complicates assessment).
No products indexed under this heading.

Valproate Sodium (Co-administration of temozolomide with valproic acid may decreases oral clearance of temozolomide by about 5%. The clinical implication of this effect is not known).
No products indexed under this heading.

Valproic Acid (Co-administration of temozolomide with valproic acid may decreases oral clearance of temozolomide by about 5%. The clinical implication of this effect is not known).
No products indexed under this heading.

Food Interactions

Food, unspecified (Temozolomide is rapidly and completely absorbed after oral administration with a peak plasma concentration (C_{max}) achieved in a median T_{max} of 1 hour. Food reduces the rate and extent of temozolomide absorption. Mean peak plasma concentration and AUC decreased by 32% and 9%, respectively, and median T_{max} increased by 2-fold (from 1 to 2.25 hours) when temozolomide was administered after a modified high-fat breakfast).

Meal, unspecified (Temozolomide is rapidly and completely absorbed after oral administration with a peak plasma concentration (C_{max}) achieved in a median T_{max} of 1 hour. Food reduces the rate and extent of temozolomide absorption. Mean peak plasma concentration and AUC decreased by 32% and 9%, respectively, and median T_{max} increased by 2-fold (from 1 to 2.25 hours) when temozolomide was administered after a modified high-fat breakfast).

TEMODAR INJECTION

(Temozolomide) 3230
May interact with corticosteroids, phenytoin, valproate, and certain other agents. Compounds in these categories include:

Alclometasone Dipropionate (All patients receiving temozolomide, particularly patients receiving steroids, should be observed closely for the development of PCP regardless of the regimen).
No products indexed under this heading.

Beclomethasone Dipropionate (All patients receiving temozolomide, particularly patients receiving steroids, should be observed closely for the development of PCP regardless of the regimen). Products include:

Qvar	3398

Beclomethasone Dipropionate Monohydrate (All patients receiving temozolomide, particularly patients receiving steroids, should be observed closely for the development of PCP regardless of the regimen). Products include:

Beconase AQ	1386

Betamethasone (All patients receiving temozolomide, particularly patients receiving steroids, should be observed closely for the development of PCP regardless of the regimen).
No products indexed under this heading.

Betamethasone Acetate (All patients receiving temozolomide, particularly patients receiving steroids, should be observed closely for the development of PCP regardless of the regimen).
No products indexed under this heading.

Betamethasone Benzoate (All patients receiving temozolomide, particularly patients receiving steroids, should be observed closely for the development of PCP regardless of the regimen).
No products indexed under this heading.

Betamethasone Dipropionate (All patients receiving temozolomide, particularly patients receiving steroids, should be observed closely for the development of PCP regardless of the regimen). Products include:

Diprolene Lotion 0.05%	3108
Diprolene Ointment 0.05%	3109
Diprolene AF Cream 0.05%	3107
Lotrisone	3163

Betamethasone Sodium Phosphate (All patients receiving temozolomide, particularly patients receiving steroids, should be observed closely for the development of PCP regardless of the regimen).
No products indexed under this heading.

Betamethasone Valerate (All patients receiving temozolomide, particularly patients receiving steroids, should be observed closely for the development of PCP regardless of the regimen). Products include:

Luxíq	3321

Budesonide (All patients receiving temozolomide, particularly patients receiving steroids, should be observed closely for the development of PCP regardless of the regimen). Products include:

Pulmicort Flexhaler	714
Symbicort 80/4.5	720
Symbicort 160/4.5	720

Carbamazepine (Temozolomide may cause myelosuppression, including prolonged pancytopenia, which may result in aplastic anemia. Exposure to concomitant medications associated with aplastic anemia, including carbamazepine, complicates assessment). Products include:

Carbatrol	3280
Equetro	3477

Ciclesonide (All patients receiving temozolomide, particularly patients receiving steroids, should be observed closely for the development of PCP regardless of the regimen).
No products indexed under this heading.

Cortisone Acetate (All patients receiving temozolomide, particularly patients receiving steroids, should be observed closely for the development of PCP regardless of the regimen).
No products indexed under this heading.

Desoximetasone (All patients receiving temozolomide, particularly patients receiving steroids, should be observed closely for the development of PCP regardless of the regimen).
No products indexed under this heading.

Dexamethasone (All patients receiving temozolomide, particularly patients receiving steroids, should be observed closely for the development of PCP regardless of the regimen). Products include:

Ciprodex	583
Ozurdex	☉223
Tobramycin and Dexamethasone Ophthalmic Suspension	☉251

Dexamethasone Acetate (All patients receiving temozolomide, particularly patients receiving steroids, should be observed closely for the development of PCP regardless of the regimen).
No products indexed under this heading.

Dexamethasone Phosphate (All patients receiving temozolomide, particularly patients receiving steroids, should be observed closely for the development of PCP regardless of the regimen).
No products indexed under this heading.

Dexamethasone Sodium (All patients receiving temozolomide, particularly patients receiving steroids, should be observed closely for the development of PCP regardless of the regimen).
No products indexed under this heading.

Dexamethasone Sodium Phosphate (All patients receiving temozolomide, particularly patients receiving steroids, should be observed closely for the development of PCP regardless of the regimen).
No products indexed under this heading.

IMPORTANT NOTE: Always consult each drug listing in the patient's regimen for possible interactions.

(⊙ Described in PDR® for Ophthalmic Medicines)

1869 Interactions Index Teveten HCT

Ketoprofen (Nonsteroidal anti-inflammatory agents can reduce the natriuretic, diuretic, and antihypertensive effects).
No products indexed under this heading.

Ketorolac Tromethamine (Nonsteroidal anti-inflammatory agents can reduce the natriuretic, diuretic, and antihypertensive effects). Products include:
Acuvail .... ⊙209

Labetalol Hydrochloride (Co-administration of thiazides with other antihypertensive agents may lead to additive effects or potentiation).
No products indexed under this heading.

Levorphanol Tartrate (Narcotics may potentiate orthostatic hypotension).
No products indexed under this heading.

Lisinopril (Co-administration of thiazides with other antihypertensive agents may lead to additive effects or potentiation). Products include:
Prinivil 2241
Prinzide 2246

Lithium (Diuretics reduce the renal clearance of lithium and add a high risk of lithium toxicity).
No products indexed under this heading.

Lithium Carbonate (Diuretics reduce the renal clearance of lithium and add a high risk of lithium toxicity).
No products indexed under this heading.

Lithium Citrate (Diuretics reduce the renal clearance of lithium and add a high risk of lithium toxicity).
No products indexed under this heading.

Losartan Potassium (Co-administration of thiazides with other antihypertensive agents may lead to additive effects or potentiation). Products include:
Cozaar 2106
Hyzaar 2162
Hyzaar 100-12.5 2162

Mecamylamine Hydrochloride (Co-administration of thiazides with other antihypertensive agents may lead to additive effects or potentiation).
No products indexed under this heading.

Meclofenamate Sodium (Nonsteroidal anti-inflammatory agents can reduce the natriuretic, diuretic, and antihypertensive effects).
No products indexed under this heading.

Mefenamic Acid (Nonsteroidal anti-inflammatory agents can reduce the natriuretic, diuretic, and antihypertensive effects).
No products indexed under this heading.

Meloxicam (Nonsteroidal anti-inflammatory agents can reduce the natriuretic, diuretic, and antihypertensive effects).
No products indexed under this heading.

Meperidine Hydrochloride (Narcotics may potentiate orthostatic hypotension).
No products indexed under this heading.

Mephobarbital (Barbiturates may potentiate orthostatic hypotension).
No products indexed under this heading.

Metformin Hydrochloride (Hyperglycemia may occur with thiazide diuretics; oral hypoglycemic dosage may need to be adjusted). Products include:
ActoPlus 3338
Avandamet 1345
Janumet 2188

Methadone Hydrochloride (Narcotics may potentiate orthostatic hypotension).
No products indexed under this heading.

Methyclothiazide (Co-administration of thiazides with other antihypertensive agents may lead to additive effects or potentiation).
No products indexed under this heading.

Methyldopa (Co-administration of thiazides with other antihypertensive agents may lead to additive effects or potentiation).
No products indexed under this heading.

Methyldopate Hydrochloride (Co-administration of thiazides with other antihypertensive agents may lead to additive effects or potentiation).
No products indexed under this heading.

Methylprednisolone (Corticosteroids intensify the electrolyte imbalance, particularly hypokalemia).
No products indexed under this heading.

Methylprednisolone Acetate (Corticosteroids intensify the electrolyte imbalance, particularly hypokalemia).
No products indexed under this heading.

Methylprednisolone Sodium Succinate (Corticosteroids intensify the electrolyte imbalance, particularly hypokalemia).
No products indexed under this heading.

Metocurine Iodide (Possible increased responsiveness to muscle relaxants).
No products indexed under this heading.

Metolazone (Co-administration of thiazides with other antihypertensive agents may lead to additive effects or potentiation).
No products indexed under this heading.

Metoprolol Succinate (Co-administration of thiazides with other antihypertensive agents may lead to additive effects or potentiation). Products include:
Toprol XL 732

Metoprolol Tartrate (Co-administration of thiazides with other antihypertensive agents may lead to additive effects or potentiation).
No products indexed under this heading.

Metyrosine (Co-administration of thiazides with other antihypertensive agents may lead to additive effects or potentiation).
No products indexed under this heading.

Mibefradil Dihydrochloride (Co-administration of thiazides with other antihypertensive agents may lead to additive effects or potentiation).
No products indexed under this heading.

Miglitol (Hyperglycemia may occur with thiazide diuretics; oral hypoglycemic dosage may need to be adjusted).
No products indexed under this heading.

Minoxidil (Co-administration of thiazides with other antihypertensive agents may lead to additive effects or potentiation).
No products indexed under this heading.

Mivacurium Chloride (Possible increased responsiveness to muscle relaxants).
No products indexed under this heading.

Moexipril Hydrochloride (Co-administration of thiazides with other antihypertensive agents may lead to additive effects or potentiation).
No products indexed under this heading.

Mometasone Furoate (Corticosteroids intensify the electrolyte imbalance, particularly hypokalemia). Products include:
Asmanex 3058
Elocon Cream 3111
Elocon Lotion 3112
Elocon Ointment 3114

Mometasone Furoate Monohydrate (Corticosteroids intensify the electrolyte imbalance, particularly hypokalemia). Products include:
Nasonex 3166

Morphine Sulfate (Narcotics may potentiate orthostatic hypotension). Products include:
Avinza 1822
Embeda 1831
MS Contin 2803

Morphine Sulfate, Liposomal (Narcotics may potentiate orthostatic hypotension).
No products indexed under this heading.

Nabumetone (Nonsteroidal anti-inflammatory agents can reduce the natriuretic, diuretic, and antihypertensive effects).
No products indexed under this heading.

Nadolol (Co-administration of thiazides with other antihypertensive agents may lead to additive effects or potentiation). Products include:
Nadolol 2359

Naproxen (Nonsteroidal anti-inflammatory agents can reduce the natriuretic, diuretic, and antihypertensive effects). Products include:
EC-Naprosyn 2850
Naprosyn 2850
Anaprox/Naprosyn 2850

Naproxen Sodium (Nonsteroidal anti-inflammatory agents can reduce the natriuretic, diuretic, and antihypertensive effects). Products include:
Anaprox 2850
Anaprox DS 2850
Treximet 1681

Nateglinide (Hyperglycemia may occur with thiazide diuretics; oral hypoglycemic dosage may need to be adjusted).
No products indexed under this heading.

Nebivolol (Co-administration of thiazides with other antihypertensive agents may lead to additive effects or potentiation). Products include:
Bystolic 1147

Nicardipine Hydrochloride (Co-administration of thiazides with other antihypertensive agents may lead to additive effects or potentiation).
No products indexed under this heading.

Nifedipine (Co-administration of thiazides with other antihypertensive agents may lead to additive effects or potentiation).
No products indexed under this heading.

Nisoldipine (Co-administration of thiazides with other antihypertensive agents may lead to additive effects or potentiation).
No products indexed under this heading.

Nitroglycerin (Co-administration of thiazides with other antihypertensive agents may lead to additive effects or potentiation). Products include:
Nitro-Dur 3170
Nitrolingual 3266

Norepinephrine Bitartrate (Possible decreased response to pressor amines).
No products indexed under this heading.

Oxaprozin (Nonsteroidal anti-inflammatory agents can reduce the natriuretic, diuretic, and antihypertensive effects).
No products indexed under this heading.

Oxycodone Hydrochloride (Narcotics may potentiate orthostatic hypotension). Products include:
OxyContin 2807
Percocet 1121
Percodan 1124

Oxycodone Terephthalate (Narcotics may potentiate orthostatic hypotension).
No products indexed under this heading.

Oxymorphone Hydrochloride (Narcotics may potentiate orthostatic hypotension). Products include:
Opana 1110
Opana ER 1114

Pancuronium Bromide (Possible increased responsiveness to muscle relaxants).
No products indexed under this heading.

Penbutolol Sulfate (Co-administration of thiazides with other antihypertensive agents may lead to additive effects or potentiation).
No products indexed under this heading.

Pentobarbital (Barbiturates may potentiate orthostatic hypotension).
No products indexed under this heading.

Pentobarbital Sodium (Barbiturates may potentiate orthostatic hypotension). Products include:
Nembutal 2012

Perindopril Erbumine (Co-administration of thiazides with other antihypertensive agents may lead to additive effects or potentiation).
No products indexed under this heading.

Phenobarbital (Barbiturates may potentiate orthostatic hypotension). Products include:
Donnatal 2711

Phenobarbital Sodium (Barbiturates may potentiate orthostatic hypotension).
No products indexed under this heading.

Phenoxybenzamine Hydrochloride (Co-administration of thiazides with other antihypertensive agents may lead to additive effects or potentiation). Products include:
Dibenzyline 3495

Phentolamine Mesylate (Co-administration of thiazides with other antihypertensive agents may lead to additive effects or potentiation).
No products indexed under this heading.

Phenylbutazone (Nonsteroidal anti-inflammatory agents can reduce the natriuretic, diuretic, and antihypertensive effects).
No products indexed under this heading.

Pindolol (Co-administration of thiazides with other antihypertensive agents may lead to additive effects or potentiation).
No products indexed under this heading.

Pioglitazone Hydrochloride (Hyperglycemia may occur with thiazide diuretics; oral hypoglycemic dosage may need to be adjusted). Products include:
ActoPlus 3338
Actos 3345
Duetact 3354

Pipecuronium Bromide (Possible increased responsiveness to muscle relaxants).
No products indexed under this heading.

Piroxicam (Nonsteroidal anti-inflammatory agents can reduce the natriuretic, diuretic, and antihypertensive effects).
No products indexed under this heading.

Polythiazide (Co-administration of thiazides with other antihypertensive agents may lead to additive effects or potentiation).
No products indexed under this heading.

Potassium Acid Phosphate (Concomitant use of potassium supplements with eprosartan may lead to hyperkalemia). Products include:
K-Phos Original 874

Potassium Bicarbonate (Concomitant use of potassium supplements with eprosartan may lead to hyperkalemia).
No products indexed under this heading.

Potassium Chloride (Concomitant use of potassium supplements with eprosartan may lead to hyperkalemia). Products include:
MoviPrep Oral Solution 2905

Potassium Citrate (Concomitant use of potassium supplements with eprosartan may lead to hyperkalemia). Products include:
Urocit-K 2333

Potassium Gluconate (Concomitant use of potassium supplements with eprosartan may lead to hyperkalemia).
No products indexed under this heading.

IMPORTANT NOTE: Always consult each drug listing in the patient's regimen for possible interactions.

1871 **Interactions Index** **Tev-Tropin**

Exforge 2443
Exforge HCT 2449

Amoxapine (Somatropin administration may alter the clearance of compounds known to be metabolized by CYP450).
No products indexed under this heading.

Amphetamine Aspartate (Somatropin administration may alter the clearance of compounds known to be metabolized by CYP450).
No products indexed under this heading.

Amphetamine Aspartate Monohydrate (Somatropin administration may alter the clearance of compounds known to be metabolized by CYP450).
No products indexed under this heading.

Amphetamine Sulfate (Somatropin administration may alter the clearance of compounds known to be metabolized by CYP450).
No products indexed under this heading.

Anagrelide Hydrochloride (Somatropin administration may alter the clearance of compounds known to be metabolized by CYP450).
No products indexed under this heading.

Aprepitant (Somatropin administration may alter the clearance of compounds known to be metabolized by CYP450). Products include:
Emend 2124

Astemizole (Somatropin administration may alter the clearance of compounds known to be metabolized by CYP450).
No products indexed under this heading.

Atomoxetine Hydrochloride (Somatropin administration may alter the clearance of compounds known to be metabolized by CYP450). Products include:
Strattera 1957

Atorvastatin Calcium (Somatropin administration may alter the clearance of compounds known to be metabolized by CYP450). Products include:
Lipitor 2703

Belladonna Ergotamine (Somatropin administration may alter the clearance of compounds known to be metabolized by CYP450).
No products indexed under this heading.

Benzphetamine Hydrochloride (Somatropin administration may alter the clearance of compounds known to be metabolized by CYP450).
No products indexed under this heading.

Betamethasone Acetate (Glucocorticoid therapy may inhibit the growth-promoting effect of human growth hormone. Patients with co-existing ACTH deficiency should have their glucocorticoid replacement dose carefully adjusted to avoid an inhibitory effect on growth).
No products indexed under this heading.

Betamethasone Sodium Phosphate (Glucocorticoid therapy may inhibit the growth-promoting effect of human growth hormone. Patients with co-existing ACTH deficiency should have their glucocorticoid replacement dose carefully adjusted to avoid an inhibitory effect on growth).
No products indexed under this heading.

Bisoprolol Fumarate (Somatropin administration may alter the clearance of compounds known to be metabolized by CYP450).
No products indexed under this heading.

Bromocriptine Mesylate (Somatropin administration may alter the clearance of compounds known to be metabolized by CYP450).
No products indexed under this heading.

Budesonide (Glucocorticoid therapy may inhibit the growth-promoting effect of human growth hormone. Patients with co-existing ACTH deficiency should have their glucocorticoid replacement dose carefully adjusted to avoid an inhibitory effect on growth). Products include:
Pulmicort Flexhaler 714
Symbicort 80/4.5 720
Symbicort 160/4.5 720

Buspirone Hydrochloride (Somatropin administration may alter the clearance of compounds known to be metabolized by CYP450).
No products indexed under this heading.

Busulfan (Somatropin administration may alter the clearance of compounds known to be metabolized by CYP450). Products include:
Myleran 1581

Caffeine (Somatropin administration may alter the clearance of compounds known to be metabolized by CYP450).
No products indexed under this heading.

Caffeine Anhydrous (Somatropin administration may alter the clearance of compounds known to be metabolized by CYP450).
No products indexed under this heading.

Caffeine Citrate (Somatropin administration may alter the clearance of compounds known to be metabolized by CYP450).
No products indexed under this heading.

Caffeine-containing medications (Somatropin administration may alter the clearance of compounds known to be metabolized by CYP450).
No products indexed under this heading.

Caffeine Sodium Benzoate (Somatropin administration may alter the clearance of compounds known to be metabolized by CYP450).
No products indexed under this heading.

Candesartan Cilexetil (Somatropin administration may alter the clearance of compounds known to be metabolized by CYP450). Products include:
Atacand 697
Atacand HCT 700

Captopril (Somatropin administration may alter the clearance of compounds known to be metabolized by CYP450). Products include:
Captopril 2341

Carbamazepine (Somatropin administration may alter the clearance of compounds known to be metabolized by CYP450). Products include:
Carbatrol 3280
Equetro 3477

Carisoprodol (Somatropin administration may alter the clearance of compounds known to be metabolized by CYP450).
No products indexed under this heading.

Carvedilol (Somatropin administration may alter the clearance of compounds known to be metabolized by CYP450). Products include:
Coreg 1409

Celecoxib (Somatropin administration may alter the clearance of compounds known to be metabolized by CYP450). Products include:
Celebrex 3272

Cerivastatin Sodium (Somatropin administration may alter the clearance of compounds known to be metabolized by CYP450).
No products indexed under this heading.

Cevimeline Hydrochloride (Somatropin administration may alter the clearance of compounds known to be metabolized by CYP450). Products include:
Evoxac 1027

Chlordiazepoxide (Somatropin administration may alter the clearance of compounds known to be metabolized by CYP450).
No products indexed under this heading.

Chlordiazepoxide Hydrochloride (Somatropin administration may alter the clearance of compounds known to be metabolized by CYP450).
No products indexed under this heading.

Chlorpheniramine (Somatropin administration may alter the clearance of compounds known to be metabolized by CYP450).
No products indexed under this heading.

Chlorpheniramine Maleate (Somatropin administration may alter the clearance of compounds known to be metabolized by CYP450).
No products indexed under this heading.

Chlorpheniramine Polistirex (Somatropin administration may alter the clearance of compounds known to be metabolized by CYP450). Products include:
Tussionex 3443

Chlorpheniramine Tannate (Somatropin administration may alter the clearance of compounds known to be metabolized by CYP450).
No products indexed under this heading.

Chlorpromazine (Somatropin administration may alter the clearance of compounds known to be metabolized by CYP450).
No products indexed under this heading.

Chlorpromazine Hydrochloride (Somatropin administration may alter the clearance of compounds known to be metabolized by CYP450).
No products indexed under this heading.

Chlorpropamide (Somatropin administration may alter the clearance of compounds known to be metabolized by CYP450).
No products indexed under this heading.

Cilostazol (Somatropin administration may alter the clearance of compounds known to be metabolized by CYP450).
No products indexed under this heading.

Cimetidine Hydrochloride (Somatropin administration may alter the clearance of compounds known to be metabolized by CYP450).
No products indexed under this heading.

Ciprofloxacin (Somatropin administration may alter the clearance of compounds known to be metabolized by CYP450). Products include:
Cipro I.V. 3082
Cipro 3073
Cipro XR 3091
Ciprodex 583

Ciprofloxacin Hydrochloride (Somatropin administration may alter the clearance of compounds known to be metabolized by CYP450). Products include:
Cipro 3073

Cisapride (Somatropin administration may alter the clearance of compounds known to be metabolized by CYP450).
No products indexed under this heading.

Citalopram Hydrobromide (Somatropin administration may alter the clearance of compounds known to be metabolized by CYP450). Products include:
Celexa 1153

Clarithromycin (Somatropin administration may alter the clearance of compounds known to be metabolized by CYP450). Products include:
Biaxin/Biaxin XL 412

Clomipramine Hydrochloride (Somatropin administration may alter the clearance of compounds known to be metabolized by CYP450).
No products indexed under this heading.

Clopidogrel Bisulfate (Somatropin administration may alter the clearance of compounds known to be metabolized by CYP450). Products include:
Plavix 3027

Clopidogrel Hydrogen Sulfate (Somatropin administration may alter the clearance of compounds known to be metabolized by CYP450).
No products indexed under this heading.

Clozapine (Somatropin administration may alter the clearance of compounds known to be metabolized by CYP450).
No products indexed under this heading.

Codeine Phosphate (Somatropin administration may alter the clearance of compounds known to be metabolized by CYP450). Products include:
Tylenol with Codeine 2691

Codeine Sulfate (Somatropin administration may alter the clearance of compounds known to be metabolized by CYP450).
No products indexed under this heading.

Cortisone Acetate (Glucocorticoid therapy may inhibit the growth-promoting effect of human growth hormone. Patients with co-existing ACTH deficiency should have their glucocorticoid replacement dose carefully adjusted to avoid an inhibitory effect on growth).
No products indexed under this heading.

Cyclobenzaprine (Somatropin administration may alter the clearance of compounds known to be metabolized by CYP450).
No products indexed under this heading.

Cyclobenzaprine Hydrochloride (Somatropin administration may alter the clearance of compounds known to be metabolized by CYP450). Products include:
Amrix 964

Cyclophosphamide (Somatropin administration may alter the clearance of compounds known to be metabolized by CYP450).
No products indexed under this heading.

Cyclosporine (Somatropin administration may alter the clearance of compounds known to be metabolized by CYP450). Products include:
Gengraf 440
Neoral Oral Solution 2496
Neoral Capsules 2496
Restasis 605

Desipramine Hydrochloride (Somatropin administration may alter the clearance of compounds known to be metabolized by CYP450).
No products indexed under this heading.

Desogestrel (Somatropin administration may alter the clearance of compounds known to be metabolized by CYP450).
No products indexed under this heading.

Dexamethasone (Glucocorticoid therapy may inhibit the growth-promoting effect of human growth hormone. Patients with co-existing ACTH deficiency should have their glucocorticoid replacement dose carefully adjusted to avoid an inhibitory effect on growth). Products include:
Ciprodex 583
Ozurdex .... ⊙223
Tobramycin and Dexamethasone Ophthalmic Suspension .... ⊙251

Dexamethasone Acetate (Glucocorticoid therapy may inhibit the growth-promoting effect of human growth hormone. Patients with co-existing ACTH deficiency should have their glucocorticoid replacement dose carefully adjusted to avoid an inhibitory effect on growth).
No products indexed under this heading.

Dexamethasone Phosphate (Somatropin administration may alter the clearance of compounds known to be metabolized by CYP450).
No products indexed under this heading.

Fluticasone Propionate (Somatropin administration may alter the clearance of compounds known to be metabolized by CYP450). Products include:

Fluvastatin Sodium (Somatropin administration may alter the clearance of compounds known to be metabolized by CYP450).
No products indexed under this heading.

Fluvoxamine Maleate (Somatropin administration may alter the clearance of compounds known to be metabolized by CYP450).
No products indexed under this heading.

Formoterol Fumarate (Somatropin administration may alter the clearance of compounds known to be metabolized by CYP450). Products include:

Fosphenytoin (Somatropin administration may alter the clearance of compounds known to be metabolized by CYP450).
No products indexed under this heading.

Fosphenytoin Sodium (Somatropin administration may alter the clearance of compounds known to be metabolized by CYP450).
No products indexed under this heading.

Gabapentin (Somatropin administration may alter the clearance of compounds known to be metabolized by CYP450).
No products indexed under this heading.

Galantamine Hydrobromide (Somatropin administration may alter the clearance of compounds known to be metabolized by CYP450).
No products indexed under this heading.

Glimepiride (Somatropin administration may alter the clearance of compounds known to be metabolized by CYP450). Products include:

Glipizide (Somatropin administration may alter the clearance of compounds known to be metabolized by CYP450).
No products indexed under this heading.

Glyburide (Somatropin administration may alter the clearance of compounds known to be metabolized by CYP450).
No products indexed under this heading.

Grepafloxacin Hydrochloride (Somatropin administration may alter the clearance of compounds known to be metabolized by CYP450).
No products indexed under this heading.

Haloperidol (Somatropin administration may alter the clearance of compounds known to be metabolized by CYP450).
No products indexed under this heading.

Haloperidol Decanoate (Somatropin administration may alter the clearance of compounds known to be metabolized by CYP450).
No products indexed under this heading.

Haloperidol Lactate (Somatropin administration may alter the clearance of compounds known to be metabolized by CYP450).
No products indexed under this heading.

Hexobarbital (Somatropin administration may alter the clearance of compounds known to be metabolized by CYP450).
No products indexed under this heading.

Hydrocodone Bitartrate (Somatropin administration may alter the clearance of compounds known to be metabolized by CYP450). Products include:

Hydrocortisone (Glucocorticoid therapy may inhibit the growth-promoting effect of human growth hormone. Patients with co-existing ACTH deficiency should have their glucocorticoid replacement dose carefully adjusted to avoid an inhibitory effect on growth).
No products indexed under this heading.

Hydrocortisone Acetate (Glucocorticoid therapy may inhibit the growth-promoting effect of human growth hormone. Patients with co-existing ACTH deficiency should have their glucocorticoid replacement dose carefully adjusted to avoid an inhibitory effect on growth).
No products indexed under this heading.

Hydrocortisone Sodium Phosphate (Glucocorticoid therapy may inhibit the growth-promoting effect of human growth hormone. Patients with co-existing ACTH deficiency should have their glucocorticoid replacement dose carefully adjusted to avoid an inhibitory effect on growth).
No products indexed under this heading.

Hydrocortisone Sodium Succinate (Glucocorticoid therapy may inhibit the growth-promoting effect of human growth hormone. Patients with co-existing ACTH deficiency should have their glucocorticoid replacement dose carefully adjusted to avoid an inhibitory effect on growth).
No products indexed under this heading.

Ibuprofen (Somatropin administration may alter the clearance of compounds known to be metabolized by CYP450). Products include:

Imipramine Hydrochloride (Somatropin administration may alter the clearance of compounds known to be metabolized by CYP450).
No products indexed under this heading.

Imipramine Pamoate (Somatropin administration may alter the clearance of compounds known to be metabolized by CYP450).
No products indexed under this heading.

Indinavir Sulfate (Somatropin administration may alter the clearance of compounds known to be metabolized by CYP450). Products include:

Indomethacin (Somatropin administration may alter the clearance of compounds known to be metabolized by CYP450). Products include:

Indomethacin Sodium Trihydrate (Somatropin administration may alter the clearance of compounds known to be metabolized by CYP450). Products include:

Indoramin Hydrochloride (Somatropin administration may alter the clearance of compounds known to be metabolized by CYP450).
No products indexed under this heading.

Irbesartan (Somatropin administration may alter the clearance of compounds known to be metabolized by CYP450). Products include:

Isotretinoin (Somatropin administration may alter the clearance of compounds known to be metabolized by CYP450). Products include:

Isradipine (Somatropin administration may alter the clearance of compounds known to be metabolized by CYP450). Products include:

Itraconazole (Somatropin administration may alter the clearance of compounds known to be metabolized by CYP450).
No products indexed under this heading.

Ixabepilone (Somatropin administration may alter the clearance of compounds known to be metabolized by CYP450).
No products indexed under this heading.

Ketoconazole (Somatropin administration may alter the clearance of compounds known to be metabolized by CYP450). Products include:

Ketoprofen (Somatropin administration may alter the clearance of compounds known to be metabolized by CYP450).
No products indexed under this heading.

Ketorolac Tromethamine (Somatropin administration may alter the clearance of compounds known to be metabolized by CYP450). Products include:

Labetalol Hydrochloride (Somatropin administration may alter the clearance of compounds known to be metabolized by CYP450).
No products indexed under this heading.

Lamotrigine (Somatropin administration may alter the clearance of compounds known to be metabolized by CYP450). Products include:

Lansoprazole (Somatropin administration may alter the clearance of compounds known to be metabolized by CYP450).
No products indexed under this heading.

Levetiracetam (Somatropin administration may alter the clearance of compounds known to be metabolized by CYP450). Products include:

Levobupivacaine Hydrochloride (Somatropin administration may alter the clearance of compounds known to be metabolized by CYP450).
No products indexed under this heading.

Levonorgestrel (Somatropin administration may alter the clearance of compounds known to be metabolized by CYP450). Products include:

Lidocaine (Somatropin administration may alter the clearance of compounds known to be metabolized by CYP450). Products include:

Lidocaine Base (Somatropin administration may alter the clearance of compounds known to be metabolized by CYP450).
No products indexed under this heading.

Lidocaine Hydrochloride (Somatropin administration may alter the clearance of compounds known to be metabolized by CYP450).
No products indexed under this heading.

Lomefloxacin Hydrochloride (Somatropin administration may alter the clearance of compounds known to be metabolized by CYP450).
No products indexed under this heading.

Losartan Potassium (Somatropin administration may alter the clearance of compounds known to be metabolized by CYP450). Products include:

Lovastatin (Somatropin administration may alter the clearance of compounds known to be metabolized by CYP450). Products include:

Maprotiline Hydrochloride (Somatropin administration may alter the clearance of compounds known to be metabolized by CYP450).
No products indexed under this heading.

Meclofenamate Sodium (Somatropin administration may alter the clearance of compounds known to be metabolized by CYP450).
No products indexed under this heading.

Mefenamic Acid (Somatropin administration may alter the clearance of compounds known to be metabolized by CYP450).
No products indexed under this heading.

Meloxicam (Somatropin administration may alter the clearance of compounds known to be metabolized by CYP450).
No products indexed under this heading.

Meperidine Hydrochloride (Somatropin administration may alter the clearance of compounds known to be metabolized by CYP450).
No products indexed under this heading.

Mephenytoin (Somatropin administration may alter the clearance of compounds known to be metabolized by CYP450).
No products indexed under this heading.

Mephobarbital (Somatropin administration may alter the clearance of compounds known to be metabolized by CYP450).
No products indexed under this heading.

Meprobamate (Somatropin administration may alter the clearance of compounds known to be metabolized by CYP450).
No products indexed under this heading.

Mestranol (Somatropin administration may alter the clearance of compounds known to be metabolized by CYP450).
No products indexed under this heading.

Metformin Hydrochloride (Somatropin administration may alter the clearance of compounds known to be metabolized by CYP450). Products include:

Methadone Hydrochloride (Somatropin administration may alter the clearance of compounds known to be metabolized by CYP450).
No products indexed under this heading.

Methamphetamine Hydrochloride (Somatropin administration may alter the clearance of compounds known to be metabolized by CYP450).
No products indexed under this heading.

Methsuximide (Somatropin administration may alter the clearance of compounds known to be metabolized by CYP450).
No products indexed under this heading.

(⊙ Described in PDR® for Ophthalmic Medicines)

IMPORTANT NOTE: Always consult each drug listing in the patient's regimen for possible interactions.

Tev-Tropin Interactions Index 1876

Triamcinolone (Glucocorticoid therapy may inhibit the growth-promoting effect of human growth hormone. Patients with co-existing ACTH deficiency should have their glucocorticoid replacement dose carefully adjusted to avoid an inhibitory effect on growth).
No products indexed under this heading.

Triamcinolone Acetonide (Glucocorticoid therapy may inhibit the growth-promoting effect of human growth hormone. Patients with co-existing ACTH deficiency should have their glucocorticoid replacement dose carefully adjusted to avoid an inhibitory effect on growth). Products include:
Azmacort ... 408
Nasacort AQ ... 3019

Triamcinolone Diacetate (Glucocorticoid therapy may inhibit the growth-promoting effect of human growth hormone. Patients with co-existing ACTH deficiency should have their glucocorticoid replacement dose carefully adjusted to avoid an inhibitory effect on growth).
No products indexed under this heading.

Triamcinolone Hexacetonide (Glucocorticoid therapy may inhibit the growth-promoting effect of human growth hormone. Patients with co-existing ACTH deficiency should have their glucocorticoid replacement dose carefully adjusted to avoid an inhibitory effect on growth).
No products indexed under this heading.

Triazolam (Somatropin administration may alter the clearance of compounds known to be metabolized by CYP450).
No products indexed under this heading.

Trimethadione (Somatropin administration may alter the clearance of compounds known to be metabolized by CYP450).
No products indexed under this heading.

Trimethaphan Camsylate (Somatropin administration may alter the clearance of compounds known to be metabolized by CYP450).
No products indexed under this heading.

Trimipramine Maleate (Somatropin administration may alter the clearance of compounds known to be metabolized by CYP450).
No products indexed under this heading.

Troglitazone (Somatropin administration may alter the clearance of compounds known to be metabolized by CYP450).
No products indexed under this heading.

Trovafloxacin Mesylate (Somatropin administration may alter the clearance of compounds known to be metabolized by CYP450).
No products indexed under this heading.

Valdecoxib (Somatropin administration may alter the clearance of compounds known to be metabolized by CYP450).
No products indexed under this heading.

Valproate Sodium (Somatropin administration may alter the clearance of compounds known to be metabolized by CYP450).
No products indexed under this heading.

Valproic Acid (Somatropin administration may alter the clearance of compounds known to be metabolized by CYP450).
No products indexed under this heading.

Valsartan (Somatropin administration may alter the clearance of compounds known to be metabolized by CYP450). Products include:
Diovan ... 2413
Diovan HCT ... 2419
Exforge ... 2443
Exforge HCT ... 2449
Valturna ... 3637

Vardenafil Hydrochloride (Somatropin administration may alter the clearance of compounds known to be metabolized by CYP450). Products include:
Levitra ... 3157

Venlafaxine Hydrochloride (Somatropin administration may alter the clearance of compounds known to be metabolized by CYP450). Products include:
Effexor XR ... 3504
Venlafaxine Hydrochloride Tablets ... 2388

Verapamil Hydrochloride (Somatropin administration may alter the clearance of compounds known to be metabolized by CYP450). Products include:
Tarka ... 534

Vinblastine Sulfate (Somatropin administration may alter the clearance of compounds known to be metabolized by CYP450).
No products indexed under this heading.

Vincristine Sulfate (Somatropin administration may alter the clearance of compounds known to be metabolized by CYP450).
No products indexed under this heading.

Vitamin A (Somatropin administration may alter the clearance of compounds known to be metabolized by CYP450). Products include:
Cardio Basics ... 3455
Heplive ... 607
Norwegian Cod Liver Oil ... 919

Vitamin A Acetate (Somatropin administration may alter the clearance of compounds known to be metabolized by CYP450).
No products indexed under this heading.

Voriconazole (Somatropin administration may alter the clearance of compounds known to be metabolized by CYP450).
No products indexed under this heading.

Warfarin Sodium (Somatropin administration may alter the clearance of compounds known to be metabolized by CYP450).
No products indexed under this heading.

Zafirlukast (Somatropin administration may alter the clearance of compounds known to be metabolized by CYP450). Products include:
Accolate ... 3612

Zileuton (Somatropin administration may alter the clearance of compounds known to be metabolized by CYP450).
No products indexed under this heading.

Zolmitriptan (Somatropin administration may alter the clearance of compounds known to be metabolized by CYP450). Products include:
Zomig Tablets ... 773
Zomig Nasal Spray ... 768
Zomig-ZMT Tablets ... 773

Zonisamide (Somatropin administration may alter the clearance of compounds known to be metabolized by CYP450). Products include:
Zonegran ... 1081

Zopiclone (Somatropin administration may alter the clearance of compounds known to be metabolized by CYP450).
No products indexed under this heading.

Food Interactions

Beverages, caffeine-containing (Somatropin administration may alter the clearance of compounds known to be metabolized by CYP450).

Food, caffeine-containing (Somatropin administration may alter the clearance of compounds known to be metabolized by CYP450).

THIORIDAZINE HYDROCHLORIDE TABLETS

(Thioridazine Hydrochloride) ... 2384
May interact with alcohols, central nervous system depressants, erythromycin, potassium-depleting diuretics, quinidine, and certain other agents. Compounds in these categories include:

Alfentanil Hydrochloride (Thioridazine is capable of potentiating CNS depressants).
No products indexed under this heading.

Alprazolam (Thioridazine is capable of potentiating CNS depressants).
No products indexed under this heading.

Amiodarone Hydrochloride (Thioridazine has been shown to prolong QTc interval in a dose-related manner; drugs with this potential have been associated with Torsade de pointes-type arrhythmias and sudden death; co-administration with other drugs that are known to prolong QTc interval is contraindicated).
No products indexed under this heading.

Amobarbital (Thioridazine is capable of potentiating CNS depressants).
No products indexed under this heading.

Amobarbital Sodium (Thioridazine is capable of potentiating CNS depressants).
No products indexed under this heading.

Aprobarbital (Thioridazine is capable of potentiating CNS depressants).
No products indexed under this heading.

Arsenic Trioxide (Thioridazine has been shown to prolong QTc interval in a dose-related manner; drugs with this potential have been associated with torsade de pointes-type arrhythmias and sudden death; co-administration with other drugs that are known to prolong QTc interval is contraindicated). Products include:
Trisenox ... 994

Atropine Sulfate (Thioridazine is capable of potentiating atropine). Products include:
Donnatal ... 2711

Bendroflumethiazide (Hypokalemia may result from diuretic therapy and this may increase the risk of QT prolongation and arrhythmias; co-administration may increase the risk of serious, potentially fatal, cardiac arrhythmias).
No products indexed under this heading.

Bepridil Hydrochloride (Thioridazine has been shown to prolong QTc interval in a dose-related manner; drugs with this potential have been associated with torsade de pointes-type arrhythmias and sudden death; co-administration with other drugs that are known to prolong QTc interval is contraindicated).
No products indexed under this heading.

Bumetanide (Hypokalemia may result from diuretic therapy and this may increase the risk of QT prolongation and arrhythmias; co-administration may increase the risk of serious, potentially fatal, cardiac arrhythmias).
No products indexed under this heading.

Buprenorphine Hydrochloride (Thioridazine is capable of potentiating CNS depressants).
No products indexed under this heading.

Buspirone Hydrochloride (Thioridazine is capable of potentiating CNS depressants).
No products indexed under this heading.

Butabarbital (Thioridazine is capable of potentiating CNS depressants).
No products indexed under this heading.

Butabarbital Sodium (Thioridazine is capable of potentiating CNS depressants).
No products indexed under this heading.

Butalbital (Thioridazine is capable of potentiating CNS depressants).
No products indexed under this heading.

Chlordiazepoxide (Thioridazine is capable of potentiating CNS depressants).
No products indexed under this heading.

Chlordiazepoxide Hydrochloride (Thioridazine is capable of potentiating CNS depressants).
No products indexed under this heading.

Chlorothiazide (Hypokalemia may result from diuretic therapy and this may increase the risk of QT prolongation and arrhythmias; co-administration may increase the risk of serious, potentially fatal, cardiac arrhythmias).
No products indexed under this heading.

Chlorothiazide Sodium (Hypokalemia may result from diuretic therapy and this may increase the risk of QT prolongation and arrhythmias; co-administration may increase the risk of serious, potentially fatal, cardiac arrhythmias). Products include:
Diuril Intravenous ... 2009

Chlorpromazine (Thioridazine is capable of potentiating CNS depressants).
No products indexed under this heading.

Chlorpromazine Hydrochloride (Thioridazine is capable of potentiating CNS depressants).
No products indexed under this heading.

Chlorprothixene (Thioridazine is capable of potentiating CNS depressants).
No products indexed under this heading.

Chlorprothixene Hydrochloride (Thioridazine is capable of potentiating CNS depressants).
No products indexed under this heading.

Chlorprothixene Lactate (Thioridazine is capable of potentiating CNS depressants).
No products indexed under this heading.

Clonazepam (Thioridazine is capable of potentiating CNS depressants). Products include:
Klonopin ... 2855

Clorazepate Dipotassium (Thioridazine is capable of potentiating CNS depressants).
No products indexed under this heading.

Clozapine (Thioridazine is capable of potentiating CNS depressants).
No products indexed under this heading.

Codeine Phosphate (Thioridazine is capable of potentiating CNS depressants). Products include:
Tylenol with Codeine ... 2691

Codeine Sulfate (Thioridazine is capable of potentiating CNS depressants).
No products indexed under this heading.

Desflurane (Thioridazine is capable of potentiating CNS depressants).
No products indexed under this heading.

Desipramine Hydrochloride (Thioridazine has been shown to prolong QTc interval in a dose-related manner; drugs with this potential have been associated with torsade de pointes-type arrhythmias and sudden death; co-administration with other drugs that are known to prolong QTc interval is contraindicated).
No products indexed under this heading.

Dezocine (Thioridazine is capable of potentiating CNS depressants).
No products indexed under this heading.

Diazepam (Thioridazine is capable of potentiating CNS depressants). Products include:
Valium Tablets ... 2880

Disopyramide Phosphate (Thioridazine has been shown to prolong QTc interval in a dose-related manner; drugs with this potential have been associated with torsade de pointes-type arrhythmias and sudden death; co-administration with other drugs that are known to prolong QTc interval is contraindicated).
No products indexed under this heading.

Dofetilide (Thioridazine has been shown to prolong QTc interval in a dose-related manner; drugs with this potential have been associated with Torsade de pointes-type arrhythmias and sudden death; co-administration with other drugs that are known to prolong QTc interval is contraindicated).
No products indexed under this heading.

Dolasetron Mesylate (Thioridazine has been shown to prolong QTc interval in a dose-related manner; drugs with this potential have been associated with Torsade de pointes-type arrhythmias and sudden death; co-administration with other drugs that are known to prolong QTc interval is contraindicated). Products include:

Droperidol (Thioridazine has been shown to prolong QTc interval in a dose-related manner; drugs with this potential have been associated with torsade de pointes-type arrhythmias and sudden death; co-administration with other drugs that are known to prolong QTc interval is contraindicated).
No products indexed under this heading.

Enflurane (Thioridazine is capable of potentiating CNS depressants).
No products indexed under this heading.

Epinephrine (Thioridazine causes orthostatic hypotension, especially in female patients; use of epinephrine should be avoided in view of the fact that phenothiazines may induce a reversed epinephrine effect). Products include:

Epinephrine Hydrochloride (Thioridazine causes orthostatic hypotension, especially in female patients; use of epinephrine should be avoided in view of the fact that phenothiazines may induce a reversed epinephrine effect).
No products indexed under this heading.

Erythromycin (Thioridazine has been shown to prolong QTc interval in a dose-related manner; drugs with this potential have been associated with torsade de pointes-type arrhythmias and sudden death; co-administration with other drugs that are known to prolong QTc interval is contraindicated).
No products indexed under this heading.

Erythromycin, Topical (Thioridazine has been shown to prolong QTc interval in a dose-related manner; drugs with this potential have been associated with torsade de pointes-type arrhythmias and sudden death; co-administration with other drugs that are known to prolong QTc interval is contraindicated).
No products indexed under this heading.

Erythromycin Estolate (Thioridazine has been shown to prolong QTc interval in a dose-related manner; drugs with this potential have been associated with torsade de pointes-type arrhythmias and sudden death; co-administration with other drugs that are known to prolong QTc interval is contraindicated).
No products indexed under this heading.

Erythromycin Ethylsuccinate (Thioridazine has been shown to prolong QTc interval in a dose-related manner; drugs with this potential have been associated with torsade de pointes-type arrhythmias and sudden death; co-

administration with other drugs that are known to prolong QTc interval is contraindicated). Products include:

Erythromycin Gluceptate (Thioridazine has been shown to prolong QTc interval in a dose-related manner; drugs with this potential have been associated with torsade de pointes-type arrhythmias and sudden death; co-administration with other drugs that are known to prolong QTc interval is contraindicated).
No products indexed under this heading.

Erythromycin Lactobionate (Thioridazine has been shown to prolong QTc interval in a dose-related manner; drugs with this potential have been associated with torsade de pointes-type arrhythmias and sudden death; co-administration with other drugs that are known to prolong QTc interval is contraindicated).
No products indexed under this heading.

Erythromycin Stearate (Thioridazine has been shown to prolong QTc interval in a dose-related manner; drugs with this potential have been associated with torsade de pointes-type arrhythmias and sudden death; co-administration with other drugs that are known to prolong QTc interval is contraindicated).
No products indexed under this heading.

Estazolam (Thioridazine is capable of potentiating CNS depressants).
No products indexed under this heading.

Ethacrynic Acid (Hypokalemia may result from diuretic therapy and this may increase the risk of QT prolongation and arrhythmias; co-administration may increase the risk of serious, potentially fatal, cardiac arrhythmias).
No products indexed under this heading.

Ethanol (Thioridazine is capable of potentiating CNS depressants).
No products indexed under this heading.

Ethchlorvynol (Thioridazine is capable of potentiating CNS depressants).
No products indexed under this heading.

Ethinamate (Thioridazine is capable of potentiating CNS depressants).
No products indexed under this heading.

Ethyl Alcohol (Thioridazine is capable of potentiating CNS depressants).
No products indexed under this heading.

Fentanyl (Thioridazine is capable of potentiating CNS depressants). Products include:

Fentanyl Citrate (Thioridazine is capable of potentiating CNS depressants). Products include:

Flecainide Acetate (Thioridazine has been shown to prolong QTc interval in a dose-related manner; drugs with this potential have been associated with Torsade de pointes-type arrhythmias and sudden death; co-administration with other drugs that are known to prolong QTc interval is contraindicated).
No products indexed under this heading.

Fluoxetine Hydrochloride (Co-administration with drugs that inhibit CYP450 2D6 isoenzyme will appreciably inhibit metabolism of thioridazine and resulting elevated levels of thioridazine would be expected to augment the prolongation of QTc interval and may increase the risk of serious, potentially fatal, cardiac arrhythmias; concurrent use is contraindicated). Products include:

Fluphenazine Decanoate (Thioridazine is capable of potentiating CNS depressants).
No products indexed under this heading.

Fluphenazine Enanthate (Thioridazine is capable of potentiating CNS depressants).
No products indexed under this heading.

Fluphenazine Hydrochloride (Thioridazine is capable of potentiating CNS depressants).
No products indexed under this heading.

Flurazepam Hydrochloride (Thioridazine is capable of potentiating CNS depressants).
No products indexed under this heading.

Fluvoxamine Maleate (Co-administration with drugs that inhibit CYP450 2D6 isoenzyme will appreciably inhibit metabolism of thioridazine and resulting elevated levels of thioridazine would be expected to augment the prolongation of QTc interval and may increase the risk of serious, potentially fatal, cardiac arrhythmias; concurrent use is contraindicated).
No products indexed under this heading.

Furosemide (Hypokalemia may result from diuretic therapy and this may increase the risk of QT prolongation and arrhythmias; co-administration may increase the risk of serious, potentially fatal, cardiac arrhythmias). Products include:

Gatifloxacin (Thioridazine has been shown to prolong QTc interval in a dose-related manner; drugs with this potential have been associated with torsade de pointes-type arrhythmias and sudden death; co-administration with other drugs that are known to prolong QTc interval is contraindicated).
No products indexed under this heading.

Glutethimide (Thioridazine is capable of potentiating CNS depressants).
No products indexed under this heading.

Halazepam (Thioridazine is capable of potentiating CNS depressants).
No products indexed under this heading.

Halofantrine (Thioridazine has been shown to prolong QTc interval in a dose-related manner; drugs with this potential have been associated with Torsade de pointes-type arrhythmias and sudden death; co-administration with other drugs that are known to prolong QTc interval is contraindicated).
No products indexed under this heading.

Haloperidol (Thioridazine is capable of potentiating CNS depressants).
No products indexed under this heading.

Haloperidol Decanoate (Thioridazine is capable of potentiating CNS depressants).
No products indexed under this heading.

Haloperidol Lactate (Thioridazine is capable of potentiating CNS depressants).
No products indexed under this heading.

Hexobarbital (Thioridazine is capable of potentiating CNS depressants).
No products indexed under this heading.

Hydrochlorothiazide (Hypokalemia may result from diuretic therapy and this may increase the risk of QT prolongation and arrhythmias; co-administration may increase the risk of serious, potentially fatal, cardiac arrhythmias). Products include:

Hydrocodone Bitartrate (Thioridazine is capable of potentiating CNS depressants). Products include:

Hydrocodone Polistirex (Thioridazine is capable of potentiating CNS depressants). Products include:

Hydroflumethiazide (Hypokalemia may result from diuretic therapy and this may increase the risk of QT prolongation and arrhythmias; co-administration may increase the risk of serious, potentially fatal, cardiac arrhythmias).
No products indexed under this heading.

Hydromorphone (Thioridazine is capable of potentiating CNS depressants).
No products indexed under this heading.

Hydromorphone Hydrochloride (Thioridazine is capable of potentiating CNS depressants). Products include:

Hydroxyzine Hydrochloride (Thioridazine is capable of potentiating CNS depressants).
No products indexed under this heading.

Ibutilide Fumarate (Thioridazine has been shown to prolong QTc interval in a dose-related manner; drugs with this potential have been associated with torsade de pointes-type arrhythmias and sudden death; co-administration with other drugs that are known to prolong QTc interval is contraindicated).
No products indexed under this heading.

Isoflurane (Thioridazine is capable of potentiating CNS depressants).
No products indexed under this heading.

Ketamine Hydrochloride (Thioridazine is capable of potentiating CNS depressants).
No products indexed under this heading.

Levomethadyl Acetate Hydrochloride (Thioridazine has been shown to prolong QTc interval in a dose-related manner; drugs with this potential have been associated with torsade de pointes-type arrhythmias and sudden death; co-administration with other drugs that are known to prolong QTc interval is contraindicated).
No products indexed under this heading.

Levorphanol Tartrate (Thioridazine is capable of potentiating CNS depressants).
No products indexed under this heading.

Lorazepam (Thioridazine is capable of potentiating CNS depressants).
No products indexed under this heading.

Loxapine Hydrochloride (Thioridazine is capable of potentiating CNS depressants).
No products indexed under this heading.

Loxapine Succinate (Thioridazine is capable of potentiating CNS depressants).
No products indexed under this heading.

Mefloquine Hydrochloride (Thioridazine has been shown to prolong QTc interval in a dose-related manner; drugs with this potential have been associated with Torsade de pointes-type arrhythmias and sudden death; co-administration with other drugs that are known to prolong QTc interval is contraindicated).
No products indexed under this heading.

Meperidine Hydrochloride (Thioridazine is capable of potentiating CNS depressants).
No products indexed under this heading.

Mephobarbital (Thioridazine is capable of potentiating CNS depressants).
No products indexed under this heading.

Meprobamate (Thioridazine is capable of potentiating CNS depressants).
No products indexed under this heading.

Mesoridazine Besylate (Thioridazine is capable of potentiating CNS depressants).
No products indexed under this heading.

Methadone Hydrochloride (Thioridazine is capable of potentiating CNS depressants).
No products indexed under this heading.

Methohexital Sodium (Thioridazine is capable of potentiating CNS depressants).
No products indexed under this heading.

Methotrimeprazine (Thioridazine is capable of potentiating CNS depressants).
No products indexed under this heading.

Methoxyflurane (Thioridazine is capable of potentiating CNS depressants).
No products indexed under this heading.

Methyclothiazide (Hypokalemia may result from diuretic therapy and this may increase the risk of QT prolongation and arrhythmias; co-administration may increase the risk of serious, potentially fatal, cardiac arrhythmias).
No products indexed under this heading.

Midazolam Hydrochloride (Thioridazine is capable of potentiating CNS depressants).
No products indexed under this heading.

Molindone Hydrochloride (Thioridazine is capable of potentiating CNS depressants). Products include:

Morphine Sulfate (Thioridazine is capable of potentiating CNS depressants). Products include:

Morphine Sulfate, Liposomal (Thioridazine is capable of potentiating CNS depressants).
No products indexed under this heading.

Moxifloxacin Hydrochloride (Thioridazine has been shown to prolong QTc interval in a dose-related manner; drugs with this potential have been associated with torsade de pointes-type arrhythmias and sudden death; co-administration with other drugs that are known to prolong QTc interval is contraindicated). Products include:

Olanzapine (Thioridazine is capable of potentiating CNS depressants). Products include:

Oxazepam (Thioridazine is capable of potentiating CNS depressants).
No products indexed under this heading.

Oxycodone Hydrochloride (Thioridazine is capable of potentiating CNS depressants). Products include:

Oxycodone Terephthalate (Thioridazine is capable of potentiating CNS depressants).
No products indexed under this heading.

Oxymorphone Hydrochloride (Thioridazine is capable of potentiating CNS depressants). Products include:

Paroxetine Hydrochloride (Co-administration with drugs that inhibit CYP450 2D6 isoenzyme will appreciably inhibit metabolism of thioridazine and resulting elevated levels of thioridazine would be expected to augment the prolongation of QTc interval and may increase the risk of serious, potentially fatal, cardiac arrhythmias; concurrent use is contraindicated). Products include:

Pentamidine Isethionate (Thioridazine has been shown to prolong QTc interval in a dose-related manner; drugs with this potential have been associated with torsade de pointes-type arrhythmias and sudden death; co-administration with other drugs that are known to prolong QTc interval is contraindicated).
No products indexed under this heading.

Pentobarbital (Thioridazine is capable of potentiating CNS depressants).
No products indexed under this heading.

Pentobarbital Sodium (Thioridazine is capable of potentiating CNS depressants). Products include:

Perphenazine (Thioridazine is capable of potentiating CNS depressants).
No products indexed under this heading.

Phenobarbital (Thioridazine is capable of potentiating CNS depressants). Products include:

Phenobarbital Sodium (Thioridazine is capable of potentiating CNS depressants).
No products indexed under this heading.

Pimozide (Thioridazine has been shown to prolong QTc interval in a dose-related manner; drugs with this potential have been associated with torsade de pointes-type arrhythmias and sudden death; co-administration with other drugs that are known to prolong QTc interval is contraindicated).
No products indexed under this heading.

Pindolol (Co-administration with drugs that inhibit CYP450 2D6 isoenzyme will appreciably inhibit metabolism of thioridazine and resulting elevated levels of thioridazine would be expected to augment the prolongation of QTc interval and may increase the risk of serious, potentially fatal, cardiac arrhythmias; concurrent use is contraindicated).
No products indexed under this heading.

Polythiazide (Hypokalemia may result from diuretic therapy and this may increase the risk of QT prolongation and arrhythmias; co-administration may increase the risk of serious, potentially fatal, cardiac arrhythmias).
No products indexed under this heading.

Prazepam (Thioridazine is capable of potentiating CNS depressants).
No products indexed under this heading.

Procainamide Hydrochloride (Thioridazine has been shown to prolong QTc interval in a dose-related manner; drugs with this potential have been associated with torsade de pointes-type arrhythmias and sudden death; co-administration with other drugs that are known to prolong QTc interval is contraindicated).
No products indexed under this heading.

Prochlorperazine (Thioridazine is capable of potentiating CNS depressants).
No products indexed under this heading.

Prochlorperazine Edisylate (Thioridazine is capable of potentiating CNS depressants).
No products indexed under this heading.

Prochlorperazine Maleate (Thioridazine is capable of potentiating CNS depressants).
No products indexed under this heading.

Promethazine (Thioridazine is capable of potentiating CNS depressants).
No products indexed under this heading.

Promethazine Hydrochloride (Thioridazine is capable of potentiating CNS depressants).
No products indexed under this heading.

Propofol (Thioridazine is capable of potentiating CNS depressants).
No products indexed under this heading.

Propoxyphene Hydrochloride (Thioridazine is capable of potentiating CNS depressants).
No products indexed under this heading.

Propoxyphene Napsylate (Thioridazine is capable of potentiating CNS depressants).
No products indexed under this heading.

Propranolol Hydrochloride (Co-administration with drugs that inhibit CYP450 2D6 isoenzyme will appreciably inhibit metabolism of thioridazine and resulting elevated levels of thioridazine would be expected to augment the prolongation of QTc interval and may increase the risk of serious, potentially fatal, cardiac arrhythmias; concurrent use is contraindicated). Products include:

Quazepam (Thioridazine is capable of potentiating CNS depressants).
No products indexed under this heading.

Quetiapine Fumarate (Thioridazine is capable of potentiating CNS depressants). Products include:

Quinidine (Thioridazine has been shown to prolong QTc interval in a dose-related manner; drugs with this potential have been associated with torsade de pointes-type arrhythmias and sudden death; co-administration with other drugs that are known to prolong QTc interval is contraindicated).
No products indexed under this heading.

Quinidine Gluconate (Thioridazine has been shown to prolong QTc interval in a dose-related manner; drugs with this potential have been associated with torsade de pointes-type arrhythmias and sudden death; co-administration with other drugs that are known to prolong QTc interval is contraindicated).
No products indexed under this heading.

Quinidine Hydrochloride (Thioridazine has been shown to prolong QTc interval in a dose-related manner; drugs with this potential have been associated with torsade de pointes-type arrhythmias and sudden death; co-administration with other drugs that are known to prolong QTc interval is contraindicated).
No products indexed under this heading.

Quinidine Polygalacturonate (Thioridazine has been shown to prolong QTc interval in a dose-related manner; drugs with this potential have been associated with torsade de pointes-type arrhythmias and sudden death; co-administration with other drugs that are known to prolong QTc interval is contraindicated).
No products indexed under this heading.

Quinidine Sulfate (Thioridazine has been shown to prolong QTc interval in a dose-related manner; drugs with this potential have been associated with torsade de pointes-type arrhythmias and sudden death; co-administration with other drugs that are known to prolong QTc interval is contraindicated).
No products indexed under this heading.

Remifentanil Hydrochloride (Thioridazine is capable of potentiating CNS depressants).
No products indexed under this heading.

Risperidone (Thioridazine is capable of potentiating CNS depressants). Products include:

Secobarbital Sodium (Thioridazine is capable of potentiating CNS depressants).
No products indexed under this heading.

Sevoflurane (Thioridazine is capable of potentiating CNS depressants). Products include:

Sodium Butabarbital (Thioridazine is capable of potentiating CNS depressants).
No products indexed under this heading.

Sodium Oxybate (Thioridazine is capable of potentiating CNS depressants).
No products indexed under this heading.

Sodium Pentobarbital (Thioridazine is capable of potentiating CNS depressants).
No products indexed under this heading.

Sotalol Hydrochloride (Thioridazine has been shown to prolong QTc interval in a dose-related manner; drugs with this potential have been associated with torsade de pointes-type arrhythmias and sudden death; co-administration with other drugs that are known to prolong QTc interval is contraindicated).
No products indexed under this heading.

Sparfloxacin (Thioridazine has been shown to prolong QTc interval in a dose-related manner; drugs with this potential have been associated with torsade de pointes-type arrhythmias and sudden death; co-administration with other drugs that are known to prolong QTc interval is contraindicated).
No products indexed under this heading.

Sufentanil Citrate (Thioridazine is capable of potentiating CNS depressants).
No products indexed under this heading.

Tacrolimus (Thioridazine has been shown to prolong QTc interval in a dose-related manner; drugs with this potential have been associated with torsade de pointes-type arrhythmias and sudden death; co-administration with other drugs that are known to prolong QTc interval is contraindicated). Products include:

Talbutal (Thioridazine is capable of potentiating CNS depressants).
No products indexed under this heading.

Temazepam (Thioridazine is capable of potentiating CNS depressants).
No products indexed under this heading.

Thiamylal Sodium (Thioridazine is capable of potentiating CNS depressants).
No products indexed under this heading.

Thioridazine (Thioridazine is capable of potentiating CNS depressants).
No products indexed under this heading.

Thiothixene (Thioridazine is capable of potentiating CNS depressants). Products include:

1879 Interactions Index Thiothixene

Thiothixene Hydrochloride (Thioridazine is capable of potentiating CNS depressants).
No products indexed under this heading.

Torsemide (Hypokalemia may result from diuretic therapy and this may increase the risk of QT prolongation and arrhythmias; co-administration may increase the risk of serious, potentially fatal, cardiac arrhythmias).
No products indexed under this heading.

Triazolam (Thioridazine is capable of potentiating CNS depressants).
No products indexed under this heading.

Trifluoperazine Hydrochloride (Thioridazine is capable of potentiating CNS depressants).
No products indexed under this heading.

Zaleplon (Thioridazine is capable of potentiating CNS depressants).
No products indexed under this heading.

Ziprasidone Hydrochloride (Thioridazine has been shown to prolong QTc interval in a dose-related manner; drugs with this potential have been associated with torsade de pointes-type arrhythmias and sudden death; co-administration with other drugs that are known to prolong QTc interval is contraindicated). Products include:
Geodon 2723

Ziprasidone Mesylate (Thioridazine has been shown to prolong QTc interval in a dose-related manner; drugs with this potential have been associated with torsade de pointes-type arrhythmias and sudden death; co-administration with other drugs that are known to prolong QTc interval is contraindicated). Products include:
Geodon 2723

Zolpidem Tartrate (Thioridazine is capable of potentiating CNS depressants). Products include:
Ambien 2920
Ambien CR 2925

Food Interactions

Alcohol (Thioridazine is capable of potentiating CNS depressants).

Beer, reduced-alcohol (Thioridazine is capable of potentiating CNS depressants).

Beer, unspecified (Thioridazine is capable of potentiating CNS depressants).

Wine, Chianti (Thioridazine is capable of potentiating CNS depressants).

Wine, Red (Thioridazine is capable of potentiating CNS depressants).

Wine, unspecified (Thioridazine is capable of potentiating CNS depressants).

Wine products (Thioridazine is capable of potentiating CNS depressants).

THIOTHIXENE CAPSULES

(Thiothixene) 2386
May interact with alcohols, anticholinergics, antihypertensives, atropines, barbiturates, central nervous system depressants, hepatic microsomal enzyme inducers, and certain other agents. Compounds in these categories include:

Acebutolol Hydrochloride (Co-administration of thiothixene with antihypertensive agents may lead to excessive hypotension due to a possible additive effect. Patients receiving these drugs should be observed closely for signs of excessive hypotension when thiothixene is added to their drug regimen).
No products indexed under this heading.

Alfentanil Hydrochloride (Patients receiving thiothixene should be cautioned about the possible additive effects (which may include hypotension) with CNS depressants. Caution as well as careful adjustment of the dosages is indicated when thiothixene is used in conjunction with other CNS depressants and with alcohol).
No products indexed under this heading.

Aliskiren (Co-administration of thiothixene with antihypertensive agents may lead to excessive hypotension due to a possible additive effect. Patients receiving these drugs should be observed closely for signs of excessive hypotension when thiothixene is added to their drug regimen). Products include:
Tekturna 2538
Tekturna HCT 2541
Valturna 3637

Allium sativum (Co-administration of thiothixene with hepatic microsomal enzyme inducing agents such as carbamazepine may increase the clearance of thiothixene. Patients receiving these drugs should be observed for signs of reduced thiothixene effectiveness).
No products indexed under this heading.

Alprazolam (Patients receiving thiothixene should be cautioned about the possible additive effects (which may include hypotension) with CNS depressants. Caution as well as careful adjustment of the dosages is indicated when thiothixene is used in conjunction with other CNS depressants and with alcohol).
No products indexed under this heading.

Aminoglutethimide (Co-administration of thiothixene with hepatic microsomal enzyme inducing agents such as carbamazepine may increase the clearance of thiothixene. Patients receiving these drugs should be observed for signs of reduced thiothixene effectiveness).
No products indexed under this heading.

Amlodipine Besylate (Co-administration of thiothixene with antihypertensive agents may lead to excessive hypotension due to a possible additive effect. Patients receiving these drugs should be observed closely for signs of excessive hypotension when thiothixene is added to their drug regimen). Products include:
Azor 1010
Exforge 2443
Exforge HCT 2449

Amobarbital (Although thiothixene potentiates the actions of the barbiturates, the dosage of the anticonvulsant therapy should not be reduced when thiothixene is administered concurrently).
No products indexed under this heading.

Amobarbital Sodium (Although thiothixene potentiates the actions of the barbiturates, the dosage of the anticonvulsant therapy should not be reduced when thiothixene is administered concurrently).
No products indexed under this heading.

Aprepitant (Co-administration of thiothixene with hepatic microsomal enzyme inducing agents such as carbamazepine may increase the clearance of thiothixene. Patients receiving these drugs should be observed for signs of reduced thiothixene effectiveness). Products include:
Emend 2124

Aprobarbital (Although thiothixene potentiates the actions of the barbiturates, the dosage of the anticonvulsant therapy should not be reduced when thiothixene is administered concurrently).
No products indexed under this heading.

Atenolol (Co-administration of thiothixene with antihypertensive agents may lead to excessive hypotension due to a possible additive effect. Patients receiving these drugs should be observed closely for signs of excessive hypotension when thiothixene is added to their drug regimen).
No products indexed under this heading.

Atropine Derivatives (Though exhibiting rather weak anticholinergic properties, thiothixene should be used with caution in patients who might be exposed to extreme heat or who are receiving atropine related drugs).
No products indexed under this heading.

Atropine Nitrate, Methyl (Though exhibiting rather weak anticholinergic properties, thiothixene should be used with caution in patients who might be exposed to extreme heat or who are receiving atropine related drugs).
No products indexed under this heading.

Atropine Sulfate (Though exhibiting rather weak anticholinergic properties, thiothixene should be used with caution in patients who might be exposed to extreme heat or who are receiving atropine related drugs). Products include:
Donnatal 2711

Belladonna Alkaloids (Though exhibiting rather weak anticholinergic properties, thiothixene should be used with caution in patients who might be exposed to extreme heat or who are receiving atropine or related drugs). Products include:
Hyland's Teething Tablets 3316

Benazepril Hydrochloride (Co-administration of thiothixene with antihypertensive agents may lead to excessive hypotension due to a possible additive effect. Patients receiving these drugs should be observed closely for signs of excessive hypotension when thiothixene is added to their drug regimen).
No products indexed under this heading.

Bendroflumethiazide (Co-administration of thiothixene with antihypertensive agents may lead to excessive hypotension due to a possible additive effect. Patients receiving these drugs should be observed closely for signs of excessive hypotension when thiothixene is added to their drug regimen).
No products indexed under this heading.

Benztropine Mesylate (Though exhibiting rather weak anticholinergic properties, thiothixene should be used with caution in patients who might be exposed to extreme heat or who are receiving atropine or related drugs).
No products indexed under this heading.

Betamethasone (Co-administration of thiothixene with hepatic microsomal enzyme inducing agents such as carbamazepine may increase the clearance of thiothixene. Patients receiving these drugs should be observed for signs of reduced thiothixene effectiveness).
No products indexed under this heading.

Betamethasone Sodium Phosphate (Co-administration of thiothixene with hepatic microsomal enzyme inducing agents such as carbamazepine may increase the clearance of thiothixene. Patients receiving these drugs should be observed for signs of reduced thiothixene effectiveness).
No products indexed under this heading.

Betaxolol Hydrochloride (Co-administration of thiothixene with antihypertensive agents may lead to excessive hypotension due to a possible additive effect. Patients receiving these drugs should be observed closely for signs of excessive hypotension when thiothixene is added to their drug regimen).
No products indexed under this heading.

Biperiden Hydrochloride (Though exhibiting rather weak anticholinergic properties, thiothixene should be used with caution in patients who might be exposed to extreme heat or who are receiving atropine or related drugs).
No products indexed under this heading.

Bisoprolol Fumarate (Co-administration of thiothixene with antihypertensive agents may lead to excessive hypotension due to a possible additive effect. Patients receiving these drugs should be observed closely for signs of excessive hypotension when thiothixene is added to their drug regimen).
No products indexed under this heading.

Bosentan (Co-administration of thiothixene with hepatic microsomal enzyme inducing agents such as carbamazepine may increase the clearance of thiothixene. Patients receiving these drugs should be observed for signs of reduced thiothixene effectiveness). Products include:
Tracleer 573

Buprenorphine Hydrochloride (Patients receiving thiothixene should be cautioned about the possible additive effects (which may include hypotension) with CNS depressants. Caution as well as careful adjustment of the dosages is indicated when thiothixene is used in conjunction with other CNS depressants and with alcohol).
No products indexed under this heading.

Buspirone Hydrochloride (Patients receiving thiothixene should be cautioned about the possible additive effects (which may include hypotension) with CNS depressants. Caution as well as careful adjustment of the dosages is indicated when thiothixene is used in conjunction with other CNS depressants and with alcohol).
No products indexed under this heading.

Butabarbital (Although thiothixene potentiates the actions of the barbiturates, the dosage of the anticonvulsant therapy should not be reduced when thiothixene is administered concurrently).
No products indexed under this heading.

Butabarbital Sodium (Although thiothixene potentiates the actions of the barbiturates, the dosage of the anticonvulsant therapy should not be reduced when thiothixene is administered concurrently).
No products indexed under this heading.

Butalbital (Although thiothixene potentiates the actions of the barbiturates, the dosage of the anticonvulsant therapy should not be reduced when thiothixene is administered concurrently).
No products indexed under this heading.

Candesartan Cilexetil (Co-administration of thiothixene with antihypertensive agents may lead to excessive hypotension due to a possible additive effect. Patients receiving these drugs should be observed closely for signs of excessive hypotension when thiothixene is added to their drug regimen). Products include:
Atacand 697
Atacand HCT 700

Captopril (Co-administration of thiothixene with antihypertensive agents may lead to excessive hypotension due to a possible additive effect. Patients

IMPORTANT NOTE: Always consult each drug listing in the patient's regimen for possible interactions.

receiving these drugs should be observed closely for signs of excessive hypotension when thiothixene is added to their drug regimen). Products include:

Carbamazepine (Co-administration of thiothixene with hepatic microsomal enzyme inducing agents such as carbamazepine may increase the clearance of thiothixene. Patients receiving these drugs should be observed for signs of reduced thiothixene effectiveness). Products include:

Carteolol Hydrochloride (Co-administration of thiothixene with antihypertensive agents may lead to excessive hypotension due to a possible additive effect. Patients receiving these drugs should be observed closely for signs of excessive hypotension when thiothixene is added to their drug regimen).

No products indexed under this heading.

Carvedilol (Co-administration of thiothixene with antihypertensive agents may lead to excessive hypotension due to a possible additive effect. Patients receiving these drugs should be observed closely for signs of excessive hypotension when thiothixene is added to their drug regimen). Products include:

Carvedilol Phosphate (Co-administration of thiothixene with antihypertensive agents may lead to excessive hypotension due to a possible additive effect. Patients receiving these drugs should be observed closely for signs of excessive hypotension when thiothixene is added to their drug regimen). Products include:

Chlordiazepoxide (Patients receiving thiothixene should be cautioned about the possible additive effects (which may include hypotension) with CNS depressants. Caution as well as careful adjustment of the dosages is indicated when thiothixene is used in conjunction with other CNS depressants and with alcohol).

No products indexed under this heading.

Chlordiazepoxide Hydrochloride (Patients receiving thiothixene should be cautioned about the possible additive effects (which may include hypotension) with CNS depressants. Caution as well as careful adjustment of the dosages is indicated when thiothixene is used in conjunction with other CNS depressants and with alcohol).

No products indexed under this heading.

Chlorothiazide (Co-administration of thiothixene with antihypertensive agents may lead to excessive hypotension due to a possible additive effect. Patients receiving these drugs should be observed closely for signs of excessive hypotension when thiothixene is added to their drug regimen).

No products indexed under this heading.

Chlorothiazide Sodium (Co-administration of thiothixene with antihypertensive agents may lead to excessive hypotension due to a possible additive effect. Patients receiving these drugs should be observed closely for signs of excessive hypotension when thiothixene is added to their drug regimen). Products include:

Chlorpromazine (Patients receiving thiothixene should be cautioned about the possible additive effects (which may include hypotension) with CNS depressants. Caution as well as careful adjustment of the dosages is indicated when thiothixene is used in conjunction with other CNS depressants and with alcohol).

No products indexed under this heading.

Chlorpromazine Hydrochloride (Patients receiving thiothixene should be cautioned about the possible additive effects (which may include hypotension) with CNS depressants. Caution as well as careful adjustment of the dosages is indicated when thiothixene is used in conjunction with other CNS depressants and with alcohol).

No products indexed under this heading.

Chlorpropamide (Co-administration of thiothixene with hepatic microsomal enzyme inducing agents such as carbamazepine may increase the clearance of thiothixene. Patients receiving these drugs should be observed for signs of reduced thiothixene effectiveness).

No products indexed under this heading.

Chlorprothixene (Patients receiving thiothixene should be cautioned about the possible additive effects (which may include hypotension) with CNS depressants. Caution as well as careful adjustment of the dosages is indicated when thiothixene is used in conjunction with other CNS depressants and with alcohol).

No products indexed under this heading.

Chlorprothixene Hydrochloride (Patients receiving thiothixene should be cautioned about the possible additive effects (which may include hypotension) with CNS depressants. Caution as well as careful adjustment of the dosages is indicated when thiothixene is used in conjunction with other CNS depressants and with alcohol).

No products indexed under this heading.

Chlorprothixene Lactate (Patients receiving thiothixene should be cautioned about the possible additive effects (which may include hypotension) with CNS depressants. Caution as well as careful adjustment of the dosages is indicated when thiothixene is used in conjunction with other CNS depressants and with alcohol).

No products indexed under this heading.

Chlorthalidone (Co-administration of thiothixene with antihypertensive agents may lead to excessive hypotension due to a possible additive effect. Patients receiving these drugs should be observed closely for signs of excessive hypotension when thiothixene is added to their drug regimen). Products include:

Ciprofloxacin (Co-administration of thiothixene with hepatic microsomal enzyme inducing agents such as carbamazepine may increase the clearance of thiothixene. Patients receiving these drugs should be observed for signs of reduced thiothixene effectiveness). Products include:

Ciprofloxacin Hydrochloride (Co-administration of thiothixene with hepatic microsomal enzyme inducing agents such as carbamazepine may increase the clearance of thiothixene. Patients receiving these drugs should be observed for signs of reduced thiothixene effectiveness). Products include:

Cisplatin (Co-administration of thiothixene with hepatic microsomal enzyme inducing agents such as carbamazepine may increase the clearance of thiothixene. Patients receiving these drugs should be observed for signs of reduced thiothixene effectiveness).

No products indexed under this heading.

Citalopram Hydrobromide (Co-administration of thiothixene with hepatic microsomal enzyme inducing agents such as carbamazepine may increase the clearance of thiothixene. Patients receiving these drugs should be observed for signs of reduced thiothixene effectiveness). Products include:

Clidinium Bromide (Though exhibiting rather weak anticholinergic properties, thiothixene should be used with caution in patients who might be exposed to extreme heat or who are receiving atropine or related drugs).

No products indexed under this heading.

Clonazepam (Patients receiving thiothixene should be cautioned about the possible additive effects (which may include hypotension) with CNS depressants. Caution as well as careful adjustment of the dosages is indicated when thiothixene is used in conjunction with other CNS depressants and with alcohol). Products include:

Clonidine (Co-administration of thiothixene with antihypertensive agents may lead to excessive hypotension due to a possible additive effect. Patients receiving these drugs should be observed closely for signs of excessive hypotension when thiothixene is added to their drug regimen). Products include:

Clonidine Hydrochloride (Co-administration of thiothixene with antihypertensive agents may lead to excessive hypotension due to a possible additive effect. Patients receiving these drugs should be observed closely for signs of excessive hypotension when thiothixene is added to their drug regimen). Products include:

Clorazepate Dipotassium (Patients receiving thiothixene should be cautioned about the possible additive effects (which may include hypotension) with CNS depressants. Caution as well as careful adjustment of the dosages is indicated when thiothixene is used in conjunction with other CNS depressants and with alcohol).

No products indexed under this heading.

Clozapine (Patients receiving thiothixene should be cautioned about the possible additive effects (which may include hypotension) with CNS depressants. Caution as well as careful adjustment of the dosages is indicated when thiothixene is used in conjunction with other CNS depressants and with alcohol).

No products indexed under this heading.

Codeine Phosphate (Patients receiving thiothixene should be cautioned about the possible additive effects (which may include hypotension) with CNS depressants. Caution as well as careful adjustment of the dosages is indicated when thiothixene is used in conjunction with other CNS depressants and with alcohol). Products include:

Codeine Sulfate (Patients receiving thiothixene should be cautioned about the possible additive effects (which may include hypotension) with CNS depressants. Caution as well as careful adjustment of the dosages is indicated when thiothixene is used in conjunction with other CNS depressants and with alcohol).

No products indexed under this heading.

Cortisone Acetate (Co-administration of thiothixene with hepatic microsomal enzyme inducing agents such as carbamazepine may increase the clearance of thiothixene. Patients receiving these drugs should be observed for signs of reduced thiothixene effectiveness).

No products indexed under this heading.

Deserpidine (Co-administration of thiothixene with antihypertensive agents may lead to excessive hypotension due to a possible additive effect. Patients receiving these drugs should be observed closely for signs of excessive hypotension when thiothixene is added to their drug regimen).

No products indexed under this heading.

Desflurane (Patients receiving thiothixene should be cautioned about the possible additive effects (which may include hypotension) with CNS depressants. Caution as well as careful adjustment of the dosages is indicated when thiothixene is used in conjunction with other CNS depressants and with alcohol).

No products indexed under this heading.

Dexamethasone (Co-administration of thiothixene with hepatic microsomal enzyme inducing agents such as carbamazepine may increase the clearance of thiothixene. Patients receiving these drugs should be observed for signs of reduced thiothixene effectiveness). Products include:

Dexamethasone Acetate (Co-administration of thiothixene with hepatic microsomal enzyme inducing agents such as carbamazepine may increase the clearance of thiothixene. Patients receiving these drugs should be observed for signs of reduced thiothixene effectiveness).

No products indexed under this heading.

Dexamethasone Phosphate (Co-administration of thiothixene with hepatic microsomal enzyme inducing agents such as carbamazepine may increase the clearance of thiothixene. Patients receiving these drugs should be observed for signs of reduced thiothixene effectiveness).

No products indexed under this heading.

Dexamethasone Sodium (Co-administration of thiothixene with hepatic microsomal enzyme inducing agents such as carbamazepine may increase the clearance of thiothixene. Patients receiving these drugs should be observed for signs of reduced thiothixene effectiveness).

No products indexed under this heading.

Dexamethasone Sodium Phosphate (Co-administration of thiothixene with hepatic microsomal enzyme inducing agents such as carbamazepine may increase the clearance of thiothixene. Patients receiving these drugs should be observed for signs of reduced thiothixene effectiveness).

No products indexed under this heading.

1881 Interactions Index Thiothixene

Dezocine (Patients receiving thiothixene should be cautioned about the possible additive effects (which may include hypotension) with CNS depressants. Caution as well as careful adjustment of the dosages is indicated when thiothixene is used in conjunction with other CNS depressants and with alcohol).
No products indexed under this heading.

Diazepam (Patients receiving thiothixene should be cautioned about the possible additive effects (which may include hypotension) with CNS depressants. Caution as well as careful adjustment of the dosages is indicated when thiothixene is used in conjunction with other CNS depressants and with alcohol). Products include:
Valium Tablets 2880

Diazoxide (Co-administration of thiothixene with antihypertensive agents may lead to excessive hypotension due to a possible additive effect. Patients receiving these drugs should be observed closely for signs of excessive hypotension when thiothixene is added to their drug regimen). Products include:
Proglycem 1179
Proglycem Suspension 1179

Dicyclomine Hydrochloride (Though exhibiting rather weak anticholinergic properties, thiothixene should be used with caution in patients who might be exposed to extreme heat or who are receiving atropine or related drugs). Products include:
Bentyl Capsules 780
Bentyl Injection 780
Bentyl Syrup 780
Bentyl Tablets 780

Diltiazem Hydrochloride (Co-administration of thiothixene with antihypertensive agents may lead to excessive hypotension due to a possible additive effect. Patients receiving these drugs should be observed closely for signs of excessive hypotension when thiothixene is added to their drug regimen). Products include:
Cardizem LA 423

Diltiazem Maleate (Co-administration of thiothixene with antihypertensive agents may lead to excessive hypotension due to a possible additive effect. Patients receiving these drugs should be observed closely for signs of excessive hypotension when thiothixene is added to their drug regimen).
No products indexed under this heading.

Doxazosin Mesylate (Co-administration of thiothixene with antihypertensive agents may lead to excessive hypotension due to a possible additive effect. Patients receiving these drugs should be observed closely for signs of excessive hypotension when thiothixene is added to their drug regimen).
No products indexed under this heading.

Doxorubicin Hydrochloride (Co-administration of thiothixene with hepatic microsomal enzyme inducing agents such as carbamazepine may increase the clearance of thiothixene. Patients receiving these drugs should be observed for signs of reduced thiothixene effectiveness).
No products indexed under this heading.

Droperidol (Patients receiving thiothixene should be cautioned about the possible additive effects (which may include hypotension) with CNS depressants. Caution as well as careful adjustment of the dosages is indicated when thiothixene is used in conjunction with other CNS depressants and with alcohol).
No products indexed under this heading.

Efavirenz (Co-administration of thiothixene with hepatic microsomal enzyme inducing agents such as carbamazepine may increase the clearance of thiothixene. Patients receiving these drugs should be observed for signs of reduced thiothixene effectiveness). Products include:
Atripla 906

Enalapril Maleate (Co-administration of thiothixene with antihypertensive agents may lead to excessive hypotension due to a possible additive effect. Patients receiving these drugs should be observed closely for signs of excessive hypotension when thiothixene is added to their drug regimen).
No products indexed under this heading.

Enalaprilat (Co-administration of thiothixene with antihypertensive agents may lead to excessive hypotension due to a possible additive effect. Patients receiving these drugs should be observed closely for signs of excessive hypotension when thiothixene is added to their drug regimen).
No products indexed under this heading.

Enflurane (Patients receiving thiothixene should be cautioned about the possible additive effects (which may include hypotension) with CNS depressants. Caution as well as careful adjustment of the dosages is indicated when thiothixene is used in conjunction with other CNS depressants and with alcohol).
No products indexed under this heading.

Epinephrine (In the event hypotension occurs, epinephrine should not be used as a pressor agent since a paradoxical further lowering of blood pressure may result). Products include:
EpiPen 3631
Twinject 3268

Eprosartan Mesylate (Co-administration of thiothixene with antihypertensive agents may lead to excessive hypotension due to a possible additive effect. Patients receiving these drugs should be observed closely for signs of excessive hypotension when thiothixene is added to their drug regimen). Products include:
Teveten 538
Teveten HCT 541

Erythromycin (Co-administration of thiothixene with hepatic microsomal enzyme inducing agents such as carbamazepine may increase the clearance of thiothixene. Patients receiving these drugs should be observed for signs of reduced thiothixene effectiveness).
No products indexed under this heading.

Erythromycin, Topical (Co-administration of thiothixene with hepatic microsomal enzyme inducing agents such as carbamazepine may increase the clearance of thiothixene. Patients receiving these drugs should be observed for signs of reduced thiothixene effectiveness).
No products indexed under this heading.

Erythromycin Estolate (Co-administration of thiothixene with hepatic microsomal enzyme inducing agents such as carbamazepine may increase the clearance of thiothixene. Patients receiving these drugs should be observed for signs of reduced thiothixene effectiveness).
No products indexed under this heading.

Erythromycin Ethylsuccinate (Co-administration of thiothixene with hepatic microsomal enzyme inducing agents such as carbamazepine may increase the clearance of thiothixene. Patients receiving these drugs should be observed for signs of reduced thiothixene effectiveness). Products include:
E.E.S. 437
EryPed 435

Erythromycin Gluceptate (Co-administration of thiothixene with hepatic microsomal enzyme inducing agents such as carbamazepine may increase the clearance of thiothixene. Patients receiving these drugs should be observed for signs of reduced thiothixene effectiveness).
No products indexed under this heading.

Erythromycin Lactobionate (Co-administration of thiothixene with hepatic microsomal enzyme inducing agents such as carbamazepine may increase the clearance of thiothixene. Patients receiving these drugs should be observed for signs of reduced thiothixene effectiveness).
No products indexed under this heading.

Erythromycin Stearate (Co-administration of thiothixene with hepatic microsomal enzyme inducing agents such as carbamazepine may increase the clearance of thiothixene. Patients receiving these drugs should be observed for signs of reduced thiothixene effectiveness).
No products indexed under this heading.

Escitalopram Oxalate (Co-administration of thiothixene with hepatic microsomal enzyme inducing agents such as carbamazepine may increase the clearance of thiothixene. Patients receiving these drugs should be observed for signs of reduced thiothixene effectiveness). Products include:
Lexapro Oral Suspension 1160
Lexapro Tablets 1160

Esmolol Hydrochloride (Co-administration of thiothixene with antihypertensive agents may lead to excessive hypotension due to a possible additive effect. Patients receiving these drugs should be observed closely for signs of excessive hypotension when thiothixene is added to their drug regimen).
No products indexed under this heading.

Esomeprazole Magnesium (Co-administration of thiothixene with hepatic microsomal enzyme inducing agents such as carbamazepine may increase the clearance of thiothixene. Patients receiving these drugs should be observed for signs of reduced thiothixene effectiveness). Products include:
Nexium Capsules 704
Nexium Oral Suspension 704

Esomeprazole Sodium (Co-administration of thiothixene with hepatic microsomal enzyme inducing agents such as carbamazepine may increase the clearance of thiothixene. Patients receiving these drugs should be observed for signs of reduced thiothixene effectiveness). Products include:
Nexium I.V. 712

Estazolam (Patients receiving thiothixene should be cautioned about the possible additive effects (which may include hypotension) with CNS depressants. Caution as well as careful adjustment of the dosages is indicated when thiothixene is used in conjunction with other CNS depressants and with alcohol).
No products indexed under this heading.

Ethanol (Patients receiving thiothixene should be cautioned about the possible additive effects (which may include hypotension) with CNS depressants and with alcohol. Extreme caution should be used in patients with a history of convulsive disorders or those in a state of alcohol withdrawal, since it may lower the convulsive threshold).
No products indexed under this heading.

Ethchlorvynol (Patients receiving thiothixene should be cautioned about the possible additive effects (which may include hypotension) with CNS depressants. Caution as well as careful adjustment of the dosages is indicated when thiothixene is used in conjunction with other CNS depressants and with alcohol).
No products indexed under this heading.

Ethinamate (Patients receiving thiothixene should be cautioned about the possible additive effects (which may include hypotension) with CNS depressants. Caution as well as careful adjustment of the dosages is indicated when thiothixene is used in conjunction with other CNS depressants and with alcohol).
No products indexed under this heading.

Ethosuximide (Co-administration of thiothixene with hepatic microsomal enzyme inducing agents such as carbamazepine may increase the clearance of thiothixene. Patients receiving these drugs should be observed for signs of reduced thiothixene effectiveness).
No products indexed under this heading.

Ethyl Alcohol (Patients receiving thiothixene should be cautioned about the possible additive effects (which may include hypotension) with CNS depressants and with alcohol. Extreme caution should be used in patients with a history of convulsive disorders or those in a state of alcohol withdrawal, since it may lower the convulsive threshold).
No products indexed under this heading.

Felbamate (Co-administration of thiothixene with hepatic microsomal enzyme inducing agents such as carbamazepine may increase the clearance of thiothixene. Patients receiving these drugs should be observed for signs of reduced thiothixene effectiveness).
No products indexed under this heading.

Felodipine (Co-administration of thiothixene with antihypertensive agents may lead to excessive hypotension due to a possible additive effect. Patients receiving these drugs should be observed closely for signs of excessive hypotension when thiothixene is added to their drug regimen).
No products indexed under this heading.

Fentanyl (Patients receiving thiothixene should be cautioned about the possible additive effects (which may include hypotension) with CNS depressants. Caution as well as careful adjustment of the dosages is indicated when thiothixene is used in conjunction with other CNS depressants and with alcohol). Products include:
Duragesic 2604
Fentanyl Transdermal System 2346
Onsolis 2054

Fentanyl Citrate (Patients receiving thiothixene should be cautioned about the possible additive effects (which may include hypotension) with CNS depressants. Caution as well as careful adjustment of the dosages is indicated when thiothixene is used in conjunction with other CNS depressants and with alcohol). Products include:
Fentora 966

Fludrocortisone Acetate (Co-administration of thiothixene with hepatic microsomal enzyme inducing agents such as carbamazepine may increase the clearance of thiothixene. Patients receiving these drugs should be observed for signs of reduced thiothixene effectiveness).
No products indexed under this heading.

IMPORTANT NOTE: Always consult each drug listing in the patient's regimen for possible interactions.

Thiothixene | Interactions Index | 1882

Fluphenazine Decanoate (Patients receiving thiothixene should be cautioned about the possible additive effects (which may include hypotension) with CNS depressants. Caution as well as careful adjustment of the dosages is indicated when thiothixene is used in conjunction with other CNS depressants and with alcohol).
No products indexed under this heading.

Fluphenazine Enanthate (Patients receiving thiothixene should be cautioned about the possible additive effects (which may include hypotension) with CNS depressants. Caution as well as careful adjustment of the dosages is indicated when thiothixene is used in conjunction with other CNS depressants and with alcohol).
No products indexed under this heading.

Fluphenazine Hydrochloride (Patients receiving thiothixene should be cautioned about the possible additive effects (which may include hypotension) with CNS depressants. Caution as well as careful adjustment of the dosages is indicated when thiothixene is used in conjunction with other CNS depressants and with alcohol).
No products indexed under this heading.

Flurazepam Hydrochloride (Patients receiving thiothixene should be cautioned about the possible additive effects (which may include hypotension) with CNS depressants. Caution as well as careful adjustment of the dosages is indicated when thiothixene is used in conjunction with other CNS depressants and with alcohol).
No products indexed under this heading.

Fluvoxamine (Co-administration of thiothixene with hepatic microsomal enzyme inducing agents such as carbamazepine may increase the clearance of thiothixene. Patients receiving these drugs should be observed for signs of reduced thiothixene effectiveness).
No products indexed under this heading.

Fluvoxamine Maleate (Co-administration of thiothixene with hepatic microsomal enzyme inducing agents such as carbamazepine may increase the clearance of thiothixene. Patients receiving these drugs should be observed for signs of reduced thiothixene effectiveness).
No products indexed under this heading.

Fosinopril Sodium (Co-administration of thiothixene with antihypertensive agents may lead to excessive hypotension due to a possible additive effect. Patients receiving these drugs should be observed closely for signs of excessive hypotension when thiothixene is added to their drug regimen).
No products indexed under this heading.

Fosphenytoin (Co-administration of thiothixene with hepatic microsomal enzyme inducing agents such as carbamazepine may increase the clearance of thiothixene. Patients receiving these drugs should be observed for signs of reduced thiothixene effectiveness).
No products indexed under this heading.

Fosphenytoin Sodium (Co-administration of thiothixene with hepatic microsomal enzyme inducing agents such as carbamazepine may increase the clearance of thiothixene. Patients receiving these drugs should be observed for signs of reduced thiothixene effectiveness).
No products indexed under this heading.

Furosemide (Co-administration of thiothixene with antihypertensive agents may lead to excessive hypotension due to a possible additive effect. Patients receiving these drugs should be observed closely for signs of excessive hypotension when thiothixene is added to their drug regimen). Products include:
Furosemide 2354

Garlic Extract (Co-administration of thiothixene with hepatic microsomal enzyme inducing agents such as carbamazepine may increase the clearance of thiothixene. Patients receiving these drugs should be observed for signs of reduced thiothixene effectiveness).
No products indexed under this heading.

Garlic Oil (Co-administration of thiothixene with hepatic microsomal enzyme inducing agents such as carbamazepine may increase the clearance of thiothixene. Patients receiving these drugs should be observed for signs of reduced thiothixene effectiveness).
No products indexed under this heading.

Glipizide (Co-administration of thiothixene with hepatic microsomal enzyme inducing agents such as carbamazepine may increase the clearance of thiothixene. Patients receiving these drugs should be observed for signs of reduced thiothixene effectiveness).
No products indexed under this heading.

Glutethimide (Patients receiving thiothixene should be cautioned about the possible additive effects (which may include hypotension) with CNS depressants. Caution as well as careful adjustment of the dosages is indicated when thiothixene is used in conjunction with other CNS depressants and with alcohol).
No products indexed under this heading.

Glyburide (Co-administration of thiothixene with hepatic microsomal enzyme inducing agents such as carbamazepine may increase the clearance of thiothixene. Patients receiving these drugs should be observed for signs of reduced thiothixene effectiveness).
No products indexed under this heading.

Glycopyrrolate (Though exhibiting rather weak anticholinergic properties, thiothixene should be used with caution in patients who might be exposed to extreme heat or who are receiving atropine or related drugs).
No products indexed under this heading.

Guanabenz Acetate (Co-administration of thiothixene with antihypertensive agents may lead to excessive hypotension due to a possible additive effect. Patients receiving these drugs should be observed closely for signs of excessive hypotension when thiothixene is added to their drug regimen).
No products indexed under this heading.

Guanethidine (Co-administration of thiothixene with antihypertensive agents may lead to excessive hypotension due to a possible additive effect. Patients receiving these drugs should be observed closely for signs of excessive hypotension when thiothixene is added to their drug regimen).
No products indexed under this heading.

Guanethidine Monosulfate (Co-administration of thiothixene with antihypertensive agents may lead to excessive hypotension due to a possible additive effect. Patients receiving these drugs should be observed closely for signs of excessive hypotension when thiothixene is added to their drug regimen).
No products indexed under this heading.

Guanethidine Sulfate (Co-administration of thiothixene with antihypertensive agents may lead to excessive hypotension due to a possible additive effect. Patients receiving these drugs should be observed closely for signs of excessive hypotension when thiothixene is added to their drug regimen).
No products indexed under this heading.

Halazepam (Patients receiving thiothixene should be cautioned about the possible additive effects (which may include hypotension) with CNS depressants. Caution as well as careful adjustment of the dosages is indicated when thiothixene is used in conjunction with other CNS depressants and with alcohol).
No products indexed under this heading.

Haloperidol (Patients receiving thiothixene should be cautioned about the possible additive effects (which may include hypotension) with CNS depressants. Caution as well as careful adjustment of the dosages is indicated when thiothixene is used in conjunction with other CNS depressants and with alcohol).
No products indexed under this heading.

Haloperidol Decanoate (Patients receiving thiothixene should be cautioned about the possible additive effects (which may include hypotension) with CNS depressants. Caution as well as careful adjustment of the dosages is indicated when thiothixene is used in conjunction with other CNS depressants and with alcohol).
No products indexed under this heading.

Haloperidol Lactate (Patients receiving thiothixene should be cautioned about the possible additive effects (which may include hypotension) with CNS depressants. Caution as well as careful adjustment of the dosages is indicated when thiothixene is used in conjunction with other CNS depressants and with alcohol).
No products indexed under this heading.

Hepatic Enzyme-Inducing Agents (Co-administration of thiothixene with hepatic microsomal enzyme inducing agents such as carbamazepine may increase the clearance of thiothixene. Patients receiving these drugs should be observed for signs of reduced thiothixene effectiveness).
No products indexed under this heading.

Hexobarbital (Although thiothixene potentiates the actions of the barbiturates, the dosage of the anticonvulsant therapy should not be reduced when thiothixene is administered concurrently).
No products indexed under this heading.

Hydralazine Hydrochloride (Co-administration of thiothixene with antihypertensive agents may lead to excessive hypotension due to a possible additive effect. Patients receiving these drugs should be observed closely for signs of excessive hypotension when thiothixene is added to their drug regimen).
No products indexed under this heading.

Hydrochlorothiazide (Co-administration of thiothixene with antihypertensive agents may lead to excessive hypotension due to a possible additive effect. Patients receiving these drugs should be observed closely for signs of excessive hypotension when thiothixene is added to their drug regimen). Products include:
Atacand HCT 700
Avalide 2956
Benicar HCT 1017
Diovan HCT 2419
Dyazide 1429
Exforge HCT 2449
Hyzaar 2162
Hyzaar 100-12.5 2162
Micardis HCT 889
Prinzide 2246
Tekturna HCT 2541
Teveten HCT 541

Hydrocodone Bitartrate (Patients receiving thiothixene should be cautioned about the possible additive effects (which may include hypotension) with CNS depressants. Caution as well as careful adjustment of the dosages is indicated when thiothixene is used in conjunction with other CNS depressants and with alcohol). Products include:
Vicodin 560
Vicodin ES 561
Vicodin HP 563
Vicoprofen 564
Zydone 1138

Hydrocodone Polistirex (Patients receiving thiothixene should be cautioned about the possible additive effects (which may include hypotension) with CNS depressants. Caution as well as careful adjustment of the dosages is indicated when thiothixene is used in conjunction with other CNS depressants and with alcohol). Products include:
Tussionex 3443

Hydrocortisone (Alcohol) (Co-administration of thiothixene with hepatic microsomal enzyme inducing agents such as carbamazepine may increase the clearance of thiothixene. Patients receiving these drugs should be observed for signs of reduced thiothixene effectiveness).
No products indexed under this heading.

Hydrocortisone Acetate (Co-administration of thiothixene with hepatic microsomal enzyme inducing agents such as carbamazepine may increase the clearance of thiothixene. Patients receiving these drugs should be observed for signs of reduced thiothixene effectiveness).
No products indexed under this heading.

Hydrocortisone Butyrate (Co-administration of thiothixene with hepatic microsomal enzyme inducing agents such as carbamazepine may increase the clearance of thiothixene. Patients receiving these drugs should be observed for signs of reduced thiothixene effectiveness).
No products indexed under this heading.

Hydrocortisone Cypionate (Co-administration of thiothixene with hepatic microsomal enzyme inducing agents such as carbamazepine may increase the clearance of thiothixene. Patients receiving these drugs should be observed for signs of reduced thiothixene effectiveness).
No products indexed under this heading.

Hydrocortisone Hemisuccinate (Co-administration of thiothixene with hepatic microsomal enzyme inducing agents such as carbamazepine may increase the clearance of thiothixene. Patients receiving these drugs should be observed for signs of reduced thiothixene effectiveness).
No products indexed under this heading.

Hydrocortisone Probutate (Co-administration of thiothixene with hepatic microsomal enzyme inducing agents such as carbamazepine may increase the clearance of thiothixene. Patients receiving these drugs should be observed for signs of reduced thiothixene effectiveness).
No products indexed under this heading.

1883 Interactions Index Thiothixene

Hydrocortisone Sodium Phosphate (Co-administration of thiothixene with hepatic microsomal enzyme inducing agents such as carbamazepine may increase the clearance of thiothixene. Patients receiving these drugs should be observed for signs of reduced thiothixene effectiveness).
No products indexed under this heading.

Hydrocortisone Sodium Succinate (Co-administration of thiothixene with hepatic microsomal enzyme inducing agents such as carbamazepine may increase the clearance of thiothixene. Patients receiving these drugs should be observed for signs of reduced thiothixene effectiveness).
No products indexed under this heading.

Hydrocortisone Valerate (Co-administration of thiothixene with hepatic microsomal enzyme inducing agents such as carbamazepine may increase the clearance of thiothixene. Patients receiving these drugs should be observed for signs of reduced thiothixene effectiveness).
No products indexed under this heading.

Hydroflumethiazide (Co-administration of thiothixene with antihypertensive agents may lead to excessive hypotension due to a possible additive effect. Patients receiving these drugs should be observed closely for signs of excessive hypotension when thiothixene is added to their drug regimen).
No products indexed under this heading.

Hydromorphone (Patients receiving thiothixene should be cautioned about the possible additive effects (which may include hypotension) with CNS depressants. Caution as well as careful adjustment of the dosages is indicated when thiothixene is used in conjunction with other CNS depressants and with alcohol).
No products indexed under this heading.

Hydromorphone Hydrochloride (Patients receiving thiothixene should be cautioned about the possible additive effects (which may include hypotension) with CNS depressants. Caution as well as careful adjustment of the dosages is indicated when thiothixene is used in conjunction with other CNS depressants and with alcohol). Products include:
Dilaudid Injection 2800
Dilaudid Oral 2797
Dilaudid Tablets 2797
Dilaudid-HP 2800

Hydroxyzine Hydrochloride (Patients receiving thiothixene should be cautioned about the possible additive effects (which may include hypotension) with CNS depressants. Caution as well as careful adjustment of the dosages is indicated when thiothixene is used in conjunction with other CNS depressants and with alcohol).
No products indexed under this heading.

Hyoscyamine (Though exhibiting rather weak anticholinergic properties, thiothixene should be used with caution in patients who might be exposed to extreme heat or who are receiving atropine or related drugs).
No products indexed under this heading.

Hyoscyamine Sulfate (Though exhibiting rather weak anticholinergic properties, thiothixene should be used with caution in patients who might be exposed to extreme heat or who are receiving atropine or related drugs). Products include:
Donnatal 2711

Hypericum (Co-administration of thiothixene with hepatic microsomal enzyme inducing agents such as carbamazepine may increase the clearance of thiothixene. Patients receiving these drugs should be observed for signs of reduced thiothixene effectiveness).
No products indexed under this heading.

Hypericum Perforatum (Co-administration of thiothixene with hepatic microsomal enzyme inducing agents such as carbamazepine may increase the clearance of thiothixene. Patients receiving these drugs should be observed for signs of reduced thiothixene effectiveness). Products include:
Traumeel 1800

Indapamide (Co-administration of thiothixene with antihypertensive agents may lead to excessive hypotension due to a possible additive effect. Patients receiving these drugs should be observed closely for signs of excessive hypotension when thiothixene is added to their drug regimen). Products include:
Indapamide 2356

Insulin (Co-administration of thiothixene with hepatic microsomal enzyme inducing agents such as carbamazepine may increase the clearance of thiothixene. Patients receiving these drugs should be observed for signs of reduced thiothixene effectiveness).
No products indexed under this heading.

Insulin, Human, Zinc Suspension (Co-administration of thiothixene with hepatic microsomal enzyme inducing agents such as carbamazepine may increase the clearance of thiothixene. Patients receiving these drugs should be observed for signs of reduced thiothixene effectiveness).
No products indexed under this heading.

Insulin, Human (rDNA origin) (Co-administration of thiothixene with hepatic microsomal enzyme inducing agents such as carbamazepine may increase the clearance of thiothixene. Patients receiving these drugs should be observed for signs of reduced thiothixene effectiveness). Products include:
Exubera 2717

Insulin, Human NPH (Co-administration of thiothixene with hepatic microsomal enzyme inducing agents such as carbamazepine may increase the clearance of thiothixene. Patients receiving these drugs should be observed for signs of reduced thiothixene effectiveness). Products include:
Humulin N Vial 1934

Insulin, Human Regular (Co-administration of thiothixene with hepatic microsomal enzyme inducing agents such as carbamazepine may increase the clearance of thiothixene. Patients receiving these drugs should be observed for signs of reduced thiothixene effectiveness). Products include:
Humulin R 1937
Humulin R (U-500) 1939

Insulin, Human Regular and Human NPH Mixture (Co-administration of thiothixene with hepatic microsomal enzyme inducing agents such as carbamazepine may increase the clearance of thiothixene. Patients receiving these drugs should be observed for signs of reduced thiothixene effectiveness). Products include:
Humulin 50/50 1930
Humulin 70/30 Vial 1931

Insulin, NPH (Co-administration of thiothixene with hepatic microsomal enzyme inducing agents such as carbamazepine may increase the clearance of thiothixene. Patients receiving these drugs should be observed for signs of reduced thiothixene effectiveness).
No products indexed under this heading.

Insulin, Regular (Co-administration of thiothixene with hepatic microsomal enzyme inducing agents such as carbamazepine may increase the clearance of thiothixene. Patients receiving these drugs should be observed for signs of reduced thiothixene effectiveness).
No products indexed under this heading.

Insulin, Regular and NPH mixture (Co-administration of thiothixene with hepatic microsomal enzyme inducing agents such as carbamazepine may increase the clearance of thiothixene. Patients receiving these drugs should be observed for signs of reduced thiothixene effectiveness).
No products indexed under this heading.

Insulin, Zinc Crystals (Co-administration of thiothixene with hepatic microsomal enzyme inducing agents such as carbamazepine may increase the clearance of thiothixene. Patients receiving these drugs should be observed for signs of reduced thiothixene effectiveness).
No products indexed under this heading.

Insulin, Zinc Suspension (Co-administration of thiothixene with hepatic microsomal enzyme inducing agents such as carbamazepine may increase the clearance of thiothixene. Patients receiving these drugs should be observed for signs of reduced thiothixene effectiveness).
No products indexed under this heading.

Insulin Aspart (Co-administration of thiothixene with hepatic microsomal enzyme inducing agents such as carbamazepine may increase the clearance of thiothixene. Patients receiving these drugs should be observed for signs of reduced thiothixene effectiveness).
No products indexed under this heading.

Insulin Aspart, Human (Co-administration of thiothixene with hepatic microsomal enzyme inducing agents such as carbamazepine may increase the clearance of thiothixene. Patients receiving these drugs should be observed for signs of reduced thiothixene effectiveness). Products include:
NovoLog Mix 70/30 2581

Insulin Aspart, Human Regular (Co-administration of thiothixene with hepatic microsomal enzyme inducing agents such as carbamazepine may increase the clearance of thiothixene. Patients receiving these drugs should be observed for signs of reduced thiothixene effectiveness). Products include:
NovoLog 2575

Insulin Aspart Protamine, Human (Co-administration of thiothixene with hepatic microsomal enzyme inducing agents such as carbamazepine may increase the clearance of thiothixene. Patients receiving these drugs should be observed for signs of reduced thiothixene effectiveness). Products include:
NovoLog Mix 70/30 2581

Insulin Detemir (rDNA Origin) (Co-administration of thiothixene with hepatic microsomal enzyme inducing agents such as carbamazepine may increase the clearance of thiothixene. Patients receiving these drugs should be observed for signs of reduced thiothixene effectiveness). Products include:
Levemir 2566

Insulin Glargine (Co-administration of thiothixene with hepatic microsomal enzyme inducing agents such as carbamazepine may increase the clearance of thiothixene. Patients receiving these drugs should be observed for signs of reduced thiothixene effectiveness). Products include:
Lantus 2996

Insulin Glulisine (Co-administration of thiothixene with hepatic microsomal enzyme inducing agents such as carbamazepine may increase the clearance of thiothixene. Patients receiving these drugs should be observed for signs of reduced thiothixene effectiveness). Products include:
Apidra 2937
Apidra SoloStar 2937

Insulin Lispro, Human (Co-administration of thiothixene with hepatic microsomal enzyme inducing agents such as carbamazepine may increase the clearance of thiothixene. Patients receiving these drugs should be observed for signs of reduced thiothixene effectiveness). Products include:
Humalog 1910
Humalog Mix 1914
Humalog Mix75/25 1917

Insulin Lispro Protamine, Human (Co-administration of thiothixene with hepatic microsomal enzyme inducing agents such as carbamazepine may increase the clearance of thiothixene. Patients receiving these drugs should be observed for signs of reduced thiothixene effectiveness). Products include:
Humalog Mix 1914
Humalog Mix75/25 1917

Ipratropium Bromide (Though exhibiting rather weak anticholinergic properties, thiothixene should be used with caution in patients who might be exposed to extreme heat or who are receiving atropine or related drugs).
No products indexed under this heading.

Irbesartan (Co-administration of thiothixene with antihypertensive agents may lead to excessive hypotension due to a possible additive effect. Patients receiving these drugs should be observed closely for signs of excessive hypotension when thiothixene is added to their drug regimen). Products include:
Avalide 2956
Avapro 2962

Isoflurane (Patients receiving thiothixene should be cautioned about the possible additive effects (which may include hypotension) with CNS depressants. Caution as well as careful adjustment of the dosages is indicated when thiothixene is used in conjunction with other CNS depressants and with alcohol).
No products indexed under this heading.

Isradipine (Co-administration of thiothixene with antihypertensive agents may lead to excessive hypotension due to a possible additive effect. Patients receiving these drugs should be observed closely for signs of excessive hypotension when thiothixene is added to their drug regimen). Products include:
DynaCirc CR 1432

IMPORTANT NOTE: Always consult each drug listing in the patient's regimen for possible interactions.

Thiothixene Interactions Index 1884

Ketamine Hydrochloride (Patients receiving thiothixene should be cautioned about the possible additive effects (which may include hypotension) with CNS depressants. Caution as well as careful adjustment of the dosages is indicated when thiothixene is used in conjunction with other CNS depressants and with alcohol).
No products indexed under this heading.

Labetalol Hydrochloride (Co-administration of thiothixene with antihypertensive agents may lead to excessive hypotension due to a possible additive effect. Patients receiving these drugs should be observed closely for signs of excessive hypotension when thiothixene is added to their drug regimen).
No products indexed under this heading.

Lansoprazole (Co-administration of thiothixene with hepatic microsomal enzyme inducing agents such as carbamazepine may increase the clearance of thiothixene. Patients receiving these drugs should be observed for signs of reduced thiothixene effectiveness).
No products indexed under this heading.

Levomethadyl Acetate Hydrochloride (Patients receiving thiothixene should be cautioned about the possible additive effects (which may include hypotension) with CNS depressants. Caution as well as careful adjustment of the dosages is indicated when thiothixene is used in conjunction with other CNS depressants and with alcohol).
No products indexed under this heading.

Levorphanol Tartrate (Patients receiving thiothixene should be cautioned about the possible additive effects (which may include hypotension) with CNS depressants. Caution as well as careful adjustment of the dosages is indicated when thiothixene is used in conjunction with other CNS depressants and with alcohol).
No products indexed under this heading.

Lisinopril (Co-administration of thiothixene with antihypertensive agents may lead to excessive hypotension due to a possible additive effect. Patients receiving these drugs should be observed closely for signs of excessive hypotension when thiothixene is added to their drug regimen). Products include:
Prinivil 2241
Prinzide 2246

Lorazepam (Patients receiving thiothixene should be cautioned about the possible additive effects (which may include hypotension) with CNS depressants. Caution as well as careful adjustment of the dosages is indicated when thiothixene is used in conjunction with other CNS depressants and with alcohol).
No products indexed under this heading.

Losartan Potassium (Co-administration of thiothixene with antihypertensive agents may lead to excessive hypotension due to a possible additive effect. Patients receiving these drugs should be observed closely for signs of excessive hypotension when thiothixene is added to their drug regimen). Products include:
Cozaar 2106
Hyzaar 2162
Hyzaar 100-12.5 2162

Loxapine Hydrochloride (Patients receiving thiothixene should be cautioned about the possible additive effects (which may include hypotension) with CNS depressants. Caution as well as careful adjustment of the dosages is indicated when thiothixene is used in conjunction with other CNS depressants and with alcohol).
No products indexed under this heading.

Loxapine Succinate (Patients receiving thiothixene should be cautioned about the possible additive effects (which may include hypotension) with CNS depressants. Caution as well as careful adjustment of the dosages is indicated when thiothixene is used in conjunction with other CNS depressants and with alcohol).
No products indexed under this heading.

Mecamylamine Hydrochloride (Co-administration of thiothixene with antihypertensive agents may lead to excessive hypotension due to a possible additive effect. Patients receiving these drugs should be observed closely for signs of excessive hypotension when thiothixene is added to their drug regimen).
No products indexed under this heading.

Mepenzolate Bromide (Though exhibiting rather weak anticholinergic properties, thiothixene should be used with caution in patients who might be exposed to extreme heat or who are receiving atropine or related drugs).
No products indexed under this heading.

Meperidine Hydrochloride (Patients receiving thiothixene should be cautioned about the possible additive effects (which may include hypotension) with CNS depressants. Caution as well as careful adjustment of the dosages is indicated when thiothixene is used in conjunction with other CNS depressants and with alcohol).
No products indexed under this heading.

Mephenytoin (Co-administration of thiothixene with hepatic microsomal enzyme inducing agents such as carbamazepine may increase the clearance of thiothixene. Patients receiving these drugs should be observed for signs of reduced thiothixene effectiveness).
No products indexed under this heading.

Mephobarbital (Although thiothixene potentiates the actions of the barbiturates, the dosage of the anticonvulsant therapy should not be reduced when thiothixene is administered concurrently).
No products indexed under this heading.

Meprobamate (Patients receiving thiothixene should be cautioned about the possible additive effects (which may include hypotension) with CNS depressants. Caution as well as careful adjustment of the dosages is indicated when thiothixene is used in conjunction with other CNS depressants and with alcohol).
No products indexed under this heading.

Mesoridazine Besylate (Patients receiving thiothixene should be cautioned about the possible additive effects (which may include hypotension) with CNS depressants. Caution as well as careful adjustment of the dosages is indicated when thiothixene is used in conjunction with other CNS depressants and with alcohol).
No products indexed under this heading.

Methadone Hydrochloride (Patients receiving thiothixene should be cautioned about the possible additive effects (which may include hypotension) with CNS depressants. Caution as well as careful adjustment of the dosages is indicated when thiothixene is used in conjunction with other CNS depressants and with alcohol).
No products indexed under this heading.

Methohexital Sodium (Patients receiving thiothixene should be cautioned about the possible additive effects (which may include hypotension) with CNS depressants. Caution as well as careful adjustment of the dosages is indicated when thiothixene is used in conjunction with other CNS depressants and with alcohol).
No products indexed under this heading.

Methotrimeprazine (Patients receiving thiothixene should be cautioned about the possible additive effects (which may include hypotension) with CNS depressants. Caution as well as careful adjustment of the dosages is indicated when thiothixene is used in conjunction with other CNS depressants and with alcohol).
No products indexed under this heading.

Methoxyflurane (Patients receiving thiothixene should be cautioned about the possible additive effects (which may include hypotension) with CNS depressants. Caution as well as careful adjustment of the dosages is indicated when thiothixene is used in conjunction with other CNS depressants and with alcohol).
No products indexed under this heading.

Methsuximide (Co-administration of thiothixene with hepatic microsomal enzyme inducing agents such as carbamazepine may increase the clearance of thiothixene. Patients receiving these drugs should be observed for signs of reduced thiothixene effectiveness).
No products indexed under this heading.

Methyclothiazide (Co-administration of thiothixene with antihypertensive agents may lead to excessive hypotension due to a possible additive effect. Patients receiving these drugs should be observed closely for signs of excessive hypotension when thiothixene is added to their drug regimen).
No products indexed under this heading.

Methyldopa (Co-administration of thiothixene with antihypertensive agents may lead to excessive hypotension due to a possible additive effect. Patients receiving these drugs should be observed closely for signs of excessive hypotension when thiothixene is added to their drug regimen).
No products indexed under this heading.

Methyldopate Hydrochloride (Co-administration of thiothixene with antihypertensive agents may lead to excessive hypotension due to a possible additive effect. Patients receiving these drugs should be observed closely for signs of excessive hypotension when thiothixene is added to their drug regimen).
No products indexed under this heading.

Methylprednisolone (Co-administration of thiothixene with hepatic microsomal enzyme inducing agents such as carbamazepine may increase the clearance of thiothixene. Patients receiving these drugs should be observed for signs of reduced thiothixene effectiveness).
No products indexed under this heading.

Methylprednisolone Acetate (Co-administration of thiothixene with hepatic microsomal enzyme inducing agents such as carbamazepine may increase the clearance of thiothixene. Patients receiving these drugs should be observed for signs of reduced thiothixene effectiveness).
No products indexed under this heading.

Methylprednisolone Sodium Succinate (Co-administration of thiothixene with hepatic microsomal enzyme inducing agents such as carbamazepine may increase the clearance of thiothixene. Patients receiving these drugs should be observed for signs of reduced thiothixene effectiveness).
No products indexed under this heading.

Metolazone (Co-administration of thiothixene with antihypertensive agents may lead to excessive hypotension due to a possible additive effect. Patients receiving these drugs should be observed closely for signs of excessive hypotension when thiothixene is added to their drug regimen).
No products indexed under this heading.

Metoprolol Succinate (Co-administration of thiothixene with antihypertensive agents may lead to excessive hypotension due to a possible additive effect. Patients receiving these drugs should be observed closely for signs of excessive hypotension when thiothixene is added to their drug regimen). Products include:
Toprol XL 732

Metoprolol Tartrate (Co-administration of thiothixene with antihypertensive agents may lead to excessive hypotension due to a possible additive effect. Patients receiving these drugs should be observed closely for signs of excessive hypotension when thiothixene is added to their drug regimen).
No products indexed under this heading.

Metyrosine (Co-administration of thiothixene with antihypertensive agents may lead to excessive hypotension due to a possible additive effect. Patients receiving these drugs should be observed closely for signs of excessive hypotension when thiothixene is added to their drug regimen).
No products indexed under this heading.

Mibefradil Dihydrochloride (Co-administration of thiothixene with antihypertensive agents may lead to excessive hypotension due to a possible additive effect. Patients receiving these drugs should be observed closely for signs of excessive hypotension when thiothixene is added to their drug regimen).
No products indexed under this heading.

Midazolam Hydrochloride (Patients receiving thiothixene should be cautioned about the possible additive effects (which may include hypotension) with CNS depressants. Caution as well as careful adjustment of the dosages is indicated when thiothixene is used in conjunction with other CNS depressants and with alcohol).
No products indexed under this heading.

Minoxidil (Co-administration of thiothixene with antihypertensive agents may lead to excessive hypotension due to a possible additive effect. Patients receiving these drugs should be observed closely for signs of excessive hypotension when thiothixene is added to their drug regimen).
No products indexed under this heading.

Modafinil (Co-administration of thiothixene with hepatic microsomal enzyme inducing agents such as carbamazepine may increase the clearance of thiothixene. Patients receiving these drugs should be observed for signs of reduced thiothixene effectiveness). Products include:
Provigil 983

(⊙ Described in PDR® for Ophthalmic Medicines)

1885 Interactions Index Thiothixene

Moexipril Hydrochloride (Co-administration of thiothixene with antihypertensive agents may lead to excessive hypotension due to a possible additive effect. Patients receiving these drugs should be observed closely for signs of excessive hypotension when thiothixene is added to their drug regimen).
No products indexed under this heading.

Molindone Hydrochloride (Patients receiving thiothixene should be cautioned about the possible additive effects (which may include hypotension) with CNS depressants. Caution as well as careful adjustment of the dosages is indicated when thiothixene is used in conjunction with other CNS depressants and with alcohol). Products include:
Moban 1108

Morphine Sulfate (Patients receiving thiothixene should be cautioned about the possible additive effects (which may include hypotension) with CNS depressants. Caution as well as careful adjustment of the dosages is indicated when thiothixene is used in conjunction with other CNS depressants and with alcohol). Products include:
Avinza 1822
Embeda 1831
MS Contin 2803

Morphine Sulfate, Liposomal (Patients receiving thiothixene should be cautioned about the possible additive effects (which may include hypotension) with CNS depressants. Caution as well as careful adjustment of the dosages is indicated when thiothixene is used in conjunction with other CNS depressants and with alcohol).
No products indexed under this heading.

Nadolol (Co-administration of thiothixene with antihypertensive agents may lead to excessive hypotension due to a possible additive effect. Patients receiving these drugs should be observed closely for signs of excessive hypotension when thiothixene is added to their drug regimen). Products include:
Nadolol 2359

Nafcillin Sodium (Co-administration of thiothixene with hepatic microsomal enzyme inducing agents such as carbamazepine may increase the clearance of thiothixene. Patients receiving these drugs should be observed for signs of reduced thiothixene effectiveness).
No products indexed under this heading.

Nebivolol (Co-administration of thiothixene with antihypertensive agents may lead to excessive hypotension due to a possible additive effect. Patients receiving these drugs should be observed closely for signs of excessive hypotension when thiothixene is added to their drug regimen). Products include:
Bystolic 1147

Nevirapine (Co-administration of thiothixene with hepatic microsomal enzyme inducing agents such as carbamazepine may increase the clearance of thiothixene. Patients receiving these drugs should be observed for signs of reduced thiothixene effectiveness). Products include:
Viramune Oral Suspension 897
Viramune Tablets 897

Nicardipine Hydrochloride (Co-administration of thiothixene with antihypertensive agents may lead to excessive hypotension due to a possible additive effect. Patients receiving these drugs should be observed closely for signs of excessive hypotension when thiothixene is added to their drug regimen).
No products indexed under this heading.

Nicotine (Co-administration of thiothixene with hepatic microsomal enzyme inducing agents such as carbamazepine may increase the clearance of thiothixene. Patients receiving these drugs should be observed for signs of reduced thiothixene effectiveness).
No products indexed under this heading.

Nicotine Polacrilex (Co-administration of thiothixene with hepatic microsomal enzyme inducing agents such as carbamazepine may increase the clearance of thiothixene. Patients receiving these drugs should be observed for signs of reduced thiothixene effectiveness).
No products indexed under this heading.

Nicotine Salicylate (Co-administration of thiothixene with hepatic microsomal enzyme inducing agents such as carbamazepine may increase the clearance of thiothixene. Patients receiving these drugs should be observed for signs of reduced thiothixene effectiveness).
No products indexed under this heading.

Nicotine Sulfate (Co-administration of thiothixene with hepatic microsomal enzyme inducing agents such as carbamazepine may increase the clearance of thiothixene. Patients receiving these drugs should be observed for signs of reduced thiothixene effectiveness).
No products indexed under this heading.

Nifedipine (Co-administration of thiothixene with antihypertensive agents may lead to excessive hypotension due to a possible additive effect. Patients receiving these drugs should be observed closely for signs of excessive hypotension when thiothixene is added to their drug regimen).
No products indexed under this heading.

Nisoldipine (Co-administration of thiothixene with antihypertensive agents may lead to excessive hypotension due to a possible additive effect. Patients receiving these drugs should be observed closely for signs of excessive hypotension when thiothixene is added to their drug regimen).
No products indexed under this heading.

Nitroglycerin (Co-administration of thiothixene with antihypertensive agents may lead to excessive hypotension due to a possible additive effect. Patients receiving these drugs should be observed closely for signs of excessive hypotension when thiothixene is added to their drug regimen). Products include:
Nitro-Dur 3170
Nitrolingual 3266

Norethindrone (Co-administration of thiothixene with hepatic microsomal enzyme inducing agents such as carbamazepine may increase the clearance of thiothixene. Patients receiving these drugs should be observed for signs of reduced thiothixene effectiveness). Products include:
Ortho Micronor 2660

Norethindrone Acetate (Co-administration of thiothixene with hepatic microsomal enzyme inducing agents such as carbamazepine may increase the clearance of thiothixene. Patients receiving these drugs should be observed for signs of reduced thiothixene effectiveness). Products include:
Activella 2561

Olanzapine (Patients receiving thiothixene should be cautioned about the possible additive effects (which may include hypotension) with CNS depressants. Caution as well as careful adjustment of the dosages is indicated when thiothixene is used in conjunction with other CNS depressants and with alcohol). Products include:
Symbyax 1965
Zyprexa 1984
Zyprexa IntraMuscular 1984
Zyprexa ZYDIS 1984

Omeprazole (Co-administration of thiothixene with hepatic microsomal enzyme inducing agents such as carbamazepine may increase the clearance of thiothixene. Patients receiving these drugs should be observed for signs of reduced thiothixene effectiveness).
No products indexed under this heading.

Omeprazole Magnesium (Co-administration of thiothixene with hepatic microsomal enzyme inducing agents such as carbamazepine may increase the clearance of thiothixene. Patients receiving these drugs should be observed for signs of reduced thiothixene effectiveness).
No products indexed under this heading.

Oxazepam (Patients receiving thiothixene should be cautioned about the possible additive effects (which may include hypotension) with CNS depressants. Caution as well as careful adjustment of the dosages is indicated when thiothixene is used in conjunction with other CNS depressants and with alcohol).
No products indexed under this heading.

Oxcarbazepine (Co-administration of thiothixene with hepatic microsomal enzyme inducing agents such as carbamazepine may increase the clearance of thiothixene. Patients receiving these drugs should be observed for signs of reduced thiothixene effectiveness).
No products indexed under this heading.

Oxybutynin Chloride (Though exhibiting rather weak anticholinergic properties, thiothixene should be used with caution in patients who might be exposed to extreme heat or who are receiving atropine or related drugs).
No products indexed under this heading.

Oxycodone Hydrochloride (Patients receiving thiothixene should be cautioned about the possible additive effects (which may include hypotension) with CNS depressants. Caution as well as careful adjustment of the dosages is indicated when thiothixene is used in conjunction with other CNS depressants and with alcohol). Products include:
OxyContin 2807
Percocet 1121
Percodan 1124

Oxycodone Terephthalate (Patients receiving thiothixene should be cautioned about the possible additive effects (which may include hypotension) with CNS depressants. Caution as well as careful adjustment of the dosages is indicated when thiothixene is used in conjunction with other CNS depressants and with alcohol).
No products indexed under this heading.

Oxymorphone Hydrochloride (Patients receiving thiothixene should be cautioned about the possible additive effects (which may include hypotension) with CNS depressants. Caution as well as careful adjustment of the dosages is indicated when thiothixene is used in conjunction with other CNS depressants and with alcohol). Products include:
Opana 1110
Opana ER 1114

Penbutolol Sulfate (Co-administration of thiothixene with antihypertensive agents may lead to excessive hypotension due to a possible additive effect. Patients receiving these drugs should be observed closely for signs of excessive hypotension when thiothixene is added to their drug regimen).
No products indexed under this heading.

Pentobarbital (Although thiothixene potentiates the actions of the barbiturates, the dosage of the anticonvulsant therapy should not be reduced when thiothixene is administered concurrently).
No products indexed under this heading.

Pentobarbital Sodium (Although thiothixene potentiates the actions of the barbiturates, the dosage of the anticonvulsant therapy should not be reduced when thiothixene is administered concurrently). Products include:
Nembutal 2012

Perindopril Erbumine (Co-administration of thiothixene with antihypertensive agents may lead to excessive hypotension due to a possible additive effect. Patients receiving these drugs should be observed closely for signs of excessive hypotension when thiothixene is added to their drug regimen).
No products indexed under this heading.

Perphenazine (Patients receiving thiothixene should be cautioned about the possible additive effects (which may include hypotension) with CNS depressants. Caution as well as careful adjustment of the dosages is indicated when thiothixene is used in conjunction with other CNS depressants and with alcohol).
No products indexed under this heading.

Phenobarbital (Although thiothixene potentiates the actions of the barbiturates, the dosage of the anticonvulsant therapy should not be reduced when thiothixene is administered concurrently). Products include:
Donnatal 2711

Phenobarbital Sodium (Although thiothixene potentiates the actions of the barbiturates, the dosage of the anticonvulsant therapy should not be reduced when thiothixene is administered concurrently).
No products indexed under this heading.

Phenoxybenzamine Hydrochloride (Co-administration of thiothixene with antihypertensive agents may lead to excessive hypotension due to a possible additive effect. Patients receiving these drugs should be observed closely for signs of excessive hypotension when thiothixene is added to their drug regimen). Products include:
Dibenzyline 3495

Phentolamine Mesylate (Co-administration of thiothixene with antihypertensive agents may lead to excessive hypotension due to a possible additive effect. Patients receiving these drugs should be observed closely for signs of excessive hypotension when thiothixene is added to their drug regimen).
No products indexed under this heading.

Phenylbutazone (Co-administration of thiothixene with hepatic microsomal enzyme inducing agents such as carbamazepine may increase the clearance of thiothixene. Patients receiving these drugs should be observed for signs of reduced thiothixene effectiveness).
No products indexed under this heading.

Phenytoin (Co-administration of thiothixene with hepatic microsomal enzyme inducing agents such as carbamazepine may increase the clearance of thiothixene. Patients receiving these drugs should be observed for signs of reduced thiothixene effectiveness).
No products indexed under this heading.

Phenytoin Sodium (Co-administration of thiothixene with hepatic microsomal enzyme inducing agents such as carbamazepine may increase the clearance of thiothixene. Patients receiving

IMPORTANT NOTE: Always consult each drug listing in the patient's regimen for possible interactions.

these drugs should be observed for signs of reduced thiothixene effectiveness). Products include:

Phenytek Capsules 2380

Pindolol (Co-administration of thiothixene with antihypertensive agents may lead to excessive hypotension due to a possible additive effect. Patients receiving these drugs should be observed closely for signs of excessive hypotension when thiothixene is added to their drug regimen).

No products indexed under this heading.

Polythiazide (Co-administration of thiothixene with antihypertensive agents may lead to excessive hypotension due to a possible additive effect. Patients receiving these drugs should be observed closely for signs of excessive hypotension when thiothixene is added to their drug regimen).

No products indexed under this heading.

Prazepam (Patients receiving thiothixene should be cautioned about the possible additive effects (which may include hypotension) with CNS depressants. Caution as well as careful adjustment of the dosages is indicated when thiothixene is used in conjunction with other CNS depressants and with alcohol).

No products indexed under this heading.

Prazosin Hydrochloride (Co-administration of thiothixene with antihypertensive agents may lead to excessive hypotension due to a possible additive effect. Patients receiving these drugs should be observed closely for signs of excessive hypotension when thiothixene is added to their drug regimen).

No products indexed under this heading.

Prednisolone (Co-administration of thiothixene with hepatic microsomal enzyme inducing agents such as carbamazepine may increase the clearance of thiothixene. Patients receiving these drugs should be observed for signs of reduced thiothixene effectiveness).

No products indexed under this heading.

Prednisolone Acetate (Co-administration of thiothixene with hepatic microsomal enzyme inducing agents such as carbamazepine may increase the clearance of thiothixene. Patients receiving these drugs should be observed for signs of reduced thiothixene effectiveness). Products include:

Blephamide .... ⊙ 212, ⊙ 214
Pred Forte .... ⊙ 225
Pred Mild .... ⊙ 230
Pred-G .... ⊙ 226, ⊙ 227

Prednisolone Sodium Phosphate (Co-administration of thiothixene with hepatic microsomal enzyme inducing agents such as carbamazepine may increase the clearance of thiothixene. Patients receiving these drugs should be observed for signs of reduced thiothixene effectiveness).

No products indexed under this heading.

Prednisolone Tebutate (Co-administration of thiothixene with hepatic microsomal enzyme inducing agents such as carbamazepine may increase the clearance of thiothixene. Patients receiving these drugs should be observed for signs of reduced thiothixene effectiveness).

No products indexed under this heading.

Prednisone (Co-administration of thiothixene with hepatic microsomal enzyme inducing agents such as carbamazepine may increase the clearance of thiothixene. Patients receiving these drugs should be observed for signs of reduced thiothixene effectiveness).

No products indexed under this heading.

Prednisone sodium phosphate (Co-administration of thiothixene with hepatic microsomal enzyme inducing agents such as carbamazepine may increase the clearance of thiothixene. Patients receiving these drugs should be observed for signs of reduced thiothixene effectiveness).

No products indexed under this heading.

Primidone (Co-administration of thiothixene with hepatic microsomal enzyme inducing agents such as carbamazepine may increase the clearance of thiothixene. Patients receiving these drugs should be observed for signs of reduced thiothixene effectiveness).

No products indexed under this heading.

Prochlorperazine (Patients receiving thiothixene should be cautioned about the possible additive effects (which may include hypotension) with CNS depressants. Caution as well as careful adjustment of the dosages is indicated when thiothixene is used in conjunction with other CNS depressants and with alcohol).

No products indexed under this heading.

Prochlorperazine Edisylate (Patients receiving thiothixene should be cautioned about the possible additive effects (which may include hypotension) with CNS depressants. Caution as well as careful adjustment of the dosages is indicated when thiothixene is used in conjunction with other CNS depressants and with alcohol).

No products indexed under this heading.

Prochlorperazine Maleate (Patients receiving thiothixene should be cautioned about the possible additive effects (which may include hypotension) with CNS depressants. Caution as well as careful adjustment of the dosages is indicated when thiothixene is used in conjunction with other CNS depressants and with alcohol).

No products indexed under this heading.

Procyclidine Hydrochloride (Though exhibiting rather weak anticholinergic properties, thiothixene should be used with caution in patients who might be exposed to extreme heat or who are receiving atropine or related drugs).

No products indexed under this heading.

Promethazine (Patients receiving thiothixene should be cautioned about the possible additive effects (which may include hypotension) with CNS depressants. Caution as well as careful adjustment of the dosages is indicated when thiothixene is used in conjunction with other CNS depressants and with alcohol).

No products indexed under this heading.

Promethazine Hydrochloride (Patients receiving thiothixene should be cautioned about the possible additive effects (which may include hypotension) with CNS depressants. Caution as well as careful adjustment of the dosages is indicated when thiothixene is used in conjunction with other CNS depressants and with alcohol).

No products indexed under this heading.

Propantheline Bromide (Though exhibiting rather weak anticholinergic properties, thiothixene should be used with caution in patients who might be exposed to extreme heat or who are receiving atropine or related drugs).

No products indexed under this heading.

Propofol (Patients receiving thiothixene should be cautioned about the possible additive effects (which may include hypotension) with CNS depressants. Caution as well as careful adjustment of the dosages is indicated when thiothixene is used in conjunction with other CNS depressants and with alcohol).

No products indexed under this heading.

Propoxyphene Hydrochloride (Patients receiving thiothixene should be cautioned about the possible additive effects (which may include hypotension) with CNS depressants. Caution as well as careful adjustment of the dosages is indicated when thiothixene is used in conjunction with other CNS depressants and with alcohol).

No products indexed under this heading.

Propoxyphene Napsylate (Patients receiving thiothixene should be cautioned about the possible additive effects (which may include hypotension) with CNS depressants. Caution as well as careful adjustment of the dosages is indicated when thiothixene is used in conjunction with other CNS depressants and with alcohol).

No products indexed under this heading.

Propranolol Hydrochloride (Co-administration of thiothixene with antihypertensive agents may lead to excessive hypotension due to a possible additive effect. Patients receiving these drugs should be observed closely for signs of excessive hypotension when thiothixene is added to their drug regimen). Products include:

InnoPran XL 1517

Quazepam (Patients receiving thiothixene should be cautioned about the possible additive effects (which may include hypotension) with CNS depressants. Caution as well as careful adjustment of the dosages is indicated when thiothixene is used in conjunction with other CNS depressants and with alcohol).

No products indexed under this heading.

Quetiapine Fumarate (Patients receiving thiothixene should be cautioned about the possible additive effects (which may include hypotension) with CNS depressants. Caution as well as careful adjustment of the dosages is indicated when thiothixene is used in conjunction with other CNS depressants and with alcohol). Products include:

Seroquel 750
Seroquel XR 759

Quinapril Hydrochloride (Co-administration of thiothixene with antihypertensive agents may lead to excessive hypotension due to a possible additive effect. Patients receiving these drugs should be observed closely for signs of excessive hypotension when thiothixene is added to their drug regimen).

No products indexed under this heading.

Ramipril (Co-administration of thiothixene with antihypertensive agents may lead to excessive hypotension due to a possible additive effect. Patients receiving these drugs should be observed closely for signs of excessive hypotension when thiothixene is added to their drug regimen).

No products indexed under this heading.

Rauwolfia Serpentina (Co-administration of thiothixene with antihypertensive agents may lead to excessive hypotension due to a possible additive effect. Patients receiving these drugs should be observed closely for signs of excessive hypotension when thiothixene is added to their drug regimen).

No products indexed under this heading.

Remifentanil Hydrochloride (Patients receiving thiothixene should be cautioned about the possible additive effects (which may include hypotension) with CNS depressants. Caution as well as careful adjustment of the dosages is indicated when thiothixene is used in conjunction with other CNS depressants and with alcohol).

No products indexed under this heading.

Rescinnamine (Co-administration of thiothixene with antihypertensive agents may lead to excessive hypotension due to a possible additive effect. Patients receiving these drugs should be observed closely for signs of excessive hypotension when thiothixene is added to their drug regimen).

No products indexed under this heading.

Reserpine (Co-administration of thiothixene with antihypertensive agents may lead to excessive hypotension due to a possible additive effect. Patients receiving these drugs should be observed closely for signs of excessive hypotension when thiothixene is added to their drug regimen).

No products indexed under this heading.

Rifabutin (Co-administration of thiothixene with hepatic microsomal enzyme inducing agents such as carbamazepine may increase the clearance of thiothixene. Patients receiving these drugs should be observed for signs of reduced thiothixene effectiveness).

No products indexed under this heading.

Rifampicin (Co-administration of thiothixene with hepatic microsomal enzyme inducing agents such as carbamazepine may increase the clearance of thiothixene. Patients receiving these drugs should be observed for signs of reduced thiothixene effectiveness).

No products indexed under this heading.

Rifampin (Co-administration of thiothixene with hepatic microsomal enzyme inducing agents such as carbamazepine may increase the clearance of thiothixene. Patients receiving these drugs should be observed for signs of reduced thiothixene effectiveness).

No products indexed under this heading.

Rifapentine (Co-administration of thiothixene with hepatic microsomal enzyme inducing agents such as carbamazepine may increase the clearance of thiothixene. Patients receiving these drugs should be observed for signs of reduced thiothixene effectiveness).

No products indexed under this heading.

Risperidone (Patients receiving thiothixene should be cautioned about the possible additive effects (which may include hypotension) with CNS depressants. Caution as well as careful adjustment of the dosages is indicated when thiothixene is used in conjunction with other CNS depressants and with alcohol). Products include:

Risperdal Consta 2682

Ritonavir (Co-administration of thiothixene with hepatic microsomal enzyme inducing agents such as carbamazepine may increase the clearance of thiothixene. Patients receiving these drugs should be observed for signs of reduced thiothixene effectiveness). Products include:

Kaletra 458
Norvir 509

Scopolamine (Though exhibiting rather weak anticholinergic properties, thiothixene should be used with caution in patients who might be exposed to extreme heat or who are receiving atropine or related drugs). Products include:

Transderm Scōp 2397

Scopolamine Hydrobromide (Though exhibiting rather weak anticholinergic properties, thiothixene should be used with caution in patients who might be exposed to extreme heat or who are receiving atropine or related drugs). Products include:

Donnatal 2711

(⊙ Described in PDR® for Ophthalmic Medicines)

1887 Interactions Index Thiothixene

Secobarbital Sodium (Although thiothixene potentiates the actions of the barbiturates, the dosage of the anticonvulsant therapy should not be reduced when thiothixene is administered concurrently).
No products indexed under this heading.

Sevoflurane (Patients receiving thiothixene should be cautioned about the possible additive effects (which may include hypotension) with CNS depressants. Caution as well as careful adjustment of the dosages is indicated when thiothixene is used in conjunction with other CNS depressants and with alcohol). Products include:
Ultane 554

Sodium Butabarbital (Although thiothixene potentiates the actions of the barbiturates, the dosage of the anticonvulsant therapy should not be reduced when thiothixene is administered concurrently).
No products indexed under this heading.

Sodium Nitroprusside (Co-administration of thiothixene with antihypertensive agents may lead to excessive hypotension due to a possible additive effect. Patients receiving these drugs should be observed closely for signs of excessive hypotension when thiothixene is added to their drug regimen).
No products indexed under this heading.

Sodium Oxybate (Patients receiving thiothixene should be cautioned about the possible additive effects (which may include hypotension) with CNS depressants. Caution as well as careful adjustment of the dosages is indicated when thiothixene is used in conjunction with other CNS depressants and with alcohol).
No products indexed under this heading.

Sodium Pentobarbital (Although thiothixene potentiates the actions of the barbiturates, the dosage of the anticonvulsant therapy should not be reduced when thiothixene is administered concurrently).
No products indexed under this heading.

Sotalol Hydrochloride (Co-administration of thiothixene with antihypertensive agents may lead to excessive hypotension due to a possible additive effect. Patients receiving these drugs should be observed closely for signs of excessive hypotension when thiothixene is added to their drug regimen).
No products indexed under this heading.

Spirapril Hydrochloride (Co-administration of thiothixene with antihypertensive agents may lead to excessive hypotension due to a possible additive effect. Patients receiving these drugs should be observed closely for signs of excessive hypotension when thiothixene is added to their drug regimen).
No products indexed under this heading.

Sufentanil Citrate (Patients receiving thiothixene should be cautioned about the possible additive effects (which may include hypotension) with CNS depressants. Caution as well as careful adjustment of the dosages is indicated when thiothixene is used in conjunction with other CNS depressants and with alcohol).
No products indexed under this heading.

Talbutal (Patients receiving thiothixene should be cautioned about the possible additive effects (which may include hypotension) with CNS depressants. Caution as well as careful adjustment of the dosages is indicated when thiothixene is used in conjunction with other CNS depressants and with alcohol).
No products indexed under this heading.

Telmisartan (Co-administration of thiothixene with antihypertensive agents may lead to excessive hypotension due to a possible additive effect. Patients receiving these drugs should be observed closely for signs of excessive hypotension when thiothixene is added to their drug regimen). Products include:
Micardis 887
Micardis HCT 889

Temazepam (Patients receiving thiothixene should be cautioned about the possible additive effects (which may include hypotension) with CNS depressants. Caution as well as careful adjustment of the dosages is indicated when thiothixene is used in conjunction with other CNS depressants and with alcohol).
No products indexed under this heading.

Terazosin Hydrochloride (Co-administration of thiothixene with antihypertensive agents may lead to excessive hypotension due to a possible additive effect. Patients receiving these drugs should be observed closely for signs of excessive hypotension when thiothixene is added to their drug regimen).
No products indexed under this heading.

Theophylline (Co-administration of thiothixene with hepatic microsomal enzyme inducing agents such as carbamazepine may increase the clearance of thiothixene. Patients receiving these drugs should be observed for signs of reduced thiothixene effectiveness).
No products indexed under this heading.

Theophylline Anhydrous (Co-administration of thiothixene with hepatic microsomal enzyme inducing agents such as carbamazepine may increase the clearance of thiothixene. Patients receiving these drugs should be observed for signs of reduced thiothixene effectiveness). Products include:
Uniphyl 2817

Theophylline Calcium Salicylate (Co-administration of thiothixene with hepatic microsomal enzyme inducing agents such as carbamazepine may increase the clearance of thiothixene. Patients receiving these drugs should be observed for signs of reduced thiothixene effectiveness).
No products indexed under this heading.

Theophylline Dihydroxypropyl (Glyceryl) (Co-administration of thiothixene with hepatic microsomal enzyme inducing agents such as carbamazepine may increase the clearance of thiothixene. Patients receiving these drugs should be observed for signs of reduced thiothixene effectiveness).
No products indexed under this heading.

Theophylline Ethylenediamine (Co-administration of thiothixene with hepatic microsomal enzyme inducing agents such as carbamazepine may increase the clearance of thiothixene. Patients receiving these drugs should be observed for signs of reduced thiothixene effectiveness).
No products indexed under this heading.

Theophylline Sodium Glycinate (Co-administration of thiothixene with hepatic microsomal enzyme inducing agents such as carbamazepine may increase the clearance of thiothixene. Patients receiving these drugs should be observed for signs of reduced thiothixene effectiveness).
No products indexed under this heading.

Thiamylal Sodium (Although thiothixene potentiates the actions of the barbiturates, the dosage of the anticonvulsant therapy should not be reduced when thiothixene is administered concurrently).
No products indexed under this heading.

Thioridazine (Patients receiving thiothixene should be cautioned about the possible additive effects (which may include hypotension) with CNS depressants. Caution as well as careful adjustment of the dosages is indicated when thiothixene is used in conjunction with other CNS depressants and with alcohol).
No products indexed under this heading.

Thioridazine Hydrochloride (Patients receiving thiothixene should be cautioned about the possible additive effects (which may include hypotension) with CNS depressants. Caution as well as careful adjustment of the dosages is indicated when thiothixene is used in conjunction with other CNS depressants and with alcohol). Products include:
Thioridazine Hydrochloride 2384

Thiothixene Hydrochloride (Patients receiving thiothixene should be cautioned about the possible additive effects (which may include hypotension) with CNS depressants. Caution as well as careful adjustment of the dosages is indicated when thiothixene is used in conjunction with other CNS depressants and with alcohol).
No products indexed under this heading.

Timolol Maleate (Co-administration of thiothixene with antihypertensive agents may lead to excessive hypotension due to a possible additive effect. Patients receiving these drugs should be observed closely for signs of excessive hypotension when thiothixene is added to their drug regimen). Products include:
Combigan 601
Dorzolamide Hydrochloride/Timolol Maleate Ophthalmic Solution .... ⊙243
Timoptic in Ocudose .... ⊙231

Tobacco (Co-administration of thiothixene with hepatic microsomal enzyme inducing agents such as carbamazepine may increase the clearance of thiothixene. Patients receiving these drugs should be observed for signs of reduced thiothixene effectiveness).
No products indexed under this heading.

Tolazamide (Co-administration of thiothixene with hepatic microsomal enzyme inducing agents such as carbamazepine may increase the clearance of thiothixene. Patients receiving these drugs should be observed for signs of reduced thiothixene effectiveness).
No products indexed under this heading.

Tolbutamide (Co-administration of thiothixene with hepatic microsomal enzyme inducing agents such as carbamazepine may increase the clearance of thiothixene. Patients receiving these drugs should be observed for signs of reduced thiothixene effectiveness).
No products indexed under this heading.

Tolterodine Tartrate (Though exhibiting rather weak anticholinergic properties, thiothixene should be used with caution in patients who might be exposed to extreme heat or who are receiving atropine or related drugs).
No products indexed under this heading.

Torsemide (Co-administration of thiothixene with antihypertensive agents may lead to excessive hypotension due to a possible additive effect. Patients receiving these drugs should be observed closely for signs of excessive hypotension when thiothixene is added to their drug regimen).
No products indexed under this heading.

Trandolapril (Co-administration of thiothixene with antihypertensive agents may lead to excessive hypotension due to a possible additive effect. Patients receiving these drugs should be observed closely for signs of excessive hypotension when thiothixene is added to their drug regimen). Products include:
Mavik 489
Tarka 534

Triamcinolone (Co-administration of thiothixene with hepatic microsomal enzyme inducing agents such as carbamazepine may increase the clearance of thiothixene. Patients receiving these drugs should be observed for signs of reduced thiothixene effectiveness).
No products indexed under this heading.

Triamcinolone Acetonide (Co-administration of thiothixene with hepatic microsomal enzyme inducing agents such as carbamazepine may increase the clearance of thiothixene. Patients receiving these drugs should be observed for signs of reduced thiothixene effectiveness). Products include:
Azmacort 408
Nasacort AQ 3019

Triamcinolone Diacetate (Co-administration of thiothixene with hepatic microsomal enzyme inducing agents such as carbamazepine may increase the clearance of thiothixene. Patients receiving these drugs should be observed for signs of reduced thiothixene effectiveness).
No products indexed under this heading.

Triamcinolone Hexacetonide (Co-administration of thiothixene with hepatic microsomal enzyme inducing agents such as carbamazepine may increase the clearance of thiothixene. Patients receiving these drugs should be observed for signs of reduced thiothixene effectiveness).
No products indexed under this heading.

Triazolam (Patients receiving thiothixene should be cautioned about the possible additive effects (which may include hypotension) with CNS depressants. Caution as well as careful adjustment of the dosages is indicated when thiothixene is used in conjunction with other CNS depressants and with alcohol).
No products indexed under this heading.

Tridihexethyl Chloride (Though exhibiting rather weak anticholinergic properties, thiothixene should be used with caution in patients who might be exposed to extreme heat or who are receiving atropine or related drugs).
No products indexed under this heading.

Trifluoperazine Hydrochloride (Patients receiving thiothixene should be cautioned about the possible additive effects (which may include hypotension) with CNS depressants. Caution as well as careful adjustment of the dosages is indicated when thiothixene is used in conjunction with other CNS depressants and with alcohol).
No products indexed under this heading.

Trihexyphenidyl Hydrochloride (Though exhibiting rather weak anticholinergic properties, thiothixene should be used with caution in patients who might be exposed to extreme heat or who are receiving atropine or related drugs).
No products indexed under this heading.

Trimethaphan Camsylate (Co-administration of thiothixene with antihypertensive agents may lead to excessive hypotension due to a possible additive effect. Patients receiving these drugs should be observed closely for signs of excessive hypotension when thiothixene is added to their drug regimen).
No products indexed under this heading.

IMPORTANT NOTE: Always consult each drug listing in the patient's regimen for possible interactions.

Troglitazone (Co-administration of thiothixene with hepatic microsomal enzyme inducing agents such as carbamazepine may increase the clearance of thiothixene. Patients receiving these drugs should be observed for signs of reduced thiothixene effectiveness).

No products indexed under this heading.

Valsartan (Co-administration of thiothixene with antihypertensive agents may lead to excessive hypotension due to a possible additive effect. Patients receiving these drugs should be observed closely for signs of excessive hypotension when thiothixene is added to their drug regimen). Products include:

Verapamil Hydrochloride (Co-administration of thiothixene with antihypertensive agents may lead to excessive hypotension due to a possible additive effect. Patients receiving these drugs should be observed closely for signs of excessive hypotension when thiothixene is added to their drug regimen). Products include:

Zaleplon (Patients receiving thiothixene should be cautioned about the possible additive effects (which may include hypotension) with CNS depressants. Caution as well as careful adjustment of the dosages is indicated when thiothixene is used in conjunction with other CNS depressants and with alcohol).

No products indexed under this heading.

Ziprasidone Hydrochloride (Patients receiving thiothixene should be cautioned about the possible additive effects (which may include hypotension) with CNS depressants. Caution as well as careful adjustment of the dosages is indicated when thiothixene is used in conjunction with other CNS depressants and with alcohol). Products include:

Zolpidem Tartrate (Patients receiving thiothixene should be cautioned about the possible additive effects (which may include hypotension) with CNS depressants. Caution as well as careful adjustment of the dosages is indicated when thiothixene is used in conjunction with other CNS depressants and with alcohol). Products include:

Food Interactions

Alcohol (Patients receiving thiothixene should be cautioned about the possible additive effects (which may include hypotension) with CNS depressants and with alcohol. Extreme caution should be used in patients with a history of convulsive disorders or those in a state of alcohol withdrawal, since it may lower the convulsive threshold).

Beer, reduced-alcohol (Patients receiving thiothixene should be cautioned about the possible additive effects (which may include hypotension) with CNS depressants and with alcohol. Extreme caution should be used in patients with a history of convulsive disorders or those in a state of alcohol withdrawal, since it may lower the convulsive threshold).

Beer, unspecified (Patients receiving thiothixene should be cautioned about the possible additive effects (which may include hypotension) with CNS depressants and with alcohol. Extreme caution should be used in patients with a history of convulsive disorders or those in a

state of alcohol withdrawal, since it may lower the convulsive threshold).

Broccoli (Co-administration of thiothixene with hepatic microsomal enzyme inducing agents such as carbamazepine may increase the clearance of thiothixene. Patients receiving these drugs should be observed for signs of reduced thiothixene effectiveness).

Brussel Sprouts (Co-administration of thiothixene with hepatic microsomal enzyme inducing agents such as carbamazepine may increase the clearance of thiothixene. Patients receiving these drugs should be observed for signs of reduced thiothixene effectiveness).

Charbroiled Food (Co-administration of thiothixene with hepatic microsomal enzyme inducing agents such as carbamazepine may increase the clearance of thiothixene. Patients receiving these drugs should be observed for signs of reduced thiothixene effectiveness).

Wine, Chianti (Patients receiving thiothixene should be cautioned about the possible additive effects (which may include hypotension) with CNS depressants and with alcohol. Extreme caution should be used in patients with a history of convulsive disorders or those in a state of alcohol withdrawal, since it may lower the convulsive threshold).

Wine, Red (Patients receiving thiothixene should be cautioned about the possible additive effects (which may include hypotension) with CNS depressants and with alcohol. Extreme caution should be used in patients with a history of convulsive disorders or those in a state of alcohol withdrawal, since it may lower the convulsive threshold).

Wine, unspecified (Patients receiving thiothixene should be cautioned about the possible additive effects (which may include hypotension) with CNS depressants and with alcohol. Extreme caution should be used in patients with a history of convulsive disorders or those in a state of alcohol withdrawal, since it may lower the convulsive threshold).

Wine products (Patients receiving thiothixene should be cautioned about the possible additive effects (which may include hypotension) with CNS depressants and with alcohol. Extreme caution should be used in patients with a history of convulsive disorders or those in a state of alcohol withdrawal, since it may lower the convulsive threshold).

TICE BCG

May interact with agents associated with myelosuppression, antibiotics, antituberculosis drugs, corticosteroids, cytotoxic drugs, immunosuppressive agents, and certain other agents. Compounds in these categories include:

Alatrofloxacin Mesylate (Co-administration of BCG, live with antimicrobial therapy for other infections may interfere with the effectiveness of BCG, live).

No products indexed under this heading.

Alclometasone Dipropionate (BCG, live is contraindicated in immunosuppressed patients or persons with congenital or acquired immune deficiencies, whether due to concurrent disease (eg, AIDS, leukemia, lymphoma), cancer therapy (eg, cytotoxic drugs, radiation), or immunosuppressive therapy (eg, corticosteroids)).

No products indexed under this heading.

Altretamine (Drug combinations containing immunosuppressants and/or bone marrow depressants and/or radiation interfere with the development of

the immune response and should not be used in combination with BCG, live). Products include:

Amikacin Sulfate (Co-administration of BCG, live with antimicrobial therapy for other infections may interfere with the effectiveness of BCG, live).

No products indexed under this heading.

Aminosalicylic Acid (Antituberculosis drugs (eg, isoniazid) should not be used to prevent or treat the local, irritative toxicities of BCG, live). Products include:

p-Aminosalicylic Acid (Antituberculosis drugs (eg, isoniazid) should not be used to prevent or treat the local, irritative toxicities of BCG, live).

No products indexed under this heading.

Amoxicillin (Co-administration of BCG, live with antimicrobial therapy for other infections may interfere with the effectiveness of BCG, live). Products include:

Amoxicillin Trihydrate (Co-administration of BCG, live with antimicrobial therapy for other infections may interfere with the effectiveness of BCG, live).

No products indexed under this heading.

Ampicillin (Co-administration of BCG, live with antimicrobial therapy for other infections may interfere with the effectiveness of BCG, live).

No products indexed under this heading.

Ampicillin Sodium (Co-administration of BCG, live with antimicrobial therapy for other infections may interfere with the effectiveness of BCG, live).

No products indexed under this heading.

Ampicillin Trihydrate (Co-administration of BCG, live with antimicrobial therapy for other infections may interfere with the effectiveness of BCG, live).

No products indexed under this heading.

Antibiotics, non-penicillin, unspecified (Co-administration of BCG, live with antimicrobial therapy for other infections may interfere with the effectiveness of BCG, live).

No products indexed under this heading.

Azathioprine (BCG, live is contraindicated in immunosuppressed patients or persons with congenital or acquired immune deficiencies, whether due to concurrent disease (eg, AIDS, leukemia, lymphoma), cancer therapy (eg, cytotoxic drugs, radiation), or immunosuppressive therapy (eg, corticosteroids)).

No products indexed under this heading.

Azithromycin Dihydrate (Co-administration of BCG, live with antimicrobial therapy for other infections may interfere with the effectiveness of BCG, live).

No products indexed under this heading.

Azlocillin Sodium (Co-administration of BCG, live with antimicrobial therapy for other infections may interfere with the effectiveness of BCG, live).

No products indexed under this heading.

Aztreonam (Co-administration of BCG, live with antimicrobial therapy for other infections may interfere with the effectiveness of BCG, live).

No products indexed under this heading.

Bacampicillin Hydrochloride (Co-administration of BCG, live with antimicrobial therapy for other infections may interfere with the effectiveness of BCG, live).

No products indexed under this heading.

Basiliximab (BCG, live is contraindicated in immunosuppressed patients or persons with congenital or acquired immune deficiencies, whether due to concurrent disease (eg, AIDS, leukemia, lymphoma), cancer therapy (eg, cytotoxic drugs, radiation), or immunosuppressive therapy (eg, corticosteroids)). Products include:

Beclomethasone Dipropionate (BCG, live is contraindicated in immunosuppressed patients or persons with congenital or acquired immune deficiencies, whether due to concurrent disease (eg, AIDS, leukemia, lymphoma), cancer therapy (eg, cytotoxic drugs, radiation), or immunosuppressive therapy (eg, corticosteroids)). Products include:

Beclomethasone Dipropionate Monohydrate (BCG, live is contraindicated in immunosuppressed patients or persons with congenital or acquired immune deficiencies, whether due to concurrent disease (eg, AIDS, leukemia, lymphoma), cancer therapy (eg, cytotoxic drugs, radiation), or immunosuppressive therapy (eg, corticosteroids)). Products include:

Betamethasone (BCG, live is contraindicated in immunosuppressed patients or persons with congenital or acquired immune deficiencies, whether due to concurrent disease (eg, AIDS, leukemia, lymphoma), cancer therapy (eg, cytotoxic drugs, radiation), or immunosuppressive therapy (eg, corticosteroids)).

No products indexed under this heading.

Betamethasone Acetate (BCG, live is contraindicated in immunosuppressed patients or persons with congenital or acquired immune deficiencies, whether due to concurrent disease (eg, AIDS, leukemia, lymphoma), cancer therapy (eg, cytotoxic drugs, radiation), or immunosuppressive therapy (eg, corticosteroids)).

No products indexed under this heading.

Betamethasone Benzoate (BCG, live is contraindicated in immunosuppressed patients or persons with congenital or acquired immune deficiencies, whether due to concurrent disease (eg, AIDS, leukemia, lymphoma), cancer therapy (eg, cytotoxic drugs, radiation), or immunosuppressive therapy (eg, corticosteroids)).

No products indexed under this heading.

Betamethasone Dipropionate (BCG, live is contraindicated in immunosuppressed patients or persons with congenital or acquired immune deficiencies, whether due to concurrent disease (eg, AIDS, leukemia, lymphoma), cancer therapy (eg, cytotoxic drugs, radiation), or immunosuppressive therapy (eg, corticosteroids)). Products include:

Betamethasone Sodium Phosphate (BCG, live is contraindicated in immunosuppressed patients or persons with congenital or acquired immune deficiencies, whether due to concurrent disease (eg, AIDS, leukemia, lymphoma), cancer therapy (eg, cytotoxic drugs, radiation), or immunosuppressive therapy (eg, corticosteroids)).

No products indexed under this heading.

1889 Interactions Index Tice BCG

Betamethasone Valerate (BCG, live is contraindicated in immunosuppressed patients or persons with congenital or acquired immune deficiencies, whether due to concurrent disease (eg, AIDS, leukemia, lymphoma), cancer therapy (eg, cytotoxic drugs, radiation), or immunosuppressive therapy (eg, corticosteroids)). Products include:
Luxíq 3321

Bleomycin Sulfate (BCG, live is contraindicated in immunosuppressed patients or persons with congenital or acquired immune deficiencies, whether due to concurrent disease (eg, AIDS, leukemia, lymphoma), cancer therapy (eg, cytotoxic drugs, radiation), or immunosuppressive therapy (eg, corticosteroids)).
No products indexed under this heading.

Bone Marrow Depressants, unspecified (Drug combinations containing immunosuppressants and/or bone marrow depressants and/or radiation interfere with the development of the immune response and should not be used in combination with BCG live).
No products indexed under this heading.

Budesonide (BCG, live is contraindicated in immunosuppressed patients or persons with congenital or acquired immune deficiencies, whether due to concurrent disease (eg, AIDS, leukemia, lymphoma), cancer therapy (eg, cytotoxic drugs, radiation), or immunosuppressive therapy (eg, corticosteroids)). Products include:
Pulmicort Flexhaler 714
Symbicort 80/4.5 720
Symbicort 160/4.5 720

Busulfan (Drug combinations containing immunosuppressants and/or bone marrow depressants and/or radiation interfere with the development of the immune response and should not be used in combination with BCG, live). Products include:
Myleran 1581

Carbenicillin Disodium (Co-administration of BCG, live with antimicrobial therapy for other infections may interfere with the effectiveness of BCG, live).
No products indexed under this heading.

Carbenicillin Indanyl Sodium (Co-administration of BCG, live with antimicrobial therapy for other infections may interfere with the effectiveness of BCG, live).
No products indexed under this heading.

Cefaclor (Co-administration of BCG, live with antimicrobial therapy for other infections may interfere with the effectiveness of BCG, live).
No products indexed under this heading.

Cefadroxil (Co-administration of BCG, live with antimicrobial therapy for other infections may interfere with the effectiveness of BCG, live).
No products indexed under this heading.

Cefamandole Nafate (Co-administration of BCG, live with antimicrobial therapy for other infections may interfere with the effectiveness of BCG, live).
No products indexed under this heading.

Cefazolin Sodium (Co-administration of BCG, live with antimicrobial therapy for other infections may interfere with the effectiveness of BCG, live).
No products indexed under this heading.

Cefixime (Co-administration of BCG, live with antimicrobial therapy for other infections may interfere with the effectiveness of BCG, live). Products include:
Suprax for Oral Suspension 2038
Suprax Tablets 2038

Cefmetazole Sodium (Co-administration of BCG, live with antimicrobial therapy for other infections may interfere with the effectiveness of BCG, live).
No products indexed under this heading.

Cefonicid Sodium (Co-administration of BCG, live with antimicrobial therapy for other infections may interfere with the effectiveness of BCG, live).
No products indexed under this heading.

Cefoperazone Sodium (Co-administration of BCG, live with antimicrobial therapy for other infections may interfere with the effectiveness of BCG, live).
No products indexed under this heading.

Ceforanide (Co-administration of BCG, live with antimicrobial therapy for other infections may interfere with the effectiveness of BCG, live).
No products indexed under this heading.

Cefotaxime Sodium (Co-administration of BCG, live with antimicrobial therapy for other infections may interfere with the effectiveness of BCG, live).
No products indexed under this heading.

Cefotetan (Co-administration of BCG, live with antimicrobial therapy for other infections may interfere with the effectiveness of BCG, live).
No products indexed under this heading.

Cefoxitin Sodium (Co-administration of BCG, live with antimicrobial therapy for other infections may interfere with the effectiveness of BCG, live).
No products indexed under this heading.

Cefpodoxime Proxetil (Co-administration of BCG, live with antimicrobial therapy for other infections may interfere with the effectiveness of BCG, live).
No products indexed under this heading.

Cefprozil (Co-administration of BCG, live with antimicrobial therapy for other infections may interfere with the effectiveness of BCG, live).
No products indexed under this heading.

Ceftazidime (Co-administration of BCG, live with antimicrobial therapy for other infections may interfere with the effectiveness of BCG, live). Products include:
Fortaz 1481

Ceftizoxime Sodium (Co-administration of BCG, live with antimicrobial therapy for other infections may interfere with the effectiveness of BCG, live).
No products indexed under this heading.

Ceftriaxone Sodium (Co-administration of BCG, live with antimicrobial therapy for other infections may interfere with the effectiveness of BCG, live). Products include:
Rocephin 2859

Cefuroxime Axetil (Co-administration of BCG, live with antimicrobial therapy for other infections may interfere with the effectiveness of BCG, live). Products include:
Ceftin 1399

Cefuroxime Sodium (Co-administration of BCG, live with antimicrobial therapy for other infections may interfere with the effectiveness of BCG, live).
No products indexed under this heading.

Cephalexin (Co-administration of BCG, live with antimicrobial therapy for other infections may interfere with the effectiveness of BCG, live).
No products indexed under this heading.

Cephalothin Sodium (Co-administration of BCG, live with antimicrobial therapy for other infections may interfere with the effectiveness of BCG, live).
No products indexed under this heading.

Cephapirin Sodium (Co-administration of BCG, live with antimicrobial therapy for other infections may interfere with the effectiveness of BCG, live).
No products indexed under this heading.

Cephradine (Co-administration of BCG, live with antimicrobial therapy for other infections may interfere with the effectiveness of BCG, live).
No products indexed under this heading.

Chlorambucil (Drug combinations containing immunosuppressants and/or bone marrow depressants and/or radiation interfere with the development of the immune response and should not be used in combination with BCG, live). Products include:
Leukeran 1557

Chloramphenicol (Drug combinations containing immunosuppressants and/or bone marrow depressants and/or radiation interfere with the development of the immune response and should not be used in combination with BCG, live).
No products indexed under this heading.

Chloramphenicol Palmitate (Drug combinations containing immunosuppressants and/or bone marrow depressants and/or radiation interfere with the development of the immune response and should not be used in combination with BCG, live).
No products indexed under this heading.

Chloramphenicol Sodium Succinate (Drug combinations containing immunosuppressants and/or bone marrow depressants and/or radiation interfere with the development of the immune response and should not be used in combination with BCG, live).
No products indexed under this heading.

Ciclesonide (BCG, live is contraindicated in immunosuppressed patients or persons with congenital or acquired immune deficiencies, whether due to concurrent disease (eg, AIDS, leukemia, lymphoma), cancer therapy (eg, cytotoxic drugs, radiation), or immunosuppressive therapy (eg, corticosteroids)).
No products indexed under this heading.

Cilastatin Sodium (Co-administration of BCG, live with antimicrobial therapy for other infections may interfere with the effectiveness of BCG, live). Products include:
Primaxin I.M. 2232
Primaxin I.V. 2235

Ciprofloxacin (Co-administration of BCG, live with antimicrobial therapy for other infections may interfere with the effectiveness of BCG, live). Products include:
Cipro I.V. 3082
Cipro 3073
Cipro XR 3091
Ciprodex 583

Ciprofloxacin Hydrochloride (Co-administration of BCG, live with antimicrobial therapy for other infections may interfere with the effectiveness of BCG, live). Products include:
Cipro 3073

Cladribine (Drug combinations containing immunosuppressants and/or bone marrow depressants and/or radiation interfere with the development of the immune response and should not be used in combination with BCG, live). Products include:
Leustatin 946

Clarithromycin (Co-administration of BCG, live with antimicrobial therapy for other infections may interfere with the effectiveness of BCG, live). Products include:
Biaxin/Biaxin XL 412

Clotrimazole (Co-administration of BCG, live with antimicrobial therapy for other infections may interfere with the effectiveness of BCG, live). Products include:
Lotrisone 3163

Cloxacillin (Co-administration of BCG, live with antimicrobial therapy for other infections may interfere with the effectiveness of BCG, live).
No products indexed under this heading.

Cloxacillin Sodium (Co-administration of BCG, live with antimicrobial therapy for other infections may interfere with the effectiveness of BCG, live).
No products indexed under this heading.

Cloxacillin Sodium Monohydrate (Co-administration of BCG, live with antimicrobial therapy for other infections may interfere with the effectiveness of BCG, live).
No products indexed under this heading.

Cortisone Acetate (BCG, live is contraindicated in immunosuppressed patients or persons with congenital or acquired immune deficiencies, whether due to concurrent disease (eg, AIDS, leukemia, lymphoma), cancer therapy (eg, cytotoxic drugs, radiation), or immunosuppressive therapy (eg, corticosteroids)).
No products indexed under this heading.

Cyclophosphamide (BCG, live is contraindicated in immunosuppressed patients or persons with congenital or acquired immune deficiencies, whether due to concurrent disease (eg, AIDS, leukemia, lymphoma), cancer therapy (eg, cytotoxic drugs, radiation), or immunosuppressive therapy (eg, corticosteroids)).
No products indexed under this heading.

Cycloserine (Antituberculosis drugs (eg, isoniazid) should not be used to prevent or treat the local, irritative toxicities of BCG, live). Products include:
Seromycin 1956

Cyclosporine (BCG, live is contraindicated in immunosuppressed patients or persons with congenital or acquired immune deficiencies, whether due to concurrent disease (eg, AIDS, leukemia, lymphoma), cancer therapy (eg, cytotoxic drugs, radiation), or immunosuppressive therapy (eg, corticosteroids)). Products include:
Gengraf 440
Neoral Oral Solution 2496
Neoral Capsules 2496
Restasis 605

Daunorubicin Citrate Liposome (Drug combinations containing immunosuppressants and/or bone marrow depressants and/or radiation interfere with the development of the immune response and should not be used in combination with BCG, live).
No products indexed under this heading.

Daunorubicin Hydrochloride (BCG, live is contraindicated in immunosuppressed patients or persons with congenital or acquired immune deficiencies, whether due to concurrent disease (eg, AIDS, leukemia, lymphoma), cancer therapy (eg, cytotoxic drugs, radiation), or immunosuppressive therapy (eg, corticosteroids)).
No products indexed under this heading.

Demeclocycline Hydrochloride (Co-administration of BCG, live with antimicrobial therapy for other infections may interfere with the effectiveness of BCG, live).
No products indexed under this heading.

IMPORTANT NOTE: Always consult each drug listing in the patient's regimen for possible interactions.

Tice BCG Interactions Index 1890

Desoximetasone (BCG, live is contraindicated in immunosuppressed patients or persons with congenital or acquired immune deficiencies, whether due to concurrent disease (eg, AIDS, leukemia, lymphoma), cancer therapy (eg, cytotoxic drugs, radiation), or immunosuppressive therapy (eg, corticosteroids)).
No products indexed under this heading.

Dexamethasone (BCG, live is contraindicated in immunosuppressed patients or persons with congenital or acquired immune deficiencies, whether due to concurrent disease (eg, AIDS, leukemia, lymphoma), cancer therapy (eg, cytotoxic drugs, radiation), or immunosuppressive therapy (eg, corticosteroids)). Products include:
Ciprodex 583
Ozurdex .... ⊙223
Tobramycin and Dexamethasone Ophthalmic Suspension .... ⊙251

Dexamethasone Acetate (BCG, live is contraindicated in immunosuppressed patients or persons with congenital or acquired immune deficiencies, whether due to concurrent disease (eg, AIDS, leukemia, lymphoma), cancer therapy (eg, cytotoxic drugs, radiation), or immunosuppressive therapy (eg, corticosteroids)).
No products indexed under this heading.

Dexamethasone Phosphate (BCG, live is contraindicated in immunosuppressed patients or persons with congenital or acquired immune deficiencies, whether due to concurrent disease (eg, AIDS, leukemia, lymphoma), cancer therapy (eg, cytotoxic drugs, radiation), or immunosuppressive therapy (eg, corticosteroids)).
No products indexed under this heading.

Dexamethasone Sodium (BCG, live is contraindicated in immunosuppressed patients or persons with congenital or acquired immune deficiencies, whether due to concurrent disease (eg, AIDS, leukemia, lymphoma), cancer therapy (eg, cytotoxic drugs, radiation), or immunosuppressive therapy (eg, corticosteroids)).
No products indexed under this heading.

Dexamethasone Sodium Phosphate (BCG, live is contraindicated in immunosuppressed patients or persons with congenital or acquired immune deficiencies, whether due to concurrent disease (eg, AIDS, leukemia, lymphoma), cancer therapy (eg, cytotoxic drugs, radiation), or immunosuppressive therapy (eg, corticosteroids)).
No products indexed under this heading.

Dexamethasone Sodium Phosphate Injection (BCG, live is contraindicated in immunosuppressed patients or persons with congenital or acquired immune deficiencies, whether due to concurrent disease (eg, AIDS, leukemia, lymphoma), cancer therapy (eg, cytotoxic drugs, radiation), or immunosuppressive therapy (eg, corticosteroids)).
No products indexed under this heading.

Dexrazoxane (Drug combinations containing immunosuppressants and/or bone marrow depressants and/or radiation interfere with the development of the immune response and should not be used in combination with BCG, live).
No products indexed under this heading.

Dicloxacillin (Co-administration of BCG, live with antimicrobial therapy for other infections may interfere with the effectiveness of BCG, live).
No products indexed under this heading.

Dicloxacillin Sodium (Co-administration of BCG, live with antimicrobial therapy for other infections may interfere with the effectiveness of BCG, live).
No products indexed under this heading.

Diflorasone Diacetate (BCG, live is contraindicated in immunosuppressed patients or persons with congenital or acquired immune deficiencies, whether due to concurrent disease (eg, AIDS, leukemia, lymphoma), cancer therapy (eg, cytotoxic drugs, radiation), or immunosuppressive therapy (eg, corticosteroids)).
No products indexed under this heading.

Dirithromycin (Co-administration of BCG, live with antimicrobial therapy for other infections may interfere with the effectiveness of BCG, live).
No products indexed under this heading.

Disodium Carbenicillin (Co-administration of BCG, live with antimicrobial therapy for other infections may interfere with the effectiveness of BCG, live).
No products indexed under this heading.

Doxorubicin Hydrochloride (BCG, live is contraindicated in immunosuppressed patients or persons with congenital or acquired immune deficiencies, whether due to concurrent disease (eg, AIDS, leukemia, lymphoma), cancer therapy (eg, cytotoxic drugs, radiation), or immunosuppressive therapy (eg, corticosteroids)).
No products indexed under this heading.

Doxorubicin Hydrochloride Liposome (Drug combinations containing immunosuppressants and/or bone marrow depressants and/or radiation interfere with the development of the immune response and should not be used in combination with BCG, live). Products include:
Doxil 939

Doxycycline Calcium (Co-administration of BCG, live with antimicrobial therapy for other infections may interfere with the effectiveness of BCG, live).
No products indexed under this heading.

Doxycycline Hyclate (Co-administration of BCG, live with antimicrobial therapy for other infections may interfere with the effectiveness of BCG, live).
No products indexed under this heading.

Doxycycline Monohydrate (Co-administration of BCG, live with antimicrobial therapy for other infections may interfere with the effectiveness of BCG, live).
No products indexed under this heading.

Enoxacin (Co-administration of BCG, live with antimicrobial therapy for other infections may interfere with the effectiveness of BCG, live).
No products indexed under this heading.

Epirubicin Hydrochloride (BCG, live is contraindicated in immunosuppressed patients or persons with congenital or acquired immune deficiencies, whether due to concurrent disease (eg, AIDS, leukemia, lymphoma), cancer therapy (eg, cytotoxic drugs, radiation), or immunosuppressive therapy (eg, corticosteroids)).
No products indexed under this heading.

Erythromycin (Co-administration of BCG, live with antimicrobial therapy for other infections may interfere with the effectiveness of BCG, live).
No products indexed under this heading.

Erythromycin, Topical (Co-administration of BCG, live with antimicrobial therapy for other infections may interfere with the effectiveness of BCG, live).
No products indexed under this heading.

Erythromycin Estolate (Co-administration of BCG, live with antimicrobial therapy for other infections may interfere with the effectiveness of BCG, live).
No products indexed under this heading.

Erythromycin Ethylsuccinate (Co-administration of BCG, live with antimicrobial therapy for other infections may interfere with the effectiveness of BCG, live). Products include:
E.E.S. 437
EryPed 435

Erythromycin Gluceptate (Co-administration of BCG, live with antimicrobial therapy for other infections may interfere with the effectiveness of BCG, live).
No products indexed under this heading.

Erythromycin Lactobionate (Co-administration of BCG, live with antimicrobial therapy for other infections may interfere with the effectiveness of BCG, live).
No products indexed under this heading.

Erythromycin Stearate (Co-administration of BCG, live with antimicrobial therapy for other infections may interfere with the effectiveness of BCG, live).
No products indexed under this heading.

Ethambutol Hydrochloride (Antituberculosis drugs (eg, isoniazid) should not be used to prevent or treat the local, irritative toxicities of BCG, live).
No products indexed under this heading.

Fludarabine Phosphate (Drug combinations containing immunosuppressants and/or bone marrow depressants and/or radiation interfere with the development of the immune response and should not be used in combination with BCG, live). Products include:
Oforta 3023

Fludrocortisone Acetate (BCG, live is contraindicated in immunosuppressed patients or persons with congenital or acquired immune deficiencies, whether due to concurrent disease (eg, AIDS, leukemia, lymphoma), cancer therapy (eg, cytotoxic drugs, radiation), or immunosuppressive therapy (eg, corticosteroids)).
No products indexed under this heading.

Flumethasone Pivalate (BCG, live is contraindicated in immunosuppressed patients or persons with congenital or acquired immune deficiencies, whether due to concurrent disease (eg, AIDS, leukemia, lymphoma), cancer therapy (eg, cytotoxic drugs, radiation), or immunosuppressive therapy (eg, corticosteroids)).
No products indexed under this heading.

Flunisolide Hemihydrate (BCG, live is contraindicated in immunosuppressed patients or persons with congenital or acquired immune deficiencies, whether due to concurrent disease (eg, AIDS, leukemia, lymphoma), cancer therapy (eg, cytotoxic drugs, radiation), or immunosuppressive therapy (eg, corticosteroids)).
No products indexed under this heading.

Fluorouracil (BCG, live is contraindicated in immunosuppressed patients or persons with congenital or acquired immune deficiencies, whether due to concurrent disease (eg, AIDS, leukemia, lymphoma), cancer therapy (eg, cytotoxic drugs, radiation), or immunosuppressive therapy (eg, corticosteroids)). Products include:
Carac 2966

Fluticasone Furoate (BCG, live is contraindicated in immunosuppressed patients or persons with congenital or acquired immune deficiencies, whether due to concurrent disease (eg, AIDS, leukemia, lymphoma), cancer therapy (eg, cytotoxic drugs, radiation), or immunosuppressive therapy (eg, corticosteroids)). Products include:
Veramyst 1713

Fluticasone Propionate (BCG, live is contraindicated in immunosuppressed patients or persons with congenital or acquired immune deficiencies, whether due to concurrent disease (eg, AIDS, leukemia, lymphoma), cancer therapy (eg, cytotoxic drugs, radiation), or immunosuppressive therapy (eg, corticosteroids)). Products include:
Advair 100/50 1275
Advair 250/50 1275
Advair 500/50 1275
Advair HFA 45/21 1288
Advair HFA 115/21 1288
Advair HFA 230/21 1288
Flonase 1459
Flovent Diskus 1463
Flovent HFA 1470

Gatifloxacin (Co-administration of BCG, live with antimicrobial therapy for other infections may interfere with the effectiveness of BCG, live).
No products indexed under this heading.

Gemcitabine Hydrochloride (Drug combinations containing immunosuppressants and/or bone marrow depressants and/or radiation interfere with the development of the immune response and should not be used in combination with BCG, live). Products include:
Gemzar 1900

Gemifloxacin Mesylate (Co-administration of BCG, live with antimicrobial therapy for other infections may interfere with the effectiveness of BCG, live).
No products indexed under this heading.

Gemtuzumab Ozogamicin (Drug combinations containing immunosuppressants and/or bone marrow depressants and/or radiation interfere with the development of the immune response and should not be used in combination with BCG, live). Products include:
Mylotarg 3524

Gentamicin Sulfate (Co-administration of BCG, live with antimicrobial therapy for other infections may interfere with the effectiveness of BCG, live). Products include:
Pred-G .... ⊙226, ⊙227

Grepafloxacin Hydrochloride (Co-administration of BCG, live with antimicrobial therapy for other infections may interfere with the effectiveness of BCG, live).
No products indexed under this heading.

Griseofulvin (Co-administration of BCG, live with antimicrobial therapy for other infections may interfere with the effectiveness of BCG, live).
No products indexed under this heading.

Hydrocortisone (BCG, live is contraindicated in immunosuppressed patients or persons with congenital or acquired immune deficiencies, whether due to concurrent disease (eg, AIDS, leukemia, lymphoma), cancer therapy (eg, cytotoxic drugs, radiation), or immunosuppressive therapy (eg, corticosteroids)).
No products indexed under this heading.

Hydrocortisone (Alcohol) (BCG, live is contraindicated in immunosuppressed patients or persons with congenital or acquired immune deficiencies, whether due to concurrent disease (eg, AIDS, leukemia, lymphoma), cancer therapy (eg, cytotoxic drugs, radiation), or immunosuppressive therapy (eg, corticosteroids)).
No products indexed under this heading.

Hydrocortisone Acetate (BCG, live is contraindicated in immunosuppressed patients or persons with congenital or acquired immune deficiencies, whether due to concurrent disease (eg, AIDS, leukemia, lymphoma), cancer therapy (eg, cytotoxic drugs, radiation), or immunosuppressive therapy (eg, corticosteroids)).
No products indexed under this heading.

1891 Interactions Index Tice BCG

Hydrocortisone Butyrate (BCG, live is contraindicated in immunosuppressed patients or persons with congenital or acquired immune deficiencies, whether due to concurrent disease (eg, AIDS, leukemia, lymphoma), cancer therapy (eg, cytotoxic drugs, radiation), or immunosuppressive therapy (eg, corticosteroids)).
No products indexed under this heading.

Hydrocortisone Cypionate (BCG, live is contraindicated in immunosuppressed patients or persons with congenital or acquired immune deficiencies, whether due to concurrent disease (eg, AIDS, leukemia, lymphoma), cancer therapy (eg, cytotoxic drugs, radiation), or immunosuppressive therapy (eg, corticosteroids)).
No products indexed under this heading.

Hydrocortisone Hemisuccinate (BCG, live is contraindicated in immunosuppressed patients or persons with congenital or acquired immune deficiencies, whether due to concurrent disease (eg, AIDS, leukemia, lymphoma), cancer therapy (eg, cytotoxic drugs, radiation), or immunosuppressive therapy (eg, corticosteroids)).
No products indexed under this heading.

Hydrocortisone Probutate (BCG, live is contraindicated in immunosuppressed patients or persons with congenital or acquired immune deficiencies, whether due to concurrent disease (eg, AIDS, leukemia, lymphoma), cancer therapy (eg, cytotoxic drugs, radiation), or immunosuppressive therapy (eg, corticosteroids)).
No products indexed under this heading.

Hydrocortisone Sodium Phosphate (BCG, live is contraindicated in immunosuppressed patients or persons with congenital or acquired immune deficiencies, whether due to concurrent disease (eg, AIDS, leukemia, lymphoma), cancer therapy (eg, cytotoxic drugs, radiation), or immunosuppressive therapy (eg, corticosteroids)).
No products indexed under this heading.

Hydrocortisone Sodium Succinate (BCG, live is contraindicated in immunosuppressed patients or persons with congenital or acquired immune deficiencies, whether due to concurrent disease (eg, AIDS, leukemia, lymphoma), cancer therapy (eg, cytotoxic drugs, radiation), or immunosuppressive therapy (eg, corticosteroids)).
No products indexed under this heading.

Hydrocortisone Valerate (BCG, live is contraindicated in immunosuppressed patients or persons with congenital or acquired immune deficiencies, whether due to concurrent disease (eg, AIDS, leukemia, lymphoma), cancer therapy (eg, cytotoxic drugs, radiation), or immunosuppressive therapy (eg, corticosteroids)).
No products indexed under this heading.

Hydroxyurea (BCG, live is contraindicated in immunosuppressed patients or persons with congenital or acquired immune deficiencies, whether due to concurrent disease (eg, AIDS, leukemia, lymphoma), cancer therapy (eg, cytotoxic drugs, radiation), or immunosuppressive therapy (eg, corticosteroids)).
No products indexed under this heading.

Idarubicin Hydrochloride (Drug combinations containing immunosuppressants and/or bone marrow depressants and/or radiation interfere with the development of the immune response and should not be used in combination with BCG, live).
No products indexed under this heading.

Imipenem (Co-administration of BCG, live with antimicrobial therapy for other infections may interfere with the effectiveness of BCG, live). Products include:
Primaxin I.M. 2232
Primaxin I.V. 2235

Interferon alfa-2a, Recombinant (Drug combinations containing immunosuppressants and/or bone marrow depressants and/or radiation interfere with the development of the immune response and should not be used in combination with BCG, live).
No products indexed under this heading.

Irinotecan Hydrochloride (Drug combinations containing immunosuppressants and/or bone marrow depressants and/or radiation interfere with the development of the immune response and should not be used in combination with BCG, live).
No products indexed under this heading.

Isoniazid (Antituberculosis drugs (eg, isoniazid) should not be used to prevent or treat the local, irritative toxicities of BCG, live).
No products indexed under this heading.

Kanamycin Sulfate (Co-administration of BCG, live with antimicrobial therapy for other infections may interfere with the effectiveness of BCG, live).
No products indexed under this heading.

Levofloxacin (Co-administration of BCG, live with antimicrobial therapy for other infections may interfere with the effectiveness of BCG, live). Products include:
Iquix 3492
Levaquin 2629
Levaquin in 5% Dextrose 2629
Quixin 3493

Lomefloxacin Hydrochloride (Co-administration of BCG, live with antimicrobial therapy for other infections may interfere with the effectiveness of BCG, live).
No products indexed under this heading.

Loracarbef (Co-administration of BCG, live with antimicrobial therapy for other infections may interfere with the effectiveness of BCG, live).
No products indexed under this heading.

Melphalan Hydrochloride (Drug combinations containing immunosuppressants and/or bone marrow depressants and/or radiation interfere with the development of the immune response and should not be used in combination with BCG, live). Products include:
Alkeran for Injection 1300

Mercaptopurine (Drug combinations containing immunosuppressants and/or bone marrow depressants and/or radiation interfere with the development of the immune response and should not be used in combination with BCG, live).
No products indexed under this heading.

Methacycline Hydrochloride (Co-administration of BCG, live with antimicrobial therapy for other infections may interfere with the effectiveness of BCG, live).
No products indexed under this heading.

Methicillin Sodium (Co-administration of BCG, live with antimicrobial therapy for other infections may interfere with the effectiveness of BCG, live).
No products indexed under this heading.

Methotrexate Sodium (BCG, live is contraindicated in immunosuppressed patients or persons with congenital or acquired immune deficiencies, whether due to concurrent disease (eg, AIDS, leukemia, lymphoma), cancer therapy (eg, cytotoxic drugs, radiation), or immunosuppressive therapy (eg, corticosteroids)).
No products indexed under this heading.

Methylprednisolone (BCG, live is contraindicated in immunosuppressed patients or persons with congenital or acquired immune deficiencies, whether due to concurrent disease (eg, AIDS, leukemia, lymphoma), cancer therapy (eg, cytotoxic drugs, radiation), or immunosuppressive therapy (eg, corticosteroids)).
No products indexed under this heading.

Methylprednisolone Acetate (BCG, live is contraindicated in immunosuppressed patients or persons with congenital or acquired immune deficiencies, whether due to concurrent disease (eg, AIDS, leukemia, lymphoma), cancer therapy (eg, cytotoxic drugs, radiation), or immunosuppressive therapy (eg, corticosteroids)).
No products indexed under this heading.

Methylprednisolone Sodium Succinate (BCG, live is contraindicated in immunosuppressed patients or persons with congenital or acquired immune deficiencies, whether due to concurrent disease (eg, AIDS, leukemia, lymphoma), cancer therapy (eg, cytotoxic drugs, radiation), or immunosuppressive therapy (eg, corticosteroids)).
No products indexed under this heading.

Mezlocillin Sodium (Co-administration of BCG, live with antimicrobial therapy for other infections may interfere with the effectiveness of BCG, live).
No products indexed under this heading.

Minocycline Hydrochloride (Co-administration of BCG, live with antimicrobial therapy for other infections may interfere with the effectiveness of BCG, live). Products include:
Solodyn 2073

Mitotane (BCG, live is contraindicated in immunosuppressed patients or persons with congenital or acquired immune deficiencies, whether due to concurrent disease (eg, AIDS, leukemia, lymphoma), cancer therapy (eg, cytotoxic drugs, radiation), or immunosuppressive therapy (eg, corticosteroids)).
No products indexed under this heading.

Mitoxantrone Hydrochloride (BCG, live is contraindicated in immunosuppressed patients or persons with congenital or acquired immune deficiencies, whether due to concurrent disease (eg, AIDS, leukemia, lymphoma), cancer therapy (eg, cytotoxic drugs, radiation), or immunosuppressive therapy (eg, corticosteroids)). Products include:
Novantrone 1088

Mometasone Furoate (BCG, live is contraindicated in immunosuppressed patients or persons with congenital or acquired immune deficiencies, whether due to concurrent disease (eg, AIDS, leukemia, lymphoma), cancer therapy (eg, cytotoxic drugs, radiation), or immunosuppressive therapy (eg, corticosteroids)). Products include:
Asmanex 3058
Elocon Cream 3111
Elocon Lotion 3112
Elocon Ointment 3114

Mometasone Furoate Monohydrate (BCG, live is contraindicated in immunosuppressed patients or persons with congenital or acquired immune deficiencies, whether due to concurrent disease (eg, AIDS, leukemia, lymphoma), cancer therapy (eg, cytotoxic drugs, radiation), or immunosuppressive therapy (eg, corticosteroids)). Products include:
Nasonex 3166

Moxifloxacin Hydrochloride (Co-administration of BCG, live with antimicrobial therapy for other infections may interfere with the effectiveness of BCG, live). Products include:
Avelox 3064
Vigamox 589

Muromonab-CD3 (BCG, live is contraindicated in immunosuppressed patients or persons with congenital or acquired immune deficiencies, whether due to concurrent disease (eg, AIDS, leukemia, lymphoma), cancer therapy (eg, cytotoxic drugs, radiation), or immunosuppressive therapy (eg, corticosteroids)). Products include:
Orthoclone OKT3 949

Mycophenolate Mofetil (BCG, live is contraindicated in immunosuppressed patients or persons with congenital or acquired immune deficiencies, whether due to concurrent disease (eg, AIDS, leukemia, lymphoma), cancer therapy (eg, cytotoxic drugs, radiation), or immunosuppressive therapy (eg, corticosteroids)).
No products indexed under this heading.

Nafcillin Sodium (Co-administration of BCG, live with antimicrobial therapy for other infections may interfere with the effectiveness of BCG, live).
No products indexed under this heading.

Norfloxacin (Co-administration of BCG, live with antimicrobial therapy for other infections may interfere with the effectiveness of BCG, live). Products include:
Noroxin 2220

Ofloxacin (Co-administration of BCG, live with antimicrobial therapy for other infections may interfere with the effectiveness of BCG, live).
No products indexed under this heading.

Oxacillin (Co-administration of BCG, live with antimicrobial therapy for other infections may interfere with the effectiveness of BCG, live).
No products indexed under this heading.

Oxacillin Sodium (Co-administration of BCG, live with antimicrobial therapy for other infections may interfere with the effectiveness of BCG, live).
No products indexed under this heading.

Oxytetracycline Hydrochloride (Co-administration of BCG, live with antimicrobial therapy for other infections may interfere with the effectiveness of BCG, live).
No products indexed under this heading.

Penicillin, Potassium Phenoxymethyl (Co-administration of BCG, live with antimicrobial therapy for other infections may interfere with the effectiveness of BCG, live).
No products indexed under this heading.

Penicillin G Benzathine (Co-administration of BCG, live with antimicrobial therapy for other infections may interfere with the effectiveness of BCG, live). Products include:
Bicillin C-R Injectable Suspension 1826
Bicillin L-A 1828

Penicillin G Dibenzylethyenediamine (Co-administration of BCG, live with antimicrobial therapy for other infections may interfere with the effectiveness of BCG, live).
No products indexed under this heading.

Penicillin G Potassium (Co-administration of BCG, live with antimicrobial therapy for other infections may interfere with the effectiveness of BCG, live).
No products indexed under this heading.

Penicillin G Procaine (Co-administration of BCG, live with antimicrobial therapy for other infections may interfere with the effectiveness of BCG, live). Products include:
Bicillin C-R Injectable Suspension 1826
Bicillin L-A 1828

IMPORTANT NOTE: Always consult each drug listing in the patient's regimen for possible interactions.

Penicillin G Sodium (Co-administration of BCG, live with antimicrobial therapy for other infections may interfere with the effectiveness of BCG, live).
No products indexed under this heading.

Penicillin V (Co-administration of BCG, live with antimicrobial therapy for other infections may interfere with the effectiveness of BCG, live).
No products indexed under this heading.

Penicillin V Potassium (Co-administration of BCG, live with antimicrobial therapy for other infections may interfere with the effectiveness of BCG, live).
No products indexed under this heading.

Penicillins (Co-administration of BCG, live with antimicrobial therapy for other infections may interfere with the effectiveness of BCG, live).
No products indexed under this heading.

Piperacillin Sodium (Co-administration of BCG, live with antimicrobial therapy for other infections may interfere with the effectiveness of BCG, live). Products include:
Zosyn 3607

Prednisolone (BCG, live is contraindicated in immunosuppressed patients or persons with congenital or acquired immune deficiencies, whether due to concurrent disease (eg, AIDS, leukemia, lymphoma), cancer therapy (eg, cytotoxic drugs, radiation), or immunosuppressive therapy (eg, corticosteroids)).
No products indexed under this heading.

Prednisolone Acetate (BCG, live is contraindicated in immunosuppressed patients or persons with congenital or acquired immune deficiencies, whether due to concurrent disease (eg, AIDS, leukemia, lymphoma), cancer therapy (eg, cytotoxic drugs, radiation), or immunosuppressive therapy (eg, corticosteroids)). Products include:
Blephamide .... ⊙212, ⊙214
Pred Forte .... ⊙225
Pred Mild .... ⊙230
Pred-G .... ⊙226, ⊙227

Prednisolone Sodium Phosphate (BCG, live is contraindicated in immunosuppressed patients or persons with congenital or acquired immune deficiencies, whether due to concurrent disease (eg, AIDS, leukemia, lymphoma), cancer therapy (eg, cytotoxic drugs, radiation), or immunosuppressive therapy (eg, corticosteroids)).
No products indexed under this heading.

Prednisolone Tebutate (BCG, live is contraindicated in immunosuppressed patients or persons with congenital or acquired immune deficiencies, whether due to concurrent disease (eg, AIDS, leukemia, lymphoma), cancer therapy (eg, cytotoxic drugs, radiation), or immunosuppressive therapy (eg, corticosteroids)).
No products indexed under this heading.

Prednisone (BCG, live is contraindicated in immunosuppressed patients or persons with congenital or acquired immune deficiencies, whether due to concurrent disease (eg, AIDS, leukemia, lymphoma), cancer therapy (eg, cytotoxic drugs, radiation), or immunosuppressive therapy (eg, corticosteroids)).
No products indexed under this heading.

Prednisone sodium phosphate (BCG, live is contraindicated in immunosuppressed patients or persons with congenital or acquired immune deficiencies, whether due to concurrent disease (eg, AIDS, leukemia, lymphoma), cancer therapy (eg, cytotoxic drugs, radiation), or immunosuppressive therapy (eg, corticosteroids)).
No products indexed under this heading.

Procarbazine Hydrochloride (BCG, live is contraindicated in immunosuppressed patients or persons with congenital or acquired immune deficiencies, whether due to concurrent disease (eg, AIDS, leukemia, lymphoma), cancer therapy (eg, cytotoxic drugs, radiation), or immunosuppressive therapy (eg, corticosteroids)).
No products indexed under this heading.

Pyrazinamide (Antituberculosis drugs (eg, isoniazid) should not be used to prevent or treat the local, irritative toxicities of BCG, live).
No products indexed under this heading.

Radiation (BCG, live is contraindicated in immunosuppressed patients or persons with congenital or acquired immune deficiencies, whether due to concurrent disease (eg, AIDS, leukemia, lymphoma), cancer therapy (eg, cytotoxic drugs, radiation), or immunosuppressive therapy (eg, corticosteroids)).
No products indexed under this heading.

Rapamycin (BCG, live is contraindicated in immunosuppressed patients or persons with congenital or acquired immune deficiencies, whether due to concurrent disease (eg, AIDS, leukemia, lymphoma), cancer therapy (eg, cytotoxic drugs, radiation), or immunosuppressive therapy (eg, corticosteroids)).
No products indexed under this heading.

Rifampin (Antituberculosis drugs (eg, isoniazid) should not be used to prevent or treat the local, irritative toxicities of BCG, live).
No products indexed under this heading.

Rifapentine (Antituberculosis drugs (eg, isoniazid) should not be used to prevent or treat the local, irritative toxicities of BCG, live).
No products indexed under this heading.

Sirolimus (BCG, live is contraindicated in immunosuppressed patients or persons with congenital or acquired immune deficiencies, whether due to concurrent disease (eg, AIDS, leukemia, lymphoma), cancer therapy (eg, cytotoxic drugs, radiation), or immunosuppressive therapy (eg, corticosteroids)). Products include:
Rapamune 3579

Sodium Cloxacillin Monohydrate (Co-administration of BCG, live with antimicrobial therapy for other infections may interfere with the effectiveness of BCG, live).
No products indexed under this heading.

Sparfloxacin (Co-administration of BCG, live with antimicrobial therapy for other infections may interfere with the effectiveness of BCG, live).
No products indexed under this heading.

Streptomycin Sulfate (Co-administration of BCG, live with antimicrobial therapy for other infections may interfere with the effectiveness of BCG, live).
No products indexed under this heading.

Sulfamethizole (Co-administration of BCG, live with antimicrobial therapy for other infections may interfere with the effectiveness of BCG, live).
No products indexed under this heading.

Sulfamethoxazole (Co-administration of BCG, live with antimicrobial therapy for other infections may interfere with the effectiveness of BCG, live).
No products indexed under this heading.

Sulfisoxazole Acetyl (Co-administration of BCG, live with antimicrobial therapy for other infections may interfere with the effectiveness of BCG, live).
No products indexed under this heading.

Sulfisoxazole Diolamine (Co-administration of BCG, live with antimicrobial therapy for other infections may interfere with the effectiveness of BCG, live).
No products indexed under this heading.

Tacrolimus (BCG, live is contraindicated in immunosuppressed patients or persons with congenital or acquired immune deficiencies, whether due to concurrent disease (eg, AIDS, leukemia, lymphoma), cancer therapy (eg, cytotoxic drugs, radiation), or immunosuppressive therapy (eg, corticosteroids)). Products include:
Prograf Capsules 677
Prograf Injection 677
Protopic 685

Tamoxifen Citrate (BCG, live is contraindicated in immunosuppressed patients or persons with congenital or acquired immune deficiencies, whether due to concurrent disease (eg, AIDS, leukemia, lymphoma), cancer therapy (eg, cytotoxic drugs, radiation), or immunosuppressive therapy (eg, corticosteroids)).
No products indexed under this heading.

Temozolomide (Drug combinations containing immunosuppressants and/or bone marrow depressants and/or radiation interfere with the development of the immune response and should not be used in combination with BCG, live). Products include:
Temodar 3230
Temodar Injection 3230

Tetracycline Hydrochloride (Co-administration of BCG, live with antimicrobial therapy for other infections may interfere with the effectiveness of BCG, live). Products include:
Pylera 793

Thioguanine (Drug combinations containing immunosuppressants and/or bone marrow depressants and/or radiation interfere with the development of the immune response and should not be used in combination with BCG, live). Products include:
Tabloid 1664

Ticarcillin Disodium (Co-administration of BCG, live with antimicrobial therapy for other infections may interfere with the effectiveness of BCG, live). Products include:
Timentin ADD-Vantage 1670
Timentin Galaxy 1674
Timentin 1666
Timentin Pharmacy 1678

Tobramycin (Co-administration of BCG, live with antimicrobial therapy for other infections may interfere with the effectiveness of BCG, live). Products include:
Tobi Nebulizer 2546
Tobramycin and Dexamethasone
Ophthalmic Suspension .... ⊙251
Zylet .... ⊙252

Tobramycin Sulfate (Co-administration of BCG, live with antimicrobial therapy for other infections may interfere with the effectiveness of BCG, live).
No products indexed under this heading.

Triamcinolone (BCG, live is contraindicated in immunosuppressed patients or persons with congenital or acquired immune deficiencies, whether due to concurrent disease (eg, AIDS, leukemia, lymphoma), cancer therapy (eg, cytotoxic drugs, radiation), or immunosuppressive therapy (eg, corticosteroids)).
No products indexed under this heading.

Triamcinolone Acetonide (BCG, live is contraindicated in immunosuppressed patients or persons with congenital or acquired immune deficiencies, whether due to concurrent disease (eg, AIDS, leukemia, lymphoma), cancer therapy (eg, cytotoxic

drugs, radiation), or immunosuppressive therapy (eg, corticosteroids)). Products include:
Azmacort 408
Nasacort AQ 3019

Triamcinolone Diacetate (BCG, live is contraindicated in immunosuppressed patients or persons with congenital or acquired immune deficiencies, whether due to concurrent disease (eg, AIDS, leukemia, lymphoma), cancer therapy (eg, cytotoxic drugs, radiation), or immunosuppressive therapy (eg, corticosteroids)).
No products indexed under this heading.

Triamcinolone Hexacetonide (BCG, live is contraindicated in immunosuppressed patients or persons with congenital or acquired immune deficiencies, whether due to concurrent disease (eg, AIDS, leukemia, lymphoma), cancer therapy (eg, cytotoxic drugs, radiation), or immunosuppressive therapy (eg, corticosteroids)).
No products indexed under this heading.

Troleandomycin (Co-administration of BCG, live with antimicrobial therapy for other infections may interfere with the effectiveness of BCG, live).
No products indexed under this heading.

Trovafloxacin Mesylate (Co-administration of BCG, live with antimicrobial therapy for other infections may interfere with the effectiveness of BCG, live).
No products indexed under this heading.

Vinblastine Sulfate (BCG, live is contraindicated in immunosuppressed patients or persons with congenital or acquired immune deficiencies, whether due to concurrent disease (eg, AIDS, leukemia, lymphoma), cancer therapy (eg, cytotoxic drugs, radiation), or immunosuppressive therapy (eg, corticosteroids)).
No products indexed under this heading.

Vincristine Sulfate (BCG, live is contraindicated in immunosuppressed patients or persons with congenital or acquired immune deficiencies, whether due to concurrent disease (eg, AIDS, leukemia, lymphoma), cancer therapy (eg, cytotoxic drugs, radiation), or immunosuppressive therapy (eg, corticosteroids)).
No products indexed under this heading.

Vinorelbine Tartrate (BCG, live is contraindicated in immunosuppressed patients or persons with congenital or acquired immune deficiencies, whether due to concurrent disease (eg, AIDS, leukemia, lymphoma), cancer therapy (eg, cytotoxic drugs, radiation), or immunosuppressive therapy (eg, corticosteroids)).
No products indexed under this heading.

TIMENTIN ADD-VANTAGE
(Clavulanate Potassium, Ticarcillin Disodium) 1670
See Timentin IV Infusion

TIMENTIN INJECTION GALAXY CONTAINER
(Clavulanate Potassium, Ticarcillin Disodium) 1674
See Timentin IV Infusion

TIMENTIN IV INFUSION
(Clavulanate Potassium, Ticarcillin Disodium) 1666
May interact with oral contraceptives, and certain other agents. Compounds in these categories include:

Desogestrel (Timentin may affect the gut flora, leading to lower estrogen reabsorption and reduced efficacy of combined oral estrogen/progesterone contraceptives).
No products indexed under this heading.

Ethinyl Estradiol (Timentin may affect the gut flora, leading to lower estrogen

(⊙ Described in PDR® for Ophthalmic Medicines)

IMPORTANT NOTE: Always consult each drug listing in the patient's regimen for possible interactions.

Insulin Lispro, Human (Beta blocking agents, usually systemic, may mask the sign and symptoms of acute hypoglycemia). Products include:
Humalog 1910
Humalog Mix 1914
Humalog Mix75/25 1917

Insulin Lispro Protamine, Human (Beta blocking agents, usually systemic, may mask the sign and symptoms of acute hypoglycemia). Products include:
Humalog Mix 1914
Humalog Mix75/25 1917

Isradipine (Possible atrioventricular conduction disturbances, left ventricular failure, or hypotension when used concurrently). Products include:
DynaCirc CR 1432

Labetalol Hydrochloride (Concurrent use with systemic beta blocker may have additive effects of beta blockade, both systemic and on intraocular pressure).
No products indexed under this heading.

Levobunolol Hydrochloride (Concurrent use of two topical beta blockers is not recommended).
No products indexed under this heading.

Metformin Hydrochloride (Beta blocking agents, usually systemic, may mask the sign and symptoms of acute hypoglycemia). Products include:
ActoPlus 3338
Avandamet 1345
Janumet 2188

Metipranolol Hydrochloride (Concurrent use of two topical beta blockers is not recommended).
No products indexed under this heading.

Metoprolol Succinate (Concurrent use with systemic beta blocker may have additive effects of beta blockade, both systemic and on intraocular pressure). Products include:
Toprol XL 732

Metoprolol Tartrate (Concurrent use with systemic beta blocker may have additive effects of beta blockade, both systemic and on intraocular pressure).
No products indexed under this heading.

Mibefradil Dihydrochloride (Possible atrioventricular conduction disturbances, left ventricular failure, or hypotension when used concurrently).
No products indexed under this heading.

Miglitol (Beta blocking agents, usually systemic, may mask the sign and symptoms of acute hypoglycemia).
No products indexed under this heading.

Nadolol (Concurrent use with systemic beta blocker may have additive effects of beta blockade, both systemic and on intraocular pressure). Products include:
Nadolol 2359

Nateglinide (Beta blocking agents, usually systemic, may mask the sign and symptoms of acute hypoglycemia).
No products indexed under this heading.

Nebivolol (Concurrent use with systemic beta blocker may have additive effects of beta blockade, both systemic and on intraocular pressure). Products include:
Bystolic 1147

Nicardipine (Possible atrioventricular conduction disturbances, left ventricular failure, or hypotension when used concurrently).
No products indexed under this heading.

Nicardipine Hydrochloride (Possible atrioventricular conduction disturbances, left ventricular failure, or hypotension when used concurrently).
No products indexed under this heading.

Nifedipine (Possible atrioventricular conduction disturbances, left ventricular failure, or hypotension when used concurrently).
No products indexed under this heading.

Nimodipine (Possible atrioventricular conduction disturbances, left ventricular failure, or hypotension when used concurrently).
No products indexed under this heading.

Nisoldipine (Possible atrioventricular conduction disturbances, left ventricular failure, or hypotension when used concurrently).
No products indexed under this heading.

Penbutolol Sulfate (Concurrent use with systemic beta blocker may have additive effects of beta blockade, both systemic and on intraocular pressure).
No products indexed under this heading.

Pindolol (Concurrent use with systemic beta blocker may have additive effects of beta blockade, both systemic and on intraocular pressure).
No products indexed under this heading.

Pioglitazone Hydrochloride (Beta blocking agents, usually systemic, may mask the sign and symptoms of acute hypoglycemia). Products include:
ActoPlus 3338
Actos 3345
Duetact 3354

Propranolol Hydrochloride (Concurrent use with systemic beta blocker may have additive effects of beta blockade, both systemic and on intraocular pressure). Products include:
InnoPran XL 1517

Quinidine (Co-administration has resulted in potentiated systemic beta-blockade, eg, decreased heart rate).
No products indexed under this heading.

Quinidine Gluconate (Co-administration has resulted in potentiated systemic beta-blockade, eg, decreased heart rate).
No products indexed under this heading.

Quinidine Hydrochloride (Co-administration has resulted in potentiated systemic beta-blockade, eg, decreased heart rate).
No products indexed under this heading.

Quinidine Polygalacturonate (Co-administration has resulted in potentiated systemic beta-blockade, eg, decreased heart rate).
No products indexed under this heading.

Quinidine Sulfate (Co-administration has resulted in potentiated systemic beta-blockade, eg, decreased heart rate).
No products indexed under this heading.

Rauwolfia Serpentina (Possible additive effects and the production of hypotension and/or bradycardia).
No products indexed under this heading.

Repaglinide (Beta blocking agents, usually systemic, may mask the sign and symptoms of acute hypoglycemia).
No products indexed under this heading.

Rescinnamine (Possible additive effects and the production of hypotension and/or bradycardia).
No products indexed under this heading.

Reserpine (Possible additive effects and the production of hypotension and/or bradycardia).
No products indexed under this heading.

Rosiglitazone Maleate (Beta blocking agents, usually systemic, may mask the sign and symptoms of acute hypoglycemia). Products include:
Avandamet 1345
Avandaryl 1356
Avandia 1366

Sitagliptin Phosphate (Beta blocking agents, usually systemic, may mask the sign and symptoms of acute hypoglycemia). Products include:
Janumet 2188
Januvia 2196

Sotalol Hydrochloride (Concurrent use with systemic beta blocker may have additive effects of beta blockade, both systemic and on intraocular pressure).
No products indexed under this heading.

Timolol Hemihydrate (Concurrent use of two topical beta blockers is not recommended). Products include:
Betimol 3490

Tolazamide (Beta blocking agents, usually systemic, may mask the sign and symptoms of acute hypoglycemia).
No products indexed under this heading.

Tolbutamide (Beta blocking agents, usually systemic, may mask the sign and symptoms of acute hypoglycemia).
No products indexed under this heading.

Troglitazone (Beta blocking agents, usually systemic, may mask the sign and symptoms of acute hypoglycemia).
No products indexed under this heading.

Verapamil Hydrochloride (Possible atrioventricular conduction disturbances, left ventricular failure, or hypotension when used concurrently). Products include:
Tarka 534

TNKASE
(Tenecteplase) 1228
May interact with anticoagulants, platelet inhibitors, vitamin K antagonists, and certain other agents. Compounds in these categories include:

Abciximab (Drugs that alter platelet function, such as abciximab, may increase the risk of bleeding if administered prior to or after tenecteplase therapy). Products include:
ReoPro 1952

Anisindione (Anticoagulants may increase the risk of bleeding if administered prior to, during, or after tenecteplase therapy).
No products indexed under this heading.

Ardeparin Sodium (Anticoagulants may increase the risk of bleeding if administered prior to, during, or after tenecteplase therapy).
No products indexed under this heading.

Aspirin (Drugs that alter platelet function, such as aspirin, may increase the risk of bleeding if administered prior to or after tenecteplase therapy). Products include:
Aggrenox 880
Bayer Aspirin 829
Percodan 1124
St. Joseph Aspirin 2045

Aspirin, Enteric Coated (Drugs that alter platelet function may increase the risk of bleeding if administered prior to, during, or after tenecteplase therapy).
No products indexed under this heading.

Aspirin Buffered (Drugs that alter platelet function may increase the risk of bleeding if administered prior to, during, or after tenecteplase therapy).
No products indexed under this heading.

Azlocillin Sodium (Drugs that alter platelet function may increase the risk of bleeding if administered prior to, during, or after tenecteplase therapy).
No products indexed under this heading.

Carbenicillin Indanyl Sodium (Drugs that alter platelet function may increase the risk of bleeding if administered prior to, during, or after tenecteplase therapy).
No products indexed under this heading.

Choline Magnesium Trisalicylate (Drugs that alter platelet function may increase the risk of bleeding if administered prior to, during, or after tenecteplase therapy).
No products indexed under this heading.

Clopidogrel Bisulfate (Drugs that alter platelet function, such as clopi-

dogrel, may increase the risk of bleeding if administered prior to or after tenecteplase therapy). Products include:
Plavix 3027

Dalteparin Sodium (Anticoagulants may increase the risk of bleeding if administered prior to, during, or after tenecteplase therapy). Products include:
Fragmin 1058

Danaparoid Sodium (Anticoagulants may increase the risk of bleeding if administered prior to, during, or after tenecteplase therapy).
No products indexed under this heading.

Dextran (Drugs that alter platelet function may increase the risk of bleeding if administered prior to, during, or after tenecteplase therapy).
No products indexed under this heading.

Dextran 40 (Drugs that alter platelet function may increase the risk of bleeding if administered prior to, during, or after tenecteplase therapy).
No products indexed under this heading.

Dextran 70 (Drugs that alter platelet function may increase the risk of bleeding if administered prior to, during, or after tenecteplase therapy).
No products indexed under this heading.

Dextran I (Drugs that alter platelet function may increase the risk of bleeding if administered prior to, during, or after tenecteplase therapy).
No products indexed under this heading.

Dextrans (Low Molecular Weight) (Drugs that alter platelet function may increase the risk of bleeding if administered prior to, during, or after tenecteplase therapy).
No products indexed under this heading.

Diclofenac Potassium (Drugs that alter platelet function may increase the risk of bleeding if administered prior to, during, or after tenecteplase therapy).
No products indexed under this heading.

Diclofenac Sodium (Drugs that alter platelet function may increase the risk of bleeding if administered prior to, during, or after tenecteplase therapy).
No products indexed under this heading.

Dicumarol (Co-administration increases the risk of bleeding).
No products indexed under this heading.

Diflunisal (Drugs that alter platelet function may increase the risk of bleeding if administered prior to, during, or after tenecteplase therapy).
No products indexed under this heading.

Dipyridamole (Drugs that alter platelet function, such as dipyridamole, may increase the risk of bleeding if administered prior to or after tenecteplase therapy). Products include:
Aggrenox 880

Enoxaparin Sodium (Anticoagulants may increase the risk of bleeding if administered prior to, during, or after tenecteplase therapy). Products include:
Lovenox 3005

Epitifibatide (Drugs that alter platelet function, such as epitifibatide, may increase the risk of bleeding if administered prior to or after tenecteplase therapy).
No products indexed under this heading.

Eptifibatide (Drugs that alter platelet function may increase the risk of bleeding if administered prior to, during, or after tenecteplase therapy). Products include:
Integrilin 3135

Fenoprofen Calcium (Drugs that alter platelet function may increase the risk of bleeding if administered prior to, during, or after tenecteplase therapy).
No products indexed under this heading.

(⊙ Described in PDR® for Ophthalmic Medicines)

Flurbiprofen (Drugs that alter platelet function may increase the risk of bleeding if administered prior to, during, or after tenecteplase therapy).
No products indexed under this heading.

Fondaparinux Sodium (Anticoagulants may increase the risk of bleeding if administered prior to, during, or after tenecteplase therapy). Products include:
Arixtra 1320

Heparin Calcium (Anticoagulants may increase the risk of bleeding if administered prior to, during, or after tenecteplase therapy).
No products indexed under this heading.

Heparin Sodium (Anticoagulants may increase the risk of bleeding if administered prior to, during, or after tenecteplase therapy).
No products indexed under this heading.

Hydroxychloroquine Sulfate (Drugs that alter platelet function may increase the risk of bleeding if administered prior to, during, or after tenecteplase therapy).
No products indexed under this heading.

Ibuprofen (Drugs that alter platelet function may increase the risk of bleeding if administered prior to, during, or after tenecteplase therapy). Products include:
Motrin IB 2043
Children's Motrin 2044
Children's Motrin Non-Staining
   Dye-Free 2044
Infants' Motrin 2044
Infants' Motrin Dye-Free 2044
Junior Strength Motrin 2044
Vicoprofen 564

Indomethacin (Drugs that alter platelet function may increase the risk of bleeding if administered prior to, during, or after tenecteplase therapy). Products include:
Indocin 2167

Indomethacin Sodium Trihydrate (Drugs that alter platelet function may increase the risk of bleeding if administered prior to, during, or after tenecteplase therapy). Products include:
Indocin I.V. 2007

Ketoprofen (Drugs that alter platelet function may increase the risk of bleeding if administered prior to, during, or after tenecteplase therapy).
No products indexed under this heading.

Low Molecular Weight Heparins (Anticoagulants may increase the risk of bleeding if administered prior to, during, or after tenecteplase therapy).
No products indexed under this heading.

Magnesium Salicylate (Drugs that alter platelet function may increase the risk of bleeding if administered prior to, during, or after tenecteplase therapy).
No products indexed under this heading.

Meclofenamate Sodium (Drugs that alter platelet function may increase the risk of bleeding if administered prior to, during, or after tenecteplase therapy).
No products indexed under this heading.

Mefenamic Acid (Drugs that alter platelet function may increase the risk of bleeding if administered prior to, during, or after tenecteplase therapy).
No products indexed under this heading.

Mezlocillin Sodium (Drugs that alter platelet function may increase the risk of bleeding if administered prior to, during, or after tenecteplase therapy).
No products indexed under this heading.

Nafcillin Sodium (Drugs that alter platelet function may increase the risk of bleeding if administered prior to, during, or after tenecteplase therapy).
No products indexed under this heading.

Naproxen (Drugs that alter platelet function may increase the risk of bleed-

ing if administered prior to, during, or after tenecteplase therapy). Products include:
EC-Naprosyn 2850
Naprosyn 2850
Anaprox/Naprosyn 2850

Naproxen Sodium (Drugs that alter platelet function may increase the risk of bleeding if administered prior to, during, or after tenecteplase therapy). Products include:
Anaprox 2850
Anaprox DS 2850
Treximet 1681

Penicillin G Benzathine (Drugs that alter platelet function may increase the risk of bleeding if administered prior to, during, or after tenecteplase therapy). Products include:
Bicillin C-R Injectable Suspension 1826
Bicillin L-A 1828

Penicillin G Procaine (Drugs that alter platelet function may increase the risk of bleeding if administered prior to, during, or after tenecteplase therapy). Products include:
Bicillin C-R Injectable Suspension 1826
Bicillin L-A 1828

Phenylbutazone (Drugs that alter platelet function may increase the risk of bleeding if administered prior to, during, or after tenecteplase therapy).
No products indexed under this heading.

Piroxicam (Drugs that alter platelet function may increase the risk of bleeding if administered prior to, during, or after tenecteplase therapy).
No products indexed under this heading.

Salsalate (Drugs that alter platelet function may increase the risk of bleeding if administered prior to, during, or after tenecteplase therapy).
No products indexed under this heading.

Sulindac (Drugs that alter platelet function may increase the risk of bleeding if administered prior to, during, or after tenecteplase therapy). Products include:
Clinoril 2098

Ticarcillin Disodium (Drugs that alter platelet function may increase the risk of bleeding if administered prior to, during, or after tenecteplase therapy). Products include:
Timentin ADD-Vantage 1670
Timentin Galaxy 1674
Timentin 1666
Timentin Pharmacy 1678

Ticlopidine Hydrochloride (Drugs that alter platelet function, such as ticlopidine, may increase the risk of bleeding if administered prior to or after tenecteplase therapy).
No products indexed under this heading.

Tinzaparin Sodium (Anticoagulants may increase the risk of bleeding if administered prior to, during, or after tenecteplase therapy).
No products indexed under this heading.

Tirofiban Hydrochloride (Drugs that alter platelet function, such as tirofiban, may increase the risk of bleeding if administered prior to or after tenecteplase therapy).
No products indexed under this heading.

Tolmetin Sodium (Drugs that alter platelet function may increase the risk of bleeding if administered prior to, during, or after tenecteplase therapy).
No products indexed under this heading.

Warfarin Sodium (Co-administration increases the risk of bleeding).
No products indexed under this heading.

TOBI NEBULIZER SOLUTION FOR INHALATION

(Tobramycin) 2546
May interact with diuretics, neurotoxic

drugs, ototoxic drugs, and certain other agents. Compounds in these categories include:

Altretamine (Concurrent and/or sequential use of tobramycin solution with other drugs with neurotoxic potential should be avoided). Products include:
Hexalen 1066

Amikacin Sulfate (Concurrent and/or sequential use of tobramycin solution with other drugs with neurotoxic potential should be avoided).
No products indexed under this heading.

Amiloride Hydrochloride (Some diuretics can enhance aminoglycoside toxicity by altering antibiotic concentrations in serum and tissue).
No products indexed under this heading.

Amiodarone Hydrochloride (Concurrent and/or sequential use of tobramycin solution with other drugs with neurotoxic potential should be avoided).
No products indexed under this heading.

Amphotericin B (Concurrent and/or sequential use of tobramycin solution with other drugs with neurotoxic potential should be avoided).
No products indexed under this heading.

Amphotericin B, liposomal (Concurrent and/or sequential use of tobramycin solution with other drugs with neurotoxic potential should be avoided). Products include:
AmBisome 659

Amphotericin B Lipid Complex (Concurrent and/or sequential use of tobramycin solution with other drugs with neurotoxic potential should be avoided).
No products indexed under this heading.

Asparaginase (Concurrent and/or sequential use of tobramycin solution with other drugs with neurotoxic potential should be avoided). Products include:
Elspar 2005, 2122

Bendroflumethiazide (Some diuretics can enhance aminoglycoside toxicity by altering antibiotic concentrations in serum and tissue).
No products indexed under this heading.

Bumetanide (Some diuretics can enhance aminoglycoside toxicity by altering antibiotic concentrations in serum and tissue).
No products indexed under this heading.

Butyrophenone (Concurrent and/or sequential use of tobramycin solution with other drugs with neurotoxic potential should be avoided).
No products indexed under this heading.

Carboplatin (Concurrent and/or sequential use of tobramycin solution with other drugs with ototoxic potential should be avoided).
No products indexed under this heading.

Cephaloridine (Concurrent and/or sequential use of tobramycin solution with other drugs with neurotoxic potential should be avoided).
No products indexed under this heading.

Chloramphenicol (Concurrent and/or sequential use of tobramycin solution with other drugs with neurotoxic potential should be avoided).
No products indexed under this heading.

Chloramphenicol Palmitate (Concurrent and/or sequential use of tobramycin solution with other drugs with neurotoxic potential should be avoided).
No products indexed under this heading.

Chloramphenicol Sodium Succinate (Concurrent and/or sequential use of tobramycin solution with other drugs with neurotoxic potential should be avoided).
No products indexed under this heading.

Chloroquine (Concurrent and/or sequential use of tobramycin solution with other drugs with neurotoxic potential should be avoided).
No products indexed under this heading.

Chlorothiazide (Some diuretics can enhance aminoglycoside toxicity by altering antibiotic concentrations in serum and tissue).
No products indexed under this heading.

Chlorothiazide Sodium (Some diuretics can enhance aminoglycoside toxicity by altering antibiotic concentrations in serum and tissue). Products include:
Diuril Intravenous 2009

Chlorpromazine (Concurrent and/or sequential use of tobramycin solution with other drugs with neurotoxic potential should be avoided).
No products indexed under this heading.

Chlorpromazine Hydrochloride (Concurrent and/or sequential use of tobramycin solution with other drugs with neurotoxic potential should be avoided).
No products indexed under this heading.

Chlorthalidone (Some diuretics can enhance aminoglycoside toxicity by altering antibiotic concentrations in serum and tissue). Products include:
Clorpres 2344

Cisplatin (Concurrent and/or sequential use of tobramycin solution with other drugs with neurotoxic potential should be avoided).
No products indexed under this heading.

Cladribine (Concurrent and/or sequential use of tobramycin solution with other drugs with neurotoxic potential should be avoided). Products include:
Leustatin 946

Clioquinol (Concurrent and/or sequential use of tobramycin solution with other drugs with neurotoxic potential should be avoided).
No products indexed under this heading.

Colistin Sulfate (Concurrent and/or sequential use of tobramycin solution with other drugs with neurotoxic potential should be avoided).
No products indexed under this heading.

Cytarabine Liposome (Concurrent and/or sequential use of tobramycin solution with other drugs with neurotoxic potential should be avoided).
No products indexed under this heading.

Digoxin (Concurrent and/or sequential use of tobramycin solution with other drugs with neurotoxic potential should be avoided). Products include:
Lanoxin Injection 1546
Lanoxin Injection Pediatric 1549
Lanoxin Tablets 1553

Digoxin Immune Fab (Ovine) (Concurrent and/or sequential use of tobramycin solution with other drugs with neurotoxic potential should be avoided). Products include:
Digibind 1427

Disulfiram (Concurrent and/or sequential use of tobramycin solution with other drugs with neurotoxic potential should be avoided).
No products indexed under this heading.

Ethacrynic Acid (Tobramycin solution should not be administered concomitantly with ethacrynic acid).
No products indexed under this heading.

Ethambutol Hydrochloride (Concurrent and/or sequential use of tobramycin solution with other drugs with neurotoxic potential should be avoided).
No products indexed under this heading.

Fludarabine Phosphate (Concurrent and/or sequential use of tobramycin solution with other drugs with neurotoxic potential should be avoided). Products include:

IMPORTANT NOTE: Always consult each drug listing in the patient's regimen for possible interactions.

Tobi Interactions Index 1896

Oforta 3023
Fluphenazine Decanoate (Concurrent and/or sequential use of tobramycin solution with other drugs with neurotoxic potential should be avoided).
No products indexed under this heading.
Fluphenazine Enanthate (Concurrent and/or sequential use of tobramycin solution with other drugs with neurotoxic potential should be avoided).
No products indexed under this heading.
Fluphenazine Hydrochloride (Concurrent and/or sequential use of tobramycin solution with other drugs with neurotoxic potential should be avoided).
No products indexed under this heading.
Furosemide (Tobramycin solution should not be administered concomitantly with furosemide). Products include:
Furosemide 2354
Gentamicin Sulfate (Concurrent and/or sequential use of tobramycin solution with other drugs with neurotoxic potential should be avoided). Products include:
Pred-G .... ⊙226, ⊙227
Haloperidol (Concurrent and/or sequential use of tobramycin solution with other drugs with neurotoxic potential should be avoided).
No products indexed under this heading.
Haloperidol Decanoate (Concurrent and/or sequential use of tobramycin solution with other drugs with neurotoxic potential should be avoided).
No products indexed under this heading.
Hydrochlorothiazide (Some diuretics can enhance aminoglycoside toxicity by altering antibiotic concentrations in serum and tissue). Products include:
Atacand HCT 700
Avalide 2956
Benicar HCT 1017
Diovan HCT 2419
Dyazide 1429
Exforge HCT 2449
Hyzaar 2162
Hyzaar 100-12.5 2162
Micardis HCT 889
Prinzide 2246
Tekturna HCT 2541
Teveten HCT 541
Hydroflumethiazide (Some diuretics can enhance aminoglycoside toxicity by altering antibiotic concentrations in serum and tissue).
No products indexed under this heading.
Indapamide (Some diuretics can enhance aminoglycoside toxicity by altering antibiotic concentrations in serum and tissue). Products include:
Indapamide 2356
Isoniazid (Concurrent and/or sequential use of tobramycin solution with other drugs with neurotoxic potential should be avoided).
No products indexed under this heading.
Kanamycin Sulfate (Concurrent and/or sequential use of tobramycin solution with other drugs with neurotoxic potential should be avoided).
No products indexed under this heading.
Lithium (Concurrent and/or sequential use of tobramycin solution with other drugs with neurotoxic potential should be avoided).
No products indexed under this heading.
Lithium Carbonate (Concurrent and/or sequential use of tobramycin solution with other drugs with neurotoxic potential should be avoided).
No products indexed under this heading.
Lithium Citrate (Concurrent and/or sequential use of tobramycin solution with other drugs with neurotoxic potential should be avoided).
No products indexed under this heading.
Mannitol (Tobramycin solution should not be administered concomitantly with mannitol).
No products indexed under this heading.
Methotrimeprazine (Concurrent and/or sequential use of tobramycin solution with other drugs with neurotoxic potential should be avoided).
No products indexed under this heading.
Methyclothiazide (Some diuretics can enhance aminoglycoside toxicity by altering antibiotic concentrations in serum and tissue).
No products indexed under this heading.
Metolazone (Some diuretics can enhance aminoglycoside toxicity by altering antibiotic concentrations in serum and tissue).
No products indexed under this heading.
Metronidazole (Concurrent and/or sequential use of tobramycin solution with other drugs with neurotoxic potential should be avoided). Products include:
Pylera 793
Metronidazole Hydrochloride (Concurrent and/or sequential use of tobramycin solution with other drugs with neurotoxic potential should be avoided).
No products indexed under this heading.
Metronidazole Sodium (Concurrent and/or sequential use of tobramycin solution with other drugs with neurotoxic potential should be avoided).
No products indexed under this heading.
Nalidixic Acid (Concurrent and/or sequential use of tobramycin solution with other drugs with neurotoxic potential should be avoided).
No products indexed under this heading.
Neostigmine Bromide (Concurrent and/or sequential use of tobramycin solution with other drugs with neurotoxic potential should be avoided).
No products indexed under this heading.
Neostigmine Methylsulfate (Concurrent and/or sequential use of tobramycin solution with other drugs with neurotoxic potential should be avoided).
No products indexed under this heading.
Nitrofurantoin (Concurrent and/or sequential use of tobramycin solution with other drugs with neurotoxic potential should be avoided).
No products indexed under this heading.
Nitrofurantoin Macrocrystals (Concurrent and/or sequential use of tobramycin solution with other drugs with neurotoxic potential should be avoided).
No products indexed under this heading.
Nitrofurantoin Monohydrate (Concurrent and/or sequential use of tobramycin solution with other drugs with neurotoxic potential should be avoided).
No products indexed under this heading.
Nitrofurantoin Sodium (Concurrent and/or sequential use of tobramycin solution with other drugs with neurotoxic potential should be avoided).
No products indexed under this heading.
Oxaliplatin (Concurrent and/or sequential use of tobramycin solution with other drugs with neurotoxic potential should be avoided). Products include:
Eloxatin 2975
Paclitaxel (Concurrent and/or sequential use of tobramycin solution with other drugs with neurotoxic potential should be avoided).
No products indexed under this heading.
Paromomycin Sulfate (Concurrent and/or sequential use of tobramycin solution with other drugs with neurotoxic potential should be avoided).
No products indexed under this heading.
Perphenazine (Concurrent and/or sequential use of tobramycin solution with other drugs with neurotoxic potential should be avoided).
No products indexed under this heading.
Physostigmine Salicylate (Concurrent and/or sequential use of tobramycin solution with other drugs with neurotoxic potential should be avoided).
No products indexed under this heading.
Polymyxin (Concurrent and/or sequential use of tobramycin solution with other drugs with neurotoxic potential should be avoided).
No products indexed under this heading.
Polymyxin Preparations (Concurrent and/or sequential use of tobramycin solution with other drugs with neurotoxic potential should be avoided).
No products indexed under this heading.
Polythiazide (Some diuretics can enhance aminoglycoside toxicity by altering antibiotic concentrations in serum and tissue).
No products indexed under this heading.
Prochlorperazine (Concurrent and/or sequential use of tobramycin solution with other drugs with neurotoxic potential should be avoided).
No products indexed under this heading.
Promethazine Hydrochloride (Concurrent and/or sequential use of tobramycin solution with other drugs with neurotoxic potential should be avoided).
No products indexed under this heading.
Propranolol (Concurrent and/or sequential use of tobramycin solution with other drugs with neurotoxic potential should be avoided).
No products indexed under this heading.
Reserpine (Concurrent and/or sequential use of tobramycin solution with other drugs with neurotoxic potential should be avoided).
No products indexed under this heading.
Spironolactone (Some diuretics can enhance aminoglycoside toxicity by altering antibiotic concentrations in serum and tissue).
No products indexed under this heading.
Streptomycin Sulfate (Concurrent and/or sequential use of tobramycin solution with other drugs with neurotoxic potential should be avoided).
No products indexed under this heading.
Thioridazine Hydrochloride (Concurrent and/or sequential use of tobramycin solution with other drugs with neurotoxic potential should be avoided). Products include:
Thioridazine Hydrochloride 2384
Tobramycin Sulfate (Concurrent and/or sequential use of tobramycin solution with other drugs with neurotoxic potential should be avoided).
No products indexed under this heading.
Torsemide (Some diuretics can enhance aminoglycoside toxicity by altering antibiotic concentrations in serum and tissue).
No products indexed under this heading.
Triamterene (Some diuretics can enhance aminoglycoside toxicity by altering antibiotic concentrations in serum and tissue). Products include:
Dyazide 1429
Dyrenium 3495
Trifluoperazine Hydrochloride (Concurrent and/or sequential use of tobramycin solution with other drugs with neurotoxic potential should be avoided).
No products indexed under this heading.
Urea (Tobramycin solution should not be administered concomitantly with urea).
No products indexed under this heading.
Urea Peroxide (Tobramycin solution should not be administered concomitantly with urea).
No products indexed under this heading.
Vancomycin Hydrochloride (Concurrent and/or sequential use of tobramycin solution with other drugs with ototoxic potential should be avoided).
No products indexed under this heading.
Vincristine Sulfate (Concurrent and/or sequential use of tobramycin solution with other drugs with neurotoxic potential should be avoided).
No products indexed under this heading.
Viomycin (Concurrent and/or sequential use of tobramycin solution with other drugs with neurotoxic potential should be avoided).
No products indexed under this heading.

TOBRAMYCIN AND DEXAMETHASONE OPHTHALMIC SUSPENSION USP

(Dexamethasone, Tobramycin) .... ⊙251
May interact with aminoglycosides. Compounds in these categories include:
Amikacin Sulfate (If topical ocular tobramycin is administered concomitantly with systemic aminoglycoide antibiotics, care should be taken to monitor the total serum concentration).
No products indexed under this heading.
Dihydrostreptomycin (If topical ocular tobramycin is administered concomitantly with systemic aminoglycoide antibiotics, care should be taken to monitor the total serum concentration).
No products indexed under this heading.
Gentamicin (If topical ocular tobramycin is administered concomitantly with systemic aminoglycoide antibiotics, care should be taken to monitor the total serum concentration).
No products indexed under this heading.
Gentamicin Sulfate (If topical ocular tobramycin is administered concomitantly with systemic aminoglycoide antibiotics, care should be taken to monitor the total serum concentration). Products include:
Pred-G .... ⊙226, ⊙227
Kanamycin Sulfate (If topical ocular tobramycin is administered concomitantly with systemic aminoglycoide antibiotics, care should be taken to monitor the total serum concentration).
No products indexed under this heading.
Neomycin (If topical ocular tobramycin is administered concomitantly with systemic aminoglycoide antibiotics, care should be taken to monitor the total serum concentration).
No products indexed under this heading.
Neomycin, oral (If topical ocular tobramycin is administered concomitantly with systemic aminoglycoide antibiotics, care should be taken to monitor the total serum concentration).
No products indexed under this heading.
Neomycin Sulfate (If topical ocular tobramycin is administered concomitantly with systemic aminoglycoide antibiotics, care should be taken to monitor the total serum concentration).
No products indexed under this heading.
Streptomycin Sulfate (If topical ocular tobramycin is administered concomitantly with systemic aminoglycoide antibiotics, care should be taken to monitor the total serum concentration).
No products indexed under this heading.
Tobramycin Sulfate (If topical ocular tobramycin is administered concomitantly with systemic aminoglycoide antibiotics, care should be taken to monitor the total serum concentration).
No products indexed under this heading.

(⊙ Described in PDR® for Ophthalmic Medicines)

TOPRICIN FOOT THERAPY CREAM
(Homeopathic Formulations) 3426
None cited in PDR database.

TOPRICIN JUNIOR
(Homeopathic Formulations) 3426
None cited in PDR database.

TOPRICIN PAIN RELIEF AND HEALING CREAM
(Homeopathic Formulations) 3426
None cited in PDR database.

TOPROL-XL TABLETS
(Metoprolol Succinate) 732
May interact with cardiac glycosides, catecholamine-depleting drugs, cytochrome p450 2d6 inhibitors (selected), epinephrine-containing products, general anesthetics, monoamine oxidase inhibitors, quinidine, and certain other agents. Compounds in these categories include:

Amiodarone Hydrochloride (Co-administration of metoprolol with drugs that inhibit CYP2D6 is likely to increase metoprolol concentration; this increase in plasma concentration would decrease the cardioselectivity of metoprolol).
No products indexed under this heading.

Amitriptyline Hydrochloride (Co-administration of metoprolol with drugs that inhibit CYP2D6 is likely to increase metoprolol concentration; this increase in plasma concentration would decrease the cardioselectivity of metoprolol).
No products indexed under this heading.

Amoxapine (Co-administration of metoprolol with drugs that inhibit CYP2D6 is likely to increase metoprolol concentration; this increase in plasma concentration would decrease the cardioselectivity of metoprolol).
No products indexed under this heading.

Bupropion Hydrochloride (Co-administration of metoprolol with drugs that inhibit CYP2D6 is likely to increase metoprolol concentration; this increase in plasma concentration would decrease the cardioselectivity of metoprolol). Products include:
Aplenzin 2948
Wellbutrin 1719
Wellbutrin SR 1725
Zyban 1762

Celecoxib (Co-administration of metoprolol with drugs that inhibit CYP2D6 is likely to increase metoprolol concentration; this increase in plasma concentration would decrease the cardioselectivity of metoprolol). Products include:
Celebrex 3272

Chloroquine (Co-administration of metoprolol with drugs that inhibit CYP2D6 is likely to increase metoprolol concentration; this increase in plasma concentration would decrease the cardioselectivity of metoprolol).
No products indexed under this heading.

Chloroquine Hydrochloride (Co-administration of metoprolol with drugs that inhibit CYP2D6 is likely to increase metoprolol concentration; this increase in plasma concentration would decrease the cardioselectivity of metoprolol).
No products indexed under this heading.

Chloroquine Phosphate (Co-administration of metoprolol with drugs that inhibit CYP2D6 is likely to increase metoprolol concentration; this increase in plasma concentration would decrease the cardioselectivity of metoprolol).
No products indexed under this heading.

Chlorpheniramine (Co-administration of metoprolol with drugs that inhibit CYP2D6 is likely to increase metoprolol concentration; this increase in plasma concentration would decrease the cardioselectivity of metoprolol).
No products indexed under this heading.

Chlorpheniramine Maleate (Co-administration of metoprolol with drugs that inhibit CYP2D6 is likely to increase metoprolol concentration; this increase in plasma concentration would decrease the cardioselectivity of metoprolol).
No products indexed under this heading.

Chlorpheniramine Polistirex (Co-administration of metoprolol with drugs that inhibit CYP2D6 is likely to increase metoprolol concentration; this increase in plasma concentration would decrease the cardioselectivity of metoprolol). Products include:
Tussionex 3443

Chlorpheniramine Tannate (Co-administration of metoprolol with drugs that inhibit CYP2D6 is likely to increase metoprolol concentration; this increase in plasma concentration would decrease the cardioselectivity of metoprolol).
No products indexed under this heading.

Cimetidine (Co-administration of metoprolol with drugs that inhibit CYP2D6 is likely to increase metoprolol concentration; this increase in plasma concentration would decrease the cardioselectivity of metoprolol).
No products indexed under this heading.

Cimetidine Hydrochloride (Co-administration of metoprolol with drugs that inhibit CYP2D6 is likely to increase metoprolol concentration; this increase in plasma concentration would decrease the cardioselectivity of metoprolol).
No products indexed under this heading.

Citalopram Hydrobromide (Co-administration of metoprolol with drugs that inhibit CYP2D6 is likely to increase metoprolol concentration; this increase in plasma concentration would decrease the cardioselectivity of metoprolol). Products include:
Celexa 1153

Clomipramine Hydrochloride (Co-administration of metoprolol with drugs that inhibit CYP2D6 is likely to increase metoprolol concentration; this increase in plasma concentration would decrease the cardioselectivity of metoprolol).
No products indexed under this heading.

Clonidine (β-blockers may exacerbate the rebound hypertension which can follow the withdrawal of clonidine. If co-administered, withdraw β-blockers several days before the gradual withdrawal of clonidine. If replacing clonidine by β-blocker therapy, delay start of β-blockers for several days after clonidine administration has stopped). Products include:
Catapres-TTS 884

Cocaine Hydrochloride (Co-administration of metoprolol with drugs that inhibit CYP2D6 is likely to increase metoprolol concentration; this increase in plasma concentration would decrease the cardioselectivity of metoprolol).
No products indexed under this heading.

Deserpidine (Catecholamine-depleting drugs may have an additive effect when given with β-blocking agents; monitor closely for signs of hypotension or marked bradycardia).
No products indexed under this heading.

Desflurane (The necessity or desirability of withdrawing β-blocking therapy prior to major surgery is controversial; the impaired ability of the heart to respond to reflex adrenergic stimuli may augment the risks of general anesthesia and surgical procedures).
No products indexed under this heading.

Desipramine Hydrochloride (Co-administration of metoprolol with drugs that inhibit CYP2D6 is likely to increase metoprolol concentration; this increase in plasma concentration would decrease the cardioselectivity of metoprolol).
No products indexed under this heading.

Deslanoside (Both digitalis glycosides and β-blockers slow atrioventricular conduction and decrease heart rate. Concomitant use can increase the risk of bradycardia).
No products indexed under this heading.

Digitalis Glycoside Preparations (Both digitalis glycosides and β-blockers slow atrioventricular conduction and decrease heart rate. Concomitant use can increase the risk of bradycardia).
No products indexed under this heading.

Digitalis Lanata (Both digitalis glycosides and β-blockers slow atrioventricular conduction and decrease heart rate. Concomitant use can increase the risk of bradycardia).
No products indexed under this heading.

Digitalis Purpurea (Both digitalis glycosides and β-blockers slow atrioventricular conduction and decrease heart rate. Concomitant use can increase the risk of bradycardia).
No products indexed under this heading.

Digitoxin (Both digitalis glycosides and β-blockers slow atrioventricular conduction and decrease heart rate. Concomitant use can increase the risk of bradycardia).
No products indexed under this heading.

Digoxin (Both digitalis glycosides and β-blockers slow atrioventricular conduction and decrease heart rate. Concomitant use can increase the risk of bradycardia). Products include:
Lanoxin Injection 1546
Lanoxin Injection Pediatric 1549
Lanoxin Tablets 1553

Diltiazem Hydrochloride (Because of significant inotropic and chronotropic effects in patients treated with β-blockers and calcium-channel blockers of the diltiazem type, caution should be exercised in patients treated with these agents concomitantly). Products include:
Cardizem LA 423

Diphenhydramine (Co-administration of metoprolol with drugs that inhibit CYP2D6 is likely to increase metoprolol concentration; this increase in plasma concentration would decrease the cardioselectivity of metoprolol).
No products indexed under this heading.

Diphenhydramine Hydrochloride (Co-administration of metoprolol with drugs that inhibit CYP2D6 is likely to increase metoprolol concentration; this increase in plasma concentration would decrease the cardioselectivity of metoprolol). Products include:
Benadryl Allergy Ultratab 2042
Children's Benadryl Allergy Liquid 2042

Doxepin Hydrochloride (Co-administration of metoprolol with drugs that inhibit CYP2D6 is likely to increase metoprolol concentration; this increase in plasma concentration would decrease the cardioselectivity of metoprolol).
No products indexed under this heading.

Enflurane (The necessity or desirability of withdrawing β-blocking therapy prior to major surgery is controversial; the impaired ability of the heart to respond to reflex adrenergic stimuli may augment the risks of general anesthesia and surgical procedures).
No products indexed under this heading.

Epinephrine (While taking β-blockers, patients with a history of severe anaphylactic reactions to a variety of allergens may be more reactive to repeated challenge, either accidental, diagnostic, or therapeutic. Such patients may be unresponsive to the usual doses of epinephrine used to treat allergic reaction). Products include:
EpiPen 3631
Twinject 3268

Epinephrine, Racemic (While taking β-blockers, patients with a history of severe anaphylactic reactions to a variety of allergens may be more reactive to repeated challenge, either accidental, diagnostic, or therapeutic. Such patients may be unresponsive to the usual doses of epinephrine used to treat allergic reaction).
No products indexed under this heading.

Epinephrine Bitartrate (While taking β-blockers, patients with a history of severe anaphylactic reactions to a variety of allergens may be more reactive to repeated challenge, either accidental, diagnostic, or therapeutic. Such patients may be unresponsive to the usual doses of epinephrine used to treat allergic reaction).
No products indexed under this heading.

Epinephrine Hydrochloride (Potential unresponsiveness to the usual dose of epinephrine to treat allergic reactions in certain patients).
No products indexed under this heading.

Escitalopram Oxalate (Co-administration of metoprolol with drugs that inhibit CYP2D6 is likely to increase metoprolol concentration; this increase in plasma concentration would decrease the cardioselectivity of metoprolol). Products include:
Lexapro Oral Suspension 1160
Lexapro Tablets 1160

Fluoxetine (Co-administration of metoprolol with drugs that inhibit CYP2D6 is likely to increase metoprolol concentration; this increase in plasma concentration would decrease the cardioselectivity of metoprolol).
No products indexed under this heading.

Fluoxetine Hydrochloride (Co-administration with drugs that inhibit CYP2D6, such as fluoxetine, are likely to increase metoprolol concentrations; these increases in plasma concentration would decrease the cardioselectivity of metoprolol). Products include:
Prozac Weekly 1941
Prozac Pulvules 1941
Symbyax 1965

Fluphenazine Decanoate (Co-administration of metoprolol with drugs that inhibit CYP2D6 is likely to increase metoprolol concentration; this increase in plasma concentration would decrease the cardioselectivity of metoprolol).
No products indexed under this heading.

Fluphenazine Enanthate (Co-administration of metoprolol with drugs that inhibit CYP2D6 is likely to increase metoprolol concentration; this increase in plasma concentration would decrease the cardioselectivity of metoprolol).
No products indexed under this heading.

IMPORTANT NOTE: Always consult each drug listing in the patient's regimen for possible interactions.

Toprol-XL Interactions Index 1898

Fluphenazine Hydrochloride (Co-administration of metoprolol with drugs that inhibit CYP2D6 is likely to increase metoprolol concentration; this increase in plasma concentration would decrease the cardioselectivity of metoprolol).
No products indexed under this heading.

Fluvoxamine Maleate (Co-administration of metoprolol with drugs that inhibit CYP2D6 is likely to increase metoprolol concentration; this increase in plasma concentration would decrease the cardioselectivity of metoprolol).
No products indexed under this heading.

Guanethidine (Catecholamine-depleting drugs may have an additive effect when given with β-blocking agents; monitor closely for signs of hypotension or marked bradycardia).
No products indexed under this heading.

Guanethidine Monosulfate (Catecholamine-depleting drugs may have an additive effect when given with β-blocking agents; monitor closely for signs of hypotension or marked bradycardia).
No products indexed under this heading.

Guanethidine Sulfate (Catecholamine-depleting drugs may have an additive effect when given with β-blocking agents; monitor closely for signs of hypotension or marked bradycardia).
No products indexed under this heading.

Halofantrine Hydrochloride (Co-administration of metoprolol with drugs that inhibit CYP2D6 is likely to increase metoprolol concentration; this increase in plasma concentration would decrease the cardioselectivity of metoprolol).
No products indexed under this heading.

Haloperidol (Co-administration of metoprolol with drugs that inhibit CYP2D6 is likely to increase metoprolol concentration; this increase in plasma concentration would decrease the cardioselectivity of metoprolol).
No products indexed under this heading.

Haloperidol Decanoate (Co-administration of metoprolol with drugs that inhibit CYP2D6 is likely to increase metoprolol concentration; this increase in plasma concentration would decrease the cardioselectivity of metoprolol).
No products indexed under this heading.

Haloperidol Lactate (Co-administration of metoprolol with drugs that inhibit CYP2D6 is likely to increase metoprolol concentration; this increase in plasma concentration would decrease the cardioselectivity of metoprolol).
No products indexed under this heading.

Halothane (The necessity or desirability of withdrawing β-blocking therapy prior to major surgery is controversial; the impaired ability of the heart to respond to reflex adrenergic stimuli may augment the risks of general anesthesia and surgical procedures).
No products indexed under this heading.

Hydroxychloroquine Sulfate (Co-administration of metoprolol with drugs that inhibit CYP2D6 is likely to increase metoprolol concentration; this increase in plasma concentration would decrease the cardioselectivity of metoprolol).
No products indexed under this heading.

Imatinib Mesylate (Co-administration of metoprolol with drugs that inhibit CYP2D6 is likely to increase metoprolol concentration; this increase in plasma concentration would decrease the cardioselectivity of metoprolol). Products include:
Gleevec 2477

Imipramine Hydrochloride (Co-administration of metoprolol with drugs that inhibit CYP2D6 is likely to increase metoprolol concentration; this increase in plasma concentration would decrease the cardioselectivity of metoprolol).
No products indexed under this heading.

Imipramine Pamoate (Co-administration of metoprolol with drugs that inhibit CYP2D6 is likely to increase metoprolol concentration; this increase in plasma concentration would decrease the cardioselectivity of metoprolol).
No products indexed under this heading.

Isocarboxazid (Catecholamine-depleting drugs may have an additive effect when given with β-blocking agents; monitor closely for signs of hypotension or marked bradycardia).
Products include:
Marplan 3481

Isoflurane (The necessity or desirability of withdrawing β-blocking therapy prior to major surgery is controversial; the impaired ability of the heart to respond to reflex adrenergic stimuli may augment the risks of general anesthesia and surgical procedures).
No products indexed under this heading.

Ketamine Hydrochloride (The necessity or desirability of withdrawing β-blocking therapy prior to major surgery is controversial; the impaired ability of the heart to respond to reflex adrenergic stimuli may augment the risks of general anesthesia and surgical procedures).
No products indexed under this heading.

Maprotiline Hydrochloride (Co-administration of metoprolol with drugs that inhibit CYP2D6 is likely to increase metoprolol concentration; this increase in plasma concentration would decrease the cardioselectivity of metoprolol).
No products indexed under this heading.

Methadone Hydrochloride (Co-administration of metoprolol with drugs that inhibit CYP2D6 is likely to increase metoprolol concentration; this increase in plasma concentration would decrease the cardioselectivity of metoprolol).
No products indexed under this heading.

Methohexital Sodium (The necessity or desirability of withdrawing β-blocking therapy prior to major surgery is controversial; the impaired ability of the heart to respond to reflex adrenergic stimuli may augment the risks of general anesthesia and surgical procedures).
No products indexed under this heading.

Methoxyflurane (The necessity or desirability of withdrawing β-blocking therapy prior to major surgery is controversial; the impaired ability of the heart to respond to reflex adrenergic stimuli may augment the risks of general anesthesia and surgical procedures).
No products indexed under this heading.

Mibefradil Dihydrochloride (Co-administration of metoprolol with drugs that inhibit CYP2D6 is likely to increase metoprolol concentration; this increase in plasma concentration would decrease the cardioselectivity of metoprolol).
No products indexed under this heading.

Moclobemide (Catecholamine-depleting drugs may have an additive effect when given with β-blocking agents; monitor closely for signs of hypotension or marked bradycardia).
No products indexed under this heading.

Nitrous Oxide (The necessity or desirability of withdrawing β-blocking therapy prior to major surgery is controversial; the impaired ability of the heart to respond to reflex adrenergic stimuli may augment the risks of general anesthesia and surgical procedures).
No products indexed under this heading.

Norepinephrine Bitartrate (While taking β-blockers, patients with a history of severe anaphylactic reactions to a variety of allergens may be more reactive to repeated challenge, either accidental, diagnostic, or therapeutic. Such patients may be unresponsive to the usual doses of epinephrine used to treat allergic reaction).
No products indexed under this heading.

Norepinephrine Hydrochloride (While taking β-blockers, patients with a history of severe anaphylactic reactions to a variety of allergens may be more reactive to repeated challenge, either accidental, diagnostic, or therapeutic. Such patients may be unresponsive to the usual doses of epinephrine used to treat allergic reaction).
No products indexed under this heading.

Nortriptyline Hydrochloride (Co-administration of metoprolol with drugs that inhibit CYP2D6 is likely to increase metoprolol concentration; this increase in plasma concentration would decrease the cardioselectivity of metoprolol).
No products indexed under this heading.

Pargyline Hydrochloride (Catecholamine-depleting drugs may have an additive effect when given with β-blocking agents; monitor closely for signs of hypotension or marked bradycardia).
No products indexed under this heading.

Paroxetine Hydrochloride (Co-administration with drugs that inhibit CYP2D6, such as paroxetine, are likely to increase metoprolol concentrations; these increases in plasma concentration would decrease the cardioselectivity of metoprolol). Products include:
Paroxetine CR 2361
Paroxetine ER 2371
Paxil 1586
Paxil CR 1596

Perphenazine (Co-administration of metoprolol with drugs that inhibit CYP2D6 is likely to increase metoprolol concentration; this increase in plasma concentration would decrease the cardioselectivity of metoprolol).
No products indexed under this heading.

Phenelzine Sulfate (Catecholamine-depleting drugs may have an additive effect when given with β-blocking agents; monitor closely for signs of hypotension or marked bradycardia).
No products indexed under this heading.

Procarbazine Hydrochloride (Catecholamine-depleting drugs may have an additive effect when given with β-blocking agents; monitor closely for signs of hypotension or marked bradycardia).
No products indexed under this heading.

Propafenone Hydrochloride (Co-administration with drugs that inhibit CYP2D6, such as propafenone, are likely to increase metoprolol concentrations; these increases in plasma concentration would decrease the cardioselectivity of metoprolol).
Products include:
Rythmol 1648
Rythmol SR 1652

Propofol (The necessity or desirability of withdrawing β-blocking therapy prior to major surgery is controversial; the impaired ability of the heart to respond to reflex adrenergic stimuli may augment the risks of general anesthesia and surgical procedures).
No products indexed under this heading.

Propoxyphene Hydrochloride (Co-administration of metoprolol with drugs that inhibit CYP2D6 is likely to increase metoprolol concentration; this increase in plasma concentration would decrease the cardioselectivity of metoprolol).
No products indexed under this heading.

Propoxyphene Napsylate (Co-administration of metoprolol with drugs that inhibit CYP2D6 is likely to increase metoprolol concentration; this increase in plasma concentration would decrease the cardioselectivity of metoprolol).
No products indexed under this heading.

Protriptyline Hydrochloride (Co-administration of metoprolol with drugs that inhibit CYP2D6 is likely to increase metoprolol concentration; this increase in plasma concentration would decrease the cardioselectivity of metoprolol).
No products indexed under this heading.

Quinacrine Hydrochloride (Co-administration of metoprolol with drugs that inhibit CYP2D6 is likely to increase metoprolol concentration; this increase in plasma concentration would decrease the cardioselectivity of metoprolol).
No products indexed under this heading.

Quinidine (Drugs that inhibit CYP2D6, such as quinidine, fluoxetine, paroxetine, and propafenone are likely to increase metoprolol concentration. These increases in plasma concentration would decrease the cardioselectivity of metoprolol).
No products indexed under this heading.

Quinidine Gluconate (Drugs that inhibit CYP2D6, such as quinidine, fluoxetine, paroxetine, and propafenone are likely to increase metoprolol concentration. These increases in plasma concentration would decrease the cardioselectivity of metoprolol).
No products indexed under this heading.

Quinidine Hydrochloride (Drugs that inhibit CYP2D6, such as quinidine, fluoxetine, paroxetine, and propafenone are likely to increase metoprolol concentration. These increases in plasma concentration would decrease the cardioselectivity of metoprolol).
No products indexed under this heading.

Quinidine Polygalacturonate (Drugs that inhibit CYP2D6, such as quinidine, fluoxetine, paroxetine, and propafenone are likely to increase metoprolol concentration. These increases in plasma concentration would decrease the cardioselectivity of metoprolol).
No products indexed under this heading.

Quinidine Sulfate (Drugs that inhibit CYP2D6, such as quinidine, fluoxetine, paroxetine, and propafenone are likely to increase metoprolol concentration. These increases in plasma concentration would decrease the cardioselectivity of metoprolol).
No products indexed under this heading.

Ranitidine Bismuth Citrate (Co-administration of metoprolol with drugs that inhibit CYP2D6 is likely to increase metoprolol concentration; this increase in plasma concentration would decrease the cardioselectivity of metoprolol).
No products indexed under this heading.

Ranitidine Hydrochloride (Co-administration of metoprolol with drugs

that inhibit CYP2D6 is likely to increase metoprolol concentration; this increase in plasma concentration would decrease the cardioselectivity of metoprolol). Products include:

Zantac 1737
Zantac Injection 1732
Zantac Pharmacy 1735

Rasagiline Mesylate (Catecholamine-depleting drugs may have an additive effect when given with β-blocking agents; monitor closely for signs of hypotension or marked bradycardia). Products include:

Azilect 3383

Rauwolfia Serpentina (Catecholamine-depleting drugs may have an additive effect when given with β-blocking agents; monitor closely for signs of hypotension or marked bradycardia).

No products indexed under this heading.

Rescinnamine (Catecholamine-depleting drugs may have an additive effect when given with β-blocking agents; monitor closely for signs of hypotension or marked bradycardia).

No products indexed under this heading.

Reserpine (Catecholamine-depleting drugs may have an additive effect when given with β-blocking agents; monitor closely for signs of hypotension or marked bradycardia).

No products indexed under this heading.

Ritonavir (Co-administration of metoprolol with drugs that inhibit CYP2D6 is likely to increase metoprolol concentration; this increase in plasma concentration would decrease the cardioselectivity of metoprolol). Products include:

Kaletra 458
Norvir 509

Selegiline (Catecholamine-depleting drugs may have an additive effect when given with β-blocking agents; monitor closely for signs of hypotension or marked bradycardia). Products include:

Emsam 3623

Selegiline Hydrochloride (Catecholamine-depleting drugs may have an additive effect when given with β-blocking agents; monitor closely for signs of hypotension or marked bradycardia). Products include:

Eldepryl 3312

Sertraline Hydrochloride (Co-administration of metoprolol with drugs that inhibit CYP2D6 is likely to increase metoprolol concentration; this increase in plasma concentration would decrease the cardioselectivity of metoprolol).

No products indexed under this heading.

Sevoflurane (The necessity or desirability of withdrawing β-blocking therapy prior to major surgery is controversial; the impaired ability of the heart to respond to reflex adrenergic stimuli may augment the risks of general anesthesia and surgical procedures). Products include:

Ultane 554

Sildenafil Citrate (Co-administration of metoprolol with drugs that inhibit CYP2D6 is likely to increase metoprolol concentration; this increase in plasma concentration would decrease the cardioselectivity of metoprolol).

No products indexed under this heading.

Terbinafine Hydrochloride (Co-administration of metoprolol with drugs that inhibit CYP2D6 is likely to increase metoprolol concentration; this increase in plasma concentration would decrease the cardioselectivity of metoprolol).

No products indexed under this heading.

Thioridazine Hydrochloride (Co-administration of metoprolol with drugs that inhibit CYP2D6 is likely to increase metoprolol concentration; this increase

in plasma concentration would decrease the cardioselectivity of metoprolol). Products include:

Thioridazine Hydrochloride 2384

Tranylcypromine Sulfate (Catecholamine-depleting drugs may have an additive effect when given with β-blocking agents; monitor closely for signs of hypotension or marked bradycardia). Products include:

Parnate 1584

Trimipramine Maleate (Co-administration of metoprolol with drugs that inhibit CYP2D6 is likely to increase metoprolol concentration; this increase in plasma concentration would decrease the cardioselectivity of metoprolol).

No products indexed under this heading.

Vardenafil Hydrochloride (Co-administration of metoprolol with drugs that inhibit CYP2D6 is likely to increase metoprolol concentration; this increase in plasma concentration would decrease the cardioselectivity of metoprolol). Products include:

Levitra 3157

Verapamil Hydrochloride (Because of significant inotropic and chronotropic effects in patients treated with β-blockers and calcium-channel blockers of the verapamil type, caution should be exercised in patients treated with these agents concomitantly). Products include:

Tarka 534

TORISEL INJECTION

(Temsirolimus) 3592
May interact with ACE inhibitors, anticoagulants, cytochrome p450 3a inducers (selected), cytochrome p450 3a4 inducers (selected), cytochrome p450 3a4 inhibitors, potent (selected), dexamethasones, insulin, lipid-lowering drugs, oral hypoglycemic agents, phenytoin, vaccines, live, and certain other agents. Compounds in these categories include:

Acarbose (The use of temsirolimus is likely to result in increases in serum glucose. In a clinical trial, 89% of patients receiving temsirolimus had at least one elevated serum glucose while on treatment, and 26% of patients reported hyperglycemia as an adverse event. This may result in the need for an increase in the dose of, or initiation of, insulin and/or oral hypoglycemic agent therapy. Serum glucose should be tested before and during treatment with temsirolimus).

No products indexed under this heading.

Allium sativum (Strong inducers of CYP3A4/5 such as dexamethasone, carbamazepine, phenytoin, phenobarbital, rifampin, rifabutin, and rifampicin may decrease exposure of the active metabolite (of temsirolimus), sirolimus, and should be avoided. If alternative treatment cannot be administered, a dose adjustment should be considered. St. John's Wort may decrease temsirolimus plasma concentrations unpredictably. Patients receiving temsirolimus should not take St. John's Wort concomitantly).

No products indexed under this heading.

Aminoglutethimide (Strong inducers of CYP3A4/5 such as dexamethasone, carbamazepine, phenytoin, phenobarbital, rifampin, rifabutin, and rifampicin may decrease exposure of the active metabolite (of temsirolimus), sirolimus, and should be avoided. If alternative treatment cannot be administered, a dose adjustment should be considered. St. John's Wort may decrease temsirolimus plasma concentrations unpredictably. Patients receiving temsirolimus should not take St. John's Wort concomitantly).

No products indexed under this heading.

Amprenavir (Strong CYP3A4 inhibitors such as atazanavir, clarithromycin, indinavir, itraconazole, ketoconazole, nefazodone, nelfinavir, ritonavir, saquinavir, and telithromycin may increase blood concentrations of the active metabolite (of temsirolimus), sirolimus, and should be avoided. If alternative treatments cannot be administered, a dose adjustment should be considered).

No products indexed under this heading.

Anisindione (Patients with central nervous system tumors (primary CNS tumor or metastases) and/or receiving anticoagulation therapy may be at an increased risk of developing intracerebral bleeding (including fatal outcomes) while receiving temsirolimus).

No products indexed under this heading.

Aprepitant (Strong inducers of CYP3A4/5 such as dexamethasone, carbamazepine, phenytoin, phenobarbital, rifampin, rifabutin, and rifampicin may decrease exposure of the active metabolite (of temsirolimus), sirolimus, and should be avoided. If alternative treatment cannot be administered, a dose adjustment should be considered. St. John's Wort may decrease temsirolimus plasma concentrations unpredictably. Patients receiving temsirolimus should not take St. John's Wort concomitantly). Products include:

Emend 2124

Ardeparin Sodium (Patients with central nervous system tumors (primary CNS tumor or metastases) and/or receiving anticoagulation therapy may be at an increased risk of developing intracerebral bleeding (including fatal outcomes) while receiving temsirolimus).

No products indexed under this heading.

Atazanavir (Strong CYP3A4 inhibitors such as atazanavir, clarithromycin, indinavir, itraconazole, ketoconazole, nefazodone, nelfinavir, ritonavir, saquinavir, and telithromycin may increase blood concentrations of the active metabolite (of temsirolimus), sirolimus, and should be avoided. If alternative treatments cannot be administered, a dose adjustment should be considered).

No products indexed under this heading.

Atazanavir Sulfate (Strong CYP3A4 inhibitors such as atazanavir, clarithromycin, indinavir, itraconazole, ketoconazole, nefazodone, nelfinavir, ritonavir, saquinavir, and telithromycin may increase blood concentrations of the active metabolite (of temsirolimus), sirolimus, and should be avoided. If alternative treatments cannot be administered, a dose adjustment should be considered).

No products indexed under this heading.

Atorvastatin Calcium (The use of temsirolimus is likely to result in increases in serum triglycerides and cholesterol. In a clinical trial, 87% of patients receiving temsirolimus had at least one elevated serum cholesterol value and 83% had at least one elevated serum triglyceride value. This may require initiation, or increase in the dose, of lipid-lowering agents). Products include:

Lipitor 2703

BCG Vaccine (The use of live vaccines (eg, intranasal influenza, measles, mumps, rubella, oral polio, BCG, yellow fever, varicella, and TY21a typhoid vaccines) and close contact with those who have received live vaccines should be avoided during treatment with temsirolimus).

No products indexed under this heading.

Benazepril Hydrochloride (Angioneurotic edema-type reactions have been observed in some patients who received temsirolimus and ACE inhibitors concomitantly).

No products indexed under this heading.

Betamethasone (Strong inducers of CYP3A4/5 such as dexamethasone, carbamazepine, phenytoin, phenobarbital, rifampin, rifabutin, and rifampicin may decrease exposure of the active metabolite (of temsirolimus), sirolimus, and should be avoided. If alternative treatment cannot be administered, a dose adjustment should be considered. St. John's Wort may decrease temsirolimus plasma concentrations unpredictably. Patients receiving temsirolimus should not take St. John's Wort concomitantly).

No products indexed under this heading.

Betamethasone Acetate (Strong inducers of CYP3A4/5 such as dexamethasone, carbamazepine, phenytoin, phenobarbital, rifampin, rifabutin, and rifampicin may decrease exposure of the active metabolite (of temsirolimus), sirolimus, and should be avoided. If alternative treatment cannot be administered, a dose adjustment should be considered. St. John's Wort may decrease temsirolimus plasma concentrations unpredictably. Patients receiving temsirolimus should not take St. John's Wort concomitantly).

No products indexed under this heading.

Betamethasone Benzoate (Strong inducers of CYP3A4/5 such as dexamethasone, carbamazepine, phenytoin, phenobarbital, rifampin, rifabutin, and rifampicin may decrease exposure of the active metabolite (of temsirolimus), sirolimus, and should be avoided. If alternative treatment cannot be administered, a dose adjustment should be considered. St. John's Wort may decrease temsirolimus plasma concentrations unpredictably. Patients receiving temsirolimus should not take St. John's Wort concomitantly).

No products indexed under this heading.

Betamethasone Dipropionate (Strong inducers of CYP3A4/5 such as dexamethasone, carbamazepine, phenytoin, phenobarbital, rifampin, rifabutin, and rifampicin may decrease exposure of the active metabolite (of temsirolimus), sirolimus, and should be avoided. If alternative treatment cannot be administered, a dose adjustment should be considered. St. John's Wort may decrease temsirolimus plasma concentrations unpredictably. Patients receiving temsirolimus should not take St. John's Wort concomitantly). Products include:

Diprolene Lotion 0.05% 3108
Diprolene Ointment 0.05% 3109
Diprolene AF Cream 0.05% 3107
Lotrisone 3163

Betamethasone Sodium Phosphate (Strong inducers of CYP3A4/5 such as dexamethasone, carbamazepine, phenytoin, phenobarbital, rifampin, rifabutin, and rifampicin may decrease exposure of the active metabolite (of temsirolimus), sirolimus, and should be avoided. If alternative treatment cannot be administered, a dose adjustment should be considered. St. John's Wort may decrease temsirolimus plasma concentrations unpredictably. Patients receiving temsirolimus should not take St. John's Wort concomitantly).

No products indexed under this heading.

Betamethasone Valerate (Strong inducers of CYP3A4/5 such as dexamethasone, carbamazepine, phenytoin, phenobarbital, rifampin, rifabutin, and rifampicin may decrease exposure of the active metabolite (of temsirolimus), sirolimus, and should be avoided. If alternative treatment cannot be adminis-

Torisel Interactions Index 1900

tered, a dose adjustment should be considered. St. John's Wort may decrease temsirolimus plasma concentrations unpredictably. Patients receiving temsirolimus should not take St. John's Wort concomitantly). Products include:
Luxiq 3321

Bosentan (Strong inducers of CYP3A4/5 such as dexamethasone, carbamazepine, phenytoin, phenobarbital, rifampin, rifabutin, and rifampicin may decrease exposure of the active metabolite (of temsirolimus), sirolimus, and should be avoided. If alternative treatment cannot be administered, a dose adjustment should be considered. St. John's Wort may decrease temsirolimus plasma concentrations unpredictably. Patients receiving temsirolimus should not take St. John's Wort concomitantly). Products include:
Tracleer 573

Captopril (Angioneurotic edema-type reactions have been observed in some patients who received temsirolimus and ACE inhibitors concomitantly). Products include:
Captopril 2341

Carbamazepine (Strong inducers of CYP3A4/5 such as dexamethasone, carbamazepine, phenytoin, phenobarbital, rifampin, rifabutin, and rifampicin may decrease exposure of the active metabolite (of temsirolimus), sirolimus, and should be avoided. If alternative treatment cannot be administered, a dose adjustment should be considered). Products include:
Carbatrol 3280
Equetro 3477

Cerivastatin Sodium (The use of temsirolimus is likely to result in increases in serum triglycerides and cholesterol. In a clinical trial, 87% of patients receiving temsirolimus had at least one elevated serum cholesterol value and 83% had at least one elevated serum triglyceride value. This may require initiation, or increase in the dose, of lipid-lowering agents).
No products indexed under this heading.

Chlorpropamide (The use of temsirolimus is likely to result in increases in serum glucose. In a clinical trial, 89% of patients receiving temsirolimus had at least one elevated serum glucose while on treatment, and 26% of patients reported hyperglycemia as an adverse event. This may result in the need for an increase in the dose of, or initiation of, insulin and/or oral hypoglycemic agent therapy. Serum glucose should be tested before and during treatment with temsirolimus).
No products indexed under this heading.

Cholestyramine (The use of temsirolimus is likely to result in increases in serum triglycerides and cholesterol. In a clinical trial, 87% of patients receiving temsirolimus had at least one elevated serum cholesterol value and 83% had at least one elevated serum triglyceride value. This may require initiation, or increase in the dose, of lipid-lowering agents).
No products indexed under this heading.

Ciprofloxacin (Strong inducers of CYP3A4/5 such as dexamethasone, carbamazepine, phenytoin, phenobarbital, rifampin, rifabutin, and rifampicin may decrease exposure of the active metabolite (of temsirolimus), sirolimus, and should be avoided. If alternative treatment cannot be administered, a dose adjustment should be considered. St. John's Wort may decrease temsirolimus plasma concentrations unpredictably. Patients receiving temsirolimus should not take St. John's Wort concomitantly). Products include:
Cipro I.V. 3082
Cipro 3073
Cipro XR 3091
Ciprodex 583

Ciprofloxacin Hydrochloride (Strong inducers of CYP3A4/5 such as dexamethasone, carbamazepine, phenytoin, phenobarbital, rifampin, rifabutin, and rifampicin may decrease exposure of the active metabolite (of temsirolimus), sirolimus, and should be avoided. If alternative treatment cannot be administered, a dose adjustment should be considered. St. John's Wort may decrease temsirolimus plasma concentrations unpredictably. Patients receiving temsirolimus should not take St. John's Wort concomitantly). Products include:
Cipro 3073

Cisplatin (Strong inducers of CYP3A4/5 such as dexamethasone, carbamazepine, phenytoin, phenobarbital, rifampin, rifabutin, and rifampicin may decrease exposure of the active metabolite (of temsirolimus), sirolimus, and should be avoided. If alternative treatment cannot be administered, a dose adjustment should be considered. St. John's Wort may decrease temsirolimus plasma concentrations unpredictably. Patients receiving temsirolimus should not take St. John's Wort concomitantly).
No products indexed under this heading.

Clarithromycin (Strong CYP3A4 inhibitors such as atazanavir, clarithromycin, indinavir, itraconazole, ketoconazole, nefazodone, nelfinavir, ritonavir, saquinavir, and telithromycin may increase blood concentrations of the active metabolite (of temsirolimus), sirolimus, and should be avoided. If alternative treatments cannot be administered, a dose adjustment should be considered). Products include:
Biaxin/Biaxin XL 412

Clofibrate (The use of temsirolimus is likely to result in increases in serum triglycerides and cholesterol. In a clinical trial, 87% of patients receiving temsirolimus had at least one elevated serum cholesterol value and 83% had at least one elevated serum triglyceride value. This may require initiation, or increase in the dose, of lipid-lowering agents).
No products indexed under this heading.

Colestipol Hydrochloride (The use of temsirolimus is likely to result in increases in serum triglycerides and cholesterol. In a clinical trial, 87% of patients receiving temsirolimus had at least one elevated serum cholesterol value and 83% had at least one elevated serum triglyceride value. This may require initiation, or increase in the dose, of lipid-lowering agents).
No products indexed under this heading.

Cortisone Acetate (Strong inducers of CYP3A4/5 such as dexamethasone, carbamazepine, phenytoin, phenobarbital, rifampin, rifabutin, and rifampicin may decrease exposure of the active metabolite (of temsirolimus), sirolimus, and should be avoided. If alternative treatment cannot be administered, a dose adjustment should be considered. St. John's Wort may decrease temsirolimus plasma concentrations unpredictably. Patients receiving temsirolimus should not take St. John's Wort concomitantly).
No products indexed under this heading.

Dalteparin Sodium (Patients with central nervous system tumors (primary CNS tumor or metastases) and/or receiving anticoagulation therapy may be at an increased risk of developing intracerebral bleeding (including fatal outcomes) while receiving temsirolimus). Products include:
Fragmin 1058

Danaparoid Sodium (Patients with central nervous system tumors (primary CNS tumor or metastases) and/or receiving anticoagulation therapy may be at an increased risk of developing intracerebral bleeding (including fatal outcomes) while receiving temsirolimus).
No products indexed under this heading.

Delavirdine Mesylate (Strong CYP3A4 inhibitors such as atazanavir, clarithromycin, indinavir, itraconazole, ketoconazole, nefazodone, nelfinavir, ritonavir, saquinavir, and telithromycin may increase blood concentrations of the active metabolite (of temsirolimus), sirolimus, and should be avoided. If alternative treatments cannot be administered, a dose adjustment should be considered).
No products indexed under this heading.

Delavirine (Strong CYP3A4 inhibitors such as atazanavir, clarithromycin, indinavir, itraconazole, ketoconazole, nefazodone, nelfinavir, ritonavir, saquinavir, and telithromycin may increase blood concentrations of the active metabolite (of temsirolimus), sirolimus, and should be avoided. If alternative treatments cannot be administered, a dose adjustment should be considered).
No products indexed under this heading.

Dexamethasone (Strong inducers of CYP3A4/5 such as dexamethasone may decrease exposure of the active metabolite (of temsirolimus), sirolimus, and should be avoided. If alternative treatment cannot be administered, a dose adjustment should be considered). Products include:
Ciprodex 583
Ozurdex .... ⊙223
Tobramycin and Dexamethasone Ophthalmic Suspension .... ⊙251

Dexamethasone Acetate (Strong inducers of CYP3A4/5 such as dexamethasone may decrease exposure of the active metabolite (of temsirolimus), sirolimus, and should be avoided. If alternative treatment cannot be administered, a dose adjustment should be considered).
No products indexed under this heading.

Dexamethasone Phosphate (Strong inducers of CYP3A4/5 such as dexamethasone may decrease exposure of the active metabolite (of temsirolimus), sirolimus, and should be avoided. If alternative treatment cannot be administered, a dose adjustment should be considered).
No products indexed under this heading.

Dexamethasone Sodium (Strong inducers of CYP3A4/5 such as dexamethasone may decrease exposure of the active metabolite (of temsirolimus), sirolimus, and should be avoided. If alternative treatment cannot be administered, a dose adjustment should be considered).
No products indexed under this heading.

Dexamethasone Sodium Phosphate (Strong inducers of CYP3A4/5 such as dexamethasone may decrease exposure of the active metabolite (of temsirolimus), sirolimus, and should be avoided. If alternative treatment cannot be administered, a dose adjustment should be considered).
No products indexed under this heading.

Dexamethasone Sodium Phosphate Injection (Strong inducers of CYP3A4/5 such as dexamethasone may decrease exposure of the active metabolite (of temsirolimus), sirolimus, and should be avoided. If alternative treatment cannot be administered, a dose adjustment should be considered).
No products indexed under this heading.

Dicumarol (Patients with central nervous system tumors (primary CNS tumor or metastases) and/or receiving anticoagulation therapy may be at an increased risk of developing intracerebral bleeding (including fatal outcomes) while receiving temsirolimus).
No products indexed under this heading.

Doxorubicin Hydrochloride (Strong inducers of CYP3A4/5 such as dexamethasone, carbamazepine, phenytoin, phenobarbital, rifampin, rifabutin, and rifampicin may decrease exposure of the active metabolite (of temsirolimus), sirolimus, and should be avoided. If alternative treatment cannot be administered, a dose adjustment should be considered. St. John's Wort may decrease temsirolimus plasma concentrations unpredictably. Patients receiving temsirolimus should not take St. John's Wort concomitantly).
No products indexed under this heading.

Efavirenz (Strong inducers of CYP3A4/5 such as dexamethasone, carbamazepine, phenytoin, phenobarbital, rifampin, rifabutin, and rifampicin may decrease exposure of the active metabolite (of temsirolimus), sirolimus, and should be avoided. If alternative treatment cannot be administered, a dose adjustment should be considered. St. John's Wort may decrease temsirolimus plasma concentrations unpredictably. Patients receiving temsirolimus should not take St. John's Wort concomitantly). Products include:
Atripla 906

Enalapril Maleate (Angioneurotic edema-type reactions have been observed in some patients who received temsirolimus and ACE inhibitors concomitantly).
No products indexed under this heading.

Enalaprilat (Angioneurotic edema-type reactions have been observed in some patients who received temsirolimus and ACE inhibitors concomitantly).
No products indexed under this heading.

Enoxaparin Sodium (Patients with central nervous system tumors (primary CNS tumor or metastases) and/or receiving anticoagulation therapy may be at an increased risk of developing intracerebral bleeding (including fatal outcomes) while receiving temsirolimus). Products include:
Lovenox 3005

Ethosuximide (Strong inducers of CYP3A4/5 such as dexamethasone, carbamazepine, phenytoin, phenobarbital, rifampin, rifabutin, and rifampicin may decrease exposure of the active metabolite (of temsirolimus), sirolimus, and should be avoided. If alternative treatment cannot be administered, a dose adjustment should be considered. St. John's Wort may decrease temsirolimus plasma concentrations unpredictably. Patients receiving temsirolimus should not take St. John's Wort concomitantly).
No products indexed under this heading.

Felbamate (Strong inducers of CYP3A4/5 such as dexamethasone, carbamazepine, phenytoin, phenobarbital, rifampin, rifabutin, and rifampicin may decrease exposure of the active metabolite (of temsirolimus), sirolimus, and should be avoided. If alternative treatment cannot be administered, a dose adjustment should be considered. St. John's Wort may decrease temsirolimus plasma concentrations unpredictably. Patients receiving temsirolimus should not take St. John's Wort concomitantly).
No products indexed under this heading.

Fenofibrate (The use of temsirolimus is likely to result in increases in serum triglycerides and cholesterol. In a clinical trial, 87% of patients receiving tem-

1901 Interactions Index Torisel

sirolimus had at least one elevated serum cholesterol value and 83% had at least one elevated serum triglyceride value. This may require initiation, or increase in the dose, of lipid-lowering agents). Products include:
Fenoglide 3263
Tricor 544
Trilipix 548

Fludrocortisone Acetate (Strong inducers of CYP3A4/5 such as dexamethasone, carbamazepine, phenytoin, phenobarbital, rifampin, rifabutin, and rifampicin may decrease exposure of the active metabolite (of temsirolimus), sirolimus, and should be avoided. If alternative treatment cannot be administered, a dose adjustment should be considered. St. John's Wort may decrease temsirolimus plasma concentrations unpredictably. Patients receiving temsirolimus should not take St. John's Wort concomitantly).
No products indexed under this heading.

Fluvastatin Sodium (The use of temsirolimus is likely to result in increases in serum triglycerides and cholesterol. In a clinical trial, 87% of patients receiving temsirolimus had at least one elevated serum cholesterol value and 83% had at least one elevated serum triglyceride value. This may require initiation, or increase in the dose, of lipid-lowering agents).
No products indexed under this heading.

Fondaparinux Sodium (Patients with central nervous system tumors (primary CNS tumor or metastases) and/or receiving anticoagulation therapy may be at an increased risk of developing intracerebral bleeding (including fatal outcomes) while receiving temsirolimus). Products include:
Arixtra 1320

Fosamprenavir Calcium (Strong CYP3A4 inhibitors such as atazanavir, clarithromycin, indinavir, itraconazole, ketoconazole, nefazodone, nelfinavir, ritonavir, saquinavir, and telithromycin may increase blood concentrations of the active metabolite (of temsirolimus), sirolimus, and should be avoided. If alternative treatments cannot be administered, a dose adjustment should be considered). Products include:
Lexiva Oral Suspension 1558
Lexiva 1558

Fosinopril Sodium (Angioneurotic edema-type reactions have been observed in some patients who received temsirolimus and ACE inhibitors concomitantly).
No products indexed under this heading.

Fosphenytoin (Strong inducers of CYP3A4/5 such as phenytoin may decrease exposure of the active metabolite (of temsirolimus), sirolimus, and should be avoided. If alternative treatment cannot be administered, a dose adjustment should be considered).
No products indexed under this heading.

Fosphenytoin Sodium (Strong inducers of CYP3A4/5 such as phenytoin may decrease exposure of the active metabolite (of temsirolimus), sirolimus, and should be avoided. If alternative treatment cannot be administered, a dose adjustment should be considered).
No products indexed under this heading.

Garlic Extract (Strong inducers of CYP3A4/5 such as dexamethasone, carbamazepine, phenytoin, phenobarbital, rifampin, rifabutin, and rifampicin may decrease exposure of the active metabolite (of temsirolimus), sirolimus, and should be avoided. If alternative treatment cannot be administered, a dose adjustment should be considered. St. John's Wort may decrease temsirolimus plasma concentrations unpredictably. Patients receiving temsirolimus should not take St. John's Wort concomitantly).
No products indexed under this heading.

Garlic Oil (Strong inducers of CYP3A4/5 such as dexamethasone, carbamazepine, phenytoin, phenobarbital, rifampin, rifabutin, and rifampicin may decrease exposure of the active metabolite (of temsirolimus), sirolimus, and should be avoided. If alternative treatment cannot be administered, a dose adjustment should be considered. St. John's Wort may decrease temsirolimus plasma concentrations unpredictably. Patients receiving temsirolimus should not take St. John's Wort concomitantly).
No products indexed under this heading.

Gemfibrozil (The use of temsirolimus is likely to result in increases in serum triglycerides and cholesterol. In a clinical trial, 87% of patients receiving temsirolimus had at least one elevated serum cholesterol value and 83% had at least one elevated serum triglyceride value. This may require initiation, or increase in the dose, of lipid-lowering agents).
No products indexed under this heading.

Glibenclamide (The use of temsirolimus is likely to result in increases in serum glucose. In a clinical trial, 89% of patients receiving temsirolimus had at least one elevated serum glucose while on treatment, and 26% of patients reported hyperglycemia as an adverse event. This may result in the need for an increase in the dose of, or initiation of, insulin and/or oral hypoglycemic agent therapy. Serum glucose should be tested before and during treatment with temsirolimus).
No products indexed under this heading.

Glimepiride (The use of temsirolimus is likely to result in increases in serum glucose. In a clinical trial, 89% of patients receiving temsirolimus had at least one elevated serum glucose while on treatment, and 26% of patients reported hyperglycemia as an adverse event. This may result in the need for an increase in the dose of, or initiation of, insulin and/or oral hypoglycemic agent therapy. Serum glucose should be tested before and during treatment with temsirolimus). Products include:
Avandaryl 1356
Duetact 3354

Glipizide (The use of temsirolimus is likely to result in increases in serum glucose. In a clinical trial, 89% of patients receiving temsirolimus had at least one elevated serum glucose while on treatment, and 26% of patients reported hyperglycemia as an adverse event. This may result in the need for an increase in the dose of, or initiation of, insulin and/or oral hypoglycemic agent therapy. Serum glucose should be tested before and during treatment with temsirolimus).
No products indexed under this heading.

Glyburide (The use of temsirolimus is likely to result in increases in serum glucose. In a clinical trial, 89% of patients receiving temsirolimus had at least one elevated serum glucose while on treatment, and 26% of patients reported hyperglycemia as an adverse event. This may result in the need for an increase in the dose of, or initiation of, insulin and/or oral hypoglycemic agent therapy. Serum glucose should be tested before and during treatment with temsirolimus).
No products indexed under this heading.

Heparin Calcium (Patients with central nervous system tumors (primary CNS tumor or metastases) and/or receiving anticoagulation therapy may be at an increased risk of developing intracerebral bleeding (including fatal outcomes) while receiving temsirolimus).
No products indexed under this heading.

Heparin Sodium (Patients with central nervous system tumors (primary CNS tumor or metastases) and/or receiving anticoagulation therapy may be at an increased risk of developing intracerebral bleeding (including fatal outcomes) while receiving temsirolimus).
No products indexed under this heading.

Hydrocortisone (Strong inducers of CYP3A4/5 such as dexamethasone, carbamazepine, phenytoin, phenobarbital, rifampin, rifabutin, and rifampicin may decrease exposure of the active metabolite (of temsirolimus), sirolimus, and should be avoided. If alternative treatment cannot be administered, a dose adjustment should be considered. St. John's Wort may decrease temsirolimus plasma concentrations unpredictably. Patients receiving temsirolimus should not take St. John's Wort concomitantly).
No products indexed under this heading.

Hydrocortisone (Alcohol) (Strong inducers of CYP3A4/5 such as dexamethasone, carbamazepine, phenytoin, phenobarbital, rifampin, rifabutin, and rifampicin may decrease exposure of the active metabolite (of temsirolimus), sirolimus, and should be avoided. If alternative treatment cannot be administered, a dose adjustment should be considered. St. John's Wort may decrease temsirolimus plasma concentrations unpredictably. Patients receiving temsirolimus should not take St. John's Wort concomitantly).
No products indexed under this heading.

Hydrocortisone Acetate (Strong inducers of CYP3A4/5 such as dexamethasone, carbamazepine, phenytoin, phenobarbital, rifampin, rifabutin, and rifampicin may decrease exposure of the active metabolite (of temsirolimus), sirolimus, and should be avoided. If alternative treatment cannot be administered, a dose adjustment should be considered. St. John's Wort may decrease temsirolimus plasma concentrations unpredictably. Patients receiving temsirolimus should not take St. John's Wort concomitantly).
No products indexed under this heading.

Hydrocortisone Butyrate (Strong inducers of CYP3A4/5 such as dexamethasone, carbamazepine, phenytoin, phenobarbital, rifampin, rifabutin, and rifampicin may decrease exposure of the active metabolite (of temsirolimus), sirolimus, and should be avoided. If alternative treatment cannot be administered, a dose adjustment should be considered. St. John's Wort may decrease temsirolimus plasma concentrations unpredictably. Patients receiving temsirolimus should not take St. John's Wort concomitantly).
No products indexed under this heading.

Hydrocortisone Cypionate (Strong inducers of CYP3A4/5 such as dexamethasone, carbamazepine, phenytoin, phenobarbital, rifampin, rifabutin, and rifampicin may decrease exposure of the active metabolite (of temsirolimus), sirolimus, and should be avoided. If alternative treatment cannot be administered, a dose adjustment should be considered. St. John's Wort may decrease temsirolimus plasma concentrations unpredictably. Patients receiving temsirolimus should not take St. John's Wort concomitantly).
No products indexed under this heading.

Hydrocortisone Hemisuccinate (Strong inducers of CYP3A4/5 such as dexamethasone, carbamazepine, phenytoin, phenobarbital, rifampin, rifabutin, and rifampicin may decrease exposure of the active metabolite (of temsirolimus), sirolimus, and should be avoided. If alternative treatment cannot be administered, a dose adjustment should be considered. St. John's Wort may decrease temsirolimus plasma concentrations unpredictably. Patients receiving temsirolimus should not take St. John's Wort concomitantly).
No products indexed under this heading.

Hydrocortisone Probutate (Strong inducers of CYP3A4/5 such as dexamethasone, carbamazepine, phenytoin, phenobarbital, rifampin, rifabutin, and rifampicin may decrease exposure of the active metabolite (of temsirolimus), sirolimus, and should be avoided. If alternative treatment cannot be administered, a dose adjustment should be considered. St. John's Wort may decrease temsirolimus plasma concentrations unpredictably. Patients receiving temsirolimus should not take St. John's Wort concomitantly).
No products indexed under this heading.

Hydrocortisone Sodium Phosphate (Strong inducers of CYP3A4/5 such as dexamethasone, carbamazepine, phenytoin, phenobarbital, rifampin, rifabutin, and rifampicin may decrease exposure of the active metabolite (of temsirolimus), sirolimus, and should be avoided. If alternative treatment cannot be administered, a dose adjustment should be considered. St. John's Wort may decrease temsirolimus plasma concentrations unpredictably. Patients receiving temsirolimus should not take St. John's Wort concomitantly).
No products indexed under this heading.

Hydrocortisone Sodium Succinate (Strong inducers of CYP3A4/5 such as dexamethasone, carbamazepine, phenytoin, phenobarbital, rifampin, rifabutin, and rifampicin may decrease exposure of the active metabolite (of temsirolimus), sirolimus, and should be avoided. If alternative treatment cannot be administered, a dose adjustment should be considered. St. John's Wort may decrease temsirolimus plasma concentrations unpredictably. Patients receiving temsirolimus should not take St. John's Wort concomitantly).
No products indexed under this heading.

Hydrocortisone Valerate (Strong inducers of CYP3A4/5 such as dexamethasone, carbamazepine, phenytoin, phenobarbital, rifampin, rifabutin, and rifampicin may decrease exposure of the active metabolite (of temsirolimus), sirolimus, and should be avoided. If alternative treatment cannot be administered, a dose adjustment should be considered. St. John's Wort may decrease temsirolimus plasma concentrations unpredictably. Patients receiving temsirolimus should not take St. John's Wort concomitantly).
No products indexed under this heading.

Hypericum (Strong inducers of CYP3A4/5 such as dexamethasone, carbamazepine, phenytoin, phenobarbital, rifampin, rifabutin, and rifampicin may decrease exposure of the active metabolite (of temsirolimus), sirolimus, and should be avoided. If alternative treatment cannot be administered, a dose adjustment should be considered. St. John's Wort may decrease temsirolimus plasma concentrations unpredictably. Patients receiving temsirolimus should not take St. John's Wort concomitantly).
No products indexed under this heading.

Hypericum Perforatum (Strong inducers of CYP3A4/5 such as dexamethasone, carbamazepine, phenytoin,

IMPORTANT NOTE: Always consult each drug listing in the patient's regimen for possible interactions.

phenobarbital, rifampin, rifabutin, and rifampacin may decrease exposure of the active metabolite (of temsirolimus), sirolimus, and should be avoided. If alternative treatment cannot be administered, a dose adjustment should be considered. St. John's Wort may decrease temsirolimus plasma concentrations unpredictably. Patients receiving temsirolimus should not take St. John's Wort concomitantly). Products include:

Traumeel **1800**

Indinavir Sulfate (Strong CYP3A4 inhibitors such as atazanavir, clarithromycin, indinavir, itraconazole, ketoconazole, nefazodone, nelfinavir, ritonavir, saquinavir, and telithromycin may increase blood concentrations of the active metabolite (of temsirolimus), sirolimus, and should be avoided. If alternative treatments cannot be administered, a dose adjustment should be considered). Products include:

Crixivan **2113**

Influenza Vaccine, Live Attenuated (The use of live vaccines (eg, intranasal influenza, measles, mumps, rubella, oral polio, BCG, yellow fever, varicella, and TY21a typhoid vaccines) and close contact with those who have received live vaccines should be avoided during treatment with temsirolimus).

No products indexed under this heading.

Influenza Virus Vaccine Live, Intranasal (The use of live vaccines (eg, intranasal influenza, measles, mumps, rubella, oral polio, BCG, yellow fever, varicella, and TY21a typhoid vaccines) and close contact with those who have received live vaccines should be avoided during treatment with temsirolimus). Products include:

FluMist **2078**

Insulin (The use of temsirolimus is likely to result in increases in serum glucose. In a clinical trial, 89% of patients receiving temsirolimus had at least one elevated serum glucose while on treatment, and 26% of patients reported hyperglycemia as an adverse event. This may result in the need for an increase in the dose of, or initiation of, insulin and/or oral hypoglycemic agent therapy. Serum glucose should be tested before and during treatment with temsirolimus).

No products indexed under this heading.

Insulin, Human, Zinc Suspension (The use of temsirolimus is likely to result in increases in serum glucose. In a clinical trial, 89% of patients receiving temsirolimus had at least one elevated serum glucose while on treatment, and 26% of patients reported hyperglycemia as an adverse event. This may result in the need for an increase in the dose of, or initiation of, insulin and/or oral hypoglycemic agent therapy. Serum glucose should be tested before and during treatment with temsirolimus).

No products indexed under this heading.

Insulin, Human (rDNA origin) (The use of temsirolimus is likely to result in increases in serum glucose. In a clinical trial, 89% of patients receiving temsirolimus had at least one elevated serum glucose while on treatment, and 26% of patients reported hyperglycemia as an adverse event. This may result in the need for an increase in the dose of, or initiation of, insulin and/or oral hypoglycemic agent therapy. Serum glucose should be tested before and during treatment with temsirolimus). Products include:

Exubera **2717**

Insulin, Human NPH (The use of temsirolimus is likely to result in increases in serum glucose. In a clinical trial, 89% of patients receiving temsirolimus had at least one elevated serum glucose while on treatment, and 26% of patients reported hyperglycemia as an adverse event. This may result in the need for an increase in the dose of, or initiation of, insulin and/or oral hypoglycemic agent therapy. Serum glucose should be tested before and during treatment with temsirolimus). Products include:

Humulin N Vial **1934**

Insulin, Human Regular (The use of temsirolimus is likely to result in increases in serum glucose. In a clinical trial, 89% of patients receiving temsirolimus had at least one elevated serum glucose while on treatment, and 26% of patients reported hyperglycemia as an adverse event. This may result in the need for an increase in the dose of, or initiation of, insulin and/or oral hypoglycemic agent therapy. Serum glucose should be tested before and during treatment with temsirolimus). Products include:

Humulin R **1937**
Humulin R (U-500) **1939**

Insulin, Human Regular and Human NPH Mixture (The use of temsirolimus is likely to result in increases in serum glucose. In a clinical trial, 89% of patients receiving temsirolimus had at least one elevated serum glucose while on treatment, and 26% of patients reported hyperglycemia as an adverse event. This may result in the need for an increase in the dose of, or initiation of, insulin and/or oral hypoglycemic agent therapy. Serum glucose should be tested before and during treatment with temsirolimus). Products include:

Humulin 50/50 .... **1930**
Humulin 70/30 Vial **1931**

Insulin, NPH (The use of temsirolimus is likely to result in increases in serum glucose. In a clinical trial, 89% of patients receiving temsirolimus had at least one elevated serum glucose while on treatment, and 26% of patients reported hyperglycemia as an adverse event. This may result in the need for an increase in the dose of, or initiation of, insulin and/or oral hypoglycemic agent therapy. Serum glucose should be tested before and during treatment with temsirolimus).

No products indexed under this heading.

Insulin, Regular (The use of temsirolimus is likely to result in increases in serum glucose. In a clinical trial, 89% of patients receiving temsirolimus had at least one elevated serum glucose while on treatment, and 26% of patients reported hyperglycemia as an adverse event. This may result in the need for an increase in the dose of, or initiation of, insulin and/or oral hypoglycemic agent therapy. Serum glucose should be tested before and during treatment with temsirolimus).

No products indexed under this heading.

Insulin, Regular and NPH mixture (The use of temsirolimus is likely to result in increases in serum glucose. In a clinical trial, 89% of patients receiving temsirolimus had at least one elevated serum glucose while on treatment, and 26% of patients reported hyperglycemia as an adverse event. This may result in the need for an increase in the dose of, or initiation of, insulin and/or oral hypoglycemic agent therapy. Serum glucose should be tested before and during treatment with temsirolimus).

No products indexed under this heading.

Insulin, Zinc Crystals (The use of temsirolimus is likely to result in increases in serum glucose. In a clinical trial, 89% of patients receiving temsirolimus had at least one elevated serum glucose while on treatment, and 26% of patients reported hyperglycemia as an adverse event. This may result in the need for an increase in the dose of, or initiation of, insulin and/or oral hypoglycemic agent therapy. Serum glucose should be tested before and during treatment with temsirolimus).

No products indexed under this heading.

Insulin, Zinc Suspension (The use of temsirolimus is likely to result in increases in serum glucose. In a clinical trial, 89% of patients receiving temsirolimus had at least one elevated serum glucose while on treatment, and 26% of patients reported hyperglycemia as an adverse event. This may result in the need for an increase in the dose of, or initiation of, insulin and/or oral hypoglycemic agent therapy. Serum glucose should be tested before and during treatment with temsirolimus).

No products indexed under this heading.

Insulin Aspart (The use of temsirolimus is likely to result in increases in serum glucose. In a clinical trial, 89% of patients receiving temsirolimus had at least one elevated serum glucose while on treatment, and 26% of patients reported hyperglycemia as an adverse event. This may result in the need for an increase in the dose of, or initiation of, insulin and/or oral hypoglycemic agent therapy. Serum glucose should be tested before and during treatment with temsirolimus).

No products indexed under this heading.

Insulin Aspart, Human (The use of temsirolimus is likely to result in increases in serum glucose. In a clinical trial, 89% of patients receiving temsirolimus had at least one elevated serum glucose while on treatment, and 26% of patients reported hyperglycemia as an adverse event. This may result in the need for an increase in the dose of, or initiation of, insulin and/or oral hypoglycemic agent therapy. Serum glucose should be tested before and during treatment with temsirolimus). Products include:

NovoLog Mix 70/30 .... **2581**

Insulin Aspart, Human Regular (The use of temsirolimus is likely to result in increases in serum glucose. In a clinical trial, 89% of patients receiving temsirolimus had at least one elevated serum glucose while on treatment, and 26% of patients reported hyperglycemia as an adverse event. This may result in the need for an increase in the dose of, or initiation of, insulin and/or oral hypoglycemic agent therapy. Serum glucose should be tested before and during treatment with temsirolimus). Products include:

NovoLog **2575**

Insulin Aspart Protamine, Human (The use of temsirolimus is likely to result in increases in serum glucose. In a clinical trial, 89% of patients receiving temsirolimus had at least one elevated serum glucose while on treatment, and 26% of patients reported hyperglycemia as an adverse event. This may result in the need for an increase in the dose of, or initiation of, insulin and/or oral hypoglycemic agent therapy. Serum glucose should be tested before and during treatment with temsirolimus). Products include:

NovoLog Mix 70/30 .... **2581**

Insulin Detemir (rDNA Origin) (The use of temsirolimus is likely to result in increases in serum glucose. In a clinical trial, 89% of patients receiving temsirolimus had at least one elevated serum glucose while on treatment, and 26% of patients reported hyperglycemia as an adverse event. This may result in the need for an increase in the dose of, or initiation of, insulin and/or oral hypoglycemic agent therapy. Serum glucose should be tested before and during treatment with temsirolimus). Products include:

Levemir **2566**

Insulin Glargine (The use of temsirolimus is likely to result in increases in serum glucose. In a clinical trial, 89% of patients receiving temsirolimus had at least one elevated serum glucose while on treatment, and 26% of patients reported hyperglycemia as an adverse event. This may result in the need for an increase in the dose of, or initiation of, insulin and/or oral hypoglycemic agent therapy. Serum glucose should be tested before and during treatment with temsirolimus). Products include:

Lantus **2996**

Insulin Glulisine (The use of temsirolimus is likely to result in increases in serum glucose. In a clinical trial, 89% of patients receiving temsirolimus had at least one elevated serum glucose while on treatment, and 26% of patients reported hyperglycemia as an adverse event. This may result in the need for an increase in the dose of, or initiation of, insulin and/or oral hypoglycemic agent therapy. Serum glucose should be tested before and during treatment with temsirolimus). Products include:

Apidra **2937**
Apidra SoloStar **2937**

Insulin Lispro, Human (The use of temsirolimus is likely to result in increases in serum glucose. In a clinical trial, 89% of patients receiving temsirolimus had at least one elevated serum glucose while on treatment, and 26% of patients reported hyperglycemia as an adverse event. This may result in the need for an increase in the dose of, or initiation of, insulin and/or oral hypoglycemic agent therapy. Serum glucose should be tested before and during treatment with temsirolimus). Products include:

Humalog **1910**
Humalog Mix **1914**
Humalog Mix75/25 .... **1917**

Insulin Lispro Protamine, Human (The use of temsirolimus is likely to result in increases in serum glucose. In a clinical trial, 89% of patients receiving temsirolimus had at least one elevated serum glucose while on treatment, and 26% of patients reported hyperglycemia as an adverse event. This may result in the need for an increase in the dose of, or initiation of, insulin and/or oral hypoglycemic agent therapy. Serum glucose should be tested before and during treatment with temsirolimus). Products include:

Humalog Mix **1914**
Humalog Mix75/25 .... **1917**

Itraconazole (Strong CYP3A4 inhibitors such as atazanavir, clarithromycin, indinavir, itraconazole, ketoconazole, nefazodone, nelfinavir, ritonavir, saquinavir, and telithromycin may increase blood concentrations of the active metabolite (of temsirolimus), sirolimus, and should be avoided. If alternative treatments cannot be administered, a dose adjustment should be considered).

No products indexed under this heading.

Ketoconazole (Co-administration of temsirolimus with ketoconazole, a potent CYP3A4 inhibitor, had no significant effect on temsirolimus C_{max} or AUC; however, sirolimus AUC increased 3.1-fold, and C_{max} increased 2.2-fold compared to temsirolimus alone. If alternative treatment cannot be administered, a dose adjustment should be considered). Products include:

Extina **3319**
Xolegel **3337**

Lisinopril (Angioneurotic edema-type reactions have been observed in some patients who received temsirolimus and ACE inhibitors concomitantly). Products include:

Prinivil **2241**

1903 Interactions Index Torisel

Prinzide 2246

Lopinavir (Strong CYP3A4 inhibitors such as atazanavir, clarithromycin, indinavir, itraconazole, ketoconazole, nefazodone, nelfinavir, ritonavir, saquinavir, and telithromycin may increase blood concentrations of the active metabolite (of temsirolimus), sirolimus, and should be avoided. If alternative treatments cannot be administered, a dose adjustment should be considered). Products include:

Kaletra 458

Lovastatin (The use of temsirolimus is likely to result in increases in serum triglycerides and cholesterol. In a clinical trial, 87% of patients receiving temsirolimus had at least one elevated serum cholesterol value and 83% had at least one elevated serum triglyceride value. This may require initiation, or increase in the dose, of lipid-lowering agents). Products include:

Advicor 402
Mevacor 2212

Low Molecular Weight Heparins (Patients with central nervous system tumors (primary CNS tumor or metastases) and/or receiving anticoagulation therapy may be at an increased risk of developing intracerebral bleeding (including fatal outcomes) while receiving temsirolimus).

No products indexed under this heading.

Measles, Mumps, Rubella and Varicella Virus Vaccine Live (The use of live vaccines (eg, intranasal influenza, measles, mumps, rubella, oral polio, BCG, yellow fever, varicella, and TY21a typhoid vaccines) and close contact with those who have received live vaccines should be avoided during treatment with temsirolimus). Products include:

ProQuad 2254

Measles, Mumps & Rubella Virus Vaccine, Live (The use of live vaccines (eg, intranasal influenza, measles, mumps, rubella, oral polio, BCG, yellow fever, varicella, and TY21a typhoid vaccines) and close contact with those who have received live vaccines should be avoided during treatment with temsirolimus). Products include:

M-M-R II 2203
ProQuad 2254

Measles & Rubella Virus Vaccine Live (The use of live vaccines (eg, intranasal influenza, measles, mumps, rubella, oral polio, BCG, yellow fever, varicella, and TY21a typhoid vaccines) and close contact with those who have received live vaccines should be avoided during treatment with temsirolimus).

No products indexed under this heading.

Measles Virus Vaccine Live (The use of live vaccines (eg, intranasal influenza, measles, mumps, rubella, oral polio, BCG, yellow fever, varicella, and TY21a typhoid vaccines) and close contact with those who have received live vaccines should be avoided during treatment with temsirolimus). Products include:

Attenuvax 2086

Mephenytoin (Strong inducers of CYP3A4/5 such as dexamethasone, carbamazepine, phenytoin, phenobarbital, rifampin, rifabutin, and rifampicin may decrease exposure of the active metabolite (of temsirolimus), sirolimus, and should be avoided. If alternative treatment cannot be administered, a dose adjustment should be considered. St. John's Wort may decrease temsirolimus plasma concentrations unpredictably. Patients receiving temsirolimus should not take St. John's Wort concomitantly).

No products indexed under this heading.

Metformin Hydrochloride (The use of temsirolimus is likely to result in increases in serum glucose. In a clinical trial, 89% of patients receiving temsirolimus had at least one elevated serum glucose while on treatment, and 26% of patients reported hyperglycemia as an adverse event. This may result in the need for an increase in the dose of, or initiation of, insulin and/or oral hypoglycemic agent therapy. Serum glucose should be tested before and during treatment with temsirolimus). Products include:

ActoPlus 3338
Avandamet 1345
Janumet 2188

Methsuximide (Strong inducers of CYP3A4/5 such as dexamethasone, carbamazepine, phenytoin, phenobarbital, rifampin, rifabutin, and rifampicin may decrease exposure of the active metabolite (of temsirolimus), sirolimus, and should be avoided. If alternative treatment cannot be administered, a dose adjustment should be considered. St. John's Wort may decrease temsirolimus plasma concentrations unpredictably. Patients receiving temsirolimus should not take St. John's Wort concomitantly).

No products indexed under this heading.

Methylprednisolone (Strong inducers of CYP3A4/5 such as dexamethasone, carbamazepine, phenytoin, phenobarbital, rifampin, rifabutin, and rifampicin may decrease exposure of the active metabolite (of temsirolimus), sirolimus, and should be avoided. If alternative treatment cannot be administered, a dose adjustment should be considered. St. John's Wort may decrease temsirolimus plasma concentrations unpredictably. Patients receiving temsirolimus should not take St. John's Wort concomitantly).

No products indexed under this heading.

Methylprednisolone Acetate (Strong inducers of CYP3A4/5 such as dexamethasone, carbamazepine, phenytoin, phenobarbital, rifampin, rifabutin, and rifampicin may decrease exposure of the active metabolite (of temsirolimus), sirolimus, and should be avoided. If alternative treatment cannot be administered, a dose adjustment should be considered. St. John's Wort may decrease temsirolimus plasma concentrations unpredictably. Patients receiving temsirolimus should not take St. John's Wort concomitantly).

No products indexed under this heading.

Methylprednisolone Sodium Succinate (Strong inducers of CYP3A4/5 such as dexamethasone, carbamazepine, phenytoin, phenobarbital, rifampin, rifabutin, and rifampicin may decrease exposure of the active metabolite (of temsirolimus), sirolimus, and should be avoided. If alternative treatment cannot be administered, a dose adjustment should be considered. St. John's Wort may decrease temsirolimus plasma concentrations unpredictably. Patients receiving temsirolimus should not take St. John's Wort concomitantly).

No products indexed under this heading.

Miglitol (The use of temsirolimus is likely to result in increases in serum glucose. In a clinical trial, 89% of patients receiving temsirolimus had at least one elevated serum glucose while on treatment, and 26% of patients reported hyperglycemia as an adverse event. This may result in the need for an increase in the dose of, or initiation of, insulin and/or oral hypoglycemic agent therapy. Serum glucose should be tested before and during treatment with temsirolimus).

No products indexed under this heading.

Modafinil (Strong inducers of CYP3A4/5 such as dexamethasone, carbamazepine, phenytoin, phenobarbital, rifampin, rifabutin, and rifampicin may decrease exposure of the active metabolite (of temsirolimus), sirolimus, and should be avoided. If alternative treatment cannot be administered, a dose adjustment should be considered. St. John's Wort may decrease temsirolimus plasma concentrations unpredictably. Patients receiving temsirolimus should not take St. John's Wort concomitantly). Products include:

Provigil 983

Moexipril Hydrochloride (Angioneurotic edema-type reactions have been observed in some patients who received temsirolimus and ACE inhibitors concomitantly).

No products indexed under this heading.

Mumps Virus Vaccine, Live (The use of live vaccines (eg, intranasal influenza, measles, mumps, rubella, oral polio, BCG, yellow fever, varicella, and TY21a typhoid vaccines) and close contact with those who have received live vaccines should be avoided during treatment with temsirolimus). Products include:

Mumpsvax 2218

Nafcillin Sodium (Strong inducers of CYP3A4/5 such as dexamethasone, carbamazepine, phenytoin, phenobarbital, rifampin, rifabutin, and rifampicin may decrease exposure of the active metabolite (of temsirolimus), sirolimus, and should be avoided. If alternative treatment cannot be administered, a dose adjustment should be considered. St. John's Wort may decrease temsirolimus plasma concentrations unpredictably. Patients receiving temsirolimus should not take St. John's Wort concomitantly).

No products indexed under this heading.

Nateglinide (The use of temsirolimus is likely to result in increases in serum glucose. In a clinical trial, 89% of patients receiving temsirolimus had at least one elevated serum glucose while on treatment, and 26% of patients reported hyperglycemia as an adverse event. This may result in the need for an increase in the dose of, or initiation of, insulin and/or oral hypoglycemic agent therapy. Serum glucose should be tested before and during treatment with temsirolimus).

No products indexed under this heading.

Nefazodone Hydrochloride (Strong CYP3A4 inhibitors such as atazanavir, clarithromycin, indinavir, itraconazole, ketoconazole, nefazodone, nelfinavir, ritonavir, saquinavir, and telithromycin may increase blood concentrations of the active metabolite (of temsirolimus), sirolimus, and should be avoided. If alternative treatments cannot be administered, a dose adjustment should be considered).

No products indexed under this heading.

Nelfinavir Mesylate (Strong CYP3A4 inhibitors such as atazanavir, clarithromycin, indinavir, itraconazole, ketoconazole, nefazodone, nelfinavir, ritonavir, saquinavir, and telithromycin may increase blood concentrations of the active metabolite (of temsirolimus), sirolimus, and should be avoided. If alternative treatments cannot be administered, a dose adjustment should be considered).

No products indexed under this heading.

Nevirapine (Strong inducers of CYP3A4/5 such as dexamethasone, carbamazepine, phenytoin, phenobarbital, rifampin, rifabutin, and rifampicin may decrease exposure of the active metabolite (of temsirolimus), sirolimus, and should be avoided. If alternative treatment cannot be administered, a dose adjustment should be considered. St. John's Wort may decrease temsirolimus plasma concentrations unpredictably. Patients receiving temsirolimus should not take St. John's Wort concomitantly). Products include:

Viramune Oral Suspension 897
Viramune Tablets 897

Oxcarbazepine (Strong inducers of CYP3A4/5 such as dexamethasone, carbamazepine, phenytoin, phenobarbital, rifampin, rifabutin, and rifampicin may decrease exposure of the active metabolite (of temsirolimus), sirolimus, and should be avoided. If alternative treatment cannot be administered, a dose adjustment should be considered. St. John's Wort may decrease temsirolimus plasma concentrations unpredictably. Patients receiving temsirolimus should not take St. John's Wort concomitantly).

No products indexed under this heading.

Perindopril Erbumine (Angioneurotic edema-type reactions have been observed in some patients who received temsirolimus and ACE inhibitors concomitantly).

No products indexed under this heading.

Phenobarbital (Strong inducers of CYP3A4/5 such as dexamethasone, carbamazepine, phenytoin, phenobarbital, rifampin, rifabutin, and rifampicin may decrease exposure of the active metabolite (of temsirolimus), sirolimus, and should be avoided. If alternative treatment cannot be administered, a dose adjustment should be considered). Products include:

Donnatal 2711

Phenobarbital Sodium (Strong inducers of CYP3A4/5 such as dexamethasone, carbamazepine, phenytoin, phenobarbital, rifampin, rifabutin, and rifampicin may decrease exposure of the active metabolite (of temsirolimus), sirolimus, and should be avoided. If alternative treatment cannot be administered, a dose adjustment should be considered).

No products indexed under this heading.

Phenytoin (Strong inducers of CYP3A4/5 such as phenytoin may decrease exposure of the active metabolite (of temsirolimus), sirolimus, and should be avoided. If alternative treatment cannot be administered, a dose adjustment should be considered).

No products indexed under this heading.

Phenytoin Sodium (Strong inducers of CYP3A4/5 such as phenytoin may decrease exposure of the active metabolite (of temsirolimus), sirolimus, and should be avoided. If alternative treatment cannot be administered, a dose adjustment should be considered). Products include:

Phenytek Capsules 2380

Pioglitazone Hydrochloride (The use of temsirolimus is likely to result in increases in serum glucose. In a clinical trial, 89% of patients receiving temsirolimus had at least one elevated serum glucose while on treatment, and 26% of patients reported hyperglycemia as an adverse event. This may result in the need for an increase in the dose of, or initiation of, insulin and/or oral hypoglycemic agent therapy. Serum glucose should be tested before and during treatment with temsirolimus). Products include:

ActoPlus 3338
Actos 3345
Duetact 3354

Poliovirus Vaccine, Live, Oral, Trivalent, Types 1,2,3 (Sabin) (The use of live vaccines (eg, intranasal influenza, measles, mumps, rubella, oral polio, BCG, yellow fever, varicella, and TY21a typhoid vaccines) and close contact with those who have received live vaccines should be avoided during treatment with temsirolimus).

No products indexed under this heading.

Pravastatin Sodium (The use of temsirolimus is likely to result in increases in serum triglycerides and cholesterol. In a clinical trial, 87% of patients receiving temsirolimus had at least one elevated serum cholesterol value and 83% had at least one elevated serum triglyceride value. This may require initiation, or increase in the dose, of lipid-lowering agents).

No products indexed under this heading.

Prednisolone (Strong inducers of CYP3A4/5 such as dexamethasone, carbamazepine, phenytoin, phenobarbital, rifampin, rifabutin, and rifampicin may decrease exposure of the active metabolite (of temsirolimus), sirolimus, and should be avoided. If alternative treatment cannot be administered, a dose adjustment should be considered. St. John's Wort may decrease temsirolimus plasma concentrations unpredictably. Patients receiving temsirolimus should not take St. John's Wort concomitantly).

No products indexed under this heading.

Prednisolone Acetate (Strong inducers of CYP3A4/5 such as dexamethasone, carbamazepine, phenytoin, phenobarbital, rifampin, rifabutin, and rifampicin may decrease exposure of the active metabolite (of temsirolimus), sirolimus, and should be avoided. If alternative treatment cannot be administered, a dose adjustment should be considered. St. John's Wort may decrease temsirolimus plasma concentrations unpredictably. Patients receiving temsirolimus should not take St. John's Wort concomitantly). Products include:

Blephamide	⊙212, ⊙214
Pred Forte	⊙225
Pred Mild	⊙230
Pred-G	⊙226, ⊙227

Prednisolone Sodium Phosphate (Strong inducers of CYP3A4/5 such as dexamethasone, carbamazepine, phenytoin, phenobarbital, rifampin, rifabutin, and rifampicin may decrease exposure of the active metabolite (of temsirolimus), sirolimus, and should be avoided. If alternative treatment cannot be administered, a dose adjustment should be considered. St. John's Wort may decrease temsirolimus plasma concentrations unpredictably. Patients receiving temsirolimus should not take St. John's Wort concomitantly).

No products indexed under this heading.

Prednisolone Tebutate (Strong inducers of CYP3A4/5 such as dexamethasone, carbamazepine, phenytoin, phenobarbital, rifampin, rifabutin, and rifampicin may decrease exposure of the active metabolite (of temsirolimus), sirolimus, and should be avoided. If alternative treatment cannot be administered, a dose adjustment should be considered. St. John's Wort may decrease temsirolimus plasma concentrations unpredictably. Patients receiving temsirolimus should not take St. John's Wort concomitantly).

No products indexed under this heading.

Prednisone (Strong inducers of CYP3A4/5 such as dexamethasone, carbamazepine, phenytoin, phenobarbital, rifampin, rifabutin, and rifampicin may decrease exposure of the active metabolite (of temsirolimus), sirolimus, and should be avoided. If alternative treatment cannot be administered, a dose adjustment should be considered. St. John's Wort may decrease temsirolimus plasma concentrations unpredictably. Patients receiving temsirolimus should not take St. John's Wort concomitantly).

No products indexed under this heading.

Prednisone sodium phosphate (Strong inducers of CYP3A4/5 such as dexamethasone, carbamazepine, phen-

ytoin, phenobarbital, rifampin, rifabutin, and rifampicin may decrease exposure of the active metabolite (of temsirolimus), sirolimus, and should be avoided. If alternative treatment cannot be administered, a dose adjustment should be considered. St. John's Wort may decrease temsirolimus plasma concentrations unpredictably. Patients receiving temsirolimus should not take St. John's Wort concomitantly).

No products indexed under this heading.

Primidone (Strong inducers of CYP3A4/5 such as dexamethasone, carbamazepine, phenytoin, phenobarbital, rifampin, rifabutin, and rifampicin may decrease exposure of the active metabolite (of temsirolimus), sirolimus, and should be avoided. If alternative treatment cannot be administered, a dose adjustment should be considered. St. John's Wort may decrease temsirolimus plasma concentrations unpredictably. Patients receiving temsirolimus should not take St. John's Wort concomitantly).

No products indexed under this heading.

Probucol (The use of temsirolimus is likely to result in increases in serum triglycerides and cholesterol. In a clinical trial, 87% of patients receiving temsirolimus had at least one elevated serum cholesterol value and 83% had at least one elevated serum triglyceride value. This may require initiation, or increase in the dose, of lipid-lowering agents).

No products indexed under this heading.

Quinapril Hydrochloride (Angioneurotic edema-type reactions have been observed in some patients who received temsirolimus and ACE inhibitors concomitantly).

No products indexed under this heading.

Ramipril (Angioneurotic edema-type reactions have been observed in some patients who received temsirolimus and ACE inhibitors concomitantly).

No products indexed under this heading.

Repaglinide (The use of temsirolimus is likely to result in increases in serum glucose. In a clinical trial, 89% of patients receiving temsirolimus had at least one elevated serum glucose while on treatment, and 26% of patients reported hyperglycemia as an adverse event. This may result in the need for an increase in the dose of, or initiation of, insulin and/or oral hypoglycemic agent therapy. Serum glucose should be tested before and during treatment with temsirolimus).

No products indexed under this heading.

Rifabutin (Strong inducers of CYP3A4/5 such as dexamethasone, carbamazepine, phenytoin, phenobarbital, rifampin, rifabutin, and rifampicin may decrease exposure of the active metabolite (of temsirolimus), sirolimus, and should be avoided. If alternative treatment cannot be administered, a dose adjustment should be considered).

No products indexed under this heading.

Rifampicin (Strong inducers of CYP3A4/5 such as dexamethasone, carbamazepine, phenytoin, phenobarbital, rifampin, rifabutin, and rifampicin may decrease exposure of the active metabolite (of temsirolimus), sirolimus, and should be avoided. If alternative treatment cannot be administered, a dose adjustment should be considered).

No products indexed under this heading.

Rifampin (Co-administration of temsirolimus with rifampin, a potent CYP3A4/5 inducer, had no significant effect on temsirolimus C_{max} (maximum concentration) and AUC (area under the concentration versus the time curve) after intravenous administration, but decreased sirolimus C_{max} by 65% and AUC by 56% compared to temsirolimus

treatment alone. If alternative treatment cannot be administered, a dose adjustment should be considered).

No products indexed under this heading.

Rifapentine (Strong inducers of CYP3A4/5 such as dexamethasone, carbamazepine, phenytoin, phenobarbital, rifampin, rifabutin, and rifampicin may decrease exposure of the active metabolite (of temsirolimus), sirolimus, and should be avoided. If alternative treatment cannot be administered, a dose adjustment should be considered. St. John's Wort may decrease temsirolimus plasma concentrations unpredictably. Patients receiving temsirolimus should not take St. John's Wort concomitantly).

No products indexed under this heading.

Ritonavir (Strong CYP3A4 inhibitors such as atazanavir, clarithromycin, indinavir, itraconazole, ketoconazole, nefazodone, nelfinavir, ritonavir, saquinavir, and telithromycin may increase blood concentrations of the active metabolite (of temsirolimus), sirolimus, and should be avoided. If alternative treatments cannot be administered, a dose adjustment should be considered). Products include:

| Kaletra | 458 |
| Norvir | 509 |

Rosiglitazone Maleate (The use of temsirolimus is likely to result in increases in serum glucose. In a clinical trial, 89% of patients receiving temsirolimus had at least one elevated serum glucose while on treatment, and 26% of patients reported hyperglycemia as an adverse event. This may result in the need for an increase in the dose of, or initiation of, insulin and/or oral hypoglycemic agent therapy. Serum glucose should be tested before and during treatment with temsirolimus). Products include:

Avandamet	1345
Avandaryl	1356
Avandia	1366

Rotavirus Vaccine, Live, Oral, Tetravalent (The use of live vaccines (eg, intranasal influenza, measles, mumps, rubella, oral polio, BCG, yellow fever, varicella, and TY21a typhoid vaccines) and close contact with those who have received live vaccines should be avoided during treatment with temsirolimus).

No products indexed under this heading.

Rubella & Mumps Virus Vaccine Live (The use of live vaccines (eg, intranasal influenza, measles, mumps, rubella, oral polio, BCG, yellow fever, varicella, and TY21a typhoid vaccines) and close contact with those who have received live vaccines should be avoided during treatment with temsirolimus).

No products indexed under this heading.

Rubella Virus Vaccine Live (The use of live vaccines (eg, intranasal influenza, measles, mumps, rubella, oral polio, BCG, yellow fever, varicella, and TY21a typhoid vaccines) and close contact with those who have received live vaccines should be avoided during treatment with temsirolimus). Products include:

| Meruvax II | 2210 |

Saquinavir (Strong CYP3A4 inhibitors such as atazanavir, clarithromycin, indinavir, itraconazole, ketoconazole, nefazodone, nelfinavir, ritonavir, saquinavir, and telithromycin may increase blood concentrations of the active metabolite (of temsirolimus), sirolimus, and should be avoided. If alternative treatments cannot be administered, a dose adjustment should be considered).

No products indexed under this heading.

Saquinavir Mesylate (Strong CYP3A4 inhibitors such as atazanavir, clarithromycin, indinavir, itraconazole, ketoconazole, nefazodone, nelfinavir, ritonavir, saquinavir, and telithromycin may increase blood concentrations of the active metabolite (of temsirolimus), sirolimus, and should be avoided. If alternative treatments cannot be administered, a dose adjustment should be considered).

No products indexed under this heading.

Simvastatin (The use of temsirolimus is likely to result in increases in serum triglycerides and cholesterol. In a clinical trial, 87% of patients receiving temsirolimus had at least one elevated serum cholesterol value and 83% had at least one elevated serum triglyceride value. This may require initiation, or increase in the dose, of lipid-lowering agents). Products include:

Simcor	524
Vytorin 10/10	2303, 3240
Vytorin 10/20	2303, 3240
Vytorin 10/40	2303, 3240
Vytorin 10/80	2303, 3240
Zocor	2289

Sitagliptin Phosphate (The use of temsirolimus is likely to result in increases in serum glucose. In a clinical trial, 89% of patients receiving temsirolimus had at least one elevated serum glucose while on treatment, and 26% of patients reported hyperglycemia as an adverse event. This may result in the need for an increase in the dose of, or initiation of, insulin and/or oral hypoglycemic agent therapy. Serum glucose should be tested before and during treatment with temsirolimus). Products include:

| Janumet | 2188 |
| Januvia | 2196 |

Smallpox Vaccine (The use of live vaccines (eg, intranasal influenza, measles, mumps, rubella, oral polio, BCG, yellow fever, varicella, and TY21a typhoid vaccines) and close contact with those who have received live vaccines should be avoided during treatment with temsirolimus).

No products indexed under this heading.

Spirapril Hydrochloride (Angioneurotic edema-type reactions have been observed in some patients who received temsirolimus and ACE inhibitors concomitantly).

No products indexed under this heading.

Sulfinpyrazone (Strong inducers of CYP3A4/5 such as dexamethasone, carbamazepine, phenytoin, phenobarbital, rifampin, rifabutin, and rifampicin may decrease exposure of the active metabolite (of temsirolimus), sirolimus, and should be avoided. If alternative treatment cannot be administered, a dose adjustment should be considered. St. John's Wort may decrease temsirolimus plasma concentrations unpredictably. Patients receiving temsirolimus should not take St. John's Wort concomitantly).

No products indexed under this heading.

Sunitinib (The combination of temsirolimus and sunitinib resulted in dose-limiting toxicity. Dose-limiting toxicities (Grade 3/4 erythematous maculopapular rash, and gout/cellulitis requiring hospitalization) were observed in two out of three patients treated in the first cohort of a phase 1 study at doses of temsirolimus 15 mg IV per week and sunitinib 25 mg oral per day (Days 1-28 followed by a 2-week rest)).

No products indexed under this heading.

Telithromycin (Strong CYP3A4 inhibitors such as atazanavir, clarithromycin, indinavir, itraconazole, ketoconazole, nefazodone, nelfinavir, ritonavir, saquinavir, and telithromycin may increase blood concentrations of the

active metabolite (of temsirolimus), sirolimus, and should be avoided. If alternative treatments cannot be administered, a dose adjustment should be considered). Products include:
Ketek 2991

Theophyllinate (Strong inducers of CYP3A4/5 such as dexamethasone, carbamazepine, phenytoin, phenobarbital, rifampin, rifabutin, and rifampicin may decrease exposure of the active metabolite (of temsirolimus), sirolimus, and should be avoided. If alternative treatment cannot be administered, a dose adjustment should be considered. St. John's Wort may decrease temsirolimus plasma concentrations unpredictably. Patients receiving temsirolimus should not take St. John's Wort concomitantly).
No products indexed under this heading.

Theophylline (Strong inducers of CYP3A4/5 such as dexamethasone, carbamazepine, phenytoin, phenobarbital, rifampin, rifabutin, and rifampicin may decrease exposure of the active metabolite (of temsirolimus), sirolimus, and should be avoided. If alternative treatment cannot be administered, a dose adjustment should be considered. St. John's Wort may decrease temsirolimus plasma concentrations unpredictably. Patients receiving temsirolimus should not take St. John's Wort concomitantly).
No products indexed under this heading.

Theophylline Anhydrous (Strong inducers of CYP3A4/5 such as dexamethasone, carbamazepine, phenytoin, phenobarbital, rifampin, rifabutin, and rifampicin may decrease exposure of the active metabolite (of temsirolimus), sirolimus, and should be avoided. If alternative treatment cannot be administered, a dose adjustment should be considered. St. John's Wort may decrease temsirolimus plasma concentrations unpredictably. Patients receiving temsirolimus should not take St. John's Wort concomitantly). Products include:
Uniphyl 2817

Theophylline Calcium Salicylate (Strong inducers of CYP3A4/5 such as dexamethasone, carbamazepine, phenytoin, phenobarbital, rifampin, rifabutin, and rifampicin may decrease exposure of the active metabolite (of temsirolimus), sirolimus, and should be avoided. If alternative treatment cannot be administered, a dose adjustment should be considered. St. John's Wort may decrease temsirolimus plasma concentrations unpredictably. Patients receiving temsirolimus should not take St. John's Wort concomitantly).
No products indexed under this heading.

Theophylline Dihydroxypropyl (Glyceryl) (Strong inducers of CYP3A4/5 such as dexamethasone, carbamazepine, phenytoin, phenobarbital, rifampin, rifabutin, and rifampicin may decrease exposure of the active metabolite (of temsirolimus), sirolimus, and should be avoided. If alternative treatment cannot be administered, a dose adjustment should be considered. St. John's Wort may decrease temsirolimus plasma concentrations unpredictably. Patients receiving temsirolimus should not take St. John's Wort concomitantly).
No products indexed under this heading.

Theophylline Ethylenediamine (Strong inducers of CYP3A4/5 such as dexamethasone, carbamazepine, phenytoin, phenobarbital, rifampin, rifabutin, and rifampicin may decrease exposure of the active metabolite (of temsirolimus), sirolimus, and should be avoided. If alternative treatment cannot be administered, a dose adjustment should be considered. St. John's Wort may decrease temsirolimus plasma concentrations unpredictably. Patients receiving temsirolimus should not take St. John's Wort concomitantly).
No products indexed under this heading.

Theophylline Sodium Glycinate (Strong inducers of CYP3A4/5 such as dexamethasone, carbamazepine, phenytoin, phenobarbital, rifampin, rifabutin, and rifampicin may decrease exposure of the active metabolite (of temsirolimus), sirolimus, and should be avoided. If alternative treatment cannot be administered, a dose adjustment should be considered. St. John's Wort may decrease temsirolimus plasma concentrations unpredictably. Patients receiving temsirolimus should not take St. John's Wort concomitantly).
No products indexed under this heading.

Tinzaparin Sodium (Patients with central nervous system tumors (primary CNS tumor or metastases) and/or receiving anticoagulation therapy may be at an increased risk of developing intracerebral bleeding (including fatal outcomes) while receiving temsirolimus).
No products indexed under this heading.

Tolazamide (The use of temsirolimus is likely to result in increases in serum glucose. In a clinical trial, 89% of patients receiving temsirolimus had at least one elevated serum glucose while on treatment, and 26% of patients reported hyperglycemia as an adverse event. This may result in the need for an increase in the dose of, or initiation of, insulin and/or oral hypoglycemic agent therapy. Serum glucose should be tested before and during treatment with temsirolimus).
No products indexed under this heading.

Tolbutamide (The use of temsirolimus is likely to result in increases in serum glucose. In a clinical trial, 89% of patients receiving temsirolimus had at least one elevated serum glucose while on treatment, and 26% of patients reported hyperglycemia as an adverse event. This may result in the need for an increase in the dose of, or initiation of, insulin and/or oral hypoglycemic agent therapy. Serum glucose should be tested before and during treatment with temsirolimus).
No products indexed under this heading.

Trandolapril (Angioneurotic edema-type reactions have been observed in some patients who received temsirolimus and ACE inhibitors concomitantly). Products include:
Mavik 489
Tarka 534

Triamcinolone (Strong inducers of CYP3A4/5 such as dexamethasone, carbamazepine, phenytoin, phenobarbital, rifampin, rifabutin, and rifampicin may decrease exposure of the active metabolite (of temsirolimus), sirolimus, and should be avoided. If alternative treatment cannot be administered, a dose adjustment should be considered. St. John's Wort may decrease temsirolimus plasma concentrations unpredictably. Patients receiving temsirolimus should not take St. John's Wort concomitantly).
No products indexed under this heading.

Triamcinolone Acetonide (Strong inducers of CYP3A4/5 such as dexamethasone, carbamazepine, phenytoin, phenobarbital, rifampin, rifabutin, and rifampicin may decrease exposure of the active metabolite (of temsirolimus), sirolimus, and should be avoided. If alternative treatment cannot be administered, a dose adjustment should be considered. St. John's Wort may decrease temsirolimus plasma concentrations unpredictably. Patients receiving temsirolimus should not take St. John's Wort concomitantly). Products include:
Azmacort 408
Nasacort AQ 3019

Triamcinolone Diacetate (Strong inducers of CYP3A4/5 such as dexamethasone, carbamazepine, phenytoin, phenobarbital, rifampin, rifabutin, and rifampicin may decrease exposure of the active metabolite (of temsirolimus), sirolimus, and should be avoided. If alternative treatment cannot be administered, a dose adjustment should be considered. St. John's Wort may decrease temsirolimus plasma concentrations unpredictably. Patients receiving temsirolimus should not take St. John's Wort concomitantly).
No products indexed under this heading.

Triamcinolone Hexacetonide (Strong inducers of CYP3A4/5 such as dexamethasone, carbamazepine, phenytoin, phenobarbital, rifampin, rifabutin, and rifampicin may decrease exposure of the active metabolite (of temsirolimus), sirolimus, and should be avoided. If alternative treatment cannot be administered, a dose adjustment should be considered. St. John's Wort may decrease temsirolimus plasma concentrations unpredictably. Patients receiving temsirolimus should not take St. John's Wort concomitantly).
No products indexed under this heading.

Troglitazone (Strong inducers of CYP3A4/5 such as dexamethasone, carbamazepine, phenytoin, phenobarbital, rifampin, rifabutin, and rifampicin may decrease exposure of the active metabolite (of temsirolimus), sirolimus, and should be avoided. If alternative treatment cannot be administered, a dose adjustment should be considered. St. John's Wort may decrease temsirolimus plasma concentrations unpredictably. Patients receiving temsirolimus should not take St. John's Wort concomitantly).
No products indexed under this heading.

Troleandomycin (Strong CYP3A4 inhibitors such as atazanavir, clarithromycin, indinavir, itraconazole, ketoconazole, nefazodone, nelfinavir, ritonavir, saquinavir, and telithromycin may increase blood concentrations of the active metabolite (of temsirolimus), sirolimus, and should be avoided. If alternative treatments cannot be administered, a dose adjustment should be considered).
No products indexed under this heading.

Typhoid Vaccine (The use of live vaccines (eg, intranasal influenza, measles, mumps, rubella, oral polio, BCG, yellow fever, varicella, and TY21a typhoid vaccines) and close contact with those who have received live vaccines should be avoided during treatment with temsirolimus).
No products indexed under this heading.

Varicella Virus Vaccine, Live (The use of live vaccines (eg, intranasal influenza, measles, mumps, rubella, oral polio, BCG, yellow fever, varicella, and TY21a typhoid vaccines) and close contact with those who have received live vaccines should be avoided during treatment with temsirolimus). Products include:
Varivax 2285

Voriconazole (Strong CYP3A4 inhibitors such as voriconazole may increase blood concentrations of the active metabolite (of temsirolimus), sirolimus, and should be avoided. If alternative treatments cannot be administered, a dose adjustment should be considered).
No products indexed under this heading.

Warfarin Sodium (Patients with central nervous system tumors (primary CNS tumor or metastases) and/or receiving anticoagulation therapy may be at an increased risk of developing intracerebral bleeding (including fatal outcomes) while receiving temsirolimus).
No products indexed under this heading.

Yellow Fever Vaccine (The use of live vaccines (eg, intranasal influenza, measles, mumps, rubella, oral polio, BCG, yellow fever, varicella, and TY21a typhoid vaccines) and close contact with those who have received live vaccines should be avoided during treatment with temsirolimus).
No products indexed under this heading.

Zoster Vaccine Live (The use of live vaccines (eg, intranasal influenza, measles, mumps, rubella, oral polio, BCG, yellow fever, varicella, and TY21a typhoid vaccines) and close contact with those who have received live vaccines should be avoided during treatment with temsirolimus). Products include:
Zostavax 2299

Food Interactions

Grapefruit Juice (Grapefruit juice may increase plasma concentrations of sirolimus (a major metabolite of temsirolimus) and should be avoided).

TOVIAZ EXTENDED-RELEASE TABLETS

(Fesoterodine Fumarate) 2753
May interact with alcohols, antimuscarinic drugs, cytochrome p450 2d6 inhibitors (selected), cytochrome p450 3a4 inducers (selected), cytochrome p450 3a4 inhibitors (selected), cytochrome p450 3a4 inhibitors, potent (selected), erythromycin, and certain other agents. Compounds in these categories include:

Acetazolamide (In patients taking weak or moderate CYP3A4 inhibitors, careful assessment of tolerability at the 4 mg daily dose is advised prior to increasing the daily dose to 8 mg. While this specific interaction potential was not examined by clinical study, some pharmacokinetic interaction is expected).
No products indexed under this heading.

Acetazolamide Sodium (In patients taking weak or moderate CYP3A4 inhibitors, careful assessment of tolerability at the 4 mg daily dose is advised prior to increasing the daily dose to 8 mg. While this specific interaction potential was not examined by clinical study, some pharmacokinetic interaction is expected).
No products indexed under this heading.

Allium sativum (Induction of CYP3A4 may lead to reduced plasma levels. No dosing adjustments are recommended in the presence of CYP3A4 inducers).
No products indexed under this heading.

Aminoglutethimide (Induction of CYP3A4 may lead to reduced plasma levels. No dosing adjustments are recommended in the presence of CYP3A4 inducers).
No products indexed under this heading.

Amiodarone Hydrochloride (In patients taking weak or moderate CYP3A4 inhibitors, careful assessment of tolerability at the 4 mg daily dose is advised prior to increasing the daily dose to 8 mg. While this specific interaction potential was not examined by clinical study, some pharmacokinetic interaction is expected).
No products indexed under this heading.

Amitriptyline Hydrochloride (The interaction with CYP2D6 inhibitors was not tested clinically. In poor metabolizers for CYP2D6, representing a maximum CYP2D6 inhibition, C_{max} and AUC of active metabolite are increased at 1.7 and 2-fold, respectively. No dosing adjustments are recommended in the presence of CYP2D6 inhibitors).
No products indexed under this heading.

Amoxapine (The interaction with CYP2D6 inhibitors was not tested clinically. In poor metabolizers for CYP2D6, representing a maximum CYP2D6 inhibition, C_{max} and AUC of active metabolite are increased at 1.7 and 2-fold, respectively. No dosing adjustments are recommended in the presence of CYP2D6 inhibitors).
No products indexed under this heading.

Amprenavir (Following blockade of CYP3A4 by co-administration of the potent CYP3A4 inhibitor ketoconazole 200 mg bid for 5 days, C_{max} and AUC of the active metabolite of fesoterodine increased 2.0- and 2.3-fold, respectively, after oral administration of fesoterodine 8 mg to CYP2D6 extensive metabolizers. In CYP2D6 poor metabolizers, C_{max} and AUC of the active metabolite of fesoterodine increased 2.1- and 2.5-fold, respectively, during co-administration of ketoconazole 200 mg bid for 5 days. C_{max} and AUC were 4.5- and 5.7-fold higher, respectively, in subjects who were CYP2D6 poor metabolizers and taking ketoconazole compared to subjects who were CYP2D6 extensive metabolizers and not taking ketoconazole. Therefore, doses of fesoterodine greater than 4 mg are not recommended in patients taking potent CYP3A4 inhibitors).
No products indexed under this heading.

Anastrozole (In patients taking weak or moderate CYP3A4 inhibitors, careful assessment of tolerability at the 4 mg daily dose is advised prior to increasing the daily dose to 8 mg. While this specific interaction potential was not examined by clinical study, some pharmacokinetic interaction is expected).
No products indexed under this heading.

Aprepitant (In patients taking weak or moderate CYP3A4 inhibitors, careful assessment of tolerability at the 4 mg daily dose is advised prior to increasing the daily dose to 8 mg. While this specific interaction potential was not examined by clinical study, some pharmacokinetic interaction is expected).
Products include:
Emend 2124

Atazanavir (Following blockade of CYP3A4 by co-administration of the potent CYP3A4 inhibitor ketoconazole 200 mg bid for 5 days, C_{max} and AUC of the active metabolite of fesoterodine increased 2.0- and 2.3-fold, respectively, after oral administration of fesoterodine 8 mg to CYP2D6 extensive metabolizers. In CYP2D6 poor metabolizers, C_{max} and AUC of the active metabolite of fesoterodine increased 2.1- and 2.5-fold, respectively, during co-administration of ketoconazole 200 mg bid for 5 days. C_{max} and AUC were 4.5- and 5.7-fold higher, respectively, in subjects who were CYP2D6 poor metabolizers and taking ketoconazole compared to subjects who were CYP2D6 extensive metabolizers and not taking ketoconazole. Therefore, doses of fesoterodine greater than 4 mg are not recommended in patients taking potent CYP3A4 inhibitors).
No products indexed under this heading.

Atazanavir Sulfate (Following blockade of CYP3A4 by co-administration of the potent CYP3A4 inhibitor ketoconazole 200 mg bid for 5 days, C_{max} and AUC of the active metabolite of fesoterodine increased 2.0- and 2.3-fold, respectively, after oral administration of fesoterodine 8 mg to CYP2D6 extensive metabolizers. In CYP2D6 poor metabolizers, C_{max} and AUC of the active metabolite of fesoterodine increased 2.1- and 2.5-fold, respectively, during co-administration of ketoconazole 200 mg bid for 5 days. C_{max} and AUC were 4.5- and 5.7-fold higher, respectively, in subjects who were CYP2D6 poor metabolizers and taking ketoconazole compared to subjects who were CYP2D6 extensive metabolizers and not taking ketoconazole. Therefore, doses of fesoterodine greater than 4 mg are not recommended in patients taking potent CYP3A4 inhibitors).
No products indexed under this heading.

Atropine Sulfate (Co-administration of fesoterodine with other antimuscarinic agents that produce dry mouth, constipation, urinary retention, and other anticholinergic pharmacological effects may increase the frequency and/or severity of such effects). Products include:
Donnatal 2711

Belladonna Alkaloids (Co-administration of fesoterodine with other antimuscarinic agents that produce dry mouth, constipation, urinary retention, and other anticholinergic pharmacological effects may increase the frequency and/or severity of such effects).
Products include:
Hyland's Teething Tablets 3316

Betamethasone (Induction of CYP3A4 may lead to reduced plasma levels. No dosing adjustments are recommended in the presence of CYP3A4 inducers).
No products indexed under this heading.

Betamethasone Acetate (Induction of CYP3A4 may lead to reduced plasma levels. No dosing adjustments are recommended in the presence of CYP3A4 inducers).
No products indexed under this heading.

Betamethasone Benzoate (Induction of CYP3A4 may lead to reduced plasma levels. No dosing adjustments are recommended in the presence of CYP3A4 inducers).
No products indexed under this heading.

Betamethasone Dipropionate (Induction of CYP3A4 may lead to reduced plasma levels. No dosing adjustments are recommended in the presence of CYP3A4 inducers).
Products include:
Diprolene Lotion 0.05% 3108
Diprolene Ointment 0.05% 3109
Diprolene AF Cream 0.05% 3107
Lotrisone 3163

Betamethasone Sodium Phosphate (Induction of CYP3A4 may lead to reduced plasma levels. No dosing adjustments are recommended in the presence of CYP3A4 inducers).
No products indexed under this heading.

Betamethasone Valerate (Induction of CYP3A4 may lead to reduced plasma levels. No dosing adjustments are recommended in the presence of CYP3A4 inducers). Products include:
Luxíq 3321

Bosentan (Induction of CYP3A4 may lead to reduced plasma levels. No dosing adjustments are recommended in the presence of CYP3A4 inducers).
Products include:
Tracleer 573

Bupropion Hydrochloride (The interaction with CYP2D6 inhibitors was not tested clinically. In poor metabolizers for CYP2D6, representing a maximum CYP2D6 inhibition, C_{max} and AUC of active metabolite are increased at 1.7 and 2-fold, respectively. No dosing adjustments are recommended in the presence of CYP2D6 inhibitors).
Products include:
Aplenzin 2948
Wellbutrin 1719
Wellbutrin SR 1725
Zyban 1762

Carbamazepine (Induction of CYP3A4 may lead to reduced plasma levels. No dosing adjustments are recommended in the presence of CYP3A4 inducers). Products include:
Carbatrol 3280
Equetro 3477

Celecoxib (The interaction with CYP2D6 inhibitors was not tested clinically. In poor metabolizers for CYP2D6, representing a maximum CYP2D6 inhibition, C_{max} and AUC of active metabolite are increased at 1.7 and 2-fold, respectively. No dosing adjustments are recommended in the presence of CYP2D6 inhibitors). Products include:
Celebrex 3272

Chloroquine (The interaction with CYP2D6 inhibitors was not tested clinically. In poor metabolizers for CYP2D6, representing a maximum CYP2D6 inhibition, C_{max} and AUC of active metabolite are increased at 1.7 and 2-fold, respectively. No dosing adjustments are recommended in the presence of CYP2D6 inhibitors).
No products indexed under this heading.

Chloroquine Hydrochloride (The interaction with CYP2D6 inhibitors was not tested clinically. In poor metabolizers for CYP2D6, representing a maximum CYP2D6 inhibition, C_{max} and AUC of active metabolite are increased at 1.7 and 2-fold, respectively. No dosing adjustments are recommended in the presence of CYP2D6 inhibitors).
No products indexed under this heading.

Chloroquine Phosphate (The interaction with CYP2D6 inhibitors was not tested clinically. In poor metabolizers for CYP2D6, representing a maximum CYP2D6 inhibition, C_{max} and AUC of active metabolite are increased at 1.7 and 2-fold, respectively. No dosing adjustments are recommended in the presence of CYP2D6 inhibitors).
No products indexed under this heading.

Chlorpheniramine (The interaction with CYP2D6 inhibitors was not tested clinically. In poor metabolizers for CYP2D6, representing a maximum CYP2D6 inhibition, C_{max} and AUC of active metabolite are increased at 1.7 and 2-fold, respectively. No dosing adjustments are recommended in the presence of CYP2D6 inhibitors).
No products indexed under this heading.

Chlorpheniramine Maleate (The interaction with CYP2D6 inhibitors was not tested clinically. In poor metabolizers for CYP2D6, representing a maximum CYP2D6 inhibition, C_{max} and AUC of active metabolite are increased at 1.7 and 2-fold, respectively. No dosing adjustments are recommended in the presence of CYP2D6 inhibitors).
No products indexed under this heading.

Chlorpheniramine Polistirex (The interaction with CYP2D6 inhibitors was not tested clinically. In poor metabolizers for CYP2D6, representing a maximum CYP2D6 inhibition, C_{max} and AUC of active metabolite are increased at 1.7 and 2-fold, respectively. No dosing adjustments are recommended in the presence of CYP2D6 inhibitors).
Products include:
Tussionex 3443

Chlorpheniramine Tannate (The interaction with CYP2D6 inhibitors was not tested clinically. In poor metabolizers for CYP2D6, representing a maximum CYP2D6 inhibition, C_{max} and AUC of active metabolite are increased at 1.7 and 2-fold, respectively. No dosing adjustments are recommended in the presence of CYP2D6 inhibitors).
No products indexed under this heading.

Cimetidine (In patients taking weak or moderate CYP3A4 inhibitors, careful assessment of tolerability at the 4 mg daily dose is advised prior to increasing the daily dose to 8 mg. While this specific interaction potential was not examined by clinical study, some pharmacokinetic interaction is expected).
No products indexed under this heading.

Cimetidine Hydrochloride (In patients taking weak or moderate CYP3A4 inhibitors, careful assessment of tolerability at the 4 mg daily dose is advised prior to increasing the daily dose to 8 mg. While this specific interaction potential was not examined by clinical study, some pharmacokinetic interaction is expected).
No products indexed under this heading.

Ciprofloxacin (In patients taking weak or moderate CYP3A4 inhibitors, careful assessment of tolerability at the 4 mg daily dose is advised prior to increasing the daily dose to 8 mg. While this specific interaction potential was not examined by clinical study, some pharmacokinetic interaction is expected).
Products include:
Cipro I.V. 3082
Cipro 3073
Cipro XR 3091
Ciprodex 583

Ciprofloxacin Hydrochloride (Induction of CYP3A4 may lead to reduced plasma levels. No dosing adjustments are recommended in the presence of CYP3A4 inducers). Products include:
Cipro 3073

Cisplatin (Induction of CYP3A4 may lead to reduced plasma levels. No dosing adjustments are recommended in the presence of CYP3A4 inducers).
No products indexed under this heading.

Citalopram Hydrobromide (The interaction with CYP2D6 inhibitors was not tested clinically. In poor metabolizers for CYP2D6, representing a maximum CYP2D6 inhibition, C_{max} and AUC of active metabolite are increased at 1.7 and 2-fold, respectively. No dosing adjustments are recommended in the presence of CYP2D6 inhibitors).
Products include:
Celexa 1153

Clarithromycin (Following blockade of CYP3A4 by co-administration of the potent CYP3A4 inhibitor ketoconazole 200 mg bid for 5 days, C_{max} and AUC of the active metabolite of fesoterodine increased 2.0- and 2.3-fold, respectively, after oral administration of fesoterodine 8 mg to CYP2D6 extensive metabolizers. In CYP2D6 poor metabolizers, C_{max} and AUC of the active metabolite of fesoterodine increased 2.1- and 2.5-fold, respectively, during co-administration of ketoconazole 200 mg bid for 5 days. C_{max} and AUC were 4.5- and 5.7-fold higher, respectively, in subjects who were CYP2D6 poor metabolizers and taking ketoconazole compared to subjects who were CYP2D6 extensive metabolizers and not taking ketoconazole. Therefore, doses of fesoterodine greater than 4 mg are not recommended in patients taking potent CYP3A4 inhibitors such as clarithromycin). Products include:
Biaxin/Biaxin XL 412

1907 Interactions Index Toviaz

Clidinium Bromide (Co-administration of fesoterodine with other antimuscarinic agents that produce dry mouth, constipation, urinary retention, and other anticholinergic pharmacological effects may increase the frequency and/or severity of such effects).
No products indexed under this heading.

Clomipramine Hydrochloride (The interaction with CYP2D6 inhibitors was not tested clinically. In poor metabolizers for CYP2D6, representing a maximum CYP2D6 inhibition, C_{max} and AUC of active metabolite are increased at 1.7 and 2-fold, respectively. No dosing adjustments are recommended in the presence of CYP2D6 inhibitors).
No products indexed under this heading.

Clotrimazole (In patients taking weak or moderate CYP3A4 inhibitors, careful assessment of tolerability at the 4 mg daily dose is advised prior to increasing the daily dose to 8 mg. While this specific interaction potential was not examined by clinical study, some pharmacokinetic interaction is expected). Products include:
Lotrisone 3163

Cocaine Hydrochloride (The interaction with CYP2D6 inhibitors was not tested clinically. In poor metabolizers for CYP2D6, representing a maximum CYP2D6 inhibition, C_{max} and AUC of active metabolite are increased at 1.7 and 2-fold, respectively. No dosing adjustments are recommended in the presence of CYP2D6 inhibitors).
No products indexed under this heading.

Conivaptan Hydrochloride (In patients taking weak or moderate CYP3A4 inhibitors, careful assessment of tolerability at the 4 mg daily dose is advised prior to increasing the daily dose to 8 mg. While this specific interaction potential was not examined by clinical study, some pharmacokinetic interaction is expected). Products include:
Vaprisol 689

Cortisone Acetate (Induction of CYP3A4 may lead to reduced plasma levels. No dosing adjustments are recommended in the presence of CYP3A4 inducers).
No products indexed under this heading.

Cyclosporine (In patients taking weak or moderate CYP3A4 inhibitors, careful assessment of tolerability at the 4 mg daily dose is advised prior to increasing the daily dose to 8 mg. While this specific interaction potential was not examined by clinical study, some pharmacokinetic interaction is expected).
Products include:
Gengraf 440
Neoral Oral Solution 2496
Neoral Capsules 2496
Restasis 605

Dalfopristin (In patients taking weak or moderate CYP3A4 inhibitors, careful assessment of tolerability at the 4 mg daily dose is advised prior to increasing the daily dose to 8 mg. While this specific interaction potential was not examined by clinical study, some pharmacokinetic interaction is expected).
No products indexed under this heading.

Danazol (In patients taking weak or moderate CYP3A4 inhibitors, careful assessment of tolerability at the 4 mg daily dose is advised prior to increasing the daily dose to 8 mg. While this specific interaction potential was not examined by clinical study, some pharmacokinetic interaction is expected).
No products indexed under this heading.

Darunavir (In patients taking weak or moderate CYP3A4 inhibitors, careful assessment of tolerability at the 4 mg daily dose is advised prior to increasing the daily dose to 8 mg. While this specific interaction potential was not examined by clinical study, some pharmacokinetic interaction is expected).
No products indexed under this heading.

Dasatinib (In patients taking weak or moderate CYP3A4 inhibitors, careful assessment of tolerability at the 4 mg daily dose is advised prior to increasing the daily dose to 8 mg. While this specific interaction potential was not examined by clinical study, some pharmacokinetic interaction is expected).
No products indexed under this heading.

Delavirdine Mesylate (Following blockade of CYP3A4 by co-administration of the potent CYP3A4 inhibitor ketoconazole 200 mg bid for 5 days, C_{max} and AUC of the active metabolite of fesoterodine increased 2.0- and 2.3-fold, respectively, after oral administration of fesoterodine 8 mg to CYP2D6 extensive metabolizers. In CYP2D6 poor metabolizers, C_{max} and AUC of the active metabolite of fesoterodine increased 2.1- and 2.5-fold, respectively, during co-administration of ketoconazole 200 mg bid for 5 days. C_{max} and AUC were 4.5- and 5.7-fold higher, respectively, in subjects who were CYP2D6 poor metabolizers and taking ketoconazole compared to subjects who were CYP2D6 extensive metabolizers and not taking ketoconazole. Therefore, doses of fesoterodine greater than 4 mg are not recommended in patients taking potent CYP3A4 inhibitors).
No products indexed under this heading.

Delavirine (Following blockade of CYP3A4 by co-administration of the potent CYP3A4 inhibitor ketoconazole 200 mg bid for 5 days, C_{max} and AUC of the active metabolite of fesoterodine increased 2.0- and 2.3-fold, respectively, after oral administration of fesoterodine 8 mg to CYP2D6 extensive metabolizers. In CYP2D6 poor metabolizers, C_{max} and AUC of the active metabolite of fesoterodine increased 2.1- and 2.5-fold, respectively, during co-administration of ketoconazole 200 mg bid for 5 days. C_{max} and AUC were 4.5- and 5.7-fold higher, respectively, in subjects who were CYP2D6 poor metabolizers and taking ketoconazole compared to subjects who were CYP2D6 extensive metabolizers and not taking ketoconazole. Therefore, doses of fesoterodine greater than 4 mg are not recommended in patients taking potent CYP3A4 inhibitors).
No products indexed under this heading.

Desipramine Hydrochloride (The interaction with CYP2D6 inhibitors was not tested clinically. In poor metabolizers for CYP2D6, representing a maximum CYP2D6 inhibition, C_{max} and AUC of active metabolite are increased at 1.7 and 2-fold, respectively. No dosing adjustments are recommended in the presence of CYP2D6 inhibitors).
No products indexed under this heading.

Desloratadine (In patients taking weak or moderate CYP3A4 inhibitors, careful assessment of tolerability at the 4 mg daily dose is advised prior to increasing the daily dose to 8 mg. While this specific interaction potential was not examined by clinical study, some pharmacokinetic interaction is expected). Products include:
Clarinex Syrup 3098
Clarinex 3098
Clarinex Reditabs 3098
Clarinex-D 12-Hour 3101
Clarinex-D 3104

Dexamethasone (Induction of CYP3A4 may lead to reduced plasma levels. No dosing adjustments are recommended in the presence of CYP3A4 inducers). Products include:
Ciprodex 583
Ozurdex .... ⊙223
Tobramycin and Dexamethasone Ophthalmic Suspension .... ⊙251

Dexamethasone Acetate (Induction of CYP3A4 may lead to reduced plasma levels. No dosing adjustments are recommended in the presence of CYP3A4 inducers).
No products indexed under this heading.

Dexamethasone Phosphate (Induction of CYP3A4 may lead to reduced plasma levels. No dosing adjustments are recommended in the presence of CYP3A4 inducers).
No products indexed under this heading.

Dexamethasone Sodium (Induction of CYP3A4 may lead to reduced plasma levels. No dosing adjustments are recommended in the presence of CYP3A4 inducers).
No products indexed under this heading.

Dexamethasone Sodium Phosphate (Induction of CYP3A4 may lead to reduced plasma levels. No dosing adjustments are recommended in the presence of CYP3A4 inducers).
No products indexed under this heading.

Dexamethasone Sodium Phosphate Injection (Induction of CYP3A4 may lead to reduced plasma levels. No dosing adjustments are recommended in the presence of CYP3A4 inducers).
No products indexed under this heading.

Dicyclomine Hydrochloride (Co-administration of fesoterodine with other antimuscarinic agents that produce dry mouth, constipation, urinary retention, and other anticholinergic pharmacological effects may increase the frequency and/or severity of such effects).
Products include:
Bentyl Capsules 780
Bentyl Injection 780
Bentyl Syrup 780
Bentyl Tablets 780

Diltiazem Hydrochloride (In patients taking weak or moderate CYP3A4 inhibitors, careful assessment of tolerability at the 4 mg daily dose is advised prior to increasing the daily dose to 8 mg. While this specific interaction potential was not examined by clinical study, some pharmacokinetic interaction is expected). Products include:
Cardizem LA 423

Diltiazem Maleate (In patients taking weak or moderate CYP3A4 inhibitors, careful assessment of tolerability at the 4 mg daily dose is advised prior to increasing the daily dose to 8 mg. While this specific interaction potential was not examined by clinical study, some pharmacokinetic interaction is expected).
No products indexed under this heading.

Diphenhydramine (The interaction with CYP2D6 inhibitors was not tested clinically. In poor metabolizers for CYP2D6, representing a maximum CYP2D6 inhibition, C_{max} and AUC of active metabolite are increased at 1.7 and 2-fold, respectively. No dosing adjustments are recommended in the presence of CYP2D6 inhibitors).
No products indexed under this heading.

Diphenhydramine Hydrochloride (The interaction with CYP2D6 inhibitors was not tested clinically. In poor metabolizers for CYP2D6, representing a maximum CYP2D6 inhibition, C_{max} and AUC of active metabolite are increased at 1.7 and 2-fold, respectively. No dosing adjustments are recommended in the presence of CYP2D6 inhibitors). Products include:
Benadryl Allergy Ultratab 2042
Children's Benadryl Allergy Liquid 2042

Doxepin Hydrochloride (The interaction with CYP2D6 inhibitors was not tested clinically. In poor metabolizers for CYP2D6, representing a maximum CYP2D6 inhibition, C_{max} and AUC of active metabolite are increased at 1.7 and 2-fold, respectively. No dosing adjustments are recommended in the presence of CYP2D6 inhibitors).
No products indexed under this heading.

Doxorubicin Hydrochloride (Induction of CYP3A4 may lead to reduced plasma levels. No dosing adjustments are recommended in the presence of CYP3A4 inducers).
No products indexed under this heading.

Drugs, unspecified (Anticholinergic agents may potentially alter the absorption of some concomitantly administered drugs due to anticholinergic effects on gastrointestinal motility).
No products indexed under this heading.

Efavirenz (In patients taking weak or moderate CYP3A4 inhibitors, careful assessment of tolerability at the 4 mg daily dose is advised prior to increasing the daily dose to 8 mg. While this specific interaction potential was not examined by clinical study, some pharmacokinetic interaction is expected).
Products include:
Atripla 906

Erythromycin (In patients taking weak or moderate CYP3A4 inhibitors (eg, erythromycin), careful assessment of tolerability at the 4 mg daily dose is advised prior to increasing the daily dose to 8 mg. While this specific interaction potential was not examined by clinical study, some pharmacokinetic interaction is expected).
No products indexed under this heading.

Erythromycin, Topical (In patients taking weak or moderate CYP3A4 inhibitors (eg, erythromycin), careful assessment of tolerability at the 4 mg daily dose is advised prior to increasing the daily dose to 8 mg. While this specific interaction potential was not examined by clinical study, some pharmacokinetic interaction is expected).
No products indexed under this heading.

Erythromycin Estolate (In patients taking weak or moderate CYP3A4 inhibitors (eg, erythromycin), careful assessment of tolerability at the 4 mg daily dose is advised prior to increasing the daily dose to 8 mg. While this specific interaction potential was not examined by clinical study, some pharmacokinetic interaction is expected).
No products indexed under this heading.

Erythromycin Ethylsuccinate (In patients taking weak or moderate CYP3A4 inhibitors (eg, erythromycin), careful assessment of tolerability at the 4 mg daily dose is advised prior to increasing the daily dose to 8 mg. While this specific interaction potential was not examined by clinical study, some pharmacokinetic interaction is expected). Products include:
E.E.S. 437
EryPed 435

Erythromycin Gluceptate (In patients taking weak or moderate CYP3A4 inhibitors (eg, erythromycin), careful assessment of tolerability at the 4 mg daily dose is advised prior to increasing the daily dose to 8 mg. While this specific interaction potential was not examined by clinical study, some pharmacokinetic interaction is expected).
No products indexed under this heading.

IMPORTANT NOTE: Always consult each drug listing in the patient's regimen for possible interactions.

Erythromycin Lactobionate (In patients taking weak or moderate CYP3A4 inhibitors (eg, erythromycin), careful assessment of tolerability at the 4 mg daily dose is advised prior to increasing the daily dose to 8 mg. While this specific interaction potential was not examined by clinical study, some pharmacokinetic interaction is expected).
No products indexed under this heading.

Erythromycin Stearate (In patients taking weak or moderate CYP3A4 inhibitors (eg, erythromycin), careful assessment of tolerability at the 4 mg daily dose is advised prior to increasing the daily dose to 8 mg. While this specific interaction potential was not examined by clinical study, some pharmacokinetic interaction is expected).
No products indexed under this heading.

Escitalopram Oxalate (The interaction with CYP2D6 inhibitors was not tested clinically. In poor metabolizers for CYP2D6, representing a maximum CYP2D6 inhibition, C_{max} and AUC of active metabolite are increased at 1.7 and 2-fold, respectively. No dosing adjustments are recommended in the presence of CYP2D6 inhibitors).
Products include:
Lexapro Oral Suspension 1160
Lexapro Tablets 1160

Esomeprazole Magnesium (In patients taking weak or moderate CYP3A4 inhibitors, careful assessment of tolerability at the 4 mg daily dose is advised prior to increasing the daily dose to 8 mg. While this specific interaction potential was not examined by clinical study, some pharmacokinetic interaction is expected). Products include:
Nexium Capsules 704
Nexium Oral Suspension 704

Esomeprazole Sodium (In patients taking weak or moderate CYP3A4 inhibitors, careful assessment of tolerability at the 4 mg daily dose is advised prior to increasing the daily dose to 8 mg. While this specific interaction potential was not examined by clinical study, some pharmacokinetic interaction is expected). Products include:
Nexium I.V. 712

Ethanol (Concomitant use with alcohol may enhance the drowsiness caused by fesoterodine).
No products indexed under this heading.

Ethosuximide (Induction of CYP3A4 may lead to reduced plasma levels. No dosing adjustments are recommended in the presence of CYP3A4 inducers).
No products indexed under this heading.

Ethyl Alcohol (Concomitant use with alcohol may enhance the drowsiness caused by fesoterodine).
No products indexed under this heading.

Felbamate (Induction of CYP3A4 may lead to reduced plasma levels. No dosing adjustments are recommended in the presence of CYP3A4 inducers).
No products indexed under this heading.

Fluconazole (In patients taking weak or moderate CYP3A4 inhibitors, careful assessment of tolerability at the 4 mg daily dose is advised prior to increasing the daily dose to 8 mg. While this specific interaction potential was not examined by clinical study, some pharmacokinetic interaction is expected).
No products indexed under this heading.

Fludrocortisone Acetate (Induction of CYP3A4 may lead to reduced plasma levels. No dosing adjustments are recommended in the presence of CYP3A4 inducers).
No products indexed under this heading.

Fluoxetine (In patients taking weak or moderate CYP3A4 inhibitors, careful assessment of tolerability at the 4 mg daily dose is advised prior to increasing the daily dose to 8 mg. While this specific interaction potential was not examined by clinical study, some pharmacokinetic interaction is expected).
No products indexed under this heading.

Fluoxetine Hydrochloride (In patients taking weak or moderate CYP3A4 inhibitors, careful assessment of tolerability at the 4 mg daily dose is advised prior to increasing the daily dose to 8 mg. While this specific interaction potential was not examined by clinical study, some pharmacokinetic interaction is expected). Products include:
Prozac Weekly 1941
Prozac Pulvules 1941
Symbyax 1965

Fluphenazine Decanoate (The interaction with CYP2D6 inhibitors was not tested clinically. In poor metabolizers for CYP2D6, representing a maximum CYP2D6 inhibition, C_{max} and AUC of active metabolite are increased at 1.7 and 2-fold, respectively. No dosing adjustments are recommended in the presence of CYP2D6 inhibitors).
No products indexed under this heading.

Fluphenazine Enanthate (The interaction with CYP2D6 inhibitors was not tested clinically. In poor metabolizers for CYP2D6, representing a maximum CYP2D6 inhibition, C_{max} and AUC of active metabolite are increased at 1.7 and 2-fold, respectively. No dosing adjustments are recommended in the presence of CYP2D6 inhibitors).
No products indexed under this heading.

Fluphenazine Hydrochloride (The interaction with CYP2D6 inhibitors was not tested clinically. In poor metabolizers for CYP2D6, representing a maximum CYP2D6 inhibition, C_{max} and AUC of active metabolite are increased at 1.7 and 2-fold, respectively. No dosing adjustments are recommended in the presence of CYP2D6 inhibitors).
No products indexed under this heading.

Fluvoxamine Maleate (In patients taking weak or moderate CYP3A4 inhibitors, careful assessment of tolerability at the 4 mg daily dose is advised prior to increasing the daily dose to 8 mg. While this specific interaction potential was not examined by clinical study, some pharmacokinetic interaction is expected).
No products indexed under this heading.

Fosamprenavir Calcium (Following blockade of CYP3A4 by co-administration of the potent CYP3A4 inhibitor ketoconazole 200 mg bid for 5 days, C_{max} and AUC of the active metabolite of fesoterodine increased 2.0- and 2.3-fold, respectively, after oral administration of fesoterodine 8 mg to CYP2D6 extensive metabolizers. In CYP2D6 poor metabolizers, C_{max} and AUC of the active metabolite of fesoterodine increased 2.1- and 2.5-fold, respectively, during co-administration of ketoconazole 200 mg bid for 5 days. C_{max} and AUC were 4.5- and 5.7-fold higher, respectively, in subjects who were CYP2D6 poor metabolizers and taking ketoconazole compared to subjects who were CYP2D6 extensive metabolizers and not taking ketoconazole. Therefore, doses of fesoterodine greater than 4 mg are not recommended in patients taking potent CYP3A4 inhibitors). Products include:
Lexiva Oral Suspension 1558
Lexiva 1558

Fosphenytoin Sodium (Induction of CYP3A4 may lead to reduced plasma levels. No dosing adjustments are recommended in the presence of CYP3A4 inducers).
No products indexed under this heading.

Garlic Extract (Induction of CYP3A4 may lead to reduced plasma levels. No dosing adjustments are recommended in the presence of CYP3A4 inducers).
No products indexed under this heading.

Garlic Oil (Induction of CYP3A4 may lead to reduced plasma levels. No dosing adjustments are recommended in the presence of CYP3A4 inducers).
No products indexed under this heading.

Glycopyrrolate (Co-administration of fesoterodine with other antimuscarinic agents that produce dry mouth, constipation, urinary retention, and other anticholinergic pharmacological effects may increase the frequency and/or severity of such effects).
No products indexed under this heading.

Halofantrine Hydrochloride (The interaction with CYP2D6 inhibitors was not tested clinically. In poor metabolizers for CYP2D6, representing a maximum CYP2D6 inhibition, C_{max} and AUC of active metabolite are increased at 1.7 and 2-fold, respectively. No dosing adjustments are recommended in the presence of CYP2D6 inhibitors).
No products indexed under this heading.

Haloperidol (The interaction with CYP2D6 inhibitors was not tested clinically. In poor metabolizers for CYP2D6, representing a maximum CYP2D6 inhibition, C_{max} and AUC of active metabolite are increased at 1.7 and 2-fold, respectively. No dosing adjustments are recommended in the presence of CYP2D6 inhibitors).
No products indexed under this heading.

Haloperidol Decanoate (The interaction with CYP2D6 inhibitors was not tested clinically. In poor metabolizers for CYP2D6, representing a maximum CYP2D6 inhibition, C_{max} and AUC of active metabolite are increased at 1.7 and 2-fold, respectively. No dosing adjustments are recommended in the presence of CYP2D6 inhibitors).
No products indexed under this heading.

Haloperidol Lactate (The interaction with CYP2D6 inhibitors was not tested clinically. In poor metabolizers for CYP2D6, representing a maximum CYP2D6 inhibition, C_{max} and AUC of active metabolite are increased at 1.7 and 2-fold, respectively. No dosing adjustments are recommended in the presence of CYP2D6 inhibitors).
No products indexed under this heading.

Hydrocortisone (Induction of CYP3A4 may lead to reduced plasma levels. No dosing adjustments are recommended in the presence of CYP3A4 inducers).
No products indexed under this heading.

Hydrocortisone (Alcohol) (Induction of CYP3A4 may lead to reduced plasma levels. No dosing adjustments are recommended in the presence of CYP3A4 inducers).
No products indexed under this heading.

Hydrocortisone Acetate (Induction of CYP3A4 may lead to reduced plasma levels. No dosing adjustments are recommended in the presence of CYP3A4 inducers).
No products indexed under this heading.

Hydrocortisone Butyrate (Induction of CYP3A4 may lead to reduced plasma levels. No dosing adjustments are recommended in the presence of CYP3A4 inducers).
No products indexed under this heading.

Hydrocortisone Cypionate (Induction of CYP3A4 may lead to reduced plasma levels. No dosing adjustments are recommended in the presence of CYP3A4 inducers).
No products indexed under this heading.

Hydrocortisone Hemisuccinate (Induction of CYP3A4 may lead to reduced plasma levels. No dosing adjustments are recommended in the presence of CYP3A4 inducers).
No products indexed under this heading.

Hydrocortisone Probutate (Induction of CYP3A4 may lead to reduced plasma levels. No dosing adjustments are recommended in the presence of CYP3A4 inducers).
No products indexed under this heading.

Hydrocortisone Sodium Phosphate (Induction of CYP3A4 may lead to reduced plasma levels. No dosing adjustments are recommended in the presence of CYP3A4 inducers).
No products indexed under this heading.

Hydrocortisone Sodium Succinate (Induction of CYP3A4 may lead to reduced plasma levels. No dosing adjustments are recommended in the presence of CYP3A4 inducers).
No products indexed under this heading.

Hydrocortisone Valerate (Induction of CYP3A4 may lead to reduced plasma levels. No dosing adjustments are recommended in the presence of CYP3A4 inducers).
No products indexed under this heading.

Hydroxychloroquine Sulfate (The interaction with CYP2D6 inhibitors was not tested clinically. In poor metabolizers for CYP2D6, representing a maximum CYP2D6 inhibition, C_{max} and AUC of active metabolite are increased at 1.7 and 2-fold, respectively. No dosing adjustments are recommended in the presence of CYP2D6 inhibitors).
No products indexed under this heading.

Hyoscyamine (Co-administration of fesoterodine with other antimuscarinic agents that produce dry mouth, constipation, urinary retention, and other anticholinergic pharmacological effects may increase the frequency and/or severity of such effects).
No products indexed under this heading.

Hyoscyamine Sulfate (Co-administration of fesoterodine with other antimuscarinic agents that produce dry mouth, constipation, urinary retention, and other anticholinergic pharmacological effects may increase the frequency and/or severity of such effects).
Products include:
Donnatal 2711

Hypericum (Induction of CYP3A4 may lead to reduced plasma levels. No dosing adjustments are recommended in the presence of CYP3A4 inducers).
No products indexed under this heading.

Hypericum Perforatum (Induction of CYP3A4 may lead to reduced plasma levels. No dosing adjustments are recommended in the presence of CYP3A4 inducers). Products include:
Traumeel 1800

Imatinib Mesylate (In patients taking weak or moderate CYP3A4 inhibitors, careful assessment of tolerability at the 4 mg daily dose is advised prior to increasing the daily dose to 8 mg. While this specific interaction potential was not examined by clinical study, some pharmacokinetic interaction is expected). Products include:
Gleevec 2477

1909 **Interactions Index** **Toviaz**

Imipramine Hydrochloride (The interaction with CYP2D6 inhibitors was not tested clinically. In poor metabolizers for CYP2D6, representing a maximum CYP2D6 inhibition, C_{max} and AUC of active metabolite are increased at 1.7 and 2-fold, respectively. No dosing adjustments are recommended in the presence of CYP2D6 inhibitors).
No products indexed under this heading.

Imipramine Pamoate (The interaction with CYP2D6 inhibitors was not tested clinically. In poor metabolizers for CYP2D6, representing a maximum CYP2D6 inhibition, C_{max} and AUC of active metabolite are increased at 1.7 and 2-fold, respectively. No dosing adjustments are recommended in the presence of CYP2D6 inhibitors).
No products indexed under this heading.

Indinavir Sulfate (Following blockade of CYP3A4 by co-administration of the potent CYP3A4 inhibitor ketoconazole 200 mg bid for 5 days, C_{max} and AUC of the active metabolite of fesoterodine increased 2.0- and 2.3-fold, respectively, after oral administration of fesoterodine 8 mg to CYP2D6 extensive metabolizers. In CYP2D6 poor metabolizers, C_{max} and AUC of the active metabolite of fesoterodine increased 2.1- and 2.5-fold, respectively, during co-administration of ketoconazole 200 mg bid for 5 days. C_{max} and AUC were 4.5- and 5.7-fold higher, respectively, in subjects who were CYP2D6 poor metabolizers and taking ketoconazole compared to subjects who were CYP2D6 extensive metabolizers and not taking ketoconazole. Therefore, doses of fesoterodine greater than 4 mg are not recommended in patients taking potent CYP3A4 inhibitors). Products include:
Crixivan **2113**

Ipratropium Bromide (Co-administration of fesoterodine with other antimuscarinic agents that produce dry mouth, constipation, urinary retention, and other anticholinergic pharmacological effects may increase the frequency and/or severity of such effects).
No products indexed under this heading.

Isoniazid (In patients taking weak or moderate CYP3A4 inhibitors, careful assessment of tolerability at the 4 mg daily dose is advised prior to increasing the daily dose to 8 mg. While this specific interaction potential was not examined by clinical study, some pharmacokinetic interaction is expected).
No products indexed under this heading.

Itraconazole (Following blockade of CYP3A4 by co-administration of the potent CYP3A4 inhibitor ketoconazole 200 mg bid for 5 days, C_{max} and AUC of the active metabolite of fesoterodine increased 2.0- and 2.3-fold, respectively, after oral administration of fesoterodine 8 mg to CYP2D6 extensive metabolizers. In CYP2D6 poor metabolizers, C_{max} and AUC of the active metabolite of fesoterodine increased 2.1- and 2.5-fold, respectively, during co-administration of ketoconazole 200 mg bid for 5 days. C_{max} and AUC were 4.5- and 5.7-fold higher, respectively, in subjects who were CYP2D6 poor metabolizers and taking ketoconazole compared to subjects who were CYP2D6 extensive metabolizers and not taking ketoconazole. Therefore, doses of fesoterodine greater than 4 mg are not recommended in patients taking potent CYP3A4 inhibitors such as itraconazole).
No products indexed under this heading.

Ketoconazole (Following blockade of CYP3A4 by co-administration of the potent CYP3A4 inhibitor ketoconazole 200 mg bid for 5 days, C_{max} and AUC of the active metabolite of fesoterodine increased 2.0- and 2.3-fold, respectively, after oral administration of fesoterodine 8 mg to CYP2D6 extensive metabolizers. In CYP2D6 poor metabolizers, C_{max} and AUC of the active metabolite of fesoterodine increased 2.1- and 2.5-fold, respectively, during co-administration of ketoconazole 200 mg bid for 5 days. C_{max} and AUC were 4.5- and 5.7-fold higher, respectively, in subjects who were CYP2D6 poor metabolizers and taking ketoconazole compared to subjects who were CYP2D6 extensive metabolizers and not taking ketoconazole. Therefore, doses of fesoterodine greater than 4mg are not recommended in patients taking potent CYP3A4 inhibitors such as ketoconazole). Products include:
Extina **3319**
Xolegel **3337**

Lapatinib (In patients taking weak or moderate CYP3A4 inhibitors, careful assessment of tolerability at the 4 mg daily dose is advised prior to increasing the daily dose to 8 mg. While this specific interaction potential was not examined by clinical study, some pharmacokinetic interaction is expected). Products include:
Tykerb **1698**

Lopinavir (Following blockade of CYP3A4 by co-administration of the potent CYP3A4 inhibitor ketoconazole 200 mg bid for 5 days, C_{max} and AUC of the active metabolite of fesoterodine increased 2.0- and 2.3-fold, respectively, after oral administration of fesoterodine 8 mg to CYP2D6 extensive metabolizers. In CYP2D6 poor metabolizers, C_{max} and AUC of the active metabolite of fesoterodine increased 2.1- and 2.5-fold, respectively, during co-administration of ketoconazole 200 mg bid for 5 days. C_{max} and AUC were 4.5- and 5.7-fold higher, respectively, in subjects who were CYP2D6 poor metabolizers and taking ketoconazole compared to subjects who were CYP2D6 extensive metabolizers and not taking ketoconazole. Therefore, doses of fesoterodine greater than 4 mg are not recommended in patients taking potent CYP3A4 inhibitors). Products include:
Kaletra **458**

Loratadine (In patients taking weak or moderate CYP3A4 inhibitors, careful assessment of tolerability at the 4 mg daily dose is advised prior to increasing the daily dose to 8 mg. While this specific interaction potential was not examined by clinical study, some pharmacokinetic interaction is expected).
No products indexed under this heading.

Maprotiline Hydrochloride (The interaction with CYP2D6 inhibitors was not tested clinically. In poor metabolizers for CYP2D6, representing a maximum CYP2D6 inhibition, C_{max} and AUC of active metabolite are increased at 1.7 and 2-fold, respectively. No dosing adjustments are recommended in the presence of CYP2D6 inhibitors).
No products indexed under this heading.

Mepenzolate Bromide (Co-administration of fesoterodine with other antimuscarinic agents that produce dry mouth, constipation, urinary retention, and other anticholinergic pharmacological effects may increase the frequency and/or severity of such effects).
No products indexed under this heading.

Mephenytoin (Induction of CYP3A4 may lead to reduced plasma levels. No dosing adjustments are recommended in the presence of CYP3A4 inducers).
No products indexed under this heading.

Methadone Hydrochloride (The interaction with CYP2D6 inhibitors was not tested clinically. In poor metabolizers for CYP2D6, representing a maximum CYP2D6 inhibition, C_{max} and AUC of active metabolite are increased at 1.7 and 2-fold, respectively. No dosing adjustments are recommended in the presence of CYP2D6 inhibitors).
No products indexed under this heading.

Methsuximide (Induction of CYP3A4 may lead to reduced plasma levels. No dosing adjustments are recommended in the presence of CYP3A4 inducers).
No products indexed under this heading.

Methylprednisolone (Induction of CYP3A4 may lead to reduced plasma levels. No dosing adjustments are recommended in the presence of CYP3A4 inducers).
No products indexed under this heading.

Methylprednisolone Acetate (Induction of CYP3A4 may lead to reduced plasma levels. No dosing adjustments are recommended in the presence of CYP3A4 inducers).
No products indexed under this heading.

Methylprednisolone Sodium Succinate (Induction of CYP3A4 may lead to reduced plasma levels. No dosing adjustments are recommended in the presence of CYP3A4 inducers).
No products indexed under this heading.

Metronidazole (In patients taking weak or moderate CYP3A4 inhibitors, careful assessment of tolerability at the 4 mg daily dose is advised prior to increasing the daily dose to 8 mg. While this specific interaction potential was not examined by clinical study, some pharmacokinetic interaction is expected). Products include:
Pylera **793**

Metronidazole Benzoate (In patients taking weak or moderate CYP3A4 inhibitors, careful assessment of tolerability at the 4 mg daily dose is advised prior to increasing the daily dose to 8 mg. While this specific interaction potential was not examined by clinical study, some pharmacokinetic interaction is expected).
No products indexed under this heading.

Metronidazole Hydrochloride (In patients taking weak or moderate CYP3A4 inhibitors, careful assessment of tolerability at the 4 mg daily dose is advised prior to increasing the daily dose to 8 mg. While this specific interaction potential was not examined by clinical study, some pharmacokinetic interaction is expected).
No products indexed under this heading.

Metronidazole Sodium (In patients taking weak or moderate CYP3A4 inhibitors, careful assessment of tolerability at the 4 mg daily dose is advised prior to increasing the daily dose to 8 mg. While this specific interaction potential was not examined by clinical study, some pharmacokinetic interaction is expected).
No products indexed under this heading.

Mibefradil Dihydrochloride (The interaction with CYP2D6 inhibitors was not tested clinically. In poor metabolizers for CYP2D6, representing a maximum CYP2D6 inhibition, C_{max} and AUC of active metabolite are increased at 1.7 and 2-fold, respectively. No dosing adjustments are recommended in the presence of CYP2D6 inhibitors).
No products indexed under this heading.

Miconazole (In patients taking weak or moderate CYP3A4 inhibitors, careful assessment of tolerability at the 4 mg daily dose is advised prior to increasing the daily dose to 8 mg. While this specific interaction potential was not examined by clinical study, some pharmacokinetic interaction is expected).
No products indexed under this heading.

Miconazole Nitrate (In patients taking weak or moderate CYP3A4 inhibitors, careful assessment of tolerability at the 4 mg daily dose is advised prior to increasing the daily dose to 8 mg. While this specific interaction potential was not examined by clinical study, some pharmacokinetic interaction is expected). Products include:
Vusion Ointment **3335**

Mifepristone (In patients taking weak or moderate CYP3A4 inhibitors, careful assessment of tolerability at the 4 mg daily dose is advised prior to increasing the daily dose to 8 mg. While this specific interaction potential was not examined by clinical study, some pharmacokinetic interaction is expected).
No products indexed under this heading.

Moclobemide (The interaction with CYP2D6 inhibitors was not tested clinically. In poor metabolizers for CYP2D6, representing a maximum CYP2D6 inhibition, C_{max} and AUC of active metabolite are increased at 1.7 and 2-fold, respectively. No dosing adjustments are recommended in the presence of CYP2D6 inhibitors).
No products indexed under this heading.

Modafinil (Induction of CYP3A4 may lead to reduced plasma levels. No dosing adjustments are recommended in the presence of CYP3A4 inducers). Products include:
Provigil **983**

Nafcillin Sodium (Induction of CYP3A4 may lead to reduced plasma levels. No dosing adjustments are recommended in the presence of CYP3A4 inducers).
No products indexed under this heading.

Nefazodone Hydrochloride (Following blockade of CYP3A4 by co-administration of the potent CYP3A4 inhibitor ketoconazole 200 mg bid for 5 days, C_{max} and AUC of the active metabolite of fesoterodine increased 2.0- and 2.3-fold, respectively, after oral administration of fesoterodine 8 mg to CYP2D6 extensive metabolizers. In CYP2D6 poor metabolizers, C_{max} and AUC of the active metabolite of fesoterodine increased 2.1- and 2.5-fold, respectively, during co-administration of ketoconazole 200 mg bid for 5 days. C_{max} and AUC were 4.5- and 5.7-fold higher, respectively, in subjects who were CYP2D6 poor metabolizers and taking ketoconazole compared to subjects who were CYP2D6 extensive metabolizers and not taking ketoconazole. Therefore, doses of fesoterodine greater than 4 mg are not recommended in patients taking potent CYP3A4 inhibitors).
No products indexed under this heading.

Nelfinavir Mesylate (Following blockade of CYP3A4 by co-administration of the potent CYP3A4 inhibitor ketoconazole 200 mg bid for 5 days, C_{max} and AUC of the active metabolite of fesoterodine increased 2.0- and 2.3-fold, respectively, after oral administration of fesoterodine 8 mg to CYP2D6 extensive metabolizers. In CYP2D6 poor metabolizers, C_{max} and AUC of the active metabolite of fesoterodine increased 2.1- and 2.5-fold, respectively, during co-administration of ketoconazole 200 mg bid for 5 days. C_{max} and AUC were 4.5- and 5.7-fold higher, respectively, in subjects who were CYP2D6 poor metabolizers and taking ketoconazole compared to subjects who were CYP2D6 extensive metabolizers and not taking ketoconazole. Therefore, doses of fesoterodine greater than 4 mg are not recommended in patients taking potent CYP3A4 inhibitors).
No products indexed under this heading.

Nevirapine (In patients taking weak or moderate CYP3A4 inhibitors, careful assessment of tolerability at the 4 mg

Toviaz Interactions Index 1910

daily dose is advised prior to increasing the daily dose to 8 mg. While this specific interaction potential was not examined by clinical study, some pharmacokinetic interaction is expected). Products include:
- Viramune Oral Suspension 897
- Viramune Tablets 897

Niacin (In patients taking weak or moderate CYP3A4 inhibitors, careful assessment of tolerability at the 4 mg daily dose is advised prior to increasing the daily dose to 8 mg. While this specific interaction potential was not examined by clinical study, some pharmacokinetic interaction is expected). Products include:
- Advicor 402
- Cardio Basics 3455
- Niaspan 497
- Simcor 524

Niacinamide (In patients taking weak or moderate CYP3A4 inhibitors, careful assessment of tolerability at the 4 mg daily dose is advised prior to increasing the daily dose to 8 mg. While this specific interaction potential was not examined by clinical study, some pharmacokinetic interaction is expected). Products include:
- CitraNatal 90 DHA Capsules 2332
- CitraNatal Assure 2332
- CitraNatal Rx 2332
- Heplive 607

Niacinamide Hydroiodide (In patients taking weak or moderate CYP3A4 inhibitors, careful assessment of tolerability at the 4 mg daily dose is advised prior to increasing the daily dose to 8 mg. While this specific interaction potential was not examined by clinical study, some pharmacokinetic interaction is expected).
No products indexed under this heading.

Nicotinamide (In patients taking weak or moderate CYP3A4 inhibitors, careful assessment of tolerability at the 4 mg daily dose is advised prior to increasing the daily dose to 8 mg. While this specific interaction potential was not examined by clinical study, some pharmacokinetic interaction is expected).
No products indexed under this heading.

Nifedipine (In patients taking weak or moderate CYP3A4 inhibitors, careful assessment of tolerability at the 4 mg daily dose is advised prior to increasing the daily dose to 8 mg. While this specific interaction potential was not examined by clinical study, some pharmacokinetic interaction is expected).
No products indexed under this heading.

Norfloxacin (In patients taking weak or moderate CYP3A4 inhibitors, careful assessment of tolerability at the 4 mg daily dose is advised prior to increasing the daily dose to 8 mg. While this specific interaction potential was not examined by clinical study, some pharmacokinetic interaction is expected). Products include:
- Noroxin 2220

Nortriptyline Hydrochloride (The interaction with CYP2D6 inhibitors was not tested clinically. In poor metabolizers for CYP2D6, representing a maximum CYP2D6 inhibition, C_{max} and AUC of active metabolite are increased at 1.7 and 2-fold, respectively. No dosing adjustments are recommended in the presence of CYP2D6 inhibitors).
No products indexed under this heading.

Omeprazole (In patients taking weak or moderate CYP3A4 inhibitors, careful assessment of tolerability at the 4 mg daily dose is advised prior to increasing the daily dose to 8 mg. While this specific interaction potential was not examined by clinical study, some pharmacokinetic interaction is expected).
No products indexed under this heading.

Oxcarbazepine (Induction of CYP3A4 may lead to reduced plasma levels. No dosing adjustments are recommended in the presence of CYP3A4 inducers).
No products indexed under this heading.

Oxyphenonium Bromide (Co-administration of fesoterodine with other antimuscarinic agents that produce dry mouth, constipation, urinary retention, and other anticholinergic pharmacological effects may increase the frequency and/or severity of such effects).
No products indexed under this heading.

Paroxetine Hydrochloride (In patients taking weak or moderate CYP3A4 inhibitors, careful assessment of tolerability at the 4 mg daily dose is advised prior to increasing the daily dose to 8 mg. While this specific interaction potential was not examined by clinical study, some pharmacokinetic interaction is expected). Products include:
- Paroxetine CR 2361
- Paroxetine ER 2371
- Paxil 1586
- Paxil CR 1596

Perphenazine (The interaction with CYP2D6 inhibitors was not tested clinically. In poor metabolizers for CYP2D6, representing a maximum CYP2D6 inhibition, C_{max} and AUC of active metabolite are increased at 1.7 and 2-fold, respectively. No dosing adjustments are recommended in the presence of CYP2D6 inhibitors).
No products indexed under this heading.

Phenobarbital (Induction of CYP3A4 may lead to reduced plasma levels. No dosing adjustments are recommended in the presence of CYP3A4 inducers). Products include:
- Donnatal 2711

Phenobarbital Sodium (Induction of CYP3A4 may lead to reduced plasma levels. No dosing adjustments are recommended in the presence of CYP3A4 inducers).
No products indexed under this heading.

Phenytoin (Induction of CYP3A4 may lead to reduced plasma levels. No dosing adjustments are recommended in the presence of CYP3A4 inducers).
No products indexed under this heading.

Phenytoin Sodium (Induction of CYP3A4 may lead to reduced plasma levels. No dosing adjustments are recommended in the presence of CYP3A4 inducers). Products include:
- Phenytek Capsules 2380

Posaconazole (In patients taking weak or moderate CYP3A4 inhibitors, careful assessment of tolerability at the 4 mg daily dose is advised prior to increasing the daily dose to 8 mg. While this specific interaction potential was not examined by clinical study, some pharmacokinetic interaction is expected). Products include:
- Noxafil 3172

Prednisolone (Induction of CYP3A4 may lead to reduced plasma levels. No dosing adjustments are recommended in the presence of CYP3A4 inducers).
No products indexed under this heading.

Prednisolone Acetate (Induction of CYP3A4 may lead to reduced plasma levels. No dosing adjustments are recommended in the presence of CYP3A4 inducers). Products include:
- Blephamide .... ⊙212, ⊙214
- Pred Forte .... ⊙225
- Pred Mild .... ⊙230
- Pred-G .... ⊙226, ⊙227

Prednisolone Sodium Phosphate (Induction of CYP3A4 may lead to reduced plasma levels. No dosing adjustments are recommended in the presence of CYP3A4 inducers).
No products indexed under this heading.

Prednisolone Tebutate (Induction of CYP3A4 may lead to reduced plasma levels. No dosing adjustments are recommended in the presence of CYP3A4 inducers).
No products indexed under this heading.

Prednisone (Induction of CYP3A4 may lead to reduced plasma levels. No dosing adjustments are recommended in the presence of CYP3A4 inducers).
No products indexed under this heading.

Prednisone sodium phosphate (Induction of CYP3A4 may lead to reduced plasma levels. No dosing adjustments are recommended in the presence of CYP3A4 inducers).
No products indexed under this heading.

Primidone (Induction of CYP3A4 may lead to reduced plasma levels. No dosing adjustments are recommended in the presence of CYP3A4 inducers).
No products indexed under this heading.

Propafenone Hydrochloride (The interaction with CYP2D6 inhibitors was not tested clinically. In poor metabolizers for CYP2D6, representing a maximum CYP2D6 inhibition, C_{max} and AUC of active metabolite are increased at 1.7 and 2-fold, respectively. No dosing adjustments are recommended in the presence of CYP2D6 inhibitors). Products include:
- Rythmol 1648
- Rythmol SR 1652

Propantheline Bromide (Co-administration of fesoterodine with other antimuscarinic agents that produce dry mouth, constipation, urinary retention, and other anticholinergic pharmacological effects may increase the frequency and/or severity of such effects).
No products indexed under this heading.

Propoxyphene Hydrochloride (In patients taking weak or moderate CYP3A4 inhibitors, careful assessment of tolerability at the 4 mg daily dose is advised prior to increasing the daily dose to 8 mg. While this specific interaction potential was not examined by clinical study, some pharmacokinetic interaction is expected).
No products indexed under this heading.

Propoxyphene Napsylate (In patients taking weak or moderate CYP3A4 inhibitors, careful assessment of tolerability at the 4 mg daily dose is advised prior to increasing the daily dose to 8 mg. While this specific interaction potential was not examined by clinical study, some pharmacokinetic interaction is expected).
No products indexed under this heading.

Protriptyline Hydrochloride (The interaction with CYP2D6 inhibitors was not tested clinically. In poor metabolizers for CYP2D6, representing a maximum CYP2D6 inhibition, C_{max} and AUC of active metabolite are increased at 1.7 and 2-fold, respectively. No dosing adjustments are recommended in the presence of CYP2D6 inhibitors).
No products indexed under this heading.

Quinacrine Hydrochloride (The interaction with CYP2D6 inhibitors was not tested clinically. In poor metabolizers for CYP2D6, representing a maximum CYP2D6 inhibition, C_{max} and AUC of active metabolite are increased at 1.7 and 2-fold, respectively. No dosing adjustments are recommended in the presence of CYP2D6 inhibitors).
No products indexed under this heading.

Quinidine (In patients taking weak or moderate CYP3A4 inhibitors, careful assessment of tolerability at the 4 mg daily dose is advised prior to increasing the daily dose to 8 mg. While this specific interaction potential was not examined by clinical study, some pharmacokinetic interaction is expected).
No products indexed under this heading.

Quinidine Gluconate (The interaction with CYP2D6 inhibitors was not tested clinically. In poor metabolizers for CYP2D6, representing a maximum CYP2D6 inhibition, C_{max} and AUC of active metabolite are increased at 1.7 and 2-fold, respectively. No dosing adjustments are recommended in the presence of CYP2D6 inhibitors).
No products indexed under this heading.

Quinidine Hydrochloride (In patients taking weak or moderate CYP3A4 inhibitors, careful assessment of tolerability at the 4 mg daily dose is advised prior to increasing the daily dose to 8 mg. While this specific interaction potential was not examined by clinical study, some pharmacokinetic interaction is expected).
No products indexed under this heading.

Quinidine Polygalacturonate (In patients taking weak or moderate CYP3A4 inhibitors, careful assessment of tolerability at the 4 mg daily dose is advised prior to increasing the daily dose to 8 mg. While this specific interaction potential was not examined by clinical study, some pharmacokinetic interaction is expected).
No products indexed under this heading.

Quinidine Sulfate (In patients taking weak or moderate CYP3A4 inhibitors, careful assessment of tolerability at the 4 mg daily dose is advised prior to increasing the daily dose to 8 mg. While this specific interaction potential was not examined by clinical study, some pharmacokinetic interaction is expected).
No products indexed under this heading.

Quinine (In patients taking weak or moderate CYP3A4 inhibitors, careful assessment of tolerability at the 4 mg daily dose is advised prior to increasing the daily dose to 8 mg. While this specific interaction potential was not examined by clinical study, some pharmacokinetic interaction is expected). Products include:
- Hyland's Leg Cramps PM with Quinine 3315

Quinine Sulfate (In patients taking weak or moderate CYP3A4 inhibitors, careful assessment of tolerability at the 4 mg daily dose is advised prior to increasing the daily dose to 8 mg. While this specific interaction potential was not examined by clinical study, some pharmacokinetic interaction is expected).
No products indexed under this heading.

Quinupristin (In patients taking weak or moderate CYP3A4 inhibitors, careful assessment of tolerability at the 4 mg daily dose is advised prior to increasing the daily dose to 8 mg. While this specific interaction potential was not examined by clinical study, some pharmacokinetic interaction is expected).
No products indexed under this heading.

Ranitidine Bismuth Citrate (In patients taking weak or moderate CYP3A4 inhibitors, careful assessment of tolerability at the 4 mg daily dose is advised prior to increasing the daily dose to 8 mg. While this specific interaction potential was not examined by clinical study, some pharmacokinetic interaction is expected).
No products indexed under this heading.

Ranitidine Hydrochloride (In patients taking weak or moderate CYP3A4 inhibitors, careful assessment of tolerability at the 4 mg daily dose is advised prior to increasing the daily dose to 8 mg. While this specific interaction potential was not examined by clinical study, some pharmacokinetic interaction is expected). Products include:
- Zantac 1737

1911 **Interactions Index** Toviaz

Zantac Injection 1732
Zantac Pharmacy 1735

Rifabutin (Induction of CYP3A4 may lead to reduced plasma levels. No dosing adjustments are recommended in the presence of CYP3A4 inducers).
No products indexed under this heading.

Rifampicin (Induction of CYP3A4 by co-administration of rifampicin 600 mg qd, C_{max} and AUC of the active metabolite of fesoterodine decreased approximately 70% and 75%, respectively, after oral administration of fesoterodine 8 mg. CYP3A4 induction may lead to reduced plasma levels. No dosing adjustments are recommended in the presence of CYP3A4 inducers).
No products indexed under this heading.

Rifampin (Induction of CYP3A4 may lead to reduced plasma levels. No dosing adjustments are recommended in the presence of CYP3A4 inducers).
No products indexed under this heading.

Rifapentine (Induction of CYP3A4 may lead to reduced plasma levels. No dosing adjustments are recommended in the presence of CYP3A4 inducers).
No products indexed under this heading.

Ritonavir (Following blockade of CYP3A4 by co-administration of the potent CYP3A4 inhibitor ketoconazole 200 mg bid for 5 days, C_{max} and AUC of the active metabolite of fesoterodine increased 2.0- and 2.3-fold, respectively, after oral administration of fesoterodine 8 mg to CYP2D6 extensive metabolizers. In CYP2D6 poor metabolizers, C_{max} and AUC of the active metabolite of fesoterodine increased 2.1- and 2.5-fold, respectively, during co-administration of ketoconazole 200 mg bid for 5 days. C_{max} and AUC were 4.5- and 5.7-fold higher, respectively, in subjects who were CYP2D6 poor metabolizers and taking ketoconazole compared to subjects who were CYP2D6 extensive metabolizers and not taking ketoconazole. Therefore, doses of fesoterodine greater than 4 mg are not recommended in patients taking potent CYP3A4 inhibitors). Products include:
Kaletra 458
Norvir 509

Saquinavir (Following blockade of CYP3A4 by co-administration of the potent CYP3A4 inhibitor ketoconazole 200 mg bid for 5 days, C_{max} and AUC of the active metabolite of fesoterodine increased 2.0- and 2.3-fold, respectively, after oral administration of fesoterodine 8 mg to CYP2D6 extensive metabolizers. In CYP2D6 poor metabolizers, C_{max} and AUC of the active metabolite of fesoterodine increased 2.1- and 2.5-fold, respectively, during co-administration of ketoconazole 200 mg bid for 5 days. C_{max} and AUC were 4.5- and 5.7-fold higher, respectively, in subjects who were CYP2D6 poor metabolizers and taking ketoconazole compared to subjects who were CYP2D6 extensive metabolizers and not taking ketoconazole. Therefore, doses of fesoterodine greater than 4 mg are not recommended in patients taking potent CYP3A4 inhibitors).
No products indexed under this heading.

Saquinavir Mesylate (Following blockade of CYP3A4 by co-administration of the potent CYP3A4 inhibitor ketoconazole 200 mg bid for 5 days, C_{max} and AUC of the active metabolite of fesoterodine increased 2.0- and 2.3-fold, respectively, after oral administration of fesoterodine 8 mg to CYP2D6 extensive metabolizers. In CYP2D6 poor metabolizers, C_{max} and AUC of the active metabolite of fesoterodine increased 2.1- and 2.5-fold, respectively, during co-administration of ketoconazole 200 mg bid for 5 days. C_{max} and AUC were 4.5- and 5.7-fold higher, respectively, in subjects who were CYP2D6 poor metabolizers and taking ketoconazole compared to subjects who were CYP2D6 extensive metabolizers and not taking ketoconazole. Therefore, doses of fesoterodine greater than 4 mg are not recommended in patients taking potent CYP3A4 inhibitors).
No products indexed under this heading.

Scopolamine (Co-administration of fesoterodine with other antimuscarinic agents that produce dry mouth, constipation, urinary retention, and other anticholinergic pharmacological effects may increase the frequency and/or severity of such effects). Products include:
Transderm Scōp 2397

Scopolamine Hydrobromide (Co-administration of fesoterodine with other antimuscarinic agents that produce dry mouth, constipation, urinary retention, and other anticholinergic pharmacological effects may increase the frequency and/or severity of such effects). Products include:
Donnatal 2711

Sertraline Hydrochloride (In patients taking weak or moderate CYP3A4 inhibitors, careful assessment of tolerability at the 4 mg daily dose is advised prior to increasing the daily dose to 8 mg. While this specific interaction potential was not examined by clinical study, some pharmacokinetic interaction is expected).
No products indexed under this heading.

Sildenafil Citrate (In patients taking weak or moderate CYP3A4 inhibitors, careful assessment of tolerability at the 4 mg daily dose is advised prior to increasing the daily dose to 8 mg. While this specific interaction potential was not examined by clinical study, some pharmacokinetic interaction is expected).
No products indexed under this heading.

Sulfinpyrazone (Induction of CYP3A4 may lead to reduced plasma levels. No dosing adjustments are recommended in the presence of CYP3A4 inducers).
No products indexed under this heading.

Telithromycin (Following blockade of CYP3A4 by co-administration of the potent CYP3A4 inhibitor ketoconazole 200 mg bid for 5 days, C_{max} and AUC of the active metabolite of fesoterodine increased 2.0- and 2.3-fold, respectively, after oral administration of fesoterodine 8 mg to CYP2D6 extensive metabolizers. In CYP2D6 poor metabolizers, C_{max} and AUC of the active metabolite of fesoterodine increased 2.1- and 2.5-fold, respectively, during co-administration of ketoconazole 200 mg bid for 5 days. C_{max} and AUC were 4.5- and 5.7-fold higher, respectively, in subjects who were CYP2D6 poor metabolizers and taking ketoconazole compared to subjects who were CYP2D6 extensive metabolizers and not taking ketoconazole. Therefore, doses of fesoterodine greater than 4 mg are not recommended in patients taking potent CYP3A4 inhibitors). Products include:
Ketek 2991

Terbinafine Hydrochloride (The interaction with CYP2D6 inhibitors was not tested clinically. In poor metabolizers for CYP2D6, representing a maximum CYP2D6 inhibition, C_{max} and AUC of active metabolite are increased at 1.7 and 2-fold, respectively. No dosing adjustments are recommended in the presence of CYP2D6 inhibitors).
No products indexed under this heading.

Theophyllinate (Induction of CYP3A4 may lead to reduced plasma levels. No dosing adjustments are recommended in the presence of CYP3A4 inducers).
No products indexed under this heading.

Theophylline (Induction of CYP3A4 may lead to reduced plasma levels. No dosing adjustments are recommended in the presence of CYP3A4 inducers).
No products indexed under this heading.

Theophylline Anhydrous (Induction of CYP3A4 may lead to reduced plasma levels. No dosing adjustments are recommended in the presence of CYP3A4 inducers). Products include:
Uniphyl 2817

Theophylline Calcium Salicylate (Induction of CYP3A4 may lead to reduced plasma levels. No dosing adjustments are recommended in the presence of CYP3A4 inducers).
No products indexed under this heading.

Theophylline Dihydroxypropyl (Glyceryl) (Induction of CYP3A4 may lead to reduced plasma levels. No dosing adjustments are recommended in the presence of CYP3A4 inducers).
No products indexed under this heading.

Theophylline Ethylenediamine (Induction of CYP3A4 may lead to reduced plasma levels. No dosing adjustments are recommended in the presence of CYP3A4 inducers).
No products indexed under this heading.

Theophylline Sodium Glycinate (Induction of CYP3A4 may lead to reduced plasma levels. No dosing adjustments are recommended in the presence of CYP3A4 inducers).
No products indexed under this heading.

Thioridazine Hydrochloride (The interaction with CYP2D6 inhibitors was not tested clinically. In poor metabolizers for CYP2D6, representing a maximum CYP2D6 inhibition, C_{max} and AUC of active metabolite are increased at 1.7 and 2-fold, respectively. No dosing adjustments are recommended in the presence of CYP2D6 inhibitors). Products include:
Thioridazine Hydrochloride 2384

Tolterodine Tartrate (Co-administration of fesoterodine with other antimuscarinic agents that produce dry mouth, constipation, urinary retention, and other anticholinergic pharmacological effects may increase the frequency and/or severity of such effects).
No products indexed under this heading.

Triamcinolone (Induction of CYP3A4 may lead to reduced plasma levels. No dosing adjustments are recommended in the presence of CYP3A4 inducers).
No products indexed under this heading.

Triamcinolone Acetonide (Induction of CYP3A4 may lead to reduced plasma levels. No dosing adjustments are recommended in the presence of CYP3A4 inducers). Products include:
Azmacort 408
Nasacort AQ 3019

Triamcinolone Diacetate (Induction of CYP3A4 may lead to reduced plasma levels. No dosing adjustments are recommended in the presence of CYP3A4 inducers).
No products indexed under this heading.

Triamcinolone Hexacetonide (Induction of CYP3A4 may lead to reduced plasma levels. No dosing adjustments are recommended in the presence of CYP3A4 inducers).
No products indexed under this heading.

Tridihexethyl Chloride (Co-administration of fesoterodine with other antimuscarinic agents that produce dry mouth, constipation, urinary retention, and other anticholinergic pharmacological effects may increase the frequency and/or severity of such effects).
No products indexed under this heading.

Trimipramine Maleate (The interaction with CYP2D6 inhibitors was not tested clinically. In poor metabolizers for CYP2D6, representing a maximum CYP2D6 inhibition, C_{max} and AUC of active metabolite are increased at 1.7 and 2-fold, respectively. No dosing adjustments are recommended in the presence of CYP2D6 inhibitors).
No products indexed under this heading.

Troglitazone (In patients taking weak or moderate CYP3A4 inhibitors, careful assessment of tolerability at the 4 mg daily dose is advised prior to increasing the daily dose to 8 mg. While this specific interaction potential was not examined by clinical study, some pharmacokinetic interaction is expected).
No products indexed under this heading.

Troleandomycin (Following blockade of CYP3A4 by co-administration of the potent CYP3A4 inhibitor ketoconazole 200 mg bid for 5 days, C_{max} and AUC of the active metabolite of fesoterodine increased 2.0- and 2.3-fold, respectively, after oral administration of fesoterodine 8 mg to CYP2D6 extensive metabolizers. In CYP2D6 poor metabolizers, C_{max} and AUC of the active metabolite of fesoterodine increased 2.1- and 2.5-fold, respectively, during co-administration of ketoconazole 200 mg bid for 5 days. C_{max} and AUC were 4.5- and 5.7-fold higher, respectively, in subjects who were CYP2D6 poor metabolizers and taking ketoconazole compared to subjects who were CYP2D6 extensive metabolizers and not taking ketoconazole. Therefore, doses of fesoterodine greater than 4 mg are not recommended in patients taking potent CYP3A4 inhibitors).
No products indexed under this heading.

Valproate Sodium (In patients taking weak or moderate CYP3A4 inhibitors, careful assessment of tolerability at the 4 mg daily dose is advised prior to increasing the daily dose to 8 mg. While this specific interaction potential was not examined by clinical study, some pharmacokinetic interaction is expected).
No products indexed under this heading.

Vardenafil Hydrochloride (In patients taking weak or moderate CYP3A4 inhibitors, careful assessment of tolerability at the 4 mg daily dose is advised prior to increasing the daily dose to 8 mg. While this specific interaction potential was not examined by clinical study, some pharmacokinetic interaction is expected). Products include:
Levitra 3157

Verapamil Hydrochloride (In patients taking weak or moderate CYP3A4 inhibitors, careful assessment of tolerability at the 4 mg daily dose is advised prior to increasing the daily dose to 8 mg. While this specific interaction potential was not examined by clinical study, some pharmacokinetic interaction is expected). Products include:
Tarka 534

Voriconazole (Following blockade of CYP3A4 by co-administration of the potent CYP3A4 inhibitor ketoconazole 200 mg bid for 5 days, C_{max} and AUC of the active metabolite of fesoterodine increased 2.0- and 2.3-fold, respectively, after oral administration of fesoterodine 8 mg to CYP2D6 extensive metabolizers. In CYP2D6 poor metabolizers, C_{max} and AUC of the active metabolite of fesoterodine increased 2.1- and 2.5-fold, respectively, during co-administration of ketoconazole 200 mg bid for 5 days. C_{max} and AUC were 4.5- and 5.7-fold higher, respectively, in subjects who were CYP2D6 poor metabolizers and taking ketoconazole compared to subjects who were CYP2D6

Toviaz Interactions Index 1912

extensive metabolizers and not taking ketoconazole. Therefore, doses of fesoterodine greater than 4 mg are not recommended in patients taking potent CYP3A4 inhibitors).

No products indexed under this heading.

Zafirlukast (In patients taking weak or moderate CYP3A4 inhibitors, careful assessment of tolerability at the 4 mg daily dose is advised prior to increasing the daily dose to 8 mg. While this specific interaction potential was not examined by clinical study, some pharmacokinetic interaction is expected). Products include:

Accolate 3612

Zileuton (In patients taking weak or moderate CYP3A4 inhibitors, careful assessment of tolerability at the 4 mg daily dose is advised prior to increasing the daily dose to 8 mg. While this specific interaction potential was not examined by clinical study, some pharmacokinetic interaction is expected).

No products indexed under this heading.

Food Interactions

Alcohol (Concomitant use with alcohol may enhance the drowsiness caused by fesoterodine).

Beer, reduced-alcohol (Concomitant use with alcohol may enhance the drowsiness caused by fesoterodine).

Beer, unspecified (Concomitant use with alcohol may enhance the drowsiness caused by fesoterodine).

Grapefruit (In patients taking weak or moderate CYP3A4 inhibitors, careful assessment of tolerability at the 4 mg daily dose is advised prior to increasing the daily dose to 8 mg. While this specific interaction potential was not examined by clinical study, some pharmacokinetic interaction is expected).

Grapefruit Juice (In patients taking weak or moderate CYP3A4 inhibitors, careful assessment of tolerability at the 4 mg daily dose is advised prior to increasing the daily dose to 8 mg. While this specific interaction potential was not examined by clinical study, some pharmacokinetic interaction is expected).

Wine, Chianti (Concomitant use with alcohol may enhance the drowsiness caused by fesoterodine).

Wine, Red (Concomitant use with alcohol may enhance the drowsiness caused by fesoterodine).

Wine, unspecified (Concomitant use with alcohol may enhance the drowsiness caused by fesoterodine).

Wine products (Concomitant use with alcohol may enhance the drowsiness caused by fesoterodine).

TRACLEER TABLETS

(Bosentan) 573

May interact with cytochrome p450 2c9 inhibitors (selected), cytochrome p450 2c9 substrates (selected), cytochrome p450 3a inhibitors (selected), cytochrome p450 3a substrates (selected), erythromycin, estrogens, oral contraceptives, oral hypoglycemic agents, progestins, statins that are metabolized by CYP3A4, and certain other agents. Compounds in these categories include:

Acarbose (Co-administration of bosentan decreased the plasma concentrations of glyburide by approximately 40%. The plasma concentrations of bosentan were also decreased by approximately 30%. Bosentan is also expected to reduce plasma concentrations of other oral hypoglycemic agents that are predominantly metabolized by CYP2C9 or CYP3A. The possibility of worsened glucose control in patients using these agents should be considered).

No products indexed under this heading.

Alfentanil Hydrochloride (Bosentan is an inducer of CYP3A and CYP2C9. Consequently plasma concentrations of drugs metabolized by these two isozymes will be decreased when bosentan is co-administered).

No products indexed under this heading.

Alprazolam (Bosentan is an inducer of CYP3A and CYP2C9. Consequently plasma concentrations of drugs metabolized by these two isozymes will be decreased when bosentan is co-administered).

No products indexed under this heading.

Aminophylline (Bosentan is an inducer of CYP3A and CYP2C9. Consequently plasma concentrations of drugs metabolized by these two isozymes will be decreased when bosentan is co-administered).

No products indexed under this heading.

Amiodarone Hydrochloride (Bosentan is metabolized by CYP2C9 and CYP3A. Inhibition of these enzymes may increase the plasma concentration of bosentan. Concomitant administration of both a CYP2C9 inhibitor (such as fluconazole or amiodarone) and a strong CYP3A inhibitor (eg, ketoconazole, itraconazole) or a moderate CYP3A inhibitor (eg, amprenavir, erythromycin, fluconazole, diltiazem) with bosentan will likely lead to large increases in plasma concentrations of bosentan. Co-administration of such combinations of a CYP2C9 inhibitor plus a strong or moderate CYP3A inhibitor with bosentan is not recommended).

No products indexed under this heading.

Amitriptyline Hydrochloride (Bosentan is an inducer of CYP3A and CYP2C9. Consequently plasma concentrations of drugs metabolized by these two isozymes will be decreased when bosentan is co-administered).

No products indexed under this heading.

Amlodipine Besylate (Bosentan is an inducer of CYP3A and CYP2C9. Consequently plasma concentrations of drugs metabolized by these two isozymes will be decreased when bosentan is co-administered). Products include:

Azor 1010

Exforge 2443

Exforge HCT 2449

Amprenavir (Bosentan is metabolized by CYP2C9 and CYP3A. Inhibition of these enzymes may increase the plasma concentration of bosentan. Concomitant administration of both a CYP2C9 inhibitor (such as fluconazole or amiodarone) and a strong CYP3A inhibitor (eg, ketoconazole, itraconazole) or a moderate CYP3A inhibitor (eg, amprenavir, erythromycin, fluconazole, diltiazem) with bosentan will likely lead to large increases in plasma concentrations of bosentan. Co-administration of such combinations of a CYP2C9 inhibitor plus a strong or moderate CYP3A inhibitor with bosentan is not recommended).

No products indexed under this heading.

Anastrozole (Bosentan is metabolized by CYP2C9 and CYP3A. Inhibition of these enzymes may increase the plasma concentration of bosentan. Concomitant administration of both a CYP2C9 inhibitor (such as fluconazole or amiodarone) and a strong CYP3A inhibitor (eg, ketoconazole, itraconazole) or a moderate CYP3A inhibitor (eg, amprenavir, erythromycin, fluconazole, diltiazem) with bosentan will likely lead to large increases in plasma concentrations of bosentan. Co-administration of such combinations of a CYP2C9 inhibitor plus a strong or moderate CYP3A inhibitor with bosentan is not recommended).

No products indexed under this heading.

Aprepitant (Bosentan is metabolized by CYP2C9 and CYP3A. Inhibition of these enzymes may increase the plasma concentration of bosentan. Concomitant administration of both a CYP2C9 inhibitor (such as fluconazole or amiodarone) and a strong CYP3A inhibitor (eg, ketoconazole, itraconazole) or a moderate CYP3A inhibitor (eg, amprenavir, erythromycin, fluconazole, diltiazem) with bosentan will likely lead to large increases in plasma concentrations of bosentan. Co-administration of such combinations of a CYP2C9 inhibitor plus a strong or moderate CYP3A inhibitor with bosentan is not recommended). Products include:

Emend 2124

Astemizole (Bosentan is an inducer of CYP3A and CYP2C9. Consequently plasma concentrations of drugs metabolized by these two isozymes will be decreased when bosentan is co-administered).

No products indexed under this heading.

Atorvastatin Calcium (Co-administration of bosentan decreased the plasma concentrations of simvastatin (a CYP3A substrate), and its active β-hydroxy acid metabolite, by approximately 50%. The plasma concentrations of bosentan were not affected. Bosentan is also expected to reduce plasma concentrations of other statins that are significantly metabolized by CYP3A, such as lovastatin and atorvastatin. The possibility of reduced statin efficacy should be considered. Patients using CYP3A-metabolized statins should have cholesterol levels monitored after bosentan is initiated to see whether the statin dose needs adjustment). Products include:

Lipitor 2703

Bendroflumethiazide (Bosentan is metabolized by CYP2C9 and CYP3A. Inhibition of these enzymes may increase the plasma concentration of bosentan. Concomitant administration of both a CYP2C9 inhibitor (such as fluconazole or amiodarone) and a strong CYP3A inhibitor (eg, ketoconazole, itraconazole) or a moderate CYP3A inhibitor (eg, amprenavir, erythromycin, fluconazole, diltiazem) with bosentan will likely lead to large increases in plasma concentrations of bosentan. Co-administration of such combinations of a CYP2C9 inhibitor plus a strong or moderate CYP3A inhibitor with bosentan is not recommended).

No products indexed under this heading.

Bromocriptine Mesylate (Bosentan is an inducer of CYP3A and CYP2C9. Consequently plasma concentrations of drugs metabolized by these two isozymes will be decreased when bosentan is co-administered).

No products indexed under this heading.

Buspirone Hydrochloride (Bosentan is an inducer of CYP3A and CYP2C9. Consequently plasma concentrations of drugs metabolized by these two isozymes will be decreased when bosentan is co-administered).

No products indexed under this heading.

Busulfan (Bosentan is an inducer of CYP3A and CYP2C9. Consequently plasma concentrations of drugs metabolized by these two isozymes will be decreased when bosentan is co-administered). Products include:

Myleran 1581

Candesartan Cilexetil (Bosentan is an inducer of CYP3A and CYP2C9. Consequently plasma concentrations of drugs metabolized by these two isozymes will be decreased when bosentan is co-administered). Products include:

Atacand 697

Atacand HCT 700

Carbamazepine (Bosentan is an inducer of CYP3A and CYP2C9. Consequently plasma concentrations of drugs metabolized by these two isozymes will be decreased when bosentan is co-administered). Products include:

Carbatrol 3280

Equetro 3477

Carvedilol (Bosentan is an inducer of CYP3A and CYP2C9. Consequently plasma concentrations of drugs metabolized by these two isozymes will be decreased when bosentan is co-administered). Products include:

Coreg 1409

Celecoxib (Bosentan is an inducer of CYP3A and CYP2C9. Consequently plasma concentrations of drugs metabolized by these two isozymes will be decreased when bosentan is co-administered). Products include:

Celebrex 3272

Cerivastatin Sodium (Bosentan is an inducer of CYP3A and CYP2C9. Consequently plasma concentrations of drugs metabolized by these two isozymes will be decreased when bosentan is co-administered).

No products indexed under this heading.

Chloramphenicol (Bosentan is metabolized by CYP2C9 and CYP3A. Inhibition of these enzymes may increase the plasma concentration of bosentan. Concomitant administration of both a CYP2C9 inhibitor (such as fluconazole or amiodarone) and a strong CYP3A inhibitor (eg, ketoconazole, itraconazole) or a moderate CYP3A inhibitor (eg, amprenavir, erythromycin, fluconazole, diltiazem) with bosentan will likely lead to large increases in plasma concentrations of bosentan. Co-administration of such combinations of a CYP2C9 inhibitor plus a strong or moderate CYP3A inhibitor with bosentan is not recommended).

No products indexed under this heading.

Chloramphenicol Palmitate (Bosentan is metabolized by CYP2C9 and CYP3A. Inhibition of these enzymes may increase the plasma concentration of bosentan. Concomitant administration of both a CYP2C9 inhibitor (such as fluconazole or amiodarone) and a strong CYP3A inhibitor (eg, ketoconazole, itraconazole) or a moderate CYP3A inhibitor (eg, amprenavir, erythromycin, fluconazole, diltiazem) with bosentan will likely lead to large increases in plasma concentrations of bosentan. Co-administration of such combinations of a CYP2C9 inhibitor plus a strong or moderate CYP3A inhibitor with bosentan is not recommended).

No products indexed under this heading.

Chloramphenicol Sodium Succinate (Bosentan is metabolized by CYP2C9 and CYP3A. Inhibition of these enzymes may increase the plasma concentration of bosentan. Concomitant administration of both a CYP2C9 inhibitor (such as fluconazole or amiodarone) and a strong CYP3A inhibitor (eg, ketoconazole, itraconazole) or a moderate CYP3A inhibitor (eg, amprenavir, erythromycin, fluconazole, diltiazem) with bosentan will likely lead to large increases in plasma concentrations of bosentan. Co-administration of such combinations of a CYP2C9 inhibitor plus a strong or moderate CYP3A inhibitor with bosentan is not recommended).

No products indexed under this heading.

Chlorothiazide (Bosentan is metabolized by CYP2C9 and CYP3A. Inhibition of these enzymes may increase the plasma concentration of bosentan. Concomitant administration of both a CYP2C9 inhibitor (such as fluconazole or amiodarone) and a strong CYP3A inhibitor (eg, ketoconazole, itraconazole) or a moderate CYP3A inhibitor (eg, amprenavir, erythromycin, flucona-

zole, diltiazem) with bosentan will likely lead to large increases in plasma concentrations of bosentan. Co-administration of such combinations of a CYP2C9 inhibitor plus a strong or moderate CYP3A inhibitor with bosentan is not recommended.

No products indexed under this heading.

Chlorothiazide Sodium (Bosentan is metabolized by CYP2C9 and CYP3A. Inhibition of these enzymes may increase the plasma concentration of bosentan. Concomitant administration of both a CYP2C9 inhibitor (such as fluconazole or amiodarone) and a strong CYP3A inhibitor (eg, ketoconazole, itraconazole) or a moderate CYP3A inhibitor (eg, amprenavir, erythromycin, fluconazole, diltiazem) with bosentan will likely lead to large increases in plasma concentrations of bosentan. Co-administration of such combinations of a CYP2C9 inhibitor plus a strong or moderate CYP3A inhibitor with bosentan is not recommended). Products include:

Diuril Intravenous 2009

Chlorotrianisene (Hormonal contraceptives, including oral, injectable, transdermal, and implantable forms, may not be reliable when bosentan is co-administered. Females should practice additional methods of contraception and not rely on hormonal contraception alone when taking bosentan. An interaction study demonstrated that co-administration of bosentan and a combination oral hormonal contraceptive produced average decreases of norethindrone and ethinyl estradiol levels of 14% and 31%, respectively. However, decreases in exposure were as much as 56% and 66%, respectively, in individual subjects).

No products indexed under this heading.

Chlorpheniramine (Bosentan is an inducer of CYP3A and CYP2C9. Consequently plasma concentrations of drugs metabolized by these two isozymes will be decreased when bosentan is co-administered).

No products indexed under this heading.

Chlorpheniramine Maleate (Bosentan is an inducer of CYP3A and CYP2C9. Consequently plasma concentrations of drugs metabolized by these two isozymes will be decreased when bosentan is co-administered).

No products indexed under this heading.

Chlorpheniramine Polistirex (Bosentan is an inducer of CYP3A and CYP2C9. Consequently plasma concentrations of drugs metabolized by these two isozymes will be decreased when bosentan is co-administered). Products include:

Tussionex 3443

Chlorpheniramine Tannate (Bosentan is an inducer of CYP3A and CYP2C9. Consequently plasma concentrations of drugs metabolized by these two isozymes will be decreased when bosentan is co-administered).

No products indexed under this heading.

Chlorpropamide (Co-administration of bosentan decreased the plasma concentrations of glyburide by approximately 40%. The plasma concentrations of bosentan were also decreased by approximately 30%. Bosentan is also expected to reduce plasma concentrations of other oral hypoglycemic agents that are predominantly metabolized by CYP2C9 or CYP3A. The possibility of worsened glucose control in patients using these agents should be considered).

No products indexed under this heading.

Cilostazol (Bosentan is an inducer of CYP3A and CYP2C9. Consequently plasma concentrations of drugs metabolized by these two isozymes will be decreased when bosentan is co-administered).

No products indexed under this heading.

Cimetidine (Bosentan is metabolized by CYP2C9 and CYP3A. Inhibition of these enzymes may increase the plasma concentration of bosentan. Concomitant administration of both a CYP2C9 inhibitor (such as fluconazole or amiodarone) and a strong CYP3A inhibitor (eg, ketoconazole, itraconazole) or a moderate CYP3A inhibitor (eg, amprenavir, erythromycin, fluconazole, diltiazem) with bosentan will likely lead to large increases in plasma concentrations of bosentan. Co-administration of such combinations of a CYP2C9 inhibitor plus a strong or moderate CYP3A inhibitor with bosentan is not recommended).

No products indexed under this heading.

Cimetidine Hydrochloride (Bosentan is metabolized by CYP2C9 and CYP3A. Inhibition of these enzymes may increase the plasma concentration of bosentan. Concomitant administration of both a CYP2C9 inhibitor (such as fluconazole or amiodarone) and a strong CYP3A inhibitor (eg, ketoconazole, itraconazole) or a moderate CYP3A inhibitor (eg, amprenavir, erythromycin, fluconazole, diltiazem) with bosentan will likely lead to large increases in plasma concentrations of bosentan. Co-administration of such combinations of a CYP2C9 inhibitor plus a strong or moderate CYP3A inhibitor with bosentan is not recommended).

No products indexed under this heading.

Ciprofloxacin (Bosentan is metabolized by CYP2C9 and CYP3A. Inhibition of these enzymes may increase the plasma concentration of bosentan. Concomitant administration of both a CYP2C9 inhibitor (such as fluconazole or amiodarone) and a strong CYP3A inhibitor (eg, ketoconazole, itraconazole) or a moderate CYP3A inhibitor (eg, amprenavir, erythromycin, fluconazole, diltiazem) with bosentan will likely lead to large increases in plasma concentrations of bosentan. Co-administration of such combinations of a CYP2C9 inhibitor plus a strong or moderate CYP3A inhibitor with bosentan is not recommended). Products include:

Cipro I.V. 3082
Cipro 3073
Cipro XR 3091
Ciprodex 583

Ciprofloxacin Hydrochloride (Bosentan is metabolized by CYP2C9 and CYP3A. Inhibition of these enzymes may increase the plasma concentration of bosentan. Concomitant administration of both a CYP2C9 inhibitor (such as fluconazole or amiodarone) and a strong CYP3A inhibitor (eg, ketoconazole, itraconazole) or a moderate CYP3A inhibitor (eg, amprenavir, erythromycin, fluconazole, diltiazem) with bosentan will likely lead to large increases in plasma concentrations of bosentan. Co-administration of such combinations of a CYP2C9 inhibitor plus a strong or moderate CYP3A inhibitor with bosentan is not recommended). Products include:

Cipro 3073

Cisapride (Bosentan is an inducer of CYP3A and CYP2C9. Consequently plasma concentrations of drugs metabolized by these two isozymes will be decreased when bosentan is co-administered).

No products indexed under this heading.

Clarithromycin (Bosentan is metabolized by CYP2C9 and CYP3A. Inhibition

of these enzymes may increase the plasma concentration of bosentan. Concomitant administration of both a CYP2C9 inhibitor (such as fluconazole or amiodarone) and a strong CYP3A inhibitor (eg, ketoconazole, itraconazole) or a moderate CYP3A inhibitor (eg, amprenavir, erythromycin, fluconazole, diltiazem) with bosentan will likely lead to large increases in plasma concentrations of bosentan. Co-administration of such combinations of a CYP2C9 inhibitor plus a strong or moderate CYP3A inhibitor with bosentan is not recommended). Products include:

Biaxin/Biaxin XL 412

Clomipramine Hydrochloride (Bosentan is an inducer of CYP3A and CYP2C9. Consequently plasma concentrations of drugs metabolized by these two isozymes will be decreased when bosentan is co-administered).

No products indexed under this heading.

Clopidogrel Bisulfate (Bosentan is metabolized by CYP2C9 and CYP3A. Inhibition of these enzymes may increase the plasma concentration of bosentan. Concomitant administration of both a CYP2C9 inhibitor (such as fluconazole or amiodarone) and a strong CYP3A inhibitor (eg, ketoconazole, itraconazole) or a moderate CYP3A inhibitor (eg, amprenavir, erythromycin, fluconazole, diltiazem) with bosentan will likely lead to large increases in plasma concentrations of bosentan. Co-administration of such combinations of a CYP2C9 inhibitor plus a strong or moderate CYP3A inhibitor with bosentan is not recommended). Products include:

Plavix 3027

Clopidogrel Hydrogen Sulfate (Bosentan is metabolized by CYP2C9 and CYP3A. Inhibition of these enzymes may increase the plasma concentration of bosentan. Concomitant administration of both a CYP2C9 inhibitor (such as fluconazole or amiodarone) and a strong CYP3A inhibitor (eg, ketoconazole, itraconazole) or a moderate CYP3A inhibitor (eg, amprenavir, erythromycin, fluconazole, diltiazem) with bosentan will likely lead to large increases in plasma concentrations of bosentan. Co-administration of such combinations of a CYP2C9 inhibitor plus a strong or moderate CYP3A inhibitor with bosentan is not recommended).

No products indexed under this heading.

Clotrimazole (Bosentan is metabolized by CYP2C9 and CYP3A. Inhibition of these enzymes may increase the plasma concentration of bosentan. Concomitant administration of both a CYP2C9 inhibitor (such as fluconazole or amiodarone) and a strong CYP3A inhibitor (eg, ketoconazole, itraconazole) or a moderate CYP3A inhibitor (eg, amprenavir, erythromycin, fluconazole, diltiazem) with bosentan will likely lead to large increases in plasma concentrations of bosentan. Co-administration of such combinations of a CYP2C9 inhibitor plus a strong or moderate CYP3A inhibitor with bosentan is not recommended). Products include:

Lotrisone 3163

Cyclosporine (The concomitant administration of bosentan and cyclosporine A is contraindicated. During the first day of concomitant administration, trough concentrations of bosentan were increased by about 30-fold. The mechanism of this interaction is most likely inhibition of transport protein-mediated uptake of bosentan into hepatocytes by cyclosporine. Steady-state bosentan plasma concentrations were 3- to 4-fold higher than in the absence of cyclosporine A. Co-

administration of bosentan decreased the plasma concentrations of cyclosporine A (a CYP3A substrate) by approximately 50%). Products include:

Gengraf 440
Neoral Oral Solution 2496
Neoral Capsules 2496
Restasis 605

Delavirdine Mesylate (Bosentan is metabolized by CYP2C9 and CYP3A. Inhibition of these enzymes may increase the plasma concentration of bosentan. Concomitant administration of both a CYP2C9 inhibitor (such as fluconazole or amiodarone) and a strong CYP3A inhibitor (eg, ketoconazole, itraconazole) or a moderate CYP3A inhibitor (eg, amprenavir, erythromycin, fluconazole, diltiazem) with bosentan will likely lead to large increases in plasma concentrations of bosentan. Co-administration of such combinations of a CYP2C9 inhibitor plus a strong or moderate CYP3A inhibitor with bosentan is not recommended).

No products indexed under this heading.

Desogestrel (Hormonal contraceptives, including oral, injectable, transdermal, and implantable forms, may not be reliable when bosentan is co-administered. Females should practice additional methods of contraception and not rely on hormonal contraception alone when taking bosentan. An interaction study demonstrated that co-administration of bosentan and a combination oral hormonal contraceptive produced average decreases of norethindrone and ethinyl estradiol levels of 14% and 31%, respectively. However, decreases in exposure were as much as 56% and 66%, respectively, in individual subjects).

No products indexed under this heading.

Dexamethasone (Bosentan is an inducer of CYP3A and CYP2C9. Consequently plasma concentrations of drugs metabolized by these two isozymes will be decreased when bosentan is co-administered). Products include:

Ciprodex 583
Ozurdex .... ☉223
Tobramycin and Dexamethasone Ophthalmic Suspension .... ☉251

Dexamethasone Acetate (Bosentan is an inducer of CYP3A and CYP2C9. Consequently plasma concentrations of drugs metabolized by these two isozymes will be decreased when bosentan is co-administered).

No products indexed under this heading.

Dexamethasone Phosphate (Bosentan is an inducer of CYP3A and CYP2C9. Consequently plasma concentrations of drugs metabolized by these two isozymes will be decreased when bosentan is co-administered).

No products indexed under this heading.

Dexamethasone Sodium (Bosentan is an inducer of CYP3A and CYP2C9. Consequently plasma concentrations of drugs metabolized by these two isozymes will be decreased when bosentan is co-administered).

No products indexed under this heading.

Dexamethasone Sodium Phosphate (Bosentan is an inducer of CYP3A and CYP2C9. Consequently plasma concentrations of drugs metabolized by these two isozymes will be decreased when bosentan is co-administered).

No products indexed under this heading.

Dextromethorphan (Bosentan is an inducer of CYP3A and CYP2C9. Consequently plasma concentrations of drugs metabolized by these two isozymes will be decreased when bosentan is co-administered).

No products indexed under this heading.

Diazepam (Bosentan is an inducer of CYP3A and CYP2C9. Consequently

Tracleer Interactions Index 1914

plasma concentrations of drugs metabolized by these two isozymes will be decreased when bosentan is co-administered). Products include:
Valium Tablets 2880

Diclofenac Epolamine (Bosentan is metabolized by CYP2C9 and CYP3A. Inhibition of these enzymes may increase the plasma concentration of bosentan. Concomitant administration of both a CYP2C9 inhibitor (such as fluconazole or amiodarone) and a strong CYP3A inhibitor (eg, ketoconazole, itraconazole) or a moderate CYP3A inhibitor (eg, amprenavir, erythromycin, fluconazole, diltiazem) with bosentan will likely lead to large increases in plasma concentrations of bosentan. Co-administration of such combinations of a CYP2C9 inhibitor plus a strong or moderate CYP3A inhibitor with bosentan is not recommended). Products include:
Flector 1839

Diclofenac Potassium (Bosentan is metabolized by CYP2C9 and CYP3A. Inhibition of these enzymes may increase the plasma concentration of bosentan. Concomitant administration of both a CYP2C9 inhibitor (such as fluconazole or amiodarone) and a strong CYP3A inhibitor (eg, ketoconazole, itraconazole) or a moderate CYP3A inhibitor (eg, amprenavir, erythromycin, fluconazole, diltiazem) with bosentan will likely lead to large increases in plasma concentrations of bosentan. Co-administration of such combinations of a CYP2C9 inhibitor plus a strong or moderate CYP3A inhibitor with bosentan is not recommended).
No products indexed under this heading.

Diclofenac Sodium (Bosentan is metabolized by CYP2C9 and CYP3A. Inhibition of these enzymes may increase the plasma concentration of bosentan. Concomitant administration of both a CYP2C9 inhibitor (such as fluconazole or amiodarone) and a strong CYP3A inhibitor (eg, ketoconazole, itraconazole) or a moderate CYP3A inhibitor (eg, amprenavir, erythromycin, fluconazole, diltiazem) with bosentan will likely lead to large increases in plasma concentrations of bosentan. Co-administration of such combinations of a CYP2C9 inhibitor plus a strong or moderate CYP3A inhibitor with bosentan is not recommended).
No products indexed under this heading.

Dienestrol (Hormonal contraceptives, including oral, injectable, transdermal, and implantable forms, may not be reliable when bosentan is co-administered. Females should practice additional methods of contraception and not rely on hormonal contraception alone when taking bosentan. An interaction study demonstrated that co-administration of bosentan and a combination oral hormonal contraceptive produced average decreases of norethindrone and ethinyl estradiol levels of 14% and 31%, respectively. However, decreases in exposure were as much as 56% and 66%, respectively, in individual subjects).
No products indexed under this heading.

Diethylstilbestrol (Hormonal contraceptives, including oral, injectable, transdermal, and implantable forms, may not be reliable when bosentan is co-administered. Females should practice additional methods of contraception and not rely on hormonal contraception alone when taking bosentan. An interaction study demonstrated that co-administration of bosentan and a combination oral hormonal contraceptive produced average decreases of norethindrone and ethinyl estradiol levels of 14% and 31%, respectively. However, decreases in exposure were as much as 56% and 66%, respectively, in individual subjects).
No products indexed under this heading.

Dihydroergotamine Mesylate (Bosentan is an inducer of CYP3A and CYP2C9. Consequently plasma concentrations of drugs metabolized by these two isozymes will be decreased when bosentan is co-administered).
No products indexed under this heading.

Diltiazem Hydrochloride (Bosentan is metabolized by CYP2C9 and CYP3A. Inhibition of these enzymes may increase the plasma concentration of bosentan. Concomitant administration of both a CYP2C9 inhibitor (such as fluconazole or amiodarone) and a strong CYP3A inhibitor (eg, ketoconazole, itraconazole) or a moderate CYP3A inhibitor (eg, amprenavir, erythromycin, fluconazole, diltiazem) with bosentan will likely lead to large increases in plasma concentrations of bosentan. Co-administration of such combinations of a CYP2C9 inhibitor plus a strong or moderate CYP3A inhibitor with bosentan is not recommended). Products include:
Cardizem LA 423

Diltiazem Maleate (Bosentan is metabolized by CYP2C9 and CYP3A. Inhibition of these enzymes may increase the plasma concentration of bosentan. Concomitant administration of both a CYP2C9 inhibitor (such as fluconazole or amiodarone) and a strong CYP3A inhibitor (eg, ketoconazole, itraconazole) or a moderate CYP3A inhibitor (eg, amprenavir, erythromycin, fluconazole, diltiazem) with bosentan will likely lead to large increases in plasma concentrations of bosentan. Co-administration of such combinations of a CYP2C9 inhibitor plus a strong or moderate CYP3A inhibitor with bosentan is not recommended).
No products indexed under this heading.

Disopyramide Phosphate (Bosentan is an inducer of CYP3A and CYP2C9. Consequently plasma concentrations of drugs metabolized by these two isozymes will be decreased when bosentan is co-administered).
No products indexed under this heading.

Disulfiram (Bosentan is metabolized by CYP2C9 and CYP3A. Inhibition of these enzymes may increase the plasma concentration of bosentan. Concomitant administration of both a CYP2C9 inhibitor (such as fluconazole or amiodarone) and a strong CYP3A inhibitor (eg, ketoconazole, itraconazole) or a moderate CYP3A inhibitor (eg, amprenavir, erythromycin, fluconazole, diltiazem) with bosentan will likely lead to large increases in plasma concentrations of bosentan. Co-administration of such combinations of a CYP2C9 inhibitor plus a strong or moderate CYP3A inhibitor with bosentan is not recommended).
No products indexed under this heading.

Doxorubicin Hydrochloride (Bosentan is an inducer of CYP3A and CYP2C9. Consequently plasma concentrations of drugs metabolized by these two isozymes will be decreased when bosentan is co-administered).
No products indexed under this heading.

Dronabinol (Bosentan is an inducer of CYP3A and CYP2C9. Consequently plasma concentrations of drugs metabolized by these two isozymes will be decreased when bosentan is co-administered).
No products indexed under this heading.

Dyphylline (Bosentan is an inducer of CYP3A and CYP2C9. Consequently plasma concentrations of drugs metabolized by these two isozymes will be decreased when bosentan is co-administered).
No products indexed under this heading.

Efavirenz (Bosentan is metabolized by CYP2C9 and CYP3A. Inhibition of these enzymes may increase the plasma concentration of bosentan. Concomitant administration of both a CYP2C9 inhibitor (such as fluconazole or amiodarone) and a strong CYP3A inhibitor (eg, ketoconazole, itraconazole) or a moderate CYP3A inhibitor (eg, amprenavir, erythromycin, fluconazole, diltiazem) with bosentan will likely lead to large increases in plasma concentrations of bosentan. Co-administration of such combinations of a CYP2C9 inhibitor plus a strong or moderate CYP3A inhibitor with bosentan is not recommended). Products include:
Atripla 906

Eprosartan Mesylate (Bosentan is an inducer of CYP3A and CYP2C9. Consequently plasma concentrations of drugs metabolized by these two isozymes will be decreased when bosentan is co-administered). Products include:
Teveten 538
Teveten HCT 541

Ergotamine Tartrate (Bosentan is an inducer of CYP3A and CYP2C9. Consequently plasma concentrations of drugs metabolized by these two isozymes will be decreased when bosentan is co-administered).
No products indexed under this heading.

Erythromycin (Bosentan is metabolized by CYP2C9 and CYP3A. Inhibition of these enzymes may increase the plasma concentration of bosentan. Concomitant administration of both a CYP2C9 inhibitor (such as fluconazole or amiodarone) and a strong CYP3A inhibitor (eg, ketoconazole, itraconazole) or a moderate CYP3A inhibitor (eg, amprenavir, erythromycin, fluconazole, diltiazem) with bosentan will likely lead to large increases in plasma concentrations of bosentan. Co-administration of such combinations of a CYP2C9 inhibitor plus a strong or moderate CYP3A inhibitor with bosentan is not recommended).
No products indexed under this heading.

Erythromycin, Topical (Bosentan is metabolized by CYP2C9 and CYP3A. Inhibition of these enzymes may increase the plasma concentration of bosentan. Concomitant administration of both a CYP2C9 inhibitor (such as fluconazole or amiodarone) and a strong CYP3A inhibitor (eg, ketoconazole, itraconazole) or a moderate CYP3A inhibitor (eg, amprenavir, erythromycin, fluconazole, diltiazem) with bosentan will likely lead to large increases in plasma concentrations of bosentan. Co-administration of such combinations of a CYP2C9 inhibitor plus a strong or moderate CYP3A inhibitor with bosentan is not recommended).
No products indexed under this heading.

Erythromycin Estolate (Bosentan is metabolized by CYP2C9 and CYP3A. Inhibition of these enzymes may increase the plasma concentration of bosentan. Concomitant administration of both a CYP2C9 inhibitor (such as fluconazole or amiodarone) and a strong CYP3A inhibitor (eg, ketoconazole, itraconazole) or a moderate CYP3A inhibitor (eg, amprenavir, erythromycin, fluconazole, diltiazem) with bosentan will likely lead to large increases in plasma concentrations of bosentan. Co-administration of such combinations of a CYP2C9 inhibitor plus a strong or moderate CYP3A inhibitor with bosentan is not recommended).
No products indexed under this heading.

Erythromycin Ethylsuccinate (Bosentan is metabolized by CYP2C9 and CYP3A. Inhibition of these enzymes may increase the plasma concentration of bosentan. Concomitant administration of both a CYP2C9 inhibitor (such as fluconazole or amiodarone) and a strong CYP3A inhibitor (eg, ketoconazole, itraconazole) or a moderate CYP3A inhibitor (eg, amprenavir, erythromycin, fluconazole, diltiazem) with bosentan will likely lead to large increases in plasma concentrations of bosentan. Co-administration of such combinations of a CYP2C9 inhibitor plus a strong or moderate CYP3A inhibitor with bosentan is not recommended). Products include:
E.E.S. 437
EryPed 435

Erythromycin Gluceptate (Bosentan is metabolized by CYP2C9 and CYP3A. Inhibition of these enzymes may increase the plasma concentration of bosentan. Concomitant administration of both a CYP2C9 inhibitor (such as fluconazole or amiodarone) and a strong CYP3A inhibitor (eg, ketoconazole, itraconazole) or a moderate CYP3A inhibitor (eg, amprenavir, erythromycin, fluconazole, diltiazem) with bosentan will likely lead to large increases in plasma concentrations of bosentan. Co-administration of such combinations of a CYP2C9 inhibitor plus a strong or moderate CYP3A inhibitor with bosentan is not recommended).
No products indexed under this heading.

Erythromycin Lactobionate (Bosentan is metabolized by CYP2C9 and CYP3A. Inhibition of these enzymes may increase the plasma concentration of bosentan. Concomitant administration of both a CYP2C9 inhibitor (such as fluconazole or amiodarone) and a strong CYP3A inhibitor (eg, ketoconazole, itraconazole) or a moderate CYP3A inhibitor (eg, amprenavir, erythromycin, fluconazole, diltiazem) with bosentan will likely lead to large increases in plasma concentrations of bosentan. Co-administration of such combinations of a CYP2C9 inhibitor plus a strong or moderate CYP3A inhibitor with bosentan is not recommended).
No products indexed under this heading.

Erythromycin Stearate (Bosentan is metabolized by CYP2C9 and CYP3A. Inhibition of these enzymes may increase the plasma concentration of bosentan. Concomitant administration of both a CYP2C9 inhibitor (such as fluconazole or amiodarone) and a strong CYP3A inhibitor (eg, ketoconazole, itraconazole) or a moderate CYP3A inhibitor (eg, amprenavir, erythromycin, fluconazole, diltiazem) with bosentan will likely lead to large increases in plasma concentrations of bosentan. Co-administration of such combinations of a CYP2C9 inhibitor plus a strong or moderate CYP3A inhibitor with bosentan is not recommended).
No products indexed under this heading.

Estradiol (Hormonal contraceptives, including oral, injectable, transdermal, and implantable forms, may not be reliable when bosentan is co-administered. Females should practice additional methods of contraception and not rely on hormonal contraception alone when taking bosentan. An interaction study demonstrated that co-administration of bosentan and a combination oral hormonal contraceptive produced average decreases of norethindrone and ethinyl estradiol levels of 14% and 31%, respectively. However, decreases in

exposure were as much as 56% and 66%, respectively, in individual subjects). Products include:

Estrogen (Bosentan is an inducer of CYP3A and CYP2C9. Consequently plasma concentrations of drugs metabolized by these two isozymes will be decreased when bosentan is co-administered).

No products indexed under this heading.

Estrogens, Conjugated (Hormonal contraceptives, including oral, injectable, transdermal, and implantable forms, may not be reliable when bosentan is co-administered. Females should practice additional methods of contraception and not rely on hormonal contraception alone when taking bosentan. An interaction study demonstrated that co-administration of bosentan and a combination oral hormonal contraceptive produced average decreases of norethindrone and ethinyl estradiol levels of 14% and 31%, respectively. However, decreases in exposure were as much as 56% and 66%, respectively, in individual subjects). Products include:

Estrogens, Conjugated, Synthetic A (Bosentan is an inducer of CYP3A and CYP2C9. Consequently plasma concentrations of drugs metabolized by these two isozymes will be decreased when bosentan is co-administered).

No products indexed under this heading.

Estrogens, Esterified (Hormonal contraceptives, including oral, injectable, transdermal, and implantable forms, may not be reliable when bosentan is co-administered. Females should practice additional methods of contraception and not rely on hormonal contraception alone when taking bosentan. An interaction study demonstrated that co-administration of bosentan and a combination oral hormonal contraceptive produced average decreases of norethindrone and ethinyl estradiol levels of 14% and 31%, respectively. However, decreases in exposure were as much as 56% and 66%, respectively, in individual subjects).

No products indexed under this heading.

Estropipate (Hormonal contraceptives, including oral, injectable, transdermal, and implantable forms, may not be reliable when bosentan is co-administered. Females should practice additional methods of contraception and not rely on hormonal contraception alone when taking bosentan. An interaction study demonstrated that co-administration of bosentan and a combination oral hormonal contraceptive produced average decreases of norethindrone and ethinyl estradiol levels of 14% and 31%, respectively. However, decreases in exposure were as much as 56% and 66%, respectively, in individual subjects).

No products indexed under this heading.

Ethinyl Estradiol (Hormonal contraceptives, including oral, injectable, transdermal, and implantable forms, may not be reliable when bosentan is co-administered. Females should practice additional methods of contraception and not rely on hormonal contraception alone when taking bosentan. An interaction study demonstrated that co-administration of bosentan and a combination oral hormonal contracep-

tive produced average decreases of norethindrone and ethinyl estradiol levels of 14% and 31%, respectively. However, decreases in exposure were as much as 56% and 66%, respectively, in individual subjects). Products include:

Ethosuximide (Bosentan is an inducer of CYP3A and CYP2C9. Consequently plasma concentrations of drugs metabolized by these two isozymes will be decreased when bosentan is co-administered).

No products indexed under this heading.

Ethynodiol Diacetate (Hormonal contraceptives, including oral, injectable, transdermal, and implantable forms, may not be reliable when bosentan is co-administered. Females should practice additional methods of contraception and not rely on hormonal contraception alone when taking bosentan. An interaction study demonstrated that co-administration of bosentan and a combination oral hormonal contraceptive produced average decreases of norethindrone and ethinyl estradiol levels of 14% and 31%, respectively. However, decreases in exposure were as much as 56% and 66%, respectively, in individual subjects).

No products indexed under this heading.

Etodolac (Bosentan is an inducer of CYP3A and CYP2C9. Consequently plasma concentrations of drugs metabolized by these two isozymes will be decreased when bosentan is co-administered).

No products indexed under this heading.

Etoposide (Bosentan is an inducer of CYP3A and CYP2C9. Consequently plasma concentrations of drugs metabolized by these two isozymes will be decreased when bosentan is co-administered).

No products indexed under this heading.

Etoposide Phosphate (Bosentan is an inducer of CYP3A and CYP2C9. Consequently plasma concentrations of drugs metabolized by these two isozymes will be decreased when bosentan is co-administered).

No products indexed under this heading.

Felodipine (Bosentan is an inducer of CYP3A and CYP2C9. Consequently plasma concentrations of drugs metabolized by these two isozymes will be decreased when bosentan is co-administered).

No products indexed under this heading.

Fenofibrate (Bosentan is metabolized by CYP2C9 and CYP3A. Inhibition of these enzymes may increase the plasma concentration of bosentan. Concomitant administration of both a CYP2C9 inhibitor (such as fluconazole or amiodarone) and a strong CYP3A inhibitor (eg, ketoconazole, itraconazole) or a moderate CYP3A inhibitor (eg, amprenavir, erythromycin, fluconazole, diltiazem) with bosentan will likely lead to large increases in plasma concentrations of bosentan. Co-administration of such combinations of a CYP2C9 inhibitor plus a strong or moderate CYP3A inhibitor with bosentan is not recommended). Products include:

Fenoprofen Calcium (Bosentan is an inducer of CYP3A and CYP2C9. Consequently plasma concentrations of drugs metabolized by these two isozymes will be decreased when bosentan is co-administered).

No products indexed under this heading.

Fentanyl (Bosentan is an inducer of CYP3A and CYP2C9. Consequently plasma concentrations of drugs metabolized by these two isozymes will be decreased when bosentan is co-administered). Products include:

Fentanyl Citrate (Bosentan is an inducer of CYP3A and CYP2C9. Consequently plasma concentrations of drugs metabolized by these two isozymes will be decreased when bosentan is co-administered). Products include:

Fluconazole (Bosentan is metabolized by CYP2C9 and CYP3A. Inhibition of these enzymes may increase the plasma concentration of bosentan. Concomitant administration of both a CYP2C9 inhibitor (such as fluconazole or amiodarone) and a strong CYP3A inhibitor (eg, ketoconazole, itraconazole) or a moderate CYP3A inhibitor (eg, amprenavir, erythromycin, fluconazole, diltiazem) with bosentan will likely lead to large increases in plasma concentrations of bosentan. Co-administration of such combinations of a CYP2C9 inhibitor plus a strong or moderate CYP3A inhibitor with bosentan is not recommended).

No products indexed under this heading.

Fluorouracil (Bosentan is metabolized by CYP2C9 and CYP3A. Inhibition of these enzymes may increase the plasma concentration of bosentan. Concomitant administration of both a CYP2C9 inhibitor (such as fluconazole or amiodarone) and a strong CYP3A inhibitor (eg, ketoconazole, itraconazole) or a moderate CYP3A inhibitor (eg, amprenavir, erythromycin, fluconazole, diltiazem) with bosentan will likely lead to large increases in plasma concentrations of bosentan. Co-administration of such combinations of a CYP2C9 inhibitor plus a strong or moderate CYP3A inhibitor with bosentan is not recommended). Products include:

Fluoxetine (Bosentan is metabolized by CYP2C9 and CYP3A. Inhibition of these enzymes may increase the plasma concentration of bosentan. Concomitant administration of both a CYP2C9 inhibitor (such as fluconazole or amiodarone) and a strong CYP3A inhibitor (eg, ketoconazole, itraconazole) or a moderate CYP3A inhibitor (eg, amprenavir, erythromycin, fluconazole, diltiazem) with bosentan will likely lead to large increases in plasma concentrations of bosentan. Co-administration of such combinations of a CYP2C9 inhibitor plus a strong or moderate CYP3A inhibitor with bosentan is not recommended).

No products indexed under this heading.

Fluoxetine Hydrochloride (Bosentan is metabolized by CYP2C9 and CYP3A. Inhibition of these enzymes may increase the plasma concentration of bosentan. Concomitant administration of both a CYP2C9 inhibitor (such as fluconazole or amiodarone) and a strong CYP3A inhibitor (eg, ketoconazole, itraconazole) or a moderate CYP3A inhibitor (eg, amprenavir, erythromycin, fluconazole, diltiazem) with bosentan will likely lead to large increases in plasma concentrations of bosentan. Co-administration of such combinations of a CYP2C9 inhibitor plus

a strong or moderate CYP3A inhibitor with bosentan is not recommended). Products include:

Flurbiprofen (Bosentan is metabolized by CYP2C9 and CYP3A. Inhibition of these enzymes may increase the plasma concentration of bosentan. Concomitant administration of both a CYP2C9 inhibitor (such as fluconazole or amiodarone) and a strong CYP3A inhibitor (eg, ketoconazole, itraconazole) or a moderate CYP3A inhibitor (eg, amprenavir, erythromycin, fluconazole, diltiazem) with bosentan will likely lead to large increases in plasma concentrations of bosentan. Co-administration of such combinations of a CYP2C9 inhibitor plus a strong or moderate CYP3A inhibitor with bosentan is not recommended).

No products indexed under this heading.

Flurbiprofen Sodium (Bosentan is metabolized by CYP2C9 and CYP3A. Inhibition of these enzymes may increase the plasma concentration of bosentan. Concomitant administration of both a CYP2C9 inhibitor (such as fluconazole or amiodarone) and a strong CYP3A inhibitor (eg, ketoconazole, itraconazole) or a moderate CYP3A inhibitor (eg, amprenavir, erythromycin, fluconazole, diltiazem) with bosentan will likely lead to large increases in plasma concentrations of bosentan. Co-administration of such combinations of a CYP2C9 inhibitor plus a strong or moderate CYP3A inhibitor with bosentan is not recommended).

No products indexed under this heading.

Fluvastatin Sodium (Bosentan is metabolized by CYP2C9 and CYP3A. Inhibition of these enzymes may increase the plasma concentration of bosentan. Concomitant administration of both a CYP2C9 inhibitor (such as fluconazole or amiodarone) and a strong CYP3A inhibitor (eg, ketoconazole, itraconazole) or a moderate CYP3A inhibitor (eg, amprenavir, erythromycin, fluconazole, diltiazem) with bosentan will likely lead to large increases in plasma concentrations of bosentan. Co-administration of such combinations of a CYP2C9 inhibitor plus a strong or moderate CYP3A inhibitor with bosentan is not recommended).

No products indexed under this heading.

Fluvoxamine Maleate (Bosentan is metabolized by CYP2C9 and CYP3A. Inhibition of these enzymes may increase the plasma concentration of bosentan. Concomitant administration of both a CYP2C9 inhibitor (such as fluconazole or amiodarone) and a strong CYP3A inhibitor (eg, ketoconazole, itraconazole) or a moderate CYP3A inhibitor (eg, amprenavir, erythromycin, fluconazole, diltiazem) with bosentan will likely lead to large increases in plasma concentrations of bosentan. Co-administration of such combinations of a CYP2C9 inhibitor plus a strong or moderate CYP3A inhibitor with bosentan is not recommended).

No products indexed under this heading.

Gemfibrozil (Bosentan is metabolized by CYP2C9 and CYP3A. Inhibition of these enzymes may increase the plasma concentration of bosentan. Concomitant administration of both a CYP2C9 inhibitor (such as fluconazole or amiodarone) and a strong CYP3A inhibitor (eg, ketoconazole, itraconazole) or a moderate CYP3A inhibitor (eg, amprenavir, erythromycin, fluconazole, diltiazem) with bosentan will likely lead to large increases in plasma concentrations of bosentan. Co-administration of such combinations of a CYP2C9 inhibi-

tor plus a strong or moderate CYP3A inhibitor with bosentan is not recommended).

No products indexed under this heading.

Glibenclamide (Co-administration of bosentan decreased the plasma concentrations of glyburide by approximately 40%. The plasma concentrations of bosentan were also decreased by approximately 30%. Bosentan is also expected to reduce plasma concentrations of other oral hypoglycemic agents that are predominantly metabolized by CYP2C9 or CYP3A. The possibility of worsened glucose control in patients using these agents should be considered.)

No products indexed under this heading.

Glimepiride (Co-administration of bosentan decreased the plasma concentrations of glyburide by approximately 40%. The plasma concentrations of bosentan were also decreased by approximately 30%. Bosentan is also expected to reduce plasma concentrations of other oral hypoglycemic agents that are predominantly metabolized by CYP2C9 or CYP3A. The possibility of worsened glucose control in patients using these agents should be considered). Products include:

Glipizide (Co-administration of bosentan decreased the plasma concentrations of glyburide by approximately 40%. The plasma concentrations of bosentan were also decreased by approximately 30%. Bosentan is also expected to reduce plasma concentrations of other oral hypoglycemic agents that are predominantly metabolized by CYP2C9 or CYP3A. The possibility of worsened glucose control in patients using these agents should be considered).

No products indexed under this heading.

Glyburide (The concomitant administration of bosentan and glyburide is contraindicated. An increased risk of elevated liver aminotransferases was observed in patients receiving concomitant therapy with glyburide. Therefore, alternative hypoglycemic agents should be considered. Co-administration of bosentan decreased the plasma concentrations of glyburide by approximately 40%. The plasma concentrations of bosentan were also decreased by approximately 30%. Bosentan is also expected to reduce plasma concentrations of other oral hypoglycemic agents that are predominantly metabolized by CYP2C9 or CYP3A. The possibility of worsened glucose control in patients using these agents should be considered).

No products indexed under this heading.

Haloperidol (Bosentan is an inducer of CYP3A and CYP2C9. Consequently plasma concentrations of drugs metabolized by these two isozymes will be decreased when bosentan is co-administered.)

No products indexed under this heading.

Haloperidol Decanoate (Bosentan is an inducer of CYP3A and CYP2C9. Consequently plasma concentrations of drugs metabolized by these two isozymes will be decreased when bosentan is co-administered.)

No products indexed under this heading.

Hydrochlorothiazide (Bosentan is metabolized by CYP2C9 and CYP3A. Inhibition of these enzymes may increase the plasma concentration of bosentan. Concomitant administration of both a CYP2C9 inhibitor (such as fluconazole or amiodarone) and a strong CYP3A inhibitor (eg, ketoconazole, itraconazole) or a moderate CYP3A inhibitor (eg, amprenavir, eryth-

romycin, fluconazole, diltiazem) with bosentan will likely lead to large increases in plasma concentrations of bosentan. Co-administration of such combinations of a CYP2C9 inhibitor plus a strong or moderate CYP3A inhibitor with bosentan is not recommended). Products include:

Hydrochlorothiazide Hydrochloride (Bosentan is metabolized by CYP2C9 and CYP3A. Inhibition of these enzymes may increase the plasma concentration of bosentan. Concomitant administration of both a CYP2C9 inhibitor (such as fluconazole or amiodarone) and a strong CYP3A inhibitor (eg, ketoconazole, itraconazole) or a moderate CYP3A inhibitor (eg, amprenavir, erythromycin, fluconazole, diltiazem) with bosentan will likely lead to large increases in plasma concentrations of bosentan. Co-administration of such combinations of a CYP2C9 inhibitor plus a strong or moderate CYP3A inhibitor with bosentan is not recommended).

No products indexed under this heading.

Hydroflumethiazide (Bosentan is metabolized by CYP2C9 and CYP3A. Inhibition of these enzymes may increase the plasma concentration of bosentan. Concomitant administration of both a CYP2C9 inhibitor (such as fluconazole or amiodarone) and a strong CYP3A inhibitor (eg, ketoconazole, itraconazole) or a moderate CYP3A inhibitor (eg, amprenavir, erythromycin, fluconazole, diltiazem) with bosentan will likely lead to large increases in plasma concentrations of bosentan. Co-administration of such combinations of a CYP2C9 inhibitor plus a strong or moderate CYP3A inhibitor with bosentan is not recommended).

No products indexed under this heading.

Ibuprofen (Bosentan is an inducer of CYP3A and CYP2C9. Consequently plasma concentrations of drugs metabolized by these two isozymes will be decreased when bosentan is co-administered). Products include:

Imatinib Mesylate (Bosentan is metabolized by CYP2C9 and CYP3A. Inhibition of these enzymes may increase the plasma concentration of bosentan. Concomitant administration of both a CYP2C9 inhibitor (such as fluconazole or amiodarone) and a strong CYP3A inhibitor (eg, ketoconazole, itraconazole) or a moderate CYP3A inhibitor (eg, amprenavir, erythromycin, fluconazole, diltiazem) with bosentan will likely lead to large increases in plasma concentrations of bosentan. Co-administration of such combinations of a CYP2C9 inhibitor plus a strong or moderate CYP3A inhibitor with bosentan is not recommended). Products include:

Imipramine Hydrochloride (Bosentan is an inducer of CYP3A and CYP2C9. Consequently plasma concentrations of drugs metabolized by these two isozymes will be decreased when bosentan is co-administered.)

No products indexed under this heading.

Imipramine Pamoate (Bosentan is an inducer of CYP3A and CYP2C9. Consequently plasma concentrations of drugs metabolized by these two isozymes will be decreased when bosentan is co-administered.)

No products indexed under this heading.

Indinavir Sulfate (Bosentan is metabolized by CYP2C9 and CYP3A. Inhibition of these enzymes may increase the plasma concentration of bosentan. Concomitant administration of both a CYP2C9 inhibitor (such as fluconazole or amiodarone) and a strong CYP3A inhibitor (eg, ketoconazole, itraconazole) or a moderate CYP3A inhibitor (eg, amprenavir, erythromycin, fluconazole, diltiazem) with bosentan will likely lead to large increases in plasma concentrations of bosentan. Co-administration of such combinations of a CYP2C9 inhibitor plus a strong or moderate CYP3A inhibitor with bosentan is not recommended). Products include:

Indomethacin (Bosentan is an inducer of CYP3A and CYP2C9. Consequently plasma concentrations of drugs metabolized by these two isozymes will be decreased when bosentan is co-administered). Products include:

Indomethacin Sodium Trihydrate (Bosentan is an inducer of CYP3A and CYP2C9. Consequently plasma concentrations of drugs metabolized by these two isozymes will be decreased when bosentan is co-administered). Products include:

Irbesartan (Bosentan is an inducer of CYP3A and CYP2C9. Consequently plasma concentrations of drugs metabolized by these two isozymes will be decreased when bosentan is co-administered). Products include:

Isoniazid (Bosentan is metabolized by CYP2C9 and CYP3A. Inhibition of these enzymes may increase the plasma concentration of bosentan. Concomitant administration of both a CYP2C9 inhibitor (such as fluconazole or amiodarone) and a strong CYP3A inhibitor (eg, ketoconazole, itraconazole) or a moderate CYP3A inhibitor (eg, amprenavir, erythromycin, fluconazole, diltiazem) with bosentan will likely lead to large increases in plasma concentrations of bosentan. Co-administration of such combinations of a CYP2C9 inhibitor plus a strong or moderate CYP3A inhibitor with bosentan is not recommended).

No products indexed under this heading.

Isradipine (Bosentan is an inducer of CYP3A and CYP2C9. Consequently plasma concentrations of drugs metabolized by these two isozymes will be decreased when bosentan is co-administered). Products include:

Itraconazole (Bosentan is metabolized by CYP2C9 and CYP3A. Inhibition of these enzymes may increase the plasma concentration of bosentan. Concomitant administration of both a CYP2C9 inhibitor (such as fluconazole or amiodarone) and a strong CYP3A inhibitor (eg, ketoconazole, itraconazole) or a moderate CYP3A inhibitor (eg, amprenavir, erythromycin, fluconazole, diltiazem) with bosentan will likely lead to large increases in plasma con-

centrations of bosentan. Co-administration of such combinations of a CYP2C9 inhibitor plus a strong or moderate CYP3A inhibitor with bosentan is not recommended).

No products indexed under this heading.

Ketoconazole (Co-administration of bosentan 125 mg bid and ketoconazole, a potent CYP3A inhibitor, increased the plasma concentrations of bosentan by approximately 2-fold in normal volunteers. No dosage adjustment of bosentan is necessary, but increased effects of bosentan should be considered. In addition, concomitant administration of both a CYP2C9 inhibitor (eg, fluconazole, amiodarone) and a strong CYP3A inhibitor (eg, ketoconazole, itraconazole) or a moderate CYP3A inhibitor (eg, amprenavir, erythromycin, fluconazole, diltiazem) with bosentan will likely lead to large increases in plasma concentrations of bosentan. Co-administration of such combinations of a CYP2C9 inhibitor plus a strong or moderate CYP3A inhibitor with bosentan is not recommended). Products include:

Ketoprofen (Bosentan is metabolized by CYP2C9 and CYP3A. Inhibition of these enzymes may increase the plasma concentration of bosentan. Concomitant administration of both a CYP2C9 inhibitor (such as fluconazole or amiodarone) and a strong CYP3A inhibitor (eg, ketoconazole, itraconazole) or a moderate CYP3A inhibitor (eg, amprenavir, erythromycin, fluconazole, diltiazem) with bosentan will likely lead to large increases in plasma concentrations of bosentan. Co-administration of such combinations of a CYP2C9 inhibitor plus a strong or moderate CYP3A inhibitor with bosentan is not recommended).

No products indexed under this heading.

Ketorolac Tromethamine (Bosentan is an inducer of CYP3A and CYP2C9. Consequently plasma concentrations of drugs metabolized by these two isozymes will be decreased when bosentan is co-administered). Products include:

Lansoprazole (Bosentan is an inducer of CYP3A and CYP2C9. Consequently plasma concentrations of drugs metabolized by these two isozymes will be decreased when bosentan is co-administered.)

No products indexed under this heading.

Leflunomide (Bosentan is metabolized by CYP2C9 and CYP3A. Inhibition of these enzymes may increase the plasma concentration of bosentan. Concomitant administration of both a CYP2C9 inhibitor (such as fluconazole or amiodarone) and a strong CYP3A inhibitor (eg, ketoconazole, itraconazole) or a moderate CYP3A inhibitor (eg, amprenavir, erythromycin, fluconazole, diltiazem) with bosentan will likely lead to large increases in plasma concentrations of bosentan. Co-administration of such combinations of a CYP2C9 inhibitor plus a strong or moderate CYP3A inhibitor with bosentan is not recommended).

No products indexed under this heading.

Levonorgestrel (Hormonal contraceptives, including oral, injectable, transdermal, and implantable forms, may not be reliable when bosentan is co-administered. Females should practice additional methods of contraception and not rely on hormonal contraception alone when taking bosentan. An interaction study demonstrated that co-administration of bosentan and a combination oral hormonal contraceptive produced average decreases of noreth-

1917 Interactions Index Tracleer

indrone and ethinyl estradiol levels of 14% and 31%, respectively. However, decreases in exposure were as much as 56% and 66%, respectively, in individual subjects). Products include:
Climara Pro 847
LoSeasonique 3407
Lybrel 3514
Mirena 854
Plan B 3416
Seasonique 3418

Lidocaine (Bosentan is an inducer of CYP3A and CYP2C9. Consequently plasma concentrations of drugs metabolized by these two isozymes will be decreased when bosentan is co-administered). Products include:
Lidoderm 1107

Lidocaine Hydrochloride (Bosentan is an inducer of CYP3A and CYP2C9. Consequently plasma concentrations of drugs metabolized by these two isozymes will be decreased when bosentan is co-administered).
No products indexed under this heading.

Lopinavir (*In vitro* data indicates that bosentan is a substrate of the Organic Anion Transport Protein (OATP), CYP3A, and CYP2C9. Ritonavir inhibits OATP and inhibits and induces CYP3A. However, the impact of ritonavir on the pharmacokinetics of bosentan may largely result from its effect on OATP. In normal volunteers, co-administration of bosentan 125 mg bid and lopinavir/ritonavir 400/100 mg bid increased the trough concentrations of bosentan on Days 4 and 10 approximately 48-fold and 5-fold, respectively, compared with those measured after bosentan administered alone. Therefore, the dose of bosentan should be adjusted when initiating lopinavir/ritonavir). Products include:
Kaletra 458

Losartan Potassium (Bosentan is an inducer of CYP3A and CYP2C9. Consequently plasma concentrations of drugs metabolized by these two isozymes will be decreased when bosentan is co-administered). Products include:
Cozaar 2106
Hyzaar 2162
Hyzaar 100-12.5 2162

Lovastatin (Co-administration of bosentan decreased the plasma concentrations of simvastatin (a CYP3A substrate), and its active β-hydroxy acid metabolite, by approximately 50%. The plasma concentrations of bosentan were not affected. Bosentan is also expected to reduce plasma concentrations of other statins that are significantly metabolized by CYP3A, such as lovastatin and atorvastatin. The possibility of reduced statin efficacy should be considered. Patients using CYP3A-metabolized statins should have cholesterol levels monitored after bosentan is initiated to see whether the statin dose needs adjustment). Products include:
Advicor 402
Mevacor 2212

Meclofenamate Sodium (Bosentan is an inducer of CYP3A and CYP2C9. Consequently plasma concentrations of drugs metabolized by these two isozymes will be decreased when bosentan is co-administered).
No products indexed under this heading.

Medroxyprogesterone Acetate (Hormonal contraceptives, including oral, injectable, transdermal, and implantable forms, may not be reliable when bosentan is co-administered. Females should practice additional methods of contraception and not rely on hormonal contraception alone when taking bosentan. An interaction study demonstrated that co-administration of bosentan and a combination oral hormonal contraceptive produced average decreases of norethindrone and ethinyl estradiol levels of 14% and 31%, respectively. However, decreases in exposure were as much as 56% and 66%, respectively, in individual subjects). Products include:
Premphase 3549
Prempro 3549

Mefenamic Acid (Bosentan is an inducer of CYP3A and CYP2C9. Consequently plasma concentrations of drugs metabolized by these two isozymes will be decreased when bosentan is co-administered).
No products indexed under this heading.

Megestrol Acetate (Hormonal contraceptives, including oral, injectable, transdermal, and implantable forms, may not be reliable when bosentan is co-administered. Females should practice additional methods of contraception and not rely on hormonal contraception alone when taking bosentan. An interaction study demonstrated that co-administration of bosentan and a combination oral hormonal contraceptive produced average decreases of norethindrone and ethinyl estradiol levels of 14% and 31%, respectively. However, decreases in exposure were as much as 56% and 66%, respectively, in individual subjects). Products include:
Megace ES 2698

Meloxicam (Bosentan is an inducer of CYP3A and CYP2C9. Consequently plasma concentrations of drugs metabolized by these two isozymes will be decreased when bosentan is co-administered).
No products indexed under this heading.

Mestranol (Hormonal contraceptives, including oral, injectable, transdermal, and implantable forms, may not be reliable when bosentan is co-administered. Females should practice additional methods of contraception and not rely on hormonal contraception alone when taking bosentan. An interaction study demonstrated that co-administration of bosentan and a combination oral hormonal contraceptive produced average decreases of norethindrone and ethinyl estradiol levels of 14% and 31%, respectively. However, decreases in exposure were as much as 56% and 66%, respectively, in individual subjects).
No products indexed under this heading.

Metformin Hydrochloride (Co-administration of bosentan decreased the plasma concentrations of glyburide by approximately 40%. The plasma concentrations of bosentan were also decreased by approximately 30%. Bosentan is also expected to reduce plasma concentrations of other oral hypoglycemic agents that are predominantly metabolized by CYP2C9 or CYP3A. The possibility of worsened glucose control in patients using these agents should be considered). Products include:
ActoPlus 3338
Avandamet 1345
Janumet 2188

Methadone Hydrochloride (Bosentan is an inducer of CYP3A and CYP2C9. Consequently plasma concentrations of drugs metabolized by these two isozymes will be decreased when bosentan is co-administered).
No products indexed under this heading.

Methyclothiazide (Bosentan is metabolized by CYP2C9 and CYP3A. Inhibition of these enzymes may increase the plasma concentration of bosentan. Concomitant administration of both a CYP2C9 inhibitor (such as fluconazole or amiodarone) and a strong CYP3A inhibitor (eg, ketoconazole, itraconazole) or a moderate CYP3A inhibitor (eg, amprenavir, erythromycin, fluconazole, diltiazem) with bosentan will likely lead to large increases in plasma concentrations of bosentan. Co-administration of such combinations of a CYP2C9 inhibitor plus a strong or moderate CYP3A inhibitor with bosentan is not recommended).
No products indexed under this heading.

Methylprednisolone (Bosentan is an inducer of CYP3A and CYP2C9. Consequently plasma concentrations of drugs metabolized by these two isozymes will be decreased when bosentan is co-administered).
No products indexed under this heading.

Methylprednisolone Acetate (Bosentan is an inducer of CYP3A and CYP2C9. Consequently plasma concentrations of drugs metabolized by these two isozymes will be decreased when bosentan is co-administered).
No products indexed under this heading.

Methylprednisolone Sodium Succinate (Bosentan is an inducer of CYP3A and CYP2C9. Consequently plasma concentrations of drugs metabolized by these two isozymes will be decreased when bosentan is co-administered).
No products indexed under this heading.

Metronidazole (Bosentan is metabolized by CYP2C9 and CYP3A. Inhibition of these enzymes may increase the plasma concentration of bosentan. Concomitant administration of both a CYP2C9 inhibitor (such as fluconazole or amiodarone) and a strong CYP3A inhibitor (eg, ketoconazole, itraconazole) or a moderate CYP3A inhibitor (eg, amprenavir, erythromycin, fluconazole, diltiazem) with bosentan will likely lead to large increases in plasma concentrations of bosentan. Co-administration of such combinations of a CYP2C9 inhibitor plus a strong or moderate CYP3A inhibitor with bosentan is not recommended). Products include:
Pylera 793

Metronidazole Benzoate (Bosentan is metabolized by CYP2C9 and CYP3A. Inhibition of these enzymes may increase the plasma concentration of bosentan. Concomitant administration of both a CYP2C9 inhibitor (such as fluconazole or amiodarone) and a strong CYP3A inhibitor (eg, ketoconazole, itraconazole) or a moderate CYP3A inhibitor (eg, amprenavir, erythromycin, fluconazole, diltiazem) with bosentan will likely lead to large increases in plasma concentrations of bosentan. Co-administration of such combinations of a CYP2C9 inhibitor plus a strong or moderate CYP3A inhibitor with bosentan is not recommended).
No products indexed under this heading.

Metronidazole Hydrochloride (Bosentan is metabolized by CYP2C9 and CYP3A. Inhibition of these enzymes may increase the plasma concentration of bosentan. Concomitant administration of both a CYP2C9 inhibitor (such as fluconazole or amiodarone) and a strong CYP3A inhibitor (eg, ketoconazole, itraconazole) or a moderate CYP3A inhibitor (eg, amprenavir, erythromycin, fluconazole, diltiazem) with bosentan will likely lead to large increases in plasma concentrations of bosentan. Co-administration of such combinations of a CYP2C9 inhibitor plus a strong or moderate CYP3A inhibitor with bosentan is not recommended).
No products indexed under this heading.

Metronidazole Sodium (Bosentan is metabolized by CYP2C9 and CYP3A. Inhibition of these enzymes may increase the plasma concentration of bosentan. Concomitant administration of both a CYP2C9 inhibitor (such as fluconazole or amiodarone) and a strong CYP3A inhibitor (eg, ketoconazole, itraconazole) or a moderate CYP3A inhibitor (eg, amprenavir, erythromycin, fluconazole, diltiazem) with bosentan will likely lead to large increases in plasma concentrations of bosentan. Co-administration of such combinations of a CYP2C9 inhibitor plus a strong or moderate CYP3A inhibitor with bosentan is not recommended).
No products indexed under this heading.

Miconazole (Bosentan is metabolized by CYP2C9 and CYP3A. Inhibition of these enzymes may increase the plasma concentration of bosentan. Concomitant administration of both a CYP2C9 inhibitor (such as fluconazole or amiodarone) and a strong CYP3A inhibitor (eg, ketoconazole, itraconazole) or a moderate CYP3A inhibitor (eg, amprenavir, erythromycin, fluconazole, diltiazem) with bosentan will likely lead to large increases in plasma concentrations of bosentan. Co-administration of such combinations of a CYP2C9 inhibitor plus a strong or moderate CYP3A inhibitor with bosentan is not recommended).
No products indexed under this heading.

Miconazole Nitrate (Bosentan is metabolized by CYP2C9 and CYP3A. Inhibition of these enzymes may increase the plasma concentration of bosentan. Concomitant administration of both a CYP2C9 inhibitor (such as fluconazole or amiodarone) and a strong CYP3A inhibitor (eg, ketoconazole, itraconazole) or a moderate CYP3A inhibitor (eg, amprenavir, erythromycin, fluconazole, diltiazem) with bosentan will likely lead to large increases in plasma concentrations of bosentan. Co-administration of such combinations of a CYP2C9 inhibitor plus a strong or moderate CYP3A inhibitor with bosentan is not recommended). Products include:
Vusion Ointment 3335

Midazolam Hydrochloride (Bosentan is an inducer of CYP3A and CYP2C9. Consequently plasma concentrations of drugs metabolized by these two isozymes will be decreased when bosentan is co-administered).
No products indexed under this heading.

Miglitol (Co-administration of bosentan decreased the plasma concentrations of glyburide by approximately 40%. The plasma concentrations of bosentan were also decreased by approximately 30%. Bosentan is also expected to reduce plasma concentrations of other oral hypoglycemic agents that are predominantly metabolized by CYP2C9 or CYP3A. The possibility of worsened glucose control in patients using these agents should be considered).
No products indexed under this heading.

Mirtazapine (Bosentan is an inducer of CYP3A and CYP2C9. Consequently plasma concentrations of drugs metabolized by these two isozymes will be decreased when bosentan is co-administered). Products include:
Remeron Tablets 3214
RemeronSolTab Tablets 3219

Modafinil (Bosentan is metabolized by CYP2C9 and CYP3A. Inhibition of these enzymes may increase the plasma concentration of bosentan. Concomitant administration of both a CYP2C9 inhibitor (such as fluconazole or amiodarone) and a strong CYP3A inhibitor (eg, ketoconazole, itraconazole) or a moderate CYP3A inhibitor (eg, amprenavir, erythromycin, fluconazole, diltiazem) with bosentan will likely lead to large increases in plasma concentrations of bosentan. Co-administration of such combinations of a CYP2C9 inhibitor plus a strong or moderate CYP3A inhibitor with bosentan is not recommended). Products include:

Tracleer Interactions Index 1918

Provigil ... 983

Montelukast Sodium (Bosentan is an inducer of CYP3A and CYP2C9. Consequently plasma concentrations of drugs metabolized by these two isozymes will be decreased when bosentan is co-administered). Products include:

Singulair ... 2270

Nabumetone (Bosentan is an inducer of CYP3A and CYP2C9. Consequently plasma concentrations of drugs metabolized by these two isozymes will be decreased when bosentan is co-administered).

No products indexed under this heading.

Naproxen (Bosentan is an inducer of CYP3A and CYP2C9. Consequently plasma concentrations of drugs metabolized by these two isozymes will be decreased when bosentan is co-administered). Products include:

EC-Naprosyn ... 2850
Naprosyn ... 2850
Anaprox/Naprosyn ... 2850

Naproxen Sodium (Bosentan is an inducer of CYP3A and CYP2C9. Consequently plasma concentrations of drugs metabolized by these two isozymes will be decreased when bosentan is co-administered). Products include:

Anaprox ... 2850
Anaprox DS ... 2850
Treximet ... 1681

Nateglinide (Co-administration of bosentan decreased the plasma concentrations of glyburide by approximately 40%. The plasma concentrations of bosentan were also decreased by approximately 30%. Bosentan is also expected to reduce plasma concentrations of other oral hypoglycemic agents that are predominantly metabolized by CYP2C9 or CYP3A. The possibility of worsened glucose control in patients using these agents should be considered).

No products indexed under this heading.

Nefazodone Hydrochloride (Bosentan is metabolized by CYP2C9 and CYP3A. Inhibition of these enzymes may increase the plasma concentration of bosentan. Concomitant administration of both a CYP2C9 inhibitor (such as fluconazole or amiodarone) and a strong CYP3A inhibitor (eg, ketoconazole, itraconazole) or a moderate CYP3A inhibitor (eg, amprenavir, erythromycin, fluconazole, diltiazem) with bosentan will likely lead to large increases in plasma concentrations of bosentan. Co-administration of such combinations of a CYP2C9 inhibitor plus a strong or moderate CYP3A inhibitor with bosentan is not recommended).

No products indexed under this heading.

Nelfinavir Mesylate (Bosentan is metabolized by CYP2C9 and CYP3A. Inhibition of these enzymes may increase the plasma concentration of bosentan. Concomitant administration of both a CYP2C9 inhibitor (such as fluconazole or amiodarone) and a strong CYP3A inhibitor (eg, ketoconazole, itraconazole) or a moderate CYP3A inhibitor (eg, amprenavir, erythromycin, fluconazole, diltiazem) with bosentan will likely lead to large increases in plasma concentrations of bosentan. Co-administration of such combinations of a CYP2C9 inhibitor plus a strong or moderate CYP3A inhibitor with bosentan is not recommended).

No products indexed under this heading.

Nicardipine (Bosentan is an inducer of CYP3A and CYP2C9. Consequently plasma concentrations of drugs metabolized by these two isozymes will be decreased when bosentan is co-administered).

No products indexed under this heading.

Nicardipine Hydrochloride (Bosentan is an inducer of CYP3A and CYP2C9. Consequently plasma concentrations of drugs metabolized by these two isozymes will be decreased when bosentan is co-administered).

No products indexed under this heading.

Nifedipine (Bosentan is metabolized by CYP2C9 and CYP3A. Inhibition of these enzymes may increase the plasma concentration of bosentan. Concomitant administration of both a CYP2C9 inhibitor (such as fluconazole or amiodarone) and a strong CYP3A inhibitor (eg, ketoconazole, itraconazole) or a moderate CYP3A inhibitor (eg, amprenavir, erythromycin, fluconazole, diltiazem) with bosentan will likely lead to large increases in plasma concentrations of bosentan. Co-administration of such combinations of a CYP2C9 inhibitor plus a strong or moderate CYP3A inhibitor with bosentan is not recommended).

No products indexed under this heading.

Nimodipine (Bosentan is an inducer of CYP3A and CYP2C9. Consequently plasma concentrations of drugs metabolized by these two isozymes will be decreased when bosentan is co-administered).

No products indexed under this heading.

Nisoldipine (Bosentan is an inducer of CYP3A and CYP2C9. Consequently plasma concentrations of drugs metabolized by these two isozymes will be decreased when bosentan is co-administered).

No products indexed under this heading.

Norethindrone (Hormonal contraceptives, including oral, injectable, transdermal, and implantable forms, may not be reliable when bosentan is co-administered. Females should practice additional methods of contraception and not rely on hormonal contraception alone when taking bosentan. An interaction study demonstrated that co-administration of bosentan and a combination oral hormonal contraceptive produced average decreases of norethindrone and ethinyl estradiol levels of 14% and 31%, respectively. However, decreases in exposure were as much as 56% and 66%, respectively, in individual subjects). Products include:

Ortho Micronor ... 2660

Norethindrone Acetate (Hormonal contraceptives, including oral, injectable, transdermal, and implantable forms, may not be reliable when bosentan is co-administered. Females should practice additional methods of contraception and not rely on hormonal contraception alone when taking bosentan. An interaction study demonstrated that co-administration of bosentan and a combination oral hormonal contraceptive produced average decreases of norethindrone and ethinyl estradiol levels of 14% and 31%, respectively. However, decreases in exposure were as much as 56% and 66%, respectively, in individual subjects). Products include:

Activella ... 2561

Norethynodrel (Hormonal contraceptives, including oral, injectable, transdermal, and implantable forms, may not be reliable when bosentan is co-administered. Females should practice additional methods of contraception and not rely on hormonal contraception alone when taking bosentan. An interaction study demonstrated that co-administration of bosentan and a combination oral hormonal contraceptive produced average decreases of norethindrone and ethinyl estradiol levels of 14% and 31%, respectively. However, decreases in exposure were as much as 56% and 66%, respectively, in individual subjects).

No products indexed under this heading.

Norfloxacin (Bosentan is metabolized by CYP2C9 and CYP3A. Inhibition of these enzymes may increase the plasma concentration of bosentan. Concomitant administration of both a CYP2C9 inhibitor (such as fluconazole or amiodarone) and a strong CYP3A inhibitor (eg, ketoconazole, itraconazole) or a moderate CYP3A inhibitor (eg, amprenavir, erythromycin, fluconazole, diltiazem) with bosentan will likely lead to large increases in plasma concentrations of bosentan. Co-administration of such combinations of a CYP2C9 inhibitor plus a strong or moderate CYP3A inhibitor with bosentan is not recommended). Products include:

Noroxin ... 2220

Norgestimate (Hormonal contraceptives, including oral, injectable, transdermal, and implantable forms, may not be reliable when bosentan is co-administered. Females should practice additional methods of contraception and not rely on hormonal contraception alone when taking bosentan. An interaction study demonstrated that co-administration of bosentan and a combination oral hormonal contraceptive produced average decreases of norethindrone and ethinyl estradiol levels of 14% and 31%, respectively. However, decreases in exposure were as much as 56% and 66%, respectively, in individual subjects). Products include:

Ortho-Cyclen/Ortho Tri-Cyclen ... 2663
Ortho Tri-Cyclen Lo Tablets ... 2673

Norgestrel (Hormonal contraceptives, including oral, injectable, transdermal, and implantable forms, may not be reliable when bosentan is co-administered. Females should practice additional methods of contraception and not rely on hormonal contraception alone when taking bosentan. An interaction study demonstrated that co-administration of bosentan and a combination oral hormonal contraceptive produced average decreases of norethindrone and ethinyl estradiol levels of 14% and 31%, respectively. However, decreases in exposure were as much as 56% and 66%, respectively, in individual subjects).

No products indexed under this heading.

Omeprazole (Bosentan is metabolized by CYP2C9 and CYP3A. Inhibition of these enzymes may increase the plasma concentration of bosentan. Concomitant administration of both a CYP2C9 inhibitor (such as fluconazole or amiodarone) and a strong CYP3A inhibitor (eg, ketoconazole, itraconazole) or a moderate CYP3A inhibitor (eg, amprenavir, erythromycin, fluconazole, diltiazem) with bosentan will likely lead to large increases in plasma concentrations of bosentan. Co-administration of such combinations of a CYP2C9 inhibitor plus a strong or moderate CYP3A inhibitor with bosentan is not recommended).

No products indexed under this heading.

Ondansetron Hydrochloride (Bosentan is an inducer of CYP3A and CYP2C9. Consequently plasma concentrations of drugs metabolized by these two isozymes will be decreased when bosentan is co-administered). Products include:

Zofran Injection ... 1750
Zofran ... 1756
Zofran ODT ... 1756

Oxaprozin (Bosentan is an inducer of CYP3A and CYP2C9. Consequently plasma concentrations of drugs metabolized by these two isozymes will be decreased when bosentan is co-administered).

No products indexed under this heading.

Oxiconazole Nitrate (Bosentan is metabolized by CYP2C9 and CYP3A. Inhibition of these enzymes may increase the plasma concentration of bosentan. Concomitant administration of both a CYP2C9 inhibitor (such as fluconazole or amiodarone) and a strong CYP3A inhibitor (eg, ketoconazole, itraconazole) or a moderate CYP3A inhibitor (eg, amprenavir, erythromycin, fluconazole, diltiazem) with bosentan will likely lead to large increases in plasma concentrations of bosentan. Co-administration of such combinations of a CYP2C9 inhibitor plus a strong or moderate CYP3A inhibitor with bosentan is not recommended).

No products indexed under this heading.

Paclitaxel (Bosentan is an inducer of CYP3A and CYP2C9. Consequently plasma concentrations of drugs metabolized by these two isozymes will be decreased when bosentan is co-administered).

No products indexed under this heading.

Paroxetine Hydrochloride (Bosentan is metabolized by CYP2C9 and CYP3A. Inhibition of these enzymes may increase the plasma concentration of bosentan. Concomitant administration of both a CYP2C9 inhibitor (such as fluconazole or amiodarone) and a strong CYP3A inhibitor (eg, ketoconazole, itraconazole) or a moderate CYP3A inhibitor (eg, amprenavir, erythromycin, fluconazole, diltiazem) with bosentan will likely lead to large increases in plasma concentrations of bosentan. Co-administration of such combinations of a CYP2C9 inhibitor plus a strong or moderate CYP3A inhibitor with bosentan is not recommended). Products include:

Paroxetine CR ... 2361
Paroxetine ER ... 2371
Paxil ... 1586
Paxil CR ... 1596

Phenylbutazone (Bosentan is metabolized by CYP2C9 and CYP3A. Inhibition of these enzymes may increase the plasma concentration of bosentan. Concomitant administration of both a CYP2C9 inhibitor (such as fluconazole or amiodarone) and a strong CYP3A inhibitor (eg, ketoconazole, itraconazole) or a moderate CYP3A inhibitor (eg, amprenavir, erythromycin, fluconazole, diltiazem) with bosentan will likely lead to large increases in plasma concentrations of bosentan. Co-administration of such combinations of a CYP2C9 inhibitor plus a strong or moderate CYP3A inhibitor with bosentan is not recommended).

No products indexed under this heading.

Phenytoin (Bosentan is an inducer of CYP3A and CYP2C9. Consequently plasma concentrations of drugs metabolized by these two isozymes will be decreased when bosentan is co-administered).

No products indexed under this heading.

Phenytoin Sodium (Bosentan is an inducer of CYP3A and CYP2C9. Consequently plasma concentrations of drugs metabolized by these two isozymes will be decreased when bosentan is co-administered). Products include:

Phenytek Capsules ... 2380

Pimozide (Bosentan is an inducer of CYP3A and CYP2C9. Consequently plasma concentrations of drugs metabolized by these two isozymes will be decreased when bosentan is co-administered).

No products indexed under this heading.

Pioglitazone Hydrochloride (Co-administration of bosentan decreased the plasma concentrations of glyburide by approximately 40%. The plasma concentrations of bosentan were also decreased by approximately 30%. Bosentan is also expected to reduce plasma concentrations of other oral hypoglycemic agents that are predomi-

1919 Interactions Index Tracleer

nantly metabolized by CYP2C9 or CYP3A. The possibility of worsened glucose control in patients using these agents should be considered). Products include:

ActoPlus 3338
Actos 3345
Duetact 3354

Piroxicam (Bosentan is an inducer of CYP3A and CYP2C9. Consequently plasma concentrations of drugs metabolized by these two isozymes will be decreased when bosentan is co-administered).
No products indexed under this heading.

Polyestradiol Phosphate (Hormonal contraceptives, including oral, injectable, transdermal, and implantable forms, may not be reliable when bosentan is co-administered. Females should practice additional methods of contraception and not rely on hormonal contraception alone when taking bosentan. An interaction study demonstrated that co-administration of bosentan and a combination oral hormonal contraceptive produced average decreases of norethindrone and ethinyl estradiol levels of 14% and 31%, respectively. However, decreases in exposure were as much as 56% and 66%, respectively, in individual subjects).
No products indexed under this heading.

Polythiazide (Bosentan is metabolized by CYP2C9 and CYP3A. Inhibition of these enzymes may increase the plasma concentration of bosentan. Concomitant administration of both a CYP2C9 inhibitor (such as fluconazole or amiodarone) and a strong CYP3A inhibitor (eg, ketoconazole, itraconazole) or a moderate CYP3A inhibitor (eg, amprenavir, erythromycin, fluconazole, diltiazem) with bosentan will likely lead to large increases in plasma concentrations of bosentan. Co-administration of such combinations of a CYP2C9 inhibitor plus a strong or moderate CYP3A inhibitor with bosentan is not recommended).
No products indexed under this heading.

Quinestrol (Hormonal contraceptives, including oral, injectable, transdermal, and implantable forms, may not be reliable when bosentan is co-administered. Females should practice additional methods of contraception and not rely on hormonal contraception alone when taking bosentan. An interaction study demonstrated that co-administration of bosentan and a combination oral hormonal contraceptive produced average decreases of norethindrone and ethinyl estradiol levels of 14% and 31%, respectively. However, decreases in exposure were as much as 56% and 66%, respectively, in individual subjects).
No products indexed under this heading.

Quinidine Gluconate (Bosentan is an inducer of CYP3A and CYP2C9. Consequently plasma concentrations of drugs metabolized by these two isozymes will be decreased when bosentan is co-administered).
No products indexed under this heading.

Quinidine Polygalacturonate (Bosentan is an inducer of CYP3A and CYP2C9. Consequently plasma concentrations of drugs metabolized by these two isozymes will be decreased when bosentan is co-administered).
No products indexed under this heading.

Quinidine Sulfate (Bosentan is an inducer of CYP3A and CYP2C9. Consequently plasma concentrations of drugs metabolized by these two isozymes will be decreased when bosentan is co-administered).
No products indexed under this heading.

Quinine (Bosentan is metabolized by CYP2C9 and CYP3A. Inhibition of these enzymes may increase the plasma concentration of bosentan. Concomitant administration of both a CYP2C9 inhibitor (such as fluconazole or amiodarone) and a strong CYP3A inhibitor (eg, ketoconazole, itraconazole) or a moderate CYP3A inhibitor (eg, amprenavir, erythromycin, fluconazole, diltiazem) with bosentan will likely lead to large increases in plasma concentrations of bosentan. Co-administration of such combinations of a CYP2C9 inhibitor plus a strong or moderate CYP3A inhibitor with bosentan is not recommended). Products include:

Hyland's Leg Cramps PM with Quinine 3315

Quinine Sulfate (Bosentan is metabolized by CYP2C9 and CYP3A. Inhibition of these enzymes may increase the plasma concentration of bosentan. Concomitant administration of both a CYP2C9 inhibitor (such as fluconazole or amiodarone) and a strong CYP3A inhibitor (eg, ketoconazole, itraconazole) or a moderate CYP3A inhibitor (eg, amprenavir, erythromycin, fluconazole, diltiazem) with bosentan will likely lead to large increases in plasma concentrations of bosentan. Co-administration of such combinations of a CYP2C9 inhibitor plus a strong or moderate CYP3A inhibitor with bosentan is not recommended).
No products indexed under this heading.

Repaglinide (Co-administration of bosentan decreased the plasma concentrations of glyburide by approximately 40%. The plasma concentrations of bosentan were also decreased by approximately 30%. Bosentan is also expected to reduce plasma concentrations of other oral hypoglycemic agents that are predominantly metabolized by CYP2C9 or CYP3A. The possibility of worsened glucose control in patients using these agents should be considered).
No products indexed under this heading.

Rifabutin (Bosentan is an inducer of CYP3A and CYP2C9. Consequently plasma concentrations of drugs metabolized by these two isozymes will be decreased when bosentan is co-administered).
No products indexed under this heading.

Rifampin (Co-administration of bosentan and rifampin in normal volunteers resulted in a mean 6-fold increase in bosentan trough levels after the first concomitant dose (likely due to inhibition of OATP by rifampin), but about a 60% decrease in bosentan levels at steady-state. The effect of bosentan on rifampin levels has not been assessed. When consideration of the potential benefits and known and unknown risks leads to concomitant use, measure liver function weekly for the first 4 weeks before reverting to normal monitoring).
No products indexed under this heading.

Ritonavir (*In vitro* data indicates that bosentan is a substrate of the Organic Anion Transport Protein (OATP), CYP3A, and CYP2C9. Ritonavir inhibits OATP and inhibits and induces CYP3A. However, the impact of ritonavir on the pharmacokinetics of bosentan may largely result from its effect on OATP. In normal volunteers, co-administration of bosentan 125 mg bid and lopinavir/ritonavir 400/100 mg bid increased the trough concentrations of bosentan on Days 4 and 10 approximately 48-fold and 5-fold, respectively, compared with those measured after bosentan administered alone. Therefore, the dose of bosentan should be adjusted when initiating lopinavir/ritonavir). Products include:

Kaletra 458
Norvir 509

Rofecoxib (Bosentan is an inducer of CYP3A and CYP2C9. Consequently plasma concentrations of drugs metabolized by these two isozymes will be decreased when bosentan is co-administered).
No products indexed under this heading.

Rosiglitazone Maleate (Co-administration of bosentan decreased the plasma concentrations of glyburide by approximately 40%. The plasma concentrations of bosentan were also decreased by approximately 30%. Bosentan is also expected to reduce plasma concentrations of other oral hypoglycemic agents that are predominantly metabolized by CYP2C9 or CYP3A. The possibility of worsened glucose control in patients using these agents should be considered). Products include:

Avandamet 1345
Avandaryl 1356
Avandia 1366

Saquinavir (Bosentan is metabolized by CYP2C9 and CYP3A. Inhibition of these enzymes may increase the plasma concentration of bosentan. Concomitant administration of both a CYP2C9 inhibitor (such as fluconazole or amiodarone) and a strong CYP3A inhibitor (eg, ketoconazole, itraconazole) or a moderate CYP3A inhibitor (eg, amprenavir, erythromycin, fluconazole, diltiazem) with bosentan will likely lead to large increases in plasma concentrations of bosentan. Co-administration of such combinations of a CYP2C9 inhibitor plus a strong or moderate CYP3A inhibitor with bosentan is not recommended).
No products indexed under this heading.

Saquinavir Mesylate (Bosentan is metabolized by CYP2C9 and CYP3A. Inhibition of these enzymes may increase the plasma concentration of bosentan. Concomitant administration of both a CYP2C9 inhibitor (such as fluconazole or amiodarone) and a strong CYP3A inhibitor (eg, ketoconazole, itraconazole) or a moderate CYP3A inhibitor (eg, amprenavir, erythromycin, fluconazole, diltiazem) with bosentan will likely lead to large increases in plasma concentrations of bosentan. Co-administration of such combinations of a CYP2C9 inhibitor plus a strong or moderate CYP3A inhibitor with bosentan is not recommended).
No products indexed under this heading.

Sertraline Hydrochloride (Bosentan is metabolized by CYP2C9 and CYP3A. Inhibition of these enzymes may increase the plasma concentration of bosentan. Concomitant administration of both a CYP2C9 inhibitor (such as fluconazole or amiodarone) and a strong CYP3A inhibitor (eg, ketoconazole, itraconazole) or a moderate CYP3A inhibitor (eg, amprenavir, erythromycin, fluconazole, diltiazem) with bosentan will likely lead to large increases in plasma concentrations of bosentan. Co-administration of such combinations of a CYP2C9 inhibitor plus a strong or moderate CYP3A inhibitor with bosentan is not recommended).
No products indexed under this heading.

Sildenafil Citrate (In normal volunteers, co-administration of multiple doses of 125 mg bid bosentan and 80 mg tid sildenafil resulted in a reduction of sildenafil plasma concentrations by 63% and increased bosentan plasma concentrations by 50%. The changes in plasma concentrations were not considered clinically relevant and dose adjustments are not necessary. This recommendation holds true when sildenafil is used for the treatment of pulmonary arterial hypertension or erectile dysfunction).
No products indexed under this heading.

Simvastatin (Co-administration of bosentan decreased the plasma concentrations of simvastatin (a CYP3A substrate), and its active β-hydroxy acid metabolite, by approximately 50%. The plasma concentrations of bosentan were not affected. Bosentan is also expected to reduce plasma concentrations of other statins that are significantly metabolized by CYP3A, such as lovastatin and atorvastatin. The possibility of reduced statin efficacy should be considered. Patients using CYP3A-metabolized statins should have cholesterol levels monitored after bosentan is initiated to see whether the statin dose needs adjustment). Products include:

Simcor 524
Vytorin 10/10 .... 2303, 3240
Vytorin 10/20 .... 2303, 3240
Vytorin 10/40 .... 2303, 3240
Vytorin 10/80 .... 2303, 3240
Zocor 2289

Sirolimus (Bosentan is an inducer of CYP3A and CYP2C9. Consequently plasma concentrations of drugs metabolized by these two isozymes will be decreased when bosentan is co-administered). Products include:

Rapamune 3579

Sitagliptin Phosphate (Co-administration of bosentan decreased the plasma concentrations of glyburide by approximately 40%. The plasma concentrations of bosentan were also decreased by approximately 30%. Bosentan is also expected to reduce plasma concentrations of other oral hypoglycemic agents that are predominantly metabolized by CYP2C9 or CYP3A. The possibility of worsened glucose control in patients using these agents should be considered). Products include:

Janumet 2188
Januvia 2196

Sulfacytine (Bosentan is metabolized by CYP2C9 and CYP3A. Inhibition of these enzymes may increase the plasma concentration of bosentan. Concomitant administration of both a CYP2C9 inhibitor (such as fluconazole or amiodarone) and a strong CYP3A inhibitor (eg, ketoconazole, itraconazole) or a moderate CYP3A inhibitor (eg, amprenavir, erythromycin, fluconazole, diltiazem) with bosentan will likely lead to large increases in plasma concentrations of bosentan. Co-administration of such combinations of a CYP2C9 inhibitor plus a strong or moderate CYP3A inhibitor with bosentan is not recommended).
No products indexed under this heading.

Sulfamethizole (Bosentan is metabolized by CYP2C9 and CYP3A. Inhibition of these enzymes may increase the plasma concentration of bosentan. Concomitant administration of both a CYP2C9 inhibitor (such as fluconazole or amiodarone) and a strong CYP3A inhibitor (eg, ketoconazole, itraconazole) or a moderate CYP3A inhibitor (eg, amprenavir, erythromycin, fluconazole, diltiazem) with bosentan will likely lead to large increases in plasma concentrations of bosentan. Co-administration of such combinations of a CYP2C9 inhibitor plus a strong or moderate CYP3A inhibitor with bosentan is not recommended).
No products indexed under this heading.

Sulfamethoxazole (Bosentan is metabolized by CYP2C9 and CYP3A. Inhibition of these enzymes may increase the plasma concentration of bosentan. Concomitant administration of both a CYP2C9 inhibitor (such as fluconazole or amiodarone) and a strong CYP3A inhibitor (eg, ketoconazole, itraconazole) or a moderate CYP3A inhibitor (eg, amprenavir, eryth-

IMPORTANT NOTE: Always consult each drug listing in the patient's regimen for possible interactions.

romycin, fluconazole, diltiazem) with bosentan will likely lead to large increases in plasma concentrations of bosentan. Co-administration of such combinations of a CYP2C9 inhibitor plus a strong or moderate CYP3A inhibitor with bosentan is not recommended).
No products indexed under this heading.

Sulfasalazine (Bosentan is metabolized by CYP2C9 and CYP3A. Inhibition of these enzymes may increase the plasma concentration of bosentan. Concomitant administration of both a CYP2C9 inhibitor (such as fluconazole or amiodarone) and a strong CYP3A inhibitor (eg, ketoconazole, itraconazole) or a moderate CYP3A inhibitor (eg, amprenavir, erythromycin, fluconazole, diltiazem) with bosentan will likely lead to large increases in plasma concentrations of bosentan. Co-administration of such combinations of a CYP2C9 inhibitor plus a strong or moderate CYP3A inhibitor with bosentan is not recommended).
No products indexed under this heading.

Sulfinpyrazone (Bosentan is metabolized by CYP2C9 and CYP3A. Inhibition of these enzymes may increase the plasma concentration of bosentan. Concomitant administration of both a CYP2C9 inhibitor (such as fluconazole or amiodarone) and a strong CYP3A inhibitor (eg, ketoconazole, itraconazole) or a moderate CYP3A inhibitor (eg, amprenavir, erythromycin, fluconazole, diltiazem) with bosentan will likely lead to large increases in plasma concentrations of bosentan. Co-administration of such combinations of a CYP2C9 inhibitor plus a strong or moderate CYP3A inhibitor with bosentan is not recommended).
No products indexed under this heading.

Sulfisoxazole Acetyl (Bosentan is metabolized by CYP2C9 and CYP3A. Inhibition of these enzymes may increase the plasma concentration of bosentan. Concomitant administration of both a CYP2C9 inhibitor (such as fluconazole or amiodarone) and a strong CYP3A inhibitor (eg, ketoconazole, itraconazole) or a moderate CYP3A inhibitor (eg, amprenavir, erythromycin, fluconazole, diltiazem) with bosentan will likely lead to large increases in plasma concentrations of bosentan. Co-administration of such combinations of a CYP2C9 inhibitor plus a strong or moderate CYP3A inhibitor with bosentan is not recommended).
No products indexed under this heading.

Sulfisoxazole Diolamine (Bosentan is metabolized by CYP2C9 and CYP3A. Inhibition of these enzymes may increase the plasma concentration of bosentan. Concomitant administration of both a CYP2C9 inhibitor (such as fluconazole or amiodarone) and a strong CYP3A inhibitor (eg, ketoconazole, itraconazole) or a moderate CYP3A inhibitor (eg, amprenavir, erythromycin, fluconazole, diltiazem) with bosentan will likely lead to large increases in plasma concentrations of bosentan. Co-administration of such combinations of a CYP2C9 inhibitor plus a strong or moderate CYP3A inhibitor with bosentan is not recommended).
No products indexed under this heading.

Sulindac (Bosentan is an inducer of CYP3A and CYP2C9. Consequently plasma concentrations of drugs metabolized by these two isozymes will be decreased when bosentan is co-administered). Products include:
Clinoril 2098

Suprofen (Bosentan is an inducer of CYP3A and CYP2C9. Consequently plasma concentrations of drugs metabolized by these two isozymes will be decreased when bosentan is co-administered).
No products indexed under this heading.

Tacrolimus (Co-administration of tacrolimus and bosentan has not been studied in humans. Co-administration of tacrolimus and bosentan resulted in markedly increased plasma concentrations of bosentan in animals. Caution should be exercised if tacrolimus and bosentan are used together). Products include:
Prograf Capsules 677
Prograf Injection 677
Protopic 685

Tamoxifen Citrate (Bosentan is an inducer of CYP3A and CYP2C9. Consequently plasma concentrations of drugs metabolized by these two isozymes will be decreased when bosentan is co-administered).
No products indexed under this heading.

Telmisartan (Bosentan is an inducer of CYP3A and CYP2C9. Consequently plasma concentrations of drugs metabolized by these two isozymes will be decreased when bosentan is co-administered). Products include:
Micardis 887
Micardis HCT 889

Terconazole (Bosentan is metabolized by CYP2C9 and CYP3A. Inhibition of these enzymes may increase the plasma concentration of bosentan. Concomitant administration of both a CYP2C9 inhibitor (such as fluconazole or amiodarone) and a strong CYP3A inhibitor (eg, ketoconazole, itraconazole) or a moderate CYP3A inhibitor (eg, amprenavir, erythromycin, fluconazole, diltiazem) with bosentan will likely lead to large increases in plasma concentrations of bosentan. Co-administration of such combinations of a CYP2C9 inhibitor plus a strong or moderate CYP3A inhibitor with bosentan is not recommended).
No products indexed under this heading.

Terfenadine (Bosentan is an inducer of CYP3A and CYP2C9. Consequently plasma concentrations of drugs metabolized by these two isozymes will be decreased when bosentan is co-administered).
No products indexed under this heading.

Testosterone (Bosentan is an inducer of CYP3A and CYP2C9. Consequently plasma concentrations of drugs metabolized by these two isozymes will be decreased when bosentan is co-administered). Products include:
AndroGel 3456

Testosterone Cypionate (Bosentan is an inducer of CYP3A and CYP2C9. Consequently plasma concentrations of drugs metabolized by these two isozymes will be decreased when bosentan is co-administered).
No products indexed under this heading.

Testosterone Enanthate (Bosentan is an inducer of CYP3A and CYP2C9. Consequently plasma concentrations of drugs metabolized by these two isozymes will be decreased when bosentan is co-administered). Products include:
Delatestryl 1102

Testosterone Propionate (Bosentan is an inducer of CYP3A and CYP2C9. Consequently plasma concentrations of drugs metabolized by these two isozymes will be decreased when bosentan is co-administered).
No products indexed under this heading.

Theophylline (Bosentan is an inducer of CYP3A and CYP2C9. Consequently plasma concentrations of drugs metabolized by these two isozymes will be decreased when bosentan is co-administered).
No products indexed under this heading.

Theophylline Anhydrous (Bosentan is an inducer of CYP3A and CYP2C9. Consequently plasma concentrations of drugs metabolized by these two isozymes will be decreased when bosentan is co-administered). Products include:
Uniphyl 2817

Theophylline Calcium Salicylate (Bosentan is an inducer of CYP3A and CYP2C9. Consequently plasma concentrations of drugs metabolized by these two isozymes will be decreased when bosentan is co-administered).
No products indexed under this heading.

Theophylline Sodium Glycinate (Bosentan is an inducer of CYP3A and CYP2C9. Consequently plasma concentrations of drugs metabolized by these two isozymes will be decreased when bosentan is co-administered).
No products indexed under this heading.

Tiagabine Hydrochloride (Bosentan is an inducer of CYP3A and CYP2C9. Consequently plasma concentrations of drugs metabolized by these two isozymes will be decreased when bosentan is co-administered). Products include:
Gabitril 972

Ticlopidine Hydrochloride (Bosentan is metabolized by CYP2C9 and CYP3A. Inhibition of these enzymes may increase the plasma concentration of bosentan. Concomitant administration of both a CYP2C9 inhibitor (such as fluconazole or amiodarone) and a strong CYP3A inhibitor (eg, ketoconazole, itraconazole) or a moderate CYP3A inhibitor (eg, amprenavir, erythromycin, fluconazole, diltiazem) with bosentan will likely lead to large increases in plasma concentrations of bosentan. Co-administration of such combinations of a CYP2C9 inhibitor plus a strong or moderate CYP3A inhibitor with bosentan is not recommended).
No products indexed under this heading.

Tolazamide (Co-administration of bosentan decreased the plasma concentrations of glyburide by approximately 40%. The plasma concentrations of bosentan were also decreased by approximately 30%. Bosentan is also expected to reduce plasma concentrations of other oral hypoglycemic agents that are predominantly metabolized by CYP2C9 or CYP3A. The possibility of worsened glucose control in patients using these agents should be considered).
No products indexed under this heading.

Tolbutamide (Co-administration of bosentan decreased the plasma concentrations of glyburide by approximately 40%. The plasma concentrations of bosentan were also decreased by approximately 30%. Bosentan is also expected to reduce plasma concentrations of other oral hypoglycemic agents that are predominantly metabolized by CYP2C9 or CYP3A. The possibility of worsened glucose control in patients using these agents should be considered).
No products indexed under this heading.

Tolbutamide Sodium (Bosentan is metabolized by CYP2C9 and CYP3A. Inhibition of these enzymes may increase the plasma concentration of bosentan. Concomitant administration of both a CYP2C9 inhibitor (such as fluconazole or amiodarone) and a strong CYP3A inhibitor (eg, ketoconazole, itraconazole) or a moderate CYP3A inhibitor (eg, amprenavir, erythromycin, fluconazole, diltiazem) with bosentan will likely lead to large increases in plasma concentrations of bosentan. Co-administration of such combinations of a CYP2C9 inhibitor plus a strong or moderate CYP3A inhibitor with bosentan is not recommended).
No products indexed under this heading.

Tolmetin Sodium (Bosentan is an inducer of CYP3A and CYP2C9. Consequently plasma concentrations of drugs metabolized by these two isozymes will be decreased when bosentan is co-administered).
No products indexed under this heading.

Tolterodine Tartrate (Bosentan is an inducer of CYP3A and CYP2C9. Consequently plasma concentrations of drugs metabolized by these two isozymes will be decreased when bosentan is co-administered).
No products indexed under this heading.

Torsemide (Bosentan is an inducer of CYP3A and CYP2C9. Consequently plasma concentrations of drugs metabolized by these two isozymes will be decreased when bosentan is co-administered).
No products indexed under this heading.

Trazodone Hydrochloride (Bosentan is an inducer of CYP3A and CYP2C9. Consequently plasma concentrations of drugs metabolized by these two isozymes will be decreased when bosentan is co-administered).
No products indexed under this heading.

Triazolam (Bosentan is an inducer of CYP3A and CYP2C9. Consequently plasma concentrations of drugs metabolized by these two isozymes will be decreased when bosentan is co-administered).
No products indexed under this heading.

Troglitazone (Co-administration of bosentan decreased the plasma concentrations of glyburide by approximately 40%. The plasma concentrations of bosentan were also decreased by approximately 30%. Bosentan is also expected to reduce plasma concentrations of other oral hypoglycemic agents that are predominantly metabolized by CYP2C9 or CYP3A. The possibility of worsened glucose control in patients using these agents should be considered).
No products indexed under this heading.

Troleandomycin (Bosentan is metabolized by CYP2C9 and CYP3A. Inhibition of these enzymes may increase the plasma concentration of bosentan. Concomitant administration of both a CYP2C9 inhibitor (such as fluconazole or amiodarone) and a strong CYP3A inhibitor (eg, ketoconazole, itraconazole) or a moderate CYP3A inhibitor (eg, amprenavir, erythromycin, fluconazole, diltiazem) with bosentan will likely lead to large increases in plasma concentrations of bosentan. Co-administration of such combinations of a CYP2C9 inhibitor plus a strong or moderate CYP3A inhibitor with bosentan is not recommended).
No products indexed under this heading.

Valdecoxib (Bosentan is an inducer of CYP3A and CYP2C9. Consequently plasma concentrations of drugs metabolized by these two isozymes will be decreased when bosentan is co-administered).
No products indexed under this heading.

Valsartan (Bosentan is an inducer of CYP3A and CYP2C9. Consequently plasma concentrations of drugs metabolized by these two isozymes will be decreased when bosentan is co-administered). Products include:
Diovan 2413
Diovan HCT 2419

Exforge 2443
Exforge HCT 2449
Valturna 3637

Vardenafil Hydrochloride (Bosentan is metabolized by CYP2C9 and CYP3A. Inhibition of these enzymes may increase the plasma concentration of bosentan. Concomitant administration of both a CYP2C9 inhibitor (such as fluconazole or amiodarone) and a strong CYP3A inhibitor (eg, ketoconazole, itraconazole) or a moderate CYP3A inhibitor (eg, amprenavir, erythromycin, fluconazole, diltiazem) with bosentan will likely lead to large increases in plasma concentrations of bosentan. Co-administration of such combinations of a CYP2C9 inhibitor plus a strong or moderate CYP3A inhibitor with bosentan is not recommended). Products include:
Levitra 3157

Venlafaxine Hydrochloride (Bosentan is metabolized by CYP2C9 and CYP3A. Inhibition of these enzymes may increase the plasma concentration of bosentan. Concomitant administration of both a CYP2C9 inhibitor (such as fluconazole or amiodarone) and a strong CYP3A inhibitor (eg, ketoconazole, itraconazole) or a moderate CYP3A inhibitor (eg, amprenavir, erythromycin, fluconazole, diltiazem) with bosentan will likely lead to large increases in plasma concentrations of bosentan. Co-administration of such combinations of a CYP2C9 inhibitor plus a strong or moderate CYP3A inhibitor with bosentan is not recommended). Products include:
Effexor XR 3504
Venlafaxine Hydrochloride Tablets ... 2388

Verapamil Hydrochloride (Bosentan is metabolized by CYP2C9 and CYP3A. Inhibition of these enzymes may increase the plasma concentration of bosentan. Concomitant administration of both a CYP2C9 inhibitor (such as fluconazole or amiodarone) and a strong CYP3A inhibitor (eg, ketoconazole, itraconazole) or a moderate CYP3A inhibitor (eg, amprenavir, erythromycin, fluconazole, diltiazem) with bosentan will likely lead to large increases in plasma concentrations of bosentan. Co-administration of such combinations of a CYP2C9 inhibitor plus a strong or moderate CYP3A inhibitor with bosentan is not recommended). Products include:
Tarka 534

Vinblastine Sulfate (Bosentan is an inducer of CYP3A and CYP2C9. Consequently plasma concentrations of drugs metabolized by these two isozymes will be decreased when bosentan is co-administered).
No products indexed under this heading.

Vincristine Sulfate (Bosentan is an inducer of CYP3A and CYP2C9. Consequently plasma concentrations of drugs metabolized by these two isozymes will be decreased when bosentan is co-administered).
No products indexed under this heading.

Voriconazole (Bosentan is metabolized by CYP2C9 and CYP3A. Inhibition of these enzymes may increase the plasma concentration of bosentan. Concomitant administration of both a CYP2C9 inhibitor (such as fluconazole or amiodarone) and a strong CYP3A inhibitor (eg, ketoconazole, itraconazole) or a moderate CYP3A inhibitor (eg, amprenavir, erythromycin, fluconazole, diltiazem) with bosentan will likely lead to large increases in plasma concentrations of bosentan. Co-administration of such combinations of a CYP2C9 inhibitor plus a strong or moderate CYP3A inhibitor with bosentan is not recommended).
No products indexed under this heading.

Warfarin Sodium (Co-administration of bosentan 500 mg bid for 6 days in normal volunteers, decreased the plasma concentrations of both S-warfarin (a CYP2C9 substrate) and R-warfarin (a CYP3A substrate) by 29 and 38%, respectively. Clinical experience with concomitant administration of bosentan and warfarin in patients with pulmonary arterial hypertension did not show clinically relevant changes in INR or warfarin dose (baseline vs. end of the clinical studies), and the need to change the warfarin dose during the trials due to changes in INR or due to adverse events was similar among bosentan- and placebo-treated patients).
No products indexed under this heading.

Zafirlukast (Bosentan is metabolized by CYP2C9 and CYP3A. Inhibition of these enzymes may increase the plasma concentration of bosentan. Concomitant administration of both a CYP2C9 inhibitor (such as fluconazole or amiodarone) and a strong CYP3A inhibitor (eg, ketoconazole, itraconazole) or a moderate CYP3A inhibitor (eg, amprenavir, erythromycin, fluconazole, diltiazem) with bosentan will likely lead to large increases in plasma concentrations of bosentan. Co-administration of such combinations of a CYP2C9 inhibitor plus a strong or moderate CYP3A inhibitor with bosentan is not recommended). Products include:
Accolate 3612

Zileuton (Bosentan is metabolized by CYP2C9 and CYP3A. Inhibition of these enzymes may increase the plasma concentration of bosentan. Concomitant administration of both a CYP2C9 inhibitor (such as fluconazole or amiodarone) and a strong CYP3A inhibitor (eg, ketoconazole, itraconazole) or a moderate CYP3A inhibitor (eg, amprenavir, erythromycin, fluconazole, diltiazem) with bosentan will likely lead to large increases in plasma concentrations of bosentan. Co-administration of such combinations of a CYP2C9 inhibitor plus a strong or moderate CYP3A inhibitor with bosentan is not recommended).
No products indexed under this heading.

Food Interactions

Grapefruit (Bosentan is metabolized by CYP2C9 and CYP3A. Inhibition of these enzymes may increase the plasma concentration of bosentan. Concomitant administration of both a CYP2C9 inhibitor (such as fluconazole or amiodarone) and a strong CYP3A inhibitor (eg, ketoconazole, itraconazole) or a moderate CYP3A inhibitor (eg, amprenavir, erythromycin, fluconazole, diltiazem) with bosentan will likely lead to large increases in plasma concentrations of bosentan. Co-administration of such combinations of a CYP2C9 inhibitor plus a strong or moderate CYP3A inhibitor with bosentan is not recommended).

Grapefruit Juice (Bosentan is metabolized by CYP2C9 and CYP3A. Inhibition of these enzymes may increase the plasma concentration of bosentan. Concomitant administration of both a CYP2C9 inhibitor (such as fluconazole or amiodarone) and a strong CYP3A inhibitor (eg, ketoconazole, itraconazole) or a moderate CYP3A inhibitor (eg, amprenavir, erythromycin, fluconazole, diltiazem) with bosentan will likely lead to large increases in plasma concentrations of bosentan. Co-administration of such combinations of a CYP2C9 inhibitor plus a strong or moderate CYP3A inhibitor with bosentan is not recommended).

TRANSDERM SCŌP TRANSDERMAL THERAPEUTIC SYSTEM

(Scopolamine) 2397

May interact with alcohols, anticholinergics, antihistamines, central nervous system depressants, hypnotics and sedatives, skeletal muscle relaxants, tranquilizers, tricyclic antidepressants, and certain other agents. Compounds in these categories include:

Acrivastine (Antihistamines have anticholinergic properties and co-administration may result in additive effects).
No products indexed under this heading.

Alfentanil Hydrochloride (Scopolamine is an anticholinergic agent and causes certain CNS effects, such as drowsiness and dizziness, and hence it should be used with care in patients on concomitant therapy).
No products indexed under this heading.

Alprazolam (Scopolamine is an anticholinergic agent and causes certain CNS effects, such as drowsiness and dizziness, and hence it should be used with care in patients on concomitant therapy).
No products indexed under this heading.

Amitriptyline Hydrochloride (Tricyclic antidepressants have anticholinergic properties and co-administration may result in additive effects).
No products indexed under this heading.

Amobarbital (Scopolamine is an anticholinergic agent and causes certain CNS effects, such as drowsiness and dizziness, and hence it should be used with care in patients on concomitant therapy).
No products indexed under this heading.

Amobarbital Sodium (Scopolamine is an anticholinergic agent and causes certain CNS effects, such as drowsiness and dizziness, and hence it should be used with care in patients on concomitant therapy).
No products indexed under this heading.

Amoxapine (Tricyclic antidepressants have anticholinergic properties and co-administration may result in additive effects).
No products indexed under this heading.

Aprobarbital (Scopolamine is an anticholinergic agent and causes certain CNS effects, such as drowsiness and dizziness, and hence it should be used with care in patients on concomitant therapy).
No products indexed under this heading.

Astemizole (Antihistamines have anticholinergic properties and co-administration may result in additive effects).
No products indexed under this heading.

Atracurium Besylate (Co-administration may result in addititve anticholinergic effects).
No products indexed under this heading.

Atropine Sulfate (Co-administration may result in additive anticholinergic effects). Products include:
Donnatal 2711

Azatadine Maleate (Antihistamines have anticholinergic properties and co-administration may result in additive effects).
No products indexed under this heading.

Baclofen (Co-administration may result in addititve anticholinergic effects).
No products indexed under this heading.

Belladonna Alkaloids (Co-administration may result in additive anticholinergic effects). Products include:
Hyland's Teething Tablets 3316

Benztropine Mesylate (Co-administration may result in additive anticholinergic effects).
No products indexed under this heading.

Biperiden Hydrochloride (Co-administration may result in additive anticholinergic effects).
No products indexed under this heading.

Bromodiphenhydramine Hydrochloride (Antihistamines have anticholinergic properties and co-administration may result in additive effects).
No products indexed under this heading.

Brompheniramine Maleate (Antihistamines have anticholinergic properties and co-administration may result in additive effects).
No products indexed under this heading.

Buprenorphine Hydrochloride (Scopolamine is an anticholinergic agent and causes certain CNS effects, such as drowsiness and dizziness, and hence it should be used with care in patients on concomitant therapy).
No products indexed under this heading.

Buspirone Hydrochloride (Scopolamine is an anticholinergic agent and causes certain CNS effects, such as drowsiness and dizziness, and hence it should be used with care in patients on concomitant therapy).
No products indexed under this heading.

Butabarbital (Scopolamine is an anticholinergic agent and causes certain CNS effects, such as drowsiness and dizziness, and hence it should be used with care in patients on concomitant therapy).
No products indexed under this heading.

Butabarbital Sodium (Scopolamine is an anticholinergic agent and causes certain CNS effects, such as drowsiness and dizziness, and hence it should be used with care in patients on concomitant therapy).
No products indexed under this heading.

Butalbital (Scopolamine is an anticholinergic agent and causes certain CNS effects, such as drowsiness and dizziness, and hence it should be used with care in patients on concomitant therapy).
No products indexed under this heading.

Carisoprodol (Co-administration may result in addititve anticholinergic effects).
No products indexed under this heading.

Cetirizine Hydrochloride (Antihistamines have anticholinergic properties and co-administration may result in additive effects). Products include:
Zyrtec Allergy 2052
Children's Zyrtec Allergy Syrup 2053
Children's Zyrtec Allergy 2053
Children's Zyrtec Hives Relief 2053
Zyrtec-D Allergy & Congestion 2054

Chloral Hydrate (Scopolamine is an anticholinergic agent and causes certain CNS effects, such as drowsiness and dizziness, and hence it should be used with care in patients on concomitant therapy).
No products indexed under this heading.

Chlordiazepoxide (Scopolamine is an anticholinergic agent and causes certain CNS effects, such as drowsiness and dizziness, and hence it should be used with care in patients on concomitant therapy).
No products indexed under this heading.

Chlordiazepoxide Hydrochloride (Scopolamine is an anticholinergic agent and causes certain CNS effects, such as drowsiness and dizziness, and hence it should be used with care in patients on concomitant therapy).
No products indexed under this heading.

Chlorpheniramine Maleate (Antihistamines have anticholinergic properties and co-administration may result in additive effects).
No products indexed under this heading.

IMPORTANT NOTE: Always consult each drug listing in the patient's regimen for possible interactions.

Transderm Scōp | Interactions Index | 1922

Chlorpheniramine Polistirex (Antihistamines have anticholinergic properties and co-administration may result in additive effects). Products include:
Tussionex 3443

Chlorpheniramine Tannate (Antihistamines have anticholinergic properties and co-administration may result in additive effects).
No products indexed under this heading.

Chlorpromazine (Scopolamine is an anticholinergic agent and causes certain CNS effects, such as drowsiness and dizziness, and hence it should be used with care in patients on concomitant therapy).
No products indexed under this heading.

Chlorpromazine Hydrochloride (Scopolamine is an anticholinergic agent and causes certain CNS effects, such as drowsiness and dizziness, and hence it should be used with care in patients on concomitant therapy).
No products indexed under this heading.

Chlorprothixene (Scopolamine is an anticholinergic agent and causes certain CNS effects, such as drowsiness and dizziness, and hence it should be used with care in patients on concomitant therapy).
No products indexed under this heading.

Chlorprothixene Hydrochloride (Scopolamine is an anticholinergic agent and causes certain CNS effects, such as drowsiness and dizziness, and hence it should be used with care in patients on concomitant therapy).
No products indexed under this heading.

Chlorprothixene Lactate (Scopolamine is an anticholinergic agent and causes certain CNS effects, such as drowsiness and dizziness, and hence it should be used with care in patients on concomitant therapy).
No products indexed under this heading.

Chlorzoxazone (Co-administration may result in additive anticholinergic effects).
No products indexed under this heading.

Cisatracurium Besylate (Co-administration may result in addititve anticholinergic effects). Products include:
Nimbex 503

Clemastine Fumarate (Antihistamines have anticholinergic properties and co-administration may result in additive effects).
No products indexed under this heading.

Clidinium Bromide (Co-administration may result in additive anticholinergic effects).
No products indexed under this heading.

Clomipramine Hydrochloride (Tricyclic antidepressants have anticholinergic properties and co-administration may result in additive effects).
No products indexed under this heading.

Clonazepam (Scopolamine is an anticholinergic agent and causes certain CNS effects, such as drowsiness and dizziness, and hence it should be used with care in patients on concomitant therapy). Products include:
Klonopin 2855

Clorazepate Dipotassium (Scopolamine is an anticholinergic agent and causes certain CNS effects, such as drowsiness and dizziness, and hence it should be used with care in patients on concomitant therapy).
No products indexed under this heading.

Clozapine (Scopolamine is an anticholinergic agent and causes certain CNS effects, such as drowsiness and dizziness, and hence it should be used with care in patients on concomitant therapy).
No products indexed under this heading.

Codeine Phosphate (Scopolamine is an anticholinergic agent and causes certain CNS effects, such as drowsiness and dizziness, and hence it should be used with care in patients on concomitant therapy). Products include:
Tylenol with Codeine 2691

Codeine Sulfate (Scopolamine is an anticholinergic agent and causes certain CNS effects, such as drowsiness and dizziness, and hence it should be used with care in patients on concomitant therapy).
No products indexed under this heading.

Cyclobenzaprine Hydrochloride (Co-administration may result in addititve anticholinergic effects). Products include:
Amrix 964

Cyproheptadine Hydrochloride (Antihistamines have anticholinergic properties and co-administration may result in additive effects).
No products indexed under this heading.

Dantrolene Sodium (Co-administration may result in addititve anticholinergic effects).
No products indexed under this heading.

Desflurane (Scopolamine is an anticholinergic agent and causes certain CNS effects, such as drowsiness and dizziness, and hence it should be used with care in patients on concomitant therapy).
No products indexed under this heading.

Desipramine Hydrochloride (Tricyclic antidepressants have anticholinergic properties and co-administration may result in additive effects).
No products indexed under this heading.

Dexchlorpheniramine Maleate (Antihistamines have anticholinergic properties and co-administration may result in additive effects).
No products indexed under this heading.

Dezocine (Scopolamine is an anticholinergic agent and causes certain CNS effects, such as drowsiness and dizziness, and hence it should be used with care in patients on concomitant therapy).
No products indexed under this heading.

Diazepam (Scopolamine is an anticholinergic agent and causes certain CNS effects, such as drowsiness and dizziness, and hence it should be used with care in patients on concomitant therapy). Products include:
Valium Tablets 2880

Dicyclomine Hydrochloride (Co-administration may result in additive anticholinergic effects). Products include:
Bentyl Capsules 780
Bentyl Injection 780
Bentyl Syrup 780
Bentyl Tablets 780

Diphenhydramine Hydrochloride (Antihistamines have anticholinergic properties and co-administration may result in additive effects). Products include:
Benadryl Allergy Ultratab 2042
Children's Benadryl Allergy Liquid 2042

Diphenylpyraline Hydrochloride (Antihistamines have anticholinergic properties and co-administration may result in additive effects).
No products indexed under this heading.

Doxacurium Chloride (Co-administration may result in addititve anticholinergic effects).
No products indexed under this heading.

Doxepin Hydrochloride (Tricyclic antidepressants have anticholinergic properties and co-administration may result in additive effects).
No products indexed under this heading.

Droperidol (Scopolamine is an anticholinergic agent and causes certain CNS effects, such as drowsiness and dizziness, and hence it should be used with care in patients on concomitant therapy).
No products indexed under this heading.

d-Tubocurarine (Co-administration may result in addititve anticholinergic effects).
No products indexed under this heading.

Enflurane (Scopolamine is an anticholinergic agent and causes certain CNS effects, such as drowsiness and dizziness, and hence it should be used with care in patients on concomitant therapy).
No products indexed under this heading.

Estazolam (Scopolamine is an anticholinergic agent and causes certain CNS effects, such as drowsiness and dizziness, and hence it should be used with care in patients on concomitant therapy).
No products indexed under this heading.

Ethanol (Scopolamine is an anticholinergic agent and causes certain CNS effects, such as drowsiness and dizziness, and hence it should be used with care in patients on concomitant therapy).
No products indexed under this heading.

Ethchlorvynol (Scopolamine is an anticholinergic agent and causes certain CNS effects, such as drowsiness and dizziness, and hence it should be used with care in patients on concomitant therapy).
No products indexed under this heading.

Ethinamate (Scopolamine is an anticholinergic agent and causes certain CNS effects, such as drowsiness and dizziness, and hence it should be used with care in patients on concomitant therapy).
No products indexed under this heading.

Ethyl Alcohol (Scopolamine is an anticholinergic agent and causes certain CNS effects, such as drowsiness and dizziness, and hence it should be used with care in patients on concomitant therapy).
No products indexed under this heading.

Fentanyl (Scopolamine is an anticholinergic agent and causes certain CNS effects, such as drowsiness and dizziness, and hence it should be used with care in patients on concomitant therapy). Products include:
Duragesic 2604
Fentanyl Transdermal System 2346
Onsolis 2054

Fentanyl Citrate (Scopolamine is an anticholinergic agent and causes certain CNS effects, such as drowsiness and dizziness, and hence it should be used with care in patients on concomitant therapy). Products include:
Fentora 966

Fexofenadine Hydrochloride (Antihistamines have anticholinergic properties and co-administration may result in additive effects). Products include:
Allegra ODT 2911
Allegra Oral Solution 2911
Allegra 2911
Allegra-D 2915
Allegra-D 24 2918

Fluphenazine Decanoate (Scopolamine is an anticholinergic agent and causes certain CNS effects, such as drowsiness and dizziness, and hence it should be used with care in patients on concomitant therapy).
No products indexed under this heading.

Fluphenazine Enanthate (Scopolamine is an anticholinergic agent and causes certain CNS effects, such as drowsiness and dizziness, and hence it should be used with care in patients on concomitant therapy).
No products indexed under this heading.

Fluphenazine Hydrochloride (Scopolamine is an anticholinergic agent and causes certain CNS effects, such as drowsiness and dizziness, and hence it should be used with care in patients on concomitant therapy).
No products indexed under this heading.

Flurazepam Hydrochloride (Scopolamine is an anticholinergic agent and causes certain CNS effects, such as drowsiness and dizziness, and hence it should be used with care in patients on concomitant therapy).
No products indexed under this heading.

Gallamine (Co-administration may result in addititve anticholinergic effects).
No products indexed under this heading.

Gallamine Triethiodide (Co-administration may result in addititve anticholinergic effects).
No products indexed under this heading.

Glutethimide (Scopolamine is an anticholinergic agent and causes certain CNS effects, such as drowsiness and dizziness, and hence it should be used with care in patients on concomitant therapy).
No products indexed under this heading.

Glycopyrrolate (Co-administration may result in additive anticholinergic effects).
No products indexed under this heading.

Halazepam (Scopolamine is an anticholinergic agent and causes certain CNS effects, such as drowsiness and dizziness, and hence it should be used with care in patients on concomitant therapy).
No products indexed under this heading.

Haloperidol (Scopolamine is an anticholinergic agent and causes certain CNS effects, such as drowsiness and dizziness, and hence it should be used with care in patients on concomitant therapy).
No products indexed under this heading.

Haloperidol Decanoate (Scopolamine is an anticholinergic agent and causes certain CNS effects, such as drowsiness and dizziness, and hence it should be used with care in patients on concomitant therapy).
No products indexed under this heading.

Haloperidol Lactate (Scopolamine is an anticholinergic agent and causes certain CNS effects, such as drowsiness and dizziness, and hence it should be used with care in patients on concomitant therapy).
No products indexed under this heading.

Hexobarbital (Scopolamine is an anticholinergic agent and causes certain CNS effects, such as drowsiness and dizziness, and hence it should be used with care in patients on concomitant therapy).
No products indexed under this heading.

Hydrocodone Bitartrate (Scopolamine is an anticholinergic agent and causes certain CNS effects, such as drowsiness and dizziness, and hence it should be used with care in patients on concomitant therapy). Products include:
Vicodin 560
Vicodin ES 561
Vicodin HP 563
Vicoprofen 564
Zydone 1138

Hydrocodone Polistirex (Scopolamine is an anticholinergic agent and causes certain CNS effects, such as

1923 Interactions Index Transderm Scōp

drowsiness and dizziness, and hence it should be used with care in patients on concomitant therapy). Products include:
Tussionex 3443

Hydromorphone (Scopolamine is an anticholinergic agent and causes certain CNS effects, such as drowsiness and dizziness, and hence it should be used with care in patients on concomitant therapy).
No products indexed under this heading.

Hydromorphone Hydrochloride (Scopolamine is an anticholinergic agent and causes certain CNS effects, such as drowsiness and dizziness, and hence it should be used with care in patients on concomitant therapy).
Products include:
Dilaudid Injection 2800
Dilaudid Oral 2797
Dilaudid Tablets 2797
Dilaudid-HP 2800

Hydroxyzine Hydrochloride (Scopolamine is an anticholinergic agent and causes certain CNS effects, such as drowsiness and dizziness, and hence it should be used with care in patients on concomitant therapy).
No products indexed under this heading.

Hyoscyamine (Co-administration may result in additive anticholinergic effects).
No products indexed under this heading.

Hyoscyamine Sulfate (Co-administration may result in additive anticholinergic effects). Products include:
Donnatal 2711

Imipramine Hydrochloride (Tricyclic antidepressants have anticholinergic properties and co-administration may result in additive effects).
No products indexed under this heading.

Imipramine Pamoate (Tricyclic antidepressants have anticholinergic properties and co-administration may result in additive effects).
No products indexed under this heading.

Ipratropium Bromide (Co-administration may result in additive anticholinergic effects).
No products indexed under this heading.

Isoflurane (Scopolamine is an anticholinergic agent and causes certain CNS effects, such as drowsiness and dizziness, and hence it should be used with care in patients on concomitant therapy).
No products indexed under this heading.

Ketamine Hydrochloride (Scopolamine is an anticholinergic agent and causes certain CNS effects, such as drowsiness and dizziness, and hence it should be used with care in patients on concomitant therapy).
No products indexed under this heading.

Levomethadyl Acetate Hydrochloride (Scopolamine is an anticholinergic agent and causes certain CNS effects, such as drowsiness and dizziness, and hence it should be used with care in patients on concomitant therapy).
No products indexed under this heading.

Levorphanol Tartrate (Scopolamine is an anticholinergic agent and causes certain CNS effects, such as drowsiness and dizziness, and hence it should be used with care in patients on concomitant therapy).
No products indexed under this heading.

Loratadine (Antihistamines have anticholinergic properties and co-administration may result in additive effects).
No products indexed under this heading.

Lorazepam (Scopolamine is an anticholinergic agent and causes certain CNS effects, such as drowsiness and dizziness, and hence it should be used with care in patients on concomitant therapy).
No products indexed under this heading.

Loxapine Hydrochloride (Scopolamine is an anticholinergic agent and causes certain CNS effects, such as drowsiness and dizziness, and hence it should be used with care in patients on concomitant therapy).
No products indexed under this heading.

Loxapine Succinate (Scopolamine is an anticholinergic agent and causes certain CNS effects, such as drowsiness and dizziness, and hence it should be used with care in patients on concomitant therapy).
No products indexed under this heading.

Maprotiline Hydrochloride (Tricyclic antidepressants have anticholinergic properties and co-administration may result in additive effects).
No products indexed under this heading.

Meclizine Hydrochloride (Antihistamines have anticholinergic properties and co-administration may result in additive effects).
No products indexed under this heading.

Mepenzolate Bromide (Co-administration may result in additive anticholinergic effects).
No products indexed under this heading.

Meperidine Hydrochloride (Scopolamine is an anticholinergic agent and causes certain CNS effects, such as drowsiness and dizziness, and hence it should be used with care in patients on concomitant therapy).
No products indexed under this heading.

Mephobarbital (Scopolamine is an anticholinergic agent and causes certain CNS effects, such as drowsiness and dizziness, and hence it should be used with care in patients on concomitant therapy).
No products indexed under this heading.

Meprobamate (Scopolamine is an anticholinergic agent and causes certain CNS effects, such as drowsiness and dizziness, and hence it should be used with care in patients on concomitant therapy).
No products indexed under this heading.

Mesoridazine Besylate (Scopolamine is an anticholinergic agent and causes certain CNS effects, such as drowsiness and dizziness, and hence it should be used with care in patients on concomitant therapy).
No products indexed under this heading.

Metaxalone (Co-administration may result in addititve anticholinergic effects). Products include:
Skelaxin 1848

Methadone Hydrochloride (Scopolamine is an anticholinergic agent and causes certain CNS effects, such as drowsiness and dizziness, and hence it should be used with care in patients on concomitant therapy).
No products indexed under this heading.

Methdilazine Hydrochloride (Antihistamines have anticholinergic properties and co-administration may result in additive effects).
No products indexed under this heading.

Methocarbamol (Co-administration may result in addititve anticholinergic effects).
No products indexed under this heading.

Methohexital Sodium (Scopolamine is an anticholinergic agent and causes certain CNS effects, such as drowsiness and dizziness, and hence it should be used with care in patients on concomitant therapy).
No products indexed under this heading.

Methotrimeprazine (Scopolamine is an anticholinergic agent and causes certain CNS effects, such as drowsiness and dizziness, and hence it should be used with care in patients on concomitant therapy).
No products indexed under this heading.

Methoxyflurane (Scopolamine is an anticholinergic agent and causes certain CNS effects, such as drowsiness and dizziness, and hence it should be used with care in patients on concomitant therapy).
No products indexed under this heading.

Metocurine Iodide (Co-administration may result in addititve anticholinergic effects).
No products indexed under this heading.

Midazolam Hydrochloride (Scopolamine is an anticholinergic agent and causes certain CNS effects, such as drowsiness and dizziness, and hence it should be used with care in patients on concomitant therapy).
No products indexed under this heading.

Mivacurium Chloride (Co-administration may result in addititve anticholinergic effects).
No products indexed under this heading.

Molindone Hydrochloride (Scopolamine is an anticholinergic agent and causes certain CNS effects, such as drowsiness and dizziness, and hence it should be used with care in patients on concomitant therapy). Products include:
Moban 1108

Morphine Sulfate (Scopolamine is an anticholinergic agent and causes certain CNS effects, such as drowsiness and dizziness, and hence it should be used with care in patients on concomitant therapy). Products include:
Avinza 1822
Embeda 1831
MS Contin 2803

Morphine Sulfate, Liposomal (Scopolamine is an anticholinergic agent and causes certain CNS effects, such as drowsiness and dizziness, and hence it should be used with care in patients on concomitant therapy).
No products indexed under this heading.

Nortriptyline Hydrochloride (Tricyclic antidepressants have anticholinergic properties and co-administration may result in additive effects).
No products indexed under this heading.

Olanzapine (Scopolamine is an anticholinergic agent and causes certain CNS effects, such as drowsiness and dizziness, and hence it should be used with care in patients on concomitant therapy). Products include:
Symbyax 1965
Zyprexa 1984
Zyprexa IntraMuscular 1984
Zyprexa ZYDIS 1984

Oral Medications, unspecified (The absorption of oral medications may be decreased during the concurrent use of scopolamine because of decreased gastric motility and delayed gastric emptying).
No products indexed under this heading.

Orphenadrine Citrate (Co-administration may result in addititve anticholinergic effects).
No products indexed under this heading.

Oxazepam (Scopolamine is an anticholinergic agent and causes certain CNS effects, such as drowsiness and dizziness, and hence it should be used with care in patients on concomitant therapy).
No products indexed under this heading.

Oxybutynin Chloride (Co-administration may result in additive anticholinergic effects).
No products indexed under this heading.

Oxycodone Hydrochloride (Scopolamine is an anticholinergic agent and causes certain CNS effects, such as drowsiness and dizziness, and hence it should be used with care in patients on concomitant therapy). Products include:
OxyContin 2807
Percocet 1121
Percodan 1124

Oxycodone Terephthalate (Scopolamine is an anticholinergic agent and causes certain CNS effects, such as drowsiness and dizziness, and hence it should be used with care in patients on concomitant therapy).
No products indexed under this heading.

Oxymorphone Hydrochloride (Scopolamine is an anticholinergic agent and causes certain CNS effects, such as drowsiness and dizziness, and hence it should be used with care in patients on concomitant therapy). Products include:
Opana 1110
Opana ER 1114

Pancuronium Bromide (Co-administration may result in addititve anticholinergic effects).
No products indexed under this heading.

Pentobarbital (Scopolamine is an anticholinergic agent and causes certain CNS effects, such as drowsiness and dizziness, and hence it should be used with care in patients on concomitant therapy).
No products indexed under this heading.

Pentobarbital Sodium (Scopolamine is an anticholinergic agent and causes certain CNS effects, such as drowsiness and dizziness, and hence it should be used with care in patients on concomitant therapy). Products include:
Nembutal 2012

Perphenazine (Scopolamine is an anticholinergic agent and causes certain CNS effects, such as drowsiness and dizziness, and hence it should be used with care in patients on concomitant therapy).
No products indexed under this heading.

Phenobarbital (Scopolamine is an anticholinergic agent and causes certain CNS effects, such as drowsiness and dizziness, and hence it should be used with care in patients on concomitant therapy). Products include:
Donnatal 2711

Phenobarbital Sodium (Scopolamine is an anticholinergic agent and causes certain CNS effects, such as drowsiness and dizziness, and hence it should be used with care in patients on concomitant therapy).
No products indexed under this heading.

Pipecuronium Bromide (Co-administration may result in addititve anticholinergic effects).
No products indexed under this heading.

Prazepam (Scopolamine is an anticholinergic agent and causes certain CNS effects, such as drowsiness and dizziness, and hence it should be used with care in patients on concomitant therapy).
No products indexed under this heading.

Prochlorperazine (Scopolamine is an anticholinergic agent and causes certain CNS effects, such as drowsiness and dizziness, and hence it should be used with care in patients on concomitant therapy).
No products indexed under this heading.

Prochlorperazine Edisylate (Scopolamine is an anticholinergic agent and causes certain CNS effects, such as drowsiness and dizziness, and hence it should be used with care in patients on concomitant therapy).
No products indexed under this heading.

IMPORTANT NOTE: Always consult each drug listing in the patient's regimen for possible interactions.

Transderm Scōp Interactions Index 1924

Prochlorperazine Maleate (Scopolamine is an anticholinergic agent and causes certain CNS effects, such as drowsiness and dizziness, and hence it should be used with care in patients on concomitant therapy).
No products indexed under this heading.

Procyclidine Hydrochloride (Co-administration may result in additive anticholinergic effects).
No products indexed under this heading.

Promethazine (Scopolamine is an anticholinergic agent and causes certain CNS effects, such as drowsiness and dizziness, and hence it should be used with care in patients on concomitant therapy).
No products indexed under this heading.

Promethazine Hydrochloride (Antihistamines have anticholinergic properties and co-administration may result in additive effects).
No products indexed under this heading.

Propantheline Bromide (Co-administration may result in additive anticholinergic effects).
No products indexed under this heading.

Propofol (Scopolamine is an anticholinergic agent and causes certain CNS effects, such as drowsiness and dizziness, and hence it should be used with care in patients on concomitant therapy).
No products indexed under this heading.

Propoxyphene Hydrochloride (Scopolamine is an anticholinergic agent and causes certain CNS effects, such as drowsiness and dizziness, and hence it should be used with care in patients on concomitant therapy).
No products indexed under this heading.

Propoxyphene Napsylate (Scopolamine is an anticholinergic agent and causes certain CNS effects, such as drowsiness and dizziness, and hence it should be used with care in patients on concomitant therapy).
No products indexed under this heading.

Protriptyline Hydrochloride (Tricyclic antidepressants have anticholinergic properties and co-administration may result in additive effects).
No products indexed under this heading.

Pyrilamine Maleate (Antihistamines have anticholinergic properties and co-administration may result in additive effects).
No products indexed under this heading.

Pyrilamine Tannate (Antihistamines have anticholinergic properties and co-administration may result in additive effects).
No products indexed under this heading.

Quazepam (Scopolamine is an anticholinergic agent and causes certain CNS effects, such as drowsiness and dizziness, and hence it should be used with care in patients on concomitant therapy).
No products indexed under this heading.

Quetiapine Fumarate (Scopolamine is an anticholinergic agent and causes certain CNS effects, such as drowsiness and dizziness, and hence it should be used with care in patients on concomitant therapy). Products include:
Seroquel 750
Seroquel XR 759

Ramelteon (Scopolamine is an anticholinergic agent and causes certain CNS effects, such as drowsiness and dizziness, and hence it should be used with care in patients on concomitant therapy). Products include:
Rozerem 3366

Rapacuronium Bromide (Co-administration may result in additive anticholinergic effects).
No products indexed under this heading.

Remifentanil Hydrochloride (Scopolamine is an anticholinergic agent and causes certain CNS effects, such as drowsiness and dizziness, and hence it should be used with care in patients on concomitant therapy).
No products indexed under this heading.

Risperidone (Scopolamine is an anticholinergic agent and causes certain CNS effects, such as drowsiness and dizziness, and hence it should be used with care in patients on concomitant therapy). Products include:
Risperdal Consta 2682

Rocuronium Bromide (Co-administration may result in addititve anticholinergic effects). Products include:
Zemuron 3249

Scopolamine Hydrobromide (Co-administration may result in additive anticholinergic effects). Products include:
Donnatal 2711

Secobarbital Sodium (Scopolamine is an anticholinergic agent and causes certain CNS effects, such as drowsiness and dizziness, and hence it should be used with care in patients on concomitant therapy).
No products indexed under this heading.

Sevoflurane (Scopolamine is an anticholinergic agent and causes certain CNS effects, such as drowsiness and dizziness, and hence it should be used with care in patients on concomitant therapy). Products include:
Ultane 554

Sodium Butabarbital (Scopolamine is an anticholinergic agent and causes certain CNS effects, such as drowsiness and dizziness, and hence it should be used with care in patients on concomitant therapy).
No products indexed under this heading.

Sodium Oxybate (Scopolamine is an anticholinergic agent and causes certain CNS effects, such as drowsiness and dizziness, and hence it should be used with care in patients on concomitant therapy).
No products indexed under this heading.

Sodium Pentobarbital (Scopolamine is an anticholinergic agent and causes certain CNS effects, such as drowsiness and dizziness, and hence it should be used with care in patients on concomitant therapy).
No products indexed under this heading.

Succinylcholine Chloride (Co-administration may result in addititve anticholinergic effects).
No products indexed under this heading.

Sufentanil Citrate (Scopolamine is an anticholinergic agent and causes certain CNS effects, such as drowsiness and dizziness, and hence it should be used with care in patients on concomitant therapy).
No products indexed under this heading.

Talbutal (Scopolamine is an anticholinergic agent and causes certain CNS effects, such as drowsiness and dizziness, and hence it should be used with care in patients on concomitant therapy).
No products indexed under this heading.

Temazepam (Scopolamine is an anticholinergic agent and causes certain CNS effects, such as drowsiness and dizziness, and hence it should be used with care in patients on concomitant therapy).
No products indexed under this heading.

Terfenadine (Antihistamines have anticholinergic properties and co-administration may result in additive effects).
No products indexed under this heading.

Thiamylal Sodium (Scopolamine is an anticholinergic agent and causes certain CNS effects, such as drowsiness and dizziness, and hence it should be used with care in patients on concomitant therapy).
No products indexed under this heading.

Thioridazine (Scopolamine is an anticholinergic agent and causes certain CNS effects, such as drowsiness and dizziness, and hence it should be used with care in patients on concomitant therapy).
No products indexed under this heading.

Thioridazine Hydrochloride (Scopolamine is an anticholinergic agent and causes certain CNS effects, such as drowsiness and dizziness, and hence it should be used with care in patients on concomitant therapy). Products include:
Thioridazine Hydrochloride 2384

Thiothixene (Scopolamine is an anticholinergic agent and causes certain CNS effects, such as drowsiness and dizziness, and hence it should be used with care in patients on concomitant therapy). Products include:
Thiothixene 2386

Thiothixene Hydrochloride (Scopolamine is an anticholinergic agent and causes certain CNS effects, such as drowsiness and dizziness, and hence it should be used with care in patients on concomitant therapy).
No products indexed under this heading.

Tizanidine (Co-administration may result in addititve anticholinergic effects).
No products indexed under this heading.

Tizanidine Hydrochloride (Co-administration may result in addititve anticholinergic effects).
No products indexed under this heading.

Tolterodine Tartrate (Co-administration may result in additive anticholinergic effects).
No products indexed under this heading.

Triazolam (Scopolamine is an anticholinergic agent and causes certain CNS effects, such as drowsiness and dizziness, and hence it should be used with care in patients on concomitant therapy).
No products indexed under this heading.

Tridihexethyl Chloride (Co-administration may result in additive anticholinergic effects).
No products indexed under this heading.

Trifluoperazine Hydrochloride (Scopolamine is an anticholinergic agent and causes certain CNS effects, such as drowsiness and dizziness, and hence it should be used with care in patients on concomitant therapy).
No products indexed under this heading.

Trihexyphenidyl Hydrochloride (Co-administration may result in additive anticholinergic effects).
No products indexed under this heading.

Trimeprazine Tartrate (Antihistamines have anticholinergic properties and co-administration may result in additive effects).
No products indexed under this heading.

Trimipramine Maleate (Tricyclic antidepressants have anticholinergic properties and co-administration may result in additive effects).
No products indexed under this heading.

Tripelennamine Hydrochloride (Antihistamines have anticholinergic properties and co-administration may result in additive effects).
No products indexed under this heading.

Triprolidine Hydrochloride (Antihistamines have anticholinergic properties and co-administration may result in additive effects).
No products indexed under this heading.

Tubocurarine Chloride (Co-administration may result in addititve anticholinergic effects).
No products indexed under this heading.

Vecuronium Bromide (Co-administration may result in addititve anticholinergic effects).
No products indexed under this heading.

Zaleplon (Scopolamine is an anticholinergic agent and causes certain CNS effects, such as drowsiness and dizziness, and hence it should be used with care in patients on concomitant therapy).
No products indexed under this heading.

Ziprasidone Hydrochloride (Scopolamine is an anticholinergic agent and causes certain CNS effects, such as drowsiness and dizziness, and hence it should be used with care in patients on concomitant therapy). Products include:
Geodon 2723

Zolpidem Tartrate (Scopolamine is an anticholinergic agent and causes certain CNS effects, such as drowsiness and dizziness, and hence it should be used with care in patients on concomitant therapy). Products include:
Ambien 2920
Ambien CR 2925

Food Interactions

Alcohol (Scopolamine is an anticholinergic agent and causes certain CNS effects, such as drowsiness and dizziness, and hence it should be used with care in patients on concomitant therapy).

Beer, reduced-alcohol (Scopolamine is an anticholinergic agent and causes certain CNS effects, such as drowsiness and dizziness, and hence it should be used with care in patients on concomitant therapy).

Beer, unspecified (Scopolamine is an anticholinergic agent and causes certain CNS effects, such as drowsiness and dizziness, and hence it should be used with care in patients on concomitant therapy).

Wine, Chianti (Scopolamine is an anticholinergic agent and causes certain CNS effects, such as drowsiness and dizziness, and hence it should be used with care in patients on concomitant therapy).

Wine, Red (Scopolamine is an anticholinergic agent and causes certain CNS effects, such as drowsiness and dizziness, and hence it should be used with care in patients on concomitant therapy).

Wine, unspecified (Scopolamine is an anticholinergic agent and causes certain CNS effects, such as drowsiness and dizziness, and hence it should be used with care in patients on concomitant therapy).

Wine products (Scopolamine is an anticholinergic agent and causes certain CNS effects, such as drowsiness and dizziness, and hence it should be used with care in patients on concomitant therapy).

TRAUMEEL INJECTION SOLUTION

(Achillea millefolium, Aconitum napellus, Arnica montana, Belladonna, Bellis perennis, Calendula officinalis, Chamomilla, Echinacea angustifolia, Echinacea purpurea, Hamamelis virginiana, Hypericum Perforatum, Symphytum officinale) 1800
None cited in PDR database.

TRAVATAN Z OPHTHALMIC SOLUTION

(Travoprost) 587
None cited in PDR database.

(⊙ Described in PDR® for Ophthalmic Medicines)

TREANDA FOR INJECTION

(Bendamustine Hydrochloride) 989

May interact with cytochrome p450 1a2 inducers (selected), cytochrome p450 1a2 inhibitors (selected), and certain other agents. Compounds in these categories include:

Alatrofloxacin Mesylate (Inhibitors of CYP1A2 (eg, fluvoxamine, ciprofloxacin) have the potential to increase plasma concentrations of bendamustine and decrease plasma concentrations of active metabolites. Caution should be used, or alternative treatments considered, if concomitant treatment with CYP1A2 inhibitors is needed).

No products indexed under this heading.

Allopurinol (Cases of Stevens-Johnson syndrome (SJS) and toxic epidermal necrolysis (TEN), some fatal, have been reported when bendamustine was administered concomitantly with allopurinol and other medications known to cause these syndromes. The relationship to bendamustine cannot be determined).

No products indexed under this heading.

Allopurinol Sodium (Cases of Stevens-Johnson syndrome (SJS) and toxic epidermal necrolysis (TEN), some fatal, have been reported when bendamustine was administered concomitantly with allopurinol and other medications known to cause these syndromes. The relationship to bendamustine cannot be determined).

No products indexed under this heading.

Amiodarone Hydrochloride (Inhibitors of CYP1A2 (eg, fluvoxamine, ciprofloxacin) have the potential to increase plasma concentrations of bendamustine and decrease plasma concentrations of active metabolites. Caution should be used, or alternative treatments considered, if concomitant treatment with CYP1A2 inhibitors is needed).

No products indexed under this heading.

Anastrozole (Inhibitors of CYP1A2 (eg, fluvoxamine, ciprofloxacin) have the potential to increase plasma concentrations of bendamustine and decrease plasma concentrations of active metabolites. Caution should be used, or alternative treatments considered, if concomitant treatment with CYP1A2 inhibitors is needed).

No products indexed under this heading.

Carbamazepine (Inducers of CYP1A2 (eg, omeprazole, smoking) have the potential to decrease plasma concentrations of bendamustine and increase plasma concentrations of its active metabolites. Caution should be used, or alternative treatments considered, if concomitant treatment with CYP1A2 inducers is needed). Products include:

Carbatrol 3280
Equetro 3477

Cimetidine (Inhibitors of CYP1A2 (eg, fluvoxamine, ciprofloxacin) have the potential to increase plasma concentrations of bendamustine and decrease plasma concentrations of active metabolites. Caution should be used, or alternative treatments considered, if concomitant treatment with CYP1A2 inhibitors is needed).

No products indexed under this heading.

Cimetidine Hydrochloride (Inhibitors of CYP1A2 (eg, fluvoxamine, ciprofloxacin) have the potential to increase plasma concentrations of bendamustine and decrease plasma concentrations of active metabolites. Caution should be used, or alternative treatments considered, if concomitant treatment with CYP1A2 inhibitors is needed).

No products indexed under this heading.

Ciprofloxacin (Inhibitors of CYP1A2 (eg, fluvoxamine, ciprofloxacin) have the potential to increase plasma concentra-

tions of bendamustine and decrease plasma concentrations of active metabolites. Caution should be used, or alternative treatments considered, if concomitant treatment with CYP1A2 inhibitors is needed). Products include:

Cipro I.V. 3082
Cipro 3073
Cipro XR 3091
Ciprodex 583

Ciprofloxacin Hydrochloride (Inhibitors of CYP1A2 (eg, fluvoxamine, ciprofloxacin) have the potential to increase plasma concentrations of bendamustine and decrease plasma concentrations of active metabolites. Caution should be used, or alternative treatments considered, if concomitant treatment with CYP1A2 inhibitors is needed). Products include:

Cipro 3073

Citalopram Hydrobromide (Inducers of CYP1A2 (eg, omeprazole, smoking) have the potential to decrease plasma concentrations of bendamustine and increase plasma concentrations of its active metabolites. Caution should be used, or alternative treatments considered, if concomitant treatment with CYP1A2 inducers is needed). Products include:

Celexa 1153

Clarithromycin (Inhibitors of CYP1A2 (eg, fluvoxamine, ciprofloxacin) have the potential to increase plasma concentrations of bendamustine and decrease plasma concentrations of active metabolites. Caution should be used, or alternative treatments considered, if concomitant treatment with CYP1A2 inhibitors is needed). Products include:

Biaxin/Biaxin XL 412

Desogestrel (Inhibitors of CYP1A2 (eg, fluvoxamine, ciprofloxacin) have the potential to increase plasma concentrations of bendamustine and decrease plasma concentrations of active metabolites. Caution should be used, or alternative treatments considered, if concomitant treatment with CYP1A2 inhibitors is needed).

No products indexed under this heading.

Diltiazem Hydrochloride (Inducers of CYP1A2 (eg, omeprazole, smoking) have the potential to decrease plasma concentrations of bendamustine and increase plasma concentrations of its active metabolites. Caution should be used, or alternative treatments considered, if concomitant treatment with CYP1A2 inducers is needed). Products include:

Cardizem LA 423

Diltiazem Maleate (Inducers of CYP1A2 (eg, omeprazole, smoking) have the potential to decrease plasma concentrations of bendamustine and increase plasma concentrations of its active metabolites. Caution should be used, or alternative treatments considered, if concomitant treatment with CYP1A2 inducers is needed).

No products indexed under this heading.

Enoxacin (Inhibitors of CYP1A2 (eg, fluvoxamine, ciprofloxacin) have the potential to increase plasma concentrations of bendamustine and decrease plasma concentrations of active metabolites. Caution should be used, or alternative treatments considered, if concomitant treatment with CYP1A2 inhibitors is needed).

No products indexed under this heading.

Erythromycin (Inducers of CYP1A2 (eg, omeprazole, smoking) have the potential to decrease plasma concentrations of bendamustine and increase plasma concentrations of its active metabolites. Caution should be used, or alternative treatments considered, if concomitant treatment with CYP1A2 inducers is needed).

No products indexed under this heading.

Erythromycin, Topical (Inducers of CYP1A2 (eg, omeprazole, smoking) have the potential to decrease plasma concentrations of bendamustine and increase plasma concentrations of its active metabolites. Caution should be used, or alternative treatments considered, if concomitant treatment with CYP1A2 inducers is needed).

No products indexed under this heading.

Erythromycin Estolate (Inducers of CYP1A2 (eg, omeprazole, smoking) have the potential to decrease plasma concentrations of bendamustine and increase plasma concentrations of its active metabolites. Caution should be used, or alternative treatments considered, if concomitant treatment with CYP1A2 inducers is needed).

No products indexed under this heading.

Erythromycin Ethylsuccinate (Inducers of CYP1A2 (eg, omeprazole, smoking) have the potential to decrease plasma concentrations of bendamustine and increase plasma concentrations of its active metabolites. Caution should be used, or alternative treatments considered, if concomitant treatment with CYP1A2 inducers is needed). Products include:

E.E.S. 437
EryPed 435

Erythromycin Gluceptate (Inducers of CYP1A2 (eg, omeprazole, smoking) have the potential to decrease plasma concentrations of bendamustine and increase plasma concentrations of its active metabolites. Caution should be used, or alternative treatments considered, if concomitant treatment with CYP1A2 inducers is needed).

No products indexed under this heading.

Erythromycin Lactobionate (Inducers of CYP1A2 (eg, omeprazole, smoking) have the potential to decrease plasma concentrations of bendamustine and increase plasma concentrations of its active metabolites. Caution should be used, or alternative treatments considered, if concomitant treatment with CYP1A2 inducers is needed).

No products indexed under this heading.

Erythromycin Stearate (Inducers of CYP1A2 (eg, omeprazole, smoking) have the potential to decrease plasma concentrations of bendamustine and increase plasma concentrations of its active metabolites. Caution should be used, or alternative treatments considered, if concomitant treatment with CYP1A2 inducers is needed).

No products indexed under this heading.

Escitalopram Oxalate (Inducers of CYP1A2 (eg, omeprazole, smoking) have the potential to decrease plasma concentrations of bendamustine and increase plasma concentrations of its active metabolites. Caution should be used, or alternative treatments considered, if concomitant treatment with CYP1A2 inducers is needed). Products include:

Lexapro Oral Suspension 1160
Lexapro Tablets 1160

Esomeprazole Magnesium (Inhibitors of CYP1A2 (eg, fluvoxamine, ciprofloxacin) have the potential to increase plasma concentrations of bendamustine and decrease plasma concentrations of active metabolites. Caution should be used, or alternative treatments considered, if concomitant treatment with CYP1A2 inhibitors is needed). Products include:

Nexium Capsules 704
Nexium Oral Suspension 704

Esomeprazole Sodium (Inhibitors of CYP1A2 (eg, fluvoxamine, ciprofloxacin) have the potential to increase plasma concentrations of bendamustine and decrease plasma concentrations of active metabolites. Caution should be

used, or alternative treatments considered, if concomitant treatment with CYP1A2 inhibitors is needed). Products include:

Nexium I.V. 712

Ethinyl Estradiol (Inhibitors of CYP1A2 (eg, fluvoxamine, ciprofloxacin) have the potential to increase plasma concentrations of bendamustine and decrease plasma concentrations of active metabolites. Caution should be used, or alternative treatments considered, if concomitant treatment with CYP1A2 inhibitors is needed). Products include:

LoSeasonique 3407
Lybrel 3514
NuvaRing 3181
Ortho Evra 2648
Ortho-Cyclen/Ortho Tri-Cyclen 2663
Ortho Tri-Cyclen Lo Tablets 2673
Seasonique 3418
Yaz 864

Fluvoxamine (Inhibitors of CYP1A2 (eg, fluvoxamine, ciprofloxacin) have the potential to increase plasma concentrations of bendamustine and decrease plasma concentrations of active metabolites. Caution should be used, or alternative treatments considered, if concomitant treatment with CYP1A2 inhibitors is needed).

No products indexed under this heading.

Fluvoxamine Maleate (Inhibitors of CYP1A2 (eg, fluvoxamine, ciprofloxacin) have the potential to increase plasma concentrations of bendamustine and decrease plasma concentrations of active metabolites. Caution should be used, or alternative treatments considered, if concomitant treatment with CYP1A2 inhibitors is needed).

No products indexed under this heading.

Gatifloxacin (Inhibitors of CYP1A2 (eg, fluvoxamine, ciprofloxacin) have the potential to increase plasma concentrations of bendamustine and decrease plasma concentrations of active metabolites. Caution should be used, or alternative treatments considered, if concomitant treatment with CYP1A2 inhibitors is needed).

No products indexed under this heading.

Gemifloxacin Mesylate (Inhibitors of CYP1A2 (eg, fluvoxamine, ciprofloxacin) have the potential to increase plasma concentrations of bendamustine and decrease plasma concentrations of active metabolites. Caution should be used, or alternative treatments considered, if concomitant treatment with CYP1A2 inhibitors is needed).

No products indexed under this heading.

Grepafloxacin Hydrochloride (Inhibitors of CYP1A2 (eg, fluvoxamine, ciprofloxacin) have the potential to increase plasma concentrations of bendamustine and decrease plasma concentrations of active metabolites. Caution should be used, or alternative treatments considered, if concomitant treatment with CYP1A2 inhibitors is needed).

No products indexed under this heading.

Hypericum (Inducers of CYP1A2 (eg, omeprazole, smoking) have the potential to decrease plasma concentrations of bendamustine and increase plasma concentrations of its active metabolites. Caution should be used, or alternative treatments considered, if concomitant treatment with CYP1A2 inducers is needed).

No products indexed under this heading.

Hypericum Perforatum (Inducers of CYP1A2 (eg, omeprazole, smoking) have the potential to decrease plasma concentrations of bendamustine and increase plasma concentrations of its active metabolites. Caution should be used, or alternative treatments consid-

ered, if concomitant treatment with CYP1A2 inducers is needed). Products include:

Insulin (Inducers of CYP1A2 (eg, omeprazole, smoking) have the potential to decrease plasma concentrations of bendamustine and increase plasma concentrations of its active metabolites. Caution should be used, or alternative treatments considered, if concomitant treatment with CYP1A2 inducers is needed).

No products indexed under this heading.

Insulin, Human, Zinc Suspension (Inducers of CYP1A2 (eg, omeprazole, smoking) have the potential to decrease plasma concentrations of bendamustine and increase plasma concentrations of its active metabolites. Caution should be used, or alternative treatments considered, if concomitant treatment with CYP1A2 inducers is needed).

No products indexed under this heading.

Insulin, Human (rDNA origin) (Inducers of CYP1A2 (eg, omeprazole, smoking) have the potential to decrease plasma concentrations of bendamustine and increase plasma concentrations of its active metabolites. Caution should be used, or alternative treatments considered, if concomitant treatment with CYP1A2 inducers is needed). Products include:

Insulin, Human NPH (Inducers of CYP1A2 (eg, omeprazole, smoking) have the potential to decrease plasma concentrations of bendamustine and increase plasma concentrations of its active metabolites. Caution should be used, or alternative treatments considered, if concomitant treatment with CYP1A2 inducers is needed). Products include:

Insulin, Human Regular (Inducers of CYP1A2 (eg, omeprazole, smoking) have the potential to decrease plasma concentrations of bendamustine and increase plasma concentrations of its active metabolites. Caution should be used, or alternative treatments considered, if concomitant treatment with CYP1A2 inducers is needed). Products include:

Insulin, Human Regular and Human NPH Mixture (Inducers of CYP1A2 (eg, omeprazole, smoking) have the potential to decrease plasma concentrations of bendamustine and increase plasma concentrations of its active metabolites. Caution should be used, or alternative treatments considered, if concomitant treatment with CYP1A2 inducers is needed). Products include:

Insulin, NPH (Inducers of CYP1A2 (eg, omeprazole, smoking) have the potential to decrease plasma concentrations of bendamustine and increase plasma concentrations of its active metabolites. Caution should be used, or alternative treatments considered, if concomitant treatment with CYP1A2 inducers is needed).

No products indexed under this heading.

Insulin, Regular (Inducers of CYP1A2 (eg, omeprazole, smoking) have the potential to decrease plasma concentrations of bendamustine and increase plasma concentrations of its active metabolites. Caution should be used, or alternative treatments considered, if concomitant treatment with CYP1A2 inducers is needed).

No products indexed under this heading.

Insulin, Regular and NPH mixture (Inducers of CYP1A2 (eg, omeprazole, smoking) have the potential to decrease plasma concentrations of bendamustine and increase plasma concentrations of its active metabolites. Caution should be used, or alternative treatments considered, if concomitant treatment with CYP1A2 inducers is needed).

No products indexed under this heading.

Insulin, Zinc Crystals (Inducers of CYP1A2 (eg, omeprazole, smoking) have the potential to decrease plasma concentrations of bendamustine and increase plasma concentrations of its active metabolites. Caution should be used, or alternative treatments considered, if concomitant treatment with CYP1A2 inducers is needed).

No products indexed under this heading.

Insulin, Zinc Suspension (Inducers of CYP1A2 (eg, omeprazole, smoking) have the potential to decrease plasma concentrations of bendamustine and increase plasma concentrations of its active metabolites. Caution should be used, or alternative treatments considered, if concomitant treatment with CYP1A2 inducers is needed).

No products indexed under this heading.

Insulin Aspart (Inducers of CYP1A2 (eg, omeprazole, smoking) have the potential to decrease plasma concentrations of bendamustine and increase plasma concentrations of its active metabolites. Caution should be used, or alternative treatments considered, if concomitant treatment with CYP1A2 inducers is needed).

No products indexed under this heading.

Insulin Aspart, Human (Inducers of CYP1A2 (eg, omeprazole, smoking) have the potential to decrease plasma concentrations of bendamustine and increase plasma concentrations of its active metabolites. Caution should be used, or alternative treatments considered, if concomitant treatment with CYP1A2 inducers is needed). Products include:

Insulin Aspart, Human Regular (Inducers of CYP1A2 (eg, omeprazole, smoking) have the potential to decrease plasma concentrations of bendamustine and increase plasma concentrations of its active metabolites. Caution should be used, or alternative treatments considered, if concomitant treatment with CYP1A2 inducers is needed). Products include:

Insulin Aspart Protamine, Human (Inducers of CYP1A2 (eg, omeprazole, smoking) have the potential to decrease plasma concentrations of bendamustine and increase plasma concentrations of its active metabolites. Caution should be used, or alternative treatments considered, if concomitant treatment with CYP1A2 inducers is needed). Products include:

Insulin Detemir (rDNA Origin) (Inducers of CYP1A2 (eg, omeprazole, smoking) have the potential to decrease plasma concentrations of bendamustine and increase plasma concentrations of its active metabolites. Caution should be used, or alternative treatments considered, if concomitant treatment with CYP1A2 inducers is needed). Products include:

Insulin Glargine (Inducers of CYP1A2 (eg, omeprazole, smoking) have the potential to decrease plasma concentrations of bendamustine and increase plasma concentrations of its active metabolites. Caution should be used, or alternative treatments considered, if

concomitant treatment with CYP1A2 inducers is needed). Products include:

Insulin Glulisine (Inducers of CYP1A2 (eg, omeprazole, smoking) have the potential to decrease plasma concentrations of bendamustine and increase plasma concentrations of its active metabolites. Caution should be used, or alternative treatments considered, if concomitant treatment with CYP1A2 inducers is needed). Products include:

Insulin Lispro, Human (Inducers of CYP1A2 (eg, omeprazole, smoking) have the potential to decrease plasma concentrations of bendamustine and increase plasma concentrations of its active metabolites. Caution should be used, or alternative treatments considered, if concomitant treatment with CYP1A2 inducers is needed). Products include:

Insulin Lispro Protamine, Human (Inducers of CYP1A2 (eg, omeprazole, smoking) have the potential to decrease plasma concentrations of bendamustine and increase plasma concentrations of its active metabolites. Caution should be used, or alternative treatments considered, if concomitant treatment with CYP1A2 inducers is needed). Products include:

Isoniazid (Inhibitors of CYP1A2 (eg, fluvoxamine, ciprofloxacin) have the potential to increase plasma concentrations of bendamustine and decrease plasma concentrations of active metabolites. Caution should be used, or alternative treatments considered, if concomitant treatment with CYP1A2 inhibitors is needed).

No products indexed under this heading.

Ketoconazole (Inhibitors of CYP1A2 (eg, fluvoxamine, ciprofloxacin) have the potential to increase plasma concentrations of bendamustine and decrease plasma concentrations of active metabolites. Caution should be used, or alternative treatments considered, if concomitant treatment with CYP1A2 inhibitors is needed). Products include:

Lansoprazole (Inducers of CYP1A2 (eg, omeprazole, smoking) have the potential to decrease plasma concentrations of bendamustine and increase plasma concentrations of its active metabolites. Caution should be used, or alternative treatments considered, if concomitant treatment with CYP1A2 inducers is needed).

No products indexed under this heading.

Levofloxacin (Inhibitors of CYP1A2 (eg, fluvoxamine, ciprofloxacin) have the potential to increase plasma concentrations of bendamustine and decrease plasma concentrations of active metabolites. Caution should be used, or alternative treatments considered, if concomitant treatment with CYP1A2 inhibitors is needed). Products include:

Levonorgestrel (Inhibitors of CYP1A2 (eg, fluvoxamine, ciprofloxacin) have the potential to increase plasma concentrations of bendamustine and decrease plasma concentrations of active metabolites. Caution should be used, or alternative treatments considered, if concomitant treatment with CYP1A2 inhibitors is needed). Products include:

Lomefloxacin Hydrochloride (Inhibitors of CYP1A2 (eg, fluvoxamine, ciprofloxacin) have the potential to increase plasma concentrations of bendamustine and decrease plasma concentrations of active metabolites. Caution should be used, or alternative treatments considered, if concomitant treatment with CYP1A2 inhibitors is needed).

No products indexed under this heading.

Mestranol (Inhibitors of CYP1A2 (eg, fluvoxamine, ciprofloxacin) have the potential to increase plasma concentrations of bendamustine and decrease plasma concentrations of active metabolites. Caution should be used, or alternative treatments considered, if concomitant treatment with CYP1A2 inhibitors is needed).

No products indexed under this heading.

Methoxsalen (Inhibitors of CYP1A2 (eg, fluvoxamine, ciprofloxacin) have the potential to increase plasma concentrations of bendamustine and decrease plasma concentrations of active metabolites. Caution should be used, or alternative treatments considered, if concomitant treatment with CYP1A2 inhibitors is needed).

No products indexed under this heading.

Mexiletine Hydrochloride (Inhibitors of CYP1A2 (eg, fluvoxamine, ciprofloxacin) have the potential to increase plasma concentrations of bendamustine and decrease plasma concentrations of active metabolites. Caution should be used, or alternative treatments considered, if concomitant treatment with CYP1A2 inhibitors is needed).

No products indexed under this heading.

Mibefradil Dihydrochloride (Inhibitors of CYP1A2 (eg, fluvoxamine, ciprofloxacin) have the potential to increase plasma concentrations of bendamustine and decrease plasma concentrations of active metabolites. Caution should be used, or alternative treatments considered, if concomitant treatment with CYP1A2 inhibitors is needed).

No products indexed under this heading.

Moxifloxacin Hydrochloride (Inhibitors of CYP1A2 (eg, fluvoxamine, ciprofloxacin) have the potential to increase plasma concentrations of bendamustine and decrease plasma concentrations of active metabolites. Caution should be used, or alternative treatments considered, if concomitant treatment with CYP1A2 inhibitors is needed). Products include:

Nafcillin Sodium (Inducers of CYP1A2 (eg, omeprazole, smoking) have the potential to decrease plasma concentrations of bendamustine and increase plasma concentrations of its active metabolites. Caution should be used, or alternative treatments considered, if concomitant treatment with CYP1A2 inducers is needed).

No products indexed under this heading.

Nalidixic Acid (Inhibitors of CYP1A2 (eg, fluvoxamine, ciprofloxacin) have the potential to increase plasma concentrations of bendamustine and decrease plasma concentrations of active metabolites. Caution should be used, or alternative treatments considered, if concomitant treatment with CYP1A2 inhibitors is needed).

No products indexed under this heading.

Nicotine (Inducers of CYP1A2 (eg, omeprazole, smoking) have the potential to decrease plasma concentrations of bendamustine and increase plasma concentrations of its active metabolites. Caution should be used, or alternative treatments considered, if concomitant treatment with CYP1A2 inducers is needed).

No products indexed under this heading.

Nicotine Polacrilex (Inducers of CYP1A2 (eg, omeprazole, smoking) have the potential to decrease plasma concentrations of bendamustine and increase plasma concentrations of its active metabolites. Caution should be used, or alternative treatments considered, if concomitant treatment with CYP1A2 inducers is needed).

No products indexed under this heading.

Nicotine Salicylate (Inducers of CYP1A2 (eg, omeprazole, smoking) have the potential to decrease plasma concentrations of bendamustine and increase plasma concentrations of its active metabolites. Caution should be used, or alternative treatments considered, if concomitant treatment with CYP1A2 inducers is needed).

No products indexed under this heading.

Nicotine Sulfate (Inducers of CYP1A2 (eg, omeprazole, smoking) have the potential to decrease plasma concentrations of bendamustine and increase plasma concentrations of its active metabolites. Caution should be used, or alternative treatments considered, if concomitant treatment with CYP1A2 inducers is needed).

No products indexed under this heading.

Norethindrone (Inhibitors of CYP1A2 (eg, fluvoxamine, ciprofloxacin) have the potential to increase plasma concentrations of bendamustine and decrease plasma concentrations of active metabolites. Caution should be used, or alternative treatments considered, if concomitant treatment with CYP1A2 inhibitors is needed). Products include:
Ortho Micronor 2660

Norethindrone Acetate (Inhibitors of CYP1A2 (eg, fluvoxamine, ciprofloxacin) have the potential to increase plasma concentrations of bendamustine and decrease plasma concentrations of active metabolites. Caution should be used, or alternative treatments considered, if concomitant treatment with CYP1A2 inhibitors is needed). Products include:
Activella 2561

Norfloxacin (Inhibitors of CYP1A2 (eg, fluvoxamine, ciprofloxacin) have the potential to increase plasma concentrations of bendamustine and decrease plasma concentrations of active metabolites. Caution should be used, or alternative treatments considered, if concomitant treatment with CYP1A2 inhibitors is needed). Products include:
Noroxin 2220

Norgestrel (Inhibitors of CYP1A2 (eg, fluvoxamine, ciprofloxacin) have the potential to increase plasma concentrations of bendamustine and decrease plasma concentrations of active metabolites. Caution should be used, or alternative treatments considered, if concomitant treatment with CYP1A2 inhibitors is needed).

No products indexed under this heading.

Ofloxacin (Inhibitors of CYP1A2 (eg, fluvoxamine, ciprofloxacin) have the potential to increase plasma concentrations of bendamustine and decrease plasma concentrations of active metabolites. Caution should be used, or alternative treatments considered, if concomitant treatment with CYP1A2 inhibitors is needed).

No products indexed under this heading.

Omeprazole (Inducers of CYP1A2 (eg, omeprazole) have the potential to decrease plasma concentrations of bendamustine and increase plasma concentrations of its active metabolites. Caution should be used, or alternative treatments considered if concomitant treatment with CYP1A2 inducers is needed).

No products indexed under this heading.

Omeprazole Magnesium (Inducers of CYP1A2 (eg, omeprazole) have the potential to decrease plasma concentrations of bendamustine and increase plasma concentrations of its active metabolites. Caution should be used, or alternative treatments considered if concomitant treatment with CYP1A2 inducers is needed).

No products indexed under this heading.

Paroxetine (Inhibitors of CYP1A2 (eg, fluvoxamine, ciprofloxacin) have the potential to increase plasma concentrations of bendamustine and decrease plasma concentrations of active metabolites. Caution should be used, or alternative treatments considered, if concomitant treatment with CYP1A2 inhibitors is needed).

No products indexed under this heading.

Paroxetine Hydrochloride (Inhibitors of CYP1A2 (eg, fluvoxamine, ciprofloxacin) have the potential to increase plasma concentrations of bendamustine and decrease plasma concentrations of active metabolites. Caution should be used, or alternative treatments considered, if concomitant treatment with CYP1A2 inhibitors is needed). Products include:
Paroxetine CR 2361
Paroxetine ER 2371
Paxil 1586
Paxil CR 1596

Paroxetine Mesylate (Inhibitors of CYP1A2 (eg, fluvoxamine, ciprofloxacin) have the potential to increase plasma concentrations of bendamustine and decrease plasma concentrations of active metabolites. Caution should be used, or alternative treatments considered, if concomitant treatment with CYP1A2 inhibitors is needed).

No products indexed under this heading.

Phenobarbital (Inducers of CYP1A2 (eg, omeprazole, smoking) have the potential to decrease plasma concentrations of bendamustine and increase plasma concentrations of its active metabolites. Caution should be used, or alternative treatments considered, if concomitant treatment with CYP1A2 inducers is needed). Products include:
Donnatal 2711

Phenobarbital Sodium (Inducers of CYP1A2 (eg, omeprazole, smoking) have the potential to decrease plasma concentrations of bendamustine and increase plasma concentrations of its active metabolites. Caution should be used, or alternative treatments considered, if concomitant treatment with CYP1A2 inducers is needed).

No products indexed under this heading.

Phenytoin (Inducers of CYP1A2 (eg, omeprazole, smoking) have the potential to decrease plasma concentrations of bendamustine and increase plasma concentrations of its active metabolites. Caution should be used, or alternative treatments considered, if concomitant treatment with CYP1A2 inducers is needed).

No products indexed under this heading.

Phenytoin Sodium (Inducers of CYP1A2 (eg, omeprazole, smoking) have the potential to decrease plasma concentrations of bendamustine and increase plasma concentrations of its active metabolites. Caution should be used, or alternative treatments consid-

ered, if concomitant treatment with CYP1A2 inducers is needed). Products include:
Phenytek Capsules 2380

Primidone (Inducers of CYP1A2 (eg, omeprazole, smoking) have the potential to decrease plasma concentrations of bendamustine and increase plasma concentrations of its active metabolites. Caution should be used, or alternative treatments considered, if concomitant treatment with CYP1A2 inducers is needed).

No products indexed under this heading.

Ranitidine Bismuth Citrate (Inhibitors of CYP1A2 (eg, fluvoxamine, ciprofloxacin) have the potential to increase plasma concentrations of bendamustine and decrease plasma concentrations of active metabolites. Caution should be used, or alternative treatments considered, if concomitant treatment with CYP1A2 inhibitors is needed).

No products indexed under this heading.

Ranitidine Hydrochloride (Inhibitors of CYP1A2 (eg, fluvoxamine, ciprofloxacin) have the potential to increase plasma concentrations of bendamustine and decrease plasma concentrations of active metabolites. Caution should be used, or alternative treatments considered, if concomitant treatment with CYP1A2 inhibitors is needed). Products include:
Zantac 1737
Zantac Injection 1732
Zantac Pharmacy 1735

Rifampicin (Inducers of CYP1A2 (eg, omeprazole, smoking) have the potential to decrease plasma concentrations of bendamustine and increase plasma concentrations of its active metabolites. Caution should be used, or alternative treatments considered, if concomitant treatment with CYP1A2 inducers is needed).

No products indexed under this heading.

Rifampin (Inducers of CYP1A2 (eg, omeprazole, smoking) have the potential to decrease plasma concentrations of bendamustine and increase plasma concentrations of its active metabolites. Caution should be used, or alternative treatments considered, if concomitant treatment with CYP1A2 inducers is needed).

No products indexed under this heading.

Ritonavir (Inhibitors of CYP1A2 (eg, fluvoxamine, ciprofloxacin) have the potential to increase plasma concentrations of bendamustine and decrease plasma concentrations of active metabolites. Caution should be used, or alternative treatments considered, if concomitant treatment with CYP1A2 inhibitors is needed). Products include:
Kaletra 458
Norvir 509

Sildenafil Citrate (Inhibitors of CYP1A2 (eg, fluvoxamine, ciprofloxacin) have the potential to increase plasma concentrations of bendamustine and decrease plasma concentrations of active metabolites. Caution should be used, or alternative treatments considered, if concomitant treatment with CYP1A2 inhibitors is needed).

No products indexed under this heading.

Sparfloxacin (Inhibitors of CYP1A2 (eg, fluvoxamine, ciprofloxacin) have the potential to increase plasma concentrations of bendamustine and decrease plasma concentrations of active metabolites. Caution should be used, or alternative treatments considered, if concomitant treatment with CYP1A2 inhibitors is needed).

No products indexed under this heading.

Tacrine Hydrochloride (Inhibitors of CYP1A2 (eg, fluvoxamine, ciprofloxacin) have the potential to increase plasma concentrations of bendamustine and decrease plasma concentrations of active metabolites. Caution should be used, or alternative treatments considered, if concomitant treatment with CYP1A2 inhibitors is needed).

No products indexed under this heading.

Ticlopidine Hydrochloride (Inhibitors of CYP1A2 (eg, fluvoxamine, ciprofloxacin) have the potential to increase plasma concentrations of bendamustine and decrease plasma concentrations of active metabolites. Caution should be used, or alternative treatments considered, if concomitant treatment with CYP1A2 inhibitors is needed).

No products indexed under this heading.

Tobacco (Inducers of CYP1A2 (eg, omeprazole, smoking) have the potential to decrease plasma concentrations of bendamustine and increase plasma concentrations of its active metabolites. Caution should be used, or alternative treatments considered, if concomitant treatment with CYP1A2 inducers is needed).

No products indexed under this heading.

Troleandomycin (Inhibitors of CYP1A2 (eg, fluvoxamine, ciprofloxacin) have the potential to increase plasma concentrations of bendamustine and decrease plasma concentrations of active metabolites. Caution should be used, or alternative treatments considered, if concomitant treatment with CYP1A2 inhibitors is needed).

No products indexed under this heading.

Trovafloxacin Mesylate (Inhibitors of CYP1A2 (eg, fluvoxamine, ciprofloxacin) have the potential to increase plasma concentrations of bendamustine and decrease plasma concentrations of active metabolites. Caution should be used, or alternative treatments considered, if concomitant treatment with CYP1A2 inhibitors is needed).

No products indexed under this heading.

Vardenafil Hydrochloride (Inhibitors of CYP1A2 (eg, fluvoxamine, ciprofloxacin) have the potential to increase plasma concentrations of bendamustine and decrease plasma concentrations of active metabolites. Caution should be used, or alternative treatments considered, if concomitant treatment with CYP1A2 inhibitors is needed). Products include:
Levitra 3157

Zileuton (Inhibitors of CYP1A2 (eg, fluvoxamine, ciprofloxacin) have the potential to increase plasma concentrations of bendamustine and decrease plasma concentrations of active metabolites. Caution should be used, or alternative treatments considered, if concomitant treatment with CYP1A2 inhibitors is needed).

No products indexed under this heading.

Food Interactions

Broccoli (Inducers of CYP1A2 (eg, omeprazole, smoking) have the potential to decrease plasma concentrations of bendamustine and increase plasma concentrations of its active metabolites. Caution should be used, or alternative treatments considered, if concomitant treatment with CYP1A2 inducers is needed).

Brussel Sprouts (Inducers of CYP1A2 (eg, omeprazole, smoking) have the potential to decrease plasma concentrations of bendamustine and increase plasma concentrations of its active metabolites. Caution should be used, or alternative treatments considered, if concomitant treatment with CYP1A2 inducers is needed).

IMPORTANT NOTE: Always consult each drug listing in the patient's regimen for possible interactions.

Charbroiled Food (Inducers of CYP1A2 (eg, omeprazole, smoking) have the potential to decrease plasma concentrations of bendamustine and increase plasma concentrations of its active metabolites. Caution should be used, or alternative treatments considered, if concomitant treatment with CYP1A2 inducers is needed).

Grapefruit (Inhibitors of CYP1A2 (eg, fluvoxamine, ciprofloxacin) have the potential to increase plasma concentrations of bendamustine and decrease plasma concentrations of active metabolites. Caution should be used, or alternative treatments considered, if concomitant treatment with CYP1A2 inhibitors is needed).

Grapefruit Juice (Inhibitors of CYP1A2 (eg, fluvoxamine, ciprofloxacin) have the potential to increase plasma concentrations of bendamustine and decrease plasma concentrations of active metabolites. Caution should be used, or alternative treatments considered, if concomitant treatment with CYP1A2 inhibitors is needed).

TREXIMET TABLETS

(Naproxen Sodium, Sumatriptan Succinate) 1681
May interact with ACE inhibitors, alcohols, anticoagulants, aspirin-acetylsalicylic acid, beta-blockers, corticosteroids, diuretics, ergot-containing drugs, lithium preparations, loop diuretics, monoamine oxidase inhibitors, selective serotonin reuptake inhibitors, serotonin and norepinephrine reuptake inhibitors, thiazides, triptans, and certain other agents. Compounds in these categories include:

Acebutolol Hydrochloride
(Naproxen and other NSAIDs can reduce the antihypertensive effect of propranolol and other β-blockers).
No products indexed under this heading.

Alclometasone Dipropionate (Other factors that increase the risk for gastrointestinal bleeding in patients treated with NSAIDs include concomitant use of oral corticosteroids or anticoagulants).
No products indexed under this heading.

Almotriptan Malate (Cases of life-threatening serotonin syndrome have been reported during combined use of triptans with Treximet). Products include:
Axert 2593

Amiloride Hydrochloride (Concomitant use of NSAIDs with diuretics may increase risk of renal decompensation).
No products indexed under this heading.

Anisindione (Other factors that increase the risk for gastrointestinal bleeding in patients treated with NSAIDs include concomitant use of oral corticosteroids or anticoagulants).
No products indexed under this heading.

Ardeparin Sodium (Other factors that increase the risk for gastrointestinal bleeding in patients treated with NSAIDs include concomitant use of oral corticosteroids or anticoagulants).
No products indexed under this heading.

Aspirin (When naproxen is administered with aspirin/aspirin-acetylsalicylic acid, its protein binding is reduced, although the clearance of free naproxen is not altered. The clinical significance of this interaction is not known, however, as with other NSAID-containing products, concomitant administration of Treximet and aspirin/aspirin-acetylsalicylic acid is not generally recommended because of the potential of increased adverse side effects). Products include:
Aggrenox 880
Bayer Aspirin 829

Percodan 1124
St. Joseph Aspirin 2045

Aspirin, Enteric Coated (When naproxen is administered with aspirin/aspirin-acetylsalicylic acid, its protein binding is reduced, although the clearance of free naproxen is not altered. The clinical significance of this interaction is not known, however, as with other NSAID-containing products, concomitant administration of Treximet and aspirin/aspirin-acetylsalicylic acid is not generally recommended because of the potential of increased adverse side effects).
No products indexed under this heading.

Aspirin Buffered (When naproxen is administered with aspirin/aspirin-acetylsalicylic acid, its protein binding is reduced, although the clearance of free naproxen is not altered. The clinical significance of this interaction is not known, however, as with other NSAID-containing products, concomitant administration of Treximet and aspirin/aspirin-acetylsalicylic acid is not generally recommended because of the potential of increased adverse side effects).
No products indexed under this heading.

Atenolol (Naproxen and other NSAIDs can reduce the antihypertensive effect of propranolol and other β-blockers).
No products indexed under this heading.

Beclomethasone Dipropionate (Other factors that increase the risk for gastrointestinal bleeding in patients treated with NSAIDs include concomitant use of oral corticosteroids or anticoagulants). Products include:
Qvar 3398

Beclomethasone Dipropionate Monohydrate (Other factors that increase the risk for gastrointestinal bleeding in patients treated with NSAIDs include concomitant use of oral corticosteroids or anticoagulants). Products include:
Beconase AQ 1386

Benazepril Hydrochloride (Reports suggest that NSAIDs may diminish the antihypertensive effect of ACE inhibitors. The use of Treximet in patients who are receiving ACE inhibitors may potentiate renal disease states).
No products indexed under this heading.

Bendroflumethiazide (Concomitant use of NSAIDs with diuretics may increase risk of renal decompensation).
No products indexed under this heading.

Betamethasone (Other factors that increase the risk for gastrointestinal bleeding in patients treated with NSAIDs include concomitant use of oral corticosteroids or anticoagulants).
No products indexed under this heading.

Betamethasone Acetate (Other factors that increase the risk for gastrointestinal bleeding in patients treated with NSAIDs include concomitant use of oral corticosteroids or anticoagulants).
No products indexed under this heading.

Betamethasone Benzoate (Other factors that increase the risk for gastrointestinal bleeding in patients treated with NSAIDs include concomitant use of oral corticosteroids or anticoagulants).
No products indexed under this heading.

Betamethasone Dipropionate (Other factors that increase the risk for gastrointestinal bleeding in patients treated with NSAIDs include concomitant use of oral corticosteroids or anticoagulants). Products include:
Diprolene Lotion 0.05% 3108
Diprolene Ointment 0.05% 3109
Diprolene AF Cream 0.05% 3107
Lotrisone 3163

Betamethasone Sodium Phosphate (Other factors that increase the risk for gastrointestinal bleeding in patients treated with NSAIDs include concomitant use of oral corticosteroids or anticoagulants).
No products indexed under this heading.

Betamethasone Valerate (Other factors that increase the risk for gastrointestinal bleeding in patients treated with NSAIDs include concomitant use of oral corticosteroids or anticoagulants). Products include:
Luxiq 3321

Betaxolol Hydrochloride (Naproxen and other NSAIDs can reduce the antihypertensive effect of propranolol and other β-blockers).
No products indexed under this heading.

Bisoprolol Fumarate (Naproxen and other NSAIDs can reduce the antihypertensive effect of propranolol and other β-blockers).
No products indexed under this heading.

Budesonide (Other factors that increase the risk for gastrointestinal bleeding in patients treated with NSAIDs include concomitant use of oral corticosteroids or anticoagulants). Products include:
Pulmicort Flexhaler 714
Symbicort 80/4.5 720
Symbicort 160/4.5 720

Bumetanide (Concomitant use of NSAIDs with diuretics may increase risk of renal decompensation).
No products indexed under this heading.

Captopril (Reports suggest that NSAIDs may diminish the antihypertensive effect of ACE inhibitors. The use of Treximet in patients who are receiving ACE inhibitors may potentiate renal disease states). Products include:
Captopril 2341

Carteolol Hydrochloride (Naproxen and other NSAIDs can reduce the antihypertensive effect of propranolol and other β-blockers).
No products indexed under this heading.

Carvedilol (Naproxen and other NSAIDs can reduce the antihypertensive effect of propranolol and other β-blockers). Products include:
Coreg 1409

Carvedilol Phosphate (Naproxen and other NSAIDs can reduce the antihypertensive effect of propranolol and other β-blockers). Products include:
Coreg CR 1416

Chlorothiazide (Concomitant use of NSAIDs with diuretics may increase risk of renal decompensation).
No products indexed under this heading.

Chlorothiazide Sodium (Concomitant use of NSAIDs with diuretics may increase risk of renal decompensation). Products include:
Diuril Intravenous 2009

Chlorthalidone (Concomitant use of NSAIDs with diuretics may increase risk of renal decompensation). Products include:
Clorpres 2344

Ciclesonide (Other factors that increase the risk for gastrointestinal bleeding in patients treated with NSAIDs include concomitant use of oral corticosteroids or anticoagulants).
No products indexed under this heading.

Citalopram Hydrobromide (Cases of life-threatening serotonin syndrome have been reported during combined use of selective serotonin reuptake inhibitors with Treximet). Products include:
Celexa 1153

Cortisone Acetate (Other factors that increase the risk for gastrointestinal bleeding in patients treated with NSAIDs include concomitant use of oral corticosteroids or anticoagulants).
No products indexed under this heading.

Dalteparin Sodium (Other factors that increase the risk for gastrointestinal bleeding in patients treated with NSAIDs include concomitant use of oral corticosteroids or anticoagulants). Products include:
Fragmin 1058

Danaparoid Sodium (Other factors that increase the risk for gastrointestinal bleeding in patients treated with NSAIDs include concomitant use of oral corticosteroids or anticoagulants).
No products indexed under this heading.

Desoximetasone (Other factors that increase the risk for gastrointestinal bleeding in patients treated with NSAIDs include concomitant use of oral corticosteroids or anticoagulants).
No products indexed under this heading.

Desvenlafaxine Succinate (Cases of life-threatening serotonin syndrome have been reported during combined use of serotonin and norepinephrine reuptake inhibitors with Treximet). Products include:
Pristiq 3564

Dexamethasone (Other factors that increase the risk for gastrointestinal bleeding in patients treated with NSAIDs include concomitant use of oral corticosteroids or anticoagulants). Products include:
Ciprodex 583
Ozurdex .... ⊙223
Tobramycin and Dexamethasone Ophthalmic Suspension .... ⊙251

Dexamethasone Acetate (Other factors that increase the risk for gastrointestinal bleeding in patients treated with NSAIDs include concomitant use of oral corticosteroids or anticoagulants).
No products indexed under this heading.

Dexamethasone Phosphate (Other factors that increase the risk for gastrointestinal bleeding in patients treated with NSAIDs include concomitant use of oral corticosteroids or anticoagulants).
No products indexed under this heading.

Dexamethasone Sodium (Other factors that increase the risk for gastrointestinal bleeding in patients treated with NSAIDs include concomitant use of oral corticosteroids or anticoagulants).
No products indexed under this heading.

Dexamethasone Sodium Phosphate (Other factors that increase the risk for gastrointestinal bleeding in patients treated with NSAIDs include concomitant use of oral corticosteroids or anticoagulants).
No products indexed under this heading.

Dexamethasone Sodium Phosphate Injection (Other factors that increase the risk for gastrointestinal bleeding in patients treated with NSAIDs include concomitant use of oral corticosteroids or anticoagulants).
No products indexed under this heading.

Dicumarol (Other factors that increase the risk for gastrointestinal bleeding in patients treated with NSAIDs include concomitant use of oral corticosteroids or anticoagulants).
No products indexed under this heading.

Diflorasone Diacetate (Other factors that increase the risk for gastrointestinal bleeding in patients treated with NSAIDs include concomitant use of oral corticosteroids or anticoagulants).
No products indexed under this heading.

1929 Interactions Index Treximet

Dihydroergotamine Mesylate (Ergot-containing drugs may cause prolonged vasospastic reactions. The use of ergot-type or ergot-containing medications (eg, dihydroergotamine, methysergide) and Treximet within 24 hours of each other should be avoided).
No products indexed under this heading.

Duloxetine Hydrochloride (Cases of life-threatening serotonin syndrome have been reported during combined use of serotonin and norepinephrine reuptake inhibitors with Treximet). Products include:
Cymbalta 1871

Eletriptan Hydrobromide (Cases of life-threatening serotonin syndrome have been reported during combined use of triptans with Treximet).
No products indexed under this heading.

Enalapril Maleate (Reports suggest that NSAIDs may diminish the antihypertensive effect of ACE inhibitors. The use of Treximet in patients who are receiving ACE inhibitors may potentiate renal disease states).
No products indexed under this heading.

Enalaprilat (Reports suggest that NSAIDs may diminish the antihypertensive effect of ACE inhibitors. The use of Treximet in patients who are receiving ACE inhibitors may potentiate renal disease states).
No products indexed under this heading.

Enoxaparin Sodium (Other factors that increase the risk for gastrointestinal bleeding in patients treated with NSAIDs include concomitant use of oral corticosteroids or anticoagulants). Products include:
Lovenox 3005

Ergonovine Maleate (Ergot-containing drugs may cause prolonged vasospastic reactions. The use of ergot-type or ergot-containing medications (eg, dihydroergotamine, methysergide) and Treximet within 24 hours of each other should be avoided).
No products indexed under this heading.

Ergotamine Tartrate (Ergot-containing drugs may cause prolonged vasospastic reactions. The use of ergot-type or ergot-containing medications (eg, dihydroergotamine, methysergide) and Treximet within 24 hours of each other should be avoided).
No products indexed under this heading.

Escitalopram Oxalate (Cases of life-threatening serotonin syndrome have been reported during combined use of selective serotonin reuptake inhibitors with Treximet). Products include:
Lexapro Oral Suspension 1160
Lexapro Tablets 1160

Esmolol Hydrochloride (Naproxen and other NSAIDs can reduce the antihypertensive effect of propranolol and other β-blockers).
No products indexed under this heading.

Ethacrynic Acid (Concomitant use of NSAIDs with diuretics may increase risk of renal decompensation).
No products indexed under this heading.

Ethanol (Other factors that increase the risk for gastrointestinal bleeding in patients treated with NSAIDs include concomitant use of alcohol).
No products indexed under this heading.

Ethyl Alcohol (Other factors that increase the risk for gastrointestinal bleeding in patients treated with NSAIDs include concomitant use of alcohol).
No products indexed under this heading.

Fludrocortisone Acetate (Other factors that increase the risk for gastrointestinal bleeding in patients treated with NSAIDs include concomitant use of oral corticosteroids or anticoagulants).
No products indexed under this heading.

Flumethasone Pivalate (Other factors that increase the risk for gastrointestinal bleeding in patients treated with NSAIDs include concomitant use of oral corticosteroids or anticoagulants).
No products indexed under this heading.

Flunisolide Hemihydrate (Other factors that increase the risk for gastrointestinal bleeding in patients treated with NSAIDs include concomitant use of oral corticosteroids or anticoagulants).
No products indexed under this heading.

Fluoxetine (Cases of life-threatening serotonin syndrome have been reported during combined use of selective serotonin reuptake inhibitors with Treximet).
No products indexed under this heading.

Fluoxetine Hydrochloride (Cases of life-threatening serotonin syndrome have been reported during combined use of selective serotonin reuptake inhibitors with Treximet). Products include:
Prozac Weekly 1941
Prozac Pulvules 1941
Symbyax 1965

Fluticasone Furoate (Other factors that increase the risk for gastrointestinal bleeding in patients treated with NSAIDs include concomitant use of oral corticosteroids or anticoagulants). Products include:
Veramyst 1713

Fluticasone Propionate (Other factors that increase the risk for gastrointestinal bleeding in patients treated with NSAIDs include concomitant use of oral corticosteroids or anticoagulants). Products include:
Advair 100/50 1275
Advair 250/50 1275
Advair 500/50 1275
Advair HFA 45/21 1288
Advair HFA 115/21 1288
Advair HFA 230/21 1288
Flonase 1459
Flovent Diskus 1463
Flovent HFA 1470

Fluvoxamine (Cases of life-threatening serotonin syndrome have been reported during combined use of selective serotonin reuptake inhibitors with Treximet).
No products indexed under this heading.

Fluvoxamine Maleate (Cases of life-threatening serotonin syndrome have been reported during combined use of selective serotonin reuptake inhibitors with Treximet).
No products indexed under this heading.

Fondaparinux Sodium (Other factors that increase the risk for gastrointestinal bleeding in patients treated with NSAIDs include concomitant use of oral corticosteroids or anticoagulants). Products include:
Arixtra 1320

Fosinopril Sodium (Reports suggest that NSAIDs may diminish the antihypertensive effect of ACE inhibitors. The use of Treximet in patients who are receiving ACE inhibitors may potentiate renal disease states).
No products indexed under this heading.

Frovatriptan Succinate (Cases of life-threatening serotonin syndrome have been reported during combined use of triptans with Treximet). Products include:
Frova 1103

Furosemide (Studies and post-marketing observations have shown that NSAIDs can reduce the natriuretic effect of furosemide and thiazides in some patients. During concomitant therapy with NSAIDs, the patient should be observed closely for signs of renal failure, as well as to assure diuretic efficacy). Products include:
Furosemide 2354

Heparin Calcium (Other factors that increase the risk for gastrointestinal bleeding in patients treated with NSAIDs include concomitant use of oral corticosteroids or anticoagulants).
No products indexed under this heading.

Heparin Sodium (Other factors that increase the risk for gastrointestinal bleeding in patients treated with NSAIDs include concomitant use of oral corticosteroids or anticoagulants).
No products indexed under this heading.

Hydrochlorothiazide (Concomitant use of NSAIDs with diuretics may increase risk of renal decompensation). Products include:
Atacand HCT 700
Avalide 2956
Benicar HCT 1017
Diovan HCT 2419
Dyazide 1429
Exforge HCT 2449
Hyzaar 2162
Hyzaar 100-12.5 2162
Micardis HCT 889
Prinzide 2246
Tekturna HCT 2541
Teveten HCT 541

Hydrocortisone (Other factors that increase the risk for gastrointestinal bleeding in patients treated with NSAIDs include concomitant use of oral corticosteroids or anticoagulants).
No products indexed under this heading.

Hydrocortisone (Alcohol) (Other factors that increase the risk for gastrointestinal bleeding in patients treated with NSAIDs include concomitant use of oral corticosteroids or anticoagulants).
No products indexed under this heading.

Hydrocortisone Acetate (Other factors that increase the risk for gastrointestinal bleeding in patients treated with NSAIDs include concomitant use of oral corticosteroids or anticoagulants).
No products indexed under this heading.

Hydrocortisone Butyrate (Other factors that increase the risk for gastrointestinal bleeding in patients treated with NSAIDs include concomitant use of oral corticosteroids or anticoagulants).
No products indexed under this heading.

Hydrocortisone Cypionate (Other factors that increase the risk for gastrointestinal bleeding in patients treated with NSAIDs include concomitant use of oral corticosteroids or anticoagulants).
No products indexed under this heading.

Hydrocortisone Hemisuccinate (Other factors that increase the risk for gastrointestinal bleeding in patients treated with NSAIDs include concomitant use of oral corticosteroids or anticoagulants).
No products indexed under this heading.

Hydrocortisone Probutate (Other factors that increase the risk for gastrointestinal bleeding in patients treated with NSAIDs include concomitant use of oral corticosteroids or anticoagulants).
No products indexed under this heading.

Hydrocortisone Sodium Phosphate (Other factors that increase the risk for gastrointestinal bleeding in patients treated with NSAIDs include concomitant use of oral corticosteroids or anticoagulants).
No products indexed under this heading.

Hydrocortisone Sodium Succinate (Other factors that increase the risk for gastrointestinal bleeding in patients treated with NSAIDs include concomitant use of oral corticosteroids or anticoagulants).
No products indexed under this heading.

Hydrocortisone Valerate (Other factors that increase the risk for gastrointestinal bleeding in patients treated with NSAIDs include concomitant use of oral corticosteroids or anticoagulants).
No products indexed under this heading.

Hydroflumethiazide (Concomitant use of NSAIDs with diuretics may increase risk of renal decompensation).
No products indexed under this heading.

Indapamide (Concomitant use of NSAIDs with diuretics may increase risk of renal decompensation). Products include:
Indapamide 2356

Isocarboxazid (The use of Treximet in patients receiving monoamine oxidase inhibitors is contraindicated. MAIOs reduce sumatriptan clearance, significantly increasing systemic exposure). Products include:
Marplan 3481

Labetalol Hydrochloride (Naproxen and other NSAIDs can reduce the antihypertensive effect of propranolol and other β-blockers).
No products indexed under this heading.

Levobunolol Hydrochloride (Naproxen and other NSAIDs can reduce the antihypertensive effect of propranolol and other β-blockers).
No products indexed under this heading.

Lisinopril (Reports suggest that NSAIDs may diminish the antihypertensive effect of ACE inhibitors. The use of Treximet in patients who are receiving ACE inhibitors may potentiate renal disease states). Products include:
Prinivil 2241
Prinzide 2246

Lithium (NSAIDs have produced an elevation of plasma lithium levels and a reduction in renal lithium clearance. The mean minimum lithium concentration increased 15% and the renal clearance was decreased by approximately 20%. These effects have been attributed to inhibition of renal prostaglandin synthesis by the NSAID. When Treximet and lithium are administered concurrently, patients should be observed carefully for signs of lithium toxicity).
No products indexed under this heading.

Lithium Carbonate (NSAIDs have produced an elevation of plasma lithium levels and a reduction in renal lithium clearance. The mean minimum lithium concentration increased 15% and the renal clearance was decreased by approximately 20%. These effects have been attributed to inhibition of renal prostaglandin synthesis by the NSAID. When Treximet and lithium are administered concurrently, patients should be observed carefully for signs of lithium toxicity).
No products indexed under this heading.

Lithium Citrate (NSAIDs have produced an elevation of plasma lithium levels and a reduction in renal lithium clearance. The mean minimum lithium concentration increased 15% and the renal clearance was decreased by approximately 20%. These effects have been attributed to inhibition of renal prostaglandin synthesis by the NSAID. When Treximet and lithium are administered concurrently, patients should be observed carefully for signs of lithium toxicity).
No products indexed under this heading.

Low Molecular Weight Heparins (Other factors that increase the risk for gastrointestinal bleeding in patients treated with NSAIDs include concomitant use of oral corticosteroids or anticoagulants).
No products indexed under this heading.

Methotrexate Sodium (Caution should be used if Treximet is administered concomitantly with methotrexate. Concomitant administration of some NSAIDs with high-dose methotrexate therapy has been reported to elevate and prolong serum methotrexate levels, resulting in deaths from severe hematologic and gastrointestinal toxicity).
No products indexed under this heading.

IMPORTANT NOTE: Always consult each drug listing in the patient's regimen for possible interactions.

Treximet Interactions Index 1930

Methyclothiazide (Concomitant use of NSAIDs with diuretics may increase risk of renal decompensation).
No products indexed under this heading.

Methylergonovine Maleate (Ergot-containing drugs may cause prolonged vasospastic reactions. The use of ergot-type or ergot-containing medications (eg, dihydroergotamine, methysergide) and Treximet within 24 hours of each other should be avoided).
No products indexed under this heading.

Methylprednisolone (Other factors that increase the risk for gastrointestinal bleeding in patients treated with NSAIDs include concomitant use of oral corticosteroids or anticoagulants).
No products indexed under this heading.

Methylprednisolone Acetate (Other factors that increase the risk for gastrointestinal bleeding in patients treated with NSAIDs include concomitant use of oral corticosteroids or anticoagulants).
No products indexed under this heading.

Methylprednisolone Sodium Succinate (Other factors that increase the risk for gastrointestinal bleeding in patients treated with NSAIDs include concomitant use of oral corticosteroids or anticoagulants).
No products indexed under this heading.

Methysergide Maleate (Ergot-containing drugs may cause prolonged vasospastic reactions. The use of ergot-type or ergot-containing medications (eg, dihydroergotamine, methysergide) and Treximet within 24 hours of each other should be avoided).
No products indexed under this heading.

Metipranolol Hydrochloride (Naproxen and other NSAIDs can reduce the antihypertensive effect of propranolol and other β-blockers).
No products indexed under this heading.

Metolazone (Concomitant use of NSAIDs with diuretics may increase risk of renal decompensation).
No products indexed under this heading.

Metoprolol Succinate (Naproxen and other NSAIDs can reduce the antihypertensive effect of propranolol and other β-blockers). Products include:
Toprol XL 732

Metoprolol Tartrate (Naproxen and other NSAIDs can reduce the antihypertensive effect of propranolol and other β-blockers).
No products indexed under this heading.

Moclobemide (The use of Treximet in patients receiving monoamine oxidase inhibitors is contraindicated. MAIOs reduce sumatriptan clearance, significantly increasing systemic exposure).
No products indexed under this heading.

Moexipril Hydrochloride (Reports suggest that NSAIDs may diminish the antihypertensive effect of ACE inhibitors. The use of Treximet in patients who are receiving ACE inhibitors may potentiate renal disease states).
No products indexed under this heading.

Mometasone Furoate (Other factors that increase the risk for gastrointestinal bleeding in patients treated with NSAIDs include concomitant use of oral corticosteroids or anticoagulants). Products include:
Asmanex 3058
Elocon Cream 3111
Elocon Lotion 3112
Elocon Ointment 3114

Mometasone Furoate Monohydrate (Other factors that increase the risk for gastrointestinal bleeding in patients treated with NSAIDs include concomitant use of oral corticosteroids or anticoagulants). Products include:
Nasonex 3166

Nadolol (Naproxen and other NSAIDs can reduce the antihypertensive effect of propranolol and other β-blockers). Products include:
Nadolol 2359

Naratriptan Hydrochloride (Cases of life-threatening serotonin syndrome have been reported during combined use of triptans with Treximet). Products include:
Amerge 1306

Nebivolol (Naproxen and other NSAIDs can reduce the antihypertensive effect of propranolol and other β-blockers). Products include:
Bystolic 1147

Nefazodone Hydrochloride (Cases of life-threatening serotonin syndrome have been reported during combined use of serotonin and norepinephrine reuptake inhibitors with Treximet).
No products indexed under this heading.

Pargyline Hydrochloride (The use of Treximet in patients receiving monoamine oxidase inhibitors is contraindicated. MAIOs reduce sumatriptan clearance, significantly increasing systemic exposure).
No products indexed under this heading.

Paroxetine (Cases of life-threatening serotonin syndrome have been reported during combined use of selective serotonin reuptake inhibitors with Treximet).
No products indexed under this heading.

Paroxetine Hydrochloride (Cases of life-threatening serotonin syndrome have been reported during combined use of selective serotonin reuptake inhibitors with Treximet). Products include:
Paroxetine CR 2361
Paroxetine ER 2371
Paxil 1586
Paxil CR 1596

Paroxetine Mesylate (Cases of life-threatening serotonin syndrome have been reported during combined use of selective serotonin reuptake inhibitors with Treximet).
No products indexed under this heading.

Penbutolol Sulfate (Naproxen and other NSAIDs can reduce the antihypertensive effect of propranolol and other β-blockers).
No products indexed under this heading.

Perindopril Erbumine (Reports suggest that NSAIDs may diminish the antihypertensive effect of ACE inhibitors. The use of Treximet in patients who are receiving ACE inhibitors may potentiate renal disease states).
No products indexed under this heading.

Phenelzine Sulfate (The use of Treximet in patients receiving monoamine oxidase inhibitors is contraindicated. MAIOs reduce sumatriptan clearance, significantly increasing systemic exposure).
No products indexed under this heading.

Pindolol (Naproxen and other NSAIDs can reduce the antihypertensive effect of propranolol and other β-blockers).
No products indexed under this heading.

Polythiazide (Concomitant use of NSAIDs with diuretics may increase risk of renal decompensation).
No products indexed under this heading.

Prednisolone (Other factors that increase the risk for gastrointestinal bleeding in patients treated with NSAIDs include concomitant use of oral corticosteroids or anticoagulants).
No products indexed under this heading.

Prednisolone Acetate (Other factors that increase the risk for gastrointestinal bleeding in patients treated with NSAIDs include concomitant use of oral corticosteroids or anticoagulants). Products include:
Blephamide .... ⊙212, ⊙214
Pred Forte .... ⊙225
Pred Mild .... ⊙230
Pred-G .... ⊙226, ⊙227

Prednisolone Sodium Phosphate (Other factors that increase the risk for gastrointestinal bleeding in patients treated with NSAIDs include concomitant use of oral corticosteroids or anticoagulants).
No products indexed under this heading.

Prednisolone Tebutate (Other factors that increase the risk for gastrointestinal bleeding in patients treated with NSAIDs include concomitant use of oral corticosteroids or anticoagulants).
No products indexed under this heading.

Prednisone (Other factors that increase the risk for gastrointestinal bleeding in patients treated with NSAIDs include concomitant use of oral corticosteroids or anticoagulants).
No products indexed under this heading.

Prednisone sodium phosphate (Other factors that increase the risk for gastrointestinal bleeding in patients treated with NSAIDs include concomitant use of oral corticosteroids or anticoagulants).
No products indexed under this heading.

Probenecid (Concurrent use of probenecid with Treximet increases naproxen anion plasma levels and extends its plasma half-life significantly).
No products indexed under this heading.

Procarbazine Hydrochloride (The use of Treximet in patients receiving monoamine oxidase inhibitors is contraindicated. MAIOs reduce sumatriptan clearance, significantly increasing systemic exposure).
No products indexed under this heading.

Propranolol Hydrochloride (Naproxen and other NSAIDs can reduce the antihypertensive effect of propranolol and other β-blockers). Products include:
InnoPran XL 1517

Quinapril Hydrochloride (Reports suggest that NSAIDs may diminish the antihypertensive effect of ACE inhibitors. The use of Treximet in patients who are receiving ACE inhibitors may potentiate renal disease states).
No products indexed under this heading.

Ramipril (Reports suggest that NSAIDs may diminish the antihypertensive effect of ACE inhibitors. The use of Treximet in patients who are receiving ACE inhibitors may potentiate renal disease states).
No products indexed under this heading.

Rasagiline Mesylate (The use of Treximet in patients receiving monoamine oxidase inhibitors is contraindicated. MAIOs reduce sumatriptan clearance, significantly increasing systemic exposure). Products include:
Azilect 3383

Rizatriptan Benzoate (Cases of life-threatening serotonin syndrome have been reported during combined use of triptans with Treximet). Products include:
Maxalt 2206
Maxalt-MLT 2206

Selegiline (The use of Treximet in patients receiving monoamine oxidase inhibitors is contraindicated. MAIOs reduce sumatriptan clearance, significantly increasing systemic exposure). Products include:
Emsam 3623

Selegiline Hydrochloride (The use of Treximet in patients receiving monoamine oxidase inhibitors is contraindicated. MAIOs reduce sumatriptan clearance, significantly increasing systemic exposure). Products include:
Eldepryl 3312

Sertraline Hydrochloride (Cases of life-threatening serotonin syndrome have been reported during combined use of selective serotonin reuptake inhibitors with Treximet).
No products indexed under this heading.

Sotalol Hydrochloride (Naproxen and other NSAIDs can reduce the antihypertensive effect of propranolol and other β-blockers).
No products indexed under this heading.

Spirapril Hydrochloride (Reports suggest that NSAIDs may diminish the antihypertensive effect of ACE inhibitors. The use of Treximet in patients who are receiving ACE inhibitors may potentiate renal disease states).
No products indexed under this heading.

Spironolactone (Concomitant use of NSAIDs with diuretics may increase risk of renal decompensation).
No products indexed under this heading.

Sumatriptan (Cases of life-threatening serotonin syndrome have been reported during combined use of triptans with Treximet). Products include:
Imitrex Nasal 1503

Timolol Hemihydrate (Naproxen and other NSAIDs can reduce the antihypertensive effect of propranolol and other β-blockers). Products include:
Betimol 3490

Timolol Maleate (Naproxen and other NSAIDs can reduce the antihypertensive effect of propranolol and other β-blockers). Products include:
Combigan 601
Dorzolamide Hydrochloride/Timolol Maleate Ophthalmic Solution .... ⊙243
Timoptic in Ocudose .... ⊙231

Tinzaparin Sodium (Other factors that increase the risk for gastrointestinal bleeding in patients treated with NSAIDs include concomitant use of oral corticosteroids or anticoagulants).
No products indexed under this heading.

Torsemide (Concomitant use of NSAIDs with diuretics may increase risk of renal decompensation).
No products indexed under this heading.

Trandolapril (Reports suggest that NSAIDs may diminish the antihypertensive effect of ACE inhibitors. The use of Treximet in patients who are receiving ACE inhibitors may potentiate renal disease states). Products include:
Mavik 489
Tarka 534

Tranylcypromine Sulfate (The use of Treximet in patients receiving monoamine oxidase inhibitors is contraindicated. MAIOs reduce sumatriptan clearance, significantly increasing systemic exposure). Products include:
Parnate 1584

Triamcinolone (Other factors that increase the risk for gastrointestinal bleeding in patients treated with NSAIDs include concomitant use of oral corticosteroids or anticoagulants).
No products indexed under this heading.

Triamcinolone Acetonide (Other factors that increase the risk for gastrointestinal bleeding in patients treated with NSAIDs include concomitant use of oral corticosteroids or anticoagulants). Products include:
Azmacort 408
Nasacort AQ 3019

Triamcinolone Diacetate (Other factors that increase the risk for gastrointestinal bleeding in patients treated with NSAIDs include concomitant use of oral corticosteroids or anticoagulants).
No products indexed under this heading.

(⊙ Described in PDR® for Ophthalmic Medicines)

Triamcinolone Hexacetonide (Other factors that increase the risk for gastrointestinal bleeding in patients treated with NSAIDs include concomitant use of oral corticosteroids or anticoagulants).
No products indexed under this heading.

Triamterene (Concomitant use of NSAIDs with diuretics may increase risk of renal decompensation). Products include:
Dyazide 1429
Dyrenium 3495

Venlafaxine Hydrochloride (Cases of life-threatening serotonin syndrome have been reported during combined use of serotonin and norepinephrine reuptake inhibitors with Treximet). Products include:
Effexor XR 3504
Venlafaxine Hydrochloride Tablets ... 2388

Warfarin Sodium (The effects of warfarin and NSAIDs on gastrointestinal bleeding are synergistic, such that patients taking both drugs have a higher risk of serious gastrointestinal bleeding than patients taking each drug alone).
No products indexed under this heading.

Zolmitriptan (Cases of life-threatening serotonin syndrome have been reported during combined use of triptans with Treximet). Products include:
Zomig Tablets 773
Zomig Nasal Spray 768
Zomig-ZMT Tablets 773

Food Interactions

Alcohol (Other factors that increase the risk for gastrointestinal bleeding in patients treated with NSAIDs include concomitant use of alcohol).

Beer, reduced-alcohol (Other factors that increase the risk for gastrointestinal bleeding in patients treated with NSAIDs include concomitant use of alcohol).

Beer, unspecified (Other factors that increase the risk for gastrointestinal bleeding in patients treated with NSAIDs include concomitant use of alcohol).

Wine, Chianti (Other factors that increase the risk for gastrointestinal bleeding in patients treated with NSAIDs include concomitant use of alcohol).

Wine, Red (Other factors that increase the risk for gastrointestinal bleeding in patients treated with NSAIDs include concomitant use of alcohol).

Wine, unspecified (Other factors that increase the risk for gastrointestinal bleeding in patients treated with NSAIDs include concomitant use of alcohol).

Wine products (Other factors that increase the risk for gastrointestinal bleeding in patients treated with NSAIDs include concomitant use of alcohol).

TRICOR TABLETS

(Fenofibrate) 544
May interact with bile acid sequestering agents, HMG-CoA reductase inhibitors, immunosuppressive agents, nephrotoxic agents, oral anticoagulants, and certain other agents. Compounds in these categories include:

Abacavir Sulfate (The benefits and risks of using fenofibrate tablets with immunosuppressants and other potentially nephrotoxic agents should be carefully considered and the lowest effective dose employed). Products include:
Epzicom 1448
Trizivir 1688
Ziagen 1740

Acyclovir (The benefits and risks of using fenofibrate tablets with immunosuppressants and other potentially nephrotoxic agents should be carefully considered and the lowest effective dose employed). Products include:
Zovirax 1760

Acyclovir Sodium (The benefits and risks of using fenofibrate tablets with immunosuppressants and other potentially nephrotoxic agents should be carefully considered and the lowest effective dose employed).
No products indexed under this heading.

Alatrofloxacin Mesylate (The benefits and risks of using fenofibrate tablets with immunosuppressants and other potentially nephrotoxic agents should be carefully considered and the lowest effective dose employed).
No products indexed under this heading.

Aldesleukin (The benefits and risks of using fenofibrate tablets with immunosuppressants and other potentially nephrotoxic agents should be carefully considered and the lowest effective dose employed). Products include:
Proleukin 2504

Amikacin Sulfate (The benefits and risks of using fenofibrate tablets with immunosuppressants and other potentially nephrotoxic agents should be carefully considered and the lowest effective dose employed).
No products indexed under this heading.

Amoxicillin (The benefits and risks of using fenofibrate tablets with immunosuppressants and other potentially nephrotoxic agents should be carefully considered and the lowest effective dose employed). Products include:
Amoxil Capsules 1311
Amoxil Chewable Tablets 1311
Amoxil 1311
Amoxil Powder 1311
Augmentin 1331
Augmentin Tablets 1335
Augmentin ES-600 1338
Augmentin XR 1342
Moxatag 2321

Amoxicillin Trihydrate (The benefits and risks of using fenofibrate tablets with immunosuppressants and other potentially nephrotoxic agents should be carefully considered and the lowest effective dose employed).
No products indexed under this heading.

Amphotericin B (The benefits and risks of using fenofibrate tablets with immunosuppressants and other potentially nephrotoxic agents should be carefully considered and the lowest effective dose employed).
No products indexed under this heading.

Amphotericin B, liposomal (The benefits and risks of using fenofibrate tablets with immunosuppressants and other potentially nephrotoxic agents should be carefully considered and the lowest effective dose employed). Products include:
AmBisome 659

Amphotericin B Cholesteryl Sulfate (The benefits and risks of using fenofibrate tablets with immunosuppressants and other potentially nephrotoxic agents should be carefully considered and the lowest effective dose employed).
No products indexed under this heading.

Amphotericin B Lipid Complex (The benefits and risks of using fenofibrate tablets with immunosuppressants and other potentially nephrotoxic agents should be carefully considered and the lowest effective dose employed).
No products indexed under this heading.

Ampicillin (The benefits and risks of using fenofibrate tablets with immunosuppressants and other potentially nephrotoxic agents should be carefully considered and the lowest effective dose employed).
No products indexed under this heading.

Ampicillin Sodium (The benefits and risks of using fenofibrate tablets with immunosuppressants and other potentially nephrotoxic agents should be carefully considered and the lowest effective dose employed).
No products indexed under this heading.

Ampicillin Trihydrate (The benefits and risks of using fenofibrate tablets with immunosuppressants and other potentially nephrotoxic agents should be carefully considered and the lowest effective dose employed).
No products indexed under this heading.

Amprenavir (The benefits and risks of using fenofibrate tablets with immunosuppressants and other potentially nephrotoxic agents should be carefully considered and the lowest effective dose employed).
No products indexed under this heading.

Anisindione (Caution should be exercised when anticoagulants are given in conjunction with fenofibrate because of the potentiation of coumarin-type anticoagulants in prolonging the PT/INR. The dosage of the anticoagulant should be reduced to maintain the PT/INR at the desired level to prevent bleeding complications. Frequent PT/INR determinations are advisable until it has been definitely determined that the PT/INR has stabilized).
No products indexed under this heading.

Aspirin (The benefits and risks of using fenofibrate tablets with immunosuppressants and other potentially nephrotoxic agents should be carefully considered and the lowest effective dose employed). Products include:
Aggrenox 880
Bayer Aspirin 829
Percodan 1124
St. Joseph Aspirin 2045

Atazanavir (The benefits and risks of using fenofibrate tablets with immunosuppressants and other potentially nephrotoxic agents should be carefully considered and the lowest effective dose employed).
No products indexed under this heading.

Atorvastatin Calcium (Co-administration of fibric acid derivatives and HMG-CoA reductase inhibitors has been associated with rhabdomyolysis, markedly elevated creatine kinase levels and myoglobulinuria, leading in a high proportion of cases to acute renal failure; the combined use should be avoided unless the benefit of further alterations in lipid levels is likely to outweigh the increased risk of this combination). Products include:
Lipitor 2703

Azathioprine (The benefits and risks of using fenofibrate tablets with immunosuppressants and other potentially nephrotoxic agents should be carefully considered and the lowest effective dose employed).
No products indexed under this heading.

Azithromycin Dihydrate (The benefits and risks of using fenofibrate tablets with immunosuppressants and other potentially nephrotoxic agents should be carefully considered and the lowest effective dose employed).
No products indexed under this heading.

Azlocillin Sodium (The benefits and risks of using fenofibrate tablets with immunosuppressants and other potentially nephrotoxic agents should be carefully considered and the lowest effective dose employed).
No products indexed under this heading.

Aztreonam (The benefits and risks of using fenofibrate tablets with immunosuppressants and other potentially nephrotoxic agents should be carefully considered and the lowest effective dose employed).
No products indexed under this heading.

Bacampicillin Hydrochloride (The benefits and risks of using fenofibrate tablets with immunosuppressants and other potentially nephrotoxic agents should be carefully considered and the lowest effective dose employed).
No products indexed under this heading.

Bacitracin (The benefits and risks of using fenofibrate tablets with immunosuppressants and other potentially nephrotoxic agents should be carefully considered and the lowest effective dose employed).
No products indexed under this heading.

Bacitracin Zinc (The benefits and risks of using fenofibrate tablets with immunosuppressants and other potentially nephrotoxic agents should be carefully considered and the lowest effective dose employed).
No products indexed under this heading.

Balsalazide Disodium (The benefits and risks of using fenofibrate tablets with immunosuppressants and other potentially nephrotoxic agents should be carefully considered and the lowest effective dose employed).
No products indexed under this heading.

Basiliximab (The benefits and risks of using fenofibrate tablets with immunosuppressants and other potentially nephrotoxic agents should be carefully considered and the lowest effective dose employed). Products include:
Simulect 2524

Benazepril Hydrochloride (The benefits and risks of using fenofibrate tablets with immunosuppressants and other potentially nephrotoxic agents should be carefully considered and the lowest effective dose employed).
No products indexed under this heading.

Bendroflumethiazide (The benefits and risks of using fenofibrate tablets with immunosuppressants and other potentially nephrotoxic agents should be carefully considered and the lowest effective dose employed).
No products indexed under this heading.

Caffeine (The benefits and risks of using fenofibrate tablets with immunosuppressants and other potentially nephrotoxic agents should be carefully considered and the lowest effective dose employed).
No products indexed under this heading.

Captopril (The benefits and risks of using fenofibrate tablets with immunosuppressants and other potentially nephrotoxic agents should be carefully considered and the lowest effective dose employed). Products include:
Captopril 2341

Carbenicillin Disodium (The benefits and risks of using fenofibrate tablets with immunosuppressants and other potentially nephrotoxic agents should be carefully considered and the lowest effective dose employed).
No products indexed under this heading.

Carbenicillin Indanyl Sodium (The benefits and risks of using fenofibrate tablets with immunosuppressants and other potentially nephrotoxic agents should be carefully considered and the lowest effective dose employed).
No products indexed under this heading.

Carboplatin (The benefits and risks of using fenofibrate tablets with immunosuppressants and other potentially nephrotoxic agents should be carefully considered and the lowest effective dose employed).
No products indexed under this heading.

Carmustine (BCNU) (The benefits and risks of using fenofibrate tablets with immunosuppressants and other potentially nephrotoxic agents should be carefully considered and the lowest effective dose employed).
No products indexed under this heading.

IMPORTANT NOTE: Always consult each drug listing in the patient's regimen for possible interactions.

Tricor Interactions Index 1932

Cefaclor (The benefits and risks of using fenofibrate tablets with immunosuppressants and other potentially nephrotoxic agents should be carefully considered and the lowest effective dose employed).
No products indexed under this heading.

Cefadroxil (The benefits and risks of using fenofibrate tablets with immunosuppressants and other potentially nephrotoxic agents should be carefully considered and the lowest effective dose employed).
No products indexed under this heading.

Cefamandole Nafate (The benefits and risks of using fenofibrate tablets with immunosuppressants and other potentially nephrotoxic agents should be carefully considered and the lowest effective dose employed).
No products indexed under this heading.

Cefazolin Sodium (The benefits and risks of using fenofibrate tablets with immunosuppressants and other potentially nephrotoxic agents should be carefully considered and the lowest effective dose employed).
No products indexed under this heading.

Cefdinir (The benefits and risks of using fenofibrate tablets with immunosuppressants and other potentially nephrotoxic agents should be carefully considered and the lowest effective dose employed). Products include:
Omnicef Capsules 518
Omnicef Oral Suspension 518

Cefepime Hydrochloride (The benefits and risks of using fenofibrate tablets with immunosuppressants and other potentially nephrotoxic agents should be carefully considered and the lowest effective dose employed).
No products indexed under this heading.

Cefixime (The benefits and risks of using fenofibrate tablets with immunosuppressants and other potentially nephrotoxic agents should be carefully considered and the lowest effective dose employed). Products include:
Suprax for Oral Suspension 2038
Suprax Tablets 2038

Cefmetazole Sodium (The benefits and risks of using fenofibrate tablets with immunosuppressants and other potentially nephrotoxic agents should be carefully considered and the lowest effective dose employed).
No products indexed under this heading.

Cefonicid Sodium (The benefits and risks of using fenofibrate tablets with immunosuppressants and other potentially nephrotoxic agents should be carefully considered and the lowest effective dose employed).
No products indexed under this heading.

Cefoperazone Sodium (The benefits and risks of using fenofibrate tablets with immunosuppressants and other potentially nephrotoxic agents should be carefully considered and the lowest effective dose employed).
No products indexed under this heading.

Ceforanide (The benefits and risks of using fenofibrate tablets with immunosuppressants and other potentially nephrotoxic agents should be carefully considered and the lowest effective dose employed).
No products indexed under this heading.

Cefotaxime Sodium (The benefits and risks of using fenofibrate tablets with immunosuppressants and other potentially nephrotoxic agents should be carefully considered and the lowest effective dose employed).
No products indexed under this heading.

Cefotetan (The benefits and risks of using fenofibrate tablets with immunosuppressants and other potentially nephrotoxic agents should be carefully considered and the lowest effective dose employed).
No products indexed under this heading.

Cefoxitin Sodium (The benefits and risks of using fenofibrate tablets with immunosuppressants and other potentially nephrotoxic agents should be carefully considered and the lowest effective dose employed).
No products indexed under this heading.

Cefpodoxime Proxetil (The benefits and risks of using fenofibrate tablets with immunosuppressants and other potentially nephrotoxic agents should be carefully considered and the lowest effective dose employed).
No products indexed under this heading.

Cefprozil (The benefits and risks of using fenofibrate tablets with immunosuppressants and other potentially nephrotoxic agents should be carefully considered and the lowest effective dose employed).
No products indexed under this heading.

Ceftazidime (The benefits and risks of using fenofibrate tablets with immunosuppressants and other potentially nephrotoxic agents should be carefully considered and the lowest effective dose employed). Products include:
Fortaz 1481

Ceftizoxime Sodium (The benefits and risks of using fenofibrate tablets with immunosuppressants and other potentially nephrotoxic agents should be carefully considered and the lowest effective dose employed).
No products indexed under this heading.

Ceftriaxone Sodium (The benefits and risks of using fenofibrate tablets with immunosuppressants and other potentially nephrotoxic agents should be carefully considered and the lowest effective dose employed). Products include:
Rocephin 2859

Cefuroxime Axetil (The benefits and risks of using fenofibrate tablets with immunosuppressants and other potentially nephrotoxic agents should be carefully considered and the lowest effective dose employed). Products include:
Ceftin 1399

Cefuroxime Sodium (The benefits and risks of using fenofibrate tablets with immunosuppressants and other potentially nephrotoxic agents should be carefully considered and the lowest effective dose employed).
No products indexed under this heading.

Celecoxib (The benefits and risks of using fenofibrate tablets with immunosuppressants and other potentially nephrotoxic agents should be carefully considered and the lowest effective dose employed). Products include:
Celebrex 3272

Cephalexin (The benefits and risks of using fenofibrate tablets with immunosuppressants and other potentially nephrotoxic agents should be carefully considered and the lowest effective dose employed).
No products indexed under this heading.

Cephalothin Sodium (The benefits and risks of using fenofibrate tablets with immunosuppressants and other potentially nephrotoxic agents should be carefully considered and the lowest effective dose employed).
No products indexed under this heading.

Cephapirin Sodium (The benefits and risks of using fenofibrate tablets with immunosuppressants and other potentially nephrotoxic agents should be carefully considered and the lowest effective dose employed).
No products indexed under this heading.

Cephradine (The benefits and risks of using fenofibrate tablets with immunosuppressants and other potentially nephrotoxic agents should be carefully considered and the lowest effective dose employed).
No products indexed under this heading.

Cerivastatin Sodium (Co-administration of fibric acid derivatives and HMG-CoA reductase inhibitors has been associated with rhabdomyolysis, markedly elevated creatine kinase levels and myoglobulinuria, leading in a high proportion of cases to acute renal failure; the combined use should be avoided unless the benefit of further alterations in lipid levels is likely to outweigh the increased risk of this combination).
No products indexed under this heading.

Chlorothiazide (The benefits and risks of using fenofibrate tablets with immunosuppressants and other potentially nephrotoxic agents should be carefully considered and the lowest effective dose employed).
No products indexed under this heading.

Chlorothiazide Sodium (The benefits and risks of using fenofibrate tablets with immunosuppressants and other potentially nephrotoxic agents should be carefully considered and the lowest effective dose employed). Products include:
Diuril Intravenous 2009

Chlorpropamide (The benefits and risks of using fenofibrate tablets with immunosuppressants and other potentially nephrotoxic agents should be carefully considered and the lowest effective dose employed).
No products indexed under this heading.

Cholestyramine (Bile acid sequestrants may bind fenofibrate; fenofibrate should be taken at least 1 hour before or 4-6 hours after a bile acid binding resin to avoid impeding its absorption).
No products indexed under this heading.

Cidofovir (The benefits and risks of using fenofibrate tablets with immunosuppressants and other potentially nephrotoxic agents should be carefully considered and the lowest effective dose employed).
No products indexed under this heading.

Cilastatin Sodium (The benefits and risks of using fenofibrate tablets with immunosuppressants and other potentially nephrotoxic agents should be carefully considered and the lowest effective dose employed). Products include:
Primaxin I.M. 2232
Primaxin I.V. 2235

Cimetidine (The benefits and risks of using fenofibrate tablets with immunosuppressants and other potentially nephrotoxic agents should be carefully considered and the lowest effective dose employed).
No products indexed under this heading.

Cimetidine Hydrochloride (The benefits and risks of using fenofibrate tablets with immunosuppressants and other potentially nephrotoxic agents should be carefully considered and the lowest effective dose employed).
No products indexed under this heading.

Cisplatin (The benefits and risks of using fenofibrate tablets with immunosuppressants and other potentially nephrotoxic agents should be carefully considered and the lowest effective dose employed).
No products indexed under this heading.

Cladribine (The benefits and risks of using fenofibrate tablets with immunosuppressants and other potentially nephrotoxic agents should be carefully considered and the lowest effective dose employed). Products include:
Leustatin 946

Clozapine (The benefits and risks of using fenofibrate tablets with immunosuppressants and other potentially nephrotoxic agents should be carefully considered and the lowest effective dose employed).
No products indexed under this heading.

Colesevelam Hydrochloride (Bile acid sequestrants may bind fenofibrate; fenofibrate should be taken at least 1 hour before or 4-6 hours after a bile acid binding resin to avoid impeding its absorption). Products include:
Welchol 1029

Colestipol Hydrochloride (Bile acid sequestrants may bind fenofibrate; fenofibrate should be taken at least 1 hour before or 4-6 hours after a bile acid binding resin to avoid impeding its absorption).
No products indexed under this heading.

Colistimethate Sodium (The benefits and risks of using fenofibrate tablets with immunosuppressants and other potentially nephrotoxic agents should be carefully considered and the lowest effective dose employed).
No products indexed under this heading.

Colistin Sulfate (The benefits and risks of using fenofibrate tablets with immunosuppressants and other potentially nephrotoxic agents should be carefully considered and the lowest effective dose employed).
No products indexed under this heading.

Cyclophosphamide (The benefits and risks of using fenofibrate tablets with immunosuppressants and other potentially nephrotoxic agents should be carefully considered and the lowest effective dose employed).
No products indexed under this heading.

Cyclosporine (Because cyclosporine can produce nephrotoxicity with decreases in creatinine clearance and rises in serum creatinine, and because renal excretion is the primary elimination route of fibrate drugs including fenofibrate, there is a risk that an interaction will lead to deterioration. The benefits and risks of using fenofibrate tablets with immunosuppressants and other potentially nephrotoxic agents should be carefully considered and the lowest effective dose employed).
Products include:
Gengraf 440
Neoral Oral Solution 2496
Neoral Capsules 2496
Restasis 605

Cytarabine (The benefits and risks of using fenofibrate tablets with immunosuppressants and other potentially nephrotoxic agents should be carefully considered and the lowest effective dose employed).
No products indexed under this heading.

Cytarabine Liposome (The benefits and risks of using fenofibrate tablets with immunosuppressants and other potentially nephrotoxic agents should be carefully considered and the lowest effective dose employed).
No products indexed under this heading.

Delavirdine Mesylate (The benefits and risks of using fenofibrate tablets with immunosuppressants and other potentially nephrotoxic agents should be carefully considered and the lowest effective dose employed).
   No products indexed under this heading.

Diatrizoate Meglumine (The benefits and risks of using fenofibrate tablets with immunosuppressants and other potentially nephrotoxic agents should be carefully considered and the lowest effective dose employed).
   No products indexed under this heading.

Diatrizoate Sodium (The benefits and risks of using fenofibrate tablets with immunosuppressants and other potentially nephrotoxic agents should be carefully considered and the lowest effective dose employed).
   No products indexed under this heading.

Diclofenac Potassium (The benefits and risks of using fenofibrate tablets with immunosuppressants and other potentially nephrotoxic agents should be carefully considered and the lowest effective dose employed).
   No products indexed under this heading.

Diclofenac Sodium (The benefits and risks of using fenofibrate tablets with immunosuppressants and other potentially nephrotoxic agents should be carefully considered and the lowest effective dose employed).
   No products indexed under this heading.

Dicloxacillin Sodium (The benefits and risks of using fenofibrate tablets with immunosuppressants and other potentially nephrotoxic agents should be carefully considered and the lowest effective dose employed).
   No products indexed under this heading.

Dicumarol (Caution should be exercised when anticoagulants are given in conjunction with fenofibrate because of the potentiation of coumarin-type anticoagulants in prolonging the PT/INR. The dosage of the anticoagulant should be reduced to maintain the PT/INR at the desired level to prevent bleeding complications. Frequent PT/INR determinations are advisable until it has been definitely determined that the PT/INR has stabilized).
   No products indexed under this heading.

Didanosine (The benefits and risks of using fenofibrate tablets with immunosuppressants and other potentially nephrotoxic agents should be carefully considered and the lowest effective dose employed).
   No products indexed under this heading.

Efavirenz (The benefits and risks of using fenofibrate tablets with immunosuppressants and other potentially nephrotoxic agents should be carefully considered and the lowest effective dose employed). Products include:
   Atripla 906

Emtricitabine (The benefits and risks of using fenofibrate tablets with immunosuppressants and other potentially nephrotoxic agents should be carefully considered and the lowest effective dose employed). Products include:
   Atripla 906
   Emtriva 1238
   Emtriva Oral Solution 1238
   Truvada 1258

Enalapril Maleate (The benefits and risks of using fenofibrate tablets with immunosuppressants and other potentially nephrotoxic agents should be carefully considered and the lowest effective dose employed).
   No products indexed under this heading.

Enalaprilat (The benefits and risks of using fenofibrate tablets with immunosuppressants and other potentially nephrotoxic agents should be carefully considered and the lowest effective dose employed).
   No products indexed under this heading.

Enfuvirtide (The benefits and risks of using fenofibrate tablets with immunosuppressants and other potentially nephrotoxic agents should be carefully considered and the lowest effective dose employed).
   No products indexed under this heading.

Ethiodized Oil (The benefits and risks of using fenofibrate tablets with immunosuppressants and other potentially nephrotoxic agents should be carefully considered and the lowest effective dose employed).
   No products indexed under this heading.

Etodolac (The benefits and risks of using fenofibrate tablets with immunosuppressants and other potentially nephrotoxic agents should be carefully considered and the lowest effective dose employed).
   No products indexed under this heading.

Fenoprofen Calcium (The benefits and risks of using fenofibrate tablets with immunosuppressants and other potentially nephrotoxic agents should be carefully considered and the lowest effective dose employed).
   No products indexed under this heading.

Filgrastim (The benefits and risks of using fenofibrate tablets with immunosuppressants and other potentially nephrotoxic agents should be carefully considered and the lowest effective dose employed). Products include:
   Neupogen 631

Fluorouracil (The benefits and risks of using fenofibrate tablets with immunosuppressants and other potentially nephrotoxic agents should be carefully considered and the lowest effective dose employed). Products include:
   Carac 2966

Flurbiprofen (The benefits and risks of using fenofibrate tablets with immunosuppressants and other potentially nephrotoxic agents should be carefully considered and the lowest effective dose employed).
   No products indexed under this heading.

Fluvastatin Sodium (Co-administration of fibric acid derivatives and HMG-CoA reductase inhibitors has been associated with rhabdomyolysis, markedly elevated creatine kinase levels and myoglobulinuria, leading in a high proportion of cases to acute renal failure; the combined use should be avoided unless the benefit of further alterations in lipid levels is likely to outweigh the increased risk of this combination).
   No products indexed under this heading.

Foscarnet Sodium (The benefits and risks of using fenofibrate tablets with immunosuppressants and other potentially nephrotoxic agents should be carefully considered and the lowest effective dose employed).
   No products indexed under this heading.

Fosinopril Sodium (The benefits and risks of using fenofibrate tablets with immunosuppressants and other potentially nephrotoxic agents should be carefully considered and the lowest effective dose employed).
   No products indexed under this heading.

Furosemide (The benefits and risks of using fenofibrate tablets with immunosuppressants and other potentially nephrotoxic agents should be carefully considered and the lowest effective dose employed). Products include:
   Furosemide 2354

Gadopentetate Dimeglumine (The benefits and risks of using fenofibrate tablets with immunosuppressants and other potentially nephrotoxic agents should be carefully considered and the lowest effective dose employed).
   No products indexed under this heading.

Gentamicin (The benefits and risks of using fenofibrate tablets with immunosuppressants and other potentially nephrotoxic agents should be carefully considered and the lowest effective dose employed).
   No products indexed under this heading.

Gentamicin Sulfate (The benefits and risks of using fenofibrate tablets with immunosuppressants and other potentially nephrotoxic agents should be carefully considered and the lowest effective dose employed). Products include:
   Pred-G ....⊙**226**, ⊙**227**

Glipizide (The benefits and risks of using fenofibrate tablets with immunosuppressants and other potentially nephrotoxic agents should be carefully considered and the lowest effective dose employed).
   No products indexed under this heading.

Globulin, Immune (Human) (The benefits and risks of using fenofibrate tablets with immunosuppressants and other potentially nephrotoxic agents should be carefully considered and the lowest effective dose employed). Products include:

Glyburide (The benefits and risks of using fenofibrate tablets with immunosuppressants and other potentially nephrotoxic agents should be carefully considered and the lowest effective dose employed).
   No products indexed under this heading.

Gold Therapy (The benefits and risks of using fenofibrate tablets with immunosuppressants and other potentially nephrotoxic agents should be carefully considered and the lowest effective dose employed).
   No products indexed under this heading.

HMG-CoA Reductase Inhibitors (The benefits and risks of using fenofibrate tablets with immunosuppressants and other potentially nephrotoxic agents should be carefully considered and the lowest effective dose employed).
   No products indexed under this heading.

Hydrochlorothiazide (The benefits and risks of using fenofibrate tablets with immunosuppressants and other potentially nephrotoxic agents should be carefully considered and the lowest effective dose employed). Products include:
   Atacand HCT 700
   Avalide 2956
   Benicar HCT 1017
   Diovan HCT 2419
   Dyazide 1429
   Exforge HCT 2449
   Hyzaar 2162
   Hyzaar 100-12.5 2162
   Micardis HCT 889
   Prinzide 2246
   Tekturna HCT 2541
   Teveten HCT 541

Hydroflumethiazide (The benefits and risks of using fenofibrate tablets with immunosuppressants and other potentially nephrotoxic agents should be carefully considered and the lowest effective dose employed).
   No products indexed under this heading.

Ibuprofen (The benefits and risks of using fenofibrate tablets with immunosuppressants and other potentially nephrotoxic agents should be carefully considered and the lowest effective dose employed). Products include:
   Motrin IB 2043

Children's Motrin 2044
Children's Motrin Non-Staining
   Dye-Free 2044
Infants' Motrin 2044
Infants' Motrin Dye-Free 2044
Junior Strength Motrin 2044
Vicoprofen 564

Idarubicin Hydrochloride (The benefits and risks of using fenofibrate tablets with immunosuppressants and other potentially nephrotoxic agents should be carefully considered and the lowest effective dose employed).
   No products indexed under this heading.

Ifosfamide (The benefits and risks of using fenofibrate tablets with immunosuppressants and other potentially nephrotoxic agents should be carefully considered and the lowest effective dose employed).
   No products indexed under this heading.

Imipenem (The benefits and risks of using fenofibrate tablets with immunosuppressants and other potentially nephrotoxic agents should be carefully considered and the lowest effective dose employed). Products include:
   Primaxin I.M. 2232
   Primaxin I.V. 2235

Immune Globulin Intravenous (Human) (The benefits and risks of using fenofibrate tablets with immunosuppressants and other potentially nephrotoxic agents should be carefully considered and the lowest effective dose employed). Products include:
   Flebogamma 5% DIF 1794
   Gammagard 812, 815
   Gamunex 3374

Indinavir Sulfate (The benefits and risks of using fenofibrate tablets with immunosuppressants and other potentially nephrotoxic agents should be carefully considered and the lowest effective dose employed). Products include:
   Crixivan 2113

Indomethacin (The benefits and risks of using fenofibrate tablets with immunosuppressants and other potentially nephrotoxic agents should be carefully considered and the lowest effective dose employed). Products include:
   Indocin 2167

Indomethacin Sodium Trihydrate (The benefits and risks of using fenofibrate tablets with immunosuppressants and other potentially nephrotoxic agents should be carefully considered and the lowest effective dose employed). Products include:
   Indocin I.V. 2007

Interferon Beta-1b (The benefits and risks of using fenofibrate tablets with immunosuppressants and other potentially nephrotoxic agents should be carefully considered and the lowest effective dose employed). Products include:
   Betaseron 836
   Extavia 2459

Interleuken-2 (The benefits and risks of using fenofibrate tablets with immunosuppressants and other potentially nephrotoxic agents should be carefully considered and the lowest effective dose employed).
   No products indexed under this heading.

Iodamide Meglumine (The benefits and risks of using fenofibrate tablets with immunosuppressants and other potentially nephrotoxic agents should be carefully considered and the lowest effective dose employed).
   No products indexed under this heading.

Iohexol (The benefits and risks of using fenofibrate tablets with immunosuppressants and other potentially nephrotoxic agents should be carefully considered and the lowest effective dose employed).
   No products indexed under this heading.

IMPORTANT NOTE: Always consult each drug listing in the patient's regimen for possible interactions.

Iopamidol (The benefits and risks of using fenofibrate tablets with immunosuppressants and other potentially nephrotoxic agents should be carefully considered and the lowest effective dose employed).
  No products indexed under this heading.

Iopanoic Acid (The benefits and risks of using fenofibrate tablets with immunosuppressants and other potentially nephrotoxic agents should be carefully considered and the lowest effective dose employed).
  No products indexed under this heading.

Iothalamate Meglumine (The benefits and risks of using fenofibrate tablets with immunosuppressants and other potentially nephrotoxic agents should be carefully considered and the lowest effective dose employed).
  No products indexed under this heading.

Ioxaglate Meglumine (The benefits and risks of using fenofibrate tablets with immunosuppressants and other potentially nephrotoxic agents should be carefully considered and the lowest effective dose employed).
  No products indexed under this heading.

Ioxaglate Sodium (The benefits and risks of using fenofibrate tablets with immunosuppressants and other potentially nephrotoxic agents should be carefully considered and the lowest effective dose employed).
  No products indexed under this heading.

Kanamycin Sulfate (The benefits and risks of using fenofibrate tablets with immunosuppressants and other potentially nephrotoxic agents should be carefully considered and the lowest effective dose employed).
  No products indexed under this heading.

Ketoprofen (The benefits and risks of using fenofibrate tablets with immunosuppressants and other potentially nephrotoxic agents should be carefully considered and the lowest effective dose employed).
  No products indexed under this heading.

Ketorolac Tromethamine (The benefits and risks of using fenofibrate tablets with immunosuppressants and other potentially nephrotoxic agents should be carefully considered and the lowest effective dose employed). Products include:
  Acuvail ....⊙ 209

Lamium album (The benefits and risks of using fenofibrate tablets with immunosuppressants and other potentially nephrotoxic agents should be carefully considered and the lowest effective dose employed).
  No products indexed under this heading.

Lisinopril (The benefits and risks of using fenofibrate tablets with immunosuppressants and other potentially nephrotoxic agents should be carefully considered and the lowest effective dose employed). Products include:
  Prinivil 2241
  Prinzide 2246

Lithium (The benefits and risks of using fenofibrate tablets with immunosuppressants and other potentially nephrotoxic agents should be carefully considered and the lowest effective dose employed).
  No products indexed under this heading.

Lithium Carbonate (The benefits and risks of using fenofibrate tablets with immunosuppressants and other potentially nephrotoxic agents should be carefully considered and the lowest effective dose employed).
  No products indexed under this heading.

Lithium Citrate (The benefits and risks of using fenofibrate tablets with immunosuppressants and other potentially nephrotoxic agents should be carefully considered and the lowest effective dose employed).
  No products indexed under this heading.

Lopinavir (The benefits and risks of using fenofibrate tablets with immunosuppressants and other potentially nephrotoxic agents should be carefully considered and the lowest effective dose employed). Products include:
  Kaletra 458

Loracarbef (The benefits and risks of using fenofibrate tablets with immunosuppressants and other potentially nephrotoxic agents should be carefully considered and the lowest effective dose employed).
  No products indexed under this heading.

Lovastatin (Co-administration of fibric acid derivatives and HMG-CoA reductase inhibitors has been associated with rhabdomyolysis, markedly elevated creatine kinase levels and myoglobulinuria, leading in a high proportion of cases to acute renal failure; the combined use should be avoided unless the benefit of further alterations in lipid levels is likely to outweigh the increased risk of this combination). Products include:
  Advicor **402**
  Mevacor 2212

Meclofenamate Sodium (The benefits and risks of using fenofibrate tablets with immunosuppressants and other potentially nephrotoxic agents should be carefully considered and the lowest effective dose employed).
  No products indexed under this heading.

Mefenamic Acid (The benefits and risks of using fenofibrate tablets with immunosuppressants and other potentially nephrotoxic agents should be carefully considered and the lowest effective dose employed).
  No products indexed under this heading.

Meloxicam (The benefits and risks of using fenofibrate tablets with immunosuppressants and other potentially nephrotoxic agents should be carefully considered and the lowest effective dose employed).
  No products indexed under this heading.

Melphalan Hydrochloride (The benefits and risks of using fenofibrate tablets with immunosuppressants and other potentially nephrotoxic agents should be carefully considered and the lowest effective dose employed). Products include:
  Alkeran for Injection 1300

Mesalamine (The benefits and risks of using fenofibrate tablets with immunosuppressants and other potentially nephrotoxic agents should be carefully considered and the lowest effective dose employed). Products include:
  Apriso **2899**
  Asacol 2786
  Asacol HD 2787
  Canasa 782
  Lialda 3295
  Pentasa 3297

Methimazole (The benefits and risks of using fenofibrate tablets with immunosuppressants and other potentially nephrotoxic agents should be carefully considered and the lowest effective dose employed).
  No products indexed under this heading.

Methotrexate (The benefits and risks of using fenofibrate tablets with immunosuppressants and other potentially nephrotoxic agents should be carefully considered and the lowest effective dose employed).
  No products indexed under this heading.

Methotrexate Sodium (The benefits and risks of using fenofibrate tablets with immunosuppressants and other potentially nephrotoxic agents should be carefully considered and the lowest effective dose employed).
  No products indexed under this heading.

Methyclothiazide (The benefits and risks of using fenofibrate tablets with immunosuppressants and other potentially nephrotoxic agents should be carefully considered and the lowest effective dose employed).
  No products indexed under this heading.

Mezlocillin Sodium (The benefits and risks of using fenofibrate tablets with immunosuppressants and other potentially nephrotoxic agents should be carefully considered and the lowest effective dose employed).
  No products indexed under this heading.

Minocycline Hydrochloride (The benefits and risks of using fenofibrate tablets with immunosuppressants and other potentially nephrotoxic agents should be carefully considered and the lowest effective dose employed). Products include:
  Solodyn 2073

Mitomycin (Mitomycin-C) (The benefits and risks of using fenofibrate tablets with immunosuppressants and other potentially nephrotoxic agents should be carefully considered and the lowest effective dose employed).
  No products indexed under this heading.

Moexipril Hydrochloride (The benefits and risks of using fenofibrate tablets with immunosuppressants and other potentially nephrotoxic agents should be carefully considered and the lowest effective dose employed).
  No products indexed under this heading.

Muromonab-CD3 (The benefits and risks of using fenofibrate tablets with immunosuppressants and other potentially nephrotoxic agents should be carefully considered and the lowest effective dose employed). Products include:
  Orthoclone OKT3 .... **949**

Mycophenolate Mofetil (The benefits and risks of using fenofibrate tablets with immunosuppressants and other potentially nephrotoxic agents should be carefully considered and the lowest effective dose employed).
  No products indexed under this heading.

Nabumetone (The benefits and risks of using fenofibrate tablets with immunosuppressants and other potentially nephrotoxic agents should be carefully considered and the lowest effective dose employed).
  No products indexed under this heading.

Nafcillin Sodium (The benefits and risks of using fenofibrate tablets with immunosuppressants and other potentially nephrotoxic agents should be carefully considered and the lowest effective dose employed).
  No products indexed under this heading.

Naproxen (The benefits and risks of using fenofibrate tablets with immunosuppressants and other potentially nephrotoxic agents should be carefully considered and the lowest effective dose employed). Products include:
  EC-Naprosyn 2850
  Naprosyn 2850
  Anaprox/Naprosyn 2850

Naproxen Sodium (The benefits and risks of using fenofibrate tablets with immunosuppressants and other potentially nephrotoxic agents should be carefully considered and the lowest effective dose employed). Products include:
  Anaprox 2850
  Anaprox DS 2850

Treximet **1681**

Nelfinavir Mesylate (The benefits and risks of using fenofibrate tablets with immunosuppressants and other potentially nephrotoxic agents should be carefully considered and the lowest effective dose employed).
  No products indexed under this heading.

Neomycin (The benefits and risks of using fenofibrate tablets with immunosuppressants and other potentially nephrotoxic agents should be carefully considered and the lowest effective dose employed).
  No products indexed under this heading.

Neomycin, oral (The benefits and risks of using fenofibrate tablets with immunosuppressants and other potentially nephrotoxic agents should be carefully considered and the lowest effective dose employed).
  No products indexed under this heading.

Neomycin Sulfate (The benefits and risks of using fenofibrate tablets with immunosuppressants and other potentially nephrotoxic agents should be carefully considered and the lowest effective dose employed).
  No products indexed under this heading.

Nevirapine (The benefits and risks of using fenofibrate tablets with immunosuppressants and other potentially nephrotoxic agents should be carefully considered and the lowest effective dose employed). Products include:
  Viramune Oral Suspension **897**
  Viramune Tablets **897**

Norfloxacin (The benefits and risks of using fenofibrate tablets with immunosuppressants and other potentially nephrotoxic agents should be carefully considered and the lowest effective dose employed). Products include:
  Noroxin 2220

Olsalazine Sodium (The benefits and risks of using fenofibrate tablets with immunosuppressants and other potentially nephrotoxic agents should be carefully considered and the lowest effective dose employed).
  No products indexed under this heading.

Omeprazole (The benefits and risks of using fenofibrate tablets with immunosuppressants and other potentially nephrotoxic agents should be carefully considered and the lowest effective dose employed).
  No products indexed under this heading.

Oxaprozin (The benefits and risks of using fenofibrate tablets with immunosuppressants and other potentially nephrotoxic agents should be carefully considered and the lowest effective dose employed).
  No products indexed under this heading.

Pamidronate Disodium (The benefits and risks of using fenofibrate tablets with immunosuppressants and other potentially nephrotoxic agents should be carefully considered and the lowest effective dose employed).
  No products indexed under this heading.

Paroxetine Hydrochloride (The benefits and risks of using fenofibrate tablets with immunosuppressants and other potentially nephrotoxic agents should be carefully considered and the lowest effective dose employed). Products include:
  Paroxetine CR 2361
  Paroxetine ER 2371
  Paxil 1586
  Paxil CR 1596

Penicillamine (The benefits and risks of using fenofibrate tablets with immunosuppressants and other potentially nephrotoxic agents should be carefully considered and the lowest effective dose employed).
  No products indexed under this heading.

IMPORTANT NOTE: Always consult each drug listing in the patient's regimen for possible interactions.

Tolazamide (The benefits and risks of using fenofibrate tablets with immuno-suppressants and other potentially nephrotoxic agents should be carefully considered and the lowest effective dose employed).

No products indexed under this heading.

Tolbutamide (The benefits and risks of using fenofibrate tablets with immunosuppressants and other potentially nephrotoxic agents should be carefully considered and the lowest effective dose employed).

No products indexed under this heading.

Tolmetin Sodium (The benefits and risks of using fenofibrate tablets with immunosuppressants and other potentially nephrotoxic agents should be carefully considered and the lowest effective dose employed).

No products indexed under this heading.

Trandolapril (The benefits and risks of using fenofibrate tablets with immuno-suppressants and other potentially nephrotoxic agents should be carefully considered and the lowest effective dose employed). Products include:

Mavik **489**
Tarka **534**

Triamterene (The benefits and risks of using fenofibrate tablets with immu-nosuppressants and other potentially nephrotoxic agents should be carefully considered and the lowest effective dose employed). Products include:

Dyazide **1429**
Dyrenium **3495**

Trimethadione (The benefits and risks of using fenofibrate tablets with immu-nosuppressants and other potentially nephrotoxic agents should be carefully considered and the lowest effective dose employed).

No products indexed under this heading.

Trovafloxacin Mesylate (The ben-efits and risks of using fenofibrate tab-lets with immunosuppressants and oth-er potentially nephrotoxic agents should be carefully considered and the lowest effective dose employed).

No products indexed under this heading.

Tyropanoate Sodium (The benefits and risks of using fenofibrate tablets with immunosuppressants and other potentially nephrotoxic agents should be carefully considered and the lowest effective dose employed).

No products indexed under this heading.

Valacyclovir Hydrochloride (The benefits and risks of using fenofibrate tablets with immunosuppressants and other potentially nephrotoxic agents should be carefully considered and the lowest effective dose employed). Products include:

Valtrex 1702

Valdecoxib (The benefits and risks of using fenofibrate tablets with immuno-suppressants and other potentially nephrotoxic agents should be carefully considered and the lowest effective dose employed).

No products indexed under this heading.

Vancomycin Hydrochloride (The benefits and risks of using fenofibrate tablets with immunosuppressants and other potentially nephrotoxic agents should be carefully considered and the lowest effective dose employed).

No products indexed under this heading.

Voriconazole (The benefits and risks of using fenofibrate tablets with immu-nosuppressants and other potentially nephrotoxic agents should be carefully considered and the lowest effective dose employed).

No products indexed under this heading.

Warfarin Sodium (Caution should be exercised when anticoagulants are giv-en in conjunction with fenofibrate because of the potentiation of

coumarin-type anticoagulants in pro-longing the PT/INR. The dosage of the anticoagulant should be reduced to maintain the PT/INR at the desired level to prevent bleeding complications. Fre-quent PT/INR determinations are advis-able until it has been definitely deter-mined that the PT/INR has stabilized).

No products indexed under this heading.

Zalcitabine (The benefits and risks of using fenofibrate tablets with immuno-suppressants and other potentially nephrotoxic agents should be carefully considered and the lowest effective dose employed).

No products indexed under this heading.

Zidovudine (The benefits and risks of using fenofibrate tablets with immuno-suppressants and other potentially nephrotoxic agents should be carefully considered and the lowest effective dose employed). Products include:

Combivir **1404**
Retrovir **1634**
Retrovir IV **1640**
Trizivir **1688**

Zoledronic Acid (The benefits and risks of using fenofibrate tablets with immunosuppressants and other poten-tially nephrotoxic agents should be carefully considered and the lowest effective dose employed). Products include:

Reclast **2509**
Zometa **2554**

Food Interactions

Food, unspecified (The absorption of fenofibrate is increased when adminis-tered with food; Tricor should be given with meals).

TRILIPIX DELAYED RELEASE CAPSULES

(Fenofibrate) 548
May interact with alcohols, beta-block-ers, bile acid sequestering agents, cy-tochrome p450 2a6 substrates (se-lected), cytochrome p450 2c19 sub-strates (selected), cytochrome p450 2c8 substrates (selected), cytochrome p450 2c9 substrates (selected), estro-gens, HMG-CoA reductase inhibitors, oral anticoagulants, thiazides, and cer-tain other agents. Compounds in these categories include:

Acarbose (Fenofibric acid is a mild-to-moderate inhibitor of CYP2C9 at thera-peutic concentrations).

No products indexed under this heading.

Acebutolol Hydrochloride (Medica-tions known to exacerbate hypertriglyc-eridemia (eg, β-blockers) should be dis-continued or changed if possible, before triglyceride-lowering drug thera-py, such as fenofibric acid, is consid-ered. If the decision is made to use lipid-altering drugs, the patient should be instructed that this does not reduce the importance of adhering to diet).

No products indexed under this heading.

Amiodarone Hydrochloride (Fenofibric acid is a weak inhibitor of CYP2C8 at therapeutic concentrations).

No products indexed under this heading.

Amitriptyline Hydrochloride (Fenofibric acid is a weak inhibitor of CYP2C8 at therapeutic concentrations).

No products indexed under this heading.

Amoxapine (Fenofibric acid is a weak inhibitor of CYP2C8 at therapeutic con-centrations).

No products indexed under this heading.

Anisindione (Caution should be exer-cised when oral coumarin anticoagu-lants are given in conjunction with fenofibric acid. Fenofibric acid may potentiate the anticoagulant effects of these agents, resulting in prolongation of the prothrombin time/INR. Frequent monitoring of prothrombin time/INR and

dose adjustment of the oral anticoagu-lant are recommended until the pro-thrombin time/INR has stabilized in order to prevent bleeding complica-tions).

No products indexed under this heading.

Atenolol (Medications known to exac-erbate hypertriglyceridemia (eg, β-blockers) should be discontinued or changed if possible, before triglyceride-lowering drug therapy, such as fenofibric acid, is considered. If the decision is made to use lipid-altering drugs, the patient should be instructed that this does not reduce the impor-tance of adhering to diet).

No products indexed under this heading.

Atorvastatin Calcium (Atorvastatin decreases fenofibric acid AUC and C_{max} by 2% and 4%, respectively, while fenofibric acid decreases atorvastatin AUC 17%). Products include:

Lipitor 2703

Bendroflumethiazide (Medications known to exacerbate hypertriglyceride-mia (eg, thiazides) should be discontin-ued or changed if possible, before triglyceride-lowering drug therapy, such as fenofibric acid, is considered. If the decision is made to use lipid-altering drugs, the patient should be instructed that this does not reduce the impor-tance of adhering to diet).

No products indexed under this heading.

Benzphetamine Hydrochloride (Fenofibric acid is a weak inhibitor of CYP2C8 at therapeutic concentrations).

No products indexed under this heading.

Betaxolol Hydrochloride (Medica-tions known to exacerbate hypertriglyc-eridemia (eg, β-blockers) should be dis-continued or changed if possible, before triglyceride-lowering drug thera-py, such as fenofibric acid, is consid-ered. If the decision is made to use lipid-altering drugs, the patient should be instructed that this does not reduce the importance of adhering to diet).

No products indexed under this heading.

Bisoprolol Fumarate (Medications known to exacerbate hypertriglyceride-mia (eg, β-blockers) should be discon-tinued or changed if possible, before triglyceride-lowering drug therapy, such as fenofibric acid, is considered. If the decision is made to use lipid-altering drugs, the patient should be instructed that this does not reduce the importance of adhering to diet).

No products indexed under this heading.

Candesartan Cilexetil (Fenofibric acid is a mild-to-moderate inhibitor of CYP2C9 at therapeutic concentrations). Products include:

Atacand **697**
Atacand HCT **700**

Carbamazepine (Fenofibric acid is a weak inhibitor of CYP2C8 at therapeutic concentrations). Products include:

Carbatrol 3280
Equetro 3477

Carisoprodol (Fenofibric acid is a weak inhibitor of CYP2C19 at therapeu-tic concentrations).

No products indexed under this heading.

Carteolol Hydrochloride (Medica-tions known to exacerbate hypertriglyc-eridemia (eg, β-blockers) should be dis-continued or changed if possible, before triglyceride-lowering drug thera-py, such as fenofibric acid, is consid-ered. If the decision is made to use lipid-altering drugs, the patient should be instructed that this does not reduce the importance of adhering to diet).

No products indexed under this heading.

Carvedilol (Medications known to exacerbate hypertriglyceridemia (eg, β-blockers) should be discontinued or changed if possible, before triglyceride-lowering drug therapy, such as

fenofibric acid, is considered. If the decision is made to use lipid-altering drugs, the patient should be instructed that this does not reduce the impor-tance of adhering to diet). Products include:

Coreg 1409

Carvedilol Phosphate (Medications known to exacerbate hypertriglyceride-mia (eg, β-blockers) should be discon-tinued or changed if possible, before triglyceride-lowering drug therapy, such as fenofibric acid, is considered. If the decision is made to use lipid-altering drugs, the patient should be instructed that this does not reduce the impor-tance of adhering to diet). Products include:

Coreg CR 1416

Celecoxib (Fenofibric acid is a mild-to-moderate inhibitor of CYP2C9 at thera-peutic concentrations). Products include:

Celebrex 3272

Cerivastatin Sodium (Fibrate and statin monotherapy increase the risk of myositis or myopathy, and have been associated with rhabdomyolysis. Data from observational studies suggest that the risk for rhabdomyolysis is increased when fibrates are co-administered with a statin (with a significantly higher rate observed for gemfibrozil). Reversible elevations in serum creatinine have been reported in patients receiving fenofibric acid as monotherapy or co-administered with statins).

No products indexed under this heading.

Chlorothiazide (Medications known to exacerbate hypertriglyceridemia (eg, thiazides) should be discontinued or changed if possible, before triglyceride-lowering drug therapy, such as fenofibric acid, is considered. If the decision is made to use lipid-altering drugs, the patient should be instructed that this does not reduce the impor-tance of adhering to diet).

No products indexed under this heading.

Chlorothiazide Sodium (Medications known to exacerbate hypertriglyceride-mia (eg, thiazides) should be discontin-ued or changed if possible, before triglyceride-lowering drug therapy, such as fenofibric acid, is considered. If the decision is made to use lipid-altering drugs, the patient should be instructed that this does not reduce the impor-tance of adhering to diet). Products include:

Diuril Intravenous 2009

Chlorotrianisene (Medications known to exacerbate hypertriglyceridemia (eg, estrogens) should be discontinued or changed if possible, before triglyceride-lowering drug therapy, such as fenofibric acid, is considered. If the decision is made to use lipid-altering drugs, the patient should be instructed that this does not reduce the impor-tance of adhering to diet).

No products indexed under this heading.

Chlorpropamide (Fenofibric acid is a mild-to-moderate inhibitor of CYP2C9 at therapeutic concentrations).

No products indexed under this heading.

Cholestyramine (Since bile acid res-ins may bind other drugs given concur-rently, patients should take fenofibric acid at least 1 hour before or 4-6 hours after a bile acid resin to avoid impeding its absorption).

No products indexed under this heading.

Cilostazol (Fenofibric acid is a weak inhibitor of CYP2C19 at therapeutic concentrations).

No products indexed under this heading.

Citalopram Hydrobromide (Fenofibric acid is a weak inhibitor of CYP2C19 at therapeutic concentra-tions). Products include:

IMPORTANT NOTE: Always consult each drug listing in the patient's regimen for possible interactions.

(⊙ Described in PDR® for Ophthalmic Medicines)

Paramethadione (Fenofibric acid is a weak inhibitor of CYP2C19 at therapeutic concentrations).
No products indexed under this heading.

Penbutolol Sulfate (Medications known to exacerbate hypertriglyceridemia (eg, β-blockers) should be discontinued or changed if possible, before triglyceride-lowering drug therapy, such as fenofibric acid, is considered. If the decision is made to use lipid-altering drugs, the patient should be instructed that this does not reduce the importance of adhering to diet).
No products indexed under this heading.

Pentamidine Isethionate (Fenofibric acid is a weak inhibitor of CYP2C19 at therapeutic concentrations).
No products indexed under this heading.

Phenacemide (Fenofibric acid is a weak inhibitor of CYP2C19 at therapeutic concentrations).
No products indexed under this heading.

Phenobarbital (Fenofibric acid is a weak inhibitor of CYP2C19 at therapeutic concentrations). Products include:
Donnatal **2711**

Phenobarbital Sodium (Fenofibric acid is a weak inhibitor of CYP2C19 at therapeutic concentrations).
No products indexed under this heading.

Phensuximide (Fenofibric acid is a weak inhibitor of CYP2C19 at therapeutic concentrations).
No products indexed under this heading.

Phenylbutazone (Fenofibric acid is a mild-to-moderate inhibitor of CYP2C9 at therapeutic concentrations).
No products indexed under this heading.

Phenytoin (Fenofibric acid is a weak inhibitor of CYP2C8 at therapeutic concentrations).
No products indexed under this heading.

Phenytoin Sodium (Fenofibric acid is a weak inhibitor of CYP2C8 at therapeutic concentrations). Products include:
Phenytek Capsules **2380**

Pindolol (Medications known to exacerbate hypertriglyceridemia (eg, β-blockers) should be discontinued or changed if possible, before triglyceride-lowering drug therapy, such as fenofibric acid, is considered. If the decision is made to use lipid-altering drugs, the patient should be instructed that this does not reduce the importance of adhering to diet).
No products indexed under this heading.

Pioglitazone Hydrochloride (Fenofibric acid is a weak inhibitor of CYP2C8 at therapeutic concentrations). Products include:
ActoPlus **3338**
Actos **3345**
Duetact **3354**

Piroxicam (Fenofibric acid is a mild-to-moderate inhibitor of CYP2C9 at therapeutic concentrations).
No products indexed under this heading.

Polyestradiol Phosphate (Medications known to exacerbate hypertriglyceridemia (eg, estrogens) should be discontinued or changed if possible, before triglyceride-lowering drug therapy, such as fenofibric acid, is considered. If the decision is made to use lipid-altering drugs, the patient should be instructed that this does not reduce the importance of adhering to diet).
No products indexed under this heading.

Polythiazide (Medications known to exacerbate hypertriglyceridemia (eg, thiazides) should be discontinued or changed if possible, before triglyceride-lowering drug therapy, such as fenofibric acid, is considered. If the decision is made to use lipid-altering drugs, the patient should be instructed that this does not reduce the importance of adhering to diet).
No products indexed under this heading.

Pravastatin Sodium (Pravastatin decreases fenofibric acid AUC and C_{max} by 1% and 2%, respectively, while fenofibric acid increases pravastatin AUC 13% to 39% and C_{max} by 13% to 55%).
No products indexed under this heading.

Primidone (Fenofibric acid is a weak inhibitor of CYP2C19 at therapeutic concentrations).
No products indexed under this heading.

Progesterone (Fenofibric acid is a weak inhibitor of CYP2C19 at therapeutic concentrations). Products include:
Crinone 4% **996**
Crinone 8% **996**
Prometrium **3307**

Proguanil Hydrochloride (Fenofibric acid is a weak inhibitor of CYP2C19 at therapeutic concentrations). Products include:
Malarone Pediatric Tablets **1572**
Malarone **1572**

Propranolol Hydrochloride (Medications known to exacerbate hypertriglyceridemia (eg, β-blockers) should be discontinued or changed if possible, before triglyceride-lowering drug therapy, such as fenofibric acid, is considered. If the decision is made to use lipid-altering drugs, the patient should be instructed that this does not reduce the importance of adhering to diet). Products include:
InnoPran XL **1517**

Protriptyline Hydrochloride (Fenofibric acid is a weak inhibitor of CYP2C8 at therapeutic concentrations).
No products indexed under this heading.

Quinestrol (Medications known to exacerbate hypertriglyceridemia (eg, estrogens) should be discontinued or changed if possible, before triglyceride-lowering drug therapy, such as fenofibric acid, is considered. If the decision is made to use lipid-altering drugs, the patient should be instructed that this does not reduce the importance of adhering to diet).
No products indexed under this heading.

Rabeprazole Sodium (Fenofibric acid is a weak inhibitor of CYP2C19 at therapeutic concentrations). Products include:
Aciphex **1035**

Repaglinide (Fenofibric acid is a weak inhibitor of CYP2C8 at therapeutic concentrations).
No products indexed under this heading.

Rofecoxib (Fenofibric acid is a mild-to-moderate inhibitor of CYP2C9 at therapeutic concentrations).
No products indexed under this heading.

Rosiglitazone (Rosiglitazone increases fenofibric acid AUC and C_{max} by 10% and 3%, respectively, while fenofibric acid increases rosiglitazone AUC by 6% and decreases its C_{max} by 1%).
No products indexed under this heading.

Rosiglitazone Maleate (Rosiglitazone increases fenofibric acid AUC and C_{max} by 10% and 3%, respectively, while fenofibric acid increases rosiglitazone AUC by 6% and decreases its C_{max} by 1%). Products include:
Avandamet **1345**
Avandaryl **1356**
Avandia **1366**

Rosiglitazone/Metformin (Fenofibric acid is a weak inhibitor of CYP2C8 at therapeutic concentrations).
No products indexed under this heading.

Rosuvastatin Calcium (Rosuvastatin decreases fenofibric acid AUC and C_{max} by 2%, while fenofibric acid increases rosuvastatin AUC and C_{max} by 6% and 20%, respectively). Products include:
Crestor **736**

Sertraline Hydrochloride (Fenofibric acid is a weak inhibitor of CYP2C19 at therapeutic concentrations).
No products indexed under this heading.

Sildenafil Citrate (Fenofibric acid is a mild-to-moderate inhibitor of CYP2C9 at therapeutic concentrations).
No products indexed under this heading.

Simvastatin (Simvastatin decreases fenofibric acid AUC and C_{max} by 5% and 11%, respectively, while fenofibric acid decreases simvastatin AUC by 8% to 36% and C_{max} by 1% to 17%). Products include:
Simcor **524**
Vytorin 10/10 .... **2303, 3240**
Vytorin 10/20 .... **2303, 3240**
Vytorin 10/40 .... **2303, 3240**
Vytorin 10/80 .... **2303, 3240**
Zocor **2289**

Sotalol Hydrochloride (Medications known to exacerbate hypertriglyceridemia (eg, β-blockers) should be discontinued or changed if possible, before triglyceride-lowering drug therapy, such as fenofibric acid, is considered. If the decision is made to use lipid-altering drugs, the patient should be instructed that this does not reduce the importance of adhering to diet).
No products indexed under this heading.

Sulfamethoxazole (Fenofibric acid is a mild-to-moderate inhibitor of CYP2C9 at therapeutic concentrations).
No products indexed under this heading.

Sulindac (Fenofibric acid is a mild-to-moderate inhibitor of CYP2C9 at therapeutic concentrations). Products include:
Clinoril **2098**

Suprofen (Fenofibric acid is a mild-to-moderate inhibitor of CYP2C9 at therapeutic concentrations).
No products indexed under this heading.

Tamoxifen Citrate (Fenofibric acid is a mild-to-moderate inhibitor of CYP2C9 at therapeutic concentrations).
No products indexed under this heading.

Telmisartan (Fenofibric acid is a mild-to-moderate inhibitor of CYP2C9 at therapeutic concentrations). Products include:
Micardis **887**
Micardis HCT **889**

Teniposide (Fenofibric acid is a weak inhibitor of CYP2C19 at therapeutic concentrations).
No products indexed under this heading.

Thioridazine (Fenofibric acid is a weak inhibitor of CYP2C19 at therapeutic concentrations).
No products indexed under this heading.

Thioridazine Hydrochloride (Fenofibric acid is a weak inhibitor of CYP2C19 at therapeutic concentrations). Products include:
Thioridazine Hydrochloride **2384**

Tiagabine Hydrochloride (Fenofibric acid is a weak inhibitor of CYP2C19 at therapeutic concentrations). Products include:
Gabitril **972**

Timolol Hemihydrate (Medications known to exacerbate hypertriglyceridemia (eg, β-blockers) should be discontinued or changed if possible, before triglyceride-lowering drug therapy, such as fenofibric acid, is considered. If the decision is made to use lipid-altering drugs, the patient should be instructed that this does not reduce the importance of adhering to diet). Products include:
Betimol **3490**

Timolol Maleate (Medications known to exacerbate hypertriglyceridemia (eg, β-blockers) should be discontinued or changed if possible, before triglyceride-lowering drug therapy, such as fenofibric acid, is considered. If the decision is made to use lipid-altering drugs, the patient should be instructed that this does not reduce the importance of adhering to diet). Products include:
Combigan **601**
Dorzolamide Hydrochloride/Timolol Maleate Ophthalmic Solution .... ⊙ **243**
Timoptic in Ocudose .... ⊙ **231**

Tolazamide (Fenofibric acid is a mild-to-moderate inhibitor of CYP2C9 at therapeutic concentrations).
No products indexed under this heading.

Tolbutamide (Fenofibric acid is a weak inhibitor of CYP2C8 at therapeutic concentrations).
No products indexed under this heading.

Tolbutamide Sodium (Fenofibric acid is a weak inhibitor of CYP2C8 at therapeutic concentrations).
No products indexed under this heading.

Tolmetin Sodium (Fenofibric acid is a mild-to-moderate inhibitor of CYP2C9 at therapeutic concentrations).
No products indexed under this heading.

Topiramate (Fenofibric acid is a weak inhibitor of CYP2C19 at therapeutic concentrations).
No products indexed under this heading.

Torsemide (Fenofibric acid is a mild-to-moderate inhibitor of CYP2C9 at therapeutic concentrations).
No products indexed under this heading.

Tretinoin (Fenofibric acid is a weak inhibitor of CYP2C8 at therapeutic concentrations).
No products indexed under this heading.

Trimethadione (Fenofibric acid is a weak inhibitor of CYP2C19 at therapeutic concentrations).
No products indexed under this heading.

Trimipramine Maleate (Fenofibric acid is a weak inhibitor of CYP2C8 at therapeutic concentrations).
No products indexed under this heading.

Troglitazone (Fenofibric acid is a mild-to-moderate inhibitor of CYP2C9 at therapeutic concentrations).
No products indexed under this heading.

Valdecoxib (Fenofibric acid is a mild-to-moderate inhibitor of CYP2C9 at therapeutic concentrations).
No products indexed under this heading.

Valproate Sodium (Fenofibric acid is a weak inhibitor of CYP2C19 at therapeutic concentrations).
No products indexed under this heading.

Valproic Acid (Fenofibric acid is a weak inhibitor of CYP2C19 at therapeutic concentrations).
No products indexed under this heading.

Valsartan (Fenofibric acid is a mild-to-moderate inhibitor of CYP2C9 at therapeutic concentrations). Products include:
Diovan **2413**
Diovan HCT **2419**
Exforge **2443**
Exforge HCT **2449**
Valturna **3637**

Vardenafil Hydrochloride (Fenofibric acid is a mild-to-moderate inhibitor of CYP2C9 at therapeutic concentrations). Products include:
Levitra **3157**

Trilipix Interactions Index 1940

Verapamil Hydrochloride (Fenofibric acid is a weak inhibitor of CYP2C8 at therapeutic concentrations). Products include:
Tarka 534

Vitamin A (Fenofibric acid is a weak inhibitor of CYP2C8 at therapeutic concentrations). Products include:
Cardio Basics 3455
Heplive 607
Norwegian Cod Liver Oil 919

Vitamin A Acetate (Fenofibric acid is a weak inhibitor of CYP2C8 at therapeutic concentrations).
No products indexed under this heading.

Voriconazole (Fenofibric acid is a weak inhibitor of CYP2C19 at therapeutic concentrations).
No products indexed under this heading.

Warfarin Sodium (Caution should be exercised when oral coumarin anticoagulants are given in conjunction with fenofibric acid. Fenofibric acid may potentiate the anticoagulant effects of these agents, resulting in prolongation of the prothrombin time/INR. Frequent monitoring of prothrombin time/INR and dose adjustment of the oral anticoagulant are recommended until the prothrombin time/INR has stabilized in order to prevent bleeding complications).
No products indexed under this heading.

Zafirlukast (Fenofibric acid is a mild-to-moderate inhibitor of CYP2C9 at therapeutic concentrations). Products include:
Accolate 3612

Zileuton (Fenofibric acid is a mild-to-moderate inhibitor of CYP2C9 at therapeutic concentrations).
No products indexed under this heading.

Zonisamide (Fenofibric acid is a weak inhibitor of CYP2C19 at therapeutic concentrations). Products include:
Zonegran 1081

Zopiclone (Fenofibric acid is a weak inhibitor of CYP2C8 at therapeutic concentrations).
No products indexed under this heading.

Food Interactions

Alcohol (Excessive alcohol intake should be addressed before triglyceride-lowering drug therapy, such as fenofibric acid, is considered. If the decision is made to use lipid-altering drugs, the patient should be instructed that this does not reduce the importance of adhering to diet).

Beer, reduced-alcohol (Excessive alcohol intake should be addressed before triglyceride-lowering drug therapy, such as fenofibric acid, is considered. If the decision is made to use lipid-altering drugs, the patient should be instructed that this does not reduce the importance of adhering to diet).

Beer, unspecified (Excessive alcohol intake should be addressed before triglyceride-lowering drug therapy, such as fenofibric acid, is considered. If the decision is made to use lipid-altering drugs, the patient should be instructed that this does not reduce the importance of adhering to diet).

Wine, Chianti (Excessive alcohol intake should be addressed before triglyceride-lowering drug therapy, such as fenofibric acid, is considered. If the decision is made to use lipid-altering drugs, the patient should be instructed that this does not reduce the importance of adhering to diet).

Wine, Red (Excessive alcohol intake should be addressed before triglyceride-lowering drug therapy, such as fenofibric acid, is considered. If the decision is made to use lipid-altering drugs, the patient should be instructed that this does not reduce the importance of adhering to diet).

Wine, unspecified (Excessive alcohol intake should be addressed before triglyceride-lowering drug therapy, such as fenofibric acid, is considered. If the decision is made to use lipid-altering drugs, the patient should be instructed that this does not reduce the importance of adhering to diet).

Wine products (Excessive alcohol intake should be addressed before triglyceride-lowering drug therapy, such as fenofibric acid, is considered. If the decision is made to use lipid-altering drugs, the patient should be instructed that this does not reduce the importance of adhering to diet).

TRISENOX INJECTION

(Arsenic Trioxide) 994

May interact with antiarrhythmics, diuretics, drugs that prolong the QT interval, potassium-depleting diuretics, and certain other agents. Compounds in these categories include:

Acebutolol Hydrochloride (Arsenic trioxide can cause QT interval prolongation and complete atrioventricular block. Caution is advised when arsenic trioxide is co-administered with other medications that can prolong the QT interval (eg, certain antiarrhythmics or thioridazine) or lead to electrolyte abnormalities (such as diuretics or amphotericin B)).
No products indexed under this heading.

Adenosine (Arsenic trioxide can cause QT interval prolongation and complete atrioventricular block. Caution is advised when arsenic trioxide is co-administered with other medications that can prolong the QT interval (eg, certain antiarrhythmics or thioridazine) or lead to electrolyte abnormalities (such as diuretics or amphotericin B)). Products include:
Adenocard 656
Adenoscan 657

Alprazolam (Arsenic trioxide can cause QT interval prolongation and complete atrioventricular block. Caution is advised when arsenic trioxide is co-administered with other medications that can prolong the QT interval (eg, certain antiarrhythmics or thioridazine) or lead to electrolyte abnormalities (such as diuretics or amphotericin B)).
No products indexed under this heading.

Amiloride Hydrochloride (Arsenic trioxide can cause QT interval prolongation and complete atrioventricular block. Caution is advised when arsenic trioxide is co-administered with other medications that can prolong the QT interval (eg, certain antiarrhythmics or thioridazine) or lead to electrolyte abnormalities (such as diuretics or amphotericin B)).
No products indexed under this heading.

Amiodarone Hydrochloride (Arsenic trioxide can cause QT interval prolongation and complete atrioventricular block. Caution is advised when arsenic trioxide is co-administered with other medications that can prolong the QT interval (eg, certain antiarrhythmics or thioridazine) or lead to electrolyte abnormalities (such as diuretics or amphotericin B)).
No products indexed under this heading.

Amitriptyline Hydrochloride (Arsenic trioxide can cause QT interval prolongation and complete atrioventricular block. Caution is advised when arsenic trioxide is co-administered with other medications that can prolong the QT interval (eg, certain antiarrhythmics or thioridazine) or lead to electrolyte abnormalities (such as diuretics or amphotericin B)).
No products indexed under this heading.

Amoxapine (Arsenic trioxide can cause QT interval prolongation and complete atrioventricular block. Caution is advised when arsenic trioxide is co-administered with other medications that can prolong the QT interval (eg, certain antiarrhythmics or thioridazine) or lead to electrolyte abnormalities (such as diuretics or amphotericin B)).
No products indexed under this heading.

Amphotericin B (Arsenic trioxide can cause QT interval prolongation and complete atrioventricular block. Hence, caution is advised when arsenic trioxide is co-administered with other medications that can prolong the QT interval (eg, certain antiarrhythmics or thioridazine) or lead to electrolyte abnormalities (such as diuretics or amphotericin B)).
No products indexed under this heading.

Astemizole (Arsenic trioxide can cause QT interval prolongation and complete atrioventricular block. Caution is advised when arsenic trioxide is co-administered with other medications that can prolong the QT interval (eg, certain antiarrhythmics or thioridazine) or lead to electrolyte abnormalities (such as diuretics or amphotericin B)).
No products indexed under this heading.

Bendroflumethiazide (Arsenic trioxide can cause QT interval prolongation and complete atrioventricular block. Concomitant administration of potassium wasting diuretic can increase the risk of QT prolongation).
No products indexed under this heading.

Bretylium Tosylate (Arsenic trioxide can cause QT interval prolongation and complete atrioventricular block. Caution is advised when arsenic trioxide is co-administered with other medications that can prolong the QT interval (eg, certain antiarrhythmics or thioridazine) or lead to electrolyte abnormalities (such as diuretics or amphotericin B)).
No products indexed under this heading.

Bumetanide (Arsenic trioxide can cause QT interval prolongation and complete atrioventricular block. Concomitant administration of potassium wasting diuretic can increase the risk of QT prolongation).
No products indexed under this heading.

Buspirone Hydrochloride (Arsenic trioxide can cause QT interval prolongation and complete atrioventricular block. Caution is advised when arsenic trioxide is co-administered with other medications that can prolong the QT interval (eg, certain antiarrhythmics or thioridazine) or lead to electrolyte abnormalities (such as diuretics or amphotericin B)).
No products indexed under this heading.

Chlordiazepoxide (Arsenic trioxide can cause QT interval prolongation and complete atrioventricular block. Caution is advised when arsenic trioxide is co-administered with other medications that can prolong the QT interval (eg, certain antiarrhythmics or thioridazine) or lead to electrolyte abnormalities (such as diuretics or amphotericin B)).
No products indexed under this heading.

Chlordiazepoxide Hydrochloride (Arsenic trioxide can cause QT interval prolongation and complete atrioventricular block. Caution is advised when arsenic trioxide is co-administered with other medications that can prolong the QT interval (eg, certain antiarrhythmics or thioridazine) or lead to electrolyte abnormalities (such as diuretics or amphotericin B)).
No products indexed under this heading.

Chlorothiazide (Arsenic trioxide can cause QT interval prolongation and complete atrioventricular block. Concomitant administration of potassium wasting diuretic can increase the risk of QT prolongation).
No products indexed under this heading.

Chlorothiazide Sodium (Arsenic trioxide can cause QT interval prolongation and complete atrioventricular block. Concomitant administration of potassium wasting diuretic can increase the risk of QT prolongation). Products include:
Diuril Intravenous 2009

Chlorpromazine (Arsenic trioxide can cause QT interval prolongation and complete atrioventricular block. Caution is advised when arsenic trioxide is co-administered with other medications that can prolong the QT interval (eg, certain antiarrhythmics or thioridazine) or lead to electrolyte abnormalities (such as diuretics or amphotericin B)).
No products indexed under this heading.

Chlorpromazine Hydrochloride (Arsenic trioxide can cause QT interval prolongation and complete atrioventricular block. Caution is advised when arsenic trioxide is co-administered with other medications that can prolong the QT interval (eg, certain antiarrhythmics or thioridazine) or lead to electrolyte abnormalities (such as diuretics or amphotericin B)).
No products indexed under this heading.

Chlorprothixene (Arsenic trioxide can cause QT interval prolongation and complete atrioventricular block. Caution is advised when arsenic trioxide is co-administered with other medications that can prolong the QT interval (eg, certain antiarrhythmics or thioridazine) or lead to electrolyte abnormalities (such as diuretics or amphotericin B)).
No products indexed under this heading.

Chlorprothixene Hydrochloride (Arsenic trioxide can cause QT interval prolongation and complete atrioventricular block. Caution is advised when arsenic trioxide is co-administered with other medications that can prolong the QT interval (eg, certain antiarrhythmics or thioridazine) or lead to electrolyte abnormalities (such as diuretics or amphotericin B)).
No products indexed under this heading.

Chlorthalidone (Arsenic trioxide can cause QT interval prolongation and complete atrioventricular block. Caution is advised when arsenic trioxide is co-administered with other medications that can prolong the QT interval (eg, certain antiarrhythmics or thioridazine) or lead to electrolyte abnormalities (such as diuretics or amphotericin B)). Products include:
Clorpres 2344

Clomipramine Hydrochloride (Arsenic trioxide can cause QT interval prolongation and complete atrioventricular block. Caution is advised when arsenic trioxide is co-administered with other medications that can prolong the QT interval (eg, certain antiarrhythmics or thioridazine) or lead to electrolyte abnormalities (such as diuretics or amphotericin B)).
No products indexed under this heading.

1941 Interactions Index Trisenox

Clorazepate Dipotassium (Arsenic trioxide can cause QT interval prolongation and complete atrioventricular block. Caution is advised when arsenic trioxide is co-administered with other medications that can prolong the QT interval (eg, certain antiarrhythmics or thioridazine) or lead to electrolyte abnormalities (such as diuretics or amphotericin B)).
No products indexed under this heading.

Clozapine (Arsenic trioxide can cause QT interval prolongation and complete atrioventricular block. Caution is advised when arsenic trioxide is co-administered with other medications that can prolong the QT interval (eg, certain antiarrhythmics or thioridazine) or lead to electrolyte abnormalities (such as diuretics or amphotericin B)).
No products indexed under this heading.

Desipramine Hydrochloride (Arsenic trioxide can cause QT interval prolongation and complete atrioventricular block. Caution is advised when arsenic trioxide is co-administered with other medications that can prolong the QT interval (eg, certain antiarrhythmics or thioridazine) or lead to electrolyte abnormalities (such as diuretics or amphotericin B)).
No products indexed under this heading.

Diazepam (Arsenic trioxide can cause QT interval prolongation and complete atrioventricular block. Caution is advised when arsenic trioxide is co-administered with other medications that can prolong the QT interval (eg, certain antiarrhythmics or thioridazine) or lead to electrolyte abnormalities (such as diuretics or amphotericin B)). Products include:
Valium Tablets 2880

Disopyramide (Arsenic trioxide can cause QT interval prolongation and complete atrioventricular block. Caution is advised when arsenic trioxide is co-administered with other medications that can prolong the QT interval (eg, certain antiarrhythmics or thioridazine) or lead to electrolyte abnormalities (such as diuretics or amphotericin B)).
No products indexed under this heading.

Disopyramide Phosphate (Arsenic trioxide can cause QT interval prolongation and complete atrioventricular block. Caution is advised when arsenic trioxide is co-administered with other medications that can prolong the QT interval (eg, certain antiarrhythmics or thioridazine) or lead to electrolyte abnormalities (such as diuretics or amphotericin B)).
No products indexed under this heading.

Dofetilide (Arsenic trioxide can cause QT interval prolongation and complete atrioventricular block. Caution is advised when arsenic trioxide is co-administered with other medications that can prolong the QT interval (eg, certain antiarrhythmics or thioridazine) or lead to electrolyte abnormalities (such as diuretics or amphotericin B)).
No products indexed under this heading.

Doxepin Hydrochloride (Arsenic trioxide can cause QT interval prolongation and complete atrioventricular block. Caution is advised when arsenic trioxide is co-administered with other medications that can prolong the QT interval (eg, certain antiarrhythmics or thioridazine) or lead to electrolyte abnormalities (such as diuretics or amphotericin B)).
No products indexed under this heading.

Droperidol (Arsenic trioxide can cause QT interval prolongation and complete atrioventricular block. Caution is advised when arsenic trioxide is co-administered with other medications that can prolong the QT interval (eg, certain antiarrhythmics or thioridazine) or lead to electrolyte abnormalities (such as diuretics or amphotericin B)).
No products indexed under this heading.

Erythromycin (Arsenic trioxide can cause QT interval prolongation and complete atrioventricular block. Caution is advised when arsenic trioxide is co-administered with other medications that can prolong the QT interval (eg, certain antiarrhythmics or thioridazine) or lead to electrolyte abnormalities (such as diuretics or amphotericin B)).
No products indexed under this heading.

Erythromycin Estolate (Arsenic trioxide can cause QT interval prolongation and complete atrioventricular block. Caution is advised when arsenic trioxide is co-administered with other medications that can prolong the QT interval (eg, certain antiarrhythmics or thioridazine) or lead to electrolyte abnormalities (such as diuretics or amphotericin B)).
No products indexed under this heading.

Erythromycin Ethylsuccinate (Arsenic trioxide can cause QT interval prolongation and complete atrioventricular block. Caution is advised when arsenic trioxide is co-administered with other medications that can prolong the QT interval (eg, certain antiarrhythmics or thioridazine) or lead to electrolyte abnormalities (such as diuretics or amphotericin B)). Products include:
E.E.S. 437
EryPed 435

Erythromycin Gluceptate (Arsenic trioxide can cause QT interval prolongation and complete atrioventricular block. Caution is advised when arsenic trioxide is co-administered with other medications that can prolong the QT interval (eg, certain antiarrhythmics or thioridazine) or lead to electrolyte abnormalities (such as diuretics or amphotericin B)).
No products indexed under this heading.

Erythromycin Lactobionate (Arsenic trioxide can cause QT interval prolongation and complete atrioventricular block. Caution is advised when arsenic trioxide is co-administered with other medications that can prolong the QT interval (eg, certain antiarrhythmics or thioridazine) or lead to electrolyte abnormalities (such as diuretics or amphotericin B)).
No products indexed under this heading.

Erythromycin Stearate (Arsenic trioxide can cause QT interval prolongation and complete atrioventricular block. Caution is advised when arsenic trioxide is co-administered with other medications that can prolong the QT interval (eg, certain antiarrhythmics or thioridazine) or lead to electrolyte abnormalities (such as diuretics or amphotericin B)).
No products indexed under this heading.

Ethacrynic Acid (Arsenic trioxide can cause QT interval prolongation and complete atrioventricular block. Concomitant administration of potassium wasting diuretic can increase the risk of QT prolongation).
No products indexed under this heading.

Flecainide Acetate (Arsenic trioxide can cause QT interval prolongation and complete atrioventricular block. Caution is advised when arsenic trioxide is co-administered with other medications that can prolong the QT interval (eg, certain antiarrhythmics or thioridazine) or lead to electrolyte abnormalities (such as diuretics or amphotericin B)).
No products indexed under this heading.

Fluphenazine Decanoate (Arsenic trioxide can cause QT interval prolongation and complete atrioventricular block. Caution is advised when arsenic trioxide is co-administered with other medications that can prolong the QT interval (eg, certain antiarrhythmics or thioridazine) or lead to electrolyte abnormalities (such as diuretics or amphotericin B)).
No products indexed under this heading.

Fluphenazine Enanthate (Arsenic trioxide can cause QT interval prolongation and complete atrioventricular block. Caution is advised when arsenic trioxide is co-administered with other medications that can prolong the QT interval (eg, certain antiarrhythmics or thioridazine) or lead to electrolyte abnormalities (such as diuretics or amphotericin B)).
No products indexed under this heading.

Fluphenazine Hydrochloride (Arsenic trioxide can cause QT interval prolongation and complete atrioventricular block. Caution is advised when arsenic trioxide is co-administered with other medications that can prolong the QT interval (eg, certain antiarrhythmics or thioridazine) or lead to electrolyte abnormalities (such as diuretics or amphotericin B)).
No products indexed under this heading.

Furosemide (Arsenic trioxide can cause QT interval prolongation and complete atrioventricular block. Concomitant administration of potassium wasting diuretic can increase the risk of QT prolongation). Products include:
Furosemide 2354

Haloperidol (Arsenic trioxide can cause QT interval prolongation and complete atrioventricular block. Caution is advised when arsenic trioxide is co-administered with other medications that can prolong the QT interval (eg, certain antiarrhythmics or thioridazine) or lead to electrolyte abnormalities (such as diuretics or amphotericin B)).
No products indexed under this heading.

Haloperidol Decanoate (Arsenic trioxide can cause QT interval prolongation and complete atrioventricular block. Caution is advised when arsenic trioxide is co-administered with other medications that can prolong the QT interval (eg, certain antiarrhythmics or thioridazine) or lead to electrolyte abnormalities (such as diuretics or amphotericin B)).
No products indexed under this heading.

Haloperidol Lactate (Arsenic trioxide can cause QT interval prolongation and complete atrioventricular block. Caution is advised when arsenic trioxide is co-administered with other medications that can prolong the QT interval (eg, certain antiarrhythmics or thioridazine) or lead to electrolyte abnormalities (such as diuretics or amphotericin B)).
No products indexed under this heading.

Hydrochlorothiazide (Arsenic trioxide can cause QT interval prolongation and complete atrioventricular block. Concomitant administration of potassium wasting diuretic can increase the risk of QT prolongation). Products include:
Atacand HCT 700
Avalide 2956
Benicar HCT 1017
Diovan HCT 2419
Dyazide 1429
Exforge HCT 2449
Hyzaar 2162
Hyzaar 100-12.5 2162
Micardis HCT 889
Prinzide 2246
Tekturna HCT 2541
Teveten HCT 541

Hydroflumethiazide (Arsenic trioxide can cause QT interval prolongation and complete atrioventricular block. Concomitant administration of potassium wasting diuretic can increase the risk of QT prolongation).
No products indexed under this heading.

Hydroxyzine Hydrochloride (Arsenic trioxide can cause QT interval prolongation and complete atrioventricular block. Caution is advised when arsenic trioxide is co-administered with other medications that can prolong the QT interval (eg, certain antiarrhythmics or thioridazine) or lead to electrolyte abnormalities (such as diuretics or amphotericin B)).
No products indexed under this heading.

Imipramine Hydrochloride (Arsenic trioxide can cause QT interval prolongation and complete atrioventricular block. Caution is advised when arsenic trioxide is co-administered with other medications that can prolong the QT interval (eg, certain antiarrhythmics or thioridazine) or lead to electrolyte abnormalities (such as diuretics or amphotericin B)).
No products indexed under this heading.

Imipramine Pamoate (Arsenic trioxide can cause QT interval prolongation and complete atrioventricular block. Caution is advised when arsenic trioxide is co-administered with other medications that can prolong the QT interval (eg, certain antiarrhythmics or thioridazine) or lead to electrolyte abnormalities (such as diuretics or amphotericin B)).
No products indexed under this heading.

Indapamide (Arsenic trioxide can cause QT interval prolongation and complete atrioventricular block. Caution is advised when arsenic trioxide is co-administered with other medications that can prolong the QT interval (eg, certain antiarrhythmics or thioridazine) or lead to electrolyte abnormalities (such as diuretics or amphotericin B)). Products include:
Indapamide 2356

Isocarboxazid (Arsenic trioxide can cause QT interval prolongation and complete atrioventricular block. Caution is advised when arsenic trioxide is co-administered with other medications that can prolong the QT interval (eg, certain antiarrhythmics or thioridazine) or lead to electrolyte abnormalities (such as diuretics or amphotericin B)). Products include:
Marplan 3481

Lidocaine (Arsenic trioxide can cause QT interval prolongation and complete atrioventricular block. Caution is advised when arsenic trioxide is co-administered with other medications that can prolong the QT interval (eg, certain antiarrhythmics or thioridazine) or lead to electrolyte abnormalities (such as diuretics or amphotericin B)). Products include:
Lidoderm 1107

Lidocaine Hydrochloride (Arsenic trioxide can cause QT interval prolongation and complete atrioventricular block. Caution is advised when arsenic trioxide is co-administered with other medications that can prolong the QT interval (eg, certain antiarrhythmics or thioridazine) or lead to electrolyte abnormalities (such as diuretics or amphotericin B)).
No products indexed under this heading.

IMPORTANT NOTE: Always consult each drug listing in the patient's regimen for possible interactions.

Lithium Carbonate (Arsenic trioxide can cause QT interval prolongation and complete atrioventricular block. Caution is advised when arsenic trioxide is co-administered with other medications that can prolong the QT interval (eg, certain antiarrhythmics or thioridazine) or lead to electrolyte abnormalities (such as diuretics or amphotericin B)).
No products indexed under this heading.

Lithium Citrate (Arsenic trioxide can cause QT interval prolongation and complete atrioventricular block. Caution is advised when arsenic trioxide is co-administered with other medications that can prolong the QT interval (eg, certain antiarrhythmics or thioridazine) or lead to electrolyte abnormalities (such as diuretics or amphotericin B)).
No products indexed under this heading.

Lorazepam (Arsenic trioxide can cause QT interval prolongation and complete atrioventricular block. Caution is advised when arsenic trioxide is co-administered with other medications that can prolong the QT interval (eg, certain antiarrhythmics or thioridazine) or lead to electrolyte abnormalities (such as diuretics or amphotericin B)).
No products indexed under this heading.

Loxapine Hydrochloride (Arsenic trioxide can cause QT interval prolongation and complete atrioventricular block. Caution is advised when arsenic trioxide is co-administered with other medications that can prolong the QT interval (eg, certain antiarrhythmics or thioridazine) or lead to electrolyte abnormalities (such as diuretics or amphotericin B)).
No products indexed under this heading.

Loxapine Succinate (Arsenic trioxide can cause QT interval prolongation and complete atrioventricular block. Caution is advised when arsenic trioxide is co-administered with other medications that can prolong the QT interval (eg, certain antiarrhythmics or thioridazine) or lead to electrolyte abnormalities (such as diuretics or amphotericin B)).
No products indexed under this heading.

Maprotiline Hydrochloride (Arsenic trioxide can cause QT interval prolongation and complete atrioventricular block. Caution is advised when arsenic trioxide is co-administered with other medications that can prolong the QT interval (eg, certain antiarrhythmics or thioridazine) or lead to electrolyte abnormalities (such as diuretics or amphotericin B)).
No products indexed under this heading.

Meprobamate (Arsenic trioxide can cause QT interval prolongation and complete atrioventricular block. Caution is advised when arsenic trioxide is co-administered with other medications that can prolong the QT interval (eg, certain antiarrhythmics or thioridazine) or lead to electrolyte abnormalities (such as diuretics or amphotericin B)).
No products indexed under this heading.

Mesoridazine Besylate (Arsenic trioxide can cause QT interval prolongation and complete atrioventricular block. Caution is advised when arsenic trioxide is co-administered with other medications that can prolong the QT interval (eg, certain antiarrhythmics or thioridazine) or lead to electrolyte abnormalities (such as diuretics or amphotericin B)).
No products indexed under this heading.

Methyclothiazide (Arsenic trioxide can cause QT interval prolongation and complete atrioventricular block. Concomitant administration of potassium wasting diuretic can increase the risk of QT prolongation).
No products indexed under this heading.

Metolazone (Arsenic trioxide can cause QT interval prolongation and complete atrioventricular block. Caution is advised when arsenic trioxide is co-administered with other medications that can prolong the QT interval (eg, certain antiarrhythmics or thioridazine) or lead to electrolyte abnormalities (such as diuretics or amphotericin B)).
No products indexed under this heading.

Mexiletine Hydrochloride (Arsenic trioxide can cause QT interval prolongation and complete atrioventricular block. Caution is advised when arsenic trioxide is co-administered with other medications that can prolong the QT interval (eg, certain antiarrhythmics or thioridazine) or lead to electrolyte abnormalities (such as diuretics or amphotericin B)).
No products indexed under this heading.

Midazolam Hydrochloride (Arsenic trioxide can cause QT interval prolongation and complete atrioventricular block. Caution is advised when arsenic trioxide is co-administered with other medications that can prolong the QT interval (eg, certain antiarrhythmics or thioridazine) or lead to electrolyte abnormalities (such as diuretics or amphotericin B)).
No products indexed under this heading.

Molindone Hydrochloride (Arsenic trioxide can cause QT interval prolongation and complete atrioventricular block. Caution is advised when arsenic trioxide is co-administered with other medications that can prolong the QT interval (eg, certain antiarrhythmics or thioridazine) or lead to electrolyte abnormalities (such as diuretics or amphotericin B)). Products include:
Moban 1108

Moricizine Hydrochloride (Arsenic trioxide can cause QT interval prolongation and complete atrioventricular block. Caution is advised when arsenic trioxide is co-administered with other medications that can prolong the QT interval (eg, certain antiarrhythmics or thioridazine) or lead to electrolyte abnormalities (such as diuretics or amphotericin B)).
No products indexed under this heading.

Nortriptyline Hydrochloride (Arsenic trioxide can cause QT interval prolongation and complete atrioventricular block. Caution is advised when arsenic trioxide is co-administered with other medications that can prolong the QT interval (eg, certain antiarrhythmics or thioridazine) or lead to electrolyte abnormalities (such as diuretics or amphotericin B)).
No products indexed under this heading.

Olanzapine (Arsenic trioxide can cause QT interval prolongation and complete atrioventricular block. Caution is advised when arsenic trioxide is co-administered with other medications that can prolong the QT interval (eg, certain antiarrhythmics or thioridazine) or lead to electrolyte abnormalities (such as diuretics or amphotericin B)). Products include:
Symbyax 1965
Zyprexa 1984
Zyprexa IntraMuscular 1984
Zyprexa ZYDIS 1984

Oxazepam (Arsenic trioxide can cause QT interval prolongation and complete atrioventricular block. Caution is advised when arsenic trioxide is co-administered with other medications that can prolong the QT interval (eg, certain antiarrhythmics or thioridazine) or lead to electrolyte abnormalities (such as diuretics or amphotericin B)).
No products indexed under this heading.

Perphenazine (Arsenic trioxide can cause QT interval prolongation and complete atrioventricular block. Caution is advised when arsenic trioxide is co-administered with other medications that can prolong the QT interval (eg, certain antiarrhythmics or thioridazine) or lead to electrolyte abnormalities (such as diuretics or amphotericin B)).
No products indexed under this heading.

Phenelzine Sulfate (Arsenic trioxide can cause QT interval prolongation and complete atrioventricular block. Caution is advised when arsenic trioxide is co-administered with other medications that can prolong the QT interval (eg, certain antiarrhythmics or thioridazine) or lead to electrolyte abnormalities (such as diuretics or amphotericin B)).
No products indexed under this heading.

Polythiazide (Arsenic trioxide can cause QT interval prolongation and complete atrioventricular block. Concomitant administration of potassium wasting diuretic can increase the risk of QT prolongation).
No products indexed under this heading.

Prazepam (Arsenic trioxide can cause QT interval prolongation and complete atrioventricular block. Caution is advised when arsenic trioxide is co-administered with other medications that can prolong the QT interval (eg, certain antiarrhythmics or thioridazine) or lead to electrolyte abnormalities (such as diuretics or amphotericin B)).
No products indexed under this heading.

Procainamide Hydrochloride (Arsenic trioxide can cause QT interval prolongation and complete atrioventricular block. Caution is advised when arsenic trioxide is co-administered with other medications that can prolong the QT interval (eg, certain antiarrhythmics or thioridazine) or lead to electrolyte abnormalities (such as diuretics or amphotericin B)).
No products indexed under this heading.

Prochlorperazine (Arsenic trioxide can cause QT interval prolongation and complete atrioventricular block. Caution is advised when arsenic trioxide is co-administered with other medications that can prolong the QT interval (eg, certain antiarrhythmics or thioridazine) or lead to electrolyte abnormalities (such as diuretics or amphotericin B)).
No products indexed under this heading.

Promethazine Hydrochloride (Arsenic trioxide can cause QT interval prolongation and complete atrioventricular block. Caution is advised when arsenic trioxide is co-administered with other medications that can prolong the QT interval (eg, certain antiarrhythmics or thioridazine) or lead to electrolyte abnormalities (such as diuretics or amphotericin B)).
No products indexed under this heading.

Propafenone Hydrochloride (Arsenic trioxide can cause QT interval prolongation and complete atrioventricular block. Caution is advised when arsenic trioxide is co-administered with other medications that can prolong the QT interval (eg, certain antiarrhythmics or thioridazine) or lead to electrolyte abnormalities (such as diuretics or amphotericin B)). Products include:
Rythmol 1648
Rythmol SR 1652

Propranolol Hydrochloride (Arsenic trioxide can cause QT interval prolongation and complete atrioventricular block. Caution is advised when arsenic trioxide is co-administered with other medications that can prolong the QT interval (eg, certain antiarrhythmics or thioridazine) or lead to electrolyte abnormalities (such as diuretics or amphotericin B)). Products include:
InnoPran XL 1517

Protriptyline Hydrochloride (Arsenic trioxide can cause QT interval prolongation and complete atrioventricular block. Caution is advised when arsenic trioxide is co-administered with other medications that can prolong the QT interval (eg, certain antiarrhythmics or thioridazine) or lead to electrolyte abnormalities (such as diuretics or amphotericin B)).
No products indexed under this heading.

Quetiapine Fumarate (Arsenic trioxide can cause QT interval prolongation and complete atrioventricular block. Caution is advised when arsenic trioxide is co-administered with other medications that can prolong the QT interval (eg, certain antiarrhythmics or thioridazine) or lead to electrolyte abnormalities (such as diuretics or amphotericin B)). Products include:
Seroquel 750
Seroquel XR 759

Quinidine (Arsenic trioxide can cause QT interval prolongation and complete atrioventricular block. Caution is advised when arsenic trioxide is co-administered with other medications that can prolong the QT interval (eg, certain antiarrhythmics or thioridazine) or lead to electrolyte abnormalities (such as diuretics or amphotericin B)).
No products indexed under this heading.

Quinidine Gluconate (Arsenic trioxide can cause QT interval prolongation and complete atrioventricular block. Caution is advised when arsenic trioxide is co-administered with other medications that can prolong the QT interval (eg, certain antiarrhythmics or thioridazine) or lead to electrolyte abnormalities (such as diuretics or amphotericin B)).
No products indexed under this heading.

Quinidine Hydrochloride (Arsenic trioxide can cause QT interval prolongation and complete atrioventricular block. Caution is advised when arsenic trioxide is co-administered with other medications that can prolong the QT interval (eg, certain antiarrhythmics or thioridazine) or lead to electrolyte abnormalities (such as diuretics or amphotericin B)).
No products indexed under this heading.

Quinidine Polygalacturonate (Arsenic trioxide can cause QT interval prolongation and complete atrioventricular block. Caution is advised when arsenic trioxide is co-administered with other medications that can prolong the QT interval (eg, certain antiarrhythmics or thioridazine) or lead to electrolyte abnormalities (such as diuretics or amphotericin B)).
No products indexed under this heading.

Quinidine Sulfate (Arsenic trioxide can cause QT interval prolongation and complete atrioventricular block. Caution is advised when arsenic trioxide is co-administered with other medications that can prolong the QT interval (eg, certain antiarrhythmics or thioridazine) or lead to electrolyte abnormalities (such as diuretics or amphotericin B)).
No products indexed under this heading.

Risperidone (Arsenic trioxide can cause QT interval prolongation and complete atrioventricular block. Caution is advised when arsenic trioxide is co-administered with other medications that can prolong the QT interval (eg, certain antiarrhythmics or thioridazine) or lead to electrolyte abnormalities (such as diuretics or amphotericin B)). Products include:
Risperdal Consta 2682

Sotalol Hydrochloride (Arsenic trioxide can cause QT interval prolongation and complete atrioventricular block. Caution is advised when arsenic trioxide is co-administered with other medications that can prolong the QT interval (eg, certain antiarrhythmics or thioridazine) or lead to electrolyte abnormalities (such as diuretics or amphotericin B)).
No products indexed under this heading.

Spironolactone (Arsenic trioxide can cause QT interval prolongation and complete atrioventricular block. Caution is advised when arsenic trioxide is co-administered with other medications that can prolong the QT interval (eg, certain antiarrhythmics or thioridazine) or lead to electrolyte abnormalities (such as diuretics or amphotericin B)).
No products indexed under this heading.

Thioridazine Hydrochloride (Arsenic trioxide can cause QT interval prolongation and complete atrioventricular block. Hence, caution is advised when arsenic trioxide is co-administered with other medications that can prolong the QT interval (eg, certain antiarrhythmics or thioridazine) or lead to electrolyte abnormalities (such as diuretics or amphotericin B)). Products include:

Thiothixene (Arsenic trioxide can cause QT interval prolongation and complete atrioventricular block. Caution is advised when arsenic trioxide is co-administered with other medications that can prolong the QT interval (eg, certain antiarrhythmics or thioridazine) or lead to electrolyte abnormalities (such as diuretics or amphotericin B)). Products include:

Tocainide Hydrochloride (Arsenic trioxide can cause QT interval prolongation and complete atrioventricular block. Caution is advised when arsenic trioxide is co-administered with other medications that can prolong the QT interval (eg, certain antiarrhythmics or thioridazine) or lead to electrolyte abnormalities (such as diuretics or amphotericin B)).
No products indexed under this heading.

Torsemide (Arsenic trioxide can cause QT interval prolongation and complete atrioventricular block. Concomitant administration of potassium wasting diuretic can increase the risk of QT prolongation).
No products indexed under this heading.

Tranylcypromine Sulfate (Arsenic trioxide can cause QT interval prolongation and complete atrioventricular block. Caution is advised when arsenic trioxide is co-administered with other medications that can prolong the QT interval (eg, certain antiarrhythmics or thioridazine) or lead to electrolyte abnormalities (such as diuretics or amphotericin B)). Products include:

Triamterene (Arsenic trioxide can cause QT interval prolongation and complete atrioventricular block. Caution is advised when arsenic trioxide is co-administered with other medications that can prolong the QT interval (eg, certain antiarrhythmics or thioridazine) or lead to electrolyte abnormalities (such as diuretics or amphotericin B)). Products include:

Trifluoperazine Hydrochloride (Arsenic trioxide can cause QT interval prolongation and complete atrioventricular block. Caution is advised when arsenic trioxide is co-administered with other medications that can prolong the QT interval (eg, certain antiarrhythmics or thioridazine) or lead to electrolyte abnormalities (such as diuretics or amphotericin B)).
No products indexed under this heading.

Trimipramine Maleate (Arsenic trioxide can cause QT interval prolongation and complete atrioventricular block. Caution is advised when arsenic trioxide is co-administered with other medications that can prolong the QT interval (eg, certain antiarrhythmics or thioridazine) or lead to electrolyte abnormalities (such as diuretics or amphotericin B)).
No products indexed under this heading.

Verapamil Hydrochloride (Arsenic trioxide can cause QT interval prolongation and complete atrioventricular block. Caution is advised when arsenic trioxide is co-administered with other medications that can prolong the QT interval (eg, certain antiarrhythmics or thioridazine) or lead to electrolyte abnormalities (such as diuretics or amphotericin B)). Products include:

Ziprasidone Hydrochloride (Arsenic trioxide can cause QT interval prolongation and complete atrioventricular block. Caution is advised when arsenic trioxide is co-administered with other medications that can prolong the QT interval (eg, certain antiarrhythmics or thioridazine) or lead to electrolyte abnormalities (such as diuretics or amphotericin B)). Products include:

TRIZIVIR TABLETS

(Abacavir Sulfate, Lamivudine, Zidovudine) 1688
May interact with agents associated with myelosuppression, alcohols, cytotoxic drugs, valproate, and certain other agents. Compounds in these categories include:

Altretamine (Co-administration with bone marrow suppressive agents may increase the hematologic toxicity of zidovudine). Products include:

Atovaquone (Co-administration may alter zidovudine blood concentrations; routine dose modification is not warranted). Products include:

Bleomycin Sulfate (Co-administration with cytotoxic agents may increase the hematologic toxicity of zidovudine).
No products indexed under this heading.

Busulfan (Co-administration with bone marrow suppressive agents may increase the hematologic toxicity of zidovudine). Products include:

Chlorambucil (Co-administration with bone marrow suppressive agents may increase the hematologic toxicity of zidovudine). Products include:

Chloramphenicol (Co-administration with bone marrow suppressive agents may increase the hematologic toxicity of zidovudine).
No products indexed under this heading.

Chloramphenicol Palmitate (Co-administration with bone marrow suppressive agents may increase the hematologic toxicity of zidovudine).
No products indexed under this heading.

Chloramphenicol Sodium Succinate (Co-administration with bone marrow suppressive agents may increase the hematologic toxicity of zidovudine).
No products indexed under this heading.

Cladribine (Co-administration with bone marrow suppressive agents may increase the hematologic toxicity of zidovudine). Products include:

Cyclophosphamide (Co-administration with cytotoxic agents may increase the hematologic toxicity of zidovudine).
No products indexed under this heading.

Daunorubicin Citrate Liposome (Co-administration with bone marrow suppressive agents may increase the hematologic toxicity of zidovudine).
No products indexed under this heading.

Daunorubicin Hydrochloride (Co-administration with cytotoxic agents may increase the hematologic toxicity of zidovudine).
No products indexed under this heading.

Dexrazoxane (Co-administration with bone marrow suppressive agents may increase the hematologic toxicity of zidovudine).
No products indexed under this heading.

Divalproex Sodium (Co-administration with valproic acid may alter zidovudine blood concentrations; routine dose modification is not warranted). Products include:

Doxorubicin Hydrochloride (Co-administration with cytotoxic agents may increase the hematologic toxicity of zidovudine).
No products indexed under this heading.

Doxorubicin Hydrochloride Liposome (Co-administration with bone marrow suppressive agents may increase the hematologic toxicity of zidovudine). Products include:

Emtricitabine (Trizivir should not be administered concomitantly with emtricitabine). Products include:

Epirubicin Hydrochloride (Co-administration with cytotoxic agents may increase the hematologic toxicity of zidovudine).
No products indexed under this heading.

Ethanol (Concurrent use with ethanol decreases the elimination of abacavir causing an increase in overall exposure).
No products indexed under this heading.

Ethyl Alcohol (Concurrent use with ethanol decreases the elimination of abacavir causing an increase in overall exposure).
No products indexed under this heading.

Fluconazole (Co-administration may alter zidovudine blood concentrations; routine dose modification is not warranted).
No products indexed under this heading.

Fludarabine Phosphate (Co-administration with bone marrow suppressive agents may increase the hematologic toxicity of zidovudine). Products include:

Fluorouracil (Co-administration with cytotoxic agents may increase the hematologic toxicity of zidovudine). Products include:

Ganciclovir (Co-administration may increase the hematologic toxicity of zidovudine).
No products indexed under this heading.

Ganciclovir Sodium (Co-administration may increase the hematologic toxicity of zidovudine).
No products indexed under this heading.

Gemcitabine Hydrochloride (Co-administration with bone marrow suppressive agents may increase the hematologic toxicity of zidovudine). Products include:

Gemtuzumab Ozogamicin (Co-administration with bone marrow suppressive agents may increase the hematologic toxicity of zidovudine). Products include:

Hydroxyurea (Co-administration with cytotoxic agents may increase the hematologic toxicity of zidovudine).
No products indexed under this heading.

Idarubicin Hydrochloride (Co-administration with bone marrow suppressive agents may increase the hematologic toxicity of zidovudine).
No products indexed under this heading.

Interferon alfa-2a, Recombinant (Hepatic decompensation (some fatal) has occurred in HIV-1/HCV co-infected patients receiving combination antiretroviral therapy for HIV-1 and interferon alfa with or without ribavirin. Patients receiving interferon alfa with or without ribavirin and Trizivir should be closely monitored for treatment-associated toxicities, especially hepatic decompensation, neutropenia, and anemia. Discontinuation of Trizivir should be considered as medically appropriate. Dose reduction or discontinuation of interferon alfa, ribavirin, or both should also be considered if worsening clinical toxicities are observed, including hepatic decompensation).
No products indexed under this heading.

Interferon Alfacon-1 (Hepatic decompensation (some fatal) has occurred in HIV-1/HCV co-infected patients receiving combination antiretroviral therapy for HIV-1 and interferon alfa with or without ribavirin. Patients receiving interferon alfa with or without ribavirin and Trizivir should be closely monitored for treatment-associated toxicities, especially hepatic decompensation, neutropenia, and anemia. Discontinuation of Trizivir should be considered as medically appropriate. Dose reduction or discontinuation of interferon alfa, ribavirin, or both should also be considered if worsening clinical toxicities are observed, including hepatic decompensation).
No products indexed under this heading.

Interferon alfa-N3 (Human Leukocyte Derived) (Hepatic decompensation (some fatal) has occurred in HIV-1/HCV co-infected patients receiving combination antiretroviral therapy for HIV-1 and interferon alfa with or without ribavirin. Patients receiving interferon alfa with or without ribavirin and Trizivir should be closely monitored for treatment-associated toxicities, especially hepatic decompensation, neutropenia, and anemia. Discontinuation of Trizivir should be considered as medically appropriate. Dose reduction or discontinuation of interferon alfa, ribavirin, or both should also be considered if worsening clinical toxicities are observed, including hepatic decompensation). Products include:

Irinotecan Hydrochloride (Co-administration with bone marrow suppressive agents may increase the hematologic toxicity of zidovudine).
No products indexed under this heading.

Melphalan Hydrochloride (Co-administration with bone marrow sup-

pressive agents may increase the hematologic toxicity of zidovudine). Products include:
Alkeran for Injection 1300

Mercaptopurine (Co-administration with bone marrow suppressive agents may increase the hematologic toxicity of zidovudine).
No products indexed under this heading.

Methadone Hydrochloride (In a study of 11 HIV-1-infected patients receiving methadone-maintenance therapy (40 mg and 90 mg daily), with 600 mg of Ziagen twice daily (twice the currently recommended dose), oral methadone clearance increased 22%. This alteration will not result in a methadone dose modification in the majority of patients; however, an increased methadone dose may be required in a small number of patients).
No products indexed under this heading.

Methotrexate Sodium (Co-administration with cytotoxic agents may increase the hematologic toxicity of zidovudine).
No products indexed under this heading.

Mitotane (Co-administration with cytotoxic agents may increase the hematologic toxicity of zidovudine).
No products indexed under this heading.

Mitoxantrone Hydrochloride (Co-administration with cytotoxic agents may increase the hematologic toxicity of zidovudine). Products include:
Novantrone 1088

Nelfinavir Mesylate (Co-administration may alter lamivudine and zidovudine blood concentrations; routine dose modification is not warranted).
No products indexed under this heading.

Probenecid (Co-administration may alter zidovudine blood concentrations; routine dose modification is not warranted).
No products indexed under this heading.

Procarbazine Hydrochloride (Co-administration with cytotoxic agents may increase the hematologic toxicity of zidovudine).
No products indexed under this heading.

Ribavirin (*In vitro* studies have shown ribavirin can reduce the phosphorylation of pyrimidine nucleoside analogues, such as lamivudine and zidovudine, components of Trizivir. Although no evidence of a pharmacokinetic or pharmacodynamic interaction was seen when ribavirin was co-administered with lamivudine or zidovudine in HIV-1/HCV co-infected patients, hepatic decompensation (some fatal) has occurred in HIV-1/HCV co-infected patients receiving combination antiretroviral therapy for HIV-1 and interferon alfa with or without ribavirin. Patients receiving interferon alfa with or without ribavirin and Trizivir should be closely monitored for treatment-associated toxicities. Discontinuation of Trizivir should be considered as medically appropriate. Dose reduction or discontinuation of interferon alfa, ribavirin, or both should also be considered if worsening clinical toxicities are observed, including hepatic decompensation). Products include:
Rebetol 3207

Ritonavir (Co-administration may alter zidovudine blood concentrations; routine dose modification is not warranted). Products include:
Kaletra 458
Norvir 509

Stavudine (Co-administration of zidovudine with stavudine should be avoided since an antagonistic relationship has been demonstrated *in vitro*).
No products indexed under this heading.

Sulfamethoxazole (Co-administration with trimethoprim (TMP) 160 mg/sulfamethoxazole (SMX) 800 mg once daily has been shown to increase lamivudine exposure (AUC). The effect of higher doses of TMP/SMX on lamivudine pharmacokinetics has not been investigated; routine dose modification is not warranted).
No products indexed under this heading.

Tamoxifen Citrate (Co-administration with cytotoxic agents may increase the hematologic toxicity of zidovudine).
No products indexed under this heading.

Temozolomide (Co-administration with bone marrow suppressive agents may increase the hematologic toxicity of zidovudine). Products include:
Temodar 3230
Temodar Injection 3230

Tenofovir Disoproxil Fumarate (Trizivir should not be administered concomitantly with the fixed-dose combination drugs emtricitabine and tenofovir). Products include:
Atripla 906
Truvada 1258
Viread 1266

Thioguanine (Co-administration with bone marrow suppressive agents may increase the hematologic toxicity of zidovudine). Products include:
Tabloid 1664

Trimethoprim (Co-administration with trimethoprim (TMP) 160 mg/sulfamethoxazole (SMX) 800 mg once daily has been shown to increase lamivudine exposure (AUC). The effect of higher doses of TMP/SMX on lamivudine pharmacokinetics has not been investigated; routine dose modification is not warranted).
No products indexed under this heading.

Valproate Sodium (Co-administration with valproic acid may alter zidovudine blood concentrations; routine dose modification is not warranted).
No products indexed under this heading.

Valproic Acid (Co-administration with valproic acid may alter zidovudine blood concentrations; routine dose modification is not warranted).
No products indexed under this heading.

Vinblastine Sulfate (Co-administration with cytotoxic agents may increase the hematologic toxicity of zidovudine).
No products indexed under this heading.

Vincristine Sulfate (Co-administration with cytotoxic agents may increase the hematologic toxicity of zidovudine).
No products indexed under this heading.

Vinorelbine Tartrate (Co-administration with cytotoxic agents may increase the hematologic toxicity of zidovudine).
No products indexed under this heading.

Zalacitabine (Lamivudine and zalcitabine may inhibit the intracellular phosphorylation of one another. Therefore, use of Trizivir in combination with zalcitabine is not recommended).
No products indexed under this heading.

Food Interactions

Alcohol (Concurrent use with ethanol decreases the elimination of abacavir causing an increase in overall exposure).

Beer, reduced-alcohol (Concurrent use with ethanol decreases the elimination of abacavir causing an increase in overall exposure).

Beer, unspecified (Concurrent use with ethanol decreases the elimination of abacavir causing an increase in overall exposure).

Wine, Chianti (Concurrent use with ethanol decreases the elimination of abacavir causing an increase in overall exposure).

Wine, Red (Concurrent use with ethanol decreases the elimination of abacavir causing an increase in overall exposure).

Wine, unspecified (Concurrent use with ethanol decreases the elimination of abacavir causing an increase in overall exposure).

Wine products (Concurrent use with ethanol decreases the elimination of abacavir causing an increase in overall exposure).

TRUSOPT STERILE OPHTHALMIC SOLUTION

(Dorzolamide Hydrochloride) 2279
May interact with carbonic anhydrase inhibitors, salicylates. Compounds in these categories include:

Acetazolamide (There is a potential for an additive effect on the known systemic effects of carbonic anhydrase inhibition in patients receiving an oral carbonic anhydrase inhibitor and dorzolamide hydrochloride. The concomitant administration of dorzolamide hydrochloride and oral carbonic anhydrase inhibitors is not recommended).
No products indexed under this heading.

Aspirin (Although acid-base and electrolyte disturbances were not reported in the clinical trials with dorzolamide hydrochloride, these disturbances have been reported with oral carbonic anhydrase inhibitors and have, in some instances, resulted in drug interactions (eg, toxicity associated with high dose salicylate therapy). Therefore, the potential for such drug interactions should be considered in patients receiving dorzolamide hydrochloride). Products include:
Aggrenox 880
Bayer Aspirin 829
Percodan 1124
St. Joseph Aspirin 2045

Aspirin, Enteric Coated (Although acid-base and electrolyte disturbances were not reported in the clinical trials with dorzolamide hydrochloride, these disturbances have been reported with oral carbonic anhydrase inhibitors and have, in some instances, resulted in drug interactions (eg, toxicity associated with high dose salicylate therapy). Therefore, the potential for such drug interactions should be considered in patients receiving dorzolamide hydrochloride).
No products indexed under this heading.

Aspirin Buffered (Although acid-base and electrolyte disturbances were not reported in the clinical trials with dorzolamide hydrochloride, these disturbances have been reported with oral carbonic anhydrase inhibitors and have, in some instances, resulted in drug interactions (eg, toxicity associated with high dose salicylate therapy). Therefore, the potential for such drug interactions should be considered in patients receiving dorzolamide hydrochloride).
No products indexed under this heading.

Choline Magnesium Trisalicylate (Although acid-base and electrolyte disturbances were not reported in the clinical trials with dorzolamide hydrochloride, these disturbances have been reported with oral carbonic anhydrase inhibitors and have, in some instances, resulted in drug interactions (eg, toxicity associated with high dose salicylate therapy). Therefore, the potential for such drug interactions should be considered in patients receiving dorzolamide hydrochloride).
No products indexed under this heading.

Dichlorphenamide (There is a potential for an additive effect on the known systemic effects of carbonic anhydrase inhibition in patients receiving an oral carbonic anhydrase inhibitor and dorzolamide hydrochloride. The concomitant administration of dorzolamide hydrochloride and oral carbonic anhydrase inhibitors is not recommended).
No products indexed under this heading.

Diflunisal (Although acid-base and electrolyte disturbances were not reported in the clinical trials with dorzolamide hydrochloride, these disturbances have been reported with oral carbonic anhydrase inhibitors and have, in some instances, resulted in drug interactions (eg, toxicity associated with high dose salicylate therapy). Therefore, the potential for such drug interactions should be considered in patients receiving dorzolamide hydrochloride).
No products indexed under this heading.

Magnesium Salicylate (Although acid-base and electrolyte disturbances were not reported in the clinical trials with dorzolamide hydrochloride, these disturbances have been reported with oral carbonic anhydrase inhibitors and have, in some instances, resulted in drug interactions (eg, toxicity associated with high dose salicylate therapy). Therefore, the potential for such drug interactions should be considered in patients receiving dorzolamide hydrochloride).
No products indexed under this heading.

Methazolamide (There is a potential for an additive effect on the known systemic effects of carbonic anhydrase inhibition in patients receiving an oral carbonic anhydrase inhibitor and dorzolamide hydrochloride. The concomitant administration of dorzolamide hydrochloride and oral carbonic anhydrase inhibitors is not recommended).
No products indexed under this heading.

Salsalate (Although acid-base and electrolyte disturbances were not reported in the clinical trials with dorzolamide hydrochloride, these disturbances have been reported with oral carbonic anhydrase inhibitors and have, in some instances, resulted in drug interactions (eg, toxicity associated with high dose salicylate therapy). Therefore, the potential for such drug interactions should be considered in patients receiving dorzolamide hydrochloride).
No products indexed under this heading.

Torsemide (There is a potential for an additive effect on the known systemic effects of carbonic anhydrase inhibition in patients receiving an oral carbonic anhydrase inhibitor and dorzolamide hydrochloride. The concomitant administration of dorzolamide hydrochloride and oral carbonic anhydrase inhibitors is not recommended).
No products indexed under this heading.

TRUVADA TABLETS

(Emtricitabine, Tenofovir Disoproxil Fumarate) 1258
May interact with cationic drugs that are eliminated by renal tubular, nephrotoxic agents, and certain other agents. Compounds in these categories include:

Abacavir Sulfate (There was no clinically significant drug interaction seen between tenofovir and abacavir. However, co-administration of abacavir (300 mg once) with tenofovir resulted on average in an increase in abacavir C_{max} by 12%). Products include:
Epzicom 1448
Trizivir 1688
Ziagen 1740

Acyclovir (Emtricitabine and tenofovir are primarily excreted by the kidneys by a combination of glomerular filtration

1945 Interactions Index Truvada

and active tubular secretion. No drug-drug interactions due to competition for renal excretion have been observed; however, co-administraiton of Truvada with drugs that are eliminated by active tubular secretion may increase concentrations of emtricitabine, tenofovir, and/or the co-administered drug. Some examples include, but are not limited to acyclovir, adefovir dipivoxil, cidofovir, ganciclovir, valacyclovir, and valganciclovir. Truvada should be avoided with concurrent or recent use of a nephrotoxic agent). Products include:
Zovirax 1760

Acyclovir Sodium (Emtricitabine and tenofovir are primarily excreted by the kidneys by a combination of glomerular filtration and active tubular secretion. No drug-drug interactions due to competition for renal excretion have been observed; however, co-administraiton of Truvada with drugs that are eliminated by active tubular secretion may increase concentrations of emtricitabine, tenofovir, and/or the co-administered drug. Some examples include, but are not limited to acyclovir, adefovir dipivoxil, cidofovir, ganciclovir, valacyclovir, and valganciclovir. Truvada should be avoided with concurrent or recent use of a nephrotoxic agent).
No products indexed under this heading.

Adefovir dipivoxil (Truvada should not be administered with adefovir dipivoxil. Emtricitabine and tenofovir are primarily excretion by the kidneys by a combination of glomerular filtration and active tubular secretion. No drug-drug interactions due to competition for renal excretion have been observed; however, co-administration of Truvada with drugs that are eliminated by active tubular secretion may increase concentrations of emtricitabine tenofovir, and/or the co-administered drug. Some examples include, but are not limited to acyclovir, adefovir dipivoxil, cidofovir, ganciclovir, valacyclovir, and valganciclovir). Products include:
Hepsera 1244

Alatrofloxacin Mesylate (Emtricitabine and tenofovir are primarily excreted by the kidneys by a combination of glomerular filtation and active tubular secretion. Drugs that decrease renal function may increase concentration of emtricitabine and/or tenofovir. Truvada should be avoided with concurrent or recent use of a nephrotoxic agents).
No products indexed under this heading.

Aldesleukin (Emtricitabine and tenofovir are primarily excreted by the kidneys by a combination of glomerular filtation and active tubular secretion. Drugs that decrease renal function may increase concentration of emtricitabine and/or tenofovir. Truvada should be avoided with concurrent or recent use of a nephrotoxic agents). Products include:
Proleukin 2504

Amikacin Sulfate (Emtricitabine and tenofovir are primarily excreted by the kidneys by a combination of glomerular filtation and active tubular secretion. Drugs that decrease renal function may increase concentration of emtricitabine and/or tenofovir. Truvada should be avoided with concurrent or recent use of a nephrotoxic agents).
No products indexed under this heading.

Amiloride Hydrochloride (Emtricitabine and tenofovir are primarily excreted by the kidneys by a combination of glomerular filtration and active tubular secretion. No drug-drug interactions due to competition for renal excretion have been observed; however, co-administration of Truvada with drugs that are eliminated by active tubular secretion may increase concentrations of emtricitabine, tenofovir, and/or the co-administered drug).
No products indexed under this heading.

Amoxicillin (Emtricitabine and tenofovir are primarily excreted by the kidneys by a combination of glomerular filtation and active tubular secretion. Drugs that decrease renal function may increase concentration of emtricitabine and/or tenofovir. Truvada should be avoided with concurrent or recent use of a nephrotoxic agents). Products include:
Amoxil Capsules 1311
Amoxil Chewable Tablets 1311
Amoxil 1311
Amoxil Powder 1311
Augmentin 1331
Augmentin Tablets 1335
Augmentin ES-600 1338
Augmentin XR 1342
Moxatag 2321

Amoxicillin Trihydrate (Emtricitabine and tenofovir are primarily excreted by the kidneys by a combination of glomerular filtation and active tubular secretion. Drugs that decrease renal function may increase concentration of emtricitabine and/or tenofovir. Truvada should be avoided with concurrent or recent use of a nephrotoxic agents).
No products indexed under this heading.

Amphotericin B (Emtricitabine and tenofovir are primarily excreted by the kidneys by a combination of glomerular filtation and active tubular secretion. Drugs that decrease renal function may increase concentration of emtricitabine and/or tenofovir. Truvada should be avoided with concurrent or recent use of a nephrotoxic agents).
No products indexed under this heading.

Amphotericin B, liposomal (Emtricitabine and tenofovir are primarily excreted by the kidneys by a combination of glomerular filtation and active tubular secretion. Drugs that decrease renal function may increase concentration of emtricitabine and/or tenofovir. Truvada should be avoided with concurrent or recent use of a nephrotoxic agents). Products include:
AmBisome 659

Amphotericin B Cholesteryl Sulfate (Emtricitabine and tenofovir are primarily excreted by the kidneys by a combination of glomerular filtation and active tubular secretion. Drugs that decrease renal function may increase concentration of emtricitabine and/or tenofovir. Truvada should be avoided with concurrent or recent use of a nephrotoxic agents).
No products indexed under this heading.

Amphotericin B Lipid Complex (Emtricitabine and tenofovir are primarily excreted by the kidneys by a combination of glomerular filtation and active tubular secretion. Drugs that decrease renal function may increase concentration of emtricitabine and/or tenofovir. Truvada should be avoided with concurrent or recent use of a nephrotoxic agents).
No products indexed under this heading.

Ampicillin (Emtricitabine and tenofovir are primarily excreted by the kidneys by a combination of glomerular filtation and active tubular secretion. Drugs that decrease renal function may increase concentration of emtricitabine and/or tenofovir. Truvada should be avoided with concurrent or recent use of a nephrotoxic agents).
No products indexed under this heading.

Ampicillin Sodium (Emtricitabine and tenofovir are primarily excreted by the kidneys by a combination of glomerular filtation and active tubular secretion. Drugs that decrease renal function may increase concentration of emtricitabine and/or tenofovir. Truvada should be avoided with concurrent or recent use of a nephrotoxic agents).
No products indexed under this heading.

Ampicillin Trihydrate (Emtricitabine and tenofovir are primarily excreted by the kidneys by a combination of glomerular filtation and active tubular secretion. Drugs that decrease renal function may increase concentration of emtricitabine and/or tenofovir. Truvada should be avoided with concurrent or recent use of a nephrotoxic agents).
No products indexed under this heading.

Amprenavir (Emtricitabine and tenofovir are primarily excreted by the kidneys by a combination of glomerular filtation and active tubular secretion. Drugs that decrease renal function may increase concentration of emtricitabine and/or tenofovir. Truvada should be avoided with concurrent or recent use of a nephrotoxic agents).
No products indexed under this heading.

Aspirin (Emtricitabine and tenofovir are primarily excreted by the kidneys by a combination of glomerular filtation and active tubular secretion. Drugs that decrease renal function may increase concentration of emtricitabine and/or tenofovir. Truvada should be avoided with concurrent or recent use of a nephrotoxic agents). Products include:
Aggrenox 880
Bayer Aspirin 829
Percodan 1124
St. Joseph Aspirin 2045

Atazanavir (Atazanavir has been shown to increase tenofovir concentrations. Patients receiving atazanavir and Truvada should be monitored for Truvada-associated adverse reactions. Truvada should be discontinued if Truvada-associated adverse reactions occur. Tenofovir decreases the AUC and C_{min} of atazanavir. When co-administered with Truvada, it is recommended that atazanavir 300 mg is given with ritonavir 100 mg. Atazanavir without ritonavir should not be co-administered with Truvada).
No products indexed under this heading.

Atazanavir Sulfate (Atazanavir has been shown to increase tenofovir concentrations. Patients receiving atazanavir and Truvada should be monitored for Truvada-associated adverse reactions. Truvada should be discontinued if Truvada-associated adverse reactions occur. Tenofovir decreases the AUC and C_{min} of atazanavir. When co-administered with Truvada, it is recommended that atazanavir 300 mg is given with ritonavir 100 mg. Atazanavir without ritonavir should not be co-administered with Truvada).
No products indexed under this heading.

Atorvastatin Calcium (Emtricitabine and tenofovir are primarily excreted by the kidneys by a combination of glomerular filtation and active tubular secretion. Drugs that decrease renal function may increase concentration of emtricitabine and/or tenofovir. Truvada should be avoided with concurrent or recent use of a nephrotoxic agents). Products include:
Lipitor 2703

Azithromycin Dihydrate (Emtricitabine and tenofovir are primarily excreted by the kidneys by a combination of glomerular filtation and active tubular secretion. Drugs that decrease renal function may increase concentration of emtricitabine and/or tenofovir. Truvada should be avoided with concurrent or recent use of a nephrotoxic agents).
No products indexed under this heading.

Azlocillin Sodium (Emtricitabine and tenofovir are primarily excreted by the kidneys by a combination of glomerular filtation and active tubular secretion. Drugs that decrease renal function may increase concentration of emtricitabine and/or tenofovir. Truvada should be avoided with concurrent or recent use of a nephrotoxic agents).
No products indexed under this heading.

Aztreonam (Emtricitabine and tenofovir are primarily excreted by the kidneys by a combination of glomerular filtation and active tubular secretion. Drugs that decrease renal function may increase concentration of emtricitabine and/or tenofovir. Truvada should be avoided with concurrent or recent use of a nephrotoxic agents).
No products indexed under this heading.

Bacampicillin Hydrochloride (Emtricitabine and tenofovir are primarily excreted by the kidneys by a combination of glomerular filtation and active tubular secretion. Drugs that decrease renal function may increase concentration of emtricitabine and/or tenofovir. Truvada should be avoided with concurrent or recent use of a nephrotoxic agents).
No products indexed under this heading.

Bacitracin (Emtricitabine and tenofovir are primarily excreted by the kidneys by a combination of glomerular filtation and active tubular secretion. Drugs that decrease renal function may increase concentration of emtricitabine and/or tenofovir. Truvada should be avoided with concurrent or recent use of a nephrotoxic agents).
No products indexed under this heading.

Bacitracin Zinc (Emtricitabine and tenofovir are primarily excreted by the kidneys by a combination of glomerular filtation and active tubular secretion. Drugs that decrease renal function may increase concentration of emtricitabine and/or tenofovir. Truvada should be avoided with concurrent or recent use of a nephrotoxic agents).
No products indexed under this heading.

Balsalazide Disodium (Emtricitabine and tenofovir are primarily excreted by the kidneys by a combination of glomerular filtation and active tubular secretion. Drugs that decrease renal function may increase concentration of emtricitabine and/or tenofovir. Truvada should be avoided with concurrent or recent use of a nephrotoxic agents).
No products indexed under this heading.

Benazepril Hydrochloride (Emtricitabine and tenofovir are primarily excreted by the kidneys by a combination of glomerular filtation and active tubular secretion. Drugs that decrease renal function may increase concentration of emtricitabine and/or tenofovir. Truvada should be avoided with concurrent or recent use of a nephrotoxic agents).
No products indexed under this heading.

Bendroflumethiazide (Emtricitabine and tenofovir are primarily excreted by the kidneys by a combination of glomerular filtation and active tubular secretion. Drugs that decrease renal function may increase concentration of emtricitabine and/or tenofovir. Truvada should be avoided with concurrent or recent use of a nephrotoxic agents).
No products indexed under this heading.

IMPORTANT NOTE: Always consult each drug listing in the patient's regimen for possible interactions.

Caffeine (Emtricitabine and tenofovir are primarily excreted by the kidneys by a combination of glomerular filtation and active tubular secretion. Drugs that decrease renal function may increase concentration of emtricitabine and/or tenofovir. Truvada should be avoided with concurrent or recent use of a nephrotoxic agents).
    No products indexed under this heading.

Captopril (Emtricitabine and tenofovir are primarily excreted by the kidneys by a combination of glomerular filtation and active tubular secretion. Drugs that decrease renal function may increase concentration of emtricitabine and/or tenofovir. Truvada should be avoided with concurrent or recent use of a nephrotoxic agents). Products include:
Captopril 2341

Carbenicillin Disodium (Emtricitabine and tenofovir are primarily excreted by the kidneys by a combination of glomerular filtation and active tubular secretion. Drugs that decrease renal function may increase concentration of emtricitabine and/or tenofovir. Truvada should be avoided with concurrent or recent use of a nephrotoxic agents).
    No products indexed under this heading.

Carbenicillin Indanyl Sodium (Emtricitabine and tenofovir are primarily excreted by the kidneys by a combination of glomerular filtation and active tubular secretion. Drugs that decrease renal function may increase concentration of emtricitabine and/or tenofovir. Truvada should be avoided with concurrent or recent use of a nephrotoxic agents).
    No products indexed under this heading.

Carboplatin (Emtricitabine and tenofovir are primarily excreted by the kidneys by a combination of glomerular filtation and active tubular secretion. Drugs that decrease renal function may increase concentration of emtricitabine and/or tenofovir. Truvada should be avoided with concurrent or recent use of a nephrotoxic agents).
    No products indexed under this heading.

Carmustine (BCNU) (Emtricitabine and tenofovir are primarily excreted by the kidneys by a combination of glomerular filtation and active tubular secretion. Drugs that decrease renal function may increase concentration of emtricitabine and/or tenofovir. Truvada should be avoided with concurrent or recent use of a nephrotoxic agents).
    No products indexed under this heading.

Cefaclor (Emtricitabine and tenofovir are primarily excreted by the kidneys by a combination of glomerular filtation and active tubular secretion. Drugs that decrease renal function may increase concentration of emtricitabine and/or tenofovir. Truvada should be avoided with concurrent or recent use of a nephrotoxic agents).
    No products indexed under this heading.

Cefadroxil (Emtricitabine and tenofovir are primarily excreted by the kidneys by a combination of glomerular filtation and active tubular secretion. Drugs that decrease renal function may increase concentration of emtricitabine and/or tenofovir. Truvada should be avoided with concurrent or recent use of a nephrotoxic agents).
    No products indexed under this heading.

Cefamandole Nafate (Emtricitabine and tenofovir are primarily excreted by the kidneys by a combination of glomerular filtation and active tubular secretion. Drugs that decrease renal function may increase concentration of emtricitabine and/or tenofovir. Truvada should be avoided with concurrent or recent use of a nephrotoxic agents).
    No products indexed under this heading.

Cefazolin Sodium (Emtricitabine and tenofovir are primarily excreted by the kidneys by a combination of glomerular filtation and active tubular secretion. Drugs that decrease renal function may increase concentration of emtricitabine and/or tenofovir. Truvada should be avoided with concurrent or recent use of a nephrotoxic agents).
    No products indexed under this heading.

Cefdinir (Emtricitabine and tenofovir are primarily excreted by the kidneys by a combination of glomerular filtation and active tubular secretion. Drugs that decrease renal function may increase concentration of emtricitabine and/or tenofovir. Truvada should be avoided with concurrent or recent use of a nephrotoxic agents). Products include:
Omnicef Capsules 518
Omnicef Oral Suspension 518

Cefepime Hydrochloride (Emtricitabine and tenofovir are primarily excreted by the kidneys by a combination of glomerular filtation and active tubular secretion. Drugs that decrease renal function may increase concentration of emtricitabine and/or tenofovir. Truvada should be avoided with concurrent or recent use of a nephrotoxic agents).
    No products indexed under this heading.

Cefixime (Emtricitabine and tenofovir are primarily excreted by the kidneys by a combination of glomerular filtation and active tubular secretion. Drugs that decrease renal function may increase concentration of emtricitabine and/or tenofovir. Truvada should be avoided with concurrent or recent use of a nephrotoxic agents). Products include:
Suprax for Oral Suspension 2038
Suprax Tablets 2038

Cefmetazole Sodium (Emtricitabine and tenofovir are primarily excreted by the kidneys by a combination of glomerular filtation and active tubular secretion. Drugs that decrease renal function may increase concentration of emtricitabine and/or tenofovir. Truvada should be avoided with concurrent or recent use of a nephrotoxic agents).
    No products indexed under this heading.

Cefonicid Sodium (Emtricitabine and tenofovir are primarily excreted by the kidneys by a combination of glomerular filtation and active tubular secretion. Drugs that decrease renal function may increase concentration of emtricitabine and/or tenofovir. Truvada should be avoided with concurrent or recent use of a nephrotoxic agents).
    No products indexed under this heading.

Cefoperazone Sodium (Emtricitabine and tenofovir are primarily excreted by the kidneys by a combination of glomerular filtation and active tubular secretion. Drugs that decrease renal function may increase concentration of emtricitabine and/or tenofovir. Truvada should be avoided with concurrent or recent use of a nephrotoxic agents).
    No products indexed under this heading.

Ceforanide (Emtricitabine and tenofovir are primarily excreted by the kidneys by a combination of glomerular filtation and active tubular secretion. Drugs that decrease renal function may increase concentration of emtricitabine and/or tenofovir. Truvada should be avoided with concurrent or recent use of a nephrotoxic agents).
    No products indexed under this heading.

Cefotaxime Sodium (Emtricitabine and tenofovir are primarily excreted by the kidneys by a combination of glomerular filtation and active tubular secretion. Drugs that decrease renal function may increase concentration of emtricitabine and/or tenofovir. Truvada should be avoided with concurrent or recent use of a nephrotoxic agents).
    No products indexed under this heading.

Cefotetan (Emtricitabine and tenofovir are primarily excreted by the kidneys by a combination of glomerular filtation and active tubular secretion. Drugs that decrease renal function may increase concentration of emtricitabine and/or tenofovir. Truvada should be avoided with concurrent or recent use of a nephrotoxic agents).
    No products indexed under this heading.

Cefoxitin Sodium (Emtricitabine and tenofovir are primarily excreted by the kidneys by a combination of glomerular filtation and active tubular secretion. Drugs that decrease renal function may increase concentration of emtricitabine and/or tenofovir. Truvada should be avoided with concurrent or recent use of a nephrotoxic agents).
    No products indexed under this heading.

Cefpodoxime Proxetil (Emtricitabine and tenofovir are primarily excreted by the kidneys by a combination of glomerular filtation and active tubular secretion. Drugs that decrease renal function may increase concentration of emtricitabine and/or tenofovir. Truvada should be avoided with concurrent or recent use of a nephrotoxic agents).
    No products indexed under this heading.

Cefprozil (Emtricitabine and tenofovir are primarily excreted by the kidneys by a combination of glomerular filtation and active tubular secretion. Drugs that decrease renal function may increase concentration of emtricitabine and/or tenofovir. Truvada should be avoided with concurrent or recent use of a nephrotoxic agents).
    No products indexed under this heading.

Ceftazidime (Emtricitabine and tenofovir are primarily excreted by the kidneys by a combination of glomerular filtation and active tubular secretion. Drugs that decrease renal function may increase concentration of emtricitabine and/or tenofovir. Truvada should be avoided with concurrent or recent use of a nephrotoxic agents). Products include:
Fortaz 1481

Ceftizoxime Sodium (Emtricitabine and tenofovir are primarily excreted by the kidneys by a combination of glomerular filtation and active tubular secretion. Drugs that decrease renal function may increase concentration of emtricitabine and/or tenofovir. Truvada should be avoided with concurrent or recent use of a nephrotoxic agents).
    No products indexed under this heading.

Ceftriaxone Sodium (Emtricitabine and tenofovir are primarily excreted by the kidneys by a combination of glomerular filtation and active tubular secretion. Drugs that decrease renal function may increase concentration of emtricitabine and/or tenofovir. Truvada should be avoided with concurrent or recent use of a nephrotoxic agents). Products include:
Rocephin 2859

Cefuroxime Axetil (Emtricitabine and tenofovir are primarily excreted by the kidneys by a combination of glomerular filtation and active tubular secretion. Drugs that decrease renal function may increase concentration of emtricitabine and/or tenofovir. Truvada should be avoided with concurrent or recent use of a nephrotoxic agents). Products include:
Ceftin 1399

Cefuroxime Sodium (Emtricitabine and tenofovir are primarily excreted by the kidneys by a combination of glomerular filtation and active tubular secretion. Drugs that decrease renal function may increase concentration of emtricitabine and/or tenofovir. Truvada should be avoided with concurrent or recent use of a nephrotoxic agents).
    No products indexed under this heading.

Celecoxib (Emtricitabine and tenofovir are primarily excreted by the kidneys by a combination of glomerular filtation and active tubular secretion. Drugs that decrease renal function may increase concentration of emtricitabine and/or tenofovir. Truvada should be avoided with concurrent or recent use of a nephrotoxic agents). Products include:
Celebrex 3272

Cephalexin (Emtricitabine and tenofovir are primarily excreted by the kidneys by a combination of glomerular filtation and active tubular secretion. Drugs that decrease renal function may increase concentration of emtricitabine and/or tenofovir. Truvada should be avoided with concurrent or recent use of a nephrotoxic agents).
    No products indexed under this heading.

Cephalothin Sodium (Emtricitabine and tenofovir are primarily excreted by the kidneys by a combination of glomerular filtation and active tubular secretion. Drugs that decrease renal function may increase concentration of emtricitabine and/or tenofovir. Truvada should be avoided with concurrent or recent use of a nephrotoxic agents).
    No products indexed under this heading.

Cephapirin Sodium (Emtricitabine and tenofovir are primarily excreted by the kidneys by a combination of glomerular filtation and active tubular secretion. Drugs that decrease renal function may increase concentration of emtricitabine and/or tenofovir. Truvada should be avoided with concurrent or recent use of a nephrotoxic agents).
    No products indexed under this heading.

Cephradine (Emtricitabine and tenofovir are primarily excreted by the kidneys by a combination of glomerular filtation and active tubular secretion. Drugs that decrease renal function may increase concentration of emtricitabine and/or tenofovir. Truvada should be avoided with concurrent or recent use of a nephrotoxic agents).
    No products indexed under this heading.

Cerivastatin Sodium (Emtricitabine and tenofovir are primarily excreted by the kidneys by a combination of glomerular filtation and active tubular secretion. Drugs that decrease renal function may increase concentration of emtricitabine and/or tenofovir. Truvada should be avoided with concurrent or recent use of a nephrotoxic agents).
    No products indexed under this heading.

Chlorothiazide (Emtricitabine and tenofovir are primarily excreted by the kidneys by a combination of glomerular filtation and active tubular secretion. Drugs that decrease renal function may increase concentration of emtricitabine and/or tenofovir, Truvada should be avoided with concurrent or recent use of a nephrotoxic agents).
    No products indexed under this heading.

Chlorothiazide Sodium (Emtricitabine and tenofovir are primarily excreted by the kidneys by a combination of glomerular filtation and active tubular secretion. Drugs that decrease renal function may increase concentration of emtricitabine and/or tenofovir. Truvada should be avoided with concurrent or recent use of a nephrotoxic agents). Products include:
Diuril Intravenous 2009

Chlorpropamide (Emtricitabine and tenofovir are primarily excreted by the kidneys by a combination of glomerular filtation and active tubular secretion. Drugs that decrease renal function may increase concentration of emtricitabine and/or tenofovir. Truvada should be avoided with concurrent or recent use of a nephrotoxic agents).
    No products indexed under this heading.

Cidofovir (Emtricitabine and tenofovir are primarily excreted by the kidneys by a combination of glomerular filtration and active tubular secretion. No drug-drug interactions due to competition for renal excretion have been observed; however, co-administration of Truvada with drugs that are eliminated by active tubular secretion may increase concentrations of emtricitabine, tenofovir, and/or the co-administered drug. Some examples include, but are not limited to acyclovir, adefovir dipivoxil, cidofovir, ganciclovir, valacyclovir, and valganciclovir. Truvada should be avoided with concurrent or recent use of a nephrotoxic agent).
No products indexed under this heading.

Cilastatin Sodium (Emtricitabine and tenofovir are primarily excreted by the kidneys by a combination of glomerular filtation and active tubular secretion. Drugs that decrease renal function may increase concentration of emtricitabine and/or tenofovir. Truvada should be avoided with concurrent or recent use of a nephrotoxic agents). Products include:
Primaxin I.M. 2232
Primaxin I.V. 2235

Cimetidine (Emtricitabine and tenofovir are primarily excreted by the kidneys by a combination of glomerular filtation and active tubular secretion. Drugs that decrease renal function may increase concentration of emtricitabine and/or tenofovir. Truvada should be avoided with concurrent or recent use of a nephrotoxic agents).
No products indexed under this heading.

Cimetidine Hydrochloride (Emtricitabine and tenofovir are primarily excreted by the kidneys by a combination of glomerular filtation and active tubular secretion. Drugs that decrease renal function may increase concentration of emtricitabine and/or tenofovir. Truvada should be avoided with concurrent or recent use of a nephrotoxic agents).
No products indexed under this heading.

Cisplatin (Emtricitabine and tenofovir are primarily excreted by the kidneys by a combination of glomerular filtation and active tubular secretion. Drugs that decrease renal function may increase concentration of emtricitabine and/or tenofovir. Truvada should be avoided with concurrent or recent use of a nephrotoxic agents).
No products indexed under this heading.

Cladribine (Emtricitabine and tenofovir are primarily excreted by the kidneys by a combination of glomerular filtation and active tubular secretion. Drugs that decrease renal function may increase concentration of emtricitabine and/or tenofovir. Truvada should be avoided with concurrent or recent use of a nephrotoxic agents). Products include:
Leustatin 946

Clozapine (Emtricitabine and tenofovir are primarily excreted by the kidneys by a combination of glomerular filtation and active tubular secretion. Drugs that decrease renal function may increase concentration of emtricitabine and/or tenofovir. Truvada should be avoided with concurrent or recent use of a nephrotoxic agents).
No products indexed under this heading.

Colistimethate Sodium (Emtricitabine and tenofovir are primarily excreted by the kidneys by a combination of glomerular filtation and active tubular secretion. Drugs that decrease renal function may increase concentration of emtricitabine and/or tenofovir. Truvada should be avoided with concurrent or recent use of a nephrotoxic agents).
No products indexed under this heading.

Colistin Sulfate (Emtricitabine and tenofovir are primarily excreted by the kidneys by a combination of glomerular filtation and active tubular secretion. Drugs that decrease renal function may increase concentration of emtricitabine and/or tenofovir. Truvada should be avoided with concurrent or recent use of a nephrotoxic agents).
No products indexed under this heading.

Cyclophosphamide (Emtricitabine and tenofovir are primarily excreted by the kidneys by a combination of glomerular filtation and active tubular secretion. Drugs that decrease renal function may increase concentration of emtricitabine and/or tenofovir. Truvada should be avoided with concurrent or recent use of a nephrotoxic agents).
No products indexed under this heading.

Cyclosporine (Emtricitabine and tenofovir are primarily excreted by the kidneys by a combination of glomerular filtation and active tubular secretion. Drugs that decrease renal function may increase concentration of emtricitabine and/or tenofovir. Truvada should be avoided with concurrent or recent use of a nephrotoxic agents). Products include:
Gengraf 440
Neoral Oral Solution 2496
Neoral Capsules 2496
Restasis 605

Cytarabine (Emtricitabine and tenofovir are primarily excreted by the kidneys by a combination of glomerular filtation and active tubular secretion. Drugs that decrease renal function may increase concentration of emtricitabine and/or tenofovir. Truvada should be avoided with concurrent or recent use of a nephrotoxic agents).
No products indexed under this heading.

Cytarabine Liposome (Emtricitabine and tenofovir are primarily excreted by the kidneys by a combination of glomerular filtation and active tubular secretion. Drugs that decrease renal function may increase concentration of emtricitabine and/or tenofovir. Truvada should be avoided with concurrent or recent use of a nephrotoxic agents).
No products indexed under this heading.

Delavirdine Mesylate (Emtricitabine and tenofovir are primarily excreted by the kidneys by a combination of glomerular filtation and active tubular secretion. Drugs that decrease renal function may increase concentration of emtricitabine and/or tenofovir. Truvada should be avoided with concurrent or recent use of a nephrotoxic agents).
No products indexed under this heading.

Diatrizoate Meglumine (Emtricitabine and tenofovir are primarily excreted by the kidneys by a combination of glomerular filtation and active tubular secretion. Drugs that decrease renal function may increase concentration of emtricitabine and/or tenofovir. Truvada should be avoided with concurrent or recent use of a nephrotoxic agents).
No products indexed under this heading.

Diatrizoate Sodium (Emtricitabine and tenofovir are primarily excreted by the kidneys by a combination of glomerular filtation and active tubular secretion. Drugs that decrease renal function may increase concentration of emtricitabine and/or tenofovir. Truvada should be avoided with concurrent or recent use of a nephrotoxic agents).
No products indexed under this heading.

Diclofenac Potassium (Emtricitabine and tenofovir are primarily excreted by the kidneys by a combination of glomerular filtation and active tubular secretion. Drugs that decrease renal function may increase concentration of emtricitabine and/or tenofovir. Truvada should be avoided with concurrent or recent use of a nephrotoxic agents).
No products indexed under this heading.

Diclofenac Sodium (Emtricitabine and tenofovir are primarily excreted by the kidneys by a combination of glomerular filtation and active tubular secretion. Drugs that decrease renal function may increase concentration of emtricitabine and/or tenofovir. Truvada should be avoided with concurrent or recent use of a nephrotoxic agents).
No products indexed under this heading.

Dicloxacillin Sodium (Emtricitabine and tenofovir are primarily excreted by the kidneys by a combination of glomerular filtation and active tubular secretion. Drugs that decrease renal function may increase concentration of emtricitabine and/or tenofovir. Truvada should be avoided with concurrent or recent use of a nephrotoxic agents).
No products indexed under this heading.

Didanosine (When tenofovir disoproxil fumarate was administered with didanosine the C_{max} and AUC of didanosine increased significantly. Higher didanosine concentrations could potentiate didanosine-associated adverse reactions (eg, pancreatitis, neuropathy). Suppression of CD4 cell counts has been observed in patients receiving tenofovir DF with didanosine 400 mg daily.. Co-administration of Truvada and didanosine should be undertaken with caution and patients receiving this combination should be monitored closely for didanosine-associated adverse reations. Didanosine should be discontinued in patients who develop didanosine-associated adverse reactions. In adult weighing> 60 kg, the didanosine dose should be reduced to 250 mg when it is co-administered with Truvada. Data is not available to recommend a dose adjustment of didanosine for patients weighing < 60 kg).
No products indexed under this heading.

Digoxin (Emtricitabine and tenofovir are primarily excreted by the kidneys by a combination of glomerular filtration and active tubular secretion. No drug-drug interactions due to competition for renal excretion have been observed; however, co-administration of Truvada with drugs that are eliminated by active tubular secretion may increase concentrations of emtricitabine, tenofovir, and/or the co-administered drug). Products include:
Lanoxin Injection 1546
Lanoxin Injection Pediatric 1549
Lanoxin Tablets 1553

Efavirenz (Emtricitabine and tenofovir are primarily excreted by the kidneys by a combination of glomerular filtation and active tubular secretion. Drugs that decrease renal function may increase concentration of emtricitabine and/or tenofovir. Truvada should be avoided with concurrent or recent use of a nephrotoxic agents). Products include:
Atripla 906

Enalapril Maleate (Emtricitabine and tenofovir are primarily excreted by the kidneys by a combination of glomerular filtation and active tubular secretion. Drugs that decrease renal function may increase concentration of emtricitabine and/or tenofovir. Truvada should be avoided with concurrent or recent use of a nephrotoxic agents).
No products indexed under this heading.

Enalaprilat (Emtricitabine and tenofovir are primarily excreted by the kidneys by a combination of glomerular filtation and active tubular secretion. Drugs that decrease renal function may increase concentration of emtricitabine and/or tenofovir. Truvada should be avoided with concurrent or recent use of a nephrotoxic agents).
No products indexed under this heading.

Enfuvirtide (Emtricitabine and tenofovir are primarily excreted by the kidneys by a combination of glomerular filtation and active tubular secretion. Drugs that decrease renal function may increase concentration of emtricitabine and/or tenofovir. Truvada should be avoided with concurrent or recent use of a nephrotoxic agents).
No products indexed under this heading.

Entecavir (There was no clinically significant drug interaction seen between tenofovir and entecavir. However, co-administration of tenofovir with entecavir (1 mg once daily for 10 days) increased the AUC of entecavir on average by 13%).
No products indexed under this heading.

Ethiodized Oil (Emtricitabine and tenofovir are primarily excreted by the kidneys by a combination of glomerular filtation and active tubular secretion. Drugs that decrease renal function may increase concentration of emtricitabine and/or tenofovir. Truvada should be avoided with concurrent or recent use of a nephrotoxic agents).
No products indexed under this heading.

Etodolac (Emtricitabine and tenofovir are primarily excreted by the kidneys by a combination of glomerular filtation and active tubular secretion. Drugs that decrease renal function may increase concentration of emtricitabine and/or tenofovir. Truvada should be avoided with concurrent or recent use of a nephrotoxic agents).
No products indexed under this heading.

Fenoprofen Calcium (Emtricitabine and tenofovir are primarily excreted by the kidneys by a combination of glomerular filtation and active tubular secretion. Drugs that decrease renal function may increase concentration of emtricitabine and/or tenofovir. Truvada should be avoided with concurrent or recent use of a nephrotoxic agents).
No products indexed under this heading.

Filgrastim (Emtricitabine and tenofovir are primarily excreted by the kidneys by a combination of glomerular filtation and active tubular secretion. Drugs that decrease renal function may increase concentration of emtricitabine and/or tenofovir. Truvada should be avoided with concurrent or recent use of a nephrotoxic agents). Products include:
Neupogen 631

Fluorouracil (Emtricitabine and tenofovir are primarily excreted by the kidneys by a combination of glomerular filtation and active tubular secretion. Drugs that decrease renal function may increase concentration of emtricitabine and/or tenofovir. Truvada should be avoided with concurrent or recent use of a nephrotoxic agents). Products include:
Carac 2966

Flurbiprofen (Emtricitabine and tenofovir are primarily excreted by the kidneys by a combination of glomerular filtation and active tubular secretion. Drugs that decrease renal function may increase concentration of emtricitabine and/or tenofovir. Truvada should be avoided with concurrent or recent use of a nephrotoxic agents).
No products indexed under this heading.

IMPORTANT NOTE: Always consult each drug listing in the patient's regimen for possible interactions.

Fluvastatin Sodium (Emtricitabine and tenofovir are primarily excreted by the kidneys by a combination of glomerular filtration and active tubular secretion. Drugs that decrease renal function may increase concentration of emtricitabine and/or tenofovir. Truvada should be avoided with concurrent or recent use of a nephrotoxic agents).

No products indexed under this heading.

Foscarnet Sodium (Emtricitabine and tenofovir are primarily excreted by the kidneys by a combination of glomerular filtration and active tubular secretion. Drugs that decrease renal function may increase concentration of emtricitabine and/or tenofovir. Truvada should be avoided with concurrent or recent use of a nephrotoxic agents).

No products indexed under this heading.

Fosinopril Sodium (Emtricitabine and tenofovir are primarily excreted by the kidneys by a combination of glomerular filtration and active tubular secretion. Drugs that decrease renal function may increase concentration of emtricitabine and/or tenofovir. Truvada should be avoided with concurrent or recent use of a nephrotoxic agents).

No products indexed under this heading.

Furosemide (Emtricitabine and tenofovir are primarily excreted by the kidneys by a combination of glomerular filtration and active tubular secretion. Drugs that decrease renal function may increase concentration of emtricitabine and/or tenofovir. Truvada should be avoided with concurrent or recent use of a nephrotoxic agents). Products include:

Furosemide 2354

Gadopentetate Dimeglumine (Emtricitabine and tenofovir are primarily excreted by the kidneys by a combination of glomerular filtration and active tubular secretion. Drugs that decrease renal function may increase concentration of emtricitabine and/or tenofovir. Truvada should be avoided with concurrent or recent use of a nephrotoxic agents).

No products indexed under this heading.

Ganciclovir (Emtricitabine and tenofovir are primarily excreted by the kidneys by a combination of glomerular filtration and active tubular secretion. No drug-drug interactions due to competition for renal excretion have been observed; however, co-administration of Truvada with drugs that are eliminated by active tubular secretion may increase concentrations of emtricitabine, tenofovir, and/or the co-administered drug. Some examples include, but are not limited to acyclovir, adefovir dipivoxil, cidofovir, ganciclovir, valacyclovir, and valganciclovir).

No products indexed under this heading.

Ganciclovir Sodium (Emtricitabine and tenofovir are primarily excreted by the kidneys by a combination of glomerular filtration and active tubular secretion. No drug-drug interactions due to competition for renal excretion have been observed; however, co-administration of Truvada with drugs that are eliminated by active tubular secretion may increase concentrations of emtricitabine, tenofovir, and/or the co-administered drug. Some examples include, but are not limited to acyclovir, adefovir dipivoxil, cidofovir, ganciclovir, valacyclovir, and valganciclovir).

No products indexed under this heading.

Gentamicin (Emtricitabine and tenofovir are primarily excreted by the kidneys by a combination of glomerular filtration and active tubular secretion. Drugs that decrease renal function may increase concentration of emtricitabine and/or tenofovir. Truvada should be avoided with concurrent or recent use of a nephrotoxic agents).

No products indexed under this heading.

Gentamicin Sulfate (Emtricitabine and tenofovir are primarily excreted by the kidneys by a combination of glomerular filtration and active tubular secretion. Drugs that decrease renal function may increase concentration of emtricitabine and/or tenofovir. Truvada should be avoided with concurrent or recent use of a nephrotoxic agents). Products include:

Pred-G ....⊙226, ⊙227

Glipizide (Emtricitabine and tenofovir are primarily excreted by the kidneys by a combination of glomerular filtration and active tubular secretion. Drugs that decrease renal function may increase concentration of emtricitabine and/or tenofovir. Truvada should be avoided with concurrent or recent use of a nephrotoxic agents).

No products indexed under this heading.

Globulin, Immune (Human) (Emtricitabine and tenofovir are primarily excreted by the kidneys by a combination of glomerular filtration and active tubular secretion. Drugs that decrease renal function may increase concentration of emtricitabine and/or tenofovir. Truvada should be avoided with concurrent or recent use of a nephrotoxic agents). Products include:

Glyburide (Emtricitabine and tenofovir are primarily excreted by the kidneys by a combination of glomerular filtration and active tubular secretion. Drugs that decrease renal function may increase concentration of emtricitabine and/or tenofovir. Truvada should be avoided with concurrent or recent use of a nephrotoxic agents).

No products indexed under this heading.

Gold Therapy (Emtricitabine and tenofovir are primarily excreted by the kidneys by a combination of glomerular filtration and active tubular secretion. Drugs that decrease renal function may increase concentration of emtricitabine and/or tenofovir. Truvada should be avoided with concurrent or recent use of a nephrotoxic agents).

No products indexed under this heading.

HMG-CoA Reductase Inhibitors (Emtricitabine and tenofovir are primarily excreted by the kidneys by a combination of glomerular filtration and active tubular secretion. Drugs that decrease renal function may increase concentration of emtricitabine and/or tenofovir. Truvada should be avoided with concurrent or recent use of a nephrotoxic agents).

No products indexed under this heading.

Hydrochlorothiazide (Emtricitabine and tenofovir are primarily excreted by the kidneys by a combination of glomerular filtration and active tubular secretion. Drugs that decrease renal function may increase concentration of emtricitabine and/or tenofovir. Truvada should be avoided with concurrent or recent use of a nephrotoxic agents). Products include:

Atacand HCT	700
Avalide	2956
Benicar HCT	1017
Diovan HCT	2419
Dyazide	1429
Exforge HCT	2449
Hyzaar	2162
Hyzaar 100-12.5	2162
Micardis HCT	889
Prinzide	2246

Tekturna HCT	2541
Teveten HCT	541

Hydroflumethiazide (Emtricitabine and tenofovir are primarily excreted by the kidneys by a combination of glomerular filtration and active tubular secretion. Drugs that decrease renal function may increase concentration of emtricitabine and/or tenofovir. Truvada should be avoided with concurrent or recent use of a nephrotoxic agents).

No products indexed under this heading.

Ibuprofen (Emtricitabine and tenofovir are primarily excreted by the kidneys by a combination of glomerular filtration and active tubular secretion. Drugs that decrease renal function may increase concentration of emtricitabine and/or tenofovir. Truvada should be avoided with concurrent or recent use of a nephrotoxic agents). Products include:

Motrin IB	2043
Children's Motrin	2044
Children's Motrin Non-Staining Dye-Free	2044
Infants' Motrin	2044
Infants' Motrin Dye-Free	2044
Junior Strength Motrin	2044
Vicoprofen	564

Idarubicin Hydrochloride (Emtricitabine and tenofovir are primarily excreted by the kidneys by a combination of glomerular filtration and active tubular secretion. Drugs that decrease renal function may increase concentration of emtricitabine and/or tenofovir. Truvada should be avoided with concurrent or recent use of a nephrotoxic agents).

No products indexed under this heading.

Ifosfamide (Emtricitabine and tenofovir are primarily excreted by the kidneys by a combination of glomerular filtration and active tubular secretion. Drugs that decrease renal function may increase concentration of emtricitabine and/or tenofovir. Truvada should be avoided with concurrent or recent use of a nephrotoxic agents).

No products indexed under this heading.

Imipenem (Emtricitabine and tenofovir are primarily excreted by the kidneys by a combination of glomerular filtration and active tubular secretion. Drugs that decrease renal function may increase concentration of emtricitabine and/or tenofovir. Truvada should be avoided with concurrent or recent use of a nephrotoxic agents). Products include:

Primaxin I.M.	2232
Primaxin I.V.	2235

Immune Globulin Intravenous (Human) (Emtricitabine and tenofovir are primarily excreted by the kidneys by a combination of glomerular filtration and active tubular secretion. Drugs that decrease renal function may increase concentration of emtricitabine and/or tenofovir. Truvada should be avoided with concurrent or recent use of a nephrotoxic agents). Products include:

Flebogamma 5% DIF	1794
Gammagard	812, 815
Gamunex	3374

Indinavir Sulfate (There was no clinically significant drug interaction seen between tenofovir and indinavir. However, co-administration of tenofovir (300 mg QD) with indinavir (800 mg three times a day for seven days) has resulted on average in an increase in tenofovir C_{max} by 14%. In addition, when tenofovir was co-administered with indinavir (800 mg three times daily for seven days), a decrease in C_{max} of indinavir was decreased on average by 11%). Products include:

Crixivan 2113

Indomethacin (Emtricitabine and tenofovir are primarily excreted by the kidneys by a combination of glomerular filtration and active tubular secretion. Drugs that decrease renal function may

increase concentration of emtricitabine and/or tenofovir. Truvada should be avoided with concurrent or recent use of a nephrotoxic agents). Products include:

Indocin 2167

Indomethacin Sodium Trihydrate (Emtricitabine and tenofovir are primarily excreted by the kidneys by a combination of glomerular filtration and active tubular secretion. Drugs that decrease renal function may increase concentration of emtricitabine and/or tenofovir. Truvada should be avoided with concurrent or recent use of a nephrotoxic agents). Products include:

Indocin I.V. 2007

Interferon Beta-1b (Emtricitabine and tenofovir are primarily excreted by the kidneys by a combination of glomerular filtration and active tubular secretion. Drugs that decrease renal function may increase concentration of emtricitabine and/or tenofovir. Truvada should be avoided with concurrent or recent use of a nephrotoxic agents). Products include:

Betaseron	836
Extavia	2459

Interleukin-2 (Emtricitabine and tenofovir are primarily excreted by the kidneys by a combination of glomerular filtration and active tubular secretion. Drugs that decrease renal function may increase concentration of emtricitabine and/or tenofovir. Truvada should be avoided with concurrent or recent use of a nephrotoxic agents).

No products indexed under this heading.

Iodamide Meglumine (Emtricitabine and tenofovir are primarily excreted by the kidneys by a combination of glomerular filtration and active tubular secretion. Drugs that decrease renal function may increase concentration of emtricitabine and/or tenofovir. Truvada should be avoided with concurrent or recent use of a nephrotoxic agents).

No products indexed under this heading.

Iohexol (Emtricitabine and tenofovir are primarily excreted by the kidneys by a combination of glomerular filtration and active tubular secretion. Drugs that decrease renal function may increase concentration of emtricitabine and/or tenofovir. Truvada should be avoided with concurrent or recent use of a nephrotoxic agents).

No products indexed under this heading.

Iopamidol (Emtricitabine and tenofovir are primarily excreted by the kidneys by a combination of glomerular filtration and active tubular secretion. Drugs that decrease renal function may increase concentration of emtricitabine and/or tenofovir. Truvada should be avoided with concurrent or recent use of a nephrotoxic agents).

No products indexed under this heading.

Iopanoic Acid (Emtricitabine and tenofovir are primarily excreted by the kidneys by a combination of glomerular filtration and active tubular secretion. Drugs that decrease renal function may increase concentration of emtricitabine and/or tenofovir. Truvada should be avoided with concurrent or recent use of a nephrotoxic agents).

No products indexed under this heading.

Iothalamate Meglumine (Emtricitabine and tenofovir are primarily excreted by the kidneys by a combination of glomerular filtration and active tubular secretion. Drugs that decrease renal function may increase concentration of emtricitabine and/or tenofovir. Truvada should be avoided with concurrent or recent use of a nephrotoxic agents).

No products indexed under this heading.

Ioxaglate Meglumine (Emtricitabine and tenofovir are primarily excreted by the kidneys by a combination of glomerular filtation and active tubular secretion. Drugs that decrease renal function may increase concentration of emtricitabine and/or tenofovir. Truvada should be avoided with concurrent or recent use of a nephrotoxic agents).
No products indexed under this heading.

Ioxaglate Sodium (Emtricitabine and tenofovir are primarily excreted by the kidneys by a combination of glomerular filtation and active tubular secretion. Drugs that decrease renal function may increase concentration of emtricitabine and/or tenofovir. Truvada should be avoided with concurrent or recent use of a nephrotoxic agents).
No products indexed under this heading.

Kanamycin Sulfate (Emtricitabine and tenofovir are primarily excreted by the kidneys by a combination of glomerular filtation and active tubular secretion. Drugs that decrease renal function may increase concentration of emtricitabine and/or tenofovir. Truvada should be avoided with concurrent or recent use of a nephrotoxic agents).
No products indexed under this heading.

Ketoprofen (Emtricitabine and tenofovir are primarily excreted by the kidneys by a combination of glomerular filtation and active tubular secretion. Drugs that decrease renal function may increase concentration of emtricitabine and/or tenofovir. Truvada should be avoided with concurrent or recent use of a nephrotoxic agents).
No products indexed under this heading.

Ketorolac Tromethamine (Emtricitabine and tenofovir are primarily excreted by the kidneys by a combination of glomerular filtation and active tubular secretion. Drugs that decrease renal function may increase concentration of emtricitabine and/or tenofovir. Truvada should be avoided with concurrent or recent use of a nephrotoxic agents). Products include:
Acuvail .... ⊙ 209

Lamium album (Emtricitabine and tenofovir are primarily excreted by the kidneys by a combination of glomerular filtation and active tubular secretion. Drugs that decrease renal function may increase concentration of emtricitabine and/or tenofovir. Truvada should be avoided with concurrent or recent use of a nephrotoxic agents).
No products indexed under this heading.

Lamivudine (Due to similarities between emtricitabine and lamivudine, Truvada should not be co-administered with other drugs containing lamivudine. There was no clinically significant drug interaction seen between tenofovir and lamivudine. However, co-administration of tenofovir with lamivudine (150 mg twice daily for seven days) decreased, on average the C_{max} of lamivudine by 24%). Products include:
Combivir 1404
Epivir 1437
Epivir-HBV 1443
Epzicom 1448
Trizivir 1688

Lisinopril (Emtricitabine and tenofovir are primarily excreted by the kidneys by a combination of glomerular filtation and active tubular secretion. Drugs that decrease renal function may increase concentration of emtricitabine and/or tenofovir. Truvada should be avoided with concurrent or recent use of a nephrotoxic agents). Products include:
Prinivil 2241
Prinzide 2246

Lithium (Emtricitabine and tenofovir are primarily excreted by the kidneys by a combination of glomerular filtation and active tubular secretion. Drugs that decrease renal function may increase concentration of emtricitabine and/or tenofovir. Truvada should be avoided with concurrent or recent use of a nephrotoxic agents).
No products indexed under this heading.

Lithium Carbonate (Emtricitabine and tenofovir are primarily excreted by the kidneys by a combination of glomerular filtation and active tubular secretion. Drugs that decrease renal function may increase concentration of emtricitabine and/or tenofovir. Truvada should be avoided with concurrent or recent use of a nephrotoxic agents).
No products indexed under this heading.

Lithium Citrate (Emtricitabine and tenofovir are primarily excreted by the kidneys by a combination of glomerular filtation and active tubular secretion. Drugs that decrease renal function may increase concentration of emtricitabine and/or tenofovir. Truvada should be avoided with concurrent or recent use of a nephrotoxic agents).
No products indexed under this heading.

Lopinavir (Lopinavir/ritonavir has been shown to increase tenofovir concentrations. Patients receiving lopinavir/ritonavir and Truvada should be monitored for Truvada-associated adverse reactions. Truvada should be discontinued in patients who develop Truvada-associated adverse reactions). Products include:
Kaletra 458

Loracarbef (Emtricitabine and tenofovir are primarily excreted by the kidneys by a combination of glomerular filtation and active tubular secretion. Drugs that decrease renal function may increase concentration of emtricitabine and/or tenofovir. Truvada should be avoided with concurrent or recent use of a nephrotoxic agents).
No products indexed under this heading.

Lovastatin (Emtricitabine and tenofovir are primarily excreted by the kidneys by a combination of glomerular filtation and active tubular secretion. Drugs that decrease renal function may increase concentration of emtricitabine and/or tenofovir. Truvada should be avoided with concurrent or recent use of a nephrotoxic agents). Products include:
Advicor 402
Mevacor 2212

Meclofenamate Sodium (Emtricitabine and tenofovir are primarily excreted by the kidneys by a combination of glomerular filtation and active tubular secretion. Drugs that decrease renal function may increase concentration of emtricitabine and/or tenofovir. Truvada should be avoided with concurrent or recent use of a nephrotoxic agents).
No products indexed under this heading.

Mefenamic Acid (Emtricitabine and tenofovir are primarily excreted by the kidneys by a combination of glomerular filtation and active tubular secretion. Drugs that decrease renal function may increase concentration of emtricitabine and/or tenofovir. Truvada should be avoided with concurrent or recent use of a nephrotoxic agents).
No products indexed under this heading.

Meloxicam (Emtricitabine and tenofovir are primarily excreted by the kidneys by a combination of glomerular filtation and active tubular secretion. Drugs that decrease renal function may increase concentration of emtricitabine and/or tenofovir. Truvada should be avoided with concurrent or recent use of a nephrotoxic agents).
No products indexed under this heading.

Melphalan Hydrochloride (Emtricitabine and tenofovir are primarily excreted by the kidneys by a combination of glomerular filtation and active tubular secretion. Drugs that decrease renal function may increase concentration of emtricitabine and/or tenofovir. Truvada should be avoided with concurrent or recent use of a nephrotoxic agents). Products include:
Alkeran for Injection 1300

Mesalamine (Emtricitabine and tenofovir are primarily excreted by the kidneys by a combination of glomerular filtation and active tubular secretion. Drugs that decrease renal function may increase concentration of emtricitabine and/or tenofovir. Truvada should be avoided with concurrent or recent use of a nephrotoxic agents). Products include:
Apriso 2899
Asacol 2786
Asacol HD 2787
Canasa 782
Lialda 3295
Pentasa 3297

Methimazole (Emtricitabine and tenofovir are primarily excreted by the kidneys by a combination of glomerular filtation and active tubular secretion. Drugs that decrease renal function may increase concentration of emtricitabine and/or tenofovir. Truvada should be avoided with concurrent or recent use of a nephrotoxic agents).
No products indexed under this heading.

Methotrexate (Emtricitabine and tenofovir are primarily excreted by the kidneys by a combination of glomerular filtation and active tubular secretion. Drugs that decrease renal function may increase concentration of emtricitabine and/or tenofovir. Truvada should be avoided with concurrent or recent use of a nephrotoxic agents).
No products indexed under this heading.

Methotrexate Sodium (Emtricitabine and tenofovir are primarily excreted by the kidneys by a combination of glomerular filtation and active tubular secretion. Drugs that decrease renal function may increase concentration of emtricitabine and/or tenofovir. Truvada should be avoided with concurrent or recent use of a nephrotoxic agents).
No products indexed under this heading.

Methyclothiazide (Emtricitabine and tenofovir are primarily excreted by the kidneys by a combination of glomerular filtation and active tubular secretion. Drugs that decrease renal function may increase concentration of emtricitabine and/or tenofovir. Truvada should be avoided with concurrent or recent use of a nephrotoxic agents).
No products indexed under this heading.

Mezlocillin Sodium (Emtricitabine and tenofovir are primarily excreted by the kidneys by a combination of glomerular filtation and active tubular secretion. Drugs that decrease renal function may increase concentration of emtricitabine and/or tenofovir. Truvada should be avoided with concurrent or recent use of a nephrotoxic agents).
No products indexed under this heading.

Minocycline Hydrochloride (Emtricitabine and tenofovir are primarily excreted by the kidneys by a combination of glomerular filtation and active tubular secretion. Drugs that decrease renal function may increase concentration of emtricitabine and/or tenofovir. Truvada should be avoided with concurrent or recent use of a nephrotoxic agents). Products include:
Solodyn 2073

Mitomycin (Mitomycin-C) (Emtricitabine and tenofovir are primarily excreted by the kidneys by a combination of glomerular filtation and active tubular secretion. Drugs that decrease renal function may increase concentration of emtricitabine and/or tenofovir. Truvada should be avoided with concurrent or recent use of a nephrotoxic agents).
No products indexed under this heading.

Moexipril Hydrochloride (Emtricitabine and tenofovir are primarily excreted by the kidneys by a combination of glomerular filtation and active tubular secretion. Drugs that decrease renal function may increase concentration of emtricitabine and/or tenofovir. Truvada should be avoided with concurrent or recent use of a nephrotoxic agents).
No products indexed under this heading.

Morphine Sulfate (Emtricitabine and tenofovir are primarily excreted by the kidneys by a combination of glomerular filtration and active tubular secretion. No drug-drug interactions due to competition for renal excretion have been observed; however, co-administration of Truvada with drugs that are eliminated by active tubular secretion may increase concentrations of emtricitabine, tenofovir, and/or the co-administered drug). Products include:
Avinza 1822
Embeda 1831
MS Contin 2803

Muromonab-CD3 (Emtricitabine and tenofovir are primarily excreted by the kidneys by a combination of glomerular filtation and active tubular secretion. Drugs that decrease renal function may increase concentration of emtricitabine and/or tenofovir. Truvada should be avoided with concurrent or recent use of a nephrotoxic agents). Products include:
Orthoclone OKT3 949

Nabumetone (Emtricitabine and tenofovir are primarily excreted by the kidneys by a combination of glomerular filtation and active tubular secretion. Drugs that decrease renal function may increase concentration of emtricitabine and/or tenofovir. Truvada should be avoided with concurrent or recent use of a nephrotoxic agents).
No products indexed under this heading.

Nafcillin Sodium (Emtricitabine and tenofovir are primarily excreted by the kidneys by a combination of glomerular filtation and active tubular secretion. Drugs that decrease renal function may increase concentration of emtricitabine and/or tenofovir. Truvada should be avoided with concurrent or recent use of a nephrotoxic agents).
No products indexed under this heading.

Naproxen (Emtricitabine and tenofovir are primarily excreted by the kidneys by a combination of glomerular filtation and active tubular secretion. Drugs that decrease renal function may increase concentration of emtricitabine and/or tenofovir. Truvada should be avoided with concurrent or recent use of a nephrotoxic agents). Products include:
EC-Naprosyn 2850
Naprosyn 2850
Anaprox/Naprosyn 2850

Naproxen Sodium (Emtricitabine and tenofovir are primarily excreted by the kidneys by a combination of glomerular filtation and active tubular secretion. Drugs that decrease renal function may increase concentration of emtricitabine and/or tenofovir. Truvada should be avoided with concurrent or recent use of a nephrotoxic agents). Products include:
Anaprox 2850
Anaprox DS 2850
Treximet 1681

IMPORTANT NOTE: Always consult each drug listing in the patient's regimen for possible interactions.

Truvada Interactions Index 1950

Nelfinavir Mesylate (Emtricitabine and tenofovir are primarily excreted by the kidneys by a combination of glomerular filtation and active tubular secretion. Drugs that decrease renal function may increase concentration of emtricitabine and/or tenofovir. Truvada should be avoided with concurrent or recent use of a nephrotoxic agents).
No products indexed under this heading.

Neomycin (Emtricitabine and tenofovir are primarily excreted by the kidneys by a combination of glomerular filtation and active tubular secretion. Drugs that decrease renal function may increase concentration of emtricitabine and/or tenofovir. Truvada should be avoided with concurrent or recent use of a nephrotoxic agents).
No products indexed under this heading.

Neomycin, oral (Emtricitabine and tenofovir are primarily excreted by the kidneys by a combination of glomerular filtation and active tubular secretion. Drugs that decrease renal function may increase concentration of emtricitabine and/or tenofovir. Truvada should be avoided with concurrent or recent use of a nephrotoxic agents).
No products indexed under this heading.

Neomycin Sulfate (Emtricitabine and tenofovir are primarily excreted by the kidneys by a combination of glomerular filtation and active tubular secretion. Drugs that decrease renal function may increase concentration of emtricitabine and/or tenofovir. Truvada should be avoided with concurrent or recent use of a nephrotoxic agents).
No products indexed under this heading.

Nevirapine (Emtricitabine and tenofovir are primarily excreted by the kidneys by a combination of glomerular filtation and active tubular secretion. Drugs that decrease renal function may increase concentration of emtricitabine and/or tenofovir. Truvada should be avoided with concurrent or recent use of a nephrotoxic agents). Products include:
Viramune Oral Suspension 897
Viramune Tablets 897

Norfloxacin (Emtricitabine and tenofovir are primarily excreted by the kidneys by a combination of glomerular filtation and active tubular secretion. Drugs that decrease renal function may increase concentration of emtricitabine and/or tenofovir. Truvada should be avoided with concurrent or recent use of a nephrotoxic agents). Products include:
Noroxin 2220

Olsalazine Sodium (Emtricitabine and tenofovir are primarily excreted by the kidneys by a combination of glomerular filtation and active tubular secretion. Drugs that decrease renal function may increase concentration of emtricitabine and/or tenofovir. Truvada should be avoided with concurrent or recent use of a nephrotoxic agents).
No products indexed under this heading.

Omeprazole (Emtricitabine and tenofovir are primarily excreted by the kidneys by a combination of glomerular filtation and active tubular secretion. Drugs that decrease renal function may increase concentration of emtricitabine and/or tenofovir. Truvada should be avoided with concurrent or recent use of a nephrotoxic agents).
No products indexed under this heading.

Oxaprozin (Emtricitabine and tenofovir are primarily excreted by the kidneys by a combination of glomerular filtation and active tubular secretion. Drugs that decrease renal function may increase concentration of emtricitabine and/or tenofovir. Truvada should be avoided with concurrent or recent use of a nephrotoxic agents).
No products indexed under this heading.

Pamidronate Disodium (Emtricitabine and tenofovir are primarily excreted by the kidneys by a combination of glomerular filtation and active tubular secretion. Drugs that decrease renal function may increase concentration of emtricitabine and/or tenofovir. Truvada should be avoided with concurrent or recent use of a nephrotoxic agents).
No products indexed under this heading.

Paroxetine Hydrochloride (Emtricitabine and tenofovir are primarily excreted by the kidneys by a combination of glomerular filtation and active tubular secretion. Drugs that decrease renal function may increase concentration of emtricitabine and/or tenofovir. Truvada should be avoided with concurrent or recent use of a nephrotoxic agents). Products include:
Paroxetine CR 2361
Paroxetine ER 2371
Paxil 1586
Paxil CR 1596

Penicillamine (Emtricitabine and tenofovir are primarily excreted by the kidneys by a combination of glomerular filtation and active tubular secretion. Drugs that decrease renal function may increase concentration of emtricitabine and/or tenofovir. Truvada should be avoided with concurrent or recent use of a nephrotoxic agents).
No products indexed under this heading.

Penicillin G Benzathine (Emtricitabine and tenofovir are primarily excreted by the kidneys by a combination of glomerular filtation and active tubular secretion. Drugs that decrease renal function may increase concentration of emtricitabine and/or tenofovir. Truvada should be avoided with concurrent or recent use of a nephrotoxic agents). Products include:
Bicillin C-R Injectable Suspension 1826
Bicillin L-A 1828

Penicillin G Potassium (Emtricitabine and tenofovir are primarily excreted by the kidneys by a combination of glomerular filtation and active tubular secretion. Drugs that decrease renal function may increase concentration of emtricitabine and/or tenofovir. Truvada should be avoided with concurrent or recent use of a nephrotoxic agents).
No products indexed under this heading.

Penicillin G Procaine (Emtricitabine and tenofovir are primarily excreted by the kidneys by a combination of glomerular filtation and active tubular secretion. Drugs that decrease renal function may increase concentration of emtricitabine and/or tenofovir. Truvada should be avoided with concurrent or recent use of a nephrotoxic agents). Products include:
Bicillin C-R Injectable Suspension 1826
Bicillin L-A 1828

Penicillin G Sodium (Emtricitabine and tenofovir are primarily excreted by the kidneys by a combination of glomerular filtation and active tubular secretion. Drugs that decrease renal function may increase concentration of emtricitabine and/or tenofovir. Truvada should be avoided with concurrent or recent use of a nephrotoxic agents).
No products indexed under this heading.

Penicillin V Potassium (Emtricitabine and tenofovir are primarily excreted by the kidneys by a combination of glomerular filtation and active tubular secretion. Drugs that decrease renal function may increase concentration of emtricitabine and/or tenofovir. Truvada should be avoided with concurrent or recent use of a nephrotoxic agents).
No products indexed under this heading.

Pentamidine Isethionate (Emtricitabine and tenofovir are primarily excreted by the kidneys by a combination of glomerular filtation and active tubular secretion. Drugs that decrease renal function may increase concentration of emtricitabine and/or tenofovir. Truvada should be avoided with concurrent or recent use of a nephrotoxic agents).
No products indexed under this heading.

Perindopril Erbumine (Emtricitabine and tenofovir are primarily excreted by the kidneys by a combination of glomerular filtation and active tubular secretion. Drugs that decrease renal function may increase concentration of emtricitabine and/or tenofovir. Truvada should be avoided with concurrent or recent use of a nephrotoxic agents).
No products indexed under this heading.

Phenylbutazone (Emtricitabine and tenofovir are primarily excreted by the kidneys by a combination of glomerular filtation and active tubular secretion. Drugs that decrease renal function may increase concentration of emtricitabine and/or tenofovir. Truvada should be avoided with concurrent or recent use of a nephrotoxic agents).
No products indexed under this heading.

Piroxicam (Emtricitabine and tenofovir are primarily excreted by the kidneys by a combination of glomerular filtation and active tubular secretion. Drugs that decrease renal function may increase concentration of emtricitabine and/or tenofovir. Truvada should be avoided with concurrent or recent use of a nephrotoxic agents).
No products indexed under this heading.

Plicamycin (Emtricitabine and tenofovir are primarily excreted by the kidneys by a combination of glomerular filtation and active tubular secretion. Drugs that decrease renal function may increase concentration of emtricitabine and/or tenofovir. Truvada should be avoided with concurrent or recent use of a nephrotoxic agents).
No products indexed under this heading.

Polymyxin (Emtricitabine and tenofovir are primarily excreted by the kidneys by a combination of glomerular filtation and active tubular secretion. Drugs that decrease renal function may increase concentration of emtricitabine and/or tenofovir. Truvada should be avoided with concurrent or recent use of a nephrotoxic agents).
No products indexed under this heading.

Polymyxin B Sulfate (Emtricitabine and tenofovir are primarily excreted by the kidneys by a combination of glomerular filtation and active tubular secretion. Drugs that decrease renal function may increase concentration of emtricitabine and/or tenofovir. Truvada should be avoided with concurrent or recent use of a nephrotoxic agents).
No products indexed under this heading.

Polythiazide (Emtricitabine and tenofovir are primarily excreted by the kidneys by a combination of glomerular filtation and active tubular secretion. Drugs that decrease renal function may increase concentration of emtricitabine and/or tenofovir. Truvada should be avoided with concurrent or recent use of a nephrotoxic agents).
No products indexed under this heading.

Pravastatin Sodium (Emtricitabine and tenofovir are primarily excreted by the kidneys by a combination of glomerular filtation and active tubular secretion. Drugs that decrease renal function may increase concentration of emtricitabine and/or tenofovir. Truvada should be avoided with concurrent or recent use of a nephrotoxic agents).
No products indexed under this heading.

Procainamide Hydrochloride (Emtricitabine and tenofovir are primarily excreted by the kidneys by a combination of glomerular filtration and active tubular secretion. No drug-drug interactions due to competition for renal excretion have been observed; however, co-administration of Truvada with drugs that are eliminated by active tubular secretion may increase concentrations of emtricitabine, tenofovir, and/or the co-administered drug).
No products indexed under this heading.

Quinapril Hydrochloride (Emtricitabine and tenofovir are primarily excreted by the kidneys by a combination of glomerular filtation and active tubular secretion. Drugs that decrease renal function may increase concentration of emtricitabine and/or tenofovir. Truvada should be avoided with concurrent or recent use of a nephrotoxic agents).
No products indexed under this heading.

Quinidine Gluconate (Emtricitabine and tenofovir are primarily excreted by the kidneys by a combination of glomerular filtation and active tubular secretion. No drug-drug interactions due to competition for renal excretion have been observed; however, co-administration of Truvada with drugs that are eliminated by active tubular secretion may increase concentrations of emtricitabine, tenofovir, and/or the co-administered drug).
No products indexed under this heading.

Quinidine Polygalacturonate (Emtricitabine and tenofovir are primarily excreted by the kidneys by a combination of glomerular filtration and active tubular secretion. No drug-drug interactions due to competition for renal excretion have been observed; however, co-administration of Truvada with drugs that are eliminated by active tubular secretion may increase concentrations of emtricitabine, tenofovir, and/or the co-administered drug).
No products indexed under this heading.

Quinidine Sulfate (Emtricitabine and tenofovir are primarily excreted by the kidneys by a combination of glomerular filtration and active tubular secretion. No drug-drug interactions due to competition for renal excretion have been observed; however, co-administration of Truvada with drugs that are eliminated by active tubular secretion may increase concentrations of emtricitabine, tenofovir, and/or the co-administered drug).
No products indexed under this heading.

Quinine Sulfate (Emtricitabine and tenofovir are primarily excreted by the kidneys by a combination of glomerular filtration and active tubular secretion. No drug-drug interactions due to competition for renal excretion have been observed; however, co-administration of Truvada with drugs that are eliminated by active tubular secretion may increase concentrations of emtricitabine, tenofovir, and/or the co-administered drug).
No products indexed under this heading.

Rabeprazole Sodium (Emtricitabine and tenofovir are primarily excreted by the kidneys by a combination of glomerular filtation and active tubular secretion. Drugs that decrease renal function may increase concentration of emtricitabine and/or tenofovir. Truvada should

be avoided with concurrent or recent use of a nephrotoxic agents). Products include:

Aciphex 1035

Ramipril (Emtricitabine and tenofovir are primarily excreted by the kidneys by a combination of glomerular filtation and active tubular secretion. Drugs that decrease renal function may increase concentration of emtricitabine and/or tenofovir. Truvada should be avoided with concurrent or recent use of a nephrotoxic agents).

No products indexed under this heading.

Ranitidine Hydrochloride (Emtricitabine and tenofovir are primarily excreted by the kidneys by a combination of glomerular filtration and active tubular secretion. No drug-drug interactions due to competition for renal excretion have been observed; however, co-administration of Truvada with drugs that are eliminated by active tubular secretion may increase concentrations of emtricitabine, tenofovir, and/or the co-administered drug). Products include:

Zantac 1737
Zantac Injection 1732
Zantac Pharmacy 1735

Rifampin (Emtricitabine and tenofovir are primarily excreted by the kidneys by a combination of glomerular filtation and active tubular secretion. Drugs that decrease renal function may increase concentration of emtricitabine and/or tenofovir. Truvada should be avoided with concurrent or recent use of a nephrotoxic agents).

No products indexed under this heading.

Riluzole (Emtricitabine and tenofovir are primarily excreted by the kidneys by a combination of glomerular filtation and active tubular secretion. Drugs that decrease renal function may increase concentration of emtricitabine and/or tenofovir. Truvada should be avoided with concurrent or recent use of a nephrotoxic agents). Products include:

Rilutek 3032

Ritonavir (Lopinavir/ritonavir has been shown to increase tenofovir concentrations. Patients receiving lopinavir/ritonavir and Truvada should be monitored for Truvada-associated adverse reactions. Truvada should be discontinued in patients who develop Truvada-associated adverse reactions. In addition, there was no clinically significant drug interaction seen between tenofovir and saquinavir/ritonavir. However, co-administered of tenofovir (300 mg QD) with saquinavir/ritonavir (1000 mg/100 mg twice daily for 14 days) has resulted on average in an increase in tenofivir C_{min} by 23% and an increase on average in ritonavir C_{min} by 23%). Products include:

Kaletra 458
Norvir 509

Rofecoxib (Emtricitabine and tenofovir are primarily excreted by the kidneys by a combination of glomerular filtation and active tubular secretion. Drugs that decrease renal function may increase concentration of emtricitabine and/or tenofovir. Truvada should be avoided with concurrent or recent use of a nephrotoxic agents).

No products indexed under this heading.

Saquinavir (There was no clinically significant drug interaction seen between tenofovir and saquinavir/ritonavir. However, co-administration of tenofovir (300 mg QD) with saquinavir/ritonavir (1000 mg/100 mg twice daily for 14 days) has resulted on average in an increase in tenofovir C_{min} by 23% and an increase on average in saquinavir C_{max} by 22%, saquinavir AUC by 29% and on average an increase in saquinavir C_{min} by 47%).

No products indexed under this heading.

Saquinavir Mesylate (There was no clinically significant drug interaction seen between tenofovir and saquinavir/ritonavir. However, co-administration of tenofovir (300 mg QD) with saquinavir/ritonavir (1000 mg/100 mg twice daily for 14 days) has resulted on average in an increase in tenofovir C_{min} by 23% and an increase on average in saquinavir C_{max} by 22%, saquinavir AUC by 29% and on average an increase in saquinavir C_{min} by 47%).

No products indexed under this heading.

Sibutramine Hydrochloride Monohydrate (Emtricitabine and tenofovir are primarily excreted by the kidneys by a combination of glomerular filtation and active tubular secretion. Drugs that decrease renal function may increase concentration of emtricitabine and/or tenofovir. Truvada should be avoided with concurrent or recent use of a nephrotoxic agents). Products include:

Meridia 492

Simvastatin (Emtricitabine and tenofovir are primarily excreted by the kidneys by a combination of glomerular filtation and active tubular secretion. Drugs that decrease renal function may increase concentration of emtricitabine and/or tenofovir. Truvada should be avoided with concurrent or recent use of a nephrotoxic agents). Products include:

Simcor 524
Vytorin 10/10 .... 2303, 3240
Vytorin 10/20 .... 2303, 3240
Vytorin 10/40 .... 2303, 3240
Vytorin 10/80 .... 2303, 3240
Zocor 2289

Spirapril Hydrochloride (Emtricitabine and tenofovir are primarily excreted by the kidneys by a combination of glomerular filtation and active tubular secretion. Drugs that decrease renal function may increase concentration of emtricitabine and/or tenofovir. Truvada should be avoided with concurrent or recent use of a nephrotoxic agents).

No products indexed under this heading.

Stavudine (Emtricitabine and tenofovir are primarily excreted by the kidneys by a combination of glomerular filtation and active tubular secretion. Drugs that decrease renal function may increase concentration of emtricitabine and/or tenofovir. Truvada should be avoided with concurrent or recent use of a nephrotoxic agents).

No products indexed under this heading.

Streptomycin Sulfate (Emtricitabine and tenofovir are primarily excreted by the kidneys by a combination of glomerular filtation and active tubular secretion. Drugs that decrease renal function may increase concentration of emtricitabine and/or tenofovir. Truvada should be avoided with concurrent or recent use of a nephrotoxic agents).

No products indexed under this heading.

Streptozocin (Emtricitabine and tenofovir are primarily excreted by the kidneys by a combination of glomerular filtation and active tubular secretion. Drugs that decrease renal function may increase concentration of emtricitabine and/or tenofovir. Truvada should be avoided with concurrent or recent use of a nephrotoxic agents).

No products indexed under this heading.

Sulfacytine (Emtricitabine and tenofovir are primarily excreted by the kidneys by a combination of glomerular filtation and active tubular secretion. Drugs that decrease renal function may increase concentration of emtricitabine and/or tenofovir. Truvada should be avoided with concurrent or recent use of a nephrotoxic agents).

No products indexed under this heading.

Sulfamethizole (Emtricitabine and tenofovir are primarily excreted by the kidneys by a combination of glomerular filtation and active tubular secretion. Drugs that decrease renal function may increase concentration of emtricitabine and/or tenofovir. Truvada should be avoided with concurrent or recent use of a nephrotoxic agents).

No products indexed under this heading.

Sulfamethoxazole (Emtricitabine and tenofovir are primarily excreted by the kidneys by a combination of glomerular filtation and active tubular secretion. Drugs that decrease renal function may increase concentration of emtricitabine and/or tenofovir. Truvada should be avoided with concurrent or recent use of a nephrotoxic agents).

No products indexed under this heading.

Sulfasalazine (Emtricitabine and tenofovir are primarily excreted by the kidneys by a combination of glomerular filtation and active tubular secretion. Drugs that decrease renal function may increase concentration of emtricitabine and/or tenofovir. Truvada should be avoided with concurrent or recent use of a nephrotoxic agents).

No products indexed under this heading.

Sulfinpyrazone (Emtricitabine and tenofovir are primarily excreted by the kidneys by a combination of glomerular filtation and active tubular secretion. Drugs that decrease renal function may increase concentration of emtricitabine and/or tenofovir. Truvada should be avoided with concurrent or recent use of a nephrotoxic agents).

No products indexed under this heading.

Sulfisoxazole Acetyl (Emtricitabine and tenofovir are primarily excreted by the kidneys by a combination of glomerular filtation and active tubular secretion. Drugs that decrease renal function may increase concentration of emtricitabine and/or tenofovir. Truvada should be avoided with concurrent or recent use of a nephrotoxic agents).

No products indexed under this heading.

Sulfisoxazole Diolamine (Emtricitabine and tenofovir are primarily excreted by the kidneys by a combination of glomerular filtation and active tubular secretion. Drugs that decrease renal function may increase concentration of emtricitabine and/or tenofovir. Truvada should be avoided with concurrent or recent use of a nephrotoxic agents).

No products indexed under this heading.

Sulindac (Emtricitabine and tenofovir are primarily excreted by the kidneys by a combination of glomerular filtation and active tubular secretion. Drugs that decrease renal function may increase concentration of emtricitabine and/or tenofovir. Truvada should be avoided with concurrent or recent use of a nephrotoxic agents). Products include:

Clinoril 2098

Tacrolimus (There was no clinically significant drug interaction seen between tenofovir and tacrolimus. However, co-administration of tenofovir (300 mg QD) with tacrolimus (0.05 mg/kg twice daily for seven days) resulted on average in an increase in C_{max} by 13%). Products include:

Prograf Capsules 677
Prograf Injection 677
Protopic 685

Thioguanine (Emtricitabine and tenofovir are primarily excreted by the kidneys by a combination of glomerular filtation and active tubular secretion. Drugs that decrease renal function may increase concentration of emtricitabine and/or tenofovir. Truvada should be avoided with concurrent or recent use of a nephrotoxic agents). Products include:

Tabloid 1664

Ticarcillin Disodium (Emtricitabine and tenofovir are primarily excreted by the kidneys by a combination of glomerular filtation and active tubular secretion. Drugs that decrease renal function may increase concentration of emtricitabine and/or tenofovir. Truvada should be avoided with concurrent or recent use of a nephrotoxic agents). Products include:

Timentin ADD-Vantage 1670
Timentin Galaxy 1674
Timentin 1666
Timentin Pharmacy 1678

Tobramycin (Emtricitabine and tenofovir are primarily excreted by the kidneys by a combination of glomerular filtation and active tubular secretion. Drugs that decrease renal function may increase concentration of emtricitabine and/or tenofovir. Truvada should be avoided with concurrent or recent use of a nephrotoxic agents). Products include:

Tobi Nebulizer 2546
Tobramycin and Dexamethasone Ophthalmic Suspension .... ⊙251
Zylet .... ⊙252

Tobramycin Sulfate (Emtricitabine and tenofovir are primarily excreted by the kidneys by a combination of glomerular filtation and active tubular secretion. Drugs that decrease renal function may increase concentration of emtricitabine and/or tenofovir. Truvada should be avoided with concurrent or recent use of a nephrotoxic agents).

No products indexed under this heading.

Tolazamide (Emtricitabine and tenofovir are primarily excreted by the kidneys by a combination of glomerular filtation and active tubular secretion. Drugs that decrease renal function may increase concentration of emtricitabine and/or tenofovir. Truvada should be avoided with concurrent or recent use of a nephrotoxic agents).

No products indexed under this heading.

Tolbutamide (Emtricitabine and tenofovir are primarily excreted by the kidneys by a combination of glomerular filtation and active tubular secretion. Drugs that decrease renal function may increase concentration of emtricitabine and/or tenofovir. Truvada should be avoided with concurrent or recent use of a nephrotoxic agents).

No products indexed under this heading.

Tolmetin Sodium (Emtricitabine and tenofovir are primarily excreted by the kidneys by a combination of glomerular filtation and active tubular secretion. Drugs that decrease renal function may increase concentration of emtricitabine and/or tenofovir. Truvada should be avoided with concurrent or recent use of a nephrotoxic agents).

No products indexed under this heading.

Trandolapril (Emtricitabine and tenofovir are primarily excreted by the kidneys by a combination of glomerular filtation and active tubular secretion. Drugs that decrease renal function may increase concentration of emtricitabine and/or tenofovir. Truvada should be avoided with concurrent or recent use of a nephrotoxic agents). Products include:

Mavik 489
Tarka 534

Triamterene (Emtricitabine and tenofovir are primarily excreted by the kidneys by a combination of glomerular filtation and active tubular secretion. Drugs that decrease renal function may increase concentration of emtricitabine and/or tenofovir. Truvada should be avoided with concurrent or recent use of a nephrotoxic agents). Products include:

Dyazide 1429
Dyrenium 3495

IMPORTANT NOTE: Always consult each drug listing in the patient's regimen for possible interactions.

Trimethadione (Emtricitabine and tenofovir are primarily excreted by the kidneys by a combination of glomerular filtation and active tubular secretion. Drugs that decrease renal function may increase concentration of emtricitabine and/or tenofovir. Truvada should be avoided with concurrent or recent use of a nephrotoxic agents).
No products indexed under this heading.

Trimethoprim (Emtricitabine and tenofovir are primarily excreted by the kidneys by a combination of glomerular filtration and active tubular secretion. No drug-drug interactions due to competition for renal excretion have been observed; however, co-administration of Truvada with drugs that are eliminated by active tubular secretion may increase concentrations of emtricitabine, tenofovir, and/or the co-administered drug).
No products indexed under this heading.

Trimethoprim Sulfate (Emtricitabine and tenofovir are primarily excreted by the kidneys by a combination of glomerular filtration and active tubular secretion. No drug-drug interactions due to competition for renal excretion have been observed; however, co-administration of Truvada with drugs that are eliminated by active tubular secretion may increase concentrations of emtricitabine, tenofovir, and/or the co-administered drug).
No products indexed under this heading.

Trovafloxacin Mesylate (Emtricitabine and tenofovir are primarily excreted by the kidneys by a combination of glomerular filtation and active tubular secretion. Drugs that decrease renal function may increase concentration of emtricitabine and/or tenofovir. Truvada should be avoided with concurrent or recent use of a nephrotoxic agents).
No products indexed under this heading.

Tyropanoate Sodium (Emtricitabine and tenofovir are primarily excreted by the kidneys by a combination of glomerular filtration and active tubular secretion. Drugs that decrease renal function may increase concentration of emtricitabine and/or tenofovir. Truvada should be avoided with concurrent or recent use of a nephrotoxic agents).
No products indexed under this heading.

Valacyclovir Hydrochloride (Emtricitabine and tenofovir are primarily excreted by the kidneys by a combination of glomerular filtration and active tubular secretion. No drug-drug interactions due to competition for renal excretion have been observed; however, co-administration of Truvada with drugs that are eliminated by active tubular secretion may increase concentrations of emtricitabine, tenofovir, and/or the co-administered drug. Some examples include, but are not limited to acyclovir, adefovir dipivoxil, cidofovir, ganciclovir, valacyclovir, and valganciclovir. Truvada should be avoided with concurrent or recent use of a nephrotoxic agent). Products include:
Valtrex 1702

Valdecoxib (Emtricitabine and tenofovir are primarily excreted by the kidneys by a combination of glomerular filtation and active tubular secretion. Drugs that decrease renal function may increase concentration of emtricitabine and/or tenofovir. Truvada should be avoided with concurrent or recent use of a nephrotoxic agents).
No products indexed under this heading.

Valganciclovir Hydrochloride (Emtricitabine and tenofovir are primarily excreted by the kidneys by a combination of glomerular filtration and active tubular secretion. No drug-drug interactions due to competition for renal excretion have been observed; however, co-

administration of Truvada with drugs that are eliminated by active tubular secretion may increase concentrations of emtricitabine, tenofovir, and/or the co-administered drug. Some examples include, but are not limited to acyclovir, adefovir dipivoxil, cidofovir, ganciclovir, valacyclovir, and valganciclovir). Products include:
Valcyte 2872

Vancomycin Hydrochloride (Emtricitabine and tenofovir are primarily excreted by the kidneys by a combination of glomerular filtation and active tubular secretion. Drugs that decrease renal function may increase concentration of emtricitabine and/or tenofovir. Truvada should be avoided with concurrent or recent use of a nephrotoxic agents).
No products indexed under this heading.

Voriconazole (Emtricitabine and tenofovir are primarily excreted by the kidneys by a combination of glomerular filtation and active tubular secretion. Drugs that decrease renal function may increase concentration of emtricitabine and/or tenofovir. Truvada should be avoided with concurrent or recent use of a nephrotoxic agents).
No products indexed under this heading.

Zalcitabine (Emtricitabine and tenofovir are primarily excreted by the kidneys by a combination of glomerular filtation and active tubular secretion. Drugs that decrease renal function may increase concentration of emtricitabine and/or tenofovir. Truvada should be avoided with concurrent or recent use of a nephrotoxic agents).
No products indexed under this heading.

Zidovudine (There was no clinically significant drug interaction seen between emtricitabine and zidovudine. However, co-administration of emtricitabine (200 mg QD for seven days) with zidovudine (300 mg twice daily for seven days) has resulted on average, in a 17% increase in zidovudine C_{max} and a 13% increase in zidovudine AUC). Products include:
Combivir 1404
Retrovir 1634
Retrovir IV 1640
Trizivir 1688

Zoledronic Acid (Emtricitabine and tenofovir are primarily excreted by the kidneys by a combination of glomerular filtation and active tubular secretion. Drugs that decrease renal function may increase concentration of emtricitabine and/or tenofovir. Truvada should be avoided with concurrent or recent use of a nephrotoxic agents). Products include:
Reclast 2509
Zometa 2554

Food Interactions

Food, unspecified (Truvada may be administered with or without food. Administration of Truvada following a high fat meal or a light meal delayed the time of tenofovir C_{max} by approximately 0.75 hour. The mean increases in tenofovir AUC and C_{max} were approximately 35% and 15%, respectively, when administered with a high fat or light meal, compared to administration in the fasted state. In previous safety and efficacy studies, tenofovir was taken under fed conditions. Emtricitabine systemic exposures (AUC and C_{max}) were unaffected when Truvada was administered with either a high fat or a light meal).

Meal, unspecified (Truvada may be administered with or without food. Administration of Truvada following a high fat meal or a light meal delayed the time of tenofovir C_{max} by approximately 0.75 hour. The mean increases in tenofovir AUC and C_{max} were approximately

35% and 15%, respectively, when administered with a high fat or light meal, compared to administration in the fasted state. In previous safety and efficacy studies, tenofovir was taken under fed conditions. Emtricitabine systemic exposures (AUC and C_{max}) were unaffected when Truvada was administered with either a high fat or a light meal).

TUSSIONEX PENNKINETIC EXTENDED-RELEASE SUSPENSION

(Chlorpheniramine Polistirex, Hydrocodone Polistirex)...................... 3443
May interact with alcohols, anticholinergics, antihistamines, central nervous system depressants, monoamine oxidase inhibitors, tricyclic antidepressants, and certain other agents. Compounds in these categories include:

Acrivastine (Combined therapy may result in additive CNS depression).
No products indexed under this heading.

Alfentanil Hydrochloride (Combined therapy may result in additive CNS depression).
No products indexed under this heading.

Alprazolam (Combined therapy may result in additive CNS depression).
No products indexed under this heading.

Amitriptyline Hydrochloride (Co-administration of hydrocodone with MAO inhibitors may increase the effect of tricyclic antidepressant or hydrocodone).
No products indexed under this heading.

Amobarbital (Combined therapy may result in additive CNS depression).
No products indexed under this heading.

Amobarbital Sodium (Combined therapy may result in additive CNS depression).
No products indexed under this heading.

Amoxapine (Co-administration of hydrocodone with MAO inhibitors may increase the effect of tricyclic antidepressant or hydrocodone).
No products indexed under this heading.

Aprobarbital (Combined therapy may result in additive CNS depression).
No products indexed under this heading.

Astemizole (Combined therapy may result in additive CNS depression).
No products indexed under this heading.

Atropine Sulfate (Concurrent use of other anticholinergic agents with hydrocodone may produce paralytic ileus). Products include:
Donnatal 2711

Azatadine Maleate (Combined therapy may result in additive CNS depression).
No products indexed under this heading.

Belladonna Alkaloids (Concurrent use of other anticholinergic agents with hydrocodone may produce paralytic ileus). Products include:
Hyland's Teething Tablets 3316

Benztropine Mesylate (Concurrent use of other anticholinergic agents with hydrocodone may produce paralytic ileus).
No products indexed under this heading.

Biperiden Hydrochloride (Concurrent use of other anticholinergic agents with hydrocodone may produce paralytic ileus).
No products indexed under this heading.

Bromodiphenhydramine Hydrochloride (Combined therapy may result in additive CNS depression).
No products indexed under this heading.

Brompheniramine Maleate (Combined therapy may result in additive CNS depression).
No products indexed under this heading.

Buprenorphine Hydrochloride (Combined therapy may result in additive CNS depression).
No products indexed under this heading.

Buspirone Hydrochloride (Combined therapy may result in additive CNS depression).
No products indexed under this heading.

Butabarbital (Combined therapy may result in additive CNS depression).
No products indexed under this heading.

Butabarbital Sodium (Combined therapy may result in additive CNS depression).
No products indexed under this heading.

Butalbital (Combined therapy may result in additive CNS depression).
No products indexed under this heading.

Cetirizine Hydrochloride (Combined therapy may result in additive CNS depression). Products include:
Zyrtec Allergy 2052
Children's Zyrtec Allergy Syrup 2053
Children's Zyrtec Allergy 2053
Children's Zyrtec Hives Relief 2053
Zyrtec-D Allergy & Congestion 2054

Chlordiazepoxide (Combined therapy may result in additive CNS depression).
No products indexed under this heading.

Chlordiazepoxide Hydrochloride (Combined therapy may result in additive CNS depression).
No products indexed under this heading.

Chlorpheniramine Maleate (Combined therapy may result in additive CNS depression).
No products indexed under this heading.

Chlorpheniramine Tannate (Combined therapy may result in additive CNS depression).
No products indexed under this heading.

Chlorpromazine (Combined therapy may result in additive CNS depression).
No products indexed under this heading.

Chlorpromazine Hydrochloride (Combined therapy may result in additive CNS depression).
No products indexed under this heading.

Chlorprothixene (Combined therapy may result in additive CNS depression).
No products indexed under this heading.

Chlorprothixene Hydrochloride (Combined therapy may result in additive CNS depression).
No products indexed under this heading.

Chlorprothixene Lactate (Combined therapy may result in additive CNS depression).
No products indexed under this heading.

Clemastine Fumarate (Combined therapy may result in additive CNS depression).
No products indexed under this heading.

Clidinium Bromide (Concurrent use of other anticholinergic agents with hydrocodone may produce paralytic ileus).
No products indexed under this heading.

Clomipramine Hydrochloride (Co-administration of hydrocodone with MAO inhibitors may increase the effect of tricyclic antidepressant or hydrocodone).
No products indexed under this heading.

Clonazepam (Combined therapy may result in additive CNS depression). Products include:
Klonopin 2855

Clorazepate Dipotassium (Combined therapy may result in additive CNS depression).
No products indexed under this heading.

Clozapine (Combined therapy may result in additive CNS depression).
No products indexed under this heading.

Codeine Phosphate (Combined therapy may result in additive CNS depression). Products include:

Tylenol with Codeine 2691

Codeine Sulfate (Combined therapy may result in additive CNS depression).
No products indexed under this heading.

Cyproheptadine Hydrochloride (Combined therapy may result in additive CNS depression).
No products indexed under this heading.

Desflurane (Combined therapy may result in additive CNS depression).
No products indexed under this heading.

Desipramine Hydrochloride (Co-administration of hydrocodone with MAO inhibitors may increase the effect of tricyclic antidepressant or hydrocodone).
No products indexed under this heading.

Dexchlorpheniramine Maleate (Combined therapy may result in additive CNS depression).
No products indexed under this heading.

Dezocine (Combined therapy may result in additive CNS depression).
No products indexed under this heading.

Diazepam (Combined therapy may result in additive CNS depression). Products include:
Valium Tablets 2880

Dicyclomine Hydrochloride (Concurrent use of other anticholinergic agents with hydrocodone may produce paralytic ileus). Products include:
Bentyl Capsules 780
Bentyl Injection 780
Bentyl Syrup 780
Bentyl Tablets 780

Diphenhydramine Hydrochloride (Combined therapy may result in additive CNS depression). Products include:
Benadryl Allergy Ultratab 2042
Children's Benadryl Allergy Liquid 2042

Diphenylpyraline Hydrochloride (Combined therapy may result in additive CNS depression).
No products indexed under this heading.

Doxepin Hydrochloride (Co-administration of hydrocodone with MAO inhibitors may increase the effect of tricyclic antidepressant or hydrocodone).
No products indexed under this heading.

Droperidol (Combined therapy may result in additive CNS depression).
No products indexed under this heading.

Enflurane (Combined therapy may result in additive CNS depression).
No products indexed under this heading.

Estazolam (Combined therapy may result in additive CNS depression).
No products indexed under this heading.

Ethanol (Combined therapy may result in additive CNS depression).
No products indexed under this heading.

Ethchlorvynol (Combined therapy may result in additive CNS depression).
No products indexed under this heading.

Ethinamate (Combined therapy may result in additive CNS depression).
No products indexed under this heading.

Ethyl Alcohol (Combined therapy may result in additive CNS depression).
No products indexed under this heading.

Fentanyl (Combined therapy may result in additive CNS depression). Products include:
Duragesic 2604
Fentanyl Transdermal System 2346
Onsolis 2054

Fentanyl Citrate (Combined therapy may result in additive CNS depression). Products include:
Fentora 966

Fexofenadine Hydrochloride (Combined therapy may result in additive CNS depression). Products include:
Allegra ODT 2911
Allegra Oral Solution 2911
Allegra 2911
Allegra-D 2915
Allegra-D 24 2918

Fluphenazine Decanoate (Combined therapy may result in additive CNS depression).
No products indexed under this heading.

Fluphenazine Enanthate (Combined therapy may result in additive CNS depression).
No products indexed under this heading.

Fluphenazine Hydrochloride (Combined therapy may result in additive CNS depression).
No products indexed under this heading.

Flurazepam Hydrochloride (Combined therapy may result in additive CNS depression).
No products indexed under this heading.

Glutethimide (Combined therapy may result in additive CNS depression).
No products indexed under this heading.

Glycopyrrolate (Concurrent use of other anticholinergic agents with hydrocodone may produce paralytic ileus).
No products indexed under this heading.

Halazepam (Combined therapy may result in additive CNS depression).
No products indexed under this heading.

Haloperidol (Combined therapy may result in additive CNS depression).
No products indexed under this heading.

Haloperidol Decanoate (Combined therapy may result in additive CNS depression).
No products indexed under this heading.

Haloperidol Lactate (Combined therapy may result in additive CNS depression).
No products indexed under this heading.

Hexobarbital (Combined therapy may result in additive CNS depression).
No products indexed under this heading.

Hydrocodone Bitartrate (Combined therapy may result in additive CNS depression). Products include:
Vicodin 560
Vicodin ES 561
Vicodin HP 563
Vicoprofen 564
Zydone 1138

Hydromorphone (Combined therapy may result in additive CNS depression).
No products indexed under this heading.

Hydromorphone Hydrochloride (Combined therapy may result in additive CNS depression). Products include:
Dilaudid Injection 2800
Dilaudid Oral 2797
Dilaudid Tablets 2797
Dilaudid-HP 2800

Hydroxyzine Hydrochloride (Combined therapy may result in additive CNS depression).
No products indexed under this heading.

Hyoscyamine (Concurrent use of other anticholinergic agents with hydrocodone may produce paralytic ileus).
No products indexed under this heading.

Hyoscyamine Sulfate (Concurrent use of other anticholinergic agents with hydrocodone may produce paralytic ileus). Products include:
Donnatal 2711

Imipramine Hydrochloride (Co-administration of hydrocodone with MAO inhibitors may increase the effect of tricyclic antidepressant or hydrocodone).
No products indexed under this heading.

Imipramine Pamoate (Co-administration of hydrocodone with MAO inhibitors may increase the effect of tricyclic antidepressant or hydrocodone).
No products indexed under this heading.

Ipratropium Bromide (Concurrent use of other anticholinergic agents with hydrocodone may produce paralytic ileus).
No products indexed under this heading.

Isocarboxazid (Co-administration of hydrocodone with MAO inhibitors may increase the effect of MAOI or hydrocodone). Products include:
Marplan 3481

Isoflurane (Combined therapy may result in additive CNS depression).
No products indexed under this heading.

Ketamine Hydrochloride (Combined therapy may result in additive CNS depression).
No products indexed under this heading.

Levomethadyl Acetate Hydrochloride (Combined therapy may result in additive CNS depression).
No products indexed under this heading.

Levorphanol Tartrate (Combined therapy may result in additive CNS depression).
No products indexed under this heading.

Loratadine (Combined therapy may result in additive CNS depression).
No products indexed under this heading.

Lorazepam (Combined therapy may result in additive CNS depression).
No products indexed under this heading.

Loxapine Hydrochloride (Combined therapy may result in additive CNS depression).
No products indexed under this heading.

Loxapine Succinate (Combined therapy may result in additive CNS depression).
No products indexed under this heading.

Maprotiline Hydrochloride (Co-administration of hydrocodone with MAO inhibitors may increase the effect of tricyclic antidepressant or hydrocodone).
No products indexed under this heading.

Mepenzolate Bromide (Concurrent use of other anticholinergic agents with hydrocodone may produce paralytic ileus).
No products indexed under this heading.

Meperidine Hydrochloride (Combined therapy may result in additive CNS depression).
No products indexed under this heading.

Mephobarbital (Combined therapy may result in additive CNS depression).
No products indexed under this heading.

Meprobamate (Combined therapy may result in additive CNS depression).
No products indexed under this heading.

Mesoridazine Besylate (Combined therapy may result in additive CNS depression).
No products indexed under this heading.

Methadone Hydrochloride (Combined therapy may result in additive CNS depression).
No products indexed under this heading.

Methdilazine Hydrochloride (Combined therapy may result in additive CNS depression).
No products indexed under this heading.

Methohexital Sodium (Combined therapy may result in additive CNS depression).
No products indexed under this heading.

Methotrimeprazine (Combined therapy may result in additive CNS depression).
No products indexed under this heading.

Methoxyflurane (Combined therapy may result in additive CNS depression).
No products indexed under this heading.

Midazolam Hydrochloride (Combined therapy may result in additive CNS depression).
No products indexed under this heading.

Moclobemide (Co-administration of hydrocodone with MAO inhibitors may increase the effect of MAOI or hydrocodone).
No products indexed under this heading.

Molindone Hydrochloride (Combined therapy may result in additive CNS depression). Products include:
Moban 1108

Morphine Sulfate (Combined therapy may result in additive CNS depression). Products include:
Avinza 1822
Embeda 1831
MS Contin 2803

Morphine Sulfate, Liposomal (Combined therapy may result in additive CNS depression).
No products indexed under this heading.

Nortriptyline Hydrochloride (Co-administration of hydrocodone with MAO inhibitors may increase the effect of tricyclic antidepressant or hydrocodone).
No products indexed under this heading.

Olanzapine (Combined therapy may result in additive CNS depression). Products include:
Symbyax 1965
Zyprexa 1984
Zyprexa IntraMuscular 1984
Zyprexa ZYDIS 1984

Oxazepam (Combined therapy may result in additive CNS depression).
No products indexed under this heading.

Oxybutynin Chloride (Concurrent use of other anticholinergic agents with hydrocodone may produce paralytic ileus).
No products indexed under this heading.

Oxycodone Hydrochloride (Combined therapy may result in additive CNS depression). Products include:
OxyContin 2807
Percocet 1121
Percodan 1124

Oxycodone Terephthalate (Combined therapy may result in additive CNS depression).
No products indexed under this heading.

Oxymorphone Hydrochloride (Combined therapy may result in additive CNS depression). Products include:
Opana 1110
Opana ER 1114

Pargyline Hydrochloride (Co-administration of hydrocodone with MAO inhibitors may increase the effect of MAOI or hydrocodone).
No products indexed under this heading.

Pentobarbital (Combined therapy may result in additive CNS depression).
No products indexed under this heading.

Pentobarbital Sodium (Combined therapy may result in additive CNS depression). Products include:
Nembutal 2012

Perphenazine (Combined therapy may result in additive CNS depression).
No products indexed under this heading.

Phenelzine Sulfate (Co-administration of hydrocodone with MAO inhibitors may increase the effect of MAOI or hydrocodone).
No products indexed under this heading.

Phenobarbital (Combined therapy may result in additive CNS depression). Products include:
Donnatal 2711

Phenobarbital Sodium (Combined therapy may result in additive CNS depression).
No products indexed under this heading.

Prazepam (Combined therapy may result in additive CNS depression).
No products indexed under this heading.

IMPORTANT NOTE: Always consult each drug listing in the patient's regimen for possible interactions.

Procarbazine Hydrochloride (Co-administration of hydrocodone with MAO inhibitors may increase the effect of MAOI or hydrocodone).
No products indexed under this heading.

Prochlorperazine (Combined therapy may result in additive CNS depression).
No products indexed under this heading.

Prochlorperazine Edisylate (Combined therapy may result in additive CNS depression).
No products indexed under this heading.

Prochlorperazine Maleate (Combined therapy may result in additive CNS depression).
No products indexed under this heading.

Procyclidine Hydrochloride (Concurrent use of other anticholinergic agents with hydrocodone may produce paralytic ileus).
No products indexed under this heading.

Promethazine (Combined therapy may result in additive CNS depression).
No products indexed under this heading.

Promethazine Hydrochloride (Combined therapy may result in additive CNS depression).
No products indexed under this heading.

Propantheline Bromide (Concurrent use of other anticholinergic agents with hydrocodone may produce paralytic ileus).
No products indexed under this heading.

Propofol (Combined therapy may result in additive CNS depression).
No products indexed under this heading.

Propoxyphene Hydrochloride (Combined therapy may result in additive CNS depression).
No products indexed under this heading.

Propoxyphene Napsylate (Combined therapy may result in additive CNS depression).
No products indexed under this heading.

Protriptyline Hydrochloride (Co-administration of hydrocodone with MAO inhibitors may increase the effect of tricyclic antidepressant or hydrocodone).
No products indexed under this heading.

Pyrilamine Maleate (Combined therapy may result in additive CNS depression).
No products indexed under this heading.

Pyrilamine Tannate (Combined therapy may result in additive CNS depression).
No products indexed under this heading.

Quazepam (Combined therapy may result in additive CNS depression).
No products indexed under this heading.

Quetiapine Fumarate (Combined therapy may result in additive CNS depression). Products include:

Rasagiline Mesylate (Co-administration of hydrocodone with MAO inhibitors may increase the effect of MAOI or hydrocodone). Products include:

Remifentanil Hydrochloride (Combined therapy may result in additive CNS depression).
No products indexed under this heading.

Risperidone (Combined therapy may result in additive CNS depression). Products include:

Scopolamine (Concurrent use of other anticholinergic agents with hydrocodone may produce paralytic ileus). Products include:

Scopolamine Hydrobromide (Concurrent use of other anticholinergic agents with hydrocodone may produce paralytic ileus). Products include:

Secobarbital Sodium (Combined therapy may result in additive CNS depression).
No products indexed under this heading.

Selegiline (Co-administration of hydrocodone with MAO inhibitors may increase the effect of MAOI or hydrocodone). Products include:

Selegiline Hydrochloride (Co-administration of hydrocodone with MAO inhibitors may increase the effect of MAOI or hydrocodone). Products include:

Sevoflurane (Combined therapy may result in additive CNS depression). Products include:

Sodium Butabarbital (Combined therapy may result in additive CNS depression).
No products indexed under this heading.

Sodium Oxybate (Combined therapy may result in additive CNS depression).
No products indexed under this heading.

Sodium Pentobarbital (Combined therapy may result in additive CNS depression).
No products indexed under this heading.

Sufentanil Citrate (Combined therapy may result in additive CNS depression).
No products indexed under this heading.

Talbutal (Combined therapy may result in additive CNS depression).
No products indexed under this heading.

Temazepam (Combined therapy may result in additive CNS depression).
No products indexed under this heading.

Terfenadine (Combined therapy may result in additive CNS depression).
No products indexed under this heading.

Thiamylal Sodium (Combined therapy may result in additive CNS depression).
No products indexed under this heading.

Thioridazine (Combined therapy may result in additive CNS depression).
No products indexed under this heading.

Thioridazine Hydrochloride (Combined therapy may result in additive CNS depression). Products include:

Thiothixene (Combined therapy may result in additive CNS depression). Products include:

Thiothixene Hydrochloride (Combined therapy may result in additive CNS depression).
No products indexed under this heading.

Tolterodine Tartrate (Concurrent use of other anticholinergic agents with hydrocodone may produce paralytic ileus).
No products indexed under this heading.

Tranylcypromine Sulfate (Co-administration of hydrocodone with MAO inhibitors may increase the effect of MAOI or hydrocodone). Products include:

Triazolam (Combined therapy may result in additive CNS depression).
No products indexed under this heading.

Tridihexethyl Chloride (Concurrent use of other anticholinergic agents with hydrocodone may produce paralytic ileus).
No products indexed under this heading.

Trifluoperazine Hydrochloride (Combined therapy may result in additive CNS depression).
No products indexed under this heading.

Trihexyphenidyl Hydrochloride (Concurrent use of other anticholinergic agents with hydrocodone may produce paralytic ileus).
No products indexed under this heading.

Trimeprazine Tartrate (Combined therapy may result in additive CNS depression).
No products indexed under this heading.

Trimipramine Maleate (Co-administration of hydrocodone with MAO inhibitors may increase the effect of tricyclic antidepressant or hydrocodone).
No products indexed under this heading.

Tripelennamine Hydrochloride (Combined therapy may result in additive CNS depression).
No products indexed under this heading.

Triprolidine Hydrochloride (Combined therapy may result in additive CNS depression).
No products indexed under this heading.

Zaleplon (Combined therapy may result in additive CNS depression).
No products indexed under this heading.

Ziprasidone Hydrochloride (Combined therapy may result in additive CNS depression). Products include:

Zolpidem Tartrate (Combined therapy may result in additive CNS depression). Products include:

Food Interactions

Alcohol (Combined therapy may result in additive CNS depression).

Beer, reduced-alcohol (Combined use may result in additive CNS depression).

Beer, unspecified (Combined use may result in additive CNS depression).

Wine, Chianti (Combined use may result in additive CNS depression).

Wine, Red (Combined use may result in additive CNS depression).

Wine, unspecified (Combined use may result in additive CNS depression).

Wine products (Combined use may result in additive CNS depression).

TWINJECT AUTO-INJECTOR

May interact with alpha adrenergic blockers, antiarrhythmics, antihistamines, beta-blockers, cardiac glycosides, diuretics, ergot-containing drugs, monoamine oxidase inhibitors, phenothiazines, tricyclic antidepressants, and certain other agents. Compounds in these categories include:

Acebutolol Hydrochloride (Epinephrine should be used with caution in patients who are on medications that may sensitize the heart to arrhythmias, (eg, digitalis, diuretics, or anti-arrhythmics). In such patients, epinephrine may precipitate or aggravate angina pectoris as well as produce ventricular arrhythmias).
No products indexed under this heading.

Acrivastine (The effects of epinephrine may be potentiated by certain antihistamines, notably chlorpheniramine, tripelennamine, and diphenhydramine).
No products indexed under this heading.

Adenosine (Epinephrine should be used with caution in patients who are on medications that may sensitize the heart to arrhythmias, (eg, digitalis, diuretics, or anti-arrhythmics). In such patients, epinephrine may precipitate or aggravate angina pectoris as well as produce ventricular arrhythmias).
Products include:

Alfuzosin Hydrochloride (The vasoconstricting and hypertensive effects are antagonized by alpha-adrenergic blocking drugs, such as phentolamine). Products include:

Amiloride Hydrochloride (Patients who receive epinephrine while concomitantly taking cardiac glycosides or diuretics should be observed carefully for the development of cardiac arrhythmias).
No products indexed under this heading.

Amiodarone Hydrochloride (Epinephrine should be used with caution in patients who are on medications that may sensitize the heart to arrhythmias, (eg, digitalis, diuretics, or anti-arrhythmics). In such patients, epinephrine may precipitate or aggravate angina pectoris as well as produce ventricular arrhythmias).
No products indexed under this heading.

Amitriptyline Hydrochloride (The effects of epinephrine may be potentiated by tricyclic antidepressants).
No products indexed under this heading.

Amoxapine (The effects of epinephrine may be potentiated by tricyclic antidepressants).
No products indexed under this heading.

Apraclonidine Hydrochloride (The vasoconstricting and hypertensive effects are antagonized by alpha-adrenergic blocking drugs, such as phentolamine).
No products indexed under this heading.

Astemizole (The effects of epinephrine may be potentiated by certain antihistamines, notably chlorpheniramine, tripelennamine, and diphenhydramine).
No products indexed under this heading.

Atenolol (The cardiostimulating and bronchodilating effects of epinephrine are antagonized by beta-adrenergic blocking drugs, such as propranolol).
No products indexed under this heading.

Azatadine Maleate (The effects of epinephrine may be potentiated by certain antihistamines, notably chlorpheniramine, tripelennamine, and diphenhydramine).
No products indexed under this heading.

Bendroflumethiazide (Patients who receive epinephrine while concomitantly taking cardiac glycosides or diuretics should be observed carefully for the development of cardiac arrhythmias).
No products indexed under this heading.

Betaxolol Hydrochloride (The cardiostimulating and bronchodilating effects of epinephrine are antagonized by beta-adrenergic blocking drugs, such as propranolol).
No products indexed under this heading.

Bisoprolol Fumarate (The cardiostimulating and bronchodilating effects of epinephrine are antagonized by beta-adrenergic blocking drugs, such as propranolol).
No products indexed under this heading.

Bretylium Tosylate (Epinephrine should be used with caution in patients who are on medications that may sensitize the heart to arrhythmias, (eg, digitalis, diuretics, or anti-arrhythmics). In such patients, epinephrine may precipitate or aggravate angina pectoris as well as produce ventricular arrhythmias).
No products indexed under this heading.

1955 Interactions Index Twinject

Bromodiphenhydramine Hydrochloride (The effects of epinephrine may be potentiated by certain antihistamines, notably chlorpheniramine, tripelennamine, and diphenhydramine).
No products indexed under this heading.

Brompheniramine Maleate (The effects of epinephrine may be potentiated by certain antihistamines, notably chlorpheniramine, tripelennamine, and diphenhydramine).
No products indexed under this heading.

Bumetanide (Patients who receive epinephrine while concomitantly taking cardiac glycosides or diuretics should be observed carefully for the development of cardiac arrhythmias).
No products indexed under this heading.

Carteolol Hydrochloride (The cardiostimulating and bronchodilating effects of epinephrine are antagonized by beta-adrenergic blocking drugs, such as propranolol).
No products indexed under this heading.

Carvedilol (The cardiostimulating and bronchodilating effects of epinephrine are antagonized by beta-adrenergic blocking drugs, such as propranolol). Products include:
Coreg **1409**

Carvedilol Phosphate (The cardiostimulating and bronchodilating effects of epinephrine are antagonized by beta-adrenergic blocking drugs, such as propranolol). Products include:
Coreg CR **1416**

Cetirizine Hydrochloride (The effects of epinephrine may be potentiated by certain antihistamines, notably chlorpheniramine, tripelennamine, and diphenhydramine). Products include:
Zyrtec Allergy **2052**
Children's Zyrtec Allergy Syrup **2053**
Children's Zyrtec Allergy **2053**
Children's Zyrtec Hives Relief **2053**
Zyrtec-D Allergy & Congestion **2054**

Chlorothiazide (Patients who receive epinephrine while concomitantly taking cardiac glycosides or diuretics should be observed carefully for the development of cardiac arrhythmias).
No products indexed under this heading.

Chlorothiazide Sodium (Patients who receive epinephrine while concomitantly taking cardiac glycosides or diuretics should be observed carefully for the development of cardiac arrhythmias). Products include:
Diuril Intravenous **2009**

Chlorpheniramine (The effects of epinephrine may be potentiated by certain antihistamines, notably chlorpheniramine, tripelennamine, and diphenhydramine).
No products indexed under this heading.

Chlorpheniramine Maleate (The effects of epinephrine may be potentiated by certain antihistamines, notably chlorpheniramine, tripelennamine, and diphenhydramine).
No products indexed under this heading.

Chlorpheniramine Polistirex (The effects of epinephrine may be potentiated by certain antihistamines, notably chlorpheniramine, tripelennamine, and diphenhydramine). Products include:
Tussionex **3443**

Chlorpheniramine Preparations (The effects of epinephrine may be potentiated by certain antihistamines, notably chlorpheniramine, tripelennamine, and diphenhydramine).
No products indexed under this heading.

Chlorpheniramine Tannate (The effects of epinephrine may be potentiated by certain antihistamines, notably chlorpheniramine, tripelennamine, and diphenhydramine).
No products indexed under this heading.

Chlorpromazine (Ergot alkaloids and phenothiazines may also reverse the pressor effects of epinephrine).
No products indexed under this heading.

Chlorpromazine Hydrochloride (Ergot alkaloids and phenothiazines may also reverse the pressor effects of epinephrine).
No products indexed under this heading.

Chlorthalidone (Patients who receive epinephrine while concomitantly taking cardiac glycosides or diuretics should be observed carefully for the development of cardiac arrhythmias). Products include:
Clorpres **2344**

Clemastine Fumarate (The effects of epinephrine may be potentiated by certain antihistamines, notably chlorpheniramine, tripelennamine, and diphenhydramine).
No products indexed under this heading.

Clomipramine Hydrochloride (The effects of epinephrine may be potentiated by tricyclic antidepressants).
No products indexed under this heading.

Clonidine (The vasoconstricting and hypertensive efffects are antagonized by alpha-adrenergic blocking drugs, such as phentolamine). Products include:
Catapres-TTS **884**

Clonidine Hydrochloride (The vasoconstricting and hypertensive efffects are antagonized by alpha-adrenergic blocking drugs, such as phentolamine). Products include:
Clorpres **2344**

Cyproheptadine Hydrochloride (The effects of epinephrine may be potentiated by certain antihistamines, notably chlorpheniramine, tripelennamine, and diphenhydramine).
No products indexed under this heading.

Desipramine Hydrochloride (The effects of epinephrine may be potentiated by tricyclic antidepressants).
No products indexed under this heading.

Deslanoside (Patients who receive epinephrine while concomitantly taking cardiac glycosides or diuretics should be observed carefully for the development of cardiac arrhythmias).
No products indexed under this heading.

Dexchlorpheniramine Maleate (The effects of epinephrine may be potentiated by certain antihistamines, notably chlorpheniramine, tripelennamine, and diphenhydramine).
No products indexed under this heading.

Digitalis Glycoside Preparations (Patients who receive epinephrine while concomitantly taking cardiac glycosides or diuretics should be observed carefully for the development of cardiac arrhythmias).
No products indexed under this heading.

Digitalis Lanata (Patients who receive epinephrine while concomitantly taking cardiac glycosides or diuretics should be observed carefully for the development of cardiac arrhythmias).
No products indexed under this heading.

Digitalis Purpurea (Patients who receive epinephrine while concomitantly taking cardiac glycosides or diuretics should be observed carefully for the development of cardiac arrhythmias).
No products indexed under this heading.

Digitoxin (Patients who receive epinephrine while concomitantly taking cardiac glycosides or diuretics should be observed carefully for the development of cardiac arrhythmias).
No products indexed under this heading.

Digoxin (Patients who receive epinephrine while concomitantly taking cardiac glycosides or diuretics should be observed carefully for the development of cardiac arrhythmias). Products include:
Lanoxin Injection **1546**
Lanoxin Injection Pediatric **1549**
Lanoxin Tablets **1553**

Dihydroergotamine Mesylate (Ergot alkaloids and phenothiazines may also reverse the pressor effects of epinephrine).
No products indexed under this heading.

Diphenhydramine (The effects of epinephrine may be potentiated by certain antihistamines, notably chlorpheniramine, tripelennamine, and diphenhydramine).
No products indexed under this heading.

Diphenhydramine Hydrochloride (The effects of epinephrine may be potentiated by certain antihistamines, notably chlorpheniramine, tripelennamine, and diphenhydramine). Products include:
Benadryl Allergy Ultratab **2042**
Children's Benadryl Allergy Liquid **2042**

Diphenylpyraline Hydrochloride (The effects of epinephrine may be potentiated by certain antihistamines, notably chlorpheniramine, tripelennamine, and diphenhydramine).
No products indexed under this heading.

Disopyramide Phosphate (Epinephrine should be used with caution in patients who are on medications that may sensitize the heart to arrhythmias, (eg, digitalis, diuretics, or anti-arrhythmics). In such patients, epinephrine may precipitate or aggravate angina pectoris as well as produce ventricular arrhythmias).
No products indexed under this heading.

Dofetilide (Epinephrine should be used with caution in patients who are on medications that may sensitize the heart to arrhythmias, (eg, digitalis, diuretics, or anti-arrhythmics). In such patients, epinephrine may precipitate or aggravate angina pectoris as well as produce ventricular arrhythmias).
No products indexed under this heading.

Doxazosin Mesylate (The vasoconstricting and hypertensive efffects are antagonized by alpha-adrenergic blocking drugs, such as phentolamine).
No products indexed under this heading.

Doxepin Hydrochloride (The effects of epinephrine may be potentiated by tricyclic antidepressants).
No products indexed under this heading.

Ergonovine Maleate (Ergot alkaloids and phenothiazines may also reverse the pressor effects of epinephrine).
No products indexed under this heading.

Ergotamine Tartrate (Ergot alkaloids and phenothiazines may also reverse the pressor effects of epinephrine).
No products indexed under this heading.

Esmolol Hydrochloride (The cardiostimulating and bronchodilating effects of epinephrine are antagonized by beta-adrenergic blocking drugs, such as propranolol).
No products indexed under this heading.

Ethacrynic Acid (Patients who receive epinephrine while concomitantly taking cardiac glycosides or diuretics should be observed carefully for the development of cardiac arrhythmias).
No products indexed under this heading.

Fexofenadine Hydrochloride (The effects of epinephrine may be potentiated by certain antihistamines, notably chlorpheniramine, tripelennamine, and diphenhydramine). Products include:
Allegra ODT **2911**
Allegra Oral Solution **2911**
Allegra **2911**
Allegra-D **2915**
Allegra-D 24 .... **2918**

Flecainide Acetate (Epinephrine should be used with caution in patients who are on medications that may sensitize the heart to arrhythmias, (eg, digitalis, diuretics, or anti-arrhythmics). In such patients, epinephrine may precipitate or aggravate angina pectoris as well as produce ventricular arrhythmias).
No products indexed under this heading.

Fluphenazine Decanoate (Ergot alkaloids and phenothiazines may also reverse the pressor effects of epinephrine).
No products indexed under this heading.

Fluphenazine Enanthate (Ergot alkaloids and phenothiazines may also reverse the pressor effects of epinephrine).
No products indexed under this heading.

Fluphenazine Hydrochloride (Ergot alkaloids and phenothiazines may also reverse the pressor effects of epinephrine).
No products indexed under this heading.

Furosemide (Patients who receive epinephrine while concomitantly taking cardiac glycosides or diuretics should be observed carefully for the development of cardiac arrhythmias). Products include:
Furosemide **2354**

Hydrochlorothiazide (Patients who receive epinephrine while concomitantly taking cardiac glycosides or diuretics should be observed carefully for the development of cardiac arrhythmias). Products include:
Atacand HCT **700**
Avalide **2956**
Benicar HCT **1017**
Diovan HCT **2419**
Dyazide **1429**
Exforge HCT **2449**
Hyzaar **2162**
Hyzaar 100-12.5 .... **2162**
Micardis HCT **889**
Prinzide **2246**
Tekturna HCT **2541**
Teveten HCT **541**

Hydroflumethiazide (Patients who receive epinephrine while concomitantly taking cardiac glycosides or diuretics should be observed carefully for the development of cardiac arrhythmias).
No products indexed under this heading.

Imipramine Hydrochloride (The effects of epinephrine may be potentiated by tricyclic antidepressants).
No products indexed under this heading.

Imipramine Pamoate (The effects of epinephrine may be potentiated by tricyclic antidepressants).
No products indexed under this heading.

Indapamide (Patients who receive epinephrine while concomitantly taking cardiac glycosides or diuretics should be observed carefully for the development of cardiac arrhythmias). Products include:
Indapamide **2356**

Isocarboxazid (The effects of epinephrine may be potentiated by monoamine oxidase inhibitors). Products include:
Marplan **3481**

Labetalol Hydrochloride (The cardiostimulating and bronchodilating effects of epinephrine are antagonized by beta-adrenergic blocking drugs, such as propranolol).
No products indexed under this heading.

Levobunolol Hydrochloride (The cardiostimulating and bronchodilating effects of epinephrine are antagonized by beta-adrenergic blocking drugs, such as propranolol).
No products indexed under this heading.

IMPORTANT NOTE: Always consult each drug listing in the patient's regimen for possible interactions.

Levothyroxine Sodium (The effects of epinephrine may be potentiated by sodium levothyroxine). Products include:
Levoxyl Tablets 1843
Synthroid 529

Lidocaine Hydrochloride (Epinephrine should be used with caution in patients who are on medications that may sensitize the heart to arrhythmias, (eg, digitalis, diuretics, or anti-arrhythmics). In such patients, epinephrine may precipitate or aggravate angina pectoris as well as produce ventricular arrhythmias).
No products indexed under this heading.

Loratadine (The effects of epinephrine may be potentiated by certain antihistamines, notably chlorpheniramine, tripelennamine, and diphenhydramine).
No products indexed under this heading.

Maprotiline Hydrochloride (The effects of epinephrine may be potentiated by tricyclic antidepressants).
No products indexed under this heading.

Mesoridazine Besylate (Ergot alkaloids and phenothiazines may also reverse the pressor effects of epinephrine).
No products indexed under this heading.

Methdilazine Hydrochloride (The effects of epinephrine may be potentiated by certain antihistamines, notably chlorpheniramine, tripelennamine, and diphenhydramine).
No products indexed under this heading.

Methotrimeprazine (Ergot alkaloids and phenothiazines may also reverse the pressor effects of epinephrine).
No products indexed under this heading.

Methyclothiazide (Patients who receive epinephrine while concomitantly taking cardiac glycosides or diuretics should be observed carefully for the development of cardiac arrhythmias).
No products indexed under this heading.

Methylergonovine Maleate (Ergot alkaloids and phenothiazines may also reverse the pressor effects of epinephrine).
No products indexed under this heading.

Methysergide Maleate (Ergot alkaloids and phenothiazines may also reverse the pressor effects of epinephrine).
No products indexed under this heading.

Metipranolol Hydrochloride (The cardiostimulating and bronchodilating effects of epinephrine are antagonized by beta-adrenergic blocking drugs, such as propranolol).
No products indexed under this heading.

Metolazone (Patients who receive epinephrine while concomitantly taking cardiac glycosides or diuretics should be observed carefully for the development of cardiac arrhythmias).
No products indexed under this heading.

Metoprolol Succinate (The cardiostimulating and bronchodilating effects of epinephrine are antagonized by beta-adrenergic blocking drugs, such as propranolol). Products include:
Toprol XL 732

Metoprolol Tartrate (The cardiostimulating and bronchodilating effects of epinephrine are antagonized by beta-adrenergic blocking drugs, such as propranolol).
No products indexed under this heading.

Mexiletine Hydrochloride (Epinephrine should be used with caution in patients who are on medications that may sensitize the heart to arrhythmias, (eg, digitalis, diuretics, or anti-arrhythmics). In such patients, epinephrine may precipitate or aggravate angina pectoris as well as produce ventricular arrhythmias).
No products indexed under this heading.

Moclobemide (The effects of epinephrine may be potentiated by monoamine oxidase inhibitors).
No products indexed under this heading.

Moricizine Hydrochloride (Epinephrine should be used with caution in patients who are on medications that may sensitize the heart to arrhythmias, (eg, digitalis, diuretics, or anti-arrhythmics). In such patients, epinephrine may precipitate or aggravate angina pectoris as well as produce ventricular arrhythmias).
No products indexed under this heading.

Nadolol (The cardiostimulating and bronchodilating effects of epinephrine are antagonized by beta-adrenergic blocking drugs, such as propranolol). Products include:
Nadolol 2359

Nebivolol (The cardiostimulating and bronchodilating effects of epinephrine are antagonized by beta-adrenergic blocking drugs, such as propranolol). Products include:
Bystolic 1147

Nortriptyline Hydrochloride (The effects of epinephrine may be potentiated by tricyclic antidepressants).
No products indexed under this heading.

Pargyline Hydrochloride (The effects of epinephrine may be potentiated by monoamine oxidase inhibitors).
No products indexed under this heading.

Penbutolol Sulfate (The cardiostimulating and bronchodilating effects of epinephrine are antagonized by beta-adrenergic blocking drugs, such as propranolol).
No products indexed under this heading.

Perphenazine (Ergot alkaloids and phenothiazines may also reverse the pressor effects of epinephrine).
No products indexed under this heading.

Phenelzine Sulfate (The effects of epinephrine may be potentiated by monoamine oxidase inhibitors).
No products indexed under this heading.

Phenothiazine Derivatives (Ergot alkaloids and phenothiazines may also reverse the pressor effects of epinephrine).
No products indexed under this heading.

Phenothiazines (Ergot alkaloids and phenothiazines may also reverse the pressor effects of epinephrine).
No products indexed under this heading.

Pindolol (The cardiostimulating and bronchodilating effects of epinephrine are antagonized by beta-adrenergic blocking drugs, such as propranolol).
No products indexed under this heading.

Polythiazide (Patients who receive epinephrine while concomitantly taking cardiac glycosides or diuretics should be observed carefully for the development of cardiac arrhythmias).
No products indexed under this heading.

Prazosin Hydrochloride (The vasoconstricting and hypertensive efffects are antagonized by alpha-adrenergic blocking drugs, such as phentolamine).
No products indexed under this heading.

Procainamide Hydrochloride (Epinephrine should be used with caution in patients who are on medications that may sensitize the heart to arrhythmias, (eg, digitalis, diuretics, or anti-arrhythmics). In such patients, epinephrine may precipitate or aggravate angina pectoris as well as produce ventricular arrhythmias).
No products indexed under this heading.

Procarbazine Hydrochloride (The effects of epinephrine may be potentiated by monoamine oxidase inhibitors).
No products indexed under this heading.

Prochlorperazine (Ergot alkaloids and phenothiazines may also reverse the pressor effects of epinephrine).
No products indexed under this heading.

Prochlorperazine Edisylate (Ergot alkaloids and phenothiazines may also reverse the pressor effects of epinephrine).
No products indexed under this heading.

Prochlorperazine Maleate (Ergot alkaloids and phenothiazines may also reverse the pressor effects of epinephrine).
No products indexed under this heading.

Promethazine (Ergot alkaloids and phenothiazines may also reverse the pressor effects of epinephrine).
No products indexed under this heading.

Promethazine Hydrochloride (The effects of epinephrine may be potentiated by certain antihistamines, notably chlorpheniramine, tripelennamine, and diphenhydramine).
No products indexed under this heading.

Propafenone Hydrochloride (Epinephrine should be used with caution in patients who are on medications that may sensitize the heart to arrhythmias, (eg, digitalis, diuretics, or anti-arrhythmics). In such patients, epinephrine may precipitate or aggravate angina pectoris as well as produce ventricular arrhythmias). Products include:
Rythmol 1648
Rythmol SR 1652

Propranolol Hydrochloride (Epinephrine should be used with caution in patients who are on medications that may sensitize the heart to arrhythmias, (eg, digitalis, diuretics, or anti-arrhythmics). In such patients, epinephrine may precipitate or aggravate angina pectoris as well as produce ventricular arrhythmias). Products include:
InnoPran XL 1517

Protriptyline Hydrochloride (The effects of epinephrine may be potentiated by tricyclic antidepressants).
No products indexed under this heading.

Pyrilamine Maleate (The effects of epinephrine may be potentiated by certain antihistamines, notably chlorpheniramine, tripelennamine, and diphenhydramine).
No products indexed under this heading.

Pyrilamine Tannate (The effects of epinephrine may be potentiated by certain antihistamines, notably chlorpheniramine, tripelennamine, and diphenhydramine).
No products indexed under this heading.

Quinidine Gluconate (Epinephrine should be used with caution in patients who are on medications that may sensitize the heart to arrhythmias, (eg, digitalis, diuretics, or anti-arrhythmics). In such patients, epinephrine may precipitate or aggravate angina pectoris as well as produce ventricular arrhythmias).
No products indexed under this heading.

Quinidine Polygalacturonate (Epinephrine should be used with caution in patients who are on medications that may sensitize the heart to arrhythmias, (eg, digitalis, diuretics, or anti-arrhythmics). In such patients, epinephrine may precipitate or aggravate angina pectoris as well as produce ventricular arrhythmias).
No products indexed under this heading.

Quinidine Sulfate (Epinephrine should be used with caution in patients who are on medications that may sensitize the heart to arrhythmias, (eg, digitalis, diuretics, or anti-arrhythmics). In such patients, epinephrine may precipitate or aggravate angina pectoris as well as produce ventricular arrhythmias).
No products indexed under this heading.

Rasagiline Mesylate (The effects of epinephrine may be potentiated by monoamine oxidase inhibitors). Products include:
Azilect 3383

Selegiline (The effects of epinephrine may be potentiated by monoamine oxidase inhibitors). Products include:
Emsam 3623

Selegiline Hydrochloride (The effects of epinephrine may be potentiated by monoamine oxidase inhibitors). Products include:
Eldepryl 3312

Sotalol Hydrochloride (Epinephrine should be used with caution in patients who are on medications that may sensitize the heart to arrhythmias, (eg, digitalis, diuretics, or anti-arrhythmics). In such patients, epinephrine may precipitate or aggravate angina pectoris as well as produce ventricular arrhythmias).
No products indexed under this heading.

Spironolactone (Patients who receive epinephrine while concomitantly taking cardiac glycosides or diuretics should be observed carefully for the development of cardiac arrhythmias).
No products indexed under this heading.

Tamsulosin Hydrochloride (The vasoconstricting and hypertensive effects are antagonized by alpha-adrenergic blocking drugs, such as phentolamine).
No products indexed under this heading.

Terazosin Hydrochloride (The vasoconstricting and hypertensive efffects are antagonized by alpha-adrenergic blocking drugs, such as phentolamine).
No products indexed under this heading.

Terfenadine (The effects of epinephrine may be potentiated by certain antihistamines, notably chlorpheniramine, tripelennamine, and diphenhydramine).
No products indexed under this heading.

Thioridazine (Ergot alkaloids and phenothiazines may also reverse the pressor effects of epinephrine).
No products indexed under this heading.

Thioridazine Hydrochloride (Ergot alkaloids and phenothiazines may also reverse the pressor effects of epinephrine). Products include:
Thioridazine Hydrochloride 2384

Timolol Hemihydrate (The cardiostimulating and bronchodilating effects of epinephrine are antagonized by beta-adrenergic blocking drugs, such as propranolol). Products include:
Betimol 3490

Timolol Maleate (The cardiostimulating and bronchodilating effects of epinephrine are antagonized by beta-adrenergic blocking drugs, such as propranolol). Products include:
Combigan 601
Dorzolamide Hydrochloride/Timolol Maleate Ophthalmic Solution .... ⊙243
Timoptic in Ocudose .... ⊙231

Tocainide Hydrochloride (Epinephrine should be used with caution in patients who are on medications that may sensitize the heart to arrhythmias, (eg, digitalis, diuretics, or anti-arrhythmics). In such patients, epinephrine may precipitate or aggravate angina pectoris as well as produce ventricular arrhythmias).
No products indexed under this heading.

(⊙ Described in PDR® for Ophthalmic Medicines)

Torsemide (Patients who receive epinephrine while concomitantly taking cardiac glycosides or diuretics should be observed carefully for the development of cardiac arrhythmias).
No products indexed under this heading.

Tranylcypromine Sulfate (The effects of epinephrine may be potentiated by monoamine oxidase inhibitors). Products include:
Parnate 1584

Triamterene (Patients who receive epinephrine while concomitantly taking cardiac glycosides or diuretics should be observed carefully for the development of cardiac arrhythmias). Products include:
Dyazide 1429
Dyrenium 3495

Trifluoperazine Hydrochloride (Ergot alkaloids and phenothiazines may also reverse the pressor effects of epinephrine).
No products indexed under this heading.

Trimeprazine Tartrate (The effects of epinephrine may be potentiated by certain antihistamines, notably chlorpheniramine, tripelennamine, and diphenhydramine).
No products indexed under this heading.

Trimipramine Maleate (The effects of epinephrine may be potentiated by tricyclic antidepressants).
No products indexed under this heading.

Tripelennamine Hydrochloride (The effects of epinephrine may be potentiated by certain antihistamines, notably chlorpheniramine, tripelennamine, and diphenhydramine).
No products indexed under this heading.

Triprolidine Hydrochloride (The effects of epinephrine may be potentiated by certain antihistamines, notably chlorpheniramine, tripelennamine, and diphenhydramine).
No products indexed under this heading.

Verapamil Hydrochloride (Epinephrine should be used with caution in patients who are on medications that may sensitize the heart to arrhythmias, (eg, digitalis, diuretics, or antiarrhythmics). In such patients, epinephrine may precipitate or aggravate angina pectoris as well as produce ventricular arrhythmias). Products include:
Tarka 534

TWINRIX VACCINE

(Hepatitis A Vaccine, Inactivated, Hepatitis B Vaccine, Recombinant) 1694
None cited in PDR database.

TYGACIL FOR INJECTION

(Tigecycline) 3596
May interact with oral contraceptives, and certain other agents. Compounds in these categories include:

Desogestrel (Concurrent use of antibacterial drugs with oral contraceptives may render oral contraceptives less effective).
No products indexed under this heading.

Ethinyl Estradiol (Concurrent use of antibacterial drugs with oral contraceptives may render oral contraceptives less effective). Products include:
LoSeasonique 3407
Lybrel 3514
NuvaRing 3181
Ortho Evra 2648
Ortho-Cyclen/Ortho Tri-Cyclen 2663
Ortho Tri-Cyclen Lo Tablets 2673
Seasonique 3418
Yaz 864

Ethynodiol Diacetate (Concurrent use of antibacterial drugs with oral contraceptives may render oral contraceptives less effective).
No products indexed under this heading.

Levonorgestrel (Concurrent use of antibacterial drugs with oral contraceptives may render oral contraceptives less effective). Products include:
Climara Pro 847
LoSeasonique 3407
Lybrel 3514
Mirena 854
Plan B 3416
Seasonique 3418

Mestranol (Concurrent use of antibacterial drugs with oral contraceptives may render oral contraceptives less effective).
No products indexed under this heading.

Norethindrone (Concurrent use of antibacterial drugs with oral contraceptives may render oral contraceptives less effective). Products include:
Ortho Micronor 2660

Norethynodrel (Concurrent use of antibacterial drugs with oral contraceptives may render oral contraceptives less effective).
No products indexed under this heading.

Norgestimate (Concurrent use of antibacterial drugs with oral contraceptives may render oral contraceptives less effective). Products include:
Ortho-Cyclen/Ortho Tri-Cyclen 2663
Ortho Tri-Cyclen Lo Tablets 2673

Norgestrel (Concurrent use of antibacterial drugs with oral contraceptives may render oral contraceptives less effective).
No products indexed under this heading.

Warfarin Sodium (Prothrombin time or other suitable anticoagulation test should be monitored if tigecycline is administered with warfarin).
No products indexed under this heading.

TYKERB TABLETS

(Lapatinib) 1698
May interact with cytochrome p450 2c8 substrates (selected), cytochrome p450 3a4 inducers (selected), cytochrome p450 3a4 inhibitors, potent (selected), cytochrome p450 3a4 substrates (selected), dexamethasones, glycoprotein (GP) IIb/IIIa inhibitors, and certain other agents. Compounds in these categories include:

Abciximab (Lapatinib is a subtrate of the efflux transporter P-glycoprotein (Pgp, ABCB1). If lapatinib is administered with drugs that inhibit Pgp, increased concentrations of lapatinib are likely, and caution should be exercised). Products include:
ReoPro 1952

Alfentanil Hydrochloride (Lapatinib inhibits CYP3A4 *in vitro* at clinically relevant concentrations. Caution should be exercised and dose reduction of the concomitant substrate drug should be considered when dosing lapatinib concurrently with medications with narrow therapeutic windows that are substrates of CYP3A4).
No products indexed under this heading.

Allium sativum (Lapatinib undergoes extensive metabolism by CYP3A4; concomitant administration of strong inducers of CYP3A4 alter lapatinib concentrations significantly and should be avoided. Dose adjustment of lapatinib should be considered for patients who must receive concomitant strong inducers of CYP3A4 enzymes. Lapatinib inhibits CYP3A4 *in vitro* at clinically relevant concentrations. Caution should be exercised and dose reduction of the concomitant substrate drug should be considered when dosing lapatinib concurrently with medications with narrow therapeutic windows that are substrates of CYP3A4).
No products indexed under this heading.

Alprazolam (Lapatinib inhibits CYP3A4 *in vitro* at clinically relevant concentrations. Caution should be exercised and dose reduction of the concomitant substrate drug should be considered when dosing lapatinib concurrently with medications with narrow therapeutic windows that are substrates of CYP3A4).
No products indexed under this heading.

Aminoglutethimide (Lapatinib undergoes extensive metabolism by CYP3A4; concomitant administration of strong inducers of CYP3A4 alter lapatinib concentrations significantly and should be avoided. Dose adjustment of lapatinib should be considered for patients who must receive concomitant strong inducers of CYP3A4 enzymes. Lapatinib inhibits CYP3A4 *in vitro* at clinically relevant concentrations. Caution should be exercised and dose reduction of the concomitant substrate drug should be considered when dosing lapatinib concurrently with medications with narrow therapeutic windows that are substrates of CYP3A4).
No products indexed under this heading.

Amiodarone Hydrochloride (Lapatinib inhibits CYP2C8 *in vitro* at clinically relevant concentrations. Caution should be exercised and dose reduction of the concomitant substrate drug should be considered when dosing lapatinib concurrently with medications with narrow therapeutic windows that are substrates of CYP2C8).
No products indexed under this heading.

Amitriptyline Hydrochloride (Lapatinib inhibits CYP2C8 *in vitro* at clinically relevant concentrations. Caution should be exercised and dose reduction of the concomitant substrate drug should be considered when dosing lapatinib concurrently with medications with narrow therapeutic windows that are substrates of CYP2C8).
No products indexed under this heading.

Amlodipine Besylate (Lapatinib inhibits CYP3A4 *in vitro* at clinically relevant concentrations. Caution should be exercised and dose reduction of the concomitant substrate drug should be considered when dosing lapatinib concurrently with medications with narrow therapeutic windows that are substrates of CYP3A4). Products include:
Azor 1010
Exforge 2443
Exforge HCT 2449

Amoxapine (Lapatinib inhibits CYP2C8 *in vitro* at clinically relevant concentrations. Caution should be exercised and dose reduction of the concomitant substrate drug should be considered when dosing lapatinib concurrently with medications with narrow therapeutic windows that are substrates of CYP2C8).
No products indexed under this heading.

Amprenavir (Lapatinib undergoes extensive metabolism by CYP3A4; concomitant administration of strong inhibitors of CYP3A4 alter lapatinib concentrations significantly and should be avoided. Dose adjustment of lapatinib should be considered for patients who must receive concomitant strong inhibitors of CYP3A4 enzymes. Lapatinib inhibits CYP3A4 *in vitro* at clinically relevant concentrations. Caution should be exercised and dose reduction of the concomitant substrate drug should be considered when dosing lapatinib concurrently with medications with narrow therapeutic windows that are substrates of CYP3A4).
No products indexed under this heading.

Aprepitant (Lapatinib undergoes extensive metabolism by CYP3A4; concomitant administration of strong inducers of CYP3A4 alter lapatinib concentrations significantly and should be avoided. Dose adjustment of lapatinib should be considered for patients who must receive concomitant strong inducers of CYP3A4 enzymes. Lapatinib inhibits CYP3A4 *in vitro* at clinically relevant concentrations. Caution should be exercised and dose reduction of the concomitant substrate drug should be considered when dosing lapatinib concurrently with medications with narrow therapeutic windows that are substrates of CYP3A4). Products include:
Emend 2124

Astemizole (Lapatinib inhibits CYP3A4 *in vitro* at clinically relevant concentrations. Caution should be exercised and dose reduction of the concomitant substrate drug should be considered when dosing lapatinib concurrently with medications with narrow therapeutic windows that are substrates of CYP3A4).
No products indexed under this heading.

Atazanavir (The concomitant use of strong CYP3A4 inhibitors should be avoided (eg, atazanavir). If patients must be co-administered a strong CYP3A4 inhibitor, based on pharmacokinetic studies, a dose reduction to 500 mg/day of lapatinib is predicted to adjust the lapatinib AUC to the range observed without inhibitors and should be considered).
No products indexed under this heading.

Atazanavir Sulfate (The concomitant use of strong CYP3A4 inhibitors should be avoided (eg, atazanavir). If patients must be co-administered a strong CYP3A4 inhibitor, based on pharmacokinetic studies, a dose reduction to 500 mg/day of lapatinib is predicted to adjust the lapatinib AUC to the range observed without inhibitors and should be considered).
No products indexed under this heading.

Atorvastatin Calcium (Lapatinib inhibits CYP3A4 *in vitro* at clinically relevant concentrations. Caution should be exercised and dose reduction of the concomitant substrate drug should be considered when dosing lapatinib concurrently with medications with narrow therapeutic windows that are substrates of CYP3A4). Products include:
Lipitor 2703

Belladonna Ergotamine (Lapatinib inhibits CYP3A4 *in vitro* at clinically relevant concentrations. Caution should be exercised and dose reduction of the concomitant substrate drug should be considered when dosing lapatinib concurrently with medications with narrow therapeutic windows that are substrates of CYP3A4).
No products indexed under this heading.

Benzphetamine Hydrochloride (Lapatinib inhibits CYP2C8 *in vitro* at clinically relevant concentrations. Caution should be exercised and dose reduction of the concomitant substrate drug should be considered when dosing lapatinib concurrently with medications with narrow therapeutic windows that are substrates of CYP2C8).
No products indexed under this heading.

Betamethasone (Lapatinib undergoes extensive metabolism by CYP3A4; concomitant administration of strong inducers of CYP3A4 alter lapatinib concentrations significantly and should be avoided. Dose adjustment of lapatinib should be considered for patients who must receive concomitant strong inducers of CYP3A4 enzymes. Lapatinib inhibits CYP3A4 *in vitro* at clinically relevant concentrations. Caution should be exercised and dose reduction of the concomitant substrate drug should be considered when dosing lapatinib concurrently with medications with narrow therapeutic windows that are substrates of CYP3A4).
No products indexed under this heading.

Betamethasone Acetate (Lapatinib undergoes extensive metabolism by CYP3A4; concomitant administration of strong inducers of CYP3A4 alter lapatinib concentrations significantly and should be avoided. Dose adjustment of lapatinib should be considered for patients who must receive concomitant strong inducers of CYP3A4 enzymes. Lapatinib inhibits CYP3A4 *in vitro* at clinically relevant concentrations. Caution should be exercised and dose reduction of the concomitant substrate drug should be considered when dosing lapatinib concurrently with medications with narrow therapeutic windows that are substrates of CYP3A4).
No products indexed under this heading.

Betamethasone Benzoate (Lapatinib undergoes extensive metabolism by CYP3A4; concomitant administration of strong inducers of CYP3A4 alter lapatinib concentrations significantly and should be avoided. Dose adjustment of lapatinib should be considered for patients who must receive concomitant strong inducers of CYP3A4 enzymes. Lapatinib inhibits CYP3A4 *in vitro* at clinically relevant concentrations. Caution should be exercised and dose reduction of the concomitant substrate drug should be considered when dosing lapatinib concurrently with medications with narrow therapeutic windows that are substrates of CYP3A4).
No products indexed under this heading.

Betamethasone Dipropionate (Lapatinib undergoes extensive metabolism by CYP3A4; concomitant administration of strong inducers of CYP3A4 alter lapatinib concentrations significantly and should be avoided. Dose adjustment of lapatinib should be considered for patients who must receive concomitant strong inducers of CYP3A4 enzymes. Lapatinib inhibits CYP3A4 *in vitro* at clinically relevant concentrations. Caution should be exercised and dose reduction of the concomitant substrate drug should be considered when dosing lapatinib concurrently with medications with narrow therapeutic windows that are substrates of CYP3A4). Products include:
Diprolene Lotion 0.05% 3108
Diprolene Ointment 0.05% 3109
Diprolene AF Cream 0.05% 3107
Lotrisone 3163

Betamethasone Sodium Phosphate (Lapatinib undergoes extensive metabolism by CYP3A4; concomitant administration of strong inducers of CYP3A4 alter lapatinib concentrations significantly and should be avoided. Dose adjustment of lapatinib should be considered for patients who must receive concomitant strong inducers of CYP3A4 enzymes. Lapatinib inhibits CYP3A4 *in vitro* at clinically relevant concentrations. Caution should be exercised and dose reduction of the concomitant substrate drug should be considered when dosing lapatinib concurrently with medications with narrow therapeutic windows that are substrates of CYP3A4).
No products indexed under this heading.

Betamethasone Valerate (Lapatinib undergoes extensive metabolism by CYP3A4; concomitant administration of strong inducers of CYP3A4 alter lapatinib concentrations significantly and should be avoided. Dose adjustment of lapatinib should be considered for patients who must receive concomitant strong inducers of CYP3A4 enzymes. Lapatinib inhibits CYP3A4 *in vitro* at clinically relevant concentrations. Caution should be exercised and dose reduction of the concomitant substrate drug should be considered when dosing lapatinib concurrently with medications with narrow therapeutic windows that are substrates of CYP3A4). Products include:
Luxíq 3321

Bosentan (Lapatinib undergoes extensive metabolism by CYP3A4; concomitant administration of strong inducers of CYP3A4 alter lapatinib concentrations significantly and should be avoided. Dose adjustment of lapatinib should be considered for patients who must receive concomitant strong inducers of CYP3A4 enzymes. Lapatinib inhibits CYP3A4 *in vitro* at clinically relevant concentrations. Caution should be exercised and dose reduction of the concomitant substrate drug should be considered when dosing lapatinib concurrently with medications with narrow therapeutic windows that are substrates of CYP3A4). Products include:
Tracleer 573

Buspirone Hydrochloride (Lapatinib inhibits CYP3A4 *in vitro* at clinically relevant concentrations. Caution should be exercised and dose reduction of the concomitant substrate drug should be considered when dosing lapatinib concurrently with medications with narrow therapeutic windows that are substrates of CYP3A4).
No products indexed under this heading.

Busulfan (Lapatinib inhibits CYP3A4 *in vitro* at clinically relevant concentrations. Caution should be exercised and dose reduction of the concomitant substrate drug should be considered when dosing lapatinib concurrently with medications with narrow therapeutic windows that are substrates of CYP3A4). Products include:
Myleran 1581

Carbamazepine (The concomitant use of strong CYP3A4 inducers should be avoided (eg, carbamazepine). If patients must be co-administered a strong CYP3A4 inducer, based on pharmacokinetic studies, the dose of lapatinib should be titrated gradually from 1,250 mg/day up to 4,500 mg/day based on tolerability). Products include:
Carbatrol 3280
Equetro 3477

Cerivastatin Sodium (Lapatinib inhibits CYP3A4 *in vitro* at clinically relevant concentrations. Caution should be exercised and dose reduction of the concomitant substrate drug should be considered when dosing lapatinib concurrently with medications with narrow therapeutic windows that are substrates of CYP3A4).
No products indexed under this heading.

Chlorpheniramine (Lapatinib inhibits CYP3A4 *in vitro* at clinically relevant concentrations. Caution should be exercised and dose reduction of the concomitant substrate drug should be considered when dosing lapatinib concurrently with medications with narrow therapeutic windows that are substrates of CYP3A4).
No products indexed under this heading.

Chlorpheniramine Maleate (Lapatinib inhibits CYP3A4 *in vitro* at clinically relevant concentrations. Caution should be exercised and dose reduction of the concomitant substrate drug should be considered when dosing lapatinib concurrently with medications with narrow therapeutic windows that are substrates of CYP3A4).
No products indexed under this heading.

Chlorpheniramine Polistirex (Lapatinib inhibits CYP3A4 *in vitro* at clinically relevant concentrations. Caution should be exercised and dose reduction of the concomitant substrate drug should be considered when dosing lapatinib concurrently with medications with narrow therapeutic windows that are substrates of CYP3A4). Products include:
Tussionex 3443

Chlorpheniramine Tannate (Lapatinib inhibits CYP3A4 *in vitro* at clinically relevant concentrations. Caution should be exercised and dose reduction of the concomitant substrate drug should be considered when dosing lapatinib concurrently with medications with narrow therapeutic windows that are substrates of CYP3A4).
No products indexed under this heading.

Ciprofloxacin (Lapatinib undergoes extensive metabolism by CYP3A4; concomitant administration of strong inducers of CYP3A4 alter lapatinib concentrations significantly and should be avoided. Dose adjustment of lapatinib should be considered for patients who must receive concomitant strong inducers of CYP3A4 enzymes. Lapatinib inhibits CYP3A4 *in vitro* at clinically relevant concentrations. Caution should be exercised and dose reduction of the concomitant substrate drug should be considered when dosing lapatinib concurrently with medications with narrow therapeutic windows that are substrates of CYP3A4). Products include:
Cipro I.V. 3082
Cipro 3073
Cipro XR 3091
Ciprodex 583

Ciprofloxacin Hydrochloride (Lapatinib undergoes extensive metabolism by CYP3A4; concomitant administration of strong inducers of CYP3A4 alter lapatinib concentrations significantly and should be avoided. Dose adjustment of lapatinib should be considered for patients who must receive concomitant strong inducers of CYP3A4 enzymes. Lapatinib inhibits CYP3A4 *in vitro* at clinically relevant concentrations. Caution should be exercised and dose reduction of the concomitant substrate drug should be considered when dosing lapatinib concurrently with medications with narrow therapeutic windows that are substrates of CYP3A4). Products include:
Cipro 3073

Cisapride (Lapatinib inhibits CYP3A4 *in vitro* at clinically relevant concentrations. Caution should be exercised and dose reduction of the concomitant substrate drug should be considered when dosing lapatinib concurrently with medications with narrow therapeutic windows that are substrates of CYP3A4).
No products indexed under this heading.

Cisplatin (Lapatinib undergoes extensive metabolism by CYP3A4; concomitant administration of strong inducers of CYP3A4 alter lapatinib concentrations significantly and should be avoided. Dose adjustment of lapatinib should be considered for patients who must receive concomitant strong inducers of CYP3A4 enzymes. Lapatinib inhibits CYP3A4 *in vitro* at clinically relevant concentrations. Caution should be exercised and dose reduction of the concomitant substrate drug should be considered when dosing lapatinib concurrently with medications with narrow therapeutic windows that are substrates of CYP3A4).
No products indexed under this heading.

Clarithromycin (The concomitant use of strong CYP3A4 inhibitors should be avoided (eg, clarithromycin). If patients must be co-administered a strong CYP3A4 inhibitor, based on pharmacokinetic studies, a dose reduction to 500 mg/day of lapatinib is predicted to adjust the lapatinib AUC to the range observed without inhibitors and should be considered). Products include:
Biaxin/Biaxin XL 412

Clomipramine Hydrochloride (Lapatinib inhibits CYP2C8 *in vitro* at clinically relevant concentrations. Caution should be exercised and dose reduction of the concomitant substrate drug should be considered when dosing lapatinib concurrently with medications with narrow therapeutic windows that are substrates of CYP2C8).
No products indexed under this heading.

Cortisone Acetate (Lapatinib undergoes extensive metabolism by CYP3A4; concomitant administration of strong inducers of CYP3A4 alter lapatinib concentrations significantly and should be avoided. Dose adjustment of lapatinib should be considered for patients who must receive concomitant strong inducers of CYP3A4 enzymes. Lapatinib inhibits CYP3A4 *in vitro* at clinically relevant concentrations. Caution should be exercised and dose reduction of the concomitant substrate drug should be considered when dosing lapatinib concurrently with medications with narrow therapeutic windows that are substrates of CYP3A4).
No products indexed under this heading.

Cyclosporine (Lapatinib inhibits CYP3A4 *in vitro* at clinically relevant concentrations. Caution should be exercised and dose reduction of the concomitant substrate drug should be considered when dosing lapatinib concurrently with medications with narrow therapeutic windows that are substrates of CYP3A4). Products include:
Gengraf 440
Neoral Oral Solution 2496
Neoral Capsules 2496
Restasis 605

Delavirdine Mesylate (Lapatinib undergoes extensive metabolism by CYP3A4; concomitant administration of strong inhibitors of CYP3A4 alter lapatinib concentrations significantly and should be avoided. Dose adjustment of lapatinib should be considered for patients who must receive concomitant strong inhibitors of CYP3A4 enzymes. Lapatinib inhibits CYP3A4 *in vitro* at clinically relevant concentrations. Caution should be exercised and dose reduction of the concomitant substrate drug should be considered when dosing lapatinib concurrently with medications with narrow therapeutic windows that are substrates of CYP3A4).
No products indexed under this heading.

Delavirine (Lapatinib undergoes extensive metabolism by CYP3A4; concomitant administration of strong inhibitors of CYP3A4 alter lapatinib concentrations significantly and should be avoided. Dose adjustment of lapatinib should be considered for patients who must receive concomitant strong inhibitors of CYP3A4 enzymes. Lapatinib inhibits CYP3A4 *in vitro* at clinically relevant concentrations. Caution should be exercised and dose reduction of the concomitant substrate drug should be considered when dosing lapatinib concurrently with medications with narrow therapeutic windows that are substrates of CYP3A4).
No products indexed under this heading.

Desipramine Hydrochloride (Lapatinib inhibits CYP2C8 *in vitro* at clinically relevant concentrations. Caution should be exercised and dose reduction of the concomitant substrate drug should be considered when dosing lapatinib concurrently with medications with narrow therapeutic windows that are substrates of CYP2C8).
No products indexed under this heading.

Desogestrel (Lapatinib inhibits CYP3A4 *in vitro* at clinically relevant concentrations. Caution should be exercised and dose reduction of the concomitant substrate drug should be considered when dosing lapatinib concurrently with medications with narrow therapeutic windows that are substrates of CYP3A4).
No products indexed under this heading.

Dexamethasone (Lapatinib undergoes extensive metabolism by CYP3A4; concomitant administration of strong inducers of CYP3A4 alter lapatinib concentrations significantly and should be avoided. Dose adjustment of lapatinib should be considered for patients who must receive concomitant strong inducers of CYP3A4 enzymes. Lapatinib inhibits CYP3A4 *in vitro* at clinically relevant concentrations. Caution should be exercised and dose reduction of the concomitant substrate drug should be considered when dosing lapatinib concurrently with medications with narrow therapeutic windows that are substrates of CYP3A4). Products include:
Ciprodex 583
Ozurdex .... ⊙ 223
Tobramycin and Dexamethasone Ophthalmic Suspension .... ⊙ 251

Dexamethasone Acetate (Lapatinib undergoes extensive metabolism by CYP3A4; concomitant administration of strong inducers of CYP3A4 alter lapatinib concentrations significantly and should be avoided. Dose adjustment of lapatinib should be considered for patients who must receive concomitant strong inducers of CYP3A4 enzymes. Lapatinib inhibits CYP3A4 *in vitro* at clinically relevant concentrations. Caution should be exercised and dose reduction of the concomitant substrate drug should be considered when dosing lapatinib concurrently with medications with narrow therapeutic windows that are substrates of CYP3A4).
No products indexed under this heading.

Dexamethasone Phosphate (Lapatinib undergoes extensive metabolism by CYP3A4; concomitant administration of strong inducers of CYP3A4 alter lapatinib concentrations significantly and should be avoided. Dose adjustment of lapatinib should be considered for patients who must receive concomitant strong inducers of CYP3A4 enzymes. Lapatinib inhibits CYP3A4 *in vitro* at clinically relevant concentrations. Caution should be exercised and dose reduction of the concomitant substrate drug should be considered when dosing lapatinib concurrently with medications with narrow therapeutic windows that are substrates of CYP3A4).
No products indexed under this heading.

Dexamethasone Sodium (Lapatinib undergoes extensive metabolism by CYP3A4; concomitant administration of strong inducers of CYP3A4 alter lapatinib concentrations significantly and should be avoided. Dose adjustment of lapatinib should be considered for patients who must receive concomitant strong inducers of CYP3A4 enzymes. Lapatinib inhibits CYP3A4 *in vitro* at clinically relevant concentrations. Caution should be exercised and dose reduction of the concomitant substrate drug should be considered when dosing lapatinib concurrently with medications with narrow therapeutic windows that are substrates of CYP3A4).
No products indexed under this heading.

Dexamethasone Sodium Phosphate (Lapatinib undergoes extensive metabolism by CYP3A4; concomitant administration of strong inducers of CYP3A4 alter lapatinib concentrations significantly and should be avoided. Dose adjustment of lapatinib should be considered for patients who must receive concomitant strong inducers of CYP3A4 enzymes. Lapatinib inhibits CYP3A4 *in vitro* at clinically relevant concentrations. Caution should be exercised and dose reduction of the concomitant substrate drug should be considered when dosing lapatinib concurrently with medications with narrow therapeutic windows that are substrates of CYP3A4).
No products indexed under this heading.

Dexamethasone Sodium Phosphate Injection (Lapatinib undergoes extensive metabolism by CYP3A4; concomitant administration of strong inducers of CYP3A4 alter lapatinib concentrations significantly and should be avoided. Dose adjustment of lapatinib should be considered for patients who must receive concomitant strong inducers of CYP3A4 enzymes. Lapatinib inhibits CYP3A4 *in vitro* at clinically relevant concentrations. Caution should be exercised and dose reduction of the concomitant substrate drug should be considered when dosing lapatinib concurrently with medications with narrow therapeutic windows that are substrates of CYP3A4).
No products indexed under this heading.

Diazepam (Lapatinib inhibits CYP2C8 *in vitro* at clinically relevant concentrations. Caution should be exercised and dose reduction of the concomitant substrate drug should be considered when dosing lapatinib concurrently with medications with narrow therapeutic windows that are substrates of CYP2C8). Products include:
Valium Tablets 2880

Diclofenac Potassium (Lapatinib inhibits CYP2C8 *in vitro* at clinically relevant concentrations. Caution should be exercised and dose reduction of the concomitant substrate drug should be considered when dosing lapatinib concurrently with medications with narrow therapeutic windows that are substrates of CYP2C8).
No products indexed under this heading.

Diclofenac Sodium (Lapatinib inhibits CYP2C8 *in vitro* at clinically relevant concentrations. Caution should be exercised and dose reduction of the concomitant substrate drug should be considered when dosing lapatinib concurrently with medications with narrow therapeutic windows that are substrates of CYP2C8).
No products indexed under this heading.

Dihydroergotamine Mesylate (Lapatinib inhibits CYP3A4 *in vitro* at clinically relevant concentrations. Caution should be exercised and dose reduction of the concomitant substrate drug should be considered when dosing lapatinib concurrently with medications with narrow therapeutic windows that are substrates of CYP3A4).
No products indexed under this heading.

Diltiazem Hydrochloride (Lapatinib inhibits CYP3A4 *in vitro* at clinically relevant concentrations. Caution should be exercised and dose reduction of the concomitant substrate drug should be considered when dosing lapatinib concurrently with medications with narrow therapeutic windows that are substrates of CYP3A4). Products include:
Cardizem LA 423

Diltiazem Maleate (Lapatinib inhibits CYP3A4 *in vitro* at clinically relevant concentrations. Caution should be exercised and dose reduction of the concomitant substrate drug should be considered when dosing lapatinib concurrently with medications with narrow therapeutic windows that are substrates of CYP3A4).
No products indexed under this heading.

Disopyramide (Lapatinib inhibits CYP3A4 *in vitro* at clinically relevant concentrations. Caution should be exercised and dose reduction of the concomitant substrate drug should be considered when dosing lapatinib concurrently with medications with narrow therapeutic windows that are substrates of CYP3A4).
No products indexed under this heading.

Disopyramide Phosphate (Lapatinib inhibits CYP3A4 *in vitro* at clinically relevant concentrations. Caution should be exercised and dose reduction of the concomitant substrate drug should be considered when dosing lapatinib concurrently with medications with narrow therapeutic windows that are substrates of CYP3A4).
No products indexed under this heading.

Disulfiram (Lapatinib inhibits CYP3A4 *in vitro* at clinically relevant concentrations. Caution should be exercised and dose reduction of the concomitant substrate drug should be considered when dosing lapatinib concurrently with medications with narrow therapeutic windows that are substrates of CYP3A4).
No products indexed under this heading.

Docetaxel (Lapatinib inhibits CYP2C8 *in vitro* at clinically relevant concentrations. Caution should be exercised and dose reduction of the concomitant substrate drug should be considered when dosing lapatinib concurrently with medications with narrow therapeutic windows that are substrates of CYP2C8). Products include:
Taxotere 3035

Doxepin Hydrochloride (Lapatinib inhibits CYP2C8 *in vitro* at clinically relevant concentrations. Caution should be exercised and dose reduction of the concomitant substrate drug should be considered when dosing lapatinib concurrently with medications with narrow therapeutic windows that are substrates of CYP2C8).
No products indexed under this heading.

Doxorubicin Hydrochloride (Lapatinib undergoes extensive metabolism by CYP3A4; concomitant administration of strong inducers of CYP3A4 alter lapatinib concentrations significantly and should be avoided. Dose adjustment of lapatinib should be considered for patients who must receive concomitant strong inducers of CYP3A4 enzymes. Lapatinib inhibits CYP3A4 *in vitro* at clinically relevant concentrations. Caution should be exercised and dose reduction of the concomitant substrate drug should be considered when dosing lapatinib concurrently with medications with narrow therapeutic windows that are substrates of CYP3A4).
No products indexed under this heading.

Dronabinol (Lapatinib inhibits CYP3A4 *in vitro* at clinically relevant concentrations. Caution should be exercised and dose reduction of the concomitant substrate drug should be considered when dosing lapatinib concurrently with medications with narrow therapeutic windows that are substrates of CYP3A4).
No products indexed under this heading.

Efavirenz (Lapatinib undergoes extensive metabolism by CYP3A4; concomitant administration of strong inducers of CYP3A4 alter lapatinib concentrations significantly and should be avoided. Dose adjustment of lapatinib should be considered for patients who must receive concomitant strong inducers of CYP3A4 enzymes. Lapatinib inhibits CYP3A4 *in vitro* at clinically relevant concentrations. Caution should be exercised and dose reduction of the concomitant substrate drug should be considered when dosing lapatinib concurrently with medications with narrow therapeutic windows that are substrates of CYP3A4). Products include:
Atripla 906

Eptifibatide (Lapatinib is a subtrate of the efflux transporter P-glycoprotein (Pgp, ABCB1). If lapatinib is administered with drugs that inhibit Pgp, increased concentrations of lapatinib are likely, and caution should be exercised). Products include:
Integrilin 3135

Ergotamine Tartrate (Lapatinib inhibits CYP3A4 *in vitro* at clinically relevant concentrations. Caution should be exercised and dose reduction of the concomitant substrate drug should be considered when dosing lapatinib concurrently with medications with narrow therapeutic windows that are substrates of CYP3A4).
No products indexed under this heading.

Erythromycin (Lapatinib inhibits CYP3A4 *in vitro* at clinically relevant concentrations. Caution should be exercised and dose reduction of the concomitant substrate drug should be considered when dosing lapatinib concurrently with medications with narrow therapeutic windows that are substrates of CYP3A4).
No products indexed under this heading.

Erythromycin Estolate (Lapatinib inhibits CYP3A4 *in vitro* at clinically relevant concentrations. Caution should be exercised and dose reduction of the concomitant substrate drug should be considered when dosing lapatinib concurrently with medications with narrow therapeutic windows that are substrates of CYP3A4).
No products indexed under this heading.

Erythromycin Ethylsuccinate (Lapatinib inhibits CYP3A4 *in vitro* at clinically relevant concentrations. Caution should be exercised and dose reduction of the concomitant substrate drug should be considered when dosing lapatinib concurrently with medications with narrow therapeutic windows that are substrates of CYP3A4). Products include:
E.E.S. 437
EryPed 435

Erythromycin Gluceptate (Lapatinib inhibits CYP3A4 *in vitro* at clinically relevant concentrations. Caution should be exercised and dose reduction of the concomitant substrate drug should be considered when dosing lapatinib concurrently with medications with narrow therapeutic windows that are substrates of CYP3A4).
No products indexed under this heading.

Erythromycin Lactobionate (Lapatinib inhibits CYP3A4 *in vitro* at clinically relevant concentrations. Caution should be exercised and dose reduction of the concomitant substrate drug should be considered when dosing lapatinib concurrently with medications with narrow therapeutic windows that are substrates of CYP3A4).
No products indexed under this heading.

Erythromycin Stearate (Lapatinib inhibits CYP3A4 *in vitro* at clinically relevant concentrations. Caution should be exercised and dose reduction of the concomitant substrate drug should be considered when dosing lapatinib concurrently with medications with narrow therapeutic windows that are substrates of CYP3A4).
No products indexed under this heading.

Estradiol (Lapatinib inhibits CYP3A4 *in vitro* at clinically relevant concentrations. Caution should be exercised and dose reduction of the concomitant substrate drug should be considered when dosing lapatinib concurrently with medi-

cations with narrow therapeutic windows that are substrates of CYP3A4). Products include:
Activella 2561
Angeliq 831
Climara 841
Climara Pro 847
Divigel 3467
Estrasorb 1777
Vagifem 2589

Estradiol Benzoate (Lapatinib inhibits CYP3A4 *in vitro* at clinically relevant concentrations. Caution should be exercised and dose reduction of the concomitant substrate drug should be considered when dosing lapatinib concurrently with medications with narrow therapeutic windows that are substrates of CYP3A4).
No products indexed under this heading.

Estradiol Cypionate (Lapatinib inhibits CYP3A4 *in vitro* at clinically relevant concentrations. Caution should be exercised and dose reduction of the concomitant substrate drug should be considered when dosing lapatinib concurrently with medications with narrow therapeutic windows that are substrates of CYP3A4).
No products indexed under this heading.

Estradiol Valerate (Lapatinib inhibits CYP3A4 *in vitro* at clinically relevant concentrations. Caution should be exercised and dose reduction of the concomitant substrate drug should be considered when dosing lapatinib concurrently with medications with narrow therapeutic windows that are substrates of CYP3A4).
No products indexed under this heading.

Ethinyl Estradiol (Lapatinib inhibits CYP3A4 *in vitro* at clinically relevant concentrations. Caution should be exercised and dose reduction of the concomitant substrate drug should be considered when dosing lapatinib concurrently with medications with narrow therapeutic windows that are substrates of CYP3A4). Products include:
LoSeasonique 3407
Lybrel 3514
NuvaRing 3181
Ortho Evra 2648
Ortho-Cyclen/Ortho Tri-Cyclen 2663
Ortho Tri-Cyclen Lo Tablets 2673
Seasonique 3418
Yaz 864

Ethosuximide (Lapatinib undergoes extensive metabolism by CYP3A4; concomitant administration of strong inducers of CYP3A4 alter lapatinib concentrations significantly and should be avoided. Dose adjustment of lapatinib should be considered for patients who must receive concomitant strong inducers of CYP3A4 enzymes. Lapatinib inhibits CYP3A4 *in vitro* at clinically relevant concentrations. Caution should be exercised and dose reduction of the concomitant substrate drug should be considered when dosing lapatinib concurrently with medications with narrow therapeutic windows that are substrates of CYP3A4).
No products indexed under this heading.

Ethynodiol Diacetate (Lapatinib inhibits CYP3A4 *in vitro* at clinically relevant concentrations. Caution should be exercised and dose reduction of the concomitant substrate drug should be considered when dosing lapatinib concurrently with medications with narrow therapeutic windows that are substrates of CYP3A4).
No products indexed under this heading.

Etoposide (Lapatinib inhibits CYP3A4 *in vitro* at clinically relevant concentrations. Caution should be exercised and dose reduction of the concomitant substrate drug should be considered when dosing lapatinib concurrently with medications with narrow therapeutic windows that are substrates of CYP3A4).
No products indexed under this heading.

Etoposide Phosphate (Lapatinib inhibits CYP3A4 *in vitro* at clinically relevant concentrations. Caution should be exercised and dose reduction of the concomitant substrate drug should be considered when dosing lapatinib concurrently with medications with narrow therapeutic windows that are substrates of CYP3A4).
No products indexed under this heading.

Felbamate (Lapatinib undergoes extensive metabolism by CYP3A4; concomitant administration of strong inducers of CYP3A4 alter lapatinib concentrations significantly and should be avoided. Dose adjustment of lapatinib should be considered for patients who must receive concomitant strong inducers of CYP3A4 enzymes. Lapatinib inhibits CYP3A4 *in vitro* at clinically relevant concentrations. Caution should be exercised and dose reduction of the concomitant substrate drug should be considered when dosing lapatinib concurrently with medications with narrow therapeutic windows that are substrates of CYP3A4).
No products indexed under this heading.

Felodipine (Lapatinib inhibits CYP3A4 *in vitro* at clinically relevant concentrations. Caution should be exercised and dose reduction of the concomitant substrate drug should be considered when dosing lapatinib concurrently with medications with narrow therapeutic windows that are substrates of CYP3A4).
No products indexed under this heading.

Fentanyl (Lapatinib inhibits CYP3A4 *in vitro* at clinically relevant concentrations. Caution should be exercised and dose reduction of the concomitant substrate drug should be considered when dosing lapatinib concurrently with medications with narrow therapeutic windows that are substrates of CYP3A4). Products include:
Duragesic 2604
Fentanyl Transdermal System 2346
Onsolis 2054

Fentanyl Citrate (Lapatinib inhibits CYP3A4 *in vitro* at clinically relevant concentrations. Caution should be exercised and dose reduction of the concomitant substrate drug should be considered when dosing lapatinib concurrently with medications with narrow therapeutic windows that are substrates of CYP3A4). Products include:
Fentora 966

Fludrocortisone Acetate (Lapatinib undergoes extensive metabolism by CYP3A4; concomitant administration of strong inducers of CYP3A4 alter lapatinib concentrations significantly and should be avoided. Dose adjustment of lapatinib should be considered for patients who must receive concomitant strong inducers of CYP3A4 enzymes. Lapatinib inhibits CYP3A4 *in vitro* at clinically relevant concentrations. Caution should be exercised and dose reduction of the concomitant substrate drug should be considered when dosing lapatinib concurrently with medications with narrow therapeutic windows that are substrates of CYP3A4).
No products indexed under this heading.

Fluvastatin Sodium (Lapatinib inhibits CYP2C8 *in vitro* at clinically relevant concentrations. Caution should be exercised and dose reduction of the concomitant substrate drug should be considered when dosing lapatinib concurrently with medications with narrow therapeutic windows that are substrates of CYP2C8).
No products indexed under this heading.

Fosamprenavir Calcium (Lapatinib undergoes extensive metabolism by CYP3A4; concomitant administration of strong inhibitors of CYP3A4 alter lapatinib concentrations significantly and should be avoided. Dose adjustment of lapatinib should be considered for patients who must receive concomitant strong inhibitors of CYP3A4 enzymes. Lapatinib inhibits CYP3A4 *in vitro* at clinically relevant concentrations. Caution should be exercised and dose reduction of the concomitant substrate drug should be considered when dosing lapatinib concurrently with medications with narrow therapeutic windows that are substrates of CYP3A4). Products include:
Lexiva Oral Suspension 1558
Lexiva 1558

Fosphenytoin Sodium (Lapatinib undergoes extensive metabolism by CYP3A4; concomitant administration of strong inducers of CYP3A4 alter lapatinib concentrations significantly and should be avoided. Dose adjustment of lapatinib should be considered for patients who must receive concomitant strong inducers of CYP3A4 enzymes. Lapatinib inhibits CYP3A4 *in vitro* at clinically relevant concentrations. Caution should be exercised and dose reduction of the concomitant substrate drug should be considered when dosing lapatinib concurrently with medications with narrow therapeutic windows that are substrates of CYP3A4).
No products indexed under this heading.

Garlic Extract (Lapatinib undergoes extensive metabolism by CYP3A4; concomitant administration of strong inducers of CYP3A4 alter lapatinib concentrations significantly and should be avoided. Dose adjustment of lapatinib should be considered for patients who must receive concomitant strong inducers of CYP3A4 enzymes. Lapatinib inhibits CYP3A4 *in vitro* at clinically relevant concentrations. Caution should be exercised and dose reduction of the concomitant substrate drug should be considered when dosing lapatinib concurrently with medications with narrow therapeutic windows that are substrates of CYP3A4).
No products indexed under this heading.

Garlic Oil (Lapatinib undergoes extensive metabolism by CYP3A4; concomitant administration of strong inducers of CYP3A4 alter lapatinib concentrations significantly and should be avoided. Dose adjustment of lapatinib should be considered for patients who must receive concomitant strong inducers of CYP3A4 enzymes. Lapatinib inhibits CYP3A4 *in vitro* at clinically relevant concentrations. Caution should be exercised and dose reduction of the concomitant substrate drug should be considered when dosing lapatinib concurrently with medications with narrow therapeutic windows that are substrates of CYP3A4).
No products indexed under this heading.

Haloperidol (Lapatinib inhibits CYP3A4 *in vitro* at clinically relevant concentrations. Caution should be exercised and dose reduction of the concomitant substrate drug should be considered when dosing lapatinib concurrently with medications with narrow therapeutic windows that are substrates of CYP3A4).
No products indexed under this heading.

Haloperidol Decanoate (Lapatinib inhibits CYP3A4 *in vitro* at clinically relevant concentrations. Caution should be exercised and dose reduction of the concomitant substrate drug should be considered when dosing lapatinib concurrently with medications with narrow therapeutic windows that are substrates of CYP3A4).
No products indexed under this heading.

Haloperidol Lactate (Lapatinib inhibits CYP3A4 *in vitro* at clinically relevant concentrations. Caution should be exercised and dose reduction of the concomitant substrate drug should be considered when dosing lapatinib concurrently with medications with narrow therapeutic windows that are substrates of CYP3A4).
No products indexed under this heading.

Hydrocortisone (Lapatinib undergoes extensive metabolism by CYP3A4; concomitant administration of strong inducers of CYP3A4 alter lapatinib concentrations significantly and should be avoided. Dose adjustment of lapatinib should be considered for patients who must receive concomitant strong inducers of CYP3A4 enzymes. Lapatinib inhibits CYP3A4 *in vitro* at clinically relevant concentrations. Caution should be exercised and dose reduction of the concomitant substrate drug should be considered when dosing lapatinib concurrently with medications with narrow therapeutic windows that are substrates of CYP3A4).
No products indexed under this heading.

Hydrocortisone (Alcohol) (Lapatinib undergoes extensive metabolism by CYP3A4; concomitant administration of strong inducers of CYP3A4 alter lapatinib concentrations significantly and should be avoided. Dose adjustment of lapatinib should be considered for patients who must receive concomitant strong inducers of CYP3A4 enzymes. Lapatinib inhibits CYP3A4 *in vitro* at clinically relevant concentrations. Caution should be exercised and dose reduction of the concomitant substrate drug should be considered when dosing lapatinib concurrently with medications with narrow therapeutic windows that are substrates of CYP3A4).
No products indexed under this heading.

Hydrocortisone Acetate (Lapatinib undergoes extensive metabolism by CYP3A4; concomitant administration of strong inducers of CYP3A4 alter lapatinib concentrations significantly and should be avoided. Dose adjustment of lapatinib should be considered for patients who must receive concomitant strong inducers of CYP3A4 enzymes. Lapatinib inhibits CYP3A4 *in vitro* at clinically relevant concentrations. Caution should be exercised and dose reduction of the concomitant substrate drug should be considered when dosing lapatinib concurrently with medications with narrow therapeutic windows that are substrates of CYP3A4).
No products indexed under this heading.

Hydrocortisone Butyrate (Lapatinib undergoes extensive metabolism by CYP3A4; concomitant administration of strong inducers of CYP3A4 alter lapatinib concentrations significantly and should be avoided. Dose adjustment of lapatinib should be considered for patients who must receive concomitant strong inducers of CYP3A4 enzymes. Lapatinib inhibits CYP3A4 *in vitro* at clinically relevant concentrations. Caution should be exercised and dose reduction of the concomitant substrate drug should be considered when dosing lapatinib concurrently with medications with narrow therapeutic windows that are substrates of CYP3A4).
No products indexed under this heading.

Hydrocortisone Cypionate (Lapatinib undergoes extensive metabolism by CYP3A4; concomitant administration of strong inducers of CYP3A4 alter lapatinib concentrations significantly and should be avoided. Dose adjustment of lapatinib should be considered for patients who must receive concomitant strong inducers of CYP3A4 enzymes. Lapatinib inhibits CYP3A4 *in vitro* at clinically relevant concentrations. Caution should be exercised and dose reduction of the concomitant substrate drug should be considered when dosing lapatinib concurrently with medications with narrow therapeutic windows that are substrates of CYP3A4).
No products indexed under this heading.

Hydrocortisone Hemisuccinate (Lapatinib undergoes extensive metabolism by CYP3A4; concomitant administration of strong inducers of CYP3A4 alter lapatinib concentrations significantly and should be avoided. Dose adjustment of lapatinib should be considered for patients who must receive concomitant strong inducers of CYP3A4 enzymes. Lapatinib inhibits CYP3A4 *in vitro* at clinically relevant concentrations. Caution should be exercised and dose reduction of the concomitant substrate drug should be considered when dosing lapatinib concurrently with medications with narrow therapeutic windows that are substrates of CYP3A4).
No products indexed under this heading.

Hydrocortisone Probutate (Lapatinib undergoes extensive metabolism by CYP3A4; concomitant administration of strong inducers of CYP3A4 alter lapatinib concentrations significantly and should be avoided. Dose adjustment of lapatinib should be considered for patients who must receive concomitant strong inducers of CYP3A4 enzymes. Lapatinib inhibits CYP3A4 *in vitro* at clinically relevant concentrations. Caution should be exercised and dose reduction of the concomitant substrate drug should be considered when dosing lapatinib concurrently with medications with narrow therapeutic windows that are substrates of CYP3A4).
No products indexed under this heading.

Hydrocortisone Sodium Phosphate (Lapatinib undergoes extensive metabolism by CYP3A4; concomitant administration of strong inducers of CYP3A4 alter lapatinib concentrations significantly and should be avoided. Dose adjustment of lapatinib should be considered for patients who must receive concomitant strong inducers of CYP3A4 enzymes. Lapatinib inhibits CYP3A4 *in vitro* at clinically relevant concentrations. Caution should be exercised and dose reduction of the concomitant substrate drug should be considered when dosing lapatinib concurrently with medications with narrow therapeutic windows that are substrates of CYP3A4).
No products indexed under this heading.

Hydrocortisone Sodium Succinate (Lapatinib undergoes extensive metabolism by CYP3A4; concomitant administration of strong inducers of CYP3A4 alter lapatinib concentrations significantly and should be avoided. Dose adjustment of lapatinib should be considered for patients who must receive concomitant strong inducers of CYP3A4 enzymes. Lapatinib inhibits CYP3A4 *in vitro* at clinically relevant concentrations. Caution should be exercised and dose reduction of the concomitant substrate drug should be considered when dosing lapatinib concurrently with medications with narrow therapeutic windows that are substrates of CYP3A4).
No products indexed under this heading.

Hydrocortisone Valerate (Lapatinib undergoes extensive metabolism by CYP3A4; concomitant administration of strong inducers of CYP3A4 alter lapatinib concentrations significantly and should be avoided. Dose adjustment of lapatinib should be considered for patients who must receive concomitant strong inducers of CYP3A4 enzymes. Lapatinib inhibits CYP3A4 *in vitro* at clinically relevant concentrations. Caution should be exercised and dose reduction of the concomitant substrate drug should be considered when dosing lapatinib concurrently with medications with narrow therapeutic windows that are substrates of CYP3A4).
No products indexed under this heading.

Hypericum (The concomitant use of strong CYP3A4 inducers should be avoided (eg St. John's Wort). If patients must be co-administered a strong CYP3A4 inducer, based on pharmacokinetic studies, the dose of lapatinib should be titrated gradually from 1,250 mg/day up to 4,500 mg/day based on tolerability).
No products indexed under this heading.

Hypericum Perforatum (The concomitant use of strong CYP3A4 inducers should be avoided (eg, St. John's Wort). If patients must be co-administered a strong CYP3A4 inducer, based on pharmacokinetic studies, the dose of lapatinib should be titrated gradually from 1,250 mg/day up to 4,500 mg/day based on tolerability). Products include:
Traumeel 1800

Imipramine Hydrochloride (Lapatinib inhibits CYP2C8 *in vitro* at clinically relevant concentrations. Caution should be exercised and dose reduction of the concomitant substrate drug should be considered when dosing lapatinib concurrently with medications with narrow therapeutic windows that are substrates of CYP2C8).
No products indexed under this heading.

Imipramine Pamoate (Lapatinib inhibits CYP2C8 *in vitro* at clinically relevant concentrations. Caution should be exercised and dose reduction of the concomitant substrate drug should be considered when dosing lapatinib concurrently with medications with narrow therapeutic windows that are substrates of CYP2C8).
No products indexed under this heading.

Indinavir Sulfate (The concomitant use of strong CYP3A4 inhibitors should be avoided (eg, indinavir). If patients must be co-administered a strong CYP3A4 inhibitor, based on pharmacokinetic studies, a dose reduction to 500 mg/day of lapatinib is predicted to adjust the lapatinib AUC to the range observed without inhibitors and should be considered). Products include:
Crixivan 2113

Isotretinoin (Lapatinib inhibits CYP2C8 *in vitro* at clinically relevant concentrations. Caution should be exercised and dose reduction of the concomitant substrate drug should be considered when dosing lapatinib concurrently with medications with narrow therapeutic windows that are substrates of CYP2C8). Products include:
Accutane 2832

Isradipine (Lapatinib inhibits CYP3A4 *in vitro* at clinically relevant concentrations. Caution should be exercised and dose reduction of the concomitant substrate drug should be considered when dosing lapatinib concurrently with medications with narrow therapeutic windows that are substrates of CYP3A4). Products include:
DynaCirc CR 1432

Itraconazole (The concomitant use of strong CYP3A4 inhibitors should be avoided (eg, itraconazole). If patients must be co-administered a strong CYP3A4 inhibitor, based on pharmacokinetic studies, a dose reduction to 500 mg/day of lapatinib is predicted to adjust the lapatinib AUC to the range observed without inhibitors and should be considered).
No products indexed under this heading.

Ixabepilone (Lapatinib inhibits CYP3A4 *in vitro* at clinically relevant concentrations. Caution should be exercised and dose reduction of the concomitant substrate drug should be considered when dosing lapatinib concurrently with medications with narrow therapeutic windows that are substrates of CYP3A4).
No products indexed under this heading.

Ketoconazole (The concomitant use of strong CYP3A4 inhibitors should be avoided (eg, ketoconazole). If patients must be co-administered a strong CYP3A4 inhibitor, based on pharmacokinetic studies, a dose reduction to 500 mg/day of lapatinib is predicted to adjust the lapatinib AUC to the range observed without inhibitors and should be considered). Products include:
Extina 3319
Xolegel 3337

Levonorgestrel (Lapatinib inhibits CYP3A4 *in vitro* at clinically relevant concentrations. Caution should be exercised and dose reduction of the concomitant substrate drug should be considered when dosing lapatinib concurrently with medications with narrow therapeutic windows that are substrates of CYP3A4). Products include:
Climara Pro 847
LoSeasonique 3407
Lybrel 3514
Mirena 854
Plan B 3416
Seasonique 3418

Lidocaine (Lapatinib inhibits CYP3A4 *in vitro* at clinically relevant concentrations. Caution should be exercised and dose reduction of the concomitant substrate drug should be considered when dosing lapatinib concurrently with medications with narrow therapeutic windows that are substrates of CYP3A4). Products include:
Lidoderm 1107

Lidocaine Hydrochloride (Lapatinib inhibits CYP3A4 *in vitro* at clinically relevant concentrations. Caution should be exercised and dose reduction of the concomitant substrate drug should be considered when dosing lapatinib concurrently with medications with narrow therapeutic windows that are substrates of CYP3A4).
No products indexed under this heading.

Lopinavir (Lapatinib undergoes extensive metabolism by CYP3A4; concomitant administration of strong inhibitors of CYP3A4 alter lapatinib concentrations significantly and should be avoided. Dose adjustment of lapatinib should be considered for patients who must receive concomitant strong inhibitors of CYP3A4 enzymes. Lapatinib inhibits CYP3A4 *in vitro* at clinically relevant concentrations. Caution should be exercised and dose reduction of the concomitant substrate drug should be considered when dosing lapatinib concurrently with medications with narrow therapeutic windows that are substrates of CYP3A4). Products include:
Kaletra 458

Lovastatin (Lapatinib inhibits CYP3A4 *in vitro* at clinically relevant concentrations. Caution should be exercised and dose reduction of the concomitant substrate drug should be considered when dosing lapatinib concurrently with medi-

cations with narrow therapeutic windows that are substrates of CYP3A4). Products include:
Advicor 402
Mevacor 2212

Maprotiline Hydrochloride (Lapatinib inhibits CYP2C8 *in vitro* at clinically relevant concentrations. Caution should be exercised and dose reduction of the concomitant substrate drug should be considered when dosing lapatinib concurrently with medications with narrow therapeutic windows that are substrates of CYP2C8).
No products indexed under this heading.

Mephenytoin (Lapatinib undergoes extensive metabolism by CYP3A4; concomitant administration of strong inducers of CYP3A4 alter lapatinib concentrations significantly and should be avoided. Dose adjustment of lapatinib should be considered for patients who must receive concomitant strong inducers of CYP3A4 enzymes. Lapatinib inhibits CYP3A4 *in vitro* at clinically relevant concentrations. Caution should be exercised and dose reduction of the concomitant substrate drug should be considered when dosing lapatinib concurrently with medications with narrow therapeutic windows that are substrates of CYP3A4).
No products indexed under this heading.

Mephobarbital (Lapatinib inhibits CYP2C8 *in vitro* at clinically relevant concentrations. Caution should be exercised and dose reduction of the concomitant substrate drug should be considered when dosing lapatinib concurrently with medications with narrow therapeutic windows that are substrates of CYP2C8).
No products indexed under this heading.

Mestranol (Lapatinib inhibits CYP3A4 *in vitro* at clinically relevant concentrations. Caution should be exercised and dose reduction of the concomitant substrate drug should be considered when dosing lapatinib concurrently with medications with narrow therapeutic windows that are substrates of CYP3A4).
No products indexed under this heading.

Methadone Hydrochloride (Lapatinib inhibits CYP3A4 *in vitro* at clinically relevant concentrations. Caution should be exercised and dose reduction of the concomitant substrate drug should be considered when dosing lapatinib concurrently with medications with narrow therapeutic windows that are substrates of CYP3A4).
No products indexed under this heading.

Methsuximide (Lapatinib undergoes extensive metabolism by CYP3A4; concomitant administration of strong inducers of CYP3A4 alter lapatinib concentrations significantly and should be avoided. Dose adjustment of lapatinib should be considered for patients who must receive concomitant strong inducers of CYP3A4 enzymes. Lapatinib inhibits CYP3A4 *in vitro* at clinically relevant concentrations. Caution should be exercised and dose reduction of the concomitant substrate drug should be considered when dosing lapatinib concurrently with medications with narrow therapeutic windows that are substrates of CYP3A4).
No products indexed under this heading.

Methylprednisolone (Lapatinib undergoes extensive metabolism by CYP3A4; concomitant administration of strong inducers of CYP3A4 alter lapatinib concentrations significantly and should be avoided. Dose adjustment of lapatinib should be considered for patients who must receive concomitant strong inducers of CYP3A4 enzymes. Lapatinib inhibits CYP3A4 *in vitro* at clinically relevant concentrations. Caution should be exercised and dose

reduction of the concomitant substrate drug should be considered when dosing lapatinib concurrently with medications with narrow therapeutic windows that are substrates of CYP3A4).
No products indexed under this heading.

Methylprednisolone Acetate (Lapatinib undergoes extensive metabolism by CYP3A4; concomitant administration of strong inducers of CYP3A4 alter lapatinib concentrations significantly and should be avoided. Dose adjustment of lapatinib should be considered for patients who must receive concomitant strong inducers of CYP3A4 enzymes. Lapatinib inhibits CYP3A4 *in vitro* at clinically relevant concentrations. Caution should be exercised and dose reduction of the concomitant substrate drug should be considered when dosing lapatinib concurrently with medications with narrow therapeutic windows that are substrates of CYP3A4).
No products indexed under this heading.

Methylprednisolone Sodium Succinate (Lapatinib undergoes extensive metabolism by CYP3A4; concomitant administration of strong inducers of CYP3A4 alter lapatinib concentrations significantly and should be avoided. Dose adjustment of lapatinib should be considered for patients who must receive concomitant strong inducers of CYP3A4 enzymes. Lapatinib inhibits CYP3A4 *in vitro* at clinically relevant concentrations. Caution should be exercised and dose reduction of the concomitant substrate drug should be considered when dosing lapatinib concurrently with medications with narrow therapeutic windows that are substrates of CYP3A4).
No products indexed under this heading.

Midazolam Hydrochloride (Lapatinib inhibits CYP3A4 *in vitro* at clinically relevant concentrations. Caution should be exercised and dose reduction of the concomitant substrate drug should be considered when dosing lapatinib concurrently with medications with narrow therapeutic windows that are substrates of CYP3A4).
No products indexed under this heading.

Modafinil (Lapatinib undergoes extensive metabolism by CYP3A4; concomitant administration of strong inducers of CYP3A4 alter lapatinib concentrations significantly and should be avoided. Dose adjustment of lapatinib should be considered for patients who must receive concomitant strong inducers of CYP3A4 enzymes. Lapatinib inhibits CYP3A4 *in vitro* at clinically relevant concentrations. Caution should be exercised and dose reduction of the concomitant substrate drug should be considered when dosing lapatinib concurrently with medications with narrow therapeutic windows that are substrates of CYP3A4). Products include:
Provigil 983

Nafcillin Sodium (Lapatinib undergoes extensive metabolism by CYP3A4; concomitant administration of strong inducers of CYP3A4 alter lapatinib concentrations significantly and should be avoided. Dose adjustment of lapatinib should be considered for patients who must receive concomitant strong inducers of CYP3A4 enzymes. Lapatinib inhibits CYP3A4 *in vitro* at clinically relevant concentrations. Caution should be exercised and dose reduction of the concomitant substrate drug should be considered when dosing lapatinib concurrently with medications with narrow therapeutic windows that are substrates of CYP3A4).
No products indexed under this heading.

Nefazodone Hydrochloride (The concomitant use of strong CYP3A4 inhibitors should be avoided (eg, nefazodone). If patients must be co-administered a strong CYP3A4 inhibitor, based on pharmacokinetic studies, a dose reduction to 500 mg/day of lapatinib is predicted to adjust the lapatinib AUC to the range observed without inhibitors and should be considered).
No products indexed under this heading.

Nelfinavir Mesylate (The concomitant use of strong CYP3A4 inhibitors should be avoided (eg, nelfinavir). If patients must be co-administered a strong CYP3A4 inhibitor, based on pharmacokinetic studies, a dose reduction to 500 mg/day of lapatinib is predicted to adjust the lapatinib AUC to the range observed without inhibitors and should be considered).
No products indexed under this heading.

Nevirapine (Lapatinib undergoes extensive metabolism by CYP3A4; concomitant administration of strong inducers of CYP3A4 alter lapatinib concentrations significantly and should be avoided. Dose adjustment of lapatinib should be considered for patients who must receive concomitant strong inducers of CYP3A4 enzymes. Lapatinib inhibits CYP3A4 *in vitro* at clinically relevant concentrations. Caution should be exercised and dose reduction of the concomitant substrate drug should be considered when dosing lapatinib concurrently with medications with narrow therapeutic windows that are substrates of CYP3A4). Products include:
Viramune Oral Suspension 897
Viramune Tablets 897

Nicardipine (Lapatinib inhibits CYP3A4 *in vitro* at clinically relevant concentrations. Caution should be exercised and dose reduction of the concomitant substrate drug should be considered when dosing lapatinib concurrently with medications with narrow therapeutic windows that are substrates of CYP3A4).
No products indexed under this heading.

Nicardipine Hydrochloride (Lapatinib inhibits CYP3A4 *in vitro* at clinically relevant concentrations. Caution should be exercised and dose reduction of the concomitant substrate drug should be considered when dosing lapatinib concurrently with medications with narrow therapeutic windows that are substrates of CYP3A4).
No products indexed under this heading.

Nifedipine (Lapatinib inhibits CYP3A4 *in vitro* at clinically relevant concentrations. Caution should be exercised and dose reduction of the concomitant substrate drug should be considered when dosing lapatinib concurrently with medications with narrow therapeutic windows that are substrates of CYP3A4).
No products indexed under this heading.

Nimodipine (Lapatinib inhibits CYP3A4 *in vitro* at clinically relevant concentrations. Caution should be exercised and dose reduction of the concomitant substrate drug should be considered when dosing lapatinib concurrently with medications with narrow therapeutic windows that are substrates of CYP3A4).
No products indexed under this heading.

Nisoldipine (Lapatinib inhibits CYP3A4 *in vitro* at clinically relevant concentrations. Caution should be exercised and dose reduction of the concomitant substrate drug should be considered when dosing lapatinib concurrently with medications with narrow therapeutic windows that are substrates of CYP3A4).
No products indexed under this heading.

Nitrendipine (Lapatinib inhibits CYP3A4 *in vitro* at clinically relevant concentrations. Caution should be exercised and dose reduction of the concomitant substrate drug should be considered when dosing lapatinib concurrently with medications with narrow therapeutic windows that are substrates of CYP3A4).
No products indexed under this heading.

Norethindrone (Lapatinib inhibits CYP3A4 *in vitro* at clinically relevant concentrations. Caution should be exercised and dose reduction of the concomitant substrate drug should be considered when dosing lapatinib concurrently with medications with narrow therapeutic windows that are substrates of CYP3A4). Products include:
Ortho Micronor 2660

Norethindrone Acetate (Lapatinib inhibits CYP3A4 *in vitro* at clinically relevant concentrations. Caution should be exercised and dose reduction of the concomitant substrate drug should be considered when dosing lapatinib concurrently with medications with narrow therapeutic windows that are substrates of CYP3A4). Products include:
Activella 2561

Norgestrel (Lapatinib inhibits CYP3A4 *in vitro* at clinically relevant concentrations. Caution should be exercised and dose reduction of the concomitant substrate drug should be considered when dosing lapatinib concurrently with medications with narrow therapeutic windows that are substrates of CYP3A4).
No products indexed under this heading.

Nortriptyline Hydrochloride (Lapatinib inhibits CYP2C8 *in vitro* at clinically relevant concentrations. Caution should be exercised and dose reduction of the concomitant substrate drug should be considered when dosing lapatinib concurrently with medications with narrow therapeutic windows that are substrates of CYP2C8).
No products indexed under this heading.

Omeprazole (Lapatinib inhibits CYP2C8 *in vitro* at clinically relevant concentrations. Caution should be exercised and dose reduction of the concomitant substrate drug should be considered when dosing lapatinib concurrently with medications with narrow therapeutic windows that are substrates of CYP2C8).
No products indexed under this heading.

Ondansetron (Lapatinib inhibits CYP3A4 *in vitro* at clinically relevant concentrations. Caution should be exercised and dose reduction of the concomitant substrate drug should be considered when dosing lapatinib concurrently with medications with narrow therapeutic windows that are substrates of CYP3A4).
No products indexed under this heading.

Ondansetron Hydrochloride (Lapatinib inhibits CYP3A4 *in vitro* at clinically relevant concentrations. Caution should be exercised and dose reduction of the concomitant substrate drug should be considered when dosing lapatinib concurrently with medications with narrow therapeutic windows that are substrates of CYP3A4). Products include:
Zofran Injection 1750
Zofran 1756
Zofran ODT 1756

Oxcarbazepine (Lapatinib undergoes extensive metabolism by CYP3A4; concomitant administration of strong inducers of CYP3A4 alter lapatinib concentrations significantly and should be avoided. Dose adjustment of lapatinib should be considered for patients who must receive concomitant strong inducers of CYP3A4 enzymes. Lapatinib inhibits CYP3A4 *in vitro* at clinically relevant concentrations. Caution should be exercised and dose reduction of the concomitant substrate drug should be considered when dosing lapatinib concurrently with medications with narrow therapeutic windows that are substrates of CYP3A4).
No products indexed under this heading.

Paclitaxel (Lapatinib inhibits CYP2C8 *in vitro* at clinically relevant concentrations. Caution should be exercised and dose reduction of the concomitant substrate drug should be considered when dosing lapatinib concurrently with medications with narrow therapeutic windows that are substrates of CYP2C8).
No products indexed under this heading.

Phenobarbital (The concomitant use of strong CYP3A4 inducers should be avoided (eg, phenobarbital). If patients must be co-administered a strong CYP3A4 inducer, based on pharmacokinetic studies, the dose of lapatinib should be titrated gradually from 1,250 mg/day up to 4,500 mg/day based on tolerability). Products include:
Donnatal 2711

Phenobarbital Sodium (The concomitant use of strong CYP3A4 inducers should be avoided (eg, phenobarbital). If patients must be co-administered a strong CYP3A4 inducer, based on pharmacokinetic studies, the dose of lapatinib should be titrated gradually from 1,250 mg/day up to 4,500 mg/day based on tolerability).
No products indexed under this heading.

Phenytoin (The concomitant use of strong CYP3A4 inducers should be avoided (eg, phenytoin). If patients must be co-administered a strong CYP3A4 inducer, based on pharmacokinetic studies, the dose of lapatinib should be titrated gradually from 1,250 mg/day up to 4,500 mg/day based on tolerability).
No products indexed under this heading.

Phenytoin Sodium (The concomitant use of strong CYP3A4 inducers should be avoided (eg, phenytoin). If patients must be co-administered a strong CYP3A4 inducer, based on pharmacokinetic studies, the dose of lapatinib should be titrated gradually from 1,250 mg/day up to 4,500 mg/day based on tolerability). Products include:
Phenytek Capsules 2380

Pimozide (Lapatinib inhibits CYP3A4 *in vitro* at clinically relevant concentrations. Caution should be exercised and dose reduction of the concomitant substrate drug should be considered when dosing lapatinib concurrently with medications with narrow therapeutic windows that are substrates of CYP3A4).
No products indexed under this heading.

Pioglitazone Hydrochloride (Lapatinib inhibits CYP2C8 *in vitro* at clinically relevant concentrations. Caution should be exercised and dose reduction of the concomitant substrate drug should be considered when dosing lapatinib concurrently with medications with narrow therapeutic windows that are substrates of CYP2C8). Products include:
ActoPlus 3338
Actos 3345
Duetact 3354

Polyestradiol Phosphate (Lapatinib inhibits CYP3A4 *in vitro* at clinically relevant concentrations. Caution should be exercised and dose reduction of the concomitant substrate drug should be considered when dosing lapatinib concurrently with medications with narrow therapeutic windows that are substrates of CYP3A4).
No products indexed under this heading.

Prednisolone (Lapatinib undergoes extensive metabolism by CYP3A4; concomitant administration of strong inducers of CYP3A4 alter lapatinib concentrations significantly and should be

avoided. Dose adjustment of lapatinib should be considered for patients who must receive concomitant strong inducers of CYP3A4 enzymes. Lapatinib inhibits CYP3A4 *in vitro* at clinically relevant concentrations. Caution should be exercised and dose reduction of the concomitant substrate drug should be considered when dosing lapatinib concurrently with medications with narrow therapeutic windows that are substrates of CYP3A4).
No products indexed under this heading.

Prednisolone Acetate (Lapatinib undergoes extensive metabolism by CYP3A4; concomitant administration of strong inducers of CYP3A4 alter lapatinib concentrations significantly and should be avoided. Dose adjustment of lapatinib should be considered for patients who must receive concomitant strong inducers of CYP3A4 enzymes. Lapatinib inhibits CYP3A4 *in vitro* at clinically relevant concentrations. Caution should be exercised and dose reduction of the concomitant substrate drug should be considered when dosing lapatinib concurrently with medications with narrow therapeutic windows that are substrates of CYP3A4). Products include:
Blephamide .... ⊙**212**, ⊙**214**
Pred Forte .... ⊙**225**
Pred Mild .... ⊙**230**
Pred-G .... ⊙**226**, ⊙**227**

Prednisolone Sodium Phosphate (Lapatinib undergoes extensive metabolism by CYP3A4; concomitant administration of strong inducers of CYP3A4 alter lapatinib concentrations significantly and should be avoided. Dose adjustment of lapatinib should be considered for patients who must receive concomitant strong inducers of CYP3A4 enzymes. Lapatinib inhibits CYP3A4 *in vitro* at clinically relevant concentrations. Caution should be exercised and dose reduction of the concomitant substrate drug should be considered when dosing lapatinib concurrently with medications with narrow therapeutic windows that are substrates of CYP3A4).
No products indexed under this heading.

Prednisolone Tebutate (Lapatinib undergoes extensive metabolism by CYP3A4; concomitant administration of strong inducers of CYP3A4 alter lapatinib concentrations significantly and should be avoided. Dose adjustment of lapatinib should be considered for patients who must receive concomitant strong inducers of CYP3A4 enzymes. Lapatinib inhibits CYP3A4 *in vitro* at clinically relevant concentrations. Caution should be exercised and dose reduction of the concomitant substrate drug should be considered when dosing lapatinib concurrently with medications with narrow therapeutic windows that are substrates of CYP3A4).
No products indexed under this heading.

Prednisone (Lapatinib undergoes extensive metabolism by CYP3A4; concomitant administration of strong inducers of CYP3A4 alter lapatinib concentrations significantly and should be avoided. Dose adjustment of lapatinib should be considered for patients who must receive concomitant strong inducers of CYP3A4 enzymes. Lapatinib inhibits CYP3A4 *in vitro* at clinically relevant concentrations. Caution should be exercised and dose reduction of the concomitant substrate drug should be considered when dosing lapatinib concurrently with medications with narrow therapeutic windows that are substrates of CYP3A4).
No products indexed under this heading.

Prednisone sodium phosphate (Lapatinib undergoes extensive metabolism by CYP3A4; concomitant administration of strong inducers of CYP3A4 alter lapatinib concentrations significantly and should be avoided. Dose adjustment of lapatinib should be considered for patients who must receive concomitant strong inducers of CYP3A4 enzymes. Lapatinib inhibits CYP3A4 *in vitro* at clinically relevant concentrations. Caution should be exercised and dose reduction of the concomitant substrate drug should be considered when dosing lapatinib concurrently with medications with narrow therapeutic windows that are substrates of CYP3A4).
No products indexed under this heading.

Primidone (Lapatinib undergoes extensive metabolism by CYP3A4; concomitant administration of strong inducers of CYP3A4 alter lapatinib concentrations significantly and should be avoided. Dose adjustment of lapatinib should be considered for patients who must receive concomitant strong inducers of CYP3A4 enzymes. Lapatinib inhibits CYP3A4 *in vitro* at clinically relevant concentrations. Caution should be exercised and dose reduction of the concomitant substrate drug should be considered when dosing lapatinib concurrently with medications with narrow therapeutic windows that are substrates of CYP3A4).
No products indexed under this heading.

Protriptyline Hydrochloride (Lapatinib inhibits CYP2C8 *in vitro* at clinically relevant concentrations. Caution should be exercised and dose reduction of the concomitant substrate drug should be considered when dosing lapatinib concurrently with medications with narrow therapeutic windows that are substrates of CYP2C8).
No products indexed under this heading.

Quinidine Gluconate (Lapatinib inhibits CYP3A4 *in vitro* at clinically relevant concentrations. Caution should be exercised and dose reduction of the concomitant substrate drug should be considered when dosing lapatinib concurrently with medications with narrow therapeutic windows that are substrates of CYP3A4).
No products indexed under this heading.

Quinidine Polygalacturonate (Lapatinib inhibits CYP3A4 *in vitro* at clinically relevant concentrations. Caution should be exercised and dose reduction of the concomitant substrate drug should be considered when dosing lapatinib concurrently with medications with narrow therapeutic windows that are substrates of CYP3A4).
No products indexed under this heading.

Quinidine Sulfate (Lapatinib inhibits CYP3A4 *in vitro* at clinically relevant concentrations. Caution should be exercised and dose reduction of the concomitant substrate drug should be considered when dosing lapatinib concurrently with medications with narrow therapeutic windows that are substrates of CYP3A4).
No products indexed under this heading.

Repaglinide (Lapatinib inhibits CYP2C8 *in vitro* at clinically relevant concentrations. Caution should be exercised and dose reduction of the concomitant substrate drug should be considered when dosing lapatinib concurrently with medications with narrow therapeutic windows that are substrates of CYP2C8).
No products indexed under this heading.

Rifabutin (The concomitant use of strong CYP3A4 inducers should be avoided (eg, rifabutin). If patients must be co-administered a strong CYP3A4 inducer, based on pharmacokinetic studies, the dose of lapatinib should be titrated gradually from 1,250 mg/day up to 4,500 mg/day based on tolerability).
No products indexed under this heading.

Rifampicin (Lapatinib undergoes extensive metabolism by CYP3A4; concomitant administration of strong inducers of CYP3A4 alter lapatinib concentrations significantly and should be avoided. Dose adjustment of lapatinib should be considered for patients who must receive concomitant strong inducers of CYP3A4 enzymes. Lapatinib inhibits CYP3A4 *in vitro* at clinically relevant concentrations. Caution should be exercised and dose reduction of the concomitant substrate drug should be considered when dosing lapatinib concurrently with medications with narrow therapeutic windows that are substrates of CYP3A4).
No products indexed under this heading.

Rifampin (The concomitant use of strong CYP3A4 inducers should be avoided (eg, rifampin). If patients must be co-administered a strong CYP3A4 inducer, based on pharmacokinetic studies, the dose of lapatinib should be titrated gradually from 1,250 mg/day up to 4,500 mg/day based on tolerability).
No products indexed under this heading.

Rifapentine (The concomitant use of strong CYP3A4 inducers should be avoided (eg, rifapentine). If patients must be co-administered a strong CYP3A4 inducer, based on pharmacokinetic studies, the dose of lapatinib should be titrated gradually from 1,250 mg/day up to 4,500 mg/day based on tolerability).
No products indexed under this heading.

Ritonavir (The concomitant use of strong CYP3A4 inhibitors should be avoided (eg, ritonavir). If patients must be co-administered a strong CYP3A4 inhibitor, based on pharmacokinetic studies, a dose reduction to 500 mg/day of lapatinib is predicted to adjust the lapatinib AUC to the range observed without inhibitors and should be considered). Products include:
Kaletra **458**
Norvir **509**

Rosiglitazone Maleate (Lapatinib inhibits CYP2C8 *in vitro* at clinically relevant concentrations. Caution should be exercised and dose reduction of the concomitant substrate drug should be considered when dosing lapatinib concurrently with medications with narrow therapeutic windows that are substrates of CYP2C8). Products include:
Avandamet **1345**
Avandaryl **1356**
Avandia **1366**

Rosiglitazone/Metformin (Lapatinib inhibits CYP2C8 *in vitro* at clinically relevant concentrations. Caution should be exercised and dose reduction of the concomitant substrate drug should be considered when dosing lapatinib concurrently with medications with narrow therapeutic windows that are substrates of CYP2C8).
No products indexed under this heading.

Saquinavir (The concomitant use of strong CYP3A4 inhibitors should be avoided (eg, saquinavir). If patients must be co-administered a strong CYP3A4 inhibitor, based on pharmacokinetic studies, a dose reduction to 500 mg/day of lapatinib is predicted to adjust the lapatinib AUC to the range observed without inhibitors and should be considered).
No products indexed under this heading.

Saquinavir Mesylate (The concomitant use of strong CYP3A4 inhibitors should be avoided (eg, saquinavir). If patients must be co-administered a strong CYP3A4 inhibitor, based on pharmacokinetic studies, a dose reduction to 500 mg/day of lapatinib is predicted to adjust the lapatinib AUC to the range observed without inhibitors and should be considered).
No products indexed under this heading.

Sertraline Hydrochloride (Lapatinib inhibits CYP3A4 *in vitro* at clinically relevant concentrations. Caution should be exercised and dose reduction of the concomitant substrate drug should be considered when dosing lapatinib concurrently with medications with narrow therapeutic windows that are substrates of CYP3A4).
No products indexed under this heading.

Sildenafil Citrate (Lapatinib inhibits CYP3A4 *in vitro* at clinically relevant concentrations. Caution should be exercised and dose reduction of the concomitant substrate drug should be considered when dosing lapatinib concurrently with medications with narrow therapeutic windows that are substrates of CYP3A4).
No products indexed under this heading.

Simvastatin (Lapatinib inhibits CYP3A4 *in vitro* at clinically relevant concentrations. Caution should be exercised and dose reduction of the concomitant substrate drug should be considered when dosing lapatinib concurrently with medications with narrow therapeutic windows that are substrates of CYP3A4). Products include:
Simcor **524**
Vytorin 10/10 .... **2303, 3240**
Vytorin 10/20 .... **2303, 3240**
Vytorin 10/40 .... **2303, 3240**
Vytorin 10/80 .... **2303, 3240**
Zocor **2289**

Sirolimus (Lapatinib inhibits CYP3A4 *in vitro* at clinically relevant concentrations. Caution should be exercised and dose reduction of the concomitant substrate drug should be considered when dosing lapatinib concurrently with medications with narrow therapeutic windows that are substrates of CYP3A4). Products include:
Rapamune **3579**

Sulfinpyrazone (Lapatinib undergoes extensive metabolism by CYP3A4; concomitant administration of strong inducers of CYP3A4 alter lapatinib concentrations significantly and should be avoided. Dose adjustment of lapatinib should be considered for patients who must receive concomitant strong inducers of CYP3A4 enzymes. Lapatinib inhibits CYP3A4 *in vitro* at clinically relevant concentrations. Caution should be exercised and dose reduction of the concomitant substrate drug should be considered when dosing lapatinib concurrently with medications with narrow therapeutic windows that are substrates of CYP3A4).
No products indexed under this heading.

Tacrolimus (Lapatinib inhibits CYP3A4 *in vitro* at clinically relevant concentrations. Caution should be exercised and dose reduction of the concomitant substrate drug should be considered when dosing lapatinib concurrently with medications with narrow therapeutic windows that are substrates of CYP3A4). Products include:
Prograf Capsules **677**
Prograf Injection **677**
Protopic **685**

Tadalafil (Lapatinib inhibits CYP3A4 *in vitro* at clinically relevant concentrations. Caution should be exercised and dose reduction of the concomitant substrate drug should be considered when dosing lapatinib concurrently with medi-

IMPORTANT NOTE: Always consult each drug listing in the patient's regimen for possible interactions.

cations with narrow therapeutic windows that are substrates of CYP3A4). Products include:
Adcirca 3461
Cialis 1861

Tamoxifen Citrate (Lapatinib inhibits CYP3A4 *in vitro* at clinically relevant concentrations. Caution should be exercised and dose reduction of the concomitant substrate drug should be considered when dosing lapatinib concurrently with medications with narrow therapeutic windows that are substrates of CYP3A4).
No products indexed under this heading.

Telithromycin (The concomitant use of strong CYP3A4 inhibitors should be avoided (eg, telithromycin). If patients must be co-administered a strong CYP3A4 inhibitor, based on pharmacokinetic studies, a dose reduction to 500 mg/day of lapatinib is predicted to adjust the lapatinib AUC to the range observed without inhibitors and should be considered). Products include:
Ketek 2991

Terfenadine (Lapatinib inhibits CYP3A4 *in vitro* at clinically relevant concentrations. Caution should be exercised and dose reduction of the concomitant substrate drug should be considered when dosing lapatinib concurrently with medications with narrow therapeutic windows that are substrates of CYP3A4).
No products indexed under this heading.

Theophyllinate (Lapatinib undergoes extensive metabolism by CYP3A4; concomitant administration of strong inducers of CYP3A4 alter lapatinib concentrations significantly and should be avoided. Dose adjustment of lapatinib should be considered for patients who must receive concomitant strong inducers of CYP3A4 enzymes. Lapatinib inhibits CYP3A4 *in vitro* at clinically relevant concentrations. Caution should be exercised and dose reduction of the concomitant substrate drug should be considered when dosing lapatinib concurrently with medications with narrow therapeutic windows that are substrates of CYP3A4).
No products indexed under this heading.

Theophylline (Lapatinib undergoes extensive metabolism by CYP3A4; concomitant administration of strong inducers of CYP3A4 alter lapatinib concentrations significantly and should be avoided. Dose adjustment of lapatinib should be considered for patients who must receive concomitant strong inducers of CYP3A4 enzymes. Lapatinib inhibits CYP3A4 *in vitro* at clinically relevant concentrations. Caution should be exercised and dose reduction of the concomitant substrate drug should be considered when dosing lapatinib concurrently with medications with narrow therapeutic windows that are substrates of CYP3A4).
No products indexed under this heading.

Theophylline Anhydrous (Lapatinib undergoes extensive metabolism by CYP3A4; concomitant administration of strong inducers of CYP3A4 alter lapatinib concentrations significantly and should be avoided. Dose adjustment of lapatinib should be considered for patients who must receive concomitant strong inducers of CYP3A4 enzymes. Lapatinib inhibits CYP3A4 *in vitro* at clinically relevant concentrations. Caution should be exercised and dose reduction of the concomitant substrate drug should be considered when dosing lapatinib concurrently with medications with narrow therapeutic windows that are substrates of CYP3A4). Products include:
Uniphyl 2817

Theophylline Calcium Salicylate (Lapatinib undergoes extensive metabolism by CYP3A4; concomitant administration of strong inducers of CYP3A4 alter lapatinib concentrations significantly and should be avoided. Dose adjustment of lapatinib should be considered for patients who must receive concomitant strong inducers of CYP3A4 enzymes. Lapatinib inhibits CYP3A4 *in vitro* at clinically relevant concentrations. Caution should be exercised and dose reduction of the concomitant substrate drug should be considered when dosing lapatinib concurrently with medications with narrow therapeutic windows that are substrates of CYP3A4).
No products indexed under this heading.

Theophylline Dihydroxypropyl (Glyceryl) (Lapatinib undergoes extensive metabolism by CYP3A4; concomitant administration of strong inducers of CYP3A4 alter lapatinib concentrations significantly and should be avoided. Dose adjustment of lapatinib should be considered for patients who must receive concomitant strong inducers of CYP3A4 enzymes. Lapatinib inhibits CYP3A4 *in vitro* at clinically relevant concentrations. Caution should be exercised and dose reduction of the concomitant substrate drug should be considered when dosing lapatinib concurrently with medications with narrow therapeutic windows that are substrates of CYP3A4).
No products indexed under this heading.

Theophylline Ethylenediamine (Lapatinib undergoes extensive metabolism by CYP3A4; concomitant administration of strong inducers of CYP3A4 alter lapatinib concentrations significantly and should be avoided. Dose adjustment of lapatinib should be considered for patients who must receive concomitant strong inducers of CYP3A4 enzymes. Lapatinib inhibits CYP3A4 *in vitro* at clinically relevant concentrations. Caution should be exercised and dose reduction of the concomitant substrate drug should be considered when dosing lapatinib concurrently with medications with narrow therapeutic windows that are substrates of CYP3A4).
No products indexed under this heading.

Theophylline Sodium Glycinate (Lapatinib undergoes extensive metabolism by CYP3A4; concomitant administration of strong inducers of CYP3A4 alter lapatinib concentrations significantly and should be avoided. Dose adjustment of lapatinib should be considered for patients who must receive concomitant strong inducers of CYP3A4 enzymes. Lapatinib inhibits CYP3A4 *in vitro* at clinically relevant concentrations. Caution should be exercised and dose reduction of the concomitant substrate drug should be considered when dosing lapatinib concurrently with medications with narrow therapeutic windows that are substrates of CYP3A4).
No products indexed under this heading.

Tiagabine Hydrochloride (Lapatinib inhibits CYP3A4 *in vitro* at clinically relevant concentrations. Caution should be exercised and dose reduction of the concomitant substrate drug should be considered when dosing lapatinib concurrently with medications with narrow therapeutic windows that are substrates of CYP3A4). Products include:
Gabitril 972

Tirofiban Hydrochloride (Lapatinib is a subtrate of the efflux transporter P-glycoprotein (Pgp, ABCB1). If lapatinib is administered with drugs that inhibit Pgp, increased concentrations of lapatinib are likely, and caution should be exercised).
No products indexed under this heading.

Tolbutamide (Lapatinib inhibits CYP2C8 *in vitro* at clinically relevant concentrations. Caution should be exercised and dose reduction of the concomitant substrate drug should be considered when dosing lapatinib concurrently with medications with narrow therapeutic windows that are substrates of CYP2C8).
No products indexed under this heading.

Tolbutamide Sodium (Lapatinib inhibits CYP2C8 *in vitro* at clinically relevant concentrations. Caution should be exercised and dose reduction of the concomitant substrate drug should be considered when dosing lapatinib concurrently with medications with narrow therapeutic windows that are substrates of CYP2C8).
No products indexed under this heading.

Tolterodine Tartrate (Lapatinib inhibits CYP3A4 *in vitro* at clinically relevant concentrations. Caution should be exercised and dose reduction of the concomitant substrate drug should be considered when dosing lapatinib concurrently with medications with narrow therapeutic windows that are substrates of CYP3A4).
No products indexed under this heading.

Trazodone Hydrochloride (Lapatinib inhibits CYP3A4 *in vitro* at clinically relevant concentrations. Caution should be exercised and dose reduction of the concomitant substrate drug should be considered when dosing lapatinib concurrently with medications with narrow therapeutic windows that are substrates of CYP3A4).
No products indexed under this heading.

Tretinoin (Lapatinib inhibits CYP2C8 *in vitro* at clinically relevant concentrations. Caution should be exercised and dose reduction of the concomitant substrate drug should be considered when dosing lapatinib concurrently with medications with narrow therapeutic windows that are substrates of CYP2C8).
No products indexed under this heading.

Triamcinolone (Lapatinib undergoes extensive metabolism by CYP3A4; concomitant administration of strong inducers of CYP3A4 alter lapatinib concentrations significantly and should be avoided. Dose adjustment of lapatinib should be considered for patients who must receive concomitant strong inducers of CYP3A4 enzymes. Lapatinib inhibits CYP3A4 *in vitro* at clinically relevant concentrations. Caution should be exercised and dose reduction of the concomitant substrate drug should be considered when dosing lapatinib concurrently with medications with narrow therapeutic windows that are substrates of CYP3A4).
No products indexed under this heading.

Triamcinolone Acetonide (Lapatinib undergoes extensive metabolism by CYP3A4; concomitant administration of strong inducers of CYP3A4 alter lapatinib concentrations significantly and should be avoided. Dose adjustment of lapatinib should be considered for patients who must receive concomitant strong inducers of CYP3A4 enzymes. Lapatinib inhibits CYP3A4 *in vitro* at clinically relevant concentrations. Caution should be exercised and dose reduction of the concomitant substrate drug should be considered when dosing lapatinib concurrently with medications with narrow therapeutic windows that are substrates of CYP3A4). Products include:
Azmacort 408
Nasacort AQ 3019

Triamcinolone Diacetate (Lapatinib undergoes extensive metabolism by CYP3A4; concomitant administration of strong inducers of CYP3A4 alter lapatinib concentrations significantly and should be avoided. Dose adjustment of lapatinib should be considered for patients who must receive concomitant strong inducers of CYP3A4 enzymes. Lapatinib inhibits CYP3A4 *in vitro* at clinically relevant concentrations. Caution should be exercised and dose reduction of the concomitant substrate drug should be considered when dosing lapatinib concurrently with medications with narrow therapeutic windows that are substrates of CYP3A4).
No products indexed under this heading.

Triamcinolone Hexacetonide (Lapatinib undergoes extensive metabolism by CYP3A4; concomitant administration of strong inducers of CYP3A4 alter lapatinib concentrations significantly and should be avoided. Dose adjustment of lapatinib should be considered for patients who must receive concomitant strong inducers of CYP3A4 enzymes. Lapatinib inhibits CYP3A4 *in vitro* at clinically relevant concentrations. Caution should be exercised and dose reduction of the concomitant substrate drug should be considered when dosing lapatinib concurrently with medications with narrow therapeutic windows that are substrates of CYP3A4).
No products indexed under this heading.

Triazolam (Lapatinib inhibits CYP3A4 *in vitro* at clinically relevant concentrations. Caution should be exercised and dose reduction of the concomitant substrate drug should be considered when dosing lapatinib concurrently with medications with narrow therapeutic windows that are substrates of CYP3A4).
No products indexed under this heading.

Trimipramine Maleate (Lapatinib inhibits CYP2C8 *in vitro* at clinically relevant concentrations. Caution should be exercised and dose reduction of the concomitant substrate drug should be considered when dosing lapatinib concurrently with medications with narrow therapeutic windows that are substrates of CYP2C8).
No products indexed under this heading.

Troglitazone (Lapatinib undergoes extensive metabolism by CYP3A4; concomitant administration of strong inducers of CYP3A4 alter lapatinib concentrations significantly and should be avoided. Dose adjustment of lapatinib should be considered for patients who must receive concomitant strong inducers of CYP3A4 enzymes. Lapatinib inhibits CYP3A4 *in vitro* at clinically relevant concentrations. Caution should be exercised and dose reduction of the concomitant substrate drug should be considered when dosing lapatinib concurrently with medications with narrow therapeutic windows that are substrates of CYP3A4).
No products indexed under this heading.

Troleandomycin (Lapatinib undergoes extensive metabolism by CYP3A4; concomitant administration of strong inhibitors of CYP3A4 alter lapatinib concentrations significantly and should be avoided. Dose adjustment of lapatinib should be considered for patients who must receive concomitant strong inhibitors of CYP3A4 enzymes. Lapatinib inhibits CYP3A4 *in vitro* at clinically relevant concentrations. Caution should be exercised and dose reduction of the concomitant substrate drug should be considered when dosing lapatinib concurrently with medications with narrow therapeutic windows that are substrates of CYP3A4).
No products indexed under this heading.

Vardenafil Hydrochloride (Lapatinib inhibits CYP3A4 *in vitro* at clinically relevant concentrations. Caution should be exercised and dose reduction of the concomitant substrate drug should be considered when dosing lapatinib con-

currently with medications with narrow therapeutic windows that are substrates of CYP3A4). Products include:
Levitra 3157

Verapamil Hydrochloride (Lapatinib inhibits CYP2C8 *in vitro* at clinically relevant concentrations. Caution should be exercised and dose reduction of the concomitant substrate drug should be considered when dosing lapatinib concurrently with medications with narrow therapeutic windows that are substrates of CYP2C8). Products include:
Tarka 534

Vinblastine Sulfate (Lapatinib inhibits CYP3A4 *in vitro* at clinically relevant concentrations. Caution should be exercised and dose reduction of the concomitant substrate drug should be considered when dosing lapatinib concurrently with medications with narrow therapeutic windows that are substrates of CYP3A4).
No products indexed under this heading.

Vincristine Sulfate (Lapatinib inhibits CYP3A4 *in vitro* at clinically relevant concentrations. Caution should be exercised and dose reduction of the concomitant substrate drug should be considered when dosing lapatinib concurrently with medications with narrow therapeutic windows that are substrates of CYP3A4).
No products indexed under this heading.

Vitamin A (Lapatinib inhibits CYP2C8 *in vitro* at clinically relevant concentrations. Caution should be exercised and dose reduction of the concomitant substrate drug should be considered when dosing lapatinib concurrently with medications with narrow therapeutic windows that are substrates of CYP2C8). Products include:
Cardio Basics 3455
Heplive 607
Norwegian Cod Liver Oil 919

Vitamin A Acetate (Lapatinib inhibits CYP2C8 *in vitro* at clinically relevant concentrations. Caution should be exercised and dose reduction of the concomitant substrate drug should be considered when dosing lapatinib concurrently with medications with narrow therapeutic windows that are substrates of CYP2C8).
No products indexed under this heading.

Voriconazole (The concomitant use of strong CYP3A4 inhibitors should be avoided (eg, voriconazole). If patients must be co-administered a strong CYP3A4 inhibitor, based on pharmacokinetic studies, a dose reduction to 500 mg/day of lapatinib is predicted to adjust the lapatinib AUC to the range observed without inhibitors and should be considered).
No products indexed under this heading.

Warfarin Sodium (Lapatinib inhibits CYP2C8 *in vitro* at clinically relevant concentrations. Caution should be exercised and dose reduction of the concomitant substrate drug should be considered when dosing lapatinib concurrently with medications with narrow therapeutic windows that are substrates of CYP2C8).
No products indexed under this heading.

Zopiclone (Lapatinib inhibits CYP2C8 *in vitro* at clinically relevant concentrations. Caution should be exercised and dose reduction of the concomitant substrate drug should be considered when dosing lapatinib concurrently with medications with narrow therapeutic windows that are substrates of CYP2C8).
No products indexed under this heading.

Food Interactions

Grapefruit (Grapefruit may also increase plasma concentrations of lapatinib and should be avoided).

Grapefruit Juice (Grapefruit may also increase plasma concentrations of lapatinib and should be avoided).

REGULAR STRENGTH TYLENOL TABLETS
(Acetaminophen) 2049
May interact with alcohols, and certain other agents. Compounds in these categories include:

Ethanol (Severe liver damage may occur if an adult has 3 or more alcoholic drinks every day while using this product).
No products indexed under this heading.

Ethyl Alcohol (Severe liver damage may occur if an adult has 3 or more alcoholic drinks every day while using this product).
No products indexed under this heading.

Warfarin Sodium (Co-administration with warfarin should be monitored).
No products indexed under this heading.

Food Interactions

Alcohol (Severe liver damage may occur if an adult has 3 or more alcoholic drinks every day while using this product).

Beer, reduced-alcohol (Severe liver damage may occur if an adult has 3 or more alcoholic drinks every day while using this product).

Beer, unspecified (Severe liver damage may occur if an adult has 3 or more alcoholic drinks every day while using this product).

Wine, Chianti (Severe liver damage may occur if an adult has 3 or more alcoholic drinks every day while using this product).

Wine, Red (Severe liver damage may occur if an adult has 3 or more alcoholic drinks every day while using this product).

Wine, unspecified (Severe liver damage may occur if an adult has 3 or more alcoholic drinks every day while using this product).

Wine products (Severe liver damage may occur if an adult has 3 or more alcoholic drinks every day while using this product).

TYLENOL 8 HOUR EXTENDED RELEASE CAPLETS
(Acetaminophen) 2049
See Regular Strength Tylenol Tablets

EXTRA STRENGTH TYLENOL CAPLETS, COOL CAPLETS, AND EZ TABS
(Acetaminophen) 2049
See Regular Strength Tylenol Tablets

EXTRA STRENGTH TYLENOL ADULT RAPID BLAST LIQUID
(Acetaminophen) 2049
See Regular Strength Tylenol Tablets

EXTRA STRENGTH TYLENOL RAPID RELEASE GELS
(Acetaminophen) 2049
See Regular Strength Tylenol Tablets

TYLENOL WITH CODEINE TABLETS
(Acetaminophen, Codeine Phosphate) 2691
May interact with alcohols, central nervous system depressants, general anesthetics, hypnotics and sedatives, narcotic analgesics, tranquilizers, and certain other agents. Compounds in these categories include:

Alfentanil Hydrochloride (Concomitant use with other CNS depressants may produce an additive CNS depression and should be avoided).
No products indexed under this heading.

Alprazolam (Concomitant use with other CNS depressants may produce an additive CNS depression and should be avoided).
No products indexed under this heading.

Amobarbital (Concomitant use with other CNS depressants may produce an additive CNS depression and should be avoided).
No products indexed under this heading.

Amobarbital Sodium (Concomitant use with other CNS depressants may produce an additive CNS depression and should be avoided).
No products indexed under this heading.

Apomorphine (Concomitant use may enhance the effects of other narcotic analgesics, causing increased CNS depression).
No products indexed under this heading.

Apomorphine Hydrochloride (Concomitant use may enhance the effects of other narcotic analgesics, causing increased CNS depression).
No products indexed under this heading.

Aprobarbital (Concomitant use with other CNS depressants may produce an additive CNS depression and should be avoided).
No products indexed under this heading.

Buprenorphine Hydrochloride (Concomitant use with other CNS depressants may produce an additive CNS depression and should be avoided).
No products indexed under this heading.

Buspirone Hydrochloride (Concomitant use with other CNS depressants may produce an additive CNS depression and should be avoided).
No products indexed under this heading.

Butabarbital (Concomitant use with other CNS depressants may produce an additive CNS depression and should be avoided).
No products indexed under this heading.

Butabarbital Sodium (Concomitant use with other CNS depressants may produce an additive CNS depression and should be avoided).
No products indexed under this heading.

Butalbital (Concomitant use with other CNS depressants may produce an additive CNS depression and should be avoided).
No products indexed under this heading.

Chloral Hydrate (Concomitant use may enhance the effects of sedative-hypnotics, causing increased CNS depression).
No products indexed under this heading.

Chlordiazepoxide (Concomitant use may enhance the effects of tranquilizers such as chlordiazepoxide, causing increased CNS depression).
No products indexed under this heading.

Chlordiazepoxide Hydrochloride (Concomitant use may enhance the effects of tranquilizers such as chlordiazepoxide, causing increased CNS depression).
No products indexed under this heading.

Chlorpromazine (Concomitant use with other CNS depressants may produce an additive CNS depression and should be avoided).
No products indexed under this heading.

Chlorpromazine Hydrochloride (Concomitant use with other CNS depressants may produce an additive CNS depression and should be avoided).
No products indexed under this heading.

Chlorprothixene (Concomitant use with other CNS depressants may produce an additive CNS depression and should be avoided).
No products indexed under this heading.

Chlorprothixene Hydrochloride (Concomitant use with other CNS depressants may produce an additive CNS depression and should be avoided).
No products indexed under this heading.

Chlorprothixene Lactate (Concomitant use with other CNS depressants may produce an additive CNS depression and should be avoided).
No products indexed under this heading.

Clonazepam (Concomitant use with other CNS depressants may produce an additive CNS depression and should be avoided). Products include:
Klonopin 2855

Clorazepate Dipotassium (Concomitant use with other CNS depressants may produce an additive CNS depression and should be avoided).
No products indexed under this heading.

Clozapine (Concomitant use with other CNS depressants may produce an additive CNS depression and should be avoided).
No products indexed under this heading.

Codeine Sulfate (Concomitant use with other CNS depressants may produce an additive CNS depression and should be avoided).
No products indexed under this heading.

Desflurane (Concomitant use with other CNS depressants may produce an additive CNS depression and should be avoided).
No products indexed under this heading.

Dezocine (Concomitant use with other CNS depressants may produce an additive CNS depression and should be avoided).
No products indexed under this heading.

Diazepam (Concomitant use with other CNS depressants may produce an additive CNS depression and should be avoided). Products include:
Valium Tablets 2880

Dihydrocodeine Bitartrate (Concomitant use may enhance the effects of other narcotic analgesics, causing increased CNS depression).
No products indexed under this heading.

Dihydrocodeinone Bitartrate (Concomitant use may enhance the effects of other narcotic analgesics, causing increased CNS depression).
No products indexed under this heading.

Droperidol (Concomitant use with other CNS depressants may produce an additive CNS depression and should be avoided).
No products indexed under this heading.

Enflurane (Concomitant use with other CNS depressants may produce an additive CNS depression and should be avoided).
No products indexed under this heading.

Estazolam (Concomitant use with other CNS depressants may produce an additive CNS depression and should be avoided).
No products indexed under this heading.

Ethanol (Concomitant use with other CNS depressants may produce an additive CNS depression and should be avoided).
No products indexed under this heading.

Ethchlorvynol (Concomitant use with other CNS depressants may produce an additive CNS depression and should be avoided).
No products indexed under this heading.

IMPORTANT NOTE: Always consult each drug listing in the patient's regimen for possible interactions.

Ethinamate (Concomitant use with other CNS depressants may produce an additive CNS depression and should be avoided).
 No products indexed under this heading.

Ethyl Alcohol (Concomitant use with other CNS depressants may produce an additive CNS depression and should be avoided).
 No products indexed under this heading.

Fentanyl (Concomitant use with other CNS depressants may produce an additive CNS depression and should be avoided). Products include:

Fentanyl Citrate (Concomitant use with other CNS depressants may produce an additive CNS depression and should be avoided). Products include:

Fluphenazine Decanoate (Concomitant use with other CNS depressants may produce an additive CNS depression and should be avoided).
 No products indexed under this heading.

Fluphenazine Enanthate (Concomitant use with other CNS depressants may produce an additive CNS depression and should be avoided).
 No products indexed under this heading.

Fluphenazine Hydrochloride (Concomitant use with other CNS depressants may produce an additive CNS depression and should be avoided).
 No products indexed under this heading.

Flurazepam Hydrochloride (Concomitant use with other CNS depressants may produce an additive CNS depression and should be avoided).
 No products indexed under this heading.

Glutethimide (Concomitant use with other CNS depressants may produce an additive CNS depression and should be avoided).
 No products indexed under this heading.

Halazepam (Concomitant use with other CNS depressants may produce an additive CNS depression and should be avoided).
 No products indexed under this heading.

Haloperidol (Concomitant use with other CNS depressants may produce an additive CNS depression and should be avoided).
 No products indexed under this heading.

Haloperidol Decanoate (Concomitant use with other CNS depressants may produce an additive CNS depression and should be avoided).
 No products indexed under this heading.

Haloperidol Lactate (Concomitant use with other CNS depressants may produce an additive CNS depression and should be avoided).
 No products indexed under this heading.

Halothane (Concomitant use may enhance the effects of general anesthetics, causing increased CNS depression).
 No products indexed under this heading.

Hexobarbital (Concomitant use with other CNS depressants may produce an additive CNS depression and should be avoided).
 No products indexed under this heading.

Hydrocodone Bitartrate (Concomitant use with other CNS depressants may produce an additive CNS depression and should be avoided). Products include:

Hydrocodone Polistirex (Concomitant use with other CNS depressants

may produce an additive CNS depression and should be avoided). Products include:

Hydromorphone (Concomitant use with other CNS depressants may produce an additive CNS depression and should be avoided).
 No products indexed under this heading.

Hydromorphone Hydrochloride (Concomitant use with other CNS depressants may produce an additive CNS depression and should be avoided). Products include:

Hydroxyzine Hydrochloride (Concomitant use with other CNS depressants may produce an additive CNS depression and should be avoided).
 No products indexed under this heading.

Isoflurane (Concomitant use with other CNS depressants may produce an additive CNS depression and should be avoided).
 No products indexed under this heading.

Ketamine Hydrochloride (Concomitant use with other CNS depressants may produce an additive CNS depression and should be avoided).
 No products indexed under this heading.

Levomethadyl Acetate Hydrochloride (Concomitant use with other CNS depressants may produce an additive CNS depression and should be avoided).
 No products indexed under this heading.

Levorphanol Tartrate (Concomitant use with other CNS depressants may produce an additive CNS depression and should be avoided).
 No products indexed under this heading.

Lorazepam (Concomitant use with other CNS depressants may produce an additive CNS depression and should be avoided).
 No products indexed under this heading.

Loxapine Hydrochloride (Concomitant use with other CNS depressants may produce an additive CNS depression and should be avoided).
 No products indexed under this heading.

Loxapine Succinate (Concomitant use with other CNS depressants may produce an additive CNS depression and should be avoided).
 No products indexed under this heading.

Meperidine Hydrochloride (Concomitant use with other CNS depressants may produce an additive CNS depression and should be avoided).
 No products indexed under this heading.

Mephobarbital (Concomitant use with other CNS depressants may produce an additive CNS depression and should be avoided).
 No products indexed under this heading.

Meprobamate (Concomitant use with other CNS depressants may produce an additive CNS depression and should be avoided).
 No products indexed under this heading.

Mesoridazine Besylate (Concomitant use with other CNS depressants may produce an additive CNS depression and should be avoided).
 No products indexed under this heading.

Methadone Hydrochloride (Concomitant use with other CNS depressants may produce an additive CNS depression and should be avoided).
 No products indexed under this heading.

Methohexital Sodium (Concomitant use with other CNS depressants may produce an additive CNS depression and should be avoided).
 No products indexed under this heading.

Methotrimeprazine (Concomitant use with other CNS depressants may produce an additive CNS depression and should be avoided).
 No products indexed under this heading.

Methoxyflurane (Concomitant use with other CNS depressants may produce an additive CNS depression and should be avoided).
 No products indexed under this heading.

Midazolam Hydrochloride (Concomitant use with other CNS depressants may produce an additive CNS depression and should be avoided).
 No products indexed under this heading.

Molindone Hydrochloride (Concomitant use with other CNS depressants may produce an additive CNS depression and should be avoided). Products include:

Morphine Sulfate (Concomitant use with other CNS depressants may produce an additive CNS depression and should be avoided). Products include:

Morphine Sulfate, Liposomal (Concomitant use with other CNS depressants may produce an additive CNS depression and should be avoided).
 No products indexed under this heading.

Nitrous Oxide (Concomitant use may enhance the effects of general anesthetics, causing increased CNS depression).
 No products indexed under this heading.

Olanzapine (Concomitant use with other CNS depressants may produce an additive CNS depression and should be avoided). Products include:

Oxazepam (Concomitant use with other CNS depressants may produce an additive CNS depression and should be avoided).
 No products indexed under this heading.

Oxycodone Hydrochloride (Concomitant use with other CNS depressants may produce an additive CNS depression and should be avoided). Products include:

Oxycodone Terephthalate (Concomitant use with other CNS depressants may produce an additive CNS depression and should be avoided).
 No products indexed under this heading.

Oxymorphone Hydrochloride (Concomitant use with other CNS depressants may produce an additive CNS depression and should be avoided). Products include:

Pentobarbital (Concomitant use with other CNS depressants may produce an additive CNS depression and should be avoided).
 No products indexed under this heading.

Pentobarbital Sodium (Concomitant use with other CNS depressants may produce an additive CNS depression and should be avoided). Products include:

Perphenazine (Concomitant use with other CNS depressants may produce an additive CNS depression and should be avoided).
 No products indexed under this heading.

Phenobarbital (Concomitant use with other CNS depressants may produce an additive CNS depression and should be avoided). Products include:

Phenobarbital Sodium (Concomitant use with other CNS depressants may produce an additive CNS depression and should be avoided).
 No products indexed under this heading.

Prazepam (Concomitant use with other CNS depressants may produce an additive CNS depression and should be avoided).
 No products indexed under this heading.

Prochlorperazine (Concomitant use with other CNS depressants may produce an additive CNS depression and should be avoided).
 No products indexed under this heading.

Prochlorperazine Edisylate (Concomitant use with other CNS depressants may produce an additive CNS depression and should be avoided).
 No products indexed under this heading.

Prochlorperazine Maleate (Concomitant use with other CNS depressants may produce an additive CNS depression and should be avoided).
 No products indexed under this heading.

Promethazine (Concomitant use with other CNS depressants may produce an additive CNS depression and should be avoided).
 No products indexed under this heading.

Promethazine Hydrochloride (Concomitant use with other CNS depressants may produce an additive CNS depression and should be avoided).
 No products indexed under this heading.

Propofol (Concomitant use with other CNS depressants may produce an additive CNS depression and should be avoided).
 No products indexed under this heading.

Propoxyphene Hydrochloride (Concomitant use with other CNS depressants may produce an additive CNS depression and should be avoided).
 No products indexed under this heading.

Propoxyphene Napsylate (Concomitant use with other CNS depressants may produce an additive CNS depression and should be avoided).
 No products indexed under this heading.

Quazepam (Concomitant use with other CNS depressants may produce an additive CNS depression and should be avoided).
 No products indexed under this heading.

Quetiapine Fumarate (Concomitant use with other CNS depressants may produce an additive CNS depression and should be avoided). Products include:

Ramelteon (Concomitant use may enhance the effects of sedative-hypnotics, causing increased CNS depression). Products include:

Remifentanil Hydrochloride (Concomitant use with other CNS depressants may produce an additive CNS depression and should be avoided).
 No products indexed under this heading.

Risperidone (Concomitant use with other CNS depressants may produce an additive CNS depression and should be avoided). Products include:

Secobarbital Sodium (Concomitant use with other CNS depressants may produce an additive CNS depression and should be avoided).
 No products indexed under this heading.

(⊙ Described in PDR® for Ophthalmic Medicines)

Sevoflurane (Concomitant use with other CNS depressants may produce an additive CNS depression and should be avoided). Products include:

Sodium Butabarbital (Concomitant use with other CNS depressants may produce an additive CNS depression and should be avoided).
No products indexed under this heading.

Sodium Oxybate (Concomitant use with other CNS depressants may produce an additive CNS depression and should be avoided).
No products indexed under this heading.

Sodium Pentobarbital (Concomitant use with other CNS depressants may produce an additive CNS depression and should be avoided).
No products indexed under this heading.

Sufentanil Citrate (Concomitant use with other CNS depressants may produce an additive CNS depression and should be avoided).
No products indexed under this heading.

Talbutal (Concomitant use with other CNS depressants may produce an additive CNS depression and should be avoided).
No products indexed under this heading.

Temazepam (Concomitant use with other CNS depressants may produce an additive CNS depression and should be avoided).
No products indexed under this heading.

Thiamylal Sodium (Concomitant use with other CNS depressants may produce an additive CNS depression and should be avoided).
No products indexed under this heading.

Thioridazine (Concomitant use with other CNS depressants may produce an additive CNS depression and should be avoided).
No products indexed under this heading.

Thioridazine Hydrochloride (Concomitant use with other CNS depressants may produce an additive CNS depression and should be avoided). Products include:

Thiothixene (Concomitant use with other CNS depressants may produce an additive CNS depression and should be avoided). Products include:

Thiothixene Hydrochloride (Concomitant use with other CNS depressants may produce an additive CNS depression and should be avoided).
No products indexed under this heading.

Triazolam (Concomitant use with other CNS depressants may produce an additive CNS depression and should be avoided).
No products indexed under this heading.

Trifluoperazine Hydrochloride (Concomitant use with other CNS depressants may produce an additive CNS depression and should be avoided).
No products indexed under this heading.

Zaleplon (Concomitant use with other CNS depressants may produce an additive CNS depression and should be avoided).
No products indexed under this heading.

Ziprasidone Hydrochloride (Concomitant use with other CNS depressants may produce an additive CNS depression and should be avoided). Products include:

Zolpidem Tartrate (Concomitant use with other CNS depressants may produce an additive CNS depression and should be avoided). Products include:

Food Interactions

Alcohol (Concomitant use with other CNS depressants may produce an additive CNS depression and should be avoided).

Beer, reduced-alcohol (Concomitant use with alcohol may produce an additive CNS depression and should be avoided).

Beer, unspecified (Concomitant use with alcohol may produce an additive CNS depression and should be avoided).

Wine, Chianti (Concomitant use with alcohol may produce an additive CNS depression and should be avoided).

Wine, Red (Concomitant use with alcohol may produce an additive CNS depression and should be avoided).

Wine, unspecified (Concomitant use with alcohol may produce an additive CNS depression and should be avoided).

Wine products (Concomitant use with alcohol may produce an additive CNS depression and should be avoided).

TYLENOL ARTHRITIS PAIN EXTENDED RELEASE GELTABS/ CAPLETS
See Regular Strength Tylenol Tablets

CHILDREN'S TYLENOL DOSING CHART

CHILDREN'S TYLENOL SUSPENSION LIQUID

Warfarin Sodium (Co-administration with warfarin should be monitored).
No products indexed under this heading.

CHILDREN'S TYLENOL MELTAWAYS
See Children's Tylenol Suspension Liquid

CONCENTRATED TYLENOL INFANTS' DROPS
See Children's Tylenol Suspension Liquid

JR. TYLENOL MELTAWAYS
See Children's Tylenol Suspension Liquid

ULESFIA LOTION
None cited in PDR database.

ULORIC TABLETS
May interact with antacids containing aluminum, calcium and magnesium, cytotoxic drugs, theophyllines, and certain other agents. Compounds in these categories include:

Aluminum Carbonate (Concomitant ingestion of an antacid containing magnesium hydroxide and aluminum hydroxide with an 80 mg single dose of febuxostat has been shown to delay absorption of febuxostat (approximately 1 hour) and to cause a 31% decrease in C_{max} and a 15% decrease in AUC. As AUC rather than C_{max} was related to drug effect, change observed in AUC was not considered clinically significant. Therefore, febuxostat may be taken without regard to antacid use).
No products indexed under this heading.

Aluminum Hydroxide (Concomitant ingestion of an antacid containing magnesium hydroxide and aluminum hydroxide with an 80 mg single dose of febuxostat has been shown to delay absorption of febuxostat (approximately 1 hour) and to cause a 31% decrease in C_{max} and a 15% decrease in AUC. As AUC rather than C_{max} was related to drug effect, change observed in AUC was not considered clinically significant. Therefore, febuxostat may be taken without regard to antacid use).
No products indexed under this heading.

Azathioprine (Concomitant administration of febuxostat with azathioprine is contraindicated as it could increase plasma concentrations of azathioprine resulting in severe toxicity).
No products indexed under this heading.

Azathioprine Sodium (Concomitant administration of febuxostat with azathioprine is contraindicated as it could increase plasma concentrations of azathioprine resulting in severe toxicity).
No products indexed under this heading.

Bleomycin Sulfate (Drug interaction studies of febuxostat with cytotoxic chemotherapy have not been conducted. No data are available regarding the safety of Uloric during cytotoxic chemotherapy).
No products indexed under this heading.

Calcium Carbonate (Concomitant ingestion of an antacid containing magnesium hydroxide and aluminum hydroxide with an 80 mg single dose of febuxostat has been shown to delay absorption of febuxostat (approximately 1 hour) and to cause a 31% decrease in C_{max} and a 15% decrease in AUC. As AUC rather than C_{max} was related to drug effect, change observed in AUC was not considered clinically significant. Therefore, febuxostat may be taken without regard to antacid use). Products include:

Cyclophosphamide (Drug interaction studies of febuxostat with cytotoxic chemotherapy have not been conducted. No data are available regarding the safety of Uloric during cytotoxic chemotherapy).
No products indexed under this heading.

Daunorubicin Hydrochloride (Drug interaction studies of febuxostat with cytotoxic chemotherapy have not been conducted. No data are available regarding the safety of Uloric during cytotoxic chemotherapy).
No products indexed under this heading.

Doxorubicin Hydrochloride (Drug interaction studies of febuxostat with cytotoxic chemotherapy have not been conducted. No data are available regarding the safety of Uloric during cytotoxic chemotherapy).
No products indexed under this heading.

Epirubicin Hydrochloride (Drug interaction studies of febuxostat with cytotoxic chemotherapy have not been conducted. No data are available regarding the safety of Uloric during cytotoxic chemotherapy).
No products indexed under this heading.

Fat (Following multiple 80 mg once daily doses with a high fat meal, there was a 49% decrease in C_{max} and an 18% decrease in AUC, respectively. However, no clinically significant change in the percent decrease in serum uric acid concentration was observed (58% fed vs. 51% fasting). Thus, febuxostat may be taken without regard to food).
No products indexed under this heading.

Fluorouracil (Drug interaction studies of febuxostat with cytotoxic chemotherapy have not been conducted. No data are available regarding the safety of Uloric during cytotoxic chemotherapy). Products include:

Hydroxyurea (Drug interaction studies of febuxostat with cytotoxic chemotherapy have not been conducted. No data are available regarding the safety of Uloric during cytotoxic chemotherapy).
No products indexed under this heading.

Magaldrate (Concomitant ingestion of an antacid containing magnesium hydroxide and aluminum hydroxide with an 80 mg single dose of febuxostat has been shown to delay absorption of febuxostat (approximately 1 hour) and to cause a 31% decrease in C_{max} and a 15% decrease in AUC. As AUC rather than C_{max} was related to drug effect, change observed in AUC was not considered clinically significant. Therefore, febuxostat may be taken without regard to antacid use).
No products indexed under this heading.

Magnesium Carbonate (Concomitant ingestion of an antacid containing magnesium hydroxide and aluminum hydroxide with an 80 mg single dose of febuxostat has been shown to delay absorption of febuxostat (approximately 1 hour) and to cause a 31% decrease in C_{max} and a 15% decrease in AUC. As AUC rather than C_{max} was related to drug effect, change observed in AUC was not considered clinically significant. Therefore, febuxostat may be taken without regard to antacid use).
No products indexed under this heading.

Magnesium Hydroxide (Concomitant ingestion of an antacid containing magnesium hydroxide and aluminum hydroxide with an 80 mg single dose of febuxostat has been shown to delay absorption of febuxostat (approximately 1 hour) and to cause a 31% decrease in C_{max} and a 15% decrease in AUC. As AUC rather than C_{max} was related to drug effect, change observed in AUC was not considered clinically significant. Therefore, febuxostat may be taken without regard to antacid use). Products include:

Magnesium Oxide (Concomitant ingestion of an antacid containing magnesium hydroxide and aluminum hydroxide with an 80 mg single dose of febuxostat has been shown to delay absorption of febuxostat (approximately 1 hour) and to cause a 31% decrease in C_{max} and a 15% decrease in AUC. As AUC rather than C_{max} was related to drug effect, change observed in AUC was not considered clinically significant. Therefore, febuxostat may be taken without regard to antacid use). Products include:

Magnesium Trisilicate (Concomitant ingestion of an antacid containing magnesium hydroxide and aluminum hydroxide with an 80 mg single dose of febuxostat has been shown to delay absorption of febuxostat (approximately 1 hour) and to cause a 31% decrease in C_{max} and a 15% decrease in AUC. As AUC rather than C_{max} was related to drug effect, change observed in AUC was not considered clinically significant. Therefore, febuxostat may be taken without regard to antacid use).
No products indexed under this heading.

Mercaptopurine (Concomitant administration of febuxostat with mercaptopurine is contraindicated as it could increase plasma concentrations of mercaptopurine resulting in severe toxicity).
No products indexed under this heading.

IMPORTANT NOTE: Always consult each drug listing in the patient's regimen for possible interactions.

Methotrexate Sodium (Drug interaction studies of febuxostat with cytotoxic chemotherapy have not been conducted. No data are available regarding the safety of Uloric during cytotoxic chemotherapy.

No products indexed under this heading.

Mitotane (Drug interaction studies of febuxostat with cytotoxic chemotherapy have not been conducted. No data are available regarding the safety of Uloric during cytotoxic chemotherapy).

No products indexed under this heading.

Mitoxantrone Hydrochloride (Drug interaction studies of febuxostat with cytotoxic chemotherapy have not been conducted. No data are available regarding the safety of Uloric during cytotoxic chemotherapy). Products include:

Novantrone 1088

Procarbazine Hydrochloride (Drug interaction studies of febuxostat with cytotoxic chemotherapy have not been conducted. No data are available regarding the safety of Uloric during cytotoxic chemotherapy).

No products indexed under this heading.

Tamoxifen Citrate (Drug interaction studies of febuxostat with cytotoxic chemotherapy have not been conducted. No data are available regarding the safety of Uloric during cytotoxic chemotherapy).

No products indexed under this heading.

Theophylline (Concomitant administration of febuxostat with theophylline is contraindicated as it could increase plasma concentrations of theophylline resulting in severe toxicity).

No products indexed under this heading.

Theophylline Anhydrous (Concomitant administration of febuxostat with theophylline is contraindicated as it could increase plasma concentrations of theophylline resulting in severe toxicity). Products include:

Uniphyl 2817

Theophylline Calcium Salicylate (Concomitant administration of febuxostat with theophylline is contraindicated as it could increase plasma concentrations of theophylline resulting in severe toxicity).

No products indexed under this heading.

Theophylline Dihydroxypropyl (Glyceryl) (Concomitant administration of febuxostat with theophylline is contraindicated as it could increase plasma concentrations of theophylline resulting in severe toxicity).

No products indexed under this heading.

Theophylline Ethylenediamine (Concomitant administration of febuxostat with theophylline is contraindicated as it could increase plasma concentrations of theophylline resulting in severe toxicity).

No products indexed under this heading.

Theophylline Sodium Glycinate (Concomitant administration of febuxostat with theophylline is contraindicated as it could increase plasma concentrations of theophylline resulting in severe toxicity).

No products indexed under this heading.

Vinblastine Sulfate (Drug interaction studies of febuxostat with cytotoxic chemotherapy have not been conducted. No data are available regarding the safety of Uloric during cytotoxic chemotherapy).

No products indexed under this heading.

Vincristine Sulfate (Drug interaction studies of febuxostat with cytotoxic chemotherapy have not been conducted. No data are available regarding the safety of Uloric during cytotoxic chemotherapy).

No products indexed under this heading.

Vinorelbine Tartrate (Drug interaction studies of febuxostat with cytotoxic chemotherapy have not been conducted. No data are available regarding the safety of Uloric during cytotoxic chemotherapy).

No products indexed under this heading.

Food Interactions

Food, unspecified (Following multiple 80 mg once daily doses with a high fat meal, there was a 49% decrease in C_{max} and an 18% decrease in AUC, respectively. However, no clinically significant change in the percent decrease in serum uric acid concentration was observed (58% fed vs. 51% fasting). Thus, febuxostat may be taken without regard to food.

Meal, unspecified (Following multiple 80 mg once daily doses with a high fat meal, there was a 49% decrease in C_{max} and an 18% decrease in AUC, respectively. However, no clinically significant change in the percent decrease in serum uric acid concentration was observed (58% fed vs. 51% fasting). Thus, febuxostat may be taken without regard to food.)

ULTANE LIQUID FOR INHALATION

(Sevoflurane) **554**
May interact with benzodiazepines, narcotic analgesics, nondepolarizing neuromuscular blocking agents, and certain other agents. Compounds in these categories include:

Alfentanil Hydrochloride (Benzodiazepines and opioids would be expected to decrease the MAC of sevoflurane in the same manner as with other inhalational anesthetics. Sevoflurane administration is compatible with benzodiazepines and opioids as commonly used in surgical practice).

No products indexed under this heading.

Alprazolam (Benzodiazepines and opioids would be expected to decrease the MAC of sevoflurane in the same manner as with other inhalational anesthetics. Sevoflurane administration is compatible with benzodiazepines and opioids as commonly used in surgical practice).

No products indexed under this heading.

Apomorphine (Benzodiazepines and opioids would be expected to decrease the MAC of sevoflurane in the same manner as with other inhalational anesthetics. Sevoflurane administration is compatible with benzodiazepines and opioids as commonly used in surgical practice).

No products indexed under this heading.

Apomorphine Hydrochloride (Benzodiazepines and opioids would be expected to decrease the MAC of sevoflurane in the same manner as with other inhalational anesthetics. Sevoflurane administration is compatible with benzodiazepines and opioids as commonly used in surgical practice).

No products indexed under this heading.

Atracurium Besylate (Sevoflurane increases both the intensity and duration of neuromuscular blockade induced by non-depolarizing muscle relaxants. When used to supplement alfentanil-nitrous oxide anesthesia, sevoflurane and isoflurane equally potentiate neuromuscular block induced with pancuronium, vecuronium or atracurium. Among available non-depolarizing agents, only vecuronium, pancuronium and atracurium interactions have been studied during sevoflurane anesthesia. In the absence of specific guidelines: 1) For endotracheal intubation, do not reduce the dose of non-depolarizing muscle relaxants. 2) During maintenance of

anesthesia, the required dose of non-depolarizing muscle relaxants is likely to be reduced compared to that during nitrous oxide/opioid anesthesia).

No products indexed under this heading.

Buprenorphine Hydrochloride (Benzodiazepines and opioids would be expected to decrease the MAC of sevoflurane in the same manner as with other inhalational anesthetics. Sevoflurane administration is compatible with benzodiazepines and opioids as commonly used in surgical practice).

No products indexed under this heading.

Chlordiazepoxide (Benzodiazepines and opioids would be expected to decrease the MAC of sevoflurane in the same manner as with other inhalational anesthetics. Sevoflurane administration is compatible with benzodiazepines and opioids as commonly used in surgical practice).

No products indexed under this heading.

Chlordiazepoxide Hydrochloride (Benzodiazepines and opioids would be expected to decrease the MAC of sevoflurane in the same manner as with other inhalational anesthetics. Sevoflurane administration is compatible with benzodiazepines and opioids as commonly used in surgical practice).

No products indexed under this heading.

Cisatracurium Besylate (Sevoflurane increases both the intensity and duration of neuromuscular blockade induced by non-depolarizing muscle relaxants. When used to supplement alfentanil-nitrous oxide anesthesia, sevoflurane and isoflurane equally potentiate neuromuscular block induced with pancuronium, vecuronium or atracurium. Among available non-depolarizing agents, only vecuronium, pancuronium and atracurium interactions have been studied during sevoflurane anesthesia. In the absence of specific guidelines: 1) For endotracheal intubation, do not reduce the dose of non-depolarizing muscle relaxants. 2) During maintenance of anesthesia, the required dose of non-depolarizing muscle relaxants is likely to be reduced compared to that during nitrous oxide/opioid anesthesia). Products include:

Nimbex **503**

Clorazepate Dipotassium (Benzodiazepines and opioids would be expected to decrease the MAC of sevoflurane in the same manner as with other inhalational anesthetics. Sevoflurane administration is compatible with benzodiazepines and opioids as commonly used in surgical practice).

No products indexed under this heading.

Codeine Phosphate (Benzodiazepines and opioids would be expected to decrease the MAC of sevoflurane in the same manner as with other inhalational anesthetics. Sevoflurane administration is compatible with benzodiazepines and opioids as commonly used in surgical practice). Products include:

Tylenol with Codeine **2691**

Codeine Sulfate (Benzodiazepines and opioids would be expected to decrease the MAC of sevoflurane in the same manner as with other inhalational anesthetics. Sevoflurane administration is compatible with benzodiazepines and opioids as commonly used in surgical practice).

No products indexed under this heading.

Dezocine (Benzodiazepines and opioids would be expected to decrease the MAC of sevoflurane in the same manner as with other inhalational anesthetics. Sevoflurane administration is compatible with benzodiazepines and opioids as commonly used in surgical practice).

No products indexed under this heading.

Diazepam (Benzodiazepines and opioids would be expected to decrease the

MAC of sevoflurane in the same manner as with other inhalational anesthetics. Sevoflurane administration is compatible with benzodiazepines and opioids as commonly used in surgical practice). Products include:

Valium Tablets **2880**

Dihydrocodeine Bitartrate (Benzodiazepines and opioids would be expected to decrease the MAC of sevoflurane in the same manner as with other inhalational anesthetics. Sevoflurane administration is compatible with benzodiazepines and opioids as commonly used in surgical practice).

No products indexed under this heading.

Dihydrocodeinone Bitartrate (Benzodiazepines and opioids would be expected to decrease the MAC of sevoflurane in the same manner as with other inhalational anesthetics. Sevoflurane administration is compatible with benzodiazepines and opioids as commonly used in surgical practice).

No products indexed under this heading.

Doxacurium Chloride (Sevoflurane increases both the intensity and duration of neuromuscular blockade induced by non-depolarizing muscle relaxants. When used to supplement alfentanil-nitrous oxide anesthesia, sevoflurane and isoflurane equally potentiate neuromuscular block induced with pancuronium, vecuronium or atracurium. Among available non-depolarizing agents, only vecuronium, pancuronium and atracurium interactions have been studied during sevoflurane anesthesia. In the absence of specific guidelines: 1) For endotracheal intubation, do not reduce the dose of non-depolarizing muscle relaxants. 2) During maintenance of anesthesia, the required dose of non-depolarizing muscle relaxants is likely to be reduced compared to that during nitrous oxide/opioid anesthesia).

No products indexed under this heading.

d-Tubocurarine (Sevoflurane increases both the intensity and duration of neuromuscular blockade induced by non-depolarizing muscle relaxants. When used to supplement alfentanil-nitrous oxide anesthesia, sevoflurane and isoflurane equally potentiate neuromuscular block induced with pancuronium, vecuronium or atracurium. Among available non-depolarizing agents, only vecuronium, pancuronium and atracurium interactions have been studied during sevoflurane anesthesia. In the absence of specific guidelines: 1) For endotracheal intubation, do not reduce the dose of non-depolarizing muscle relaxants. 2) During maintenance of anesthesia, the required dose of non-depolarizing muscle relaxants is likely to be reduced compared to that during nitrous oxide/opioid anesthesia).

No products indexed under this heading.

Estazolam (Benzodiazepines and opioids would be expected to decrease the MAC of sevoflurane in the same manner as with other inhalational anesthetics. Sevoflurane administration is compatible with benzodiazepines and opioids as commonly used in surgical practice).

No products indexed under this heading.

Fentanyl (Benzodiazepines and opioids would be expected to decrease the MAC of sevoflurane in the same manner as with other inhalational anesthetics. Sevoflurane administration is compatible with benzodiazepines and opioids as commonly used in surgical practice). Products include:

Duragesic **2604**
Fentanyl Transdermal System **2346**
Onsolis **2054**

Fentanyl Citrate (Benzodiazepines and opioids would be expected to decrease the MAC of sevoflurane in the same manner as with other inhalational

1969 Interactions Index Ultane

anesthetics. Sevoflurane administration is compatible with benzodiazepines and opioids as commonly used in surgical practice). Products include:

Fentora 966

Flurazepam Hydrochloride (Benzodiazepines and opioids would be expected to decrease the MAC of sevoflurane in the same manner as with other inhalational anesthetics. Sevoflurane administration is compatible with benzodiazepines and opioids as commonly used in surgical practice).

No products indexed under this heading.

Gallamine (Sevoflurane increases both the intensity and duration of neuromuscular blockade induced by non-depolarizing muscle relaxants. When used to supplement alfentanil-nitrous oxide anesthesia, sevoflurane and isoflurane equally potentiate neuromuscular block induced with pancuronium, vecuronium or atracurium. Among available non-depolarizing agents, only vecuronium, pancuronium and atracurium interactions have been studied during sevoflurane anesthesia. In the absence of specific guidelines: 1) For endotracheal intubation, do not reduce the dose of non-depolarizing muscle relaxants. 2) During maintenance of anesthesia, the required dose of non-depolarizing muscle relaxants is likely to be reduced compared to that during nitrous oxide/opioid anesthesia).

No products indexed under this heading.

Gallamine Triethiodide (Sevoflurane increases both the intensity and duration of neuromuscular blockade induced by non-depolarizing muscle relaxants. When used to supplement alfentanil-nitrous oxide anesthesia, sevoflurane and isoflurane equally potentiate neuromuscular block induced with pancuronium, vecuronium or atracurium. Among available non-depolarizing agents, only vecuronium, pancuronium and atracurium interactions have been studied during sevoflurane anesthesia. In the absence of specific guidelines: 1) For endotracheal intubation, do not reduce the dose of non-depolarizing muscle relaxants. 2) During maintenance of anesthesia, the required dose of non-depolarizing muscle relaxants is likely to be reduced compared to that during nitrous oxide/opioid anesthesia).

No products indexed under this heading.

Halazepam (Benzodiazepines and opioids would be expected to decrease the MAC of sevoflurane in the same manner as with other inhalational anesthetics. Sevoflurane administration is compatible with benzodiazepines and opioids as commonly used in surgical practice).

No products indexed under this heading.

Hydrocodone Bitartrate (Benzodiazepines and opioids would be expected to decrease the MAC of sevoflurane in the same manner as with other inhalational anesthetics. Sevoflurane administration is compatible with benzodiazepines and opioids as commonly used in surgical practice). Products include:

Vicodin 560
Vicodin ES 561
Vicodin HP 563
Vicoprofen 564
Zydone 1138

Hydrocodone Polistirex (Benzodiazepines and opioids would be expected to decrease the MAC of sevoflurane in the same manner as with other inhalational anesthetics. Sevoflurane administration is compatible with benzodiazepines and opioids as commonly used in surgical practice). Products include:

Tussionex 3443

Hydromorphone (Benzodiazepines and opioids would be expected to decrease the MAC of sevoflurane in the same manner as with other inhalational anesthetics. Sevoflurane administration is compatible with benzodiazepines and opioids as commonly used in surgical practice).

No products indexed under this heading.

Hydromorphone Hydrochloride (Benzodiazepines and opioids would be expected to decrease the MAC of sevoflurane in the same manner as with other inhalational anesthetics. Sevoflurane administration is compatible with benzodiazepines and opioids as commonly used in surgical practice). Products include:

Dilaudid Injection 2800
Dilaudid Oral 2797
Dilaudid Tablets 2797
Dilaudid-HP 2800

Levorphanol Tartrate (Benzodiazepines and opioids would be expected to decrease the MAC of sevoflurane in the same manner as with other inhalational anesthetics. Sevoflurane administration is compatible with benzodiazepines and opioids as commonly used in surgical practice).

No products indexed under this heading.

Lorazepam (Benzodiazepines and opioids would be expected to decrease the MAC of sevoflurane in the same manner as with other inhalational anesthetics. Sevoflurane administration is compatible with benzodiazepines and opioids as commonly used in surgical practice).

No products indexed under this heading.

Meperidine Hydrochloride (Benzodiazepines and opioids would be expected to decrease the MAC of sevoflurane in the same manner as with other inhalational anesthetics. Sevoflurane administration is compatible with benzodiazepines and opioids as commonly used in surgical practice).

No products indexed under this heading.

Methadone Hydrochloride (Benzodiazepines and opioids would be expected to decrease the MAC of sevoflurane in the same manner as with other inhalational anesthetics. Sevoflurane administration is compatible with benzodiazepines and opioids as commonly used in surgical practice).

No products indexed under this heading.

Metocurine Iodide (Sevoflurane increases both the intensity and duration of neuromuscular blockade induced by non-depolarizing muscle relaxants. When used to supplement alfentanil-nitrous oxide anesthesia, sevoflurane and isoflurane equally potentiate neuromuscular block induced with pancuronium, vecuronium or atracurium. Among available non-depolarizing agents, only vecuronium, pancuronium and atracurium interactions have been studied during sevoflurane anesthesia. In the absence of specific guidelines: 1) For endotracheal intubation, do not reduce the dose of non-depolarizing muscle relaxants. 2) During maintenance of anesthesia, the required dose of non-depolarizing muscle relaxants is likely to be reduced compared to that during nitrous oxide/opioid anesthesia).

No products indexed under this heading.

Midazolam Hydrochloride (Benzodiazepines and opioids would be expected to decrease the MAC of sevoflurane in the same manner as with other inhalational anesthetics. Sevoflurane administration is compatible with benzodiazepines and opioids as commonly used in surgical practice).

No products indexed under this heading.

Mivacurium Chloride (Sevoflurane increases both the intensity and duration of neuromuscular blockade induced by non-depolarizing muscle relaxants. When used to supplement alfentanil-nitrous oxide anesthesia, sevoflurane and isoflurane equally potentiate neuromuscular block induced with pancuronium, vecuronium or atracurium. Among available non-depolarizing agents, only vecuronium, pancuronium and atracurium interactions have been studied during sevoflurane anesthesia. In the absence of specific guidelines: 1) For endotracheal intubation, do not reduce the dose of non-depolarizing muscle relaxants. 2) During maintenance of anesthesia, the required dose of non-depolarizing muscle relaxants is likely to be reduced compared to that during nitrous oxide/opioid anesthesia).

No products indexed under this heading.

Morphine Sulfate (Benzodiazepines and opioids would be expected to decrease the MAC of sevoflurane in the same manner as with other inhalational anesthetics. Sevoflurane administration is compatible with benzodiazepines and opioids as commonly used in surgical practice). Products include:

Avinza 1822
Embeda 1831
MS Contin 2803

Morphine Sulfate, Liposomal (Benzodiazepines and opioids would be expected to decrease the MAC of sevoflurane in the same manner as with other inhalational anesthetics. Sevoflurane administration is compatible with benzodiazepines and opioids as commonly used in surgical practice).

No products indexed under this heading.

Nitrous Oxide (As with other halogenated volatile anesthetics, the anesthetic requirement for sevoflurane is decreased when administered in combination with nitrous oxide. Using 50% nitrous oxide, the MAC equivalent dose requirement is reduced approximately 50% in adults and approximately 25% in pediatrics patients).

No products indexed under this heading.

Oxazepam (Benzodiazepines and opioids would be expected to decrease the MAC of sevoflurane in the same manner as with other inhalational anesthetics. Sevoflurane administration is compatible with benzodiazepines and opioids as commonly used in surgical practice).

No products indexed under this heading.

Oxycodone Hydrochloride (Benzodiazepines and opioids would be expected to decrease the MAC of sevoflurane in the same manner as with other inhalational anesthetics. Sevoflurane administration is compatible with benzodiazepines and opioids as commonly used in surgical practice). Products include:

OxyContin 2807
Percocet 1121
Percodan 1124

Oxycodone Terephthalate (Benzodiazepines and opioids would be expected to decrease the MAC of sevoflurane in the same manner as with other inhalational anesthetics. Sevoflurane administration is compatible with benzodiazepines and opioids as commonly used in surgical practice).

No products indexed under this heading.

Oxymorphone Hydrochloride (Benzodiazepines and opioids would be expected to decrease the MAC of sevoflurane in the same manner as with other inhalational anesthetics. Sevoflurane administration is compatible with benzodiazepines and opioids as commonly used in surgical practice). Products include:

Opana 1110
Opana ER 1114

Pancuronium Bromide (Sevoflurane increases both the intensity and duration of neuromuscular blockade induced by non-depolarizing muscle relaxants. When used to supplement alfentanil-nitrous oxide anesthesia, sevoflurane and isoflurane equally potentiate neuromuscular block induced with pancuronium, vecuronium or atracurium. Among available non-depolarizing agents, only vecuronium, pancuronium and atracurium interactions have been studied during sevoflurane anesthesia. In the absence of specific guidelines: 1) For endotracheal intubation, do not reduce the dose of non-depolarizing muscle relaxants. 2) During maintenance of anesthesia, the required dose of non-depolarizing muscle relaxants is likely to be reduced compared to that during nitrous oxide/opioid anesthesia).

No products indexed under this heading.

Pipecuronium Bromide (Sevoflurane increases both the intensity and duration of neuromuscular blockade induced by non-depolarizing muscle relaxants. When used to supplement alfentanil-nitrous oxide anesthesia, sevoflurane and isoflurane equally potentiate neuromuscular block induced with pancuronium, vecuronium or atracurium. Among available non-depolarizing agents, only vecuronium, pancuronium and atracurium interactions have been studied during sevoflurane anesthesia. In the absence of specific guidelines: 1) For endotracheal intubation, do not reduce the dose of non-depolarizing muscle relaxants. 2) During maintenance of anesthesia, the required dose of non-depolarizing muscle relaxants is likely to be reduced compared to that during nitrous oxide/opioid anesthesia).

No products indexed under this heading.

Prazepam (Benzodiazepines and opioids would be expected to decrease the MAC of sevoflurane in the same manner as with other inhalational anesthetics. Sevoflurane administration is compatible with benzodiazepines and opioids as commonly used in surgical practice).

No products indexed under this heading.

Propoxyphene Hydrochloride (Benzodiazepines and opioids would be expected to decrease the MAC of sevoflurane in the same manner as with other inhalational anesthetics. Sevoflurane administration is compatible with benzodiazepines and opioids as commonly used in surgical practice).

No products indexed under this heading.

Propoxyphene Napsylate (Benzodiazepines and opioids would be expected to decrease the MAC of sevoflurane in the same manner as with other inhalational anesthetics. Sevoflurane administration is compatible with benzodiazepines and opioids as commonly used in surgical practice).

No products indexed under this heading.

Quazepam (Benzodiazepines and opioids would be expected to decrease the MAC of sevoflurane in the same manner as with other inhalational anesthetics. Sevoflurane administration is compatible with benzodiazepines and opioids as commonly used in surgical practice).

No products indexed under this heading.

Rapacuronium Bromide (Sevoflurane increases both the intensity and duration of neuromuscular blockade induced by non-depolarizing muscle relaxants. When used to supplement alfentanil-nitrous oxide anesthesia, sevoflurane and isoflurane equally potentiate neuromuscular block induced with pancuronium, vecuronium or atracurium. Among available non-depolarizing agents, only vecuronium, pancuronium and atracurium interactions have been studied during sevoflurane anesthesia. In the absence of specific guidelines: 1) For endotracheal intubation, do not reduce the dose of

Ultane Interactions Index 1970

non-depolarizing muscle relaxants. 2) During maintenance of anesthesia, the required dose of non-depolarizing muscle relaxants is likely to be reduced compared to that during nitrous oxide/opioid anesthesia).
No products indexed under this heading.

Remifentanil Hydrochloride (Benzodiazepines and opioids would be expected to decrease the MAC of sevoflurane in the same manner as with other inhalational anesthetics. Sevoflurane administration is compatible with benzodiazepines and opioids as commonly used in surgical practice).
No products indexed under this heading.

Rocuronium Bromide (Sevoflurane increases both the intensity and duration of neuromuscular blockade induced by non-depolarizing muscle relaxants. When used to supplement alfentanil-nitrous oxide anesthesia, sevoflurane and isoflurane equally potentiate neuromuscular block induced with pancuronium, vecuronium or atracurium. Among available non-depolarizing agents, only vecuronium, pancuronium and atracurium interactions have been studied during sevoflurane anesthesia. In the absence of specific guidelines: 1) For endotracheal intubation, do not reduce the dose of non-depolarizing muscle relaxants. 2) During maintenance of anesthesia, the required dose of non-depolarizing muscle relaxants is likely to be reduced compared to that during nitrous oxide/opioid anesthesia). Products include:
Zemuron 3249

Sufentanil Citrate (Benzodiazepines and opioids would be expected to decrease the MAC of sevoflurane in the same manner as with other inhalational anesthetics. Sevoflurane administration is compatible with benzodiazepines and opioids as commonly used in surgical practice).
No products indexed under this heading.

Temazepam (Benzodiazepines and opioids would be expected to decrease the MAC of sevoflurane in the same manner as with other inhalational anesthetics. Sevoflurane administration is compatible with benzodiazepines and opioids as commonly used in surgical practice).
No products indexed under this heading.

Triazolam (Benzodiazepines and opioids would be expected to decrease the MAC of sevoflurane in the same manner as with other inhalational anesthetics. Sevoflurane administration is compatible with benzodiazepines and opioids as commonly used in surgical practice).
No products indexed under this heading.

Tubocurarine Chloride (Sevoflurane increases both the intensity and duration of neuromuscular blockade induced by non-depolarizing muscle relaxants. When used to supplement alfentanil-nitrous oxide anesthesia, sevoflurane and isoflurane equally potentiate neuromuscular block induced with pancuronium, vecuronium or atracurium. Among available non-depolarizing agents, only vecuronium, pancuronium and atracurium interactions have been studied during sevoflurane anesthesia. In the absence of specific guidelines: 1) For endotracheal intubation, do not reduce the dose of non-depolarizing muscle relaxants. 2) During maintenance of anesthesia, the required dose of non-depolarizing muscle relaxants is likely to be reduced compared to that during nitrous oxide/opioid anesthesia).
No products indexed under this heading.

Vecuronium Bromide (Sevoflurane increases both the intensity and duration of neuromuscular blockade induced by non-depolarizing muscle relaxants. When used to supplement alfentanil-nitrous oxide anesthesia, sevoflurane and isoflurane equally potentiate neuromuscular block induced with pancuronium, vecuronium or atracurium. Among available non-depolarizing agents, only vecuronium, pancuronium and atracurium interactions have been studied during sevoflurane anesthesia. In the absence of specific guidelines: 1) For endotracheal intubation, do not reduce the dose of non-depolarizing muscle relaxants. 2) During maintenance of anesthesia, the required dose of non-depolarizing muscle relaxants is likely to be reduced compared to that during nitrous oxide/opioid anesthesia).
No products indexed under this heading.

ULTRAM ER EXTENDED-RELEASE TABLETS

(Tramadol Hydrochloride) 2693
May interact with alcohols, anesthetics, antipsychotic agents, central nervous system depressants, cytochrome p450 2d6 inhibitors (selected), cytochrome p450 3a4 inducers (selected), cytochrome p450 3a4 inhibitors (selected), hypnotics and sedatives, monoamine oxidase inhibitors, narcotic analgesics, phenothiazines, psychotropics, quinidine, selective serotonin reuptake inhibitors, serotonin and norepinephrine reuptake inhibitors, tranquilizers, tricyclic antidepressants, triptans, and certain other agents. Compounds in these categories include:

Acetazolamide (Administration of CYP3A4 inhibitors, such as ketoconazole and erythromycin, with tramadol hydrochloride may effect the metabolism of tramadol leading to altered tramadol exposure).
No products indexed under this heading.

Acetazolamide Sodium (Administration of CYP3A4 inhibitors, such as ketoconazole and erythromycin, with tramadol hydrochloride may effect the metabolism of tramadol leading to altered tramadol exposure).
No products indexed under this heading.

Alfentanil Hydrochloride (Tramadol hydrochloride is contraindicated in acute intoxication with narcotics, opioids, and centrally-acting analgesics. Concomitant use of tramadol increases the seizure risk in patients taking opioids. Tramadol hydrochloride should be used with caution and in reduced dosages when administered to patients receiving CNS depressants, such as opioids or narcotics. Tramadol hydrochloride increases the risk of CNS and respiratory depression. Tramadol may be expected to have additive effects when used in conjunction with other opioids).
No products indexed under this heading.

Allium sativum (Administration of CYP3A4 inducers, such as rifampin or St. John's Wort, with tramadol hydrochloride may effect the metabolism of tramadol leading to altered tramadol exposure).
No products indexed under this heading.

Almotriptan Malate (Concomitant use of tramadol increases the seizure risk in patients taking triptans. Concomitant use of tramadol with triptans increases the risk of adverse events, including seizure and serotonin syndrome. If concomitant treatment of tramadol with a drug affecting the serotonergic neurotransmitter system is clinically warranted, careful observation of the patient is advised, particularly during treatment initiation and dose increases). Products include:
Axert 2593

Alprazolam (Tramadol hydrochloride is contraindicated in acute intoxication with psychotropic drugs).
No products indexed under this heading.

Aminoglutethimide (Administration of CYP3A4 inducers, such as rifampin or St. John's Wort, with tramadol hydrochloride may effect the metabolism of tramadol leading to altered tramadol exposure).
No products indexed under this heading.

Amiodarone Hydrochloride (In vitro drug interaction studies in human liver microsomes indicate that concomitant administration with inhibitors of CYP2D6 could result in some inhibition of the metabolism of tramadol).
No products indexed under this heading.

Amitriptyline Hydrochloride (Tramadol hydrochloride is contraindicated in acute intoxication with psychotropic drugs).
No products indexed under this heading.

Amobarbital (Tramadol hydrochloride should be used with caution and in reduced dosages when administered to patients receiving CNS depressants, such as alcohol, opioids, anesthetic agents, narcotics, phenothiazines, tranquilizers, or sedative hypnotics. Tramadol hydrochloride increases the risk of CNS and respiratory depression).
No products indexed under this heading.

Amobarbital Sodium (Tramadol hydrochloride should be used with caution and in reduced dosages when administered to patients receiving CNS depressants, such as alcohol, opioids, anesthetic agents, narcotics, phenothiazines, tranquilizers, or sedative hypnotics. Tramadol hydrochloride increases the risk of CNS and respiratory depression).
No products indexed under this heading.

Amoxapine (Tramadol hydrochloride is contraindicated in acute intoxication with psychotropic drugs).
No products indexed under this heading.

Amprenavir (Administration of CYP3A4 inhibitors, such as ketoconazole and erythromycin, with tramadol hydrochloride may effect the metabolism of tramadol leading to altered tramadol exposure).
No products indexed under this heading.

Anastrozole (Administration of CYP3A4 inhibitors, such as ketoconazole and erythromycin, with tramadol hydrochloride may effect the metabolism of tramadol leading to altered tramadol exposure).
No products indexed under this heading.

Apomorphine (Tramadol hydrochloride is contraindicated in acute intoxication with narcotics, opioids, and centrally-acting analgesics. Concomitant use of tramadol increases the seizure risk in patients taking opioids. Tramadol hydrochloride should be used with caution and in reduced dosages when administered to patients receiving CNS depressants, such as opioids or narcotics. Tramadol hydrochloride increases the risk of CNS and respiratory depression. Tramadol may be expected to have additive effects when used in conjunction with other opioids).
No products indexed under this heading.

Apomorphine Hydrochloride (Tramadol hydrochloride is contraindicated in acute intoxication with narcotics, opioids, and centrally-acting analgesics. Concomitant use of tramadol increases the seizure risk in patients taking opioids. Tramadol hydrochloride should be used with caution and in reduced dosages when administered to patients receiving CNS depressants, such as opioids or narcotics. Tramadol hydrochloride increases the risk of CNS and respiratory depression. Tramadol may be expected to have additive effects when used in conjunction with other opioids).
No products indexed under this heading.

Aprepitant (Administration of CYP3A4 inhibitors, such as ketoconazole and erythromycin, with tramadol hydrochloride may effect the metabolism of tramadol leading to altered tramadol exposure). Products include:
Emend 2124

Aprobarbital (Tramadol hydrochloride should be used with caution and in reduced dosages when administered to patients receiving CNS depressants, such as alcohol, opioids, anesthetic agents, narcotics, phenothiazines, tranquilizers, or sedative hypnotics. Tramadol hydrochloride increases the risk of CNS and respiratory depression).
No products indexed under this heading.

Aripiprazole (Administration of tramadol may increase the seizure risk in patients taking neuroleptics or other drugs that reduce the seizure threshold).
No products indexed under this heading.

Articaine Hydrochloride (Tramadol hydrochloride should be used with caution and in reduced dosages when administered to patients receiving CNS depressants, such as anesthetic agents. Tramadol hydrochloride increases the risk of CNS and respiratory depression).
No products indexed under this heading.

Atazanavir (Administration of CYP3A4 inhibitors, such as ketoconazole and erythromycin, with tramadol hydrochloride may effect the metabolism of tramadol leading to altered tramadol exposure).
No products indexed under this heading.

Atazanavir Sulfate (Administration of CYP3A4 inhibitors, such as ketoconazole and erythromycin, with tramadol hydrochloride may effect the metabolism of tramadol leading to altered tramadol exposure).
No products indexed under this heading.

Benzocaine (Tramadol hydrochloride should be used with caution and in reduced dosages when administered to patients receiving CNS depressants, such as anesthetic agents. Tramadol hydrochloride increases the risk of CNS and respiratory depression).
No products indexed under this heading.

Betamethasone (Administration of CYP3A4 inducers, such as rifampin or St. John's Wort, with tramadol hydrochloride may effect the metabolism of tramadol leading to altered tramadol exposure).
No products indexed under this heading.

Betamethasone Acetate (Administration of CYP3A4 inducers, such as rifampin or St. John's Wort, with tramadol hydrochloride may effect the metabolism of tramadol leading to altered tramadol exposure).
No products indexed under this heading.

Betamethasone Benzoate (Administration of CYP3A4 inducers, such as rifampin or St. John's Wort, with tramadol hydrochloride may effect the metabolism of tramadol leading to altered tramadol exposure).
No products indexed under this heading.

Betamethasone Dipropionate (Administration of CYP3A4 inducers, such as rifampin or St. John's Wort, with tramadol hydrochloride may effect the metabolism of tramadol leading to altered tramadol exposure). Products include:
Diprolene Lotion 0.05% 3108
Diprolene Ointment 0.05% 3109
Diprolene AF Cream 0.05% 3107
Lotrisone 3163

Betamethasone Sodium Phosphate (Administration of CYP3A4 inducers, such as rifampin or St. John's Wort, with tramadol hydrochloride may effect the metabolism of tramadol leading to altered tramadol exposure).
No products indexed under this heading.

Betamethasone Valerate (Administration of CYP3A4 inducers, such as rifampin or St. John's Wort, with tramadol hydrochloride may effect the metabolism of tramadol leading to altered tramadol exposure). Products include:
Luxiq 3321

Bosentan (Administration of CYP3A4 inducers, such as rifampin or St. John's Wort, with tramadol hydrochloride may effect the metabolism of tramadol leading to altered tramadol exposure). Products include:
Tracleer 573

Bupivacaine Hydrochloride (Tramadol hydrochloride should be used with caution and in reduced dosages when administered to patients receiving CNS depressants, such as anesthetic agents. Tramadol hydrochloride increases the risk of CNS and respiratory depression).
No products indexed under this heading.

Buprenorphine Hydrochloride (Tramadol hydrochloride is contraindicated in acute intoxication with narcotics, opioids, and centrally-acting analgesics. Concomitant use of tramadol increases the seizure risk in patients taking opioids. Tramadol hydrochloride should be used with caution and in reduced dosages when administered to patients receiving CNS depressants, such as opioids or narcotics. Tramadol hydrochloride increases the risk of CNS and respiratory depression. Tramadol may be expected to have additive effects when used in conjunction with other opioids).
No products indexed under this heading.

Bupropion Hydrochloride (In vitro drug interaction studies in human liver microsomes indicate that concomitant administration with inhibitors of CYP2D6 could result in some inhibition of the metabolism of tramadol). Products include:
Aplenzin 2948
Wellbutrin 1719
Wellbutrin SR 1725
Zyban 1762

Buspirone Hydrochloride (Tramadol hydrochloride is contraindicated in acute intoxication with psychotropic drugs).
No products indexed under this heading.

Butabarbital (Tramadol hydrochloride is contraindicated in acute intoxication with hypnotics. Tramadol hydrochloride should be used with caution and in reduced dosages when administered to patients receiving CNS depressants, such as sedative hypnotics. Tramadol hydrochloride increases the risk of CNS and respiratory depression).
No products indexed under this heading.

Butabarbital Sodium (Tramadol hydrochloride is contraindicated in acute intoxication with hypnotics. Tramadol hydrochloride should be used with caution and in reduced dosages when administered to patients receiving CNS depressants, such as sedative hypnotics. Tramadol hydrochloride increases the risk of CNS and respiratory depression).
No products indexed under this heading.

Butalbital (Tramadol hydrochloride is contraindicated in acute intoxication with hypnotics. Tramadol hydrochloride should be used with caution and in reduced dosages when administered to patients receiving CNS depressants, such as sedative hypnotics. Tramadol hydrochloride increases the risk of CNS and respiratory depression).
No products indexed under this heading.

Carbamazepine (Patients taking carbamazepine, a CYP3A4 inducer, may have a significantly reduced analgesic effect of tramadol. Because carbamazepine increases tramadol metabolism and because of the seizure risk associated with tramadol, concomitant administration of tramadol hydrochloride and carbamazepine is not recommended). Products include:
Carbatrol 3280
Equetro 3477

Celecoxib (In vitro drug interaction studies in human liver microsomes indicate that concomitant administration with inhibitors of CYP2D6 could result in some inhibition of the metabolism of tramadol). Products include:
Celebrex 3272

Chloral Hydrate (Tramadol hydrochloride is contraindicated in acute intoxication with hypnotics. Tramadol hydrochloride should be used with caution and in reduced dosages when administered to patients receiving CNS depressants, such as sedative hypnotics. Tramadol hydrochloride increases the risk of CNS and respiratory depression).
No products indexed under this heading.

Chlordiazepoxide (Tramadol hydrochloride is contraindicated in acute intoxication with psychotropic drugs).
No products indexed under this heading.

Chlordiazepoxide Hydrochloride (Tramadol hydrochloride is contraindicated in acute intoxication with psychotropic drugs).
No products indexed under this heading.

Chloroprocaine Hydrochloride (Tramadol hydrochloride should be used with caution and in reduced dosages when administered to patients receiving CNS depressants, such as anesthetic agents. Tramadol hydrochloride increases the risk of CNS and respiratory depression).
No products indexed under this heading.

Chloroquine (In vitro drug interaction studies in human liver microsomes indicate that concomitant administration with inhibitors of CYP2D6 could result in some inhibition of the metabolism of tramadol).
No products indexed under this heading.

Chloroquine Hydrochloride (In vitro drug interaction studies in human liver microsomes indicate that concomitant administration with inhibitors of CYP2D6 could result in some inhibition of the metabolism of tramadol).
No products indexed under this heading.

Chloroquine Phosphate (In vitro drug interaction studies in human liver microsomes indicate that concomitant administration with inhibitors of CYP2D6 could result in some inhibition of the metabolism of tramadol).
No products indexed under this heading.

Chlorpheniramine (In vitro drug interaction studies in human liver microsomes indicate that concomitant administration with inhibitors of CYP2D6 could result in some inhibition of the metabolism of tramadol).
No products indexed under this heading.

Chlorpheniramine Maleate (In vitro drug interaction studies in human liver microsomes indicate that concomitant administration with inhibitors of CYP2D6 could result in some inhibition of the metabolism of tramadol).
No products indexed under this heading.

Chlorpheniramine Polistirex (In vitro drug interaction studies in human liver microsomes indicate that concomitant administration with inhibitors of CYP2D6 could result in some inhibition of the metabolism of tramadol). Products include:
Tussionex 3443

Chlorpheniramine Tannate (In vitro drug interaction studies in human liver microsomes indicate that concomitant administration with inhibitors of CYP2D6 could result in some inhibition of the metabolism of tramadol).
No products indexed under this heading.

Chlorpromazine (Tramadol hydrochloride is contraindicated in acute intoxication with psychotropic drugs).
No products indexed under this heading.

Chlorpromazine Hydrochloride (Tramadol hydrochloride is contraindicated in acute intoxication with psychotropic drugs).
No products indexed under this heading.

Chlorprothixene (Tramadol hydrochloride is contraindicated in acute intoxication with psychotropic drugs).
No products indexed under this heading.

Chlorprothixene Hydrochloride (Tramadol hydrochloride is contraindicated in acute intoxication with psychotropic drugs).
No products indexed under this heading.

Chlorprothixene Lactate (Administration of tramadol may increase the seizure risk in patients taking neuroleptics or other drugs that reduce the seizure threshold).
No products indexed under this heading.

Cimetidine (In vitro drug interaction studies in human liver microsomes indicate that concomitant administration with inhibitors of CYP2D6 could result in some inhibition of the metabolism of tramadol).
No products indexed under this heading.

Cimetidine Hydrochloride (In vitro drug interaction studies in human liver microsomes indicate that concomitant administration with inhibitors of CYP2D6 could result in some inhibition of the metabolism of tramadol).
No products indexed under this heading.

Ciprofloxacin (Administration of CYP3A4 inhibitors, such as ketoconazole and erythromycin, with tramadol hydrochloride may effect the metabolism of tramadol leading to altered tramadol exposure). Products include:
Cipro I.V. 3082
Cipro 3073
Cipro XR 3091
Ciprodex 583

Ciprofloxacin Hydrochloride (Administration of CYP3A4 inducers, such as rifampin or St. John's Wort, with tramadol hydrochloride may effect the metabolism of tramadol leading to altered tramadol exposure). Products include:
Cipro 3073

Cisplatin (Administration of CYP3A4 inducers, such as rifampin or St. John's Wort, with tramadol hydrochloride may effect the metabolism of tramadol leading to altered tramadol exposure).
No products indexed under this heading.

Citalopram Hydrobromide (Concomitant use of tramadol increases the seizure risk in patients taking selective serotonin re-uptake inhibitors. Concomitant use of tramadol with SSRIs increases the risk of adverse events, including seizure and serotonin syndrome). Products include:
Celexa 1153

Clarithromycin (Administration of CYP3A4 inhibitors, such as ketoconazole and erythromycin, with tramadol hydrochloride may effect the metabolism of tramadol leading to altered tramadol exposure). Products include:
Biaxin/Biaxin XL 412

Clomipramine Hydrochloride (Concomitant use of tramadol increases the seizure risk in patients taking tricyclic antidepressants).
No products indexed under this heading.

Clonazepam (Tramadol hydrochloride should be used with caution and in reduced dosages when administered to patients receiving CNS depressants, such as alcohol, opioids, anesthetic agents, narcotics, phenothiazines, tranquilizers, or sedative hypnotics. Tramadol hydrochloride increases the risk of CNS and respiratory depression). Products include:
Klonopin 2855

Clorazepate Dipotassium (Tramadol hydrochloride is contraindicated in acute intoxication with psychotropic drugs).
No products indexed under this heading.

Clotrimazole (Administration of CYP3A4 inhibitors, such as ketoconazole and erythromycin, with tramadol hydrochloride may effect the metabolism of tramadol leading to altered tramadol exposure). Products include:
Lotrisone 3163

Clozapine (Tramadol hydrochloride is contraindicated in acute intoxication with psychotropic drugs).
No products indexed under this heading.

Cocaine Hydrochloride (Tramadol hydrochloride should be used with caution and in reduced dosages when administered to patients receiving CNS depressants, such as anesthetic agents. Tramadol hydrochloride increases the risk of CNS and respiratory depression).
No products indexed under this heading.

Codeine Phosphate (Tramadol hydrochloride is contraindicated in acute intoxication with narcotics, opioids, and centrally-acting analgesics. Concomitant use of tramadol increases the seizure risk in patients taking opioids. Tramadol hydrochloride should be used with caution and in reduced dosages when administered to patients receiving CNS depressants, such as opioids or narcotics. Tramadol hydrochloride increases the risk of CNS and respiratory depression. Tramadol may be expected to have additive effects when used in conjunction with other opioids). Products include:
Tylenol with Codeine 2691

Codeine Sulfate (Tramadol hydrochloride is contraindicated in acute intoxication with narcotics, opioids, and centrally-acting analgesics. Concomitant use of tramadol increases the seizure risk in patients taking opioids. Tramadol hydrochloride should be used with caution and in reduced dosages when administered to patients receiving CNS depressants, such as opioids or narcotics. Tramadol hydrochloride increases the risk of CNS and respiratory depression. Tramadol may be expected to have additive effects when used in conjunction with other opioids).
No products indexed under this heading.

Conivaptan Hydrochloride (Administration of CYP3A4 inhibitors, such as ketoconazole and erythromycin, with tramadol hydrochloride may effect the metabolism of tramadol leading to altered tramadol exposure). Products include:

IMPORTANT NOTE: Always consult each drug listing in the patient's regimen for possible interactions.

Erythromycin Lactobionate (Administration of CYP3A4 inhibitors, such as ketoconazole and erythromycin, with tramadol hydrochloride may effect the metabolism of tramadol leading to altered tramadol exposure).
No products indexed under this heading.

Erythromycin Stearate (Administration of CYP3A4 inhibitors, such as ketoconazole and erythromycin, with tramadol hydrochloride may effect the metabolism of tramadol leading to altered tramadol exposure).
No products indexed under this heading.

Escitalopram Oxalate (Concomitant use of tramadol increases the seizure risk in patients taking selective serotonin re-uptake inhibitors. Concomitant use of tramadol with SSRIs increases the risk of adverse events, including seizure and serotonin syndrome).
Products include:
Lexapro Oral Suspension 1160
Lexapro Tablets 1160

Esomeprazole Magnesium (Administration of CYP3A4 inhibitors, such as ketoconazole and erythromycin, with tramadol hydrochloride may effect the metabolism of tramadol leading to altered tramadol exposure). Products include:
Nexium Capsules 704
Nexium Oral Suspension 704

Esomeprazole Sodium (Administration of CYP3A4 inhibitors, such as ketoconazole and erythromycin, with tramadol hydrochloride may effect the metabolism of tramadol leading to altered tramadol exposure). Products include:
Nexium I.V. 712

Estazolam (Tramadol hydrochloride is contraindicated in acute intoxication with hypnotics. Tramadol hydrochloride should be used with caution and in reduced dosages when administered to patients receiving CNS depressants, such as sedative hypnotics. Tramadol hydrochloride increases the risk of CNS and respiratory depression).
No products indexed under this heading.

Ethanol (Tramadol hydrochloride should be used with caution and in reduced dosages when administered to patients receiving CNS depressants, such as alcohol, opioids, anesthetic agents, narcotics, phenothiazines, tranquilizers, or sedative hypnotics. Tramadol hydrochloride increases the risk of CNS and respiratory depression).
No products indexed under this heading.

Ethchlorvynol (Tramadol hydrochloride is contraindicated in acute intoxication with hypnotics. Tramadol hydrochloride should be used with caution and in reduced dosages when administered to patients receiving CNS depressants, such as sedative hypnotics. Tramadol hydrochloride increases the risk of CNS and respiratory depression).
No products indexed under this heading.

Ethinamate (Tramadol hydrochloride is contraindicated in acute intoxication with hypnotics. Tramadol hydrochloride should be used with caution and in reduced dosages when administered to patients receiving CNS depressants, such as sedative hypnotics. Tramadol hydrochloride increases the risk of CNS and respiratory depression).
No products indexed under this heading.

Ethosuximide (Administration of CYP3A4 inducers, such as rifampin or St. John's Wort, with tramadol hydrochloride may effect the metabolism of tramadol leading to altered tramadol exposure).
No products indexed under this heading.

Ethyl Alcohol (Tramadol hydrochloride should be used with caution and in reduced dosages when administered to patients receiving CNS depressants, such as alcohol, opioids, anesthetic agents, narcotics, phenothiazines, tranquilizers, or sedative hypnotics. Tramadol hydrochloride increases the risk of CNS and respiratory depression).
No products indexed under this heading.

Etidocaine Hydrochloride (Tramadol hydrochloride should be used with caution and in reduced dosages when administered to patients receiving CNS depressants, such as anesthetic agents. Tramadol hydrochloride increases the risk of CNS and respiratory depression).
No products indexed under this heading.

Felbamate (Administration of CYP3A4 inducers, such as rifampin or St. John's Wort, with tramadol hydrochloride may effect the metabolism of tramadol leading to altered tramadol exposure).
No products indexed under this heading.

Fentanyl (Tramadol hydrochloride is contraindicated in acute intoxication with narcotics, opioids, and centrally-acting analgesics. Concomitant use of tramadol increases the seizure risk in patients taking opioids. Tramadol hydrochloride should be used with caution and in reduced dosages when administered to patients receiving CNS depressants, such as opioids or narcotics. Tramadol hydrochloride increases the risk of CNS and respiratory depression. Tramadol may be expected to have additive effects when used in conjunction with other opioids). Products include:
Duragesic 2604
Fentanyl Transdermal System 2346
Onsolis 2054

Fentanyl Citrate (Tramadol hydrochloride is contraindicated in acute intoxication with narcotics, opioids, and centrally-acting analgesics. Concomitant use of tramadol increases the seizure risk in patients taking opioids. Tramadol hydrochloride should be used with caution and in reduced dosages when administered to patients receiving CNS depressants, such as opioids or narcotics. Tramadol hydrochloride increases the risk of CNS and respiratory depression. Tramadol may be expected to have additive effects when used in conjunction with other opioids). Products include:
Fentora 966

Fluconazole (Administration of CYP3A4 inhibitors, such as ketoconazole and erythromycin, with tramadol hydrochloride may effect the metabolism of tramadol leading to altered tramadol exposure).
No products indexed under this heading.

Fludrocortisone Acetate (Administration of CYP3A4 inducers, such as rifampin or St. John's Wort, with tramadol hydrochloride may effect the metabolism of tramadol leading to altered tramadol exposure).
No products indexed under this heading.

Fluoxetine (Concomitant use of tramadol increases the seizure risk in patients taking selective serotonin re-uptake inhibitors. Concomitant use of tramadol with SSRIs increases the risk of adverse events, including seizure and serotonin syndrome).
No products indexed under this heading.

Fluoxetine Hydrochloride (Concomitant use of tramadol increases the seizure risk in patients taking selective serotonin re-uptake inhibitors. Concomitant use of tramadol with SSRIs increases the risk of adverse events, including seizure and serotonin syndrome). Products include:
Prozac Weekly 1941
Prozac Pulvules 1941
Symbyax 1965

Fluphenazine Decanoate (Tramadol hydrochloride is contraindicated in acute intoxication with psychotropic drugs).
No products indexed under this heading.

Fluphenazine Enanthate (Tramadol hydrochloride is contraindicated in acute intoxication with psychotropic drugs).
No products indexed under this heading.

Fluphenazine Hydrochloride (Tramadol hydrochloride is contraindicated in acute intoxication with psychotropic drugs).
No products indexed under this heading.

Flurazepam Hydrochloride (Tramadol hydrochloride is contraindicated in acute intoxication with hypnotics. Tramadol hydrochloride should be used with caution and in reduced dosages when administered to patients receiving CNS depressants, such as sedative hypnotics. Tramadol hydrochloride increases the risk of CNS and respiratory depression).
No products indexed under this heading.

Fluvoxamine (Concomitant use of tramadol increases the seizure risk in patients taking selective serotonin re-uptake inhibitors. Concomitant use of tramadol with SSRIs increases the risk of adverse events, including seizure and serotonin syndrome).
No products indexed under this heading.

Fluvoxamine Maleate (Concomitant use of tramadol increases the seizure risk in patients taking selective serotonin re-uptake inhibitors. Concomitant use of tramadol with SSRIs increases the risk of adverse events, including seizure and serotonin syndrome).
No products indexed under this heading.

Fosamprenavir Calcium (Administration of CYP3A4 inhibitors, such as ketoconazole and erythromycin, with tramadol hydrochloride may effect the metabolism of tramadol leading to altered tramadol exposure). Products include:
Lexiva Oral Suspension 1558
Lexiva 1558

Fosphenytoin Sodium (Administration of CYP3A4 inducers, such as rifampin or St. John's Wort, with tramadol hydrochloride may effect the metabolism of tramadol leading to altered tramadol exposure).
No products indexed under this heading.

Frovatriptan Succinate (Concomitant use of tramadol increases the seizure risk in patients taking triptans. Concomitant use of tramadol with triptans increases the risk of adverse events, including seizure and serotonin syndrome. If concomitant treatment of tramadol with a drug affecting the serotonergic neurotransmitter system is clinically warranted, careful observation of the patient is advised, particularly during treatment initiation and dose increases). Products include:
Frova 1103

Garlic Extract (Administration of CYP3A4 inducers, such as rifampin or St. John's Wort, with tramadol hydrochloride may effect the metabolism of tramadol leading to altered tramadol exposure).
No products indexed under this heading.

Garlic Oil (Administration of CYP3A4 inducers, such as rifampin or St. John's Wort, with tramadol hydrochloride may effect the metabolism of tramadol leading to altered tramadol exposure).
No products indexed under this heading.

Glutethimide (Tramadol hydrochloride is contraindicated in acute intoxication with hypnotics. Tramadol hydrochloride should be used with caution and in reduced dosages when administered to patients receiving CNS depressants, such as sedative hypnotics. Tramadol hydrochloride increases the risk of CNS and respiratory depression).
No products indexed under this heading.

Halazepam (Tramadol hydrochloride should be used with caution and in reduced dosages when administered to patients receiving CNS depressants, such as alcohol, opioids, anesthetic agents, narcotics, phenothiazines, tranquilizers, or sedative hypnotics. Tramadol hydrochloride increases the risk of CNS and respiratory depression).
No products indexed under this heading.

Halofantrine Hydrochloride (In vitro drug interaction studies in human liver microsomes indicate that concomitant administration with inhibitors of CYP2D6 could result in some inhibition of the metabolism of tramadol).
No products indexed under this heading.

Haloperidol (Tramadol hydrochloride is contraindicated in acute intoxication with psychotropic drugs).
No products indexed under this heading.

Haloperidol Decanoate (Tramadol hydrochloride is contraindicated in acute intoxication with psychotropic drugs).
No products indexed under this heading.

Haloperidol Lactate (Administration of tramadol may increase the seizure risk in patients taking neuroleptics or other drugs that reduce the seizure threshold).
No products indexed under this heading.

Halothane (Tramadol hydrochloride should be used with caution and in reduced dosages when administered to patients receiving CNS depressants, such as anesthetic agents. Tramadol hydrochloride increases the risk of CNS and respiratory depression).
No products indexed under this heading.

Hexobarbital (Tramadol hydrochloride should be used with caution and in reduced dosages when administered to patients receiving CNS depressants, such as alcohol, opioids, anesthetic agents, narcotics, phenothiazines, tranquilizers, or sedative hypnotics. Tramadol hydrochloride increases the risk of CNS and respiratory depression).
No products indexed under this heading.

Hydrocodone Bitartrate (Tramadol hydrochloride is contraindicated in acute intoxication with narcotics, opioids, and centrally-acting analgesics. Concomitant use of tramadol increases the seizure risk in patients taking opioids. Tramadol hydrochloride should be used with caution and in reduced dosages when administered to patients receiving CNS depressants, such as opioids or narcotics. Tramadol hydrochloride increases the risk of CNS and respiratory depression. Tramadol may be expected to have additive effects when used in conjunction with other opioids). Products include:
Vicodin 560
Vicodin ES 561
Vicodin HP 563
Vicoprofen 564
Zydone 1138

Hydrocodone Polistirex (Tramadol hydrochloride is contraindicated in acute intoxication with narcotics, opioids, and centrally-acting analgesics. Concomitant use of tramadol increases the seizure risk in patients taking opioids. Tramadol hydrochloride should be used with caution and in reduced dosages when administered to patients receiving CNS depressants, such as

Ultram Interactions Index 1974

opioids or narcotics. Tramadol hydrochloride increases the risk of CNS and respiratory depression. Tramadol may be expected to have additive effects when used in conjunction with other opioids). Products include:
Tussionex 3443

Hydrocortisone (Administration of CYP3A4 inducers, such as rifampin or St. John's Wort, with tramadol hydrochloride may effect the metabolism of tramadol leading to altered tramadol exposure).
No products indexed under this heading.

Hydrocortisone (Alcohol) (Administration of CYP3A4 inducers, such as rifampin or St. John's Wort, with tramadol hydrochloride may effect the metabolism of tramadol leading to altered tramadol exposure).
No products indexed under this heading.

Hydrocortisone Acetate (Administration of CYP3A4 inducers, such as rifampin or St. John's Wort, with tramadol hydrochloride may effect the metabolism of tramadol leading to altered tramadol exposure).
No products indexed under this heading.

Hydrocortisone Butyrate (Administration of CYP3A4 inducers, such as rifampin or St. John's Wort, with tramadol hydrochloride may effect the metabolism of tramadol leading to altered tramadol exposure).
No products indexed under this heading.

Hydrocortisone Cypionate (Administration of CYP3A4 inducers, such as rifampin or St. John's Wort, with tramadol hydrochloride may effect the metabolism of tramadol leading to altered tramadol exposure).
No products indexed under this heading.

Hydrocortisone Hemisuccinate (Administration of CYP3A4 inducers, such as rifampin or St. John's Wort, with tramadol hydrochloride may effect the metabolism of tramadol leading to altered tramadol exposure).
No products indexed under this heading.

Hydrocortisone Probutate (Administration of CYP3A4 inducers, such as rifampin or St. John's Wort, with tramadol hydrochloride may effect the metabolism of tramadol leading to altered tramadol exposure).
No products indexed under this heading.

Hydrocortisone Sodium Phosphate (Administration of CYP3A4 inducers, such as rifampin or St. John's Wort, with tramadol hydrochloride may effect the metabolism of tramadol leading to altered tramadol exposure).
No products indexed under this heading.

Hydrocortisone Sodium Succinate (Administration of CYP3A4 inducers, such as rifampin or St. John's Wort, with tramadol hydrochloride may effect the metabolism of tramadol leading to altered tramadol exposure).
No products indexed under this heading.

Hydrocortisone Valerate (Administration of CYP3A4 inducers, such as rifampin or St. John's Wort, with tramadol hydrochloride may effect the metabolism of tramadol leading to altered tramadol exposure).
No products indexed under this heading.

Hydromorphone (Tramadol hydrochloride is contraindicated in acute intoxication with narcotics, opioids, and centrally-acting analgesics. Concomitant use of tramadol increases the seizure risk in patients taking opioids. Tramadol hydrochloride should be used with caution and in reduced dosages when administered to patients receiving CNS depressants, such as opioids or narcotics. Tramadol hydrochloride increases the risk of CNS and respiratory depression. Tramadol may be expected to have additive effects when used in conjunction with other opioids).
No products indexed under this heading.

Hydromorphone Hydrochloride (Tramadol hydrochloride is contraindicated in acute intoxication with narcotics, opioids, and centrally-acting analgesics. Concomitant use of tramadol increases the seizure risk in patients taking opioids. Tramadol hydrochloride should be used with caution and in reduced dosages when administered to patients receiving CNS depressants, such as opioids or narcotics. Tramadol hydrochloride increases the risk of CNS and respiratory depression. Tramadol may be expected to have additive effects when used in conjunction with other opioids). Products include:
Dilaudid Injection 2800
Dilaudid Oral 2797
Dilaudid Tablets 2797
Dilaudid-HP 2800

Hydroxychloroquine Sulfate (In vitro drug interaction studies in human liver microsomes indicate that concomitant administration with inhibitors of CYP2D6 could result in some inhibition of the metabolism of tramadol).
No products indexed under this heading.

Hydroxyzine Hydrochloride (Tramadol hydrochloride is contraindicated in acute intoxication with psychotropic drugs).
No products indexed under this heading.

Hypericum (Administration of CYP3A4 inducers, such as rifampin or St. John's Wort, with tramadol hydrochloride may effect the metabolism of tramadol leading to altered tramadol exposure).
No products indexed under this heading.

Hypericum Perforatum (Administration of CYP3A4 inducers, such as rifampin or St. John's Wort, with tramadol hydrochloride may effect the metabolism of tramadol leading to altered tramadol exposure). Products include:
Traumeel 1800

Imatinib Mesylate (In vitro drug interaction studies in human liver microsomes indicate that concomitant administration with inhibitors of CYP2D6 could result in some inhibition of the metabolism of tramadol). Products include:
Gleevec 2477

Imipramine Hydrochloride (Tramadol hydrochloride is contraindicated in acute intoxication with psychotropic drugs).
No products indexed under this heading.

Imipramine Pamoate (Tramadol hydrochloride is contraindicated in acute intoxication with psychotropic drugs).
No products indexed under this heading.

Indinavir Sulfate (Administration of CYP3A4 inhibitors, such as ketoconazole and erythromycin, with tramadol hydrochloride may effect the metabolism of tramadol leading to altered tramadol exposure). Products include:
Crixivan 2113

Isocarboxazid (Tramadol hydrochloride is contraindicated in acute intoxication with psychotropic drugs). Products include:
Marplan 3481

Isoflurane (Tramadol hydrochloride should be used with caution and in reduced dosages when administered to patients receiving CNS depressants, such as alcohol, opioids, anesthetic agents, narcotics, phenothiazines, tranquilizers, or sedative hypnotics. Tramadol hydrochloride increases the risk of CNS and respiratory depression).
No products indexed under this heading.

Isoniazid (Administration of CYP3A4 inhibitors, such as ketoconazole and erythromycin, with tramadol hydrochloride may effect the metabolism of tramadol leading to altered tramadol exposure).
No products indexed under this heading.

Itraconazole (Administration of CYP3A4 inhibitors, such as ketoconazole and erythromycin, with tramadol hydrochloride may effect the metabolism of tramadol leading to altered tramadol exposure).
No products indexed under this heading.

Ketamine Hydrochloride (Tramadol hydrochloride should be used with caution and in reduced dosages when administered to patients receiving CNS depressants, such as alcohol, opioids, anesthetic agents, narcotics, phenothiazines, tranquilizers, or sedative hypnotics. Tramadol hydrochloride increases the risk of CNS and respiratory depression).
No products indexed under this heading.

Ketoconazole (Administration of CYP3A4 inhibitors, such as ketoconazole and erythromycin, with tramadol hydrochloride may effect the metabolism of tramadol leading to altered tramadol exposure). Products include:
Extina 3319
Xolegel 3337

Lapatinib (Administration of CYP3A4 inhibitors, such as ketoconazole and erythromycin, with tramadol hydrochloride may effect the metabolism of tramadol leading to altered tramadol exposure). Products include:
Tykerb 1698

Levobupivacaine Hydrochloride (Tramadol hydrochloride should be used with caution and in reduced dosages when administered to patients receiving CNS depressants, such as anesthetic agents. Tramadol hydrochloride increases the risk of CNS and respiratory depression).
No products indexed under this heading.

Levomethadyl Acetate Hydrochloride (Tramadol hydrochloride should be used with caution and in reduced dosages when administered to patients receiving CNS depressants, such as alcohol, opioids, anesthetic agents, narcotics, phenothiazines, tranquilizers, or sedative hypnotics. Tramadol hydrochloride increases the risk of CNS and respiratory depression).
No products indexed under this heading.

Levorphanol Tartrate (Tramadol hydrochloride is contraindicated in acute intoxication with narcotics, opioids, and centrally-acting analgesics. Concomitant use of tramadol increases the seizure risk in patients taking opioids. Tramadol hydrochloride should be used with caution and in reduced dosages when administered to patients receiving CNS depressants, such as opioids or narcotics. Tramadol hydrochloride increases the risk of CNS and respiratory depression. Tramadol may be expected to have additive effects when used in conjunction with other opioids).
No products indexed under this heading.

Lidocaine (Tramadol hydrochloride should be used with caution and in reduced dosages when administered to patients receiving CNS depressants, such as anesthetic agents. Tramadol hydrochloride increases the risk of CNS and respiratory depression). Products include:
Lidoderm 1107

Lidocaine Base (Tramadol hydrochloride should be used with caution and in reduced dosages when administered to patients receiving CNS depressants, such as anesthetic agents. Tramadol hydrochloride increases the risk of CNS and respiratory depression).
No products indexed under this heading.

Lidocaine Hydrochloride (Tramadol hydrochloride should be used with caution and in reduced dosages when administered to patients receiving CNS depressants, such as anesthetic agents. Tramadol hydrochloride increases the risk of CNS and respiratory depression).
No products indexed under this heading.

Lithium (Administration of tramadol may increase the seizure risk in patients taking neuroleptics or other drugs that reduce the seizure threshold).
No products indexed under this heading.

Lithium Carbonate (Tramadol hydrochloride is contraindicated in acute intoxication with psychotropic drugs).
No products indexed under this heading.

Lithium Citrate (Tramadol hydrochloride is contraindicated in acute intoxication with psychotropic drugs).
No products indexed under this heading.

Lopinavir (Administration of CYP3A4 inhibitors, such as ketoconazole and erythromycin, with tramadol hydrochloride may effect the metabolism of tramadol leading to altered tramadol exposure). Products include:
Kaletra 458

Loratadine (Administration of CYP3A4 inhibitors, such as ketoconazole and erythromycin, with tramadol hydrochloride may effect the metabolism of tramadol leading to altered tramadol exposure).
No products indexed under this heading.

Lorazepam (Tramadol hydrochloride is contraindicated in acute intoxication with hypnotics. Tramadol hydrochloride should be used with caution and in reduced dosages when administered to patients receiving CNS depressants, such as sedative hypnotics. Tramadol hydrochloride increases the risk of CNS and respiratory depression).
No products indexed under this heading.

Loxapine Hydrochloride (Tramadol hydrochloride is contraindicated in acute intoxication with psychotropic drugs).
No products indexed under this heading.

Loxapine Succinate (Tramadol hydrochloride is contraindicated in acute intoxication with psychotropic drugs).
No products indexed under this heading.

Maprotiline Hydrochloride (Tramadol hydrochloride is contraindicated in acute intoxication with psychotropic drugs).
No products indexed under this heading.

Meperidine Hydrochloride (Tramadol hydrochloride is contraindicated in acute intoxication with narcotics, opioids, and centrally-acting analgesics. Concomitant use of tramadol increases the seizure risk in patients taking opioids. Tramadol hydrochloride should be used with caution and in reduced dosages when administered to patients receiving CNS depressants, such as opioids or narcotics. Tramadol hydrochloride increases the risk of CNS and respiratory depression. Tramadol may be expected to have additive effects when used in conjunction with other opioids).
No products indexed under this heading.

Mephenytoin (Administration of CYP3A4 inducers, such as rifampin or St. John's Wort, with tramadol hydrochloride may effect the metabolism of tramadol leading to altered tramadol exposure).

No products indexed under this heading.

Mephobarbital (Tramadol hydrochloride should be used with caution and in reduced dosages when administered to patients receiving CNS depressants, such as alcohol, opioids, anesthetic agents, narcotics, phenothiazines, tranquilizers, or sedative hypnotics. Tramadol hydrochloride increases the risk of CNS and respiratory depression).

No products indexed under this heading.

Mepivacaine Hydrochloride (Tramadol hydrochloride should be used with caution and in reduced dosages when administered to patients receiving CNS depressants, such as anesthetic agents. Tramadol hydrochloride increases the risk of CNS and respiratory depression).

No products indexed under this heading.

Meprobamate (Tramadol hydrochloride is contraindicated in acute intoxication with psychotropic drugs).

No products indexed under this heading.

Mesoridazine Besylate (Tramadol hydrochloride is contraindicated in acute intoxication with psychotropic drugs).

No products indexed under this heading.

Methadone Hydrochloride (Tramadol hydrochloride is contraindicated in acute intoxication with narcotics, opioids, and centrally-acting analgesics. Concomitant use of tramadol increases the seizure risk in patients taking opioids. Tramadol hydrochloride should be used with caution and in reduced dosages when administered to patients receiving CNS depressants, such as opioids or narcotics. Tramadol hydrochloride increases the risk of CNS and respiratory depression. Tramadol may be expected to have additive effects when used in conjunction with other opioids).

No products indexed under this heading.

Methohexital Sodium (Tramadol hydrochloride should be used with caution and in reduced dosages when administered to patients receiving CNS depressants, such as alcohol, opioids, anesthetic agents, narcotics, phenothiazines, tranquilizers, or sedative hypnotics. Tramadol hydrochloride increases the risk of CNS and respiratory depression).

No products indexed under this heading.

Methotrimeprazine (Administration of tramadol may increase the seizure risk in patients taking neuroleptics or other drugs that reduce the seizure threshold).

No products indexed under this heading.

Methoxyflurane (Tramadol hydrochloride should be used with caution and in reduced dosages when administered to patients receiving CNS depressants, such as alcohol, opioids, anesthetic agents, narcotics, phenothiazines, tranquilizers, or sedative hypnotics. Tramadol hydrochloride increases the risk of CNS and respiratory depression).

No products indexed under this heading.

Methsuximide (Administration of CYP3A4 inducers, such as rifampin or St. John's Wort, with tramadol hydrochloride may effect the metabolism of tramadol leading to altered tramadol exposure).

No products indexed under this heading.

Methylprednisolone (Administration of CYP3A4 inducers, such as rifampin or St. John's Wort, with tramadol hydrochloride may effect the metabolism of tramadol leading to altered tramadol exposure).

No products indexed under this heading.

Methylprednisolone Acetate (Administration of CYP3A4 inducers, such as rifampin or St. John's Wort, with tramadol hydrochloride may effect the metabolism of tramadol leading to altered tramadol exposure).

No products indexed under this heading.

Methylprednisolone Sodium Succinate (Administration of CYP3A4 inducers, such as rifampin or St. John's Wort, with tramadol hydrochloride may effect the metabolism of tramadol leading to altered tramadol exposure).

No products indexed under this heading.

Metronidazole (Administration of CYP3A4 inhibitors, such as ketoconazole and erythromycin, with tramadol hydrochloride may effect the metabolism of tramadol leading to altered tramadol exposure). Products include:
Pylera 793

Metronidazole Benzoate (Administration of CYP3A4 inhibitors, such as ketoconazole and erythromycin, with tramadol hydrochloride may effect the metabolism of tramadol leading to altered tramadol exposure).

No products indexed under this heading.

Metronidazole Hydrochloride (Administration of CYP3A4 inhibitors, such as ketoconazole and erythromycin, with tramadol hydrochloride may effect the metabolism of tramadol leading to altered tramadol exposure).

No products indexed under this heading.

Metronidazole Sodium (Administration of CYP3A4 inhibitors, such as ketoconazole and erythromycin, with tramadol hydrochloride may effect the metabolism of tramadol leading to altered tramadol exposure).

No products indexed under this heading.

Mibefradil Dihydrochloride (In vitro drug interaction studies in human liver microsomes indicate that concomitant administration with inhibitors of CYP2D6 could result in some inhibition of the metabolism of tramadol).

No products indexed under this heading.

Miconazole (Administration of CYP3A4 inhibitors, such as ketoconazole and erythromycin, with tramadol hydrochloride may effect the metabolism of tramadol leading to altered tramadol exposure).

No products indexed under this heading.

Miconazole Nitrate (Administration of CYP3A4 inhibitors, such as ketoconazole and erythromycin, with tramadol hydrochloride may effect the metabolism of tramadol leading to altered tramadol exposure). Products include:
Vusion Ointment 3335

Midazolam Hydrochloride (Tramadol hydrochloride is contraindicated in acute intoxication with hypnotics. Tramadol hydrochloride should be used with caution and in reduced dosages when administered to patients receiving CNS depressants, such as sedative hypnotics. Tramadol hydrochloride increases the risk of CNS and respiratory depression).

No products indexed under this heading.

Mifepristone (Administration of CYP3A4 inhibitors, such as ketoconazole and erythromycin, with tramadol hydrochloride may effect the metabolism of tramadol leading to altered tramadol exposure).

No products indexed under this heading.

Moclobemide (Administration of tramadol may increase the seizure risk in patients taking monoamine oxidase inhibitors or other drugs that reduce the seizure threshold. Use tramadol with great caution in patients taking MAO inhibitors. Concomitant use of tramadol with MAO inhibitors increases the risk of adverse events, including seizure and serotonin syndrome).

No products indexed under this heading.

Modafinil (Administration of CYP3A4 inducers, such as rifampin or St. John's Wort, with tramadol hydrochloride may effect the metabolism of tramadol leading to altered tramadol exposure). Products include:
Provigil 983

Molindone Hydrochloride (Tramadol hydrochloride is contraindicated in acute intoxication with psychotropic drugs). Products include:
Moban 1108

Morphine Sulfate (Tramadol hydrochloride is contraindicated in acute intoxication with narcotics, opioids, and centrally-acting analgesics. Concomitant use of tramadol increases the seizure risk in patients taking opioids. Tramadol hydrochloride should be used with caution and in reduced dosages when administered to patients receiving CNS depressants, such as opioids or narcotics. Tramadol hydrochloride increases the risk of CNS and respiratory depression. Tramadol may be expected to have additive effects when used in conjunction with other opioids). Products include:
Avinza 1822
Embeda 1831
MS Contin 2803

Morphine Sulfate, Liposomal (Tramadol hydrochloride is contraindicated in acute intoxication with narcotics, opioids, and centrally-acting analgesics. Concomitant use of tramadol increases the seizure risk in patients taking opioids. Tramadol hydrochloride should be used with caution and in reduced dosages when administered to patients receiving CNS depressants, such as opioids or narcotics. Tramadol hydrochloride increases the risk of CNS and respiratory depression. Tramadol may be expected to have additive effects when used in conjunction with other opioids).

No products indexed under this heading.

Nafcillin Sodium (Administration of CYP3A4 inducers, such as rifampin or St. John's Wort, with tramadol hydrochloride may effect the metabolism of tramadol leading to altered tramadol exposure).

No products indexed under this heading.

Naratriptan Hydrochloride (Concomitant use of tramadol increases the seizure risk in patients taking triptans. Concomitant use of tramadol with triptans increases the risk of adverse events, including seizure and serotonin syndrome. If concomitant treatment of tramadol with a drug affecting the serotonergic neurotransmitter system is clinically warranted, careful observation of the patient is advised, particularly during treatment initiation and dose increases). Products include:
Amerge 1306

Nefazodone Hydrochloride (Administration of CYP3A4 inhibitors, such as ketoconazole and erythromycin, with tramadol hydrochloride may effect the metabolism of tramadol leading to altered tramadol exposure).

No products indexed under this heading.

Nelfinavir Mesylate (Administration of CYP3A4 inhibitors, such as ketoconazole and erythromycin, with tramadol hydrochloride may effect the metabolism of tramadol leading to altered tramadol exposure).

No products indexed under this heading.

Nevirapine (Administration of CYP3A4 inhibitors, such as ketoconazole and erythromycin, with tramadol hydrochloride may effect the metabolism of tramadol leading to altered tramadol exposure). Products include:
Viramune Oral Suspension 897
Viramune Tablets 897

Niacin (Administration of CYP3A4 inhibitors, such as ketoconazole and erythromycin, with tramadol hydrochloride may effect the metabolism of tramadol leading to altered tramadol exposure). Products include:
Advicor 402
Cardio Basics 3455
Niaspan 497
Simcor 524

Niacinamide (Administration of CYP3A4 inhibitors, such as ketoconazole and erythromycin, with tramadol hydrochloride may effect the metabolism of tramadol leading to altered tramadol exposure). Products include:
CitraNatal 90 DHA Capsules 2332
CitraNatal Assure 2332
CitraNatal Rx 2332
Heplive 607

Niacinamide Hydroiodide (Administration of CYP3A4 inhibitors, such as ketoconazole and erythromycin, with tramadol hydrochloride may effect the metabolism of tramadol leading to altered tramadol exposure).

No products indexed under this heading.

Nicotinamide (Administration of CYP3A4 inhibitors, such as ketoconazole and erythromycin, with tramadol hydrochloride may effect the metabolism of tramadol leading to altered tramadol exposure).

No products indexed under this heading.

Nifedipine (Administration of CYP3A4 inhibitors, such as ketoconazole and erythromycin, with tramadol hydrochloride may effect the metabolism of tramadol leading to altered tramadol exposure).

No products indexed under this heading.

Norfloxacin (Administration of CYP3A4 inhibitors, such as ketoconazole and erythromycin, with tramadol hydrochloride may effect the metabolism of tramadol leading to altered tramadol exposure). Products include:
Noroxin 2220

Nortriptyline Hydrochloride (Tramadol hydrochloride is contraindicated in acute intoxication with psychotropic drugs).

No products indexed under this heading.

Olanzapine (Tramadol hydrochloride is contraindicated in acute intoxication with psychotropic drugs). Products include:
Symbyax 1965
Zyprexa 1984
Zyprexa IntraMuscular 1984
Zyprexa ZYDIS 1984

Omeprazole (Administration of CYP3A4 inhibitors, such as ketoconazole and erythromycin, with tramadol hydrochloride may effect the metabolism of tramadol leading to altered tramadol exposure).

No products indexed under this heading.

Oxazepam (Tramadol hydrochloride is contraindicated in acute intoxication with psychotropic drugs).

No products indexed under this heading.

IMPORTANT NOTE: Always consult each drug listing in the patient's regimen for possible interactions.

Ultram **Interactions Index** 1976

Oxcarbazepine (Administration of CYP3A4 inducers, such as rifampin or St. John's Wort, with tramadol hydrochloride may effect the metabolism of tramadol leading to altered tramadol exposure).
No products indexed under this heading.

Oxycodone Hydrochloride (Tramadol hydrochloride is contraindicated in acute intoxication with narcotics, opioids, and centrally-acting analgesics. Concomitant use of tramadol increases the seizure risk in patients taking opioids. Tramadol hydrochloride should be used with caution and in reduced dosages when administered to patients receiving CNS depressants, such as opioids or narcotics. Tramadol hydrochloride increases the risk of CNS and respiratory depression. Tramadol may be expected to have additive effects when used in conjunction with other opioids). Products include:
OxyContin 2807
Percocet 1121
Percodan 1124

Oxycodone Terephthalate (Tramadol hydrochloride is contraindicated in acute intoxication with narcotics, opioids, and centrally-acting analgesics. Concomitant use of tramadol increases the seizure risk in patients taking opioids. Tramadol hydrochloride should be used with caution and in reduced dosages when administered to patients receiving CNS depressants, such as opioids or narcotics. Tramadol hydrochloride increases the risk of CNS and respiratory depression. Tramadol may be expected to have additive effects when used in conjunction with other opioids).
No products indexed under this heading.

Oxymorphone Hydrochloride (Tramadol hydrochloride is contraindicated in acute intoxication with narcotics, opioids, and centrally-acting analgesics. Concomitant use of tramadol increases the seizure risk in patients taking opioids. Tramadol hydrochloride should be used with caution and in reduced dosages when administered to patients receiving CNS depressants, such as opioids or narcotics. Tramadol hydrochloride increases the risk of CNS and respiratory depression. Tramadol may be expected to have additive effects when used in conjunction with other opioids). Products include:
Opana 1110
Opana ER 1114

Paliperidone (Tramadol hydrochloride is contraindicated in acute intoxication with psychotropic drugs). Products include:
Invega 2613
Invega Sustenna 2621

Pargyline Hydrochloride (Administration of tramadol may increase the seizure risk in patients taking monoamine oxidase inhibitors or other drugs that reduce the seizure threshold. Use tramadol with great caution in patients taking MAO inhibitors. Concomitant use of tramadol with MAO inhibitors increases the risk of adverse events, including seizure and serotonin syndrome).
No products indexed under this heading.

Paroxetine (Concomitant use of tramadol increases the seizure risk in patients taking selective serotonin reuptake inhibitors. Concomitant use of tramadol with SSRIs increases the risk of adverse events, including seizure and serotonin syndrome).
No products indexed under this heading.

Paroxetine Hydrochloride (Concomitant use of tramadol increases the seizure risk in patients taking selective serotonin re-uptake inhibitors. Concomitant use of tramadol with SSRIs increases the risk of adverse events, including seizure and serotonin syndrome). Products include:
Paroxetine CR 2361
Paroxetine ER 2371
Paxil 1586
Paxil CR 1596

Paroxetine Mesylate (Concomitant use of tramadol increases the seizure risk in patients taking selective serotonin re-uptake inhibitors. Concomitant use of tramadol with SSRIs increases the risk of adverse events, including seizure and serotonin syndrome).
No products indexed under this heading.

Pentobarbital (Tramadol hydrochloride should be used with caution and in reduced dosages when administered to patients receiving CNS depressants, such as alcohol, opioids, anesthetic agents, narcotics, phenothiazines, tranquilizers, or sedative hypnotics. Tramadol hydrochloride increases the risk of CNS and respiratory depression).
No products indexed under this heading.

Pentobarbital Sodium (Tramadol hydrochloride should be used with caution and in reduced dosages when administered to patients receiving CNS depressants, such as alcohol, opioids, anesthetic agents, narcotics, phenothiazines, tranquilizers, or sedative hypnotics. Tramadol hydrochloride increases the risk of CNS and respiratory depression). Products include:
Nembutal 2012

Perphenazine (Tramadol hydrochloride is contraindicated in acute intoxication with psychotropic drugs).
No products indexed under this heading.

Phenelzine Sulfate (Tramadol hydrochloride is contraindicated in acute intoxication with psychotropic drugs).
No products indexed under this heading.

Phenobarbital (Tramadol hydrochloride should be used with caution and in reduced dosages when administered to patients receiving CNS depressants, such as alcohol, opioids, anesthetic agents, narcotics, phenothiazines, tranquilizers, or sedative hypnotics. Tramadol hydrochloride increases the risk of CNS and respiratory depression). Products include:
Donnatal 2711

Phenobarbital Sodium (Tramadol hydrochloride should be used with caution and in reduced dosages when administered to patients receiving CNS depressants, such as alcohol, opioids, anesthetic agents, narcotics, phenothiazines, tranquilizers, or sedative hypnotics. Tramadol hydrochloride increases the risk of CNS and respiratory depression).
No products indexed under this heading.

Phenothiazine Derivatives (Tramadol hydrochloride should be used with caution and in reduced dosages when administered to patients receiving CNS depressants, such as phenothiazines. Tramadol hydrochloride increases the risk of CNS and respiratory depression).
No products indexed under this heading.

Phenothiazines (Tramadol hydrochloride should be used with caution and in reduced dosages when administered to patients receiving CNS depressants, such as phenothiazines. Tramadol hydrochloride increases the risk of CNS and respiratory depression).
No products indexed under this heading.

Phenytoin (Administration of CYP3A4 inducers, such as rifampin or St. John's Wort, with tramadol hydrochloride may effect the metabolism of tramadol leading to altered tramadol exposure).
No products indexed under this heading.

Phenytoin Sodium (Administration of CYP3A4 inducers, such as rifampin or St. John's Wort, with tramadol hydrochloride may effect the metabolism of tramadol leading to altered tramadol exposure). Products include:
Phenytek Capsules 2380

Pimozide (Administration of tramadol may increase the seizure risk in patients taking neuroleptics or other drugs that reduce the seizure threshold).
No products indexed under this heading.

Posaconazole (Administration of CYP3A4 inhibitors, such as ketoconazole and erythromycin, with tramadol hydrochloride may effect the metabolism of tramadol leading to altered tramadol exposure). Products include:
Noxafil 3172

Prazepam (Tramadol hydrochloride is contraindicated in acute intoxication with psychotropic drugs).
No products indexed under this heading.

Prednisolone (Administration of CYP3A4 inducers, such as rifampin or St. John's Wort, with tramadol hydrochloride may effect the metabolism of tramadol leading to altered tramadol exposure).
No products indexed under this heading.

Prednisolone Acetate (Administration of CYP3A4 inducers, such as rifampin or St. John's Wort, with tramadol hydrochloride may effect the metabolism of tramadol leading to altered tramadol exposure). Products include:
Blephamide .... ⊙212, ⊙214
Pred Forte .... ⊙225
Pred Mild .... ⊙230
Pred-G .... ⊙226, ⊙227

Prednisolone Sodium Phosphate (Administration of CYP3A4 inducers, such as rifampin or St. John's Wort, with tramadol hydrochloride may effect the metabolism of tramadol leading to altered tramadol exposure).
No products indexed under this heading.

Prednisolone Tebutate (Administration of CYP3A4 inducers, such as rifampin or St. John's Wort, with tramadol hydrochloride may effect the metabolism of tramadol leading to altered tramadol exposure).
No products indexed under this heading.

Prednisone (Administration of CYP3A4 inducers, such as rifampin or St. John's Wort, with tramadol hydrochloride may effect the metabolism of tramadol leading to altered tramadol exposure).
No products indexed under this heading.

Prednisone sodium phosphate (Administration of CYP3A4 inducers, such as rifampin or St. John's Wort, with tramadol hydrochloride may effect the metabolism of tramadol leading to altered tramadol exposure).
No products indexed under this heading.

Prilocaine (Tramadol hydrochloride should be used with caution and in reduced dosages when administered to patients receiving CNS depressants, such as anesthetic agents. Tramadol hydrochloride increases the risk of CNS and respiratory depression).
No products indexed under this heading.

Prilocaine Hydrochloride (Tramadol hydrochloride should be used with caution and in reduced dosages when administered to patients receiving CNS depressants, such as anesthetic agents. Tramadol hydrochloride increases the risk of CNS and respiratory depression).
No products indexed under this heading.

Primidone (Administration of CYP3A4 inducers, such as rifampin or St. John's Wort, with tramadol hydrochloride may effect the metabolism of tramadol leading to altered tramadol exposure).
No products indexed under this heading.

Procaine (Tramadol hydrochloride should be used with caution and in reduced dosages when administered to patients receiving CNS depressants, such as anesthetic agents. Tramadol hydrochloride increases the risk of CNS and respiratory depression).
No products indexed under this heading.

Procaine Hydrochloride (Tramadol hydrochloride should be used with caution and in reduced dosages when administered to patients receiving CNS depressants, such as anesthetic agents. Tramadol hydrochloride increases the risk of CNS and respiratory depression).
No products indexed under this heading.

Procarbazine Hydrochloride (Administration of tramadol may increase the seizure risk in patients taking monoamine oxidase inhibitors or other drugs that reduce the seizure threshold. Use tramadol with great caution in patients taking MAO inhibitors. Concomitant use of tramadol with MAO inhibitors increases the risk of adverse events, including seizure and serotonin syndrome).
No products indexed under this heading.

Prochlorperazine (Tramadol hydrochloride is contraindicated in acute intoxication with psychotropic drugs).
No products indexed under this heading.

Prochlorperazine Edisylate (Tramadol hydrochloride should be used with caution and in reduced dosages when administered to patients receiving CNS depressants, such as alcohol, opioids, anesthetic agents, narcotics, phenothiazines, tranquilizers, or sedative hypnotics. Tramadol hydrochloride increases the risk of CNS and respiratory depression).
No products indexed under this heading.

Prochlorperazine Maleate (Tramadol hydrochloride should be used with caution and in reduced dosages when administered to patients receiving CNS depressants, such as alcohol, opioids, anesthetic agents, narcotics, phenothiazines, tranquilizers, or sedative hypnotics. Tramadol hydrochloride increases the risk of CNS and respiratory depression).
No products indexed under this heading.

Promethazine (Concomitant use of tramadol increases the seizure risk in patients taking tricyclic compounds, such as promethazine).
No products indexed under this heading.

Promethazine Hydrochloride (Concomitant use of tramadol increases the seizure risk in patients taking tricyclic compounds, such as promethazine).
No products indexed under this heading.

Propafenone Hydrochloride (In vitro drug interaction studies in human liver microsomes indicate that concomitant administration with inhibitors of CYP2D6 could result in some inhibition of the metabolism of tramadol). Products include:
Rythmol 1648
Rythmol SR 1652

Proparacaine Hydrochloride (Tramadol hydrochloride should be used with caution and in reduced dosages when administered to patients receiving CNS depressants, such as anesthetic agents. Tramadol hydrochloride increases the risk of CNS and respiratory depression).
No products indexed under this heading.

1977 Interactions Index Ultram

Propofol (Tramadol hydrochloride is contraindicated in acute intoxication with hypnotics. Tramadol hydrochloride should be used with caution and in reduced dosages when administered to patients receiving CNS depressants, such as sedative hypnotics. Tramadol hydrochloride increases the risk of CNS and respiratory depression).
No products indexed under this heading.

Propoxyphene Hydrochloride (Tramadol hydrochloride is contraindicated in acute intoxication with narcotics, opioids, and centrally-acting analgesics. Concomitant use of tramadol increases the seizure risk in patients taking opioids. Tramadol hydrochloride should be used with caution and in reduced dosages when administered to patients receiving CNS depressants, such as opioids or narcotics. Tramadol hydrochloride increases the risk of CNS and respiratory depression. Tramadol may be expected to have additive effects when used in conjunction with other opioids).
No products indexed under this heading.

Propoxyphene Napsylate (Tramadol hydrochloride is contraindicated in acute intoxication with narcotics, opioids, and centrally-acting analgesics. Concomitant use of tramadol increases the seizure risk in patients taking opioids. Tramadol hydrochloride should be used with caution and in reduced dosages when administered to patients receiving CNS depressants, such as opioids or narcotics. Tramadol hydrochloride increases the risk of CNS and respiratory depression. Tramadol may be expected to have additive effects when used in conjunction with other opioids).
No products indexed under this heading.

Protriptyline Hydrochloride (Tramadol hydrochloride is contraindicated in acute intoxication with psychotropic drugs).
No products indexed under this heading.

Quazepam (Tramadol hydrochloride is contraindicated in acute intoxication with hypnotics. Tramadol hydrochloride should be used with caution and in reduced dosages when administered to patients receiving CNS depressants, such as sedative hypnotics. Tramadol hydrochloride increases the risk of CNS and respiratory depression).
No products indexed under this heading.

Quetiapine Fumarate (Tramadol hydrochloride is contraindicated in acute intoxication with psychotropic drugs). Products include:
Seroquel 750
Seroquel XR 759

Quinacrine Hydrochloride (In vitro drug interaction studies in human liver microsomes indicate that concomitant administration with inhibitors of CYP2D6 could result in some inhibition of the metabolism of tramadol).
No products indexed under this heading.

Quinidine (In vitro drug interaction studies in human liver microsomes indicate that concomitant administration with inhibitors of CYP2D6 could result in some inhibition of the metabolism of tramadol).
No products indexed under this heading.

Quinidine Gluconate (In vitro drug interaction studies in human liver microsomes indicate that concomitant administration with inhibitors of CYP2D6 could result in some inhibition of the metabolism of tramadol).
No products indexed under this heading.

Quinidine Hydrochloride (In vitro drug interaction studies in human liver microsomes indicate that concomitant administration with inhibitors of CYP2D6 could result in some inhibition of the metabolism of tramadol).
No products indexed under this heading.

Quinidine Polygalacturonate (In vitro drug interaction studies in human liver microsomes indicate that concomitant administration with inhibitors of CYP2D6 could result in some inhibition of the metabolism of tramadol).
No products indexed under this heading.

Quinidine Sulfate (In vitro drug interaction studies in human liver microsomes indicate that concomitant administration with inhibitors of CYP2D6 could result in some inhibition of the metabolism of tramadol).
No products indexed under this heading.

Quinine (Administration of CYP3A4 inhibitors, such as ketoconazole and erythromycin, with tramadol hydrochloride may effect the metabolism of tramadol leading to altered tramadol exposure). Products include:
Hyland's Leg Cramps PM with Quinine 3315

Quinine Sulfate (Administration of CYP3A4 inhibitors, such as ketoconazole and erythromycin, with tramadol hydrochloride may effect the metabolism of tramadol leading to altered tramadol exposure).
No products indexed under this heading.

Quinupristin (Administration of CYP3A4 inhibitors, such as ketoconazole and erythromycin, with tramadol hydrochloride may effect the metabolism of tramadol leading to altered tramadol exposure).
No products indexed under this heading.

Ramelteon (Tramadol hydrochloride is contraindicated in acute intoxication with hypnotics. Tramadol hydrochloride should be used with caution and in reduced dosages when administered to patients receiving CNS depressants, such as sedative hypnotics. Tramadol hydrochloride increases the risk of CNS and respiratory depression). Products include:
Rozerem 3366

Ranitidine Bismuth Citrate (In vitro drug interaction studies in human liver microsomes indicate that concomitant administration with inhibitors of CYP2D6 could result in some inhibition of the metabolism of tramadol).
No products indexed under this heading.

Ranitidine Hydrochloride (In vitro drug interaction studies in human liver microsomes indicate that concomitant administration with inhibitors of CYP2D6 could result in some inhibition of the metabolism of tramadol). Products include:
Zantac 1737
Zantac Injection 1732
Zantac Pharmacy 1735

Rasagiline Mesylate (Administration of tramadol may increase the seizure risk in patients taking monoamine oxidase inhibitors or other drugs that reduce the seizure threshold. Use tramadol with great caution in patients taking MAO inhibitors. Concomitant use of tramadol with MAO inhibitors increases the risk of adverse events, including seizure and serotonin syndrome). Products include:
Azilect 3383

Remifentanil Hydrochloride (Tramadol hydrochloride is contraindicated in acute intoxication with narcotics, opioids, and centrally-acting analgesics. Concomitant use of tramadol increases the seizure risk in patients taking opioids. Tramadol hydrochloride should be used with caution and in reduced dosages when administered to patients receiving CNS depressants, such as opioids or narcotics. Tramadol hydrochloride increases the risk of CNS and respiratory depression. Tramadol may be expected to have additive effects when used in conjunction with other opioids).
No products indexed under this heading.

Rifabutin (Administration of CYP3A4 inducers, such as rifampin or St. John's Wort, with tramadol hydrochloride may effect the metabolism of tramadol leading to altered tramadol exposure).
No products indexed under this heading.

Rifampicin (Administration of CYP3A4 inducers, such as rifampin or St. John's Wort, with tramadol hydrochloride may effect the metabolism of tramadol leading to altered tramadol exposure).
No products indexed under this heading.

Rifampin (Administration of CYP3A4 inducers, such as rifampin or St. John's Wort, with tramadol hydrochloride may effect the metabolism of tramadol leading to altered tramadol exposure).
No products indexed under this heading.

Rifapentine (Administration of CYP3A4 inducers, such as rifampin or St. John's Wort, with tramadol hydrochloride may effect the metabolism of tramadol leading to altered tramadol exposure).
No products indexed under this heading.

Risperidone (Tramadol hydrochloride is contraindicated in acute intoxication with psychotropic drugs). Products include:
Risperdal Consta 2682

Ritonavir (In vitro drug interaction studies in human liver microsomes indicate that concomitant administration with inhibitors of CYP2D6 could result in some inhibition of the metabolism of tramadol). Products include:
Kaletra 458
Norvir 509

Rizatriptan Benzoate (Concomitant use of tramadol increases the seizure risk in patients taking triptans. Concomitant use of tramadol with triptans increases the risk of adverse events, including seizure and serotonin syndrome. If concomitant treatment of tramadol with a drug affecting the serotonergic neurotransmitter system is clinically warranted, careful observation of the patient is advised, particularly during treatment initiation and dose increases). Products include:
Maxalt 2206
Maxalt-MLT 2206

Ropivacaine Hydrochloride (Tramadol hydrochloride should be used with caution and in reduced dosages when administered to patients receiving CNS depressants, such as anesthetic agents. Tramadol hydrochloride increases the risk of CNS and respiratory depression).
No products indexed under this heading.

Saquinavir (Administration of CYP3A4 inhibitors, such as ketoconazole and erythromycin, with tramadol hydrochloride may effect the metabolism of tramadol leading to altered tramadol exposure).
No products indexed under this heading.

Saquinavir Mesylate (Administration of CYP3A4 inhibitors, such as ketoconazole and erythromycin, with tramadol hydrochloride may effect the metabolism of tramadol leading to altered tramadol exposure).
No products indexed under this heading.

Secobarbital Sodium (Tramadol hydrochloride is contraindicated in acute intoxication with hypnotics. Tramadol hydrochloride should be used with caution and in reduced dosages when administered to patients receiving CNS depressants, such as sedative hypnotics. Tramadol hydrochloride increases the risk of CNS and respiratory depression).
No products indexed under this heading.

Selegiline (Administration of tramadol may increase the seizure risk in patients taking monoamine oxidase inhibitors or other drugs that reduce the seizure threshold. Use tramadol with great caution in patients taking MAO inhibitors. Concomitant use of tramadol with MAO inhibitors increases the risk of adverse events, including seizure and serotonin syndrome). Products include:
Emsam 3623

Selegiline Hydrochloride (Administration of tramadol may increase the seizure risk in patients taking monoamine oxidase inhibitors or other drugs that reduce the seizure threshold. Use tramadol with great caution in patients taking MAO inhibitors. Concomitant use of tramadol with MAO inhibitors increases the risk of adverse events, including seizure and serotonin syndrome). Products include:
Eldepryl 3312

Sertraline Hydrochloride (Concomitant use of tramadol increases the seizure risk in patients taking selective serotonin re-uptake inhibitors. Concomitant use of tramadol with SSRIs increases the risk of adverse events, including seizure and serotonin syndrome).
No products indexed under this heading.

Sevoflurane (Tramadol hydrochloride should be used with caution and in reduced dosages when administered to patients receiving CNS depressants, such as alcohol, opioids, anesthetic agents, narcotics, phenothiazines, tranquilizers, or sedative hypnotics. Tramadol hydrochloride increases the risk of CNS and respiratory depression). Products include:
Ultane 554

Sildenafil Citrate (In vitro drug interaction studies in human liver microsomes indicate that concomitant administration with inhibitors of CYP2D6 could result in some inhibition of the metabolism of tramadol).
No products indexed under this heading.

Sodium Butabarbital (Tramadol hydrochloride is contraindicated in acute intoxication with hypnotics. Tramadol hydrochloride should be used with caution and in reduced dosages when administered to patients receiving CNS depressants, such as sedative hypnotics. Tramadol hydrochloride increases the risk of CNS and respiratory depression).
No products indexed under this heading.

Sodium Oxybate (Tramadol hydrochloride should be used with caution and in reduced dosages when administered to patients receiving CNS depressants, such as alcohol, opioids, anesthetic agents, narcotics, phenothiazines, tranquilizers, or sedative hypnotics. Tramadol hydrochloride increases the risk of CNS and respiratory depression).
No products indexed under this heading.

IMPORTANT NOTE: Always consult each drug listing in the patient's regimen for possible interactions.

Ultram Interactions Index 1978

Sodium Pentobarbital (Tramadol hydrochloride should be used with caution and in reduced dosages when administered to patients receiving CNS depressants, such as alcohol, opioids, anesthetic agents, narcotics, phenothiazines, tranquilizers, or sedative hypnotics. Tramadol hydrochloride increases the risk of CNS and respiratory depression).
No products indexed under this heading.

Sufentanil Citrate (Tramadol hydrochloride is contraindicated in acute intoxication with narcotics, opioids, and centrally-acting analgesics. Concomitant use of tramadol increases the seizure risk in patients taking opioids. Tramadol hydrochloride should be used with caution and in reduced dosages when administered to patients receiving CNS depressants, such as opioids or narcotics. Tramadol hydrochloride increases the risk of CNS and respiratory depression. Tramadol may be expected to have additive effects when used in conjunction with other opioids).
No products indexed under this heading.

Sulfinpyrazone (Administration of CYP3A4 inducers, such as rifampin or St. John's Wort, with tramadol hydrochloride may effect the metabolism of tramadol leading to altered tramadol exposure).
No products indexed under this heading.

Sumatriptan (Concomitant use of tramadol increases the seizure risk in patients taking triptans. Concomitant use of tramadol with triptans increases the risk of adverse events, including seizure and serotonin syndrome. If concomitant treatment of tramadol with a drug affecting the serotonergic neurotransmitter system is clinically warranted, careful observation of the patient is advised, particularly during treatment initiation and dose increases). Products include:
Imitrex Nasal 1503

Sumatriptan Succinate (Concomitant use of tramadol increases the seizure risk in patients taking triptans. Concomitant use of tramadol with triptans increases the risk of adverse events, including seizure and serotonin syndrome. If concomitant treatment of tramadol with a drug affecting the serotonergic neurotransmitter system is clinically warranted, careful observation of the patient is advised, particularly during treatment initiation and dose increases). Products include:
Imitrex 1497
Imitrex Tablets 1508
Treximet 1681

Talbutal (Tramadol hydrochloride should be used with caution and in reduced dosages when administered to patients receiving CNS depressants, such as alcohol, opioids, anesthetic agents, narcotics, phenothiazines, tranquilizers, or sedative hypnotics. Tramadol hydrochloride increases the risk of CNS and respiratory depression).
No products indexed under this heading.

Telithromycin (Administration of CYP3A4 inhibitors, such as ketoconazole and erythromycin, with tramadol hydrochloride may effect the metabolism of tramadol leading to altered tramadol exposure). Products include:
Ketek 2991

Temazepam (Tramadol hydrochloride is contraindicated in acute intoxication with hypnotics. Tramadol hydrochloride should be used with caution and in reduced dosages when administered to patients receiving CNS depressants, such as sedative hypnotics. Tramadol hydrochloride increases the risk of CNS and respiratory depression).
No products indexed under this heading.

Terbinafine Hydrochloride (In vitro drug interaction studies in human liver microsomes indicate that concomitant administration with inhibitors of CYP2D6 could result in some inhibition of the metabolism of tramadol).
No products indexed under this heading.

Tetracaine (Tramadol hydrochloride should be used with caution and in reduced dosages when administered to patients receiving CNS depressants, such as anesthetic agents. Tramadol hydrochloride increases the risk of CNS and respiratory depression).
No products indexed under this heading.

Tetracaine Hydrochloride (Tramadol hydrochloride should be used with caution and in reduced dosages when administered to patients receiving CNS depressants, such as anesthetic agents. Tramadol hydrochloride increases the risk of CNS and respiratory depression).
No products indexed under this heading.

Theophyllinate (Administration of CYP3A4 inducers, such as rifampin or St. John's Wort, with tramadol hydrochloride may effect the metabolism of tramadol leading to altered tramadol exposure).
No products indexed under this heading.

Theophylline (Administration of CYP3A4 inducers, such as rifampin or St. John's Wort, with tramadol hydrochloride may effect the metabolism of tramadol leading to altered tramadol exposure).
No products indexed under this heading.

Theophylline Anhydrous (Administration of CYP3A4 inducers, such as rifampin or St. John's Wort, with tramadol hydrochloride may effect the metabolism of tramadol leading to altered tramadol exposure). Products include:
Uniphyl 2817

Theophylline Calcium Salicylate (Administration of CYP3A4 inducers, such as rifampin or St. John's Wort, with tramadol hydrochloride may effect the metabolism of tramadol leading to altered tramadol exposure).
No products indexed under this heading.

Theophylline Dihydroxypropyl (Glyceryl) (Administration of CYP3A4 inducers, such as rifampin or St. John's Wort, with tramadol hydrochloride may effect the metabolism of tramadol leading to altered tramadol exposure).
No products indexed under this heading.

Theophylline Ethylenediamine (Administration of CYP3A4 inducers, such as rifampin or St. John's Wort, with tramadol hydrochloride may effect the metabolism of tramadol leading to altered tramadol exposure).
No products indexed under this heading.

Theophylline Sodium Glycinate (Administration of CYP3A4 inducers, such as rifampin or St. John's Wort, with tramadol hydrochloride may effect the metabolism of tramadol leading to altered tramadol exposure).
No products indexed under this heading.

Thiamylal Sodium (Tramadol hydrochloride should be used with caution and in reduced dosages when administered to patients receiving CNS depressants, such as alcohol, opioids, anesthetic agents, narcotics, phenothiazines, tranquilizers, or sedative hypnotics. Tramadol hydrochloride increases the risk of CNS and respiratory depression).
No products indexed under this heading.

Thioridazine (Tramadol hydrochloride should be used with caution and in reduced dosages when administered to patients receiving CNS depressants, such as alcohol, opioids, anesthetic agents, narcotics, phenothiazines, tranquilizers, or sedative hypnotics. Tramadol hydrochloride increases the risk of CNS and respiratory depression).
No products indexed under this heading.

Thioridazine Hydrochloride (Tramadol hydrochloride is contraindicated in acute intoxication with psychotropic drugs). Products include:
Thioridazine Hydrochloride 2384

Thiothixene (Tramadol hydrochloride is contraindicated in acute intoxication with psychotropic drugs). Products include:
Thiothixene 2386

Thiothixene Hydrochloride (Tramadol hydrochloride should be used with caution and in reduced dosages when administered to patients receiving CNS depressants, such as alcohol, opioids, anesthetic agents, narcotics, phenothiazines, tranquilizers, or sedative hypnotics. Tramadol hydrochloride increases the risk of CNS and respiratory depression).
No products indexed under this heading.

Tranylcypromine Sulfate (Tramadol hydrochloride is contraindicated in acute intoxication with psychotropic drugs). Products include:
Parnate 1584

Triamcinolone (Administration of CYP3A4 inducers, such as rifampin or St. John's Wort, with tramadol hydrochloride may effect the metabolism of tramadol leading to altered tramadol exposure).
No products indexed under this heading.

Triamcinolone Acetonide (Administration of CYP3A4 inducers, such as rifampin or St. John's Wort, with tramadol hydrochloride may effect the metabolism of tramadol leading to altered tramadol exposure). Products include:
Azmacort 408
Nasacort AQ 3019

Triamcinolone Diacetate (Administration of CYP3A4 inducers, such as rifampin or St. John's Wort, with tramadol hydrochloride may effect the metabolism of tramadol leading to altered tramadol exposure).
No products indexed under this heading.

Triamcinolone Hexacetonide (Administration of CYP3A4 inducers, such as rifampin or St. John's Wort, with tramadol hydrochloride may effect the metabolism of tramadol leading to altered tramadol exposure).
No products indexed under this heading.

Triazolam (Tramadol hydrochloride is contraindicated in acute intoxication with hypnotics. Tramadol hydrochloride should be used with caution and in reduced dosages when administered to patients receiving CNS depressants, such as sedative hypnotics. Tramadol hydrochloride increases the risk of CNS and respiratory depression).
No products indexed under this heading.

Trifluoperazine Hydrochloride (Tramadol hydrochloride is contraindicated in acute intoxication with psychotropic drugs).
No products indexed under this heading.

Trimipramine Maleate (Tramadol hydrochloride is contraindicated in acute intoxication with psychotropic drugs).
No products indexed under this heading.

Troglitazone (Administration of CYP3A4 inhibitors, such as ketoconazole and erythromycin, with tramadol hydrochloride may effect the metabolism of tramadol leading to altered tramadol exposure).
No products indexed under this heading.

Troleandomycin (Administration of CYP3A4 inhibitors, such as ketoconazole and erythromycin, with tramadol hydrochloride may effect the metabolism of tramadol leading to altered tramadol exposure).
No products indexed under this heading.

Valproate Sodium (Administration of CYP3A4 inhibitors, such as ketoconazole and erythromycin, with tramadol hydrochloride may effect the metabolism of tramadol leading to altered tramadol exposure).
No products indexed under this heading.

Vardenafil Hydrochloride (In vitro drug interaction studies in human liver microsomes indicate that concomitant administration with inhibitors of CYP2D6 could result in some inhibition of the metabolism of tramadol). Products include:
Levitra 3157

Venlafaxine Hydrochloride (Concomitant use of tramadol increases the seizure risk in patients taking serotonin and norepinephrine reuptake inhibitors. Concomitant use of tramadol with SNRIs increases the risk of adverse events, including seizure and serotonin syndrome. If concomitant treatment of tramadol with a drug affecting the serotonergic neurotransmitter system is clinically warranted, careful observation of the patient is advised, particularly during treatment initiation and dose increases). Products include:
Effexor XR 3504
Venlafaxine Hydrochloride Tablets ... 2388

Verapamil Hydrochloride (Administration of CYP3A4 inhibitors, such as ketoconazole and erythromycin, with tramadol hydrochloride may effect the metabolism of tramadol leading to altered tramadol exposure). Products include:
Tarka 534

Voriconazole (Administration of CYP3A4 inhibitors, such as ketoconazole and erythromycin, with tramadol hydrochloride may effect the metabolism of tramadol leading to altered tramadol exposure).
No products indexed under this heading.

Warfarin Sodium (Post-marketing surveillance of tramadol has revealed rare reports of alteration of warfarin effect, including elevation of prothrombin times).
No products indexed under this heading.

Zafirlukast (Administration of CYP3A4 inhibitors, such as ketoconazole and erythromycin, with tramadol hydrochloride may effect the metabolism of tramadol leading to altered tramadol exposure). Products include:
Accolate 3612

Zaleplon (Tramadol hydrochloride is contraindicated in acute intoxication with hypnotics. Tramadol hydrochloride should be used with caution and in reduced dosages when administered to patients receiving CNS depressants, such as sedative hypnotics. Tramadol hydrochloride increases the risk of CNS and respiratory depression).
No products indexed under this heading.

Zileuton (Administration of CYP3A4 inhibitors, such as ketoconazole and erythromycin, with tramadol hydrochloride may effect the metabolism of tramadol leading to altered tramadol exposure).
No products indexed under this heading.

1979 Interactions Index Uniphyl

Ziprasidone Hydrochloride (Tramadol hydrochloride is contraindicated in acute intoxication with psychotropic drugs). Products include:
Geodon ... 2723

Zolmitriptan (Concomitant use of tramadol increases the seizure risk in patients taking triptans. Concomitant use of tramadol with triptans increases the risk of adverse events, including seizure and serotonin syndrome. If concomitant treatment of tramadol with a drug affecting the serotonergic neurotransmitter system is clinically warranted, careful observation of the patient is advised, particularly during treatment initiation and dose increases). Products include:
Zomig Tablets ... 773
Zomig Nasal Spray ... 768
Zomig-ZMT Tablets ... 773

Zolpidem Tartrate (Tramadol hydrochloride is contraindicated in acute intoxication with hypnotics. Tramadol hydrochloride should be used with caution and in reduced dosages when administered to patients receiving CNS depressants, such as sedative hypnotics. Tramadol hydrochloride increases the risk of CNS and respiratory depression). Products include:
Ambien ... 2920
Ambien CR ... 2925

Food Interactions

Alcohol (Tramadol hydrochloride should be used with caution and in reduced dosages when administered to patients receiving CNS depressants, such as alcohol, opioids, anesthetic agents, narcotics, phenothiazines, tranquilizers, or sedative hypnotics. Tramadol hydrochloride increases the risk of CNS and respiratory depression).

Beer, reduced-alcohol (Tramadol hydrochloride is contraindicated in acute intoxication with alcohol. Tramadol hydrochloride should be used with caution and in reduced dosages when administered to patients receiving CNS depressants, such as alcohol. Tramadol may be expected to have additive effects when used in conjunction with alcohol).

Beer, unspecified (Tramadol hydrochloride is contraindicated in acute intoxication with alcohol. Tramadol hydrochloride should be used with caution and in reduced dosages when administered to patients receiving CNS depressants, such as alcohol. Tramadol may be expected to have additive effects when used in conjunction with alcohol).

Grapefruit (Administration of CYP3A4 inhibitors, such as ketoconazole and erythromycin, with tramadol hydrochloride may effect the metabolism of tramadol leading to altered tramadol exposure).

Grapefruit Juice (Administration of CYP3A4 inhibitors, such as ketoconazole and erythromycin, with tramadol hydrochloride may effect the metabolism of tramadol leading to altered tramadol exposure).

Wine, Chianti (Tramadol hydrochloride is contraindicated in acute intoxication with alcohol. Tramadol hydrochloride should be used with caution and in reduced dosages when administered to patients receiving CNS depressants, such as alcohol. Tramadol may be expected to have additive effects when used in conjunction with alcohol).

Wine, Red (Tramadol hydrochloride is contraindicated in acute intoxication with alcohol. Tramadol hydrochloride should be used with caution and in reduced dosages when administered to patients receiving CNS depressants, such as alcohol. Tramadol may be expected to have additive effects when used in conjunction with alcohol).

Wine, unspecified (Tramadol hydrochloride is contraindicated in acute intoxication with alcohol. Tramadol hydrochloride should be used with caution and in reduced dosages when administered to patients receiving CNS depressants, such as alcohol. Tramadol may be expected to have additive effects when used in conjunction with alcohol).

Wine products (Tramadol hydrochloride is contraindicated in acute intoxication with alcohol. Tramadol hydrochloride should be used with caution and in reduced dosages when administered to patients receiving CNS depressants, such as alcohol. Tramadol may be expected to have additive effects when used in conjunction with alcohol).

ULTRASE CAPSULES

(Pancrelipase) ... 797

Food Interactions

Food having a pH greater than 5.5 (Can dissolve the protective coating resulting in early release of enzymes, irritation of oral mucosa, and/or loss of enzyme activity).

ULTRASE MT CAPSULES

(Pancrelipase) ... 798

Food Interactions

Food having a pH greater than 5.5 (Can dissolve the protective enteric shell).

UNIPHYL TABLETS

(Theophylline Anhydrous) ... 2817
May interact with alcohols, erythromycin, lithium preparations, and certain other agents. Compounds in these categories include:

Adenosine (Theophylline blocks adenosine receptors; higher doses of adenosine may be required to achieve desired effect). Products include:
Adenocard ... 656
Adenoscan ... 657

Allopurinol (Decreases theophylline clearance at allopurinol doses greater than or equal to 600 mg/day).
No products indexed under this heading.

Aminoglutethimide (Increases theophylline clearance by induction of microsomal enzyme).
No products indexed under this heading.

Carbamazepine (Increases theophylline clearance by induction of microsomal enzyme). Products include:
Carbatrol ... 3280
Equetro ... 3477

Cimetidine (Decreases theophylline clearance by inhibiting cytochrome P450 1A2).
No products indexed under this heading.

Cimetidine Hydrochloride (Decreases theophylline clearance by inhibiting cytochrome P450 1A2).
No products indexed under this heading.

Ciprofloxacin (Decreases theophylline clearance by inhibiting cytochrome P450 1A2). Products include:
Cipro I.V. ... 3082
Cipro ... 3073
Cipro XR ... 3091
Ciprodex ... 583

Ciprofloxacin Hydrochloride (Decreases theophylline clearance by inhibiting cytochrome P450 1A2). Products include:
Cipro ... 3073

Clarithromycin (Decreases theophylline clearance by inhibiting cytochrome P450 3A3). Products include:
Biaxin/Biaxin XL ... 412

Diazepam (Benzodiazepines increase CNS concentrations of adenosine, a potent CNS depressant, while theophylline blocks adenosine receptors; larger diazepam doses may be required to produce desired level of sedation; discontinuation of theophylline without reduction of diazepam dose may result in respiratory depression). Products include:
Valium Tablets ... 2880

Disulfiram (Decreases theophylline clearance by inhibiting hydroxylation and demethylation).
No products indexed under this heading.

Enoxacin (Decreases theophylline clearance by inhibiting cytochrome P450 1A2).
No products indexed under this heading.

Ephedrine Hydrochloride (Co-administration results in synergistic CNS effects resulting in increased frequency of nausea, nervousness, and insomnia).
No products indexed under this heading.

Ephedrine Sulfate (Co-administration results in synergistic CNS effects resulting in increased frequency of nausea, nervousness, and insomnia).
No products indexed under this heading.

Ephedrine Tannate (Co-administration results in synergistic CNS effects resulting in increased frequency of nausea, nervousness, and insomnia).
No products indexed under this heading.

Erythromycin (Erythromycin metabolite decreases theophylline clearance by inhibiting cytochrome P450 3A3; decreased erythromycin steady-state serum concentrations).
No products indexed under this heading.

Erythromycin, Topical (Erythromycin metabolite decreases theophylline clearance by inhibiting cytochrome P450 3A3; decreased erythromycin steady-state serum concentrations).
No products indexed under this heading.

Erythromycin Estolate (Erythromycin metabolite decreases theophylline clearance by inhibiting cytochrome P450 3A3; decreased erythromycin steady-state serum concentrations).
No products indexed under this heading.

Erythromycin Ethylsuccinate (Erythromycin metabolite decreases theophylline clearance by inhibiting cytochrome P450 3A3; decreased erythromycin steady-state serum concentrations). Products include:
E.E.S. ... 437
EryPed ... 435

Erythromycin Gluceptate (Erythromycin metabolite decreases theophylline clearance by inhibiting cytochrome P450 3A3; decreased erythromycin steady-state serum concentrations).
No products indexed under this heading.

Erythromycin Lactobionate (Erythromycin metabolite decreases theophylline clearance by inhibiting cytochrome P450 3A3; decreased erythromycin steady-state serum concentrations).
No products indexed under this heading.

Erythromycin Stearate (Erythromycin metabolite decreases theophylline clearance by inhibiting cytochrome P450 3A3; decreased erythromycin steady-state serum concentrations).
No products indexed under this heading.

Ethanol (Concurrent use with a single dose of alcohol (3mL/kg of whiskey) decreases theophylline clearance for up to 24 hours).
No products indexed under this heading.

Ethinyl Estradiol (Estrogen containing oral contraceptives decreases theophylline clearance in dose dependent fashion). Products include:
LoSeasonique ... 3407
Lybrel ... 3514
NuvaRing ... 3181
Ortho Evra ... 2648
Ortho-Cyclen/Ortho Tri-Cyclen ... 2663
Ortho Tri-Cyclen Lo Tablets ... 2673
Seasonique ... 3418
Yaz ... 864

Ethyl Alcohol (Concurrent use with a single dose of alcohol (3mL/kg of whiskey) decreases theophylline clearance for up to 24 hours).
No products indexed under this heading.

Flurazepam Hydrochloride (Benzodiazepines increase CNS concentrations of adenosine, a potent CNS depressant, while theophylline blocks adenosine receptors; larger flurazepam doses may be required to produce desired level of sedation; discontinuation of theophylline without reduction of flurazepam dose may result in respiratory depression).
No products indexed under this heading.

Fluvoxamine Maleate (Decreases theophylline clearance by inhibiting cytochrome P450 1A2).
No products indexed under this heading.

Halothane (Halothane sensitizes the myocardium to catecholamines; theophylline increases release of endogenous catecholamines resulting in increased risk of ventricular arrhythmias).
No products indexed under this heading.

Hypericum (Increases theophylline clearance; higher doses of theophylline may be required to achieve desired effect; stopping St. John's Wort may result in theophylline toxicity).
No products indexed under this heading.

Interferon alfa-2a, Recombinant (Decreases theophylline clearance).
No products indexed under this heading.

Isoproterenol Hydrochloride (Co-administration with intravenous isoproterenol decreases theophylline clearance).
No products indexed under this heading.

Ketamine Hydrochloride (May lower theophylline seizure threshold).
No products indexed under this heading.

Lithium (Theophylline increases renal lithium clearance; increase in lithium dose may be required to achieve a therapeutic serum concentration).
No products indexed under this heading.

Lithium Carbonate (Theophylline increases renal lithium clearance; increase in lithium dose may be required to achieve a therapeutic serum concentration).
No products indexed under this heading.

Lithium Citrate (Theophylline increases renal lithium clearance; increase in lithium dose may be required to achieve a therapeutic serum concentration).
No products indexed under this heading.

Lorazepam (Benzodiazepines increase CNS concentrations of adenosine, a potent CNS depressant, while theophylline blocks adenosine receptors; larger lorazepam doses may be required to produce desired level of sedation; discontinuation of theophylline without reduction of lorazepam dose may result in respiratory depression).
No products indexed under this heading.

Mestranol (Estrogen containing oral contraceptives decreases theophylline clearance in dose dependent fashion).
No products indexed under this heading.

Methotrexate Sodium (Decreases theophylline clearance).
No products indexed under this heading.

Mexiletine Hydrochloride (Decreases theophylline clearance by inhibiting hydroxylation and demethylation).
No products indexed under this heading.

Midazolam Hydrochloride (Benzodiazepines increase CNS concentrations of adenosine, a potent CNS depressant, while theophylline blocks adenosine receptors; larger midazolam doses may be required to produce desired level of sedation; discontinuation of theophylline without reduction of midazolam dose may result in respiratory depression).
No products indexed under this heading.

Moricizine Hydrochloride (Increases theophylline clearance).
No products indexed under this heading.

Pancuronium Bromide (Theophylline may antagonize non-depolarizing neuromuscular blocking effects; possibly due to phosphodiesterase inhibition; larger pancuronium doses may be required to achieve neuromuscular blockade).
No products indexed under this heading.

Pentoxifylline (Decreases theophylline clearance).
No products indexed under this heading.

Phenobarbital (Increases theophylline clearance by induction of microsomal enzyme). Products include:
Donnatal 2711

Phenytoin (Phenytoin increases theophylline clearance by increasing microsomal enzyme activity; theophylline decreases phenytoin absorption).
No products indexed under this heading.

Phenytoin Sodium (Phenytoin increases theophylline clearance by increasing microsomal enzyme activity; theophylline decreases phenytoin absorption). Products include:
Phenytek Capsules 2380

Propafenone Hydrochloride (Decreases theophylline clearance). Products include:
Rythmol 1648
Rythmol SR 1652

Propranolol Hydrochloride (Decreases theophylline clearance by inhibiting cytochrome P450 1A2). Products include:
InnoPran XL 1517

Rifampin (Increases theophylline clearance by increasing cytochrome P450 1A2 and 3A3 activity).
No products indexed under this heading.

Sulfinpyrazone (Increases theophylline clearance by increasing demethylation and hydroxylation; decreases renal clearance of theophylline).
No products indexed under this heading.

Tacrine Hydrochloride (Decreases theophylline clearance by inhibiting cytochrome P450 1A2 and also increases renal clearance of theophylline).
No products indexed under this heading.

Thiabendazole (Decreases theophylline clearance).
No products indexed under this heading.

Ticlopidine Hydrochloride (Decreases theophylline clearance).
No products indexed under this heading.

Troleandomycin (Decreases theophylline clearance by inhibiting cytochrome P450 3A3).
No products indexed under this heading.

Verapamil Hydrochloride (Decreases theophylline clearance by inhibiting hydroxylation and demethylation). Products include:
Tarka 534

Food Interactions

Alcohol (Concurrent use with a single dose of alcohol (3mL/kg of whiskey) decreases theophylline clearance for up to 24 hours).

Beer, reduced-alcohol (Concurrent use with a single dose of alcohol (3mL/kg of whiskey) decreases theophylline clearance for up to 24 hours).

Beer, unspecified (Concurrent use with a single dose of alcohol (3mL/kg of whiskey) decreases theophylline clearance for up to 24 hours).

Diet, high-lipid (Co-administration with a standardized high-fat meal results in increased peak plasma concentration and bioavailability; however, a precipitous increase in the rate and extent of absorption was not evident; the dosing should be ideally administered consistently either with or without food).

Wine, Chianti (Concurrent use with a single dose of alcohol (3mL/kg of whiskey) decreases theophylline clearance for up to 24 hours).

Wine, Red (Concurrent use with a single dose of alcohol (3mL/kg of whiskey) decreases theophylline clearance for up to 24 hours).

Wine, unspecified (Concurrent use with a single dose of alcohol (3mL/kg of whiskey) decreases theophylline clearance for up to 24 hours).

Wine products (Concurrent use with a single dose of alcohol (3mL/kg of whiskey) decreases theophylline clearance for up to 24 hours).

UROCIT-K TABLETS

(Potassium Citrate) 2333
May interact with anticholinergics, potassium sparing diuretics, and certain other agents. Compounds in these categories include:

Amiloride Hydrochloride (Concomitant administration of potassium citrate with potassium-sparing diuretics is contraindicated. They should be avoided since the simultaneous administration of these agents can produce severe hyperkalemia).
No products indexed under this heading.

Atropine Sulfate (Concomitant administration of potassium citrate with drugs that slow gastrointestinal transit time (anticholinergics) is contraindicated. They may increase the gastrointestinal irritation produced by potassium salts). Products include:
Donnatal 2711

Belladonna Alkaloids (Concomitant administration of potassium citrate with drugs that slow gastrointestinal transit time (anticholinergics) is contraindicated. They may increase the gastrointestinal irritation produced by potassium salts). Products include:
Hyland's Teething Tablets 3316

Benztropine Mesylate (Concomitant administration of potassium citrate with drugs that slow gastrointestinal transit time (anticholinergics) is contraindicated. They may increase the gastrointestinal irritation produced by potassium salts).
No products indexed under this heading.

Biperiden Hydrochloride (Concomitant administration of potassium citrate with drugs that slow gastrointestinal transit time (anticholinergics) is contraindicated. They may increase the gastrointestinal irritation produced by potassium salts).
No products indexed under this heading.

Clidinium Bromide (Concomitant administration of potassium citrate with drugs that slow gastrointestinal transit time (anticholinergics) is contraindicated. They may increase the gastrointestinal irritation produced by potassium salts).
No products indexed under this heading.

Dicyclomine Hydrochloride (Concomitant administration of potassium citrate with drugs that slow gastrointestinal transit time (anticholinergics) is contraindicated. They may increase the gastrointestinal irritation produced by potassium salts). Products include:
Bentyl Capsules 780
Bentyl Injection 780
Bentyl Syrup 780
Bentyl Tablets 780

Glycopyrrolate (Concomitant administration of potassium citrate with drugs that slow gastrointestinal transit time (anticholinergics) is contraindicated. They may increase the gastrointestinal irritation produced by potassium salts).
No products indexed under this heading.

Hyoscyamine (Concomitant administration of potassium citrate with drugs that slow gastrointestinal transit time (anticholinergics) is contraindicated. They may increase the gastrointestinal irritation produced by potassium salts).
No products indexed under this heading.

Hyoscyamine Sulfate (Concomitant administration of potassium citrate with drugs that slow gastrointestinal transit time (anticholinergics) is contraindicated. They may increase the gastrointestinal irritation produced by potassium salts). Products include:
Donnatal 2711

Ipratropium Bromide (Concomitant administration of potassium citrate with drugs that slow gastrointestinal transit time (anticholinergics) is contraindicated. They may increase the gastrointestinal irritation produced by potassium salts).
No products indexed under this heading.

Mepenzolate Bromide (Concomitant administration of potassium citrate with drugs that slow gastrointestinal transit time (anticholinergics) is contraindicated. They may increase the gastrointestinal irritation produced by potassium salts).
No products indexed under this heading.

Oxybutynin Chloride (Concomitant administration of potassium citrate with drugs that slow gastrointestinal transit time (anticholinergics) is contraindicated. They may increase the gastrointestinal irritation produced by potassium salts).
No products indexed under this heading.

Procyclidine Hydrochloride (Concomitant administration of potassium citrate with drugs that slow gastrointestinal transit time (anticholinergics) is contraindicated. They may increase the gastrointestinal irritation produced by potassium salts).
No products indexed under this heading.

Propantheline Bromide (Concomitant administration of potassium citrate with drugs that slow gastrointestinal transit time (anticholinergics) is contraindicated. They may increase the gastrointestinal irritation produced by potassium salts).
No products indexed under this heading.

Scopolamine (Concomitant administration of potassium citrate with drugs that slow gastrointestinal transit time (anticholinergics) is contraindicated. They may increase the gastrointestinal irritation produced by potassium salts). Products include:
Transderm Scōp 2397

Scopolamine Hydrobromide (Concomitant administration of potassium citrate with drugs that slow gastrointestinal transit time (anticholinergics) is contraindicated. They may increase the gastrointestinal irritation produced by potassium salts). Products include:
Donnatal 2711

Spironolactone (Concomitant administration of potassium citrate with potassium-sparing diuretics is contraindicated. They should be avoided since the simultaneous administration of these agents can produce severe hyperkalemia).
No products indexed under this heading.

Tolterodine Tartrate (Concomitant administration of potassium citrate with drugs that slow gastrointestinal transit time (anticholinergics) is contraindicated. They may increase the gastrointestinal irritation produced by potassium salts).
No products indexed under this heading.

Triamterene (Concomitant administration of potassium citrate with potassium-sparing diuretics is contraindicated. They should be avoided since the simultaneous administration of these agents can produce severe hyperkalemia). Products include:
Dyazide 1429
Dyrenium 3495

Tridihexethyl Chloride (Concomitant administration of potassium citrate with drugs that slow gastrointestinal transit time (anticholinergics) is contraindicated. They may increase the gastrointestinal irritation produced by potassium salts).
No products indexed under this heading.

Trihexyphenidyl Hydrochloride (Concomitant administration of potassium citrate with drugs that slow gastrointestinal transit time (anticholinergics) is contraindicated. They may increase the gastrointestinal irritation produced by potassium salts).
No products indexed under this heading.

Food Interactions

Food, unspecified (A dose of potassium citrate taken with meals or snacks may alleviate minor gastrointestinal complaints such as abdominal discomfort, vomiting, diarrhea, loose bowel movements or nausea in some patients).

Meal, unspecified (A dose of potassium citrate taken with meals or snacks may alleviate minor gastrointestinal complaints such as abdominal discomfort, vomiting, diarrhea, loose bowel movements or nausea in some patients).

UROQID-ACID NO. 2 TABLETS

(Methenamine Mandelate, Sodium Acid Phosphate) 874

Acetazolamide (Reduces the effectiveness of methenamine by causing urine to become alkaline).
No products indexed under this heading.

ACTH (Concurrent use with sodium phosphate may result in hypernatremia).
No products indexed under this heading.

Aluminum Carbonate (Reduces the effectiveness of methenamine by causing urine to become alkaline).
No products indexed under this heading.

Aluminum Hydroxide (Reduces the effectiveness of methenamine by causing urine to become alkaline).
No products indexed under this heading.

Aspirin (Concurrent use may lead to increased serum salicylate levels since excretion of salicylates is reduced in acidic urine). Products include:
Aggrenox 880
Bayer Aspirin 829
Percodan 1124
St. Joseph Aspirin 2045

Bendroflumethiazide (Reduces the effectiveness of methenamine by causing urine to become alkaline).
No products indexed under this heading.

Betamethasone Acetate (Concurrent use with sodium phosphate may result in hypernatremia).
No products indexed under this heading.

Betamethasone Sodium Phosphate (Concurrent use with sodium phosphate may result in hypernatremia).
No products indexed under this heading.

Chlorothiazide (Reduces the effectiveness of methenamine by causing urine to become alkaline).
No products indexed under this heading.

Chlorothiazide Sodium (Reduces the effectiveness of methenamine by causing urine to become alkaline). Products include:
Diuril Intravenous 2009

Choline Magnesium Trisalicylate (Concurrent use may lead to increased serum salicylate levels since excretion of salicylates is reduced in acidic urine).
No products indexed under this heading.

Cortisone Acetate (Concurrent use with sodium phosphate may result in hypernatremia).
No products indexed under this heading.

Deserpidine (Concurrent use with sodium phosphate may result in hypernatremia).
No products indexed under this heading.

Desoxycorticosterone Acetate (Concurrent use with sodium phosphate may result in hypernatremia).
No products indexed under this heading.

Desoxycorticosterone Pivalate (Concurrent use with sodium phosphate may result in hypernatremia).
No products indexed under this heading.

Dexamethasone (Concurrent use with sodium phosphate may result in hypernatremia). Products include:
Ciprodex **583**
Ozurdex ....⊙**223**
Tobramycin and Dexamethasone Ophthalmic Suspension ....⊙**251**

Dexamethasone Acetate (Concurrent use with sodium phosphate may result in hypernatremia).
No products indexed under this heading.

Dexamethasone Sodium Phosphate (Concurrent use with sodium phosphate may result in hypernatremia).
No products indexed under this heading.

Diazoxide (Concurrant use with sodium phosphate may result in hypernatremia). Products include:
Proglycem 1179
Proglycem Suspension 1179

Dichlorphenamide (Reduces the effectiveness of methenamine by causing urine to become alkaline).
No products indexed under this heading.

Diflunisal (Concurrent use may lead to increased serum salicylate levels since excretion of salicylates is reduced in acidic urine).
No products indexed under this heading.

Fludrocortisone Acetate (Concurrent use with sodium phosphate may result in hypernatremia).
No products indexed under this heading.

Guanethidine Monosulfate (Concurrent use with sodium phosphate may result in hypernatremia).
No products indexed under this heading.

Hydralazine Hydrochloride (Concurrent use with sodium phosphate may result in hypernatremia).
No products indexed under this heading.

Hydrochlorothiazide (Reduces the effectiveness of methenamine by causing urine to become alkaline). Products include:
Atacand HCT **700**
Avalide 2956
Benicar HCT 1017
Diovan HCT 2419
Dyazide 1429

Exforge HCT **2449**
Hyzaar 2162
Hyzaar 100-12.5 2162
Micardis HCT **889**
Prinzide 2246
Tekturna HCT 2541
Teveten HCT 541

Hydrocortisone (Concurrent use with sodium phosphate may result in hypernatremia).
No products indexed under this heading.

Hydrocortisone Acetate (Concurrent use with sodium phosphate may result in hypernatremia).
No products indexed under this heading.

Hydrocortisone Sodium Phosphate (Concurrent use with sodium phosphate may result in hypernatremia).
No products indexed under this heading.

Hydrocortisone Sodium Succinate (Concurrent use with sodium phosphate may result in hypernatremia).
No products indexed under this heading.

Hydroflumethiazide (Reduces the effectiveness of methenamine by causing urine to become alkaline).
No products indexed under this heading.

Magaldrate (Reduces the effectiveness of methenamine by causing urine to become alkaline).
No products indexed under this heading.

Magnesium Hydroxide (Reduces the effectiveness of methenamine by causing urine to become alkaline). Products include:
Fleet Pedia-Lax Chewable Tablets 1144
Pepcid Complete 1822

Magnesium Oxide (Reduces the effectiveness of methenamine by causing urine to become alkaline). Products include:
Beelith 873

Magnesium Salicylate (Concurrent use may lead to increased serum salicylate levels since excretion of salicylates is reduced in acidic urine).
No products indexed under this heading.

Methazolamide (Reduces the effectiveness of methenamine by causing urine to become alkaline).
No products indexed under this heading.

Methyclothiazide (Reduces the effectiveness of methenamine by causing urine to become alkaline).
No products indexed under this heading.

Methyldopa (Concurrent use with sodium phosphate may result in hypernatremia).
No products indexed under this heading.

Methylprednisolone Acetate (Concurrent use with sodium phosphate may result in hypernatremia).
No products indexed under this heading.

Methylprednisolone Sodium Succinate (Concurrent use with sodium phosphate may result in hypernatremia).
No products indexed under this heading.

Polythiazide (Reduces the effectiveness of methenamine by causing urine to become alkaline).
No products indexed under this heading.

Potassium Citrate (Reduces the effectiveness of methenamine by causing urine to become alkaline). Products include:
Urocit-K 2333

Prednisolone Acetate (Concurrent use with sodium phosphate may result in hypernatremia). Products include:
Blephamide ....⊙**212,**⊙**214**
Pred Forte ....⊙**225**
Pred Mild ....⊙**230**
Pred-G ....⊙**226,**⊙**227**

Prednisolone Sodium Phosphate (Concurrent use with sodium phosphate may result in hypernatremia).
No products indexed under this heading.

Prednisolone Tebutate (Concurrent use with sodium phosphate may result in hypernatremia).
No products indexed under this heading.

Prednisone (Concurrent use with sodium phosphate may result in hypernatremia).
No products indexed under this heading.

Rauwolfia Serpentina (Concurrent use with sodium phosphate may result in hypernatremia).
No products indexed under this heading.

Rescinnamine (Concurrent use with sodium phosphate may result in hypernatremia).
No products indexed under this heading.

Reserpine (Concurrent use with sodium phosphate may result in hypernatremia).
No products indexed under this heading.

Salsalate (Concurrent use may lead to increased serum salicylate levels since excretion of salicylates is reduced in acidic urine).
No products indexed under this heading.

Sodium Bicarbonate (Reduces the effectiveness of methenamine by causing urine to become alkaline).
No products indexed under this heading.

Sodium Citrate (Reduces the effectiveness of methenamine by causing urine to become alkaline).
No products indexed under this heading.

Sulfamethizole (Concurrent use with sulfamethizole and formaldehyde forms an insoluble precipitate in acid urine and increases the risk of crystaluria).
No products indexed under this heading.

Triamcinolone (Concurrent use with sodium phosphate may result in hypernatremia).
No products indexed under this heading.

Triamcinolone Acetonide (Concurrent use with sodium phosphate may result in hypernatremia). Products include:
Azmacort **408**
Nasacort AQ 3019

Triamcinolone Diacetate (Concurrent use with sodium phosphate may result in hypernatremia).
No products indexed under this heading.

Triamcinolone Hexacetonide (Concurrent use with sodium phosphate may result in hypernatremia).
No products indexed under this heading.

UROXATRAL TABLETS
(Alfuzosin Hydrochloride) 3050
May interact with alpha adrenergic blockers, antihypertensives, cytochrome p450 3a4 inhibitors, potent (selected), drugs that prolong the QT interval, nitrates and nitrites, and certain other agents. Compounds in these categories include:

Acebutolol Hydrochloride (There may be an increased risk of hypotension/postural hypotension and syncope when taking alfuzosin concomitantly with anti-hypertensive medication and nitrates. Care should be taken when alfuzosin is administered to patients with symptomatic hypotension or patients who have had a hypotensive response to other medications).
No products indexed under this heading.

Aliskiren (There may be an increased risk of hypotension/postural hypotension and syncope when taking alfuzosin concomitantly with anti-hypertensive medication and nitrates. Care should be taken when alfuzosin is administered to patients with symptomatic hypotension or patients who have had a hypotensive response to other medications).
Products include:
Tekturna 2538
Tekturna HCT 2541

Valturna 3637

Alprazolam (A post-marketing study evaluating the effect of combining alfuzosin hydrochloride with another drug of comparable QT effect showed an increased effect when compared to either drug alone. Although this study was not designed to make direct statistical comparisons between drugs, the QT increase with both drugs was no more than additive and was lower than that of the active control moxifloxacin. These observations should be considered in clinical decisions when prescribing alfuzosin hydrochloride for patients with a known history of QT prolongation or patients who are taking medications which prolong the QT interval).
No products indexed under this heading.

Amiodarone Hydrochloride (A post-marketing study evaluating the effect of combining alfuzosin hydrochloride with another drug of comparable QT effect showed an increased effect when compared to either drug alone. Although this study was not designed to make direct statistical comparisons between drugs, the QT increase with both drugs was no more than additive and was lower than that of the active control moxifloxacin. These observations should be considered in clinical decisions when prescribing alfuzosin hydrochloride for patients with a known history of QT prolongation or patients who are taking medications which prolong the QT interval).
No products indexed under this heading.

Amitriptyline Hydrochloride (A post-marketing study evaluating the effect of combining alfuzosin hydrochloride with another drug of comparable QT effect showed an increased effect when compared to either drug alone. Although this study was not designed to make direct statistical comparisons between drugs, the QT increase with both drugs was no more than additive and was lower than that of the active control moxifloxacin. These observations should be considered in clinical decisions when prescribing alfuzosin hydrochloride for patients with a known history of QT prolongation or patients who are taking medications which prolong the QT interval).
No products indexed under this heading.

Amlodipine Besylate (There may be an increased risk of hypotension/postural hypotension and syncope when taking alfuzosin concomitantly with anti-hypertensive medication and nitrates. Care should be taken when alfuzosin is administered to patients with symptomatic hypotension or patients who have had a hypotensive response to other medications). Products include:
Azor 1010
Exforge 2443
Exforge HCT 2449

Amoxapine (A post-marketing study evaluating the effect of combining alfuzosin hydrochloride with another drug of comparable QT effect showed an increased effect when compared to either drug alone. Although this study was not designed to make direct statistical comparisons between drugs, the QT increase with both drugs was no more than additive and was lower than that of the active control moxifloxacin. These observations should be considered in clinical decisions when prescribing alfuzosin hydrochloride for patients with a known history of QT prolongation or patients who are taking medications which prolong the QT interval).
No products indexed under this heading.

IMPORTANT NOTE: Always consult each drug listing in the patient's regimen for possible interactions.

Amprenavir (Co-administration of alfuzosin with potent CYP3A4 inhibitors, such as ketoconazole, itraconazole, and ritonavir, is contraindicated, since alfuzosin blood levels are increased).
No products indexed under this heading.

Amyl Nitrite (There may be an increased risk of hypotension/postural hypotension and syncope when taking alfuzosin concomitantly with anti-hypertensive medication and nitrates. Care should be taken when alfuzosin is administered to patients with symptomatic hypotension or patients who have had a hypotensive response to other medications).
No products indexed under this heading.

Apraclonidine Hydrochloride (The pharmacokinetic and pharmacodynamic interactions between alfuzosin and other α-blockers have not been determined. However, interactions may be expected, and alfuzosin should not be used in combination with other α-blockers).
No products indexed under this heading.

Astemizole (A post-marketing study evaluating the effect of combining alfuzosin hydrochloride with another drug of comparable QT effect showed an increased effect when compared to either drug alone. Although this study was not designed to make direct statistical comparisons between drugs, the QT increase with both drugs was no more than additive and was lower than that of the active control moxifloxacin. These observations should be considered in clinical decisions when prescribing alfuzosin hydrochloride for patients with a known history of QT prolongation or patients who are taking medications which prolong the QT interval).
No products indexed under this heading.

Atazanavir (Co-administration of alfuzosin with potent CYP3A4 inhibitors, such as ketoconazole, itraconazole, and ritonavir, is contraindicated, since alfuzosin blood levels are increased).
No products indexed under this heading.

Atazanavir Sulfate (Co-administration of alfuzosin with potent CYP3A4 inhibitors, such as ketoconazole, itraconazole, and ritonavir, is contraindicated, since alfuzosin blood levels are increased).
No products indexed under this heading.

Atenolol (Single administration of 100 mg atenolol with a single dose of 2.5 mg of an immediate release alfuzosin tablet in eight healthy young male volunteers increased alfuzosin C_{max} and AUC values by 28% and 21%, respectively. Alfuzosin increased atenolol C_{max} and AUC values by 26% and 14%, respectively. In this study, the combination of alfuzosin with atenolol caused significant reductions in mean blood pressure and in mean heart rate).
No products indexed under this heading.

Benazepril Hydrochloride (There may be an increased risk of hypotension/postural hypotension and syncope when taking alfuzosin concomitantly with anti-hypertensive medication and nitrates. Care should be taken when alfuzosin is administered to patients with symptomatic hypotension or patients who have had a hypotensive response to other medications).
No products indexed under this heading.

Bendroflumethiazide (There may be an increased risk of hypotension/postural hypotension and syncope when taking alfuzosin concomitantly with anti-hypertensive medication and nitrates. Care should be taken when alfuzosin is administered to patients with symptomatic hypotension or patients who have had a hypotensive response to other medications).
No products indexed under this heading.

Betaxolol Hydrochloride (There may be an increased risk of hypotension/postural hypotension and syncope when taking alfuzosin concomitantly with anti-hypertensive medication and nitrates. Care should be taken when alfuzosin is administered to patients with symptomatic hypotension or patients who have had a hypotensive response to other medications).
No products indexed under this heading.

Bisoprolol Fumarate (There may be an increased risk of hypotension/postural hypotension and syncope when taking alfuzosin concomitantly with anti-hypertensive medication and nitrates. Care should be taken when alfuzosin is administered to patients with symptomatic hypotension or patients who have had a hypotensive response to other medications).
No products indexed under this heading.

Bretylium Tosylate (A post-marketing study evaluating the effect of combining alfuzosin hydrochloride with another drug of comparable QT effect showed an increased effect when compared to either drug alone. Although this study was not designed to make direct statistical comparisons between drugs, the QT increase with both drugs was no more than additive and was lower than that of the active control moxifloxacin. These observations should be considered in clinical decisions when prescribing alfuzosin hydrochloride for patients with a known history of QT prolongation or patients who are taking medications which prolong the QT interval).
No products indexed under this heading.

Buspirone Hydrochloride (A post-marketing study evaluating the effect of combining alfuzosin hydrochloride with another drug of comparable QT effect showed an increased effect when compared to either drug alone. Although this study was not designed to make direct statistical comparisons between drugs, the QT increase with both drugs was no more than additive and was lower than that of the active control moxifloxacin. These observations should be considered in clinical decisions when prescribing alfuzosin hydrochloride for patients with a known history of QT prolongation or patients who are taking medications which prolong the QT interval).
No products indexed under this heading.

Candesartan Cilexetil (There may be an increased risk of hypotension/postural hypotension and syncope when taking alfuzosin concomitantly with anti-hypertensive medication and nitrates. Care should be taken when alfuzosin is administered to patients with symptomatic hypotension or patients who have had a hypotensive response to other medications). Products include:
Atacand 697
Atacand HCT 700

Captopril (There may be an increased risk of hypotension/postural hypotension and syncope when taking alfuzosin concomitantly with anti-hypertensive medication and nitrates. Care should be taken when alfuzosin is administered to patients with symptomatic hypotension or patients who have had a hypotensive response to other medications). Products include:
Captopril 2341

Carteolol Hydrochloride (There may be an increased risk of hypotension/postural hypotension and syncope when taking alfuzosin concomitantly with anti-hypertensive medication and nitrates. Care should be taken when alfuzosin is administered to patients with symptomatic hypotension or patients who have had a hypotensive response to other medications).
No products indexed under this heading.

Carvedilol (There may be an increased risk of hypotension/postural hypotension and syncope when taking alfuzosin concomitantly with anti-hypertensive medication and nitrates. Care should be taken when alfuzosin is administered to patients with symptomatic hypotension or patients who have had a hypotensive response to other medications). Products include:
Coreg 1409

Carvedilol Phosphate (There may be an increased risk of hypotension/postural hypotension and syncope when taking alfuzosin concomitantly with anti-hypertensive medication and nitrates. Care should be taken when alfuzosin is administered to patients with symptomatic hypotension or patients who have had a hypotensive response to other medications). Products include:
Coreg CR 1416

Chlordiazepoxide (A post-marketing study evaluating the effect of combining alfuzosin hydrochloride with another drug of comparable QT effect showed an increased effect when compared to either drug alone. Although this study was not designed to make direct statistical comparisons between drugs, the QT increase with both drugs was no more than additive and was lower than that of the active control moxifloxacin. These observations should be considered in clinical decisions when prescribing alfuzosin hydrochloride for patients with a known history of QT prolongation or patients who are taking medications which prolong the QT interval).
No products indexed under this heading.

Chlordiazepoxide Hydrochloride (A post-marketing study evaluating the effect of combining alfuzosin hydrochloride with another drug of comparable QT effect showed an increased effect when compared to either drug alone. Although this study was not designed to make direct statistical comparisons between drugs, the QT increase with both drugs was no more than additive and was lower than that of the active control moxifloxacin. These observations should be considered in clinical decisions when prescribing alfuzosin hydrochloride for patients with a known history of QT prolongation or patients who are taking medications which prolong the QT interval).
No products indexed under this heading.

Chlorothiazide (There may be an increased risk of hypotension/postural hypotension and syncope when taking alfuzosin concomitantly with anti-hypertensive medication and nitrates. Care should be taken when alfuzosin is administered to patients with symptomatic hypotension or patients who have had a hypotensive response to other medications).
No products indexed under this heading.

Chlorothiazide Sodium (There may be an increased risk of hypotension/postural hypotension and syncope when taking alfuzosin concomitantly with anti-hypertensive medication and nitrates. Care should be taken when alfuzosin is administered to patients with symptomatic hypotension or patients who have had a hypotensive response to other medications). Products include:
Diuril Intravenous 2009

Chlorpromazine (A post-marketing study evaluating the effect of combining alfuzosin hydrochloride with another drug of comparable QT effect showed an increased effect when compared to either drug alone. Although this study was not designed to make direct statistical comparisons between drugs, the QT increase with both drugs was no more than additive and was lower than that of the active control moxifloxacin. These observations should be consid-

ered in clinical decisions when prescribing alfuzosin hydrochloride for patients with a known history of QT prolongation or patients who are taking medications which prolong the QT interval).
No products indexed under this heading.

Chlorpromazine Hydrochloride (A post-marketing study evaluating the effect of combining alfuzosin hydrochloride with another drug of comparable QT effect showed an increased effect when compared to either drug alone. Although this study was not designed to make direct statistical comparisons between drugs, the QT increase with both drugs was no more than additive and was lower than that of the active control moxifloxacin. These observations should be considered in clinical decisions when prescribing alfuzosin hydrochloride for patients with a known history of QT prolongation or patients who are taking medications which prolong the QT interval).
No products indexed under this heading.

Chlorprothixene (A post-marketing study evaluating the effect of combining alfuzosin hydrochloride with another drug of comparable QT effect showed an increased effect when compared to either drug alone. Although this study was not designed to make direct statistical comparisons between drugs, the QT increase with both drugs was no more than additive and was lower than that of the active control moxifloxacin. These observations should be considered in clinical decisions when prescribing alfuzosin hydrochloride for patients with a known history of QT prolongation or patients who are taking medications which prolong the QT interval).
No products indexed under this heading.

Chlorprothixene Hydrochloride (A post-marketing study evaluating the effect of combining alfuzosin hydrochloride with another drug of comparable QT effect showed an increased effect when compared to either drug alone. Although this study was not designed to make direct statistical comparisons between drugs, the QT increase with both drugs was no more than additive and was lower than that of the active control moxifloxacin. These observations should be considered in clinical decisions when prescribing alfuzosin hydrochloride for patients with a known history of QT prolongation or patients who are taking medications which prolong the QT interval).
No products indexed under this heading.

Chlorthalidone (There may be an increased risk of hypotension/postural hypotension and syncope when taking alfuzosin concomitantly with anti-hypertensive medication and nitrates. Care should be taken when alfuzosin is administered to patients with symptomatic hypotension or patients who have had a hypotensive response to other medications). Products include:
Clorpres 2344

Cimetidine (Repeated administration of 1 g/day cimetidine increased both alfuzosin C_{max} and AUC values by 20%).
No products indexed under this heading.

Cimetidine Hydrochloride (Repeated administration of 1 g/day cimetidine increased both alfuzosin C_{max} and AUC values by 20%).
No products indexed under this heading.

Clarithromycin (Co-administration of alfuzosin with potent CYP3A4 inhibitors, such as ketoconazole, itraconazole, and ritonavir, is contraindicated, since alfuzosin blood levels are increased). Products include:
Biaxin/Biaxin XL 412

Clomipramine Hydrochloride (A post-marketing study evaluating the effect of combining alfuzosin hydrochlo-

ride with another drug of comparable QT effect showed an increased effect when compared to either drug alone. Although this study was not designed to make direct statistical comparisons between drugs, the QT increase with both drugs was no more than additive and was lower than that of the active control moxifloxacin. These observations should be considered in clinical decisions when prescribing alfuzosin hydrochloride for patients with a known history of QT prolongation or patients who are taking medications which prolong the QT interval).

No products indexed under this heading.

Clonidine (The pharmacokinetic and pharmacodynamic interactions between alfuzosin and other α-blockers have not been determined. However, interactions may be expected, and alfuzosin should not be used in combination with other α-blockers). Products include:

Catapres-TTS 884

Clonidine Hydrochloride (The pharmacokinetic and pharmacodynamic interactions between alfuzosin and other α-blockers have not been determined. However, interactions may be expected, and alfuzosin should not be used in combination with other α-blockers). Products include:

Clorpres 2344

Clorazepate Dipotassium (A post-marketing study evaluating the effect of combining alfuzosin hydrochloride with another drug of comparable QT effect showed an increased effect when compared to either drug alone. Although this study was not designed to make direct statistical comparisons between drugs, the QT increase with both drugs was no more than additive and was lower than that of the active control moxifloxacin. These observations should be considered in clinical decisions when prescribing alfuzosin hydrochloride for patients with a known history of QT prolongation or patients who are taking medications which prolong the QT interval).

No products indexed under this heading.

Clozapine (A post-marketing study evaluating the effect of combining alfuzosin hydrochloride with another drug of comparable QT effect showed an increased effect when compared to either drug alone. Although this study was not designed to make direct statistical comparisons between drugs, the QT increase with both drugs was no more than additive and was lower than that of the active control moxifloxacin. These observations should be considered in clinical decisions when prescribing alfuzosin hydrochloride for patients with a known history of QT prolongation or patients who are taking medications which prolong the QT interval).

No products indexed under this heading.

Delavirdine Mesylate (Co-administration of alfuzosin with potent CYP3A4 inhibitors, such as ketoconazole, itraconazole, and ritonavir, is contraindicated, since alfuzosin blood levels are increased).

No products indexed under this heading.

Delavirine (Co-administration of alfuzosin with potent CYP3A4 inhibitors, such as ketoconazole, itraconazole, and ritonavir, is contraindicated, since alfuzosin blood levels are increased).

No products indexed under this heading.

Deserpidine (There may be an increased risk of hypotension/postural hypotension and syncope when taking alfuzosin concomitantly with anti-hypertensive medication and nitrates. Care should be taken when alfuzosin is administered to patients with symptomatic hypotension or patients who have had a hypotensive response to other medications).

No products indexed under this heading.

Desipramine Hydrochloride (A post-marketing study evaluating the effect of combining alfuzosin hydrochloride with another drug of comparable QT effect showed an increased effect when compared to either drug alone. Although this study was not designed to make direct statistical comparisons between drugs, the QT increase with both drugs was no more than additive and was lower than that of the active control moxifloxacin. These observations should be considered in clinical decisions when prescribing alfuzosin hydrochloride for patients with a known history of QT prolongation or patients who are taking medications which prolong the QT interval).

No products indexed under this heading.

Diazepam (A post-marketing study evaluating the effect of combining alfuzosin hydrochloride with another drug of comparable QT effect showed an increased effect when compared to either drug alone. Although this study was not designed to make direct statistical comparisons between drugs, the QT increase with both drugs was no more than additive and was lower than that of the active control moxifloxacin. These observations should be considered in clinical decisions when prescribing alfuzosin hydrochloride for patients with a known history of QT prolongation or patients who are taking medications which prolong the QT interval). Products include:

Valium Tablets 2880

Diazoxide (There may be an increased risk of hypotension/postural hypotension and syncope when taking alfuzosin concomitantly with anti-hypertensive medication and nitrates. Care should be taken when alfuzosin is administered to patients with symptomatic hypotension or patients who have had a hypotensive response to other medications). Products include:

Proglycem 1179
Proglycem Suspension 1179

Diltiazem Hydrochloride (Repeated co-administration of 240 mg/day of diltiazem, a moderately-potent inhibitor of CYP3A4, with 7.5 mg/day (2.5 mg three times daily) alfuzosin increased the C_{max} and AUC_{0-24} of alfuzosin 1.5- and 1.3-fold, respectively. Alfuzosin increased the C_{max} and AUC_{0-12} of diltiazem 1.4-fold. Although no changes in blood pressure were observed in this study, diltiazem is an antihypertensive medication and the combination of alfuzosin and antihypertensive medications has the potential to cause hypotension in some patients). Products include:

Cardizem LA 423

Diltiazem Maleate (Repeated co-administration of 240 mg/day of diltiazem, a moderately-potent inhibitor of CYP3A4, with 7.5 mg/day (2.5 mg three times daily) alfuzosin increased the C_{max} and AUC_{0-24} of alfuzosin 1.5- and 1.3-fold, respectively. Alfuzosin increased the C_{max} and AUC_{0-12} of diltiazem 1.4-fold. Although no changes in blood pressure were observed in this study, diltiazem is an antihypertensive medication and the combination of alfuzosin and antihypertensive medications has the potential to cause hypotension in some patients).

No products indexed under this heading.

Disopyramide (A post-marketing study evaluating the effect of combining alfuzosin hydrochloride with another drug of comparable QT effect showed an increased effect when compared to either drug alone. Although this study was not designed to make direct statistical comparisons between drugs, the QT increase with both drugs was no more than additive and was lower than that of the active control moxifloxacin. These observations should be considered in clinical decisions when prescribing alfuzosin hydrochloride for patients with a known history of QT prolongation or patients who are taking medications which prolong the QT interval).

No products indexed under this heading.

Disopyramide Phosphate (A post-marketing study evaluating the effect of combining alfuzosin hydrochloride with another drug of comparable QT effect showed an increased effect when compared to either drug alone. Although this study was not designed to make direct statistical comparisons between drugs, the QT increase with both drugs was no more than additive and was lower than that of the active control moxifloxacin. These observations should be considered in clinical decisions when prescribing alfuzosin hydrochloride for patients with a known history of QT prolongation or patients who are taking medications which prolong the QT interval).

No products indexed under this heading.

Dofetilide (A post-marketing study evaluating the effect of combining alfuzosin hydrochloride with another drug of comparable QT effect showed an increased effect when compared to either drug alone. Although this study was not designed to make direct statistical comparisons between drugs, the QT increase with both drugs was no more than additive and was lower than that of the active control moxifloxacin. These observations should be considered in clinical decisions when prescribing alfuzosin hydrochloride for patients with a known history of QT prolongation or patients who are taking medications which prolong the QT interval).

No products indexed under this heading.

Doxazosin Mesylate (The pharmacokinetic and pharmacodynamic interactions between alfuzosin and other α-blockers have not been determined. However, interactions may be expected, and alfuzosin should not be used in combination with other α-blockers).

No products indexed under this heading.

Doxepin Hydrochloride (A post-marketing study evaluating the effect of combining alfuzosin hydrochloride with another drug of comparable QT effect showed an increased effect when compared to either drug alone. Although this study was not designed to make direct statistical comparisons between drugs, the QT increase with both drugs was no more than additive and was lower than that of the active control moxifloxacin. These observations should be considered in clinical decisions when prescribing alfuzosin hydrochloride for patients with a known history of QT prolongation or patients who are taking medications which prolong the QT interval).

No products indexed under this heading.

Droperidol (A post-marketing study evaluating the effect of combining alfuzosin hydrochloride with another drug of comparable QT effect showed an increased effect when compared to either drug alone. Although this study was not designed to make direct statistical comparisons between drugs, the QT increase with both drugs was no more than additive and was lower than

that of the active control moxifloxacin. These observations should be considered in clinical decisions when prescribing alfuzosin hydrochloride for patients with a known history of QT prolongation or patients who are taking medications which prolong the QT interval).

No products indexed under this heading.

Enalapril Maleate (There may be an increased risk of hypotension/postural hypotension and syncope when taking alfuzosin concomitantly with anti-hypertensive medication and nitrates. Care should be taken when alfuzosin is administered to patients with symptomatic hypotension or patients who have had a hypotensive response to other medications).

No products indexed under this heading.

Enalaprilat (There may be an increased risk of hypotension/postural hypotension and syncope when taking alfuzosin concomitantly with anti-hypertensive medication and nitrates. Care should be taken when alfuzosin is administered to patients with symptomatic hypotension or patients who have had a hypotensive response to other medications).

No products indexed under this heading.

Eprosartan Mesylate (There may be an increased risk of hypotension/postural hypotension and syncope when taking alfuzosin concomitantly with anti-hypertensive medication and nitrates. Care should be taken when alfuzosin is administered to patients with symptomatic hypotension or patients who have had a hypotensive response to other medications). Products include:

Teveten 538
Teveten HCT 541

Erythrityl Tetranitrate (There may be an increased risk of hypotension/postural hypotension and syncope when taking alfuzosin concomitantly with anti-hypertensive medication and nitrates. Care should be taken when alfuzosin is administered to patients with symptomatic hypotension or patients who have had a hypotensive response to other medications).

No products indexed under this heading.

Erythromycin (A post-marketing study evaluating the effect of combining alfuzosin hydrochloride with another drug of comparable QT effect showed an increased effect when compared to either drug alone. Although this study was not designed to make direct statistical comparisons between drugs, the QT increase with both drugs was no more than additive and was lower than that of the active control moxifloxacin. These observations should be considered in clinical decisions when prescribing alfuzosin hydrochloride for patients with a known history of QT prolongation or patients who are taking medications which prolong the QT interval).

No products indexed under this heading.

Erythromycin Estolate (A post-marketing study evaluating the effect of combining alfuzosin hydrochloride with another drug of comparable QT effect showed an increased effect when compared to either drug alone. Although this study was not designed to make direct statistical comparisons between drugs, the QT increase with both drugs was no more than additive and was lower than that of the active control moxifloxacin. These observations should be considered in clinical decisions when prescribing alfuzosin hydrochloride for patients with a known history of QT prolongation or patients who are taking medications which prolong the QT interval).

No products indexed under this heading.

Erythromycin Ethylsuccinate (A post-marketing study evaluating the

Uroxatral Interactions Index 1984

effect of combining alfuzosin hydrochloride with another drug of comparable QT effect showed an increased effect when compared to either drug alone. Although this study was not designed to make direct statistical comparisons between drugs, the QT increase with both drugs was no more than additive and was lower than that of the active control moxifloxacin. These observations should be considered in clinical decisions when prescribing alfuzosin hydrochloride for patients with a known history of QT prolongation or patients who are taking medications which prolong the QT interval). Products include:
E.E.S. 437
EryPed 435

Erythromycin Gluceptate (A post-marketing study evaluating the effect of combining alfuzosin hydrochloride with another drug of comparable QT effect showed an increased effect when compared to either drug alone. Although this study was not designed to make direct statistical comparisons between drugs, the QT increase with both drugs was no more than additive and was lower than that of the active control moxifloxacin. These observations should be considered in clinical decisions when prescribing alfuzosin hydrochloride for patients with a known history of QT prolongation or patients who are taking medications which prolong the QT interval).
No products indexed under this heading.

Erythromycin Lactobionate (A post-marketing study evaluating the effect of combining alfuzosin hydrochloride with another drug of comparable QT effect showed an increased effect when compared to either drug alone. Although this study was not designed to make direct statistical comparisons between drugs, the QT increase with both drugs was no more than additive and was lower than that of the active control moxifloxacin. These observations should be considered in clinical decisions when prescribing alfuzosin hydrochloride for patients with a known history of QT prolongation or patients who are taking medications which prolong the QT interval).
No products indexed under this heading.

Erythromycin Stearate (A post-marketing study evaluating the effect of combining alfuzosin hydrochloride with another drug of comparable QT effect showed an increased effect when compared to either drug alone. Although this study was not designed to make direct statistical comparisons between drugs, the QT increase with both drugs was no more than additive and was lower than that of the active control moxifloxacin. These observations should be considered in clinical decisions when prescribing alfuzosin hydrochloride for patients with a known history of QT prolongation or patients who are taking medications which prolong the QT interval).
No products indexed under this heading.

Esmolol Hydrochloride (There may be an increased risk of hypotension/postural hypotension and syncope when taking alfuzosin concomitantly with anti-hypertensive medication and nitrates. Care should be taken when alfuzosin is administered to patients with symptomatic hypotension or patients who have had a hypotensive response to other medications).
No products indexed under this heading.

Felodipine (There may be an increased risk of hypotension/postural hypotension and syncope when taking alfuzosin concomitantly with anti-hypertensive medication and nitrates. Care should be taken when alfuzosin is administered to patients with symptomatic hypotension or patients who have had a hypotensive response to other medications).
No products indexed under this heading.

Flecainide Acetate (A post-marketing study evaluating the effect of combining alfuzosin hydrochloride with another drug of comparable QT effect showed an increased effect when compared to either drug alone. Although this study was not designed to make direct statistical comparisons between drugs, the QT increase with both drugs was no more than additive and was lower than that of the active control moxifloxacin. These observations should be considered in clinical decisions when prescribing alfuzosin hydrochloride for patients with a known history of QT prolongation or patients who are taking medications which prolong the QT interval).
No products indexed under this heading.

Fluphenazine Decanoate (A post-marketing study evaluating the effect of combining alfuzosin hydrochloride with another drug of comparable QT effect showed an increased effect when compared to either drug alone. Although this study was not designed to make direct statistical comparisons between drugs, the QT increase with both drugs was no more than additive and was lower than that of the active control moxifloxacin. These observations should be considered in clinical decisions when prescribing alfuzosin hydrochloride for patients with a known history of QT prolongation or patients who are taking medications which prolong the QT interval).
No products indexed under this heading.

Fluphenazine Enanthate (A post-marketing study evaluating the effect of combining alfuzosin hydrochloride with another drug of comparable QT effect showed an increased effect when compared to either drug alone. Although this study was not designed to make direct statistical comparisons between drugs, the QT increase with both drugs was no more than additive and was lower than that of the active control moxifloxacin. These observations should be considered in clinical decisions when prescribing alfuzosin hydrochloride for patients with a known history of QT prolongation or patients who are taking medications which prolong the QT interval).
No products indexed under this heading.

Fluphenazine Hydrochloride (A post-marketing study evaluating the effect of combining alfuzosin hydrochloride with another drug of comparable QT effect showed an increased effect when compared to either drug alone. Although this study was not designed to make direct statistical comparisons between drugs, the QT increase with both drugs was no more than additive and was lower than that of the active control moxifloxacin. These observations should be considered in clinical decisions when prescribing alfuzosin hydrochloride for patients with a known history of QT prolongation or patients who are taking medications which prolong the QT interval).
No products indexed under this heading.

Fosamprenavir Calcium (Co-administration of alfuzosin with potent CYP3A4 inhibitors, such as ketoconazole, itraconazole, and ritonavir, is contraindicated, since alfuzosin blood levels are increased). Products include:
Lexiva Oral Suspension 1558
Lexiva 1558

Fosinopril Sodium (There may be an increased risk of hypotension/postural hypotension and syncope when taking alfuzosin concomitantly with anti-hypertensive medication and nitrates. Care should be taken when alfuzosin is administered to patients with symptomatic hypotension or patients who have had a hypotensive response to other medications).
No products indexed under this heading.

Furosemide (There may be an increased risk of hypotension/postural hypotension and syncope when taking alfuzosin concomitantly with anti-hypertensive medication and nitrates. Care should be taken when alfuzosin is administered to patients with symptomatic hypotension or patients who have had a hypotensive response to other medications). Products include:
Furosemide 2354

Glyceryl Trinitrate (There may be an increased risk of hypotension/postural hypotension and syncope when taking alfuzosin concomitantly with anti-hypertensive medication and nitrates. Care should be taken when alfuzosin is administered to patients with symptomatic hypotension or patients who have had a hypotensive response to other medications).
No products indexed under this heading.

Guanabenz Acetate (There may be an increased risk of hypotension/postural hypotension and syncope when taking alfuzosin concomitantly with anti-hypertensive medication and nitrates. Care should be taken when alfuzosin is administered to patients with symptomatic hypotension or patients who have had a hypotensive response to other medications).
No products indexed under this heading.

Guanethidine (There may be an increased risk of hypotension/postural hypotension and syncope when taking alfuzosin concomitantly with anti-hypertensive medication and nitrates. Care should be taken when alfuzosin is administered to patients with symptomatic hypotension or patients who have had a hypotensive response to other medications).
No products indexed under this heading.

Guanethidine Monosulfate (There may be an increased risk of hypotension/postural hypotension and syncope when taking alfuzosin concomitantly with anti-hypertensive medication and nitrates. Care should be taken when alfuzosin is administered to patients with symptomatic hypotension or patients who have had a hypotensive response to other medications).
No products indexed under this heading.

Guanethidine Sulfate (There may be an increased risk of hypotension/postural hypotension and syncope when taking alfuzosin concomitantly with anti-hypertensive medication and nitrates. Care should be taken when alfuzosin is administered to patients with symptomatic hypotension or patients who have had a hypotensive response to other medications).
No products indexed under this heading.

Haloperidol (A post-marketing study evaluating the effect of combining alfuzosin hydrochloride with another drug of comparable QT effect showed an increased effect when compared to either drug alone. Although this study was not designed to make direct statistical comparisons between drugs, the QT increase with both drugs was no more than additive and was lower than that of the active control moxifloxacin. These observations should be considered in clinical decisions when prescribing alfuzosin hydrochloride for patients with a known history of QT prolongation or patients who are taking medications which prolong the QT interval).
No products indexed under this heading.

Haloperidol Decanoate (A post-marketing study evaluating the effect of combining alfuzosin hydrochloride with another drug of comparable QT effect showed an increased effect when compared to either drug alone. Although this study was not designed to make direct statistical comparisons between drugs, the QT increase with both drugs was no more than additive and was lower than that of the active control moxifloxacin. These observations should be considered in clinical decisions when prescribing alfuzosin hydrochloride for patients with a known history of QT prolongation or patients who are taking medications which prolong the QT interval).
No products indexed under this heading.

Haloperidol Lactate (A post-marketing study evaluating the effect of combining alfuzosin hydrochloride with another drug of comparable QT effect showed an increased effect when compared to either drug alone. Although this study was not designed to make direct statistical comparisons between drugs, the QT increase with both drugs was no more than additive and was lower than that of the active control moxifloxacin. These observations should be considered in clinical decisions when prescribing alfuzosin hydrochloride for patients with a known history of QT prolongation or patients who are taking medications which prolong the QT interval).
No products indexed under this heading.

Hydralazine Hydrochloride (There may be an increased risk of hypotension/postural hypotension and syncope when taking alfuzosin concomitantly with anti-hypertensive medication and nitrates. Care should be taken when alfuzosin is administered to patients with symptomatic hypotension or patients who have had a hypotensive response to other medications).
No products indexed under this heading.

Hydrochlorothiazide (There may be an increased risk of hypotension/postural hypotension and syncope when taking alfuzosin concomitantly with anti-hypertensive medication and nitrates. Care should be taken when alfuzosin is administered to patients with symptomatic hypotension or patients who have had a hypotensive response to other medications). Products include:
Atacand HCT 700
Avalide 2956
Benicar HCT 1017
Diovan HCT 2419
Dyazide 1429
Exforge HCT 2449
Hyzaar 2162
Hyzaar 100-12.5 2162
Micardis HCT 889
Prinzide 2246
Tekturna HCT 2541
Teveten HCT 541

Hydroflumethiazide (There may be an increased risk of hypotension/postural hypotension and syncope when taking alfuzosin concomitantly with anti-hypertensive medication and nitrates. Care should be taken when alfuzosin is administered to patients with symptomatic hypotension or patients who have had a hypotensive response to other medications).
No products indexed under this heading.

Hydroxyzine Hydrochloride (A post-marketing study evaluating the effect of combining alfuzosin hydrochloride with another drug of comparable QT effect showed an increased effect when com-

1985 Interactions Index Uroxatral

pared to either drug alone. Although this study was not designed to make direct statistical comparisons between drugs, the QT increase with both drugs was no more than additive and was lower than that of the active control moxifloxacin. These observations should be considered in clinical decisions when prescribing alfuzosin hydrochloride for patients with a known history of QT prolongation or patients who are taking medications which prolong the QT interval).

No products indexed under this heading.

Imipramine Hydrochloride (A post-marketing study evaluating the effect of combining alfuzosin hydrochloride with another drug of comparable QT effect showed an increased effect when compared to either drug alone. Although this study was not designed to make direct statistical comparisons between drugs, the QT increase with both drugs was no more than additive and was lower than that of the active control moxifloxacin. These observations should be considered in clinical decisions when prescribing alfuzosin hydrochloride for patients with a known history of QT prolongation or patients who are taking medications which prolong the QT interval).

No products indexed under this heading.

Imipramine Pamoate (A post-marketing study evaluating the effect of combining alfuzosin hydrochloride with another drug of comparable QT effect showed an increased effect when compared to either drug alone. Although this study was not designed to make direct statistical comparisons between drugs, the QT increase with both drugs was no more than additive and was lower than that of the active control moxifloxacin. These observations should be considered in clinical decisions when prescribing alfuzosin hydrochloride for patients with a known history of QT prolongation or patients who are taking medications which prolong the QT interval).

No products indexed under this heading.

Indapamide (There may be an increased risk of hypotension/postural hypotension and syncope when taking alfuzosin concomitantly with anti-hypertensive medication and nitrates. Care should be taken when alfuzosin is administered to patients with symptomatic hypotension or patients who have had a hypotensive response to other medications). Products include:

Indapamide 2356

Indinavir Sulfate (Co-administration of alfuzosin with potent CYP3A4 inhibitors, such as ketoconazole, itraconazole, and ritonavir, is contraindicated, since alfuzosin blood levels are increased). Products include:

Crixivan 2113

Irbesartan (There may be an increased risk of hypotension/postural hypotension and syncope when taking alfuzosin concomitantly with anti-hypertensive medication and nitrates. Care should be taken when alfuzosin is administered to patients with symptomatic hypotension or patients who have had a hypotensive response to other medications). Products include:

Avalide 2956

Avapro 2962

Isocarboxazid (A post-marketing study evaluating the effect of combining alfuzosin hydrochloride with another drug of comparable QT effect showed an increased effect when compared to either drug alone. Although this study was not designed to make direct statistical comparisons between drugs, the QT increase with both drugs was no more than additive and was lower than that of the active control moxifloxacin. These observations should be considered in clinical decisions when prescribing alfuzosin hydrochloride for patients with a known history of QT prolongation or patients who are taking medications which prolong the QT interval). Products include:

Marplan 3481

Isosorbide Dinitrate (There may be an increased risk of hypotension/postural hypotension and syncope when taking alfuzosin concomitantly with anti-hypertensive medication and nitrates. Care should be taken when alfuzosin is administered to patients with symptomatic hypotension or patients who have had a hypotensive response to other medications).

No products indexed under this heading.

Isosorbide Mononitrate (There may be an increased risk of hypotension/postural hypotension and syncope when taking alfuzosin concomitantly with anti-hypertensive medication and nitrates. Care should be taken when alfuzosin is administered to patients with symptomatic hypotension or patients who have had a hypotensive response to other medications).

No products indexed under this heading.

Isradipine (There may be an increased risk of hypotension/postural hypotension and syncope when taking alfuzosin concomitantly with anti-hypertensive medication and nitrates. Care should be taken when alfuzosin is administered to patients with symptomatic hypotension or patients who have had a hypotensive response to other medications). Products include:

DynaCirc CR 1432

Itraconazole (Co-administration of alfuzosin with potent CYP3A4 inhibitors, such as itraconazole, is contraindicated, since alfuzosin blood levels are increased).

No products indexed under this heading.

Ketoconazole (Co-administration of alfuzosin with potent CYP3A4 inhibitors, such as ketoconazole, is contraindicated, since alfuzosin blood levels are increased. Repeated administration of 200 and 400 mg of ketoconazole, a potent inhibitor of CYP3A4, increased alfuzosin C_{max} 2.1- and 2.3- fold, respectively, and AUC_{last} 2.5- and 3.2-fold, respectively, following a single 10 mg dose of alfuzosin. Therefore, alfuzosin should not be co-administered with potent inhibitors of CYP3A4 because exposure is increased (eg, with ketoconazole)). Products include:

Extina 3319

Xolegel 3337

Labetalol Hydrochloride (There may be an increased risk of hypotension/postural hypotension and syncope when taking alfuzosin concomitantly with anti-hypertensive medication and nitrates. Care should be taken when alfuzosin is administered to patients with symptomatic hypotension or patients who have had a hypotensive response to other medications).

No products indexed under this heading.

Lidocaine (A post-marketing study evaluating the effect of combining alfuzosin hydrochloride with another drug of comparable QT effect showed an increased effect when compared to either drug alone. Although this study was not designed to make direct statistical comparisons between drugs, the QT increase with both drugs was no more than additive and was lower than that of the active control moxifloxacin. These observations should be considered in clinical decisions when prescribing alfuzosin hydrochloride for patients with a known history of QT prolongation or patients who are taking medications which prolong the QT interval). Products include:

Lidoderm 1107

Lidocaine Hydrochloride (A post-marketing study evaluating the effect of combining alfuzosin hydrochloride with another drug of comparable QT effect showed an increased effect when compared to either drug alone. Although this study was not designed to make direct statistical comparisons between drugs, the QT increase with both drugs was no more than additive and was lower than that of the active control moxifloxacin. These observations should be considered in clinical decisions when prescribing alfuzosin hydrochloride for patients with a known history of QT prolongation or patients who are taking medications which prolong the QT interval).

No products indexed under this heading.

Lisinopril (There may be an increased risk of hypotension/postural hypotension and syncope when taking alfuzosin concomitantly with anti-hypertensive medication and nitrates. Care should be taken when alfuzosin is administered to patients with symptomatic hypotension or patients who have had a hypotensive response to other medications). Products include:

Prinivil 2241

Prinzide 2246

Lithium Carbonate (A post-marketing study evaluating the effect of combining alfuzosin hydrochloride with another drug of comparable QT effect showed an increased effect when compared to either drug alone. Although this study was not designed to make direct statistical comparisons between drugs, the QT increase with both drugs was no more than additive and was lower than that of the active control moxifloxacin. These observations should be considered in clinical decisions when prescribing alfuzosin hydrochloride for patients with a known history of QT prolongation or patients who are taking medications which prolong the QT interval).

No products indexed under this heading.

Lithium Citrate (A post-marketing study evaluating the effect of combining alfuzosin hydrochloride with another drug of comparable QT effect showed an increased effect when compared to either drug alone. Although this study was not designed to make direct statistical comparisons between drugs, the QT increase with both drugs was no more than additive and was lower than that of the active control moxifloxacin. These observations should be considered in clinical decisions when prescribing alfuzosin hydrochloride for patients with a known history of QT prolongation or patients who are taking medications which prolong the QT interval).

No products indexed under this heading.

Lopinavir (Co-administration of alfuzosin with potent CYP3A4 inhibitors, such as ketoconazole, itraconazole, and ritonavir, is contraindicated, since alfuzosin blood levels are increased). Products include:

Kaletra 458

Lorazepam (A post-marketing study evaluating the effect of combining alfuzosin hydrochloride with another drug of comparable QT effect showed an increased effect when compared to either drug alone. Although this study was not designed to make direct statistical comparisons between drugs, the QT increase with both drugs was no more than additive and was lower than that of the active control moxifloxacin. These observations should be considered in clinical decisions when prescribing alfuzosin hydrochloride for patients with a known history of QT prolongation or patients who are taking medications which prolong the QT interval).

No products indexed under this heading.

Losartan Potassium (There may be an increased risk of hypotension/postural hypotension and syncope when taking alfuzosin concomitantly with anti-hypertensive medication and nitrates. Care should be taken when alfuzosin is administered to patients with symptomatic hypotension or patients who have had a hypotensive response to other medications). Products include:

Cozaar 2106

Hyzaar 2162

Hyzaar 100-12.5 2162

Loxapine Hydrochloride (A post-marketing study evaluating the effect of combining alfuzosin hydrochloride with another drug of comparable QT effect showed an increased effect when compared to either drug alone. Although this study was not designed to make direct statistical comparisons between drugs, the QT increase with both drugs was no more than additive and was lower than that of the active control moxifloxacin. These observations should be considered in clinical decisions when prescribing alfuzosin hydrochloride for patients with a known history of QT prolongation or patients who are taking medications which prolong the QT interval).

No products indexed under this heading.

Loxapine Succinate (A post-marketing study evaluating the effect of combining alfuzosin hydrochloride with another drug of comparable QT effect showed an increased effect when compared to either drug alone. Although this study was not designed to make direct statistical comparisons between drugs, the QT increase with both drugs was no more than additive and was lower than that of the active control moxifloxacin. These observations should be considered in clinical decisions when prescribing alfuzosin hydrochloride for patients with a known history of QT prolongation or patients who are taking medications which prolong the QT interval).

No products indexed under this heading.

Maprotiline Hydrochloride (A post-marketing study evaluating the effect of combining alfuzosin hydrochloride with another drug of comparable QT effect showed an increased effect when compared to either drug alone. Although this study was not designed to make direct statistical comparisons between drugs, the QT increase with both drugs was no more than additive and was lower than that of the active control moxifloxacin. These observations should be considered in clinical decisions when prescribing alfuzosin hydrochloride for patients with a known history of QT prolongation or patients who are taking medications which prolong the QT interval).

No products indexed under this heading.

Mecamylamine Hydrochloride (There may be an increased risk of hypotension/postural hypotension and syncope when taking alfuzosin concomitantly with anti-hypertensive medication and nitrates. Care should be taken when alfuzosin is administered to patients with symptomatic hypotension or patients who have had a hypotensive response to other medications).

No products indexed under this heading.

Meprobamate (A post-marketing study evaluating the effect of combining alfuzosin hydrochloride with another drug of comparable QT effect showed an increased effect when compared to either drug alone. Although this study was not designed to make direct statistical comparisons between drugs, the QT increase with both drugs was no more than additive and was lower than that of the active control moxifloxacin. These observations should be consid-

IMPORTANT NOTE: Always consult each drug listing in the patient's regimen for possible interactions.

Uroxatral Interactions Index 1986

ered in clinical decisions when prescribing alfuzosin hydrochloride for patients with a known history of QT prolongation or patients who are taking medications which prolong the QT interval).
No products indexed under this heading.

Mesoridazine Besylate (A post-marketing study evaluating the effect of combining alfuzosin hydrochloride with another drug of comparable QT effect showed an increased effect when compared to either drug alone. Although this study was not designed to make direct statistical comparisons between drugs, the QT increase with both drugs was no more than additive and was lower than that of the active control moxifloxacin. These observations should be considered in clinical decisions when prescribing alfuzosin hydrochloride for patients with a known history of QT prolongation or patients who are taking medications which prolong the QT interval).
No products indexed under this heading.

Methyclothiazide (There may be an increased risk of hypotension/postural hypotension and syncope when taking alfuzosin concomitantly with anti-hypertensive medication and nitrates. Care should be taken when alfuzosin is administered to patients with symptomatic hypotension or patients who have had a hypotensive response to other medications).
No products indexed under this heading.

Methyldopa (There may be an increased risk of hypotension/postural hypotension and syncope when taking alfuzosin concomitantly with anti-hypertensive medication and nitrates. Care should be taken when alfuzosin is administered to patients with symptomatic hypotension or patients who have had a hypotensive response to other medications).
No products indexed under this heading.

Methyldopate Hydrochloride (There may be an increased risk of hypotension/postural hypotension and syncope when taking alfuzosin concomitantly with anti-hypertensive medication and nitrates. Care should be taken when alfuzosin is administered to patients with symptomatic hypotension or patients who have had a hypotensive response to other medications).
No products indexed under this heading.

Metolazone (There may be an increased risk of hypotension/postural hypotension and syncope when taking alfuzosin concomitantly with anti-hypertensive medication and nitrates. Care should be taken when alfuzosin is administered to patients with symptomatic hypotension or patients who have had a hypotensive response to other medications).
No products indexed under this heading.

Metoprolol Succinate (There may be an increased risk of hypotension/postural hypotension and syncope when taking alfuzosin concomitantly with anti-hypertensive medication and nitrates. Care should be taken when alfuzosin is administered to patients with symptomatic hypotension or patients who have had a hypotensive response to other medications). Products include:
Toprol XL **732**

Metoprolol Tartrate (There may be an increased risk of hypotension/postural hypotension and syncope when taking alfuzosin concomitantly with anti-hypertensive medication and nitrates. Care should be taken when alfuzosin is administered to patients with symptomatic hypotension or patients who have had a hypotensive response to other medications).
No products indexed under this heading.

Metyrosine (There may be an increased risk of hypotension/postural hypotension and syncope when taking alfuzosin concomitantly with anti-hypertensive medication and nitrates. Care should be taken when alfuzosin is administered to patients with symptomatic hypotension or patients who have had a hypotensive response to other medications).
No products indexed under this heading.

Mexiletine Hydrochloride (A post-marketing study evaluating the effect of combining alfuzosin hydrochloride with another drug of comparable QT effect showed an increased effect when compared to either drug alone. Although this study was not designed to make direct statistical comparisons between drugs, the QT increase with both drugs was no more than additive and was lower than that of the active control moxifloxacin. These observations should be considered in clinical decisions when prescribing alfuzosin hydrochloride for patients with a known history of QT prolongation or patients who are taking medications which prolong the QT interval).
No products indexed under this heading.

Mibefradil Dihydrochloride (There may be an increased risk of hypotension/postural hypotension and syncope when taking alfuzosin concomitantly with anti-hypertensive medication and nitrates. Care should be taken when alfuzosin is administered to patients with symptomatic hypotension or patients who have had a hypotensive response to other medications).
No products indexed under this heading.

Midazolam Hydrochloride (A post-marketing study evaluating the effect of combining alfuzosin hydrochloride with another drug of comparable QT effect showed an increased effect when compared to either drug alone. Although this study was not designed to make direct statistical comparisons between drugs, the QT increase with both drugs was no more than additive and was lower than that of the active control moxifloxacin. These observations should be considered in clinical decisions when prescribing alfuzosin hydrochloride for patients with a known history of QT prolongation or patients who are taking medications which prolong the QT interval).
No products indexed under this heading.

Minoxidil (There may be an increased risk of hypotension/postural hypotension and syncope when taking alfuzosin concomitantly with anti-hypertensive medication and nitrates. Care should be taken when alfuzosin is administered to patients with symptomatic hypotension or patients who have had a hypotensive response to other medications).
No products indexed under this heading.

Moexipril Hydrochloride (There may be an increased risk of hypotension/postural hypotension and syncope when taking alfuzosin concomitantly with anti-hypertensive medication and nitrates. Care should be taken when alfuzosin is administered to patients with symptomatic hypotension or patients who have had a hypotensive response to other medications).
No products indexed under this heading.

Molindone Hydrochloride (A post-marketing study evaluating the effect of combining alfuzosin hydrochloride with another drug of comparable QT effect showed an increased effect when compared to either drug alone. Although this study was not designed to make direct statistical comparisons between drugs, the QT increase with both drugs was no more than additive and was lower than that of the active control moxifloxacin. These observations should be considered in clinical decisions when prescribing alfuzosin hydrochloride for patients with a known history of QT prolongation or patients who are taking medications which prolong the QT interval). Products include:
Moban **1108**

Nadolol (There may be an increased risk of hypotension/postural hypotension and syncope when taking alfuzosin concomitantly with anti-hypertensive medication and nitrates. Care should be taken when alfuzosin is administered to patients with symptomatic hypotension or patients who have had a hypotensive response to other medications).
Products include:
Nadolol **2359**

Nebivolol (There may be an increased risk of hypotension/postural hypotension and syncope when taking alfuzosin concomitantly with anti-hypertensive medication and nitrates. Care should be taken when alfuzosin is administered to patients with symptomatic hypotension or patients who have had a hypotensive response to other medications).
Products include:
Bystolic **1147**

Nefazodone Hydrochloride (Co-administration of alfuzosin with potent CYP3A4 inhibitors, such as ketoconazole, itraconazole, and ritonavir, is contraindicated, since alfuzosin blood levels are increased).
No products indexed under this heading.

Nelfinavir Mesylate (Co-administration of alfuzosin with potent CYP3A4 inhibitors, such as ketoconazole, itraconazole, and ritonavir, is contraindicated, since alfuzosin blood levels are increased).
No products indexed under this heading.

Nicardipine Hydrochloride (There may be an increased risk of hypotension/postural hypotension and syncope when taking alfuzosin concomitantly with anti-hypertensive medication and nitrates. Care should be taken when alfuzosin is administered to patients with symptomatic hypotension or patients who have had a hypotensive response to other medications).
No products indexed under this heading.

Nifedipine (There may be an increased risk of hypotension/postural hypotension and syncope when taking alfuzosin concomitantly with anti-hypertensive medication and nitrates. Care should be taken when alfuzosin is administered to patients with symptomatic hypotension or patients who have had a hypotensive response to other medications).
No products indexed under this heading.

Nisoldipine (There may be an increased risk of hypotension/postural hypotension and syncope when taking alfuzosin concomitantly with anti-hypertensive medication and nitrates. Care should be taken when alfuzosin is administered to patients with symptomatic hypotension or patients who have had a hypotensive response to other medications).
No products indexed under this heading.

Nitrate & Nitrite Preparations (There may be an increased risk of hypotension/postural hypotension and syncope when taking alfuzosin concomitantly with anti-hypertensive medication and nitrates. Care should be taken when alfuzosin is administered to patients with symptomatic hypotension or patients who have had a hypotensive response to other medications).
No products indexed under this heading.

Nitrates, organic (There may be an increased risk of hypotension/postural hypotension and syncope when taking alfuzosin concomitantly with anti-hypertensive medication and nitrates. Care should be taken when alfuzosin is administered to patients with symptomatic hypotension or patients who have had a hypotensive response to other medications).
No products indexed under this heading.

Nitrates and Nitrites (There may be an increased risk of hypotension/postural hypotension and syncope when taking alfuzosin concomitantly with anti-hypertensive medication and nitrates. Care should be taken when alfuzosin is administered to patients with symptomatic hypotension or patients who have had a hypotensive response to other medications).
No products indexed under this heading.

Nitroglycerin (There may be an increased risk of hypotension/postural hypotension and syncope when taking alfuzosin concomitantly with anti-hypertensive medication and nitrates. Care should be taken when alfuzosin is administered to patients with symptomatic hypotension or patients who have had a hypotensive response to other medications). Products include:
Nitro-Dur **3170**
Nitrolingual **3266**

Nitroglycerin, long-acting formulations (There may be an increased risk of hypotension/postural hypotension and syncope when taking alfuzosin concomitantly with anti-hypertensive medication and nitrates. Care should be taken when alfuzosin is administered to patients with symptomatic hypotension or patients who have had a hypotensive response to other medications).
No products indexed under this heading.

Nitroglycerin Intravenous (There may be an increased risk of hypotension/postural hypotension and syncope when taking alfuzosin concomitantly with anti-hypertensive medication and nitrates. Care should be taken when alfuzosin is administered to patients with symptomatic hypotension or patients who have had a hypotensive response to other medications).
No products indexed under this heading.

Nortriptyline Hydrochloride (A post-marketing study evaluating the effect of combining alfuzosin hydrochloride with another drug of comparable QT effect showed an increased effect when compared to either drug alone. Although this study was not designed to make direct statistical comparisons between drugs, the QT increase with both drugs was no more than additive and was lower than that of the active control moxifloxacin. These observations should be considered in clinical decisions when prescribing alfuzosin hydrochloride for patients with a known history of QT prolongation or patients who are taking medications which prolong the QT interval).
No products indexed under this heading.

Olanzapine (A post-marketing study evaluating the effect of combining alfuzosin hydrochloride with another drug of comparable QT effect showed an increased effect when compared to either drug alone. Although this study was not designed to make direct statistical comparisons between drugs, the QT increase with both drugs was no more than additive and was lower than that of the active control moxifloxacin. These observations should be considered in clinical decisions when prescribing alfuzosin hydrochloride for patients with a known history of QT prolongation or patients who are taking medications which prolong the QT interval). Products include:

1987 **Interactions Index** **Uroxatral**

Symbyax **1965**
Zyprexa **1984**
Zyprexa IntraMuscular **1984**
Zyprexa ZYDIS **1984**

Oxazepam (A post-marketing study evaluating the effect of combining alfuzosin hydrochloride with another drug of comparable QT effect showed an increased effect when compared to either drug alone. Although this study was not designed to make direct statistical comparisons between drugs, the QT increase with both drugs was no more than additive and was lower than that of the active control moxifloxacin. These observations should be considered in clinical decisions when prescribing alfuzosin hydrochloride for patients with a known history of QT prolongation or patients who are taking medications which prolong the QT interval).
No products indexed under this heading.

Penbutolol Sulfate (There may be an increased risk of hypotension/postural hypotension and syncope when taking alfuzosin concomitantly with anti-hypertensive medication and nitrates. Care should be taken when alfuzosin is administered to patients with symptomatic hypotension or patients who have had a hypotensive response to other medications).
No products indexed under this heading.

Pentaerythritol Tetranitrate (There may be an increased risk of hypotension/postural hypotension and syncope when taking alfuzosin concomitantly with anti-hypertensive medication and nitrates. Care should be taken when alfuzosin is administered to patients with symptomatic hypotension or patients who have had a hypotensive response to other medications).
No products indexed under this heading.

Perindopril Erbumine (There may be an increased risk of hypotension/postural hypotension and syncope when taking alfuzosin concomitantly with anti-hypertensive medication and nitrates. Care should be taken when alfuzosin is administered to patients with symptomatic hypotension or patients who have had a hypotensive response to other medications).
No products indexed under this heading.

Perphenazine (A post-marketing study evaluating the effect of combining alfuzosin hydrochloride with another drug of comparable QT effect showed an increased effect when compared to either drug alone. Although this study was not designed to make direct statistical comparisons between drugs, the QT increase with both drugs was no more than additive and was lower than that of the active control moxifloxacin. These observations should be considered in clinical decisions when prescribing alfuzosin hydrochloride for patients with a known history of QT prolongation or patients who are taking medications which prolong the QT interval).
No products indexed under this heading.

Phenelzine Sulfate (A post-marketing study evaluating the effect of combining alfuzosin hydrochloride with another drug of comparable QT effect showed an increased effect when compared to either drug alone. Although this study was not designed to make direct statistical comparisons between drugs, the QT increase with both drugs was no more than additive and was lower than that of the active control moxifloxacin. These observations should be considered in clinical decisions when prescribing alfuzosin hydrochloride for patients with a known history of QT prolongation or patients who are taking medications which prolong the QT interval).
No products indexed under this heading.

Phenoxybenzamine Hydrochloride (There may be an increased risk of hypotension/postural hypotension and syncope when taking alfuzosin concomitantly with anti-hypertensive medication and nitrates. Care should be taken when alfuzosin is administered to patients with symptomatic hypotension or patients who have had a hypotensive response to other medications). Products include:
Dibenzyline **3495**

Phentolamine Mesylate (There may be an increased risk of hypotension/postural hypotension and syncope when taking alfuzosin concomitantly with anti-hypertensive medication and nitrates. Care should be taken when alfuzosin is administered to patients with symptomatic hypotension or patients who have had a hypotensive response to other medications).
No products indexed under this heading.

Pindolol (There may be an increased risk of hypotension/postural hypotension and syncope when taking alfuzosin concomitantly with anti-hypertensive medication and nitrates. Care should be taken when alfuzosin is administered to patients with symptomatic hypotension or patients who have had a hypotensive response to other medications).
No products indexed under this heading.

Polythiazide (There may be an increased risk of hypotension/postural hypotension and syncope when taking alfuzosin concomitantly with anti-hypertensive medication and nitrates. Care should be taken when alfuzosin is administered to patients with symptomatic hypotension or patients who have had a hypotensive response to other medications).
No products indexed under this heading.

Prazepam (A post-marketing study evaluating the effect of combining alfuzosin hydrochloride with another drug of comparable QT effect showed an increased effect when compared to either drug alone. Although this study was not designed to make direct statistical comparisons between drugs, the QT increase with both drugs was no more than additive and was lower than that of the active control moxifloxacin. These observations should be considered in clinical decisions when prescribing alfuzosin hydrochloride for patients with a known history of QT prolongation or patients who are taking medications which prolong the QT interval).
No products indexed under this heading.

Prazosin Hydrochloride (The pharmacokinetic and pharmacodynamic interactions between alfuzosin and other α-blockers have not been determined. However, interactions may be expected, and alfuzosin should not be used in combination with other α-blockers).
No products indexed under this heading.

Procainamide Hydrochloride (A post-marketing study evaluating the effect of combining alfuzosin hydrochloride with another drug of comparable QT effect showed an increased effect when compared to either drug alone. Although this study was not designed to make direct statistical comparisons between drugs, the QT increase with both drugs was no more than additive and was lower than that of the active control moxifloxacin. These observations should be considered in clinical decisions when prescribing alfuzosin hydrochloride for patients with a known history of QT prolongation or patients who are taking medications which prolong the QT interval).
No products indexed under this heading.

Prochlorperazine (A post-marketing study evaluating the effect of combining alfuzosin hydrochloride with another drug of comparable QT effect showed an increased effect when compared to either drug alone. Although this study was not designed to make direct statistical comparisons between drugs, the QT increase with both drugs was no more than additive and was lower than that of the active control moxifloxacin. These observations should be considered in clinical decisions when prescribing alfuzosin hydrochloride for patients with a known history of QT prolongation or patients who are taking medications which prolong the QT interval).
No products indexed under this heading.

Promethazine Hydrochloride (A post-marketing study evaluating the effect of combining alfuzosin hydrochloride with another drug of comparable QT effect showed an increased effect when compared to either drug alone. Although this study was not designed to make direct statistical comparisons between drugs, the QT increase with both drugs was no more than additive and was lower than that of the active control moxifloxacin. These observations should be considered in clinical decisions when prescribing alfuzosin hydrochloride for patients with a known history of QT prolongation or patients who are taking medications which prolong the QT interval).
No products indexed under this heading.

Propafenone Hydrochloride (A post-marketing study evaluating the effect of combining alfuzosin hydrochloride with another drug of comparable QT effect showed an increased effect when compared to either drug alone. Although this study was not designed to make direct statistical comparisons between drugs, the QT increase with both drugs was no more than additive and was lower than that of the active control moxifloxacin. These observations should be considered in clinical decisions when prescribing alfuzosin hydrochloride for patients with a known history of QT prolongation or patients who are taking medications which prolong the QT interval). Products include:
Rythmol **1648**
Rythmol SR **1652**

Propranolol Hydrochloride (There may be an increased risk of hypotension/postural hypotension and syncope when taking alfuzosin concomitantly with anti-hypertensive medication and nitrates. Care should be taken when alfuzosin is administered to patients with symptomatic hypotension or patients who have had a hypotensive response to other medications). Products include:
InnoPran XL **1517**

Protriptyline Hydrochloride (A post-marketing study evaluating the effect of combining alfuzosin hydrochloride with another drug of comparable QT effect showed an increased effect when compared to either drug alone. Although this study was not designed to make direct statistical comparisons between drugs, the QT increase with both drugs was no more than additive and was lower than that of the active control moxifloxacin. These observations should be considered in clinical decisions when prescribing alfuzosin hydrochloride for patients with a known history of QT prolongation or patients who are taking medications which prolong the QT interval).
No products indexed under this heading.

Quetiapine Fumarate (A post-marketing study evaluating the effect of combining alfuzosin hydrochloride with another drug of comparable QT effect showed an increased effect when compared to either drug alone. Although this study was not designed to make direct statistical comparisons between drugs, the QT increase with both drugs was no more than additive and was lower than that of the active control moxifloxacin. These observations should be considered in clinical decisions when prescribing alfuzosin hydrochloride for patients with a known history of QT prolongation or patients who are taking medications which prolong the QT interval). Products include:
Seroquel **750**
Seroquel XR **759**

Quinapril Hydrochloride (There may be an increased risk of hypotension/postural hypotension and syncope when taking alfuzosin concomitantly with anti-hypertensive medication and nitrates. Care should be taken when alfuzosin is administered to patients with symptomatic hypotension or patients who have had a hypotensive response to other medications).
No products indexed under this heading.

Quinidine (A post-marketing study evaluating the effect of combining alfuzosin hydrochloride with another drug of comparable QT effect showed an increased effect when compared to either drug alone. Although this study was not designed to make direct statistical comparisons between drugs, the QT increase with both drugs was no more than additive and was lower than that of the active control moxifloxacin. These observations should be considered in clinical decisions when prescribing alfuzosin hydrochloride for patients with a known history of QT prolongation or patients who are taking medications which prolong the QT interval).
No products indexed under this heading.

Quinidine Gluconate (A post-marketing study evaluating the effect of combining alfuzosin hydrochloride with another drug of comparable QT effect showed an increased effect when compared to either drug alone. Although this study was not designed to make direct statistical comparisons between drugs, the QT increase with both drugs was no more than additive and was lower than that of the active control moxifloxacin. These observations should be considered in clinical decisions when prescribing alfuzosin hydrochloride for patients with a known history of QT prolongation or patients who are taking medications which prolong the QT interval).
No products indexed under this heading.

Quinidine Hydrochloride (A post-marketing study evaluating the effect of combining alfuzosin hydrochloride with another drug of comparable QT effect showed an increased effect when compared to either drug alone. Although this study was not designed to make direct statistical comparisons between drugs, the QT increase with both drugs was no more than additive and was lower than that of the active control moxifloxacin. These observations should be considered in clinical decisions when prescribing alfuzosin hydrochloride for patients with a known history of QT prolongation or patients who are taking medications which prolong the QT interval).
No products indexed under this heading.

Quinidine Polygalacturonate (A post-marketing study evaluating the effect of combining alfuzosin hydrochloride with another drug of comparable QT effect showed an increased effect when compared to either drug alone. Although this study was not designed to make direct statistical comparisons between drugs, the QT increase with both drugs was no more than additive and was lower than that of the active control moxifloxacin. These observations should be considered in clinical decisions when prescribing alfuzosin hydrochloride for patients with a known

IMPORTANT NOTE: Always consult each drug listing in the patient's regimen for possible interactions.

history of QT prolongation or patients who are taking medications which prolong the QT interval).
No products indexed under this heading.

Quinidine Sulfate (A post-marketing study evaluating the effect of combining alfuzosin hydrochloride with another drug of comparable QT effect showed an increased effect when compared to either drug alone. Although this study was not designed to make direct statistical comparisons between drugs, the QT increase with both drugs was no more than additive and was lower than that of the active control moxifloxacin. These observations should be considered in clinical decisions when prescribing alfuzosin hydrochloride for patients with a known history of QT prolongation or patients who are taking medications which prolong the QT interval).
No products indexed under this heading.

Ramipril (There may be an increased risk of hypotension/postural hypotension and syncope when taking alfuzosin concomitantly with anti-hypertensive medication and nitrates. Care should be taken when alfuzosin is administered to patients with symptomatic hypotension or patients who have had a hypotensive response to other medications).
No products indexed under this heading.

Rauwolfia Serpentina (There may be an increased risk of hypotension/postural hypotension and syncope when taking alfuzosin concomitantly with anti-hypertensive medication and nitrates. Care should be taken when alfuzosin is administered to patients with symptomatic hypotension or patients who have had a hypotensive response to other medications).
No products indexed under this heading.

Rescinnamine (There may be an increased risk of hypotension/postural hypotension and syncope when taking alfuzosin concomitantly with anti-hypertensive medication and nitrates. Care should be taken when alfuzosin is administered to patients with symptomatic hypotension or patients who have had a hypotensive response to other medications).
No products indexed under this heading.

Reserpine (There may be an increased risk of hypotension/postural hypotension and syncope when taking alfuzosin concomitantly with anti-hypertensive medication and nitrates. Care should be taken when alfuzosin is administered to patients with symptomatic hypotension or patients who have had a hypotensive response to other medications).
No products indexed under this heading.

Risperidone (A post-marketing study evaluating the effect of combining alfuzosin hydrochloride with another drug of comparable QT effect showed an increased effect when compared to either drug alone. Although this study was not designed to make direct statistical comparisons between drugs, the QT increase with both drugs was no more than additive and was lower than that of the active control moxifloxacin. These observations should be considered in clinical decisions when prescribing alfuzosin hydrochloride for patients with a known history of QT prolongation or patients who are taking medications which prolong the QT interval). Products include:
Risperdal Consta 2682

Ritonavir (Co-administration of alfuzosin with potent CYP3A4 inhibitors, such as ritonavir, is contraindicated, since alfuzosin blood levels are increased). Products include:
Kaletra 458
Norvir 509

Saquinavir (Co-administration of alfuzosin with potent CYP3A4 inhibitors, such as ketoconazole, itraconazole, and ritonavir, is contraindicated, since alfuzosin blood levels are increased).
No products indexed under this heading.

Saquinavir Mesylate (Co-administration of alfuzosin with potent CYP3A4 inhibitors, such as ketoconazole, itraconazole, and ritonavir, is contraindicated, since alfuzosin blood levels are increased).
No products indexed under this heading.

Sodium Nitroprusside (There may be an increased risk of hypotension/postural hypotension and syncope when taking alfuzosin concomitantly with anti-hypertensive medication and nitrates. Care should be taken when alfuzosin is administered to patients with symptomatic hypotension or patients who have had a hypotensive response to other medications).
No products indexed under this heading.

Sotalol Hydrochloride (There may be an increased risk of hypotension/postural hypotension and syncope when taking alfuzosin concomitantly with anti-hypertensive medication and nitrates. Care should be taken when alfuzosin is administered to patients with symptomatic hypotension or patients who have had a hypotensive response to other medications).
No products indexed under this heading.

Spirapril Hydrochloride (There may be an increased risk of hypotension/postural hypotension and syncope when taking alfuzosin concomitantly with anti-hypertensive medication and nitrates. Care should be taken when alfuzosin is administered to patients with symptomatic hypotension or patients who have had a hypotensive response to other medications).
No products indexed under this heading.

Tamsulosin Hydrochloride (The pharmacokinetic and pharmacodynamic interactions between alfuzosin and other α-blockers have not been determined. However, interactions may be expected, and alfuzosin should not be used in combination with other α-blockers).
No products indexed under this heading.

Telithromycin (Co-administration of alfuzosin with potent CYP3A4 inhibitors, such as ketoconazole, itraconazole, and ritonavir, is contraindicated, since alfuzosin blood levels are increased). Products include:
Ketek 2991

Telmisartan (There may be an increased risk of hypotension/postural hypotension and syncope when taking alfuzosin concomitantly with anti-hypertensive medication and nitrates. Care should be taken when alfuzosin is administered to patients with symptomatic hypotension or patients who have had a hypotensive response to other medications). Products include:
Micardis 887
Micardis HCT 889

Terazosin Hydrochloride (The pharmacokinetic and pharmacodynamic interactions between alfuzosin and other α-blockers have not been determined. However, interactions may be expected, and alfuzosin should not be used in combination with other α-blockers).
No products indexed under this heading.

Thioridazine Hydrochloride (A post-marketing study evaluating the effect of combining alfuzosin hydrochloride with another drug of comparable QT effect showed an increased effect when compared to either drug alone. Although this study was not designed to make direct statistical comparisons between drugs, the QT increase with both drugs

was no more than additive and was lower than that of the active control moxifloxacin. These observations should be considered in clinical decisions when prescribing alfuzosin hydrochloride for patients with a known history of QT prolongation or patients who are taking medications which prolong the QT interval). Products include:
Thioridazine Hydrochloride 2384

Thiothixene (A post-marketing study evaluating the effect of combining alfuzosin hydrochloride with another drug of comparable QT effect showed an increased effect when compared to either drug alone. Although this study was not designed to make direct statistical comparisons between drugs, the QT increase with both drugs was no more than additive and was lower than that of the active control moxifloxacin. These observations should be considered in clinical decisions when prescribing alfuzosin hydrochloride for patients with a known history of QT prolongation or patients who are taking medications which prolong the QT interval). Products include:
Thiothixene 2386

Timolol Maleate (There may be an increased risk of hypotension/postural hypotension and syncope when taking alfuzosin concomitantly with anti-hypertensive medication and nitrates. Care should be taken when alfuzosin is administered to patients with symptomatic hypotension or patients who have had a hypotensive response to other medications). Products include:
Combigan 601
Dorzolamide Hydrochloride/Timolol Maleate Ophthalmic Solution .... ⊙243
Timoptic in Ocudose .... ⊙231

Tocainide Hydrochloride (A post-marketing study evaluating the effect of combining alfuzosin hydrochloride with another drug of comparable QT effect showed an increased effect when compared to either drug alone. Although this study was not designed to make direct statistical comparisons between drugs, the QT increase with both drugs was no more than additive and was lower than that of the active control moxifloxacin. These observations should be considered in clinical decisions when prescribing alfuzosin hydrochloride for patients with a known history of QT prolongation or patients who are taking medications which prolong the QT interval).
No products indexed under this heading.

Torsemide (There may be an increased risk of hypotension/postural hypotension and syncope when taking alfuzosin concomitantly with anti-hypertensive medication and nitrates. Care should be taken when alfuzosin is administered to patients with symptomatic hypotension or patients who have had a hypotensive response to other medications).
No products indexed under this heading.

Trandolapril (There may be an increased risk of hypotension/postural hypotension and syncope when taking alfuzosin concomitantly with anti-hypertensive medication and nitrates. Care should be taken when alfuzosin is administered to patients with symptomatic hypotension or patients who have had a hypotensive response to other medications). Products include:
Mavik 489
Tarka 534

Tranylcypromine Sulfate (A post-marketing study evaluating the effect of combining alfuzosin hydrochloride with another drug of comparable QT effect showed an increased effect when compared to either drug alone. Although this study was not designed to make

direct statistical comparisons between drugs, the QT increase with both drugs was no more than additive and was lower than that of the active control moxifloxacin. These observations should be considered in clinical decisions when prescribing alfuzosin hydrochloride for patients with a known history of QT prolongation or patients who are taking medications which prolong the QT interval). Products include:
Parnate 1584

Trifluoperazine Hydrochloride (A post-marketing study evaluating the effect of combining alfuzosin hydrochloride with another drug of comparable QT effect showed an increased effect when compared to either drug alone. Although this study was not designed to make direct statistical comparisons between drugs, the QT increase with both drugs was no more than additive and was lower than that of the active control moxifloxacin. These observations should be considered in clinical decisions when prescribing alfuzosin hydrochloride for patients with a known history of QT prolongation or patients who are taking medications which prolong the QT interval).
No products indexed under this heading.

Trimethaphan Camsylate (There may be an increased risk of hypotension/postural hypotension and syncope when taking alfuzosin concomitantly with anti-hypertensive medication and nitrates. Care should be taken when alfuzosin is administered to patients with symptomatic hypotension or patients who have had a hypotensive response to other medications).
No products indexed under this heading.

Trimipramine Maleate (A post-marketing study evaluating the effect of combining alfuzosin hydrochloride with another drug of comparable QT effect showed an increased effect when compared to either drug alone. Although this study was not designed to make direct statistical comparisons between drugs, the QT increase with both drugs was no more than additive and was lower than that of the active control moxifloxacin. These observations should be considered in clinical decisions when prescribing alfuzosin hydrochloride for patients with a known history of QT prolongation or patients who are taking medications which prolong the QT interval).
No products indexed under this heading.

Troleandomycin (Co-administration of alfuzosin with potent CYP3A4 inhibitors, such as ketoconazole, itraconazole, and ritonavir, is contraindicated, since alfuzosin blood levels are increased).
No products indexed under this heading.

Valsartan (There may be an increased risk of hypotension/postural hypotension and syncope when taking alfuzosin concomitantly with anti-hypertensive medication and nitrates. Care should be taken when alfuzosin is administered to patients with symptomatic hypotension or patients who have had a hypotensive response to other medications). Products include:
Diovan 2413
Diovan HCT 2419
Exforge 2443
Exforge HCT 2449
Valturna 3637

Verapamil Hydrochloride (There may be an increased risk of hypotension/postural hypotension and syncope when taking alfuzosin concomitantly with anti-hypertensive medication and nitrates. Care should be taken when alfuzosin is administered to patients with symptomatic hypotension or

patients who have had a hypotensive response to other medications). Products include:

Tarka 534

Voriconazole (Co-administration of alfuzosin with potent CYP3A4 inhibitors, such as ketoconazole, itraconazole, and ritonavir, is contraindicated, since alfuzosin blood levels are increased).
No products indexed under this heading.

Ziprasidone Hydrochloride (A post-marketing study evaluating the effect of combining alfuzosin hydrochloride with another drug of comparable QT effect showed an increased effect when compared to either drug alone. Although this study was not designed to make direct statistical comparisons between drugs, the QT increase with both drugs was no more than additive and was lower than that of the active control moxifloxacin. These observations should be considered in clinical decisions when prescribing alfuzosin hydrochloride for patients with a known history of QT prolongation or patients who are taking medications which prolong the QT interval). Products include:

Geodon 2723

Food Interactions

Food, unspecified (The extent of absorption of alfuzosin is 50% lower under fasting conditions. Therefore, alfuzosin should be taken immediately following a meal).

Meal, unspecified (The extent of absorption of alfuzosin is 50% lower under fasting conditions. Therefore, alfuzosin should be taken immediately following a meal).

URSO 250 TABLETS

(Ursodiol) 799

May interact with bile acid sequestering agents, estrogens, lipid-lowering drugs, oral contraceptives, and certain other agents. Compounds in these categories include:

Aluminum Hydroxide (Aluminum-based antacids have been shown to adsorb bile acid *in vitro* and may be expected to interfere with ursodiol in the same manner as the bile acid sequestering agents).
No products indexed under this heading.

Atorvastatin Calcium (Lipid-lowering drugs increase hepatic cholesterol secretion and encourage cholesterol gallstone formation and hence may counteract the effectiveness of ursodiol). Products include:

Lipitor 2703

Cerivastatin Sodium (Lipid-lowering drugs increase hepatic cholesterol secretion and encourage cholesterol gallstone formation and hence may counteract the effectiveness of ursodiol).
No products indexed under this heading.

Chlorotrianisene (Estrogens and oral contraceptives increase hepatic cholesterol excretion and encourage cholesterol gallstone formation and hence may counteract the effectiveness of ursodiol).
No products indexed under this heading.

Cholestyramine (Lipid-lowering drugs increase hepatic cholesterol secretion and encourage cholesterol gallstone formation and hence may counteract the effectiveness of ursodiol).
No products indexed under this heading.

Clofibrate (Lipid-lowering drugs increase hepatic cholesterol secretion and encourage cholesterol gallstone formation and hence may counteract the effectiveness of ursodiol).
No products indexed under this heading.

Colesevelam Hydrochloride (Bile sequestering agents may interfere with the action of ursodiol by reducing its absorption). Products include:

Welchol 1029

Colestipol Hydrochloride (Lipid-lowering drugs increase hepatic cholesterol secretion and encourage cholesterol gallstone formation and hence may counteract the effectiveness of ursodiol).
No products indexed under this heading.

Desogestrel (Estrogens and oral contraceptives increase hepatic cholesterol secretion and encourage cholesterol gallstone formation and hence may counteract the effectiveness of ursodiol).
No products indexed under this heading.

Dienestrol (Estrogens and oral contraceptives increase hepatic cholesterol excretion and encourage cholesterol gallstone formation and hence may counteract the effectiveness of ursodiol).
No products indexed under this heading.

Diethylstilbestrol (Estrogens and oral contraceptives increase hepatic cholesterol excretion and encourage cholesterol gallstone formation and hence may counteract the effectiveness of ursodiol).
No products indexed under this heading.

Estradiol (Estrogens and oral contraceptives increase hepatic cholesterol excretion and encourage cholesterol gallstone formation and hence may counteract the effectiveness of ursodiol). Products include:

Activella 2561
Angeliq 831
Climara 841
Climara Pro 847
Divigel 3467
Estrasorb 1777
Vagifem 2589

Estrogens, Conjugated (Estrogens and oral contraceptives increase hepatic cholesterol excretion and encourage cholesterol gallstone formation and hence may counteract the effectiveness of ursodiol). Products include:

Premarin Intravenous 3528
Premarin Tablets 3533
Premarin Vaginal Cream 3540
Premphase 3549
Prempro 3549

Estrogens, Esterified (Estrogens and oral contraceptives increase hepatic cholesterol excretion and encourage cholesterol gallstone formation and hence may counteract the effectiveness of ursodiol).
No products indexed under this heading.

Estropipate (Estrogens and oral contraceptives increase hepatic cholesterol excretion and encourage cholesterol gallstone formation and hence may counteract the effectiveness of ursodiol).
No products indexed under this heading.

Ethinyl Estradiol (Estrogens and oral contraceptives increase hepatic cholesterol secretion and encourage cholesterol gallstone formation and hence may counteract the effectiveness of ursodiol). Products include:

LoSeasonique 3407
Lybrel 3514
NuvaRing 3181
Ortho Evra 2648
Ortho-Cyclen/Ortho Tri-Cyclen 2663
Ortho Tri-Cyclen Lo Tablets 2673
Seasonique 3418
Yaz 864

Ethynodiol Diacetate (Estrogens and oral contraceptives increase hepatic cholesterol secretion and encourage cholesterol gallstone formation and hence may counteract the effectiveness of ursodiol).
No products indexed under this heading.

Fenofibrate (Lipid-lowering drugs increase hepatic cholesterol secretion and encourage cholesterol gallstone formation and hence may counteract the effectiveness of ursodiol). Products include:

Fenoglide 3263
Tricor 544
Trilipix 548

Fluvastatin Sodium (Lipid-lowering drugs increase hepatic cholesterol secretion and encourage cholesterol gallstone formation and hence may counteract the effectiveness of ursodiol).
No products indexed under this heading.

Gemfibrozil (Lipid-lowering drugs increase hepatic cholesterol secretion and encourage cholesterol gallstone formation and hence may counteract the effectiveness of ursodiol).
No products indexed under this heading.

Levonorgestrel (Estrogens and oral contraceptives increase hepatic cholesterol secretion and encourage cholesterol gallstone formation and hence may counteract the effectiveness of ursodiol). Products include:

Climara Pro 847
LoSeasonique 3407
Lybrel 3514
Mirena 854
Plan B 3416
Seasonique 3418

Lovastatin (Lipid-lowering drugs increase hepatic cholesterol secretion and encourage cholesterol gallstone formation and hence may counteract the effectiveness of ursodiol). Products include:

Advicor 402
Mevacor 2212

Mestranol (Estrogens and oral contraceptives increase hepatic cholesterol secretion and encourage cholesterol gallstone formation and hence may counteract the effectiveness of ursodiol).
No products indexed under this heading.

Norethindrone (Estrogens and oral contraceptives increase hepatic cholesterol secretion and encourage cholesterol gallstone formation and hence may counteract the effectiveness of ursodiol). Products include:

Ortho Micronor 2660

Norethynodrel (Estrogens and oral contraceptives increase hepatic cholesterol secretion and encourage cholesterol gallstone formation and hence may counteract the effectiveness of ursodiol).
No products indexed under this heading.

Norgestimate (Estrogens and oral contraceptives increase hepatic cholesterol secretion and encourage cholesterol gallstone formation and hence may counteract the effectiveness of ursodiol). Products include:

Ortho-Cyclen/Ortho Tri-Cyclen 2663
Ortho Tri-Cyclen Lo Tablets 2673

Norgestrel (Estrogens and oral contraceptives increase hepatic cholesterol secretion and encourage cholesterol gallstone formation and hence may counteract the effectiveness of ursodiol).
No products indexed under this heading.

Polyestradiol Phosphate (Estrogens and oral contraceptives increase hepatic cholesterol excretion and encourage cholesterol gallstone formation and hence may counteract the effectiveness of ursodiol).
No products indexed under this heading.

Pravastatin Sodium (Lipid-lowering drugs increase hepatic cholesterol secretion and encourage cholesterol gallstone formation and hence may counteract the effectiveness of ursodiol).
No products indexed under this heading.

Probucol (Lipid-lowering drugs increase hepatic cholesterol secretion and encourage cholesterol gallstone formation and hence may counteract the effectiveness of ursodiol).
No products indexed under this heading.

Quinestrol (Estrogens and oral contraceptives increase hepatic cholesterol excretion and encourage cholesterol gallstone formation and hence may counteract the effectiveness of ursodiol).
No products indexed under this heading.

Simvastatin (Lipid-lowering drugs increase hepatic cholesterol secretion and encourage cholesterol gallstone formation and hence may counteract the effectiveness of ursodiol). Products include:

Simcor 524
Vytorin 10/10 .... 2303, 3240
Vytorin 10/20 .... 2303, 3240
Vytorin 10/40 .... 2303, 3240
Vytorin 10/80 .... 2303, 3240
Zocor 2289

URSO FORTE TABLETS

(Ursodiol) 799

See Urso 250 Tablets

VAGIFEM TABLETS

(Estradiol) 2589

None cited in PDR database.

VALCYTE TABLETS

(Valganciclovir Hydrochloride) 2872

May interact with agents associated with myelosuppression, drugs inhibiting replication of cell populations of bone marrow, spermatogonia, and germinal layers, nephrotoxic agents, and certain other agents. Compounds in these categories include:

Abacavir Sulfate (Acute renal failure may occur in patients receiving potential nephrotoxic drugs. Caution should be exercised when administering valganciclovir to patients receiving potential nephrotoxic drugs). Products include:

Epzicom 1448
Trizivir 1688
Ziagen 1740

Acyclovir (Acute renal failure may occur in patients receiving potential nephrotoxic drugs. Caution should be exercised when administering valganciclovir to patients receiving potential nephrotoxic drugs). Products include:

Zovirax 1760

Acyclovir Sodium (Acute renal failure may occur in patients receiving potential nephrotoxic drugs. Caution should be exercised when administering valganciclovir to patients receiving potential nephrotoxic drugs).
No products indexed under this heading.

Alatrofloxacin Mesylate (Acute renal failure may occur in patients receiving potential nephrotoxic drugs. Caution should be exercised when administering valganciclovir to patients receiving potential nephrotoxic drugs).
No products indexed under this heading.

Aldesleukin (Acute renal failure may occur in patients receiving potential nephrotoxic drugs. Caution should be

exercised when administering valganciclovir to patients receiving potential nephrotoxic drugs). Products include:
Proleukin 2504

Altretamine (Valganciclovir should also be used with caution in patients with pre-existing cytopenias, or who have received or who are receiving myelosuppressive drugs or irradiation). Products include:
Hexalen 1066

Amikacin Sulfate (Acute renal failure may occur in patients receiving potential nephrotoxic drugs. Caution should be exercised when administering valganciclovir to patients receiving potential nephrotoxic drugs).
No products indexed under this heading.

Amoxicillin (Acute renal failure may occur in patients receiving potential nephrotoxic drugs. Caution should be exercised when administering valganciclovir to patients receiving potential nephrotoxic drugs). Products include:
Amoxil Capsules 1311
Amoxil Chewable Tablets 1311
Amoxil 1311
Amoxil Powder 1311
Augmentin 1331
Augmentin Tablets 1335
Augmentin ES-600 1338
Augmentin XR 1342
Moxatag 2321

Amoxicillin Trihydrate (Acute renal failure may occur in patients receiving potential nephrotoxic drugs. Caution should be exercised when administering valganciclovir to patients receiving potential nephrotoxic drugs).
No products indexed under this heading.

Amphotericin B (Acute renal failure may occur in patients receiving potential nephrotoxic drugs. Caution should be exercised when administering valganciclovir to patients receiving potential nephrotoxic drugs).
No products indexed under this heading.

Amphotericin B, liposomal (Acute renal failure may occur in patients receiving potential nephrotoxic drugs. Caution should be exercised when administering valganciclovir to patients receiving potential nephrotoxic drugs). Products include:
AmBisome 659

Amphotericin B Cholesteryl Sulfate (Acute renal failure may occur in patients receiving potential nephrotoxic drugs. Caution should be exercised when administering valganciclovir to patients receiving potential nephrotoxic drugs).
No products indexed under this heading.

Amphotericin B Lipid Complex (Acute renal failure may occur in patients receiving potential nephrotoxic drugs. Caution should be exercised when administering valganciclovir to patients receiving potential nephrotoxic drugs).
No products indexed under this heading.

Ampicillin (Acute renal failure may occur in patients receiving potential nephrotoxic drugs. Caution should be exercised when administering valganciclovir to patients receiving potential nephrotoxic drugs).
No products indexed under this heading.

Ampicillin Sodium (Acute renal failure may occur in patients receiving potential nephrotoxic drugs. Caution should be exercised when administering valganciclovir to patients receiving potential nephrotoxic drugs).
No products indexed under this heading.

Ampicillin Trihydrate (Acute renal failure may occur in patients receiving potential nephrotoxic drugs. Caution should be exercised when administering valganciclovir to patients receiving potential nephrotoxic drugs).
No products indexed under this heading.

Amprenavir (Acute renal failure may occur in patients receiving potential nephrotoxic drugs. Caution should be exercised when administering valganciclovir to patients receiving potential nephrotoxic drugs).
No products indexed under this heading.

Aspirin (Acute renal failure may occur in patients receiving potential nephrotoxic drugs. Caution should be exercised when administering valganciclovir to patients receiving potential nephrotoxic drugs). Products include:
Aggrenox 880
Bayer Aspirin 829
Percodan 1124
St. Joseph Aspirin 2045

Atazanavir (Acute renal failure may occur in patients receiving potential nephrotoxic drugs. Caution should be exercised when administering valganciclovir to patients receiving potential nephrotoxic drugs).
No products indexed under this heading.

Atorvastatin Calcium (Acute renal failure may occur in patients receiving potential nephrotoxic drugs. Caution should be exercised when administering valganciclovir to patients receiving potential nephrotoxic drugs). Products include:
Lipitor 2703

Azithromycin Dihydrate (Acute renal failure may occur in patients receiving potential nephrotoxic drugs. Caution should be exercised when administering valganciclovir to patients receiving potential nephrotoxic drugs).
No products indexed under this heading.

Azlocillin Sodium (Acute renal failure may occur in patients receiving potential nephrotoxic drugs. Caution should be exercised when administering valganciclovir to patients receiving potential nephrotoxic drugs).
No products indexed under this heading.

Aztreonam (Acute renal failure may occur in patients receiving potential nephrotoxic drugs. Caution should be exercised when administering valganciclovir to patients receiving potential nephrotoxic drugs).
No products indexed under this heading.

Bacampicillin Hydrochloride (Acute renal failure may occur in patients receiving potential nephrotoxic drugs. Caution should be exercised when administering valganciclovir to patients receiving potential nephrotoxic drugs).
No products indexed under this heading.

Bacitracin (Acute renal failure may occur in patients receiving potential nephrotoxic drugs. Caution should be exercised when administering valganciclovir to patients receiving potential nephrotoxic drugs).
No products indexed under this heading.

Bacitracin Zinc (Acute renal failure may occur in patients receiving potential nephrotoxic drugs. Caution should be exercised when administering valganciclovir to patients receiving potential nephrotoxic drugs).
No products indexed under this heading.

Balsalazide Disodium (Acute renal failure may occur in patients receiving potential nephrotoxic drugs. Caution should be exercised when administering valganciclovir to patients receiving potential nephrotoxic drugs).
No products indexed under this heading.

Benazepril Hydrochloride (Acute renal failure may occur in patients receiving potential nephrotoxic drugs. Caution should be exercised when administering valganciclovir to patients receiving potential nephrotoxic drugs).
No products indexed under this heading.

Bendroflumethiazide (Acute renal failure may occur in patients receiving potential nephrotoxic drugs. Caution should be exercised when administering valganciclovir to patients receiving potential nephrotoxic drugs).
No products indexed under this heading.

Busulfan (Valganciclovir should also be used with caution in patients with pre-existing cytopenias, or who have received or who are receiving myelosuppressive drugs or irradiation). Products include:
Myleran 1581

Caffeine (Acute renal failure may occur in patients receiving potential nephrotoxic drugs. Caution should be exercised when administering valganciclovir to patients receiving potential nephrotoxic drugs).
No products indexed under this heading.

Captopril (Acute renal failure may occur in patients receiving potential nephrotoxic drugs. Caution should be exercised when administering valganciclovir to patients receiving potential nephrotoxic drugs). Products include:
Captopril 2341

Carbenicillin Disodium (Acute renal failure may occur in patients receiving potential nephrotoxic drugs. Caution should be exercised when administering valganciclovir to patients receiving potential nephrotoxic drugs).
No products indexed under this heading.

Carbenicillin Indanyl Sodium (Acute renal failure may occur in patients receiving potential nephrotoxic drugs. Caution should be exercised when administering valganciclovir to patients receiving potential nephrotoxic drugs).
No products indexed under this heading.

Carboplatin (Acute renal failure may occur in patients receiving potential nephrotoxic drugs. Caution should be exercised when administering valganciclovir to patients receiving potential nephrotoxic drugs).
No products indexed under this heading.

Carmustine (BCNU) (Acute renal failure may occur in patients receiving potential nephrotoxic drugs. Caution should be exercised when administering valganciclovir to patients receiving potential nephrotoxic drugs).
No products indexed under this heading.

Cefaclor (Acute renal failure may occur in patients receiving potential nephrotoxic drugs. Caution should be exercised when administering valganciclovir to patients receiving potential nephrotoxic drugs).
No products indexed under this heading.

Cefadroxil (Acute renal failure may occur in patients receiving potential nephrotoxic drugs. Caution should be exercised when administering valganciclovir to patients receiving potential nephrotoxic drugs).
No products indexed under this heading.

Cefamandole Nafate (Acute renal failure may occur in patients receiving potential nephrotoxic drugs. Caution should be exercised when administering valganciclovir to patients receiving potential nephrotoxic drugs).
No products indexed under this heading.

Cefazolin Sodium (Acute renal failure may occur in patients receiving potential nephrotoxic drugs. Caution should be exercised when administering valganciclovir to patients receiving potential nephrotoxic drugs).
No products indexed under this heading.

Cefdinir (Acute renal failure may occur in patients receiving potential nephrotoxic drugs. Caution should be exercised when administering valganciclovir to patients receiving potential nephrotoxic drugs). Products include:

Omnicef Capsules 518
Omnicef Oral Suspension 518

Cefepime Hydrochloride (Acute renal failure may occur in patients receiving potential nephrotoxic drugs. Caution should be exercised when administering valganciclovir to patients receiving potential nephrotoxic drugs).
No products indexed under this heading.

Cefixime (Acute renal failure may occur in patients receiving potential nephrotoxic drugs. Caution should be exercised when administering valganciclovir to patients receiving potential nephrotoxic drugs). Products include:
Suprax for Oral Suspension 2038
Suprax Tablets 2038

Cefmetazole Sodium (Acute renal failure may occur in patients receiving potential nephrotoxic drugs. Caution should be exercised when administering valganciclovir to patients receiving potential nephrotoxic drugs).
No products indexed under this heading.

Cefonicid Sodium (Acute renal failure may occur in patients receiving potential nephrotoxic drugs. Caution should be exercised when administering valganciclovir to patients receiving potential nephrotoxic drugs).
No products indexed under this heading.

Cefoperazone Sodium (Acute renal failure may occur in patients receiving potential nephrotoxic drugs. Caution should be exercised when administering valganciclovir to patients receiving potential nephrotoxic drugs).
No products indexed under this heading.

Ceforanide (Acute renal failure may occur in patients receiving potential nephrotoxic drugs. Caution should be exercised when administering valganciclovir to patients receiving potential nephrotoxic drugs).
No products indexed under this heading.

Cefotaxime Sodium (Acute renal failure may occur in patients receiving potential nephrotoxic drugs. Caution should be exercised when administering valganciclovir to patients receiving potential nephrotoxic drugs).
No products indexed under this heading.

Cefotetan (Acute renal failure may occur in patients receiving potential nephrotoxic drugs. Caution should be exercised when administering valganciclovir to patients receiving potential nephrotoxic drugs).
No products indexed under this heading.

Cefoxitin Sodium (Acute renal failure may occur in patients receiving potential nephrotoxic drugs. Caution should be exercised when administering valganciclovir to patients receiving potential nephrotoxic drugs).
No products indexed under this heading.

Cefpodoxime Proxetil (Acute renal failure may occur in patients receiving potential nephrotoxic drugs. Caution should be exercised when administering valganciclovir to patients receiving potential nephrotoxic drugs).
No products indexed under this heading.

Cefprozil (Acute renal failure may occur in patients receiving potential nephrotoxic drugs. Caution should be exercised when administering valganciclovir to patients receiving potential nephrotoxic drugs).
No products indexed under this heading.

Ceftazidime (Acute renal failure may occur in patients receiving potential nephrotoxic drugs. Caution should be exercised when administering valganciclovir to patients receiving potential nephrotoxic drugs). Products include:
Fortaz 1481

Ceftizoxime Sodium (Acute renal failure may occur in patients receiving potential nephrotoxic drugs. Caution should be exercised when administering valganciclovir to patients receiving potential nephrotoxic drugs).
No products indexed under this heading.

Ceftriaxone Sodium (Acute renal failure may occur in patients receiving potential nephrotoxic drugs. Caution should be exercised when administering valganciclovir to patients receiving potential nephrotoxic drugs). Products include:
Rocephin 2859

Cefuroxime Axetil (Acute renal failure may occur in patients receiving potential nephrotoxic drugs. Caution should be exercised when administering valganciclovir to patients receiving potential nephrotoxic drugs). Products include:
Ceftin 1399

Cefuroxime Sodium (Acute renal failure may occur in patients receiving potential nephrotoxic drugs. Caution should be exercised when administering valganciclovir to patients receiving potential nephrotoxic drugs).
No products indexed under this heading.

Celecoxib (Acute renal failure may occur in patients receiving potential nephrotoxic drugs. Caution should be exercised when administering valganciclovir to patients receiving potential nephrotoxic drugs). Products include:
Celebrex 3272

Cephalexin (Acute renal failure may occur in patients receiving potential nephrotoxic drugs. Caution should be exercised when administering valganciclovir to patients receiving potential nephrotoxic drugs).
No products indexed under this heading.

Cephalothin Sodium (Acute renal failure may occur in patients receiving potential nephrotoxic drugs. Caution should be exercised when administering valganciclovir to patients receiving potential nephrotoxic drugs).
No products indexed under this heading.

Cephapirin Sodium (Acute renal failure may occur in patients receiving potential nephrotoxic drugs. Caution should be exercised when administering valganciclovir to patients receiving potential nephrotoxic drugs).
No products indexed under this heading.

Cephradine (Acute renal failure may occur in patients receiving potential nephrotoxic drugs. Caution should be exercised when administering valganciclovir to patients receiving potential nephrotoxic drugs).
No products indexed under this heading.

Cerivastatin Sodium (Acute renal failure may occur in patients receiving potential nephrotoxic drugs. Caution should be exercised when administering valganciclovir to patients receiving potential nephrotoxic drugs).
No products indexed under this heading.

Chlorambucil (Valganciclovir should also be used with caution in patients with pre-existing cytopenias, or who have received or who are receiving myelosuppressive drugs or irradiation). Products include:
Leukeran 1557

Chloramphenicol (Valganciclovir should also be used with caution in patients with pre-existing cytopenias, or who have received or who are receiving myelosuppressive drugs or irradiation).
No products indexed under this heading.

Chloramphenicol Palmitate (Valganciclovir should also be used with caution in patients with pre-existing cytopenias, or who have received or who are receiving myelosuppressive drugs or irradiation).
No products indexed under this heading.

Chloramphenicol Sodium Succinate (Valganciclovir should also be used with caution in patients with pre-existing cytopenias, or who have received or who are receiving myelosuppressive drugs or irradiation).
No products indexed under this heading.

Chlorothiazide (Acute renal failure may occur in patients receiving potential nephrotoxic drugs. Caution should be exercised when administering valganciclovir to patients receiving potential nephrotoxic drugs).
No products indexed under this heading.

Chlorothiazide Sodium (Acute renal failure may occur in patients receiving potential nephrotoxic drugs. Caution should be exercised when administering valganciclovir to patients receiving potential nephrotoxic drugs). Products include:
Diuril Intravenous 2009

Chlorpropamide (Acute renal failure may occur in patients receiving potential nephrotoxic drugs. Caution should be exercised when administering valganciclovir to patients receiving potential nephrotoxic drugs).
No products indexed under this heading.

Cidofovir (Acute renal failure may occur in patients receiving potential nephrotoxic drugs. Caution should be exercised when administering valganciclovir to patients receiving potential nephrotoxic drugs).
No products indexed under this heading.

Cilastatin Sodium (Acute renal failure may occur in patients receiving potential nephrotoxic drugs. Caution should be exercised when administering valganciclovir to patients receiving potential nephrotoxic drugs). Products include:
Primaxin I.M. 2232
Primaxin I.V. 2235

Cimetidine (Acute renal failure may occur in patients receiving potential nephrotoxic drugs. Caution should be exercised when administering valganciclovir to patients receiving potential nephrotoxic drugs).
No products indexed under this heading.

Cimetidine Hydrochloride (Acute renal failure may occur in patients receiving potential nephrotoxic drugs. Caution should be exercised when administering valganciclovir to patients receiving potential nephrotoxic drugs).
No products indexed under this heading.

Cisplatin (Acute renal failure may occur in patients receiving potential nephrotoxic drugs. Caution should be exercised when administering valganciclovir to patients receiving potential nephrotoxic drugs).
No products indexed under this heading.

Cladribine (Acute renal failure may occur in patients receiving potential nephrotoxic drugs. Caution should be exercised when administering valganciclovir to patients receiving potential nephrotoxic drugs). Products include:
Leustatin 946

Clozapine (Acute renal failure may occur in patients receiving potential nephrotoxic drugs. Caution should be exercised when administering valganciclovir to patients receiving potential nephrotoxic drugs).
No products indexed under this heading.

Colistimethate Sodium (Acute renal failure may occur in patients receiving potential nephrotoxic drugs. Caution should be exercised when administering valganciclovir to patients receiving potential nephrotoxic drugs).
No products indexed under this heading.

Colistin Sulfate (Acute renal failure may occur in patients receiving potential nephrotoxic drugs. Caution should be exercised when administering valganciclovir to patients receiving potential nephrotoxic drugs).
No products indexed under this heading.

Cyclophosphamide (Acute renal failure may occur in patients receiving potential nephrotoxic drugs. Caution should be exercised when administering valganciclovir to patients receiving potential nephrotoxic drugs).
No products indexed under this heading.

Cyclosporine (Acute renal failure may occur in patients receiving potential nephrotoxic drugs. Caution should be exercised when administering valganciclovir to patients receiving potential nephrotoxic drugs). Products include:
Gengraf 440
Neoral Oral Solution 2496
Neoral Capsules 2496
Restasis 605

Cytarabine (Acute renal failure may occur in patients receiving potential nephrotoxic drugs. Caution should be exercised when administering valganciclovir to patients receiving potential nephrotoxic drugs).
No products indexed under this heading.

Cytarabine Liposome (Acute renal failure may occur in patients receiving potential nephrotoxic drugs. Caution should be exercised when administering valganciclovir to patients receiving potential nephrotoxic drugs).
No products indexed under this heading.

Dapsone (Valganciclovir should also be used with caution in patients with pre-existing cytopenias, or who have received or who are receiving myelosuppressive drugs or irradiation). Products include:
Aczone 593
Dapsone 1819

Daunorubicin Citrate Liposome (Valganciclovir should also be used with caution in patients with pre-existing cytopenias, or who have received or who are receiving myelosuppressive drugs or irradiation).
No products indexed under this heading.

Daunorubicin Hydrochloride (Valganciclovir should also be used with caution in patients with pre-existing cytopenias, or who have received or who are receiving myelosuppressive drugs or irradiation).
No products indexed under this heading.

Delavirdine Mesylate (Acute renal failure may occur in patients receiving potential nephrotoxic drugs. Caution should be exercised when administering valganciclovir to patients receiving potential nephrotoxic drugs).
No products indexed under this heading.

Dexrazoxane (Valganciclovir should also be used with caution in patients with pre-existing cytopenias, or who have received or who are receiving myelosuppressive drugs or irradiation).
No products indexed under this heading.

Diatrizoate Meglumine (Acute renal failure may occur in patients receiving potential nephrotoxic drugs. Caution should be exercised when administering valganciclovir to patients receiving potential nephrotoxic drugs).
No products indexed under this heading.

Diatrizoate Sodium (Acute renal failure may occur in patients receiving potential nephrotoxic drugs. Caution should be exercised when administering valganciclovir to patients receiving potential nephrotoxic drugs).
No products indexed under this heading.

Diclofenac Potassium (Acute renal failure may occur in patients receiving potential nephrotoxic drugs. Caution should be exercised when administering valganciclovir to patients receiving potential nephrotoxic drugs).
No products indexed under this heading.

Diclofenac Sodium (Acute renal failure may occur in patients receiving potential nephrotoxic drugs. Caution should be exercised when administering valganciclovir to patients receiving potential nephrotoxic drugs).
No products indexed under this heading.

Dicloxacillin Sodium (Acute renal failure may occur in patients receiving potential nephrotoxic drugs. Caution should be exercised when administering valganciclovir to patients receiving potential nephrotoxic drugs).
No products indexed under this heading.

Didanosine (Valganciclovir is extensively converted to ganciclovir; coadministration of ganciclovir with didanosine has resulted in decreased AUC of ganciclovir and increased AUC of didanosine; patients should be monitored for didanosine toxicity).
No products indexed under this heading.

Doxorubicin Hydrochloride (Valganciclovir should also be used with caution in patients with pre-existing cytopenias, or who have received or who are receiving myelosuppressive drugs or irradiation).
No products indexed under this heading.

Doxorubicin Hydrochloride Liposome (Valganciclovir should also be used with caution in patients with pre-existing cytopenias, or who have received or who are receiving myelosuppressive drugs or irradiation). Products include:
Doxil 939

Efavirenz (Acute renal failure may occur in patients receiving potential nephrotoxic drugs. Caution should be exercised when administering valganciclovir to patients receiving potential nephrotoxic drugs). Products include:
Atripla 906

Emtricitabine (Acute renal failure may occur in patients receiving potential nephrotoxic drugs. Caution should be exercised when administering valganciclovir to patients receiving potential nephrotoxic drugs). Products include:
Atripla 906
Emtriva 1238
Emtriva Oral Solution 1238
Truvada 1258

Enalapril Maleate (Acute renal failure may occur in patients receiving potential nephrotoxic drugs. Caution should be exercised when administering valganciclovir to patients receiving potential nephrotoxic drugs).
No products indexed under this heading.

Enalaprilat (Acute renal failure may occur in patients receiving potential nephrotoxic drugs. Caution should be exercised when administering valganciclovir to patients receiving potential nephrotoxic drugs).
No products indexed under this heading.

Enfuvirtide (Acute renal failure may occur in patients receiving potential nephrotoxic drugs. Caution should be exercised when administering valganciclovir to patients receiving potential nephrotoxic drugs).
No products indexed under this heading.

IMPORTANT NOTE: Always consult each drug listing in the patient's regimen for possible interactions.

Valcyte
Interactions Index
1992

Ethiodized Oil (Acute renal failure may occur in patients receiving potential nephrotoxic drugs. Caution should be exercised when administering valganciclovir to patients receiving potential nephrotoxic drugs).
No products indexed under this heading.

Etodolac (Acute renal failure may occur in patients receiving potential nephrotoxic drugs. Caution should be exercised when administering valganciclovir to patients receiving potential nephrotoxic drugs).
No products indexed under this heading.

Fat (Co-administration with high fat meals has resulted in increased steady-state ganciclovir AUC and C_{max} without any prolongation in time to peak plasma concentrations; Valcyte should be administered with food).
No products indexed under this heading.

Fenoprofen Calcium (Acute renal failure may occur in patients receiving potential nephrotoxic drugs. Caution should be exercised when administering valganciclovir to patients receiving potential nephrotoxic drugs).
No products indexed under this heading.

Filgrastim (Acute renal failure may occur in patients receiving potential nephrotoxic drugs. Caution should be exercised when administering valganciclovir to patients receiving potential nephrotoxic drugs). Products include:
Neupogen 631

Flucytosine (Valganciclovir should also be used with caution in patients with pre-existing cytopenias, or who have received or who are receiving myelosuppressive drugs or irradiation).
No products indexed under this heading.

Fludarabine Phosphate (Valganciclovir should also be used with caution in patients with pre-existing cytopenias, or who have received or who are receiving myelosuppressive drugs or irradiation). Products include:
Oforta 3023

Fluorouracil (Acute renal failure may occur in patients receiving potential nephrotoxic drugs. Caution should be exercised when administering valganciclovir to patients receiving potential nephrotoxic drugs). Products include:
Carac 2966

Flurbiprofen (Acute renal failure may occur in patients receiving potential nephrotoxic drugs. Caution should be exercised when administering valganciclovir to patients receiving potential nephrotoxic drugs).
No products indexed under this heading.

Fluvastatin Sodium (Acute renal failure may occur in patients receiving potential nephrotoxic drugs. Caution should be exercised when administering valganciclovir to patients receiving potential nephrotoxic drugs).
No products indexed under this heading.

Foscarnet Sodium (Acute renal failure may occur in patients receiving potential nephrotoxic drugs. Caution should be exercised when administering valganciclovir to patients receiving potential nephrotoxic drugs).
No products indexed under this heading.

Fosinopril Sodium (Acute renal failure may occur in patients receiving potential nephrotoxic drugs. Caution should be exercised when administering valganciclovir to patients receiving potential nephrotoxic drugs).
No products indexed under this heading.

Furosemide (Acute renal failure may occur in patients receiving potential nephrotoxic drugs. Caution should be exercised when administering valganciclovir to patients receiving potential nephrotoxic drugs). Products include:
Furosemide 2354

Gadopentetate Dimeglumine (Acute renal failure may occur in patients receiving potential nephrotoxic drugs. Caution should be exercised when administering valganciclovir to patients receiving potential nephrotoxic drugs).
No products indexed under this heading.

Gemcitabine Hydrochloride (Valganciclovir should also be used with caution in patients with pre-existing cytopenias, or who have received or who are receiving myelosuppressive drugs or irradiation). Products include:
Gemzar 1900

Gemtuzumab Ozogamicin (Valganciclovir should also be used with caution in patients with pre-existing cytopenias, or who have received or who are receiving myelosuppressive drugs or irradiation). Products include:
Mylotarg 3524

Gentamicin (Acute renal failure may occur in patients receiving potential nephrotoxic drugs. Caution should be exercised when administering valganciclovir to patients receiving potential nephrotoxic drugs).
No products indexed under this heading.

Gentamicin Sulfate (Acute renal failure may occur in patients receiving potential nephrotoxic drugs. Caution should be exercised when administering valganciclovir to patients receiving potential nephrotoxic drugs). Products include:
Pred-G .... ⊙226, ⊙227

Glipizide (Acute renal failure may occur in patients receiving potential nephrotoxic drugs. Caution should be exercised when administering valganciclovir to patients receiving potential nephrotoxic drugs).
No products indexed under this heading.

Globulin, Immune (Human) (Acute renal failure may occur in patients receiving potential nephrotoxic drugs. Caution should be exercised when administering valganciclovir to patients receiving potential nephrotoxic drugs). Products include:

Glyburide (Acute renal failure may occur in patients receiving potential nephrotoxic drugs. Caution should be exercised when administering valganciclovir to patients receiving potential nephrotoxic drugs).
No products indexed under this heading.

Gold Therapy (Acute renal failure may occur in patients receiving potential nephrotoxic drugs. Caution should be exercised when administering valganciclovir to patients receiving potential nephrotoxic drugs).
No products indexed under this heading.

HMG-CoA Reductase Inhibitors (Acute renal failure may occur in patients receiving potential nephrotoxic drugs. Caution should be exercised when administering valganciclovir to patients receiving potential nephrotoxic drugs).
No products indexed under this heading.

Hydrochlorothiazide (Acute renal failure may occur in patients receiving potential nephrotoxic drugs. Caution should be exercised when administering valganciclovir to patients receiving potential nephrotoxic drugs). Products include:
Atacand HCT 700
Avalide 2956
Benicar HCT 1017
Diovan HCT 2419
Dyazide 1429
Exforge HCT 2449
Hyzaar 2162
Hyzaar 100-12.5 2162
Micardis HCT 889
Prinzide 2246
Tekturna HCT 2541
Teveten HCT 541

Hydroflumethiazide (Acute renal failure may occur in patients receiving potential nephrotoxic drugs. Caution should be exercised when administering valganciclovir to patients receiving potential nephrotoxic drugs).
No products indexed under this heading.

Ibuprofen (Acute renal failure may occur in patients receiving potential nephrotoxic drugs. Caution should be exercised when administering valganciclovir to patients receiving potential nephrotoxic drugs). Products include:
Motrin IB 2043
Children's Motrin 2044
Children's Motrin Non-Staining Dye-Free 2044
Infants' Motrin 2044
Infants' Motrin Dye-Free 2044
Junior Strength Motrin 2044
Vicoprofen 564

Idarubicin Hydrochloride (Acute renal failure may occur in patients receiving potential nephrotoxic drugs. Caution should be exercised when administering valganciclovir to patients receiving potential nephrotoxic drugs).
No products indexed under this heading.

Ifosfamide (Acute renal failure may occur in patients receiving potential nephrotoxic drugs. Caution should be exercised when administering valganciclovir to patients receiving potential nephrotoxic drugs).
No products indexed under this heading.

Imipenem (Acute renal failure may occur in patients receiving potential nephrotoxic drugs. Caution should be exercised when administering valganciclovir to patients receiving potential nephrotoxic drugs). Products include:
Primaxin I.M. 2232
Primaxin I.V. 2235

Immune Globulin Intravenous (Human) (Acute renal failure may occur in patients receiving potential nephrotoxic drugs. Caution should be exercised when administering valganciclovir to patients receiving potential nephrotoxic drugs). Products include:
Flebogamma 5% DIF 1794
Gammagard 812, 815
Gamunex 3374

Indinavir Sulfate (Acute renal failure may occur in patients receiving potential nephrotoxic drugs. Caution should be exercised when administering valganciclovir to patients receiving potential nephrotoxic drugs). Products include:
Crixivan 2113

Indomethacin (Acute renal failure may occur in patients receiving potential nephrotoxic drugs. Caution should be exercised when administering valganciclovir to patients receiving potential nephrotoxic drugs). Products include:
Indocin 2167

Indomethacin Sodium Trihydrate (Acute renal failure may occur in patients receiving potential nephrotoxic drugs. Caution should be exercised when administering valganciclovir to patients receiving potential nephrotoxic drugs). Products include:
Indocin I.V. 2007

Interferon alfa-2a, Recombinant (Valganciclovir should also be used with caution in patients with pre-existing cytopenias, or who have received or who are receiving myelosuppressive drugs or irradiation).
No products indexed under this heading.

Interferon Beta-1b (Acute renal failure may occur in patients receiving potential nephrotoxic drugs. Caution should be exercised when administering valganciclovir to patients receiving potential nephrotoxic drugs). Products include:
Betaseron 836
Extavia 2459

Interleuken-2 (Acute renal failure may occur in patients receiving potential nephrotoxic drugs. Caution should be exercised when administering valganciclovir to patients receiving potential nephrotoxic drugs).
No products indexed under this heading.

Iodamide Meglumine (Acute renal failure may occur in patients receiving potential nephrotoxic drugs. Caution should be exercised when administering valganciclovir to patients receiving potential nephrotoxic drugs).
No products indexed under this heading.

Iohexol (Acute renal failure may occur in patients receiving potential nephrotoxic drugs. Caution should be exercised when administering valganciclovir to patients receiving potential nephrotoxic drugs).
No products indexed under this heading.

Iopamidol (Acute renal failure may occur in patients receiving potential nephrotoxic drugs. Caution should be exercised when administering valganciclovir to patients receiving potential nephrotoxic drugs).
No products indexed under this heading.

Iopanoic Acid (Acute renal failure may occur in patients receiving potential nephrotoxic drugs. Caution should be exercised when administering valganciclovir to patients receiving potential nephrotoxic drugs).
No products indexed under this heading.

Iothalamate Meglumine (Acute renal failure may occur in patients receiving potential nephrotoxic drugs. Caution should be exercised when administering valganciclovir to patients receiving potential nephrotoxic drugs).
No products indexed under this heading.

Ioxaglate Meglumine (Acute renal failure may occur in patients receiving potential nephrotoxic drugs. Caution should be exercised when administering valganciclovir to patients receiving potential nephrotoxic drugs).
No products indexed under this heading.

Ioxaglate Sodium (Acute renal failure may occur in patients receiving potential nephrotoxic drugs. Caution should be exercised when administering valganciclovir to patients receiving potential nephrotoxic drugs).
No products indexed under this heading.

Irinotecan Hydrochloride (Valganciclovir should also be used with caution in patients with pre-existing cytopenias, or who have received or who are receiving myelosuppressive drugs or irradiation).
No products indexed under this heading.

Kanamycin Sulfate (Acute renal failure may occur in patients receiving potential nephrotoxic drugs. Caution should be exercised when administering valganciclovir to patients receiving potential nephrotoxic drugs).
No products indexed under this heading.

Ketoprofen (Acute renal failure may occur in patients receiving potential nephrotoxic drugs. Caution should be exercised when administering valganciclovir to patients receiving potential nephrotoxic drugs).
No products indexed under this heading.

Ketorolac Tromethamine (Acute renal failure may occur in patients receiving potential nephrotoxic drugs. Caution should be exercised when administering valganciclovir to patients receiving potential nephrotoxic drugs). Products include:
Acuvail .... ⊙209

IMPORTANT NOTE: Always consult each drug listing in the patient's regimen for possible interactions.

Tyropanoate Sodium (Acute renal failure may occur in patients receiving potential nephrotoxic drugs. Caution should be exercised when administering valganciclovir to patients receiving potential nephrotoxic drugs).
No products indexed under this heading.

Valacyclovir Hydrochloride (Acute renal failure may occur in patients receiving potential nephrotoxic drugs. Caution should be exercised when administering valganciclovir to patients receiving potential nephrotoxic drugs). Products include:
Valtrex 1702

Valdecoxib (Acute renal failure may occur in patients receiving potential nephrotoxic drugs. Caution should be exercised when administering valganciclovir to patients receiving potential nephrotoxic drugs).
No products indexed under this heading.

Vancomycin Hydrochloride (Acute renal failure may occur in patients receiving potential nephrotoxic drugs. Caution should be exercised when administering valganciclovir to patients receiving potential nephrotoxic drugs).
No products indexed under this heading.

Vinblastine Sulfate (Valganciclovir should also be used with caution in patients with pre-existing cytopenias, or who have received or who are receiving myelosuppressive drugs or irradiation).
No products indexed under this heading.

Vincristine Sulfate (Valganciclovir should also be used with caution in patients with pre-existing cytopenias, or who have received or who are receiving myelosuppressive drugs or irradiation).
No products indexed under this heading.

Vinorelbine Tartrate (Valganciclovir should also be used with caution in patients with pre-existing cytopenias, or who have received or who are receiving myelosuppressive drugs or irradiation).
No products indexed under this heading.

Voriconazole (Acute renal failure may occur in patients receiving potential nephrotoxic drugs. Caution should be exercised when administering valganciclovir to patients receiving potential nephrotoxic drugs).
No products indexed under this heading.

Zalcitabine (Acute renal failure may occur in patients receiving potential nephrotoxic drugs. Caution should be exercised when administering valganciclovir to patients receiving potential nephrotoxic drugs).
No products indexed under this heading.

Zidovudine (Valganciclovir is extensively converted to ganciclovir; co-administration of ganciclovir with zidovudine has resulted in decreased AUC of ganciclovir and increased AUC of zidovudine; zidovudine and valganciclovir each have the potential to cause neutropenia and anemia; some patients may not tolerate concomitant therapy at full dosage). Products include:
Combivir 1404
Retrovir 1634
Retrovir IV 1640
Trizivir 1688

Zoledronic Acid (Acute renal failure may occur in patients receiving potential nephrotoxic drugs. Caution should be exercised when administering valganciclovir to patients receiving potential nephrotoxic drugs). Products include:
Reclast 2509
Zometa 2554

Food Interactions

Food, unspecified (Co-administration with high fat meals has resulted in increased steady-state ganciclovir AUC and C_{max} without any prolongation in time to peak plasma concentrations;

Valcyte should be administered with food).

Meal, unspecified (Co-administration with high fat meals has resulted in increased steady-state ganciclovir AUC and C_{max} without any prolongation in time to peak plasma concentrations; Valcyte should be administered with food).

VALCYTE FOR ORAL SOLUTION
(Valganciclovir Hydrochloride) 2872
See Valcyte Tablets

VALIUM TABLETS
(Diazepam) 2880
May interact with alcohols, anesthetics, antacids, anticonvulsants, antidepressant drugs, antipsychotic agents, barbiturates, cytochrome p450 2c19 inhibitors (selected), cytochrome p450 3a4 inhibitors (selected), hypnotics and sedatives, monoamine oxidase inhibitors, narcotic analgesics, phenothiazines, sedating antihistamines, and certain other agents. Compounds in these categories include:

Acetazolamide (There is a potentially relevant interaction between diazepam and certain hepatic enzyme inhibitors such as CYP450 3A4. It has been shown that these compounds influence the pharmacokinetics of diazepam and may lead to increased and prolonged sedation).
No products indexed under this heading.

Acetazolamide Sodium (There is a potentially relevant interaction between diazepam and certain hepatic enzyme inhibitors such as CYP450 3A4. It has been shown that these compounds influence the pharmacokinetics of diazepam and may lead to increased and prolonged sedation).
No products indexed under this heading.

Acrivastine (Careful considerations should be given to the pharmacology of other centrally acting agents (eg, sedating antihistamines) if used concomitantly with diazepam).
No products indexed under this heading.

Alfentanil Hydrochloride (Careful considerations should be given to the pharmacology of other centrally acting agents (eg, narcotics) if used concomitantly with diazepam).
No products indexed under this heading.

Aluminum Carbonate (Diazepam peak concentrations are lower when antacids are administered concurrently. The peak concentrations appear to be lower due to a slower rate of absorption, with the time required to achieve peak concentration on average 20 to 25 minutes greater in the presence of antacids).
No products indexed under this heading.

Aluminum Hydroxide (Diazepam peak concentrations are lower when antacids are administered concurrently. The peak concentrations appear to be lower due to a slower rate of absorption, with the time required to achieve peak concentration on average 20 to 25 minutes greater in the presence of antacids).
No products indexed under this heading.

Amiodarone Hydrochloride (There is a potentially relevant interaction between diazepam and certain hepatic enzyme inhibitors such as CYP450 3A4. It has been shown that these compounds influence the pharmacokinetics of diazepam and may lead to increased and prolonged sedation).
No products indexed under this heading.

Amitriptyline Hydrochloride (Careful considerations should be given to the pharmacology of other centrally acting agents (eg, antidepressants) if used concomitantly with diazepam).
No products indexed under this heading.

Amobarbital (Careful considerations should be given to the pharmacology of other centrally acting agents (eg, barbiturates) if used concomitantly with diazepam).
No products indexed under this heading.

Amobarbital Sodium (Careful considerations should be given to the pharmacology of other centrally acting agents (eg, barbiturates) if used concomitantly with diazepam).
No products indexed under this heading.

Amoxapine (Careful considerations should be given to the pharmacology of other centrally acting agents (eg, antidepressants) if used concomitantly with diazepam).
No products indexed under this heading.

Amprenavir (There is a potentially relevant interaction between diazepam and certain hepatic enzyme inhibitors such as CYP450 3A4. It has been shown that these compounds influence the pharmacokinetics of diazepam and may lead to increased and prolonged sedation).
No products indexed under this heading.

Anastrozole (There is a potentially relevant interaction between diazepam and certain hepatic enzyme inhibitors such as CYP450 3A4. It has been shown that these compounds influence the pharmacokinetics of diazepam and may lead to increased and prolonged sedation).
No products indexed under this heading.

Apomorphine (Careful considerations should be given to the pharmacology of other centrally acting agents (eg, narcotics) if used concomitantly with diazepam).
No products indexed under this heading.

Apomorphine Hydrochloride (Careful considerations should be given to the pharmacology of other centrally acting agents (eg, narcotics) if used concomitantly with diazepam).
No products indexed under this heading.

Aprepitant (There is a potentially relevant interaction between diazepam and certain hepatic enzyme inhibitors such as CYP450 3A4. It has been shown that these compounds influence the pharmacokinetics of diazepam and may lead to increased and prolonged sedation). Products include:
Emend 2124

Aprobarbital (Careful considerations should be given to the pharmacology of other centrally acting agents (eg, barbiturates) if used concomitantly with diazepam).
No products indexed under this heading.

Aripiprazole (Careful considerations should be given to the pharmacology of other centrally acting agents (eg, antipsychotics) if used concomitantly with diazepam).
No products indexed under this heading.

Articaine Hydrochloride (Careful considerations should be given to the pharmacology of other centrally acting agents (eg, anesthetics) if used concomitantly with diazepam).
No products indexed under this heading.

Atazanavir (There is a potentially relevant interaction between diazepam and certain hepatic enzyme inhibitors such as CYP450 3A4. It has been shown that these compounds influence the pharmacokinetics of diazepam and may lead to increased and prolonged sedation).
No products indexed under this heading.

Atazanavir Sulfate (There is a potentially relevant interaction between diazepam and certain hepatic enzyme inhibitors such as CYP450 3A4. It has been shown that these compounds influence the pharmacokinetics of diazepam and may lead to increased and prolonged sedation).
No products indexed under this heading.

Azatadine Maleate (Careful considerations should be given to the pharmacology of other centrally acting agents (eg, sedating antihistamines) if used concomitantly with diazepam).
No products indexed under this heading.

Benzocaine (Careful considerations should be given to the pharmacology of other centrally acting agents (eg, anesthetics) if used concomitantly with diazepam).
No products indexed under this heading.

Bromodiphenhydramine Hydrochloride (Careful considerations should be given to the pharmacology of other centrally acting agents (eg, sedating antihistamines) if used concomitantly with diazepam).
No products indexed under this heading.

Brompheniramine Maleate (Careful considerations should be given to the pharmacology of other centrally acting agents (eg, sedating antihistamines) if used concomitantly with diazepam).
No products indexed under this heading.

Bupivacaine Hydrochloride (Careful considerations should be given to the pharmacology of other centrally acting agents (eg, anesthetics) if used concomitantly with diazepam).
No products indexed under this heading.

Buprenorphine Hydrochloride (Careful considerations should be given to the pharmacology of other centrally acting agents (eg, narcotics) if used concomitantly with diazepam).
No products indexed under this heading.

Bupropion Hydrochloride (Careful considerations should be given to the pharmacology of other centrally acting agents (eg, antidepressants) if used concomitantly with diazepam). Products include:
Aplenzin 2948
Wellbutrin 1719
Wellbutrin SR 1725
Zyban 1762

Butabarbital (Careful considerations should be given to the pharmacology of other centrally acting agents (eg, sedatives and hypnotics) if used concomitantly with diazepam).
No products indexed under this heading.

Butabarbital Sodium (Careful considerations should be given to the pharmacology of other centrally acting agents (eg, sedatives and hypnotics) if used concomitantly with diazepam).
No products indexed under this heading.

Butalbital (Careful considerations should be given to the pharmacology of other centrally acting agents (eg, sedatives and hypnotics) if used concomitantly with diazepam).
No products indexed under this heading.

Calcium Carbonate (Diazepam peak concentrations are lower when antacids are administered concurrently. The peak concentrations appear to be lower due to a slower rate of absorption, with the time required to achieve peak concentration on average 20 to 25 minutes greater in the presence of antacids). Products include:
Chelated Mineral 3476
Pepcid Complete 1822
Extra Strength Rolaids Softchews
Vanilla Creme 2045

Carbamazepine (Careful considerations should be given to the pharmacology of other centrally acting agents

Valium Interactions Index 1996

(eg, anticonvulsants) if used concomitantly with diazepam). Products include:
Carbatrol 3280
Equetro 3477

Chloral Hydrate (Careful considerations should be given to the pharmacology of other centrally acting agents (eg, sedatives and hypnotics) if used concomitantly with diazepam).
No products indexed under this heading.

Chloroprocaine Hydrochloride (Careful considerations should be given to the pharmacology of other centrally acting agents (eg, anesthetics) if used concomitantly with diazepam).
No products indexed under this heading.

Chlorpheniramine Maleate (Careful considerations should be given to the pharmacology of other centrally acting agents (eg, sedating antihistamines) if used concomitantly with diazepam).
No products indexed under this heading.

Chlorpheniramine Polistirex (Careful considerations should be given to the pharmacology of other centrally acting agents (eg, sedating antihistamines) if used concomitantly with diazepam). Products include:
Tussionex 3443

Chlorpheniramine Tannate (Careful considerations should be given to the pharmacology of other centrally acting agents (eg, sedating antihistamines) if used concomitantly with diazepam).
No products indexed under this heading.

Chlorpromazine (Careful considerations should be given to the pharmacology of other centrally acting agents (eg, phenothiazines) if used concomitantly with diazepam).
No products indexed under this heading.

Chlorpromazine Hydrochloride (Careful considerations should be given to the pharmacology of other centrally acting agents (eg, phenothiazines) if used concomitantly with diazepam).
No products indexed under this heading.

Chlorprothixene (Careful considerations should be given to the pharmacology of other centrally acting agents (eg, antipsychotics) if used concomitantly with diazepam).
No products indexed under this heading.

Chlorprothixene Hydrochloride (Careful considerations should be given to the pharmacology of other centrally acting agents (eg, antipsychotics) if used concomitantly with diazepam).
No products indexed under this heading.

Chlorprothixene Lactate (Careful considerations should be given to the pharmacology of other centrally acting agents (eg, antipsychotics) if used concomitantly with diazepam).
No products indexed under this heading.

Cimetidine (There is a potentially relevant interaction between diazepam and certain hepatic enzyme inhibitors such as cimetidine. It has been shown that these compounds influence the pharmacokinetics of diazepam and may lead to increased and prolonged sedation).
No products indexed under this heading.

Cimetidine Hydrochloride (There is a potentially relevant interaction between diazepam and certain hepatic enzyme inhibitors such as cimetidine. It has been shown that these compounds influence the pharmacokinetics of diazepam and may lead to increased and prolonged sedation).
No products indexed under this heading.

Ciprofloxacin (There is a potentially relevant interaction between diazepam and certain hepatic enzyme inhibitors such as CYP450 3A4. It has been shown that these compounds influence the pharmacokinetics of diazepam and may lead to increased and prolonged sedation). Products include:
Cipro I.V. 3082
Cipro 3073
Cipro XR 3091
Ciprodex 583

Citalopram Hydrobromide (Careful considerations should be given to the pharmacology of other centrally acting agents (eg, antidepressants) if used concomitantly with diazepam). Products include:
Celexa 1153

Clarithromycin (There is a potentially relevant interaction between diazepam and certain hepatic enzyme inhibitors such as CYP450 3A4. It has been shown that these compounds influence the pharmacokinetics of diazepam and may lead to increased and prolonged sedation). Products include:
Biaxin/Biaxin XL 412

Clemastine Fumarate (Careful considerations should be given to the pharmacology of other centrally acting agents (eg, sedating antihistamines) if used concomitantly with diazepam).
No products indexed under this heading.

Clonazepam (Co-administration of diazepam as an adjunct in treating convulsive disorders results in possibility of an increase in the frequency and/or severity of grand mal seizures which may require an increase in the dosage of standard anticonvulsant agent; may potentiate the CNS depression caused by diazepam). Products include:
Klonopin 2855

Clotrimazole (There is a potentially relevant interaction between diazepam and certain hepatic enzyme inhibitors such as CYP450 3A4. It has been shown that these compounds influence the pharmacokinetics of diazepam and may lead to increased and prolonged sedation). Products include:
Lotrisone 3163

Clozapine (Careful considerations should be given to the pharmacology of other centrally acting agents (eg, antipsychotics) if used concomitantly with diazepam).
No products indexed under this heading.

Cocaine Hydrochloride (Careful considerations should be given to the pharmacology of other centrally acting agents (eg, anesthetics) if used concomitantly with diazepam).
No products indexed under this heading.

Codeine Phosphate (Careful considerations should be given to the pharmacology of other centrally acting agents (eg, narcotics) if used concomitantly with diazepam). Products include:
Tylenol with Codeine 2691

Codeine Sulfate (Careful considerations should be given to the pharmacology of other centrally acting agents (eg, narcotics) if used concomitantly with diazepam).
No products indexed under this heading.

Conivaptan Hydrochloride (There is a potentially relevant interaction between diazepam and certain hepatic enzyme inhibitors such as CYP450 3A4. It has been shown that these compounds influence the pharmacokinetics of diazepam and may lead to increased and prolonged sedation). Products include:
Vaprisol 689

Cyclosporine (There is a potentially relevant interaction between diazepam and certain hepatic enzyme inhibitors such as CYP450 3A4. It has been shown that these compounds influence the pharmacokinetics of diazepam and may lead to increased and prolonged sedation). Products include:
Gengraf 440
Neoral Oral Solution 2496
Neoral Capsules 2496
Restasis 605

Cyproheptadine Hydrochloride (Careful considerations should be given to the pharmacology of other centrally acting agents (eg, sedating antihistamines) if used concomitantly with diazepam).
No products indexed under this heading.

Dalfopristin (There is a potentially relevant interaction between diazepam and certain hepatic enzyme inhibitors such as CYP450 3A4. It has been shown that these compounds influence the pharmacokinetics of diazepam and may lead to increased and prolonged sedation).
No products indexed under this heading.

Danazol (There is a potentially relevant interaction between diazepam and certain hepatic enzyme inhibitors such as CYP450 3A4. It has been shown that these compounds influence the pharmacokinetics of diazepam and may lead to increased and prolonged sedation).
No products indexed under this heading.

Darunavir (There is a potentially relevant interaction between diazepam and certain hepatic enzyme inhibitors such as CYP450 3A4. It has been shown that these compounds influence the pharmacokinetics of diazepam and may lead to increased and prolonged sedation).
No products indexed under this heading.

Dasatinib (There is a potentially relevant interaction between diazepam and certain hepatic enzyme inhibitors such as CYP450 3A4. It has been shown that these compounds influence the pharmacokinetics of diazepam and may lead to increased and prolonged sedation).
No products indexed under this heading.

Delavirdine Mesylate (There is a potentially relevant interaction between diazepam and certain hepatic enzyme inhibitors such as CYP450 3A4. It has been shown that these compounds influence the pharmacokinetics of diazepam and may lead to increased and prolonged sedation).
No products indexed under this heading.

Delavirine (There is a potentially relevant interaction between diazepam and certain hepatic enzyme inhibitors such as CYP450 3A4. It has been shown that these compounds influence the pharmacokinetics of diazepam and may lead to increased and prolonged sedation).
No products indexed under this heading.

Desipramine Hydrochloride (Careful considerations should be given to the pharmacology of other centrally acting agents (eg, antidepressants) if used concomitantly with diazepam).
No products indexed under this heading.

Desloratadine (There is a potentially relevant interaction between diazepam and certain hepatic enzyme inhibitors such as CYP450 3A4. It has been shown that these compounds influence the pharmacokinetics of diazepam and may lead to increased and prolonged sedation). Products include:
Clarinex Syrup 3098
Clarinex 3098
Clarinex Reditabs 3098
Clarinex-D 12-Hour 3101
Clarinex-D 3104

Desogestrel (There is a potentially relevant interaction between diazepam and certain hepatic enzyme inhibitors such as CYP450 2C19. It has been shown that these compounds influence the pharmacokinetics of diazepam and may lead to increased and prolonged sedation).
No products indexed under this heading.

Dexchlorpheniramine Maleate (Careful considerations should be given to the pharmacology of other centrally acting agents (eg, sedating antihistamines) if used concomitantly with diazepam).
No products indexed under this heading.

Dezocine (Careful considerations should be given to the pharmacology of other centrally acting agents (eg, narcotics) if used concomitantly with diazepam).
No products indexed under this heading.

Dibucaine (Careful considerations should be given to the pharmacology of other centrally acting agents (eg, anesthetics) if used concomitantly with diazepam).
No products indexed under this heading.

Dibucaine Hydrochloride (Careful considerations should be given to the pharmacology of other centrally acting agents (eg, anesthetics) if used concomitantly with diazepam).
No products indexed under this heading.

Dihydrocodeine Bitartrate (Careful considerations should be given to the pharmacology of other centrally acting agents (eg, narcotics) if used concomitantly with diazepam).
No products indexed under this heading.

Dihydrocodeinone Bitartrate (Careful considerations should be given to the pharmacology of other centrally acting agents (eg, narcotics) if used concomitantly with diazepam).
No products indexed under this heading.

Diltiazem Hydrochloride (There is a potentially relevant interaction between diazepam and certain hepatic enzyme inhibitors such as CYP450 3A4. It has been shown that these compounds influence the pharmacokinetics of diazepam and may lead to increased and prolonged sedation). Products include:
Cardizem LA 423

Diltiazem Maleate (There is a potentially relevant interaction between diazepam and certain hepatic enzyme inhibitors such as CYP450 3A4. It has been shown that these compounds influence the pharmacokinetics of diazepam and may lead to increased and prolonged sedation).
No products indexed under this heading.

Diphenhydramine Hydrochloride (Careful considerations should be given to the pharmacology of other centrally acting agents (eg, sedating antihistamines) if used concomitantly with diazepam). Products include:
Benadryl Allergy Ultratab 2042
Children's Benadryl Allergy Liquid 2042

Diphenylpyraline Hydrochloride (Careful considerations should be given to the pharmacology of other centrally acting agents (eg, sedating antihistamines) if used concomitantly with diazepam).
No products indexed under this heading.

Divalproex Sodium (Careful considerations should be given to the pharmacology of other centrally acting agents (eg, anticonvulsants) if used concomitantly with diazepam). Products include:
Depakote ER 426

Doxepin Hydrochloride (Careful considerations should be given to the pharmacology of other centrally acting agents (eg, antidepressants) if used concomitantly with diazepam).
No products indexed under this heading.

Efavirenz (There is a potentially relevant interaction between diazepam and certain hepatic enzyme inhibitors such as CYP450 3A4. It has been shown that these compounds influence the pharmacokinetics of diazepam and may lead to increased and prolonged sedation). Products include:

(⊙ Described in PDR® for Ophthalmic Medicines)

1997 Interactions Index Valium

Atripla 906

Enflurane (Careful considerations should be given to the pharmacology of other centrally acting agents (eg, anesthetics) if used concomitantly with diazepam).
No products indexed under this heading.

Erythromycin (There is a potentially relevant interaction between diazepam and certain hepatic enzyme inhibitors such as CYP450 3A4. It has been shown that these compounds influence the pharmacokinetics of diazepam and may lead to increased and prolonged sedation).
No products indexed under this heading.

Erythromycin Estolate (There is a potentially relevant interaction between diazepam and certain hepatic enzyme inhibitors such as CYP450 3A4. It has been shown that these compounds influence the pharmacokinetics of diazepam and may lead to increased and prolonged sedation).
No products indexed under this heading.

Erythromycin Ethylsuccinate (There is a potentially relevant interaction between diazepam and certain hepatic enzyme inhibitors such as CYP450 3A4. It has been shown that these compounds influence the pharmacokinetics of diazepam and may lead to increased and prolonged sedation). Products include:
E.E.S. 437
EryPed 435

Erythromycin Gluceptate (There is a potentially relevant interaction between diazepam and certain hepatic enzyme inhibitors such as CYP450 3A4. It has been shown that these compounds influence the pharmacokinetics of diazepam and may lead to increased and prolonged sedation).
No products indexed under this heading.

Erythromycin Lactobionate (There is a potentially relevant interaction between diazepam and certain hepatic enzyme inhibitors such as CYP450 3A4. It has been shown that these compounds influence the pharmacokinetics of diazepam and may lead to increased and prolonged sedation).
No products indexed under this heading.

Erythromycin Stearate (There is a potentially relevant interaction between diazepam and certain hepatic enzyme inhibitors such as CYP450 3A4. It has been shown that these compounds influence the pharmacokinetics of diazepam and may lead to increased and prolonged sedation).
No products indexed under this heading.

Escitalopram Oxalate (Careful considerations should be given to the pharmacology of other centrally acting agents (eg, antidepressants) if used concomitantly with diazepam). Products include:
Lexapro Oral Suspension 1160
Lexapro Tablets 1160

Esomeprazole Magnesium (There is a potentially relevant interaction between diazepam and certain hepatic enzyme inhibitors such as CYP450 3A4. It has been shown that these compounds influence the pharmacokinetics of diazepam and may lead to increased and prolonged sedation). Products include:
Nexium Capsules 704
Nexium Oral Suspension 704

Esomeprazole Sodium (There is a potentially relevant interaction between diazepam and certain hepatic enzyme inhibitors such as CYP450 3A4. It has been shown that these compounds influence the pharmacokinetics of diazepam and may lead to increased and prolonged sedation). Products include:
Nexium I.V. 712

Estazolam (Careful considerations should be given to the pharmacology of other centrally acting agents (eg, sedatives and hypnotics) if used concomitantly with diazepam).
No products indexed under this heading.

Ethanol (Concomitant use with alcohol is not recommended due to enhancement of the sedative effect).
No products indexed under this heading.

Ethchlorvynol (Careful considerations should be given to the pharmacology of other centrally acting agents (eg, sedatives and hypnotics) if used concomitantly with diazepam).
No products indexed under this heading.

Ethinamate (Careful considerations should be given to the pharmacology of other centrally acting agents (eg, sedatives and hypnotics) if used concomitantly with diazepam).
No products indexed under this heading.

Ethinyl Estradiol (There is a potentially relevant interaction between diazepam and certain hepatic enzyme inhibitors such as CYP450 2C19. It has been shown that these compounds influence the pharmacokinetics of diazepam and may lead to increased and prolonged sedation). Products include:
LoSeasonique 3407
Lybrel 3514
NuvaRing 3181
Ortho Evra 2648
Ortho-Cyclen/Ortho Tri-Cyclen 2663
Ortho Tri-Cyclen Lo Tablets 2673
Seasonique 3418
Yaz 864

Ethosuximide (Careful considerations should be given to the pharmacology of other centrally acting agents (eg, anticonvulsants) if used concomitantly with diazepam).
No products indexed under this heading.

Ethotoin (Careful considerations should be given to the pharmacology of other centrally acting agents (eg, anticonvulsants) if used concomitantly with diazepam).
No products indexed under this heading.

Ethyl Alcohol (Concomitant use with alcohol is not recommended due to enhancement of the sedative effect).
No products indexed under this heading.

Ethynodiol Diacetate (There is a potentially relevant interaction between diazepam and certain hepatic enzyme inhibitors such as CYP450 2C19. It has been shown that these compounds influence the pharmacokinetics of diazepam and may lead to increased and prolonged sedation).
No products indexed under this heading.

Etidocaine Hydrochloride (Careful considerations should be given to the pharmacology of other centrally acting agents (eg, anesthetics) if used concomitantly with diazepam).
No products indexed under this heading.

Felbamate (Careful considerations should be given to the pharmacology of other centrally acting agents (eg, anticonvulsants) if used concomitantly with diazepam).
No products indexed under this heading.

Fentanyl (Careful considerations should be given to the pharmacology of other centrally acting agents (eg, narcotics) if used concomitantly with diazepam). Products include:
Duragesic 2604
Fentanyl Transdermal System 2346
Onsolis 2054

Fentanyl Citrate (Careful considerations should be given to the pharmacology of other centrally acting agents (eg, narcotics) if used concomitantly with diazepam). Products include:
Fentora 966

Fluconazole (There is a potentially relevant interaction between diazepam and certain hepatic enzyme inhibitors such as CYP450 3A4. It has been shown that these compounds influence the pharmacokinetics of diazepam and may lead to increased and prolonged sedation).
No products indexed under this heading.

Fluoxetine (There is a potentially relevant interaction between diazepam and certain hepatic enzyme inhibitors such as fluoxetine. It has been shown that these compounds influence the pharmacokinetics of diazepam and may lead to increased and prolonged sedation).
No products indexed under this heading.

Fluoxetine Hydrochloride (There is a potentially relevant interaction between diazepam and certain hepatic enzyme inhibitors such as fluoxetine. It has been shown that these compounds influence the pharmacokinetics of diazepam and may lead to increased and prolonged sedation). Products include:
Prozac Weekly 1941
Prozac Pulvules 1941
Symbyax 1965

Fluphenazine Decanoate (Careful considerations should be given to the pharmacology of other centrally acting agents (eg, phenothiazines) if used concomitantly with diazepam).
No products indexed under this heading.

Fluphenazine Enanthate (Careful considerations should be given to the pharmacology of other centrally acting agents (eg, phenothiazines) if used concomitantly with diazepam).
No products indexed under this heading.

Fluphenazine Hydrochloride (Careful considerations should be given to the pharmacology of other centrally acting agents (eg, phenothiazines) if used concomitantly with diazepam).
No products indexed under this heading.

Flurazepam Hydrochloride (Careful considerations should be given to the pharmacology of other centrally acting agents (eg, sedatives and hypnotics) if used concomitantly with diazepam).
No products indexed under this heading.

Fluvastatin Sodium (There is a potentially relevant interaction between diazepam and certain hepatic enzyme inhibitors such as CYP450 2C19. It has been shown that these compounds influence the pharmacokinetics of diazepam and may lead to increased and prolonged sedation).
No products indexed under this heading.

Fluvoxamine (There is a potentially relevant interaction between diazepam and certain hepatic enzyme inhibitors such as fluvoxamine. It has been shown that these compounds influence the pharmacokinetics of diazepam and may lead to increased and prolonged sedation).
No products indexed under this heading.

Fluvoxamine Maleate (There is a potentially relevant interaction between diazepam and certain hepatic enzyme inhibitors such as fluvoxamine. It has been shown that these compounds influence the pharmacokinetics of diazepam and may lead to increased and prolonged sedation).
No products indexed under this heading.

Fosamprenavir Calcium (There is a potentially relevant interaction between diazepam and certain hepatic enzyme inhibitors such as CYP450 3A4. It has been shown that these compounds influence the pharmacokinetics of diazepam and may lead to increased and prolonged sedation). Products include:
Lexiva Oral Suspension 1558
Lexiva 1558

Fosphenytoin (Careful considerations should be given to the pharmacology of other centrally acting agents (eg, anticonvulsants) if used concomitantly with diazepam).
No products indexed under this heading.

Fosphenytoin Sodium (Careful considerations should be given to the pharmacology of other centrally acting agents (eg, anticonvulsants) if used concomitantly with diazepam).
No products indexed under this heading.

Gabapentin (Careful considerations should be given to the pharmacology of other centrally acting agents (eg, anticonvulsants) if used concomitantly with diazepam).
No products indexed under this heading.

Glutethimide (Careful considerations should be given to the pharmacology of other centrally acting agents (eg, sedatives and hypnotics) if used concomitantly with diazepam).
No products indexed under this heading.

Haloperidol (Careful considerations should be given to the pharmacology of other centrally acting agents (eg, antipsychotics) if used concomitantly with diazepam).
No products indexed under this heading.

Haloperidol Decanoate (Careful considerations should be given to the pharmacology of other centrally acting agents (eg, antipsychotics) if used concomitantly with diazepam).
No products indexed under this heading.

Haloperidol Lactate (Careful considerations should be given to the pharmacology of other centrally acting agents (eg, antipsychotics) if used concomitantly with diazepam).
No products indexed under this heading.

Halothane (Careful considerations should be given to the pharmacology of other centrally acting agents (eg, anesthetics) if used concomitantly with diazepam).
No products indexed under this heading.

Hexobarbital (Careful considerations should be given to the pharmacology of other centrally acting agents (eg, barbiturates) if used concomitantly with diazepam).
No products indexed under this heading.

Hydrocodone Bitartrate (Careful considerations should be given to the pharmacology of other centrally acting agents (eg, narcotics) if used concomitantly with diazepam). Products include:
Vicodin 560
Vicodin ES 561
Vicodin HP 563
Vicoprofen 564
Zydone 1138

Hydrocodone Polistirex (Careful considerations should be given to the pharmacology of other centrally acting agents (eg, narcotics) if used concomitantly with diazepam). Products include:
Tussionex 3443

Hydromorphone (Careful considerations should be given to the pharmacology of other centrally acting agents (eg, narcotics) if used concomitantly with diazepam).
No products indexed under this heading.

Hydromorphone Hydrochloride (Careful considerations should be given to the pharmacology of other centrally acting agents (eg, narcotics) if used concomitantly with diazepam). Products include:
Dilaudid Injection 2800
Dilaudid Oral 2797
Dilaudid Tablets 2797
Dilaudid-HP 2800

Imatinib Mesylate (There is a potentially relevant interaction between diazepam and certain hepatic enzyme inhibitors such as CYP450 3A4. It has been

IMPORTANT NOTE: Always consult each drug listing in the patient's regimen for possible interactions.

Valium Interactions Index 1998

shown that these compounds influence the pharmacokinetics of diazepam and may lead to increased and prolonged sedation). Products include:
Gleevec 2477

Imipramine Hydrochloride (Careful considerations should be given to the pharmacology of other centrally acting agents (eg, antidepressants) if used concomitantly with diazepam).
No products indexed under this heading.

Imipramine Pamoate (Careful considerations should be given to the pharmacology of other centrally acting agents (eg, antidepressants) if used concomitantly with diazepam).
No products indexed under this heading.

Indinavir Sulfate (There is a potentially relevant interaction between diazepam and certain hepatic enzyme inhibitors such as CYP450 3A4. It has been shown that these compounds influence the pharmacokinetics of diazepam and may lead to increased and prolonged sedation). Products include:
Crixivan 2113

Indomethacin (There is a potentially relevant interaction between diazepam and certain hepatic enzyme inhibitors such as CYP450 2C19. It has been shown that these compounds influence the pharmacokinetics of diazepam and may lead to increased and prolonged sedation). Products include:
Indocin 2167

Indomethacin Sodium Trihydrate (There is a potentially relevant interaction between diazepam and certain hepatic enzyme inhibitors such as CYP450 2C19. It has been shown that these compounds influence the pharmacokinetics of diazepam and may lead to increased and prolonged sedation). Products include:
Indocin I.V. 2007

Isocarboxazid (Careful considerations should be given to the pharmacology of other centrally acting agents (eg, MAO inhibitors) if used concomitantly with diazepam). Products include:
Marplan 3481

Isoflurane (Careful considerations should be given to the pharmacology of other centrally acting agents (eg, anesthetics) if used concomitantly with diazepam).
No products indexed under this heading.

Isoniazid (There is a potentially relevant interaction between diazepam and certain hepatic enzyme inhibitors such as CYP450 3A4. It has been shown that these compounds influence the pharmacokinetics of diazepam and may lead to increased and prolonged sedation).
No products indexed under this heading.

Isopropyl Alcohol (Concomitant use with alcohol is not recommended due to enhancement of the sedative effect).
No products indexed under this heading.

Itraconazole (There is a potentially relevant interaction between diazepam and certain hepatic enzyme inhibitors such as CYP450 3A4. It has been shown that these compounds influence the pharmacokinetics of diazepam and may lead to increased and prolonged sedation).
No products indexed under this heading.

Ketamine Hydrochloride (Careful considerations should be given to the pharmacology of other centrally acting agents (eg, anesthetics) if used concomitantly with diazepam).
No products indexed under this heading.

Ketoconazole (There is a potentially relevant interaction between diazepam and certain hepatic enzyme inhibitors such as ketoconazole. It has been shown that these compounds influence the pharmacokinetics of diazepam and may lead to increased and prolonged sedation). Products include:
Extina 3319
Xolegel 3337

Lamotrigine (Careful considerations should be given to the pharmacology of other centrally acting agents (eg, anticonvulsants) if used concomitantly with diazepam). Products include:
Lamictal 1522
Lamictal ODT 1522
Lamictal XR 1536

Lansoprazole (There is a potentially relevant interaction between diazepam and certain hepatic enzyme inhibitors such as CYP450 2C19. It has been shown that these compounds influence the pharmacokinetics of diazepam and may lead to increased and prolonged sedation).
No products indexed under this heading.

Lapatinib (There is a potentially relevant interaction between diazepam and certain hepatic enzyme inhibitors such as CYP450 3A4. It has been shown that these compounds influence the pharmacokinetics of diazepam and may lead to increased and prolonged sedation). Products include:
Tykerb 1698

Letrozole (There is a potentially relevant interaction between diazepam and certain hepatic enzyme inhibitors such as CYP450 2C19. It has been shown that these compounds influence the pharmacokinetics of diazepam and may lead to increased and prolonged sedation). Products include:
Femara 2466

Levetiracetam (Careful considerations should be given to the pharmacology of other centrally acting agents (eg, anticonvulsants) if used concomitantly with diazepam). Products include:
Keppra XR 3434

Levobupivacaine Hydrochloride (Careful considerations should be given to the pharmacology of other centrally acting agents (eg, anesthetics) if used concomitantly with diazepam).
No products indexed under this heading.

Levonorgestrel (There is a potentially relevant interaction between diazepam and certain hepatic enzyme inhibitors such as CYP450 2C19. It has been shown that these compounds influence the pharmacokinetics of diazepam and may lead to increased and prolonged sedation). Products include:
Climara Pro 847
LoSeasonique 3407
Lybrel 3514
Mirena 854
Plan B 3416
Seasonique 3418

Levorphanol Tartrate (Careful considerations should be given to the pharmacology of other centrally acting agents (eg, narcotics) if used concomitantly with diazepam).
No products indexed under this heading.

Lidocaine (Careful considerations should be given to the pharmacology of other centrally acting agents (eg, anesthetics) if used concomitantly with diazepam). Products include:
Lidoderm 1107

Lidocaine Base (Careful considerations should be given to the pharmacology of other centrally acting agents (eg, anesthetics) if used concomitantly with diazepam).
No products indexed under this heading.

Lidocaine Hydrochloride (Careful considerations should be given to the pharmacology of other centrally acting agents (eg, anesthetics) if used concomitantly with diazepam).
No products indexed under this heading.

Lithium (Careful considerations should be given to the pharmacology of other centrally acting agents (eg, antipsychotics) if used concomitantly with diazepam).
No products indexed under this heading.

Lithium Carbonate (Careful considerations should be given to the pharmacology of other centrally acting agents (eg, antipsychotics) if used concomitantly with diazepam).
No products indexed under this heading.

Lithium Citrate (Careful considerations should be given to the pharmacology of other centrally acting agents (eg, antipsychotics) if used concomitantly with diazepam).
No products indexed under this heading.

Lopinavir (There is a potentially relevant interaction between diazepam and certain hepatic enzyme inhibitors such as CYP450 3A4. It has been shown that these compounds influence the pharmacokinetics of diazepam and may lead to increased and prolonged sedation). Products include:
Kaletra 458

Loratadine (There is a potentially relevant interaction between diazepam and certain hepatic enzyme inhibitors such as CYP450 3A4. It has been shown that these compounds influence the pharmacokinetics of diazepam and may lead to increased and prolonged sedation).
No products indexed under this heading.

Lorazepam (Careful considerations should be given to the pharmacology of other centrally acting agents (eg, sedatives and hypnotics) if used concomitantly with diazepam).
No products indexed under this heading.

Loxapine Hydrochloride (Careful considerations should be given to the pharmacology of other centrally acting agents (eg, antipsychotics) if used concomitantly with diazepam).
No products indexed under this heading.

Loxapine Succinate (Careful considerations should be given to the pharmacology of other centrally acting agents (eg, antipsychotics) if used concomitantly with diazepam).
No products indexed under this heading.

Magaldrate (Diazepam peak concentrations are lower when antacids are administered concurrently. The peak concentrations appear to be lower due to a slower rate of absorption, with the time required to achieve peak concentration on average 20 to 25 minutes greater in the presence of antacids).
No products indexed under this heading.

Magnesium Carbonate (Diazepam peak concentrations are lower when antacids are administered concurrently. The peak concentrations appear to be lower due to a slower rate of absorption, with the time required to achieve peak concentration on average 20 to 25 minutes greater in the presence of antacids).
No products indexed under this heading.

Magnesium Hydroxide (Diazepam peak concentrations are lower when antacids are administered concurrently. The peak concentrations appear to be lower due to a slower rate of absorption, with the time required to achieve peak concentration on average 20 to 25 minutes greater in the presence of antacids). Products include:
Fleet Pedia-Lax Chewable Tablets 1144
Pepcid Complete 1822

Magnesium Oxide (Diazepam peak concentrations are lower when antacids are administered concurrently. The peak concentrations appear to be lower due to a slower rate of absorption, with the time required to achieve peak concentration on average 20 to 25 minutes greater in the presence of antacids). Products include:
Beelith 873

Magnesium Trisilicate (Diazepam peak concentrations are lower when antacids are administered concurrently. The peak concentrations appear to be lower due to a slower rate of absorption, with the time required to achieve peak concentration on average 20 to 25 minutes greater in the presence of antacids).
No products indexed under this heading.

Maprotiline Hydrochloride (Careful considerations should be given to the pharmacology of other centrally acting agents (eg, antidepressants) if used concomitantly with diazepam).
No products indexed under this heading.

Meperidine Hydrochloride (Careful considerations should be given to the pharmacology of other centrally acting agents (eg, narcotics) if used concomitantly with diazepam).
No products indexed under this heading.

Mephenytoin (Careful considerations should be given to the pharmacology of other centrally acting agents (eg, anticonvulsants) if used concomitantly with diazepam).
No products indexed under this heading.

Mephobarbital (Careful considerations should be given to the pharmacology of other centrally acting agents (eg, barbiturates) if used concomitantly with diazepam).
No products indexed under this heading.

Mepivacaine Hydrochloride (Careful considerations should be given to the pharmacology of other centrally acting agents (eg, anesthetics) if used concomitantly with diazepam).
No products indexed under this heading.

Mesoridazine Besylate (Careful considerations should be given to the pharmacology of other centrally acting agents (eg, phenothiazines) if used concomitantly with diazepam).
No products indexed under this heading.

Mestranol (There is a potentially relevant interaction between diazepam and certain hepatic enzyme inhibitors such as CYP450 2C19. It has been shown that these compounds influence the pharmacokinetics of diazepam and may lead to increased and prolonged sedation).
No products indexed under this heading.

Methadone Hydrochloride (Careful considerations should be given to the pharmacology of other centrally acting agents (eg, narcotics) if used concomitantly with diazepam).
No products indexed under this heading.

Methdilazine Hydrochloride (Careful considerations should be given to the pharmacology of other centrally acting agents (eg, sedating antihistamines) if used concomitantly with diazepam).
No products indexed under this heading.

Methohexital Sodium (Careful considerations should be given to the pharmacology of other centrally acting agents (eg, anesthetics) if used concomitantly with diazepam).
No products indexed under this heading.

Methotrimeprazine (Careful considerations should be given to the pharmacology of other centrally acting agents (eg, phenothiazines) if used concomitantly with diazepam).
No products indexed under this heading.

Methsuximide (Careful considerations should be given to the pharmacology of other centrally acting agents (eg, anticonvulsants) if used concomitantly with diazepam).
No products indexed under this heading.

(⊙ Described in PDR® for Ophthalmic Medicines)

1999 Interactions Index Valium

Metronidazole (There is a potentially relevant interaction between diazepam and certain hepatic enzyme inhibitors such as CYP450 3A4. It has been shown that these compounds influence the pharmacokinetics of diazepam and may lead to increased and prolonged sedation). Products include:
Pylera 793

Metronidazole Benzoate (There is a potentially relevant interaction between diazepam and certain hepatic enzyme inhibitors such as CYP450 3A4. It has been shown that these compounds influence the pharmacokinetics of diazepam and may lead to increased and prolonged sedation).
No products indexed under this heading.

Metronidazole Hydrochloride (There is a potentially relevant interaction between diazepam and certain hepatic enzyme inhibitors such as CYP450 3A4. It has been shown that these compounds influence the pharmacokinetics of diazepam and may lead to increased and prolonged sedation).
No products indexed under this heading.

Metronidazole Sodium (There is a potentially relevant interaction between diazepam and certain hepatic enzyme inhibitors such as CYP450 3A4. It has been shown that these compounds influence the pharmacokinetics of diazepam and may lead to increased and prolonged sedation).
No products indexed under this heading.

Miconazole (There is a potentially relevant interaction between diazepam and certain hepatic enzyme inhibitors such as CYP450 3A4. It has been shown that these compounds influence the pharmacokinetics of diazepam and may lead to increased and prolonged sedation).
No products indexed under this heading.

Miconazole Nitrate (There is a potentially relevant interaction between diazepam and certain hepatic enzyme inhibitors such as CYP450 3A4. It has been shown that these compounds influence the pharmacokinetics of diazepam and may lead to increased and prolonged sedation). Products include:
Vusion Ointment 3335

Midazolam Hydrochloride (Careful considerations should be given to the pharmacology of other centrally acting agents (eg, sedatives and hypnotics) if used concomitantly with diazepam).
No products indexed under this heading.

Mifepristone (There is a potentially relevant interaction between diazepam and certain hepatic enzyme inhibitors such as CYP450 3A4. It has been shown that these compounds influence the pharmacokinetics of diazepam and may lead to increased and prolonged sedation).
No products indexed under this heading.

Mirtazapine (Careful considerations should be given to the pharmacology of other centrally acting agents (eg, antidepressants) if used concomitantly with diazepam). Products include:
Remeron Tablets 3214
RemeronSolTab Tablets 3219

Moclobemide (Careful considerations should be given to the pharmacology of other centrally acting agents (eg, MAO inhibitors) if used concomitantly with diazepam).
No products indexed under this heading.

Modafinil (There is a potentially relevant interaction between diazepam and certain hepatic enzyme inhibitors such as CYP450 2C19. It has been shown that these compounds influence the pharmacokinetics of diazepam and may lead to increased and prolonged sedation). Products include:
Provigil 983

Molindone Hydrochloride (Careful considerations should be given to the pharmacology of other centrally acting agents (eg, antipsychotics) if used concomitantly with diazepam). Products include:
Moban 1108

Morphine Sulfate (Careful considerations should be given to the pharmacology of other centrally acting agents (eg, narcotics) if used concomitantly with diazepam). Products include:
Avinza 1822
Embeda 1831
MS Contin 2803

Morphine Sulfate, Liposomal (Careful considerations should be given to the pharmacology of other centrally acting agents (eg, narcotics) if used concomitantly with diazepam).
No products indexed under this heading.

Nefazodone Hydrochloride (Careful considerations should be given to the pharmacology of other centrally acting agents (eg, antidepressants) if used concomitantly with diazepam).
No products indexed under this heading.

Nelfinavir Mesylate (There is a potentially relevant interaction between diazepam and certain hepatic enzyme inhibitors such as CYP450 3A4. It has been shown that these compounds influence the pharmacokinetics of diazepam and may lead to increased and prolonged sedation).
No products indexed under this heading.

Nevirapine (There is a potentially relevant interaction between diazepam and certain hepatic enzyme inhibitors such as CYP450 3A4. It has been shown that these compounds influence the pharmacokinetics of diazepam and may lead to increased and prolonged sedation). Products include:
Viramune Oral Suspension 897
Viramune Tablets 897

Niacin (There is a potentially relevant interaction between diazepam and certain hepatic enzyme inhibitors such as CYP450 3A4. It has been shown that these compounds influence the pharmacokinetics of diazepam and may lead to increased and prolonged sedation). Products include:
Advicor 402
Cardio Basics 3455
Niaspan 497
Simcor 524

Niacinamide (There is a potentially relevant interaction between diazepam and certain hepatic enzyme inhibitors such as CYP450 3A4. It has been shown that these compounds influence the pharmacokinetics of diazepam and may lead to increased and prolonged sedation). Products include:
CitraNatal 90 DHA Capsules 2332
CitraNatal Assure 2332
CitraNatal Rx 2332
Heplive 607

Niacinamide Hydroiodide (There is a potentially relevant interaction between diazepam and certain hepatic enzyme inhibitors such as CYP450 3A4. It has been shown that these compounds influence the pharmacokinetics of diazepam and may lead to increased and prolonged sedation).
No products indexed under this heading.

Nicotinamide (There is a potentially relevant interaction between diazepam and certain hepatic enzyme inhibitors such as CYP450 3A4. It has been shown that these compounds influence the pharmacokinetics of diazepam and may lead to increased and prolonged sedation).
No products indexed under this heading.

Nifedipine (There is a potentially relevant interaction between diazepam and certain hepatic enzyme inhibitors such as CYP450 3A4. It has been shown that these compounds influence the pharmacokinetics of diazepam and may lead to increased and prolonged sedation).
No products indexed under this heading.

Norethindrone (There is a potentially relevant interaction between diazepam and certain hepatic enzyme inhibitors such as CYP450 2C19. It has been shown that these compounds influence the pharmacokinetics of diazepam and may lead to increased and prolonged sedation). Products include:
Ortho Micronor 2660

Norethynodrel (There is a potentially relevant interaction between diazepam and certain hepatic enzyme inhibitors such as CYP450 2C19. It has been shown that these compounds influence the pharmacokinetics of diazepam and may lead to increased and prolonged sedation).
No products indexed under this heading.

Norfloxacin (There is a potentially relevant interaction between diazepam and certain hepatic enzyme inhibitors such as CYP450 3A4. It has been shown that these compounds influence the pharmacokinetics of diazepam and may lead to increased and prolonged sedation). Products include:
Noroxin 2220

Norgestimate (There is a potentially relevant interaction between diazepam and certain hepatic enzyme inhibitors such as CYP450 2C19. It has been shown that these compounds influence the pharmacokinetics of diazepam and may lead to increased and prolonged sedation). Products include:
Ortho-Cyclen/Ortho Tri-Cyclen 2663
Ortho Tri-Cyclen Lo Tablets 2673

Norgestrel (There is a potentially relevant interaction between diazepam and certain hepatic enzyme inhibitors such as CYP450 2C19. It has been shown that these compounds influence the pharmacokinetics of diazepam and may lead to increased and prolonged sedation).
No products indexed under this heading.

Nortriptyline Hydrochloride (Careful considerations should be given to the pharmacology of other centrally acting agents (eg, antidepressants) if used concomitantly with diazepam).
No products indexed under this heading.

Olanzapine (Careful considerations should be given to the pharmacology of other centrally acting agents (eg, antipsychotics) if used concomitantly with diazepam). Products include:
Symbyax 1965
Zyprexa 1984
Zyprexa IntraMuscular 1984
Zyprexa ZYDIS 1984

Omeprazole (There is a potentially relevant interaction between diazepam and certain hepatic enzyme inhibitors such as omeprazole. It has been shown that these compounds influence the pharmacokinetics of diazepam and may lead to increased and prolonged sedation).
No products indexed under this heading.

Omeprazole Magnesium (There is a potentially relevant interaction between diazepam and certain hepatic enzyme inhibitors such as omeprazole. It has been shown that these compounds influence the pharmacokinetics of diazepam and may lead to increased and prolonged sedation).
No products indexed under this heading.

Oxcarbazepine (Careful considerations should be given to the pharmacology of other centrally acting agents (eg, anticonvulsants) if used concomitantly with diazepam).
No products indexed under this heading.

Oxycodone Hydrochloride (Careful considerations should be given to the pharmacology of other centrally acting agents (eg, narcotics) if used concomitantly with diazepam). Products include:
OxyContin 2807
Percocet 1121
Percodan 1124

Oxycodone Terephthalate (Careful considerations should be given to the pharmacology of other centrally acting agents (eg, narcotics) if used concomitantly with diazepam).
No products indexed under this heading.

Oxymorphone Hydrochloride (Careful considerations should be given to the pharmacology of other centrally acting agents (eg, narcotics) if used concomitantly with diazepam). Products include:
Opana 1110
Opana ER 1114

Paliperidone (Careful considerations should be given to the pharmacology of other centrally acting agents (eg, antipsychotics) if used concomitantly with diazepam). Products include:
Invega 2613
Invega Sustenna 2621

Paramethadione (Careful considerations should be given to the pharmacology of other centrally acting agents (eg, anticonvulsants) if used concomitantly with diazepam).
No products indexed under this heading.

Pargyline Hydrochloride (Careful considerations should be given to the pharmacology of other centrally acting agents (eg, MAO inhibitors) if used concomitantly with diazepam).
No products indexed under this heading.

Paroxetine (Careful considerations should be given to the pharmacology of other centrally acting agents (eg, antidepressants) if used concomitantly with diazepam).
No products indexed under this heading.

Paroxetine Hydrochloride (Careful considerations should be given to the pharmacology of other centrally acting agents (eg, antidepressants) if used concomitantly with diazepam). Products include:
Paroxetine CR 2361
Paroxetine ER 2371
Paxil 1586
Paxil CR 1596

Paroxetine Mesylate (Careful considerations should be given to the pharmacology of other centrally acting agents (eg, antidepressants) if used concomitantly with diazepam).
No products indexed under this heading.

Pentobarbital (Careful considerations should be given to the pharmacology of other centrally acting agents (eg, barbiturates) if used concomitantly with diazepam).
No products indexed under this heading.

Pentobarbital Sodium (Careful considerations should be given to the pharmacology of other centrally acting agents (eg, barbiturates) if used concomitantly with diazepam). Products include:
Nembutal 2012

Perphenazine (Careful considerations should be given to the pharmacology of other centrally acting agents (eg, phenothiazines) if used concomitantly with diazepam).
No products indexed under this heading.

Valium **Interactions Index** **2000**

Phenacemide (Careful considerations should be given to the pharmacology of other centrally acting agents (eg, anticonvulsants) if used concomitantly with diazepam).
No products indexed under this heading.

Phenelzine Sulfate (Careful considerations should be given to the pharmacology of other centrally acting agents (eg, MAO inhibitors) if used concomitantly with diazepam).
No products indexed under this heading.

Phenobarbital (Co-administration of diazepam as an adjunct in treating convulsive disorders results in possibility of an increase in the frequency and/or severity of grand mal seizures which may require an increase in the dosage of standard anticonvulsant agent; may potentiate the CNS depression caused by diazepam). Products include:
Donnatal ... **2711**

Phenobarbital Sodium (Careful considerations should be given to the pharmacology of other centrally acting agents (eg, anticonvulsants) if used concomitantly with diazepam).
No products indexed under this heading.

Phenothiazine Derivatives (Careful considerations should be given to the pharmacology of other centrally acting agents (eg, phenothiazines) if used concomitantly with diazepam).
No products indexed under this heading.

Phenothiazines (Careful considerations should be given to the pharmacology of other centrally acting agents (eg, phenothiazines) if used concomitantly with diazepam).
No products indexed under this heading.

Phensuximide (Careful considerations should be given to the pharmacology of other centrally acting agents (eg, anticonvulsants) if used concomitantly with diazepam).
No products indexed under this heading.

Phenytoin (There have been reports that the metabolic elimination of phenytoin is decreased by diazepam).
No products indexed under this heading.

Phenytoin Sodium (There have been reports that the metabolic elimination of phenytoin is decreased by diazepam). Products include:
Phenytek Capsules ... **2380**

Pimozide (Careful considerations should be given to the pharmacology of other centrally acting agents (eg, antipsychotics) if used concomitantly with diazepam).
No products indexed under this heading.

Posaconazole (There is a potentially relevant interaction between diazepam and certain hepatic enzyme inhibitors such as CYP450 3A4. It has been shown that these compounds influence the pharmacokinetics of diazepam and may lead to increased and prolonged sedation). Products include:
Noxafil ... **3172**

Prilocaine (Careful considerations should be given to the pharmacology of other centrally acting agents (eg, anesthetics) if used concomitantly with diazepam).
No products indexed under this heading.

Prilocaine Hydrochloride (Careful considerations should be given to the pharmacology of other centrally acting agents (eg, anesthetics) if used concomitantly with diazepam).
No products indexed under this heading.

Primidone (Careful considerations should be given to the pharmacology of other centrally acting agents (eg, anticonvulsants) if used concomitantly with diazepam).
No products indexed under this heading.

Procaine (Careful considerations should be given to the pharmacology of other centrally acting agents (eg, anesthetics) if used concomitantly with diazepam).
No products indexed under this heading.

Procaine Hydrochloride (Careful considerations should be given to the pharmacology of other centrally acting agents (eg, anesthetics) if used concomitantly with diazepam).
No products indexed under this heading.

Procarbazine Hydrochloride (Careful considerations should be given to the pharmacology of other centrally acting agents (eg, MAO inhibitors) if used concomitantly with diazepam).
No products indexed under this heading.

Prochlorperazine (Careful considerations should be given to the pharmacology of other centrally acting agents (eg, phenothiazines) if used concomitantly with diazepam).
No products indexed under this heading.

Prochlorperazine Edisylate (Careful considerations should be given to the pharmacology of other centrally acting agents (eg, phenothiazines) if used concomitantly with diazepam).
No products indexed under this heading.

Prochlorperazine Maleate (Careful considerations should be given to the pharmacology of other centrally acting agents (eg, phenothiazines) if used concomitantly with diazepam).
No products indexed under this heading.

Promethazine (Careful considerations should be given to the pharmacology of other centrally acting agents (eg, phenothiazines) if used concomitantly with diazepam).
No products indexed under this heading.

Promethazine Hydrochloride (Careful considerations should be given to the pharmacology of other centrally acting agents (eg, phenothiazines) if used concomitantly with diazepam).
No products indexed under this heading.

Proparacaine Hydrochloride (Careful considerations should be given to the pharmacology of other centrally acting agents (eg, anesthetics) if used concomitantly with diazepam).
No products indexed under this heading.

Propofol (Careful considerations should be given to the pharmacology of other centrally acting agents (eg, sedatives and hypnotics) if used concomitantly with diazepam).
No products indexed under this heading.

Propoxyphene Hydrochloride (Careful considerations should be given to the pharmacology of other centrally acting agents (eg, narcotics) if used concomitantly with diazepam).
No products indexed under this heading.

Propoxyphene Napsylate (Careful considerations should be given to the pharmacology of other centrally acting agents (eg, narcotics) if used concomitantly with diazepam).
No products indexed under this heading.

Protriptyline Hydrochloride (Careful considerations should be given to the pharmacology of other centrally acting agents (eg, antidepressants) if used concomitantly with diazepam).
No products indexed under this heading.

Pyrilamine Maleate (Careful considerations should be given to the pharmacology of other centrally acting agents (eg, sedating antihistamines) if used concomitantly with diazepam).
No products indexed under this heading.

Pyrilamine Tannate (Careful considerations should be given to the pharmacology of other centrally acting agents (eg, sedating antihistamines) if used concomitantly with diazepam).
No products indexed under this heading.

Quazepam (Careful considerations should be given to the pharmacology of other centrally acting agents (eg, sedatives and hypnotics) if used concomitantly with diazepam).
No products indexed under this heading.

Quetiapine Fumarate (Careful considerations should be given to the pharmacology of other centrally acting agents (eg, antipsychotics) if used concomitantly with diazepam). Products include:
Seroquel ... **750**
Seroquel XR ... **759**

Quinidine (There is a potentially relevant interaction between diazepam and certain hepatic enzyme inhibitors such as CYP450 3A4. It has been shown that these compounds influence the pharmacokinetics of diazepam and may lead to increased and prolonged sedation).
No products indexed under this heading.

Quinidine Gluconate (There is a potentially relevant interaction between diazepam and certain hepatic enzyme inhibitors such as CYP450 2C19. It has been shown that these compounds influence the pharmacokinetics of diazepam and may lead to increased and prolonged sedation).
No products indexed under this heading.

Quinidine Hydrochloride (There is a potentially relevant interaction between diazepam and certain hepatic enzyme inhibitors such as CYP450 3A4. It has been shown that these compounds influence the pharmacokinetics of diazepam and may lead to increased and prolonged sedation).
No products indexed under this heading.

Quinidine Polygalacturonate (There is a potentially relevant interaction between diazepam and certain hepatic enzyme inhibitors such as CYP450 3A4. It has been shown that these compounds influence the pharmacokinetics of diazepam and may lead to increased and prolonged sedation).
No products indexed under this heading.

Quinidine Sulfate (There is a potentially relevant interaction between diazepam and certain hepatic enzyme inhibitors such as CYP450 3A4. It has been shown that these compounds influence the pharmacokinetics of diazepam and may lead to increased and prolonged sedation).
No products indexed under this heading.

Quinine (There is a potentially relevant interaction between diazepam and certain hepatic enzyme inhibitors such as CYP450 3A4. It has been shown that these compounds influence the pharmacokinetics of diazepam and may lead to increased and prolonged sedation). Products include:
Hyland's Leg Cramps PM with Quinine ... **3315**

Quinine Sulfate (There is a potentially relevant interaction between diazepam and certain hepatic enzyme inhibitors such as CYP450 3A4. It has been shown that these compounds influence the pharmacokinetics of diazepam and may lead to increased and prolonged sedation).
No products indexed under this heading.

Quinupristin (There is a potentially relevant interaction between diazepam and certain hepatic enzyme inhibitors such as CYP450 3A4. It has been shown that these compounds influence the pharmacokinetics of diazepam and may lead to increased and prolonged sedation).
No products indexed under this heading.

Ramelteon (Careful considerations should be given to the pharmacology of other centrally acting agents (eg, sedatives and hypnotics) if used concomitantly with diazepam). Products include:
Rozerem ... **3366**

Ranitidine Bismuth Citrate (There is a potentially relevant interaction between diazepam and certain hepatic enzyme inhibitors such as CYP450 3A4. It has been shown that these compounds influence the pharmacokinetics of diazepam and may lead to increased and prolonged sedation).
No products indexed under this heading.

Ranitidine Hydrochloride (There is a potentially relevant interaction between diazepam and certain hepatic enzyme inhibitors such as CYP450 3A4. It has been shown that these compounds influence the pharmacokinetics of diazepam and may lead to increased and prolonged sedation). Products include:
Zantac ... **1737**
Zantac Injection ... **1732**
Zantac Pharmacy ... **1735**

Rasagiline Mesylate (Careful considerations should be given to the pharmacology of other centrally acting agents (eg, MAO inhibitors) if used concomitantly with diazepam). Products include:
Azilect ... **3383**

Remifentanil Hydrochloride (Careful considerations should be given to the pharmacology of other centrally acting agents (eg, narcotics) if used concomitantly with diazepam).
No products indexed under this heading.

Risperidone (Careful considerations should be given to the pharmacology of other centrally acting agents (eg, antipsychotics) if used concomitantly with diazepam). Products include:
Risperdal Consta ... **2682**

Ritonavir (There is a potentially relevant interaction between diazepam and certain hepatic enzyme inhibitors such as CYP450 3A4. It has been shown that these compounds influence the pharmacokinetics of diazepam and may lead to increased and prolonged sedation). Products include:
Kaletra ... **458**
Norvir ... **509**

Ropivacaine Hydrochloride (Careful considerations should be given to the pharmacology of other centrally acting agents (eg, anesthetics) if used concomitantly with diazepam).
No products indexed under this heading.

Rufinamide (Careful considerations should be given to the pharmacology of other centrally acting agents (eg, anticonvulsants) if used concomitantly with diazepam). Products include:
Banzel ... **1050**

Saquinavir (There is a potentially relevant interaction between diazepam and certain hepatic enzyme inhibitors such as CYP450 3A4. It has been shown that these compounds influence the pharmacokinetics of diazepam and may lead to increased and prolonged sedation).
No products indexed under this heading.

Saquinavir Mesylate (There is a potentially relevant interaction between diazepam and certain hepatic enzyme inhibitors such as CYP450 3A4. It has been shown that these compounds influence the pharmacokinetics of diazepam and may lead to increased and prolonged sedation).
No products indexed under this heading.

Secobarbital Sodium (Careful considerations should be given to the pharmacology of other centrally acting agents (eg, sedatives and hypnotics) if used concomitantly with diazepam).
No products indexed under this heading.

Selegiline (Careful considerations should be given to the pharmacology of other centrally acting agents (eg, MAO inhibitors) if used concomitantly with diazepam). Products include:
Emsam ... **3623**

Food Interactions

Alcohol (Concomitant use with alcohol is not recommended due to enhancement of the sedative effect).

Beer, reduced-alcohol (Concomitant use with alcohol is not recommended due to enhancement of the sedative effect).

Beer, unspecified (Concomitant use with alcohol is not recommended due to enhancement of the sedative effect).

Grapefruit (There is a potentially relevant interaction between diazepam and certain hepatic enzyme inhibitors such as CYP450 3A4. It has been shown that these compounds influence the pharmacokinetics of diazepam and may lead to increased and prolonged sedation).

Grapefruit Juice (There is a potentially relevant interaction between diazepam and certain hepatic enzyme inhibitors such as CYP450 3A4. It has been shown that these compounds influence the pharmacokinetics of diazepam and may lead to increased and prolonged sedation).

Wine, Chianti (Concomitant use with alcohol is not recommended due to enhancement of the sedative effect).

Wine, Red (Concomitant use with alcohol is not recommended due to enhancement of the sedative effect).

IMPORTANT NOTE: Always consult each drug listing in the patient's regimen for possible interactions.

Wine, unspecified (Concomitant use with alcohol is not recommended due to enhancement of the sedative effect).

Wine products (Concomitant use with alcohol is not recommended due to enhancement of the sedative effect).

VALSTAR STERILE SOLUTION FOR INTRAVESICAL INSTILLATION

(Valrubicin) 1131
None cited in PDR database.

VALTREX CAPLETS

(Valacyclovir Hydrochloride) 1702
May interact with nephrotoxic agents, and certain other agents. Compounds in these categories include:

Abacavir Sulfate (Cases of acute renal failure have been reported in patients receiving other nephrotoxic drugs. Caution should be exercised when administering valacyclovir to patients receiving potentially nephrotoxic drugs). Products include:

Acyclovir (Cases of acute renal failure have been reported in patients receiving other nephrotoxic drugs. Caution should be exercised when administering valacyclovir to patients receiving potentially nephrotoxic drugs). Products include:

Acyclovir Sodium (Cases of acute renal failure have been reported in patients receiving other nephrotoxic drugs. Caution should be exercised when administering valacyclovir to patients receiving potentially nephrotoxic drugs).
No products indexed under this heading.

Alatrofloxacin Mesylate (Cases of acute renal failure have been reported in patients receiving other nephrotoxic drugs. Caution should be exercised when administering valacyclovir to patients receiving potentially nephrotoxic drugs).
No products indexed under this heading.

Aldesleukin (Cases of acute renal failure have been reported in patients receiving other nephrotoxic drugs. Caution should be exercised when administering valacyclovir to patients receiving potentially nephrotoxic drugs). Products include:

Amikacin Sulfate (Cases of acute renal failure have been reported in patients receiving other nephrotoxic drugs. Caution should be exercised when administering valacyclovir to patients receiving potentially nephrotoxic drugs).
No products indexed under this heading.

Amoxicillin (Cases of acute renal failure have been reported in patients receiving other nephrotoxic drugs. Caution should be exercised when administering valacyclovir to patients receiving potentially nephrotoxic drugs). Products include:

Amoxicillin Trihydrate (Cases of acute renal failure have been reported in patients receiving other nephrotoxic drugs. Caution should be exercised when administering valacyclovir to patients receiving potentially nephrotoxic drugs).
No products indexed under this heading.

Amphotericin B (Cases of acute renal failure have been reported in patients receiving other nephrotoxic drugs. Caution should be exercised when administering valacyclovir to patients receiving potentially nephrotoxic drugs).
No products indexed under this heading.

Amphotericin B, liposomal (Cases of acute renal failure have been reported in patients receiving other nephrotoxic drugs. Caution should be exercised when administering valacyclovir to patients receiving potentially nephrotoxic drugs). Products include:

Amphotericin B Cholesteryl Sulfate (Cases of acute renal failure have been reported in patients receiving other nephrotoxic drugs. Caution should be exercised when administering valacyclovir to patients receiving potentially nephrotoxic drugs).
No products indexed under this heading.

Amphotericin B Lipid Complex (Cases of acute renal failure have been reported in patients receiving other nephrotoxic drugs. Caution should be exercised when administering valacyclovir to patients receiving potentially nephrotoxic drugs).
No products indexed under this heading.

Ampicillin (Cases of acute renal failure have been reported in patients receiving other nephrotoxic drugs. Caution should be exercised when administering valacyclovir to patients receiving potentially nephrotoxic drugs).
No products indexed under this heading.

Ampicillin Sodium (Cases of acute renal failure have been reported in patients receiving other nephrotoxic drugs. Caution should be exercised when administering valacyclovir to patients receiving potentially nephrotoxic drugs).
No products indexed under this heading.

Ampicillin Trihydrate (Cases of acute renal failure have been reported in patients receiving other nephrotoxic drugs. Caution should be exercised when administering valacyclovir to patients receiving potentially nephrotoxic drugs).
No products indexed under this heading.

Amprenavir (Cases of acute renal failure have been reported in patients receiving other nephrotoxic drugs. Caution should be exercised when administering valacyclovir to patients receiving potentially nephrotoxic drugs).
No products indexed under this heading.

Aspirin (Cases of acute renal failure have been reported in patients receiving other nephrotoxic drugs. Caution should be exercised when administering valacyclovir to patients receiving potentially nephrotoxic drugs). Products include:

Atazanavir (Cases of acute renal failure have been reported in patients receiving other nephrotoxic drugs. Caution should be exercised when administering valacyclovir to patients receiving potentially nephrotoxic drugs).
No products indexed under this heading.

Atorvastatin Calcium (Cases of acute renal failure have been reported in patients receiving other nephrotoxic drugs. Caution should be exercised when administering valacyclovir to patients receiving potentially nephrotoxic drugs). Products include:

Azithromycin Dihydrate (Cases of acute renal failure have been reported in patients receiving other nephrotoxic drugs. Caution should be exercised when administering valacyclovir to patients receiving potentially nephrotoxic drugs).
No products indexed under this heading.

Azlocillin Sodium (Cases of acute renal failure have been reported in patients receiving other nephrotoxic drugs. Caution should be exercised when administering valacyclovir to patients receiving potentially nephrotoxic drugs).
No products indexed under this heading.

Aztreonam (Cases of acute renal failure have been reported in patients receiving other nephrotoxic drugs. Caution should be exercised when administering valacyclovir to patients receiving potentially nephrotoxic drugs).
No products indexed under this heading.

Bacampicillin Hydrochloride (Cases of acute renal failure have been reported in patients receiving other nephrotoxic drugs. Caution should be exercised when administering valacyclovir to patients receiving potentially nephrotoxic drugs).
No products indexed under this heading.

Bacitracin (Cases of acute renal failure have been reported in patients receiving other nephrotoxic drugs. Caution should be exercised when administering valacyclovir to patients receiving potentially nephrotoxic drugs).
No products indexed under this heading.

Bacitracin Zinc (Cases of acute renal failure have been reported in patients receiving other nephrotoxic drugs. Caution should be exercised when administering valacyclovir to patients receiving potentially nephrotoxic drugs).
No products indexed under this heading.

Balsalazide Disodium (Cases of acute renal failure have been reported in patients receiving other nephrotoxic drugs. Caution should be exercised when administering valacyclovir to patients receiving potentially nephrotoxic drugs).
No products indexed under this heading.

Benazepril Hydrochloride (Cases of acute renal failure have been reported in patients receiving other nephrotoxic drugs. Caution should be exercised when administering valacyclovir to patients receiving potentially nephrotoxic drugs).
No products indexed under this heading.

Bendroflumethiazide (Cases of acute renal failure have been reported in patients receiving other nephrotoxic drugs. Caution should be exercised when administering valacyclovir to patients receiving potentially nephrotoxic drugs).
No products indexed under this heading.

Caffeine (Cases of acute renal failure have been reported in patients receiving other nephrotoxic drugs. Caution should be exercised when administering valacyclovir to patients receiving potentially nephrotoxic drugs).
No products indexed under this heading.

Captopril (Cases of acute renal failure have been reported in patients receiving other nephrotoxic drugs. Caution should be exercised when administering valacyclovir to patients receiving potentially nephrotoxic drugs). Products include:

Carbenicillin Disodium (Cases of acute renal failure have been reported in patients receiving other nephrotoxic drugs. Caution should be exercised when administering valacyclovir to patients receiving potentially nephrotoxic drugs).
No products indexed under this heading.

Carbenicillin Indanyl Sodium (Cases of acute renal failure have been reported in patients receiving other nephrotoxic drugs. Caution should be exercised when administering valacyclovir to patients receiving potentially nephrotoxic drugs).
No products indexed under this heading.

Carboplatin (Cases of acute renal failure have been reported in patients receiving other nephrotoxic drugs. Caution should be exercised when administering valacyclovir to patients receiving potentially nephrotoxic drugs).
No products indexed under this heading.

Carmustine (BCNU) (Cases of acute renal failure have been reported in patients receiving other nephrotoxic drugs. Caution should be exercised when administering valacyclovir to patients receiving potentially nephrotoxic drugs).
No products indexed under this heading.

Cefaclor (Cases of acute renal failure have been reported in patients receiving other nephrotoxic drugs. Caution should be exercised when administering valacyclovir to patients receiving potentially nephrotoxic drugs).
No products indexed under this heading.

Cefadroxil (Cases of acute renal failure have been reported in patients receiving other nephrotoxic drugs. Caution should be exercised when administering valacyclovir to patients receiving potentially nephrotoxic drugs).
No products indexed under this heading.

Cefamandole Nafate (Cases of acute renal failure have been reported in patients receiving other nephrotoxic drugs. Caution should be exercised when administering valacyclovir to patients receiving potentially nephrotoxic drugs).
No products indexed under this heading.

Cefazolin Sodium (Cases of acute renal failure have been reported in patients receiving other nephrotoxic drugs. Caution should be exercised when administering valacyclovir to patients receiving potentially nephrotoxic drugs).
No products indexed under this heading.

Cefdinir (Cases of acute renal failure have been reported in patients receiving other nephrotoxic drugs. Caution should be exercised when administering valacyclovir to patients receiving potentially nephrotoxic drugs). Products include:

Cefepime Hydrochloride (Cases of acute renal failure have been reported in patients receiving other nephrotoxic drugs. Caution should be exercised when administering valacyclovir to patients receiving potentially nephrotoxic drugs).
No products indexed under this heading.

Cefixime (Cases of acute renal failure have been reported in patients receiving other nephrotoxic drugs. Caution should be exercised when administering valacyclovir to patients receiving potentially nephrotoxic drugs). Products include:

(⊙ Described in PDR® for Ophthalmic Medicines)

Cefmetazole Sodium (Cases of acute renal failure have been reported in patients receiving other nephrotoxic drugs. Caution should be exercised when administering valacyclovir to patients receiving potentially nephrotoxic drugs).
No products indexed under this heading.

Cefonicid Sodium (Cases of acute renal failure have been reported in patients receiving other nephrotoxic drugs. Caution should be exercised when administering valacyclovir to patients receiving potentially nephrotoxic drugs).
No products indexed under this heading.

Cefoperazone Sodium (Cases of acute renal failure have been reported in patients receiving other nephrotoxic drugs. Caution should be exercised when administering valacyclovir to patients receiving potentially nephrotoxic drugs).
No products indexed under this heading.

Ceforanide (Cases of acute renal failure have been reported in patients receiving other nephrotoxic drugs. Caution should be exercised when administering valacyclovir to patients receiving potentially nephrotoxic drugs).
No products indexed under this heading.

Cefotaxime Sodium (Cases of acute renal failure have been reported in patients receiving other nephrotoxic drugs. Caution should be exercised when administering valacyclovir to patients receiving potentially nephrotoxic drugs).
No products indexed under this heading.

Cefotetan (Cases of acute renal failure have been reported in patients receiving other nephrotoxic drugs. Caution should be exercised when administering valacyclovir to patients receiving potentially nephrotoxic drugs).
No products indexed under this heading.

Cefoxitin Sodium (Cases of acute renal failure have been reported in patients receiving other nephrotoxic drugs. Caution should be exercised when administering valacyclovir to patients receiving potentially nephrotoxic drugs).
No products indexed under this heading.

Cefpodoxime Proxetil (Cases of acute renal failure have been reported in patients receiving other nephrotoxic drugs. Caution should be exercised when administering valacyclovir to patients receiving potentially nephrotoxic drugs).
No products indexed under this heading.

Cefprozil (Cases of acute renal failure have been reported in patients receiving other nephrotoxic drugs. Caution should be exercised when administering valacyclovir to patients receiving potentially nephrotoxic drugs).
No products indexed under this heading.

Ceftazidime (Cases of acute renal failure have been reported in patients receiving other nephrotoxic drugs. Caution should be exercised when administering valacyclovir to patients receiving potentially nephrotoxic drugs). Products include:
Fortaz 1481

Ceftizoxime Sodium (Cases of acute renal failure have been reported in patients receiving other nephrotoxic drugs. Caution should be exercised when administering valacyclovir to patients receiving potentially nephrotoxic drugs).
No products indexed under this heading.

Ceftriaxone Sodium (Cases of acute renal failure have been reported in patients receiving other nephrotoxic drugs. Caution should be exercised

when administering valacyclovir to patients receiving potentially nephrotoxic drugs). Products include:
Rocephin............................ 2859

Cefuroxime Axetil (Cases of acute renal failure have been reported in patients receiving other nephrotoxic drugs. Caution should be exercised when administering valacyclovir to patients receiving potentially nephrotoxic drugs). Products include:
Ceftin 1399

Cefuroxime Sodium (Cases of acute renal failure have been reported in patients receiving other nephrotoxic drugs. Caution should be exercised when administering valacyclovir to patients receiving potentially nephrotoxic drugs).
No products indexed under this heading.

Celecoxib (Cases of acute renal failure have been reported in patients receiving other nephrotoxic drugs. Caution should be exercised when administering valacyclovir to patients receiving potentially nephrotoxic drugs). Products include:
Celebrex 3272

Cephalexin (Cases of acute renal failure have been reported in patients receiving other nephrotoxic drugs. Caution should be exercised when administering valacyclovir to patients receiving potentially nephrotoxic drugs).
No products indexed under this heading.

Cephalothin Sodium (Cases of acute renal failure have been reported in patients receiving other nephrotoxic drugs. Caution should be exercised when administering valacyclovir to patients receiving potentially nephrotoxic drugs).
No products indexed under this heading.

Cephapirin Sodium (Cases of acute renal failure have been reported in patients receiving other nephrotoxic drugs. Caution should be exercised when administering valacyclovir to patients receiving potentially nephrotoxic drugs).
No products indexed under this heading.

Cephradine (Cases of acute renal failure have been reported in patients receiving other nephrotoxic drugs. Caution should be exercised when administering valacyclovir to patients receiving potentially nephrotoxic drugs).
No products indexed under this heading.

Cerivastatin Sodium (Cases of acute renal failure have been reported in patients receiving other nephrotoxic drugs. Caution should be exercised when administering valacyclovir to patients receiving potentially nephrotoxic drugs).
No products indexed under this heading.

Chlorothiazide (Cases of acute renal failure have been reported in patients receiving other nephrotoxic drugs. Caution should be exercised when administering valacyclovir to patients receiving potentially nephrotoxic drugs).
No products indexed under this heading.

Chlorothiazide Sodium (Cases of acute renal failure have been reported in patients receiving other nephrotoxic drugs. Caution should be exercised when administering valacyclovir to patients receiving potentially nephrotoxic drugs). Products include:
Diuril Intravenous 2009

Chlorpropamide (Cases of acute renal failure have been reported in patients receiving other nephrotoxic drugs. Caution should be exercised when administering valacyclovir to patients receiving potentially nephrotoxic drugs).
No products indexed under this heading.

Cidofovir (Cases of acute renal failure have been reported in patients receiving other nephrotoxic drugs. Caution should be exercised when administering valacyclovir to patients receiving potentially nephrotoxic drugs).
No products indexed under this heading.

Cilastatin Sodium (Cases of acute renal failure have been reported in patients receiving other nephrotoxic drugs. Caution should be exercised when administering valacyclovir to patients receiving potentially nephrotoxic drugs). Products include:
Primaxin I.M. 2232
Primaxin I.V. 2235

Cimetidine (Acyclovir C_{max} and AUC following a single dose of valacyclovir (1 gram) increased by 8% and 32%, respectively, after a single dose of cimetidine (800 mg). When cimetidine plus probenecid were co-administered with a single dose of valacyclovir (1 gram) the C_{max} and AUC of acyclovir were increased by 30% and 78%, respectively, primarily due to a reduction in renal clearance of acyclovir. These effects are not considered to be of clinical significance in subjects with normal renal function).
No products indexed under this heading.

Cimetidine Hydrochloride (Acyclovir C_{max} and AUC following a single dose of valacyclovir (1 gram) increased by 8% and 32%, respectively, after a single dose of cimetidine (800 mg). When cimetidine plus probenecid were co-administered with a single dose of valacyclovir (1 gram) the C_{max} and AUC of acyclovir were increased by 30% and 78%, respectively, primarily due to a reduction in renal clearance of acyclovir. These effects are not considered to be of clinical significance in subjects with normal renal function).
No products indexed under this heading.

Cisplatin (Cases of acute renal failure have been reported in patients receiving other nephrotoxic drugs. Caution should be exercised when administering valacyclovir to patients receiving potentially nephrotoxic drugs).
No products indexed under this heading.

Cladribine (Cases of acute renal failure have been reported in patients receiving other nephrotoxic drugs. Caution should be exercised when administering valacyclovir to patients receiving potentially nephrotoxic drugs). Products include:
Leustatin 946

Clozapine (Cases of acute renal failure have been reported in patients receiving other nephrotoxic drugs. Caution should be exercised when administering valacyclovir to patients receiving potentially nephrotoxic drugs).
No products indexed under this heading.

Colistimethate Sodium (Cases of acute renal failure have been reported in patients receiving other nephrotoxic drugs. Caution should be exercised when administering valacyclovir to patients receiving potentially nephrotoxic drugs).
No products indexed under this heading.

Colistin Sulfate (Cases of acute renal failure have been reported in patients receiving other nephrotoxic drugs. Caution should be exercised when administering valacyclovir to patients receiving potentially nephrotoxic drugs).
No products indexed under this heading.

Cyclophosphamide (Cases of acute renal failure have been reported in patients receiving other nephrotoxic drugs. Caution should be exercised when administering valacyclovir to patients receiving potentially nephrotoxic drugs).
No products indexed under this heading.

Cyclosporine (Cases of acute renal failure have been reported in patients receiving other nephrotoxic drugs. Caution should be exercised when administering valacyclovir to patients receiving potentially nephrotoxic drugs). Products include:
Gengraf 440
Neoral Oral Solution 2496
Neoral Capsules 2496
Restasis 605

Cytarabine (Cases of acute renal failure have been reported in patients receiving other nephrotoxic drugs. Caution should be exercised when administering valacyclovir to patients receiving potentially nephrotoxic drugs).
No products indexed under this heading.

Cytarabine Liposome (Cases of acute renal failure have been reported in patients receiving other nephrotoxic drugs. Caution should be exercised when administering valacyclovir to patients receiving potentially nephrotoxic drugs).
No products indexed under this heading.

Delavirdine Mesylate (Cases of acute renal failure have been reported in patients receiving other nephrotoxic drugs. Caution should be exercised when administering valacyclovir to patients receiving potentially nephrotoxic drugs).
No products indexed under this heading.

Diatrizoate Meglumine (Cases of acute renal failure have been reported in patients receiving other nephrotoxic drugs. Caution should be exercised when administering valacyclovir to patients receiving potentially nephrotoxic drugs).
No products indexed under this heading.

Diatrizoate Sodium (Cases of acute renal failure have been reported in patients receiving other nephrotoxic drugs. Caution should be exercised when administering valacyclovir to patients receiving potentially nephrotoxic drugs).
No products indexed under this heading.

Diclofenac Potassium (Cases of acute renal failure have been reported in patients receiving other nephrotoxic drugs. Caution should be exercised when administering valacyclovir to patients receiving potentially nephrotoxic drugs).
No products indexed under this heading.

Diclofenac Sodium (Cases of acute renal failure have been reported in patients receiving other nephrotoxic drugs. Caution should be exercised when administering valacyclovir to patients receiving potentially nephrotoxic drugs).
No products indexed under this heading.

Dicloxacillin Sodium (Cases of acute renal failure have been reported in patients receiving other nephrotoxic drugs. Caution should be exercised when administering valacyclovir to patients receiving potentially nephrotoxic drugs).
No products indexed under this heading.

Didanosine (Cases of acute renal failure have been reported in patients receiving other nephrotoxic drugs. Caution should be exercised when administering valacyclovir to patients receiving potentially nephrotoxic drugs).
No products indexed under this heading.

Efavirenz (Cases of acute renal failure have been reported in patients receiving other nephrotoxic drugs. Caution should be exercised when administering valacyclovir to patients receiving potentially nephrotoxic drugs). Products include:
Atripla 906

Emtricitabine (Cases of acute renal failure have been reported in patients receiving other nephrotoxic drugs. Cau-

(⊙ Described in PDR® for Ophthalmic Medicines)

IMPORTANT NOTE: Always consult each drug listing in the patient's regimen for possible interactions.

Valtrex Interactions Index 2006

Piroxicam (Cases of acute renal failure have been reported in patients receiving other nephrotoxic drugs. Caution should be exercised when administering valacyclovir to patients receiving potentially nephrotoxic drugs).
No products indexed under this heading.

Plicamycin (Cases of acute renal failure have been reported in patients receiving other nephrotoxic drugs. Caution should be exercised when administering valacyclovir to patients receiving potentially nephrotoxic drugs).
No products indexed under this heading.

Polymyxin (Cases of acute renal failure have been reported in patients receiving other nephrotoxic drugs. Caution should be exercised when administering valacyclovir to patients receiving potentially nephrotoxic drugs).
No products indexed under this heading.

Polymyxin B Sulfate (Cases of acute renal failure have been reported in patients receiving other nephrotoxic drugs. Caution should be exercised when administering valacyclovir to patients receiving potentially nephrotoxic drugs).
No products indexed under this heading.

Polythiazide (Cases of acute renal failure have been reported in patients receiving other nephrotoxic drugs. Caution should be exercised when administering valacyclovir to patients receiving potentially nephrotoxic drugs).
No products indexed under this heading.

Pravastatin Sodium (Cases of acute renal failure have been reported in patients receiving other nephrotoxic drugs. Caution should be exercised when administering valacyclovir to patients receiving potentially nephrotoxic drugs).
No products indexed under this heading.

Probenecid (Acyclovir C_{max} and AUC following a single dose of valacyclovir (1 gram) increased by 8% and 32%, respectively, after a single dose of cimetidine (800 mg). Acyclovir C_{max} and AUC following a single dose of valacyclovir (1 gram) increased by 30% and 78%, respectively after a combination of cimetidine and probenecid, primarily due to a reduction in renal clearance of acyclovir. These effects are not considered to be of clinical significance in patients with normal renal function).
No products indexed under this heading.

Quinapril Hydrochloride (Cases of acute renal failure have been reported in patients receiving other nephrotoxic drugs. Caution should be exercised when administering valacyclovir to patients receiving potentially nephrotoxic drugs).
No products indexed under this heading.

Rabeprazole Sodium (Cases of acute renal failure have been reported in patients receiving other nephrotoxic drugs. Caution should be exercised when administering valacyclovir to patients receiving potentially nephrotoxic drugs). Products include:
Aciphex **1035**

Ramipril (Cases of acute renal failure have been reported in patients receiving other nephrotoxic drugs. Caution should be exercised when administering valacyclovir to patients receiving potentially nephrotoxic drugs).
No products indexed under this heading.

Rifampin (Cases of acute renal failure have been reported in patients receiving other nephrotoxic drugs. Caution should be exercised when administering valacyclovir to patients receiving potentially nephrotoxic drugs).
No products indexed under this heading.

Riluzole (Cases of acute renal failure have been reported in patients receiving other nephrotoxic drugs. Caution should be exercised when administering valacyclovir to patients receiving potentially nephrotoxic drugs). Products include:
Rilutek **3032**

Ritonavir (Cases of acute renal failure have been reported in patients receiving other nephrotoxic drugs. Caution should be exercised when administering valacyclovir to patients receiving potentially nephrotoxic drugs). Products include:
Kaletra **458**
Norvir **509**

Rofecoxib (Cases of acute renal failure have been reported in patients receiving other nephrotoxic drugs. Caution should be exercised when administering valacyclovir to patients receiving potentially nephrotoxic drugs).
No products indexed under this heading.

Saquinavir (Cases of acute renal failure have been reported in patients receiving other nephrotoxic drugs. Caution should be exercised when administering valacyclovir to patients receiving potentially nephrotoxic drugs).
No products indexed under this heading.

Sibutramine Hydrochloride Monohydrate (Cases of acute renal failure have been reported in patients receiving other nephrotoxic drugs. Caution should be exercised when administering valacyclovir to patients receiving potentially nephrotoxic drugs). Products include:
Meridia **492**

Simvastatin (Cases of acute renal failure have been reported in patients receiving other nephrotoxic drugs. Caution should be exercised when administering valacyclovir to patients receiving potentially nephrotoxic drugs). Products include:
Simcor **524**
Vytorin 10/10 .... **2303, 3240**
Vytorin 10/20 .... **2303, 3240**
Vytorin 10/40 .... **2303, 3240**
Vytorin 10/80 .... **2303, 3240**
Zocor **2289**

Spirapril Hydrochloride (Cases of acute renal failure have been reported in patients receiving other nephrotoxic drugs. Caution should be exercised when administering valacyclovir to patients receiving potentially nephrotoxic drugs).
No products indexed under this heading.

Stavudine (Cases of acute renal failure have been reported in patients receiving other nephrotoxic drugs. Caution should be exercised when administering valacyclovir to patients receiving potentially nephrotoxic drugs).
No products indexed under this heading.

Streptomycin Sulfate (Cases of acute renal failure have been reported in patients receiving other nephrotoxic drugs. Caution should be exercised when administering valacyclovir to patients receiving potentially nephrotoxic drugs).
No products indexed under this heading.

Streptozocin (Cases of acute renal failure have been reported in patients receiving other nephrotoxic drugs. Caution should be exercised when administering valacyclovir to patients receiving potentially nephrotoxic drugs).
No products indexed under this heading.

Sulfacytine (Cases of acute renal failure have been reported in patients receiving other nephrotoxic drugs. Caution should be exercised when administering valacyclovir to patients receiving potentially nephrotoxic drugs).
No products indexed under this heading.

Sulfamethizole (Cases of acute renal failure have been reported in patients receiving other nephrotoxic drugs. Caution should be exercised when administering valacyclovir to patients receiving potentially nephrotoxic drugs).
No products indexed under this heading.

Sulfamethoxazole (Cases of acute renal failure have been reported in patients receiving other nephrotoxic drugs. Caution should be exercised when administering valacyclovir to patients receiving potentially nephrotoxic drugs).
No products indexed under this heading.

Sulfasalazine (Cases of acute renal failure have been reported in patients receiving other nephrotoxic drugs. Caution should be exercised when administering valacyclovir to patients receiving potentially nephrotoxic drugs).
No products indexed under this heading.

Sulfinpyrazone (Cases of acute renal failure have been reported in patients receiving other nephrotoxic drugs. Caution should be exercised when administering valacyclovir to patients receiving potentially nephrotoxic drugs).
No products indexed under this heading.

Sulfisoxazole Acetyl (Cases of acute renal failure have been reported in patients receiving other nephrotoxic drugs. Caution should be exercised when administering valacyclovir to patients receiving potentially nephrotoxic drugs).
No products indexed under this heading.

Sulfisoxazole Diolamine (Cases of acute renal failure have been reported in patients receiving other nephrotoxic drugs. Caution should be exercised when administering valacyclovir to patients receiving potentially nephrotoxic drugs).
No products indexed under this heading.

Sulindac (Cases of acute renal failure have been reported in patients receiving other nephrotoxic drugs. Caution should be exercised when administering valacyclovir to patients receiving potentially nephrotoxic drugs). Products include:
Clinoril **2098**

Tacrolimus (Cases of acute renal failure have been reported in patients receiving other nephrotoxic drugs. Caution should be exercised when administering valacyclovir to patients receiving potentially nephrotoxic drugs). Products include:
Prograf Capsules **677**
Prograf Injection **677**
Protopic **685**

Tenofovir Disoproxil Fumarate (Cases of acute renal failure have been reported in patients receiving other nephrotoxic drugs. Caution should be exercised when administering valacyclovir to patients receiving potentially nephrotoxic drugs). Products include:
Atripla **906**
Truvada **1258**
Viread **1266**

Thioguanine (Cases of acute renal failure have been reported in patients receiving other nephrotoxic drugs. Caution should be exercised when administering valacyclovir to patients receiving potentially nephrotoxic drugs). Products include:
Tabloid **1664**

Ticarcillin Disodium (Cases of acute renal failure have been reported in patients receiving other nephrotoxic drugs. Caution should be exercised when administering valacyclovir to patients receiving potentially nephrotoxic drugs). Products include:
Timentin ADD-Vantage **1670**
Timentin Galaxy **1674**
Timentin **1666**
Timentin Pharmacy **1678**

Tobramycin (Cases of acute renal failure have been reported in patients receiving other nephrotoxic drugs. Caution should be exercised when administering valacyclovir to patients receiving potentially nephrotoxic drugs). Products include:
Tobi Nebulizer **2546**
Tobramycin and Dexamethasone Ophthalmic Suspension .... ⊙**251**
Zylet .... ⊙**252**

Tobramycin Sulfate (Cases of acute renal failure have been reported in patients receiving other nephrotoxic drugs. Caution should be exercised when administering valacyclovir to patients receiving potentially nephrotoxic drugs).
No products indexed under this heading.

Tolazamide (Cases of acute renal failure have been reported in patients receiving other nephrotoxic drugs. Caution should be exercised when administering valacyclovir to patients receiving potentially nephrotoxic drugs).
No products indexed under this heading.

Tolbutamide (Cases of acute renal failure have been reported in patients receiving other nephrotoxic drugs. Caution should be exercised when administering valacyclovir to patients receiving potentially nephrotoxic drugs).
No products indexed under this heading.

Tolmetin Sodium (Cases of acute renal failure have been reported in patients receiving other nephrotoxic drugs. Caution should be exercised when administering valacyclovir to patients receiving potentially nephrotoxic drugs).
No products indexed under this heading.

Trandolapril (Cases of acute renal failure have been reported in patients receiving other nephrotoxic drugs. Caution should be exercised when administering valacyclovir to patients receiving potentially nephrotoxic drugs). Products include:
Mavik **489**
Tarka **534**

Triamterene (Cases of acute renal failure have been reported in patients receiving other nephrotoxic drugs. Caution should be exercised when administering valacyclovir to patients receiving potentially nephrotoxic drugs). Products include:
Dyazide **1429**
Dyrenium **3495**

Trimethadione (Cases of acute renal failure have been reported in patients receiving other nephrotoxic drugs. Caution should be exercised when administering valacyclovir to patients receiving potentially nephrotoxic drugs).
No products indexed under this heading.

Trovafloxacin Mesylate (Cases of acute renal failure have been reported in patients receiving other nephrotoxic drugs. Caution should be exercised when administering valacyclovir to patients receiving potentially nephrotoxic drugs).
No products indexed under this heading.

Tyropanoate Sodium (Cases of acute renal failure have been reported in patients receiving other nephrotoxic drugs. Caution should be exercised when administering valacyclovir to patients receiving potentially nephrotoxic drugs).
No products indexed under this heading.

Valdecoxib (Cases of acute renal failure have been reported in patients receiving other nephrotoxic drugs. Caution should be exercised when administering valacyclovir to patients receiving potentially nephrotoxic drugs).
No products indexed under this heading.

Vancomycin Hydrochloride (Cases of acute renal failure have been reported in patients receiving other nephrotoxic drugs. Caution should be exercised when administering valacyclovir to patients receiving potentially nephrotoxic drugs).
No products indexed under this heading.

(⊙ Described in PDR® for Ophthalmic Medicines)

Voriconazole (Cases of acute renal failure have been reported in patients receiving other nephrotoxic drugs. Caution should be exercised when administering valacyclovir to patients receiving potentially nephrotoxic drugs).

No products indexed under this heading.

Zalcitabine (Cases of acute renal failure have been reported in patients receiving other nephrotoxic drugs. Caution should be exercised when administering valacyclovir to patients receiving potentially nephrotoxic drugs).

No products indexed under this heading.

Zidovudine (Cases of acute renal failure have been reported in patients receiving other nephrotoxic drugs. Caution should be exercised when administering valacyclovir to patients receiving potentially nephrotoxic drugs). Products include:

Zoledronic Acid (Cases of acute renal failure have been reported in patients receiving other nephrotoxic drugs. Caution should be exercised when administering valacyclovir to patients receiving potentially nephrotoxic drugs). Products include:

VALTURNA TABLETS

May interact with diuretics, potassium preparations, potassium sparing diuretics, and certain other agents. Compounds in these categories include:

Amiloride Hydrochloride (Caution is advised when concomitant use of Valturna with potassium sparing diuretics (eg, spironolactone, triamterene, amiloride) may lead to increases in serum potassium and in heart failure patients to increases in serum creatinine).

No products indexed under this heading.

Atorvastatin Calcium (Co-administration of atorvastatin with aliskiren has resulted in about a 50% increase in aliskiren C_{max} and AUC after multiple dosing). Products include:

Bendroflumethiazide (In patients with an activated renin-angiotensin system, such as volume- and/or salt-depleted patients receiving high doses of diuretics, symptomatic hypotension may occur).

No products indexed under this heading.

Bumetanide (In patients with an activated renin-angiotensin system, such as volume- and/or salt-depleted patients receiving high doses of diuretics, symptomatic hypotension may occur).

No products indexed under this heading.

Chlorothiazide (In patients with an activated renin-angiotensin system, such as volume- and/or salt-depleted patients receiving high doses of diuretics, symptomatic hypotension may occur).

No products indexed under this heading.

Chlorothiazide Sodium (In patients with an activated renin-angiotensin system, such as volume- and/or salt-depleted patients receiving high doses of diuretics, symptomatic hypotension may occur). Products include:

Chlorthalidone (In patients with an activated renin-angiotensin system, such as volume- and/or salt-depleted patients receiving high doses of diuretics, symptomatic hypotension may occur). Products include:

Cyclosporine (Co-administration of 200 mg and 600 mg cyclosporine, a highly potent Pgp inhibitor, with 75 mg aliskiren resulted in an approximately 2.5-fold increase in C_{max} and 5-fold increase in AUC of aliskiren. Concomitant use of aliskiren with cyclosporine is not recommended. The results from an *in vitro* study with human liver tissue indicate that valsartan is a substrate of the hepatic uptake transporter OATP1B1 and the hepatic efflux transporter MRP2. Co-administration of inhibitors of the uptake transporter (eg, rifampin, cyclosporine) or efflux transporter (eg, ritonavir) may increase the systemic exposure to valsartan). Products include:

Ethacrynic Acid (In patients with an activated renin-angiotensin system, such as volume- and/or salt-depleted patients receiving high doses of diuretics, symptomatic hypotension may occur).

No products indexed under this heading.

Furosemide (When aliskiren was co-administered with furosemide, the AUC and C_{max} of furosemide were reduced by about 30% and 50%, respectively. Patients receiving furosemide could find its effect diminished after starting aliskiren). Products include:

Hydrochlorothiazide (In patients with an activated renin-angiotensin system, such as volume- and/or salt-depleted patients receiving high doses of diuretics, symptomatic hypotension may occur). Products include:

Hydroflumethiazide (In patients with an activated renin-angiotensin system, such as volume- and/or salt-depleted patients receiving high doses of diuretics, symptomatic hypotension may occur).

No products indexed under this heading.

Indapamide (In patients with an activated renin-angiotensin system, such as volume- and/or salt-depleted patients receiving high doses of diuretics, symptomatic hypotension may occur). Products include:

Irbesartan (Co-administration of irbesartan with aliskiren has reduced aliskiren C_{max} up to 50% after multiple dosing). Products include:

Ketoconazole (Co-administration of 200 mg twice-daily ketoconazole, a potent Pgp inhibitor, with aliskiren resulted in approximate 80% increase in plasma levels of aliskiren. A 400 mg once-daily dose was not studied but would be expected to increase aliskiren blood levels further). Products include:

Methyclothiazide (In patients with an activated renin-angiotensin system, such as volume- and/or salt-depleted patients receiving high doses of diuretics, symptomatic hypotension may occur).

No products indexed under this heading.

Metolazone (In patients with an activated renin-angiotensin system, such as volume- and/or salt-depleted patients receiving high doses of diuretics, symptomatic hypotension may occur).

No products indexed under this heading.

Polythiazide (In patients with an activated renin-angiotensin system, such as volume- and/or salt-depleted patients receiving high doses of diuretics, symptomatic hypotension may occur).

No products indexed under this heading.

Potassium Acid Phosphate (Caution is advised when concomitant use of Valturna with potassium supplements may lead to increases in serum potassium and in heart failure patients to increases in serum creatinine). Products include:

Potassium Bicarbonate (Caution is advised when concomitant use of Valturna with potassium supplements may lead to increases in serum potassium and in heart failure patients to increases in serum creatinine).

No products indexed under this heading.

Potassium Chloride (Caution is advised when concomitant use of Valturna with potassium supplements may lead to increases in serum potassium and in heart failure patients to increases in serum creatinine). Products include:

Potassium Citrate (Caution is advised when concomitant use of Valturna with potassium supplements may lead to increases in serum potassium and in heart failure patients to increases in serum creatinine). Products include:

Potassium Gluconate (Caution is advised when concomitant use of Valturna with potassium supplements may lead to increases in serum potassium and in heart failure patients to increases in serum creatinine).

No products indexed under this heading.

Potassium Phosphate (Caution is advised when concomitant use of Valturna with potassium supplements may lead to increases in serum potassium and in heart failure patients to increases in serum creatinine). Products include:

Rifampin (The results from an *in vitro* study with human liver tissue indicate that valsartan is a substrate of the hepatic uptake transporter OATP1B1 and the hepatic efflux transporter MRP2. Co-administration of inhibitors of the uptake transporter (eg, rifampin, cyclosporine) or efflux transporter (eg, ritonavir) may increase the systemic exposure to valsartan).

No products indexed under this heading.

Ritonavir (The results from an *in vitro* study with human liver tissue indicate that valsartan is a substrate of the hepatic uptake transporter OATP1B1 and the hepatic efflux transporter MRP2. Co-administration of inhibitors of the uptake transporter (eg, rifampin, cyclosporine) or efflux transporter (eg, ritonavir) may increase the systemic exposure to valsartan). Products include:

Spironolactone (Caution is advised when concomitant use of Valturna with potassium sparing diuretics (eg, spironolactone, triamterene, amiloride) may lead to increases in serum potassium and in heart failure patients to increases in serum creatinine).

No products indexed under this heading.

Torsemide (In patients with an activated renin-angiotensin system, such as volume- and/or salt-depleted patients receiving high doses of diuretics, symptomatic hypotension may occur).

No products indexed under this heading.

Triamterene (Caution is advised when concomitant use of Valturna with potassium sparing diuretics (eg, spironolactone, triamterene, amiloride) may lead to increases in serum potassium and in heart failure patients to increases in serum creatinine). Products include:

Food Interactions

Food, unspecified (When taken with food, mean AUC and C_{max} of aliskiren are decreased by 76% and 88%, respectively; mean AUC and C_{max} of valsartan were not significantly affected. In clinical trials of Valturna, it was administered without requiring a fixed relation of administration to meals. High-fat meals decrease absorption of Valturna substantially).

Meal, unspecified (When taken with food, mean AUC and C_{max} of aliskiren are decreased by 76% and 88%, respectively; mean AUC and C_{max} of valsartan were not significantly affected. In clinical trials of Valturna, it was administered without requiring a fixed relation of administration to meals. High-fat meals decrease absorption of Valturna substantially).

Salt Substitutes, Potassium-Containing (Caution is advised when concomitant use of Valturna with salt substitute containing potassium may lead to increases in serum potassium and in heart failure patients to increases in serum creatinine).

VANOS CREAM

None cited in PDR database.

VANTAS IMPLANT

None cited in PDR database.

VAPRISOL

May interact with cytochrome p450 3a4 inhibitors (selected), cytochrome p450 3a4 inhibitors, potent (selected), cytochrome p450 3a4 substrates (selected), HMG-CoA reductase inhibitors, and certain other agents. Compounds in these categories include:

Acetazolamide (The co-administration of conivaptan with potent CYP3A4 inhibitors, such as ketoconazole, itraconazole, clarithromycin, ritonavir and indinavir, is contraindicated. Conivaptan is a substrate of CYP3A4. Co-administration of conivaptan with CYP3A4 inhibitors could lead to an increase in conivaptan concentrations).

No products indexed under this heading.

Acetazolamide Sodium (The co-administration of conivaptan with potent CYP3A4 inhibitors, such as ketoconazole, itraconazole, clarithromycin, ritonavir and indinavir, is contraindicated. Conivaptan is a substrate of CYP3A4. Co-administration of conivaptan with CYP3A4 inhibitors could lead to an increase in conivaptan concentrations).

No products indexed under this heading.

Alfentanil Hydrochloride (Conivaptan is a potent inhibitor of CYP3A4. Conivaptan may increase plasma concentrations of co-administered drugs that are primarily metabolized by

CYP3A4. In clinical trials of oral conivaptan hydrochloride, two cases of rhabdomyolysis occurred in patients who were also receiving a CYP3A4-metabolized HMG-CoA reductase inhibitor. Concomitant use of conivaptan hydrochloride with drugs that are primarily metabolized by CYP3A4 should be closely monitored or the combination should be avoided. If a clinical decision is made to discontinue concomitant medications at recommended doses, an appropriate amount of time (at least 24 hours) following the end of conivaptan hydrochloride administration should be allowed before resuming these medications).
No products indexed under this heading.

Alprazolam (Conivaptan is a potent inhibitor of CYP3A4. Conivaptan may increase plasma concentrations of co-administered drugs that are primarily metabolized by CYP3A4. In clinical trials of oral conivaptan hydrochloride, two cases of rhabdomyolysis occurred in patients who were also receiving a CYP3A4-metabolized HMG-CoA reductase inhibitor. Concomitant use of conivaptan hydrochloride with drugs that are primarily metabolized by CYP3A4 should be closely monitored or the combination should be avoided. If a clinical decision is made to discontinue concomitant medications at recommended doses, an appropriate amount of time (at least 24 hours) following the end of conivaptan hydrochloride administration should be allowed before resuming these medications).
No products indexed under this heading.

Amiodarone Hydrochloride (The co-administration of conivaptan with potent CYP3A4 inhibitors, such as ketoconazole, itraconazole, clarithromycin, ritonavir and indinavir, is contraindicated. Conivaptan is a substrate of CYP3A4. Co-administration of conivaptan with CYP3A4 inhibitors could lead to an increase in conivaptan concentrations).
No products indexed under this heading.

Amitriptyline Hydrochloride (Conivaptan is a potent inhibitor of CYP3A4. Conivaptan may increase plasma concentrations of co-administered drugs that are primarily metabolized by CYP3A4. In clinical trials of oral conivaptan hydrochloride, two cases of rhabdomyolysis occurred in patients who were also receiving a CYP3A4-metabolized HMG-CoA reductase inhibitor. Concomitant use of conivaptan hydrochloride with drugs that are primarily metabolized by CYP3A4 should be closely monitored or the combination should be avoided. If a clinical decision is made to discontinue concomitant medications at recommended doses, an appropriate amount of time (at least 24 hours) following the end of conivaptan hydrochloride administration should be allowed before resuming these medications).
No products indexed under this heading.

Amlodipine Besylate (Oral conivaptan hydrochloride 40 mg twice daily resulted in a 2-fold increase in the AUC and half-life of amlodipine). Products include:
Azor 1010
Exforge 2443
Exforge HCT 2449

Amprenavir (The co-administration of conivaptan with potent CYP3A4 inhibitors, such as ketoconazole, itraconazole, clarithromycin, ritonavir and indinavir, is contraindicated. Conivaptan is a substrate of CYP3A4. Co-administration of conivaptan with CYP3A4 inhibitors could lead to an increase in conivaptan concentrations).
No products indexed under this heading.

Anastrozole (The co-administration of conivaptan with potent CYP3A4 inhibitors, such as ketoconazole, itraconazole, clarithromycin, ritonavir and indinavir, is contraindicated. Conivaptan is a substrate of CYP3A4. Co-administration of conivaptan with CYP3A4 inhibitors could lead to an increase in conivaptan concentrations).
No products indexed under this heading.

Aprepitant (The co-administration of conivaptan with potent CYP3A4 inhibitors, such as ketoconazole, itraconazole, clarithromycin, ritonavir and indinavir, is contraindicated. Conivaptan is a substrate of CYP3A4. Co-administration of conivaptan with CYP3A4 inhibitors could lead to an increase in conivaptan concentrations). Products include:
Emend 2124

Astemizole (Conivaptan is a potent inhibitor of CYP3A4. Conivaptan may increase plasma concentrations of co-administered drugs that are primarily metabolized by CYP3A4. In clinical trials of oral conivaptan hydrochloride, two cases of rhabdomyolysis occurred in patients who were also receiving a CYP3A4-metabolized HMG-CoA reductase inhibitor. Concomitant use of conivaptan hydrochloride with drugs that are primarily metabolized by CYP3A4 should be closely monitored or the combination should be avoided. If a clinical decision is made to discontinue concomitant medications at recommended doses, an appropriate amount of time (at least 24 hours) following the end of conivaptan hydrochloride administration should be allowed before resuming these medications).
No products indexed under this heading.

Atazanavir (The co-administration of conivaptan with potent CYP3A4 inhibitors, such as ketoconazole, itraconazole, clarithromycin, ritonavir and indinavir, is contraindicated. Conivaptan is a substrate of CYP3A4. Co-administration of conivaptan with CYP3A4 inhibitors could lead to an increase in conivaptan concentrations).
No products indexed under this heading.

Atazanavir Sulfate (The co-administration of conivaptan with potent CYP3A4 inhibitors, such as ketoconazole, itraconazole, clarithromycin, ritonavir and indinavir, is contraindicated. Conivaptan is a substrate of CYP3A4. Co-administration of conivaptan with CYP3A4 inhibitors could lead to an increase in conivaptan concentrations).
No products indexed under this heading.

Atorvastatin Calcium (Conivaptan is a potent inhibitor of CYP3A4. Conivaptan may increase plasma concentrations of co-administered drugs that are primarily metabolized by CYP3A4. In clinical trials of oral conivaptan hydrochloride, two cases of rhabdomyolysis occurred in patients who were also receiving a CYP3A4-metabolized HMG-CoA reductase inhibitor. Concomitant use of conivaptan hydrochloride with drugs that are primarily metabolized by CYP3A4 should be closely monitored or the combination should be avoided. If a clinical decision is made to discontinue concomitant medications at recommended doses, an appropriate amount of time (at least 24 hours) following the end of conivaptan hydrochloride administration should be allowed before resuming these medications). Products include:
Lipitor 2703

Belladonna Ergotamine (Conivaptan is a potent inhibitor of CYP3A4. Conivaptan may increase plasma concentrations of co-administered drugs that are primarily metabolized by CYP3A4. In clinical trials of oral conivaptan hydrochloride, two cases of rhabdomyolysis occurred in patients who were also receiving a CYP3A4-metabolized HMG-CoA reductase inhibitor. Concomitant use of conivaptan hydrochloride with drugs that are primarily metabolized by CYP3A4 should be closely monitored or the combination should be avoided. If a clinical decision is made to discontinue concomitant medications at recommended doses, an appropriate amount of time (at least 24 hours) following the end of conivaptan hydrochloride administration should be allowed before resuming these medications).
No products indexed under this heading.

Buspirone Hydrochloride (Conivaptan is a potent inhibitor of CYP3A4. Conivaptan may increase plasma concentrations of co-administered drugs that are primarily metabolized by CYP3A4. In clinical trials of oral conivaptan hydrochloride, two cases of rhabdomyolysis occurred in patients who were also receiving a CYP3A4-metabolized HMG-CoA reductase inhibitor. Concomitant use of conivaptan hydrochloride with drugs that are primarily metabolized by CYP3A4 should be closely monitored or the combination should be avoided. If a clinical decision is made to discontinue concomitant medications at recommended doses, an appropriate amount of time (at least 24 hours) following the end of conivaptan hydrochloride administration should be allowed before resuming these medications).
No products indexed under this heading.

Busulfan (Conivaptan is a potent inhibitor of CYP3A4. Conivaptan may increase plasma concentrations of co-administered drugs that are primarily metabolized by CYP3A4. In clinical trials of oral conivaptan hydrochloride, two cases of rhabdomyolysis occurred in patients who were also receiving a CYP3A4-metabolized HMG-CoA reductase inhibitor. Concomitant use of conivaptan hydrochloride with drugs that are primarily metabolized by CYP3A4 should be closely monitored or the combination should be avoided. If a clinical decision is made to discontinue concomitant medications at recommended doses, an appropriate amount of time (at least 24 hours) following the end of conivaptan hydrochloride administration should be allowed before resuming these medications). Products include:
Myleran 1581

Carbamazepine (Conivaptan is a potent inhibitor of CYP3A4. Conivaptan may increase plasma concentrations of co-administered drugs that are primarily metabolized by CYP3A4. In clinical trials of oral conivaptan hydrochloride, two cases of rhabdomyolysis occurred in patients who were also receiving a CYP3A4-metabolized HMG-CoA reductase inhibitor. Concomitant use of conivaptan hydrochloride with drugs that are primarily metabolized by CYP3A4 should be closely monitored or the combination should be avoided. If a clinical decision is made to discontinue concomitant medications at recommended doses, an appropriate amount of time (at least 24 hours) following the end of conivaptan hydrochloride administration should be allowed before resuming these medications). Products include:
Carbatrol 3280
Equetro 3477

Cerivastatin Sodium (Conivaptan is a potent inhibitor of CYP3A4. Conivaptan may increase plasma concentrations of co-administered drugs that are primarily metabolized by CYP3A4. In clinical trials of oral conivaptan hydrochloride, two cases of rhabdomyolysis occurred in patients who were also receiving a CYP3A4-metabolized HMG-CoA reductase inhibitor. Concomitant use of conivaptan hydrochloride with drugs that are primarily metabolized by CYP3A4 should be closely monitored or the combination should be avoided. If a clinical decision is made to discontinue concomitant medications at recommended doses, an appropriate amount of time (at least 24 hours) following the end of conivaptan hydrochloride administration should be allowed before resuming these medications).
No products indexed under this heading.

Chlorpheniramine (Conivaptan is a potent inhibitor of CYP3A4. Conivaptan may increase plasma concentrations of co-administered drugs that are primarily metabolized by CYP3A4. In clinical trials of oral conivaptan hydrochloride, two cases of rhabdomyolysis occurred in patients who were also receiving a CYP3A4-metabolized HMG-CoA reductase inhibitor. Concomitant use of conivaptan hydrochloride with drugs that are primarily metabolized by CYP3A4 should be closely monitored or the combination should be avoided. If a clinical decision is made to discontinue concomitant medications at recommended doses, an appropriate amount of time (at least 24 hours) following the end of conivaptan hydrochloride administration should be allowed before resuming these medications).
No products indexed under this heading.

Chlorpheniramine Maleate (Conivaptan is a potent inhibitor of CYP3A4. Conivaptan may increase plasma concentrations of co-administered drugs that are primarily metabolized by CYP3A4. In clinical trials of oral conivaptan hydrochloride, two cases of rhabdomyolysis occurred in patients who were also receiving a CYP3A4-metabolized HMG-CoA reductase inhibitor. Concomitant use of conivaptan hydrochloride with drugs that are primarily metabolized by CYP3A4 should be closely monitored or the combination should be avoided. If a clinical decision is made to discontinue concomitant medications at recommended doses, an appropriate amount of time (at least 24 hours) following the end of conivaptan hydrochloride administration should be allowed before resuming these medications).
No products indexed under this heading.

Chlorpheniramine Polistirex (Conivaptan is a potent inhibitor of CYP3A4. Conivaptan may increase plasma concentrations of co-administered drugs that are primarily metabolized by CYP3A4. In clinical trials of oral conivaptan hydrochloride, two cases of rhabdomyolysis occurred in patients who were also receiving a CYP3A4-metabolized HMG-CoA reductase inhibitor. Concomitant use of conivaptan hydrochloride with drugs that are primarily metabolized by CYP3A4 should be closely monitored or the combination should be avoided. If a clinical decision is made to discontinue concomitant medications at recommended doses, an appropriate amount of time (at least 24 hours) following the end of conivaptan hydrochloride administration should be allowed before resuming these medications). Products include:
Tussionex 3443

Chlorpheniramine Tannate (Conivaptan is a potent inhibitor of CYP3A4. Conivaptan may increase plasma concentrations of co-administered drugs that are primarily metabolized by CYP3A4. In clinical trials of oral conivaptan hydrochloride, two cases of rhabdomyolysis occurred in patients who were also receiving a CYP3A4-metabolized HMG-CoA reductase inhibitor. Concomitant use of conivaptan hydrochloride with drugs that are primarily metabo-

lized by CYP3A4 should be closely monitored or the combination should be avoided. If a clinical decision is made to discontinue concomitant medications at recommended doses, an appropriate amount of time (at least 24 hours) following the end of conivaptan hydrochloride administration should be allowed before resuming these medications).
No products indexed under this heading.

Cimetidine (The co-administration of conivaptan with potent CYP3A4 inhibitors, such as ketoconazole, itraconazole, clarithromycin, ritonavir and indinavir, is contraindicated. Conivaptan is a substrate of CYP3A4. Co-administration of conivaptan with CYP3A4 inhibitors could lead to an increase in conivaptan concentrations).
No products indexed under this heading.

Cimetidine Hydrochloride (The co-administration of conivaptan with potent CYP3A4 inhibitors, such as ketoconazole, itraconazole, clarithromycin, ritonavir and indinavir, is contraindicated. Conivaptan is a substrate of CYP3A4. Co-administration of conivaptan with CYP3A4 inhibitors could lead to an increase in conivaptan concentrations).
No products indexed under this heading.

Ciprofloxacin (The co-administration of conivaptan with potent CYP3A4 inhibitors, such as ketoconazole, itraconazole, clarithromycin, ritonavir and indinavir, is contraindicated. Conivaptan is a substrate of CYP3A4. Co-administration of conivaptan with CYP3A4 inhibitors could lead to an increase in conivaptan concentrations). Products include:
Cipro I.V. **3082**
Cipro **3073**
Cipro XR **3091**
Ciprodex **583**

Cisapride (Conivaptan is a potent inhibitor of CYP3A4. Conivaptan may increase plasma concentrations of co-administered drugs that are primarily metabolized by CYP3A4. In clinical trials of oral conivaptan hydrochloride, two cases of rhabdomyolysis occurred in patients who were also receiving a CYP3A4-metabolized HMG-CoA reductase inhibitor. Concomitant use of conivaptan hydrochloride with drugs that are primarily metabolized by CYP3A4 should be closely monitored or the combination should be avoided. If a clinical decision is made to discontinue concomitant medications at recommended doses, an appropriate amount of time (at least 24 hours) following the end of conivaptan hydrochloride administration should be allowed before resuming these medications).
No products indexed under this heading.

Clarithromycin (The co-administration of conivaptan with potent CYP3A4 inhibitors, such as clarithromycin, is contraindicated. Conivaptan is a substrate of CYP3A4. Co-administration of conivaptan with CYP3A4 inhibitors could lead to an increase in conivaptan concentrations). Products include:
Biaxin/Biaxin XL **412**

Clotrimazole (The co-administration of conivaptan with potent CYP3A4 inhibitors, such as ketoconazole, itraconazole, clarithromycin, ritonavir and indinavir, is contraindicated. Conivaptan is a substrate of CYP3A4. Co-administration of conivaptan with CYP3A4 inhibitors could lead to an increase in conivaptan concentrations). Products include:
Lotrisone **3163**

Cyclosporine (The co-administration of conivaptan with potent CYP3A4 inhibitors, such as ketoconazole, itraconazole, clarithromycin, ritonavir and indinavir, is contraindicated. Conivaptan is a substrate of CYP3A4. Co-administration of conivaptan with CYP3A4 inhibitors could lead to an increase in conivaptan concentrations). Products include:
Gengraf **440**
Neoral Oral Solution **2496**
Neoral Capsules **2496**
Restasis **605**

Dalfopristin (The co-administration of conivaptan with potent CYP3A4 inhibitors, such as ketoconazole, itraconazole, clarithromycin, ritonavir and indinavir, is contraindicated. Conivaptan is a substrate of CYP3A4. Co-administration of conivaptan with CYP3A4 inhibitors could lead to an increase in conivaptan concentrations).
No products indexed under this heading.

Danazol (The co-administration of conivaptan with potent CYP3A4 inhibitors, such as ketoconazole, itraconazole, clarithromycin, ritonavir and indinavir, is contraindicated. Conivaptan is a substrate of CYP3A4. Co-administration of conivaptan with CYP3A4 inhibitors could lead to an increase in conivaptan concentrations).
No products indexed under this heading.

Darunavir (The co-administration of conivaptan with potent CYP3A4 inhibitors, such as ketoconazole, itraconazole, clarithromycin, ritonavir and indinavir, is contraindicated. Conivaptan is a substrate of CYP3A4. Co-administration of conivaptan with CYP3A4 inhibitors could lead to an increase in conivaptan concentrations).
No products indexed under this heading.

Dasatinib (The co-administration of conivaptan with potent CYP3A4 inhibitors, such as ketoconazole, itraconazole, clarithromycin, ritonavir and indinavir, is contraindicated. Conivaptan is a substrate of CYP3A4. Co-administration of conivaptan with CYP3A4 inhibitors could lead to an increase in conivaptan concentrations).
No products indexed under this heading.

Delavirdine Mesylate (The co-administration of conivaptan with potent CYP3A4 inhibitors, such as ketoconazole, itraconazole, clarithromycin, ritonavir and indinavir, is contraindicated. Conivaptan is a substrate of CYP3A4. Co-administration of conivaptan with CYP3A4 inhibitors could lead to an increase in conivaptan concentrations).
No products indexed under this heading.

Delavirine (The co-administration of conivaptan with potent CYP3A4 inhibitors, such as ketoconazole, itraconazole, clarithromycin, ritonavir and indinavir, is contraindicated. Conivaptan is a substrate of CYP3A4. Co-administration of conivaptan with CYP3A4 inhibitors could lead to an increase in conivaptan concentrations).
No products indexed under this heading.

Desloratadine (The co-administration of conivaptan with potent CYP3A4 inhibitors, such as ketoconazole, itraconazole, clarithromycin, ritonavir and indinavir, is contraindicated. Conivaptan is a substrate of CYP3A4. Co-administration of conivaptan with CYP3A4 inhibitors could lead to an increase in conivaptan concentrations). Products include:
Clarinex Syrup **3098**
Clarinex **3098**
Clarinex Reditabs **3098**
Clarinex-D 12-Hour **3101**
Clarinex-D **3104**

Desogestrel (Conivaptan is a potent inhibitor of CYP3A4. Conivaptan may increase plasma concentrations of co-administered drugs that are primarily metabolized by CYP3A4. In clinical trials of oral conivaptan hydrochloride, two cases of rhabdomyolysis occurred in patients who were also receiving a CYP3A4-metabolized HMG-CoA reductase inhibitor. Concomitant use of conivaptan hydrochloride with drugs that are primarily metabolized by CYP3A4 should be closely monitored or the combination should be avoided. If a clinical decision is made to discontinue concomitant medications at recommended doses, an appropriate amount of time (at least 24 hours) following the end of conivaptan hydrochloride administration should be allowed before resuming these medications).
No products indexed under this heading.

Diazepam (Conivaptan is a potent inhibitor of CYP3A4. Conivaptan may increase plasma concentrations of co-administered drugs that are primarily metabolized by CYP3A4. In clinical trials of oral conivaptan hydrochloride, two cases of rhabdomyolysis occurred in patients who were also receiving a CYP3A4-metabolized HMG-CoA reductase inhibitor. Concomitant use of conivaptan hydrochloride with drugs that are primarily metabolized by CYP3A4 should be closely monitored or the combination should be avoided. If a clinical decision is made to discontinue concomitant medications at recommended doses, an appropriate amount of time (at least 24 hours) following the end of conivaptan hydrochloride administration should be allowed before resuming these medications). Products include:
Valium Tablets **2880**

Digoxin (Co-administration of a 0.5-mg dose of digoxin, a P-glycoprotein substrate, with oral conivaptan hydrochloride 40 mg twice daily resulted in a 30% reduction in clearance and 79% and 43% increases in digoxin C_{max} and AUC values, respectively. Therefore, if digoxin is administered with conivaptan hydrochloride, the clinician should be alert to the possibility of increases in digoxin levels). Products include:
Lanoxin Injection **1546**
Lanoxin Injection Pediatric **1549**
Lanoxin Tablets **1553**

Dihydroergotamine Mesylate (Conivaptan is a potent inhibitor of CYP3A4. Conivaptan may increase plasma concentrations of co-administered drugs that are primarily metabolized by CYP3A4. In clinical trials of oral conivaptan hydrochloride, two cases of rhabdomyolysis occurred in patients who were also receiving a CYP3A4-metabolized HMG-CoA reductase inhibitor. Concomitant use of conivaptan hydrochloride with drugs that are primarily metabolized by CYP3A4 should be closely monitored or the combination should be avoided. If a clinical decision is made to discontinue concomitant medications at recommended doses, an appropriate amount of time (at least 24 hours) following the end of conivaptan hydrochloride administration should be allowed before resuming these medications).
No products indexed under this heading.

Diltiazem Hydrochloride (The co-administration of conivaptan with potent CYP3A4 inhibitors, such as ketoconazole, itraconazole, clarithromycin, ritonavir and indinavir, is contraindicated. Conivaptan is a substrate of CYP3A4. Co-administration of conivaptan with CYP3A4 inhibitors could lead to an increase in conivaptan concentrations). Products include:
Cardizem LA **423**

Diltiazem Maleate (The co-administration of conivaptan with potent CYP3A4 inhibitors, such as ketoconazole, itraconazole, clarithromycin, ritonavir and indinavir, is contraindicated. Conivaptan is a substrate of CYP3A4. Co-administration of conivaptan with CYP3A4 inhibitors could lead to an increase in conivaptan concentrations).
No products indexed under this heading.

Disopyramide (Conivaptan is a potent inhibitor of CYP3A4. Conivaptan may increase plasma concentrations of co-administered drugs that are primarily metabolized by CYP3A4. In clinical trials of oral conivaptan hydrochloride, two cases of rhabdomyolysis occurred in patients who were also receiving a CYP3A4-metabolized HMG-CoA reductase inhibitor. Concomitant use of conivaptan hydrochloride with drugs that are primarily metabolized by CYP3A4 should be closely monitored or the combination should be avoided. If a clinical decision is made to discontinue concomitant medications at recommended doses, an appropriate amount of time (at least 24 hours) following the end of conivaptan hydrochloride administration should be allowed before resuming these medications).
No products indexed under this heading.

Disopyramide Phosphate (Conivaptan is a potent inhibitor of CYP3A4. Conivaptan may increase plasma concentrations of co-administered drugs that are primarily metabolized by CYP3A4. In clinical trials of oral conivaptan hydrochloride, two cases of rhabdomyolysis occurred in patients who were also receiving a CYP3A4-metabolized HMG-CoA reductase inhibitor. Concomitant use of conivaptan hydrochloride with drugs that are primarily metabolized by CYP3A4 should be closely monitored or the combination should be avoided. If a clinical decision is made to discontinue concomitant medications at recommended doses, an appropriate amount of time (at least 24 hours) following the end of conivaptan hydrochloride administration should be allowed before resuming these medications).
No products indexed under this heading.

Disulfiram (Conivaptan is a potent inhibitor of CYP3A4. Conivaptan may increase plasma concentrations of co-administered drugs that are primarily metabolized by CYP3A4. In clinical trials of oral conivaptan hydrochloride, two cases of rhabdomyolysis occurred in patients who were also receiving a CYP3A4-metabolized HMG-CoA reductase inhibitor. Concomitant use of conivaptan hydrochloride with drugs that are primarily metabolized by CYP3A4 should be closely monitored or the combination should be avoided. If a clinical decision is made to discontinue concomitant medications at recommended doses, an appropriate amount of time (at least 24 hours) following the end of conivaptan hydrochloride administration should be allowed before resuming these medications).
No products indexed under this heading.

Doxorubicin Hydrochloride (Conivaptan is a potent inhibitor of CYP3A4. Conivaptan may increase plasma concentrations of co-administered drugs that are primarily metabolized by CYP3A4. In clinical trials of oral conivaptan hydrochloride, two cases of rhabdomyolysis occurred in patients who were also receiving a CYP3A4-metabolized HMG-CoA reductase inhibitor. Concomitant use of conivaptan hydrochloride with drugs that are primarily metabolized by CYP3A4 should be closely monitored or the combination should be avoided. If a clinical decision is made to discontinue concomitant medications at

IMPORTANT NOTE: Always consult each drug listing in the patient's regimen for possible interactions.

recommended doses, an appropriate amount of time (at least 24 hours) following the end of conivaptan hydrochloride administration should be allowed before resuming these medications).

No products indexed under this heading.

Dronabinol (Conivaptan is a potent inhibitor of CYP3A4. Conivaptan may increase plasma concentrations of co-administered drugs that are primarily metabolized by CYP3A4. In clinical trials of oral conivaptan hydrochloride, two cases of rhabdomyolysis occurred in patients who were also receiving a CYP3A4-metabolized HMG-CoA reductase inhibitor. Concomitant use of conivaptan hydrochloride with drugs that are primarily metabolized by CYP3A4 should be closely monitored or the combination should be avoided. If a clinical decision is made to discontinue concomitant medications at recommended doses, an appropriate amount of time (at least 24 hours) following the end of conivaptan hydrochloride administration should be allowed before resuming these medications).

No products indexed under this heading.

Efavirenz (The co-administration of conivaptan with potent CYP3A4 inhibitors, such as ketoconazole, itraconazole, clarithromycin, ritonavir and indinavir, is contraindicated. Conivaptan is a substrate of CYP3A4. Co-administration of conivaptan with CYP3A4 inhibitors could lead to an increase in conivaptan concentrations). Products include:

Atripla 906

Ergotamine Tartrate (Conivaptan is a potent inhibitor of CYP3A4. Conivaptan may increase plasma concentrations of co-administered drugs that are primarily metabolized by CYP3A4. In clinical trials of oral conivaptan hydrochloride, two cases of rhabdomyolysis occurred in patients who were also receiving a CYP3A4-metabolized HMG-CoA reductase inhibitor. Concomitant use of conivaptan hydrochloride with drugs that are primarily metabolized by CYP3A4 should be closely monitored or the combination should be avoided. If a clinical decision is made to discontinue concomitant medications at recommended doses, an appropriate amount of time (at least 24 hours) following the end of conivaptan hydrochloride administration should be allowed before resuming these medications).

No products indexed under this heading.

Erythromycin (The co-administration of conivaptan with potent CYP3A4 inhibitors, such as ketoconazole, itraconazole, clarithromycin, ritonavir and indinavir, is contraindicated. Conivaptan is a substrate of CYP3A4. Co-administration of conivaptan with CYP3A4 inhibitors could lead to an increase in conivaptan concentrations).

No products indexed under this heading.

Erythromycin Estolate (The co-administration of conivaptan with potent CYP3A4 inhibitors, such as ketoconazole, itraconazole, clarithromycin, ritonavir and indinavir, is contraindicated. Conivaptan is a substrate of CYP3A4. Co-administration of conivaptan with CYP3A4 inhibitors could lead to an increase in conivaptan concentrations).

No products indexed under this heading.

Erythromycin Ethylsuccinate (The co-administration of conivaptan with potent CYP3A4 inhibitors, such as ketoconazole, itraconazole, clarithromycin, ritonavir and indinavir, is contraindicated. Conivaptan is a substrate of CYP3A4. Co-administration of conivaptan with CYP3A4 inhibitors could lead to an increase in conivaptan concentrations). Products include:

E.E.S. 437
EryPed 435

Erythromycin Gluceptate (The co-administration of conivaptan with potent CYP3A4 inhibitors, such as ketoconazole, itraconazole, clarithromycin, ritonavir and indinavir, is contraindicated. Conivaptan is a substrate of CYP3A4. Co-administration of conivaptan with CYP3A4 inhibitors could lead to an increase in conivaptan concentrations).

No products indexed under this heading.

Erythromycin Lactobionate (The co-administration of conivaptan with potent CYP3A4 inhibitors, such as ketoconazole, itraconazole, clarithromycin, ritonavir and indinavir, is contraindicated. Conivaptan is a substrate of CYP3A4. Co-administration of conivaptan with CYP3A4 inhibitors could lead to an increase in conivaptan concentrations).

No products indexed under this heading.

Erythromycin Stearate (The co-administration of conivaptan with potent CYP3A4 inhibitors, such as ketoconazole, itraconazole, clarithromycin, ritonavir and indinavir, is contraindicated. Conivaptan is a substrate of CYP3A4. Co-administration of conivaptan with CYP3A4 inhibitors could lead to an increase in conivaptan concentrations).

No products indexed under this heading.

Esomeprazole Magnesium (The co-administration of conivaptan with potent CYP3A4 inhibitors, such as ketoconazole, itraconazole, clarithromycin, ritonavir and indinavir, is contraindicated. Conivaptan is a substrate of CYP3A4. Co-administration of conivaptan with CYP3A4 inhibitors could lead to an increase in conivaptan concentrations). Products include:

Nexium Capsules 704
Nexium Oral Suspension 704

Esomeprazole Sodium (The co-administration of conivaptan with potent CYP3A4 inhibitors, such as ketoconazole, itraconazole, clarithromycin, ritonavir and indinavir, is contraindicated. Conivaptan is a substrate of CYP3A4. Co-administration of conivaptan with CYP3A4 inhibitors could lead to an increase in conivaptan concentrations). Products include:

Nexium I.V. 712

Estradiol (Conivaptan is a potent inhibitor of CYP3A4. Conivaptan may increase plasma concentrations of co-administered drugs that are primarily metabolized by CYP3A4. In clinical trials of oral conivaptan hydrochloride, two cases of rhabdomyolysis occurred in patients who were also receiving a CYP3A4-metabolized HMG-CoA reductase inhibitor. Concomitant use of conivaptan hydrochloride with drugs that are primarily metabolized by CYP3A4 should be closely monitored or the combination should be avoided. If a clinical decision is made to discontinue concomitant medications at recommended doses, an appropriate amount of time (at least 24 hours) following the end of conivaptan hydrochloride administration should be allowed before resuming these medications). Products include:

Activella 2561
Angeliq 831
Climara 841
Climara Pro 847
Divigel 3467
Estrasorb 1777
Vagifem 2589

Estradiol Benzoate (Conivaptan is a potent inhibitor of CYP3A4. Conivaptan may increase plasma concentrations of co-administered drugs that are primarily metabolized by CYP3A4. In clinical trials of oral conivaptan hydrochloride, two cases of rhabdomyolysis occurred in patients who were also receiving a CYP3A4-metabolized HMG-CoA reductase inhibitor. Concomitant use of conivaptan hydrochloride with drugs that are primarily metabolized by CYP3A4 should be closely monitored or the combination should be avoided. If a clinical decision is made to discontinue concomitant medications at recommended doses, an appropriate amount of time (at least 24 hours) following the end of conivaptan hydrochloride administration should be allowed before resuming these medications).

No products indexed under this heading.

Estradiol Cypionate (Conivaptan is a potent inhibitor of CYP3A4. Conivaptan may increase plasma concentrations of co-administered drugs that are primarily metabolized by CYP3A4. In clinical trials of oral conivaptan hydrochloride, two cases of rhabdomyolysis occurred in patients who were also receiving a CYP3A4-metabolized HMG-CoA reductase inhibitor. Concomitant use of conivaptan hydrochloride with drugs that are primarily metabolized by CYP3A4 should be closely monitored or the combination should be avoided. If a clinical decision is made to discontinue concomitant medications at recommended doses, an appropriate amount of time (at least 24 hours) following the end of conivaptan hydrochloride administration should be allowed before resuming these medications).

No products indexed under this heading.

Estradiol Valerate (Conivaptan is a potent inhibitor of CYP3A4. Conivaptan may increase plasma concentrations of co-administered drugs that are primarily metabolized by CYP3A4. In clinical trials of oral conivaptan hydrochloride, two cases of rhabdomyolysis occurred in patients who were also receiving a CYP3A4-metabolized HMG-CoA reductase inhibitor. Concomitant use of conivaptan hydrochloride with drugs that are primarily metabolized by CYP3A4 should be closely monitored or the combination should be avoided. If a clinical decision is made to discontinue concomitant medications at recommended doses, an appropriate amount of time (at least 24 hours) following the end of conivaptan hydrochloride administration should be allowed before resuming these medications).

No products indexed under this heading.

Ethinyl Estradiol (Conivaptan is a potent inhibitor of CYP3A4. Conivaptan may increase plasma concentrations of co-administered drugs that are primarily metabolized by CYP3A4. In clinical trials of oral conivaptan hydrochloride, two cases of rhabdomyolysis occurred in patients who were also receiving a CYP3A4-metabolized HMG-CoA reductase inhibitor. Concomitant use of conivaptan hydrochloride with drugs that are primarily metabolized by CYP3A4 should be closely monitored or the combination should be avoided. If a clinical decision is made to discontinue concomitant medications at recommended doses, an appropriate amount of time (at least 24 hours) following the end of conivaptan hydrochloride administration should be allowed before resuming these medications). Products include:

LoSeasonique 3407
Lybrel 3514
NuvaRing 3181
Ortho Evra 2648
Ortho-Cyclen/Ortho Tri-Cyclen 2663
Ortho Tri-Cyclen Lo Tablets 2673
Seasonique 3418
Yaz 864

Ethosuximide (Conivaptan is a potent inhibitor of CYP3A4. Conivaptan may increase plasma concentrations of co-administered drugs that are primarily metabolized by CYP3A4. In clinical trials of oral conivaptan hydrochloride, two cases of rhabdomyolysis occurred in patients who were also receiving a CYP3A4-metabolized HMG-CoA reductase inhibitor. Concomitant use of conivaptan hydrochloride with drugs that are primarily metabolized by CYP3A4 should be closely monitored or the combination should be avoided. If a clinical decision is made to discontinue concomitant medications at recommended doses, an appropriate amount of time (at least 24 hours) following the end of conivaptan hydrochloride administration should be allowed before resuming these medications).

No products indexed under this heading.

Ethynodiol Diacetate (Conivaptan is a potent inhibitor of CYP3A4. Conivaptan may increase plasma concentrations of co-administered drugs that are primarily metabolized by CYP3A4. In clinical trials of oral conivaptan hydrochloride, two cases of rhabdomyolysis occurred in patients who were also receiving a CYP3A4-metabolized HMG-CoA reductase inhibitor. Concomitant use of conivaptan hydrochloride with drugs that are primarily metabolized by CYP3A4 should be closely monitored or the combination should be avoided. If a clinical decision is made to discontinue concomitant medications at recommended doses, an appropriate amount of time (at least 24 hours) following the end of conivaptan hydrochloride administration should be allowed before resuming these medications).

No products indexed under this heading.

Etoposide (Conivaptan is a potent inhibitor of CYP3A4. Conivaptan may increase plasma concentrations of co-administered drugs that are primarily metabolized by CYP3A4. In clinical trials of oral conivaptan hydrochloride, two cases of rhabdomyolysis occurred in patients who were also receiving a CYP3A4-metabolized HMG-CoA reductase inhibitor. Concomitant use of conivaptan hydrochloride with drugs that are primarily metabolized by CYP3A4 should be closely monitored or the combination should be avoided. If a clinical decision is made to discontinue concomitant medications at recommended doses, an appropriate amount of time (at least 24 hours) following the end of conivaptan hydrochloride administration should be allowed before resuming these medications).

No products indexed under this heading.

Etoposide Phosphate (Conivaptan is a potent inhibitor of CYP3A4. Conivaptan may increase plasma concentrations of co-administered drugs that are primarily metabolized by CYP3A4. In clinical trials of oral conivaptan hydrochloride, two cases of rhabdomyolysis occurred in patients who were also receiving a CYP3A4-metabolized HMG-CoA reductase inhibitor. Concomitant use of conivaptan hydrochloride with drugs that are primarily metabolized by CYP3A4 should be closely monitored or the combination should be avoided. If a clinical decision is made to discontinue concomitant medications at recommended doses, an appropriate amount of time (at least 24 hours) following the end of conivaptan hydrochloride administration should be allowed before resuming these medications).

No products indexed under this heading.

Felodipine (Conivaptan is a potent inhibitor of CYP3A4. Conivaptan may increase plasma concentrations of co-administered drugs that are primarily metabolized by CYP3A4. In clinical trials of oral conivaptan hydrochloride, two cases of rhabdomyolysis occurred in

patients who were also receiving a CYP3A4-metabolized HMG-CoA reductase inhibitor. Concomitant use of conivaptan hydrochloride with drugs that are primarily metabolized by CYP3A4 should be closely monitored or the combination should be avoided. If a clinical decision is made to discontinue concomitant medications at recommended doses, an appropriate amount of time (at least 24 hours) following the end of conivaptan hydrochloride administration should be allowed before resuming these medications).

No products indexed under this heading.

Fentanyl (Conivaptan is a potent inhibitor of CYP3A4. Conivaptan may increase plasma concentrations of co-administered drugs that are primarily metabolized by CYP3A4. In clinical trials of oral conivaptan hydrochloride, two cases of rhabdomyolysis occurred in patients who were also receiving a CYP3A4-metabolized HMG-CoA reductase inhibitor. Concomitant use of conivaptan hydrochloride with drugs that are primarily metabolized by CYP3A4 should be closely monitored or the combination should be avoided. If a clinical decision is made to discontinue concomitant medications at recommended doses, an appropriate amount of time (at least 24 hours) following the end of conivaptan hydrochloride administration should be allowed before resuming these medications). Products include:

Duragesic **2604**
Fentanyl Transdermal System **2346**
Onsolis **2054**

Fentanyl Citrate (Conivaptan is a potent inhibitor of CYP3A4. Conivaptan may increase plasma concentrations of co-administered drugs that are primarily metabolized by CYP3A4. In clinical trials of oral conivaptan hydrochloride, two cases of rhabdomyolysis occurred in patients who were also receiving a CYP3A4-metabolized HMG-CoA reductase inhibitor. Concomitant use of conivaptan hydrochloride with drugs that are primarily metabolized by CYP3A4 should be closely monitored or the combination should be avoided. If a clinical decision is made to discontinue concomitant medications at recommended doses, an appropriate amount of time (at least 24 hours) following the end of conivaptan hydrochloride administration should be allowed before resuming these medications). Products include:

Fentora **966**

Fluconazole (The co-administration of conivaptan with potent CYP3A4 inhibitors, such as ketoconazole, itraconazole, clarithromycin, ritonavir and indinavir, is contraindicated. Conivaptan is a substrate of CYP3A4. Co-administration of conivaptan with CYP3A4 inhibitors could lead to an increase in conivaptan concentrations).

No products indexed under this heading.

Fluoxetine (The co-administration of conivaptan with potent CYP3A4 inhibitors, such as ketoconazole, itraconazole, clarithromycin, ritonavir and indinavir, is contraindicated. Conivaptan is a substrate of CYP3A4. Co-administration of conivaptan with CYP3A4 inhibitors could lead to an increase in conivaptan concentrations).

No products indexed under this heading.

Fluoxetine Hydrochloride (The co-administration of conivaptan with potent CYP3A4 inhibitors, such as ketoconazole, itraconazole, clarithromycin, ritonavir and indinavir, is contraindicated. Conivaptan is a substrate of CYP3A4. Co-administration of conivaptan with CYP3A4 inhibitors could lead to an increase in conivaptan concentrations). Products include:

Prozac Weekly **1941**
Prozac Pulvules **1941**
Symbyax **1965**

Fluvastatin Sodium (Conivaptan is a potent inhibitor of CYP3A4. Conivaptan may increase plasma concentrations of co-administered drugs that are primarily metabolized by CYP3A4. In clinical trials of oral conivaptan hydrochloride, two cases of rhabdomyolysis occurred in patients who were also receiving a CYP3A4-metabolized HMG-CoA reductase inhibitor. Concomitant use of conivaptan hydrochloride with drugs that are primarily metabolized by CYP3A4 should be closely monitored or the combination should be avoided. If a clinical decision is made to discontinue concomitant medications at recommended doses, an appropriate amount of time (at least 24 hours) following the end of conivaptan hydrochloride administration should be allowed before resuming these medications).

No products indexed under this heading.

Fluvoxamine Maleate (The co-administration of conivaptan with potent CYP3A4 inhibitors, such as ketoconazole, itraconazole, clarithromycin, ritonavir and indinavir, is contraindicated. Conivaptan is a substrate of CYP3A4. Co-administration of conivaptan with CYP3A4 inhibitors could lead to an increase in conivaptan concentrations).

No products indexed under this heading.

Fosamprenavir Calcium (The co-administration of conivaptan with potent CYP3A4 inhibitors, such as ketoconazole, itraconazole, clarithromycin, ritonavir and indinavir, is contraindicated. Conivaptan is a substrate of CYP3A4. Co-administration of conivaptan with CYP3A4 inhibitors could lead to an increase in conivaptan concentrations). Products include:

Lexiva Oral Suspension **1558**
Lexiva **1558**

Haloperidol (Conivaptan is a potent inhibitor of CYP3A4. Conivaptan may increase plasma concentrations of co-administered drugs that are primarily metabolized by CYP3A4. In clinical trials of oral conivaptan hydrochloride, two cases of rhabdomyolysis occurred in patients who were also receiving a CYP3A4-metabolized HMG-CoA reductase inhibitor. Concomitant use of conivaptan hydrochloride with drugs that are primarily metabolized by CYP3A4 should be closely monitored or the combination should be avoided. If a clinical decision is made to discontinue concomitant medications at recommended doses, an appropriate amount of time (at least 24 hours) following the end of conivaptan hydrochloride administration should be allowed before resuming these medications).

No products indexed under this heading.

Haloperidol Decanoate (Conivaptan is a potent inhibitor of CYP3A4. Conivaptan may increase plasma concentrations of co-administered drugs that are primarily metabolized by CYP3A4. In clinical trials of oral conivaptan hydrochloride, two cases of rhabdomyolysis occurred in patients who were also receiving a CYP3A4-metabolized HMG-CoA reductase inhibitor. Concomitant use of conivaptan hydrochloride with drugs that are primarily metabolized by CYP3A4 should be closely monitored or the combination should be avoided. If a clinical decision is made to discontinue concomitant medications at recommended doses, an appropriate amount of time (at least 24 hours) following the end of conivaptan hydrochloride administration should be allowed before resuming these medications).

No products indexed under this heading.

Haloperidol Lactate (Conivaptan is a potent inhibitor of CYP3A4. Conivaptan may increase plasma concentrations of co-administered drugs that are primarily metabolized by CYP3A4. In clinical trials of oral conivaptan hydrochloride, two cases of rhabdomyolysis occurred in patients who were also receiving a CYP3A4-metabolized HMG-CoA reductase inhibitor. Concomitant use of conivaptan hydrochloride with drugs that are primarily metabolized by CYP3A4 should be closely monitored or the combination should be avoided. If a clinical decision is made to discontinue concomitant medications at recommended doses, an appropriate amount of time (at least 24 hours) following the end of conivaptan hydrochloride administration should be allowed before resuming these medications).

No products indexed under this heading.

Imatinib Mesylate (The co-administration of conivaptan with potent CYP3A4 inhibitors, such as ketoconazole, itraconazole, clarithromycin, ritonavir and indinavir, is contraindicated. Conivaptan is a substrate of CYP3A4. Co-administration of conivaptan with CYP3A4 inhibitors could lead to an increase in conivaptan concentrations). Products include:

Gleevec **2477**

Indinavir Sulfate (The co-administration of conivaptan with potent CYP3A4 inhibitors, such as indinavir, is contraindicated. Conivaptan is a substrate of CYP3A4. Co-administration of conivaptan with CYP3A4 inhibitors could lead to an increase in conivaptan concentrations). Products include:

Crixivan **2113**

Isoniazid (The co-administration of conivaptan with potent CYP3A4 inhibitors, such as ketoconazole, itraconazole, clarithromycin, ritonavir and indinavir, is contraindicated. Conivaptan is a substrate of CYP3A4. Co-administration of conivaptan with CYP3A4 inhibitors could lead to an increase in conivaptan concentrations).

No products indexed under this heading.

Isradipine (Conivaptan is a potent inhibitor of CYP3A4. Conivaptan may increase plasma concentrations of co-administered drugs that are primarily metabolized by CYP3A4. In clinical trials of oral conivaptan hydrochloride, two cases of rhabdomyolysis occurred in patients who were also receiving a CYP3A4-metabolized HMG-CoA reductase inhibitor. Concomitant use of conivaptan hydrochloride with drugs that are primarily metabolized by CYP3A4 should be closely monitored or the combination should be avoided. If a clinical decision is made to discontinue concomitant medications at recommended doses, an appropriate amount of time (at least 24 hours) following the end of conivaptan hydrochloride administration should be allowed before resuming these medications). Products include:

DynaCirc CR **1432**

Itraconazole (The co-administration of conivaptan with potent CYP3A4 inhibitors, such as itraconazole, is contraindicated. Conivaptan is a substrate of CYP3A4. Co-administration of conivaptan with CYP3A4 inhibitors could lead to an increase in conivaptan concentrations).

No products indexed under this heading.

Ixabepilone (Conivaptan is a potent inhibitor of CYP3A4. Conivaptan may increase plasma concentrations of co-administered drugs that are primarily metabolized by CYP3A4. In clinical trials of oral conivaptan hydrochloride, two cases of rhabdomyolysis occurred in patients who were also receiving a CYP3A4-metabolized HMG-CoA reductase inhibitor. Concomitant use of conivaptan hydrochloride with drugs that are primarily metabolized by CYP3A4 should be closely monitored or the combination should be avoided. If a clinical decision is made to discontinue concomitant medications at recommended doses, an appropriate amount of time (at least 24 hours) following the end of conivaptan hydrochloride administration should be allowed before resuming these medications).

No products indexed under this heading.

Ketoconazole (The co-administration of conivaptan with potent CYP3A4 inhibitors, such as ketoconazole, is contraindicated. Co-administration of oral conivaptan hydrochloride 10 mg with ketoconazole 200 mg resulted in 4- and 11-fold increases in C_{max} and AUC of conivaptan, respectively). Products include:

Extina **3319**
Xolegel **3337**

Lapatinib (The co-administration of conivaptan with potent CYP3A4 inhibitors, such as ketoconazole, itraconazole, clarithromycin, ritonavir and indinavir, is contraindicated. Conivaptan is a substrate of CYP3A4. Co-administration of conivaptan with CYP3A4 inhibitors could lead to an increase in conivaptan concentrations). Products include:

Tykerb **1698**

Levonorgestrel (Conivaptan is a potent inhibitor of CYP3A4. Conivaptan may increase plasma concentrations of co-administered drugs that are primarily metabolized by CYP3A4. In clinical trials of oral conivaptan hydrochloride, two cases of rhabdomyolysis occurred in patients who were also receiving a CYP3A4-metabolized HMG-CoA reductase inhibitor. Concomitant use of conivaptan hydrochloride with drugs that are primarily metabolized by CYP3A4 should be closely monitored or the combination should be avoided. If a clinical decision is made to discontinue concomitant medications at recommended doses, an appropriate amount of time (at least 24 hours) following the end of conivaptan hydrochloride administration should be allowed before resuming these medications). Products include:

Climara Pro **847**
LoSeasonique **3407**
Lybrel **3514**
Mirena **854**
Plan B **3416**
Seasonique **3418**

Lidocaine (Conivaptan is a potent inhibitor of CYP3A4. Conivaptan may increase plasma concentrations of co-administered drugs that are primarily metabolized by CYP3A4. In clinical trials of oral conivaptan hydrochloride, two cases of rhabdomyolysis occurred in patients who were also receiving a CYP3A4-metabolized HMG-CoA reductase inhibitor. Concomitant use of conivaptan hydrochloride with drugs that are primarily metabolized by CYP3A4 should be closely monitored or the combination should be avoided. If a clinical decision is made to discontinue concomitant medications at recommended doses, an appropriate amount of time (at least 24 hours) following the end of conivaptan hydrochloride administration should be allowed before resuming these medications). Products include:

Lidoderm **1107**

Lidocaine Hydrochloride (Conivaptan is a potent inhibitor of CYP3A4. Conivaptan may increase plasma concentrations of co-administered drugs that are primarily metabolized by CYP3A4. In clinical trials of oral conivaptan hydrochloride, two cases of rhabdo-

myolysis occurred in patients who were also receiving a CYP3A4-metabolized HMG-CoA reductase inhibitor. Concomitant use of conivaptan hydrochloride with drugs that are primarily metabolized by CYP3A4 should be closely monitored or the combination should be avoided. If a clinical decision is made to discontinue concomitant medications at recommended doses, an appropriate amount of time (at least 24 hours) following the end of conivaptan hydrochloride administration should be allowed before resuming these medications).
No products indexed under this heading.

Lopinavir (The co-administration of conivaptan with potent CYP3A4 inhibitors, such as ketoconazole, itraconazole, clarithromycin, ritonavir and indinavir, is contraindicated. Conivaptan is a substrate of CYP3A4. Co-administration of conivaptan with CYP3A4 inhibitors could lead to an increase in conivaptan concentrations). Products include:
Kaletra 458

Loratadine (The co-administration of conivaptan with potent CYP3A4 inhibitors, such as ketoconazole, itraconazole, clarithromycin, ritonavir and indinavir, is contraindicated. Conivaptan is a substrate of CYP3A4. Co-administration of conivaptan with CYP3A4 inhibitors could lead to an increase in conivaptan concentrations).
No products indexed under this heading.

Lovastatin (Conivaptan is a potent inhibitor of CYP3A4. Conivaptan may increase plasma concentrations of co-administered drugs that are primarily metabolized by CYP3A4. In clinical trials of oral conivaptan hydrochloride, two cases of rhabdomyolysis occurred in patients who were also receiving a CYP3A4-metabolized HMG-CoA reductase inhibitor. Concomitant use of conivaptan hydrochloride with drugs that are primarily metabolized by CYP3A4 should be closely monitored or the combination should be avoided. If a clinical decision is made to discontinue concomitant medications at recommended doses, an appropriate amount of time (at least 24 hours) following the end of conivaptan hydrochloride administration should be allowed before resuming these medications). Products include:
Advicor 402
Mevacor 2212

Mestranol (Conivaptan is a potent inhibitor of CYP3A4. Conivaptan may increase plasma concentrations of co-administered drugs that are primarily metabolized by CYP3A4. In clinical trials of oral conivaptan hydrochloride, two cases of rhabdomyolysis occurred in patients who were also receiving a CYP3A4-metabolized HMG-CoA reductase inhibitor. Concomitant use of conivaptan hydrochloride with drugs that are primarily metabolized by CYP3A4 should be closely monitored or the combination should be avoided. If a clinical decision is made to discontinue concomitant medications at recommended doses, an appropriate amount of time (at least 24 hours) following the end of conivaptan hydrochloride administration should be allowed before resuming these medications).
No products indexed under this heading.

Methadone Hydrochloride (Conivaptan is a potent inhibitor of CYP3A4. Conivaptan may increase plasma concentrations of co-administered drugs that are primarily metabolized by CYP3A4. In clinical trials of oral conivaptan hydrochloride, two cases of rhabdomyolysis occurred in patients who were also receiving a CYP3A4-metabolized HMG-CoA reductase inhibitor. Concomitant use of conivaptan hydrochloride with drugs that are primarily metabolized by CYP3A4 should be closely monitored or the combination should be avoided. If a clinical decision is made to discontinue concomitant medications at recommended doses, an appropriate amount of time (at least 24 hours) following the end of conivaptan hydrochloride administration should be allowed before resuming these medications).
No products indexed under this heading.

Metronidazole (The co-administration of conivaptan with potent CYP3A4 inhibitors, such as ketoconazole, itraconazole, clarithromycin, ritonavir and indinavir, is contraindicated. Conivaptan is a substrate of CYP3A4. Co-administration of conivaptan with CYP3A4 inhibitors could lead to an increase in conivaptan concentrations). Products include:
Pylera 793

Metronidazole Benzoate (The co-administration of conivaptan with potent CYP3A4 inhibitors, such as ketoconazole, itraconazole, clarithromycin, ritonavir and indinavir, is contraindicated. Conivaptan is a substrate of CYP3A4. Co-administration of conivaptan with CYP3A4 inhibitors could lead to an increase in conivaptan concentrations).
No products indexed under this heading.

Metronidazole Hydrochloride (The co-administration of conivaptan with potent CYP3A4 inhibitors, such as ketoconazole, itraconazole, clarithromycin, ritonavir and indinavir, is contraindicated. Conivaptan is a substrate of CYP3A4. Co-administration of conivaptan with CYP3A4 inhibitors could lead to an increase in conivaptan concentrations).
No products indexed under this heading.

Metronidazole Sodium (The co-administration of conivaptan with potent CYP3A4 inhibitors, such as ketoconazole, itraconazole, clarithromycin, ritonavir and indinavir, is contraindicated. Conivaptan is a substrate of CYP3A4. Co-administration of conivaptan with CYP3A4 inhibitors could lead to an increase in conivaptan concentrations).
No products indexed under this heading.

Miconazole (The co-administration of conivaptan with potent CYP3A4 inhibitors, such as ketoconazole, itraconazole, clarithromycin, ritonavir and indinavir, is contraindicated. Conivaptan is a substrate of CYP3A4. Co-administration of conivaptan with CYP3A4 inhibitors could lead to an increase in conivaptan concentrations).
No products indexed under this heading.

Miconazole Nitrate (The co-administration of conivaptan with potent CYP3A4 inhibitors, such as ketoconazole, itraconazole, clarithromycin, ritonavir and indinavir, is contraindicated. Conivaptan is a substrate of CYP3A4. Co-administration of conivaptan with CYP3A4 inhibitors could lead to an increase in conivaptan concentrations). Products include:
Vusion Ointment 3335

Midazolam Hydrochloride (Intravenous conivaptan hydrochloride 40 mg/day increased the mean AUC values by approximately 2- and 3-fold for 1 mg intravenous or 2 mg oral doses of midazolam, respectively).
No products indexed under this heading.

Mifepristone (The co-administration of conivaptan with potent CYP3A4 inhibitors, such as ketoconazole, itraconazole, clarithromycin, ritonavir and indinavir, is contraindicated. Conivaptan is a substrate of CYP3A4. Co-administration of conivaptan with CYP3A4 inhibitors could lead to an increase in conivaptan concentrations).
No products indexed under this heading.

Nefazodone Hydrochloride (The co-administration of conivaptan with potent CYP3A4 inhibitors, such as ketoconazole, itraconazole, clarithromycin, ritonavir and indinavir, is contraindicated. Conivaptan is a substrate of CYP3A4. Co-administration of conivaptan with CYP3A4 inhibitors could lead to an increase in conivaptan concentrations).
No products indexed under this heading.

Nelfinavir Mesylate (The co-administration of conivaptan with potent CYP3A4 inhibitors, such as ketoconazole, itraconazole, clarithromycin, ritonavir and indinavir, is contraindicated. Conivaptan is a substrate of CYP3A4. Co-administration of conivaptan with CYP3A4 inhibitors could lead to an increase in conivaptan concentrations).
No products indexed under this heading.

Nevirapine (The co-administration of conivaptan with potent CYP3A4 inhibitors, such as ketoconazole, itraconazole, clarithromycin, ritonavir and indinavir, is contraindicated. Conivaptan is a substrate of CYP3A4. Co-administration of conivaptan with CYP3A4 inhibitors could lead to an increase in conivaptan concentrations). Products include:
Viramune Oral Suspension 897
Viramune Tablets 897

Niacin (The co-administration of conivaptan with potent CYP3A4 inhibitors, such as ketoconazole, itraconazole, clarithromycin, ritonavir and indinavir, is contraindicated. Conivaptan is a substrate of CYP3A4. Co-administration of conivaptan with CYP3A4 inhibitors could lead to an increase in conivaptan concentrations). Products include:
Advicor 402
Cardio Basics 3455
Niaspan 497
Simcor 524

Niacinamide (The co-administration of conivaptan with potent CYP3A4 inhibitors, such as ketoconazole, itraconazole, clarithromycin, ritonavir and indinavir, is contraindicated. Conivaptan is a substrate of CYP3A4. Co-administration of conivaptan with CYP3A4 inhibitors could lead to an increase in conivaptan concentrations). Products include:
CitraNatal 90 DHA Capsules 2332
CitraNatal Assure 2332
CitraNatal Rx 2332
Heplive 607

Niacinamide Hydroiodide (The co-administration of conivaptan with potent CYP3A4 inhibitors, such as ketoconazole, itraconazole, clarithromycin, ritonavir and indinavir, is contraindicated. Conivaptan is a substrate of CYP3A4. Co-administration of conivaptan with CYP3A4 inhibitors could lead to an increase in conivaptan concentrations).
No products indexed under this heading.

Nicardipine (Conivaptan is a potent inhibitor of CYP3A4. Conivaptan may increase plasma concentrations of co-administered drugs that are primarily metabolized by CYP3A4. In clinical trials of oral conivaptan hydrochloride, two cases of rhabdomyolysis occurred in patients who were also receiving a CYP3A4-metabolized HMG-CoA reductase inhibitor. Concomitant use of conivaptan hydrochloride with drugs that are primarily metabolized by CYP3A4 should be closely monitored or the combination should be avoided. If a clinical decision is made to discontinue concomitant medications at recommended doses, an appropriate amount of time (at least 24 hours) following the end of conivaptan hydrochloride administration should be allowed before resuming these medications).
No products indexed under this heading.

Nicardipine Hydrochloride (Conivaptan is a potent inhibitor of CYP3A4. Conivaptan may increase plasma concentrations of co-administered drugs that are primarily metabolized by CYP3A4. In clinical trials of oral conivaptan hydrochloride, two cases of rhabdomyolysis occurred in patients who were also receiving a CYP3A4-metabolized HMG-CoA reductase inhibitor. Concomitant use of conivaptan hydrochloride with drugs that are primarily metabolized by CYP3A4 should be closely monitored or the combination should be avoided. If a clinical decision is made to discontinue concomitant medications at recommended doses, an appropriate amount of time (at least 24 hours) following the end of conivaptan hydrochloride administration should be allowed before resuming these medications).
No products indexed under this heading.

Nicotinamide (The co-administration of conivaptan with potent CYP3A4 inhibitors, such as ketoconazole, itraconazole, clarithromycin, ritonavir and indinavir, is contraindicated. Conivaptan is a substrate of CYP3A4. Co-administration of conivaptan with CYP3A4 inhibitors could lead to an increase in conivaptan concentrations).
No products indexed under this heading.

Nifedipine (The co-administration of conivaptan with potent CYP3A4 inhibitors, such as ketoconazole, itraconazole, clarithromycin, ritonavir and indinavir, is contraindicated. Conivaptan is a substrate of CYP3A4. Co-administration of conivaptan with CYP3A4 inhibitors could lead to an increase in conivaptan concentrations).
No products indexed under this heading.

Nimodipine (Conivaptan is a potent inhibitor of CYP3A4. Conivaptan may increase plasma concentrations of co-administered drugs that are primarily metabolized by CYP3A4. In clinical trials of oral conivaptan hydrochloride, two cases of rhabdomyolysis occurred in patients who were also receiving a CYP3A4-metabolized HMG-CoA reductase inhibitor. Concomitant use of conivaptan hydrochloride with drugs that are primarily metabolized by CYP3A4 should be closely monitored or the combination should be avoided. If a clinical decision is made to discontinue concomitant medications at recommended doses, an appropriate amount of time (at least 24 hours) following the end of conivaptan hydrochloride administration should be allowed before resuming these medications).
No products indexed under this heading.

Nisoldipine (Conivaptan is a potent inhibitor of CYP3A4. Conivaptan may increase plasma concentrations of co-administered drugs that are primarily metabolized by CYP3A4. In clinical trials of oral conivaptan hydrochloride, two cases of rhabdomyolysis occurred in patients who were also receiving a CYP3A4-metabolized HMG-CoA reductase inhibitor. Concomitant use of conivaptan hydrochloride with drugs that are primarily metabolized by CYP3A4 should be closely monitored or the combination should be avoided. If a clinical decision is made to discontinue concomitant medications at recom-

mended doses, an appropriate amount of time (at least 24 hours) following the end of conivaptan hydrochloride administration should be allowed before resuming these medications).
No products indexed under this heading.

Nitrendipine (Conivaptan is a potent inhibitor of CYP3A4. Conivaptan may increase plasma concentrations of co-administered drugs that are primarily metabolized by CYP3A4. In clinical trials of oral conivaptan hydrochloride, two cases of rhabdomyolysis occurred in patients who were also receiving a CYP3A4-metabolized HMG-CoA reductase inhibitor. Concomitant use of conivaptan hydrochloride with drugs that are primarily metabolized by CYP3A4 should be closely monitored or the combination should be avoided. If a clinical decision is made to discontinue concomitant medications at recommended doses, an appropriate amount of time (at least 24 hours) following the end of conivaptan hydrochloride administration should be allowed before resuming these medications).
No products indexed under this heading.

Norethindrone (Conivaptan is a potent inhibitor of CYP3A4. Conivaptan may increase plasma concentrations of co-administered drugs that are primarily metabolized by CYP3A4. In clinical trials of oral conivaptan hydrochloride, two cases of rhabdomyolysis occurred in patients who were also receiving a CYP3A4-metabolized HMG-CoA reductase inhibitor. Concomitant use of conivaptan hydrochloride with drugs that are primarily metabolized by CYP3A4 should be closely monitored or the combination should be avoided. If a clinical decision is made to discontinue concomitant medications at recommended doses, an appropriate amount of time (at least 24 hours) following the end of conivaptan hydrochloride administration should be allowed before resuming these medications). Products include:
Ortho Micronor 2660

Norethindrone Acetate (Conivaptan is a potent inhibitor of CYP3A4. Conivaptan may increase plasma concentrations of co-administered drugs that are primarily metabolized by CYP3A4. In clinical trials of oral conivaptan hydrochloride, two cases of rhabdomyolysis occurred in patients who were also receiving a CYP3A4-metabolized HMG-CoA reductase inhibitor. Concomitant use of conivaptan hydrochloride with drugs that are primarily metabolized by CYP3A4 should be closely monitored or the combination should be avoided. If a clinical decision is made to discontinue concomitant medications at recommended doses, an appropriate amount of time (at least 24 hours) following the end of conivaptan hydrochloride administration should be allowed before resuming these medications). Products include:
Activella 2561

Norfloxacin (The co-administration of conivaptan with potent CYP3A4 inhibitors, such as ketoconazole, itraconazole, clarithromycin, ritonavir and indinavir, is contraindicated. Conivaptan is a substrate of CYP3A4. Co-administration of conivaptan with CYP3A4 inhibitors could lead to an increase in conivaptan concentrations). Products include:
Noroxin 2220

Norgestrel (Conivaptan is a potent inhibitor of CYP3A4. Conivaptan may increase plasma concentrations of co-administered drugs that are primarily metabolized by CYP3A4. In clinical trials of oral conivaptan hydrochloride, two cases of rhabdomyolysis occurred in patients who were also receiving a CYP3A4-metabolized HMG-CoA reductase inhibitor. Concomitant use of conivaptan hydrochloride with drugs that are primarily metabolized by CYP3A4 should be closely monitored or the combination should be avoided. If a clinical decision is made to discontinue concomitant medications at recommended doses, an appropriate amount of time (at least 24 hours) following the end of conivaptan hydrochloride administration should be allowed before resuming these medications).
No products indexed under this heading.

Omeprazole (The co-administration of conivaptan with potent CYP3A4 inhibitors, such as ketoconazole, itraconazole, clarithromycin, ritonavir and indinavir, is contraindicated. Conivaptan is a substrate of CYP3A4. Co-administration of conivaptan with CYP3A4 inhibitors could lead to an increase in conivaptan concentrations).
No products indexed under this heading.

Ondansetron (Conivaptan is a potent inhibitor of CYP3A4. Conivaptan may increase plasma concentrations of co-administered drugs that are primarily metabolized by CYP3A4. In clinical trials of oral conivaptan hydrochloride, two cases of rhabdomyolysis occurred in patients who were also receiving a CYP3A4-metabolized HMG-CoA reductase inhibitor. Concomitant use of conivaptan hydrochloride with drugs that are primarily metabolized by CYP3A4 should be closely monitored or the combination should be avoided. If a clinical decision is made to discontinue concomitant medications at recommended doses, an appropriate amount of time (at least 24 hours) following the end of conivaptan hydrochloride administration should be allowed before resuming these medications).
No products indexed under this heading.

Ondansetron Hydrochloride (Conivaptan is a potent inhibitor of CYP3A4. Conivaptan may increase plasma concentrations of co-administered drugs that are primarily metabolized by CYP3A4. In clinical trials of oral conivaptan hydrochloride, two cases of rhabdomyolysis occurred in patients who were also receiving a CYP3A4-metabolized HMG-CoA reductase inhibitor. Concomitant use of conivaptan hydrochloride with drugs that are primarily metabolized by CYP3A4 should be closely monitored or the combination should be avoided. If a clinical decision is made to discontinue concomitant medications at recommended doses, an appropriate amount of time (at least 24 hours) following the end of conivaptan hydrochloride administration should be allowed before resuming these medications). Products include:
Zofran Injection 1750
Zofran 1756
Zofran ODT 1756

Paclitaxel (Conivaptan is a potent inhibitor of CYP3A4. Conivaptan may increase plasma concentrations of co-administered drugs that are primarily metabolized by CYP3A4. In clinical trials of oral conivaptan hydrochloride, two cases of rhabdomyolysis occurred in patients who were also receiving a CYP3A4-metabolized HMG-CoA reductase inhibitor. Concomitant use of conivaptan hydrochloride with drugs that are primarily metabolized by CYP3A4 should be closely monitored or the combination should be avoided. If a clinical decision is made to discontinue concomitant medications at recommended doses, an appropriate amount of time (at least 24 hours) following the end of conivaptan hydrochloride administration should be allowed before resuming these medications).
No products indexed under this heading.

Paroxetine Hydrochloride (The co-administration of conivaptan with potent CYP3A4 inhibitors, such as ketoconazole, itraconazole, clarithromycin, ritonavir and indinavir, is contraindicated. Conivaptan is a substrate of CYP3A4. Co-administration of conivaptan with CYP3A4 inhibitors could lead to an increase in conivaptan concentrations). Products include:
Paroxetine CR 2361
Paroxetine ER 2371
Paxil 1586
Paxil CR 1596

Pimozide (Conivaptan is a potent inhibitor of CYP3A4. Conivaptan may increase plasma concentrations of co-administered drugs that are primarily metabolized by CYP3A4. In clinical trials of oral conivaptan hydrochloride, two cases of rhabdomyolysis occurred in patients who were also receiving a CYP3A4-metabolized HMG-CoA reductase inhibitor. Concomitant use of conivaptan hydrochloride with drugs that are primarily metabolized by CYP3A4 should be closely monitored or the combination should be avoided. If a clinical decision is made to discontinue concomitant medications at recommended doses, an appropriate amount of time (at least 24 hours) following the end of conivaptan hydrochloride administration should be allowed before resuming these medications).
No products indexed under this heading.

Polyestradiol Phosphate (Conivaptan is a potent inhibitor of CYP3A4. Conivaptan may increase plasma concentrations of co-administered drugs that are primarily metabolized by CYP3A4. In clinical trials of oral conivaptan hydrochloride, two cases of rhabdomyolysis occurred in patients who were also receiving a CYP3A4-metabolized HMG-CoA reductase inhibitor. Concomitant use of conivaptan hydrochloride with drugs that are primarily metabolized by CYP3A4 should be closely monitored or the combination should be avoided. If a clinical decision is made to discontinue concomitant medications at recommended doses, an appropriate amount of time (at least 24 hours) following the end of conivaptan hydrochloride administration should be allowed before resuming these medications).
No products indexed under this heading.

Posaconazole (The co-administration of conivaptan with potent CYP3A4 inhibitors, such as ketoconazole, itraconazole, clarithromycin, ritonavir and indinavir, is contraindicated. Conivaptan is a substrate of CYP3A4. Co-administration of conivaptan with CYP3A4 inhibitors could lead to an increase in conivaptan concentrations). Products include:
Noxafil 3172

Pravastatin Sodium (Conivaptan is a potent inhibitor of CYP3A4. Conivaptan may increase plasma concentrations of co-administered drugs that are primarily metabolized by CYP3A4. In clinical trials of oral conivaptan hydrochloride, two cases of rhabdomyolysis occurred in patients who were also receiving a CYP3A4-metabolized HMG-CoA reductase inhibitor. Concomitant use of conivaptan hydrochloride with drugs that are primarily metabolized by CYP3A4 should be closely monitored or the combination should be avoided. If a clinical decision is made to discontinue concomitant medications at recommended doses, an appropriate amount of time (at least 24 hours) following the end of conivaptan hydrochloride administration should be allowed before resuming these medications).
No products indexed under this heading.

Propoxyphene Hydrochloride (The co-administration of conivaptan with potent CYP3A4 inhibitors, such as ketoconazole, itraconazole, clarithromycin, ritonavir and indinavir, is contraindicated. Conivaptan is a substrate of CYP3A4. Co-administration of conivaptan with CYP3A4 inhibitors could lead to an increase in conivaptan concentrations).
No products indexed under this heading.

Propoxyphene Napsylate (The co-administration of conivaptan with potent CYP3A4 inhibitors, such as ketoconazole, itraconazole, clarithromycin, ritonavir and indinavir, is contraindicated. Conivaptan is a substrate of CYP3A4. Co-administration of conivaptan with CYP3A4 inhibitors could lead to an increase in conivaptan concentrations).
No products indexed under this heading.

Quinidine (The co-administration of conivaptan with potent CYP3A4 inhibitors, such as ketoconazole, itraconazole, clarithromycin, ritonavir and indinavir, is contraindicated. Conivaptan is a substrate of CYP3A4. Co-administration of conivaptan with CYP3A4 inhibitors could lead to an increase in conivaptan concentrations).
No products indexed under this heading.

Quinidine Gluconate (Conivaptan is a potent inhibitor of CYP3A4. Conivaptan may increase plasma concentrations of co-administered drugs that are primarily metabolized by CYP3A4. In clinical trials of oral conivaptan hydrochloride, two cases of rhabdomyolysis occurred in patients who were also receiving a CYP3A4-metabolized HMG-CoA reductase inhibitor. Concomitant use of conivaptan hydrochloride with drugs that are primarily metabolized by CYP3A4 should be closely monitored or the combination should be avoided. If a clinical decision is made to discontinue concomitant medications at recommended doses, an appropriate amount of time (at least 24 hours) following the end of conivaptan hydrochloride administration should be allowed before resuming these medications).
No products indexed under this heading.

Quinidine Hydrochloride (The co-administration of conivaptan with potent CYP3A4 inhibitors, such as ketoconazole, itraconazole, clarithromycin, ritonavir and indinavir, is contraindicated. Conivaptan is a substrate of CYP3A4. Co-administration of conivaptan with CYP3A4 inhibitors could lead to an increase in conivaptan concentrations).
No products indexed under this heading.

Quinidine Polygalacturonate (The co-administration of conivaptan with potent CYP3A4 inhibitors, such as ketoconazole, itraconazole, clarithromycin, ritonavir and indinavir, is contraindicated. Conivaptan is a substrate of CYP3A4. Co-administration of conivaptan with CYP3A4 inhibitors could lead to an increase in conivaptan concentrations).
No products indexed under this heading.

Quinidine Sulfate (The co-administration of conivaptan with potent CYP3A4 inhibitors, such as ketoconazole, itraconazole, clarithromycin, ritonavir and indinavir, is contraindicated. Conivaptan is a substrate of CYP3A4. Co-administration of conivaptan with CYP3A4 inhibitors could lead to an increase in conivaptan concentrations).
No products indexed under this heading.

Quinine (The co-administration of conivaptan with potent CYP3A4 inhibitors, such as ketoconazole, itraconazole, clarithromycin, ritonavir and indinavir, is contraindicated. Conivaptan is

a substrate of CYP3A4. Co-administration of conivaptan with CYP3A4 inhibitors could lead to an increase in conivaptan concentrations). Products include:
Hyland's Leg Cramps PM with Quinine 3315

Quinine Sulfate (The co-administration of conivaptan with potent CYP3A4 inhibitors, such as ketoconazole, itraconazole, clarithromycin, ritonavir and indinavir, is contraindicated. Conivaptan is a substrate of CYP3A4. Co-administration of conivaptan with CYP3A4 inhibitors could lead to an increase in conivaptan concentrations).
No products indexed under this heading.

Quinupristin (The co-administration of conivaptan with potent CYP3A4 inhibitors, such as ketoconazole, itraconazole, clarithromycin, ritonavir and indinavir, is contraindicated. Conivaptan is a substrate of CYP3A4. Co-administration of conivaptan with CYP3A4 inhibitors could lead to an increase in conivaptan concentrations).
No products indexed under this heading.

Ranitidine Bismuth Citrate (The co-administration of conivaptan with potent CYP3A4 inhibitors, such as ketoconazole, itraconazole, clarithromycin, ritonavir and indinavir, is contraindicated. Conivaptan is a substrate of CYP3A4. Co-administration of conivaptan with CYP3A4 inhibitors could lead to an increase in conivaptan concentrations).
No products indexed under this heading.

Ranitidine Hydrochloride (The co-administration of conivaptan with potent CYP3A4 inhibitors, such as ketoconazole, itraconazole, clarithromycin, ritonavir and indinavir, is contraindicated. Conivaptan is a substrate of CYP3A4. Co-administration of conivaptan with CYP3A4 inhibitors could lead to an increase in conivaptan concentrations). Products include:
Zantac 1737
Zantac Injection 1732
Zantac Pharmacy 1735

Rifabutin (Conivaptan is a potent inhibitor of CYP3A4. Conivaptan may increase plasma concentrations of co-administered drugs that are primarily metabolized by CYP3A4. In clinical trials of oral conivaptan hydrochloride, two cases of rhabdomyolysis occurred in patients who were also receiving a CYP3A4-metabolized HMG-CoA reductase inhibitor. Concomitant use of conivaptan hydrochloride with drugs that are primarily metabolized by CYP3A4 should be closely monitored or the combination should be avoided. If a clinical decision is made to discontinue concomitant medications at recommended doses, an appropriate amount of time (at least 24 hours) following the end of conivaptan hydrochloride administration should be allowed before resuming these medications).
No products indexed under this heading.

Ritonavir (The co-administration of conivaptan with potent CYP3A4 inhibitors, such as ritonavir, is contraindicated. Conivaptan is a substrate of CYP3A4. Co-administration of conivaptan with CYP3A4 inhibitors could lead to an increase in conivaptan concentrations). Products include:
Kaletra 458
Norvir 509

Rosuvastatin Calcium (Conivaptan is a potent inhibitor of CYP3A4. Conivaptan may increase plasma concentrations of co-administered drugs that are primarily metabolized by CYP3A4. In clinical trials of oral conivaptan hydrochloride, two cases of rhabdomyolysis occurred in patients who were also receiving a CYP3A4-metabolized HMG-CoA reductase inhibitor. Concomitant use of conivaptan hydrochloride with drugs that are primarily metabolized by CYP3A4 should be closely monitored or the combination should be avoided. If a clinical decision is made to discontinue concomitant medications at recommended doses, an appropriate amount of time (at least 24 hours) following the end of conivaptan hydrochloride administration should be allowed before resuming these medications). Products include:
Crestor 736

Saquinavir (The co-administration of conivaptan with potent CYP3A4 inhibitors, such as ketoconazole, itraconazole, clarithromycin, ritonavir and indinavir, is contraindicated. Conivaptan is a substrate of CYP3A4. Co-administration of conivaptan with CYP3A4 inhibitors could lead to an increase in conivaptan concentrations).
No products indexed under this heading.

Saquinavir Mesylate (The co-administration of conivaptan with potent CYP3A4 inhibitors, such as ketoconazole, itraconazole, clarithromycin, ritonavir and indinavir, is contraindicated. Conivaptan is a substrate of CYP3A4. Co-administration of conivaptan with CYP3A4 inhibitors could lead to an increase in conivaptan concentrations).
No products indexed under this heading.

Sertraline Hydrochloride (The co-administration of conivaptan with potent CYP3A4 inhibitors, such as ketoconazole, itraconazole, clarithromycin, ritonavir and indinavir, is contraindicated. Conivaptan is a substrate of CYP3A4. Co-administration of conivaptan with CYP3A4 inhibitors could lead to an increase in conivaptan concentrations).
No products indexed under this heading.

Sildenafil Citrate (The co-administration of conivaptan with potent CYP3A4 inhibitors, such as ketoconazole, itraconazole, clarithromycin, ritonavir and indinavir, is contraindicated. Conivaptan is a substrate of CYP3A4. Co-administration of conivaptan with CYP3A4 inhibitors could lead to an increase in conivaptan concentrations).
No products indexed under this heading.

Simvastatin (Intravenous conivaptan hydrochloride 30 mg/day resulted in a 3-fold increase in the AUC of simvastatin). Products include:
Simcor 524
Vytorin 10/10 .... 2303, 3240
Vytorin 10/20 .... 2303, 3240
Vytorin 10/40 .... 2303, 3240
Vytorin 10/80 .... 2303, 3240
Zocor 2289

Sirolimus (Conivaptan is a potent inhibitor of CYP3A4. Conivaptan may increase plasma concentrations of co-administered drugs that are primarily metabolized by CYP3A4. In clinical trials of oral conivaptan hydrochloride, two cases of rhabdomyolysis occurred in patients who were also receiving a CYP3A4-metabolized HMG-CoA reductase inhibitor. Concomitant use of conivaptan hydrochloride with drugs that are primarily metabolized by CYP3A4 should be closely monitored or the combination should be avoided. If a clinical decision is made to discontinue concomitant medications at recommended doses, an appropriate amount of time (at least 24 hours) following the end of conivaptan hydrochloride administration should be allowed before resuming these medications). Products include:
Rapamune 3579

Tacrolimus (Conivaptan is a potent inhibitor of CYP3A4. Conivaptan may increase plasma concentrations of co-administered drugs that are primarily metabolized by CYP3A4. In clinical trials of oral conivaptan hydrochloride, two cases of rhabdomyolysis occurred in patients who were also receiving a CYP3A4-metabolized HMG-CoA reductase inhibitor. Concomitant use of conivaptan hydrochloride with drugs that are primarily metabolized by CYP3A4 should be closely monitored or the combination should be avoided. If a clinical decision is made to discontinue concomitant medications at recommended doses, an appropriate amount of time (at least 24 hours) following the end of conivaptan hydrochloride administration should be allowed before resuming these medications). Products include:
Prograf Capsules 677
Prograf Injection 677
Protopic 685

Tadalafil (Conivaptan is a potent inhibitor of CYP3A4. Conivaptan may increase plasma concentrations of co-administered drugs that are primarily metabolized by CYP3A4. In clinical trials of oral conivaptan hydrochloride, two cases of rhabdomyolysis occurred in patients who were also receiving a CYP3A4-metabolized HMG-CoA reductase inhibitor. Concomitant use of conivaptan hydrochloride with drugs that are primarily metabolized by CYP3A4 should be closely monitored or the combination should be avoided. If a clinical decision is made to discontinue concomitant medications at recommended doses, an appropriate amount of time (at least 24 hours) following the end of conivaptan hydrochloride administration should be allowed before resuming these medications). Products include:
Adcirca 3461
Cialis 1861

Tamoxifen Citrate (Conivaptan is a potent inhibitor of CYP3A4. Conivaptan may increase plasma concentrations of co-administered drugs that are primarily metabolized by CYP3A4. In clinical trials of oral conivaptan hydrochloride, two cases of rhabdomyolysis occurred in patients who were also receiving a CYP3A4-metabolized HMG-CoA reductase inhibitor. Concomitant use of conivaptan hydrochloride with drugs that are primarily metabolized by CYP3A4 should be closely monitored or the combination should be avoided. If a clinical decision is made to discontinue concomitant medications at recommended doses, an appropriate amount of time (at least 24 hours) following the end of conivaptan hydrochloride administration should be allowed before resuming these medications).
No products indexed under this heading.

Telithromycin (The co-administration of conivaptan with potent CYP3A4 inhibitors, such as ketoconazole, itraconazole, clarithromycin, ritonavir and indinavir, is contraindicated. Conivaptan is a substrate of CYP3A4. Co-administration of conivaptan with CYP3A4 inhibitors could lead to an increase in conivaptan concentrations). Products include:
Ketek 2991

Terfenadine (Conivaptan is a potent inhibitor of CYP3A4. Conivaptan may increase plasma concentrations of co-administered drugs that are primarily metabolized by CYP3A4. In clinical trials of oral conivaptan hydrochloride, two cases of rhabdomyolysis occurred in patients who were also receiving a CYP3A4-metabolized HMG-CoA reductase inhibitor. Concomitant use of conivaptan hydrochloride with drugs that are primarily metabolized by CYP3A4 should be closely monitored or the combination should be avoided. If a clinical decision is made to discontinue concomitant medications at recommended doses, an appropriate amount of time (at least 24 hours) following the end of conivaptan hydrochloride administration should be allowed before resuming these medications).
No products indexed under this heading.

Theophylline (Conivaptan is a potent inhibitor of CYP3A4. Conivaptan may increase plasma concentrations of co-administered drugs that are primarily metabolized by CYP3A4. In clinical trials of oral conivaptan hydrochloride, two cases of rhabdomyolysis occurred in patients who were also receiving a CYP3A4-metabolized HMG-CoA reductase inhibitor. Concomitant use of conivaptan hydrochloride with drugs that are primarily metabolized by CYP3A4 should be closely monitored or the combination should be avoided. If a clinical decision is made to discontinue concomitant medications at recommended doses, an appropriate amount of time (at least 24 hours) following the end of conivaptan hydrochloride administration should be allowed before resuming these medications).
No products indexed under this heading.

Theophylline Anhydrous (Conivaptan is a potent inhibitor of CYP3A4. Conivaptan may increase plasma concentrations of co-administered drugs that are primarily metabolized by CYP3A4. In clinical trials of oral conivaptan hydrochloride, two cases of rhabdomyolysis occurred in patients who were also receiving a CYP3A4-metabolized HMG-CoA reductase inhibitor. Concomitant use of conivaptan hydrochloride with drugs that are primarily metabolized by CYP3A4 should be closely monitored or the combination should be avoided. If a clinical decision is made to discontinue concomitant medications at recommended doses, an appropriate amount of time (at least 24 hours) following the end of conivaptan hydrochloride administration should be allowed before resuming these medications). Products include:
Uniphyl 2817

Theophylline Calcium Salicylate (Conivaptan is a potent inhibitor of CYP3A4. Conivaptan may increase plasma concentrations of co-administered drugs that are primarily metabolized by CYP3A4. In clinical trials of oral conivaptan hydrochloride, two cases of rhabdomyolysis occurred in patients who were also receiving a CYP3A4-metabolized HMG-CoA reductase inhibitor. Concomitant use of conivaptan hydrochloride with drugs that are primarily metabolized by CYP3A4 should be closely monitored or the combination should be avoided. If a clinical decision is made to discontinue concomitant medications at recommended doses, an appropriate amount of time (at least 24 hours) following the end of conivaptan hydrochloride administration should be allowed before resuming these medications).
No products indexed under this heading.

Theophylline Dihydroxypropyl (Glyceryl) (Conivaptan is a potent inhibitor of CYP3A4. Conivaptan may increase plasma concentrations of co-administered drugs that are primarily metabolized by CYP3A4. In clinical trials of oral conivaptan hydrochloride, two cases of rhabdomyolysis occurred in patients who were also receiving a CYP3A4-metabolized HMG-CoA reductase inhibitor. Concomitant use of conivaptan hydrochloride with drugs that are primarily metabolized by CYP3A4 should be closely monitored or the combination should be avoided. If a clinical decision is made to discontinue

concomitant medications at recommended doses, an appropriate amount of time (at least 24 hours) following the end of conivaptan hydrochloride administration should be allowed before resuming these medications).
No products indexed under this heading.

Theophylline Ethylenediamine (Conivaptan is a potent inhibitor of CYP3A4. Conivaptan may increase plasma concentrations of co-administered drugs that are primarily metabolized by CYP3A4. In clinical trials of oral conivaptan hydrochloride, two cases of rhabdomyolysis occurred in patients who were also receiving a CYP3A4-metabolized HMG-CoA reductase inhibitor. Concomitant use of conivaptan hydrochloride with drugs that are primarily metabolized by CYP3A4 should be closely monitored or the combination should be avoided. If a clinical decision is made to discontinue concomitant medications at recommended doses, an appropriate amount of time (at least 24 hours) following the end of conivaptan hydrochloride administration should be allowed before resuming these medications).
No products indexed under this heading.

Theophylline Sodium Glycinate (Conivaptan is a potent inhibitor of CYP3A4. Conivaptan may increase plasma concentrations of co-administered drugs that are primarily metabolized by CYP3A4. In clinical trials of oral conivaptan hydrochloride, two cases of rhabdomyolysis occurred in patients who were also receiving a CYP3A4-metabolized HMG-CoA reductase inhibitor. Concomitant use of conivaptan hydrochloride with drugs that are primarily metabolized by CYP3A4 should be closely monitored or the combination should be avoided. If a clinical decision is made to discontinue concomitant medications at recommended doses, an appropriate amount of time (at least 24 hours) following the end of conivaptan hydrochloride administration should be allowed before resuming these medications).
No products indexed under this heading.

Tiagabine Hydrochloride (Conivaptan is a potent inhibitor of CYP3A4. Conivaptan may increase plasma concentrations of co-administered drugs that are primarily metabolized by CYP3A4. In clinical trials of oral conivaptan hydrochloride, two cases of rhabdomyolysis occurred in patients who were also receiving a CYP3A4-metabolized HMG-CoA reductase inhibitor. Concomitant use of conivaptan hydrochloride with drugs that are primarily metabolized by CYP3A4 should be closely monitored or the combination should be avoided. If a clinical decision is made to discontinue concomitant medications at recommended doses, an appropriate amount of time (at least 24 hours) following the end of conivaptan hydrochloride administration should be allowed before resuming these medications). Products include:
Gabitril 972

Tolterodine Tartrate (Conivaptan is a potent inhibitor of CYP3A4. Conivaptan may increase plasma concentrations of co-administered drugs that are primarily metabolized by CYP3A4. In clinical trials of oral conivaptan hydrochloride, two cases of rhabdomyolysis occurred in patients who were also receiving a CYP3A4-metabolized HMG-CoA reductase inhibitor. Concomitant use of conivaptan hydrochloride with drugs that are primarily metabolized by CYP3A4 should be closely monitored or the combination should be avoided. If a clinical decision is made to discontinue concomitant medications at recommended doses, an appropriate amount of time (at least 24 hours) following the end of conivaptan hydrochloride administration should be allowed before resuming these medications).
No products indexed under this heading.

Trazodone Hydrochloride (Conivaptan is a potent inhibitor of CYP3A4. Conivaptan may increase plasma concentrations of co-administered drugs that are primarily metabolized by CYP3A4. In clinical trials of oral conivaptan hydrochloride, two cases of rhabdomyolysis occurred in patients who were also receiving a CYP3A4-metabolized HMG-CoA reductase inhibitor. Concomitant use of conivaptan hydrochloride with drugs that are primarily metabolized by CYP3A4 should be closely monitored or the combination should be avoided. If a clinical decision is made to discontinue concomitant medications at recommended doses, an appropriate amount of time (at least 24 hours) following the end of conivaptan hydrochloride administration should be allowed before resuming these medications).
No products indexed under this heading.

Triazolam (Conivaptan is a potent inhibitor of CYP3A4. Conivaptan may increase plasma concentrations of co-administered drugs that are primarily metabolized by CYP3A4. In clinical trials of oral conivaptan hydrochloride, two cases of rhabdomyolysis occurred in patients who were also receiving a CYP3A4-metabolized HMG-CoA reductase inhibitor. Concomitant use of conivaptan hydrochloride with drugs that are primarily metabolized by CYP3A4 should be closely monitored or the combination should be avoided. If a clinical decision is made to discontinue concomitant medications at recommended doses, an appropriate amount of time (at least 24 hours) following the end of conivaptan hydrochloride administration should be allowed before resuming these medications).
No products indexed under this heading.

Troglitazone (The co-administration of conivaptan with potent CYP3A4 inhibitors, such as ketoconazole, itraconazole, clarithromycin, ritonavir and indinavir, is contraindicated. Conivaptan is a substrate of CYP3A4. Co-administration of conivaptan with CYP3A4 inhibitors could lead to an increase in conivaptan concentrations).
No products indexed under this heading.

Troleandomycin (The co-administration of conivaptan with potent CYP3A4 inhibitors, such as ketoconazole, itraconazole, clarithromycin, ritonavir and indinavir, is contraindicated. Conivaptan is a substrate of CYP3A4. Co-administration of conivaptan with CYP3A4 inhibitors could lead to an increase in conivaptan concentrations).
No products indexed under this heading.

Valproate Sodium (The co-administration of conivaptan with potent CYP3A4 inhibitors, such as ketoconazole, itraconazole, clarithromycin, ritonavir and indinavir, is contraindicated. Conivaptan is a substrate of CYP3A4. Co-administration of conivaptan with CYP3A4 inhibitors could lead to an increase in conivaptan concentrations).
No products indexed under this heading.

Vardenafil Hydrochloride (The co-administration of conivaptan with potent CYP3A4 inhibitors, such as ketoconazole, itraconazole, clarithromycin, ritonavir and indinavir, is contraindicated. Conivaptan is a substrate of CYP3A4. Co-administration of conivaptan with CYP3A4 inhibitors could lead to an increase in conivaptan concentrations). Products include:
Levitra 3157

Verapamil Hydrochloride (The co-administration of conivaptan with potent CYP3A4 inhibitors, such as ketoconazole, itraconazole, clarithromycin, ritonavir and indinavir, is contraindicated. Conivaptan is a substrate of CYP3A4. Co-administration of conivaptan with CYP3A4 inhibitors could lead to an increase in conivaptan concentrations). Products include:
Tarka 534

Vinblastine Sulfate (Conivaptan is a potent inhibitor of CYP3A4. Conivaptan may increase plasma concentrations of co-administered drugs that are primarily metabolized by CYP3A4. In clinical trials of oral conivaptan hydrochloride, two cases of rhabdomyolysis occurred in patients who were also receiving a CYP3A4-metabolized HMG-CoA reductase inhibitor. Concomitant use of conivaptan hydrochloride with drugs that are primarily metabolized by CYP3A4 should be closely monitored or the combination should be avoided. If a clinical decision is made to discontinue concomitant medications at recommended doses, an appropriate amount of time (at least 24 hours) following the end of conivaptan hydrochloride administration should be allowed before resuming these medications).
No products indexed under this heading.

Vincristine Sulfate (Conivaptan is a potent inhibitor of CYP3A4. Conivaptan may increase plasma concentrations of co-administered drugs that are primarily metabolized by CYP3A4. In clinical trials of oral conivaptan hydrochloride, two cases of rhabdomyolysis occurred in patients who were also receiving a CYP3A4-metabolized HMG-CoA reductase inhibitor. Concomitant use of conivaptan hydrochloride with drugs that are primarily metabolized by CYP3A4 should be closely monitored or the combination should be avoided. If a clinical decision is made to discontinue concomitant medications at recommended doses, an appropriate amount of time (at least 24 hours) following the end of conivaptan hydrochloride administration should be allowed before resuming these medications).
No products indexed under this heading.

Voriconazole (The co-administration of conivaptan with potent CYP3A4 inhibitors, such as ketoconazole, itraconazole, clarithromycin, ritonavir and indinavir, is contraindicated. Conivaptan is a substrate of CYP3A4. Co-administration of conivaptan with CYP3A4 inhibitors could lead to an increase in conivaptan concentrations).
No products indexed under this heading.

Warfarin Sodium (The effects of oral conivaptan hydrochloride 40 mg twice daily on prothrombin time was assessed in patients receiving stable oral warfarin therapy. After 10 days of oral conivaptan administration, the S- and R-warfarin concentrations were 90% and 98%, respectively, of those prior to conivaptan administration. The corresponding prothrombin time values after 10 days of oral conivaptan administration were 95% of baseline. No effect of oral conivaptan on the pharmacokinetics or pharmacodynamics of warfarin was observed).
No products indexed under this heading.

Zafirlukast (The co-administration of conivaptan with potent CYP3A4 inhibitors, such as ketoconazole, itraconazole, clarithromycin, ritonavir and indinavir, is contraindicated. Conivaptan is a substrate of CYP3A4. Co-administration of conivaptan with CYP3A4 inhibitors could lead to an increase in conivaptan concentrations). Products include:
Accolate 3612

Zileuton (The co-administration of conivaptan with potent CYP3A4 inhibitors, such as ketoconazole, itraconazole, clarithromycin, ritonavir and indinavir, is contraindicated. Conivaptan is a substrate of CYP3A4. Co-administration of conivaptan with CYP3A4 inhibitors could lead to an increase in conivaptan concentrations).
No products indexed under this heading.

Food Interactions

Grapefruit (The co-administration of conivaptan with potent CYP3A4 inhibitors, such as ketoconazole, itraconazole, clarithromycin, ritonavir and indinavir, is contraindicated. Conivaptan is a substrate of CYP3A4. Co-administration of conivaptan with CYP3A4 inhibitors could lead to an increase in conivaptan concentrations).

Grapefruit Juice (The co-administration of conivaptan with potent CYP3A4 inhibitors, such as ketoconazole, itraconazole, clarithromycin, ritonavir and indinavir, is contraindicated. Conivaptan is a substrate of CYP3A4. Co-administration of conivaptan with CYP3A4 inhibitors could lead to an increase in conivaptan concentrations).

VAQTA

(Hepatitis A Vaccine, Inactivated) 2281
May interact with typhoid vaccine, and certain other agents. Compounds in these categories include:

Typhoid Vaccine (Co-administration of Vaqta, typhoid and yellow fever vaccines has resulted in reduced GMTs for hepatitis A compared to Vaqta alone; however, following the receipt of the booster dose of Vaqta the GMTs for hepatits A in these two groups were observed to be comparable).
No products indexed under this heading.

Typhoid Vaccine Live Oral TY21a (Co-administration of Vaqta, typhoid and yellow fever vaccines has resulted in reduced GMTs for hepatitis A compared to Vaqta alone; however, following the receipt of the booster dose of Vaqta the GMTs for hepatits A in these two groups were observed to be comparable).
No products indexed under this heading.

Typhoid Vi Polysaccharide Vaccine (Co-administration of Vaqta, typhoid and yellow fever vaccines has resulted in reduced GMTs for hepatitis A compared to Vaqta alone; however, following the receipt of the booster dose of Vaqta the GMTs for hepatits A in these two groups were observed to be comparable).
No products indexed under this heading.

Yellow Fever Vaccine (Co-administration of Vaqta, typhoid and yellow fever vaccines has resulted in reduced GMTs for hepatitis A compared to Vaqta alone; however, following the receipt of the booster dose of Vaqta the GMTs for hepatitis A in these two groups were observed to be comparable).
No products indexed under this heading.

VARIVAX

(Varicella Virus Vaccine, Live) 2285
May interact with corticosteroids, salicylates, and certain other agents. Compounds in these categories include:

Alclometasone Dipropionate (Co-administration in individuals on immunosuppressant doses of corticosteroids can result in more extensive vaccine-associated rash or disseminated disease. Vaccine administration in immunosuppressed individuals in contraindicated).
No products indexed under this heading.

Aspirin (Vaccine recipients should avoid use of salicylates for 6 weeks

IMPORTANT NOTE: Always consult each drug listing in the patient's regimen for possible interactions.

Varivax Interactions Index 2016

after vaccination with Varivax because of the potential for Reye's syndrome). Products include:
Aggrenox 880
Bayer Aspirin 829
Percodan 1124
St. Joseph Aspirin 2045

Aspirin, Enteric Coated (Vaccine recipients should avoid use of salicylates for 6 weeks after vaccination with Varivax because of the potential for Reye's syndrome).
No products indexed under this heading.

Aspirin Buffered (Vaccine recipients should avoid use of salicylates for 6 weeks after vaccination with Varivax because of the potential for Reye's syndrome).
No products indexed under this heading.

Azathioprine (Concurrent use in individuals who are on immunosuppressant drugs can result in greater susceptibility to infections; co-administration is contraindicated).
No products indexed under this heading.

Beclomethasone Dipropionate (Co-administration in individuals on immunosuppressant doses of corticosteroids can result in more extensive vaccine-associated rash or disseminated disease. Vaccine administration in immunosuppressed individuals in contraindicated). Products include:
Qvar 3398

Beclomethasone Dipropionate Monohydrate (Co-administration in individuals on immunosuppressant doses of corticosteroids can result in more extensive vaccine-associated rash or disseminated disease. Vaccine administration in immunosuppressed individuals in contraindicated). Products include:
Beconase AQ 1386

Betamethasone (Co-administration in individuals on immunosuppressant doses of corticosteroids can result in more extensive vaccine-associated rash or disseminated disease. Vaccine administration in immunosuppressed individuals in contraindicated).
No products indexed under this heading.

Betamethasone Acetate (Co-administration in individuals on immunosuppressant doses of corticosteroids can result in more extensive vaccine-associated rash or disseminated disease. Vaccine administration in immunosuppressed individuals in contraindicated).
No products indexed under this heading.

Betamethasone Benzoate (Co-administration in individuals on immunosuppressant doses of corticosteroids can result in more extensive vaccine-associated rash or disseminated disease. Vaccine administration in immunosuppressed individuals in contraindicated).
No products indexed under this heading.

Betamethasone Dipropionate (Co-administration in individuals on immunosuppressant doses of corticosteroids can result in more extensive vaccine-associated rash or disseminated disease. Vaccine administration in immunosuppressed individuals in contraindicated). Products include:
Diprolene Lotion 0.05% 3108
Diprolene Ointment 0.05% 3109
Diprolene AF Cream 0.05% 3107
Lotrisone 3163

Betamethasone Sodium Phosphate (Co-administration in individuals on immunosuppressant doses of corticosteroids can result in more extensive vaccine-associated rash or disseminated disease. Vaccine administration in immunosuppressed individuals in contraindicated).
No products indexed under this heading.

Betamethasone Valerate (Co-administration in individuals on immunosuppressant doses of corticosteroids can result in more extensive vaccine-associated rash or disseminated disease. Vaccine administration in immunosuppressed individuals in contraindicated). Products include:
Luxiq 3321

Budesonide (Co-administration in individuals on immunosuppressant doses of corticosteroids can result in more extensive vaccine-associated rash or disseminated disease. Vaccine administration in immunosuppressed individuals in contraindicated). Products include:
Pulmicort Flexhaler 714
Symbicort 80/4.5 720
Symbicort 160/4.5 720

Choline Magnesium Trisalicylate (Vaccine recipients should avoid use of salicylates for 6 weeks after vaccination with Varivax because of the potential for Reye's syndrome).
No products indexed under this heading.

Ciclesonide (Co-administration in individuals on immunosuppressant doses of corticosteroids can result in more extensive vaccine-associated rash or disseminated disease. Vaccine administration in immunosuppressed individuals in contraindicated).
No products indexed under this heading.

Cortisone Acetate (Co-administration in individuals on immunosuppressant doses of corticosteroids can result in more extensive vaccine-associated rash or disseminated disease. Vaccine administration in immunosuppressed individuals in contraindicated).
No products indexed under this heading.

Cyclosporine (Concurrent use in individuals who are on immunosuppressant drugs can result in greater susceptibility to infections; co-administration is contraindicated). Products include:
Gengraf 440
Neoral Oral Solution 2496
Neoral Capsules 2496
Restasis 605

Desoximetasone (Co-administration in individuals on immunosuppressant doses of corticosteroids can result in more extensive vaccine-associated rash or disseminated disease. Vaccine administration in immunosuppressed individuals in contraindicated).
No products indexed under this heading.

Dexamethasone (Co-administration in individuals on immunosuppressant doses of corticosteroids can result in more extensive vaccine-associated rash or disseminated disease. Vaccine administration in immunosuppressed individuals in contraindicated). Products include:
Ciprodex 583
Ozurdex .... ⊙ 223
Tobramycin and Dexamethasone Ophthalmic Suspension .... ⊙ 251

Dexamethasone Acetate (Co-administration in individuals on immunosuppressant doses of corticosteroids can result in more extensive vaccine-associated rash or disseminated disease. Vaccine administration in immunosuppressed individuals in contraindicated).
No products indexed under this heading.

Dexamethasone Phosphate (Co-administration in individuals on immunosuppressant doses of corticosteroids can result in more extensive vaccine-associated rash or disseminated disease. Vaccine administration in immunosuppressed individuals in contraindicated).
No products indexed under this heading.

Dexamethasone Sodium (Co-administration in individuals on immunosuppressant doses of corticosteroids can result in more extensive vaccine-associated rash or disseminated disease. Vaccine administration in immunosuppressed individuals in contraindicated).
No products indexed under this heading.

Dexamethasone Sodium Phosphate (Co-administration in individuals on immunosuppressant doses of corticosteroids can result in more extensive vaccine-associated rash or disseminated disease. Vaccine administration in immunosuppressed individuals in contraindicated).
No products indexed under this heading.

Dexamethasone Sodium Phosphate Injection (Co-administration in individuals on immunosuppressant doses of corticosteroids can result in more extensive vaccine-associated rash or disseminated disease. Vaccine administration in immunosuppressed individuals in contraindicated).
No products indexed under this heading.

Diflorasone Diacetate (Co-administration in individuals on immunosuppressant doses of corticosteroids can result in more extensive vaccine-associated rash or disseminated disease. Vaccine administration in immunosuppressed individuals in contraindicated).
No products indexed under this heading.

Diflunisal (Vaccine recipients should avoid use of salicylates for 6 weeks after vaccination with Varivax because of the potential for Reye's syndrome).
No products indexed under this heading.

Fludrocortisone Acetate (Co-administration in individuals on immunosuppressant doses of corticosteroids can result in more extensive vaccine-associated rash or disseminated disease. Vaccine administration in immunosuppressed individuals in contraindicated).
No products indexed under this heading.

Flumethasone Pivalate (Co-administration in individuals on immunosuppressant doses of corticosteroids can result in more extensive vaccine-associated rash or disseminated disease. Vaccine administration in immunosuppressed individuals in contraindicated).
No products indexed under this heading.

Flunisolide Hemihydrate (Co-administration in individuals on immunosuppressant doses of corticosteroids can result in more extensive vaccine-associated rash or disseminated disease. Vaccine administration in immunosuppressed individuals in contraindicated).
No products indexed under this heading.

Fluticasone Furoate (Co-administration in individuals on immunosuppressant doses of corticosteroids can result in more extensive vaccine-associated rash or disseminated disease. Vaccine administration in immunosuppressed individuals in contraindicated). Products include:
Veramyst 1713

Fluticasone Propionate (Co-administration in individuals on immunosuppressant doses of corticosteroids can result in more extensive vaccine-associated rash or disseminated disease. Vaccine administration in immunosuppressed individuals in contraindicated). Products include:
Advair 100/50 1275
Advair 250/50 1275
Advair 500/50 1275
Advair HFA 45/21 1288
Advair HFA 115/21 1288
Advair HFA 230/21 1288
Flonase 1459
Flovent Diskus 1463
Flovent HFA 1470

Globulin, Immune (Human) (Vaccination should be deferred for at least 5 months following immune globulin administration; following administration of Varivax, immune globulin should not be given for 2 months). Products include:

Hydrocortisone (Co-administration in individuals on immunosuppressant doses of corticosteroids can result in more extensive vaccine-associated rash or disseminated disease. Vaccine administration in immunosuppressed individuals in contraindicated).
No products indexed under this heading.

Hydrocortisone (Alcohol) (Co-administration in individuals on immunosuppressant doses of corticosteroids can result in more extensive vaccine-associated rash or disseminated disease. Vaccine administration in immunosuppressed individuals in contraindicated).
No products indexed under this heading.

Hydrocortisone Acetate (Co-administration in individuals on immunosuppressant doses of corticosteroids can result in more extensive vaccine-associated rash or disseminated disease. Vaccine administration in immunosuppressed individuals in contraindicated).
No products indexed under this heading.

Hydrocortisone Butyrate (Co-administration in individuals on immunosuppressant doses of corticosteroids can result in more extensive vaccine-associated rash or disseminated disease. Vaccine administration in immunosuppressed individuals in contraindicated).
No products indexed under this heading.

Hydrocortisone Cypionate (Co-administration in individuals on immunosuppressant doses of corticosteroids can result in more extensive vaccine-associated rash or disseminated disease. Vaccine administration in immunosuppressed individuals in contraindicated).
No products indexed under this heading.

Hydrocortisone Hemisuccinate (Co-administration in individuals on immunosuppressant doses of corticosteroids can result in more extensive vaccine-associated rash or disseminated disease. Vaccine administration in immunosuppressed individuals in contraindicated).
No products indexed under this heading.

Hydrocortisone Probutate (Co-administration in individuals on immunosuppressant doses of corticosteroids can result in more extensive vaccine-associated rash or disseminated disease. Vaccine administration in immunosuppressed individuals in contraindicated).
No products indexed under this heading.

Hydrocortisone Sodium Phosphate (Co-administration in individuals on immunosuppressant doses of corticosteroids can result in more extensive vaccine-associated rash or disseminated disease. Vaccine administration in immunosuppressed individuals in contraindicated).
No products indexed under this heading.

Hydrocortisone Sodium Succinate (Co-administration in individuals on immunosuppressant doses of corticosteroids can result in more extensive vaccine-associated rash or disseminated disease. Vaccine administration in immunosuppressed individuals in contraindicated).
No products indexed under this heading.

(⊙ Described in PDR® for Ophthalmic Medicines)

2017 **Interactions Index** **Vectibix**

Hydrocortisone Valerate (Co-administration in individuals on immunosuppressant doses of corticosteroids can result in more extensive vaccine-associated rash or disseminated disease. Vaccine administration in immunosuppressed individuals in contraindicated).
No products indexed under this heading.

Magnesium Salicylate (Vaccine recipients should avoid use of salicylates for 6 weeks after vaccination with Varivax because of the potential for Reye's syndrome).
No products indexed under this heading.

Methylprednisolone (Co-administration in individuals on immunosuppressant doses of corticosteroids can result in more extensive vaccine-associated rash or disseminated disease. Vaccine administration in immunosuppressed individuals in contraindicated).
No products indexed under this heading.

Methylprednisolone Acetate (Co-administration in individuals on immunosuppressant doses of corticosteroids can result in more extensive vaccine-associated rash or disseminated disease. Vaccine administration in immunosuppressed individuals in contraindicated).
No products indexed under this heading.

Methylprednisolone Sodium Succinate (Co-administration in individuals on immunosuppressant doses of corticosteroids can result in more extensive vaccine-associated rash or disseminated disease. Vaccine administration in immunosuppressed individuals in contraindicated).
No products indexed under this heading.

Mometasone Furoate (Co-administration in individuals on immunosuppressant doses of corticosteroids can result in more extensive vaccine-associated rash or disseminated disease. Vaccine administration in immunosuppressed individuals in contraindicated). Products include:
Asmanex 3058
Elocon Cream 3111
Elocon Lotion 3112
Elocon Ointment 3114

Mometasone Furoate Monohydrate (Co-administration in individuals on immunosuppressant doses of corticosteroids can result in more extensive vaccine-associated rash or disseminated disease. Vaccine administration in immunosuppressed individuals in contraindicated). Products include:
Nasonex 3166

Muromonab-CD3 (Concurrent use in individuals who are on immunosuppressant drugs can result in greater susceptibility to infections; co-administration is contraindicated). Products include:
Orthoclone OKT3 949

Mycophenolate Mofetil (Concurrent use in individuals who are on immunosuppressant drugs can result in greater susceptibility to infections; co-administration is contraindicated).
No products indexed under this heading.

Prednisolone (Co-administration in individuals on immunosuppressant doses of corticosteroids can result in more extensive vaccine-associated rash or disseminated disease. Vaccine administration in immunosuppressed individuals in contraindicated).
No products indexed under this heading.

Prednisolone Acetate (Co-administration in individuals on immunosuppressant doses of corticosteroids can result in more extensive vaccine-associated rash or disseminated disease. Vaccine administration in immunosuppressed individuals in contraindicated). Products include:
Blephamide .... ⊙212, ⊙214
Pred Forte .... ⊙225
Pred Mild .... ⊙230
Pred-G .... ⊙226, ⊙227

Prednisolone Sodium Phosphate (Co-administration in individuals on immunosuppressant doses of corticosteroids can result in more extensive vaccine-associated rash or disseminated disease. Vaccine administration in immunosuppressed individuals in contraindicated).
No products indexed under this heading.

Prednisolone Tebutate (Co-administration in individuals on immunosuppressant doses of corticosteroids can result in more extensive vaccine-associated rash or disseminated disease. Vaccine administration in immunosuppressed individuals in contraindicated).
No products indexed under this heading.

Prednisone (Co-administration in individuals on immunosuppressant doses of corticosteroids can result in more extensive vaccine-associated rash or disseminated disease. Vaccine administration in immunosuppressed individuals in contraindicated).
No products indexed under this heading.

Prednisone sodium phosphate (Co-administration in individuals on immunosuppressant doses of corticosteroids can result in more extensive vaccine-associated rash or disseminated disease. Vaccine administration in immunosuppressed individuals in contraindicated).
No products indexed under this heading.

Salsalate (Vaccine recipients should avoid use of salicylates for 6 weeks after vaccination with Varivax because of the potential for Reye's syndrome).
No products indexed under this heading.

Tacrolimus (Concurrent use in individuals who are on immunosuppressant drugs can result in greater susceptibility to infections; co-administration is contraindicated). Products include:
Prograf Capsules 677
Prograf Injection 677
Protopic 685

Triamcinolone (Co-administration in individuals on immunosuppressant doses of corticosteroids can result in more extensive vaccine-associated rash or disseminated disease. Vaccine administration in immunosuppressed individuals in contraindicated).
No products indexed under this heading.

Triamcinolone Acetonide (Co-administration in individuals on immunosuppressant doses of corticosteroids can result in more extensive vaccine-associated rash or disseminated disease. Vaccine administration in immunosuppressed individuals in contraindicated). Products include:
Azmacort 408
Nasacort AQ 3019

Triamcinolone Diacetate (Co-administration in individuals on immunosuppressant doses of corticosteroids can result in more extensive vaccine-associated rash or disseminated disease. Vaccine administration in immunosuppressed individuals in contraindicated).
No products indexed under this heading.

Triamcinolone Hexacetonide (Co-administration in individuals on immunosuppressant doses of corticosteroids can result in more extensive vaccine-associated rash or disseminated disease. Vaccine administration in immunosuppressed individuals in contraindicated).
No products indexed under this heading.

VECTIBIX INJECTION FOR INTRAVENOUS USE
(Panitumumab) 643

May interact with antineoplastics, and certain other agents. Compounds in these categories include:

Altretamine (The addition of panitumumab to the combination of bevacizumab and chemotherapy resulted in decreased overall survival and increased incidence of NCI-CTC grade 3-5 (87% vs 72%) adverse reactions. In a single-arm study of 19 patients receiving panitumumab in combination with IFL (Irinotecan, Leucovorin and Fluorouracil), the incidence of NCI-CTC grade 3–4 diarrhea was 58%; in addition, grade 5 diarrhea occurred in one patient. In a single-arm study of 24 patients receiving panitumumab plus FOLFIRI (Leucovorin, Fluorouracil and Irinotecan), the incidence of NCI-CTC grade 3 diarrhea was 25%). Products include:
Hexalen 1066

Anastrozole (The addition of panitumumab to the combination of bevacizumab and chemotherapy resulted in decreased overall survival and increased incidence of NCI-CTC grade 3-5 (87% vs 72%) adverse reactions. In a single-arm study of 19 patients receiving panitumumab in combination with IFL (Irinotecan, Leucovorin and Fluorouracil), the incidence of NCI-CTC grade 3–4 diarrhea was 58%; in addition, grade 5 diarrhea occurred in one patient. In a single-arm study of 24 patients receiving panitumumab plus FOLFIRI (Leucovorin, Fluorouracil and Irinotecan), the incidence of NCI-CTC grade 3 diarrhea was 25%).
No products indexed under this heading.

Asparaginase (The addition of panitumumab to the combination of bevacizumab and chemotherapy resulted in decreased overall survival and increased incidence of NCI-CTC grade 3-5 (87% vs 72%) adverse reactions. In a single-arm study of 19 patients receiving panitumumab in combination with IFL (Irinotecan, Leucovorin and Fluorouracil), the incidence of NCI-CTC grade 3–4 diarrhea was 58%; in addition, grade 5 diarrhea occurred in one patient. In a single-arm study of 24 patients receiving panitumumab plus FOLFIRI (Leucovorin, Fluorouracil and Irinotecan), the incidence of NCI-CTC grade 3 diarrhea was 25%). Products include:
Elspar 2005, 2122

Bevacizumab (The addition of panitumumab to the combination of bevacizumab and chemotherapy resulted in decreased overall survival and increased incidence of NCI-CTC grade 3-5 (87% vs 72%) adverse reactions). Products include:
Avastin 1187

Bicalutamide (The addition of panitumumab to the combination of bevacizumab and chemotherapy resulted in decreased overall survival and increased incidence of NCI-CTC grade 3-5 (87% vs 72%) adverse reactions. In a single-arm study of 19 patients receiving panitumumab in combination with IFL (Irinotecan, Leucovorin and Fluorouracil), the incidence of NCI-CTC grade 3–4 diarrhea was 58%; in addition, grade 5 diarrhea occurred in one patient. In a single-arm study of 24 patients receiving panitumumab plus FOLFIRI (Leucovorin, Fluorouracil and Irinotecan), the incidence of NCI-CTC grade 3 diarrhea was 25%).
No products indexed under this heading.

Bleomycin Sulfate (The addition of panitumumab to the combination of bevacizumab and chemotherapy resulted in decreased overall survival and increased incidence of NCI-CTC grade 3-5 (87% vs 72%) adverse reactions. In a single-arm study of 19 patients receiving panitumumab in combination with IFL (Irinotecan, Leucovorin and Fluorouracil), the incidence of NCI-CTC grade 3–4 diarrhea was 58%; in addition, grade 5 diarrhea occurred in one patient. In a single-arm study of 24 patients receiving panitumumab plus FOLFIRI (Leucovorin, Fluorouracil and Irinotecan), the incidence of NCI-CTC grade 3 diarrhea was 25%).
No products indexed under this heading.

Busulfan (The addition of panitumumab to the combination of bevacizumab and chemotherapy resulted in decreased overall survival and increased incidence of NCI-CTC grade 3-5 (87% vs 72%) adverse reactions. In a single-arm study of 19 patients receiving panitumumab in combination with IFL (Irinotecan, Leucovorin and Fluorouracil), the incidence of NCI-CTC grade 3–4 diarrhea was 58%; in addition, grade 5 diarrhea occurred in one patient. In a single-arm study of 24 patients receiving panitumumab plus FOLFIRI (Leucovorin, Fluorouracil and Irinotecan), the incidence of NCI-CTC grade 3 diarrhea was 25%). Products include:
Myleran 1581

Carboplatin (The addition of panitumumab to the combination of bevacizumab and chemotherapy resulted in decreased overall survival and increased incidence of NCI-CTC grade 3-5 (87% vs 72%) adverse reactions. In a single-arm study of 19 patients receiving panitumumab in combination with IFL (Irinotecan, Leucovorin and Fluorouracil), the incidence of NCI-CTC grade 3–4 diarrhea was 58%; in addition, grade 5 diarrhea occurred in one patient. In a single-arm study of 24 patients receiving panitumumab plus FOLFIRI (Leucovorin, Fluorouracil and Irinotecan), the incidence of NCI-CTC grade 3 diarrhea was 25%).
No products indexed under this heading.

Carmustine (BCNU) (The addition of panitumumab to the combination of bevacizumab and chemotherapy resulted in decreased overall survival and increased incidence of NCI-CTC grade 3-5 (87% vs 72%) adverse reactions. In a single-arm study of 19 patients receiving panitumumab in combination with IFL (Irinotecan, Leucovorin and Fluorouracil), the incidence of NCI-CTC grade 3–4 diarrhea was 58%; in addition, grade 5 diarrhea occurred in one patient. In a single-arm study of 24 patients receiving panitumumab plus FOLFIRI (Leucovorin, Fluorouracil and Irinotecan), the incidence of NCI-CTC grade 3 diarrhea was 25%).
No products indexed under this heading.

Chlorambucil (The addition of panitumumab to the combination of bevacizumab and chemotherapy resulted in decreased overall survival and increased incidence of NCI-CTC grade 3-5 (87% vs 72%) adverse reactions. In a single-arm study of 19 patients receiving panitumumab in combination with IFL (Irinotecan, Leucovorin and Fluorouracil), the incidence of NCI-CTC grade 3–4 diarrhea was 58%; in addition, grade 5 diarrhea occurred in one patient. In a single-arm study of 24 patients receiving panitumumab plus FOLFIRI (Leucovorin, Fluorouracil and Irinotecan), the incidence of NCI-CTC grade 3 diarrhea was 25%). Products include:
Leukeran 1557

Cisplatin (The addition of panitumumab to the combination of bevacizumab and chemotherapy resulted in decreased overall survival and increased incidence of NCI-CTC grade 3-5 (87% vs 72%) adverse reactions. In a single-arm study of 19 patients receiving panitumumab in combination with IFL (Irinotecan, Leucovorin and Fluoro-

uracil), the incidence of NCI-CTC grade 3–4 diarrhea was 58%; in addition, grade 5 diarrhea occurred in one patient. In a single-arm study of 24 patients receiving panitumumab plus FOLFIRI (Leucovorin, Fluorouracil and Irinotecan), the incidence of NCI-CTC grade 3 diarrhea was 25%).
No products indexed under this heading.

Cyclophosphamide (The addition of panitumumab to the combination of bevacizumab and chemotherapy resulted in decreased overall survival and increased incidence of NCI-CTC grade 3-5 (87% vs 72%) adverse reactions. In a single-arm study of 19 patients receiving panitumumab in combination with IFL (Irinotecan, Leucovorin and Fluorouracil), the incidence of NCI-CTC grade 3–4 diarrhea was 58%; in addition, grade 5 diarrhea occurred in one patient. In a single-arm study of 24 patients receiving panitumumab plus FOLFIRI (Leucovorin, Fluorouracil and Irinotecan), the incidence of NCI-CTC grade 3 diarrhea was 25%).
No products indexed under this heading.

Dacarbazine (The addition of panitumumab to the combination of bevacizumab and chemotherapy resulted in decreased overall survival and increased incidence of NCI-CTC grade 3-5 (87% vs 72%) adverse reactions. In a single-arm study of 19 patients receiving panitumumab in combination with IFL (Irinotecan, Leucovorin and Fluorouracil), the incidence of NCI-CTC grade 3–4 diarrhea was 58%; in addition, grade 5 diarrhea occurred in one patient. In a single-arm study of 24 patients receiving panitumumab plus FOLFIRI (Leucovorin, Fluorouracil and Irinotecan), the incidence of NCI-CTC grade 3 diarrhea was 25%).
No products indexed under this heading.

Daunorubicin Citrate (The addition of panitumumab to the combination of bevacizumab and chemotherapy resulted in decreased overall survival and increased incidence of NCI-CTC grade 3-5 (87% vs 72%) adverse reactions. In a single-arm study of 19 patients receiving panitumumab in combination with IFL (Irinotecan, Leucovorin and Fluorouracil), the incidence of NCI-CTC grade 3–4 diarrhea was 58%; in addition, grade 5 diarrhea occurred in one patient. In a single-arm study of 24 patients receiving panitumumab plus FOLFIRI (Leucovorin, Fluorouracil and Irinotecan), the incidence of NCI-CTC grade 3 diarrhea was 25%).
No products indexed under this heading.

Daunorubicin Hydrochloride (The addition of panitumumab to the combination of bevacizumab and chemotherapy resulted in decreased overall survival and increased incidence of NCI-CTC grade 3-5 (87% vs 72%) adverse reactions. In a single-arm study of 19 patients receiving panitumumab in combination with IFL (Irinotecan, Leucovorin and Fluorouracil), the incidence of NCI-CTC grade 3–4 diarrhea was 58%; in addition, grade 5 diarrhea occurred in one patient. In a single-arm study of 24 patients receiving panitumumab plus FOLFIRI (Leucovorin, Fluorouracil and Irinotecan), the incidence of NCI-CTC grade 3 diarrhea was 25%).
No products indexed under this heading.

Denileukin Diftitox (The addition of panitumumab to the combination of bevacizumab and chemotherapy resulted in decreased overall survival and increased incidence of NCI-CTC grade 3-5 (87% vs 72%) adverse reactions. In a single-arm study of 19 patients receiving panitumumab in combination with IFL (Irinotecan, Leucovorin and Fluorouracil), the incidence of NCI-CTC grade 3–4 diarrhea was 58%; in addition, grade 5 diarrhea occurred in one patient. In a single-arm study of 24 patients receiving panitumumab plus FOLFIRI (Leucovorin, Fluorouracil and Irinotecan), the incidence of NCI-CTC grade 3 diarrhea was 25%). Products include:
Ontak 1068

Docetaxel (The addition of panitumumab to the combination of bevacizumab and chemotherapy resulted in decreased overall survival and increased incidence of NCI-CTC grade 3-5 (87% vs 72%) adverse reactions. In a single-arm study of 19 patients receiving panitumumab in combination with IFL (Irinotecan, Leucovorin and Fluorouracil), the incidence of NCI-CTC grade 3–4 diarrhea was 58%; in addition, grade 5 diarrhea occurred in one patient. In a single-arm study of 24 patients receiving panitumumab plus FOLFIRI (Leucovorin, Fluorouracil and Irinotecan), the incidence of NCI-CTC grade 3 diarrhea was 25%). Products include:
Taxotere 3035

Doxorubicin Hydrochloride (The addition of panitumumab to the combination of bevacizumab and chemotherapy resulted in decreased overall survival and increased incidence of NCI-CTC grade 3-5 (87% vs 72%) adverse reactions. In a single-arm study of 19 patients receiving panitumumab in combination with IFL (Irinotecan, Leucovorin and Fluorouracil), the incidence of NCI-CTC grade 3–4 diarrhea was 58%; in addition, grade 5 diarrhea occurred in one patient. In a single-arm study of 24 patients receiving panitumumab plus FOLFIRI (Leucovorin, Fluorouracil and Irinotecan), the incidence of NCI-CTC grade 3 diarrhea was 25%).
No products indexed under this heading.

Epirubicin Hydrochloride (The addition of panitumumab to the combination of bevacizumab and chemotherapy resulted in decreased overall survival and increased incidence of NCI-CTC grade 3-5 (87% vs 72%) adverse reactions. In a single-arm study of 19 patients receiving panitumumab in combination with IFL (Irinotecan, Leucovorin and Fluorouracil), the incidence of NCI-CTC grade 3–4 diarrhea was 58%; in addition, grade 5 diarrhea occurred in one patient. In a single-arm study of 24 patients receiving panitumumab plus FOLFIRI (Leucovorin, Fluorouracil and Irinotecan), the incidence of NCI-CTC grade 3 diarrhea was 25%).
No products indexed under this heading.

Estramustine Phosphate Sodium (The addition of panitumumab to the combination of bevacizumab and chemotherapy resulted in decreased overall survival and increased incidence of NCI-CTC grade 3-5 (87% vs 72%) adverse reactions. In a single-arm study of 19 patients receiving panitumumab in combination with IFL (Irinotecan, Leucovorin and Fluorouracil), the incidence of NCI-CTC grade 3–4 diarrhea was 58%; in addition, grade 5 diarrhea occurred in one patient. In a single-arm study of 24 patients receiving panitumumab plus FOLFIRI (Leucovorin, Fluorouracil and Irinotecan), the incidence of NCI-CTC grade 3 diarrhea was 25%).
No products indexed under this heading.

Etoposide (The addition of panitumumab to the combination of bevacizumab and chemotherapy resulted in decreased overall survival and increased incidence of NCI-CTC grade 3-5 (87% vs 72%) adverse reactions. In a single-arm study of 19 patients receiving panitumumab in combination with IFL (Irinotecan, Leucovorin and Fluorouracil), the incidence of NCI-CTC grade 3–4 diarrhea was 58%; in addition, grade 5 diarrhea occurred in one patient. In a single-arm study of 24 patients receiving panitumumab plus FOLFIRI (Leucovorin, Fluorouracil and Irinotecan), the incidence of NCI-CTC grade 3 diarrhea was 25%).
No products indexed under this heading.

Exemestane (The addition of panitumumab to the combination of bevacizumab and chemotherapy resulted in decreased overall survival and increased incidence of NCI-CTC grade 3-5 (87% vs 72%) adverse reactions. In a single-arm study of 19 patients receiving panitumumab in combination with IFL (Irinotecan, Leucovorin and Fluorouracil), the incidence of NCI-CTC grade 3–4 diarrhea was 58%; in addition, grade 5 diarrhea occurred in one patient. In a single-arm study of 24 patients receiving panitumumab plus FOLFIRI (Leucovorin, Fluorouracil and Irinotecan), the incidence of NCI-CTC grade 3 diarrhea was 25%). Products include:
Aromasin 2758

Floxuridine (The addition of panitumumab to the combination of bevacizumab and chemotherapy resulted in decreased overall survival and increased incidence of NCI-CTC grade 3-5 (87% vs 72%) adverse reactions. In a single-arm study of 19 patients receiving panitumumab in combination with IFL (Irinotecan, Leucovorin and Fluorouracil), the incidence of NCI-CTC grade 3–4 diarrhea was 58%; in addition, grade 5 diarrhea occurred in one patient. In a single-arm study of 24 patients receiving panitumumab plus FOLFIRI (Leucovorin, Fluorouracil and Irinotecan), the incidence of NCI-CTC grade 3 diarrhea was 25%).
No products indexed under this heading.

Fluorouracil (The addition of panitumumab to the combination of bevacizumab and chemotherapy resulted in decreased overall survival and increased incidence of NCI-CTC grade 3-5 (87% vs 72%) adverse reactions. In a single-arm study of 19 patients receiving panitumumab in combination with IFL (Irinotecan, Leucovorin and Fluorouracil), the incidence of NCI-CTC grade 3–4 diarrhea was 58%; in addition, grade 5 diarrhea occurred in one patient. In a single-arm study of 24 patients receiving panitumumab plus FOLFIRI (Leucovorin, Fluorouracil and Irinotecan), the incidence of NCI-CTC grade 3 diarrhea was 25%). Products include:
Carac 2966

Fluorouracil, Topical (The addition of panitumumab to the combination of bevacizumab and chemotherapy resulted in decreased overall survival and increased incidence of NCI-CTC grade 3-5 (87% vs 72%) adverse reactions. In a single-arm study of 19 patients receiving panitumumab in combination with IFL (Irinotecan, Leucovorin and Fluorouracil), the incidence of NCI-CTC grade 3–4 diarrhea was 58%; in addition, grade 5 diarrhea occurred in one patient. In a single-arm study of 24 patients receiving panitumumab plus FOLFIRI (Leucovorin, Fluorouracil and Irinotecan), the incidence of NCI-CTC grade 3 diarrhea was 25%).
No products indexed under this heading.

Flutamide (The addition of panitumumab to the combination of bevacizumab and chemotherapy resulted in decreased overall survival and increased incidence of NCI-CTC grade 3-5 (87% vs 72%) adverse reactions. In a single-arm study of 19 patients receiving panitumumab in combination with IFL (Irinotecan, Leucovorin and Fluorouracil), the incidence of NCI-CTC grade 3–4 diarrhea was 58%; in addition, grade 5 diarrhea occurred in one patient. In a single-arm study of 24 patients receiving panitumumab plus FOLFIRI (Leucovorin, Fluorouracil and Irinotecan), the incidence of NCI-CTC grade 3 diarrhea was 25%).
No products indexed under this heading.

Gemcitabine Hydrochloride (The addition of panitumumab to the combination of bevacizumab and chemotherapy resulted in decreased overall survival and increased incidence of NCI-CTC grade 3-5 (87% vs 72%) adverse reactions. In a single-arm study of 19 patients receiving panitumumab in combination with IFL (Irinotecan, Leucovorin and Fluorouracil), the incidence of NCI-CTC grade 3–4 diarrhea was 58%; in addition, grade 5 diarrhea occurred in one patient. In a single-arm study of 24 patients receiving panitumumab plus FOLFIRI (Leucovorin, Fluorouracil and Irinotecan), the incidence of NCI-CTC grade 3 diarrhea was 25%). Products include:
Gemzar 1900

Hydroxyurea (The addition of panitumumab to the combination of bevacizumab and chemotherapy resulted in decreased overall survival and increased incidence of NCI-CTC grade 3-5 (87% vs 72%) adverse reactions. In a single-arm study of 19 patients receiving panitumumab in combination with IFL (Irinotecan, Leucovorin and Fluorouracil), the incidence of NCI-CTC grade 3–4 diarrhea was 58%; in addition, grade 5 diarrhea occurred in one patient. In a single-arm study of 24 patients receiving panitumumab plus FOLFIRI (Leucovorin, Fluorouracil and Irinotecan), the incidence of NCI-CTC grade 3 diarrhea was 25%).
No products indexed under this heading.

Idarubicin Hydrochloride (The addition of panitumumab to the combination of bevacizumab and chemotherapy resulted in decreased overall survival and increased incidence of NCI-CTC grade 3-5 (87% vs 72%) adverse reactions. In a single-arm study of 19 patients receiving panitumumab in combination with IFL (Irinotecan, Leucovorin and Fluorouracil), the incidence of NCI-CTC grade 3–4 diarrhea was 58%; in addition, grade 5 diarrhea occurred in one patient. In a single-arm study of 24 patients receiving panitumumab plus FOLFIRI (Leucovorin, Fluorouracil and Irinotecan), the incidence of NCI-CTC grade 3 diarrhea was 25%).
No products indexed under this heading.

Ifosfamide (The addition of panitumumab to the combination of bevacizumab and chemotherapy resulted in decreased overall survival and increased incidence of NCI-CTC grade 3-5 (87% vs 72%) adverse reactions. In a single-arm study of 19 patients receiving panitumumab in combination with IFL (Irinotecan, Leucovorin and Fluorouracil), the incidence of NCI-CTC grade 3–4 diarrhea was 58%; in addition, grade 5 diarrhea occurred in one patient. In a single-arm study of 24 patients receiving panitumumab plus FOLFIRI (Leucovorin, Fluorouracil and Irinotecan), the incidence of NCI-CTC grade 3 diarrhea was 25%).
No products indexed under this heading.

Interferon alfa-2a, Recombinant (The addition of panitumumab to the combination of bevacizumab and chemotherapy resulted in decreased overall survival and increased incidence of NCI-CTC grade 3-5 (87% vs 72%) adverse reactions. In a single-arm study of 19 patients receiving panitumumab in combination with IFL (Irinotecan, Leucovorin and Fluorouracil), the incidence of NCI-CTC grade 3–4 diarrhea was 58%; in addition, grade 5 diarrhea occurred in one patient. In a single-arm study of 24 patients receiving panitumumab plus

2019 Interactions Index Vectibix

FOLFIRI (Leucovorin, Fluorouracil and Irinotecan), the incidence of NCI-CTC grade 3 diarrhea was 25%).
No products indexed under this heading.

Interferon alfa-2b, Recombinant (The addition of panitumumab to the combination of bevacizumab and chemotherapy resulted in decreased overall survival and increased incidence of NCI-CTC grade 3-5 (87% vs 72%) adverse reactions. In a single-arm study of 19 patients receiving panitumumab in combination with IFL (Irinotecan, Leucovorin and Fluorouracil), the incidence of NCI-CTC grade 3–4 diarrhea was 58%; in addition, grade 5 diarrhea occurred in one patient. In a single-arm study of 24 patients receiving panitumumab plus FOLFIRI (Leucovorin, Fluorouracil and Irinotecan), the incidence of NCI-CTC grade 3 diarrhea was 25%). Products include:
Intron A 3140

Irinotecan Hydrochloride (The addition of panitumumab to the combination of bevacizumab and chemotherapy resulted in decreased overall survival and increased incidence of NCI-CTC grade 3-5 (87% vs 72%) adverse reactions. In a single-arm study of 19 patients receiving panitumumab in combination with IFL (Irinotecan, Leucovorin and Fluorouracil), the incidence of NCI-CTC grade 3–4 diarrhea was 58%; in addition, grade 5 diarrhea occurred in one patient. In a single-arm study of 24 patients receiving panitumumab plus FOLFIRI (Leucovorin, Fluorouracil and Irinotecan), the incidence of NCI-CTC grade 3 diarrhea was 25%).
No products indexed under this heading.

Leucovorin Calcium (The addition of panitumumab to the combination of bevacizumab and chemotherapy resulted in decreased overall survival and increased incidence of NCI-CTC grade 3-5 (87% vs 72%) adverse reactions. In a single-arm study of 19 patients receiving panitumumab in combination with IFL (Irinotecan, Leucovorin and Fluorouracil), the incidence of NCI-CTC grade 3–4 diarrhea was 58%; in addition, grade 5 diarrhea occurred in one patient. In a single-arm study of 24 patients receiving panitumumab plus FOLFIRI (Leucovorin, Fluorouracil and Irinotecan), the incidence of NCI-CTC grade 3 diarrhea was 25%).
No products indexed under this heading.

Levamisole Hydrochloride (The addition of panitumumab to the combination of bevacizumab and chemotherapy resulted in decreased overall survival and increased incidence of NCI-CTC grade 3-5 (87% vs 72%) adverse reactions. In a single-arm study of 19 patients receiving panitumumab in combination with IFL (Irinotecan, Leucovorin and Fluorouracil), the incidence of NCI-CTC grade 3–4 diarrhea was 58%; in addition, grade 5 diarrhea occurred in one patient. In a single-arm study of 24 patients receiving panitumumab plus FOLFIRI (Leucovorin, Fluorouracil and Irinotecan), the incidence of NCI-CTC grade 3 diarrhea was 25%).
No products indexed under this heading.

Lomustine (CCNU) (The addition of panitumumab to the combination of bevacizumab and chemotherapy resulted in decreased overall survival and increased incidence of NCI-CTC grade 3-5 (87% vs 72%) adverse reactions. In a single-arm study of 19 patients receiving panitumumab in combination with IFL (Irinotecan, Leucovorin and Fluorouracil), the incidence of NCI-CTC grade 3–4 diarrhea was 58%; in addition, grade 5 diarrhea occurred in one patient. In a single-arm study of 24 patients receiving panitumumab plus FOLFIRI (Leucovorin, Fluorouracil and Irinotecan), the incidence of NCI-CTC grade 3 diarrhea was 25%).
No products indexed under this heading.

Mechlorethamine Hydrochloride (The addition of panitumumab to the combination of bevacizumab and chemotherapy resulted in decreased overall survival and increased incidence of NCI-CTC grade 3-5 (87% vs 72%) adverse reactions. In a single-arm study of 19 patients receiving panitumumab in combination with IFL (Irinotecan, Leucovorin and Fluorouracil), the incidence of NCI-CTC grade 3–4 diarrhea was 58%; in addition, grade 5 diarrhea occurred in one patient. In a single-arm study of 24 patients receiving panitumumab plus FOLFIRI (Leucovorin, Fluorouracil and Irinotecan), the incidence of NCI-CTC grade 3 diarrhea was 25%). Products include:
Mustargen 2010

Megestrol Acetate (The addition of panitumumab to the combination of bevacizumab and chemotherapy resulted in decreased overall survival and increased incidence of NCI-CTC grade 3-5 (87% vs 72%) adverse reactions. In a single-arm study of 19 patients receiving panitumumab in combination with IFL (Irinotecan, Leucovorin and Fluorouracil), the incidence of NCI-CTC grade 3–4 diarrhea was 58%; in addition, grade 5 diarrhea occurred in one patient. In a single-arm study of 24 patients receiving panitumumab plus FOLFIRI (Leucovorin, Fluorouracil and Irinotecan), the incidence of NCI-CTC grade 3 diarrhea was 25%). Products include:
Megace ES 2698

Melphalan (The addition of panitumumab to the combination of bevacizumab and chemotherapy resulted in decreased overall survival and increased incidence of NCI-CTC grade 3-5 (87% vs 72%) adverse reactions. In a single-arm study of 19 patients receiving panitumumab in combination with IFL (Irinotecan, Leucovorin and Fluorouracil), the incidence of NCI-CTC grade 3–4 diarrhea was 58%; in addition, grade 5 diarrhea occurred in one patient. In a single-arm study of 24 patients receiving panitumumab plus FOLFIRI (Leucovorin, Fluorouracil and Irinotecan), the incidence of NCI-CTC grade 3 diarrhea was 25%). Products include:
Alkeran 1302

Mercaptopurine (The addition of panitumumab to the combination of bevacizumab and chemotherapy resulted in decreased overall survival and increased incidence of NCI-CTC grade 3-5 (87% vs 72%) adverse reactions. In a single-arm study of 19 patients receiving panitumumab in combination with IFL (Irinotecan, Leucovorin and Fluorouracil), the incidence of NCI-CTC grade 3–4 diarrhea was 58%; in addition, grade 5 diarrhea occurred in one patient. In a single-arm study of 24 patients receiving panitumumab plus FOLFIRI (Leucovorin, Fluorouracil and Irinotecan), the incidence of NCI-CTC grade 3 diarrhea was 25%).
No products indexed under this heading.

Methotrexate (The addition of panitumumab to the combination of bevacizumab and chemotherapy resulted in decreased overall survival and increased incidence of NCI-CTC grade 3-5 (87% vs 72%) adverse reactions. In a single-arm study of 19 patients receiving panitumumab in combination with IFL (Irinotecan, Leucovorin and Fluorouracil), the incidence of NCI-CTC grade 3–4 diarrhea was 58%; in addition, grade 5 diarrhea occurred in one patient. In a single-arm study of 24 patients receiving panitumumab plus FOLFIRI (Leucovorin, Fluorouracil and Irinotecan), the incidence of NCI-CTC grade 3 diarrhea was 25%).
No products indexed under this heading.

Methotrexate Sodium (The addition of panitumumab to the combination of bevacizumab and chemotherapy resulted in decreased overall survival and increased incidence of NCI-CTC grade 3-5 (87% vs 72%) adverse reactions. In a single-arm study of 19 patients receiving panitumumab in combination with IFL (Irinotecan, Leucovorin and Fluorouracil), the incidence of NCI-CTC grade 3–4 diarrhea was 58%; in addition, grade 5 diarrhea occurred in one patient. In a single-arm study of 24 patients receiving panitumumab plus FOLFIRI (Leucovorin, Fluorouracil and Irinotecan), the incidence of NCI-CTC grade 3 diarrhea was 25%).
No products indexed under this heading.

Mitomycin (Mitomycin-C) (The addition of panitumumab to the combination of bevacizumab and chemotherapy resulted in decreased overall survival and increased incidence of NCI-CTC grade 3-5 (87% vs 72%) adverse reactions. In a single-arm study of 19 patients receiving panitumumab in combination with IFL (Irinotecan, Leucovorin and Fluorouracil), the incidence of NCI-CTC grade 3–4 diarrhea was 58%; in addition, grade 5 diarrhea occurred in one patient. In a single-arm study of 24 patients receiving panitumumab plus FOLFIRI (Leucovorin, Fluorouracil and Irinotecan), the incidence of NCI-CTC grade 3 diarrhea was 25%).
No products indexed under this heading.

Mitotane (The addition of panitumumab to the combination of bevacizumab and chemotherapy resulted in decreased overall survival and increased incidence of NCI-CTC grade 3-5 (87% vs 72%) adverse reactions. In a single-arm study of 19 patients receiving panitumumab in combination with IFL (Irinotecan, Leucovorin and Fluorouracil), the incidence of NCI-CTC grade 3–4 diarrhea was 58%; in addition, grade 5 diarrhea occurred in one patient. In a single-arm study of 24 patients receiving panitumumab plus FOLFIRI (Leucovorin, Fluorouracil and Irinotecan), the incidence of NCI-CTC grade 3 diarrhea was 25%).
No products indexed under this heading.

Mitoxantrone Hydrochloride (The addition of panitumumab to the combination of bevacizumab and chemotherapy resulted in decreased overall survival and increased incidence of NCI-CTC grade 3-5 (87% vs 72%) adverse reactions. In a single-arm study of 19 patients receiving panitumumab in combination with IFL (Irinotecan, Leucovorin and Fluorouracil), the incidence of NCI-CTC grade 3–4 diarrhea was 58%; in addition, grade 5 diarrhea occurred in one patient. In a single-arm study of 24 patients receiving panitumumab plus FOLFIRI (Leucovorin, Fluorouracil and Irinotecan), the incidence of NCI-CTC grade 3 diarrhea was 25%). Products include:
Novantrone 1088

Oxaliplatin (The addition of panitumumab to the combination of bevacizumab and chemotherapy resulted in decreased overall survival and increased incidence of NCI-CTC grade 3-5 (87% vs 72%) adverse reactions. In a single-arm study of 19 patients receiving panitumumab in combination with IFL (Irinotecan, Leucovorin and Fluorouracil), the incidence of NCI-CTC grade 3–4 diarrhea was 58%; in addition, grade 5 diarrhea occurred in one patient. In a single-arm study of 24 patients receiving panitumumab plus FOLFIRI (Leucovorin, Fluorouracil and Irinotecan), the incidence of NCI-CTC grade 3 diarrhea was 25%). Products include:
Eloxatin 2975

Paclitaxel (The addition of panitumumab to the combination of bevacizumab and chemotherapy resulted in decreased overall survival and increased incidence of NCI-CTC grade 3-5 (87% vs 72%) adverse reactions. In a single-arm study of 19 patients receiving panitumumab in combination with IFL (Irinotecan, Leucovorin and Fluorouracil), the incidence of NCI-CTC grade 3–4 diarrhea was 58%; in addition, grade 5 diarrhea occurred in one patient. In a single-arm study of 24 patients receiving panitumumab plus FOLFIRI (Leucovorin, Fluorouracil and Irinotecan), the incidence of NCI-CTC grade 3 diarrhea was 25%).
No products indexed under this heading.

Procarbazine Hydrochloride (The addition of panitumumab to the combination of bevacizumab and chemotherapy resulted in decreased overall survival and increased incidence of NCI-CTC grade 3-5 (87% vs 72%) adverse reactions. In a single-arm study of 19 patients receiving panitumumab in combination with IFL (Irinotecan, Leucovorin and Fluorouracil), the incidence of NCI-CTC grade 3–4 diarrhea was 58%; in addition, grade 5 diarrhea occurred in one patient. In a single-arm study of 24 patients receiving panitumumab plus FOLFIRI (Leucovorin, Fluorouracil and Irinotecan), the incidence of NCI-CTC grade 3 diarrhea was 25%).
No products indexed under this heading.

Streptozocin (The addition of panitumumab to the combination of bevacizumab and chemotherapy resulted in decreased overall survival and increased incidence of NCI-CTC grade 3-5 (87% vs 72%) adverse reactions. In a single-arm study of 19 patients receiving panitumumab in combination with IFL (Irinotecan, Leucovorin and Fluorouracil), the incidence of NCI-CTC grade 3–4 diarrhea was 58%; in addition, grade 5 diarrhea occurred in one patient. In a single-arm study of 24 patients receiving panitumumab plus FOLFIRI (Leucovorin, Fluorouracil and Irinotecan), the incidence of NCI-CTC grade 3 diarrhea was 25%).
No products indexed under this heading.

Tamoxifen Citrate (The addition of panitumumab to the combination of bevacizumab and chemotherapy resulted in decreased overall survival and increased incidence of NCI-CTC grade 3-5 (87% vs 72%) adverse reactions. In a single-arm study of 19 patients receiving panitumumab in combination with IFL (Irinotecan, Leucovorin and Fluorouracil), the incidence of NCI-CTC grade 3–4 diarrhea was 58%; in addition, grade 5 diarrhea occurred in one patient. In a single-arm study of 24 patients receiving panitumumab plus FOLFIRI (Leucovorin, Fluorouracil and Irinotecan), the incidence of NCI-CTC grade 3 diarrhea was 25%).
No products indexed under this heading.

Teniposide (The addition of panitumumab to the combination of bevacizumab and chemotherapy resulted in decreased overall survival and increased incidence of NCI-CTC grade 3-5 (87% vs 72%) adverse reactions. In a single-arm study of 19 patients receiving panitumumab in combination with IFL (Irinotecan, Leucovorin and Fluorouracil), the incidence of NCI-CTC grade 3–4 diarrhea was 58%; in addition, grade 5 diarrhea occurred in one patient. In a single-arm study of 24 patients receiving panitumumab plus

IMPORTANT NOTE: Always consult each drug listing in the patient's regimen for possible interactions.

FOLFIRI (Leucovorin, Fluorouracil and Irinotecan), the incidence of NCI-CTC grade 3 diarrhea was 25%).
No products indexed under this heading.

Thioguanine (The addition of panitumumab to the combination of bevacizumab and chemotherapy resulted in decreased overall survival and increased incidence of NCI-CTC grade 3-5 (87% vs 72%) adverse reactions. In a single-arm study of 19 patients receiving panitumumab in combination with IFL (Irinotecan, Leucovorin and Fluorouracil), the incidence of NCI-CTC grade 3–4 diarrhea was 58%; in addition, grade 5 diarrhea occurred in one patient. In a single-arm study of 24 patients receiving panitumumab plus FOLFIRI (Leucovorin, Fluorouracil and Irinotecan), the incidence of NCI-CTC grade 3 diarrhea was 25%). Products include:
Tabloid 1664

Thiotepa (The addition of panitumumab to the combination of bevacizumab and chemotherapy resulted in decreased overall survival and increased incidence of NCI-CTC grade 3-5 (87% vs 72%) adverse reactions. In a single-arm study of 19 patients receiving panitumumab in combination with IFL (Irinotecan, Leucovorin and Fluorouracil), the incidence of NCI-CTC grade 3–4 diarrhea was 58%; in addition, grade 5 diarrhea occurred in one patient. In a single-arm study of 24 patients receiving panitumumab plus FOLFIRI (Leucovorin, Fluorouracil and Irinotecan), the incidence of NCI-CTC grade 3 diarrhea was 25%).
No products indexed under this heading.

Topotecan Hydrochloride (The addition of panitumumab to the combination of bevacizumab and chemotherapy resulted in decreased overall survival and increased incidence of NCI-CTC grade 3-5 (87% vs 72%) adverse reactions. In a single-arm study of 19 patients receiving panitumumab in combination with IFL (Irinotecan, Leucovorin and Fluorouracil), the incidence of NCI-CTC grade 3–4 diarrhea was 58%; in addition, grade 5 diarrhea occurred in one patient. In a single-arm study of 24 patients receiving panitumumab plus FOLFIRI (Leucovorin, Fluorouracil and Irinotecan), the incidence of NCI-CTC grade 3 diarrhea was 25%). Products include:
Hycamtin 1491
Hycamtin Capsules 1488

Toremifene Citrate (The addition of panitumumab to the combination of bevacizumab and chemotherapy resulted in decreased overall survival and increased incidence of NCI-CTC grade 3-5 (87% vs 72%) adverse reactions. In a single-arm study of 19 patients receiving panitumumab in combination with IFL (Irinotecan, Leucovorin and Fluorouracil), the incidence of NCI-CTC grade 3–4 diarrhea was 58%; in addition, grade 5 diarrhea occurred in one patient. In a single-arm study of 24 patients receiving panitumumab plus FOLFIRI (Leucovorin, Fluorouracil and Irinotecan), the incidence of NCI-CTC grade 3 diarrhea was 25%).
No products indexed under this heading.

Valrubicin (The addition of panitumumab to the combination of bevacizumab and chemotherapy resulted in decreased overall survival and increased incidence of NCI-CTC grade 3-5 (87% vs 72%) adverse reactions. In a single-arm study of 19 patients receiving panitumumab in combination with IFL (Irinotecan, Leucovorin and Fluorouracil), the incidence of NCI-CTC grade 3–4 diarrhea was 58%; in addition, grade 5 diarrhea occurred in one patient. In a single-arm study of 24 patients receiving panitumumab plus

FOLFIRI (Leucovorin, Fluorouracil and Irinotecan), the incidence of NCI-CTC grade 3 diarrhea was 25%). Products include:
Valstar 1131

Vincristine Sulfate (The addition of panitumumab to the combination of bevacizumab and chemotherapy resulted in decreased overall survival and increased incidence of NCI-CTC grade 3-5 (87% vs 72%) adverse reactions. In a single-arm study of 19 patients receiving panitumumab in combination with IFL (Irinotecan, Leucovorin and Fluorouracil), the incidence of NCI-CTC grade 3–4 diarrhea was 58%; in addition, grade 5 diarrhea occurred in one patient. In a single-arm study of 24 patients receiving panitumumab plus FOLFIRI (Leucovorin, Fluorouracil and Irinotecan), the incidence of NCI-CTC grade 3 diarrhea was 25%).
No products indexed under this heading.

Vinorelbine Tartrate (The addition of panitumumab to the combination of bevacizumab and chemotherapy resulted in decreased overall survival and increased incidence of NCI-CTC grade 3-5 (87% vs 72%) adverse reactions. In a single-arm study of 19 patients receiving panitumumab in combination with IFL (Irinotecan, Leucovorin and Fluorouracil), the incidence of NCI-CTC grade 3–4 diarrhea was 58%; in addition, grade 5 diarrhea occurred in one patient. In a single-arm study of 24 patients receiving panitumumab plus FOLFIRI (Leucovorin, Fluorouracil and Irinotecan), the incidence of NCI-CTC grade 3 diarrhea was 25%).
No products indexed under this heading.

VELCADE FOR INJECTION

(Bortezomib) 2324
May interact with cytochrome p450 2c19 substrates (selected), cytochrome p450 3a4 inducers (selected), cytochrome p450 3a4 inhibitors (selected), oral hypoglycemic agents, and certain other agents. Compounds in these categories include:

Acarbose (During clinical trials, hypoglycemia and hyperglycemia were reported in diabetic patients receiving oral hypoglycemics. Patients on oral antidiabetic agents receiving bortezomib treatment may require close monitoring of their blood glucose levels and adjustment of the dose of their antidiabetic medication).
No products indexed under this heading.

Acetazolamide (Patients who are concomitantly receiving bortezomib and drugs that are inhibitors or inducers of cytochrome P450 3A4 should be closely monitored for either toxicities or reduced efficacy).
No products indexed under this heading.

Acetazolamide Sodium (Patients who are concomitantly receiving bortezomib and drugs that are inhibitors or inducers of cytochrome P450 3A4 should be closely monitored for either toxicities or reduced efficacy).
No products indexed under this heading.

Allium sativum (Patients who are concomitantly receiving bortezomib and drugs that are inhibitors or inducers of cytochrome P450 3A4 should be closely monitored for either toxicities or reduced efficacy).
No products indexed under this heading.

Aminoglutethimide (Patients who are concomitantly receiving bortezomib and drugs that are inhibitors or inducers of cytochrome P450 3A4 should be closely monitored for either toxicities or reduced efficacy).
No products indexed under this heading.

Amiodarone Hydrochloride (Patients who are concomitantly receiving bortezomib and drugs that are inhibitors or inducers of cytochrome P450 3A4 should be closely monitored for either toxicities or reduced efficacy).
No products indexed under this heading.

Amitriptyline Hydrochloride (Bortezomib may inhibit 2C19 activity and increase exposure to drugs that are substrates for this enzyme).
No products indexed under this heading.

Amoxapine (Bortezomib may inhibit 2C19 activity and increase exposure to drugs that are substrates for this enzyme).
No products indexed under this heading.

Amprenavir (Patients who are concomitantly receiving bortezomib and drugs that are inhibitors or inducers of cytochrome P450 3A4 should be closely monitored for either toxicities or reduced efficacy).
No products indexed under this heading.

Anastrozole (Patients who are concomitantly receiving bortezomib and drugs that are inhibitors or inducers of cytochrome P450 3A4 should be closely monitored for either toxicities or reduced efficacy).
No products indexed under this heading.

Aprepitant (Patients who are concomitantly receiving bortezomib and drugs that are inhibitors or inducers of cytochrome P450 3A4 should be closely monitored for either toxicities or reduced efficacy). Products include:
Emend 2124

Atazanavir (Patients who are concomitantly receiving bortezomib and drugs that are inhibitors or inducers of cytochrome P450 3A4 should be closely monitored for either toxicities or reduced efficacy).
No products indexed under this heading.

Atazanavir Sulfate (Patients who are concomitantly receiving bortezomib and drugs that are inhibitors or inducers of cytochrome P450 3A4 should be closely monitored for either toxicities or reduced efficacy).
No products indexed under this heading.

Betamethasone (Patients who are concomitantly receiving bortezomib and drugs that are inhibitors or inducers of cytochrome P450 3A4 should be closely monitored for either toxicities or reduced efficacy).
No products indexed under this heading.

Betamethasone Acetate (Patients who are concomitantly receiving bortezomib and drugs that are inhibitors or inducers of cytochrome P450 3A4 should be closely monitored for either toxicities or reduced efficacy).
No products indexed under this heading.

Betamethasone Benzoate (Patients who are concomitantly receiving bortezomib and drugs that are inhibitors or inducers of cytochrome P450 3A4 should be closely monitored for either toxicities or reduced efficacy).
No products indexed under this heading.

Betamethasone Dipropionate (Patients who are concomitantly receiving bortezomib and drugs that are inhibitors or inducers of cytochrome P450 3A4 should be closely monitored for either toxicities or reduced efficacy). Products include:
Diprolene Lotion 0.05% 3108
Diprolene Ointment 0.05% 3109
Diprolene AF Cream 0.05% 3107
Lotrisone 3163

Betamethasone Sodium Phosphate (Patients who are concomitantly receiving bortezomib and drugs that are inhibitors or inducers of cytochrome P450 3A4 should be closely monitored for either toxicities or reduced efficacy).
No products indexed under this heading.

Betamethasone Valerate (Patients who are concomitantly receiving bortezomib and drugs that are inhibitors or inducers of cytochrome P450 3A4 should be closely monitored for either toxicities or reduced efficacy). Products include:
Luxiq 3321

Bosentan (Patients who are concomitantly receiving bortezomib and drugs that are inhibitors or inducers of cytochrome P450 3A4 should be closely monitored for either toxicities or reduced efficacy). Products include:
Tracleer 573

Carbamazepine (Patients who are concomitantly receiving bortezomib and drugs that are inhibitors or inducers of cytochrome P450 3A4 should be closely monitored for either toxicities or reduced efficacy). Products include:
Carbatrol 3280
Equetro 3477

Carisoprodol (Bortezomib may inhibit 2C19 activity and increase exposure to drugs that are substrates for this enzyme).
No products indexed under this heading.

Chlorpropamide (During clinical trials, hypoglycemia and hyperglycemia were reported in diabetic patients receiving oral hypoglycemics. Patients on oral antidiabetic agents receiving bortezomib treatment may require close monitoring of their blood glucose levels and adjustment of the dose of their antidiabetic medication).
No products indexed under this heading.

Cilostazol (Bortezomib may inhibit 2C19 activity and increase exposure to drugs that are substrates for this enzyme).
No products indexed under this heading.

Cimetidine (Patients who are concomitantly receiving bortezomib and drugs that are inhibitors or inducers of cytochrome P450 3A4 should be closely monitored for either toxicities or reduced efficacy).
No products indexed under this heading.

Cimetidine Hydrochloride (Patients who are concomitantly receiving bortezomib and drugs that are inhibitors or inducers of cytochrome P450 3A4 should be closely monitored for either toxicities or reduced efficacy).
No products indexed under this heading.

Ciprofloxacin (Patients who are concomitantly receiving bortezomib and drugs that are inhibitors or inducers of cytochrome P450 3A4 should be closely monitored for either toxicities or reduced efficacy). Products include:
Cipro I.V. 3082
Cipro 3073
Cipro XR 3091
Ciprodex 583

Ciprofloxacin Hydrochloride (Patients who are concomitantly receiving bortezomib and drugs that are inhibitors or inducers of cytochrome P450 3A4 should be closely monitored for either toxicities or reduced efficacy). Products include:
Cipro 3073

Cisplatin (Patients who are concomitantly receiving bortezomib and drugs that are inhibitors or inducers of cytochrome P450 3A4 should be closely monitored for either toxicities or reduced efficacy).
No products indexed under this heading.

Citalopram Hydrobromide (Bortezomib may inhibit 2C19 activity and

increase exposure to drugs that are substrates for this enzyme). Products include:
Celexa **1153**

Clarithromycin (Patients who are concomitantly receiving bortezomib and drugs that are inhibitors or inducers of cytochrome P450 3A4 should be closely monitored for either toxicities or reduced efficacy). Products include:
Biaxin/Biaxin XL **412**

Clomipramine Hydrochloride (Bortezomib may inhibit 2C19 activity and increase exposure to drugs that are substrates for this enzyme).
No products indexed under this heading.

Clotrimazole (Patients who are concomitantly receiving bortezomib and drugs that are inhibitors or inducers of cytochrome P450 3A4 should be closely monitored for either toxicities or reduced efficacy). Products include:
Lotrisone **3163**

Conivaptan Hydrochloride (Patients who are concomitantly receiving bortezomib and drugs that are inhibitors or inducers of cytochrome P450 3A4 should be closely monitored for either toxicities or reduced efficacy). Products include:
Vaprisol **689**

Cortisone Acetate (Patients who are concomitantly receiving bortezomib and drugs that are inhibitors or inducers of cytochrome P450 3A4 should be closely monitored for either toxicities or reduced efficacy).
No products indexed under this heading.

Cyclophosphamide (Bortezomib may inhibit 2C19 activity and increase exposure to drugs that are substrates for this enzyme).
No products indexed under this heading.

Cyclosporine (Patients who are concomitantly receiving bortezomib and drugs that are inhibitors or inducers of cytochrome P450 3A4 should be closely monitored for either toxicities or reduced efficacy). Products include:
Gengraf **440**
Neoral Oral Solution **2496**
Neoral Capsules **2496**
Restasis **605**

Dalfopristin (Patients who are concomitantly receiving bortezomib and drugs that are inhibitors or inducers of cytochrome P450 3A4 should be closely monitored for either toxicities or reduced efficacy).
No products indexed under this heading.

Danazol (Patients who are concomitantly receiving bortezomib and drugs that are inhibitors or inducers of cytochrome P450 3A4 should be closely monitored for either toxicities or reduced efficacy).
No products indexed under this heading.

Darunavir (Patients who are concomitantly receiving bortezomib and drugs that are inhibitors or inducers of cytochrome P450 3A4 should be closely monitored for either toxicities or reduced efficacy).
No products indexed under this heading.

Dasatinib (Patients who are concomitantly receiving bortezomib and drugs that are inhibitors or inducers of cytochrome P450 3A4 should be closely monitored for either toxicities or reduced efficacy).
No products indexed under this heading.

Delavirdine Mesylate (Patients who are concomitantly receiving bortezomib and drugs that are inhibitors or inducers of cytochrome P450 3A4 should be closely monitored for either toxicities or reduced efficacy).
No products indexed under this heading.

Delavirine (Patients who are concomitantly receiving bortezomib and drugs that are inhibitors or inducers of cytochrome P450 3A4 should be closely monitored for either toxicities or reduced efficacy).
No products indexed under this heading.

Desipramine Hydrochloride (Bortezomib may inhibit 2C19 activity and increase exposure to drugs that are substrates for this enzyme).
No products indexed under this heading.

Desloratadine (Patients who are concomitantly receiving bortezomib and drugs that are inhibitors or inducers of cytochrome P450 3A4 should be closely monitored for either toxicities or reduced efficacy). Products include:
Clarinex Syrup **3098**
Clarinex **3098**
Clarinex Reditabs **3098**
Clarinex-D 12-Hour **3101**
Clarinex-D **3104**

Dexamethasone (Patients who are concomitantly receiving bortezomib and drugs that are inhibitors or inducers of cytochrome P450 3A4 should be closely monitored for either toxicities or reduced efficacy). Products include:
Ciprodex **583**
Ozurdex .... ⊙**223**
Tobramycin and Dexamethasone Ophthalmic Suspension .... ⊙**251**

Dexamethasone Acetate (Patients who are concomitantly receiving bortezomib and drugs that are inhibitors or inducers of cytochrome P450 3A4 should be closely monitored for either toxicities or reduced efficacy).
No products indexed under this heading.

Dexamethasone Phosphate (Patients who are concomitantly receiving bortezomib and drugs that are inhibitors or inducers of cytochrome P450 3A4 should be closely monitored for either toxicities or reduced efficacy).
No products indexed under this heading.

Dexamethasone Sodium (Patients who are concomitantly receiving bortezomib and drugs that are inhibitors or inducers of cytochrome P450 3A4 should be closely monitored for either toxicities or reduced efficacy).
No products indexed under this heading.

Dexamethasone Sodium Phosphate (Patients who are concomitantly receiving bortezomib and drugs that are inhibitors or inducers of cytochrome P450 3A4 should be closely monitored for either toxicities or reduced efficacy).
No products indexed under this heading.

Dexamethasone Sodium Phosphate Injection (Patients who are concomitantly receiving bortezomib and drugs that are inhibitors or inducers of cytochrome P450 3A4 should be closely monitored for either toxicities or reduced efficacy).
No products indexed under this heading.

Dextromethorphan (Bortezomib may inhibit 2C19 activity and increase exposure to drugs that are substrates for this enzyme).
No products indexed under this heading.

Dextromethorphan Hydrobromide (Bortezomib may inhibit 2C19 activity and increase exposure to drugs that are substrates for this enzyme).
No products indexed under this heading.

Diazepam (Bortezomib may inhibit 2C19 activity and increase exposure to drugs that are substrates for this enzyme). Products include:
Valium Tablets **2880**

Diltiazem Hydrochloride (Patients who are concomitantly receiving bortezomib and drugs that are inhibitors or inducers of cytochrome P450 3A4 should be closely monitored for either toxicities or reduced efficacy). Products include:

Cardizem LA **423**

Diltiazem Maleate (Patients who are concomitantly receiving bortezomib and drugs that are inhibitors or inducers of cytochrome P450 3A4 should be closely monitored for either toxicities or reduced efficacy).
No products indexed under this heading.

Divalproex Sodium (Bortezomib may inhibit 2C19 activity and increase exposure to drugs that are substrates for this enzyme). Products include:
Depakote ER **426**

Doxepin Hydrochloride (Bortezomib may inhibit 2C19 activity and increase exposure to drugs that are substrates for this enzyme).
No products indexed under this heading.

Doxorubicin Hydrochloride (Patients who are concomitantly receiving bortezomib and drugs that are inhibitors or inducers of cytochrome P450 3A4 should be closely monitored for either toxicities or reduced efficacy).
No products indexed under this heading.

Efavirenz (Patients who are concomitantly receiving bortezomib and drugs that are inhibitors or inducers of cytochrome P450 3A4 should be closely monitored for either toxicities or reduced efficacy). Products include:
Atripla **906**

Erythromycin (Patients who are concomitantly receiving bortezomib and drugs that are inhibitors or inducers of cytochrome P450 3A4 should be closely monitored for either toxicities or reduced efficacy).
No products indexed under this heading.

Erythromycin Estolate (Patients who are concomitantly receiving bortezomib and drugs that are inhibitors or inducers of cytochrome P450 3A4 should be closely monitored for either toxicities or reduced efficacy).
No products indexed under this heading.

Erythromycin Ethylsuccinate (Patients who are concomitantly receiving bortezomib and drugs that are inhibitors or inducers of cytochrome P450 3A4 should be closely monitored for either toxicities or reduced efficacy). Products include:
E.E.S. **437**
EryPed **435**

Erythromycin Gluceptate (Patients who are concomitantly receiving bortezomib and drugs that are inhibitors or inducers of cytochrome P450 3A4 should be closely monitored for either toxicities or reduced efficacy).
No products indexed under this heading.

Erythromycin Lactobionate (Patients who are concomitantly receiving bortezomib and drugs that are inhibitors or inducers of cytochrome P450 3A4 should be closely monitored for either toxicities or reduced efficacy).
No products indexed under this heading.

Erythromycin Stearate (Patients who are concomitantly receiving bortezomib and drugs that are inhibitors or inducers of cytochrome P450 3A4 should be closely monitored for either toxicities or reduced efficacy).
No products indexed under this heading.

Esomeprazole Magnesium (Patients who are concomitantly receiving bortezomib and drugs that are inhibitors or inducers of cytochrome P450 3A4 should be closely monitored for either toxicities or reduced efficacy). Products include:
Nexium Capsules **704**
Nexium Oral Suspension **704**

Esomeprazole Sodium (Patients who are concomitantly receiving bortezomib and drugs that are inhibitors or inducers of cytochrome P450 3A4

should be closely monitored for either toxicities or reduced efficacy). Products include:
Nexium I.V. **712**

Ethosuximide (Patients who are concomitantly receiving bortezomib and drugs that are inhibitors or inducers of cytochrome P450 3A4 should be closely monitored for either toxicities or reduced efficacy).
No products indexed under this heading.

Ethotoin (Bortezomib may inhibit 2C19 activity and increase exposure to drugs that are substrates for this enzyme).
No products indexed under this heading.

Felbamate (Patients who are concomitantly receiving bortezomib and drugs that are inhibitors or inducers of cytochrome P450 3A4 should be closely monitored for either toxicities or reduced efficacy).
No products indexed under this heading.

Fluconazole (Patients who are concomitantly receiving bortezomib and drugs that are inhibitors or inducers of cytochrome P450 3A4 should be closely monitored for either toxicities or reduced efficacy).
No products indexed under this heading.

Fludrocortisone Acetate (Patients who are concomitantly receiving bortezomib and drugs that are inhibitors or inducers of cytochrome P450 3A4 should be closely monitored for either toxicities or reduced efficacy).
No products indexed under this heading.

Fluoxetine (Patients who are concomitantly receiving bortezomib and drugs that are inhibitors or inducers of cytochrome P450 3A4 should be closely monitored for either toxicities or reduced efficacy).
No products indexed under this heading.

Fluoxetine Hydrochloride (Patients who are concomitantly receiving bortezomib and drugs that are inhibitors or inducers of cytochrome P450 3A4 should be closely monitored for either toxicities or reduced efficacy). Products include:
Prozac Weekly **1941**
Prozac Pulvules **1941**
Symbyax **1965**

Fluvoxamine Maleate (Patients who are concomitantly receiving bortezomib and drugs that are inhibitors or inducers of cytochrome P450 3A4 should be closely monitored for either toxicities or reduced efficacy).
No products indexed under this heading.

Formoterol Fumarate (Bortezomib may inhibit 2C19 activity and increase exposure to drugs that are substrates for this enzyme). Products include:
Foradil **3121**
Perforomist **3634**

Fosamprenavir Calcium (Patients who are concomitantly receiving bortezomib and drugs that are inhibitors or inducers of cytochrome P450 3A4 should be closely monitored for either toxicities or reduced efficacy). Products include:
Lexiva Oral Suspension **1558**
Lexiva **1558**

Fosphenytoin (Bortezomib may inhibit 2C19 activity and increase exposure to drugs that are substrates for this enzyme).
No products indexed under this heading.

Fosphenytoin Sodium (Patients who are concomitantly receiving bortezomib and drugs that are inhibitors or inducers of cytochrome P450 3A4 should be closely monitored for either toxicities or reduced efficacy).
No products indexed under this heading.

IMPORTANT NOTE: Always consult each drug listing in the patient's regimen for possible interactions.

Gabapentin (Bortezomib may inhibit 2C19 activity and increase exposure to drugs that are substrates for this enzyme).

No products indexed under this heading.

Garlic Extract (Patients who are concomitantly receiving bortezomib and drugs that are inhibitors or inducers of cytochrome P450 3A4 should be closely monitored for either toxicities or reduced efficacy).

No products indexed under this heading.

Garlic Oil (Patients who are concomitantly receiving bortezomib and drugs that are inhibitors or inducers of cytochrome P450 3A4 should be closely monitored for either toxicities or reduced efficacy).

No products indexed under this heading.

Glibenclamide (During clinical trials, hypoglycemia and hyperglycemia were reported in diabetic patients receiving oral hypoglycemics. Patients on oral antidiabetic agents receiving bortezomib treatment may require close monitoring of their blood glucose levels and adjustment of the dose of their antidiabetic medication).

No products indexed under this heading.

Glimepiride (During clinical trials, hypoglycemia and hyperglycemia were reported in diabetic patients receiving oral hypoglycemics. Patients on oral antidiabetic agents receiving bortezomib treatment may require close monitoring of their blood glucose levels and adjustment of the dose of their antidiabetic medication). Products include:

Avandaryl 1356
Duetact 3354

Glipizide (During clinical trials, hypoglycemia and hyperglycemia were reported in diabetic patients receiving oral hypoglycemics. Patients on oral antidiabetic agents receiving bortezomib treatment may require close monitoring of their blood glucose levels and adjustment of the dose of their antidiabetic medication).

No products indexed under this heading.

Glyburide (During clinical trials, hypoglycemia and hyperglycemia were reported in diabetic patients receiving oral hypoglycemics. Patients on oral antidiabetic agents receiving bortezomib treatment may require close monitoring of their blood glucose levels and adjustment of the dose of their antidiabetic medication).

No products indexed under this heading.

Hydrocortisone (Patients who are concomitantly receiving bortezomib and drugs that are inhibitors or inducers of cytochrome P450 3A4 should be closely monitored for either toxicities or reduced efficacy).

No products indexed under this heading.

Hydrocortisone (Alcohol) (Patients who are concomitantly receiving bortezomib and drugs that are inhibitors or inducers of cytochrome P450 3A4 should be closely monitored for either toxicities or reduced efficacy).

No products indexed under this heading.

Hydrocortisone Acetate (Patients who are concomitantly receiving bortezomib and drugs that are inhibitors or inducers of cytochrome P450 3A4 should be closely monitored for either toxicities or reduced efficacy).

No products indexed under this heading.

Hydrocortisone Butyrate (Patients who are concomitantly receiving bortezomib and drugs that are inhibitors or inducers of cytochrome P450 3A4 should be closely monitored for either toxicities or reduced efficacy).

No products indexed under this heading.

Hydrocortisone Cypionate (Patients who are concomitantly receiving bortezomib and drugs that are inhibitors or inducers of cytochrome P450 3A4 should be closely monitored for either toxicities or reduced efficacy).

No products indexed under this heading.

Hydrocortisone Hemisuccinate (Patients who are concomitantly receiving bortezomib and drugs that are inhibitors or inducers of cytochrome P450 3A4 should be closely monitored for either toxicities or reduced efficacy).

No products indexed under this heading.

Hydrocortisone Probutate (Patients who are concomitantly receiving bortezomib and drugs that are inhibitors or inducers of cytochrome P450 3A4 should be closely monitored for either toxicities or reduced efficacy).

No products indexed under this heading.

Hydrocortisone Sodium Phosphate (Patients who are concomitantly receiving bortezomib and drugs that are inhibitors or inducers of cytochrome P450 3A4 should be closely monitored for either toxicities or reduced efficacy).

No products indexed under this heading.

Hydrocortisone Sodium Succinate (Patients who are concomitantly receiving bortezomib and drugs that are inhibitors or inducers of cytochrome P450 3A4 should be closely monitored for either toxicities or reduced efficacy).

No products indexed under this heading.

Hydrocortisone Valerate (Patients who are concomitantly receiving bortezomib and drugs that are inhibitors or inducers of cytochrome P450 3A4 should be closely monitored for either toxicities or reduced efficacy).

No products indexed under this heading.

Hypericum (Patients who are concomitantly receiving bortezomib and drugs that are inhibitors or inducers of cytochrome P450 3A4 should be closely monitored for either toxicities or reduced efficacy).

No products indexed under this heading.

Hypericum Perforatum (Patients who are concomitantly receiving bortezomib and drugs that are inhibitors or inducers of cytochrome P450 3A4 should be closely monitored for either toxicities or reduced efficacy). Products include:

Traumeel 1800

Imatinib Mesylate (Patients who are concomitantly receiving bortezomib and drugs that are inhibitors or inducers of cytochrome P450 3A4 should be closely monitored for either toxicities or reduced efficacy). Products include:

Gleevec 2477

Imipramine Hydrochloride (Bortezomib may inhibit 2C19 activity and increase exposure to drugs that are substrates for this enzyme).

No products indexed under this heading.

Imipramine Pamoate (Bortezomib may inhibit 2C19 activity and increase exposure to drugs that are substrates for this enzyme).

No products indexed under this heading.

Indinavir Sulfate (Patients who are concomitantly receiving bortezomib and drugs that are inhibitors or inducers of cytochrome P450 3A4 should be closely monitored for either toxicities or reduced efficacy). Products include:

Crixivan 2113

Indomethacin (Bortezomib may inhibit 2C19 activity and increase exposure to drugs that are substrates for this enzyme). Products include:

Indocin 2167

Indomethacin Sodium Trihydrate (Bortezomib may inhibit 2C19 activity and increase exposure to drugs that are substrates for this enzyme). Products include:

Indocin I.V. 2007

Isoniazid (Patients who are concomitantly receiving bortezomib and drugs that are inhibitors or inducers of cytochrome P450 3A4 should be closely monitored for either toxicities or reduced efficacy).

No products indexed under this heading.

Itraconazole (Patients who are concomitantly receiving bortezomib and drugs that are inhibitors or inducers of cytochrome P450 3A4 should be closely monitored for either toxicities or reduced efficacy).

No products indexed under this heading.

Ketoconazole (Co-administration of ketoconazole, a potent CYP3A inhibitor, showed a 35% increase in mean bortezomib AUC, based on data from 12 patients. Therefore, patients should be closely monitored when given bortezomib in combination with potent CYP3A4 inhibitors (eg, ketoconazole)). Products include:

Extina 3319
Xolegel 3337

Lamotrigine (Bortezomib may inhibit 2C19 activity and increase exposure to drugs that are substrates for this enzyme). Products include:

Lamictal 1522
Lamictal ODT 1522
Lamictal XR 1536

Lansoprazole (Bortezomib may inhibit 2C19 activity and increase exposure to drugs that are substrates for this enzyme).

No products indexed under this heading.

Lapatinib (Patients who are concomitantly receiving bortezomib and drugs that are inhibitors or inducers of cytochrome P450 3A4 should be closely monitored for either toxicities or reduced efficacy). Products include:

Tykerb 1698

Levetiracetam (Bortezomib may inhibit 2C19 activity and increase exposure to drugs that are substrates for this enzyme). Products include:

Keppra XR 3434

Lopinavir (Patients who are concomitantly receiving bortezomib and drugs that are inhibitors or inducers of cytochrome P450 3A4 should be closely monitored for either toxicities or reduced efficacy). Products include:

Kaletra 458

Loratadine (Patients who are concomitantly receiving bortezomib and drugs that are inhibitors or inducers of cytochrome P450 3A4 should be closely monitored for either toxicities or reduced efficacy).

No products indexed under this heading.

Maprotiline Hydrochloride (Bortezomib may inhibit 2C19 activity and increase exposure to drugs that are substrates for this enzyme).

No products indexed under this heading.

Melphalan (Co-administration of melphalan-prednisone on bortezomib showed a 17% increase in mean bortezomib AUC based on data from 21 patients. This increase is unlikely to be clinically relevant). Products include:

Alkeran 1302

Melphalan Hydrochloride (Co-administration of melphalan-prednisone on bortezomib showed a 17% increase in mean bortezomib AUC based on data from 21 patients. This increase is unlikely to be clinically relevant). Products include:

Alkeran for Injection 1300

Mephenytoin (Patients who are concomitantly receiving bortezomib and drugs that are inhibitors or inducers of cytochrome P450 3A4 should be closely monitored for either toxicities or reduced efficacy).

No products indexed under this heading.

Mephobarbital (Bortezomib may inhibit 2C19 activity and increase exposure to drugs that are substrates for this enzyme).

No products indexed under this heading.

Meprobamate (Bortezomib may inhibit 2C19 activity and increase exposure to drugs that are substrates for this enzyme).

No products indexed under this heading.

Metformin Hydrochloride (During clinical trials, hypoglycemia and hyperglycemia were reported in diabetic patients receiving oral hypoglycemics. Patients on oral antidiabetic agents receiving bortezomib treatment may require close monitoring of their blood glucose levels and adjustment of the dose of their antidiabetic medication). Products include:

ActoPlus 3338
Avandamet 1345
Janumet 2188

Methsuximide (Patients who are concomitantly receiving bortezomib and drugs that are inhibitors or inducers of cytochrome P450 3A4 should be closely monitored for either toxicities or reduced efficacy).

No products indexed under this heading.

Methylprednisolone (Patients who are concomitantly receiving bortezomib and drugs that are inhibitors or inducers of cytochrome P450 3A4 should be closely monitored for either toxicities or reduced efficacy).

No products indexed under this heading.

Methylprednisolone Acetate (Patients who are concomitantly receiving bortezomib and drugs that are inhibitors or inducers of cytochrome P450 3A4 should be closely monitored for either toxicities or reduced efficacy).

No products indexed under this heading.

Methylprednisolone Sodium Succinate (Patients who are concomitantly receiving bortezomib and drugs that are inhibitors or inducers of cytochrome P450 3A4 should be closely monitored for either toxicities or reduced efficacy).

No products indexed under this heading.

Metronidazole (Patients who are concomitantly receiving bortezomib and drugs that are inhibitors or inducers of cytochrome P450 3A4 should be closely monitored for either toxicities or reduced efficacy). Products include:

Pylera 793

Metronidazole Benzoate (Patients who are concomitantly receiving bortezomib and drugs that are inhibitors or inducers of cytochrome P450 3A4 should be closely monitored for either toxicities or reduced efficacy).

No products indexed under this heading.

Metronidazole Hydrochloride (Patients who are concomitantly receiving bortezomib and drugs that are inhibitors or inducers of cytochrome P450 3A4 should be closely monitored for either toxicities or reduced efficacy).

No products indexed under this heading.

Metronidazole Sodium (Patients who are concomitantly receiving bortezomib and drugs that are inhibitors or inducers of cytochrome P450 3A4 should be closely monitored for either toxicities or reduced efficacy).

No products indexed under this heading.

Miconazole (Patients who are concomitantly receiving bortezomib and drugs that are inhibitors or inducers of cytochrome P450 3A4 should be closely monitored for either toxicities or reduced efficacy).

No products indexed under this heading.

Miconazole Nitrate (Patients who are concomitantly receiving bortezomib and drugs that are inhibitors or inducers

IMPORTANT NOTE: Always consult each drug listing in the patient's regimen for possible interactions.

Quinine Sulfate (Patients who are concomitantly receiving bortezomib and drugs that are inhibitors or inducers of cytochrome P450 3A4 should be closely monitored for either toxicities or reduced efficacy).
    No products indexed under this heading.

Quinupristin (Patients who are concomitantly receiving bortezomib and drugs that are inhibitors or inducers of cytochrome P450 3A4 should be closely monitored for either toxicities or reduced efficacy).
    No products indexed under this heading.

Rabeprazole Sodium (Bortezomib may inhibit 2C19 activity and increase exposure to drugs that are substrates for this enzyme). Products include:
    Aciphex 1035

Ranitidine Bismuth Citrate (Patients who are concomitantly receiving bortezomib and drugs that are inhibitors or inducers of cytochrome P450 3A4 should be closely monitored for either toxicities or reduced efficacy).
    No products indexed under this heading.

Ranitidine Hydrochloride (Patients who are concomitantly receiving bortezomib and drugs that are inhibitors or inducers of cytochrome P450 3A4 should be closely monitored for either toxicities or reduced efficacy). Products include:
    Zantac 1737
    Zantac Injection 1732
    Zantac Pharmacy 1735

Repaglinide (During clinical trials, hypoglycemia and hyperglycemia were reported in diabetic patients receiving oral hypoglycemics. Patients on oral antidiabetic agents receiving bortezomib treatment may require close monitoring of their blood glucose levels and adjustment of the dose of their antidiabetic medication).
    No products indexed under this heading.

Rifabutin (Patients who are concomitantly receiving bortezomib and drugs that are inhibitors or inducers of cytochrome P450 3A4 should be closely monitored for either toxicities or reduced efficacy).
    No products indexed under this heading.

Rifampicin (Patients who are concomitantly receiving bortezomib and drugs that are inhibitors or inducers of cytochrome P450 3A4 should be closely monitored for either toxicities or reduced efficacy).
    No products indexed under this heading.

Rifampin (Patients who are concomitantly receiving bortezomib and drugs that are inhibitors or inducers of cytochrome P450 3A4 should be closely monitored for either toxicities or reduced efficacy).
    No products indexed under this heading.

Rifapentine (Patients who are concomitantly receiving bortezomib and drugs that are inhibitors or inducers of cytochrome P450 3A4 should be closely monitored for either toxicities or reduced efficacy).
    No products indexed under this heading.

Ritonavir (Patients who are concomitantly receiving bortezomib and drugs that are inhibitors or inducers of cytochrome P450 3A4 should be closely monitored for either toxicities or reduced efficacy). Products include:
    Kaletra 458
    Norvir 509

Rosiglitazone Maleate (During clinical trials, hypoglycemia and hyperglycemia were reported in diabetic patients receiving oral hypoglycemics. Patients on oral antidiabetic agents receiving bortezomib treatment may require close monitoring of their blood glucose

levels and adjustment of the dose of their antidiabetic medication). Products include:
    Avandamet 1345
    Avandaryl 1356
    Avandia 1366

Saquinavir (Patients who are concomitantly receiving bortezomib and drugs that are inhibitors or inducers of cytochrome P450 3A4 should be closely monitored for either toxicities or reduced efficacy).
    No products indexed under this heading.

Saquinavir Mesylate (Patients who are concomitantly receiving bortezomib and drugs that are inhibitors or inducers of cytochrome P450 3A4 should be closely monitored for either toxicities or reduced efficacy).
    No products indexed under this heading.

Sertraline Hydrochloride (Patients who are concomitantly receiving bortezomib and drugs that are inhibitors or inducers of cytochrome P450 3A4 should be closely monitored for either toxicities or reduced efficacy).
    No products indexed under this heading.

Sildenafil Citrate (Patients who are concomitantly receiving bortezomib and drugs that are inhibitors or inducers of cytochrome P450 3A4 should be closely monitored for either toxicities or reduced efficacy).
    No products indexed under this heading.

Sitagliptin Phosphate (During clinical trials, hypoglycemia and hyperglycemia were reported in diabetic patients receiving oral hypoglycemics. Patients on oral antidiabetic agents receiving bortezomib treatment may require close monitoring of their blood glucose levels and adjustment of the dose of their antidiabetic medication). Products include:
    Janumet 2188
    Januvia 2196

Sulfinpyrazone (Patients who are concomitantly receiving bortezomib and drugs that are inhibitors or inducers of cytochrome P450 3A4 should be closely monitored for either toxicities or reduced efficacy).
    No products indexed under this heading.

Telithromycin (Patients who are concomitantly receiving bortezomib and drugs that are inhibitors or inducers of cytochrome P450 3A4 should be closely monitored for either toxicities or reduced efficacy). Products include:
    Ketek 2991

Teniposide (Bortezomib may inhibit 2C19 activity and increase exposure to drugs that are substrates for this enzyme).
    No products indexed under this heading.

Theophyllinate (Patients who are concomitantly receiving bortezomib and drugs that are inhibitors or inducers of cytochrome P450 3A4 should be closely monitored for either toxicities or reduced efficacy).
    No products indexed under this heading.

Theophylline (Patients who are concomitantly receiving bortezomib and drugs that are inhibitors or inducers of cytochrome P450 3A4 should be closely monitored for either toxicities or reduced efficacy).
    No products indexed under this heading.

Theophylline Anhydrous (Patients who are concomitantly receiving bortezomib and drugs that are inhibitors or inducers of cytochrome P450 3A4 should be closely monitored for either toxicities or reduced efficacy). Products include:
    Uniphyl 2817

Theophylline Calcium Salicylate (Patients who are concomitantly receiving bortezomib and drugs that are inhibitors or inducers of cytochrome P450 3A4 should be closely monitored for either toxicities or reduced efficacy).
    No products indexed under this heading.

Theophylline Dihydroxypropyl (Glyceryl) (Patients who are concomitantly receiving bortezomib and drugs that are inhibitors or inducers of cytochrome P450 3A4 should be closely monitored for either toxicities or reduced efficacy).
    No products indexed under this heading.

Theophylline Ethylenediamine (Patients who are concomitantly receiving bortezomib and drugs that are inhibitors or inducers of cytochrome P450 3A4 should be closely monitored for either toxicities or reduced efficacy).
    No products indexed under this heading.

Theophylline Sodium Glycinate (Patients who are concomitantly receiving bortezomib and drugs that are inhibitors or inducers of cytochrome P450 3A4 should be closely monitored for either toxicities or reduced efficacy).
    No products indexed under this heading.

Thioridazine (Bortezomib may inhibit 2C19 activity and increase exposure to drugs that are substrates for this enzyme).
    No products indexed under this heading.

Thioridazine Hydrochloride (Bortezomib may inhibit 2C19 activity and increase exposure to drugs that are substrates for this enzyme). Products include:
    Thioridazine Hydrochloride 2384

Tiagabine Hydrochloride (Bortezomib may inhibit 2C19 activity and increase exposure to drugs that are substrates for this enzyme). Products include:
    Gabitril 972

Tolazamide (During clinical trials, hypoglycemia and hyperglycemia were reported in diabetic patients receiving oral hypoglycemics. Patients on oral antidiabetic agents receiving bortezomib treatment may require close monitoring of their blood glucose levels and adjustment of the dose of their antidiabetic medication).
    No products indexed under this heading.

Tolbutamide (During clinical trials, hypoglycemia and hyperglycemia were reported in diabetic patients receiving oral hypoglycemics. Patients on oral antidiabetic agents receiving bortezomib treatment may require close monitoring of their blood glucose levels and adjustment of the dose of their antidiabetic medication).
    No products indexed under this heading.

Tolbutamide Sodium (Bortezomib may inhibit 2C19 activity and increase exposure to drugs that are substrates for this enzyme).
    No products indexed under this heading.

Topiramate (Bortezomib may inhibit 2C19 activity and increase exposure to drugs that are substrates for this enzyme).
    No products indexed under this heading.

Triamcinolone (Patients who are concomitantly receiving bortezomib and drugs that are inhibitors or inducers of cytochrome P450 3A4 should be closely monitored for either toxicities or reduced efficacy).
    No products indexed under this heading.

Triamcinolone Acetonide (Patients who are concomitantly receiving bortezomib and drugs that are inhibitors or inducers of cytochrome P450 3A4 should be closely monitored for either toxicities or reduced efficacy). Products include:

    Azmacort 408
    Nasacort AQ 3019

Triamcinolone Diacetate (Patients who are concomitantly receiving bortezomib and drugs that are inhibitors or inducers of cytochrome P450 3A4 should be closely monitored for either toxicities or reduced efficacy).
    No products indexed under this heading.

Triamcinolone Hexacetonide (Patients who are concomitantly receiving bortezomib and drugs that are inhibitors or inducers of cytochrome P450 3A4 should be closely monitored for either toxicities or reduced efficacy).
    No products indexed under this heading.

Trimethadione (Bortezomib may inhibit 2C19 activity and increase exposure to drugs that are substrates for this enzyme).
    No products indexed under this heading.

Trimipramine Maleate (Bortezomib may inhibit 2C19 activity and increase exposure to drugs that are substrates for this enzyme).
    No products indexed under this heading.

Troglitazone (During clinical trials, hypoglycemia and hyperglycemia were reported in diabetic patients receiving oral hypoglycemics. Patients on oral antidiabetic agents receiving bortezomib treatment may require close monitoring of their blood glucose levels and adjustment of the dose of their antidiabetic medication).
    No products indexed under this heading.

Troleandomycin (Patients who are concomitantly receiving bortezomib and drugs that are inhibitors or inducers of cytochrome P450 3A4 should be closely monitored for either toxicities or reduced efficacy).
    No products indexed under this heading.

Valproate Sodium (Patients who are concomitantly receiving bortezomib and drugs that are inhibitors or inducers of cytochrome P450 3A4 should be closely monitored for either toxicities or reduced efficacy).
    No products indexed under this heading.

Valproic Acid (Bortezomib may inhibit 2C19 activity and increase exposure to drugs that are substrates for this enzyme).
    No products indexed under this heading.

Vardenafil Hydrochloride (Patients who are concomitantly receiving bortezomib and drugs that are inhibitors or inducers of cytochrome P450 3A4 should be closely monitored for either toxicities or reduced efficacy). Products include:
    Levitra 3157

Verapamil Hydrochloride (Patients who are concomitantly receiving bortezomib and drugs that are inhibitors or inducers of cytochrome P450 3A4 should be closely monitored for either toxicities or reduced efficacy). Products include:
    Tarka 534

Voriconazole (Patients who are concomitantly receiving bortezomib and drugs that are inhibitors or inducers of cytochrome P450 3A4 should be closely monitored for either toxicities or reduced efficacy).
    No products indexed under this heading.

Warfarin Sodium (Bortezomib may inhibit 2C19 activity and increase exposure to drugs that are substrates for this enzyme).
    No products indexed under this heading.

Zafirlukast (Patients who are concomitantly receiving bortezomib and drugs that are inhibitors or inducers of cytochrome P450 3A4 should be closely monitored for either toxicities or reduced efficacy). Products include:
    Accolate 3612

2025 Interactions Index Venlafaxine

Zileuton (Patients who are concomitantly receiving bortezomib and drugs that are inhibitors or inducers of cytochrome P450 3A4 should be closely monitored for either toxicities or reduced efficacy).
No products indexed under this heading.

Zonisamide (Bortezomib may inhibit 2C19 activity and increase exposure to drugs that are substrates for this enzyme). Products include:
Zonegran 1081

Food Interactions

Grapefruit (Patients who are concomitantly receiving bortezomib and drugs that are inhibitors or inducers of cytochrome P450 3A4 should be closely monitored for either toxicities or reduced efficacy).

Grapefruit Juice (Patients who are concomitantly receiving bortezomib and drugs that are inhibitors or inducers of cytochrome P450 3A4 should be closely monitored for either toxicities or reduced efficacy).

VENLAFAXINE HYDROCHLORIDE TABLETS

(Venlafaxine Hydrochloride) 2388
May interact with alcohols, anticoagulants, aspirin-acetylsalicylic acid, centrally-acting drugs, cytochrome p450 2d6 inhibitors (selected), cytochrome p450 2d6 substrates (selected), cytochrome p450 3a4 inhibitors (selected), diuretics, haloperidols, lithium preparations, monoamine oxidase inhibitors, non-steroidal anti-inflammatory agents, selective serotonin reuptake inhibitors, serotonin and norepinephrine reuptake inhibitors, serotoninergic agents, triptans, and certain other agents. Compounds in these categories include:

5-hydroxytryptophan (Patients should be cautioned about the risk of serotonin syndrome with the concomitant use of venlafaxine and tryptophan supplements. The concomitant use of venlafaxine with serotonin precursors (such as tryptophan) is not recommended).
No products indexed under this heading.

Acetazolamide (Concomitant use of CYP3A4 inhibitors and venlafaxine may increase levels of venlafaxine and ODV. Therefore, caution is advised if a patient's therapy includes a CYP3A4 inhibitor and venlafaxine concomitantly. The concomitant use of venlafaxine with a drug treatment(s) that potently inhibits both CYP2D6 and CYP3A4, the primary metabolizing enzymes for venlafaxine, has not been studied. Therefore, caution is advised should a patient's therapy include venlafaxine and any agent(s) that produce potent simultaneous inhibition of these two enzyme systems).
No products indexed under this heading.

Acetazolamide Sodium (Concomitant use of CYP3A4 inhibitors and venlafaxine may increase levels of venlafaxine and ODV. Therefore, caution is advised if a patient's therapy includes a CYP3A4 inhibitor and venlafaxine concomitantly. The concomitant use of venlafaxine with a drug treatment(s) that potently inhibits both CYP2D6 and CYP3A4, the primary metabolizing enzymes for venlafaxine, has not been studied. Therefore, caution is advised should a patient's therapy include venlafaxine and any agent(s) that produce potent simultaneous inhibition of these two enzyme systems).
No products indexed under this heading.

Alfentanil Hydrochloride (The risk of using venlafaxine in combination with other CNS active drugs has not been systematically evaluated. Consequently, caution is advised if the concomitant administration of venlafaxine and such drugs is required).
No products indexed under this heading.

Almotriptan Malate (There have been rare post-marketing reports of serotonin syndrome with use of an SSRI and a triptan. If concomitant treatment of venlafaxine with a triptan is clinically warranted, careful observation of the patient is advised, particularly during treatment initiation and dose increases. Patients should be cautioned about the risk of serotonin syndrome with the concomitant use of venlafaxine and triptans, tramadol, tryptophan supplements or other serotonergic agents). Products include:
Axert 2593

Alprazolam (The risk of using venlafaxine in combination with other CNS active drugs has not been systematically evaluated. Consequently, caution is advised if the concomitant administration of venlafaxine and such drugs is required).
No products indexed under this heading.

Amiloride Hydrochloride (Elderly patients may be at greater risk of developing hyponatremia with SSRIs and SNRIs. Also patients taking diuretics or who are otherwise volume depleted may be at greater risk. Discontinuation of venlafaxine should be considered in patients with symptomatic hyponatremia and appropriate medical intervention should be instituted).
No products indexed under this heading.

Amiodarone Hydrochloride (Studies indicate that venlafaxine is metabolized to its active metabolite, ODV, by CYP2D6. Thus the potential exists for a drug interaction between drugs that inhibit CYP2D6-mediated metabolism and venlafaxine. However, although imipramine partially inhibited the CYP2D6-mediated metabolism of venlafaxine, resulting in higher plasma concentrations of venlafaxine and lower plasma concentrations of ODV, the total concentration of active compounds (venlafaxine plus ODV) was not affected. Also, in a clinical study involving CYP2D6 poor and extensive metabolizers, the total concentration of active compounds (venlafaxine plus ODV), was similar in both groups. No dosage adjustment is required when venlafaxine is co-administered with a CYP2D6 inhibitor. Caution is advised should a patient's therapy include venlafaxine and CYP2D6 inhibitor).
No products indexed under this heading.

Amitriptyline Hydrochloride (Studies indicate that venlafaxine is metabolized to its active metabolite, ODV, by CYP2D6. Thus the potential exists for a drug interaction between drugs that inhibit CYP2D6-mediated metabolism and venlafaxine. However, although imipramine partially inhibited the CYP2D6-mediated metabolism of venlafaxine, resulting in higher plasma concentrations of venlafaxine and lower plasma concentrations of ODV, the total concentration of active compounds (venlafaxine plus ODV) was not affected. Also, in a clinical study involving CYP2D6 poor and extensive metabolizers, the total concentration of active compounds (venlafaxine plus ODV), was similar in both groups. No dosage adjustment is required when venlafaxine is co-administered with a CYP2D6 inhibitor. Caution is advised should a patient's therapy include venlafaxine and CYP2D6 inhibitor).
No products indexed under this heading.

Amoxapine (Studies indicate that venlafaxine is metabolized to its active metabolite, ODV, by CYP2D6. Thus the potential exists for a drug interaction between drugs that inhibit CYP2D6-mediated metabolism and venlafaxine. However, although imipramine partially inhibited the CYP2D6-mediated metabolism of venlafaxine, resulting in higher plasma concentrations of venlafaxine and lower plasma concentrations of ODV, the total concentration of active compounds (venlafaxine plus ODV) was not affected. Also, in a clinical study involving CYP2D6 poor and extensive metabolizers, the total concentration of active compounds (venlafaxine plus ODV), was similar in both groups. No dosage adjustment is required when venlafaxine is co-administered with a CYP2D6 inhibitor. Caution is advised should a patient's therapy include venlafaxine and CYP2D6 inhibitor).
No products indexed under this heading.

Amphetamine Aspartate (The risk of using venlafaxine in combination with other CNS active drugs has not been systematically evaluated. Consequently, caution is advised if the concomitant administration of venlafaxine and such drugs is required).
No products indexed under this heading.

Amphetamine Aspartate Monohydrate (The risk of using venlafaxine in combination with other CNS active drugs has not been systematically evaluated. Consequently, caution is advised if the concomitant administration of venlafaxine and such drugs is required).
No products indexed under this heading.

Amphetamine Resins (The risk of using venlafaxine in combination with other CNS active drugs has not been systematically evaluated. Consequently, caution is advised if the concomitant administration of venlafaxine and such drugs is required).
No products indexed under this heading.

Amphetamine Sulfate (The risk of using venlafaxine in combination with other CNS active drugs has not been systematically evaluated. Consequently, caution is advised if the concomitant administration of venlafaxine and such drugs is required).
No products indexed under this heading.

Amprenavir (Concomitant use of CYP3A4 inhibitors and venlafaxine may increase levels of venlafaxine and ODV. Therefore, caution is advised if a patient's therapy includes a CYP3A4 inhibitor and venlafaxine concomitantly. The concomitant use of venlafaxine with a drug treatment(s) that potently inhibits both CYP2D6 and CYP3A4, the primary metabolizing enzymes for venlafaxine, has not been studied. Therefore, caution is advised should a patient's therapy include venlafaxine and any agent(s) that produce potent simultaneous inhibition of these two enzyme systems).
No products indexed under this heading.

Anastrozole (Concomitant use of CYP3A4 inhibitors and venlafaxine may increase levels of venlafaxine and ODV. Therefore, caution is advised if a patient's therapy includes a CYP3A4 inhibitor and venlafaxine concomitantly. The concomitant use of venlafaxine with a drug treatment(s) that potently inhibits both CYP2D6 and CYP3A4, the primary metabolizing enzymes for venlafaxine, has not been studied. Therefore, caution is advised should a patient's therapy include venlafaxine and any agent(s) that produce potent simultaneous inhibition of these two enzyme systems).
No products indexed under this heading.

Anisindione (Patients should be cautioned about the concomitant use of venlafaxine and anti-coagulants since combined use of psychotropic drugs that interfere with serotonin reuptake and this agent has been associated with an increased risk of bleeding. SSRIs and SNRIs, including venlafaxine, may increase the risk of bleeding events. Concomitant use of anti-coagulants may add to this risk. Case reports and epidemiological studies (case-control and cohort design) have demonstrated an association between use of drugs that interfere with serotonin reuptake and the occurrence of gastrointestinal bleeding).
No products indexed under this heading.

Aprepitant (Concomitant use of CYP3A4 inhibitors and venlafaxine may increase levels of venlafaxine and ODV. Therefore, caution is advised if a patient's therapy includes a CYP3A4 inhibitor and venlafaxine concomitantly. The concomitant use of venlafaxine with a drug treatment(s) that potently inhibits both CYP2D6 and CYP3A4, the primary metabolizing enzymes for venlafaxine, has not been studied. Therefore, caution is advised should a patient's therapy include venlafaxine and any agent(s) that produce potent simultaneous inhibition of these two enzyme systems). Products include:
Emend 2124

Aprobarbital (The risk of using venlafaxine in combination with other CNS active drugs has not been systematically evaluated. Consequently, caution is advised if the concomitant administration of venlafaxine and such drugs is required).
No products indexed under this heading.

Ardeparin Sodium (Patients should be cautioned about the concomitant use of venlafaxine and anti-coagulants since combined use of psychotropic drugs that interfere with serotonin reuptake and this agent has been associated with an increased risk of bleeding. SSRIs and SNRIs, including venlafaxine, may increase the risk of bleeding events. Concomitant use of anti-coagulants may add to this risk. Case reports and epidemiological studies (case-control and cohort design) have demonstrated an association between use of drugs that interfere with serotonin reuptake and the occurrence of gastrointestinal bleeding).
No products indexed under this heading.

Aspirin (Patients should be cautioned about the concomitant use of venlafaxine and aspirin since combined use of psychotropic drugs that interfere with serotonin reuptake and this agent has been associated with an increased risk of bleeding. SSRIs and SNRIs, including venlafaxine, may increase the risk of bleeding events. Concomitant use of aspirin may add to this risk. Case reports and epidemiological studies (case-control and cohort design) have demonstrated an association between use of drugs that interfere with serotonin reuptake and the occurrence of gastrointestinal bleeding). Products include:
Aggrenox 880
Bayer Aspirin 829
Percodan 1124
St. Joseph Aspirin 2045

Aspirin, Enteric Coated (Patients should be cautioned about the concomitant use of venlafaxine and aspirin since combined use of psychotropic drugs that interfere with serotonin reuptake and this agent has been associated with an increased risk of bleeding. SSRIs and SNRIs, including venlafaxine, may increase the risk of bleeding events. Concomitant use of aspirin may add to this risk. Case reports and epidemiological studies (case-control and cohort design) have demonstrated an associa-

IMPORTANT NOTE: Always consult each drug listing in the patient's regimen for possible interactions.

Venlafaxine Interactions Index 2026

tion between use of drugs that interfere with serotonin reuptake and the occurrence of gastrointestinal bleeding).
No products indexed under this heading.

Aspirin Buffered (Patients should be cautioned about the concomitant use of venlafaxine and aspirin since combined use of psychotropic drugs that interfere with serotonin reuptake and this agent has been associated with an increased risk of bleeding. SSRIs and SNRIs, including venlafaxine, may increase the risk of bleeding events. Concomitant use of aspirin may add to this risk. Case reports and epidemiological studies (case-control and cohort design) have demonstrated an association between use of drugs that interfere with serotonin reuptake and the occurrence of gastrointestinal bleeding).
No products indexed under this heading.

Atazanavir (Concomitant use of CYP3A4 inhibitors and venlafaxine may increase levels of venlafaxine and ODV. Therefore, caution is advised if a patient's therapy includes a CYP3A4 inhibitor and venlafaxine concomitantly. The concomitant use of venlafaxine with a drug treatment(s) that potently inhibits both CYP2D6 and CYP3A4, the primary metabolizing enzymes for venlafaxine, has not been studied. Therefore, caution is advised should a patient's therapy include venlafaxine and any agent(s) that produce potent simultaneous inhibition of these two enzyme systems).
No products indexed under this heading.

Atazanavir Sulfate (Concomitant use of CYP3A4 inhibitors and venlafaxine may increase levels of venlafaxine and ODV. Therefore, caution is advised if a patient's therapy includes a CYP3A4 inhibitor and venlafaxine concomitantly. The concomitant use of venlafaxine with a drug treatment(s) that potently inhibits both CYP2D6 and CYP3A4, the primary metabolizing enzymes for venlafaxine, has not been studied. Therefore, caution is advised should a patient's therapy include venlafaxine and any agent(s) that produce potent simultaneous inhibition of these two enzyme systems).
No products indexed under this heading.

Atomoxetine Hydrochloride (*In vitro* studies indicate that venlafaxine is a relatively weak inhibitor of CYP2D6. These findings have been confirmed in a clinical drug interaction study comparing the effect of venlafaxine to that of fluoxetine on the CYP2D6-mediated metabolism of dextrometrophan to dextrophan). Products include:
Strattera 1957

Bendroflumethiazide (Elderly patients may be at greater risk of developing hyponatremia with SSRIs and SNRIs. Also patients taking diuretics or who are otherwise volume depleted may be at greater risk. Discontinuation of venlafaxine should be considered in patients with symptomatic hyponatremia and appropriate medical intervention should be instituted).
No products indexed under this heading.

Bisoprolol Fumarate (*In vitro* studies indicate that venlafaxine is a relatively weak inhibitor of CYP2D6. These findings have been confirmed in a clinical drug interaction study comparing the effect of venlafaxine to that of fluoxetine on the CYP2D6-mediated metabolism of dextrometrophan to dextrophan).
No products indexed under this heading.

Bumetanide (Elderly patients may be at greater risk of developing hyponatremia with SSRIs and SNRIs. Also patients taking diuretics or who are otherwise volume depleted may be at greater risk. Discontinuation of venlafaxine should be considered in patients with symptomatic hyponatremia and appropriate medical intervention should be instituted).
No products indexed under this heading.

Buprenorphine Hydrochloride (The risk of using venlafaxine in combination with other CNS active drugs has not been systematically evaluated. Consequently, caution is advised if the concomitant administration of venlafaxine and such drugs is required).
No products indexed under this heading.

Bupropion Hydrochloride (Studies indicate that venlafaxine is metabolized to its active metabolite, ODV, by CYP2D6. Thus the potential exists for a drug interaction between drugs that inhibit CYP2D6-mediated metabolism and venlafaxine. However, although imipramine partially inhibited the CYP2D6-mediated metabolism of venlafaxine, resulting in higher plasma concentrations of venlafaxine and lower plasma concentrations of ODV, the total concentration of active compounds (venlafaxine plus ODV) was not affected. Also, in a clinical study involving CYP2D6 poor and extensive metabolizers, the total concentration of active compounds (venlafaxine plus ODV), was similar in both groups. No dosage adjustment is required when venlafaxine is co-administered with a CYP2D6 inhibitor. Caution is advised should a patient's therapy include venlafaxine and CYP2D6 inhibitor). Products include:
Aplenzin 2948
Wellbutrin 1719
Wellbutrin SR 1725
Zyban 1762

Buspirone Hydrochloride (The risk of using venlafaxine in combination with other CNS active drugs has not been systematically evaluated. Consequently, caution is advised if the concomitant administration of venlafaxine and such drugs is required).
No products indexed under this heading.

Butabarbital (The risk of using venlafaxine in combination with other CNS active drugs has not been systematically evaluated. Consequently, caution is advised if the concomitant administration of venlafaxine and such drugs is required).
No products indexed under this heading.

Butalbital (The risk of using venlafaxine in combination with other CNS active drugs has not been systematically evaluated. Consequently, caution is advised if the concomitant administration of venlafaxine and such drugs is required).
No products indexed under this heading.

Captopril (*In vitro* studies indicate that venlafaxine is a relatively weak inhibitor of CYP2D6. These findings have been confirmed in a clinical drug interaction study comparing the effect of venlafaxine to that of fluoxetine on the CYP2D6-mediated metabolism of dextrometrophan to dextrophan). Products include:
Captopril 2341

Carvedilol (*In vitro* studies indicate that venlafaxine is a relatively weak inhibitor of CYP2D6. These findings have been confirmed in a clinical drug interaction study comparing the effect of venlafaxine to that of fluoxetine on the CYP2D6-mediated metabolism of dextrometrophan to dextrophan). Products include:
Coreg 1409

Celecoxib (Patients should be cautioned about the concomitant use of venlafaxine and NSAIDs since combined use of psychotropic drugs that interfere with serotonin reuptake and this agent has been associated with an increased risk of bleeding. SSRIs and SNRIs, including venlafaxine, may increase the risk of bleeding events. Concomitant use of nonsteroidal anti-inflammatory drugs may add to this risk. Case reports and epidemiological studies (case-control and cohort design) have demonstrated an association between use of drugs that interfere with serotonin reuptake and the occurrence of gastrointestinal bleeding). Products include:
Celebrex 3272

Cevimeline Hydrochloride (*In vitro* studies indicate that venlafaxine is a relatively weak inhibitor of CYP2D6. These findings have been confirmed in a clinical drug interaction study comparing the effect of venlafaxine to that of fluoxetine on the CYP2D6-mediated metabolism of dextrometrophan to dextrophan). Products include:
Evoxac 1027

Chlordiazepoxide (The risk of using venlafaxine in combination with other CNS active drugs has not been systematically evaluated. Consequently, caution is advised if the concomitant administration of venlafaxine and such drugs is required).
No products indexed under this heading.

Chlordiazepoxide Hydrochloride (The risk of using venlafaxine in combination with other CNS active drugs has not been systematically evaluated. Consequently, caution is advised if the concomitant administration of venlafaxine and such drugs is required).
No products indexed under this heading.

Chloroquine (Studies indicate that venlafaxine is metabolized to its active metabolite, ODV, by CYP2D6. Thus the potential exists for a drug interaction between drugs that inhibit CYP2D6-mediated metabolism and venlafaxine. However, although imipramine partially inhibited the CYP2D6-mediated metabolism of venlafaxine, resulting in higher plasma concentrations of venlafaxine and lower plasma concentrations of ODV, the total concentration of active compounds (venlafaxine plus ODV) was not affected. Also, in a clinical study involving CYP2D6 poor and extensive metabolizers, the total concentration of active compounds (venlafaxine plus ODV), was similar in both groups. No dosage adjustment is required when venlafaxine is co-administered with a CYP2D6 inhibitor. Caution is advised should a patient's therapy include venlafaxine and CYP2D6 inhibitor).
No products indexed under this heading.

Chloroquine Hydrochloride (Studies indicate that venlafaxine is metabolized to its active metabolite, ODV, by CYP2D6. Thus the potential exists for a drug interaction between drugs that inhibit CYP2D6-mediated metabolism and venlafaxine. However, although imipramine partially inhibited the CYP2D6-mediated metabolism of venlafaxine, resulting in higher plasma concentrations of venlafaxine and lower plasma concentrations of ODV, the total concentration of active compounds (venlafaxine plus ODV) was not affected. Also, in a clinical study involving CYP2D6 poor and extensive metabolizers, the total concentration of active compounds (venlafaxine plus ODV), was similar in both groups. No dosage adjustment is required when venlafaxine is co-administered with a CYP2D6 inhibitor. Caution is advised should a patient's therapy include venlafaxine and CYP2D6 inhibitor).
No products indexed under this heading.

Chloroquine Phosphate (Studies indicate that venlafaxine is metabolized to its active metabolite, ODV, by CYP2D6. Thus the potential exists for a drug interaction between drugs that inhibit CYP2D6-mediated metabolism and venlafaxine. However, although imipramine partially inhibited the CYP2D6-mediated metabolism of venlafaxine, resulting in higher plasma concentrations of venlafaxine and lower plasma concentrations of ODV, the total concentration of active compounds (venlafaxine plus ODV) was not affected. Also, in a clinical study involving CYP2D6 poor and extensive metabolizers, the total concentration of active compounds (venlafaxine plus ODV), was similar in both groups. No dosage adjustment is required when venlafaxine is co-administered with a CYP2D6 inhibitor. Caution is advised should a patient's therapy include venlafaxine and CYP2D6 inhibitor).
No products indexed under this heading.

Chlorothiazide (Elderly patients may be at greater risk of developing hyponatremia with SSRIs and SNRIs. Also patients taking diuretics or who are otherwise volume depleted may be at greater risk. Discontinuation of venlafaxine should be considered in patients with symptomatic hyponatremia and appropriate medical intervention should be instituted).
No products indexed under this heading.

Chlorothiazide Sodium (Elderly patients may be at greater risk of developing hyponatremia with SSRIs and SNRIs. Also patients taking diuretics or who are otherwise volume depleted may be at greater risk. Discontinuation of venlafaxine should be considered in patients with symptomatic hyponatremia and appropriate medical intervention should be instituted). Products include:
Diuril Intravenous 2009

Chlorpheniramine (Studies indicate that venlafaxine is metabolized to its active metabolite, ODV, by CYP2D6. Thus the potential exists for a drug interaction between drugs that inhibit CYP2D6-mediated metabolism and venlafaxine. However, although imipramine partially inhibited the CYP2D6-mediated metabolism of venlafaxine, resulting in higher plasma concentrations of venlafaxine and lower plasma concentrations of ODV, the total concentration of active compounds (venlafaxine plus ODV) was not affected. Also, in a clinical study involving CYP2D6 poor and extensive metabolizers, the total concentration of active compounds (venlafaxine plus ODV), was similar in both groups. No dosage adjustment is required when venlafaxine is co-administered with a CYP2D6 inhibitor. Caution is advised should a patient's therapy include venlafaxine and CYP2D6 inhibitor).
No products indexed under this heading.

Chlorpheniramine Maleate (Studies indicate that venlafaxine is metabolized to its active metabolite, ODV, by CYP2D6. Thus the potential exists for a drug interaction between drugs that inhibit CYP2D6-mediated metabolism and venlafaxine. However, although imipramine partially inhibited the CYP2D6-mediated metabolism of venlafaxine, resulting in higher plasma concentrations of venlafaxine and lower plasma concentrations of ODV, the total concentration of active compounds (venlafaxine plus ODV) was not affected. Also, in a clinical study involving CYP2D6 poor and extensive metabolizers, the total concentration of active compounds (venlafaxine plus ODV), was similar in both groups. No dosage adjustment is required when venlafaxine is co-administered with a CYP2D6 inhibitor. Caution is advised should a patient's therapy include venlafaxine and CYP2D6 inhibitor).
No products indexed under this heading.

Chlorpheniramine Polistirex (Studies indicate that venlafaxine is metabolized to its active metabolite, ODV, by CYP2D6. Thus the potential exists for a drug interaction between drugs that inhibit CYP2D6-mediated metabolism and venlafaxine. However, although

2027 Interactions Index Venlafaxine

imipramine partially inhibited the CYP2D6-mediated metabolism of venlafaxine, resulting in higher plasma concentrations of venlafaxine and lower plasma concentrations of ODV, the total concentration of active compounds (venlafaxine plus ODV) was not affected. Also, in a clinical study involving CYP2D6 poor and extensive metabolizers, the total concentration of active compounds (venlafaxine plus ODV), was similar in both groups. No dosage adjustment is required when venlafaxine is co-administered with a CYP2D6 inhibitor. Caution is advised should a patient's therapy include venlafaxine and CYP2D6 inhibitor). Products include:

Tussionex 3443

Chlorpheniramine Tannate (Studies indicate that venlafaxine is metabolized to its active metabolite, ODV, by CYP2D6. Thus the potential exists for a drug interaction between drugs that inhibit CYP2D6-mediated metabolism and venlafaxine. However, although imipramine partially inhibited the CYP2D6-mediated metabolism of venlafaxine, resulting in higher plasma concentrations of venlafaxine and lower plasma concentrations of ODV, the total concentration of active compounds (venlafaxine plus ODV) was not affected. Also, in a clinical study involving CYP2D6 poor and extensive metabolizers, the total concentration of active compounds (venlafaxine plus ODV), was similar in both groups. No dosage adjustment is required when venlafaxine is co-administered with a CYP2D6 inhibitor. Caution is advised should a patient's therapy include venlafaxine and CYP2D6 inhibitor).

No products indexed under this heading.

Chlorpromazine (The risk of using venlafaxine in combination with other CNS active drugs has not been systematically evaluated. Consequently, caution is advised if the concomitant administration of venlafaxine and such drugs is required).

No products indexed under this heading.

Chlorpromazine Hydrochloride (The risk of using venlafaxine in combination with other CNS active drugs has not been systematically evaluated. Consequently, caution is advised if the concomitant administration of venlafaxine and such drugs is required).

No products indexed under this heading.

Chlorpropamide (*In vitro* studies indicate that venlafaxine is a relatively weak inhibitor of CYP2D6. These findings have been confirmed in a clinical drug interaction study comparing the effect of venlafaxine to that of fluoxetine on the CYP2D6-mediated metabolism of dextrometrophan to dextrophan).

No products indexed under this heading.

Chlorprothixene (The risk of using venlafaxine in combination with other CNS active drugs has not been systematically evaluated. Consequently, caution is advised if the concomitant administration of venlafaxine and such drugs is required).

No products indexed under this heading.

Chlorprothixene Hydrochloride (The risk of using venlafaxine in combination with other CNS active drugs has not been systematically evaluated. Consequently, caution is advised if the concomitant administration of venlafaxine and such drugs is required).

No products indexed under this heading.

Chlorprothixene Lactate (The risk of using venlafaxine in combination with other CNS active drugs has not been systematically evaluated. Consequently, caution is advised if the concomitant administration of venlafaxine and such drugs is required).

No products indexed under this heading.

Chlorthalidone (Elderly patients may be at greater risk of developing hyponatremia with SSRIs and SNRIs. Also patients taking diuretics or who are otherwise volume depleted may be at greater risk. Discontinuation of venlafaxine should be considered in patients with symptomatic hyponatremia and appropriate medical intervention should be instituted). Products include:

Clorpres 2344

Cimetidine (Concomitant administration of cimetidine and venlafaxine resulted in inhibition of first-pass metabolism of venlafaxine. The oral clearance of venlafaxine was reduced by about 43%, and the exposure (AUC) and maximum concentration (C_{max}) of the drug were increased by about 60%. However, co-administration of cimetidine had no apparent effect on the pharmacokinetics of O-desmethylvenlafaxine (ODV). The overall pharmacological activity of venlafaxine plus ODV is expected to increase only slightly, and no dosage adjustment should be necessary for most normal adults. However, in elderly patients, patients with pre-existing hypertension or hepatic dysfunction, the interaction of venlafaxine and cimetidine is not known and potentially could be more pronounced).

No products indexed under this heading.

Cimetidine Hydrochloride (Concomitant administration of cimetidine and venlafaxine resulted in inhibition of first-pass metabolism of venlafaxine. The oral clearance of venlafaxine was reduced by about 43%, and the exposure (AUC) and maximum concentration (C_{max}) of the drug were increased by about 60%. However, co-administration of cimetidine had no apparent effect on the pharmacokinetics of O-desmethylvenlafaxine (ODV). The overall pharmacological activity of venlafaxine plus ODV is expected to increase only slightly, and no dosage adjustment should be necessary for most normal adults. However, in elderly patients, patients with pre-existing hypertension or hepatic dysfunction, the interaction of venlafaxine and cimetidine is not known and potentially could be more pronounced).

No products indexed under this heading.

Ciprofloxacin (Concomitant use of CYP3A4 inhibitors and venlafaxine may increase levels of venlafaxine and ODV. Therefore, caution is advised if a patient's therapy includes a CYP3A4 inhibitor and venlafaxine concomitantly. The concomitant use of venlafaxine with a drug treatment(s) that potently inhibits both CYP2D6 and CYP3A4, the primary metabolizing enzymes for venlafaxine, has not been studied. Therefore, caution is advised should a patient's therapy include venlafaxine and any agent(s) that produce potent simultaneous inhibition of these two enzyme systems). Products include:

Cipro I.V. 3082
Cipro 3073
Cipro XR 3091
Ciprodex 583

Citalopram Hydrobromide (Based on the mechanism of action of venlafaxine and the potential for serotonin syndrome, caution is advised when venlafaxine is co-administered with other drugs that may affect the serotonergic neurotransmitter systems, such as SSRIs. If concomitant treatment of venlafaxine with an SSRI is clinically warranted, careful observation of the patient is advised, particularly during treatment initiation and dose increases). Products include:

Celexa 1153

Clarithromycin (Concomitant use of CYP3A4 inhibitors and venlafaxine may increase levels of venlafaxine and ODV. Therefore, caution is advised if a patient's therapy includes a CYP3A4 inhibitor and venlafaxine concomitantly. The concomitant use of venlafaxine with a drug treatment(s) that potently inhibits both CYP2D6 and CYP3A4, the primary metabolizing enzymes for venlafaxine, has not been studied. Therefore, caution is advised should a patient's therapy include venlafaxine and any agent(s) that produce potent simultaneous inhibition of these two enzyme systems). Products include:

Biaxin/Biaxin XL 412

Clomipramine Hydrochloride (Studies indicate that venlafaxine is metabolized to its active metabolite, ODV, by CYP2D6. Thus the potential exists for a drug interaction between drugs that inhibit CYP2D6-mediated metabolism and venlafaxine. However, although imipramine partially inhibited the CYP2D6-mediated metabolism of venlafaxine, resulting in higher plasma concentrations of venlafaxine and lower plasma concentrations of ODV, the total concentration of active compounds (venlafaxine plus ODV) was not affected. Also, in a clinical study involving CYP2D6 poor and extensive metabolizers, the total concentration of active compounds (venlafaxine plus ODV), was similar in both groups. No dosage adjustment is required when venlafaxine is co-administered with a CYP2D6 inhibitor. Caution is advised should a patient's therapy include venlafaxine and CYP2D6 inhibitor).

No products indexed under this heading.

Clorazepate Dipotassium (The risk of using venlafaxine in combination with other CNS active drugs has not been systematically evaluated. Consequently, caution is advised if the concomitant administration of venlafaxine and such drugs is required).

No products indexed under this heading.

Clotrimazole (Concomitant use of CYP3A4 inhibitors and venlafaxine may increase levels of venlafaxine and ODV. Therefore, caution is advised if a patient's therapy includes a CYP3A4 inhibitor and venlafaxine concomitantly. The concomitant use of venlafaxine with a drug treatment(s) that potently inhibits both CYP2D6 and CYP3A4, the primary metabolizing enzymes for venlafaxine, has not been studied. Therefore, caution is advised should a patient's therapy include venlafaxine and any agent(s) that produce potent simultaneous inhibition of these two enzyme systems). Products include:

Lotrisone 3163

Clozapine (There have been reports of elevated clozapine levels that were temporally associated with adverse events, including seizures, following the addition of venlafaxine).

No products indexed under this heading.

Cocaine Hydrochloride (Studies indicate that venlafaxine is metabolized to its active metabolite, ODV, by CYP2D6. Thus the potential exists for a drug interaction between drugs that inhibit CYP2D6-mediated metabolism and venlafaxine. However, although imipramine partially inhibited the CYP2D6-mediated metabolism of venlafaxine, resulting in higher plasma concentrations of venlafaxine and lower plasma concentrations of ODV, the total concentration of active compounds (venlafaxine plus ODV) was not affected. Also, in a clinical study involving CYP2D6 poor and extensive metabolizers, the total concentration of active compounds (venlafaxine plus ODV), was similar in both groups. No dosage adjustment is required when venlafaxine is co-administered with a CYP2D6 inhibitor. Caution is advised should a patient's therapy include venlafaxine and CYP2D6 inhibitor).

No products indexed under this heading.

Codeine Phosphate (The risk of using venlafaxine in combination with other CNS active drugs has not been systematically evaluated. Consequently, caution is advised if the concomitant administration of venlafaxine and such drugs is required). Products include:

Tylenol with Codeine 2691

Codeine Sulfate (The risk of using venlafaxine in combination with other CNS active drugs has not been systematically evaluated. Consequently, caution is advised if the concomitant administration of venlafaxine and such drugs is required).

No products indexed under this heading.

Conivaptan Hydrochloride (Concomitant use of CYP3A4 inhibitors and venlafaxine may increase levels of venlafaxine and ODV. Therefore, caution is advised if a patient's therapy includes a CYP3A4 inhibitor and venlafaxine concomitantly. The concomitant use of venlafaxine with a drug treatment(s) that potently inhibits both CYP2D6 and CYP3A4, the primary metabolizing enzymes for venlafaxine, has not been studied. Therefore, caution is advised should a patient's therapy include venlafaxine and any agent(s) that produce potent simultaneous inhibition of these two enzyme systems). Products include:

Vaprisol 689

Cyclobenzaprine Hydrochloride (*In vitro* studies indicate that venlafaxine is a relatively weak inhibitor of CYP2D6. These findings have been confirmed in a clinical drug interaction study comparing the effect of venlafaxine to that of fluoxetine on the CYP2D6-mediated metabolism of dextrometrophan to dextrophan). Products include:

Amrix 964

Cyclosporine (Concomitant use of CYP3A4 inhibitors and venlafaxine may increase levels of venlafaxine and ODV. Therefore, caution is advised if a patient's therapy includes a CYP3A4 inhibitor and venlafaxine concomitantly. The concomitant use of venlafaxine with a drug treatment(s) that potently inhibits both CYP2D6 and CYP3A4, the primary metabolizing enzymes for venlafaxine, has not been studied. Therefore, caution is advised should a patient's therapy include venlafaxine and any agent(s) that produce potent simultaneous inhibition of these two enzyme systems). Products include:

Gengraf 440
Neoral Oral Solution 2496
Neoral Capsules 2496
Restasis 605

Dalfopristin (Concomitant use of CYP3A4 inhibitors and venlafaxine may increase levels of venlafaxine and ODV. Therefore, caution is advised if a patient's therapy includes a CYP3A4 inhibitor and venlafaxine concomitantly. The concomitant use of venlafaxine with a drug treatment(s) that potently inhibits both CYP2D6 and CYP3A4, the primary metabolizing enzymes for venlafaxine, has not been studied. Therefore, caution is advised should a patient's therapy include venlafaxine and any agent(s) that produce potent simultaneous inhibition of these two enzyme systems).

No products indexed under this heading.

Dalteparin Sodium (Patients should be cautioned about the concomitant use of venlafaxine and anti-coagulants since combined use of psychotropic drugs that interfere with serotonin reuptake and this agent has been associated with an increased risk of bleeding. SSRIs and SNRIs, including venlafaxine, may increase the risk of

IMPORTANT NOTE: Always consult each drug listing in the patient's regimen for possible interactions.

bleeding events. Concomitant use of anti-coagulants may add to this risk. Case reports and epidemiological studies (case-control and cohort design) have demonstrated an association between use of drugs that interfere with serotonin reuptake and the occurrence of gastrointestinal bleeding). Products include:

Fragmin 1058

Danaparoid Sodium (Patients should be cautioned about the concomitant use of venlafaxine and anti-coagulants since combined use of psychotropic drugs that interfere with serotonin reuptake and this agent has been associated with an increased risk of bleeding. SSRIs and SNRIs, including venlafaxine, may increase the risk of bleeding events. Concomitant use of anti-coagulants may add to this risk. Case reports and epidemiological studies (case-control and cohort design) have demonstrated an association between use of drugs that interfere with serotonin reuptake and the occurrence of gastrointestinal bleeding).

No products indexed under this heading.

Danazol (Concomitant use of CYP3A4 inhibitors and venlafaxine may increase levels of venlafaxine and ODV. Therefore, caution is advised if a patient's therapy includes a CYP3A4 inhibitor and venlafaxine concomitantly. The concomitant use of venlafaxine with a drug treatment(s) that potently inhibits both CYP2D6 and CYP3A4, the primary metabolizing enzymes for venlafaxine, has not been studied. Therefore, caution is advised should a patient's therapy include venlafaxine and any agent(s) that produce potent simultaneous inhibition of these two enzyme systems).

No products indexed under this heading.

Darunavir (Concomitant use of CYP3A4 inhibitors and venlafaxine may increase levels of venlafaxine and ODV. Therefore, caution is advised if a patient's therapy includes a CYP3A4 inhibitor and venlafaxine concomitantly. The concomitant use of venlafaxine with a drug treatment(s) that potently inhibits both CYP2D6 and CYP3A4, the primary metabolizing enzymes for venlafaxine, has not been studied. Therefore, caution is advised should a patient's therapy include venlafaxine and any agent(s) that produce potent simultaneous inhibition of these two enzyme systems).

No products indexed under this heading.

Dasatinib (Concomitant use of CYP3A4 inhibitors and venlafaxine may increase levels of venlafaxine and ODV. Therefore, caution is advised if a patient's therapy includes a CYP3A4 inhibitor and venlafaxine concomitantly. The concomitant use of venlafaxine with a drug treatment(s) that potently inhibits both CYP2D6 and CYP3A4, the primary metabolizing enzymes for venlafaxine, has not been studied. Therefore, caution is advised should a patient's therapy include venlafaxine and any agent(s) that produce potent simultaneous inhibition of these two enzyme systems).

No products indexed under this heading.

Debrisoquine (*In vitro* studies indicate that venlafaxine is a relatively weak inhibitor of CYP2D6. These findings have been confirmed in a clinical drug interaction study comparing the effect of venlafaxine to that of fluoxetine on the CYP2D6-mediated metabolism of dextrometrophan to dextrophan).

No products indexed under this heading.

Delavirdine Mesylate (Concomitant use of CYP3A4 inhibitors and venlafaxine may increase levels of venlafaxine and ODV. Therefore, caution is advised if a patient's therapy includes a CYP3A4 inhibitor and venlafaxine concomitantly. The concomitant use of venlafaxine with a drug treatment(s) that potently inhibits both CYP2D6 and CYP3A4, the primary metabolizing enzymes for venlafaxine, has not been studied. Therefore, caution is advised should a patient's therapy include venlafaxine and any agent(s) that produce potent simultaneous inhibition of these two enzyme systems).

No products indexed under this heading.

Delavirine (Concomitant use of CYP3A4 inhibitors and venlafaxine may increase levels of venlafaxine and ODV. Therefore, caution is advised if a patient's therapy includes a CYP3A4 inhibitor and venlafaxine concomitantly. The concomitant use of venlafaxine with a drug treatment(s) that potently inhibits both CYP2D6 and CYP3A4, the primary metabolizing enzymes for venlafaxine, has not been studied. Therefore, caution is advised should a patient's therapy include venlafaxine and any agent(s) that produce potent simultaneous inhibition of these two enzyme systems).

No products indexed under this heading.

Desflurane (The risk of using venlafaxine in combination with other CNS active drugs has not been systematically evaluated. Consequently, caution is advised if the concomitant administration of venlafaxine and such drugs is required).

No products indexed under this heading.

Desipramine Hydrochloride (Desipramine AUC, C_{max}, and C_{min} increased by about 35% in the presence of venlafaxine. The 2-OH-desipramine AUCs increased by at least 2.5 fold (with venlafaxine 37.5 mg q12h) and by 4.5 fold (with venlafaxine 75 mg q12h)).

No products indexed under this heading.

Desloratadine (Concomitant use of CYP3A4 inhibitors and venlafaxine may increase levels of venlafaxine and ODV. Therefore, caution is advised if a patient's therapy includes a CYP3A4 inhibitor and venlafaxine concomitantly. The concomitant use of venlafaxine with a drug treatment(s) that potently inhibits both CYP2D6 and CYP3A4, the primary metabolizing enzymes for venlafaxine, has not been studied. Therefore, caution is advised should a patient's therapy include venlafaxine and any agent(s) that produce potent simultaneous inhibition of these two enzyme systems). Products include:

Clarinex Syrup 3098
Clarinex 3098
Clarinex Reditabs 3098
Clarinex-D 12-Hour 3101
Clarinex-D 3104

Desvenlafaxine Succinate (Based on the mechanism of action of venlafaxine and the potential for serotonin syndrome, caution is advised when venlafaxine is co-administered with other drugs that may affect the serotonergic neurotransmitter systems, such as other SNRIs. If concomitant treatment of venlafaxine with another SNRI is clinically warranted, careful observation of the patient is advised, particularly during treatment initiation and dose increases). Products include:

Pristiq 3564

Dexfenfluramine Hydrochloride (*In vitro* studies indicate that venlafaxine is a relatively weak inhibitor of CYP2D6. These findings have been confirmed in a clinical drug interaction study comparing the effect of venlafaxine to that of fluoxetine on the CYP2D6-mediated metabolism of dextrometrophan to dextrophan).

No products indexed under this heading.

Dexmethylphenidate Hydrochloride (The risk of using venlafaxine in combination with other CNS active drugs has not been systematically evaluated. Consequently, caution is advised if the concomitant administration of venlafaxine and such drugs is required). Products include:

Focalin XR 2472

Dextroamphetamine (The risk of using venlafaxine in combination with other CNS active drugs has not been systematically evaluated. Consequently, caution is advised if the concomitant administration of venlafaxine and such drugs is required).

No products indexed under this heading.

Dextroamphetamine Saccharate (The risk of using venlafaxine in combination with other CNS active drugs has not been systematically evaluated. Consequently, caution is advised if the concomitant administration of venlafaxine and such drugs is required).

No products indexed under this heading.

Dextroamphetamine Sulfate (The risk of using venlafaxine in combination with other CNS active drugs has not been systematically evaluated. Consequently, caution is advised if the concomitant administration of venlafaxine and such drugs is required). Products include:

Dexedrine 1425

Dextromethorphan Hydrobromide (*In vitro* studies indicate that venlafaxine is a relatively weak inhibitor of CYP2D6. These findings have been confirmed in a clinical drug interaction study comparing the effect of venlafaxine to that of fluoxetine on the CYP2D6-mediated metabolism of dextrometrophan to dextrophan).

No products indexed under this heading.

Dextromethorphan Polistirex (*In vitro* studies indicate that venlafaxine is a relatively weak inhibitor of CYP2D6. These findings have been confirmed in a clinical drug interaction study comparing the effect of venlafaxine to that of fluoxetine on the CYP2D6-mediated metabolism of dextrometrophan to dextrophan).

No products indexed under this heading.

Dezocine (The risk of using venlafaxine in combination with other CNS active drugs has not been systematically evaluated. Consequently, caution is advised if the concomitant administration of venlafaxine and such drugs is required).

No products indexed under this heading.

Diazepam (The risk of using venlafaxine in combination with other CNS active drugs has not been systematically evaluated. Consequently, caution is advised if the concomitant administration of venlafaxine and such drugs is required). Products include:

Valium Tablets 2880

Diclofenac Epolamine (Patients should be cautioned about the concomitant use of venlafaxine and NSAIDs since combined use of psychotropic drugs that interfere with serotonin reuptake and this agent has been associated with an increased risk of bleeding. SSRIs and SNRIs, including venlafaxine, may increase the risk of bleeding events. Concomitant use of nonsteroidal anti-inflammatory drugs may add to this risk. Case reports and epidemiological studies (case-control and cohort design) have demonstrated an association between use of drugs that interfere with serotonin reuptake and the occurrence of gastrointestinal bleeding). Products include:

Flector 1839

Diclofenac Potassium (Patients should be cautioned about the concomitant use of venlafaxine and NSAIDs since combined use of psychotropic drugs that interfere with serotonin reuptake and this agent has been associated with an increased risk of bleeding. SSRIs and SNRIs, including venlafaxine, may increase the risk of bleeding events. Concomitant use of nonsteroidal anti-inflammatory drugs may add to this risk. Case reports and epidemiological studies (case-control and cohort design) have demonstrated an association between use of drugs that interfere with serotonin reuptake and the occurrence of gastrointestinal bleeding).

No products indexed under this heading.

Diclofenac Sodium (Patients should be cautioned about the concomitant use of venlafaxine and NSAIDs since combined use of psychotropic drugs that interfere with serotonin reuptake and this agent has been associated with an increased risk of bleeding. SSRIs and SNRIs, including venlafaxine, may increase the risk of bleeding events. Concomitant use of nonsteroidal anti-inflammatory drugs may add to this risk. Case reports and epidemiological studies (case-control and cohort design) have demonstrated an association between use of drugs that interfere with serotonin reuptake and the occurrence of gastrointestinal bleeding).

No products indexed under this heading.

Dicumarol (Patients should be cautioned about the concomitant use of venlafaxine and anti-coagulants since combined use of psychotropic drugs that interfere with serotonin reuptake and this agent has been associated with an increased risk of bleeding. SSRIs and SNRIs, including venlafaxine, may increase the risk of bleeding events. Concomitant use of anti-coagulants may add to this risk. Case reports and epidemiological studies (case-control and cohort design) have demonstrated an association between use of drugs that interfere with serotonin reuptake and the occurrence of gastrointestinal bleeding).

No products indexed under this heading.

Diltiazem Hydrochloride (Concomitant use of CYP3A4 inhibitors and venlafaxine may increase levels of venlafaxine and ODV. Therefore, caution is advised if a patient's therapy includes a CYP3A4 inhibitor and venlafaxine concomitantly. The concomitant use of venlafaxine with a drug treatment(s) that potently inhibits both CYP2D6 and CYP3A4, the primary metabolizing enzymes for venlafaxine, has not been studied. Therefore, caution is advised should a patient's therapy include venlafaxine and any agent(s) that produce potent simultaneous inhibition of these two enzyme systems). Products include:

Cardizem LA 423

Diltiazem Maleate (Concomitant use of CYP3A4 inhibitors and venlafaxine may increase levels of venlafaxine and ODV. Therefore, caution is advised if a patient's therapy includes a CYP3A4 inhibitor and venlafaxine concomitantly. The concomitant use of venlafaxine with a drug treatment(s) that potently inhibits both CYP2D6 and CYP3A4, the primary metabolizing enzymes for venlafaxine, has not been studied. Therefore, caution is advised should a patient's therapy include venlafaxine and any agent(s) that produce potent simultaneous inhibition of these two enzyme systems).

No products indexed under this heading.

Diphenhydramine (Studies indicate that venlafaxine is metabolized to its active metabolite, ODV, by CYP2D6. Thus the potential exists for a drug interaction between drugs that inhibit CYP2D6-mediated metabolism and venlafaxine. However, although imipramine partially inhibited the CYP2D6-mediated metabolism of venlafaxine, resulting in higher plasma concentrations of venlafaxine and lower plasma concentrations of ODV, the total concentration of

2029 Interactions Index Venlafaxine

active compounds (venlafaxine plus ODV) was not affected. Also, in a clinical study involving CYP2D6 poor and extensive metabolizers, the total concentration of active compounds (venlafaxine plus ODV), was similar in both groups. No dosage adjustment is required when venlafaxine is co-administered with a CYP2D6 inhibitor. Caution is advised should a patient's therapy include venlafaxine and CYP2D6 inhibitor).
No products indexed under this heading.

Diphenhydramine Hydrochloride (Studies indicate that venlafaxine is metabolized to its active metabolite, ODV, by CYP2D6. Thus the potential exists for a drug interaction between drugs that inhibit CYP2D6-mediated metabolism and venlafaxine. However, although imipramine partially inhibited the CYP2D6-mediated metabolism of venlafaxine, resulting in higher plasma concentrations of venlafaxine and lower plasma concentrations of ODV, the total concentration of active compounds (venlafaxine plus ODV) was not affected. Also, in a clinical study involving CYP2D6 poor and extensive metabolizers, the total concentration of active compounds (venlafaxine plus ODV), was similar in both groups. No dosage adjustment is required when venlafaxine is co-administered with a CYP2D6 inhibitor. Caution is advised should a patient's therapy include venlafaxine and CYP2D6 inhibitor). Products include:
Benadryl Allergy Ultratab 2042
Children's Benadryl Allergy Liquid 2042

Dolasetron Mesylate (*In vitro* studies indicate that venlafaxine is a relatively weak inhibitor of CYP2D6. These findings have been confirmed in a clinical drug interaction study comparing the effect of venlafaxine to that of fluoxetine on the CYP2D6-mediated metabolism of dextrometrophan to dextrophan). Products include:
Anzemet Injection 2931
Anzemet Tablets 2934

Donepezil Hydrochloride (*In vitro* studies indicate that venlafaxine is a relatively weak inhibitor of CYP2D6. These findings have been confirmed in a clinical drug interaction study comparing the effect of venlafaxine to that of fluoxetine on the CYP2D6-mediated metabolism of dextrometrophan to dextrophan). Products include:
Aricept 1045
Aricept ODT 1045

Doxepin Hydrochloride (Studies indicate that venlafaxine is metabolized to its active metabolite, ODV, by CYP2D6. Thus the potential exists for a drug interaction between drugs that inhibit CYP2D6-mediated metabolism and venlafaxine. However, although imipramine partially inhibited the CYP2D6-mediated metabolism of venlafaxine, resulting in higher plasma concentrations of venlafaxine and lower plasma concentrations of ODV, the total concentration of active compounds (venlafaxine plus ODV) was not affected. Also, in a clinical study involving CYP2D6 poor and extensive metabolizers, the total concentration of active compounds (venlafaxine plus ODV), was similar in both groups. No dosage adjustment is required when venlafaxine is co-administered with a CYP2D6 inhibitor. Caution is advised should a patient's therapy include venlafaxine and CYP2D6 inhibitor).
No products indexed under this heading.

Droperidol (The risk of using venlafaxine in combination with other CNS active drugs has not been systematically evaluated. Consequently, caution is advised if the concomitant administration of venlafaxine and such drugs is required).
No products indexed under this heading.

Duloxetine Hydrochloride (Based on the mechanism of action of venlafaxine and the potential for serotonin syndrome, caution is advised when venlafaxine is co-administered with other drugs that may affect the serotonergic neurotransmitter systems, such as other SNRIs. If concomitant treatment of venlafaxine with another SNRI is clinically warranted, careful observation of the patient is advised, particularly during treatment initiation and dose increases). Products include:
Cymbalta 1871

Efavirenz (Concomitant use of CYP3A4 inhibitors and venlafaxine may increase levels of venlafaxine and ODV. Therefore, caution is advised if a patient's therapy includes a CYP3A4 inhibitor and venlafaxine concomitantly. The concomitant use of venlafaxine with a drug treatment(s) that potently inhibits both CYP2D6 and CYP3A4, the primary metabolizing enzymes for venlafaxine, has not been studied. Therefore, caution is advised should a patient's therapy include venlafaxine and any agent(s) that produce potent simultaneous inhibition of these two enzyme systems). Products include:
Atripla 906

Eletriptan Hydrobromide (There have been rare post-marketing reports of serotonin syndrome with use of an SSRI and a triptan. If concomitant treatment of venlafaxine with a triptan is clinically warranted, careful observation of the patient is advised, particularly during treatment initiation and dose increases. Patients should be cautioned about the risk of serotonin syndrome with the concomitant use of venlafaxine and triptans, tramadol, tryptophan supplements or other serotonergic agents).
No products indexed under this heading.

Encainide Hydrochloride (*In vitro* studies indicate that venlafaxine is a relatively weak inhibitor of CYP2D6. These findings have been confirmed in a clinical drug interaction study comparing the effect of venlafaxine to that of fluoxetine on the CYP2D6-mediated metabolism of dextrometrophan to dextrophan).
No products indexed under this heading.

Enflurane (The risk of using venlafaxine in combination with other CNS active drugs has not been systematically evaluated. Consequently, caution is advised if the concomitant administration of venlafaxine and such drugs is required).
No products indexed under this heading.

Enoxaparin Sodium (Patients should be cautioned about the concomitant use of venlafaxine and anti-coagulants since combined use of psychotropic drugs that interfere with serotonin reuptake and this agent has been associated with an increased risk of bleeding. SSRIs and SNRIs, including venlafaxine, may increase the risk of bleeding events. Concomitant use of anti-coagulants may add to this risk. Case reports and epidemiological studies (case-control and cohort design) have demonstrated an association between use of drugs that interfere with serotonin reuptake and the occurrence of gastrointestinal bleeding). Products include:
Lovenox 3005

Erythromycin (Concomitant use of CYP3A4 inhibitors and venlafaxine may increase levels of venlafaxine and ODV. Therefore, caution is advised if a patient's therapy includes a CYP3A4 inhibitor and venlafaxine concomitantly. The concomitant use of venlafaxine with a drug treatment(s) that potently inhibits both CYP2D6 and CYP3A4, the primary metabolizing enzymes for venlafaxine, has not been studied. Therefore, caution is advised should a patient's therapy include venlafaxine and any agent(s) that produce potent simultaneous inhibition of these two enzyme systems).
No products indexed under this heading.

Erythromycin Estolate (Concomitant use of CYP3A4 inhibitors and venlafaxine may increase levels of venlafaxine and ODV. Therefore, caution is advised if a patient's therapy includes a CYP3A4 inhibitor and venlafaxine concomitantly. The concomitant use of venlafaxine with a drug treatment(s) that potently inhibits both CYP2D6 and CYP3A4, the primary metabolizing enzymes for venlafaxine, has not been studied. Therefore, caution is advised should a patient's therapy include venlafaxine and any agent(s) that produce potent simultaneous inhibition of these two enzyme systems).
No products indexed under this heading.

Erythromycin Ethylsuccinate (Concomitant use of CYP3A4 inhibitors and venlafaxine may increase levels of venlafaxine and ODV. Therefore, caution is advised if a patient's therapy includes a CYP3A4 inhibitor and venlafaxine concomitantly. The concomitant use of venlafaxine with a drug treatment(s) that potently inhibits both CYP2D6 and CYP3A4, the primary metabolizing enzymes for venlafaxine, has not been studied. Therefore, caution is advised should a patient's therapy include venlafaxine and any agent(s) that produce potent simultaneous inhibition of these two enzyme systems). Products include:
E.E.S. 437
EryPed 435

Erythromycin Gluceptate (Concomitant use of CYP3A4 inhibitors and venlafaxine may increase levels of venlafaxine and ODV. Therefore, caution is advised if a patient's therapy includes a CYP3A4 inhibitor and venlafaxine concomitantly. The concomitant use of venlafaxine with a drug treatment(s) that potently inhibits both CYP2D6 and CYP3A4, the primary metabolizing enzymes for venlafaxine, has not been studied. Therefore, caution is advised should a patient's therapy include venlafaxine and any agent(s) that produce potent simultaneous inhibition of these two enzyme systems).
No products indexed under this heading.

Erythromycin Lactobionate (Concomitant use of CYP3A4 inhibitors and venlafaxine may increase levels of venlafaxine and ODV. Therefore, caution is advised if a patient's therapy includes a CYP3A4 inhibitor and venlafaxine concomitantly. The concomitant use of venlafaxine with a drug treatment(s) that potently inhibits both CYP2D6 and CYP3A4, the primary metabolizing enzymes for venlafaxine, has not been studied. Therefore, caution is advised should a patient's therapy include venlafaxine and any agent(s) that produce potent simultaneous inhibition of these two enzyme systems).
No products indexed under this heading.

Erythromycin Stearate (Concomitant use of CYP3A4 inhibitors and venlafaxine may increase levels of venlafaxine and ODV. Therefore, caution is advised if a patient's therapy includes a CYP3A4 inhibitor and venlafaxine concomitantly. The concomitant use of venlafaxine with a drug treatment(s) that potently inhibits both CYP2D6 and CYP3A4, the primary metabolizing enzymes for venlafaxine, has not been studied. Therefore, caution is advised should a patient's therapy include venlafaxine and any agent(s) that produce potent simultaneous inhibition of these two enzyme systems).
No products indexed under this heading.

Escitalopram Oxalate (Based on the mechanism of action of venlafaxine and the potential for serotonin syndrome, caution is advised when venlafaxine is co-administered with other drugs that may affect the serotonergic neurotransmitter systems, such as SSRIs. If concomitant treatment of venlafaxine with an SSRI is clinically warranted, careful observation of the patient is advised, particularly during treatment initiation and dose increases). Products include:
Lexapro Oral Suspension 1160
Lexapro Tablets 1160

Esomeprazole Magnesium (Concomitant use of CYP3A4 inhibitors and venlafaxine may increase levels of venlafaxine and ODV. Therefore, caution is advised if a patient's therapy includes a CYP3A4 inhibitor and venlafaxine concomitantly. The concomitant use of venlafaxine with a drug treatment(s) that potently inhibits both CYP2D6 and CYP3A4, the primary metabolizing enzymes for venlafaxine, has not been studied. Therefore, caution is advised should a patient's therapy include venlafaxine and any agent(s) that produce potent simultaneous inhibition of these two enzyme systems). Products include:
Nexium Capsules 704
Nexium Oral Suspension 704

Esomeprazole Sodium (Concomitant use of CYP3A4 inhibitors and venlafaxine may increase levels of venlafaxine and ODV. Therefore, caution is advised if a patient's therapy includes a CYP3A4 inhibitor and venlafaxine concomitantly. The concomitant use of venlafaxine with a drug treatment(s) that potently inhibits both CYP2D6 and CYP3A4, the primary metabolizing enzymes for venlafaxine, has not been studied. Therefore, caution is advised should a patient's therapy include venlafaxine and any agent(s) that produce potent simultaneous inhibition of these two enzyme systems). Products include:
Nexium I.V. 712

Estazolam (The risk of using venlafaxine in combination with other CNS active drugs has not been systematically evaluated. Consequently, caution is advised if the concomitant administration of venlafaxine and such drugs is required).
No products indexed under this heading.

Ethacrynic Acid (Elderly patients may be at greater risk of developing hyponatremia with SSRIs and SNRIs. Also patients taking diuretics or who are otherwise volume depleted may be at greater risk. Discontinuation of venlafaxine should be considered in patients with symptomatic hyponatremia and appropriate medical intervention should be instituted).
No products indexed under this heading.

Ethanol (Although venlafaxine has not been shown to increase the impairment of mental and motor skills caused by alcohol, patients should be advised to avoid alcohol while taking venlafaxine).
No products indexed under this heading.

Ethchlorvynol (The risk of using venlafaxine in combination with other CNS active drugs has not been systematically evaluated. Consequently, caution is advised if the concomitant administration of venlafaxine and such drugs is required).
No products indexed under this heading.

Ethinamate (The risk of using venlafaxine in combination with other CNS active drugs has not been systematically evaluated. Consequently, caution is advised if the concomitant administration of venlafaxine and such drugs is required).
No products indexed under this heading.

IMPORTANT NOTE: Always consult each drug listing in the patient's regimen for possible interactions.

Ethyl Alcohol (Although venlafaxine has not been shown to increase the impairment of mental and motor skills caused by alcohol, patients should be advised to avoid alcohol while taking venlafaxine).

No products indexed under this heading.

Etodolac (Patients should be cautioned about the concomitant use of venlafaxine and NSAIDs since combined use of psychotropic drugs that interfere with serotonin reuptake and this agent has been associated with an increased risk of bleeding. SSRIs and SNRIs, including venlafaxine, may increase the risk of bleeding events. Concomitant use of nonsteroidal anti-inflammatory drugs may add to this risk. Case reports and epidemiological studies (case-control and cohort design) have demonstrated an association between use of drugs that interfere with serotonin reuptake and the occurrence of gastrointestinal bleeding).

No products indexed under this heading.

Fenoprofen Calcium (Patients should be cautioned about the concomitant use of venlafaxine and NSAIDs since combined use of psychotropic drugs that interfere with serotonin reuptake and this agent has been associated with an increased risk of bleeding. SSRIs and SNRIs, including venlafaxine, may increase the risk of bleeding events. Concomitant use of nonsteroidal anti-inflammatory drugs may add to this risk. Case reports and epidemiological studies (case-control and cohort design) have demonstrated an association between use of drugs that interfere with serotonin reuptake and the occurrence of gastrointestinal bleeding).

No products indexed under this heading.

Fentanyl (The risk of using venlafaxine in combination with other CNS active drugs has not been systematically evaluated. Consequently, caution is advised if the concomitant administration of venlafaxine and such drugs is required). Products include:

Duragesic	2604
Fentanyl Transdermal System	2346
Onsolis	2054

Fentanyl Citrate (The risk of using venlafaxine in combination with other CNS active drugs has not been systematically evaluated. Consequently, caution is advised if the concomitant administration of venlafaxine and such drugs is required). Products include:

Fentora	966

Flecainide Acetate (*In vitro* studies indicate that venlafaxine is a relatively weak inhibitor of CYP2D6. These findings have been confirmed in a clinical drug interaction study comparing the effect of venlafaxine to that of fluoxetine on the CYP2D6-mediated metabolism of dextrometrophan to dextrophan).

No products indexed under this heading.

Fluconazole (Concomitant use of CYP3A4 inhibitors and venlafaxine may increase levels of venlafaxine and ODV. Therefore, caution is advised if a patient's therapy includes a CYP3A4 inhibitor and venlafaxine concomitantly. The concomitant use of venlafaxine with a drug treatment(s) that potently inhibits both CYP2D6 and CYP3A4, the primary metabolizing enzymes for venlafaxine, has not been studied. Therefore, caution is advised should a patient's therapy include venlafaxine and any agent(s) that produce potent simultaneous inhibition of these two enzyme systems).

No products indexed under this heading.

Fluoxetine (Based on the mechanism of action of venlafaxine and the potential for serotonin syndrome, caution is advised when venlafaxine is co-administered with other drugs that may affect the serotonergic neurotransmitter systems, such as SSRIs. If concomitant treatment of venlafaxine with an SSRI is clinically warranted, careful observation of the patient is advised, particularly during treatment initiation and dose increases).

No products indexed under this heading.

Fluoxetine Hydrochloride (Based on the mechanism of action of venlafaxine and the potential for serotonin syndrome, caution is advised when venlafaxine is co-administered with other drugs that may affect the serotonergic neurotransmitter systems, such as SSRIs. If concomitant treatment of venlafaxine with an SSRI is clinically warranted, careful observation of the patient is advised, particularly during treatment initiation and dose increases). Products include:

Prozac Weekly	1941
Prozac Pulvules	1941
Symbyax	1965

Fluphenazine Decanoate (The risk of using venlafaxine in combination with other CNS active drugs has not been systematically evaluated. Consequently, caution is advised if the concomitant administration of venlafaxine and such drugs is required).

No products indexed under this heading.

Fluphenazine Enanthate (The risk of using venlafaxine in combination with other CNS active drugs has not been systematically evaluated. Consequently, caution is advised if the concomitant administration of venlafaxine and such drugs is required).

No products indexed under this heading.

Fluphenazine Hydrochloride (The risk of using venlafaxine in combination with other CNS active drugs has not been systematically evaluated. Consequently, caution is advised if the concomitant administration of venlafaxine and such drugs is required).

No products indexed under this heading.

Flurazepam Hydrochloride (The risk of using venlafaxine in combination with other CNS active drugs has not been systematically evaluated. Consequently, caution is advised if the concomitant administration of venlafaxine and such drugs is required).

No products indexed under this heading.

Flurbiprofen (Patients should be cautioned about the concomitant use of venlafaxine and NSAIDs since combined use of psychotropic drugs that interfere with serotonin reuptake and this agent has been associated with an increased risk of bleeding. SSRIs and SNRIs, including venlafaxine, may increase the risk of bleeding events. Concomitant use of nonsteroidal anti-inflammatory drugs may add to this risk. Case reports and epidemiological studies (case-control and cohort design) have demonstrated an association between use of drugs that interfere with serotonin reuptake and the occurrence of gastrointestinal bleeding).

No products indexed under this heading.

Fluvoxamine (Based on the mechanism of action of venlafaxine and the potential for serotonin syndrome, caution is advised when venlafaxine is co-administered with other drugs that may affect the serotonergic neurotransmitter systems, such as SSRIs. If concomitant treatment of venlafaxine with an SSRI is clinically warranted, careful observation of the patient is advised, particularly during treatment initiation and dose increases).

No products indexed under this heading.

Fluvoxamine Maleate (Based on the mechanism of action of venlafaxine and the potential for serotonin syndrome, caution is advised when venlafaxine is co-administered with other drugs that may affect the serotonergic neurotrans-mitter systems, such as SSRIs. If concomitant treatment of venlafaxine with an SSRI is clinically warranted, careful observation of the patient is advised, particularly during treatment initiation and dose increases).

No products indexed under this heading.

Fondaparinux Sodium (Patients should be cautioned about the concomitant use of venlafaxine and anti-coagulants since combined use of psychotropic drugs that interfere with serotonin reuptake and this agent has been associated with an increased risk of bleeding. SSRIs and SNRIs, including venlafaxine, may increase the risk of bleeding events. Concomitant use of anti-coagulants may add to this risk. Case reports and epidemiological studies (case-control and cohort design) have demonstrated an association between use of drugs that interfere with serotonin reuptake and the occurrence of gastrointestinal bleeding). Products include:

Arixtra	1320

Formoterol Fumarate (*In vitro* studies indicate that venlafaxine is a relatively weak inhibitor of CYP2D6. These findings have been confirmed in a clinical drug interaction study comparing the effect of venlafaxine to that of fluoxetine on the CYP2D6-mediated metabolism of dextrometrophan to dextrophan). Products include:

Foradil	3121
Perforomist	3634

Fosamprenavir Calcium (Concomitant use of CYP3A4 inhibitors and venlafaxine may increase levels of venlafaxine and ODV. Therefore, caution is advised if a patient's therapy includes a CYP3A4 inhibitor and venlafaxine concomitantly. The concomitant use of venlafaxine with a drug treatment(s) that potently inhibits both CYP2D6 and CYP3A4, the primary metabolizing enzymes for venlafaxine, has not been studied. Therefore, caution is advised should a patient's therapy include venlafaxine and any agent(s) that produce potent simultaneous inhibition of these two enzyme systems). Products include:

Lexiva Oral Suspension	1558
Lexiva	1558

Frovatriptan Succinate (There have been rare post-marketing reports of serotonin syndrome with use of an SSRI and a triptan. If concomitant treatment of venlafaxine with a triptan is clinically warranted, careful observation of the patient is advised, particularly during treatment initiation and dose increases. Patients should be cautioned about the risk of serotonin syndrome with the concomitant use of venlafaxine and triptans, tramadol, tryptophan supplements or other serotonergic agents). Products include:

Frova	1103

Furosemide (Elderly patients may be at greater risk of developing hyponatremia with SSRIs and SNRIs. Also patients taking diuretics or who are otherwise volume depleted may be at greater risk. Discontinuation of venlafaxine should be considered in patients with symptomatic hyponatremia and appropriate medical intervention should be instituted). Products include:

Furosemide	2354

Galantamine Hydrobromide (*In vitro* studies indicate that venlafaxine is a relatively weak inhibitor of CYP2D6. These findings have been confirmed in a clinical drug interaction study comparing the effect of venlafaxine to that of fluoxetine on the CYP2D6-mediated metabolism of dextrometrophan to dextrophan).

No products indexed under this heading.

Glutethimide (The risk of using venlafaxine in combination with other CNS active drugs has not been systematically evaluated. Consequently, caution is advised if the concomitant administration of venlafaxine and such drugs is required).

No products indexed under this heading.

Halofantrine Hydrochloride (Studies indicate that venlafaxine is metabolized to its active metabolite, ODV, by CYP2D6. Thus the potential exists for a drug interaction between drugs that inhibit CYP2D6-mediated metabolism and venlafaxine. However, although imipramine partially inhibited the CYP2D6-mediated metabolism of venlafaxine, resulting in higher plasma concentrations of venlafaxine and lower plasma concentrations of ODV, the total concentration of active compounds (venlafaxine plus ODV) was not affected. Also, in a clinical study involving CYP2D6 poor and extensive metabolizers, the total concentration of active compounds (venlafaxine plus ODV), was similar in both groups. No dosage adjustment is required when venlafaxine is co-administered with a CYP2D6 inhibitor. Caution is advised should a patient's therapy include venlafaxine and CYP2D6 inhibitor).

No products indexed under this heading.

Haloperidol (The risk of using venlafaxine in combination with other CNS active drugs has not been systematically evaluated. Consequently, caution is advised if the concomitant administration of venlafaxine and such drugs is required).

No products indexed under this heading.

Haloperidol Decanoate (The risk of using venlafaxine in combination with other CNS active drugs has not been systematically evaluated. Consequently, caution is advised if the concomitant administration of venlafaxine and such drugs is required).

No products indexed under this heading.

Haloperidol Lactate (Venlafaxine administered under steady-state conditions at 150 mg/day in 24 healthy subjects decreased total oral-dose clearance (Cl/F) of a single 2 mg dose of haloperidol by 42%, which resulted in a 70% increase in haloperidol AUC. In addition, the haloperidol C_{max} increased 88% when co-administered with venlafaxine, but the haloperidol elimination half-life ($t_{1/2}$) was unchanged. The mechanism explaining this finding is unknown).

No products indexed under this heading.

Heparin Calcium (Patients should be cautioned about the concomitant use of venlafaxine and anti-coagulants since combined use of psychotropic drugs that interfere with serotonin reuptake and this agent has been associated with an increased risk of bleeding. SSRIs and SNRIs, including venlafaxine, may increase the risk of bleeding events. Concomitant use of anti-coagulants may add to this risk. Case reports and epidemiological studies (case-control and cohort design) have demonstrated an association between use of drugs that interfere with serotonin reuptake and the occurrence of gastrointestinal bleeding).

No products indexed under this heading.

Heparin Sodium (Patients should be cautioned about the concomitant use of venlafaxine and anti-coagulants since combined use of psychotropic drugs that interfere with serotonin reuptake and this agent has been associated with an increased risk of bleeding. SSRIs and SNRIs, including venlafaxine, may increase the risk of bleeding events. Concomitant use of anti-coagulants may add to this risk. Case reports and epidemiological studies (case-control and

2031 Interactions Index Venlafaxine

cohort design) have demonstrated an association between use of drugs that interfere with serotonin reuptake and the occurrence of gastrointestinal bleeding).
No products indexed under this heading.

Hydrochlorothiazide (Elderly patients may be at greater risk of developing hyponatremia with SSRIs and SNRIs. Also patients taking diuretics or who are otherwise volume depleted may be at greater risk. Discontinuation of venlafaxine should be considered in patients with symptomatic hyponatremia and appropriate medical intervention should be instituted). Products include:
Atacand HCT ... 700
Avalide ... 2956
Benicar HCT ... 1017
Diovan HCT ... 2419
Dyazide ... 1429
Exforge HCT ... 2449
Hyzaar ... 2162
Hyzaar 100-12.5 ... 2162
Micardis HCT ... 889
Prinzide ... 2246
Tekturna HCT ... 2541
Teveten HCT ... 541

Hydrocodone Bitartrate (The risk of using venlafaxine in combination with other CNS active drugs has not been systematically evaluated. Consequently, caution is advised if the concomitant administration of venlafaxine and such drugs is required). Products include:
Vicodin ... 560
Vicodin ES ... 561
Vicodin HP ... 563
Vicoprofen ... 564
Zydone ... 1138

Hydrocodone Polistirex (The risk of using venlafaxine in combination with other CNS active drugs has not been systematically evaluated. Consequently, caution is advised if the concomitant administration of venlafaxine and such drugs is required). Products include:
Tussionex ... 3443

Hydroflumethiazide (Elderly patients may be at greater risk of developing hyponatremia with SSRIs and SNRIs. Also patients taking diuretics or who are otherwise volume depleted may be at greater risk. Discontinuation of venlafaxine should be considered in patients with symptomatic hyponatremia and appropriate medical intervention should be instituted).
No products indexed under this heading.

Hydromorphone Hydrochloride (The risk of using venlafaxine in combination with other CNS active drugs has not been systematically evaluated. Consequently, caution is advised if the concomitant administration of venlafaxine and such drugs is required). Products include:
Dilaudid Injection ... 2800
Dilaudid Oral ... 2797
Dilaudid Tablets ... 2797
Dilaudid-HP ... 2800

Hydroxyamphetamine Hydrobromide (The risk of using venlafaxine in combination with other CNS active drugs has not been systematically evaluated. Consequently, caution is advised if the concomitant administration of venlafaxine and such drugs is required).
No products indexed under this heading.

Hydroxychloroquine Sulfate (Studies indicate that venlafaxine is metabolized to its active metabolite, ODV, by CYP2D6. Thus the potential exists for a drug interaction between drugs that inhibit CYP2D6-mediated metabolism and venlafaxine. However, although imipramine partially inhibited the CYP2D6-mediated metabolism of venlafaxine, resulting in higher plasma concentrations of venlafaxine and lower plasma concentrations of ODV, the total concentration of active compounds (venlafaxine plus ODV) was not affected. Also, in a clinical study involving CYP2D6 poor and extensive metabolizers, the total concentration of active compounds (venlafaxine plus ODV), was similar in both groups. No dosage adjustment is required when venlafaxine is co-administered with a CYP2D6 inhibitor. Caution is advised should a patient's therapy include venlafaxine and CYP2D6 inhibitor).
No products indexed under this heading.

Hydroxyzine Hydrochloride (The risk of using venlafaxine in combination with other CNS active drugs has not been systematically evaluated. Consequently, caution is advised if the concomitant administration of venlafaxine and such drugs is required).
No products indexed under this heading.

Hypericum (Based on the mechanism of action of venlafaxine and the potential for serotonin syndrome, caution is advised when venlafaxine is co-administered with other drugs that may affect the serotonergic neurotransmitter systems, such as St. John's Wort. If concomitant treatment of venlafaxine with St. John's Wort is clinically warranted, careful observation of the patient is advised, particularly during treatment initiation and dose increases).
No products indexed under this heading.

Hypericum Perforatum (Based on the mechanism of action of venlafaxine and the potential for serotonin syndrome, caution is advised when venlafaxine is co-administered with other drugs that may affect the serotonergic neurotransmitter systems, such as St. John's Wort. If concomitant treatment of venlafaxine with St. John's Wort is clinically warranted, careful observation of the patient is advised, particularly during treatment initiation and dose increases). Products include:
Traumeel ... 1800

Ibuprofen (Patients should be cautioned about the concomitant use of venlafaxine and NSAIDs since combined use of psychotropic drugs that interfere with serotonin reuptake and this agent has been associated with an increased risk of bleeding. SSRIs and SNRIs, including venlafaxine, may increase the risk of bleeding events. Concomitant use of nonsteroidal anti-inflammatory drugs may add to this risk. Case reports and epidemiological studies (case-control and cohort design) have demonstrated an association between use of drugs that interfere with serotonin reuptake and the occurrence of gastrointestinal bleeding). Products include:
Motrin IB ... 2043
Children's Motrin ... 2044
Children's Motrin Non-Staining Dye-Free ... 2044
Infants' Motrin ... 2044
Infants' Motrin Dye-Free ... 2044
Junior Strength Motrin ... 2044
Vicoprofen ... 564

Imatinib Mesylate (Studies indicate that venlafaxine is metabolized to its active metabolite, ODV, by CYP2D6. Thus the potential exists for a drug interaction between drugs that inhibit CYP2D6-mediated metabolism and venlafaxine. However, although imipramine partially inhibited the CYP2D6-mediated metabolism of venlafaxine, resulting in higher plasma concentrations of venlafaxine and lower plasma concentrations of ODV, the total concentration of active compounds (venlafaxine plus ODV) was not affected. Also, in a clinical study involving CYP2D6 poor and extensive metabolizers, the total concentration of active compounds (venlafaxine plus ODV), was similar in both groups. No dosage adjustment is required when venlafaxine is co-administered with a CYP2D6 inhibitor. Caution is advised should a patient's therapy include venlafaxine and CYP2D6 inhibitor). Products include:
Gleevec ... 2477

Imipramine Hydrochloride (Venlafaxine did not affect the pharmacokinetics of imipramine and 2-OH-imipramine. However, desipramine AUC, C_{max}, and C_{min} increased by about 35% in the presence of venlafaxine. The 2-OH-desipramine AUCs increased by at least 2.5-fold (with venlafaxine 37.5 mg q 12h) and 4.5-fold (with venlafaxine 75 mg q 12h). Imipramine did not affect the pharmacokinetics of venlafaxine and ODV. The clinical significance of elevated 2-OH-desipramine levels is unknown).
No products indexed under this heading.

Imipramine Pamoate (Venlafaxine did not affect the pharmacokinetics of imipramine and 2-OH-imipramine. However, desipramine AUC, C_{max}, and C_{min} increased by about 35% in the presence of venlafaxine. The 2-OH-desipramine AUCs increased by at least 2.5-fold (with venlafaxine 37.5 mg q 12h) and 4.5-fold (with venlafaxine 75 mg q 12h). Imipramine did not affect the pharmacokinetics of venlafaxine and ODV. The clinical significance of elevated 2-OH-desipramine levels is unknown).
No products indexed under this heading.

Indapamide (Elderly patients may be at greater risk of developing hyponatremia with SSRIs and SNRIs. Also patients taking diuretics or who are otherwise volume depleted may be at greater risk. Discontinuation of venlafaxine should be considered in patients with symptomatic hyponatremia and appropriate medical intervention should be instituted). Products include:
Indapamide ... 2356

Indinavir Sulfate (In a study of nine healthy volunteers, venlafaxine administered under steady-state conditions at 150 mg/day resulted in a 28% decrease in the AUC of a single 800 mg dose of indinavir and a 36% decrease in indinavir C_{max}. Indinavir did not affect the pharmacokinetics of venlafaxine and ODV. The clinical significance of this finding is unknown). Products include:
Crixivan ... 2113

Indomethacin (Patients should be cautioned about the concomitant use of venlafaxine and NSAIDs since combined use of psychotropic drugs that interfere with serotonin reuptake and this agent has been associated with an increased risk of bleeding. SSRIs and SNRIs, including venlafaxine, may increase the risk of bleeding events. Concomitant use of nonsteroidal anti-inflammatory drugs may add to this risk. Case reports and epidemiological studies (case-control and cohort design) have demonstrated an association between use of drugs that interfere with serotonin reuptake and the occurrence of gastrointestinal bleeding). Products include:
Indocin ... 2167

Indomethacin Sodium Trihydrate (Patients should be cautioned about the concomitant use of venlafaxine and NSAIDs since combined use of psychotropic drugs that interfere with serotonin reuptake and this agent has been associated with an increased risk of bleeding. SSRIs and SNRIs, including venlafaxine, may increase the risk of bleeding events. Concomitant use of nonsteroidal anti-inflammatory drugs may add to this risk. Case reports and epidemiological studies (case-control and cohort design) have demonstrated an association between use of drugs that interfere with serotonin reuptake and the occurrence of gastrointestinal bleeding). Products include:
Indocin I.V. ... 2007

Indoramin Hydrochloride (*In vitro* studies indicate that venlafaxine is a relatively weak inhibitor of CYP2D6. These findings have been confirmed in a clinical drug interaction study comparing the effect of venlafaxine to that of fluoxetine on the CYP2D6-mediated metabolism of dextrometrophan to dextrophan).
No products indexed under this heading.

Isocarboxazid (Concomitant use in patients taking monoamine oxidase inhibitors (MAOIs) is contraindicated. Adverse reactions, some of which were serious, have been reported in patients who have recently been discontinued from a monoamine oxidase inhibitor (MAOI) and started on venlafaxine hydrochloride, or who have recently had venlafaxine hydrochloride therapy discontinued prior to initiation of a MAOI. It is recommended that venlafaxine hydrochloride not be used in combination with a MAOI, or within at least 14 days of discontinuing treatment with a MAOI. Based on the half-life of venlafaxine hydrochloride, at least 7 days should be allowed after stopping venlafaxine hydrochloride before starting an MAOI). Products include:
Marplan ... 3481

Isoflurane (The risk of using venlafaxine in combination with other CNS active drugs has not been systematically evaluated. Consequently, caution is advised if the concomitant administration of venlafaxine and such drugs is required).
No products indexed under this heading.

Isoniazid (Concomitant use of CYP3A4 inhibitors and venlafaxine may increase levels of venlafaxine and ODV. Therefore, caution is advised if a patient's therapy includes a CYP3A4 inhibitor and venlafaxine concomitantly. The concomitant use of venlafaxine with a drug treatment(s) that potently inhibits both CYP2D6 and CYP3A4, the primary metabolizing enzymes for venlafaxine, has not been studied. Therefore, caution is advised should a patient's therapy include venlafaxine and any agent(s) that produce potent simultaneous inhibition of these two enzyme systems).
No products indexed under this heading.

Itraconazole (Concomitant use of CYP3A4 inhibitors and venlafaxine may increase levels of venlafaxine and ODV. Therefore, caution is advised if a patient's therapy includes a CYP3A4 inhibitor and venlafaxine concomitantly. The concomitant use of venlafaxine with a drug treatment(s) that potently inhibits both CYP2D6 and CYP3A4, the primary metabolizing enzymes for venlafaxine, has not been studied. Therefore, caution is advised should a patient's therapy include venlafaxine and any agent(s) that produce potent simultaneous inhibition of these two enzyme systems).
No products indexed under this heading.

Ketamine Hydrochloride (The risk of using venlafaxine in combination with other CNS active drugs has not been systematically evaluated. Consequently, caution is advised if the concomitant administration of venlafaxine and such drugs is required).
No products indexed under this heading.

Ketoconazole (A study of ketoconazole 100 mg b.i.d. with a single dose of venlafaxine 50 mg in extensive metabolizers and 25 mg in poor metabolizers of CYP2D6 resulted in higher plasma concentrations of both venlafaxine and O-desvenlafaxine (ODV) in most subjects following administration of ketoconazole. Venlafaxine C_{max} increased by 26% in EM subjects and 48% in PM subjects. C_{max} values for ODV increased by 14% and 29% in EM and PM subjects, respectively. Venlafaxine AUC increased by 21% in EM subjects and 70% in PM

IMPORTANT NOTE: Always consult each drug listing in the patient's regimen for possible interactions.

subjects, and AUC values for ODV increased by 23% and 141% in EM and PM subjects, respectively. Combined AUCs of venlafaxine and ODV increased on an average of approximately 23% in EMs and 53% in PMs). Products include:

Extina 3319
Xolegel 3337

Ketoprofen (Patients should be cautioned about the concomitant use of venlafaxine and NSAIDs since combined use of psychotropic drugs that interfere with serotonin reuptake and this agent has been associated with an increased risk of bleeding. SSRIs and SNRIs, including venlafaxine, may increase the risk of bleeding events. Concomitant use of nonsteroidal anti-inflammatory drugs may add to this risk. Case reports and epidemiological studies (case-control and cohort design) have demonstrated an association between use of drugs that interfere with serotonin reuptake and the occurrence of gastrointestinal bleeding).

No products indexed under this heading.

Ketorolac Tromethamine (Patients should be cautioned about the concomitant use of venlafaxine and NSAIDs since combined use of psychotropic drugs that interfere with serotonin reuptake and this agent has been associated with an increased risk of bleeding. SSRIs and SNRIs, including venlafaxine, may increase the risk of bleeding events. Concomitant use of nonsteroidal anti-inflammatory drugs may add to this risk. Case reports and epidemiological studies (case-control and cohort design) have demonstrated an association between use of drugs that interfere with serotonin reuptake and the occurrence of gastrointestinal bleeding). Products include:

Acuvail .... ⊙ 209

Labetalol Hydrochloride (In vitro studies indicate that venlafaxine is a relatively weak inhibitor of CYP2D6. These findings have been confirmed in a clinical drug interaction study comparing the effect of venlafaxine to that of fluoxetine on the CYP2D6-mediated metabolism of dextrometrophan to dextrophan).

No products indexed under this heading.

Lapatinib (Concomitant use of CYP3A4 inhibitors and venlafaxine may increase levels of venlafaxine and ODV. Therefore, caution is advised if a patient's therapy includes a CYP3A4 inhibitor and venlafaxine concomitantly. The concomitant use of venlafaxine with a drug treatment(s) that potently inhibits both CYP2D6 and CYP3A4, the primary metabolizing enzymes for venlafaxine, has not been studied. Therefore, caution is advised should a patient's therapy include venlafaxine and any agent(s) that produce potent simultaneous inhibition of these two enzyme systems). Products include:

Tykerb 1698

Levomethadyl Acetate Hydrochloride (The risk of using venlafaxine in combination with other CNS active drugs has not been systematically evaluated. Consequently, caution is advised if the concomitant administration of venlafaxine and such drugs is required).

No products indexed under this heading.

Levorphanol Tartrate (The risk of using venlafaxine in combination with other CNS active drugs has not been systematically evaluated. Consequently, caution is advised if the concomitant administration of venlafaxine and such drugs is required).

No products indexed under this heading.

Lidocaine (In vitro studies indicate that venlafaxine is a relatively weak inhibitor of CYP2D6. These findings have been confirmed in a clinical drug interaction study comparing the effect of venlafax-

ine to that of fluoxetine on the CYP2D6-mediated metabolism of dextrometrophan to dextrophan). Products include:

Lidoderm 1107

Lidocaine Hydrochloride (In vitro studies indicate that venlafaxine is a relatively weak inhibitor of CYP2D6. These findings have been confirmed in a clinical drug interaction study comparing the effect of venlafaxine to that of fluoxetine on the CYP2D6-mediated metabolism of dextrometrophan to dextrophan).

No products indexed under this heading.

Linezolid (Based on the mechanism of action of venlafaxine and the potential for serotonin syndrome, caution is advised when venlafaxine is co-administered with other drugs that may affect the serotonergic neurotransmitter systems, such as linezolid (an antibiotic which is a reversible non-selective MAOI). If concomitant treatment of venlafaxine with linezolid is clinically warranted, careful observation of the patient is advised, particularly during treatment initiation and dose increases). Products include:

Zyvox 2769

Lisdexamfetamine Dimesylate (The risk of using venlafaxine in combination with other CNS active drugs has not been systematically evaluated. Consequently, caution is advised if the concomitant administration of venlafaxine and such drugs is required). Products include:

Vyvanse 3298

Lithium (Based on the mechanism of action of venlafaxine and the potential for serotonin syndrome, caution is advised when venlafaxine is co-administered with other drugs that may affect the serotonergic neurotransmitter systems, such as lithium. If concomitant treatment of venlafaxine with lithium is clinically warranted, careful observation of the patient is advised, particularly during treatment initiation and dose increases).

No products indexed under this heading.

Lithium Carbonate (Based on the mechanism of action of venlafaxine and the potential for serotonin syndrome, caution is advised when venlafaxine is co-administered with other drugs that may affect the serotonergic neurotransmitter systems, such as lithium. If concomitant treatment of venlafaxine with lithium is clinically warranted, careful observation of the patient is advised, particularly during treatment initiation and dose increases).

No products indexed under this heading.

Lithium Citrate (Based on the mechanism of action of venlafaxine and the potential for serotonin syndrome, caution is advised when venlafaxine is co-administered with other drugs that may affect the serotonergic neurotransmitter systems, such as lithium. If concomitant treatment of venlafaxine with lithium is clinically warranted, careful observation of the patient is advised, particularly during treatment initiation and dose increases).

No products indexed under this heading.

Lopinavir (Concomitant use of CYP3A4 inhibitors and venlafaxine may increase levels of venlafaxine and ODV. Therefore, caution is advised if a patient's therapy includes a CYP3A4 inhibitor and venlafaxine concomitantly. The concomitant use of venlafaxine with a drug treatment(s) that potently inhibits both CYP2D6 and CYP3A4, the primary metabolizing enzymes for venlafaxine, has not been studied. Therefore, caution is advised should a patient's therapy include venlafaxine and any agent(s)

that produce potent simultaneous inhibition of these two enzyme systems). Products include:

Kaletra 458

Loratadine (Concomitant use of CYP3A4 inhibitors and venlafaxine may increase levels of venlafaxine and ODV. Therefore, caution is advised if a patient's therapy includes a CYP3A4 inhibitor and venlafaxine concomitantly. The concomitant use of venlafaxine with a drug treatment(s) that potently inhibits both CYP2D6 and CYP3A4, the primary metabolizing enzymes for venlafaxine, has not been studied. Therefore, caution is advised should a patient's therapy include venlafaxine and any agent(s) that produce potent simultaneous inhibition of these two enzyme systems).

No products indexed under this heading.

Lorazepam (The risk of using venlafaxine in combination with other CNS active drugs has not been systematically evaluated. Consequently, caution is advised if the concomitant administration of venlafaxine and such drugs is required).

No products indexed under this heading.

Low Molecular Weight Heparins (Patients should be cautioned about the concomitant use of venlafaxine and anti-coagulants since combined use of psychotropic drugs that interfere with serotonin reuptake and this agent has been associated with an increased risk of bleeding. SSRIs and SNRIs, including venlafaxine, may increase the risk of bleeding events. Concomitant use of anti-coagulants may add to this risk. Case reports and epidemiological studies (case-control and cohort design) have demonstrated an association between use of drugs that interfere with serotonin reuptake and the occurrence of gastrointestinal bleeding).

No products indexed under this heading.

Loxapine Hydrochloride (The risk of using venlafaxine in combination with other CNS active drugs has not been systematically evaluated. Consequently, caution is advised if the concomitant administration of venlafaxine and such drugs is required).

No products indexed under this heading.

Loxapine Succinate (The risk of using venlafaxine in combination with other CNS active drugs has not been systematically evaluated. Consequently, caution is advised if the concomitant administration of venlafaxine and such drugs is required).

No products indexed under this heading.

Maprotiline Hydrochloride (Studies indicate that venlafaxine is metabolized to its active metabolite, ODV, by CYP2D6. Thus the potential exists for a drug interaction between drugs that inhibit CYP2D6-mediated metabolism and venlafaxine. However, although imipramine partially inhibited the CYP2D6-mediated metabolism of venlafaxine, resulting in higher plasma concentrations of venlafaxine and lower plasma concentrations of ODV, the total concentration of active compounds (venlafaxine plus ODV) was not affected. Also, in a clinical study involving CYP2D6 poor and extensive metabolizers, the total concentration of active compounds (venlafaxine plus ODV), was similar in both groups. No dosage adjustment is required when venlafaxine is co-administered with a CYP2D6 inhibitor. Caution is advised should a patient's therapy include venlafaxine and CYP2D6 inhibitor).

No products indexed under this heading.

Meclofenamate Sodium (Patients should be cautioned about the concomitant use of venlafaxine and NSAIDs since combined use of psychotropic drugs that interfere with serotonin

reuptake and this agent has been associated with an increased risk of bleeding. SSRIs and SNRIs, including venlafaxine, may increase the risk of bleeding events. Concomitant use of nonsteroidal anti-inflammatory drugs may add to this risk. Case reports and epidemiological studies (case-control and cohort design) have demonstrated an association between use of drugs that interfere with serotonin reuptake and the occurrence of gastrointestinal bleeding).

No products indexed under this heading.

Mefenamic Acid (Patients should be cautioned about the concomitant use of venlafaxine and NSAIDs since combined use of psychotropic drugs that interfere with serotonin reuptake and this agent has been associated with an increased risk of bleeding. SSRIs and SNRIs, including venlafaxine, may increase the risk of bleeding events. Concomitant use of nonsteroidal anti-inflammatory drugs may add to this risk. Case reports and epidemiological studies (case-control and cohort design) have demonstrated an association between use of drugs that interfere with serotonin reuptake and the occurrence of gastrointestinal bleeding).

No products indexed under this heading.

Meloxicam (Patients should be cautioned about the concomitant use of venlafaxine and NSAIDs since combined use of psychotropic drugs that interfere with serotonin reuptake and this agent has been associated with an increased risk of bleeding. SSRIs and SNRIs, including venlafaxine, may increase the risk of bleeding events. Concomitant use of nonsteroidal anti-inflammatory drugs may add to this risk. Case reports and epidemiological studies (case-control and cohort design) have demonstrated an association between use of drugs that interfere with serotonin reuptake and the occurrence of gastrointestinal bleeding).

No products indexed under this heading.

Meperidine Hydrochloride (The risk of using venlafaxine in combination with other CNS active drugs has not been systematically evaluated. Consequently, caution is advised if the concomitant administration of venlafaxine and such drugs is required).

No products indexed under this heading.

Mephobarbital (The risk of using venlafaxine in combination with other CNS active drugs has not been systematically evaluated. Consequently, caution is advised if the concomitant administration of venlafaxine and such drugs is required).

No products indexed under this heading.

Meprobamate (The risk of using venlafaxine in combination with other CNS active drugs has not been systematically evaluated. Consequently, caution is advised if the concomitant administration of venlafaxine and such drugs is required).

No products indexed under this heading.

Mesoridazine Besylate (The risk of using venlafaxine in combination with other CNS active drugs has not been systematically evaluated. Consequently, caution is advised if the concomitant administration of venlafaxine and such drugs is required).

No products indexed under this heading.

Methadone Hydrochloride (The risk of using venlafaxine in combination with other CNS active drugs has not been systematically evaluated. Consequently, caution is advised if the concomitant administration of venlafaxine and such drugs is required).

No products indexed under this heading.

2033 Interactions Index Venlafaxine

Methamphetamine Hydrochloride (The risk of using venlafaxine in combination with other CNS active drugs has not been systematically evaluated. Consequently, caution is advised if the concomitant administration of venlafaxine and such drugs is required).
No products indexed under this heading.

Methohexital Sodium (The risk of using venlafaxine in combination with other CNS active drugs has not been systematically evaluated. Consequently, caution is advised if the concomitant administration of venlafaxine and such drugs is required).
No products indexed under this heading.

Methotrimeprazine (The risk of using venlafaxine in combination with other CNS active drugs has not been systematically evaluated. Consequently, caution is advised if the concomitant administration of venlafaxine and such drugs is required).
No products indexed under this heading.

Methoxyflurane (The risk of using venlafaxine in combination with other CNS active drugs has not been systematically evaluated. Consequently, caution is advised if the concomitant administration of venlafaxine and such drugs is required).
No products indexed under this heading.

Methoxyphenamine (*In vitro* studies indicate that venlafaxine is a relatively weak inhibitor of CYP2D6. These findings have been confirmed in a clinical drug interaction study comparing the effect of venlafaxine to that of fluoxetine on the CYP2D6-mediated metabolism of dextrometrophan to dextrophan).
No products indexed under this heading.

Methyclothiazide (Elderly patients may be at greater risk of developing hyponatremia with SSRIs and SNRIs. Also patients taking diuretics or who are otherwise volume depleted may be at greater risk. Discontinuation of venlafaxine should be considered in patients with symptomatic hyponatremia and appropriate medical intervention should be instituted).
No products indexed under this heading.

Methylphenidate (The risk of using venlafaxine in combination with other CNS active drugs has not been systematically evaluated. Consequently, caution is advised if the concomitant administration of venlafaxine and such drugs is required). Products include:
Daytrana 3283

Methylphenidate Hydrochloride (The risk of using venlafaxine in combination with other CNS active drugs has not been systematically evaluated. Consequently, caution is advised if the concomitant administration of venlafaxine and such drugs is required). Products include:
Concerta 2598
Metadate CD 3439

Metolazone (Elderly patients may be at greater risk of developing hyponatremia with SSRIs and SNRIs. Also patients taking diuretics or who are otherwise volume depleted may be at greater risk. Discontinuation of venlafaxine should be considered in patients with symptomatic hyponatremia and appropriate medical intervention should be instituted).
No products indexed under this heading.

Metoprolol Succinate (Concomitant administration of venlafaxine (50 mg every 8 hours for 5 days) and metoprolol (100 mg every 24 hours for 5 days) to 18 healthy male subjects in a pharmacokinetic interaction study for both drugs resulted in an increase of plasma concentrations of metoprolol by approximately 30% to 40% without altering the plasma concentrations of its active metabolite, alpha-hydroxymetoprolol. Metoprolol did not alter the pharmacokinetic profile of venlafaxine or its active metabolite, O-desmethylvenlafaxine. Venlafaxine appeared to reduce the blood pressure-lowering effect of metoprolol in this study. The clinical relevance of this finding for hypertensive patients is unknown. Caution should be exercised with co-administration of venlafaxine and metoprolol. It is recommended that patients receiving venlafaxine hydrochloride have regular monitoring of blood pressure). Products include:
Toprol XL 732

Metoprolol Tartrate (Concomitant administration of venlafaxine (50 mg every 8 hours for 5 days) and metoprolol (100 mg every 24 hours for 5 days) to 18 healthy male subjects in a pharmacokinetic interaction study for both drugs resulted in an increase of plasma concentrations of metoprolol by approximately 30% to 40% without altering the plasma concentrations of its active metabolite, alpha-hydroxymetoprolol. Metoprolol did not alter the pharmacokinetic profile of venlafaxine or its active metabolite, O-desmethylvenlafaxine. Venlafaxine appeared to reduce the blood pressure-lowering effect of metoprolol in this study. The clinical relevance of this finding for hypertensive patients is unknown. Caution should be exercised with co-administration of venlafaxine and metoprolol. It is recommended that patients receiving venlafaxine hydrochloride have regular monitoring of blood pressure).
No products indexed under this heading.

Metronidazole (Concomitant use of CYP3A4 inhibitors and venlafaxine may increase levels of venlafaxine and ODV. Therefore, caution is advised if a patient's therapy includes a CYP3A4 inhibitor and venlafaxine concomitantly. The concomitant use of venlafaxine with a drug treatment(s) that potently inhibits both CYP2D6 and CYP3A4, the primary metabolizing enzymes for venlafaxine, has not been studied. Therefore, caution is advised should a patient's therapy include venlafaxine and any agent(s) that produce potent simultaneous inhibition of these two enzyme systems). Products include:
Pylera 793

Metronidazole Benzoate (Concomitant use of CYP3A4 inhibitors and venlafaxine may increase levels of venlafaxine and ODV. Therefore, caution is advised if a patient's therapy includes a CYP3A4 inhibitor and venlafaxine concomitantly. The concomitant use of venlafaxine with a drug treatment(s) that potently inhibits both CYP2D6 and CYP3A4, the primary metabolizing enzymes for venlafaxine, has not been studied. Therefore, caution is advised should a patient's therapy include venlafaxine and any agent(s) that produce potent simultaneous inhibition of these two enzyme systems).
No products indexed under this heading.

Metronidazole Hydrochloride (Concomitant use of CYP3A4 inhibitors and venlafaxine may increase levels of venlafaxine and ODV. Therefore, caution is advised if a patient's therapy includes a CYP3A4 inhibitor and venlafaxine concomitantly. The concomitant use of venlafaxine with a drug treatment(s) that potently inhibits both CYP2D6 and CYP3A4, the primary metabolizing enzymes for venlafaxine, has not been studied. Therefore, caution is advised should a patient's therapy include venlafaxine and any agent(s) that produce potent simultaneous inhibition of these two enzyme systems).
No products indexed under this heading.

Metronidazole Sodium (Concomitant use of CYP3A4 inhibitors and venlafaxine may increase levels of venlafaxine and ODV. Therefore, caution is advised if a patient's therapy includes a CYP3A4 inhibitor and venlafaxine concomitantly. The concomitant use of venlafaxine with a drug treatment(s) that potently inhibits both CYP2D6 and CYP3A4, the primary metabolizing enzymes for venlafaxine, has not been studied. Therefore, caution is advised should a patient's therapy include venlafaxine and any agent(s) that produce potent simultaneous inhibition of these two enzyme systems).
No products indexed under this heading.

Mexiletine Hydrochloride (*In vitro* studies indicate that venlafaxine is a relatively weak inhibitor of CYP2D6. These findings have been confirmed in a clinical drug interaction study comparing the effect of venlafaxine to that of fluoxetine on the CYP2D6-mediated metabolism of dextrometrophan to dextrophan).
No products indexed under this heading.

Mibefradil Dihydrochloride (Studies indicate that venlafaxine is metabolized to its active metabolite, ODV, by CYP2D6. Thus the potential exists for a drug interaction between drugs that inhibit CYP2D6-mediated metabolism and venlafaxine. However, although imipramine partially inhibited the CYP2D6-mediated metabolism of venlafaxine, resulting in higher plasma concentrations of venlafaxine and lower plasma concentrations of ODV, the total concentration of active compounds (venlafaxine plus ODV) was not affected. Also, in a clinical study involving CYP2D6 poor and extensive metabolizers, the total concentration of active compounds (venlafaxine plus ODV), was similar in both groups. No dosage adjustment is required when venlafaxine is co-administered with a CYP2D6 inhibitor. Caution is advised should a patient's therapy include venlafaxine and CYP2D6 inhibitor).
No products indexed under this heading.

Miconazole (Concomitant use of CYP3A4 inhibitors and venlafaxine may increase levels of venlafaxine and ODV. Therefore, caution is advised if a patient's therapy includes a CYP3A4 inhibitor and venlafaxine concomitantly. The concomitant use of venlafaxine with a drug treatment(s) that potently inhibits both CYP2D6 and CYP3A4, the primary metabolizing enzymes for venlafaxine, has not been studied. Therefore, caution is advised should a patient's therapy include venlafaxine and any agent(s) that produce potent simultaneous inhibition of these two enzyme systems).
No products indexed under this heading.

Miconazole Nitrate (Concomitant use of CYP3A4 inhibitors and venlafaxine may increase levels of venlafaxine and ODV. Therefore, caution is advised if a patient's therapy includes a CYP3A4 inhibitor and venlafaxine concomitantly. The concomitant use of venlafaxine with a drug treatment(s) that potently inhibits both CYP2D6 and CYP3A4, the primary metabolizing enzymes for venlafaxine, has not been studied. Therefore, caution is advised should a patient's therapy include venlafaxine and any agent(s) that produce potent simultaneous inhibition of these two enzyme systems). Products include:
Vusion Ointment 3335

Midazolam Hydrochloride (The risk of using venlafaxine in combination with other CNS active drugs has not been systematically evaluated. Consequently, caution is advised if the concomitant administration of venlafaxine and such drugs is required).
No products indexed under this heading.

Mifepristone (Concomitant use of CYP3A4 inhibitors and venlafaxine may increase levels of venlafaxine and ODV. Therefore, caution is advised if a patient's therapy includes a CYP3A4 inhibitor and venlafaxine concomitantly. The concomitant use of venlafaxine with a drug treatment(s) that potently inhibits both CYP2D6 and CYP3A4, the primary metabolizing enzymes for venlafaxine, has not been studied. Therefore, caution is advised should a patient's therapy include venlafaxine and any agent(s) that produce potent simultaneous inhibition of these two enzyme systems).
No products indexed under this heading.

Mirtazapine (*In vitro* studies indicate that venlafaxine is a relatively weak inhibitor of CYP2D6. These findings have been confirmed in a clinical drug interaction study comparing the effect of venlafaxine to that of fluoxetine on the CYP2D6-mediated metabolism of dextrometrophan to dextrophan). Products include:
Remeron Tablets 3214
RemeronSolTab Tablets 3219

Moclobemide (Concomitant use in patients taking monoamine oxidase inhibitors (MAOIs) is contraindicated. Adverse reactions, some of which were serious, have been reported in patients who have recently been discontinued from a monoamine oxidase inhibitor (MAOI) and started on venlafaxine hydrochloride, or who have recently had venlafaxine hydrochloride therapy discontinued prior to initiation of a MAOI. It is recommended that venlafaxine hydrochloride not be used in combination with a MAOI, or within at least 14 days of discontinuing treatment with a MAOI. Based on the half-life of venlafaxine hydrochloride, at least 7 days should be allowed after stopping venlafaxine hydrochloride before starting an MAOI).
No products indexed under this heading.

Molindone Hydrochloride (The risk of using venlafaxine in combination with other CNS active drugs has not been systematically evaluated. Consequently, caution is advised if the concomitant administration of venlafaxine and such drugs is required). Products include:
Moban 1108

Morphine Sulfate (The risk of using venlafaxine in combination with other CNS active drugs has not been systematically evaluated. Consequently, caution is advised if the concomitant administration of venlafaxine and such drugs is required). Products include:
Avinza 1822
Embeda 1831
MS Contin 2803

Nabumetone (Patients should be cautioned about the concomitant use of venlafaxine and NSAIDs since combined use of psychotropic drugs that interfere with serotonin reuptake and this agent has been associated with an increased risk of bleeding. SSRIs and SNRIs, including venlafaxine, may increase the risk of bleeding events. Concomitant use of nonsteroidal anti-inflammatory drugs may add to this risk. Case reports and epidemiological studies (case-control and cohort design) have demonstrated an association between use of drugs that interfere with serotonin reuptake and the occurrence of gastrointestinal bleeding).
No products indexed under this heading.

Naproxen (Patients should be cautioned about the concomitant use of venlafaxine and NSAIDs since combined use of psychotropic drugs that interfere with serotonin reuptake and this agent has been associated with an increased risk of bleeding. SSRIs and SNRIs, including venlafaxine, may increase the risk of bleeding events. Concomitant use of nonsteroidal anti-inflammatory drugs may add to this risk. Case reports and epidemiological studies

IMPORTANT NOTE: Always consult each drug listing in the patient's regimen for possible interactions.

Venlafaxine | Interactions Index | 2034

(case-control and cohort design) have demonstrated an association between use of drugs that interfere with serotonin reuptake and the occurrence of gastrointestinal bleeding). Products include:
EC-Naprosyn 2850
Naprosyn 2850
Anaprox/Naprosyn 2850

Naproxen Sodium (Patients should be cautioned about the concomitant use of venlafaxine and NSAIDs since combined use of psychotropic drugs that interfere with serotonin reuptake and this agent has been associated with an increased risk of bleeding. SSRIs and SNRIs, including venlafaxine, may increase the risk of bleeding events. Concomitant use of nonsteroidal anti-inflammatory drugs may add to this risk. Case reports and epidemiological studies (case-control and cohort design) have demonstrated an association between use of drugs that interfere with serotonin reuptake and the occurrence of gastrointestinal bleeding). Products include:
Anaprox 2850
Anaprox DS 2850
Treximet 1681

Naratriptan Hydrochloride (There have been rare post-marketing reports of serotonin syndrome with use of an SSRI and a triptan. If concomitant treatment of venlafaxine with a triptan is clinically warranted, careful observation of the patient is advised, particularly during treatment initiation and dose increases. Patients should be cautioned about the risk of serotonin syndrome with the concomitant use of venlafaxine and triptans, tramadol, tryptophan supplements or other serotonergic agents). Products include:
Amerge 1306

Nefazodone Hydrochloride (Based on the mechanism of action of venlafaxine and the potential for serotonin syndrome, caution is advised when venlafaxine is co-administered with other drugs that may affect the serotonergic neurotransmitter systems, such as other SNRIs. If concomitant treatment of venlafaxine with another SNRI is clinically warranted, careful observation of the patient is advised, particularly during treatment initiation and dose increases).
No products indexed under this heading.

Nelfinavir Mesylate (Concomitant use of CYP3A4 inhibitors and venlafaxine may increase levels of venlafaxine and ODV. Therefore, caution is advised if a patient's therapy includes a CYP3A4 inhibitor and venlafaxine concomitantly. The concomitant use of venlafaxine with a drug treatment(s) that potently inhibits both CYP2D6 and CYP3A4, the primary metabolizing enzymes for venlafaxine, has not been studied. Therefore, caution is advised should a patient's therapy include venlafaxine and any agent(s) that produce potent simultaneous inhibition of these two enzyme systems).
No products indexed under this heading.

Nevirapine (Concomitant use of CYP3A4 inhibitors and venlafaxine may increase levels of venlafaxine and ODV. Therefore, caution is advised if a patient's therapy includes a CYP3A4 inhibitor and venlafaxine concomitantly. The concomitant use of venlafaxine with a drug treatment(s) that potently inhibits both CYP2D6 and CYP3A4, the primary metabolizing enzymes for venlafaxine, has not been studied. Therefore, caution is advised should a patient's therapy include venlafaxine and any agent(s) that produce potent simultaneous inhibition of these two enzyme systems). Products include:
Viramune Oral Suspension 897
Viramune Tablets 897

Niacin (Concomitant use of CYP3A4 inhibitors and venlafaxine may increase levels of venlafaxine and ODV. Therefore, caution is advised if a patient's therapy includes a CYP3A4 inhibitor and venlafaxine concomitantly. The concomitant use of venlafaxine with a drug treatment(s) that potently inhibits both CYP2D6 and CYP3A4, the primary metabolizing enzymes for venlafaxine, has not been studied. Therefore, caution is advised should a patient's therapy include venlafaxine and any agent(s) that produce potent simultaneous inhibition of these two enzyme systems). Products include:
Advicor 402
Cardio Basics 3455
Niaspan 497
Simcor 524

Niacinamide (Concomitant use of CYP3A4 inhibitors and venlafaxine may increase levels of venlafaxine and ODV. Therefore, caution is advised if a patient's therapy includes a CYP3A4 inhibitor and venlafaxine concomitantly. The concomitant use of venlafaxine with a drug treatment(s) that potently inhibits both CYP2D6 and CYP3A4, the primary metabolizing enzymes for venlafaxine, has not been studied. Therefore, caution is advised should a patient's therapy include venlafaxine and any agent(s) that produce potent simultaneous inhibition of these two enzyme systems). Products include:
CitraNatal 90 DHA Capsules 2332
CitraNatal Assure 2332
CitraNatal Rx 2332
Heplive 607

Niacinamide Hydroiodide (Concomitant use of CYP3A4 inhibitors and venlafaxine may increase levels of venlafaxine and ODV. Therefore, caution is advised if a patient's therapy includes a CYP3A4 inhibitor and venlafaxine concomitantly. The concomitant use of venlafaxine with a drug treatment(s) that potently inhibits both CYP2D6 and CYP3A4, the primary metabolizing enzymes for venlafaxine, has not been studied. Therefore, caution is advised should a patient's therapy include venlafaxine and any agent(s) that produce potent simultaneous inhibition of these two enzyme systems).
No products indexed under this heading.

Nicotinamide (Concomitant use of CYP3A4 inhibitors and venlafaxine may increase levels of venlafaxine and ODV. Therefore, caution is advised if a patient's therapy includes a CYP3A4 inhibitor and venlafaxine concomitantly. The concomitant use of venlafaxine with a drug treatment(s) that potently inhibits both CYP2D6 and CYP3A4, the primary metabolizing enzymes for venlafaxine, has not been studied. Therefore, caution is advised should a patient's therapy include venlafaxine and any agent(s) that produce potent simultaneous inhibition of these two enzyme systems).
No products indexed under this heading.

Nifedipine (Concomitant use of CYP3A4 inhibitors and venlafaxine may increase levels of venlafaxine and ODV. Therefore, caution is advised if a patient's therapy includes a CYP3A4 inhibitor and venlafaxine concomitantly. The concomitant use of venlafaxine with a drug treatment(s) that potently inhibits both CYP2D6 and CYP3A4, the primary metabolizing enzymes for venlafaxine, has not been studied. Therefore, caution is advised should a patient's therapy include venlafaxine and any agent(s) that produce potent simultaneous inhibition of these two enzyme systems).
No products indexed under this heading.

Norfloxacin (Concomitant use of CYP3A4 inhibitors and venlafaxine may increase levels of venlafaxine and ODV. Therefore, caution is advised if a patient's therapy includes a CYP3A4 inhibitor and venlafaxine concomitantly. The concomitant use of venlafaxine with a drug treatment(s) that potently inhibits both CYP2D6 and CYP3A4, the primary metabolizing enzymes for venlafaxine, has not been studied. Therefore, caution is advised should a patient's therapy include venlafaxine and any agent(s) that produce potent simultaneous inhibition of these two enzyme systems). Products include:
Noroxin 2220

Nortriptyline Hydrochloride (Studies indicate that venlafaxine is metabolized to its active metabolite, ODV, by CYP2D6. Thus the potential exists for a drug interaction between drugs that inhibit CYP2D6-mediated metabolism and venlafaxine. However, although imipramine partially inhibited the CYP2D6-mediated metabolism of venlafaxine, resulting in higher plasma concentrations of venlafaxine and lower plasma concentrations of ODV, the total concentration of active compounds (venlafaxine plus ODV) was not affected. Also, in a clinical study involving CYP2D6 poor and extensive metabolizers, the total concentration of active compounds (venlafaxine plus ODV), was similar in both groups. No dosage adjustment is required when venlafaxine is co-administered with a CYP2D6 inhibitor. Caution is advised should a patient's therapy include venlafaxine and CYP2D6 inhibitor).
No products indexed under this heading.

Olanzapine (The risk of using venlafaxine in combination with other CNS active drugs has not been systematically evaluated. Consequently, caution is advised if the concomitant administration of venlafaxine and such drugs is required). Products include:
Symbyax 1965
Zyprexa 1984
Zyprexa IntraMuscular 1984
Zyprexa ZYDIS 1984

Omeprazole (Concomitant use of CYP3A4 inhibitors and venlafaxine may increase levels of venlafaxine and ODV. Therefore, caution is advised if a patient's therapy includes a CYP3A4 inhibitor and venlafaxine concomitantly. The concomitant use of venlafaxine with a drug treatment(s) that potently inhibits both CYP2D6 and CYP3A4, the primary metabolizing enzymes for venlafaxine, has not been studied. Therefore, caution is advised should a patient's therapy include venlafaxine and any agent(s) that produce potent simultaneous inhibition of these two enzyme systems).
No products indexed under this heading.

Ondansetron (*In vitro* studies indicate that venlafaxine is a relatively weak inhibitor of CYP2D6. These findings have been confirmed in a clinical drug interaction study comparing the effect of venlafaxine to that of fluoxetine on the CYP2D6-mediated metabolism of dextromethorphan to dextrophan).
No products indexed under this heading.

Ondansetron Hydrochloride (*In vitro* studies indicate that venlafaxine is a relatively weak inhibitor of CYP2D6. These findings have been confirmed in a clinical drug interaction study comparing the effect of venlafaxine to that of fluoxetine on the CYP2D6-mediated metabolism of dextromethorphan to dextrophan). Products include:
Zofran Injection 1750
Zofran 1756
Zofran ODT 1756

Oxaprozin (Patients should be cautioned about the concomitant use of venlafaxine and NSAIDs since combined use of psychotropic drugs that interfere with serotonin reuptake and this agent has been associated with an increased risk of bleeding. SSRIs and SNRIs, including venlafaxine, may increase the risk of bleeding events. Concomitant use of nonsteroidal anti-inflammatory drugs may add to this risk. Case reports and epidemiological studies (case-control and cohort design) have demonstrated an association between use of drugs that interfere with serotonin reuptake and the occurrence of gastrointestinal bleeding).
No products indexed under this heading.

Oxazepam (The risk of using venlafaxine in combination with other CNS active drugs has not been systematically evaluated. Consequently, caution is advised if the concomitant administration of venlafaxine and such drugs is required).
No products indexed under this heading.

Oxycodone Hydrochloride (The risk of using venlafaxine in combination with other CNS active drugs has not been systematically evaluated. Consequently, caution is advised if the concomitant administration of venlafaxine and such drugs is required). Products include:
OxyContin 2807
Percocet 1121
Percodan 1124

Paclitaxel (*In vitro* studies indicate that venlafaxine is a relatively weak inhibitor of CYP2D6. These findings have been confirmed in a clinical drug interaction study comparing the effect of venlafaxine to that of fluoxetine on the CYP2D6-mediated metabolism of dextromethorphan to dextrophan).
No products indexed under this heading.

Pargyline Hydrochloride (Concomitant use in patients taking monoamine oxidase inhibitors (MAOIs) is contraindicated. Adverse reactions, some of which were serious, have been reported in patients who have recently been discontinued from a monoamine oxidase inhibitor (MAOI) and started on venlafaxine hydrochloride, or who have recently had venlafaxine hydrochloride therapy discontinued prior to initiation of a MAOI. It is recommended that venlafaxine hydrochloride not be used in combination with a MAOI, or within at least 14 days of discontinuing treatment with a MAOI. Based on the half-life of venlafaxine hydrochloride, at least 7 days should be allowed after stopping venlafaxine hydrochloride before starting an MAOI).
No products indexed under this heading.

Paroxetine (Based on the mechanism of action of venlafaxine and the potential for serotonin syndrome, caution is advised when venlafaxine is co-administered with other drugs that may affect the serotonergic neurotransmitter systems, such as SSRIs. If concomitant treatment of venlafaxine with an SSRI is clinically warranted, careful observation of the patient is advised, particularly during treatment initiation and dose increases).
No products indexed under this heading.

Paroxetine Hydrochloride (Based on the mechanism of action of venlafaxine and the potential for serotonin syndrome, caution is advised when venlafaxine is co-administered with other drugs that may affect the serotonergic neurotransmitter systems, such as SSRIs. If concomitant treatment of venlafaxine with an SSRI is clinically warranted, careful observation of the patient is advised, particularly during treatment initiation and dose increases). Products include:
Paroxetine CR 2361
Paroxetine ER 2371
Paxil 1586
Paxil CR 1596

Paroxetine Mesylate (Based on the mechanism of action of venlafaxine and the potential for serotonin syndrome, caution is advised when venlafaxine is co-administered with other drugs that

2035 Interactions Index Venlafaxine

may affect the serotonergic neurotransmitter systems, such as SSRIs. If concomitant treatment of venlafaxine with an SSRI is clinically warranted, careful observation of the patient is advised, particularly during treatment initiation and dose increases).
No products indexed under this heading.

Pemoline (The risk of using venlafaxine in combination with other CNS active drugs has not been systematically evaluated. Consequently, caution is advised if the concomitant administration of venlafaxine and such drugs is required).
No products indexed under this heading.

Pentobarbital Sodium (The risk of using venlafaxine in combination with other CNS active drugs has not been systematically evaluated. Consequently, caution is advised if the concomitant administration of venlafaxine and such drugs is required). Products include:
Nembutal 2012

Perphenazine (The risk of using venlafaxine in combination with other CNS active drugs has not been systematically evaluated. Consequently, caution is advised if the concomitant administration of venlafaxine and such drugs is required).
No products indexed under this heading.

Phenelzine Sulfate (Concomitant use in patients taking monoamine oxidase inhibitors (MAOIs) is contraindicated. Adverse reactions, some of which were serious, have been reported in patients who have recently been discontinued from a monoamine oxidase inhibitor (MAOI) and started on venlafaxine hydrochloride, or who have recently had venlafaxine hydrochloride therapy discontinued prior to initiation of a MAOI. It is recommended that venlafaxine hydrochloride not be used in combination with a MAOI, or within at least 14 days of discontinuing treatment with a MAOI. Based on the half-life of venlafaxine hydrochloride, at least 7 days should be allowed after stopping venlafaxine hydrochloride before starting an MAOI).
No products indexed under this heading.

Phenobarbital (The risk of using venlafaxine in combination with other CNS active drugs has not been systematically evaluated. Consequently, caution is advised if the concomitant administration of venlafaxine and such drugs is required). Products include:
Donnatal 2711

Phenobarbital Sodium (The risk of using venlafaxine in combination with other CNS active drugs has not been systematically evaluated. Consequently, caution is advised if the concomitant administration of venlafaxine and such drugs is required).
No products indexed under this heading.

Phentermine Hydrochloride (The safety and efficacy of venlafaxine therapy in combination with weight loss agents, including phentermine, have not been established. Co-administration of venlafaxine and weight loss agents is not recommended). Products include:
Adipex-P 1178

Phenylbutazone (Patients should be cautioned about the concomitant use of venlafaxine and NSAIDs since combined use of psychotropic drugs that interfere with serotonin reuptake and this agent has been associated with an increased risk of bleeding. SSRIs and SNRIs, including venlafaxine, may increase the risk of bleeding events. Concomitant use of nonsteroidal anti-inflammatory drugs may add to this risk. Case reports and epidemiological studies (case-control and cohort design) have demonstrated an association between use of drugs that interfere with serotonin reuptake and the occurrence of gastrointestinal bleeding).
No products indexed under this heading.

Pindolol (*In vitro* studies indicate that venlafaxine is a relatively weak inhibitor of CYP2D6. These findings have been confirmed in a clinical drug interaction study comparing the effect of venlafaxine to that of fluoxetine on the CYP2D6-mediated metabolism of dextrometrophan to dextrophan).
No products indexed under this heading.

Piroxicam (Patients should be cautioned about the concomitant use of venlafaxine and NSAIDs since combined use of psychotropic drugs that interfere with serotonin reuptake and this agent has been associated with an increased risk of bleeding. SSRIs and SNRIs, including venlafaxine, may increase the risk of bleeding events. Concomitant use of nonsteroidal anti-inflammatory drugs may add to this risk. Case reports and epidemiological studies (case-control and cohort design) have demonstrated an association between use of drugs that interfere with serotonin reuptake and the occurrence of gastrointestinal bleeding).
No products indexed under this heading.

Polythiazide (Elderly patients may be at greater risk of developing hyponatremia with SSRIs and SNRIs. Also patients taking diuretics or who are otherwise volume depleted may be at greater risk. Discontinuation of venlafaxine should be considered in patients with symptomatic hyponatremia and appropriate medical intervention should be instituted).
No products indexed under this heading.

Posaconazole (Concomitant use of CYP3A4 inhibitors and venlafaxine may increase levels of venlafaxine and ODV. Therefore, caution is advised if a patient's therapy includes a CYP3A4 inhibitor and venlafaxine concomitantly. The concomitant use of venlafaxine with a drug treatment(s) that potently inhibits both CYP2D6 and CYP3A4, the primary metabolizing enzymes for venlafaxine, has not been studied. Therefore, caution is advised should a patient's therapy include venlafaxine and any agent(s) that produce potent simultaneous inhibition of these two enzyme systems). Products include:
Noxafil 3172

Prazepam (The risk of using venlafaxine in combination with other CNS active drugs has not been systematically evaluated. Consequently, caution is advised if the concomitant administration of venlafaxine and such drugs is required).
No products indexed under this heading.

Procarbazine Hydrochloride (Concomitant use in patients taking monoamine oxidase inhibitors (MAOIs) is contraindicated. Adverse reactions, some of which were serious, have been reported in patients who have recently been discontinued from a monoamine oxidase inhibitor (MAOI) and started on venlafaxine hydrochloride, or who have recently had venlafaxine hydrochloride therapy discontinued prior to initiation of a MAOI. It is recommended that venlafaxine hydrochloride not be used in combination with a MAOI, or within at least 14 days of discontinuing treatment with a MAOI. Based on the half-life of venlafaxine hydrochloride, at least 7 days should be allowed after stopping venlafaxine hydrochloride before starting an MAOI).
No products indexed under this heading.

Prochlorperazine (The risk of using venlafaxine in combination with other CNS active drugs has not been systematically evaluated. Consequently, caution is advised if the concomitant administration of venlafaxine and such drugs is required).
No products indexed under this heading.

Promethazine Hydrochloride (The risk of using venlafaxine in combination with other CNS active drugs has not been systematically evaluated. Consequently, caution is advised if the concomitant administration of venlafaxine and such drugs is required).
No products indexed under this heading.

Propafenone Hydrochloride (Studies indicate that venlafaxine is metabolized to its active metabolite, ODV, by CYP2D6. Thus the potential exists for a drug interaction between drugs that inhibit CYP2D6-mediated metabolism and venlafaxine. However, although imipramine partially inhibited the CYP2D6-mediated metabolism of venlafaxine, resulting in higher plasma concentrations of venlafaxine and lower plasma concentrations of ODV, the total concentration of active compounds (venlafaxine plus ODV) was not affected. Also, in a clinical study involving CYP2D6 poor and extensive metabolizers, the total concentration of active compounds (venlafaxine plus ODV), was similar in both groups. No dosage adjustment is required when venlafaxine is co-administered with a CYP2D6 inhibitor. Caution is advised should a patient's therapy include venlafaxine and CYP2D6 inhibitor). Products include:
Rythmol 1648
Rythmol SR 1652

Propofol (The risk of using venlafaxine in combination with other CNS active drugs has not been systematically evaluated. Consequently, caution is advised if the concomitant administration of venlafaxine and such drugs is required).
No products indexed under this heading.

Propoxyphene Hydrochloride (The risk of using venlafaxine in combination with other CNS active drugs has not been systematically evaluated. Consequently, caution is advised if the concomitant administration of venlafaxine and such drugs is required).
No products indexed under this heading.

Propoxyphene Napsylate (The risk of using venlafaxine in combination with other CNS active drugs has not been systematically evaluated. Consequently, caution is advised if the concomitant administration of venlafaxine and such drugs is required).
No products indexed under this heading.

Propranolol Hydrochloride (*In vitro* studies indicate that venlafaxine is a relatively weak inhibitor of CYP2D6. These findings have been confirmed in a clinical drug interaction study comparing the effect of venlafaxine to that of fluoxetine on the CYP2D6-mediated metabolism of dextrometrophan to dextrophan). Products include:
InnoPran XL 1517

Protriptyline Hydrochloride (Studies indicate that venlafaxine is metabolized to its active metabolite, ODV, by CYP2D6. Thus the potential exists for a drug interaction between drugs that inhibit CYP2D6-mediated metabolism and venlafaxine. However, although imipramine partially inhibited the CYP2D6-mediated metabolism of venlafaxine, resulting in higher plasma concentrations of venlafaxine and lower plasma concentrations of ODV, the total concentration of active compounds (venlafaxine plus ODV) was not affected. Also, in a clinical study involving CYP2D6 poor and extensive metabolizers, the total concentration of active compounds (venlafaxine plus ODV), was similar in both groups. No dosage adjustment is required when venlafaxine is co-administered with a CYP2D6 inhibitor. Caution is advised should a patient's therapy include venlafaxine and CYP2D6 inhibitor).
No products indexed under this heading.

Quazepam (The risk of using venlafaxine in combination with other CNS active drugs has not been systematically evaluated. Consequently, caution is advised if the concomitant administration of venlafaxine and such drugs is required).
No products indexed under this heading.

Quetiapine Fumarate (The risk of using venlafaxine in combination with other CNS active drugs has not been systematically evaluated. Consequently, caution is advised if the concomitant administration of venlafaxine and such drugs is required). Products include:
Seroquel 750
Seroquel XR 759

Quinacrine Hydrochloride (Studies indicate that venlafaxine is metabolized to its active metabolite, ODV, by CYP2D6. Thus the potential exists for a drug interaction between drugs that inhibit CYP2D6-mediated metabolism and venlafaxine. However, although imipramine partially inhibited the CYP2D6-mediated metabolism of venlafaxine, resulting in higher plasma concentrations of venlafaxine and lower plasma concentrations of ODV, the total concentration of active compounds (venlafaxine plus ODV) was not affected. Also, in a clinical study involving CYP2D6 poor and extensive metabolizers, the total concentration of active compounds (venlafaxine plus ODV), was similar in both groups. No dosage adjustment is required when venlafaxine is co-administered with a CYP2D6 inhibitor. Caution is advised should a patient's therapy include venlafaxine and CYP2D6 inhibitor).
No products indexed under this heading.

Quinidine (Studies indicate that venlafaxine is metabolized to its active metabolite, ODV, by CYP2D6. Thus the potential exists for a drug interaction between drugs that inhibit CYP2D6-mediated metabolism and venlafaxine. However, although imipramine partially inhibited the CYP2D6-mediated metabolism of venlafaxine, resulting in higher plasma concentrations of venlafaxine and lower plasma concentrations of ODV, the total concentration of active compounds (venlafaxine plus ODV) was not affected. Also, in a clinical study involving CYP2D6 poor and extensive metabolizers, the total concentration of active compounds (venlafaxine plus ODV), was similar in both groups. No dosage adjustment is required when venlafaxine is co-administered with a CYP2D6 inhibitor. Caution is advised should a patient's therapy include venlafaxine and CYP2D6 inhibitor).
No products indexed under this heading.

Quinidine Gluconate (Studies indicate that venlafaxine is metabolized to its active metabolite, ODV, by CYP2D6. Thus the potential exists for a drug interaction between drugs that inhibit CYP2D6-mediated metabolism and venlafaxine. However, although imipramine partially inhibited the CYP2D6-mediated metabolism of venlafaxine, resulting in higher plasma concentrations of venlafaxine and lower plasma concentrations of ODV, the total concentration of active compounds (venlafaxine plus ODV) was not affected. Also, in a clinical study involving CYP2D6 poor and extensive metabolizers, the total concentration of active compounds (venlafaxine plus ODV), was similar in both groups.

IMPORTANT NOTE: Always consult each drug listing in the patient's regimen for possible interactions.

Venlafaxine Interactions Index 2036

No dosage adjustment is required when venlafaxine is co-administered with a CYP2D6 inhibitor. Caution is advised should a patient's therapy include venlafaxine and CYP2D6 inhibitor).
No products indexed under this heading.

Quinidine Hydrochloride (Studies indicate that venlafaxine is metabolized to its active metabolite, ODV, by CYP2D6. Thus the potential exists for a drug interaction between drugs that inhibit CYP2D6-mediated metabolism and venlafaxine. However, although imipramine partially inhibited the CYP2D6-mediated metabolism of venlafaxine, resulting in higher plasma concentrations of venlafaxine and lower plasma concentrations of ODV, the total concentration of active compounds (venlafaxine plus ODV) was not affected. Also, in a clinical study involving CYP2D6 poor and extensive metabolizers, the total concentration of active compounds (venlafaxine plus ODV), was similar in both groups. No dosage adjustment is required when venlafaxine is co-administered with a CYP2D6 inhibitor. Caution is advised should a patient's therapy include venlafaxine and CYP2D6 inhibitor).
No products indexed under this heading.

Quinidine Polygalacturonate (Studies indicate that venlafaxine is metabolized to its active metabolite, ODV, by CYP2D6. Thus the potential exists for a drug interaction between drugs that inhibit CYP2D6-mediated metabolism and venlafaxine. However, although imipramine partially inhibited the CYP2D6-mediated metabolism of venlafaxine, resulting in higher plasma concentrations of venlafaxine and lower plasma concentrations of ODV, the total concentration of active compounds (venlafaxine plus ODV) was not affected. Also, in a clinical study involving CYP2D6 poor and extensive metabolizers, the total concentration of active compounds (venlafaxine plus ODV), was similar in both groups. No dosage adjustment is required when venlafaxine is co-administered with a CYP2D6 inhibitor. Caution is advised should a patient's therapy include venlafaxine and CYP2D6 inhibitor).
No products indexed under this heading.

Quinidine Sulfate (Studies indicate that venlafaxine is metabolized to its active metabolite, ODV, by CYP2D6. Thus the potential exists for a drug interaction between drugs that inhibit CYP2D6-mediated metabolism and venlafaxine. However, although imipramine partially inhibited the CYP2D6-mediated metabolism of venlafaxine, resulting in higher plasma concentrations of venlafaxine and lower plasma concentrations of ODV, the total concentration of active compounds (venlafaxine plus ODV) was not affected. Also, in a clinical study involving CYP2D6 poor and extensive metabolizers, the total concentration of active compounds (venlafaxine plus ODV), was similar in both groups. No dosage adjustment is required when venlafaxine is co-administered with a CYP2D6 inhibitor. Caution is advised should a patient's therapy include venlafaxine and CYP2D6 inhibitor).
No products indexed under this heading.

Quinine (Concomitant use of CYP3A4 inhibitors and venlafaxine may increase levels of venlafaxine and ODV. Therefore, caution is advised if a patient's therapy includes a CYP3A4 inhibitor and venlafaxine concomitantly. The concomitant use of venlafaxine with a drug treatment(s) that potently inhibits both CYP2D6 and CYP3A4, the primary metabolizing enzymes for venlafaxine, has not been studied. Therefore, caution is advised should a patient's therapy include venlafaxine and any agent(s) that produce potent simultaneous inhibition of these two enzyme systems). Products include:
Hyland's Leg Cramps PM with Quinine 3315

Quinine Sulfate (Concomitant use of CYP3A4 inhibitors and venlafaxine may increase levels of venlafaxine and ODV. Therefore, caution is advised if a patient's therapy includes a CYP3A4 inhibitor and venlafaxine concomitantly. The concomitant use of venlafaxine with a drug treatment(s) that potently inhibits both CYP2D6 and CYP3A4, the primary metabolizing enzymes for venlafaxine, has not been studied. Therefore, caution is advised should a patient's therapy include venlafaxine and any agent(s) that produce potent simultaneous inhibition of these two enzyme systems).
No products indexed under this heading.

Quinupristin (Concomitant use of CYP3A4 inhibitors and venlafaxine may increase levels of venlafaxine and ODV. Therefore, caution is advised if a patient's therapy includes a CYP3A4 inhibitor and venlafaxine concomitantly. The concomitant use of venlafaxine with a drug treatment(s) that potently inhibits both CYP2D6 and CYP3A4, the primary metabolizing enzymes for venlafaxine, has not been studied. Therefore, caution is advised should a patient's therapy include venlafaxine and any agent(s) that produce potent simultaneous inhibition of these two enzyme systems).
No products indexed under this heading.

Ranitidine Bismuth Citrate (Studies indicate that venlafaxine is metabolized to its active metabolite, ODV, by CYP2D6. Thus the potential exists for a drug interaction between drugs that inhibit CYP2D6-mediated metabolism and venlafaxine. However, although imipramine partially inhibited the CYP2D6-mediated metabolism of venlafaxine, resulting in higher plasma concentrations of venlafaxine and lower plasma concentrations of ODV, the total concentration of active compounds (venlafaxine plus ODV) was not affected. Also, in a clinical study involving CYP2D6 poor and extensive metabolizers, the total concentration of active compounds (venlafaxine plus ODV), was similar in both groups. No dosage adjustment is required when venlafaxine is co-administered with a CYP2D6 inhibitor. Caution is advised should a patient's therapy include venlafaxine and CYP2D6 inhibitor).
No products indexed under this heading.

Ranitidine Hydrochloride (Studies indicate that venlafaxine is metabolized to its active metabolite, ODV, by CYP2D6. Thus the potential exists for a drug interaction between drugs that inhibit CYP2D6-mediated metabolism and venlafaxine. However, although imipramine partially inhibited the CYP2D6-mediated metabolism of venlafaxine, resulting in higher plasma concentrations of venlafaxine and lower plasma concentrations of ODV, the total concentration of active compounds (venlafaxine plus ODV) was not affected. Also, in a clinical study involving CYP2D6 poor and extensive metabolizers, the total concentration of active compounds (venlafaxine plus ODV), was similar in both groups. No dosage adjustment is required when venlafaxine is co-administered with a CYP2D6 inhibitor. Caution is advised should a patient's therapy include venlafaxine and CYP2D6 inhibitor). Products include:
Zantac 1737
Zantac Injection 1732
Zantac Pharmacy 1735

Rasagiline Mesylate (Concomitant use in patients taking monoamine oxidase inhibitors (MAOIs) is contraindicated. Adverse reactions, some of which were serious, have been reported in patients who have recently been discontinued from a monoamine oxidase inhibitor (MAOI) and started on venlafaxine hydrochloride, or who have recently had venlafaxine hydrochloride therapy discontinued prior to initiation of a MAOI. It is recommended that venlafaxine hydrochloride not be used in combination with a MAOI, or within at least 14 days of discontinuing treatment with a MAOI. Based on the half-life of venlafaxine hydrochloride, at least 7 days should be allowed after stopping venlafaxine hydrochloride before starting an MAOI). Products include:
Azilect 3383

Remifentanil Hydrochloride (The risk of using venlafaxine in combination with other CNS active drugs has not been systematically evaluated. Consequently, caution is advised if the concomitant administration of venlafaxine and such drugs is required).
No products indexed under this heading.

Risperidone (Venlafaxine administered under steady-state conditions at 150 mg/day slightly inhibited the CYP2D6-mediated metabolism of risperidone (administered as a single 1 mg oral dose) to its active metabolite, 9-hydroxyrisperidone, resulting in an approximately 32% increase in risperidone AUC. However, venlafaxine coadministration did not significantly alter the pharmacokinetic profile of the total active moiety (risperidone plus 9-hydroxyrisperidone)). Products include:
Risperdal Consta 2682

Ritonavir (Studies indicate that venlafaxine is metabolized to its active metabolite, ODV, by CYP2D6. Thus the potential exists for a drug interaction between drugs that inhibit CYP2D6-mediated metabolism and venlafaxine. However, although imipramine partially inhibited the CYP2D6-mediated metabolism of venlafaxine, resulting in higher plasma concentrations of venlafaxine and lower plasma concentrations of ODV, the total concentration of active compounds (venlafaxine plus ODV) was not affected. Also, in a clinical study involving CYP2D6 poor and extensive metabolizers, the total concentration of active compounds (venlafaxine plus ODV), was similar in both groups. No dosage adjustment is required when venlafaxine is co-administered with a CYP2D6 inhibitor. Caution is advised should a patient's therapy include venlafaxine and CYP2D6 inhibitor). Products include:
Kaletra 458
Norvir 509

Rizatriptan Benzoate (There have been rare post-marketing reports of serotonin syndrome with use of an SSRI and a triptan. If concomitant treatment of venlafaxine with a triptan is clinically warranted, careful observation of the patient is advised, particularly during treatment initiation and dose increases. Patients should be cautioned about the risk of serotonin syndrome with the concomitant use of venlafaxine and triptans, tramadol, tryptophan supplements or other serotonergic agents). Products include:
Maxalt 2206
Maxalt-MLT 2206

Rofecoxib (Patients should be cautioned about the concomitant use of venlafaxine and NSAIDs since combined use of psychotropic drugs that interfere with serotonin reuptake and this agent has been associated with an increased risk of bleeding. SSRIs and SNRIs, including venlafaxine, may increase the risk of bleeding events. Concomitant use of nonsteroidal anti-inflammatory drugs may add to this risk. Case reports and epidemiological studies (case-control and cohort design) have demonstrated an association between use of drugs that interfere with serotonin reuptake and the occurrence of gastrointestinal bleeding).
No products indexed under this heading.

Saquinavir (Concomitant use of CYP3A4 inhibitors and venlafaxine may increase levels of venlafaxine and ODV. Therefore, caution is advised if a patient's therapy includes a CYP3A4 inhibitor and venlafaxine concomitantly. The concomitant use of venlafaxine with a drug treatment(s) that potently inhibits both CYP2D6 and CYP3A4, the primary metabolizing enzymes for venlafaxine, has not been studied. Therefore, caution is advised should a patient's therapy include venlafaxine and any agent(s) that produce potent simultaneous inhibition of these two enzyme systems).
No products indexed under this heading.

Saquinavir Mesylate (Concomitant use of CYP3A4 inhibitors and venlafaxine may increase levels of venlafaxine and ODV. Therefore, caution is advised if a patient's therapy includes a CYP3A4 inhibitor and venlafaxine concomitantly. The concomitant use of venlafaxine with a drug treatment(s) that potently inhibits both CYP2D6 and CYP3A4, the primary metabolizing enzymes for venlafaxine, has not been studied. Therefore, caution is advised should a patient's therapy include venlafaxine and any agent(s) that produce potent simultaneous inhibition of these two enzyme systems).
No products indexed under this heading.

Secobarbital Sodium (The risk of using venlafaxine in combination with other CNS active drugs has not been systematically evaluated. Consequently, caution is advised if the concomitant administration of venlafaxine and such drugs is required).
No products indexed under this heading.

Selegiline (Concomitant use in patients taking monoamine oxidase inhibitors (MAOIs) is contraindicated. Adverse reactions, some of which were serious, have been reported in patients who have recently been discontinued from a monoamine oxidase inhibitor (MAOI) and started on venlafaxine hydrochloride, or who have recently had venlafaxine hydrochloride therapy discontinued prior to initiation of a MAOI. It is recommended that venlafaxine hydrochloride not be used in combination with a MAOI, or within at least 14 days of discontinuing treatment with a MAOI. Based on the half-life of venlafaxine hydrochloride, at least 7 days should be allowed after stopping venlafaxine hydrochloride before starting an MAOI). Products include:
Emsam 3623

Selegiline Hydrochloride (Concomitant use in patients taking monoamine oxidase inhibitors (MAOIs) is contraindicated. Adverse reactions, some of which were serious, have been reported in patients who have recently been discontinued from a monoamine oxidase inhibitor (MAOI) and started on venlafaxine hydrochloride, or who have recently had venlafaxine hydrochloride therapy discontinued prior to initiation of a MAOI. It is recommended that venlafaxine hydrochloride not be used in combination with a MAOI, or within at least 14 days of discontinuing treatment with a MAOI. Based on the half-life of venlafaxine hydrochloride, at least 7 days should be allowed after stopping venlafaxine hydrochloride before starting an MAOI). Products include:
Eldepryl 3312

Sertraline Hydrochloride (Based on the mechanism of action of venlafaxine and the potential for serotonin syn-

drome, caution is advised when venlafaxine is co-administered with other drugs that may affect the serotonergic neurotransmitter systems, such as SSRIs. If concomitant treatment of venlafaxine with an SSRI is clinically warranted, careful observation of the patient is advised, particularly during treatment initiation and dose increases).
No products indexed under this heading.

Sevoflurane (The risk of using venlafaxine in combination with other CNS active drugs has not been systematically evaluated. Consequently, caution is advised if the concomitant administration of venlafaxine and such drugs is required). Products include:
Ultane **554**

Sildenafil Citrate (Studies indicate that venlafaxine is metabolized to its active metabolite, ODV, by CYP2D6. Thus the potential exists for a drug interaction between drugs that inhibit CYP2D6-mediated metabolism and venlafaxine. However, although imipramine partially inhibited the CYP2D6-mediated metabolism of venlafaxine, resulting in higher plasma concentrations of venlafaxine and lower plasma concentrations of ODV, the total concentration of active compounds (venlafaxine plus ODV), was not affected. Also, in a clinical study involving CYP2D6 poor and extensive metabolizers, the total concentration of active compounds (venlafaxine plus ODV), was similar in both groups. No dosage adjustment is required when venlafaxine is co-administered with a CYP2D6 inhibitor. Caution is advised should a patient's therapy include venlafaxine and CYP2D6 inhibitor).
No products indexed under this heading.

Sodium Oxybate (The risk of using venlafaxine in combination with other CNS active drugs has not been systematically evaluated. Consequently, caution is advised if the concomitant administration of venlafaxine and such drugs is required).
No products indexed under this heading.

Spironolactone (Elderly patients may be at greater risk of developing hyponatremia with SSRIs and SNRIs. Also patients taking diuretics or who are otherwise volume depleted may be at greater risk. Discontinuation of venlafaxine should be considered in patients with symptomatic hyponatremia and appropriate medical intervention should be instituted).
No products indexed under this heading.

Sufentanil Citrate (The risk of using venlafaxine in combination with other CNS active drugs has not been systematically evaluated. Consequently, caution is advised if the concomitant administration of venlafaxine and such drugs is required).
No products indexed under this heading.

Sulindac (Patients should be cautioned about the concomitant use of venlafaxine and NSAIDs since combined use of psychotropic drugs that interfere with serotonin reuptake and this agent has been associated with an increased risk of bleeding. SSRIs and SNRIs, including venlafaxine, may increase the risk of bleeding events. Concomitant use of nonsteroidal anti-inflammatory drugs may add to this risk. Case reports and epidemiological studies (case-control and cohort design) have demonstrated an association between use of drugs that interfere with serotonin reuptake and the occurrence of gastrointestinal bleeding). Products include:
Clinoril **2098**

Sumatriptan (There have been rare post-marketing reports of serotonin syndrome with use of an SSRI and a triptan. If concomitant treatment of venlafaxine with a triptan is clinically war-

ranted, careful observation of the patient is advised, particularly during treatment initiation and dose increases. Patients should be cautioned about the risk of serotonin syndrome with the concomitant use of venlafaxine and triptans, tramadol, tryptophan supplements or other serotonergic agents). Products include:
Imitrex Nasal **1503**

Sumatriptan Succinate (There have been rare post-marketing reports of serotonin syndrome with use of an SSRI and a triptan. If concomitant treatment of venlafaxine with a triptan is clinically warranted, careful observation of the patient is advised, particularly during treatment initiation and dose increases. Patients should be cautioned about the risk of serotonin syndrome with the concomitant use of venlafaxine and triptans, tramadol, tryptophan supplements or other serotonergic agents). Products include:
Imitrex **1497**
Imitrex Tablets **1508**
Treximet **1681**

Tamoxifen Citrate (In vitro studies indicate that venlafaxine is a relatively weak inhibitor of CYP2D6. These findings have been confirmed in a clinical drug interaction study comparing the effect of venlafaxine to that of fluoxetine on the CYP2D6-mediated metabolism of dextrometrophan to dextrophan).
No products indexed under this heading.

Telithromycin (Concomitant use of CYP3A4 inhibitors and venlafaxine may increase levels of venlafaxine and ODV. Therefore, caution is advised if a patient's therapy includes a CYP3A4 inhibitor and venlafaxine concomitantly. The concomitant use of venlafaxine with a drug treatment(s) that potently inhibits both CYP2D6 and CYP3A4, the primary metabolizing enzymes for venlafaxine, has not been studied. Therefore, caution is advised should a patient's therapy include venlafaxine and any agent(s) that produce potent simultaneous inhibition of these two enzyme systems). Products include:
Ketek **2991**

Temazepam (The risk of using venlafaxine in combination with other CNS active drugs has not been systematically evaluated. Consequently, caution is advised if the concomitant administration of venlafaxine and such drugs is required).
No products indexed under this heading.

Teniposide (In vitro studies indicate that venlafaxine is a relatively weak inhibitor of CYP2D6. These findings have been confirmed in a clinical drug interaction study comparing the effect of venlafaxine to that of fluoxetine on the CYP2D6-mediated metabolism of dextrometrophan to dextrophan).
No products indexed under this heading.

Terbinafine Hydrochloride (Studies indicate that venlafaxine is metabolized to its active metabolite, ODV, by CYP2D6. Thus the potential exists for a drug interaction between drugs that inhibit CYP2D6-mediated metabolism and venlafaxine. However, although imipramine partially inhibited the CYP2D6-mediated metabolism of venlafaxine, resulting in higher plasma concentrations of venlafaxine and lower plasma concentrations of ODV, the total concentration of active compounds (venlafaxine plus ODV) was not affected. Also, in a clinical study involving CYP2D6 poor and extensive metabolizers, the total concentration of active compounds (venlafaxine plus ODV), was similar in both groups. No dosage adjustment is required when venlafaxine is co-administered with a CYP2D6 inhibi-

tor. Caution is advised should a patient's therapy include venlafaxine and CYP2D6 inhibitor).
No products indexed under this heading.

Testosterone (In vitro studies indicate that venlafaxine is a relatively weak inhibitor of CYP2D6. These findings have been confirmed in a clinical drug interaction study comparing the effect of venlafaxine to that of fluoxetine on the CYP2D6-mediated metabolism of dextrometrophan to dextrophan). Products include:
AndroGel **3456**

Testosterone Cypionate (In vitro studies indicate that venlafaxine is a relatively weak inhibitor of CYP2D6. These findings have been confirmed in a clinical drug interaction study comparing the effect of venlafaxine to that of fluoxetine on the CYP2D6-mediated metabolism of dextrometrophan to dextrophan).
No products indexed under this heading.

Testosterone Enanthate (In vitro studies indicate that venlafaxine is a relatively weak inhibitor of CYP2D6. These findings have been confirmed in a clinical drug interaction study comparing the effect of venlafaxine to that of fluoxetine on the CYP2D6-mediated metabolism of dextrometrophan to dextrophan). Products include:
Delatestryl **1102**

Testosterone Propionate (In vitro studies indicate that venlafaxine is a relatively weak inhibitor of CYP2D6. These findings have been confirmed in a clinical drug interaction study comparing the effect of venlafaxine to that of fluoxetine on the CYP2D6-mediated metabolism of dextrometrophan to dextrophan).
No products indexed under this heading.

Thiamylal Sodium (The risk of using venlafaxine in combination with other CNS active drugs has not been systematically evaluated. Consequently, caution is advised if the concomitant administration of venlafaxine and such drugs is required).
No products indexed under this heading.

Thioridazine (In vitro studies indicate that venlafaxine is a relatively weak inhibitor of CYP2D6. These findings have been confirmed in a clinical drug interaction study comparing the effect of venlafaxine to that of fluoxetine on the CYP2D6-mediated metabolism of dextrometrophan to dextrophan).
No products indexed under this heading.

Thioridazine Hydrochloride (The risk of using venlafaxine in combination with other CNS active drugs has not been systematically evaluated. Consequently, caution is advised if the concomitant administration of venlafaxine and such drugs is required). Products include:
Thioridazine Hydrochloride **2384**

Thiothixene (The risk of using venlafaxine in combination with other CNS active drugs has not been systematically evaluated. Consequently, caution is advised if the concomitant administration of venlafaxine and such drugs is required). Products include:
Thiothixene **2386**

Timolol Maleate (In vitro studies indicate that venlafaxine is a relatively weak inhibitor of CYP2D6. These findings have been confirmed in a clinical drug interaction study comparing the effect of venlafaxine to that of fluoxetine on the CYP2D6-mediated metabolism of dextrometrophan to dextrophan). Products include:
Combigan **601**
Dorzolamide
 Hydrochloride/Timolol Maleate
 Ophthalmic Solution .... ⊙**243**
Timoptic in Ocudose .... ⊙**231**

Tinzaparin Sodium (Patients should be cautioned about the concomitant use of venlafaxine and anti-coagulants since combined use of psychotropic drugs that interfere with serotonin reuptake and this agent has been associated with an increased risk of bleeding. SSRIs and SNRIs, including venlafaxine, may increase the risk of bleeding events. Concomitant use of anti-coagulants may add to this risk. Case reports and epidemiological studies (case-control and cohort design) have demonstrated an association between use of drugs that interfere with serotonin reuptake and the occurrence of gastrointestinal bleeding).
No products indexed under this heading.

Tolmetin Sodium (Patients should be cautioned about the concomitant use of venlafaxine and NSAIDs since combined use of psychotropic drugs that interfere with serotonin reuptake and this agent has been associated with an increased risk of bleeding. SSRIs and SNRIs, including venlafaxine, may increase the risk of bleeding events. Concomitant use of nonsteroidal anti-inflammatory drugs may add to this risk. Case reports and epidemiological studies (case-control and cohort design) have demonstrated an association between use of drugs that interfere with serotonin reuptake and the occurrence of gastrointestinal bleeding).
No products indexed under this heading.

Tolterodine Tartrate (In vitro studies indicate that venlafaxine is a relatively weak inhibitor of CYP2D6. These findings have been confirmed in a clinical drug interaction study comparing the effect of venlafaxine to that of fluoxetine on the CYP2D6-mediated metabolism of dextrometrophan to dextrophan).
No products indexed under this heading.

Torsemide (Elderly patients may be at greater risk of developing hyponatremia with SSRIs and SNRIs. Also patients taking diuretics or who are otherwise volume depleted may be at greater risk. Discontinuation of venlafaxine should be considered in patients with symptomatic hyponatremia and appropriate medical intervention should be instituted).
No products indexed under this heading.

Tramadol Hydrochloride (Based on the mechanism of action of venlafaxine and the potential for serotonin syndrome, caution is advised when venlafaxine is co-administered with other drugs that may affect the serotonergic neurotransmitter systems, such as tramadol. If concomitant treatment of venlafaxine with tramadol is clinically warranted, careful observation of the patient is advised, particularly during treatment initiation and dose increases). Products include:
Ryzolt **2813**
Ultram ER **2693**

Tranylcypromine Sulfate (Concomitant use in patients taking monoamine oxidase inhibitors (MAOIs) is contraindicated. Adverse reactions, some of which were serious, have been reported in patients who have recently been discontinued from a monoamine oxidase inhibitor (MAOI) and started on venlafaxine hydrochloride, or who have recently had venlafaxine hydrochloride therapy discontinued prior to initiation of a MAOI. It is recommended that venlafaxine hydrochloride not be used in combination with a MAOI, or within at least 14 days of discontinuing treatment with a MAOI. Based on the half-life of venlafaxine hydrochloride, at least 7 days should be allowed after stopping venlafaxine hydrochloride before starting an MAOI). Products include:
Parnate **1584**

IMPORTANT NOTE: Always consult each drug listing in the patient's regimen for possible interactions.

Trazodone Hydrochloride (*In vitro* studies indicate that venlafaxine is a relatively weak inhibitor of CYP2D6. These findings have been confirmed in a clinical drug interaction study comparing the effect of venlafaxine to that of fluoxetine on the CYP2D6-mediated metabolism of dextrometrophan to dextrophan).
No products indexed under this heading.

Triamterene (Elderly patients may be at greater risk of developing hyponatremia with SSRIs and SNRIs. Also patients taking diuretics or who are otherwise volume depleted may be at greater risk. Discontinuation of venlafaxine should be considered in patients with symptomatic hyponatremia and appropriate medical intervention should be instituted). Products include:
Dyazide 1429
Dyrenium 3495

Triazolam (The risk of using venlafaxine in combination with other CNS active drugs has not been systematically evaluated. Consequently, caution is advised if the concomitant administration of venlafaxine and such drugs is required).
No products indexed under this heading.

Trifluoperazine Hydrochloride (The risk of using venlafaxine in combination with other CNS active drugs has not been systematically evaluated. Consequently, caution is advised if the concomitant administration of venlafaxine and such drugs is required).
No products indexed under this heading.

Trimipramine Maleate (Studies indicate that venlafaxine is metabolized to its active metabolite, ODV, by CYP2D6. Thus the potential exists for a drug interaction between drugs that inhibit CYP2D6-mediated metabolism and venlafaxine. However, although imipramine partially inhibited the CYP2D6-mediated metabolism of venlafaxine, resulting in higher plasma concentrations of venlafaxine and lower plasma concentrations of ODV, the total concentration of active compounds (venlafaxine plus ODV) was not affected. Also, in a clinical study involving CYP2D6 poor and extensive metabolizers, the total concentration of active compounds (venlafaxine plus ODV), was similar in both groups. No dosage adjustment is required when venlafaxine is co-administered with a CYP2D6 inhibitor. Caution is advised should a patient's therapy include venlafaxine and CYP2D6 inhibitor).
No products indexed under this heading.

Troglitazone (Concomitant use of CYP3A4 inhibitors and venlafaxine may increase levels of venlafaxine and ODV. Therefore, caution is advised if a patient's therapy includes a CYP3A4 inhibitor and venlafaxine concomitantly. The concomitant use of venlafaxine with a drug treatment(s) that potently inhibits both CYP2D6 and CYP3A4, the primary metabolizing enzymes for venlafaxine, has not been studied. Therefore, caution is advised should a patient's therapy include venlafaxine and any agent(s) that produce potent simultaneous inhibition of these two enzyme systems).
No products indexed under this heading.

Troleandomycin (Concomitant use of CYP3A4 inhibitors and venlafaxine may increase levels of venlafaxine and ODV. Therefore, caution is advised if a patient's therapy includes a CYP3A4 inhibitor and venlafaxine concomitantly. The concomitant use of venlafaxine with a drug treatment(s) that potently inhibits both CYP2D6 and CYP3A4, the primary metabolizing enzymes for venlafaxine, has not been studied. Therefore, caution is advised should a patient's therapy include venlafaxine and any agent(s) that produce potent simultaneous inhibition of these two enzyme systems).
No products indexed under this heading.

Tryptophan (Patients should be cautioned about the risk of serotonin syndrome with the concomitant use of venlafaxine and tryptophan supplements. The concomitant use of venlafaxine with serotonin precursors (such as tryptophan) is not recommended).
No products indexed under this heading.

L-Tryptophan (Patients should be cautioned about the risk of serotonin syndrome with the concomitant use of venlafaxine and tryptophan supplements. The concomitant use of venlafaxine with serotonin precursors (such as tryptophan) is not recommended).
No products indexed under this heading.

Valdecoxib (Patients should be cautioned about the concomitant use of venlafaxine and NSAIDs since combined use of psychotropic drugs that interfere with serotonin reuptake and this agent has been associated with an increased risk of bleeding. SSRIs and SNRIs, including venlafaxine, may increase the risk of bleeding events. Concomitant use of nonsteroidal anti-inflammatory drugs may add to this risk. Case reports and epidemiological studies (case-control and cohort design) have demonstrated an association between use of drugs that interfere with serotonin reuptake and the occurrence of gastrointestinal bleeding).
No products indexed under this heading.

Valproate Sodium (Concomitant use of CYP3A4 inhibitors and venlafaxine may increase levels of venlafaxine and ODV. Therefore, caution is advised if a patient's therapy includes a CYP3A4 inhibitor and venlafaxine concomitantly. The concomitant use of venlafaxine with a drug treatment(s) that potently inhibits both CYP2D6 and CYP3A4, the primary metabolizing enzymes for venlafaxine, has not been studied. Therefore, caution is advised should a patient's therapy include venlafaxine and any agent(s) that produce potent simultaneous inhibition of these two enzyme systems).
No products indexed under this heading.

Vardenafil Hydrochloride (Studies indicate that venlafaxine is metabolized to its active metabolite, ODV, by CYP2D6. Thus the potential exists for a drug interaction between drugs that inhibit CYP2D6-mediated metabolism and venlafaxine. However, although imipramine partially inhibited the CYP2D6-mediated metabolism of venlafaxine, resulting in higher plasma concentrations of venlafaxine and lower plasma concentrations of ODV, the total concentration of active compounds (venlafaxine plus ODV) was not affected. Also, in a clinical study involving CYP2D6 poor and extensive metabolizers, the total concentration of active compounds (venlafaxine plus ODV), was similar in both groups. No dosage adjustment is required when venlafaxine is co-administered with a CYP2D6 inhibitor. Caution is advised should a patient's therapy include venlafaxine and CYP2D6 inhibitor). Products include:
Levitra 3157

Verapamil Hydrochloride (Concomitant use of CYP3A4 inhibitors and venlafaxine may increase levels of venlafaxine and ODV. Therefore, caution is advised if a patient's therapy includes a CYP3A4 inhibitor and venlafaxine concomitantly. The concomitant use of venlafaxine with a drug treatment(s) that potently inhibits both CYP2D6 and CYP3A4, the primary metabolizing enzymes for venlafaxine, has not been studied. Therefore, caution is advised should a patient's therapy include venlafaxine and any agent(s) that produce potent simultaneous inhibition of these two enzyme systems). Products include:
Tarka 534

Vinblastine Sulfate (*In vitro* studies indicate that venlafaxine is a relatively weak inhibitor of CYP2D6. These findings have been confirmed in a clinical drug interaction study comparing the effect of venlafaxine to that of fluoxetine on the CYP2D6-mediated metabolism of dextrometrophan to dextrophan).
No products indexed under this heading.

Voriconazole (Concomitant use of CYP3A4 inhibitors and venlafaxine may increase levels of venlafaxine and ODV. Therefore, caution is advised if a patient's therapy includes a CYP3A4 inhibitor and venlafaxine concomitantly. The concomitant use of venlafaxine with a drug treatment(s) that potently inhibits both CYP2D6 and CYP3A4, the primary metabolizing enzymes for venlafaxine, has not been studied. Therefore, caution is advised should a patient's therapy include venlafaxine and any agent(s) that produce potent simultaneous inhibition of these two enzyme systems).
No products indexed under this heading.

Warfarin Sodium (Patients should be cautioned about the concomitant use of venlafaxine and warfarin since combined use of psychotropic drugs that interfere with serotonin reuptake and this agent has been associated with an increased risk of bleeding. SSRIs and SNRIs, including venlafaxine, may increase the risk of bleeding events. Concomitant use of warfarin may add to this risk. Case reports and epidemiological studies (case-control and cohort design) have demonstrated an association between use of drugs that interfere with serotonin reuptake and the occurrence of gastrointestinal bleeding. Altered anticoagulant effects, including increased bleeding, have been reported when SSRIs and SNRIs are co-administered with warfarin. Patients receiving warfarin therapy should be carefully monitored when venlafaxine is initiated or discontinued).
No products indexed under this heading.

Zafirlukast (Concomitant use of CYP3A4 inhibitors and venlafaxine may increase levels of venlafaxine and ODV. Therefore, caution is advised if a patient's therapy includes a CYP3A4 inhibitor and venlafaxine concomitantly. The concomitant use of venlafaxine with a drug treatment(s) that potently inhibits both CYP2D6 and CYP3A4, the primary metabolizing enzymes for venlafaxine, has not been studied. Therefore, caution is advised should a patient's therapy include venlafaxine and any agent(s) that produce potent simultaneous inhibition of these two enzyme systems). Products include:
Accolate 3612

Zaleplon (The risk of using venlafaxine in combination with other CNS active drugs has not been systematically evaluated. Consequently, caution is advised if the concomitant administration of venlafaxine and such drugs is required).
No products indexed under this heading.

Zileuton (Concomitant use of CYP3A4 inhibitors and venlafaxine may increase levels of venlafaxine and ODV. Therefore, caution is advised if a patient's therapy includes a CYP3A4 inhibitor and venlafaxine concomitantly. The concomitant use of venlafaxine with a drug treatment(s) that potently inhibits both CYP2D6 and CYP3A4, the primary metabolizing enzymes for venlafaxine, has not been studied. Therefore, caution is advised should a patient's therapy include venlafaxine and any agent(s) that produce potent simultaneous inhibition of these two enzyme systems).
No products indexed under this heading.

Ziprasidone Hydrochloride (The risk of using venlafaxine in combination with other CNS active drugs has not been systematically evaluated. Consequently, caution is advised if the concomitant administration of venlafaxine and such drugs is required). Products include:
Geodon 2723

Zolmitriptan (There have been rare post-marketing reports of serotonin syndrome with use of an SSRI and a triptan. If concomitant treatment of venlafaxine with a triptan is clinically warranted, careful observation of the patient is advised, particularly during treatment initiation and dose increases. Patients should be cautioned about the risk of serotonin syndrome with the concomitant use of venlafaxine and triptans, tramadol, tryptophan supplements or other serotonergic agents). Products include:
Zomig Tablets 773
Zomig Nasal Spray 768
Zomig-ZMT Tablets 773

Zolpidem Tartrate (The risk of using venlafaxine in combination with other CNS active drugs has not been systematically evaluated. Consequently, caution is advised if the concomitant administration of venlafaxine and such drugs is required). Products include:
Ambien 2920
Ambien CR 2925

Zonisamide (*In vitro* studies indicate that venlafaxine is a relatively weak inhibitor of CYP2D6. These findings have been confirmed in a clinical drug interaction study comparing the effect of venlafaxine to that of fluoxetine on the CYP2D6-mediated metabolism of dextrometrophan to dextrophan). Products include:
Zonegran 1081

Food Interactions

Alcohol (Although venlafaxine has not been shown to increase the impairment of mental and motor skills caused by alcohol, patients should be advised to avoid alcohol while taking venlafaxine).

Beer, reduced-alcohol (Although venlafaxine has not been shown to increase the impairment of mental and motor skills caused by alcohol, patients should be advised to avoid alcohol while taking venlafaxine).

Beer, unspecified (Although venlafaxine has not been shown to increase the impairment of mental and motor skills caused by alcohol, patients should be advised to avoid alcohol while taking venlafaxine).

Grapefruit (Concomitant use of CYP3A4 inhibitors and venlafaxine may increase levels of venlafaxine and ODV. Therefore, caution is advised if a patient's therapy includes a CYP3A4 inhibitor and venlafaxine concomitantly. The concomitant use of venlafaxine with a drug treatment(s) that potently inhibits both CYP2D6 and CYP3A4, the primary metabolizing enzymes for venlafaxine, has not been studied. Therefore, caution is advised should a patient's therapy include venlafaxine and any agent(s) that produce potent simultaneous inhibition of these two enzyme systems).

Grapefruit Juice (Concomitant use of CYP3A4 inhibitors and venlafaxine may increase levels of venlafaxine and ODV. Therefore, caution is advised if a patient's therapy includes a CYP3A4 inhibitor and venlafaxine concomitantly. The concomitant use of venlafaxine with

a drug treatment(s) that potently inhibits both CYP2D6 and CYP3A4, the primary metabolizing enzymes for venlafaxine, has not been studied. Therefore, caution is advised should a patient's therapy include venlafaxine and any agent(s) that produce potent simultaneous inhibition of these two enzyme systems.

Wine, Chianti (Although venlafaxine has not been shown to increase the impairment of mental and motor skills caused by alcohol, patients should be advised to avoid alcohol while taking venlafaxine).

Wine, Red (Although venlafaxine has not been shown to increase the impairment of mental and motor skills caused by alcohol, patients should be advised to avoid alcohol while taking venlafaxine).

Wine, unspecified (Although venlafaxine has not been shown to increase the impairment of mental and motor skills caused by alcohol, patients should be advised to avoid alcohol while taking venlafaxine).

Wine products (Although venlafaxine has not been shown to increase the impairment of mental and motor skills caused by alcohol, patients should be advised to avoid alcohol while taking venlafaxine).

VENTOLIN HFA INHALATION AEROSOL

(Albuterol Sulfate) 1708
May interact with beta-blockers, monoamine oxidase inhibitors, nonpotassium-sparing diuretics, sympathomimetic bronchodilators, sympathomimetics, tricyclic antidepressants, and certain other agents. Compounds in these categories include:

Acebutolol Hydrochloride
(β-adrenergic receptor blocking agents not only block the pulmonary effect of β-agonists such as albuterol sulfate inhalation aerosol, but may produce severe bronchospasm in patients with asthma. Therefore, patients with asthma should not normally be treated with β-blockers. However, under certain circumstances, (eg, as prophylaxis after myocardial infarction), there may be no acceptable alternatives to the use of β-adrenergic blocking agents in patients with asthma. In this setting, cardioselective β-blockers should be considered, although they should be administered with caution).
No products indexed under this heading.

Albuterol (Other short-acting sympathomimetic aerosol bronchodilators should not be used concomitantly with albuterol).
No products indexed under this heading.

Amitriptyline Hydrochloride
(Albuterol sulfate inhalation aerosol should be administered with extreme caution to patients being treated with tricyclic antidepressants, or within 2 weeks of discontinuation of such agents, because the action of albuterol on the vascular system may be potentiated. Consider alternative therapy in patients taking tricyclic antidepressants).
No products indexed under this heading.

Amoxapine (Albuterol sulfate inhalation aerosol should be administered with extreme caution to patients being treated with tricyclic antidepressants, or within 2 weeks of discontinuation of such agents, because the action of albuterol on the vascular system may be potentiated. Consider alternative therapy in patients taking tricyclic antidepressants).
No products indexed under this heading.

Atenolol (β-adrenergic receptor blocking agents not only block the pulmonary effect of β-agonists such as albuterol

sulfate inhalation aerosol, but may produce severe bronchospasm in patients with asthma. Therefore, patients with asthma should not normally be treated with β-blockers. However, under certain circumstances, (eg, as prophylaxis after myocardial infarction), there may be no acceptable alternatives to the use of β-adrenergic blocking agents in patients with asthma. In this setting, cardioselective β-blockers should be considered, although they should be administered with caution).
No products indexed under this heading.

Bendroflumethiazide (The ECG changes and/or hypokalemia that may result from the administration of nonpotassium-sparing diuretics (eg, loop or thiazide diuretics) can be acutely worsened by β-agonists, especially when the recommended dose of the β-agonist is exceeded. Although the clinical relevance of these effects is not known, caution is advised in the co-administration of β-agonists with nonpotassium-sparing diuretics. Consider monitoring potassium levels).
No products indexed under this heading.

Betaxolol Hydrochloride
(β-adrenergic receptor blocking agents not only block the pulmonary effect of β-agonists such as albuterol sulfate inhalation aerosol, but may produce severe bronchospasm in patients with asthma. Therefore, patients with asthma should not normally be treated with β-blockers. However, under certain circumstances, (eg, as prophylaxis after myocardial infarction), there may be no acceptable alternatives to the use of β-adrenergic blocking agents in patients with asthma. In this setting, cardioselective β-blockers should be considered, although they should be administered with caution).
No products indexed under this heading.

Bisoprolol Fumarate (β-adrenergic receptor blocking agents not only block the pulmonary effect of β-agonists such as albuterol sulfate inhalation aerosol, but may produce severe bronchospasm in patients with asthma. Therefore, patients with asthma should not normally be treated with β-blockers. However, under certain circumstances, (eg, as prophylaxis after myocardial infarction), there may be no acceptable alternatives to the use of β-adrenergic blocking agents in patients with asthma. In this setting, cardioselective β-blockers should be considered, although they should be administered with caution).
No products indexed under this heading.

Bitolterol Mesylate (Other short-acting sympathomimetic aerosol bronchodilators should not be used concomitantly with albuterol).
No products indexed under this heading.

Bumetanide (The ECG changes and/or hypokalemia that may result from the administration of nonpotassium-sparing diuretics (eg, loop or thiazide diuretics) can be acutely worsened by β-agonists, especially when the recommended dose of the β-agonist is exceeded. Although the clinical relevance of these effects is not known, caution is advised in the co-administration of β-agonists with nonpotassium-sparing diuretics. Consider monitoring potassium levels).
No products indexed under this heading.

Carteolol Hydrochloride
(β-adrenergic receptor blocking agents not only block the pulmonary effect of β-agonists such as albuterol sulfate inhalation aerosol, but may produce severe bronchospasm in patients with asthma. Therefore, patients with asthma should not normally be treated with β-blockers. However, under certain circumstances, (eg, as prophylaxis after myocardial infarction), there may be no acceptable alternatives to the use of

β-adrenergic blocking agents in patients with asthma. In this setting, cardioselective β-blockers should be considered, although they should be administered with caution).
No products indexed under this heading.

Carvedilol (β-adrenergic receptor blocking agents not only block the pulmonary effect of β-agonists such as albuterol sulfate inhalation aerosol, but may produce severe bronchospasm in patients with asthma. Therefore, patients with asthma should not normally be treated with β-blockers. However, under certain circumstances, (eg, as prophylaxis after myocardial infarction), there may be no acceptable alternatives to the use of β-adrenergic blocking agents in patients with asthma. In this setting, cardioselective β-blockers should be considered, although they should be administered with caution).
Products include:
Coreg 1409

Carvedilol Phosphate (β-adrenergic receptor blocking agents not only block the pulmonary effect of β-agonists such as albuterol sulfate inhalation aerosol, but may produce severe bronchospasm in patients with asthma. Therefore, patients with asthma should not normally be treated with β-blockers. However, under certain circumstances, (eg, as prophylaxis after myocardial infarction), there may be no acceptable alternatives to the use of β-adrenergic blocking agents in patients with asthma. In this setting, cardioselective β-blockers should be considered, although they should be administered with caution).
Products include:
Coreg CR 1416

Chlorothiazide (The ECG changes and/or hypokalemia that may result from the administration of nonpotassium-sparing diuretics (eg, loop or thiazide diuretics) can be acutely worsened by β-agonists, especially when the recommended dose of the β-agonist is exceeded. Although the clinical relevance of these effects is not known, caution is advised in the co-administration of β-agonists with nonpotassium-sparing diuretics. Consider monitoring potassium levels).
No products indexed under this heading.

Chlorothiazide Sodium (The ECG changes and/or hypokalemia that may result from the administration of nonpotassium-sparing diuretics (eg, loop or thiazide diuretics) can be acutely worsened by β-agonists, especially when the recommended dose of the β-agonist is exceeded. Although the clinical relevance of these effects is not known, caution is advised in the co-administration of β-agonists with nonpotassium-sparing diuretics. Consider monitoring potassium levels).
Products include:
Diuril Intravenous 2009

Clomipramine Hydrochloride
(Albuterol sulfate inhalation aerosol should be administered with extreme caution to patients being treated with tricyclic antidepressants, or within 2 weeks of discontinuation of such agents, because the action of albuterol on the vascular system may be potentiated. Consider alternative therapy in patients taking tricyclic antidepressants).
No products indexed under this heading.

Desipramine Hydrochloride
(Albuterol sulfate inhalation aerosol should be administered with extreme caution to patients being treated with tricyclic antidepressants, or within 2 weeks of discontinuation of such agents, because the action of albuterol on the vascular system may be potentiated. Consider alternative therapy in patients taking tricyclic antidepressants).
No products indexed under this heading.

Digoxin (Mean decreases of 16% to 22% in serum digoxin levels were demonstrated after single dose intravenous and oral administration of albuterol, respectively, to normal volunteers who had received digoxin for 10 days. The clinical relevance of these findings for patients with obstructive airway disease who are receiving inhaled albuterol and digoxin on a chronic basis is unclear. Nevertheless it would be prudent to carefully evaluate the serum digoxin levels in patients who are currently receiving digoxin and albuterol).
Products include:
Lanoxin Injection 1546
Lanoxin Injection Pediatric 1549
Lanoxin Tablets 1553

Dobutamine Hydrochloride (If additional adrenergic drugs are to be administered by any route, they should be used with caution to avoid deleterious cardiovascular effects).
No products indexed under this heading.

Dopamine Hydrochloride (If additional adrenergic drugs are to be administered by any route, they should be used with caution to avoid deleterious cardiovascular effects).
No products indexed under this heading.

Doxepin Hydrochloride (Albuterol sulfate inhalation aerosol should be administered with extreme caution to patients being treated with tricyclic antidepressants, or within 2 weeks of discontinuation of such agents, because the action of albuterol on the vascular system may be potentiated. Consider alternative therapy in patients taking tricyclic antidepressants).
No products indexed under this heading.

Ephedrine Hydrochloride (Other short-acting sympathomimetic aerosol bronchodilators should not be used concomitantly with albuterol).
No products indexed under this heading.

Ephedrine Sulfate (Other short-acting sympathomimetic aerosol bronchodilators should not be used concomitantly with albuterol).
No products indexed under this heading.

Ephedrine Tannate (Other short-acting sympathomimetic aerosol bronchodilators should not be used concomitantly with albuterol).
No products indexed under this heading.

Epinephrine (Other short-acting sympathomimetic aerosol bronchodilators should not be used concomitantly with albuterol). Products include:
EpiPen 3631
Twinject 3268

Epinephrine Bitartrate (If additional adrenergic drugs are to be administered by any route, they should be used with caution to avoid deleterious cardiovascular effects).
No products indexed under this heading.

Epinephrine Hydrochloride (Other short-acting sympathomimetic aerosol bronchodilators should not be used concomitantly with albuterol).
No products indexed under this heading.

Esmolol Hydrochloride
(β-adrenergic receptor blocking agents not only block the pulmonary effect of β-agonists such as albuterol sulfate inhalation aerosol, but may produce severe bronchospasm in patients with

asthma. Therefore, patients with asthma should not normally be treated with β-blockers. However, under certain circumstances, (eg, as prophylaxis after myocardial infarction), there may be no acceptable alternatives to the use of β-adrenergic blocking agents in patients with asthma. In this setting, cardioselective β-blockers should be considered, although they should be administered with caution).
No products indexed under this heading.

Ethacrynic Acid (The ECG changes and/or hypokalemia that may result from the administration of nonpotassium-sparing diuretics (eg, loop or thiazide diuretics) can be acutely worsened by β-agonists, especially when the recommended dose of the β-agonist is exceeded. Although the clinical relevance of these effects is not known, caution is advised in the co-administration of β-agonists with nonpotassium-sparing diuretics. Consider monitoring potassium levels).
No products indexed under this heading.

Furosemide (The ECG changes and/or hypokalemia that may result from the administration of nonpotassium-sparing diuretics (eg, loop or thiazide diuretics) can be acutely worsened by β-agonists, especially when the recommended dose of the β-agonist is exceeded. Although the clinical relevance of these effects is not known, caution is advised in the co-administration of β-agonists with nonpotassium-sparing diuretics. Consider monitoring potassium levels). Products include:
Furosemide 2354

Hydrochlorothiazide (The ECG changes and/or hypokalemia that may result from the administration of nonpotassium-sparing diuretics (eg, loop or thiazide diuretics) can be acutely worsened by β-agonists, especially when the recommended dose of the β-agonist is exceeded. Although the clinical relevance of these effects is not known, caution is advised in the co-administration of β-agonists with nonpotassium-sparing diuretics. Consider monitoring potassium levels).
Products include:
Atacand HCT 700
Avalide 2956
Benicar HCT 1017
Diovan HCT 2419
Dyazide 1429
Exforge HCT 2449
Hyzaar 2162
Hyzaar 100-12.5 2162
Micardis HCT 889
Prinzide 2246
Tekturna HCT 2541
Teveten HCT 541

Hydroflumethiazide (The ECG changes and/or hypokalemia that may result from the administration of nonpotassium-sparing diuretics (eg, loop or thiazide diuretics) can be acutely worsened by β-agonists, especially when the recommended dose of the β-agonist is exceeded. Although the clinical relevance of these effects is not known, caution is advised in the co-administration of β-agonists with nonpotassium-sparing diuretics. Consider monitoring potassium levels).
No products indexed under this heading.

Imipramine Hydrochloride (Albuterol sulfate inhalation aerosol should be administered with extreme caution to patients being treated with tricyclic antidepressants, or within 2 weeks of discontinuation of such agents, because the action of albuterol on the vascular system may be potentiated. Consider alternative therapy in patients taking tricyclic antidepressants).
No products indexed under this heading.

Imipramine Pamoate (Albuterol sulfate inhalation aerosol should be administered with extreme caution to patients being treated with tricyclic antidepressants, or within 2 weeks of discontinuation of such agents, because the action of albuterol on the vascular system may be potentiated. Consider alternative therapy in patients taking tricyclic antidepressants).
No products indexed under this heading.

Isocarboxazid (Albuterol sulfate inhalation aerosol should be administered with extreme caution to patients being treated with monoamine oxidase inhibitors, or within 2 weeks of discontinuation of such agents, because the action of albuterol on the vascular system may be potentiated. Consider alternative therapy in patients taking MAO inhibitors). Products include:
Marplan 3481

Isoetharine (Other short-acting sympathomimetic aerosol bronchodilators should not be used concomitantly with albuterol).
No products indexed under this heading.

Isoproterenol Hydrochloride (Other short-acting sympathomimetic aerosol bronchodilators should not be used concomitantly with albuterol).
No products indexed under this heading.

Isoproterenol Sulfate (Other short-acting sympathomimetic aerosol bronchodilators should not be used concomitantly with albuterol).
No products indexed under this heading.

Labetalol Hydrochloride (β-adrenergic receptor blocking agents not only block the pulmonary effect of β-agonists such as albuterol sulfate inhalation aerosol, but may produce severe bronchospasm in patients with asthma. Therefore, patients with asthma should not normally be treated with β-blockers. However, under certain circumstances, (eg, as prophylaxis after myocardial infarction), there may be no acceptable alternatives to the use of β-adrenergic blocking agents in patients with asthma. In this setting, cardioselective β-blockers should be considered, although they should be administered with caution).
No products indexed under this heading.

Levalbuterol Hydrochloride (Other short-acting sympathomimetic aerosol bronchodilators should not be used concomitantly with albuterol).
No products indexed under this heading.

Levobunolol Hydrochloride (β-adrenergic receptor blocking agents not only block the pulmonary effect of β-agonists such as albuterol sulfate inhalation aerosol, but may produce severe bronchospasm in patients with asthma. Therefore, patients with asthma should not normally be treated with β-blockers. However, under certain circumstances, (eg, as prophylaxis after myocardial infarction), there may be no acceptable alternatives to the use of β-adrenergic blocking agents in patients with asthma. In this setting, cardioselective β-blockers should be considered, although they should be administered with caution).
No products indexed under this heading.

Maprotiline Hydrochloride (Albuterol sulfate inhalation aerosol should be administered with extreme caution to patients being treated with tricyclic antidepressants, or within 2 weeks of discontinuation of such agents, because the action of albuterol on the vascular system may be potentiated. Consider alternative therapy in patients taking tricyclic antidepressants).
No products indexed under this heading.

Metaproterenol Sulfate (Other short-acting sympathomimetic aerosol bronchodilators should not be used concomitantly with albuterol).
No products indexed under this heading.

Metaraminol Bitartrate (If additional adrenergic drugs are to be administered by any route, they should be used with caution to avoid deleterious cardiovascular effects).
No products indexed under this heading.

Methoxamine Hydrochloride (If additional adrenergic drugs are to be administered by any route, they should be used with caution to avoid deleterious cardiovascular effects).
No products indexed under this heading.

Methyclothiazide (The ECG changes and/or hypokalemia that may result from the administration of nonpotassium-sparing diuretics (eg, loop or thiazide diuretics) can be acutely worsened by β-agonists, especially when the recommended dose of the β-agonist is exceeded. Although the clinical relevance of these effects is not known, caution is advised in the co-administration of β-agonists with nonpotassium-sparing diuretics. Consider monitoring potassium levels).
No products indexed under this heading.

Metipranolol Hydrochloride (β-adrenergic receptor blocking agents not only block the pulmonary effect of β-agonists such as albuterol sulfate inhalation aerosol, but may produce severe bronchospasm in patients with asthma. Therefore, patients with asthma should not normally be treated with β-blockers. However, under certain circumstances, (eg, as prophylaxis after myocardial infarction), there may be no acceptable alternatives to the use of β-adrenergic blocking agents in patients with asthma. In this setting, cardioselective β-blockers should be considered, although they should be administered with caution).
No products indexed under this heading.

Metoprolol Succinate (β-adrenergic receptor blocking agents not only block the pulmonary effect of β-agonists such as albuterol sulfate inhalation aerosol, but may produce severe bronchospasm in patients with asthma. Therefore, patients with asthma should not normally be treated with β-blockers. However, under certain circumstances, (eg, as prophylaxis after myocardial infarction), there may be no acceptable alternatives to the use of β-adrenergic blocking agents in patients with asthma. In this setting, cardioselective β-blockers should be considered, although they should be administered with caution).
Products include:
Toprol XL 732

Metoprolol Tartrate (β-adrenergic receptor blocking agents not only block the pulmonary effect of β-agonists such as albuterol sulfate inhalation aerosol, but may produce severe bronchospasm in patients with asthma. Therefore, patients with asthma should not normally be treated with β-blockers. However, under certain circumstances, (eg, as prophylaxis after myocardial infarction), there may be no acceptable alternatives to the use of β-adrenergic blocking agents in patients with asthma. In this setting, cardioselective β-blockers should be considered, although they should be administered with caution).
No products indexed under this heading.

Moclobemide (Albuterol sulfate inhalation aerosol should be administered with extreme caution to patients being treated with monoamine oxidase inhibitors, or within 2 weeks of discontinuation of such agents, because the action of albuterol on the vascular system may be potentiated. Consider alternative therapy in patients taking MAO inhibitors).
No products indexed under this heading.

Nadolol (β-adrenergic receptor blocking agents not only block the pulmonary effect of β-agonists such as albuterol sulfate inhalation aerosol, but may produce severe bronchospasm in patients with asthma. Therefore, patients with asthma should not normally be treated with β-blockers. However, under certain circumstances, (eg, as prophylaxis after myocardial infarction), there may be no acceptable alternatives to the use of β-adrenergic blocking agents in patients with asthma. In this setting, cardioselective β-blockers should be considered, although they should be administered with caution). Products include:
Nadolol 2359

Nebivolol (β-adrenergic receptor blocking agents not only block the pulmonary effect of β-agonists such as albuterol sulfate inhalation aerosol, but may produce severe bronchospasm in patients with asthma. Therefore, patients with asthma should not normally be treated with β-blockers. However, under certain circumstances, (eg, as prophylaxis after myocardial infarction), there may be no acceptable alternatives to the use of β-adrenergic blocking agents in patients with asthma. In this setting, cardioselective β-blockers should be considered, although they should be administered with caution).
Products include:
Bystolic 1147

Norepinephrine Bitartrate (If additional adrenergic drugs are to be administered by any route, they should be used with caution to avoid deleterious cardiovascular effects).
No products indexed under this heading.

Nortriptyline Hydrochloride (Albuterol sulfate inhalation aerosol should be administered with extreme caution to patients being treated with tricyclic antidepressants, or within 2 weeks of discontinuation of such agents, because the action of albuterol on the vascular system may be potentiated. Consider alternative therapy in patients taking tricyclic antidepressants).
No products indexed under this heading.

Pargyline Hydrochloride (Albuterol sulfate inhalation aerosol should be administered with extreme caution to patients being treated with monoamine oxidase inhibitors, or within 2 weeks of discontinuation of such agents, because the action of albuterol on the vascular system may be potentiated. Consider alternative therapy in patients taking MAO inhibitors).
No products indexed under this heading.

Penbutolol Sulfate (β-adrenergic receptor blocking agents not only block the pulmonary effect of β-agonists such as albuterol sulfate inhalation aerosol, but may produce severe bronchospasm in patients with asthma. Therefore, patients with asthma should not normally be treated with β-blockers. However, under certain circumstances, (eg, as prophylaxis after myocardial infarction), there may be no acceptable alternatives to the use of β-adrenergic blocking agents in patients with asthma. In this setting, cardioselective β-blockers should be considered, although they should be administered with caution).
No products indexed under this heading.

Phenelzine Sulfate (Albuterol sulfate inhalation aerosol should be administered with extreme caution to patients being treated with monoamine oxidase inhibitors, or within 2 weeks of discontinuation of such agents, because the action of albuterol on the vascular system may be potentiated. Consider alternative therapy in patients taking MAO inhibitors).
No products indexed under this heading.

Phenylephrine Bitartrate (If additional adrenergic drugs are to be administered by any route, they should be used with caution to avoid deleterious cardiovascular effects).
No products indexed under this heading.

Phenylephrine Hydrochloride (If additional adrenergic drugs are to be administered by any route, they should be used with caution to avoid deleterious cardiovascular effects). Products include:
Sudafed PE Nasal Decongestant **2048**
Children's Sudafed PE Nasal Decongestant **2047**

Phenylephrine Tannate (If additional adrenergic drugs are to be administered by any route, they should be used with caution to avoid deleterious cardiovascular effects).
No products indexed under this heading.

Phenylpropanolamine Hydrochloride (If additional adrenergic drugs are to be administered by any route, they should be used with caution to avoid deleterious cardiovascular effects).
No products indexed under this heading.

Pindolol (β-adrenergic receptor blocking agents not only block the pulmonary effect of β-agonists such as albuterol sulfate inhalation aerosol, but may produce severe bronchospasm in patients with asthma. Therefore, patients with asthma should not normally be treated with β-blockers. However, under certain circumstances, (eg, as prophylaxis after myocardial infarction), there may be no acceptable alternatives to the use of β-adrenergic blocking agents in patients with asthma. In this setting, cardioselective β-blockers should be considered, although they should be administered with caution).
No products indexed under this heading.

Pirbuterol Acetate (Other short-acting sympathomimetic aerosol bronchodilators should not be used concomitantly with albuterol). Products include:
Maxair Autohaler **1782**

Polythiazide (The ECG changes and/or hypokalemia that may result from the administration of nonpotassium-sparing diuretics (eg, loop or thiazide diuretics) can be acutely worsened by β-agonists, especially when the recommended dose of the β-agonist is exceeded. Although the clinical relevance of these effects is not known, caution is advised in the co-administration of β-agonists with nonpotassium-sparing diuretics. Consider monitoring potassium levels).
No products indexed under this heading.

Procarbazine Hydrochloride (Albuterol sulfate inhalation aerosol should be administered with extreme caution to patients being treated with monoamine oxidase inhibitors, or within 2 weeks of discontinuation of such agents, because the action of albuterol on the vascular system may be potentiated. Consider alternative therapy in patients taking MAO inhibitors).
No products indexed under this heading.

Propranolol Hydrochloride (β-adrenergic receptor blocking agents not only block the pulmonary effect of β-agonists such as albuterol sulfate inhalation aerosol, but may produce severe bronchospasm in patients with asthma. Therefore, patients with asthma should not normally be treated with β-blockers. However, under certain circumstances, (eg, as prophylaxis after myocardial infarction), there may be no acceptable alternatives to the use of β-adrenergic blocking agents in patients with asthma. In this setting, cardioselective β-blockers should be considered, although they should be administered with caution). Products include:
InnoPran XL **1517**

Protriptyline Hydrochloride (Albuterol sulfate inhalation aerosol should be administered with extreme caution to patients being treated with tricyclic antidepressants, or within 2 weeks of discontinuation of such agents, because the action of albuterol on the vascular system may be potentiated. Consider alternative therapy in patients taking tricyclic antidepressants).
No products indexed under this heading.

Pseudoephedrine Hydrochloride (If additional adrenergic drugs are to be administered by any route, they should be used with caution to avoid deleterious cardiovascular effects). Products include:
Allegra-D **2915**
Allegra-D 24 .... **2918**
Sudafed 12 Hour Nasal Decongestant Non-Drowsy **2048**
Sudafed 24 Hour **2048**
Sudafed Nasal Decongestant **2047**
Children's Sudafed Nasal Decongestant Liquid **2047**
Zyrtec-D Allergy & Congestion **2054**

Pseudoephedrine Sulfate (If additional adrenergic drugs are to be administered by any route, they should be used with caution to avoid deleterious cardiovascular effects). Products include:
Clarinex-D 12-Hour **3101**
Clarinex-D **3104**

Rasagiline Mesylate (Albuterol sulfate inhalation aerosol should be administered with extreme caution to patients being treated with monoamine oxidase inhibitors, or within 2 weeks of discontinuation of such agents, because the action of albuterol on the vascular system may be potentiated. Consider alternative therapy in patients taking MAO inhibitors). Products include:
Azilect **3383**

Salmeterol Xinafoate (Other short-acting sympathomimetic aerosol bronchodilators should not be used concomitantly with albuterol). Products include:
Advair 100/50 .... **1275**
Advair 250/50 .... **1275**
Advair 500/50 .... **1275**
Advair HFA 45/21 .... **1288**
Advair HFA 115/21 .... **1288**
Advair HFA 230/21 .... **1288**
Serevent Diskus **1656**

Selegiline (Albuterol sulfate inhalation aerosol should be administered with extreme caution to patients being treated with monoamine oxidase inhibitors, or within 2 weeks of discontinuation of such agents, because the action of albuterol on the vascular system may be potentiated. Consider alternative therapy in patients taking MAO inhibitors). Products include:
Emsam **3623**

Selegiline Hydrochloride (Albuterol sulfate inhalation aerosol should be administered with extreme caution to patients being treated with monoamine oxidase inhibitors, or within 2 weeks of discontinuation of such agents, because the action of albuterol on the vascular system may be potentiated. Consider alternative therapy in patients taking MAO inhibitors). Products include:
Eldepryl **3312**

Sotalol Hydrochloride (β-adrenergic receptor blocking agents not only block the pulmonary effect of β-agonists such as albuterol sulfate inhalation aerosol, but may produce severe bronchospasm in patients with asthma. Therefore, patients with asthma should not normally be treated with β-blockers. However, under certain circumstances, (eg, as prophylaxis after myocardial infarction), there may be no acceptable alternatives to the use of β-adrenergic blocking agents in patients with asthma. In this setting, cardioselective β-blockers should be considered, although they should be administered with caution).
No products indexed under this heading.

Terbutaline Sulfate (Other short-acting sympathomimetic aerosol bronchodilators should not be used concomitantly with albuterol).
No products indexed under this heading.

Timolol Hemihydrate (β-adrenergic receptor blocking agents not only block the pulmonary effect of β-agonists such as albuterol sulfate inhalation aerosol, but may produce severe bronchospasm in patients with asthma. Therefore, patients with asthma should not normally be treated with β-blockers. However, under certain circumstances, (eg, as prophylaxis after myocardial infarction), there may be no acceptable alternatives to the use of β-adrenergic blocking agents in patients with asthma. In this setting, cardioselective β-blockers should be considered, although they should be administered with caution). Products include:
Betimol **3490**

Timolol Maleate (β-adrenergic receptor blocking agents not only block the pulmonary effect of β-agonists such as albuterol sulfate inhalation aerosol, but may produce severe bronchospasm in patients with asthma. Therefore, patients with asthma should not normally be treated with β-blockers. However, under certain circumstances, (eg, as prophylaxis after myocardial infarction), there may be no acceptable alternatives to the use of β-adrenergic blocking agents in patients with asthma. In this setting, cardioselective β-blockers should be considered, although they should be administered with caution). Products include:
Combigan **601**
Dorzolamide Hydrochloride/Timolol Maleate Ophthalmic Solution .... ⊙ **243**
Timoptic in Ocudose .... ⊙ **231**

Torsemide (The ECG changes and/or hypokalemia that may result from the administration of nonpotassium-sparing diuretics (eg, loop or thiazide diuretics) can be acutely worsened by β-agonists, especially when the recommended dose of the β-agonist is exceeded. Although the clinical relevance of these effects is not known, caution is advised in the co-administration of β-agonists with nonpotassium-sparing diuretics. Consider monitoring potassium levels).
No products indexed under this heading.

Tranylcypromine Sulfate (Albuterol sulfate inhalation aerosol should be administered with extreme caution to patients being treated with monoamine oxidase inhibitors, or within 2 weeks of discontinuation of such agents, because the action of albuterol on the vascular system may be potentiated. Consider alternative therapy in patients taking MAO inhibitors). Products include:
Parnate **1584**

Trimipramine Maleate (Albuterol sulfate inhalation aerosol should be administered with extreme caution to patients being treated with tricyclic antidepressants, or within 2 weeks of discontinuation of such agents, because the action of albuterol on the vascular system may be potentiated. Consider alternative therapy in patients taking tricyclic antidepressants).
No products indexed under this heading.

VERAMYST NASAL SPRAY

(Fluticasone Furoate) **1713**
May interact with cytochrome p450 3a4 inhibitors, potent (selected), and certain other agents. Compounds in these categories include:

Amprenavir (Use caution with the co-administration of fluticasone furoate and other potent cytochrome P450 3A4 (CYP3A4) inhibitors, such as ketoconazole. Fluticasone furoate is cleared by extensive first-pass metabolism mediated by CYP3A4. Co-administration of fluticasone furoate and ketoconazole or other potent CYP3A4 inhibitors had measurable but low levels of fluticasone furoate. There was a 5% reduction in 24-hour serum cortisol levels with ketoconazole).
No products indexed under this heading.

Atazanavir (Use caution with the co-administration of fluticasone furoate and other potent cytochrome P450 3A4 (CYP3A4) inhibitors, such as ketoconazole. Fluticasone furoate is cleared by extensive first-pass metabolism mediated by CYP3A4. Co-administration of fluticasone furoate and ketoconazole or other potent CYP3A4 inhibitors had measurable but low levels of fluticasone furoate. There was a 5% reduction in 24-hour serum cortisol levels with ketoconazole).
No products indexed under this heading.

Atazanavir Sulfate (Use caution with the co-administration of fluticasone furoate and other potent cytochrome P450 3A4 (CYP3A4) inhibitors, such as ketoconazole. Fluticasone furoate is cleared by extensive first-pass metabolism mediated by CYP3A4. Co-administration of fluticasone furoate and ketoconazole or other potent CYP3A4 inhibitors had measurable but low levels of fluticasone furoate. There was a 5% reduction in 24-hour serum cortisol levels with ketoconazole).
No products indexed under this heading.

Clarithromycin (Use caution with the co-administration of fluticasone furoate and other potent cytochrome P450 3A4 (CYP3A4) inhibitors, such as ketoconazole. Fluticasone furoate is cleared by extensive first-pass metabolism mediated by CYP3A4. Co-administration of fluticasone furoate and ketoconazole or other potent CYP3A4 inhibitors had measurable but low levels of fluticasone furoate. There was a 5% reduction in 24-hour serum cortisol levels with ketoconazole). Products include:
Biaxin/Biaxin XL **412**

Delavirdine Mesylate (Use caution with the co-administration of fluticasone furoate and other potent cytochrome P450 3A4 (CYP3A4) inhibitors, such as ketoconazole. Fluticasone furoate is cleared by extensive first-pass metabolism mediated by CYP3A4. Co-administration of fluticasone furoate and ketoconazole or other potent CYP3A4 inhibitors had measurable but low levels of fluticasone furoate. There was a 5% reduction in 24-hour serum cortisol levels with ketoconazole).
No products indexed under this heading.

Delavirine (Use caution with the co-administration of fluticasone furoate and other potent cytochrome P450 3A4 (CYP3A4) inhibitors, such as ketocona-

Veramyst Interactions Index 2042

zole. Fluticasone furoate is cleared by extensive first-pass metabolism mediated by CYP3A4. Co-administration of fluticasone furoate and ketoconazole or other potent CYP3A4 inhibitors had measurable but low levels of fluticasone furoate. There was a 5% reduction in 24-hour serum cortisol levels with ketoconazole).
No products indexed under this heading.

Fosamprenavir Calcium (Use caution with the co-administration of fluticasone furoate and other potent cytochrome P450 3A4 (CYP3A4) inhibitors, such as ketoconazole. Fluticasone furoate is cleared by extensive first-pass metabolism mediated by CYP3A4. Co-administration of fluticasone furoate and ketoconazole or other potent CYP3A4 inhibitors had measurable but low levels of fluticasone furoate. There was a 5% reduction in 24-hour serum cortisol levels with ketoconazole). Products include:
Lexiva Oral Suspension 1558
Lexiva 1558

Indinavir Sulfate (Use caution with the co-administration of fluticasone furoate and other potent cytochrome P450 3A4 (CYP3A4) inhibitors, such as ketoconazole. Fluticasone furoate is cleared by extensive first-pass metabolism mediated by CYP3A4. Co-administration of fluticasone furoate and ketoconazole or other potent CYP3A4 inhibitors had measurable but low levels of fluticasone furoate. There was a 5% reduction in 24-hour serum cortisol levels with ketoconazole). Products include:
Crixivan 2113

Itraconazole (Use caution with the co-administration of fluticasone furoate and other potent cytochrome P450 3A4 (CYP3A4) inhibitors, such as ketoconazole. Fluticasone furoate is cleared by extensive first-pass metabolism mediated by CYP3A4. Co-administration of fluticasone furoate and ketoconazole or other potent CYP3A4 inhibitors had measurable but low levels of fluticasone furoate. There was a 5% reduction in 24-hour serum cortisol levels with ketoconazole).
No products indexed under this heading.

Ketoconazole (Use caution with the co-administration of fluticasone furoate and other potent cytochrome P450 3A4 (CYP3A4) inhibitors, such as ketoconazole. Fluticasone furoate is cleared by extensive first-pass metabolism mediated by CYP3A4. Co-administration of fluticasone furoate and ketoconazole or other potent CYP3A4 inhibitors had measurable but low levels of fluticasone furoate. There was a 5% reduction in 24-hour serum cortisol levels with ketoconazole; therefore, caution is required with the co-administration of fluticasone furoate and ketoconazole or other potent CYP3A4 inhibitors). Products include:
Extina 3319
Xolegel 3337

Lopinavir (Use caution with the co-administration of fluticasone furoate and other potent cytochrome P450 3A4 (CYP3A4) inhibitors, such as ketoconazole. Fluticasone furoate is cleared by extensive first-pass metabolism mediated by CYP3A4. Co-administration of fluticasone furoate and ketoconazole or other potent CYP3A4 inhibitors had measurable but low levels of fluticasone furoate. There was a 5% reduction in 24-hour serum cortisol levels with ketoconazole). Products include:
Kaletra 458

Nefazodone Hydrochloride (Use caution with the co-administration of fluticasone furoate and other potent cytochrome P450 3A4 (CYP3A4) inhibitors, such as ketoconazole. Fluticasone furoate is cleared by extensive first-pass metabolism mediated by CYP3A4. Co-administration of fluticasone furoate and ketoconazole or other potent CYP3A4 inhibitors had measurable but low levels of fluticasone furoate. There was a 5% reduction in 24-hour serum cortisol levels with ketoconazole).
No products indexed under this heading.

Nelfinavir Mesylate (Use caution with the co-administration of fluticasone furoate and other potent cytochrome P450 3A4 (CYP3A4) inhibitors, such as ketoconazole. Fluticasone furoate is cleared by extensive first-pass metabolism mediated by CYP3A4. Co-administration of fluticasone furoate and ketoconazole or other potent CYP3A4 inhibitors had measurable but low levels of fluticasone furoate. There was a 5% reduction in 24-hour serum cortisol levels with ketoconazole).
No products indexed under this heading.

Ritonavir (Based on data with another glucocorticoid, fluticasone propionate, metabolized by CYP3A4, co-administration of fluticasone furoate with the potent CYP3A4 inhibitor ritonavir is not recommended because of the risk of systemic effects secondary to increased exposure to fluticasone furoate. High exposure to corticosteroids increases the potential for systemic side effects, such as cortisol suppression). Products include:
Kaletra 458
Norvir 509

Saquinavir (Use caution with the co-administration of fluticasone furoate and other potent cytochrome P450 3A4 (CYP3A4) inhibitors, such as ketoconazole. Fluticasone furoate is cleared by extensive first-pass metabolism mediated by CYP3A4. Co-administration of fluticasone furoate and ketoconazole or other potent CYP3A4 inhibitors had measurable but low levels of fluticasone furoate. There was a 5% reduction in 24-hour serum cortisol levels with ketoconazole).
No products indexed under this heading.

Saquinavir Mesylate (Use caution with the co-administration of fluticasone furoate and other potent cytochrome P450 3A4 (CYP3A4) inhibitors, such as ketoconazole. Fluticasone furoate is cleared by extensive first-pass metabolism mediated by CYP3A4. Co-administration of fluticasone furoate and ketoconazole or other potent CYP3A4 inhibitors had measurable but low levels of fluticasone furoate. There was a 5% reduction in 24-hour serum cortisol levels with ketoconazole).
No products indexed under this heading.

Telithromycin (Use caution with the co-administration of fluticasone furoate and other potent cytochrome P450 3A4 (CYP3A4) inhibitors, such as ketoconazole. Fluticasone furoate is cleared by extensive first-pass metabolism mediated by CYP3A4. Co-administration of fluticasone furoate and ketoconazole or other potent CYP3A4 inhibitors had measurable but low levels of fluticasone furoate. There was a 5% reduction in 24-hour serum cortisol levels with ketoconazole). Products include:
Ketek 2991

Troleandomycin (Use caution with the co-administration of fluticasone furoate and other potent cytochrome P450 3A4 (CYP3A4) inhibitors, such as ketoconazole. Fluticasone furoate is cleared by extensive first-pass metabolism mediated by CYP3A4. Co-administration of fluticasone furoate and ketoconazole or other potent CYP3A4 inhibitors had measurable but low levels of fluticasone furoate. There was a 5% reduction in 24-hour serum cortisol levels with ketoconazole).
No products indexed under this heading.

Voriconazole (Use caution with the co-administration of fluticasone furoate and other potent cytochrome P450 3A4 (CYP3A4) inhibitors, such as ketoconazole. Fluticasone furoate is cleared by extensive first-pass metabolism mediated by CYP3A4. Co-administration of fluticasone furoate and ketoconazole or other potent CYP3A4 inhibitors had measurable but low levels of fluticasone furoate. There was a 5% reduction in 24-hour serum cortisol levels with ketoconazole).
No products indexed under this heading.

VERDESO FOAM

(Desonide) 3334
None cited in PDR database.

VESICARE TABLETS

(Solifenacin Succinate) 694
May interact with cytochrome p450 3a4 inducers (selected), cytochrome p450 3a4 inhibitors (selected), cytochrome p450 3a4 inhibitors, potent (selected), drugs that prolong the QT interval, and certain other agents. Compounds in these categories include:

Acetazolamide (Inhibitors of CYP3A4 may alter solifenacin pharmacokinetics. Following the administration of 10 mg of solifenacin in the presence of 400 mg of ketoconazole, a potent inhibitor of CYP3A4, the mean C_{max} and AUC of solifenacin increased by 1.5 and 2.7-fold, respectively. Therefore, it is recommended not to exceed a 5 mg daily dose of solifenacin when administered with therapeutic doses of ketoconazole or other potent CYP3A4 inhibitors).
No products indexed under this heading.

Acetazolamide Sodium (Inhibitors of CYP3A4 may alter solifenacin pharmacokinetics. Following the administration of 10 mg of solifenacin in the presence of 400 mg of ketoconazole, a potent inhibitor of CYP3A4, the mean C_{max} and AUC of solifenacin increased by 1.5 and 2.7-fold, respectively. Therefore, it is recommended not to exceed a 5 mg daily dose of solifenacin when administered with therapeutic doses of ketoconazole or other potent CYP3A4 inhibitors).
No products indexed under this heading.

Allium sativum (Inducers of CYP3A4 may alter solifenacin pharmacokinetics).
No products indexed under this heading.

Alprazolam (In a study of the effect of solifenacin on the QT interval in 76 healthy women, the QT prolonging effect appeared less with solifenacin 10 mg than with 30 mg (three times the maximum recommended dose), and the effect of solifenacin 30 mg did not appear as large as that of the positive control moxifloxacin at its therapeutic dose. This observation should be considered in clinical decisions to prescribe solifenacin succinate for patients with a known history of QT prolongation or patients who are taking medications known to prolong the QT interval).
No products indexed under this heading.

Aminoglutethimide (Inducers of CYP3A4 may alter solifenacin pharmacokinetics).
No products indexed under this heading.

Amiodarone Hydrochloride (In a study of the effect of solifenacin on the QT interval in 76 healthy women, the QT prolonging effect appeared less with solifenacin 10 mg than with 30 mg (three times the maximum recommended dose), and the effect of solifenacin 30 mg did not appear as large as that of the positive control moxifloxacin at its therapeutic dose. This observation should be considered in clinical decisions to prescribe solifenacin succinate for patients with a known history of QT prolongation or patients who are taking medications known to prolong the QT interval).
No products indexed under this heading.

Amitriptyline Hydrochloride (In a study of the effect of solifenacin on the QT interval in 76 healthy women, the QT prolonging effect appeared less with solifenacin 10 mg than with 30 mg (three times the maximum recommended dose), and the effect of solifenacin 30 mg did not appear as large as that of the positive control moxifloxacin at its therapeutic dose. This observation should be considered in clinical decisions to prescribe solifenacin succinate for patients with a known history of QT prolongation or patients who are taking medications known to prolong the QT interval).
No products indexed under this heading.

Amoxapine (In a study of the effect of solifenacin on the QT interval in 76 healthy women, the QT prolonging effect appeared less with solifenacin 10 mg than with 30 mg (three times the maximum recommended dose), and the effect of solifenacin 30 mg did not appear as large as that of the positive control moxifloxacin at its therapeutic dose. This observation should be considered in clinical decisions to prescribe solifenacin succinate for patients with a known history of QT prolongation or patients who are taking medications known to prolong the QT interval).
No products indexed under this heading.

Amprenavir (Following the administration of 10 mg of solifenacin in the presence of 400 mg of ketoconazole, a potent inhibitor of CYP3A4, the mean C_{max} and AUC of solifenacin increased by 1.5 and 2.7-fold, respectively. Therefore, it is recommended not to exceed a 5 mg daily dose of solifenacin when administered with therapeutic doses of ketoconazole or other potent CYP3A4 inhibitors).
No products indexed under this heading.

Anastrozole (Inhibitors of CYP3A4 may alter solifenacin pharmacokinetics. Following the administration of 10 mg of solifenacin in the presence of 400 mg of ketoconazole, a potent inhibitor of CYP3A4, the mean C_{max} and AUC of solifenacin increased by 1.5 and 2.7-fold, respectively. Therefore, it is recommended not to exceed a 5 mg daily dose of solifenacin when administered with therapeutic doses of ketoconazole or other potent CYP3A4 inhibitors).
No products indexed under this heading.

Aprepitant (Inhibitors of CYP3A4 may alter solifenacin pharmacokinetics. Following the administration of 10 mg of solifenacin in the presence of 400 mg of ketoconazole, a potent inhibitor of CYP3A4, the mean C_{max} and AUC of solifenacin increased by 1.5 and 2.7-fold, respectively. Therefore, it is recommended not to exceed a 5 mg daily dose of solifenacin when administered with therapeutic doses of ketoconazole or other potent CYP3A4 inhibitors). Products include:
Emend 2124

Astemizole (In a study of the effect of solifenacin on the QT interval in 76 healthy women, the QT prolonging effect appeared less with solifenacin 10 mg than with 30 mg (three times the maximum recommended dose), and the effect of solifenacin 30 mg did not appear as large as that of the positive control moxifloxacin at its therapeutic dose. This observation should be considered in clinical decisions to prescribe solifenacin succinate for patients with a

(⊙ Described in PDR® for Ophthalmic Medicines)

known history of QT prolongation or patients who are taking medications known to prolong the QT interval).
No products indexed under this heading.

Atazanavir (Following the administration of 10 mg of solifenacin in the presence of 400 mg of ketoconazole, a potent inhibitor of CYP3A4, the mean C_{max} and AUC of solifenacin increased by 1.5 and 2.7-fold, respectively. Therefore, it is recommended not to exceed a 5 mg daily dose of solifenacin when administered with therapeutic doses of ketoconazole or other potent CYP3A4 inhibitors).
No products indexed under this heading.

Atazanavir Sulfate (Following the administration of 10 mg of solifenacin in the presence of 400 mg of ketoconazole, a potent inhibitor of CYP3A4, the mean C_{max} and AUC of solifenacin increased by 1.5 and 2.7-fold, respectively. Therefore, it is recommended not to exceed a 5 mg daily dose of solifenacin when administered with therapeutic doses of ketoconazole or other potent CYP3A4 inhibitors).
No products indexed under this heading.

Betamethasone (Inducers of CYP3A4 may alter solifenacin pharmacokinetics).
No products indexed under this heading.

Betamethasone Acetate (Inducers of CYP3A4 may alter solifenacin pharmacokinetics).
No products indexed under this heading.

Betamethasone Benzoate (Inducers of CYP3A4 may alter solifenacin pharmacokinetics).
No products indexed under this heading.

Betamethasone Dipropionate (Inducers of CYP3A4 may alter solifenacin pharmacokinetics). Products include:
Diprolene Lotion 0.05% 3108
Diprolene Ointment 0.05% 3109
Diprolene AF Cream 0.05% 3107
Lotrisone 3163

Betamethasone Sodium Phosphate (Inducers of CYP3A4 may alter solifenacin pharmacokinetics).
No products indexed under this heading.

Betamethasone Valerate (Inducers of CYP3A4 may alter solifenacin pharmacokinetics). Products include:
Luxíq 3321

Bosentan (Inducers of CYP3A4 may alter solifenacin pharmacokinetics). Products include:
Tracleer 573

Bretylium Tosylate (In a study of the effect of solifenacin on the QT interval in 76 healthy women, the QT prolonging effect appeared less with solifenacin 10 mg than with 30 mg (three times the maximum recommended dose), and the effect of solifenacin 30 mg did not appear as large as that of the positive control moxifloxacin at its therapeutic dose. This observation should be considered in clinical decisions to prescribe solifenacin succinate for patients with a known history of QT prolongation or patients who are taking medications known to prolong the QT interval).
No products indexed under this heading.

Buspirone Hydrochloride (In a study of the effect of solifenacin on the QT interval in 76 healthy women, the QT prolonging effect appeared less with solifenacin 10 mg than with 30 mg (three times the maximum recommended dose), and the effect of solifenacin 30 mg did not appear as large as that of the positive control moxifloxacin at its therapeutic dose. This observation should be considered in clinical decisions to prescribe solifenacin succinate for patients with a known history of QT prolongation or patients who are taking medications known to prolong the QT interval).
No products indexed under this heading.

Carbamazepine (Inducers of CYP3A4 may alter solifenacin pharmacokinetics). Products include:
Carbatrol 3280
Equetro 3477

Chlordiazepoxide (In a study of the effect of solifenacin on the QT interval in 76 healthy women, the QT prolonging effect appeared less with solifenacin 10 mg than with 30 mg (three times the maximum recommended dose), and the effect of solifenacin 30 mg did not appear as large as that of the positive control moxifloxacin at its therapeutic dose. This observation should be considered in clinical decisions to prescribe solifenacin succinate for patients with a known history of QT prolongation or patients who are taking medications known to prolong the QT interval).
No products indexed under this heading.

Chlordiazepoxide Hydrochloride (In a study of the effect of solifenacin on the QT interval in 76 healthy women, the QT prolonging effect appeared less with solifenacin 10 mg than with 30 mg (three times the maximum recommended dose), and the effect of solifenacin 30 mg did not appear as large as that of the positive control moxifloxacin at its therapeutic dose. This observation should be considered in clinical decisions to prescribe solifenacin succinate for patients with a known history of QT prolongation or patients who are taking medications known to prolong the QT interval).
No products indexed under this heading.

Chlorpromazine (In a study of the effect of solifenacin on the QT interval in 76 healthy women, the QT prolonging effect appeared less with solifenacin 10 mg than with 30 mg (three times the maximum recommended dose), and the effect of solifenacin 30 mg did not appear as large as that of the positive control moxifloxacin at its therapeutic dose. This observation should be considered in clinical decisions to prescribe solifenacin succinate for patients with a known history of QT prolongation or patients who are taking medications known to prolong the QT interval).
No products indexed under this heading.

Chlorpromazine Hydrochloride (In a study of the effect of solifenacin on the QT interval in 76 healthy women, the QT prolonging effect appeared less with solifenacin 10 mg than with 30 mg (three times the maximum recommended dose), and the effect of solifenacin 30 mg did not appear as large as that of the positive control moxifloxacin at its therapeutic dose. This observation should be considered in clinical decisions to prescribe solifenacin succinate for patients with a known history of QT prolongation or patients who are taking medications known to prolong the QT interval).
No products indexed under this heading.

Chlorprothixene (In a study of the effect of solifenacin on the QT interval in 76 healthy women, the QT prolonging effect appeared less with solifenacin 10 mg than with 30 mg (three times the maximum recommended dose), and the effect of solifenacin 30 mg did not appear as large as that of the positive control moxifloxacin at its therapeutic dose. This observation should be considered in clinical decisions to prescribe solifenacin succinate for patients with a known history of QT prolongation or patients who are taking medications known to prolong the QT interval).
No products indexed under this heading.

Chlorprothixene Hydrochloride (In a study of the effect of solifenacin on the QT interval in 76 healthy women, the QT prolonging effect appeared less with solifenacin 10 mg than with 30 mg (three times the maximum recommended dose), and the effect of solifenacin 30 mg did not appear as large as that of the positive control moxifloxacin at its therapeutic dose. This observation should be considered in clinical decisions to prescribe solifenacin succinate for patients with a known history of QT prolongation or patients who are taking medications known to prolong the QT interval).
No products indexed under this heading.

Cimetidine (Inhibitors of CYP3A4 may alter solifenacin pharmacokinetics. Following the administration of 10 mg of solifenacin in the presence of 400 mg of ketoconazole, a potent inhibitor of CYP3A4, the mean C_{max} and AUC of solifenacin increased by 1.5 and 2.7-fold, respectively. Therefore, it is recommended not to exceed a 5 mg daily dose of solifenacin when administered with therapeutic doses of ketoconazole or other potent CYP3A4 inhibitors).
No products indexed under this heading.

Cimetidine Hydrochloride (Inhibitors of CYP3A4 may alter solifenacin pharmacokinetics. Following the administration of 10 mg of solifenacin in the presence of 400 mg of ketoconazole, a potent inhibitor of CYP3A4, the mean C_{max} and AUC of solifenacin increased by 1.5 and 2.7-fold, respectively. Therefore, it is recommended not to exceed a 5 mg daily dose of solifenacin when administered with therapeutic doses of ketoconazole or other potent CYP3A4 inhibitors).
No products indexed under this heading.

Ciprofloxacin (Inhibitors of CYP3A4 may alter solifenacin pharmacokinetics. Following the administration of 10 mg of solifenacin in the presence of 400 mg of ketoconazole, a potent inhibitor of CYP3A4, the mean C_{max} and AUC of solifenacin increased by 1.5 and 2.7-fold, respectively. Therefore, it is recommended not to exceed a 5 mg daily dose of solifenacin when administered with therapeutic doses of ketoconazole or other potent CYP3A4 inhibitors). Products include:
Cipro I.V. 3082
Cipro 3073
Cipro XR 3091
Ciprodex 583

Ciprofloxacin Hydrochloride (Inducers of CYP3A4 may alter solifenacin pharmacokinetics). Products include:
Cipro 3073

Cisplatin (Inducers of CYP3A4 may alter solifenacin pharmacokinetics).
No products indexed under this heading.

Clarithromycin (Following the administration of 10 mg of solifenacin in the presence of 400 mg of ketoconazole, a potent inhibitor of CYP3A4, the mean C_{max} and AUC of solifenacin increased by 1.5 and 2.7-fold, respectively. Therefore, it is recommended not to exceed a 5 mg daily dose of solifenacin when administered with therapeutic doses of ketoconazole or other potent CYP3A4 inhibitors). Products include:
Biaxin/Biaxin XL 412

Clomipramine Hydrochloride (In a study of the effect of solifenacin on the QT interval in 76 healthy women, the QT prolonging effect appeared less with solifenacin 10 mg than with 30 mg (three times the maximum recommended dose), and the effect of solifenacin 30 mg did not appear as large as that of the positive control moxifloxacin at its therapeutic dose. This observation should be considered in clinical decisions to prescribe solifenacin succinate for patients with a known history of QT prolongation or patients who are taking medications known to prolong the QT interval).
No products indexed under this heading.

Clorazepate Dipotassium (In a study of the effect of solifenacin on the QT interval in 76 healthy women, the QT prolonging effect appeared less with solifenacin 10 mg than with 30 mg (three times the maximum recommended dose), and the effect of solifenacin 30 mg did not appear as large as that of the positive control moxifloxacin at its therapeutic dose. This observation should be considered in clinical decisions to prescribe solifenacin succinate for patients with a known history of QT prolongation or patients who are taking medications known to prolong the QT interval).
No products indexed under this heading.

Clotrimazole (Inhibitors of CYP3A4 may alter solifenacin pharmacokinetics. Following the administration of 10 mg of solifenacin in the presence of 400 mg of ketoconazole, a potent inhibitor of CYP3A4, the mean C_{max} and AUC of solifenacin increased by 1.5 and 2.7-fold, respectively. Therefore, it is recommended not to exceed a 5 mg daily dose of solifenacin when administered with therapeutic doses of ketoconazole or other potent CYP3A4 inhibitors). Products include:
Lotrisone 3163

Clozapine (In a study of the effect of solifenacin on the QT interval in 76 healthy women, the QT prolonging effect appeared less with solifenacin 10 mg than with 30 mg (three times the maximum recommended dose), and the effect of solifenacin 30 mg did not appear as large as that of the positive control moxifloxacin at its therapeutic dose. This observation should be considered in clinical decisions to prescribe solifenacin succinate for patients with a known history of QT prolongation or patients who are taking medications known to prolong the QT interval).
No products indexed under this heading.

Conivaptan Hydrochloride (Inhibitors of CYP3A4 may alter solifenacin pharmacokinetics. Following the administration of 10 mg of solifenacin in the presence of 400 mg of ketoconazole, a potent inhibitor of CYP3A4, the mean C_{max} and AUC of solifenacin increased by 1.5 and 2.7-fold, respectively. Therefore, it is recommended not to exceed a 5 mg daily dose of solifenacin when administered with therapeutic doses of ketoconazole or other potent CYP3A4 inhibitors). Products include:
Vaprisol 689

Cortisone Acetate (Inducers of CYP3A4 may alter solifenacin pharmacokinetics).
No products indexed under this heading.

Cyclosporine (Inhibitors of CYP3A4 may alter solifenacin pharmacokinetics. Following the administration of 10 mg of solifenacin in the presence of 400 mg of ketoconazole, a potent inhibitor of CYP3A4, the mean C_{max} and AUC of solifenacin increased by 1.5 and 2.7-fold, respectively. Therefore, it is recommended not to exceed a 5 mg daily dose of solifenacin when administered with therapeutic doses of ketoconazole or other potent CYP3A4 inhibitors). Products include:
Gengraf 440
Neoral Oral Solution 2496
Neoral Capsules 2496
Restasis 605

Dalfopristin (Inhibitors of CYP3A4 may alter solifenacin pharmacokinetics. Following the administration of 10 mg of solifenacin in the presence of 400 mg of ketoconazole, a potent inhibitor of CYP3A4, the mean C_{max} and AUC

of solifenacin increased by 1.5 and 2.7-fold, respectively. Therefore, it is recommended not to exceed a 5 mg daily dose of solifenacin when administered with therapeutic doses of ketoconazole or other potent CYP3A4 inhibitors).

No products indexed under this heading.

Danazol (Inhibitors of CYP3A4 may alter solifenacin pharmacokinetics. Following the administration of 10 mg of solifenacin in the presence of 400 mg of ketoconazole, a potent inhibitor of CYP3A4, the mean C_{max} and AUC of solifenacin increased by 1.5 and 2.7-fold, respectively. Therefore, it is recommended not to exceed a 5 mg daily dose of solifenacin when administered with therapeutic doses of ketoconazole or other potent CYP3A4 inhibitors).

No products indexed under this heading.

Darunavir (Inhibitors of CYP3A4 may alter solifenacin pharmacokinetics. Following the administration of 10 mg of solifenacin in the presence of 400 mg of ketoconazole, a potent inhibitor of CYP3A4, the mean C_{max} and AUC of solifenacin increased by 1.5 and 2.7-fold, respectively. Therefore, it is recommended not to exceed a 5 mg daily dose of solifenacin when administered with therapeutic doses of ketoconazole or other potent CYP3A4 inhibitors).

No products indexed under this heading.

Dasatinib (Inhibitors of CYP3A4 may alter solifenacin pharmacokinetics. Following the administration of 10 mg of solifenacin in the presence of 400 mg of ketoconazole, a potent inhibitor of CYP3A4, the mean C_{max} and AUC of solifenacin increased by 1.5 and 2.7-fold, respectively. Therefore, it is recommended not to exceed a 5 mg daily dose of solifenacin when administered with therapeutic doses of ketoconazole or other potent CYP3A4 inhibitors).

No products indexed under this heading.

Delavirdine Mesylate (Following the administration of 10 mg of solifenacin in the presence of 400 mg of ketoconazole, a potent inhibitor of CYP3A4, the mean C_{max} and AUC of solifenacin increased by 1.5 and 2.7-fold, respectively. Therefore, it is recommended not to exceed a 5 mg daily dose of solifenacin when administered with therapeutic doses of ketoconazole or other potent CYP3A4 inhibitors).

No products indexed under this heading.

Delavirine (Following the administration of 10 mg of solifenacin in the presence of 400 mg of ketoconazole, a potent inhibitor of CYP3A4, the mean C_{max} and AUC of solifenacin increased by 1.5 and 2.7-fold, respectively. Therefore, it is recommended not to exceed a 5 mg daily dose of solifenacin when administered with therapeutic doses of ketoconazole or other potent CYP3A4 inhibitors).

No products indexed under this heading.

Desipramine Hydrochloride (In a study of the effect of solifenacin on the QT interval in 76 healthy women, the QT prolonging effect appeared less with solifenacin 10 mg than with 30 mg (three times the maximum recommended dose), and the effect of solifenacin 30 mg did not appear as large as that of the positive control moxifloxacin at its therapeutic dose. This observation should be considered in clinical decisions to prescribe solifenacin succinate for patients with a known history of QT prolongation or patients who are taking medications known to prolong the QT interval).

No products indexed under this heading.

Desloratadine (Inhibitors of CYP3A4 may alter solifenacin pharmacokinetics. Following the administration of 10 mg of solifenacin in the presence of 400 mg of ketoconazole, a potent inhibitor of CYP3A4, the mean C_{max} and AUC of solifenacin increased by 1.5 and 2.7-fold, respectively. Therefore, it is recommended not to exceed a 5 mg daily dose of solifenacin when administered with therapeutic doses of ketoconazole or other potent CYP3A4 inhibitors). Products include:

Clarinex Syrup 3098
Clarinex 3098
Clarinex Reditabs 3098
Clarinex-D 12-Hour 3101
Clarinex-D 3104

Dexamethasone (Inducers of CYP3A4 may alter solifenacin pharmacokinetics). Products include:

Ciprodex 583
Ozurdex .... ⊙ 223
Tobramycin and Dexamethasone Ophthalmic Suspension .... ⊙ 251

Dexamethasone Acetate (Inducers of CYP3A4 may alter solifenacin pharmacokinetics).

No products indexed under this heading.

Dexamethasone Phosphate (Inducers of CYP3A4 may alter solifenacin pharmacokinetics).

No products indexed under this heading.

Dexamethasone Sodium (Inducers of CYP3A4 may alter solifenacin pharmacokinetics).

No products indexed under this heading.

Dexamethasone Sodium Phosphate (Inducers of CYP3A4 may alter solifenacin pharmacokinetics).

No products indexed under this heading.

Dexamethasone Sodium Phosphate Injection (Inducers of CYP3A4 may alter solifenacin pharmacokinetics).

No products indexed under this heading.

Diazepam (In a study of the effect of solifenacin on the QT interval in 76 healthy women, the QT prolonging effect appeared less with solifenacin 10 mg than with 30 mg (three times the maximum recommended dose), and the effect of solifenacin 30 mg did not appear as large as that of the positive control moxifloxacin at its therapeutic dose. This observation should be considered in clinical decisions to prescribe solifenacin succinate for patients with a known history of QT prolongation or patients who are taking medications known to prolong the QT interval). Products include:

Valium Tablets 2880

Diltiazem Hydrochloride (Inhibitors of CYP3A4 may alter solifenacin pharmacokinetics. Following the administration of 10 mg of solifenacin in the presence of 400 mg of ketoconazole, a potent inhibitor of CYP3A4, the mean C_{max} and AUC of solifenacin increased by 1.5 and 2.7-fold, respectively. Therefore, it is recommended not to exceed a 5 mg daily dose of solifenacin when administered with therapeutic doses of ketoconazole or other potent CYP3A4 inhibitors). Products include:

Cardizem LA 423

Diltiazem Maleate (Inhibitors of CYP3A4 may alter solifenacin pharmacokinetics. Following the administration of 10 mg of solifenacin in the presence of 400 mg of ketoconazole, a potent inhibitor of CYP3A4, the mean C_{max} and AUC of solifenacin increased by 1.5 and 2.7-fold, respectively. Therefore, it is recommended not to exceed a 5 mg daily dose of solifenacin when administered with therapeutic doses of ketoconazole or other potent CYP3A4 inhibitors).

No products indexed under this heading.

Disopyramide (In a study of the effect of solifenacin on the QT interval in 76 healthy women, the QT prolonging effect appeared less with solifenacin 10 mg than with 30 mg (three times the maximum recommended dose), and the effect of solifenacin 30 mg did not appear as large as that of the positive control moxifloxacin at its therapeutic dose. This observation should be considered in clinical decisions to prescribe solifenacin succinate for patients with a known history of QT prolongation or patients who are taking medications known to prolong the QT interval).

No products indexed under this heading.

Disopyramide Phosphate (In a study of the effect of solifenacin on the QT interval in 76 healthy women, the QT prolonging effect appeared less with solifenacin 10 mg than with 30 mg (three times the maximum recommended dose), and the effect of solifenacin 30 mg did not appear as large as that of the positive control moxifloxacin at its therapeutic dose. This observation should be considered in clinical decisions to prescribe solifenacin succinate for patients with a known history of QT prolongation or patients who are taking medications known to prolong the QT interval).

No products indexed under this heading.

Dofetilide (In a study of the effect of solifenacin on the QT interval in 76 healthy women, the QT prolonging effect appeared less with solifenacin 10 mg than with 30 mg (three times the maximum recommended dose), and the effect of solifenacin 30 mg did not appear as large as that of the positive control moxifloxacin at its therapeutic dose. This observation should be considered in clinical decisions to prescribe solifenacin succinate for patients with a known history of QT prolongation or patients who are taking medications known to prolong the QT interval).

No products indexed under this heading.

Doxepin Hydrochloride (In a study of the effect of solifenacin on the QT interval in 76 healthy women, the QT prolonging effect appeared less with solifenacin 10 mg than with 30 mg (three times the maximum recommended dose), and the effect of solifenacin 30 mg did not appear as large as that of the positive control moxifloxacin at its therapeutic dose. This observation should be considered in clinical decisions to prescribe solifenacin succinate for patients with a known history of QT prolongation or patients who are taking medications known to prolong the QT interval).

No products indexed under this heading.

Doxorubicin Hydrochloride (Inducers of CYP3A4 may alter solifenacin pharmacokinetics).

No products indexed under this heading.

Droperidol (In a study of the effect of solifenacin on the QT interval in 76 healthy women, the QT prolonging effect appeared less with solifenacin 10 mg than with 30 mg (three times the maximum recommended dose), and the effect of solifenacin 30 mg did not appear as large as that of the positive control moxifloxacin at its therapeutic dose. This observation should be considered in clinical decisions to prescribe solifenacin succinate for patients with a known history of QT prolongation or patients who are taking medications known to prolong the QT interval).

No products indexed under this heading.

Efavirenz (Inhibitors of CYP3A4 may alter solifenacin pharmacokinetics. Following the administration of 10 mg of solifenacin in the presence of 400 mg of ketoconazole, a potent inhibitor of CYP3A4, the mean C_{max} and AUC of solifenacin increased by 1.5 and 2.7-fold, respectively. Therefore, it is recommended not to exceed a 5 mg daily dose of solifenacin when administered with therapeutic doses of ketoconazole or other potent CYP3A4 inhibitors). Products include:

Atripla 906

Erythromycin (In a study of the effect of solifenacin on the QT interval in 76 healthy women, the QT prolonging effect appeared less with solifenacin 10 mg than with 30 mg (three times the maximum recommended dose), and the effect of solifenacin 30 mg did not appear as large as that of the positive control moxifloxacin at its therapeutic dose. This observation should be considered in clinical decisions to prescribe solifenacin succinate for patients with a known history of QT prolongation or patients who are taking medications known to prolong the QT interval).

No products indexed under this heading.

Erythromycin Estolate (In a study of the effect of solifenacin on the QT interval in 76 healthy women, the QT prolonging effect appeared less with solifenacin 10 mg than with 30 mg (three times the maximum recommended dose), and the effect of solifenacin 30 mg did not appear as large as that of the positive control moxifloxacin at its therapeutic dose. This observation should be considered in clinical decisions to prescribe solifenacin succinate for patients with a known history of QT prolongation or patients who are taking medications known to prolong the QT interval).

No products indexed under this heading.

Erythromycin Ethylsuccinate (In a study of the effect of solifenacin on the QT interval in 76 healthy women, the QT prolonging effect appeared less with solifenacin 10 mg than with 30 mg (three times the maximum recommended dose), and the effect of solifenacin 30 mg did not appear as large as that of the positive control moxifloxacin at its therapeutic dose. This observation should be considered in clinical decisions to prescribe solifenacin succinate for patients with a known history of QT prolongation or patients who are taking medications known to prolong the QT interval). Products include:

E.E.S. 437
EryPed 435

Erythromycin Gluceptate (In a study of the effect of solifenacin on the QT interval in 76 healthy women, the QT prolonging effect appeared less with solifenacin 10 mg than with 30 mg (three times the maximum recommended dose), and the effect of solifenacin 30 mg did not appear as large as that of the positive control moxifloxacin at its therapeutic dose. This observation should be considered in clinical decisions to prescribe solifenacin succinate for patients with a known history of QT prolongation or patients who are taking medications known to prolong the QT interval).

No products indexed under this heading.

Erythromycin Lactobionate (In a study of the effect of solifenacin on the QT interval in 76 healthy women, the QT prolonging effect appeared less with solifenacin 10 mg than with 30 mg (three times the maximum recommended dose), and the effect of solifenacin 30 mg did not appear as large as that of the positive control moxifloxacin at its therapeutic dose. This observation should be considered in clinical decisions to prescribe solifenacin succinate for patients with a known history of QT prolongation or patients who are taking medications known to prolong the QT interval).

No products indexed under this heading.

Erythromycin Stearate (In a study of the effect of solifenacin on the QT interval in 76 healthy women, the QT prolonging effect appeared less with solif-

2045 Interactions Index VESIcare

enacin 10 mg than with 30 mg (three times the maximum recommended dose), and the effect of solifenacin 30 mg did not appear as large as that of the positive control moxifloxacin at its therapeutic dose. This observation should be considered in clinical decisions to prescribe solifenacin succinate for patients with a known history of QT prolongation or patients who are taking medications known to prolong the QT interval).
No products indexed under this heading.

Esomeprazole Magnesium (Inhibitors of CYP3A4 may alter solifenacin pharmacokinetics. Following the administration of 10 mg of solifenacin in the presence of 400 mg of ketoconazole, a potent inhibitor of CYP3A4, the mean C_{max} and AUC of solifenacin increased by 1.5 and 2.7-fold, respectively. Therefore, it is recommended not to exceed a 5 mg daily dose of solifenacin when administered with therapeutic doses of ketoconazole or other potent CYP3A4 inhibitors). Products include:
Nexium Capsules 704
Nexium Oral Suspension 704

Esomeprazole Sodium (Inhibitors of CYP3A4 may alter solifenacin pharmacokinetics. Following the administration of 10 mg of solifenacin in the presence of 400 mg of ketoconazole, a potent inhibitor of CYP3A4, the mean C_{max} and AUC of solifenacin increased by 1.5 and 2.7-fold, respectively. Therefore, it is recommended not to exceed a 5 mg daily dose of solifenacin when administered with therapeutic doses of ketoconazole or other potent CYP3A4 inhibitors). Products include:
Nexium I.V. 712

Ethosuximide (Inducers of CYP3A4 may alter solifenacin pharmacokinetics).
No products indexed under this heading.

Felbamate (Inducers of CYP3A4 may alter solifenacin pharmacokinetics).
No products indexed under this heading.

Flecainide Acetate (In a study of the effect of solifenacin on the QT interval in 76 healthy women, the QT prolonging effect appeared less with solifenacin 10 mg than with 30 mg (three times the maximum recommended dose), and the effect of solifenacin 30 mg did not appear as large as that of the positive control moxifloxacin at its therapeutic dose. This observation should be considered in clinical decisions to prescribe solifenacin succinate for patients with a known history of QT prolongation or patients who are taking medications known to prolong the QT interval).
No products indexed under this heading.

Fluconazole (Inhibitors of CYP3A4 may alter solifenacin pharmacokinetics. Following the administration of 10 mg of solifenacin in the presence of 400 mg of ketoconazole, a potent inhibitor of CYP3A4, the mean C_{max} and AUC of solifenacin increased by 1.5 and 2.7-fold, respectively. Therefore, it is recommended not to exceed a 5 mg daily dose of solifenacin when administered with therapeutic doses of ketoconazole or other potent CYP3A4 inhibitors).
No products indexed under this heading.

Fludrocortisone Acetate (Inducers of CYP3A4 may alter solifenacin pharmacokinetics).
No products indexed under this heading.

Fluoxetine (Inhibitors of CYP3A4 may alter solifenacin pharmacokinetics. Following the administration of 10 mg of solifenacin in the presence of 400 mg of ketoconazole, a potent inhibitor of CYP3A4, the mean C_{max} and AUC of solifenacin increased by 1.5 and 2.7-fold, respectively. Therefore, it is recommended not to exceed a 5 mg daily dose of solifenacin when administered with therapeutic doses of ketoconazole or other potent CYP3A4 inhibitors).
No products indexed under this heading.

Fluoxetine Hydrochloride (Inhibitors of CYP3A4 may alter solifenacin pharmacokinetics. Following the administration of 10 mg of solifenacin in the presence of 400 mg of ketoconazole, a potent inhibitor of CYP3A4, the mean C_{max} and AUC of solifenacin increased by 1.5 and 2.7-fold, respectively. Therefore, it is recommended not to exceed a 5 mg daily dose of solifenacin when administered with therapeutic doses of ketoconazole or other potent CYP3A4 inhibitors). Products include:
Prozac Weekly 1941
Prozac Pulvules 1941
Symbyax 1965

Fluphenazine Decanoate (In a study of the effect of solifenacin on the QT interval in 76 healthy women, the QT prolonging effect appeared less with solifenacin 10 mg than with 30 mg (three times the maximum recommended dose), and the effect of solifenacin 30 mg did not appear as large as that of the positive control moxifloxacin at its therapeutic dose. This observation should be considered in clinical decisions to prescribe solifenacin succinate for patients with a known history of QT prolongation or patients who are taking medications known to prolong the QT interval).
No products indexed under this heading.

Fluphenazine Enanthate (In a study of the effect of solifenacin on the QT interval in 76 healthy women, the QT prolonging effect appeared less with solifenacin 10 mg than with 30 mg (three times the maximum recommended dose), and the effect of solifenacin 30 mg did not appear as large as that of the positive control moxifloxacin at its therapeutic dose. This observation should be considered in clinical decisions to prescribe solifenacin succinate for patients with a known history of QT prolongation or patients who are taking medications known to prolong the QT interval).
No products indexed under this heading.

Fluphenazine Hydrochloride (In a study of the effect of solifenacin on the QT interval in 76 healthy women, the QT prolonging effect appeared less with solifenacin 10 mg than with 30 mg (three times the maximum recommended dose), and the effect of solifenacin 30 mg did not appear as large as that of the positive control moxifloxacin at its therapeutic dose. This observation should be considered in clinical decisions to prescribe solifenacin succinate for patients with a known history of QT prolongation or patients who are taking medications known to prolong the QT interval).
No products indexed under this heading.

Fluvoxamine Maleate (Inhibitors of CYP3A4 may alter solifenacin pharmacokinetics. Following the administration of 10 mg of solifenacin in the presence of 400 mg of ketoconazole, a potent inhibitor of CYP3A4, the mean C_{max} and AUC of solifenacin increased by 1.5 and 2.7-fold, respectively. Therefore, it is recommended not to exceed a 5 mg daily dose of solifenacin when administered with therapeutic doses of ketoconazole or other potent CYP3A4 inhibitors).
No products indexed under this heading.

Fosamprenavir Calcium (Following the administration of 10 mg of solifenacin in the presence of 400 mg of ketoconazole, a potent inhibitor of CYP3A4, the mean C_{max} and AUC of solifenacin increased by 1.5 and 2.7-fold, respectively. Therefore, it is recommended not to exceed a 5 mg daily dose of solifenacin when administered with therapeutic doses of ketoconazole or other potent CYP3A4 inhibitors). Products include:
Lexiva Oral Suspension 1558
Lexiva 1558

Fosphenytoin Sodium (Inducers of CYP3A4 may alter solifenacin pharmacokinetics).
No products indexed under this heading.

Garlic Extract (Inducers of CYP3A4 may alter solifenacin pharmacokinetics).
No products indexed under this heading.

Garlic Oil (Inducers of CYP3A4 may alter solifenacin pharmacokinetics).
No products indexed under this heading.

Haloperidol (In a study of the effect of solifenacin on the QT interval in 76 healthy women, the QT prolonging effect appeared less with solifenacin 10 mg than with 30 mg (three times the maximum recommended dose), and the effect of solifenacin 30 mg did not appear as large as that of the positive control moxifloxacin at its therapeutic dose. This observation should be considered in clinical decisions to prescribe solifenacin succinate for patients with a known history of QT prolongation or patients who are taking medications known to prolong the QT interval).
No products indexed under this heading.

Haloperidol Decanoate (In a study of the effect of solifenacin on the QT interval in 76 healthy women, the QT prolonging effect appeared less with solifenacin 10 mg than with 30 mg (three times the maximum recommended dose), and the effect of solifenacin 30 mg did not appear as large as that of the positive control moxifloxacin at its therapeutic dose. This observation should be considered in clinical decisions to prescribe solifenacin succinate for patients with a known history of QT prolongation or patients who are taking medications known to prolong the QT interval).
No products indexed under this heading.

Haloperidol Lactate (In a study of the effect of solifenacin on the QT interval in 76 healthy women, the QT prolonging effect appeared less with solifenacin 10 mg than with 30 mg (three times the maximum recommended dose), and the effect of solifenacin 30 mg did not appear as large as that of the positive control moxifloxacin at its therapeutic dose. This observation should be considered in clinical decisions to prescribe solifenacin succinate for patients with a known history of QT prolongation or patients who are taking medications known to prolong the QT interval).
No products indexed under this heading.

Hydrocortisone (Inducers of CYP3A4 may alter solifenacin pharmacokinetics).
No products indexed under this heading.

Hydrocortisone (Alcohol) (Inducers of CYP3A4 may alter solifenacin pharmacokinetics).
No products indexed under this heading.

Hydrocortisone Acetate (Inducers of CYP3A4 may alter solifenacin pharmacokinetics).
No products indexed under this heading.

Hydrocortisone Butyrate (Inducers of CYP3A4 may alter solifenacin pharmacokinetics).
No products indexed under this heading.

Hydrocortisone Cypionate (Inducers of CYP3A4 may alter solifenacin pharmacokinetics).
No products indexed under this heading.

Hydrocortisone Hemisuccinate (Inducers of CYP3A4 may alter solifenacin pharmacokinetics).
No products indexed under this heading.

Hydrocortisone Probutate (Inducers of CYP3A4 may alter solifenacin pharmacokinetics).
No products indexed under this heading.

Hydrocortisone Sodium Phosphate (Inducers of CYP3A4 may alter solifenacin pharmacokinetics).
No products indexed under this heading.

Hydrocortisone Sodium Succinate (Inducers of CYP3A4 may alter solifenacin pharmacokinetics).
No products indexed under this heading.

Hydrocortisone Valerate (Inducers of CYP3A4 may alter solifenacin pharmacokinetics).
No products indexed under this heading.

Hydroxyzine Hydrochloride (In a study of the effect of solifenacin on the QT interval in 76 healthy women, the QT prolonging effect appeared less with solifenacin 10 mg than with 30 mg (three times the maximum recommended dose), and the effect of solifenacin 30 mg did not appear as large as that of the positive control moxifloxacin at its therapeutic dose. This observation should be considered in clinical decisions to prescribe solifenacin succinate for patients with a known history of QT prolongation or patients who are taking medications known to prolong the QT interval).
No products indexed under this heading.

Hypericum (Inducers of CYP3A4 may alter solifenacin pharmacokinetics).
No products indexed under this heading.

Hypericum Perforatum (Inducers of CYP3A4 may alter solifenacin pharmacokinetics). Products include:
Traumeel 1800

Imatinib Mesylate (Inhibitors of CYP3A4 may alter solifenacin pharmacokinetics. Following the administration of 10 mg of solifenacin in the presence of 400 mg of ketoconazole, a potent inhibitor of CYP3A4, the mean C_{max} and AUC of solifenacin increased by 1.5 and 2.7-fold, respectively. Therefore, it is recommended not to exceed a 5 mg daily dose of solifenacin when administered with therapeutic doses of ketoconazole or other potent CYP3A4 inhibitors). Products include:
Gleevec 2477

Imipramine Hydrochloride (In a study of the effect of solifenacin on the QT interval in 76 healthy women, the QT prolonging effect appeared less with solifenacin 10 mg than with 30 mg (three times the maximum recommended dose), and the effect of solifenacin 30 mg did not appear as large as that of the positive control moxifloxacin at its therapeutic dose. This observation should be considered in clinical decisions to prescribe solifenacin succinate for patients with a known history of QT prolongation or patients who are taking medications known to prolong the QT interval).
No products indexed under this heading.

Imipramine Pamoate (In a study of the effect of solifenacin on the QT interval in 76 healthy women, the QT prolonging effect appeared less with solifenacin 10 mg than with 30 mg (three times the maximum recommended dose), and the effect of solifenacin 30 mg did not appear as large as that of the positive control moxifloxacin at its therapeutic dose. This observation should be considered in clinical decisions to prescribe solifenacin succinate for patients with a known history of QT prolongation or patients who are taking medications known to prolong the QT interval).
No products indexed under this heading.

Indinavir Sulfate (Following the administration of 10 mg of solifenacin in the presence of 400 mg of ketocona-

zole, a potent inhibitor of CYP3A4, the mean C_{max} and AUC of solifenacin increased by 1.5 and 2.7-fold, respectively. Therefore, it is recommended not to exceed a 5 mg daily dose of solifenacin when administered with therapeutic doses of ketoconazole or other potent CYP3A4 inhibitors). Products include:

Crixivan 2113

Isocarboxazid (In a study of the effect of solifenacin on the QT interval in 76 healthy women, the QT prolonging effect appeared less with solifenacin 10 mg than with 30 mg (three times the maximum recommended dose), and the effect of solifenacin 30 mg did not appear as large as that of the positive control moxifloxacin at its therapeutic dose. This observation should be considered in clinical decisions to prescribe solifenacin succinate for patients with a known history of QT prolongation or patients who are taking medications known to prolong the QT interval). Products include:

Marplan 3481

Isoniazid (Inhibitors of CYP3A4 may alter solifenacin pharmacokinetics. Following the administration of 10 mg of solifenacin in the presence of 400 mg of ketoconazole, a potent inhibitor of CYP3A4, the mean C_{max} and AUC of solifenacin increased by 1.5 and 2.7-fold, respectively. Therefore, it is recommended not to exceed a 5 mg daily dose of solifenacin when administered with therapeutic doses of ketoconazole or other potent CYP3A4 inhibitors).

No products indexed under this heading.

Itraconazole (Following the administration of 10 mg of solifenacin in the presence of 400 mg of ketoconazole, a potent inhibitor of CYP3A4, the mean C_{max} and AUC of solifenacin increased by 1.5 and 2.7-fold, respectively. Therefore, it is recommended not to exceed a 5 mg daily dose of solifenacin when administered with therapeutic doses of ketoconazole or other potent CYP3A4 inhibitors).

No products indexed under this heading.

Ketoconazole (Following the administration of 10 mg of solifenacin in the presence of 400 mg of ketoconazole, a potent inhibitor of CYP3A4, the mean C_{max} and AUC of solifenacin increased by 1.5 and 2.7-fold, respectively. Therefore, it is recommended not to exceed a 5 mg daily dose of solifenacin when administered with therapeutic doses of ketoconazole or other potent CYP3A4 inhibitors). Products include:

Extina 3319
Xolegel 3337

Lapatinib (Inhibitors of CYP3A4 may alter solifenacin pharmacokinetics. Following the administration of 10 mg of solifenacin in the presence of 400 mg of ketoconazole, a potent inhibitor of CYP3A4, the mean C_{max} and AUC of solifenacin increased by 1.5 and 2.7-fold, respectively. Therefore, it is recommended not to exceed a 5 mg daily dose of solifenacin when administered with therapeutic doses of ketoconazole or other potent CYP3A4 inhibitors). Products include:

Tykerb 1698

Lidocaine (In a study of the effect of solifenacin on the QT interval in 76 healthy women, the QT prolonging effect appeared less with solifenacin 10 mg than with 30 mg (three times the maximum recommended dose), and the effect of solifenacin 30 mg did not appear as large as that of the positive control moxifloxacin at its therapeutic dose. This observation should be considered in clinical decisions to prescribe solifenacin succinate for patients with a known history of QT prolongation or patients who are taking medications known to prolong the QT interval). Products include:

Lidoderm 1107

Lidocaine Hydrochloride (In a study of the effect of solifenacin on the QT interval in 76 healthy women, the QT prolonging effect appeared less with solifenacin 10 mg than with 30 mg (three times the maximum recommended dose), and the effect of solifenacin 30 mg did not appear as large as that of the positive control moxifloxacin at its therapeutic dose. This observation should be considered in clinical decisions to prescribe solifenacin succinate for patients with a known history of QT prolongation or patients who are taking medications known to prolong the QT interval).

No products indexed under this heading.

Lithium Carbonate (In a study of the effect of solifenacin on the QT interval in 76 healthy women, the QT prolonging effect appeared less with solifenacin 10 mg than with 30 mg (three times the maximum recommended dose), and the effect of solifenacin 30 mg did not appear as large as that of the positive control moxifloxacin at its therapeutic dose. This observation should be considered in clinical decisions to prescribe solifenacin succinate for patients with a known history of QT prolongation or patients who are taking medications known to prolong the QT interval).

No products indexed under this heading.

Lithium Citrate (In a study of the effect of solifenacin on the QT interval in 76 healthy women, the QT prolonging effect appeared less with solifenacin 10 mg than with 30 mg (three times the maximum recommended dose), and the effect of solifenacin 30 mg did not appear as large as that of the positive control moxifloxacin at its therapeutic dose. This observation should be considered in clinical decisions to prescribe solifenacin succinate for patients with a known history of QT prolongation or patients who are taking medications known to prolong the QT interval).

No products indexed under this heading.

Lopinavir (Following the administration of 10 mg of solifenacin in the presence of 400 mg of ketoconazole, a potent inhibitor of CYP3A4, the mean C_{max} and AUC of solifenacin increased by 1.5 and 2.7-fold, respectively. Therefore, it is recommended not to exceed a 5 mg daily dose of solifenacin when administered with therapeutic doses of ketoconazole or other potent CYP3A4 inhibitors). Products include:

Kaletra 458

Loratadine (Inhibitors of CYP3A4 may alter solifenacin pharmacokinetics. Following the administration of 10 mg of solifenacin in the presence of 400 mg of ketoconazole, a potent inhibitor of CYP3A4, the mean C_{max} and AUC of solifenacin increased by 1.5 and 2.7-fold, respectively. Therefore, it is recommended not to exceed a 5 mg daily dose of solifenacin when administered with therapeutic doses of ketoconazole or other potent CYP3A4 inhibitors).

No products indexed under this heading.

Lorazepam (In a study of the effect of solifenacin on the QT interval in 76 healthy women, the QT prolonging effect appeared less with solifenacin 10 mg than with 30 mg (three times the maximum recommended dose), and the effect of solifenacin 30 mg did not appear as large as that of the positive control moxifloxacin at its therapeutic dose. This observation should be considered in clinical decisions to prescribe solifenacin succinate for patients with a known history of QT prolongation or patients who are taking medications known to prolong the QT interval).

No products indexed under this heading.

Loxapine Hydrochloride (In a study of the effect of solifenacin on the QT interval in 76 healthy women, the QT prolonging effect appeared less with solifenacin 10 mg than with 30 mg (three times the maximum recommended dose), and the effect of solifenacin 30 mg did not appear as large as that of the positive control moxifloxacin at its therapeutic dose. This observation should be considered in clinical decisions to prescribe solifenacin succinate for patients with a known history of QT prolongation or patients who are taking medications known to prolong the QT interval).

No products indexed under this heading.

Loxapine Succinate (In a study of the effect of solifenacin on the QT interval in 76 healthy women, the QT prolonging effect appeared less with solifenacin 10 mg than with 30 mg (three times the maximum recommended dose), and the effect of solifenacin 30 mg did not appear as large as that of the positive control moxifloxacin at its therapeutic dose. This observation should be considered in clinical decisions to prescribe solifenacin succinate for patients with a known history of QT prolongation or patients who are taking medications known to prolong the QT interval).

No products indexed under this heading.

Maprotiline Hydrochloride (In a study of the effect of solifenacin on the QT interval in 76 healthy women, the QT prolonging effect appeared less with solifenacin 10 mg than with 30 mg (three times the maximum recommended dose), and the effect of solifenacin 30 mg did not appear as large as that of the positive control moxifloxacin at its therapeutic dose. This observation should be considered in clinical decisions to prescribe solifenacin succinate for patients with a known history of QT prolongation or patients who are taking medications known to prolong the QT interval).

No products indexed under this heading.

Mephenytoin (Inducers of CYP3A4 may alter solifenacin pharmacokinetics).

No products indexed under this heading.

Meprobamate (In a study of the effect of solifenacin on the QT interval in 76 healthy women, the QT prolonging effect appeared less with solifenacin 10 mg than with 30 mg (three times the maximum recommended dose), and the effect of solifenacin 30 mg did not appear as large as that of the positive control moxifloxacin at its therapeutic dose. This observation should be considered in clinical decisions to prescribe solifenacin succinate for patients with a known history of QT prolongation or patients who are taking medications known to prolong the QT interval).

No products indexed under this heading.

Mesoridazine Besylate (In a study of the effect of solifenacin on the QT interval in 76 healthy women, the QT prolonging effect appeared less with solifenacin 10 mg than with 30 mg (three times the maximum recommended dose), and the effect of solifenacin 30 mg did not appear as large as that of the positive control moxifloxacin at its therapeutic dose. This observation should be considered in clinical decisions to prescribe solifenacin succinate for patients with a known history of QT prolongation or patients who are taking medications known to prolong the QT interval).

No products indexed under this heading.

Methsuximide (Inducers of CYP3A4 may alter solifenacin pharmacokinetics).

No products indexed under this heading.

Methylprednisolone (Inducers of CYP3A4 may alter solifenacin pharmacokinetics).

No products indexed under this heading.

Methylprednisolone Acetate (Inducers of CYP3A4 may alter solifenacin pharmacokinetics).

No products indexed under this heading.

Methylprednisolone Sodium Succinate (Inducers of CYP3A4 may alter solifenacin pharmacokinetics).

No products indexed under this heading.

Metronidazole (Inhibitors of CYP3A4 may alter solifenacin pharmacokinetics. Following the administration of 10 mg of solifenacin in the presence of 400 mg of ketoconazole, a potent inhibitor of CYP3A4, the mean C_{max} and AUC of solifenacin increased by 1.5 and 2.7-fold, respectively. Therefore, it is recommended not to exceed a 5 mg daily dose of solifenacin when administered with therapeutic doses of ketoconazole or other potent CYP3A4 inhibitors). Products include:

Pylera 793

Metronidazole Benzoate (Inhibitors of CYP3A4 may alter solifenacin pharmacokinetics. Following the administration of 10 mg of solifenacin in the presence of 400 mg of ketoconazole, a potent inhibitor of CYP3A4, the mean C_{max} and AUC of solifenacin increased by 1.5 and 2.7-fold, respectively. Therefore, it is recommended not to exceed a 5 mg daily dose of solifenacin when administered with therapeutic doses of ketoconazole or other potent CYP3A4 inhibitors).

No products indexed under this heading.

Metronidazole Hydrochloride (Inhibitors of CYP3A4 may alter solifenacin pharmacokinetics. Following the administration of 10 mg of solifenacin in the presence of 400 mg of ketoconazole, a potent inhibitor of CYP3A4, the mean C_{max} and AUC of solifenacin increased by 1.5 and 2.7-fold, respectively. Therefore, it is recommended not to exceed a 5 mg daily dose of solifenacin when administered with therapeutic doses of ketoconazole or other potent CYP3A4 inhibitors).

No products indexed under this heading.

Metronidazole Sodium (Inhibitors of CYP3A4 may alter solifenacin pharmacokinetics. Following the administration of 10 mg of solifenacin in the presence of 400 mg of ketoconazole, a potent inhibitor of CYP3A4, the mean C_{max} and AUC of solifenacin increased by 1.5 and 2.7-fold, respectively. Therefore, it is recommended not to exceed a 5 mg daily dose of solifenacin when administered with therapeutic doses of ketoconazole or other potent CYP3A4 inhibitors).

No products indexed under this heading.

Mexiletine Hydrochloride (In a study of the effect of solifenacin on the QT interval in 76 healthy women, the QT prolonging effect appeared less with solifenacin 10 mg than with 30 mg (three times the maximum recommended dose), and the effect of solifenacin 30 mg did not appear as large as that of the positive control moxifloxacin at its therapeutic dose. This observation should be considered in clinical decisions to prescribe solifenacin succinate for patients with a known history of QT prolongation or patients who are taking medications known to prolong the QT interval).

No products indexed under this heading.

Miconazole (Inhibitors of CYP3A4 may alter solifenacin pharmacokinetics. Following the administration of 10 mg

2047 Interactions Index VESIcare

of solifenacin in the presence of 400 mg of ketoconazole, a potent inhibitor of CYP3A4, the mean C_{max} and AUC of solifenacin increased by 1.5 and 2.7-fold, respectively. Therefore, it is recommended not to exceed a 5 mg daily dose of solifenacin when administered with therapeutic doses of ketoconazole or other potent CYP3A4 inhibitors).
No products indexed under this heading.

Miconazole Nitrate (Inhibitors of CYP3A4 may alter solifenacin pharmacokinetics. Following the administration of 10 mg of solifenacin in the presence of 400 mg of ketoconazole, a potent inhibitor of CYP3A4, the mean C_{max} and AUC of solifenacin increased by 1.5 and 2.7-fold, respectively. Therefore, it is recommended not to exceed a 5 mg daily dose of solifenacin when administered with therapeutic doses of ketoconazole or other potent CYP3A4 inhibitors). Products include:
Vusion Ointment 3335

Midazolam Hydrochloride (In a study of the effect of solifenacin on the QT interval in 76 healthy women, the QT prolonging effect appeared less with solifenacin 10 mg than with 30 mg (three times the maximum recommended dose), and the effect of solifenacin 30 mg did not appear as large as that of the positive control moxifloxacin at its therapeutic dose. This observation should be considered in clinical decisions to prescribe solifenacin succinate for patients with a known history of QT prolongation or patients who are taking medications known to prolong the QT interval).
No products indexed under this heading.

Mifepristone (Inhibitors of CYP3A4 may alter solifenacin pharmacokinetics. Following the administration of 10 mg of solifenacin in the presence of 400 mg of ketoconazole, a potent inhibitor of CYP3A4, the mean C_{max} and AUC of solifenacin increased by 1.5 and 2.7-fold, respectively. Therefore, it is recommended not to exceed a 5 mg daily dose of solifenacin when administered with therapeutic doses of ketoconazole or other potent CYP3A4 inhibitors).
No products indexed under this heading.

Modafinil (Inducers of CYP3A4 may alter solifenacin pharmacokinetics). Products include:
Provigil 983

Molindone Hydrochloride (In a study of the effect of solifenacin on the QT interval in 76 healthy women, the QT prolonging effect appeared less with solifenacin 10 mg than with 30 mg (three times the maximum recommended dose), and the effect of solifenacin 30 mg did not appear as large as that of the positive control moxifloxacin at its therapeutic dose. This observation should be considered in clinical decisions to prescribe solifenacin succinate for patients with a known history of QT prolongation or patients who are taking medications known to prolong the QT interval). Products include:
Moban 1108

Nafcillin Sodium (Inducers of CYP3A4 may alter solifenacin pharmacokinetics).
No products indexed under this heading.

Nefazodone Hydrochloride (Following the administration of 10 mg of solifenacin in the presence of 400 mg of ketoconazole, a potent inhibitor of CYP3A4, the mean C_{max} and AUC of solifenacin increased by 1.5 and 2.7-fold, respectively. Therefore, it is recommended not to exceed a 5 mg daily dose of solifenacin when administered with therapeutic doses of ketoconazole or other potent CYP3A4 inhibitors).
No products indexed under this heading.

Nelfinavir Mesylate (Following the administration of 10 mg of solifenacin in the presence of 400 mg of ketoconazole, a potent inhibitor of CYP3A4, the mean C_{max} and AUC of solifenacin increased by 1.5 and 2.7-fold, respectively. Therefore, it is recommended not to exceed a 5 mg daily dose of solifenacin when administered with therapeutic doses of ketoconazole or other potent CYP3A4 inhibitors).
No products indexed under this heading.

Nevirapine (Inhibitors of CYP3A4 may alter solifenacin pharmacokinetics. Following the administration of 10 mg of solifenacin in the presence of 400 mg of ketoconazole, a potent inhibitor of CYP3A4, the mean C_{max} and AUC of solifenacin increased by 1.5 and 2.7-fold, respectively. Therefore, it is recommended not to exceed a 5 mg daily dose of solifenacin when administered with therapeutic doses of ketoconazole or other potent CYP3A4 inhibitors). Products include:
Viramune Oral Suspension 897
Viramune Tablets 897

Niacin (Inhibitors of CYP3A4 may alter solifenacin pharmacokinetics. Following the administration of 10 mg of solifenacin in the presence of 400 mg of ketoconazole, a potent inhibitor of CYP3A4, the mean C_{max} and AUC of solifenacin increased by 1.5 and 2.7-fold, respectively. Therefore, it is recommended not to exceed a 5 mg daily dose of solifenacin when administered with therapeutic doses of ketoconazole or other potent CYP3A4 inhibitors). Products include:
Advicor 402
Cardio Basics 3455
Niaspan 497
Simcor 524

Niacinamide (Inhibitors of CYP3A4 may alter solifenacin pharmacokinetics. Following the administration of 10 mg of solifenacin in the presence of 400 mg of ketoconazole, a potent inhibitor of CYP3A4, the mean C_{max} and AUC of solifenacin increased by 1.5 and 2.7-fold, respectively. Therefore, it is recommended not to exceed a 5 mg daily dose of solifenacin when administered with therapeutic doses of ketoconazole or other potent CYP3A4 inhibitors). Products include:
CitraNatal 90 DHA Capsules 2332
CitraNatal Assure 2332
CitraNatal Rx 2332
Heplive 607

Niacinamide Hydroiodide (Inhibitors of CYP3A4 may alter solifenacin pharmacokinetics. Following the administration of 10 mg of solifenacin in the presence of 400 mg of ketoconazole, a potent inhibitor of CYP3A4, the mean C_{max} and AUC of solifenacin increased by 1.5 and 2.7-fold, respectively. Therefore, it is recommended not to exceed a 5 mg daily dose of solifenacin when administered with therapeutic doses of ketoconazole or other potent CYP3A4 inhibitors).
No products indexed under this heading.

Nicotinamide (Inhibitors of CYP3A4 may alter solifenacin pharmacokinetics. Following the administration of 10 mg of solifenacin in the presence of 400 mg of ketoconazole, a potent inhibitor of CYP3A4, the mean C_{max} and AUC of solifenacin increased by 1.5 and 2.7-fold, respectively. Therefore, it is recommended not to exceed a 5 mg daily dose of solifenacin when administered with therapeutic doses of ketoconazole or other potent CYP3A4 inhibitors).
No products indexed under this heading.

Nifedipine (Inhibitors of CYP3A4 may alter solifenacin pharmacokinetics. Following the administration of 10 mg of solifenacin in the presence of 400 mg of ketoconazole, a potent inhibitor of CYP3A4, the mean C_{max} and AUC of solifenacin increased by 1.5 and 2.7-fold, respectively. Therefore, it is recommended not to exceed a 5 mg daily dose of solifenacin when administered with therapeutic doses of ketoconazole or other potent CYP3A4 inhibitors).
No products indexed under this heading.

Norfloxacin (Inhibitors of CYP3A4 may alter solifenacin pharmacokinetics. Following the administration of 10 mg of solifenacin in the presence of 400 mg of ketoconazole, a potent inhibitor of CYP3A4, the mean C_{max} and AUC of solifenacin increased by 1.5 and 2.7-fold, respectively. Therefore, it is recommended not to exceed a 5 mg daily dose of solifenacin when administered with therapeutic doses of ketoconazole or other potent CYP3A4 inhibitors). Products include:
Noroxin 2220

Nortriptyline Hydrochloride (In a study of the effect of solifenacin on the QT interval in 76 healthy women, the QT prolonging effect appeared less with solifenacin 10 mg than with 30 mg (three times the maximum recommended dose), and the effect of solifenacin 30 mg did not appear as large as that of the positive control moxifloxacin at its therapeutic dose. This observation should be considered in clinical decisions to prescribe solifenacin succinate for patients with a known history of QT prolongation or patients who are taking medications known to prolong the QT interval).
No products indexed under this heading.

Olanzapine (In a study of the effect of solifenacin on the QT interval in 76 healthy women, the QT prolonging effect appeared less with solifenacin 10 mg than with 30 mg (three times the maximum recommended dose), and the effect of solifenacin 30 mg did not appear as large as that of the positive control moxifloxacin at its therapeutic dose. This observation should be considered in clinical decisions to prescribe solifenacin succinate for patients with a known history of QT prolongation or patients who are taking medications known to prolong the QT interval). Products include:
Symbyax 1965
Zyprexa 1984
Zyprexa IntraMuscular 1984
Zyprexa ZYDIS 1984

Omeprazole (Inhibitors of CYP3A4 may alter solifenacin pharmacokinetics. Following the administration of 10 mg of solifenacin in the presence of 400 mg of ketoconazole, a potent inhibitor of CYP3A4, the mean C_{max} and AUC of solifenacin increased by 1.5 and 2.7-fold, respectively. Therefore, it is recommended not to exceed a 5 mg daily dose of solifenacin when administered with therapeutic doses of ketoconazole or other potent CYP3A4 inhibitors).
No products indexed under this heading.

Oxazepam (In a study of the effect of solifenacin on the QT interval in 76 healthy women, the QT prolonging effect appeared less with solifenacin 10 mg than with 30 mg (three times the maximum recommended dose), and the effect of solifenacin 30 mg did not appear as large as that of the positive control moxifloxacin at its therapeutic dose. This observation should be considered in clinical decisions to prescribe solifenacin succinate for patients with a known history of QT prolongation or patients who are taking medications known to prolong the QT interval).
No products indexed under this heading.

Oxcarbazepine (Inducers of CYP3A4 may alter solifenacin pharmacokinetics).
No products indexed under this heading.

Paroxetine Hydrochloride (Inhibitors of CYP3A4 may alter solifenacin pharmacokinetics. Following the administration of 10 mg of solifenacin in the presence of 400 mg of ketoconazole, a potent inhibitor of CYP3A4, the mean C_{max} and AUC of solifenacin increased by 1.5 and 2.7-fold, respectively. Therefore, it is recommended not to exceed a 5 mg daily dose of solifenacin when administered with therapeutic doses of ketoconazole or other potent CYP3A4 inhibitors). Products include:
Paroxetine CR 2361
Paroxetine ER 2371
Paxil 1586
Paxil CR 1596

Perphenazine (In a study of the effect of solifenacin on the QT interval in 76 healthy women, the QT prolonging effect appeared less with solifenacin 10 mg than with 30 mg (three times the maximum recommended dose), and the effect of solifenacin 30 mg did not appear as large as that of the positive control moxifloxacin at its therapeutic dose. This observation should be considered in clinical decisions to prescribe solifenacin succinate for patients with a known history of QT prolongation or patients who are taking medications known to prolong the QT interval).
No products indexed under this heading.

Phenelzine Sulfate (In a study of the effect of solifenacin on the QT interval in 76 healthy women, the QT prolonging effect appeared less with solifenacin 10 mg than with 30 mg (three times the maximum recommended dose), and the effect of solifenacin 30 mg did not appear as large as that of the positive control moxifloxacin at its therapeutic dose. This observation should be considered in clinical decisions to prescribe solifenacin succinate for patients with a known history of QT prolongation or patients who are taking medications known to prolong the QT interval).
No products indexed under this heading.

Phenobarbital (Inducers of CYP3A4 may alter solifenacin pharmacokinetics). Products include:
Donnatal 2711

Phenobarbital Sodium (Inducers of CYP3A4 may alter solifenacin pharmacokinetics).
No products indexed under this heading.

Phenytoin (Inducers of CYP3A4 may alter solifenacin pharmacokinetics).
No products indexed under this heading.

Phenytoin Sodium (Inducers of CYP3A4 may alter solifenacin pharmacokinetics). Products include:
Phenytek Capsules 2380

Posaconazole (Inhibitors of CYP3A4 may alter solifenacin pharmacokinetics. Following the administration of 10 mg of solifenacin in the presence of 400 mg of ketoconazole, a potent inhibitor of CYP3A4, the mean C_{max} and AUC of solifenacin increased by 1.5 and 2.7-fold, respectively. Therefore, it is recommended not to exceed a 5 mg daily dose of solifenacin when administered with therapeutic doses of ketoconazole or other potent CYP3A4 inhibitors). Products include:
Noxafil 3172

Prazepam (In a study of the effect of solifenacin on the QT interval in 76 healthy women, the QT prolonging effect appeared less with solifenacin 10 mg than with 30 mg (three times the maximum recommended dose), and the

IMPORTANT NOTE: Always consult each drug listing in the patient's regimen for possible interactions.

effect of solifenacin 30 mg did not appear as large as that of the positive control moxifloxacin at its therapeutic dose. This observation should be considered in clinical decisions to prescribe solifenacin succinate for patients with a known history of QT prolongation or patients who are taking medications known to prolong the QT interval).

No products indexed under this heading.

Prednisolone (Inducers of CYP3A4 may alter solifenacin pharmacokinetics).

No products indexed under this heading.

Prednisolone Acetate (Inducers of CYP3A4 may alter solifenacin pharmacokinetics). Products include:

Blephamide .... ⊙**212,** ⊙**214**
Pred Forte .... ⊙**225**
Pred Mild .... ⊙**230**
Pred-G .... ⊙**226,** ⊙**227**

Prednisolone Sodium Phosphate (Inducers of CYP3A4 may alter solifenacin pharmacokinetics).

No products indexed under this heading.

Prednisolone Tebutate (Inducers of CYP3A4 may alter solifenacin pharmacokinetics).

No products indexed under this heading.

Prednisone (Inducers of CYP3A4 may alter solifenacin pharmacokinetics).

No products indexed under this heading.

Prednisone sodium phosphate (Inducers of CYP3A4 may alter solifenacin pharmacokinetics).

No products indexed under this heading.

Primidone (Inducers of CYP3A4 may alter solifenacin pharmacokinetics).

No products indexed under this heading.

Procainamide Hydrochloride (In a study of the effect of solifenacin on the QT interval in 76 healthy women, the QT prolonging effect appeared less with solifenacin 10 mg than with 30 mg (three times the maximum recommended dose), and the effect of solifenacin 30 mg did not appear as large as that of the positive control moxifloxacin at its therapeutic dose. This observation should be considered in clinical decisions to prescribe solifenacin succinate for patients with a known history of QT prolongation or patients who are taking medications known to prolong the QT interval).

No products indexed under this heading.

Prochlorperazine (In a study of the effect of solifenacin on the QT interval in 76 healthy women, the QT prolonging effect appeared less with solifenacin 10 mg than with 30 mg (three times the maximum recommended dose), and the effect of solifenacin 30 mg did not appear as large as that of the positive control moxifloxacin at its therapeutic dose. This observation should be considered in clinical decisions to prescribe solifenacin succinate for patients with a known history of QT prolongation or patients who are taking medications known to prolong the QT interval).

No products indexed under this heading.

Promethazine Hydrochloride (In a study of the effect of solifenacin on the QT interval in 76 healthy women, the QT prolonging effect appeared less with solifenacin 10 mg than with 30 mg (three times the maximum recommended dose), and the effect of solifenacin 30 mg did not appear as large as that of the positive control moxifloxacin at its therapeutic dose. This observation should be considered in clinical decisions to prescribe solifenacin succinate for patients with a known history of QT prolongation or patients who are taking medications known to prolong the QT interval).

No products indexed under this heading.

Propafenone Hydrochloride (In a study of the effect of solifenacin on the

QT interval in 76 healthy women, the QT prolonging effect appeared less with solifenacin 10 mg than with 30 mg (three times the maximum recommended dose), and the effect of solifenacin 30 mg did not appear as large as that of the positive control moxifloxacin at its therapeutic dose. This observation should be considered in clinical decisions to prescribe solifenacin succinate for patients with a known history of QT prolongation or patients who are taking medications known to prolong the QT interval). Products include:

Rythmol **1648**
Rythmol SR **1652**

Propoxyphene Hydrochloride (Inhibitors of CYP3A4 may alter solifenacin pharmacokinetics. Following the administration of 10 mg of solifenacin in the presence of 400 mg of ketoconazole, a potent inhibitor of CYP3A4, the mean C_{max} and AUC of solifenacin increased by 1.5 and 2.7-fold, respectively. Therefore, it is recommended not to exceed a 5 mg daily dose of solifenacin when administered with therapeutic doses of ketoconazole or other potent CYP3A4 inhibitors).

No products indexed under this heading.

Propoxyphene Napsylate (Inhibitors of CYP3A4 may alter solifenacin pharmacokinetics. Following the administration of 10 mg of solifenacin in the presence of 400 mg of ketoconazole, a potent inhibitor of CYP3A4, the mean C_{max} and AUC of solifenacin increased by 1.5 and 2.7-fold, respectively. Therefore, it is recommended not to exceed a 5 mg daily dose of solifenacin when administered with therapeutic doses of ketoconazole or other potent CYP3A4 inhibitors).

No products indexed under this heading.

Protriptyline Hydrochloride (In a study of the effect of solifenacin on the QT interval in 76 healthy women, the QT prolonging effect appeared less with solifenacin 10 mg than with 30 mg (three times the maximum recommended dose), and the effect of solifenacin 30 mg did not appear as large as that of the positive control moxifloxacin at its therapeutic dose. This observation should be considered in clinical decisions to prescribe solifenacin succinate for patients with a known history of QT prolongation or patients who are taking medications known to prolong the QT interval).

No products indexed under this heading.

Quetiapine Fumarate (In a study of the effect of solifenacin on the QT interval in 76 healthy women, the QT prolonging effect appeared less with solifenacin 10 mg than with 30 mg (three times the maximum recommended dose), and the effect of solifenacin 30 mg did not appear as large as that of the positive control moxifloxacin at its therapeutic dose. This observation should be considered in clinical decisions to prescribe solifenacin succinate for patients with a known history of QT prolongation or patients who are taking medications known to prolong the QT interval). Products include:

Seroquel **750**
Seroquel XR **759**

Quinidine (In a study of the effect of solifenacin on the QT interval in 76 healthy women, the QT prolonging effect appeared less with solifenacin 10 mg than with 30 mg (three times the maximum recommended dose), and the effect of solifenacin 30 mg did not appear as large as that of the positive control moxifloxacin at its therapeutic dose. This observation should be considered in clinical decisions to prescribe solifenacin succinate for patients with a

known history of QT prolongation or patients who are taking medications known to prolong the QT interval).

No products indexed under this heading.

Quinidine Gluconate (In a study of the effect of solifenacin on the QT interval in 76 healthy women, the QT prolonging effect appeared less with solifenacin 10 mg than with 30 mg (three times the maximum recommended dose), and the effect of solifenacin 30 mg did not appear as large as that of the positive control moxifloxacin at its therapeutic dose. This observation should be considered in clinical decisions to prescribe solifenacin succinate for patients with a known history of QT prolongation or patients who are taking medications known to prolong the QT interval).

No products indexed under this heading.

Quinidine Hydrochloride (In a study of the effect of solifenacin on the QT interval in 76 healthy women, the QT prolonging effect appeared less with solifenacin 10 mg than with 30 mg (three times the maximum recommended dose), and the effect of solifenacin 30 mg did not appear as large as that of the positive control moxifloxacin at its therapeutic dose. This observation should be considered in clinical decisions to prescribe solifenacin succinate for patients with a known history of QT prolongation or patients who are taking medications known to prolong the QT interval).

No products indexed under this heading.

Quinidine Polygalacturonate (In a study of the effect of solifenacin on the QT interval in 76 healthy women, the QT prolonging effect appeared less with solifenacin 10 mg than with 30 mg (three times the maximum recommended dose), and the effect of solifenacin 30 mg did not appear as large as that of the positive control moxifloxacin at its therapeutic dose. This observation should be considered in clinical decisions to prescribe solifenacin succinate for patients with a known history of QT prolongation or patients who are taking medications known to prolong the QT interval).

No products indexed under this heading.

Quinidine Sulfate (In a study of the effect of solifenacin on the QT interval in 76 healthy women, the QT prolonging effect appeared less with solifenacin 10 mg than with 30 mg (three times the maximum recommended dose), and the effect of solifenacin 30 mg did not appear as large as that of the positive control moxifloxacin at its therapeutic dose. This observation should be considered in clinical decisions to prescribe solifenacin succinate for patients with a known history of QT prolongation or patients who are taking medications known to prolong the QT interval).

No products indexed under this heading.

Quinine (Inhibitors of CYP3A4 may alter solifenacin pharmacokinetics. Following the administration of 10 mg of solifenacin in the presence of 400 mg of ketoconazole, a potent inhibitor of CYP3A4, the mean C_{max} and AUC of solifenacin increased by 1.5 and 2.7-fold, respectively. Therefore, it is recommended not to exceed a 5 mg daily dose of solifenacin when administered with therapeutic doses of ketoconazole or other potent CYP3A4 inhibitors). Products include:

Hyland's Leg Cramps PM with
  Quinine **3315**

Quinine Sulfate (Inhibitors of CYP3A4 may alter solifenacin pharmacokinetics. Following the administration of 10 mg of solifenacin in the presence of 400 mg of ketoconazole, a potent inhibitor of CYP3A4, the mean C_{max} and AUC of solifenacin increased by 1.5 and

2.7-fold, respectively. Therefore, it is recommended not to exceed a 5 mg daily dose of solifenacin when administered with therapeutic doses of ketoconazole or other potent CYP3A4 inhibitors).

No products indexed under this heading.

Quinupristin (Inhibitors of CYP3A4 may alter solifenacin pharmacokinetics. Following the administration of 10 mg of solifenacin in the presence of 400 mg of ketoconazole, a potent inhibitor of CYP3A4, the mean C_{max} and AUC of solifenacin increased by 1.5 and 2.7-fold, respectively. Therefore, it is recommended not to exceed a 5 mg daily dose of solifenacin when administered with therapeutic doses of ketoconazole or other potent CYP3A4 inhibitors).

No products indexed under this heading.

Ranitidine Bismuth Citrate (Inhibitors of CYP3A4 may alter solifenacin pharmacokinetics. Following the administration of 10 mg of solifenacin in the presence of 400 mg of ketoconazole, a potent inhibitor of CYP3A4, the mean C_{max} and AUC of solifenacin increased by 1.5 and 2.7-fold, respectively. Therefore, it is recommended not to exceed a 5 mg daily dose of solifenacin when administered with therapeutic doses of ketoconazole or other potent CYP3A4 inhibitors).

No products indexed under this heading.

Ranitidine Hydrochloride (Inhibitors of CYP3A4 may alter solifenacin pharmacokinetics. Following the administration of 10 mg of solifenacin in the presence of 400 mg of ketoconazole, a potent inhibitor of CYP3A4, the mean C_{max} and AUC of solifenacin increased by 1.5 and 2.7-fold, respectively. Therefore, it is recommended not to exceed a 5 mg daily dose of solifenacin when administered with therapeutic doses of ketoconazole or other potent CYP3A4 inhibitors). Products include:

Zantac **1737**
Zantac Injection **1732**
Zantac Pharmacy **1735**

Rifabutin (Inducers of CYP3A4 may alter solifenacin pharmacokinetics).
No products indexed under this heading.

Rifampicin (Inducers of CYP3A4 may alter solifenacin pharmacokinetics).
No products indexed under this heading.

Rifampin (Inducers of CYP3A4 may alter solifenacin pharmacokinetics).
No products indexed under this heading.

Rifapentine (Inducers of CYP3A4 may alter solifenacin pharmacokinetics).
No products indexed under this heading.

Risperidone (In a study of the effect of solifenacin on the QT interval in 76 healthy women, the QT prolonging effect appeared less with solifenacin 10 mg than with 30 mg (three times the maximum recommended dose), and the effect of solifenacin 30 mg did not appear as large as that of the positive control moxifloxacin at its therapeutic dose. This observation should be considered in clinical decisions to prescribe solifenacin succinate for patients with a known history of QT prolongation or patients who are taking medications known to prolong the QT interval). Products include:

Risperdal Consta **2682**

Ritonavir (Following the administration of 10 mg of solifenacin in the presence of 400 mg of ketoconazole, a potent inhibitor of CYP3A4, the mean C_{max} and AUC of solifenacin increased by 1.5 and 2.7-fold, respectively. Therefore, it is recommended not to exceed a 5 mg daily dose of solifenacin when administered with therapeutic doses of ketoconazole or other potent CYP3A4 inhibitors). Products include:

Kaletra 458
Norvir 509

Saquinavir (Following the administration of 10 mg of solifenacin in the presence of 400 mg of ketoconazole, a potent inhibitor of CYP3A4, the mean C_{max} and AUC of solifenacin increased by 1.5 and 2.7-fold, respectively. Therefore, it is recommended not to exceed a 5 mg daily dose of solifenacin when administered with therapeutic doses of ketoconazole or other potent CYP3A4 inhibitors).
No products indexed under this heading.

Saquinavir Mesylate (Following the administration of 10 mg of solifenacin in the presence of 400 mg of ketoconazole, a potent inhibitor of CYP3A4, the mean C_{max} and AUC of solifenacin increased by 1.5 and 2.7-fold, respectively. Therefore, it is recommended not to exceed a 5 mg daily dose of solifenacin when administered with therapeutic doses of ketoconazole or other potent CYP3A4 inhibitors).
No products indexed under this heading.

Sertraline Hydrochloride (Inhibitors of CYP3A4 may alter solifenacin pharmacokinetics. Following the administration of 10 mg of solifenacin in the presence of 400 mg of ketoconazole, a potent inhibitor of CYP3A4, the mean C_{max} and AUC of solifenacin increased by 1.5 and 2.7-fold, respectively. Therefore, it is recommended not to exceed a 5 mg daily dose of solifenacin when administered with therapeutic doses of ketoconazole or other potent CYP3A4 inhibitors).
No products indexed under this heading.

Sildenafil Citrate (Inhibitors of CYP3A4 may alter solifenacin pharmacokinetics. Following the administration of 10 mg of solifenacin in the presence of 400 mg of ketoconazole, a potent inhibitor of CYP3A4, the mean C_{max} and AUC of solifenacin increased by 1.5 and 2.7-fold, respectively. Therefore, it is recommended not to exceed a 5 mg daily dose of solifenacin when administered with therapeutic doses of ketoconazole or other potent CYP3A4 inhibitors).
No products indexed under this heading.

Sulfinpyrazone (Inducers of CYP3A4 may alter solifenacin pharmacokinetics).
No products indexed under this heading.

Telithromycin (Following the administration of 10 mg of solifenacin in the presence of 400 mg of ketoconazole, a potent inhibitor of CYP3A4, the mean C_{max} and AUC of solifenacin increased by 1.5 and 2.7-fold, respectively. Therefore, it is recommended not to exceed a 5 mg daily dose of solifenacin when administered with therapeutic doses of ketoconazole or other potent CYP3A4 inhibitors). Products include:
Ketek 2991

Theophyllinate (Inducers of CYP3A4 may alter solifenacin pharmacokinetics).
No products indexed under this heading.

Theophylline (Inducers of CYP3A4 may alter solifenacin pharmacokinetics).
No products indexed under this heading.

Theophylline Anhydrous (Inducers of CYP3A4 may alter solifenacin pharmacokinetics). Products include:
Uniphyl 2817

Theophylline Calcium Salicylate (Inducers of CYP3A4 may alter solifenacin pharmacokinetics).
No products indexed under this heading.

Theophylline Dihydroxypropyl (Glyceryl) (Inducers of CYP3A4 may alter solifenacin pharmacokinetics).
No products indexed under this heading.

Theophylline Ethylenediamine (Inducers of CYP3A4 may alter solifenacin pharmacokinetics).
No products indexed under this heading.

Theophylline Sodium Glycinate (Inducers of CYP3A4 may alter solifenacin pharmacokinetics).
No products indexed under this heading.

Thioridazine Hydrochloride (In a study of the effect of solifenacin on the QT interval in 76 healthy women, the QT prolonging effect appeared less with solifenacin 10 mg than with 30 mg (three times the maximum recommended dose), and the effect of solifenacin 30 mg did not appear as large as that of the positive control moxifloxacin at its therapeutic dose. This observation should be considered in clinical decisions to prescribe solifenacin succinate for patients with a known history of QT prolongation or patients who are taking medications known to prolong the QT interval). Products include:
Thioridazine Hydrochloride 2384

Thiothixene (In a study of the effect of solifenacin on the QT interval in 76 healthy women, the QT prolonging effect appeared less with solifenacin 10 mg than with 30 mg (three times the maximum recommended dose), and the effect of solifenacin 30 mg did not appear as large as that of the positive control moxifloxacin at its therapeutic dose. This observation should be considered in clinical decisions to prescribe solifenacin succinate for patients with a known history of QT prolongation or patients who are taking medications known to prolong the QT interval). Products include:
Thiothixene 2386

Tocainide Hydrochloride (In a study of the effect of solifenacin on the QT interval in 76 healthy women, the QT prolonging effect appeared less with solifenacin 10 mg than with 30 mg (three times the maximum recommended dose), and the effect of solifenacin 30 mg did not appear as large as that of the positive control moxifloxacin at its therapeutic dose. This observation should be considered in clinical decisions to prescribe solifenacin succinate for patients with a known history of QT prolongation or patients who are taking medications known to prolong the QT interval).
No products indexed under this heading.

Tranylcypromine Sulfate (In a study of the effect of solifenacin on the QT interval in 76 healthy women, the QT prolonging effect appeared less with solifenacin 10 mg than with 30 mg (three times the maximum recommended dose), and the effect of solifenacin 30 mg did not appear as large as that of the positive control moxifloxacin at its therapeutic dose. This observation should be considered in clinical decisions to prescribe solifenacin succinate for patients with a known history of QT prolongation or patients who are taking medications known to prolong the QT interval). Products include:
Parnate 1584

Triamcinolone (Inducers of CYP3A4 may alter solifenacin pharmacokinetics).
No products indexed under this heading.

Triamcinolone Acetonide (Inducers of CYP3A4 may alter solifenacin pharmacokinetics). Products include:
Azmacort 408
Nasacort AQ 3019

Triamcinolone Diacetate (Inducers of CYP3A4 may alter solifenacin pharmacokinetics).
No products indexed under this heading.

Triamcinolone Hexacetonide (Inducers of CYP3A4 may alter solifenacin pharmacokinetics).
No products indexed under this heading.

Trifluoperazine Hydrochloride (In a study of the effect of solifenacin on the QT interval in 76 healthy women, the QT prolonging effect appeared less with solifenacin 10 mg than with 30 mg (three times the maximum recommended dose), and the effect of solifenacin 30 mg did not appear as large as that of the positive control moxifloxacin at its therapeutic dose. This observation should be considered in clinical decisions to prescribe solifenacin succinate for patients with a known history of QT prolongation or patients who are taking medications known to prolong the QT interval).
No products indexed under this heading.

Trimipramine Maleate (In a study of the effect of solifenacin on the QT interval in 76 healthy women, the QT prolonging effect appeared less with solifenacin 10 mg than with 30 mg (three times the maximum recommended dose), and the effect of solifenacin 30 mg did not appear as large as that of the positive control moxifloxacin at its therapeutic dose. This observation should be considered in clinical decisions to prescribe solifenacin succinate for patients with a known history of QT prolongation or patients who are taking medications known to prolong the QT interval).
No products indexed under this heading.

Troglitazone (Inhibitors of CYP3A4 may alter solifenacin pharmacokinetics. Following the administration of 10 mg of solifenacin in the presence of 400 mg of ketoconazole, a potent inhibitor of CYP3A4, the mean C_{max} and AUC of solifenacin increased by 1.5 and 2.7-fold, respectively. Therefore, it is recommended not to exceed a 5 mg daily dose of solifenacin when administered with therapeutic doses of ketoconazole or other potent CYP3A4 inhibitors).
No products indexed under this heading.

Troleandomycin (Following the administration of 10 mg of solifenacin in the presence of 400 mg of ketoconazole, a potent inhibitor of CYP3A4, the mean C_{max} and AUC of solifenacin increased by 1.5 and 2.7-fold, respectively. Therefore, it is recommended not to exceed a 5 mg daily dose of solifenacin when administered with therapeutic doses of ketoconazole or other potent CYP3A4 inhibitors).
No products indexed under this heading.

Valproate Sodium (Inhibitors of CYP3A4 may alter solifenacin pharmacokinetics. Following the administration of 10 mg of solifenacin in the presence of 400 mg of ketoconazole, a potent inhibitor of CYP3A4, the mean C_{max} and AUC of solifenacin increased by 1.5 and 2.7-fold, respectively. Therefore, it is recommended not to exceed a 5 mg daily dose of solifenacin when administered with therapeutic doses of ketoconazole or other potent CYP3A4 inhibitors).
No products indexed under this heading.

Vardenafil Hydrochloride (Inhibitors of CYP3A4 may alter solifenacin pharmacokinetics. Following the administration of 10 mg of solifenacin in the presence of 400 mg of ketoconazole, a potent inhibitor of CYP3A4, the mean C_{max} and AUC of solifenacin increased by 1.5 and 2.7-fold, respectively. Therefore, it is recommended not to exceed a 5 mg daily dose of solifenacin when administered with therapeutic doses of ketoconazole or other potent CYP3A4 inhibitors). Products include:
Levitra 3157

Verapamil Hydrochloride (Inhibitors of CYP3A4 may alter solifenacin pharmacokinetics. Following the administration of 10 mg of solifenacin in the presence of 400 mg of ketoconazole, a potent inhibitor of CYP3A4, the mean C_{max} and AUC of solifenacin increased by 1.5 and 2.7-fold, respectively. Therefore, it is recommended not to exceed a 5 mg daily dose of solifenacin when administered with therapeutic doses of ketoconazole or other potent CYP3A4 inhibitors). Products include:
Tarka 534

Voriconazole (Following the administration of 10 mg of solifenacin in the presence of 400 mg of ketoconazole, a potent inhibitor of CYP3A4, the mean C_{max} and AUC of solifenacin increased by 1.5 and 2.7-fold, respectively. Therefore, it is recommended not to exceed a 5 mg daily dose of solifenacin when administered with therapeutic doses of ketoconazole or other potent CYP3A4 inhibitors).
No products indexed under this heading.

Zafirlukast (Inhibitors of CYP3A4 may alter solifenacin pharmacokinetics. Following the administration of 10 mg of solifenacin in the presence of 400 mg of ketoconazole, a potent inhibitor of CYP3A4, the mean C_{max} and AUC of solifenacin increased by 1.5 and 2.7-fold, respectively. Therefore, it is recommended not to exceed a 5 mg daily dose of solifenacin when administered with therapeutic doses of ketoconazole or other potent CYP3A4 inhibitors). Products include:
Accolate 3612

Zileuton (Inhibitors of CYP3A4 may alter solifenacin pharmacokinetics. Following the administration of 10 mg of solifenacin in the presence of 400 mg of ketoconazole, a potent inhibitor of CYP3A4, the mean C_{max} and AUC of solifenacin increased by 1.5 and 2.7-fold, respectively. Therefore, it is recommended not to exceed a 5 mg daily dose of solifenacin when administered with therapeutic doses of ketoconazole or other potent CYP3A4 inhibitors).
No products indexed under this heading.

Ziprasidone Hydrochloride (In a study of the effect of solifenacin on the QT interval in 76 healthy women, the QT prolonging effect appeared less with solifenacin 10 mg than with 30 mg (three times the maximum recommended dose), and the effect of solifenacin 30 mg did not appear as large as that of the positive control moxifloxacin at its therapeutic dose. This observation should be considered in clinical decisions to prescribe solifenacin succinate for patients with a known history of QT prolongation or patients who are taking medications known to prolong the QT interval). Products include:
Geodon 2723

Food Interactions

Grapefruit (Inhibitors of CYP3A4 may alter solifenacin pharmacokinetics. Following the administration of 10 mg of solifenacin in the presence of 400 mg of ketoconazole, a potent inhibitor of CYP3A4, the mean C_{max} and AUC of solifenacin increased by 1.5 and 2.7-fold, respectively. Therefore, it is recommended not to exceed a 5 mg daily dose of solifenacin when administered with therapeutic doses of ketoconazole or other potent CYP3A4 inhibitors).

Grapefruit Juice (Inhibitors of CYP3A4 may alter solifenacin pharmacokinetics. Following the administration of 10 mg of solifenacin in the presence of 400 mg of ketoconazole, a potent inhibitor of CYP3A4, the mean C_{max} and AUC of

solifenacin increased by 1.5 and 2.7-fold, respectively. Therefore, it is recommended not to exceed a 5 mg daily dose of solifenacin when administered with therapeutic doses of ketoconazole or other potent CYP3A4 inhibitors).

VICODIN TABLETS

(Acetaminophen, Hydrocodone Bitartrate) 560
May interact with alcohols, antihistamines, antipsychotic agents, central nervous system depressants, monoamine oxidase inhibitors, narcotic analgesics, tricyclic antidepressants. Compounds in these categories include:

Acrivastine (May exhibit an additive CNS depression).
No products indexed under this heading.

Alfentanil Hydrochloride (May exhibit an additive CNS depression).
No products indexed under this heading.

Alprazolam (May exhibit an additive CNS depression).
No products indexed under this heading.

Amitriptyline Hydrochloride (Co-administration may increase the effect of either antidepressant or hydrocodone).
No products indexed under this heading.

Amobarbital (May exhibit an additive CNS depression).
No products indexed under this heading.

Amobarbital Sodium (May exhibit an additive CNS depression).
No products indexed under this heading.

Amoxapine (Co-administration may increase the effect of either antidepressant or hydrocodone).
No products indexed under this heading.

Apomorphine (May exhibit an additive CNS depression).
No products indexed under this heading.

Apomorphine Hydrochloride (May exhibit an additive CNS depression).
No products indexed under this heading.

Aprobarbital (May exhibit an additive CNS depression).
No products indexed under this heading.

Aripiprazole (May exhibit an additive CNS depression).
No products indexed under this heading.

Astemizole (May exhibit an additive CNS depression).
No products indexed under this heading.

Azatadine Maleate (May exhibit an additive CNS depression).
No products indexed under this heading.

Bromodiphenhydramine Hydrochloride (May exhibit an additive CNS depression).
No products indexed under this heading.

Brompheniramine Maleate (May exhibit an additive CNS depression).
No products indexed under this heading.

Buprenorphine Hydrochloride (May exhibit an additive CNS depression).
No products indexed under this heading.

Buspirone Hydrochloride (May exhibit an additive CNS depression).
No products indexed under this heading.

Butabarbital (May exhibit an additive CNS depression).
No products indexed under this heading.

Butabarbital Sodium (May exhibit an additive CNS depression).
No products indexed under this heading.

Butalbital (May exhibit an additive CNS depression).
No products indexed under this heading.

Cetirizine Hydrochloride (May exhibit an additive CNS depression). Products include:
Zyrtec Allergy 2052

Children's Zyrtec Allergy Syrup 2053
Children's Zyrtec Allergy 2053
Children's Zyrtec Hives Relief 2053
Zyrtec-D Allergy & Congestion 2054

Chlordiazepoxide (May exhibit an additive CNS depression).
No products indexed under this heading.

Chlordiazepoxide Hydrochloride (May exhibit an additive CNS depression).
No products indexed under this heading.

Chlorpheniramine Maleate (May exhibit an additive CNS depression).
No products indexed under this heading.

Chlorpheniramine Polistirex (May exhibit an additive CNS depression). Products include:
Tussionex 3443

Chlorpheniramine Tannate (May exhibit an additive CNS depression).
No products indexed under this heading.

Chlorpromazine (May exhibit an additive CNS depression).
No products indexed under this heading.

Chlorpromazine Hydrochloride (May exhibit an additive CNS depression).
No products indexed under this heading.

Chlorprothixene (May exhibit an additive CNS depression).
No products indexed under this heading.

Chlorprothixene Hydrochloride (May exhibit an additive CNS depression).
No products indexed under this heading.

Chlorprothixene Lactate (May exhibit an additive CNS depression).
No products indexed under this heading.

Clemastine Fumarate (May exhibit an additive CNS depression).
No products indexed under this heading.

Clomipramine Hydrochloride (Co-administration may increase the effect of either antidepressant or hydrocodone).
No products indexed under this heading.

Clonazepam (May exhibit an additive CNS depression). Products include:
Klonopin 2855

Clorazepate Dipotassium (May exhibit an additive CNS depression).
No products indexed under this heading.

Clozapine (May exhibit an additive CNS depression).
No products indexed under this heading.

Codeine Phosphate (May exhibit an additive CNS depression). Products include:
Tylenol with Codeine 2691

Codeine Sulfate (May exhibit an additive CNS depression).
No products indexed under this heading.

Cyproheptadine Hydrochloride (May exhibit an additive CNS depression).
No products indexed under this heading.

Desflurane (May exhibit an additive CNS depression).
No products indexed under this heading.

Desipramine Hydrochloride (Co-administration may increase the effect of either antidepressant or hydrocodone).
No products indexed under this heading.

Dexchlorpheniramine Maleate (May exhibit an additive CNS depression).
No products indexed under this heading.

Dezocine (May exhibit an additive CNS depression).
No products indexed under this heading.

Diazepam (May exhibit an additive CNS depression). Products include:
Valium Tablets 2880

Dihydrocodeine Bitartrate (May exhibit an additive CNS depression).
No products indexed under this heading.

Dihydrocodeinone Bitartrate (May exhibit an additive CNS depression).
No products indexed under this heading.

Diphenhydramine Hydrochloride (May exhibit an additive CNS depression). Products include:
Benadryl Allergy Ultratab 2042
Children's Benadryl Allergy Liquid 2042

Diphenylpyraline Hydrochloride (May exhibit an additive CNS depression).
No products indexed under this heading.

Doxepin Hydrochloride (Co-administration may increase the effect of either antidepressant or hydrocodone).
No products indexed under this heading.

Droperidol (May exhibit an additive CNS depression).
No products indexed under this heading.

Enflurane (May exhibit an additive CNS depression).
No products indexed under this heading.

Estazolam (May exhibit an additive CNS depression).
No products indexed under this heading.

Ethanol (May exhibit an additive CNS depression).
No products indexed under this heading.

Ethchlorvynol (May exhibit an additive CNS depression).
No products indexed under this heading.

Ethinamate (May exhibit an additive CNS depression).
No products indexed under this heading.

Ethyl Alcohol (May exhibit an additive CNS depression).
No products indexed under this heading.

Fentanyl (May exhibit an additive CNS depression). Products include:
Duragesic 2604
Fentanyl Transdermal System 2346
Onsolis 2054

Fentanyl Citrate (May exhibit an additive CNS depression). Products include:
Fentora 966

Fexofenadine Hydrochloride (May exhibit an additive CNS depression). Products include:
Allegra ODT 2911
Allegra Oral Solution 2911
Allegra 2911
Allegra-D 2915
Allegra-D 24 2918

Fluphenazine Decanoate (May exhibit an additive CNS depression).
No products indexed under this heading.

Fluphenazine Enanthate (May exhibit an additive CNS depression).
No products indexed under this heading.

Fluphenazine Hydrochloride (May exhibit an additive CNS depression).
No products indexed under this heading.

Flurazepam Hydrochloride (May exhibit an additive CNS depression).
No products indexed under this heading.

Glutethimide (May exhibit an additive CNS depression).
No products indexed under this heading.

Halazepam (May exhibit an additive CNS depression).
No products indexed under this heading.

Haloperidol (May exhibit an additive CNS depression).
No products indexed under this heading.

Haloperidol Decanoate (May exhibit an additive CNS depression).
No products indexed under this heading.

Haloperidol Lactate (May exhibit an additive CNS depression).
No products indexed under this heading.

Hexobarbital (May exhibit an additive CNS depression).
No products indexed under this heading.

Hydrocodone Polistirex (May exhibit an additive CNS depression). Products include:

Tussionex 3443

Hydromorphone (May exhibit an additive CNS depression).
No products indexed under this heading.

Hydromorphone Hydrochloride (May exhibit an additive CNS depression). Products include:
Dilaudid Injection 2800
Dilaudid Oral 2797
Dilaudid Tablets 2797
Dilaudid-HP 2800

Hydroxyzine Hydrochloride (May exhibit an additive CNS depression).
No products indexed under this heading.

Imipramine Hydrochloride (Co-administration may increase the effect of either antidepressant or hydrocodone).
No products indexed under this heading.

Imipramine Pamoate (Co-administration may increase the effect of either antidepressant or hydrocodone).
No products indexed under this heading.

Isocarboxazid (Co-administration may increase the effect of either the MAO inhibitor or hydrocodone). Products include:
Marplan 3481

Isoflurane (May exhibit an additive CNS depression).
No products indexed under this heading.

Ketamine Hydrochloride (May exhibit an additive CNS depression).
No products indexed under this heading.

Levomethadyl Acetate Hydrochloride (May exhibit an additive CNS depression).
No products indexed under this heading.

Levorphanol Tartrate (May exhibit an additive CNS depression).
No products indexed under this heading.

Lithium (May exhibit an additive CNS depression).
No products indexed under this heading.

Lithium Carbonate (May exhibit an additive CNS depression).
No products indexed under this heading.

Lithium Citrate (May exhibit an additive CNS depression).
No products indexed under this heading.

Loratadine (May exhibit an additive CNS depression).
No products indexed under this heading.

Lorazepam (May exhibit an additive CNS depression).
No products indexed under this heading.

Loxapine Hydrochloride (May exhibit an additive CNS depression).
No products indexed under this heading.

Loxapine Succinate (May exhibit an additive CNS depression).
No products indexed under this heading.

Maprotiline Hydrochloride (Co-administration may increase the effect of either antidepressant or hydrocodone).
No products indexed under this heading.

Meperidine Hydrochloride (May exhibit an additive CNS depression).
No products indexed under this heading.

Mephobarbital (May exhibit an additive CNS depression).
No products indexed under this heading.

Meprobamate (May exhibit an additive CNS depression).
No products indexed under this heading.

Mesoridazine Besylate (May exhibit an additive CNS depression).
No products indexed under this heading.

Methadone Hydrochloride (May exhibit an additive CNS depression).
No products indexed under this heading.

Methdilazine Hydrochloride (May exhibit an additive CNS depression).
No products indexed under this heading.

Methohexital Sodium (May exhibit an additive CNS depression).
No products indexed under this heading.

Methotrimeprazine (May exhibit an additive CNS depression).
No products indexed under this heading.

Methoxyflurane (May exhibit an additive CNS depression).
No products indexed under this heading.

Midazolam Hydrochloride (May exhibit an additive CNS depression).
No products indexed under this heading.

Moclobemide (Co-administration may increase the effect of either the MAO inhibitor or hydrocodone).
No products indexed under this heading.

Molindone Hydrochloride (May exhibit an additive CNS depression). Products include:
Moban 1108

Morphine Sulfate (May exhibit an additive CNS depression). Products include:
Avinza 1822
Embeda 1831
MS Contin 2803

Morphine Sulfate, Liposomal (May exhibit an additive CNS depression).
No products indexed under this heading.

Nortriptyline Hydrochloride (Co-administration may increase the effect of either antidepressant or hydrocodone).
No products indexed under this heading.

Olanzapine (May exhibit an additive CNS depression). Products include:
Symbyax 1965
Zyprexa 1984
Zyprexa IntraMuscular 1984
Zyprexa ZYDIS 1984

Oxazepam (May exhibit an additive CNS depression).
No products indexed under this heading.

Oxycodone Hydrochloride (May exhibit an additive CNS depression). Products include:
OxyContin 2807
Percocet 1121
Percodan 1124

Oxycodone Terephthalate (May exhibit an additive CNS depression).
No products indexed under this heading.

Oxymorphone Hydrochloride (May exhibit an additive CNS depression). Products include:
Opana 1110
Opana ER 1114

Paliperidone (May exhibit an additive CNS depression). Products include:
Invega 2613
Invega Sustenna 2621

Pargyline Hydrochloride (Co-administration may increase the effect of either the MAO inhibitor or hydrocodone).
No products indexed under this heading.

Pentobarbital (May exhibit an additive CNS depression).
No products indexed under this heading.

Pentobarbital Sodium (May exhibit an additive CNS depression). Products include:
Nembutal 2012

Perphenazine (May exhibit an additive CNS depression).
No products indexed under this heading.

Phenelzine Sulfate (Co-administration may increase the effect of either the MAO inhibitor or hydrocodone).
No products indexed under this heading.

Phenobarbital (May exhibit an additive CNS depression). Products include:
Donnatal 2711

Phenobarbital Sodium (May exhibit an additive CNS depression).
No products indexed under this heading.

Pimozide (May exhibit an additive CNS depression).
No products indexed under this heading.

Prazepam (May exhibit an additive CNS depression).
No products indexed under this heading.

Procarbazine Hydrochloride (Co-administration may increase the effect of either the MAO inhibitor or hydrocodone).
No products indexed under this heading.

Prochlorperazine (May exhibit an additive CNS depression).
No products indexed under this heading.

Prochlorperazine Edisylate (May exhibit an additive CNS depression).
No products indexed under this heading.

Prochlorperazine Maleate (May exhibit an additive CNS depression).
No products indexed under this heading.

Promethazine (May exhibit an additive CNS depression).
No products indexed under this heading.

Promethazine Hydrochloride (May exhibit an additive CNS depression).
No products indexed under this heading.

Propofol (May exhibit an additive CNS depression).
No products indexed under this heading.

Propoxyphene Hydrochloride (May exhibit an additive CNS depression).
No products indexed under this heading.

Propoxyphene Napsylate (May exhibit an additive CNS depression).
No products indexed under this heading.

Protriptyline Hydrochloride (Co-administration may increase the effect of either antidepressant or hydrocodone).
No products indexed under this heading.

Pyrilamine Maleate (May exhibit an additive CNS depression).
No products indexed under this heading.

Pyrilamine Tannate (May exhibit an additive CNS depression).
No products indexed under this heading.

Quazepam (May exhibit an additive CNS depression).
No products indexed under this heading.

Quetiapine Fumarate (May exhibit an additive CNS depression). Products include:
Seroquel 750
Seroquel XR 759

Rasagiline Mesylate (Co-administration may increase the effect of either the MAO inhibitor or hydrocodone). Products include:
Azilect 3383

Remifentanil Hydrochloride (May exhibit an additive CNS depression).
No products indexed under this heading.

Risperidone (May exhibit an additive CNS depression). Products include:
Risperdal Consta 2682

Secobarbital Sodium (May exhibit an additive CNS depression).
No products indexed under this heading.

Selegiline (Co-administration may increase the effect of either the MAO inhibitor or hydrocodone). Products include:
Emsam 3623

Selegiline Hydrochloride (Co-administration may increase the effect of either the MAO inhibitor or hydrocodone). Products include:
Eldepryl 3312

Sevoflurane (May exhibit an additive CNS depression). Products include:
Ultane 554

Sodium Butabarbital (May exhibit an additive CNS depression).
No products indexed under this heading.

Sodium Oxybate (May exhibit an additive CNS depression).
No products indexed under this heading.

Sodium Pentobarbital (May exhibit an additive CNS depression).
No products indexed under this heading.

Sufentanil Citrate (May exhibit an additive CNS depression).
No products indexed under this heading.

Talbutal (May exhibit an additive CNS depression).
No products indexed under this heading.

Temazepam (May exhibit an additive CNS depression).
No products indexed under this heading.

Terfenadine (May exhibit an additive CNS depression).
No products indexed under this heading.

Thiamylal Sodium (May exhibit an additive CNS depression).
No products indexed under this heading.

Thioridazine (May exhibit an additive CNS depression).
No products indexed under this heading.

Thioridazine Hydrochloride (May exhibit an additive CNS depression). Products include:
Thioridazine Hydrochloride 2384

Thiothixene (May exhibit an additive CNS depression). Products include:
Thiothixene 2386

Thiothixene Hydrochloride (May exhibit an additive CNS depression).
No products indexed under this heading.

Tranylcypromine Sulfate (Co-administration may increase the effect of either the MAO inhibitor or hydrocodone). Products include:
Parnate 1584

Triazolam (May exhibit an additive CNS depression).
No products indexed under this heading.

Trifluoperazine Hydrochloride (May exhibit an additive CNS depression).
No products indexed under this heading.

Trimeprazine Tartrate (May exhibit an additive CNS depression).
No products indexed under this heading.

Trimipramine Maleate (Co-administration may increase the effect of either antidepressant or hydrocodone).
No products indexed under this heading.

Tripelennamine Hydrochloride (May exhibit an additive CNS depression).
No products indexed under this heading.

Triprolidine Hydrochloride (May exhibit an additive CNS depression).
No products indexed under this heading.

Zaleplon (May exhibit an additive CNS depression).
No products indexed under this heading.

Ziprasidone Hydrochloride (May exhibit an additive CNS depression). Products include:
Geodon 2723

Zolpidem Tartrate (May exhibit an additive CNS depression). Products include:
Ambien 2920
Ambien CR 2925

Food Interactions

Alcohol (May exhibit an additive CNS depression).

Beer, reduced-alcohol (May exhibit an additive CNS depression).

Beer, unspecified (May exhibit an additive CNS depression).

Wine, Chianti (May exhibit an additive CNS depression).

Wine, Red (May exhibit an additive CNS depression).

Wine, unspecified (May exhibit an additive CNS depression).

Wine products (May exhibit an additive CNS depression).

VICODIN ES TABLETS
(Acetaminophen, Hydrocodone Bitartrate)... 561
May interact with alcohols, anticholinergics, central nervous system depressants, narcotic analgesics, psychotropics, tranquilizers, tricyclic antidepressants, and certain other agents. Compounds in these categories include:

Alfentanil Hydrochloride (Additive CNS depression; the dose of one or both agents should be reduced).
No products indexed under this heading.

Alprazolam (Additive CNS depression; the dose of one or both agents should be reduced).
No products indexed under this heading.

Amitriptyline Hydrochloride (Concurrent use of tricyclic antidepressants and hydrocodone preparations may increase the effect of either the antidepressant or hydrocodone).
No products indexed under this heading.

Amobarbital (Additive CNS depression; the dose of one or both agents should be reduced).
No products indexed under this heading.

Amobarbital Sodium (Additive CNS depression; the dose of one or both agents should be reduced).
No products indexed under this heading.

Amoxapine (Concurrent use of tricyclic antidepressants and hydrocodone preparations may increase the effect of either the antidepressant or hydrocodone).
No products indexed under this heading.

Apomorphine (Additive CNS depression; the dose of one or both agents should be reduced).
No products indexed under this heading.

Apomorphine Hydrochloride (Additive CNS depression; the dose of one or both agents should be reduced).
No products indexed under this heading.

Aprobarbital (Additive CNS depression; the dose of one or both agents should be reduced).
No products indexed under this heading.

Atropine Sulfate (May produce paralytic ileus). Products include:
Donnatal 2711

Belladonna Alkaloids (May produce paralytic ileus). Products include:
Hyland's Teething Tablets 3316

Benztropine Mesylate (May produce paralytic ileus).
No products indexed under this heading.

Biperiden Hydrochloride (May produce paralytic ileus).
No products indexed under this heading.

Buprenorphine Hydrochloride (Additive CNS depression; the dose of one or both agents should be reduced).
No products indexed under this heading.

Buspirone Hydrochloride (Additive CNS depression; the dose of one or both agents should be reduced).
No products indexed under this heading.

Butabarbital (Additive CNS depression; the dose of one or both agents should be reduced).
No products indexed under this heading.

Butabarbital Sodium (Additive CNS depression; the dose of one or both agents should be reduced).
No products indexed under this heading.

Butalbital (Additive CNS depression; the dose of one or both agents should be reduced).
No products indexed under this heading.

Chlordiazepoxide (Additive CNS depression; the dose of one or both agents should be reduced).
No products indexed under this heading.

IMPORTANT NOTE: Always consult each drug listing in the patient's regimen for possible interactions.

(⊙ Described in PDR® for Ophthalmic Medicines)

Oxycodone Terephthalate (Additive CNS depression; the dose of one or both agents should be reduced).
No products indexed under this heading.

Oxymorphone Hydrochloride (Additive CNS depression; the dose of one or both agents should be reduced). Products include:
Opana 1110
Opana ER 1114

Paliperidone (Additive CNS depression; the dose of one or both agents should be reduced). Products include:
Invega 2613
Invega Sustenna 2621

Pentobarbital (Additive CNS depression; the dose of one or both agents should be reduced).
No products indexed under this heading.

Pentobarbital Sodium (Additive CNS depression; the dose of one or both agents should be reduced). Products include:
Nembutal 2012

Perphenazine (Additive CNS depression; the dose of one or both agents should be reduced).
No products indexed under this heading.

Phenelzine Sulfate (Concurrent use of MAO inhibitor and hydrocodone preparations may increase the effect of either the MAO inhibitor or hydrocodone).
No products indexed under this heading.

Phenobarbital (Additive CNS depression; the dose of one or both agents should be reduced). Products include:
Donnatal 2711

Phenobarbital Sodium (Additive CNS depression; the dose of one or both agents should be reduced).
No products indexed under this heading.

Prazepam (Additive CNS depression; the dose of one or both agents should be reduced).
No products indexed under this heading.

Prochlorperazine (Additive CNS depression; the dose of one or both agents should be reduced).
No products indexed under this heading.

Prochlorperazine Edisylate (Additive CNS depression; the dose of one or both agents should be reduced).
No products indexed under this heading.

Prochlorperazine Maleate (Additive CNS depression; the dose of one or both agents should be reduced).
No products indexed under this heading.

Procyclidine Hydrochloride (May produce paralytic ileus).
No products indexed under this heading.

Promethazine (Additive CNS depression; the dose of one or both agents should be reduced).
No products indexed under this heading.

Promethazine Hydrochloride (Additive CNS depression; the dose of one or both agents should be reduced).
No products indexed under this heading.

Propantheline Bromide (May produce paralytic ileus).
No products indexed under this heading.

Propofol (Additive CNS depression; the dose of one or both agents should be reduced).
No products indexed under this heading.

Propoxyphene Hydrochloride (Additive CNS depression; the dose of one or both agents should be reduced).
No products indexed under this heading.

Propoxyphene Napsylate (Additive CNS depression; the dose of one or both agents should be reduced).
No products indexed under this heading.

Protriptyline Hydrochloride (Concurrent use of tricyclic antidepressants and hydrocodone preparations may increase the effect of either the antidepressant or hydrocodone).
No products indexed under this heading.

Quazepam (Additive CNS depression; the dose of one or both agents should be reduced).
No products indexed under this heading.

Quetiapine Fumarate (Additive CNS depression; the dose of one or both agents should be reduced). Products include:
Seroquel 750
Seroquel XR 759

Remifentanil Hydrochloride (Additive CNS depression; the dose of one or both agents should be reduced).
No products indexed under this heading.

Risperidone (Additive CNS depression; the dose of one or both agents should be reduced). Products include:
Risperdal Consta 2682

Scopolamine (May produce paralytic ileus). Products include:
Transderm Scōp 2397

Scopolamine Hydrobromide (May produce paralytic ileus). Products include:
Donnatal 2711

Secobarbital Sodium (Additive CNS depression; the dose of one or both agents should be reduced).
No products indexed under this heading.

Selegiline Hydrochloride (Concurrent use of MAO inhibitor and hydrocodone preparations may increase the effect of either the MAO inhibitor or hydrocodone). Products include:
Eldepryl 3312

Sevoflurane (Additive CNS depression; the dose of one or both agents should be reduced). Products include:
Ultane 554

Sodium Butabarbital (Additive CNS depression; the dose of one or both agents should be reduced).
No products indexed under this heading.

Sodium Oxybate (Additive CNS depression; the dose of one or both agents should be reduced).
No products indexed under this heading.

Sodium Pentobarbital (Additive CNS depression; the dose of one or both agents should be reduced).
No products indexed under this heading.

Sufentanil Citrate (Additive CNS depression; the dose of one or both agents should be reduced).
No products indexed under this heading.

Talbutal (Additive CNS depression; the dose of one or both agents should be reduced).
No products indexed under this heading.

Temazepam (Additive CNS depression; the dose of one or both agents should be reduced).
No products indexed under this heading.

Thiamylal Sodium (Additive CNS depression; the dose of one or both agents should be reduced).
No products indexed under this heading.

Thioridazine (Additive CNS depression; the dose of one or both agents should be reduced).
No products indexed under this heading.

Thioridazine Hydrochloride (Additive CNS depression; the dose of one or both agents should be reduced). Products include:
Thioridazine Hydrochloride 2384

Thiothixene (Additive CNS depression; the dose of one or both agents should be reduced). Products include:
Thiothixene 2386

Thiothixene Hydrochloride (Additive CNS depression; the dose of one or both agents should be reduced).
No products indexed under this heading.

Tolterodine Tartrate (May produce paralytic ileus).
No products indexed under this heading.

Tranylcypromine Sulfate (Concurrent use of MAO inhibitor and hydrocodone preparations may increase the effect of either the MAO inhibitor or hydrocodone). Products include:
Parnate 1584

Triazolam (Additive CNS depression; the dose of one or both agents should be reduced).
No products indexed under this heading.

Tridihexethyl Chloride (May produce paralytic ileus).
No products indexed under this heading.

Trifluoperazine Hydrochloride (Additive CNS depression; the dose of one or both agents should be reduced).
No products indexed under this heading.

Trihexyphenidyl Hydrochloride (May produce paralytic ileus).
No products indexed under this heading.

Trimipramine Maleate (Concurrent use of tricyclic antidepressants and hydrocodone preparations may increase the effect of either the antidepressant or hydrocodone).
No products indexed under this heading.

Zaleplon (Additive CNS depression; the dose of one or both agents should be reduced).
No products indexed under this heading.

Ziprasidone Hydrochloride (Additive CNS depression; the dose of one or both agents should be reduced). Products include:
Geodon 2723

Zolpidem Tartrate (Additive CNS depression; the dose of one or both agents should be reduced). Products include:
Ambien 2920
Ambien CR 2925

Food Interactions

Alcohol (Additive CNS depression; the dose of one or both agents should be reduced).

Beer, reduced-alcohol (Additive CNS depression).

Beer, unspecified (Additive CNS depression).

Wine, Chianti (Additive CNS depression).

Wine, Red (Additive CNS depression).

Wine, unspecified (Additive CNS depression).

Wine products (Additive CNS depression).

VICODIN HP TABLETS

(Acetaminophen, Hydrocodone Bitartrate)............................. 563
May interact with alcohols, antihistamines, central nervous system depressants, monoamine oxidase inhibitors, narcotic analgesics, tranquilizers, tricyclic antidepressants. Compounds in these categories include:

Acrivastine (Co-administration may result in an additive CNS depression).
No products indexed under this heading.

Alfentanil Hydrochloride (Co-administration may result in an additive CNS depression).
No products indexed under this heading.

Alprazolam (Co-administration may result in an additive CNS depression).
No products indexed under this heading.

Amitriptyline Hydrochloride (Co-administration with tricyclic antidepressants may increase the effect of either hydrocodone or the tricyclic antidepressant).
No products indexed under this heading.

Amobarbital (Co-administration may result in an additive CNS depression).
No products indexed under this heading.

Amobarbital Sodium (Co-administration may result in an additive CNS depression).
No products indexed under this heading.

Amoxapine (Co-administration with tricyclic antidepressants may increase the effect of either hydrocodone or the tricyclic antidepressant).
No products indexed under this heading.

Apomorphine (Co-administration may result in an additive CNS depression).
No products indexed under this heading.

Apomorphine Hydrochloride (Co-administration may result in an additive CNS depression).
No products indexed under this heading.

Aprobarbital (Co-administration may result in an additive CNS depression).
No products indexed under this heading.

Astemizole (Co-administration may result in an additive CNS depression).
No products indexed under this heading.

Azatadine Maleate (Co-administration may result in an additive CNS depression).
No products indexed under this heading.

Bromodiphenhydramine Hydrochloride (Co-administration may result in an additive CNS depression).
No products indexed under this heading.

Brompheniramine Maleate (Co-administration may result in an additive CNS depression).
No products indexed under this heading.

Buprenorphine Hydrochloride (Co-administration may result in an additive CNS depression).
No products indexed under this heading.

Buspirone Hydrochloride (Co-administration may result in an additive CNS depression).
No products indexed under this heading.

Butabarbital (Co-administration may result in an additive CNS depression).
No products indexed under this heading.

Butabarbital Sodium (Co-administration may result in an additive CNS depression).
No products indexed under this heading.

Butalbital (Co-administration may result in an additive CNS depression).
No products indexed under this heading.

Cetirizine Hydrochloride (Co-administration may result in an additive CNS depression). Products include:
Zyrtec Allergy 2052
Children's Zyrtec Allergy Syrup 2053
Children's Zyrtec Allergy 2053
Children's Zyrtec Hives Relief 2053
Zyrtec-D Allergy & Congestion 2054

Chlordiazepoxide (Co-administration may result in an additive CNS depression).
No products indexed under this heading.

Chlordiazepoxide Hydrochloride (Co-administration may result in an additive CNS depression).
No products indexed under this heading.

Chlorpheniramine Maleate (Co-administration may result in an additive CNS depression).
No products indexed under this heading.

Chlorpheniramine Polistirex (Co-administration may result in an additive CNS depression). Products include:
Tussionex 3443

IMPORTANT NOTE: Always consult each drug listing in the patient's regimen for possible interactions.

Chlorpheniramine Tannate (Co-administration may result in an additive CNS depression).
No products indexed under this heading.

Chlorpromazine (Co-administration may result in an additive CNS depression).
No products indexed under this heading.

Chlorpromazine Hydrochloride (Co-administration may result in an additive CNS depression).
No products indexed under this heading.

Chlorprothixene (Co-administration may result in an additive CNS depression).
No products indexed under this heading.

Chlorprothixene Hydrochloride (Co-administration may result in an additive CNS depression).
No products indexed under this heading.

Chlorprothixene Lactate (Co-administration may result in an additive CNS depression).
No products indexed under this heading.

Clemastine Fumarate (Co-administration may result in an additive CNS depression).
No products indexed under this heading.

Clomipramine Hydrochloride (Co-administration with tricyclic antidepressants may increase the effect of either hydrocodone or the tricyclic antidepressant).
No products indexed under this heading.

Clonazepam (Co-administration may result in an additive CNS depression). Products include:
Klonopin 2855

Clorazepate Dipotassium (Co-administration may result in an additive CNS depression).
No products indexed under this heading.

Clozapine (Co-administration may result in an additive CNS depression).
No products indexed under this heading.

Codeine Phosphate (Co-administration may result in an additive CNS depression). Products include:
Tylenol with Codeine 2691

Codeine Sulfate (Co-administration may result in an additive CNS depression).
No products indexed under this heading.

Cyproheptadine Hydrochloride (Co-administration may result in an additive CNS depression).
No products indexed under this heading.

Desflurane (Co-administration may result in an additive CNS depression).
No products indexed under this heading.

Desipramine Hydrochloride (Co-administration with tricyclic antidepressants may increase the effect of either hydrocodone or the tricyclic antidepressant).
No products indexed under this heading.

Dexchlorpheniramine Maleate (Co-administration may result in an additive CNS depression).
No products indexed under this heading.

Dezocine (Co-administration may result in an additive CNS depression).
No products indexed under this heading.

Diazepam (Co-administration may result in an additive CNS depression). Products include:
Valium Tablets 2880

Dihydrocodeine Bitartrate (Co-administration may result in an additive CNS depression).
No products indexed under this heading.

Dihydrocodeinone Bitartrate (Co-administration may result in an additive CNS depression).
No products indexed under this heading.

Diphenhydramine Hydrochloride (Co-administration may result in an additive CNS depression). Products include:

Benadryl Allergy Ultratab 2042
Children's Benadryl Allergy Liquid 2042

Diphenylpyraline Hydrochloride (Co-administration may result in an additive CNS depression).
No products indexed under this heading.

Doxepin Hydrochloride (Co-administration with tricyclic antidepressants may increase the effect of either hydrocodone or the tricyclic antidepressant).
No products indexed under this heading.

Droperidol (Co-administration may result in an additive CNS depression).
No products indexed under this heading.

Enflurane (Co-administration may result in an additive CNS depression).
No products indexed under this heading.

Estazolam (Co-administration may result in an additive CNS depression).
No products indexed under this heading.

Ethanol (Co-administration may result in an additive CNS depression).
No products indexed under this heading.

Ethchlorvynol (Co-administration may result in an additive CNS depression).
No products indexed under this heading.

Ethinamate (Co-administration may result in an additive CNS depression).
No products indexed under this heading.

Ethyl Alcohol (Co-administration may result in an additive CNS depression).
No products indexed under this heading.

Fentanyl (Co-administration may result in an additive CNS depression).
Products include:
Duragesic 2604
Fentanyl Transdermal System 2346
Onsolis 2054

Fentanyl Citrate (Co-administration may result in an additive CNS depression). Products include:
Fentora 966

Fexofenadine Hydrochloride (Co-administration may result in an additive CNS depression). Products include:
Allegra ODT 2911
Allegra Oral Solution 2911
Allegra 2911
Allegra-D 2915
Allegra-D 24 2918

Fluphenazine Decanoate (Co-administration may result in an additive CNS depression).
No products indexed under this heading.

Fluphenazine Enanthate (Co-administration may result in an additive CNS depression).
No products indexed under this heading.

Fluphenazine Hydrochloride (Co-administration may result in an additive CNS depression).
No products indexed under this heading.

Flurazepam Hydrochloride (Co-administration may result in an additive CNS depression).
No products indexed under this heading.

Glutethimide (Co-administration may result in an additive CNS depression).
No products indexed under this heading.

Halazepam (Co-administration may result in an additive CNS depression).
No products indexed under this heading.

Haloperidol (Co-administration may result in an additive CNS depression).
No products indexed under this heading.

Haloperidol Decanoate (Co-administration may result in an additive CNS depression).
No products indexed under this heading.

Haloperidol Lactate (Co-administration may result in an additive CNS depression).
No products indexed under this heading.

Hexobarbital (Co-administration may result in an additive CNS depression).
No products indexed under this heading.

Hydrocodone Polistirex (Co-administration may result in an additive CNS depression). Products include:
Tussionex 3443

Hydromorphone (Co-administration may result in an additive CNS depression).
No products indexed under this heading.

Hydromorphone Hydrochloride (Co-administration may result in an additive CNS depression). Products include:
Dilaudid Injection 2800
Dilaudid Oral 2797
Dilaudid Tablets 2797
Dilaudid-HP 2800

Hydroxyzine Hydrochloride (Co-administration may result in an additive CNS depression).
No products indexed under this heading.

Imipramine Hydrochloride (Co-administration with tricyclic antidepressants may increase the effect of either hydrocodone or the tricyclic antidepressant).
No products indexed under this heading.

Imipramine Pamoate (Co-administration with tricyclic antidepressants may increase the effect of either hydrocodone or the tricyclic antidepressant).
No products indexed under this heading.

Isocarboxazid (Co-administration with an MAO inhibitor may increase the effect of either hydrocodone or the MAO inhibitor). Products include:
Marplan 3481

Isoflurane (Co-administration may result in an additive CNS depression).
No products indexed under this heading.

Ketamine Hydrochloride (Co-administration may result in an additive CNS depression).
No products indexed under this heading.

Levomethadyl Acetate Hydrochloride (Co-administration may result in an additive CNS depression).
No products indexed under this heading.

Levorphanol Tartrate (Co-administration may result in an additive CNS depression).
No products indexed under this heading.

Loratadine (Co-administration may result in an additive CNS depression).
No products indexed under this heading.

Lorazepam (Co-administration may result in an additive CNS depression).
No products indexed under this heading.

Loxapine Hydrochloride (Co-administration may result in an additive CNS depression).
No products indexed under this heading.

Loxapine Succinate (Co-administration may result in an additive CNS depression).
No products indexed under this heading.

Maprotiline Hydrochloride (Co-administration with tricyclic antidepressants may increase the effect of either hydrocodone or the tricyclic antidepressant).
No products indexed under this heading.

Meperidine Hydrochloride (Co-administration may result in an additive CNS depression).
No products indexed under this heading.

Mephobarbital (Co-administration may result in an additive CNS depression).
No products indexed under this heading.

Meprobamate (Co-administration may result in an additive CNS depression).
No products indexed under this heading.

Mesoridazine Besylate (Co-administration may result in an additive CNS depression).
No products indexed under this heading.

Methadone Hydrochloride (Co-administration may result in an additive CNS depression).
No products indexed under this heading.

Methdilazine Hydrochloride (Co-administration may result in an additive CNS depression).
No products indexed under this heading.

Methohexital Sodium (Co-administration may result in an additive CNS depression).
No products indexed under this heading.

Methotrimeprazine (Co-administration may result in an additive CNS depression).
No products indexed under this heading.

Methoxyflurane (Co-administration may result in an additive CNS depression).
No products indexed under this heading.

Midazolam Hydrochloride (Co-administration may result in an additive CNS depression).
No products indexed under this heading.

Moclobemide (Co-administration with an MAO inhibitor may increase the effect of either hydrocodone or the MAO inhibitor).
No products indexed under this heading.

Molindone Hydrochloride (Co-administration may result in an additive CNS depression). Products include:
Moban 1108

Morphine Sulfate (Co-administration may result in an additive CNS depression). Products include:
Avinza 1822
Embeda 1831
MS Contin 2803

Morphine Sulfate, Liposomal (Co-administration may result in an additive CNS depression).
No products indexed under this heading.

Nortriptyline Hydrochloride (Co-administration with tricyclic antidepressants may increase the effect of either hydrocodone or the tricyclic antidepressant).
No products indexed under this heading.

Olanzapine (Co-administration may result in an additive CNS depression). Products include:
Symbyax 1965
Zyprexa 1984
Zyprexa IntraMuscular 1984
Zyprexa ZYDIS 1984

Oxazepam (Co-administration may result in an additive CNS depression).
No products indexed under this heading.

Oxycodone Hydrochloride (Co-administration may result in an additive CNS depression). Products include:
OxyContin 2807
Percocet 1121
Percodan 1124

Oxycodone Terephthalate (Co-administration may result in an additive CNS depression).
No products indexed under this heading.

Oxymorphone Hydrochloride (Co-administration may result in an additive CNS depression). Products include:
Opana 1110
Opana ER 1114

Pargyline Hydrochloride (Co-administration with an MAO inhibitor may increase the effect of either hydrocodone or the MAO inhibitor).
No products indexed under this heading.

Pentobarbital (Co-administration may result in an additive CNS depression).
No products indexed under this heading.

Pentobarbital Sodium (Co-administration may result in an additive CNS depression). Products include:
Nembutal 2012

(⊙ Described in PDR® for Ophthalmic Medicines)

Perphenazine (Co-administration may result in an additive CNS depression).
No products indexed under this heading.

Phenelzine Sulfate (Co-administration with an MAO inhibitor may increase the effect of either hydrocodone or the MAO inhibitor).
No products indexed under this heading.

Phenobarbital (Co-administration may result in an additive CNS depression). Products include:
Donnatal 2711

Phenobarbital Sodium (Co-administration may result in an additive CNS depression).
No products indexed under this heading.

Prazepam (Co-administration may result in an additive CNS depression).
No products indexed under this heading.

Procarbazine Hydrochloride (Co-administration with an MAO inhibitor may increase the effect of either hydrocodone or the MAO inhibitor).
No products indexed under this heading.

Prochlorperazine (Co-administration may result in an additive CNS depression).
No products indexed under this heading.

Prochlorperazine Edisylate (Co-administration may result in an additive CNS depression).
No products indexed under this heading.

Prochlorperazine Maleate (Co-administration may result in an additive CNS depression).
No products indexed under this heading.

Promethazine (Co-administration may result in an additive CNS depression).
No products indexed under this heading.

Promethazine Hydrochloride (Co-administration may result in an additive CNS depression).
No products indexed under this heading.

Propofol (Co-administration may result in an additive CNS depression).
No products indexed under this heading.

Propoxyphene Hydrochloride (Co-administration may result in an additive CNS depression).
No products indexed under this heading.

Propoxyphene Napsylate (Co-administration may result in an additive CNS depression).
No products indexed under this heading.

Protriptyline Hydrochloride (Co-administration with tricyclic antidepressants may increase the effect of either hydrocodone or the tricyclic antidepressant).
No products indexed under this heading.

Pyrilamine Maleate (Co-administration may result in an additive CNS depression).
No products indexed under this heading.

Pyrilamine Tannate (Co-administration may result in an additive CNS depression).
No products indexed under this heading.

Quazepam (Co-administration may result in an additive CNS depression).
No products indexed under this heading.

Quetiapine Fumarate (Co-administration may result in an additive CNS depression). Products include:
Seroquel 750
Seroquel XR 759

Rasagiline Mesylate (Co-administration with an MAO inhibitor may increase the effect of either hydrocodone or the MAO inhibitor). Products include:
Azilect 3383

Remifentanil Hydrochloride (Co-administration may result in an additive CNS depression).
No products indexed under this heading.

Risperidone (Co-administration may result in an additive CNS depression). Products include:
Risperdal Consta 2682

Secobarbital Sodium (Co-administration may result in an additive CNS depression).
No products indexed under this heading.

Selegiline (Co-administration with an MAO inhibitor may increase the effect of either hydrocodone or the MAO inhibitor). Products include:
Emsam 3623

Selegiline Hydrochloride (Co-administration with an MAO inhibitor may increase the effect of either hydrocodone or the MAO inhibitor). Products include:
Eldepryl 3312

Sevoflurane (Co-administration may result in an additive CNS depression). Products include:
Ultane 554

Sodium Butabarbital (Co-administration may result in an additive CNS depression).
No products indexed under this heading.

Sodium Oxybate (Co-administration may result in an additive CNS depression).
No products indexed under this heading.

Sodium Pentobarbital (Co-administration may result in an additive CNS depression).
No products indexed under this heading.

Sufentanil Citrate (Co-administration may result in an additive CNS depression).
No products indexed under this heading.

Talbutal (Co-administration may result in an additive CNS depression).
No products indexed under this heading.

Temazepam (Co-administration may result in an additive CNS depression).
No products indexed under this heading.

Terfenadine (Co-administration may result in an additive CNS depression).
No products indexed under this heading.

Thiamylal Sodium (Co-administration may result in an additive CNS depression).
No products indexed under this heading.

Thioridazine (Co-administration may result in an additive CNS depression).
No products indexed under this heading.

Thioridazine Hydrochloride (Co-administration may result in an additive CNS depression). Products include:
Thioridazine Hydrochloride 2384

Thiothixene (Co-administration may result in an additive CNS depression). Products include:
Thiothixene 2386

Thiothixene Hydrochloride (Co-administration may result in an additive CNS depression).
No products indexed under this heading.

Tranylcypromine Sulfate (Co-administration with an MAO inhibitor may increase the effect of either hydrocodone or the MAO inhibitor). Products include:
Parnate 1584

Triazolam (Co-administration may result in an additive CNS depression).
No products indexed under this heading.

Trifluoperazine Hydrochloride (Co-administration may result in an additive CNS depression).
No products indexed under this heading.

Trimeprazine Tartrate (Co-administration may result in an additive CNS depression).
No products indexed under this heading.

Trimipramine Maleate (Co-administration with tricyclic antidepressants may increase the effect of either hydrocodone or the tricyclic antidepressant).
No products indexed under this heading.

Tripelennamine Hydrochloride (Co-administration may result in an additive CNS depression).
No products indexed under this heading.

Triprolidine Hydrochloride (Co-administration may result in an additive CNS depression).
No products indexed under this heading.

Zaleplon (Co-administration may result in an additive CNS depression).
No products indexed under this heading.

Ziprasidone Hydrochloride (Co-administration may result in an additive CNS depression). Products include:
Geodon 2723

Zolpidem Tartrate (Co-administration may result in an additive CNS depression). Products include:
Ambien 2920
Ambien CR 2925

Food Interactions

Alcohol (Co-administration may result in an additive CNS depression).

Beer, reduced-alcohol (Concurrent use results in an additive CNS depression).

Beer, unspecified (Concurrent use results in an additive CNS depression).

Wine, Chianti (Concurrent use results in an additive CNS depression).

Wine, Red (Concurrent use results in an additive CNS depression).

Wine, unspecified (Concurrent use results in an additive CNS depression).

Wine products (Concurrent use results in an additive CNS depression).

VICOPROFEN TABLETS

(Hydrocodone Bitartrate, Ibuprofen) 564
May interact with ACE inhibitors, alcohols, anticholinergics, aspirin-acetylsalicylic acid, central nervous system depressants, diuretics, lithium preparations, monoamine oxidase inhibitors, neuromuscular blocking agents, thiazides, tricyclic antidepressants, and certain other agents. Compounds in these categories include:

Alfentanil Hydrochloride (May exhibit additive CNS depression).
No products indexed under this heading.

Alprazolam (May exhibit additive CNS depression).
No products indexed under this heading.

Amiloride Hydrochloride (Ibuprofen has been shown to reduce the natriuretic effect of furosemide and thiazides in some patients. This response has been attributed to inhibition of renal prostaglandin synthesis. During concomitant therapy with Vicoprofen the patient should be observed closely for signs of renal failure).
No products indexed under this heading.

Amitriptyline Hydrochloride (Co-administration of tricyclic antidepressants with hydrocodone preparations may increase the effect of either the antidepressant or hydrocodone).
No products indexed under this heading.

Amobarbital (May exhibit additive CNS depression).
No products indexed under this heading.

Amobarbital Sodium (May exhibit additive CNS depression).
No products indexed under this heading.

Amoxapine (Co-administration of tricyclic antidepressants with hydrocodone preparations may increase the effect of either the antidepressant or hydrocodone).
No products indexed under this heading.

Aprobarbital (May exhibit additive CNS depression).
No products indexed under this heading.

Aspirin (Co-administration of Vicoprofen and aspirin may increase the risk of adverse effects; concurrent use should be avoided). Products include:
Aggrenox 880
Bayer Aspirin 829
Percodan 1124
St. Joseph Aspirin 2045

Aspirin, Enteric Coated (Co-administration of Vicoprofen and aspirin may increase the risk of adverse effects; concurrent use should be avoided).
No products indexed under this heading.

Aspirin Buffered (Co-administration of Vicoprofen and aspirin may increase the risk of adverse effects; concurrent use should be avoided).
No products indexed under this heading.

Atracurium Besylate (Hydrocodone as well as other opioid analgesics may enhance the neuromuscular blocking action of skeletal muscle relaxants and produce an increased degree of respiratory depression).
No products indexed under this heading.

Atropine Sulfate (Concurrent use of anticholinergics with hydrocodone preparations may produce paralytic ileus). Products include:
Donnatal 2711

Belladonna Alkaloids (Concurrent use of anticholinergics with hydrocodone preparations may produce paralytic ileus). Products include:
Hyland's Teething Tablets 3316

Benazepril Hydrochloride (NSAIDs may diminish the antihypertensive effect of ACE inhibitors).
No products indexed under this heading.

Bendroflumethiazide (Ibuprofen has been shown to reduce the natriuretic effect of thiazides in some patients).
No products indexed under this heading.

Benztropine Mesylate (Concurrent use of anticholinergics with hydrocodone preparations may produce paralytic ileus).
No products indexed under this heading.

Biperiden Hydrochloride (Concurrent use of anticholinergics with hydrocodone preparations may produce paralytic ileus).
No products indexed under this heading.

Bumetanide (Ibuprofen has been shown to reduce the natriuretic effect of furosemide and thiazides in some patients. This response has been attributed to inhibition of renal prostaglandin synthesis. During concomitant therapy with Vicoprofen the patient should be observed closely for signs of renal failure).
No products indexed under this heading.

Buprenorphine Hydrochloride (May exhibit additive CNS depression).
No products indexed under this heading.

Buspirone Hydrochloride (May exhibit additive CNS depression).
No products indexed under this heading.

Butabarbital (May exhibit additive CNS depression).
No products indexed under this heading.

Butabarbital Sodium (May exhibit additive CNS depression).
No products indexed under this heading.

Butalbital (May exhibit additive CNS depression).
No products indexed under this heading.

(⊙ Described in PDR® for Ophthalmic Medicines)

2057 Interactions Index Vicoprofen

Lithium Carbonate (Ibuprofen has been shown to elevate plasma lithium concentration and reduce renal clearance. The mean minimum lithium concentration is increased 15% and the renal clearance is decreased by approximately 20%. Patients should be observed for signs of lithium toxicity when Vicoprofen and lithium are administered concurrently).
No products indexed under this heading.

Lithium Citrate (Ibuprofen has been shown to elevate plasma lithium concentration and reduce renal clearance. The mean minimum lithium concentration is increased 15% and the renal clearance is decreased by approximately 20%. Patients should be observed for signs of lithium toxicity when Vicoprofen and lithium are administered concurrently).
No products indexed under this heading.

Lorazepam (May exhibit additive CNS depression).
No products indexed under this heading.

Loxapine Hydrochloride (May exhibit additive CNS depression).
No products indexed under this heading.

Loxapine Succinate (May exhibit additive CNS depression).
No products indexed under this heading.

Maprotiline Hydrochloride (Co-administration of tricyclic antidepressants with hydrocodone preparations may increase the effect of either the antidepressant or hydrocodone).
No products indexed under this heading.

Mepenzolate Bromide (Concurrent use of anticholinergics with hydrocodone preparations may produce paralytic ileus).
No products indexed under this heading.

Meperidine Hydrochloride (May exhibit additive CNS depression).
No products indexed under this heading.

Mephobarbital (May exhibit additive CNS depression).
No products indexed under this heading.

Meprobamate (May exhibit additive CNS depression).
No products indexed under this heading.

Mesoridazine Besylate (May exhibit additive CNS depression).
No products indexed under this heading.

Methadone Hydrochloride (May exhibit additive CNS depression).
No products indexed under this heading.

Methohexital Sodium (May exhibit additive CNS depression).
No products indexed under this heading.

Methotrexate Sodium (Ibuprofen, in animal studies, has been reported to competitively inhibit methotrexate accumulation; this could lead to enhanced toxicity of methotrexate).
No products indexed under this heading.

Methotrimeprazine (May exhibit additive CNS depression).
No products indexed under this heading.

Methoxyflurane (May exhibit additive CNS depression).
No products indexed under this heading.

Methyclothiazide (Ibuprofen has been shown to reduce the natriuretic effect of thiazides in some patients).
No products indexed under this heading.

Metocurine Iodide (Hydrocodone as well as other opioid analgesics may enhance the neuromuscular blocking action of skeletal muscle relaxants and produce an increased degree of respiratory depression).
No products indexed under this heading.

Metolazone (Ibuprofen has been shown to reduce the natriuretic effect of furosemide and thiazides in some patients. This response has been attributed to inhibition of renal prostaglandin synthesis. During concomitant therapy with Vicoprofen the patient should be observed closely for signs of renal failure).
No products indexed under this heading.

Midazolam Hydrochloride (May exhibit additive CNS depression).
No products indexed under this heading.

Mivacurium Chloride (Hydrocodone as well as other opioid analgesics may enhance the neuromuscular blocking action of skeletal muscle relaxants and produce an increased degree of respiratory depression).
No products indexed under this heading.

Moclobemide (Co-administration of MAO inhibitors with hydrocodone preparations may increase the effect of either the MAO inhibitors or hydrocodone. The use of hydrocodone is not recommended for patients taking MAOIs or within 14 days of stopping such treatment).
No products indexed under this heading.

Moexipril Hydrochloride (NSAIDs may diminish the antihypertensive effect of ACE inhibitors).
No products indexed under this heading.

Molindone Hydrochloride (May exhibit additive CNS depression). Products include:
Moban 1108

Morphine Sulfate (May exhibit additive CNS depression). Products include:
Avinza 1822
Embeda 1831
MS Contin 2803

Morphine Sulfate, Liposomal (May exhibit additive CNS depression).
No products indexed under this heading.

Nortriptyline Hydrochloride (Co-administration of tricyclic antidepressants with hydrocodone preparations may increase the effect of either the antidepressant or hydrocodone).
No products indexed under this heading.

Olanzapine (May exhibit additive CNS depression). Products include:
Symbyax 1965
Zyprexa 1984
Zyprexa IntraMuscular 1984
Zyprexa ZYDIS 1984

Oxazepam (May exhibit additive CNS depression).
No products indexed under this heading.

Oxybutynin Chloride (Concurrent use of anticholinergics with hydrocodone preparations may produce paralytic ileus).
No products indexed under this heading.

Oxycodone Hydrochloride (May exhibit additive CNS depression). Products include:
OxyContin 2807
Percocet 1121
Percodan 1124

Oxycodone Terephthalate (May exhibit additive CNS depression).
No products indexed under this heading.

Oxymorphone Hydrochloride (May exhibit additive CNS depression). Products include:
Opana 1110
Opana ER 1114

Pancuronium Bromide (Hydrocodone as well as other opioid analgesics may enhance the neuromuscular blocking action of skeletal muscle relaxants and produce an increased degree of respiratory depression).
No products indexed under this heading.

Pargyline Hydrochloride (Co-administration of MAO inhibitors with hydrocodone preparations may increase the effect of either the MAO inhibitors or hydrocodone. The use of hydrocodone is not recommended for patients taking MAOIs or within 14 days of stopping such treatment).
No products indexed under this heading.

Pentobarbital (May exhibit additive CNS depression).
No products indexed under this heading.

Pentobarbital Sodium (May exhibit additive CNS depression). Products include:
Nembutal 2012

Perindopril Erbumine (NSAIDs may diminish the antihypertensive effect of ACE inhibitors).
No products indexed under this heading.

Perphenazine (May exhibit additive CNS depression).
No products indexed under this heading.

Phenelzine Sulfate (Co-administration of MAO inhibitors with hydrocodone preparations may increase the effect of either the MAO inhibitors or hydrocodone. The use of hydrocodone is not recommended for patients taking MAOIs or within 14 days of stopping such treatment).
No products indexed under this heading.

Phenobarbital (May exhibit additive CNS depression). Products include:
Donnatal 2711

Phenobarbital Sodium (May exhibit additive CNS depression).
No products indexed under this heading.

Polythiazide (Ibuprofen has been shown to reduce the natriuretic effect of thiazides in some patients).
No products indexed under this heading.

Prazepam (May exhibit additive CNS depression).
No products indexed under this heading.

Procarbazine Hydrochloride (Co-administration of MAO inhibitors with hydrocodone preparations may increase the effect of either the MAO inhibitors or hydrocodone. The use of hydrocodone is not recommended for patients taking MAOIs or within 14 days of stopping such treatment).
No products indexed under this heading.

Prochlorperazine (May exhibit additive CNS depression).
No products indexed under this heading.

Prochlorperazine Edisylate (May exhibit additive CNS depression).
No products indexed under this heading.

Prochlorperazine Maleate (May exhibit additive CNS depression).
No products indexed under this heading.

Procyclidine Hydrochloride (Concurrent use of anticholinergics with hydrocodone preparations may produce paralytic ileus).
No products indexed under this heading.

Promethazine (May exhibit additive CNS depression).
No products indexed under this heading.

Promethazine Hydrochloride (May exhibit additive CNS depression).
No products indexed under this heading.

Propantheline Bromide (Concurrent use of anticholinergics with hydrocodone preparations may produce paralytic ileus).
No products indexed under this heading.

Propofol (May exhibit additive CNS depression).
No products indexed under this heading.

Propoxyphene Hydrochloride (May exhibit additive CNS depression).
No products indexed under this heading.

Propoxyphene Napsylate (May exhibit additive CNS depression).
No products indexed under this heading.

Protriptyline Hydrochloride (Co-administration of tricyclic antidepressants with hydrocodone preparations may increase the effect of either the antidepressant or hydrocodone).
No products indexed under this heading.

Quazepam (May exhibit additive CNS depression).
No products indexed under this heading.

Quetiapine Fumarate (May exhibit additive CNS depression). Products include:
Seroquel 750
Seroquel XR 759

Quinapril Hydrochloride (NSAIDs may diminish the antihypertensive effect of ACE inhibitors).
No products indexed under this heading.

Ramipril (NSAIDs may diminish the antihypertensive effect of ACE inhibitors).
No products indexed under this heading.

Rapacuronium Bromide (Hydrocodone as well as other opioid analgesics may enhance the neuromuscular blocking action of skeletal muscle relaxants and produce an increased degree of respiratory depression).
No products indexed under this heading.

Rasagiline Mesylate (Co-administration of MAO inhibitors with hydrocodone preparations may increase the effect of either the MAO inhibitors or hydrocodone. The use of hydrocodone is not recommended for patients taking MAOIs or within 14 days of stopping such treatment). Products include:
Azilect 3383

Remifentanil Hydrochloride (May exhibit additive CNS depression).
No products indexed under this heading.

Risperidone (May exhibit additive CNS depression). Products include:
Risperdal Consta 2682

Rocuronium Bromide (Hydrocodone as well as other opioid analgesics may enhance the neuromuscular blocking action of skeletal muscle relaxants and produce an increased degree of respiratory depression). Products include:
Zemuron 3249

Scopolamine (Concurrent use of anticholinergics with hydrocodone preparations may produce paralytic ileus). Products include:
Transderm Scōp 2397

Scopolamine Hydrobromide (Concurrent use of anticholinergics with hydrocodone preparations may produce paralytic ileus). Products include:
Donnatal 2711

Secobarbital Sodium (May exhibit additive CNS depression).
No products indexed under this heading.

Selegiline (Co-administration of MAO inhibitors with hydrocodone preparations may increase the effect of either the MAO inhibitors or hydrocodone. The use of hydrocodone is not recommended for patients taking MAOIs or within 14 days of stopping such treatment). Products include:
Emsam 3623

Selegiline Hydrochloride (Co-administration of MAO inhibitors with hydrocodone preparations may increase the effect of either the MAO inhibitors or hydrocodone. The use of hydrocodone is not recommended for patients taking MAOIs or within 14 days of stopping such treatment). Products include:
Eldepryl 3312

Sevoflurane (May exhibit additive CNS depression). Products include:
Ultane 554

Sodium Butabarbital (May exhibit additive CNS depression).
No products indexed under this heading.

IMPORTANT NOTE: Always consult each drug listing in the patient's regimen for possible interactions.

Sodium Oxybate (May exhibit additive CNS depression).
No products indexed under this heading.

Sodium Pentobarbital (May exhibit additive CNS depression).
No products indexed under this heading.

Spirapril Hydrochloride (NSAIDs may diminish the antihypertensive effect of ACE inhibitors).
No products indexed under this heading.

Spironolactone (Ibuprofen has been shown to reduce the natriuretic effect of furosemide and thiazides in some patients. This response has been attributed to inhibition of renal prostaglandin synthesis. During concomitant therapy with Vicoprofen the patient should be observed closely for signs of renal failure.
No products indexed under this heading.

Succinylcholine Chloride (Hydrocodone as well as other opioid analgesics may enhance the neuromuscular blocking action of skeletal muscle relaxants and produce an increased degree of respiratory depression).
No products indexed under this heading.

Sufentanil Citrate (May exhibit additive CNS depression).
No products indexed under this heading.

Talbutal (May exhibit additive CNS depression).
No products indexed under this heading.

Temazepam (May exhibit additive CNS depression).
No products indexed under this heading.

Thiamylal Sodium (May exhibit additive CNS depression).
No products indexed under this heading.

Thioridazine (May exhibit additive CNS depression).
No products indexed under this heading.

Thioridazine Hydrochloride (May exhibit additive CNS depression). Products include:
Thioridazine Hydrochloride 2384

Thiothixene (May exhibit additive CNS depression). Products include:
Thiothixene 2386

Thiothixene Hydrochloride (May exhibit additive CNS depression).
No products indexed under this heading.

Tolterodine Tartrate (Concurrent use of anticholinergics with hydrocodone preparations may produce paralytic ileus).
No products indexed under this heading.

Torsemide (Ibuprofen has been shown to reduce the natriuretic effect of furosemide and thiazides in some patients. This response has been attributed to inhibition of renal prostaglandin synthesis. During concomitant therapy with Vicoprofen the patient should be observed closely for signs of renal failure).
No products indexed under this heading.

Trandolapril (NSAIDs may diminish the antihypertensive effect of ACE inhibitors). Products include:
Mavik **489**
Tarka **534**

Tranylcypromine Sulfate (Co-administration of MAO inhibitors with hydrocodone preparations may increase the effect of either the MAO inhibitors or hydrocodone. The use of hydrocodone is not recommended for patients taking MAOIs or within 14 days of stopping such treatment. Products include:
Parnate **1584**

Triamterene (Ibuprofen has been shown to reduce the natriuretic effect of furosemide and thiazides in some patients. This response has been attributed to inhibition of renal prostaglandin synthesis. During concomitant therapy

with Vicoprofen the patient should be observed closely for signs of renal failure). Products include:
Dyazide **1429**
Dyrenium **3495**

Triazolam (May exhibit additive CNS depression).
No products indexed under this heading.

Tridihexethyl Chloride (Concurrent use of anticholinergics with hydrocodone preparations may produce paralytic ileus).
No products indexed under this heading.

Trifluoperazine Hydrochloride (May exhibit additive CNS depression).
No products indexed under this heading.

Trihexyphenidyl Hydrochloride (Concurrent use of anticholinergics with hydrocodone preparations may produce paralytic ileus).
No products indexed under this heading.

Trimipramine Maleate (Co-administration of tricyclic antidepressants with hydrocodone preparations may increase the effect of either the antidepressant or hydrocodone).
No products indexed under this heading.

Tubocurarine Chloride (Hydrocodone as well as other opioid analgesics may enhance the neuromuscular blocking action of skeletal muscle relaxants and produce an increased degree of respiratory depression).
No products indexed under this heading.

Vecuronium Bromide (Hydrocodone as well as other opioid analgesics may enhance the neuromuscular blocking action of skeletal muscle relaxants and produce an increased degree of respiratory depression).
No products indexed under this heading.

Warfarin Sodium (The effects of warfarin and NSAIDs on GI bleeding are synergistic).
No products indexed under this heading.

Zaleplon (May exhibit additive CNS depression).
No products indexed under this heading.

Ziprasidone Hydrochloride (May exhibit additive CNS depression). Products include:
Geodon **2723**

Zolpidem Tartrate (May exhibit additive CNS depression). Products include:
Ambien **2920**
Ambien CR **2925**

Food Interactions
Alcohol (May exhibit additive CNS depression).

Beer, reduced-alcohol (May exhibit additive CNS depression).

Beer, unspecified (May exhibit additive CNS depression).

Wine, Chianti (May exhibit additive CNS depression).

Wine, Red (May exhibit additive CNS depression).

Wine, unspecified (May exhibit additive CNS depression).

Wine products (May exhibit additive CNS depression).

VIGAMOX OPHTHALMIC SOLUTION
(Moxifloxacin Hydrochloride) **589**
None cited in PDR database.

VIMPAT INJECTION
(Lacosamide) **3444**
May interact with agents known affect cardiac contractility and/or sa or av node conduction (selected), beta-blockers, cytochrome p450 2c19 substrates (selected), drugs that prolong the PR interval, phenytoin, and certain other agents. Compounds in these categories include:

Acebutolol Hydrochloride (One case of profound bradycardia (26 bpm: BP 100/60 mmHg) was observed in a patient during a 15 minute infusion of 150 mg lacosamide. The patient was on a β-blocker).
No products indexed under this heading.

Alfentanil Hydrochloride (The lack of pharmacokinetic interaction does not rule out the possibility of pharmacodynamic interactions, particularly among drugs that affect the heart conduction system).
No products indexed under this heading.

Amitriptyline Hydrochloride (In vitro data suggest that lacosamide has the potential to inhibit CYP2C19 at therapeutic concentrations. However, an in vivo study with omeprazole did not show an inhibitory effect on omeprazole pharmacokinetics).
No products indexed under this heading.

Amoxapine (In vitro data suggest that lacosamide has the potential to inhibit CYP2C19 at therapeutic concentrations. However, an in vivo study with omeprazole did not show an inhibitory effect on omeprazole pharmacokinetics).
No products indexed under this heading.

Atenolol (One case of profound bradycardia (26 bpm: BP 100/60 mmHg) was observed in a patient during a 15 minute infusion of 150 mg lacosamide. The patient was on a β-blocker).
No products indexed under this heading.

Betaxolol Hydrochloride (One case of profound bradycardia (26 bpm: BP 100/60 mmHg) was observed in a patient during a 15 minute infusion of 150 mg lacosamide. The patient was on a β-blocker).
No products indexed under this heading.

Bisoprolol Fumarate (One case of profound bradycardia (26 bpm: BP 100/60 mmHg) was observed in a patient during a 15 minute infusion of 150 mg lacosamide. The patient was on a β-blocker).
No products indexed under this heading.

Carbamazepine (Population pharmacokinetics results in patients with partial-onset seizures showed small reductions (15% to 20% lower) in lacosamide plasma concentrations when lacosamide was co-administered with carbamazepine, phenobarbital, or phenytoin). Products include:
Carbatrol **3280**
Equetro **3477**

Carisoprodol (In vitro data suggest that lacosamide has the potential to inhibit CYP2C19 at therapeutic concentrations. However, an in vivo study with omeprazole did not show an inhibitory effect on omeprazole pharmacokinetics).
No products indexed under this heading.

Carteolol Hydrochloride (One case of profound bradycardia (26 bpm: BP 100/60 mmHg) was observed in a patient during a 15 minute infusion of 150 mg lacosamide. The patient was on a β-blocker).
No products indexed under this heading.

Carvedilol (One case of profound bradycardia (26 bpm: BP 100/60 mmHg) was observed in a patient during a 15 minute infusion of 150 mg lacosamide. The patient was on a β-blocker). Products include:
Coreg **1409**

Carvedilol Phosphate (One case of profound bradycardia (26 bpm: BP 100/60 mmHg) was observed in a patient during a 15 minute infusion of 150 mg lacosamide. The patient was on a β-blocker). Products include:
Coreg CR **1416**

Cilostazol (In vitro data suggest that lacosamide has the potential to inhibit CYP2C19 at therapeutic concentrations. However, an in vivo study with omeprazole did not show an inhibitory effect on omeprazole pharmacokinetics).
No products indexed under this heading.

Citalopram Hydrobromide (In vitro data suggest that lacosamide has the potential to inhibit CYP2C19 at therapeutic concentrations. However, an in vivo study with omeprazole did not show an inhibitory effect on omeprazole pharmacokinetics). Products include:
Celexa **1153**

Clomipramine Hydrochloride (In vitro data suggest that lacosamide has the potential to inhibit CYP2C19 at therapeutic concentrations. However, an in vivo study with omeprazole did not show an inhibitory effect on omeprazole pharmacokinetics).
No products indexed under this heading.

Cyclophosphamide (In vitro data suggest that lacosamide has the potential to inhibit CYP2C19 at therapeutic concentrations. However, an in vivo study with omeprazole did not show an inhibitory effect on omeprazole pharmacokinetics).
No products indexed under this heading.

Desipramine Hydrochloride (In vitro data suggest that lacosamide has the potential to inhibit CYP2C19 at therapeutic concentrations. However, an in vivo study with omeprazole did not show an inhibitory effect on omeprazole pharmacokinetics).
No products indexed under this heading.

Deslanoside (The lack of pharmacokinetic interaction does not rule out the possibility of pharmacodynamic interactions, particularly among drugs that affect the heart conduction system).
No products indexed under this heading.

Dextromethorphan (In vitro data suggest that lacosamide has the potential to inhibit CYP2C19 at therapeutic concentrations. However, an in vivo study with omeprazole did not show an inhibitory effect on omeprazole pharmacokinetics).
No products indexed under this heading.

Dextromethorphan Hydrobromide (In vitro data suggest that lacosamide has the potential to inhibit CYP2C19 at therapeutic concentrations. However, an in vivo study with omeprazole did not show an inhibitory effect on omeprazole pharmacokinetics).
No products indexed under this heading.

Diazepam (In vitro data suggest that lacosamide has the potential to inhibit CYP2C19 at therapeutic concentrations. However, an in vivo study with omeprazole did not show an inhibitory effect on omeprazole pharmacokinetics). Products include:
Valium Tablets **2880**

Digitoxin (The lack of pharmacokinetic interaction does not rule out the possibility of pharmacodynamic interactions, particularly among drugs that affect the heart conduction system).
No products indexed under this heading.

Digoxin (The lack of pharmacokinetic interaction does not rule out the possibility of pharmacodynamic interactions, particularly among drugs that affect the heart conduction system). Products include:
Lanoxin Injection **1546**
Lanoxin Injection Pediatric **1549**
Lanoxin Tablets **1553**

Diltiazem Hydrochloride (Dose-dependent prolongations in PR interval with lacosamide have been observed in clinical studies in patients and in healthy volunteers. When lacosamide is given

with other drugs that prolong the PR interval, further PR prolongation is possible). Products include:

Diltiazem Maleate (Dose-dependent prolongations in PR interval with lacosamide have been observed in clinical studies in patients and in healthy volunteers. When lacosamide is given with other drugs that prolong the PR interval, further PR prolongation is possible).

No products indexed under this heading.

Divalproex Sodium (In vitro data suggest that lacosamide has the potential to inhibit CYP2C19 at therapeutic concentrations. However, an in vivo study with omeprazole did not show an inhibitory effect on omeprazole pharmacokinetics). Products include:

Doxepin Hydrochloride (In vitro data suggest that lacosamide has the potential to inhibit CYP2C19 at therapeutic concentrations. However, an in vivo study with omeprazole did not show an inhibitory effect on omeprazole pharmacokinetics).

No products indexed under this heading.

Enflurane (The lack of pharmacokinetic interaction does not rule out the possibility of pharmacodynamic interactions, particularly among drugs that affect the heart conduction system).

No products indexed under this heading.

Esmolol Hydrochloride (One case of profound bradycardia (26 bpm: BP 100/60 mmHg) was observed in a patient during a 15 minute infusion of 150 mg lacosamide. The patient was on a β-blocker).

No products indexed under this heading.

Esomeprazole Magnesium (In vitro data suggest that lacosamide has the potential to inhibit CYP2C19 at therapeutic concentrations. However, an in vivo study with omeprazole did not show an inhibitory effect on omeprazole pharmacokinetics). Products include:

Esomeprazole Sodium (In vitro data suggest that lacosamide has the potential to inhibit CYP2C19 at therapeutic concentrations. However, an in vivo study with omeprazole did not show an inhibitory effect on omeprazole pharmacokinetics). Products include:

Ethinyl Estradiol (There was no influence of lacosamide (400 mg/day) on the pharmacodynamics and pharmacokinetics of an oral contraceptive containing 0.03 mg ethinyl estradiol and 0.15 mg levonorgestrel in healthy subjects, except that a 20% increase in ethinyl estradiol C_{max} was observed). Products include:

Ethosuximide (In vitro data suggest that lacosamide has the potential to inhibit CYP2C19 at therapeutic concentrations. However, an in vivo study with omeprazole did not show an inhibitory effect on omeprazole pharmacokinetics).

No products indexed under this heading.

Ethotoin (In vitro data suggest that lacosamide has the potential to inhibit CYP2C19 at therapeutic concentrations. However, an in vivo study with omeprazole did not show an inhibitory effect on omeprazole pharmacokinetics).

No products indexed under this heading.

Felbamate (In vitro data suggest that lacosamide has the potential to inhibit CYP2C19 at therapeutic concentrations. However, an in vivo study with omeprazole did not show an inhibitory effect on omeprazole pharmacokinetics).

No products indexed under this heading.

Fentanyl Citrate (The lack of pharmacokinetic interaction does not rule out the possibility of pharmacodynamic interactions, particularly among drugs that affect the heart conduction system). Products include:

Flecainide Acetate (Dose-dependent prolongations in PR interval with lacosamide have been observed in clinical studies in patients and in healthy volunteers. When lacosamide is given with other drugs that prolong the PR interval, further PR prolongation is possible).

No products indexed under this heading.

Formoterol Fumarate (In vitro data suggest that lacosamide has the potential to inhibit CYP2C19 at therapeutic concentrations. However, an in vivo study with omeprazole did not show an inhibitory effect on omeprazole pharmacokinetics). Products include:

Fosphenytoin (Population pharmacokinetics results in patients with partial-onset seizures showed small reductions (15% to 20% lower) in lacosamide plasma concentrations when lacosamide was co-administered with carbamazepine, phenobarbital, or phenytoin).

No products indexed under this heading.

Fosphenytoin Sodium (Population pharmacokinetics results in patients with partial-onset seizures showed small reductions (15% to 20% lower) in lacosamide plasma concentrations when lacosamide was co-administered with carbamazepine, phenobarbital, or phenytoin).

No products indexed under this heading.

Gabapentin (In vitro data suggest that lacosamide has the potential to inhibit CYP2C19 at therapeutic concentrations. However, an in vivo study with omeprazole did not show an inhibitory effect on omeprazole pharmacokinetics).

No products indexed under this heading.

Halothane (The lack of pharmacokinetic interaction does not rule out the possibility of pharmacodynamic interactions, particularly among drugs that affect the heart conduction system).

No products indexed under this heading.

Imipramine Hydrochloride (In vitro data suggest that lacosamide has the potential to inhibit CYP2C19 at therapeutic concentrations. However, an in vivo study with omeprazole did not show an inhibitory effect on omeprazole pharmacokinetics).

No products indexed under this heading.

Imipramine Pamoate (In vitro data suggest that lacosamide has the potential to inhibit CYP2C19 at therapeutic concentrations. However, an in vivo study with omeprazole did not show an inhibitory effect on omeprazole pharmacokinetics).

No products indexed under this heading.

Indomethacin (In vitro data suggest that lacosamide has the potential to inhibit CYP2C19 at therapeutic concentrations. However, an in vivo study with omeprazole did not show an inhibitory effect on omeprazole pharmacokinetics). Products include:

Indomethacin Sodium Trihydrate (In vitro data suggest that lacosamide has the potential to inhibit CYP2C19 at therapeutic concentrations. However,

an in vivo study with omeprazole did not show an inhibitory effect on omeprazole pharmacokinetics). Products include:

Isoflurane (The lack of pharmacokinetic interaction does not rule out the possibility of pharmacodynamic interactions, particularly among drugs that affect the heart conduction system).

No products indexed under this heading.

Ketamine Hydrochloride (The lack of pharmacokinetic interaction does not rule out the possibility of pharmacodynamic interactions, particularly among drugs that affect the heart conduction system).

No products indexed under this heading.

Labetalol Hydrochloride (One case of profound bradycardia (26 bpm: BP 100/60 mmHg) was observed in a patient during a 15 minute infusion of 150 mg lacosamide. The patient was on a β-blocker).

No products indexed under this heading.

Lamotrigine (In vitro data suggest that lacosamide has the potential to inhibit CYP2C19 at therapeutic concentrations. However, an in vivo study with omeprazole did not show an inhibitory effect on omeprazole pharmacokinetics). Products include:

Lansoprazole (In vitro data suggest that lacosamide has the potential to inhibit CYP2C19 at therapeutic concentrations. However, an in vivo study with omeprazole did not show an inhibitory effect on omeprazole pharmacokinetics).

No products indexed under this heading.

Levetiracetam (In vitro data suggest that lacosamide has the potential to inhibit CYP2C19 at therapeutic concentrations. However, an in vivo study with omeprazole did not show an inhibitory effect on omeprazole pharmacokinetics). Products include:

Levobunolol Hydrochloride (One case of profound bradycardia (26 bpm: BP 100/60 mmHg) was observed in a patient during a 15 minute infusion of 150 mg lacosamide. The patient was on a β-blocker).

No products indexed under this heading.

Maprotiline Hydrochloride (In vitro data suggest that lacosamide has the potential to inhibit CYP2C19 at therapeutic concentrations. However, an in vivo study with omeprazole did not show an inhibitory effect on omeprazole pharmacokinetics).

No products indexed under this heading.

Mephenytoin (In vitro data suggest that lacosamide has the potential to inhibit CYP2C19 at therapeutic concentrations. However, an in vivo study with omeprazole did not show an inhibitory effect on omeprazole pharmacokinetics).

No products indexed under this heading.

Mephobarbital (In vitro data suggest that lacosamide has the potential to inhibit CYP2C19 at therapeutic concentrations. However, an in vivo study with omeprazole did not show an inhibitory effect on omeprazole pharmacokinetics).

No products indexed under this heading.

Meprobamate (In vitro data suggest that lacosamide has the potential to inhibit CYP2C19 at therapeutic concentrations. However, an in vivo study with omeprazole did not show an inhibitory effect on omeprazole pharmacokinetics).

No products indexed under this heading.

Methohexital Sodium (The lack of pharmacokinetic interaction does not rule out the possibility of pharmacodynamic interactions, particularly among drugs that affect the heart conduction system).

No products indexed under this heading.

Methsuximide (In vitro data suggest that lacosamide has the potential to inhibit CYP2C19 at therapeutic concentrations. However, an in vivo study with omeprazole did not show an inhibitory effect on omeprazole pharmacokinetics).

No products indexed under this heading.

Metipranolol Hydrochloride (One case of profound bradycardia (26 bpm: BP 100/60 mmHg) was observed in a patient during a 15 minute infusion of 150 mg lacosamide. The patient was on a β-blocker).

No products indexed under this heading.

Metoprolol Succinate (Dose-dependent prolongations in PR interval with lacosamide have been observed in clinical studies in patients and in healthy volunteers. When lacosamide is given with other drugs that prolong the PR interval, further PR prolongation is possible). Products include:

Metoprolol Tartrate (Dose-dependent prolongations in PR interval with lacosamide have been observed in clinical studies in patients and in healthy volunteers. When lacosamide is given with other drugs that prolong the PR interval, further PR prolongation is possible).

No products indexed under this heading.

Midazolam Hydrochloride (The lack of pharmacokinetic interaction does not rule out the possibility of pharmacodynamic interactions, particularly among drugs that affect the heart conduction system).

No products indexed under this heading.

Nadolol (One case of profound bradycardia (26 bpm: BP 100/60 mmHg) was observed in a patient during a 15 minute infusion of 150 mg lacosamide. The patient was on a β-blocker). Products include:

Nebivolol (One case of profound bradycardia (26 bpm: BP 100/60 mmHg) was observed in a patient during a 15 minute infusion of 150 mg lacosamide. The patient was on a β-blocker). Products include:

Nelfinavir Mesylate (In vitro data suggest that lacosamide has the potential to inhibit CYP2C19 at therapeutic concentrations. However, an in vivo study with omeprazole did not show an inhibitory effect on omeprazole pharmacokinetics).

No products indexed under this heading.

Nilutamide (In vitro data suggest that lacosamide has the potential to inhibit CYP2C19 at therapeutic concentrations. However, an in vivo study with omeprazole did not show an inhibitory effect on omeprazole pharmacokinetics).

No products indexed under this heading.

Nortriptyline Hydrochloride (In vitro data suggest that lacosamide has the potential to inhibit CYP2C19 at therapeutic concentrations. However, an in vivo study with omeprazole did not show an inhibitory effect on omeprazole pharmacokinetics).

No products indexed under this heading.

IMPORTANT NOTE: Always consult each drug listing in the patient's regimen for possible interactions.

(⊙ Described in PDR® for Ophthalmic Medicines)

May interact with agents known affect cardiac contractility and/or sa or av node conduction (selected), cytochrome p450 2c19 substrates (selected), drugs that prolong the PR interval, phenytoin, and certain other agents. Compounds in these categories include:

Alfentanil Hydrochloride (The lack of pharmacokinetic interaction between lacosamide and other drugs does not rule out the possibility of pharmacodynamic interactions, particularly among drugs that affect the heart conduction system).
No products indexed under this heading.

Amitriptyline Hydrochloride (*In vitro* data suggest that lacosamide has the potential to inhibit CYP2C19 at therapeutic concentrations. However, an *in vivo* study with omeprazole did not show an inhibitory effect on omeprazole pharmacokinetics).
No products indexed under this heading.

Amoxapine (*In vitro* data suggest that lacosamide has the potential to inhibit CYP2C19 at therapeutic concentrations. However, an *in vivo* study with omeprazole did not show an inhibitory effect on omeprazole pharmacokinetics).
No products indexed under this heading.

Carbamazepine (Population pharmacokinetics results in patients with partial-onset seizures showed small reductions (15% to 20% lower) in lacosamide plasma concentrations when lacosamide was co-administered with carbamazepine, phenobarbital, or phenytoin). Products include:
Carbatrol 3280
Equetro 3477

Carisoprodol (*In vitro* data suggest that lacosamide has the potential to inhibit CYP2C19 at therapeutic concentrations. However, an *in vivo* study with omeprazole did not show an inhibitory effect on omeprazole pharmacokinetics).
No products indexed under this heading.

Cilostazol (*In vitro* data suggest that lacosamide has the potential to inhibit CYP2C19 at therapeutic concentrations. However, an *in vivo* study with omeprazole did not show an inhibitory effect on omeprazole pharmacokinetics).
No products indexed under this heading.

Citalopram Hydrobromide (*In vitro* data suggest that lacosamide has the potential to inhibit CYP2C19 at therapeutic concentrations. However, an *in vivo* study with omeprazole did not show an inhibitory effect on omeprazole pharmacokinetics). Products include:
Celexa 1153

Clomipramine Hydrochloride (*In vitro* data suggest that lacosamide has the potential to inhibit CYP2C19 at therapeutic concentrations. However, an *in vivo* study with omeprazole did not show an inhibitory effect on omeprazole pharmacokinetics).
No products indexed under this heading.

Cyclophosphamide (*In vitro* data suggest that lacosamide has the potential to inhibit CYP2C19 at therapeutic concentrations. However, an *in vivo* study with omeprazole did not show an inhibitory effect on omeprazole pharmacokinetics).
No products indexed under this heading.

Desipramine Hydrochloride (*In vitro* data suggest that lacosamide has the potential to inhibit CYP2C19 at therapeutic concentrations. However, an *in vivo* study with omeprazole did not show an inhibitory effect on omeprazole pharmacokinetics).
No products indexed under this heading.

Deslanoside (The lack of pharmacokinetic interaction between lacosamide and other drugs does not rule out the possibility of pharmacodynamic interactions, particularly among drugs that affect the heart conduction system).
No products indexed under this heading.

Dextromethorphan (*In vitro* data suggest that lacosamide has the potential to inhibit CYP2C19 at therapeutic concentrations. However, an *in vivo* study with omeprazole did not show an inhibitory effect on omeprazole pharmacokinetics).
No products indexed under this heading.

Dextromethorphan Hydrobromide (*In vitro* data suggest that lacosamide has the potential to inhibit CYP2C19 at therapeutic concentrations. However, an *in vivo* study with omeprazole did not show an inhibitory effect on omeprazole pharmacokinetics).
No products indexed under this heading.

Diazepam (*In vitro* data suggest that lacosamide has the potential to inhibit CYP2C19 at therapeutic concentrations. However, an *in vivo* study with omeprazole did not show an inhibitory effect on omeprazole pharmacokinetics). Products include:
Valium Tablets 2880

Digitoxin (The lack of pharmacokinetic interaction between lacosamide and other drugs does not rule out the possibility of pharmacodynamic interactions, particularly among drugs that affect the heart conduction system).
No products indexed under this heading.

Digoxin (The lack of pharmacokinetic interaction between lacosamide and other drugs does not rule out the possibility of pharmacodynamic interactions, particularly among drugs that affect the heart conduction system). Products include:
Lanoxin Injection 1546
Lanoxin Injection Pediatric 1549
Lanoxin Tablets 1553

Diltiazem Hydrochloride (Dose-dependent prolongations in PR interval with lacosamide have been observed in clinical studies in patients and in healthy volunteers. When lacosamide is given with other drugs that prolong the PR interval, further PR prolongation is possible). Products include:
Cardizem LA 423

Diltiazem Maleate (Dose-dependent prolongations in PR interval with lacosamide have been observed in clinical studies in patients and in healthy volunteers. When lacosamide is given with other drugs that prolong the PR interval, further PR prolongation is possible).
No products indexed under this heading.

Divalproex Sodium (*In vitro* data suggest that lacosamide has the potential to inhibit CYP2C19 at therapeutic concentrations. However, an *in vivo* study with omeprazole did not show an inhibitory effect on omeprazole pharmacokinetics). Products include:
Depakote ER 426

Doxepin Hydrochloride (*In vitro* data suggest that lacosamide has the potential to inhibit CYP2C19 at therapeutic concentrations. However, an *in vivo* study with omeprazole did not show an inhibitory effect on omeprazole pharmacokinetics).
No products indexed under this heading.

Enflurane (The lack of pharmacokinetic interaction between lacosamide and other drugs does not rule out the possibility of pharmacodynamic interactions, particularly among drugs that affect the heart conduction system).
No products indexed under this heading.

Esomeprazole Magnesium (*In vitro* data suggest that lacosamide has the potential to inhibit CYP2C19 at therapeutic concentrations. However, an *in vivo* study with omeprazole did not show an inhibitory effect on omeprazole pharmacokinetics). Products include:
Nexium Capsules 704
Nexium Oral Suspension 704

Esomeprazole Sodium (*In vitro* data suggest that lacosamide has the potential to inhibit CYP2C19 at therapeutic concentrations. However, an *in vivo* study with omeprazole did not show an inhibitory effect on omeprazole pharmacokinetics). Products include:
Nexium I.V. 712

Ethinyl Estradiol (There was no influence of lacosamide (400 mg/day) on the pharmacodynamics and pharmacokinetics of an oral contraceptive containing 0.03 mg ethinyl estradiol and 0.15 mg levonorgestrel in healthy subjects, except that a 20% increase in ethinyl estradiol C_{max} was observed). Products include:
LoSeasonique 3407
Lybrel 3514
NuvaRing 3181
Ortho Evra 2648
Ortho-Cyclen/Ortho Tri-Cyclen 2663
Ortho Tri-Cyclen Lo Tablets 2673
Seasonique 3418
Yaz 864

Ethosuximide (*In vitro* data suggest that lacosamide has the potential to inhibit CYP2C19 at therapeutic concentrations. However, an *in vivo* study with omeprazole did not show an inhibitory effect on omeprazole pharmacokinetics).
No products indexed under this heading.

Ethotoin (*In vitro* data suggest that lacosamide has the potential to inhibit CYP2C19 at therapeutic concentrations. However, an *in vivo* study with omeprazole did not show an inhibitory effect on omeprazole pharmacokinetics).
No products indexed under this heading.

Felbamate (*In vitro* data suggest that lacosamide has the potential to inhibit CYP2C19 at therapeutic concentrations. However, an *in vivo* study with omeprazole did not show an inhibitory effect on omeprazole pharmacokinetics).
No products indexed under this heading.

Fentanyl Citrate (The lack of pharmacokinetic interaction between lacosamide and other drugs does not rule out the possibility of pharmacodynamic interactions, particularly among drugs that affect the heart conduction system). Products include:
Fentora 966

Flecainide Acetate (Dose-dependent prolongations in PR interval with lacosamide have been observed in clinical studies in patients and in healthy volunteers. When lacosamide is given with other drugs that prolong the PR interval, further PR prolongation is possible).
No products indexed under this heading.

Formoterol Fumarate (*In vitro* data suggest that lacosamide has the potential to inhibit CYP2C19 at therapeutic concentrations. However, an *in vivo* study with omeprazole did not show an inhibitory effect on omeprazole pharmacokinetics). Products include:
Foradil 3121
Perforomist 3634

Fosphenytoin (Population pharmacokinetics results in patients with partial-onset seizures showed small reductions (15% to 20% lower) in lacosamide plasma concentrations when lacosamide was co-administered with carbamazepine, phenobarbital, or phenytoin).
No products indexed under this heading.

Fosphenytoin Sodium (Population pharmacokinetics results in patients with partial-onset seizures showed small reductions (15% to 20% lower) in lacosamide plasma concentrations when lacosamide was co-administered with carbamazepine, phenobarbital, or phenytoin).
No products indexed under this heading.

Gabapentin (*In vitro* data suggest that lacosamide has the potential to inhibit CYP2C19 at therapeutic concentrations. However, an *in vivo* study with omeprazole did not show an inhibitory effect on omeprazole pharmacokinetics).
No products indexed under this heading.

Halothane (The lack of pharmacokinetic interaction between lacosamide and other drugs does not rule out the possibility of pharmacodynamic interactions, particularly among drugs that affect the heart conduction system).
No products indexed under this heading.

Imipramine Hydrochloride (*In vitro* data suggest that lacosamide has the potential to inhibit CYP2C19 at therapeutic concentrations. However, an *in vivo* study with omeprazole did not show an inhibitory effect on omeprazole pharmacokinetics).
No products indexed under this heading.

Imipramine Pamoate (*In vitro* data suggest that lacosamide has the potential to inhibit CYP2C19 at therapeutic concentrations. However, an *in vivo* study with omeprazole did not show an inhibitory effect on omeprazole pharmacokinetics).
No products indexed under this heading.

Indomethacin (*In vitro* data suggest that lacosamide has the potential to inhibit CYP2C19 at therapeutic concentrations. However, an *in vivo* study with omeprazole did not show an inhibitory effect on omeprazole pharmacokinetics). Products include:
Indocin 2167

Indomethacin Sodium Trihydrate (*In vitro* data suggest that lacosamide has the potential to inhibit CYP2C19 at therapeutic concentrations. However, an *in vivo* study with omeprazole did not show an inhibitory effect on omeprazole pharmacokinetics). Products include:
Indocin I.V. 2007

Isoflurane (The lack of pharmacokinetic interaction between lacosamide and other drugs does not rule out the possibility of pharmacodynamic interactions, particularly among drugs that affect the heart conduction system).
No products indexed under this heading.

Ketamine Hydrochloride (The lack of pharmacokinetic interaction between lacosamide and other drugs does not rule out the possibility of pharmacodynamic interactions, particularly among drugs that affect the heart conduction system).
No products indexed under this heading.

Lamotrigine (*In vitro* data suggest that lacosamide has the potential to inhibit CYP2C19 at therapeutic concentrations. However, an *in vivo* study with omeprazole did not show an inhibitory effect on omeprazole pharmacokinetics). Products include:
Lamictal 1522
Lamictal ODT 1522
Lamictal XR 1536

Lansoprazole (*In vitro* data suggest that lacosamide has the potential to inhibit CYP2C19 at therapeutic concentrations. However, an *in vivo* study with omeprazole did not show an inhibitory effect on omeprazole pharmacokinetics).
No products indexed under this heading.

Levetiracetam (*In vitro* data suggest that lacosamide has the potential to

Vimpat Interactions Index 2062

inhibit CYP2C19 at therapeutic concentrations. However, an *in vivo* study with omeprazole did not show an inhibitory effect on omeprazole pharmacokinetics). Products include:
Keppra XR 3434

Maprotiline Hydrochloride (*In vitro* data suggest that lacosamide has the potential to inhibit CYP2C19 at therapeutic concentrations. However, an *in vivo* study with omeprazole did not show an inhibitory effect on omeprazole pharmacokinetics).
No products indexed under this heading.

Mephenytoin (*In vitro* data suggest that lacosamide has the potential to inhibit CYP2C19 at therapeutic concentrations. However, an *in vivo* study with omeprazole did not show an inhibitory effect on omeprazole pharmacokinetics).
No products indexed under this heading.

Mephobarbital (*In vitro* data suggest that lacosamide has the potential to inhibit CYP2C19 at therapeutic concentrations. However, an *in vivo* study with omeprazole did not show an inhibitory effect on omeprazole pharmacokinetics).
No products indexed under this heading.

Meprobamate (*In vitro* data suggest that lacosamide has the potential to inhibit CYP2C19 at therapeutic concentrations. However, an *in vivo* study with omeprazole did not show an inhibitory effect on omeprazole pharmacokinetics).
No products indexed under this heading.

Methohexital Sodium (The lack of pharmacokinetic interaction between lacosamide and other drugs does not rule out the possibility of pharmacodynamic interactions, particularly among drugs that affect the heart conduction system).
No products indexed under this heading.

Methsuximide (*In vitro* data suggest that lacosamide has the potential to inhibit CYP2C19 at therapeutic concentrations. However, an *in vivo* study with omeprazole did not show an inhibitory effect on omeprazole pharmacokinetics).
No products indexed under this heading.

Metoprolol Succinate (Dose-dependent prolongations in PR interval with lacosamide have been observed in clinical studies in patients and in healthy volunteers. When lacosamide is given with other drugs that prolong the PR interval, further PR prolongation is possible). Products include:
Toprol XL 732

Metoprolol Tartrate (Dose-dependent prolongations in PR interval with lacosamide have been observed in clinical studies in patients and in healthy volunteers. When lacosamide is given with other drugs that prolong the PR interval, further PR prolongation is possible).
No products indexed under this heading.

Midazolam Hydrochloride (The lack of pharmacokinetic interaction between lacosamide and other drugs does not rule out the possibility of pharmacodynamic interactions, particularly among drugs that affect the heart conduction system).
No products indexed under this heading.

Nelfinavir Mesylate (*In vitro* data suggest that lacosamide has the potential to inhibit CYP2C19 at therapeutic concentrations. However, an *in vivo* study with omeprazole did not show an inhibitory effect on omeprazole pharmacokinetics).
No products indexed under this heading.

Nilutamide (*In vitro* data suggest that lacosamide has the potential to inhibit CYP2C19 at therapeutic concentrations. However, an *in vivo* study with omeprazole did not show an inhibitory effect on omeprazole pharmacokinetics).
No products indexed under this heading.

Nortriptyline Hydrochloride (*In vitro* data suggest that lacosamide has the potential to inhibit CYP2C19 at therapeutic concentrations. However, an *in vivo* study with omeprazole did not show an inhibitory effect on omeprazole pharmacokinetics).
No products indexed under this heading.

Omeprazole (Omeprazole at a dose of 40 mg once daily had no effect on the pharmacokinetics of lacosamide (300 mg single dose). However, plasma levels of the O-desmethyl metabolite were reduced about 60% in the presence of omeprazole).
No products indexed under this heading.

Omeprazole Magnesium (Omeprazole at a dose of 40 mg once daily had no effect on the pharmacokinetics of lacosamide (300 mg single dose). However, plasma levels of the O-desmethyl metabolite were reduced about 60% in the presence of omeprazole).
No products indexed under this heading.

Oxcarbazepine (*In vitro* data suggest that lacosamide has the potential to inhibit CYP2C19 at therapeutic concentrations. However, an *in vivo* study with omeprazole did not show an inhibitory effect on omeprazole pharmacokinetics).
No products indexed under this heading.

Pantoprazole Sodium (*In vitro* data suggest that lacosamide has the potential to inhibit CYP2C19 at therapeutic concentrations. However, an *in vivo* study with omeprazole did not show an inhibitory effect on omeprazole pharmacokinetics). Products include:
Protonix Tablets 3571
Protonix 3575

Paramethadione (*In vitro* data suggest that lacosamide has the potential to inhibit CYP2C19 at therapeutic concentrations. However, an *in vivo* study with omeprazole did not show an inhibitory effect on omeprazole pharmacokinetics).
No products indexed under this heading.

Pentamidine Isethionate (*In vitro* data suggest that lacosamide has the potential to inhibit CYP2C19 at therapeutic concentrations. However, an *in vivo* study with omeprazole did not show an inhibitory effect on omeprazole pharmacokinetics).
No products indexed under this heading.

Phenacemide (*In vitro* data suggest that lacosamide has the potential to inhibit CYP2C19 at therapeutic concentrations. However, an *in vivo* study with omeprazole did not show an inhibitory effect on omeprazole pharmacokinetics).
No products indexed under this heading.

Phenobarbital (Population pharmacokinetics results in patients with partial-onset seizures showed small reductions (15% to 20% lower) in lacosamide plasma concentrations when lacosamide was co-administered with carbamazepine, phenobarbital, or phenytoin). Products include:
Donnatal 2711

Phenobarbital Sodium (Population pharmacokinetics results in patients with partial-onset seizures showed small reductions (15% to 20% lower) in lacosamide plasma concentrations when lacosamide was co-administered with carbamazepine, phenobarbital, or phenytoin).
No products indexed under this heading.

Phensuximide (*In vitro* data suggest that lacosamide has the potential to inhibit CYP2C19 at therapeutic concentrations. However, an *in vivo* study with omeprazole did not show an inhibitory effect on omeprazole pharmacokinetics).
No products indexed under this heading.

Phenytoin (Population pharmacokinetics results in patients with partial-onset seizures showed small reductions (15% to 20% lower) in lacosamide plasma concentrations when lacosamide was co-administered with carbamazepine, phenobarbital, or phenytoin).
No products indexed under this heading.

Phenytoin Sodium (Population pharmacokinetics results in patients with partial-onset seizures showed small reductions (15% to 20% lower) in lacosamide plasma concentrations when lacosamide was co-administered with carbamazepine, phenobarbital, or phenytoin). Products include:
Phenytek Capsules 2380

Primidone (*In vitro* data suggest that lacosamide has the potential to inhibit CYP2C19 at therapeutic concentrations. However, an *in vivo* study with omeprazole did not show an inhibitory effect on omeprazole pharmacokinetics).
No products indexed under this heading.

Progesterone (*In vitro* data suggest that lacosamide has the potential to inhibit CYP2C19 at therapeutic concentrations. However, an *in vivo* study with omeprazole did not show an inhibitory effect on omeprazole pharmacokinetics). Products include:
Crinone 4% 996
Crinone 8% 996
Prometrium 3307

Proguanil Hydrochloride (*In vitro* data suggest that lacosamide has the potential to inhibit CYP2C19 at therapeutic concentrations. However, an *in vivo* study with omeprazole did not show an inhibitory effect on omeprazole pharmacokinetics). Products include:
Malarone Pediatric Tablets 1572
Malarone 1572

Propafenone Hydrochloride (Dose-dependent prolongations in PR interval with lacosamide have been observed in clinical studies in patients and in healthy volunteers. When lacosamide is given with other drugs that prolong the PR interval, further PR prolongation is possible). Products include:
Rythmol 1648
Rythmol SR 1652

Propofol (The lack of pharmacokinetic interaction between lacosamide and other drugs does not rule out the possibility of pharmacodynamic interactions, particularly among drugs that affect the heart conduction system).
No products indexed under this heading.

Propranolol Hydrochloride (*In vitro* data suggest that lacosamide has the potential to inhibit CYP2C19 at therapeutic concentrations. However, an *in vivo* study with omeprazole did not show an inhibitory effect on omeprazole pharmacokinetics). Products include:
InnoPran XL 1517

Protriptyline Hydrochloride (*In vitro* data suggest that lacosamide has the potential to inhibit CYP2C19 at therapeutic concentrations. However, an *in vivo* study with omeprazole did not show an inhibitory effect on omeprazole pharmacokinetics).
No products indexed under this heading.

Rabeprazole Sodium (*In vitro* data suggest that lacosamide has the potential to inhibit CYP2C19 at therapeutic concentrations. However, an *in vivo* study with omeprazole did not show an inhibitory effect on omeprazole pharmacokinetics). Products include:
Aciphex 1035

Ritonavir (Dose-dependent prolongations in PR interval with lacosamide have been observed in clinical studies in patients and in healthy volunteers. When lacosamide is given with other drugs that prolong the PR interval, further PR prolongation is possible). Products include:
Kaletra 458
Norvir 509

Sertraline Hydrochloride (*In vitro* data suggest that lacosamide has the potential to inhibit CYP2C19 at therapeutic concentrations. However, an *in vivo* study with omeprazole did not show an inhibitory effect on omeprazole pharmacokinetics).
No products indexed under this heading.

Sufentanil Citrate (The lack of pharmacokinetic interaction between lacosamide and other drugs does not rule out the possibility of pharmacodynamic interactions, particularly among drugs that affect the heart conduction system).
No products indexed under this heading.

Teniposide (*In vitro* data suggest that lacosamide has the potential to inhibit CYP2C19 at therapeutic concentrations. However, an *in vivo* study with omeprazole did not show an inhibitory effect on omeprazole pharmacokinetics).
No products indexed under this heading.

Thiamylal Sodium (The lack of pharmacokinetic interaction between lacosamide and other drugs does not rule out the possibility of pharmacodynamic interactions, particularly among drugs that affect the heart conduction system).
No products indexed under this heading.

Thioridazine (*In vitro* data suggest that lacosamide has the potential to inhibit CYP2C19 at therapeutic concentrations. However, an *in vivo* study with omeprazole did not show an inhibitory effect on omeprazole pharmacokinetics).
No products indexed under this heading.

Thioridazine Hydrochloride (*In vitro* data suggest that lacosamide has the potential to inhibit CYP2C19 at therapeutic concentrations. However, an *in vivo* study with omeprazole did not show an inhibitory effect on omeprazole pharmacokinetics). Products include:
Thioridazine Hydrochloride 2384

Tiagabine Hydrochloride (*In vitro* data suggest that lacosamide has the potential to inhibit CYP2C19 at therapeutic concentrations. However, an *in vivo* study with omeprazole did not show an inhibitory effect on omeprazole pharmacokinetics). Products include:
Gabitril 972

Tolbutamide (*In vitro* data suggest that lacosamide has the potential to inhibit CYP2C19 at therapeutic concentrations. However, an *in vivo* study with omeprazole did not show an inhibitory effect on omeprazole pharmacokinetics).
No products indexed under this heading.

Tolbutamide Sodium (*In vitro* data suggest that lacosamide has the potential to inhibit CYP2C19 at therapeutic concentrations. However, an *in vivo* study with omeprazole did not show an inhibitory effect on omeprazole pharmacokinetics).
No products indexed under this heading.

Topiramate (*In vitro* data suggest that lacosamide has the potential to inhibit CYP2C19 at therapeutic concentrations. However, an *in vivo* study with omeprazole did not show an inhibitory effect on omeprazole pharmacokinetics).
No products indexed under this heading.

Trimethadione (*In vitro* data suggest that lacosamide has the potential to inhibit CYP2C19 at therapeutic concentrations. However, an *in vivo* study with omeprazole did not show an inhibitory effect on omeprazole pharmacokinetics).
No products indexed under this heading.

Trimipramine Maleate (*In vitro* data suggest that lacosamide has the potential to inhibit CYP2C19 at therapeutic concentrations. However, an *in vivo* study with omeprazole did not show an inhibitory effect on omeprazole pharmacokinetics).
No products indexed under this heading.

Valproate Sodium (*In vitro* data suggest that lacosamide has the potential to inhibit CYP2C19 at therapeutic concentrations. However, an *in vivo* study with omeprazole did not show an inhibitory effect on omeprazole pharmacokinetics).
No products indexed under this heading.

Valproic Acid (*In vitro* data suggest that lacosamide has the potential to inhibit CYP2C19 at therapeutic concentrations. However, an *in vivo* study with omeprazole did not show an inhibitory effect on omeprazole pharmacokinetics).
No products indexed under this heading.

Verapamil Hydrochloride (Dose-dependent prolongations in PR interval with lacosamide have been observed in clinical studies in patients and in healthy volunteers. When lacosamide is given with other drugs that prolong the PR interval, further PR prolongation is possible). Products include:
Tarka 534

Voriconazole (*In vitro* data suggest that lacosamide has the potential to inhibit CYP2C19 at therapeutic concentrations. However, an *in vivo* study with omeprazole did not show an inhibitory effect on omeprazole pharmacokinetics).
No products indexed under this heading.

Warfarin Sodium (*In vitro* data suggest that lacosamide has the potential to inhibit CYP2C19 at therapeutic concentrations. However, an *in vivo* study with omeprazole did not show an inhibitory effect on omeprazole pharmacokinetics).
No products indexed under this heading.

Zonisamide (*In vitro* data suggest that lacosamide has the potential to inhibit CYP2C19 at therapeutic concentrations. However, an *in vivo* study with omeprazole did not show an inhibitory effect on omeprazole pharmacokinetics). Products include:
Zonegran 1081

VIOKASE POWDER

(Pancrelipase) 800
None cited in PDR database.

VIOKASE TABLETS

(Pancrelipase) 800
None cited in PDR database.

VIRAMUNE ORAL SUSPENSION

(Nevirapine) 897
See Viramune Tablets

VIRAMUNE TABLETS

(Nevirapine) 897
May interact with antiarrhythmics, anticoagulants, anticonvulsants, antineoplastics, azole antifungals, calcium channel blockers, cytochrome p450 3a substrates (selected), drugs affecting gastrointestinal motility, ergot-containing drugs, immunosuppressive agents, narcotic analgesics, oral contraceptives, and certain other agents. Compounds in these categories include:

Acebutolol Hydrochloride (Plasma concentrations of antiarrhythmics may be decreased with concomitant use of nevirapine).
No products indexed under this heading.

Adenosine (Plasma concentrations of antiarrhythmics may be decreased with concomitant use of nevirapine).
Products include:
Adenocard 656
Adenoscan 657

Albuterol (Plasma concentrations of motility agents may be decreased with concomitant use of nevirapine).
No products indexed under this heading.

Albuterol Sulfate (Plasma concentrations of motility agents may be decreased with concomitant use of nevirapine). Products include:
ProAir HFA 3393
Proventil HFA 3204
Ventolin HFA 1708

Alfentanil Hydrochloride (Plasma concentrations of motility agents may be decreased with concomitant use of nevirapine).
No products indexed under this heading.

Alprazolam (Nevirapine is principally metabolized by the liver via cytochrome P450 isoenzymes 3A and 2B6. Nevirapine is known to be an inducer of these enzymes. As a result, drugs that are metabolized by these enzyme systems may have lower than expected plasma levels when co-administered with nevirapine).
No products indexed under this heading.

Altretamine (Plasma concentrations of cancer chemotherapeutic agents may be decreased with concomitant use of nevirapine). Products include:
Hexalen 1066

Aminophylline (Nevirapine is principally metabolized by the liver via cytochrome P450 isoenzymes 3A and 2B6. Nevirapine is known to be an inducer of these enzymes. As a result, drugs that are metabolized by these enzyme systems may have lower than expected plasma levels when co-administered with nevirapine).
No products indexed under this heading.

Amiodarone Hydrochloride (Plasma concentrations of antiarrhythmics may be decreased with concomitant use of nevirapine).
No products indexed under this heading.

Amitriptyline Hydrochloride (Plasma concentrations of motility agents may be decreased with concomitant use of nevirapine).
No products indexed under this heading.

Amlodipine Besylate (Plasma concentrations of calcium channel blockers may be decreased with concomitant use of nevirapine). Products include:
Azor 1010
Exforge 2443
Exforge HCT 2449

Amoxapine (Plasma concentrations of motility agents may be decreased with concomitant use of nevirapine).
No products indexed under this heading.

Anastrozole (Plasma concentrations of cancer chemotherapeutic agents may be decreased with concomitant use of nevirapine).
No products indexed under this heading.

Anisindione (Plasma concentrations of antithrombotics may be increased with concomitant use of nevirapine. This may have a potential effect on anticoagulation. Monitoring of anticoagulation levels is recommended).
No products indexed under this heading.

Apomorphine (Plasma concentrations of motility agents may be decreased with concomitant use of nevirapine).
No products indexed under this heading.

Apomorphine Hydrochloride (Plasma concentrations of motility agents may be decreased with concomitant use of nevirapine).
No products indexed under this heading.

Aprepitant (Nevirapine is principally metabolized by the liver via cytochrome P450 isoenzymes 3A and 2B6. Nevirapine is known to be an inducer of these enzymes. As a result, drugs that are metabolized by these enzyme systems may have lower than expected plasma levels when co-administered with nevirapine). Products include:
Emend 2124

Ardeparin Sodium (Plasma concentrations of antithrombotics may be increased with concomitant use of nevirapine. This may have a potential effect on anticoagulation. Monitoring of anticoagulation levels is recommended).
No products indexed under this heading.

Asparaginase (Plasma concentrations of cancer chemotherapeutic agents may be decreased with concomitant use of nevirapine). Products include:
Elspar 2005, 2122

Astemizole (Plasma concentrations of motility agents may be decreased with concomitant use of nevirapine).
No products indexed under this heading.

Atorvastatin Calcium (Nevirapine is principally metabolized by the liver via cytochrome P450 isoenzymes 3A and 2B6. Nevirapine is known to be an inducer of these enzymes. As a result, drugs that are metabolized by these enzyme systems may have lower than expected plasma levels when co-administered with nevirapine). Products include:
Lipitor 2703

Atropine Sulfate (Plasma concentrations of motility agents may be decreased with concomitant use of nevirapine). Products include:
Donnatal 2711

Azatadine Maleate (Plasma concentrations of motility agents may be decreased with concomitant use of nevirapine).
No products indexed under this heading.

Azathioprine (Plasma concentrations of cancer immunosuppressants agents may be decreased with concomitant use of nevirapine).
No products indexed under this heading.

Basiliximab (Plasma concentrations of cancer immunosuppressants agents may be decreased with concomitant use of nevirapine). Products include:
Simulect 2524

Belladonna Alkaloids (Plasma concentrations of motility agents may be decreased with concomitant use of nevirapine). Products include:
Hyland's Teething Tablets 3316

Benztropine Mesylate (Plasma concentrations of motility agents may be decreased with concomitant use of nevirapine).
No products indexed under this heading.

Bepridil Hydrochloride (Plasma concentrations of calcium channel blockers may be decreased with concomitant use of nevirapine).
No products indexed under this heading.

Bethanechol Chloride (Plasma concentrations of motility agents may be decreased with concomitant use of nevirapine).
No products indexed under this heading.

Bicalutamide (Plasma concentrations of cancer chemotherapeutic agents may be decreased with concomitant use of nevirapine).
No products indexed under this heading.

Biperiden Hydrochloride (Plasma concentrations of motility agents may be decreased with concomitant use of nevirapine).
No products indexed under this heading.

Bitolterol Mesylate (Plasma concentrations of motility agents may be decreased with concomitant use of nevirapine).
No products indexed under this heading.

Bleomycin Sulfate (Plasma concentrations of cancer chemotherapeutic agents may be decreased with concomitant use of nevirapine).
No products indexed under this heading.

Bretylium Tosylate (Plasma concentrations of antiarrhythmics may be decreased with concomitant use of nevirapine).
No products indexed under this heading.

Bromocriptine Mesylate (Plasma concentrations of motility agents may be decreased with concomitant use of nevirapine).
No products indexed under this heading.

Bromodiphenhydramine Hydrochloride (Plasma concentrations of motility agents may be decreased with concomitant use of nevirapine).
No products indexed under this heading.

Brompheniramine Maleate (Plasma concentrations of motility agents may be decreased with concomitant use of nevirapine).
No products indexed under this heading.

Buprenorphine Hydrochloride (Plasma concentrations of motility agents may be decreased with concomitant use of nevirapine).
No products indexed under this heading.

Buspirone Hydrochloride (Nevirapine is principally metabolized by the liver via cytochrome P450 isoenzymes 3A and 2B6. Nevirapine is known to be an inducer of these enzymes. As a result, drugs that are metabolized by these enzyme systems may have lower than expected plasma levels when co-administered with nevirapine).
No products indexed under this heading.

Busulfan (Plasma concentrations of cancer chemotherapeutic agents may be decreased with concomitant use of nevirapine). Products include:
Myleran 1581

Butoconazole Nitrate (Plasma concentrations of antifungals may be decreased with concomitant use of nevirapine).
No products indexed under this heading.

Carbamazepine (Plasma concentrations of anticonvulsants may be decreased with concomitant use of nevirapine). Products include:
Carbatrol 3280
Equetro 3477

Carboplatin (Plasma concentrations of cancer chemotherapeutic agents may be decreased with concomitant use of nevirapine).
No products indexed under this heading.

Carmustine (BCNU) (Plasma concentrations of cancer chemotherapeutic agents may be decreased with concomitant use of nevirapine).
No products indexed under this heading.

Cerivastatin Sodium (Nevirapine is principally metabolized by the liver via cytochrome P450 isoenzymes 3A and 2B6. Nevirapine is known to be an inducer of these enzymes. As a result, drugs that are metabolized by these enzyme systems may have lower than expected plasma levels when co-administered with nevirapine).
No products indexed under this heading.

Cevimeline Hydrochloride (Plasma concentrations of motility agents may be decreased with concomitant use of nevirapine). Products include:

IMPORTANT NOTE: Always consult each drug listing in the patient's regimen for possible interactions.

(⊙ Described in PDR® for Ophthalmic Medicines)

Doxorubicin Hydrochloride (Plasma concentrations of cancer chemotherapeutic agents may be decreased with concomitant use of nevirapine).

No products indexed under this heading.

Dronabinol (Nevirapine is principally metabolized by the liver via cytochrome P450 isoenzymes 3A and 2B6. Nevirapine is known to be an inducer of these enzymes. As a result, drugs that are metabolized by these enzyme systems may have lower than expected plasma levels when co-administered with nevirapine).

No products indexed under this heading.

Dyphylline (Nevirapine is principally metabolized by the liver via cytochrome P450 isoenzymes 3A and 2B6. Nevirapine is known to be an inducer of these enzymes. As a result, drugs that are metabolized by these enzyme systems may have lower than expected plasma levels when co-administered with nevirapine).

No products indexed under this heading.

Econazole Nitrate (Plasma concentrations of antifungals may be decreased with concomitant use of nevirapine).

No products indexed under this heading.

Edrophonium Chloride (Plasma concentrations of motility agents may be decreased with concomitant use of nevirapine).

No products indexed under this heading.

Efavirenz (Efavirenz concentrations are decreased when used concomitantly with nevirapine. Appropriate doses for this combination are not established). Products include:

Atripla 906

Enoxaparin Sodium (Plasma concentrations of antithrombotics may be increased with concomitant use of nevirapine. This may have a potential effect on anticoagulation. Monitoring of anticoagulation levels is recommended). Products include:

Lovenox 3005

Ephedrine Hydrochloride (Plasma concentrations of motility agents may be decreased with concomitant use of nevirapine).

No products indexed under this heading.

Ephedrine Sulfate (Plasma concentrations of motility agents may be decreased with concomitant use of nevirapine).

No products indexed under this heading.

Ephedrine Tannate (Plasma concentrations of motility agents may be decreased with concomitant use of nevirapine).

No products indexed under this heading.

Epinephrine (Plasma concentrations of motility agents may be decreased with concomitant use of nevirapine). Products include:

EpiPen 3631
Twinject 3268

Epinephrine Hydrochloride (Plasma concentrations of motility agents may be decreased with concomitant use of nevirapine).

No products indexed under this heading.

Epirubicin Hydrochloride (Plasma concentrations of cancer chemotherapeutic agents may be decreased with concomitant use of nevirapine).

No products indexed under this heading.

Ergonovine Maleate (Plasma concentrations of ergot alkaloids may be decreased with concomitant use of nevirapine).

No products indexed under this heading.

Ergotamine Tartrate (Plasma concentrations of ergot alkaloids may be decreased with concomitant use of nevirapine).

No products indexed under this heading.

Erythromycin (Plasma concentrations of motility agents may be decreased with concomitant use of nevirapine).

No products indexed under this heading.

Erythromycin Estolate (Plasma concentrations of motility agents may be decreased with concomitant use of nevirapine).

No products indexed under this heading.

Erythromycin Ethylsuccinate (Plasma concentrations of motility agents may be decreased with concomitant use of nevirapine). Products include:

E.E.S. 437
EryPed 435

Erythromycin Gluceptate (Plasma concentrations of motility agents may be decreased with concomitant use of nevirapine).

No products indexed under this heading.

Erythromycin Lactobionate (Nevirapine is principally metabolized by the liver via cytochrome P450 isoenzymes 3A and 2B6. Nevirapine is known to be an inducer of these enzymes. As a result, drugs that are metabolized by these enzyme systems may have lower than expected plasma levels when co-administered with nevirapine).

No products indexed under this heading.

Erythromycin Stearate (Plasma concentrations of motility agents may be decreased with concomitant use of nevirapine).

No products indexed under this heading.

Estramustine Phosphate Sodium (Plasma concentrations of cancer chemotherapeutic agents may be decreased with concomitant use of nevirapine).

No products indexed under this heading.

Estrogen (Nevirapine is principally metabolized by the liver via cytochrome P450 isoenzymes 3A and 2B6. Nevirapine is known to be an inducer of these enzymes. As a result, drugs that are metabolized by these enzyme systems may have lower than expected plasma levels when co-administered with nevirapine).

No products indexed under this heading.

Estrogens, Conjugated (Nevirapine is principally metabolized by the liver via cytochrome P450 isoenzymes 3A and 2B6. Nevirapine is known to be an inducer of these enzymes. As a result, drugs that are metabolized by these enzyme systems may have lower than expected plasma levels when co-administered with nevirapine). Products include:

Premarin Intravenous 3528
Premarin Tablets 3533
Premarin Vaginal Cream 3540
Premphase 3549
Prempro 3549

Estrogens, Conjugated, Synthetic A (Nevirapine is principally metabolized by the liver via cytochrome P450 isoenzymes 3A and 2B6. Nevirapine is known to be an inducer of these enzymes. As a result, drugs that are metabolized by these enzyme systems may have lower than expected plasma levels when co-administered with nevirapine).

No products indexed under this heading.

Estrogens, Esterified (Nevirapine is principally metabolized by the liver via cytochrome P450 isoenzymes 3A and 2B6. Nevirapine is known to be an inducer of these enzymes. As a result, drugs that are metabolized by these enzyme systems may have lower than expected plasma levels when co-administered with nevirapine).

No products indexed under this heading.

Ethinyl Estradiol (Oral contraceptives and other hormonal methods of birth control should not be used as the sole method of contraception in women taking nevirapine, since nevirapine may

lower the plasma levels of these medications. An alternative or additional method of contraception is recommended). Products include:

LoSeasonique 3407
Lybrel 3514
NuvaRing 3181
Ortho Evra 2648
Ortho-Cyclen/Ortho Tri-Cyclen 2663
Ortho Tri-Cyclen Lo Tablets 2673
Seasonique 3418
Yaz 864

Ethosuximide (Plasma concentrations of anticonvulsants may be decreased with concomitant use of nevirapine).

No products indexed under this heading.

Ethotoin (Plasma concentrations of anticonvulsants may be decreased with concomitant use of nevirapine).

No products indexed under this heading.

Ethynodiol Diacetate (Oral contraceptives and other hormonal methods of birth control should not be used as the sole method of contraception in women taking nevirapine, since nevirapine may lower the plasma levels of these medications. An alternative or additional method of contraception is recommended).

No products indexed under this heading.

Etoposide (Plasma concentrations of cancer chemotherapeutic agents may be decreased with concomitant use of nevirapine).

No products indexed under this heading.

Etoposide Phosphate (Nevirapine is principally metabolized by the liver via cytochrome P450 isoenzymes 3A and 2B6. Nevirapine is known to be an inducer of these enzymes. As a result, drugs that are metabolized by these enzyme systems may have lower than expected plasma levels when co-administered with nevirapine).

No products indexed under this heading.

Exemestane (Plasma concentrations of cancer chemotherapeutic agents may be decreased with concomitant use of nevirapine). Products include:

Aromasin 2758

Felbamate (Plasma concentrations of anticonvulsants may be decreased with concomitant use of nevirapine).

No products indexed under this heading.

Felodipine (Plasma concentrations of calcium channel blockers may be decreased with concomitant use of nevirapine).

No products indexed under this heading.

Fentanyl (Plasma concentrations of motility agents may be decreased with concomitant use of nevirapine). Products include:

Duragesic 2604
Fentanyl Transdermal System 2346
Onsolis 2054

Fentanyl Citrate (Plasma concentrations of motility agents may be decreased with concomitant use of nevirapine). Products include:

Fentora 966

Flecainide Acetate (Plasma concentrations of antiarrhythmics may be decreased with concomitant use of nevirapine).

No products indexed under this heading.

Floxuridine (Plasma concentrations of cancer chemotherapeutic agents may be decreased with concomitant use of nevirapine).

No products indexed under this heading.

Fluconazole (Nevirapine concentrations are increased when used concomitantly with fluconazole. Because of the risk of increased exposure to nevirapine, caution should be used in concomitant administration and patients should be monitored closely for nevirapine-associated adverse events).

No products indexed under this heading.

Fluorouracil (Plasma concentrations of cancer chemotherapeutic agents may be decreased with concomitant use of nevirapine). Products include:

Carac 2966

Flutamide (Plasma concentrations of cancer chemotherapeutic agents may be decreased with concomitant use of nevirapine).

No products indexed under this heading.

Fondaparinux Sodium (Plasma concentrations of antithrombotics may be increased with concomitant use of nevirapine. This may have a potential effect on anticoagulation. Monitoring of anticoagulation levels is recommended). Products include:

Arixtra 1320

Fosphenytoin (Plasma concentrations of anticonvulsants may be decreased with concomitant use of nevirapine).

No products indexed under this heading.

Fosphenytoin Sodium (Plasma concentrations of anticonvulsants may be decreased with concomitant use of nevirapine).

No products indexed under this heading.

Gabapentin (Plasma concentrations of anticonvulsants may be decreased with concomitant use of nevirapine).

No products indexed under this heading.

Galantamine Hydrobromide (Plasma concentrations of motility agents may be decreased with concomitant use of nevirapine).

No products indexed under this heading.

Gemcitabine Hydrochloride (Plasma concentrations of cancer chemotherapeutic agents may be decreased with concomitant use of nevirapine). Products include:

Gemzar 1900

Glyburide (Nevirapine is principally metabolized by the liver via cytochrome P450 isoenzymes 3A and 2B6. Nevirapine is known to be an inducer of these enzymes. As a result, drugs that are metabolized by these enzyme systems may have lower than expected plasma levels when co-administered with nevirapine).

No products indexed under this heading.

Glycopyrrolate (Plasma concentrations of motility agents may be decreased with concomitant use of nevirapine).

No products indexed under this heading.

Haloperidol (Nevirapine is principally metabolized by the liver via cytochrome P450 isoenzymes 3A and 2B6. Nevirapine is known to be an inducer of these enzymes. As a result, drugs that are metabolized by these enzyme systems may have lower than expected plasma levels when co-administered with nevirapine).

No products indexed under this heading.

Haloperidol Decanoate (Nevirapine is principally metabolized by the liver via cytochrome P450 isoenzymes 3A and 2B6. Nevirapine is known to be an inducer of these enzymes. As a result, drugs that are metabolized by these enzyme systems may have lower than expected plasma levels when co-administered with nevirapine).

No products indexed under this heading.

Heparin Calcium (Plasma concentrations of antithrombotics may be increased with concomitant use of nevirapine. This may have a potential effect on anticoagulation. Monitoring of anticoagulation levels is recommended).

No products indexed under this heading.

Heparin Sodium (Plasma concentrations of antithrombotics may be increased with concomitant use of nevirapine. This may have a potential effect on anticoagulation. Monitoring of anticoagulation levels is recommended).

No products indexed under this heading.

IMPORTANT NOTE: Always consult each drug listing in the patient's regimen for possible interactions.

2067 Interactions Index Viramune

Methylprednisolone Sodium Succinate (Nevirapine is principally metabolized by the liver via cytochrome P450 isoenzymes 3A and 2B6. Nevirapine is known to be an inducer of these enzymes. As a result, drugs that are metabolized by these enzyme systems may have lower than expected plasma levels when co-administered with nevirapine).
No products indexed under this heading.

Methysergide Maleate (Plasma concentrations of ergot alkaloids may be decreased with concomitant use of nevirapine).
No products indexed under this heading.

Metoclopramide Hydrochloride (Plasma concentrations of motility agents may be decreased with concomitant use of nevirapine). Products include:
Metozolv ODT 2901

Mexiletine Hydrochloride (Plasma concentrations of antiarrhythmics may be decreased with concomitant use of nevirapine).
No products indexed under this heading.

Mibefradil Dihydrochloride (Plasma concentrations of calcium channel blockers may be decreased with concomitant use of nevirapine).
No products indexed under this heading.

Miconazole (Plasma concentrations of antifungals may be decreased with concomitant use of nevirapine).
No products indexed under this heading.

Midazolam Hydrochloride (Nevirapine is principally metabolized by the liver via cytochrome P450 isoenzymes 3A and 2B6. Nevirapine is known to be an inducer of these enzymes. As a result, drugs that are metabolized by these enzyme systems may have lower than expected plasma levels when co-administered with nevirapine).
No products indexed under this heading.

Mitomycin (Mitomycin-C) (Plasma concentrations of cancer chemotherapeutic agents may be decreased with concomitant use of nevirapine).
No products indexed under this heading.

Mitotane (Plasma concentrations of cancer chemotherapeutic agents may be decreased with concomitant use of nevirapine).
No products indexed under this heading.

Mitoxantrone Hydrochloride (Plasma concentrations of cancer chemotherapeutic agents may be decreased with concomitant use of nevirapine). Products include:
Novantrone 1088

Moricizine Hydrochloride (Plasma concentrations of antiarrhythmics may be decreased with concomitant use of nevirapine).
No products indexed under this heading.

Morphine Sulfate (Plasma concentrations of motility agents may be decreased with concomitant use of nevirapine). Products include:
Avinza 1822
Embeda 1831
MS Contin 2803

Morphine Sulfate, Liposomal (Plasma concentrations of motility agents may be decreased with concomitant use of nevirapine).
No products indexed under this heading.

Muromonab-CD3 (Plasma concentrations of cancer immunosuppressants agents may be decreased with concomitant use of nevirapine). Products include:
Orthoclone OKT3 949

Mycophenolate Mofetil (Plasma concentrations of cancer immunosuppressants agents may be decreased with concomitant use of nevirapine).
No products indexed under this heading.

Nefazodone Hydrochloride (Nevirapine is principally metabolized by the liver via cytochrome P450 isoenzymes 3A and 2B6. Nevirapine is known to be an inducer of these enzymes. As a result, drugs that are metabolized by these enzyme systems may have lower than expected plasma levels when co-administered with nevirapine).
No products indexed under this heading.

Nelfinavir Mesylate (Concomitant use with nevirapine has shown a decrease in nelfinavir M8 metabolite concentrations and a decrease in nevirapine C_{min}. The appropriate dose for nelfinavir in combination with nevirapine, with respect to safety and efficacy, has not been established).
No products indexed under this heading.

Neostigmine Bromide (Plasma concentrations of motility agents may be decreased with concomitant use of nevirapine).
No products indexed under this heading.

Neostigmine Methylsulfate (Plasma concentrations of motility agents may be decreased with concomitant use of nevirapine).
No products indexed under this heading.

Nicardipine (Plasma concentrations of calcium channel blockers may be decreased with concomitant use of nevirapine).
No products indexed under this heading.

Nicardipine Hydrochloride (Plasma concentrations of calcium channel blockers may be decreased with concomitant use of nevirapine).
No products indexed under this heading.

Nifedipine (Plasma concentrations of calcium channel blockers may be decreased with concomitant use of nevirapine).
No products indexed under this heading.

Nimodipine (Plasma concentrations of calcium channel blockers may be decreased with concomitant use of nevirapine).
No products indexed under this heading.

Nisoldipine (Plasma concentrations of calcium channel blockers may be decreased with concomitant use of nevirapine).
No products indexed under this heading.

Norethindrone (Oral contraceptives and other hormonal methods of birth control should not be used as the sole method of contraception in women taking nevirapine, since nevirapine may lower the plasma levels of these medications. An alternative or additional method of contraception is recommended). Products include:
Ortho Micronor 2660

Norethindrone Acetate (Oral contraceptives and other hormonal methods of birth control should not be used as the sole method of contraception in women taking nevirapine, since nevirapine may lower the plasma levels of these medications. An alternative or additional method of contraception is recommended). Products include:
Activella 2561

Norethynodrel (Oral contraceptives and other hormonal methods of birth control should not be used as the sole method of contraception in women taking nevirapine, since nevirapine may lower the plasma levels of these medications. An alternative or additional method of contraception is recommended).
No products indexed under this heading.

Norgestimate (Oral contraceptives and other hormonal methods of birth control should not be used as the sole method of contraception in women taking nevirapine, since nevirapine may lower the plasma levels of these medications. An alternative or additional method of contraception is recommended). Products include:
Ortho-Cyclen/Ortho Tri-Cyclen 2663
Ortho Tri-Cyclen Lo Tablets 2673

Norgestrel (Oral contraceptives and other hormonal methods of birth control should not be used as the sole method of contraception in women taking nevirapine, since nevirapine may lower the plasma levels of these medications. An alternative or additional method of contraception is recommended).
No products indexed under this heading.

Nortriptyline Hydrochloride (Plasma concentrations of motility agents may be decreased with concomitant use of nevirapine).
No products indexed under this heading.

Octreotide Acetate (Plasma concentrations of motility agents may be decreased with concomitant use of nevirapine). Products include:
Sandostatin 2517
Sandostatin LAR 2519

Ondansetron Hydrochloride (Nevirapine is principally metabolized by the liver via cytochrome P450 isoenzymes 3A and 2B6. Nevirapine is known to be an inducer of these enzymes. As a result, drugs that are metabolized by these enzyme systems may have lower than expected plasma levels when co-administered with nevirapine). Products include:
Zofran Injection 1750
Zofran 1756
Zofran ODT 1756

Oxaliplatin (Plasma concentrations of cancer chemotherapeutic agents may be decreased with concomitant use of nevirapine). Products include:
Eloxatin 2975

Oxcarbazepine (Plasma concentrations of anticonvulsants may be decreased with concomitant use of nevirapine).
No products indexed under this heading.

Oxiconazole Nitrate (Plasma concentrations of antifungals may be decreased with concomitant use of nevirapine).
No products indexed under this heading.

Oxybutynin Chloride (Plasma concentrations of motility agents may be decreased with concomitant use of nevirapine).
No products indexed under this heading.

Oxycodone Hydrochloride (Plasma concentrations of motility agents may be decreased with concomitant use of nevirapine). Products include:
OxyContin 2807
Percocet 1121
Percodan 1124

Oxycodone Terephthalate (Plasma concentrations of motility agents may be decreased with concomitant use of nevirapine).
No products indexed under this heading.

Oxymorphone Hydrochloride (Plasma concentrations of motility agents may be decreased with concomitant use of nevirapine). Products include:
Opana 1110
Opana ER 1114

Oxyphenonium Bromide (Plasma concentrations of motility agents may be decreased with concomitant use of nevirapine).
No products indexed under this heading.

Paclitaxel (Plasma concentrations of cancer chemotherapeutic agents may be decreased with concomitant use of nevirapine).
No products indexed under this heading.

Paramethadione (Plasma concentrations of anticonvulsants may be decreased with concomitant use of nevirapine).
No products indexed under this heading.

Pergolide Mesylate (Plasma concentrations of motility agents may be decreased with concomitant use of nevirapine).
No products indexed under this heading.

Phenacemide (Plasma concentrations of anticonvulsants may be decreased with concomitant use of nevirapine).
No products indexed under this heading.

Phenobarbital (Plasma concentrations of anticonvulsants may be decreased with concomitant use of nevirapine). Products include:
Donnatal 2711

Phenobarbital Sodium (Plasma concentrations of anticonvulsants may be decreased with concomitant use of nevirapine).
No products indexed under this heading.

Phensuximide (Plasma concentrations of anticonvulsants may be decreased with concomitant use of nevirapine).
No products indexed under this heading.

Phenytoin (Plasma concentrations of anticonvulsants may be decreased with concomitant use of nevirapine).
No products indexed under this heading.

Phenytoin Sodium (Plasma concentrations of anticonvulsants may be decreased with concomitant use of nevirapine). Products include:
Phenytek Capsules 2380

Pimozide (Nevirapine is principally metabolized by the liver via cytochrome P450 isoenzymes 3A and 2B6. Nevirapine is known to be an inducer of these enzymes. As a result, drugs that are metabolized by these enzyme systems may have lower than expected plasma levels when co-administered with nevirapine).
No products indexed under this heading.

Pirbuterol Acetate (Plasma concentrations of motility agents may be decreased with concomitant use of nevirapine). Products include:
Maxair Autohaler 1782

Posaconazole (Plasma concentrations of antifungals may be decreased with concomitant use of nevirapine). Products include:
Noxafil 3172

Pramipexole Dihydrochloride (Plasma concentrations of motility agents may be decreased with concomitant use of nevirapine).
No products indexed under this heading.

Primidone (Plasma concentrations of anticonvulsants may be decreased with concomitant use of nevirapine).
No products indexed under this heading.

Procainamide Hydrochloride (Plasma concentrations of antiarrhythmics may be decreased with concomitant use of nevirapine).
No products indexed under this heading.

Procarbazine Hydrochloride (Plasma concentrations of cancer chemotherapeutic agents may be decreased with concomitant use of nevirapine).
No products indexed under this heading.

Procyclidine Hydrochloride (Plasma concentrations of motility agents may be decreased with concomitant use of nevirapine).
No products indexed under this heading.

Promethazine Hydrochloride (Plasma concentrations of motility agents may be decreased with concomitant use of nevirapine).
No products indexed under this heading.

Propafenone Hydrochloride (Plasma concentrations of antiarrhythmics may be decreased with concomitant use of nevirapine). Products include:
Rythmol 1648
Rythmol SR 1652

IMPORTANT NOTE: Always consult each drug listing in the patient's regimen for possible interactions.

Viramune Interactions Index 2068

Propantheline Bromide (Plasma concentrations of motility agents may be decreased with concomitant use of nevirapine).
No products indexed under this heading.

Propoxyphene Hydrochloride (Plasma concentrations of motility agents may be decreased with concomitant use of nevirapine).
No products indexed under this heading.

Propoxyphene Napsylate (Plasma concentrations of motility agents may be decreased with concomitant use of nevirapine).
No products indexed under this heading.

Propranolol Hydrochloride (Plasma concentrations of antiarrhythmics may be decreased with concomitant use of nevirapine). Products include:
InnoPran XL 1517

Protriptyline Hydrochloride (Plasma concentrations of motility agents may be decreased with concomitant use of nevirapine).
No products indexed under this heading.

Pyridostigmine Bromide (Plasma concentrations of motility agents may be decreased with concomitant use of nevirapine).
No products indexed under this heading.

Pyrilamine Maleate (Plasma concentrations of motility agents may be decreased with concomitant use of nevirapine).
No products indexed under this heading.

Pyrilamine Tannate (Plasma concentrations of motility agents may be decreased with concomitant use of nevirapine).
No products indexed under this heading.

Quinidine Gluconate (Plasma concentrations of antiarrhythmics may be decreased with concomitant use of nevirapine).
No products indexed under this heading.

Quinidine Polygalacturonate (Plasma concentrations of antiarrhythmics may be decreased with concomitant use of nevirapine).
No products indexed under this heading.

Quinidine Sulfate (Plasma concentrations of antiarrhythmics may be decreased with concomitant use of nevirapine).
No products indexed under this heading.

Quinine (Nevirapine is principally metabolized by the liver via cytochrome P450 isoenzymes 3A and 2B6. Nevirapine is known to be an inducer of these enzymes. As a result, drugs that are metabolized by these enzyme systems may have lower than expected plasma levels when co-administered with nevirapine). Products include:
Hyland's Leg Cramps PM with Quinine 3315

Quinine Sulfate (Nevirapine is principally metabolized by the liver via cytochrome P450 isoenzymes 3A and 2B6. Nevirapine is known to be an inducer of these enzymes. As a result, drugs that are metabolized by these enzyme systems may have lower than expected plasma levels when co-administered with nevirapine).
No products indexed under this heading.

Rapamycin (Plasma concentrations of cancer immunosuppressants agents may be decreased with concomitant use of nevirapine).
No products indexed under this heading.

Remifentanil Hydrochloride (Plasma concentrations of motility agents may be decreased with concomitant use of nevirapine).
No products indexed under this heading.

Rifabutin (Rifabutin and its metabolite concentrations were moderately increased. Due to high inter-subject variability; however, some patients may experience large increases in rifabutin exposure and may be at higher risk for rifabutin toxicity. Therefore, caution should be used in concomitant administration).
No products indexed under this heading.

Rifampin (Nevirapine and rifampin should not be administered concomitantly because decreases in nevirapine plasma concentrations may reduce the efficacy of the drug. Physicians needing to treat patients co-infected with tuberculosis and using a nevirapine-containing regimen may use rifabutin instead).
No products indexed under this heading.

Ritonavir (A dose increase of lopinavir/ritonavir tablets to 100/150 mg b.i.d. may be considered when used in combination with nevirapine in treatment experienced patients where decreased susceptibility to lopinavir is suspected. A dose increase of lopinavir/ritonavir oral solution to 533/133 mg b.i.d. with food is recommended in combination with nevirapine. In children 6 months to 12 years of age, consideration should be given to increasing the dose of lopinavir/ritonavir to 12/3.25 mg/kg for those 7 to less than 15 kg; 11/2.75 mg/kg for those 15 to 45 kg; and a maximum dose of 533/133 mg for those greater than 45 kg b.i.d. when used in combination with nevirapine, particularly for patients in who reduced susceptibility to lopinavir/ritonavir is suspected).
Products include:
Kaletra 458
Norvir 509

Rivastigmine Tartrate (Plasma concentrations of motility agents may be decreased with concomitant use of nevirapine). Products include:
Exelon 2432
Exelon Oral 2432
Exelon Patch 2437

Ropinirole Hydrochloride (Plasma concentrations of motility agents may be decreased with concomitant use of nevirapine). Products include:
Requip 1620
Requip XL 1628

Rufinamide (Plasma concentrations of anticonvulsants may be decreased with concomitant use of nevirapine).
Products include:
Banzel 1050

Salmeterol Xinafoate (Plasma concentrations of motility agents may be decreased with concomitant use of nevirapine). Products include:
Advair 100/50 1275
Advair 250/50 1275
Advair 500/50 1275
Advair HFA 45/21 1288
Advair HFA 115/21 1288
Advair HFA 230/21 1288
Serevent Diskus 1656

Saquinavir (Concomitant use with nevirapine may decrease the concentrations of saquinavir. Appropriate doses for this combination are not established, but an increase in the dosage of saquinavir may be required).
No products indexed under this heading.

Saquinavir Mesylate (Concomitant use with nevirapine may decrease the concentrations of saquinavir. Appropriate doses for this combination are not established, but an increase in the dosage of saquinavir may be required).
No products indexed under this heading.

Scopolamine (Plasma concentrations of motility agents may be decreased with concomitant use of nevirapine).
Products include:
Transderm Scōp 2397

Scopolamine Hydrobromide (Plasma concentrations of motility agents may be decreased with concomitant use of nevirapine). Products include:
Donnatal 2711

Sertaconazole Nitrate (Plasma concentrations of antifungals may be decreased with concomitant use of nevirapine).
No products indexed under this heading.

Sertraline Hydrochloride (Nevirapine is principally metabolized by the liver via cytochrome P450 isoenzymes 3A and 2B6. Nevirapine is known to be an inducer of these enzymes. As a result, drugs that are metabolized by these enzyme systems may have lower than expected plasma levels when co-administered with nevirapine).
No products indexed under this heading.

Sildenafil Citrate (Nevirapine is principally metabolized by the liver via cytochrome P450 isoenzymes 3A and 2B6. Nevirapine is known to be an inducer of these enzymes. As a result, drugs that are metabolized by these enzyme systems may have lower than expected plasma levels when co-administered with nevirapine).
No products indexed under this heading.

Simvastatin (Nevirapine is principally metabolized by the liver via cytochrome P450 isoenzymes 3A and 2B6. Nevirapine is known to be an inducer of these enzymes. As a result, drugs that are metabolized by these enzyme systems may have lower than expected plasma levels when co-administered with nevirapine). Products include:
Simcor 524
Vytorin 10/10 .... 2303, 3240
Vytorin 10/20 .... 2303, 3240
Vytorin 10/40 .... 2303, 3240
Vytorin 10/80 .... 2303, 3240
Zocor 2289

Sirolimus (Plasma concentrations of cancer immunosuppressants agents may be decreased with concomitant use of nevirapine). Products include:
Rapamune 3579

Sotalol Hydrochloride (Plasma concentrations of antiarrhythmics may be decreased with concomitant use of nevirapine).
No products indexed under this heading.

Streptozocin (Plasma concentrations of cancer chemotherapeutic agents may be decreased with concomitant use of nevirapine).
No products indexed under this heading.

Sucralfate (Plasma concentrations of motility agents may be decreased with concomitant use of nevirapine).
Products include:
Carafate Suspension 784
Carafate Tablets 785

Sufentanil Citrate (Plasma concentrations of motility agents may be decreased with concomitant use of nevirapine).
No products indexed under this heading.

Tacrine Hydrochloride (Plasma concentrations of motility agents may be decreased with concomitant use of nevirapine).
No products indexed under this heading.

Tacrolimus (Plasma concentrations of cancer immunosuppressants agents may be decreased with concomitant use of nevirapine). Products include:
Prograf Capsules 677
Prograf Injection 677
Protopic 685

Tamoxifen Citrate (Plasma concentrations of cancer chemotherapeutic agents may be decreased with concomitant use of nevirapine).
No products indexed under this heading.

Teniposide (Plasma concentrations of cancer chemotherapeutic agents may be decreased with concomitant use of nevirapine).
No products indexed under this heading.

Terbutaline Sulfate (Plasma concentrations of motility agents may be decreased with concomitant use of nevirapine).
No products indexed under this heading.

Terconazole (Plasma concentrations of antifungals may be decreased with concomitant use of nevirapine).
No products indexed under this heading.

Terfenadine (Nevirapine is principally metabolized by the liver via cytochrome P450 isoenzymes 3A and 2B6. Nevirapine is known to be an inducer of these enzymes. As a result, drugs that are metabolized by these enzyme systems may have lower than expected plasma levels when co-administered with nevirapine).
No products indexed under this heading.

Testosterone (Nevirapine is principally metabolized by the liver via cytochrome P450 isoenzymes 3A and 2B6. Nevirapine is known to be an inducer of these enzymes. As a result, drugs that are metabolized by these enzyme systems may have lower than expected plasma levels when co-administered with nevirapine). Products include:
AndroGel 3456

Testosterone Cypionate (Nevirapine is principally metabolized by the liver via cytochrome P450 isoenzymes 3A and 2B6. Nevirapine is known to be an inducer of these enzymes. As a result, drugs that are metabolized by these enzyme systems may have lower than expected plasma levels when co-administered with nevirapine).
No products indexed under this heading.

Testosterone Enanthate (Nevirapine is principally metabolized by the liver via cytochrome P450 isoenzymes 3A and 2B6. Nevirapine is known to be an inducer of these enzymes. As a result, drugs that are metabolized by these enzyme systems may have lower than expected plasma levels when co-administered with nevirapine). Products include:
Delatestryl 1102

Testosterone Propionate (Nevirapine is principally metabolized by the liver via cytochrome P450 isoenzymes 3A and 2B6. Nevirapine is known to be an inducer of these enzymes. As a result, drugs that are metabolized by these enzyme systems may have lower than expected plasma levels when co-administered with nevirapine).
No products indexed under this heading.

Theophylline (Nevirapine is principally metabolized by the liver via cytochrome P450 isoenzymes 3A and 2B6. Nevirapine is known to be an inducer of these enzymes. As a result, drugs that are metabolized by these enzyme systems may have lower than expected plasma levels when co-administered with nevirapine).
No products indexed under this heading.

Theophylline Anhydrous (Nevirapine is principally metabolized by the liver via cytochrome P450 isoenzymes 3A and 2B6. Nevirapine is known to be an inducer of these enzymes. As a result, drugs that are metabolized by these enzyme systems may have lower than expected plasma levels when co-administered with nevirapine). Products include:
Uniphyl 2817

2069 Interactions Index Viread

Theophylline Calcium Salicylate (Nevirapine is principally metabolized by the liver via cytochrome P450 isoenzymes 3A and 2B6. Nevirapine is known to be an inducer of these enzymes. As a result, drugs that are metabolized by these enzyme systems may have lower than expected plasma levels when co-administered with nevirapine).
No products indexed under this heading.

Theophylline Sodium Glycinate (Nevirapine is principally metabolized by the liver via cytochrome P450 isoenzymes 3A and 2B6. Nevirapine is known to be an inducer of these enzymes. As a result, drugs that are metabolized by these enzyme systems may have lower than expected plasma levels when co-administered with nevirapine).
No products indexed under this heading.

Thioguanine (Plasma concentrations of cancer chemotherapeutic agents may be decreased with concomitant use of nevirapine). Products include:
Tabloid **1664**

Thiotepa (Plasma concentrations of cancer chemotherapeutic agents may be decreased with concomitant use of nevirapine).
No products indexed under this heading.

Tiagabine Hydrochloride (Plasma concentrations of anticonvulsants may be decreased with concomitant use of nevirapine). Products include:
Gabitril **972**

Tinzaparin Sodium (Plasma concentrations of antithrombotics may be increased with concomitant use of nevirapine. This may have a potential effect on anticoagulation. Monitoring of anticoagulation levels is recommended).
No products indexed under this heading.

Tocainide Hydrochloride (Plasma concentrations of antiarrhythmics may be decreased with concomitant use of nevirapine).
No products indexed under this heading.

Tolterodine Tartrate (Plasma concentrations of motility agents may be decreased with concomitant use of nevirapine).
No products indexed under this heading.

Topiramate (Plasma concentrations of anticonvulsants may be decreased with concomitant use of nevirapine).
No products indexed under this heading.

Topotecan Hydrochloride (Plasma concentrations of cancer chemotherapeutic agents may be decreased with concomitant use of nevirapine). Products include:
Hycamtin **1491**
Hycamtin Capsules **1488**

Toremifene Citrate (Plasma concentrations of cancer chemotherapeutic agents may be decreased with concomitant use of nevirapine).
No products indexed under this heading.

Trazodone Hydrochloride (Nevirapine is principally metabolized by the liver via cytochrome P450 isoenzymes 3A and 2B6. Nevirapine is known to be an inducer of these enzymes. As a result, drugs that are metabolized by these enzyme systems may have lower than expected plasma levels when co-administered with nevirapine).
No products indexed under this heading.

Triazolam (Nevirapine is principally metabolized by the liver via cytochrome P450 isoenzymes 3A and 2B6. Nevirapine is known to be an inducer of these enzymes. As a result, drugs that are metabolized by these enzyme systems may have lower than expected plasma levels when co-administered with nevirapine).
No products indexed under this heading.

Tridihexethyl Chloride (Plasma concentrations of motility agents may be decreased with concomitant use of nevirapine).
No products indexed under this heading.

Trihexyphenidyl Hydrochloride (Plasma concentrations of motility agents may be decreased with concomitant use of nevirapine).
No products indexed under this heading.

Trimeprazine Tartrate (Plasma concentrations of motility agents may be decreased with concomitant use of nevirapine).
No products indexed under this heading.

Trimethadione (Plasma concentrations of anticonvulsants may be decreased with concomitant use of nevirapine).
No products indexed under this heading.

Trimipramine Maleate (Plasma concentrations of motility agents may be decreased with concomitant use of nevirapine).
No products indexed under this heading.

Tripelennamine Hydrochloride (Plasma concentrations of motility agents may be decreased with concomitant use of nevirapine).
No products indexed under this heading.

Triprolidine Hydrochloride (Plasma concentrations of motility agents may be decreased with concomitant use of nevirapine).
No products indexed under this heading.

Valproate Sodium (Plasma concentrations of anticonvulsants may be decreased with concomitant use of nevirapine).
No products indexed under this heading.

Valproic Acid (Plasma concentrations of anticonvulsants may be decreased with concomitant use of nevirapine).
No products indexed under this heading.

Valrubicin (Plasma concentrations of cancer chemotherapeutic agents may be decreased with concomitant use of nevirapine). Products include:
Valstar **1131**

Venlafaxine Hydrochloride (Nevirapine is principally metabolized by the liver via cytochrome P450 isoenzymes 3A and 2B6. Nevirapine is known to be an inducer of these enzymes. As a result, drugs that are metabolized by these enzyme systems may have lower than expected plasma levels when co-administered with nevirapine). Products include:
Effexor XR **3504**
Venlafaxine Hydrochloride Tablets ... **2388**

Verapamil Hydrochloride (Plasma concentrations of antiarrhythmics may be decreased with concomitant use of nevirapine). Products include:
Tarka **534**

Vinblastine Sulfate (Nevirapine is principally metabolized by the liver via cytochrome P450 isoenzymes 3A and 2B6. Nevirapine is known to be an inducer of these enzymes. As a result, drugs that are metabolized by these enzyme systems may have lower than expected plasma levels when co-administered with nevirapine).
No products indexed under this heading.

Vincristine Sulfate (Plasma concentrations of cancer chemotherapeutic agents may be decreased with concomitant use of nevirapine).
No products indexed under this heading.

Vinorelbine Tartrate (Plasma concentrations of cancer chemotherapeutic agents may be decreased with concomitant use of nevirapine).
No products indexed under this heading.

Voriconazole (Plasma concentrations of antifungals may be decreased with concomitant use of nevirapine).
No products indexed under this heading.

Warfarin Sodium (The interaction between nevirapine and the antithrombotic agent warfarin is complex. As a result, when giving these drugs concomitantly, plasma warfarin levels may change with the potential for increases in coagulation time. When warfarin is co-administered with nevirapine, anticoagulation levels should be monitored frequently).
No products indexed under this heading.

Zidovudine (When zidovudine was co-administered with nevirapine, the AUC and C_{max} of zidovudine were decreased by 28% and 30%, respectively). Products include:
Combivir **1404**
Retrovir **1634**
Retrovir IV **1640**
Trizivir **1688**

Zonisamide (Plasma concentrations of anticonvulsants may be decreased with concomitant use of nevirapine). Products include:
Zonegran **1081**

VIREAD TABLETS

(Tenofovir Disoproxil Fumarate) **1266**

May interact with inhibitors of renal tubular secretion or resorption, nephrotoxic agents, and certain other agents. Compounds in these categories include:

Abacavir Sulfate (Since tenofovir is primarily eliminated by the kidneys, co-administration of tenofovir with drugs that reduce renal function may increase serum concentrations of tenofovir and/or increase the concentrations of other renally eliminated drugs). Products include:
Epzicom **1448**
Trizivir **1688**
Ziagen **1740**

Acyclovir (Since tenofovir is primarily eliminated by the kidneys, co-administration of tenofovir with drugs that reduce renal function or compete for active tubular secretion may increase serum concentrations of tenofovir and/or increase the concentrations of other renally eliminated drugs). Products include:
Zovirax **1760**

Acyclovir Sodium (Since tenofovir is primarily eliminated by the kidneys, co-administration of tenofovir with drugs that reduce renal function or compete for active tubular secretion may increase serum concentrations of tenofovir and/or increase the concentrations of other renally eliminated drugs).
No products indexed under this heading.

Adefovir dipivoxil (In the treatment of chronic hepatitis B, tenofovir should not be administered in combination with adefovir dipivoxil). Products include:
Hepsera **1244**

Alatrofloxacin Mesylate (Since tenofovir is primarily eliminated by the kidneys, co-administration of tenofovir with drugs that reduce renal function may increase serum concentrations of tenofovir and/or increase the concentrations of other renally eliminated drugs).
No products indexed under this heading.

Aldesleukin (Since tenofovir is primarily eliminated by the kidneys, co-administration of tenofovir with drugs that reduce renal function may increase serum concentrations of tenofovir and/or increase the concentrations of other renally eliminated drugs). Products include:
Proleukin **2504**

Amikacin Sulfate (Since tenofovir is primarily eliminated by the kidneys, co-administration of tenofovir with drugs that reduce renal function may increase serum concentrations of tenofovir and/or increase the concentrations of other renally eliminated drugs).
No products indexed under this heading.

Amoxicillin (Since tenofovir is primarily eliminated by the kidneys, co-administration of tenofovir with drugs that reduce renal function may increase serum concentrations of tenofovir and/or increase the concentrations of other renally eliminated drugs). Products include:
Amoxil Capsules **1311**
Amoxil Chewable Tablets **1311**
Amoxil **1311**
Amoxil Powder **1311**
Augmentin **1331**
Augmentin Tablets **1335**
Augmentin ES-600 .... **1338**
Augmentin XR **1342**
Moxatag **2321**

Amoxicillin Trihydrate (Since tenofovir is primarily eliminated by the kidneys, co-administration of tenofovir with drugs that reduce renal function may increase serum concentrations of tenofovir and/or increase the concentrations of other renally eliminated drugs).
No products indexed under this heading.

Amphotericin B (Since tenofovir is primarily eliminated by the kidneys, co-administration of tenofovir with drugs that reduce renal function may increase serum concentrations of tenofovir and/or increase the concentrations of other renally eliminated drugs).
No products indexed under this heading.

Amphotericin B, liposomal (Since tenofovir is primarily eliminated by the kidneys, co-administration of tenofovir with drugs that reduce renal function may increase serum concentrations of tenofovir and/or increase the concentrations of other renally eliminated drugs). Products include:
AmBisome **659**

Amphotericin B Cholesteryl Sulfate (Since tenofovir is primarily eliminated by the kidneys, co-administration of tenofovir with drugs that reduce renal function may increase serum concentrations of tenofovir and/or increase the concentrations of other renally eliminated drugs).
No products indexed under this heading.

Amphotericin B Lipid Complex (Since tenofovir is primarily eliminated by the kidneys, co-administration of tenofovir with drugs that reduce renal function may increase serum concentrations of tenofovir and/or increase the concentrations of other renally eliminated drugs).
No products indexed under this heading.

Ampicillin (Since tenofovir is primarily eliminated by the kidneys, co-administration of tenofovir with drugs that reduce renal function may increase serum concentrations of tenofovir and/or increase the concentrations of other renally eliminated drugs).
No products indexed under this heading.

Ampicillin Sodium (Since tenofovir is primarily eliminated by the kidneys, co-administration of tenofovir with drugs that reduce renal function may increase serum concentrations of tenofovir and/or increase the concentrations of other renally eliminated drugs).
No products indexed under this heading.

Ampicillin Trihydrate (Since tenofovir is primarily eliminated by the kidneys, co-administration of tenofovir with drugs that reduce renal function may increase serum concentrations of tenofovir and/or increase the concentrations of other renally eliminated drugs).
No products indexed under this heading.

IMPORTANT NOTE: Always consult each drug listing in the patient's regimen for possible interactions.

Viread Interactions Index 2070

Amprenavir (Since tenofovir is primarily eliminated by the kidneys, co-administration of tenofovir with drugs that reduce renal function may increase serum concentrations of tenofovir and/or increase the concentrations of other renally eliminated drugs).
No products indexed under this heading.

Aspirin (Since tenofovir is primarily eliminated by the kidneys, co-administration of tenofovir with drugs that reduce renal function may increase serum concentrations of tenofovir and/or increase the concentrations of other renally eliminated drugs). Products include:
Aggrenox 880
Bayer Aspirin 829
Percodan 1124
St. Joseph Aspirin 2045

Atazanavir (Atazanavir has been shown to increase tenofovir concentrations. Patients receiving atazanavir and tenofovir should be monitored for tenofovir-associated adverse reactions. Tenofovir should be discontinued in patients who develop tenofovir-associated adverse reactions. Tenofovir also decreases the AUC and C_{min} of atazanavir. When co-administered with tenofovir, it is recommended that atazanavir 300 mg is given with ritonavir 100 mg. Atazanavir without ritonavir should not be co-administered with tenofovir).
No products indexed under this heading.

Atazanavir Sulfate (Atazanavir has been shown to increase tenofovir concentrations. Patients receiving atazanavir and tenofovir should be monitored for tenofovir-associated adverse reactions. Tenofovir should be discontinued in patients who develop tenofovir-associated adverse reactions. Tenofovir also decreases the AUC and C_{min} of atazanavir. When co-administered with tenofovir, it is recommended that atazanavir 300 mg is given with ritonavir 100 mg. Atazanavir without ritonavir should not be co-administered with tenofovir).
No products indexed under this heading.

Atorvastatin Calcium (Since tenofovir is primarily eliminated by the kidneys, co-administration of tenofovir with drugs that reduce renal function may increase serum concentrations of tenofovir and/or increase the concentrations of other renally eliminated drugs). Products include:
Lipitor 2703

Azithromycin Dihydrate (Since tenofovir is primarily eliminated by the kidneys, co-administration of tenofovir with drugs that reduce renal function may increase serum concentrations of tenofovir and/or increase the concentrations of other renally eliminated drugs).
No products indexed under this heading.

Azlocillin Sodium (Since tenofovir is primarily eliminated by the kidneys, co-administration of tenofovir with drugs that reduce renal function may increase serum concentrations of tenofovir and/or increase the concentrations of other renally eliminated drugs).
No products indexed under this heading.

Aztreonam (Since tenofovir is primarily eliminated by the kidneys, co-administration of tenofovir with drugs that reduce renal function may increase serum concentrations of tenofovir and/or increase the concentrations of other renally eliminated drugs).
No products indexed under this heading.

Bacampicillin Hydrochloride (Since tenofovir is primarily eliminated by the kidneys, co-administration of tenofovir with drugs that reduce renal function may increase serum concentrations of tenofovir and/or increase the concentrations of other renally eliminated drugs).
No products indexed under this heading.

Bacitracin (Since tenofovir is primarily eliminated by the kidneys, co-administration of tenofovir with drugs that reduce renal function may increase serum concentrations of tenofovir and/or increase the concentrations of other renally eliminated drugs).
No products indexed under this heading.

Bacitracin Zinc (Since tenofovir is primarily eliminated by the kidneys, co-administration of tenofovir with drugs that reduce renal function may increase serum concentrations of tenofovir and/or increase the concentrations of other renally eliminated drugs).
No products indexed under this heading.

Balsalazide Disodium (Since tenofovir is primarily eliminated by the kidneys, co-administration of tenofovir with drugs that reduce renal function may increase serum concentrations of tenofovir and/or increase the concentrations of other renally eliminated drugs).
No products indexed under this heading.

Benazepril Hydrochloride (Since tenofovir is primarily eliminated by the kidneys, co-administration of tenofovir with drugs that reduce renal function may increase serum concentrations of tenofovir and/or increase the concentrations of other renally eliminated drugs).
No products indexed under this heading.

Bendroflumethiazide (Since tenofovir is primarily eliminated by the kidneys, co-administration of tenofovir with drugs that reduce renal function may increase serum concentrations of tenofovir and/or increase the concentrations of other renally eliminated drugs).
No products indexed under this heading.

Caffeine (Since tenofovir is primarily eliminated by the kidneys, co-administration of tenofovir with drugs that reduce renal function may increase serum concentrations of tenofovir and/or increase the concentrations of other renally eliminated drugs).
No products indexed under this heading.

Captopril (Since tenofovir is primarily eliminated by the kidneys, co-administration of tenofovir with drugs that reduce renal function may increase serum concentrations of tenofovir and/or increase the concentrations of other renally eliminated drugs). Products include:
Captopril 2341

Carbenicillin Disodium (Since tenofovir is primarily eliminated by the kidneys, co-administration of tenofovir with drugs that reduce renal function may increase serum concentrations of tenofovir and/or increase the concentrations of other renally eliminated drugs).
No products indexed under this heading.

Carbenicillin Indanyl Sodium (Since tenofovir is primarily eliminated by the kidneys, co-administration of tenofovir with drugs that reduce renal function may increase serum concentrations of tenofovir and/or increase the concentrations of other renally eliminated drugs).
No products indexed under this heading.

Carboplatin (Since tenofovir is primarily eliminated by the kidneys, co-administration of tenofovir with drugs that reduce renal function may increase serum concentrations of tenofovir and/or increase the concentrations of other renally eliminated drugs).
No products indexed under this heading.

Carmustine (BCNU) (Since tenofovir is primarily eliminated by the kidneys, co-administration of tenofovir with drugs that reduce renal function may increase serum concentrations of tenofovir and/or increase the concentrations of other renally eliminated drugs).
No products indexed under this heading.

Cefaclor (Since tenofovir is primarily eliminated by the kidneys, co-administration of tenofovir with drugs that reduce renal function may increase serum concentrations of tenofovir and/or increase the concentrations of other renally eliminated drugs).
No products indexed under this heading.

Cefadroxil (Since tenofovir is primarily eliminated by the kidneys, co-administration of tenofovir with drugs that reduce renal function may increase serum concentrations of tenofovir and/or increase the concentrations of other renally eliminated drugs).
No products indexed under this heading.

Cefamandole Nafate (Since tenofovir is primarily eliminated by the kidneys, co-administration of tenofovir with drugs that reduce renal function may increase serum concentrations of tenofovir and/or increase the concentrations of other renally eliminated drugs).
No products indexed under this heading.

Cefazolin Sodium (Since tenofovir is primarily eliminated by the kidneys, co-administration of tenofovir with drugs that reduce renal function may increase serum concentrations of tenofovir and/or increase the concentrations of other renally eliminated drugs).
No products indexed under this heading.

Cefdinir (Since tenofovir is primarily eliminated by the kidneys, co-administration of tenofovir with drugs that reduce renal function may increase serum concentrations of tenofovir and/or increase the concentrations of other renally eliminated drugs). Products include:
Omnicef Capsules 518
Omnicef Oral Suspension 518

Cefepime Hydrochloride (Since tenofovir is primarily eliminated by the kidneys, co-administration of tenofovir with drugs that reduce renal function may increase serum concentrations of tenofovir and/or increase the concentrations of other renally eliminated drugs).
No products indexed under this heading.

Cefixime (Since tenofovir is primarily eliminated by the kidneys, co-administration of tenofovir with drugs that reduce renal function may increase serum concentrations of tenofovir and/or increase the concentrations of other renally eliminated drugs). Products include:
Suprax for Oral Suspension 2038
Suprax Tablets 2038

Cefmetazole Sodium (Since tenofovir is primarily eliminated by the kidneys, co-administration of tenofovir with drugs that reduce renal function may increase serum concentrations of tenofovir and/or increase the concentrations of other renally eliminated drugs).
No products indexed under this heading.

Cefonicid Sodium (Since tenofovir is primarily eliminated by the kidneys, co-administration of tenofovir with drugs that reduce renal function may increase serum concentrations of tenofovir and/or increase the concentrations of other renally eliminated drugs).
No products indexed under this heading.

Cefoperazone Sodium (Since tenofovir is primarily eliminated by the kidneys, co-administration of tenofovir with drugs that reduce renal function may increase serum concentrations of tenofovir and/or increase the concentrations of other renally eliminated drugs).
No products indexed under this heading.

Ceforanide (Since tenofovir is primarily eliminated by the kidneys, co-administration of tenofovir with drugs that reduce renal function may increase serum concentrations of tenofovir and/or increase the concentrations of other renally eliminated drugs).
No products indexed under this heading.

Cefotaxime Sodium (Since tenofovir is primarily eliminated by the kidneys, co-administration of tenofovir with drugs that reduce renal function may increase serum concentrations of tenofovir and/or increase the concentrations of other renally eliminated drugs).
No products indexed under this heading.

Cefotetan (Since tenofovir is primarily eliminated by the kidneys, co-administration of tenofovir with drugs that reduce renal function may increase serum concentrations of tenofovir and/or increase the concentrations of other renally eliminated drugs).
No products indexed under this heading.

Cefoxitin Sodium (Since tenofovir is primarily eliminated by the kidneys, co-administration of tenofovir with drugs that reduce renal function may increase serum concentrations of tenofovir and/or increase the concentrations of other renally eliminated drugs).
No products indexed under this heading.

Cefpodoxime Proxetil (Since tenofovir is primarily eliminated by the kidneys, co-administration of tenofovir with drugs that reduce renal function may increase serum concentrations of tenofovir and/or increase the concentrations of other renally eliminated drugs).
No products indexed under this heading.

Cefprozil (Since tenofovir is primarily eliminated by the kidneys, co-administration of tenofovir with drugs that reduce renal function may increase serum concentrations of tenofovir and/or increase the concentrations of other renally eliminated drugs).
No products indexed under this heading.

Ceftazidime (Since tenofovir is primarily eliminated by the kidneys, co-administration of tenofovir with drugs that reduce renal function may increase serum concentrations of tenofovir and/or increase the concentrations of other renally eliminated drugs). Products include:
Fortaz 1481

Ceftizoxime Sodium (Since tenofovir is primarily eliminated by the kidneys, co-administration of tenofovir with drugs that reduce renal function may increase serum concentrations of tenofovir and/or increase the concentrations of other renally eliminated drugs).
No products indexed under this heading.

Ceftriaxone Sodium (Since tenofovir is primarily eliminated by the kidneys, co-administration of tenofovir with drugs that reduce renal function may increase serum concentrations of tenofovir and/or increase the concentrations of other renally eliminated drugs). Products include:
Rocephin 2859

Cefuroxime Axetil (Since tenofovir is primarily eliminated by the kidneys, co-administration of tenofovir with drugs that reduce renal function may increase serum concentrations of tenofovir and/or increase the concentrations of other renally eliminated drugs). Products include:
Ceftin 1399

Cefuroxime Sodium (Since tenofovir is primarily eliminated by the kidneys, co-administration of tenofovir with drugs that reduce renal function may increase serum concentrations of tenofovir and/or increase the concentrations of other renally eliminated drugs).
No products indexed under this heading.

Celecoxib (Since tenofovir is primarily eliminated by the kidneys, co-administration of tenofovir with drugs that reduce renal function may increase serum concentrations of tenofovir and/or increase the concentrations of other renally eliminated drugs). Products include:
Celebrex 3272

Cephalexin (Since tenofovir is primarily eliminated by the kidneys, co-administration of tenofovir with drugs that reduce renal function may increase serum concentrations of tenofovir and/or increase the concentrations of other renally eliminated drugs).
No products indexed under this heading.

Cephalothin Sodium (Since tenofovir is primarily eliminated by the kidneys, co-administration of tenofovir with drugs that reduce renal function may increase serum concentrations of tenofovir and/or increase the concentrations of other renally eliminated drugs).
No products indexed under this heading.

Cephapirin Sodium (Since tenofovir is primarily eliminated by the kidneys, co-administration of tenofovir with drugs that reduce renal function may increase serum concentrations of tenofovir and/or increase the concentrations of other renally eliminated drugs).
No products indexed under this heading.

Cephradine (Since tenofovir is primarily eliminated by the kidneys, co-administration of tenofovir with drugs that reduce renal function may increase serum concentrations of tenofovir and/or increase the concentrations of other renally eliminated drugs).
No products indexed under this heading.

Cerivastatin Sodium (Since tenofovir is primarily eliminated by the kidneys, co-administration of tenofovir with drugs that reduce renal function may increase serum concentrations of tenofovir and/or increase the concentrations of other renally eliminated drugs).
No products indexed under this heading.

Chlorothiazide (Since tenofovir is primarily eliminated by the kidneys, co-administration of tenofovir with drugs that reduce renal function may increase serum concentrations of tenofovir and/or increase the concentrations of other renally eliminated drugs).
No products indexed under this heading.

Chlorothiazide Sodium (Since tenofovir is primarily eliminated by the kidneys, co-administration of tenofovir with drugs that reduce renal function may increase serum concentrations of tenofovir and/or increase the concentrations of other renally eliminated drugs). Products include:
Diuril Intravenous 2009

Chlorpropamide (Since tenofovir is primarily eliminated by the kidneys, co-administration of tenofovir with drugs that reduce renal function may increase serum concentrations of tenofovir and/or increase the concentrations of other renally eliminated drugs).
No products indexed under this heading.

Cidofovir (Since tenofovir is primarily eliminated by the kidneys, co-administration of tenofovir with drugs that reduce renal function or compete for active tubular secretion may increase serum concentrations of tenofovir and/or increase the concentrations of other renally eliminated drugs).
No products indexed under this heading.

Cilastatin Sodium (Since tenofovir is primarily eliminated by the kidneys, co-administration of tenofovir with drugs that reduce renal function may increase serum concentrations of tenofovir and/or increase the concentrations of other renally eliminated drugs). Products include:
Primaxin I.M. 2232
Primaxin I.V. 2235

Cimetidine (Since tenofovir is primarily eliminated by the kidneys, co-administration of tenofovir with drugs that reduce renal function may increase serum concentrations of tenofovir and/or increase the concentrations of other renally eliminated drugs).
No products indexed under this heading.

Cimetidine Hydrochloride (Since tenofovir is primarily eliminated by the kidneys, co-administration of tenofovir with drugs that reduce renal function may increase serum concentrations of tenofovir and/or increase the concentrations of other renally eliminated drugs).
No products indexed under this heading.

Cisplatin (Since tenofovir is primarily eliminated by the kidneys, co-administration of tenofovir with drugs that reduce renal function may increase serum concentrations of tenofovir and/or increase the concentrations of other renally eliminated drugs).
No products indexed under this heading.

Cladribine (Since tenofovir is primarily eliminated by the kidneys, co-administration of tenofovir with drugs that reduce renal function may increase serum concentrations of tenofovir and/or increase the concentrations of other renally eliminated drugs). Products include:
Leustatin 946

Clozapine (Since tenofovir is primarily eliminated by the kidneys, co-administration of tenofovir with drugs that reduce renal function may increase serum concentrations of tenofovir and/or increase the concentrations of other renally eliminated drugs).
No products indexed under this heading.

Colistimethate Sodium (Since tenofovir is primarily eliminated by the kidneys, co-administration of tenofovir with drugs that reduce renal function may increase serum concentrations of tenofovir and/or increase the concentrations of other renally eliminated drugs).
No products indexed under this heading.

Colistin Sulfate (Since tenofovir is primarily eliminated by the kidneys, co-administration of tenofovir with drugs that reduce renal function may increase serum concentrations of tenofovir and/or increase the concentrations of other renally eliminated drugs).
No products indexed under this heading.

Cyclophosphamide (Since tenofovir is primarily eliminated by the kidneys, co-administration of tenofovir with drugs that reduce renal function may increase serum concentrations of tenofovir and/or increase the concentrations of other renally eliminated drugs).
No products indexed under this heading.

Cyclosporine (Since tenofovir is primarily eliminated by the kidneys, co-administration of tenofovir with drugs that reduce renal function may increase serum concentrations of tenofovir and/or increase the concentrations of other renally eliminated drugs). Products include:
Gengraf 440
Neoral Oral Solution 2496
Neoral Capsules 2496
Restasis 605

Cytarabine (Since tenofovir is primarily eliminated by the kidneys, co-administration of tenofovir with drugs that reduce renal function may increase serum concentrations of tenofovir and/or increase the concentrations of other renally eliminated drugs).
No products indexed under this heading.

Cytarabine Liposome (Since tenofovir is primarily eliminated by the kidneys, co-administration of tenofovir with drugs that reduce renal function may increase serum concentrations of tenofovir and/or increase the concentrations of other renally eliminated drugs).
No products indexed under this heading.

Delavirdine Mesylate (Since tenofovir is primarily eliminated by the kidneys, co-administration of tenofovir with drugs that reduce renal function may increase serum concentrations of tenofovir and/or increase the concentrations of other renally eliminated drugs).
No products indexed under this heading.

Diatrizoate Meglumine (Since tenofovir is primarily eliminated by the kidneys, co-administration of tenofovir with drugs that reduce renal function may increase serum concentrations of tenofovir and/or increase the concentrations of other renally eliminated drugs).
No products indexed under this heading.

Diatrizoate Sodium (Since tenofovir is primarily eliminated by the kidneys, co-administration of tenofovir with drugs that reduce renal function may increase serum concentrations of tenofovir and/or increase the concentrations of other renally eliminated drugs).
No products indexed under this heading.

Diclofenac Potassium (Since tenofovir is primarily eliminated by the kidneys, co-administration of tenofovir with drugs that reduce renal function may increase serum concentrations of tenofovir and/or increase the concentrations of other renally eliminated drugs).
No products indexed under this heading.

Diclofenac Sodium (Since tenofovir is primarily eliminated by the kidneys, co-administration of tenofovir with drugs that reduce renal function may increase serum concentrations of tenofovir and/or increase the concentrations of other renally eliminated drugs).
No products indexed under this heading.

Dicloxacillin Sodium (Since tenofovir is primarily eliminated by the kidneys, co-administration of tenofovir with drugs that reduce renal function may increase serum concentrations of tenofovir and/or increase the concentrations of other renally eliminated drugs).
No products indexed under this heading.

Didanosine (Co-administration results in significant increases in C_{max} and AUC of didanosine. Higher didanosine concentrations may potentiate didanosine-associated adverse reactions. Suppression of CD4+ cell counts has been observed in patients receiving tenofovir disoproxil fumarate with didanosine 400 mg daily. In adults weighing>60 kg, the didanosine dose should be reduced to 250 mg when co-administered with tenofovir disoproxil fumarate. Data is not available for patients wieghing <60 kg. Co-administration with didanosine should be undertaken with caution and patients receiving this combination should be closely monitored for didanosine-associated adverse reactions.

Didanosine should be discontinued in patients who develop didanosine-associated adverse effects).
No products indexed under this heading.

Efavirenz (Since tenofovir is primarily eliminated by the kidneys, co-administration of tenofovir with drugs that reduce renal function may increase serum concentrations of tenofovir and/or increase the concentrations of other renally eliminated drugs). Products include:
Atripla 906

Emtricitabine (Since tenofovir is primarily eliminated by the kidneys, co-administration of tenofovir with drugs that reduce renal function may increase serum concentrations of tenofovir and/or increase the concentrations of other renally eliminated drugs). Products include:
Atripla 906
Emtriva 1238
Emtriva Oral Solution 1238
Truvada 1258

Enalapril Maleate (Since tenofovir is primarily eliminated by the kidneys, co-administration of tenofovir with drugs that reduce renal function may increase serum concentrations of tenofovir and/or increase the concentrations of other renally eliminated drugs).
No products indexed under this heading.

Enalaprilat (Since tenofovir is primarily eliminated by the kidneys, co-administration of tenofovir with drugs that reduce renal function may increase serum concentrations of tenofovir and/or increase the concentrations of other renally eliminated drugs).
No products indexed under this heading.

Enfuvirtide (Since tenofovir is primarily eliminated by the kidneys, co-administration of tenofovir with drugs that reduce renal function may increase serum concentrations of tenofovir and/or increase the concentrations of other renally eliminated drugs).
No products indexed under this heading.

Ethiodized Oil (Since tenofovir is primarily eliminated by the kidneys, co-administration of tenofovir with drugs that reduce renal function may increase serum concentrations of tenofovir and/or increase the concentrations of other renally eliminated drugs).
No products indexed under this heading.

Etodolac (Since tenofovir is primarily eliminated by the kidneys, co-administration of tenofovir with drugs that reduce renal function may increase serum concentrations of tenofovir and/or increase the concentrations of other renally eliminated drugs).
No products indexed under this heading.

Fenoprofen Calcium (Since tenofovir is primarily eliminated by the kidneys, co-administration of tenofovir with drugs that reduce renal function may increase serum concentrations of tenofovir and/or increase the concentrations of other renally eliminated drugs).
No products indexed under this heading.

Filgrastim (Since tenofovir is primarily eliminated by the kidneys, co-administration of tenofovir with drugs that reduce renal function may increase serum concentrations of tenofovir and/or increase the concentrations of other renally eliminated drugs). Products include:
Neupogen 631

Fluorouracil (Since tenofovir is primarily eliminated by the kidneys, co-administration of tenofovir with drugs that reduce renal function may increase serum concentrations of tenofovir and/or increase the concentrations of other renally eliminated drugs). Products include:
Carac 2966

IMPORTANT NOTE: Always consult each drug listing in the patient's regimen for possible interactions.

Flurbiprofen (Since tenofovir is primarily eliminated by the kidneys, co-administration of tenofovir with drugs that reduce renal function may increase serum concentrations of tenofovir and/or increase the concentrations of other renally eliminated drugs).
No products indexed under this heading.

Fluvastatin Sodium (Since tenofovir is primarily eliminated by the kidneys, co-administration of tenofovir with drugs that reduce renal function may increase serum concentrations of tenofovir and/or increase the concentrations of other renally eliminated drugs).
No products indexed under this heading.

Foscarnet Sodium (Since tenofovir is primarily eliminated by the kidneys, co-administration of tenofovir with drugs that reduce renal function may increase serum concentrations of tenofovir and/or increase the concentrations of other renally eliminated drugs).
No products indexed under this heading.

Fosinopril Sodium (Since tenofovir is primarily eliminated by the kidneys, co-administration of tenofovir with drugs that reduce renal function may increase serum concentrations of tenofovir and/or increase the concentrations of other renally eliminated drugs).
No products indexed under this heading.

Furosemide (Since tenofovir is primarily eliminated by the kidneys, co-administration of tenofovir with drugs that reduce renal function may increase serum concentrations of tenofovir and/or increase the concentrations of other renally eliminated drugs). Products include:
Furosemide 2354

Gadopentetate Dimeglumine (Since tenofovir is primarily eliminated by the kidneys, co-administration of tenofovir with drugs that reduce renal function may increase serum concentrations of tenofovir and/or increase the concentrations of other renally eliminated drugs).
No products indexed under this heading.

Ganciclovir (Since tenofovir is primarily eliminated by the kidneys, co-administration of tenofovir with drugs that reduce renal function or compete for active tubular secretion may increase serum concentrations of tenofovir and/or increase the concentrations of other renally eliminated drugs).
No products indexed under this heading.

Ganciclovir Sodium (Since tenofovir is primarily eliminated by the kidneys, co-administration of tenofovir with drugs that reduce renal function or compete for active tubular secretion may increase serum concentrations of tenofovir and/or increase the concentrations of other renally eliminated drugs).
No products indexed under this heading.

Gentamicin (Since tenofovir is primarily eliminated by the kidneys, co-administration of tenofovir with drugs that reduce renal function may increase serum concentrations of tenofovir and/or increase the concentrations of other renally eliminated drugs).
No products indexed under this heading.

Gentamicin Sulfate (Since tenofovir is primarily eliminated by the kidneys, co-administration of tenofovir with drugs that reduce renal function may increase serum concentrations of tenofovir and/or increase the concentrations of other renally eliminated drugs). Products include:
Pred-G .... ⊙226, ⊙227

Glipizide (Since tenofovir is primarily eliminated by the kidneys, co-administration of tenofovir with drugs that reduce renal function may increase serum concentrations of tenofovir and/or increase the concentrations of other renally eliminated drugs).
No products indexed under this heading.

Globulin, Immune (Human) (Since tenofovir is primarily eliminated by the kidneys, co-administration of tenofovir with drugs that reduce renal function may increase serum concentrations of tenofovir and/or increase the concentrations of other renally eliminated drugs). Products include:

Glyburide (Since tenofovir is primarily eliminated by the kidneys, co-administration of tenofovir with drugs that reduce renal function may increase serum concentrations of tenofovir and/or increase the concentrations of other renally eliminated drugs).
No products indexed under this heading.

Gold Therapy (Since tenofovir is primarily eliminated by the kidneys, co-administration of tenofovir with drugs that reduce renal function may increase serum concentrations of tenofovir and/or increase the concentrations of other renally eliminated drugs).
No products indexed under this heading.

HMG-CoA Reductase Inhibitors (Since tenofovir is primarily eliminated by the kidneys, co-administration of tenofovir with drugs that reduce renal function may increase serum concentrations of tenofovir and/or increase the concentrations of other renally eliminated drugs).
No products indexed under this heading.

Hydrochlorothiazide (Since tenofovir is primarily eliminated by the kidneys, co-administration of tenofovir with drugs that reduce renal function may increase serum concentrations of tenofovir and/or increase the concentrations of other renally eliminated drugs). Products include:
Atacand HCT 700
Avalide 2956
Benicar HCT 1017
Diovan HCT 2419
Dyazide 1429
Exforge HCT 2449
Hyzaar 2162
Hyzaar 100-12.5 2162
Micardis HCT 889
Prinzide 2246
Tekturna HCT 2541
Teveten HCT 541

Hydroflumethiazide (Since tenofovir is primarily eliminated by the kidneys, co-administration of tenofovir with drugs that reduce renal function may increase serum concentrations of tenofovir and/or increase the concentrations of other renally eliminated drugs).
No products indexed under this heading.

Ibuprofen (Since tenofovir is primarily eliminated by the kidneys, co-administration of tenofovir with drugs that reduce renal function may increase serum concentrations of tenofovir and/or increase the concentrations of other renally eliminated drugs). Products include:
Motrin IB 2043
Children's Motrin 2044
Children's Motrin Non-Staining Dye-Free 2044
Infants' Motrin 2044
Infants' Motrin Dye-Free 2044
Junior Strength Motrin 2044
Vicoprofen 564

Idarubicin Hydrochloride (Since tenofovir is primarily eliminated by the kidneys, co-administration of tenofovir with drugs that reduce renal function may increase serum concentrations of tenofovir and/or increase the concentrations of other renally eliminated drugs).
No products indexed under this heading.

Ifosfamide (Since tenofovir is primarily eliminated by the kidneys, co-administration of tenofovir with drugs that reduce renal function may increase serum concentrations of tenofovir and/or increase the concentrations of other renally eliminated drugs).
No products indexed under this heading.

Imipenem (Since tenofovir is primarily eliminated by the kidneys, co-administration of tenofovir with drugs that reduce renal function may increase serum concentrations of tenofovir and/or increase the concentrations of other renally eliminated drugs). Products include:
Primaxin I.M. 2232
Primaxin I.V. 2235

Immune Globulin Intravenous (Human) (Since tenofovir is primarily eliminated by the kidneys, co-administration of tenofovir with drugs that reduce renal function may increase serum concentrations of tenofovir and/or increase the concentrations of other renally eliminated drugs). Products include:
Flebogamma 5% DIF 1794
Gammagard 812, 815
Gamunex 3374

Indinavir Sulfate (Since tenofovir is primarily eliminated by the kidneys, co-administration of tenofovir with drugs that reduce renal function may increase serum concentrations of tenofovir and/or increase the concentrations of other renally eliminated drugs). Products include:
Crixivan 2113

Indomethacin (Since tenofovir is primarily eliminated by the kidneys, co-administration of tenofovir with drugs that reduce renal function may increase serum concentrations of tenofovir and/or increase the concentrations of other renally eliminated drugs). Products include:
Indocin 2167

Indomethacin Sodium Trihydrate (Since tenofovir is primarily eliminated by the kidneys, co-administration of tenofovir with drugs that reduce renal function may increase serum concentrations of tenofovir and/or increase the concentrations of other renally eliminated drugs). Products include:
Indocin I.V. 2007

Interferon Beta-1b (Since tenofovir is primarily eliminated by the kidneys, co-administration of tenofovir with drugs that reduce renal function may increase serum concentrations of tenofovir and/or increase the concentrations of other renally eliminated drugs). Products include:
Betaseron 836
Extavia 2459

Interleuken-2 (Since tenofovir is primarily eliminated by the kidneys, co-administration of tenofovir with drugs that reduce renal function may increase serum concentrations of tenofovir and/or increase the concentrations of other renally eliminated drugs).
No products indexed under this heading.

Iodamide Meglumine (Since tenofovir is primarily eliminated by the kidneys, co-administration of tenofovir with drugs that reduce renal function may increase serum concentrations of tenofovir and/or increase the concentrations of other renally eliminated drugs).
No products indexed under this heading.

Iohexol (Since tenofovir is primarily eliminated by the kidneys, co-administration of tenofovir with drugs that reduce renal function may increase serum concentrations of tenofovir and/or increase the concentrations of other renally eliminated drugs).
No products indexed under this heading.

Iopamidol (Since tenofovir is primarily eliminated by the kidneys, co-administration of tenofovir with drugs that reduce renal function may increase serum concentrations of tenofovir and/or increase the concentrations of other renally eliminated drugs).
No products indexed under this heading.

Iopanoic Acid (Since tenofovir is primarily eliminated by the kidneys, co-administration of tenofovir with drugs that reduce renal function may increase serum concentrations of tenofovir and/or increase the concentrations of other renally eliminated drugs).
No products indexed under this heading.

Iothalamate Meglumine (Since tenofovir is primarily eliminated by the kidneys, co-administration of tenofovir with drugs that reduce renal function may increase serum concentrations of tenofovir and/or increase the concentrations of other renally eliminated drugs).
No products indexed under this heading.

Ioxaglate Meglumine (Since tenofovir is primarily eliminated by the kidneys, co-administration of tenofovir with drugs that reduce renal function may increase serum concentrations of tenofovir and/or increase the concentrations of other renally eliminated drugs).
No products indexed under this heading.

Ioxaglate Sodium (Since tenofovir is primarily eliminated by the kidneys, co-administration of tenofovir with drugs that reduce renal function may increase serum concentrations of tenofovir and/or increase the concentrations of other renally eliminated drugs).
No products indexed under this heading.

Kanamycin Sulfate (Since tenofovir is primarily eliminated by the kidneys, co-administration of tenofovir with drugs that reduce renal function may increase serum concentrations of tenofovir and/or increase the concentrations of other renally eliminated drugs).
No products indexed under this heading.

Ketoprofen (Since tenofovir is primarily eliminated by the kidneys, co-administration of tenofovir with drugs that reduce renal function may increase serum concentrations of tenofovir and/or increase the concentrations of other renally eliminated drugs).
No products indexed under this heading.

Ketorolac Tromethamine (Since tenofovir is primarily eliminated by the kidneys, co-administration of tenofovir with drugs that reduce renal function may increase serum concentrations of tenofovir and/or increase the concentrations of other renally eliminated drugs). Products include:
Acuvail .... ⊙209

Lamium album (Since tenofovir is primarily eliminated by the kidneys, co-administration of tenofovir with drugs that reduce renal function may increase serum concentrations of tenofovir and/or increase the concentrations of other renally eliminated drugs).
No products indexed under this heading.

Lisinopril (Since tenofovir is primarily eliminated by the kidneys, co-administration of tenofovir with drugs that reduce renal function may increase serum concentrations of tenofovir and/or increase the concentrations of other renally eliminated drugs). Products include:
Prinivil 2241
Prinzide 2246

(⊙ Described in PDR® for Ophthalmic Medicines)

2073 Interactions Index Viread

Lithium (Since tenofovir is primarily eliminated by the kidneys, co-administration of tenofovir with drugs that reduce renal function may increase serum concentrations of tenofovir and/or increase the concentrations of other renally eliminated drugs).
No products indexed under this heading.

Lithium Carbonate (Since tenofovir is primarily eliminated by the kidneys, co-administration of tenofovir with drugs that reduce renal function may increase serum concentrations of tenofovir and/or increase the concentrations of other renally eliminated drugs).
No products indexed under this heading.

Lithium Citrate (Since tenofovir is primarily eliminated by the kidneys, co-administration of tenofovir with drugs that reduce renal function may increase serum concentrations of tenofovir and/or increase the concentrations of other renally eliminated drugs).
No products indexed under this heading.

Lopinavir (Lopinavir has been shown to increase tenofovir concentrations. Patients receiving lopinavir and tenofovir should be monitored for tenofovir-associated adverse reactions. Tenofovir should be discontinued in patients who develop tenofovir-associated adverse reactions). Products include:
Kaletra 458

Loracarbef (Since tenofovir is primarily eliminated by the kidneys, co-administration of tenofovir with drugs that reduce renal function may increase serum concentrations of tenofovir and/or increase the concentrations of other renally eliminated drugs).
No products indexed under this heading.

Lovastatin (Since tenofovir is primarily eliminated by the kidneys, co-administration of tenofovir with drugs that reduce renal function may increase serum concentrations of tenofovir and/or increase the concentrations of other renally eliminated drugs). Products include:
Advicor 402
Mevacor 2212

Meclofenamate Sodium (Since tenofovir is primarily eliminated by the kidneys, co-administration of tenofovir with drugs that reduce renal function may increase serum concentrations of tenofovir and/or increase the concentrations of other renally eliminated drugs).
No products indexed under this heading.

Mefenamic Acid (Since tenofovir is primarily eliminated by the kidneys, co-administration of tenofovir with drugs that reduce renal function may increase serum concentrations of tenofovir and/or increase the concentrations of other renally eliminated drugs).
No products indexed under this heading.

Meloxicam (Since tenofovir is primarily eliminated by the kidneys, co-administration of tenofovir with drugs that reduce renal function may increase serum concentrations of tenofovir and/or increase the concentrations of other renally eliminated drugs).
No products indexed under this heading.

Melphalan Hydrochloride (Since tenofovir is primarily eliminated by the kidneys, co-administration of tenofovir with drugs that reduce renal function may increase serum concentrations of tenofovir and/or increase the concentrations of other renally eliminated drugs). Products include:
Alkeran for Injection 1300

Mesalamine (Since tenofovir is primarily eliminated by the kidneys, co-administration of tenofovir with drugs that reduce renal function may increase serum concentrations of tenofovir and/or increase the concentrations of other renally eliminated drugs). Products include:
Apriso 2899
Asacol 2786
Asacol HD 2787
Canasa 782
Lialda 3295
Pentasa 3297

Methimazole (Since tenofovir is primarily eliminated by the kidneys, co-administration of tenofovir with drugs that reduce renal function may increase serum concentrations of tenofovir and/or increase the concentrations of other renally eliminated drugs).
No products indexed under this heading.

Methotrexate (Since tenofovir is primarily eliminated by the kidneys, co-administration of tenofovir with drugs that reduce renal function may increase serum concentrations of tenofovir and/or increase the concentrations of other renally eliminated drugs).
No products indexed under this heading.

Methotrexate Sodium (Since tenofovir is primarily eliminated by the kidneys, co-administration of tenofovir with drugs that reduce renal function may increase serum concentrations of tenofovir and/or increase the concentrations of other renally eliminated drugs).
No products indexed under this heading.

Methyclothiazide (Since tenofovir is primarily eliminated by the kidneys, co-administration of tenofovir with drugs that reduce renal function may increase serum concentrations of tenofovir and/or increase the concentrations of other renally eliminated drugs).
No products indexed under this heading.

Mezlocillin Sodium (Since tenofovir is primarily eliminated by the kidneys, co-administration of tenofovir with drugs that reduce renal function may increase serum concentrations of tenofovir and/or increase the concentrations of other renally eliminated drugs).
No products indexed under this heading.

Minocycline Hydrochloride (Since tenofovir is primarily eliminated by the kidneys, co-administration of tenofovir with drugs that reduce renal function may increase serum concentrations of tenofovir and/or increase the concentrations of other renally eliminated drugs). Products include:
Solodyn 2073

Mitomycin (Mitomycin-C) (Since tenofovir is primarily eliminated by the kidneys, co-administration of tenofovir with drugs that reduce renal function may increase serum concentrations of tenofovir and/or increase the concentrations of other renally eliminated drugs).
No products indexed under this heading.

Moexipril Hydrochloride (Since tenofovir is primarily eliminated by the kidneys, co-administration of tenofovir with drugs that reduce renal function may increase serum concentrations of tenofovir and/or increase the concentrations of other renally eliminated drugs).
No products indexed under this heading.

Muromonab-CD3 (Since tenofovir is primarily eliminated by the kidneys, co-administration of tenofovir with drugs that reduce renal function may increase serum concentrations of tenofovir and/or increase the concentrations of other renally eliminated drugs). Products include:
Orthoclone OKT3 949

Nabumetone (Since tenofovir is primarily eliminated by the kidneys, co-administration of tenofovir with drugs that reduce renal function may increase serum concentrations of tenofovir and/or increase the concentrations of other renally eliminated drugs).
No products indexed under this heading.

Nafcillin Sodium (Since tenofovir is primarily eliminated by the kidneys, co-administration of tenofovir with drugs that reduce renal function may increase serum concentrations of tenofovir and/or increase the concentrations of other renally eliminated drugs).
No products indexed under this heading.

Naproxen (Since tenofovir is primarily eliminated by the kidneys, co-administration of tenofovir with drugs that reduce renal function may increase serum concentrations of tenofovir and/or increase the concentrations of other renally eliminated drugs). Products include:
EC-Naprosyn 2850
Naprosyn 2850
Anaprox/Naprosyn 2850

Naproxen Sodium (Since tenofovir is primarily eliminated by the kidneys, co-administration of tenofovir with drugs that reduce renal function may increase serum concentrations of tenofovir and/or increase the concentrations of other renally eliminated drugs). Products include:
Anaprox 2850
Anaprox DS 2850
Treximet 1681

Nelfinavir Mesylate (Since tenofovir is primarily eliminated by the kidneys, co-administration of tenofovir with drugs that reduce renal function may increase serum concentrations of tenofovir and/or increase the concentrations of other renally eliminated drugs).
No products indexed under this heading.

Neomycin (Since tenofovir is primarily eliminated by the kidneys, co-administration of tenofovir with drugs that reduce renal function may increase serum concentrations of tenofovir and/or increase the concentrations of other renally eliminated drugs).
No products indexed under this heading.

Neomycin, oral (Since tenofovir is primarily eliminated by the kidneys, co-administration of tenofovir with drugs that reduce renal function may increase serum concentrations of tenofovir and/or increase the concentrations of other renally eliminated drugs).
No products indexed under this heading.

Neomycin Sulfate (Since tenofovir is primarily eliminated by the kidneys, co-administration of tenofovir with drugs that reduce renal function may increase serum concentrations of tenofovir and/or increase the concentrations of other renally eliminated drugs).
No products indexed under this heading.

Nevirapine (Since tenofovir is primarily eliminated by the kidneys, co-administration of tenofovir with drugs that reduce renal function may increase serum concentrations of tenofovir and/or increase the concentrations of other renally eliminated drugs). Products include:
Viramune Oral Suspension 897
Viramune Tablets 897

Norfloxacin (Since tenofovir is primarily eliminated by the kidneys, co-administration of tenofovir with drugs that reduce renal function may increase serum concentrations of tenofovir and/or increase the concentrations of other renally eliminated drugs). Products include:
Noroxin 2220

Olsalazine Sodium (Since tenofovir is primarily eliminated by the kidneys, co-administration of tenofovir with drugs that reduce renal function may increase serum concentrations of tenofovir and/or increase the concentrations of other renally eliminated drugs).
No products indexed under this heading.

Omeprazole (Since tenofovir is primarily eliminated by the kidneys, co-administration of tenofovir with drugs that reduce renal function may increase serum concentrations of tenofovir and/or increase the concentrations of other renally eliminated drugs).
No products indexed under this heading.

Oxaprozin (Since tenofovir is primarily eliminated by the kidneys, co-administration of tenofovir with drugs that reduce renal function may increase serum concentrations of tenofovir and/or increase the concentrations of other renally eliminated drugs).
No products indexed under this heading.

Pamidronate Disodium (Since tenofovir is primarily eliminated by the kidneys, co-administration of tenofovir with drugs that reduce renal function may increase serum concentrations of tenofovir and/or increase the concentrations of other renally eliminated drugs).
No products indexed under this heading.

Paroxetine Hydrochloride (Since tenofovir is primarily eliminated by the kidneys, co-administration of tenofovir with drugs that reduce renal function may increase serum concentrations of tenofovir and/or increase the concentrations of other renally eliminated drugs). Products include:
Paroxetine CR 2361
Paroxetine ER 2371
Paxil 1586
Paxil CR 1596

Penicillamine (Since tenofovir is primarily eliminated by the kidneys, co-administration of tenofovir with drugs that reduce renal function may increase serum concentrations of tenofovir and/or increase the concentrations of other renally eliminated drugs).
No products indexed under this heading.

Penicillin G Benzathine (Since tenofovir is primarily eliminated by the kidneys, co-administration of tenofovir with drugs that reduce renal function may increase serum concentrations of tenofovir and/or increase the concentrations of other renally eliminated drugs). Products include:
Bicillin C-R Injectable Suspension 1826
Bicillin L-A 1828

Penicillin G Potassium (Since tenofovir is primarily eliminated by the kidneys, co-administration of tenofovir with drugs that reduce renal function may increase serum concentrations of tenofovir and/or increase the concentrations of other renally eliminated drugs).
No products indexed under this heading.

Penicillin G Procaine (Since tenofovir is primarily eliminated by the kidneys, co-administration of tenofovir with drugs that reduce renal function may increase serum concentrations of tenofovir and/or increase the concentrations of other renally eliminated drugs). Products include:
Bicillin C-R Injectable Suspension 1826
Bicillin L-A 1828

Penicillin G Sodium (Since tenofovir is primarily eliminated by the kidneys, co-administration of tenofovir with drugs that reduce renal function may increase serum concentrations of tenofovir and/or increase the concentrations of other renally eliminated drugs).
No products indexed under this heading.

IMPORTANT NOTE: Always consult each drug listing in the patient's regimen for possible interactions.

or increase the concentrations of other renally eliminated drugs). Products include:

Triamterene (Since tenofovir is primarily eliminated by the kidneys, co-administration of tenofovir with drugs that reduce renal function may increase serum concentrations of tenofovir and/or increase the concentrations of other renally eliminated drugs). Products include:

Trimethadione (Since tenofovir is primarily eliminated by the kidneys, co-administration of tenofovir with drugs that reduce renal function may increase serum concentrations of tenofovir and/or increase the concentrations of other renally eliminated drugs).

No products indexed under this heading.

Trovafloxacin Mesylate (Since tenofovir is primarily eliminated by the kidneys, co-administration of tenofovir with drugs that reduce renal function may increase serum concentrations of tenofovir and/or increase the concentrations of other renally eliminated drugs).

No products indexed under this heading.

Tyropanoate Sodium (Since tenofovir is primarily eliminated by the kidneys, co-administration of tenofovir with drugs that reduce renal function may increase serum concentrations of tenofovir and/or increase the concentrations of other renally eliminated drugs).

No products indexed under this heading.

Valacyclovir Hydrochloride (Since tenofovir is primarily eliminated by the kidneys, co-administration of tenofovir with drugs that reduce renal function or compete for active tubular secretion may increase serum concentrations of tenofovir and/or increase the concentrations of other renally eliminated drugs). Products include:

Valdecoxib (Since tenofovir is primarily eliminated by the kidneys, co-administration of tenofovir with drugs that reduce renal function may increase serum concentrations of tenofovir and/or increase the concentrations of other renally eliminated drugs).

No products indexed under this heading.

Valganciclovir Hydrochloride (Since tenofovir is primarily eliminated by the kidneys, co-administration of tenofovir with drugs that reduce renal function or compete for active tubular secretion may increase serum concentrations of tenofovir and/or increase the concentrations of other renally eliminated drugs). Products include:

Vancomycin Hydrochloride (Since tenofovir is primarily eliminated by the kidneys, co-administration of tenofovir with drugs that reduce renal function may increase serum concentrations of tenofovir and/or increase the concentrations of other renally eliminated drugs).

No products indexed under this heading.

Voriconazole (Since tenofovir is primarily eliminated by the kidneys, co-administration of tenofovir with drugs that reduce renal function may increase serum concentrations of tenofovir and/or increase the concentrations of other renally eliminated drugs).

No products indexed under this heading.

Zalcitabine (Since tenofovir is primarily eliminated by the kidneys, co-administration of tenofovir with drugs that reduce renal function may increase serum concentrations of tenofovir and/or increase the concentrations of other renally eliminated drugs).

No products indexed under this heading.

Zidovudine (Since tenofovir is primarily eliminated by the kidneys, co-administration of tenofovir with drugs that reduce renal function may increase serum concentrations of tenofovir and/or increase the concentrations of other renally eliminated drugs). Products include:

Zoledronic Acid (Since tenofovir is primarily eliminated by the kidneys, co-administration of tenofovir with drugs that reduce renal function may increase serum concentrations of tenofovir and/or increase the concentrations of other renally eliminated drugs). Products include:

VISINE TEARS LUBRICANT EYE DROPS

None cited in PDR database.

VISINE PURE TEARS DRY EYE RELIEF LUBRICANT EYE DROPS

None cited in PDR database.

VISINE-A EYE ALLERGY RELIEF EYE DROPS

None cited in PDR database.

VISUDYNE FOR INJECTION

May interact with alcohols, anticoagulants, calcium channel blockers, phenothiazines, sulfonamides, sulfonylureas, tetracyclines, thiazides, and certain other agents. Compounds in these categories include:

Amlodipine Besylate (Co-administration with calcium channel blockers could enhance the rate of verteporfin's uptake by the vascular endothelium). Products include:

Anisindione (Co-administration with drugs that decrease clotting would be expected to decrease verteporfin activity).

No products indexed under this heading.

Ardeparin Sodium (Co-administration with drugs that decrease clotting would be expected to decrease verteporfin activity).

No products indexed under this heading.

Aspirin (Co-administration with drugs that decrease platelet aggregation would be expected to decrease verteporfin activity). Products include:

Bendroflumethiazide (Co-administration with other photosensitizing agents, such as thiazide diuretics, could increase the potential for skin photosensitivity reactions).

No products indexed under this heading.

Bepridil Hydrochloride (Co-administration with calcium channel blockers could enhance the rate of verteporfin's uptake by the vascular endothelium).

No products indexed under this heading.

Chlorothiazide (Co-administration with other photosensitizing agents, such as thiazide diuretics, could increase the potential for skin photosensitivity reactions).

No products indexed under this heading.

Chlorothiazide Sodium (Co-administration with other photosensitizing agents, such as thiazide diuretics, could increase the potential for skin photosensitivity reactions). Products include:

Chlorpromazine (Co-administration with other photosensitizing agents, such as phenothiazines, could increase the potential for skin photosensitivity reactions).

No products indexed under this heading.

Chlorpromazine Hydrochloride (Co-administration with other photosensitizing agents, such as phenothiazines, could increase the potential for skin photosensitivity reactions).

No products indexed under this heading.

Chlorpropamide (Co-administration with other photosensitizing agents, such as sulfonylurea hypoglycemic agents, could increase the potential for skin photosensitivity reactions).

No products indexed under this heading.

Clopidogrel Bisulfate (Co-administration with drugs that decrease platelet aggregation would be expected to decrease verteporfin activity). Products include:

Dalteparin Sodium (Co-administration with drugs that decrease clotting would be expected to decrease verteporfin activity). Products include:

Danaparoid Sodium (Co-administration with drugs that decrease clotting would be expected to decrease verteporfin activity).

No products indexed under this heading.

Demeclocycline Hydrochloride (Co-administration with other photosensitizing agents, such as tetracyclines, could increase the potential for skin photosensitivity reactions).

No products indexed under this heading.

Dicumarol (Co-administration with drugs that decrease clotting would be expected to decrease verteporfin activity).

No products indexed under this heading.

Diltiazem Hydrochloride (Co-administration with calcium channel blockers could enhance the rate of verteporfin's uptake by the vascular endothelium). Products include:

Dimethyl Sulfoxide (Co-administration with compounds that quench active oxygen species or scavenge radicals, such as dimethyl sulfoxide, would be expected to decrease verteporfin activity).

No products indexed under this heading.

Dipyridamole (Co-administration with drugs that decrease platelet aggregation would be expected to decrease verteporfin activity). Products include:

Doxycycline (Co-administration with other photosensitizing agents, such as tetracyclines, could increase the potential for skin photosensitivity reactions).

No products indexed under this heading.

Doxycycline Calcium (Co-administration with other photosensitizing agents, such as tetracyclines, could increase the potential for skin photosensitivity reactions).

No products indexed under this heading.

Doxycycline Hyclate (Co-administration with other photosensitizing agents, such as tetracyclines, could increase the potential for skin photosensitivity reactions).

No products indexed under this heading.

Doxycycline Monohydrate (Co-administration with other photosensitizing agents, such as tetracyclines, could increase the potential for skin photosensitivity reactions).

No products indexed under this heading.

Enoxaparin Sodium (Co-administration with drugs that decrease clotting would be expected to decrease verteporfin activity). Products include:

Ethanol (Co-administration with compounds that quench active oxygen species or scavenge radicals, such as ethanol, would be expected to decrease verteporfin activity).

No products indexed under this heading.

Ethyl Alcohol (Co-administration with compounds that quench active oxygen species or scavenge radicals, such as ethanol, would be expected to decrease verteporfin activity).

No products indexed under this heading.

Felodipine (Co-administration with calcium channel blockers could enhance the rate of verteporfin's uptake by the vascular endothelium).

No products indexed under this heading.

Fluphenazine Decanoate (Co-administration with other photosensitizing agents, such as phenothiazines, could increase the potential for skin photosensitivity reactions).

No products indexed under this heading.

Fluphenazine Enanthate (Co-administration with other photosensitizing agents, such as phenothiazines, could increase the potential for skin photosensitivity reactions).

No products indexed under this heading.

Fluphenazine Hydrochloride (Co-administration with other photosensitizing agents, such as phenothiazines, could increase the potential for skin photosensitivity reactions).

No products indexed under this heading.

Fondaparinux Sodium (Co-administration with drugs that decrease clotting would be expected to decrease verteporfin activity). Products include:

Glimepiride (Co-administration with other photosensitizing agents, such as sulfonylurea hypoglycemic agents, could increase the potential for skin photosensitivity reactions). Products include:

Glipizide (Co-administration with other photosensitizing agents, such as sulfonylurea hypoglycemic agents, could increase the potential for skin photosensitivity reactions).

No products indexed under this heading.

Glyburide (Co-administration with other photosensitizing agents, such as sulfonylurea hypoglycemic agents, could increase the potential for skin photosensitivity reactions).

No products indexed under this heading.

Griseofulvin (Co-administration with other photosensitizing agents, such as griseofulvin, could increase the potential for skin photosensitivity reactions).

No products indexed under this heading.

Heparin Calcium (Co-administration with drugs that decrease clotting would be expected to decrease verteporfin activity).

No products indexed under this heading.

IMPORTANT NOTE: Always consult each drug listing in the patient's regimen for possible interactions.

Heparin Sodium (Co-administration with drugs that decrease clotting would be expected to decrease verteporfin activity).
No products indexed under this heading.

Hydrochlorothiazide (Co-administration with other photosensitizing agents, such as thiazide diuretics, could increase the potential for skin photosensitivity reactions). Products include:

Hydroflumethiazide (Co-administration with other photosensitizing agents, such as thiazide diuretics, could increase the potential for skin photosensitivity reactions).
No products indexed under this heading.

Isradipine (Co-administration with calcium channel blockers could enhance the rate of verteporfin's uptake by the vascular endothelium). Products include:

Low Molecular Weight Heparins (Co-administration with drugs that decrease clotting would be expected to decrease verteporfin activity).
No products indexed under this heading.

Mannitol (Co-administration with compounds that quench active oxygen species or scavenge radicals, such as mannitol, would be expected to decrease verteporfin activity).
No products indexed under this heading.

Mesoridazine Besylate (Co-administration with other photosensitizing agents, such as phenothiazines, could increase the potential for skin photosensitivity reactions).
No products indexed under this heading.

Methacycline Hydrochloride (Co-administration with other photosensitizing agents, such as tetracyclines, could increase the potential for skin photosensitivity reactions).
No products indexed under this heading.

Methotrimeprazine (Co-administration with other photosensitizing agents, such as phenothiazines, could increase the potential for skin photosensitivity reactions).
No products indexed under this heading.

Methyclothiazide (Co-administration with other photosensitizing agents, such as thiazide diuretics, could increase the potential for skin photosensitivity reactions).
No products indexed under this heading.

Mibefradil Dihydrochloride (Co-administration with calcium channel blockers could enhance the rate of verteporfin's uptake by the vascular endothelium).
No products indexed under this heading.

Minocycline Hydrochloride (Co-administration with other photosensitizing agents, such as tetracyclines, could increase the potential for skin photosensitivity reactions). Products include:

Nicardipine (Co-administration with calcium channel blockers could enhance the rate of verteporfin's uptake by the vascular endothelium).
No products indexed under this heading.

Nicardipine Hydrochloride (Co-administration with calcium channel blockers could enhance the rate of verteporfin's uptake by the vascular endothelium).
No products indexed under this heading.

Nifedipine (Co-administration with calcium channel blockers could enhance the rate of verteporfin's uptake by the vascular endothelium).
No products indexed under this heading.

Nimodipine (Co-administration with calcium channel blockers could enhance the rate of verteporfin's uptake by the vascular endothelium).
No products indexed under this heading.

Nisoldipine (Co-administration with calcium channel blockers could enhance the rate of verteporfin's uptake by the vascular endothelium).
No products indexed under this heading.

Oxytetracycline (Co-administration with other photosensitizing agents, such as tetracyclines, could increase the potential for skin photosensitivity reactions).
No products indexed under this heading.

Oxytetracycline Hydrochloride (Co-administration with other photosensitizing agents, such as tetracyclines, could increase the potential for skin photosensitivity reactions).
No products indexed under this heading.

Perphenazine (Co-administration with other photosensitizing agents, such as phenothiazines, could increase the potential for skin photosensitivity reactions).
No products indexed under this heading.

Phenothiazine Derivatives (Co-administration with other photosensitizing agents, such as phenothiazines, could increase the potential for skin photosensitivity reactions).
No products indexed under this heading.

Phenothiazines (Co-administration with other photosensitizing agents, such as phenothiazines, could increase the potential for skin photosensitivity reactions).
No products indexed under this heading.

Polymyxin B Sulfate (Co-administration with polymyxin B could enhance the rate of verteporfin's uptake by the vascular endothelium).
No products indexed under this heading.

Polythiazide (Co-administration with other photosensitizing agents, such as thiazide diuretics, could increase the potential for skin photosensitivity reactions).
No products indexed under this heading.

Prochlorperazine (Co-administration with other photosensitizing agents, such as phenothiazines, could increase the potential for skin photosensitivity reactions).
No products indexed under this heading.

Prochlorperazine Edisylate (Co-administration with other photosensitizing agents, such as phenothiazines, could increase the potential for skin photosensitivity reactions).
No products indexed under this heading.

Prochlorperazine Maleate (Co-administration with other photosensitizing agents, such as phenothiazines, could increase the potential for skin photosensitivity reactions).
No products indexed under this heading.

Promethazine (Co-administration with other photosensitizing agents, such as phenothiazines, could increase the potential for skin photosensitivity reactions).
No products indexed under this heading.

Promethazine Hydrochloride (Co-administration with other photosensitizing agents, such as phenothiazines, could increase the potential for skin photosensitivity reactions).
No products indexed under this heading.

Sulfacytine (Co-administration with other photosensitizing agents, such as sulfonamides, could increase the potential for skin photosensitivity reactions).
No products indexed under this heading.

Sulfamethizole (Co-administration with other photosensitizing agents, such as sulfonamides, could increase the potential for skin photosensitivity reactions).
No products indexed under this heading.

Sulfamethoxazole (Co-administration with other photosensitizing agents, such as sulfonamides, could increase the potential for skin photosensitivity reactions).
No products indexed under this heading.

Sulfasalazine (Co-administration with other photosensitizing agents, such as sulfonamides, could increase the potential for skin photosensitivity reactions).
No products indexed under this heading.

Sulfinpyrazone (Co-administration with other photosensitizing agents, such as sulfonamides, could increase the potential for skin photosensitivity reactions).
No products indexed under this heading.

Sulfisoxazole Acetyl (Co-administration with other photosensitizing agents, such as sulfonamides, could increase the potential for skin photosensitivity reactions).
No products indexed under this heading.

Sulfisoxazole Diolamine (Co-administration with other photosensitizing agents, such as sulfonamides, could increase the potential for skin photosensitivity reactions).
No products indexed under this heading.

Tetracycline Hydrochloride (Co-administration with other photosensitizing agents, such as tetracyclines, could increase the potential for skin photosensitivity reactions). Products include:

Tetracycline Phosphate Complex (Co-administration with other photosensitizing agents, such as tetracyclines, could increase the potential for skin photosensitivity reactions).
No products indexed under this heading.

Thioridazine (Co-administration with other photosensitizing agents, such as phenothiazines, could increase the potential for skin photosensitivity reactions).
No products indexed under this heading.

Thioridazine Hydrochloride (Co-administration with other photosensitizing agents, such as phenothiazines, could increase the potential for skin photosensitivity reactions). Products include:

Tinzaparin Sodium (Co-administration with drugs that decrease clotting would be expected to decrease verteporfin activity).
No products indexed under this heading.

Tolazamide (Co-administration with other photosensitizing agents, such as sulfonylurea hypoglycemic agents, could increase the potential for skin photosensitivity reactions).
No products indexed under this heading.

Tolbutamide (Co-administration with other photosensitizing agents, such as sulfonylurea hypoglycemic agents, could increase the potential for skin photosensitivity reactions).
No products indexed under this heading.

Trifluoperazine Hydrochloride (Co-administration with other photosensitizing agents, such as phenothiazines, could increase the potential for skin photosensitivity reactions).
No products indexed under this heading.

Verapamil Hydrochloride (Co-administration with calcium channel blockers could enhance the rate of verteporfin's uptake by the vascular endothelium). Products include:

Warfarin Sodium (Co-administration with drugs that decrease clotting would be expected to decrease verteporfin activity).
No products indexed under this heading.

Food Interactions

Alcohol (Co-administration with compounds that quench active oxygen species or scavenge radicals, such as ethanol, would be expected to decrease verteporfin activity).

Beer, reduced-alcohol (Co-administration with compounds that quench active oxygen species or scavenge radicals, such as ethanol, would be expected to decrease verteporfin activity).

Beer, unspecified (Co-administration with compounds that quench active oxygen species or scavenge radicals, such as ethanol, would be expected to decrease verteporfin activity).

Wine, Chianti (Co-administration with compounds that quench active oxygen species or scavenge radicals, such as ethanol, would be expected to decrease verteporfin activity).

Wine, Red (Co-administration with compounds that quench active oxygen species or scavenge radicals, such as ethanol, would be expected to decrease verteporfin activity).

Wine, unspecified (Co-administration with compounds that quench active oxygen species or scavenge radicals, such as ethanol, would be expected to decrease verteporfin activity).

Wine products (Co-administration with compounds that quench active oxygen species or scavenge radicals, such as ethanol, would be expected to decrease verteporfin activity).

VISUTEIN CAPSULES

(Acetylcysteine, Carotenoids, Lutein, Vitamin B2, Zinc) 3456
None cited in PDR database.

VUSION OINTMENT

(Miconazole Nitrate, Petrolatum, White, Zinc Oxide) 3335

Warfarin Sodium (Women who take a warfarin anticoagulant and use a miconazole intravaginal cream, or suppository may be at risk for developing an increased prothrombin time, INR and bleeding; the potential for this interaction to occur between warfarin and Vusion is unknown).
No products indexed under this heading.

VYTORIN 10/10 TABLETS

(Ezetimibe, Simvastatin) 2303
May interact with alcohols, azole antifungals, bile acid sequestering agents, cytochrome p450 3a4 inhibitors (selected), cytochrome p450 3a4 inhibitors, potent (selected), erythromycin, fibrates, lipid-lowering drugs, macrolide antibiotics, protease inhibitors, vitamin K antagonists, and certain other agents. Compounds in these categories include:

Acetazolamide (Simvastatin is metabolized by the cytochrome P450 isoform 3A4. Certain drugs that inhibit this met-

abolic pathway can raise the plasma levels of simvastatin and may increase the risk of myopathy. These include itraconazole, ketoconazole, and other antifungal azoles, the macrolide antibiotics erythromycin and clarithromycin, and the ketolide antibiotic telithromycin, HIV protease inhibitors, the antidepressant nefazodone, or large quantities of grapefruit juice (>1 quart daily). The use of Vytorin concomitantly with these CYP3A4 inhibitors should be avoided. If treatment with itraconazole, ketoconazole, erythromycin, clarithromycin or telithromycin is unavoidable, therapy with Vytorin should be suspended during the course of treatment).
No products indexed under this heading.

Acetazolamide Sodium (Simvastatin is metabolized by the cytochrome P450 isoform 3A4. Certain drugs that inhibit this metabolic pathway can raise the plasma levels of simvastatin and may increase the risk of myopathy. These include itraconazole, ketoconazole, and other antifungal azoles, the macrolide antibiotics erythromycin and clarithromycin, and the ketolide antibiotic telithromycin, HIV protease inhibitors, the antidepressant nefazodone, or large quantities of grapefruit juice (>1 quart daily). The use of Vytorin concomitantly with these CYP3A4 inhibitors should be avoided. If treatment with itraconazole, ketoconazole, erythromycin, clarithromycin or telithromycin is unavoidable, therapy with Vytorin should be suspended during the course of treatment).
No products indexed under this heading.

Aluminum Hydroxide (Aluminum and magnesium hydroxide combination antacid decreases ezetimibe AUC by 4% and ezetimibe C_{max} by 30%).
No products indexed under this heading.

Amiodarone Hydrochloride (The risk of myopathy/rhabdomyolysis is increased by concomitant administration of amiodarone with higher doses of Vytorin. In patients taking amiodarone concomitantly with Vytorin, the dose of Vytorin should not exceed 10/20 mg/day).
No products indexed under this heading.

Amlodipine Besylate (Concomitant administration of amlodipine and simvastatin leads to a geometric mean ratio of simvastatin acid and simvastatin as follows - AUC: 1.58 and 1.77 and C_{max}: 1.56 and 1.47). Products include:
Azor 1010
Exforge 2443
Exforge HCT 2449

Amprenavir (Simvastatin is metabolized by the cytochrome P450 isoform 3A4. Certain drugs that inhibit this metabolic pathway can raise plasma levels of simvastatin and may increase the risk of myopathy. These drugs include HIV protease inhibitors. The use of Vytorin concomitantly with these CYP3A4 inhibitors should be avoided).
No products indexed under this heading.

Anastrozole (Simvastatin is metabolized by the cytochrome P450 isoform 3A4. Certain drugs that inhibit this metabolic pathway can raise the plasma levels of simvastatin and may increase the risk of myopathy. These include itraconazole, ketoconazole, and other antifungal azoles, the macrolide antibiotics erythromycin and clarithromycin, and the ketolide antibiotic telithromycin, HIV protease inhibitors, the antidepressant nefazodone, or large quantities of grapefruit juice (>1 quart daily). The use of Vytorin concomitantly with these CYP3A4 inhibitors should be avoided. If treatment with itraconazole, ketoconazole, erythromycin, clarithromycin or telithromycin is unavoidable, therapy with Vytorin should be suspended during the course of treatment).
No products indexed under this heading.

Aprepitant (Simvastatin is metabolized by the cytochrome P450 isoform 3A4. Certain drugs that inhibit this metabolic pathway can raise the plasma levels of simvastatin and may increase the risk of myopathy. These include itraconazole, ketoconazole, and other antifungal azoles, the macrolide antibiotics erythromycin and clarithromycin, and the ketolide antibiotic telithromycin, HIV protease inhibitors, the antidepressant nefazodone, or large quantities of grapefruit juice (>1 quart daily). The use of Vytorin concomitantly with these CYP3A4 inhibitors should be avoided. If treatment with itraconazole, ketoconazole, erythromycin, clarithromycin or telithromycin is unavoidable, therapy with Vytorin should be suspended during the course of treatment). Products include:
Emend 2124

Atazanavir (Simvastatin is metabolized by the cytochrome P450 isoform 3A4. Certain drugs that inhibit this metabolic pathway can raise plasma levels of simvastatin and may increase the risk of myopathy. These drugs include HIV protease inhibitors. The use of Vytorin concomitantly with these CYP3A4 inhibitors should be avoided).
No products indexed under this heading.

Atazanavir Sulfate (Simvastatin is metabolized by the cytochrome P450 isoform 3A4. Certain drugs that inhibit this metabolic pathway can raise plasma levels of simvastatin and may increase the risk of myopathy. These drugs include HIV protease inhibitors. The use of Vytorin concomitantly with these CYP3A4 inhibitors should be avoided).
No products indexed under this heading.

Atorvastatin Calcium (Atorvastatin decreases ezetimibe AUC by 2% and increases ezetimibe C_{max} by 12%. Ezetimibe decreases atorvastatin AUC by 4% and increases atorvastatin C_{max} by 7%). Products include:
Lipitor 2703

Azithromycin Dihydrate (Simvastatin is metabolized by the cytochrome P450 isoform 3A4. Certain drugs that inhibit this metabolic pathway can raise plasma levels of simvastatin and may increase the risk of myopathy. These drugs include the macrolide antibiotics erythromycin and clarithromycin. The use of Vytorin concomitantly with these CYP3A4 inhibitors should be avoided. If treatment with erythromycin or clarithromycin is unavoidable, therapy with Vytorin should be suspended during the course of treatment).
No products indexed under this heading.

Butoconazole Nitrate (Simvastatin is metabolized by the cytochrome P450 isoform 3A4. Certain drugs that inhibit this metabolic pathway can raise plasma levels of simvastatin and may increase the risk of myopathy. These drugs include itraconazole, ketoconazole, and other antifungal azoles. The use of Vytorin concomitantly with these CYP3A4 inhibitors should be avoided).
No products indexed under this heading.

Cerivastatin Sodium (The benefits of the combined use of Vytorin with the following drugs should be carefully weighed against the potential risks of combinations: gemfibrozil, other lipid-lowering drugs (other fibrates or>/= 1 g/day of niacin), cyclosporine, danazol, amiodarone, or verapamil. Caution should be used when prescribing other fibrates or lipid-lowering doses (>/= 1 g/day) of niacin with Vytorin, as these agents can cause myopathy when given alone).
No products indexed under this heading.

Cholestyramine (Concomitant cholestyramine administration decreased the mean AUC of total ezetimibe approximately 55%. The incremental LDL-C reduction due to adding Vytorin to cholestyramine may be reduced by this interaction. Dosing of Vytorin should occur either greater than or equal to 2 hours before or greater than or equal to 4 hours after administration of a bile acid sequestrant).
No products indexed under this heading.

Cimetidine (Cimetidine increases ezetimibe AUC by 6% and ezetimibe C_{max} by 22%).
No products indexed under this heading.

Cimetidine Hydrochloride (Cimetidine increases ezetimibe AUC by 6% and ezetimibe C_{max} by 22%).
No products indexed under this heading.

Ciprofloxacin (Simvastatin is metabolized by the cytochrome P450 isoform 3A4. Certain drugs that inhibit this metabolic pathway can raise the plasma levels of simvastatin and may increase the risk of myopathy. These include itraconazole, ketoconazole, and other antifungal azoles, the macrolide antibiotics erythromycin and clarithromycin, and the ketolide antibiotic telithromycin, HIV protease inhibitors, the antidepressant nefazodone, or large quantities of grapefruit juice (>1 quart daily). The use of Vytorin concomitantly with these CYP3A4 inhibitors should be avoided. If treatment with itraconazole, ketoconazole, erythromycin, clarithromycin or telithromycin is unavoidable, therapy with Vytorin should be suspended during the course of treatment). Products include:
Cipro I.V. 3082
Cipro 3073
Cipro XR 3091
Ciprodex 583

Clarithromycin (Simvastatin is metabolized by the cytochrome P450 isoform 3A4. Certain drugs that inhibit this metabolic pathway can raise plasma levels of simvastatin and may increase the risk of myopathy. These drugs include the macrolide antibiotic clarithromycin. The use of Vytorin concomitantly with this CYP3A4 inhibitor should be avoided. If treatment with clarithromycin is unavoidable, therapy with Vytorin should be suspended during the course of treatment). Products include:
Biaxin/Biaxin XL 412

Clofibrate (The safety and effectiveness of Vytorin administered with fibrates have not been established. Fibrates may increase cholesterol excretion into the bile, leading to cholelithiasis. Therefore, the combination of Vytorin and fibrates should be avoided. There is an increased risk of myopathy when simvastatin is used concomitantly with fibrates. Rhabdomyolysis has been reported very rarely with the addition of ezetimibe to agents known to be associated with increased risk of rhabdomyolysis, such as fibrates).
No products indexed under this heading.

Clotrimazole (Simvastatin is metabolized by the cytochrome P450 isoform 3A4. Certain drugs that inhibit this metabolic pathway can raise plasma levels of simvastatin and may increase the risk of myopathy. These drugs include itraconazole, ketoconazole, and other antifungal azoles. The use of Vytorin concomitantly with these CYP3A4 inhibitors should be avoided). Products include:
Lotrisone 3163

Colesevelam Hydrochloride (Fibrates may increase cholesterol excretion into the bile, leading to cholelithiasis. Ezetimibe may increase cholesterol in the gallbladder bile. Co-administration of Vytorin with fibrates is not recommended until use in patients is studied. Dosing of Vytorin should occur either greater than or equal to 2 hours before or greater than or equal to 4 hours after administration of a bile acid sequestrant). Products include:
Welchol 1029

Colestipol Hydrochloride (The benefits of the combined use of Vytorin with the following drugs should be carefully weighed against the potential risks of combinations: gemfibrozil, other lipid-lowering drugs (other fibrates or>/= 1 g/day of niacin), cyclosporine, danazol, amiodarone, or verapamil. Caution should be used when prescribing other fibrates or lipid-lowering doses (>/= 1 g/day) of niacin with Vytorin, as these agents can cause myopathy when given alone).
No products indexed under this heading.

Conivaptan Hydrochloride (Simvastatin is metabolized by the cytochrome P450 isoform 3A4. Certain drugs that inhibit this metabolic pathway can raise the plasma levels of simvastatin and may increase the risk of myopathy. These include itraconazole, ketoconazole, and other antifungal azoles, the macrolide antibiotics erythromycin and clarithromycin, and the ketolide antibiotic telithromycin, HIV protease inhibitors, the antidepressant nefazodone, or large quantities of grapefruit juice (>1 quart daily). The use of Vytorin concomitantly with these CYP3A4 inhibitors should be avoided. If treatment with itraconazole, ketoconazole, erythromycin, clarithromycin or telithromycin is unavoidable, therapy with Vytorin should be suspended during the course of treatment). Products include:
Vaprisol 689

Cyclosporine (Caution should be exercised when using Vytorin and cyclosporine concurrently due to increased exposure to both ezetimibe and cyclosporine. The risk of myopathy/rhabdomyolysis is increased by concomitant administration of cyclosporine with Vytorin. Cyclosporine concentrations should be monitored if using Vytorin concomitantly. In patients treated with cyclosporine, the potential effects of the increased exposure to ezetimibe from concomitant use should be carefully weighed against the benefits of alterations in lipid levels provided by ezetimibe. In patients taking cyclosporine, Vytorin should not be started unless the patient has already tolerated treatment with simvastatin at a dose of 5 mg or higher. The dose of Vytorin should not exceed 10/10 mg/day). Products include:
Gengraf 440
Neoral Oral Solution 2496
Neoral Capsules 2496
Restasis 605

Dalfopristin (Simvastatin is metabolized by the cytochrome P450 isoform 3A4. Certain drugs that inhibit this metabolic pathway can raise the plasma levels of simvastatin and may increase the risk of myopathy. These include itraconazole, ketoconazole, and other antifungal azoles, the macrolide antibiotics erythromycin and clarithromycin, and the ketolide antibiotic telithromycin, HIV protease inhibitors, the antidepressant nefazodone, or large quantities of grapefruit juice (>1 quart daily). The use of Vytorin concomitantly with these CYP3A4 inhibitors should be avoided. If treatment with itraconazole, ketoconazole, erythromycin, clarithromycin or telithromycin is unavoidable, therapy with Vytorin should be suspended during the course of treatment).
No products indexed under this heading.

IMPORTANT NOTE: Always consult each drug listing in the patient's regimen for possible interactions.

Danazol (The risk of myopathy/rhabdomyolysis is increased by concomitant administration of danazol particularly with higher doses of Vytorin. In patients taking danazol, Vytorin should not be started unless the patient has already tolerated treatment with simvastatin at a dose of 5 mg or higher. The dose of Vytorin should not exceed 10/10 mg/day).

No products indexed under this heading.

Darunavir (Simvastatin is metabolized by the cytochrome P450 isoform 3A4. Certain drugs that inhibit this metabolic pathway can raise plasma levels of simvastatin and may increase the risk of myopathy. These drugs include HIV protease inhibitors. The use of Vytorin concomitantly with these CYP3A4 inhibitors should be avoided).

No products indexed under this heading.

Dasatinib (Simvastatin is metabolized by the cytochrome P450 isoform 3A4. Certain drugs that inhibit this metabolic pathway can raise the plasma levels of simvastatin and may increase the risk of myopathy. These include itraconazole, ketoconazole, and other antifungal azoles, the macrolide antibiotics erythromycin and clarithromycin, and the ketolide antibiotic telithromycin, HIV protease inhibitors, the antidepressant nefazodone, or large quantities of grapefruit juice (>1 quart daily). The use of Vytorin concomitantly with these CYP3A4 inhibitors should be avoided. If treatment with itraconazole, ketoconazole, erythromycin, clarithromycin or telithromycin is unavoidable, therapy with Vytorin should be suspended during the course of treatment).

No products indexed under this heading.

Delavirdine Mesylate (Simvastatin is metabolized by the cytochrome P450 isoform 3A4. Certain drugs that inhibit this metabolic pathway can raise the plasma levels of simvastatin and may increase the risk of myopathy. These include itraconazole, ketoconazole, and other antifungal azoles, the macrolide antibiotics erythromycin and clarithromycin, and the ketolide antibiotic telithromycin, HIV protease inhibitors, the antidepressant nefazodone, or large quantities of grapefruit juice (>1 quart daily). The use of Vytorin concomitantly with these CYP3A4 inhibitors should be avoided. If treatment with itraconazole, ketoconazole, erythromycin, clarithromycin or telithromycin is unavoidable, therapy with Vytorin should be suspended during the course of treatment).

No products indexed under this heading.

Delavirine (Simvastatin is metabolized by the cytochrome P450 isoform 3A4. Certain drugs that inhibit this metabolic pathway can raise the plasma levels of simvastatin and may increase the risk of myopathy. These include itraconazole, ketoconazole, and other antifungal azoles, the macrolide antibiotics erythromycin and clarithromycin, and the ketolide antibiotic telithromycin, HIV protease inhibitors, the antidepressant nefazodone, or large quantities of grapefruit juice (>1 quart daily). The use of Vytorin concomitantly with these CYP3A4 inhibitors should be avoided. If treatment with itraconazole, ketoconazole, erythromycin, clarithromycin or telithromycin is unavoidable, therapy with Vytorin should be suspended during the course of treatment).

No products indexed under this heading.

Desloratadine (Simvastatin is metabolized by the cytochrome P450 isoform 3A4. Certain drugs that inhibit this metabolic pathway can raise the plasma levels of simvastatin and may increase the risk of myopathy. These include itraconazole, ketoconazole, and other antifungal azoles, the macrolide antibiotics erythromycin and clarithromycin,

and the ketolide antibiotic telithromycin, HIV protease inhibitors, the antidepressant nefazodone, or large quantities of grapefruit juice (>1 quart daily). The use of Vytorin concomitantly with these CYP3A4 inhibitors should be avoided. If treatment with itraconazole, ketoconazole, erythromycin, clarithromycin or telithromycin is unavoidable, therapy with Vytorin should be suspended during the course of treatment). Products include:

Dicumarol (Simvastatin 20-40 mg/day modestly potentiated the effect of coumarin anticoagulants: the prothrombin time, reported as International Normalized Ratio (INR), increased from a baseline of 1.7 to 1.8 and from 2.6 to 3.4 in a normal volunteer study and in a hypercholesterolemic patient study, respectively. Prothrombin time should be determined before starting Vytorin and frequently enough during early therapy to ensure that no significant alteration of prothrombin time occurs. Once a stable prothrombin time has been documented, prothrombin times can be monitored at the intervals usually recommended for patients on coumarin anticoagulants. If the dose of Vytorin is changed or discontinued, the same procedure should be repeated).

No products indexed under this heading.

Digoxin (In one study, concomitant administration of digoxin with simvastatin resulted in a slight elevation of plasma digoxin concentrations. Patients taking digoxin should be monitored appropriately when Vytorin is initiated). Products include:

Diltiazem Hydrochloride (Concomitant administration of diltiazem and simvastatin leads to a geometric mean ratio of simvastatin acid and simvastatin as follows - AUC: 2.69 and 3.10 and C_{max}: 2.69 and 2.88). Products include:

Diltiazem Maleate (Concomitant administration of diltiazem and simvastatin leads to a geometric mean ratio of simvastatin acid and simvastatin as follows - AUC: 2.69 and 3.10 and C_{max}: 2.69 and 2.88).

No products indexed under this heading.

Dirithromycin (Simvastatin is metabolized by the cytochrome P450 isoform 3A4. Certain drugs that inhibit this metabolic pathway can raise plasma levels of simvastatin and may increase the risk of myopathy. These drugs include the macrolide antibiotics erythromycin and clarithromycin. The use of Vytorin concomitantly with these CYP3A4 inhibitors should be avoided. If treatment with erythromycin or clarithromycin is unavoidable, therapy with Vytorin should be suspended during the course of treatment).

No products indexed under this heading.

Econazole Nitrate (Simvastatin is metabolized by the cytochrome P450 isoform 3A4. Certain drugs that inhibit this metabolic pathway can raise plasma levels of simvastatin and may increase the risk of myopathy. These drugs include itraconazole, ketoconazole, and other antifungal azoles. The use of Vytorin concomitantly with these CYP3A4 inhibitors should be avoided).

No products indexed under this heading.

Efavirenz (Simvastatin is metabolized by the cytochrome P450 isoform 3A4. Certain drugs that inhibit this metabolic pathway can raise the plasma levels of simvastatin and may increase the risk

of myopathy. These include itraconazole, ketoconazole, and other antifungal azoles, the macrolide antibiotics erythromycin and clarithromycin, and the ketolide antibiotic telithromycin, HIV protease inhibitors, the antidepressant nefazodone, or large quantities of grapefruit juice (>1 quart daily). The use of Vytorin concomitantly with these CYP3A4 inhibitors should be avoided. If treatment with itraconazole, ketoconazole, erythromycin, clarithromycin or telithromycin is unavoidable, therapy with Vytorin should be suspended during the course of treatment). Products include:

Erythromycin (Simvastatin is metabolized by the cytochrome P450 isoform 3A4. Certain drugs that inhibit this metabolic pathway can raise plasma levels of simvastatin and may increase the risk of myopathy. These drugs include the macrolide antibiotic erythromycin. The use of Vytorin concomitantly with this CYP3A4 inhibitor should be avoided. If treatment with erythromycin is unavoidable, therapy with Vytorin should be suspended during the course of treatment).

No products indexed under this heading.

Erythromycin, Topical (Simvastatin is metabolized by the cytochrome P450 isoform 3A4. Certain drugs that inhibit this metabolic pathway can raise plasma levels of simvastatin and may increase the risk of myopathy. These drugs include the macrolide antibiotic erythromycin. The use of Vytorin concomitantly with this CYP3A4 inhibitor should be avoided. If treatment with erythromycin is unavoidable, therapy with Vytorin should be suspended during the course of treatment).

No products indexed under this heading.

Erythromycin Estolate (Simvastatin is metabolized by the cytochrome P450 isoform 3A4. Certain drugs that inhibit this metabolic pathway can raise plasma levels of simvastatin and may increase the risk of myopathy. These drugs include the macrolide antibiotic erythromycin. The use of Vytorin concomitantly with this CYP3A4 inhibitor should be avoided. If treatment with erythromycin is unavoidable, therapy with Vytorin should be suspended during the course of treatment).

No products indexed under this heading.

Erythromycin Ethylsuccinate (Simvastatin is metabolized by the cytochrome P450 isoform 3A4. Certain drugs that inhibit this metabolic pathway can raise plasma levels of simvastatin and may increase the risk of myopathy. These drugs include the macrolide antibiotic erythromycin. The use of Vytorin concomitantly with this CYP3A4 inhibitor should be avoided. If treatment with erythromycin is unavoidable, therapy with Vytorin should be suspended during the course of treatment). Products include:

Erythromycin Gluceptate (Simvastatin is metabolized by the cytochrome P450 isoform 3A4. Certain drugs that inhibit this metabolic pathway can raise plasma levels of simvastatin and may increase the risk of myopathy. These drugs include the macrolide antibiotic erythromycin. The use of Vytorin concomitantly with this CYP3A4 inhibitor should be avoided. If treatment with erythromycin is unavoidable, therapy with Vytorin should be suspended during the course of treatment).

No products indexed under this heading.

Erythromycin Lactobionate (Simvastatin is metabolized by the cytochrome P450 isoform 3A4. Certain drugs that inhibit this metabolic path-

way can raise plasma levels of simvastatin and may increase the risk of myopathy. These drugs include the macrolide antibiotic erythromycin. The use of Vytorin concomitantly with this CYP3A4 inhibitor should be avoided. If treatment with erythromycin is unavoidable, therapy with Vytorin should be suspended during the course of treatment).

No products indexed under this heading.

Erythromycin Stearate (Simvastatin is metabolized by the cytochrome P450 isoform 3A4. Certain drugs that inhibit this metabolic pathway can raise plasma levels of simvastatin and may increase the risk of myopathy. These drugs include the macrolide antibiotic erythromycin. The use of Vytorin concomitantly with this CYP3A4 inhibitor should be avoided. If treatment with erythromycin is unavoidable, therapy with Vytorin should be suspended during the course of treatment).

No products indexed under this heading.

Esomeprazole Magnesium (Simvastatin is metabolized by the cytochrome P450 isoform 3A4. Certain drugs that inhibit this metabolic pathway can raise the plasma levels of simvastatin and may increase the risk of myopathy. These include itraconazole, ketoconazole, and other antifungal azoles, the macrolide antibiotics erythromycin and clarithromycin, and the ketolide antibiotic telithromycin, HIV protease inhibitors, the antidepressant nefazodone, or large quantities of grapefruit juice (>1 quart daily). The use of Vytorin concomitantly with these CYP3A4 inhibitors should be avoided. If treatment with itraconazole, ketoconazole, erythromycin, clarithromycin or telithromycin is unavoidable, therapy with Vytorin should be suspended during the course of treatment). Products include:

Esomeprazole Sodium (Simvastatin is metabolized by the cytochrome P450 isoform 3A4. Certain drugs that inhibit this metabolic pathway can raise the plasma levels of simvastatin and may increase the risk of myopathy. These include itraconazole, ketoconazole, and other antifungal azoles, the macrolide antibiotics erythromycin and clarithromycin, and the ketolide antibiotic telithromycin, HIV protease inhibitors, the antidepressant nefazodone, or large quantities of grapefruit juice (>1 quart daily). The use of Vytorin concomitantly with these CYP3A4 inhibitors should be avoided. If treatment with itraconazole, ketoconazole, erythromycin, clarithromycin or telithromycin is unavoidable, therapy with Vytorin should be suspended during the course of treatment). Products include:

Ethanol (Vytorin should be used with caution in patients who consume substantial quantities of alcohol and/or have a past history of liver disease).

No products indexed under this heading.

Ethinyl Estradiol (During concomitant use with ethinyl estradiol and levonorgestrel, ezetimibe decreases ethinyl estradiol C_{max} by 9% and levonorgestrel C_{max} by 5%). Products include:

Ethyl Alcohol (Vytorin should be used with caution in patients who consume substantial quantities of alcohol and/or have a past history of liver disease).

No products indexed under this heading.

Fat (Concomitant food administration (high-fat or non-fat meals) had no effect on the extent of absorption of ezetimibe when administered as 10-mg tablets. The C_{max} value of ezetimibe was increased by 38% with consumption of high-fat meals).

No products indexed under this heading.

Fenofibrate (Fenofibrate increases ezetimibe AUC by 48% and ezetimibe C_{max} by 64%. Ezetimibe increases fenofibrate AUC by 11% and fenofibrate C_{max} by 7%). Products include:

Fenoglide	**3263**
Tricor	**544**
Trilipix	**548**

Fluconazole (Simvastatin is metabolized by the cytochrome P450 isoform 3A4. Certain drugs that inhibit this metabolic pathway can raise plasma levels of simvastatin and may increase the risk of myopathy. These drugs include itraconazole, ketoconazole, and other antifungal azoles. The use of Vytorin concomitantly with these CYP3A4 inhibitors should be avoided.)

No products indexed under this heading.

Fluoxetine (Simvastatin is metabolized by the cytochrome P450 isoform 3A4. Certain drugs that inhibit this metabolic pathway can raise the plasma levels of simvastatin and may increase the risk of myopathy. These include itraconazole, ketoconazole, and other antifungal azoles, the macrolide antibiotics erythromycin and clarithromycin, and the ketolide antibiotic telithromycin, HIV protease inhibitors, the antidepressant nefazodone, or large quantities of grapefruit juice (>1 quart daily). The use of Vytorin concomitantly with these CYP3A4 inhibitors should be avoided. If treatment with itraconazole, ketoconazole, erythromycin, clarithromycin or telithromycin is unavoidable, therapy with Vytorin should be suspended during the course of treatment).

No products indexed under this heading.

Fluoxetine Hydrochloride (Simvastatin is metabolized by the cytochrome P450 isoform 3A4. Certain drugs that inhibit this metabolic pathway can raise the plasma levels of simvastatin and may increase the risk of myopathy. These include itraconazole, ketoconazole, and other antifungal azoles, the macrolide antibiotics erythromycin and clarithromycin, and the ketolide antibiotic telithromycin, HIV protease inhibitors, the antidepressant nefazodone, or large quantities of grapefruit juice (>1 quart daily). The use of Vytorin concomitantly with these CYP3A4 inhibitors should be avoided. If treatment with itraconazole, ketoconazole, erythromycin, clarithromycin or telithromycin is unavoidable, therapy with Vytorin should be suspended during the course of treatment). Products include:

Prozac Weekly	**1941**
Prozac Pulvules	**1941**
Symbyax	**1965**

Fluvastatin Sodium (Fluvastatin decreases ezetimibe AUC by 19% and increases ezetimibe C_{max} by 7%. Ezetimibe decreases fluvastatin AUC by 39% and fluvastatin C_{max} by 27%).

No products indexed under this heading.

Fluvoxamine Maleate (Simvastatin is metabolized by the cytochrome P450 isoform 3A4. Certain drugs that inhibit this metabolic pathway can raise the plasma levels of simvastatin and may increase the risk of myopathy. These include itraconazole, ketoconazole, and other antifungal azoles, the macrolide antibiotics erythromycin and clarithromycin, and the ketolide antibiotic telithromycin, HIV protease inhibitors, the antidepressant nefazodone, or large quantities of grapefruit juice (>1 quart daily). The use of Vytorin concomitantly with these CYP3A4 inhibitors should be avoided. If treatment with itraconazole, ketoconazole, erythromycin, clarithromycin or telithromycin is unavoidable, therapy with Vytorin should be suspended during the course of treatment).

No products indexed under this heading.

Fosamprenavir Calcium (Simvastatin is metabolized by the cytochrome P450 isoform 3A4. Certain drugs that inhibit this metabolic pathway can raise plasma levels of simvastatin and may increase the risk of myopathy. These drugs include HIV protease inhibitors. The use of Vytorin concomitantly with these CYP3A4 inhibitors should be avoided). Products include:

Lexiva Oral Suspension	**1558**
Lexiva	**1558**

Gemfibrozil (The safety and effectiveness of Vytorin administered with fibrates have not been established. Therefore, the combination of Vytorin and fibrates should be avoided. There is an increased risk of myopathy when simvastatin is used concomitantly with fibrates (especially gemfibrozil). Combination therapy with gemfibrozil should be avoided because of an increase in simvastatin exposure with concomitant use).

No products indexed under this heading.

Glipizide (Glipizide increases ezetimibe AUC by 4% and decreases ezetimibe C_{max} by 8%. Ezetimibe decreases glipizide AUC by 3% and glipizide C_{max} by 5%).

No products indexed under this heading.

Imatinib Mesylate (Simvastatin is metabolized by the cytochrome P450 isoform 3A4. Certain drugs that inhibit this metabolic pathway can raise the plasma levels of simvastatin and may increase the risk of myopathy. These include itraconazole, ketoconazole, and other antifungal azoles, the macrolide antibiotics erythromycin and clarithromycin, and the ketolide antibiotic telithromycin, HIV protease inhibitors, the antidepressant nefazodone, or large quantities of grapefruit juice (>1 quart daily). The use of Vytorin concomitantly with these CYP3A4 inhibitors should be avoided. If treatment with itraconazole, ketoconazole, erythromycin, clarithromycin or telithromycin is unavoidable, therapy with Vytorin should be suspended during the course of treatment). Products include:

Gleevec	**2477**

Indinavir Sulfate (Simvastatin is metabolized by the cytochrome P450 isoform 3A4. Certain drugs that inhibit this metabolic pathway can raise plasma levels of simvastatin and may increase the risk of myopathy. These drugs include HIV protease inhibitors. The use of Vytorin concomitantly with these CYP3A4 inhibitors should be avoided). Products include:

Crixivan	**2113**

Isoniazid (Simvastatin is metabolized by the cytochrome P450 isoform 3A4. Certain drugs that inhibit this metabolic pathway can raise the plasma levels of simvastatin and may increase the risk of myopathy. These include itraconazole, ketoconazole, and other antifungal azoles, the macrolide antibiotics erythromycin and clarithromycin, and the ketolide antibiotic telithromycin, HIV protease inhibitors, the antidepressant nefazodone, or large quantities of grapefruit juice (>1 quart daily). The use of Vytorin concomitantly with these CYP3A4 inhibitors should be avoided. If treatment with itraconazole, ketoconazole, erythromycin, clarithromycin or telithromycin is unavoidable, therapy with Vytorin should be suspended during the course of treatment).

No products indexed under this heading.

Itraconazole (Simvastatin is metabolized by the cytochrome P450 isoform 3A4. Certain drugs that inhibit this metabolic pathway can raise plasma levels of simvastatin and may increase the risk of myopathy. These drugs include itraconazole. The use of Vytorin concomitantly with this CYP3A4 inhibitor should be avoided. If treatment with itraconazole is unavoidable, therapy with Vytorin should be suspended during the course of treatment).

No products indexed under this heading.

Ketoconazole (Simvastatin is metabolized by the cytochrome P450 isoform 3A4. Certain drugs that inhibit this metabolic pathway can raise plasma levels of simvastatin and may increase the risk of myopathy. These drugs include ketoconazole. The use of Vytorin concomitantly with this CYP3A4 inhibitor should be avoided. If treatment with ketoconazole is unavoidable, therapy with Vytorin should be suspended during the course of treatment). Products include:

Extina	**3319**
Xolegel	**3337**

Lapatinib (Simvastatin is metabolized by the cytochrome P450 isoform 3A4. Certain drugs that inhibit this metabolic pathway can raise the plasma levels of simvastatin and may increase the risk of myopathy. These include itraconazole, ketoconazole, and other antifungal azoles, the macrolide antibiotics erythromycin and clarithromycin, and the ketolide antibiotic telithromycin, HIV protease inhibitors, the antidepressant nefazodone, or large quantities of grapefruit juice (>1 quart daily). The use of Vytorin concomitantly with these CYP3A4 inhibitors should be avoided. If treatment with itraconazole, ketoconazole, erythromycin, clarithromycin or telithromycin is unavoidable, therapy with Vytorin should be suspended during the course of treatment). Products include:

Tykerb	**1698**

Levonorgestrel (During concomitant use with ethinyl estradiol and levonorgestrel, ezetimibe decreases ethinyl estradiol C_{max} by 9% and levonorgestrel C_{max} by 5%). Products include:

Climara Pro	**847**
LoSeasonique	**3407**
Lybrel	**3514**
Mirena	**854**
Plan B	**3416**
Seasonique	**3418**

Lopinavir (Simvastatin is metabolized by the cytochrome P450 isoform 3A4. Certain drugs that inhibit this metabolic pathway can raise plasma levels of simvastatin and may increase the risk of myopathy. These drugs include HIV protease inhibitors. The use of Vytorin concomitantly with these CYP3A4 inhibitors should be avoided). Products include:

Kaletra	**458**

Loratadine (Simvastatin is metabolized by the cytochrome P450 isoform 3A4. Certain drugs that inhibit this metabolic pathway can raise the plasma levels of simvastatin and may increase the risk of myopathy. These include itraconazole, ketoconazole, and other antifungal azoles, the macrolide antibiotics erythromycin and clarithromycin, and the ketolide antibiotic telithromycin, HIV protease inhibitors, the antidepressant nefazodone, or large quantities of grapefruit juice (>1 quart daily). The use of Vytorin concomitantly with these CYP3A4 inhibitors should be avoided. If treatment with itraconazole, ketoconazole, erythromycin, clarithromycin or telithromycin is unavoidable, therapy with Vytorin should be suspended during the course of treatment).

No products indexed under this heading.

Lovastatin (Lovastatin increases ezetimibe AUC by 9% and ezetimibe

C_{max} by 3%. Ezetimibe increases lovastatin AUC by 19% and lovastatin C_{max} by 3%). Products include:

Advicor	**402**
Mevacor	**2212**

Magnesium Hydroxide (Aluminium and magnesium hydroxide combination antacid decreases ezetimibe AUC by 4% and ezetimibe C_{max} by 30%). Products include:

Fleet Pedia-Lax Chewable Tablets	**1144**
Pepcid Complete	**1822**

Metronidazole (Simvastatin is metabolized by the cytochrome P450 isoform 3A4. Certain drugs that inhibit this metabolic pathway can raise the plasma levels of simvastatin and may increase the risk of myopathy. These include itraconazole, ketoconazole, and other antifungal azoles, the macrolide antibiotics erythromycin and clarithromycin, and the ketolide antibiotic telithromycin, HIV protease inhibitors, the antidepressant nefazodone, or large quantities of grapefruit juice (>1 quart daily). The use of Vytorin concomitantly with these CYP3A4 inhibitors should be avoided. If treatment with itraconazole, ketoconazole, erythromycin, clarithromycin or telithromycin is unavoidable, therapy with Vytorin should be suspended during the course of treatment). Products include:

Pylera	**793**

Metronidazole Benzoate (Simvastatin is metabolized by the cytochrome P450 isoform 3A4. Certain drugs that inhibit this metabolic pathway can raise the plasma levels of simvastatin and may increase the risk of myopathy. These include itraconazole, ketoconazole, and other antifungal azoles, the macrolide antibiotics erythromycin and clarithromycin, and the ketolide antibiotic telithromycin, HIV protease inhibitors, the antidepressant nefazodone, or large quantities of grapefruit juice (>1 quart daily). The use of Vytorin concomitantly with these CYP3A4 inhibitors should be avoided. If treatment with itraconazole, ketoconazole, erythromycin, clarithromycin or telithromycin is unavoidable, therapy with Vytorin should be suspended during the course of treatment).

No products indexed under this heading.

Metronidazole Hydrochloride (Simvastatin is metabolized by the cytochrome P450 isoform 3A4. Certain drugs that inhibit this metabolic pathway can raise the plasma levels of simvastatin and may increase the risk of myopathy. These include itraconazole, ketoconazole, and other antifungal azoles, the macrolide antibiotics erythromycin and clarithromycin, and the ketolide antibiotic telithromycin, HIV protease inhibitors, the antidepressant nefazodone, or large quantities of grapefruit juice (>1 quart daily). The use of Vytorin concomitantly with these CYP3A4 inhibitors should be avoided. If treatment with itraconazole, ketoconazole, erythromycin, clarithromycin or telithromycin is unavoidable, therapy with Vytorin should be suspended during the course of treatment).

No products indexed under this heading.

Metronidazole Sodium (Simvastatin is metabolized by the cytochrome P450 isoform 3A4. Certain drugs that inhibit this metabolic pathway can raise the plasma levels of simvastatin and may increase the risk of myopathy. These include itraconazole, ketoconazole, and other antifungal azoles, the macrolide antibiotics erythromycin and clarithromycin, and the ketolide antibiotic telithromycin, HIV protease inhibitors, the antidepressant nefazodone, or large quantities of grapefruit juice (>1 quart daily). The use of Vytorin concomitantly with these CYP3A4 inhibitors should be avoided. If treatment with itraconazole,

Vytorin Interactions Index 2080

ketoconazole, erythromycin, clarithromycin or telithromycin is unavoidable, therapy with Vytorin should be suspended during the course of treatment).
No products indexed under this heading.

Miconazole (Simvastatin is metabolized by the cytochrome P450 isoform 3A4. Certain drugs that inhibit this metabolic pathway can raise plasma levels of simvastatin and may increase the risk of myopathy. These drugs include itraconazole, ketoconazole, and other antifungal azoles. The use of Vytorin concomitantly with these CYP3A4 inhibitors should be avoided).
No products indexed under this heading.

Miconazole Nitrate (Simvastatin is metabolized by the cytochrome P450 isoform 3A4. Certain drugs that inhibit this metabolic pathway can raise the plasma levels of simvastatin and may increase the risk of myopathy. These include itraconazole, ketoconazole, and other antifungal azoles, the macrolide antibiotics erythromycin and clarithromycin, and the ketolide antibiotic telithromycin, HIV protease inhibitors, the antidepressant nefazodone, or large quantities of grapefruit juice (>1 quart daily). The use of Vytorin concomitantly with these CYP3A4 inhibitors should be avoided. If treatment with itraconazole, ketoconazole, erythromycin, clarithromycin or telithromycin is unavoidable, therapy with Vytorin should be suspended during the course of treatment). Products include:
Vusion Ointment 3335

Mifepristone (Simvastatin is metabolized by the cytochrome P450 isoform 3A4. Certain drugs that inhibit this metabolic pathway can raise the plasma levels of simvastatin and may increase the risk of myopathy. These include itraconazole, ketoconazole, and other antifungal azoles, the macrolide antibiotics erythromycin and clarithromycin, and the ketolide antibiotic telithromycin, HIV protease inhibitors, the antidepressant nefazodone, or large quantities of grapefruit juice (>1 quart daily). The use of Vytorin concomitantly with these CYP3A4 inhibitors should be avoided. If treatment with itraconazole, ketoconazole, erythromycin, clarithromycin or telithromycin is unavoidable, therapy with Vytorin should be suspended during the course of treatment).
No products indexed under this heading.

Nefazodone Hydrochloride (Simvastatin is metabolized by the cytochrome P450 isoform 3A4. Certain drugs that inhibit this metabolic pathway can raise plasma levels of simvastatin and may increase the risk of myopathy. These drugs include the antidepressant nefazodone. The use of Vytorin concomitantly with this CYP3A4 inhibitor should be avoided).
No products indexed under this heading.

Nelfinavir Mesylate (Concomitant administration of nelfinavir and simvastatin leads to a geometric mean ratio of simvastatin acid and simvastatin as follows - AUC: 6 and C_{max}: 6.2. Concomitant administration of nelfinavir and simvastatin should be avoided).
No products indexed under this heading.

Nevirapine (Simvastatin is metabolized by the cytochrome P450 isoform 3A4. Certain drugs that inhibit this metabolic pathway can raise the plasma levels of simvastatin and may increase the risk of myopathy. These include itraconazole, ketoconazole, and other antifungal azoles, the macrolide antibiotics erythromycin and clarithromycin, and the ketolide antibiotic telithromycin, HIV protease inhibitors, the antidepressant nefazodone, or large quantities of grapefruit juice (>1 quart daily). The use of Vytorin concomitantly with these CYP3A4 inhibitors should be avoided. If treatment with itraconazole, ketoconazole, erythromycin, clarithromycin or telithromycin is unavoidable, therapy with Vytorin should be suspended during the course of treatment). Products include:
Viramune Oral Suspension 897
Viramune Tablets 897

Niacin (The effect of Vytorin (10/20 mg daily for 7 days) on the pharmacokinetics ofniacin extended-release tablets (1000 mg for 2 days and 2000 mg for 5 days following a low-fat breakfast) was studied in healthy subjects. The mean C_{max} and AUC of niacin increased 9% and 22%, respectively. The mean C_{max} and AUC of nicotinuric acid increased 10% and 19%, respectively (N=13). In the same study, the effect of niacin on the pharmacokinetics of Vytorin was evaluated (N=15). While concomitant niacin decreased the mean C_{max} of total ezetimibe (1%), and simvastatin (2%), it increased the mean C_{max} of simvastatin acid (18%). In addition, concomitant niacin increased the mean AUC of total ezetimibe (26%), simvastatin (20%), and simvastatin acid (35%)). Products include:
Advicor 402
Cardio Basics 3455
Niaspan 497
Simcor 524

Niacinamide (Simvastatin is metabolized by the cytochrome P450 isoform 3A4. Certain drugs that inhibit this metabolic pathway can raise the plasma levels of simvastatin and may increase the risk of myopathy. These include itraconazole, ketoconazole, and other antifungal azoles, the macrolide antibiotics erythromycin and clarithromycin, and the ketolide antibiotic telithromycin, HIV protease inhibitors, the antidepressant nefazodone, or large quantities of grapefruit juice (>1 quart daily). The use of Vytorin concomitantly with these CYP3A4 inhibitors should be avoided. If treatment with itraconazole, ketoconazole, erythromycin, clarithromycin or telithromycin is unavoidable, therapy with Vytorin should be suspended during the course of treatment). Products include:
CitraNatal 90 DHA Capsules 2332
CitraNatal Assure 2332
CitraNatal Rx 2332
Heplive 607

Niacinamide Hydroiodide (Simvastatin is metabolized by the cytochrome P450 isoform 3A4. Certain drugs that inhibit this metabolic pathway can raise the plasma levels of simvastatin and may increase the risk of myopathy. These include itraconazole, ketoconazole, and other antifungal azoles, the macrolide antibiotics erythromycin and clarithromycin, and the ketolide antibiotic telithromycin, HIV protease inhibitors, the antidepressant nefazodone, or large quantities of grapefruit juice (>1 quart daily). The use of Vytorin concomitantly with these CYP3A4 inhibitors should be avoided. If treatment with itraconazole, ketoconazole, erythromycin, clarithromycin or telithromycin is unavoidable, therapy with Vytorin should be suspended during the course of treatment).
No products indexed under this heading.

Nicotinamide (Simvastatin is metabolized by the cytochrome P450 isoform 3A4. Certain drugs that inhibit this metabolic pathway can raise the plasma levels of simvastatin and may increase the risk of myopathy. These include itraconazole, ketoconazole, and other antifungal azoles, the macrolide antibiotics erythromycin and clarithromycin, and the ketolide antibiotic telithromycin, HIV protease inhibitors, the antidepressant nefazodone, or large quantities of grapefruit juice (>1 quart daily). The use of Vytorin concomitantly with these CYP3A4 inhibitors should be avoided. If treatment with itraconazole, ketoconazole, erythromycin, clarithromycin or telithromycin is unavoidable, therapy with Vytorin should be suspended during the course of treatment).
No products indexed under this heading.

Nifedipine (Simvastatin is metabolized by the cytochrome P450 isoform 3A4. Certain drugs that inhibit this metabolic pathway can raise the plasma levels of simvastatin and may increase the risk of myopathy. These include itraconazole, ketoconazole, and other antifungal azoles, the macrolide antibiotics erythromycin and clarithromycin, and the ketolide antibiotic telithromycin, HIV protease inhibitors, the antidepressant nefazodone, or large quantities of grapefruit juice (>1 quart daily). The use of Vytorin concomitantly with these CYP3A4 inhibitors should be avoided. If treatment with itraconazole, ketoconazole, erythromycin, clarithromycin or telithromycin is unavoidable, therapy with Vytorin should be suspended during the course of treatment).
No products indexed under this heading.

Norfloxacin (Simvastatin is metabolized by the cytochrome P450 isoform 3A4. Certain drugs that inhibit this metabolic pathway can raise the plasma levels of simvastatin and may increase the risk of myopathy. These include itraconazole, ketoconazole, and other antifungal azoles, the macrolide antibiotics erythromycin and clarithromycin, and the ketolide antibiotic telithromycin, HIV protease inhibitors, the antidepressant nefazodone, or large quantities of grapefruit juice (>1 quart daily). The use of Vytorin concomitantly with these CYP3A4 inhibitors should be avoided. If treatment with itraconazole, ketoconazole, erythromycin, clarithromycin or telithromycin is unavoidable, therapy with Vytorin should be suspended during the course of treatment). Products include:
Noroxin 2220

Omeprazole (Simvastatin is metabolized by the cytochrome P450 isoform 3A4. Certain drugs that inhibit this metabolic pathway can raise the plasma levels of simvastatin and may increase the risk of myopathy. These include itraconazole, ketoconazole, and other antifungal azoles, the macrolide antibiotics erythromycin and clarithromycin, and the ketolide antibiotic telithromycin, HIV protease inhibitors, the antidepressant nefazodone, or large quantities of grapefruit juice (>1 quart daily). The use of Vytorin concomitantly with these CYP3A4 inhibitors should be avoided. If treatment with itraconazole, ketoconazole, erythromycin, clarithromycin or telithromycin is unavoidable, therapy with Vytorin should be suspended during the course of treatment).
No products indexed under this heading.

Oxiconazole Nitrate (Simvastatin is metabolized by the cytochrome P450 isoform 3A4. Certain drugs that inhibit this metabolic pathway can raise plasma levels of simvastatin and may increase the risk of myopathy. These drugs include itraconazole, ketoconazole, and other antifungal azoles. The use of Vytorin concomitantly with these CYP3A4 inhibitors should be avoided).
No products indexed under this heading.

Paroxetine Hydrochloride (Simvastatin is metabolized by the cytochrome P450 isoform 3A4. Certain drugs that inhibit this metabolic pathway can raise the plasma levels of simvastatin and may increase the risk of myopathy. These include itraconazole, ketoconazole, and other antifungal azoles, the macrolide antibiotics erythromycin and clarithromycin, and the ketolide antibiotic telithromycin, HIV protease inhibitors, the antidepressant nefazodone, or large quantities of grapefruit juice (>1 quart daily). The use of Vytorin concomitantly with these CYP3A4 inhibitors should be avoided. If treatment with itraconazole, ketoconazole, erythromycin, clarithromycin or telithromycin is unavoidable, therapy with Vytorin should be suspended during the course of treatment). Products include:
Paroxetine CR 2361
Paroxetine ER 2371
Paxil 1586
Paxil CR 1596

Posaconazole (Simvastatin is metabolized by the cytochrome P450 isoform 3A4. Certain drugs that inhibit this metabolic pathway can raise plasma levels of simvastatin and may increase the risk of myopathy. These drugs include itraconazole, ketoconazole, and other antifungal azoles. The use of Vytorin concomitantly with these CYP3A4 inhibitors should be avoided). Products include:
Noxafil 3172

Pravastatin Sodium (Pravastatin increases ezetimibe AUC by 7% and ezetimibe C_{max} by 23%. Ezetimibe decreases pravastatin AUC by 20% and pravastatin C_{max} by 24%).
No products indexed under this heading.

Probucol (The benefits of the combined use of Vytorin with the following drugs should be carefully weighed against the potential risks of combinations: gemfibrozil, other lipid-lowering drugs (other fibrates or>/= 1 g/day of niacin), cyclosporine, danazol, amiodarone, or verapamil. Caution should be used when prescribing other fibrates or lipid-lowering doses (>/= 1 g/day) of niacin with Vytorin, as these agents can cause myopathy when given alone).
No products indexed under this heading.

Propoxyphene Hydrochloride (Simvastatin is metabolized by the cytochrome P450 isoform 3A4. Certain drugs that inhibit this metabolic pathway can raise the plasma levels of simvastatin and may increase the risk of myopathy. These include itraconazole, ketoconazole, and other antifungal azoles, the macrolide antibiotics erythromycin and clarithromycin, and the ketolide antibiotic telithromycin, HIV protease inhibitors, the antidepressant nefazodone, or large quantities of grapefruit juice (>1 quart daily). The use of Vytorin concomitantly with these CYP3A4 inhibitors should be avoided. If treatment with itraconazole, ketoconazole, erythromycin, clarithromycin or telithromycin is unavoidable, therapy with Vytorin should be suspended during the course of treatment).
No products indexed under this heading.

Propoxyphene Napsylate (Simvastatin is metabolized by the cytochrome P450 isoform 3A4. Certain drugs that inhibit this metabolic pathway can raise the plasma levels of simvastatin and may increase the risk of myopathy. These include itraconazole, ketoconazole, and other antifungal azoles, the macrolide antibiotics erythromycin and clarithromycin, and the ketolide antibiotic telithromycin, HIV protease inhibitors, the antidepressant nefazodone, or large quantities of grapefruit juice (>1 quart daily). The use of Vytorin concomitantly with these CYP3A4 inhibitors should be avoided. If treatment with itraconazole, ketoconazole, erythromycin, clarithromycin or telithromycin is unavoidable, therapy with Vytorin should be suspended during the course of treatment).
No products indexed under this heading.

Propranolol (Concomitant administration of propranolol and simvastatin leads to a geometric mean ratio of total inhibitor and active inhibitor as follows - AUC: 0.79 and 0.79).
No products indexed under this heading.

2081 Interactions Index Vytorin

Propranolol Hydrochloride (Concomitant administration of propranolol and simvastatin leads to a geometric mean ratio of total inhibitor and active inhibitor as follows - AUC: 0.79 and 0.79). Products include:
InnoPran XL 1517

Quinidine (Simvastatin is metabolized by the cytochrome P450 isoform 3A4. Certain drugs that inhibit this metabolic pathway can raise the plasma levels of simvastatin and may increase the risk of myopathy. These include itraconazole, ketoconazole, and other antifungal azoles, the macrolide antibiotics erythromycin and clarithromycin, and the ketolide antibiotic telithromycin, HIV protease inhibitors, the antidepressant nefazodone, or large quantities of grapefruit juice (>1 quart daily). The use of Vytorin concomitantly with these CYP3A4 inhibitors should be avoided. If treatment with itraconazole, ketoconazole, erythromycin, clarithromycin or telithromycin is unavoidable, therapy with Vytorin should be suspended during the course of treatment).
No products indexed under this heading.

Quinidine Hydrochloride (Simvastatin is metabolized by the cytochrome P450 isoform 3A4. Certain drugs that inhibit this metabolic pathway can raise the plasma levels of simvastatin and may increase the risk of myopathy. These include itraconazole, ketoconazole, and other antifungal azoles, the macrolide antibiotics erythromycin and clarithromycin, and the ketolide antibiotic telithromycin, HIV protease inhibitors, the antidepressant nefazodone, or large quantities of grapefruit juice (>1 quart daily). The use of Vytorin concomitantly with these CYP3A4 inhibitors should be avoided. If treatment with itraconazole, ketoconazole, erythromycin, clarithromycin or telithromycin is unavoidable, therapy with Vytorin should be suspended during the course of treatment).
No products indexed under this heading.

Quinidine Polygalacturonate (Simvastatin is metabolized by the cytochrome P450 isoform 3A4. Certain drugs that inhibit this metabolic pathway can raise the plasma levels of simvastatin and may increase the risk of myopathy. These include itraconazole, ketoconazole, and other antifungal azoles, the macrolide antibiotics erythromycin and clarithromycin, and the ketolide antibiotic telithromycin, HIV protease inhibitors, the antidepressant nefazodone, or large quantities of grapefruit juice (>1 quart daily). The use of Vytorin concomitantly with these CYP3A4 inhibitors should be avoided. If treatment with itraconazole, ketoconazole, erythromycin, clarithromycin or telithromycin is unavoidable, therapy with Vytorin should be suspended during the course of treatment).
No products indexed under this heading.

Quinidine Sulfate (Simvastatin is metabolized by the cytochrome P450 isoform 3A4. Certain drugs that inhibit this metabolic pathway can raise the plasma levels of simvastatin and may increase the risk of myopathy. These include itraconazole, ketoconazole, and other antifungal azoles, the macrolide antibiotics erythromycin and clarithromycin, and the ketolide antibiotic telithromycin, HIV protease inhibitors, the antidepressant nefazodone, or large quantities of grapefruit juice (>1 quart daily). The use of Vytorin concomitantly with these CYP3A4 inhibitors should be avoided. If treatment with itraconazole, ketoconazole, erythromycin, clarithromycin or telithromycin is unavoidable, therapy with Vytorin should be suspended during the course of treatment).
No products indexed under this heading.

Quinine (Simvastatin is metabolized by the cytochrome P450 isoform 3A4. Certain drugs that inhibit this metabolic pathway can raise the plasma levels of simvastatin and may increase the risk of myopathy. These include itraconazole, ketoconazole, and other antifungal azoles, the macrolide antibiotics erythromycin and clarithromycin, and the ketolide antibiotic telithromycin, HIV protease inhibitors, the antidepressant nefazodone, or large quantities of grapefruit juice (>1 quart daily). The use of Vytorin concomitantly with these CYP3A4 inhibitors should be avoided. If treatment with itraconazole, ketoconazole, erythromycin, clarithromycin or telithromycin is unavoidable, therapy with Vytorin should be suspended during the course of treatment). Products include:
Hyland's Leg Cramps PM with Quinine 3315

Quinine Sulfate (Simvastatin is metabolized by the cytochrome P450 isoform 3A4. Certain drugs that inhibit this metabolic pathway can raise the plasma levels of simvastatin and may increase the risk of myopathy. These include itraconazole, ketoconazole, and other antifungal azoles, the macrolide antibiotics erythromycin and clarithromycin, and the ketolide antibiotic telithromycin, HIV protease inhibitors, the antidepressant nefazodone, or large quantities of grapefruit juice (>1 quart daily). The use of Vytorin concomitantly with these CYP3A4 inhibitors should be avoided. If treatment with itraconazole, ketoconazole, erythromycin, clarithromycin or telithromycin is unavoidable, therapy with Vytorin should be suspended during the course of treatment).
No products indexed under this heading.

Quinupristin (Simvastatin is metabolized by the cytochrome P450 isoform 3A4. Certain drugs that inhibit this metabolic pathway can raise the plasma levels of simvastatin and may increase the risk of myopathy. These include itraconazole, ketoconazole, and other antifungal azoles, the macrolide antibiotics erythromycin and clarithromycin, and the ketolide antibiotic telithromycin, HIV protease inhibitors, the antidepressant nefazodone, or large quantities of grapefruit juice (>1 quart daily). The use of Vytorin concomitantly with these CYP3A4 inhibitors should be avoided. If treatment with itraconazole, ketoconazole, erythromycin, clarithromycin or telithromycin is unavoidable, therapy with Vytorin should be suspended during the course of treatment).
No products indexed under this heading.

Ranitidine Bismuth Citrate (Simvastatin is metabolized by the cytochrome P450 isoform 3A4. Certain drugs that inhibit this metabolic pathway can raise the plasma levels of simvastatin and may increase the risk of myopathy. These include itraconazole, ketoconazole, and other antifungal azoles, the macrolide antibiotics erythromycin and clarithromycin, and the ketolide antibiotic telithromycin, HIV protease inhibitors, the antidepressant nefazodone, or large quantities of grapefruit juice (>1 quart daily). The use of Vytorin concomitantly with these CYP3A4 inhibitors should be avoided. If treatment with itraconazole, ketoconazole, erythromycin, clarithromycin or telithromycin is unavoidable, therapy with Vytorin should be suspended during the course of treatment).
No products indexed under this heading.

Ranitidine Hydrochloride (Simvastatin is metabolized by the cytochrome P450 isoform 3A4. Certain drugs that inhibit this metabolic pathway can raise the plasma levels of simvastatin and may increase the risk of myopathy. These include itraconazole, ketoconazole, and other antifungal azoles, the macrolide antibiotics erythromycin and clarithromycin, and the ketolide antibiotic telithromycin, HIV protease inhibitors, the antidepressant nefazodone, or large quantities of grapefruit juice (>1 quart daily). The use of Vytorin concomitantly with these CYP3A4 inhibitors should be avoided. If treatment with itraconazole, ketoconazole, erythromycin, clarithromycin or telithromycin is unavoidable, therapy with Vytorin should be suspended during the course of treatment). Products include:
Zantac 1737
Zantac Injection 1732
Zantac Pharmacy 1735

Ritonavir (Simvastatin is metabolized by the cytochrome P450 isoform 3A4. Certain drugs that inhibit this metabolic pathway can raise plasma levels of simvastatin and may increase the risk of myopathy. These drugs include HIV protease inhibitors. The use of Vytorin concomitantly with these CYP3A4 inhibitors should be avoided). Products include:
Kaletra 458
Norvir 509

Rosuvastatin Calcium (Rosuvastatin increases ezetimibe AUC by 13% and ezetimibe C_{max} by 18%. Ezetimibe increases rosuvastatin AUC by 19% and rosuvastatin C_{max} by 17%). Products include:
Crestor 736

Saquinavir (Simvastatin is metabolized by the cytochrome P450 isoform 3A4. Certain drugs that inhibit this metabolic pathway can raise plasma levels of simvastatin and may increase the risk of myopathy. These drugs include HIV protease inhibitors. The use of Vytorin concomitantly with these CYP3A4 inhibitors should be avoided).
No products indexed under this heading.

Saquinavir Mesylate (Simvastatin is metabolized by the cytochrome P450 isoform 3A4. Certain drugs that inhibit this metabolic pathway can raise plasma levels of simvastatin and may increase the risk of myopathy. These drugs include HIV protease inhibitors. The use of Vytorin concomitantly with these CYP3A4 inhibitors should be avoided).
No products indexed under this heading.

Sertaconazole Nitrate (Simvastatin is metabolized by the cytochrome P450 isoform 3A4. Certain drugs that inhibit this metabolic pathway can raise plasma levels of simvastatin and may increase the risk of myopathy. These drugs include itraconazole, ketoconazole, and other antifungal azoles. The use of Vytorin concomitantly with these CYP3A4 inhibitors should be avoided).
No products indexed under this heading.

Sertraline Hydrochloride (Simvastatin is metabolized by the cytochrome P450 isoform 3A4. Certain drugs that inhibit this metabolic pathway can raise the plasma levels of simvastatin and may increase the risk of myopathy. These include itraconazole, ketoconazole, and other antifungal azoles, the macrolide antibiotics erythromycin and clarithromycin, and the ketolide antibiotic telithromycin, HIV protease inhibitors, the antidepressant nefazodone, or large quantities of grapefruit juice (>1 quart daily). The use of Vytorin concomitantly with these CYP3A4 inhibitors should be avoided. If treatment with itraconazole, ketoconazole, erythromycin, clarithromycin or telithromycin is unavoidable, therapy with Vytorin should be suspended during the course of treatment).
No products indexed under this heading.

Sildenafil Citrate (Simvastatin is metabolized by the cytochrome P450 isoform 3A4. Certain drugs that inhibit this metabolic pathway can raise the plasma levels of simvastatin and may increase the risk of myopathy. These include itraconazole, ketoconazole, and other antifungal azoles, the macrolide antibiotics erythromycin and clarithromycin, and the ketolide antibiotic telithromycin, HIV protease inhibitors, the antidepressant nefazodone, or large quantities of grapefruit juice (>1 quart daily). The use of Vytorin concomitantly with these CYP3A4 inhibitors should be avoided. If treatment with itraconazole, ketoconazole, erythromycin, clarithromycin or telithromycin is unavoidable, therapy with Vytorin should be suspended during the course of treatment).
No products indexed under this heading.

Telithromycin (Simvastatin is metabolized by the cytochrome P450 isoform 3A4. Certain drugs that inhibit this metabolic pathway can raise plasma levels of simvastatin and may increase the risk of myopathy. These drugs include the ketolide antibiotic telithromycin. The use of Vytorin concomitantly with this CYP3A4 inhibitor should be avoided. If treatment with telithromycin is unavoidable, therapy with Vytorin should be suspended during the course of treatment). Products include:
Ketek 2991

Terconazole (Simvastatin is metabolized by the cytochrome P450 isoform 3A4. Certain drugs that inhibit this metabolic pathway can raise plasma levels of simvastatin and may increase the risk of myopathy. These drugs include itraconazole, ketoconazole, and other antifungal azoles. The use of Vytorin concomitantly with these CYP3A4 inhibitors should be avoided).
No products indexed under this heading.

Tipranavir (Simvastatin is metabolized by the cytochrome P450 isoform 3A4. Certain drugs that inhibit this metabolic pathway can raise plasma levels of simvastatin and may increase the risk of myopathy. These drugs include HIV protease inhibitors. The use of Vytorin concomitantly with these CYP3A4 inhibitors should be avoided).
No products indexed under this heading.

Troglitazone (Simvastatin is metabolized by the cytochrome P450 isoform 3A4. Certain drugs that inhibit this metabolic pathway can raise the plasma levels of simvastatin and may increase the risk of myopathy. These include itraconazole, ketoconazole, and other antifungal azoles, the macrolide antibiotics erythromycin and clarithromycin, and the ketolide antibiotic telithromycin, HIV protease inhibitors, the antidepressant nefazodone, or large quantities of grapefruit juice (>1 quart daily). The use of Vytorin concomitantly with these CYP3A4 inhibitors should be avoided. If treatment with itraconazole, ketoconazole, erythromycin, clarithromycin or telithromycin is unavoidable, therapy with Vytorin should be suspended during the course of treatment).
No products indexed under this heading.

Troleandomycin (Simvastatin is metabolized by the cytochrome P450 isoform 3A4. Certain drugs that inhibit this metabolic pathway can raise plasma levels of simvastatin and may increase the risk of myopathy. These drugs include the macrolide antibiotics erythromycin and clarithromycin. The use of Vytorin concomitantly with these CYP3A4 inhibitors should be avoided. If treatment with erythromycin or clarithromycin is unavoidable, therapy with Vytorin should be suspended during the course of treatment).
No products indexed under this heading.

Valproate Sodium (Simvastatin is metabolized by the cytochrome P450 isoform 3A4. Certain drugs that inhibit this metabolic pathway can raise the plasma levels of simvastatin and may increase the risk of myopathy. These include itraconazole, ketoconazole, and

other antifungal azoles, the macrolide antibiotics erythromycin and clarithromycin, and the ketolide antibiotic telithromycin, HIV protease inhibitors, the antidepressant nefazodone, or large quantities of grapefruit juice (>1 quart daily). The use of Vytorin concomitantly with these CYP3A4 inhibitors should be avoided. If treatment with itraconazole, ketoconazole, erythromycin, clarithromycin or telithromycin is unavoidable, therapy with Vytorin should be suspended during the course of treatment).
No products indexed under this heading.

Vardenafil Hydrochloride (Simvastatin is metabolized by the cytochrome P450 isoform 3A4. Certain drugs that inhibit this metabolic pathway can raise the plasma levels of simvastatin and may increase the risk of myopathy. These include itraconazole, ketoconazole, and other antifungal azoles, the macrolide antibiotics erythromycin and clarithromycin, and the ketolide antibiotic telithromycin, HIV protease inhibitors, the antidepressant nefazodone, or large quantities of grapefruit juice (>1 quart daily). The use of Vytorin concomitantly with these CYP3A4 inhibitors should be avoided. If treatment with itraconazole, ketoconazole, erythromycin, clarithromycin or telithromycin is unavoidable, therapy with Vytorin should be suspended during the course of treatment). Products include:
Levitra 3157

Verapamil Hydrochloride (The risk of myopathy/rhabdomyolysis is increased by concomitant administration of verapamil with higher doses of Vytorin. In patients taking verapamil concomitantly with Vytorin, the dose of Vytorin should not exceed 10/20 mg/day). Products include:
Tarka 534

Voriconazole (Simvastatin is metabolized by the cytochrome P450 isoform 3A4. Certain drugs that inhibit this metabolic pathway can raise plasma levels of simvastatin and may increase the risk of myopathy. These drugs include itraconazole, ketoconazole, and other antifungal azoles. The use of Vytorin concomitantly with these CYP3A4 inhibitors should be avoided).
No products indexed under this heading.

Warfarin Sodium (Co-administration of warfarin and ezetimibe decreases R-warfarin AUC by 2% and S-warfarin AUC by 4% and also increases R-warfarin C_{max} by 3% and S-warfarin C_{max} by 1%).
No products indexed under this heading.

Zafirlukast (Simvastatin is metabolized by the cytochrome P450 isoform 3A4. Certain drugs that inhibit this metabolic pathway can raise the plasma levels of simvastatin and may increase the risk of myopathy. These include itraconazole, ketoconazole, and other antifungal azoles, the macrolide antibiotics erythromycin and clarithromycin, and the ketolide antibiotic telithromycin, HIV protease inhibitors, the antidepressant nefazodone, or large quantities of grapefruit juice (>1 quart daily). The use of Vytorin concomitantly with these CYP3A4 inhibitors should be avoided. If treatment with itraconazole, ketoconazole, erythromycin, clarithromycin or telithromycin is unavoidable, therapy with Vytorin should be suspended during the course of treatment). Products include:
Accolate 3612

Zileuton (Simvastatin is metabolized by the cytochrome P450 isoform 3A4. Certain drugs that inhibit this metabolic pathway can raise the plasma levels of simvastatin and may increase the risk of myopathy. These include itraconazole, ketoconazole, and other antifungal azoles, the macrolide antibiotics erythromycin and clarithromycin, and the ketolide antibiotic telithromycin, HIV protease inhibitors, the antidepressant nefazodone, or large quantities of grapefruit juice (>1 quart daily). The use of Vytorin concomitantly with these CYP3A4 inhibitors should be avoided. If treatment with itraconazole, ketoconazole, erythromycin, clarithromycin or telithromycin is unavoidable, therapy with Vytorin should be suspended during the course of treatment).
No products indexed under this heading.

Food Interactions

Alcohol (Vytorin should be used with caution in patients who consume substantial quantities of alcohol and/or have a past history of liver disease).

Beer, reduced-alcohol (Vytorin should be used with caution in patients who consume substantial quantities of alcohol and/or have a past history of liver disease).

Beer, unspecified (Vytorin should be used with caution in patients who consume substantial quantities of alcohol and/or have a past history of liver disease).

Food, unspecified (Concomitant food administration (high-fat or non-fat meals) had no effect on the extent of absorption of ezetimibe when administered as 10-mg tablets. The C_{max} value of ezetimibe was increased by 38% with consumption of high-fat meals).

Grapefruit (Simvastatin is metabolized by the cytochrome P450 isoform 3A4. Certain agents that inhibit this metabolic pathway can raise plasma levels of simvastatin and may increase the risk of myopathy. These agents include large quantities of grapefruit juice (greater than 1 quart daily). The use of Vytorin concomitantly with this CYP3A4 inhibitor should be avoided).

Grapefruit Juice (Simvastatin is metabolized by the cytochrome P450 isoform 3A4. Certain agents that inhibit this metabolic pathway can raise plasma levels of simvastatin and may increase the risk of myopathy. These agents include large quantities of grapefruit juice (greater than 1 quart daily). The use of Vytorin concomitantly with this CYP3A4 inhibitor should be avoided).

Meal, unspecified (Concomitant food administration (high-fat or non-fat meals) had no effect on the extent of absorption of ezetimibe when administered as 10-mg tablets. The C_{max} value of ezetimibe was increased by 38% with consumption of high-fat meals).

Wine, Chianti (Vytorin should be used with caution in patients who consume substantial quantities of alcohol and/or have a past history of liver disease).

Wine, Red (Vytorin should be used with caution in patients who consume substantial quantities of alcohol and/or have a past history of liver disease).

Wine, unspecified (Vytorin should be used with caution in patients who consume substantial quantities of alcohol and/or have a past history of liver disease).

Wine products (Vytorin should be used with caution in patients who consume substantial quantities of alcohol and/or have a past history of liver disease).

VYTORIN 10/10 TABLETS

(Ezetimibe, Simvastatin) 3240
May interact with alcohols, azole antifungals, bile acid sequestering agents, cytochrome p450 3a4 inhibitors (selected), cytochrome p450 3a4 inhibitors, potent (selected), erythromycin, fibrates, lipid-lowering drugs, macrolide antibiotics, oral anticoagulants, protease inhibitors, and certain other agents. Compounds in these categories include:

Acetazolamide (The risk of myopathy is increased by reducing the elimination of the simvastatin component of Vytorin. Hence when Vytorin is used with an inhibitor of CYP3A4, elevated plasma levels of HMG-CoA reductase inhibitory activity can increase the risk of myopathy and rhabdomyolysis, particularly with higher doses of Vytorin. Concomitant use of any medication labeled as having a strong inhibitory effect on CYP3A4 should be avoided unless the benefits of combined therapy outweigh the increased risk).
No products indexed under this heading.

Acetazolamide Sodium (The risk of myopathy is increased by reducing the elimination of the simvastatin component of Vytorin. Hence when Vytorin is used with an inhibitor of CYP3A4, elevated plasma levels of HMG-CoA reductase inhibitory activity can increase the risk of myopathy and rhabdomyolysis, particularly with higher doses of Vytorin. Concomitant use of any medication labeled as having a strong inhibitory effect on CYP3A4 should be avoided unless the benefits of combined therapy outweigh the increased risk).
No products indexed under this heading.

Aluminum Hydroxide (Concomitant use with aluminum and magnesium hydroxide combination antacid may decrease total ezetimibe AUC by 4% and total ezetimibe C_{max} by 30%).
No products indexed under this heading.

Amiodarone Hydrochloride (The risk of myopathy/rhabdomyolysis is increased by concomitant administration of amiodarone with higher doses of Vytorin. The combined use of Vytorin at doses higher than 10/20 mg daily with amiodarone should be avoided unless the clinical benefit is likely to outweigh the increased risk of myopathy).
No products indexed under this heading.

Amlodipine Besylate (Concomitant administration of amlodipine and simvastatin leads to a geometric mean ratio of simvastatin acid and simvastatin as follows - AUC: 1.58 and 1.77 and C_{max}: 1.56 and 1.47. No dosing adjustments are required). Products include:
Azor 1010
Exforge 2443
Exforge HCT 2449

Amprenavir (Simvastatin is metabolized by the cytochrome P450 isoform 3A4. The risk of myopathy is increased by reducing the elimination of the simvastatin component of Vytorin. Hence when Vytorin is used with an inhibitor of CYP3A4 (eg, HIV protease inhibitors), elevated plasma levels of HMG-CoA reductase inhibitory activity can increase the risk of myopathy and rhabdomyolysis, particularly with higher doses of Vytorin. The use of Vytorin concomitantly with HIV protease inhibitors should be avoided).
No products indexed under this heading.

Anastrozole (The risk of myopathy is increased by reducing the elimination of the simvastatin component of Vytorin. Hence when Vytorin is used with an inhibitor of CYP3A4, elevated plasma levels of HMG-CoA reductase inhibitory activity can increase the risk of myopathy and rhabdomyolysis, particularly with higher doses of Vytorin. Concomitant use of any medication labeled as having a strong inhibitory effect on CYP3A4 should be avoided unless the benefits of combined therapy outweigh the increased risk).
No products indexed under this heading.

Anisindione (Simvastatin 20-40 mg/day modestly potentiated the effect of coumarin anticoagulants: the prothrombin time, reported as International Normalized Ratio (INR), increased from a baseline of 1.7 to 1.8 and from 2.6 to 3.4 in a normal volunteer study and in a hypercholesterolemic patient study, respectively. Prothrombin time should be determined before starting Vytorin and frequently enough during early therapy to ensure that no significant alteration of prothrombin time occurs. Once a stable prothrombin time has been documented, prothrombin times can be monitored at the intervals usually recommended for patients on coumarin anticoagulants. If the dose of Vytorin is changed or discontinued, the same procedure should be repeated).
No products indexed under this heading.

Aprepitant (The risk of myopathy is increased by reducing the elimination of the simvastatin component of Vytorin. Hence when Vytorin is used with an inhibitor of CYP3A4, elevated plasma levels of HMG-CoA reductase inhibitory activity can increase the risk of myopathy and rhabdomyolysis, particularly with higher doses of Vytorin. Concomitant use of any medication labeled as having a strong inhibitory effect on CYP3A4 should be avoided unless the benefits of combined therapy outweigh the increased risk). Products include:
Emend 2124

Atazanavir (Simvastatin is metabolized by the cytochrome P450 isoform 3A4. The risk of myopathy is increased by reducing the elimination of the simvastatin component of Vytorin. Hence when Vytorin is used with an inhibitor of CYP3A4 (eg, HIV protease inhibitors), elevated plasma levels of HMG-CoA reductase inhibitory activity can increase the risk of myopathy and rhabdomyolysis, particularly with higher doses of Vytorin. The use of Vytorin concomitantly with HIV protease inhibitors should be avoided).
No products indexed under this heading.

Atazanavir Sulfate (Simvastatin is metabolized by the cytochrome P450 isoform 3A4. The risk of myopathy is increased by reducing the elimination of the simvastatin component of Vytorin. Hence when Vytorin is used with an inhibitor of CYP3A4 (eg, HIV protease inhibitors), elevated plasma levels of HMG-CoA reductase inhibitory activity can increase the risk of myopathy and rhabdomyolysis, particularly with higher doses of Vytorin. The use of Vytorin concomitantly with HIV protease inhibitors should be avoided).
No products indexed under this heading.

Atorvastatin Calcium (Concomitant use with atorvastatin may decrease total ezetimibe AUC by 2% and increase total ezetimibe C_{max} by 12%. In addition, concomitant use with ezetimibe may decrease atorvastatin AUC by 4% and increase atorvastatin C_{max} by 7%). Products include:
Lipitor 2703

Azithromycin Dihydrate (The risk of myopathy and rhabdomyolysis is increased by high levels of statin activity in plasma. Simvastatin is metabolized by the cytochrome P450 isoform 3A4. Certain drugs that inhibit this metabolic pathway can raise the plasma levels of simvastatin and may increase the risk of myopathy. These include the macrolide antibiotics erythromycin and clarithromycin. The use of Vytorin concomitantly with these CYP3A4 inhibitors should be avoided. If treatment with erythromycin or clarithromycin is unavoidable, therapy with Vytorin should be suspended during the course of treatment).
No products indexed under this heading.

Butoconazole Nitrate (The risk of myopathy and rhabdomyolysis is increased by high levels of statin activity in plasma. Simvastatin is metabolized by the cytochrome P450 isoform 3A4. Certain drugs that inhibit this metabolic pathway can raise the plasma levels of simvastatin and may increase the risk of myopathy. These include itraconazole, ketoconazole, and other antifungal azoles. The use of Vytorin concomitantly with these CYP3A4 inhibitors should be avoided. If treatment with itraconazole or ketoconazole or other antifungal azoles is unavoidable, therapy with Vytorin should be suspended during the course of treatment).
No products indexed under this heading.

Cerivastatin Sodium (The benefits of the combined use of Vytorin with the following drugs should be carefully weighed against the potential risks of combinations: gemfibrozil, other lipid-lowering drugs (other fibrates or ≥1 g/day of niacin), cyclosporine, danazol, amiodarone, or verapamil. Caution should be used when prescribing other fibrates or lipid-lowering doses (≥1 g/day) of niacin with Vytorin, as these agents can cause myopathy when given alone).
No products indexed under this heading.

Cholestyramine (Concomitant use with cholestyramine may decrease the mean AUC of total ezetimibe by approximately 55% and may decrease the C_{max} of ezetimibe by 4%. The incremental LDL-C reduction due to adding Vytorin to cholestyramine may be reduced by this interaction. Dosing of Vytorin should occur either ≥2 hours before or ≥4 hours after administration of a bile acid sequestrant).
No products indexed under this heading.

Cimetidine (Concomitant use with cimetidine 400 mg bid for 7 days may increase total ezetimibe AUC by 6% and total ezetimibe C_{max} by 22%).
No products indexed under this heading.

Cimetidine Hydrochloride (Concomitant use with cimetidine 400 mg bid for 7 days may increase total ezetimibe AUC by 6% and total ezetimibe C_{max} by 22%).
No products indexed under this heading.

Ciprofloxacin (The risk of myopathy is increased by reducing the elimination of the simvastatin component of Vytorin. Hence when Vytorin is used with an inhibitor of CYP3A4, elevated plasma levels of HMG-CoA reductase inhibitory activity can increase the risk of myopathy and rhabdomyolysis, particularly with higher doses of Vytorin. Concomitant use of any medication labeled as having a strong inhibitory effect on CYP3A4 should be avoided unless the benefits of combined therapy outweigh the increased risk). Products include:
Cipro I.V. 3082
Cipro 3073
Cipro XR 3091
Ciprodex 583

Clarithromycin (Simvastatin is metabolized by the cytochrome P450 isoform 3A4. The risk of myopathy is increased by reducing the elimination of the simvastatin component of Vytorin. Hence when Vytorin is used with an inhibitor of CYP3A4 (eg, clarithromycin), elevated plasma levels of HMG-CoA reductase inhibitory activity can increase the risk of myopathy and rhabdomyolysis, particularly with higher doses of Vytorin. If treatment with clarithromycin is unavoidable, therapy with Vytorin should be suspended during the course of treatment). Products include:
Biaxin/Biaxin XL 412

Clofibrate (The safety and effectiveness of Vytorin administered with fibrates have not been established. Fibrates may increase cholesterol excretion into the bile, leading to cholelithiasis. There is an increased risk of myopathy when simvastatin is used concomitantly with fibrates. The benefits of the combined use of Vytorin with fibrates should be carefully weighed against the risks. Combination therapy with fibrates should be avoided).
No products indexed under this heading.

Clotrimazole (The risk of myopathy and rhabdomyolysis is increased by high levels of statin activity in plasma. Simvastatin is metabolized by the cytochrome P450 isoform 3A4. Certain drugs that inhibit this metabolic pathway can raise the plasma levels of simvastatin and may increase the risk of myopathy. These include itraconazole, ketoconazole, and other antifungal azoles. The use of Vytorin concomitantly with these CYP3A4 inhibitors should be avoided. If treatment with itraconazole or ketoconazole or other antifungal azoles is unavoidable, therapy with Vytorin should be suspended during the course of treatment). Products include:
Lotrisone 3163

Colesevelam Hydrochloride (Dosing of Vytorin should occur either ≥2 hours before or ≥4 hours after administration of a bile acid sequestrant). Products include:
Welchol 1029

Colestipol Hydrochloride (Dosing of Vytorin should occur either ≥2 hours before or ≥4 hours after administration of a bile acid sequestrant).
No products indexed under this heading.

Conivaptan Hydrochloride (The risk of myopathy is increased by reducing the elimination of the simvastatin component of Vytorin. Hence when Vytorin is used with an inhibitor of CYP3A4, elevated plasma levels of HMG-CoA reductase inhibitory activity can increase the risk of myopathy and rhabdomyolysis, particularly with higher doses of Vytorin. Concomitant use of any medication labeled as having a strong inhibitory effect on CYP3A4 should be avoided unless the benefits of combined therapy outweigh the increased risk). Products include:
Vaprisol 689

Cyclosporine (Caution should be exercised when using Vytorin and cyclosporine concurrently due to increased exposure to both ezetimibe and cyclosporine. The degree of increase in ezetimibe exposure may be greater in patients with severe renal impairment. The risk of myopathy/rhabdomyolysis is increased by concomitant administration of cyclosporine with Vytorin. Cyclosporine concentrations should be monitored if using Vytorin concomitantly. In patients treated with cyclosporine, the potential effects of the increased exposure to ezetimibe from concomitant use should be carefully weighed against the benefits of alterations in lipid levels provided by ezetimibe. In patients taking cyclosporine, Vytorin should not be started unless the patient has already tolerated treatment with simvastatin at a dose of 5 mg or higher. The dose of Vytorin should not exceed 10/10 mg/day). Products include:
Gengraf 440
Neoral Oral Solution 2496
Neoral Capsules 2496
Restasis 605

Dalfopristin (The risk of myopathy is increased by reducing the elimination of the simvastatin component of Vytorin. Hence when Vytorin is used with an inhibitor of CYP3A4, elevated plasma levels of HMG-CoA reductase inhibitory activity can increase the risk of myopathy and rhabdomyolysis, particularly with higher doses of Vytorin. Concomitant use of any medication labeled as having a strong inhibitory effect on CYP3A4 should be avoided unless the benefits of combined therapy outweigh the increased risk).
No products indexed under this heading.

Danazol (The risk of myopathy/rhabdomyolysis is increased by concomitant administration of danazol particularly with higher doses of Vytorin. The benefits of the combined use of Vytorin with danazol should be carefully weighed against the potential risks. In patients taking danazol, Vytorin should not be started unless the patient has already tolerated treatment with simvastatin at a dose of 5 mg or higher. The dose of Vytorin should not exceed 10/10 mg/day).
No products indexed under this heading.

Darunavir (Simvastatin is metabolized by the cytochrome P450 isoform 3A4. The risk of myopathy is increased by reducing the elimination of the simvastatin component of Vytorin. Hence when Vytorin is used with an inhibitor of CYP3A4 (eg, HIV protease inhibitors), elevated plasma levels of HMG-CoA reductase inhibitory activity can increase the risk of myopathy and rhabdomyolysis, particularly with higher doses of Vytorin. The use of Vytorin concomitantly with HIV protease inhibitors should be avoided).
No products indexed under this heading.

Dasatinib (The risk of myopathy is increased by reducing the elimination of the simvastatin component of Vytorin. Hence when Vytorin is used with an inhibitor of CYP3A4, elevated plasma levels of HMG-CoA reductase inhibitory activity can increase the risk of myopathy and rhabdomyolysis, particularly with higher doses of Vytorin. Concomitant use of any medication labeled as having a strong inhibitory effect on CYP3A4 should be avoided unless the benefits of combined therapy outweigh the increased risk).
No products indexed under this heading.

Delavirdine Mesylate (The risk of myopathy is increased by reducing the elimination of the simvastatin component of Vytorin. Hence when Vytorin is used with an inhibitor of CYP3A4, elevated plasma levels of HMG-CoA reductase inhibitory activity can increase the risk of myopathy and rhabdomyolysis, particularly with higher doses of Vytorin. Concomitant use of any medication labeled as having a strong inhibitory effect on CYP3A4 should be avoided unless the benefits of combined therapy outweigh the increased risk).
No products indexed under this heading.

Delavirine (The risk of myopathy is increased by reducing the elimination of the simvastatin component of Vytorin. Hence when Vytorin is used with an inhibitor of CYP3A4, elevated plasma levels of HMG-CoA reductase inhibitory activity can increase the risk of myopathy and rhabdomyolysis, particularly with higher doses of Vytorin. Concomitant use of any medication labeled as having a strong inhibitory effect on CYP3A4 should be avoided unless the benefits of combined therapy outweigh the increased risk).
No products indexed under this heading.

Desloratadine (The risk of myopathy is increased by reducing the elimination of the simvastatin component of Vytorin. Hence when Vytorin is used with an inhibitor of CYP3A4, elevated plasma levels of HMG-CoA reductase inhibitory activity can increase the risk of myopathy and rhabdomyolysis, particularly with higher doses of Vytorin. Concomitant use of any medication labeled as having a strong inhibitory effect on CYP3A4 should be avoided unless the benefits of combined therapy outweigh the increased risk). Products include:
Clarinex Syrup 3098
Clarinex 3098
Clarinex Reditabs 3098
Clarinex-D 12-Hour 3101
Clarinex-D 3104

Dicumarol (Simvastatin 20-40 mg/day modestly potentiated the effect of coumarin anticoagulants: the prothrombin time, reported as International Normalized Ratio (INR), increased from a baseline of 1.7 to 1.8 and from 2.6 to 3.4 in a normal volunteer study and in a hypercholesterolemic patient study, respectively. Prothrombin time should be determined before starting Vytorin and frequently enough during early therapy to ensure that no significant alteration of prothrombin time occurs. Once a stable prothrombin time has been documented, prothrombin times can be monitored at the intervals usually recommended for patients on coumarin anticoagulants. If the dose of Vytorin is changed or discontinued, the same procedure should be repeated).
No products indexed under this heading.

Digoxin (In one study, concomitant administration of digoxin with simvastatin resulted in a slight elevation in plasma digoxin concentrations. Patients taking digoxin should be monitored appropriately when Vytorin is initiated). Products include:
Lanoxin Injection 1546
Lanoxin Injection Pediatric 1549
Lanoxin Tablets 1553

Diltiazem Hydrochloride (Concomitant administration of diltiazem and simvastatin leads to a geometric mean ratio of simvastatin acid and simvastatin as follows - AUC: 2.69 and 3.10 and C_{max}: 2.69 and 2.88. No dosing adjustments are required). Products include:
Cardizem LA 423

Diltiazem Maleate (Concomitant administration of diltiazem and simvastatin leads to a geometric mean ratio of simvastatin acid and simvastatin as follows - AUC: 2.69 and 3.10 and C_{max}: 2.69 and 2.88. No dosing adjustments are required).
No products indexed under this heading.

Dirithromycin (The risk of myopathy and rhabdomyolysis is increased by high levels of statin activity in plasma. Simvastatin is metabolized by the cytochrome P450 isoform 3A4. Certain drugs that inhibit this metabolic pathway can raise the plasma levels of simvastatin and may increase the risk of myopathy. These include the macrolide antibiotics erythromycin and clarithromycin. The use of Vytorin concomitantly with these CYP3A4 inhibitors should be avoided. If treatment with erythromycin or clarithromycin is unavoidable, therapy with Vytorin should be suspended during the course of treatment).
No products indexed under this heading.

Econazole Nitrate (The risk of myopathy and rhabdomyolysis is increased by high levels of statin activity in plasma. Simvastatin is metabolized by the cytochrome P450 isoform 3A4. Certain drugs that inhibit this metabolic pathway can raise the plasma levels of simvastatin and may increase the risk of myopathy. These include itraconazole, ketoconazole, and other antifungal azoles. The use of Vytorin concomitantly with these CYP3A4 inhibitors should be avoided. If treatment with itraconazole or ketoconazole or other antifungal azoles is unavoidable, therapy with Vytorin should be suspended during the course of treatment).
No products indexed under this heading.

Efavirenz (The risk of myopathy is increased by reducing the elimination of the simvastatin component of Vytorin.

IMPORTANT NOTE: Always consult each drug listing in the patient's regimen for possible interactions.

Hence when Vytorin is used with an inhibitor of CYP3A4, elevated plasma levels of HMG-CoA reductase inhibitory activity can increase the risk of myopathy and rhabdomyolysis, particularly with higher doses of Vytorin. Concomitant use of any medication labeled as having a strong inhibitory effect on CYP3A4 should be avoided unless the benefits of combined therapy outweigh the increased risk). Products include:

Atripla 906

Erythromycin (Simvastatin is metabolized by the cytochrome P450 isoform 3A4. The risk of myopathy is increased by reducing the elimination of the simvastatin component of Vytorin. Hence when Vytorin is used with an inhibitor of CYP3A4 (eg, erythromycin), elevated plasma levels of HMG-CoA reductase inhibitory activity can increase the risk of myopathy and rhabdomyolysis, particularly with higher doses of Vytorin. If treatment with erythromycin is unavoidable, therapy with Vytorin should be suspended during the course of treatment).

No products indexed under this heading.

Erythromycin, Topical (Simvastatin is metabolized by the cytochrome P450 isoform 3A4. The risk of myopathy is increased by reducing the elimination of the simvastatin component of Vytorin. Hence when Vytorin is used with an inhibitor of CYP3A4 (eg, erythromycin), elevated plasma levels of HMG-CoA reductase inhibitory activity can increase the risk of myopathy and rhabdomyolysis, particularly with higher doses of Vytorin. If treatment with erythromycin is unavoidable, therapy with Vytorin should be suspended during the course of treatment).

No products indexed under this heading.

Erythromycin Estolate (Simvastatin is metabolized by the cytochrome P450 isoform 3A4. The risk of myopathy is increased by reducing the elimination of the simvastatin component of Vytorin. Hence when Vytorin is used with an inhibitor of CYP3A4 (eg, erythromycin), elevated plasma levels of HMG-CoA reductase inhibitory activity can increase the risk of myopathy and rhabdomyolysis, particularly with higher doses of Vytorin. If treatment with erythromycin is unavoidable, therapy with Vytorin should be suspended during the course of treatment).

No products indexed under this heading.

Erythromycin Ethylsuccinate (Simvastatin is metabolized by the cytochrome P450 isoform 3A4. The risk of myopathy is increased by reducing the elimination of the simvastatin component of Vytorin. Hence when Vytorin is used with an inhibitor of CYP3A4 (eg, erythromycin), elevated plasma levels of HMG-CoA reductase inhibitory activity can increase the risk of myopathy and rhabdomyolysis, particularly with higher doses of Vytorin. If treatment with erythromycin is unavoidable, therapy with Vytorin should be suspended during the course of treatment). Products include:

E.E.S. 437
EryPed 435

Erythromycin Gluceptate (Simvastatin is metabolized by the cytochrome P450 isoform 3A4. The risk of myopathy is increased by reducing the elimination of the simvastatin component of Vytorin. Hence when Vytorin is used with an inhibitor of CYP3A4 (eg, erythromycin), elevated plasma levels of HMG-CoA reductase inhibitory activity can increase the risk of myopathy and rhabdomyolysis, particularly with higher doses of Vytorin. If treatment with erythromycin is unavoidable, therapy with Vytorin should be suspended during the course of treatment).

No products indexed under this heading.

Erythromycin Lactobionate (Simvastatin is metabolized by the cytochrome P450 isoform 3A4. The risk of myopathy is increased by reducing the elimination of the simvastatin component of Vytorin. Hence when Vytorin is used with an inhibitor of CYP3A4 (eg, erythromycin), elevated plasma levels of HMG-CoA reductase inhibitory activity can increase the risk of myopathy and rhabdomyolysis, particularly with higher doses of Vytorin. If treatment with erythromycin is unavoidable, therapy with Vytorin should be suspended during the course of treatment).

No products indexed under this heading.

Erythromycin Stearate (Simvastatin is metabolized by the cytochrome P450 isoform 3A4. The risk of myopathy is increased by reducing the elimination of the simvastatin component of Vytorin. Hence when Vytorin is used with an inhibitor of CYP3A4 (eg, erythromycin), elevated plasma levels of HMG-CoA reductase inhibitory activity can increase the risk of myopathy and rhabdomyolysis, particularly with higher doses of Vytorin. If treatment with erythromycin is unavoidable, therapy with Vytorin should be suspended during the course of treatment).

No products indexed under this heading.

Esomeprazole Magnesium (The risk of myopathy is increased by reducing the elimination of the simvastatin component of Vytorin. Hence when Vytorin is used with an inhibitor of CYP3A4, elevated plasma levels of HMG-CoA reductase inhibitory activity can increase the risk of myopathy and rhabdomyolysis, particularly with higher doses of Vytorin. Concomitant use of any medication labeled as having a strong inhibitory effect on CYP3A4 should be avoided unless the benefits of combined therapy outweigh the increased risk). Products include:

Nexium Capsules 704
Nexium Oral Suspension 704

Esomeprazole Sodium (The risk of myopathy is increased by reducing the elimination of the simvastatin component of Vytorin. Hence when Vytorin is used with an inhibitor of CYP3A4, elevated plasma levels of HMG-CoA reductase inhibitory activity can increase the risk of myopathy and rhabdomyolysis, particularly with higher doses of Vytorin. Concomitant use of any medication labeled as having a strong inhibitory effect on CYP3A4 should be avoided unless the benefits of combined therapy outweigh the increased risk). Products include:

Nexium I.V. 712

Ethanol (Vytorin should be used with caution in patients who consume substantial quantities of alcohol and/or have a past history of liver disease).

No products indexed under this heading.

Ethinyl Estradiol (During concomitant use with ethinyl estradiol and levonorgestrel, ezetimibe may decrease ethinyl estradiol C_{max} by 9% and levonorgestrel C_{max} by 5%). Products include:

LoSeasonique 3407
Lybrel 3514
NuvaRing 3181
Ortho Evra 2648
Ortho-Cyclen/Ortho Tri-Cyclen 2663
Ortho Tri-Cyclen Lo Tablets 2673
Seasonique 3418
Yaz 864

Ethyl Alcohol (Vytorin should be used with caution in patients who consume substantial quantities of alcohol and/or have a past history of liver disease).

No products indexed under this heading.

Fat (Concomitant food administration (high-fat or non-fat meals) had no effect on the extent of absorption of ezetimibe when administered as 10-mg tablets. The C_{max} value of ezetimibe was increased by 38% with consumption of high-fat meals).

No products indexed under this heading.

Fenofibrate (Concurrent use with fenofibrate may increase total ezetimibe AUC by 48% and total ezetimibe C_{max} by 64%. Ezetimibe may increase fenofibrate AUC by 11% and fenofibrate C_{max} by 7%. The safety and effectiveness of Vytorin administered with fibrates have not been established. Fibrates may increase cholesterol excretion into the bile, leading to cholelithiasis. There is an increased risk of myopathy when simvastatin is used concomitantly with fibrates. The benefits of the combined use of Vytorin with fibrates should be carefully weighed against the risks. Combination therapy with fibrates should be avoided). Products include:

Fenoglide 3263
Tricor 544
Trilipix 548

Fluconazole (The risk of myopathy and rhabdomyolysis is increased by high levels of statin activity in plasma. Simvastatin is metabolized by the cytochrome P450 isoform 3A4. Certain drugs that inhibit this metabolic pathway can raise the plasma levels of simvastatin and may increase the risk of myopathy. These include itraconazole, ketoconazole, and other antifungal azoles. The use of Vytorin concomitantly with these CYP3A4 inhibitors should be avoided. If treatment with itraconazole or ketoconazole or other antifungal azoles is unavoidable, therapy with Vytorin should be suspended during the course of treatment).

No products indexed under this heading.

Fluoxetine (The risk of myopathy is increased by reducing the elimination of the simvastatin component of Vytorin. Hence when Vytorin is used with an inhibitor of CYP3A4, elevated plasma levels of HMG-CoA reductase inhibitory activity can increase the risk of myopathy and rhabdomyolysis, particularly with higher doses of Vytorin. Concomitant use of any medication labeled as having a strong inhibitory effect on CYP3A4 should be avoided unless the benefits of combined therapy outweigh the increased risk).

No products indexed under this heading.

Fluoxetine Hydrochloride (The risk of myopathy is increased by reducing the elimination of the simvastatin component of Vytorin. Hence when Vytorin is used with an inhibitor of CYP3A4, elevated plasma levels of HMG-CoA reductase inhibitory activity can increase the risk of myopathy and rhabdomyolysis, particularly with higher doses of Vytorin. Concomitant use of any medication labeled as having a strong inhibitory effect on CYP3A4 should be avoided unless the benefits of combined therapy outweigh the increased risk). Products include:

Prozac Weekly 1941
Prozac Pulvules 1941
Symbyax 1965

Fluvastatin Sodium (Concomitant use with fluvastatin may decrease total ezetimibe AUC by 19% and increase total ezetimibe C_{max} by 7%. In addition, concomitant use with ezetimibe may decrease fluvastatin AUC by 39% and fluvastatin C_{max} by 27%).

No products indexed under this heading.

Fluvoxamine Maleate (The risk of myopathy is increased by reducing the elimination of the simvastatin component of Vytorin. Hence when Vytorin is used with an inhibitor of CYP3A4, elevated plasma levels of HMG-CoA reductase inhibitory activity can increase the risk of myopathy and rhabdomyolysis, particularly with higher doses of Vytorin. Concomitant use of any medication labeled as having a strong inhibitory effect on CYP3A4 should be avoided unless the benefits of combined therapy outweigh the increased risk).

No products indexed under this heading.

Fosamprenavir Calcium (Simvastatin is metabolized by the cytochrome P450 isoform 3A4. The risk of myopathy is increased by reducing the elimination of the simvastatin component of Vytorin. Hence when Vytorin is used with an inhibitor of CYP3A4 (eg, HIV protease inhibitors), elevated plasma levels of HMG-CoA reductase inhibitory activity can increase the risk of myopathy and rhabdomyolysis, particularly with higher doses of Vytorin. The use of Vytorin concomitantly with HIV protease inhibitors should be avoided). Products include:

Lexiva Oral Suspension 1558
Lexiva 1558

Gemfibrozil (Concomitant use with gemfibrozil may increase the AUC of total ezetimibe by 64%, increase the C_{max} of total ezetimibe by 91%, decrease the AUC of gemfibrozil by 1%, and decrease the C_{max} of gemfibrozil by 11%. The safety and effectiveness of Vytorin administered with fibrates have not been established. Fibrates may increase cholesterol excretion into the bile, leading to cholelithiasis. There is an increased risk of myopathy when simvastatin is used concomitantly with fibrates (especially gemfibrozil). The benefits of the combined use of Vytorin with gemfibrozil should be carefully weighed against the risks. Combination therapy with fibrates should be avoided; however although not recommended, if Vytorin is used in combination with gemfibrozil, the dose should not exceed 10/10 mg daily).

No products indexed under this heading.

Glipizide (Concomitant use with glipizide 10 mg single dose may increase total ezetimibe AUC by 4% and decrease total ezetimibe C_{max} by 8%. Also, concomitant use with ezetimibe may decrease glipizide AUC by 3% and glipizide C_{max} by 5%).

No products indexed under this heading.

Imatinib Mesylate (The risk of myopathy is increased by reducing the elimination of the simvastatin component of Vytorin. Hence when Vytorin is used with an inhibitor of CYP3A4, elevated plasma levels of HMG-CoA reductase inhibitory activity can increase the risk of myopathy and rhabdomyolysis, particularly with higher doses of Vytorin. Concomitant use of any medication labeled as having a strong inhibitory effect on CYP3A4 should be avoided unless the benefits of combined therapy outweigh the increased risk). Products include:

Gleevec 2477

Indinavir Sulfate (Simvastatin is metabolized by the cytochrome P450 isoform 3A4. The risk of myopathy is increased by reducing the elimination of the simvastatin component of Vytorin. Hence when Vytorin is used with an inhibitor of CYP3A4 (eg, HIV protease inhibitors), elevated plasma levels of HMG-CoA reductase inhibitory activity can increase the risk of myopathy and rhabdomyolysis, particularly with higher doses of Vytorin. The use of Vytorin concomitantly with HIV protease inhibitors should be avoided). Products include:

Crixivan 2113

Isoniazid (The risk of myopathy is increased by reducing the elimination of the simvastatin component of Vytorin.

2085 Interactions Index Vytorin

Hence when Vytorin is used with an inhibitor of CYP3A4, elevated plasma levels of HMG-CoA reductase inhibitory activity can increase the risk of myopathy and rhabdomyolysis, particularly with higher doses of Vytorin. Concomitant use of any medication labeled as having a strong inhibitory effect on CYP3A4 should be avoided unless the benefits of combined therapy outweigh the increased risk).
No products indexed under this heading.

Itraconazole (Simvastatin is metabolized by the cytochrome P450 isoform 3A4. The risk of myopathy is increased by reducing the elimination of the simvastatin component of Vytorin. Hence when Vytorin is used with an inhibitor of CYP3A4 (eg, itraconazole), elevated plasma levels of HMG-CoA reductase inhibitory activity can increase the risk of myopathy and rhabdomyolysis, particularly with higher doses of Vytorin. If treatment with itraconazole is unavoidable, therapy with Vytorin should be suspended during the course of treatment).
No products indexed under this heading.

Ketoconazole (Simvastatin is metabolized by the cytochrome P450 isoform 3A4. The risk of myopathy is increased by reducing the elimination of the simvastatin component of Vytorin. Hence when Vytorin is used with an inhibitor of CYP3A4 (eg, ketoconazole), elevated plasma levels of HMG-CoA reductase inhibitory activity can increase the risk of myopathy and rhabdomyolysis, particularly with higher doses of Vytorin. If treatment with ketoconazole is unavoidable, therapy with Vytorin should be suspended during the course of treatment). Products include:
Extina 3319
Xolegel 3337

Lapatinib (The risk of myopathy is increased by reducing the elimination of the simvastatin component of Vytorin. Hence when Vytorin is used with an inhibitor of CYP3A4, elevated plasma levels of HMG-CoA reductase inhibitory activity can increase the risk of myopathy and rhabdomyolysis, particularly with higher doses of Vytorin. Concomitant use of any medication labeled as having a strong inhibitory effect on CYP3A4 should be avoided unless the benefits of combined therapy outweigh the increased risk). Products include:
Tykerb 1698

Levonorgestrel (During concomitant use with ethinyl estradiol and levonorgestrel, ezetimibe may decrease ethinyl estradiol C_{max} by 9% and levonorgestrel C_{max} by 5%). Products include:
Climara Pro 847
LoSeasonique 3407
Lybrel 3514
Mirena 854
Plan B 3416
Seasonique 3418

Lopinavir (Simvastatin is metabolized by the cytochrome P450 isoform 3A4. The risk of myopathy is increased by reducing the elimination of the simvastatin component of Vytorin. Hence when Vytorin is used with an inhibitor of CYP3A4 (eg, HIV protease inhibitors), elevated plasma levels of HMG-CoA reductase inhibitory activity can increase the risk of myopathy and rhabdomyolysis, particularly with higher doses of Vytorin. The use of Vytorin concomitantly with HIV protease inhibitors should be avoided). Products include:
Kaletra 458

Loratadine (The risk of myopathy is increased by reducing the elimination of the simvastatin component of Vytorin. Hence when Vytorin is used with an inhibitor of CYP3A4, elevated plasma levels of HMG-CoA reductase inhibitory activity can increase the risk of myopathy and rhabdomyolysis, particularly with higher doses of Vytorin. Concomitant use of any medication labeled as having a strong inhibitory effect on CYP3A4 should be avoided unless the benefits of combined therapy outweigh the increased risk).
No products indexed under this heading.

Lovastatin (Concomitant use with lovastatin may increase total ezetimibe AUC by 9% and total ezetimibe C_{max} by 3%. Also, concomitant use with ezetimibe may increase lovastatin AUC by 19% and lovastatin C_{max} by 3%). Products include:
Advicor 402
Mevacor 2212

Magnesium Hydroxide (Concomitant use with aluminium and magnesium hydroxide combination antacid may decrease total ezetimibe AUC by 4% and total ezetimibe C_{max} by 30%). Products include:
Fleet Pedia-Lax Chewable Tablets 1144
Pepcid Complete 1822

Metronidazole (The risk of myopathy is increased by reducing the elimination of the simvastatin component of Vytorin. Hence when Vytorin is used with an inhibitor of CYP3A4, elevated plasma levels of HMG-CoA reductase inhibitory activity can increase the risk of myopathy and rhabdomyolysis, particularly with higher doses of Vytorin. Concomitant use of any medication labeled as having a strong inhibitory effect on CYP3A4 should be avoided unless the benefits of combined therapy outweigh the increased risk). Products include:
Pylera 793

Metronidazole Benzoate (The risk of myopathy is increased by reducing the elimination of the simvastatin component of Vytorin. Hence when Vytorin is used with an inhibitor of CYP3A4, elevated plasma levels of HMG-CoA reductase inhibitory activity can increase the risk of myopathy and rhabdomyolysis, particularly with higher doses of Vytorin. Concomitant use of any medication labeled as having a strong inhibitory effect on CYP3A4 should be avoided unless the benefits of combined therapy outweigh the increased risk).
No products indexed under this heading.

Metronidazole Hydrochloride (The risk of myopathy is increased by reducing the elimination of the simvastatin component of Vytorin. Hence when Vytorin is used with an inhibitor of CYP3A4, elevated plasma levels of HMG-CoA reductase inhibitory activity can increase the risk of myopathy and rhabdomyolysis, particularly with higher doses of Vytorin. Concomitant use of any medication labeled as having a strong inhibitory effect on CYP3A4 should be avoided unless the benefits of combined therapy outweigh the increased risk).
No products indexed under this heading.

Metronidazole Sodium (The risk of myopathy is increased by reducing the elimination of the simvastatin component of Vytorin. Hence when Vytorin is used with an inhibitor of CYP3A4, elevated plasma levels of HMG-CoA reductase inhibitory activity can increase the risk of myopathy and rhabdomyolysis, particularly with higher doses of Vytorin. Concomitant use of any medication labeled as having a strong inhibitory effect on CYP3A4 should be avoided unless the benefits of combined therapy outweigh the increased risk).
No products indexed under this heading.

Miconazole (The risk of myopathy and rhabdomyolysis is increased by high levels of statin activity in plasma. Simvastatin is metabolized by the cytochrome P450 isoform 3A4. Certain drugs that inhibit this metabolic pathway can raise the plasma levels of simvastatin and may increase the risk of myopathy. These include itraconazole, ketoconazole, and other antifungal azoles. The use of Vytorin concomitantly with these CYP3A4 inhibitors should be avoided. If treatment with itraconazole or ketoconazole or other antifungal azoles is unavoidable, therapy with Vytorin should be suspended during the course of treatment).
No products indexed under this heading.

Miconazole Nitrate (The risk of myopathy is increased by reducing the elimination of the simvastatin component of Vytorin. Hence when Vytorin is used with an inhibitor of CYP3A4, elevated plasma levels of HMG-CoA reductase inhibitory activity can increase the risk of myopathy and rhabdomyolysis, particularly with higher doses of Vytorin. Concomitant use of any medication labeled as having a strong inhibitory effect on CYP3A4 should be avoided unless the benefits of combined therapy outweigh the increased risk). Products include:
Vusion Ointment 3335

Mifepristone (The risk of myopathy is increased by reducing the elimination of the simvastatin component of Vytorin. Hence when Vytorin is used with an inhibitor of CYP3A4, elevated plasma levels of HMG-CoA reductase inhibitory activity can increase the risk of myopathy and rhabdomyolysis, particularly with higher doses of Vytorin. Concomitant use of any medication labeled as having a strong inhibitory effect on CYP3A4 should be avoided unless the benefits of combined therapy outweigh the increased risk).
No products indexed under this heading.

Nefazodone Hydrochloride (Simvastatin is metabolized by the cytochrome P450 isoform 3A4. The risk of myopathy is increased by reducing the elimination of the simvastatin component of Vytorin. Hence when Vytorin is used with an inhibitor of CYP3A4 (eg, nefazodone), elevated plasma levels of HMG-CoA reductase inhibitory activity can increase the risk of myopathy and rhabdomyolysis, particularly with higher doses of Vytorin. The use of Vytorin concomitantly with the CYP3A4 inhibitor nefazodone should be avoided).
No products indexed under this heading.

Nelfinavir Mesylate (Concomitant administration of nelfinavir and simvastatin leads to a geometric mean ratio of simvastatin acid and simvastatin as follows- AUC: 6 and C_{max}: 6.2. Concomitant administration of nelfinavir and simvastatin should be avoided).
No products indexed under this heading.

Nevirapine (The risk of myopathy is increased by reducing the elimination of the simvastatin component of Vytorin. Hence when Vytorin is used with an inhibitor of CYP3A4, elevated plasma levels of HMG-CoA reductase inhibitory activity can increase the risk of myopathy and rhabdomyolysis, particularly with higher doses of Vytorin. Concomitant use of any medication labeled as having a strong inhibitory effect on CYP3A4 should be avoided unless the benefits of combined therapy outweigh the increased risk). Products include:
Viramune Oral Suspension 897
Viramune Tablets 897

Niacin (The effect of Vytorin (10/20 mg daily for 7 days) on the pharmacokinetics of niacin extended-release tablets (1000 mg for 2 days and 2000 mg for 5 days following a low-fat breakfast) was studied in healthy subjects. The mean C_{max} and AUC of niacin increased 9% and 22%, respectively. The mean C_{max} and AUC of nicotinuric acid increased 10% and 19%, respectively (N=13). In the same study, the effect of niacin on the pharmacokinetics of Vytorin was evaluated (N=15). While concomitant niacin decreased the mean C_{max} of total ezetimibe (1%), and simvastatin (2%), it increased the mean C_{max} of simvastatin acid (18%). In addition, concomitant niacin increased the mean AUC of total ezetimibe (26%), simvastatin (20%), and simvastatin acid (35%). Caution should be used when prescribing lipid lowering doses (≥1 g/day) of niacin with Vytorin, as these agents can cause myopathy when given alone). Products include:
Advicor 402
Cardio Basics 3455
Niaspan 497
Simcor 524

Niacinamide (The risk of myopathy is increased by reducing the elimination of the simvastatin component of Vytorin. Hence when Vytorin is used with an inhibitor of CYP3A4, elevated plasma levels of HMG-CoA reductase inhibitory activity can increase the risk of myopathy and rhabdomyolysis, particularly with higher doses of Vytorin. Concomitant use of any medication labeled as having a strong inhibitory effect on CYP3A4 should be avoided unless the benefits of combined therapy outweigh the increased risk). Products include:
CitraNatal 90 DHA Capsules 2332
CitraNatal Assure 2332
CitraNatal Rx 2332
Heplive 607

Niacinamide Hydroiodide (The risk of myopathy is increased by reducing the elimination of the simvastatin component of Vytorin. Hence when Vytorin is used with an inhibitor of CYP3A4, elevated plasma levels of HMG-CoA reductase inhibitory activity can increase the risk of myopathy and rhabdomyolysis, particularly with higher doses of Vytorin. Concomitant use of any medication labeled as having a strong inhibitory effect on CYP3A4 should be avoided unless the benefits of combined therapy outweigh the increased risk).
No products indexed under this heading.

Nicotinamide (The risk of myopathy is increased by reducing the elimination of the simvastatin component of Vytorin. Hence when Vytorin is used with an inhibitor of CYP3A4, elevated plasma levels of HMG-CoA reductase inhibitory activity can increase the risk of myopathy and rhabdomyolysis, particularly with higher doses of Vytorin. Concomitant use of any medication labeled as having a strong inhibitory effect on CYP3A4 should be avoided unless the benefits of combined therapy outweigh the increased risk).
No products indexed under this heading.

Nifedipine (The risk of myopathy is increased by reducing the elimination of the simvastatin component of Vytorin. Hence when Vytorin is used with an inhibitor of CYP3A4, elevated plasma levels of HMG-CoA reductase inhibitory activity can increase the risk of myopathy and rhabdomyolysis, particularly with higher doses of Vytorin. Concomitant use of any medication labeled as having a strong inhibitory effect on CYP3A4 should be avoided unless the benefits of combined therapy outweigh the increased risk).
No products indexed under this heading.

Norfloxacin (The risk of myopathy is increased by reducing the elimination of the simvastatin component of Vytorin. Hence when Vytorin is used with an inhibitor of CYP3A4, elevated plasma levels of HMG-CoA reductase inhibitory activity can increase the risk of myopathy and rhabdomyolysis, particularly

with higher doses of Vytorin. Concomitant use of any medication labeled as having a strong inhibitory effect on CYP3A4 should be avoided unless the benefits of combined therapy outweigh the increased risk). Products include:

Noroxin 2220

Omeprazole (The risk of myopathy is increased by reducing the elimination of the simvastatin component of Vytorin. Hence when Vytorin is used with an inhibitor of CYP3A4, elevated plasma levels of HMG-CoA reductase inhibitory activity can increase the risk of myopathy and rhabdomyolysis, particularly with higher doses of Vytorin. Concomitant use of any medication labeled as having a strong inhibitory effect on CYP3A4 should be avoided unless the benefits of combined therapy outweigh the increased risk).

No products indexed under this heading.

Oxiconazole Nitrate (The risk of myopathy and rhabdomyolysis is increased by high levels of statin activity in plasma. Simvastatin is metabolized by the cytochrome P450 isoform 3A4. Certain drugs that inhibit this metabolic pathway can raise the plasma levels of simvastatin and may increase the risk of myopathy. These include itraconazole, ketoconazole, and other antifungal azoles. The use of Vytorin concomitantly with these CYP3A4 inhibitors should be avoided. If treatment with itraconazole or ketoconazole or other antifungal azoles is unavoidable, therapy with Vytorin should be suspended during the course of treatment).

No products indexed under this heading.

Paroxetine Hydrochloride (The risk of myopathy is increased by reducing the elimination of the simvastatin component of Vytorin. Hence when Vytorin is used with an inhibitor of CYP3A4, elevated plasma levels of HMG-CoA reductase inhibitory activity can increase the risk of myopathy and rhabdomyolysis, particularly with higher doses of Vytorin. Concomitant use of any medication labeled as having a strong inhibitory effect on CYP3A4 should be avoided unless the benefits of combined therapy outweigh the increased risk). Products include:

Paroxetine CR 2361
Paroxetine ER 2371
Paxil 1586
Paxil CR 1596

Posaconazole (The risk of myopathy and rhabdomyolysis is increased by high levels of statin activity in plasma. Simvastatin is metabolized by the cytochrome P450 isoform 3A4. Certain drugs that inhibit this metabolic pathway can raise the plasma levels of simvastatin and may increase the risk of myopathy. These include itraconazole, ketoconazole, and other antifungal azoles. The use of Vytorin concomitantly with these CYP3A4 inhibitors should be avoided. If treatment with itraconazole or ketoconazole or other antifungal azoles is unavoidable, therapy with Vytorin should be suspended during the course of treatment). Products include:

Noxafil 3172

Pravastatin Sodium (Concomitant use with pravastatin may increase total ezetimibe AUC by 7% and total ezetimibe C_{max} by 23%. In addition, concomitant use with ezetimibe may decrease pravastatin AUC by 20% and pravastatin C_{max} by 24%).

No products indexed under this heading.

Probucol (The benefits of the combined use of Vytorin with the following drugs should be carefully weighed against the potential risks of combinations: gemfibrozil, other lipid-lowering drugs (other fibrates or ≥1 g/day of niacin), cyclosporine, danazol, amiodarone, or verapamil. Caution should be used when prescribing other fibrates or lipid-lowering doses (≥1 g/day) of niacin with Vytorin, as these agents can cause myopathy when given alone).

No products indexed under this heading.

Propoxyphene Hydrochloride (The risk of myopathy is increased by reducing the elimination of the simvastatin component of Vytorin. Hence when Vytorin is used with an inhibitor of CYP3A4, elevated plasma levels of HMG-CoA reductase inhibitory activity can increase the risk of myopathy and rhabdomyolysis, particularly with higher doses of Vytorin. Concomitant use of any medication labeled as having a strong inhibitory effect on CYP3A4 should be avoided unless the benefits of combined therapy outweigh the increased risk).

No products indexed under this heading.

Propoxyphene Napsylate (The risk of myopathy is increased by reducing the elimination of the simvastatin component of Vytorin. Hence when Vytorin is used with an inhibitor of CYP3A4, elevated plasma levels of HMG-CoA reductase inhibitory activity can increase the risk of myopathy and rhabdomyolysis, particularly with higher doses of Vytorin. Concomitant use of any medication labeled as having a strong inhibitory effect on CYP3A4 should be avoided unless the benefits of combined therapy outweigh the increased risk).

No products indexed under this heading.

Propranolol (Concomitant administration of propranolol and simvastatin leads to a geometric mean ratio of total inhibitor and active inhibitor as follows - AUC: 0.79 and 0.79. No dosing adjustments are required).

No products indexed under this heading.

Propranolol Hydrochloride (Concomitant administration of propranolol and simvastatin leads to a geometric mean ratio of total inhibitor and active inhibitor as follows - AUC: 0.79 and 0.79. No dosing adjustments are required). Products include:

InnoPran XL 1517

Quinidine (The risk of myopathy is increased by reducing the elimination of the simvastatin component of Vytorin. Hence when Vytorin is used with an inhibitor of CYP3A4, elevated plasma levels of HMG-CoA reductase inhibitory activity can increase the risk of myopathy and rhabdomyolysis, particularly with higher doses of Vytorin. Concomitant use of any medication labeled as having a strong inhibitory effect on CYP3A4 should be avoided unless the benefits of combined therapy outweigh the increased risk).

No products indexed under this heading.

Quinidine Hydrochloride (The risk of myopathy is increased by reducing the elimination of the simvastatin component of Vytorin. Hence when Vytorin is used with an inhibitor of CYP3A4, elevated plasma levels of HMG-CoA reductase inhibitory activity can increase the risk of myopathy and rhabdomyolysis, particularly with higher doses of Vytorin. Concomitant use of any medication labeled as having a strong inhibitory effect on CYP3A4 should be avoided unless the benefits of combined therapy outweigh the increased risk).

No products indexed under this heading.

Quinidine Polygalacturonate (The risk of myopathy is increased by reducing the elimination of the simvastatin component of Vytorin. Hence when Vytorin is used with an inhibitor of CYP3A4, elevated plasma levels of HMG-CoA reductase inhibitory activity can increase the risk of myopathy and rhabdomyolysis, particularly with higher doses of Vytorin. Concomitant use of any medication labeled as having a strong inhibitory effect on CYP3A4 should be avoided unless the benefits of combined therapy outweigh the increased risk).

No products indexed under this heading.

Quinidine Sulfate (The risk of myopathy is increased by reducing the elimination of the simvastatin component of Vytorin. Hence when Vytorin is used with an inhibitor of CYP3A4, elevated plasma levels of HMG-CoA reductase inhibitory activity can increase the risk of myopathy and rhabdomyolysis, particularly with higher doses of Vytorin. Concomitant use of any medication labeled as having a strong inhibitory effect on CYP3A4 should be avoided unless the benefits of combined therapy outweigh the increased risk).

No products indexed under this heading.

Quinine (The risk of myopathy is increased by reducing the elimination of the simvastatin component of Vytorin. Hence when Vytorin is used with an inhibitor of CYP3A4, elevated plasma levels of HMG-CoA reductase inhibitory activity can increase the risk of myopathy and rhabdomyolysis, particularly with higher doses of Vytorin. Concomitant use of any medication labeled as having a strong inhibitory effect on CYP3A4 should be avoided unless the benefits of combined therapy outweigh the increased risk). Products include:

Hyland's Leg Cramps PM with Quinine 3315

Quinine Sulfate (The risk of myopathy is increased by reducing the elimination of the simvastatin component of Vytorin. Hence when Vytorin is used with an inhibitor of CYP3A4, elevated plasma levels of HMG-CoA reductase inhibitory activity can increase the risk of myopathy and rhabdomyolysis, particularly with higher doses of Vytorin. Concomitant use of any medication labeled as having a strong inhibitory effect on CYP3A4 should be avoided unless the benefits of combined therapy outweigh the increased risk).

No products indexed under this heading.

Quinupristin (The risk of myopathy is increased by reducing the elimination of the simvastatin component of Vytorin. Hence when Vytorin is used with an inhibitor of CYP3A4, elevated plasma levels of HMG-CoA reductase inhibitory activity can increase the risk of myopathy and rhabdomyolysis, particularly with higher doses of Vytorin. Concomitant use of any medication labeled as having a strong inhibitory effect on CYP3A4 should be avoided unless the benefits of combined therapy outweigh the increased risk).

No products indexed under this heading.

Ranitidine Bismuth Citrate (The risk of myopathy is increased by reducing the elimination of the simvastatin component of Vytorin. Hence when Vytorin is used with an inhibitor of CYP3A4, elevated plasma levels of HMG-CoA reductase inhibitory activity can increase the risk of myopathy and rhabdomyolysis, particularly with higher doses of Vytorin. Concomitant use of any medication labeled as having a strong inhibitory effect on CYP3A4 should be avoided unless the benefits of combined therapy outweigh the increased risk).

No products indexed under this heading.

Ranitidine Hydrochloride (The risk of myopathy is increased by reducing the elimination of the simvastatin component of Vytorin. Hence when Vytorin is used with an inhibitor of CYP3A4, elevated plasma levels of HMG-CoA reductase inhibitory activity can increase the risk of myopathy and rhabdomyolysis, particularly with higher doses of Vytorin. Concomitant use of any medication labeled as having a strong inhibitory effect on CYP3A4 should be avoided unless the benefits of combined therapy outweigh the increased risk). Products include:

Zantac 1737
Zantac Injection 1732
Zantac Pharmacy 1735

Ritonavir (Simvastatin is metabolized by the cytochrome P450 isoform 3A4. The risk of myopathy is increased by reducing the elimination of the simvastatin component of Vytorin. Hence when Vytorin is used with an inhibitor of CYP3A4 (eg, HIV protease inhibitors), elevated plasma levels of HMG-CoA reductase inhibitory activity can increase the risk of myopathy and rhabdomyolysis, particularly with higher doses of Vytorin. The use of Vytorin concomitantly with HIV protease inhibitors should be avoided). Products include:

Kaletra 458
Norvir 509

Rosuvastatin Calcium (Concomitant use with rosuvastatin may increase total ezetimibe AUC by 13% and total ezetimibe C_{max} by 18%. In addition, concomitant use with ezetimibe may increase rosuvastatin AUC by 19% and rosuvastatin C_{max} by 17%). Products include:

Crestor 736

Saquinavir (Simvastatin is metabolized by the cytochrome P450 isoform 3A4. The risk of myopathy is increased by reducing the elimination of the simvastatin component of Vytorin. Hence when Vytorin is used with an inhibitor of CYP3A4 (eg, HIV protease inhibitors), elevated plasma levels of HMG-CoA reductase inhibitory activity can increase the risk of myopathy and rhabdomyolysis, particularly with higher doses of Vytorin. The use of Vytorin concomitantly with HIV protease inhibitors should be avoided).

No products indexed under this heading.

Saquinavir Mesylate (Simvastatin is metabolized by the cytochrome P450 isoform 3A4. The risk of myopathy is increased by reducing the elimination of the simvastatin component of Vytorin. Hence when Vytorin is used with an inhibitor of CYP3A4 (eg, HIV protease inhibitors), elevated plasma levels of HMG-CoA reductase inhibitory activity can increase the risk of myopathy and rhabdomyolysis, particularly with higher doses of Vytorin. The use of Vytorin concomitantly with HIV protease inhibitors should be avoided).

No products indexed under this heading.

Sertaconazole Nitrate (The risk of myopathy and rhabdomyolysis is increased by high levels of statin activity in plasma. Simvastatin is metabolized by the cytochrome P450 isoform 3A4. Certain drugs that inhibit this metabolic pathway can raise the plasma levels of simvastatin and may increase the risk of myopathy. These include itraconazole, ketoconazole, and other antifungal azoles. The use of Vytorin concomitantly with these CYP3A4 inhibitors should be avoided. If treatment with itraconazole or ketoconazole or other antifungal azoles is unavoidable, therapy with Vytorin should be suspended during the course of treatment).

No products indexed under this heading.

Sertraline Hydrochloride (The risk of myopathy is increased by reducing the elimination of the simvastatin component of Vytorin. Hence when Vytorin is used with an inhibitor of CYP3A4, elevated plasma levels of HMG-CoA reductase inhibitory activity can increase the risk of myopathy and rhabdomyolysis, particularly with higher doses of Vytorin. Concomitant use of

any medication labeled as having a strong inhibitory effect on CYP3A4 should be avoided unless the benefits of combined therapy outweigh the increased risk).
No products indexed under this heading.

Sildenafil Citrate (The risk of myopathy is increased by reducing the elimination of the simvastatin component of Vytorin. Hence when Vytorin is used with an inhibitor of CYP3A4, elevated plasma levels of HMG-CoA reductase inhibitory activity can increase the risk of myopathy and rhabdomyolysis, particularly with higher doses of Vytorin. Concomitant use of any medication labeled as having a strong inhibitory effect on CYP3A4 should be avoided unless the benefits of combined therapy outweigh the increased risk).
No products indexed under this heading.

Telithromycin (Simvastatin is metabolized by the cytochrome P450 isoform 3A4. The risk of myopathy is increased by reducing the elimination of the simvastatin component of Vytorin. Hence when Vytorin is used with an inhibitor of CYP3A4 (eg, telithromycin), elevated plasma levels of HMG-CoA reductase inhibitory activity can increase the risk of myopathy and rhabdomyolysis, particularly with higher doses of Vytorin. If treatment with telithromycin is unavoidable, therapy with Vytorin should be suspended during the course of treatment). Products include:

Terconazole (The risk of myopathy and rhabdomyolysis is increased by high levels of statin activity in plasma. Simvastatin is metabolized by the cytochrome P450 isoform 3A4. Certain drugs that inhibit this metabolic pathway can raise the plasma levels of simvastatin and may increase the risk of myopathy. These include itraconazole, ketoconazole, and other antifungal azoles. The use of Vytorin concomitantly with these CYP3A4 inhibitors should be avoided. If treatment with itraconazole or ketoconazole or other antifungal azoles is unavoidable, therapy with Vytorin should be suspended during the course of treatment).
No products indexed under this heading.

Tipranavir (Simvastatin is metabolized by the cytochrome P450 isoform 3A4. The risk of myopathy is increased by reducing the elimination of the simvastatin component of Vytorin. Hence when Vytorin is used with an inhibitor of CYP3A4 (eg, HIV protease inhibitors), elevated plasma levels of HMG-CoA reductase inhibitory activity can increase the risk of myopathy and rhabdomyolysis, particularly with higher doses of Vytorin. The use of Vytorin concomitantly with HIV protease inhibitors should be avoided).
No products indexed under this heading.

Troglitazone (The risk of myopathy is increased by reducing the elimination of the simvastatin component of Vytorin. Hence when Vytorin is used with an inhibitor of CYP3A4, elevated plasma levels of HMG-CoA reductase inhibitory activity can increase the risk of myopathy and rhabdomyolysis, particularly with higher doses of Vytorin. Concomitant use of any medication labeled as having a strong inhibitory effect on CYP3A4 should be avoided unless the benefits of combined therapy outweigh the increased risk).
No products indexed under this heading.

Troleandomycin (The risk of myopathy and rhabdomyolysis is increased by high levels of statin activity in plasma. Simvastatin is metabolized by the cytochrome P450 isoform 3A4. Certain drugs that inhibit this metabolic pathway can raise the plasma levels of simvastatin and may increase the risk of

myopathy. These include the macrolide antibiotics erythromycin and clarithromycin. The use of Vytorin concomitantly with these CYP3A4 inhibitors should be avoided. If treatment with erythromycin or clarithromycin is unavailable, therapy with Vytorin should be suspended during the course of treatment).
No products indexed under this heading.

Valproate Sodium (The risk of myopathy is increased by reducing the elimination of the simvastatin component of Vytorin. Hence when Vytorin is used with an inhibitor of CYP3A4, elevated plasma levels of HMG-CoA reductase inhibitory activity can increase the risk of myopathy and rhabdomyolysis, particularly with higher doses of Vytorin. Concomitant use of any medication labeled as having a strong inhibitory effect on CYP3A4 should be avoided unless the benefits of combined therapy outweigh the increased risk).
No products indexed under this heading.

Vardenafil Hydrochloride (The risk of myopathy is increased by reducing the elimination of the simvastatin component of Vytorin. Hence when Vytorin is used with an inhibitor of CYP3A4, elevated plasma levels of HMG-CoA reductase inhibitory activity can increase the risk of myopathy and rhabdomyolysis, particularly with higher doses of Vytorin. Concomitant use of any medication labeled as having a strong inhibitory effect on CYP3A4 should be avoided unless the benefits of combined therapy outweigh the increased risk). Products include:

Verapamil Hydrochloride (The risk of myopathy/rhabdomyolysis is increased by concomitant administration of verapamil with higher doses of Vytorin. The combined use of Vytorin at doses higher than 10/20 mg daily with verapamil should be avoided unless the clinical benefit is likely to outweigh the increased risk of myopathy). Products include:

Voriconazole (The risk of myopathy and rhabdomyolysis is increased by high levels of statin activity in plasma. Simvastatin is metabolized by the cytochrome P450 isoform 3A4. Certain drugs that inhibit this metabolic pathway can raise the plasma levels of simvastatin and may increase the risk of myopathy. These include itraconazole, ketoconazole, and other antifungal azoles. The use of Vytorin concomitantly with these CYP3A4 inhibitors should be avoided. If treatment with itraconazole or ketoconazole or other antifungal azoles is unavoidable, therapy with Vytorin should be suspended during the course of treatment).
No products indexed under this heading.

Warfarin Sodium (Co-administration of warfarin and ezetimibe may decrease R-warfarin AUC by 2% and S-warfarin AUC by 4%, and also may increase R-warfarin C_{max} by 3% and S-warfarin C_{max} by 1%. Simvastatin 20-40 mg/day modestly potentiated the effect of coumarin anticoagulants: the prothrombin time, reported as International Normalized Ratio (INR), increased from a baseline of 1.7 to 1.8 and from 2.6 to 3.4 in a normal volunteer study and in a hypercholesterolemic patient study, respectively. Prothrombin time should be determined before starting Vytorin and frequently enough during early therapy to ensure that no significant alteration of prothrombin time occurs. Once a stable prothrombin time has been documented, prothrombin times can be monitored at the intervals usually recommended for patients on coumarin

anticoagulants. If the dose of Vytorin is changed or discontinued, the same procedure should be repeated).
No products indexed under this heading.

Zafirlukast (The risk of myopathy is increased by reducing the elimination of the simvastatin component of Vytorin. Hence when Vytorin is used with an inhibitor of CYP3A4, elevated plasma levels of HMG-CoA reductase inhibitory activity can increase the risk of myopathy and rhabdomyolysis, particularly with higher doses of Vytorin. Concomitant use of any medication labeled as having a strong inhibitory effect on CYP3A4 should be avoided unless the benefits of combined therapy outweigh the increased risk). Products include:

Zileuton (The risk of myopathy is increased by reducing the elimination of the simvastatin component of Vytorin. Hence when Vytorin is used with an inhibitor of CYP3A4, elevated plasma levels of HMG-CoA reductase inhibitory activity can increase the risk of myopathy and rhabdomyolysis, particularly with higher doses of Vytorin. Concomitant use of any medication labeled as having a strong inhibitory effect on CYP3A4 should be avoided unless the benefits of combined therapy outweigh the increased risk).
No products indexed under this heading.

Food Interactions

Alcohol (Vytorin should be used with caution in patients who consume substantial quantities of alcohol and/or have a past history of liver disease).

Beer, reduced-alcohol (Vytorin should be used with caution in patients who consume substantial quantities of alcohol and/or have a past history of liver disease).

Beer, unspecified (Vytorin should be used with caution in patients who consume substantial quantities of alcohol and/or have a past history of liver disease).

Food, unspecified (Concomitant food administration (high-fat or non-fat meals) had no effect on the extent of absorption of ezetimibe when administered as 10-mg tablets. The C_{max} value of ezetimibe was increased by 38% with consumption of high-fat meals).

Grapefruit (Simvastatin is metabolized by the cytochrome P450 isoform 3A4. The risk of myopathy is increased by reducing the elimination of the simvastatin component of Vytorin. Hence when Vytorin is used with an inhibitor of CYP3A4 (eg, grapefruit juice), elevated plasma levels of HMG-CoA reductase inhibitory activity can increase the risk of myopathy and rhabdomyolysis, particularly with higher doses of Vytorin. Avoid large quantities of grapefruit juice (>1 quart daily)).

Grapefruit Juice (Simvastatin is metabolized by the cytochrome P450 isoform 3A4. The risk of myopathy is increased by reducing the elimination of the simvastatin component of Vytorin. Hence when Vytorin is used with an inhibitor of CYP3A4 (eg, grapefruit juice), elevated plasma levels of HMG-CoA reductase inhibitory activity can increase the risk of myopathy and rhabdomyolysis, particularly with higher doses of Vytorin. Avoid large quantities of grapefruit juice (>1 quart daily)).

Meal, unspecified (Concomitant food administration (high-fat or non-fat meals) had no effect on the extent of absorption of ezetimibe when administered as 10-mg tablets. The C_{max} value of ezetimibe was increased by 38% with consumption of high-fat meals).

Wine, Chianti (Vytorin should be used with caution in patients who consume substantial quantities of alcohol and/or have a past history of liver disease).

Wine, Red (Vytorin should be used with caution in patients who consume substantial quantities of alcohol and/or have a past history of liver disease).

Wine, unspecified (Vytorin should be used with caution in patients who consume substantial quantities of alcohol and/or have a past history of liver disease).

Wine products (Vytorin should be used with caution in patients who consume substantial quantities of alcohol and/or have a past history of liver disease).

May interact with alpha adrenergic blockers, antihistamines, antihypertensives, beta-blockers, monoamine oxidase inhibitors, phenytoin, sympathomimetics, thiazides, tricyclic antidepressants, urinary alkalinizing agents, veratrum alkaloids, and certain other agents. Compounds in these categories include:

Acebutolol Hydrochloride (Adrenergic blockers are inhibited by amphetamines).
No products indexed under this heading.

Acetazolamide (Urinary alkalinizing agents such as acetazolamide increase the concentration of the non-ionized species of the amphetamine molecule, thereby decreasing urinary excretion).
No products indexed under this heading.

Acrivastine (Amphetamines may counteract the sedative effect of antihistamines).
No products indexed under this heading.

Albuterol (Amphetamines may enhance the activity of sympathomimetic agents).
No products indexed under this heading.

Albuterol Sulfate (Amphetamines may enhance the activity of sympathomimetic agents). Products include:

Alfuzosin Hydrochloride (Adrenergic blockers are inhibited by amphetamines). Products include:

Aliskiren (Amphetamines may antagonize the hypotensive effects of antihypertensives). Products include:

IMPORTANT NOTE: Always consult each drug listing in the patient's regimen for possible interactions.

(⊙ Described in PDR® for Ophthalmic Medicines)

Haloperidol Lactate (Haloperidol blocks dopamine receptors, thus inhibiting the central stimulant effects of amphetamines).
No products indexed under this heading.

Hydralazine Hydrochloride (Amphetamines may enhance the hypotensive effects of antihypertensives).
No products indexed under this heading.

Hydrochlorothiazide (Urinary alkalinizing agents including some thiazides, increase the concentration of the nonionized species of the amphetamine molecule, thereby decreasing urinary excretion). Products include:

Hydroflumethiazide (Urinary alkalinizing agents including some thiazides, increase the concentration of the nonionized species of the amphetamine molecule, thereby decreasing urinary excretion).
No products indexed under this heading.

Imipramine Hydrochloride (Amphetamines may enhance the activity of tricyclic antidepressants; d-amphetamine with desipramine or protriptyline and possibly other tricyclics cause striking and sustained increases in the concentration of d-amphetamine in the brain; cardiovascular effects can be potentiated).
No products indexed under this heading.

Imipramine Pamoate (Amphetamines may enhance the activity of tricyclic antidepressants; d-amphetamine with desipramine or protriptyline and possibly other tricyclics cause striking and sustained increases in the concentration of d-amphetamine in the brain; cardiovascular effects can be potentiated).
No products indexed under this heading.

Indapamide (Amphetamines may antagonize the hypotensive effects of antihypertensives). Products include:

Irbesartan (Amphetamines may antagonize the hypotensive effects of antihypertensives). Products include:

Isocarboxazid (Monoamine oxidase inhibitors (MAIO) antidepressants slow amphetamine metabolism. This slowing potentiates amphetamines, increasing their effect on the release of norepinephrine and other monoamines from adrenergic nerve endings; this can cause headachesand other signs of hypertensive crisis. A variety of toxic neurological effects and malignant hyperpyrexia can occur, sometimes with fatal results. Use of lisdexamfetamine is contraindicated during or within the 14 days following the administration of MAOIs). Products include:

Isoproterenol Hydrochloride (Amphetamines may enhance the activity of sympathomimetic agents).
No products indexed under this heading.

Isoproterenol Sulfate (Amphetamines may enhance the activity of sympathomimetic agents).
No products indexed under this heading.

Isradipine (Amphetamines may antagonize the hypotensive effects of antihypertensives). Products include:

Labetalol Hydrochloride (Adrenergic blockers are inhibited by amphetamines).
No products indexed under this heading.

Levalbuterol Hydrochloride (Amphetamines may enhance the activity of sympathomimetic agents).
No products indexed under this heading.

Levobunolol Hydrochloride (Adrenergic blockers are inhibited by amphetamines).
No products indexed under this heading.

Lisinopril (Amphetamines may antagonize the hypotensive effects of antihypertensives). Products include:

Lithium Carbonate (The anorectic and stimulatory effects of amphetamines may be inhibited by lithium carbonate).
No products indexed under this heading.

Loratadine (Amphetamines may counteract the sedative effect of antihistamines).
No products indexed under this heading.

Losartan Potassium (Amphetamines may antagonize the hypotensive effects of antihypertensives). Products include:

Maprotiline Hydrochloride (Amphetamines may enhance the activity of tricyclic antidepressants; d-amphetamine with desipramine or protriptyline and possibly other tricyclics cause striking and sustained increases in the concentration of d-amphetamine in the brain; cardiovascular effects can be potentiated).
No products indexed under this heading.

Mecamylamine Hydrochloride (Amphetamines may antagonize the hypotensive effects of antihypertensives).
No products indexed under this heading.

Meperidine Hydrochloride (Amphetamines potentiate the analgesic effect of meperidine).
No products indexed under this heading.

Metaproterenol Sulfate (Amphetamines may enhance the activity of sympathomimetic agents).
No products indexed under this heading.

Metaraminol Bitartrate (Amphetamines may enhance the activity of sympathomimetic agents).
No products indexed under this heading.

Methdilazine Hydrochloride (Amphetamines may counteract the sedative effect of antihistamines).
No products indexed under this heading.

Methenamine (Urinary excretion of amphetamines is increased and efficacy is reduced by acidifying agents used in methenamine therapy).
No products indexed under this heading.

Methenamine Hippurate (Urinary excretion of amphetamines is increased and efficacy is reduced by acidifying agents used in methenamine therapy).
No products indexed under this heading.

Methenamine Mandelate (Urinary excretion of amphetamines is increased and efficacy is reduced by acidifying agents used in methenamine therapy). Products include:

Methoxamine Hydrochloride (Amphetamines may enhance the activity of sympathomimetic agents).
No products indexed under this heading.

Methyclothiazide (Urinary alkalinizing agents including some thiazides, increase the concentration of the nonionized species of the amphetamine molecule, thereby decreasing urinary excretion).
No products indexed under this heading.

Methyldopa (Amphetamines may antagonize the hypotensive effects of antihypertensives).
No products indexed under this heading.

Methyldopate Hydrochloride (Amphetamines may antagonize the hypotensive effects of antihypertensives).
No products indexed under this heading.

Metipranolol Hydrochloride (Adrenergic blockers are inhibited by amphetamines).
No products indexed under this heading.

Metolazone (Amphetamines may antagonize the hypotensive effects of antihypertensives).
No products indexed under this heading.

Metoprolol Succinate (Adrenergic blockers are inhibited by amphetamines). Products include:

Metoprolol Tartrate (Adrenergic blockers are inhibited by amphetamines).
No products indexed under this heading.

Metyrosine (Amphetamines may antagonize the hypotensive effects of antihypertensives).
No products indexed under this heading.

Mibefradil Dihydrochloride (Amphetamines may antagonize the hypotensive effects of antihypertensives).
No products indexed under this heading.

Minoxidil (Amphetamines may antagonize the hypotensive effects of antihypertensives).
No products indexed under this heading.

Moclobemide (Monoamine oxidase inhibitors (MAIO) antidepressants slow amphetamine metabolism. This slowing potentiates amphetamines, increasing their effect on the release of norepinephrine and other monoamines from adrenergic nerve endings; this can cause headachesand other signs of hypertensive crisis. A variety of toxic neurological effects and malignant hyperpyrexia can occur, sometimes with fatal results. Use of lisdexamfetamine is contraindicated during or within the 14 days following the administration of MAOIs).
No products indexed under this heading.

Moexipril Hydrochloride (Amphetamines may antagonize the hypotensive effects of antihypertensives).
No products indexed under this heading.

Nadolol (Adrenergic blockers are inhibited by amphetamines). Products include:

Nebivolol (Adrenergic blockers are inhibited by amphetamines). Products include:

Nicardipine Hydrochloride (Amphetamines may antagonize the hypotensive effects of antihypertensives).
No products indexed under this heading.

Nifedipine (Amphetamines may antagonize the hypotensive effects of antihypertensives).
No products indexed under this heading.

Nisoldipine (Amphetamines may antagonize the hypotensive effects of antihypertensives).
No products indexed under this heading.

Nitroglycerin (Amphetamines may antagonize the hypotensive effects of antihypertensives). Products include:

Norepinephrine Bitartrate (Amphetamines enhance the adrenergic effect of norepinephrine).
No products indexed under this heading.

Norepinephrine Hydrochloride (Amphetamines enhance the adrenergic effect of norepinephrine).
No products indexed under this heading.

Nortriptyline Hydrochloride (Amphetamines may enhance the activity of tricyclic antidepressants; d-amphetamine with desipramine or protriptyline and possibly other tricyclics cause striking and sustained increases in the concentration of d-amphetamine in the brain; cardiovascular effects can be potentiated).
No products indexed under this heading.

Pargyline Hydrochloride (Monoamine oxidase inhibitors (MAIO) antidepressants slow amphetamine metabolism. This slowing potentiates amphetamines, increasing their effect on the release of norepinephrine and other monoamines from adrenergic nerve endings; this can cause headachesand other signs of hypertensive crisis. A variety of toxic neurological effects and malignant hyperpyrexia can occur, sometimes with fatal results. Use of lisdexamfetamine is contraindicated during or within the 14 days following the administration of MAOIs).
No products indexed under this heading.

Penbutolol Sulfate (Adrenergic blockers are inhibited by amphetamines).
No products indexed under this heading.

Perindopril Erbumine (Amphetamines may antagonize the hypotensive effects of antihypertensives).
No products indexed under this heading.

Phenelzine Sulfate (Monoamine oxidase inhibitors (MAIO) antidepressants slow amphetamine metabolism. This slowing potentiates amphetamines, increasing their effect on the release of norepinephrine and other monoamines from adrenergic nerve endings; this can cause headachesand other signs of hypertensive crisis. A variety of toxic neurological effects and malignant hyperpyrexia can occur, sometimes with fatal results. Use of lisdexamfetamine is contraindicated during or within the 14 days following the administration of MAOIs).
No products indexed under this heading.

Phenobarbital (Amphetamines may delay intestinal absorption of phenobarbital; co-administration of phenobarbital may produce a synergistic anticonvulsant action). Products include:

Phenobarbital Sodium (Amphetamines may delay intestinal absorption of phenobarbital; co-administration of phenobarbital may produce a synergistic anticonvulsant action).
No products indexed under this heading.

Phenoxybenzamine Hydrochloride (Amphetamines may antagonize the hypotensive effects of antihypertensives). Products include:

Phentolamine Mesylate (Amphetamines may antagonize the hypotensive effects of antihypertensives).
No products indexed under this heading.

Phenylephrine Bitartrate (Amphetamines may enhance the activity of sympathomimetic agents).
No products indexed under this heading.

Phenylephrine Hydrochloride (Amphetamines may enhance the activity of sympathomimetic agents). Products include:

IMPORTANT NOTE: Always consult each drug listing in the patient's regimen for possible interactions.

Vyvanse Interactions Index 2090

Children's Sudafed PE Nasal Decongestant 2047

Phenylephrine Tannate (Amphetamines may enhance the activity of sympathomimetic agents).
No products indexed under this heading.

Phenylpropanolamine Hydrochloride (Amphetamines may enhance the activity of sympathomimetic agents).
No products indexed under this heading.

Phenytoin (Amphetamines may delay intestinal absorption of phenytoin; co-administration of phenytoin may produce a synergistic anticonvulsant action).
No products indexed under this heading.

Phenytoin Sodium (Amphetamines may delay intestinal absorption of phenytoin; co-administration of phenytoin may produce a synergistic anticonvulsant action). Products include:
Phenytek Capsules 2380

Pindolol (Adrenergic blockers are inhibited by amphetamines).
No products indexed under this heading.

Pirbuterol Acetate (Amphetamines may enhance the activity of sympathomimetic agents). Products include:
Maxair Autohaler 1782

Polythiazide (Urinary alkalinizing agents including some thiazides, increase the concentration of the non-ionized species of the amphetamine molecule, thereby decreasing urinary excretion).
No products indexed under this heading.

Potassium Citrate (Urinary alkalinizing agents increase the concentration of the non-ionized species of the amphetamine molecule, thereby decreasing urinary excretion). Products include:
Urocit-K 2333

Prazosin Hydrochloride (Adrenergic blockers are inhibited by amphetamines).
No products indexed under this heading.

Procarbazine Hydrochloride (Monoamine oxidase inhibitors (MAIO) antidepressants slow amphetamine metabolism. This slowing potentiates amphetamines, increasing their effect on the release of norepinephrine and other monoamines from adrenergic nerve endings; this can cause headachesand other signs of hypertensive crisis. A variety of toxic neurological effects and malignant hyperpyrexia can occur, sometimes with fatal results. Use of lisdexamfetamine is contraindicated during or within the 14 days following the administration of MAOIs).
No products indexed under this heading.

Promethazine Hydrochloride (Amphetamines may counteract the sedative effect of antihistamines).
No products indexed under this heading.

Propoxyphene Hydrochloride (In cases of propoxyphene overdosage, amphetamine CNS stimulation is potentiated and fatal convulsions can occur).
No products indexed under this heading.

Propoxyphene Napsylate (In cases of propoxyphene overdosage, amphetamine CNS stimulation is potentiated and fatal convulsions can occur).
No products indexed under this heading.

Propranolol Hydrochloride (Adrenergic blockers are inhibited by amphetamines). Products include:
InnoPran XL 1517

Protriptyline Hydrochloride (Amphetamines may enhance the activity of tricyclic antidepressants; d-amphetamine with desipramine or protriptyline and possibly other tricyclics cause striking and sustained increases in the concentration of d-amphetamine in the brain; cardiovascular effects can be potentiated).
No products indexed under this heading.

Pseudoephedrine Hydrochloride (Amphetamines may enhance the activity of sympathomimetic agents). Products include:
Allegra-D 2915
Allegra-D 24 2918
Sudafed 12 Hour Nasal Decongestant Non-Drowsy 2048
Sudafed 24 Hour 2048
Sudafed Nasal Decongestant 2047
Children's Sudafed Nasal Decongestant Liquid 2047
Zyrtec-D Allergy & Congestion 2054

Pseudoephedrine Sulfate (Amphetamines may enhance the activity of sympathomimetic agents). Products include:
Clarinex-D 12-Hour 3101
Clarinex-D 3104

Pyrilamine Maleate (Amphetamines may counteract the sedative effect of antihistamines).
No products indexed under this heading.

Pyrilamine Tannate (Amphetamines may counteract the sedative effect of antihistamines).
No products indexed under this heading.

Quinapril Hydrochloride (Amphetamines may antagonize the hypotensive effects of antihypertensives).
No products indexed under this heading.

Ramipril (Amphetamines may antagonize the hypotensive effects of antihypertensives).
No products indexed under this heading.

Rasagiline Mesylate (Monoamine oxidase inhibitors (MAIO) antidepressants slow amphetamine metabolism. This slowing potentiates amphetamines, increasing their effect on the release of norepinephrine and other monoamines from adrenergic nerve endings; this can cause headachesand other signs of hypertensive crisis. A variety of toxic neurological effects and malignant hyperpyrexia can occur, sometimes with fatal results. Use of lisdexamfetamine is contraindicated during or within the 14 days following the administration of MAOIs). Products include:
Azilect 3383

Rauwolfia Serpentina (Amphetamines may antagonize the hypotensive effects of antihypertensives).
No products indexed under this heading.

Rescinnamine (Amphetamines may antagonize the hypotensive effects of antihypertensives).
No products indexed under this heading.

Reserpine (Amphetamines may antagonize the hypotensive effects of antihypertensives).
No products indexed under this heading.

Salmeterol Xinafoate (Amphetamines may enhance the activity of sympathomimetic agents). Products include:
Advair 100/50 1275
Advair 250/50 1275
Advair 500/50 1275
Advair HFA 45/21 1288
Advair HFA 115/21 1288
Advair HFA 230/21 1288
Serevent Diskus 1656

Selegiline (Monoamine oxidase inhibitors (MAIO) antidepressants slow amphetamine metabolism. This slowing potentiates amphetamines, increasing their effect on the release of norepinephrine and other monoamines from adrenergic nerve endings; this can cause headachesand other signs of hypertensive crisis. A variety of toxic neurological effects and malignant hyperpyrexia can occur, sometimes with fatal results. Use of lisdexamfetamine is contraindicated during or within the 14 days following the administration of MAOIs). Products include:
Emsam 3623

Selegiline Hydrochloride (Monoamine oxidase inhibitors (MAIO) antidepressants slow amphetamine metabolism. This slowing potentiates amphetamines, increasing their effect on the release of norepinephrine and other monoamines from adrenergic nerve endings; this can cause headachesand other signs of hypertensive crisis. A variety of toxic neurological effects and malignant hyperpyrexia can occur, sometimes with fatal results. Use of lisdexamfetamine is contraindicated during or within the 14 days following the administration of MAOIs). Products include:
Eldepryl 3312

Sodium Acid Phosphate (Amphetamines inhibit the hypotensive effect of veratrum alkaloids). Products include:
Uroqid-Acid 874

Sodium Bicarbonate (Urinary alkalinizing agents increase the concentration of the non-ionized species of the amphetamine molecule, thereby decreasing urinary excretion).
No products indexed under this heading.

Sodium Citrate (Urinary alkalinizing agents increase the concentration of the non-ionized species of the amphetamine molecule, thereby decreasing urinary excretion).
No products indexed under this heading.

Sodium Nitroprusside (Amphetamines may antagonize the hypotensive effects of antihypertensives).
No products indexed under this heading.

Sotalol Hydrochloride (Adrenergic blockers are inhibited by amphetamines).
No products indexed under this heading.

Spirapril Hydrochloride (Amphetamines may antagonize the hypotensive effects of antihypertensives).
No products indexed under this heading.

Tamsulosin Hydrochloride (Adrenergic blockers are inhibited by amphetamines).
No products indexed under this heading.

Telmisartan (Amphetamines may antagonize the hypotensive effects of antihypertensives). Products include:
Micardis 887
Micardis HCT 889

Terazosin Hydrochloride (Adrenergic blockers are inhibited by amphetamines).
No products indexed under this heading.

Terbutaline Sulfate (Amphetamines may enhance the activity of sympathomimetic agents).
No products indexed under this heading.

Terfenadine (Amphetamines may counteract the sedative effect of antihistamines).
No products indexed under this heading.

Timolol Hemihydrate (Adrenergic blockers are inhibited by amphetamines). Products include:
Betimol 3490

Timolol Maleate (Adrenergic blockers are inhibited by amphetamines). Products include:
Combigan 601
Dorzolamide Hydrochloride/Timolol Maleate Ophthalmic Solution .... ⊙243
Timoptic in Ocudose .... ⊙231

Torsemide (Amphetamines may antagonize the hypotensive effects of antihypertensives).
No products indexed under this heading.

Trandolapril (Amphetamines may antagonize the hypotensive effects of antihypertensives). Products include:
Mavik 489
Tarka 534

Tranylcypromine Sulfate (Monoamine oxidase inhibitors (MAIO) antidepressants slow amphetamine metabolism. This slowing potentiates amphetamines, increasing their effect on the release of norepinephrine and other monoamines from adrenergic nerve endings; this can cause headachesand other signs of hypertensive crisis. A variety of toxic neurological effects and malignant hyperpyrexia can occur, sometimes with fatal results. Use of lisdexamfetamine is contraindicated during or within the 14 days following the administration of MAOIs). Products include:
Parnate 1584

Trimeprazine Tartrate (Amphetamines may counteract the sedative effect of antihistamines).
No products indexed under this heading.

Trimethaphan Camsylate (Amphetamines may antagonize the hypotensive effects of antihypertensives).
No products indexed under this heading.

Trimipramine Maleate (Amphetamines may enhance the activity of tricyclic antidepressants; d-amphetamine with desipramine or protriptyline and possibly other tricyclics cause striking and sustained increases in the concentration of d-amphetamine in the brain; cardiovascular effects can be potentiated).
No products indexed under this heading.

Tripelennamine Hydrochloride (Amphetamines may counteract the sedative effect of antihistamines).
No products indexed under this heading.

Triprolidine Hydrochloride (Amphetamines may counteract the sedative effect of antihistamines).
No products indexed under this heading.

Valsartan (Amphetamines may antagonize the hypotensive effects of antihypertensives). Products include:
Diovan 2413
Diovan HCT 2419
Exforge 2443
Exforge HCT 2449
Valturna 3637

Verapamil Hydrochloride (Amphetamines may antagonize the hypotensive effects of antihypertensives). Products include:
Tarka 534

WELCHOL TABLETS

(Colesevelam Hydrochloride) 1029
May interact with oral contraceptives, phenytoin, and certain other agents. Compounds in these categories include:

Desogestrel (In drug interaction studies, colesevelam hydrochloride reduced levels of oral contraceptives containing ethinyl estradiol and norethindrone).
No products indexed under this heading.

Drugs, unspecified (When administering a drug with a narrow therapeutic index or margin of safety that has not been evaluated in formal drug-drug interaction studies, the drug should be administered at least 1 hr before or 4 hrs after colesevelam hydrochloride).
No products indexed under this heading.

Ethinyl Estradiol (In drug interaction studies, colesevelam hydrochloride reduced levels of oral contraceptives containing ethinyl estradiol and norethindrone). Products include:

(⊙ Described in PDR® for Ophthalmic Medicines)

Ethynodiol Diacetate (In drug interaction studies, colesevelam hydrochloride reduced levels of oral contraceptives containing ethinyl estradiol and norethindrone).
No products indexed under this heading.

Fosphenytoin (There have been postmarketing reports of decreases in phenytoin levels in patients receiving phenytoin concomitantly with colesevelam hydrochloride).
No products indexed under this heading.

Fosphenytoin Sodium (There have been postmarketing reports of decreases in phenytoin levels in patients receiving phenytoin concomitantly with colesevelam hydrochloride).
No products indexed under this heading.

Glyburide (In drug interaction studies, colesevelam reduced levels of glyburide).
No products indexed under this heading.

Levonorgestrel (In drug interaction studies, colesevelam hydrochloride reduced levels of oral contraceptives containing ethinyl estradiol and norethindrone). Products include:

Levothyroxine (In drug interaction studies, colesevelam reduced levels of levothyroxine).
No products indexed under this heading.

Levothyroxine Sodium (In drug interaction studies, colesevelam reduced levels of levothyroxine). Products include:

Mestranol (In drug interaction studies, colesevelam hydrochloride reduced levels of oral contraceptives containing ethinyl estradiol and norethindrone).
No products indexed under this heading.

Norethindrone (In drug interaction studies, colesevelam hydrochloride reduced levels of oral contraceptives containing ethinyl estradiol and norethindrone). Products include:

Norethynodrel (In drug interaction studies, colesevelam hydrochloride reduced levels of oral contraceptives containing ethinyl estradiol and norethindrone).
No products indexed under this heading.

Norgestimate (In drug interaction studies, colesevelam hydrochloride reduced levels of oral contraceptives containing ethinyl estradiol and norethindrone). Products include:

Norgestrel (In drug interaction studies, colesevelam hydrochloride reduced levels of oral contraceptives containing ethinyl estradiol and norethindrone).
No products indexed under this heading.

Phenytoin (There have been postmarketing reports of decreases in phenytoin levels in patients receiving phenytoin concomitantly with colesevelam hydrochloride).
No products indexed under this heading.

Phenytoin Sodium (There have been postmarketing reports of decreases in phenytoin levels in patients receiving phenytoin concomitantly with colesevelam hydrochloride). Products include:

Warfarin Sodium (There have been postmarketing reports of decreases in INR in patients receiving warfarin concomitantly with colesevelam hydrochloride).
No products indexed under this heading.

WELLBUTRIN TABLETS
May interact with alcohols, anorexiants, antiarrhythmics, antidepressant drugs, antipsychotic agents, benzodiazepines, beta-blockers, central nervous system stimulants, class IC antiarrhythmics, corticosteroids, cytochrome p450 2b6 inhibitors (selected), cytochrome p450 2b6 substrates (selected), cytochrome p450 2d6 substrates (selected), drugs which lower seizure threshold, haloperidols, hypnotics and sedatives, insulin, monoamine oxidase inhibitors, narcotic analgesics, nicotines, oral hypoglycemic agents, phenytoin, selective serotonin reuptake inhibitors, theophyllines, tricyclic antidepressants, and certain other agents. Compounds in these categories include:

Acarbose (Concomitant use of oral hypoglycemics with bupropion is associated with an increased seizure risk).
No products indexed under this heading.

Acebutolol Hydrochloride (Co-administration of bupropion with drugs that are metabolized by the CYP2D6 isoenzyme, including β-blockers (eg, metoprolol) should be approached with caution and should be initiated at the lower end of the dose range of the concomitant medication. If bupropion is added to the treatment regimen of a patient already receiving a drug metabolized by CYP2D6, the need to decrease the dose of the original medication should be considered, particularly for those concomitant medications with a narrow therapeutic index).
No products indexed under this heading.

Adenosine (Co-administration of bupropion with drugs that are metabolized by the CYP2D6 isoenzyme, including antiarrhythmics should be approached with caution and should be initiated at the lower end of the dose range of the concomitant medication. If bupropion is added to the treatment regimen of a patient already receiving a drug metabolized by CYP2D6, the need to decrease the dose of the original medication should be considered, particularly for those concomitant medications with a narrow therapeutic index). Products include:

Alclometasone Dipropionate (Concurrent administration of bupropion and agents that lower seizure threshold, such as systemic steroids, should be undertaken with extreme caution. Low initial dosing and gradual dose increases should be employed).
No products indexed under this heading.

Alfentanil Hydrochloride (An addiction to opiates and concomitant use of bupropion has been associated with an increased seizure risk).
No products indexed under this heading.

Alprazolam (Bupropion is contraindicated in patients undergoing abrupt discontinuation of sedatives (including benzodiazepines). Patients should be told that the excessive use or abrupt discontinuation of sedatives (including benzodiazepines) may alter the seizure threshold).
No products indexed under this heading.

Amantadine Hydrochloride (Limited clinical data suggest a higher incidence of adverse experiences in patients receiving bupropion concurrently with amantadine. Administration of bupropion tablets to patients receiving amantadine concurrently should be undertaken with caution, using small initial doses and small gradual dose increases).
No products indexed under this heading.

Amiodarone Hydrochloride (In vitro studies indicate that bupropion is primarily metabolized to hydroxybupropion by the CYP2B6 isoenzyme. Therefore, co-administration of bupropion with CYP2B6 substrates or inhibitors (eg, orphenadrine, thiotepa, and cyclophosphamide) may result in a drug interaction).
No products indexed under this heading.

Amitriptyline Hydrochloride (Concurrent administration of bupropion and agents (eg, other antidepressants) that lower seizure threshold should be undertaken only with extreme caution. Low initial dosing and small gradual dose increases should be employed. In addition, many drugs, including most antidepressants (many tricyclics), are metabolized by the CYP2D6 isoenzyme. Co-administration of bupropion with drugs that are metabolized by CYP2D6 isoenzyme should be approached with caution and should be initiated at the lower end of the dose range of the concomitant medication. If bupropion is added to the treatment regimen of a patient already receiving a drug metabolized by CYP2D6, the need to decrease the dose of the original medication should be considered, particularly for those concomitant medications with a narrow therapeutic index).
No products indexed under this heading.

Amlodipine Besylate (In vitro studies indicate that bupropion is primarily metabolized to hydroxybupropion by the CYP2B6 isoenzyme. Therefore, co-administration of bupropion with CYP2B6 substrates or inhibitors (eg, orphenadrine, thiotepa, and cyclophosphamide) may result in a drug interaction). Products include:

Amoxapine (Concurrent administration of bupropion and agents (eg, other antidepressants) that lower seizure threshold should be undertaken only with extreme caution. Low initial dosing and small gradual dose increases should be employed. In addition, many drugs, including most antidepressants (many tricyclics), are metabolized by the CYP2D6 isoenzyme. Co-administration of bupropion with drugs that are metabolized by CYP2D6 isoenzyme should be approached with caution and should be initiated at the lower end of the dose range of the concomitant medication. If bupropion is added to the treatment regimen of a patient already receiving a drug metabolized by CYP2D6, the need to decrease the dose of the original medication should be considered, particularly for those concomitant medications with a narrow therapeutic index).
No products indexed under this heading.

Amphetamine Aspartate (Concomitant use of anorectics with bupropion is associated with an increased seizure risk).
No products indexed under this heading.

Amphetamine Aspartate Monohydrate (Concomitant use of anorectics with bupropion is associated with an increased seizure risk).
No products indexed under this heading.

Amphetamine Resins (Concomitant use of anorectics with bupropion is associated with an increased seizure risk).
No products indexed under this heading.

Amphetamine Sulfate (Concomitant use of anorectics with bupropion is associated with an increased seizure risk).
No products indexed under this heading.

Apomorphine (An addiction to opiates and concomitant use of bupropion has been associated with an increased seizure risk).
No products indexed under this heading.

Apomorphine Hydrochloride (An addiction to opiates and concomitant use of bupropion has been associated with an increased seizure risk).
No products indexed under this heading.

Aripiprazole (Concurrent administration of bupropion and agents that lower seizure threshold, such as antipsychotics, should be undertaken with extreme caution. Low initial dosing and gradual dose increases should be employed. Co-administration of bupropion with drugs that are metabolized by the CYP2D6 isoenzyme including antipsychotics (eg, haloperidol, risperidone, thioridazine) should be approached with caution and should be initiated at the lower end of the dose range of the concomitant medication. If bupropion is added to the treatment regimen of a patient already receiving a drug metabolized by CYP2D6, the need to decrease the dose of the original medication should be considered, particularly for those concomitant medications with a narrow therapeutic index).
No products indexed under this heading.

Atenolol (Co-administration of bupropion with drugs that are metabolized by the CYP2D6 isoenzyme, including β-blockers (eg, metoprolol) should be approached with caution and should be initiated at the lower end of the dose range of the concomitant medication. If bupropion is added to the treatment regimen of a patient already receiving a drug metabolized by CYP2D6, the need to decrease the dose of the original medication should be considered, particularly for those concomitant medications with a narrow therapeutic index).
No products indexed under this heading.

Atomoxetine Hydrochloride (Co-administration of bupropion with drugs that are metabolized by the CYP2D6 isoenzyme should be approached with caution and should be initiated at the lower end of the dose range of the concomitant medication. If bupropion is added to the treatment regimen of a patient already receiving a drug metabolized by CYP2D6, the need to decrease the dose of the original medication should be considered, particularly for those concomitant medications with a narrow therapeutic index). Products include:

Azelastine Hydrochloride (In vitro studies indicate that bupropion is primarily metabolized to hydroxybupropion by the CYP2B6 isoenzyme. Therefore, co-administration of bupropion with CYP2B6 substrates or inhibitors (eg, orphenadrine, thiotepa, and cyclophosphamide) may result in a drug interaction).
No products indexed under this heading.

Beclomethasone Dipropionate (Concurrent administration of bupropion and agents that lower seizure threshold, such as systemic steroids, should be undertaken with extreme caution. Low initial dosing and gradual dose increases should be employed). Products include:

IMPORTANT NOTE: Always consult each drug listing in the patient's regimen for possible interactions.

Qvar 3398

Beclomethasone Dipropionate Monohydrate (Concurrent administration of bupropion and agents that lower seizure threshold, such as systemic steroids, should be undertaken with extreme caution. Low initial dosing and gradual dose increases should be employed). Products include:
Beconase AQ 1386

Benzphetamine Hydrochloride (Concomitant use of anorectics with bupropion is associated with an increased seizure risk).
No products indexed under this heading.

Betamethasone (Concurrent administration of bupropion and agents that lower seizure threshold, such as systemic steroids, should be undertaken with extreme caution. Low initial dosing and gradual dose increases should be employed).
No products indexed under this heading.

Betamethasone Acetate (Concurrent administration of bupropion and agents that lower seizure threshold, such as systemic steroids, should be undertaken with extreme caution. Low initial dosing and gradual dose increases should be employed).
No products indexed under this heading.

Betamethasone Benzoate (Concurrent administration of bupropion and agents that lower seizure threshold, such as systemic steroids, should be undertaken with extreme caution. Low initial dosing and gradual dose increases should be employed).
No products indexed under this heading.

Betamethasone Dipropionate (Concurrent administration of bupropion and agents that lower seizure threshold, such as systemic steroids, should be undertaken with extreme caution. Low initial dosing and gradual dose increases should be employed). Products include:
Diprolene Lotion 0.05% 3108
Diprolene Ointment 0.05% 3109
Diprolene AF Cream 0.05% 3107
Lotrisone 3163

Betamethasone Sodium Phosphate (Concurrent administration of bupropion and agents that lower seizure threshold, such as systemic steroids, should be undertaken with extreme caution. Low initial dosing and gradual dose increases should be employed).
No products indexed under this heading.

Betamethasone Valerate (Concurrent administration of bupropion and agents that lower seizure threshold, such as systemic steroids, should be undertaken with extreme caution. Low initial dosing and gradual dose increases should be employed). Products include:
Luxíq 3321

Betaxolol Hydrochloride (Co-administration of bupropion with drugs that are metabolized by the CYP2D6 isoenzyme, including β-blockers (eg, metoprolol) should be approached with caution and should be initiated at the lower end of the dose range of the concomitant medication. If bupropion is added to the treatment regimen of a patient already receiving a drug metabolized by CYP2D6, the need to decrease the dose of the original medication should be considered, particularly for those concomitant medications with a narrow therapeutic index).
No products indexed under this heading.

Bisoprolol Fumarate (Co-administration of bupropion with drugs that are metabolized by the CYP2D6 isoenzyme, including β-blockers (eg, metoprolol) should be approached with caution and should be initiated at the lower end of the dose range of the concomitant medication. If bupropion is added to the treatment regimen of a patient already receiving a drug metabolized by CYP2D6, the need to decrease the dose of the original medication should be considered, particularly for those concomitant medications with a narrow therapeutic index).
No products indexed under this heading.

Bretylium Tosylate (Co-administration of bupropion with drugs that are metabolized by the CYP2D6 isoenzyme, including antiarrhythmics should be approached with caution and should be initiated at the lower end of the dose range of the concomitant medication. If bupropion is added to the treatment regimen of a patient already receiving a drug metabolized by CYP2D6, the need to decrease the dose of the original medication should be considered, particularly for those concomitant medications with a narrow therapeutic index).
No products indexed under this heading.

Budesonide (Concurrent administration of bupropion and agents that lower seizure threshold, such as systemic steroids, should be undertaken with extreme caution. Low initial dosing and gradual dose increases should be employed). Products include:
Pulmicort Flexhaler 714
Symbicort 80/4.5 720
Symbicort 160/4.5 720

Buprenorphine Hydrochloride (An addiction to opiates and concomitant use of bupropion has been associated with an increased seizure risk).
No products indexed under this heading.

Bupropion (Concomitant use with any other medication that contains bupropion is contraindicated because the incidence of seizure is dose dependent).
No products indexed under this heading.

Butabarbital (Bupropion is contraindicated in patients undergoing abrupt discontinuation of sedatives (including benzodiazepines). Patients should be told that the excessive use or abrupt discontinuation of sedatives (including benzodiazepines) may alter the seizure threshold).
No products indexed under this heading.

Butabarbital Sodium (Bupropion is contraindicated in patients undergoing abrupt discontinuation of sedatives (including benzodiazepines). Patients should be told that the excessive use or abrupt discontinuation of sedatives (including benzodiazepines) may alter the seizure threshold).
No products indexed under this heading.

Butalbital (Bupropion is contraindicated in patients undergoing abrupt discontinuation of sedatives (including benzodiazepines). Patients should be told that the excessive use or abrupt discontinuation of sedatives (including benzodiazepines) may alter the seizure threshold).
No products indexed under this heading.

Captopril (Co-administration of bupropion with drugs that are metabolized by the CYP2D6 isoenzyme should be approached with caution and should be initiated at the lower end of the dose range of the concomitant medication. If bupropion is added to the treatment regimen of a patient already receiving a drug metabolized by CYP2D6, the need to decrease the dose of the original medication should be considered, particularly for those concomitant medications with a narrow therapeutic index). Products include:
Captopril 2341

Carbamazepine (While not systematically studied, certain drugs may induce the metabolism of bupropion (eg, carbamazepine)). Products include:
Carbatrol 3280
Equetro 3477

Carteolol Hydrochloride (Co-administration of bupropion with drugs that are metabolized by the CYP2D6 isoenzyme, including β-blockers (eg, metoprolol) should be approached with caution and should be initiated at the lower end of the dose range of the concomitant medication. If bupropion is added to the treatment regimen of a patient already receiving a drug metabolized by CYP2D6, the need to decrease the dose of the original medication should be considered, particularly for those concomitant medications with a narrow therapeutic index).
No products indexed under this heading.

Carvedilol (Co-administration of bupropion with drugs that are metabolized by the CYP2D6 isoenzyme, including β-blockers (eg, metoprolol) should be approached with caution and should be initiated at the lower end of the dose range of the concomitant medication. If bupropion is added to the treatment regimen of a patient already receiving a drug metabolized by CYP2D6, the need to decrease the dose of the original medication should be considered, particularly for those concomitant medications with a narrow therapeutic index). Products include:
Coreg 1409

Carvedilol Phosphate (Co-administration of bupropion with drugs that are metabolized by the CYP2D6 isoenzyme, including β-blockers (eg, metoprolol) should be approached with caution and should be initiated at the lower end of the dose range of the concomitant medication. If bupropion is added to the treatment regimen of a patient already receiving a drug metabolized by CYP2D6, the need to decrease the dose of the original medication should be considered, particularly for those concomitant medications with a narrow therapeutic index). Products include:
Coreg CR 1416

Cevimeline Hydrochloride (Co-administration of bupropion with drugs that are metabolized by the CYP2D6 isoenzyme should be approached with caution and should be initiated at the lower end of the dose range of the concomitant medication. If bupropion is added to the treatment regimen of a patient already receiving a drug metabolized by CYP2D6, the need to decrease the dose of the original medication should be considered, particularly for those concomitant medications with a narrow therapeutic index). Products include:
Evoxac 1027

Chloral Hydrate (Bupropion is contraindicated in patients undergoing abrupt discontinuation of sedatives (including benzodiazepines). Patients should be told that the excessive use or abrupt discontinuation of sedatives (including benzodiazepines) may alter the seizure threshold).
No products indexed under this heading.

Chlordiazepoxide (Bupropion is contraindicated in patients undergoing abrupt discontinuation of sedatives (including benzodiazepines). Patients should be told that the excessive use or abrupt discontinuation of sedatives (including benzodiazepines) may alter the seizure threshold).
No products indexed under this heading.

Chlordiazepoxide Hydrochloride (Bupropion is contraindicated in patients undergoing abrupt discontinuation of sedatives (including benzodiazepines). Patients should be told that the excessive use or abrupt discontinuation of sedatives (including benzodiazepines) may alter the seizure threshold).
No products indexed under this heading.

Chlorpromazine (Concurrent administration of bupropion and agents that lower seizure threshold, such as antipsychotics, should be undertaken with extreme caution. Low initial dosing and gradual dose increases should be employed. Co-administration of bupropion with drugs that are metabolized by the CYP2D6 isoenzyme including antipsychotics (eg, haloperidol, risperidone, thioridazine) should be approached with caution and should be initiated at the lower end of the dose range of the concomitant medication. If bupropion is added to the treatment regimen of a patient already receiving a drug metabolized by CYP2D6, the need to decrease the dose of the original medication should be considered, particularly for those concomitant medications with a narrow therapeutic index).
No products indexed under this heading.

Chlorpromazine Hydrochloride (Concurrent administration of bupropion and agents that lower seizure threshold, such as antipsychotics, should be undertaken with extreme caution. Low initial dosing and gradual dose increases should be employed. Co-administration of bupropion with drugs that are metabolized by the CYP2D6 isoenzyme including antipsychotics (eg, haloperidol, risperidone, thioridazine) should be approached with caution and should be initiated at the lower end of the dose range of the concomitant medication. If bupropion is added to the treatment regimen of a patient already receiving a drug metabolized by CYP2D6, the need to decrease the dose of the original medication should be considered, particularly for those concomitant medications with a narrow therapeutic index).
No products indexed under this heading.

Chlorpropamide (Concomitant use of oral hypoglycemics with bupropion is associated with an increased seizure risk).
No products indexed under this heading.

Chlorprothixene (Concurrent administration of bupropion and agents that lower seizure threshold, such as antipsychotics, should be undertaken with extreme caution. Low initial dosing and gradual dose increases should be employed. Co-administration of bupropion with drugs that are metabolized by the CYP2D6 isoenzyme including antipsychotics (eg, haloperidol, risperidone, thioridazine) should be approached with caution and should be initiated at the lower end of the dose range of the concomitant medication. If bupropion is added to the treatment regimen of a patient already receiving a drug metabolized by CYP2D6, the need to decrease the dose of the original medication should be considered, particularly for those concomitant medications with a narrow therapeutic index).
No products indexed under this heading.

Chlorprothixene Hydrochloride (Concurrent administration of bupropion and agents that lower seizure threshold, such as antipsychotics, should be undertaken with extreme caution. Low initial dosing and gradual dose increases should be employed. Co-administration of bupropion with drugs that are metabolized by the CYP2D6 isoenzyme including antipsychotics (eg, haloperidol, risperidone, thioridazine) should be approached with caution and

2093 Interactions Index Wellbutrin

should be initiated at the lower end of the dose range of the concomitant medication. If bupropion is added to the treatment regimen of a patient already receiving a drug metabolized by CYP2D6, the need to decrease the dose of the original medication should be considered, particularly for those concomitant medications with a narrow therapeutic index).
No products indexed under this heading.

Chlorprothixene Lactate (Concurrent administration of bupropion and agents that lower seizure threshold, such as antipsychotics, should be undertaken with extreme caution. Low initial dosing and gradual dose increases should be employed. Co-administration of bupropion with drugs that are metabolized by the CYP2D6 isoenzyme including antipsychotics (eg, haloperidol, risperidone, thioridazine) should be approached with caution and should be initiated at the lower end of the dose range of the concomitant medication. If bupropion is added to the treatment regimen of a patient already receiving a drug metabolized by CYP2D6, the need to decrease the dose of the original medication should be considered, particularly for those concomitant medications with a narrow therapeutic index).
No products indexed under this heading.

Ciclesonide (Concurrent administration of bupropion and agents that lower seizure threshold, such as systemic steroids, should be undertaken with extreme caution. Low initial dosing and gradual dose increases should be employed).
No products indexed under this heading.

Cimetidine (The effects of concomitant administration of cimetidine on the pharmacokinetics of bupropion and its active metabolites were studied in 24 healthy young male volunteers. Following oral administration of two 150 mg sustained-release tablets with and without 800 mg of cimetidine, the pharmacokinetics of bupropion and hydroxybupropion were unaffected. However, there were 16% and 32% increases in the AUC and C_{max}, respectively, of the combined moieties of threohydrobupropion and erythrohydrobupropion).
No products indexed under this heading.

Cimetidine Hydrochloride (The effects of concomitant administration of cimetidine on the pharmacokinetics of bupropion and its active metabolites were studied in 24 healthy young male volunteers. Following oral administration of two 150 mg sustained-release tablets with and without 800 mg of cimetidine, the pharmacokinetics of bupropion and hydroxybupropion were unaffected. However, there were 16% and 32% increases in the AUC and C_{max}, respectively, of the combined moieties of threohydrobupropion and erythrohydrobupropion).
No products indexed under this heading.

Cisapride (*In vitro* studies indicate that bupropion is primarily metabolized to hydroxybupropion by the CYP2B6 isoenzyme. Therefore, co-administration of bupropion with CYP2B6 substrates or inhibitors (eg, orphenadrine, thiotepa, and cyclophosphamide) may result in a drug interaction).
No products indexed under this heading.

Citalopram Hydrobromide (Concurrent administration of bupropion and agents (eg, other antidepressants) that lower seizure threshold should be undertaken only with extreme caution. Low initial dosing and small gradual dose increases should be employed. In addition, many drugs, including most antidepressants (SSRIs), are metabolized by the CYP2D6 isoenzyme. Co-administration of bupropion with drugs that are metabolized by CYP2D6 isoenzyme should be approached with caution and should be initiated at the lower end of the dose range of the concomitant medication. If bupropion is added to the treatment regimen of a patient already receiving a drug metabolized by CYP2D6, the need to decrease the dose of the original medication should be considered, particularly for those concomitant medications with a narrow therapeutic index). Products include:
Celexa 1153

Clomipramine Hydrochloride (Concurrent administration of bupropion and agents (eg, other antidepressants) that lower seizure threshold should be undertaken only with extreme caution. Low initial dosing and small gradual dose increases should be employed. In addition, many drugs, including most antidepressants (many tricyclics), are metabolized by the CYP2D6 isoenzyme. Co-administration of bupropion with drugs that are metabolized by CYP2D6 isoenzyme should be approached with caution and should be initiated at the lower end of the dose range of the concomitant medication. If bupropion is added to the treatment regimen of a patient already receiving a drug metabolized by CYP2D6, the need to decrease the dose of the original medication should be considered, particularly for those concomitant medications with a narrow therapeutic index).
No products indexed under this heading.

Clorazepate Dipotassium (Bupropion is contraindicated in patients undergoing abrupt discontinuation of sedatives (including benzodiazepines). Patients should be told that the excessive use or abrupt discontinuation of sedatives (including benzodiazepines) may alter the seizure threshold).
No products indexed under this heading.

Clotrimazole (*In vitro* studies indicate that bupropion is primarily metabolized to hydroxybupropion by the CYP2B6 isoenzyme. Therefore, co-administration of bupropion with CYP2B6 substrates or inhibitors (eg, orphenadrine, thiotepa, and cyclophosphamide) may result in a drug interaction). Products include:
Lotrisone 3163

Clotrimazole, Topical (*In vitro* studies indicate that bupropion is primarily metabolized to hydroxybupropion by the CYP2B6 isoenzyme. Therefore, co-administration of bupropion with CYP2B6 substrates or inhibitors (eg, orphenadrine, thiotepa, and cyclophosphamide) may result in a drug interaction).
No products indexed under this heading.

Clozapine (Concurrent administration of bupropion and agents that lower seizure threshold, such as antipsychotics, should be undertaken with extreme caution. Low initial dosing and gradual dose increases should be employed. Co-administration of bupropion with drugs that are metabolized by the CYP2D6 isoenzyme including antipsychotics (eg, haloperidol, risperidone, thioridazine) should be approached with caution and should be initiated at the lower end of the dose range of the concomitant medication. If bupropion is added to the treatment regimen of a patient already receiving a drug metabolized by CYP2D6, the need to decrease the dose of the original medication should be considered, particularly for those concomitant medications with a narrow therapeutic index).
No products indexed under this heading.

Cocaine Hydrochloride (Concomitant use of cocaine with bupropion is associated with an increased seizure risk).
No products indexed under this heading.

Codeine Phosphate (An addiction to opiates and concomitant use of bupropion has been associated with an increased seizure risk). Products include:
Tylenol with Codeine 2691

Codeine Sulfate (An addiction to opiates and concomitant use of bupropion has been associated with an increased seizure risk).
No products indexed under this heading.

Cortisone Acetate (Concurrent administration of bupropion and agents that lower seizure threshold, such as systemic steroids, should be undertaken with extreme caution. Low initial dosing and gradual dose increases should be employed).
No products indexed under this heading.

Cyclobenzaprine Hydrochloride (Co-administration of bupropion with drugs that are metabolized by the CYP2D6 isoenzyme should be approached with caution and should be initiated at the lower end of the dose range of the concomitant medication. If bupropion is added to the treatment regimen of a patient already receiving a drug metabolized by CYP2D6, the need to decrease the dose of the original medication should be considered, particularly for those concomitant medications with a narrow therapeutic index). Products include:
Amrix 964

Cyclophosphamide (*In vitro* studies indicate that bupropion is primarily metabolized to hydroxybupropion by the CYP2B6 isoenzyme. Therefore, co-administration of bupropion with CYP2B6 substrates or inhibitors (eg, orphenadrine, thiotepa, and cyclophosphamide) may result in a drug interaction).
No products indexed under this heading.

Debrisoquine (Co-administration of bupropion with drugs that are metabolized by the CYP2D6 isoenzyme should be approached with caution and should be initiated at the lower end of the dose range of the concomitant medication. If bupropion is added to the treatment regimen of a patient already receiving a drug metabolized by CYP2D6, the need to decrease the dose of the original medication should be considered, particularly for those concomitant medications with a narrow therapeutic index).
No products indexed under this heading.

Desipramine Hydrochloride (Concurrent administration of bupropion and agents that lower seizure threshold, such as antidepressants, should be undertaken with extreme caution. Low initial dosing and gradual dose increases should be employed. In a study of 15 males who were extensive metabolizers of the CYP2D6 isoenzyme, daily doses of bupropion given as 150 mg twice daily followed by a single dose of 50 mg desipramine increased the C_{max}, AUC, and $t_{1/2}$ of desipramine by an average of approximately 2-, 5- and 2-fold, respectively. Co-administration of bupropion with drugs that are metabolized by the CYP2D6 isoenzyme including antidepressants (eg, desipramine) should be approached with caution and should be initiated at the lower end of the dose range of the concomitant medication. If bupropion is added to the treatment regimen of a patient already receiving a drug metabolized by CYP2D6, the need to decrease the dose of the original medication should be considered, particularly for those concomitant medications with a narrow therapeutic index).
No products indexed under this heading.

Desoximetasone (Concurrent administration of bupropion and agents that lower seizure threshold, such as systemic steroids, should be undertaken with extreme caution. Low initial dosing and gradual dose increases should be employed).
No products indexed under this heading.

Desvenlafaxine (*In vitro* studies indicate that bupropion is primarily metabolized to hydroxybupropion by the CYP2B6 isoenzyme. Therefore, co-administration of bupropion with CYP2B6 substrates or inhibitors (eg, orphenadrine, thiotepa, and cyclophosphamide) may result in a drug interaction).
No products indexed under this heading.

Desvenlafaxine Succinate (*In vitro* studies indicate that bupropion is primarily metabolized to hydroxybupropion by the CYP2B6 isoenzyme. Therefore, co-administration of bupropion with CYP2B6 substrates or inhibitors (eg, orphenadrine, thiotepa, and cyclophosphamide) may result in a drug interaction). Products include:
Pristiq 3564

Dexamethasone (Concurrent administration of bupropion and agents that lower seizure threshold, such as systemic steroids, should be undertaken with extreme caution. Low initial dosing and gradual dose increases should be employed). Products include:
Ciprodex 583
Ozurdex .... ⊙ 223
Tobramycin and Dexamethasone Ophthalmic Suspension .... ⊙ 251

Dexamethasone Acetate (Concurrent administration of bupropion and agents that lower seizure threshold, such as systemic steroids, should be undertaken with extreme caution. Low initial dosing and gradual dose increases should be employed).
No products indexed under this heading.

Dexamethasone Phosphate (Concurrent administration of bupropion and agents that lower seizure threshold, such as systemic steroids, should be undertaken with extreme caution. Low initial dosing and gradual dose increases should be employed).
No products indexed under this heading.

Dexamethasone Sodium (Concurrent administration of bupropion and agents that lower seizure threshold, such as systemic steroids, should be undertaken with extreme caution. Low initial dosing and gradual dose increases should be employed).
No products indexed under this heading.

Dexamethasone Sodium Phosphate (Concurrent administration of bupropion and agents that lower seizure threshold, such as systemic steroids, should be undertaken with extreme caution. Low initial dosing and gradual dose increases should be employed).
No products indexed under this heading.

Dexamethasone Sodium Phosphate Injection (Concurrent administration of bupropion and agents that lower seizure threshold, such as systemic steroids, should be undertaken with extreme caution. Low initial dosing and gradual dose increases should be employed).
No products indexed under this heading.

Dexfenfluramine Hydrochloride (Concomitant use of anorectics with bupropion is associated with an increased seizure risk).
No products indexed under this heading.

Dexmethylphenidate Hydrochloride (Concomitant use of over-the-counter stimulants with bupropion is associated with an increased seizure risk). Products include:
Focalin XR 2472

IMPORTANT NOTE: Always consult each drug listing in the patient's regimen for possible interactions.

Wellbutrin Interactions Index 2094

Dextroamphetamine (Concomitant use of anorectics with bupropion is associated with an increased seizure risk).
No products indexed under this heading.

Dextroamphetamine Saccharate (Concomitant use of anorectics with bupropion is associated with an increased seizure risk).
No products indexed under this heading.

Dextroamphetamine Sulfate (Concomitant use of anorectics with bupropion is associated with an increased seizure risk). Products include:
Dexedrine 1425

Dextromethorphan Hydrobromide (Co-administration of bupropion with drugs that are metabolized by the CYP2D6 isoenzyme should be approached with caution and should be initiated at the lower end of the dose range of the concomitant medication. If bupropion is added to the treatment regimen of a patient already receiving a drug metabolized by CYP2D6, the need to decrease the dose of the original medication should be considered, particularly for those concomitant medications with a narrow therapeutic index).
No products indexed under this heading.

Dextromethorphan Polistirex (Co-administration of bupropion with drugs that are metabolized by the CYP2D6 isoenzyme should be approached with caution and should be initiated at the lower end of the dose range of the concomitant medication. If bupropion is added to the treatment regimen of a patient already receiving a drug metabolized by CYP2D6, the need to decrease the dose of the original medication should be considered, particularly for those concomitant medications with a narrow therapeutic index).
No products indexed under this heading.

Dezocine (An addiction to opiates and concomitant use of bupropion has been associated with an increased seizure risk).
No products indexed under this heading.

Diazepam (Bupropion is contraindicated in patients undergoing abrupt discontinuation of sedatives (including benzodiazepines). Patients should be told that the excessive use or abrupt discontinuation of sedatives (including benzodiazepines) may alter the seizure threshold). Products include:
Valium Tablets 2880

Diclofenac Epolamine (*In vitro* studies indicate that bupropion is primarily metabolized to hydroxybupropion by the CYP2B6 isoenzyme. Therefore, co-administration of bupropion with CYP2B6 substrates or inhibitors (eg, orphenadrine, thiotepa, and cyclophosphamide) may result in a drug interaction). Products include:
Flector 1839

Diclofenac Potassium (*In vitro* studies indicate that bupropion is primarily metabolized to hydroxybupropion by the CYP2B6 isoenzyme. Therefore, co-administration of bupropion with CYP2B6 substrates or inhibitors (eg, orphenadrine, thiotepa, and cyclophosphamide) may result in a drug interaction).
No products indexed under this heading.

Diclofenac Sodium (*In vitro* studies indicate that bupropion is primarily metabolized to hydroxybupropion by the CYP2B6 isoenzyme. Therefore, co-administration of bupropion with CYP2B6 substrates or inhibitors (eg, orphenadrine, thiotepa, and cyclophosphamide) may result in a drug interaction).
No products indexed under this heading.

Diethylpropion Hydrochloride (Concomitant use of anorectics with bupropion is associated with an increased seizure risk).
No products indexed under this heading.

Diflorasone Diacetate (Concurrent administration of bupropion and agents that lower seizure threshold, such as systemic steroids, should be undertaken with extreme caution. Low initial dosing and gradual dose increases should be employed).
No products indexed under this heading.

Dihydrocodeine Bitartrate (An addiction to opiates and concomitant use of bupropion has been associated with an increased seizure risk).
No products indexed under this heading.

Dihydrocodeinone Bitartrate (An addiction to opiates and concomitant use of bupropion has been associated with an increased seizure risk).
No products indexed under this heading.

Disopyramide Phosphate (Co-administration of bupropion with drugs that are metabolized by the CYP2D6 isoenzyme, including antiarrhythmics should be approached with caution and should be initiated at the lower end of the dose range of the concomitant medication. If bupropion is added to the treatment regimen of a patient already receiving a drug metabolized by CYP2D6, the need to decrease the dose of the original medication should be considered, particularly for those concomitant medications with a narrow therapeutic index).
No products indexed under this heading.

Disulfiram (*In vitro* studies indicate that bupropion is primarily metabolized to hydroxybupropion by the CYP2B6 isoenzyme. Therefore, co-administration of bupropion with CYP2B6 substrates or inhibitors (eg, orphenadrine, thiotepa, and cyclophosphamide) may result in a drug interaction).
No products indexed under this heading.

Divalproex Sodium (*In vitro* studies indicate that bupropion is primarily metabolized to hydroxybupropion by the CYP2B6 isoenzyme. Therefore, co-administration of bupropion with CYP2B6 substrates or inhibitors (eg, orphenadrine, thiotepa, and cyclophosphamide) may result in a drug interaction). Products include:
Depakote ER 426

Dofetilide (Co-administration of bupropion with drugs that are metabolized by the CYP2D6 isoenzyme, including antiarrhythmics should be approached with caution and should be initiated at the lower end of the dose range of the concomitant medication. If bupropion is added to the treatment regimen of a patient already receiving a drug metabolized by CYP2D6, the need to decrease the dose of the original medication should be considered, particularly for those concomitant medications with a narrow therapeutic index).
No products indexed under this heading.

Dolasetron Mesylate (Co-administration of bupropion with drugs that are metabolized by the CYP2D6 isoenzyme should be approached with caution and should be initiated at the lower end of the dose range of the concomitant medication. If bupropion is added to the treatment regimen of a patient already receiving a drug metabolized by CYP2D6, the need to decrease the dose of the original medication should be considered, particularly for those concomitant medications with a narrow therapeutic index).
Products include:
Anzemet Injection 2931
Anzemet Tablets 2934

Donepezil Hydrochloride (Co-administration of bupropion with drugs that are metabolized by the CYP2D6 isoenzyme should be approached with caution and should be initiated at the lower end of the dose range of the concomitant medication. If bupropion is added to the treatment regimen of a patient already receiving a drug metabolized by CYP2D6, the need to decrease the dose of the original medication should be considered, particularly for those concomitant medications with a narrow therapeutic index).
Products include:
Aricept 1045
Aricept ODT 1045

Doxepin Hydrochloride (Concurrent administration of bupropion and agents (eg, other antidepressants) that lower seizure threshold should be undertaken only with extreme caution. Low initial dosing and small gradual dose increases should be employed. In addition, many drugs, including most antidepressants (many tricyclics), are metabolized by the CYP2D6 isoenzyme. Co-administration of bupropion with drugs that are metabolized by CYP2D6 isoenzyme should be approached with caution and should be initiated at the lower end of the dose range of the concomitant medication. If bupropion is added to the treatment regimen of a patient already receiving a drug metabolized by CYP2D6, the need to decrease the dose of the original medication should be considered, particularly for those concomitant medications with a narrow therapeutic index).
No products indexed under this heading.

Doxorubicin Hydrochloride (*In vitro* studies indicate that bupropion is primarily metabolized to hydroxybupropion by the CYP2B6 isoenzyme. Therefore, co-administration of bupropion with CYP2B6 substrates or inhibitors (eg, orphenadrine, thiotepa, and cyclophosphamide) may result in a drug interaction).
No products indexed under this heading.

Doxorubicin Hydrochloride Liposome (*In vitro* studies indicate that bupropion is primarily metabolized to hydroxybupropion by the CYP2B6 isoenzyme. Therefore, co-administration of bupropion with CYP2B6 substrates or inhibitors (eg, orphenadrine, thiotepa, and cyclophosphamide) may result in a drug interaction). Products include:
Doxil 939

Efavirenz (*In vitro* studies suggest that efavirenz inhibits the hydroxylation of bupropion). Products include:
Atripla 906

Encainide Hydrochloride (Co-administration of bupropion with drugs that are metabolized by the CYP2D6 isoenzyme including Type 1C antiarrhythmics (eg, propafenone and flecainide) should be approached with caution and should be initiated at the lower end of the dose range of the concomitant medication. If bupropion is added to the treatment regimen of a patient already receiving a drug metabolized by CYP2D6, the need to decrease the dose of the original medication should be considered, particularly for those concomitant medications with a narrow therapeutic index).
No products indexed under this heading.

Erythromycin (*In vitro* studies indicate that bupropion is primarily metabolized to hydroxybupropion by the CYP2B6 isoenzyme. Therefore, co-administration of bupropion with CYP2B6 substrates or inhibitors (eg, orphenadrine, thiotepa, and cyclophosphamide) may result in a drug interaction).
No products indexed under this heading.

Erythromycin, Topical (*In vitro* studies indicate that bupropion is primarily metabolized to hydroxybupropion by the CYP2B6 isoenzyme. Therefore, co-administration of bupropion with CYP2B6 substrates or inhibitors (eg, orphenadrine, thiotepa, and cyclophosphamide) may result in a drug interaction).
No products indexed under this heading.

Erythromycin Estolate (*In vitro* studies indicate that bupropion is primarily metabolized to hydroxybupropion by the CYP2B6 isoenzyme. Therefore, co-administration of bupropion with CYP2B6 substrates or inhibitors (eg, orphenadrine, thiotepa, and cyclophosphamide) may result in a drug interaction).
No products indexed under this heading.

Erythromycin Ethylsuccinate (*In vitro* studies indicate that bupropion is primarily metabolized to hydroxybupropion by the CYP2B6 isoenzyme. Therefore, co-administration of bupropion with CYP2B6 substrates or inhibitors (eg, orphenadrine, thiotepa, and cyclophosphamide) may result in a drug interaction). Products include:
E.E.S. 437
EryPed 435

Erythromycin Gluceptate (*In vitro* studies indicate that bupropion is primarily metabolized to hydroxybupropion by the CYP2B6 isoenzyme. Therefore, co-administration of bupropion with CYP2B6 substrates or inhibitors (eg, orphenadrine, thiotepa, and cyclophosphamide) may result in a drug interaction).
No products indexed under this heading.

Erythromycin Lactobionate (*In vitro* studies indicate that bupropion is primarily metabolized to hydroxybupropion by the CYP2B6 isoenzyme. Therefore, co-administration of bupropion with CYP2B6 substrates or inhibitors (eg, orphenadrine, thiotepa, and cyclophosphamide) may result in a drug interaction).
No products indexed under this heading.

Erythromycin Stearate (*In vitro* studies indicate that bupropion is primarily metabolized to hydroxybupropion by the CYP2B6 isoenzyme. Therefore, co-administration of bupropion with CYP2B6 substrates or inhibitors (eg, orphenadrine, thiotepa, and cyclophosphamide) may result in a drug interaction).
No products indexed under this heading.

Escitalopram Oxalate (Concurrent administration of bupropion and agents (eg, other antidepressants) that lower seizure threshold should be undertaken only with extreme caution. Low initial dosing and small gradual dose increases should be employed. In addition, many drugs, including most antidepressants (SSRIs), are metabolized by the CYP2D6 isoenzyme. Co-administration of bupropion with drugs that are metabolized by CYP2D6 isoenzyme should be approached with caution and should be initiated at the lower end of the dose range of the concomitant medication. If bupropion is added to the treatment regimen of a patient already receiving a drug metabolized by CYP2D6, the need to decrease the dose of the original medication should be considered, particularly for those concomitant medications with a narrow therapeutic index). Products include:
Lexapro Oral Suspension 1160
Lexapro Tablets 1160

Esmolol Hydrochloride (Co-administration of bupropion with drugs that are metabolized by the CYP2D6 isoenzyme, including β-blockers (eg, metoprolol) should be approached with caution and should be initiated at the

2095 Interactions Index Wellbutrin

lower end of the dose range of the concomitant medication. If bupropion is added to the treatment regimen of a patient already receiving a drug metabolized by CYP2D6, the need to decrease the dose of the original medication should be considered, particularly for those concomitant medications with a narrow therapeutic index).
No products indexed under this heading.

Estazolam (Bupropion is contraindicated in patients undergoing abrupt discontinuation of sedatives (including benzodiazepines). Patients should be told that the excessive use or abrupt discontinuation of sedatives (including benzodiazepines) may alter the seizure threshold).
No products indexed under this heading.

Estradiol (*In vitro* studies indicate that bupropion is primarily metabolized to hydroxybupropion by the CYP2B6 isoenzyme. Therefore, co-administration of bupropion with CYP2B6 substrates or inhibitors (eg, orphenadrine, thiotepa, and cyclophosphamide) may result in a drug interaction). Products include:
Activella 2561
Angeliq 831
Climara 841
Climara Pro 847
Divigel 3467
Estrasorb 1777
Vagifem 2589

Estradiol Acetate (*In vitro* studies indicate that bupropion is primarily metabolized to hydroxybupropion by the CYP2B6 isoenzyme. Therefore, co-administration of bupropion with CYP2B6 substrates or inhibitors (eg, orphenadrine, thiotepa, and cyclophosphamide) may result in a drug interaction).
No products indexed under this heading.

Estradiol Benzoate (*In vitro* studies indicate that bupropion is primarily metabolized to hydroxybupropion by the CYP2B6 isoenzyme. Therefore, co-administration of bupropion with CYP2B6 substrates or inhibitors (eg, orphenadrine, thiotepa, and cyclophosphamide) may result in a drug interaction).
No products indexed under this heading.

Estradiol Cypionate (*In vitro* studies indicate that bupropion is primarily metabolized to hydroxybupropion by the CYP2B6 isoenzyme. Therefore, co-administration of bupropion with CYP2B6 substrates or inhibitors (eg, orphenadrine, thiotepa, and cyclophosphamide) may result in a drug interaction).
No products indexed under this heading.

Estradiol Valerate (*In vitro* studies indicate that bupropion is primarily metabolized to hydroxybupropion by the CYP2B6 isoenzyme. Therefore, co-administration of bupropion with CYP2B6 substrates or inhibitors (eg, orphenadrine, thiotepa, and cyclophosphamide) may result in a drug interaction).
No products indexed under this heading.

Estrogen (*In vitro* studies indicate that bupropion is primarily metabolized to hydroxybupropion by the CYP2B6 isoenzyme. Therefore, co-administration of bupropion with CYP2B6 substrates or inhibitors (eg, orphenadrine, thiotepa, and cyclophosphamide) may result in a drug interaction).
No products indexed under this heading.

Estrogens, Conjugated (*In vitro* studies indicate that bupropion is primarily metabolized to hydroxybupropion by the CYP2B6 isoenzyme. Therefore, co-administration of bupropion with CYP2B6 substrates or inhibitors (eg, orphenadrine, thiotepa, and cyclophosphamide) may result in a drug interaction). Products include:
Premarin Intravenous 3528
Premarin Tablets 3533
Premarin Vaginal Cream 3540
Premphase 3549
Prempro 3549

Estrogens, Conjugated, Synthetic A (*In vitro* studies indicate that bupropion is primarily metabolized to hydroxybupropion by the CYP2B6 isoenzyme. Therefore, co-administration of bupropion with CYP2B6 substrates or inhibitors (eg, orphenadrine, thiotepa, and cyclophosphamide) may result in a drug interaction).
No products indexed under this heading.

Estrogens, Conjugated, Synthetic B (*In vitro* studies indicate that bupropion is primarily metabolized to hydroxybupropion by the CYP2B6 isoenzyme. Therefore, co-administration of bupropion with CYP2B6 substrates or inhibitors (eg, orphenadrine, thiotepa, and cyclophosphamide) may result in a drug interaction). Products include:
Enjuvia 3401

Estrogens, Esterified (*In vitro* studies indicate that bupropion is primarily metabolized to hydroxybupropion by the CYP2B6 isoenzyme. Therefore, co-administration of bupropion with CYP2B6 substrates or inhibitors (eg, orphenadrine, thiotepa, and cyclophosphamide) may result in a drug interaction).
No products indexed under this heading.

Estrone (*In vitro* studies indicate that bupropion is primarily metabolized to hydroxybupropion by the CYP2B6 isoenzyme. Therefore, co-administration of bupropion with CYP2B6 substrates or inhibitors (eg, orphenadrine, thiotepa, and cyclophosphamide) may result in a drug interaction).
No products indexed under this heading.

Estropipate (*In vitro* studies indicate that bupropion is primarily metabolized to hydroxybupropion by the CYP2B6 isoenzyme. Therefore, co-administration of bupropion with CYP2B6 substrates or inhibitors (eg, orphenadrine, thiotepa, and cyclophosphamide) may result in a drug interaction).
No products indexed under this heading.

Ethanol (Bupropion is contraindicated in patients undergoing abrupt discontinuation of alcohol. In post-marketing experience, there have been rare reports of adverse neuropsychiatric events or reduced alcohol tolerance in patients who were drinking during treatment with bupropion. The consumption of alcohol should be minimized or avoided).
No products indexed under this heading.

Ethchlorvynol (Bupropion is contraindicated in patients undergoing abrupt discontinuation of sedatives (including benzodiazepines). Patients should be told that the excessive use or abrupt discontinuation of sedatives (including benzodiazepines) may alter the seizure threshold).
No products indexed under this heading.

Ethinamate (Bupropion is contraindicated in patients undergoing abrupt discontinuation of sedatives (including benzodiazepines). Patients should be told that the excessive use or abrupt discontinuation of sedatives (including benzodiazepines) may alter the seizure threshold).
No products indexed under this heading.

Ethinyl Estradiol (*In vitro* studies indicate that bupropion is primarily metabolized to hydroxybupropion by the CYP2B6 isoenzyme. Therefore, co-administration of bupropion with CYP2B6 substrates or inhibitors (eg, orphenadrine, thiotepa, and cyclophosphamide) may result in a drug interaction). Products include:
LoSeasonique 3407
Lybrel 3514
NuvaRing 3181
Ortho Evra 2648
Ortho-Cyclen/Ortho Tri-Cyclen 2663
Ortho Tri-Cyclen Lo Tablets 2673
Seasonique 3418
Yaz 864

Ethyl Alcohol (Bupropion is contraindicated in patients undergoing abrupt discontinuation of alcohol. In post-marketing experience, there have been rare reports of adverse neuropsychiatric events or reduced alcohol tolerance in patients who were drinking during treatment with bupropion. The consumption of alcohol should be minimized or avoided).
No products indexed under this heading.

Fenfluramine Hydrochloride (Concomitant use of anorectics with bupropion is associated with an increased seizure risk).
No products indexed under this heading.

Fentanyl (An addiction to opiates and concomitant use of bupropion has been associated with an increased seizure risk). Products include:
Duragesic 2604
Fentanyl Transdermal System 2346
Onsolis 2054

Fentanyl Citrate (An addiction to opiates and concomitant use of bupropion has been associated with an increased seizure risk). Products include:
Fentora 966

Flecainide Acetate (Co-administration of bupropion with drugs that are metabolized by the CYP2D6 isoenzyme including Type 1C antiarrhythmics (eg, flecainide) should be approached with caution and should be initiated at the lower end of the dose range of the concomitant medication. If bupropion is added to the treatment regimen of a patient already receiving a drug metabolized by CYP2D6, the need to decrease the dose of the original medication should be considered, particularly for those concomitant medications with a narrow therapeutic index).
No products indexed under this heading.

Fludrocortisone Acetate (Concurrent administration of bupropion and agents that lower seizure threshold, such as systemic steroids, should be undertaken with extreme caution. Low initial dosing and gradual dose increases should be employed).
No products indexed under this heading.

Flumethasone Pivalate (Concurrent administration of bupropion and agents that lower seizure threshold, such as systemic steroids, should be undertaken with extreme caution. Low initial dosing and gradual dose increases should be employed).
No products indexed under this heading.

Flunisolide Hemihydrate (Concurrent administration of bupropion and agents that lower seizure threshold, such as systemic steroids, should be undertaken with extreme caution. Low initial dosing and gradual dose increases should be employed).
No products indexed under this heading.

Fluoxetine (Concurrent administration of bupropion and agents that lower seizure threshold, such as antidepressants, should be undertaken with extreme caution. Low initial dosing and gradual dose increases should be employed. Co-administration of bupropion with drugs that are metabolized by the CYP2D6 isoenzyme including antidepressants (eg, fluoxetine) should be approached with caution and should be initiated at the lower end of the dose range of the concomitant medication. If bupropion is added to the treatment regimen of a patient already receiving a drug metabolized by CYP2D6, the need to decrease the dose of the original medication should be considered, particularly for those concomitant medications with a narrow therapeutic index).
No products indexed under this heading.

Fluoxetine Hydrochloride (Concurrent administration of bupropion and agents that lower seizure threshold, such as antidepressants, should be undertaken with extreme caution. Low initial dosing and gradual dose increases should be employed. Co-administration of bupropion with drugs that are metabolized by the CYP2D6 isoenzyme including antidepressants (eg, fluoxetine) should be approached with caution and should be initiated at the lower end of the dose range of the concomitant medication. If bupropion is added to the treatment regimen of a patient already receiving a drug metabolized by CYP2D6, the need to decrease the dose of the original medication should be considered, particularly for those concomitant medications with a narrow therapeutic index).
Products include:
Prozac Weekly 1941
Prozac Pulvules 1941
Symbyax 1965

Fluphenazine Decanoate (Concurrent administration of bupropion and agents that lower seizure threshold, such as antipsychotics, should be undertaken with extreme caution. Low initial dosing and gradual dose increases should be employed. Co-administration of bupropion with drugs that are metabolized by the CYP2D6 isoenzyme including antipsychotics (eg, haloperidol, risperidone, thioridazine) should be approached with caution and should be initiated at the lower end of the dose range of the concomitant medication. If bupropion is added to the treatment regimen of a patient already receiving a drug metabolized by CYP2D6, the need to decrease the dose of the original medication should be considered, particularly for those concomitant medications with a narrow therapeutic index).
No products indexed under this heading.

Fluphenazine Enanthate (Concurrent administration of bupropion and agents that lower seizure threshold, such as antipsychotics, should be undertaken with extreme caution. Low initial dosing and gradual dose increases should be employed. Co-administration of bupropion with drugs that are metabolized by the CYP2D6 isoenzyme including antipsychotics (eg, haloperidol, risperidone, thioridazine) should be approached with caution and should be initiated at the lower end of the dose range of the concomitant medication. If bupropion is added to the treatment regimen of a patient already receiving a drug metabolized by CYP2D6, the need to decrease the dose of the original medication should be considered, particularly for those concomitant medications with a narrow therapeutic index).
No products indexed under this heading.

Fluphenazine Hydrochloride (Concurrent administration of bupropion and agents that lower seizure threshold, such as antipsychotics, should be undertaken with extreme caution. Low initial dosing and gradual dose increases should be employed. Co-administration of bupropion with drugs that are metabolized by the CYP2D6 isoenzyme including antipsychotics (eg, haloperidol, risperidone, thioridazine) should be approached with caution and should be initiated at the lower end of the dose range of the concomitant medication. If bupropion is added to the treatment regimen of a patient already receiving a drug metabolized by

IMPORTANT NOTE: Always consult each drug listing in the patient's regimen for possible interactions.

CYP2D6, the need to decrease the dose of the original medication should be considered, particularly for those concomitant medications with a narrow therapeutic index).

No products indexed under this heading.

Flurazepam Hydrochloride (Bupropion is contraindicated in patients undergoing abrupt discontinuation of sedatives (including benzodiazepines). Patients should be told that the excessive use or abrupt discontinuation of sedatives (including benzodiazepines) may alter the seizure threshold).

No products indexed under this heading.

Fluticasone Furoate (Concurrent administration of bupropion and agents that lower seizure threshold, such as systemic steroids, should be undertaken with extreme caution. Low initial dosing and gradual dose increases should be employed). Products include:

Fluticasone Propionate (Concurrent administration of bupropion and agents that lower seizure threshold, such as systemic steroids, should be undertaken with extreme caution. Low initial dosing and gradual dose increases should be employed). Products include:

Fluvoxamine (Concurrent administration of bupropion and agents (eg, other antidepressants) that lower seizure threshold should be undertaken only with extreme caution. Low initial dosing and small gradual dose increases should be employed. In addition, many drugs, including most antidepressants (SSRIs), are metabolized by the CYP2D6 isoenzyme. Co-administration of bupropion with drugs that are metabolized by CYP2D6 isoenzyme should be approached with caution and should be initiated at the lower end of the dose range of the concomitant medication. If bupropion is added to the treatment regimen of a patient already receiving a drug metabolized by CYP2D6, the need to decrease the dose of the original medication should be considered, particularly for those concomitant medications with a narrow therapeutic index).

No products indexed under this heading.

Fluvoxamine Maleate (Concurrent administration of bupropion and agents (eg, other antidepressants) that lower seizure threshold should be undertaken only with extreme caution. Low initial dosing and small gradual dose increases should be employed. In addition, many drugs, including most antidepressants (SSRIs), are metabolized by the CYP2D6 isoenzyme. Co-administration of bupropion with drugs that are metabolized by CYP2D6 isoenzyme should be approached with caution and should be initiated at the lower end of the dose range of the concomitant medication. If bupropion is added to the treatment regimen of a patient already receiving a drug metabolized by CYP2D6, the need to decrease the dose of the original medication should be considered, particularly for those concomitant medications with a narrow therapeutic index).

No products indexed under this heading.

Formoterol Fumarate (Co-administration of bupropion with drugs that are metabolized by the CYP2D6 isoenzyme should be approached with caution and should be initiated at the lower end of the dose range of the concomitant medication. If bupropion is

added to the treatment regimen of a patient already receiving a drug metabolized by CYP2D6, the need to decrease the dose of the original medication should be considered, particularly for those concomitant medications with a narrow therapeutic index). Products include:

Fosphenytoin (While not systematically studied, certain drugs may induce the metabolism of bupropion (eg, phenytoin)).

No products indexed under this heading.

Fosphenytoin Sodium (While not systematically studied, certain drugs may induce the metabolism of bupropion (eg, phenytoin)).

No products indexed under this heading.

Galantamine Hydrobromide (Co-administration of bupropion with drugs that are metabolized by the CYP2D6 isoenzyme should be approached with caution and should be initiated at the lower end of the dose range of the concomitant medication. If bupropion is added to the treatment regimen of a patient already receiving a drug metabolized by CYP2D6, the need to decrease the dose of the original medication should be considered, particularly for those concomitant medications with a narrow therapeutic index).

No products indexed under this heading.

Glibenclamide (Concomitant use of oral hypoglycemics with bupropion is associated with an increased seizure risk).

No products indexed under this heading.

Glimepiride (Concomitant use of oral hypoglycemics with bupropion is associated with an increased seizure risk). Products include:

Glipizide (Concomitant use of oral hypoglycemics with bupropion is associated with an increased seizure risk).

No products indexed under this heading.

Glutethimide (Bupropion is contraindicated in patients undergoing abrupt discontinuation of sedatives (including benzodiazepines). Patients should be told that the excessive use or abrupt discontinuation of sedatives (including benzodiazepines) may alter the seizure threshold).

No products indexed under this heading.

Glyburide (Concomitant use of oral hypoglycemics with bupropion is associated with an increased seizure risk).

No products indexed under this heading.

Halazepam (Bupropion is contraindicated in patients undergoing abrupt discontinuation of sedatives (including benzodiazepines). Patients should be told that the excessive use or abrupt discontinuation of sedatives (including benzodiazepines) may alter the seizure threshold).

No products indexed under this heading.

Haloperidol (Concurrent administration of bupropion and agents that lower seizure threshold, such as antipsychotics, should be undertaken with extreme caution. Low initial dosing and gradual dose increases should be employed. Co-administration of bupropion with drugs that are metabolized by the CYP2D6 isoenzyme including antipsychotics (eg, haloperidol) should be approached with caution and should be initiated at the lower end of the dose range of the concomitant medication. If bupropion is added to the treatment regimen of a patient already receiving a drug metabolized by CYP2D6, the need to decrease the dose of the original

medication should be considered, particularly for those concomitant medications with a narrow therapeutic index).

No products indexed under this heading.

Haloperidol Decanoate (Concurrent administration of bupropion and agents that lower seizure threshold, such as antipsychotics, should be undertaken with extreme caution. Low initial dosing and gradual dose increases should be employed. Co-administration of bupropion with drugs that are metabolized by the CYP2D6 isoenzyme including antipsychotics (eg, haloperidol) should be approached with caution and should be initiated at the lower end of the dose range of the concomitant medication. If bupropion is added to the treatment regimen of a patient already receiving a drug metabolized by CYP2D6, the need to decrease the dose of the original medication should be considered, particularly for those concomitant medications with a narrow therapeutic index).

No products indexed under this heading.

Haloperidol Lactate (Concurrent administration of bupropion and agents that lower seizure threshold, such as antipsychotics, should be undertaken with extreme caution. Low initial dosing and gradual dose increases should be employed. Co-administration of bupropion with drugs that are metabolized by the CYP2D6 isoenzyme including antipsychotics (eg, haloperidol) should be approached with caution and should be initiated at the lower end of the dose range of the concomitant medication. If bupropion is added to the treatment regimen of a patient already receiving a drug metabolized by CYP2D6, the need to decrease the dose of the original medication should be considered, particularly for those concomitant medications with a narrow therapeutic index).

No products indexed under this heading.

Halothane (*In vitro* studies indicate that bupropion is primarily metabolized to hydroxybupropion by the CYP2B6 isoenzyme. Therefore, co-administration of bupropion with CYP2B6 substrates or inhibitors (eg, orphenadrine, thiotepa, and cyclophosphamide) may result in a drug interaction).

No products indexed under this heading.

Hydrocodone Bitartrate (An addiction to opiates and concomitant use of bupropion has been associated with an increased seizure risk). Products include:

Hydrocodone Polistirex (An addiction to opiates and concomitant use of bupropion has been associated with an increased seizure risk). Products include:

Hydrocortisone (Concurrent administration of bupropion and agents that lower seizure threshold, such as systemic steroids, should be undertaken with extreme caution. Low initial dosing and gradual dose increases should be employed).

No products indexed under this heading.

Hydrocortisone (Alcohol) (Concurrent administration of bupropion and agents that lower seizure threshold, such as systemic steroids, should be undertaken with extreme caution. Low initial dosing and gradual dose increases should be employed).

No products indexed under this heading.

Hydrocortisone Acetate (Concurrent administration of bupropion and agents that lower seizure threshold, such as systemic steroids, should be undertaken with extreme caution. Low initial dosing and gradual dose increases should be employed).

No products indexed under this heading.

Hydrocortisone Butyrate (Concurrent administration of bupropion and agents that lower seizure threshold, such as systemic steroids, should be undertaken with extreme caution. Low initial dosing and gradual dose increases should be employed).

No products indexed under this heading.

Hydrocortisone Cypionate (Concurrent administration of bupropion and agents that lower seizure threshold, such as systemic steroids, should be undertaken with extreme caution. Low initial dosing and gradual dose increases should be employed).

No products indexed under this heading.

Hydrocortisone Hemisuccinate (Concurrent administration of bupropion and agents that lower seizure threshold, such as systemic steroids, should be undertaken with extreme caution. Low initial dosing and gradual dose increases should be employed).

No products indexed under this heading.

Hydrocortisone Probutate (Concurrent administration of bupropion and agents that lower seizure threshold, such as systemic steroids, should be undertaken with extreme caution. Low initial dosing and gradual dose increases should be employed).

No products indexed under this heading.

Hydrocortisone Sodium Phosphate (Concurrent administration of bupropion and agents that lower seizure threshold, such as systemic steroids, should be undertaken with extreme caution. Low initial dosing and gradual dose increases should be employed).

No products indexed under this heading.

Hydrocortisone Sodium Succinate (Concurrent administration of bupropion and agents that lower seizure threshold, such as systemic steroids, should be undertaken with extreme caution. Low initial dosing and gradual dose increases should be employed).

No products indexed under this heading.

Hydrocortisone Valerate (Concurrent administration of bupropion and agents that lower seizure threshold, such as systemic steroids, should be undertaken with extreme caution. Low initial dosing and gradual dose increases should be employed).

No products indexed under this heading.

Hydromorphone (An addiction to opiates and concomitant use of bupropion has been associated with an increased seizure risk).

No products indexed under this heading.

Hydromorphone Hydrochloride (An addiction to opiates and concomitant use of bupropion has been associated with an increased seizure risk). Products include:

Hydroxyamphetamine Hydrobromide (Concomitant use of anorectics with bupropion is associated with an increased seizure risk).

No products indexed under this heading.

2097 Interactions Index Wellbutrin

Ifosfamide (*In vitro* studies indicate that bupropion is primarily metabolized to hydroxybupropion by the CYP2B6 isoenzyme. Therefore, co-administration of bupropion with CYP2B6 substrates or inhibitors (eg, orphenadrine, thiotepa, and cyclophosphamide) may result in a drug interaction).
No products indexed under this heading.

Imipramine Hydrochloride (Concurrent administration of bupropion and agents that lower seizure threshold, such as antidepressants, should be undertaken with extreme caution. Low initial dosing and gradual dose increases should be employed. Co-administration of bupropion with drugs that are metabolized by the CYP2D6 isoenzyme including antidepressants (eg, imipramine) should be approached with caution and should be initiated at the lower end of the dose range of the concomitant medication. If bupropion is added to the treatment regimen of a patient already receiving a drug metabolized by CYP2D6, the need to decrease the dose of the original medication should be considered, particularly for those concomitant medications with a narrow therapeutic index).
No products indexed under this heading.

Imipramine Pamoate (Concurrent administration of bupropion and agents that lower seizure threshold, such as antidepressants, should be undertaken with extreme caution. Low initial dosing and gradual dose increases should be employed. Co-administration of bupropion with drugs that are metabolized by the CYP2D6 isoenzyme including antidepressants (eg, imipramine) should be approached with caution and should be initiated at the lower end of the dose range of the concomitant medication. If bupropion is added to the treatment regimen of a patient already receiving a drug metabolized by CYP2D6, the need to decrease the dose of the original medication should be considered, particularly for those concomitant medications with a narrow therapeutic index).
No products indexed under this heading.

Indoramin Hydrochloride (Co-administration of bupropion with drugs that are metabolized by the CYP2D6 isoenzyme should be approached with caution and should be initiated at the lower end of the dose range of the concomitant medication. If bupropion is added to the treatment regimen of a patient already receiving a drug metabolized by CYP2D6, the need to decrease the dose of the original medication should be considered, particularly for those concomitant medications with a narrow therapeutic index).
No products indexed under this heading.

Insulin (Concomitant use of insulin with bupropion is associated with an increased seizure risk).
No products indexed under this heading.

Insulin, Human, Zinc Suspension (Concomitant use of insulin with bupropion is associated with an increased seizure risk).
No products indexed under this heading.

Insulin, Human (rDNA origin) (Concomitant use of insulin with bupropion is associated with an increased seizure risk). Products include:
Exubera 2717

Insulin, Human NPH (Concomitant use of insulin with bupropion is associated with an increased seizure risk). Products include:
Humulin N Vial 1934

Insulin, Human Regular (Concomitant use of insulin with bupropion is associated with an increased seizure risk). Products include:
Humulin R 1937
Humulin R (U-500) 1939

Insulin, Human Regular and Human NPH Mixture (Concomitant use of insulin with bupropion is associated with an increased seizure risk). Products include:
Humulin 50/50 1930
Humulin 70/30 Vial 1931

Insulin, NPH (Concomitant use of insulin with bupropion is associated with an increased seizure risk).
No products indexed under this heading.

Insulin, Regular (Concomitant use of insulin with bupropion is associated with an increased seizure risk).
No products indexed under this heading.

Insulin, Regular and NPH mixture (Concomitant use of insulin with bupropion is associated with an increased seizure risk).
No products indexed under this heading.

Insulin, Zinc Crystals (Concomitant use of insulin with bupropion is associated with an increased seizure risk).
No products indexed under this heading.

Insulin, Zinc Suspension (Concomitant use of insulin with bupropion is associated with an increased seizure risk).
No products indexed under this heading.

Insulin Aspart (Concomitant use of insulin with bupropion is associated with an increased seizure risk).
No products indexed under this heading.

Insulin Aspart, Human (Concomitant use of insulin with bupropion is associated with an increased seizure risk). Products include:
NovoLog Mix 70/30 2581

Insulin Aspart, Human Regular (Concomitant use of insulin with bupropion is associated with an increased seizure risk). Products include:
NovoLog 2575

Insulin Aspart Protamine, Human (Concomitant use of insulin with bupropion is associated with an increased seizure risk). Products include:
NovoLog Mix 70/30 2581

Insulin Detemir (rDNA Origin) (Concomitant use of insulin with bupropion is associated with an increased seizure risk). Products include:
Levemir 2566

Insulin Glargine (Concomitant use of insulin with bupropion is associated with an increased seizure risk). Products include:
Lantus 2996

Insulin Glulisine (Concomitant use of insulin with bupropion is associated with an increased seizure risk). Products include:
Apidra 2937
Apidra SoloStar 2937

Insulin Lispro, Human (Concomitant use of insulin with bupropion is associated with an increased seizure risk). Products include:
Humalog 1910
Humalog Mix 1914
Humalog Mix75/25 1917

Insulin Lispro Protamine, Human (Concomitant use of insulin with bupropion is associated with an increased seizure risk). Products include:
Humalog Mix 1914
Humalog Mix75/25 1917

Irinotecan Hydrochloride (*In vitro* studies indicate that bupropion is primarily metabolized to hydroxybupropion by the CYP2B6 isoenzyme. Therefore, co-administration of bupropion with CYP2B6 substrates or inhibitors (eg, orphenadrine, thiotepa, and cyclophosphamide) may result in a drug interaction).
No products indexed under this heading.

Isocarboxazid (Concurrent administration of bupropion and a monoamine oxidase (MAO) inhibitor is contraindicated. At least 14 days should elapse between discontinuation of a MAO inhibitor and initiation of treatment with bupropion). Products include:
Marplan 3481

Isoflurane (*In vitro* studies indicate that bupropion is primarily metabolized to hydroxybupropion by the CYP2B6 isoenzyme. Therefore, co-administration of bupropion with CYP2B6 substrates or inhibitors (eg, orphenadrine, thiotepa, and cyclophosphamide) may result in a drug interaction).
No products indexed under this heading.

Isotretinoin (*In vitro* studies indicate that bupropion is primarily metabolized to hydroxybupropion by the CYP2B6 isoenzyme. Therefore, co-administration of bupropion with CYP2B6 substrates or inhibitors (eg, orphenadrine, thiotepa, and cyclophosphamide) may result in a drug interaction). Products include:
Accutane 2832

Ketamine (*In vitro* studies indicate that bupropion is primarily metabolized to hydroxybupropion by the CYP2B6 isoenzyme. Therefore, co-administration of bupropion with CYP2B6 substrates or inhibitors (eg, orphenadrine, thiotepa, and cyclophosphamide) may result in a drug interaction).
No products indexed under this heading.

Ketamine Hydrochloride (*In vitro* studies indicate that bupropion is primarily metabolized to hydroxybupropion by the CYP2B6 isoenzyme. Therefore, co-administration of bupropion with CYP2B6 substrates or inhibitors (eg, orphenadrine, thiotepa, and cyclophosphamide) may result in a drug interaction).
No products indexed under this heading.

Ketoconazole (*In vitro* studies indicate that bupropion is primarily metabolized to hydroxybupropion by the CYP2B6 isoenzyme. Therefore, co-administration of bupropion with CYP2B6 substrates or inhibitors (eg, orphenadrine, thiotepa, and cyclophosphamide) may result in a drug interaction). Products include:
Extina 3319
Xolegel 3337

Labetalol Hydrochloride (Co-administration of bupropion with drugs that are metabolized by the CYP2D6 isoenzyme, including β-blockers (eg, metoprolol) should be approached with caution and should be initiated at the lower end of the dose range of the concomitant medication. If bupropion is added to the treatment regimen of a patient already receiving a drug metabolized by CYP2D6, the need to decrease the dose of the original medication should be considered, particularly for those concomitant medications with a narrow therapeutic index).
No products indexed under this heading.

Levobunolol Hydrochloride (Co-administration of bupropion with drugs that are metabolized by the CYP2D6 isoenzyme, including β-blockers (eg, metoprolol) should be approached with caution and should be initiated at the lower end of the dose range of the concomitant medication. If bupropion is added to the treatment regimen of a patient already receiving a drug metabolized by CYP2D6, the need to decrease the dose of the original medication should be considered, particularly for those concomitant medications with a narrow therapeutic index).
No products indexed under this heading.

Levodopa (Limited clinical data suggest a higher incidence of adverse experiences in patients receiving bupropion concurrently with levodopa. Administration of bupropion tablets to patients receiving levodopa concurrently should be undertaken with caution, using small initial doses and small gradual dose increases). Products include:
Stalevo 2526

Levorphanol Tartrate (An addiction to opiates and concomitant use of bupropion has been associated with an increased seizure risk).
No products indexed under this heading.

Lidocaine (Co-administration of bupropion with drugs that are metabolized by the CYP2D6 isoenzyme should be approached with caution and should be initiated at the lower end of the dose range of the concomitant medication. If bupropion is added to the treatment regimen of a patient already receiving a drug metabolized by CYP2D6, the need to decrease the dose of the original medication should be considered, particularly for those concomitant medications with a narrow therapeutic index). Products include:
Lidoderm 1107

Lidocaine Base (*In vitro* studies indicate that bupropion is primarily metabolized to hydroxybupropion by the CYP2B6 isoenzyme. Therefore, co-administration of bupropion with CYP2B6 substrates or inhibitors (eg, orphenadrine, thiotepa, and cyclophosphamide) may result in a drug interaction).
No products indexed under this heading.

Lidocaine Hydrochloride (Co-administration of bupropion with drugs that are metabolized by the CYP2D6 isoenzyme should be approached with caution and should be initiated at the lower end of the dose range of the concomitant medication. If bupropion is added to the treatment regimen of a patient already receiving a drug metabolized by CYP2D6, the need to decrease the dose of the original medication should be considered, particularly for those concomitant medications with a narrow therapeutic index).
No products indexed under this heading.

Lisdexamfetamine Dimesylate (Concomitant use of over-the-counter stimulants with bupropion is associated with an increased seizure risk). Products include:
Vyvanse 3298

Lithium (Concurrent administration of bupropion and agents that lower seizure threshold, such as antipsychotics, should be undertaken with extreme caution. Low initial dosing and gradual dose increases should be employed. Co-administration of bupropion with drugs that are metabolized by the CYP2D6 isoenzyme including antipsychotics (eg, haloperidol, risperidone, thioridazine) should be approached with caution and should be initiated at the lower end of the dose range of the concomitant medication. If bupropion is added to the treatment regimen of a patient already receiving a drug metabolized by CYP2D6, the need to decrease the dose of the original medication should be considered, particularly for those concomitant medications with a narrow therapeutic index).
No products indexed under this heading.

Lithium Carbonate (Concurrent administration of bupropion and agents that lower seizure threshold, such as antipsychotics, should be undertaken with extreme caution. Low initial dosing and gradual dose increases should be employed. Co-administration of bupropion with drugs that are metabolized by the CYP2D6 isoenzyme including antipsychotics (eg, haloperidol, risperidone, thioridazine) should be approached with caution and should be initiated at the lower end of the dose range of the concomitant medication. If bupropion is added to the treatment regimen of a patient already receiving a drug metab-

IMPORTANT NOTE: Always consult each drug listing in the patient's regimen for possible interactions.

Wellbutrin Interactions Index 2098

olized by CYP2D6, the need to decrease the dose of the original medication should be considered, particularly for those concomitant medications with a narrow therapeutic index).
No products indexed under this heading.

Lithium Citrate (Concurrent administration of bupropion and agents that lower seizure threshold, such as antipsychotics, should be undertaken with extreme caution. Low initial dosing and gradual dose increases should be employed. Co-administration of bupropion with drugs that are metabolized by the CYP2D6 isoenzyme including antipsychotics (eg, haloperidol, risperidone, thioridazine) should be approached with caution and should be initiated at the lower end of the dose range of the concomitant medication. If bupropion is added to the treatment regimen of a patient already receiving a drug metabolized by CYP2D6, the need to decrease the dose of the original medication should be considered, particularly for those concomitant medications with a narrow therapeutic index).
No products indexed under this heading.

Lorazepam (Bupropion is contraindicated in patients undergoing abrupt discontinuation of sedatives (including benzodiazepines). Patients should be told that the excessive use or abrupt discontinuation of sedatives (including benzodiazepines) may alter the seizure threshold).
No products indexed under this heading.

Loxapine Hydrochloride (Concurrent administration of bupropion and agents that lower seizure threshold, such as antipsychotics, should be undertaken with extreme caution. Low initial dosing and gradual dose increases should be employed. Co-administration of bupropion with drugs that are metabolized by the CYP2D6 isoenzyme including antipsychotics (eg, haloperidol, risperidone, thioridazine) should be approached with caution and should be initiated at the lower end of the dose range of the concomitant medication. If bupropion is added to the treatment regimen of a patient already receiving a drug metabolized by CYP2D6, the need to decrease the dose of the original medication should be considered, particularly for those concomitant medications with a narrow therapeutic index).
No products indexed under this heading.

Loxapine Succinate (Concurrent administration of bupropion and agents that lower seizure threshold, such as antipsychotics, should be undertaken with extreme caution. Low initial dosing and gradual dose increases should be employed. Co-administration of bupropion with drugs that are metabolized by the CYP2D6 isoenzyme including antipsychotics (eg, haloperidol, risperidone, thioridazine) should be approached with caution and should be initiated at the lower end of the dose range of the concomitant medication. If bupropion is added to the treatment regimen of a patient already receiving a drug metabolized by CYP2D6, the need to decrease the dose of the original medication should be considered, particularly for those concomitant medications with a narrow therapeutic index).
No products indexed under this heading.

Maprotiline Hydrochloride (Concurrent administration of bupropion and agents (eg, other antidepressants) that lower seizure threshold should be undertaken only with extreme caution. Low initial dosing and small gradual dose increases should be employed. In addition, many drugs, including most antidepressants (many tricyclics), are metabolized by the CYP2D6 isoenzyme. Co-administration of bupropion with drugs that are metabolized by CYP2D6 isoenzyme should be approached with caution and should be initiated at the lower end of the dose range of the concomitant medication. If bupropion is added to the treatment regimen of a patient already receiving a drug metabolized by CYP2D6, the need to decrease the dose of the original medication should be considered, particularly for those concomitant medications with a narrow therapeutic index).
No products indexed under this heading.

Mazindol (Concomitant use of anorectics with bupropion is associated with an increased seizure risk).
No products indexed under this heading.

Meperidine Hydrochloride (An addiction to opiates and concomitant use of bupropion has been associated with an increased seizure risk).
No products indexed under this heading.

Mephenytoin (*In vitro* studies indicate that bupropion is primarily metabolized to hydroxybupropion by the CYP2B6 isoenzyme. Therefore, co-administration of bupropion with CYP2B6 substrates or inhibitors (eg, orphenadrine, thiotepa, and cyclophosphamide) may result in a drug interaction).
No products indexed under this heading.

Mephobarbital (*In vitro* studies indicate that bupropion is primarily metabolized to hydroxybupropion by the CYP2B6 isoenzyme. Therefore, co-administration of bupropion with CYP2B6 substrates or inhibitors (eg, orphenadrine, thiotepa, and cyclophosphamide) may result in a drug interaction).
No products indexed under this heading.

Mesoridazine Besylate (Concurrent administration of bupropion and agents that lower seizure threshold, such as antipsychotics, should be undertaken with extreme caution. Low initial dosing and gradual dose increases should be employed. Co-administration of bupropion with drugs that are metabolized by the CYP2D6 isoenzyme including antipsychotics (eg, haloperidol, risperidone, thioridazine) should be approached with caution and should be initiated at the lower end of the dose range of the concomitant medication. If bupropion is added to the treatment regimen of a patient already receiving a drug metabolized by CYP2D6, the need to decrease the dose of the original medication should be considered, particularly for those concomitant medications with a narrow therapeutic index).
No products indexed under this heading.

Metformin Hydrochloride (Concomitant use of oral hypoglycemics with bupropion is associated with an increased seizure risk). Products include:
ActoPlus 3338
Avandamet 1345
Janumet 2188

Methadone Hydrochloride (An addiction to opiates and concomitant use of bupropion has been associated with an increased seizure risk).
No products indexed under this heading.

Methamphetamine Hydrochloride (Concomitant use of anorectics with bupropion is associated with an increased seizure risk).
No products indexed under this heading.

Methimazole (*In vitro* studies indicate that bupropion is primarily metabolized to hydroxybupropion by the CYP2B6 isoenzyme. Therefore, co-administration of bupropion with CYP2B6 substrates or inhibitors (eg, orphenadrine, thiotepa, and cyclophosphamide) may result in a drug interaction).
No products indexed under this heading.

Methotrimeprazine (Concurrent administration of bupropion and agents that lower seizure threshold, such as antipsychotics, should be undertaken with extreme caution. Low initial dosing and gradual dose increases should be employed. Co-administration of bupropion with drugs that are metabolized by the CYP2D6 isoenzyme including antipsychotics (eg, haloperidol, risperidone, thioridazine) should be approached with caution and should be initiated at the lower end of the dose range of the concomitant medication. If bupropion is added to the treatment regimen of a patient already receiving a drug metabolized by CYP2D6, the need to decrease the dose of the original medication should be considered, particularly for those concomitant medications with a narrow therapeutic index).
No products indexed under this heading.

Methoxyphenamine (Co-administration of bupropion with drugs that are metabolized by the CYP2D6 isoenzyme should be approached with caution and should be initiated at the lower end of the dose range of the concomitant medication. If bupropion is added to the treatment regimen of a patient already receiving a drug metabolized by CYP2D6, the need to decrease the dose of the original medication should be considered, particularly for those concomitant medications with a narrow therapeutic index).
No products indexed under this heading.

Methylphenidate (Concomitant use of over-the-counter stimulants with bupropion is associated with an increased seizure risk). Products include:
Daytrana 3283

Methylphenidate Hydrochloride (Concomitant use of over-the-counter stimulants with bupropion is associated with an increased seizure risk). Products include:
Concerta 2598
Metadate CD 3439

Methylprednisolone (Concurrent administration of bupropion and agents that lower seizure threshold, such as systemic steroids, should be undertaken with extreme caution. Low initial dosing and gradual dose increases should be employed).
No products indexed under this heading.

Methylprednisolone Acetate (Concurrent administration of bupropion and agents that lower seizure threshold, such as systemic steroids, should be undertaken with extreme caution. Low initial dosing and gradual dose increases should be employed).
No products indexed under this heading.

Methylprednisolone Sodium Succinate (Concurrent administration of bupropion and agents that lower seizure threshold, such as systemic steroids, should be undertaken with extreme caution. Low initial dosing and gradual dose increases should be employed).
No products indexed under this heading.

Methyltestosterone (*In vitro* studies indicate that bupropion is primarily metabolized to hydroxybupropion by the CYP2B6 isoenzyme. Therefore, co-administration of bupropion with CYP2B6 substrates or inhibitors (eg, orphenadrine, thiotepa, and cyclophosphamide) may result in a drug interaction).
No products indexed under this heading.

Metipranolol Hydrochloride (Co-administration of bupropion with drugs that are metabolized by the CYP2D6 isoenzyme, including β-blockers (eg, metoprolol) should be approached with caution and should be initiated at the lower end of the dose range of the concomitant medication. If bupropion is added to the treatment regimen of a patient already receiving a drug metabolized by CYP2D6, the need to decrease the dose of the original medication should be considered, particularly for those concomitant medications with a narrow therapeutic index).
No products indexed under this heading.

Metoprolol Succinate (Co-administration of bupropion with drugs that are metabolized by the CYP2D6 isoenzyme, including β-blockers (eg, metoprolol) should be approached with caution and should be initiated at the lower end of the dose range of the concomitant medication. If bupropion is added to the treatment regimen of a patient already receiving a drug metabolized by CYP2D6, the need to decrease the dose of the original medication should be considered, particularly for those concomitant medications with a narrow therapeutic index).
Products include:
Toprol XL 732

Metoprolol Tartrate (Co-administration of bupropion with drugs that are metabolized by the CYP2D6 isoenzyme, including β-blockers (eg, metoprolol) should be approached with caution and should be initiated at the lower end of the dose range of the concomitant medication. If bupropion is added to the treatment regimen of a patient already receiving a drug metabolized by CYP2D6, the need to decrease the dose of the original medication should be considered, particularly for those concomitant medications with a narrow therapeutic index).
No products indexed under this heading.

Mexiletine Hydrochloride (Co-administration of bupropion with drugs that are metabolized by the CYP2D6 isoenzyme should be approached with caution and should be initiated at the lower end of the dose range of the concomitant medication. If bupropion is added to the treatment regimen of a patient already receiving a drug metabolized by CYP2D6, the need to decrease the dose of the original medication should be considered, particularly for those concomitant medications with a narrow therapeutic index).
No products indexed under this heading.

Miconazole (*In vitro* studies indicate that bupropion is primarily metabolized to hydroxybupropion by the CYP2B6 isoenzyme. Therefore, co-administration of bupropion with CYP2B6 substrates or inhibitors (eg, orphenadrine, thiotepa, and cyclophosphamide) may result in a drug interaction).
No products indexed under this heading.

Miconazole Nitrate (*In vitro* studies indicate that bupropion is primarily metabolized to hydroxybupropion by the CYP2B6 isoenzyme. Therefore, co-administration of bupropion with CYP2B6 substrates or inhibitors (eg, orphenadrine, thiotepa, and cyclophosphamide) may result in a drug interaction). Products include:
Vusion Ointment 3335

Midazolam Hydrochloride (Bupropion is contraindicated in patients undergoing abrupt discontinuation of sedatives (including benzodiazepines). Patients should be told that the excessive use or abrupt discontinuation of sedatives (including benzodiazepines) may alter the seizure threshold).
No products indexed under this heading.

Miglitol (Concomitant use of oral hypoglycemics with bupropion is associated with an increased seizure risk).
No products indexed under this heading.

Mirtazapine (Concurrent administration of bupropion and agents that lower seizure threshold, such as antidepressants, should be undertaken with

2099 Interactions Index Wellbutrin

extreme caution. Low initial dosing and gradual dose increases should be employed. Co-administration of bupropion with drugs that are metabolized by the CYP2D6 isoenzyme including antidepressants (eg, nortriptyline, imipramine, desipramine, paroxentine, fluoxetine, sertraline) should be approached with caution and should be initiated at the lower end of the dose range of the concomitant medication. If bupropion is added to the treatment regimen of a patient already receiving a drug metabolized by CYP2D6, the need to decrease the dose of the original medication should be considered, particularly for those concomitant medications with a narrow therapeutic index). Products include:

Remeron Tablets 3214
RemeronSolTab Tablets 3219

Moclobemide (Concurrent administration of bupropion and a monoamine oxidase (MAO) inhibitor is contraindicated. At least 14 days should elapse between discontinuation of a MAO inhibitor and initiation of treatment with bupropion).
No products indexed under this heading.

Molindone Hydrochloride (Concurrent administration of bupropion and agents that lower seizure threshold, such as antipsychotics, should be undertaken with extreme caution. Low initial dosing and gradual dose increases should be employed. Co-administration of bupropion with drugs that are metabolized by the CYP2D6 isoenzyme including antipsychotics (eg, haloperidol, risperidone, thioridazine) should be approached with caution and should be initiated at the lower end of the dose range of the concomitant medication. If bupropion is added to the treatment regimen of a patient already receiving a drug metabolized by CYP2D6, the need to decrease the dose of the original medication should be considered, particularly for those concomitant medications with a narrow therapeutic index). Products include:

Moban 1108

Mometasone Furoate (Concurrent administration of bupropion and agents that lower seizure threshold, such as systemic steroids, should be undertaken with extreme caution. Low initial dosing and gradual dose increases should be employed). Products include:

Asmanex 3058
Elocon Cream 3111
Elocon Lotion 3112
Elocon Ointment 3114

Mometasone Furoate Monohydrate (Concurrent administration of bupropion and agents that lower seizure threshold, such as systemic steroids, should be undertaken with extreme caution. Low initial dosing and gradual dose increases should be employed).
Products include:

Nasonex 3166

Moricizine Hydrochloride (Co-administration of bupropion with drugs that are metabolized by the CYP2D6 isoenzyme, including antiarrhythmics should be approached with caution and should be initiated at the lower end of the dose range of the concomitant medication. If bupropion is added to the treatment regimen of a patient already receiving a drug metabolized by CYP2D6, the need to decrease the dose of the original medication should be considered, particularly for those concomitant medications with a narrow therapeutic index).
No products indexed under this heading.

Morphine Sulfate (An addiction to opiates and concomitant use of bupropion has been associated with an increased seizure risk). Products include:

Avinza 1822
Embeda 1831
MS Contin 2803

Morphine Sulfate, Liposomal (An addiction to opiates and concomitant use of bupropion has been associated with an increased seizure risk).
No products indexed under this heading.

Nadolol (Co-administration of bupropion with drugs that are metabolized by the CYP2D6 isoenzyme, including β-blockers (eg, metoprolol) should be approached with caution and should be initiated at the lower end of the dose range of the concomitant medication. If bupropion is added to the treatment regimen of a patient already receiving a drug metabolized by CYP2D6, the need to decrease the dose of the original medication should be considered, particularly for those concomitant medications with a narrow therapeutic index).
Products include:

Nadolol 2359

Nateglinide (Concomitant use of oral hypoglycemics with bupropion is associated with an increased seizure risk).
No products indexed under this heading.

Nebivolol (Co-administration of bupropion with drugs that are metabolized by the CYP2D6 isoenzyme, including β-blockers (eg, metoprolol) should be approached with caution and should be initiated at the lower end of the dose range of the concomitant medication. If bupropion is added to the treatment regimen of a patient already receiving a drug metabolized by CYP2D6, the need to decrease the dose of the original medication should be considered, particularly for those concomitant medications with a narrow therapeutic index).
Products include:

Bystolic 1147

Nefazodone Hydrochloride (Concurrent administration of bupropion and agents that lower seizure threshold, such as antidepressants, should be undertaken with extreme caution. Low initial dosing and gradual dose increases should be employed. Co-administration of bupropion with drugs that are metabolized by the CYP2D6 isoenzyme including antidepressants (eg, nortriptyline, imipramine, desipramine, paroxentine, fluoxetine, sertraline) should be approached with caution and should be initiated at the lower end of the dose range of the concomitant medication. If bupropion is added to the treatment regimen of a patient already receiving a drug metabolized by CYP2D6, the need to decrease the dose of the original medication should be considered, particularly for those concomitant medications with a narrow therapeutic index).
No products indexed under this heading.

Nelfinavir Mesylate (*In vitro* studies suggest that nelfinavir inhibits the hydroxylation of bupropion).
No products indexed under this heading.

Nevirapine (*In vitro* studies indicate that bupropion is primarily metabolized to hydroxybupropion by the CYP2B6 isoenzyme. Therefore, co-administration of bupropion with CYP2B6 substrates or inhibitors (eg, orphenadrine, thiotepa, and cyclophosphamide) may result in a drug interaction). Products include:

Viramune Oral Suspension 897
Viramune Tablets 897

Nicotine (In clinical practice, hypertension, in some cases severe, requiring acute treatment, has been reported in patients receiving bupropion alone and in combination with nicotine replacement therapy. These events have been observed in both patients with and without evidence of preexisting hypertension. Monitoring of blood pressure is recommended in patients who receive the combination of bupropion and nicotine replacement).
No products indexed under this heading.

Nicotine Polacrilex (In clinical practice, hypertension, in some cases severe, requiring acute treatment, has been reported in patients receiving bupropion alone and in combination with nicotine replacement therapy. These events have been observed in both patients with and without evidence of preexisting hypertension. Monitoring of blood pressure is recommended in patients who receive the combination of bupropion and nicotine replacement).
No products indexed under this heading.

Nicotine Salicylate (In clinical practice, hypertension, in some cases severe, requiring acute treatment, has been reported in patients receiving bupropion alone and in combination with nicotine replacement therapy. These events have been observed in both patients with and without evidence of preexisting hypertension. Monitoring of blood pressure is recommended in patients who receive the combination of bupropion and nicotine replacement).
No products indexed under this heading.

Nicotine Sulfate (In clinical practice, hypertension, in some cases severe, requiring acute treatment, has been reported in patients receiving bupropion alone and in combination with nicotine replacement therapy. These events have been observed in both patients with and without evidence of preexisting hypertension. Monitoring of blood pressure is recommended in patients who receive the combination of bupropion and nicotine replacement).
No products indexed under this heading.

Norfluoxetine (*In vitro* studies indicate that bupropion is primarily metabolized to hydroxybupropion by the CYP2B6 isoenzyme. Therefore, co-administration of bupropion with CYP2B6 substrates or inhibitors (eg, orphenadrine, thiotepa, and cyclophosphamide) may result in a drug interaction).
No products indexed under this heading.

Nortriptyline Hydrochloride (Concurrent administration of bupropion and agents that lower seizure threshold, such as antidepressants, should be undertaken with extreme caution. Low initial dosing and gradual dose increases should be employed. Co-administration of bupropion with drugs that are metabolized by the CYP2D6 isoenzyme including antidepressants (eg, nortriptyline) should be approached with caution and should be initiated at the lower end of the dose range of the concomitant medication. If bupropion is added to the treatment regimen of a patient already receiving a drug metabolized by CYP2D6, the need to decrease the dose of the original medication should be considered, particularly for those concomitant medications with a narrow therapeutic index).
No products indexed under this heading.

Olanzapine (Concurrent administration of bupropion and agents that lower seizure threshold, such as antipsychotics, should be undertaken with extreme caution. Low initial dosing and gradual dose increases should be employed. Co-administration of bupropion with drugs that are metabolized by the CYP2D6 isoenzyme including antipsychotics (eg, haloperidol, risperidone, thioridazine) should be approached with caution and should be initiated at the lower end of the dose range of the concomitant medication. If bupropion is added to the treatment regimen of a patient already receiving a drug metabolized by CYP2D6, the need to decrease the dose of the original medication should be considered, particularly for those concomitant medications with a narrow therapeutic index).
Products include:

Symbyax 1965
Zyprexa 1984
Zyprexa IntraMuscular 1984
Zyprexa ZYDIS 1984

Omeprazole (Co-administration of bupropion with drugs that are metabolized by the CYP2D6 isoenzyme should be approached with caution and should be initiated at the lower end of the dose range of the concomitant medication. If bupropion is added to the treatment regimen of a patient already receiving a drug metabolized by CYP2D6, the need to decrease the dose of the original medication should be considered, particularly for those concomitant medications with a narrow therapeutic index).
No products indexed under this heading.

Ondansetron (Co-administration of bupropion with drugs that are metabolized by the CYP2D6 isoenzyme should be approached with caution and should be initiated at the lower end of the dose range of the concomitant medication. If bupropion is added to the treatment regimen of a patient already receiving a drug metabolized by CYP2D6, the need to decrease the dose of the original medication should be considered, particularly for those concomitant medications with a narrow therapeutic index).
No products indexed under this heading.

Ondansetron Hydrochloride (Co-administration of bupropion with drugs that are metabolized by the CYP2D6 isoenzyme should be approached with caution and should be initiated at the lower end of the dose range of the concomitant medication. If bupropion is added to the treatment regimen of a patient already receiving a drug metabolized by CYP2D6, the need to decrease the dose of the original medication should be considered, particularly for those concomitant medications with a narrow therapeutic index).
Products include:

Zofran Injection 1750
Zofran 1756
Zofran ODT 1756

Orphenadrine Citrate (*In vitro* studies indicate that bupropion is primarily metabolized to hydroxybupropion by the CYP2B6 isoenzyme. Therefore, co-administration of bupropion with CYP2B6 substrates or inhibitors (eg, orphenadrine, thiotepa, and cyclophosphamide) may result in a drug interaction).
No products indexed under this heading.

Orphenadrine Hydrochloride (*In vitro* studies indicate that bupropion is primarily metabolized to hydroxybupropion by the CYP2B6 isoenzyme. Therefore, co-administration of bupropion with CYP2B6 substrates or inhibitors (eg, orphenadrine, thiotepa, and cyclophosphamide) may result in a drug interaction).
No products indexed under this heading.

Oxazepam (Bupropion is contraindicated in patients undergoing abrupt discontinuation of sedatives (including benzodiazepines). Patients should be told that the excessive use or abrupt discontinuation of sedatives (including benzodiazepines) may alter the seizure threshold).
No products indexed under this heading.

Oxycodone Hydrochloride (An addiction to opiates and concomitant use of bupropion has been associated with an increased seizure risk).
Products include:

OxyContin 2807
Percocet 1121
Percodan 1124

IMPORTANT NOTE: Always consult each drug listing in the patient's regimen for possible interactions.

Oxycodone Terephthalate (An addiction to opiates and concomitant use of bupropion has been associated with an increased seizure risk).

No products indexed under this heading.

Oxymorphone Hydrochloride (An addiction to opiates and concomitant use of bupropion has been associated with an increased seizure risk). Products include:

Opana 1110
Opana ER 1114

Paclitaxel (Co-administration of bupropion with drugs that are metabolized by the CYP2D6 isoenzyme should be approached with caution and should be initiated at the lower end of the dose range of the concomitant medication. If bupropion is added to the treatment regimen of a patient already receiving a drug metabolized by CYP2D6, the need to decrease the dose of the original medication should be considered, particularly for those concomitant medications with a narrow therapeutic index).

No products indexed under this heading.

Paliperidone (Concurrent administration of bupropion and agents that lower seizure threshold, such as antipsychotics, should be undertaken with extreme caution. Low initial dosing and gradual dose increases should be employed. Co-administration of bupropion with drugs that are metabolized by the CYP2D6 isoenzyme including antipsychotics (eg, haloperidol, risperidone, thioridazine) should be approached with caution and should be initiated at the lower end of the dose range of the concomitant medication. If bupropion is added to the treatment regimen of a patient already receiving a drug metabolized by CYP2D6, the need to decrease the dose of the original medication should be considered, particularly for those concomitant medications with a narrow therapeutic index). Products include:

Invega 2613
Invega Sustenna 2621

Pargyline Hydrochloride (Concurrent administration of bupropion and a monoamine oxidase (MAO) inhibitor is contraindicated. At least 14 days should elapse between discontinuation of a MAO inhibitor and initiation of treatment with bupropion).

No products indexed under this heading.

Paroxetine (Concurrent administration of bupropion and agents that lower seizure threshold (eg, antidepressants) should be approached with caution. Co-administration of bupropion with drugs that are metabolized by CYP2D6 isoenzyme including certain antidepressants (eg, paroxetine) should be approached with caution and should be initiated at the lower end of the dose range of the concomitant medication. If bupropion is added to the treatment regimen of a patient already receiving a drug metabolized by CYP2D6, the need to decrease the dose of the original medication should be considered, particularly for those concomitant medications with a narrow therapeutic index).

No products indexed under this heading.

Paroxetine Hydrochloride (Concurrent administration of bupropion and agents that lower seizure threshold (eg, antidepressants) should be approached with caution. Co-administration of bupropion with drugs that are metabolized by CYP2D6 isoenzyme including certain antidepressants (eg, paroxetine) should be approached with caution and should be initiated at the lower end of the dose range of the concomitant medication. If bupropion is added to the treatment regimen of a patient already receiving a drug metabolized by CYP2D6, the need to decrease the dose of the original medication should be considered, par-

ticularly for those concomitant medications with a narrow therapeutic index). Products include:

Paroxetine CR 2361
Paroxetine ER 2371
Paxil 1586
Paxil CR 1596

Paroxetine Mesylate (Concurrent administration of bupropion and agents that lower seizure threshold (eg, antidepressants) should be approached with caution. Co-administration of bupropion with drugs that are metabolized by CYP2D6 isoenzyme including certain antidepressants (eg, paroxetine) should be approached with caution and should be initiated at the lower end of the dose range of the concomitant medication. If bupropion is added to the treatment regimen of a patient already receiving a drug metabolized by CYP2D6, the need to decrease the dose of the original medication should be considered, particularly for those concomitant medications with a narrow therapeutic index).

No products indexed under this heading.

Pemoline (Concomitant use of over-the-counter stimulants with bupropion is associated with an increased seizure risk).

No products indexed under this heading.

Penbutolol Sulfate (Co-administration of bupropion with drugs that are metabolized by the CYP2D6 isoenzyme, including β-blockers (eg, metoprolol) should be approached with caution and should be initiated at the lower end of the dose range of the concomitant medication. If bupropion is added to the treatment regimen of a patient already receiving a drug metabolized by CYP2D6, the need to decrease the dose of the original medication should be considered, particularly for those concomitant medications with a narrow therapeutic index).

No products indexed under this heading.

Perphenazine (Concurrent administration of bupropion and agents that lower seizure threshold, such as antipsychotics, should be undertaken with extreme caution. Low initial dosing and gradual dose increases should be employed. Co-administration of bupropion with drugs that are metabolized by the CYP2D6 isoenzyme including antipsychotics (eg, haloperidol, risperidone, thioridazine) should be approached with caution and should be initiated at the lower end of the dose range of the concomitant medication. If bupropion is added to the treatment regimen of a patient already receiving a drug metabolized by CYP2D6, the need to decrease the dose of the original medication should be considered, particularly for those concomitant medications with a narrow therapeutic index).

No products indexed under this heading.

Phendimetrazine Tartrate (Concomitant use of anorectics with bupropion is associated with an increased seizure risk).

No products indexed under this heading.

Phenelzine Sulfate (Concurrent administration of bupropion and a monoamine oxidase (MAO) inhibitor is contraindicated. At least 14 days should elapse between discontinuation of a MAO inhibitor and initiation of treatment with bupropion).

No products indexed under this heading.

Phenmetrazine Hydrochloride (Concomitant use of anorectics with bupropion is associated with an increased seizure risk).

No products indexed under this heading.

Phenobarbital (While not systematically studied, certain drugs may induce the metabolism of bupropion (eg, phenobarbital)). Products include:

Donnatal 2711

Phenobarbital Sodium (While not systematically studied, certain drugs may induce the metabolism of bupropion (eg, phenobarbital)).

No products indexed under this heading.

Phenytoin (While not systematically studied, certain drugs may induce the metabolism of bupropion (eg, phenytoin)).

No products indexed under this heading.

Phenytoin Sodium (While not systematically studied, certain drugs may induce the metabolism of bupropion (eg, phenytoin)). Products include:

Phenytek Capsules 2380

Pimozide (Concurrent administration of bupropion and agents that lower seizure threshold, such as antipsychotics, should be undertaken with extreme caution. Low initial dosing and gradual dose increases should be employed. Co-administration of bupropion with drugs that are metabolized by the CYP2D6 isoenzyme including antipsychotics (eg, haloperidol, risperidone, thioridazine) should be approached with caution and should be initiated at the lower end of the dose range of the concomitant medication. If bupropion is added to the treatment regimen of a patient already receiving a drug metabolized by CYP2D6, the need to decrease the dose of the original medication should be considered, particularly for those concomitant medications with a narrow therapeutic index).

No products indexed under this heading.

Pindolol (Co-administration of bupropion with drugs that are metabolized by the CYP2D6 isoenzyme, including β-blockers (eg, metoprolol) should be approached with caution and should be initiated at the lower end of the dose range of the concomitant medication. If bupropion is added to the treatment regimen of a patient already receiving a drug metabolized by CYP2D6, the need to decrease the dose of the original medication should be considered, particularly for those concomitant medications with a narrow therapeutic index).

No products indexed under this heading.

Pioglitazone Hydrochloride (Concomitant use of oral hypoglycemics with bupropion is associated with an increased seizure risk). Products include:

ActoPlus 3338
Actos 3345
Duetact 3354

Polyestradiol Phosphate (*In vitro* studies indicate that bupropion is primarily metabolized to hydroxybupropion by the CYP2B6 isoenzyme. Therefore, co-administration of bupropion with CYP2B6 substrates or inhibitors (eg, orphenadrine, thiotepa, and cyclophosphamide) may result in a drug interaction).

No products indexed under this heading.

Prazepam (Bupropion is contraindicated in patients undergoing abrupt discontinuation of sedatives (including benzodiazepines). Patients should be told that the excessive use or abrupt discontinuation of sedatives (including benzodiazepines) may alter the seizure threshold).

No products indexed under this heading.

Prednisolone (Concurrent administration of bupropion and agents that lower seizure threshold, such as systemic steroids, should be undertaken with extreme caution. Low initial dosing and gradual dose increases should be employed).

No products indexed under this heading.

Prednisolone Acetate (Concurrent administration of bupropion and agents that lower seizure threshold, such as systemic steroids, should be undertak-

en with extreme caution. Low initial dosing and gradual dose increases should be employed). Products include:

Blephamide .... ⊙212, ⊙214
Pred Forte .... ⊙225
Pred Mild .... ⊙230
Pred-G .... ⊙226, ⊙227

Prednisolone Sodium Phosphate (Concurrent administration of bupropion and agents that lower seizure threshold, such as systemic steroids, should be undertaken with extreme caution. Low initial dosing and gradual dose increases should be employed).

No products indexed under this heading.

Prednisolone Tebutate (Concurrent administration of bupropion and agents that lower seizure threshold, such as systemic steroids, should be undertaken with extreme caution. Low initial dosing and gradual dose increases should be employed).

No products indexed under this heading.

Prednisone (Concurrent administration of bupropion and agents that lower seizure threshold, such as systemic steroids, should be undertaken with extreme caution. Low initial dosing and gradual dose increases should be employed).

No products indexed under this heading.

Prednisone sodium phosphate (Concurrent administration of bupropion and agents that lower seizure threshold, such as systemic steroids, should be undertaken with extreme caution. Low initial dosing and gradual dose increases should be employed).

No products indexed under this heading.

Procainamide Hydrochloride (Co-administration of bupropion with drugs that are metabolized by the CYP2D6 isoenzyme, including antiarrhythmics should be approached with caution and should be initiated at the lower end of the dose range of the concomitant medication. If bupropion is added to the treatment regimen of a patient already receiving a drug metabolized by CYP2D6, the need to decrease the dose of the original medication should be considered, particularly for those concomitant medications with a narrow therapeutic index).

No products indexed under this heading.

Procarbazine Hydrochloride (Concurrent administration of bupropion and a monoamine oxidase (MAO) inhibitor is contraindicated. At least 14 days should elapse between discontinuation of a MAO inhibitor and initiation of treatment with bupropion).

No products indexed under this heading.

Prochlorperazine (Concurrent administration of bupropion and agents that lower seizure threshold, such as antipsychotics, should be undertaken with extreme caution. Low initial dosing and gradual dose increases should be employed. Co-administration of bupropion with drugs that are metabolized by the CYP2D6 isoenzyme including antipsychotics (eg, haloperidol, risperidone, thioridazine) should be approached with caution and should be initiated at the lower end of the dose range of the concomitant medication. If bupropion is added to the treatment regimen of a patient already receiving a drug metabolized by CYP2D6, the need to decrease the dose of the original medication should be considered, particularly for those concomitant medications with a narrow therapeutic index).

No products indexed under this heading.

Promethazine (*In vitro* studies indicate that bupropion is primarily metabolized to hydroxybupropion by the CYP2B6 isoenzyme. Therefore, co-administration of bupropion with CYP2B6 substrates or inhibitors (eg, orphenadrine, thiotepa, and cyclophosphamide) may result in a drug interaction).

No products indexed under this heading.

Promethazine Hydrochloride (Concurrent administration of bupropion and agents that lower seizure threshold should be undertaken with extreme caution. Low initial dosing and gradual dose increases should be employed).

No products indexed under this heading.

Propafenone Hydrochloride (Co-administration of bupropion with drugs that are metabolized by the CYP2D6 isoenzyme including Type 1C antiarrhythmics (eg, propafenone) should be approached with caution and should be initiated at the lower end of the dose range of the concomitant medication. If bupropion is added to the treatment regimen of a patient already receiving a drug metabolized by CYP2D6, the need to decrease the dose of the original medication should be considered, particularly for those concomitant medications with a narrow therapeutic index). Products include:

Rythmol 1648
Rythmol SR 1652

Propofol (Bupropion is contraindicated in patients undergoing abrupt discontinuation of sedatives (including benzodiazepines). Patients should be told that the excessive use or abrupt discontinuation of sedatives (including benzodiazepines) may alter the seizure threshold).

No products indexed under this heading.

Propoxyphene Hydrochloride (An addiction to opiates and concomitant use of bupropion has been associated with an increased seizure risk).

No products indexed under this heading.

Propoxyphene Napsylate (An addiction to opiates and concomitant use of bupropion has been associated with an increased seizure risk).

No products indexed under this heading.

Propranolol Hydrochloride (Co-administration of bupropion with drugs that are metabolized by the CYP2D6 isoenzyme, including β-blockers (eg, metoprolol) should be approached with caution and should be initiated at the lower end of the dose range of the concomitant medication. If bupropion is added to the treatment regimen of a patient already receiving a drug metabolized by CYP2D6, the need to decrease the dose of the original medication should be considered, particularly for those concomitant medications with a narrow therapeutic index). Products include:

InnoPran XL 1517

Protriptyline Hydrochloride (Concurrent administration of bupropion and agents (eg, other antidepressants) that lower seizure threshold should be undertaken only with extreme caution. Low initial dosing and small gradual dose increases should be employed. In addition, many drugs, including most antidepressants (many tricyclics), are metabolized by the CYP2D6 isoenzyme. Co-administration of bupropion with drugs that are metabolized by CYP2D6 isoenzyme should be approached with caution and should be initiated at the lower end of the dose range of the concomitant medication. If bupropion is added to the treatment regimen of a patient already receiving a drug metabolized by CYP2D6, the need to decrease the dose of the original medi-

cation should be considered, particularly for those concomitant medications with a narrow therapeutic index).

No products indexed under this heading.

Quazepam (Bupropion is contraindicated in patients undergoing abrupt discontinuation of sedatives (including benzodiazepines). Patients should be told that the excessive use or abrupt discontinuation of sedatives (including benzodiazepines) may alter the seizure threshold).

No products indexed under this heading.

Quetiapine Fumarate (Concurrent administration of bupropion and agents that lower seizure threshold, such as antipsychotics, should be undertaken with extreme caution. Low initial dosing and gradual dose increases should be employed. Co-administration of bupropion with drugs that are metabolized by the CYP2D6 isoenzyme including antipsychotics (eg, haloperidol, risperidone, thioridazine) should be approached with caution and should be initiated at the lower end of the dose range of the concomitant medication. If bupropion is added to the treatment regimen of a patient already receiving a drug metabolized by CYP2D6, the need to decrease the dose of the original medication should be considered, particularly for those concomitant medications with a narrow therapeutic index). Products include:

Seroquel 750
Seroquel XR 759

Quinidine Gluconate (Co-administration of bupropion with drugs that are metabolized by the CYP2D6 isoenzyme should be approached with caution and should be initiated at the lower end of the dose range of the concomitant medication. If bupropion is added to the treatment regimen of a patient already receiving a drug metabolized by CYP2D6, the need to decrease the dose of the original medication should be considered, particularly for those concomitant medications with a narrow therapeutic index).

No products indexed under this heading.

Quinidine Hydrochloride (Co-administration of bupropion with drugs that are metabolized by the CYP2D6 isoenzyme should be approached with caution and should be initiated at the lower end of the dose range of the concomitant medication. If bupropion is added to the treatment regimen of a patient already receiving a drug metabolized by CYP2D6, the need to decrease the dose of the original medication should be considered, particularly for those concomitant medications with a narrow therapeutic index).

No products indexed under this heading.

Quinidine Polygalacturonate (Co-administration of bupropion with drugs that are metabolized by the CYP2D6 isoenzyme should be approached with caution and should be initiated at the lower end of the dose range of the concomitant medication. If bupropion is added to the treatment regimen of a patient already receiving a drug metabolized by CYP2D6, the need to decrease the dose of the original medication should be considered, particularly for those concomitant medications with a narrow therapeutic index).

No products indexed under this heading.

Quinidine Sulfate (Co-administration of bupropion with drugs that are metabolized by the CYP2D6 isoenzyme should be approached with caution and should be initiated at the lower end of the dose range of the concomitant medication. If bupropion is added to the treatment regimen of a patient already receiving a drug metabolized by CYP2D6, the need to decrease the dose of the original medication should

be considered, particularly for those concomitant medications with a narrow therapeutic index).

No products indexed under this heading.

Ramelteon (Bupropion is contraindicated in patients undergoing abrupt discontinuation of sedatives (including benzodiazepines). Patients should be told that the excessive use or abrupt discontinuation of sedatives (including benzodiazepines) may alter the seizure threshold). Products include:

Rozerem 3366

Rasagiline Mesylate (Concurrent administration of bupropion and a monoamine oxidase (MAO) inhibitor is contraindicated. At least 14 days should elapse between discontinuation of a MAO inhibitor and initiation of treatment with bupropion). Products include:

Azilect 3383

Remifentanil Hydrochloride (An addiction to opiates and concomitant use of bupropion has been associated with an increased seizure risk).

No products indexed under this heading.

Repaglinide (Concomitant use of oral hypoglycemics with bupropion is associated with an increased seizure risk).

No products indexed under this heading.

Risperidone (Concurrent administration of bupropion and agents that lower seizure threshold, such as antipsychotics, should be undertaken with extreme caution. Low initial dosing and gradual dose increases should be employed. Co-administration of bupropion with drugs that are metabolized by the CYP2D6 isoenzyme including antipsychotics (eg, risperidone) should be approached with caution and should be initiated at the lower end of the dose range of the concomitant medication. If bupropion is added to the treatment regimen of a patient already receiving a drug metabolized by CYP2D6, the need to decrease the dose of the original medication should be considered, particularly for those concomitant medications with a narrow therapeutic index). Products include:

Risperdal Consta 2682

Ritonavir (*In vitro* studies suggest that ritonavir inhibits the hydroxylation of bupropion). Products include:

Kaletra 458
Norvir 509

Ropivacaine Hydrochloride (*In vitro* studies indicate that bupropion is primarily metabolized to hydroxybupropion by the CYP2B6 isoenzyme. Therefore, co-administration of bupropion with CYP2B6 substrates or inhibitors (eg, orphenadrine, thiotepa, and cyclophosphamide) may result in a drug interaction).

No products indexed under this heading.

Rosiglitazone Maleate (Concomitant use of oral hypoglycemics with bupropion is associated with an increased seizure risk). Products include:

Avandamet 1345
Avandaryl 1356
Avandia 1366

Secobarbital Sodium (Bupropion is contraindicated in patients undergoing abrupt discontinuation of sedatives (including benzodiazepines). Patients should be told that the excessive use or abrupt discontinuation of sedatives (including benzodiazepines) may alter the seizure threshold).

No products indexed under this heading.

Selegiline (Concurrent administration of bupropion and a monoamine oxidase (MAO) inhibitor is contraindicated. At least 14 days should elapse between discontinuation of a MAO inhibitor and initiation of treatment with bupropion). Products include:

Emsam 3623

Selegiline Hydrochloride (Concurrent administration of bupropion and a monoamine oxidase (MAO) inhibitor is contraindicated. At least 14 days should elapse between discontinuation of a MAO inhibitor and initiation of treatment with bupropion). Products include:

Eldepryl 3312

Sertraline Hydrochloride (Concurrent administration of bupropion and agents that lower seizure threshold (eg, antidepressants) should be approached with caution. Co-administration of bupropion with drugs that are metabolized by CYP2D6 isoenzyme including certain antidepressants (eg, sertraline) should be approached with caution and should be initiated at the lower end of the dose range of the concomitant medication. If bupropion is added to the treatment regimen of a patient already receiving a drug metabolized by CYP2D6, the need to decrease the dose of the original medication should be considered, particularly for those concomitant medications with a narrow therapeutic index).

No products indexed under this heading.

Sevoflurane (*In vitro* studies indicate that bupropion is primarily metabolized to hydroxybupropion by the CYP2B6 isoenzyme. Therefore, co-administration of bupropion with CYP2B6 substrates or inhibitors (eg, orphenadrine, thiotepa, and cyclophosphamide) may result in a drug interaction). Products include:

Ultane 554

Sibutramine Hydrochloride Monohydrate (Concomitant use of anorectics with bupropion is associated with an increased seizure risk). Products include:

Meridia 492

Sitagliptin Phosphate (Concomitant use of oral hypoglycemics with bupropion is associated with an increased seizure risk). Products include:

Janumet 2188
Januvia 2196

Sodium Butabarbital (Bupropion is contraindicated in patients undergoing abrupt discontinuation of sedatives (including benzodiazepines). Patients should be told that the excessive use or abrupt discontinuation of sedatives (including benzodiazepines) may alter the seizure threshold).

No products indexed under this heading.

Sotalol Hydrochloride (Co-administration of bupropion with drugs that are metabolized by the CYP2D6 isoenzyme, including β-blockers (eg, metoprolol) should be approached with caution and should be initiated at the lower end of the dose range of the concomitant medication. If bupropion is added to the treatment regimen of a patient already receiving a drug metabolized by CYP2D6, the need to decrease the dose of the original medication should be considered, particularly for those concomitant medications with a narrow therapeutic index).

No products indexed under this heading.

Sufentanil Citrate (An addiction to opiates and concomitant use of bupropion has been associated with an increased seizure risk).

No products indexed under this heading.

Tamoxifen Citrate (Co-administration of bupropion with drugs that are metabolized by the CYP2D6 isoenzyme should be approached with caution and should be initiated at the lower end of the dose range of the concomitant medication. If bupropion is added to the treatment regimen of a patient already receiving a drug metabolized by CYP2D6, the need to decrease the dose of the original medication should be considered, particularly for those concomitant medications with a narrow therapeutic index).

No products indexed under this heading.

IMPORTANT NOTE: Always consult each drug listing in the patient's regimen for possible interactions.

Wellbutrin Interactions Index 2102

Temazepam (Bupropion is contraindicated in patients undergoing abrupt discontinuation of sedatives (including benzodiazepines). Patients should be told that the excessive use or abrupt discontinuation of sedatives (including benzodiazepines) may alter the seizure threshold).
No products indexed under this heading.

Teniposide (Co-administration of bupropion with drugs that are metabolized by the CYP2D6 isoenzyme should be approached with caution and should be initiated at the lower end of the dose range of the concomitant medication. If bupropion is added to the treatment regimen of a patient already receiving a drug metabolized by CYP2D6, the need to decrease the dose of the original medication should be considered, particularly for those concomitant medications with a narrow therapeutic index).
No products indexed under this heading.

Testosterone (Co-administration of bupropion with drugs that are metabolized by the CYP2D6 isoenzyme should be approached with caution and should be initiated at the lower end of the dose range of the concomitant medication. If bupropion is added to the treatment regimen of a patient already receiving a drug metabolized by CYP2D6, the need to decrease the dose of the original medication should be considered, particularly for those concomitant medications with a narrow therapeutic index). Products include:
AndroGel 3456

Testosterone Cypionate (Co-administration of bupropion with drugs that are metabolized by the CYP2D6 isoenzyme should be approached with caution and should be initiated at the lower end of the dose range of the concomitant medication. If bupropion is added to the treatment regimen of a patient already receiving a drug metabolized by CYP2D6, the need to decrease the dose of the original medication should be considered, particularly for those concomitant medications with a narrow therapeutic index).
No products indexed under this heading.

Testosterone Enanthate (Co-administration of bupropion with drugs that are metabolized by the CYP2D6 isoenzyme should be approached with caution and should be initiated at the lower end of the dose range of the concomitant medication. If bupropion is added to the treatment regimen of a patient already receiving a drug metabolized by CYP2D6, the need to decrease the dose of the original medication should be considered, particularly for those concomitant medications with a narrow therapeutic index). Products include:
Delatestryl 1102

Testosterone Propionate (Co-administration of bupropion with drugs that are metabolized by the CYP2D6 isoenzyme should be approached with caution and should be initiated at the lower end of the dose range of the concomitant medication. If bupropion is added to the treatment regimen of a patient already receiving a drug metabolized by CYP2D6, the need to decrease the dose of the original medication should be considered, particularly for those concomitant medications with a narrow therapeutic index).
No products indexed under this heading.

Theophylline (Concurrent administration of bupropion and agents that lower seizure threshold, such as theophylline, should be undertaken with extreme caution. Low initial dosing and gradual dose increases should be employed).
No products indexed under this heading.

Theophylline Anhydrous (Concurrent administration of bupropion and agents that lower seizure threshold, such as theophylline, should be undertaken with extreme caution. Low initial dosing and gradual dose increases should be employed). Products include:
Uniphyl 2817

Theophylline Calcium Salicylate (Concurrent administration of bupropion and agents that lower seizure threshold, such as theophylline, should be undertaken with extreme caution. Low initial dosing and gradual dose increases should be employed).
No products indexed under this heading.

Theophylline Dihydroxypropyl (Glyceryl) (Concurrent administration of bupropion and agents that lower seizure threshold, such as theophylline, should be undertaken with extreme caution. Low initial dosing and gradual dose increases should be employed).
No products indexed under this heading.

Theophylline Ethylenediamine (Concurrent administration of bupropion and agents that lower seizure threshold, such as theophylline, should be undertaken with extreme caution. Low initial dosing and gradual dose increases should be employed).
No products indexed under this heading.

Theophylline Sodium Glycinate (Concurrent administration of bupropion and agents that lower seizure threshold, such as theophylline, should be undertaken with extreme caution. Low initial dosing and gradual dose increases should be employed).
No products indexed under this heading.

Thioridazine (Concurrent administration of bupropion and agents that lower seizure threshold, such as antipsychotics, should be undertaken with extreme caution. Low initial dosing and gradual dose increases should be employed. Co-administration of bupropion with drugs that are metabolized by the CYP2D6 isoenzyme including antipsychotics (eg, thioridazine) should be approached with caution and should be initiated at the lower end of the dose range of the concomitant medication. If bupropion is added to the treatment regimen of a patient already receiving a drug metabolized by CYP2D6, the need to decrease the dose of the original medication should be considered, particularly for those concomitant medications with a narrow therapeutic index).
No products indexed under this heading.

Thioridazine Hydrochloride (Concurrent administration of bupropion and agents that lower seizure threshold, such as antipsychotics, should be undertaken with extreme caution. Low initial dosing and gradual dose increases should be employed. Co-administration of bupropion with drugs that are metabolized by the CYP2D6 isoenzyme including antipsychotics (eg, thioridazine) should be approached with caution and should be initiated at the lower end of the dose range of the concomitant medication. If bupropion is added to the treatment regimen of a patient already receiving a drug metabolized by CYP2D6, the need to decrease the dose of the original medication should be considered, particularly for those concomitant medications with a narrow therapeutic index). Products include:
Thioridazine Hydrochloride 2384

Thiotepa (*In vitro* studies indicate that bupropion is primarily metabolized to hydroxybupropion by the CYP2B6 isoenzyme. Therefore, co-administration of bupropion with CYP2B6 substrates or inhibitors (eg, orphenadrine, thiotepa, and cyclophosphamide) may result in a drug interaction).
No products indexed under this heading.

Thiothixene (Concurrent administration of bupropion and agents that lower seizure threshold, such as antipsychotics, should be undertaken with extreme caution. Low initial dosing and gradual dose increases should be employed. Co-administration of bupropion with drugs that are metabolized by the CYP2D6 isoenzyme including antipsychotics (eg, haloperidol, risperidone, thioridazine) should be approached with caution and should be initiated at the lower end of the dose range of the concomitant medication. If bupropion is added to the treatment regimen of a patient already receiving a drug metabolized by CYP2D6, the need to decrease the dose of the original medication should be considered, particularly for those concomitant medications with a narrow therapeutic index). Products include:
Thiothixene 2386

Timolol Hemihydrate (Co-administration of bupropion with drugs that are metabolized by the CYP2D6 isoenzyme, including β-blockers (eg, metoprolol) should be approached with caution and should be initiated at the lower end of the dose range of the concomitant medication. If bupropion is added to the treatment regimen of a patient already receiving a drug metabolized by CYP2D6, the need to decrease the dose of the original medication should be considered, particularly for those concomitant medications with a narrow therapeutic index). Products include:
Betimol 3490

Timolol Maleate (Co-administration of bupropion with drugs that are metabolized by the CYP2D6 isoenzyme, including β-blockers (eg, metoprolol) should be approached with caution and should be initiated at the lower end of the dose range of the concomitant medication. If bupropion is added to the treatment regimen of a patient already receiving a drug metabolized by CYP2D6, the need to decrease the dose of the original medication should be considered, particularly for those concomitant medications with a narrow therapeutic index). Products include:
Combigan 601
Dorzolamide Hydrochloride/Timolol Maleate Ophthalmic Solution .... ⊙243
Timoptic in Ocudose .... ⊙231

Tocainide Hydrochloride (Co-administration of bupropion with drugs that are metabolized by the CYP2D6 isoenzyme, including antiarrhythmics should be approached with caution and should be initiated at the lower end of the dose range of the concomitant medication. If bupropion is added to the treatment regimen of a patient already receiving a drug metabolized by CYP2D6, the need to decrease the dose of the original medication should be considered, particularly for those concomitant medications with a narrow therapeutic index).
No products indexed under this heading.

Tolazamide (Concomitant use of oral hypoglycemics with bupropion is associated with an increased seizure risk).
No products indexed under this heading.

Tolbutamide (Concomitant use of oral hypoglycemics with bupropion is associated with an increased seizure risk).
No products indexed under this heading.

Tolterodine Tartrate (Co-administration of bupropion with drugs that are metabolized by the CYP2D6 isoenzyme should be approached with caution and should be initiated at the lower end of the dose range of the concomitant medication. If bupropion is added to the treatment regimen of a patient already receiving a drug metabolized by CYP2D6, the need to decrease the dose of the original medication should be considered, particularly for those concomitant medications with a narrow therapeutic index).
No products indexed under this heading.

Tramadol Hydrochloride (Co-administration of bupropion with drugs that are metabolized by the CYP2D6 isoenzyme should be approached with caution and should be initiated at the lower end of the dose range of the concomitant medication. If bupropion is added to the treatment regimen of a patient already receiving a drug metabolized by CYP2D6, the need to decrease the dose of the original medication should be considered, particularly for those concomitant medications with a narrow therapeutic index). Products include:
Ryzolt 2813
Ultram ER 2693

Tranylcypromine Sulfate (Concurrent administration of bupropion and a monoamine oxidase (MAO) inhibitor is contraindicated. At least 14 days should elapse between discontinuation of a MAO inhibitor and initiation of treatment with bupropion). Products include:
Parnate 1584

Trazodone Hydrochloride (Concurrent administration of bupropion and agents that lower seizure threshold, such as antidepressants, should be undertaken with extreme caution. Low initial dosing and gradual dose increases should be employed. Co-administration of bupropion with drugs that are metabolized by the CYP2D6 isoenzyme including antidepressants (eg, nortriptyline, imipramine, desipramine, paroxetine, fluoxetine, sertraline) should be approached with caution and should be initiated at the lower end of the dose range of the concomitant medication. If bupropion is added to the treatment regimen of a patient already receiving a drug metabolized by CYP2D6, the need to decrease the dose of the original medication should be considered, particularly for those concomitant medications with a narrow therapeutic index).
No products indexed under this heading.

Tretinoin (*In vitro* studies indicate that bupropion is primarily metabolized to hydroxybupropion by the CYP2B6 isoenzyme. Therefore, co-administration of bupropion with CYP2B6 substrates or inhibitors (eg, orphenadrine, thiotepa, and cyclophosphamide) may result in a drug interaction).
No products indexed under this heading.

Triamcinolone (Concurrent administration of bupropion and agents that lower seizure threshold, such as systemic steroids, should be undertaken with extreme caution. Low initial dosing and gradual dose increases should be employed).
No products indexed under this heading.

Triamcinolone Acetonide (Concurrent administration of bupropion and agents that lower seizure threshold, such as systemic steroids, should be undertaken with extreme caution. Low initial dosing and gradual dose increases should be employed). Products include:
Azmacort 408
Nasacort AQ 3019

Triamcinolone Diacetate (Concurrent administration of bupropion and agents that lower seizure threshold, such as systemic steroids, should be undertaken with extreme caution. Low initial dosing and gradual dose increases should be employed).
No products indexed under this heading.

(⊙ Described in PDR® for Ophthalmic Medicines)

Triamcinolone Hexacetonide (Concurrent administration of bupropion and agents that lower seizure threshold, such as systemic steroids, should be undertaken with extreme caution. Low initial dosing and gradual dose increases should be employed).
No products indexed under this heading.

Triazolam (Bupropion is contraindicated in patients undergoing abrupt discontinuation of sedatives (including benzodiazepines). Patients should be told that the excessive use or abrupt discontinuation of sedatives (including benzodiazepines) may alter the seizure threshold).
No products indexed under this heading.

Trifluoperazine Hydrochloride (Concurrent administration of bupropion and agents that lower seizure threshold, such as antipsychotics, should be undertaken with extreme caution. Low initial dosing and gradual dose increases should be employed. Co-administration of bupropion with drugs that are metabolized by the CYP2D6 isoenzyme including antipsychotics (eg, haloperidol, risperidone, thioridazine) should be approached with caution and should be initiated at the lower end of the dose range of the concomitant medication. If bupropion is added to the treatment regimen of a patient already receiving a drug metabolized by CYP2D6, the need to decrease the dose of the original medication should be considered, particularly for those concomitant medications with a narrow therapeutic index).
No products indexed under this heading.

Trimipramine Maleate (Concurrent administration of bupropion and agents (eg, other antidepressants) that lower seizure threshold should be undertaken only with extreme caution. Low initial dosing and small gradual dose increases should be employed. In addition, many drugs, including most antidepressants (many tricyclics), are metabolized by the CYP2D6 isoenzyme. Co-administration of bupropion with drugs that are metabolized by CYP2D6 isoenzyme should be approached with caution and should be initiated at the lower end of the dose range of the concomitant medication. If bupropion is added to the treatment regimen of a patient already receiving a drug metabolized by CYP2D6, the need to decrease the dose of the original medication should be considered, particularly for those concomitant medications with a narrow therapeutic index).
No products indexed under this heading.

Troglitazone (Concomitant use of oral hypoglycemics with bupropion is associated with an increased seizure risk).
No products indexed under this heading.

Valproate Sodium (In vitro studies indicate that bupropion is primarily metabolized to hydroxybupropion by the CYP2B6 isoenzyme. Therefore, co-administration of bupropion with CYP2B6 substrates or inhibitors (eg, orphenadrine, thiotepa, and cyclophosphamide) may result in a drug interaction).
No products indexed under this heading.

Valproic Acid (In vitro studies indicate that bupropion is primarily metabolized to hydroxybupropion by the CYP2B6 isoenzyme. Therefore, co-administration of bupropion with CYP2B6 substrates or inhibitors (eg, orphenadrine, thiotepa, and cyclophosphamide) may result in a drug interaction).
No products indexed under this heading.

Venlafaxine Hydrochloride (Concurrent administration of bupropion and agents that lower seizure threshold, such as antidepressants, should be undertaken with extreme caution. Low

initial dosing and gradual dose increases should be employed. Co-administration of bupropion with drugs that are metabolized by the CYP2D6 isoenzyme including antidepressants (eg, nortriptyline, imipramine, desipramine, paroxentine, fluoxetine, sertraline) should be approached with caution and should be initiated at the lower end of the dose range of the concomitant medication. If bupropion is added to the treatment regimen of a patient already receiving a drug metabolized by CYP2D6, the need to decrease the dose of the original medication should be considered, particularly for those concomitant medications with a narrow therapeutic index). Products include:
Effexor XR **3504**
Venlafaxine Hydrochloride Tablets ... **2388**

Verapamil Hydrochloride (In vitro studies indicate that bupropion is primarily metabolized to hydroxybupropion by the CYP2B6 isoenzyme. Therefore, co-administration of bupropion with CYP2B6 substrates or inhibitors (eg, orphenadrine, thiotepa, and cyclophosphamide) may result in a drug interaction). Products include:
Tarka **534**

Vinblastine Sulfate (Co-administration of bupropion with drugs that are metabolized by the CYP2D6 isoenzyme should be approached with caution and should be initiated at the lower end of the dose range of the concomitant medication. If bupropion is added to the treatment regimen of a patient already receiving a drug metabolized by CYP2D6, the need to decrease the dose of the original medication should be considered, particularly for those concomitant medications with a narrow therapeutic index).
No products indexed under this heading.

Warfarin Sodium (Altered PT and/or INR, infrequently associated with hemorrhagic or thrombotic complications, were observed when bupropion was co-administered with warfarin).
No products indexed under this heading.

Zaleplon (Bupropion is contraindicated in patients undergoing abrupt discontinuation of sedatives (including benzodiazepines). Patients should be told that the excessive use or abrupt discontinuation of sedatives (including benzodiazepines) may alter the seizure threshold).
No products indexed under this heading.

Ziprasidone Hydrochloride (Concurrent administration of bupropion and agents that lower seizure threshold, such as antipsychotics, should be undertaken with extreme caution. Low initial dosing and gradual dose increases should be employed. Co-administration of bupropion with drugs that are metabolized by the CYP2D6 isoenzyme including antipsychotics (eg, haloperidol, risperidone, thioridazine) should be approached with caution and should be initiated at the lower end of the dose range of the concomitant medication. If bupropion is added to the treatment regimen of a patient already receiving a drug metabolized by CYP2D6, the need to decrease the dose of the original medication should be considered, particularly for those concomitant medications with a narrow therapeutic index). Products include:
Geodon **2723**

Zolpidem Tartrate (Bupropion is contraindicated in patients undergoing abrupt discontinuation of sedatives (including benzodiazepines). Patients should be told that the excessive use or abrupt discontinuation of sedatives (including benzodiazepines) may alter the seizure threshold). Products include:
Ambien **2920**
Ambien CR **2925**

Zonisamide (Co-administration of bupropion with drugs that are metabolized by the CYP2D6 isoenzyme should be approached with caution and should be initiated at the lower end of the dose range of the concomitant medication. If bupropion is added to the treatment regimen of a patient already receiving a drug metabolized by CYP2D6, the need to decrease the dose of the original medication should be considered, particularly for those concomitant medications with a narrow therapeutic index). Products include:
Zonegran **1081**

Food Interactions

Alcohol (Bupropion is contraindicated in patients undergoing abrupt discontinuation of alcohol. In post-marketing experience, there have been rare reports of adverse neuropsychiatric events or reduced alcohol tolerance in patients who were drinking during treatment with bupropion. The consumption of alcohol should be minimized or avoided).

Beer, reduced-alcohol (Bupropion is contraindicated in patients undergoing abrupt discontinuation of alcohol. In post-marketing experience, there have been rare reports of adverse neuropsychiatric events or reduced alcohol tolerance in patients who were drinking during treatment with bupropion. The consumption of alcohol should be minimized or avoided).

Beer, unspecified (Bupropion is contraindicated in patients undergoing abrupt discontinuation of alcohol. In post-marketing experience, there have been rare reports of adverse neuropsychiatric events or reduced alcohol tolerance in patients who were drinking during treatment with bupropion. The consumption of alcohol should be minimized or avoided).

Wine, Chianti (Bupropion is contraindicated in patients undergoing abrupt discontinuation of alcohol. In post-marketing experience, there have been rare reports of adverse neuropsychiatric events or reduced alcohol tolerance in patients who were drinking during treatment with bupropion. The consumption of alcohol should be minimized or avoided).

Wine, Red (Bupropion is contraindicated in patients undergoing abrupt discontinuation of alcohol. In post-marketing experience, there have been rare reports of adverse neuropsychiatric events or reduced alcohol tolerance in patients who were drinking during treatment with bupropion. The consumption of alcohol should be minimized or avoided).

Wine, unspecified (Bupropion is contraindicated in patients undergoing abrupt discontinuation of alcohol. In post-marketing experience, there have been rare reports of adverse neuropsychiatric events or reduced alcohol tolerance in patients who were drinking during treatment with bupropion. The consumption of alcohol should be minimized or avoided).

Wine products (Bupropion is contraindicated in patients undergoing abrupt discontinuation of alcohol. In post-marketing experience, there have been rare reports of adverse neuropsychiatric events or reduced alcohol tolerance in patients who were drinking during treatment with bupropion. The consumption of alcohol should be minimized or avoided).

WELLBUTRIN SR SUSTAINED-RELEASE TABLETS
(Bupropion Hydrochloride) **1725**
See Wellbutrin Tablets

WINRHO SDF
(Rho (D) Immune Globulin (Human)) **824**
May interact with vaccines, live. Compounds in these categories include:

BCG Vaccine (Other antibodies contained in WinRho SDF may interfere with the response to live virus vaccines such as measles, mumps, polio or rubella. Therefore, immunization with live vaccines should not be given within 3 months after WinRho SDF administration).
No products indexed under this heading.

Influenza Vaccine, Live Attenuated (Other antibodies contained in WinRho SDF may interfere with the response to live virus vaccines such as measles, mumps, polio or rubella. Therefore, immunization with live vaccines should not be given within 3 months after WinRho SDF administration).
No products indexed under this heading.

Influenza Virus Vaccine Live, Intranasal (Other antibodies contained in WinRho SDF may interfere with the response to live virus vaccines such as measles, mumps, polio or rubella. Therefore, immunization with live vaccines should not be given within 3 months after WinRho SDF administration). Products include:
FluMist **2078**

Measles, Mumps, Rubella and Varicella Virus Vaccine Live (Other antibodies contained in WinRho SDF may interfere with the response to live virus vaccines such as measles, mumps, polio or rubella. Therefore, immunization with live vaccines should not be given within 3 months after WinRho SDF administration). Products include:
ProQuad **2254**

Measles, Mumps & Rubella Virus Vaccine, Live (Other antibodies contained in WinRho SDF may interfere with the response to live virus vaccines such as measles, mumps, polio or rubella. Therefore, immunization with live vaccines should not be given within 3 months after WinRho SDF administration). Products include:
M-M-R II **2203**
ProQuad **2254**

Measles & Rubella Virus Vaccine Live (Other antibodies contained in WinRho SDF may interfere with the response to live virus vaccines such as measles, mumps, polio or rubella. Therefore, immunization with live vaccines should not be given within 3 months after WinRho SDF administration).
No products indexed under this heading.

Measles Virus Vaccine Live (Other antibodies contained in WinRho SDF may interfere with the response to live virus vaccines such as measles, mumps, polio or rubella. Therefore, immunization with live vaccines should not be given within 3 months after WinRho SDF administration). Products include:
Attenuvax **2086**

Mumps Virus Vaccine, Live (Other antibodies contained in WinRho SDF may interfere with the response to live virus vaccines such as measles, mumps, polio or rubella. Therefore, immunization with live vaccines should not be given within 3 months after WinRho SDF administration). Products include:
Mumpsvax **2218**

Poliovirus Vaccine, Live, Oral, Trivalent, Types 1,2,3 (Sabin) (Other antibodies contained in WinRho SDF may interfere with the response to live virus vaccines such as measles, mumps, polio or rubella. Therefore, immunization with live vaccines should not be given within 3 months after WinRho SDF administration).
No products indexed under this heading.

Rotavirus Vaccine, Live, Oral, Tetravalent (Other antibodies contained in WinRho SDF may interfere with the response to live virus vaccines such as measles, mumps, polio or rubella. Therefore, immunization with live vaccines should not be given within 3 months after WinRho SDF administration).
No products indexed under this heading.

Rubella & Mumps Virus Vaccine Live (Other antibodies contained in WinRho SDF may interfere with the response to live virus vaccines such as measles, mumps, polio or rubella. Therefore, immunization with live vaccines should not be given within 3 months after WinRho SDF administration).
No products indexed under this heading.

Rubella Virus Vaccine Live (Other antibodies contained in WinRho SDF may interfere with the response to live virus vaccines such as measles, mumps, polio or rubella. Therefore, immunization with live vaccines should not be given within 3 months after WinRho SDF administration). Products include:
Meruvax II 2210

Smallpox Vaccine (Other antibodies contained in WinRho SDF may interfere with the response to live virus vaccines such as measles, mumps, polio or rubella. Therefore, immunization with live vaccines should not be given within 3 months after WinRho SDF administration).
No products indexed under this heading.

Typhoid Vaccine (Other antibodies contained in WinRho SDF may interfere with the response to live virus vaccines such as measles, mumps, polio or rubella. Therefore, immunization with live vaccines should not be given within 3 months after WinRho SDF administration).
No products indexed under this heading.

Varicella Virus Vaccine, Live (Other antibodies contained in WinRho SDF may interfere with the response to live virus vaccines such as measles, mumps, polio or rubella. Therefore, immunization with live vaccines should not be given within 3 months after WinRho SDF administration). Products include:
Varivax 2285

Yellow Fever Vaccine (Other antibodies contained in WinRho SDF may interfere with the response to live virus vaccines such as measles, mumps, polio or rubella. Therefore, immunization with live vaccines should not be given within 3 months after WinRho SDF administration).
No products indexed under this heading.

Zoster Vaccine Live (Other antibodies contained in WinRho SDF may interfere with the response to live virus vaccines such as measles, mumps, polio or rubella. Therefore, immunization with live vaccines should not be given within 3 months after WinRho SDF administration). Products include:
Zostavax 2299

XALATAN OPHTHALMIC SOLUTION

(Latanoprost) .... ⊙261
None cited in PDR database.

XELODA TABLETS

(Capecitabine) 2882
May interact with oral anticoagulants, phenytoin, and certain other agents. Compounds in these categories include:

Aluminum Hydroxide (Co-administration of capecitabine with aluminum hydroxide- and magnesium hydroxide-containing antacids has resulted in a small increase in plasma concentrations of capecitabine and one metabolite (5'DFCR)).
No products indexed under this heading.

Anisindione (Co-administration has resulted in altered coagulation parameters and/or bleeding).
No products indexed under this heading.

Dicumarol (Co-administration has resulted in altered coagulation parameters and/or bleeding).
No products indexed under this heading.

Fosphenytoin (Co-administration has resulted in toxicity associated with elevated phenytoin levels).
No products indexed under this heading.

Fosphenytoin Sodium (Co-administration has resulted in toxicity associated with elevated phenytoin levels).
No products indexed under this heading.

Leucovorin Calcium (The concentrations of 5-fluorouracil, capecitabine is a prodrug and it is converted to 5-FU, is increased and its toxicity may be enhanced by leucovorin; deaths from severe enterocolitis, diarrhea, and dehydration have been reported in elderly patients receiving fluorouracil and leucovorin).
No products indexed under this heading.

Magnesium Hydroxide (Co-administration of capecitabine with aluminum hydroxide- and magnesium hydroxide-containing antacids has resulted in a small increase in plasma concentrations of capecitabine and one metabolite (5'DFCR)). Products include:
Fleet Pedia-Lax Chewable Tablets 1144
Pepcid Complete 1822

Phenytoin (Co-administration has resulted in toxicity associated with elevated phenytoin levels).
No products indexed under this heading.

Phenytoin Sodium (Co-administration has resulted in toxicity associated with elevated phenytoin levels). Products include:
Phenytek Capsules 2380

Warfarin Sodium (Co-administration has resulted in altered coagulation parameters and/or bleeding).
No products indexed under this heading.

Food Interactions

Food, unspecified (Reduces both rate and extent of absorption of capecitabine and delays T_{max} of both parent and 5-FU).

XENADERM OINTMENT

(Balsam Peru, Castor Oil, Trypsin) 1800
None cited in PDR database.

XENAZINE TABLETS

(Tetrabenazine) 2033
May interact with alcohols, antipsychotic agents, atypical antipsychotics, class 1A antiarrhythmics, class III antiarrhythmics, cytochrome p450 2d6 inhibitors (selected), dopamine antagonists, drugs that prolong the QT interval, haloperidols, hypnotics and sedatives, monoamine oxidase inhibitors, quinidine, selective serotonin reuptake inhibitors, serotonin and norepinephrine reuptake inhibitors, and certain other agents. Compounds in these categories include:

Alprazolam (Tetrabenazine causes a small increase (about 8 msec) in the corrected QT (QTc) interval. QT prolongation can lead to development of torsade de pointes-type ventricular tachycardia with the risk increasing as the degree of prolongation increases. The use of tetrabenazine should be avoided in combination with other drugs that are known to prolong QTc interval, including antipsychotic medications (eg, chlorpromazine, thioridazine, ziprasidone), antibiotics (eg, moxifloxacin), Class 1A (eg, quinidine, procainamide) and Class III (eg, amiodarone, sotalol) antiarrhythmic medications, or any other medications known to prolong the QTc interval).
No products indexed under this heading.

Amiodarone Hydrochloride (Tetrabenazine causes a small increase (about 8 msec) in the corrected QT (QTc) interval. QT prolongation can lead to development of torsade de pointes-type ventricular tachycardia with the risk increasing as the degree of prolongation increases. The use of tetrabenazine should be avoided in combination with other drugs that are known to prolong QTc interval, including Class III antiarrhythmic medications (eg, amiodarone, sotalol)).
No products indexed under this heading.

Amitriptyline Hydrochloride (Tetrabenazine causes a small increase (about 8 msec) in the corrected QT (QTc) interval. QT prolongation can lead to development of torsade de pointes-type ventricular tachycardia with the risk increasing as the degree of prolongation increases. The use of tetrabenazine should be avoided in combination with other drugs that are known to prolong QTc interval, including antipsychotic medications (eg, chlorpromazine, thioridazine, ziprasidone), antibiotics (eg, moxifloxacin), Class 1A (eg, quinidine, procainamide) and Class III (eg, amiodarone, sotalol) antiarrhythmic medications, or any other medications known to prolong the QTc interval).
No products indexed under this heading.

Amoxapine (Tetrabenazine causes a small increase (about 8 msec) in the corrected QT (QTc) interval. QT prolongation can lead to development of torsade de pointes-type ventricular tachycardia with the risk increasing as the degree of prolongation increases. The use of tetrabenazine should be avoided in combination with other drugs that are known to prolong QTc interval, including antipsychotic medications (eg, chlorpromazine, thioridazine, ziprasidone), antibiotics (eg, moxifloxacin), Class 1A (eg, quinidine, procainamide) and Class III (eg, amiodarone, sotalol) antiarrhythmic medications, or any other medications known to prolong the QTc interval).
No products indexed under this heading.

Aripiprazole (Tetrabenazine causes a small increase (about 8 msec) in the corrected QT (QTc) interval. QT prolongation can lead to development of torsade de pointes-type ventricular tachycardia with the risk increasing as the degree of prolongation increases. The use of tetrabenazine should be avoided in combination with other drugs that are known to prolong QTc interval, including antipsychotic medications (eg, chlorpromazine, thioridazine, ziprasidone). Patients taking neuroleptic drugs (eg, haloperidol) were excluded from clinical studies during the tetrabenazine development program. Adverse reactions associated with tetrabenazine, such as QTc prolongation, NMS, and extrapyramidal disorders, may be exaggerated by concomitant use of dopamine antagonists).
No products indexed under this heading.

Astemizole (Tetrabenazine causes a small increase (about 8 msec) in the corrected QT (QTc) interval. QT prolongation can lead to development of torsade de pointes-type ventricular tachycardia with the risk increasing as the degree of prolongation increases. The use of tetrabenazine should be avoided in combination with other drugs that are known to prolong QTc interval, including antipsychotic medications (eg, chlorpromazine, thioridazine, ziprasidone), antibiotics (eg, moxifloxacin), Class 1A (eg, quinidine, procainamide) and Class III (eg, amiodarone, sotalol) antiarrhythmic medications, or any other medications known to prolong the QTc interval).
No products indexed under this heading.

Bretylium Tosylate (Tetrabenazine causes a small increase (about 8 msec) in the corrected QT (QTc) interval. QT prolongation can lead to development of torsade de pointes-type ventricular tachycardia with the risk increasing as the degree of prolongation increases. The use of tetrabenazine should be avoided in combination with other drugs that are known to prolong QTc interval, including Class III antiarrhythmic medications (eg, amiodarone, sotalol)).
No products indexed under this heading.

Bupropion Hydrochloride (Caution should be used when giving any strong CYP2D6 inhibitor (eg, fluoxetine, paroxetine, quinidine) to a patient already receiving a stable dose of tetrabenazine, and the daily dose of tetrabenazine should be halved). Products include:
Aplenzin 2948
Wellbutrin 1719
Wellbutrin SR 1725
Zyban 1762

Buspirone Hydrochloride (Tetrabenazine causes a small increase (about 8 msec) in the corrected QT (QTc) interval. QT prolongation can lead to development of torsade de pointes-type ventricular tachycardia with the risk increasing as the degree of prolongation increases. The use of tetrabenazine should be avoided in combination with other drugs that are known to prolong QTc interval, including antipsychotic medications (eg, chlorpromazine, thioridazine, ziprasidone), antibiotics (eg, moxifloxacin), Class 1A (eg, quinidine, procainamide) and Class III (eg, amiodarone, sotalol) antiarrhythmic medications, or any other medications known to prolong the QTc interval).
No products indexed under this heading.

Butabarbital (Patients should be advised that the concomitant use of alcohol or other sedating drugs with tetrabenazine may have additive effects and worsen sedation and somnolence).
No products indexed under this heading.

Butabarbital Sodium (Patients should be advised that the concomitant use of alcohol or other sedating drugs with tetrabenazine may have additive effects and worsen sedation and somnolence).
No products indexed under this heading.

Butalbital (Patients should be advised that the concomitant use of alcohol or other sedating drugs with tetrabenazine may have additive effects and worsen sedation and somnolence).
No products indexed under this heading.

Celecoxib (Caution should be used when giving any strong CYP2D6 inhibitor (eg, fluoxetine, paroxetine, quinidine) to a patient already receiving a stable dose of tetrabenazine, and the daily dose of tetrabenazine should be halved). Products include:
Celebrex 3272

Chloral Hydrate (Patients should be advised that the concomitant use of alcohol or other sedating drugs with tetrabenazine may have additive effects and worsen sedation and somnolence).
No products indexed under this heading.

2105 Interactions Index Xenazine

Chlordiazepoxide (Tetrabenazine causes a small increase (about 8 msec) in the corrected QT (QTc) interval. QT prolongation can lead to development of torsade de pointes-type ventricular tachycardia with the risk increasing as the degree of prolongation increases. The use of tetrabenazine should be avoided in combination with other drugs that are known to prolong QTc interval, including antipsychotic medications (eg, chlorpromazine, thioridazine, ziprasidone), antibiotics (eg, moxifloxacin), Class 1A (eg, quinidine, procainamide) and Class III (eg, amiodarone, sotalol) antiarrhythmic medications, or any other medications known to prolong the QTc interval).
No products indexed under this heading.

Chlordiazepoxide Hydrochloride (Tetrabenazine causes a small increase (about 8 msec) in the corrected QT (QTc) interval. QT prolongation can lead to development of torsade de pointes-type ventricular tachycardia with the risk increasing as the degree of prolongation increases. The use of tetrabenazine should be avoided in combination with other drugs that are known to prolong QTc interval, including antipsychotic medications (eg, chlorpromazine, thioridazine, ziprasidone), antibiotics (eg, moxifloxacin), Class 1A (eg, quinidine, procainamide) and Class III (eg, amiodarone, sotalol) antiarrhythmic medications, or any other medications known to prolong the QTc interval).
No products indexed under this heading.

Chloroquine (Caution should be used when giving any strong CYP2D6 inhibitor (eg, fluoxetine, paroxetine, quinidine) to a patient already receiving a stable dose of tetrabenazine, and the daily dose of tetrabenazine should be halved).
No products indexed under this heading.

Chloroquine Hydrochloride (Caution should be used when giving any strong CYP2D6 inhibitor (eg, fluoxetine, paroxetine, quinidine) to a patient already receiving a stable dose of tetrabenazine, and the daily dose of tetrabenazine should be halved).
No products indexed under this heading.

Chloroquine Phosphate (Caution should be used when giving any strong CYP2D6 inhibitor (eg, fluoxetine, paroxetine, quinidine) to a patient already receiving a stable dose of tetrabenazine, and the daily dose of tetrabenazine should be halved).
No products indexed under this heading.

Chlorpheniramine (Caution should be used when giving any strong CYP2D6 inhibitor (eg, fluoxetine, paroxetine, quinidine) to a patient already receiving a stable dose of tetrabenazine, and the daily dose of tetrabenazine should be halved).
No products indexed under this heading.

Chlorpheniramine Maleate (Caution should be used when giving any strong CYP2D6 inhibitor (eg, fluoxetine, paroxetine, quinidine) to a patient already receiving a stable dose of tetrabenazine, and the daily dose of tetrabenazine should be halved).
No products indexed under this heading.

Chlorpheniramine Polistirex (Caution should be used when giving any strong CYP2D6 inhibitor (eg, fluoxetine, paroxetine, quinidine) to a patient already receiving a stable dose of tetrabenazine, and the daily dose of tetrabenazine should be halved). Products include:
Tussionex 3443

Chlorpheniramine Tannate (Caution should be used when giving any strong CYP2D6 inhibitor (eg, fluoxetine, paroxetine, quinidine) to a patient already receiving a stable dose of tetrabenazine, and the daily dose of tetrabenazine should be halved).
No products indexed under this heading.

Chlorpromazine (Tetrabenazine causes a small increase (about 8 msec) in the corrected QT (QTc) interval. QT prolongation can lead to development of torsade de pointes-type ventricular tachycardia with the risk increasing as the degree of prolongation increases. The use of tetrabenazine should be avoided in combination with other drugs that are known to prolong QTc interval, including antipsychotic medications (eg, chlorpromazine, thioridazine, ziprasidone)).
No products indexed under this heading.

Chlorpromazine Hydrochloride (Tetrabenazine causes a small increase (about 8 msec) in the corrected QT (QTc) interval. QT prolongation can lead to development of torsade de pointes-type ventricular tachycardia with the risk increasing as the degree of prolongation increases. The use of tetrabenazine should be avoided in combination with other drugs that are known to prolong QTc interval, including antipsychotic medications (eg, chlorpromazine, thioridazine, ziprasidone)).
No products indexed under this heading.

Chlorprothixene (Tetrabenazine causes a small increase (about 8 msec) in the corrected QT (QTc) interval. QT prolongation can lead to development of torsade de pointes-type ventricular tachycardia with the risk increasing as the degree of prolongation increases. The use of tetrabenazine should be avoided in combination with other drugs that are known to prolong QTc interval, including antipsychotic medications (eg, chlorpromazine, thioridazine, ziprasidone). Patients taking neuroleptic drugs (eg, haloperidol) were excluded from clinical studies during the tetrabenazine development program. Adverse reactions associated with tetrabenazine, such as QTc prolongation, NMS, and extrapyramidal disorders, may be exaggerated by concomitant use of dopamine antagonists).
No products indexed under this heading.

Chlorprothixene Hydrochloride (Tetrabenazine causes a small increase (about 8 msec) in the corrected QT (QTc) interval. QT prolongation can lead to development of torsade de pointes-type ventricular tachycardia with the risk increasing as the degree of prolongation increases. The use of tetrabenazine should be avoided in combination with other drugs that are known to prolong QTc interval, including antipsychotic medications (eg, chlorpromazine, thioridazine, ziprasidone). Patients taking neuroleptic drugs (eg, haloperidol) were excluded from clinical studies during the tetrabenazine development program. Adverse reactions associated with tetrabenazine, such as QTc prolongation, NMS, and extrapyramidal disorders, may be exaggerated by concomitant use of dopamine antagonists).
No products indexed under this heading.

Chlorprothixene Lactate (Tetrabenazine causes a small increase (about 8 msec) in the corrected QT (QTc) interval. QT prolongation can lead to development of torsade de pointes-type ventricular tachycardia with the risk increasing as the degree of prolongation increases. The use of tetrabenazine should be avoided in combination with other drugs that are known to prolong QTc interval, including antipsychotic medications (eg, chlorpromazine, thioridazine, ziprasidone). Patients taking neuroleptic drugs (eg, haloperidol) were excluded from clinical studies during the tetrabenazine development program. Adverse reactions associated with tetrabenazine, such as QTc prolongation, NMS, and extrapyramidal disorders, may be exaggerated by concomitant use of dopamine antagonists).
No products indexed under this heading.

Cimetidine (Caution should be used when giving any strong CYP2D6 inhibitor (eg, fluoxetine, paroxetine, quinidine) to a patient already receiving a stable dose of tetrabenazine, and the daily dose of tetrabenazine should be halved).
No products indexed under this heading.

Cimetidine Hydrochloride (Caution should be used when giving any strong CYP2D6 inhibitor (eg, fluoxetine, paroxetine, quinidine) to a patient already receiving a stable dose of tetrabenazine, and the daily dose of tetrabenazine should be halved).
No products indexed under this heading.

Citalopram Hydrobromide (Patients taking neuroleptic drugs (eg, haloperidol) were excluded from clinical studies during the tetrabenazine development program. Adverse reactions associated with tetrabenazine, such as QTc prolongation, NMS, and extrapyramidal disorders, may be exaggerated by concomitant use of dopamine antagonists). Products include:
Celexa 1153

Clomipramine Hydrochloride (Tetrabenazine causes a small increase (about 8 msec) in the corrected QT (QTc) interval. QT prolongation can lead to development of torsade de pointes-type ventricular tachycardia with the risk increasing as the degree of prolongation increases. The use of tetrabenazine should be avoided in combination with other drugs that are known to prolong QTc interval, including antipsychotic medications (eg, chlorpromazine, thioridazine, ziprasidone), antibiotics (eg, moxifloxacin), Class 1A (eg, quinidine, procainamide) and Class III (eg, amiodarone, sotalol) antiarrhythmic medications, or any other medications known to prolong the QTc interval).
No products indexed under this heading.

Clorazepate Dipotassium (Tetrabenazine causes a small increase (about 8 msec) in the corrected QT (QTc) interval. QT prolongation can lead to development of torsade de pointes-type ventricular tachycardia with the risk increasing as the degree of prolongation increases. The use of tetrabenazine should be avoided in combination with other drugs that are known to prolong QTc interval, including antipsychotic medications (eg, chlorpromazine, thioridazine, ziprasidone), antibiotics (eg, moxifloxacin), Class 1A (eg, quinidine, procainamide) and Class III (eg, amiodarone, sotalol) antiarrhythmic medications, or any other medications known to prolong the QTc interval).
No products indexed under this heading.

Clozapine (Tetrabenazine causes a small increase (about 8 msec) in the corrected QT (QTc) interval. QT prolongation can lead to development of torsade de pointes-type ventricular tachycardia with the risk increasing as the degree of prolongation increases. The use of tetrabenazine should be avoided in combination with other drugs that are known to prolong QTc interval, including antipsychotic medications (eg, chlorpromazine, thioridazine, ziprasidone). Patients taking neuroleptic drugs (eg, haloperidol) were excluded from clinical studies during the tetrabenazine development program. Adverse reactions associated with tetrabenazine, such as QTc prolongation, NMS, and extrapyramidal disorders, may be exaggerated by concomitant use of dopamine antagonists).
No products indexed under this heading.

Cocaine Hydrochloride (Caution should be used when giving any strong CYP2D6 inhibitor (eg, fluoxetine, paroxetine, quinidine) to a patient already receiving a stable dose of tetrabenazine, and the daily dose of tetrabenazine should be halved).
No products indexed under this heading.

Desipramine Hydrochloride (Tetrabenazine causes a small increase (about 8 msec) in the corrected QT (QTc) interval. QT prolongation can lead to development of torsade de pointes-type ventricular tachycardia with the risk increasing as the degree of prolongation increases. The use of tetrabenazine should be avoided in combination with other drugs that are known to prolong QTc interval, including antipsychotic medications (eg, chlorpromazine, thioridazine, ziprasidone), antibiotics (eg, moxifloxacin), Class 1A (eg, quinidine, procainamide) and Class III (eg, amiodarone, sotalol) antiarrhythmic medications, or any other medications known to prolong the QTc interval).
No products indexed under this heading.

Desvenlafaxine Succinate (Patients taking neuroleptic drugs (eg, haloperidol) were excluded from clinical studies during the tetrabenazine development program. Adverse reactions associated with tetrabenazine, such as QTc prolongation, NMS, and extrapyramidal disorders, may be exaggerated by concomitant use of dopamine antagonists). Products include:
Pristiq 3564

Diazepam (Tetrabenazine causes a small increase (about 8 msec) in the corrected QT (QTc) interval. QT prolongation can lead to development of torsade de pointes-type ventricular tachycardia with the risk increasing as the degree of prolongation increases. The use of tetrabenazine should be avoided in combination with other drugs that are known to prolong QTc interval, including antipsychotic medications (eg, chlorpromazine, thioridazine, ziprasidone), antibiotics (eg, moxifloxacin), Class 1A (eg, quinidine, procainamide) and Class III (eg, amiodarone, sotalol) antiarrhythmic medications, or any other medications known to prolong the QTc interval). Products include:
Valium Tablets 2880

Diphenhydramine (Caution should be used when giving any strong CYP2D6 inhibitor (eg, fluoxetine, paroxetine, quinidine) to a patient already receiving a stable dose of tetrabenazine, and the daily dose of tetrabenazine should be halved).
No products indexed under this heading.

Diphenhydramine Hydrochloride (Caution should be used when giving any strong CYP2D6 inhibitor (eg, fluoxetine, paroxetine, quinidine) to a patient already receiving a stable dose of tetrabenazine, and the daily dose of tetrabenazine should be halved). Products include:
Benadryl Allergy Ultratab 2042
Children's Benadryl Allergy Liquid 2042

Disopyramide (Tetrabenazine causes a small increase (about 8 msec) in the corrected QT (QTc) interval. QT prolongation can lead to development of torsade de pointes-type ventricular tachycardia with the risk increasing as the degree of prolongation increases. The use of tetrabenazine should be avoided in combination with other drugs that are known to prolong QTc interval, including Class 1A antiarrhythmic medications (eg, quinidine, procainamide)).
No products indexed under this heading.

Xenazine Interactions Index 2106

Disopyramide Phosphate (Tetrabenazine causes a small increase (about 8 msec) in the corrected QT (QTc) interval. QT prolongation can lead to development of torsade de pointes-type ventricular tachycardia with the risk increasing as the degree of prolongation increases. The use of tetrabenazine should be avoided in combination with other drugs that are known to prolong QTc interval, including Class 1A antiarrhythmic medications (eg, quinidine, procainamide)).
No products indexed under this heading.

Dofetilide (Tetrabenazine causes a small increase (about 8 msec) in the corrected QT (QTc) interval. QT prolongation can lead to development of torsade de pointes-type ventricular tachycardia with the risk increasing as the degree of prolongation increases. The use of tetrabenazine should be avoided in combination with other drugs that are known to prolong QTc interval, including antipsychotic medications (eg, chlorpromazine, thioridazine, ziprasidone), antibiotics (eg, moxifloxacin), Class 1A (eg, quinidine, procainamide) and Class III (eg, amiodarone, sotalol) antiarrhythmic medications, or any other medications known to prolong the QTc interval).
No products indexed under this heading.

Doxepin Hydrochloride (Tetrabenazine causes a small increase (about 8 msec) in the corrected QT (QTc) interval. QT prolongation can lead to development of torsade de pointes-type ventricular tachycardia with the risk increasing as the degree of prolongation increases. The use of tetrabenazine should be avoided in combination with other drugs that are known to prolong QTc interval, including antipsychotic medications (eg, chlorpromazine, thioridazine, ziprasidone), antibiotics (eg, moxifloxacin), Class 1A (eg, quinidine, procainamide) and Class III (eg, amiodarone, sotalol) antiarrhythmic medications, or any other medications known to prolong the QTc interval).
No products indexed under this heading.

Droperidol (Tetrabenazine causes a small increase (about 8 msec) in the corrected QT (QTc) interval. QT prolongation can lead to development of torsade de pointes-type ventricular tachycardia with the risk increasing as the degree of prolongation increases. The use of tetrabenazine should be avoided in combination with other drugs that are known to prolong QTc interval, including antipsychotic medications (eg, chlorpromazine, thioridazine, ziprasidone), antibiotics (eg, moxifloxacin), Class 1A (eg, quinidine, procainamide) and Class III (eg, amiodarone, sotalol) antiarrhythmic medications, or any other medications known to prolong the QTc interval).
No products indexed under this heading.

Duloxetine Hydrochloride (Patients taking neuroleptic drugs (eg, haloperidol) were excluded from clinical studies during the tetrabenazine development program. Adverse reactions associated with tetrabenazine, such as QTc prolongation, NMS, and extrapyramidal disorders, may be exaggerated by concomitant use of dopamine antagonists). Products include:
Cymbalta 1871

Erythromycin (Tetrabenazine causes a small increase (about 8 msec) in the corrected QT (QTc) interval. QT prolongation can lead to development of torsade de pointes-type ventricular tachycardia with the risk increasing as the degree of prolongation increases. The use of tetrabenazine should be avoided in combination with other drugs that are known to prolong QTc interval, including antipsychotic medications (eg, chlorpromazine, thioridazine, ziprasidone), antibiotics (eg, moxifloxacin), Class 1A (eg, quinidine, procainamide) and Class III (eg, amiodarone, sotalol) antiarrhythmic medications, or any other medications known to prolong the QTc interval).
No products indexed under this heading.

Erythromycin Estolate (Tetrabenazine causes a small increase (about 8 msec) in the corrected QT (QTc) interval. QT prolongation can lead to development of torsade de pointes-type ventricular tachycardia with the risk increasing as the degree of prolongation increases. The use of tetrabenazine should be avoided in combination with other drugs that are known to prolong QTc interval, including antipsychotic medications (eg, chlorpromazine, thioridazine, ziprasidone), antibiotics (eg, moxifloxacin), Class 1A (eg, quinidine, procainamide) and Class III (eg, amiodarone, sotalol) antiarrhythmic medications, or any other medications known to prolong the QTc interval).
No products indexed under this heading.

Erythromycin Ethylsuccinate (Tetrabenazine causes a small increase (about 8 msec) in the corrected QT (QTc) interval. QT prolongation can lead to development of torsade de pointes-type ventricular tachycardia with the risk increasing as the degree of prolongation increases. The use of tetrabenazine should be avoided in combination with other drugs that are known to prolong QTc interval, including antipsychotic medications (eg, chlorpromazine, thioridazine, ziprasidone), antibiotics (eg, moxifloxacin), Class 1A (eg, quinidine, procainamide) and Class III (eg, amiodarone, sotalol) antiarrhythmic medications, or any other medications known to prolong the QTc interval). Products include:
E.E.S. 437
EryPed 435

Erythromycin Gluceptate (Tetrabenazine causes a small increase (about 8 msec) in the corrected QT (QTc) interval. QT prolongation can lead to development of torsade de pointes-type ventricular tachycardia with the risk increasing as the degree of prolongation increases. The use of tetrabenazine should be avoided in combination with other drugs that are known to prolong QTc interval, including antipsychotic medications (eg, chlorpromazine, thioridazine, ziprasidone), antibiotics (eg, moxifloxacin), Class 1A (eg, quinidine, procainamide) and Class III (eg, amiodarone, sotalol) antiarrhythmic medications, or any other medications known to prolong the QTc interval).
No products indexed under this heading.

Erythromycin Lactobionate (Tetrabenazine causes a small increase (about 8 msec) in the corrected QT (QTc) interval. QT prolongation can lead to development of torsade de pointes-type ventricular tachycardia with the risk increasing as the degree of prolongation increases. The use of tetrabenazine should be avoided in combination with other drugs that are known to prolong QTc interval, including antipsychotic medications (eg, chlorpromazine, thioridazine, ziprasidone), antibiotics (eg, moxifloxacin), Class 1A (eg, quinidine, procainamide) and Class III (eg, amiodarone, sotalol) antiarrhythmic medications, or any other medications known to prolong the QTc interval).
No products indexed under this heading.

Erythromycin Stearate (Tetrabenazine causes a small increase (about 8 msec) in the corrected QT (QTc) interval. QT prolongation can lead to development of torsade de pointes-type ventricular tachycardia with the risk increasing as the degree of prolongation increases. The use of tetrabenazine should be avoided in combination with other drugs that are known to prolong QTc interval, including antipsychotic medications (eg, chlorpromazine, thioridazine, ziprasidone), antibiotics (eg, moxifloxacin), Class 1A (eg, quinidine, procainamide) and Class III (eg, amiodarone, sotalol) antiarrhythmic medications, or any other medications known to prolong the QTc interval).
No products indexed under this heading.

Escitalopram Oxalate (Patients taking neuroleptic drugs (eg, haloperidol) were excluded from clinical studies during the tetrabenazine development program. Adverse reactions associated with tetrabenazine, such as QTc prolongation, NMS, and extrapyramidal disorders, may be exaggerated by concomitant use of dopamine antagonists). Products include:
Lexapro Oral Suspension 1160
Lexapro Tablets 1160

Estazolam (Patients should be advised that the concomitant use of alcohol or other sedating drugs with tetrabenazine may have additive effects and worsen sedation and somnolence).
No products indexed under this heading.

Ethanol (Patients should be advised that the concomitant use of alcohol or other sedating drugs with tetrabenazine may have additive effects and worsen sedation and somnolence).
No products indexed under this heading.

Ethchlorvynol (Patients should be advised that the concomitant use of alcohol or other sedating drugs with tetrabenazine may have additive effects and worsen sedation and somnolence).
No products indexed under this heading.

Ethinamate (Patients should be advised that the concomitant use of alcohol or other sedating drugs with tetrabenazine may have additive effects and worsen sedation and somnolence).
No products indexed under this heading.

Ethyl Alcohol (Patients should be advised that the concomitant use of alcohol or other sedating drugs with tetrabenazine may have additive effects and worsen sedation and somnolence).
No products indexed under this heading.

Flecainide Acetate (Tetrabenazine causes a small increase (about 8 msec) in the corrected QT (QTc) interval. QT prolongation can lead to development of torsade de pointes-type ventricular tachycardia with the risk increasing as the degree of prolongation increases. The use of tetrabenazine should be avoided in combination with other drugs that are known to prolong QTc interval, including antipsychotic medications (eg, chlorpromazine, thioridazine, ziprasidone), antibiotics (eg, moxifloxacin), Class 1A (eg, quinidine, procainamide) and Class III (eg, amiodarone, sotalol) antiarrhythmic medications, or any other medications known to prolong the QTc interval).
No products indexed under this heading.

Fluoxetine (*In vitro* studies indicate that α-HTBZ and β-HTBZ are substrates for CYP2D6. The effect of CYP2D6 inhibition on the pharmacokinetics of tetrabenazine and its metabolites was studied in subjects following a single 50 mg dose of tetrabenazine given after 10 days of administration of the strong CYP2D6 inhibitor paroxetine 20 mg daily. There was an approximately 30% increase in C_{max} and an approximately 3-fold increase in AUC for α-HTBZ in subjects given paroxetine prior to tetrabenazine compared to tetrabenazine given alone. For β-HTBZ, the C_{max} and AUC were increased 2.4- and 9-fold, respectively, in subjects given paroxetine prior to tetrabenazine given alone. The elimination half-life of α-HTBZ and β-HTBZ was approximately 14 hours when tetrabenazine was given with paroxetine. Caution should be used when giving any strong CYP2D6 inhibitor (eg, fluoxetine, paroxetine, quinidine) to a patient already receiving a stable dose of tetrabenazine, and the daily dose of tetrabenazine should be halved).
No products indexed under this heading.

Fluoxetine Hydrochloride (*In vitro* studies indicate that α-HTBZ and β-HTBZ are substrates for CYP2D6. The effect of CYP2D6 inhibition on the pharmacokinetics of tetrabenazine and its metabolites was studied in subjects following a single 50 mg dose of tetrabenazine given after 10 days of administration of the strong CYP2D6 inhibitor paroxetine 20 mg daily. There was an approximately 30% increase in C_{max} and an approximately 3-fold increase in AUC for α-HTBZ in subjects given paroxetine prior to tetrabenazine compared to tetrabenazine given alone. For β-HTBZ, the C_{max} and AUC were increased 2.4- and 9-fold, respectively, in subjects given paroxetine prior to tetrabenazine given alone. The elimination half-life of α-HTBZ and β-HTBZ was approximately 14 hours when tetrabenazine was given with paroxetine. Caution should be used when giving any strong CYP2D6 inhibitor (eg, fluoxetine, paroxetine, quinidine) to a patient already receiving a stable dose of tetrabenazine, and the daily dose of tetrabenazine should be halved). Products include:
Prozac Weekly 1941
Prozac Pulvules 1941
Symbyax 1965

Fluphenazine Decanoate (Tetrabenazine causes a small increase (about 8 msec) in the corrected QT (QTc) interval. QT prolongation can lead to development of torsade de pointes-type ventricular tachycardia with the risk increasing as the degree of prolongation increases. The use of tetrabenazine should be avoided in combination with other drugs that are known to prolong QTc interval, including antipsychotic medications (eg, chlorpromazine, thioridazine, ziprasidone). Patients taking neuroleptic drugs (eg, haloperidol) were excluded from clinical studies during the tetrabenazine development program. Adverse reactions associated with tetrabenazine, such as QTc prolongation, NMS, and extrapyramidal disorders, may be exaggerated by concomitant use of dopamine antagonists).
No products indexed under this heading.

Fluphenazine Enanthate (Tetrabenazine causes a small increase (about 8 msec) in the corrected QT (QTc) interval. QT prolongation can lead to development of torsade de pointes-type ventricular tachycardia with the risk increasing as the degree of prolongation increases. The use of tetrabenazine should be avoided in combination with other drugs that are known to prolong QTc interval, including antipsychotic medications (eg, chlorpromazine, thioridazine, ziprasidone). Patients taking neuroleptic drugs (eg, haloperidol) were excluded from clinical studies during the tetrabenazine development program. Adverse reactions associated with tetrabenazine, such as QTc prolongation, NMS, and extrapyramidal disorders, may be exaggerated by concomitant use of dopamine antagonists).
No products indexed under this heading.

Fluphenazine Hydrochloride (Tetrabenazine causes a small increase (about 8 msec) in the corrected QT (QTc) interval. QT prolongation can lead to development of torsade de pointes-type ventricular tachycardia with the risk increasing as the degree of prolongation increases. The use of tetrabenazine should be avoided in combination with other drugs that are known to prolong QTc interval, including antipsychot-

ic medications (eg, chlorpromazine, thioridazine, ziprasidone). Patients taking neuroleptic drugs (eg, haloperidol) were excluded from clinical studies during the tetrabenazine development program. Adverse reactions associated with tetrabenazine, such as QTc prolongation, NMS, and extrapyramidal disorders, may be exaggerated by concomitant use of dopamine antagonists).
No products indexed under this heading.

Flurazepam Hydrochloride (Patients should be advised that the concomitant use of alcohol or other sedating drugs with tetrabenazine may have additive effects and worsen sedation and somnolence).
No products indexed under this heading.

Fluvoxamine (Patients taking neuroleptic drugs (eg, haloperidol) were excluded from clinical studies during the tetrabenazine development program. Adverse reactions associated with tetrabenazine, such as QTc prolongation, NMS, and extrapyramidal disorrders, may be exaggerated by concomitant use of dopamine antagonists).
No products indexed under this heading.

Fluvoxamine Maleate (Patients taking neuroleptic drugs (eg, haloperidol) were excluded from clinical studies during the tetrabenazine development program. Adverse reactions associated with tetrabenazine, such as QTc prolongation, NMS, and extrapyramidal disorrders, may be exaggerated by concomitant use of dopamine antagonists).
No products indexed under this heading.

Glutethimide (Patients should be advised that the concomitant use of alcohol or other sedating drugs with tetrabenazine may have additive effects and worsen sedation and somnolence).
No products indexed under this heading.

Halofantrine Hydrochloride (Caution should be used when giving any strong CYP2D6 inhibitor (eg, fluoxetine, paroxetine, quinidine) to a patient already receiving a stable dose of tetrabenazine, and the daily dose of tetrabenazine should be halved).
No products indexed under this heading.

Haloperidol (Tetrabenazine causes a small increase (about 8 msec) in the corrected QT (QTc) interval. QT prolongation can lead to development of torsade de pointes-type ventricular tachycardia with the risk increasing as the degree of prolongation increases. The use of tetrabenazine should be avoided in combination with other drugs that are known to prolong QTc interval, including antipsychotic medications (eg, chlorpromazine, thioridazine, ziprasidone). Patients taking neuroleptic drugs (eg, haloperidol) were excluded from clinical studies during the tetrabenazine development program. Adverse reactions associated with tetrabenazine, such as QTc prolongation, NMS, and extrapyramidal disorders, may be exaggerated by concomitant use of dopamine antagonists).
No products indexed under this heading.

Haloperidol Decanoate (Tetrabenazine causes a small increase (about 8 msec) in the corrected QT (QTc) interval. QT prolongation can lead to development of torsade de pointes-type ventricular tachycardia with the risk increasing as the degree of prolongation increases. The use of tetrabenazine should be avoided in combination with other drugs that are known to prolong QTc interval, including antipsychotic medications (eg, chlorpromazine, thioridazine, ziprasidone). Patients taking neuroleptic drugs (eg, haloperidol) were excluded from clinical studies during the tetrabenazine development program. Adverse reactions associated with tetrabenazine, such as QTc prolongation, NMS, and extrapyramidal disorders, may be exaggerated by concomitant use of dopamine antagonists).
No products indexed under this heading.

Haloperidol Lactate (Tetrabenazine causes a small increase (about 8 msec) in the corrected QT (QTc) interval. QT prolongation can lead to development of torsade de pointes-type ventricular tachycardia with the risk increasing as the degree of prolongation increases. The use of tetrabenazine should be avoided in combination with other drugs that are known to prolong QTc interval, including antipsychotic medications (eg, chlorpromazine, thioridazine, ziprasidone). Patients taking neuroleptic drugs (eg, haloperidol) were excluded from clinical studies during the tetrabenazine development program. Adverse reactions associated with tetrabenazine, such as QTc prolongation, NMS, and extrapyramidal disorders, may be exaggerated by concomitant use of dopamine antagonists).
No products indexed under this heading.

Hydroxychloroquine Sulfate (Caution should be used when giving any strong CYP2D6 inhibitor (eg, fluoxetine, paroxetine, quinidine) to a patient already receiving a stable dose of tetrabenazine, and the daily dose of tetrabenazine should be halved).
No products indexed under this heading.

Hydroxyzine Hydrochloride (Tetrabenazine causes a small increase (about 8 msec) in the corrected QT (QTc) interval. QT prolongation can lead to development of torsade de pointes-type ventricular tachycardia with the risk increasing as the degree of prolongation increases. The use of tetrabenazine should be avoided in combination with other drugs that are known to prolong QTc interval, including antipsychotic medications (eg, chlorpromazine, thioridazine, ziprasidone), antibiotics (eg, moxifloxacin), Class 1A (eg, quinidine, procainamide) and Class III (eg, amiodarone, sotalol) antiarrhythmic medications, or any other medications known to prolong the QTc interval).
No products indexed under this heading.

Imatinib Mesylate (Caution should be used when giving any strong CYP2D6 inhibitor (eg, fluoxetine, paroxetine, quinidine) to a patient already receiving a stable dose of tetrabenazine, and the daily dose of tetrabenazine should be halved). Products include:
Gleevec 2477

Imipramine Hydrochloride (Tetrabenazine causes a small increase (about 8 msec) in the corrected QT (QTc) interval. QT prolongation can lead to development of torsade de pointes-type ventricular tachycardia with the risk increasing as the degree of prolongation increases. The use of tetrabenazine should be avoided in combination with other drugs that are known to prolong QTc interval, including antipsychotic medications (eg, chlorpromazine, thioridazine, ziprasidone), antibiotics (eg, moxifloxacin), Class 1A (eg, quinidine, procainamide) and Class III (eg, amiodarone, sotalol) antiarrhythmic medications, or any other medications known to prolong the QTc interval).
No products indexed under this heading.

Imipramine Pamoate (Tetrabenazine causes a small increase (about 8 msec) in the corrected QT (QTc) interval. QT prolongation can lead to development of torsade de pointes-type ventricular tachycardia with the risk increasing as the degree of prolongation increases. The use of tetrabenazine should be avoided in combination with other drugs that are known to prolong QTc interval, including antipsychotic medications (eg, chlorpromazine, thioridazine, ziprasidone), antibiotics (eg, moxifloxacin), Class 1A (eg, quinidine, procainamide) and Class III (eg, amiodarone, sotalol) antiarrhythmic medications, or any other medications known to prolong the QTc interval).
No products indexed under this heading.

Isocarboxazid (Tetrabenazine is contraindicated in patients taking monoamine oxidase inhibitors). Products include:
Marplan 3481

Lidocaine (Tetrabenazine causes a small increase (about 8 msec) in the corrected QT (QTc) interval. QT prolongation can lead to development of torsade de pointes-type ventricular tachycardia with the risk increasing as the degree of prolongation increases. The use of tetrabenazine should be avoided in combination with other drugs that are known to prolong QTc interval, including antipsychotic medications (eg, chlorpromazine, thioridazine, ziprasidone), antibiotics (eg, moxifloxacin), Class 1A (eg, quinidine, procainamide) and Class III (eg, amiodarone, sotalol) antiarrhythmic medications, or any other medications known to prolong the QTc interval). Products include:
Lidoderm 1107

Lidocaine Hydrochloride (Tetrabenazine causes a small increase (about 8 msec) in the corrected QT (QTc) interval. QT prolongation can lead to development of torsade de pointes-type ventricular tachycardia with the risk increasing as the degree of prolongation increases. The use of tetrabenazine should be avoided in combination with other drugs that are known to prolong QTc interval, including antipsychotic medications (eg, chlorpromazine, thioridazine, ziprasidone), antibiotics (eg, moxifloxacin), Class 1A (eg, quinidine, procainamide) and Class III (eg, amiodarone, sotalol) antiarrhythmic medications, or any other medications known to prolong the QTc interval).
No products indexed under this heading.

Lithium (Tetrabenazine causes a small increase (about 8 msec) in the corrected QT (QTc) interval. QT prolongation can lead to development of torsade de pointes-type ventricular tachycardia with the risk increasing as the degree of prolongation increases. The use of tetrabenazine should be avoided in combination with other drugs that are known to prolong QTc interval, including antipsychotic medications (eg, chlorpromazine, thioridazine, ziprasidone). Patients taking neuroleptic drugs (eg, haloperidol) were excluded from clinical studies during the tetrabenazine development program. Adverse reactions associated with tetrabenazine, such as QTc prolongation, NMS, and extrapyramidal disorders, may be exaggerated by concomitant use of dopamine antagonists).
No products indexed under this heading.

Lithium Carbonate (Tetrabenazine causes a small increase (about 8 msec) in the corrected QT (QTc) interval. QT prolongation can lead to development of torsade de pointes-type ventricular tachycardia with the risk increasing as the degree of prolongation increases. The use of tetrabenazine should be avoided in combination with other drugs that are known to prolong QTc interval, including antipsychotic medications (eg, chlorpromazine, thioridazine, ziprasidone). Patients taking neuroleptic drugs (eg, haloperidol) were excluded from clinical studies during the tetrabenazine development program. Adverse reactions associated with tetrabenazine, such as QTc prolongation, NMS, and extrapyramidal disorders, may be exaggerated by concomitant use of dopamine antagonists).
No products indexed under this heading.

Lithium Citrate (Tetrabenazine causes a small increase (about 8 msec) in the corrected QT (QTc) interval. QT prolongation can lead to development of torsade de pointes-type ventricular tachycardia with the risk increasing as the degree of prolongation increases. The use of tetrabenazine should be avoided in combination with other drugs that are known to prolong QTc interval, including antipsychotic medications (eg, chlorpromazine, thioridazine, ziprasidone). Patients taking neuroleptic drugs (eg, haloperidol) were excluded from clinical studies during the tetrabenazine development program. Adverse reactions associated with tetrabenazine, such as QTc prolongation, NMS, and extrapyramidal disorders, may be exaggerated by concomitant use of dopamine antagonists).
No products indexed under this heading.

Lorazepam (Tetrabenazine causes a small increase (about 8 msec) in the corrected QT (QTc) interval. QT prolongation can lead to development of torsade de pointes-type ventricular tachycardia with the risk increasing as the degree of prolongation increases. The use of tetrabenazine should be avoided in combination with other drugs that are known to prolong QTc interval, including antipsychotic medications (eg, chlorpromazine, thioridazine, ziprasidone), antibiotics (eg, moxifloxacin), Class 1A (eg, quinidine, procainamide) and Class III (eg, amiodarone, sotalol) antiarrhythmic medications, or any other medications known to prolong the QTc interval).
No products indexed under this heading.

Loxapine Hydrochloride (Tetrabenazine causes a small increase (about 8 msec) in the corrected QT (QTc) interval. QT prolongation can lead to development of torsade de pointes-type ventricular tachycardia with the risk increasing as the degree of prolongation increases. The use of tetrabenazine should be avoided in combination with other drugs that are known to prolong QTc interval, including antipsychotic medications (eg, chlorpromazine, thioridazine, ziprasidone). Patients taking neuroleptic drugs (eg, haloperidol) were excluded from clinical studies during the tetrabenazine development program. Adverse reactions associated with tetrabenazine, such as QTc prolongation, NMS, and extrapyramidal disorders, may be exaggerated by concomitant use of dopamine antagonists).
No products indexed under this heading.

Loxapine Succinate (Tetrabenazine causes a small increase (about 8 msec) in the corrected QT (QTc) interval. QT prolongation can lead to development of torsade de pointes-type ventricular tachycardia with the risk increasing as the degree of prolongation increases. The use of tetrabenazine should be avoided in combination with other drugs that are known to prolong QTc interval, including antipsychotic medications (eg, chlorpromazine, thioridazine, ziprasidone). Patients taking neuroleptic drugs (eg, haloperidol) were excluded from clinical studies during the tetrabenazine development program. Adverse reactions associated with tetrabenazine, such as QTc prolongation, NMS, and extrapyramidal disorders, may be exaggerated by concomitant use of dopamine antagonists).
No products indexed under this heading.

Maprotiline Hydrochloride (Tetrabenazine causes a small increase (about 8 msec) in the corrected QT (QTc) interval. QT prolongation can lead to development of torsade de pointes-type ventricular tachycardia with the risk increasing as the degree of prolongation increases. The use of tetrabenazine should be avoided in combination

Xenazine Interactions Index 2108

with other drugs that are known to prolong QTc interval, including antipsychotic medications (eg, chlorpromazine, thioridazine, ziprasidone), antibiotics (eg, moxifloxacin), Class 1A (eg, quinidine, procainamide) and Class III (eg, amiodarone, sotalol) antiarrhythmic medications, or any other medications known to prolong the QTc interval).
No products indexed under this heading.

Meprobamate (Tetrabenazine causes a small increase (about 8 msec) in the corrected QT (QTc) interval. QT prolongation can lead to development of torsade de pointes-type ventricular tachycardia with the risk increasing as the degree of prolongation increases. The use of tetrabenazine should be avoided in combination with other drugs that are known to prolong QTc interval, including antipsychotic medications (eg, chlorpromazine, thioridazine, ziprasidone), antibiotics (eg, moxifloxacin), Class 1A (eg, quinidine, procainamide) and Class III (eg, amiodarone, sotalol) antiarrhythmic medications, or any other medications known to prolong the QTc interval).
No products indexed under this heading.

Mesoridazine Besylate (Tetrabenazine causes a small increase (about 8 msec) in the corrected QT (QTc) interval. QT prolongation can lead to development of torsade de pointes-type ventricular tachycardia with the risk increasing as the degree of prolongation increases. The use of tetrabenazine should be avoided in combination with other drugs that are known to prolong QTc interval, including antipsychotic medications (eg, chlorpromazine, thioridazine, ziprasidone). Patients taking neuroleptic drugs (eg, haloperidol) were excluded from clinical studies during the tetrabenazine development program. Adverse reactions associated with tetrabenazine, such as QTc prolongation, NMS, and extrapyramidal disorders, may be exaggerated by concomitant use of dopamine antagonists).
No products indexed under this heading.

Methadone Hydrochloride (Caution should be used when giving any strong CYP2D6 inhibitor (eg, fluoxetine, paroxetine, quinidine) to a patient already receiving a stable dose of tetrabenazine, and the daily dose of tetrabenazine should be halved).
No products indexed under this heading.

Methotrimeprazine (Tetrabenazine causes a small increase (about 8 msec) in the corrected QT (QTc) interval. QT prolongation can lead to development of torsade de pointes-type ventricular tachycardia with the risk increasing as the degree of prolongation increases. The use of tetrabenazine should be avoided in combination with other drugs that are known to prolong QTc interval, including antipsychotic medications (eg, chlorpromazine, thioridazine, ziprasidone). Patients taking neuroleptic drugs (eg, haloperidol) were excluded from clinical studies during the tetrabenazine development program. Adverse reactions associated with tetrabenazine, such as QTc prolongation, NMS, and extrapyramidal disorders, may be exaggerated by concomitant use of dopamine antagonists).
No products indexed under this heading.

Metoclopramide Hydrochloride (Adverse reactions associated with tetrabenazine, such as QTc prolongation, Neuroleptic Malignant Syndrome (NMS), and extrapyramidal disorders, may be exaggerated by concomitant use of dopamine antagonists). Products include:
Metozolv ODT **2901**

Mexiletine Hydrochloride (Tetrabenazine causes a small increase (about 8 msec) in the corrected QT (QTc) interval. QT prolongation can lead to development of torsade de pointes-type ventricular tachycardia with the risk increasing as the degree of prolongation increases. The use of tetrabenazine should be avoided in combination with other drugs that are known to prolong QTc interval, including antipsychotic medications (eg, chlorpromazine, thioridazine, ziprasidone), antibiotics (eg, moxifloxacin), Class 1A (eg, quinidine, procainamide) and Class III (eg, amiodarone, sotalol) antiarrhythmic medications, or any other medications known to prolong the QTc interval).
No products indexed under this heading.

Mibefradil Dihydrochloride (Caution should be used when giving any strong CYP2D6 inhibitor (eg, fluoxetine, paroxetine, quinidine) to a patient already receiving a stable dose of tetrabenazine, and the daily dose of tetrabenazine should be halved).
No products indexed under this heading.

Midazolam Hydrochloride (Tetrabenazine causes a small increase (about 8 msec) in the corrected QT (QTc) interval. QT prolongation can lead to development of torsade de pointes-type ventricular tachycardia with the risk increasing as the degree of prolongation increases. The use of tetrabenazine should be avoided in combination with other drugs that are known to prolong QTc interval, including antipsychotic medications (eg, chlorpromazine, thioridazine, ziprasidone), antibiotics (eg, moxifloxacin), Class 1A (eg, quinidine, procainamide) and Class III (eg, amiodarone, sotalol) antiarrhythmic medications, or any other medications known to prolong the QTc interval).
No products indexed under this heading.

Moclobemide (Tetrabenazine is contraindicated in patients taking monoamine oxidase inhibitors).
No products indexed under this heading.

Molindone Hydrochloride (Tetrabenazine causes a small increase (about 8 msec) in the corrected QT (QTc) interval. QT prolongation can lead to development of torsade de pointes-type ventricular tachycardia with the risk increasing as the degree of prolongation increases. The use of tetrabenazine should be avoided in combination with other drugs that are known to prolong QTc interval, including antipsychotic medications (eg, chlorpromazine, thioridazine, ziprasidone). Patients taking neuroleptic drugs (eg, haloperidol) were excluded from clinical studies during the tetrabenazine development program. Adverse reactions associated with tetrabenazine, such as QTc prolongation, NMS, and extrapyramidal disorders, may be exaggerated by concomitant use of dopamine antagonists). Products include:
Moban **1108**

Moricizine Hydrochloride (Tetrabenazine causes a small increase (about 8 msec) in the corrected QT (QTc) interval. QT prolongation can lead to development of torsade de pointes-type ventricular tachycardia with the risk increasing as the degree of prolongation increases. The use of tetrabenazine should be avoided in combination with other drugs that are known to prolong QTc interval, including Class 1A antiarrhythmic medications (eg, quinidine, procainamide)).
No products indexed under this heading.

Moxifloxacin Hydrochloride (Tetrabenazine causes a small increase (about 8 msec) in the corrected QT (QTc) interval. QT prolongation can lead to development of torsade de pointes-type ventricular tachycardia with the risk increasing as the degree of prolongation increases. The use of tetrabenazine should be avoided in combination with other drugs that are known to prolong QTc interval, including antibiotics (eg, moxifloxacin)). Products include:
Avelox **3064**
Vigamox **589**

Nefazodone Hydrochloride (Patients taking neuroleptic drugs (eg, haloperidol) were excluded from clinical studies during the tetrabenazine development program. Adverse reactions associated with tetrabenazine, such as QTc prolongation, NMS, and extrapyramidal disorders, may be exaggerated by concomitant use of dopamine antagonists).
No products indexed under this heading.

Nortriptyline Hydrochloride (Tetrabenazine causes a small increase (about 8 msec) in the corrected QT (QTc) interval. QT prolongation can lead to development of torsade de pointes-type ventricular tachycardia with the risk increasing as the degree of prolongation increases. The use of tetrabenazine should be avoided in combination with other drugs that are known to prolong QTc interval, including antipsychotic medications (eg, chlorpromazine, thioridazine, ziprasidone), antibiotics (eg, moxifloxacin), Class 1A (eg, quinidine, procainamide) and Class III (eg, amiodarone, sotalol) antiarrhythmic medications, or any other medications known to prolong the QTc interval).
No products indexed under this heading.

Olanzapine (Tetrabenazine causes a small increase (about 8 msec) in the corrected QT (QTc) interval. QT prolongation can lead to development of torsade de pointes-type ventricular tachycardia with the risk increasing as the degree of prolongation increases. The use of tetrabenazine should be avoided in combination with other drugs that are known to prolong QTc interval, including antipsychotic medications (eg, chlorpromazine, thioridazine, ziprasidone). Patients taking neuroleptic drugs (eg, haloperidol) were excluded from clinical studies during the tetrabenazine development program. Adverse reactions associated with tetrabenazine, such as QTc prolongation, NMS, and extrapyramidal disorders, may be exaggerated by concomitant use of dopamine antagonists). Products include:
Symbyax **1965**
Zyprexa **1984**
Zyprexa IntraMuscular **1984**
Zyprexa ZYDIS **1984**

Oxazepam (Tetrabenazine causes a small increase (about 8 msec) in the corrected QT (QTc) interval. QT prolongation can lead to development of torsade de pointes-type ventricular tachycardia with the risk increasing as the degree of prolongation increases. The use of tetrabenazine should be avoided in combination with other drugs that are known to prolong QTc interval, including antipsychotic medications (eg, chlorpromazine, thioridazine, ziprasidone), antibiotics (eg, moxifloxacin), Class 1A (eg, quinidine, procainamide) and Class III (eg, amiodarone, sotalol) antiarrhythmic medications, or any other medications known to prolong the QTc interval).
No products indexed under this heading.

Paliperidone (Tetrabenazine causes a small increase (about 8 msec) in the corrected QT (QTc) interval. QT prolongation can lead to development of torsade de pointes-type ventricular tachycardia with the risk increasing as the degree of prolongation increases. The use of tetrabenazine should be avoided in combination with other drugs that are known to prolong QTc interval, including antipsychotic medications (eg, chlorpromazine, thioridazine, ziprasidone). Patients taking neuroleptic drugs (eg, haloperidol) were excluded from clinical studies during the tetrabenazine development program. Adverse reactions associated with tetrabenazine, such as QTc prolongation, NMS, and extrapyramidal disorders, may be exaggerated by concomitant use of dopamine antagonists). Products include:
Invega **2613**
Invega Sustenna **2621**

Pargyline Hydrochloride (Tetrabenazine is contraindicated in patients taking monoamine oxidase inhibitors).
No products indexed under this heading.

Paroxetine (*In vitro* studies indicate that α-HTBZ and β-HTBZ are substrates for CYP2D6. The effect of CYP2D6 inhibition on the pharmacokinetics of tetrabenazine and its metabolites was studied in subjects following a single 50 mg dose of tetrabenazine given after 10 days of administration of the strong CYP2D6 inhibitor paroxetine 20 mg daily. There was an approximately 30% increase in C_{max} and an approximately 3-fold increase in AUC for α-HTBZ in subjects given paroxetine prior to tetrabenazine compared to tetrabenazine given alone. For β-HTBZ, the C_{max} and AUC were increased 2.4- and 9-fold, respectively, in subjects given paroxetine prior to tetrabenazine given alone. The elimination half-life of α-HTBZ and β-HTBZ was approximately 14 hours when tetrabenazine was given with paroxetine. Caution should be used when giving any strong CYP2D6 inhibitor (eg, fluoxetine, paroxetine, quinidine) to a patient already receiving a stable dose of tetrabenazine, and the daily dose of tetrabenazine should be halved).
No products indexed under this heading.

Paroxetine Hydrochloride (*In vitro* studies indicate that α-HTBZ and β-HTBZ are substrates for CYP2D6. The effect of CYP2D6 inhibition on the pharmacokinetics of tetrabenazine and its metabolites was studied in subjects following a single 50 mg dose of tetrabenazine given after 10 days of administration of the strong CYP2D6 inhibitor paroxetine 20 mg daily. There was an approximately 30% increase in C_{max} and an approximately 3-fold increase in AUC for α-HTBZ in subjects given paroxetine prior to tetrabenazine compared to tetrabenazine given alone. For β-HTBZ, the C_{max} and AUC were increased 2.4- and 9-fold, respectively, in subjects given paroxetine prior to tetrabenazine given alone. The elimination half-life of α-HTBZ and β-HTBZ was approximately 14 hours when tetrabenazine was given with paroxetine. Caution should be used when giving any strong CYP2D6 inhibitor (eg, fluoxetine, paroxetine, quinidine) to a patient already receiving a stable dose of tetrabenazine, and the daily dose of tetrabenazine should be halved). Products include:
Paroxetine CR **2361**
Paroxetine ER **2371**
Paxil **1586**
Paxil CR **1596**

Paroxetine Mesylate (*In vitro* studies indicate that α-HTBZ and β-HTBZ are substrates for CYP2D6. The effect of CYP2D6 inhibition on the pharmacokinetics of tetrabenazine and its metabolites was studied in subjects following a single 50 mg dose of tetrabenazine given after 10 days of administration of the strong CYP2D6 inhibitor paroxetine 20 mg daily. There was an approximately 30% increase in C_{max} and an approximately 3-fold increase in AUC for α-HTBZ in subjects given paroxetine prior to tetrabenazine compared to tetrabenazine given alone. For β-HTBZ, the C_{max} and AUC were increased 2.4- and 9-fold, respectively, in subjects given paroxetine prior to tetrabenazine given alone. The elimination half-life of α-HTBZ and β-HTBZ was approximately 14

2109 **Interactions Index** **Xenazine**

hours when tetrabenazine was given with paroxetine. Caution should be used when giving any strong CYP2D6 inhibitor (eg, fluoxetine, paroxetine, quinidine) to a patient already receiving a stable dose of tetrabenazine, and the daily dose of tetrabenazine should be halved).
No products indexed under this heading.

Perphenazine (Tetrabenazine causes a small increase (about 8 msec) in the corrected QT (QTc) interval. QT prolongation can lead to development of torsade de pointes-type ventricular tachycardia with the risk increasing as the degree of prolongation increases. The use of tetrabenazine should be avoided in combination with other drugs that are known to prolong QTc interval, including antipsychotic medications (eg, chlorpromazine, thioridazine, ziprasidone). Patients taking neuroleptic drugs (eg, haloperidol) were excluded from clinical studies during the tetrabenazine development program. Adverse reactions associated with tetrabenazine, such as QTc prolongation, NMS, and extrapyramidal disorders, may be exaggerated by concomitant use of dopamine antagonists).
No products indexed under this heading.

Phenelzine Sulfate (Tetrabenazine is contraindicated in patients taking monoamine oxidase inhibitors).
No products indexed under this heading.

Pimozide (Tetrabenazine causes a small increase (about 8 msec) in the corrected QT (QTc) interval. QT prolongation can lead to development of torsade de pointes-type ventricular tachycardia with the risk increasing as the degree of prolongation increases. The use of tetrabenazine should be avoided in combination with other drugs that are known to prolong QTc interval, including antipsychotic medications (eg, chlorpromazine, thioridazine, ziprasidone). Patients taking neuroleptic drugs (eg, haloperidol) were excluded from clinical studies during the tetrabenazine development program. Adverse reactions associated with tetrabenazine, such as QTc prolongation, NMS, and extrapyramidal disorders, may be exaggerated by concomitant use of dopamine antagonists).
No products indexed under this heading.

Prazepam (Tetrabenazine causes a small increase (about 8 msec) in the corrected QT (QTc) interval. QT prolongation can lead to development of torsade de pointes-type ventricular tachycardia with the risk increasing as the degree of prolongation increases. The use of tetrabenazine should be avoided in combination with other drugs that are known to prolong QTc interval, including antipsychotic medications (eg, chlorpromazine, thioridazine, ziprasidone), antibiotics (eg, moxifloxacin), Class 1A (eg, quinidine, procainamide) and Class III (eg, amiodarone, sotalol) antiarrhythmic medications, or any other medications known to prolong the QTc interval).
No products indexed under this heading.

Procainamide (Tetrabenazine causes a small increase (about 8 msec) in the corrected QT (QTc) interval. QT prolongation can lead to development of torsade de pointes-type ventricular tachycardia with the risk increasing as the degree of prolongation increases. The use of tetrabenazine should be avoided in combination with other drugs that are known to prolong QTc interval, including Class 1A antiarrhythmic medications (eg, quinidine, procainamide)).
No products indexed under this heading.

Procainamide Hydrochloride (Tetrabenazine causes a small increase (about 8 msec) in the corrected QT (QTc) interval. QT prolongation can lead to development of torsade de pointes-type ventricular tachycardia with the risk increasing as the degree of prolongation increases. The use of tetrabenazine should be avoided in combination with other drugs that are known to prolong QTc interval, including Class 1A antiarrhythmic medications (eg, quinidine, procainamide)).
No products indexed under this heading.

Procarbazine Hydrochloride (Tetrabenazine is contraindicated in patients taking monoamine oxidase inhibitors).
No products indexed under this heading.

Prochlorperazine (Tetrabenazine causes a small increase (about 8 msec) in the corrected QT (QTc) interval. QT prolongation can lead to development of torsade de pointes-type ventricular tachycardia with the risk increasing as the degree of prolongation increases. The use of tetrabenazine should be avoided in combination with other drugs that are known to prolong QTc interval, including antipsychotic medications (eg, chlorpromazine, thioridazine, ziprasidone). Patients taking neuroleptic drugs (eg, haloperidol) were excluded from clinical studies during the tetrabenazine development program. Adverse reactions associated with tetrabenazine, such as QTc prolongation, NMS, and extrapyramidal disorders, may be exaggerated by concomitant use of dopamine antagonists).
No products indexed under this heading.

Promethazine (Adverse reactions associated with tetrabenazine, such as QTc prolongation, Neuroleptic Malignant Syndrome (NMS), and extrapyramidal disorders, may be exaggerated by concomitant use of dopamine antagonists).
No products indexed under this heading.

Promethazine Hydrochloride (Adverse reactions associated with tetrabenazine, such as QTc prolongation, Neuroleptic Malignant Syndrome (NMS), and extrapyramidal disorders, may be exaggerated by concomitant use of dopamine antagonists).
No products indexed under this heading.

Propafenone Hydrochloride (Tetrabenazine causes a small increase (about 8 msec) in the corrected QT (QTc) interval. QT prolongation can lead to development of torsade de pointes-type ventricular tachycardia with the risk increasing as the degree of prolongation increases. The use of tetrabenazine should be avoided in combination with other drugs that are known to prolong QTc interval, including antipsychotic medications (eg, chlorpromazine, thioridazine, ziprasidone), antibiotics (eg, moxifloxacin), Class 1A (eg, quinidine, procainamide) and Class III (eg, amiodarone, sotalol) antiarrhythmic medications, or any other medications known to prolong the QTc interval). Products include:
Rythmol **1648**
Rythmol SR **1652**

Propofol (Patients should be advised that the concomitant use of alcohol or other sedating drugs with tetrabenazine may have additive effects and worsen sedation and somnolence).
No products indexed under this heading.

Propoxyphene Hydrochloride (Caution should be used when giving any strong CYP2D6 inhibitor (eg, fluoxetine, paroxetine, quinidine) to a patient already receiving a stable dose of tetrabenazine, and the daily dose of tetrabenazine should be halved).
No products indexed under this heading.

Propoxyphene Napsylate (Caution should be used when giving any strong CYP2D6 inhibitor (eg, fluoxetine, paroxetine, quinidine) to a patient already receiving a stable dose of tetrabenazine, and the daily dose of tetrabenazine should be halved).
No products indexed under this heading.

Protriptyline Hydrochloride (Tetrabenazine causes a small increase (about 8 msec) in the corrected QT (QTc) interval. QT prolongation can lead to development of torsade de pointes-type ventricular tachycardia with the risk increasing as the degree of prolongation increases. The use of tetrabenazine should be avoided in combination with other drugs that are known to prolong QTc interval, including antipsychotic medications (eg, chlorpromazine, thioridazine, ziprasidone), antibiotics (eg, moxifloxacin), Class 1A (eg, quinidine, procainamide) and Class III (eg, amiodarone, sotalol) antiarrhythmic medications, or any other medications known to prolong the QTc interval).
No products indexed under this heading.

Quazepam (Patients should be advised that the concomitant use of alcohol or other sedating drugs with tetrabenazine may have additive effects and worsen sedation and somnolence).
No products indexed under this heading.

Quetiapine Fumarate (Tetrabenazine causes a small increase (about 8 msec) in the corrected QT (QTc) interval. QT prolongation can lead to development of torsade de pointes-type ventricular tachycardia with the risk increasing as the degree of prolongation increases. The use of tetrabenazine should be avoided in combination with other drugs that are known to prolong QTc interval, including antipsychotic medications (eg, chlorpromazine, thioridazine, ziprasidone). Patients taking neuroleptic drugs (eg, haloperidol) were excluded from clinical studies during the tetrabenazine development program. Adverse reactions associated with tetrabenazine, such as QTc prolongation, NMS, and extrapyramidal disorders, may be exaggerated by concomitant use of dopamine antagonists). Products include:
Seroquel **750**
Seroquel XR **759**

Quinacrine Hydrochloride (Caution should be used when giving any strong CYP2D6 inhibitor (eg, fluoxetine, paroxetine, quinidine) to a patient already receiving a stable dose of tetrabenazine, and the daily dose of tetrabenazine should be halved).
No products indexed under this heading.

Quinidine (Tetrabenazine causes a small increase (about 8 msec) in the corrected QT (QTc) interval. QT prolongation can lead to development of torsade de pointes-type ventricular tachycardia with the risk increasing as the degree of prolongation increases. The use of tetrabenazine should be avoided in combination with other drugs that are known to prolong QTc interval, including Class 1A antiarrhythmic medications (eg, quinidine, procainamide)).
No products indexed under this heading.

Quinidine Gluconate (Tetrabenazine causes a small increase (about 8 msec) in the corrected QT (QTc) interval. QT prolongation can lead to development of torsade de pointes-type ventricular tachycardia with the risk increasing as the degree of prolongation increases. The use of tetrabenazine should be avoided in combination with other drugs that are known to prolong QTc interval, including Class 1A antiarrhythmic medications (eg, quinidine, procainamide)).
No products indexed under this heading.

Quinidine Hydrochloride (Tetrabenazine causes a small increase (about 8 msec) in the corrected QT (QTc) interval. QT prolongation can lead to development of torsade de pointes-type ventricular tachycardia with the risk increasing as the degree of prolongation increases. The use of tetrabenazine should be avoided in combination with other drugs that are known to prolong QTc interval, including Class 1A antiarrhythmic medications (eg, quinidine, procainamide)).
No products indexed under this heading.

Quinidine Polygalacturonate (Tetrabenazine causes a small increase (about 8 msec) in the corrected QT (QTc) interval. QT prolongation can lead to development of torsade de pointes-type ventricular tachycardia with the risk increasing as the degree of prolongation increases. The use of tetrabenazine should be avoided in combination with other drugs that are known to prolong QTc interval, including Class 1A antiarrhythmic medications (eg, quinidine, procainamide)).
No products indexed under this heading.

Quinidine Sulfate (Tetrabenazine causes a small increase (about 8 msec) in the corrected QT (QTc) interval. QT prolongation can lead to development of torsade de pointes-type ventricular tachycardia with the risk increasing as the degree of prolongation increases. The use of tetrabenazine should be avoided in combination with other drugs that are known to prolong QTc interval, including Class 1A antiarrhythmic medications (eg, quinidine, procainamide)).
No products indexed under this heading.

Ramelteon (Patients should be advised that the concomitant use of alcohol or other sedating drugs with tetrabenazine may have additive effects and worsen sedation and somnolence). Products include:
Rozerem **3366**

Ranitidine Bismuth Citrate (Caution should be used when giving any strong CYP2D6 inhibitor (eg, fluoxetine, paroxetine, quinidine) to a patient already receiving a stable dose of tetrabenazine, and the daily dose of tetrabenazine should be halved).
No products indexed under this heading.

Ranitidine Hydrochloride (Caution should be used when giving any strong CYP2D6 inhibitor (eg, fluoxetine, paroxetine, quinidine) to a patient already receiving a stable dose of tetrabenazine, and the daily dose of tetrabenazine should be halved). Products include:
Zantac **1737**
Zantac Injection **1732**
Zantac Pharmacy **1735**

Rasagiline Mesylate (Tetrabenazine is contraindicated in patients taking monoamine oxidase inhibitors). Products include:
Azilect **3383**

Reserpine (Tetrabenazine is contraindicated in patients taking reserpine. Reserpine binds irreversibly to vesicular monoamine transporter type 2 (VMAT2) and the duration of its effect is several days. Caution should therefore be used when switching a patient from reserpine to tetrabenazine. The physician should wait for chorea to re-emerge before administering tetrabenazine to avoid overdosage and major depletion of serotonin and norepinephrine in the CNS. At least 20 days should elapse after stopping reserpine before starting tetrabenazine).
No products indexed under this heading.

Risperidone (Tetrabenazine causes a small increase (about 8 msec) in the corrected QT (QTc) interval. QT prolongation can lead to development of torsade de pointes-type ventricular tachycardia with the risk increasing as the

IMPORTANT NOTE: Always consult each drug listing in the patient's regimen for possible interactions.

Xenazine Interactions Index 2110

degree of prolongation increases. The use of tetrabenazine should be avoided in combination with other drugs that are known to prolong QTc interval, including antipsychotic medications (eg, chlorpromazine, thioridazine, ziprasidone). Patients taking neuroleptic drugs (eg, haloperidol) were excluded from clinical studies during the tetrabenazine development program. Adverse reactions associated with tetrabenazine, such as QTc prolongation, NMS, and extrapyramidal disorders, may be exaggerated by concomitant use of dopamine antagonists). Products include:
Risperdal Consta 2682

Ritonavir (Caution should be used when giving any strong CYP2D6 inhibitor (eg, fluoxetine, paroxetine, quinidine) to a patient already receiving a stable dose of tetrabenazine, and the daily dose of tetrabenazine should be halved). Products include:
Kaletra 458
Norvir 509

Secobarbital Sodium (Patients should be advised that the concomitant use of alcohol or other sedating drugs with tetrabenazine may have additive effects and worsen sedation and somnolence).
No products indexed under this heading.

Selegiline (Tetrabenazine is contraindicated in patients taking monoamine oxidase inhibitors). Products include:
Emsam 3623

Selegiline Hydrochloride (Tetrabenazine is contraindicated in patients taking monoamine oxidase inhibitors). Products include:
Eldepryl 3312

Sertraline Hydrochloride (Patients taking neuroleptic drugs (eg, haloperidol) were excluded from clinical studies during the tetrabenazine development program. Adverse reactions associated with tetrabenazine, such as QTc prolongation, NMS, and extrapyramidal disorders, may be exaggerated by concomitant use of dopamine antagonists).
No products indexed under this heading.

Sildenafil Citrate (Caution should be used when giving any strong CYP2D6 inhibitor (eg, fluoxetine, paroxetine, quinidine) to a patient already receiving a stable dose of tetrabenazine, and the daily dose of tetrabenazine should be halved).
No products indexed under this heading.

Sodium Butabarbital (Patients should be advised that the concomitant use of alcohol or other sedating drugs with tetrabenazine may have additive effects and worsen sedation and somnolence).
No products indexed under this heading.

Sotalol Hydrochloride (Tetrabenazine causes a small increase (about 8 msec) in the corrected QT (QTc) interval. QT prolongation can lead to development of torsade de pointes-type ventricular tachycardia with the risk increasing as the degree of prolongation increases. The use of tetrabenazine should be avoided in combination with other drugs that are known to prolong QTc interval, including Class III antiarrhythmic medications (eg, amiodarone, sotalol)).
No products indexed under this heading.

Temazepam (Patients should be advised that the concomitant use of alcohol or other sedating drugs with tetrabenazine may have additive effects and worsen sedation and somnolence).
No products indexed under this heading.

Terbinafine Hydrochloride (Caution should be used when giving any strong CYP2D6 inhibitor (eg, fluoxetine, paroxetine, quinidine) to a patient already receiving a stable dose of tetrabenazine, and the daily dose of tetrabenazine should be halved).
No products indexed under this heading.

Thioridazine (Tetrabenazine causes a small increase (about 8 msec) in the corrected QT (QTc) interval. QT prolongation can lead to development of torsade de pointes-type ventricular tachycardia with the risk increasing as the degree of prolongation increases. The use of tetrabenazine should be avoided in combination with other drugs that are known to prolong QTc interval, including antipsychotic medications (eg, chlorpromazine, thioridazine, ziprasidone)).
No products indexed under this heading.

Thioridazine Hydrochloride (Tetrabenazine causes a small increase (about 8 msec) in the corrected QT (QTc) interval. QT prolongation can lead to development of torsade de pointes-type ventricular tachycardia with the risk increasing as the degree of prolongation increases. The use of tetrabenazine should be avoided in combination with other drugs that are known to prolong QTc interval, including antipsychotic medications (eg, chlorpromazine, thioridazine, ziprasidone)). Products include:
Thioridazine Hydrochloride 2384

Thiothixene (Tetrabenazine causes a small increase (about 8 msec) in the corrected QT (QTc) interval. QT prolongation can lead to development of torsade de pointes-type ventricular tachycardia with the risk increasing as the degree of prolongation increases. The use of tetrabenazine should be avoided in combination with other drugs that are known to prolong QTc interval, including antipsychotic medications (eg, chlorpromazine, thioridazine, ziprasidone). Patients taking neuroleptic drugs (eg, haloperidol) were excluded from clinical studies during the tetrabenazine development program. Adverse reactions associated with tetrabenazine, such as QTc prolongation, NMS, and extrapyramidal disorders, may be exaggerated by concomitant use of dopamine antagonists). Products include:
Thiothixene 2386

Tocainide Hydrochloride (Tetrabenazine causes a small increase (about 8 msec) in the corrected QT (QTc) interval. QT prolongation can lead to development of torsade de pointes-type ventricular tachycardia with the risk increasing as the degree of prolongation increases. The use of tetrabenazine should be avoided in combination with other drugs that are known to prolong QTc interval, including antipsychotic medications (eg, chlorpromazine, thioridazine, ziprasidone), antibiotics (eg, moxifloxacin), Class 1A (eg, quinidine, procainamide) and Class III (eg, amiodarone, sotalol) antiarrhythmic medications, or any other medications known to prolong the QTc interval).
No products indexed under this heading.

Tranylcypromine Sulfate (Tetrabenazine is contraindicated in patients taking monoamine oxidase inhibitors). Products include:
Parnate 1584

Triazolam (Patients should be advised that the concomitant use of alcohol or other sedating drugs with tetrabenazine may have additive effects and worsen sedation and somnolence).
No products indexed under this heading.

Trifluoperazine Hydrochloride (Tetrabenazine causes a small increase (about 8 msec) in the corrected QT (QTc) interval. QT prolongation can lead to development of torsade de pointes-type ventricular tachycardia with the risk increasing as the degree of prolongation increases. The use of tetrabenazine should be avoided in combination with other drugs that are known to prolong QTc interval, including antipsychotic medications (eg, chlorpromazine, thioridazine, ziprasidone). Patients taking neuroleptic drugs (eg, haloperidol) were excluded from clinical studies during the tetrabenazine development program. Adverse reactions associated with tetrabenazine, such as QTc prolongation, NMS, and extrapyramidal disorders, may be exaggerated by concomitant use of dopamine antagonists).
No products indexed under this heading.

Trimipramine Maleate (Tetrabenazine causes a small increase (about 8 msec) in the corrected QT (QTc) interval. QT prolongation can lead to development of torsade de pointes-type ventricular tachycardia with the risk increasing as the degree of prolongation increases. The use of tetrabenazine should be avoided in combination with other drugs that are known to prolong QTc interval, including antipsychotic medications (eg, chlorpromazine, thioridazine, ziprasidone), antibiotics (eg, moxifloxacin), Class 1A (eg, quinidine, procainamide) and Class III (eg, amiodarone, sotalol) antiarrhythmic medications, or any other medications known to prolong the QTc interval).
No products indexed under this heading.

Vardenafil Hydrochloride (Caution should be used when giving any strong CYP2D6 inhibitor (eg, fluoxetine, paroxetine, quinidine) to a patient already receiving a stable dose of tetrabenazine, and the daily dose of tetrabenazine should be halved). Products include:
Levitra 3157

Venlafaxine Hydrochloride (Patients taking neuroleptic drugs (eg, haloperidol) were excluded from clinical studies during the tetrabenazine development program. Adverse reactions associated with tetrabenazine, such as QTc prolongation, NMS, and extrapyramidal disorders, may be exaggerated by concomitant use of dopamine antagonists). Products include:
Effexor XR 3504
Venlafaxine Hydrochloride Tablets ... 2388

Zaleplon (Patients should be advised that the concomitant use of alcohol or other sedating drugs with tetrabenazine may have additive effects and worsen sedation and somnolence).
No products indexed under this heading.

Ziprasidone Hydrochloride (Tetrabenazine causes a small increase (about 8 msec) in the corrected QT (QTc) interval. QT prolongation can lead to development of torsade de pointes-type ventricular tachycardia with the risk increasing as the degree of prolongation increases. The use of tetrabenazine should be avoided in combination with other drugs that are known to prolong QTc interval, including antipsychotic medications (eg, chlorpromazine, thioridazine, ziprasidone)). Products include:
Geodon 2723

Ziprasidone Mesylate (Tetrabenazine causes a small increase (about 8 msec) in the corrected QT (QTc) interval. QT prolongation can lead to development of torsade de pointes-type ventricular tachycardia with the risk increasing as the degree of prolongation increases. The use of tetrabenazine should be avoided in combination with other drugs that are known to prolong QTc interval, including antipsychotic medications (eg, chlorpromazine, thioridazine, ziprasidone)). Products include:
Geodon 2723

Zolpidem Tartrate (Patients should be advised that the concomitant use of alcohol or other sedating drugs with tetrabenazine may have additive effects and worsen sedation and somnolence). Products include:
Ambien 2920
Ambien CR 2925

Food Interactions

Alcohol (Patients should be advised that the concomitant use of alcohol or other sedating drugs with tetrabenazine may have additive effects and worsen sedation and somnolence).

Beer, reduced-alcohol (Patients should be advised that the concomitant use of alcohol or other sedating drugs with tetrabenazine may have additive effects and worsen sedation and somnolence).

Beer, unspecified (Patients should be advised that the concomitant use of alcohol or other sedating drugs with tetrabenazine may have additive effects and worsen sedation and somnolence).

Wine, Chianti (Patients should be advised that the concomitant use of alcohol or other sedating drugs with tetrabenazine may have additive effects and worsen sedation and somnolence).

Wine, Red (Patients should be advised that the concomitant use of alcohol or other sedating drugs with tetrabenazine may have additive effects and worsen sedation and somnolence).

Wine, unspecified (Patients should be advised that the concomitant use of alcohol or other sedating drugs with tetrabenazine may have additive effects and worsen sedation and somnolence).

Wine products (Patients should be advised that the concomitant use of alcohol or other sedating drugs with tetrabenazine may have additive effects and worsen sedation and somnolence).

XENICAL CAPSULES

(Orlistat) 2893

Beta-Carotene (Orlistat has been shown to reduce the absorption of some fat soluble vitamins; the vitamin supplement should be taken once a day at least 2 hours before or after the administration of orlistat). Products include:
Cardio Basics 3455
Meili Clear 607

Cyclosporine (Co-administration has resulted in reduction in cyclosporine plasma levels; concurrent use is not recommended; if used concurrently, cyclosporine should be taken at least 2 hours before or after Xenical). Products include:
Gengraf 440
Neoral Oral Solution 2496
Neoral Capsules 2496
Restasis 605

Levothyroxine (Hypothyroidism has been reported in patients treated concomitantly with orlistat and levothyroxine post-marketing. Patients treated concomitantly with orlistat and levothyroxine should be monitored for changes in thyroid function. Administer levothyroxine and orlistat at least 4 hours apart).
No products indexed under this heading.

Pravastatin Sodium (Co-administration results in additive lipid lowering effect of pravastatin; modest increases in pravastatin plasma concentrations were observed during co-administration).
No products indexed under this heading.

Vitamin A (Orlistat has been shown to reduce the absorption of some fat solu-

2111 Interactions Index Xigris

ble vitamins; the vitamin supplement should be taken once a day at least 2 hours before or after the administration of orlistat). Products include:
Cardio Basics ... 3455
Heplive ... 607
Norwegian Cod Liver Oil ... 919

Vitamin D (Orlistat has been shown to reduce the absorption of some fat soluble vitamins; the vitamin supplement should be taken once a day at least 2 hours before or after the administration of orlistat). Products include:
Active Calcium ... 3476
BoneMate Plus ... 3454
Cardio Basics ... 3455
Norwegian Cod Liver Oil ... 919

Vitamin E (Orlistat has been shown to reduce the absorption of some fat soluble vitamins; the vitamin supplement should be taken once a day at least 2 hours before or after the administration of orlistat). Products include:
Bausch & Lomb Ocuvite Adult 50+ ... ⊙238
Cardio Basics ... 3455
CitraNatal 90 DHA Capsules ... 2332
CitraNatal Assure ... 2332
CitraNatal Harmony ... 2332
CitraNatal Rx ... 2332
Heplive ... 607
MarineOmega ... 2778
Norwegian Cod Liver Oil ... 919
OmegaLife-3 ... 3456
PreNexa ... 3473

Vitamin K1 (Absorption of vitamin K may be decreased).
No products indexed under this heading.

Warfarin Sodium (Vitamin K absorption may be decreased with orlistat; patients on chronic stable doses of warfarin who are prescribed orlistat should be monitored closely for changes in coagulation parameters).
No products indexed under this heading.

Food Interactions

Food, unspecified (Gastrointestinal events may increase when orlistat is taken with a diet high in fat).

XIFAXAN TABLETS

(Rifaximin) ... 2909
None cited in PDR database.

XIGRIS POWDER FOR INTRAVENOUS INFUSION

(Drotrecogin Alfa (Activated)) ... 1980
May interact with anticoagulants, aspirin-acetylsalicylic acid, glycoprotein (GP) IIb/IIIa inhibitors, oral anticoagulants, platelet inhibitors, thrombolytics, and certain other agents. Compounds in these categories include:

Abciximab (Since there is an increased risk of bleeding with drotrecogin alfa, caution should be employed when drotrecogin alfa is used with other drugs that affect hemostasis. The increased risk of bleeding should be carefully considered when deciding whether to use drotrecogin alfa in patients who received recent administration (within 7 days) with glycoprotein IIb/IIIa inhibitors). Products include:
ReoPro ... 1952

Alteplase (Since there is an increased risk of bleeding with drotrecogin alfa, caution should be employed when drotrecogin alfa is used with other drugs that affect hemostasis. The increased risk of bleeding should be carefully considered when deciding whether to use drotrecogin alfa in patients who received recent administration (within 3 days) with thrombolytic therapy). Products include:
Activase ... 1183
Cathflo ... 1192

Anisindione (Since there is an increased risk of bleeding with drotrecogin alfa, caution should be employed when drotrecogin alfa is used with other drugs that affect hemostasis. The increased risk of bleeding should be carefully considered when deciding whether to use drotrecogin alfa in patients who received recent administration (within 7 days) with oral anticoagulants).
No products indexed under this heading.

Anistreplase (Since there is an increased risk of bleeding with drotrecogin alfa, caution should be employed when drotrecogin alfa is used with other drugs that affect hemostasis. The increased risk of bleeding should be carefully considered when deciding whether to use drotrecogin alfa in patients who received recent administration (within 3 days) with thrombolytic therapy).
No products indexed under this heading.

Ardeparin Sodium (Since there is an increased risk of bleeding with drotrecogin alfa, caution should be employed when drotrecogin alfa is used with other drugs that affect hemostasis).
No products indexed under this heading.

Aspirin (Since there is an increased risk of bleeding with drotrecogin alfa, caution should be employed when drotrecogin alfa is used with other drugs that affect hemostasis. The increased risk of bleeding should be carefully considered when deciding whether to use drotrecogin alfa in patients who received recent administration (within 7 days) with aspirin> 650 mg per day). Products include:
Aggrenox ... 880
Bayer Aspirin ... 829
Percodan ... 1124
St. Joseph Aspirin ... 2045

Aspirin, Enteric Coated (Since there is an increased risk of bleeding with drotrecogin alfa, caution should be employed when drotrecogin alfa is used with other drugs that affect hemostasis. The increased risk of bleeding should be carefully considered when deciding whether to use drotrecogin alfa in patients who received recent administration (within 7 days) with aspirin> 650 mg per day).
No products indexed under this heading.

Aspirin Buffered (Since there is an increased risk of bleeding with drotrecogin alfa, caution should be employed when drotrecogin alfa is used with other drugs that affect hemostasis. The increased risk of bleeding should be carefully considered when deciding whether to use drotrecogin alfa in patients who received recent administration (within 7 days) with aspirin> 650 mg per day).
No products indexed under this heading.

Azlocillin Sodium (Since there is an increased risk of bleeding with drotrecogin alfa, caution should be employed when drotrecogin alfa is used with other drugs that affect hemostasis. The increased risk of bleeding should be carefully considered when deciding whether to use drotrecogin alfa in patients who received recent administration (within 7 days) with platelet inhibitors).
No products indexed under this heading.

Bivalirudin (Since there is an increased risk of bleeding with drotrecogin alfa, caution should be employed when drotrecogin alfa is used with other drugs that affect hemostasis. The increased risk of bleeding should be carefully considered when deciding whether to use drotrecogin alfa in patients who received recent administration (within 3 days) with thrombolytic therapy). Products include:
Angiomax for Injection ... 2061

Carbenicillin Indanyl Sodium (Since there is an increased risk of bleeding with drotrecogin alfa, caution should be employed when drotrecogin alfa is used with other drugs that affect hemostasis. The increased risk of bleeding should be carefully considered when deciding whether to use drotrecogin alfa in patients who received recent administration (within 7 days) with platelet inhibitors).
No products indexed under this heading.

Choline Magnesium Trisalicylate (Since there is an increased risk of bleeding with drotrecogin alfa, caution should be employed when drotrecogin alfa is used with other drugs that affect hemostasis. The increased risk of bleeding should be carefully considered when deciding whether to use drotrecogin alfa in patients who received recent administration (within 7 days) with platelet inhibitors).
No products indexed under this heading.

Clopidogrel Bisulfate (Since there is an increased risk of bleeding with drotrecogin alfa, caution should be employed when drotrecogin alfa is used with other drugs that affect hemostasis. The increased risk of bleeding should be carefully considered when deciding whether to use drotrecogin alfa in patients who received recent administration (within 7 days) with platelet inhibitors). Products include:
Plavix ... 3027

Dalteparin Sodium (Since there is an increased risk of bleeding with drotrecogin alfa, caution should be employed when drotrecogin alfa is used with other drugs that affect hemostasis). Products include:
Fragmin ... 1058

Danaparoid Sodium (Since there is an increased risk of bleeding with drotrecogin alfa, caution should be employed when drotrecogin alfa is used with other drugs that affect hemostasis).
No products indexed under this heading.

Dextran (Since there is an increased risk of bleeding with drotrecogin alfa, caution should be employed when drotrecogin alfa is used with other drugs that affect hemostasis. The increased risk of bleeding should be carefully considered when deciding whether to use drotrecogin alfa in patients who received recent administration (within 7 days) with platelet inhibitors).
No products indexed under this heading.

Dextran 40 (Since there is an increased risk of bleeding with drotrecogin alfa, caution should be employed when drotrecogin alfa is used with other drugs that affect hemostasis. The increased risk of bleeding should be carefully considered when deciding whether to use drotrecogin alfa in patients who received recent administration (within 7 days) with platelet inhibitors).
No products indexed under this heading.

Dextran 70 (Since there is an increased risk of bleeding with drotrecogin alfa, caution should be employed when drotrecogin alfa is used with other drugs that affect hemostasis. The increased risk of bleeding should be carefully considered when deciding whether to use drotrecogin alfa in patients who received recent administration (within 7 days) with platelet inhibitors).
No products indexed under this heading.

Dextran I (Since there is an increased risk of bleeding with drotrecogin alfa, caution should be employed when drotrecogin alfa is used with other drugs that affect hemostasis. The increased risk of bleeding should be carefully considered when deciding whether to use drotrecogin alfa in patients who received recent administration (within 7 days) with platelet inhibitors).
No products indexed under this heading.

Dextrans (Low Molecular Weight) (Since there is an increased risk of bleeding with drotrecogin alfa, caution should be employed when drotrecogin alfa is used with other drugs that affect hemostasis. The increased risk of bleeding should be carefully considered when deciding whether to use drotrecogin alfa in patients who received recent administration (within 7 days) with platelet inhibitors).
No products indexed under this heading.

Diclofenac Potassium (Since there is an increased risk of bleeding with drotrecogin alfa, caution should be employed when drotrecogin alfa is used with other drugs that affect hemostasis. The increased risk of bleeding should be carefully considered when deciding whether to use drotrecogin alfa in patients who received recent administration (within 7 days) with platelet inhibitors).
No products indexed under this heading.

Diclofenac Sodium (Since there is an increased risk of bleeding with drotrecogin alfa, caution should be employed when drotrecogin alfa is used with other drugs that affect hemostasis. The increased risk of bleeding should be carefully considered when deciding whether to use drotrecogin alfa in patients who received recent administration (within 7 days) with platelet inhibitors).
No products indexed under this heading.

Dicumarol (Since there is an increased risk of bleeding with drotrecogin alfa, caution should be employed when drotrecogin alfa is used with other drugs that affect hemostasis. The increased risk of bleeding should be carefully considered when deciding whether to use drotrecogin alfa in patients who received recent administration (within 7 days) with oral anticoagulants).
No products indexed under this heading.

Diflunisal (Since there is an increased risk of bleeding with drotrecogin alfa, caution should be employed when drotrecogin alfa is used with other drugs that affect hemostasis. The increased risk of bleeding should be carefully considered when deciding whether to use drotrecogin alfa in patients who received recent administration (within 7 days) with platelet inhibitors).
No products indexed under this heading.

Dipyridamole (Since there is an increased risk of bleeding with drotrecogin alfa, caution should be employed when drotrecogin alfa is used with other drugs that affect hemostasis. The increased risk of bleeding should be carefully considered when deciding whether to use drotrecogin alfa in patients who received recent administration (within 7 days) with platelet inhibitors). Products include:
Aggrenox ... 880

Enoxaparin Sodium (Since there is an increased risk of bleeding with drotrecogin alfa, caution should be employed when drotrecogin alfa is used with other drugs that affect hemostasis). Products include:
Lovenox ... 3005

IMPORTANT NOTE: Always consult each drug listing in the patient's regimen for possible interactions.

Eptifibatide (Since there is an increased risk of bleeding with drotrecogin alfa, caution should be employed when drotrecogin alfa is used with other drugs that affect hemostasis. The increased risk of bleeding should be carefully considered when deciding whether to use drotrecogin alfa in patients who received recent administration (within 7 days) with glycoprotein IIb/IIIa inhibitors). Products include:
Integrilin 3135

Fenoprofen Calcium (Since there is an increased risk of bleeding with drotrecogin alfa, caution should be employed when drotrecogin alfa is used with other drugs that affect hemostasis. The increased risk of bleeding should be carefully considered when deciding whether to use drotrecogin alfa in patients who received recent administration (within 7 days) with platelet inhibitors).
No products indexed under this heading.

Flurbiprofen (Since there is an increased risk of bleeding with drotrecogin alfa, caution should be employed when drotrecogin alfa is used with other drugs that affect hemostasis. The increased risk of bleeding should be carefully considered when deciding whether to use drotrecogin alfa in patients who received recent administration (within 7 days) with platelet inhibitors).
No products indexed under this heading.

Fondaparinux Sodium (Since there is an increased risk of bleeding with drotrecogin alfa, caution should be employed when drotrecogin alfa is used with other drugs that affect hemostasis). Products include:
Arixtra 1320

Heparin Calcium (Bleeding is the most common serious adverse effect associated with drotrecogin alfa therapy; concurrent therapeutic dosing of heparin used to treat an active thrombotic or embolic event increases the risk of bleeding. Heparin for venous thromboembolism (VTE) prophylaxis may be co-administered with drotrecogin alfa. No dosage adjustment of drotrecogin alfa is recommended when co-administered with prophylactic heparin).
No products indexed under this heading.

Heparin Sodium (Bleeding is the most common serious adverse effect associated with drotrecogin alfa therapy; concurrent therapeutic dosing of heparin used to treat an active thrombotic or embolic event increases the risk of bleeding. Heparin for venous thromboembolism (VTE) prophylaxis may be co-administered with drotrecogin alfa. No dosage adjustment of drotrecogin alfa is recommended when co-administered with prophylactic heparin).
No products indexed under this heading.

Hydroxychloroquine Sulfate (Since there is an increased risk of bleeding with drotrecogin alfa, caution should be employed when drotrecogin alfa is used with other drugs that affect hemostasis. The increased risk of bleeding should be carefully considered when deciding whether to use drotrecogin alfa in patients who received recent administration (within 7 days) with platelet inhibitors).
No products indexed under this heading.

Ibuprofen (Since there is an increased risk of bleeding with drotrecogin alfa, caution should be employed when drotrecogin alfa is used with other drugs that affect hemostasis. The increased risk of bleeding should be carefully considered when deciding whether to use drotrecogin alfa in patients who received recent administration (within 7 days) with platelet inhibitors). Products include:
Motrin IB 2043
Children's Motrin 2044
Children's Motrin Non-Staining Dye-Free 2044
Infants' Motrin 2044
Infants' Motrin Dye-Free 2044
Junior Strength Motrin 2044
Vicoprofen 564

Indomethacin (Since there is an increased risk of bleeding with drotrecogin alfa, caution should be employed when drotrecogin alfa is used with other drugs that affect hemostasis. The increased risk of bleeding should be carefully considered when deciding whether to use drotrecogin alfa in patients who received recent administration (within 7 days) with platelet inhibitors). Products include:
Indocin 2167

Indomethacin Sodium Trihydrate (Since there is an increased risk of bleeding with drotrecogin alfa, caution should be employed when drotrecogin alfa is used with other drugs that affect hemostasis. The increased risk of bleeding should be carefully considered when deciding whether to use drotrecogin alfa in patients who received recent administration (within 7 days) with platelet inhibitors). Products include:
Indocin I.V. 2007

Ketoprofen (Since there is an increased risk of bleeding with drotrecogin alfa, caution should be employed when drotrecogin alfa is used with other drugs that affect hemostasis. The increased risk of bleeding should be carefully considered when deciding whether to use drotrecogin alfa in patients who received recent administration (within 7 days) with platelet inhibitors).
No products indexed under this heading.

Low Molecular Weight Heparins (Since there is an increased risk of bleeding with drotrecogin alfa, caution should be employed when drotrecogin alfa is used with other drugs that affect hemostasis).
No products indexed under this heading.

Magnesium Salicylate (Since there is an increased risk of bleeding with drotrecogin alfa, caution should be employed when drotrecogin alfa is used with other drugs that affect hemostasis. The increased risk of bleeding should be carefully considered when deciding whether to use drotrecogin alfa in patients who received recent administration (within 7 days) with platelet inhibitors).
No products indexed under this heading.

Meclofenamate Sodium (Since there is an increased risk of bleeding with drotrecogin alfa, caution should be employed when drotrecogin alfa is used with other drugs that affect hemostasis. The increased risk of bleeding should be carefully considered when deciding whether to use drotrecogin alfa in patients who received recent administration (within 7 days) with platelet inhibitors).
No products indexed under this heading.

Mefenamic Acid (Since there is an increased risk of bleeding with drotrecogin alfa, caution should be employed when drotrecogin alfa is used with other drugs that affect hemostasis. The increased risk of bleeding should be carefully considered when deciding whether to use drotrecogin alfa in patients who received recent administration (within 7 days) with platelet inhibitors).
No products indexed under this heading.

Mezlocillin Sodium (Since there is an increased risk of bleeding with drotrecogin alfa, caution should be employed when drotrecogin alfa is used with other drugs that affect hemostasis. The increased risk of bleeding should be carefully considered when deciding whether to use drotrecogin alfa in patients who received recent administration (within 7 days) with platelet inhibitors).
No products indexed under this heading.

Nafcillin Sodium (Since there is an increased risk of bleeding with drotrecogin alfa, caution should be employed when drotrecogin alfa is used with other drugs that affect hemostasis. The increased risk of bleeding should be carefully considered when deciding whether to use drotrecogin alfa in patients who received recent administration (within 7 days) with platelet inhibitors).
No products indexed under this heading.

Naproxen (Since there is an increased risk of bleeding with drotrecogin alfa, caution should be employed when drotrecogin alfa is used with other drugs that affect hemostasis. The increased risk of bleeding should be carefully considered when deciding whether to use drotrecogin alfa in patients who received recent administration (within 7 days) with platelet inhibitors). Products include:
EC-Naprosyn 2850
Naprosyn 2850
Anaprox/Naprosyn 2850

Naproxen Sodium (Since there is an increased risk of bleeding with drotrecogin alfa, caution should be employed when drotrecogin alfa is used with other drugs that affect hemostasis. The increased risk of bleeding should be carefully considered when deciding whether to use drotrecogin alfa in patients who received recent administration (within 7 days) with platelet inhibitors). Products include:
Anaprox 2850
Anaprox DS 2850
Treximet 1681

Penicillin G Benzathine (Since there is an increased risk of bleeding with drotrecogin alfa, caution should be employed when drotrecogin alfa is used with other drugs that affect hemostasis. The increased risk of bleeding should be carefully considered when deciding whether to use drotrecogin alfa in patients who received recent administration (within 7 days) with platelet inhibitors). Products include:
Bicillin C-R Injectable Suspension 1826
Bicillin L-A 1828

Penicillin G Procaine (Since there is an increased risk of bleeding with drotrecogin alfa, caution should be employed when drotrecogin alfa is used with other drugs that affect hemostasis. The increased risk of bleeding should be carefully considered when deciding whether to use drotrecogin alfa in patients who received recent administration (within 7 days) with platelet inhibitors). Products include:
Bicillin C-R Injectable Suspension 1826
Bicillin L-A 1828

Phenylbutazone (Since there is an increased risk of bleeding with drotrecogin alfa, caution should be employed when drotrecogin alfa is used with other drugs that affect hemostasis. The increased risk of bleeding should be carefully considered when deciding whether to use drotrecogin alfa in patients who received recent administration (within 7 days) with platelet inhibitors).
No products indexed under this heading.

Piroxicam (Since there is an increased risk of bleeding with drotrecogin alfa, caution should be employed when drotrecogin alfa is used with other drugs that affect hemostasis. The increased risk of bleeding should be carefully considered when deciding whether to use drotrecogin alfa in patients who received recent administration (within 7 days) with platelet inhibitors).
No products indexed under this heading.

Reteplase (Since there is an increased risk of bleeding with drotrecogin alfa, caution should be employed when drotrecogin alfa is used with other drugs that affect hemostasis. The increased risk of bleeding should be carefully considered when deciding whether to use drotrecogin alfa in patients who received recent administration (within 3 days) with thrombolytic therapy).
No products indexed under this heading.

Salsalate (Since there is an increased risk of bleeding with drotrecogin alfa, caution should be employed when drotrecogin alfa is used with other drugs that affect hemostasis. The increased risk of bleeding should be carefully considered when deciding whether to use drotrecogin alfa in patients who received recent administration (within 7 days) with platelet inhibitors).
No products indexed under this heading.

Streptokinase (Since there is an increased risk of bleeding with drotrecogin alfa, caution should be employed when drotrecogin alfa is used with other drugs that affect hemostasis. The increased risk of bleeding should be carefully considered when deciding whether to use drotrecogin alfa in patients who received recent administration (within 3 days) with thrombolytic therapy).
No products indexed under this heading.

Sulindac (Since there is an increased risk of bleeding with drotrecogin alfa, caution should be employed when drotrecogin alfa is used with other drugs that affect hemostasis. The increased risk of bleeding should be carefully considered when deciding whether to use drotrecogin alfa in patients who received recent administration (within 7 days) with platelet inhibitors). Products include:
Clinoril 2098

Ticarcillin Disodium (Since there is an increased risk of bleeding with drotrecogin alfa, caution should be employed when drotrecogin alfa is used with other drugs that affect hemostasis. The increased risk of bleeding should be carefully considered when deciding whether to use drotrecogin alfa in patients who received recent administration (within 7 days) with platelet inhibitors). Products include:
Timentin ADD-Vantage 1670
Timentin Galaxy 1674
Timentin 1666
Timentin Pharmacy 1678

Ticlopidine Hydrochloride (Since there is an increased risk of bleeding with drotrecogin alfa, caution should be employed when drotrecogin alfa is used with other drugs that affect hemostasis. The increased risk of bleeding should be carefully considered when deciding whether to use drotrecogin alfa in patients who received recent administration (within 7 days) with platelet inhibitors).
No products indexed under this heading.

Tinzaparin Sodium (Since there is an increased risk of bleeding with drotrecogin alfa, caution should be employed when drotrecogin alfa is used with other drugs that affect hemostasis).
No products indexed under this heading.

2113 Interactions Index Xyzal

Tirofiban Hydrochloride (Since there is an increased risk of bleeding with drotrecogin alfa, caution should be employed when drotrecogin alfa is used with other drugs that affect hemostasis. The increased risk of bleeding should be carefully considered when deciding whether to use drotrecogin alfa in patients who received recent administration (within 7 days) with glycoprotein IIb/IIIa inhibitors).
No products indexed under this heading.

Tolmetin Sodium (Since there is an increased risk of bleeding with drotrecogin alfa, caution should be employed when drotrecogin alfa is used with other drugs that affect hemostasis. The increased risk of bleeding should be carefully considered when deciding whether to use drotrecogin alfa in patients who received recent administration (within 7 days) with platelet inhibitors).
No products indexed under this heading.

Urokinase (Since there is an increased risk of bleeding with drotrecogin alfa, caution should be employed when drotrecogin alfa is used with other drugs that affect hemostasis. The increased risk of bleeding should be carefully considered when deciding whether to use drotrecogin alfa in patients who received recent administration (within 3 days) with thrombolytic therapy).
No products indexed under this heading.

Warfarin Sodium (Since there is an increased risk of bleeding with drotrecogin alfa, caution should be employed when drotrecogin alfa is used with other drugs that affect hemostasis. The increased risk of bleeding should be carefully considered when deciding whether to use drotrecogin alfa in patients who received recent administration (within 7 days) with oral anticoagulants).
No products indexed under this heading.

XOLAIR
(Omalizumab) 1230
None cited in PDR database. (None cited in PDR database).

XOLAIR
(Omalizumab) 2551
None cited in PDR database.

XOLEGEL GEL
(Ketoconazole) 3337
None cited in PDR database.

XYNTHA VIALS
(Antihemophilic Factor (Recombinant), Plasma/Albumin-Free) 3602
None cited in PDR database.

XYZAL ORAL SOLUTION
(Levocetirizine Dihydrochloride) 3449
May interact with alcohols, central nervous system depressants, theophyllines, and certain other agents. Compounds in these categories include:

Alfentanil Hydrochloride (Concurrent use of levocetirizine dihydrochloride with other central nervous system depressants should be avoided because additional reductions in alertness and additional impairment of central nervous system performance may occur).
No products indexed under this heading.

Alprazolam (Concurrent use of levocetirizine dihydrochloride with other central nervous system depressants should be avoided because additional reductions in alertness and additional impairment of central nervous system performance may occur).
No products indexed under this heading.

Amobarbital (Concurrent use of levocetirizine dihydrochloride with other central nervous system depressants should be avoided because additional reductions in alertness and additional impairment of central nervous system performance may occur).
No products indexed under this heading.

Amobarbital Sodium (Concurrent use of levocetirizine dihydrochloride with other central nervous system depressants should be avoided because additional reductions in alertness and additional impairment of central nervous system performance may occur).
No products indexed under this heading.

Aprobarbital (Concurrent use of levocetirizine dihydrochloride with other central nervous system depressants should be avoided because additional reductions in alertness and additional impairment of central nervous system performance may occur).
No products indexed under this heading.

Buprenorphine Hydrochloride (Concurrent use of levocetirizine dihydrochloride with other central nervous system depressants should be avoided because additional reductions in alertness and additional impairment of central nervous system performance may occur).
No products indexed under this heading.

Buspirone Hydrochloride (Concurrent use of levocetirizine dihydrochloride with other central nervous system depressants should be avoided because additional reductions in alertness and additional impairment of central nervous system performance may occur).
No products indexed under this heading.

Butabarbital (Concurrent use of levocetirizine dihydrochloride with other central nervous system depressants should be avoided because additional reductions in alertness and additional impairment of central nervous system performance may occur).
No products indexed under this heading.

Butabarbital Sodium (Concurrent use of levocetirizine dihydrochloride with other central nervous system depressants should be avoided because additional reductions in alertness and additional impairment of central nervous system performance may occur).
No products indexed under this heading.

Butalbital (Concurrent use of levocetirizine dihydrochloride with other central nervous system depressants should be avoided because additional reductions in alertness and additional impairment of central nervous system performance may occur).
No products indexed under this heading.

Chlordiazepoxide (Concurrent use of levocetirizine dihydrochloride with other central nervous system depressants should be avoided because additional reductions in alertness and additional impairment of central nervous system performance may occur).
No products indexed under this heading.

Chlordiazepoxide Hydrochloride (Concurrent use of levocetirizine dihydrochloride with other central nervous system depressants should be avoided because additional reductions in alertness and additional impairment of central nervous system performance may occur).
No products indexed under this heading.

Chlorpromazine (Concurrent use of levocetirizine dihydrochloride with other central nervous system depressants should be avoided because additional reductions in alertness and additional impairment of central nervous system performance may occur).
No products indexed under this heading.

Chlorpromazine Hydrochloride (Concurrent use of levocetirizine dihydrochloride with other central nervous system depressants should be avoided because additional reductions in alertness and additional impairment of central nervous system performance may occur).
No products indexed under this heading.

Chlorprothixene (Concurrent use of levocetirizine dihydrochloride with other central nervous system depressants should be avoided because additional reductions in alertness and additional impairment of central nervous system performance may occur).
No products indexed under this heading.

Chlorprothixene Hydrochloride (Concurrent use of levocetirizine dihydrochloride with other central nervous system depressants should be avoided because additional reductions in alertness and additional impairment of central nervous system performance may occur).
No products indexed under this heading.

Chlorprothixene Lactate (Concurrent use of levocetirizine dihydrochloride with other central nervous system depressants should be avoided because additional reductions in alertness and additional impairment of central nervous system performance may occur).
No products indexed under this heading.

Clonazepam (Concurrent use of levocetirizine dihydrochloride with other central nervous system depressants should be avoided because additional reductions in alertness and additional impairment of central nervous system performance may occur). Products include:
Klonopin 2855

Clorazepate Dipotassium (Concurrent use of levocetirizine dihydrochloride with other central nervous system depressants should be avoided because additional reductions in alertness and additional impairment of central nervous system performance may occur).
No products indexed under this heading.

Clozapine (Concurrent use of levocetirizine dihydrochloride with other central nervous system depressants should be avoided because additional reductions in alertness and additional impairment of central nervous system performance may occur).
No products indexed under this heading.

Codeine Phosphate (Concurrent use of levocetirizine dihydrochloride with other central nervous system depressants should be avoided because additional reductions in alertness and additional impairment of central nervous system performance may occur). Products include:
Tylenol with Codeine 2691

Codeine Sulfate (Concurrent use of levocetirizine dihydrochloride with other central nervous system depressants should be avoided because additional reductions in alertness and additional impairment of central nervous system performance may occur).
No products indexed under this heading.

Desflurane (Concurrent use of levocetirizine dihydrochloride with other central nervous system depressants should be avoided because additional reductions in alertness and additional impairment of central nervous system performance may occur).
No products indexed under this heading.

Dezocine (Concurrent use of levocetirizine dihydrochloride with other central nervous system depressants should be avoided because additional reductions in alertness and additional impairment of central nervous system performance may occur).
No products indexed under this heading.

Diazepam (Concurrent use of levocetirizine dihydrochloride with other central nervous system depressants should be avoided because additional reductions in alertness and additional impairment of central nervous system performance may occur). Products include:
Valium Tablets 2880

Droperidol (Concurrent use of levocetirizine dihydrochloride with other central nervous system depressants should be avoided because additional reductions in alertness and additional impairment of central nervous system performance may occur).
No products indexed under this heading.

Enflurane (Concurrent use of levocetirizine dihydrochloride with other central nervous system depressants should be avoided because additional reductions in alertness and additional impairment of central nervous system performance may occur).
No products indexed under this heading.

Estazolam (Concurrent use of levocetirizine dihydrochloride with other central nervous system depressants should be avoided because additional reductions in alertness and additional impairment of central nervous system performance may occur).
No products indexed under this heading.

Ethanol (Concurrent use of levocetirizine dihydrochloride with other central nervous system depressants should be avoided because additional reductions in alertness and additional impairment of central nervous system performance may occur).
No products indexed under this heading.

Ethchlorvynol (Concurrent use of levocetirizine dihydrochloride with other central nervous system depressants should be avoided because additional reductions in alertness and additional impairment of central nervous system performance may occur).
No products indexed under this heading.

Ethinamate (Concurrent use of levocetirizine dihydrochloride with other central nervous system depressants should be avoided because additional reductions in alertness and additional impairment of central nervous system performance may occur).
No products indexed under this heading.

Ethyl Alcohol (Concurrent use of levocetirizine dihydrochloride with other central nervous system depressants should be avoided because additional reductions in alertness and additional impairment of central nervous system performance may occur).
No products indexed under this heading.

Fentanyl (Concurrent use of levocetirizine dihydrochloride with other central nervous system depressants should be avoided because additional reductions in alertness and additional impairment of central nervous system performance may occur). Products include:
Duragesic 2604
Fentanyl Transdermal System 2346
Onsolis 2054

IMPORTANT NOTE: Always consult each drug listing in the patient's regimen for possible interactions.

Fentanyl Citrate (Concurrent use of levocetirizine dihydrochloride with other central nervous system depressants should be avoided because additional reductions in alertness and additional impairment of central nervous system performance may occur). Products include:

Fluphenazine Decanoate (Concurrent use of levocetirizine dihydrochloride with other central nervous system depressants should be avoided because additional reductions in alertness and additional impairment of central nervous system performance may occur).
No products indexed under this heading.

Fluphenazine Enanthate (Concurrent use of levocetirizine dihydrochloride with other central nervous system depressants should be avoided because additional reductions in alertness and additional impairment of central nervous system performance may occur).
No products indexed under this heading.

Fluphenazine Hydrochloride (Concurrent use of levocetirizine dihydrochloride with other central nervous system depressants should be avoided because additional reductions in alertness and additional impairment of central nervous system performance may occur).
No products indexed under this heading.

Flurazepam Hydrochloride (Concurrent use of levocetirizine dihydrochloride with other central nervous system depressants should be avoided because additional reductions in alertness and additional impairment of central nervous system performance may occur).
No products indexed under this heading.

Glutethimide (Concurrent use of levocetirizine dihydrochloride with other central nervous system depressants should be avoided because additional reductions in alertness and additional impairment of central nervous system performance may occur).
No products indexed under this heading.

Halazepam (Concurrent use of levocetirizine dihydrochloride with other central nervous system depressants should be avoided because additional reductions in alertness and additional impairment of central nervous system performance may occur).
No products indexed under this heading.

Haloperidol (Concurrent use of levocetirizine dihydrochloride with other central nervous system depressants should be avoided because additional reductions in alertness and additional impairment of central nervous system performance may occur).
No products indexed under this heading.

Haloperidol Decanoate (Concurrent use of levocetirizine dihydrochloride with other central nervous system depressants should be avoided because additional reductions in alertness and additional impairment of central nervous system performance may occur).
No products indexed under this heading.

Haloperidol Lactate (Concurrent use of levocetirizine dihydrochloride with other central nervous system depressants should be avoided because additional reductions in alertness and additional impairment of central nervous system performance may occur).
No products indexed under this heading.

Hexobarbital (Concurrent use of levocetirizine dihydrochloride with other central nervous system depressants should be avoided because additional reductions in alertness and additional impairment of central nervous system performance may occur).
No products indexed under this heading.

Hydrocodone Bitartrate (Concurrent use of levocetirizine dihydrochloride with other central nervous system depressants should be avoided because additional reductions in alertness and additional impairment of central nervous system performance may occur). Products include:

Hydrocodone Polistirex (Concurrent use of levocetirizine dihydrochloride with other central nervous system depressants should be avoided because additional reductions in alertness and additional impairment of central nervous system performance may occur). Products include:

Hydromorphone (Concurrent use of levocetirizine dihydrochloride with other central nervous system depressants should be avoided because additional reductions in alertness and additional impairment of central nervous system performance may occur).
No products indexed under this heading.

Hydromorphone Hydrochloride (Concurrent use of levocetirizine dihydrochloride with other central nervous system depressants should be avoided because additional reductions in alertness and additional impairment of central nervous system performance may occur). Products include:

Hydroxyzine Hydrochloride (Concurrent use of levocetirizine dihydrochloride with other central nervous system depressants should be avoided because additional reductions in alertness and additional impairment of central nervous system performance may occur).
No products indexed under this heading.

Isoflurane (Concurrent use of levocetirizine dihydrochloride with other central nervous system depressants should be avoided because additional reductions in alertness and additional impairment of central nervous system performance may occur).
No products indexed under this heading.

Ketamine Hydrochloride (Concurrent use of levocetirizine dihydrochloride with other central nervous system depressants should be avoided because additional reductions in alertness and additional impairment of central nervous system performance may occur).
No products indexed under this heading.

Levomethadyl Acetate Hydrochloride (Concurrent use of levocetirizine dihydrochloride with other central nervous system depressants should be avoided because additional reductions in alertness and additional impairment of central nervous system performance may occur).
No products indexed under this heading.

Levorphanol Tartrate (Concurrent use of levocetirizine dihydrochloride with other central nervous system depressants should be avoided because additional reductions in alertness and additional impairment of central nervous system performance may occur).
No products indexed under this heading.

Lorazepam (Concurrent use of levocetirizine dihydrochloride with other central nervous system depressants should be avoided because additional reductions in alertness and additional impairment of central nervous system performance may occur).
No products indexed under this heading.

Loxapine Hydrochloride (Concurrent use of levocetirizine dihydrochloride with other central nervous system depressants should be avoided because additional reductions in alertness and additional impairment of central nervous system performance may occur).
No products indexed under this heading.

Loxapine Succinate (Concurrent use of levocetirizine dihydrochloride with other central nervous system depressants should be avoided because additional reductions in alertness and additional impairment of central nervous system performance may occur).
No products indexed under this heading.

Meperidine Hydrochloride (Concurrent use of levocetirizine dihydrochloride with other central nervous system depressants should be avoided because additional reductions in alertness and additional impairment of central nervous system performance may occur).
No products indexed under this heading.

Mephobarbital (Concurrent use of levocetirizine dihydrochloride with other central nervous system depressants should be avoided because additional reductions in alertness and additional impairment of central nervous system performance may occur).
No products indexed under this heading.

Meprobamate (Concurrent use of levocetirizine dihydrochloride with other central nervous system depressants should be avoided because additional reductions in alertness and additional impairment of central nervous system performance may occur).
No products indexed under this heading.

Mesoridazine Besylate (Concurrent use of levocetirizine dihydrochloride with other central nervous system depressants should be avoided because additional reductions in alertness and additional impairment of central nervous system performance may occur).
No products indexed under this heading.

Methadone Hydrochloride (Concurrent use of levocetirizine dihydrochloride with other central nervous system depressants should be avoided because additional reductions in alertness and additional impairment of central nervous system performance may occur).
No products indexed under this heading.

Methohexital Sodium (Concurrent use of levocetirizine dihydrochloride with other central nervous system depressants should be avoided because additional reductions in alertness and additional impairment of central nervous system performance may occur).
No products indexed under this heading.

Methotrimeprazine (Concurrent use of levocetirizine dihydrochloride with other central nervous system depressants should be avoided because additional reductions in alertness and additional impairment of central nervous system performance may occur).
No products indexed under this heading.

Methoxyflurane (Concurrent use of levocetirizine dihydrochloride with other central nervous system depressants should be avoided because additional reductions in alertness and additional impairment of central nervous system performance may occur).
No products indexed under this heading.

Midazolam Hydrochloride (Concurrent use of levocetirizine dihydrochloride with other central nervous system depressants should be avoided because additional reductions in alertness and additional impairment of central nervous system performance may occur).
No products indexed under this heading.

Molindone Hydrochloride (Concurrent use of levocetirizine dihydrochloride with other central nervous system depressants should be avoided because additional reductions in alertness and additional impairment of central nervous system performance may occur). Products include:

Morphine Sulfate (Concurrent use of levocetirizine dihydrochloride with other central nervous system depressants should be avoided because additional reductions in alertness and additional impairment of central nervous system performance may occur). Products include:

Morphine Sulfate, Liposomal (Concurrent use of levocetirizine dihydrochloride with other central nervous system depressants should be avoided because additional reductions in alertness and additional impairment of central nervous system performance may occur).
No products indexed under this heading.

Olanzapine (Concurrent use of levocetirizine dihydrochloride with other central nervous system depressants should be avoided because additional reductions in alertness and additional impairment of central nervous system performance may occur). Products include:

Oxazepam (Concurrent use of levocetirizine dihydrochloride with other central nervous system depressants should be avoided because additional reductions in alertness and additional impairment of central nervous system performance may occur).
No products indexed under this heading.

Oxycodone Hydrochloride (Concurrent use of levocetirizine dihydrochloride with other central nervous system depressants should be avoided because additional reductions in alertness and additional impairment of central nervous system performance may occur). Products include:

2115 Interactions Index Xyzal

Oxycodone Terephthalate (Concurrent use of levocetirizine dihydrochloride with other central nervous system depressants should be avoided because additional reductions in alertness and additional impairment of central nervous system performance may occur).
No products indexed under this heading.

Oxymorphone Hydrochloride (Concurrent use of levocetirizine dihydrochloride with other central nervous system depressants should be avoided because additional reductions in alertness and additional impairment of central nervous system performance may occur). Products include:
Opana 1110
Opana ER 1114

Pentobarbital (Concurrent use of levocetirizine dihydrochloride with other central nervous system depressants should be avoided because additional reductions in alertness and additional impairment of central nervous system performance may occur).
No products indexed under this heading.

Pentobarbital Sodium (Concurrent use of levocetirizine dihydrochloride with other central nervous system depressants should be avoided because additional reductions in alertness and additional impairment of central nervous system performance may occur). Products include:
Nembutal 2012

Perphenazine (Concurrent use of levocetirizine dihydrochloride with other central nervous system depressants should be avoided because additional reductions in alertness and additional impairment of central nervous system performance may occur).
No products indexed under this heading.

Phenobarbital (Concurrent use of levocetirizine dihydrochloride with other central nervous system depressants should be avoided because additional reductions in alertness and additional impairment of central nervous system performance may occur). Products include:
Donnatal 2711

Phenobarbital Sodium (Concurrent use of levocetirizine dihydrochloride with other central nervous system depressants should be avoided because additional reductions in alertness and additional impairment of central nervous system performance may occur).
No products indexed under this heading.

Prazepam (Concurrent use of levocetirizine dihydrochloride with other central nervous system depressants should be avoided because additional reductions in alertness and additional impairment of central nervous system performance may occur).
No products indexed under this heading.

Prochlorperazine (Concurrent use of levocetirizine dihydrochloride with other central nervous system depressants should be avoided because additional reductions in alertness and additional impairment of central nervous system performance may occur).
No products indexed under this heading.

Prochlorperazine Edisylate (Concurrent use of levocetirizine dihydrochloride with other central nervous system depressants should be avoided because additional reductions in alertness and additional impairment of central nervous system performance may occur).
No products indexed under this heading.

Prochlorperazine Maleate (Concurrent use of levocetirizine dihydrochloride with other central nervous system depressants should be avoided because additional reductions in alertness and additional impairment of central nervous system performance may occur).
No products indexed under this heading.

Promethazine (Concurrent use of levocetirizine dihydrochloride with other central nervous system depressants should be avoided because additional reductions in alertness and additional impairment of central nervous system performance may occur).
No products indexed under this heading.

Promethazine Hydrochloride (Concurrent use of levocetirizine dihydrochloride with other central nervous system depressants should be avoided because additional reductions in alertness and additional impairment of central nervous system performance may occur).
No products indexed under this heading.

Propofol (Concurrent use of levocetirizine dihydrochloride with other central nervous system depressants should be avoided because additional reductions in alertness and additional impairment of central nervous system performance may occur).
No products indexed under this heading.

Propoxyphene Hydrochloride (Concurrent use of levocetirizine dihydrochloride with other central nervous system depressants should be avoided because additional reductions in alertness and additional impairment of central nervous system performance may occur).
No products indexed under this heading.

Propoxyphene Napsylate (Concurrent use of levocetirizine dihydrochloride with other central nervous system depressants should be avoided because additional reductions in alertness and additional impairment of central nervous system performance may occur).
No products indexed under this heading.

Quazepam (Concurrent use of levocetirizine dihydrochloride with other central nervous system depressants should be avoided because additional reductions in alertness and additional impairment of central nervous system performance may occur).
No products indexed under this heading.

Quetiapine Fumarate (Concurrent use of levocetirizine dihydrochloride with other central nervous system depressants should be avoided because additional reductions in alertness and additional impairment of central nervous system performance may occur). Products include:
Seroquel 750
Seroquel XR 759

Remifentanil Hydrochloride (Concurrent use of levocetirizine dihydrochloride with other central nervous system depressants should be avoided because additional reductions in alertness and additional impairment of central nervous system performance may occur).
No products indexed under this heading.

Risperidone (Concurrent use of levocetirizine dihydrochloride with other central nervous system depressants should be avoided because additional reductions in alertness and additional impairment of central nervous system performance may occur). Products include:
Risperdal Consta 2682

Ritonavir (Ritonavir increased the plasma AUC of cetirizine by about 42% accompanied by an increase in half-life (53%) and a decrease in clearance (29%) of cetirizine. The disposition of ritonavir was not altered by concomitant cetirizine administration). Products include:
Kaletra 458
Norvir 509

Secobarbital Sodium (Concurrent use of levocetirizine dihydrochloride with other central nervous system depressants should be avoided because additional reductions in alertness and additional impairment of central nervous system performance may occur).
No products indexed under this heading.

Sevoflurane (Concurrent use of levocetirizine dihydrochloride with other central nervous system depressants should be avoided because additional reductions in alertness and additional impairment of central nervous system performance may occur). Products include:
Ultane 554

Sodium Butabarbital (Concurrent use of levocetirizine dihydrochloride with other central nervous system depressants should be avoided because additional reductions in alertness and additional impairment of central nervous system performance may occur).
No products indexed under this heading.

Sodium Oxybate (Concurrent use of levocetirizine dihydrochloride with other central nervous system depressants should be avoided because additional reductions in alertness and additional impairment of central nervous system performance may occur).
No products indexed under this heading.

Sodium Pentobarbital (Concurrent use of levocetirizine dihydrochloride with other central nervous system depressants should be avoided because additional reductions in alertness and additional impairment of central nervous system performance may occur).
No products indexed under this heading.

Sufentanil Citrate (Concurrent use of levocetirizine dihydrochloride with other central nervous system depressants should be avoided because additional reductions in alertness and additional impairment of central nervous system performance may occur).
No products indexed under this heading.

Talbutal (Concurrent use of levocetirizine dihydrochloride with other central nervous system depressants should be avoided because additional reductions in alertness and additional impairment of central nervous system performance may occur).
No products indexed under this heading.

Temazepam (Concurrent use of levocetirizine dihydrochloride with other central nervous system depressants should be avoided because additional reductions in alertness and additional impairment of central nervous system performance may occur).
No products indexed under this heading.

Theophylline (There was a small decrease (approximately 16%) in the clearance of cetirizine caused by a 400 mg dose of theophylline. It is possible that higher theophylline doses could have a greater effect).
No products indexed under this heading.

Theophylline Anhydrous (There was a small decrease (approximately 16%) in the clearance of cetirizine caused by a 400 mg dose of theophylline. It is possible that higher theophylline doses could have a greater effect). Products include:
Uniphyl 2817

Theophylline Calcium Salicylate (There was a small decrease (approximately 16%) in the clearance of cetirizine caused by a 400 mg dose of theophylline. It is possible that higher theophylline doses could have a greater effect).
No products indexed under this heading.

Theophylline Dihydroxypropyl (Glyceryl) (There was a small decrease (approximately 16%) in the clearance of cetirizine caused by a 400 mg dose of theophylline. It is possible that higher theophylline doses could have a greater effect).
No products indexed under this heading.

Theophylline Ethylenediamine (There was a small decrease (approximately 16%) in the clearance of cetirizine caused by a 400 mg dose of theophylline. It is possible that higher theophylline doses could have a greater effect).
No products indexed under this heading.

Theophylline Sodium Glycinate (There was a small decrease (approximately 16%) in the clearance of cetirizine caused by a 400 mg dose of theophylline. It is possible that higher theophylline doses could have a greater effect).
No products indexed under this heading.

Thiamylal Sodium (Concurrent use of levocetirizine dihydrochloride with other central nervous system depressants should be avoided because additional reductions in alertness and additional impairment of central nervous system performance may occur).
No products indexed under this heading.

Thioridazine (Concurrent use of levocetirizine dihydrochloride with other central nervous system depressants should be avoided because additional reductions in alertness and additional impairment of central nervous system performance may occur).
No products indexed under this heading.

Thioridazine Hydrochloride (Concurrent use of levocetirizine dihydrochloride with other central nervous system depressants should be avoided because additional reductions in alertness and additional impairment of central nervous system performance may occur). Products include:
Thioridazine Hydrochloride 2384

Thiothixene (Concurrent use of levocetirizine dihydrochloride with other central nervous system depressants should be avoided because additional reductions in alertness and additional impairment of central nervous system performance may occur). Products include:
Thiothixene 2386

Thiothixene Hydrochloride (Concurrent use of levocetirizine dihydrochloride with other central nervous system depressants should be avoided because additional reductions in alertness and additional impairment of central nervous system performance may occur).
No products indexed under this heading.

Triazolam (Concurrent use of levocetirizine dihydrochloride with other central nervous system depressants should be avoided because additional reductions in alertness and additional impairment of central nervous system performance may occur).
No products indexed under this heading.

Trifluoperazine Hydrochloride (Concurrent use of levocetirizine dihydrochloride with other central nervous system depressants should be avoided because additional reductions in alertness and additional impairment of central nervous system performance may occur).
No products indexed under this heading.

IMPORTANT NOTE: Always consult each drug listing in the patient's regimen for possible interactions.

Zaleplon (Concurrent use of levocetirizine dihydrochloride with other central nervous system depressants should be avoided because additional reductions in alertness and additional impairment of central nervous system performance may occur).
No products indexed under this heading.

Ziprasidone Hydrochloride (Concurrent use of levocetirizine dihydrochloride with other central nervous system depressants should be avoided because additional reductions in alertness and additional impairment of central nervous system performance may occur). Products include:
Geodon 2723

Zolpidem Tartrate (Concurrent use of levocetirizine dihydrochloride with other central nervous system depressants should be avoided because additional reductions in alertness and additional impairment of central nervous system performance may occur). Products include:
Ambien 2920
Ambien CR 2925

Food Interactions

Alcohol (Concurrent use of levocetirizine dihydrochloride with other central nervous system depressants should be avoided because additional reductions in alertness and additional impairment of central nervous system performance may occur).

Beer, reduced-alcohol (Concurrent use of levocetirizine dihydrochloride with alcohol should be avoided because additional reductions in alertness and additional impairment of central nervous system performance may occur).

Beer, unspecified (Concurrent use of levocetirizine dihydrochloride with alcohol should be avoided because additional reductions in alertness and additional impairment of central nervous system performance may occur).

Wine, Chianti (Concurrent use of levocetirizine dihydrochloride with alcohol should be avoided because additional reductions in alertness and additional impairment of central nervous system performance may occur).

Wine, Red (Concurrent use of levocetirizine dihydrochloride with alcohol should be avoided because additional reductions in alertness and additional impairment of central nervous system performance may occur).

Wine, unspecified (Concurrent use of levocetirizine dihydrochloride with alcohol should be avoided because additional reductions in alertness and additional impairment of central nervous system performance may occur).

Wine products (Concurrent use of levocetirizine dihydrochloride with alcohol should be avoided because additional reductions in alertness and additional impairment of central nervous system performance may occur).

XYZAL ORAL SOLUTION
(Levocetirizine Dihydrochloride) 3053
May interact with alcohols, central nervous system depressants, theophyllines, and certain other agents. Compounds in these categories include:

Alfentanil Hydrochloride (Concurrent use of levocetirizine dihydrochloride with other central nervous system depressants should be avoided because additional reductions in alertness and additional impairment of central nervous system performance may occur).
No products indexed under this heading.

Alprazolam (Concurrent use of levocetirizine dihydrochloride with other central nervous system depressants should be avoided because additional reductions in alertness and additional impairment of central nervous system performance may occur).
No products indexed under this heading.

Amobarbital (Concurrent use of levocetirizine dihydrochloride with other central nervous system depressants should be avoided because additional reductions in alertness and additional impairment of central nervous system performance may occur).
No products indexed under this heading.

Amobarbital Sodium (Concurrent use of levocetirizine dihydrochloride with other central nervous system depressants should be avoided because additional reductions in alertness and additional impairment of central nervous system performance may occur).
No products indexed under this heading.

Aprobarbital (Concurrent use of levocetirizine dihydrochloride with other central nervous system depressants should be avoided because additional reductions in alertness and additional impairment of central nervous system performance may occur).
No products indexed under this heading.

Buprenorphine Hydrochloride (Concurrent use of levocetirizine dihydrochloride with other central nervous system depressants should be avoided because additional reductions in alertness and additional impairment of central nervous system performance may occur).
No products indexed under this heading.

Buspirone Hydrochloride (Concurrent use of levocetirizine dihydrochloride with other central nervous system depressants should be avoided because additional reductions in alertness and additional impairment of central nervous system performance may occur).
No products indexed under this heading.

Butabarbital (Concurrent use of levocetirizine dihydrochloride with other central nervous system depressants should be avoided because additional reductions in alertness and additional impairment of central nervous system performance may occur).
No products indexed under this heading.

Butabarbital Sodium (Concurrent use of levocetirizine dihydrochloride with other central nervous system depressants should be avoided because additional reductions in alertness and additional impairment of central nervous system performance may occur).
No products indexed under this heading.

Butalbital (Concurrent use of levocetirizine dihydrochloride with other central nervous system depressants should be avoided because additional reductions in alertness and additional impairment of central nervous system performance may occur).
No products indexed under this heading.

Chlordiazepoxide (Concurrent use of levocetirizine dihydrochloride with other central nervous system depressants should be avoided because additional reductions in alertness and additional impairment of central nervous system performance may occur).
No products indexed under this heading.

Chlordiazepoxide Hydrochloride (Concurrent use of levocetirizine dihydrochloride with other central nervous system depressants should be avoided because additional reductions in alertness and additional impairment of central nervous system performance may occur).
No products indexed under this heading.

Chlorpromazine (Concurrent use of levocetirizine dihydrochloride with other central nervous system depressants should be avoided because additional reductions in alertness and additional impairment of central nervous system performance may occur).
No products indexed under this heading.

Chlorpromazine Hydrochloride (Concurrent use of levocetirizine dihydrochloride with other central nervous system depressants should be avoided because additional reductions in alertness and additional impairment of central nervous system performance may occur).
No products indexed under this heading.

Chlorprothixene (Concurrent use of levocetirizine dihydrochloride with other central nervous system depressants should be avoided because additional reductions in alertness and additional impairment of central nervous system performance may occur).
No products indexed under this heading.

Chlorprothixene Hydrochloride (Concurrent use of levocetirizine dihydrochloride with other central nervous system depressants should be avoided because additional reductions in alertness and additional impairment of central nervous system performance may occur).
No products indexed under this heading.

Chlorprothixene Lactate (Concurrent use of levocetirizine dihydrochloride with other central nervous system depressants should be avoided because additional reductions in alertness and additional impairment of central nervous system performance may occur).
No products indexed under this heading.

Clonazepam (Concurrent use of levocetirizine dihydrochloride with other central nervous system depressants should be avoided because additional reductions in alertness and additional impairment of central nervous system performance may occur). Products include:
Klonopin 2855

Clorazepate Dipotassium (Concurrent use of levocetirizine dihydrochloride with other central nervous system depressants should be avoided because additional reductions in alertness and additional impairment of central nervous system performance may occur).
No products indexed under this heading.

Clozapine (Concurrent use of levocetirizine dihydrochloride with other central nervous system depressants should be avoided because additional reductions in alertness and additional impairment of central nervous system performance may occur).
No products indexed under this heading.

Codeine Phosphate (Concurrent use of levocetirizine dihydrochloride with other central nervous system depressants should be avoided because additional reductions in alertness and additional impairment of central nervous system performance may occur). Products include:
Tylenol with Codeine 2691

Codeine Sulfate (Concurrent use of levocetirizine dihydrochloride with other central nervous system depressants should be avoided because additional reductions in alertness and additional impairment of central nervous system performance may occur).
No products indexed under this heading.

Desflurane (Concurrent use of levocetirizine dihydrochloride with other central nervous system depressants should be avoided because additional reductions in alertness and additional impairment of central nervous system performance may occur).
No products indexed under this heading.

Dezocine (Concurrent use of levocetirizine dihydrochloride with other central nervous system depressants should be avoided because additional reductions in alertness and additional impairment of central nervous system performance may occur).
No products indexed under this heading.

Diazepam (Concurrent use of levocetirizine dihydrochloride with other central nervous system depressants should be avoided because additional reductions in alertness and additional impairment of central nervous system performance may occur). Products include:
Valium Tablets 2880

Droperidol (Concurrent use of levocetirizine dihydrochloride with other central nervous system depressants should be avoided because additional reductions in alertness and additional impairment of central nervous system performance may occur).
No products indexed under this heading.

Enflurane (Concurrent use of levocetirizine dihydrochloride with other central nervous system depressants should be avoided because additional reductions in alertness and additional impairment of central nervous system performance may occur).
No products indexed under this heading.

Estazolam (Concurrent use of levocetirizine dihydrochloride with other central nervous system depressants should be avoided because additional reductions in alertness and additional impairment of central nervous system performance may occur).
No products indexed under this heading.

Ethanol (Concurrent use of levocetirizine dihydrochloride with other central nervous system depressants should be avoided because additional reductions in alertness and additional impairment of central nervous system performance may occur).
No products indexed under this heading.

Ethchlorvynol (Concurrent use of levocetirizine dihydrochloride with other central nervous system depressants should be avoided because additional reductions in alertness and additional impairment of central nervous system performance may occur).
No products indexed under this heading.

Ethinamate (Concurrent use of levocetirizine dihydrochloride with other central nervous system depressants should be avoided because additional reductions in alertness and additional impairment of central nervous system performance may occur).
No products indexed under this heading.

Ethyl Alcohol (Concurrent use of levocetirizine dihydrochloride with other central nervous system depressants should be avoided because additional reductions in alertness and additional impairment of central nervous system performance may occur).
No products indexed under this heading.

Fentanyl (Concurrent use of levocetirizine dihydrochloride with other central nervous system depressants should be

avoided because additional reductions in alertness and additional impairment of central nervous system performance may occur). Products include:

Fentanyl Citrate (Concurrent use of levocetirizine dihydrochloride with other central nervous system depressants should be avoided because additional reductions in alertness and additional impairment of central nervous system performance may occur). Products include:

Fluphenazine Decanoate (Concurrent use of levocetirizine dihydrochloride with other central nervous system depressants should be avoided because additional reductions in alertness and additional impairment of central nervous system performance may occur).

No products indexed under this heading.

Fluphenazine Enanthate (Concurrent use of levocetirizine dihydrochloride with other central nervous system depressants should be avoided because additional reductions in alertness and additional impairment of central nervous system performance may occur).

No products indexed under this heading.

Fluphenazine Hydrochloride (Concurrent use of levocetirizine dihydrochloride with other central nervous system depressants should be avoided because additional reductions in alertness and additional impairment of central nervous system performance may occur).

No products indexed under this heading.

Flurazepam Hydrochloride (Concurrent use of levocetirizine dihydrochloride with other central nervous system depressants should be avoided because additional reductions in alertness and additional impairment of central nervous system performance may occur).

No products indexed under this heading.

Glutethimide (Concurrent use of levocetirizine dihydrochloride with other central nervous system depressants should be avoided because additional reductions in alertness and additional impairment of central nervous system performance may occur).

No products indexed under this heading.

Halazepam (Concurrent use of levocetirizine dihydrochloride with other central nervous system depressants should be avoided because additional reductions in alertness and additional impairment of central nervous system performance may occur).

No products indexed under this heading.

Haloperidol (Concurrent use of levocetirizine dihydrochloride with other central nervous system depressants should be avoided because additional reductions in alertness and additional impairment of central nervous system performance may occur).

No products indexed under this heading.

Haloperidol Decanoate (Concurrent use of levocetirizine dihydrochloride with other central nervous system depressants should be avoided because additional reductions in alertness and additional impairment of central nervous system performance may occur).

No products indexed under this heading.

Haloperidol Lactate (Concurrent use of levocetirizine dihydrochloride with other central nervous system depressants should be avoided because additional reductions in alertness and additional impairment of central nervous system performance may occur).

No products indexed under this heading.

Hexobarbital (Concurrent use of levocetirizine dihydrochloride with other central nervous system depressants should be avoided because additional reductions in alertness and additional impairment of central nervous system performance may occur).

No products indexed under this heading.

Hydrocodone Bitartrate (Concurrent use of levocetirizine dihydrochloride with other central nervous system depressants should be avoided because additional reductions in alertness and additional impairment of central nervous system performance may occur). Products include:

Hydrocodone Polistirex (Concurrent use of levocetirizine dihydrochloride with other central nervous system depressants should be avoided because additional reductions in alertness and additional impairment of central nervous system performance may occur). Products include:

Hydromorphone (Concurrent use of levocetirizine dihydrochloride with other central nervous system depressants should be avoided because additional reductions in alertness and additional impairment of central nervous system performance may occur).

No products indexed under this heading.

Hydromorphone Hydrochloride (Concurrent use of levocetirizine dihydrochloride with other central nervous system depressants should be avoided because additional reductions in alertness and additional impairment of central nervous system performance may occur). Products include:

Hydroxyzine Hydrochloride (Concurrent use of levocetirizine dihydrochloride with other central nervous system depressants should be avoided because additional reductions in alertness and additional impairment of central nervous system performance may occur).

No products indexed under this heading.

Isoflurane (Concurrent use of levocetirizine dihydrochloride with other central nervous system depressants should be avoided because additional reductions in alertness and additional impairment of central nervous system performance may occur).

No products indexed under this heading.

Ketamine Hydrochloride (Concurrent use of levocetirizine dihydrochloride with other central nervous system depressants should be avoided because additional reductions in alertness and additional impairment of central nervous system performance may occur).

No products indexed under this heading.

Levomethadyl Acetate Hydrochloride (Concurrent use of levocetirizine dihydrochloride with other central nervous system depressants should be avoided because additional reductions in alertness and additional impairment of central nervous system performance may occur).

No products indexed under this heading.

Levorphanol Tartrate (Concurrent use of levocetirizine dihydrochloride with other central nervous system depressants should be avoided because additional reductions in alertness and additional impairment of central nervous system performance may occur).

No products indexed under this heading.

Lorazepam (Concurrent use of levocetirizine dihydrochloride with other central nervous system depressants should be avoided because additional reductions in alertness and additional impairment of central nervous system performance may occur).

No products indexed under this heading.

Loxapine Hydrochloride (Concurrent use of levocetirizine dihydrochloride with other central nervous system depressants should be avoided because additional reductions in alertness and additional impairment of central nervous system performance may occur).

No products indexed under this heading.

Loxapine Succinate (Concurrent use of levocetirizine dihydrochloride with other central nervous system depressants should be avoided because additional reductions in alertness and additional impairment of central nervous system performance may occur).

No products indexed under this heading.

Meperidine Hydrochloride (Concurrent use of levocetirizine dihydrochloride with other central nervous system depressants should be avoided because additional reductions in alertness and additional impairment of central nervous system performance may occur).

No products indexed under this heading.

Mephobarbital (Concurrent use of levocetirizine dihydrochloride with other central nervous system depressants should be avoided because additional reductions in alertness and additional impairment of central nervous system performance may occur).

No products indexed under this heading.

Meprobamate (Concurrent use of levocetirizine dihydrochloride with other central nervous system depressants should be avoided because additional reductions in alertness and additional impairment of central nervous system performance may occur).

No products indexed under this heading.

Mesoridazine Besylate (Concurrent use of levocetirizine dihydrochloride with other central nervous system depressants should be avoided because additional reductions in alertness and additional impairment of central nervous system performance may occur).

No products indexed under this heading.

Methadone Hydrochloride (Concurrent use of levocetirizine dihydrochloride with other central nervous system depressants should be avoided because additional reductions in alertness and additional impairment of central nervous system performance may occur).

No products indexed under this heading.

Methohexital Sodium (Concurrent use of levocetirizine dihydrochloride with other central nervous system depressants should be avoided because additional reductions in alertness and additional impairment of central nervous system performance may occur).

No products indexed under this heading.

Methotrimeprazine (Concurrent use of levocetirizine dihydrochloride with other central nervous system depressants should be avoided because additional reductions in alertness and additional impairment of central nervous system performance may occur).

No products indexed under this heading.

Methoxyflurane (Concurrent use of levocetirizine dihydrochloride with other central nervous system depressants should be avoided because additional reductions in alertness and additional impairment of central nervous system performance may occur).

No products indexed under this heading.

Midazolam Hydrochloride (Concurrent use of levocetirizine dihydrochloride with other central nervous system depressants should be avoided because additional reductions in alertness and additional impairment of central nervous system performance may occur).

No products indexed under this heading.

Molindone Hydrochloride (Concurrent use of levocetirizine dihydrochloride with other central nervous system depressants should be avoided because additional reductions in alertness and additional impairment of central nervous system performance may occur). Products include:

Morphine Sulfate (Concurrent use of levocetirizine dihydrochloride with other central nervous system depressants should be avoided because additional reductions in alertness and additional impairment of central nervous system performance may occur). Products include:

Morphine Sulfate, Liposomal (Concurrent use of levocetirizine dihydrochloride with other central nervous system depressants should be avoided because additional reductions in alertness and additional impairment of central nervous system performance may occur).

No products indexed under this heading.

Olanzapine (Concurrent use of levocetirizine dihydrochloride with other central nervous system depressants should be avoided because additional reductions in alertness and additional impairment of central nervous system performance may occur). Products include:

Oxazepam (Concurrent use of levocetirizine dihydrochloride with other central nervous system depressants should be avoided because additional reductions in alertness and additional impairment of central nervous system performance may occur).

No products indexed under this heading.

Oxycodone Hydrochloride (Concurrent use of levocetirizine dihydrochloride with other central nervous system depressants should be avoided because additional reductions in alertness and additional impairment of central nervous system performance may occur). Products include:

IMPORTANT NOTE: Always consult each drug listing in the patient's regimen for possible interactions.

Xyzal Interactions Index 2118

Percocet 1121
Percodan 1124

Oxycodone Terephthalate (Concurrent use of levocetirizine dihydrochloride with other central nervous system depressants should be avoided because additional reductions in alertness and additional impairment of central nervous system performance may occur).
No products indexed under this heading.

Oxymorphone Hydrochloride (Concurrent use of levocetirizine dihydrochloride with other central nervous system depressants should be avoided because additional reductions in alertness and additional impairment of central nervous system performance may occur). Products include:
Opana 1110
Opana ER 1114

Pentobarbital (Concurrent use of levocetirizine dihydrochloride with other central nervous system depressants should be avoided because additional reductions in alertness and additional impairment of central nervous system performance may occur).
No products indexed under this heading.

Pentobarbital Sodium (Concurrent use of levocetirizine dihydrochloride with other central nervous system depressants should be avoided because additional reductions in alertness and additional impairment of central nervous system performance may occur). Products include:
Nembutal 2012

Perphenazine (Concurrent use of levocetirizine dihydrochloride with other central nervous system depressants should be avoided because additional reductions in alertness and additional impairment of central nervous system performance may occur).
No products indexed under this heading.

Phenobarbital (Concurrent use of levocetirizine dihydrochloride with other central nervous system depressants should be avoided because additional reductions in alertness and additional impairment of central nervous system performance may occur). Products include:
Donnatal 2711

Phenobarbital Sodium (Concurrent use of levocetirizine dihydrochloride with other central nervous system depressants should be avoided because additional reductions in alertness and additional impairment of central nervous system performance may occur).
No products indexed under this heading.

Prazepam (Concurrent use of levocetirizine dihydrochloride with other central nervous system depressants should be avoided because additional reductions in alertness and additional impairment of central nervous system performance may occur).
No products indexed under this heading.

Prochlorperazine (Concurrent use of levocetirizine dihydrochloride with other central nervous system depressants should be avoided because additional reductions in alertness and additional impairment of central nervous system performance may occur).
No products indexed under this heading.

Prochlorperazine Edisylate (Concurrent use of levocetirizine dihydrochloride with other central nervous system depressants should be avoided because additional reductions in alertness and additional impairment of central nervous system performance may occur).
No products indexed under this heading.

Prochlorperazine Maleate (Concurrent use of levocetirizine dihydrochloride with other central nervous system depressants should be avoided because additional reductions in alertness and additional impairment of central nervous system performance may occur).
No products indexed under this heading.

Promethazine (Concurrent use of levocetirizine dihydrochloride with other central nervous system depressants should be avoided because additional reductions in alertness and additional impairment of central nervous system performance may occur).
No products indexed under this heading.

Promethazine Hydrochloride (Concurrent use of levocetirizine dihydrochloride with other central nervous system depressants should be avoided because additional reductions in alertness and additional impairment of central nervous system performance may occur).
No products indexed under this heading.

Propofol (Concurrent use of levocetirizine dihydrochloride with other central nervous system depressants should be avoided because additional reductions in alertness and additional impairment of central nervous system performance may occur).
No products indexed under this heading.

Propoxyphene Hydrochloride (Concurrent use of levocetirizine dihydrochloride with other central nervous system depressants should be avoided because additional reductions in alertness and additional impairment of central nervous system performance may occur).
No products indexed under this heading.

Propoxyphene Napsylate (Concurrent use of levocetirizine dihydrochloride with other central nervous system depressants should be avoided because additional reductions in alertness and additional impairment of central nervous system performance may occur).
No products indexed under this heading.

Quazepam (Concurrent use of levocetirizine dihydrochloride with other central nervous system depressants should be avoided because additional reductions in alertness and additional impairment of central nervous system performance may occur).
No products indexed under this heading.

Quetiapine Fumarate (Concurrent use of levocetirizine dihydrochloride with other central nervous system depressants should be avoided because additional reductions in alertness and additional impairment of central nervous system performance may occur). Products include:
Seroquel 750
Seroquel XR 759

Remifentanil Hydrochloride (Concurrent use of levocetirizine dihydrochloride with other central nervous system depressants should be avoided because additional reductions in alertness and additional impairment of central nervous system performance may occur).
No products indexed under this heading.

Risperidone (Concurrent use of levocetirizine dihydrochloride with other central nervous system depressants should be avoided because additional reductions in alertness and additional impairment of central nervous system performance may occur). Products include:
Risperdal Consta 2682

Ritonavir (Ritonavir increased the plasma AUC of cetirizine by about 42% accompanied by an increase in half-life (53%) and a decrease in clearance (29%) of cetirizine. The disposition of ritonavir was not altered by concomitant cetirizine administration). Products include:
Kaletra 458
Norvir 509

Secobarbital Sodium (Concurrent use of levocetirizine dihydrochloride with other central nervous system depressants should be avoided because additional reductions in alertness and additional impairment of central nervous system performance may occur).
No products indexed under this heading.

Sevoflurane (Concurrent use of levocetirizine dihydrochloride with other central nervous system depressants should be avoided because additional reductions in alertness and additional impairment of central nervous system performance may occur). Products include:
Ultane 554

Sodium Butabarbital (Concurrent use of levocetirizine dihydrochloride with other central nervous system depressants should be avoided because additional reductions in alertness and additional impairment of central nervous system performance may occur).
No products indexed under this heading.

Sodium Oxybate (Concurrent use of levocetirizine dihydrochloride with other central nervous system depressants should be avoided because additional reductions in alertness and additional impairment of central nervous system performance may occur).
No products indexed under this heading.

Sodium Pentobarbital (Concurrent use of levocetirizine dihydrochloride with other central nervous system depressants should be avoided because additional reductions in alertness and additional impairment of central nervous system performance may occur).
No products indexed under this heading.

Sufentanil Citrate (Concurrent use of levocetirizine dihydrochloride with other central nervous system depressants should be avoided because additional reductions in alertness and additional impairment of central nervous system performance may occur).
No products indexed under this heading.

Talbutal (Concurrent use of levocetirizine dihydrochloride with other central nervous system depressants should be avoided because additional reductions in alertness and additional impairment of central nervous system performance may occur).
No products indexed under this heading.

Temazepam (Concurrent use of levocetirizine dihydrochloride with other central nervous system depressants should be avoided because additional reductions in alertness and additional impairment of central nervous system performance may occur).
No products indexed under this heading.

Theophylline (There was a small decrease (approximately 16%) in the clearance of cetirizine caused by a 400 mg dose of theophylline. It is possible that higher theophylline doses could have greater effect).
No products indexed under this heading.

Theophylline Anhydrous (There was a small decrease (approximately 16%) in the clearance of cetirizine caused by a 400 mg dose of theophylline. It is possible that higher theophylline doses could have greater effect). Products include:
Uniphyl 2817

Theophylline Calcium Salicylate (There was a small decrease (approximately 16%) in the clearance of cetirizine caused by a 400 mg dose of theophylline. It is possible that higher theophylline doses could have greater effect).
No products indexed under this heading.

Theophylline Dihydroxypropyl (Glyceryl) (There was a small decrease (approximately 16%) in the clearance of cetirizine caused by a 400 mg dose of theophylline. It is possible that higher theophylline doses could have greater effect).
No products indexed under this heading.

Theophylline Ethylenediamine (There was a small decrease (approximately 16%) in the clearance of cetirizine caused by a 400 mg dose of theophylline. It is possible that higher theophylline doses could have greater effect).
No products indexed under this heading.

Theophylline Sodium Glycinate (There was a small decrease (approximately 16%) in the clearance of cetirizine caused by a 400 mg dose of theophylline. It is possible that higher theophylline doses could have greater effect).
No products indexed under this heading.

Thiamylal Sodium (Concurrent use of levocetirizine dihydrochloride with other central nervous system depressants should be avoided because additional reductions in alertness and additional impairment of central nervous system performance may occur).
No products indexed under this heading.

Thioridazine (Concurrent use of levocetirizine dihydrochloride with other central nervous system depressants should be avoided because additional reductions in alertness and additional impairment of central nervous system performance may occur).
No products indexed under this heading.

Thioridazine Hydrochloride (Concurrent use of levocetirizine dihydrochloride with other central nervous system depressants should be avoided because additional reductions in alertness and additional impairment of central nervous system performance may occur). Products include:
Thioridazine Hydrochloride 2384

Thiothixene (Concurrent use of levocetirizine dihydrochloride with other central nervous system depressants should be avoided because additional reductions in alertness and additional impairment of central nervous system performance may occur). Products include:
Thiothixene 2386

Thiothixene Hydrochloride (Concurrent use of levocetirizine dihydrochloride with other central nervous system depressants should be avoided because additional reductions in alertness and additional impairment of central nervous system performance may occur).
No products indexed under this heading.

Triazolam (Concurrent use of levocetirizine dihydrochloride with other central nervous system depressants should be avoided because additional reductions in alertness and additional impairment of central nervous system performance may occur).
No products indexed under this heading.

Trifluoperazine Hydrochloride (Concurrent use of levocetirizine dihydrochloride with other central nervous system depressants should be avoided because additional reductions in alertness and additional impairment of central nervous system performance may occur).
No products indexed under this heading.

Zaleplon (Concurrent use of levocetirizine dihydrochloride with other central nervous system depressants should be avoided because additional reductions in alertness and additional impairment of central nervous system performance may occur).

No products indexed under this heading.

Ziprasidone Hydrochloride (Concurrent use of levocetirizine dihydrochloride with other central nervous system depressants should be avoided because additional reductions in alertness and additional impairment of central nervous system performance may occur). Products include:

Geodon 2723

Zolpidem Tartrate (Concurrent use of levocetirizine dihydrochloride with other central nervous system depressants should be avoided because additional reductions in alertness and additional impairment of central nervous system performance may occur). Products include:

Ambien 2920
Ambien CR 2925

Food Interactions

Alcohol (Concurrent use of levocetirizine dihydrochloride with other central nervous system depressants should be avoided because additional reductions in alertness and additional impairment of central nervous system performance may occur).

Beer, reduced-alcohol (Concurrent use of levocetirizine dihydrochloride with alcohol should be avoided because additional reductions in alertness and additional impairment of central nervous system performance may occur).

Beer, unspecified (Concurrent use of levocetirizine dihydrochloride with alcohol should be avoided because additional reductions in alertness and additional impairment of central nervous system performance may occur).

Wine, Chianti (Concurrent use of levocetirizine dihydrochloride with alcohol should be avoided because additional reductions in alertness and additional impairment of central nervous system performance may occur).

Wine, Red (Concurrent use of levocetirizine dihydrochloride with alcohol should be avoided because additional reductions in alertness and additional impairment of central nervous system performance may occur).

Wine, unspecified (Concurrent use of levocetirizine dihydrochloride with alcohol should be avoided because additional reductions in alertness and additional impairment of central nervous system performance may occur).

Wine products (Concurrent use of levocetirizine dihydrochloride with alcohol should be avoided because additional reductions in alertness and additional impairment of central nervous system performance may occur).

XYZAL TABLETS
(Levocetirizine Dihydrochloride) 3053
See Xyzal Oral Solution

XYZAL TABLETS
(Levocetirizine Dihydrochloride) 3449
See Xyzal Oral Solution

YAZ TABLETS
(Drospirenone, Ethinyl Estradiol) 864
May interact with ACE inhibitors, aldosterone-inhibiting diuretic agents, angiotensin-II receptor antagonists, anticonvulsants, non-steroidal anti-inflammatory agents, potassium preparations, potassium sparing diuretics, prednisolone, tetracyclines, theophyllines, and certain other agents. Compounds in these categories include:

Acetaminophen (Ascorbic acid and acetaminophen may increase plasma concentrations of some synthetic estrogens, possibly by inhibition of conjugation. Decreased plasma concentrations of acetaminophen have been noted when administered with oral contraceptives). Products include:

Percocet 1121
Tylenol 2049
Tylenol 8 Hour 2049
Extra Strength Tylenol Caplets, Cool Caplets, and EZ Tabs............ 2049
Extra Strength Tylenol Adult Rapid Blast Liquid.................................. 2049
Extra Strength Tylenol Rapid Release 2049
Tylenol with Codeine 2691
Tylenol Arthritis Pain Extended Release Geltabs/Caplets............ 2049
Children's Tylenol Suspension Liquid 2048
Children's Tylenol Meltaways 2048
Tylenol, Infants' Drops 2048
Junior Tylenol 2048
Vicodin 560
Vicodin ES 561
Vicodin HP 563
Zydone 1138

Amiloride Hydrochloride (YAZ has the potential to cause hyperkalemia in high-risk patients; co-administration with other drugs that have the potential to increase serum potassium, such as potassium-sparing diuretics, may increase the risk further).

No products indexed under this heading.

Ampicillin (Pregnancy while taking combined hormonal contraceptives has been reported when the combined hormonal contraceptives were administered with antimicrobials such as ampicillin).

No products indexed under this heading.

Ampicillin Sodium (Pregnancy while taking combined hormonal contraceptives has been reported when the combined hormonal contraceptives were administered with antimicrobials such as ampicillin).

No products indexed under this heading.

Ampicillin Trihydrate (Pregnancy while taking combined hormonal contraceptives has been reported when the combined hormonal contraceptives were administered with antimicrobials such as ampicillin).

No products indexed under this heading.

Ascorbic Acid (Ascorbic acid and acetaminophen may increase plasma concentrations of some synthetic estrogens, possibly by inhibition of conjugation).

No products indexed under this heading.

Atorvastatin Calcium (Co-administration of atorvastatin and an oral contraceptive increased AUC values for norethindrone and ethinyl estradiol by approximately 30% and 20%, respectively). Products include:

Lipitor 2703

Benazepril Hydrochloride (YAZ has the potential to cause hyperkalemia in high-risk patients; co-administration with other drugs that have the potential to increase serum potassium, such as ACE inhibitors, may increase the risk further).

No products indexed under this heading.

Candesartan Cilexetil (YAZ has the potential to cause hyperkalemia in high-risk patients; co-administration with other drugs that have the potential to increase serum potassium, such as angiotensin-II receptor antagonists, may increase the risk further). Products include:

Atacand 697
Atacand HCT 700

Captopril (YAZ has the potential to cause hyperkalemia in high-risk patients; co-administration with other

---

drugs that have the potential to increase serum potassium, such as ACE inhibitors, may increase the risk further). Products include:

Captopril 2341

Carbamazepine (Co-administration results in increased metabolism of ethinyl estradiol and/or some progestins which could result in a reduction of contraceptive effectiveness). Products include:

Carbatrol 3280
Equetro 3477

Celecoxib (YAZ has the potential to cause hyperkalemia in high-risk patients; co-administration with other drugs that have the potential to increase serum potassium, such as NSAIDs, may increase the risk further). Products include:

Celebrex 3272

Clofibrate (Co-administration of products containing ethinyl estradiol may increase clearance of clofibric acid).

No products indexed under this heading.

Clofibric Acid (Increased clearance of clofibric acid has been noted when administered with oral contraceptives).

No products indexed under this heading.

Cyclosporine (Increased plasma concentrations of cyclosporine have been reported with concomitant administration of oral contraceptives). Products include:

Gengraf 440
Neoral Oral Solution 2496
Neoral Capsules 2496
Restasis 605

Demeclocycline Hydrochloride (Pregnancy while taking combined hormonal contraceptives has been reported when the combined hormonal contraceptives were administered with antimicrobials such as tetracycline).

No products indexed under this heading.

Diclofenac Epolamine (YAZ has the potential to cause hyperkalemia in high-risk patients; co-administration with other drugs that have the potential to increase serum potassium, such as NSAIDs, may increase the risk further). Products include:

Flector 1839

Diclofenac Potassium (YAZ has the potential to cause hyperkalemia in high-risk patients; co-administration with other drugs that have the potential to increase serum potassium, such as NSAIDs, may increase the risk further).

No products indexed under this heading.

Diclofenac Sodium (YAZ has the potential to cause hyperkalemia in high-risk patients; co-administration with other drugs that have the potential to increase serum potassium, such as NSAIDs, may increase the risk further).

No products indexed under this heading.

Divalproex Sodium (Anticonvulsants have been shown to increase the metabolism of ethinyl estradiol and/or some progestins, which could result in a reduction of contraceptive effectiveness). Products include:

Depakote ER 426

Doxycycline (Pregnancy while taking combined hormonal contraceptives has been reported when the combined hormonal contraceptives were administered with antimicrobials such as tetracycline).

No products indexed under this heading.

Doxycycline Calcium (Pregnancy while taking combined hormonal contraceptives has been reported when the combined hormonal contraceptives were administered with antimicrobials such as tetracycline).

No products indexed under this heading.

Doxycycline Hyclate (Pregnancy while taking combined hormonal contraceptives has been reported when the combined hormonal contraceptives were administered with antimicrobials such as tetracycline).

No products indexed under this heading.

Doxycycline Monohydrate (Pregnancy while taking combined hormonal contraceptives has been reported when the combined hormonal contraceptives were administered with antimicrobials such as tetracycline).

No products indexed under this heading.

Enalapril Maleate (YAZ has the potential to cause hyperkalemia in high-risk patients; co-administration with other drugs that have the potential to increase serum potassium, such as ACE inhibitors, may increase the risk further).

No products indexed under this heading.

Enalaprilat (YAZ has the potential to cause hyperkalemia in high-risk patients; co-administration with other drugs that have the potential to increase serum potassium, such as ACE inhibitors, may increase the risk further).

No products indexed under this heading.

Eprosartan Mesylate (YAZ has the potential to cause hyperkalemia in high-risk patients; co-administration with other drugs that have the potential to increase serum potassium, such as angiotensin-II receptor antagonists, may increase the risk further). Products include:

Teveten 538
Teveten HCT 541

Ethosuximide (Anticonvulsants have been shown to increase the metabolism of ethinyl estradiol and/or some progestins, which could result in a reduction of contraceptive effectiveness).

No products indexed under this heading.

Ethotoin (Anticonvulsants have been shown to increase the metabolism of ethinyl estradiol and/or some progestins, which could result in a reduction of contraceptive effectiveness).

No products indexed under this heading.

Etodolac (YAZ has the potential to cause hyperkalemia in high-risk patients; co-administration with other drugs that have the potential to increase serum potassium, such as NSAIDs, may increase the risk further).

No products indexed under this heading.

Felbamate (Anticonvulsants have been shown to increase the metabolism of ethinyl estradiol and/or some progestins, which could result in a reduction of contraceptive effectiveness).

No products indexed under this heading.

Fenoprofen Calcium (YAZ has the potential to cause hyperkalemia in high-risk patients; co-administration with other drugs that have the potential to increase serum potassium, such as NSAIDs, may increase the risk further).

No products indexed under this heading.

Flurbiprofen (YAZ has the potential to cause hyperkalemia in high-risk patients; co-administration with other drugs that have the potential to increase serum potassium, such as NSAIDs, may increase the risk further).

No products indexed under this heading.

Fosinopril Sodium (YAZ has the potential to cause hyperkalemia in high-risk patients; co-administration with other drugs that have the potential to increase serum potassium, such as ACE inhibitors, may increase the risk further).

No products indexed under this heading.

IMPORTANT NOTE: Always consult each drug listing in the patient's regimen for possible interactions.

Yaz Interactions Index 2120

Fosphenytoin (Anticonvulsants have been shown to increase the metabolism of ethinyl estradiol and/or some progestins, which could result in a reduction of contraceptive effectiveness).
No products indexed under this heading.

Fosphenytoin Sodium (Anticonvulsants have been shown to increase the metabolism of ethinyl estradiol and/or some progestins, which could result in a reduction of contraceptive effectiveness).
No products indexed under this heading.

Gabapentin (Anticonvulsants have been shown to increase the metabolism of ethinyl estradiol and/or some progestins, which could result in a reduction of contraceptive effectiveness).
No products indexed under this heading.

Griseofulvin (Pregnancy while taking combined hormonal contraceptives has been reported when the combined hormonal contraceptives were administered with antimicrobials such as griseofulvin).
No products indexed under this heading.

Heparin Calcium (YAZ has the potential to cause hyperkalemia in high-risk patients; co-administration with other drugs that have the potential to increase serum potassium, such as heparin, may increase the risk further).
No products indexed under this heading.

Heparin Sodium (YAZ has the potential to cause hyperkalemia in high-risk patients; co-administration with other drugs that have the potential to increase serum potassium, such as heparin, may increase the risk further).
No products indexed under this heading.

Hypericum (Herbal products containing St. John's Wort may induce hepatic enzyme and p-glycoprotein transporter and may reduce the effectiveness of oral contraceptives and emergency contraceptive pills. This may also result in breakthrough bleeding).
No products indexed under this heading.

Hypericum Perforatum (Herbal products containing St. John's Wort may induce hepatic enzyme and p-glycoprotein transporter and may reduce the effectiveness of oral contraceptives and emergency contraceptive pills. This may also result in breakthrough bleeding). Products include:
Traumeel 1800

Ibuprofen (YAZ has the potential to cause hyperkalemia in high-risk patients; co-administration with other drugs that have the potential to increase serum potassium, such as NSAIDs, may increase the risk further). Products include:
Motrin IB 2043
Children's Motrin 2044
Children's Motrin Non-Staining Dye-Free 2044
Infants' Motrin 2044
Infants' Motrin Dye-Free 2044
Junior Strength Motrin 2044
Vicoprofen 564

Indomethacin (YAZ has the potential to cause hyperkalemia in high-risk patients; co-administration with other drugs that have the potential to increase serum potassium, such as NSAIDs, may increase the risk further). Products include:
Indocin 2167

Indomethacin Sodium Trihydrate (YAZ has the potential to cause hyperkalemia in high-risk patients; co-administration with other drugs that have the potential to increase serum potassium, such as NSAIDs, may increase the risk further). Products include:
Indocin I.V. 2007

Irbesartan (YAZ has the potential to cause hyperkalemia in high-risk patients; co-administration with other drugs that have the potential to increase serum potassium, such as angiotensin-II receptor antagonists, may increase the risk further). Products include:
Avalide 2956
Avapro 2962

Ketoprofen (YAZ has the potential to cause hyperkalemia in high-risk patients; co-administration with other drugs that have the potential to increase serum potassium, such as NSAIDs, may increase the risk further).
No products indexed under this heading.

Ketorolac Tromethamine (YAZ has the potential to cause hyperkalemia in high-risk patients; co-administration with other drugs that have the potential to increase serum potassium, such as NSAIDs, may increase the risk further). Products include:
Acuvail .... ⊙ 209

Lamotrigine (Anticonvulsants have been shown to increase the metabolism of ethinyl estradiol and/or some progestins, which could result in a reduction of contraceptive effectiveness). Products include:
Lamictal 1522
Lamictal ODT 1522
Lamictal XR 1536

Levetiracetam (Anticonvulsants have been shown to increase the metabolism of ethinyl estradiol and/or some progestins, which could result in a reduction of contraceptive effectiveness). Products include:
Keppra XR 3434

Lisinopril (YAZ has the potential to cause hyperkalemia in high-risk patients; co-administration with other drugs that have the potential to increase serum potassium, such as ACE inhibitors, may increase the risk further). Products include:
Prinivil 2241
Prinzide 2246

Losartan Potassium (YAZ has the potential to cause hyperkalemia in high-risk patients; co-administration with other drugs that have the potential to increase serum potassium, such as angiotensin-II receptor antagonists, may increase the risk further). Products include:
Cozaar 2106
Hyzaar 2162
Hyzaar 100-12.5 2162

Low Molecular Weight Heparins (YAZ has the potential to cause hyperkalemia in high-risk patients; co-administration with other drugs that have the potential to increase serum potassium, such as heparin, may increase the risk further).
No products indexed under this heading.

Meclofenamate Sodium (YAZ has the potential to cause hyperkalemia in high-risk patients; co-administration with other drugs that have the potential to increase serum potassium, such as NSAIDs, may increase the risk further).
No products indexed under this heading.

Mefenamic Acid (YAZ has the potential to cause hyperkalemia in high-risk patients; co-administration with other drugs that have the potential to increase serum potassium, such as NSAIDs, may increase the risk further).
No products indexed under this heading.

Meloxicam (YAZ has the potential to cause hyperkalemia in high-risk patients; co-administration with other drugs that have the potential to increase serum potassium, such as NSAIDs, may increase the risk further).
No products indexed under this heading.

Mephenytoin (Anticonvulsants have been shown to increase the metabolism of ethinyl estradiol and/or some progestins, which could result in a reduction of contraceptive effectiveness).
No products indexed under this heading.

Methacycline Hydrochloride (Pregnancy while taking combined hormonal contraceptives has been reported when the combined hormonal contraceptives were administered with antimicrobials such as tetracycline).
No products indexed under this heading.

Methsuximide (Anticonvulsants have been shown to increase the metabolism of ethinyl estradiol and/or some progestins, which could result in a reduction of contraceptive effectiveness).
No products indexed under this heading.

Minocycline Hydrochloride (Minocycline-related changes in estradiol, progesterone, FSH, and LH plasma levels, breakthrough bleeding, or contraceptive failure cannot be ruled out). Products include:
Solodyn 2073

Moexipril Hydrochloride (YAZ has the potential to cause hyperkalemia in high-risk patients; co-administration with other drugs that have the potential to increase serum potassium, such as ACE inhibitors, may increase the risk further).
No products indexed under this heading.

Morphine Sulfate (Increased clearance of morphine has been noted when administered with oral contraceptives). Products include:
Avinza 1822
Embeda 1831
MS Contin 2803

Nabumetone (YAZ has the potential to cause hyperkalemia in high-risk patients; co-administration with other drugs that have the potential to increase serum potassium, such as NSAIDs, may increase the risk further).
No products indexed under this heading.

Naproxen (YAZ has the potential to cause hyperkalemia in high-risk patients; co-administration with other drugs that have the potential to increase serum potassium, such as NSAIDs, may increase the risk further). Products include:
EC-Naprosyn 2850
Naprosyn 2850
Anaprox/Naprosyn 2850

Naproxen Sodium (YAZ has the potential to cause hyperkalemia in high-risk patients; co-administration with other drugs that have the potential to increase serum potassium, such as NSAIDs, may increase the risk further). Products include:
Anaprox 2850
Anaprox DS 2850
Treximet 1681

Oxaprozin (YAZ has the potential to cause hyperkalemia in high-risk patients; co-administration with other drugs that have the potential to increase serum potassium, such as NSAIDs, may increase the risk further).
No products indexed under this heading.

Oxcarbazepine (Anticonvulsants have been shown to increase the metabolism of ethinyl estradiol and/or some progestins, which could result in a reduction of contraceptive effectiveness).
No products indexed under this heading.

Oxytetracycline (Pregnancy while taking combined hormonal contraceptives has been reported when the combined hormonal contraceptives were administered with antimicrobials such as tetracycline).
No products indexed under this heading.

Oxytetracycline Hydrochloride (Pregnancy while taking combined hormonal contraceptives has been reported when the combined hormonal contraceptives were administered with antimicrobials such as tetracycline).
No products indexed under this heading.

Paramethadione (Anticonvulsants have been shown to increase the metabolism of ethinyl estradiol and/or some progestins, which could result in a reduction of contraceptive effectiveness).
No products indexed under this heading.

Perindopril Erbumine (YAZ has the potential to cause hyperkalemia in high-risk patients; co-administration with other drugs that have the potential to increase serum potassium, such as ACE inhibitors, may increase the risk further).
No products indexed under this heading.

Phenacemide (Anticonvulsants have been shown to increase the metabolism of ethinyl estradiol and/or some progestins, which could result in a reduction of contraceptive effectiveness).
No products indexed under this heading.

Phenobarbital (Co-administration results in increased metabolism of ethinyl estradiol and/or some progestins which could result in a reduction of contraceptive effectiveness). Products include:
Donnatal 2711

Phenobarbital Sodium (Anticonvulsants have been shown to increase the metabolism of ethinyl estradiol and/or some progestins, which could result in a reduction of contraceptive effectiveness).
No products indexed under this heading.

Phensuximide (Anticonvulsants have been shown to increase the metabolism of ethinyl estradiol and/or some progestins, which could result in a reduction of contraceptive effectiveness).
No products indexed under this heading.

Phenylbutazone (A reduction in contraceptive effectiveness and an increased incidence of menstrual irregularities has been suggested with phenylbutazone).
No products indexed under this heading.

Phenytoin (Anticonvulsants have been shown to increase the metabolism of ethinyl estradiol and/or some progestins, which could result in a reduction of contraceptive effectiveness).
No products indexed under this heading.

Phenytoin Sodium (Anticonvulsants have been shown to increase the metabolism of ethinyl estradiol and/or some progestins, which could result in a reduction of contraceptive effectiveness). Products include:
Phenytek Capsules 2380

Piroxicam (YAZ has the potential to cause hyperkalemia in high-risk patients; co-administration with other drugs that have the potential to increase serum potassium, such as NSAIDs, may increase the risk further).
No products indexed under this heading.

Potassium Acid Phosphate (YAZ has the potential to cause hyperkalemia in high-risk patients; co-administration with other drugs that have the potential to increase serum potassium, such as potassium supplementation, may increase the risk further). Products include:
K-Phos Original 874

(⊙ Described in PDR® for Ophthalmic Medicines)

Potassium Bicarbonate (YAZ has the potential to cause hyperkalemia in high-risk patients; co-administration with other drugs that have the potential to increase serum potassium, such as potassium supplementation, may increase the risk further).
No products indexed under this heading.

Potassium Chloride (YAZ has the potential to cause hyperkalemia in high-risk patients; co-administration with other drugs that have the potential to increase serum potassium, such as potassium supplementation, may increase the risk further). Products include:

MoviPrep Oral Solution 2905

Potassium Citrate (YAZ has the potential to cause hyperkalemia in high-risk patients; co-administration with other drugs that have the potential to increase serum potassium, such as potassium supplementation, may increase the risk further). Products include:

Urocit-K 2333

Potassium Gluconate (YAZ has the potential to cause hyperkalemia in high-risk patients; co-administration with other drugs that have the potential to increase serum potassium, such as potassium supplementation, may increase the risk further).
No products indexed under this heading.

Potassium Phosphate (YAZ has the potential to cause hyperkalemia in high-risk patients; co-administration with other drugs that have the potential to increase serum potassium, such as potassium supplementation, may increase the risk further). Products include:

K-Phos Neutral 873

Prednisolone (Increased plasma concentrations of prednisolone have been reported with concomitant administration of oral contraceptives).
No products indexed under this heading.

Prednisolone Acetate (Increased plasma concentrations of prednisolone have been reported with concomitant administration of oral contraceptives). Products include:

Blephamide .... ⊙212, ⊙214
Pred Forte .... ⊙225
Pred Mild .... ⊙230
Pred-G .... ⊙226, ⊙227

Prednisolone Sodium Phosphate (Increased plasma concentrations of prednisolone have been reported with concomitant administration of oral contraceptives).
No products indexed under this heading.

Prednisolone Tebutate (Increased plasma concentrations of prednisolone have been reported with concomitant administration of oral contraceptives).
No products indexed under this heading.

Primidone (Anticonvulsants have been shown to increase the metabolism of ethinyl estradiol and/or some progestins, which could result in a reduction of contraceptive effectiveness).
No products indexed under this heading.

Quinapril Hydrochloride (YAZ has the potential to cause hyperkalemia in high-risk patients; co-administration with other drugs that have the potential to increase serum potassium, such as ACE inhibitors, may increase the risk further).
No products indexed under this heading.

Ramipril (YAZ has the potential to cause hyperkalemia in high-risk patients; co-administration with other drugs that have the potential to increase serum potassium, such as ACE inhibitors, may increase the risk further).
No products indexed under this heading.

Rifampin (Co-administration results in increased metabolism of ethinyl estradiol precipitating a reduction in contraceptive effectiveness and an increase in menstrual irregularities).
No products indexed under this heading.

Rofecoxib (YAZ has the potential to cause hyperkalemia in high-risk patients; co-administration with other drugs that have the potential to increase serum potassium, such as NSAIDs, may increase the risk further).
No products indexed under this heading.

Rufinamide (Anticonvulsants have been shown to increase the metabolism of ethinyl estradiol and/or some progestins, which could result in a reduction of contraceptive effectiveness). Products include:

Banzel 1050

Salicylic Acid (Increased clearance of salicylic acid has been noted when administered with oral contraceptives).
No products indexed under this heading.

Spirapril Hydrochloride (YAZ has the potential to cause hyperkalemia in high-risk patients; co-administration with other drugs that have the potential to increase serum potassium, such as ACE inhibitors, may increase the risk further).
No products indexed under this heading.

Spironolactone (YAZ has the potential to cause hyperkalemia in high-risk patients; co-administration with other drugs that have the potential to increase serum potassium, such as aldosterone antagonists, may increase the risk further).
No products indexed under this heading.

Sulindac (YAZ has the potential to cause hyperkalemia in high-risk patients; co-administration with other drugs that have the potential to increase serum potassium, such as NSAIDs, may increase the risk further). Products include:

Clinoril 2098

Telmisartan (YAZ has the potential to cause hyperkalemia in high-risk patients; co-administration with other drugs that have the potential to increase serum potassium, such as angiotensin-II receptor antagonists, may increase the risk further). Products include:

Micardis 887
Micardis HCT 889

Temazepam (Increased clearance of temazepam has been noted when administered with oral contraceptives).
No products indexed under this heading.

Tetracycline Hydrochloride (Pregnancy while taking combined hormonal contraceptives has been reported when the combined hormonal contraceptives were administered with antimicrobials such as tetracycline). Products include:

Pylera 793

Tetracycline Phosphate Complex (Pregnancy while taking combined hormonal contraceptives has been reported when the combined hormonal contraceptives were administered with antimicrobials such as tetracycline).
No products indexed under this heading.

Theophylline (Increased plasma concentrations of theophylline have been reported with concomitant administration of oral contraceptives).
No products indexed under this heading.

Theophylline Anhydrous (Increased plasma concentrations of theophylline have been reported with concomitant administration of oral contraceptives). Products include:

Uniphyl 2817

Theophylline Calcium Salicylate (Increased plasma concentrations of theophylline have been reported with concomitant administration of oral contraceptives).
No products indexed under this heading.

Theophylline Dihydroxypropyl (Glyceryl) (Increased plasma concentrations of theophylline have been reported with concomitant administration of oral contraceptives).
No products indexed under this heading.

Theophylline Ethylenediamine (Increased plasma concentrations of theophylline have been reported with concomitant administration of oral contraceptives).
No products indexed under this heading.

Theophylline Sodium Glycinate (Increased plasma concentrations of theophylline have been reported with concomitant administration of oral contraceptives).
No products indexed under this heading.

Tiagabine Hydrochloride (Anticonvulsants have been shown to increase the metabolism of ethinyl estradiol and/or some progestins, which could result in a reduction of contraceptive effectiveness). Products include:

Gabitril 972

Tolmetin Sodium (YAZ has the potential to cause hyperkalemia in high-risk patients; co-administration with other drugs that have the potential to increase serum potassium, such as NSAIDs, may increase the risk further).
No products indexed under this heading.

Topiramate (Anticonvulsants have been shown to increase the metabolism of ethinyl estradiol and/or some progestins, which could result in a reduction of contraceptive effectiveness).
No products indexed under this heading.

Trandolapril (YAZ has the potential to cause hyperkalemia in high-risk patients; co-administration with other drugs that have the potential to increase serum potassium, such as ACE inhibitors, may increase the risk further). Products include:

Mavik 489
Tarka 534

Triamterene (YAZ has the potential to cause hyperkalemia in high-risk patients; co-administration with other drugs that have the potential to increase serum potassium, such as potassium-sparing diuretics, may increase the risk further). Products include:

Dyazide 1429
Dyrenium 3495

Trimethadione (Anticonvulsants have been shown to increase the metabolism of ethinyl estradiol and/or some progestins, which could result in a reduction of contraceptive effectiveness).
No products indexed under this heading.

Valdecoxib (YAZ has the potential to cause hyperkalemia in high-risk patients; co-administration with other drugs that have the potential to increase serum potassium, such as NSAIDs, may increase the risk further).
No products indexed under this heading.

Valproate Sodium (Anticonvulsants have been shown to increase the metabolism of ethinyl estradiol and/or some progestins, which could result in a reduction of contraceptive effectiveness).
No products indexed under this heading.

Valproic Acid (Anticonvulsants have been shown to increase the metabolism of ethinyl estradiol and/or some progestins, which could result in a reduction of contraceptive effectiveness).
No products indexed under this heading.

Valsartan (YAZ has the potential to cause hyperkalemia in high-risk patients; co-administration with other drugs that have the potential to increase serum potassium, such as angiotensin-II receptor antagonists, may increase the risk further). Products include:

Diovan 2413
Diovan HCT 2419
Exforge 2443
Exforge HCT 2449
Valturna 3637

Vitamin C (May increase plasma levels of ethinyl estradiol possibly by inhibition of conjugation). Products include:

Bausch & Lomb Ocuvite Adult
50+ .... ⊙238
Bio-C 3454
BoneMate Plus 3454
Cardio Basics 3455
CitraNatal 90 DHA Capsules 2332
CitraNatal Assure 2332
CitraNatal Rx 2332
Ferralet 2333
Heplive 607
Meili Clear 607
MoviPrep Oral Solution 2905
PreNexa 3473
Proflavanol 90 3476

Zonisamide (Anticonvulsants have been shown to increase the metabolism of ethinyl estradiol and/or some progestins, which could result in a reduction of contraceptive effectiveness). Products include:

Zonegran 1081

ZANTAC 25 EFFERDOSE TABLETS

(Ranitidine Hydrochloride) 1737
See Zantac 150 Tablets

ZANTAC 150 TABLETS

(Ranitidine Hydrochloride) 1737
May interact with absorption of drugs where gastric ph is an important determinant in their bioavailability, cationic drugs that are eliminated by renal tubular, and certain other agents. Compounds in these categories include:

Amiloride Hydrochloride (Ranitidine, a substrate of the renal organic cation transport system, may affect the clearance of other drugs eliminated by this route).
No products indexed under this heading.

Atazanavir Sulfate (Ranitidine may alter the absorption of drugs in which gastric pH is an important determinant of bioavailability. This can result in either an increase in absorption (eg, triazolam, midazolam, glipizide) or a decrease in absorption (eg, ketoconazole, atazanavir, delavirdine, gefitinib). Appropriate clinical monitoring is recommended. Atazanavir absorption may be impaired based on known interactions with other agents that increase gastric pH. Use with caution. See atazanavir label for specific recommendations).
No products indexed under this heading.

Bacampicillin Hydrochloride (Ranitidine may alter the absorption of drugs in which gastric pH is an important determinant of bioavailability. This can result in either an increase in absorption (eg, triazolam, midazolam, glipizide) or a decrease in absorption (eg, ketoconazole, atazanavir, delavirdine, gefitinib). Appropriate clinical monitoring is recommended).
No products indexed under this heading.

Delavirdine Mesylate (Ranitidine may alter the absorption of drugs in

which gastric pH is an important determinant of bioavailability. This can result in either an increase in absorption (eg, triazolam, midazolam, glipizide) or a decrease in absorption (eg, ketoconazole, atazanavir, delavirdine, gefitinib). Appropriate clinical monitoring is recommended. Delavirdine absorption may be impaired based on known interactions with other agents that increase gastric pH. Chronic use of H_2-receptor antagonists with delavirdine is not recommended).
No products indexed under this heading.

Digoxin (Ranitidine, a substrate of the renal organic cation transport system, may affect the clearance of other drugs eliminated by this route). Products include:
Lanoxin Injection 1546
Lanoxin Injection Pediatric 1549
Lanoxin Tablets 1553

Ferrous Fumarate (Ranitidine may alter the absorption of drugs in which gastric pH is an important determinant of bioavailability. This can result in either an increase in absorption (eg, triazolam, midazolam, glipizide) or a decrease in absorption (eg, ketoconazole, atazanavir, delavirdine, gefitinib). Appropriate clinical monitoring is recommended). Products include:
PreNexa 3473

Ferrous Gluconate (Ranitidine may alter the absorption of drugs in which gastric pH is an important determinant of bioavailability. This can result in either an increase in absorption (eg, triazolam, midazolam, glipizide) or a decrease in absorption (eg, ketoconazole, atazanavir, delavirdine, gefitinib). Appropriate clinical monitoring is recommended). Products include:
CitraNatal Assure 2332
CitraNatal Rx 2332

Ferrous Sulfate (Ranitidine may alter the absorption of drugs in which gastric pH is an important determinant of bioavailability. This can result in either an increase in absorption (eg, triazolam, midazolam, glipizide) or a decrease in absorption (eg, ketoconazole, atazanavir, delavirdine, gefitinib). Appropriate clinical monitoring is recommended).
No products indexed under this heading.

Gefitinib (Ranitidine may alter the absorption of drugs in which gastric pH is an important determinant of bioavailability. This can result in either an increase in absorption (eg, triazolam, midazolam, glipizide) or a decrease in absorption (eg, ketoconazole, atazanavir, delavirdine, gefitinib). Appropriate clinical monitoring is recommended. Gefitinib exposure was reduced by 44% with the co-administration of ranitidine and sodium bicarbonate (dosed to maintain gastric pH above 5.0). Use with caution).
No products indexed under this heading.

Glipizide (Ranitidine may alter the absorption of drugs in which gastric pH is an important determinant of bioavailability. This can result in either an increase in absorption (eg, triazolam, midazolam, glipizide) or a decrease in absorption (eg, ketoconazole, atazanavir, delavirdine, gefitinib). Appropriate clinical monitoring is recommended. In diabetic patients, glipizide exposure was increased by 34% following a single 150 mg dose of oral ranitidine. Use appropriate clinical monitoring when initiating or discontinuing ranitidine).
No products indexed under this heading.

Ketoconazole (Ranitidine may alter the absorption of drugs in which gastric pH is an important determinant of bioavailability. This can result in either an increase in absorption (eg, triazolam, midazolam, glipizide) or a decrease in absorption (eg, ketoconazole, atazanavir, delavirdine, gefitinib). Appropriate clinical monitoring is recommended. Oral ketoconazole exposure was reduced by up to 95% when oral ranitidine was co-administered in a regimen to maintain a gastric pH of 6 or above. The degree of interaction with usual dose of ranitidine (150 mg bid) is unknown). Products include:
Extina 3319
Xolegel 3337

Midazolam Hydrochloride (Ranitidine may alter the absorption of drugs in which gastric pH is an important determinant of bioavailability. This can result in either an increase in absorption (eg, triazolam, midazolam, glipizide) or a decrease in absorption (eg, ketoconazole, atazanavir, delavirdine, gefitinib). Appropriate clinical monitoring is recommended. Oral midazolam exposure in 5 healthy volunteers was increased by up to 65% when administered with oral ranitidine at a dose of 150 mg bid. However, in another interaction study in 8 volunteers receiving IV midazolam, a 300 mg oral dose of ranitidine increased midazolam exposure by about 9%. Monitor patients for excessive or prolonged sedation when ranitidine is co-administered with oral midazolam).
No products indexed under this heading.

Morphine Sulfate (Ranitidine, a substrate of the renal organic cation transport system, may affect the clearance of other drugs eliminated by this route). Products include:
Avinza 1822
Embeda 1831
MS Contin 2803

Procainamide Hydrochloride (Ranitidine, a substrate of the renal organic cation transport system, may affect the clearance of other drugs eliminated by this route. High doses of ranitidine (eg, such as those used in the treatment of Zollinger-Ellison syndrome) have been shown to reduce the renal excretion of procainamide and N-acetylprocainamide resulting in increased plasma levels of these drugs. Although this interaction is unlikely to be clinically relevant at usual ranitidine doses, it may be prudent to monitor for procainamide toxicity when administered with oral ranitidine at a dose exceeding 300 mg/day).
No products indexed under this heading.

Quinidine Gluconate (Ranitidine, a substrate of the renal organic cation transport system, may affect the clearance of other drugs eliminated by this route).
No products indexed under this heading.

Quinidine Polygalacturonate (Ranitidine, a substrate of the renal organic cation transport system, may affect the clearance of other drugs eliminated by this route).
No products indexed under this heading.

Quinidine Sulfate (Ranitidine, a substrate of the renal organic cation transport system, may affect the clearance of other drugs eliminated by this route).
No products indexed under this heading.

Quinine Sulfate (Ranitidine, a substrate of the renal organic cation transport system, may affect the clearance of other drugs eliminated by this route).
No products indexed under this heading.

Triamterene (Ranitidine, a substrate of the renal organic cation transport system, may affect the clearance of other drugs eliminated by this route). Products include:
Dyazide 1429
Dyrenium 3495

Triazolam (Ranitidine may alter the absorption of drugs in which gastric pH is an important determinant of bioavailability. This can result in either an increase in absorption (eg, triazolam, midazolam, glipizide) or a decrease in absorption (eg, ketoconazole, atazanavir, delavirdine, gefitinib). Appropriate clinical monitoring is recommended. Triazolam exposure in healthy volunteers was increased by approximately 30% when administered with oral ranitidine at a dose of 150 mg bid. Monitor patients for excessive or prolonged sedation).
No products indexed under this heading.

Trimethoprim (Ranitidine, a substrate of the renal organic cation transport system, may affect the clearance of other drugs eliminated by this route).
No products indexed under this heading.

Trimethoprim Sulfate (Ranitidine, a substrate of the renal organic cation transport system, may affect the clearance of other drugs eliminated by this route).
No products indexed under this heading.

Vancomycin Hydrochloride (Ranitidine, a substrate of the renal organic cation transport system, may affect the clearance of other drugs eliminated by this route).
No products indexed under this heading.

Warfarin Sodium (There have been reports of altered prothrombin time among patients on concomitant warfarin and ranitidine therapy. Due to the narrow therapeutic index, close monitoring of increased or decreased prothrombin time is recommended during concurrent treatment with ranitidine).
No products indexed under this heading.

ZANTAC 300 TABLETS

(Ranitidine Hydrochloride) 1737
See Zantac 150 Tablets

ZANTAC INJECTION

(Ranitidine Hydrochloride) 1732
May interact with absorption of drugs where gastric ph is an important determinant in their bioavailability, cationic drugs that are eliminated by renal tubular, drugs which undergo biotransformation by cytochrome p-450 mixed function oxidase, and certain other agents. Compounds in these categories include:

Acarbose (Ranitidine has been reported to affect the bioavailability of other drugs through several different mechanisms, such as competition for renal tubular secretion, alteration of gastric pH, and inhibition of cytochrome P450 enzymes).
No products indexed under this heading.

Acetaminophen (Ranitidine has been reported to affect the bioavailability of other drugs through several different mechanisms, such as competition for renal tubular secretion, alteration of gastric pH, and inhibition of cytochrome P450 enzymes). Products include:
Percocet 1121
Tylenol 2049
Tylenol 8 Hour 2049
Extra Strength Tylenol Caplets, Cool Caplets, and EZ Tabs 2049
Extra Strength Tylenol Adult Rapid Blast Liquid 2049
Extra Strength Tylenol Rapid Release 2049
Tylenol with Codeine 2691
Tylenol Arthritis Pain Extended Release Geltabs/Caplets 2049
Children's Tylenol Suspension Liquid 2048
Children's Tylenol Meltaways 2048
Tylenol, Infants' Drops 2048
Junior Tylenol 2048
Vicodin 560
Vicodin ES 561
Vicodin HP 563
Zydone 1138

Alatrofloxacin Mesylate (Ranitidine has been reported to affect the bioavailability of other drugs through several different mechanisms, such as competition for renal tubular secretion, alteration of gastric pH, and inhibition of cytochrome P450 enzymes).
No products indexed under this heading.

Alfentanil Hydrochloride (Ranitidine has been reported to affect the bioavailability of other drugs through several different mechanisms, such as competition for renal tubular secretion, alteration of gastric pH, and inhibition of cytochrome P450 enzymes).
No products indexed under this heading.

Alprazolam (Ranitidine has been reported to affect the bioavailability of other drugs through several different mechanisms, such as competition for renal tubular secretion, alteration of gastric pH, and inhibition of cytochrome P450 enzymes).
No products indexed under this heading.

Amiloride Hydrochloride (Ranitidine, a substrate of the renal organic cation transport system, may affect the clearance of other drugs eliminated by this route).
No products indexed under this heading.

Aminophylline (Ranitidine has been reported to affect the bioavailability of other drugs through several different mechanisms, such as competition for renal tubular secretion, alteration of gastric pH, and inhibition of cytochrome P450 enzymes).
No products indexed under this heading.

Amiodarone Hydrochloride (Ranitidine has been reported to affect the bioavailability of other drugs through several different mechanisms, such as competition for renal tubular secretion, alteration of gastric pH, and inhibition of cytochrome P450 enzymes).
No products indexed under this heading.

Amitriptyline Hydrochloride (Ranitidine has been reported to affect the bioavailability of other drugs through several different mechanisms, such as competition for renal tubular secretion, alteration of gastric pH, and inhibition of cytochrome P450 enzymes).
No products indexed under this heading.

Amlodipine Besylate (Ranitidine has been reported to affect the bioavailability of other drugs through several different mechanisms, such as competition for renal tubular secretion, alteration of gastric pH, and inhibition of cytochrome P450 enzymes). Products include:
Azor 1010
Exforge 2443
Exforge HCT 2449

Amoxapine (Ranitidine has been reported to affect the bioavailability of other drugs through several different mechanisms, such as competition for renal tubular secretion, alteration of gastric pH, and inhibition of cytochrome P450 enzymes).
No products indexed under this heading.

Amphetamine Aspartate (Ranitidine has been reported to affect the bioavailability of other drugs through several different mechanisms, such as competition for renal tubular secretion, alteration of gastric pH, and inhibition of cytochrome P450 enzymes).
No products indexed under this heading.

Amphetamine Aspartate Monohydrate (Ranitidine has been reported to affect the bioavailability of other drugs through several different mechanisms, such as competition for renal tubular secretion, alteration of gastric pH, and inhibition of cytochrome P450 enzymes).
No products indexed under this heading.

Amphetamine Sulfate (Ranitidine has been reported to affect the bioavailability of other drugs through several different mechanisms, such as competition for renal tubular secretion, alteration of gastric pH, and inhibition of cytochrome P450 enzymes).
No products indexed under this heading.

Anagrelide Hydrochloride (Ranitidine has been reported to affect the bioavailability of other drugs through several different mechanisms, such as competition for renal tubular secretion, alteration of gastric pH, and inhibition of cytochrome P450 enzymes).
No products indexed under this heading.

Aprepitant (Ranitidine has been reported to affect the bioavailability of other drugs through several different mechanisms, such as competition for renal tubular secretion, alteration of gastric pH, and inhibition of cytochrome P450 enzymes). Products include:
Emend 2124

Astemizole (Ranitidine has been reported to affect the bioavailability of other drugs through several different mechanisms, such as competition for renal tubular secretion, alteration of gastric pH, and inhibition of cytochrome P450 enzymes).
No products indexed under this heading.

Atazanavir (Ranitidine may alter the absorption of drugs in which gastric pH is an important determinant of bioavailability. Atazanavir absorption may be impaired based on known interactions with other agents that increase gastric pH. Use with caution. Appropriate clinical monitoring is recommended. See the atazanavir label for specific recommendations).
No products indexed under this heading.

Atazanavir Sulfate (Ranitidine may alter the absorption of drugs in which gastric pH is an important determinant of bioavailability. Atazanavir absorption may be impaired based on known interactions with other agents that increase gastric pH. Use with caution. Appropriate clinical monitoring is recommended. See the atazanavir label for specific recommendations).
No products indexed under this heading.

Atomoxetine Hydrochloride (Ranitidine has been reported to affect the bioavailability of other drugs through several different mechanisms, such as competition for renal tubular secretion, alteration of gastric pH, and inhibition of cytochrome P450 enzymes). Products include:
Strattera 1957

Atorvastatin Calcium (Ranitidine has been reported to affect the bioavailability of other drugs through several different mechanisms, such as competition for renal tubular secretion, alteration of gastric pH, and inhibition of cytochrome P450 enzymes). Products include:
Lipitor 2703

Bacampicillin Hydrochloride (Ranitidine may alter the absorption of drugs in which gastric pH is an important determinant of bioavailability. This can result in an increase in absorption (eg, triazolam, midazolam, glipizide) or a decrease in absorption (eg, ketoconazole, atazanavir, delavirdine, gefitinib). Appropriate clinical monitoring is recommended).
No products indexed under this heading.

Belladonna Ergotamine (Ranitidine has been reported to affect the bioavailability of other drugs through several different mechanisms, such as competition for renal tubular secretion, alteration of gastric pH, and inhibition of cytochrome P450 enzymes).
No products indexed under this heading.

Benzphetamine Hydrochloride (Ranitidine has been reported to affect the bioavailability of other drugs through several different mechanisms, such as competition for renal tubular secretion, alteration of gastric pH, and inhibition of cytochrome P450 enzymes).
No products indexed under this heading.

Bisoprolol Fumarate (Ranitidine has been reported to affect the bioavailability of other drugs through several different mechanisms, such as competition for renal tubular secretion, alteration of gastric pH, and inhibition of cytochrome P450 enzymes).
No products indexed under this heading.

Bromocriptine Mesylate (Ranitidine has been reported to affect the bioavailability of other drugs through several different mechanisms, such as competition for renal tubular secretion, alteration of gastric pH, and inhibition of cytochrome P450 enzymes).
No products indexed under this heading.

Buspirone Hydrochloride (Ranitidine has been reported to affect the bioavailability of other drugs through several different mechanisms, such as competition for renal tubular secretion, alteration of gastric pH, and inhibition of cytochrome P450 enzymes).
No products indexed under this heading.

Busulfan (Ranitidine has been reported to affect the bioavailability of other drugs through several different mechanisms, such as competition for renal tubular secretion, alteration of gastric pH, and inhibition of cytochrome P450 enzymes). Products include:
Myleran 1581

Caffeine (Ranitidine has been reported to affect the bioavailability of other drugs through several different mechanisms, such as competition for renal tubular secretion, alteration of gastric pH, and inhibition of cytochrome P450 enzymes).
No products indexed under this heading.

Caffeine Anhydrous (Ranitidine has been reported to affect the bioavailability of other drugs through several different mechanisms, such as competition for renal tubular secretion, alteration of gastric pH, and inhibition of cytochrome P450 enzymes).
No products indexed under this heading.

Caffeine Citrate (Ranitidine has been reported to affect the bioavailability of other drugs through several different mechanisms, such as competition for renal tubular secretion, alteration of gastric pH, and inhibition of cytochrome P450 enzymes).
No products indexed under this heading.

Caffeine-containing medications (Ranitidine has been reported to affect the bioavailability of other drugs through several different mechanisms, such as competition for renal tubular secretion, alteration of gastric pH, and inhibition of cytochrome P450 enzymes).
No products indexed under this heading.

Caffeine Sodium Benzoate (Ranitidine has been reported to affect the bioavailability of other drugs through several different mechanisms, such as competition for renal tubular secretion, alteration of gastric pH, and inhibition of cytochrome P450 enzymes).
No products indexed under this heading.

Candesartan Cilexetil (Ranitidine has been reported to affect the bioavailability of other drugs through several different mechanisms, such as competition for renal tubular secretion, alteration of gastric pH, and inhibition of cytochrome P450 enzymes). Products include:
Atacand 697

Atacand HCT 700

Captopril (Ranitidine has been reported to affect the bioavailability of other drugs through several different mechanisms, such as competition for renal tubular secretion, alteration of gastric pH, and inhibition of cytochrome P450 enzymes). Products include:
Captopril 2341

Carbamazepine (Ranitidine has been reported to affect the bioavailability of other drugs through several different mechanisms, such as competition for renal tubular secretion, alteration of gastric pH, and inhibition of cytochrome P450 enzymes). Products include:
Carbatrol 3280
Equetro 3477

Carisoprodol (Ranitidine has been reported to affect the bioavailability of other drugs through several different mechanisms, such as competition for renal tubular secretion, alteration of gastric pH, and inhibition of cytochrome P450 enzymes).
No products indexed under this heading.

Carvedilol (Ranitidine has been reported to affect the bioavailability of other drugs through several different mechanisms, such as competition for renal tubular secretion, alteration of gastric pH, and inhibition of cytochrome P450 enzymes). Products include:
Coreg 1409

Celecoxib (Ranitidine has been reported to affect the bioavailability of other drugs through several different mechanisms, such as competition for renal tubular secretion, alteration of gastric pH, and inhibition of cytochrome P450 enzymes). Products include:
Celebrex 3272

Cerivastatin Sodium (Ranitidine has been reported to affect the bioavailability of other drugs through several different mechanisms, such as competition for renal tubular secretion, alteration of gastric pH, and inhibition of cytochrome P450 enzymes).
No products indexed under this heading.

Cevimeline Hydrochloride (Ranitidine has been reported to affect the bioavailability of other drugs through several different mechanisms, such as competition for renal tubular secretion, alteration of gastric pH, and inhibition of cytochrome P450 enzymes). Products include:
Evoxac 1027

Chlordiazepoxide (Ranitidine has been reported to affect the bioavailability of other drugs through several different mechanisms, such as competition for renal tubular secretion, alteration of gastric pH, and inhibition of cytochrome P450 enzymes).
No products indexed under this heading.

Chlordiazepoxide Hydrochloride (Ranitidine has been reported to affect the bioavailability of other drugs through several different mechanisms, such as competition for renal tubular secretion, alteration of gastric pH, and inhibition of cytochrome P450 enzymes).
No products indexed under this heading.

Chlorpheniramine (Ranitidine has been reported to affect the bioavailability of other drugs through several different mechanisms, such as competition for renal tubular secretion, alteration of gastric pH, and inhibition of cytochrome P450 enzymes).
No products indexed under this heading.

Chlorpheniramine Maleate (Ranitidine has been reported to affect the bioavailability of other drugs through several different mechanisms, such as competition for renal tubular secretion, alteration of gastric pH, and inhibition of cytochrome P450 enzymes).
No products indexed under this heading.

Chlorpheniramine Polistirex (Ranitidine has been reported to affect the bioavailability of other drugs through several different mechanisms, such as competition for renal tubular secretion, alteration of gastric pH, and inhibition of cytochrome P450 enzymes). Products include:
Tussionex 3443

Chlorpheniramine Tannate (Ranitidine has been reported to affect the bioavailability of other drugs through several different mechanisms, such as competition for renal tubular secretion, alteration of gastric pH, and inhibition of cytochrome P450 enzymes).
No products indexed under this heading.

Chlorpromazine (Ranitidine has been reported to affect the bioavailability of other drugs through several different mechanisms, such as competition for renal tubular secretion, alteration of gastric pH, and inhibition of cytochrome P450 enzymes).
No products indexed under this heading.

Chlorpromazine Hydrochloride (Ranitidine has been reported to affect the bioavailability of other drugs through several different mechanisms, such as competition for renal tubular secretion, alteration of gastric pH, and inhibition of cytochrome P450 enzymes).
No products indexed under this heading.

Chlorpropamide (Ranitidine has been reported to affect the bioavailability of other drugs through several different mechanisms, such as competition for renal tubular secretion, alteration of gastric pH, and inhibition of cytochrome P450 enzymes).
No products indexed under this heading.

Cilostazol (Ranitidine has been reported to affect the bioavailability of other drugs through several different mechanisms, such as competition for renal tubular secretion, alteration of gastric pH, and inhibition of cytochrome P450 enzymes).
No products indexed under this heading.

Cimetidine Hydrochloride (Ranitidine has been reported to affect the bioavailability of other drugs through several different mechanisms, such as competition for renal tubular secretion, alteration of gastric pH, and inhibition of cytochrome P450 enzymes).
No products indexed under this heading.

Ciprofloxacin (Ranitidine has been reported to affect the bioavailability of other drugs through several different mechanisms, such as competition for renal tubular secretion, alteration of gastric pH, and inhibition of cytochrome P450 enzymes). Products include:
Cipro I.V. 3082
Cipro 3073
Cipro XR 3091
Ciprodex 583

Ciprofloxacin Hydrochloride (Ranitidine has been reported to affect the bioavailability of other drugs through several different mechanisms, such as competition for renal tubular secretion, alteration of gastric pH, and inhibition of cytochrome P450 enzymes). Products include:
Cipro 3073

Cisapride (Ranitidine has been reported to affect the bioavailability of other drugs through several different mechanisms, such as competition for renal tubular secretion, alteration of gastric pH, and inhibition of cytochrome P450 enzymes).
No products indexed under this heading.

Citalopram Hydrobromide (Ranitidine has been reported to affect the bioavailability of other drugs through several different mechanisms, such as competition for renal tubular secretion,

Zantac Injection Interactions Index 2124

alteration of gastric pH, and inhibition of cytochrome P450 enzymes). Products include:
Celexa 1153

Clarithromycin (Ranitidine has been reported to affect the bioavailability of other drugs through several different mechanisms, such as competition for renal tubular secretion, alteration of gastric pH, and inhibition of cytochrome P450 enzymes). Products include:
Biaxin/Biaxin XL 412

Clomipramine Hydrochloride (Ranitidine has been reported to affect the bioavailability of other drugs through several different mechanisms, such as competition for renal tubular secretion, alteration of gastric pH, and inhibition of cytochrome P450 enzymes).
No products indexed under this heading.

Clopidogrel Bisulfate (Ranitidine has been reported to affect the bioavailability of other drugs through several different mechanisms, such as competition for renal tubular secretion, alteration of gastric pH, and inhibition of cytochrome P450 enzymes). Products include:
Plavix 3027

Clopidogrel Hydrogen Sulfate (Ranitidine has been reported to affect the bioavailability of other drugs through several different mechanisms, such as competition for renal tubular secretion, alteration of gastric pH, and inhibition of cytochrome P450 enzymes).
No products indexed under this heading.

Clozapine (Ranitidine has been reported to affect the bioavailability of other drugs through several different mechanisms, such as competition for renal tubular secretion, alteration of gastric pH, and inhibition of cytochrome P450 enzymes).
No products indexed under this heading.

Codeine Phosphate (Ranitidine has been reported to affect the bioavailability of other drugs through several different mechanisms, such as competition for renal tubular secretion, alteration of gastric pH, and inhibition of cytochrome P450 enzymes). Products include:
Tylenol with Codeine 2691

Codeine Sulfate (Ranitidine has been reported to affect the bioavailability of other drugs through several different mechanisms, such as competition for renal tubular secretion, alteration of gastric pH, and inhibition of cytochrome P450 enzymes).
No products indexed under this heading.

Cyclobenzaprine (Ranitidine has been reported to affect the bioavailability of other drugs through several different mechanisms, such as competition for renal tubular secretion, alteration of gastric pH, and inhibition of cytochrome P450 enzymes).
No products indexed under this heading.

Cyclobenzaprine Hydrochloride (Ranitidine has been reported to affect the bioavailability of other drugs through several different mechanisms, such as competition for renal tubular secretion, alteration of gastric pH, and inhibition of cytochrome P450 enzymes). Products include:
Amrix 964

Cyclophosphamide (Ranitidine has been reported to affect the bioavailability of other drugs through several different mechanisms, such as competition for renal tubular secretion, alteration of gastric pH, and inhibition of cytochrome P450 enzymes).
No products indexed under this heading.

Cyclosporine (Ranitidine has been reported to affect the bioavailability of other drugs through several different mechanisms, such as competition for renal tubular secretion, alteration of gastric pH, and inhibition of cytochrome P450 enzymes). Products include:
Gengraf 440
Neoral Oral Solution 2496
Neoral Capsules 2496
Restasis 605

Delavirdine Mesylate (Ranitidine may alter the absorption of drugs in which gastric pH is an important determinant of bioavailability. Delavirdine absorption may be impaired based on known interactions with other agents at increase gastric pH. Appropriate clinical monitoring is recommended. Chronic use of H_2-receptor antagonists with delavirdine is not recommended).
No products indexed under this heading.

Desipramine Hydrochloride (Ranitidine has been reported to affect the bioavailability of other drugs through several different mechanisms, such as competition for renal tubular secretion, alteration of gastric pH, and inhibition of cytochrome P450 enzymes).
No products indexed under this heading.

Desogestrel (Ranitidine has been reported to affect the bioavailability of other drugs through several different mechanisms, such as competition for renal tubular secretion, alteration of gastric pH, and inhibition of cytochrome P450 enzymes).
No products indexed under this heading.

Dexamethasone (Ranitidine has been reported to affect the bioavailability of other drugs through several different mechanisms, such as competition for renal tubular secretion, alteration of gastric pH, and inhibition of cytochrome P450 enzymes). Products include:
Ciprodex 583
Ozurdex .... ⊙ 223
Tobramycin and Dexamethasone Ophthalmic Suspension .... ⊙ 251

Dexamethasone Acetate (Ranitidine has been reported to affect the bioavailability of other drugs through several different mechanisms, such as competition for renal tubular secretion, alteration of gastric pH, and inhibition of cytochrome P450 enzymes).
No products indexed under this heading.

Dexamethasone Phosphate (Ranitidine has been reported to affect the bioavailability of other drugs through several different mechanisms, such as competition for renal tubular secretion, alteration of gastric pH, and inhibition of cytochrome P450 enzymes).
No products indexed under this heading.

Dexamethasone Sodium (Ranitidine has been reported to affect the bioavailability of other drugs through several different mechanisms, such as competition for renal tubular secretion, alteration of gastric pH, and inhibition of cytochrome P450 enzymes).
No products indexed under this heading.

Dexamethasone Sodium Phosphate (Ranitidine has been reported to affect the bioavailability of other drugs through several different mechanisms, such as competition for renal tubular secretion, alteration of gastric pH, and inhibition of cytochrome P450 enzymes).
No products indexed under this heading.

Dexfenfluramine Hydrochloride (Ranitidine has been reported to affect the bioavailability of other drugs through several different mechanisms, such as competition for renal tubular secretion, alteration of gastric pH, and inhibition of cytochrome P450 enzymes).
No products indexed under this heading.

Dextromethorphan (Ranitidine has been reported to affect the bioavailability of other drugs through several different mechanisms, such as competition for renal tubular secretion, alteration of gastric pH, and inhibition of cytochrome P450 enzymes).
No products indexed under this heading.

Dextromethorphan Hydrobromide (Ranitidine has been reported to affect the bioavailability of other drugs through several different mechanisms, such as competition for renal tubular secretion, alteration of gastric pH, and inhibition of cytochrome P450 enzymes).
No products indexed under this heading.

Dextromethorphan Polistirex (Ranitidine has been reported to affect the bioavailability of other drugs through several different mechanisms, such as competition for renal tubular secretion, alteration of gastric pH, and inhibition of cytochrome P450 enzymes).
No products indexed under this heading.

Diazepam (Ranitidine has been reported to affect the bioavailability of other drugs through several different mechanisms, such as competition for renal tubular secretion, alteration of gastric pH, and inhibition of cytochrome P450 enzymes). Products include:
Valium Tablets 2880

Diclofenac Potassium (Ranitidine has been reported to affect the bioavailability of other drugs through several different mechanisms, such as competition for renal tubular secretion, alteration of gastric pH, and inhibition of cytochrome P450 enzymes).
No products indexed under this heading.

Diclofenac Sodium (Ranitidine has been reported to affect the bioavailability of other drugs through several different mechanisms, such as competition for renal tubular secretion, alteration of gastric pH, and inhibition of cytochrome P450 enzymes).
No products indexed under this heading.

Digoxin (Ranitidine, a substrate of the renal organic cation transport system, may affect the clearance of other drugs eliminated by this route). Products include:
Lanoxin Injection 1546
Lanoxin Injection Pediatric 1549
Lanoxin Tablets 1553

Dihydroergotamine Mesylate (Ranitidine has been reported to affect the bioavailability of other drugs through several different mechanisms, such as competition for renal tubular secretion, alteration of gastric pH, and inhibition of cytochrome P450 enzymes).
No products indexed under this heading.

Diltiazem Hydrochloride (Ranitidine has been reported to affect the bioavailability of other drugs through several different mechanisms, such as competition for renal tubular secretion, alteration of gastric pH, and inhibition of cytochrome P450 enzymes). Products include:
Cardizem LA 423

Diltiazem Maleate (Ranitidine has been reported to affect the bioavailability of other drugs through several different mechanisms, such as competition for renal tubular secretion, alteration of gastric pH, and inhibition of cytochrome P450 enzymes).
No products indexed under this heading.

Disopyramide (Ranitidine has been reported to affect the bioavailability of other drugs through several different mechanisms, such as competition for renal tubular secretion, alteration of gastric pH, and inhibition of cytochrome P450 enzymes).
No products indexed under this heading.

Disopyramide Phosphate (Ranitidine has been reported to affect the bioavailability of other drugs through several different mechanisms, such as competition for renal tubular secretion, alteration of gastric pH, and inhibition of cytochrome P450 enzymes).
No products indexed under this heading.

Disulfiram (Ranitidine has been reported to affect the bioavailability of other drugs through several different mechanisms, such as competition for renal tubular secretion, alteration of gastric pH, and inhibition of cytochrome P450 enzymes).
No products indexed under this heading.

Divalproex Sodium (Ranitidine has been reported to affect the bioavailability of other drugs through several different mechanisms, such as competition for renal tubular secretion, alteration of gastric pH, and inhibition of cytochrome P450 enzymes). Products include:
Depakote ER 426

Docetaxel (Ranitidine has been reported to affect the bioavailability of other drugs through several different mechanisms, such as competition for renal tubular secretion, alteration of gastric pH, and inhibition of cytochrome P450 enzymes). Products include:
Taxotere 3035

Dolasetron Mesylate (Ranitidine has been reported to affect the bioavailability of other drugs through several different mechanisms, such as competition for renal tubular secretion, alteration of gastric pH, and inhibition of cytochrome P450 enzymes). Products include:
Anzemet Injection 2931
Anzemet Tablets 2934

Donepezil Hydrochloride (Ranitidine has been reported to affect the bioavailability of other drugs through several different mechanisms, such as competition for renal tubular secretion, alteration of gastric pH, and inhibition of cytochrome P450 enzymes). Products include:
Aricept 1045
Aricept ODT 1045

Doxepin Hydrochloride (Ranitidine has been reported to affect the bioavailability of other drugs through several different mechanisms, such as competition for renal tubular secretion, alteration of gastric pH, and inhibition of cytochrome P450 enzymes).
No products indexed under this heading.

Doxorubicin Hydrochloride (Ranitidine has been reported to affect the bioavailability of other drugs through several different mechanisms, such as competition for renal tubular secretion, alteration of gastric pH, and inhibition of cytochrome P450 enzymes).
No products indexed under this heading.

Dronabinol (Ranitidine has been reported to affect the bioavailability of other drugs through several different mechanisms, such as competition for renal tubular secretion, alteration of gastric pH, and inhibition of cytochrome P450 enzymes).
No products indexed under this heading.

Drugs that Undergo Biotransformation by Cytochrome P-450 Mixed Function Oxidase (Ranitidine has been reported to affect the bioavailability of other drugs through several different mechanisms, such as competition for renal tubular secretion, alteration of gastric pH, and inhibition of cytochrome P450 enzymes).
No products indexed under this heading.

Dyphylline (Ranitidine has been reported to affect the bioavailability of other drugs through several different mechanisms, such as competition for renal tubular secretion, alteration of gastric pH, and inhibition of cytochrome P450 enzymes).
No products indexed under this heading.

(⊙ Described in PDR® for Ophthalmic Medicines)

Encainide Hydrochloride (Ranitidine has been reported to affect the bioavailability of other drugs through several different mechanisms, such as competition for renal tubular secretion, alteration of gastric pH, and inhibition of cytochrome P450 enzymes).
No products indexed under this heading.

Enoxacin (Ranitidine has been reported to affect the bioavailability of other drugs through several different mechanisms, such as competition for renal tubular secretion, alteration of gastric pH, and inhibition of cytochrome P450 enzymes).
No products indexed under this heading.

Eprosartan Mesylate (Ranitidine has been reported to affect the bioavailability of other drugs through several different mechanisms, such as competition for renal tubular secretion, alteration of gastric pH, and inhibition of cytochrome P450 enzymes). Products include:

Ergotamine Tartrate (Ranitidine has been reported to affect the bioavailability of other drugs through several different mechanisms, such as competition for renal tubular secretion, alteration of gastric pH, and inhibition of cytochrome P450 enzymes).
No products indexed under this heading.

Erythromycin (Ranitidine has been reported to affect the bioavailability of other drugs through several different mechanisms, such as competition for renal tubular secretion, alteration of gastric pH, and inhibition of cytochrome P450 enzymes).
No products indexed under this heading.

Erythromycin Estolate (Ranitidine has been reported to affect the bioavailability of other drugs through several different mechanisms, such as competition for renal tubular secretion, alteration of gastric pH, and inhibition of cytochrome P450 enzymes).
No products indexed under this heading.

Erythromycin Ethylsuccinate (Ranitidine has been reported to affect the bioavailability of other drugs through several different mechanisms, such as competition for renal tubular secretion, alteration of gastric pH, and inhibition of cytochrome P450 enzymes). Products include:

Erythromycin Gluceptate (Ranitidine has been reported to affect the bioavailability of other drugs through several different mechanisms, such as competition for renal tubular secretion, alteration of gastric pH, and inhibition of cytochrome P450 enzymes).
No products indexed under this heading.

Erythromycin Lactobionate (Ranitidine has been reported to affect the bioavailability of other drugs through several different mechanisms, such as competition for renal tubular secretion, alteration of gastric pH, and inhibition of cytochrome P450 enzymes).
No products indexed under this heading.

Erythromycin Stearate (Ranitidine has been reported to affect the bioavailability of other drugs through several different mechanisms, such as competition for renal tubular secretion, alteration of gastric pH, and inhibition of cytochrome P450 enzymes).
No products indexed under this heading.

Esomeprazole Magnesium (Ranitidine has been reported to affect the bioavailability of other drugs through several different mechanisms, such as competition for renal tubular secretion, alteration of gastric pH, and inhibition of cytochrome P450 enzymes). Products include:

Esomeprazole Sodium (Ranitidine has been reported to affect the bioavailability of other drugs through several different mechanisms, such as competition for renal tubular secretion, alteration of gastric pH, and inhibition of cytochrome P450 enzymes). Products include:

Estradiol (Ranitidine has been reported to affect the bioavailability of other drugs through several different mechanisms, such as competition for renal tubular secretion, alteration of gastric pH, and inhibition of cytochrome P450 enzymes). Products include:

Estradiol Benzoate (Ranitidine has been reported to affect the bioavailability of other drugs through several different mechanisms, such as competition for renal tubular secretion, alteration of gastric pH, and inhibition of cytochrome P450 enzymes).
No products indexed under this heading.

Estradiol Cypionate (Ranitidine has been reported to affect the bioavailability of other drugs through several different mechanisms, such as competition for renal tubular secretion, alteration of gastric pH, and inhibition of cytochrome P450 enzymes).
No products indexed under this heading.

Estradiol Valerate (Ranitidine has been reported to affect the bioavailability of other drugs through several different mechanisms, such as competition for renal tubular secretion, alteration of gastric pH, and inhibition of cytochrome P450 enzymes).
No products indexed under this heading.

Estrogen (Ranitidine has been reported to affect the bioavailability of other drugs through several different mechanisms, such as competition for renal tubular secretion, alteration of gastric pH, and inhibition of cytochrome P450 enzymes).
No products indexed under this heading.

Estrogens, Conjugated (Ranitidine has been reported to affect the bioavailability of other drugs through several different mechanisms, such as competition for renal tubular secretion, alteration of gastric pH, and inhibition of cytochrome P450 enzymes). Products include:

Estrogens, Conjugated, Synthetic A (Ranitidine has been reported to affect the bioavailability of other drugs through several different mechanisms, such as competition for renal tubular secretion, alteration of gastric pH, and inhibition of cytochrome P450 enzymes).
No products indexed under this heading.

Estrogens, Esterified (Ranitidine has been reported to affect the bioavailability of other drugs through several different mechanisms, such as competition for renal tubular secretion, alteration of gastric pH, and inhibition of cytochrome P450 enzymes).
No products indexed under this heading.

Ethinyl Estradiol (Ranitidine has been reported to affect the bioavailability of other drugs through several different mechanisms, such as competition for renal tubular secretion, alteration of gastric pH, and inhibition of cytochrome P450 enzymes). Products include:

Ethosuximide (Ranitidine has been reported to affect the bioavailability of other drugs through several different mechanisms, such as competition for renal tubular secretion, alteration of gastric pH, and inhibition of cytochrome P450 enzymes).
No products indexed under this heading.

Ethotoin (Ranitidine has been reported to affect the bioavailability of other drugs through several different mechanisms, such as competition for renal tubular secretion, alteration of gastric pH, and inhibition of cytochrome P450 enzymes).
No products indexed under this heading.

Ethynodiol Diacetate (Ranitidine has been reported to affect the bioavailability of other drugs through several different mechanisms, such as competition for renal tubular secretion, alteration of gastric pH, and inhibition of cytochrome P450 enzymes).
No products indexed under this heading.

Etodolac (Ranitidine has been reported to affect the bioavailability of other drugs through several different mechanisms, such as competition for renal tubular secretion, alteration of gastric pH, and inhibition of cytochrome P450 enzymes).
No products indexed under this heading.

Etoposide (Ranitidine has been reported to affect the bioavailability of other drugs through several different mechanisms, such as competition for renal tubular secretion, alteration of gastric pH, and inhibition of cytochrome P450 enzymes).
No products indexed under this heading.

Etoposide Phosphate (Ranitidine has been reported to affect the bioavailability of other drugs through several different mechanisms, such as competition for renal tubular secretion, alteration of gastric pH, and inhibition of cytochrome P450 enzymes).
No products indexed under this heading.

Felbamate (Ranitidine has been reported to affect the bioavailability of other drugs through several different mechanisms, such as competition for renal tubular secretion, alteration of gastric pH, and inhibition of cytochrome P450 enzymes).
No products indexed under this heading.

Felodipine (Ranitidine has been reported to affect the bioavailability of other drugs through several different mechanisms, such as competition for renal tubular secretion, alteration of gastric pH, and inhibition of cytochrome P450 enzymes).
No products indexed under this heading.

Fenoprofen Calcium (Ranitidine has been reported to affect the bioavailability of other drugs through several different mechanisms, such as competition for renal tubular secretion, alteration of gastric pH, and inhibition of cytochrome P450 enzymes).
No products indexed under this heading.

Fentanyl (Ranitidine has been reported to affect the bioavailability of other drugs through several different mechanisms, such as competition for renal tubular secretion, alteration of gastric pH, and inhibition of cytochrome P450 enzymes). Products include:

Fentanyl Citrate (Ranitidine has been reported to affect the bioavailability of other drugs through several different mechanisms, such as competition for renal tubular secretion, alteration of gastric pH, and inhibition of cytochrome P450 enzymes). Products include:

Ferrous Fumarate (Ranitidine may alter the absorption of drugs in which gastric pH is an important determinant of bioavailability. This can result in an increase in absorption (eg, triazolam, midazolam, glipizide) or a decrease in absorption (eg, ketoconazole, atazanavir, delavirdine, gefitinib). Appropriate clinical monitoring is recommended). Products include:

Ferrous Gluconate (Ranitidine may alter the absorption of drugs in which gastric pH is an important determinant of bioavailability. This can result in an increase in absorption (eg, triazolam, midazolam, glipizide) or a decrease in absorption (eg, ketoconazole, atazanavir, delavirdine, gefitinib). Appropriate clinical monitoring is recommended). Products include:

Ferrous Sulfate (Ranitidine may alter the absorption of drugs in which gastric pH is an important determinant of bioavailability. This can result in an increase in absorption (eg, triazolam, midazolam, glipizide) or a decrease in absorption (eg, ketoconazole, atazanavir, delavirdine, gefitinib). Appropriate clinical monitoring is recommended).
No products indexed under this heading.

Flecainide Acetate (Ranitidine has been reported to affect the bioavailability of other drugs through several different mechanisms, such as competition for renal tubular secretion, alteration of gastric pH, and inhibition of cytochrome P450 enzymes).
No products indexed under this heading.

Fluoxetine (Ranitidine has been reported to affect the bioavailability of other drugs through several different mechanisms, such as competition for renal tubular secretion, alteration of gastric pH, and inhibition of cytochrome P450 enzymes).
No products indexed under this heading.

Fluoxetine Hydrochloride (Ranitidine has been reported to affect the bioavailability of other drugs through several different mechanisms, such as competition for renal tubular secretion, alteration of gastric pH, and inhibition of cytochrome P450 enzymes). Products include:

Fluphenazine Decanoate (Ranitidine has been reported to affect the bioavailability of other drugs through several different mechanisms, such as competition for renal tubular secretion, alteration of gastric pH, and inhibition of cytochrome P450 enzymes).
No products indexed under this heading.

Fluphenazine Enanthate (Ranitidine has been reported to affect the bioavailability of other drugs through several different mechanisms, such as competition for renal tubular secretion, alteration of gastric pH, and inhibition of cytochrome P450 enzymes).
No products indexed under this heading.

IMPORTANT NOTE: Always consult each drug listing in the patient's regimen for possible interactions.

Fluphenazine Hydrochloride (Ranitidine has been reported to affect the bioavailability of other drugs through several different mechanisms, such as competition for renal tubular secretion, alteration of gastric pH, and inhibition of cytochrome P450 enzymes).
No products indexed under this heading.

Flurbiprofen (Ranitidine has been reported to affect the bioavailability of other drugs through several different mechanisms, such as competition for renal tubular secretion, alteration of gastric pH, and inhibition of cytochrome P450 enzymes).
No products indexed under this heading.

Flurbiprofen Sodium (Ranitidine has been reported to affect the bioavailability of other drugs through several different mechanisms, such as competition for renal tubular secretion, alteration of gastric pH, and inhibition of cytochrome P450 enzymes).
No products indexed under this heading.

Flutamide (Ranitidine has been reported to affect the bioavailability of other drugs through several different mechanisms, such as competition for renal tubular secretion, alteration of gastric pH, and inhibition of cytochrome P450 enzymes).
No products indexed under this heading.

Fluticasone Propionate (Ranitidine has been reported to affect the bioavailability of other drugs through several different mechanisms, such as competition for renal tubular secretion, alteration of gastric pH, and inhibition of cytochrome P450 enzymes). Products include:

Fluvastatin Sodium (Ranitidine has been reported to affect the bioavailability of other drugs through several different mechanisms, such as competition for renal tubular secretion, alteration of gastric pH, and inhibition of cytochrome P450 enzymes).
No products indexed under this heading.

Fluvoxamine Maleate (Ranitidine has been reported to affect the bioavailability of other drugs through several different mechanisms, such as competition for renal tubular secretion, alteration of gastric pH, and inhibition of cytochrome P450 enzymes).
No products indexed under this heading.

Formoterol Fumarate (Ranitidine has been reported to affect the bioavailability of other drugs through several different mechanisms, such as competition for renal tubular secretion, alteration of gastric pH, and inhibition of cytochrome P450 enzymes). Products include:

Fosphenytoin (Ranitidine has been reported to affect the bioavailability of other drugs through several different mechanisms, such as competition for renal tubular secretion, alteration of gastric pH, and inhibition of cytochrome P450 enzymes).
No products indexed under this heading.

Fosphenytoin Sodium (Ranitidine has been reported to affect the bioavailability of other drugs through several different mechanisms, such as competition for renal tubular secretion, alteration of gastric pH, and inhibition of cytochrome P450 enzymes).
No products indexed under this heading.

Gabapentin (Ranitidine has been reported to affect the bioavailability of other drugs through several different mechanisms, such as competition for renal tubular secretion, alteration of gastric pH, and inhibition of cytochrome P450 enzymes).
No products indexed under this heading.

Galantamine Hydrobromide (Ranitidine has been reported to affect the bioavailability of other drugs through several different mechanisms, such as competition for renal tubular secretion, alteration of gastric pH, and inhibition of cytochrome P450 enzymes).
No products indexed under this heading.

Gefitinib (Ranitidine may alter the absorption of drugs in which gastric pH is an important determinant if bioavailability. Gefitinib exposure was reduced by 44% with the co-administration of ranitidine and sodium bicarbonate (dose maintained gastric pH above 5). Use with caution. Appropriate clinical monitoring is recommended).
No products indexed under this heading.

Glimepiride (Ranitidine has been reported to affect the bioavailability of other drugs through several different mechanisms, such as competition for renal tubular secretion, alteration of gastric pH, and inhibition of cytochrome P450 enzymes). Products include:

Glipizide (Ranitidine may alter the absorption of drugs in which gastric pH is an important determinant of bioavailability. In diabetic patients, glipizide exposure was increased by 34% following a single 150 mg dose of oral ranitidine. Use appropriate clinical monitoring when initiating or discontinuing ranitidine).
No products indexed under this heading.

Glyburide (Ranitidine has been reported to affect the bioavailability of other drugs through several different mechanisms, such as competition for renal tubular secretion, alteration of gastric pH, and inhibition of cytochrome P450 enzymes).
No products indexed under this heading.

Grepafloxacin Hydrochloride (Ranitidine has been reported to affect the bioavailability of other drugs through several different mechanisms, such as competition for renal tubular secretion, alteration of gastric pH, and inhibition of cytochrome P450 enzymes).
No products indexed under this heading.

Haloperidol (Ranitidine has been reported to affect the bioavailability of other drugs through several different mechanisms, such as competition for renal tubular secretion, alteration of gastric pH, and inhibition of cytochrome P450 enzymes).
No products indexed under this heading.

Haloperidol Decanoate (Ranitidine has been reported to affect the bioavailability of other drugs through several different mechanisms, such as competition for renal tubular secretion, alteration of gastric pH, and inhibition of cytochrome P450 enzymes).
No products indexed under this heading.

Haloperidol Lactate (Ranitidine has been reported to affect the bioavailability of other drugs through several different mechanisms, such as competition for renal tubular secretion, alteration of gastric pH, and inhibition of cytochrome P450 enzymes).
No products indexed under this heading.

Hexobarbital (Ranitidine has been reported to affect the bioavailability of other drugs through several different mechanisms, such as competition for renal tubular secretion, alteration of gastric pH, and inhibition of cytochrome P450 enzymes).
No products indexed under this heading.

Hydrocodone Bitartrate (Ranitidine has been reported to affect the bioavailability of other drugs through several different mechanisms, such as competition for renal tubular secretion, alteration of gastric pH, and inhibition of cytochrome P450 enzymes). Products include:

Ibuprofen (Ranitidine has been reported to affect the bioavailability of other drugs through several different mechanisms, such as competition for renal tubular secretion, alteration of gastric pH, and inhibition of cytochrome P450 enzymes). Products include:

Imipramine Hydrochloride (Ranitidine has been reported to affect the bioavailability of other drugs through several different mechanisms, such as competition for renal tubular secretion, alteration of gastric pH, and inhibition of cytochrome P450 enzymes).
No products indexed under this heading.

Imipramine Pamoate (Ranitidine has been reported to affect the bioavailability of other drugs through several different mechanisms, such as competition for renal tubular secretion, alteration of gastric pH, and inhibition of cytochrome P450 enzymes).
No products indexed under this heading.

Indinavir Sulfate (Ranitidine has been reported to affect the bioavailability of other drugs through several different mechanisms, such as competition for renal tubular secretion, alteration of gastric pH, and inhibition of cytochrome P450 enzymes). Products include:

Indomethacin (Ranitidine has been reported to affect the bioavailability of other drugs through several different mechanisms, such as competition for renal tubular secretion, alteration of gastric pH, and inhibition of cytochrome P450 enzymes). Products include:

Indomethacin Sodium Trihydrate (Ranitidine has been reported to affect the bioavailability of other drugs through several different mechanisms, such as competition for renal tubular secretion, alteration of gastric pH, and inhibition of cytochrome P450 enzymes). Products include:

Indoramin Hydrochloride (Ranitidine has been reported to affect the bioavailability of other drugs through several different mechanisms, such as competition for renal tubular secretion, alteration of gastric pH, and inhibition of cytochrome P450 enzymes).
No products indexed under this heading.

Irbesartan (Ranitidine has been reported to affect the bioavailability of other drugs through several different mechanisms, such as competition for renal tubular secretion, alteration of gastric pH, and inhibition of cytochrome P450 enzymes). Products include:

Isotretinoin (Ranitidine has been reported to affect the bioavailability of other drugs through several different mechanisms, such as competition for renal tubular secretion, alteration of gastric pH, and inhibition of cytochrome P450 enzymes). Products include:

Isradipine (Ranitidine has been reported to affect the bioavailability of other drugs through several different mechanisms, such as competition for renal tubular secretion, alteration of gastric pH, and inhibition of cytochrome P450 enzymes). Products include:

Itraconazole (Ranitidine has been reported to affect the bioavailability of other drugs through several different mechanisms, such as competition for renal tubular secretion, alteration of gastric pH, and inhibition of cytochrome P450 enzymes).
No products indexed under this heading.

Ixabepilone (Ranitidine has been reported to affect the bioavailability of other drugs through several different mechanisms, such as competition for renal tubular secretion, alteration of gastric pH, and inhibition of cytochrome P450 enzymes).
No products indexed under this heading.

Ketoconazole (Ranitidine may alter the absorption of drugs in which gastric pH is an important determinant of bioavailability. Oral ketoconazole exposure was reduced by up to 95% when oral ranitidine was co-administered in a regimen to maintain a gastric pH of 6 or above. The degree of interaction with the usual dose of ranitidine (150 mg twice daily) is unknown. Appropriate clinical monitoring is recommended). Products include:

Ketoprofen (Ranitidine has been reported to affect the bioavailability of other drugs through several different mechanisms, such as competition for renal tubular secretion, alteration of gastric pH, and inhibition of cytochrome P450 enzymes).
No products indexed under this heading.

Ketorolac Tromethamine (Ranitidine has been reported to affect the bioavailability of other drugs through several different mechanisms, such as competition for renal tubular secretion, alteration of gastric pH, and inhibition of cytochrome P450 enzymes). Products include:

Labetalol Hydrochloride (Ranitidine has been reported to affect the bioavailability of other drugs through several different mechanisms, such as competition for renal tubular secretion, alteration of gastric pH, and inhibition of cytochrome P450 enzymes).
No products indexed under this heading.

Lamotrigine (Ranitidine has been reported to affect the bioavailability of other drugs through several different mechanisms, such as competition for renal tubular secretion, alteration of gastric pH, and inhibition of cytochrome P450 enzymes). Products include:

Lansoprazole (Ranitidine has been reported to affect the bioavailability of other drugs through several different mechanisms, such as competition for renal tubular secretion, alteration of gastric pH, and inhibition of cytochrome P450 enzymes).
No products indexed under this heading.

2127 Interactions Index Zantac Injection

Levetiracetam (Ranitidine has been reported to affect the bioavailability of other drugs through several different mechanisms, such as competition for renal tubular secretion, alteration of gastric pH, and inhibition of cytochrome P450 enzymes). Products include:
Keppra XR 3434

Levobupivacaine Hydrochloride (Ranitidine has been reported to affect the bioavailability of other drugs through several different mechanisms, such as competition for renal tubular secretion, alteration of gastric pH, and inhibition of cytochrome P450 enzymes).
No products indexed under this heading.

Levonorgestrel (Ranitidine has been reported to affect the bioavailability of other drugs through several different mechanisms, such as competition for renal tubular secretion, alteration of gastric pH, and inhibition of cytochrome P450 enzymes). Products include:
Climara Pro 847
LoSeasonique 3407
Lybrel 3514
Mirena 854
Plan B 3416
Seasonique 3418

Lidocaine (Ranitidine has been reported to affect the bioavailability of other drugs through several different mechanisms, such as competition for renal tubular secretion, alteration of gastric pH, and inhibition of cytochrome P450 enzymes). Products include:
Lidoderm 1107

Lidocaine Base (Ranitidine has been reported to affect the bioavailability of other drugs through several different mechanisms, such as competition for renal tubular secretion, alteration of gastric pH, and inhibition of cytochrome P450 enzymes).
No products indexed under this heading.

Lidocaine Hydrochloride (Ranitidine has been reported to affect the bioavailability of other drugs through several different mechanisms, such as competition for renal tubular secretion, alteration of gastric pH, and inhibition of cytochrome P450 enzymes).
No products indexed under this heading.

Lomefloxacin Hydrochloride (Ranitidine has been reported to affect the bioavailability of other drugs through several different mechanisms, such as competition for renal tubular secretion, alteration of gastric pH, and inhibition of cytochrome P450 enzymes).
No products indexed under this heading.

Losartan Potassium (Ranitidine has been reported to affect the bioavailability of other drugs through several different mechanisms, such as competition for renal tubular secretion, alteration of gastric pH, and inhibition of cytochrome P450 enzymes). Products include:
Cozaar 2106
Hyzaar 2162
Hyzaar 100-12.5 2162

Lovastatin (Ranitidine has been reported to affect the bioavailability of other drugs through several different mechanisms, such as competition for renal tubular secretion, alteration of gastric pH, and inhibition of cytochrome P450 enzymes). Products include:
Advicor 402
Mevacor 2212

Maprotiline Hydrochloride (Ranitidine has been reported to affect the bioavailability of other drugs through several different mechanisms, such as competition for renal tubular secretion, alteration of gastric pH, and inhibition of cytochrome P450 enzymes).
No products indexed under this heading.

Meclofenamate Sodium (Ranitidine has been reported to affect the bioavailability of other drugs through several different mechanisms, such as competition for renal tubular secretion, alteration of gastric pH, and inhibition of cytochrome P450 enzymes).
No products indexed under this heading.

Mefenamic Acid (Ranitidine has been reported to affect the bioavailability of other drugs through several different mechanisms, such as competition for renal tubular secretion, alteration of gastric pH, and inhibition of cytochrome P450 enzymes).
No products indexed under this heading.

Meloxicam (Ranitidine has been reported to affect the bioavailability of other drugs through several different mechanisms, such as competition for renal tubular secretion, alteration of gastric pH, and inhibition of cytochrome P450 enzymes).
No products indexed under this heading.

Meperidine Hydrochloride (Ranitidine has been reported to affect the bioavailability of other drugs through several different mechanisms, such as competition for renal tubular secretion, alteration of gastric pH, and inhibition of cytochrome P450 enzymes).
No products indexed under this heading.

Mephenytoin (Ranitidine has been reported to affect the bioavailability of other drugs through several different mechanisms, such as competition for renal tubular secretion, alteration of gastric pH, and inhibition of cytochrome P450 enzymes).
No products indexed under this heading.

Mephobarbital (Ranitidine has been reported to affect the bioavailability of other drugs through several different mechanisms, such as competition for renal tubular secretion, alteration of gastric pH, and inhibition of cytochrome P450 enzymes).
No products indexed under this heading.

Meprobamate (Ranitidine has been reported to affect the bioavailability of other drugs through several different mechanisms, such as competition for renal tubular secretion, alteration of gastric pH, and inhibition of cytochrome P450 enzymes).
No products indexed under this heading.

Mestranol (Ranitidine has been reported to affect the bioavailability of other drugs through several different mechanisms, such as competition for renal tubular secretion, alteration of gastric pH, and inhibition of cytochrome P450 enzymes).
No products indexed under this heading.

Metformin Hydrochloride (Ranitidine has been reported to affect the bioavailability of other drugs through several different mechanisms, such as competition for renal tubular secretion, alteration of gastric pH, and inhibition of cytochrome P450 enzymes). Products include:
ActoPlus 3338
Avandamet 1345
Janumet 2188

Methadone Hydrochloride (Ranitidine has been reported to affect the bioavailability of other drugs through several different mechanisms, such as competition for renal tubular secretion, alteration of gastric pH, and inhibition of cytochrome P450 enzymes).
No products indexed under this heading.

Methamphetamine Hydrochloride (Ranitidine has been reported to affect the bioavailability of other drugs through several different mechanisms, such as competition for renal tubular secretion, alteration of gastric pH, and inhibition of cytochrome P450 enzymes).
No products indexed under this heading.

Methsuximide (Ranitidine has been reported to affect the bioavailability of other drugs through several different mechanisms, such as competition for renal tubular secretion, alteration of gastric pH, and inhibition of cytochrome P450 enzymes).
No products indexed under this heading.

Metoprolol Succinate (Ranitidine has been reported to affect the bioavailability of other drugs through several different mechanisms, such as competition for renal tubular secretion, alteration of gastric pH, and inhibition of cytochrome P450 enzymes). Products include:
Toprol XL 732

Metoprolol Tartrate (Ranitidine has been reported to affect the bioavailability of other drugs through several different mechanisms, such as competition for renal tubular secretion, alteration of gastric pH, and inhibition of cytochrome P450 enzymes).
No products indexed under this heading.

Mexiletine Hydrochloride (Ranitidine has been reported to affect the bioavailability of other drugs through several different mechanisms, such as competition for renal tubular secretion, alteration of gastric pH, and inhibition of cytochrome P450 enzymes).
No products indexed under this heading.

Midazolam Hydrochloride (Ranitidine may alter the absorption of drugs in which gastric pH is an important determinant of bioavailability. Oral midazolam exposure in 5 healthy volunteers was increased by up to 65% when administered with oral ranitidine at a dose of 150 mg twice daily. However, in another interaction study in 8 volunteers receiving IV midazolam, a 300 mg oral dose of ranitidine increased midazolam exposure by about 9%. Monitor patients for excessive or prolonged sedation when ranitidine is co-administered with oral midazolam).
No products indexed under this heading.

Miglitol (Ranitidine has been reported to affect the bioavailability of other drugs through several different mechanisms, such as competition for renal tubular secretion, alteration of gastric pH, and inhibition of cytochrome P450 enzymes).
No products indexed under this heading.

Mirtazapine (Ranitidine has been reported to affect the bioavailability of other drugs through several different mechanisms, such as competition for renal tubular secretion, alteration of gastric pH, and inhibition of cytochrome P450 enzymes). Products include:
Remeron Tablets 3214
RemeronSolTab Tablets 3219

Montelukast Sodium (Ranitidine has been reported to affect the bioavailability of other drugs through several different mechanisms, such as competition for renal tubular secretion, alteration of gastric pH, and inhibition of cytochrome P450 enzymes). Products include:
Singulair 2270

Morphine Sulfate (Ranitidine, a substrate of the renal organic cation transport system, may affect the clearance of other drugs eliminated by this route). Products include:
Avinza 1822
Embeda 1831
MS Contin 2803

Moxifloxacin Hydrochloride (Ranitidine has been reported to affect the bioavailability of other drugs through several different mechanisms, such as competition for renal tubular secretion, alteration of gastric pH, and inhibition of cytochrome P450 enzymes). Products include:
Avelox 3064
Vigamox 589

Nabumetone (Ranitidine has been reported to affect the bioavailability of other drugs through several different mechanisms, such as competition for renal tubular secretion, alteration of gastric pH, and inhibition of cytochrome P450 enzymes).
No products indexed under this heading.

Nafcillin Sodium (Ranitidine has been reported to affect the bioavailability of other drugs through several different mechanisms, such as competition for renal tubular secretion, alteration of gastric pH, and inhibition of cytochrome P450 enzymes).
No products indexed under this heading.

Naproxen (Ranitidine has been reported to affect the bioavailability of other drugs through several different mechanisms, such as competition for renal tubular secretion, alteration of gastric pH, and inhibition of cytochrome P450 enzymes). Products include:
EC-Naprosyn 2850
Naprosyn 2850
Anaprox/Naprosyn 2850

Naproxen Sodium (Ranitidine has been reported to affect the bioavailability of other drugs through several different mechanisms, such as competition for renal tubular secretion, alteration of gastric pH, and inhibition of cytochrome P450 enzymes). Products include:
Anaprox 2850
Anaprox DS 2850
Treximet 1681

Nateglinide (Ranitidine has been reported to affect the bioavailability of other drugs through several different mechanisms, such as competition for renal tubular secretion, alteration of gastric pH, and inhibition of cytochrome P450 enzymes).
No products indexed under this heading.

Nefazodone Hydrochloride (Ranitidine has been reported to affect the bioavailability of other drugs through several different mechanisms, such as competition for renal tubular secretion, alteration of gastric pH, and inhibition of cytochrome P450 enzymes).
No products indexed under this heading.

Nelfinavir Mesylate (Ranitidine has been reported to affect the bioavailability of other drugs through several different mechanisms, such as competition for renal tubular secretion, alteration of gastric pH, and inhibition of cytochrome P450 enzymes).
No products indexed under this heading.

Nicardipine (Ranitidine has been reported to affect the bioavailability of other drugs through several different mechanisms, such as competition for renal tubular secretion, alteration of gastric pH, and inhibition of cytochrome P450 enzymes).
No products indexed under this heading.

Nicardipine Hydrochloride (Ranitidine has been reported to affect the bioavailability of other drugs through several different mechanisms, such as competition for renal tubular secretion, alteration of gastric pH, and inhibition of cytochrome P450 enzymes).
No products indexed under this heading.

IMPORTANT NOTE: Always consult each drug listing in the patient's regimen for possible interactions.

Zantac Injection Interactions Index 2128

Nicotine Polacrilex (Ranitidine has been reported to affect the bioavailability of other drugs through several different mechanisms, such as competition for renal tubular secretion, alteration of gastric pH, and inhibition of cytochrome P450 enzymes).
No products indexed under this heading.

Nicotine Salicylate (Ranitidine has been reported to affect the bioavailability of other drugs through several different mechanisms, such as competition for renal tubular secretion, alteration of gastric pH, and inhibition of cytochrome P450 enzymes).
No products indexed under this heading.

Nicotine Sulfate (Ranitidine has been reported to affect the bioavailability of other drugs through several different mechanisms, such as competition for renal tubular secretion, alteration of gastric pH, and inhibition of cytochrome P450 enzymes).
No products indexed under this heading.

Nifedipine (Ranitidine has been reported to affect the bioavailability of other drugs through several different mechanisms, such as competition for renal tubular secretion, alteration of gastric pH, and inhibition of cytochrome P450 enzymes).
No products indexed under this heading.

Nilutamide (Ranitidine has been reported to affect the bioavailability of other drugs through several different mechanisms, such as competition for renal tubular secretion, alteration of gastric pH, and inhibition of cytochrome P450 enzymes).
No products indexed under this heading.

Nimodipine (Ranitidine has been reported to affect the bioavailability of other drugs through several different mechanisms, such as competition for renal tubular secretion, alteration of gastric pH, and inhibition of cytochrome P450 enzymes).
No products indexed under this heading.

Nisoldipine (Ranitidine has been reported to affect the bioavailability of other drugs through several different mechanisms, such as competition for renal tubular secretion, alteration of gastric pH, and inhibition of cytochrome P450 enzymes).
No products indexed under this heading.

Nitrendipine (Ranitidine has been reported to affect the bioavailability of other drugs through several different mechanisms, such as competition for renal tubular secretion, alteration of gastric pH, and inhibition of cytochrome P450 enzymes).
No products indexed under this heading.

Norethindrone (Ranitidine has been reported to affect the bioavailability of other drugs through several different mechanisms, such as competition for renal tubular secretion, alteration of gastric pH, and inhibition of cytochrome P450 enzymes). Products include:
Ortho Micronor **2660**

Norethindrone Acetate (Ranitidine has been reported to affect the bioavailability of other drugs through several different mechanisms, such as competition for renal tubular secretion, alteration of gastric pH, and inhibition of cytochrome P450 enzymes). Products include:
Activella **2561**

Norfloxacin (Ranitidine has been reported to affect the bioavailability of other drugs through several different mechanisms, such as competition for renal tubular secretion, alteration of gastric pH, and inhibition of cytochrome P450 enzymes). Products include:
Noroxin **2220**

Norgestrel (Ranitidine has been reported to affect the bioavailability of other drugs through several different mechanisms, such as competition for renal tubular secretion, alteration of gastric pH, and inhibition of cytochrome P450 enzymes).
No products indexed under this heading.

Nortriptyline Hydrochloride (Ranitidine has been reported to affect the bioavailability of other drugs through several different mechanisms, such as competition for renal tubular secretion, alteration of gastric pH, and inhibition of cytochrome P450 enzymes).
No products indexed under this heading.

Ofloxacin (Ranitidine has been reported to affect the bioavailability of other drugs through several different mechanisms, such as competition for renal tubular secretion, alteration of gastric pH, and inhibition of cytochrome P450 enzymes).
No products indexed under this heading.

Olanzapine (Ranitidine has been reported to affect the bioavailability of other drugs through several different mechanisms, such as competition for renal tubular secretion, alteration of gastric pH, and inhibition of cytochrome P450 enzymes). Products include:
Symbyax **1965**
Zyprexa **1984**
Zyprexa IntraMuscular **1984**
Zyprexa ZYDIS **1984**

Omeprazole (Ranitidine has been reported to affect the bioavailability of other drugs through several different mechanisms, such as competition for renal tubular secretion, alteration of gastric pH, and inhibition of cytochrome P450 enzymes).
No products indexed under this heading.

Omeprazole Magnesium (Ranitidine has been reported to affect the bioavailability of other drugs through several different mechanisms, such as competition for renal tubular secretion, alteration of gastric pH, and inhibition of cytochrome P450 enzymes).
No products indexed under this heading.

Ondansetron (Ranitidine has been reported to affect the bioavailability of other drugs through several different mechanisms, such as competition for renal tubular secretion, alteration of gastric pH, and inhibition of cytochrome P450 enzymes).
No products indexed under this heading.

Ondansetron Hydrochloride (Ranitidine has been reported to affect the bioavailability of other drugs through several different mechanisms, such as competition for renal tubular secretion, alteration of gastric pH, and inhibition of cytochrome P450 enzymes). Products include:
Zofran Injection **1750**
Zofran **1756**
Zofran ODT **1756**

Oxaprozin (Ranitidine has been reported to affect the bioavailability of other drugs through several different mechanisms, such as competition for renal tubular secretion, alteration of gastric pH, and inhibition of cytochrome P450 enzymes).
No products indexed under this heading.

Oxcarbazepine (Ranitidine has been reported to affect the bioavailability of other drugs through several different mechanisms, such as competition for renal tubular secretion, alteration of gastric pH, and inhibition of cytochrome P450 enzymes).
No products indexed under this heading.

Oxycodone Hydrochloride (Ranitidine has been reported to affect the bioavailability of other drugs through several different mechanisms, such as competition for renal tubular secretion, alteration of gastric pH, and inhibition of cytochrome P450 enzymes). Products include:
OxyContin **2807**
Percocet **1121**
Percodan **1124**

Paclitaxel (Ranitidine has been reported to affect the bioavailability of other drugs through several different mechanisms, such as competition for renal tubular secretion, alteration of gastric pH, and inhibition of cytochrome P450 enzymes).
No products indexed under this heading.

Pantoprazole Sodium (Ranitidine has been reported to affect the bioavailability of other drugs through several different mechanisms, such as competition for renal tubular secretion, alteration of gastric pH, and inhibition of cytochrome P450 enzymes). Products include:
Protonix Tablets **3571**
Protonix **3575**

Paramethadione (Ranitidine has been reported to affect the bioavailability of other drugs through several different mechanisms, such as competition for renal tubular secretion, alteration of gastric pH, and inhibition of cytochrome P450 enzymes).
No products indexed under this heading.

Paroxetine Hydrochloride (Ranitidine has been reported to affect the bioavailability of other drugs through several different mechanisms, such as competition for renal tubular secretion, alteration of gastric pH, and inhibition of cytochrome P450 enzymes). Products include:
Paroxetine CR **2361**
Paroxetine ER **2371**
Paxil **1586**
Paxil CR **1596**

Pentamidine Isethionate (Ranitidine has been reported to affect the bioavailability of other drugs through several different mechanisms, such as competition for renal tubular secretion, alteration of gastric pH, and inhibition of cytochrome P450 enzymes).
No products indexed under this heading.

Phenacemide (Ranitidine has been reported to affect the bioavailability of other drugs through several different mechanisms, such as competition for renal tubular secretion, alteration of gastric pH, and inhibition of cytochrome P450 enzymes).
No products indexed under this heading.

Phenobarbital (Ranitidine has been reported to affect the bioavailability of other drugs through several different mechanisms, such as competition for renal tubular secretion, alteration of gastric pH, and inhibition of cytochrome P450 enzymes). Products include:
Donnatal **2711**

Phenobarbital Sodium (Ranitidine has been reported to affect the bioavailability of other drugs through several different mechanisms, such as competition for renal tubular secretion, alteration of gastric pH, and inhibition of cytochrome P450 enzymes).
No products indexed under this heading.

Phensuximide (Ranitidine has been reported to affect the bioavailability of other drugs through several different mechanisms, such as competition for renal tubular secretion, alteration of gastric pH, and inhibition of cytochrome P450 enzymes).
No products indexed under this heading.

Phenylbutazone (Ranitidine has been reported to affect the bioavailability of other drugs through several different mechanisms, such as competition for renal tubular secretion, alteration of gastric pH, and inhibition of cytochrome P450 enzymes).
No products indexed under this heading.

Phenytoin (Ranitidine has been reported to affect the bioavailability of other drugs through several different mechanisms, such as competition for renal tubular secretion, alteration of gastric pH, and inhibition of cytochrome P450 enzymes).
No products indexed under this heading.

Phenytoin Sodium (Ranitidine has been reported to affect the bioavailability of other drugs through several different mechanisms, such as competition for renal tubular secretion, alteration of gastric pH, and inhibition of cytochrome P450 enzymes). Products include:
Phenytek Capsules **2380**

Pimozide (Ranitidine has been reported to affect the bioavailability of other drugs through several different mechanisms, such as competition for renal tubular secretion, alteration of gastric pH, and inhibition of cytochrome P450 enzymes).
No products indexed under this heading.

Pindolol (Ranitidine has been reported to affect the bioavailability of other drugs through several different mechanisms, such as competition for renal tubular secretion, alteration of gastric pH, and inhibition of cytochrome P450 enzymes).
No products indexed under this heading.

Pioglitazone Hydrochloride (Ranitidine has been reported to affect the bioavailability of other drugs through several different mechanisms, such as competition for renal tubular secretion, alteration of gastric pH, and inhibition of cytochrome P450 enzymes). Products include:
ActoPlus **3338**
Actos **3345**
Duetact **3354**

Piroxicam (Ranitidine has been reported to affect the bioavailability of other drugs through several different mechanisms, such as competition for renal tubular secretion, alteration of gastric pH, and inhibition of cytochrome P450 enzymes).
No products indexed under this heading.

Polyestradiol Phosphate (Ranitidine has been reported to affect the bioavailability of other drugs through several different mechanisms, such as competition for renal tubular secretion, alteration of gastric pH, and inhibition of cytochrome P450 enzymes).
No products indexed under this heading.

Primidone (Ranitidine has been reported to affect the bioavailability of other drugs through several different mechanisms, such as competition for renal tubular secretion, alteration of gastric pH, and inhibition of cytochrome P450 enzymes).
No products indexed under this heading.

Procainamide (Ranitidine, a substrate of the renal organic cation transport system, may affect the clearance of other drugs eliminated by this route. High doses of ranitidine (eg, such as those used in the treatment of Zollinger-Ellison syndrome) have been shown to reduce the renal excretion of procainamide and N-acetylprocainamide, resulting in increased plasma levels of these drugs. Although this interaction is unlikely to be clinically relevant at usual ranitidine doses, it may be prudent to monitor for procainamide toxicity when administered with oral ranitidine at a dose exceeding 300 mg per day).
No products indexed under this heading.

Procainamide Hydrochloride (Ranitidine, a substrate of the renal organic cation transport system, may affect the clearance of other drugs eliminated by this route. High doses of ranitidine (eg, such as those used in the treatment of Zollinger-Ellison syndrome) have been shown to reduce the renal excretion of

(⊙ Described in PDR® for Ophthalmic Medicines)

2129 Interactions Index Zantac Injection

procainamide and N-acetylprocainamide, resulting in increased plasma levels of these drugs. Although this interaction is unlikely to be clinically relevant at usual ranitidine doses, it may be prudent to monitor for procainamide toxicity when administered with oral ranitidine at a dose exceeding 300 mg per day).
No products indexed under this heading.

Progesterone (Ranitidine has been reported to affect the bioavailability of other drugs through several different mechanisms, such as competition for renal tubular secretion, alteration of gastric pH, and inhibition of cytochrome P450 enzymes). Products include:
Crinone 4% 996
Crinone 8% 996
Prometrium 3307

Proguanil Hydrochloride (Ranitidine has been reported to affect the bioavailability of other drugs through several different mechanisms, such as competition for renal tubular secretion, alteration of gastric pH, and inhibition of cytochrome P450 enzymes). Products include:
Malarone Pediatric Tablets 1572
Malarone 1572

Propafenone Hydrochloride (Ranitidine has been reported to affect the bioavailability of other drugs through several different mechanisms, such as competition for renal tubular secretion, alteration of gastric pH, and inhibition of cytochrome P450 enzymes). Products include:
Rythmol 1648
Rythmol SR 1652

Propoxyphene Hydrochloride (Ranitidine has been reported to affect the bioavailability of other drugs through several different mechanisms, such as competition for renal tubular secretion, alteration of gastric pH, and inhibition of cytochrome P450 enzymes).
No products indexed under this heading.

Propoxyphene Napsylate (Ranitidine has been reported to affect the bioavailability of other drugs through several different mechanisms, such as competition for renal tubular secretion, alteration of gastric pH, and inhibition of cytochrome P450 enzymes).
No products indexed under this heading.

Propranolol Hydrochloride (Ranitidine has been reported to affect the bioavailability of other drugs through several different mechanisms, such as competition for renal tubular secretion, alteration of gastric pH, and inhibition of cytochrome P450 enzymes). Products include:
InnoPran XL 1517

Protriptyline Hydrochloride (Ranitidine has been reported to affect the bioavailability of other drugs through several different mechanisms, such as competition for renal tubular secretion, alteration of gastric pH, and inhibition of cytochrome P450 enzymes).
No products indexed under this heading.

Quetiapine Fumarate (Ranitidine has been reported to affect the bioavailability of other drugs through several different mechanisms, such as competition for renal tubular secretion, alteration of gastric pH, and inhibition of cytochrome P450 enzymes). Products include:
Seroquel 750
Seroquel XR 759

Quinidine Gluconate (Ranitidine, a substrate of the renal organic cation transport system, may affect the clearance of other drugs eliminated by this route).
No products indexed under this heading.

Quinidine Hydrochloride (Ranitidine has been reported to affect the bioavailability of other drugs through several different mechanisms, such as competition for renal tubular secretion, alteration of gastric pH, and inhibition of cytochrome P450 enzymes).
No products indexed under this heading.

Quinidine Polygalacturonate (Ranitidine, a substrate of the renal organic cation transport system, may affect the clearance of other drugs eliminated by this route).
No products indexed under this heading.

Quinidine Sulfate (Ranitidine, a substrate of the renal organic cation transport system, may affect the clearance of other drugs eliminated by this route).
No products indexed under this heading.

Quinine (Ranitidine has been reported to affect the bioavailability of other drugs through several different mechanisms, such as competition for renal tubular secretion, alteration of gastric pH, and inhibition of cytochrome P450 enzymes). Products include:
Hyland's Leg Cramps PM with Quinine 3315

Quinine Sulfate (Ranitidine, a substrate of the renal organic cation transport system, may affect the clearance of other drugs eliminated by this route).
No products indexed under this heading.

Rabeprazole Sodium (Ranitidine has been reported to affect the bioavailability of other drugs through several different mechanisms, such as competition for renal tubular secretion, alteration of gastric pH, and inhibition of cytochrome P450 enzymes). Products include:
Aciphex 1035

Repaglinide (Ranitidine has been reported to affect the bioavailability of other drugs through several different mechanisms, such as competition for renal tubular secretion, alteration of gastric pH, and inhibition of cytochrome P450 enzymes).
No products indexed under this heading.

Rifabutin (Ranitidine has been reported to affect the bioavailability of other drugs through several different mechanisms, such as competition for renal tubular secretion, alteration of gastric pH, and inhibition of cytochrome P450 enzymes).
No products indexed under this heading.

Riluzole (Ranitidine has been reported to affect the bioavailability of other drugs through several different mechanisms, such as competition for renal tubular secretion, alteration of gastric pH, and inhibition of cytochrome P450 enzymes). Products include:
Rilutek 3032

Risperidone (Ranitidine has been reported to affect the bioavailability of other drugs through several different mechanisms, such as competition for renal tubular secretion, alteration of gastric pH, and inhibition of cytochrome P450 enzymes). Products include:
Risperdal Consta 2682

Ritonavir (Ranitidine has been reported to affect the bioavailability of other drugs through several different mechanisms, such as competition for renal tubular secretion, alteration of gastric pH, and inhibition of cytochrome P450 enzymes). Products include:
Kaletra 458
Norvir 509

Rofecoxib (Ranitidine has been reported to affect the bioavailability of other drugs through several different mechanisms, such as competition for renal tubular secretion, alteration of gastric pH, and inhibition of cytochrome P450 enzymes).
No products indexed under this heading.

Ropinirole Hydrochloride (Ranitidine has been reported to affect the bioavailability of other drugs through several different mechanisms, such as competition for renal tubular secretion, alteration of gastric pH, and inhibition of cytochrome P450 enzymes). Products include:
Requip 1620
Requip XL 1628

Ropivacaine Hydrochloride (Ranitidine has been reported to affect the bioavailability of other drugs through several different mechanisms, such as competition for renal tubular secretion, alteration of gastric pH, and inhibition of cytochrome P450 enzymes).
No products indexed under this heading.

Rosiglitazone (Ranitidine has been reported to affect the bioavailability of other drugs through several different mechanisms, such as competition for renal tubular secretion, alteration of gastric pH, and inhibition of cytochrome P450 enzymes).
No products indexed under this heading.

Rosiglitazone Maleate (Ranitidine has been reported to affect the bioavailability of other drugs through several different mechanisms, such as competition for renal tubular secretion, alteration of gastric pH, and inhibition of cytochrome P450 enzymes). Products include:
Avandamet 1345
Avandaryl 1356
Avandia 1366

Rosiglitazone/Metformin (Ranitidine has been reported to affect the bioavailability of other drugs through several different mechanisms, such as competition for renal tubular secretion, alteration of gastric pH, and inhibition of cytochrome P450 enzymes).
No products indexed under this heading.

Saquinavir (Ranitidine has been reported to affect the bioavailability of other drugs through several different mechanisms, such as competition for renal tubular secretion, alteration of gastric pH, and inhibition of cytochrome P450 enzymes).
No products indexed under this heading.

Saquinavir Mesylate (Ranitidine has been reported to affect the bioavailability of other drugs through several different mechanisms, such as competition for renal tubular secretion, alteration of gastric pH, and inhibition of cytochrome P450 enzymes).
No products indexed under this heading.

Sertraline Hydrochloride (Ranitidine has been reported to affect the bioavailability of other drugs through several different mechanisms, such as competition for renal tubular secretion, alteration of gastric pH, and inhibition of cytochrome P450 enzymes).
No products indexed under this heading.

Sildenafil Citrate (Ranitidine has been reported to affect the bioavailability of other drugs through several different mechanisms, such as competition for renal tubular secretion, alteration of gastric pH, and inhibition of cytochrome P450 enzymes).
No products indexed under this heading.

Simvastatin (Ranitidine has been reported to affect the bioavailability of other drugs through several different mechanisms, such as competition for renal tubular secretion, alteration of gastric pH, and inhibition of cytochrome P450 enzymes). Products include:
Simcor 524
Vytorin 10/10 .... 2303, 3240
Vytorin 10/20 .... 2303, 3240
Vytorin 10/40 .... 2303, 3240
Vytorin 10/80 .... 2303, 3240
Zocor 2289

Sirolimus (Ranitidine has been reported to affect the bioavailability of other drugs through several different mechanisms, such as competition for renal tubular secretion, alteration of gastric pH, and inhibition of cytochrome P450 enzymes). Products include:
Rapamune 3579

Sulfamethoxazole (Ranitidine has been reported to affect the bioavailability of other drugs through several different mechanisms, such as competition for renal tubular secretion, alteration of gastric pH, and inhibition of cytochrome P450 enzymes).
No products indexed under this heading.

Sulindac (Ranitidine has been reported to affect the bioavailability of other drugs through several different mechanisms, such as competition for renal tubular secretion, alteration of gastric pH, and inhibition of cytochrome P450 enzymes). Products include:
Clinoril 2098

Suprofen (Ranitidine has been reported to affect the bioavailability of other drugs through several different mechanisms, such as competition for renal tubular secretion, alteration of gastric pH, and inhibition of cytochrome P450 enzymes).
No products indexed under this heading.

Tacrine Hydrochloride (Ranitidine has been reported to affect the bioavailability of other drugs through several different mechanisms, such as competition for renal tubular secretion, alteration of gastric pH, and inhibition of cytochrome P450 enzymes).
No products indexed under this heading.

Tacrolimus (Ranitidine has been reported to affect the bioavailability of other drugs through several different mechanisms, such as competition for renal tubular secretion, alteration of gastric pH, and inhibition of cytochrome P450 enzymes). Products include:
Prograf Capsules 677
Prograf Injection 677
Protopic 685

Tadalafil (Ranitidine has been reported to affect the bioavailability of other drugs through several different mechanisms, such as competition for renal tubular secretion, alteration of gastric pH, and inhibition of cytochrome P450 enzymes). Products include:
Adcirca 3461
Cialis 1861

Tamoxifen Citrate (Ranitidine has been reported to affect the bioavailability of other drugs through several different mechanisms, such as competition for renal tubular secretion, alteration of gastric pH, and inhibition of cytochrome P450 enzymes).
No products indexed under this heading.

Telmisartan (Ranitidine has been reported to affect the bioavailability of other drugs through several different mechanisms, such as competition for renal tubular secretion, alteration of gastric pH, and inhibition of cytochrome P450 enzymes). Products include:
Micardis 887
Micardis HCT 889

Teniposide (Ranitidine has been reported to affect the bioavailability of other drugs through several different mechanisms, such as competition for renal tubular secretion, alteration of gastric pH, and inhibition of cytochrome P450 enzymes).
No products indexed under this heading.

Terfenadine (Ranitidine has been reported to affect the bioavailability of other drugs through several different mechanisms, such as competition for renal tubular secretion, alteration of gastric pH, and inhibition of cytochrome P450 enzymes).
No products indexed under this heading.

IMPORTANT NOTE: Always consult each drug listing in the patient's regimen for possible interactions.

Testosterone (Ranitidine has been reported to affect the bioavailability of other drugs through several different mechanisms, such as competition for renal tubular secretion, alteration of gastric pH, and inhibition of cytochrome P450 enzymes). Products include:
AndroGel 3456

Testosterone Cypionate (Ranitidine has been reported to affect the bioavailability of other drugs through several different mechanisms, such as competition for renal tubular secretion, alteration of gastric pH, and inhibition of cytochrome P450 enzymes).
No products indexed under this heading.

Testosterone Enanthate (Ranitidine has been reported to affect the bioavailability of other drugs through several different mechanisms, such as competition for renal tubular secretion, alteration of gastric pH, and inhibition of cytochrome P450 enzymes). Products include:
Delatestryl 1102

Testosterone Propionate (Ranitidine has been reported to affect the bioavailability of other drugs through several different mechanisms, such as competition for renal tubular secretion, alteration of gastric pH, and inhibition of cytochrome P450 enzymes).
No products indexed under this heading.

Theophylline (Ranitidine has been reported to affect the bioavailability of other drugs through several different mechanisms, such as competition for renal tubular secretion, alteration of gastric pH, and inhibition of cytochrome P450 enzymes).
No products indexed under this heading.

Theophylline Anhydrous (Ranitidine has been reported to affect the bioavailability of other drugs through several different mechanisms, such as competition for renal tubular secretion, alteration of gastric pH, and inhibition of cytochrome P450 enzymes). Products include:
Uniphyl 2817

Theophylline Calcium Salicylate (Ranitidine has been reported to affect the bioavailability of other drugs through several different mechanisms, such as competition for renal tubular secretion, alteration of gastric pH, and inhibition of cytochrome P450 enzymes).
No products indexed under this heading.

Theophylline Dihydroxypropyl (Glyceryl) (Ranitidine has been reported to affect the bioavailability of other drugs through several different mechanisms, such as competition for renal tubular secretion, alteration of gastric pH, and inhibition of cytochrome P450 enzymes).
No products indexed under this heading.

Theophylline Ethylenediamine (Ranitidine has been reported to affect the bioavailability of other drugs through several different mechanisms, such as competition for renal tubular secretion, alteration of gastric pH, and inhibition of cytochrome P450 enzymes).
No products indexed under this heading.

Theophylline Sodium Glycinate (Ranitidine has been reported to affect the bioavailability of other drugs through several different mechanisms, such as competition for renal tubular secretion, alteration of gastric pH, and inhibition of cytochrome P450 enzymes).
No products indexed under this heading.

Thioridazine (Ranitidine has been reported to affect the bioavailability of other drugs through several different mechanisms, such as competition for renal tubular secretion, alteration of gastric pH, and inhibition of cytochrome P450 enzymes).
No products indexed under this heading.

Thioridazine Hydrochloride (Ranitidine has been reported to affect the bioavailability of other drugs through several different mechanisms, such as competition for renal tubular secretion, alteration of gastric pH, and inhibition of cytochrome P450 enzymes). Products include:
Thioridazine Hydrochloride 2384

Tiagabine Hydrochloride (Ranitidine has been reported to affect the bioavailability of other drugs through several different mechanisms, such as competition for renal tubular secretion, alteration of gastric pH, and inhibition of cytochrome P450 enzymes). Products include:
Gabitril 972

Timolol Maleate (Ranitidine has been reported to affect the bioavailability of other drugs through several different mechanisms, such as competition for renal tubular secretion, alteration of gastric pH, and inhibition of cytochrome P450 enzymes). Products include:
Combigan 601
Dorzolamide
Hydrochloride/Timolol Maleate
Ophthalmic Solution .... ⊙243
Timoptic in Ocudose .... ⊙231

Tolazamide (Ranitidine has been reported to affect the bioavailability of other drugs through several different mechanisms, such as competition for renal tubular secretion, alteration of gastric pH, and inhibition of cytochrome P450 enzymes).
No products indexed under this heading.

Tolbutamide (Ranitidine has been reported to affect the bioavailability of other drugs through several different mechanisms, such as competition for renal tubular secretion, alteration of gastric pH, and inhibition of cytochrome P450 enzymes).
No products indexed under this heading.

Tolbutamide Sodium (Ranitidine has been reported to affect the bioavailability of other drugs through several different mechanisms, such as competition for renal tubular secretion, alteration of gastric pH, and inhibition of cytochrome P450 enzymes).
No products indexed under this heading.

Tolmetin Sodium (Ranitidine has been reported to affect the bioavailability of other drugs through several different mechanisms, such as competition for renal tubular secretion, alteration of gastric pH, and inhibition of cytochrome P450 enzymes).
No products indexed under this heading.

Tolterodine Tartrate (Ranitidine has been reported to affect the bioavailability of other drugs through several different mechanisms, such as competition for renal tubular secretion, alteration of gastric pH, and inhibition of cytochrome P450 enzymes).
No products indexed under this heading.

Topiramate (Ranitidine has been reported to affect the bioavailability of other drugs through several different mechanisms, such as competition for renal tubular secretion, alteration of gastric pH, and inhibition of cytochrome P450 enzymes).
No products indexed under this heading.

Torsemide (Ranitidine has been reported to affect the bioavailability of other drugs through several different mechanisms, such as competition for renal tubular secretion, alteration of gastric pH, and inhibition of cytochrome P450 enzymes).
No products indexed under this heading.

Tramadol Hydrochloride (Ranitidine has been reported to affect the bioavailability of other drugs through several different mechanisms, such as competition for renal tubular secretion, alteration of gastric pH, and inhibition of cytochrome P450 enzymes). Products include:
Ryzolt 2813
Ultram ER 2693

Trazodone Hydrochloride (Ranitidine has been reported to affect the bioavailability of other drugs through several different mechanisms, such as competition for renal tubular secretion, alteration of gastric pH, and inhibition of cytochrome P450 enzymes).
No products indexed under this heading.

Tretinoin (Ranitidine has been reported to affect the bioavailability of other drugs through several different mechanisms, such as competition for renal tubular secretion, alteration of gastric pH, and inhibition of cytochrome P450 enzymes).
No products indexed under this heading.

Triamterene (Ranitidine, a substrate of the renal organic cation transport system, may affect the clearance of other drugs eliminated by this route). Products include:
Dyazide 1429
Dyrenium 3495

Triazolam (Ranitidine may alter the absorption of drugs in which gastric pH is an important determinant of bioavailability. Triazolam exposure in healthy volunteers was increased by approximately 30% when administered with oral ranitidine at a dose of 150 mg twice daily. Monitor patients for excessive or prolonged sedation).
No products indexed under this heading.

Trimethadione (Ranitidine has been reported to affect the bioavailability of other drugs through several different mechanisms, such as competition for renal tubular secretion, alteration of gastric pH, and inhibition of cytochrome P450 enzymes).
No products indexed under this heading.

Trimethaphan Camsylate (Ranitidine has been reported to affect the bioavailability of other drugs through several different mechanisms, such as competition for renal tubular secretion, alteration of gastric pH, and inhibition of cytochrome P450 enzymes).
No products indexed under this heading.

Trimethoprim (Ranitidine, a substrate of the renal organic cation transport system, may affect the clearance of other drugs eliminated by this route).
No products indexed under this heading.

Trimethoprim Sulfate (Ranitidine, a substrate of the renal organic cation transport system, may affect the clearance of other drugs eliminated by this route).
No products indexed under this heading.

Trimipramine Maleate (Ranitidine has been reported to affect the bioavailability of other drugs through several different mechanisms, such as competition for renal tubular secretion, alteration of gastric pH, and inhibition of cytochrome P450 enzymes).
No products indexed under this heading.

Troglitazone (Ranitidine has been reported to affect the bioavailability of other drugs through several different mechanisms, such as competition for renal tubular secretion, alteration of gastric pH, and inhibition of cytochrome P450 enzymes).
No products indexed under this heading.

Trovafloxacin Mesylate (Ranitidine has been reported to affect the bioavailability of other drugs through several different mechanisms, such as competition for renal tubular secretion, alteration of gastric pH, and inhibition of cytochrome P450 enzymes).
No products indexed under this heading.

Valdecoxib (Ranitidine has been reported to affect the bioavailability of other drugs through several different mechanisms, such as competition for renal tubular secretion, alteration of gastric pH, and inhibition of cytochrome P450 enzymes).
No products indexed under this heading.

Valproate Sodium (Ranitidine has been reported to affect the bioavailability of other drugs through several different mechanisms, such as competition for renal tubular secretion, alteration of gastric pH, and inhibition of cytochrome P450 enzymes).
No products indexed under this heading.

Valproic Acid (Ranitidine has been reported to affect the bioavailability of other drugs through several different mechanisms, such as competition for renal tubular secretion, alteration of gastric pH, and inhibition of cytochrome P450 enzymes).
No products indexed under this heading.

Valsartan (Ranitidine has been reported to affect the bioavailability of other drugs through several different mechanisms, such as competition for renal tubular secretion, alteration of gastric pH, and inhibition of cytochrome P450 enzymes). Products include:
Diovan 2413
Diovan HCT 2419
Exforge 2443
Exforge HCT 2449
Valturna 3637

Vancomycin Hydrochloride (Ranitidine, a substrate of the renal organic cation transport system, may affect the clearance of other drugs eliminated by this route).
No products indexed under this heading.

Vardenafil Hydrochloride (Ranitidine has been reported to affect the bioavailability of other drugs through several different mechanisms, such as competition for renal tubular secretion, alteration of gastric pH, and inhibition of cytochrome P450 enzymes). Products include:
Levitra 3157

Venlafaxine Hydrochloride (Ranitidine has been reported to affect the bioavailability of other drugs through several different mechanisms, such as competition for renal tubular secretion, alteration of gastric pH, and inhibition of cytochrome P450 enzymes). Products include:
Effexor XR 3504
Venlafaxine Hydrochloride Tablets ... 2388

Verapamil Hydrochloride (Ranitidine has been reported to affect the bioavailability of other drugs through several different mechanisms, such as competition for renal tubular secretion, alteration of gastric pH, and inhibition of cytochrome P450 enzymes). Products include:
Tarka 534

(⊙ Described in PDR® for Ophthalmic Medicines)

2131 Interactions Index Zemplar Capsules

Vinblastine Sulfate (Ranitidine has been reported to affect the bioavailability of other drugs through several different mechanisms, such as competition for renal tubular secretion, alteration of gastric pH, and inhibition of cytochrome P450 enzymes).
No products indexed under this heading.

Vincristine Sulfate (Ranitidine has been reported to affect the bioavailability of other drugs through several different mechanisms, such as competition for renal tubular secretion, alteration of gastric pH, and inhibition of cytochrome P450 enzymes).
No products indexed under this heading.

Vitamin A (Ranitidine has been reported to affect the bioavailability of other drugs through several different mechanisms, such as competition for renal tubular secretion, alteration of gastric pH, and inhibition of cytochrome P450 enzymes). Products include:
Cardio Basics 3455
Heplive 607
Norwegian Cod Liver Oil 919

Vitamin A Acetate (Ranitidine has been reported to affect the bioavailability of other drugs through several different mechanisms, such as competition for renal tubular secretion, alteration of gastric pH, and inhibition of cytochrome P450 enzymes).
No products indexed under this heading.

Voriconazole (Ranitidine has been reported to affect the bioavailability of other drugs through several different mechanisms, such as competition for renal tubular secretion, alteration of gastric pH, and inhibition of cytochrome P450 enzymes).
No products indexed under this heading.

Warfarin Sodium (There have been reports of altered prothrombin time among patients on concomitant warfarin and ranitidine therapy. Due to the narrow therapeutic index, close monitoring of increased or decreased prothrombin time is recommended during concurrent treatment with ranitidine).
No products indexed under this heading.

Zafirlukast (Ranitidine has been reported to affect the bioavailability of other drugs through several different mechanisms, such as competition for renal tubular secretion, alteration of gastric pH, and inhibition of cytochrome P450 enzymes). Products include:
Accolate 3612

Zileuton (Ranitidine has been reported to affect the bioavailability of other drugs through several different mechanisms, such as competition for renal tubular secretion, alteration of gastric pH, and inhibition of cytochrome P450 enzymes).
No products indexed under this heading.

Zolmitriptan (Ranitidine has been reported to affect the bioavailability of other drugs through several different mechanisms, such as competition for renal tubular secretion, alteration of gastric pH, and inhibition of cytochrome P450 enzymes). Products include:
Zomig Tablets 773
Zomig Nasal Spray 768
Zomig-ZMT Tablets 773

Zonisamide (Ranitidine has been reported to affect the bioavailability of other drugs through several different mechanisms, such as competition for renal tubular secretion, alteration of gastric pH, and inhibition of cytochrome P450 enzymes). Products include:
Zonegran 1081

Zopiclone (Ranitidine has been reported to affect the bioavailability of other drugs through several different mechanisms, such as competition for renal tubular secretion, alteration of gastric pH, and inhibition of cytochrome P450 enzymes).
No products indexed under this heading.

Food Interactions

Beverages, caffeine-containing (Ranitidine has been reported to affect the bioavailability of other drugs through several different mechanisms, such as competition for renal tubular secretion, alteration of gastric pH, and inhibition of cytochrome P450 enzymes).

Food, caffeine-containing (Ranitidine has been reported to affect the bioavailability of other drugs through several different mechanisms, such as competition for renal tubular secretion, alteration of gastric pH, and inhibition of cytochrome P450 enzymes).

ZANTAC INJECTION PHARMACY BULK PACKAGE

(Ranitidine Hydrochloride) 1735
See Zantac Injection

ZANTAC INJECTION PREMIXED

(Ranitidine Hydrochloride) 1732
See Zantac Injection

ZANTAC SYRUP

(Ranitidine Hydrochloride) 1737
See Zantac 150 Tablets

ZEEL INJECTION SOLUTION

(Homeopathic Formulations) 1801
None cited in PDR database.

ZEMPLAR CAPSULES

(Paricalcitol) 568
May interact with cytochrome p450 3a4 inhibitors, potent (selected), and certain other agents. Compounds in these categories include:

Amprenavir (A study has demonstrated that ketoconazole approximately doubled paricalcitol AUC. Since paricalcitol is partially metabolized by CYP3A and ketoconazole is known to be a strong inhibitor of cytochrome P450 3A enzyme, care should be taken while dosing paricalcitol with ketoconazole and other strong P450 3A inhibitors. Dose adjustment of paricalcitol capsules may be required and iPTH and serum calcium concentrations should be closely monitored if a patient initiates or discontinues therapy with a strong CYP3A4 inhibitor, such as ketoconazole).
No products indexed under this heading.

Atazanavir (A study has demonstrated that ketoconazole approximately doubled paricalcitol AUC. Since paricalcitol is partially metabolized by CYP3A and ketoconazole is known to be a strong inhibitor of cytochrome P450 3A enzyme, care should be taken while dosing paricalcitol with ketoconazole and other strong P450 3A inhibitors. Dose adjustment of paricalcitol capsules may be required and iPTH and serum calcium concentrations should be closely monitored if a patient initiates or discontinues therapy with a strong CYP3A4 inhibitor, such as ketoconazole).
No products indexed under this heading.

Atazanavir Sulfate (A study has demonstrated that ketoconazole approximately doubled paricalcitol AUC. Since paricalcitol is partially metabolized by CYP3A and ketoconazole is known to be a strong inhibitor of cytochrome P450 3A enzyme, care should be taken while dosing paricalcitol with ketoconazole and other strong P450 3A inhibitors. Dose adjustment of paricalcitol capsules may be required and iPTH and serum calcium concentrations should be closely monitored if a patient initiates or discontinues therapy with a strong CYP3A4 inhibitor, such as ketoconazole).
No products indexed under this heading.

Cholestyramine (Drugs that impair intestinal absorption of fat-soluble vitamins, such as cholestyramine, may interfere with the absorption of paricalcitol).
No products indexed under this heading.

Clarithromycin (A study has demonstrated that ketoconazole approximately doubled paricalcitol AUC. Since paricalcitol is partially metabolized by CYP3A and ketoconazole is known to be a strong inhibitor of cytochrome P450 3A enzyme, care should be taken while dosing paricalcitol with ketoconazole and other strong P450 3A inhibitors. Dose adjustment of paricalcitol capsules may be required and iPTH and serum calcium concentrations should be closely monitored if a patient initiates or discontinues therapy with a strong CYP3A4 inhibitor, such as ketoconazole). Products include:
Biaxin/Biaxin XL 412

Delavirdine Mesylate (A study has demonstrated that ketoconazole approximately doubled paricalcitol AUC. Since paricalcitol is partially metabolized by CYP3A and ketoconazole is known to be a strong inhibitor of cytochrome P450 3A enzyme, care should be taken while dosing paricalcitol with ketoconazole and other strong P450 3A inhibitors. Dose adjustment of paricalcitol capsules may be required and iPTH and serum calcium concentrations should be closely monitored if a patient initiates or discontinues therapy with a strong CYP3A4 inhibitor, such as ketoconazole).
No products indexed under this heading.

Delavirine (A study has demonstrated that ketoconazole approximately doubled paricalcitol AUC. Since paricalcitol is partially metabolized by CYP3A and ketoconazole is known to be a strong inhibitor of cytochrome P450 3A enzyme, care should be taken while dosing paricalcitol with ketoconazole and other strong P450 3A inhibitors. Dose adjustment of paricalcitol capsules may be required and iPTH and serum calcium concentrations should be closely monitored if a patient initiates or discontinues therapy with a strong CYP3A4 inhibitor, such as ketoconazole).
No products indexed under this heading.

Fosamprenavir Calcium (A study has demonstrated that ketoconazole approximately doubled paricalcitol AUC. Since paricalcitol is partially metabolized by CYP3A and ketoconazole is known to be a strong inhibitor of cytochrome P450 3A enzyme, care should be taken while dosing paricalcitol with ketoconazole and other strong P450 3A inhibitors. Dose adjustment of paricalcitol capsules may be required and iPTH and serum calcium concentrations should be closely monitored if a patient initiates or discontinues therapy with a strong CYP3A4 inhibitor, such as ketoconazole). Products include:
Lexiva Oral Suspension 1558
Lexiva 1558

Indinavir Sulfate (A study has demonstrated that ketoconazole approximately doubled paricalcitol AUC. Since paricalcitol is partially metabolized by CYP3A and ketoconazole is known to be a strong inhibitor of cytochrome P450 3A enzyme, care should be taken while dosing paricalcitol with ketoconazole and other strong P450 3A inhibitors. Dose adjustment of paricalcitol capsules may be required and iPTH and serum calcium concentrations should be closely monitored if a patient initiates or discontinues therapy with a strong CYP3A4 inhibitor, such as ketoconazole). Products include:
Crixivan 2113

Itraconazole (A study has demonstrated that ketoconazole approximately doubled paricalcitol AUC. Since paricalcitol is partially metabolized by CYP3A and ketoconazole is known to be a strong inhibitor of cytochrome P450 3A enzyme, care should be taken while dosing paricalcitol with ketoconazole and other strong P450 3A inhibitors. Dose adjustment of paricalcitol capsules may be required and iPTH and serum calcium concentrations should be closely monitored if a patient initiates or discontinues therapy with a strong CYP3A4 inhibitor, such as ketoconazole).
No products indexed under this heading.

Ketoconazole (A study has demonstrated that ketoconazole approximately doubled paricalcitol AUC. Since paricalcitol is partially metabolized by CYP3A and ketoconazole is known to be a strong inhibitor of cytochrome P450 3A enzyme, care should be taken while dosing paricalcitol with ketoconazole and other strong P450 3A inhibitors. Dose adjustment of paricalcitol capsules may be required and iPTH and serum calcium concentrations should be closely monitored if a patient initiates or discontinues therapy with a strong CYP3A4 inhibitor, such as ketoconazole). Products include:
Extina 3319
Xolegel 3337

Lopinavir (A study has demonstrated that ketoconazole approximately doubled paricalcitol AUC. Since paricalcitol is partially metabolized by CYP3A and ketoconazole is known to be a strong inhibitor of cytochrome P450 3A enzyme, care should be taken while dosing paricalcitol with ketoconazole and other strong P450 3A inhibitors. Dose adjustment of paricalcitol capsules may be required and iPTH and serum calcium concentrations should be closely monitored if a patient initiates or discontinues therapy with a strong CYP3A4 inhibitor, such as ketoconazole). Products include:
Kaletra 458

Nefazodone Hydrochloride (A study has demonstrated that ketoconazole approximately doubled paricalcitol AUC. Since paricalcitol is partially metabolized by CYP3A and ketoconazole is known to be a strong inhibitor of cytochrome P450 3A enzyme, care should be taken while dosing paricalcitol with ketoconazole and other strong P450 3A inhibitors. Dose adjustment of paricalcitol capsules may be required and iPTH and serum calcium concentrations should be closely monitored if a patient initiates or discontinues therapy with a strong CYP3A4 inhibitor, such as ketoconazole).
No products indexed under this heading.

Nelfinavir Mesylate (A study has demonstrated that ketoconazole approximately doubled paricalcitol AUC. Since paricalcitol is partially metabolized by CYP3A and ketoconazole is known to be a strong inhibitor of cytochrome P450 3A enzyme, care should be taken while dosing paricalcitol with ketoconazole and other strong P450 3A inhibitors. Dose adjustment of paricalcitol capsules may be required and iPTH and serum calcium concentrations should be closely monitored if a patient

IMPORTANT NOTE: Always consult each drug listing in the patient's regimen for possible interactions.

initiates or discontinues therapy with a strong CYP3A4 inhibitor, such as ketoconazole).

No products indexed under this heading.

Ritonavir (A study has demonstrated that ketoconazole approximately doubled paricalcitol AUC. Since paricalcitol is partially metabolized by CYP3A and ketoconazole is known to be a strong inhibitor of cytochrome P450 3A enzyme, care should be taken while dosing paricalcitol with ketoconazole and other strong P450 3A inhibitors. Dose adjustment of paricalcitol capsules may be required and iPTH and serum calcium concentrations should be closely monitored if a patient initiates or discontinues therapy with a strong CYP3A4 inhibitor, such as ketoconazole). Products include:

Kaletra 458
Norvir 509

Saquinavir (A study has demonstrated that ketoconazole approximately doubled paricalcitol AUC. Since paricalcitol is partially metabolized by CYP3A and ketoconazole is known to be a strong inhibitor of cytochrome P450 3A enzyme, care should be taken while dosing paricalcitol with ketoconazole and other strong P450 3A inhibitors. Dose adjustment of paricalcitol capsules may be required and iPTH and serum calcium concentrations should be closely monitored if a patient initiates or discontinues therapy with a strong CYP3A4 inhibitor, such as ketoconazole).

No products indexed under this heading.

Saquinavir Mesylate (A study has demonstrated that ketoconazole approximately doubled paricalcitol AUC. Since paricalcitol is partially metabolized by CYP3A and ketoconazole is known to be a strong inhibitor of cytochrome P450 3A enzyme, care should be taken while dosing paricalcitol with ketoconazole and other strong P450 3A inhibitors. Dose adjustment of paricalcitol capsules may be required and iPTH and serum calcium concentrations should be closely monitored if a patient initiates or discontinues therapy with a strong CYP3A4 inhibitor, such as ketoconazole).

No products indexed under this heading.

Telithromycin (A study has demonstrated that ketoconazole approximately doubled paricalcitol AUC. Since paricalcitol is partially metabolized by CYP3A and ketoconazole is known to be a strong inhibitor of cytochrome P450 3A enzyme, care should be taken while dosing paricalcitol with ketoconazole and other strong P450 3A inhibitors. Dose adjustment of paricalcitol capsules may be required and iPTH and serum calcium concentrations should be closely monitored if a patient initiates or discontinues therapy with a strong CYP3A4 inhibitor, such as ketoconazole). Products include:

Ketek 2991

Troleandomycin (A study has demonstrated that ketoconazole approximately doubled paricalcitol AUC. Since paricalcitol is partially metabolized by CYP3A and ketoconazole is known to be a strong inhibitor of cytochrome P450 3A enzyme, care should be taken while dosing paricalcitol with ketoconazole and other strong P450 3A inhibitors. Dose adjustment of paricalcitol capsules may be required and iPTH and serum calcium concentrations should be closely monitored if a patient initiates or discontinues therapy with a strong CYP3A4 inhibitor, such as ketoconazole).

No products indexed under this heading.

Voriconazole (A study has demonstrated that ketoconazole approximately doubled paricalcitol AUC. Since paricalcitol is partially metabolized by CYP3A and ketoconazole is known to be a strong inhibitor of cytochrome P450 3A enzyme, care should be taken while dosing paricalcitol with ketoconazole and other strong P450 3A inhibitors. Dose adjustment of paricalcitol capsules may be required and iPTH and serum calcium concentrations should be closely monitored if a patient initiates or discontinues therapy with a strong CYP3A4 inhibitor, such as ketoconazole).

No products indexed under this heading.

ZEMPLAR INJECTION

(Paricalcitol) 571

May interact with cardiac glycosides, cytochrome p450 3a inhibitors (selected), and certain other agents. Compounds in these categories include:

Amiodarone Hydrochloride (A multiple dose drug-drug interaction study with ketoconazole and paricalcitol capsule demonstrated that ketoconazole approximately doubled paricalcitol AUC since paricalcitol is partially metabolized by CYP3A and ketoconazole is known to be a strong inhibitor of cytochrome P450 3A enzyme. Care should be taken while dosing paricalcitol with ketoconazole and other strong P450 3A inhibitors including atazanavir, clarithromycin, indinavir, itraconazole, nefazodone, nelfinavir, ritonavir, saquinavir, telithromycin or voriconazole).

No products indexed under this heading.

Amprenavir (A multiple dose drug-drug interaction study with ketoconazole and paricalcitol capsule demonstrated that ketoconazole approximately doubled paricalcitol AUC since paricalcitol is partially metabolized by CYP3A and ketoconazole is known to be a strong inhibitor of cytochrome P450 3A enzyme. Care should be taken while dosing paricalcitol with ketoconazole and other strong P450 3A inhibitors including atazanavir, clarithromycin, indinavir, itraconazole, nefazodone, nelfinavir, ritonavir, saquinavir, telithromycin or voriconazole).

No products indexed under this heading.

Aprepitant (A multiple dose drug-drug interaction study with ketoconazole and paricalcitol capsule demonstrated that ketoconazole approximately doubled paricalcitol AUC since paricalcitol is partially metabolized by CYP3A and ketoconazole is known to be a strong inhibitor of cytochrome P450 3A enzyme. Care should be taken while dosing paricalcitol with ketoconazole and other strong P450 3A inhibitors including atazanavir, clarithromycin, indinavir, itraconazole, nefazodone, nelfinavir, ritonavir, saquinavir, telithromycin or voriconazole). Products include:

Emend 2124

Atazanavir (A multiple dose drug-drug interaction study with ketoconazole and paricalcitol capsule demonstrated that ketoconazole approximately doubled paricalcitol AUC since paricalcitol is partially metabolized by CYP3A and ketoconazole is known to be a strong inhibitor of cytochrome P450 3A enzyme. Care should be taken while dosing paricalcitol with ketoconazole and other strong P450 3A inhibitors including atazanavir, clarithromycin, indinavir, itraconazole, nefazodone, nelfinavir, ritonavir, saquinavir, telithromycin or voriconazole).

No products indexed under this heading.

Atazanavir Sulfate (A multiple dose drug-drug interaction study with ketoconazole and paricalcitol capsule demonstrated that ketoconazole approximately doubled paricalcitol AUC since paricalcitol is partially metabolized by CYP3A and ketoconazole is known to be a strong inhibitor of cytochrome P450 3A enzyme. Care should be taken while dosing paricalcitol with ketoconazole and other strong P450 3A inhibitors including atazanavir, clarithromycin, indinavir, itraconazole, nefazodone, nelfinavir, ritonavir, saquinavir, telithromycin or voriconazole).

No products indexed under this heading.

Calcitriol (Vitamin D-related compounds should not be taken concomitantly with paricalcitol). Products include:

Calcijex 422

Cimetidine (A multiple dose drug-drug interaction study with ketoconazole and paricalcitol capsule demonstrated that ketoconazole approximately doubled paricalcitol AUC since paricalcitol is partially metabolized by CYP3A and ketoconazole is known to be a strong inhibitor of cytochrome P450 3A enzyme. Care should be taken while dosing paricalcitol with ketoconazole and other strong P450 3A inhibitors including atazanavir, clarithromycin, indinavir, itraconazole, nefazodone, nelfinavir, ritonavir, saquinavir, telithromycin or voriconazole).

No products indexed under this heading.

Cimetidine Hydrochloride (A multiple dose drug-drug interaction study with ketoconazole and paricalcitol capsule demonstrated that ketoconazole approximately doubled paricalcitol AUC since paricalcitol is partially metabolized by CYP3A and ketoconazole is known to be a strong inhibitor of cytochrome P450 3A enzyme. Care should be taken while dosing paricalcitol with ketoconazole and other strong P450 3A inhibitors including atazanavir, clarithromycin, indinavir, itraconazole, nefazodone, nelfinavir, ritonavir, saquinavir, telithromycin or voriconazole).

No products indexed under this heading.

Ciprofloxacin (A multiple dose drug-drug interaction study with ketoconazole and paricalcitol capsule demonstrated that ketoconazole approximately doubled paricalcitol AUC since paricalcitol is partially metabolized by CYP3A and ketoconazole is known to be a strong inhibitor of cytochrome P450 3A enzyme. Care should be taken while dosing paricalcitol with ketoconazole and other strong P450 3A inhibitors including atazanavir, clarithromycin, indinavir, itraconazole, nefazodone, nelfinavir, ritonavir, saquinavir, telithromycin or voriconazole). Products include:

Cipro I.V. 3082
Cipro 3073
Cipro XR 3091
Ciprodex 583

Ciprofloxacin Hydrochloride (A multiple dose drug-drug interaction study with ketoconazole and paricalcitol capsule demonstrated that ketoconazole approximately doubled paricalcitol AUC since paricalcitol is partially metabolized by CYP3A and ketoconazole is known to be a strong inhibitor of cytochrome P450 3A enzyme. Care should be taken while dosing paricalcitol with ketoconazole and other strong P450 3A inhibitors including atazanavir, clarithromycin, indinavir, itraconazole, nefazodone, nelfinavir, ritonavir, saquinavir, telithromycin or voriconazole). Products include:

Cipro 3073

Clarithromycin (A multiple dose drug-drug interaction study with ketoconazole and paricalcitol capsule demonstrated that ketoconazole approximately doubled paricalcitol AUC since paricalcitol is partially metabolized by CYP3A and ketoconazole is known to be a strong inhibitor of cytochrome P450 3A enzyme. Care should be taken while dosing paricalcitol with ketoconazole and other strong P450 3A inhibitors including atazanavir, clarithromycin, indinavir, itraconazole, nefazodone, nelfinavir, ritonavir, saquinavir, telithromycin or voriconazole). Products include:

Biaxin/Biaxin XL 412

Cyclosporine (A multiple dose drug-drug interaction study with ketoconazole and paricalcitol capsule demonstrated that ketoconazole approximately doubled paricalcitol AUC since paricalcitol is partially metabolized by CYP3A and ketoconazole is known to be a strong inhibitor of cytochrome P450 3A enzyme. Care should be taken while dosing paricalcitol with ketoconazole and other strong P450 3A inhibitors including atazanavir, clarithromycin, indinavir, itraconazole, nefazodone, nelfinavir, ritonavir, saquinavir, telithromycin or voriconazole). Products include:

Gengraf 440
Neoral Oral Solution 2496
Neoral Capsules 2496
Restasis 605

Delavirdine Mesylate (A multiple dose drug-drug interaction study with ketoconazole and paricalcitol capsule demonstrated that ketoconazole approximately doubled paricalcitol AUC since paricalcitol is partially metabolized by CYP3A and ketoconazole is known to be a strong inhibitor of cytochrome P450 3A enzyme. Care should be taken while dosing paricalcitol with ketoconazole and other strong P450 3A inhibitors including atazanavir, clarithromycin, indinavir, itraconazole, nefazodone, nelfinavir, ritonavir, saquinavir, telithromycin or voriconazole).

No products indexed under this heading.

Deslanoside (Digitalis toxicity is potentiated by hypercalcemia of any cause, so caution should be applied when digitalis compounds are prescribed concomitantly with paricalcitol).

No products indexed under this heading.

Digitalis Glycoside Preparations (Digitalis toxicity is potentiated by hypercalcemia of any cause, so caution should be applied when digitalis compounds are prescribed concomitantly with paricalcitol).

No products indexed under this heading.

Digitalis Lanata (Digitalis toxicity is potentiated by hypercalcemia of any cause, so caution should be applied when digitalis compounds are prescribed concomitantly with paricalcitol).

No products indexed under this heading.

Digitalis Purpurea (Digitalis toxicity is potentiated by hypercalcemia of any cause, so caution should be applied when digitalis compounds are prescribed concomitantly with paricalcitol).

No products indexed under this heading.

Digitoxin (Digitalis toxicity is potentiated by hypercalcemia of any cause, so caution should be applied when digitalis compounds are prescribed concomitantly with paricalcitol).

No products indexed under this heading.

Digoxin (Digitalis toxicity is potentiated by hypercalcemia of any cause, so caution should be applied when digitalis compounds are prescribed concomitantly with paricalcitol). Products include:

Lanoxin Injection 1546
Lanoxin Injection Pediatric 1549
Lanoxin Tablets 1553

Diltiazem Hydrochloride (A multiple dose drug-drug interaction study with ketoconazole and paricalcitol capsule demonstrated that ketoconazole approximately doubled paricalcitol AUC since paricalcitol is partially metabolized by CYP3A and ketoconazole is known to be a strong inhibitor of cytochrome P450 3A enzyme. Care should

2133 Interactions Index Zemplar Injection

be taken while dosing paricalcitol with ketoconazole and other strong P450 3A inhibitors including atazanavir, clarithromycin, indinavir, itraconazole, nefazodone, nelfinavir, ritonavir, saquinavir, telithromycin or voriconazole). Products include:

Cardizem LA 423

Diltiazem Maleate (A multiple dose drug-drug interaction study with ketoconazole and paricalcitol capsule demonstrated that ketoconazole approximately doubled paricalcitol AUC since paricalcitol is partially metabolized by CYP3A and ketoconazole is known to be a strong inhibitor of cytochrome P450 3A enzyme. Care should be taken while dosing paricalcitol with ketoconazole and other strong P450 3A inhibitors including atazanavir, clarithromycin, indinavir, itraconazole, nefazodone, nelfinavir, ritonavir, saquinavir, telithromycin or voriconazole).

No products indexed under this heading.

Efavirenz (A multiple dose drug-drug interaction study with ketoconazole and paricalcitol capsule demonstrated that ketoconazole approximately doubled paricalcitol AUC since paricalcitol is partially metabolized by CYP3A and ketoconazole is known to be a strong inhibitor of cytochrome P450 3A enzyme. Care should be taken while dosing paricalcitol with ketoconazole and other strong P450 3A inhibitors including atazanavir, clarithromycin, indinavir, itraconazole, nefazodone, nelfinavir, ritonavir, saquinavir, telithromycin or voriconazole). Products include:

Atripla 906

Erythromycin (A multiple dose drug-drug interaction study with ketoconazole and paricalcitol capsule demonstrated that ketoconazole approximately doubled paricalcitol AUC since paricalcitol is partially metabolized by CYP3A and ketoconazole is known to be a strong inhibitor of cytochrome P450 3A enzyme. Care should be taken while dosing paricalcitol with ketoconazole and other strong P450 3A inhibitors including atazanavir, clarithromycin, indinavir, itraconazole, nefazodone, nelfinavir, ritonavir, saquinavir, telithromycin or voriconazole).

No products indexed under this heading.

Fluconazole (A multiple dose drug-drug interaction study with ketoconazole and paricalcitol capsule demonstrated that ketoconazole approximately doubled paricalcitol AUC since paricalcitol is partially metabolized by CYP3A and ketoconazole is known to be a strong inhibitor of cytochrome P450 3A enzyme. Care should be taken while dosing paricalcitol with ketoconazole and other strong P450 3A inhibitors including atazanavir, clarithromycin, indinavir, itraconazole, nefazodone, nelfinavir, ritonavir, saquinavir, telithromycin or voriconazole).

No products indexed under this heading.

Fluoxetine (A multiple dose drug-drug interaction study with ketoconazole and paricalcitol capsule demonstrated that ketoconazole approximately doubled paricalcitol AUC since paricalcitol is partially metabolized by CYP3A and ketoconazole is known to be a strong inhibitor of cytochrome P450 3A enzyme. Care should be taken while dosing paricalcitol with ketoconazole and other strong P450 3A inhibitors including atazanavir, clarithromycin, indinavir, itraconazole, nefazodone, nelfinavir, ritonavir, saquinavir, telithromycin or voriconazole).

No products indexed under this heading.

Fluoxetine Hydrochloride (A multiple dose drug-drug interaction study with ketoconazole and paricalcitol capsule demonstrated that ketoconazole approximately doubled paricalcitol AUC since paricalcitol is partially metabolized by CYP3A and ketoconazole is known to be a strong inhibitor of cytochrome P450 3A enzyme. Care should be taken while dosing paricalcitol with ketoconazole and other strong P450 3A inhibitors including atazanavir, clarithromycin, indinavir, itraconazole, nefazodone, nelfinavir, ritonavir, saquinavir, telithromycin or voriconazole). Products include:

Prozac Weekly 1941
Prozac Pulvules 1941
Symbyax 1965

Fluvoxamine Maleate (A multiple dose drug-drug interaction study with ketoconazole and paricalcitol capsule demonstrated that ketoconazole approximately doubled paricalcitol AUC since paricalcitol is partially metabolized by CYP3A and ketoconazole is known to be a strong inhibitor of cytochrome P450 3A enzyme. Care should be taken while dosing paricalcitol with ketoconazole and other strong P450 3A inhibitors including atazanavir, clarithromycin, indinavir, itraconazole, nefazodone, nelfinavir, ritonavir, saquinavir, telithromycin or voriconazole).

No products indexed under this heading.

Indinavir Sulfate (A multiple dose drug-drug interaction study with ketoconazole and paricalcitol capsule demonstrated that ketoconazole approximately doubled paricalcitol AUC since paricalcitol is partially metabolized by CYP3A and ketoconazole is known to be a strong inhibitor of cytochrome P450 3A enzyme. Care should be taken while dosing paricalcitol with ketoconazole and other strong P450 3A inhibitors including atazanavir, clarithromycin, indinavir, itraconazole, nefazodone, nelfinavir, ritonavir, saquinavir, telithromycin or voriconazole). Products include:

Crixivan 2113

Isoniazid (A multiple dose drug-drug interaction study with ketoconazole and paricalcitol capsule demonstrated that ketoconazole approximately doubled paricalcitol AUC since paricalcitol is partially metabolized by CYP3A and ketoconazole is known to be a strong inhibitor of cytochrome P450 3A enzyme. Care should be taken while dosing paricalcitol with ketoconazole and other strong P450 3A inhibitors including atazanavir, clarithromycin, indinavir, itraconazole, nefazodone, nelfinavir, ritonavir, saquinavir, telithromycin or voriconazole).

No products indexed under this heading.

Itraconazole (A multiple dose drug-drug interaction study with ketoconazole and paricalcitol capsule demonstrated that ketoconazole approximately doubled paricalcitol AUC since paricalcitol is partially metabolized by CYP3A and ketoconazole is known to be a strong inhibitor of cytochrome P450 3A enzyme. Care should be taken while dosing paricalcitol with ketoconazole and other strong P450 3A inhibitors including atazanavir, clarithromycin, indinavir, itraconazole, nefazodone, nelfinavir, ritonavir, saquinavir, telithromycin or voriconazole).

No products indexed under this heading.

Ketoconazole (A multiple dose drug-drug interaction study with ketoconazole and paricalcitol capsule demonstrated that ketoconazole approximately doubled paricalcitol AUC since paricalcitol is partially metabolized by CYP3A and ketoconazole is known to be a strong inhibitor of cytochrome P450 3A enzyme. Care should be taken while dosing paricalcitol with ketoconazole and other strong P450 3A inhibitors including atazanavir, clarithromycin, indinavir, itraconazole, nefazodone, nelfinavir, ritonavir, saquinavir, telithromycin or voriconazole). Products include:

Extina 3319
Xolegel 3337

Lopinavir (A multiple dose drug-drug interaction study with ketoconazole and paricalcitol capsule demonstrated that ketoconazole approximately doubled paricalcitol AUC since paricalcitol is partially metabolized by CYP3A and ketoconazole is known to be a strong inhibitor of cytochrome P450 3A enzyme. Care should be taken while dosing paricalcitol with ketoconazole and other strong P450 3A inhibitors including atazanavir, clarithromycin, indinavir, itraconazole, nefazodone, nelfinavir, ritonavir, saquinavir, telithromycin or voriconazole). Products include:

Kaletra 458

Metronidazole (A multiple dose drug-drug interaction study with ketoconazole and paricalcitol capsule demonstrated that ketoconazole approximately doubled paricalcitol AUC since paricalcitol is partially metabolized by CYP3A and ketoconazole is known to be a strong inhibitor of cytochrome P450 3A enzyme. Care should be taken while dosing paricalcitol with ketoconazole and other strong P450 3A inhibitors including atazanavir, clarithromycin, indinavir, itraconazole, nefazodone, nelfinavir, ritonavir, saquinavir, telithromycin or voriconazole). Products include:

Pylera 793

Metronidazole Benzoate (A multiple dose drug-drug interaction study with ketoconazole and paricalcitol capsule demonstrated that ketoconazole approximately doubled paricalcitol AUC since paricalcitol is partially metabolized by CYP3A and ketoconazole is known to be a strong inhibitor of cytochrome P450 3A enzyme. Care should be taken while dosing paricalcitol with ketoconazole and other strong P450 3A inhibitors including atazanavir, clarithromycin, indinavir, itraconazole, nefazodone, nelfinavir, ritonavir, saquinavir, telithromycin or voriconazole).

No products indexed under this heading.

Metronidazole Hydrochloride (A multiple dose drug-drug interaction study with ketoconazole and paricalcitol capsule demonstrated that ketoconazole approximately doubled paricalcitol AUC since paricalcitol is partially metabolized by CYP3A and ketoconazole is known to be a strong inhibitor of cytochrome P450 3A enzyme. Care should be taken while dosing paricalcitol with ketoconazole and other strong P450 3A inhibitors including atazanavir, clarithromycin, indinavir, itraconazole, nefazodone, nelfinavir, ritonavir, saquinavir, telithromycin or voriconazole).

No products indexed under this heading.

Miconazole (A multiple dose drug-drug interaction study with ketoconazole and paricalcitol capsule demonstrated that ketoconazole approximately doubled paricalcitol AUC since paricalcitol is partially metabolized by CYP3A and ketoconazole is known to be a strong inhibitor of cytochrome P450 3A enzyme. Care should be taken while dosing paricalcitol with ketoconazole and other strong P450 3A inhibitors including atazanavir, clarithromycin, indinavir, itraconazole, nefazodone, nelfinavir, ritonavir, saquinavir, telithromycin or voriconazole).

No products indexed under this heading.

Nefazodone Hydrochloride (A multiple dose drug-drug interaction study with ketoconazole and paricalcitol capsule demonstrated that ketoconazole approximately doubled paricalcitol AUC since paricalcitol is partially metabolized by CYP3A and ketoconazole is known to be a strong inhibitor of cytochrome P450 3A enzyme. Care should be taken while dosing paricalcitol with ketoconazole and other strong P450 3A inhibitors including atazanavir, clarithromycin, indinavir, itraconazole, nefazodone, nelfinavir, ritonavir, saquinavir, telithromycin or voriconazole).

No products indexed under this heading.

Nelfinavir Mesylate (A multiple dose drug-drug interaction study with ketoconazole and paricalcitol capsule demonstrated that ketoconazole approximately doubled paricalcitol AUC since paricalcitol is partially metabolized by CYP3A and ketoconazole is known to be a strong inhibitor of cytochrome P450 3A enzyme. Care should be taken while dosing paricalcitol with ketoconazole and other strong P450 3A inhibitors including atazanavir, clarithromycin, indinavir, itraconazole, nefazodone, nelfinavir, ritonavir, saquinavir, telithromycin or voriconazole).

No products indexed under this heading.

Nifedipine (A multiple dose drug-drug interaction study with ketoconazole and paricalcitol capsule demonstrated that ketoconazole approximately doubled paricalcitol AUC since paricalcitol is partially metabolized by CYP3A and ketoconazole is known to be a strong inhibitor of cytochrome P450 3A enzyme. Care should be taken while dosing paricalcitol with ketoconazole and other strong P450 3A inhibitors including atazanavir, clarithromycin, indinavir, itraconazole, nefazodone, nelfinavir, ritonavir, saquinavir, telithromycin or voriconazole).

No products indexed under this heading.

Norfloxacin (A multiple dose drug-drug interaction study with ketoconazole and paricalcitol capsule demonstrated that ketoconazole approximately doubled paricalcitol AUC since paricalcitol is partially metabolized by CYP3A and ketoconazole is known to be a strong inhibitor of cytochrome P450 3A enzyme. Care should be taken while dosing paricalcitol with ketoconazole and other strong P450 3A inhibitors including atazanavir, clarithromycin, indinavir, itraconazole, nefazodone, nelfinavir, ritonavir, saquinavir, telithromycin or voriconazole). Products include:

Noroxin 2220

Paroxetine Hydrochloride (A multiple dose drug-drug interaction study with ketoconazole and paricalcitol capsule demonstrated that ketoconazole approximately doubled paricalcitol AUC since paricalcitol is partially metabolized by CYP3A and ketoconazole is known to be a strong inhibitor of cytochrome P450 3A enzyme. Care should be taken while dosing paricalcitol with ketoconazole and other strong P450 3A inhibitors including atazanavir, clarithromycin, indinavir, itraconazole, nefazodone, nelfinavir, ritonavir, saquinavir, telithromycin or voriconazole). Products include:

Paroxetine CR 2361
Paroxetine ER 2371
Paxil 1586
Paxil CR 1596

Potassium Acid Phosphate (Phosphate compounds should not be taken concomitantly with paricalcitol). Products include:

K-Phos Original 874

Potassium Phosphate (Phosphate compounds should not be taken concomitantly with paricalcitol). Products include:

K-Phos Neutral 873

Quinine (A multiple dose drug-drug interaction study with ketoconazole and paricalcitol capsule demonstrated that

IMPORTANT NOTE: Always consult each drug listing in the patient's regimen for possible interactions.

ketoconazole approximately doubled paricalcitol AUC since paricalcitol is partially metabolized by CYP3A and ketoconazole is known to be a strong inhibitor of cytochrome P450 3A enzyme. Care should be taken while dosing paricalcitol with ketoconazole and other strong P450 3A inhibitors including atazanavir, clarithromycin, indinavir, itraconazole, nefazodone, nelfinavir, ritonavir, saquinavir, telithromycin or voriconazole). Products include:

Hyland's Leg Cramps PM with Quinine 3315

Quinine Sulfate (A multiple dose drug-drug interaction study with ketoconazole and paricalcitol capsule demonstrated that ketoconazole approximately doubled paricalcitol AUC since paricalcitol is partially metabolized by CYP3A and ketoconazole is known to be a strong inhibitor of cytochrome P450 3A enzyme. Care should be taken while dosing paricalcitol with ketoconazole and other strong P450 3A inhibitors including atazanavir, clarithromycin, indinavir, itraconazole, nefazodone, nelfinavir, ritonavir, saquinavir, telithromycin or voriconazole).

No products indexed under this heading.

Ritonavir (A multiple dose drug-drug interaction study with ketoconazole and paricalcitol capsule demonstrated that ketoconazole approximately doubled paricalcitol AUC since paricalcitol is partially metabolized by CYP3A and ketoconazole is known to be a strong inhibitor of cytochrome P450 3A enzyme. Care should be taken while dosing paricalcitol with ketoconazole and other strong P450 3A inhibitors including atazanavir, clarithromycin, indinavir, itraconazole, nefazodone, nelfinavir, ritonavir, saquinavir, telithromycin or voriconazole). Products include:

Kaletra 458
Norvir 509

Saquinavir (A multiple dose drug-drug interaction study with ketoconazole and paricalcitol capsule demonstrated that ketoconazole approximately doubled paricalcitol AUC since paricalcitol is partially metabolized by CYP3A and ketoconazole is known to be a strong inhibitor of cytochrome P450 3A enzyme. Care should be taken while dosing paricalcitol with ketoconazole and other strong P450 3A inhibitors including atazanavir, clarithromycin, indinavir, itraconazole, nefazodone, nelfinavir, ritonavir, saquinavir, telithromycin or voriconazole).

No products indexed under this heading.

Saquinavir Mesylate (A multiple dose drug-drug interaction study with ketoconazole and paricalcitol capsule demonstrated that ketoconazole approximately doubled paricalcitol AUC since paricalcitol is partially metabolized by CYP3A and ketoconazole is known to be a strong inhibitor of cytochrome P450 3A enzyme. Care should be taken while dosing paricalcitol with ketoconazole and other strong P450 3A inhibitors including atazanavir, clarithromycin, indinavir, itraconazole, nefazodone, nelfinavir, ritonavir, saquinavir, telithromycin or voriconazole).

No products indexed under this heading.

Sertraline Hydrochloride (A multiple dose drug-drug interaction study with ketoconazole and paricalcitol capsule demonstrated that ketoconazole approximately doubled paricalcitol AUC since paricalcitol is partially metabolized by CYP3A and ketoconazole is known to be a strong inhibitor of cytochrome P450 3A enzyme. Care should be taken while dosing paricalcitol with ketoconazole and other strong P450 3A inhibitors including atazanavir, clarithromycin, indinavir, itraconazole, nefazodone, nelfinavir, ritonavir, saquinavir, telithromycin or voriconazole).

No products indexed under this heading.

Telithromycin (A multiple dose drug-drug interaction study with ketoconazole and paricalcitol capsule demonstrated that ketoconazole approximately doubled paricalcitol AUC since paricalcitol is partially metabolized by CYP3A and ketoconazole is known to be a strong inhibitor of cytochrome P450 3A enzyme. Care should be taken while dosing paricalcitol with ketoconazole and other strong P450 3A inhibitors including atazanavir, clarithromycin, indinavir, itraconazole, nefazodone, nelfinavir, ritonavir, saquinavir, telithromycin or voriconazole). Products include:

Ketek 2991

Troleandomycin (A multiple dose drug-drug interaction study with ketoconazole and paricalcitol capsule demonstrated that ketoconazole approximately doubled paricalcitol AUC since paricalcitol is partially metabolized by CYP3A and ketoconazole is known to be a strong inhibitor of cytochrome P450 3A enzyme. Care should be taken while dosing paricalcitol with ketoconazole and other strong P450 3A inhibitors including atazanavir, clarithromycin, indinavir, itraconazole, nefazodone, nelfinavir, ritonavir, saquinavir, telithromycin or voriconazole).

No products indexed under this heading.

Venlafaxine Hydrochloride (A multiple dose drug-drug interaction study with ketoconazole and paricalcitol capsule demonstrated that ketoconazole approximately doubled paricalcitol AUC since paricalcitol is partially metabolized by CYP3A and ketoconazole is known to be a strong inhibitor of cytochrome P450 3A enzyme. Care should be taken while dosing paricalcitol with ketoconazole and other strong P450 3A inhibitors including atazanavir, clarithromycin, indinavir, itraconazole, nefazodone, nelfinavir, ritonavir, saquinavir, telithromycin or voriconazole). Products include:

Effexor XR 3504
Venlafaxine Hydrochloride Tablets ... 2388

Verapamil Hydrochloride (A multiple dose drug-drug interaction study with ketoconazole and paricalcitol capsule demonstrated that ketoconazole approximately doubled paricalcitol AUC since paricalcitol is partially metabolized by CYP3A and ketoconazole is known to be a strong inhibitor of cytochrome P450 3A enzyme. Care should be taken while dosing paricalcitol with ketoconazole and other strong P450 3A inhibitors including atazanavir, clarithromycin, indinavir, itraconazole, nefazodone, nelfinavir, ritonavir, saquinavir, telithromycin or voriconazole). Products include:

Tarka 534

Voriconazole (A multiple dose drug-drug interaction study with ketoconazole and paricalcitol capsule demonstrated that ketoconazole approximately doubled paricalcitol AUC since paricalcitol is partially metabolized by CYP3A and ketoconazole is known to be a strong inhibitor of cytochrome P450 3A enzyme. Care should be taken while dosing paricalcitol with ketoconazole and other strong P450 3A inhibitors including atazanavir, clarithromycin, indinavir, itraconazole, nefazodone, nelfinavir, ritonavir, saquinavir, telithromycin or voriconazole).

No products indexed under this heading.

Zafirlukast (A multiple dose drug-drug interaction study with ketoconazole and paricalcitol capsule demonstrated that ketoconazole approximately doubled paricalcitol AUC since paricalcitol is partially metabolized by CYP3A and ketoconazole is known to be a strong inhibitor of cytochrome P450 3A enzyme. Care should be taken while dosing paricalcitol with ketoconazole and other strong P450 3A inhibitors including atazanavir, clarithromycin, indinavir, itraconazole, nefazodone, nelfinavir, ritonavir, saquinavir, telithromycin or voriconazole). Products include:

Accolate 3612

Zileuton (A multiple dose drug-drug interaction study with ketoconazole and paricalcitol capsule demonstrated that ketoconazole approximately doubled paricalcitol AUC since paricalcitol is partially metabolized by CYP3A and ketoconazole is known to be a strong inhibitor of cytochrome P450 3A enzyme. Care should be taken while dosing paricalcitol with ketoconazole and other strong P450 3A inhibitors including atazanavir, clarithromycin, indinavir, itraconazole, nefazodone, nelfinavir, ritonavir, saquinavir, telithromycin or voriconazole).

No products indexed under this heading.

Food Interactions

Grapefruit (A multiple dose drug-drug interaction study with ketoconazole and paricalcitol capsule demonstrated that ketoconazole approximately doubled paricalcitol AUC since paricalcitol is partially metabolized by CYP3A and ketoconazole is known to be a strong inhibitor of cytochrome P450 3A enzyme. Care should be taken while dosing paricalcitol with ketoconazole and other strong P450 3A inhibitors including atazanavir, clarithromycin, indinavir, itraconazole, nefazodone, nelfinavir, ritonavir, saquinavir, telithromycin or voriconazole).

Grapefruit Juice (A multiple dose drug-drug interaction study with ketoconazole and paricalcitol capsule demonstrated that ketoconazole approximately doubled paricalcitol AUC since paricalcitol is partially metabolized by CYP3A and ketoconazole is known to be a strong inhibitor of cytochrome P450 3A enzyme. Care should be taken while dosing paricalcitol with ketoconazole and other strong P450 3A inhibitors including atazanavir, clarithromycin, indinavir, itraconazole, nefazodone, nelfinavir, ritonavir, saquinavir, telithromycin or voriconazole).

ZEMURON INJECTION

(Rocuronium Bromide) 3249

May interact with aminoglycosides, antibiotics, anticonvulsants, barbiturates, corticosteroids, general anesthetics, inhalant anesthetics, lithium preparations, local anesthetics, magnesium salts, nondepolarizing neuromuscular blocking agents, phenytoin, quinidine, tetracyclines, and certain other agents. Compounds in these categories include:

Alatrofloxacin Mesylate (Drugs which may enhance the neuromuscular blocking action of non-depolarizing agents such as rocuronium include certain antibiotics (eg, aminoglycosides, vancomycin, tetracyclines, bacitracin, polymyxins, colistin, and sodium colistimethate). If these antibiotics are used in conjunction with rocuronium, prolongation of neuromuscular block may occur. In patients in whom potentiation of neuromuscular block may be anticipated, a decrease from the recommended initial dose of rocuronium should be considered).

No products indexed under this heading.

Alclometasone Dipropionate (Myopathy after long-term administration of other non-depolarizing neuromuscular blocking agents in the ICU alone or in combination with corticosteroid therapy has been reported. Therefore, for patients receiving both neuromuscular blocking agents and corticosteroids, the period of use of the neuromuscular blocking agent should be limited as much as possible and only used in the setting where in the opinion of the prescribing physician, the specific advantages of the drug outweigh the risk).

No products indexed under this heading.

Alkaline Drugs (Rocuronium, which has an acid pH, should not be mixed with alkaline solutions (eg, barbiturate solutions) in the same syringe or administered simultaneously during intravenous infusion through the same needle).

No products indexed under this heading.

Amikacin Sulfate (Drugs which may enhance the neuromuscular blocking action of rocuronium include certain antibiotics, such as aminoglyosides. If aminoglycosides are used in conjunction with rocuronium, prolongation of neuromuscular block may occur. In patients in whom potentiation of neuromuscular block may be anticipated, a decrease from the recommended initial dose of rocuronium should be considered).

No products indexed under this heading.

Amobarbital (Rocuronium, which has an acid pH, should not be mixed with alkaline solutions (eg, barbiturate solutions) in the same syringe or administered simultaneously during intravenous infusion through the same needle).

No products indexed under this heading.

Amobarbital Sodium (Rocuronium, which has an acid pH, should not be mixed with alkaline solutions (eg, barbiturate solutions) in the same syringe or administered simultaneously during intravenous infusion through the same needle).

No products indexed under this heading.

Amoxicillin (Drugs which may enhance the neuromuscular blocking action of non-depolarizing agents such as rocuronium include certain antibiotics (eg, aminoglycosides, vancomycin, tetracyclines, bacitracin, polymyxins, colistin, and sodium colistimethate). If these antibiotics are used in conjunction with rocuronium, prolongation of neuromuscular block may occur. In patients in whom potentiation of neuromuscular block may be anticipated, a decrease from the recommended initial dose of rocuronium should be considered). Products include:

Amoxil Capsules 1311
Amoxil Chewable Tablets 1311
Amoxil 1311
Amoxil Powder 1311
Augmentin 1331
Augmentin Tablets 1335
Augmentin ES-600 1338
Augmentin XR 1342
Moxatag 2321

Amoxicillin Trihydrate (Drugs which may enhance the neuromuscular blocking action of non-depolarizing agents such as rocuronium include certain antibiotics (eg, aminoglycosides, vancomycin, tetracyclines, bacitracin, polymyxins, colistin, and sodium colistimethate). If these antibiotics are used in conjunction with rocuronium, prolongation of neuromuscular block may occur. In patients in whom potentiation of neuromuscular block may be anticipated, a decrease from the recommended initial dose of rocuronium should be considered).

No products indexed under this heading.

Ampicillin (Drugs which may enhance the neuromuscular blocking action of non-depolarizing agents such as rocuronium include certain antibiotics (eg, aminoglycosides, vancomycin, tetracy-

2135 Interactions Index Zemuron

clines, bacitracin, polymyxins, colistin, and sodium colistimethate). If these antibiotics are used in conjunction with rocuronium, prolongation of neuromuscular block may occur. In patients in whom potentiation of neuromuscular block may be anticipated, a decrease from the recommended initial dose of rocuronium should be considered).
No products indexed under this heading.

Ampicillin Sodium (Drugs which may enhance the neuromuscular blocking action of non-depolarizing agents such as rocuronium include certain antibiotics (eg, aminoglycosides, vancomycin, tetracyclines, bacitracin, polymyxins, colistin, and sodium colistimethate). If these antibiotics are used in conjunction with rocuronium, prolongation of neuromuscular block may occur. In patients in whom potentiation of neuromuscular block may be anticipated, a decrease from the recommended initial dose of rocuronium should be considered).
No products indexed under this heading.

Ampicillin Trihydrate (Drugs which may enhance the neuromuscular blocking action of non-depolarizing agents such as rocuronium include certain antibiotics (eg, aminoglycosides, vancomycin, tetracyclines, bacitracin, polymyxins, colistin, and sodium colistimethate). If these antibiotics are used in conjunction with rocuronium, prolongation of neuromuscular block may occur. In patients in whom potentiation of neuromuscular block may be anticipated, a decrease from the recommended initial dose of rocuronium should be considered).
No products indexed under this heading.

Antibiotics, non-penicillin, unspecified (Drugs which may enhance the neuromuscular blocking action of non-depolarizing agents such as rocuronium include certain antibiotics (eg, aminoglycosides, vancomycin, tetracyclines, bacitracin, polymyxins, colistin, and sodium colistimethate). If these antibiotics are used in conjunction with rocuronium, prolongation of neuromuscular block may occur. In patients in whom potentiation of neuromuscular block may be anticipated, a decrease from the recommended initial dose of rocuronium should be considered).
No products indexed under this heading.

Aprobarbital (Rocuronium, which has an acid pH, should not be mixed with alkaline solutions (eg, barbiturate solutions) in the same syringe or administered simultaneously during intravenous infusion through the same needle).
No products indexed under this heading.

Articaine Hydrochloride (Local anesthetics have been shown to increase the duration of neuromuscular block and decrease infusion requirements of other neuromuscular blocking agents. In patients in whom potentiation of neuromuscular block may be anticipated, a decrease from the recommended initial dose of rocuronium should be considered).
No products indexed under this heading.

Atracurium Besylate (There are no controlled studies documenting the use of rocuronium before or after other non-depolarizing muscle relaxants. Interactions have been observed when other non-depolarizing muscle relaxants have been administered in succession).
No products indexed under this heading.

Azithromycin Dihydrate (Drugs which may enhance the neuromuscular blocking action of non-depolarizing agents such as rocuronium include certain antibiotics (eg, aminoglycosides, vancomycin, tetracyclines, bacitracin, polymyxins, colistin, and sodium colistimethate). If these antibiotics are used in conjunction with rocuronium, prolongation of neuromuscular block may occur. In patients in whom potentiation of neuromuscular block may be anticipated, a decrease from the recommended initial dose of rocuronium should be considered).
No products indexed under this heading.

Azlocillin Sodium (Drugs which may enhance the neuromuscular blocking action of non-depolarizing agents such as rocuronium include certain antibiotics (eg, aminoglycosides, vancomycin, tetracyclines, bacitracin, polymyxins, colistin, and sodium colistimethate). If these antibiotics are used in conjunction with rocuronium, prolongation of neuromuscular block may occur. In patients in whom potentiation of neuromuscular block may be anticipated, a decrease from the recommended initial dose of rocuronium should be considered).
No products indexed under this heading.

Aztreonam (Drugs which may enhance the neuromuscular blocking action of non-depolarizing agents such as rocuronium include certain antibiotics (eg, aminoglycosides, vancomycin, tetracyclines, bacitracin, polymyxins, colistin, and sodium colistimethate). If these antibiotics are used in conjunction with rocuronium, prolongation of neuromuscular block may occur. In patients in whom potentiation of neuromuscular block may be anticipated, a decrease from the recommended initial dose of rocuronium should be considered).
No products indexed under this heading.

Bacampicillin Hydrochloride (Drugs which may enhance the neuromuscular blocking action of non-depolarizing agents such as rocuronium include certain antibiotics (eg, aminoglycosides, vancomycin, tetracyclines, bacitracin, polymyxins, colistin, and sodium colistimethate). If these antibiotics are used in conjunction with rocuronium, prolongation of neuromuscular block may occur. In patients in whom potentiation of neuromuscular block may be anticipated, a decrease from the recommended initial dose of rocuronium should be considered).
No products indexed under this heading.

Bacitracin (Drugs which may enhance the neuromuscular blocking action of nondepolarizing agents such as rocuronium include certain antibiotics (eg, bacitracin). If bacitracin is used in conjunction with rocuronium, prolongation of neuromuscular block may occur. In patients in whom potentiation of neuromuscular block may be anticipated, a decrease from the recommended initial dose of rocuronium should be considered).
No products indexed under this heading.

Beclomethasone Dipropionate (Myopathy after long-term administration of other non-depolarizing neuromuscular blocking agents in the ICU alone or in combination with corticosteroid therapy has been reported. Therefore, for patients receiving both neuromuscular blocking agents and corticosteroids, the period of use of the neuromuscular blocking agent should be limited as much as possible and only used in the setting where in the opinion of the prescribing physician, the specific advantages of the drug outweigh the risk). Products include:
Qvar 3398

Beclomethasone Dipropionate Monohydrate (Myopathy after long-term administration of other non-depolarizing neuromuscular blocking agents in the ICU alone or in combination with corticosteroid therapy has been reported. Therefore, for patients receiving both neuromuscular blocking agents and corticosteroids, the period of use of the neuromuscular blocking agent should be limited as much as possible and only used in the setting where in the opinion of the prescribing physician, the specific advantages of the drug outweigh the risk). Products include:
Beconase AQ 1386

Betamethasone (Myopathy after long-term administration of other non-depolarizing neuromuscular blocking agents in the ICU alone or in combination with corticosteroid therapy has been reported. Therefore, for patients receiving both neuromuscular blocking agents and corticosteroids, the period of use of the neuromuscular blocking agent should be limited as much as possible and only used in the setting where in the opinion of the prescribing physician, the specific advantages of the drug outweigh the risk).
No products indexed under this heading.

Betamethasone Acetate (Myopathy after long-term administration of other non-depolarizing neuromuscular blocking agents in the ICU alone or in combination with corticosteroid therapy has been reported. Therefore, for patients receiving both neuromuscular blocking agents and corticosteroids, the period of use of the neuromuscular blocking agent should be limited as much as possible and only used in the setting where in the opinion of the prescribing physician, the specific advantages of the drug outweigh the risk).
No products indexed under this heading.

Betamethasone Benzoate (Myopathy after long-term administration of other non-depolarizing neuromuscular blocking agents in the ICU alone or in combination with corticosteroid therapy has been reported. Therefore, for patients receiving both neuromuscular blocking agents and corticosteroids, the period of use of the neuromuscular blocking agent should be limited as much as possible and only used in the setting where in the opinion of the prescribing physician, the specific advantages of the drug outweigh the risk).
No products indexed under this heading.

Betamethasone Dipropionate (Myopathy after long-term administration of other non-depolarizing neuromuscular blocking agents in the ICU alone or in combination with corticosteroid therapy has been reported. Therefore, for patients receiving both neuromuscular blocking agents and corticosteroids, the period of use of the neuromuscular blocking agent should be limited as much as possible and only used in the setting where in the opinion of the prescribing physician, the specific advantages of the drug outweigh the risk). Products include:
Diprolene Lotion 0.05% 3108
Diprolene Ointment 0.05% 3109
Diprolene AF Cream 0.05% 3107
Lotrisone 3163

Betamethasone Sodium Phosphate (Myopathy after long-term administration of other non-depolarizing neuromuscular blocking agents in the ICU alone or in combination with corticosteroid therapy has been reported. Therefore, for patients receiving both neuromuscular blocking agents and corticosteroids, the period of use of the neuromuscular blocking agent should be limited as much as possible and only used in the setting where in the opinion of the prescribing physician, the specific advantages of the drug outweigh the risk).
No products indexed under this heading.

Betamethasone Valerate (Myopathy after long-term administration of other non-depolarizing neuromuscular blocking agents in the ICU alone or in combination with corticosteroid therapy has been reported. Therefore, for patients receiving both neuromuscular blocking agents and corticosteroids, the period of use of the neuromuscular blocking agent should be limited as much as possible and only used in the setting where in the opinion of the prescribing physician, the specific advantages of the drug outweigh the risk). Products include:
Luxiq 3321

Budesonide (Myopathy after long-term administration of other non-depolarizing neuromuscular blocking agents in the ICU alone or in combination with corticosteroid therapy has been reported. Therefore, for patients receiving both neuromuscular blocking agents and corticosteroids, the period of use of the neuromuscular blocking agent should be limited as much as possible and only used in the setting where in the opinion of the prescribing physician, the specific advantages of the drug outweigh the risk). Products include:
Pulmicort Flexhaler 714
Symbicort 80/4.5 720
Symbicort 160/4.5 720

Bupivacaine Hydrochloride (Local anesthetics have been shown to increase the duration of neuromuscular block and decrease infusion requirements of other neuromuscular blocking agents. In patients in whom potentiation of neuromuscular block may be anticipated, a decrease from the recommended initial dose of rocuronium should be considered).
No products indexed under this heading.

Butabarbital (Rocuronium, which has an acid pH, should not be mixed with alkaline solutions (eg, barbiturate solutions) in the same syringe or administered simultaneously during intravenous infusion through the same needle).
No products indexed under this heading.

Butabarbital Sodium (Rocuronium, which has an acid pH, should not be mixed with alkaline solutions (eg, barbiturate solutions) in the same syringe or administered simultaneously during intravenous infusion through the same needle).
No products indexed under this heading.

Butalbital (Rocuronium, which has an acid pH, should not be mixed with alkaline solutions (eg, barbiturate solutions) in the same syringe or administered simultaneously during intravenous infusion through the same needle).
No products indexed under this heading.

Carbamazepine (In two out of four patients receiving chronic anticonvulsant therapy, apparent resistance to the effects of rocuronium was observed in the form of diminished magnitude of neuromuscular block, or shortened clinical duration. As with other non-depolarizing neuromuscular blocking drugs, if rocuronium is administered to patients chronically receiving anticonvulsant agents, such as carbamazepine, shorter durations of neuromuscular block may occur and infusion rates may be higher due to the development of resistance to non-depolarizing muscle relaxants. While the mechanism for development of this resistance is not known, receptor upregulation may be a contributing factor). Products include:
Carbatrol 3280
Equetro 3477

Carbenicillin Disodium (Drugs which may enhance the neuromuscular blocking action of non-depolarizing agents such as rocuronium include certain antibiotics (eg, aminoglycosides, vancomycin, tetracyclines, bacitracin, polymyxins, colistin, and sodium colistimethate). If these antibiotics are used in conjunction with rocuronium, prolongation of neuromuscular block may occur. In patients in whom potentiation of neuromuscular block may be anticipated, a

IMPORTANT NOTE: Always consult each drug listing in the patient's regimen for possible interactions.

Zemuron Interactions Index 2136

decrease from the recommended initial dose of rocuronium should be considered).
No products indexed under this heading.

Carbenicillin Indanyl Sodium (Drugs which may enhance the neuromuscular blocking action of non-depolarizing agents such as rocuronium include certain antibiotics (eg, aminoglycosides, vancomycin, tetracyclines, bacitracin, polymyxins, colistin, and sodium colistimethate). If these antibiotics are used in conjunction with rocuronium, prolongation of neuromuscular block may occur. In patients in whom potentiation of neuromuscular block may be anticipated, a decrease from the recommended initial dose of rocuronium should be considered).
No products indexed under this heading.

Cefaclor (Drugs which may enhance the neuromuscular blocking action of non-depolarizing agents such as rocuronium include certain antibiotics (eg, aminoglycosides, vancomycin, tetracyclines, bacitracin, polymyxins, colistin, and sodium colistimethate). If these antibiotics are used in conjunction with rocuronium, prolongation of neuromuscular block may occur. In patients in whom potentiation of neuromuscular block may be anticipated, a decrease from the recommended initial dose of rocuronium should be considered).
No products indexed under this heading.

Cefadroxil (Drugs which may enhance the neuromuscular blocking action of non-depolarizing agents such as rocuronium include certain antibiotics (eg, aminoglycosides, vancomycin, tetracyclines, bacitracin, polymyxins, colistin, and sodium colistimethate). If these antibiotics are used in conjunction with rocuronium, prolongation of neuromuscular block may occur. In patients in whom potentiation of neuromuscular block may be anticipated, a decrease from the recommended initial dose of rocuronium should be considered).
No products indexed under this heading.

Cefamandole Nafate (Drugs which may enhance the neuromuscular blocking action of non-depolarizing agents such as rocuronium include certain antibiotics (eg, aminoglycosides, vancomycin, tetracyclines, bacitracin, polymyxins, colistin, and sodium colistimethate). If these antibiotics are used in conjunction with rocuronium, prolongation of neuromuscular block may occur. In patients in whom potentiation of neuromuscular block may be anticipated, a decrease from the recommended initial dose of rocuronium should be considered).
No products indexed under this heading.

Cefazolin Sodium (Drugs which may enhance the neuromuscular blocking action of non-depolarizing agents such as rocuronium include certain antibiotics (eg, aminoglycosides, vancomycin, tetracyclines, bacitracin, polymyxins, colistin, and sodium colistimethate). If these antibiotics are used in conjunction with rocuronium, prolongation of neuromuscular block may occur. In patients in whom potentiation of neuromuscular block may be anticipated, a decrease from the recommended initial dose of rocuronium should be considered).
No products indexed under this heading.

Cefixime (Drugs which may enhance the neuromuscular blocking action of non-depolarizing agents such as rocuronium include certain antibiotics (eg, aminoglycosides, vancomycin, tetracyclines, bacitracin, polymyxins, colistin, and sodium colistimethate). If these antibiotics are used in conjunction with rocuronium, prolongation of neuromuscular block may occur. In patients in whom potentiation of neuromuscular block may be anticipated, a decrease from the recommended initial dose of rocuronium should be considered). Products include:
Suprax for Oral Suspension 2038
Suprax Tablets 2038

Cefmetazole Sodium (Drugs which may enhance the neuromuscular blocking action of non-depolarizing agents such as rocuronium include certain antibiotics (eg, aminoglycosides, vancomycin, tetracyclines, bacitracin, polymyxins, colistin, and sodium colistimethate). If these antibiotics are used in conjunction with rocuronium, prolongation of neuromuscular block may occur. In patients in whom potentiation of neuromuscular block may be anticipated, a decrease from the recommended initial dose of rocuronium should be considered).
No products indexed under this heading.

Cefonicid Sodium (Drugs which may enhance the neuromuscular blocking action of non-depolarizing agents such as rocuronium include certain antibiotics (eg, aminoglycosides, vancomycin, tetracyclines, bacitracin, polymyxins, colistin, and sodium colistimethate). If these antibiotics are used in conjunction with rocuronium, prolongation of neuromuscular block may occur. In patients in whom potentiation of neuromuscular block may be anticipated, a decrease from the recommended initial dose of rocuronium should be considered).
No products indexed under this heading.

Cefoperazone Sodium (Drugs which may enhance the neuromuscular blocking action of non-depolarizing agents such as rocuronium include certain antibiotics (eg, aminoglycosides, vancomycin, tetracyclines, bacitracin, polymyxins, colistin, and sodium colistimethate). If these antibiotics are used in conjunction with rocuronium, prolongation of neuromuscular block may occur. In patients in whom potentiation of neuromuscular block may be anticipated, a decrease from the recommended initial dose of rocuronium should be considered).
No products indexed under this heading.

Ceforanide (Drugs which may enhance the neuromuscular blocking action of non-depolarizing agents such as rocuronium include certain antibiotics (eg, aminoglycosides, vancomycin, tetracyclines, bacitracin, polymyxins, colistin, and sodium colistimethate). If these antibiotics are used in conjunction with rocuronium, prolongation of neuromuscular block may occur. In patients in whom potentiation of neuromuscular block may be anticipated, a decrease from the recommended initial dose of rocuronium should be considered).
No products indexed under this heading.

Cefotaxime Sodium (Drugs which may enhance the neuromuscular blocking action of non-depolarizing agents such as rocuronium include certain antibiotics (eg, aminoglycosides, vancomycin, tetracyclines, bacitracin, polymyxins, colistin, and sodium colistimethate). If these antibiotics are used in conjunction with rocuronium, prolongation of neuromuscular block may occur. In patients in whom potentiation of neuromuscular block may be anticipated, a decrease from the recommended initial dose of rocuronium should be considered).
No products indexed under this heading.

Cefotetan (Drugs which may enhance the neuromuscular blocking action of non-depolarizing agents such as rocuronium include certain antibiotics (eg, aminoglycosides, vancomycin, tetracyclines, bacitracin, polymyxins, colistin, and sodium colistimethate). If these antibiotics are used in conjunction with rocuronium, prolongation of neuromuscular block may occur. In patients in whom potentiation of neuromuscular block may be anticipated, a decrease from the recommended initial dose of rocuronium should be considered).
No products indexed under this heading.

Cefoxitin Sodium (Drugs which may enhance the neuromuscular blocking action of non-depolarizing agents such as rocuronium include certain antibiotics (eg, aminoglycosides, vancomycin, tetracyclines, bacitracin, polymyxins, colistin, and sodium colistimethate). If these antibiotics are used in conjunction with rocuronium, prolongation of neuromuscular block may occur. In patients in whom potentiation of neuromuscular block may be anticipated, a decrease from the recommended initial dose of rocuronium should be considered).
No products indexed under this heading.

Cefpodoxime Proxetil (Drugs which may enhance the neuromuscular blocking action of non-depolarizing agents such as rocuronium include certain antibiotics (eg, aminoglycosides, vancomycin, tetracyclines, bacitracin, polymyxins, colistin, and sodium colistimethate). If these antibiotics are used in conjunction with rocuronium, prolongation of neuromuscular block may occur. In patients in whom potentiation of neuromuscular block may be anticipated, a decrease from the recommended initial dose of rocuronium should be considered).
No products indexed under this heading.

Cefprozil (Drugs which may enhance the neuromuscular blocking action of non-depolarizing agents such as rocuronium include certain antibiotics (eg, aminoglycosides, vancomycin, tetracyclines, bacitracin, polymyxins, colistin, and sodium colistimethate). If these antibiotics are used in conjunction with rocuronium, prolongation of neuromuscular block may occur. In patients in whom potentiation of neuromuscular block may be anticipated, a decrease from the recommended initial dose of rocuronium should be considered).
No products indexed under this heading.

Ceftazidime (Drugs which may enhance the neuromuscular blocking action of non-depolarizing agents such as rocuronium include certain antibiotics (eg, aminoglycosides, vancomycin, tetracyclines, bacitracin, polymyxins, colistin, and sodium colistimethate). If these antibiotics are used in conjunction with rocuronium, prolongation of neuromuscular block may occur. In patients in whom potentiation of neuromuscular block may be anticipated, a decrease from the recommended initial dose of rocuronium should be considered). Products include:
Fortaz 1481

Ceftizoxime Sodium (Drugs which may enhance the neuromuscular blocking action of non-depolarizing agents such as rocuronium include certain antibiotics (eg, aminoglycosides, vancomycin, tetracyclines, bacitracin, polymyxins, colistin, and sodium colistimethate). If these antibiotics are used in conjunction with rocuronium, prolongation of neuromuscular block may occur. In patients in whom potentiation of neuromuscular block may be anticipated, a decrease from the recommended initial dose of rocuronium should be considered).
No products indexed under this heading.

Ceftriaxone Sodium (Drugs which may enhance the neuromuscular blocking action of non-depolarizing agents such as rocuronium include certain antibiotics (eg, aminoglycosides, vancomycin, tetracyclines, bacitracin, polymyxins, colistin, and sodium colistimethate). If these antibiotics are used in conjunction with rocuronium, prolongation of neuromuscular block may occur. In patients in whom potentiation of neuromuscular block may be anticipated, a decrease from the recommended initial dose of rocuronium should be considered). Products include:
Rocephin 2859

Cefuroxime Axetil (Drugs which may enhance the neuromuscular blocking action of non-depolarizing agents such as rocuronium include certain antibiotics (eg, aminoglycosides, vancomycin, tetracyclines, bacitracin, polymyxins, colistin, and sodium colistimethate). If these antibiotics are used in conjunction with rocuronium, prolongation of neuromuscular block may occur. In patients in whom potentiation of neuromuscular block may be anticipated, a decrease from the recommended initial dose of rocuronium should be considered). Products include:
Ceftin 1399

Cefuroxime Sodium (Drugs which may enhance the neuromuscular blocking action of non-depolarizing agents such as rocuronium include certain antibiotics (eg, aminoglycosides, vancomycin, tetracyclines, bacitracin, polymyxins, colistin, and sodium colistimethate). If these antibiotics are used in conjunction with rocuronium, prolongation of neuromuscular block may occur. In patients in whom potentiation of neuromuscular block may be anticipated, a decrease from the recommended initial dose of rocuronium should be considered).
No products indexed under this heading.

Cephalexin (Drugs which may enhance the neuromuscular blocking action of non-depolarizing agents such as rocuronium include certain antibiotics (eg, aminoglycosides, vancomycin, tetracyclines, bacitracin, polymyxins, colistin, and sodium colistimethate). If these antibiotics are used in conjunction with rocuronium, prolongation of neuromuscular block may occur. In patients in whom potentiation of neuromuscular block may be anticipated, a decrease from the recommended initial dose of rocuronium should be considered).
No products indexed under this heading.

Cephalothin Sodium (Drugs which may enhance the neuromuscular blocking action of non-depolarizing agents such as rocuronium include certain antibiotics (eg, aminoglycosides, vancomycin, tetracyclines, bacitracin, polymyxins, colistin, and sodium colistimethate). If these antibiotics are used in conjunction with rocuronium, prolongation of neuromuscular block may occur. In patients in whom potentiation of neuromuscular block may be anticipated, a decrease from the recommended initial dose of rocuronium should be considered).
No products indexed under this heading.

Cephapirin Sodium (Drugs which may enhance the neuromuscular blocking action of non-depolarizing agents such as rocuronium include certain antibiotics (eg, aminoglycosides, vancomycin, tetracyclines, bacitracin, polymyxins, colistin, and sodium colistimethate). If these antibiotics are used in conjunction with rocuronium, prolongation of neuromuscular block may occur. In patients in whom potentiation of neuromuscular block may be anticipated, a decrease from the recommended initial dose of rocuronium should be considered).
No products indexed under this heading.

Cephradine (Drugs which may enhance the neuromuscular blocking action of non-depolarizing agents such as rocuronium include certain antibiotics (eg, aminoglycosides, vancomycin, tetracyclines, bacitracin, polymyxins, colistin, and sodium colistimethate). If these antibiotics are used in conjunction

with rocuronium, prolongation of neuromuscular block may occur. In patients in whom potentiation of neuromuscular block may be anticipated, a decrease from the recommended initial dose of rocuronium should be considered).
No products indexed under this heading.

Chloramphenicol (Drugs which may enhance the neuromuscular blocking action of non-depolarizing agents such as rocuronium include certain antibiotics (eg, aminoglycosides, vancomycin, tetracyclines, bacitracin, polymyxins, colistin, and sodium colistimethate). If these antibiotics are used in conjunction with rocuronium, prolongation of neuromuscular block may occur. In patients in whom potentiation of neuromuscular block may be anticipated, a decrease from the recommended initial dose of rocuronium should be considered).
No products indexed under this heading.

Chloramphenicol Palmitate (Drugs which may enhance the neuromuscular blocking action of non-depolarizing agents such as rocuronium include certain antibiotics (eg, aminoglycosides, vancomycin, tetracyclines, bacitracin, polymyxins, colistin, and sodium colistimethate). If these antibiotics are used in conjunction with rocuronium, prolongation of neuromuscular block may occur. In patients in whom potentiation of neuromuscular block may be anticipated, a decrease from the recommended initial dose of rocuronium should be considered).
No products indexed under this heading.

Chloramphenicol Sodium Succinate (Drugs which may enhance the neuromuscular blocking action of non-depolarizing agents such as rocuronium include certain antibiotics (eg, aminoglycosides, vancomycin, tetracyclines, bacitracin, polymyxins, colistin, and sodium colistimethate). If these antibiotics are used in conjunction with rocuronium, prolongation of neuromuscular block may occur. In patients in whom potentiation of neuromuscular block may be anticipated, a decrease from the recommended initial dose of rocuronium should be considered).
No products indexed under this heading.

Chloroprocaine Hydrochloride (Local anesthetics have been shown to increase the duration of neuromuscular block and decrease infusion requirements of other neuromuscular blocking agents. In patients in whom potentiation of neuromuscular block may be anticipated, a decrease from the recommended initial dose of rocuronium should be considered).
No products indexed under this heading.

Ciclesonide (Myopathy after long-term administration of other non-depolarizing neuromuscular blocking agents in the ICU alone or in combination with corticosteroid therapy has been reported. Therefore, for patients receiving both neuromuscular blocking agents and corticosteroids, the period of use of the neuromuscular blocking agent should be limited as much as possible and only used in the setting where in the opinion of the prescribing physician, the specific advantages of the drug outweigh the risk).
No products indexed under this heading.

Cilastatin Sodium (Drugs which may enhance the neuromuscular blocking action of non-depolarizing agents such as rocuronium include certain antibiotics (eg, aminoglycosides, vancomycin, tetracyclines, bacitracin, polymyxins, colistin, and sodium colistimethate). If these antibiotics are used in conjunction with rocuronium, prolongation of neuromuscular block may occur. In patients in whom potentiation of neuromuscular block may be anticipated, a decrease from the recommended initial dose of rocuronium should be considered).
Products include:
Primaxin I.M. 2232
Primaxin I.V. 2235

Ciprofloxacin (Drugs which may enhance the neuromuscular blocking action of non-depolarizing agents such as rocuronium include certain antibiotics (eg, aminoglycosides, vancomycin, tetracyclines, bacitracin, polymyxins, colistin, and sodium colistimethate). If these antibiotics are used in conjunction with rocuronium, prolongation of neuromuscular block may occur. In patients in whom potentiation of neuromuscular block may be anticipated, a decrease from the recommended initial dose of rocuronium should be considered).
Products include:
Cipro I.V. 3082
Cipro 3073
Cipro XR 3091
Ciprodex 583

Ciprofloxacin Hydrochloride (Drugs which may enhance the neuromuscular blocking action of non-depolarizing agents such as rocuronium include certain antibiotics (eg, aminoglycosides, vancomycin, tetracyclines, bacitracin, polymyxins, colistin, and sodium colistimethate). If these antibiotics are used in conjunction with rocuronium, prolongation of neuromuscular block may occur. In patients in whom potentiation of neuromuscular block may be anticipated, a decrease from the recommended initial dose of rocuronium should be considered). Products include:
Cipro 3073

Cisatracurium Besylate (There are no controlled studies documenting the use of rocuronium before or after other non-depolarizing muscle relaxants. Interactions have been observed when other non-depolarizing muscle relaxants have been administered in succession).
Products include:
Nimbex 503

Clarithromycin (Drugs which may enhance the neuromuscular blocking action of non-depolarizing agents such as rocuronium include certain antibiotics (eg, aminoglycosides, vancomycin, tetracyclines, bacitracin, polymyxins, colistin, and sodium colistimethate). If these antibiotics are used in conjunction with rocuronium, prolongation of neuromuscular block may occur. In patients in whom potentiation of neuromuscular block may be anticipated, a decrease from the recommended initial dose of rocuronium should be considered).
Products include:
Biaxin/Biaxin XL 412

Clotrimazole (Drugs which may enhance the neuromuscular blocking action of non-depolarizing agents such as rocuronium include certain antibiotics (eg, aminoglycosides, vancomycin, tetracyclines, bacitracin, polymyxins, colistin, and sodium colistimethate). If these antibiotics are used in conjunction with rocuronium, prolongation of neuromuscular block may occur. In patients in whom potentiation of neuromuscular block may be anticipated, a decrease from the recommended initial dose of rocuronium should be considered).
Products include:
Lotrisone 3163

Cloxacillin (Drugs which may enhance the neuromuscular blocking action of non-depolarizing agents such as rocuronium include certain antibiotics (eg, aminoglycosides, vancomycin, tetracyclines, bacitracin, polymyxins, colistin, and sodium colistimethate). If these antibiotics are used in conjunction with rocuronium, prolongation of neuromuscular block may occur. In patients in whom potentiation of neuromuscular block may be anticipated, a decrease from the recommended initial dose of rocuronium should be considered).
No products indexed under this heading.

Cloxacillin Sodium (Drugs which may enhance the neuromuscular blocking action of non-depolarizing agents such as rocuronium include certain antibiotics (eg, aminoglycosides, vancomycin, tetracyclines, bacitracin, polymyxins, colistin, and sodium colistimethate). If these antibiotics are used in conjunction with rocuronium, prolongation of neuromuscular block may occur. In patients in whom potentiation of neuromuscular block may be anticipated, a decrease from the recommended initial dose of rocuronium should be considered).
No products indexed under this heading.

Cloxacillin Sodium Monohydrate (Drugs which may enhance the neuromuscular blocking action of non-depolarizing agents such as rocuronium include certain antibiotics (eg, aminoglycosides, vancomycin, tetracyclines, bacitracin, polymyxins, colistin, and sodium colistimethate). If these antibiotics are used in conjunction with rocuronium, prolongation of neuromuscular block may occur. In patients in whom potentiation of neuromuscular block may be anticipated, a decrease from the recommended initial dose of rocuronium should be considered).
No products indexed under this heading.

Cocaine Hydrochloride (Local anesthetics have been shown to increase the duration of neuromuscular block and decrease infusion requirements of other neuromuscular blocking agents. In patients in whom potentiation of neuromuscular block may be anticipated, a decrease from the recommended initial dose of rocuronium should be considered).
No products indexed under this heading.

Colistimethate Sodium (Drugs which may enhance the neuromuscular blocking action of rocuronium include certain antibiotics, such as colistimethate sodium. If colistimethate sodium is used in conjunction with rocuronium, prolongation of neuromuscular block may occur. In patients in whom potentiation of neuromuscular block may be anticipated, a decrease from the recommended initial dose of rocuronium should be considered).
No products indexed under this heading.

Colistin Sulfate (Drugs which may enhance the neuromuscular blocking action of rocuronium include certain antibiotics, such as colistin. If colistin is used in conjunction with rocuronium, prolongation of neuromuscular block may occur. In patients in whom potentiation of neuromuscular block may be anticipated, a decrease from the recommended initial dose of rocuronium should be considered).
No products indexed under this heading.

Cortisone Acetate (Myopathy after long-term administration of other non-depolarizing neuromuscular blocking agents in the ICU alone or in combination with corticosteroid therapy has been reported. Therefore, for patients receiving both neuromuscular blocking agents and corticosteroids, the period of use of the neuromuscular blocking agent should be limited as much as possible and only used in the setting where in the opinion of the prescribing physician, the specific advantages of the drug outweigh the risk).
No products indexed under this heading.

Daunorubicin Hydrochloride (Drugs which may enhance the neuromuscular blocking action of non-depolarizing agents such as rocuronium include certain antibiotics (eg, aminoglycosides, vancomycin, tetracyclines, bacitracin, polymyxins, colistin, and sodium colistimethate). If these antibiotics are used in conjunction with rocuronium, prolongation of neuromuscular block may occur. In patients in whom potentiation of neuromuscular block may be anticipated, a decrease from the recommended initial dose of rocuronium should be considered).
No products indexed under this heading.

Demeclocycline Hydrochloride (Drugs which may enhance the neuromuscular blocking action of rocuronium include certain antibiotics, such as tetracyclines. If tetracyclines are used in conjunction with rocuronium, prolongation of neuromuscular block may occur. In patients in whom potentiation of neuromuscular block may be anticipated, a decrease from the recommended initial dose of rocuronium should be considered).
No products indexed under this heading.

Desflurane (Use of inhalation anesthetics as been shown to enhance the activity of other neuromuscular blocking agents. In patients in whom potentiation of neuromuscular block may be anticipated, a decrease from the recommended initial dose of rocuronium should be considered).
No products indexed under this heading.

Desoximetasone (Myopathy after long-term administration of other non-depolarizing neuromuscular blocking agents in the ICU alone or in combination with corticosteroid therapy has been reported. Therefore, for patients receiving both neuromuscular blocking agents and corticosteroids, the period of use of the neuromuscular blocking agent should be limited as much as possible and only used in the setting where in the opinion of the prescribing physician, the specific advantages of the drug outweigh the risk).
No products indexed under this heading.

Dexamethasone (Myopathy after long-term administration of other non-depolarizing neuromuscular blocking agents in the ICU alone or in combination with corticosteroid therapy has been reported. Therefore, for patients receiving both neuromuscular blocking agents and corticosteroids, the period of use of the neuromuscular blocking agent should be limited as much as possible and only used in the setting where in the opinion of the prescribing physician, the specific advantages of the drug outweigh the risk). Products include:
Ciprodex 583
Ozurdex .... ⊙ 223
Tobramycin and Dexamethasone Ophthalmic Suspension .... ⊙ 251

Dexamethasone Acetate (Myopathy after long-term administration of other non-depolarizing neuromuscular blocking agents in the ICU alone or in combination with corticosteroid therapy has been reported. Therefore, for patients receiving both neuromuscular blocking agents and corticosteroids, the period of use of the neuromuscular blocking agent should be limited as much as possible and only used in the setting where in the opinion of the prescribing physician, the specific advantages of the drug outweigh the risk).
No products indexed under this heading.

Dexamethasone Phosphate (Myopathy after long-term administration of other non-depolarizing neuromuscular blocking agents in the ICU alone or in combination with corticosteroid therapy has been reported. Therefore, for patients receiving both neuromuscular blocking agents and corticosteroids, the period of use of the neuromuscular blocking agent should be limited as much as possible and only used in the

Zemuron Interactions Index 2138

setting where in the opinion of the prescribing physician, the specific advantages of the drug outweigh the risk).
No products indexed under this heading.

Dexamethasone Sodium (Myopathy after long-term administration of other non-depolarizing neuromuscular blocking agents in the ICU alone or in combination with corticosteroid therapy has been reported. Therefore, for patients receiving both neuromuscular blocking agents and corticosteroids, the period of use of the neuromuscular blocking agent should be limited as much as possible and only used in the setting where in the opinion of the prescribing physician, the specific advantages of the drug outweigh the risk).
No products indexed under this heading.

Dexamethasone Sodium Phosphate (Myopathy after long-term administration of other non-depolarizing neuromuscular blocking agents in the ICU alone or in combination with corticosteroid therapy has been reported. Therefore, for patients receiving both neuromuscular blocking agents and corticosteroids, the period of use of the neuromuscular blocking agent should be limited as much as possible and only used in the setting where in the opinion of the prescribing physician, the specific advantages of the drug outweigh the risk).
No products indexed under this heading.

Dexamethasone Sodium Phosphate Injection (Myopathy after long-term administration of other non-depolarizing neuromuscular blocking agents in the ICU alone or in combination with corticosteroid therapy has been reported. Therefore, for patients receiving both neuromuscular blocking agents and corticosteroids, the period of use of the neuromuscular blocking agent should be limited as much as possible and only used in the setting where in the opinion of the prescribing physician, the specific advantages of the drug outweigh the risk).
No products indexed under this heading.

Dicloxacillin (Drugs which may enhance the neuromuscular blocking action of non-depolarizing agents such as rocuronium include certain antibiotics (eg, aminoglycosides, vancomycin, tetracyclines, bacitracin, polymyxins, colistin, and sodium colistimethate). If these antibiotics are used in conjunction with rocuronium, prolongation of neuromuscular block may occur. In patients in whom potentiation of neuromuscular block may be anticipated, a decrease from the recommended initial dose of rocuronium should be considered).
No products indexed under this heading.

Dicloxacillin Sodium (Drugs which may enhance the neuromuscular blocking action of non-depolarizing agents such as rocuronium include certain antibiotics (eg, aminoglycosides, vancomycin, tetracyclines, bacitracin, polymyxins, colistin, and sodium colistimethate). If these antibiotics are used in conjunction with rocuronium, prolongation of neuromuscular block may occur. In patients in whom potentiation of neuromuscular block may be anticipated, a decrease from the recommended initial dose of rocuronium should be considered).
No products indexed under this heading.

Diflorasone Diacetate (Myopathy after long-term administration of other non-depolarizing neuromuscular blocking agents in the ICU alone or in combination with corticosteroid therapy has been reported. Therefore, for patients receiving both neuromuscular blocking agents and corticosteroids, the period of use of the neuromuscular blocking agent should be limited as much as possible and only used in the setting where in the opinion of the prescribing physician, the specific advantages of the drug outweigh the risk).
No products indexed under this heading.

Dihydrostreptomycin (Drugs which may enhance the neuromuscular blocking action of rocuronium include certain antibiotics, such as aminoglyosides. If aminoglycosides are used in conjunction with rocuronium, prolongation of neuromuscular block may occur. In patients in whom potentiation of neuromuscular block may be anticipated, a decrease from the recommended initial dose of rocuronium should be considered).
No products indexed under this heading.

Dirithromycin (Drugs which may enhance the neuromuscular blocking action of non-depolarizing agents such as rocuronium include certain antibiotics (eg, aminoglycosides, vancomycin, tetracyclines, bacitracin, polymyxins, colistin, and sodium colistimethate). If these antibiotics are used in conjunction with rocuronium, prolongation of neuromuscular block may occur. In patients in whom potentiation of neuromuscular block may be anticipated, a decrease from the recommended initial dose of rocuronium should be considered).
No products indexed under this heading.

Disodium Carbenicillin (Drugs which may enhance the neuromuscular blocking action of non-depolarizing agents such as rocuronium include certain antibiotics (eg, aminoglycosides, vancomycin, tetracyclines, bacitracin, polymyxins, colistin, and sodium colistimethate). If these antibiotics are used in conjunction with rocuronium, prolongation of neuromuscular block may occur. In patients in whom potentiation of neuromuscular block may be anticipated, a decrease from the recommended initial dose of rocuronium should be considered).
No products indexed under this heading.

Divalproex Sodium (In two out of four patients receiving chronic anticonvulsant therapy, apparent resistance to the effects of rocuronium was observed in the form of diminished magnitude of neuromuscular block, or shortened clinical duration. As with other non-depolarizing neuromuscular blocking drugs, if rocuronium is administered to patients chronically receiving anticonvulsant agents, shorter durations of neuromuscular block may occur and infusion rates may be higher due to the development of resistance to non-depolarizing muscle relaxants. While the mechanism for development of this resistance is not known, receptor upregulation may be a contributing factor). Products include:
Depakote ER **426**

Doxacurium Chloride (There are no controlled studies documenting the use of rocuronium before or after other non-depolarizing muscle relaxants. Interactions have been observed when other non-depolarizing muscle relaxants have been administered in succession).
No products indexed under this heading.

Doxycycline (Drugs which may enhance the neuromuscular blocking action of rocuronium include certain antibiotics, such as tetracyclines. If tetracyclines are used in conjunction with rocuronium, prolongation of neuromuscular block may occur. In patients in whom potentiation of neuromuscular block may be anticipated, a decrease from the recommended initial dose of rocuronium should be considered).
No products indexed under this heading.

Doxycycline Calcium (Drugs which may enhance the neuromuscular blocking action of rocuronium include certain antibiotics, such as tetracyclines. If tetracyclines are used in conjunction with rocuronium, prolongation of neuromuscular block may occur. In patients in whom potentiation of neuromuscular block may be anticipated, a decrease from the recommended initial dose of rocuronium should be considered).
No products indexed under this heading.

Doxycycline Hyclate (Drugs which may enhance the neuromuscular blocking action of rocuronium include certain antibiotics, such as tetracyclines. If tetracyclines are used in conjunction with rocuronium, prolongation of neuromuscular block may occur. In patients in whom potentiation of neuromuscular block may be anticipated, a decrease from the recommended initial dose of rocuronium should be considered).
No products indexed under this heading.

Doxycycline Monohydrate (Drugs which may enhance the neuromuscular blocking action of rocuronium include certain antibiotics, such as tetracyclines. If tetracyclines are used in conjunction with rocuronium, prolongation of neuromuscular block may occur. In patients in whom potentiation of neuromuscular block may be anticipated, a decrease from the recommended initial dose of rocuronium should be considered).
No products indexed under this heading.

d-Tubocurarine (There are no controlled studies documenting the use of rocuronium before or after other non-depolarizing muscle relaxants. Interactions have been observed when other non-depolarizing muscle relaxants have been administered in succession).
No products indexed under this heading.

Enflurane (Use of inhalation anesthetics has been shown to enhance the activity of other neuromuscular blocking agents (enflurane> isoflurane> halothane). Enflurane may also prolong the duration of action of initial and maintenance doses of rocuronium and decrease the average infusion requirement of rocuronium by 40% compared to opioid/nitrous oxide/oxygen anesthesia. The clinical duration of initial doses of rocuronium of 0.57 to 0.85 mg/kg under enflurane anesthesia was increased by 11%. The duration of maintenance doses was increased by 30% to 50% under enflurane. Potentiation by enflurane is also seen with the infusion rates of rocuronium required to maintain 95% neuromuscular block. Infusion rates are decreased by 40% compared to opioid/nitrous oxide/oxygen anesthesia. The median spontaneous recovery time is prolonged by enflurane (15% longer). In patients in whom potentiation of neuromuscular block may be anticipated, a decrease from the recommended initial dose of rocuronium should be considered).
No products indexed under this heading.

Enoxacin (Drugs which may enhance the neuromuscular blocking action of non-depolarizing agents such as rocuronium include certain antibiotics (eg, aminoglycosides, vancomycin, tetracyclines, bacitracin, polymyxins, colistin, and sodium colistimethate). If these antibiotics are used in conjunction with rocuronium, prolongation of neuromuscular block may occur. In patients in whom potentiation of neuromuscular block may be anticipated, a decrease from the recommended initial dose of rocuronium should be considered).
No products indexed under this heading.

Epirubicin Hydrochloride (Drugs which may enhance the neuromuscular blocking action of non-depolarizing agents such as rocuronium include certain antibiotics (eg, aminoglycosides, vancomycin, tetracyclines, bacitracin, polymyxins, colistin, and sodium colistimethate). If these antibiotics are used in conjunction with rocuronium, prolongation of neuromuscular block may occur. In patients in whom potentiation of neuromuscular block may be anticipated, a decrease from the recommended initial dose of rocuronium should be considered).
No products indexed under this heading.

Erythromycin (Drugs which may enhance the neuromuscular blocking action of non-depolarizing agents such as rocuronium include certain antibiotics (eg, aminoglycosides, vancomycin, tetracyclines, bacitracin, polymyxins, colistin, and sodium colistimethate). If these antibiotics are used in conjunction with rocuronium, prolongation of neuromuscular block may occur. In patients in whom potentiation of neuromuscular block may be anticipated, a decrease from the recommended initial dose of rocuronium should be considered).
No products indexed under this heading.

Erythromycin, Topical (Drugs which may enhance the neuromuscular blocking action of non-depolarizing agents such as rocuronium include certain antibiotics (eg, aminoglycosides, vancomycin, tetracyclines, bacitracin, polymyxins, colistin, and sodium colistimethate). If these antibiotics are used in conjunction with rocuronium, prolongation of neuromuscular block may occur. In patients in whom potentiation of neuromuscular block may be anticipated, a decrease from the recommended initial dose of rocuronium should be considered).
No products indexed under this heading.

Erythromycin Estolate (Drugs which may enhance the neuromuscular blocking action of non-depolarizing agents such as rocuronium include certain antibiotics (eg, aminoglycosides, vancomycin, tetracyclines, bacitracin, polymyxins, colistin, and sodium colistimethate). If these antibiotics are used in conjunction with rocuronium, prolongation of neuromuscular block may occur. In patients in whom potentiation of neuromuscular block may be anticipated, a decrease from the recommended initial dose of rocuronium should be considered).
No products indexed under this heading.

Erythromycin Ethylsuccinate (Drugs which may enhance the neuromuscular blocking action of non-depolarizing agents such as rocuronium include certain antibiotics (eg, aminoglycosides, vancomycin, tetracyclines, bacitracin, polymyxins, colistin, and sodium colistimethate). If these antibiotics are used in conjunction with rocuronium, prolongation of neuromuscular block may occur. In patients in whom potentiation of neuromuscular block may be anticipated, a decrease from the recommended initial dose of rocuronium should be considered). Products include:
E.E.S. **437**
EryPed **435**

Erythromycin Gluceptate (Drugs which may enhance the neuromuscular blocking action of non-depolarizing agents such as rocuronium include certain antibiotics (eg, aminoglycosides, vancomycin, tetracyclines, bacitracin, polymyxins, colistin, and sodium colistimethate). If these antibiotics are used in conjunction with rocuronium, prolongation of neuromuscular block may occur. In patients in whom potentiation of neuromuscular block may be anticipated, a decrease from the recommended initial dose of rocuronium should be considered).
No products indexed under this heading.

Erythromycin Lactobionate (Drugs which may enhance the neuromuscular blocking action of non-depolarizing agents such as rocuronium include cer-

2139 Interactions Index Zemuron

tain antibiotics (eg, aminoglycosides, vancomycin, tetracyclines, bacitracin, polymyxins, colistin, and sodium colistimethate). If these antibiotics are used in conjunction with rocuronium, prolongation of neuromuscular block may occur. In patients in whom potentiation of neuromuscular block may be anticipated, a decrease from the recommended initial dose of rocuronium should be considered).
No products indexed under this heading.

Erythromycin Stearate (Drugs which may enhance the neuromuscular blocking action of non-depolarizing agents such as rocuronium include certain antibiotics (eg, aminoglycosides, vancomycin, tetracyclines, bacitracin, polymyxins, colistin, and sodium colistimethate). If these antibiotics are used in conjunction with rocuronium, prolongation of neuromuscular block may occur. In patients in whom potentiation of neuromuscular block may be anticipated, a decrease from the recommended initial dose of rocuronium should be considered).
No products indexed under this heading.

Ethosuximide (In two out of four patients receiving chronic anticonvulsant therapy, apparent resistance to the effects of rocuronium was observed in the form of diminished magnitude of neuromuscular block, or shortened clinical duration. As with other non-depolarizing neuromuscular blocking drugs, if rocuronium is administered to patients chronically receiving anticonvulsant agents, shorter durations of neuromuscular block may occur and infusion rates may be higher due to the development of resistance to non-depolarizing muscle relaxants. While the mechanism for development of this resistance is not known, receptor upregulation may be a contributing factor).
No products indexed under this heading.

Ethotoin (In two out of four patients receiving chronic anticonvulsant therapy, apparent resistance to the effects of rocuronium was observed in the form of diminished magnitude of neuromuscular block, or shortened clinical duration. As with other non-depolarizing neuromuscular blocking drugs, if rocuronium is administered to patients chronically receiving anticonvulsant agents, shorter durations of neuromuscular block may occur and infusion rates may be higher due to the development of resistance to non-depolarizing muscle relaxants. While the mechanism for development of this resistance is not known, receptor upregulation may be a contributing factor).
No products indexed under this heading.

Etidocaine Hydrochloride (Local anesthetics have been shown to increase the duration of neuromuscular block and decrease infusion requirements of other neuromuscular blocking agents. In patients in whom potentiation of neuromuscular block may be anticipated, a decrease from the recommended initial dose of rocuronium should be considered).
No products indexed under this heading.

Felbamate (In two out of four patients receiving chronic anticonvulsant therapy, apparent resistance to the effects of rocuronium was observed in the form of diminished magnitude of neuromuscular block, or shortened clinical duration. As with other non-depolarizing neuromuscular blocking drugs, if rocuronium is administered to patients chronically receiving anticonvulsant agents, shorter durations of neuromuscular block may occur and infusion rates may be higher due to the development of resistance to non-depolarizing muscle relaxants. While the mechanism for development of this resistance is not known, receptor upregulation may be a contributing factor).
No products indexed under this heading.

Fludrocortisone Acetate (Myopathy after long-term administration of other non-depolarizing neuromuscular blocking agents in the ICU alone or in combination with corticosteroid therapy has been reported. Therefore, for patients receiving both neuromuscular blocking agents and corticosteroids, the period of use of the neuromuscular blocking agent should be limited as much as possible and only used in the setting where in the opinion of the prescribing physician, the specific advantages of the drug outweigh the risk).
No products indexed under this heading.

Flumethasone Pivalate (Myopathy after long-term administration of other non-depolarizing neuromuscular blocking agents in the ICU alone or in combination with corticosteroid therapy has been reported. Therefore, for patients receiving both neuromuscular blocking agents and corticosteroids, the period of use of the neuromuscular blocking agent should be limited as much as possible and only used in the setting where in the opinion of the prescribing physician, the specific advantages of the drug outweigh the risk).
No products indexed under this heading.

Flunisolide Hemihydrate (Myopathy after long-term administration of other non-depolarizing neuromuscular blocking agents in the ICU alone or in combination with corticosteroid therapy has been reported. Therefore, for patients receiving both neuromuscular blocking agents and corticosteroids, the period of use of the neuromuscular blocking agent should be limited as much as possible and only used in the setting where in the opinion of the prescribing physician, the specific advantages of the drug outweigh the risk).
No products indexed under this heading.

Fluticasone Furoate (Myopathy after long-term administration of other non-depolarizing neuromuscular blocking agents in the ICU alone or in combination with corticosteroid therapy has been reported. Therefore, for patients receiving both neuromuscular blocking agents and corticosteroids, the period of use of the neuromuscular blocking agent should be limited as much as possible and only used in the setting where in the opinion of the prescribing physician, the specific advantages of the drug outweigh the risk). Products include:
Veramyst 1713

Fluticasone Propionate (Myopathy after long-term administration of other non-depolarizing neuromuscular blocking agents in the ICU alone or in combination with corticosteroid therapy has been reported. Therefore, for patients receiving both neuromuscular blocking agents and corticosteroids, the period of use of the neuromuscular blocking agent should be limited as much as possible and only used in the setting where in the opinion of the prescribing physician, the specific advantages of the drug outweigh the risk). Products include:
Advair 100/50 1275
Advair 250/50 1275
Advair 500/50 1275
Advair HFA 45/21 1288
Advair HFA 115/21 1288
Advair HFA 230/21 1288
Flonase 1459
Flovent Diskus 1463
Flovent HFA 1470

Fosphenytoin (In two out of four patients receiving chronic anticonvulsant therapy, apparent resistance to the effects of rocuronium was observed in the form of diminished magnitude of neuromuscular block, or shortened clinical duration. As with other non-depolarizing neuromuscular blocking drugs, if rocuronium is administered to patients chronically receiving anticonvulsant agents, such as phenytoin, shorter durations of neuromuscular block may occur and infusion rates may be higher due to the development of resistance to non-depolarizing muscle relaxants. While the mechanism for development of this resistance is not known, receptor upregulation may be a contributing factor).
No products indexed under this heading.

Fosphenytoin Sodium (In two out of four patients receiving chronic anticonvulsant therapy, apparent resistance to the effects of rocuronium was observed in the form of diminished magnitude of neuromuscular block, or shortened clinical duration. As with other non-depolarizing neuromuscular blocking drugs, if rocuronium is administered to patients chronically receiving anticonvulsant agents, such as phenytoin, shorter durations of neuromuscular block may occur and infusion rates may be higher due to the development of resistance to non-depolarizing muscle relaxants. While the mechanism for development of this resistance is not known, receptor upregulation may be a contributing factor).
No products indexed under this heading.

Gabapentin (In two out of four patients receiving chronic anticonvulsant therapy, apparent resistance to the effects of rocuronium was observed in the form of diminished magnitude of neuromuscular block, or shortened clinical duration. As with other non-depolarizing neuromuscular blocking drugs, if rocuronium is administered to patients chronically receiving anticonvulsant agents, shorter durations of neuromuscular block may occur and infusion rates may be higher due to the development of resistance to non-depolarizing muscle relaxants. While the mechanism for development of this resistance is not known, receptor upregulation may be a contributing factor).
No products indexed under this heading.

Gallamine (There are no controlled studies documenting the use of rocuronium before or after other non-depolarizing muscle relaxants. Interactions have been observed when other non-depolarizing muscle relaxants have been administered in succession).
No products indexed under this heading.

Gallamine Triethiodide (There are no controlled studies documenting the use of rocuronium before or after other non-depolarizing muscle relaxants. Interactions have been observed when other non-depolarizing muscle relaxants have been administered in succession).
No products indexed under this heading.

Gatifloxacin (Drugs which may enhance the neuromuscular blocking action of non-depolarizing agents such as rocuronium include certain antibiotics (eg, aminoglycosides, vancomycin, tetracyclines, bacitracin, polymyxins, colistin, and sodium colistimethate). If these antibiotics are used in conjunction with rocuronium, prolongation of neuromuscular block may occur. In patients in whom potentiation of neuromuscular block may be anticipated, a decrease from the recommended initial dose of rocuronium should be considered).
No products indexed under this heading.

Gemifloxacin Mesylate (Drugs which may enhance the neuromuscular blocking action of non-depolarizing agents such as rocuronium include certain antibiotics (eg, aminoglycosides, vancomycin, tetracyclines, bacitracin, polymyxins, colistin, and sodium colistimethate). If these antibiotics are used in conjunction with rocuronium, prolongation of neuromuscular block may occur. In patients in whom potentiation of neuromuscular block may be anticipated, a decrease from the recommended initial dose of rocuronium should be considered).
No products indexed under this heading.

Gentamicin (Drugs which may enhance the neuromuscular blocking action of rocuronium include certain antibiotics, such as aminoglyosides. If aminoglycosides are used in conjunction with rocuronium, prolongation of neuromuscular block may occur. In patients in whom potentiation of neuromuscular block may be anticipated, a decrease from the recommended initial dose of rocuronium should be considered).
No products indexed under this heading.

Gentamicin Sulfate (Drugs which may enhance the neuromuscular blocking action of rocuronium include certain antibiotics, such as aminoglyosides. If aminoglycosides are used in conjunction with rocuronium, prolongation of neuromuscular block may occur. In patients in whom potentiation of neuromuscular block may be anticipated, a decrease from the recommended initial dose of rocuronium should be considered). Products include:
Pred-G .... ⊙ 226, ⊙ 227

Grepafloxacin Hydrochloride (Drugs which may enhance the neuromuscular blocking action of non-depolarizing agents such as rocuronium include certain antibiotics (eg, aminoglycosides, vancomycin, tetracyclines, bacitracin, polymyxins, colistin, and sodium colistimethate). If these antibiotics are used in conjunction with rocuronium, prolongation of neuromuscular block may occur. In patients in whom potentiation of neuromuscular block may be anticipated, a decrease from the recommended initial dose of rocuronium should be considered).
No products indexed under this heading.

Griseofulvin (Drugs which may enhance the neuromuscular blocking action of non-depolarizing agents such as rocuronium include certain antibiotics (eg, aminoglycosides, vancomycin, tetracyclines, bacitracin, polymyxins, colistin, and sodium colistimethate). If these antibiotics are used in conjunction with rocuronium, prolongation of neuromuscular block may occur. In patients in whom potentiation of neuromuscular block may be anticipated, a decrease from the recommended initial dose of rocuronium should be considered).
No products indexed under this heading.

Halothane (Use of inhalation anesthetics has been shown to enhance the activity of other neuromuscular blocking agents (enflurane> isoflurane> halothane). However, there has been no definite interaction demonstrated between rocuronium and halothane).
No products indexed under this heading.

Hexobarbital (Rocuronium, which has an acid pH, should not be mixed with alkaline solutions (eg, barbiturate solutions) in the same syringe or administered simultaneously during intravenous infusion through the same needle).
No products indexed under this heading.

Hydrocortisone (Myopathy after long-term administration of other non-depolarizing neuromuscular blocking agents in the ICU alone or in combination with corticosteroid therapy has been reported. Therefore, for patients receiving both neuromuscular blocking agents and corticosteroids, the period of use of the neuromuscular blocking agent should be limited as much as

IMPORTANT NOTE: Always consult each drug listing in the patient's regimen for possible interactions.

possible and only used in the setting where in the opinion of the prescribing physician, the specific advantages of the drug outweigh the risk).
No products indexed under this heading.

Hydrocortisone (Alcohol) (Myopathy after long-term administration of other non-depolarizing neuromuscular blocking agents in the ICU alone or in combination with corticosteroid therapy has been reported. Therefore, for patients receiving both neuromuscular blocking agents and corticosteroids, the period of use of the neuromuscular blocking agent should be limited as much as possible and only used in the setting where in the opinion of the prescribing physician, the specific advantages of the drug outweigh the risk).
No products indexed under this heading.

Hydrocortisone Acetate (Myopathy after long-term administration of other non-depolarizing neuromuscular blocking agents in the ICU alone or in combination with corticosteroid therapy has been reported. Therefore, for patients receiving both neuromuscular blocking agents and corticosteroids, the period of use of the neuromuscular blocking agent should be limited as much as possible and only used in the setting where in the opinion of the prescribing physician, the specific advantages of the drug outweigh the risk).
No products indexed under this heading.

Hydrocortisone Butyrate (Myopathy after long-term administration of other non-depolarizing neuromuscular blocking agents in the ICU alone or in combination with corticosteroid therapy has been reported. Therefore, for patients receiving both neuromuscular blocking agents and corticosteroids, the period of use of the neuromuscular blocking agent should be limited as much as possible and only used in the setting where in the opinion of the prescribing physician, the specific advantages of the drug outweigh the risk).
No products indexed under this heading.

Hydrocortisone Cypionate (Myopathy after long-term administration of other non-depolarizing neuromuscular blocking agents in the ICU alone or in combination with corticosteroid therapy has been reported. Therefore, for patients receiving both neuromuscular blocking agents and corticosteroids, the period of use of the neuromuscular blocking agent should be limited as much as possible and only used in the setting where in the opinion of the prescribing physician, the specific advantages of the drug outweigh the risk).
No products indexed under this heading.

Hydrocortisone Hemisuccinate (Myopathy after long-term administration of other non-depolarizing neuromuscular blocking agents in the ICU alone or in combination with corticosteroid therapy has been reported. Therefore, for patients receiving both neuromuscular blocking agents and corticosteroids, the period of use of the neuromuscular blocking agent should be limited as much as possible and only used in the setting where in the opinion of the prescribing physician, the specific advantages of the drug outweigh the risk).
No products indexed under this heading.

Hydrocortisone Probutate (Myopathy after long-term administration of other non-depolarizing neuromuscular blocking agents in the ICU alone or in combination with corticosteroid therapy has been reported. Therefore, for patients receiving both neuromuscular blocking agents and corticosteroids, the period of use of the neuromuscular blocking agent should be limited as much as possible and only used in the setting where in the opinion of the prescribing physician, the specific advantages of the drug outweigh the risk).
No products indexed under this heading.

Hydrocortisone Sodium Phosphate (Myopathy after long-term administration of other non-depolarizing neuromuscular blocking agents in the ICU alone or in combination with corticosteroid therapy has been reported. Therefore, for patients receiving both neuromuscular blocking agents and corticosteroids, the period of use of the neuromuscular blocking agent should be limited as much as possible and only used in the setting where in the opinion of the prescribing physician, the specific advantages of the drug outweigh the risk).
No products indexed under this heading.

Hydrocortisone Sodium Succinate (Myopathy after long-term administration of other non-depolarizing neuromuscular blocking agents in the ICU alone or in combination with corticosteroid therapy has been reported. Therefore, for patients receiving both neuromuscular blocking agents and corticosteroids, the period of use of the neuromuscular blocking agent should be limited as much as possible and only used in the setting where in the opinion of the prescribing physician, the specific advantages of the drug outweigh the risk).
No products indexed under this heading.

Hydrocortisone Valerate (Myopathy after long-term administration of other non-depolarizing neuromuscular blocking agents in the ICU alone or in combination with corticosteroid therapy has been reported. Therefore, for patients receiving both neuromuscular blocking agents and corticosteroids, the period of use of the neuromuscular blocking agent should be limited as much as possible and only used in the setting where in the opinion of the prescribing physician, the specific advantages of the drug outweigh the risk).
No products indexed under this heading.

Idarubicin Hydrochloride (Drugs which may enhance the neuromuscular blocking action of non-depolarizing agents such as rocuronium include certain antibiotics (eg, aminoglycosides, vancomycin, tetracyclines, bacitracin, polymyxins, colistin, and sodium colistimethate). If these antibiotics are used in conjunction with rocuronium, prolongation of neuromuscular block may occur. In patients in whom potentiation of neuromuscular block may be anticipated, a decrease from the recommended initial dose of rocuronium should be considered).
No products indexed under this heading.

Imipenem (Drugs which may enhance the neuromuscular blocking action of non-depolarizing agents such as rocuronium include certain antibiotics (eg, aminoglycosides, vancomycin, tetracyclines, bacitracin, polymyxins, colistin, and sodium colistimethate). If these antibiotics are used in conjunction with rocuronium, prolongation of neuromuscular block may occur. In patients in whom potentiation of neuromuscular block may be anticipated, a decrease from the recommended initial dose of rocuronium should be considered). Products include:
Primaxin I.M. **2232**
Primaxin I.V. **2235**

Isoflurane (Use of inhalation anesthetics has been shown to enhance the activity of other neuromuscular blocking agents (enflurane> isoflurane> halothane). Isoflurane may also prolong the duration of action of initial and maintenance doses of rocuronium and decrease the average infusion requirement of rocuronium by 40% compared to opioid/nitrous oxide/oxygen anesthesia. The clinical duration of initial doses of rocuronium of 0.57 to 0.85 mg/kg under isoflurane anesthesia was increased by 23%. The duration of maintenance doses was increased by 30% to 50% under isoflurane. Potentiation by isoflurane is also seen with the infusion rates of rocuronium required to maintain 95% neuromuscular block. Infusion rates are decreased by 40% compared to opioid/nitrous oxide/oxygen anesthesia. The median spontaneous recovery time is prolonged by isoflurane (62% longer). In patients in whom potentiation of neuromuscular block may be anticipated, a decrease from the recommended initial dose of rocuronium should be considered).
No products indexed under this heading.

Kanamycin Sulfate (Drugs which may enhance the neuromuscular blocking action of rocuronium include certain antibiotics, such as aminoglyosides. If aminoglycosides are used in conjunction with rocuronium, prolongation of neuromuscular block may occur. In patients in whom potentiation of neuromuscular block may be anticipated, a decrease from the recommended initial dose of rocuronium should be considered).
No products indexed under this heading.

Ketamine Hydrochloride (The overall analysis of ECG data in pediatric patients indicates that the concomitant use of rocuronium with general anesthetic agents can prolong the QTc interval).
No products indexed under this heading.

Lamotrigine (In two out of four patients receiving chronic anticonvulsant therapy, apparent resistance to the effects of rocuronium was observed in the form of diminished magnitude of neuromuscular block, or shortened clinical duration. As with other non-depolarizing neuromuscular blocking drugs, if rocuronium is administered to patients chronically receiving anticonvulsant agents, shorter durations of neuromuscular block may occur and infusion rates may be higher due to the development of resistance to non-depolarizing muscle relaxants. While the mechanism for development of this resistance is not known, receptor upregulation may be a contributing factor). Products include:
Lamictal **1522**
Lamictal ODT **1522**
Lamictal XR **1536**

Levetiracetam (In two out of four patients receiving chronic anticonvulsant therapy, apparent resistance to the effects of rocuronium was observed in the form of diminished magnitude of neuromuscular block, or shortened clinical duration. As with other non-depolarizing neuromuscular blocking drugs, if rocuronium is administered to patients chronically receiving anticonvulsant agents, shorter durations of neuromuscular block may occur and infusion rates may be higher due to the development of resistance to non-depolarizing muscle relaxants. While the mechanism for development of this resistance is not known, receptor upregulation may be a contributing factor). Products include:
Keppra XR **3434**

Levobupivacaine Hydrochloride (Local anesthetics have been shown to increase the duration of neuromuscular block and decrease infusion requirements of other neuromuscular blocking agents. In patients in whom potentiation of neuromuscular block may be anticipated, a decrease from the recommended initial dose of rocuronium should be considered).
No products indexed under this heading.

Levofloxacin (Drugs which may enhance the neuromuscular blocking action of non-depolarizing agents such as rocuronium include certain antibiotics (eg, aminoglycosides, vancomycin, tetracyclines, bacitracin, polymyxins, colistin, and sodium colistimethate). If these antibiotics are used in conjunction with rocuronium, prolongation of neuromuscular block may occur. In patients in whom potentiation of neuromuscular block may be anticipated, a decrease from the recommended initial dose of rocuronium should be considered).
Products include:
Iquix **3492**
Levaquin **2629**
Levaquin in 5% Dextrose **2629**
Quixin **3493**

Lidocaine Hydrochloride (Local anesthetics have been shown to increase the duration of neuromuscular block and decrease infusion requirements of other neuromuscular blocking agents. In patients in whom potentiation of neuromuscular block may be anticipated, a decrease from the recommended initial dose of rocuronium should be considered).
No products indexed under this heading.

Lithium (Lithium has been shown to increase the duration of neuromuscular block and decrease infusion requirements of other neuromuscular blocking agents. In patients in whom potentiation of neuromuscular block may be anticipated, a decrease from the recommended initial dose of rocuronium should be considered).
No products indexed under this heading.

Lithium Carbonate (Lithium has been shown to increase the duration of neuromuscular block and decrease infusion requirements of other neuromuscular blocking agents. In patients in whom potentiation of neuromuscular block may be anticipated, a decrease from the recommended initial dose of rocuronium should be considered).
No products indexed under this heading.

Lithium Citrate (Lithium has been shown to increase the duration of neuromuscular block and decrease infusion requirements of other neuromuscular blocking agents. In patients in whom potentiation of neuromuscular block may be anticipated, a decrease from the recommended initial dose of rocuronium should be considered).
No products indexed under this heading.

Lomefloxacin Hydrochloride (Drugs which may enhance the neuromuscular blocking action of non-depolarizing agents such as rocuronium include certain antibiotics (eg, aminoglycosides, vancomycin, tetracyclines, bacitracin, polymyxins, colistin, and sodium colistimethate). If these antibiotics are used in conjunction with rocuronium, prolongation of neuromuscular block may occur. In patients in whom potentiation of neuromuscular block may be anticipated, a decrease from the recommended initial dose of rocuronium should be considered).
No products indexed under this heading.

Loracarbef (Drugs which may enhance the neuromuscular blocking action of non-depolarizing agents such as rocuronium include certain antibiotics (eg, aminoglycosides, vancomycin, tetracyclines, bacitracin, polymyxins, colistin, and sodium colistimethate). If these antibiotics are used in conjunction with rocuronium, prolongation of neuromuscular block may occur. In patients in whom potentiation of neuromuscular block may be anticipated, a decrease from the recommended initial dose of rocuronium should be considered).
No products indexed under this heading.

Magnesium (Magnesium salts administered for the management of toxemia

2141 Interactions Index Zemuron

of pregnancy may enhance neuromuscular blockade. In patients in whom potentiation of neuromuscular block may be anticipated, a decrease from the recommended initial dose of rocuronium should be considered). Products include:

BoneMate Plus 3454
Cardio Basics 3455
Chelated Mineral 3476

Magnesium Aluminum Silicate (Magnesium salts administered for the management of toxemia of pregnancy may enhance neuromuscular blockade. In patients in whom potentiation of neuromuscular block may be anticipated, a decrease from the recommended initial dose of rocuronium should be considered).
No products indexed under this heading.

Magnesium Carbonate (Magnesium salts administered for the management of toxemia of pregnancy may enhance neuromuscular blockade. In patients in whom potentiation of neuromuscular block may be anticipated, a decrease from the recommended initial dose of rocuronium should be considered).
No products indexed under this heading.

Magnesium Chloride (Magnesium salts administered for the management of toxemia of pregnancy may enhance neuromuscular blockade. In patients in whom potentiation of neuromuscular block may be anticipated, a decrease from the recommended initial dose of rocuronium should be considered).
No products indexed under this heading.

Magnesium Citrate (Magnesium salts administered for the management of toxemia of pregnancy may enhance neuromuscular blockade. In patients in whom potentiation of neuromuscular block may be anticipated, a decrease from the recommended initial dose of rocuronium should be considered). Products include:

Chelated Mineral 3476

Magnesium Gluconate (Magnesium salts administered for the management of toxemia of pregnancy may enhance neuromuscular blockade. In patients in whom potentiation of neuromuscular block may be anticipated, a decrease from the recommended initial dose of rocuronium should be considered).
No products indexed under this heading.

Magnesium Hydroxide (Magnesium salts administered for the management of toxemia of pregnancy may enhance neuromuscular blockade. In patients in whom potentiation of neuromuscular block may be anticipated, a decrease from the recommended initial dose of rocuronium should be considered). Products include:

Fleet Pedia-Lax Chewable Tablets 1144
Pepcid Complete 1822

Magnesium Lactate (Magnesium salts administered for the management of toxemia of pregnancy may enhance neuromuscular blockade. In patients in whom potentiation of neuromuscular block may be anticipated, a decrease from the recommended initial dose of rocuronium should be considered).
No products indexed under this heading.

Magnesium Oxide (Magnesium salts administered for the management of toxemia of pregnancy may enhance neuromuscular blockade. In patients in whom potentiation of neuromuscular block may be anticipated, a decrease from the recommended initial dose of rocuronium should be considered). Products include:

Beelith 873

Magnesium Salicylate (Magnesium salts administered for the management of toxemia of pregnancy may enhance neuromuscular blockade. In patients in whom potentiation of neuromuscular block may be anticipated, a decrease from the recommended initial dose of rocuronium should be considered).
No products indexed under this heading.

Magnesium Salicylate Tetrahydrate (Magnesium salts administered for the management of toxemia of pregnancy may enhance neuromuscular blockade. In patients in whom potentiation of neuromuscular block may be anticipated, a decrease from the recommended initial dose of rocuronium should be considered).
No products indexed under this heading.

Magnesium Salts (Magnesium salts have been shown to increase the duration of neuromuscular block and decrease infusion requirements of other neuromuscular blocking agents. In patients in whom potentiation of neuromuscular block may be anticipated, a decrease from the recommended initial dose should be considered).
No products indexed under this heading.

Magnesium Sulfate (Magnesium salts administered for the management of toxemia of pregnancy may enhance neuromuscular blockade. In patients in whom potentiation of neuromuscular block may be anticipated, a decrease from the recommended initial dose of rocuronium should be considered).
No products indexed under this heading.

Magnesium Trisilicate (Magnesium salts administered for the management of toxemia of pregnancy may enhance neuromuscular blockade. In patients in whom potentiation of neuromuscular block may be anticipated, a decrease from the recommended initial dose of rocuronium should be considered).
No products indexed under this heading.

Mephenytoin (In two out of four patients receiving chronic anticonvulsant therapy, apparent resistance to the effects of rocuronium was observed in the form of diminished magnitude of neuromuscular block, or shortened clinical duration. As with other non-depolarizing neuromuscular blocking drugs, if rocuronium is administered to patients chronically receiving anticonvulsant agents, shorter durations of neuromuscular block may occur and infusion rates may be higher due to the development of resistance to non-depolarizing muscle relaxants. While the mechanism for development of this resistance is not known, receptor upregulation may be a contributing factor).
No products indexed under this heading.

Mephobarbital (Rocuronium, which has an acid pH, should not be mixed with alkaline solutions (eg, barbiturate solutions) in the same syringe or administered simultaneously during intravenous infusion through the same needle).
No products indexed under this heading.

Mepivacaine Hydrochloride (Local anesthetics have been shown to increase the duration of neuromuscular block and decrease infusion requirements of other neuromuscular blocking agents. In patients in whom potentiation of neuromuscular block may be anticipated, a decrease from the recommended initial dose of rocuronium should be considered).
No products indexed under this heading.

Methacycline Hydrochloride (Drugs which may enhance the neuromuscular blocking action of rocuronium include certain antibiotics, such as tetracyclines. If tetracyclines are used in conjunction with rocuronium, prolongation of neuromuscular block may occur. In patients in whom potentiation of neuromuscular block may be anticipated, a decrease from the recommended initial dose of rocuronium should be considered).
No products indexed under this heading.

Methicillin Sodium (Drugs which may enhance the neuromuscular blocking action of non-depolarizing agents such as rocuronium include certain antibiotics (eg, aminoglycosides, vancomycin, tetracyclines, bacitracin, polymyxins, colistin, and sodium colistimethate). If these antibiotics are used in conjunction with rocuronium, prolongation of neuromuscular block may occur. In patients in whom potentiation of neuromuscular block may be anticipated, a decrease from the recommended initial dose of rocuronium should be considered).
No products indexed under this heading.

Methohexital Sodium (The overall analysis of ECG data in pediatric patients indicates that the concomitant use of rocuronium with general anesthetic agents can prolong the QTc interval).
No products indexed under this heading.

Methoxyflurane (Use of inhalation anesthetics as been shown to enhance the activity of other neuromuscular blocking agents. In patients in whom potentiation of neuromuscular block may be anticipated, a decrease from the recommended initial dose of rocuronium should be considered).
No products indexed under this heading.

Methsuximide (In two out of four patients receiving chronic anticonvulsant therapy, apparent resistance to the effects of rocuronium was observed in the form of diminished magnitude of neuromuscular block, or shortened clinical duration. As with other non-depolarizing neuromuscular blocking drugs, if rocuronium is administered to patients chronically receiving anticonvulsant agents, shorter durations of neuromuscular block may occur and infusion rates may be higher due to the development of resistance to non-depolarizing muscle relaxants. While the mechanism for development of this resistance is not known, receptor upregulation may be a contributing factor).
No products indexed under this heading.

Methylprednisolone (Myopathy after long-term administration of other non-depolarizing neuromuscular blocking agents in the ICU alone or in combination with corticosteroid therapy has been reported. Therefore, for patients receiving both neuromuscular blocking agents and corticosteroids, the period of use of the neuromuscular blocking agent should be limited as much as possible and only used in the setting where in the opinion of the prescribing physician, the specific advantages of the drug outweigh the risk).
No products indexed under this heading.

Methylprednisolone Acetate (Myopathy after long-term administration of other non-depolarizing neuromuscular blocking agents in the ICU alone or in combination with corticosteroid therapy has been reported. Therefore, for patients receiving both neuromuscular blocking agents and corticosteroids, the period of use of the neuromuscular blocking agent should be limited as much as possible and only used in the setting where in the opinion of the prescribing physician, the specific advantages of the drug outweigh the risk).
No products indexed under this heading.

Methylprednisolone Sodium Succinate (Myopathy after long-term administration of other non-depolarizing neuromuscular blocking agents in the ICU alone or in combination with corticosteroid therapy has been reported. Therefore, for patients receiving both neuromuscular blocking agents and corticosteroids, the period of use of the neuromuscular blocking agent should be limited as much as possible and only used in the setting where in the opinion of the prescribing physician, the specific advantages of the drug outweigh the risk).
No products indexed under this heading.

Metocurine Iodide (There are no controlled studies documenting the use of rocuronium before or after other non-depolarizing muscle relaxants. Interactions have been observed when other non-depolarizing muscle relaxants have been administered in succession).
No products indexed under this heading.

Mezlocillin Sodium (Drugs which may enhance the neuromuscular blocking action of non-depolarizing agents such as rocuronium include certain antibiotics (eg, aminoglycosides, vancomycin, tetracyclines, bacitracin, polymyxins, colistin, and sodium colistimethate). If these antibiotics are used in conjunction with rocuronium, prolongation of neuromuscular block may occur. In patients in whom potentiation of neuromuscular block may be anticipated, a decrease from the recommended initial dose of rocuronium should be considered).
No products indexed under this heading.

Minocycline Hydrochloride (Drugs which may enhance the neuromuscular blocking action of rocuronium include certain antibiotics, such as tetracyclines. If tetracyclines are used in conjunction with rocuronium, prolongation of neuromuscular block may occur. In patients in whom potentiation of neuromuscular block may be anticipated, a decrease from the recommended initial dose of rocuronium should be considered). Products include:

Solodyn 2073

Mivacurium Chloride (There are no controlled studies documenting the use of rocuronium before or after other non-depolarizing muscle relaxants. Interactions have been observed when other non-depolarizing muscle relaxants have been administered in succession).
No products indexed under this heading.

Mometasone Furoate (Myopathy after long-term administration of other non-depolarizing neuromuscular blocking agents in the ICU alone or in combination with corticosteroid therapy has been reported. Therefore, for patients receiving both neuromuscular blocking agents and corticosteroids, the period of use of the neuromuscular blocking agent should be limited as much as possible and only used in the setting where in the opinion of the prescribing physician, the specific advantages of the drug outweigh the risk). Products include:

Asmanex 3058
Elocon Cream 3111
Elocon Lotion 3112
Elocon Ointment 3114

Mometasone Furoate Monohydrate (Myopathy after long-term administration of other non-depolarizing neuromuscular blocking agents in the ICU alone or in combination with corticosteroid therapy has been reported. Therefore, for patients receiving both neuromuscular blocking agents and corticosteroids, the period of use of the neuromuscular blocking agent should be limited as much as possible and only used in the setting where in the opinion of the prescribing physician, the specific advantages of the drug outweigh the risk). Products include:

Nasonex 3166

Moxifloxacin Hydrochloride (Drugs which may enhance the neuromuscular blocking action of non-depolarizing

IMPORTANT NOTE: Always consult each drug listing in the patient's regimen for possible interactions.

Zemuron Interactions Index 2142

agents such as rocuronium include certain antibiotics (eg, aminoglycosides, vancomycin, tetracyclines, bacitracin, polymyxins, colistin, and sodium colistimethate). If these antibiotics are used in conjunction with rocuronium, prolongation of neuromuscular block may occur. In patients in whom potentiation of neuromuscular block may be anticipated, a decrease from the recommended initial dose of rocuronium should be considered). Products include:

Avelox 3064
Vigamox 589

Nafcillin Sodium (Drugs which may enhance the neuromuscular blocking action of non-depolarizing agents such as rocuronium include certain antibiotics (eg, aminoglycosides, vancomycin, tetracyclines, bacitracin, polymyxins, colistin, and sodium colistimethate). If these antibiotics are used in conjunction with rocuronium, prolongation of neuromuscular block may occur. In patients in whom potentiation of neuromuscular block may be anticipated, a decrease from the recommended initial dose of rocuronium should be considered).
No products indexed under this heading.

Neomycin (Drugs which may enhance the neuromuscular blocking action of rocuronium include certain antibiotics, such as aminoglyosides. If aminoglycosides are used in conjunction with rocuronium, prolongation of neuromuscular block may occur. In patients in whom potentiation of neuromuscular block may be anticipated, a decrease from the recommended initial dose of rocuronium should be considered).
No products indexed under this heading.

Neomycin, oral (Drugs which may enhance the neuromuscular blocking action of rocuronium include certain antibiotics, such as aminoglyosides. If aminoglycosides are used in conjunction with rocuronium, prolongation of neuromuscular block may occur. In patients in whom potentiation of neuromuscular block may be anticipated, a decrease from the recommended initial dose of rocuronium should be considered).
No products indexed under this heading.

Neomycin Sulfate (Drugs which may enhance the neuromuscular blocking action of rocuronium include certain antibiotics, such as aminoglyosides. If aminoglycosides are used in conjunction with rocuronium, prolongation of neuromuscular block may occur. In patients in whom potentiation of neuromuscular block may be anticipated, a decrease from the recommended initial dose of rocuronium should be considered).
No products indexed under this heading.

Nitrous Oxide (The overall analysis of ECG data in pediatric patients indicates that the concomitant use of rocuronium with general anesthetic agents can prolong the QTc interval).
No products indexed under this heading.

Norfloxacin (Drugs which may enhance the neuromuscular blocking action of non-depolarizing agents such as rocuronium include certain antibiotics (eg, aminoglycosides, vancomycin, tetracyclines, bacitracin, polymyxins, colistin, and sodium colistimethate). If these antibiotics are used in conjunction with rocuronium, prolongation of neuromuscular block may occur. In patients in whom potentiation of neuromuscular block may be anticipated, a decrease from the recommended initial dose of rocuronium should be considered). Products include:

Noroxin 2220

Ofloxacin (Drugs which may enhance the neuromuscular blocking action of non-depolarizing agents such as rocuronium include certain antibiotics (eg, aminoglycosides, vancomycin, tetracyclines, bacitracin, polymyxins, colistin, and sodium colistimethate). If these antibiotics are used in conjunction with rocuronium, prolongation of neuromuscular block may occur. In patients in whom potentiation of neuromuscular block may be anticipated, a decrease from the recommended initial dose of rocuronium should be considered).
No products indexed under this heading.

Oxacillin (Drugs which may enhance the neuromuscular blocking action of non-depolarizing agents such as rocuronium include certain antibiotics (eg, aminoglycosides, vancomycin, tetracyclines, bacitracin, polymyxins, colistin, and sodium colistimethate). If these antibiotics are used in conjunction with rocuronium, prolongation of neuromuscular block may occur. In patients in whom potentiation of neuromuscular block may be anticipated, a decrease from the recommended initial dose of rocuronium should be considered).
No products indexed under this heading.

Oxacillin Sodium (Drugs which may enhance the neuromuscular blocking action of non-depolarizing agents such as rocuronium include certain antibiotics (eg, aminoglycosides, vancomycin, tetracyclines, bacitracin, polymyxins, colistin, and sodium colistimethate). If these antibiotics are used in conjunction with rocuronium, prolongation of neuromuscular block may occur. In patients in whom potentiation of neuromuscular block may be anticipated, a decrease from the recommended initial dose of rocuronium should be considered).
No products indexed under this heading.

Oxcarbazepine (In two out of four patients receiving chronic anticonvulsant therapy, apparent resistance to the effects of rocuronium was observed in the form of diminished magnitude of neuromuscular block, or shortened clinical duration. As with other non-depolarizing neuromuscular blocking drugs, if rocuronium is administered to patients chronically receiving anticonvulsant agents, shorter durations of neuromuscular block may occur and infusion rates may be higher due to the development of resistance to non-depolarizing muscle relaxants. While the mechanism for development of this resistance is not known, receptor upregulation may be a contributing factor).
No products indexed under this heading.

Oxytetracycline (Drugs which may enhance the neuromuscular blocking action of rocuronium include certain antibiotics, such as tetracyclines. If tetracyclines are used in conjunction with rocuronium, prolongation of neuromuscular block may occur. In patients in whom potentiation of neuromuscular block may be anticipated, a decrease from the recommended initial dose of rocuronium should be considered).
No products indexed under this heading.

Oxytetracycline Hydrochloride (Drugs which may enhance the neuromuscular blocking action of rocuronium include certain antibiotics, such as tetracyclines. If tetracyclines are used in conjunction with rocuronium, prolongation of neuromuscular block may occur. In patients in whom potentiation of neuromuscular block may be anticipated, a decrease from the recommended initial dose of rocuronium should be considered).
No products indexed under this heading.

Pancuronium Bromide (There are no controlled studies documenting the use of rocuronium before or after other non-depolarizing muscle relaxants. Interactions have been observed when other non-depolarizing muscle relaxants have been administered in succession).
No products indexed under this heading.

Paramethadione (In two out of four patients receiving chronic anticonvulsant therapy, apparent resistance to the effects of rocuronium was observed in the form of diminished magnitude of neuromuscular block, or shortened clinical duration. As with other non-depolarizing neuromuscular blocking drugs, if rocuronium is administered to patients chronically receiving anticonvulsant agents, shorter durations of neuromuscular block may occur and infusion rates may be higher due to the development of resistance to non-depolarizing muscle relaxants. While the mechanism for development of this resistance is not known, receptor upregulation may be a contributing factor).
No products indexed under this heading.

Penicillin, Potassium Phenoxymethyl (Drugs which may enhance the neuromuscular blocking action of non-depolarizing agents such as rocuronium include certain antibiotics (eg, aminoglycosides, vancomycin, tetracyclines, bacitracin, polymyxins, colistin, and sodium colistimethate). If these antibiotics are used in conjunction with rocuronium, prolongation of neuromuscular block may occur. In patients in whom potentiation of neuromuscular block may be anticipated, a decrease from the recommended initial dose of rocuronium should be considered).
No products indexed under this heading.

Penicillin G Benzathine (Drugs which may enhance the neuromuscular blocking action of non-depolarizing agents such as rocuronium include certain antibiotics (eg, aminoglycosides, vancomycin, tetracyclines, bacitracin, polymyxins, colistin, and sodium colistimethate). If these antibiotics are used in conjunction with rocuronium, prolongation of neuromuscular block may occur. In patients in whom potentiation of neuromuscular block may be anticipated, a decrease from the recommended initial dose of rocuronium should be considered). Products include:

Bicillin C-R Injectable Suspension 1826
Bicillin L-A 1828

Penicillin G Dibenzylethyenediamine (Drugs which may enhance the neuromuscular blocking action of non-depolarizing agents such as rocuronium include certain antibiotics (eg, aminoglycosides, vancomycin, tetracyclines, bacitracin, polymyxins, colistin, and sodium colistimethate). If these antibiotics are used in conjunction with rocuronium, prolongation of neuromuscular block may occur. In patients in whom potentiation of neuromuscular block may be anticipated, a decrease from the recommended initial dose of rocuronium should be considered).
No products indexed under this heading.

Penicillin G Potassium (Drugs which may enhance the neuromuscular blocking action of non-depolarizing agents such as rocuronium include certain antibiotics (eg, aminoglycosides, vancomycin, tetracyclines, bacitracin, polymyxins, colistin, and sodium colistimethate). If these antibiotics are used in conjunction with rocuronium, prolongation of neuromuscular block may occur. In patients in whom potentiation of neuromuscular block may be anticipated, a decrease from the recommended initial dose of rocuronium should be considered).
No products indexed under this heading.

Penicillin G Procaine (Drugs which may enhance the neuromuscular blocking action of non-depolarizing agents such as rocuronium include certain antibiotics (eg, aminoglycosides, vancomycin, tetracyclines, bacitracin, polymyxins, colistin, and sodium colistimethate). If these antibiotics are used in conjunction with rocuronium, prolongation of neuromuscular block may occur. In patients in whom potentiation of neuromuscular block may be anticipated, a decrease from the recommended initial dose of rocuronium should be considered). Products include:

Bicillin C-R Injectable Suspension 1826
Bicillin L-A 1828

Penicillin G Sodium (Drugs which may enhance the neuromuscular blocking action of non-depolarizing agents such as rocuronium include certain antibiotics (eg, aminoglycosides, vancomycin, tetracyclines, bacitracin, polymyxins, colistin, and sodium colistimethate). If these antibiotics are used in conjunction with rocuronium, prolongation of neuromuscular block may occur. In patients in whom potentiation of neuromuscular block may be anticipated, a decrease from the recommended initial dose of rocuronium should be considered).
No products indexed under this heading.

Penicillin V (Drugs which may enhance the neuromuscular blocking action of non-depolarizing agents such as rocuronium include certain antibiotics (eg, aminoglycosides, vancomycin, tetracyclines, bacitracin, polymyxins, colistin, and sodium colistimethate). If these antibiotics are used in conjunction with rocuronium, prolongation of neuromuscular block may occur. In patients in whom potentiation of neuromuscular block may be anticipated, a decrease from the recommended initial dose of rocuronium should be considered).
No products indexed under this heading.

Penicillin V Potassium (Drugs which may enhance the neuromuscular blocking action of non-depolarizing agents such as rocuronium include certain antibiotics (eg, aminoglycosides, vancomycin, tetracyclines, bacitracin, polymyxins, colistin, and sodium colistimethate). If these antibiotics are used in conjunction with rocuronium, prolongation of neuromuscular block may occur. In patients in whom potentiation of neuromuscular block may be anticipated, a decrease from the recommended initial dose of rocuronium should be considered).
No products indexed under this heading.

Penicillins (Drugs which may enhance the neuromuscular blocking action of non-depolarizing agents such as rocuronium include certain antibiotics (eg, aminoglycosides, vancomycin, tetracyclines, bacitracin, polymyxins, colistin, and sodium colistimethate). If these antibiotics are used in conjunction with rocuronium, prolongation of neuromuscular block may occur. In patients in whom potentiation of neuromuscular block may be anticipated, a decrease from the recommended initial dose of rocuronium should be considered).
No products indexed under this heading.

Pentobarbital (Rocuronium, which has an acid pH, should not be mixed with alkaline solutions (eg, barbiturate solutions) in the same syringe or administered simultaneously during intravenous infusion through the same needle).
No products indexed under this heading.

Pentobarbital Sodium (Rocuronium, which has an acid pH, should not be mixed with alkaline solutions (eg, barbiturate solutions) in the same syringe or administered simultaneously during intravenous infusion through the same needle). Products include:

Nembutal 2012

Phenacemide (In two out of four patients receiving chronic anticonvulsant therapy, apparent resistance to the effects of rocuronium was observed in the form of diminished magnitude of neuromuscular block, or shortened clinical duration. As with other non-depolarizing neuromuscular blocking drugs, if rocuronium is administered to patients chronically receiving anticonvulsant agents, shorter durations of neuromuscular block may occur and infusion rates may be higher due to the development of resistance to non-depolarizing muscle relaxants. While the mechanism for development of this resistance is not known, receptor upregulation may be a contributing factor).
No products indexed under this heading.

Phenobarbital (In two out of four patients receiving chronic anticonvulsant therapy, apparent resistance to the effects of rocuronium was observed in the form of diminished magnitude of neuromuscular block, or shortened clinical duration. As with other non-depolarizing neuromuscular blocking drugs, if rocuronium is administered to patients chronically receiving anticonvulsant agents, shorter durations of neuromuscular block may occur and infusion rates may be higher due to the development of resistance to non-depolarizing muscle relaxants. While the mechanism for development of this resistance is not known, receptor upregulation may be a contributing factor). Products include:
Donnatal 2711

Phenobarbital Sodium (In two out of four patients receiving chronic anticonvulsant therapy, apparent resistance to the effects of rocuronium was observed in the form of diminished magnitude of neuromuscular block, or shortened clinical duration. As with other non-depolarizing neuromuscular blocking drugs, if rocuronium is administered to patients chronically receiving anticonvulsant agents, shorter durations of neuromuscular block may occur and infusion rates may be higher due to the development of resistance to non-depolarizing muscle relaxants. While the mechanism for development of this resistance is not known, receptor upregulation may be a contributing factor).
No products indexed under this heading.

Phensuximide (In two out of four patients receiving chronic anticonvulsant therapy, apparent resistance to the effects of rocuronium was observed in the form of diminished magnitude of neuromuscular block, or shortened clinical duration. As with other non-depolarizing neuromuscular blocking drugs, if rocuronium is administered to patients chronically receiving anticonvulsant agents, shorter durations of neuromuscular block may occur and infusion rates may be higher due to the development of resistance to non-depolarizing muscle relaxants. While the mechanism for development of this resistance is not known, receptor upregulation may be a contributing factor).
No products indexed under this heading.

Phenytoin (In two out of four patients receiving chronic anticonvulsant therapy, apparent resistance to the effects of rocuronium was observed in the form of diminished magnitude of neuromuscular block, or shortened clinical duration. As with other non-depolarizing neuromuscular blocking drugs, if rocuronium is administered to patients chronically receiving anticonvulsant agents, such as phenytoin, shorter durations of neuromuscular block may occur and infusion rates may be higher due to the development of resistance to non-depolarizing muscle relaxants. While the mechanism for development of this resistance is not known, receptor upregulation may be a contributing factor).
No products indexed under this heading.

Phenytoin Sodium (In two out of four patients receiving chronic anticonvulsant therapy, apparent resistance to the effects of rocuronium was observed in the form of diminished magnitude of neuromuscular block, or shortened clinical duration. As with other non-depolarizing neuromuscular blocking drugs, if rocuronium is administered to patients chronically receiving anticonvulsant agents, such as phenytoin, shorter durations of neuromuscular block may occur and infusion rates may be higher due to the development of resistance to non-depolarizing muscle relaxants. While the mechanism for development of this resistance is not known, receptor upregulation may be a contributing factor). Products include:
Phenytek Capsules 2380

Pipecuronium Bromide (There are no controlled studies documenting the use of rocuronium before or after other non-depolarizing muscle relaxants. Interactions have been observed when other non-depolarizing muscle relaxants have been administered in succession).
No products indexed under this heading.

Piperacillin Sodium (Drugs which may enhance the neuromuscular blocking action of non-depolarizing agents such as rocuronium include certain antibiotics (eg, aminoglycosides, vancomycin, tetracyclines, bacitracin, polymyxins, colistin, and sodium colistimethate). If these antibiotics are used in conjunction with rocuronium, prolongation of neuromuscular block may occur. In patients in whom potentiation of neuromuscular block may be anticipated, a decrease from the recommended initial dose of rocuronium should be considered). Products include:
Zosyn 3607

Polymyxin (Drugs which may enhance the neuromuscular blocking action of rocuronium include certain antibiotics, such as polymyxins. If polymyxins are used in conjunction with rocuronium, prolongation of neuromuscular block may occur and decreased infusion requirements of the neuromuscular blocking agent may be required).
No products indexed under this heading.

Polymyxin B Sulfate (Drugs which may enhance the neuromuscular blocking action of rocuronium include certain antibiotics, such as polymyxins. If polymyxins are used in conjunction with rocuronium, prolongation of neuromuscular block may occur and decreased infusion requirements of the neuromuscular blocking agent may be required).
No products indexed under this heading.

Polymyxin Preparations (Drugs which may enhance the neuromuscular blocking action of rocuronium include certain antibiotics, such as polymyxins. If polymyxins are used in conjunction with rocuronium, prolongation of neuromuscular block may occur and decreased infusion requirements of the neuromuscular blocking agent may be required).
No products indexed under this heading.

Prednisolone (Myopathy after long-term administration of other non-depolarizing neuromuscular blocking agents in the ICU alone or in combination with corticosteroid therapy has been reported. Therefore, for patients receiving both neuromuscular blocking agents and corticosteroids, the period of use of the neuromuscular blocking agent should be limited as much as possible and only used in the setting where in the opinion of the prescribing physician, the specific advantages of the drug outweigh the risk).
No products indexed under this heading.

Prednisolone Acetate (Myopathy after long-term administration of other non-depolarizing neuromuscular blocking agents in the ICU alone or in combination with corticosteroid therapy has been reported. Therefore, for patients receiving both neuromuscular blocking agents and corticosteroids, the period of use of the neuromuscular blocking agent should be limited as much as possible and only used in the setting where in the opinion of the prescribing physician, the specific advantages of the drug outweigh the risk). Products include:
Blephamide .... ⊙212, ⊙214
Pred Forte .... ⊙225
Pred Mild .... ⊙230
Pred-G .... ⊙226, ⊙227

Prednisolone Sodium Phosphate (Myopathy after long-term administration of other non-depolarizing neuromuscular blocking agents in the ICU alone or in combination with corticosteroid therapy has been reported. Therefore, for patients receiving both neuromuscular blocking agents and corticosteroids, the period of use of the neuromuscular blocking agent should be limited as much as possible and only used in the setting where in the opinion of the prescribing physician, the specific advantages of the drug outweigh the risk).
No products indexed under this heading.

Prednisolone Tebutate (Myopathy after long-term administration of other non-depolarizing neuromuscular blocking agents in the ICU alone or in combination with corticosteroid therapy has been reported. Therefore, for patients receiving both neuromuscular blocking agents and corticosteroids, the period of use of the neuromuscular blocking agent should be limited as much as possible and only used in the setting where in the opinion of the prescribing physician, the specific advantages of the drug outweigh the risk).
No products indexed under this heading.

Prednisone (Myopathy after long-term administration of other non-depolarizing neuromuscular blocking agents in the ICU alone or in combination with corticosteroid therapy has been reported. Therefore, for patients receiving both neuromuscular blocking agents and corticosteroids, the period of use of the neuromuscular blocking agent should be limited as much as possible and only used in the setting where in the opinion of the prescribing physician, the specific advantages of the drug outweigh the risk).
No products indexed under this heading.

Prednisone sodium phosphate (Myopathy after long-term administration of other non-depolarizing neuromuscular blocking agents in the ICU alone or in combination with corticosteroid therapy has been reported. Therefore, for patients receiving both neuromuscular blocking agents and corticosteroids, the period of use of the neuromuscular blocking agent should be limited as much as possible and only used in the setting where in the opinion of the prescribing physician, the specific advantages of the drug outweigh the risk).
No products indexed under this heading.

Primidone (In two out of four patients receiving chronic anticonvulsant therapy, apparent resistance to the effects of rocuronium was observed in the form of diminished magnitude of neuromuscular block, or shortened clinical duration. As with other non-depolarizing neuromuscular blocking drugs, if rocuronium is administered to patients chronically receiving anticonvulsant agents, shorter durations of neuromuscular block may occur and infusion rates may be higher due to the development of resistance to non-depolarizing muscle relaxants. While the mechanism for development of this resistance is not known, receptor upregulation may be a contributing factor).
No products indexed under this heading.

Procainamide (Procainamide has been shown to increase the duration of neuromuscular block and decrease infusion requirements of other neuromuscular blocking agents. In patients in whom potentiation of neuromuscular block may be anticipated, a decrease from the recommended initial dose of rocuronium should be considered).
No products indexed under this heading.

Procainamide Hydrochloride (Procainamide has been shown to increase the duration of neuromuscular block and decrease infusion requirements of other neuromuscular blocking agents. In patients in whom potentiation of neuromuscular block may be anticipated, a decrease from the recommended initial dose of rocuronium should be considered).
No products indexed under this heading.

Procaine Hydrochloride (Local anesthetics have been shown to increase the duration of neuromuscular block and decrease infusion requirements of other neuromuscular blocking agents. In patients in whom potentiation of neuromuscular block may be anticipated, a decrease from the recommended initial dose of rocuronium should be considered).
No products indexed under this heading.

Propofol (The overall analysis of ECG data in pediatric patients indicates that the concomitant use of rocuronium with general anesthetic agents can prolong the QTc interval).
No products indexed under this heading.

Quinidine (Injection of quinidine during recovery from use of muscle relaxants is associated with recurrent paralysis. This possibility must also be considered for rocuronium. In patients in whom potentiation of neuromuscular block may be anticipated, a decrease from the recommended initial dose of rocuronium should be considered).
No products indexed under this heading.

Quinidine Gluconate (Injection of quinidine during recovery from use of muscle relaxants is associated with recurrent paralysis. This possibility must also be considered for rocuronium. In patients in whom potentiation of neuromuscular block may be anticipated, a decrease from the recommended initial dose of rocuronium should be considered).
No products indexed under this heading.

Quinidine Hydrochloride (Injection of quinidine during recovery from use of muscle relaxants is associated with recurrent paralysis. This possibility must also be considered for rocuronium. In patients in whom potentiation of neuromuscular block may be anticipated, a decrease from the recommended initial dose of rocuronium should be considered).
No products indexed under this heading.

Quinidine Polygalacturonate (Injection of quinidine during recovery from use of muscle relaxants is associated with recurrent paralysis. This possibility must also be considered for rocuronium. In patients in whom potentiation of neuromuscular block may be anticipated, a decrease from the recommended initial dose of rocuronium should be considered).
No products indexed under this heading.

Quinidine Sulfate (Injection of quinidine during recovery from use of muscle relaxants is associated with recurrent paralysis. This possibility must also be considered for rocuronium. In patients in whom potentiation of neuromuscular block may be anticipated, a decrease from the recommended initial dose of rocuronium should be considered).
No products indexed under this heading.

Rapacuronium Bromide (There are no controlled studies documenting the use of rocuronium before or after other non-depolarizing muscle relaxants. Interactions have been observed when other non-depolarizing muscle relaxants have been administered in succession).
No products indexed under this heading.

Rufinamide (In two out of four patients receiving chronic anticonvulsant therapy, apparent resistance to the effects of rocuronium was observed in the form of diminished magnitude of neuromuscular block, or shortened clinical duration. As with other non-depolarizing neuromuscular blocking drugs, if rocuronium is administered to patients chronically receiving anticonvulsant agents, shorter durations of neuromuscular block may occur and infusion rates may be higher due to the development of resistance to non-depolarizing muscle relaxants. While the mechanism for development of this resistance is not known, receptor upregulation may be a contributing factor). Products include:
Banzel 1050

Secobarbital Sodium (Rocuronium, which has an acid pH, should not be mixed with alkaline solutions (eg, barbiturate solutions) in the same syringe or administered simultaneously during intravenous infusion through the same needle).
No products indexed under this heading.

Sevoflurane (Use of inhalation anesthetics as been shown to enhance the activity of other neuromuscular blocking agents. In patients in whom potentiation of neuromuscular block may be anticipated, a decrease from the recommended initial dose of rocuronium should be considered). Products include:
Ultane 554

Sodium Butabarbital (Rocuronium, which has an acid pH, should not be mixed with alkaline solutions (eg, barbiturate solutions) in the same syringe or administered simultaneously during intravenous infusion through the same needle).
No products indexed under this heading.

Sodium Cloxacillin Monohydrate (Drugs which may enhance the neuromuscular blocking action of non-depolarizing agents such as rocuronium include certain antibiotics (eg, aminoglycosides, vancomycin, tetracyclines, bacitracin, polymyxins, colistin, and sodium colistimethate). If these antibiotics are used in conjunction with rocuronium, prolongation of neuromuscular block may occur. In patients in whom potentiation of neuromuscular block may be anticipated, a decrease from the recommended initial dose of rocuronium should be considered).
No products indexed under this heading.

Sodium Pentobarbital (Rocuronium, which has an acid pH, should not be mixed with alkaline solutions (eg, barbiturate solutions) in the same syringe or administered simultaneously during intravenous infusion through the same needle).
No products indexed under this heading.

Sparfloxacin (Drugs which may enhance the neuromuscular blocking action of non-depolarizing agents such as rocuronium include certain antibiotics (eg, aminoglycosides, vancomycin, tetracyclines, bacitracin, polymyxins, colistin, and sodium colistimethate). If these antibiotics are used in conjunction with rocuronium, prolongation of neuromuscular block may occur. In patients in whom potentiation of neuromuscular block may be anticipated, a decrease from the recommended initial dose of rocuronium should be considered).
No products indexed under this heading.

Streptomycin Sulfate (Drugs which may enhance the neuromuscular blocking action of rocuronium include certain antibiotics, such as aminoglyosides. If aminoglycosides are used in conjunction with rocuronium, prolongation of neuromuscular block may occur. In patients in whom potentiation of neuromuscular block may be anticipated, a decrease from the recommended initial dose of rocuronium should be considered).
No products indexed under this heading.

Succinylcholine Chloride (The use of rocuronium before succinylcholine, for the purpose of attenuating some of the side effects of succinylcholine, has not been studied. If rocuronium is administered following administration of succinylcholine, it should not be given until recovery from succinylcholine has been observed. The median duration of action of rocuronium 0.6 mg/kg administered after a 1 mg/kg dose of succinylcholine when T_1 returned to 75% of control was 36 minutes (range 14 to 57, n=12) vs. 28 minutes (17 to 51, n=12) without succinylcholine).
No products indexed under this heading.

Sulfamethizole (Drugs which may enhance the neuromuscular blocking action of non-depolarizing agents such as rocuronium include certain antibiotics (eg, aminoglycosides, vancomycin, tetracyclines, bacitracin, polymyxins, colistin, and sodium colistimethate). If these antibiotics are used in conjunction with rocuronium, prolongation of neuromuscular block may occur. In patients in whom potentiation of neuromuscular block may be anticipated, a decrease from the recommended initial dose of rocuronium should be considered).
No products indexed under this heading.

Sulfamethoxazole (Drugs which may enhance the neuromuscular blocking action of non-depolarizing agents such as rocuronium include certain antibiotics (eg, aminoglycosides, vancomycin, tetracyclines, bacitracin, polymyxins, colistin, and sodium colistimethate). If these antibiotics are used in conjunction with rocuronium, prolongation of neuromuscular block may occur. In patients in whom potentiation of neuromuscular block may be anticipated, a decrease from the recommended initial dose of rocuronium should be considered).
No products indexed under this heading.

Sulfisoxazole Acetyl (Drugs which may enhance the neuromuscular blocking action of non-depolarizing agents such as rocuronium include certain antibiotics (eg, aminoglycosides, vancomycin, tetracyclines, bacitracin, polymyxins, colistin, and sodium colistimethate). If these antibiotics are used in conjunction with rocuronium, prolongation of neuromuscular block may occur. In patients in whom potentiation of neuromuscular block may be anticipated, a decrease from the recommended initial dose of rocuronium should be considered).
No products indexed under this heading.

Sulfisoxazole Diolamine (Drugs which may enhance the neuromuscular blocking action of non-depolarizing agents such as rocuronium include certain antibiotics (eg, aminoglycosides, vancomycin, tetracyclines, bacitracin, polymyxins, colistin, and sodium colistimethate). If these antibiotics are used in conjunction with rocuronium, prolongation of neuromuscular block may occur. In patients in whom potentiation of neuromuscular block may be anticipated, a decrease from the recommended initial dose of rocuronium should be considered).
No products indexed under this heading.

Tetracaine Hydrochloride (Local anesthetics have been shown to increase the duration of neuromuscular block and decrease infusion requirements of other neuromuscular blocking agents. In patients in whom potentiation of neuromuscular block may be anticipated, a decrease from the recommended initial dose of rocuronium should be considered).
No products indexed under this heading.

Tetracycline Hydrochloride (Drugs which may enhance the neuromuscular blocking action of rocuronium include certain antibiotics, such as tetracyclines. If tetracyclines are used in conjunction with rocuronium, prolongation of neuromuscular block may occur. In patients in whom potentiation of neuromuscular block may be anticipated, a decrease from the recommended initial dose of rocuronium should be considered). Products include:
Pylera 793

Tetracycline Phosphate Complex (Drugs which may enhance the neuromuscular blocking action of rocuronium include certain antibiotics, such as tetracyclines. If tetracyclines are used in conjunction with rocuronium, prolongation of neuromuscular block may occur. In patients in whom potentiation of neuromuscular block may be anticipated, a decrease from the recommended initial dose of rocuronium should be considered).
No products indexed under this heading.

Thiamylal Sodium (Rocuronium, which has an acid pH, should not be mixed with alkaline solutions (eg, barbiturate solutions) in the same syringe or administered simultaneously during intravenous infusion through the same needle).
No products indexed under this heading.

Tiagabine Hydrochloride (In two out of four patients receiving chronic anticonvulsant therapy, apparent resistance to the effects of rocuronium was observed in the form of diminished magnitude of neuromuscular block, or shortened clinical duration. As with other non-depolarizing neuromuscular blocking drugs, if rocuronium is administered to patients chronically receiving anticonvulsant agents, shorter durations of neuromuscular block may occur and infusion rates may be higher due to the development of resistance to non-depolarizing muscle relaxants. While the mechanism for development of this resistance is not known, receptor upregulation may be a contributing factor). Products include:
Gabitril 972

Ticarcillin Disodium (Drugs which may enhance the neuromuscular blocking action of non-depolarizing agents such as rocuronium include certain antibiotics (eg, aminoglycosides, vancomycin, tetracyclines, bacitracin, polymyxins, colistin, and sodium colistimethate). If these antibiotics are used in conjunction with rocuronium, prolongation of neuromuscular block may occur. In patients in whom potentiation of neuromuscular block may be anticipated, a decrease from the recommended initial dose of rocuronium should be considered). Products include:
Timentin ADD-Vantage 1670
Timentin Galaxy 1674
Timentin 1666
Timentin Pharmacy 1678

Tobramycin (Drugs which may enhance the neuromuscular blocking action of rocuronium include certain antibiotics, such as aminoglyosides. If aminoglycosides are used in conjunction with rocuronium, prolongation of neuromuscular block may occur. In patients in whom potentiation of neuromuscular block may be anticipated, a decrease from the recommended initial dose of rocuronium should be considered). Products include:
Tobi Nebulizer 2546
Tobramycin and Dexamethasone Ophthalmic Suspension .... ⊙251
Zylet .... ⊙252

Tobramycin Sulfate (Drugs which may enhance the neuromuscular blocking action of rocuronium include certain antibiotics, such as aminoglyosides. If aminoglycosides are used in conjunction with rocuronium, prolongation of neuromuscular block may occur. In patients in whom potentiation of neuromuscular block may be anticipated, a decrease from the recommended initial dose of rocuronium should be considered).
No products indexed under this heading.

Topiramate (In two out of four patients receiving chronic anticonvulsant therapy, apparent resistance to the effects of rocuronium was observed in the form of diminished magnitude of neuromuscular block, or shortened clinical duration. As with other non-depolarizing neuromuscular blocking drugs, if rocuronium is administered to patients chronically receiving anticonvulsant agents, shorter durations of neuromuscular block may occur and infusion rates may be higher due to the development of resistance to non-depolarizing muscle relaxants. While the mechanism for development of this resistance is not known, receptor upregulation may be a contributing factor).
No products indexed under this heading.

Triamcinolone (Myopathy after long-term administration of other non-depolarizing neuromuscular blocking agents in the ICU alone or in combination with corticosteroid therapy has been reported. Therefore, for patients receiving both neuromuscular blocking agents and corticosteroids, the period of use of the neuromuscular blocking agent should be limited as much as possible and only used in the setting where in the opinion of the prescribing physician, the specific advantages of the drug outweigh the risk).
No products indexed under this heading.

Triamcinolone Acetonide (Myopathy after long-term administration of other non-depolarizing neuromuscular blocking agents in the ICU alone or in combination with corticosteroid therapy has been reported. Therefore, for patients receiving both neuromuscular blocking agents and corticosteroids, the period of use of the neuromuscular blocking agent should be limited as much as possible and only used in the setting where in the opinion of the prescribing physician, the specific advantages of the drug outweigh the risk). Products include:
Azmacort 408
Nasacort AQ 3019

Triamcinolone Diacetate (Myopathy after long-term administration of other non-depolarizing neuromuscular blocking agents in the ICU alone or in combination with corticosteroid therapy has been reported. Therefore, for patients receiving both neuromuscular blocking agents and corticosteroids, the period of use of the neuromuscular blocking agent should be limited as much as possible and only used in the setting

2145 Interactions Index Zetia

where in the opinion of the prescribing physician, the specific advantages of the drug outweigh the risk).
No products indexed under this heading.

Triamcinolone Hexacetonide (Myopathy after long-term administration of other non-depolarizing neuromuscular blocking agents in the ICU alone or in combination with corticosteroid therapy has been reported. Therefore, for patients receiving both neuromuscular blocking agents and corticosteroids, the period of use of the neuromuscular blocking agent should be limited as much as possible and only used in the setting where in the opinion of the prescribing physician, the specific advantages of the drug outweigh the risk).
No products indexed under this heading.

Trimethadione (In two out of four patients receiving chronic anticonvulsant therapy, apparent resistance to the effects of rocuronium was observed in the form of diminished magnitude of neuromuscular block, or shortened clinical duration. As with other non-depolarizing neuromuscular blocking drugs, if rocuronium is administered to patients chronically receiving anticonvulsant agents, shorter durations of neuromuscular block may occur and infusion rates may be higher due to the development of resistance to non-depolarizing muscle relaxants. While the mechanism for development of this resistance is not known, receptor upregulation may be a contributing factor).
No products indexed under this heading.

Troleandomycin (Drugs which may enhance the neuromuscular blocking action of non-depolarizing agents such as rocuronium include certain antibiotics (eg, aminoglycosides, vancomycin, tetracyclines, bacitracin, polymyxins, colistin, and sodium colistimethate). If these antibiotics are used in conjunction with rocuronium, prolongation of neuromuscular block may occur. In patients in whom potentiation of neuromuscular block may be anticipated, a decrease from the recommended initial dose of rocuronium should be considered).
No products indexed under this heading.

Trovafloxacin Mesylate (Drugs which may enhance the neuromuscular blocking action of non-depolarizing agents such as rocuronium include certain antibiotics (eg, aminoglycosides, vancomycin, tetracyclines, bacitracin, polymyxins, colistin, and sodium colistimethate). If these antibiotics are used in conjunction with rocuronium, prolongation of neuromuscular block may occur. In patients in whom potentiation of neuromuscular block may be anticipated, a decrease from the recommended initial dose of rocuronium should be considered).
No products indexed under this heading.

Tubocurarine Chloride (There are no controlled studies documenting the use of rocuronium before or after other non-depolarizing muscle relaxants. Interactions have been observed when other non-depolarizing muscle relaxants have been administered in succession).
No products indexed under this heading.

Valproate Sodium (In two out of four patients receiving chronic anticonvulsant therapy, apparent resistance to the effects of rocuronium was observed in the form of diminished magnitude of neuromuscular block, or shortened clinical duration. As with other non-depolarizing neuromuscular blocking drugs, if rocuronium is administered to patients chronically receiving anticonvulsant agents, shorter durations of neuromuscular block may occur and infusion rates may be higher due to the development of resistance to non-depolarizing muscle relaxants. While the mechanism for development of this resistance is not known, receptor upregulation may be a contributing factor).
No products indexed under this heading.

Valproic Acid (In two out of four patients receiving chronic anticonvulsant therapy, apparent resistance to the effects of rocuronium was observed in the form of diminished magnitude of neuromuscular block, or shortened clinical duration. As with other non-depolarizing neuromuscular blocking drugs, if rocuronium is administered to patients chronically receiving anticonvulsant agents, shorter durations of neuromuscular block may occur and infusion rates may be higher due to the development of resistance to non-depolarizing muscle relaxants. While the mechanism for development of this resistance is not known, receptor upregulation may be a contributing factor).
No products indexed under this heading.

Vancomycin Hydrochloride (Drugs which may enhance the neuromuscular blocking action of rocuronium include certain antibiotics, such as vancomycin. If vancomycin is used in conjunction with rocuronium, prolongation of neuromuscular block may occur. In patients in whom potentiation of neuromuscular block may be anticipated, a decrease from the recommended initial dose of rocuronium should be considered).
No products indexed under this heading.

Vecuronium Bromide (There are no controlled studies documenting the use of rocuronium before or after other non-depolarizing muscle relaxants. Interactions have been observed when other non-depolarizing muscle relaxants have been administered in succession).
No products indexed under this heading.

Zonisamide (In two out of four patients receiving chronic anticonvulsant therapy, apparent resistance to the effects of rocuronium was observed in the form of diminished magnitude of neuromuscular block, or shortened clinical duration. As with other non-depolarizing neuromuscular blocking drugs, if rocuronium is administered to patients chronically receiving anticonvulsant agents, shorter durations of neuromuscular block may occur and infusion rates may be higher due to the development of resistance to non-depolarizing muscle relaxants. While the mechanism for development of this resistance is not known, receptor upregulation may be a contributing factor). Products include:
Zonegran 1081

ZETIA TABLETS

(Ezetimibe) 3256
May interact with bile acid sequestering agents, fibrates, HMG-CoA reductase inhibitors, statins that are metabolized by CYP3A4, vitamin K antagonists, and certain other agents. Compounds in these categories include:

Aluminum Hydroxide (Co-administration of ezetimibe with aluminum and magnesium hydroxide combination antacid may lead to a 4% decrease in ezetimibe AUC, and a 30% decrease in ezetimibe C_{max}).
No products indexed under this heading.

Atorvastatin Calcium (The combination of ezetimibe with a statin is contraindicated in patients with active liver disease or unexplained persistent elevations in hepatic transaminase levels, pregnant women, and in women who are nursing. Co-administration of ezetimibe and atorvastatin may lead to a 2% decrease in ezetimibe AUC, a 12% increase in ezetimibe C_{max}, a 4% decrease in atorvastatin AUC, and a 7% increase in atorvastatin C_{max}. In addition, in controlled clinical combination studies of ezetimibe initiated concurrently with a statin, the incidence of consecutive elevations in hepatic transaminase levels was 1.3% for patients treated with ezetimibe administered with statins and 0.4% for patients treated with statins alone. When ezetimibe is co-administered with a statin, liver tests should be performed at initiation of therapy and according to the recommendations of the statin. Should an increase in ALT or AST $\geq 3 \times$ ULN persist, consider withdrawal of ezetimibe and/or the statin. Also, in post-marketing experience with ezetimibe, cases of myopathy and rhabdomyolysis have been reported. Most patients who developed rhabdomyolysis were taking a statin prior to initiating ezetimibe. Ezetimibe and any statin that the patient is taking concomitantly should be immediately discontinued if myopathy is diagnosed or suspected). Products include:
Lipitor 2703

Cerivastatin Sodium (The combination of ezetimibe with a statin is contraindicated in patients with active liver disease or unexplained persistent elevations in hepatic transaminase levels, pregnant women, and in women who are nursing. In controlled clinical combination studies of ezetimibe initiated concurrently with a statin, the incidence of consecutive elevations in hepatic transaminase levels was 1.3% for patients treated with ezetimibe administered with statins and 0.4% for patients treated with statins alone. When ezetimibe is co-administered with a statin, liver tests should be performed at initiation of therapy and according to the recommendations of the statin. Should an increase in ALT or AST $\geq 3 \times$ ULN persist, consider withdrawal of ezetimibe and/or the statin. In addition, in post-marketing experience with ezetimibe, cases of myopathy and rhabdomyolysis have been reported. Most patients who developed rhabdomyolysis were taking a statin prior to initiating ezetimibe. Ezetimibe and any statin that the patient is taking concomitantly should be immediately discontinued if myopathy is diagnosed or suspected).
No products indexed under this heading.

Cholestyramine (Concomitant cholestyramine administration decreased the mean area under the curve (AUC) of total ezetimibe approximately 55% and the C_{max} by 4%. The incremental LDL-C reduction due to adding ezetimibe to cholestyramine may be reduced by this interaction).
No products indexed under this heading.

Cimetidine (Co-administration of ezetimibe and cimetidine may lead to a 6% increase in ezetimibe AUC and a 22% increase in ezetimibe C_{max}).
No products indexed under this heading.

Cimetidine Hydrochloride (Co-administration of ezetimibe and cimetidine may lead to a 6% increase in ezetimibe AUC and a 22% increase in ezetimibe C_{max}).
No products indexed under this heading.

Clofibrate (The efficacy and safety of co-administration of ezetimibe with fibrates other than fenofibrate have not been studied. Fibrates may increase cholesterol excretion into the bile, leading to cholelithiasis. In a preclinical study in dogs, ezetimibe increased cholesterol in the gallbladder bile. In addition, rhabdomyolysis has been reported with ezetimibe monotherapy and with the addition of agents known to be associated with increased risk of rhabdomyolysis, such as fibrates. Co-administration of ezetimibe with fibrates other than fenofibrate is not recommended until use in patients is adequately studied).
No products indexed under this heading.

Colesevelam Hydrochloride (Dosing of ezetimibe should occur either 2 hours or more before or 4 hours or more after administration of a bile acid sequestrant). Products include:
Welchol 1029

Colestipol Hydrochloride (Dosing of ezetimibe should occur either 2 hours or more before or 4 hours or more after administration of a bile acid sequestrant).
No products indexed under this heading.

Cyclosporine (Caution should be exercised when using ezetimibe and cyclosporine concomitantly due to increased exposure to both ezetimibe and cyclosporine. Cyclosporine concentrations should be monitored in patients receiving ezetimibe and cyclosporine. The degree of increase in ezetimibe exposure may be greater in patients with severe renal insufficiency. In patients treated with cyclosporine, the potential effects of the increased exposure to ezetimibe from concomitant use should be carefully weighed against the benefits of alterations in lipid levels provided by ezetimibe. Co-administration of ezetimibe and cyclosporine may lead to a 240% increase in ezetimibe AUC, a 290% increase in ezetimibe C_{max}, a 15% increase in cyclosporine AUC, and a 10% increase in cyclosporine C_{max}). Products include:
Gengraf 440
Neoral Oral Solution 2496
Neoral Capsules 2496
Restasis 605

Dicumarol (If ezetimibe is added to warfarin, a coumarin anticoagulant, the International Normalized Ratio (INR) should be appropriately monitored).
No products indexed under this heading.

Digoxin (Co-administration of ezetimibe and digoxin may lead to a 2% increase in digoxin AUC and a 7% decrease in digoxin C_{max}). Products include:
Lanoxin Injection 1546
Lanoxin Injection Pediatric 1549
Lanoxin Tablets 1553

Ethinyl Estradiol (Co-administration of ezetimibe with ethinyl estradiol and levonorgestrel may lead to a 9% decrease in ethinyl estradiol C_{max} and a 5% decrease in levonorgestrel C_{max}). Products include:
LoSeasonique 3407
Lybrel 3514
NuvaRing 3181
Ortho Evra 2648
Ortho-Cyclen/Ortho Tri-Cyclen 2663
Ortho Tri-Cyclen Lo Tablets 2673
Seasonique 3418
Yaz 864

Fat (The C_{max} value of ezetimibe was increased by 38% with consumption of high-fat meals. Ezetimibe can be administered with or without food).
No products indexed under this heading.

Fenofibrate (Fibrates may increase cholesterol excretion into the bile, leading to cholelithiasis. If cholelithiasis is suspected in a patient receiving ezetimibe and fenofibrate, gallbladder studies are indicated and alternative lipid-lowering therapy should be considered. In addition, rhabdomyolysis has been reported with ezetimibe monotherapy and with the addition of agents known to be associated with increased risk of rhabdomyolysis, such as fibrates. Co-administration with fenofibrate may lead to a 48% increase in AUC and a 64% increase in C_{max} of ezetimibe. Co-administration with fenofibrate may also lead to an 11% increase in AUC and a 7% increase in C_{max} of fenofibrate). Products include:
Fenoglide 3263
Tricor 544
Trilipix 548

IMPORTANT NOTE: Always consult each drug listing in the patient's regimen for possible interactions.

Fluvastatin Sodium (The combination of ezetimibe with a statin is contraindicated in patients with active liver disease or unexplained persistent elevations in hepatic transaminase levels, pregnant women, and in women who are nursing. Co-administration of ezetimibe and fluvastatin may lead to a 19% decrease in ezetimibe AUC, a 7% increase in ezetimibe C_{max}, a 39% decrease in fluvastatin AUC, and a 27% decrease in fluvastatin C_{max}. In addition, in controlled clinical combination studies of ezetimibe initiated concurrently with a statin, the incidence of consecutive elevations in hepatic transaminase levels was 1.3% for patients treated with ezetimibe administered with statins and 0.4% for patients treated with statins alone. When ezetimibe is co-administered with a statin, liver tests should be performed at initiation of therapy and according to the recommendations of the statin. Should an increase in ALT or AST $\geq3 \times$ ULN persist, consider withdrawal of ezetimibe and/or the statin. Also, in post-marketing experience with ezetimibe, cases of myopathy and rhabdomyolysis have been reported. Most patients who developed rhabdomyolysis were taking a statin prior to initiating ezetimibe. Ezetimibe and any statin that the patient is taking concomitantly should be immediately discontinued if myopathy is diagnosed or suspected.

No products indexed under this heading.

Gemfibrozil (The efficacy and safety of co-administration of ezetimibe with fibrates other than fenofibrate have not been studied. Fibrates may increase cholesterol excretion into the bile, leading to cholelithiasis. In a preclinical study in dogs, ezetimibe increased cholesterol in the gallbladder bile. In addition, rhabdomyolysis has been reported with ezetimibe monotherapy and with the addition of agents known to be associated with increased risk of rhabdomyolysis, such as fibrates. Co-administration of ezetimibe with fibrates other than fenofibrate is not recommended until use in patients is adequately studied. Co-administration of ezetimibe and gemfibrozil may lead to a 64% increase in ezetimibe AUC, a 91% increase in ezetimibe C_{max}, a 1% decrease in gemfibrozil AUC, and an 11% decrease in gemfibrozil C_{max}).
No products indexed under this heading.

Glipizide (Co-administration of ezetimibe and glipizide may lead to a 4% increase in ezetimibe AUC, an 8% decrease in ezetimibe C_{max}, a 3% decrease in glipizide AUC, and a 5% decrease in glipizide C_{max}).
No products indexed under this heading.

Levonorgestrel (Co-administration of ezetimibe with ethinyl estradiol and levonorgestrel may lead to a 9% decrease in ethinyl estradiol C_{max} and a 5% decrease in levonorgestrel C_{max}).
Products include:

Lovastatin (The combination of ezetimibe with a statin is contraindicated in patients with active liver disease or unexplained persistent elevations in hepatic transaminase levels, pregnant women, and in women who are nursing. Co-administration of ezetimibe and lovastatin may lead to a 9% increase in ezetimibe AUC, a 3% increase in ezetimibe C_{max}, a 19% increase in lovastatin AUC, and a 3% increase in lovastatin C_{max}. Also, in controlled clinical combination studies of ezetimibe initiated concurrently with a

statin, the incidence of consecutive elevations in hepatic transaminase levels was 1.3% for patients treated with ezetimibe administered with statins and 0.4% for patients treated with statins alone. When ezetimibe is co-administered with a statin, liver tests should be performed at initiation of therapy and according to the recommendations of the statin. Should an increase in ALT or AST $\geq3 \times$ ULN persist, consider withdrawal of ezetimibe and/or the statin. In addition, in post-marketing experience with ezetimibe, cases of myopathy and rhabdomyolysis have been reported. Most patients who developed rhabdomyolysis were taking a statin prior to initiating ezetimibe. Ezetimibe and any statin that the patient is taking concomitantly should be immediately discontinued if myopathy is diagnosed or suspected). Products include:

Magnesium Hydroxide (Co-administration of ezetimibe with aluminum and magnesium hydroxide combination antacid may lead to a 4% decrease in ezetimibe AUC, and a 30% decrease in ezetimibe C_{max}). Products include:

Pravastatin Sodium (The combination of ezetimibe with a statin is contraindicated in patients with active liver disease or unexplained persistent elevations in hepatic transaminase levels, pregnant women, and in women who are nursing. Co-administration of ezetimibe and pravastatin may lead to a 7% increase in ezetimibe AUC, a 23% increase in ezetimibe C_{max}, a 20% decrease in pravastatin AUC, and a 24% decrease in pravastatin C_{max}. In addition, in controlled clinical combination studies of ezetimibe initiated concurrently with a statin, the incidence of consecutive elevations in hepatic transaminase levels was 1.3% for patients treated with ezetimibe administered with statins and 0.4% for patients treated with statins alone. When ezetimibe is co-administered with a statin, liver tests should be performed at initiation of therapy and according to the recommendations of the statin. Should an increase in ALT or AST $\geq3 \times$ ULN persist, consider withdrawal of ezetimibe and/or the statin. Also, in post-marketing experience with ezetimibe, cases of myopathy and rhabdomyolysis have been reported. Most patients who developed rhabdomyolysis were taking a statin prior to initiating ezetimibe. Ezetimibe and any statin that the patient is taking concomitantly should be immediately discontinued if myopathy is diagnosed or suspected).
No products indexed under this heading.

Rosuvastatin Calcium (The combination of ezetimibe with a statin is contraindicated in patients with active liver disease or unexplained persistent elevations in hepatic transaminase levels, pregnant women, and in women who are nursing. Co-administration of ezetimibe and rosuvastatin may lead to a 13% increase in ezetimibe AUC, an 18% increase in ezetimibe C_{max}, a 19% increase in rosuvastatin AUC, and a 17% increase in rosuvastatin C_{max}. In addition, in controlled clinical combination studies of ezetimibe initiated concurrently with a statin, the incidence of consecutive elevations in hepatic transaminase levels was 1.3% for patients treated with ezetimibe administered with statins and 0.4% for patients treated with statins alone. When ezetimibe is co-administered with a statin, liver tests should be performed at initiation of therapy and according to the recommendations of the statin. Should an increase in

ALT or AST $\geq3 \times$ ULN persist, consider withdrawal of ezetimibe and/or the statin. Also, in post-marketing experience with ezetimibe, cases of myopathy and rhabdomyolysis have been reported. Most patients who developed rhabdomyolysis were taking a statin prior to initiating ezetimibe. Ezetimibe and any statin that the patient is taking concomitantly should be immediately discontinued if myopathy is diagnosed or suspected). Products include:

Simvastatin (The combination of ezetimibe with a statin is contraindicated in patients with active liver disease or unexplained persistent elevations in hepatic transaminase levels, pregnant women, and in women who are nursing. In controlled clinical combination studies of ezetimibe initiated concurrently with a statin, the incidence of consecutive elevations in hepatic transaminase levels was 1.3% for patients treated with ezetimibe administered with statins and 0.4% for patients treated with statins alone. When ezetimibe is co-administered with a statin, liver tests should be performed at initiation of therapy and according to the recommendations of the statin. Should an increase in ALT or AST $\geq3 \times$ ULN persist, consider withdrawal of ezetimibe and/or the statin. In addition, in post-marketing experience with ezetimibe, cases of myopathy and rhabdomyolysis have been reported. Most patients who developed rhabdomyolysis were taking a statin prior to initiating ezetimibe. Ezetimibe and any statin that the patient is taking concomitantly should be immediately discontinued if myopathy is diagnosed or suspected). Products include:

Warfarin Sodium (If ezetimibe is added to warfarin, a coumarin anticoagulant, the International Normalized Ratio (INR) should be appropriately monitored. Co-administration of ezetimibe and warfarin may lead to a decrease in warfarin AUC, and an increase in warfarin C_{max}).
No products indexed under this heading.

Food Interactions

Food, unspecified (The C_{max} value of ezetimibe was increased by 38% with consumption of high-fat meals. Ezetimibe can be administered with or without food).

Meal, unspecified (The C_{max} value of ezetimibe was increased by 38% with consumption of high-fat meals. Ezetimibe can be administered with or without food).

ZETIA TABLETS

May interact with bile acid sequestering agents, fibrates, HMG-CoA reductase inhibitors, lipid-lowering drugs, statins that are metabolized by CYP3A4, and certain other agents. Compounds in these categories include:

Aluminum Hydroxide (Co-administration of ezetimibe with aluminum and magnesium hydroxide combination antacid may lead to a 4% decrease in ezetimibe AUC, and a 30% decrease in ezetimibe C_{max}).
No products indexed under this heading.

Atorvastatin Calcium (Concomitant administration of ezetimibe and atorvastatin may lead to a 2% decrease in ezetimibe AUC, a 12% increase in ezetimibe C_{max}, a 4% decrease in atorvastatin AUC, and a 7% increase in atorvastatin C_{max}). Products include:

Cerivastatin Sodium (Administration of ezetimibe with a statin is effective in improving serum total-cholesterol, LDL-cholesterol, apolipoprotein B, triglycerides, and HDL-cholesterol beyond either treatment alone. Cases of myopathy and rhabdomyolysis have been reported in patients treated with ezetimibe co-administered with a statin and with ezetimibe administered alone. Risk for skeletal muscle toxicity increases with higher doses of statin).
No products indexed under this heading.

Cholestyramine (Concomitant cholestyramine administration decreased the mean AUC of total ezetimibe approximately 55%. The incremental LDL-cholesterol reduction due to adding ezetimibe to cholestyramine may be reduced by this interaction).
No products indexed under this heading.

Cimetidine (Concomitant administration of ezetimibe and cimetidine may lead to a 6% increase in ezetimibe AUC, and a 22% increase in ezetimibe C_{max}).
No products indexed under this heading.

Cimetidine Hydrochloride (Concomitant administration of ezetimibe and cimetidine may lead to a 6% increase in ezetimide AUC, and a 22% increase in ezetimibe C_{max}).
No products indexed under this heading.

Clofibrate (The efficacy and safety of co-administration of ezetimibe with fibrates other than fenofibrate have not been studied. Fibrates may increase cholesterol excretion into the bile, leading to cholelithiasis. In a preclinical study in dogs, ezetimibe increased cholesterol in the gallbladder bile. Co-administration of ezetimibe with fibrates other than fenofibrate is not recommended until use in patients is adequately studied).
No products indexed under this heading.

Colesevelam Hydrochloride (Dosing of ezetimibe should occur either>/= 2 hours before or>/= 4 hours after administration of a bile acid sequestrant). Products include:

Colestipol Hydrochloride (Dosing of ezetimibe should occur either>/= 2 hours before or>/= 4 hours after administration of a bile acid sequestrant).
No products indexed under this heading.

Cyclosporine (Caution should be exercised when using ezetimibe and cyclosporine concomitantly due to increased exposure to both ezetimibe and cyclosporine. Cyclosporine concentrations should be monitored in patients receiving ezetimibe and cyclosporine. In patients treated with cyclosporine, the potential effects of the increased exposure to ezetimibe from concomitant use should be carefully weighed against the benefits of alterations in lipid levels provided by ezetimibe. Concomitant administration of ezetimibe and cyclosporine may lead to a 240% increase in ezetimibe AUC, a 290% increase in ezetimibe C_{max}, a 15% increase in cyclosporine AUC, and a 10% increase in cyclosporine C_{max}). Products include:

Digoxin (Concomitant administration of ezetimibe and digoxin may lead to a 2% increase in digoxin AUC, and a 7% decrease in digoxin $Cmax$). Products include:

Ethinyl Estradiol (Concomitant administration of ezetimibe with ethinyl estradiol and levonorgestrel may lead to a 9% decrease in ethinyl estradiol C_{max} and a 5% decrease in levonorgestrel C_{max}). Products include:

Fat (Concomitant food administration (high-fat meals) had no effect on the extent of absorption of ezetimibe when administered as ezetimibe 10-mg tablets. The C_{max} value of ezetimibe was increased by 38% with consumption of high-fat meals. Ezetimibe can be administered with or without food.
No products indexed under this heading.

Fenofibrate (If cholelithiasis is suspected in a patient receiving ezetimibe and fenofibrate, gallbladder studies are indicated and alternative lipid-lowering therapy should be considered. Concomitant administration of ezetimibe and fenofibrate may lead to a 48% increase in ezetimibe AUC, a 64% increase in ezetimibe C_{max}, an 11% increase in fenofibrate AUC, and a 7% increase in fenofibrate C_{max}. Ezetimibe co-administered with fenofibrate significantly lowered total-cholesterol, LDL-cholesterol, apolipoprotein B, and non-HDL-cholesterol compared to fenofibrate administered alone). Products include:

Fluvastatin Sodium (Concomitant administration of ezetimibe and fluvastatin may lead to a 19% decrease in ezetimibe AUC, a 7% increase in ezetimibe C_{max}, a 39% decrease in fluvastatin AUC, and a 27% decrease in fluvastatin C_{max}).
No products indexed under this heading.

Gemfibrozil (Concomitant administration of ezetimibe and gemfibrozil may lead to a 64% increase in ezetimibe AUC, a 91% increase in ezetimibe C_{max}, a 1% decrease in gemfibrozil AUC, and an 11% decrease in gemfibrozil C_{max}).
No products indexed under this heading.

Glipizide (Concomitant administration of ezetimibe and glipizide may lead to a 4% increase in ezetimibe AUC, an 8% decrease in ezetimibe C_{max}, a 3% decrease in glipizide AUC, and a 5% decrease in glipizide C_{max}).
No products indexed under this heading.

Levonorgestrel (Concomitant administration of ezetimibe with ethinyl estradiol and levonorgestrel may lead to a 9% decrease in ethinyl estradiol C_{max} and a 5% decrease in levonorgestrel C_{max}). Products include:

Lovastatin (Concomitant administration of ezetimibe and lovastatin may lead to a 9% increase in ezetimibe AUC, a 3% increase in ezetimibe C_{max}, a 19% increase in lovastatin AUC, and a 3% increase in lovastatin C_{max}). Products include:

Magnesium Hydroxide (Co-administration of ezetimibe with aluminum and magnesium hydroxide combination antacid may lead to a 4%

decrease in ezetimibe AUC, and a 30% decrease in ezetimibe C_{max}). Products include:

Pravastatin Sodium (Concomitant administration of ezetimibe and pravastatin may lead to a 7% increase in ezetimibe AUC, a 23% increase in ezetimibe C_{max}, a 20% decrease in pravastatin AUC, and a 24% decrease in pravastatin C_{max}).
No products indexed under this heading.

Probucol (Ezetimibe may be administered with a statin (in patients with primary hyperlipidemia) or with fenofibrate (in patients with mixed hyperlipidemia) for incremental effect. For convenience, the daily dose of ezetimibe may be taken at the same time as the statin or fenofibrate, according to the dosing recommendations for the respective lipid-lowering medications).
No products indexed under this heading.

Rosuvastatin Calcium (Concomitant administration of ezetimibe and rosuvastatin may lead to a 13% increase in ezetimibe AUC, an 18% increase in ezetimibe C_{max}, a 19% increase in rosuvastatin AUC, and a 17% increase in rosuvastatin C_{max}). Products include:

Simvastatin (Administration of ezetimibe with a statin is effective in improving serum total-cholesterol, LDL-cholesterol, apolipoprotein B, triglycerides, and HDL-cholesterol beyond either treatment alone. Cases of myopathy and rhabdomyolysis have been reported in patients treated with ezetimibe co-administered with a statin and with ezetimibe administered alone. Risk for skeletal muscle toxicity increases with higher doses of statin). Products include:

Warfarin Sodium (If ezetimibe is added to warfarin, a coumarin anticoagulant, the International Normalized Ratio (INR) should be appropriately monitored).
No products indexed under this heading.

Food Interactions

Food, unspecified (Concomitant food administration (non-fat meals) had no effect on the extent of absorption of ezetimibe when administered as ezetimibe 10-mg tablets. The C_{max} value of ezetimibe was increased by 38% with consumption of high-fat meals. Ezetimibe can be administered with or without food).

Meal, unspecified (Concomitant food administration (non-fat meals) had no effect on the extent of absorption of ezetimibe when administered as ezetimibe 10-mg tablets. The C_{max} value of ezetimibe was increased by 38% with consumption of high-fat meals. Ezetimibe can be administered with or without food).

ZIAGEN ORAL SOLUTION

(Abacavir Sulfate) 1740
See Ziagen Tablets

ZIAGEN TABLETS

(Abacavir Sulfate) 1740
May interact with alcohols, and certain other agents. Compounds in these categories include:

Ethanol (Ethanol decreases the elimination of abacavir, causing an increase in overall exposure. Co-administration of ethanol and abacavir resulted in a 41% increase in abacavir AUC and a 26% increase in abacavir t1/2).
No products indexed under this heading.

Ethyl Alcohol (Ethanol decreases the elimination of abacavir, causing an increase in overall exposure. Co-administration of ethanol and abacavir resulted in a 41% increase in abacavir AUC and a 26% increase in abacavir $t_{1/2}$).
No products indexed under this heading.

Lamivudine (Due to the common metabolic pathways of abacavir and zidovudine via glucuronyl transferase, 15 HIV-infected patients were enrolled in a crossover study evaluating single doses of abacavir (600 mg), lamivudine (150 mg), and zidovudine (300 mg) alone or in combination. Analysis showed no clinically relevant changes in the pharmacokinetics of abacavir with the addition of lamivudine or zidovudine, or the combination of lamivudine and zidovudine. Lamivudine exposure (AUC decreased 15%) and zidovudine exposure (AUC increased 10%) did not show clinically relevant changes with concurrent abacavir). Products include:

Methadone Hydrochloride (The addition of methadone has no clinically significant effect on the pharmacokinetic properties of abacavir. In a study of 11 HIV infected patients receiving methadone-maintenance therapy with 600 mg of abacavir (twice the currently recommended dose), oral methadone clearance increased by 22%. This alteration will not result in a methadone dose modification in the majority of patients; however, an increased methadone dose may be required in a small number of patients).
No products indexed under this heading.

Zidovudine (Due to the common metabolic pathways of abacavir and zidovudine via glucuronyl transferase, 15 HIV-infected patients were enrolled in a crossover study evaluating single doses of abacavir (600 mg), lamivudine (150 mg), and zidovudine (300 mg) alone or in combination. Analysis showed no clinically relevant changes in the pharmacokinetics of abacavir with the addition of lamivudine or zidovudine, or the combination of lamivudine and zidovudine. Lamivudine exposure (AUC decreased 15%) and zidovudine exposure (AUC increased 10%) did not show clinically relevant changes with concurrent abacavir). Products include:

Food Interactions

Alcohol (Ethanol decreases the elimination of abacavir, causing an increase in overall exposure. Co-administration of ethanol and abacavir resulted in a 41% increase in abacavir AUC and a 26% increase in abacavir $t_{1/2}$).

Beer, reduced-alcohol (Ethanol decreases the elimination of abacavir, causing an increase in overall exposure. Co-administration of ethanol and abacavir resulted in a 41% increase in abacavir AUC and a 26% increase in abacavir $t_{1/2}$).

Beer, unspecified (Ethanol decreases the elimination of abacavir, causing an increase in overall exposure. Co-administration of ethanol and abacavir

resulted in a 41% increase in abacavir AUC and a 26% increase in abacavir $t_{1/2}$).

Wine, Chianti (Ethanol decreases the elimination of abacavir, causing an increase in overall exposure. Co-administration of ethanol and abacavir resulted in a 41% increase in abacavir AUC and a 26% increase in abacavir $t_{1/2}$).

Wine, Red (Ethanol decreases the elimination of abacavir, causing an increase in overall exposure. Co-administration of ethanol and abacavir resulted in a 41% increase in abacavir AUC and a 26% increase in abacavir $t_{1/2}$).

Wine, unspecified (Ethanol decreases the elimination of abacavir, causing an increase in overall exposure. Co-administration of ethanol and abacavir resulted in a 41% increase in abacavir AUC and a 26% increase in abacavir $t_{1/2}$).

Wine products (Ethanol decreases the elimination of abacavir, causing an increase in overall exposure. Co-administration of ethanol and abacavir resulted in a 41% increase in abacavir AUC and a 26% increase in abacavir $t_{1/2}$).

ZINACEF FOR INJECTION

(Cefuroxime) 1746
See Zinacef Injection

ZINACEF INJECTION

(Cefuroxime) 1746
May interact with aminoglycosides, oral anticoagulants, and certain other agents. Compounds in these categories include:

Amikacin Sulfate (Concomitant administration may produce nephrotoxicity).
No products indexed under this heading.

Anisindione (Cephalosporins may be associated with a fall in prothrombin activity; those at risk include patients stabilized on anticoagulants).
No products indexed under this heading.

Dicumarol (Cephalosporins may be associated with a fall in prothrombin activity; those at risk include patients stabilized on anticoagulants).
No products indexed under this heading.

Dihydrostreptomycin (Concomitant administration may produce nephrotoxicity).
No products indexed under this heading.

Gentamicin (Concomitant administration may produce nephrotoxicity).
No products indexed under this heading.

Gentamicin Sulfate (Concomitant administration may produce nephrotoxicity). Products include:

Kanamycin Sulfate (Concomitant administration may produce nephrotoxicity).
No products indexed under this heading.

Neomycin (Concomitant administration may produce nephrotoxicity).
No products indexed under this heading.

Neomycin, oral (Concomitant administration may produce nephrotoxicity).
No products indexed under this heading.

Neomycin Sulfate (Concomitant administration may produce nephrotoxicity).
No products indexed under this heading.

Probenecid (Concurrent administration of probenecid decreases renal clearance and increases peak serum levels of cefuroxime).
No products indexed under this heading.

IMPORTANT NOTE: Always consult each drug listing in the patient's regimen for possible interactions.

2149 Interactions Index Zocor

Dicumarol (Concomitant use with simvastatin may prolong INR. Achieve stable INR prior to initiation of simvastatin. Monitor INR frequently until stable upon initiation or alteration of simvastatin therapy).
No products indexed under this heading.

Digoxin (In one study, concomitant administration of digoxin with simvastatin resulted in a slight elevation of digoxin concentrations in plasma. Patients taking digoxin should be monitored appropriately when simvastatin is initiated). Products include:
Lanoxin Injection **1546**
Lanoxin Injection Pediatric **1549**
Lanoxin Tablets **1553**

Diltiazem Hydrochloride (The risk of myopathy is increased by reducing the elimination of simvastatin. Hence when simvastatin is used with an inhibitor of CYP3A4, elevated plasma levels of HMG-CoA reductase inhibitory activity can increase the risk of myopathy and rhabdomyolysis, particularly with higher doses of simvastatin). Products include:
Cardizem LA **423**

Diltiazem Maleate (The risk of myopathy is increased by reducing the elimination of simvastatin. Hence when simvastatin is used with an inhibitor of CYP3A4, elevated plasma levels of HMG-CoA reductase inhibitory activity can increase the risk of myopathy and rhabdomyolysis, particularly with higher doses of simvastatin).
No products indexed under this heading.

Dirithromycin (The risk of myopathy and rhabdomyolysis is increased by high levels of statin activity in plasma. Simvastatin is metabolized by the cytochrome P450 isoform 3A4. Certain drugs, including the macrolide antibiotics erythromycin and clarithromycin, which inhibit this metabolic pathway can raise the plasma levels of simvastatin and may increase the risk of myopathy. The use of simvastatin concomitantly with these CYP3A4 inhibitors should be avoided. If treatment with erythromycin or clarithromycin is unavoidable, therapy with simvastatin should be suspended during the course of treatment).
No products indexed under this heading.

Econazole Nitrate (The risk of myopathy and rhabdomyolysis is increased by high levels of statin activity in plasma. Simvastatin is metabolized by the cytochrome P450 isoform 3A4. Certain drugs, including itraconazole, ketoconazole, and other antifungal azoles, which inhibit this metabolic pathway can raise the plasma levels of simvastatin and may increase the risk of myopathy. The use of simvastatin concomitantly with these CYP3A4 inhibitors should be avoided. If treatment with itraconazole or ketoconazole is unavoidable, therapy with simvastatin should be suspended during the course of treatment).
No products indexed under this heading.

Efavirenz (The risk of myopathy is increased by reducing the elimination of simvastatin. Hence when simvastatin is used with an inhibitor of CYP3A4, elevated plasma levels of HMG-CoA reductase inhibitory activity can increase the risk of myopathy and rhabdomyolysis, particularly with higher doses of simvastatin). Products include:
Atripla **906**

Erythromycin (The risk of myopathy and rhabdomyolysis is increased by high levels of statin activity in plasma. Simvastatin is metabolized by the cytochrome P450 isoform 3A4. Certain drugs, including the macrolide antibiotics erythromycin and clarithromycin, which inhibit this metabolic pathway can raise the plasma levels of simvastatin and may increase the risk of myopathy. The use of simvastatin concomitantly with these CYP3A4 inhibitors should be avoided. If treatment with erythromycin or clarithromycin is unavoidable, therapy with simvastatin should be suspended during the course of treatment).
No products indexed under this heading.

Erythromycin Estolate (The risk of myopathy and rhabdomyolysis is increased by high levels of statin activity in plasma. Simvastatin is metabolized by the cytochrome P450 isoform 3A4. Certain drugs, including the macrolide antibiotics erythromycin and clarithromycin, which inhibit this metabolic pathway can raise the plasma levels of simvastatin and may increase the risk of myopathy. The use of simvastatin concomitantly with these CYP3A4 inhibitors should be avoided. If treatment with erythromycin or clarithromycin is unavoidable, therapy with simvastatin should be suspended during the course of treatment).
No products indexed under this heading.

Erythromycin Ethylsuccinate (The risk of myopathy and rhabdomyolysis is increased by high levels of statin activity in plasma. Simvastatin is metabolized by the cytochrome P450 isoform 3A4. Certain drugs, including the macrolide antibiotics erythromycin and clarithromycin, which inhibit this metabolic pathway can raise the plasma levels of simvastatin and may increase the risk of myopathy. The use of simvastatin concomitantly with these CYP3A4 inhibitors should be avoided. If treatment with erythromycin or clarithromycin is unavoidable, therapy with simvastatin should be suspended during the course of treatment). Products include:
E.E.S. **437**
EryPed **435**

Erythromycin Gluceptate (The risk of myopathy and rhabdomyolysis is increased by high levels of statin activity in plasma. Simvastatin is metabolized by the cytochrome P450 isoform 3A4. Certain drugs, including the macrolide antibiotics erythromycin and clarithromycin, which inhibit this metabolic pathway can raise the plasma levels of simvastatin and may increase the risk of myopathy. The use of simvastatin concomitantly with these CYP3A4 inhibitors should be avoided. If treatment with erythromycin or clarithromycin is unavoidable, therapy with simvastatin should be suspended during the course of treatment).
No products indexed under this heading.

Erythromycin Lactobionate (The risk of myopathy is increased by reducing the elimination of simvastatin. Hence when simvastatin is used with an inhibitor of CYP3A4, elevated plasma levels of HMG-CoA reductase inhibitory activity can increase the risk of myopathy and rhabdomyolysis, particularly with higher doses of simvastatin).
No products indexed under this heading.

Erythromycin Stearate (The risk of myopathy and rhabdomyolysis is increased by high levels of statin activity in plasma. Simvastatin is metabolized by the cytochrome P450 isoform 3A4. Certain drugs, including the macrolide antibiotics erythromycin and clarithromycin, which inhibit this metabolic pathway can raise the plasma levels of simvastatin and may increase the risk of myopathy. The use of simvastatin concomitantly with these CYP3A4 inhibitors should be avoided. If treatment with erythromycin or clarithromycin is unavoidable, therapy with simvastatin should be suspended during the course of treatment).
No products indexed under this heading.

Esomeprazole Magnesium (The risk of myopathy is increased by reducing the elimination of simvastatin. Hence when simvastatin is used with an inhibitor of CYP3A4, elevated plasma levels of HMG-CoA reductase inhibitory activity can increase the risk of myopathy and rhabdomyolysis, particularly with higher doses of simvastatin). Products include:
Nexium Capsules **704**
Nexium Oral Suspension **704**

Esomeprazole Sodium (The risk of myopathy is increased by reducing the elimination of simvastatin. Hence when simvastatin is used with an inhibitor of CYP3A4, elevated plasma levels of HMG-CoA reductase inhibitory activity can increase the risk of myopathy and rhabdomyolysis, particularly with higher doses of simvastatin). Products include:
Nexium I.V. **712**

Ethanol (Simvastatin should be used with caution in patients who consume substantial quantities of alcohol).
No products indexed under this heading.

Ethyl Alcohol (Simvastatin should be used with caution in patients who consume substantial quantities of alcohol).
No products indexed under this heading.

Fenofibrate (The risk of myopathy is increased by gemfibrozil and to a lesser extent by other fibrates. The combined use of simvastatin with gemfibrozil should be avoided, unless benefits are likely to outweight the increased risks. If concurrent use is deemed necessary, the dose of simvastatin should not exceed 10 mg daily. Caution should be used when prescribing other fibrates with simvastatin). Products include:
Fenoglide **3263**
Tricor **544**
Trilipix **548**

Fluconazole (The risk of myopathy and rhabdomyolysis is increased by high levels of statin activity in plasma. Simvastatin is metabolized by the cytochrome P450 isoform 3A4. Certain drugs, including itraconazole, ketoconazole, and other antifungal azoles, which inhibit this metabolic pathway can raise the plasma levels of simvastatin and may increase the risk of myopathy. The use of simvastatin concomitantly with these CYP3A4 inhibitors should be avoided. If treatment with itraconazole or ketoconazole is unavoidable, therapy with simvastatin should be suspended during the course of treatment).
No products indexed under this heading.

Fluoxetine (The risk of myopathy is increased by reducing the elimination of simvastatin. Hence when simvastatin is used with an inhibitor of CYP3A4, elevated plasma levels of HMG-CoA reductase inhibitory activity can increase the risk of myopathy and rhabdomyolysis, particularly with higher doses of simvastatin).
No products indexed under this heading.

Fluoxetine Hydrochloride (The risk of myopathy is increased by reducing the elimination of simvastatin. Hence when simvastatin is used with an inhibitor of CYP3A4, elevated plasma levels of HMG-CoA reductase inhibitory activity can increase the risk of myopathy and rhabdomyolysis, particularly with higher doses of simvastatin). Products include:
Prozac Weekly **1941**
Prozac Pulvules **1941**
Symbyax **1965**

Fluvoxamine Maleate (The risk of myopathy is increased by reducing the elimination of simvastatin. Hence when simvastatin is used with an inhibitor of CYP3A4, elevated plasma levels of HMG-CoA reductase inhibitory activity can increase the risk of myopathy and rhabdomyolysis, particularly with higher doses of simvastatin).
No products indexed under this heading.

Fosamprenavir Calcium (The risk of myopathy and rhabdomyolysis is increased by high levels of statin activity in plasma. Simvastatin is metabolized by the cytochrome P450 isoform 3A4. Certain drugs, including the HIV protease inhibitors, which inhibit this metabolic pathway can raise the plasma levels of simvastatin and may increase the risk of myopathy. The use of simvastatin concomitantly with these CYP3A4 inhibitors should be avoided). Products include:
Lexiva Oral Suspension **1558**
Lexiva **1558**

Gemfibrozil (The risk of myopathy is increased by gemfibrozil and to a lesser extent by other fibrates. The combined use of simvastatin with gemfibrozil should be avoided, unless benefits are likely to outweight the increased risks. If concurrent use is deemed necessary, the dose of simvastatin should not exceed 10 mg daily. Caution should be used when prescribing other fibrates with simvastatin).
No products indexed under this heading.

Imatinib Mesylate (The risk of myopathy is increased by reducing the elimination of simvastatin. Hence when simvastatin is used with an inhibitor of CYP3A4, elevated plasma levels of HMG-CoA reductase inhibitory activity can increase the risk of myopathy and rhabdomyolysis, particularly with higher doses of simvastatin). Products include:
Gleevec **2477**

Indinavir Sulfate (The risk of myopathy and rhabdomyolysis is increased by high levels of statin activity in plasma. Simvastatin is metabolized by the cytochrome P450 isoform 3A4. Certain drugs, including the HIV protease inhibitors, which inhibit this metabolic pathway can raise the plasma levels of simvastatin and may increase the risk of myopathy. The use of simvastatin concomitantly with these CYP3A4 inhibitors should be avoided). Products include:
Crixivan **2113**

Isoniazid (The risk of myopathy is increased by reducing the elimination of simvastatin. Hence when simvastatin is used with an inhibitor of CYP3A4, elevated plasma levels of HMG-CoA reductase inhibitory activity can increase the risk of myopathy and rhabdomyolysis, particularly with higher doses of simvastatin).
No products indexed under this heading.

Itraconazole (Simvastatin is metabolized by CYP3A4; co-administration with potent inhibitors of CYP3A4, such as itraconazole, increases the risk of myopathy by reducing the elimination of simvastatin; concurrent use should be avoided).
No products indexed under this heading.

Ketoconazole (Simvastatin is metabolized by CYP3A4; co-administration with potent inhibitors of CYP3A4, such as ketoconazole, increases the risk of myopathy by reducing the elimination of simvastatin; concurrent use should be avoided). Products include:
Extina **3319**
Xolegel **3337**

Lapatinib (The risk of myopathy is increased by reducing the elimination of simvastatin. Hence when simvastatin is used with an inhibitor of CYP3A4, elevated plasma levels of HMG-CoA reductase inhibitory activity can increase the risk of myopathy and rhabdomyolysis, particularly with higher doses of simvastatin). Products include:
Tykerb **1698**

Lopinavir (The risk of myopathy and rhabdomyolysis is increased by high levels of statin activity in plasma. Simvastatin is metabolized by the cytochrome P450 isoform 3A4. Certain drugs, including the HIV protease inhibitors, which inhibit this metabolic pathway can raise the plasma levels of simv-

IMPORTANT NOTE: Always consult each drug listing in the patient's regimen for possible interactions.

astatin and may increase the risk of myopathy. The use of simvastatin concomitantly with these CYP3A4 inhibitors should be avoided). Products include:
Kaletra 458

Loratadine (The risk of myopathy is increased by reducing the elimination of simvastatin. Hence when simvastatin is used with an inhibitor of CYP3A4, elevated plasma levels of HMG-CoA reductase inhibitory activity can increase the risk of myopathy and rhabdomyolysis, particularly with higher doses of simvastatin).
No products indexed under this heading.

Metronidazole (The risk of myopathy is increased by reducing the elimination of simvastatin. Hence when simvastatin is used with an inhibitor of CYP3A4, elevated plasma levels of HMG-CoA reductase inhibitory activity can increase the risk of myopathy and rhabdomyolysis, particularly with higher doses of simvastatin). Products include:
Pylera 793

Metronidazole Benzoate (The risk of myopathy is increased by reducing the elimination of simvastatin. Hence when simvastatin is used with an inhibitor of CYP3A4, elevated plasma levels of HMG-CoA reductase inhibitory activity can increase the risk of myopathy and rhabdomyolysis, particularly with higher doses of simvastatin).
No products indexed under this heading.

Metronidazole Hydrochloride (The risk of myopathy is increased by reducing the elimination of simvastatin. Hence when simvastatin is used with an inhibitor of CYP3A4, elevated plasma levels of HMG-CoA reductase inhibitory activity can increase the risk of myopathy and rhabdomyolysis, particularly with higher doses of simvastatin).
No products indexed under this heading.

Metronidazole Sodium (The risk of myopathy is increased by reducing the elimination of simvastatin. Hence when simvastatin is used with an inhibitor of CYP3A4, elevated plasma levels of HMG-CoA reductase inhibitory activity can increase the risk of myopathy and rhabdomyolysis, particularly with higher doses of simvastatin).
No products indexed under this heading.

Miconazole (The risk of myopathy and rhabdomyolysis is increased by high levels of statin activity in plasma. Simvastatin is metabolized by the cytochrome P450 isoform 3A4. Certain drugs, including itraconazole, ketoconazole, and other antifungal azoles, which inhibit this metabolic pathway can raise the plasma levels of simvastatin and may increase the risk of myopathy. The use of simvastatin concomitantly with these CYP3A4 inhibitors should be avoided. If treatment with itraconazole or ketoconazole is unavoidable, therapy with simvastatin should be suspended during the course of treatment).
No products indexed under this heading.

Miconazole Nitrate (The risk of myopathy is increased by reducing the elimination of simvastatin. Hence when simvastatin is used with an inhibitor of CYP3A4, elevated plasma levels of HMG-CoA reductase inhibitory activity can increase the risk of myopathy and rhabdomyolysis, particularly with higher doses of simvastatin). Products include:
Vusion Ointment 3335

Mifepristone (The risk of myopathy is increased by reducing the elimination of simvastatin. Hence when simvastatin is used with an inhibitor of CYP3A4, elevated plasma levels of HMG-CoA reductase inhibitory activity can increase the risk of myopathy and rhabdomyolysis, particularly with higher doses of simvastatin).
No products indexed under this heading.

Nefazodone Hydrochloride (The risk of myopathy and rhabdomyolysis is increased by high level of statin activity in plasma. Simvastatin is metabolized by the cytochrome P450 isoform 3A4. Certain drugs, including the antidepressant nefazodone, which inhibit this metabolic pathwaycan raise the plasma levels of simvastatin and may increase the risk of myopathy. The use of simvastatin concomitantly with this CYP3A4 inhibitor should be avoided).
No products indexed under this heading.

Nelfinavir Mesylate (The risk of myopathy and rhabdomyolysis is increased by high levels of statin activity in plasma. Simvastatin is metabolized by the cytochrome P450 isoform 3A4. Certain drugs, including the HIV protease inhibitors, which inhibit this metabolic pathway can raise the plasma levels of simvastatin and may increase the risk of myopathy. The use of simvastatin concomitantly with these CYP3A4 inhibitors should be avoided).
No products indexed under this heading.

Nevirapine (The risk of myopathy is increased by reducing the elimination of simvastatin. Hence when simvastatin is used with an inhibitor of CYP3A4, elevated plasma levels of HMG-CoA reductase inhibitory activity can increase the risk of myopathy and rhabdomyolysis, particularly with higher doses of simvastatin). Products include:
Viramune Oral Suspension 897
Viramune Tablets 897

Niacin (The risk of myopathy is increased by niacin (nicotinic acid) (greater or equal to 1 gm/day). Caution should be used when prescribing lipid-lowering doses (greater or equal to 1 gm/day) of niacin with simvastatin). Products include:
Advicor 402
Cardio Basics 3455
Niaspan 497
Simcor 524

Niacinamide (The risk of myopathy is increased by niacin (nicotinic acid) (greater or equal to 1 gm/day). Caution should be used when prescribing lipid-lowering doses (greater or equal to 1 gm/day) of niacin with simvastatin). Products include:
CitraNatal 90 DHA Capsules 2332
CitraNatal Assure 2332
CitraNatal Rx 2332
Heplive 607

Niacinamide Hydroiodide (The risk of myopathy is increased by reducing the elimination of simvastatin. Hence when simvastatin is used with an inhibitor of CYP3A4, elevated plasma levels of HMG-CoA reductase inhibitory activity can increase the risk of myopathy and rhabdomyolysis, particularly with higher doses of simvastatin).
No products indexed under this heading.

Nicotinamide (The risk of myopathy is increased by reducing the elimination of simvastatin. Hence when simvastatin is used with an inhibitor of CYP3A4, elevated plasma levels of HMG-CoA reductase inhibitory activity can increase the risk of myopathy and rhabdomyolysis, particularly with higher doses of simvastatin).
No products indexed under this heading.

Nifedipine (The risk of myopathy is increased by reducing the elimination of simvastatin. Hence when simvastatin is used with an inhibitor of CYP3A4, elevated plasma levels of HMG-CoA reductase inhibitory activity can increase the risk of myopathy and rhabdomyolysis, particularly with higher doses of simvastatin).
No products indexed under this heading.

Norfloxacin (The risk of myopathy is increased by reducing the elimination of simvastatin. Hence when simvastatin is

used with an inhibitor of CYP3A4, elevated plasma levels of HMG-CoA reductase inhibitory activity can increase the risk of myopathy and rhabdomyolysis, particularly with higher doses of simvastatin). Products include:
Noroxin 2220

Omeprazole (The risk of myopathy is increased by reducing the elimination of simvastatin. Hence when simvastatin is used with an inhibitor of CYP3A4, elevated plasma levels of HMG-CoA reductase inhibitory activity can increase the risk of myopathy and rhabdomyolysis, particularly with higher doses of simvastatin).
No products indexed under this heading.

Oxiconazole Nitrate (The risk of myopathy and rhabdomyolysis is increased by high levels of statin activity in plasma. Simvastatin is metabolized by the cytochrome P450 isoform 3A4. Certain drugs, including itraconazole, ketoconazole, and other antifungal azoles, which inhibit this metabolic pathway can raise the plasma levels of simvastatin and may increase the risk of myopathy. The use of simvastatin concomitantly with these CYP3A4 inhibitors should be avoided. If treatment with itraconazole or ketoconazole is unavoidable, therapy with simvastatin should be suspended during the course of treatment).
No products indexed under this heading.

Paroxetine Hydrochloride (The risk of myopathy is increased by reducing the elimination of simvastatin. Hence when simvastatin is used with an inhibitor of CYP3A4, elevated plasma levels of HMG-CoA reductase inhibitory activity can increase the risk of myopathy and rhabdomyolysis, particularly with higher doses of simvastatin). Products include:
Paroxetine CR 2361
Paroxetine ER 2371
Paxil 1586
Paxil CR 1596

Posaconazole (The risk of myopathy and rhabdomyolysis is increased by high levels of statin activity in plasma. Simvastatin is metabolized by the cytochrome P450 isoform 3A4. Certain drugs, including itraconazole, ketoconazole, and other antifungal azoles, which inhibit this metabolic pathway can raise the plasma levels of simvastatin and may increase the risk of myopathy. The use of simvastatin concomitantly with these CYP3A4 inhibitors should be avoided. If treatment with itraconazole or ketoconazole is unavoidable, therapy with simvastatin should be suspended during the course of treatment). Products include:
Noxafil 3172

Propoxyphene Hydrochloride (The risk of myopathy is increased by reducing the elimination of simvastatin. Hence when simvastatin is used with an inhibitor of CYP3A4, elevated plasma levels of HMG-CoA reductase inhibitory activity can increase the risk of myopathy and rhabdomyolysis, particularly with higher doses of simvastatin).
No products indexed under this heading.

Propoxyphene Napsylate (The risk of myopathy is increased by reducing the elimination of simvastatin. Hence when simvastatin is used with an inhibitor of CYP3A4, elevated plasma levels of HMG-CoA reductase inhibitory activity can increase the risk of myopathy and rhabdomyolysis, particularly with higher doses of simvastatin).
No products indexed under this heading.

Propranolol Hydrochloride (Significant decreases in mean C_{max}, but no change in AUC). Products include:
InnoPran XL 1517

Quinidine (The risk of myopathy is increased by reducing the elimination of simvastatin. Hence when simvastatin is used with an inhibitor of CYP3A4, elevated plasma levels of HMG-CoA reductase inhibitory activity can increase the risk of myopathy and rhabdomyolysis, particularly with higher doses of simvastatin).
No products indexed under this heading.

Quinidine Hydrochloride (The risk of myopathy is increased by reducing the elimination of simvastatin. Hence when simvastatin is used with an inhibitor of CYP3A4, elevated plasma levels of HMG-CoA reductase inhibitory activity can increase the risk of myopathy and rhabdomyolysis, particularly with higher doses of simvastatin).
No products indexed under this heading.

Quinidine Polygalacturonate (The risk of myopathy is increased by reducing the elimination of simvastatin. Hence when simvastatin is used with an inhibitor of CYP3A4, elevated plasma levels of HMG-CoA reductase inhibitory activity can increase the risk of myopathy and rhabdomyolysis, particularly with higher doses of simvastatin).
No products indexed under this heading.

Quinidine Sulfate (The risk of myopathy is increased by reducing the elimination of simvastatin. Hence when simvastatin is used with an inhibitor of CYP3A4, elevated plasma levels of HMG-CoA reductase inhibitory activity can increase the risk of myopathy and rhabdomyolysis, particularly with higher doses of simvastatin).
No products indexed under this heading.

Quinine (The risk of myopathy is increased by reducing the elimination of simvastatin. Hence when simvastatin is used with an inhibitor of CYP3A4, elevated plasma levels of HMG-CoA reductase inhibitory activity can increase the risk of myopathy and rhabdomyolysis, particularly with higher doses of simvastatin). Products include:
Hyland's Leg Cramps PM with
Quinine 3315

Quinine Sulfate (The risk of myopathy is increased by reducing the elimination of simvastatin. Hence when simvastatin is used with an inhibitor of CYP3A4, elevated plasma levels of HMG-CoA reductase inhibitory activity can increase the risk of myopathy and rhabdomyolysis, particularly with higher doses of simvastatin).
No products indexed under this heading.

Quinupristin (The risk of myopathy is increased by reducing the elimination of simvastatin. Hence when simvastatin is used with an inhibitor of CYP3A4, elevated plasma levels of HMG-CoA reductase inhibitory activity can increase the risk of myopathy and rhabdomyolysis, particularly with higher doses of simvastatin).
No products indexed under this heading.

Ranitidine Bismuth Citrate (The risk of myopathy is increased by reducing the elimination of simvastatin. Hence when simvastatin is used with an inhibitor of CYP3A4, elevated plasma levels of HMG-CoA reductase inhibitory activity can increase the risk of myopathy and rhabdomyolysis, particularly with higher doses of simvastatin).
No products indexed under this heading.

Ranitidine Hydrochloride (The risk of myopathy is increased by reducing the elimination of simvastatin. Hence when simvastatin is used with an inhibitor of CYP3A4, elevated plasma levels of HMG-CoA reductase inhibitory activity can increase the risk of myopathy and rhabdomyolysis, particularly with higher doses of simvastatin). Products include:
Zantac 1737

Zantac Injection 1732
Zantac Pharmacy 1735

Ritonavir (The risk of myopathy and rhabdomyolysis is increased by high levels of statin activity in plasma. Simvastatin is metabolized by the cytochrome P450 isoform 3A4. Certain drugs, including the HIV protease inhibitors, which inhibit this metabolic pathway can raise the plasma levels of simvastatin and may increase the risk of myopathy. The use of simvastatin concomitantly with these CYP3A4 inhibitors should be avoided). Products include:
Kaletra 458
Norvir 509

Saquinavir (The risk of myopathy and rhabdomyolysis is increased by high levels of statin activity in plasma. Simvastatin is metabolized by the cytochrome P450 isoform 3A4. Certain drugs, including the HIV protease inhibitors, which inhibit this metabolic pathway can raise the plasma levels of simvastatin and may increase the risk of myopathy. The use of simvastatin concomitantly with these CYP3A4 inhibitors should be avoided).
No products indexed under this heading.

Saquinavir Mesylate (The risk of myopathy and rhabdomyolysis is increased by high levels of statin activity in plasma. Simvastatin is metabolized by the cytochrome P450 isoform 3A4. Certain drugs, including the HIV protease inhibitors, which inhibit this metabolic pathway can raise the plasma levels of simvastatin and may increase the risk of myopathy. The use of simvastatin concomitantly with these CYP3A4 inhibitors should be avoided).
No products indexed under this heading.

Sertaconazole Nitrate (The risk of myopathy and rhabdomyolysis is increased by high levels of statin activity in plasma. Simvastatin is metabolized by the cytochrome P450 isoform 3A4. Certain drugs, including itraconazole, ketoconazole, and other antifungal azoles, which inhibit this metabolic pathway can raise the plasma levels of simvastatin and may increase the risk of myopathy. The use of simvastatin concomitantly with these CYP3A4 inhibitors should be avoided. If treatment with itraconazole or ketoconazole is unavoidable, therapy with simvastatin should be suspended during the course of treatment).
No products indexed under this heading.

Sertraline Hydrochloride (The risk of myopathy is increased by reducing the elimination of simvastatin. Hence when simvastatin is used with an inhibitor of CYP3A4, elevated plasma levels of HMG-CoA reductase inhibitory activity can increase the risk of myopathy and rhabdomyolysis, particularly with higher doses of simvastatin).
No products indexed under this heading.

Sildenafil Citrate (The risk of myopathy is increased by reducing the elimination of simvastatin. Hence when simvastatin is used with an inhibitor of CYP3A4, elevated plasma levels of HMG-CoA reductase inhibitory activity can increase the risk of myopathy and rhabdomyolysis, particularly with higher doses of simvastatin).
No products indexed under this heading.

Telithromycin (The risk of myopathy and rhabdomyolysis is increased by high level of statin activity in plasma. Simvastatin is metabolized by the cytochrome P450 isoform 3A4. Certain drugs, including telithromycin, which inhibit this metabolic pathway can raise the plasma levels of simvastatin and may increase the risk of myopathy. The use of simvastatin concomitantly with this CYP3A4 inhibitor should be avoided). Products include:
Ketek 2991

Terconazole (The risk of myopathy and rhabdomyolysis is increased by high levels of statin activity in plasma. Simvastatin is metabolized by the cytochrome P450 isoform 3A4. Certain drugs, including itraconazole, ketoconazole, and other antifungal azoles, which inhibit this metabolic pathway can raise the plasma levels of simvastatin and may increase the risk of myopathy. The use of simvastatin concomitantly with these CYP3A4 inhibitors should be avoided. If treatment with itraconazole or ketoconazole is unavoidable, therapy with simvastatin should be suspended during the course of treatment).
No products indexed under this heading.

Tipranavir (The risk of myopathy and rhabdomyolysis is increased by high levels of statin activity in plasma. Simvastatin is metabolized by the cytochrome P450 isoform 3A4. Certain drugs, including the HIV protease inhibitors, which inhibit this metabolic pathway can raise the plasma levels of simvastatin and may increase the risk of myopathy. The use of simvastatin concomitantly with these CYP3A4 inhibitors should be avoided).
No products indexed under this heading.

Troglitazone (The risk of myopathy is increased by reducing the elimination of simvastatin. Hence when simvastatin is used with an inhibitor of CYP3A4, elevated plasma levels of HMG-CoA reductase inhibitory activity can increase the risk of myopathy and rhabdomyolysis, particularly with higher doses of simvastatin).
No products indexed under this heading.

Troleandomycin (The risk of myopathy and rhabdomyolysis is increased by high levels of statin activity in plasma. Simvastatin is metabolized by the cytochrome P450 isoform 3A4. Certain drugs, including the macrolide antibiotics erythromycin and clarithromycin, which inhibit this metabolic pathway can raise the plasma levels of simvastatin and may increase the risk of myopathy. The use of simvastatin concomitantly with these CYP3A4 inhibitors should be avoided. If treatment with erythromycin or clarithromycin is unavoidable, therapy with simvastatin should be suspended during the course of treatment).
No products indexed under this heading.

Valproate Sodium (The risk of myopathy is increased by reducing the elimination of simvastatin. Hence when simvastatin is used with an inhibitor of CYP3A4, elevated plasma levels of HMG-CoA reductase inhibitory activity can increase the risk of myopathy and rhabdomyolysis, particularly with higher doses of simvastatin).
No products indexed under this heading.

Vardenafil Hydrochloride (The risk of myopathy is increased by reducing the elimination of simvastatin. Hence when simvastatin is used with an inhibitor of CYP3A4, elevated plasma levels of HMG-CoA reductase inhibitory activity can increase the risk of myopathy and rhabdomyolysis, particularly with higher doses of simvastatin). Products include:
Levitra 3157

Verapamil Hydrochloride (The risk of myopathy/rhabdomyolysis is increased by concomitant administration of verapamil with higher doses of simvastatin. The combined use of simvastatin at doses higher than 20 mg with verapamil should be avoided unless the clinical benefit is likely to outweigh the increased risk of myopathy). Products include:
Tarka 534

Voriconazole (The risk of myopathy and rhabdomyolysis is increased by high levels of statin activity in plasma. Simvastatin is metabolized by the cytochrome P450 isoform 3A4. Certain drugs, including itraconazole, ketoconazole, and other antifungal azoles, which inhibit this metabolic pathway can raise the plasma levels of simvastatin and may increase the risk of myopathy. The use of simvastatin concomitantly with these CYP3A4 inhibitors should be avoided. If treatment with itraconazole or ketoconazole is unavoidable, therapy with simvastatin should be suspended during the course of treatment).
No products indexed under this heading.

Warfarin Sodium (Concomitant use with simvastatin may prolong INR. Achieve stable INR prior to initiation of simvastatin. Monitor INR frequently until stable upon initiation or alteration of simvastatin therapy).
No products indexed under this heading.

Zafirlukast (The risk of myopathy is increased by reducing the elimination of simvastatin. Hence when simvastatin is used with an inhibitor of CYP3A4, elevated plasma levels of HMG-CoA reductase inhibitory activity can increase the risk of myopathy and rhabdomyolysis, particularly with higher doses of simvastatin). Products include:
Accolate 3612

Zileuton (The risk of myopathy is increased by reducing the elimination of simvastatin. Hence when simvastatin is used with an inhibitor of CYP3A4, elevated plasma levels of HMG-CoA reductase inhibitory activity can increase the risk of myopathy and rhabdomyolysis, particularly with higher doses of simvastatin).
No products indexed under this heading.

Food Interactions

Alcohol (Simvastatin should be used with caution in patients who consume substantial quantities of alcohol).

Beer, reduced-alcohol (Simvastatin should be used with caution in patients who consume substantial quantities of alcohol).

Beer, unspecified (Simvastatin should be used with caution in patients who consume substantial quantities of alcohol).

Grapefruit (The risk of myopathy and rhabdomyolysis is increased by high level of statin activity in plasma. Simvastatin is metabolized by the cytochrome P450 isoform 3A4. Certain drugs, including the large quantities of grapefruit juice (greater than 1 quart daily), which inhibit this metabolic pathway can raise the plasma levels of simvastatin and may increase the risk of myopathy. The use of simvastatin concomitantly with this CYP3A4 inhibitor should be avoided).

Grapefruit Juice (The risk of myopathy and rhabdomyolysis is increased by high level of statin activity in plasma. Simvastatin is metabolized by the cytochrome P450 isoform 3A4. Certain drugs, including the large quantities of grapefruit juice (greater than 1 quart daily), which inhibit this metabolic pathway can raise the plasma levels of simvastatin and may increase the risk of myopathy. The use of simvastatin concomitantly with this CYP3A4 inhibitor should be avoided).

Wine, Chianti (Simvastatin should be used with caution in patients who consume substantial quantities of alcohol).

Wine, Red (Simvastatin should be used with caution in patients who consume substantial quantities of alcohol).

Wine, unspecified (Simvastatin should be used with caution in patients who consume substantial quantities of alcohol).

Wine products (Simvastatin should be used with caution in patients who consume substantial quantities of alcohol).

ZOFRAN INJECTION

(Ondansetron Hydrochloride) 1750
See Zofran Tablets

ZOFRAN INJECTION PREMIXED

(Ondansetron Hydrochloride) 1750
See Zofran Tablets

ZOFRAN ORAL SOLUTION

(Ondansetron Hydrochloride) 1756
See Zofran Tablets

ZOFRAN TABLETS

(Ondansetron Hydrochloride) 1756
May interact with antibiotics, antineoplastics, cytochrome p450 1a2 inducers (selected), cytochrome p450 1a2 inhibitors (selected), cytochrome p450 2d6 inducers (selected), cytochrome p450 2d6 inhibitors (selected), cytochrome p450 3a4 inducers (selected), cytochrome p450 3a4 inhibitors (selected), cytochrome p450 inducers (selected), cytochrome p450 inhibitors (selected), cytotoxic drugs, phenytoin, and certain other agents. Compounds in these categories include:

Acetazolamide (Ondansetron does not itself appear to induce or inhibit the cytochrome P-450 drug metabolizing enzyme system of the liver. Because ondansetron is metabolized by hepatic cytochrome P-450 drug-metabolizing enzymes (CYP3A4, CYP2D6, CYP1A2), inducers or inhibitors of these enzymes may change the clearance and, hence, the half-life of ondansetron. On the basis of available data, no dosage adjustment is recommended for patients on these drugs).
No products indexed under this heading.

Acetazolamide Sodium (Ondansetron does not itself appear to induce or inhibit the cytochrome P-450 drug metabolizing enzyme system of the liver. Because ondansetron is metabolized by hepatic cytochrome P-450 drug-metabolizing enzymes (CYP3A4, CYP2D6, CYP1A2), inducers or inhibitors of these enzymes may change the clearance and, hence, the half-life of ondansetron. On the basis of available data, no dosage adjustment is recommended for patients on these drugs).
No products indexed under this heading.

Alatrofloxacin Mesylate (There have been reports of liver failure and death in patients with cancer receiving concurrent medications including antibiotics. The etiology of liver failure is unclear).
No products indexed under this heading.

Allium cepa (Ondansetron elimination may be affected by cytochrome P-450 inducers). Products include:
Hyland's Cold 'N Cough 3314
Mederma 2319
Mederma for Kids 2319

Allium sativum (Ondansetron does not itself appear to induce or inhibit the cytochrome P-450 drug metabolizing enzyme system of the liver. Because ondansetron is metabolized by hepatic cytochrome P-450 drug-metabolizing enzymes (CYP3A4, CYP2D6, CYP1A2), inducers or inhibitors of these enzymes may change the clearance and, hence, the half-life of ondansetron. In patients treated with potent inducers of CYP3A4 the clearance of ondansetron was significantly increased and ondansetron blood concentrations were decreased. However, on the basis of available data, no dosage adjustment for ondansetron is recommended for patients on these drugs).
No products indexed under this heading.

Zofran Interactions Index 2152

Allium schoenoprasum
(Ondansetron elimination may be affected by cytochrome P-450 inducers).
No products indexed under this heading.

Allium ursinum (Ondansetron elimination may be affected by cytochrome P-450 inducers).
No products indexed under this heading.

Altretamine (There have been reports of liver failure and death in patients with cancer receiving concurrent medications including potentially hepatotoxic cytotoxic chemotherapeutic drugs. The etiology of the liver failure is unclear). Products include:
Hexalen **1066**

Amikacin Sulfate (There have been reports of liver failure and death in patients with cancer receiving concurrent medications including antibiotics. The etiology of liver failure is unclear).
No products indexed under this heading.

Aminoglutethimide (Ondansetron does not itself appear to induce or inhibit the cytochrome P-450 drug metabolizing enzyme system of the liver. Because ondansetron is metabolized by hepatic cytochrome P-450 drug-metabolizing enzymes (CYP3A4, CYP2D6, CYP1A2), inducers or inhibitors of these enzymes may change the clearance and, hence, the half-life of ondansetron. In patients treated with potent inducers of CYP3A4 the clearance of ondansetron was significantly increased and ondansetron blood concentrations were decreased. However, on the basis of available data, no dosage adjustment for ondansetron is recommended for patients on these drugs).
No products indexed under this heading.

Amiodarone Hydrochloride
(Ondansetron does not itself appear to induce or inhibit the cytochrome P-450 drug metabolizing enzyme system of the liver. Because ondansetron is metabolized by hepatic cytochrome P-450 drug-metabolizing enzymes (CYP3A4, CYP2D6, CYP1A2), inducers or inhibitors of these enzymes may change the clearance and, hence, the half-life of ondansetron. On the basis of available data, no dosage adjustment is recommended for patients on these drugs).
No products indexed under this heading.

Amitriptyline Hydrochloride
(Ondansetron does not itself appear to induce or inhibit the cytochrome P-450 drug metabolizing enzyme system of the liver. Because ondansetron is metabolized by hepatic cytochrome P-450 drug-metabolizing enzymes (CYP3A4, CYP2D6, CYP1A2), inducers or inhibitors of these enzymes may change the clearance and, hence, the half-life of ondansetron. On the basis of available data, no dosage adjustment is recommended for patients on these drugs).
No products indexed under this heading.

Amoxapine (Ondansetron does not itself appear to induce or inhibit the cytochrome P-450 drug metabolizing enzyme system of the liver. Because ondansetron is metabolized by hepatic cytochrome P-450 drug-metabolizing enzymes (CYP3A4, CYP2D6, CYP1A2), inducers or inhibitors of these enzymes may change the clearance and, hence, the half-life of ondansetron. On the basis of available data, no dosage adjustment is recommended for patients on these drugs).
No products indexed under this heading.

Amoxicillin (There have been reports of liver failure and death in patients with cancer receiving concurrent medications including antibiotics. The etiology of liver failure is unclear). Products include:
Amoxil Capsules **1311**
Amoxil Chewable Tablets **1311**
Amoxil **1311**
Amoxil Powder **1311**
Augmentin **1331**
Augmentin Tablets **1335**
Augmentin ES-600 .... **1338**
Augmentin XR **1342**
Moxatag **2321**

Amoxicillin Trihydrate (There have been reports of liver failure and death in patients with cancer receiving concurrent medications including antibiotics. The etiology of liver failure is unclear).
No products indexed under this heading.

Ampicillin (There have been reports of liver failure and death in patients with cancer receiving concurrent medications including antibiotics. The etiology of liver failure is unclear).
No products indexed under this heading.

Ampicillin Sodium (There have been reports of liver failure and death in patients with cancer receiving concurrent medications including antibiotics. The etiology of liver failure is unclear).
No products indexed under this heading.

Ampicillin Trihydrate (There have been reports of liver failure and death in patients with cancer receiving concurrent medications including antibiotics. The etiology of liver failure is unclear).
No products indexed under this heading.

Amprenavir (Ondansetron does not itself appear to induce or inhibit the cytochrome P-450 drug metabolizing enzyme system of the liver. Because ondansetron is metabolized by hepatic cytochrome P-450 drug-metabolizing enzymes (CYP3A4, CYP2D6, CYP1A2), inducers or inhibitors of these enzymes may change the clearance and, hence, the half-life of ondansetron. On the basis of available data, no dosage adjustment is recommended for patients on these drugs).
No products indexed under this heading.

Anastrozole (There have been reports of liver failure and death in patients with cancer receiving concurrent medications including potentially hepatotoxic cytotoxic chemotherapeutic drugs. The etiology of the liver failure is unclear).
No products indexed under this heading.

Antibiotics, non-penicillin, unspecified (There have been reports of liver failure and death in patients with cancer receiving concurrent medications including antibiotics. The etiology of liver failure is unclear).
No products indexed under this heading.

Aprepitant (Ondansetron does not itself appear to induce or inhibit the cytochrome P-450 drug metabolizing enzyme system of the liver. Because ondansetron is metabolized by hepatic cytochrome P-450 drug-metabolizing enzymes (CYP3A4, CYP2D6, CYP1A2), inducers or inhibitors of these enzymes may change the clearance and, hence, the half-life of ondansetron. In patients treated with potent inducers of CYP3A4 the clearance of ondansetron was significantly increased and ondansetron blood concentrations were decreased. However, on the basis of available data, no dosage adjustment for ondansetron is recommended for patients on these drugs). Products include:
Emend **2124**

Asparaginase (There have been reports of liver failure and death in patients with cancer receiving concurrent medications including potentially hepatotoxic cytotoxic chemotherapeutic drugs. The etiology of the liver failure is unclear). Products include:
Elspar **2005, 2122**

Atazanavir (Ondansetron does not itself appear to induce or inhibit the cytochrome P-450 drug metabolizing enzyme system of the liver. Because ondansetron is metabolized by hepatic cytochrome P-450 drug-metabolizing enzymes (CYP3A4, CYP2D6, CYP1A2), inducers or inhibitors of these enzymes may change the clearance and, hence, the half-life of ondansetron. On the basis of available data, no dosage adjustment is recommended for patients on these drugs).
No products indexed under this heading.

Atazanavir Sulfate (Ondansetron does not itself appear to induce or inhibit the cytochrome P-450 drug metabolizing enzyme system of the liver. Because ondansetron is metabolized by hepatic cytochrome P-450 drug-metabolizing enzymes (CYP3A4, CYP2D6, CYP1A2), inducers or inhibitors of these enzymes may change the clearance and, hence, the half-life of ondansetron. On the basis of available data, no dosage adjustment is recommended for patients on these drugs).
No products indexed under this heading.

Azithromycin Dihydrate (There have been reports of liver failure and death in patients with cancer receiving concurrent medications including antibiotics. The etiology of liver failure is unclear).
No products indexed under this heading.

Azlocillin Sodium (There have been reports of liver failure and death in patients with cancer receiving concurrent medications including antibiotics. The etiology of liver failure is unclear).
No products indexed under this heading.

Azosulfisoxazole (*In vitro* metabolism studies have shown that ondansetron is a substrate for human hepatic cytochrome P-450 enzymes, including CYP1A2, CYP2D6, and CYP3A4. In terms of overall ondansetron turnover, CYP3A4 played the predominant role. Because of the multiplicity of metabolic enzymes capable of metabolizing ondansetron, it is likely that inhibition of one of these enzymes will be compensated by others and may result in little change in overall rates of ondansetron elimination).
No products indexed under this heading.

Aztreonam (There have been reports of liver failure and death in patients with cancer receiving concurrent medications including antibiotics. The etiology of liver failure is unclear).
No products indexed under this heading.

Bacampicillin Hydrochloride (There have been reports of liver failure and death in patients with cancer receiving concurrent medications including antibiotics. The etiology of liver failure is unclear).
No products indexed under this heading.

Bendroflumethiazide (*In vitro* metabolism studies have shown that ondansetron is a substrate for human hepatic cytochrome P-450 enzymes, including CYP1A2, CYP2D6, and CYP3A4. In terms of overall ondansetron turnover, CYP3A4 played the predominant role. Because of the multiplicity of metabolic enzymes capable of metabolizing ondansetron, it is likely that inhibition of one of these enzymes will be compensated by others and may result in little change in overall rates of ondansetron elimination).
No products indexed under this heading.

Betamethasone (Ondansetron does not itself appear to induce or inhibit the cytochrome P-450 drug metabolizing enzyme system of the liver. Because ondansetron is metabolized by hepatic cytochrome P-450 drug-metabolizing enzymes (CYP3A4, CYP2D6, CYP1A2), inducers or inhibitors of these enzymes may change the clearance and, hence, the half-life of ondansetron. In patients treated with potent inducers of CYP3A4 the clearance of ondansetron was significantly increased and ondansetron blood concentrations were decreased. However, on the basis of available data, no dosage adjustment for ondansetron is recommended for patients on these drugs).
No products indexed under this heading.

Betamethasone Acetate
(Ondansetron does not itself appear to induce or inhibit the cytochrome P-450 drug metabolizing enzyme system of the liver. Because ondansetron is metabolized by hepatic cytochrome P-450 drug-metabolizing enzymes (CYP3A4, CYP2D6, CYP1A2), inducers or inhibitors of these enzymes may change the clearance and, hence, the half-life of ondansetron. In patients treated with potent inducers of CYP3A4 the clearance of ondansetron was significantly increased and ondansetron blood concentrations were decreased. However, on the basis of available data, no dosage adjustment for ondansetron is recommended for patients on these drugs).
No products indexed under this heading.

Betamethasone Benzoate
(Ondansetron does not itself appear to induce or inhibit the cytochrome P-450 drug metabolizing enzyme system of the liver. Because ondansetron is metabolized by hepatic cytochrome P-450 drug-metabolizing enzymes (CYP3A4, CYP2D6, CYP1A2), inducers or inhibitors of these enzymes may change the clearance and, hence, the half-life of ondansetron. In patients treated with potent inducers of CYP3A4 the clearance of ondansetron was significantly increased and ondansetron blood concentrations were decreased. However, on the basis of available data, no dosage adjustment for ondansetron is recommended for patients on these drugs).
No products indexed under this heading.

Betamethasone Dipropionate
(Ondansetron does not itself appear to induce or inhibit the cytochrome P-450 drug metabolizing enzyme system of the liver. Because ondansetron is metabolized by hepatic cytochrome P-450 drug-metabolizing enzymes (CYP3A4, CYP2D6, CYP1A2), inducers or inhibitors of these enzymes may change the clearance and, hence, the half-life of ondansetron. In patients treated with potent inducers of CYP3A4 the clearance of ondansetron was significantly increased and ondansetron blood concentrations were decreased. However, on the basis of available data, no dosage adjustment for ondansetron is recommended for patients on these drugs). Products include:
Diprolene Lotion 0.05% **3108**
Diprolene Ointment 0.05% **3109**
Diprolene AF Cream 0.05% **3107**
Lotrisone **3163**

Betamethasone Sodium Phosphate (Ondansetron does not itself appear to induce or inhibit the cytochrome P-450 drug metabolizing enzyme system of the liver. Because ondansetron is metabolized by hepatic cytochrome P-450 drug-metabolizing enzymes (CYP3A4, CYP2D6, CYP1A2), inducers or inhibitors of these enzymes may change the clearance and, hence, the half-life of ondansetron. In patients treated with potent inducers of CYP3A4 the clearance of ondansetron was significantly increased and ondansetron blood concentrations were decreased. However, on the basis of available data, no dosage adjustment for ondansetron is recommended for patients on these drugs).
No products indexed under this heading.

Betamethasone Valerate
(Ondansetron does not itself appear to induce or inhibit the cytochrome P-450 drug metabolizing enzyme system of

2153 Interactions Index Zofran

the liver. Because ondansetron is metabolized by hepatic cytochrome P-450 drug-metabolizing enzymes (CYP3A4, CYP2D6, CYP1A2), inducers or inhibitors of these enzymes may change the clearance and, hence, the half-life of ondansetron. In patients treated with potent inducers of CYP3A4 the clearance of ondansetron was significantly increased and ondansetron blood concentrations were decreased. However, on the basis of available data, no dosage adjustment for ondansetron is recommended for patients on these drugs). Products include:
Luxíq 3321

Bicalutamide (There have been reports of liver failure and death in patients with cancer receiving concurrent medications including potentially hepatotoxic cytotoxic chemotherapeutic drugs. The etiology of the liver failure is unclear).
No products indexed under this heading.

Bleomycin Sulfate (There have been reports of liver failure and death in patients with cancer receiving concurrent medications including potentially hepatotoxic cytotoxic chemotherapeutic drugs. The etiology of liver failure is unclear).
No products indexed under this heading.

Bosentan (Ondansetron does not itself appear to induce or inhibit the cytochrome P-450 drug metabolizing enzyme system of the liver. Because ondansetron is metabolized by hepatic cytochrome P-450 drug-metabolizing enzymes (CYP3A4, CYP2D6, CYP1A2), inducers or inhibitors of these enzymes may change the clearance and, hence, the half-life of ondansetron. In patients treated with potent inducers of CYP3A4 the clearance of ondansetron was significantly increased and ondansetron blood concentrations were decreased. However, on the basis of available data, no dosage adjustment for ondansetron is recommended for patients on these drugs). Products include:
Tracleer 573

Bupropion Hydrochloride (Ondansetron does not itself appear to induce or inhibit the cytochrome P-450 drug metabolizing enzyme system of the liver. Because ondansetron is metabolized by hepatic cytochrome P-450 drug-metabolizing enzymes (CYP3A4, CYP2D6, CYP1A2), inducers or inhibitors of these enzymes may change the clearance and, hence, the half-life of ondansetron. On the basis of available data, no dosage adjustment is recommended for patients on these drugs). Products include:
Aplenzin 2948
Wellbutrin 1719
Wellbutrin SR 1725
Zyban 1762

Busulfan (There have been reports of liver failure and death in patients with cancer receiving concurrent medications including potentially hepatotoxic cytotoxic chemotherapeutic drugs. The etiology of the liver failure is unclear). Products include:
Myleran 1581

Carbamazepine (In patients treated with potent inducers of CYP3A4 (eg, carbamazepine), the clearance of ondansetron was significantly increased and ondansetron blood concentrations were decreased. However, on the basis of available data, no dosage adjustment for ondansetron is recommended for patients on these drugs). Products include:
Carbatrol 3280
Equetro 3477

Carbenicillin Disodium (There have been reports of liver failure and death in patients with cancer receiving concurrent medications including antibiotics. The etiology of liver failure is unclear).
No products indexed under this heading.

Carbenicillin Indanyl Sodium (There have been reports of liver failure and death in patients with cancer receiving concurrent medications including antibiotics. The etiology of liver failure is unclear).
No products indexed under this heading.

Carboplatin (There have been reports of liver failure and death in patients with cancer receiving concurrent medications including potentially hepatotoxic cytotoxic chemotherapeutic drugs. The etiology of the liver failure is unclear).
No products indexed under this heading.

Carmustine (BCNU) (There have been reports of liver failure and death in patients with cancer receiving concurrent medications including potentially hepatotoxic cytotoxic chemotherapeutic drugs. The etiology of the liver failure is unclear).
No products indexed under this heading.

Cefaclor (There have been reports of liver failure and death in patients with cancer receiving concurrent medications including antibiotics. The etiology of liver failure is unclear).
No products indexed under this heading.

Cefadroxil (There have been reports of liver failure and death in patients with cancer receiving concurrent medications including antibiotics. The etiology of liver failure is unclear).
No products indexed under this heading.

Cefamandole Nafate (There have been reports of liver failure and death in patients with cancer receiving concurrent medications including antibiotics. The etiology of liver failure is unclear).
No products indexed under this heading.

Cefazolin Sodium (There have been reports of liver failure and death in patients with cancer receiving concurrent medications including antibiotics. The etiology of liver failure is unclear).
No products indexed under this heading.

Cefixime (There have been reports of liver failure and death in patients with cancer receiving concurrent medications including antibiotics. The etiology of liver failure is unclear). Products include:
Suprax for Oral Suspension 2038
Suprax Tablets 2038

Cefmetazole Sodium (There have been reports of liver failure and death in patients with cancer receiving concurrent medications including antibiotics. The etiology of liver failure is unclear).
No products indexed under this heading.

Cefonicid Sodium (There have been reports of liver failure and death in patients with cancer receiving concurrent medications including antibiotics. The etiology of liver failure is unclear).
No products indexed under this heading.

Cefoperazone Sodium (There have been reports of liver failure and death in patients with cancer receiving concurrent medications including antibiotics. The etiology of liver failure is unclear).
No products indexed under this heading.

Ceforanide (There have been reports of liver failure and death in patients with cancer receiving concurrent medications including antibiotics. The etiology of liver failure is unclear).
No products indexed under this heading.

Cefotaxime Sodium (There have been reports of liver failure and death in patients with cancer receiving concurrent medications including antibiotics. The etiology of liver failure is unclear).
No products indexed under this heading.

Cefotetan (There have been reports of liver failure and death in patients with cancer receiving concurrent medications including antibiotics. The etiology of liver failure is unclear).
No products indexed under this heading.

Cefoxitin Sodium (There have been reports of liver failure and death in patients with cancer receiving concurrent medications including antibiotics. The etiology of liver failure is unclear).
No products indexed under this heading.

Cefpodoxime Proxetil (There have been reports of liver failure and death in patients with cancer receiving concurrent medications including antibiotics. The etiology of liver failure is unclear).
No products indexed under this heading.

Cefprozil (There have been reports of liver failure and death in patients with cancer receiving concurrent medications including antibiotics. The etiology of liver failure is unclear).
No products indexed under this heading.

Ceftazidime (There have been reports of liver failure and death in patients with cancer receiving concurrent medications including antibiotics. The etiology of liver failure is unclear). Products include:
Fortaz 1481

Ceftizoxime Sodium (There have been reports of liver failure and death in patients with cancer receiving concurrent medications including antibiotics. The etiology of liver failure is unclear).
No products indexed under this heading.

Ceftriaxone Sodium (There have been reports of liver failure and death in patients with cancer receiving concurrent medications including antibiotics. The etiology of liver failure is unclear). Products include:
Rocephin 2859

Cefuroxime Axetil (There have been reports of liver failure and death in patients with cancer receiving concurrent medications including antibiotics. The etiology of liver failure is unclear). Products include:
Ceftin 1399

Cefuroxime Sodium (There have been reports of liver failure and death in patients with cancer receiving concurrent medications including antibiotics. The etiology of liver failure is unclear).
No products indexed under this heading.

Celecoxib (Ondansetron does not itself appear to induce or inhibit the cytochrome P-450 drug metabolizing enzyme system of the liver. Because ondansetron is metabolized by hepatic cytochrome P-450 drug-metabolizing enzymes (CYP3A4, CYP2D6, CYP1A2), inducers or inhibitors of these enzymes may change the clearance and, hence, the half-life of ondansetron. On the basis of available data, no dosage adjustment is recommended for patients on these drugs). Products include:
Celebrex 3272

Cephalexin (There have been reports of liver failure and death in patients with cancer receiving concurrent medications including antibiotics. The etiology of liver failure is unclear).
No products indexed under this heading.

Cephalothin Sodium (There have been reports of liver failure and death in patients with cancer receiving concurrent medications including antibiotics. The etiology of liver failure is unclear).
No products indexed under this heading.

Cephapirin Sodium (There have been reports of liver failure and death in patients with cancer receiving concurrent medications including antibiotics. The etiology of liver failure is unclear).
No products indexed under this heading.

Cephradine (There have been reports of liver failure and death in patients with cancer receiving concurrent medications including antibiotics. The etiology of liver failure is unclear).
No products indexed under this heading.

Chlorambucil (There have been reports of liver failure and death in patients with cancer receiving concurrent medications including potentially hepatotoxic cytotoxic chemotherapeutic drugs. The etiology of the liver failure is unclear). Products include:
Leukeran 1557

Chloramphenicol (There have been reports of liver failure and death in patients with cancer receiving concurrent medications including antibiotics. The etiology of liver failure is unclear).
No products indexed under this heading.

Chloramphenicol Palmitate (There have been reports of liver failure and death in patients with cancer receiving concurrent medications including antibiotics. The etiology of liver failure is unclear).
No products indexed under this heading.

Chloramphenicol Sodium Succinate (There have been reports of liver failure and death in patients with cancer receiving concurrent medications including antibiotics. The etiology of liver failure is unclear).
No products indexed under this heading.

Chloroquine (Ondansetron does not itself appear to induce or inhibit the cytochrome P-450 drug metabolizing enzyme system of the liver. Because ondansetron is metabolized by hepatic cytochrome P-450 drug-metabolizing enzymes (CYP3A4, CYP2D6, CYP1A2), inducers or inhibitors of these enzymes may change the clearance and, hence, the half-life of ondansetron. On the basis of available data, no dosage adjustment is recommended for patients on these drugs).
No products indexed under this heading.

Chloroquine Hydrochloride (Ondansetron does not itself appear to induce or inhibit the cytochrome P-450 drug metabolizing enzyme system of the liver. Because ondansetron is metabolized by hepatic cytochrome P-450 drug-metabolizing enzymes (CYP3A4, CYP2D6, CYP1A2), inducers or inhibitors of these enzymes may change the clearance and, hence, the half-life of ondansetron. On the basis of available data, no dosage adjustment is recommended for patients on these drugs).
No products indexed under this heading.

Chloroquine Phosphate (Ondansetron does not itself appear to induce or inhibit the cytochrome P-450 drug metabolizing enzyme system of the liver. Because ondansetron is metabolized by hepatic cytochrome P-450 drug-metabolizing enzymes (CYP3A4, CYP2D6, CYP1A2), inducers or inhibitors of these enzymes may change the clearance and, hence, the half-life of ondansetron. On the basis of available data, no dosage adjustment is recommended for patients on these drugs).
No products indexed under this heading.

Chlorothiazide (*In vitro* metabolism studies have shown that ondansetron is a substrate for human hepatic cytochrome P-450 enzymes, including CYP1A2, CYP2D6, and CYP3A4. In terms of overall ondansetron turnover, CYP3A4 played the predominant role. Because of the multiplicity of metabolic enzymes capable of metabolizing ondansetron, it is likely that inhibition of one of these enzymes will be compen-

sated by others and may result in little change in overall rates of ondansetron elimination).

No products indexed under this heading.

Chlorothiazide Sodium (*In vitro* metabolism studies have shown that ondansetron is a substrate for human hepatic cytochrome P-450 enzymes, including CYP1A2, CYP2D6, and CYP3A4. In terms of overall ondansetron turnover, CYP3A4 played the predominant role. Because of the multiplicity of metabolic enzymes capable of metabolizing ondansetron, it is likely that inhibition of one of these enzymes will be compensated by others and may result in little change in overall rates of ondansetron elimination). Products include:
Diuril Intravenous 2009

Chlorpheniramine (Ondansetron does not itself appear to induce or inhibit the cytochrome P-450 drug metabolizing enzyme system of the liver. Because ondansetron is metabolized by hepatic cytochrome P-450 drug-metabolizing enzymes (CYP3A4, CYP2D6, CYP1A2), inducers or inhibitors of these enzymes may change the clearance and, hence, the half-life of ondansetron. On the basis of available data, no dosage adjustment is recommended for patients on these drugs).

No products indexed under this heading.

Chlorpheniramine Maleate (Ondansetron does not itself appear to induce or inhibit the cytochrome P-450 drug metabolizing enzyme system of the liver. Because ondansetron is metabolized by hepatic cytochrome P-450 drug-metabolizing enzymes (CYP3A4, CYP2D6, CYP1A2), inducers or inhibitors of these enzymes may change the clearance and, hence, the half-life of ondansetron. On the basis of available data, no dosage adjustment is recommended for patients on these drugs).

No products indexed under this heading.

Chlorpheniramine Polistirex (Ondansetron does not itself appear to induce or inhibit the cytochrome P-450 drug metabolizing enzyme system of the liver. Because ondansetron is metabolized by hepatic cytochrome P-450 drug-metabolizing enzymes (CYP3A4, CYP2D6, CYP1A2), inducers or inhibitors of these enzymes may change the clearance and, hence, the half-life of ondansetron. On the basis of available data, no dosage adjustment is recommended for patients on these drugs). Products include:
Tussionex 3443

Chlorpheniramine Tannate (Ondansetron does not itself appear to induce or inhibit the cytochrome P-450 drug metabolizing enzyme system of the liver. Because ondansetron is metabolized by hepatic cytochrome P-450 drug-metabolizing enzymes (CYP3A4, CYP2D6, CYP1A2), inducers or inhibitors of these enzymes may change the clearance and, hence, the half-life of ondansetron. On the basis of available data, no dosage adjustment is recommended for patients on these drugs).

No products indexed under this heading.

Chlorpropamide (*In vitro* metabolism studies have shown that ondansetron is a substrate for human hepatic cytochrome P-450 enzymes, including CYP1A2, CYP2D6, and CYP3A4. In terms of overall ondansetron turnover, CYP3A4 played the predominant role. Because of the multiplicity of metabolic enzymes capable of metabolizing ondansetron, it is likely that inhibition of one of these enzymes will be compen-

sated by others and may result in little change in overall rates of ondansetron elimination).

No products indexed under this heading.

Cilastatin Sodium (There have been reports of liver failure and death in patients with cancer receiving concurrent medications including antibiotics. The etiology of liver failure is unclear). Products include:
Primaxin I.M. 2232
Primaxin I.V. 2235

Cimetidine (Ondansetron does not itself appear to induce or inhibit the cytochrome P-450 drug metabolizing enzyme system of the liver. Because ondansetron is metabolized by hepatic cytochrome P-450 drug-metabolizing enzymes (CYP3A4, CYP2D6, CYP1A2), inducers or inhibitors of these enzymes may change the clearance and, hence, the half-life of ondansetron. On the basis of available data, no dosage adjustment is recommended for patients on these drugs).

No products indexed under this heading.

Cimetidine Hydrochloride (Ondansetron does not itself appear to induce or inhibit the cytochrome P-450 drug metabolizing enzyme system of the liver. Because ondansetron is metabolized by hepatic cytochrome P-450 drug-metabolizing enzymes (CYP3A4, CYP2D6, CYP1A2), inducers or inhibitors of these enzymes may change the clearance and, hence, the half-life of ondansetron. On the basis of available data, no dosage adjustment is recommended for patients on these drugs).

No products indexed under this heading.

Ciprofloxacin (There have been reports of liver failure and death in patients with cancer receiving concurrent medications including antibiotics. The etiology of liver failure is unclear). Products include:
Cipro I.V. 3082
Cipro 3073
Cipro XR 3091
Ciprodex 583

Ciprofloxacin Hydrochloride (There have been reports of liver failure and death in patients with cancer receiving concurrent medications including antibiotics. The etiology of liver failure is unclear). Products include:
Cipro 3073

Cisplatin (There have been reports of liver failure and death in patients with cancer receiving concurrent medications including potentially hepatotoxic cytotoxic chemotherapeutic drugs. The etiology of the liver failure is unclear).

No products indexed under this heading.

Citalopram Hydrobromide (Ondansetron does not itself appear to induce or inhibit the cytochrome P-450 drug metabolizing enzyme system of the liver. Because ondansetron is metabolized by hepatic cytochrome P-450 drug-metabolizing enzymes (CYP3A4, CYP2D6, CYP1A2), inducers or inhibitors of these enzymes may change the clearance and, hence, the half-life of ondansetron. On the basis of available data, no dosage adjustment is recommended for patients on these drugs). Products include:
Celexa 1153

Clarithromycin (There have been reports of liver failure and death in patients with cancer receiving concurrent medications including antibiotics. The etiology of liver failure is unclear). Products include:
Biaxin/Biaxin XL 412

Clomipramine Hydrochloride (Ondansetron does not itself appear to induce or inhibit the cytochrome P-450 drug metabolizing enzyme system of the liver. Because ondansetron is

metabolized by hepatic cytochrome P-450 drug-metabolizing enzymes (CYP3A4, CYP2D6, CYP1A2), inducers or inhibitors of these enzymes may change the clearance and, hence, the half-life of ondansetron. On the basis of available data, no dosage adjustment is recommended for patients on these drugs).

No products indexed under this heading.

Clopidogrel Bisulfate (*In vitro* metabolism studies have shown that ondansetron is a substrate for human hepatic cytochrome P-450 enzymes, including CYP1A2, CYP2D6, and CYP3A4. In terms of overall ondansetron turnover, CYP3A4 played the predominant role. Because of the multiplicity of metabolic enzymes capable of metabolizing ondansetron, it is likely that inhibition of one of these enzymes will be compensated by others and may result in little change in overall rates of ondansetron elimination). Products include:
Plavix 3027

Clopidogrel Hydrogen Sulfate (*In vitro* metabolism studies have shown that ondansetron is a substrate for human hepatic cytochrome P-450 enzymes, including CYP1A2, CYP2D6, and CYP3A4. In terms of overall ondansetron turnover, CYP3A4 played the predominant role. Because of the multiplicity of metabolic enzymes capable of metabolizing ondansetron, it is likely that inhibition of one of these enzymes will be compensated by others and may result in little change in overall rates of ondansetron elimination).

No products indexed under this heading.

Clotrimazole (There have been reports of liver failure and death in patients with cancer receiving concurrent medications including antibiotics. The etiology of liver failure is unclear). Products include:
Lotrisone 3163

Cloxacillin (There have been reports of liver failure and death in patients with cancer receiving concurrent medications including antibiotics. The etiology of liver failure is unclear).

No products indexed under this heading.

Cloxacillin Sodium (There have been reports of liver failure and death in patients with cancer receiving concurrent medications including antibiotics. The etiology of liver failure is unclear).

No products indexed under this heading.

Cloxacillin Sodium Monohydrate (There have been reports of liver failure and death in patients with cancer receiving concurrent medications including antibiotics. The etiology of liver failure is unclear).

No products indexed under this heading.

Cocaine Hydrochloride (Ondansetron does not itself appear to induce or inhibit the cytochrome P-450 drug metabolizing enzyme system of the liver. Because ondansetron is metabolized by hepatic cytochrome P-450 drug-metabolizing enzymes (CYP3A4, CYP2D6, CYP1A2), inducers or inhibitors of these enzymes may change the clearance and, hence, the half-life of ondansetron. On the basis of available data, no dosage adjustment is recommended for patients on these drugs).

No products indexed under this heading.

Conivaptan Hydrochloride (Ondansetron does not itself appear to induce or inhibit the cytochrome P-450 drug metabolizing enzyme system of the liver. Because ondansetron is metabolized by hepatic cytochrome P-450 drug-metabolizing enzymes (CYP3A4, CYP2D6, CYP1A2), inducers or inhibitors of these enzymes may change the clearance and, hence, the

half-life of ondansetron. On the basis of available data, no dosage adjustment is recommended for patients on these drugs). Products include:
Vaprisol 689

Cortisone Acetate (Ondansetron does not itself appear to induce or inhibit the cytochrome P-450 drug metabolizing enzyme system of the liver. Because ondansetron is metabolized by hepatic cytochrome P-450 drug-metabolizing enzymes (CYP3A4, CYP2D6, CYP1A2), inducers or inhibitors of these enzymes may change the clearance and, hence, the half-life of ondansetron. In patients treated with potent inducers of CYP3A4 the clearance of ondansetron was significantly increased and ondansetron blood concentrations were decreased. However, on the basis of available data, no dosage adjustment for ondansetron is recommended for patients on these drugs).

No products indexed under this heading.

Cyclophosphamide (There have been reports of liver failure and death in patients with cancer receiving concurrent medications including potentially hepatotoxic cytotoxic chemotherapeutic drugs. The etiology of liver failure is unclear).

No products indexed under this heading.

Cyclosporine (Ondansetron does not itself appear to induce or inhibit the cytochrome P-450 drug metabolizing enzyme system of the liver. Because ondansetron is metabolized by hepatic cytochrome P-450 drug-metabolizing enzymes (CYP3A4, CYP2D6, CYP1A2), inducers or inhibitors of these enzymes may change the clearance and, hence, the half-life of ondansetron. On the basis of available data, no dosage adjustment is recommended for patients on these drugs). Products include:
Gengraf 440
Neoral Oral Solution 2496
Neoral Capsules 2496
Restasis 605

Dacarbazine (There have been reports of liver failure and death in patients with cancer receiving concurrent medications including potentially hepatotoxic cytotoxic chemotherapeutic drugs. The etiology of the liver failure is unclear).

No products indexed under this heading.

Dalfopristin (Ondansetron does not itself appear to induce or inhibit the cytochrome P-450 drug metabolizing enzyme system of the liver. Because ondansetron is metabolized by hepatic cytochrome P-450 drug-metabolizing enzymes (CYP3A4, CYP2D6, CYP1A2), inducers or inhibitors of these enzymes may change the clearance and, hence, the half-life of ondansetron. On the basis of available data, no dosage adjustment is recommended for patients on these drugs).

No products indexed under this heading.

Danazol (Ondansetron does not itself appear to induce or inhibit the cytochrome P-450 drug metabolizing enzyme system of the liver. Because ondansetron is metabolized by hepatic cytochrome P-450 drug-metabolizing enzymes (CYP3A4, CYP2D6, CYP1A2), inducers or inhibitors of these enzymes may change the clearance and, hence, the half-life of ondansetron. On the basis of available data, no dosage adjustment is recommended for patients on these drugs).

No products indexed under this heading.

Darunavir (Ondansetron does not itself appear to induce or inhibit the cytochrome P-450 drug metabolizing enzyme system of the liver. Because ondansetron is metabolized by hepatic cytochrome P-450 drug-metabolizing

enzymes (CYP3A4, CYP2D6, CYP1A2), inducers or inhibitors of these enzymes may change the clearance and, hence, the half-life of ondansetron. On the basis of available data, no dosage adjustment is recommended for patients on these drugs).
No products indexed under this heading.

Dasatinib (Ondansetron does not itself appear to induce or inhibit the cytochrome P-450 drug metabolizing enzyme system of the liver. Because ondansetron is metabolized by hepatic cytochrome P-450 drug-metabolizing enzymes (CYP3A4, CYP2D6, CYP1A2), inducers or inhibitors of these enzymes may change the clearance and, hence, the half-life of ondansetron. On the basis of available data, no dosage adjustment is recommended for patients on these drugs).
No products indexed under this heading.

Daunorubicin Citrate (There have been reports of liver failure and death in patients with cancer receiving concurrent medications including potentially hepatotoxic cytotoxic chemotherapeutic drugs. The etiology of the liver failure is unclear).
No products indexed under this heading.

Daunorubicin Hydrochloride (There have been reports of liver failure and death in patients with cancer receiving concurrent medications including potentially hepatotoxic cytotoxic chemotherapeutic drugs. The etiology of liver failure is unclear).
No products indexed under this heading.

Delavirdine Mesylate (Ondansetron does not itself appear to induce or inhibit the cytochrome P-450 drug metabolizing enzyme system of the liver. Because ondansetron is metabolized by hepatic cytochrome P-450 drug-metabolizing enzymes (CYP3A4, CYP2D6, CYP1A2), inducers or inhibitors of these enzymes may change the clearance and, hence, the half-life of ondansetron. On the basis of available data, no dosage adjustment is recommended for patients on these drugs).
No products indexed under this heading.

Delavirine (Ondansetron does not itself appear to induce or inhibit the cytochrome P-450 drug metabolizing enzyme system of the liver. Because ondansetron is metabolized by hepatic cytochrome P-450 drug-metabolizing enzymes (CYP3A4, CYP2D6, CYP1A2), inducers or inhibitors of these enzymes may change the clearance and, hence, the half-life of ondansetron. On the basis of available data, no dosage adjustment is recommended for patients on these drugs).
No products indexed under this heading.

Demeclocycline Hydrochloride (There have been reports of liver failure and death in patients with cancer receiving concurrent medications including antibiotics. The etiology of liver failure is unclear).
No products indexed under this heading.

Denileukin Diftitox (There have been reports of liver failure and death in patients with cancer receiving concurrent medications including potentially hepatotoxic cytotoxic chemotherapeutic drugs. The etiology of the liver failure is unclear). Products include:
Ontak 1068

Desipramine Hydrochloride (Ondansetron does not itself appear to induce or inhibit the cytochrome P-450 drug metabolizing enzyme system of the liver. Because ondansetron is metabolized by hepatic cytochrome P-450 drug-metabolizing enzymes (CYP3A4, CYP2D6, CYP1A2), inducers or inhibitors of these enzymes may change the clearance and, hence, the half-life of ondansetron. On the basis of available data, no dosage adjustment is recommended for patients on these drugs).
No products indexed under this heading.

Desloratadine (Ondansetron does not itself appear to induce or inhibit the cytochrome P-450 drug metabolizing enzyme system of the liver. Because ondansetron is metabolized by hepatic cytochrome P-450 drug-metabolizing enzymes (CYP3A4, CYP2D6, CYP1A2), inducers or inhibitors of these enzymes may change the clearance and, hence, the half-life of ondansetron. On the basis of available data, no dosage adjustment is recommended for patients on these drugs). Products include:
Clarinex Syrup 3098
Clarinex 3098
Clarinex Reditabs 3098
Clarinex-D 12-Hour 3101
Clarinex-D 3104

Desogestrel (Ondansetron does not itself appear to induce or inhibit the cytochrome P-450 drug metabolizing enzyme system of the liver. Because ondansetron is metabolized by hepatic cytochrome P-450 drug-metabolizing enzymes (CYP3A4, CYP2D6, CYP1A2), inducers or inhibitors of these enzymes may change the clearance and, hence, the half-life of ondansetron. On the basis of available data, no dosage adjustment is recommended for patients on these drugs).
No products indexed under this heading.

Dexamethasone (Ondansetron does not itself appear to induce or inhibit the cytochrome P-450 drug metabolizing enzyme system of the liver. Because ondansetron is metabolized by hepatic cytochrome P-450 drug-metabolizing enzymes (CYP3A4, CYP2D6, CYP1A2), inducers or inhibitors of these enzymes may change the clearance and, hence, the half-life of ondansetron. In patients treated with potent inducers of CYP3A4 the clearance of ondansetron was significantly increased and ondansetron blood concentrations were decreased. However, on the basis of available data, no dosage adjustment for ondansetron is recommended for patients on these drugs). Products include:
Ciprodex 583
Ozurdex .... ⊙ 223
Tobramycin and Dexamethasone Ophthalmic Suspension .... ⊙ 251

Dexamethasone Acetate (Ondansetron does not itself appear to induce or inhibit the cytochrome P-450 drug metabolizing enzyme system of the liver. Because ondansetron is metabolized by hepatic cytochrome P-450 drug-metabolizing enzymes (CYP3A4, CYP2D6, CYP1A2), inducers or inhibitors of these enzymes may change the clearance and, hence, the half-life of ondansetron. In patients treated with potent inducers of CYP3A4 the clearance of ondansetron was significantly increased and ondansetron blood concentrations were decreased. However, on the basis of available data, no dosage adjustment for ondansetron is recommended for patients on these drugs).
No products indexed under this heading.

Dexamethasone Phosphate (Ondansetron does not itself appear to induce or inhibit the cytochrome P-450 drug metabolizing enzyme system of the liver. Because ondansetron is metabolized by hepatic cytochrome P-450 drug-metabolizing enzymes (CYP3A4, CYP2D6, CYP1A2), inducers or inhibitors of these enzymes may change the clearance and, hence, the half-life of ondansetron. In patients treated with potent inducers of CYP3A4 the clearance of ondansetron was significantly increased and ondansetron blood concentrations were decreased. However, on the basis of available data, no dosage adjustment for ondansetron is recommended for patients on these drugs).
No products indexed under this heading.

Dexamethasone Sodium (Ondansetron does not itself appear to induce or inhibit the cytochrome P-450 drug metabolizing enzyme system of the liver. Because ondansetron is metabolized by hepatic cytochrome P-450 drug-metabolizing enzymes (CYP3A4, CYP2D6, CYP1A2), inducers or inhibitors of these enzymes may change the clearance and, hence, the half-life of ondansetron. In patients treated with potent inducers of CYP3A4 the clearance of ondansetron was significantly increased and ondansetron blood concentrations were decreased. However, on the basis of available data, no dosage adjustment for ondansetron is recommended for patients on these drugs).
No products indexed under this heading.

Dexamethasone Sodium Phosphate (Ondansetron does not itself appear to induce or inhibit the cytochrome P-450 drug metabolizing enzyme system of the liver. Because ondansetron is metabolized by hepatic cytochrome P-450 drug-metabolizing enzymes (CYP3A4, CYP2D6, CYP1A2), inducers or inhibitors of these enzymes may change the clearance and, hence, the half-life of ondansetron. In patients treated with potent inducers of CYP3A4 the clearance of ondansetron was significantly increased and ondansetron blood concentrations were decreased. However, on the basis of available data, no dosage adjustment for ondansetron is recommended for patients on these drugs).
No products indexed under this heading.

Dexamethasone Sodium Phosphate Injection (Ondansetron does not itself appear to induce or inhibit the cytochrome P-450 drug metabolizing enzyme system of the liver. Because ondansetron is metabolized by hepatic cytochrome P-450 drug-metabolizing enzymes (CYP3A4, CYP2D6, CYP1A2), inducers or inhibitors of these enzymes may change the clearance and, hence, the half-life of ondansetron. In patients treated with potent inducers of CYP3A4 the clearance of ondansetron was significantly increased and ondansetron blood concentrations were decreased. However, on the basis of available data, no dosage adjustment for ondansetron is recommended for patients on these drugs).
No products indexed under this heading.

Diclofenac Epolamine (*In vitro* metabolism studies have shown that ondansetron is a substrate for human hepatic cytochrome P-450 enzymes, including CYP1A2, CYP2D6, and CYP3A4. In terms of overall ondansetron turnover, CYP3A4 played the predominant role. Because of the multiplicity of metabolic enzymes capable of metabolizing ondansetron, it is likely that inhibition of one of these enzymes will be compensated by others and may result in little change in overall rates of ondansetron elimination). Products include:
Flector 1839

Diclofenac Potassium (*In vitro* metabolism studies have shown that ondansetron is a substrate for human hepatic cytochrome P-450 enzymes, including CYP1A2, CYP2D6, and CYP3A4. In terms of overall ondansetron turnover, CYP3A4 played the predominant role. Because of the multiplicity of metabolic enzymes capable of metabolizing ondansetron, it is likely that inhibition of one of these enzymes will be compensated by others and may result in little change in overall rates of ondansetron elimination).
No products indexed under this heading.

Diclofenac Sodium (*In vitro* metabolism studies have shown that ondansetron is a substrate for human hepatic cytochrome P-450 enzymes, including CYP1A2, CYP2D6, and CYP3A4. In terms of overall ondansetron turnover, CYP3A4 played the predominant role. Because of the multiplicity of metabolic enzymes capable of metabolizing ondansetron, it is likely that inhibition of one of these enzymes will be compensated by others and may result in little change in overall rates of ondansetron elimination).
No products indexed under this heading.

Dicloxacillin (There have been reports of liver failure and death in patients with cancer receiving concurrent medications including antibiotics. The etiology of liver failure is unclear).
No products indexed under this heading.

Dicloxacillin Sodium (There have been reports of liver failure and death in patients with cancer receiving concurrent medications including antibiotics. The etiology of liver failure is unclear).
No products indexed under this heading.

Diltiazem Hydrochloride (Ondansetron does not itself appear to induce or inhibit the cytochrome P-450 drug metabolizing enzyme system of the liver. Because ondansetron is metabolized by hepatic cytochrome P-450 drug-metabolizing enzymes (CYP3A4, CYP2D6, CYP1A2), inducers or inhibitors of these enzymes may change the clearance and, hence, the half-life of ondansetron. On the basis of available data, no dosage adjustment is recommended for patients on these drugs). Products include:
Cardizem LA 423

Diltiazem Maleate (Ondansetron does not itself appear to induce or inhibit the cytochrome P-450 drug metabolizing enzyme system of the liver. Because ondansetron is metabolized by hepatic cytochrome P-450 drug-metabolizing enzymes (CYP3A4, CYP2D6, CYP1A2), inducers or inhibitors of these enzymes may change the clearance and, hence, the half-life of ondansetron. On the basis of available data, no dosage adjustment is recommended for patients on these drugs).
No products indexed under this heading.

Diphenhydramine (Ondansetron does not itself appear to induce or inhibit the cytochrome P-450 drug metabolizing enzyme system of the liver. Because ondansetron is metabolized by hepatic cytochrome P-450 drug-metabolizing enzymes (CYP3A4, CYP2D6, CYP1A2), inducers or inhibitors of these enzymes may change the clearance and, hence, the half-life of ondansetron. On the basis of available data, no dosage adjustment is recommended for patients on these drugs).
No products indexed under this heading.

Diphenhydramine Hydrochloride (Ondansetron does not itself appear to induce or inhibit the cytochrome P-450 drug metabolizing enzyme system of the liver. Because ondansetron is metabolized by hepatic cytochrome P-450 drug-metabolizing enzymes (CYP3A4, CYP2D6, CYP1A2), inducers or inhibitors of these enzymes may change the clearance and, hence, the half-life of ondansetron. On the basis of available data, no dosage adjustment is recommended for patients on these drugs). Products include:
Benadryl Allergy Ultratab 2042
Children's Benadryl Allergy Liquid 2042

IMPORTANT NOTE: Always consult each drug listing in the patient's regimen for possible interactions.

Zofran Interactions Index 2156

Dirithromycin (There have been reports of liver failure and death in patients with cancer receiving concurrent medications including antibiotics. The etiology of liver failure is unclear).
No products indexed under this heading.

Disodium Carbenicillin (There have been reports of liver failure and death in patients with cancer receiving concurrent medications including antibiotics. The etiology of liver failure is unclear).
No products indexed under this heading.

Disulfiram (*In vitro* metabolism studies have shown that ondansetron is a substrate for human hepatic cytochrome P-450 enzymes, including CYP1A2, CYP2D6, and CYP3A4. In terms of overall ondansetron turnover, CYP3A4 played the predominant role. Because of the multiplicity of metabolic enzymes capable of metabolizing ondansetron, it is likely that inhibition of one of these enzymes will be compensated by others and may result in little change in overall rates of ondansetron elimination).
No products indexed under this heading.

Docetaxel (There have been reports of liver failure and death in patients with cancer receiving concurrent medications including potentially hepatotoxic cytotoxic chemotherapeutic drugs. The etiology of the liver failure is unclear). Products include:
Taxotere 3035

Doxepin Hydrochloride (Ondansetron does not itself appear to induce or inhibit the cytochrome P-450 drug metabolizing enzyme system of the liver. Because ondansetron is metabolized by hepatic cytochrome P-450 drug-metabolizing enzymes (CYP3A4, CYP2D6, CYP1A2), inducers or inhibitors of these enzymes may change the clearance and, hence, the half-life of ondansetron. On the basis of available data, no dosage adjustment is recommended for patients on these drugs).
No products indexed under this heading.

Doxorubicin Hydrochloride (There have been reports of liver failure and death in patients with cancer receiving concurrent medications including potentially hepatotoxic cytotoxic chemotherapeutic drugs. The etiology of liver failure is unclear).
No products indexed under this heading.

Doxycycline Calcium (There have been reports of liver failure and death in patients with cancer receiving concurrent medications including antibiotics. The etiology of liver failure is unclear).
No products indexed under this heading.

Doxycycline Hyclate (There have been reports of liver failure and death in patients with cancer receiving concurrent medications including antibiotics. The etiology of liver failure is unclear).
No products indexed under this heading.

Doxycycline Monohydrate (There have been reports of liver failure and death in patients with cancer receiving concurrent medications including antibiotics. The etiology of liver failure is unclear).
No products indexed under this heading.

Efavirenz (Ondansetron does not itself appear to induce or inhibit the cytochrome P-450 drug metabolizing enzyme system of the liver. Because ondansetron is metabolized by hepatic cytochrome P-450 drug-metabolizing enzymes (CYP3A4, CYP2D6, CYP1A2), inducers or inhibitors of these enzymes may change the clearance and, hence, the half-life of ondansetron. In patients treated with potent inducers of CYP3A4 the clearance of ondansetron was significantly increased and ondansetron blood concentrations were decreased. However, on the basis of available data, no dosage adjustment for ondansetron is recommended for patients on these drugs). Products include:
Atripla 906

Enoxacin (There have been reports of liver failure and death in patients with cancer receiving concurrent medications including antibiotics. The etiology of liver failure is unclear).
No products indexed under this heading.

Epirubicin Hydrochloride (There have been reports of liver failure and death in patients with cancer receiving concurrent medications including potentially hepatotoxic cytotoxic chemotherapeutic drugs. The etiology of liver failure is unclear).
No products indexed under this heading.

Erythromycin (There have been reports of liver failure and death in patients with cancer receiving concurrent medications including antibiotics. The etiology of liver failure is unclear).
No products indexed under this heading.

Erythromycin, Topical (There have been reports of liver failure and death in patients with cancer receiving concurrent medications including antibiotics. The etiology of liver failure is unclear).
No products indexed under this heading.

Erythromycin Estolate (There have been reports of liver failure and death in patients with cancer receiving concurrent medications including antibiotics. The etiology of liver failure is unclear).
No products indexed under this heading.

Erythromycin Ethylsuccinate (There have been reports of liver failure and death in patients with cancer receiving concurrent medications including antibiotics. The etiology of liver failure is unclear). Products include:
E.E.S. 437
EryPed 435

Erythromycin Gluceptate (There have been reports of liver failure and death in patients with cancer receiving concurrent medications including antibiotics. The etiology of liver failure is unclear).
No products indexed under this heading.

Erythromycin Lactobionate (There have been reports of liver failure and death in patients with cancer receiving concurrent medications including antibiotics. The etiology of liver failure is unclear).
No products indexed under this heading.

Erythromycin Stearate (There have been reports of liver failure and death in patients with cancer receiving concurrent medications including antibiotics. The etiology of liver failure is unclear).
No products indexed under this heading.

Escitalopram Oxalate (Ondansetron does not itself appear to induce or inhibit the cytochrome P-450 drug metabolizing enzyme system of the liver. Because ondansetron is metabolized by hepatic cytochrome P-450 drug-metabolizing enzymes (CYP3A4, CYP2D6, CYP1A2), inducers or inhibitors of these enzymes may change the clearance and, hence, the half-life of ondansetron. On the basis of available data, no dosage adjustment is recommended for patients on these drugs). Products include:
Lexapro Oral Suspension 1160
Lexapro Tablets 1160

Esomeprazole Magnesium (Ondansetron does not itself appear to induce or inhibit the cytochrome P-450 drug metabolizing enzyme system of the liver. Because ondansetron is metabolized by hepatic cytochrome P-450 drug-metabolizing enzymes (CYP3A4, CYP2D6, CYP1A2), inducers or inhibitors of these enzymes may change the clearance and, hence, the half-life of ondansetron. On the basis of available data, no dosage adjustment is recommended for patients on these drugs). Products include:
Nexium Capsules 704
Nexium Oral Suspension 704

Esomeprazole Sodium (Ondansetron does not itself appear to induce or inhibit the cytochrome P-450 drug metabolizing enzyme system of the liver. Because ondansetron is metabolized by hepatic cytochrome P-450 drug-metabolizing enzymes (CYP3A4, CYP2D6, CYP1A2), inducers or inhibitors of these enzymes may change the clearance and, hence, the half-life of ondansetron. On the basis of available data, no dosage adjustment is recommended for patients on these drugs). Products include:
Nexium I.V. 712

Estramustine Phosphate Sodium (There have been reports of liver failure and death in patients with cancer receiving concurrent medications including potentially hepatotoxic cytotoxic chemotherapeutic drugs. The etiology of the liver failure is unclear).
No products indexed under this heading.

Ethanol (Ondansetron does not itself appear to induce or inhibit the cytochrome P-450 drug metabolizing enzyme system of the liver. Because ondansetron is metabolized by hepatic cytochrome P-450 drug-metabolizing enzymes (CYP3A4, CYP2D6, CYP1A2), inducers or inhibitors of these enzymes may change the clearance and, hence, the half-life of ondansetron. On the basis of available data, no dosage adjustment is recommended for patients on these drugs).
No products indexed under this heading.

Ethinyl Estradiol (Ondansetron does not itself appear to induce or inhibit the cytochrome P-450 drug metabolizing enzyme system of the liver. Because ondansetron is metabolized by hepatic cytochrome P-450 drug-metabolizing enzymes (CYP3A4, CYP2D6, CYP1A2), inducers or inhibitors of these enzymes may change the clearance and, hence, the half-life of ondansetron. On the basis of available data, no dosage adjustment is recommended for patients on these drugs). Products include:
LoSeasonique 3407
Lybrel 3514
NuvaRing 3181
Ortho Evra 2648
Ortho-Cyclen/Ortho Tri-Cyclen 2663
Ortho Tri-Cyclen Lo Tablets 2673
Seasonique 3418
Yaz 864

Ethosuximide (Ondansetron does not itself appear to induce or inhibit the cytochrome P-450 drug metabolizing enzyme system of the liver. Because ondansetron is metabolized by hepatic cytochrome P-450 drug-metabolizing enzymes (CYP3A4, CYP2D6, CYP1A2), inducers or inhibitors of these enzymes may change the clearance and, hence, the half-life of ondansetron. In patients treated with potent inducers of CYP3A4 the clearance of ondansetron was significantly increased and ondansetron blood concentrations were decreased. However, on the basis of available data, no dosage adjustment for ondansetron is recommended for patients on these drugs).
No products indexed under this heading.

Ethynodiol Diacetate (*In vitro* metabolism studies have shown that ondansetron is a substrate for human hepatic cytochrome P-450 enzymes, including CYP1A2, CYP2D6, and CYP3A4. In terms of overall ondansetron turnover, CYP3A4 played the predominant role. Because of the multiplicity of metabolic enzymes capable of metabolizing ondansetron, it is likely that inhibition of one of these enzymes will be compensated by others and may result in little change in overall rates of ondansetron elimination).
No products indexed under this heading.

Etoposide (There have been reports of liver failure and death in patients with cancer receiving concurrent medications including potentially hepatotoxic cytotoxic chemotherapeutic drugs. The etiology of the liver failure is unclear).
No products indexed under this heading.

Exemestane (There have been reports of liver failure and death in patients with cancer receiving concurrent medications including potentially hepatotoxic cytotoxic chemotherapeutic drugs. The etiology of the liver failure is unclear). Products include:
Aromasin 2758

Felbamate (Ondansetron does not itself appear to induce or inhibit the cytochrome P-450 drug metabolizing enzyme system of the liver. Because ondansetron is metabolized by hepatic cytochrome P-450 drug-metabolizing enzymes (CYP3A4, CYP2D6, CYP1A2), inducers or inhibitors of these enzymes may change the clearance and, hence, the half-life of ondansetron. In patients treated with potent inducers of CYP3A4 the clearance of ondansetron was significantly increased and ondansetron blood concentrations were decreased. However, on the basis of available data, no dosage adjustment for ondansetron is recommended for patients on these drugs).
No products indexed under this heading.

Fenofibrate (*In vitro* metabolism studies have shown that ondansetron is a substrate for human hepatic cytochrome P-450 enzymes, including CYP1A2, CYP2D6, and CYP3A4. In terms of overall ondansetron turnover, CYP3A4 played the predominant role. Because of the multiplicity of metabolic enzymes capable of metabolizing ondansetron, it is likely that inhibition of one of these enzymes will be compensated by others and may result in little change in overall rates of ondansetron elimination). Products include:
Fenoglide 3263
Tricor 544
Trilipix 548

Floxuridine (There have been reports of liver failure and death in patients with cancer receiving concurrent medications including potentially hepatotoxic cytotoxic chemotherapeutic drugs. The etiology of the liver failure is unclear).
No products indexed under this heading.

Fluconazole (Ondansetron does not itself appear to induce or inhibit the cytochrome P-450 drug metabolizing enzyme system of the liver. Because ondansetron is metabolized by hepatic cytochrome P-450 drug-metabolizing enzymes (CYP3A4, CYP2D6, CYP1A2), inducers or inhibitors of these enzymes may change the clearance and, hence, the half-life of ondansetron. On the basis of available data, no dosage adjustment is recommended for patients on these drugs).
No products indexed under this heading.

Fludrocortisone Acetate (Ondansetron does not itself appear to induce or inhibit the cytochrome P-450 drug metabolizing enzyme system of the liver. Because ondansetron is metabolized by hepatic cytochrome P-450 drug-metabolizing enzymes (CYP3A4, CYP2D6, CYP1A2), inducers or inhibitors of these enzymes may change the clearance and, hence, the half-life of ondansetron. In patients treated with potent inducers of CYP3A4 the clearance of ondansetron was significantly increased and ondansetron blood concentrations were decreased. However, on the basis of available data, no

2157 Interactions Index Zofran

dosage adjustment for ondansetron is recommended for patients on these drugs).
No products indexed under this heading.

Fluorouracil (There have been reports of liver failure and death in patients with cancer receiving concurrent medications including potentially hepatotoxic cytotoxic chemotherapeutic drugs. The etiology of liver failure is unclear). Products include:
Carac 2966

Fluoxetine (Ondansetron does not itself appear to induce or inhibit the cytochrome P-450 drug metabolizing enzyme system of the liver. Because ondansetron is metabolized by hepatic cytochrome P-450 drug-metabolizing enzymes (CYP3A4, CYP2D6, CYP1A2), inducers or inhibitors of these enzymes may change the clearance and, hence, the half-life of ondansetron. On the basis of available data, no dosage adjustment is recommended for patients on these drugs).
No products indexed under this heading.

Fluoxetine Hydrochloride (Ondansetron does not itself appear to induce or inhibit the cytochrome P-450 drug metabolizing enzyme system of the liver. Because ondansetron is metabolized by hepatic cytochrome P-450 drug-metabolizing enzymes (CYP3A4, CYP2D6, CYP1A2), inducers or inhibitors of these enzymes may change the clearance and, hence, the half-life of ondansetron. On the basis of available data, no dosage adjustment is recommended for patients on these drugs). Products include:
Prozac Weekly 1941
Prozac Pulvules 1941
Symbyax 1965

Fluphenazine Decanoate (Ondansetron does not itself appear to induce or inhibit the cytochrome P-450 drug metabolizing enzyme system of the liver. Because ondansetron is metabolized by hepatic cytochrome P-450 drug-metabolizing enzymes (CYP3A4, CYP2D6, CYP1A2), inducers or inhibitors of these enzymes may change the clearance and, hence, the half-life of ondansetron. On the basis of available data, no dosage adjustment is recommended for patients on these drugs).
No products indexed under this heading.

Fluphenazine Enanthate (Ondansetron does not itself appear to induce or inhibit the cytochrome P-450 drug metabolizing enzyme system of the liver. Because ondansetron is metabolized by hepatic cytochrome P-450 drug-metabolizing enzymes (CYP3A4, CYP2D6, CYP1A2), inducers or inhibitors of these enzymes may change the clearance and, hence, the half-life of ondansetron. On the basis of available data, no dosage adjustment is recommended for patients on these drugs).
No products indexed under this heading.

Fluphenazine Hydrochloride (Ondansetron does not itself appear to induce or inhibit the cytochrome P-450 drug metabolizing enzyme system of the liver. Because ondansetron is metabolized by hepatic cytochrome P-450 drug-metabolizing enzymes (CYP3A4, CYP2D6, CYP1A2), inducers or inhibitors of these enzymes may change the clearance and, hence, the half-life of ondansetron. On the basis of available data, no dosage adjustment is recommended for patients on these drugs).
No products indexed under this heading.

Flurbiprofen (*In vitro* metabolism studies have shown that ondansetron is a substrate for human hepatic cytochrome P-450 enzymes, including CYP1A2, CYP2D6, and CYP3A4. In terms of overall ondansetron turnover, CYP3A4 played the predominant role. Because of the multiplicity of metabolizing enzymes capable of metabolizing ondansetron, it is likely that inhibition of one of these enzymes will be compensated by others and may result in little change in overall rates of ondansetron elimination).
No products indexed under this heading.

Flurbiprofen Sodium (*In vitro* metabolism studies have shown that ondansetron is a substrate for human hepatic cytochrome P-450 enzymes, including CYP1A2, CYP2D6, and CYP3A4. In terms of overall ondansetron turnover, CYP3A4 played the predominant role. Because of the multiplicity of metabolic enzymes capable of metabolizing ondansetron, it is likely that inhibition of one of these enzymes will be compensated by others and may result in little change in overall rates of ondansetron elimination).
No products indexed under this heading.

Flutamide (There have been reports of liver failure and death in patients with cancer receiving concurrent medications including potentially hepatotoxic cytotoxic chemotherapeutic drugs. The etiology of the liver failure is unclear).
No products indexed under this heading.

Fluvastatin Sodium (*In vitro* metabolism studies have shown that ondansetron is a substrate for human hepatic cytochrome P-450 enzymes, including CYP1A2, CYP2D6, and CYP3A4. In terms of overall ondansetron turnover, CYP3A4 played the predominant role. Because of the multiplicity of metabolic enzymes capable of metabolizing ondansetron, it is likely that inhibition of one of these enzymes will be compensated by others and may result in little change in overall rates of ondansetron elimination).
No products indexed under this heading.

Fluvoxamine (Ondansetron does not itself appear to induce or inhibit the cytochrome P-450 drug metabolizing enzyme system of the liver. Because ondansetron is metabolized by hepatic cytochrome P-450 drug-metabolizing enzymes (CYP3A4, CYP2D6, CYP1A2), inducers or inhibitors of these enzymes may change the clearance and, hence, the half-life of ondansetron. On the basis of available data, no dosage adjustment is recommended for patients on these drugs).
No products indexed under this heading.

Fluvoxamine Maleate (Ondansetron does not itself appear to induce or inhibit the cytochrome P-450 drug metabolizing enzyme system of the liver. Because ondansetron is metabolized by hepatic cytochrome P-450 drug-metabolizing enzymes (CYP3A4, CYP2D6, CYP1A2), inducers or inhibitors of these enzymes may change the clearance and, hence, the half-life of ondansetron. On the basis of available data, no dosage adjustment is recommended for patients on these drugs).
No products indexed under this heading.

Fosamprenavir Calcium (Ondansetron does not itself appear to induce or inhibit the cytochrome P-450 drug metabolizing enzyme system of the liver. Because ondansetron is metabolized by hepatic cytochrome P-450 drug-metabolizing enzymes (CYP3A4, CYP2D6, CYP1A2), inducers or inhibitors of these enzymes may change the clearance and, hence, the half-life of ondansetron. On the basis of available data, no dosage adjustment is recommended for patients on these drugs). Products include:
Lexiva Oral Suspension 1558
Lexiva 1558

Fosphenytoin (In patients treated with potent inducers of CYP3A4 (eg, phenytoin), the clearance of ondansetron was significantly increased and ondansetron blood concentrations were decreased. However, on the basis of available data, no dosage adjustment for ondansetron is recommended for patients on these drugs).
No products indexed under this heading.

Fosphenytoin Sodium (In patients treated with potent inducers of CYP3A4 (eg, phenytoin), the clearance of ondansetron was significantly increased and ondansetron blood concentrations were decreased. However, on the basis of available data, no dosage adjustment for ondansetron is recommended for patients on these drugs).
No products indexed under this heading.

Garlic Extract (Ondansetron does not itself appear to induce or inhibit the cytochrome P-450 drug metabolizing enzyme system of the liver. Because ondansetron is metabolized by hepatic cytochrome P-450 drug-metabolizing enzymes (CYP3A4, CYP2D6, CYP1A2), inducers or inhibitors of these enzymes may change the clearance and, hence, the half-life of ondansetron. In patients treated with potent inducers of CYP3A4 the clearance of ondansetron was significantly increased and ondansetron blood concentrations were decreased. However, on the basis of available data, no dosage adjustment for ondansetron is recommended for patients on these drugs).
No products indexed under this heading.

Garlic Oil (Ondansetron does not itself appear to induce or inhibit the cytochrome P-450 drug metabolizing enzyme system of the liver. Because ondansetron is metabolized by hepatic cytochrome P-450 drug-metabolizing enzymes (CYP3A4, CYP2D6, CYP1A2), inducers or inhibitors of these enzymes may change the clearance and, hence, the half-life of ondansetron. In patients treated with potent inducers of CYP3A4 the clearance of ondansetron was significantly increased and ondansetron blood concentrations were decreased. However, on the basis of available data, no dosage adjustment for ondansetron is recommended for patients on these drugs).
No products indexed under this heading.

Gatifloxacin (There have been reports of liver failure and death in patients with cancer receiving concurrent medications including antibiotics. The etiology of liver failure is unclear).
No products indexed under this heading.

Gemcitabine Hydrochloride (There have been reports of liver failure and death in patients with cancer receiving concurrent medications including potentially hepatotoxic cytotoxic chemotherapeutic drugs. The etiology of the liver failure is unclear). Products include:
Gemzar 1900

Gemfibrozil (*In vitro* metabolism studies have shown that ondansetron is a substrate for human hepatic cytochrome P-450 enzymes, including CYP1A2, CYP2D6, and CYP3A4. In terms of overall ondansetron turnover, CYP3A4 played the predominant role. Because of the multiplicity of metabolic enzymes capable of metabolizing ondansetron, it is likely that inhibition of one of these enzymes will be compensated by others and may result in little change in overall rates of ondansetron elimination).
No products indexed under this heading.

Gemifloxacin Mesylate (There have been reports of liver failure and death in patients with cancer receiving concurrent medications including antibiotics. The etiology of liver failure is unclear).
No products indexed under this heading.

Gentamicin Sulfate (There have been reports of liver failure and death in patients with cancer receiving concurrent medications including antibiotics. The etiology of liver failure is unclear). Products include:
Pred-G .... ⊙226, ⊙227

Glipizide (*In vitro* metabolism studies have shown that ondansetron is a substrate for human hepatic cytochrome P-450 enzymes, including CYP1A2, CYP2D6, and CYP3A4. In terms of overall ondansetron turnover, CYP3A4 played the predominant role. Because of the multiplicity of metabolic enzymes capable of metabolizing ondansetron, it is likely that inhibition of one of these enzymes will be compensated by others and may result in little change in overall rates of ondansetron elimination).
No products indexed under this heading.

Glyburide (*In vitro* metabolism studies have shown that ondansetron is a substrate for human hepatic cytochrome P-450 enzymes, including CYP1A2, CYP2D6, and CYP3A4. In terms of overall ondansetron turnover, CYP3A4 played the predominant role. Because of the multiplicity of metabolic enzymes capable of metabolizing ondansetron, it is likely that inhibition of one of these enzymes will be compensated by others and may result in little change in overall rates of ondansetron elimination).
No products indexed under this heading.

Grepafloxacin Hydrochloride (There have been reports of liver failure and death in patients with cancer receiving concurrent medications including antibiotics. The etiology of liver failure is unclear).
No products indexed under this heading.

Griseofulvin (There have been reports of liver failure and death in patients with cancer receiving concurrent medications including antibiotics. The etiology of liver failure is unclear).
No products indexed under this heading.

Halofantrine Hydrochloride (Ondansetron does not itself appear to induce or inhibit the cytochrome P-450 drug metabolizing enzyme system of the liver. Because ondansetron is metabolized by hepatic cytochrome P-450 drug-metabolizing enzymes (CYP3A4, CYP2D6, CYP1A2), inducers or inhibitors of these enzymes may change the clearance and, hence, the half-life of ondansetron. On the basis of available data, no dosage adjustment is recommended for patients on these drugs).
No products indexed under this heading.

Haloperidol (Ondansetron does not itself appear to induce or inhibit the cytochrome P-450 drug metabolizing enzyme system of the liver. Because ondansetron is metabolized by hepatic cytochrome P-450 drug-metabolizing enzymes (CYP3A4, CYP2D6, CYP1A2), inducers or inhibitors of these enzymes may change the clearance and, hence, the half-life of ondansetron. On the basis of available data, no dosage adjustment is recommended for patients on these drugs).
No products indexed under this heading.

Haloperidol Decanoate (Ondansetron does not itself appear to induce or inhibit the cytochrome P-450 drug metabolizing enzyme system of the liver. Because ondansetron is metabolized by hepatic cytochrome P-450 drug-metabolizing enzymes (CYP3A4, CYP2D6, CYP1A2), inducers or inhibitors of these enzymes may

change the clearance and, hence, the half-life of ondansetron. On the basis of available data, no dosage adjustment is recommended for patients on these drugs).

No products indexed under this heading.

Haloperidol Lactate (Ondansetron does not itself appear to induce or inhibit the cytochrome P-450 drug metabolizing enzyme system of the liver. Because ondansetron is metabolized by hepatic cytochrome P-450 drug-metabolizing enzymes (CYP3A4, CYP2D6, CYP1A2), inducers or inhibitors of these enzymes may change the clearance and, hence, the half-life of ondansetron. On the basis of available data, no dosage adjustment is recommended for patients on these drugs).

No products indexed under this heading.

Hydrochlorothiazide (*In vitro* metabolism studies have shown that ondansetron is a substrate for human hepatic cytochrome P-450 enzymes, including CYP1A2, CYP2D6, and CYP3A4. In terms of overall ondansetron turnover, CYP3A4 played the predominant role. Because of the multiplicity of metabolic enzymes capable of metabolizing ondansetron, it is likely that inhibition of one of these enzymes will be compensated by others and may result in little change in overall rates of ondansetron elimination).
Products include:

Atacand HCT	700
Avalide	2956
Benicar HCT	1017
Diovan HCT	2419
Dyazide	1429
Exforge HCT	2449
Hyzaar	2162
Hyzaar 100-12.5	2162
Micardis HCT	889
Prinzide	2246
Tekturna HCT	2541
Teveten HCT	541

Hydrochlorothiazide Hydrochloride (*In vitro* metabolism studies have shown that ondansetron is a substrate for human hepatic cytochrome P-450 enzymes, including CYP1A2, CYP2D6, and CYP3A4. In terms of overall ondansetron turnover, CYP3A4 played the predominant role. Because of the multiplicity of metabolic enzymes capable of metabolizing ondansetron, it is likely that inhibition of one of these enzymes will be compensated by others and may result in little change in overall rates of ondansetron elimination).

No products indexed under this heading.

Hydrocortisone (Ondansetron does not itself appear to induce or inhibit the cytochrome P-450 drug metabolizing enzyme system of the liver. Because ondansetron is metabolized by hepatic cytochrome P-450 drug-metabolizing enzymes (CYP3A4, CYP2D6, CYP1A2), inducers or inhibitors of these enzymes may change the clearance and, hence, the half-life of ondansetron. In patients treated with potent inducers of CYP3A4 the clearance of ondansetron was significantly increased and ondansetron blood concentrations were decreased. However, on the basis of available data, no dosage adjustment for ondansetron is recommended for patients on these drugs).

No products indexed under this heading.

Hydrocortisone (Alcohol) (Ondansetron does not itself appear to induce or inhibit the cytochrome P-450 drug metabolizing enzyme system of the liver. Because ondansetron is metabolized by hepatic cytochrome P-450 drug-metabolizing enzymes (CYP3A4, CYP2D6, CYP1A2), inducers or inhibitors of these enzymes may change the clearance and, hence, the half-life of ondansetron. In patients treated with potent inducers of CYP3A4 the

clearance of ondansetron was significantly increased and ondansetron blood concentrations were decreased. However, on the basis of available data, no dosage adjustment for ondansetron is recommended for patients on these drugs).

No products indexed under this heading.

Hydrocortisone Acetate (Ondansetron does not itself appear to induce or inhibit the cytochrome P-450 drug metabolizing enzyme system of the liver. Because ondansetron is metabolized by hepatic cytochrome P-450 drug-metabolizing enzymes (CYP3A4, CYP2D6, CYP1A2), inducers or inhibitors of these enzymes may change the clearance and, hence, the half-life of ondansetron. In patients treated with potent inducers of CYP3A4 the clearance of ondansetron was significantly increased and ondansetron blood concentrations were decreased. However, on the basis of available data, no dosage adjustment for ondansetron is recommended for patients on these drugs).

No products indexed under this heading.

Hydrocortisone Butyrate (Ondansetron does not itself appear to induce or inhibit the cytochrome P-450 drug metabolizing enzyme system of the liver. Because ondansetron is metabolized by hepatic cytochrome P-450 drug-metabolizing enzymes (CYP3A4, CYP2D6, CYP1A2), inducers or inhibitors of these enzymes may change the clearance and, hence, the half-life of ondansetron. In patients treated with potent inducers of CYP3A4 the clearance of ondansetron was significantly increased and ondansetron blood concentrations were decreased. However, on the basis of available data, no dosage adjustment for ondansetron is recommended for patients on these drugs).

No products indexed under this heading.

Hydrocortisone Cypionate (Ondansetron does not itself appear to induce or inhibit the cytochrome P-450 drug metabolizing enzyme system of the liver. Because ondansetron is metabolized by hepatic cytochrome P-450 drug-metabolizing enzymes (CYP3A4, CYP2D6, CYP1A2), inducers or inhibitors of these enzymes may change the clearance and, hence, the half-life of ondansetron. In patients treated with potent inducers of CYP3A4 the clearance of ondansetron was significantly increased and ondansetron blood concentrations were decreased. However, on the basis of available data, no dosage adjustment for ondansetron is recommended for patients on these drugs).

No products indexed under this heading.

Hydrocortisone Hemisuccinate (Ondansetron does not itself appear to induce or inhibit the cytochrome P-450 drug metabolizing enzyme system of the liver. Because ondansetron is metabolized by hepatic cytochrome P-450 drug-metabolizing enzymes (CYP3A4, CYP2D6, CYP1A2), inducers or inhibitors of these enzymes may change the clearance and, hence, the half-life of ondansetron. In patients treated with potent inducers of CYP3A4 the clearance of ondansetron was significantly increased and ondansetron blood concentrations were decreased. However, on the basis of available data, no dosage adjustment for ondansetron is recommended for patients on these drugs).

No products indexed under this heading.

Hydrocortisone Probutate (Ondansetron does not itself appear to induce or inhibit the cytochrome P-450 drug metabolizing enzyme system of the liver. Because ondansetron is

metabolized by hepatic cytochrome P-450 drug-metabolizing enzymes (CYP3A4, CYP2D6, CYP1A2), inducers or inhibitors of these enzymes may change the clearance and, hence, the half-life of ondansetron. In patients treated with potent inducers of CYP3A4 the clearance of ondansetron was significantly increased and ondansetron blood concentrations were decreased. However, on the basis of available data, no dosage adjustment for ondansetron is recommended for patients on these drugs).

No products indexed under this heading.

Hydrocortisone Sodium Phosphate (Ondansetron does not itself appear to induce or inhibit the cytochrome P-450 drug metabolizing enzyme system of the liver. Because ondansetron is metabolized by hepatic cytochrome P-450 drug-metabolizing enzymes (CYP3A4, CYP2D6, CYP1A2), inducers or inhibitors of these enzymes may change the clearance and, hence, the half-life of ondansetron. In patients treated with potent inducers of CYP3A4 the clearance of ondansetron was significantly increased and ondansetron blood concentrations were decreased. However, on the basis of available data, no dosage adjustment for ondansetron is recommended for patients on these drugs).

No products indexed under this heading.

Hydrocortisone Sodium Succinate (Ondansetron does not itself appear to induce or inhibit the cytochrome P-450 drug metabolizing enzyme system of the liver. Because ondansetron is metabolized by hepatic cytochrome P-450 drug-metabolizing enzymes (CYP3A4, CYP2D6, CYP1A2), inducers or inhibitors of these enzymes may change the clearance and, hence, the half-life of ondansetron. In patients treated with potent inducers of CYP3A4 the clearance of ondansetron was significantly increased and ondansetron blood concentrations were decreased. However, on the basis of available data, no dosage adjustment for ondansetron is recommended for patients on these drugs).

No products indexed under this heading.

Hydrocortisone Valerate (Ondansetron does not itself appear to induce or inhibit the cytochrome P-450 drug metabolizing enzyme system of the liver. Because ondansetron is metabolized by hepatic cytochrome P-450 drug-metabolizing enzymes (CYP3A4, CYP2D6, CYP1A2), inducers or inhibitors of these enzymes may change the clearance and, hence, the half-life of ondansetron. In patients treated with potent inducers of CYP3A4 the clearance of ondansetron was significantly increased and ondansetron blood concentrations were decreased. However, on the basis of available data, no dosage adjustment for ondansetron is recommended for patients on these drugs).

No products indexed under this heading.

Hydroflumethiazide (*In vitro* metabolism studies have shown that ondansetron is a substrate for human hepatic cytochrome P-450 enzymes, including CYP1A2, CYP2D6, and CYP3A4. In terms of overall ondansetron turnover, CYP3A4 played the predominant role. Because of the multiplicity of metabolic enzymes capable of metabolizing ondansetron, it is likely that inhibition of one of these enzymes will be compensated by others and may result in little change in overall rates of ondansetron elimination).

No products indexed under this heading.

Hydroxychloroquine Sulfate (Ondansetron does not itself appear to induce or inhibit the cytochrome P-450

drug metabolizing enzyme system of the liver. Because ondansetron is metabolized by hepatic cytochrome P-450 drug-metabolizing enzymes (CYP3A4, CYP2D6, CYP1A2), inducers or inhibitors of these enzymes may change the clearance and, hence, the half-life of ondansetron. On the basis of available data, no dosage adjustment is recommended for patients on these drugs).

No products indexed under this heading.

Hydroxyurea (There have been reports of liver failure and death in patients with cancer receiving concurrent medications including potentially hepatotoxic cytotoxic chemotherapeutic drugs. The etiology of liver failure is unclear).

No products indexed under this heading.

Hypericum (Ondansetron does not itself appear to induce or inhibit the cytochrome P-450 drug metabolizing enzyme system of the liver. Because ondansetron is metabolized by hepatic cytochrome P-450 drug-metabolizing enzymes (CYP3A4, CYP2D6, CYP1A2), inducers or inhibitors of these enzymes may change the clearance and, hence, the half-life of ondansetron. In patients treated with potent inducers of CYP3A4 the clearance of ondansetron was significantly increased and ondansetron blood concentrations were decreased. However, on the basis of available data, no dosage adjustment for ondansetron is recommended for patients on these drugs).

No products indexed under this heading.

Hypericum Perforatum (Ondansetron does not itself appear to induce or inhibit the cytochrome P-450 drug metabolizing enzyme system of the liver. Because ondansetron is metabolized by hepatic cytochrome P-450 drug-metabolizing enzymes (CYP3A4, CYP2D6, CYP1A2), inducers or inhibitors of these enzymes may change the clearance and, hence, the half-life of ondansetron. In patients treated with potent inducers of CYP3A4 the clearance of ondansetron was significantly increased and ondansetron blood concentrations were decreased. However, on the basis of available data, no dosage adjustment for ondansetron is recommended for patients on these drugs). Products include:

Traumeel	1800

Idarubicin Hydrochloride (There have been reports of liver failure and death in patients with cancer receiving concurrent medications including potentially hepatotoxic cytotoxic chemotherapeutic drugs. The etiology of the liver failure is unclear).

No products indexed under this heading.

Ifosfamide (There have been reports of liver failure and death in patients with cancer receiving concurrent medications including potentially hepatotoxic cytotoxic chemotherapeutic drugs. The etiology of the liver failure is unclear).

No products indexed under this heading.

Imatinib Mesylate (Ondansetron does not itself appear to induce or inhibit the cytochrome P-450 drug metabolizing enzyme system of the liver. Because ondansetron is metabolized by hepatic cytochrome P-450 drug-metabolizing enzymes (CYP3A4, CYP2D6, CYP1A2), inducers or inhibitors of these enzymes may change the clearance and, hence, the half-life of ondansetron. On the basis of available data, no dosage adjustment is recommended for patients on these drugs).
Products include:

Gleevec	2477

Imipenem (There have been reports of liver failure and death in patients with cancer receiving concurrent medica-

2159 Interactions Index Zofran

tions including antibiotics. The etiology of liver failure is unclear). Products include:
Primaxin I.M. 2232
Primaxin I.V. 2235

Imipramine Hydrochloride (Ondansetron does not itself appear to induce or inhibit the cytochrome P-450 drug metabolizing enzyme system of the liver. Because ondansetron is metabolized by hepatic cytochrome P-450 drug-metabolizing enzymes (CYP3A4, CYP2D6, CYP1A2), inducers or inhibitors of these enzymes may change the clearance and, hence, the half-life of ondansetron. On the basis of available data, no dosage adjustment is recommended for patients on these drugs).
No products indexed under this heading.

Imipramine Pamoate (Ondansetron does not itself appear to induce or inhibit the cytochrome P-450 drug metabolizing enzyme system of the liver. Because ondansetron is metabolized by hepatic cytochrome P-450 drug-metabolizing enzymes (CYP3A4, CYP2D6, CYP1A2), inducers or inhibitors of these enzymes may change the clearance and, hence, the half-life of ondansetron. On the basis of available data, no dosage adjustment is recommended for patients on these drugs).
No products indexed under this heading.

Indinavir Sulfate (Ondansetron does not itself appear to induce or inhibit the cytochrome P-450 drug metabolizing enzyme system of the liver. Because ondansetron is metabolized by hepatic cytochrome P-450 drug-metabolizing enzymes (CYP3A4, CYP2D6, CYP1A2), inducers or inhibitors of these enzymes may change the clearance and, hence, the half-life of ondansetron. On the basis of available data, no dosage adjustment is recommended for patients on these drugs). Products include:
Crixivan 2113

Indomethacin (*In vitro* metabolism studies have shown that ondansetron is a substrate for human hepatic cytochrome P-450 enzymes, including CYP1A2, CYP2D6, and CYP3A4. In terms of overall ondansetron turnover, CYP3A4 played the predominant role. Because of the multiplicity of metabolic enzymes capable of metabolizing ondansetron, it is likely that inhibition of one of these enzymes will be compensated by others and may result in little change in overall rates of ondansetron elimination). Products include:
Indocin 2167

Indomethacin Sodium Trihydrate (*In vitro* metabolism studies have shown that ondansetron is a substrate for human hepatic cytochrome P-450 enzymes, including CYP1A2, CYP2D6, and CYP3A4. In terms of overall ondansetron turnover, CYP3A4 played the predominant role. Because of the multiplicity of metabolic enzymes capable of metabolizing ondansetron, it is likely that inhibition of one of these enzymes will be compensated by others and may result in little change in overall rates of ondansetron elimination). Products include:
Indocin I.V. 2007

Insulin (Ondansetron does not itself appear to induce or inhibit the cytochrome P-450 drug metabolizing enzyme system of the liver. Because ondansetron is metabolized by hepatic cytochrome P-450 drug-metabolizing enzymes (CYP3A4, CYP2D6, CYP1A2), inducers or inhibitors of these enzymes may change the clearance and, hence, the half-life of ondansetron. On the basis of available data, no dosage adjustment is recommended for patients on these drugs).
No products indexed under this heading.

Insulin, Human, Zinc Suspension (Ondansetron does not itself appear to induce or inhibit the cytochrome P-450 drug metabolizing enzyme system of the liver. Because ondansetron is metabolized by hepatic cytochrome P-450 drug-metabolizing enzymes (CYP3A4, CYP2D6, CYP1A2), inducers or inhibitors of these enzymes may change the clearance and, hence, the half-life of ondansetron. On the basis of available data, no dosage adjustment is recommended for patients on these drugs).
No products indexed under this heading.

Insulin, Human (rDNA origin) (Ondansetron does not itself appear to induce or inhibit the cytochrome P-450 drug metabolizing enzyme system of the liver. Because ondansetron is metabolized by hepatic cytochrome P-450 drug-metabolizing enzymes (CYP3A4, CYP2D6, CYP1A2), inducers or inhibitors of these enzymes may change the clearance and, hence, the half-life of ondansetron. On the basis of available data, no dosage adjustment is recommended for patients on these drugs). Products include:
Exubera 2717

Insulin, Human NPH (Ondansetron does not itself appear to induce or inhibit the cytochrome P-450 drug metabolizing enzyme system of the liver. Because ondansetron is metabolized by hepatic cytochrome P-450 drug-metabolizing enzymes (CYP3A4, CYP2D6, CYP1A2), inducers or inhibitors of these enzymes may change the clearance and, hence, the half-life of ondansetron. On the basis of available data, no dosage adjustment is recommended for patients on these drugs). Products include:
Humulin N Vial 1934

Insulin, Human Regular (Ondansetron does not itself appear to induce or inhibit the cytochrome P-450 drug metabolizing enzyme system of the liver. Because ondansetron is metabolized by hepatic cytochrome P-450 drug-metabolizing enzymes (CYP3A4, CYP2D6, CYP1A2), inducers or inhibitors of these enzymes may change the clearance and, hence, the half-life of ondansetron. On the basis of available data, no dosage adjustment is recommended for patients on these drugs). Products include:
Humulin R 1937
Humulin R (U-500) 1939

Insulin, Human Regular and Human NPH Mixture (Ondansetron does not itself appear to induce or inhibit the cytochrome P-450 drug metabolizing enzyme system of the liver. Because ondansetron is metabolized by hepatic cytochrome P-450 drug-metabolizing enzymes (CYP3A4, CYP2D6, CYP1A2), inducers or inhibitors of these enzymes may change the clearance and, hence, the half-life of ondansetron. On the basis of available data, no dosage adjustment is recommended for patients on these drugs). Products include:
Humulin 50/50 1930
Humulin 70/30 Vial 1931

Insulin, NPH (Ondansetron does not itself appear to induce or inhibit the cytochrome P-450 drug metabolizing enzyme system of the liver. Because ondansetron is metabolized by hepatic cytochrome P-450 drug-metabolizing enzymes (CYP3A4, CYP2D6, CYP1A2), inducers or inhibitors of these enzymes may change the clearance and, hence, the half-life of ondansetron. On the basis of available data, no dosage adjustment is recommended for patients on these drugs).
No products indexed under this heading.

Insulin, Regular (Ondansetron does not itself appear to induce or inhibit the cytochrome P-450 drug metabolizing enzyme system of the liver. Because ondansetron is metabolized by hepatic cytochrome P-450 drug-metabolizing enzymes (CYP3A4, CYP2D6, CYP1A2), inducers or inhibitors of these enzymes may change the clearance and, hence, the half-life of ondansetron. On the basis of available data, no dosage adjustment is recommended for patients on these drugs).
No products indexed under this heading.

Insulin, Regular and NPH mixture (Ondansetron does not itself appear to induce or inhibit the cytochrome P-450 drug metabolizing enzyme system of the liver. Because ondansetron is metabolized by hepatic cytochrome P-450 drug-metabolizing enzymes (CYP3A4, CYP2D6, CYP1A2), inducers or inhibitors of these enzymes may change the clearance and, hence, the half-life of ondansetron. On the basis of available data, no dosage adjustment is recommended for patients on these drugs).
No products indexed under this heading.

Insulin, Zinc Crystals (Ondansetron does not itself appear to induce or inhibit the cytochrome P-450 drug metabolizing enzyme system of the liver. Because ondansetron is metabolized by hepatic cytochrome P-450 drug-metabolizing enzymes (CYP3A4, CYP2D6, CYP1A2), inducers or inhibitors of these enzymes may change the clearance and, hence, the half-life of ondansetron. On the basis of available data, no dosage adjustment is recommended for patients on these drugs).
No products indexed under this heading.

Insulin, Zinc Suspension (Ondansetron does not itself appear to induce or inhibit the cytochrome P-450 drug metabolizing enzyme system of the liver. Because ondansetron is metabolized by hepatic cytochrome P-450 drug-metabolizing enzymes (CYP3A4, CYP2D6, CYP1A2), inducers or inhibitors of these enzymes may change the clearance and, hence, the half-life of ondansetron. On the basis of available data, no dosage adjustment is recommended for patients on these drugs).
No products indexed under this heading.

Insulin Aspart (Ondansetron does not itself appear to induce or inhibit the cytochrome P-450 drug metabolizing enzyme system of the liver. Because ondansetron is metabolized by hepatic cytochrome P-450 drug-metabolizing enzymes (CYP3A4, CYP2D6, CYP1A2), inducers or inhibitors of these enzymes may change the clearance and, hence, the half-life of ondansetron. On the basis of available data, no dosage adjustment is recommended for patients on these drugs).
No products indexed under this heading.

Insulin Aspart, Human (Ondansetron does not itself appear to induce or inhibit the cytochrome P-450 drug metabolizing enzyme system of the liver. Because ondansetron is metabolized by hepatic cytochrome P-450 drug-metabolizing enzymes (CYP3A4, CYP2D6, CYP1A2), inducers or inhibitors of these enzymes may change the clearance and, hence, the half-life of ondansetron. On the basis of available data, no dosage adjustment is recommended for patients on these drugs). Products include:
NovoLog Mix 70/30 2581

Insulin Aspart, Human Regular (Ondansetron does not itself appear to induce or inhibit the cytochrome P-450 drug metabolizing enzyme system of the liver. Because ondansetron is metabolized by hepatic cytochrome P-450 drug-metabolizing enzymes (CYP3A4, CYP2D6, CYP1A2), inducers or inhibitors of these enzymes may change the clearance and, hence, the half-life of ondansetron. On the basis of available data, no dosage adjustment is recommended for patients on these drugs). Products include:
NovoLog 2575

Insulin Aspart Protamine, Human (Ondansetron does not itself appear to induce or inhibit the cytochrome P-450 drug metabolizing enzyme system of the liver. Because ondansetron is metabolized by hepatic cytochrome P-450 drug-metabolizing enzymes (CYP3A4, CYP2D6, CYP1A2), inducers or inhibitors of these enzymes may change the clearance and, hence, the half-life of ondansetron. On the basis of available data, no dosage adjustment is recommended for patients on these drugs). Products include:
NovoLog Mix 70/30 2581

Insulin Detemir (rDNA Origin) (Ondansetron does not itself appear to induce or inhibit the cytochrome P-450 drug metabolizing enzyme system of the liver. Because ondansetron is metabolized by hepatic cytochrome P-450 drug-metabolizing enzymes (CYP3A4, CYP2D6, CYP1A2), inducers or inhibitors of these enzymes may change the clearance and, hence, the half-life of ondansetron. On the basis of available data, no dosage adjustment is recommended for patients on these drugs). Products include:
Levemir 2566

Insulin Glargine (Ondansetron does not itself appear to induce or inhibit the cytochrome P-450 drug metabolizing enzyme system of the liver. Because ondansetron is metabolized by hepatic cytochrome P-450 drug-metabolizing enzymes (CYP3A4, CYP2D6, CYP1A2), inducers or inhibitors of these enzymes may change the clearance and, hence, the half-life of ondansetron. On the basis of available data, no dosage adjustment is recommended for patients on these drugs). Products include:
Lantus 2996

Insulin Glulisine (Ondansetron does not itself appear to induce or inhibit the cytochrome P-450 drug metabolizing enzyme system of the liver. Because ondansetron is metabolized by hepatic cytochrome P-450 drug-metabolizing enzymes (CYP3A4, CYP2D6, CYP1A2), inducers or inhibitors of these enzymes may change the clearance and, hence, the half-life of ondansetron. On the basis of available data, no dosage adjustment is recommended for patients on these drugs). Products include:
Apidra 2937
Apidra SoloStar 2937

Insulin Lispro, Human (Ondansetron does not itself appear to induce or inhibit the cytochrome P-450 drug metabolizing enzyme system of the liver. Because ondansetron is metabolized by hepatic cytochrome P-450 drug-metabolizing enzymes (CYP3A4, CYP2D6, CYP1A2), inducers or inhibitors of these enzymes may change the clearance and, hence, the half-life of ondansetron. On the basis of available data, no dosage adjustment is recommended for patients on these drugs). Products include:
Humalog 1910
Humalog Mix 1914
Humalog Mix75/25 1917

IMPORTANT NOTE: Always consult each drug listing in the patient's regimen for possible interactions.

Zofran Interactions Index 2160

Insulin Lispro Protamine, Human (Ondansetron does not itself appear to induce or inhibit the cytochrome P-450 drug metabolizing enzyme system of the liver. Because ondansetron is metabolized by hepatic cytochrome P-450 drug-metabolizing enzymes (CYP3A4, CYP2D6, CYP1A2), inducers or inhibitors of these enzymes may change the clearance and, hence, the half-life of ondansetron. On the basis of available data, no dosage adjustment is recommended for patients on these drugs). Products include:
Humalog Mix 1914
Humalog Mix75/25 1917

Interferon alfa-2a, Recombinant (There have been reports of liver failure and death in patients with cancer receiving concurrent medications including potentially hepatotoxic cytotoxic chemotherapeutic drugs. The etiology of the liver failure is unclear).
No products indexed under this heading.

Interferon alfa-2b, Recombinant (There have been reports of liver failure and death in patients with cancer receiving concurrent medications including potentially hepatotoxic cytotoxic chemotherapeutic drugs. The etiology of the liver failure is unclear). Products include:
Intron A 3140

Irinotecan Hydrochloride (There have been reports of liver failure and death in patients with cancer receiving concurrent medications including potentially hepatotoxic cytotoxic chemotherapeutic drugs. The etiology of the liver failure is unclear).
No products indexed under this heading.

Isoniazid (Ondansetron does not itself appear to induce or inhibit the cytochrome P-450 drug metabolizing enzyme system of the liver. Because ondansetron is metabolized by hepatic cytochrome P-450 drug-metabolizing enzymes (CYP3A4, CYP2D6, CYP1A2), inducers or inhibitors of these enzymes may change the clearance and, hence, the half-life of ondansetron. On the basis of available data, no dosage adjustment is recommended for patients on these drugs).
No products indexed under this heading.

Itraconazole (Ondansetron does not itself appear to induce or inhibit the cytochrome P-450 drug metabolizing enzyme system of the liver. Because ondansetron is metabolized by hepatic cytochrome P-450 drug-metabolizing enzymes (CYP3A4, CYP2D6, CYP1A2), inducers or inhibitors of these enzymes may change the clearance and, hence, the half-life of ondansetron. On the basis of available data, no dosage adjustment is recommended for patients on these drugs).
No products indexed under this heading.

Kanamycin Sulfate (There have been reports of liver failure and death in patients with cancer receiving concurrent medications including antibiotics. The etiology of liver failure is unclear).
No products indexed under this heading.

Ketoconazole (Ondansetron does not itself appear to induce or inhibit the cytochrome P-450 drug metabolizing enzyme system of the liver. Because ondansetron is metabolized by hepatic cytochrome P-450 drug-metabolizing enzymes (CYP3A4, CYP2D6, CYP1A2), inducers or inhibitors of these enzymes may change the clearance and, hence, the half-life of ondansetron. On the basis of available data, no dosage adjustment is recommended for patients on these drugs). Products include:
Extina 3319
Xolegel 3337

Ketoprofen (*In vitro* metabolism studies have shown that ondansetron is a substrate for human hepatic cytochrome P-450 enzymes, including CYP1A2, CYP2D6, and CYP3A4. In terms of overall ondansetron turnover, CYP3A4 played the predominant role. Because of the multiplicity of metabolic enzymes capable of metabolizing ondansetron, it is likely that inhibition of one of these enzymes will be compensated by others and may result in little change in overall rates of ondansetron elimination).
No products indexed under this heading.

Lansoprazole (Ondansetron does not itself appear to induce or inhibit the cytochrome P-450 drug metabolizing enzyme system of the liver. Because ondansetron is metabolized by hepatic cytochrome P-450 drug-metabolizing enzymes (CYP3A4, CYP2D6, CYP1A2), inducers or inhibitors of these enzymes may change the clearance and, hence, the half-life of ondansetron. On the basis of available data, no dosage adjustment is recommended for patients on these drugs).
No products indexed under this heading.

Lapatinib (Ondansetron does not itself appear to induce or inhibit the cytochrome P-450 drug metabolizing enzyme system of the liver. Because ondansetron is metabolized by hepatic cytochrome P-450 drug-metabolizing enzymes (CYP3A4, CYP2D6, CYP1A2), inducers or inhibitors of these enzymes may change the clearance and, hence, the half-life of ondansetron. On the basis of available data, no dosage adjustment is recommended for patients on these drugs). Products include:
Tykerb 1698

Leflunomide (*In vitro* metabolism studies have shown that ondansetron is a substrate for human hepatic cytochrome P-450 enzymes, including CYP1A2, CYP2D6, and CYP3A4. In terms of overall ondansetron turnover, CYP3A4 played the predominant role. Because of the multiplicity of metabolic enzymes capable of metabolizing ondansetron, it is likely that inhibition of one of these enzymes will be compensated by others and may result in little change in overall rates of ondansetron elimination).
No products indexed under this heading.

Letrozole (*In vitro* metabolism studies have shown that ondansetron is a substrate for human hepatic cytochrome P-450 enzymes, including CYP1A2, CYP2D6, and CYP3A4. In terms of overall ondansetron turnover, CYP3A4 played the predominant role. Because of the multiplicity of metabolic enzymes capable of metabolizing ondansetron, it is likely that inhibition of one of these enzymes will be compensated by others and may result in little change in overall rates of ondansetron elimination). Products include:
Femara 2466

Levamisole Hydrochloride (There have been reports of liver failure and death in patients with cancer receiving concurrent medications including potentially hepatotoxic cytotoxic chemotherapeutic drugs. The etiology of the liver failure is unclear).
No products indexed under this heading.

Levofloxacin (There have been reports of liver failure and death in patients with cancer receiving concurrent medications including antibiotics. The etiology of liver failure is unclear). Products include:
Iquix 3492
Levaquin 2629
Levaquin in 5% Dextrose 2629
Quixin 3493

Levonorgestrel (Ondansetron does not itself appear to induce or inhibit the cytochrome P-450 drug metabolizing enzyme system of the liver. Because ondansetron is metabolized by hepatic cytochrome P-450 drug-metabolizing enzymes (CYP3A4, CYP2D6, CYP1A2), inducers or inhibitors of these enzymes may change the clearance and, hence, the half-life of ondansetron. On the basis of available data, no dosage adjustment is recommended for patients on these drugs). Products include:
Climara Pro 847
LoSeasonique 3407
Lybrel 3514
Mirena 854
Plan B 3416
Seasonique 3418

Lomefloxacin Hydrochloride (There have been reports of liver failure and death in patients with cancer receiving concurrent medications including antibiotics. The etiology of liver failure is unclear).
No products indexed under this heading.

Lomustine (CCNU) (There have been reports of liver failure and death in patients with cancer receiving concurrent medications including potentially hepatotoxic cytotoxic chemotherapeutic drugs. The etiology of the liver failure is unclear).
No products indexed under this heading.

Lopinavir (Ondansetron does not itself appear to induce or inhibit the cytochrome P-450 drug metabolizing enzyme system of the liver. Because ondansetron is metabolized by hepatic cytochrome P-450 drug-metabolizing enzymes (CYP3A4, CYP2D6, CYP1A2), inducers or inhibitors of these enzymes may change the clearance and, hence, the half-life of ondansetron. On the basis of available data, no dosage adjustment is recommended for patients on these drugs). Products include:
Kaletra 458

Loracarbef (There have been reports of liver failure and death in patients with cancer receiving concurrent medications including antibiotics. The etiology of liver failure is unclear).
No products indexed under this heading.

Loratadine (Ondansetron does not itself appear to induce or inhibit the cytochrome P-450 drug metabolizing enzyme system of the liver. Because ondansetron is metabolized by hepatic cytochrome P-450 drug-metabolizing enzymes (CYP3A4, CYP2D6, CYP1A2), inducers or inhibitors of these enzymes may change the clearance and, hence, the half-life of ondansetron. On the basis of available data, no dosage adjustment is recommended for patients on these drugs).
No products indexed under this heading.

Lovastatin (*In vitro* metabolism studies have shown that ondansetron is a substrate for human hepatic cytochrome P-450 enzymes, including CYP1A2, CYP2D6, and CYP3A4. In terms of overall ondansetron turnover, CYP3A4 played the predominant role. Because of the multiplicity of metabolic enzymes capable of metabolizing ondansetron, it is likely that inhibition of one of these enzymes will be compensated by others and may result in little change in overall rates of ondansetron elimination). Products include:
Advicor 402
Mevacor 2212

Maprotiline Hydrochloride (Ondansetron does not itself appear to induce or inhibit the cytochrome P-450 drug metabolizing enzyme system of the liver. Because ondansetron is metabolized by hepatic cytochrome P-450 drug-metabolizing enzymes (CYP3A4, CYP2D6, CYP1A2), inducers or inhibitors of these enzymes may change the clearance and, hence, the half-life of ondansetron. On the basis of available data, no dosage adjustment is recommended for patients on these drugs).
No products indexed under this heading.

Mechlorethamine Hydrochloride (There have been reports of liver failure and death in patients with cancer receiving concurrent medications including potentially hepatotoxic cytotoxic chemotherapeutic drugs. The etiology of the liver failure is unclear). Products include:
Mustargen 2010

Megestrol Acetate (There have been reports of liver failure and death in patients with cancer receiving concurrent medications including potentially hepatotoxic cytotoxic chemotherapeutic drugs. The etiology of the liver failure is unclear). Products include:
Megace ES 2698

Melphalan (There have been reports of liver failure and death in patients with cancer receiving concurrent medications including potentially hepatotoxic cytotoxic chemotherapeutic drugs. The etiology of the liver failure is unclear). Products include:
Alkeran 1302

Mephenytoin (Ondansetron does not itself appear to induce or inhibit the cytochrome P-450 drug metabolizing enzyme system of the liver. Because ondansetron is metabolized by hepatic cytochrome P-450 drug-metabolizing enzymes (CYP3A4, CYP2D6, CYP1A2), inducers or inhibitors of these enzymes may change the clearance and, hence, the half-life of ondansetron. In patients treated with potent inducers of CYP3A4 the clearance of ondansetron was significantly increased and ondansetron blood concentrations were decreased. However, on the basis of available data, no dosage adjustment for ondansetron is recommended for patients on these drugs).
No products indexed under this heading.

Mercaptopurine (There have been reports of liver failure and death in patients with cancer receiving concurrent medications including potentially hepatotoxic cytotoxic chemotherapeutic drugs. The etiology of the liver failure is unclear).
No products indexed under this heading.

Mestranol (Ondansetron does not itself appear to induce or inhibit the cytochrome P-450 drug metabolizing enzyme system of the liver. Because ondansetron is metabolized by hepatic cytochrome P-450 drug-metabolizing enzymes (CYP3A4, CYP2D6, CYP1A2), inducers or inhibitors of these enzymes may change the clearance and, hence, the half-life of ondansetron. On the basis of available data, no dosage adjustment is recommended for patients on these drugs).
No products indexed under this heading.

Methacycline Hydrochloride (There have been reports of liver failure and death in patients with cancer receiving concurrent medications including antibiotics. The etiology of liver failure is unclear).
No products indexed under this heading.

Methadone Hydrochloride (Ondansetron does not itself appear to induce or inhibit the cytochrome P-450 drug metabolizing enzyme system of the liver. Because ondansetron is metabolized by hepatic cytochrome P-450 drug-metabolizing enzymes (CYP3A4, CYP2D6, CYP1A2), inducers or inhibitors of these enzymes may change the clearance and, hence, the half-life of ondansetron. On the basis of

2161 **Interactions Index** **Zofran**

available data, no dosage adjustment is recommended for patients on these drugs).
No products indexed under this heading.

Methicillin Sodium (There have been reports of liver failure and death in patients with cancer receiving concurrent medications including antibiotics. The etiology of liver failure is unclear).
No products indexed under this heading.

Methotrexate (There have been reports of liver failure and death in patients with cancer receiving concurrent medications including potentially hepatotoxic cytotoxic chemotherapeutic drugs. The etiology of the liver failure is unclear).
No products indexed under this heading.

Methotrexate Sodium (There have been reports of liver failure and death in patients with cancer receiving concurrent medications including potentially hepatotoxic cytotoxic chemotherapeutic drugs. The etiology of liver failure is unclear).
No products indexed under this heading.

Methoxsalen (Ondansetron does not itself appear to induce or inhibit the cytochrome P-450 drug metabolizing enzyme system of the liver. Because ondansetron is metabolized by hepatic cytochrome P-450 drug-metabolizing enzymes (CYP3A4, CYP2D6, CYP1A2), inducers or inhibitors of these enzymes may change the clearance and, hence, the half-life of ondansetron. On the basis of available data, no dosage adjustment is recommended for patients on these drugs).
No products indexed under this heading.

Methsuximide (Ondansetron does not itself appear to induce or inhibit the cytochrome P-450 drug metabolizing enzyme system of the liver. Because ondansetron is metabolized by hepatic cytochrome P-450 drug-metabolizing enzymes (CYP3A4, CYP2D6, CYP1A2), inducers or inhibitors of these enzymes may change the clearance and, hence, the half-life of ondansetron. In patients treated with potent inducers of CYP3A4 the clearance of ondansetron was significantly increased and ondansetron blood concentrations were decreased. However, on the basis of available data, no dosage adjustment for ondansetron is recommended for patients on these drugs).
No products indexed under this heading.

Methyclothiazide (*In vitro* metabolism studies have shown that ondansetron is a substrate for human hepatic cytochrome P-450 enzymes, including CYP1A2, CYP2D6, and CYP3A4. In terms of overall ondansetron turnover, CYP3A4 played the predominant role. Because of the multiplicity of metabolic enzymes capable of metabolizing ondansetron, it is likely that inhibition of one of these enzymes will be compensated by others and may result in little change in overall rates of ondansetron elimination).
No products indexed under this heading.

Methylprednisolone (Ondansetron does not itself appear to induce or inhibit the cytochrome P-450 drug metabolizing enzyme system of the liver. Because ondansetron is metabolized by hepatic cytochrome P-450 drug-metabolizing enzymes (CYP3A4, CYP2D6, CYP1A2), inducers or inhibitors of these enzymes may change the clearance and, hence, the half-life of ondansetron. In patients treated with potent inducers of CYP3A4 the clearance of ondansetron was significantly increased and ondansetron blood concentrations were decreased. However, on the basis of available data, no dosage adjustment for ondansetron is recommended for patients on these drugs).
No products indexed under this heading.

Methylprednisolone Acetate (Ondansetron does not itself appear to induce or inhibit the cytochrome P-450 drug metabolizing enzyme system of the liver. Because ondansetron is metabolized by hepatic cytochrome P-450 drug-metabolizing enzymes (CYP3A4, CYP2D6, CYP1A2), inducers or inhibitors of these enzymes may change the clearance and, hence, the half-life of ondansetron. In patients treated with potent inducers of CYP3A4 the clearance of ondansetron was significantly increased and ondansetron blood concentrations were decreased. However, on the basis of available data, no dosage adjustment for ondansetron is recommended for patients on these drugs).
No products indexed under this heading.

Methylprednisolone Sodium Succinate (Ondansetron does not itself appear to induce or inhibit the cytochrome P-450 drug metabolizing enzyme system of the liver. Because ondansetron is metabolized by hepatic cytochrome P-450 drug-metabolizing enzymes (CYP3A4, CYP2D6, CYP1A2), inducers or inhibitors of these enzymes may change the clearance and, hence, the half-life of ondansetron. In patients treated with potent inducers of CYP3A4 the clearance of ondansetron was significantly increased and ondansetron blood concentrations were decreased. However, on the basis of available data, no dosage adjustment for ondansetron is recommended for patients on these drugs).
No products indexed under this heading.

Metronidazole (Ondansetron does not itself appear to induce or inhibit the cytochrome P-450 drug metabolizing enzyme system of the liver. Because ondansetron is metabolized by hepatic cytochrome P-450 drug-metabolizing enzymes (CYP3A4, CYP2D6, CYP1A2), inducers or inhibitors of these enzymes may change the clearance and, hence, the half-life of ondansetron. On the basis of available data, no dosage adjustment is recommended for patients on these drugs). Products include:
Pylera 793

Metronidazole Benzoate (Ondansetron does not itself appear to induce or inhibit the cytochrome P-450 drug metabolizing enzyme system of the liver. Because ondansetron is metabolized by hepatic cytochrome P-450 drug-metabolizing enzymes (CYP3A4, CYP2D6, CYP1A2), inducers or inhibitors of these enzymes may change the clearance and, hence, the half-life of ondansetron. On the basis of available data, no dosage adjustment is recommended for patients on these drugs).
No products indexed under this heading.

Metronidazole Hydrochloride (Ondansetron does not itself appear to induce or inhibit the cytochrome P-450 drug metabolizing enzyme system of the liver. Because ondansetron is metabolized by hepatic cytochrome P-450 drug-metabolizing enzymes (CYP3A4, CYP2D6, CYP1A2), inducers or inhibitors of these enzymes may change the clearance and, hence, the half-life of ondansetron. On the basis of available data, no dosage adjustment is recommended for patients on these drugs).
No products indexed under this heading.

Metronidazole Sodium (Ondansetron does not itself appear to induce or inhibit the cytochrome P-450 drug metabolizing enzyme system of the liver. Because ondansetron is metabolized by hepatic cytochrome P-450 drug-metabolizing enzymes (CYP3A4, CYP2D6, CYP1A2), inducers or inhibitors of these enzymes may change the clearance and, hence, the half-life of ondansetron. On the basis of available data, no dosage adjustment is recommended for patients on these drugs).
No products indexed under this heading.

Mexiletine Hydrochloride (Ondansetron does not itself appear to induce or inhibit the cytochrome P-450 drug metabolizing enzyme system of the liver. Because ondansetron is metabolized by hepatic cytochrome P-450 drug-metabolizing enzymes (CYP3A4, CYP2D6, CYP1A2), inducers or inhibitors of these enzymes may change the clearance and, hence, the half-life of ondansetron. On the basis of available data, no dosage adjustment is recommended for patients on these drugs).
No products indexed under this heading.

Mezlocillin Sodium (There have been reports of liver failure and death in patients with cancer receiving concurrent medications including antibiotics. The etiology of liver failure is unclear).
No products indexed under this heading.

Mibefradil Dihydrochloride (Ondansetron does not itself appear to induce or inhibit the cytochrome P-450 drug metabolizing enzyme system of the liver. Because ondansetron is metabolized by hepatic cytochrome P-450 drug-metabolizing enzymes (CYP3A4, CYP2D6, CYP1A2), inducers or inhibitors of these enzymes may change the clearance and, hence, the half-life of ondansetron. On the basis of available data, no dosage adjustment is recommended for patients on these drugs).
No products indexed under this heading.

Miconazole (Ondansetron does not itself appear to induce or inhibit the cytochrome P-450 drug metabolizing enzyme system of the liver. Because ondansetron is metabolized by hepatic cytochrome P-450 drug-metabolizing enzymes (CYP3A4, CYP2D6, CYP1A2), inducers or inhibitors of these enzymes may change the clearance and, hence, the half-life of ondansetron. On the basis of available data, no dosage adjustment is recommended for patients on these drugs).
No products indexed under this heading.

Miconazole Nitrate (Ondansetron does not itself appear to induce or inhibit the cytochrome P-450 drug metabolizing enzyme system of the liver. Because ondansetron is metabolized by hepatic cytochrome P-450 drug-metabolizing enzymes (CYP3A4, CYP2D6, CYP1A2), inducers or inhibitors of these enzymes may change the clearance and, hence, the half-life of ondansetron. On the basis of available data, no dosage adjustment is recommended for patients on these drugs). Products include:
Vusion Ointment 3335

Mifepristone (Ondansetron does not itself appear to induce or inhibit the cytochrome P-450 drug metabolizing enzyme system of the liver. Because ondansetron is metabolized by hepatic cytochrome P-450 drug-metabolizing enzymes (CYP3A4, CYP2D6, CYP1A2), inducers or inhibitors of these enzymes may change the clearance and, hence, the half-life of ondansetron. On the basis of available data, no dosage adjustment is recommended for patients on these drugs).
No products indexed under this heading.

Minocycline Hydrochloride (There have been reports of liver failure and death in patients with cancer receiving concurrent medications including antibiotics. The etiology of liver failure is unclear). Products include:
Solodyn 2073

Mitomycin (Mitomycin-C) (There have been reports of liver failure and death in patients with cancer receiving concurrent medications including potentially hepatotoxic cytotoxic chemotherapeutic drugs. The etiology of the liver failure is unclear).
No products indexed under this heading.

Mitotane (There have been reports of liver failure and death in patients with cancer receiving concurrent medications including potentially hepatotoxic cytotoxic chemotherapeutic drugs. The etiology of liver failure is unclear).
No products indexed under this heading.

Mitoxantrone Hydrochloride (There have been reports of liver failure and death in patients with cancer receiving concurrent medications including potentially hepatotoxic cytotoxic chemotherapeutic drugs. The etiology of liver failure is unclear). Products include:
Novantrone 1088

Moclobemide (Ondansetron does not itself appear to induce or inhibit the cytochrome P-450 drug metabolizing enzyme system of the liver. Because ondansetron is metabolized by hepatic cytochrome P-450 drug-metabolizing enzymes (CYP3A4, CYP2D6, CYP1A2), inducers or inhibitors of these enzymes may change the clearance and, hence, the half-life of ondansetron. On the basis of available data, no dosage adjustment is recommended for patients on these drugs).
No products indexed under this heading.

Modafinil (Ondansetron does not itself appear to induce or inhibit the cytochrome P-450 drug metabolizing enzyme system of the liver. Because ondansetron is metabolized by hepatic cytochrome P-450 drug-metabolizing enzymes (CYP3A4, CYP2D6, CYP1A2), inducers or inhibitors of these enzymes may change the clearance and, hence, the half-life of ondansetron. In patients treated with potent inducers of CYP3A4 the clearance of ondansetron was significantly increased and ondansetron blood concentrations were decreased. However, on the basis of available data, no dosage adjustment for ondansetron is recommended for patients on these drugs). Products include:
Provigil 983

Moxifloxacin Hydrochloride (There have been reports of liver failure and death in patients with cancer receiving concurrent medications including antibiotics. The etiology of liver failure is unclear). Products include:
Avelox 3064
Vigamox 589

Nafcillin Sodium (There have been reports of liver failure and death in patients with cancer receiving concurrent medications including antibiotics. The etiology of liver failure is unclear).
No products indexed under this heading.

Nalidixic Acid (Ondansetron does not itself appear to induce or inhibit the cytochrome P-450 drug metabolizing enzyme system of the liver. Because ondansetron is metabolized by hepatic cytochrome P-450 drug-metabolizing enzymes (CYP3A4, CYP2D6, CYP1A2), inducers or inhibitors of these enzymes may change the clearance and, hence, the half-life of ondansetron. On the basis of available data, no dosage adjustment is recommended for patients on these drugs).
No products indexed under this heading.

Nefazodone Hydrochloride (Ondansetron does not itself appear to induce or inhibit the cytochrome P-450

Zofran Interactions Index 2162

drug metabolizing enzyme system of the liver. Because ondansetron is metabolized by hepatic cytochrome P-450 drug-metabolizing enzymes (CYP3A4, CYP2D6, CYP1A2), inducers or inhibitors of these enzymes may change the clearance and, hence, the half-life of ondansetron. On the basis of available data, no dosage adjustment is recommended for patients on these drugs).
No products indexed under this heading.

Nelfinavir Mesylate (Ondansetron does not itself appear to induce or inhibit the cytochrome P-450 drug metabolizing enzyme system of the liver. Because ondansetron is metabolized by hepatic cytochrome P-450 drug-metabolizing enzymes (CYP3A4, CYP2D6, CYP1A2), inducers or inhibitors of these enzymes may change the clearance and, hence, the half-life of ondansetron. On the basis of available data, no dosage adjustment is recommended for patients on these drugs).
No products indexed under this heading.

Nevirapine (Ondansetron does not itself appear to induce or inhibit the cytochrome P-450 drug metabolizing enzyme system of the liver. Because ondansetron is metabolized by hepatic cytochrome P-450 drug-metabolizing enzymes (CYP3A4, CYP2D6, CYP1A2), inducers or inhibitors of these enzymes may change the clearance and, hence, the half-life of ondansetron. In patients treated with potent inducers of CYP3A4 the clearance of ondansetron was significantly increased and ondansetron blood concentrations were decreased. However, on the basis of available data, no dosage adjustment for ondansetron is recommended for patients on these drugs). Products include:
Viramune Oral Suspension 897
Viramune Tablets 897

Niacin (Ondansetron does not itself appear to induce or inhibit the cytochrome P-450 drug metabolizing enzyme system of the liver. Because ondansetron is metabolized by hepatic cytochrome P-450 drug-metabolizing enzymes (CYP3A4, CYP2D6, CYP1A2), inducers or inhibitors of these enzymes may change the clearance and, hence, the half-life of ondansetron. On the basis of available data, no dosage adjustment is recommended for patients on these drugs). Products include:
Advicor 402
Cardio Basics 3455
Niaspan 497
Simcor 524

Niacinamide (Ondansetron does not itself appear to induce or inhibit the cytochrome P-450 drug metabolizing enzyme system of the liver. Because ondansetron is metabolized by hepatic cytochrome P-450 drug-metabolizing enzymes (CYP3A4, CYP2D6, CYP1A2), inducers or inhibitors of these enzymes may change the clearance and, hence, the half-life of ondansetron. On the basis of available data, no dosage adjustment is recommended for patients on these drugs). Products include:
CitraNatal 90 DHA Capsules 2332
CitraNatal Assure 2332
CitraNatal Rx 2332
Heplive 607

Niacinamide Hydroiodide (Ondansetron does not itself appear to induce or inhibit the cytochrome P-450 drug metabolizing enzyme system of the liver. Because ondansetron is metabolized by hepatic cytochrome P-450 drug-metabolizing enzymes (CYP3A4, CYP2D6, CYP1A2), inducers or inhibitors of these enzymes may change the clearance and, hence, the half-life of ondansetron. On the basis of available data, no dosage adjustment is recommended for patients on these drugs).
No products indexed under this heading.

Nicardipine (*In vitro* metabolism studies have shown that ondansetron is a substrate for human hepatic cytochrome P-450 enzymes, including CYP1A2, CYP2D6, and CYP3A4. In terms of overall ondansetron turnover, CYP3A4 played the predominant role. Because of the multiplicity of metabolic enzymes capable of metabolizing ondansetron, it is likely that inhibition of one of these enzymes will be compensated by others and may result in little change in overall rates of ondansetron elimination).
No products indexed under this heading.

Nicardipine Hydrochloride (*In vitro* metabolism studies have shown that ondansetron is a substrate for human hepatic cytochrome P-450 enzymes, including CYP1A2, CYP2D6, and CYP3A4. In terms of overall ondansetron turnover, CYP3A4 played the predominant role. Because of the multiplicity of metabolic enzymes capable of metabolizing ondansetron, it is likely that inhibition of one of these enzymes will be compensated by others and may result in little change in overall rates of ondansetron elimination).
No products indexed under this heading.

Nicotinamide (Ondansetron does not itself appear to induce or inhibit the cytochrome P-450 drug metabolizing enzyme system of the liver. Because ondansetron is metabolized by hepatic cytochrome P-450 drug-metabolizing enzymes (CYP3A4, CYP2D6, CYP1A2), inducers or inhibitors of these enzymes may change the clearance and, hence, the half-life of ondansetron. On the basis of available data, no dosage adjustment is recommended for patients on these drugs).
No products indexed under this heading.

Nicotine (Ondansetron does not itself appear to induce or inhibit the cytochrome P-450 drug metabolizing enzyme system of the liver. Because ondansetron is metabolized by hepatic cytochrome P-450 drug-metabolizing enzymes (CYP3A4, CYP2D6, CYP1A2), inducers or inhibitors of these enzymes may change the clearance and, hence, the half-life of ondansetron. On the basis of available data, no dosage adjustment is recommended for patients on these drugs).
No products indexed under this heading.

Nicotine Polacrilex (Ondansetron does not itself appear to induce or inhibit the cytochrome P-450 drug metabolizing enzyme system of the liver. Because ondansetron is metabolized by hepatic cytochrome P-450 drug-metabolizing enzymes (CYP3A4, CYP2D6, CYP1A2), inducers or inhibitors of these enzymes may change the clearance and, hence, the half-life of ondansetron. On the basis of available data, no dosage adjustment is recommended for patients on these drugs).
No products indexed under this heading.

Nicotine Salicylate (Ondansetron does not itself appear to induce or inhibit the cytochrome P-450 drug metabolizing enzyme system of the liver. Because ondansetron is metabolized by hepatic cytochrome P-450 drug-metabolizing enzymes (CYP3A4, CYP2D6, CYP1A2), inducers or inhibitors of these enzymes may change the clearance and, hence, the half-life of ondansetron. On the basis of available data, no dosage adjustment is recommended for patients on these drugs).
No products indexed under this heading.

Nicotine Sulfate (Ondansetron does not itself appear to induce or inhibit the cytochrome P-450 drug metabolizing enzyme system of the liver. Because ondansetron is metabolized by hepatic cytochrome P-450 drug-metabolizing enzymes (CYP3A4, CYP2D6, CYP1A2), inducers or inhibitors of these enzymes may change the clearance and, hence, the half-life of ondansetron. On the basis of available data, no dosage adjustment is recommended for patients on these drugs).
No products indexed under this heading.

Nifedipine (Ondansetron does not itself appear to induce or inhibit the cytochrome P-450 drug metabolizing enzyme system of the liver. Because ondansetron is metabolized by hepatic cytochrome P-450 drug-metabolizing enzymes (CYP3A4, CYP2D6, CYP1A2), inducers or inhibitors of these enzymes may change the clearance and, hence, the half-life of ondansetron. On the basis of available data, no dosage adjustment is recommended for patients on these drugs).
No products indexed under this heading.

Norethindrone (Ondansetron does not itself appear to induce or inhibit the cytochrome P-450 drug metabolizing enzyme system of the liver. Because ondansetron is metabolized by hepatic cytochrome P-450 drug-metabolizing enzymes (CYP3A4, CYP2D6, CYP1A2), inducers or inhibitors of these enzymes may change the clearance and, hence, the half-life of ondansetron. On the basis of available data, no dosage adjustment is recommended for patients on these drugs). Products include:
Ortho Micronor 2660

Norethindrone Acetate (Ondansetron does not itself appear to induce or inhibit the cytochrome P-450 drug metabolizing enzyme system of the liver. Because ondansetron is metabolized by hepatic cytochrome P-450 drug-metabolizing enzymes (CYP3A4, CYP2D6, CYP1A2), inducers or inhibitors of these enzymes may change the clearance and, hence, the half-life of ondansetron. On the basis of available data, no dosage adjustment is recommended for patients on these drugs). Products include:
Activella 2561

Norethynodrel (*In vitro* metabolism studies have shown that ondansetron is a substrate for human hepatic cytochrome P-450 enzymes, including CYP1A2, CYP2D6, and CYP3A4. In terms of overall ondansetron turnover, CYP3A4 played the predominant role. Because of the multiplicity of metabolic enzymes capable of metabolizing ondansetron, it is likely that inhibition of one of these enzymes will be compensated by others and may result in little change in overall rates of ondansetron elimination).
No products indexed under this heading.

Norfloxacin (There have been reports of liver failure and death in patients with cancer receiving concurrent medications including antibiotics. The etiology of liver failure is unclear). Products include:
Noroxin 2220

Norgestimate (*In vitro* metabolism studies have shown that ondansetron is a substrate for human hepatic cytochrome P-450 enzymes, including CYP1A2, CYP2D6, and CYP3A4. In terms of overall ondansetron turnover, CYP3A4 played the predominant role. Because of the multiplicity of metabolic enzymes capable of metabolizing ondansetron, it is likely that inhibition of one of these enzymes will be compensated by others and may result in little change in overall rates of ondansetron elimination). Products include:
Ortho-Cyclen/Ortho Tri-Cyclen 2663
Ortho Tri-Cyclen Lo Tablets 2673

Norgestrel (Ondansetron does not itself appear to induce or inhibit the cytochrome P-450 drug metabolizing enzyme system of the liver. Because ondansetron is metabolized by hepatic cytochrome P-450 drug-metabolizing enzymes (CYP3A4, CYP2D6, CYP1A2), inducers or inhibitors of these enzymes may change the clearance and, hence, the half-life of ondansetron. On the basis of available data, no dosage adjustment is recommended for patients on these drugs).
No products indexed under this heading.

Nortriptyline Hydrochloride (Ondansetron does not itself appear to induce or inhibit the cytochrome P-450 drug metabolizing enzyme system of the liver. Because ondansetron is metabolized by hepatic cytochrome P-450 drug-metabolizing enzymes (CYP3A4, CYP2D6, CYP1A2), inducers or inhibitors of these enzymes may change the clearance and, hence, the half-life of ondansetron. On the basis of available data, no dosage adjustment is recommended for patients on these drugs).
No products indexed under this heading.

Ofloxacin (There have been reports of liver failure and death in patients with cancer receiving concurrent medications including antibiotics. The etiology of liver failure is unclear).
No products indexed under this heading.

Omeprazole (Ondansetron does not itself appear to induce or inhibit the cytochrome P-450 drug metabolizing enzyme system of the liver. Because ondansetron is metabolized by hepatic cytochrome P-450 drug-metabolizing enzymes (CYP3A4, CYP2D6, CYP1A2), inducers or inhibitors of these enzymes may change the clearance and, hence, the half-life of ondansetron. On the basis of available data, no dosage adjustment is recommended for patients on these drugs).
No products indexed under this heading.

Omeprazole Magnesium (Ondansetron does not itself appear to induce or inhibit the cytochrome P-450 drug metabolizing enzyme system of the liver. Because ondansetron is metabolized by hepatic cytochrome P-450 drug-metabolizing enzymes (CYP3A4, CYP2D6, CYP1A2), inducers or inhibitors of these enzymes may change the clearance and, hence, the half-life of ondansetron. On the basis of available data, no dosage adjustment is recommended for patients on these drugs).
No products indexed under this heading.

Oxacillin (There have been reports of liver failure and death in patients with cancer receiving concurrent medications including antibiotics. The etiology of liver failure is unclear).
No products indexed under this heading.

Oxacillin Sodium (There have been reports of liver failure and death in patients with cancer receiving concurrent medications including antibiotics. The etiology of liver failure is unclear).
No products indexed under this heading.

Oxaliplatin (There have been reports of liver failure and death in patients with cancer receiving concurrent medications including potentially hepatotoxic cytotoxic chemotherapeutic drugs. The etiology of the liver failure is unclear). Products include:
Eloxatin 2975

Oxcarbazepine (Ondansetron does not itself appear to induce or inhibit the cytochrome P-450 drug metabolizing enzyme system of the liver. Because ondansetron is metabolized by hepatic cytochrome P-450 drug-metabolizing

enzymes (CYP3A4, CYP2D6, CYP1A2), inducers or inhibitors of these enzymes may change the clearance and, hence, the half-life of ondansetron. In patients treated with potent inducers of CYP3A4 the clearance of ondansetron was significantly increased and ondansetron blood concentrations were decreased. However, on the basis of available data, no dosage adjustment for ondansetron is recommended for patients on these drugs).
No products indexed under this heading.

Oxiconazole Nitrate (*In vitro* metabolism studies have shown that ondansetron is a substrate for human hepatic cytochrome P-450 enzymes, including CYP1A2, CYP2D6, and CYP3A4. In terms of overall ondansetron turnover, CYP3A4 played the predominant role. Because of the multiplicity of metabolic enzymes capable of metabolizing ondansetron, it is likely that inhibition of one of these enzymes will be compensated by others and may result in little change in overall rates of ondansetron elimination).
No products indexed under this heading.

Oxytetracycline Hydrochloride (There have been reports of liver failure and death in patients with cancer receiving concurrent medications including antibiotics. The etiology of liver failure is unclear).
No products indexed under this heading.

Paclitaxel (There have been reports of liver failure and death in patients with cancer receiving concurrent medications including potentially hepatotoxic cytotoxic chemotherapeutic drugs. The etiology of the liver failure is unclear).
No products indexed under this heading.

Paroxetine (Ondansetron does not itself appear to induce or inhibit the cytochrome P-450 drug metabolizing enzyme system of the liver. Because ondansetron is metabolized by hepatic cytochrome P-450 drug-metabolizing enzymes (CYP3A4, CYP2D6, CYP1A2), inducers or inhibitors of these enzymes may change the clearance and, hence, the half-life of ondansetron. On the basis of available data, no dosage adjustment is recommended for patients on these drugs).
No products indexed under this heading.

Paroxetine Hydrochloride (Ondansetron does not itself appear to induce or inhibit the cytochrome P-450 drug metabolizing enzyme system of the liver. Because ondansetron is metabolized by hepatic cytochrome P-450 drug-metabolizing enzymes (CYP3A4, CYP2D6, CYP1A2), inducers or inhibitors of these enzymes may change the clearance and, hence, the half-life of ondansetron. On the basis of available data, no dosage adjustment is recommended for patients on these drugs). Products include:
Paroxetine CR 2361
Paroxetine ER 2371
Paxil 1586
Paxil CR 1596

Paroxetine Mesylate (Ondansetron does not itself appear to induce or inhibit the cytochrome P-450 drug metabolizing enzyme system of the liver. Because ondansetron is metabolized by hepatic cytochrome P-450 drug-metabolizing enzymes (CYP3A4, CYP2D6, CYP1A2), inducers or inhibitors of these enzymes may change the clearance and, hence, the half-life of ondansetron. On the basis of available data, no dosage adjustment is recommended for patients on these drugs).
No products indexed under this heading.

Penicillin, Potassium Phenoxymethyl (There have been reports of liver failure and death in patients with cancer receiving concurrent medications including antibiotics. The etiology of liver failure is unclear).
No products indexed under this heading.

Penicillin G Benzathine (There have been reports of liver failure and death in patients with cancer receiving concurrent medications including antibiotics. The etiology of liver failure is unclear). Products include:
Bicillin C-R Injectable Suspension 1826
Bicillin L-A 1828

Penicillin G Dibenzylethyenediamine (There have been reports of liver failure and death in patients with cancer receiving concurrent medications including antibiotics. The etiology of liver failure is unclear).
No products indexed under this heading.

Penicillin G Potassium (There have been reports of liver failure and death in patients with cancer receiving concurrent medications including antibiotics. The etiology of liver failure is unclear).
No products indexed under this heading.

Penicillin G Procaine (There have been reports of liver failure and death in patients with cancer receiving concurrent medications including antibiotics. The etiology of liver failure is unclear). Products include:
Bicillin C-R Injectable Suspension 1826
Bicillin L-A 1828

Penicillin G Sodium (There have been reports of liver failure and death in patients with cancer receiving concurrent medications including antibiotics. The etiology of liver failure is unclear).
No products indexed under this heading.

Penicillin V (There have been reports of liver failure and death in patients with cancer receiving concurrent medications including antibiotics. The etiology of liver failure is unclear).
No products indexed under this heading.

Penicillin V Potassium (There have been reports of liver failure and death in patients with cancer receiving concurrent medications including antibiotics. The etiology of liver failure is unclear).
No products indexed under this heading.

Penicillins (There have been reports of liver failure and death in patients with cancer receiving concurrent medications including antibiotics. The etiology of liver failure is unclear).
No products indexed under this heading.

Perphenazine (Ondansetron does not itself appear to induce or inhibit the cytochrome P-450 drug metabolizing enzyme system of the liver. Because ondansetron is metabolized by hepatic cytochrome P-450 drug-metabolizing enzymes (CYP3A4, CYP2D6, CYP1A2), inducers or inhibitors of these enzymes may change the clearance and, hence, the half-life of ondansetron. On the basis of available data, no dosage adjustment is recommended for patients on these drugs).
No products indexed under this heading.

Phenobarbital (Ondansetron does not itself appear to induce or inhibit the cytochrome P-450 drug metabolizing enzyme system of the liver. Because ondansetron is metabolized by hepatic cytochrome P-450 drug-metabolizing enzymes (CYP3A4, CYP2D6, CYP1A2), inducers or inhibitors of these enzymes may change the clearance and, hence, the half-life of ondansetron. In patients treated with potent inducers of CYP3A4 the clearance of ondansetron was significantly increased and ondansetron blood concentrations were decreased. However, on the basis of available data, no dosage adjustment for ondansetron is recommended for patients on these drugs). Products include:
Donnatal 2711

Phenobarbital Sodium (Ondansetron does not itself appear to induce or inhibit the cytochrome P-450 drug metabolizing enzyme system of the liver. Because ondansetron is metabolized by hepatic cytochrome P-450 drug-metabolizing enzymes (CYP3A4, CYP2D6, CYP1A2), inducers or inhibitors of these enzymes may change the clearance and, hence, the half-life of ondansetron. In patients treated with potent inducers of CYP3A4 the clearance of ondansetron was significantly increased and ondansetron blood concentrations were decreased. However, on the basis of available data, no dosage adjustment for ondansetron is recommended for patients on these drugs).
No products indexed under this heading.

Phenylbutazone (*In vitro* metabolism studies have shown that ondansetron is a substrate for human hepatic cytochrome P-450 enzymes, including CYP1A2, CYP2D6, and CYP3A4. In terms of overall ondansetron turnover, CYP3A4 played the predominant role. Because of the multiplicity of metabolic enzymes capable of metabolizing ondansetron, it is likely that inhibition of one of these enzymes will be compensated by others and may result in little change in overall rates of ondansetron elimination).
No products indexed under this heading.

Phenytoin (In patients treated with potent inducers of CYP3A4 (eg, phenytoin), the clearance of ondansetron was significantly increased and ondansetron blood concentrations were decreased. However, on the basis of available data, no dosage adjustment for ondansetron is recommended for patients on these drugs).
No products indexed under this heading.

Phenytoin Sodium (In patients treated with potent inducers of CYP3A4 (eg, phenytoin), the clearance of ondansetron was significantly increased and ondansetron blood concentrations were decreased. However, on the basis of available data, no dosage adjustment for ondansetron is recommended for patients on these drugs). Products include:
Phenytek Capsules 2380

Piperacillin Sodium (There have been reports of liver failure and death in patients with cancer receiving concurrent medications including antibiotics. The etiology of liver failure is unclear). Products include:
Zosyn 3607

Polythiazide (*In vitro* metabolism studies have shown that ondansetron is a substrate for human hepatic cytochrome P-450 enzymes, including CYP1A2, CYP2D6, and CYP3A4. In terms of overall ondansetron turnover, CYP3A4 played the predominant role. Because of the multiplicity of metabolic enzymes capable of metabolizing ondansetron, it is likely that inhibition of one of these enzymes will be compensated by others and may result in little change in overall rates of ondansetron elimination).
No products indexed under this heading.

Posaconazole (Ondansetron does not itself appear to induce or inhibit the cytochrome P-450 drug metabolizing enzyme system of the liver. Because ondansetron is metabolized by hepatic cytochrome P-450 drug-metabolizing enzymes (CYP3A4, CYP2D6, CYP1A2), inducers or inhibitors of these enzymes may change the clearance and, hence, the half-life of ondansetron. On the basis of available data, no dosage adjustment is recommended for patients on these drugs). Products include:
Noxafil 3172

Prednisolone (Ondansetron does not itself appear to induce or inhibit the cytochrome P-450 drug metabolizing enzyme system of the liver. Because ondansetron is metabolized by hepatic cytochrome P-450 drug-metabolizing enzymes (CYP3A4, CYP2D6, CYP1A2), inducers or inhibitors of these enzymes may change the clearance and, hence, the half-life of ondansetron. In patients treated with potent inducers of CYP3A4 the clearance of ondansetron was significantly increased and ondansetron blood concentrations were decreased. However, on the basis of available data, no dosage adjustment for ondansetron is recommended for patients on these drugs).
No products indexed under this heading.

Prednisolone Acetate (Ondansetron does not itself appear to induce or inhibit the cytochrome P-450 drug metabolizing enzyme system of the liver. Because ondansetron is metabolized by hepatic cytochrome P-450 drug-metabolizing enzymes (CYP3A4, CYP2D6, CYP1A2), inducers or inhibitors of these enzymes may change the clearance and, hence, the half-life of ondansetron. In patients treated with potent inducers of CYP3A4 the clearance of ondansetron was significantly increased and ondansetron blood concentrations were decreased. However, on the basis of available data, no dosage adjustment for ondansetron is recommended for patients on these drugs). Products include:
Blephamide .... ⊙212, ⊙214
Pred Forte .... ⊙225
Pred Mild .... ⊙230
Pred-G .... ⊙226, ⊙227

Prednisolone Sodium Phosphate (Ondansetron does not itself appear to induce or inhibit the cytochrome P-450 drug metabolizing enzyme system of the liver. Because ondansetron is metabolized by hepatic cytochrome P-450 drug-metabolizing enzymes (CYP3A4, CYP2D6, CYP1A2), inducers or inhibitors of these enzymes may change the clearance and, hence, the half-life of ondansetron. In patients treated with potent inducers of CYP3A4 the clearance of ondansetron was significantly increased and ondansetron blood concentrations were decreased. However, on the basis of available data, no dosage adjustment for ondansetron is recommended for patients on these drugs).
No products indexed under this heading.

Prednisolone Tebutate (Ondansetron does not itself appear to induce or inhibit the cytochrome P-450 drug metabolizing enzyme system of the liver. Because ondansetron is metabolized by hepatic cytochrome P-450 drug-metabolizing enzymes (CYP3A4, CYP2D6, CYP1A2), inducers or inhibitors of these enzymes may change the clearance and, hence, the half-life of ondansetron. In patients treated with potent inducers of CYP3A4 the clearance of ondansetron was significantly increased and ondansetron blood concentrations were decreased. However, on the basis of available data, no dosage adjustment for ondansetron is recommended for patients on these drugs).
No products indexed under this heading.

Prednisone (Ondansetron does not itself appear to induce or inhibit the cytochrome P-450 drug metabolizing enzyme system of the liver. Because ondansetron is metabolized by hepatic cytochrome P-450 drug-metabolizing enzymes (CYP3A4, CYP2D6, CYP1A2), inducers or inhibitors of these enzymes may change the clearance and, hence, the half-life of ondansetron. In patients

Zofran Interactions Index 2164

treated with potent inducers of CYP3A4 the clearance of ondansetron was significantly increased and ondansetron blood concentrations were decreased. However, on the basis of available data, no dosage adjustment for ondansetron is recommended for patients on these drugs).
No products indexed under this heading.

Prednisone sodium phosphate (Ondansetron does not itself appear to induce or inhibit the cytochrome P-450 drug metabolizing enzyme system of the liver. Because ondansetron is metabolized by hepatic cytochrome P-450 drug-metabolizing enzymes (CYP3A4, CYP2D6, CYP1A2), inducers or inhibitors of these enzymes may change the clearance and, hence, the half-life of ondansetron. In patients treated with potent inducers of CYP3A4 the clearance of ondansetron was significantly increased and ondansetron blood concentrations were decreased. However, on the basis of available data, no dosage adjustment for ondansetron is recommended for patients on these drugs).
No products indexed under this heading.

Primidone (Ondansetron does not itself appear to induce or inhibit the cytochrome P-450 drug metabolizing enzyme system of the liver. Because ondansetron is metabolized by hepatic cytochrome P-450 drug-metabolizing enzymes (CYP3A4, CYP2D6, CYP1A2), inducers or inhibitors of these enzymes may change the clearance and, hence, the half-life of ondansetron. In patients treated with potent inducers of CYP3A4 the clearance of ondansetron was significantly increased and ondansetron blood concentrations were decreased. However, on the basis of available data, no dosage adjustment for ondansetron is recommended for patients on these drugs).
No products indexed under this heading.

Procarbazine Hydrochloride (There have been reports of liver failure and death in patients with cancer receiving concurrent medications including potentially hepatotoxic cytotoxic chemotherapeutic drugs. The etiology of liver failure is unclear).
No products indexed under this heading.

Propafenone Hydrochloride (Ondansetron does not itself appear to induce or inhibit the cytochrome P-450 drug metabolizing enzyme system of the liver. Because ondansetron is metabolized by hepatic cytochrome P-450 drug-metabolizing enzymes (CYP3A4, CYP2D6, CYP1A2), inducers or inhibitors of these enzymes may change the clearance and, hence, the half-life of ondansetron. On the basis of available data, no dosage adjustment is recommended for patients on these drugs). Products include:
Rythmol **1648**
Rythmol SR **1652**

Propoxyphene Hydrochloride (Ondansetron does not itself appear to induce or inhibit the cytochrome P-450 drug metabolizing enzyme system of the liver. Because ondansetron is metabolized by hepatic cytochrome P-450 drug-metabolizing enzymes (CYP3A4, CYP2D6, CYP1A2), inducers or inhibitors of these enzymes may change the clearance and, hence, the half-life of ondansetron. On the basis of available data, no dosage adjustment is recommended for patients on these drugs).
No products indexed under this heading.

Propoxyphene Napsylate (Ondansetron does not itself appear to induce or inhibit the cytochrome P-450 drug metabolizing enzyme system of the liver. Because ondansetron is metabolized by hepatic cytochrome P-450 drug-metabolizing enzymes (CYP3A4, CYP2D6, CYP1A2), inducers or inhibitors of these enzymes may change the clearance and, hence, the half-life of ondansetron. On the basis of available data, no dosage adjustment is recommended for patients on these drugs).
No products indexed under this heading.

Protriptyline Hydrochloride (Ondansetron does not itself appear to induce or inhibit the cytochrome P-450 drug metabolizing enzyme system of the liver. Because ondansetron is metabolized by hepatic cytochrome P-450 drug-metabolizing enzymes (CYP3A4, CYP2D6, CYP1A2), inducers or inhibitors of these enzymes may change the clearance and, hence, the half-life of ondansetron. On the basis of available data, no dosage adjustment is recommended for patients on these drugs).
No products indexed under this heading.

Quercetin (*In vitro* metabolism studies have shown that ondansetron is a substrate for human hepatic cytochrome P-450 enzymes, including CYP1A2, CYP2D6, and CYP3A4. In terms of overall ondansetron turnover, CYP3A4 played the predominant role. Because of the multiplicity of metabolic enzymes capable of metabolizing ondansetron, it is likely that inhibition of one of these enzymes will be compensated by others and may result in little change in overall rates of ondansetron elimination).
No products indexed under this heading.

Quinacrine Hydrochloride (Ondansetron does not itself appear to induce or inhibit the cytochrome P-450 drug metabolizing enzyme system of the liver. Because ondansetron is metabolized by hepatic cytochrome P-450 drug-metabolizing enzymes (CYP3A4, CYP2D6, CYP1A2), inducers or inhibitors of these enzymes may change the clearance and, hence, the half-life of ondansetron. On the basis of available data, no dosage adjustment is recommended for patients on these drugs).
No products indexed under this heading.

Quinidine (Ondansetron does not itself appear to induce or inhibit the cytochrome P-450 drug metabolizing enzyme system of the liver. Because ondansetron is metabolized by hepatic cytochrome P-450 drug-metabolizing enzymes (CYP3A4, CYP2D6, CYP1A2), inducers or inhibitors of these enzymes may change the clearance and, hence, the half-life of ondansetron. On the basis of available data, no dosage adjustment is recommended for patients on these drugs).
No products indexed under this heading.

Quinidine Gluconate (Ondansetron does not itself appear to induce or inhibit the cytochrome P-450 drug metabolizing enzyme system of the liver. Because ondansetron is metabolized by hepatic cytochrome P-450 drug-metabolizing enzymes (CYP3A4, CYP2D6, CYP1A2), inducers or inhibitors of these enzymes may change the clearance and, hence, the half-life of ondansetron. On the basis of available data, no dosage adjustment is recommended for patients on these drugs).
No products indexed under this heading.

Quinidine Hydrochloride (Ondansetron does not itself appear to induce or inhibit the cytochrome P-450 drug metabolizing enzyme system of the liver. Because ondansetron is metabolized by hepatic cytochrome P-450 drug-metabolizing enzymes (CYP3A4, CYP2D6, CYP1A2), inducers or inhibitors of these enzymes may change the clearance and, hence, the half-life of ondansetron. On the basis of available data, no dosage adjustment is recommended for patients on these drugs).
No products indexed under this heading.

Quinidine Polygalacturonate (Ondansetron does not itself appear to induce or inhibit the cytochrome P-450 drug metabolizing enzyme system of the liver. Because ondansetron is metabolized by hepatic cytochrome P-450 drug-metabolizing enzymes (CYP3A4, CYP2D6, CYP1A2), inducers or inhibitors of these enzymes may change the clearance and, hence, the half-life of ondansetron. On the basis of available data, no dosage adjustment is recommended for patients on these drugs).
No products indexed under this heading.

Quinidine Sulfate (Ondansetron does not itself appear to induce or inhibit the cytochrome P-450 drug metabolizing enzyme system of the liver. Because ondansetron is metabolized by hepatic cytochrome P-450 drug-metabolizing enzymes (CYP3A4, CYP2D6, CYP1A2), inducers or inhibitors of these enzymes may change the clearance and, hence, the half-life of ondansetron. On the basis of available data, no dosage adjustment is recommended for patients on these drugs).
No products indexed under this heading.

Quinine (Ondansetron does not itself appear to induce or inhibit the cytochrome P-450 drug metabolizing enzyme system of the liver. Because ondansetron is metabolized by hepatic cytochrome P-450 drug-metabolizing enzymes (CYP3A4, CYP2D6, CYP1A2), inducers or inhibitors of these enzymes may change the clearance and, hence, the half-life of ondansetron. On the basis of available data, no dosage adjustment is recommended for patients on these drugs). Products include:
Hyland's Leg Cramps PM with Quinine **3315**

Quinine Sulfate (Ondansetron does not itself appear to induce or inhibit the cytochrome P-450 drug metabolizing enzyme system of the liver. Because ondansetron is metabolized by hepatic cytochrome P-450 drug-metabolizing enzymes (CYP3A4, CYP2D6, CYP1A2), inducers or inhibitors of these enzymes may change the clearance and, hence, the half-life of ondansetron. On the basis of available data, no dosage adjustment is recommended for patients on these drugs).
No products indexed under this heading.

Quinupristin (Ondansetron does not itself appear to induce or inhibit the cytochrome P-450 drug metabolizing enzyme system of the liver. Because ondansetron is metabolized by hepatic cytochrome P-450 drug-metabolizing enzymes (CYP3A4, CYP2D6, CYP1A2), inducers or inhibitors of these enzymes may change the clearance and, hence, the half-life of ondansetron. On the basis of available data, no dosage adjustment is recommended for patients on these drugs).
No products indexed under this heading.

Ranitidine Bismuth Citrate (Ondansetron does not itself appear to induce or inhibit the cytochrome P-450 drug metabolizing enzyme system of the liver. Because ondansetron is metabolized by hepatic cytochrome P-450 drug-metabolizing enzymes (CYP3A4, CYP2D6, CYP1A2), inducers or inhibitors of these enzymes may change the clearance and, hence, the half-life of ondansetron. On the basis of available data, no dosage adjustment is recommended for patients on these drugs).
No products indexed under this heading.

Ranitidine Hydrochloride (Ondansetron does not itself appear to induce or inhibit the cytochrome P-450 drug metabolizing enzyme system of the liver. Because ondansetron is metabolized by hepatic cytochrome P-450 drug-metabolizing enzymes (CYP3A4, CYP2D6, CYP1A2), inducers or inhibitors of these enzymes may change the clearance and, hence, the half-life of ondansetron. On the basis of available data, no dosage adjustment is recommended for patients on these drugs). Products include:
Zantac **1737**
Zantac Injection **1732**
Zantac Pharmacy **1735**

Rifabutin (Ondansetron does not itself appear to induce or inhibit the cytochrome P-450 drug metabolizing enzyme system of the liver. Because ondansetron is metabolized by hepatic cytochrome P-450 drug-metabolizing enzymes (CYP3A4, CYP2D6, CYP1A2), inducers or inhibitors of these enzymes may change the clearance and, hence, the half-life of ondansetron. In patients treated with potent inducers of CYP3A4 the clearance of ondansetron was significantly increased and ondansetron blood concentrations were decreased. However, on the basis of available data, no dosage adjustment for ondansetron is recommended for patients on these drugs).
No products indexed under this heading.

Rifampicin (In patients treated with potent inducers of CYP3A4 (eg, rifampicin), the clearance of ondansetron was significantly increased and ondansetron blood concentrations were decreased. However, on the basis of available data, no dosage adjustment for ondansetron is recommended for patients on these drugs).
No products indexed under this heading.

Rifampin (Ondansetron does not itself appear to induce or inhibit the cytochrome P-450 drug metabolizing enzyme system of the liver. Because ondansetron is metabolized by hepatic cytochrome P-450 drug-metabolizing enzymes (CYP3A4, CYP2D6, CYP1A2), inducers or inhibitors of these enzymes may change the clearance and, hence, the half-life of ondansetron. In patients treated with potent inducers of CYP3A4 the clearance of ondansetron was significantly increased and ondansetron blood concentrations were decreased. However, on the basis of available data, no dosage adjustment for ondansetron is recommended for patients on these drugs).
No products indexed under this heading.

Rifapentine (Ondansetron does not itself appear to induce or inhibit the cytochrome P-450 drug metabolizing enzyme system of the liver. Because ondansetron is metabolized by hepatic cytochrome P-450 drug-metabolizing enzymes (CYP3A4, CYP2D6, CYP1A2), inducers or inhibitors of these enzymes may change the clearance and, hence, the half-life of ondansetron. In patients treated with potent inducers of CYP3A4 the clearance of ondansetron was significantly increased and ondansetron blood concentrations were decreased. However, on the basis of available data, no dosage adjustment for ondansetron is recommended for patients on these drugs).
No products indexed under this heading.

Ritonavir (Ondansetron does not itself appear to induce or inhibit the cytochrome P-450 drug metabolizing enzyme system of the liver. Because ondansetron is metabolized by hepatic cytochrome P-450 drug-metabolizing enzymes (CYP3A4, CYP2D6, CYP1A2), inducers or inhibitors of these enzymes may change the clearance and, hence,

2165 Interactions Index Zofran

the half-life of ondansetron. On the basis of available data, no dosage adjustment is recommended for patients on these drugs). Products include:

Kaletra 458
Norvir 509

Saquinavir (Ondansetron does not itself appear to induce or inhibit the cytochrome P-450 drug metabolizing enzyme system of the liver. Because ondansetron is metabolized by hepatic cytochrome P-450 drug-metabolizing enzymes (CYP3A4, CYP2D6, CYP1A2), inducers or inhibitors of these enzymes may change the clearance and, hence, the half-life of ondansetron. On the basis of available data, no dosage adjustment is recommended for patients on these drugs).
No products indexed under this heading.

Saquinavir Mesylate (Ondansetron does not itself appear to induce or inhibit the cytochrome P-450 drug metabolizing enzyme system of the liver. Because ondansetron is metabolized by hepatic cytochrome P-450 drug-metabolizing enzymes (CYP3A4, CYP2D6, CYP1A2), inducers or inhibitors of these enzymes may change the clearance and, hence, the half-life of ondansetron. On the basis of available data, no dosage adjustment is recommended for patients on these drugs).
No products indexed under this heading.

Secobarbital Sodium (Ondansetron elimination may be affected by cytochrome P-450 inducers).
No products indexed under this heading.

Sertraline Hydrochloride (Ondansetron does not itself appear to induce or inhibit the cytochrome P-450 drug metabolizing enzyme system of the liver. Because ondansetron is metabolized by hepatic cytochrome P-450 drug-metabolizing enzymes (CYP3A4, CYP2D6, CYP1A2), inducers or inhibitors of these enzymes may change the clearance and, hence, the half-life of ondansetron. On the basis of available data, no dosage adjustment is recommended for patients on these drugs).
No products indexed under this heading.

Sildenafil Citrate (Ondansetron does not itself appear to induce or inhibit the cytochrome P-450 drug metabolizing enzyme system of the liver. Because ondansetron is metabolized by hepatic cytochrome P-450 drug-metabolizing enzymes (CYP3A4, CYP2D6, CYP1A2), inducers or inhibitors of these enzymes may change the clearance and, hence, the half-life of ondansetron. On the basis of available data, no dosage adjustment is recommended for patients on these drugs).
No products indexed under this heading.

Sodium Cloxacillin Monohydrate (There have been reports of liver failure and death in patients with cancer receiving concurrent medications including antibiotics. The etiology of liver failure is unclear).
No products indexed under this heading.

Sparfloxacin (There have been reports of liver failure and death in patients with cancer receiving concurrent medications including antibiotics. The etiology of liver failure is unclear).
No products indexed under this heading.

Streptomycin Sulfate (There have been reports of liver failure and death in patients with cancer receiving concurrent medications including antibiotics. The etiology of liver failure is unclear).
No products indexed under this heading.

Streptozocin (There have been reports of liver failure and death in patients with cancer receiving concurrent medications including potentially hepatotoxic cytotoxic chemotherapeutic drugs. The etiology of the liver failure is unclear).
No products indexed under this heading.

Sulfacytine (*In vitro* metabolism studies have shown that ondansetron is a substrate for human hepatic cytochrome P-450 enzymes, including CYP1A2, CYP2D6, and CYP3A4. In terms of overall ondansetron turnover, CYP3A4 played the predominant role. Because of the multiplicity of metabolic enzymes capable of metabolizing ondansetron, it is likely that inhibition of one of these enzymes will be compensated by others and may result in little change in overall rates of ondansetron elimination).
No products indexed under this heading.

Sulfamethizole (There have been reports of liver failure and death in patients with cancer receiving concurrent medications including antibiotics. The etiology of liver failure is unclear).
No products indexed under this heading.

Sulfamethoxazole (There have been reports of liver failure and death in patients with cancer receiving concurrent medications including antibiotics. The etiology of liver failure is unclear).
No products indexed under this heading.

Sulfaphenazole (*In vitro* metabolism studies have shown that ondansetron is a substrate for human hepatic cytochrome P-450 enzymes, including CYP1A2, CYP2D6, and CYP3A4. In terms of overall ondansetron turnover, CYP3A4 played the predominant role. Because of the multiplicity of metabolic enzymes capable of metabolizing ondansetron, it is likely that inhibition of one of these enzymes will be compensated by others and may result in little change in overall rates of ondansetron elimination).
No products indexed under this heading.

Sulfasalazine (*In vitro* metabolism studies have shown that ondansetron is a substrate for human hepatic cytochrome P-450 enzymes, including CYP1A2, CYP2D6, and CYP3A4. In terms of overall ondansetron turnover, CYP3A4 played the predominant role. Because of the multiplicity of metabolic enzymes capable of metabolizing ondansetron, it is likely that inhibition of one of these enzymes will be compensated by others and may result in little change in overall rates of ondansetron elimination).
No products indexed under this heading.

Sulfinpyrazone (Ondansetron does not itself appear to induce or inhibit the cytochrome P-450 drug metabolizing enzyme system of the liver. Because ondansetron is metabolized by hepatic cytochrome P-450 drug-metabolizing enzymes (CYP3A4, CYP2D6, CYP1A2), inducers or inhibitors of these enzymes may change the clearance and, hence, the half-life of ondansetron. In patients treated with potent inducers of CYP3A4 the clearance of ondansetron was significantly increased and ondansetron blood concentrations were decreased. However, on the basis of available data, no dosage adjustment for ondansetron is recommended for patients on these drugs).
No products indexed under this heading.

Sulfisoxazole Acetyl (There have been reports of liver failure and death in patients with cancer receiving concurrent medications including antibiotics. The etiology of liver failure is unclear).
No products indexed under this heading.

Sulfisoxazole Diolamine (There have been reports of liver failure and death in patients with cancer receiving concurrent medications including antibiotics. The etiology of liver failure is unclear).
No products indexed under this heading.

Tacrine Hydrochloride (Ondansetron does not itself appear to induce or inhibit the cytochrome P-450 drug metabolizing enzyme system of the liver. Because ondansetron is metabolized by hepatic cytochrome P-450 drug-metabolizing enzymes (CYP3A4, CYP2D6, CYP1A2), inducers or inhibitors of these enzymes may change the clearance and, hence, the half-life of ondansetron. On the basis of available data, no dosage adjustment is recommended for patients on these drugs).
No products indexed under this heading.

Tamoxifen Citrate (There have been reports of liver failure and death in patients with cancer receiving concurrent medications including potentially hepatotoxic cytotoxic chemotherapeutic drugs. The etiology of liver failure is unclear).
No products indexed under this heading.

Telithromycin (Ondansetron does not itself appear to induce or inhibit the cytochrome P-450 drug metabolizing enzyme system of the liver. Because ondansetron is metabolized by hepatic cytochrome P-450 drug-metabolizing enzymes (CYP3A4, CYP2D6, CYP1A2), inducers or inhibitors of these enzymes may change the clearance and, hence, the half-life of ondansetron. On the basis of available data, no dosage adjustment is recommended for patients on these drugs). Products include:

Ketek 2991

Telmisartan (*In vitro* metabolism studies have shown that ondansetron is a substrate for human hepatic cytochrome P-450 enzymes, including CYP1A2, CYP2D6, and CYP3A4. In terms of overall ondansetron turnover, CYP3A4 played the predominant role. Because of the multiplicity of metabolic enzymes capable of metabolizing ondansetron, it is likely that inhibition of one of these enzymes will be compensated by others and may result in little change in overall rates of ondansetron elimination). Products include:

Micardis 887
Micardis HCT 889

Teniposide (There have been reports of liver failure and death in patients with cancer receiving concurrent medications including potentially hepatotoxic cytotoxic chemotherapeutic drugs. The etiology of the liver failure is unclear).
No products indexed under this heading.

Terbinafine Hydrochloride (Ondansetron does not itself appear to induce or inhibit the cytochrome P-450 drug metabolizing enzyme system of the liver. Because ondansetron is metabolized by hepatic cytochrome P-450 drug-metabolizing enzymes (CYP3A4, CYP2D6, CYP1A2), inducers or inhibitors of these enzymes may change the clearance and, hence, the half-life of ondansetron. On the basis of available data, no dosage adjustment is recommended for patients on these drugs).
No products indexed under this heading.

Terconazole (*In vitro* metabolism studies have shown that ondansetron is a substrate for human hepatic cytochrome P-450 enzymes, including CYP1A2, CYP2D6, and CYP3A4. In terms of overall ondansetron turnover, CYP3A4 played the predominant role. Because of the multiplicity of metabolic enzymes capable of metabolizing ondansetron, it is likely that inhibition of one of these enzymes will be compensated by others and may result in little change in overall rates of ondansetron elimination).
No products indexed under this heading.

Tetracycline Hydrochloride (There have been reports of liver failure and death in patients with cancer receiving concurrent medications including antibiotics. The etiology of liver failure is unclear). Products include:

Pylera 793

Theophyllinate (Ondansetron does not itself appear to induce or inhibit the cytochrome P-450 drug metabolizing enzyme system of the liver. Because ondansetron is metabolized by hepatic cytochrome P-450 drug-metabolizing enzymes (CYP3A4, CYP2D6, CYP1A2), inducers or inhibitors of these enzymes may change the clearance and, hence, the half-life of ondansetron. In patients treated with potent inducers of CYP3A4 the clearance of ondansetron was significantly increased and ondansetron blood concentrations were decreased. However, on the basis of available data, no dosage adjustment for ondansetron is recommended for patients on these drugs).
No products indexed under this heading.

Theophylline (Ondansetron does not itself appear to induce or inhibit the cytochrome P-450 drug metabolizing enzyme system of the liver. Because ondansetron is metabolized by hepatic cytochrome P-450 drug-metabolizing enzymes (CYP3A4, CYP2D6, CYP1A2), inducers or inhibitors of these enzymes may change the clearance and, hence, the half-life of ondansetron. In patients treated with potent inducers of CYP3A4 the clearance of ondansetron was significantly increased and ondansetron blood concentrations were decreased. However, on the basis of available data, no dosage adjustment for ondansetron is recommended for patients on these drugs).
No products indexed under this heading.

Theophylline Anhydrous (Ondansetron does not itself appear to induce or inhibit the cytochrome P-450 drug metabolizing enzyme system of the liver. Because ondansetron is metabolized by hepatic cytochrome P-450 drug-metabolizing enzymes (CYP3A4, CYP2D6, CYP1A2), inducers or inhibitors of these enzymes may change the clearance and, hence, the half-life of ondansetron. In patients treated with potent inducers of CYP3A4 the clearance of ondansetron was significantly increased and ondansetron blood concentrations were decreased. However, on the basis of available data, no dosage adjustment for ondansetron is recommended for patients on these drugs). Products include:

Uniphyl 2817

Theophylline Calcium Salicylate (Ondansetron does not itself appear to induce or inhibit the cytochrome P-450 drug metabolizing enzyme system of the liver. Because ondansetron is metabolized by hepatic cytochrome P-450 drug-metabolizing enzymes (CYP3A4, CYP2D6, CYP1A2), inducers or inhibitors of these enzymes may change the clearance and, hence, the half-life of ondansetron. In patients treated with potent inducers of CYP3A4 the clearance of ondansetron was significantly increased and ondansetron blood concentrations were decreased. However, on the basis of available data, no dosage adjustment for ondansetron is recommended for patients on these drugs).
No products indexed under this heading.

Theophylline Dihydroxypropyl (Glyceryl) (Ondansetron does not itself appear to induce or inhibit the cytochrome P-450 drug metabolizing

Zofran Interactions Index 2166

enzyme system of the liver. Because ondansetron is metabolized by hepatic cytochrome P-450 drug-metabolizing enzymes (CYP3A4, CYP2D6, CYP1A2), inducers or inhibitors of these enzymes may change the clearance and, hence, the half-life of ondansetron. In patients treated with potent inducers of CYP3A4 the clearance of ondansetron was significantly increased and ondansetron blood concentrations were decreased. However, on the basis of available data, no dosage adjustment for ondansetron is recommended for patients on these drugs).
No products indexed under this heading.

Theophylline Ethylenediamine (Ondansetron does not itself appear to induce or inhibit the cytochrome P-450 drug metabolizing enzyme system of the liver. Because ondansetron is metabolized by hepatic cytochrome P-450 drug-metabolizing enzymes (CYP3A4, CYP2D6, CYP1A2), inducers or inhibitors of these enzymes may change the clearance and, hence, the half-life of ondansetron. In patients treated with potent inducers of CYP3A4 the clearance of ondansetron was significantly increased and ondansetron blood concentrations were decreased. However, on the basis of available data, no dosage adjustment for ondansetron is recommended for patients on these drugs).
No products indexed under this heading.

Theophylline Sodium Glycinate (Ondansetron does not itself appear to induce or inhibit the cytochrome P-450 drug metabolizing enzyme system of the liver. Because ondansetron is metabolized by hepatic cytochrome P-450 drug-metabolizing enzymes (CYP3A4, CYP2D6, CYP1A2), inducers or inhibitors of these enzymes may change the clearance and, hence, the half-life of ondansetron. In patients treated with potent inducers of CYP3A4 the clearance of ondansetron was significantly increased and ondansetron blood concentrations were decreased. However, on the basis of available data, no dosage adjustment for ondansetron is recommended for patients on these drugs).
No products indexed under this heading.

Thioguanine (There have been reports of liver failure and death in patients with cancer receiving concurrent medications including potentially hepatotoxic cytotoxic chemotherapeutic drugs. The etiology of the liver failure is unclear). Products include:
Tabloid 1664

Thioridazine Hydrochloride (Ondansetron does not itself appear to induce or inhibit the cytochrome P-450 drug metabolizing enzyme system of the liver. Because ondansetron is metabolized by hepatic cytochrome P-450 drug-metabolizing enzymes (CYP3A4, CYP2D6, CYP1A2), inducers or inhibitors of these enzymes may change the clearance and, hence, the half-life of ondansetron. On the basis of available data, no dosage adjustment is recommended for patients on these drugs). Products include:
Thioridazine Hydrochloride 2384

Thiotepa (There have been reports of liver failure and death in patients with cancer receiving concurrent medications including potentially hepatotoxic cytotoxic chemotherapeutic drugs. The etiology of the liver failure is unclear).
No products indexed under this heading.

Ticarcillin Disodium (There have been reports of liver failure and death in patients with cancer receiving concurrent medications including antibiotics. The etiology of liver failure is unclear). Products include:
Timentin ADD-Vantage 1670
Timentin Galaxy 1674
Timentin 1666
Timentin Pharmacy 1678

Ticlopidine Hydrochloride (Ondansetron does not itself appear to induce or inhibit the cytochrome P-450 drug metabolizing enzyme system of the liver. Because ondansetron is metabolized by hepatic cytochrome P-450 drug-metabolizing enzymes (CYP3A4, CYP2D6, CYP1A2), inducers or inhibitors of these enzymes may change the clearance and, hence, the half-life of ondansetron. On the basis of available data, no dosage adjustment is recommended for patients on these drugs).
No products indexed under this heading.

Tobacco (Ondansetron does not itself appear to induce or inhibit the cytochrome P-450 drug metabolizing enzyme system of the liver. Because ondansetron is metabolized by hepatic cytochrome P-450 drug-metabolizing enzymes (CYP3A4, CYP2D6, CYP1A2), inducers or inhibitors of these enzymes may change the clearance and, hence, the half-life of ondansetron. On the basis of available data, no dosage adjustment is recommended for patients on these drugs).
No products indexed under this heading.

Tobramycin (There have been reports of liver failure and death in patients with cancer receiving concurrent medications including antibiotics. The etiology of liver failure is unclear). Products include:
Tobi Nebulizer 2546
Tobramycin and Dexamethasone Ophthalmic Suspension .... ⊙ 251
Zylet .... ⊙ 252

Tobramycin Sulfate (There have been reports of liver failure and death in patients with cancer receiving concurrent medications including antibiotics. The etiology of liver failure is unclear).
No products indexed under this heading.

Tolazamide (*In vitro* metabolism studies have shown that ondansetron is a substrate for human hepatic cytochrome P-450 enzymes, including CYP1A2, CYP2D6, and CYP3A4. In terms of overall ondansetron turnover, CYP3A4 played the predominant role. Because of the multiplicity of metabolic enzymes capable of metabolizing ondansetron, it is likely that inhibition of one of these enzymes will be compensated by others and may result in little change in overall rates of ondansetron elimination).
No products indexed under this heading.

Tolbutamide (*In vitro* metabolism studies have shown that ondansetron is a substrate for human hepatic cytochrome P-450 enzymes, including CYP1A2, CYP2D6, and CYP3A4. In terms of overall ondansetron turnover, CYP3A4 played the predominant role. Because of the multiplicity of metabolic enzymes capable of metabolizing ondansetron, it is likely that inhibition of one of these enzymes will be compensated by others and may result in little change in overall rates of ondansetron elimination).
No products indexed under this heading.

Tolbutamide Sodium (*In vitro* metabolism studies have shown that ondansetron is a substrate for human hepatic cytochrome P-450 enzymes, including CYP1A2, CYP2D6, and CYP3A4. In terms of overall ondansetron turnover, CYP3A4 played the predominant role. Because of the multiplicity of metabolic enzymes capable of metabolizing ondansetron, it is likely that inhibition of one of these enzymes will be compensated by others and may result in little change in overall rates of ondansetron elimination).
No products indexed under this heading.

Topiramate (*In vitro* metabolism studies have shown that ondansetron is a substrate for human hepatic cytochrome P-450 enzymes, including CYP1A2, CYP2D6, and CYP3A4. In terms of overall ondansetron turnover, CYP3A4 played the predominant role. Because of the multiplicity of metabolic enzymes capable of metabolizing ondansetron, it is likely that inhibition of one of these enzymes will be compensated by others and may result in little change in overall rates of ondansetron elimination).
No products indexed under this heading.

Topotecan Hydrochloride (There have been reports of liver failure and death in patients with cancer receiving concurrent medications including potentially hepatotoxic cytotoxic chemotherapeutic drugs. The etiology of the liver failure is unclear). Products include:
Hycamtin 1491
Hycamtin Capsules 1488

Toremifene Citrate (There have been reports of liver failure and death in patients with cancer receiving concurrent medications including potentially hepatotoxic cytotoxic chemotherapeutic drugs. The etiology of the liver failure is unclear).
No products indexed under this heading.

Tramadol Hydrochloride (Although no pharmacokinetic drug interaction between ondansetron and tramadol has been observed, data from 2 small studies indicate that ondansetron may be associated with an increase in patient controlled administration of tramadol). Products include:
Ryzolt 2813
Ultram ER 2693

Triamcinolone (Ondansetron does not itself appear to induce or inhibit the cytochrome P-450 drug metabolizing enzyme system of the liver. Because ondansetron is metabolized by hepatic cytochrome P-450 drug-metabolizing enzymes (CYP3A4, CYP2D6, CYP1A2), inducers or inhibitors of these enzymes may change the clearance and, hence, the half-life of ondansetron. In patients treated with potent inducers of CYP3A4 the clearance of ondansetron was significantly increased and ondansetron blood concentrations were decreased. However, on the basis of available data, no dosage adjustment for ondansetron is recommended for patients on these drugs).
No products indexed under this heading.

Triamcinolone Acetonide (Ondansetron does not itself appear to induce or inhibit the cytochrome P-450 drug metabolizing enzyme system of the liver. Because ondansetron is metabolized by hepatic cytochrome P-450 drug-metabolizing enzymes (CYP3A4, CYP2D6, CYP1A2), inducers or inhibitors of these enzymes may change the clearance and, hence, the half-life of ondansetron. In patients treated with potent inducers of CYP3A4 the clearance of ondansetron was significantly increased and ondansetron blood concentrations were decreased. However, on the basis of available data, no dosage adjustment for ondansetron is recommended for patients on these drugs). Products include:
Azmacort 408
Nasacort AQ 3019

Triamcinolone Diacetate (Ondansetron does not itself appear to induce or inhibit the cytochrome P-450 drug metabolizing enzyme system of the liver. Because ondansetron is metabolized by hepatic cytochrome P-450 drug-metabolizing enzymes (CYP3A4, CYP2D6, CYP1A2), inducers or inhibitors of these enzymes may change the clearance and, hence, the half-life of ondansetron. In patients treated with potent inducers of CYP3A4 the clearance of ondansetron was significantly increased and ondansetron blood concentrations were decreased. However, on the basis of available data, no dosage adjustment for ondansetron is recommended for patients on these drugs).
No products indexed under this heading.

Triamcinolone Hexacetonide (Ondansetron does not itself appear to induce or inhibit the cytochrome P-450 drug metabolizing enzyme system of the liver. Because ondansetron is metabolized by hepatic cytochrome P-450 drug-metabolizing enzymes (CYP3A4, CYP2D6, CYP1A2), inducers or inhibitors of these enzymes may change the clearance and, hence, the half-life of ondansetron. In patients treated with potent inducers of CYP3A4 the clearance of ondansetron was significantly increased and ondansetron blood concentrations were decreased. However, on the basis of available data, no dosage adjustment for ondansetron is recommended for patients on these drugs).
No products indexed under this heading.

Trimethoprim (*In vitro* metabolism studies have shown that ondansetron is a substrate for human hepatic cytochrome P-450 enzymes, including CYP1A2, CYP2D6, and CYP3A4. In terms of overall ondansetron turnover, CYP3A4 played the predominant role. Because of the multiplicity of metabolic enzymes capable of metabolizing ondansetron, it is likely that inhibition of one of these enzymes will be compensated by others and may result in little change in overall rates of ondansetron elimination).
No products indexed under this heading.

Trimethoprim Hydrochloride (*In vitro* metabolism studies have shown that ondansetron is a substrate for human hepatic cytochrome P-450 enzymes, including CYP1A2, CYP2D6, and CYP3A4. In terms of overall ondansetron turnover, CYP3A4 played the predominant role. Because of the multiplicity of metabolic enzymes capable of metabolizing ondansetron, it is likely that inhibition of one of these enzymes will be compensated by others and may result in little change in overall rates of ondansetron elimination).
No products indexed under this heading.

Trimethoprim Sulfate (*In vitro* metabolism studies have shown that ondansetron is a substrate for human hepatic cytochrome P-450 enzymes, including CYP1A2, CYP2D6, and CYP3A4. In terms of overall ondansetron turnover, CYP3A4 played the predominant role. Because of the multiplicity of metabolic enzymes capable of metabolizing ondansetron, it is likely that inhibition of one of these enzymes will be compensated by others and may result in little change in overall rates of ondansetron elimination).
No products indexed under this heading.

Trimipramine Maleate (Ondansetron does not itself appear to induce or inhibit the cytochrome P-450 drug metabolizing enzyme system of the liver. Because ondansetron is metabolized by hepatic cytochrome P-450 drug-metabolizing enzymes (CYP3A4, CYP2D6, CYP1A2), inducers or inhibitors of these enzymes may change the clearance and, hence, the half-life of ondansetron. On the basis of available data, no dosage adjustment is recommended for patients on these drugs).
No products indexed under this heading.

Troglitazone (Ondansetron does not itself appear to induce or inhibit the cytochrome P-450 drug metabolizing enzyme system of the liver. Because ondansetron is metabolized by hepatic cytochrome P-450 drug-metabolizing enzymes (CYP3A4, CYP2D6, CYP1A2), inducers or inhibitors of these enzymes may change the clearance and, hence, the half-life of ondansetron. In patients treated with potent inducers of CYP3A4 the clearance of ondansetron was significantly increased and ondansetron blood concentrations were decreased. However, on the basis of available data, no dosage adjustment for ondansetron is recommended for patients on these drugs).
No products indexed under this heading.

Troleandomycin (There have been reports of liver failure and death in patients with cancer receiving concurrent medications including antibiotics. The etiology of liver failure is unclear).
No products indexed under this heading.

Trovafloxacin Mesylate (There have been reports of liver failure and death in patients with cancer receiving concurrent medications including antibiotics. The etiology of liver failure is unclear).
No products indexed under this heading.

Valproate Sodium (Ondansetron does not itself appear to induce or inhibit the cytochrome P-450 drug metabolizing enzyme system of the liver. Because ondansetron is metabolized by hepatic cytochrome P-450 drug-metabolizing enzymes (CYP3A4, CYP2D6, CYP1A2), inducers or inhibitors of these enzymes may change the clearance and, hence, the half-life of ondansetron. On the basis of available data, no dosage adjustment is recommended for patients on these drugs).
No products indexed under this heading.

Valrubicin (There have been reports of liver failure and death in patients with cancer receiving concurrent medications including potentially hepatotoxic cytotoxic chemotherapeutic drugs. The etiology of the liver failure is unclear). Products include:
Valstar 1131

Vardenafil Hydrochloride (Ondansetron does not itself appear to induce or inhibit the cytochrome P-450 drug metabolizing enzyme system of the liver. Because ondansetron is metabolized by hepatic cytochrome P-450 drug-metabolizing enzymes (CYP3A4, CYP2D6, CYP1A2), inducers or inhibitors of these enzymes may change the clearance and, hence, the half-life of ondansetron. On the basis of available data, no dosage adjustment is recommended for patients on these drugs). Products include:
Levitra 3157

Venlafaxine Hydrochloride (*In vitro* metabolism studies have shown that ondansetron is a substrate for human hepatic cytochrome P-450 enzymes, including CYP1A2, CYP2D6, and CYP3A4. In terms of overall ondansetron turnover, CYP3A4 played the predominant role. Because of the multiplicity of metabolic enzymes capable of metabolizing ondansetron, it is likely that inhibition of one of these enzymes will be compensated by others and may result in little change in overall rates of ondansetron elimination). Products include:
Effexor XR 3504
Venlafaxine Hydrochloride Tablets ... 2388

Verapamil Hydrochloride (Ondansetron does not itself appear to induce or inhibit the cytochrome P-450 drug metabolizing enzyme system of the liver. Because ondansetron is metabolized by hepatic cytochrome P-450 drug-metabolizing enzymes (CYP3A4, CYP2D6, CYP1A2), inducers or inhibitors of these enzymes may change the clearance and, hence, the half-life of ondansetron. On the basis of available data, no dosage adjustment is recommended for patients on these drugs). Products include:
Tarka 534

Vinblastine Sulfate (There have been reports of liver failure and death in patients with cancer receiving concurrent medications including potentially hepatotoxic cytotoxic chemotherapeutic drugs. The etiology of liver failure is unclear).
No products indexed under this heading.

Vincristine Sulfate (There have been reports of liver failure and death in patients with cancer receiving concurrent medications including potentially hepatotoxic cytotoxic chemotherapeutic drugs. The etiology of liver failure is unclear).
No products indexed under this heading.

Vinorelbine Tartrate (There have been reports of liver failure and death in patients with cancer receiving concurrent medications including potentially hepatotoxic cytotoxic chemotherapeutic drugs. The etiology of liver failure is unclear).
No products indexed under this heading.

Voriconazole (Ondansetron does not itself appear to induce or inhibit the cytochrome P-450 drug metabolizing enzyme system of the liver. Because ondansetron is metabolized by hepatic cytochrome P-450 drug-metabolizing enzymes (CYP3A4, CYP2D6, CYP1A2), inducers or inhibitors of these enzymes may change the clearance and, hence, the half-life of ondansetron. On the basis of available data, no dosage adjustment is recommended for patients on these drugs).
No products indexed under this heading.

Zafirlukast (Ondansetron does not itself appear to induce or inhibit the cytochrome P-450 drug metabolizing enzyme system of the liver. Because ondansetron is metabolized by hepatic cytochrome P-450 drug-metabolizing enzymes (CYP3A4, CYP2D6, CYP1A2), inducers or inhibitors of these enzymes may change the clearance and, hence, the half-life of ondansetron. On the basis of available data, no dosage adjustment is recommended for patients on these drugs). Products include:
Accolate 3612

Zileuton (Ondansetron does not itself appear to induce or inhibit the cytochrome P-450 drug metabolizing enzyme system of the liver. Because ondansetron is metabolized by hepatic cytochrome P-450 drug-metabolizing enzymes (CYP3A4, CYP2D6, CYP1A2), inducers or inhibitors of these enzymes may change the clearance and, hence, the half-life of ondansetron. On the basis of available data, no dosage adjustment is recommended for patients on these drugs).
No products indexed under this heading.

Food Interactions

Broccoli (Ondansetron does not itself appear to induce or inhibit the cytochrome P-450 drug metabolizing enzyme system of the liver. Because ondansetron is metabolized by hepatic cytochrome P-450 drug-metabolizing enzymes (CYP3A4, CYP2D6, CYP1A2), inducers or inhibitors of these enzymes may change the clearance and, hence, the half-life of ondansetron. On the basis of available data, no dosage adjustment is recommended for patients on these drugs).

Brussel Sprouts (Ondansetron does not itself appear to induce or inhibit the cytochrome P-450 drug metabolizing enzyme system of the liver. Because ondansetron is metabolized by hepatic cytochrome P-450 drug-metabolizing enzymes (CYP3A4, CYP2D6, CYP1A2), inducers or inhibitors of these enzymes may change the clearance and, hence, the half-life of ondansetron. On the basis of available data, no dosage adjustment is recommended for patients on these drugs).

Charbroiled Food (Ondansetron does not itself appear to induce or inhibit the cytochrome P-450 drug metabolizing enzyme system of the liver. Because ondansetron is metabolized by hepatic cytochrome P-450 drug-metabolizing enzymes (CYP3A4, CYP2D6, CYP1A2), inducers or inhibitors of these enzymes may change the clearance and, hence, the half-life of ondansetron. On the basis of available data, no dosage adjustment is recommended for patients on these drugs).

Food, unspecified (Bioavailability is slightly enhanced by food).

Grapefruit (Ondansetron does not itself appear to induce or inhibit the cytochrome P-450 drug metabolizing enzyme system of the liver. Because ondansetron is metabolized by hepatic cytochrome P-450 drug-metabolizing enzymes (CYP3A4, CYP2D6, CYP1A2), inducers or inhibitors of these enzymes may change the clearance and, hence, the half-life of ondansetron. On the basis of available data, no dosage adjustment is recommended for patients on these drugs).

Grapefruit Juice (Ondansetron does not itself appear to induce or inhibit the cytochrome P-450 drug metabolizing enzyme system of the liver. Because ondansetron is metabolized by hepatic cytochrome P-450 drug-metabolizing enzymes (CYP3A4, CYP2D6, CYP1A2), inducers or inhibitors of these enzymes may change the clearance and, hence, the half-life of ondansetron. On the basis of available data, no dosage adjustment is recommended for patients on these drugs).

Meal, unspecified (Bioavailability is slightly enhanced by food).

ZOFRAN ODT ORALLY DISINTEGRATING TABLETS

(Ondansetron Hydrochloride) 1756
See Zofran Tablets

ZOLINZA CAPSULES

(Vorinostat) 2295
May interact with oral anticoagulants, valproate. Compounds in these categories include:

Anisindione (Prolongation of PT and INR were observed in patients receiving vorinostat concomitantly with coumarin-derivative anticoagulants; carefully monitor PT and INR in patients concurrently administered vorinostat and coumarin derivatives).
No products indexed under this heading.

Dicumarol (Prolongation of PT and INR were observed in patients receiving vorinostat concomitantly with coumarin-derivative anticoagulants; carefully monitor PT and INR in patients concurrently administered vorinostat and coumarin derivatives).
No products indexed under this heading.

Divalproex Sodium (Severe thrombocytopenia and GI bleeding have been reported with concomitant use of vorinostat and other histone deacetylase inhibitors (eg, valproic acid). Monitor platelet count every two weeks for the first two months). Products include:
Depakote ER 426

Valproate Sodium (Severe thrombocytopenia and GI bleeding have been reported with concomitant use of vorinostat and other histone deacetylase inhibitors (eg, valproic acid). Monitor platelet count every two weeks for the first two months).
No products indexed under this heading.

Valproic Acid (Severe thrombocytopenia and GI bleeding have been reported with concomitant use of vorinostat and other histone deacetylase inhibitors (eg, valproic acid). Monitor platelet count every two weeks for the first two months).
No products indexed under this heading.

Warfarin Sodium (Prolongation of PT and INR were observed in patients receiving vorinostat concomitantly with coumarin-derivative anticoagulants; carefully monitor PT and INR in patients concurrently administered vorinostat and coumarin derivatives).
No products indexed under this heading.

ZOMETA FOR INTRAVENOUS INFUSION

(Zoledronic Acid) 2554
May interact with aminoglycosides, loop diuretics, nephrotoxic agents, and certain other agents. Compounds in these categories include:

Abacavir Sulfate (Caution is indicated when zoledronic acid is used with other potentially nephrotoxic drugs). Products include:
Epzicom 1448
Trizivir 1688
Ziagen 1740

Acyclovir (Caution is indicated when zoledronic acid is used with other potentially nephrotoxic drugs). Products include:
Zovirax 1760

Acyclovir Sodium (Caution is indicated when zoledronic acid is used with other potentially nephrotoxic drugs).
No products indexed under this heading.

Alatrofloxacin Mesylate (Caution is indicated when zoledronic acid is used with other potentially nephrotoxic drugs).
No products indexed under this heading.

Aldesleukin (Caution is indicated when zoledronic acid is used with other potentially nephrotoxic drugs). Products include:
Proleukin 2504

Amikacin Sulfate (Co-administration with aminoglycosides may have an additive effect to lower serum calcium for prolonged periods).
No products indexed under this heading.

Amoxicillin (Caution is indicated when zoledronic acid is used with other potentially nephrotoxic drugs). Products include:
Amoxil Capsules 1311
Amoxil Chewable Tablets 1311
Amoxil 1311
Amoxil Powder 1311
Augmentin 1331
Augmentin Tablets 1335
Augmentin ES-600 1338
Augmentin XR 1342
Moxatag 2321

Amoxicillin Trihydrate (Caution is indicated when zoledronic acid is used with other potentially nephrotoxic drugs).
No products indexed under this heading.

Amphotericin B (Caution is indicated when zoledronic acid is used with other potentially nephrotoxic drugs).
No products indexed under this heading.

IMPORTANT NOTE: Always consult each drug listing in the patient's regimen for possible interactions.

Amphotericin B, liposomal (Caution is indicated when zoledronic acid is used with other potentially nephrotoxic drugs). Products include:
AmBisome 659

Amphotericin B Cholesteryl Sulfate (Caution is indicated when zoledronic acid is used with other potentially nephrotoxic drugs).
No products indexed under this heading.

Amphotericin B Lipid Complex (Caution is indicated when zoledronic acid is used with other potentially nephrotoxic drugs).
No products indexed under this heading.

Ampicillin (Caution is indicated when zoledronic acid is used with other potentially nephrotoxic drugs).
No products indexed under this heading.

Ampicillin Sodium (Caution is indicated when zoledronic acid is used with other potentially nephrotoxic drugs).
No products indexed under this heading.

Ampicillin Trihydrate (Caution is indicated when zoledronic acid is used with other potentially nephrotoxic drugs).
No products indexed under this heading.

Amprenavir (Caution is indicated when zoledronic acid is used with other potentially nephrotoxic drugs).
No products indexed under this heading.

Aspirin (Caution is indicated when zoledronic acid is used with other potentially nephrotoxic drugs). Products include:
Aggrenox 880
Bayer Aspirin 829
Percodan 1124
St. Joseph Aspirin 2045

Atazanavir (Caution is indicated when zoledronic acid is used with other potentially nephrotoxic drugs).
No products indexed under this heading.

Atorvastatin Calcium (Caution is indicated when zoledronic acid is used with other potentially nephrotoxic drugs). Products include:
Lipitor 2703

Azithromycin Dihydrate (Caution is indicated when zoledronic acid is used with other potentially nephrotoxic drugs).
No products indexed under this heading.

Azlocillin Sodium (Caution is indicated when zoledronic acid is used with other potentially nephrotoxic drugs).
No products indexed under this heading.

Aztreonam (Caution is indicated when zoledronic acid is used with other potentially nephrotoxic drugs).
No products indexed under this heading.

Bacampicillin Hydrochloride (Caution is indicated when zoledronic acid is used with other potentially nephrotoxic drugs).
No products indexed under this heading.

Bacitracin (Caution is indicated when zoledronic acid is used with other potentially nephrotoxic drugs).
No products indexed under this heading.

Bacitracin Zinc (Caution is indicated when zoledronic acid is used with other potentially nephrotoxic drugs).
No products indexed under this heading.

Balsalazide Disodium (Caution is indicated when zoledronic acid is used with other potentially nephrotoxic drugs).
No products indexed under this heading.

Benazepril Hydrochloride (Caution is indicated when zoledronic acid is used with other potentially nephrotoxic drugs).
No products indexed under this heading.

Bendroflumethiazide (Caution is indicated when zoledronic acid is used with other potentially nephrotoxic drugs).
No products indexed under this heading.

Bumetanide (Concomitant use may increase risk of hypocalcemia).
No products indexed under this heading.

Caffeine (Caution is indicated when zoledronic acid is used with other potentially nephrotoxic drugs).
No products indexed under this heading.

Captopril (Caution is indicated when zoledronic acid is used with other potentially nephrotoxic drugs). Products include:
Captopril 2341

Carbenicillin Disodium (Caution is indicated when zoledronic acid is used with other potentially nephrotoxic drugs).
No products indexed under this heading.

Carbenicillin Indanyl Sodium (Caution is indicated when zoledronic acid is used with other potentially nephrotoxic drugs).
No products indexed under this heading.

Carboplatin (Caution is indicated when zoledronic acid is used with other potentially nephrotoxic drugs).
No products indexed under this heading.

Carmustine (BCNU) (Caution is indicated when zoledronic acid is used with other potentially nephrotoxic drugs).
No products indexed under this heading.

Cefaclor (Caution is indicated when zoledronic acid is used with other potentially nephrotoxic drugs).
No products indexed under this heading.

Cefadroxil (Caution is indicated when zoledronic acid is used with other potentially nephrotoxic drugs).
No products indexed under this heading.

Cefamandole Nafate (Caution is indicated when zoledronic acid is used with other potentially nephrotoxic drugs).
No products indexed under this heading.

Cefazolin Sodium (Caution is indicated when zoledronic acid is used with other potentially nephrotoxic drugs).
No products indexed under this heading.

Cefdinir (Caution is indicated when zoledronic acid is used with other potentially nephrotoxic drugs). Products include:
Omnicef Capsules 518
Omnicef Oral Suspension 518

Cefepime Hydrochloride (Caution is indicated when zoledronic acid is used with other potentially nephrotoxic drugs).
No products indexed under this heading.

Cefixime (Caution is indicated when zoledronic acid is used with other potentially nephrotoxic drugs). Products include:
Suprax for Oral Suspension 2038
Suprax Tablets 2038

Cefmetazole Sodium (Caution is indicated when zoledronic acid is used with other potentially nephrotoxic drugs).
No products indexed under this heading.

Cefonicid Sodium (Caution is indicated when zoledronic acid is used with other potentially nephrotoxic drugs).
No products indexed under this heading.

Cefoperazone Sodium (Caution is indicated when zoledronic acid is used with other potentially nephrotoxic drugs).
No products indexed under this heading.

Ceforanide (Caution is indicated when zoledronic acid is used with other potentially nephrotoxic drugs).
No products indexed under this heading.

Cefotaxime Sodium (Caution is indicated when zoledronic acid is used with other potentially nephrotoxic drugs).
No products indexed under this heading.

Cefotetan (Caution is indicated when zoledronic acid is used with other potentially nephrotoxic drugs).
No products indexed under this heading.

Cefoxitin Sodium (Caution is indicated when zoledronic acid is used with other potentially nephrotoxic drugs).
No products indexed under this heading.

Cefpodoxime Proxetil (Caution is indicated when zoledronic acid is used with other potentially nephrotoxic drugs).
No products indexed under this heading.

Cefprozil (Caution is indicated when zoledronic acid is used with other potentially nephrotoxic drugs).
No products indexed under this heading.

Ceftazidime (Caution is indicated when zoledronic acid is used with other potentially nephrotoxic drugs). Products include:
Fortaz 1481

Ceftizoxime Sodium (Caution is indicated when zoledronic acid is used with other potentially nephrotoxic drugs).
No products indexed under this heading.

Ceftriaxone Sodium (Caution is indicated when zoledronic acid is used with other potentially nephrotoxic drugs). Products include:
Rocephin 2859

Cefuroxime Axetil (Caution is indicated when zoledronic acid is used with other potentially nephrotoxic drugs). Products include:
Ceftin 1399

Cefuroxime Sodium (Caution is indicated when zoledronic acid is used with other potentially nephrotoxic drugs).
No products indexed under this heading.

Celecoxib (Caution is indicated when zoledronic acid is used with other potentially nephrotoxic drugs). Products include:
Celebrex 3272

Cephalexin (Caution is indicated when zoledronic acid is used with other potentially nephrotoxic drugs).
No products indexed under this heading.

Cephalothin Sodium (Caution is indicated when zoledronic acid is used with other potentially nephrotoxic drugs).
No products indexed under this heading.

Cephapirin Sodium (Caution is indicated when zoledronic acid is used with other potentially nephrotoxic drugs).
No products indexed under this heading.

Cephradine (Caution is indicated when zoledronic acid is used with other potentially nephrotoxic drugs).
No products indexed under this heading.

Cerivastatin Sodium (Caution is indicated when zoledronic acid is used with other potentially nephrotoxic drugs).
No products indexed under this heading.

Chlorothiazide (Caution is indicated when zoledronic acid is used with other potentially nephrotoxic drugs).
No products indexed under this heading.

Chlorothiazide Sodium (Caution is indicated when zoledronic acid is used with other potentially nephrotoxic drugs). Products include:
Diuril Intravenous 2009

Chlorpropamide (Caution is indicated when zoledronic acid is used with other potentially nephrotoxic drugs).
No products indexed under this heading.

Cidofovir (Caution is indicated when zoledronic acid is used with other potentially nephrotoxic drugs).
No products indexed under this heading.

Cilastatin Sodium (Caution is indicated when zoledronic acid is used with other potentially nephrotoxic drugs). Products include:
Primaxin I.M. 2232
Primaxin I.V. 2235

Cimetidine (Caution is indicated when zoledronic acid is used with other potentially nephrotoxic drugs).
No products indexed under this heading.

Cimetidine Hydrochloride (Caution is indicated when zoledronic acid is used with other potentially nephrotoxic drugs).
No products indexed under this heading.

Cisplatin (Caution is indicated when zoledronic acid is used with other potentially nephrotoxic drugs).
No products indexed under this heading.

Cladribine (Caution is indicated when zoledronic acid is used with other potentially nephrotoxic drugs). Products include:
Leustatin 946

Clozapine (Caution is indicated when zoledronic acid is used with other potentially nephrotoxic drugs).
No products indexed under this heading.

Colistimethate Sodium (Caution is indicated when zoledronic acid is used with other potentially nephrotoxic drugs).
No products indexed under this heading.

Colistin Sulfate (Caution is indicated when zoledronic acid is used with other potentially nephrotoxic drugs).
No products indexed under this heading.

Cyclophosphamide (Caution is indicated when zoledronic acid is used with other potentially nephrotoxic drugs).
No products indexed under this heading.

Cyclosporine (Caution is indicated when zoledronic acid is used with other potentially nephrotoxic drugs). Products include:
Gengraf 440
Neoral Oral Solution 2496
Neoral Capsules 2496
Restasis 605

Cytarabine (Caution is indicated when zoledronic acid is used with other potentially nephrotoxic drugs).
No products indexed under this heading.

Cytarabine Liposome (Caution is indicated when zoledronic acid is used with other potentially nephrotoxic drugs).
No products indexed under this heading.

Delavirdine Mesylate (Caution is indicated when zoledronic acid is used with other potentially nephrotoxic drugs).
No products indexed under this heading.

Diatrizoate Meglumine (Caution is indicated when zoledronic acid is used with other potentially nephrotoxic drugs).
No products indexed under this heading.

Diatrizoate Sodium (Caution is indicated when zoledronic acid is used with other potentially nephrotoxic drugs).
No products indexed under this heading.

Diclofenac Potassium (Caution is indicated when zoledronic acid is used with other potentially nephrotoxic drugs).
No products indexed under this heading.

Diclofenac Sodium (Caution is indicated when zoledronic acid is used with other potentially nephrotoxic drugs).
No products indexed under this heading.

Dicloxacillin Sodium (Caution is indicated when zoledronic acid is used with other potentially nephrotoxic drugs).
No products indexed under this heading.

Didanosine (Caution is indicated when zoledronic acid is used with other potentially nephrotoxic drugs).
No products indexed under this heading.

Dihydrostreptomycin (Co-administration with aminoglycosides may have an additive effect to lower serum calcium for prolonged periods).
No products indexed under this heading.

2169 Interactions Index Zometa

Efavirenz (Caution is indicated when zoledronic acid is used with other potentially nephrotoxic drugs). Products include:
Atripla ... 906

Emtricitabine (Caution is indicated when zoledronic acid is used with other potentially nephrotoxic drugs). Products include:
Atripla ... 906
Emtriva ... 1238
Emtriva Oral Solution ... 1238
Truvada ... 1258

Enalapril Maleate (Caution is indicated when zoledronic acid is used with other potentially nephrotoxic drugs).
No products indexed under this heading.

Enalaprilat (Caution is indicated when zoledronic acid is used with other potentially nephrotoxic drugs).
No products indexed under this heading.

Enfuvirtide (Caution is indicated when zoledronic acid is used with other potentially nephrotoxic drugs).
No products indexed under this heading.

Ethacrynic Acid (Concomitant use may increase risk of hypocalcemia).
No products indexed under this heading.

Ethiodized Oil (Caution is indicated when zoledronic acid is used with other potentially nephrotoxic drugs).
No products indexed under this heading.

Etodolac (Caution is indicated when zoledronic acid is used with other potentially nephrotoxic drugs).
No products indexed under this heading.

Fenoprofen Calcium (Caution is indicated when zoledronic acid is used with other potentially nephrotoxic drugs).
No products indexed under this heading.

Filgrastim (Caution is indicated when zoledronic acid is used with other potentially nephrotoxic drugs). Products include:
Neupogen ... 631

Fluorouracil (Caution is indicated when zoledronic acid is used with other potentially nephrotoxic drugs). Products include:
Carac ... 2966

Flurbiprofen (Caution is indicated when zoledronic acid is used with other potentially nephrotoxic drugs).
No products indexed under this heading.

Fluvastatin Sodium (Caution is indicated when zoledronic acid is used with other potentially nephrotoxic drugs).
No products indexed under this heading.

Foscarnet Sodium (Caution is indicated when zoledronic acid is used with other potentially nephrotoxic drugs).
No products indexed under this heading.

Fosinopril Sodium (Caution is indicated when zoledronic acid is used with other potentially nephrotoxic drugs).
No products indexed under this heading.

Furosemide (Concomitant use may increase risk of hypocalcemia). Products include:
Furosemide ... 2354

Gadopentetate Dimeglumine (Caution is indicated when zoledronic acid is used with other potentially nephrotoxic drugs).
No products indexed under this heading.

Gentamicin (Co-administration with aminoglycosides may have an additive effect to lower serum calcium for prolonged periods).
No products indexed under this heading.

Gentamicin Sulfate (Co-administration with aminoglycosides may have an additive effect to lower serum calcium for prolonged periods). Products include:
Pred-G ... ⊙226, ⊙227

Glipizide (Caution is indicated when zoledronic acid is used with other potentially nephrotoxic drugs).
No products indexed under this heading.

Globulin, Immune (Human) (Caution is indicated when zoledronic acid is used with other potentially nephrotoxic drugs). Products include:

Glyburide (Caution is indicated when zoledronic acid is used with other potentially nephrotoxic drugs).
No products indexed under this heading.

Gold Therapy (Caution is indicated when zoledronic acid is used with other potentially nephrotoxic drugs).
No products indexed under this heading.

HMG-CoA Reductase Inhibitors (Caution is indicated when zoledronic acid is used with other potentially nephrotoxic drugs).
No products indexed under this heading.

Hydrochlorothiazide (Caution is indicated when zoledronic acid is used with other potentially nephrotoxic drugs). Products include:
Atacand HCT ... 700
Avalide ... 2956
Benicar HCT ... 1017
Diovan HCT ... 2419
Dyazide ... 1429
Exforge HCT ... 2449
Hyzaar ... 2162
Hyzaar 100-12.5 ... 2162
Micardis HCT ... 889
Prinzide ... 2246
Tekturna HCT ... 2541
Teveten HCT ... 541

Hydroflumethiazide (Caution is indicated when zoledronic acid is used with other potentially nephrotoxic drugs).
No products indexed under this heading.

Ibuprofen (Caution is indicated when zoledronic acid is used with other potentially nephrotoxic drugs). Products include:
Motrin IB ... 2043
Children's Motrin ... 2044
Children's Motrin Non-Staining Dye-Free ... 2044
Infants' Motrin ... 2044
Infants' Motrin Dye-Free ... 2044
Junior Strength Motrin ... 2044
Vicoprofen ... 564

Idarubicin Hydrochloride (Caution is indicated when zoledronic acid is used with other potentially nephrotoxic drugs).
No products indexed under this heading.

Ifosfamide (Caution is indicated when zoledronic acid is used with other potentially nephrotoxic drugs).
No products indexed under this heading.

Imipenem (Caution is indicated when zoledronic acid is used with other potentially nephrotoxic drugs). Products include:
Primaxin I.M. ... 2232
Primaxin I.V. ... 2235

Immune Globulin Intravenous (Human) (Caution is indicated when zoledronic acid is used with other potentially nephrotoxic drugs). Products include:
Flebogamma 5% DIF ... 1794
Gammagard ... 812, 815
Gamunex ... 3374

Indinavir Sulfate (Caution is indicated when zoledronic acid is used with other potentially nephrotoxic drugs). Products include:
Crixivan ... 2113

Indomethacin (Caution is indicated when zoledronic acid is used with other potentially nephrotoxic drugs). Products include:
Indocin ... 2167

Indomethacin Sodium Trihydrate (Caution is indicated when zoledronic acid is used with other potentially nephrotoxic drugs). Products include:
Indocin I.V. ... 2007

Interferon Beta-1b (Caution is indicated when zoledronic acid is used with other potentially nephrotoxic drugs). Products include:
Betaseron ... 836
Extavia ... 2459

Interleuken-2 (Caution is indicated when zoledronic acid is used with other potentially nephrotoxic drugs).
No products indexed under this heading.

Iodamide Meglumine (Caution is indicated when zoledronic acid is used with other potentially nephrotoxic drugs).
No products indexed under this heading.

Iohexol (Caution is indicated when zoledronic acid is used with other potentially nephrotoxic drugs).
No products indexed under this heading.

Iopamidol (Caution is indicated when zoledronic acid is used with other potentially nephrotoxic drugs).
No products indexed under this heading.

Iopanoic Acid (Caution is indicated when zoledronic acid is used with other potentially nephrotoxic drugs).
No products indexed under this heading.

Iothalamate Meglumine (Caution is indicated when zoledronic acid is used with other potentially nephrotoxic drugs).
No products indexed under this heading.

Ioxaglate Meglumine (Caution is indicated when zoledronic acid is used with other potentially nephrotoxic drugs).
No products indexed under this heading.

Ioxaglate Sodium (Caution is indicated when zoledronic acid is used with other potentially nephrotoxic drugs).
No products indexed under this heading.

Kanamycin Sulfate (Co-administration with aminoglycosides may have an additive effect to lower serum calcium for prolonged periods).
No products indexed under this heading.

Ketoprofen (Caution is indicated when zoledronic acid is used with other potentially nephrotoxic drugs).
No products indexed under this heading.

Ketorolac Tromethamine (Caution is indicated when zoledronic acid is used with other potentially nephrotoxic drugs). Products include:
Acuvail ... ⊙209

Lamium album (Caution is indicated when zoledronic acid is used with other potentially nephrotoxic drugs).
No products indexed under this heading.

Lisinopril (Caution is indicated when zoledronic acid is used with other potentially nephrotoxic drugs). Products include:
Prinivil ... 2241
Prinzide ... 2246

Lithium (Caution is indicated when zoledronic acid is used with other potentially nephrotoxic drugs).
No products indexed under this heading.

Lithium Carbonate (Caution is indicated when zoledronic acid is used with other potentially nephrotoxic drugs).
No products indexed under this heading.

Lithium Citrate (Caution is indicated when zoledronic acid is used with other potentially nephrotoxic drugs).
No products indexed under this heading.

Lopinavir (Caution is indicated when zoledronic acid is used with other potentially nephrotoxic drugs). Products include:
Kaletra ... 458

Loracarbef (Caution is indicated when zoledronic acid is used with other potentially nephrotoxic drugs).
No products indexed under this heading.

Lovastatin (Caution is indicated when zoledronic acid is used with other potentially nephrotoxic drugs). Products include:
Advicor ... 402
Mevacor ... 2212

Meclofenamate Sodium (Caution is indicated when zoledronic acid is used with other potentially nephrotoxic drugs).
No products indexed under this heading.

Mefenamic Acid (Caution is indicated when zoledronic acid is used with other potentially nephrotoxic drugs).
No products indexed under this heading.

Meloxicam (Caution is indicated when zoledronic acid is used with other potentially nephrotoxic drugs).
No products indexed under this heading.

Melphalan Hydrochloride (Caution is indicated when zoledronic acid is used with other potentially nephrotoxic drugs). Products include:
Alkeran for Injection ... 1300

Mesalamine (Caution is indicated when zoledronic acid is used with other potentially nephrotoxic drugs). Products include:
Apriso ... 2899
Asacol ... 2786
Asacol HD ... 2787
Canasa ... 782
Lialda ... 3295
Pentasa ... 3297

Methimazole (Caution is indicated when zoledronic acid is used with other potentially nephrotoxic drugs).
No products indexed under this heading.

Methotrexate (Caution is indicated when zoledronic acid is used with other potentially nephrotoxic drugs).
No products indexed under this heading.

Methotrexate Sodium (Caution is indicated when zoledronic acid is used with other potentially nephrotoxic drugs).
No products indexed under this heading.

Methyclothiazide (Caution is indicated when zoledronic acid is used with other potentially nephrotoxic drugs).
No products indexed under this heading.

Mezlocillin Sodium (Caution is indicated when zoledronic acid is used with other potentially nephrotoxic drugs).
No products indexed under this heading.

Minocycline Hydrochloride (Caution is indicated when zoledronic acid is used with other potentially nephrotoxic drugs). Products include:
Solodyn ... 2073

Mitomycin (Mitomycin-C) (Caution is indicated when zoledronic acid is used with other potentially nephrotoxic drugs).
No products indexed under this heading.

Moexipril Hydrochloride (Caution is indicated when zoledronic acid is used with other potentially nephrotoxic drugs).
No products indexed under this heading.

Muromonab-CD3 (Caution is indicated when zoledronic acid is used with other potentially nephrotoxic drugs). Products include:
Orthoclone OKT3 ... 949

Nabumetone (Caution is indicated when zoledronic acid is used with other potentially nephrotoxic drugs).
No products indexed under this heading.

Nafcillin Sodium (Caution is indicated when zoledronic acid is used with other potentially nephrotoxic drugs).
No products indexed under this heading.

Naproxen (Caution is indicated when zoledronic acid is used with other potentially nephrotoxic drugs). Products include:
EC-Naprosyn ... 2850

IMPORTANT NOTE: Always consult each drug listing in the patient's regimen for possible interactions.

Naprosyn 2850
Anaprox/Naprosyn 2850

Naproxen Sodium (Caution is indicated when zoledronic acid is used with other potentially nephrotoxic drugs). Products include:
Anaprox 2850
Anaprox DS 2850
Treximet 1681

Nelfinavir Mesylate (Caution is indicated when zoledronic acid is used with other potentially nephrotoxic drugs).
No products indexed under this heading.

Neomycin (Co-administration with aminoglycosides may have an additive effect to lower serum calcium for prolonged periods).
No products indexed under this heading.

Neomycin, oral (Co-administration with aminoglycosides may have an additive effect to lower serum calcium for prolonged periods).
No products indexed under this heading.

Neomycin Sulfate (Co-administration with aminoglycosides may have an additive effect to lower serum calcium for prolonged periods).
No products indexed under this heading.

Nevirapine (Caution is indicated when zoledronic acid is used with other potentially nephrotoxic drugs). Products include:
Viramune Oral Suspension 897
Viramune Tablets 897

Norfloxacin (Caution is indicated when zoledronic acid is used with other potentially nephrotoxic drugs). Products include:
Noroxin 2220

Olsalazine Sodium (Caution is indicated when zoledronic acid is used with other potentially nephrotoxic drugs).
No products indexed under this heading.

Omeprazole (Caution is indicated when zoledronic acid is used with other potentially nephrotoxic drugs).
No products indexed under this heading.

Oxaprozin (Caution is indicated when zoledronic acid is used with other potentially nephrotoxic drugs).
No products indexed under this heading.

Pamidronate Disodium (Caution is indicated when zoledronic acid is used with other potentially nephrotoxic drugs).
No products indexed under this heading.

Paroxetine Hydrochloride (Caution is indicated when zoledronic acid is used with other potentially nephrotoxic drugs). Products include:
Paroxetine CR 2361
Paroxetine ER 2371
Paxil 1586
Paxil CR 1596

Penicillamine (Caution is indicated when zoledronic acid is used with other potentially nephrotoxic drugs).
No products indexed under this heading.

Penicillin G Benzathine (Caution is indicated when zoledronic acid is used with other potentially nephrotoxic drugs). Products include:
Bicillin C-R Injectable Suspension 1826
Bicillin L-A 1828

Penicillin G Potassium (Caution is indicated when zoledronic acid is used with other potentially nephrotoxic drugs).
No products indexed under this heading.

Penicillin G Procaine (Caution is indicated when zoledronic acid is used with other potentially nephrotoxic drugs). Products include:
Bicillin C-R Injectable Suspension 1826
Bicillin L-A 1828

Penicillin G Sodium (Caution is indicated when zoledronic acid is used with other potentially nephrotoxic drugs).
No products indexed under this heading.

Penicillin V Potassium (Caution is indicated when zoledronic acid is used with other potentially nephrotoxic drugs).
No products indexed under this heading.

Pentamidine Isethionate (Caution is indicated when zoledronic acid is used with other potentially nephrotoxic drugs).
No products indexed under this heading.

Perindopril Erbumine (Caution is indicated when zoledronic acid is used with other potentially nephrotoxic drugs).
No products indexed under this heading.

Phenylbutazone (Caution is indicated when zoledronic acid is used with other potentially nephrotoxic drugs).
No products indexed under this heading.

Piroxicam (Caution is indicated when zoledronic acid is used with other potentially nephrotoxic drugs).
No products indexed under this heading.

Plicamycin (Caution is indicated when zoledronic acid is used with other potentially nephrotoxic drugs).
No products indexed under this heading.

Polymyxin (Caution is indicated when zoledronic acid is used with other potentially nephrotoxic drugs).
No products indexed under this heading.

Polymyxin B Sulfate (Caution is indicated when zoledronic acid is used with other potentially nephrotoxic drugs).
No products indexed under this heading.

Polythiazide (Caution is indicated when zoledronic acid is used with other potentially nephrotoxic drugs).
No products indexed under this heading.

Pravastatin Sodium (Caution is indicated when zoledronic acid is used with other potentially nephrotoxic drugs).
No products indexed under this heading.

Quinapril Hydrochloride (Caution is indicated when zoledronic acid is used with other potentially nephrotoxic drugs).
No products indexed under this heading.

Rabeprazole Sodium (Caution is indicated when zoledronic acid is used with other potentially nephrotoxic drugs). Products include:
Aciphex 1035

Ramipril (Caution is indicated when zoledronic acid is used with other potentially nephrotoxic drugs).
No products indexed under this heading.

Rifampin (Caution is indicated when zoledronic acid is used with other potentially nephrotoxic drugs).
No products indexed under this heading.

Riluzole (Caution is indicated when zoledronic acid is used with other potentially nephrotoxic drugs). Products include:
Rilutek 3032

Ritonavir (Caution is indicated when zoledronic acid is used with other potentially nephrotoxic drugs). Products include:
Kaletra 458
Norvir 509

Rofecoxib (Caution is indicated when zoledronic acid is used with other potentially nephrotoxic drugs).
No products indexed under this heading.

Saquinavir (Caution is indicated when zoledronic acid is used with other potentially nephrotoxic drugs).
No products indexed under this heading.

Sibutramine Hydrochloride Monohydrate (Caution is indicated when zoledronic acid is used with other potentially nephrotoxic drugs). Products include:
Meridia 492

Simvastatin (Caution is indicated when zoledronic acid is used with other potentially nephrotoxic drugs). Products include:
Simcor 524
Vytorin 10/10 .... 2303, 3240
Vytorin 10/20 .... 2303, 3240
Vytorin 10/40 .... 2303, 3240
Vytorin 10/80 .... 2303, 3240
Zocor 2289

Spirapril Hydrochloride (Caution is indicated when zoledronic acid is used with other potentially nephrotoxic drugs).
No products indexed under this heading.

Stavudine (Caution is indicated when zoledronic acid is used with other potentially nephrotoxic drugs).
No products indexed under this heading.

Streptomycin Sulfate (Co-administration with aminoglycosides may have an additive effect to lower serum calcium for prolonged periods).
No products indexed under this heading.

Streptozocin (Caution is indicated when zoledronic acid is used with other potentially nephrotoxic drugs).
No products indexed under this heading.

Sulfacytine (Caution is indicated when zoledronic acid is used with other potentially nephrotoxic drugs).
No products indexed under this heading.

Sulfamethizole (Caution is indicated when zoledronic acid is used with other potentially nephrotoxic drugs).
No products indexed under this heading.

Sulfamethoxazole (Caution is indicated when zoledronic acid is used with other potentially nephrotoxic drugs).
No products indexed under this heading.

Sulfasalazine (Caution is indicated when zoledronic acid is used with other potentially nephrotoxic drugs).
No products indexed under this heading.

Sulfinpyrazone (Caution is indicated when zoledronic acid is used with other potentially nephrotoxic drugs).
No products indexed under this heading.

Sulfisoxazole Acetyl (Caution is indicated when zoledronic acid is used with other potentially nephrotoxic drugs).
No products indexed under this heading.

Sulfisoxazole Diolamine (Caution is indicated when zoledronic acid is used with other potentially nephrotoxic drugs).
No products indexed under this heading.

Sulindac (Caution is indicated when zoledronic acid is used with other potentially nephrotoxic drugs). Products include:
Clinoril 2098

Tacrolimus (Caution is indicated when zoledronic acid is used with other potentially nephrotoxic drugs). Products include:
Prograf Capsules 677
Prograf Injection 677
Protopic 685

Tenofovir Disoproxil Fumarate (Caution is indicated when zoledronic acid is used with other potentially nephrotoxic drugs). Products include:
Atripla 906
Truvada 1258
Viread 1266

Thalidomide (In multiple myeloma patients, the risk of renal dysfunction may be increased with zoledronic acid is used in combination with thalidomide).
No products indexed under this heading.

Thioguanine (Caution is indicated when zoledronic acid is used with other potentially nephrotoxic drugs). Products include:
Tabloid 1664

Ticarcillin Disodium (Caution is indicated when zoledronic acid is used with other potentially nephrotoxic drugs). Products include:
Timentin ADD-Vantage 1670
Timentin Galaxy 1674
Timentin 1666
Timentin Pharmacy 1678

Tobramycin (Co-administration with aminoglycosides may have an additive effect to lower serum calcium for prolonged periods). Products include:
Tobi Nebulizer 2546
Tobramycin and Dexamethasone Ophthalmic Suspension............... ⊙251
Zylet .... ⊙252

Tobramycin Sulfate (Co-administration with aminoglycosides may have an additive effect to lower serum calcium for prolonged periods).
No products indexed under this heading.

Tolazamide (Caution is indicated when zoledronic acid is used with other potentially nephrotoxic drugs).
No products indexed under this heading.

Tolbutamide (Caution is indicated when zoledronic acid is used with other potentially nephrotoxic drugs).
No products indexed under this heading.

Tolmetin Sodium (Caution is indicated when zoledronic acid is used with other potentially nephrotoxic drugs).
No products indexed under this heading.

Torsemide (Concomitant use may increase risk of hypocalcemia).
No products indexed under this heading.

Trandolapril (Caution is indicated when zoledronic acid is used with other potentially nephrotoxic drugs). Products include:
Mavik 489
Tarka 534

Triamterene (Caution is indicated when zoledronic acid is used with other potentially nephrotoxic drugs). Products include:
Dyazide 1429
Dyrenium 3495

Trimethadione (Caution is indicated when zoledronic acid is used with other potentially nephrotoxic drugs).
No products indexed under this heading.

Trovafloxacin Mesylate (Caution is indicated when zoledronic acid is used with other potentially nephrotoxic drugs).
No products indexed under this heading.

Tyropanoate Sodium (Caution is indicated when zoledronic acid is used with other potentially nephrotoxic drugs).
No products indexed under this heading.

Valacyclovir Hydrochloride (Caution is indicated when zoledronic acid is used with other potentially nephrotoxic drugs). Products include:
Valtrex 1702

Valdecoxib (Caution is indicated when zoledronic acid is used with other potentially nephrotoxic drugs).
No products indexed under this heading.

Vancomycin Hydrochloride (Caution is indicated when zoledronic acid is used with other potentially nephrotoxic drugs).
No products indexed under this heading.

Voriconazole (Caution is indicated when zoledronic acid is used with other potentially nephrotoxic drugs).
No products indexed under this heading.

Zalcitabine (Caution is indicated when zoledronic acid is used with other potentially nephrotoxic drugs).
No products indexed under this heading.

Zidovudine (Caution is indicated when zoledronic acid is used with other potentially nephrotoxic drugs). Products include:
Combivir 1404

(⊙ Described in PDR® for Ophthalmic Medicines)

ZOMIG TABLETS

(Zolmitriptan) 773
May interact with 5HT1-receptor agonists, ergot-containing drugs, monoamine oxidase inhibitors, oral contraceptives, selective serotonin reuptake
inhibitors, serotonin and norepinephrine
reuptake inhibitors, and certain other
agents. Compounds in these categories include:

Acetaminophen (A single 1 g dose of
acetaminophen does not alter the pharmacokinetics of zolmitriptan and its
N-desmethyl metabolite. However,
zolmitriptan delayed the T_{max} of acetaminophen by one hour). Products
include:

**Acetaminophen-containing prod-
ucts** (A single 1 g dose of acetaminophen does not alter the pharmacokinetics of zolmitriptan and its N-desmethyl
metabolite. However, zolmitriptan
delayed the T_{max} of acetaminophen by
one hour).
No products indexed under this heading.

Almotriptan Malate (Concomitant
use of other 5-HT$_{1B/1D}$ agonists (eg,
triptans) within 24 hours of zolmitriptan
treatment is contraindicated). Products
include:

Cimetidine (Following administration
of cimetidine, the half-life and AUC of
zolmitriptan and its active metabolites
were approximately doubled).
No products indexed under this heading.

Cimetidine Hydrochloride (Following administration of cimetidine, the
half-life and AUC of zolmitriptan and its
active metabolites were approximately
doubled).
No products indexed under this heading.

Citalopram Hydrobromide (Cases
of life-threatening serotonin syndrome
have been reported during combined
use of selective serotonin reuptake
inhibitors (SSRIs) and triptans. If concomitant treatment with zolmitriptan
and an SSRI (eg, citalopram) is clinically
warranted, careful observation of the
patient is advised, particularly during
treatment initiation and dose increases.
Serotonin syndrome symptoms may
include mental status changes, autonomic instability, neuromuscular aberrations, and/or gastrointestinal symptoms). Products include:

Desogestrel (Retrospective analysis
of pharmacokinetic data across studies
indicated that mean plasma concentrations of zolmitriptan were generally
higher in females taking oral contraceptives compared with those not taking
oral contraceptives. Mean C_{max} and
AUC of zolmitriptan were found to be
higher by 30% and 50%, respectively,
and T_{max} was delayed by one-half hour

in females taking oral contraceptives.
The effect of zolmitriptan on the pharmacokinetics of oral contraceptives has
not been studied).
No products indexed under this heading.

Desvenlafaxine Succinate (Cases
of life-threatening serotonin syndrome
have been reported during combined
use of serotonin norepinephrine
reuptake inhibitors (SNRIs) and triptans.
If concomitant treatment with zolmitriptan and a SNRI (eg, venlafaxine, duloxetine) is clinically warranted, careful
observation of the patient is advised,
particularly during treatment initiation
and dose increases. Serotonin syndrome symptoms may include mental
status changes, autonomic instability,
neuromuscular aberrations, and/or gastrointestinal symptoms). Products
include:

Dihydroergotamine Mesylate (Concomitant use and use within 24 hours of
zolmitriptan and any ergotamine containing medication, or ergot type medication (such as dihydroergotamine) is
contraindicated. Ergot-containing drugs
have been reported to cause prolonged
vasospastic reactions. There is a theoretical basis that these effects may be
additive with concurrent use).
No products indexed under this heading.

Duloxetine Hydrochloride (Cases of
life-threatening serotonin syndrome
have been reported during combined
use of serotonin norepinephrine
reuptake inhibitors (SNRIs) and triptans.
If concomitant treatment with zolmitriptan and a SNRI (eg, duloxetine) is clinically warranted, careful observation of
the patient is advised, particularly during treatment initiation and dose
increases. Serotonin syndrome symptoms may include mental status changes, autonomic instability, neuromuscular
aberrations, and/or gastrointestinal
symptoms). Products include:

Eletriptan Hydrobromide (Concomitant use of other 5-HT$_{1B/1D}$ agonists
(eg, triptans) within 24 hours of zolmitriptan treatment is contraindicated).
No products indexed under this heading.

Ergonovine Maleate (Concomitant
use and use within 24 hours of zolmitriptan and any ergotamine containing
medication, or ergot type medication
(such as dihydroergotamine or methysergide) is contraindicated. Ergot-
containing drugs have been reported to
cause prolonged vasospastic reactions.
There is a theoretical basis that these
effects may be additive with concurrent
use).
No products indexed under this heading.

Ergotamine Tartrate (Concomitant
use and use within 24 hours of zolmitriptan and any ergotamine containing
medication, or ergot type medication
(such as dihydroergotamine or methysergide) is contraindicated. Ergot-
containing drugs have been reported to
cause prolonged vasospastic reactions.
There is a theoretical basis that these
effects may be additive with concurrent
use).
No products indexed under this heading.

Escitalopram Oxalate (Cases of
life-threatening serotonin syndrome
have been reported during combined
use of selective serotonin reuptake
inhibitors (SSRIs) and triptans. If concomitant treatment with zolmitriptan
and an SSRI (eg, escitalopram) is clinically warranted, careful observation of
the patient is advised, particularly during treatment initiation and dose
increases. Serotonin syndrome symptoms may include mental status changes, autonomic instability, neuromuscular
aberrations, and/or gastrointestinal
symptoms). Products include:

Ethinyl Estradiol (Retrospective analysis of pharmacokinetic data across
studies indicated that mean plasma
concentrations of zolmitriptan were
generally higher in females taking oral
contraceptives compared with those
not taking oral contraceptives. Mean
C_{max} and AUC of zolmitriptan were
found to be higher by 30% and 50%,
respectively, and T_{max} was delayed by
one-half hour in females taking oral contraceptives. The effect of zolmitriptan
on the pharmacokinetics of oral contraceptives has not been studied).
Products include:

Ethynodiol Diacetate (Retrospective
analysis of pharmacokinetic data
across studies indicated that mean
plasma concentrations of zolmitriptan
were generally higher in females taking
oral contraceptives compared with
those not taking oral contraceptives.
Mean C_{max} and AUC of zolmitriptan
were found to be higher by 30% and
50%, respectively, and T_{max} was
delayed by one-half hour in females taking oral contraceptives. The effect of
zolmitriptan on the pharmacokinetics of
oral contraceptives has not been studied).
No products indexed under this heading.

Fluoxetine (Cases of life-threatening
serotonin syndrome have been reported
during combined use of selective serotonin reuptake inhibitors (SSRIs) and
triptans. If concomitant treatment with
zolmitriptan and an SSRI (eg, fluoxetine)
is clinically warranted, careful observation of the patient is advised, particularly during treatment initiation and dose
increases. Serotonin syndrome symptoms may include mental status changes, autonomic instability, neuromuscular
symptoms).
No products indexed under this heading.

Fluoxetine Hydrochloride (Cases of
life-threatening serotonin syndrome
have been reported during combined
use of selective serotonin reuptake
inhibitors (SSRIs) and triptans. If concomitant treatment with zolmitriptan
and an SSRI (eg, fluoxetine) is clinically
warranted, careful observation of the
patient is advised, particularly during
treatment initiation and dose increases.
Serotonin syndrome symptoms may
include mental status changes, autonomic instability, neuromuscular aberrations, and/or gastrointestinal symptoms). Products include:
Fluvoxamine (Cases of life-
threatening serotonin syndrome have
been reported during combined use of
selective serotonin reuptake inhibitors
(SSRIs) and triptans. If concomitant
treatment with zolmitriptan and an SSRI
(eg, fluvoxamine) is clinically warranted,
careful observation of the patient is
advised, particularly during treatment
initiation and dose increases. Serotonin
syndrome symptoms may include mental status changes, autonomic instability, neuromuscular aberrations, and/or
gastrointestinal symptoms).
No products indexed under this heading.

Fluvoxamine Maleate (Cases of life-
threatening serotonin syndrome have
been reported during combined use of
selective serotonin reuptake inhibitors

(SSRIs) and triptans. If concomitant
treatment with zolmitriptan and an SSRI
(eg, fluvoxamine) is clinically warranted,
careful observation of the patient is
advised, particularly during treatment
initiation and dose increases. Serotonin
syndrome symptoms may include mental status changes, autonomic instability, neuromuscular aberrations, and/or
gastrointestinal symptoms).
No products indexed under this heading.

Frovatriptan Succinate (Concomitant use of other 5-HT$_{1B/1D}$ agonists
(eg, triptans) within 24 hours of zolmitriptan treatment is contraindicated).
Products include:

Isocarboxazid (Concurrent administration of MAO-A inhibitors or use of
zolmitriptan within 2 weeks of discontinuation of MAO-A inhibitor therapy is
contraindicated. MAO-A inhibitors
increase the systemic exposure of
zolmitriptan. Therefore, the use of
zolmitriptan in patients receiving MAO-A
inhibitors is contraindicated. Following
one week of administration of 150 mg
bid moclobemide, a specific MAO-A
inhibitor, there was an increase of about
25% in both C_{max} and AUC for zolmitriptan and a 3–fold increase in the C_{max}
and AUC of the active N-desmethyl
metabolite of zolmitriptan). Products
include:

Levonorgestrel (Retrospective analysis of pharmacokinetic data across
studies indicated that mean plasma
concentrations of zolmitriptan were
generally higher in females taking oral
contraceptives compared with those
not taking oral contraceptives. Mean
C_{max} and AUC of zolmitriptan were
found to be higher by 30% and 50%,
respectively, and T_{max} was delayed by
one-half hour in females taking oral contraceptives. The effect of zolmitriptan
on the pharmacokinetics of oral contraceptives has not been studied).
Products include:

Mestranol (Retrospective analysis of
pharmacokinetic data across studies
indicated that mean plasma concentrations of zolmitriptan were generally
higher in females taking oral contraceptives compared with those not taking
oral contraceptives. Mean C_{max} and
AUC of zolmitriptan were found to be
higher by 30% and 50%, respectively,
and T_{max} was delayed by one-half hour
in females taking oral contraceptives.
The effect of zolmitriptan on the pharmacokinetics of oral contraceptives has
not been studied).
No products indexed under this heading.

Methylergonovine Maleate (Concomitant use and use within 24 hours of
zolmitriptan and any ergotamine containing medication, or ergot type medication (such as dihydroergotamine or
methysergide) is contraindicated. Ergot-
containing drugs have been reported to
cause prolonged vasospastic reactions.
There is a theoretical basis that these
effects may be additive with concurrent
use).
No products indexed under this heading.

IMPORTANT NOTE: Always consult each drug listing in the patient's regimen for possible interactions.

Methysergide Maleate (Concomitant use and use within 24 hours of zolmitriptan and any ergotamine containing medication, or ergot type medication (such as methysergide) is contraindicated. Ergot-containing drugs have been reported to cause prolonged vasospastic reactions. There is a theoretical basis that these effects may be additive with concurrent use).
No products indexed under this heading.

Moclobemide (Concurrent administration of MAO-A inhibitors or use of zolmitriptan within 2 weeks of discontinuation of MAO-A inhibitor therapy is contraindicated. MAO-A inhibitors increase the systemic exposure of zolmitriptan. Therefore, the use of zolmitriptan in patients receiving MAO-A inhibitors is contraindicated. Following one week of administration of 150 mg bid moclobemide, a specific MAO-A inhibitor, there was an increase of about 25% in both C_{max} and AUC for zolmitriptan and a 3–fold increase in the C_{max} and AUC of the active N-desmethyl metabolite of zolmitriptan).
No products indexed under this heading.

Naratriptan Hydrochloride (Concomitant use of other 5-$HT_{1B/1D}$ agonists (eg, triptans) within 24 hours of zolmitriptan treatment is contraindicated). Products include:
Amerge 1306

Nefazodone Hydrochloride (Cases of life-threatening serotonin syndrome have been reported during combined use of serotonin norepinephrine reuptake inhibitors (SNRIs) and triptans. If concomitant treatment with zolmitriptan and a SNRI (eg, venlafaxine, duloxetine) is clinically warranted, careful observation of the patient is advised, particularly during treatment initiation and dose increases. Serotonin syndrome symptoms may include mental status changes, autonomic instability, neuromuscular aberrations, and/or gastrointestinal symptoms).
No products indexed under this heading.

Norethindrone (Retrospective analysis of pharmacokinetic data across studies indicated that mean plasma concentrations of zolmitriptan were generally higher in females taking oral contraceptives compared with those not taking oral contraceptives. Mean C_{max} and AUC of zolmitriptan were found to be higher by 30% and 50%, respectively, and T_{max} was delayed by one-half hour in females taking oral contraceptives. The effect of zolmitriptan on the pharmacokinetics of oral contraceptives has not been studied). Products include:
Ortho Micronor 2660

Norethynodrel (Retrospective analysis of pharmacokinetic data across studies indicated that mean plasma concentrations of zolmitriptan were generally higher in females taking oral contraceptives compared with those not taking oral contraceptives. Mean C_{max} and AUC of zolmitriptan were found to be higher by 30% and 50%, respectively, and T_{max} was delayed by one-half hour in females taking oral contraceptives. The effect of zolmitriptan on the pharmacokinetics of oral contraceptives has not been studied).
No products indexed under this heading.

Norgestimate (Retrospective analysis of pharmacokinetic data across studies indicated that mean plasma concentrations of zolmitriptan were generally higher in females taking oral contraceptives compared with those not taking oral contraceptives. Mean C_{max} and AUC of zolmitriptan were found to be higher by 30% and 50%, respectively, and T_{max} was delayed by one-half hour in females taking oral contraceptives. The effect of zolmitriptan on the pharmacokinetics of oral contraceptives has not been studied). Products include:
Ortho-Cyclen/Ortho Tri-Cyclen 2663
Ortho Tri-Cyclen Lo Tablets 2673

Norgestrel (Retrospective analysis of pharmacokinetic data across studies indicated that mean plasma concentrations of zolmitriptan were generally higher in females taking oral contraceptives compared with those not taking oral contraceptives. Mean C_{max} and AUC of zolmitriptan were found to be higher by 30% and 50%, respectively, and T_{max} was delayed by one-half hour in females taking oral contraceptives. The effect of zolmitriptan on the pharmacokinetics of oral contraceptives has not been studied).
No products indexed under this heading.

Pargyline Hydrochloride (Concurrent administration of MAO-A inhibitors or use of zolmitriptan within 2 weeks of discontinuation of MAO-A inhibitor therapy is contraindicated. MAO-A inhibitors increase the systemic exposure of zolmitriptan. Therefore, the use of zolmitriptan in patients receiving MAO-A inhibitors is contraindicated. Following one week of administration of 150 mg bid moclobemide, a specific MAO-A inhibitor, there was an increase of about 25% in both C_{max} and AUC for zolmitriptan and a 3–fold increase in the C_{max} and AUC of the active N-desmethyl metabolite of zolmitriptan).
No products indexed under this heading.

Paroxetine (Cases of life-threatening serotonin syndrome have been reported during combined use of selective serotonin reuptake inhibitors (SSRIs) and triptans. If concomitant treatment with zolmitriptan and an SSRI (eg, paroxetine) is clinically warranted, careful observation of the patient is advised, particularly during treatment initiation and dose increases. Serotonin syndrome symptoms may include mental status changes, autonomic instability, neuromuscular aberrations, and/or gastrointestinal symptoms).
No products indexed under this heading.

Paroxetine Hydrochloride (Cases of life-threatening serotonin syndrome have been reported during combined use of selective serotonin reuptake inhibitors (SSRIs) and triptans. If concomitant treatment with zolmitriptan and an SSRI (eg, paroxetine) is clinically warranted, careful observation of the patient is advised, particularly during treatment initiation and dose increases. Serotonin syndrome symptoms may include mental status changes, autonomic instability, neuromuscular aberrations, and/or gastrointestinal symptoms). Products include:
Paroxetine CR 2361
Paroxetine ER 2371
Paxil 1586
Paxil CR 1596

Paroxetine Mesylate (Cases of life-threatening serotonin syndrome have been reported during combined use of selective serotonin reuptake inhibitors (SSRIs) and triptans. If concomitant treatment with zolmitriptan and an SSRI (eg, paroxetine) is clinically warranted, careful observation of the patient is advised, particularly during treatment initiation and dose increases. Serotonin syndrome symptoms may include mental status changes, autonomic instability, neuromuscular aberrations, and/or gastrointestinal symptoms).
No products indexed under this heading.

Phenelzine Sulfate (Concurrent administration of MAO-A inhibitors or use of zolmitriptan within 2 weeks of discontinuation of MAO-A inhibitor therapy is contraindicated. MAO-A inhibitors increase the systemic exposure of zolmitriptan. Therefore, the use of zolmitriptan in patients receiving MAO-A inhibitors is contraindicated. Following one week of administration of 150 mg bid moclobemide, a specific MAO-A inhibitor, there was an increase of about 25% in both C_{max} and AUC for zolmitriptan and a 3–fold increase in the C_{max} and AUC of the active N-desmethyl metabolite of zolmitriptan).
No products indexed under this heading.

Procarbazine Hydrochloride (Concurrent administration of MAO-A inhibitors or use of zolmitriptan within 2 weeks of discontinuation of MAO-A inhibitor therapy is contraindicated. MAO-A inhibitors increase the systemic exposure of zolmitriptan. Therefore, the use of zolmitriptan in patients receiving MAO-A inhibitors is contraindicated. Following one week of administration of 150 mg bid moclobemide, a specific MAO-A inhibitor, there was an increase of about 25% in both C_{max} and AUC for zolmitriptan and a 3–fold increase in the C_{max} and AUC of the active N-desmethyl metabolite of zolmitriptan).
No products indexed under this heading.

Propranolol (C_{max} and AUC of zolmitriptan increased 1.5-fold after one week of dosing with propranolol (160 mg/day). C_{max} and AUC of the N-desmethyl metabolite were reduced by 30% and 15%, respectively. There were no interactive effects on blood pressure or pulse rate following administration of propranolol with zolmitriptan).
No products indexed under this heading.

Propranolol Hydrochloride (C_{max} and AUC of zolmitriptan increased 1.5-fold after one week of dosing with propranolol (160 mg/day). C_{max} and AUC of the N-desmethyl metabolite were reduced by 30% and 15%, respectively. There were no interactive effects on blood pressure or pulse rate following administration of propranolol with zolmitriptan). Products include:
InnoPran XL 1517

Rasagiline Mesylate (Concurrent administration of MAO-A inhibitors or use of zolmitriptan within 2 weeks of discontinuation of MAO-A inhibitor therapy is contraindicated. MAO-A inhibitors increase the systemic exposure of zolmitriptan. Therefore, the use of zolmitriptan in patients receiving MAO-A inhibitors is contraindicated. Following one week of administration of 150 mg bid moclobemide, a specific MAO-A inhibitor, there was an increase of about 25% in both C_{max} and AUC for zolmitriptan and a 3–fold increase in the C_{max} and AUC of the active N-desmethyl metabolite of zolmitriptan). Products include:
Azilect 3383

Rizatriptan Benzoate (Concomitant use of other 5-$HT_{1B/1D}$ agonists (eg, triptans) within 24 hours of zolmitriptan treatment is contraindicated). Products include:
Maxalt 2206
Maxalt-MLT 2206

Selegiline (Concurrent administration of MAO-A inhibitors or use of zolmitriptan within 2 weeks of discontinuation of MAO-A inhibitor therapy is contraindicated. MAO-A inhibitors increase the systemic exposure of zolmitriptan. Therefore, the use of zolmitriptan in patients receiving MAO-A inhibitors is contraindicated. Following one week of administration of 150 mg bid moclobemide, a specific MAO-A inhibitor, there was an increase of about 25% in both C_{max} and AUC for zolmitriptan and a 3–fold increase in the C_{max} and AUC of the active N-desmethyl metabolite of zolmitriptan). Products include:
Emsam 3623

Selegiline Hydrochloride (Concurrent administration of MAO-A inhibitors or use of zolmitriptan within 2 weeks of discontinuation of MAO-A inhibitor therapy is contraindicated. MAO-A inhibitors increase the systemic exposure of zolmitriptan. Therefore, the use of zolmitriptan in patients receiving MAO-A inhibitors is contraindicated. Following one week of administration of 150 mg bid moclobemide, a specific MAO-A inhibitor, there was an increase of about 25% in both C_{max} and AUC for zolmitriptan and a 3–fold increase in the C_{max} and AUC of the active N-desmethyl metabolite of zolmitriptan). Products include:
Eldepryl 3312

Sertraline Hydrochloride (Cases of life-threatening serotonin syndrome have been reported during combined use of selective serotonin reuptake inhibitors (SSRIs) and triptans. If concomitant treatment with zolmitriptan and an SSRI (eg, sertraline) is clinically warranted, careful observation of the patient is advised, particularly during treatment initiation and dose increases. Serotonin syndrome symptoms may include mental status changes, autonomic instability, neuromuscular aberrations, and/or gastrointestinal symptoms).
No products indexed under this heading.

Sumatriptan (Concomitant use of other 5-$HT_{1B/1D}$ agonists (eg, triptans) within 24 hours of zolmitriptan treatment is contraindicated). Products include:
Imitrex Nasal 1503

Sumatriptan Succinate (Concomitant use of other 5-$HT_{1B/1D}$ agonists (eg, triptans) within 24 hours of zolmitriptan treatment is contraindicated). Products include:
Imitrex 1497
Imitrex Tablets 1508
Treximet 1681

Tranylcypromine Sulfate (Concurrent administration of MAO-A inhibitors or use of zolmitriptan within 2 weeks of discontinuation of MAO-A inhibitor therapy is contraindicated. MAO-A inhibitors increase the systemic exposure of zolmitriptan. Therefore, the use of zolmitriptan in patients receiving MAO-A inhibitors is contraindicated. Following one week of administration of 150 mg bid moclobemide, a specific MAO-A inhibitor, there was an increase of about 25% in both C_{max} and AUC for zolmitriptan and a 3–fold increase in the C_{max} and AUC of the active N-desmethyl metabolite of zolmitriptan). Products include:
Parnate 1584

Venlafaxine Hydrochloride (Cases of life-threatening serotonin syndrome have been reported during combined use of serotonin norepinephrine reuptake inhibitors (SNRIs) and triptans. If concomitant treatment with zolmitriptan and a SNRI (eg, venlafaxine) is clinically warranted, careful observation of the patient is advised, particularly during treatment initiation and dose increases. Serotonin syndrome symptoms may include mental status changes, autonomic instability, neuromuscular aberrations, and/or gastrointestinal symptoms). Products include:
Effexor XR 3504
Venlafaxine Hydrochloride Tablets ... 2388

ZOMIG NASAL SPRAY

(Zolmitriptan) 768
May interact with 5HT1-receptor agonists, ergot-containing drugs, monoamine oxidase inhibitors, oral contraceptives, selective serotonin reuptake inhibitors, serotonin and norepinephrine reuptake inhibitors, triptans, and certain other agents. Compounds in these categories include:

Acetaminophen-containing products (A single 1 g dose of acetaminophen does not alter the pharmacokinetics of zolmitriptan and its N-desmethyl metabolite. However, zolmitriptan delayed the T_{max} of acetaminophen by one hour).

No products indexed under this heading.

Almotriptan Malate (Concomitant use of other 5-HT1B/1D agonists (eg, triptans) within 24 hours of zolmitriptan treatment is contraindicated). Products include:

Cimetidine (Following administration of cimetidine, the half-life and AUC of zolmitriptan and its active metabolites were approximately doubled).

No products indexed under this heading.

Cimetidine Hydrochloride (Following administration of cimetidine, the half-life and AUC of zolmitriptan and its active metabolites were approximately doubled).

No products indexed under this heading.

Citalopram Hydrobromide (Cases of life-threatening serotonin syndrome have been reported during combined use of selective serotonin reuptake inhibitors (SSRIs) and triptans. If concomitant treatment with zolmitriptan and an SSRI (eg, citalopram) is clinically warranted, careful observation of the patient is advised, particularly during treatment initiation and dose increases. Serotonin syndrome symptoms may include mental status changes, autonomic instability, neuromuscular aberrations, and/or gastrointestinal symptoms). Products include:

Desogestrel (Retrospective analysis of pharmacokinetic data across studies indicated that mean plasma concentrations of zolmitriptan were generally higher in females taking oral contraceptives compared with those not taking oral contraceptives. Mean C_{max} and AUC of zolmitriptan were found to be higher by 30% and 50%, respectively, and T_{max} was delayed by one-half hour in females taking oral contraceptives. The effect of zolmitriptan on the pharmacokinetics of oral contraceptives has not been studied).

No products indexed under this heading.

Desvenlafaxine Succinate (Cases of life-threatening serotonin syndrome have been reported during combined use of serotonin norepinephrine reuptake inhibitors (SNRIs) and triptans. If concomitant treatment with zolmitriptan and a SNRI (eg, venlafaxine, duloxetine) is clinically warranted, careful observation of the patient is advised,

particularly during treatment initiation and dose increases. Serotonin syndrome symptoms may include mental status changes, autonomic instability, neuromuscular aberrations, and/or gastrointestinal symptoms). Products include:

Dihydroergotamine Mesylate (Concomitant use and use within 24 hours of zolmitriptan and any ergotamine containing medication, or ergot type medication (such as dihydroergotamine) is contraindicated. Ergot-containing drugs have been reported to cause prolonged vasospastic reactions. There is a theoretical basis that these effects may be additive with concurrent use).

No products indexed under this heading.

Duloxetine Hydrochloride (Cases of life-threatening serotonin syndrome have been reported during combined use of serotonin norepinephrine reuptake inhibitors (SNRIs) and triptans. If concomitant treatment with zolmitriptan and a SNRI (eg, duloxetine) is clinically warranted, careful observation of the patient is advised, particularly during treatment initiation and dose increases. Serotonin syndrome symptoms may include mental status changes, autonomic instability, neuromuscular aberrations, and/or gastrointestinal symptoms). Products include:

Eletriptan Hydrobromide (Concomitant use of other 5-HT1B/1D agonists (eg, triptans) within 24 hours of zolmitriptan treatment is contraindicated).

No products indexed under this heading.

Ergonovine Maleate (Concomitant use and use within 24 hours of zolmitriptan and any ergotamine containing medication, or ergot type medication (such as dihydroergotamine or methysergide) is contraindicated. Ergot-containing drugs have been reported to cause prolonged vasospastic reactions. There is a theoretical basis that these effects may be additive with concurrent use).

No products indexed under this heading.

Ergotamine Tartrate (Concomitant use and use within 24 hours of zolmitriptan and any ergotamine containing medication, or ergot type medication (such as dihydroergotamine or methysergide) is contraindicated. Ergot-containing drugs have been reported to cause prolonged vasospastic reactions. There is a theoretical basis that these effects may be additive with concurrent use).

No products indexed under this heading.

Escitalopram Oxalate (Cases of life-threatening serotonin syndrome have been reported during combined use of selective serotonin reuptake inhibitors (SSRIs) and triptans. If concomitant treatment with zolmitriptan and an SSRI (eg, escitalopram) is clinically warranted, careful observation of the patient is advised, particularly during treatment initiation and dose increases. Serotonin syndrome symptoms may include mental status changes, autonomic instability, neuromuscular aberrations, and/or gastrointestinal symptoms). Products include:

Ethinyl Estradiol (Retrospective analysis of pharmacokinetic data across studies indicated that mean plasma concentrations of zolmitriptan were generally higher in females taking oral contraceptives compared with those not taking oral contraceptives. Mean C_{max} and AUC of zolmitriptan were found to be higher by 30% and 50%, respectively, and T_{max} was delayed by one-half hour in females taking oral contraceptives. The effect of zolmitriptan

on the pharmacokinetics of oral contraceptives has not been studied). Products include:

Ethynodiol Diacetate (Retrospective analysis of pharmacokinetic data across studies indicated that mean plasma concentrations of zolmitriptan were generally higher in females taking oral contraceptives compared with those not taking oral contraceptives. Mean C_{max} and AUC of zolmitriptan were found to be higher by 30% and 50%, respectively, and T_{max} was delayed by one-half hour in females taking oral contraceptives. The effect of zolmitriptan on the pharmacokinetics of oral contraceptives has not been studied).

No products indexed under this heading.

Fluoxetine (Cases of life-threatening serotonin syndrome have been reported during combined use of selective serotonin reuptake inhibitors (SSRIs) and triptans. If concomitant treatment with zolmitriptan and an SSRI (eg, fluoxetine) is clinically warranted, careful observation of the patient is advised, particularly during treatment initiation and dose increases. Serotonin syndrome symptoms may include mental status changes, autonomic instability, neuromuscular aberrations, and/or gastrointestinal symptoms).

No products indexed under this heading.

Fluoxetine Hydrochloride (Cases of life-threatening serotonin syndrome have been reported during combined use of selective serotonin reuptake inhibitors (SSRIs) and triptans. If concomitant treatment with zolmitriptan and an SSRI (eg, fluoxetine) is clinically warranted, careful observation of the patient is advised, particularly during treatment initiation and dose increases. Serotonin syndrome symptoms may include mental status changes, autonomic instability, neuromuscular aberrations, and/or gastrointestinal symptoms). Products include:

Fluvoxamine (Cases of life-threatening serotonin syndrome have been reported during combined use of selective serotonin reuptake inhibitors (SSRIs) and triptans. If concomitant treatment with zolmitriptan and an SSRI (eg, fluvoxamine) is clinically warranted, careful observation of the patient is advised, particularly during treatment initiation and dose increases. Serotonin syndrome symptoms may include mental status changes, autonomic instability, neuromuscular aberrations, and/or gastrointestinal symptoms).

No products indexed under this heading.

Fluvoxamine Maleate (Cases of life-threatening serotonin syndrome have been reported during combined use of selective serotonin reuptake inhibitors (SSRIs) and triptans. If concomitant treatment with zolmitriptan and an SSRI (eg, fluvoxamine) is clinically warranted, careful observation of the patient is advised, particularly during treatment initiation and dose increases. Serotonin syndrome symptoms may include mental status changes, autonomic instability, neuromuscular aberrations, and/or gastrointestinal symptoms).

No products indexed under this heading.

Frovatriptan Succinate (Concomitant use of other 5-HT1B/1D agonists

(eg, triptans) within 24 hours of zolmitriptan treatment is contraindicated). Products include:

Isocarboxazid (Concurrent administration of MAO-A inhibitors or use of zolmitriptan within 2 weeks of discontinuation of MAO-A inhibitor therapy is contraindicated. MAO-A inhibitors increase the systemic exposure of zolmitriptan. Therefore, the use of zolmitriptan in patients receiving MAO-A inhibitors is contraindicated. Following one week of administration of 150 mg bid moclobemide, a specific MAO-A inhibitor, there was an increase of about 25% in both C_{max} and AUC for zolmitriptan and a 3-fold increase in the C_{max} and AUC of the active N-desmethyl metabolite of zolmitriptan). Products include:

Levonorgestrel (Retrospective analysis of pharmacokinetic data across studies indicated that mean plasma concentrations of zolmitriptan were generally higher in females taking oral contraceptives compared with those not taking oral contraceptives. Mean C_{max} and AUC of zolmitriptan were found to be higher by 30% and 50%, respectively, and T_{max} was delayed by one-half hour in females taking oral contraceptives. The effect of zolmitriptan on the pharmacokinetics of oral contraceptives has not been studied). Products include:

Mestranol (Retrospective analysis of pharmacokinetic data across studies indicated that mean plasma concentrations of zolmitriptan were generally higher in females taking oral contraceptives compared with those not taking oral contraceptives. Mean C_{max} and AUC of zolmitriptan were found to be higher by 30% and 50%, respectively, and T_{max} was delayed by one-half hour in females taking oral contraceptives. The effect of zolmitriptan on the pharmacokinetics of oral contraceptives has not been studied).

No products indexed under this heading.

Methylergonovine Maleate (Concomitant use and use within 24 hours of zolmitriptan and any ergotamine containing medication, or ergot type medication (such as dihydroergotamine or methysergide) is contraindicated. Ergot-containing drugs have been reported to cause prolonged vasospastic reactions. There is a theoretical basis that these effects may be additive with concurrent use).

No products indexed under this heading.

Methysergide Maleate (Concomitant use and use within 24 hours of zolmitriptan and any ergotamine containing medication, or ergot type medication (such as methysergide) is contraindicated. Ergot-containing drugs have been reported to cause prolonged vasospastic reactions. There is a theoretical basis that these effects may be additive with concurrent use).

No products indexed under this heading.

Moclobemide (Concurrent administration of MAO-A inhibitors or use of zolmitriptan within 2 weeks of discontinuation of MAO-A inhibitor therapy is contraindicated. MAO-A inhibitors increase the systemic exposure of zolmitriptan. Therefore, the use of zolmitriptan in patients receiving MAO-A inhibitors is contraindicated. Following one week of administration of 150 mg bid moclobemide, a specific MAO-A inhibitor, there was an increase of about 25% in both

C_{max} and AUC for zolmitriptan and a 3-fold increase in the C_{max} and AUC of the active N-desmethyl metabolite of zolmitriptan).

No products indexed under this heading.

Naratriptan Hydrochloride (Concomitant use of other 5-HT1B/1D agonists (eg, triptans) within 24 hours of zolmitriptan treatment is contraindicated). Products include:

Amerge 1306

Nefazodone Hydrochloride (Cases of life-threatening serotonin syndrome have been reported during combined use of serotonin norepinephrine reuptake inhibitors (SNRIs) and triptans. If concomitant treatment with zolmitriptan and a SNRI (eg, venlafaxine, duloxetine) is clinically warranted, careful observation of the patient is advised, particularly during treatment initiation and dose increases. Serotonin syndrome symptoms may include mental status changes, autonomic instability, neuromuscular aberrations, and/or gastrointestinal symptoms).

No products indexed under this heading.

Norethindrone (Retrospective analysis of pharmacokinetic data across studies indicated that mean plasma concentrations of zolmitriptan were generally higher in females taking oral contraceptives compared with those not taking oral contraceptives. Mean C_{max} and AUC of zolmitriptan were found to be higher by 30% and 50%, respectively, and T_{max} was delayed by one-half hour in females taking oral contraceptives. The effect of zolmitriptan on the pharmacokinetics of oral contraceptives has not been studied). Products include:

Ortho Micronor 2660

Norethynodrel (Retrospective analysis of pharmacokinetic data across studies indicated that mean plasma concentrations of zolmitriptan were generally higher in females taking oral contraceptives compared with those not taking oral contraceptives. Mean C_{max} and AUC of zolmitriptan were found to be higher by 30% and 50%, respectively, and T_{max} was delayed by one-half hour in females taking oral contraceptives. The effect of zolmitriptan on the pharmacokinetics of oral contraceptives has not been studied).

No products indexed under this heading.

Norgestimate (Retrospective analysis of pharmacokinetic data across studies indicated that mean plasma concentrations of zolmitriptan were generally higher in females taking oral contraceptives compared with those not taking oral contraceptives. Mean C_{max} and AUC of zolmitriptan were found to be higher by 30% and 50%, respectively, and T_{max} was delayed by one-half hour in females taking oral contraceptives. The effect of zolmitriptan on the pharmacokinetics of oral contraceptives has not been studied). Products include:

Ortho-Cyclen/Ortho Tri-Cyclen 2663
Ortho Tri-Cyclen Lo Tablets 2673

Norgestrel (Retrospective analysis of pharmacokinetic data across studies indicated that mean plasma concentrations of zolmitriptan were generally higher in females taking oral contraceptives compared with those not taking oral contraceptives. Mean C_{max} and AUC of zolmitriptan were found to be higher by 30% and 50%, respectively, and T_{max} was delayed by one-half hour in females taking oral contraceptives. The effect of zolmitriptan on the pharmacokinetics of oral contraceptives has not been studied).

No products indexed under this heading.

Pargyline Hydrochloride (Concurrent administration of MAO-A inhibitors or use of zolmitriptan within 2 weeks of discontinuation of MAO-A inhibitor therapy is contraindicated. MAO-A inhibitors increase the systemic exposure of zolmitriptan. Therefore, the use of zolmitriptan in patients receiving MAO-A inhibitors is contraindicated. Following one week of administration of 150 mg bid moclobemide, a specific MAO-A inhibitor, there was an increase of about 25% in both C_{max} and AUC for zolmitriptan and a 3-fold increase in the C_{max} and AUC of the active N-desmethyl metabolite of zolmitriptan).

No products indexed under this heading.

Paroxetine (Cases of life-threatening serotonin syndrome have been reported during combined use of selective serotonin reuptake inhibitors (SSRIs) and triptans. If concomitant treatment with zolmitriptan and an SSRI (eg, paroxetine) is clinically warranted, careful observation of the patient is advised, particularly during treatment initiation and dose increases. Serotonin syndrome symptoms may include mental status changes, autonomic instability, neuromuscular aberrations, and/or gastrointestinal symptoms).

No products indexed under this heading.

Paroxetine Hydrochloride (Cases of life-threatening serotonin syndrome have been reported during combined use of selective serotonin reuptake inhibitors (SSRIs) and triptans. If concomitant treatment with zolmitriptan and an SSRI (eg, paroxetine) is clinically warranted, careful observation of the patient is advised, particularly during treatment initiation and dose increases. Serotonin syndrome symptoms may include mental status changes, autonomic instability, neuromuscular aberrations, and/or gastrointestinal symptoms). Products include:

Paroxetine CR 2361
Paroxetine ER 2371
Paxil 1586
Paxil CR 1596

Paroxetine Mesylate (Cases of life-threatening serotonin syndrome have been reported during combined use of selective serotonin reuptake inhibitors (SSRIs) and triptans. If concomitant treatment with zolmitriptan and an SSRI (eg, paroxetine) is clinically warranted, careful observation of the patient is advised, particularly during treatment initiation and dose increases. Serotonin syndrome symptoms may include mental status changes, autonomic instability, neuromuscular aberrations, and/or gastrointestinal symptoms).

No products indexed under this heading.

Phenelzine Sulfate (Concurrent administration of MAO-A inhibitors or use of zolmitriptan within 2 weeks of discontinuation of MAO-A inhibitor therapy is contraindicated. MAO-A inhibitors increase the systemic exposure of zolmitriptan. Therefore, the use of zolmitriptan in patients receiving MAO-A inhibitors is contraindicated. Following one week of administration of 150 mg bid moclobemide, a specific MAO-A inhibitor, there was an increase of about 25% in both C_{max} and AUC for zolmitriptan and a 3-fold increase in the C_{max} and AUC of the active N-desmethyl metabolite of zolmitriptan).

No products indexed under this heading.

Procarbazine Hydrochloride (Concurrent administration of MAO-A inhibitors or use of zolmitriptan within 2 weeks of discontinuation of MAO-A inhibitor therapy is contraindicated. MAO-A inhibitors increase the systemic exposure of zolmitriptan. Therefore, the use of zolmitriptan in patients receiving MAO-A inhibitors is contraindicated. Following one week of administration of 150 mg bid moclobemide, a specific MAO-A inhibitor, there was an increase of about 25% in both C_{max} and AUC for zolmitriptan and a 3-fold increase in the C_{max} and AUC of the active N-desmethyl metabolite of zolmitriptan).

No products indexed under this heading.

Propranolol (C_{max} and AUC of zolmitriptan increased 1.5-fold after one week of dosing with propranolol (160 mg/day). C_{max} and AUC of the N-desmethyl metabolite were reduced by 30% and 15%, respectively. There were no interactive effects on blood pressure or pulse rate following administration of propranolol with zolmitriptan).

No products indexed under this heading.

Propranolol Hydrochloride (C_{max} and AUC of zolmitriptan increased 1.5-fold after one week of dosing with propranolol (160 mg/day). C_{max} and AUC of the N-desmethyl metabolite were reduced by 30% and 15%, respectively. There were no interactive effects on blood pressure or pulse rate following administration of propranolol with zolmitriptan). Products include:

InnoPran XL 1517

Rasagiline Mesylate (Concurrent administration of MAO-A inhibitors or use of zolmitriptan within 2 weeks of discontinuation of MAO-A inhibitor therapy is contraindicated. MAO-A inhibitors increase the systemic exposure of zolmitriptan. Therefore, the use of zolmitriptan in patients receiving MAO-A inhibitors is contraindicated. Following one week of administration of 150 mg bid moclobemide, a specific MAO-A inhibitor, there was an increase of about 25% in both C_{max} and AUC for zolmitriptan and a 3-fold increase in the C_{max} and AUC of the active N-desmethyl metabolite of zolmitriptan). Products include:

Azilect 3383

Rizatriptan Benzoate (Concomitant use of other 5-HT1B/1D agonists (eg, triptans) within 24 hours of zolmitriptan treatment is contraindicated). Products include:

Maxalt 2206
Maxalt-MLT 2206

Selegiline (Concurrent administration of MAO-A inhibitors or use of zolmitriptan within 2 weeks of discontinuation of MAO-A inhibitor therapy is contraindicated. MAO-A inhibitors increase the systemic exposure of zolmitriptan. Therefore, the use of zolmitriptan in patients receiving MAO-A inhibitors is contraindicated. Following one week of administration of 150 mg bid moclobemide, a specific MAO-A inhibitor, there was an increase of about 25% in both C_{max} and AUC for zolmitriptan and a 3-fold increase in the C_{max} and AUC of the active N-desmethyl metabolite of zolmitriptan). Products include:

Emsam 3623

Selegiline Hydrochloride (Concurrent administration of MAO-A inhibitors or use of zolmitriptan within 2 weeks of discontinuation of MAO-A inhibitor therapy is contraindicated. MAO-A inhibitors increase the systemic exposure of zolmitriptan. Therefore, the use of zolmitriptan in patients receiving MAO-A inhibitors is contraindicated. Following one week of administration of 150 mg bid moclobemide, a specific MAO-A inhibitor, there was an increase of about 25% in both C_{max} and AUC for zolmitriptan and a 3-fold increase in the C_{max} and AUC of the active N-desmethyl metabolite of zolmitriptan). Products include:

Eldepryl 3312

Sertraline Hydrochloride (Cases of life-threatening serotonin syndrome have been reported during combined use of selective serotonin reuptake inhibitors (SSRIs) and triptans. If concomitant treatment with zolmitriptan and an SSRI (eg, sertraline) is clinically warranted, careful observation of the patient is advised, particularly during treatment initiation and dose increases. Serotonin syndrome symptoms may include mental status changes, autonomic instability, neuromuscular aberrations, and/or gastrointestinal symptoms).

No products indexed under this heading.

Sumatriptan (Concomitant use of other 5-HT1B/1D agonists (eg, triptans) within 24 hours of zolmitriptan treatment is contraindicated). Products include:

Imitrex Nasal 1503

Sumatriptan Succinate (Concomitant use of other 5-HT1B/1D agonists (eg, triptans) within 24 hours of zolmitriptan treatment is contraindicated). Products include:

Imitrex 1497
Imitrex Tablets 1508
Treximet 1681

Tranylcypromine Sulfate (Concurrent administration of MAO-A inhibitors or use of zolmitriptan within 2 weeks of discontinuation of MAO-A inhibitor therapy is contraindicated. MAO-A inhibitors increase the systemic exposure of zolmitriptan. Therefore, the use of zolmitriptan in patients receiving MAO-A inhibitors is contraindicated. Following one week of administration of 150 mg bid moclobemide, a specific MAO-A inhibitor, there was an increase of about 25% in both C_{max} and AUC for zolmitriptan and a 3-fold increase in the C_{max} and AUC of the active N-desmethyl metabolite of zolmitriptan). Products include:

Parnate 1584

Venlafaxine Hydrochloride (Cases of life-threatening serotonin syndrome have been reported during combined use of serotonin norepinephrine reuptake inhibitors (SNRIs) and triptans. If concomitant treatment with zolmitriptan and a SNRI (eg, venlafaxine) is clinically warranted, careful observation of the patient is advised, particularly during treatment initiation and dose increases. Serotonin syndrome symptoms may include mental status changes, autonomic instability, neuromuscular aberrations, and/or gastrointestinal symptoms). Products include:

Effexor XR 3504
Venlafaxine Hydrochloride Tablets ... 2388

ZOMIG-ZMT TABLETS

(Zolmitriptan) 773
See Zomig Tablets

ZONEGRAN CAPSULES

(Zonisamide) 1081

May interact with alcohols, anticholinergic-type antiparkinsonism drugs, anticholinergics, carbonic anhydrase inhibitors, central nervous system depressants, cytochrome p450 3a4 inducers (selected), cytochrome p450 3a4 inhibitors (selected), hepatic microsomal enzyme inducers, phenytoin, valproate, and certain other agents. Compounds in these categories include:

Acetazolamide (Caution should be used when zonisamide is prescribed with other drugs that predispose patients to heat-related disorders; these drugs include, but are not limited to, carbonic anhydrase inhibitors and drugs with anticholinergic activity).

No products indexed under this heading.

Acetazolamide Sodium (Concurrent use with drugs that inhibit CYP3A4 may alter serum concentrations of zonisamide).

No products indexed under this heading.

IMPORTANT NOTE: Always consult each drug listing in the patient's regimen for possible interactions.

(⊙ Described in PDR® for Ophthalmic Medicines)

2177 Interactions Index Zonegran

Estazolam (Concomitant administration of zonisamide and alcohol or other CNS depressants has not been evaluated in clinical studies. Because of the potential of zonisamide to cause CNS depression, as well as other cognitive and/or neuropsychiatric adverse events, zonisamide should be used with caution if used in combination with alcohol or other CNS depressants).
No products indexed under this heading.

Ethanol (Concomitant administration of zonisamide and alcohol or other CNS depressants has not been evaluated in clinical studies. Because of the potential of zonisamide to cause CNS depression, as well as other cognitive and/or neuropsychiatric adverse events, zonisamide should be used with caution if used in combination with alcohol or other CNS depressants).
No products indexed under this heading.

Ethchlorvynol (Concomitant administration of zonisamide and alcohol or other CNS depressants has not been evaluated in clinical studies. Because of the potential of zonisamide to cause CNS depression, as well as other cognitive and/or neuropsychiatric adverse events, zonisamide should be used with caution if used in combination with alcohol or other CNS depressants).
No products indexed under this heading.

Ethinamate (Concomitant administration of zonisamide and alcohol or other CNS depressants has not been evaluated in clinical studies. Because of the potential of zonisamide to cause CNS depression, as well as other cognitive and/or neuropsychiatric adverse events, zonisamide should be used with caution if used in combination with alcohol or other CNS depressants).
No products indexed under this heading.

Ethosuximide (Drugs that induce liver enzymes increase the metabolism and clearance of zonisamide and decrease its half-life).
No products indexed under this heading.

Ethyl Alcohol (Concomitant administration of zonisamide and alcohol or other CNS depressants has not been evaluated in clinical studies. Because of the potential of zonisamide to cause CNS depression, as well as other cognitive and/or neuropsychiatric adverse events, zonisamide should be used with caution if used in combination with alcohol or other CNS depressants).
No products indexed under this heading.

Felbamate (Drugs that induce liver enzymes increase the metabolism and clearance of zonisamide and decrease its half-life).
No products indexed under this heading.

Fentanyl (Concomitant administration of zonisamide and alcohol or other CNS depressants has not been evaluated in clinical studies. Because of the potential of zonisamide to cause CNS depression, as well as other cognitive and/or neuropsychiatric adverse events, zonisamide should be used with caution if used in combination with alcohol or other CNS depressants). Products include:
Duragesic 2604
Fentanyl Transdermal System 2346
Onsolis 2054

Fentanyl Citrate (Concomitant administration of zonisamide and alcohol or other CNS depressants has not been evaluated in clinical studies. Because of the potential of zonisamide to cause CNS depression, as well as other cognitive and/or neuropsychiatric adverse events, zonisamide should be used with caution if used in combination with alcohol or other CNS depressants). Products include:
Fentora 966

Fluconazole (Concurrent use with drugs that inhibit CYP3A4 may alter serum concentrations of zonisamide).
No products indexed under this heading.

Fludrocortisone Acetate (Drugs that induce liver enzymes increase the metabolism and clearance of zonisamide and decrease its half-life).
No products indexed under this heading.

Fluoxetine (Concurrent use with drugs that inhibit CYP3A4 may alter serum concentrations of zonisamide).
No products indexed under this heading.

Fluoxetine Hydrochloride (Concurrent use with drugs that inhibit CYP3A4 may alter serum concentrations of zonisamide). Products include:
Prozac Weekly 1941
Prozac Pulvules 1941
Symbyax 1965

Fluphenazine Decanoate (Concomitant administration of zonisamide and alcohol or other CNS depressants has not been evaluated in clinical studies. Because of the potential of zonisamide to cause CNS depression, as well as other cognitive and/or neuropsychiatric adverse events, zonisamide should be used with caution if used in combination with alcohol or other CNS depressants).
No products indexed under this heading.

Fluphenazine Enanthate (Concomitant administration of zonisamide and alcohol or other CNS depressants has not been evaluated in clinical studies. Because of the potential of zonisamide to cause CNS depression, as well as other cognitive and/or neuropsychiatric adverse events, zonisamide should be used with caution if used in combination with alcohol or other CNS depressants).
No products indexed under this heading.

Fluphenazine Hydrochloride (Concomitant administration of zonisamide and alcohol or other CNS depressants has not been evaluated in clinical studies. Because of the potential of zonisamide to cause CNS depression, as well as other cognitive and/or neuropsychiatric adverse events, zonisamide should be used with caution if used in combination with alcohol or other CNS depressants).
No products indexed under this heading.

Flurazepam Hydrochloride (Concomitant administration of zonisamide and alcohol or other CNS depressants has not been evaluated in clinical studies. Because of the potential of zonisamide to cause CNS depression, as well as other cognitive and/or neuropsychiatric adverse events, zonisamide should be used with caution if used in combination with alcohol or other CNS depressants).
No products indexed under this heading.

Fluvoxamine (Drugs that induce liver enzymes increase the metabolism and clearance of zonisamide and decrease its half-life).
No products indexed under this heading.

Fluvoxamine Maleate (Drugs that induce liver enzymes increase the metabolism and clearance of zonisamide and decrease its half-life).
No products indexed under this heading.

Fosamprenavir Calcium (Concurrent use with drugs that inhibit CYP3A4 may alter serum concentrations of zonisamide). Products include:
Lexiva Oral Suspension 1558
Lexiva 1558

Fosphenytoin (Concomitant administration of phenytoin and carbamazepine increases zonisamide plasma clearance from 0.30–0.35 mL/min/kg to 0.35–0.5 mL/min/kg. The half-life of zonisamide is decreased to 27 hours by phenytoin. Plasma protein binding of phenytoin was not affected by zonisamide administration).
No products indexed under this heading.

Fosphenytoin Sodium (Concomitant administration of phenytoin and carbamazepine increases zonisamide plasma clearance from 0.30–0.35 mL/min/kg to 0.35–0.5 mL/min/kg. The half-life of zonisamide is decreased to 27 hours by phenytoin. Plasma protein binding of phenytoin was not affected by zonisamide administration).
No products indexed under this heading.

Garlic Extract (Drugs that induce liver enzymes increase the metabolism and clearance of zonisamide and decrease its half-life).
No products indexed under this heading.

Garlic Oil (Drugs that induce liver enzymes increase the metabolism and clearance of zonisamide and decrease its half-life).
No products indexed under this heading.

Glipizide (Drugs that induce liver enzymes increase the metabolism and clearance of zonisamide and decrease its half-life).
No products indexed under this heading.

Glutethimide (Concomitant administration of zonisamide and alcohol or other CNS depressants has not been evaluated in clinical studies. Because of the potential of zonisamide to cause CNS depression, as well as other cognitive and/or neuropsychiatric adverse events, zonisamide should be used with caution if used in combination with alcohol or other CNS depressants).
No products indexed under this heading.

Glyburide (Drugs that induce liver enzymes increase the metabolism and clearance of zonisamide and decrease its half-life).
No products indexed under this heading.

Glycopyrrolate (Caution should be used when zonisamide is prescribed with other drugs that predispose patients to heat-related disorders; these drugs include, but are not limited to, carbonic anhydrase inhibitors and drugs with anticholinergic activity).
No products indexed under this heading.

Halazepam (Concomitant administration of zonisamide and alcohol or other CNS depressants has not been evaluated in clinical studies. Because of the potential of zonisamide to cause CNS depression, as well as other cognitive and/or neuropsychiatric adverse events, zonisamide should be used with caution if used in combination with alcohol or other CNS depressants).
No products indexed under this heading.

Haloperidol (Concomitant administration of zonisamide and alcohol or other CNS depressants has not been evaluated in clinical studies. Because of the potential of zonisamide to cause CNS depression, as well as other cognitive and/or neuropsychiatric adverse events, zonisamide should be used with caution if used in combination with alcohol or other CNS depressants).
No products indexed under this heading.

Haloperidol Decanoate (Concomitant administration of zonisamide and alcohol or other CNS depressants has not been evaluated in clinical studies. Because of the potential of zonisamide to cause CNS depression, as well as other cognitive and/or neuropsychiatric adverse events, zonisamide should be used with caution if used in combination with alcohol or other CNS depressants).
No products indexed under this heading.

Haloperidol Lactate (Concomitant administration of zonisamide and alcohol or other CNS depressants has not been evaluated in clinical studies. Because of the potential of zonisamide to cause CNS depression, as well as other cognitive and/or neuropsychiatric adverse events, zonisamide should be used with caution if used in combination with alcohol or other CNS depressants).
No products indexed under this heading.

Hepatic Enzyme-Inducing Agents (Drugs that induce liver enzymes increase the metabolism and clearance of zonisamide and decrease its half-life).
No products indexed under this heading.

Hexobarbital (Concomitant administration of zonisamide and alcohol or other CNS depressants has not been evaluated in clinical studies. Because of the potential of zonisamide to cause CNS depression, as well as other cognitive and/or neuropsychiatric adverse events, zonisamide should be used with caution if used in combination with alcohol or other CNS depressants).
No products indexed under this heading.

Hydrocodone Bitartrate (Concomitant administration of zonisamide and alcohol or other CNS depressants has not been evaluated in clinical studies. Because of the potential of zonisamide to cause CNS depression, as well as other cognitive and/or neuropsychiatric adverse events, zonisamide should be used with caution if used in combination with alcohol or other CNS depressants). Products include:
Vicodin 560
Vicodin ES 561
Vicodin HP 563
Vicoprofen 564
Zydone 1138

Hydrocodone Polistirex (Concomitant administration of zonisamide and alcohol or other CNS depressants has not been evaluated in clinical studies. Because of the potential of zonisamide to cause CNS depression, as well as other cognitive and/or neuropsychiatric adverse events, zonisamide should be used with caution if used in combination with alcohol or other CNS depressants). Products include:
Tussionex 3443

Hydrocortisone (Concurrent use with drugs that induce CYP3A4 may alter serum concentrations of zonisamide).
No products indexed under this heading.

Hydrocortisone (Alcohol) (Drugs that induce liver enzymes increase the metabolism and clearance of zonisamide and decrease its half-life).
No products indexed under this heading.

Hydrocortisone Acetate (Drugs that induce liver enzymes increase the metabolism and clearance of zonisamide and decrease its half-life).
No products indexed under this heading.

Hydrocortisone Butyrate (Drugs that induce liver enzymes increase the metabolism and clearance of zonisamide and decrease its half-life).
No products indexed under this heading.

Hydrocortisone Cypionate (Drugs that induce liver enzymes increase the metabolism and clearance of zonisamide and decrease its half-life).
No products indexed under this heading.

IMPORTANT NOTE: Always consult each drug listing in the patient's regimen for possible interactions.

Hydrocortisone Hemisuccinate
(Drugs that induce liver enzymes increase the metabolism and clearance of zonisamide and decrease its half-life). No products indexed under this heading.

Hydrocortisone Probutate (Drugs that induce liver enzymes increase the metabolism and clearance of zonisamide and decrease its half-life). No products indexed under this heading.

Hydrocortisone Sodium Phosphate (Drugs that induce liver enzymes increase the metabolism and clearance of zonisamide and decrease its half-life). No products indexed under this heading.

Hydrocortisone Sodium Succinate (Drugs that induce liver enzymes increase the metabolism and clearance of zonisamide and decrease its half-life). No products indexed under this heading.

Hydrocortisone Valerate (Drugs that induce liver enzymes increase the metabolism and clearance of zonisamide and decrease its half-life). No products indexed under this heading.

Hydromorphone (Concomitant administration of zonisamide and alcohol or other CNS depressants has not been evaluated in clinical studies. Because of the potential of zonisamide to cause CNS depression, as well as other cognitive and/or neuropsychiatric adverse events, zonisamide should be used with caution if used in combination with alcohol or other CNS depressants). No products indexed under this heading.

Hydromorphone Hydrochloride (Concomitant administration of zonisamide and alcohol or other CNS depressants has not been evaluated in clinical studies. Because of the potential of zonisamide to cause CNS depression, as well as other cognitive and/or neuropsychiatric adverse events, zonisamide should be used with caution if used in combination with alcohol or other CNS depressants). Products include:
Dilaudid Injection 2800
Dilaudid Oral 2797
Dilaudid Tablets 2797
Dilaudid-HP 2800

Hydroxyzine Hydrochloride (Concomitant administration of zonisamide and alcohol or other CNS depressants has not been evaluated in clinical studies. Because of the potential of zonisamide to cause CNS depression, as well as other cognitive and/or neuropsychiatric adverse events, zonisamide should be used with caution if used in combination with alcohol or other CNS depressants). No products indexed under this heading.

Hyoscyamine (Caution should be used when zonisamide is prescribed with other drugs that predispose patients to heat-related disorders; these drugs include, but are not limited to, carbonic anhydrase inhibitors and drugs with anticholinergic activity). No products indexed under this heading.

Hyoscyamine Sulfate (Caution should be used when zonisamide is prescribed with other drugs that predispose patients to heat-related disorders; these drugs include, but are not limited to, carbonic anhydrase inhibitors and drugs with anticholinergic activity). Products include:
Donnatal 2711

Hypericum (Drugs that induce liver enzymes increase the metabolism and clearance of zonisamide and decrease its half-life). No products indexed under this heading.

Hypericum Perforatum (Drugs that induce liver enzymes increase the metabolism and clearance of zonisamide and decrease its half-life). Products include:

Traumeel 1800

Imatinib Mesylate (Concurrent use with drugs that inhibit CYP3A4 may alter serum concentrations of zonisamide). Products include:
Gleevec 2477

Indinavir Sulfate (Concurrent use with drugs that inhibit CYP3A4 may alter serum concentrations of zonisamide). Products include:
Crixivan 2113

Insulin (Drugs that induce liver enzymes increase the metabolism and clearance of zonisamide and decrease its half-life). No products indexed under this heading.

Insulin, Human, Zinc Suspension (Drugs that induce liver enzymes increase the metabolism and clearance of zonisamide and decrease its half-life). No products indexed under this heading.

Insulin, Human (rDNA origin) (Drugs that induce liver enzymes increase the metabolism and clearance of zonisamide and decrease its half-life). Products include:
Exubera 2717

Insulin, Human NPH (Drugs that induce liver enzymes increase the metabolism and clearance of zonisamide and decrease its half-life). Products include:
Humulin N Vial 1934

Insulin, Human Regular (Drugs that induce liver enzymes increase the metabolism and clearance of zonisamide and decrease its half-life). Products include:
Humulin R 1937
Humulin R (U-500) 1939

Insulin, Human Regular and Human NPH Mixture (Drugs that induce liver enzymes increase the metabolism and clearance of zonisamide and decrease its half-life). Products include:
Humulin 50/50 1930
Humulin 70/30 Vial 1931

Insulin, NPH (Drugs that induce liver enzymes increase the metabolism and clearance of zonisamide and decrease its half-life). No products indexed under this heading.

Insulin, Regular (Drugs that induce liver enzymes increase the metabolism and clearance of zonisamide and decrease its half-life). No products indexed under this heading.

Insulin, Regular and NPH mixture (Drugs that induce liver enzymes increase the metabolism and clearance of zonisamide and decrease its half-life). No products indexed under this heading.

Insulin, Zinc Crystals (Drugs that induce liver enzymes increase the metabolism and clearance of zonisamide and decrease its half-life). No products indexed under this heading.

Insulin, Zinc Suspension (Drugs that induce liver enzymes increase the metabolism and clearance of zonisamide and decrease its half-life). No products indexed under this heading.

Insulin Aspart (Drugs that induce liver enzymes increase the metabolism and clearance of zonisamide and decrease its half-life). No products indexed under this heading.

Insulin Aspart, Human (Drugs that induce liver enzymes increase the metabolism and clearance of zonisamide and decrease its half-life). Products include:
NovoLog Mix 70/30 2581

Insulin Aspart, Human Regular (Drugs that induce liver enzymes increase the metabolism and clearance of zonisamide and decrease its half-life). Products include:

NovoLog 2575

Insulin Aspart Protamine, Human (Drugs that induce liver enzymes increase the metabolism and clearance of zonisamide and decrease its half-life). Products include:
NovoLog Mix 70/30 2581

Insulin Detemir (rDNA Origin) (Drugs that induce liver enzymes increase the metabolism and clearance of zonisamide and decrease its half-life). Products include:
Levemir 2566

Insulin Glargine (Drugs that induce liver enzymes increase the metabolism and clearance of zonisamide and decrease its half-life). Products include:
Lantus 2996

Insulin Glulisine (Drugs that induce liver enzymes increase the metabolism and clearance of zonisamide and decrease its half-life). Products include:
Apidra 2937
Apidra SoloStar 2937

Insulin Lispro, Human (Drugs that induce liver enzymes increase the metabolism and clearance of zonisamide and decrease its half-life). Products include:
Humalog 1910
Humalog Mix 1914
Humalog Mix 75/25 1917

Insulin Lispro Protamine, Human (Drugs that induce liver enzymes increase the metabolism and clearance of zonisamide and decrease its half-life). Products include:
Humalog Mix 1914
Humalog Mix 75/25 1917

Ipratropium Bromide (Caution should be used when zonisamide is prescribed with other drugs that predispose patients to heat-related disorders; these drugs include, but are not limited to, carbonic anhydrase inhibitors and drugs with anticholinergic activity). No products indexed under this heading.

Isoflurane (Concomitant administration of zonisamide and alcohol or other CNS depressants has not been evaluated in clinical studies. Because of the potential of zonisamide to cause CNS depression, as well as other cognitive and/or neuropsychiatric adverse events, zonisamide should be used with caution if used in combination with alcohol or other CNS depressants). No products indexed under this heading.

Isoniazid (Concurrent use with drugs that inhibit CYP3A4 may alter serum concentrations of zonisamide). No products indexed under this heading.

Itraconazole (Concurrent use with drugs that inhibit CYP3A4 may alter serum concentrations of zonisamide). No products indexed under this heading.

Ketamine Hydrochloride (Concomitant administration of zonisamide and alcohol or other CNS depressants has not been evaluated in clinical studies. Because of the potential of zonisamide to cause CNS depression, as well as other cognitive and/or neuropsychiatric adverse events, zonisamide should be used with caution if used in combination with alcohol or other CNS depressants). No products indexed under this heading.

Ketoconazole (Concurrent use with drugs that inhibit CYP3A4 may alter serum concentrations of zonisamide). Products include:
Extina 3319
Xolegel 3337

Lansoprazole (Drugs that induce liver enzymes increase the metabolism and clearance of zonisamide and decrease its half-life). No products indexed under this heading.

Lapatinib (Concurrent use with drugs that inhibit CYP3A4 may alter serum concentrations of zonisamide). Products include:
Tykerb 1698

Levomethadyl Acetate Hydrochloride (Concomitant administration of zonisamide and alcohol or other CNS depressants has not been evaluated in clinical studies. Because of the potential of zonisamide to cause CNS depression, as well as other cognitive and/or neuropsychiatric adverse events, zonisamide should be used with caution if used in combination with alcohol or other CNS depressants). No products indexed under this heading.

Levorphanol Tartrate (Concomitant administration of zonisamide and alcohol or other CNS depressants has not been evaluated in clinical studies. Because of the potential of zonisamide to cause CNS depression, as well as other cognitive and/or neuropsychiatric adverse events, zonisamide should be used with caution if used in combination with alcohol or other CNS depressants). No products indexed under this heading.

Lopinavir (Concurrent use with drugs that inhibit CYP3A4 may alter serum concentrations of zonisamide). Products include:
Kaletra 458

Loratadine (Concurrent use with drugs that inhibit CYP3A4 may alter serum concentrations of zonisamide). No products indexed under this heading.

Lorazepam (Concomitant administration of zonisamide and alcohol or other CNS depressants has not been evaluated in clinical studies. Because of the potential of zonisamide to cause CNS depression, as well as other cognitive and/or neuropsychiatric adverse events, zonisamide should be used with caution if used in combination with alcohol or other CNS depressants). No products indexed under this heading.

Loxapine Hydrochloride (Concomitant administration of zonisamide and alcohol or other CNS depressants has not been evaluated in clinical studies. Because of the potential of zonisamide to cause CNS depression, as well as other cognitive and/or neuropsychiatric adverse events, zonisamide should be used with caution if used in combination with alcohol or other CNS depressants). No products indexed under this heading.

Loxapine Succinate (Concomitant administration of zonisamide and alcohol or other CNS depressants has not been evaluated in clinical studies. Because of the potential of zonisamide to cause CNS depression, as well as other cognitive and/or neuropsychiatric adverse events, zonisamide should be used with caution if used in combination with alcohol or other CNS depressants). No products indexed under this heading.

Mepenzolate Bromide (Caution should be used when zonisamide is prescribed with other drugs that predispose patients to heat-related disorders; these drugs include, but are not limited to, carbonic anhydrase inhibitors and drugs with anticholinergic activity). No products indexed under this heading.

Meperidine Hydrochloride (Concomitant administration of zonisamide and alcohol or other CNS depressants has not been evaluated in clinical studies. Because of the potential of zonisamide to cause CNS depression, as well as other cognitive and/or neuropsychiatric adverse events, zonisamide should be used with caution if used in combination with alcohol or other CNS depressants). No products indexed under this heading.

2179 Interactions Index Zonegran

Mephenytoin (Drugs that induce liver enzymes increase the metabolism and clearance of zonisamide and decrease its half-life).
No products indexed under this heading.

Mephobarbital (Concomitant administration of zonisamide and alcohol or other CNS depressants has not been evaluated in clinical studies. Because of the potential of zonisamide to cause CNS depression, as well as other cognitive and/or neuropsychiatric adverse events, zonisamide should be used with caution if used in combination with alcohol or other CNS depressants).
No products indexed under this heading.

Meprobamate (Concomitant administration of zonisamide and alcohol or other CNS depressants has not been evaluated in clinical studies. Because of the potential of zonisamide to cause CNS depression, as well as other cognitive and/or neuropsychiatric adverse events, zonisamide should be used with caution if used in combination with alcohol or other CNS depressants).
No products indexed under this heading.

Mesoridazine Besylate (Concomitant administration of zonisamide and alcohol or other CNS depressants has not been evaluated in clinical studies. Because of the potential of zonisamide to cause CNS depression, as well as other cognitive and/or neuropsychiatric adverse events, zonisamide should be used with caution if used in combination with alcohol or other CNS depressants).
No products indexed under this heading.

Methadone Hydrochloride (Concomitant administration of zonisamide and alcohol or other CNS depressants has not been evaluated in clinical studies. Because of the potential of zonisamide to cause CNS depression, as well as other cognitive and/or neuropsychiatric adverse events, zonisamide should be used with caution if used in combination with alcohol or other CNS depressants).
No products indexed under this heading.

Methazolamide (Caution should be used when zonisamide is prescribed with other drugs that predispose patients to heat-related disorders; these drugs include, but are not limited to, carbonic anhydrase inhibitors and drugs with anticholinergic activity).
No products indexed under this heading.

Methohexital Sodium (Concomitant administration of zonisamide and alcohol or other CNS depressants has not been evaluated in clinical studies. Because of the potential of zonisamide to cause CNS depression, as well as other cognitive and/or neuropsychiatric adverse events, zonisamide should be used with caution if used in combination with alcohol or other CNS depressants).
No products indexed under this heading.

Methotrimeprazine (Concomitant administration of zonisamide and alcohol or other CNS depressants has not been evaluated in clinical studies. Because of the potential of zonisamide to cause CNS depression, as well as other cognitive and/or neuropsychiatric adverse events, zonisamide should be used with caution if used in combination with alcohol or other CNS depressants).
No products indexed under this heading.

Methoxyflurane (Concomitant administration of zonisamide and alcohol or other CNS depressants has not been evaluated in clinical studies. Because of the potential of zonisamide to cause CNS depression, as well as other cognitive and/or neuropsychiatric adverse events, zonisamide should be used with caution if used in combination with alcohol or other CNS depressants).
No products indexed under this heading.

Methsuximide (Drugs that induce liver enzymes increase the metabolism and clearance of zonisamide and decrease its half-life).
No products indexed under this heading.

Methylprednisolone (Drugs that induce liver enzymes increase the metabolism and clearance of zonisamide and decrease its half-life).
No products indexed under this heading.

Methylprednisolone Acetate (Drugs that induce liver enzymes increase the metabolism and clearance of zonisamide and decrease its half-life).
No products indexed under this heading.

Methylprednisolone Sodium Succinate (Drugs that induce liver enzymes increase the metabolism and clearance of zonisamide and decrease its half-life).
No products indexed under this heading.

Metronidazole (Concurrent use with drugs that inhibit CYP3A4 may alter serum concentrations of zonisamide). Products include:
Pylera 793

Metronidazole Benzoate (Concurrent use with drugs that inhibit CYP3A4 may alter serum concentrations of zonisamide).
No products indexed under this heading.

Metronidazole Hydrochloride (Concurrent use with drugs that inhibit CYP3A4 may alter serum concentrations of zonisamide).
No products indexed under this heading.

Metronidazole Sodium (Concurrent use with drugs that inhibit CYP3A4 may alter serum concentrations of zonisamide).
No products indexed under this heading.

Miconazole (Concurrent use with drugs that inhibit CYP3A4 may alter serum concentrations of zonisamide).
No products indexed under this heading.

Miconazole Nitrate (Concurrent use with drugs that inhibit CYP3A4 may alter serum concentrations of zonisamide). Products include:
Vusion Ointment 3335

Midazolam Hydrochloride (Concomitant administration of zonisamide and alcohol or other CNS depressants has not been evaluated in clinical studies. Because of the potential of zonisamide to cause CNS depression, as well as other cognitive and/or neuropsychiatric adverse events, zonisamide should be used with caution if used in combination with alcohol or other CNS depressants).
No products indexed under this heading.

Mifepristone (Concurrent use with drugs that inhibit CYP3A4 may alter serum concentrations of zonisamide).
No products indexed under this heading.

Modafinil (Drugs that induce liver enzymes increase the metabolism and clearance of zonisamide and decrease its half-life). Products include:
Provigil 983

Molindone Hydrochloride (Concomitant administration of zonisamide and alcohol or other CNS depressants has not been evaluated in clinical studies. Because of the potential of zonisamide to cause CNS depression, as well as other cognitive and/or neuropsychiatric adverse events, zonisamide should be used with caution if used in combination with alcohol or other CNS depressants). Products include:
Moban 1108

Morphine Sulfate (Concomitant administration of zonisamide and alcohol or other CNS depressants has not been evaluated in clinical studies. Because of the potential of zonisamide to cause CNS depression, as well as other cognitive and/or neuropsychiatric adverse events, zonisamide should be used with caution if used in combination with alcohol or other CNS depressants). Products include:
Avinza 1822
Embeda 1831
MS Contin 2803

Morphine Sulfate, Liposomal (Concomitant administration of zonisamide and alcohol or other CNS depressants has not been evaluated in clinical studies. Because of the potential of zonisamide to cause CNS depression, as well as other cognitive and/or neuropsychiatric adverse events, zonisamide should be used with caution if used in combination with alcohol or other CNS depressants).
No products indexed under this heading.

Nafcillin Sodium (Drugs that induce liver enzymes increase the metabolism and clearance of zonisamide and decrease its half-life).
No products indexed under this heading.

Nefazodone Hydrochloride (Concurrent use with drugs that inhibit CYP3A4 may alter serum concentrations of zonisamide).
No products indexed under this heading.

Nelfinavir Mesylate (Concurrent use with drugs that inhibit CYP3A4 may alter serum concentrations of zonisamide).
No products indexed under this heading.

Nevirapine (Drugs that induce liver enzymes increase the metabolism and clearance of zonisamide and decrease its half-life). Products include:
Viramune Oral Suspension 897
Viramune Tablets 897

Niacin (Concurrent use with drugs that inhibit CYP3A4 may alter serum concentrations of zonisamide). Products include:
Advicor 402
Cardio Basics 3455
Niaspan 497
Simcor 524

Niacinamide (Concurrent use with drugs that inhibit CYP3A4 may alter serum concentrations of zonisamide). Products include:
CitraNatal 90 DHA Capsules 2332
CitraNatal Assure 2332
CitraNatal Rx 2332
Heplive 607

Niacinamide Hydroiodide (Concurrent use with drugs that inhibit CYP3A4 may alter serum concentrations of zonisamide).
No products indexed under this heading.

Nicotinamide (Concurrent use with drugs that inhibit CYP3A4 may alter serum concentrations of zonisamide).
No products indexed under this heading.

Nicotine (Drugs that induce liver enzymes increase the metabolism and clearance of zonisamide and decrease its half-life).
No products indexed under this heading.

Nicotine Polacrilex (Drugs that induce liver enzymes increase the metabolism and clearance of zonisamide and decrease its half-life).
No products indexed under this heading.

Nicotine Salicylate (Drugs that induce liver enzymes increase the metabolism and clearance of zonisamide and decrease its half-life).
No products indexed under this heading.

Nicotine Sulfate (Drugs that induce liver enzymes increase the metabolism and clearance of zonisamide and decrease its half-life).
No products indexed under this heading.

Nifedipine (Concurrent use with drugs that inhibit CYP3A4 may alter serum concentrations of zonisamide).
No products indexed under this heading.

Norethindrone (Drugs that induce liver enzymes increase the metabolism and clearance of zonisamide and decrease its half-life). Products include:
Ortho Micronor 2660

Norethindrone Acetate (Drugs that induce liver enzymes increase the metabolism and clearance of zonisamide and decrease its half-life). Products include:
Activella 2561

Norfloxacin (Concurrent use with drugs that inhibit CYP3A4 may alter serum concentrations of zonisamide). Products include:
Noroxin 2220

Olanzapine (Concomitant administration of zonisamide and alcohol or other CNS depressants has not been evaluated in clinical studies. Because of the potential of zonisamide to cause CNS depression, as well as other cognitive and/or neuropsychiatric adverse events, zonisamide should be used with caution if used in combination with alcohol or other CNS depressants). Products include:
Symbyax 1965
Zyprexa 1984
Zyprexa IntraMuscular 1984
Zyprexa ZYDIS 1984

Omeprazole (Drugs that induce liver enzymes increase the metabolism and clearance of zonisamide and decrease its half-life).
No products indexed under this heading.

Omeprazole Magnesium (Drugs that induce liver enzymes increase the metabolism and clearance of zonisamide and decrease its half-life).
No products indexed under this heading.

Oxazepam (Concomitant administration of zonisamide and alcohol or other CNS depressants has not been evaluated in clinical studies. Because of the potential of zonisamide to cause CNS depression, as well as other cognitive and/or neuropsychiatric adverse events, zonisamide should be used with caution if used in combination with alcohol or other CNS depressants).
No products indexed under this heading.

Oxcarbazepine (Drugs that induce liver enzymes increase the metabolism and clearance of zonisamide and decrease its half-life).
No products indexed under this heading.

Oxybutynin Chloride (Caution should be used when zonisamide is prescribed with other drugs that predispose patients to heat-related disorders; these drugs include, but are not limited to, carbonic anhydrase inhibitors and drugs with anticholinergic activity).
No products indexed under this heading.

Oxycodone Hydrochloride (Concomitant administration of zonisamide and alcohol or other CNS depressants has not been evaluated in clinical studies. Because of the potential of zonisamide to cause CNS depression, as well as other cognitive and/or neuropsychiatric adverse events, zonisamide should be used with caution if used in combination with alcohol or other CNS depressants). Products include:
OxyContin 2807
Percocet 1121
Percodan 1124

Oxycodone Terephthalate (Concomitant administration of zonisamide and alcohol or other CNS depressants has not been evaluated in clinical studies. Because of the potential of zonisamide to cause CNS depression, as well as other cognitive and/or neuropsychiatric adverse events, zonisamide should be used with caution if used in combination with alcohol or other CNS depressants).
No products indexed under this heading.

IMPORTANT NOTE: Always consult each drug listing in the patient's regimen for possible interactions.

events, zonisamide should be used with caution if used in combination with alcohol or other CNS depressants). Products include:
Risperdal Consta 2682

Ritonavir (Drugs that induce liver enzymes increase the metabolism and clearance of zonisamide and decrease its half-life). Products include:
Kaletra 458
Norvir 509

Saquinavir (Concurrent use with drugs that inhibit CYP3A4 may alter serum concentrations of zonisamide).
No products indexed under this heading.

Saquinavir Mesylate (Concurrent use with drugs that inhibit CYP3A4 may alter serum concentrations of zonisamide).
No products indexed under this heading.

Scopolamine (Caution should be used when zonisamide is prescribed with other drugs that predispose patients to heat-related disorders; these drugs include, but are not limited to, carbonic anhydrase inhibitors and drugs with anticholinergic activity). Products include:
Transderm Scōp 2397

Scopolamine Hydrobromide (Caution should be used when zonisamide is prescribed with other drugs that predispose patients to heat-related disorders; these drugs include, but are not limited to, carbonic anhydrase inhibitors and drugs with anticholinergic activity). Products include:
Donnatal 2711

Secobarbital Sodium (Concomitant administration of zonisamide and alcohol or other CNS depressants has not been evaluated in clinical studies. Because of the potential of zonisamide to cause CNS depression, as well as other cognitive and/or neuropsychiatric adverse events, zonisamide should be used with caution if used in combination with alcohol or other CNS depressants).
No products indexed under this heading.

Sertraline Hydrochloride (Concurrent use with drugs that inhibit CYP3A4 may alter serum concentrations of zonisamide).
No products indexed under this heading.

Sevoflurane (Concomitant administration of zonisamide and alcohol or other CNS depressants has not been evaluated in clinical studies. Because of the potential of zonisamide to cause CNS depression, as well as other cognitive and/or neuropsychiatric adverse events, zonisamide should be used with caution if used in combination with alcohol or other CNS depressants). Products include:
Ultane 554

Sildenafil Citrate (Concurrent use with drugs that inhibit CYP3A4 may alter serum concentrations of zonisamide).
No products indexed under this heading.

Sodium Butabarbital (Concomitant administration of zonisamide and alcohol or other CNS depressants has not been evaluated in clinical studies. Because of the potential of zonisamide to cause CNS depression, as well as other cognitive and/or neuropsychiatric adverse events, zonisamide should be used with caution if used in combination with alcohol or other CNS depressants).
No products indexed under this heading.

Sodium Oxybate (Concomitant administration of zonisamide and alcohol or other CNS depressants has not been evaluated in clinical studies. Because of the potential of zonisamide to cause CNS depression, as well as other cognitive and/or neuropsychiatric adverse events, zonisamide should be used with caution if used in combination with alcohol or other CNS depressants).
No products indexed under this heading.

Sodium Pentobarbital (Concomitant administration of zonisamide and alcohol or other CNS depressants has not been evaluated in clinical studies. Because of the potential of zonisamide to cause CNS depression, as well as other cognitive and/or neuropsychiatric adverse events, zonisamide should be used with caution if used in combination with alcohol or other CNS depressants).
No products indexed under this heading.

Sufentanil Citrate (Concomitant administration of zonisamide and alcohol or other CNS depressants has not been evaluated in clinical studies. Because of the potential of zonisamide to cause CNS depression, as well as other cognitive and/or neuropsychiatric adverse events, zonisamide should be used with caution if used in combination with alcohol or other CNS depressants).
No products indexed under this heading.

Sulfinpyrazone (Concurrent use with drugs that induce CYP3A4 may alter serum concentrations of zonisamide).
No products indexed under this heading.

Talbutal (Concomitant administration of zonisamide and alcohol or other CNS depressants has not been evaluated in clinical studies. Because of the potential of zonisamide to cause CNS depression, as well as other cognitive and/or neuropsychiatric adverse events, zonisamide should be used with caution if used in combination with alcohol or other CNS depressants).
No products indexed under this heading.

Telithromycin (Concurrent use with drugs that inhibit CYP3A4 may alter serum concentrations of zonisamide). Products include:
Ketek 2991

Temazepam (Concomitant administration of zonisamide and alcohol or other CNS depressants has not been evaluated in clinical studies. Because of the potential of zonisamide to cause CNS depression, as well as other cognitive and/or neuropsychiatric adverse events, zonisamide should be used with caution if used in combination with alcohol or other CNS depressants).
No products indexed under this heading.

Theophyllinate (Concurrent use with drugs that induce CYP3A4 may alter serum concentrations of zonisamide).
No products indexed under this heading.

Theophylline (Drugs that induce liver enzymes increase the metabolism and clearance of zonisamide and decrease its half-life).
No products indexed under this heading.

Theophylline Anhydrous (Drugs that induce liver enzymes increase the metabolism and clearance of zonisamide and decrease its half-life). Products include:
Uniphyl 2817

Theophylline Calcium Salicylate (Drugs that induce liver enzymes increase the metabolism and clearance of zonisamide and decrease its half-life).
No products indexed under this heading.

Theophylline Dihydroxypropyl (Glyceryl) (Drugs that induce liver enzymes increase the metabolism and clearance of zonisamide and decrease its half-life).
No products indexed under this heading.

Theophylline Ethylenediamine (Drugs that induce liver enzymes increase the metabolism and clearance of zonisamide and decrease its half-life).
No products indexed under this heading.

Theophylline Sodium Glycinate (Drugs that induce liver enzymes increase the metabolism and clearance of zonisamide and decrease its half-life).
No products indexed under this heading.

Thiamylal Sodium (Concomitant administration of zonisamide and alcohol or other CNS depressants has not been evaluated in clinical studies. Because of the potential of zonisamide to cause CNS depression, as well as other cognitive and/or neuropsychiatric adverse events, zonisamide should be used with caution if used in combination with alcohol or other CNS depressants).
No products indexed under this heading.

Thioridazine (Concomitant administration of zonisamide and alcohol or other CNS depressants has not been evaluated in clinical studies. Because of the potential of zonisamide to cause CNS depression, as well as other cognitive and/or neuropsychiatric adverse events, zonisamide should be used with caution if used in combination with alcohol or other CNS depressants).
No products indexed under this heading.

Thioridazine Hydrochloride (Concomitant administration of zonisamide and alcohol or other CNS depressants has not been evaluated in clinical studies. Because of the potential of zonisamide to cause CNS depression, as well as other cognitive and/or neuropsychiatric adverse events, zonisamide should be used with caution if used in combination with alcohol or other CNS depressants). Products include:
Thioridazine Hydrochloride 2384

Thiothixene (Concomitant administration of zonisamide and alcohol or other CNS depressants has not been evaluated in clinical studies. Because of the potential of zonisamide to cause CNS depression, as well as other cognitive and/or neuropsychiatric adverse events, zonisamide should be used with caution if used in combination with alcohol or other CNS depressants). Products include:
Thiothixene 2386

Thiothixene Hydrochloride (Concomitant administration of zonisamide and alcohol or other CNS depressants has not been evaluated in clinical studies. Because of the potential of zonisamide to cause CNS depression, as well as other cognitive and/or neuropsychiatric adverse events, zonisamide should be used with caution if used in combination with alcohol or other CNS depressants).
No products indexed under this heading.

Tobacco (Drugs that induce liver enzymes increase the metabolism and clearance of zonisamide and decrease its half-life).
No products indexed under this heading.

Tolazamide (Drugs that induce liver enzymes increase the metabolism and clearance of zonisamide and decrease its half-life).
No products indexed under this heading.

Tolbutamide (Drugs that induce liver enzymes increase the metabolism and clearance of zonisamide and decrease its half-life).
No products indexed under this heading.

Tolterodine Tartrate (Caution should be used when zonisamide is prescribed with other drugs that predispose patients to heat-related disorders; these drugs include, but are not limited to, carbonic anhydrase inhibitors and drugs with anticholinergic activity).
No products indexed under this heading.

Torsemide (Caution should be used when zonisamide is prescribed with other drugs that predispose patients to heat-related disorders; these drugs include, but are not limited to, carbonic anhydrase inhibitors and drugs with anticholinergic activity).
No products indexed under this heading.

Triamcinolone (Drugs that induce liver enzymes increase the metabolism and clearance of zonisamide and decrease its half-life).
No products indexed under this heading.

Triamcinolone Acetonide (Drugs that induce liver enzymes increase the metabolism and clearance of zonisamide and decrease its half-life). Products include:
Azmacort 408
Nasacort AQ 3019

Triamcinolone Diacetate (Drugs that induce liver enzymes increase the metabolism and clearance of zonisamide and decrease its half-life).
No products indexed under this heading.

Triamcinolone Hexacetonide (Drugs that induce liver enzymes increase the metabolism and clearance of zonisamide and decrease its half-life).
No products indexed under this heading.

Triazolam (Concomitant administration of zonisamide and alcohol or other CNS depressants has not been evaluated in clinical studies. Because of the potential of zonisamide to cause CNS depression, as well as other cognitive and/or neuropsychiatric adverse events, zonisamide should be used with caution if used in combination with alcohol or other CNS depressants).
No products indexed under this heading.

Tridihexethyl Chloride (Caution should be used when zonisamide is prescribed with other drugs that predispose patients to heat-related disorders; these drugs include, but are not limited to, carbonic anhydrase inhibitors and drugs with anticholinergic activity).
No products indexed under this heading.

Trifluoperazine Hydrochloride (Concomitant administration of zonisamide and alcohol or other CNS depressants has not been evaluated in clinical studies. Because of the potential of zonisamide to cause CNS depression, as well as other cognitive and/or neuropsychiatric adverse events, zonisamide should be used with caution if used in combination with alcohol or other CNS depressants).
No products indexed under this heading.

Trihexyphenidyl Hydrochloride (Caution should be used when zonisamide is prescribed with other drugs that predispose patients to heat-related disorders; these drugs include, but are not limited to, carbonic anhydrase inhibitors and drugs with anticholinergic activity).
No products indexed under this heading.

Troglitazone (Drugs that induce liver enzymes increase the metabolism and clearance of zonisamide and decrease its half-life).
No products indexed under this heading.

Troleandomycin (Concurrent use with drugs that inhibit CYP3A4 may alter serum concentrations of zonisamide).
No products indexed under this heading.

Valproate Sodium (Co-administration of zonisamide and valproate leads to a decrease in the half-life of zonisamide to 46 hours).
No products indexed under this heading.

Valproic Acid (Co-administration of zonisamide and valproate leads to a decrease in the half-life of zonisamide to 46 hours).
No products indexed under this heading.

Vardenafil Hydrochloride (Concurrent use with drugs that inhibit CYP3A4 may alter serum concentrations of zonisamide). Products include:

Verapamil Hydrochloride (Concurrent use with drugs that inhibit CYP3A4 may alter serum concentrations of zonisamide). Products include:

Voriconazole (Concurrent use with drugs that inhibit CYP3A4 may alter serum concentrations of zonisamide).
No products indexed under this heading.

Zafirlukast (Concurrent use with drugs that inhibit CYP3A4 may alter serum concentrations of zonisamide). Products include:

Zaleplon (Concomitant administration of zonisamide and alcohol or other CNS depressants has not been evaluated in clinical studies. Because of the potential of zonisamide to cause CNS depression, as well as other cognitive and/or neuropsychiatric adverse events, zonisamide should be used with caution if used in combination with alcohol or other CNS depressants).
No products indexed under this heading.

Zileuton (Concurrent use with drugs that inhibit CYP3A4 may alter serum concentrations of zonisamide).
No products indexed under this heading.

Ziprasidone Hydrochloride (Concomitant administration of zonisamide and alcohol or other CNS depressants has not been evaluated in clinical studies. Because of the potential of zonisamide to cause CNS depression, as well as other cognitive and/or neuropsychiatric adverse events, zonisamide should be used with caution if used in combination with alcohol or other CNS depressants). Products include:

Zolpidem Tartrate (Concomitant administration of zonisamide and alcohol or other CNS depressants has not been evaluated in clinical studies. Because of the potential of zonisamide to cause CNS depression, as well as other cognitive and/or neuropsychiatric adverse events, zonisamide should be used with caution if used in combination with alcohol or other CNS depressants). Products include:

Food Interactions

Alcohol (Concomitant administration of zonisamide and alcohol or other CNS depressants has not been evaluated in clinical studies. Because of the potential of zonisamide to cause CNS depression, as well as other cognitive and/or neuropsychiatric adverse events, zonisamide should be used with caution if used in combination with alcohol or other CNS depressants).

Beer, reduced-alcohol (Concomitant administration of zonisamide and alcohol or other CNS depressants has not been evaluated in clinical studies. Because of the potential of zonisamide to cause CNS depression, as well as other cognitive and/or neuropsychiatric adverse events, zonisamide should be used with caution if used in combination with alcohol or other CNS depressants).

Beer, unspecified (Concomitant administration of zonisamide and alcohol or other CNS depressants has not been evaluated in clinical studies. Because of the potential of zonisamide to cause CNS depression, as well as other cognitive and/or neuropsychiatric adverse events, zonisamide should be used with caution if used in combination with alcohol or other CNS depressants).

Broccoli (Drugs that induce liver enzymes increase the metabolism and clearance of zonisamide and decrease its half-life).

Brussel Sprouts (Drugs that induce liver enzymes increase the metabolism and clearance of zonisamide and decrease its half-life).

Charbroiled Food (Drugs that induce liver enzymes increase the metabolism and clearance of zonisamide and decrease its half-life).

Food, unspecified (Following a 200–400 mg oral zonisamide dose, peak plasma concentrations (range: 2–5 µg/mL) in normal volunteers occur within 2–6 hours. In the presence of food, the time to maximum concentration is delayed, occurring at 4–6 hours, but food has no effect on the bioavailability of zonisamide. Zonisamide can be taken with or without food).

Grapefruit (Concurrent use with drugs that inhibit CYP3A4 may alter serum concentrations of zonisamide).

Grapefruit Juice (Concurrent use with drugs that inhibit CYP3A4 may alter serum concentrations of zonisamide).

Meal, unspecified (Following a 200–400 mg oral zonisamide dose, peak plasma concentrations (range: 2–5 µg/mL) in normal volunteers occur within 2–6 hours. In the presence of food, the time to maximum concentration is delayed, occurring at 4–6 hours, but food has no effect on the bioavailability of zonisamide. Zonisamide can be taken with or without food).

Wine, Chianti (Concomitant administration of zonisamide and alcohol or other CNS depressants has not been evaluated in clinical studies. Because of the potential of zonisamide to cause CNS depression, as well as other cognitive and/or neuropsychiatric adverse events, zonisamide should be used with caution if used in combination with alcohol or other CNS depressants).

Wine, Red (Concomitant administration of zonisamide and alcohol or other CNS depressants has not been evaluated in clinical studies. Because of the potential of zonisamide to cause CNS depression, as well as other cognitive and/or neuropsychiatric adverse events, zonisamide should be used with caution if used in combination with alcohol or other CNS depressants).

Wine, unspecified (Concomitant administration of zonisamide and alcohol or other CNS depressants has not been evaluated in clinical studies. Because of the potential of zonisamide to cause CNS depression, as well as other cognitive and/or neuropsychiatric adverse events, zonisamide should be used with caution if used in combination with alcohol or other CNS depressants).

Wine products (Concomitant administration of zonisamide and alcohol or other CNS depressants has not been evaluated in clinical studies. Because of the potential of zonisamide to cause CNS depression, as well as other cognitive and/or neuropsychiatric adverse events, zonisamide should be used with caution if used in combination with alcohol or other CNS depressants).

ZOSTAVAX INJECTION

May interact with immunosuppressive agents. Compounds in these categories include:

Azathioprine (Live zoster vaccines are contraindicated in patients on immunosuppressive therapy).
No products indexed under this heading.

Basiliximab (Live zoster vaccines are contraindicated in patients on immunosuppressive therapy). Products include:

Cyclosporine (Live zoster vaccines are contraindicated in patients on immunosuppressive therapy). Products include:

Muromonab-CD3 (Live zoster vaccines are contraindicated in patients on immunosuppressive therapy). Products include:

Mycophenolate Mofetil (Live zoster vaccines are contraindicated in patients on immunosuppressive therapy).
No products indexed under this heading.

Rapamycin (Live zoster vaccines are contraindicated in patients on immunosuppressive therapy).
No products indexed under this heading.

Sirolimus (Live zoster vaccines are contraindicated in patients on immunosuppressive therapy). Products include:

Tacrolimus (Live zoster vaccines are contraindicated in patients on immunosuppressive therapy). Products include:

ZOSYN FOR INJECTION

May interact with aminoglycosides, anticoagulants, nondepolarizing neuromuscular blocking agents, and certain other agents. Compounds in these categories include:

Amikacin Sulfate (The mixing of beta-lactam antibiotics with aminoglycosides in-vitro can result in substantial inactivation of the aminoglycoside. However, amikacin and gentamicin have been shown to be compatible *in vitro* with reformulated Zosyn containing EDTA supplied in vials or bulk pharmacy containers in certain diluents at specific concentrations for a simultaneous Y-site infusion. Reformulated Zosyn containing EDTA is not compatible with tobramycin for simultaneous administration via Y-site infusion).
No products indexed under this heading.

Anisindione (Coagulation parameters should be tested more frequently and monitored regularly during simultaneous administration; effect of concurrent use is not specified).
No products indexed under this heading.

Ardeparin Sodium (Coagulation parameters should be tested more frequently and monitored regularly during simultaneous administration; effect of concurrent use is not specified).
No products indexed under this heading.

Atracurium Besylate (Due to similar mechanism of action as vecuronium, it is expected that the neuromuscular blockade produced by other non-depolarizing muscle relaxants could be prolonged in the presence of piperacillin).
No products indexed under this heading.

Cisatracurium Besylate (Due to similar mechanism of action as vecuronium, it is expected that the neuromuscular blockade produced by other non-depolarizing muscle relaxants could be prolonged in the presence of piperacillin). Products include:

Dalteparin Sodium (Coagulation parameters should be tested more frequently and monitored regularly during simultaneous administration; effect of concurrent use is not specified). Products include:

Danaparoid Sodium (Coagulation parameters should be tested more frequently and monitored regularly during simultaneous administration; effect of concurrent use is not specified).
No products indexed under this heading.

Dicumarol (Coagulation parameters should be tested more frequently and monitored regularly during simultaneous administration; effect of concurrent use is not specified).
No products indexed under this heading.

Dihydrostreptomycin (The mixing of beta-lactam antibiotics with aminoglycosides in-vitro can result in substantial inactivation of the aminoglycoside. However, amikacin and gentamicin have been shown to be compatible *in vitro* with reformulated Zosyn containing EDTA supplied in vials or bulk pharmacy containers in certain diluents at specific concentrations for a simultaneous Y-site infusion. Reformulated Zosyn containing EDTA is not compatible with tobramycin for simultaneous administration via Y-site infusion).
No products indexed under this heading.

Doxacurium Chloride (Due to similar mechanism of action as vecuronium, it is expected that the neuromuscular blockade produced by other non-depolarizing muscle relaxants could be prolonged in the presence of piperacillin).
No products indexed under this heading.

d-Tubocurarine (Due to similar mechanism of action as vecuronium, it is expected that the neuromuscular blockade produced by other non-depolarizing muscle relaxants could be prolonged in the presence of piperacillin).
No products indexed under this heading.

Enoxaparin Sodium (Coagulation parameters should be tested more frequently and monitored regularly during simultaneous administration; effect of concurrent use is not specified). Products include:

Fondaparinux Sodium (Coagulation parameters should be tested more frequently and monitored regularly during simultaneous administration; effect of concurrent use is not specified). Products include:

Gallamine (Due to similar mechanism of action as vecuronium, it is expected that the neuromuscular blockade produced by other non-depolarizing muscle relaxants could be prolonged in the presence of piperacillin).
No products indexed under this heading.

Gallamine Triethiodide (Due to similar mechanism of action as vecuronium, it is expected that the neuromuscular blockade produced by other non-depolarizing muscle relaxants could be prolonged in the presence of piperacillin).
No products indexed under this heading.

Gentamicin (The mixing of beta-lactam antibiotics with aminoglycosides in-vitro can result in substantial inactivation of the aminoglycoside. However, amikacin and gentamicin have been shown to be compatible *in vitro* with reformulated Zosyn containing EDTA supplied in vials or bulk pharmacy containers in certain diluents at specific concentrations for a simultaneous Y-site infusion. Reformulated Zosyn containing

EDTA is not compatible with tobramycin for simultaneous administration via Y-site infusion).

No products indexed under this heading.

Gentamicin Sulfate (The mixing of beta-lactam antibiotics with aminoglycosides in-vitro can result in substantial inactivation of the aminoglycoside. However, amikacin and gentamicin have been shown to be compatible *in vitro* with reformulated Zosyn containing EDTA supplied in vials or bulk pharmacy containers in certain diluents at specific concentrations for a simultaneous Y-site infusion. Reformulated Zosyn containing EDTA is not compatible with tobramycin for simultaneous administration via Y-site infusion). Products include:

Pred-G .... ☉ 226, ☉ 227

Heparin Calcium (Coagulation parameters should be tested more frequently and monitored regularly during simultaneous administration; effect of concurrent use is not specified).

No products indexed under this heading.

Heparin Sodium (Coagulation parameters should be tested more frequently and monitored regularly during simultaneous administration; effect of concurrent use is not specified).

No products indexed under this heading.

Kanamycin Sulfate (The mixing of beta-lactam antibiotics with aminoglycosides in-vitro can result in substantial inactivation of the aminoglycoside. However, amikacin and gentamicin have been shown to be compatible *in vitro* with reformulated Zosyn containing EDTA supplied in vials or bulk pharmacy containers in certain diluents at specific concentrations for a simultaneous Y-site infusion. Reformulated Zosyn containing EDTA is not compatible with tobramycin for simultaneous administration via Y-site infusion).

No products indexed under this heading.

Low Molecular Weight Heparins (Coagulation parameters should be tested more frequently and monitored regularly during simultaneous administration; effect of concurrent use is not specified).

No products indexed under this heading.

Methotrexate (Limited data suggests that co-administration of methotrexate and piperacillin may reduce the clearance of methotrexate due to competition for renal excretion).

No products indexed under this heading.

Metocurine Iodide (Due to similar mechanism of action as vecuronium, it is expected that the neuromuscular blockade produced by other non-depolarizing muscle relaxants could be prolonged in the presence of piperacillin).

No products indexed under this heading.

Mivacurium Chloride (Due to similar mechanism of action as vecuronium, it is expected that the neuromuscular blockade produced by other non-depolarizing muscle relaxants could be prolonged in the presence of piperacillin).

No products indexed under this heading.

Neomycin (The mixing of beta-lactam antibiotics with aminoglycosides in-vitro can result in substantial inactivation of the aminoglycoside. However, amikacin and gentamicin have been shown to be compatible *in vitro* with reformulated Zosyn containing EDTA supplied in vials or bulk pharmacy containers in certain diluents at specific concentrations for a simultaneous Y-site infusion. Reformulated Zosyn containing EDTA is not compatible with tobramycin for simultaneous administration via Y-site infusion).

No products indexed under this heading.

Neomycin, oral (The mixing of beta-lactam antibiotics with aminoglycosides

in-vitro can result in substantial inactivation of the aminoglycoside. However, amikacin and gentamicin have been shown to be compatible *in vitro* with reformulated Zosyn containing EDTA supplied in vials or bulk pharmacy containers in certain diluents at specific concentrations for a simultaneous Y-site infusion. Reformulated Zosyn containing EDTA is not compatible with tobramycin for simultaneous administration via Y-site infusion).

No products indexed under this heading.

Neomycin Sulfate (The mixing of beta-lactam antibiotics with aminoglycosides in-vitro can result in substantial inactivation of the aminoglycoside. However, amikacin and gentamicin have been shown to be compatible *in vitro* with reformulated Zosyn containing EDTA supplied in vials or bulk pharmacy containers in certain diluents at specific concentrations for a simultaneous Y-site infusion. Reformulated Zosyn containing EDTA is not compatible with tobramycin for simultaneous administration via Y-site infusion).

No products indexed under this heading.

Pancuronium Bromide (Due to similar mechanism of action as vecuronium, it is expected that the neuromuscular blockade produced by other non-depolarizing muscle relaxants could be prolonged in the presence of piperacillin).

No products indexed under this heading.

Pipecuronium Bromide (Due to similar mechanism of action as vecuronium, it is expected that the neuromuscular blockade produced by other non-depolarizing muscle relaxants could be prolonged in the presence of piperacillin).

No products indexed under this heading.

Probenecid (Concomitant administration prolongs half-life of piperacillin by 21% and of tazobactam by 71%).

No products indexed under this heading.

Rapacuronium Bromide (Due to similar mechanism of action as vecuronium, it is expected that the neuromuscular blockade produced by other non-depolarizing muscle relaxants could be prolonged in the presence of piperacillin).

No products indexed under this heading.

Rocuronium Bromide (Due to similar mechanism of action as vecuronium, it is expected that the neuromuscular blockade produced by other non-depolarizing muscle relaxants could be prolonged in the presence of piperacillin). Products include:

Zemuron 3249

Streptomycin Sulfate (The mixing of beta-lactam antibiotics with aminoglycosides in-vitro can result in substantial inactivation of the aminoglycoside. However, amikacin and gentamicin have been shown to be compatible *in vitro* with reformulated Zosyn containing EDTA supplied in vials or bulk pharmacy containers in certain diluents at specific concentrations for a simultaneous Y-site infusion. Reformulated Zosyn containing EDTA is not compatible with tobramycin for simultaneous administration via Y-site infusion).

No products indexed under this heading.

Tinzaparin Sodium (Coagulation parameters should be tested more frequently and monitored regularly during simultaneous administration; effect of concurrent use is not specified).

No products indexed under this heading.

Tobramycin (The mixing of beta-lactam antibiotics with aminoglycosides in-vitro can result in substantial inactivation of the aminoglycoside. However, amikacin and gentamicin have been shown to be compatible *in vitro* with reformulated Zosyn containing EDTA

supplied in vials or bulk pharmacy containers in certain diluents at specific concentrations for a simultaneous Y-site infusion. Reformulated Zosyn containing EDTA is not compatible with tobramycin for simultaneous administration via Y-site infusion). Products include:

Tobi Nebulizer **2546**
Tobramycin and Dexamethasone
  Ophthalmic Suspension............... ☉ **251**
Zylet .... ☉ **252**

Tobramycin Sulfate (Co-administration has resulted in the alteration of tobramycin pharmacokinetics which may be due to *in vitro* and *in vivo* inactivation of tobramycin).

No products indexed under this heading.

Tubocurarine Chloride (Due to similar mechanism of action as vecuronium, it is expected that the neuromuscular blockade produced by other non-depolarizing muscle relaxants could be prolonged in the presence of piperacillin).

No products indexed under this heading.

Vecuronium Bromide (Co-administration of piperacillin and vecuronium has been implicated in the prolongation of the neuromuscular blockade).

No products indexed under this heading.

Warfarin Sodium (Coagulation parameters should be tested more frequently and monitored regularly during simultaneous administration; effect of concurrent use is not specified).

No products indexed under this heading.

ZOVIRAX CAPSULES
(Acyclovir) **1760**
May interact with nephrotoxic agents, and certain other agents. Compounds in these categories include:

Abacavir Sulfate (Caution should be exercised when administering acyclovir to patients receiving potentially nephrotoxic agents since this may increase the risk of renal dysfunction and/or the risk of reversible CNS symptoms such as those that have been reported in patients treated with intravenous acyclovir. Adequate hydration should be maintained). Products include:

Epzicom **1448**
Trizivir **1688**
Ziagen **1740**

Acyclovir Sodium (Caution should be exercised when administering acyclovir to patients receiving potentially nephrotoxic agents since this may increase the risk of renal dysfunction and/or the risk of reversible CNS symptoms such as those that have been reported in patients treated with intravenous acyclovir. Adequate hydration should be maintained).

No products indexed under this heading.

Alatrofloxacin Mesylate (Caution should be exercised when administering acyclovir to patients receiving potentially nephrotoxic agents since this may increase the risk of renal dysfunction and/or the risk of reversible CNS symptoms such as those that have been reported in patients treated with intravenous acyclovir. Adequate hydration should be maintained).

No products indexed under this heading.

Aldesleukin (Caution should be exercised when administering acyclovir to patients receiving potentially nephrotoxic agents since this may increase the risk of renal dysfunction and/or the risk of reversible CNS symptoms such as those that have been reported in patients treated with intravenous acyclovir. Adequate hydration should be maintained). Products include:

Proleukin **2504**

Amikacin Sulfate (Caution should be exercised when administering acyclovir to patients receiving potentially nephrotoxic agents since this may increase the risk of renal dysfunction and/or the risk of reversible CNS symptoms such as those that have been reported in patients treated with intravenous acyclovir. Adequate hydration should be maintained).

No products indexed under this heading.

Amoxicillin (Caution should be exercised when administering acyclovir to patients receiving potentially nephrotoxic agents since this may increase the risk of renal dysfunction and/or the risk of reversible CNS symptoms such as those that have been reported in patients treated with intravenous acyclovir. Adequate hydration should be maintained). Products include:

Amoxil Capsules **1311**
Amoxil Chewable Tablets **1311**
Amoxil **1311**
Amoxil Powder **1311**
Augmentin **1331**
Augmentin Tablets **1335**
Augmentin ES-600 .... **1338**
Augmentin XR **1342**
Moxatag **2321**

Amoxicillin Trihydrate (Caution should be exercised when administering acyclovir to patients receiving potentially nephrotoxic agents since this may increase the risk of renal dysfunction and/or the risk of reversible CNS symptoms such as those that have been reported in patients treated with intravenous acyclovir. Adequate hydration should be maintained).

No products indexed under this heading.

Amphotericin B (Caution should be exercised when administering acyclovir to patients receiving potentially nephrotoxic agents since this may increase the risk of renal dysfunction and/or the risk of reversible CNS symptoms such as those that have been reported in patients treated with intravenous acyclovir. Adequate hydration should be maintained).

No products indexed under this heading.

Amphotericin B, liposomal (Caution should be exercised when administering acyclovir to patients receiving potentially nephrotoxic agents since this may increase the risk of renal dysfunction and/or the risk of reversible CNS symptoms such as those that have been reported in patients treated with intravenous acyclovir. Adequate hydration should be maintained). Products include:

AmBisome **659**

Amphotericin B Cholesteryl Sulfate (Caution should be exercised when administering acyclovir to patients receiving potentially nephrotoxic agents since this may increase the risk of renal dysfunction and/or the risk of reversible CNS symptoms such as those that have been reported in patients treated with intravenous acyclovir. Adequate hydration should be maintained).

No products indexed under this heading.

Amphotericin B Lipid Complex (Caution should be exercised when administering acyclovir to patients receiving potentially nephrotoxic agents since this may increase the risk of renal dysfunction and/or the risk of reversible CNS symptoms such as those that have been reported in patients treated with intravenous acyclovir. Adequate hydration should be maintained).

No products indexed under this heading.

IMPORTANT NOTE: Always consult each drug listing in the patient's regimen for possible interactions.

Zovirax Interactions Index 2184

Ampicillin (Caution should be exercised when administering acyclovir to patients receiving potentially nephrotoxic agents since this may increase the risk of renal dysfunction and/or the risk of reversible CNS symptoms such as those that have been reported in patients treated with intravenous acyclovir. Adequate hydration should be maintained).
No products indexed under this heading.

Ampicillin Sodium (Caution should be exercised when administering acyclovir to patients receiving potentially nephrotoxic agents since this may increase the risk of renal dysfunction and/or the risk of reversible CNS symptoms such as those that have been reported in patients treated with intravenous acyclovir. Adequate hydration should be maintained).
No products indexed under this heading.

Ampicillin Trihydrate (Caution should be exercised when administering acyclovir to patients receiving potentially nephrotoxic agents since this may increase the risk of renal dysfunction and/or the risk of reversible CNS symptoms such as those that have been reported in patients treated with intravenous acyclovir. Adequate hydration should be maintained).
No products indexed under this heading.

Amprenavir (Caution should be exercised when administering acyclovir to patients receiving potentially nephrotoxic agents since this may increase the risk of renal dysfunction and/or the risk of reversible CNS symptoms such as those that have been reported in patients treated with intravenous acyclovir. Adequate hydration should be maintained).
No products indexed under this heading.

Aspirin (Caution should be exercised when administering acyclovir to patients receiving potentially nephrotoxic agents since this may increase the risk of renal dysfunction and/or the risk of reversible CNS symptoms such as those that have been reported in patients treated with intravenous acyclovir. Adequate hydration should be maintained). Products include:
Aggrenox 880
Bayer Aspirin 829
Percodan 1124
St. Joseph Aspirin 2045

Atazanavir (Caution should be exercised when administering acyclovir to patients receiving potentially nephrotoxic agents since this may increase the risk of renal dysfunction and/or the risk of reversible CNS symptoms such as those that have been reported in patients treated with intravenous acyclovir. Adequate hydration should be maintained).
No products indexed under this heading.

Atorvastatin Calcium (Caution should be exercised when administering acyclovir to patients receiving potentially nephrotoxic agents since this may increase the risk of renal dysfunction and/or the risk of reversible CNS symptoms such as those that have been reported in patients treated with intravenous acyclovir. Adequate hydration should be maintained). Products include:
Lipitor 2703

Azithromycin Dihydrate (Caution should be exercised when administering acyclovir to patients receiving potentially nephrotoxic agents since this may increase the risk of renal dysfunction and/or the risk of reversible CNS symptoms such as those that have been reported in patients treated with intravenous acyclovir. Adequate hydration should be maintained).
No products indexed under this heading.

Azlocillin Sodium (Caution should be exercised when administering acyclovir to patients receiving potentially nephrotoxic agents since this may increase the risk of renal dysfunction and/or the risk of reversible CNS symptoms such as those that have been reported in patients treated with intravenous acyclovir. Adequate hydration should be maintained).
No products indexed under this heading.

Aztreonam (Caution should be exercised when administering acyclovir to patients receiving potentially nephrotoxic agents since this may increase the risk of renal dysfunction and/or the risk of reversible CNS symptoms such as those that have been reported in patients treated with intravenous acyclovir. Adequate hydration should be maintained).
No products indexed under this heading.

Bacampicillin Hydrochloride (Caution should be exercised when administering acyclovir to patients receiving potentially nephrotoxic agents since this may increase the risk of renal dysfunction and/or the risk of reversible CNS symptoms such as those that have been reported in patients treated with intravenous acyclovir. Adequate hydration should be maintained).
No products indexed under this heading.

Bacitracin (Caution should be exercised when administering acyclovir to patients receiving potentially nephrotoxic agents since this may increase the risk of renal dysfunction and/or the risk of reversible CNS symptoms such as those that have been reported in patients treated with intravenous acyclovir. Adequate hydration should be maintained).
No products indexed under this heading.

Bacitracin Zinc (Caution should be exercised when administering acyclovir to patients receiving potentially nephrotoxic agents since this may increase the risk of renal dysfunction and/or the risk of reversible CNS symptoms such as those that have been reported in patients treated with intravenous acyclovir. Adequate hydration should be maintained).
No products indexed under this heading.

Balsalazide Disodium (Caution should be exercised when administering acyclovir to patients receiving potentially nephrotoxic agents since this may increase the risk of renal dysfunction and/or the risk of reversible CNS symptoms such as those that have been reported in patients treated with intravenous acyclovir. Adequate hydration should be maintained).
No products indexed under this heading.

Benazepril Hydrochloride (Caution should be exercised when administering acyclovir to patients receiving potentially nephrotoxic agents since this may increase the risk of renal dysfunction and/or the risk of reversible CNS symptoms such as those that have been reported in patients treated with intravenous acyclovir. Adequate hydration should be maintained).
No products indexed under this heading.

Bendroflumethiazide (Caution should be exercised when administering acyclovir to patients receiving potentially nephrotoxic agents since this may increase the risk of renal dysfunction and/or the risk of reversible CNS symptoms such as those that have been reported in patients treated with intravenous acyclovir. Adequate hydration should be maintained).
No products indexed under this heading.

Caffeine (Caution should be exercised when administering acyclovir to patients receiving potentially nephrotoxic agents since this may increase the risk of renal dysfunction and/or the risk of reversible CNS symptoms such as those that have been reported in patients treated with intravenous acyclovir. Adequate hydration should be maintained).
No products indexed under this heading.

Captopril (Caution should be exercised when administering acyclovir to patients receiving potentially nephrotoxic agents since this may increase the risk of renal dysfunction and/or the risk of reversible CNS symptoms such as those that have been reported in patients treated with intravenous acyclovir. Adequate hydration should be maintained). Products include:
Captopril 2341

Carbenicillin Disodium (Caution should be exercised when administering acyclovir to patients receiving potentially nephrotoxic agents since this may increase the risk of renal dysfunction and/or the risk of reversible CNS symptoms such as those that have been reported in patients treated with intravenous acyclovir. Adequate hydration should be maintained).
No products indexed under this heading.

Carbenicillin Indanyl Sodium (Caution should be exercised when administering acyclovir to patients receiving potentially nephrotoxic agents since this may increase the risk of renal dysfunction and/or the risk of reversible CNS symptoms such as those that have been reported in patients treated with intravenous acyclovir. Adequate hydration should be maintained).
No products indexed under this heading.

Carboplatin (Caution should be exercised when administering acyclovir to patients receiving potentially nephrotoxic agents since this may increase the risk of renal dysfunction and/or the risk of reversible CNS symptoms such as those that have been reported in patients treated with intravenous acyclovir. Adequate hydration should be maintained).
No products indexed under this heading.

Carmustine (BCNU) (Caution should be exercised when administering acyclovir to patients receiving potentially nephrotoxic agents since this may increase the risk of renal dysfunction and/or the risk of reversible CNS symptoms such as those that have been reported in patients treated with intravenous acyclovir. Adequate hydration should be maintained).
No products indexed under this heading.

Cefaclor (Caution should be exercised when administering acyclovir to patients receiving potentially nephrotoxic agents since this may increase the risk of renal dysfunction and/or the risk of reversible CNS symptoms such as those that have been reported in patients treated with intravenous acyclovir. Adequate hydration should be maintained).
No products indexed under this heading.

Cefadroxil (Caution should be exercised when administering acyclovir to patients receiving potentially nephrotoxic agents since this may increase the risk of renal dysfunction and/or the risk of reversible CNS symptoms such as those that have been reported in patients treated with intravenous acyclovir. Adequate hydration should be maintained).
No products indexed under this heading.

Cefamandole Nafate (Caution should be exercised when administering acyclovir to patients receiving potentially nephrotoxic agents since this may increase the risk of renal dysfunction and/or the risk of reversible CNS symptoms such as those that have been reported in patients treated with intravenous acyclovir. Adequate hydration should be maintained).
No products indexed under this heading.

Cefazolin Sodium (Caution should be exercised when administering acyclovir to patients receiving potentially nephrotoxic agents since this may increase the risk of renal dysfunction and/or the risk of reversible CNS symptoms such as those that have been reported in patients treated with intravenous acyclovir. Adequate hydration should be maintained).
No products indexed under this heading.

Cefdinir (Caution should be exercised when administering acyclovir to patients receiving potentially nephrotoxic agents since this may increase the risk of renal dysfunction and/or the risk of reversible CNS symptoms such as those that have been reported in patients treated with intravenous acyclovir. Adequate hydration should be maintained). Products include:
Omnicef Capsules 518
Omnicef Oral Suspension 518

Cefepime Hydrochloride (Caution should be exercised when administering acyclovir to patients receiving potentially nephrotoxic agents since this may increase the risk of renal dysfunction and/or the risk of reversible CNS symptoms such as those that have been reported in patients treated with intravenous acyclovir. Adequate hydration should be maintained).
No products indexed under this heading.

Cefixime (Caution should be exercised when administering acyclovir to patients receiving potentially nephrotoxic agents since this may increase the risk of renal dysfunction and/or the risk of reversible CNS symptoms such as those that have been reported in patients treated with intravenous acyclovir. Adequate hydration should be maintained). Products include:
Suprax for Oral Suspension 2038
Suprax Tablets 2038

Cefmetazole Sodium (Caution should be exercised when administering acyclovir to patients receiving potentially nephrotoxic agents since this may increase the risk of renal dysfunction and/or the risk of reversible CNS symptoms such as those that have been reported in patients treated with intravenous acyclovir. Adequate hydration should be maintained).
No products indexed under this heading.

Cefonicid Sodium (Caution should be exercised when administering acyclovir to patients receiving potentially nephrotoxic agents since this may increase the risk of renal dysfunction and/or the risk of reversible CNS symptoms such as those that have been reported in patients treated with intravenous acyclovir. Adequate hydration should be maintained).
No products indexed under this heading.

Cefoperazone Sodium (Caution should be exercised when administering acyclovir to patients receiving potentially nephrotoxic agents since this may increase the risk of renal dysfunction and/or the risk of reversible CNS symptoms such as those that have been reported in patients treated with intravenous acyclovir. Adequate hydration should be maintained).
No products indexed under this heading.

(⊙ Described in PDR® for Ophthalmic Medicines)

2185 Interactions Index Zovirax

Ceforanide (Caution should be exercised when administering acyclovir to patients receiving potentially nephrotoxic agents since this may increase the risk of renal dysfunction and/or the risk of reversible CNS symptoms such as those that have been reported in patients treated with intravenous acyclovir. Adequate hydration should be maintained).
No products indexed under this heading.

Cefotaxime Sodium (Caution should be exercised when administering acyclovir to patients receiving potentially nephrotoxic agents since this may increase the risk of renal dysfunction and/or the risk of reversible CNS symptoms such as those that have been reported in patients treated with intravenous acyclovir. Adequate hydration should be maintained).
No products indexed under this heading.

Cefotetan (Caution should be exercised when administering acyclovir to patients receiving potentially nephrotoxic agents since this may increase the risk of renal dysfunction and/or the risk of reversible CNS symptoms such as those that have been reported in patients treated with intravenous acyclovir. Adequate hydration should be maintained).
No products indexed under this heading.

Cefoxitin Sodium (Caution should be exercised when administering acyclovir to patients receiving potentially nephrotoxic agents since this may increase the risk of renal dysfunction and/or the risk of reversible CNS symptoms such as those that have been reported in patients treated with intravenous acyclovir. Adequate hydration should be maintained).
No products indexed under this heading.

Cefpodoxime Proxetil (Caution should be exercised when administering acyclovir to patients receiving potentially nephrotoxic agents since this may increase the risk of renal dysfunction and/or the risk of reversible CNS symptoms such as those that have been reported in patients treated with intravenous acyclovir. Adequate hydration should be maintained).
No products indexed under this heading.

Cefprozil (Caution should be exercised when administering acyclovir to patients receiving potentially nephrotoxic agents since this may increase the risk of renal dysfunction and/or the risk of reversible CNS symptoms such as those that have been reported in patients treated with intravenous acyclovir. Adequate hydration should be maintained).
No products indexed under this heading.

Ceftazidime (Caution should be exercised when administering acyclovir to patients receiving potentially nephrotoxic agents since this may increase the risk of renal dysfunction and/or the risk of reversible CNS symptoms such as those that have been reported in patients treated with intravenous acyclovir. Adequate hydration should be maintained). Products include:
Fortaz 1481

Ceftizoxime Sodium (Caution should be exercised when administering acyclovir to patients receiving potentially nephrotoxic agents since this may increase the risk of renal dysfunction and/or the risk of reversible CNS symptoms such as those that have been reported in patients treated with intravenous acyclovir. Adequate hydration should be maintained).
No products indexed under this heading.

Ceftriaxone Sodium (Caution should be exercised when administering acyclovir to patients receiving potentially nephrotoxic agents since this may increase the risk of renal dysfunction and/or the risk of reversible CNS symptoms such as those that have been reported in patients treated with intravenous acyclovir. Adequate hydration should be maintained). Products include:
Rocephin 2859

Cefuroxime Axetil (Caution should be exercised when administering acyclovir to patients receiving potentially nephrotoxic agents since this may increase the risk of renal dysfunction and/or the risk of reversible CNS symptoms such as those that have been reported in patients treated with intravenous acyclovir. Adequate hydration should be maintained). Products include:
Ceftin 1399

Cefuroxime Sodium (Caution should be exercised when administering acyclovir to patients receiving potentially nephrotoxic agents since this may increase the risk of renal dysfunction and/or the risk of reversible CNS symptoms such as those that have been reported in patients treated with intravenous acyclovir. Adequate hydration should be maintained).
No products indexed under this heading.

Celecoxib (Caution should be exercised when administering acyclovir to patients receiving potentially nephrotoxic agents since this may increase the risk of renal dysfunction and/or the risk of reversible CNS symptoms such as those that have been reported in patients treated with intravenous acyclovir. Adequate hydration should be maintained). Products include:
Celebrex 3272

Cephalexin (Caution should be exercised when administering acyclovir to patients receiving potentially nephrotoxic agents since this may increase the risk of renal dysfunction and/or the risk of reversible CNS symptoms such as those that have been reported in patients treated with intravenous acyclovir. Adequate hydration should be maintained).
No products indexed under this heading.

Cephalothin Sodium (Caution should be exercised when administering acyclovir to patients receiving potentially nephrotoxic agents since this may increase the risk of renal dysfunction and/or the risk of reversible CNS symptoms such as those that have been reported in patients treated with intravenous acyclovir. Adequate hydration should be maintained).
No products indexed under this heading.

Cephapirin Sodium (Caution should be exercised when administering acyclovir to patients receiving potentially nephrotoxic agents since this may increase the risk of renal dysfunction and/or the risk of reversible CNS symptoms such as those that have been reported in patients treated with intravenous acyclovir. Adequate hydration should be maintained).
No products indexed under this heading.

Cephradine (Caution should be exercised when administering acyclovir to patients receiving potentially nephrotoxic agents since this may increase the risk of renal dysfunction and/or the risk of reversible CNS symptoms such as those that have been reported in patients treated with intravenous acyclovir. Adequate hydration should be maintained).
No products indexed under this heading.

Cerivastatin Sodium (Caution should be exercised when administering acyclovir to patients receiving potentially nephrotoxic agents since this may increase the risk of renal dysfunction and/or the risk of reversible CNS symptoms such as those that have been reported in patients treated with intravenous acyclovir. Adequate hydration should be maintained).
No products indexed under this heading.

Chlorothiazide (Caution should be exercised when administering acyclovir to patients receiving potentially nephrotoxic agents since this may increase the risk of renal dysfunction and/or the risk of reversible CNS symptoms such as those that have been reported in patients treated with intravenous acyclovir. Adequate hydration should be maintained).
No products indexed under this heading.

Chlorothiazide Sodium (Caution should be exercised when administering acyclovir to patients receiving potentially nephrotoxic agents since this may increase the risk of renal dysfunction and/or the risk of reversible CNS symptoms such as those that have been reported in patients treated with intravenous acyclovir. Adequate hydration should be maintained). Products include:
Diuril Intravenous 2009

Chlorpropamide (Caution should be exercised when administering acyclovir to patients receiving potentially nephrotoxic agents since this may increase the risk of renal dysfunction and/or the risk of reversible CNS symptoms such as those that have been reported in patients treated with intravenous acyclovir. Adequate hydration should be maintained).
No products indexed under this heading.

Cidofovir (Caution should be exercised when administering acyclovir to patients receiving potentially nephrotoxic agents since this may increase the risk of renal dysfunction and/or the risk of reversible CNS symptoms such as those that have been reported in patients treated with intravenous acyclovir. Adequate hydration should be maintained).
No products indexed under this heading.

Cilastatin Sodium (Caution should be exercised when administering acyclovir to patients receiving potentially nephrotoxic agents since this may increase the risk of renal dysfunction and/or the risk of reversible CNS symptoms such as those that have been reported in patients treated with intravenous acyclovir. Adequate hydration should be maintained). Products include:
Primaxin I.M. 2232
Primaxin I.V. 2235

Cimetidine (Caution should be exercised when administering acyclovir to patients receiving potentially nephrotoxic agents since this may increase the risk of renal dysfunction and/or the risk of reversible CNS symptoms such as those that have been reported in patients treated with intravenous acyclovir. Adequate hydration should be maintained).
No products indexed under this heading.

Cimetidine Hydrochloride (Caution should be exercised when administering acyclovir to patients receiving potentially nephrotoxic agents since this may increase the risk of renal dysfunction and/or the risk of reversible CNS symptoms such as those that have been reported in patients treated with intravenous acyclovir. Adequate hydration should be maintained).
No products indexed under this heading.

Cisplatin (Caution should be exercised when administering acyclovir to patients receiving potentially nephrotoxic agents since this may increase the risk of renal dysfunction and/or the risk of reversible CNS symptoms such as those that have been reported in patients treated with intravenous acyclovir. Adequate hydration should be maintained).
No products indexed under this heading.

Cladribine (Caution should be exercised when administering acyclovir to patients receiving potentially nephrotoxic agents since this may increase the risk of renal dysfunction and/or the risk of reversible CNS symptoms such as those that have been reported in patients treated with intravenous acyclovir. Adequate hydration should be maintained). Products include:
Leustatin 946

Clozapine (Caution should be exercised when administering acyclovir to patients receiving potentially nephrotoxic agents since this may increase the risk of renal dysfunction and/or the risk of reversible CNS symptoms such as those that have been reported in patients treated with intravenous acyclovir. Adequate hydration should be maintained).
No products indexed under this heading.

Colistimethate Sodium (Caution should be exercised when administering acyclovir to patients receiving potentially nephrotoxic agents since this may increase the risk of renal dysfunction and/or the risk of reversible CNS symptoms such as those that have been reported in patients treated with intravenous acyclovir. Adequate hydration should be maintained).
No products indexed under this heading.

Colistin Sulfate (Caution should be exercised when administering acyclovir to patients receiving potentially nephrotoxic agents since this may increase the risk of renal dysfunction and/or the risk of reversible CNS symptoms such as those that have been reported in patients treated with intravenous acyclovir. Adequate hydration should be maintained).
No products indexed under this heading.

Cyclophosphamide (Caution should be exercised when administering acyclovir to patients receiving potentially nephrotoxic agents since this may increase the risk of renal dysfunction and/or the risk of reversible CNS symptoms such as those that have been reported in patients treated with intravenous acyclovir. Adequate hydration should be maintained).
No products indexed under this heading.

Cyclosporine (Caution should be exercised when administering acyclovir to patients receiving potentially nephrotoxic agents since this may increase the risk of renal dysfunction and/or the risk of reversible CNS symptoms such as those that have been reported in patients treated with intravenous acyclovir. Adequate hydration should be maintained). Products include:
Gengraf 440
Neoral Oral Solution 2496
Neoral Capsules 2496
Restasis 605

Cytarabine (Caution should be exercised when administering acyclovir to patients receiving potentially nephrotoxic agents since this may increase the risk of renal dysfunction and/or the risk of reversible CNS symptoms such as those that have been reported in patients treated with intravenous acyclovir. Adequate hydration should be maintained).
No products indexed under this heading.

IMPORTANT NOTE: Always consult each drug listing in the patient's regimen for possible interactions.

Cytarabine Liposome (Caution should be exercised when administering acyclovir to patients receiving potentially nephrotoxic agents since this may increase the risk of renal dysfunction and/or the risk of reversible CNS symptoms such as those that have been reported in patients treated with intravenous acyclovir. Adequate hydration should be maintained).
No products indexed under this heading.

Delavirdine Mesylate (Caution should be exercised when administering acyclovir to patients receiving potentially nephrotoxic agents since this may increase the risk of renal dysfunction and/or the risk of reversible CNS symptoms such as those that have been reported in patients treated with intravenous acyclovir. Adequate hydration should be maintained).
No products indexed under this heading.

Diatrizoate Meglumine (Caution should be exercised when administering acyclovir to patients receiving potentially nephrotoxic agents since this may increase the risk of renal dysfunction and/or the risk of reversible CNS symptoms such as those that have been reported in patients treated with intravenous acyclovir. Adequate hydration should be maintained).
No products indexed under this heading.

Diatrizoate Sodium (Caution should be exercised when administering acyclovir to patients receiving potentially nephrotoxic agents since this may increase the risk of renal dysfunction and/or the risk of reversible CNS symptoms such as those that have been reported in patients treated with intravenous acyclovir. Adequate hydration should be maintained).
No products indexed under this heading.

Diclofenac Potassium (Caution should be exercised when administering acyclovir to patients receiving potentially nephrotoxic agents since this may increase the risk of renal dysfunction and/or the risk of reversible CNS symptoms such as those that have been reported in patients treated with intravenous acyclovir. Adequate hydration should be maintained).
No products indexed under this heading.

Diclofenac Sodium (Caution should be exercised when administering acyclovir to patients receiving potentially nephrotoxic agents since this may increase the risk of renal dysfunction and/or the risk of reversible CNS symptoms such as those that have been reported in patients treated with intravenous acyclovir. Adequate hydration should be maintained).
No products indexed under this heading.

Dicloxacillin Sodium (Caution should be exercised when administering acyclovir to patients receiving potentially nephrotoxic agents since this may increase the risk of renal dysfunction and/or the risk of reversible CNS symptoms such as those that have been reported in patients treated with intravenous acyclovir. Adequate hydration should be maintained).
No products indexed under this heading.

Didanosine (Caution should be exercised when administering acyclovir to patients receiving potentially nephrotoxic agents since this may increase the risk of renal dysfunction and/or the risk of reversible CNS symptoms such as those that have been reported in patients treated with intravenous acyclovir. Adequate hydration should be maintained).
No products indexed under this heading.

Efavirenz (Caution should be exercised when administering acyclovir to patients receiving potentially nephrotoxic agents since this may increase the risk of renal dysfunction and/or the risk of reversible CNS symptoms such as those that have been reported in patients treated with intravenous acyclovir. Adequate hydration should be maintained). Products include:
Atripla ... 906

Emtricitabine (Caution should be exercised when administering acyclovir to patients receiving potentially nephrotoxic agents since this may increase the risk of renal dysfunction and/or the risk of reversible CNS symptoms such as those that have been reported in patients treated with intravenous acyclovir. Adequate hydration should be maintained). Products include:
Atripla ... 906
Emtriva ... 1238
Emtriva Oral Solution ... 1238
Truvada ... 1258

Enalapril Maleate (Caution should be exercised when administering acyclovir to patients receiving potentially nephrotoxic agents since this may increase the risk of renal dysfunction and/or the risk of reversible CNS symptoms such as those that have been reported in patients treated with intravenous acyclovir. Adequate hydration should be maintained).
No products indexed under this heading.

Enalaprilat (Caution should be exercised when administering acyclovir to patients receiving potentially nephrotoxic agents since this may increase the risk of renal dysfunction and/or the risk of reversible CNS symptoms such as those that have been reported in patients treated with intravenous acyclovir. Adequate hydration should be maintained).
No products indexed under this heading.

Enfuvirtide (Caution should be exercised when administering acyclovir to patients receiving potentially nephrotoxic agents since this may increase the risk of renal dysfunction and/or the risk of reversible CNS symptoms such as those that have been reported in patients treated with intravenous acyclovir. Adequate hydration should be maintained).
No products indexed under this heading.

Ethiodized Oil (Caution should be exercised when administering acyclovir to patients receiving potentially nephrotoxic agents since this may increase the risk of renal dysfunction and/or the risk of reversible CNS symptoms such as those that have been reported in patients treated with intravenous acyclovir. Adequate hydration should be maintained).
No products indexed under this heading.

Etodolac (Caution should be exercised when administering acyclovir to patients receiving potentially nephrotoxic agents since this may increase the risk of renal dysfunction and/or the risk of reversible CNS symptoms such as those that have been reported in patients treated with intravenous acyclovir. Adequate hydration should be maintained).
No products indexed under this heading.

Fenoprofen Calcium (Caution should be exercised when administering acyclovir to patients receiving potentially nephrotoxic agents since this may increase the risk of renal dysfunction and/or the risk of reversible CNS symptoms such as those that have been reported in patients treated with intravenous acyclovir. Adequate hydration should be maintained).
No products indexed under this heading.

Filgrastim (Caution should be exercised when administering acyclovir to patients receiving potentially nephrotoxic agents since this may increase the risk of renal dysfunction and/or the risk of reversible CNS symptoms such as those that have been reported in patients treated with intravenous acyclovir. Adequate hydration should be maintained). Products include:
Neupogen ... 631

Fluorouracil (Caution should be exercised when administering acyclovir to patients receiving potentially nephrotoxic agents since this may increase the risk of renal dysfunction and/or the risk of reversible CNS symptoms such as those that have been reported in patients treated with intravenous acyclovir. Adequate hydration should be maintained). Products include:
Carac ... 2966

Flurbiprofen (Caution should be exercised when administering acyclovir to patients receiving potentially nephrotoxic agents since this may increase the risk of renal dysfunction and/or the risk of reversible CNS symptoms such as those that have been reported in patients treated with intravenous acyclovir. Adequate hydration should be maintained).
No products indexed under this heading.

Fluvastatin Sodium (Caution should be exercised when administering acyclovir to patients receiving potentially nephrotoxic agents since this may increase the risk of renal dysfunction and/or the risk of reversible CNS symptoms such as those that have been reported in patients treated with intravenous acyclovir. Adequate hydration should be maintained).
No products indexed under this heading.

Foscarnet Sodium (Caution should be exercised when administering acyclovir to patients receiving potentially nephrotoxic agents since this may increase the risk of renal dysfunction and/or the risk of reversible CNS symptoms such as those that have been reported in patients treated with intravenous acyclovir. Adequate hydration should be maintained).
No products indexed under this heading.

Fosinopril Sodium (Caution should be exercised when administering acyclovir to patients receiving potentially nephrotoxic agents since this may increase the risk of renal dysfunction and/or the risk of reversible CNS symptoms such as those that have been reported in patients treated with intravenous acyclovir. Adequate hydration should be maintained).
No products indexed under this heading.

Furosemide (Caution should be exercised when administering acyclovir to patients receiving potentially nephrotoxic agents since this may increase the risk of renal dysfunction and/or the risk of reversible CNS symptoms such as those that have been reported in patients treated with intravenous acyclovir. Adequate hydration should be maintained). Products include:
Furosemide ... 2354

Gadopentetate Dimeglumine (Caution should be exercised when administering acyclovir to patients receiving potentially nephrotoxic agents since this may increase the risk of renal dysfunction and/or the risk of reversible CNS symptoms such as those that have been reported in patients treated with intravenous acyclovir. Adequate hydration should be maintained).
No products indexed under this heading.

Gentamicin (Caution should be exercised when administering acyclovir to patients receiving potentially nephrotoxic agents since this may increase the risk of renal dysfunction and/or the risk of reversible CNS symptoms such as those that have been reported in patients treated with intravenous acyclovir. Adequate hydration should be maintained).
No products indexed under this heading.

Gentamicin Sulfate (Caution should be exercised when administering acyclovir to patients receiving potentially nephrotoxic agents since this may increase the risk of renal dysfunction and/or the risk of reversible CNS symptoms such as those that have been reported in patients treated with intravenous acyclovir. Adequate hydration should be maintained). Products include:
Pred-G ... ⊙226, ⊙227

Glipizide (Caution should be exercised when administering acyclovir to patients receiving potentially nephrotoxic agents since this may increase the risk of renal dysfunction and/or the risk of reversible CNS symptoms such as those that have been reported in patients treated with intravenous acyclovir. Adequate hydration should be maintained).
No products indexed under this heading.

Globulin, Immune (Human) (Caution should be exercised when administering acyclovir to patients receiving potentially nephrotoxic agents since this may increase the risk of renal dysfunction and/or the risk of reversible CNS symptoms such as those that have been reported in patients treated with intravenous acyclovir. Adequate hydration should be maintained). Products include:

Glyburide (Caution should be exercised when administering acyclovir to patients receiving potentially nephrotoxic agents since this may increase the risk of renal dysfunction and/or the risk of reversible CNS symptoms such as those that have been reported in patients treated with intravenous acyclovir. Adequate hydration should be maintained).
No products indexed under this heading.

Gold Therapy (Caution should be exercised when administering acyclovir to patients receiving potentially nephrotoxic agents since this may increase the risk of renal dysfunction and/or the risk of reversible CNS symptoms such as those that have been reported in patients treated with intravenous acyclovir. Adequate hydration should be maintained).
No products indexed under this heading.

HMG-CoA Reductase Inhibitors (Caution should be exercised when administering acyclovir to patients receiving potentially nephrotoxic agents since this may increase the risk of renal dysfunction and/or the risk of reversible CNS symptoms such as those that have been reported in patients treated with intravenous acyclovir. Adequate hydration should be maintained).
No products indexed under this heading.

Hydrochlorothiazide (Caution should be exercised when administering acyclovir to patients receiving potentially nephrotoxic agents since this may increase the risk of renal dysfunction and/or the risk of reversible CNS symptoms such as those that have been reported in patients treated with intravenous acyclovir. Adequate hydration should be maintained). Products include:
Atacand HCT ... 700
Avalide ... 2956
Benicar HCT ... 1017
Diovan HCT ... 2419
Dyazide ... 1429
Exforge HCT ... 2449
Hyzaar ... 2162
Hyzaar 100-12.5 ... 2162
Micardis HCT ... 889
Prinzide ... 2246
Tekturna HCT ... 2541
Teveten HCT ... 541

Hydroflumethiazide (Caution should be exercised when administering acyclovir to patients receiving potentially nephrotoxic agents since this may increase the risk of renal dysfunction and/or the risk of reversible CNS symptoms such as those that have been reported in patients treated with intravenous acyclovir. Adequate hydration should be maintained).
No products indexed under this heading.

Ibuprofen (Caution should be exercised when administering acyclovir to patients receiving potentially nephrotoxic agents since this may increase the risk of renal dysfunction and/or the risk of reversible CNS symptoms such as those that have been reported in patients treated with intravenous acyclovir. Adequate hydration should be maintained). Products include:
Motrin IB 2043
Children's Motrin 2044
Children's Motrin Non-Staining Dye-Free 2044
Infants' Motrin 2044
Infants' Motrin Dye-Free 2044
Junior Strength Motrin 2044
Vicoprofen 564

Idarubicin Hydrochloride (Caution should be exercised when administering acyclovir to patients receiving potentially nephrotoxic agents since this may increase the risk of renal dysfunction and/or the risk of reversible CNS symptoms such as those that have been reported in patients treated with intravenous acyclovir. Adequate hydration should be maintained).
No products indexed under this heading.

Ifosfamide (Caution should be exercised when administering acyclovir to patients receiving potentially nephrotoxic agents since this may increase the risk of renal dysfunction and/or the risk of reversible CNS symptoms such as those that have been reported in patients treated with intravenous acyclovir. Adequate hydration should be maintained).
No products indexed under this heading.

Imipenem (Caution should be exercised when administering acyclovir to patients receiving potentially nephrotoxic agents since this may increase the risk of renal dysfunction and/or the risk of reversible CNS symptoms such as those that have been reported in patients treated with intravenous acyclovir. Adequate hydration should be maintained). Products include:
Primaxin I.M. 2232
Primaxin I.V. 2235

Immune Globulin Intravenous (Human) (Caution should be exercised when administering acyclovir to patients receiving potentially nephrotoxic agents since this may increase the risk of renal dysfunction and/or the risk of reversible CNS symptoms such as those that have been reported in patients treated with intravenous acyclovir. Adequate hydration should be maintained). Products include:
Flebogamma 5% DIF 1794
Gammagard 812, 815
Gamunex 3374

Indinavir Sulfate (Caution should be exercised when administering acyclovir to patients receiving potentially nephrotoxic agents since this may increase the risk of renal dysfunction and/or the risk of reversible CNS symptoms such as those that have been reported in patients treated with intravenous acyclovir. Adequate hydration should be maintained). Products include:
Crixivan 2113

Indomethacin (Caution should be exercised when administering acyclovir to patients receiving potentially nephrotoxic agents since this may increase the risk of renal dysfunction and/or the risk of reversible CNS symptoms such as those that have been reported in patients treated with intravenous acyclovir. Adequate hydration should be maintained). Products include:
Indocin 2167

Indomethacin Sodium Trihydrate (Caution should be exercised when administering acyclovir to patients receiving potentially nephrotoxic agents since this may increase the risk of renal dysfunction and/or the risk of reversible CNS symptoms such as those that have been reported in patients treated with intravenous acyclovir. Adequate hydration should be maintained). Products include:
Indocin I.V. 2007

Interferon Beta-1b (Caution should be exercised when administering acyclovir to patients receiving potentially nephrotoxic agents since this may increase the risk of renal dysfunction and/or the risk of reversible CNS symptoms such as those that have been reported in patients treated with intravenous acyclovir. Adequate hydration should be maintained). Products include:
Betaseron 836
Extavia 2459

Interleuken-2 (Caution should be exercised when administering acyclovir to patients receiving potentially nephrotoxic agents since this may increase the risk of renal dysfunction and/or the risk of reversible CNS symptoms such as those that have been reported in patients treated with intravenous acyclovir. Adequate hydration should be maintained).
No products indexed under this heading.

Iodamide Meglumine (Caution should be exercised when administering acyclovir to patients receiving potentially nephrotoxic agents since this may increase the risk of renal dysfunction and/or the risk of reversible CNS symptoms such as those that have been reported in patients treated with intravenous acyclovir. Adequate hydration should be maintained).
No products indexed under this heading.

Iohexol (Caution should be exercised when administering acyclovir to patients receiving potentially nephrotoxic agents since this may increase the risk of renal dysfunction and/or the risk of reversible CNS symptoms such as those that have been reported in patients treated with intravenous acyclovir. Adequate hydration should be maintained).
No products indexed under this heading.

Iopamidol (Caution should be exercised when administering acyclovir to patients receiving potentially nephrotoxic agents since this may increase the risk of renal dysfunction and/or the risk of reversible CNS symptoms such as those that have been reported in patients treated with intravenous acyclovir. Adequate hydration should be maintained).
No products indexed under this heading.

Iopanoic Acid (Caution should be exercised when administering acyclovir to patients receiving potentially nephrotoxic agents since this may increase the risk of renal dysfunction and/or the risk of reversible CNS symptoms such as those that have been reported in patients treated with intravenous acyclovir. Adequate hydration should be maintained).
No products indexed under this heading.

Iothalamate Meglumine (Caution should be exercised when administering acyclovir to patients receiving potentially nephrotoxic agents since this may increase the risk of renal dysfunction and/or the risk of reversible CNS symptoms such as those that have been reported in patients treated with intravenous acyclovir. Adequate hydration should be maintained).
No products indexed under this heading.

Ioxaglate Meglumine (Caution should be exercised when administering acyclovir to patients receiving potentially nephrotoxic agents since this may increase the risk of renal dysfunction and/or the risk of reversible CNS symptoms such as those that have been reported in patients treated with intravenous acyclovir. Adequate hydration should be maintained).
No products indexed under this heading.

Ioxaglate Sodium (Caution should be exercised when administering acyclovir to patients receiving potentially nephrotoxic agents since this may increase the risk of renal dysfunction and/or the risk of reversible CNS symptoms such as those that have been reported in patients treated with intravenous acyclovir. Adequate hydration should be maintained).
No products indexed under this heading.

Kanamycin Sulfate (Caution should be exercised when administering acyclovir to patients receiving potentially nephrotoxic agents since this may increase the risk of renal dysfunction and/or the risk of reversible CNS symptoms such as those that have been reported in patients treated with intravenous acyclovir. Adequate hydration should be maintained).
No products indexed under this heading.

Ketoprofen (Caution should be exercised when administering acyclovir to patients receiving potentially nephrotoxic agents since this may increase the risk of renal dysfunction and/or the risk of reversible CNS symptoms such as those that have been reported in patients treated with intravenous acyclovir. Adequate hydration should be maintained).
No products indexed under this heading.

Ketorolac Tromethamine (Caution should be exercised when administering acyclovir to patients receiving potentially nephrotoxic agents since this may increase the risk of renal dysfunction and/or the risk of reversible CNS symptoms such as those that have been reported in patients treated with intravenous acyclovir. Adequate hydration should be maintained). Products include:
Acuvail .... ⊙ 209

Lamium album (Caution should be exercised when administering acyclovir to patients receiving potentially nephrotoxic agents since this may increase the risk of renal dysfunction and/or the risk of reversible CNS symptoms such as those that have been reported in patients treated with intravenous acyclovir. Adequate hydration should be maintained).
No products indexed under this heading.

Lisinopril (Caution should be exercised when administering acyclovir to patients receiving potentially nephrotoxic agents since this may increase the risk of renal dysfunction and/or the risk of reversible CNS symptoms such as those that have been reported in patients treated with intravenous acyclovir. Adequate hydration should be maintained). Products include:
Prinivil 2241
Prinzide 2246

Lithium (Caution should be exercised when administering acyclovir to patients receiving potentially nephrotoxic agents since this may increase the risk of renal dysfunction and/or the risk of reversible CNS symptoms such as those that have been reported in patients treated with intravenous acyclovir. Adequate hydration should be maintained).
No products indexed under this heading.

Lithium Carbonate (Caution should be exercised when administering acyclovir to patients receiving potentially nephrotoxic agents since this may increase the risk of renal dysfunction and/or the risk of reversible CNS symptoms such as those that have been reported in patients treated with intravenous acyclovir. Adequate hydration should be maintained).
No products indexed under this heading.

Lithium Citrate (Caution should be exercised when administering acyclovir to patients receiving potentially nephrotoxic agents since this may increase the risk of renal dysfunction and/or the risk of reversible CNS symptoms such as those that have been reported in patients treated with intravenous acyclovir. Adequate hydration should be maintained).
No products indexed under this heading.

Lopinavir (Caution should be exercised when administering acyclovir to patients receiving potentially nephrotoxic agents since this may increase the risk of renal dysfunction and/or the risk of reversible CNS symptoms such as those that have been reported in patients treated with intravenous acyclovir. Adequate hydration should be maintained). Products include:
Kaletra 458

Loracarbef (Caution should be exercised when administering acyclovir to patients receiving potentially nephrotoxic agents since this may increase the risk of renal dysfunction and/or the risk of reversible CNS symptoms such as those that have been reported in patients treated with intravenous acyclovir. Adequate hydration should be maintained).
No products indexed under this heading.

Lovastatin (Caution should be exercised when administering acyclovir to patients receiving potentially nephrotoxic agents since this may increase the risk of renal dysfunction and/or the risk of reversible CNS symptoms such as those that have been reported in patients treated with intravenous acyclovir. Adequate hydration should be maintained). Products include:
Advicor 402
Mevacor 2212

Meclofenamate Sodium (Caution should be exercised when administering acyclovir to patients receiving potentially nephrotoxic agents since this may increase the risk of renal dysfunction and/or the risk of reversible CNS symptoms such as those that have been reported in patients treated with intravenous acyclovir. Adequate hydration should be maintained).
No products indexed under this heading.

Mefenamic Acid (Caution should be exercised when administering acyclovir to patients receiving potentially nephrotoxic agents since this may increase the risk of renal dysfunction and/or the risk of reversible CNS symptoms such as those that have been reported in patients treated with intravenous acyclovir. Adequate hydration should be maintained).
No products indexed under this heading.

IMPORTANT NOTE: Always consult each drug listing in the patient's regimen for possible interactions.

Meloxicam (Caution should be exercised when administering acyclovir to patients receiving potentially nephrotoxic agents since this may increase the risk of renal dysfunction and/or the risk of reversible CNS symptoms such as those that have been reported in patients treated with intravenous acyclovir. Adequate hydration should be maintained).

No products indexed under this heading.

Melphalan Hydrochloride (Caution should be exercised when administering acyclovir to patients receiving potentially nephrotoxic agents since this may increase the risk of renal dysfunction and/or the risk of reversible CNS symptoms such as those that have been reported in patients treated with intravenous acyclovir. Adequate hydration should be maintained). Products include:

Mesalamine (Caution should be exercised when administering acyclovir to patients receiving potentially nephrotoxic agents since this may increase the risk of renal dysfunction and/or the risk of reversible CNS symptoms such as those that have been reported in patients treated with intravenous acyclovir. Adequate hydration should be maintained). Products include:

Methimazole (Caution should be exercised when administering acyclovir to patients receiving potentially nephrotoxic agents since this may increase the risk of renal dysfunction and/or the risk of reversible CNS symptoms such as those that have been reported in patients treated with intravenous acyclovir. Adequate hydration should be maintained).

No products indexed under this heading.

Methotrexate (Caution should be exercised when administering acyclovir to patients receiving potentially nephrotoxic agents since this may increase the risk of renal dysfunction and/or the risk of reversible CNS symptoms such as those that have been reported in patients treated with intravenous acyclovir. Adequate hydration should be maintained).

No products indexed under this heading.

Methotrexate Sodium (Caution should be exercised when administering acyclovir to patients receiving potentially nephrotoxic agents since this may increase the risk of renal dysfunction and/or the risk of reversible CNS symptoms such as those that have been reported in patients treated with intravenous acyclovir. Adequate hydration should be maintained).

No products indexed under this heading.

Methyclothiazide (Caution should be exercised when administering acyclovir to patients receiving potentially nephrotoxic agents since this may increase the risk of renal dysfunction and/or the risk of reversible CNS symptoms such as those that have been reported in patients treated with intravenous acyclovir. Adequate hydration should be maintained).

No products indexed under this heading.

Mezlocillin Sodium (Caution should be exercised when administering acyclovir to patients receiving potentially nephrotoxic agents since this may increase the risk of renal dysfunction and/or the risk of reversible CNS symptoms such as those that have been reported in patients treated with intravenous acyclovir. Adequate hydration should be maintained).

No products indexed under this heading.

Minocycline Hydrochloride (Caution should be exercised when administering acyclovir to patients receiving potentially nephrotoxic agents since this may increase the risk of renal dysfunction and/or the risk of reversible CNS symptoms such as those that have been reported in patients treated with intravenous acyclovir. Adequate hydration should be maintained). Products include:

Mitomycin (Mitomycin-C) (Caution should be exercised when administering acyclovir to patients receiving potentially nephrotoxic agents since this may increase the risk of renal dysfunction and/or the risk of reversible CNS symptoms such as those that have been reported in patients treated with intravenous acyclovir. Adequate hydration should be maintained).

No products indexed under this heading.

Moexipril Hydrochloride (Caution should be exercised when administering acyclovir to patients receiving potentially nephrotoxic agents since this may increase the risk of renal dysfunction and/or the risk of reversible CNS symptoms such as those that have been reported in patients treated with intravenous acyclovir. Adequate hydration should be maintained).

No products indexed under this heading.

Muromonab-CD3 (Caution should be exercised when administering acyclovir to patients receiving potentially nephrotoxic agents since this may increase the risk of renal dysfunction and/or the risk of reversible CNS symptoms such as those that have been reported in patients treated with intravenous acyclovir. Adequate hydration should be maintained). Products include:

Nabumetone (Caution should be exercised when administering acyclovir to patients receiving potentially nephrotoxic agents since this may increase the risk of renal dysfunction and/or the risk of reversible CNS symptoms such as those that have been reported in patients treated with intravenous acyclovir. Adequate hydration should be maintained).

No products indexed under this heading.

Nafcillin Sodium (Caution should be exercised when administering acyclovir to patients receiving potentially nephrotoxic agents since this may increase the risk of renal dysfunction and/or the risk of reversible CNS symptoms such as those that have been reported in patients treated with intravenous acyclovir. Adequate hydration should be maintained).

No products indexed under this heading.

Naproxen (Caution should be exercised when administering acyclovir to patients receiving potentially nephrotoxic agents since this may increase the risk of renal dysfunction and/or the risk of reversible CNS symptoms such as those that have been reported in patients treated with intravenous acyclovir. Adequate hydration should be maintained). Products include:

Naproxen Sodium (Caution should be exercised when administering acyclovir to patients receiving potentially nephrotoxic agents since this may increase the risk of renal dysfunction and/or the risk of reversible CNS symptoms such as those that have been reported in patients treated with intravenous acyclovir. Adequate hydration should be maintained). Products include:

Nelfinavir Mesylate (Caution should be exercised when administering acyclovir to patients receiving potentially nephrotoxic agents since this may increase the risk of renal dysfunction and/or the risk of reversible CNS symptoms such as those that have been reported in patients treated with intravenous acyclovir. Adequate hydration should be maintained).

No products indexed under this heading.

Neomycin (Caution should be exercised when administering acyclovir to patients receiving potentially nephrotoxic agents since this may increase the risk of renal dysfunction and/or the risk of reversible CNS symptoms such as those that have been reported in patients treated with intravenous acyclovir. Adequate hydration should be maintained).

No products indexed under this heading.

Neomycin, oral (Caution should be exercised when administering acyclovir to patients receiving potentially nephrotoxic agents since this may increase the risk of renal dysfunction and/or the risk of reversible CNS symptoms such as those that have been reported in patients treated with intravenous acyclovir. Adequate hydration should be maintained).

No products indexed under this heading.

Neomycin Sulfate (Caution should be exercised when administering acyclovir to patients receiving potentially nephrotoxic agents since this may increase the risk of renal dysfunction and/or the risk of reversible CNS symptoms such as those that have been reported in patients treated with intravenous acyclovir. Adequate hydration should be maintained).

No products indexed under this heading.

Nephrotoxic Drugs (Caution should be exercised when administering acyclovir to patients receiving potentially nephrotoxic agents since this may increase the risk of renal dysfunction and/or the risk of reversible CNS symptoms such as those that have been reported in patients treated with intravenous acyclovir. Adequate hydration should be maintained).

No products indexed under this heading.

Nevirapine (Caution should be exercised when administering acyclovir to patients receiving potentially nephrotoxic agents since this may increase the risk of renal dysfunction and/or the risk of reversible CNS symptoms such as those that have been reported in patients treated with intravenous acyclovir. Adequate hydration should be maintained). Products include:

Norfloxacin (Caution should be exercised when administering acyclovir to patients receiving potentially nephrotoxic agents since this may increase the risk of renal dysfunction and/or the risk of reversible CNS symptoms such as those that have been reported in patients treated with intravenous acyclovir. Adequate hydration should be maintained). Products include:

Olsalazine Sodium (Caution should be exercised when administering acyclovir to patients receiving potentially nephrotoxic agents since this may increase the risk of renal dysfunction and/or the risk of reversible CNS symptoms such as those that have been reported in patients treated with intravenous acyclovir. Adequate hydration should be maintained).

No products indexed under this heading.

Omeprazole (Caution should be exercised when administering acyclovir to patients receiving potentially nephrotoxic agents since this may increase the risk of renal dysfunction and/or the risk of reversible CNS symptoms such as those that have been reported in patients treated with intravenous acyclovir. Adequate hydration should be maintained).

No products indexed under this heading.

Oxaprozin (Caution should be exercised when administering acyclovir to patients receiving potentially nephrotoxic agents since this may increase the risk of renal dysfunction and/or the risk of reversible CNS symptoms such as those that have been reported in patients treated with intravenous acyclovir. Adequate hydration should be maintained).

No products indexed under this heading.

Pamidronate Disodium (Caution should be exercised when administering acyclovir to patients receiving potentially nephrotoxic agents since this may increase the risk of renal dysfunction and/or the risk of reversible CNS symptoms such as those that have been reported in patients treated with intravenous acyclovir. Adequate hydration should be maintained).

No products indexed under this heading.

Paroxetine Hydrochloride (Caution should be exercised when administering acyclovir to patients receiving potentially nephrotoxic agents since this may increase the risk of renal dysfunction and/or the risk of reversible CNS symptoms such as those that have been reported in patients treated with intravenous acyclovir. Adequate hydration should be maintained). Products include:

Penicillamine (Caution should be exercised when administering acyclovir to patients receiving potentially nephrotoxic agents since this may increase the risk of renal dysfunction and/or the risk of reversible CNS symptoms such as those that have been reported in patients treated with intravenous acyclovir. Adequate hydration should be maintained).

No products indexed under this heading.

Penicillin G Benzathine (Caution should be exercised when administering acyclovir to patients receiving potentially nephrotoxic agents since this may increase the risk of renal dysfunction and/or the risk of reversible CNS symptoms such as those that have been reported in patients treated with intravenous acyclovir. Adequate hydration should be maintained). Products include:

(⊙ Described in PDR® for Ophthalmic Medicines)

2189 Interactions Index Zovirax

Penicillin G Potassium (Caution should be exercised when administering acyclovir to patients receiving potentially nephrotoxic agents since this may increase the risk of renal dysfunction and/or the risk of reversible CNS symptoms such as those that have been reported in patients treated with intravenous acyclovir. Adequate hydration should be maintained).
No products indexed under this heading.

Penicillin G Procaine (Caution should be exercised when administering acyclovir to patients receiving potentially nephrotoxic agents since this may increase the risk of renal dysfunction and/or the risk of reversible CNS symptoms such as those that have been reported in patients treated with intravenous acyclovir. Adequate hydration should be maintained). Products include:
Bicillin C-R Injectable Suspension 1826
Bicillin L-A 1828

Penicillin G Sodium (Caution should be exercised when administering acyclovir to patients receiving potentially nephrotoxic agents since this may increase the risk of renal dysfunction and/or the risk of reversible CNS symptoms such as those that have been reported in patients treated with intravenous acyclovir. Adequate hydration should be maintained).
No products indexed under this heading.

Penicillin V Potassium (Caution should be exercised when administering acyclovir to patients receiving potentially nephrotoxic agents since this may increase the risk of renal dysfunction and/or the risk of reversible CNS symptoms such as those that have been reported in patients treated with intravenous acyclovir. Adequate hydration should be maintained).
No products indexed under this heading.

Pentamidine Isethionate (Caution should be exercised when administering acyclovir to patients receiving potentially nephrotoxic agents since this may increase the risk of renal dysfunction and/or the risk of reversible CNS symptoms such as those that have been reported in patients treated with intravenous acyclovir. Adequate hydration should be maintained).
No products indexed under this heading.

Perindopril Erbumine (Caution should be exercised when administering acyclovir to patients receiving potentially nephrotoxic agents since this may increase the risk of renal dysfunction and/or the risk of reversible CNS symptoms such as those that have been reported in patients treated with intravenous acyclovir. Adequate hydration should be maintained).
No products indexed under this heading.

Phenylbutazone (Caution should be exercised when administering acyclovir to patients receiving potentially nephrotoxic agents since this may increase the risk of renal dysfunction and/or the risk of reversible CNS symptoms such as those that have been reported in patients treated with intravenous acyclovir. Adequate hydration should be maintained).
No products indexed under this heading.

Piroxicam (Caution should be exercised when administering acyclovir to patients receiving potentially nephrotoxic agents since this may increase the risk of renal dysfunction and/or the risk of reversible CNS symptoms such as those that have been reported in patients treated with intravenous acyclovir. Adequate hydration should be maintained).
No products indexed under this heading.

Plicamycin (Caution should be exercised when administering acyclovir to patients receiving potentially nephrotoxic agents since this may increase the risk of renal dysfunction and/or the risk of reversible CNS symptoms such as those that have been reported in patients treated with intravenous acyclovir. Adequate hydration should be maintained).
No products indexed under this heading.

Polymyxin (Caution should be exercised when administering acyclovir to patients receiving potentially nephrotoxic agents since this may increase the risk of renal dysfunction and/or the risk of reversible CNS symptoms such as those that have been reported in patients treated with intravenous acyclovir. Adequate hydration should be maintained).
No products indexed under this heading.

Polymyxin B Sulfate (Caution should be exercised when administering acyclovir to patients receiving potentially nephrotoxic agents since this may increase the risk of renal dysfunction and/or the risk of reversible CNS symptoms such as those that have been reported in patients treated with intravenous acyclovir. Adequate hydration should be maintained).
No products indexed under this heading.

Polythiazide (Caution should be exercised when administering acyclovir to patients receiving potentially nephrotoxic agents since this may increase the risk of renal dysfunction and/or the risk of reversible CNS symptoms such as those that have been reported in patients treated with intravenous acyclovir. Adequate hydration should be maintained).
No products indexed under this heading.

Pravastatin Sodium (Caution should be exercised when administering acyclovir to patients receiving potentially nephrotoxic agents since this may increase the risk of renal dysfunction and/or the risk of reversible CNS symptoms such as those that have been reported in patients treated with intravenous acyclovir. Adequate hydration should be maintained).
No products indexed under this heading.

Probenecid (Co-administration of probenecid with intravenous acyclovir has been shown to increase acyclovir half-life and systemic exposure; urinary excretion and renal clearance were correspondingly reduced).
No products indexed under this heading.

Quinapril Hydrochloride (Caution should be exercised when administering acyclovir to patients receiving potentially nephrotoxic agents since this may increase the risk of renal dysfunction and/or the risk of reversible CNS symptoms such as those that have been reported in patients treated with intravenous acyclovir. Adequate hydration should be maintained).
No products indexed under this heading.

Rabeprazole Sodium (Caution should be exercised when administering acyclovir to patients receiving potentially nephrotoxic agents since this may increase the risk of renal dysfunction and/or the risk of reversible CNS symptoms such as those that have been reported in patients treated with intravenous acyclovir. Adequate hydration should be maintained). Products include:
Aciphex 1035

Ramipril (Caution should be exercised when administering acyclovir to patients receiving potentially nephrotoxic agents since this may increase the risk of renal dysfunction and/or the risk of reversible CNS symptoms such as those that have been reported in patients treated with intravenous acyclovir. Adequate hydration should be maintained).
No products indexed under this heading.

Rifampin (Caution should be exercised when administering acyclovir to patients receiving potentially nephrotoxic agents since this may increase the risk of renal dysfunction and/or the risk of reversible CNS symptoms such as those that have been reported in patients treated with intravenous acyclovir. Adequate hydration should be maintained).
No products indexed under this heading.

Riluzole (Caution should be exercised when administering acyclovir to patients receiving potentially nephrotoxic agents since this may increase the risk of renal dysfunction and/or the risk of reversible CNS symptoms such as those that have been reported in patients treated with intravenous acyclovir. Adequate hydration should be maintained). Products include:
Rilutek 3032

Ritonavir (Caution should be exercised when administering acyclovir to patients receiving potentially nephrotoxic agents since this may increase the risk of renal dysfunction and/or the risk of reversible CNS symptoms such as those that have been reported in patients treated with intravenous acyclovir. Adequate hydration should be maintained). Products include:
Kaletra 458
Norvir 509

Rofecoxib (Caution should be exercised when administering acyclovir to patients receiving potentially nephrotoxic agents since this may increase the risk of renal dysfunction and/or the risk of reversible CNS symptoms such as those that have been reported in patients treated with intravenous acyclovir. Adequate hydration should be maintained).
No products indexed under this heading.

Saquinavir (Caution should be exercised when administering acyclovir to patients receiving potentially nephrotoxic agents since this may increase the risk of renal dysfunction and/or the risk of reversible CNS symptoms such as those that have been reported in patients treated with intravenous acyclovir. Adequate hydration should be maintained).
No products indexed under this heading.

Sibutramine Hydrochloride Monohydrate (Caution should be exercised when administering acyclovir to patients receiving potentially nephrotoxic agents since this may increase the risk of renal dysfunction and/or the risk of reversible CNS symptoms such as those that have been reported in patients treated with intravenous acyclovir. Adequate hydration should be maintained). Products include:
Meridia 492

Simvastatin (Caution should be exercised when administering acyclovir to patients receiving potentially nephrotoxic agents since this may increase the risk of renal dysfunction and/or the risk of reversible CNS symptoms such as those that have been reported in patients treated with intravenous acyclovir. Adequate hydration should be maintained). Products include:
Simcor 524
Vytorin 10/10 ..... 2303, 3240
Vytorin 10/20 ..... 2303, 3240
Vytorin 10/40 ..... 2303, 3240
Vytorin 10/80 ..... 2303, 3240
Zocor 2289

Spirapril Hydrochloride (Caution should be exercised when administering acyclovir to patients receiving potentially nephrotoxic agents since this may increase the risk of renal dysfunction and/or the risk of reversible CNS symptoms such as those that have been reported in patients treated with intravenous acyclovir. Adequate hydration should be maintained).
No products indexed under this heading.

Stavudine (Caution should be exercised when administering acyclovir to patients receiving potentially nephrotoxic agents since this may increase the risk of renal dysfunction and/or the risk of reversible CNS symptoms such as those that have been reported in patients treated with intravenous acyclovir. Adequate hydration should be maintained).
No products indexed under this heading.

Streptomycin Sulfate (Caution should be exercised when administering acyclovir to patients receiving potentially nephrotoxic agents since this may increase the risk of renal dysfunction and/or the risk of reversible CNS symptoms such as those that have been reported in patients treated with intravenous acyclovir. Adequate hydration should be maintained).
No products indexed under this heading.

Streptozocin (Caution should be exercised when administering acyclovir to patients receiving potentially nephrotoxic agents since this may increase the risk of renal dysfunction and/or the risk of reversible CNS symptoms such as those that have been reported in patients treated with intravenous acyclovir. Adequate hydration should be maintained).
No products indexed under this heading.

Sulfacytine (Caution should be exercised when administering acyclovir to patients receiving potentially nephrotoxic agents since this may increase the risk of renal dysfunction and/or the risk of reversible CNS symptoms such as those that have been reported in patients treated with intravenous acyclovir. Adequate hydration should be maintained).
No products indexed under this heading.

Sulfamethizole (Caution should be exercised when administering acyclovir to patients receiving potentially nephrotoxic agents since this may increase the risk of renal dysfunction and/or the risk of reversible CNS symptoms such as those that have been reported in patients treated with intravenous acyclovir. Adequate hydration should be maintained).
No products indexed under this heading.

Sulfamethoxazole (Caution should be exercised when administering acyclovir to patients receiving potentially nephrotoxic agents since this may increase the risk of renal dysfunction and/or the risk of reversible CNS symptoms such as those that have been reported in patients treated with intravenous acyclovir. Adequate hydration should be maintained).
No products indexed under this heading.

Sulfasalazine (Caution should be exercised when administering acyclovir to patients receiving potentially nephrotoxic agents since this may increase the risk of renal dysfunction and/or the risk of reversible CNS symptoms such as those that have been reported in patients treated with intravenous acyclovir. Adequate hydration should be maintained).
No products indexed under this heading.

Sulfinpyrazone (Caution should be exercised when administering acyclovir to patients receiving potentially nephrotoxic agents since this may increase the risk of renal dysfunction and/or the risk of reversible CNS symptoms such as those that have been reported in patients treated with intravenous acyclovir. Adequate hydration should be maintained).
No products indexed under this heading.

Sulfisoxazole Acetyl (Caution should be exercised when administering acyclovir to patients receiving potentially nephrotoxic agents since this may increase the risk of renal dysfunction and/or the risk of reversible CNS symptoms such as those that have been reported in patients treated with intravenous acyclovir. Adequate hydration should be maintained).
No products indexed under this heading.

Sulfisoxazole Diolamine (Caution should be exercised when administering acyclovir to patients receiving potentially nephrotoxic agents since this may increase the risk of renal dysfunction and/or the risk of reversible CNS symptoms such as those that have been reported in patients treated with intravenous acyclovir. Adequate hydration should be maintained).
No products indexed under this heading.

Sulindac (Caution should be exercised when administering acyclovir to patients receiving potentially nephrotoxic agents since this may increase the risk of renal dysfunction and/or the risk of reversible CNS symptoms such as those that have been reported in patients treated with intravenous acyclovir. Adequate hydration should be maintained). Products include:

Tacrolimus (Caution should be exercised when administering acyclovir to patients receiving potentially nephrotoxic agents since this may increase the risk of renal dysfunction and/or the risk of reversible CNS symptoms such as those that have been reported in patients treated with intravenous acyclovir. Adequate hydration should be maintained). Products include:

Tenofovir Disoproxil Fumarate (Caution should be exercised when administering acyclovir to patients receiving potentially nephrotoxic agents since this may increase the risk of renal dysfunction and/or the risk of reversible CNS symptoms such as those that have been reported in patients treated with intravenous acyclovir. Adequate hydration should be maintained). Products include:

Thioguanine (Caution should be exercised when administering acyclovir to patients receiving potentially nephrotoxic agents since this may increase the risk of renal dysfunction and/or the risk of reversible CNS symptoms such as those that have been reported in patients treated with intravenous acyclovir. Adequate hydration should be maintained). Products include:

Ticarcillin Disodium (Caution should be exercised when administering acyclovir to patients receiving potentially nephrotoxic agents since this may increase the risk of renal dysfunction and/or the risk of reversible CNS symptoms such as those that have been reported in patients treated with intravenous acyclovir. Adequate hydration should be maintained). Products include:

Tobramycin (Caution should be exercised when administering acyclovir to patients receiving potentially nephrotoxic agents since this may increase the risk of renal dysfunction and/or the risk of reversible CNS symptoms such as those that have been reported in patients treated with intravenous acyclovir. Adequate hydration should be maintained). Products include:

Tobramycin Sulfate (Caution should be exercised when administering acyclovir to patients receiving potentially nephrotoxic agents since this may increase the risk of renal dysfunction and/or the risk of reversible CNS symptoms such as those that have been reported in patients treated with intravenous acyclovir. Adequate hydration should be maintained).
No products indexed under this heading.

Tolazamide (Caution should be exercised when administering acyclovir to patients receiving potentially nephrotoxic agents since this may increase the risk of renal dysfunction and/or the risk of reversible CNS symptoms such as those that have been reported in patients treated with intravenous acyclovir. Adequate hydration should be maintained).
No products indexed under this heading.

Tolbutamide (Caution should be exercised when administering acyclovir to patients receiving potentially nephrotoxic agents since this may increase the risk of renal dysfunction and/or the risk of reversible CNS symptoms such as those that have been reported in patients treated with intravenous acyclovir. Adequate hydration should be maintained).
No products indexed under this heading.

Tolmetin Sodium (Caution should be exercised when administering acyclovir to patients receiving potentially nephrotoxic agents since this may increase the risk of renal dysfunction and/or the risk of reversible CNS symptoms such as those that have been reported in patients treated with intravenous acyclovir. Adequate hydration should be maintained).
No products indexed under this heading.

Trandolapril (Caution should be exercised when administering acyclovir to patients receiving potentially nephrotoxic agents since this may increase the risk of renal dysfunction and/or the risk of reversible CNS symptoms such as those that have been reported in patients treated with intravenous acyclovir. Adequate hydration should be maintained). Products include:

Triamterene (Caution should be exercised when administering acyclovir to patients receiving potentially nephrotoxic agents since this may increase the risk of renal dysfunction and/or the risk of reversible CNS symptoms such as those that have been reported in patients treated with intravenous acyclovir. Adequate hydration should be maintained). Products include:

Trimethadione (Caution should be exercised when administering acyclovir to patients receiving potentially nephrotoxic agents since this may increase the risk of renal dysfunction and/or the risk of reversible CNS symptoms such as those that have been reported in patients treated with intravenous acyclovir. Adequate hydration should be maintained).
No products indexed under this heading.

Trovafloxacin Mesylate (Caution should be exercised when administering acyclovir to patients receiving potentially nephrotoxic agents since this may increase the risk of renal dysfunction and/or the risk of reversible CNS symptoms such as those that have been reported in patients treated with intravenous acyclovir. Adequate hydration should be maintained).
No products indexed under this heading.

Tyropanoate Sodium (Caution should be exercised when administering acyclovir to patients receiving potentially nephrotoxic agents since this may increase the risk of renal dysfunction and/or the risk of reversible CNS symptoms such as those that have been reported in patients treated with intravenous acyclovir. Adequate hydration should be maintained).
No products indexed under this heading.

Valacyclovir Hydrochloride (Caution should be exercised when administering acyclovir to patients receiving potentially nephrotoxic agents since this may increase the risk of renal dysfunction and/or the risk of reversible CNS symptoms such as those that have been reported in patients treated with intravenous acyclovir. Adequate hydration should be maintained). Products include:

Valdecoxib (Caution should be exercised when administering acyclovir to patients receiving potentially nephrotoxic agents since this may increase the risk of renal dysfunction and/or the risk of reversible CNS symptoms such as those that have been reported in patients treated with intravenous acyclovir. Adequate hydration should be maintained).
No products indexed under this heading.

Vancomycin Hydrochloride (Caution should be exercised when administering acyclovir to patients receiving potentially nephrotoxic agents since this may increase the risk of renal dysfunction and/or the risk of reversible CNS symptoms such as those that have been reported in patients treated with intravenous acyclovir. Adequate hydration should be maintained).
No products indexed under this heading.

Voriconazole (Caution should be exercised when administering acyclovir to patients receiving potentially nephrotoxic agents since this may increase the risk of renal dysfunction and/or the risk of reversible CNS symptoms such as those that have been reported in patients treated with intravenous acyclovir. Adequate hydration should be maintained).
No products indexed under this heading.

Zalcitabine (Caution should be exercised when administering acyclovir to patients receiving potentially nephrotoxic agents since this may increase the risk of renal dysfunction and/or the risk of reversible CNS symptoms such as those that have been reported in patients treated with intravenous acyclovir. Adequate hydration should be maintained).
No products indexed under this heading.

Zidovudine (Caution should be exercised when administering acyclovir to patients receiving potentially nephrotoxic agents since this may increase the risk of renal dysfunction and/or the risk of reversible CNS symptoms such as those that have been reported in patients treated with intravenous acyclovir. Adequate hydration should be maintained). Products include:

Zoledronic Acid (Caution should be exercised when administering acyclovir to patients receiving potentially nephrotoxic agents since this may increase the risk of renal dysfunction and/or the risk of reversible CNS symptoms such as those that have been reported in patients treated with intravenous acyclovir. Adequate hydration should be maintained). Products include:

ZOVIRAX SUSPENSION

See Zovirax Capsules

ZOVIRAX TABLETS

See Zovirax Capsules

ZYBAN SUSTAINED-RELEASE TABLETS

May interact with alcohols, anorexiants, antiarrhythmics, antidepressant drugs, antipsychotic agents, benzodiazepines, beta-blockers, central nervous system stimulants, class IC antiarrhythmics, corticosteroids, cytochrome p450 2b6 inhibitors (selected), cytochrome p450 2b6 substrates (selected), cytochrome p450 2d6 substrates (selected), drugs which lower seizure threshold, haloperidols, hypnotics and sedatives, insulin, monoamine oxidase inhibitors, narcotic analgesics, nicotines, oral hypoglycemic agents, phenytoin, selective serotonin reuptake inhibitors, theophyllines, tricyclic antidepressants, and certain other agents. Compounds in these categories include:

Acarbose (Concomitant use of oral hypoglycemics with bupropion is associated with an increased seizure risk).
No products indexed under this heading.

Acebutolol Hydrochloride (Co-administration of bupropion with drugs that are metabolized by the CYP2D6 isoenzyme, including beta blockers (eg, metoprolol) should be approached with caution and should be initiated at the lower end of the dose range of the concomitant medication. If bupropion is added to the treatment regimen of a patient already receiving a drug metabolized by CYP2D6, the need to decrease the dose of the original medication should be considered, particularly for those concomitant medications with a narrow therapeutic index).
No products indexed under this heading.

Adenosine (Co-administration of bupropion with drugs that are metabolized by the CYP2D6 isoenzyme, including antiarrhythmics, should be approached with caution and should be initiated at the lower end of the dose range of the concomitant medication. If bupropion is added to the treatment regimen of a patient already receiving a drug metabolized by CYP2D6, the need to decrease the dose of the original medication should be considered, particularly for those concomitant medications with a narrow therapeutic index). Products include:

2191 Interactions Index Zyban

Alclometasone Dipropionate (Concurrent administration of bupropion and agents (eg, systemic steroids) that lower seizure threshold should be undertaken only with extreme caution).
No products indexed under this heading.

Alfentanil Hydrochloride (An addiction to opiates and concomitant use of opiates is associated with an increased seizure risk).
No products indexed under this heading.

Alprazolam (Bupropion is contraindicated in patients undergoing abrupt discontinuation of sedatives (including benzodiazepines). Excessive use of sedatives (including benzodiazepines) is associated with an increased seizure risk).
No products indexed under this heading.

Amantadine Hydrochloride (Limited clinical data suggest a higher incidence of adverse experiences in patients receiving bupropion concurrently with either levodopa or amantadine. Administration of bupropion to patients receiving amantadine concurrently should be undertaken with caution, using small initial doses and gradual dose increases).
No products indexed under this heading.

Amiodarone Hydrochloride (*In vitro* studies indicate that bupropion is primarily metabolized to hydroxybupropion by the CYP2B6 isoenzyme. Therefore, the potential exists for a drug interaction between bupropion hydrochloride and drugs that are substrates or inhibitors of the CYP2B6 isoenzyme (eg, orphenadrine, thiotepa, cyclophosphamide)).
No products indexed under this heading.

Amitriptyline Hydrochloride (Concurrent administration of bupropion and agents (eg, antidepressants) that lower seizure threshold should be undertaken only with extreme caution. Many drugs, including certain antidepressants (many tricyclics), are metabolized by the CYP2D6 isoenzyme. Co-administration of bupropion with drugs that are metabolized by CYP2D6 isoenzyme should be approached with caution and should be initiated at the lower end of the dose range of the concomitant medication. If bupropion is added to the treatment regimen of a patient already receiving a drug metabolized by CYP2D6, the need to decrease the dose of the original medication should be considered, particularly for those concomitant medications with a narrow therapeutic index).
No products indexed under this heading.

Amlodipine Besylate (*In vitro* studies indicate that bupropion is primarily metabolized to hydroxybupropion by the CYP2B6 isoenzyme. Therefore, the potential exists for a drug interaction between bupropion hydrochloride and drugs that are substrates or inhibitors of the CYP2B6 isoenzyme (eg, orphenadrine, thiotepa, cyclophosphamide)). Products include:
Azor 1010
Exforge 2443
Exforge HCT 2449

Amoxapine (Concurrent administration of bupropion and agents (eg, antidepressants) that lower seizure threshold should be undertaken only with extreme caution. Many drugs, including certain antidepressants (many tricyclics), are metabolized by the CYP2D6 isoenzyme. Co-administration of bupropion with drugs that are metabolized by CYP2D6 isoenzyme should be approached with caution and should be initiated at the lower end of the dose range of the concomitant medication. If bupropion is added to the treatment regimen of a patient already receiving a drug metabolized by CYP2D6, the need to decrease the dose of the original medication should be considered, particularly for those concomitant medications with a narrow therapeutic index).
No products indexed under this heading.

Amphetamine Aspartate (Concomitant use of anorectics with bupropion is associated with an increased seizure risk).
No products indexed under this heading.

Amphetamine Aspartate Monohydrate (Concomitant use of anorectics with bupropion is associated with an increased seizure risk).
No products indexed under this heading.

Amphetamine Resins (Concomitant use of anorectics with bupropion is associated with an increased seizure risk).
No products indexed under this heading.

Amphetamine Sulfate (Concomitant use of anorectics with bupropion is associated with an increased seizure risk).
No products indexed under this heading.

Apomorphine (An addiction to opiates and concomitant use of opiates is associated with an increased seizure risk).
No products indexed under this heading.

Apomorphine Hydrochloride (An addiction to opiates and concomitant use of opiates is associated with an increased seizure risk).
No products indexed under this heading.

Aripiprazole (Concurrent administration of bupropion and agents such as antipsychotics that lower seizure threshold should be undertaken with extreme caution. Co-administration of bupropion with drugs that are metabolized by CYP2D6 isoenzyme, including antipsychotics (eg, haloperidol, risperidone, thioridazine), should be approached with caution and should be initiated at the lower end of the dose range of the concomitant medication. If bupropion is added to the treatment regimen of a patient already receiving a drug metabolized by CYP2D6, the need to decrease the dose of the original medication should be considered, particularly for those concomitant medications with a narrow therapeutic index).
No products indexed under this heading.

Atenolol (Co-administration of bupropion with drugs that are metabolized by the CYP2D6 isoenzyme, including beta blockers (eg, metoprolol) should be approached with caution and should be initiated at the lower end of the dose range of the concomitant medication. If bupropion is added to the treatment regimen of a patient already receiving a drug metabolized by CYP2D6, the need to decrease the dose of the original medication should be considered, particularly for those concomitant medications with a narrow therapeutic index).
No products indexed under this heading.

Atomoxetine Hydrochloride (Co-administration of bupropion with drugs that are metabolized by the CYP2D6 isoenzyme should be approached with caution and should be initiated at the lower end of the dose range of the concomitant medication. If bupropion is added to the treatment regimen of a patient already receiving a drug metabolized by CYP2D6, the need to decrease the dose of the original medication should be considered, particularly for those concomitant medications with a narrow therapeutic index). Products include:
Strattera 1957

Azelastine Hydrochloride (*In vitro* studies indicate that bupropion is primarily metabolized to hydroxybupropion by the CYP2B6 isoenzyme. Therefore, the potential exists for a drug interaction between bupropion hydrochloride and drugs that are substrates or inhibitors of the CYP2B6 isoenzyme (eg, orphenadrine, thiotepa, cyclophosphamide)).
No products indexed under this heading.

Beclomethasone Dipropionate (Concurrent administration of bupropion and agents (eg, systemic steroids) that lower seizure threshold should be undertaken only with extreme caution). Products include:
Qvar 3398

Beclomethasone Dipropionate Monohydrate (Concurrent administration of bupropion and agents (eg, systemic steroids) that lower seizure threshold should be undertaken only with extreme caution). Products include:
Beconase AQ 1386

Benzphetamine Hydrochloride (Concomitant use of anorectics with bupropion is associated with an increased seizure risk).
No products indexed under this heading.

Betamethasone (Concurrent administration of bupropion and agents (eg, systemic steroids) that lower seizure threshold should be undertaken only with extreme caution).
No products indexed under this heading.

Betamethasone Acetate (Concurrent administration of bupropion and agents (eg, systemic steroids) that lower seizure threshold should be undertaken only with extreme caution).
No products indexed under this heading.

Betamethasone Benzoate (Concurrent administration of bupropion and agents (eg, systemic steroids) that lower seizure threshold should be undertaken only with extreme caution).
No products indexed under this heading.

Betamethasone Dipropionate (Concurrent administration of bupropion and agents (eg, systemic steroids) that lower seizure threshold should be undertaken only with extreme caution). Products include:
Diprolene Lotion 0.05% 3108
Diprolene Ointment 0.05% 3109
Diprolene AF Cream 0.05% 3107
Lotrisone 3163

Betamethasone Sodium Phosphate (Concurrent administration of bupropion and agents (eg, systemic steroids) that lower seizure threshold should be undertaken only with extreme caution).
No products indexed under this heading.

Betamethasone Valerate (Concurrent administration of bupropion and agents (eg, systemic steroids) that lower seizure threshold should be undertaken only with extreme caution). Products include:
Luxiq 3321

Betaxolol Hydrochloride (Co-administration of bupropion with drugs that are metabolized by the CYP2D6 isoenzyme, including beta blockers (eg, metoprolol) should be approached with caution and should be initiated at the lower end of the dose range of the concomitant medication. If bupropion is added to the treatment regimen of a patient already receiving a drug metabolized by CYP2D6, the need to decrease the dose of the original medication should be considered, particularly for those concomitant medications with a narrow therapeutic index).
No products indexed under this heading.

Bisoprolol Fumarate (Co-administration of bupropion with drugs that are metabolized by the CYP2D6 isoenzyme, including beta blockers (eg, metoprolol) should be approached with caution and should be initiated at the lower end of the dose range of the concomitant medication. If bupropion is added to the treatment regimen of a patient already receiving a drug metabolized by CYP2D6, the need to decrease the dose of the original medication should be considered, particularly for those concomitant medications with a narrow therapeutic index).
No products indexed under this heading.

Bretylium Tosylate (Co-administration of bupropion with drugs that are metabolized by the CYP2D6 isoenzyme, including antiarrhythmics, should be approached with caution and should be initiated at the lower end of the dose range of the concomitant medication. If bupropion is added to the treatment regimen of a patient already receiving a drug metabolized by CYP2D6, the need to decrease the dose of the original medication should be considered, particularly for those concomitant medications with a narrow therapeutic index).
No products indexed under this heading.

Budesonide (Concurrent administration of bupropion and agents (eg, systemic steroids) that lower seizure threshold should be undertaken only with extreme caution). Products include:
Pulmicort Flexhaler 714
Symbicort 80/4.5 720
Symbicort 160/4.5 720

Buprenorphine Hydrochloride (An addiction to opiates and concomitant use of opiates is associated with an increased seizure risk).
No products indexed under this heading.

Bupropion (Concomitant use with any other medication that contains bupropion is contraindicated because the incidence of seizure is dose dependent).
No products indexed under this heading.

Butabarbital (Bupropion is contraindicated in patients undergoing abrupt discontinuation of sedatives (including benzodiazepines). Excessive use of sedatives (including benzodiazepines) is associated with an increased seizure risk).
No products indexed under this heading.

Butabarbital Sodium (Bupropion is contraindicated in patients undergoing abrupt discontinuation of sedatives (including benzodiazepines). Excessive use of sedatives (including benzodiazepines) is associated with an increased seizure risk).
No products indexed under this heading.

Butalbital (Bupropion is contraindicated in patients undergoing abrupt discontinuation of sedatives (including benzodiazepines). Excessive use of sedatives (including benzodiazepines) is associated with an increased seizure risk).
No products indexed under this heading.

Captopril (Co-administration of bupropion with drugs that are metabolized by the CYP2D6 isoenzyme should be approached with caution and should be initiated at the lower end of the dose range of the concomitant medication. If bupropion is added to the treatment regimen of a patient already receiving a drug metabolized by CYP2D6, the need to decrease the dose of the original medication should be considered, particularly for those concomitant medications with a narrow therapeutic index). Products include:
Captopril 2341

Carbamazepine (Because bupropion is extensively metabolized, the co-administration of other drugs may affect its clinical activity. In particular,

Zyban Interactions Index 2192

certain drugs may induce the metabolism of bupropion including carbamazepine). Products include:
Carbatrol 3280
Equetro 3477

Carteolol Hydrochloride (Co-administration of bupropion with drugs that are metabolized by the CYP2D6 isoenzyme, including beta blockers (eg, metoprolol) should be approached with caution and should be initiated at the lower end of the dose range of the concomitant medication. If bupropion is added to the treatment regimen of a patient already receiving a drug metabolized by CYP2D6, the need to decrease the dose of the original medication should be considered, particularly for those concomitant medications with a narrow therapeutic index).
No products indexed under this heading.

Carvedilol (Co-administration of bupropion with drugs that are metabolized by the CYP2D6 isoenzyme, including beta blockers (eg, metoprolol) should be approached with caution and should be initiated at the lower end of the dose range of the concomitant medication. If bupropion is added to the treatment regimen of a patient already receiving a drug metabolized by CYP2D6, the need to decrease the dose of the original medication should be considered, particularly for those concomitant medications with a narrow therapeutic index). Products include:
Coreg 1409

Carvedilol Phosphate (Co-administration of bupropion with drugs that are metabolized by the CYP2D6 isoenzyme, including beta blockers (eg, metoprolol) should be approached with caution and should be initiated at the lower end of the dose range of the concomitant medication. If bupropion is added to the treatment regimen of a patient already receiving a drug metabolized by CYP2D6, the need to decrease the dose of the original medication should be considered, particularly for those concomitant medications with a narrow therapeutic index). Products include:
Coreg CR 1416

Cevimeline Hydrochloride (Co-administration of bupropion with drugs that are metabolized by the CYP2D6 isoenzyme should be approached with caution and should be initiated at the lower end of the dose range of the concomitant medication. If bupropion is added to the treatment regimen of a patient already receiving a drug metabolized by CYP2D6, the need to decrease the dose of the original medication should be considered, particularly for those concomitant medications with a narrow therapeutic index). Products include:
Evoxac 1027

Chloral Hydrate (Bupropion is contraindicated in patients undergoing abrupt discontinuation of sedatives (including benzodiazepines). Excessive use of sedatives (including benzodiazepines) is associated with an increased seizure risk).
No products indexed under this heading.

Chlordiazepoxide (Bupropion is contraindicated in patients undergoing abrupt discontinuation of sedatives (including benzodiazepines). Excessive use of sedatives (including benzodiazepines) is associated with an increased seizure risk).
No products indexed under this heading.

Chlordiazepoxide Hydrochloride (Bupropion is contraindicated in patients undergoing abrupt discontinuation of sedatives (including benzodiazepines). Excessive use of sedatives (including benzodiazepines) is associated with an increased seizure risk).
No products indexed under this heading.

Chlorpromazine (Concurrent administration of bupropion and agents such as antipsychotics that lower seizure threshold should be undertaken with extreme caution. Co-administration of bupropion with drugs that are metabolized by CYP2D6 isoenzyme, including antipsychotics (eg, haloperidol, risperidone, thioridazine), should be approached with caution and should be initiated at the lower end of the dose range of the concomitant medication. If bupropion is added to the treatment regimen of a patient already receiving a drug metabolized by CYP2D6, the need to decrease the dose of the original medication should be considered, particularly for those concomitant medications with a narrow therapeutic index).
No products indexed under this heading.

Chlorpromazine Hydrochloride (Concurrent administration of bupropion and agents such as antipsychotics that lower seizure threshold should be undertaken with extreme caution. Co-administration of bupropion with drugs that are metabolized by CYP2D6 isoenzyme, including antipsychotics (eg, haloperidol, risperidone, thioridazine), should be approached with caution and should be initiated at the lower end of the dose range of the concomitant medication. If bupropion is added to the treatment regimen of a patient already receiving a drug metabolized by CYP2D6, the need to decrease the dose of the original medication should be considered, particularly for those concomitant medications with a narrow therapeutic index).
No products indexed under this heading.

Chlorpropamide (Concomitant use of oral hypoglycemics with bupropion is associated with an increased seizure risk).
No products indexed under this heading.

Chlorprothixene (Concurrent administration of bupropion and agents such as antipsychotics that lower seizure threshold should be undertaken with extreme caution. Co-administration of bupropion with drugs that are metabolized by CYP2D6 isoenzyme, including antipsychotics (eg, haloperidol, risperidone, thioridazine), should be approached with caution and should be initiated at the lower end of the dose range of the concomitant medication. If bupropion is added to the treatment regimen of a patient already receiving a drug metabolized by CYP2D6, the need to decrease the dose of the original medication should be considered, particularly for those concomitant medications with a narrow therapeutic index).
No products indexed under this heading.

Chlorprothixene Hydrochloride (Concurrent administration of bupropion and agents such as antipsychotics that lower seizure threshold should be undertaken with extreme caution. Co-administration of bupropion with drugs that are metabolized by CYP2D6 isoenzyme, including antipsychotics (eg, haloperidol, risperidone, thioridazine), should be approached with caution and should be initiated at the lower end of the dose range of the concomitant medication. If bupropion is added to the treatment regimen of a patient already receiving a drug metabolized by CYP2D6, the need to decrease the dose of the original medication should be considered, particularly for those concomitant medications with a narrow therapeutic index).
No products indexed under this heading.

Chlorprothixene Lactate (Concurrent administration of bupropion and agents such as antipsychotics that lower seizure threshold should be undertaken with extreme caution. Co-administration of bupropion with drugs that are metabolized by CYP2D6 isoenzyme, including antipsychotics (eg, haloperidol, risperidone, thioridazine), should be approached with caution and should be initiated at the lower end of the dose range of the concomitant medication. If bupropion is added to the treatment regimen of a patient already receiving a drug metabolized by CYP2D6, the need to decrease the dose of the original medication should be considered, particularly for those concomitant medications with a narrow therapeutic index).
No products indexed under this heading.

Ciclesonide (Concurrent administration of bupropion and agents (eg, systemic steroids) that lower seizure threshold should be undertaken only with extreme caution).
No products indexed under this heading.

Cimetidine (Cimetidine may inhibit the metabolism of bupropion. The effects of concomitant administration of cimetidine on the pharmacokinetics of bupropion and its active metabolites were studied in 24 healthy young male volunteers. Following oral administration of two 150 mg bupropion tablets with and without 800 mg of cimetidine, the pharmacokinetics of bupropion and its hydroxy metabolite were unaffected. However, there were 16% and 32% increases, respectively, in the AUC and C_{max} of the combined moieties of threohydro- and erythrohydrobupropion).
No products indexed under this heading.

Cimetidine Hydrochloride (Cimetidine may inhibit the metabolism of bupropion. The effects of concomitant administration of cimetidine on the pharmacokinetics of bupropion and its active metabolites were studied in 24 healthy young male volunteers. Following oral administration of two 150 mg bupropion tablets with and without 800 mg of cimetidine, the pharmacokinetics of bupropion and its hydroxy metabolite were unaffected. However, there were 16% and 32% increases, respectively, in the AUC and C_{max} of the combined moieties of threohydro- and erythrohydrobupropion).
No products indexed under this heading.

Cisapride (*In vitro* studies indicate that bupropion is primarily metabolized to hydroxybupropion by the CYP2B6 isoenzyme. Therefore, the potential exists for a drug interaction between bupropion hydrochloride and drugs that are substrates or inhibitors of the CYP2B6 isoenzyme (eg, orphenadrine, thiotepa, cyclophosphamide)).
No products indexed under this heading.

Citalopram Hydrobromide (Concurrent administration of bupropion and agents (eg, antidepressants) that lower seizure threshold should be undertaken only with caution. Many drugs, including most antidepressants (eg, SSRIs), are metabolized by the CYP2D6 isoenzyme. Co-administration of bupropion with drugs that are metabolized by CYP2D6 isoenzyme should be approached with caution and should be initiated at the lower end of the dose range of the concomitant medication. If bupropion is added to the treatment regimen of a patient already receiving a drug metabolized by CYP2D6, the need to decrease the dose of the original medication should be considered, particularly for those concomitant medications with a narrow therapeutic index). Products include:
Celexa 1153

Clomipramine Hydrochloride (Concurrent administration of bupropion and agents (eg, antidepressants) that lower seizure threshold should be undertaken only with extreme caution. Many drugs, including certain antidepressants (many tricyclics), are metabolized by the CYP2D6 isoenzyme. Co-administration of bupropion with drugs that are metabolized by CYP2D6 isoenzyme should be approached with caution and should be initiated at the lower end of the dose range of the concomitant medication. If bupropion is added to the treatment regimen of a patient already receiving a drug metabolized by CYP2D6, the need to decrease the dose of the original medication should be considered, particularly for those concomitant medications with a narrow therapeutic index).
No products indexed under this heading.

Clorazepate Dipotassium (Bupropion is contraindicated in patients undergoing abrupt discontinuation of sedatives (including benzodiazepines). Excessive use of sedatives (including benzodiazepines) is associated with an increased seizure risk).
No products indexed under this heading.

Clotrimazole (*In vitro* studies indicate that bupropion is primarily metabolized to hydroxybupropion by the CYP2B6 isoenzyme. Therefore, the potential exists for a drug interaction between bupropion hydrochloride and drugs that are substrates or inhibitors of the CYP2B6 isoenzyme (eg, orphenadrine, thiotepa, cyclophosphamide)). Products include:
Lotrisone 3163

Clotrimazole, Topical (*In vitro* studies indicate that bupropion is primarily metabolized to hydroxybupropion by the CYP2B6 isoenzyme. Therefore, the potential exists for a drug interaction between bupropion hydrochloride and drugs that are substrates or inhibitors of the CYP2B6 isoenzyme (eg, orphenadrine, thiotepa, cyclophosphamide)).
No products indexed under this heading.

Clozapine (Concurrent administration of bupropion and agents such as antipsychotics that lower seizure threshold should be undertaken with extreme caution. Co-administration of bupropion with drugs that are metabolized by CYP2D6 isoenzyme, including antipsychotics (eg, haloperidol, risperidone, thioridazine), should be approached with caution and should be initiated at the lower end of the dose range of the concomitant medication. If bupropion is added to the treatment regimen of a patient already receiving a drug metabolized by CYP2D6, the need to decrease the dose of the original medication should be considered, particularly for those concomitant medications with a narrow therapeutic index).
No products indexed under this heading.

Cocaine Hydrochloride (Concomitant use of cocaine and bupropion has been associated with an increased seizure risk).
No products indexed under this heading.

Codeine Phosphate (An addiction to opiates and concomitant use of opiates is associated with an increased seizure risk). Products include:
Tylenol with Codeine 2691

Codeine Sulfate (An addiction to opiates and concomitant use of opiates is associated with an increased seizure risk).
No products indexed under this heading.

2193 Interactions Index Zyban

Cortisone Acetate (Concurrent administration of bupropion and agents (eg, systemic steroids) that lower seizure threshold should be undertaken only with extreme caution).
No products indexed under this heading.

Cyclobenzaprine Hydrochloride (Co-administration of bupropion with drugs that are metabolized by the CYP2D6 isoenzyme should be approached with caution and should be initiated at the lower end of the dose range of the concomitant medication. If bupropion is added to the treatment regimen of a patient already receiving a drug metabolized by CYP2D6, the need to decrease the dose of the original medication should be considered, particularly for those concomitant medications with a narrow therapeutic index). Products include:
Amrix ... 964

Cyclophosphamide (*In vitro* studies indicate that bupropion is primarily metabolized to hydroxybupropion by the CYP2B6 isoenzyme. Therefore, the potential exists for a drug interaction between bupropion and drugs that are substrates or inhibitors of the CYP2B6 isoenzyme (eg, orphenadrine, thiotepa, cyclophosphamide)).
No products indexed under this heading.

Debrisoquine (Co-administration of bupropion with drugs that are metabolized by the CYP2D6 isoenzyme should be approached with caution and should be initiated at the lower end of the dose range of the concomitant medication. If bupropion is added to the treatment regimen of a patient already receiving a drug metabolized by CYP2D6, the need to decrease the dose of the original medication should be considered, particularly for those concomitant medications with a narrow therapeutic index).
No products indexed under this heading.

Desipramine Hydrochloride (Concurrent administration of bupropion and agents that lower seizure threshold, such as antidepressants, should be undertaken with extreme caution. In a study of 15 males who were extensive metabolizers of the CYP2D6 isoenzyme, daily doses of bupropion given as 150 mg twice daily followed by a single dose of 50 mg desipramine increased the C_{max}, AUC, and $t_{1/2}$ of desipramine by an average of approximately 2-, 5- and 2-fold, respectively. Co-administration of bupropion with drugs that are metabolized by the CYP2D6 isoenzyme, including antidepressants (eg, desipramine), should be approached with caution and should be initiated at the lower end of the dose range of the concomitant medication. If bupropion is added to the treatment regimen of a patient already receiving a drug metabolized by CYP2D6, the need to decrease the dose of the original medication should be considered, particularly for those concomitant medications with a narrow therapeutic index).
No products indexed under this heading.

Desoximetasone (Concurrent administration of bupropion and agents (eg, systemic steroids) that lower seizure threshold should be undertaken only with extreme caution).
No products indexed under this heading.

Desvenlafaxine (*In vitro* studies indicate that bupropion is primarily metabolized to hydroxybupropion by the CYP2B6 isoenzyme. Therefore, the potential exists for a drug interaction between bupropion hydrochloride and drugs that are substrates or inhibitors of the CYP2B6 isoenzyme (eg, orphenadrine, thiotepa, cyclophosphamide)).
No products indexed under this heading.

Desvenlafaxine Succinate (*In vitro* studies indicate that bupropion is primarily metabolized to hydroxybupropion by the CYP2B6 isoenzyme. Therefore, the potential exists for a drug interaction between bupropion hydrochloride and drugs that are substrates or inhibitors of the CYP2B6 isoenzyme (eg, orphenadrine, thiotepa, cyclophosphamide)). Products include:
Pristiq ... 3564

Dexamethasone (Concurrent administration of bupropion and agents (eg, systemic steroids) that lower seizure threshold should be undertaken only with extreme caution). Products include:
Ciprodex ... 583
Ozurdex ... ⊙223
Tobramycin and Dexamethasone Ophthalmic Suspension ... ⊙251

Dexamethasone Acetate (Concurrent administration of bupropion and agents (eg, systemic steroids) that lower seizure threshold should be undertaken only with extreme caution).
No products indexed under this heading.

Dexamethasone Phosphate (Concurrent administration of bupropion and agents (eg, systemic steroids) that lower seizure threshold should be undertaken only with extreme caution).
No products indexed under this heading.

Dexamethasone Sodium (Concurrent administration of bupropion and agents (eg, systemic steroids) that lower seizure threshold should be undertaken only with extreme caution).
No products indexed under this heading.

Dexamethasone Sodium Phosphate (Concurrent administration of bupropion and agents (eg, systemic steroids) that lower seizure threshold should be undertaken only with extreme caution).
No products indexed under this heading.

Dexamethasone Sodium Phosphate Injection (Concurrent administration of bupropion and agents (eg, systemic steroids) that lower seizure threshold should be undertaken only with extreme caution).
No products indexed under this heading.

Dexfenfluramine Hydrochloride (Concomitant use of anorectics with bupropion is associated with an increased seizure risk).
No products indexed under this heading.

Dexmethylphenidate Hydrochloride (An addiction to stimulants or use of over-the-counter stimulants with bupropion is associated with an increased seizure risk). Products include:
Focalin XR ... 2472

Dextroamphetamine (Concomitant use of anorectics with bupropion is associated with an increased seizure risk).
No products indexed under this heading.

Dextroamphetamine Saccharate (Concomitant use of anorectics with bupropion is associated with an increased seizure risk).
No products indexed under this heading.

Dextroamphetamine Sulfate (Concomitant use of anorectics with bupropion is associated with an increased seizure risk). Products include:
Dexedrine ... 1425

Dextromethorphan Hydrobromide (Co-administration of bupropion with drugs that are metabolized by the CYP2D6 isoenzyme should be approached with caution and should be initiated at the lower end of the dose range of the concomitant medication. If bupropion is added to the treatment regimen of a patient already receiving a drug metabolized by CYP2D6, the need to decrease the dose of the original medication should be considered, particularly for those concomitant medications with a narrow therapeutic index).
No products indexed under this heading.

Dextromethorphan Polistirex (Co-administration of bupropion with drugs that are metabolized by the CYP2D6 isoenzyme should be approached with caution and should be initiated at the lower end of the dose range of the concomitant medication. If bupropion is added to the treatment regimen of a patient already receiving a drug metabolized by CYP2D6, the need to decrease the dose of the original medication should be considered, particularly for those concomitant medications with a narrow therapeutic index).
No products indexed under this heading.

Dezocine (An addiction to opiates and concomitant use of opiates is associated with an increased seizure risk).
No products indexed under this heading.

Diazepam (Bupropion is contraindicated in patients undergoing abrupt discontinuation of sedatives (including benzodiazepines). Excessive use of sedatives (including benzodiazepines) is associated with an increased seizure risk). Products include:
Valium Tablets ... 2880

Diclofenac Epolamine (*In vitro* studies indicate that bupropion is primarily metabolized to hydroxybupropion by the CYP2B6 isoenzyme. Therefore, the potential exists for a drug interaction between bupropion hydrochloride and drugs that are substrates or inhibitors of the CYP2B6 isoenzyme (eg, orphenadrine, thiotepa, cyclophosphamide)). Products include:
Flector ... 1839

Diclofenac Potassium (*In vitro* studies indicate that bupropion is primarily metabolized to hydroxybupropion by the CYP2B6 isoenzyme. Therefore, the potential exists for a drug interaction between bupropion hydrochloride and drugs that are substrates or inhibitors of the CYP2B6 isoenzyme (eg, orphenadrine, thiotepa, cyclophosphamide)).
No products indexed under this heading.

Diclofenac Sodium (*In vitro* studies indicate that bupropion is primarily metabolized to hydroxybupropion by the CYP2B6 isoenzyme. Therefore, the potential exists for a drug interaction between bupropion hydrochloride and drugs that are substrates or inhibitors of the CYP2B6 isoenzyme (eg, orphenadrine, thiotepa, cyclophosphamide)).
No products indexed under this heading.

Diethylpropion Hydrochloride (Concomitant use of anorectics with bupropion is associated with an increased seizure risk).
No products indexed under this heading.

Diflorasone Diacetate (Concurrent administration of bupropion and agents (eg, systemic steroids) that lower seizure threshold should be undertaken only with extreme caution).
No products indexed under this heading.

Dihydrocodeine Bitartrate (An addiction to opiates and concomitant use of opiates is associated with an increased seizure risk).
No products indexed under this heading.

Dihydrocodeinone Bitartrate (An addiction to opiates and concomitant use of opiates is associated with an increased seizure risk).
No products indexed under this heading.

Disopyramide Phosphate (Co-administration of bupropion with drugs that are metabolized by the CYP2D6 isoenzyme, including antiarrhythmics, should be approached with caution and should be initiated at the lower end of the dose range of the concomitant medication. If bupropion is added to the treatment regimen of a patient already receiving a drug metabolized by CYP2D6, the need to decrease the dose of the original medication should be considered, particularly for those concomitant medications with a narrow therapeutic index).
No products indexed under this heading.

Disulfiram (*In vitro* studies indicate that bupropion is primarily metabolized to hydroxybupropion by the CYP2B6 isoenzyme. Therefore, the potential exists for a drug interaction between bupropion hydrochloride and drugs that are substrates or inhibitors of the CYP2B6 isoenzyme (eg, orphenadrine, thiotepa, cyclophosphamide)).
No products indexed under this heading.

Divalproex Sodium (*In vitro* studies indicate that bupropion is primarily metabolized to hydroxybupropion by the CYP2B6 isoenzyme. Therefore, the potential exists for a drug interaction between bupropion hydrochloride and drugs that are substrates or inhibitors of the CYP2B6 isoenzyme (eg, orphenadrine, thiotepa, cyclophosphamide)). Products include:
Depakote ER ... 426

Dofetilide (Co-administration of bupropion with drugs that are metabolized by the CYP2D6 isoenzyme, including antiarrhythmics, should be approached with caution and should be initiated at the lower end of the dose range of the concomitant medication. If bupropion is added to the treatment regimen of a patient already receiving a drug metabolized by CYP2D6, the need to decrease the dose of the original medication should be considered, particularly for those concomitant medications with a narrow therapeutic index).
No products indexed under this heading.

Dolasetron Mesylate (Co-administration of bupropion with drugs that are metabolized by the CYP2D6 isoenzyme should be approached with caution and should be initiated at the lower end of the dose range of the concomitant medication. If bupropion is added to the treatment regimen of a patient already receiving a drug metabolized by CYP2D6, the need to decrease the dose of the original medication should be considered, particularly for those concomitant medications with a narrow therapeutic index). Products include:
Anzemet Injection ... 2931
Anzemet Tablets ... 2934

Donepezil Hydrochloride (Co-administration of bupropion with drugs that are metabolized by the CYP2D6 isoenzyme should be approached with caution and should be initiated at the lower end of the dose range of the concomitant medication. If bupropion is added to the treatment regimen of a patient already receiving a drug metabolized by CYP2D6, the need to decrease the dose of the original medication should be considered, particularly for those concomitant medications with a narrow therapeutic index). Products include:
Aricept ... 1045
Aricept ODT ... 1045

Doxepin Hydrochloride (Concurrent administration of bupropion and agents (eg, antidepressants) that lower seizure threshold should be undertaken only with extreme caution. Many drugs, including certain antidepressants (many tricyclics), are metabolized by the CYP2D6 isoenzyme. Co-administration of bupropion with drugs that are metabolized by CYP2D6 isoenzyme should be approached with caution and should be initiated at the lower end of the dose range of the concomitant medication. If bupropion is added to the treatment regimen of a patient already receiving a

IMPORTANT NOTE: Always consult each drug listing in the patient's regimen for possible interactions.

Zyban Interactions Index 2194

drug metabolized by CYP2D6, the need to decrease the dose of the original medication should be considered, particularly for those concomitant medications with a narrow therapeutic index).
No products indexed under this heading.

Doxorubicin Hydrochloride (*In vitro* studies indicate that bupropion is primarily metabolized to hydroxybupropion by the CYP2B6 isoenzyme. Therefore, the potential exists for a drug interaction between bupropion hydrochloride and drugs that are substrates or inhibitors of the CYP2B6 isoenzyme (eg, orphenadrine, thiotepa, cyclophosphamide)).
No products indexed under this heading.

Doxorubicin Hydrochloride Liposome (*In vitro* studies indicate that bupropion is primarily metabolized to hydroxybupropion by the CYP2B6 isoenzyme. Therefore, the potential exists for a drug interaction between bupropion hydrochloride and drugs that are substrates or inhibitors of the CYP2B6 isoenzyme (eg, orphenadrine, thiotepa, cyclophosphamide)). Products include:
Doxil 939

Efavirenz (*In vitro* studies suggest that efavirenz inhibits the hydroxylation of bupropion). Products include:
Atripla 906

Encainide Hydrochloride (Co-administration of bupropion with drugs that are metabolized by the CYP2D6 isoenzyme, including Type 1C antiarrhythmics (eg, propafenone and flecainide), should be approached with caution and should be initiated at the lower end of the dose range of the concomitant medication. If bupropion is added to the treatment regimen of a patient already receiving a drug metabolized by CYP2D6, the need to decrease the dose of the original medication should be considered, particularly for those concomitant medications with a narrow therapeutic index).
No products indexed under this heading.

Erythromycin (*In vitro* studies indicate that bupropion is primarily metabolized to hydroxybupropion by the CYP2B6 isoenzyme. Therefore, the potential exists for a drug interaction between bupropion hydrochloride and drugs that are substrates or inhibitors of the CYP2B6 isoenzyme (eg, orphenadrine, thiotepa, cyclophosphamide)).
No products indexed under this heading.

Erythromycin, Topical (*In vitro* studies indicate that bupropion is primarily metabolized to hydroxybupropion by the CYP2B6 isoenzyme. Therefore, the potential exists for a drug interaction between bupropion hydrochloride and drugs that are substrates or inhibitors of the CYP2B6 isoenzyme (eg, orphenadrine, thiotepa, cyclophosphamide)).
No products indexed under this heading.

Erythromycin Estolate (*In vitro* studies indicate that bupropion is primarily metabolized to hydroxybupropion by the CYP2B6 isoenzyme. Therefore, the potential exists for a drug interaction between bupropion hydrochloride and drugs that are substrates or inhibitors of the CYP2B6 isoenzyme (eg, orphenadrine, thiotepa, cyclophosphamide)).
No products indexed under this heading.

Erythromycin Ethylsuccinate (*In vitro* studies indicate that bupropion is primarily metabolized to hydroxybupropion by the CYP2B6 isoenzyme. Therefore, the potential exists for a drug interaction between bupropion hydrochloride and drugs that are substrates or inhibitors of the CYP2B6 isoenzyme (eg, orphenadrine, thiotepa, cyclophosphamide)). Products include:
E.E.S. 437
EryPed 435

Erythromycin Gluceptate (*In vitro* studies indicate that bupropion is primarily metabolized to hydroxybupropion by the CYP2B6 isoenzyme. Therefore, the potential exists for a drug interaction between bupropion hydrochloride and drugs that are substrates or inhibitors of the CYP2B6 isoenzyme (eg, orphenadrine, thiotepa, cyclophosphamide)).
No products indexed under this heading.

Erythromycin Lactobionate (*In vitro* studies indicate that bupropion is primarily metabolized to hydroxybupropion by the CYP2B6 isoenzyme. Therefore, the potential exists for a drug interaction between bupropion hydrochloride and drugs that are substrates or inhibitors of the CYP2B6 isoenzyme (eg, orphenadrine, thiotepa, cyclophosphamide)).
No products indexed under this heading.

Erythromycin Stearate (*In vitro* studies indicate that bupropion is primarily metabolized to hydroxybupropion by the CYP2B6 isoenzyme. Therefore, the potential exists for a drug interaction between bupropion hydrochloride and drugs that are substrates or inhibitors of the CYP2B6 isoenzyme (eg, orphenadrine, thiotepa, cyclophosphamide)).
No products indexed under this heading.

Escitalopram Oxalate (Concurrent administration of bupropion and agents (eg, antidepressants) that lower seizure threshold should be undertaken only with caution. Many drugs, including most antidepressants (eg, SSRIs), are metabolized by the CYP2D6 isoenzyme. Co-administration of bupropion with drugs that are metabolized by CYP2D6 isoenzyme should be approached with caution and should be initiated at the lower end of the dose range of the concomitant medication. If bupropion is added to the treatment regimen of a patient already receiving a drug metabolized by CYP2D6, the need to decrease the dose of the original medication should be considered, particularly for those concomitant medications with a narrow therapeutic index). Products include:
Lexapro Oral Suspension 1160
Lexapro Tablets 1160

Esmolol Hydrochloride (Co-administration of bupropion with drugs that are metabolized by the CYP2D6 isoenzyme, including beta blockers (eg, metoprolol) should be approached with caution and should be initiated at the lower end of the dose range of the concomitant medication. If bupropion is added to the treatment regimen of a patient already receiving a drug metabolized by CYP2D6, the need to decrease the dose of the original medication should be considered, particularly for those concomitant medications with a narrow therapeutic index).
No products indexed under this heading.

Estazolam (Bupropion is contraindicated in patients undergoing abrupt discontinuation of sedatives (including benzodiazepines). Excessive use of sedatives (including benzodiazepines) is associated with an increased seizure risk).
No products indexed under this heading.

Estradiol (*In vitro* studies indicate that bupropion is primarily metabolized to hydroxybupropion by the CYP2B6 isoenzyme. Therefore, the potential exists for a drug interaction between bupropion hydrochloride and drugs that are substrates or inhibitors of the CYP2B6 isoenzyme (eg, orphenadrine, thiotepa, cyclophosphamide)). Products include:
Activella 2561
Angeliq 831
Climara 841
Climara Pro 847
Divigel 3467
Estrasorb 1777
Vagifem 2589

Estradiol Acetate (*In vitro* studies indicate that bupropion is primarily metabolized to hydroxybupropion by the CYP2B6 isoenzyme. Therefore, the potential exists for a drug interaction between bupropion hydrochloride and drugs that are substrates or inhibitors of the CYP2B6 isoenzyme (eg, orphenadrine, thiotepa, cyclophosphamide)).
No products indexed under this heading.

Estradiol Benzoate (*In vitro* studies indicate that bupropion is primarily metabolized to hydroxybupropion by the CYP2B6 isoenzyme. Therefore, the potential exists for a drug interaction between bupropion hydrochloride and drugs that are substrates or inhibitors of the CYP2B6 isoenzyme (eg, orphenadrine, thiotepa, cyclophosphamide)).
No products indexed under this heading.

Estradiol Cypionate (*In vitro* studies indicate that bupropion is primarily metabolized to hydroxybupropion by the CYP2B6 isoenzyme. Therefore, the potential exists for a drug interaction between bupropion hydrochloride and drugs that are substrates or inhibitors of the CYP2B6 isoenzyme (eg, orphenadrine, thiotepa, cyclophosphamide)).
No products indexed under this heading.

Estradiol Valerate (*In vitro* studies indicate that bupropion is primarily metabolized to hydroxybupropion by the CYP2B6 isoenzyme. Therefore, the potential exists for a drug interaction between bupropion hydrochloride and drugs that are substrates or inhibitors of the CYP2B6 isoenzyme (eg, orphenadrine, thiotepa, cyclophosphamide)).
No products indexed under this heading.

Estrogen (*In vitro* studies indicate that bupropion is primarily metabolized to hydroxybupropion by the CYP2B6 isoenzyme. Therefore, the potential exists for a drug interaction between bupropion hydrochloride and drugs that are substrates or inhibitors of the CYP2B6 isoenzyme (eg, orphenadrine, thiotepa, cyclophosphamide)).
No products indexed under this heading.

Estrogens, Conjugated (*In vitro* studies indicate that bupropion is primarily metabolized to hydroxybupropion by the CYP2B6 isoenzyme. Therefore, the potential exists for a drug interaction between bupropion hydrochloride and drugs that are substrates or inhibitors of the CYP2B6 isoenzyme (eg, orphenadrine, thiotepa, cyclophosphamide)). Products include:
Premarin Intravenous 3528
Premarin Tablets 3533
Premarin Vaginal Cream 3540
Premphase 3549
Prempro 3549

Estrogens, Conjugated, Synthetic A (*In vitro* studies indicate that bupropion is primarily metabolized to hydroxybupropion by the CYP2B6 isoenzyme. Therefore, the potential exists for a drug interaction between bupropion hydrochloride and drugs that are substrates or inhibitors of the CYP2B6 isoenzyme (eg, orphenadrine, thiotepa, cyclophosphamide)).
No products indexed under this heading.

Estrogens, Conjugated, Synthetic B (*In vitro* studies indicate that bupropion is primarily metabolized to hydroxybupropion by the CYP2B6 isoenzyme. Therefore, the potential exists for a drug interaction between bupropion hydrochloride and drugs that are substrates or inhibitors of the CYP2B6 isoenzyme (eg, orphenadrine, thiotepa, cyclophosphamide)). Products include:
Enjuvia 3401

Estrogens, Esterified (*In vitro* studies indicate that bupropion is primarily metabolized to hydroxybupropion by the CYP2B6 isoenzyme. Therefore, the potential exists for a drug interaction between bupropion hydrochloride and drugs that are substrates or inhibitors of the CYP2B6 isoenzyme (eg, orphenadrine, thiotepa, cyclophosphamide)).
No products indexed under this heading.

Estrone (*In vitro* studies indicate that bupropion is primarily metabolized to hydroxybupropion by the CYP2B6 isoenzyme. Therefore, the potential exists for a drug interaction between bupropion hydrochloride and drugs that are substrates or inhibitors of the CYP2B6 isoenzyme (eg, orphenadrine, thiotepa, cyclophosphamide)).
No products indexed under this heading.

Estropipate (*In vitro* studies indicate that bupropion is primarily metabolized to hydroxybupropion by the CYP2B6 isoenzyme. Therefore, the potential exists for a drug interaction between bupropion hydrochloride and drugs that are substrates or inhibitors of the CYP2B6 isoenzyme (eg, orphenadrine, thiotepa, cyclophosphamide)).
No products indexed under this heading.

Ethanol (Bupropion is contraindicated in patients undergoing abrupt discontinuation of alcohol. In post-marketing experience, there have been rare reports of adverse neuropsychiatric events or reduced alcohol tolerance in patients who were drinking alcohol during treatment with bupropion. The consumption of alcohol during treatment with bupropion should be minimized or avoided).
No products indexed under this heading.

Ethchlorvynol (Bupropion is contraindicated in patients undergoing abrupt discontinuation of sedatives (including benzodiazepines). Excessive use of sedatives (including benzodiazepines) is associated with an increased seizure risk).
No products indexed under this heading.

Ethinamate (Bupropion is contraindicated in patients undergoing abrupt discontinuation of sedatives (including benzodiazepines). Excessive use of sedatives (including benzodiazepines) is associated with an increased seizure risk).
No products indexed under this heading.

Ethinyl Estradiol (*In vitro* studies indicate that bupropion is primarily metabolized to hydroxybupropion by the CYP2B6 isoenzyme. Therefore, the potential exists for a drug interaction between bupropion hydrochloride and drugs that are substrates or inhibitors of the CYP2B6 isoenzyme (eg, orphenadrine, thiotepa, cyclophosphamide)).
Products include:
LoSeasonique 3407
Lybrel 3514
NuvaRing 3181
Ortho Evra 2648
Ortho-Cyclen/Ortho Tri-Cyclen 2663
Ortho Tri-Cyclen Lo Tablets 2673
Seasonique 3418
Yaz 864

Ethyl Alcohol (Bupropion is contraindicated in patients undergoing abrupt discontinuation of alcohol. In post-marketing experience, there have been rare reports of adverse neuropsychiatric events or reduced alcohol tolerance in patients who were drinking alcohol during treatment with bupropion. The consumption of alcohol during treatment with bupropion should be minimized or avoided).
No products indexed under this heading.

2195 Interactions Index Zyban

Fenfluramine Hydrochloride (Concomitant use of anorectics with bupropion is associated with an increased seizure risk).
No products indexed under this heading.

Fentanyl (An addiction to opiates and concomitant use of opiates is associated with an increased seizure risk).
Products include:
Duragesic 2604
Fentanyl Transdermal System 2346
Onsolis 2054

Fentanyl Citrate (An addiction to opiates and concomitant use of opiates is associated with an increased seizure risk). Products include:
Fentora 966

Flecainide Acetate (Co-administration of bupropion with drugs that are metabolized by the CYP2D6 isoenzyme including Type 1C antiarrhythmics (eg, flecainide) should be approached with caution and should be initiated at the lower end of the dose range of the concomitant medication. If bupropion is added to the treatment regimen of a patient already receiving a drug metabolized by CYP2D6, the need to decrease the dose of the original medication should be considered, particularly for those concomitant medications with a narrow therapeutic index).
No products indexed under this heading.

Fludrocortisone Acetate (Concurrent administration of bupropion and agents (eg, systemic steroids) that lower seizure threshold should be undertaken only with extreme caution).
No products indexed under this heading.

Flumethasone Pivalate (Concurrent administration of bupropion and agents (eg, systemic steroids) that lower seizure threshold should be undertaken only with extreme caution).
No products indexed under this heading.

Flunisolide Hemihydrate (Concurrent administration of bupropion and agents (eg, systemic steroids) that lower seizure threshold should be undertaken only with extreme caution).
No products indexed under this heading.

Fluoxetine (Concurrent administration of bupropion and agents that lower seizure threshold (eg, antidepressants) should be approached with caution. Co-administration of bupropion with drugs that are metabolized by CYP2D6 isoenzyme including certain antidepressants (eg, fluoxetine) should be approached with caution and should be initiated at the lower end of the dose range of the concomitant medication. If bupropion is added to the treatment regimen of a patient already receiving a drug metabolized by CYP2D6, the need to decrease the dose of the original medication should be considered, particularly for those concomitant medications with a narrow therapeutic index).
No products indexed under this heading.

Fluoxetine Hydrochloride (Concurrent administration of bupropion and agents that lower seizure threshold (eg, antidepressants) should be approached with caution. Co-administration of bupropion with drugs that are metabolized by CYP2D6 isoenzyme including certain antidepressants (eg, fluoxetine) should be approached with caution and should be initiated at the lower end of the dose range of the concomitant medication. If bupropion is added to the treatment regimen of a patient already receiving a drug metabolized by CYP2D6, the need to decrease the dose of the original medication should be considered, particularly for those concomitant medications with a narrow therapeutic index).
Products include:
Prozac Weekly 1941
Prozac Pulvules 1941
Symbyax 1965

Fluphenazine Decanoate (Concurrent administration of bupropion and agents such as antipsychotics that lower seizure threshold should be undertaken with extreme caution. Co-administration of bupropion with drugs that are metabolized by CYP2D6 isoenzyme, including antipsychotics (eg, haloperidol, risperidone, thioridazine), should be approached with caution and should be initiated at the lower end of the dose range of the concomitant medication. If bupropion is added to the treatment regimen of a patient already receiving a drug metabolized by CYP2D6, the need to decrease the dose of the original medication should be considered, particularly for those concomitant medications with a narrow therapeutic index).
No products indexed under this heading.

Fluphenazine Enanthate (Concurrent administration of bupropion and agents such as antipsychotics that lower seizure threshold should be undertaken with extreme caution. Co-administration of bupropion with drugs that are metabolized by CYP2D6 isoenzyme, including antipsychotics (eg, haloperidol, risperidone, thioridazine), should be approached with caution and should be initiated at the lower end of the dose range of the concomitant medication. If bupropion is added to the treatment regimen of a patient already receiving a drug metabolized by CYP2D6, the need to decrease the dose of the original medication should be considered, particularly for those concomitant medications with a narrow therapeutic index).
No products indexed under this heading.

Fluphenazine Hydrochloride (Concurrent administration of bupropion and agents such as antipsychotics that lower seizure threshold should be undertaken with extreme caution. Co-administration of bupropion with drugs that are metabolized by CYP2D6 isoenzyme, including antipsychotics (eg, haloperidol, risperidone, thioridazine), should be approached with caution and should be initiated at the lower end of the dose range of the concomitant medication. If bupropion is added to the treatment regimen of a patient already receiving a drug metabolized by CYP2D6, the need to decrease the dose of the original medication should be considered, particularly for those concomitant medications with a narrow therapeutic index).
No products indexed under this heading.

Flurazepam Hydrochloride (Bupropion is contraindicated in patients undergoing abrupt discontinuation of sedatives (including benzodiazepines). Excessive use of sedatives (including benzodiazepines) is associated with an increased seizure risk).
No products indexed under this heading.

Fluticasone Furoate (Concurrent administration of bupropion and agents (eg, systemic steroids) that lower seizure threshold should be undertaken only with extreme caution). Products include:
Veramyst 1713

Fluticasone Propionate (Concurrent administration of bupropion and agents (eg, systemic steroids) that lower seizure threshold should be undertaken only with extreme caution). Products include:
Advair 100/50 1275
Advair 250/50 1275
Advair 500/50 1275
Advair HFA 45/21 1288
Advair HFA 115/21 1288
Advair HFA 230/21 1288
Flonase 1459
Flovent Diskus 1463
Flovent HFA 1470

Fluvoxamine (Concurrent administration of bupropion and agents (eg, antidepressants) that lower seizure threshold should be undertaken only with caution. Many drugs, including most antidepressants (eg, SSRIs), are metabolized by the CYP2D6 isoenzyme. Co-administration of bupropion with drugs that are metabolized by CYP2D6 isoenzyme should be approached with caution and should be initiated at the lower end of the dose range of the concomitant medication. If bupropion is added to the treatment regimen of a patient already receiving a drug metabolized by CYP2D6, the need to decrease the dose of the original medication should be considered, particularly for those concomitant medications with a narrow therapeutic index).
No products indexed under this heading.

Fluvoxamine Maleate (Concurrent administration of bupropion and agents (eg, antidepressants) that lower seizure threshold should be undertaken only with caution. Many drugs, including most antidepressants (eg, SSRIs), are metabolized by the CYP2D6 isoenzyme. Co-administration of bupropion with drugs that are metabolized by CYP2D6 isoenzyme should be approached with caution and should be initiated at the lower end of the dose range of the concomitant medication. If bupropion is added to the treatment regimen of a patient already receiving a drug metabolized by CYP2D6, the need to decrease the dose of the original medication should be considered, particularly for those concomitant medications with a narrow therapeutic index).
No products indexed under this heading.

Formoterol Fumarate (Co-administration of bupropion with drugs that are metabolized by the CYP2D6 isoenzyme should be approached with caution and should be initiated at the lower end of the dose range of the concomitant medication. If bupropion is added to the treatment regimen of a patient already receiving a drug metabolized by CYP2D6, the need to decrease the dose of the original medication should be considered, particularly for those concomitant medications with a narrow therapeutic index).
Products include:
Foradil 3121
Perforomist 3634

Fosphenytoin (Because bupropion is extensively metabolized, the co-administration of other drugs may affect its clinical activity. In particular, certain drugs may induce the metabolism of bupropion including phenytoin).
No products indexed under this heading.

Fosphenytoin Sodium (Because bupropion is extensively metabolized, the co-administration of other drugs may affect its clinical activity. In particular, certain drugs may induce the metabolism of bupropion including phenytoin).
No products indexed under this heading.

Galantamine Hydrobromide (Co-administration of bupropion with drugs that are metabolized by the CYP2D6 isoenzyme should be approached with caution and should be initiated at the lower end of the dose range of the concomitant medication. If bupropion is added to the treatment regimen of a patient already receiving a drug metabolized by CYP2D6, the need to decrease the dose of the original medication should be considered, particularly for those concomitant medications with a narrow therapeutic index).
No products indexed under this heading.

Glibenclamide (Concomitant use of oral hypoglycemics with bupropion is associated with an increased seizure risk).
No products indexed under this heading.

Glimepiride (Concomitant use of oral hypoglycemics with bupropion is associated with an increased seizure risk).
Products include:
Avandaryl 1356
Duetact 3354

Glipizide (Concomitant use of oral hypoglycemics with bupropion is associated with an increased seizure risk).
No products indexed under this heading.

Glutethimide (Bupropion is contraindicated in patients undergoing abrupt discontinuation of sedatives (including benzodiazepines). Excessive use of sedatives (including benzodiazepines) is associated with an increased seizure risk).
No products indexed under this heading.

Glyburide (Concomitant use of oral hypoglycemics with bupropion is associated with an increased seizure risk).
No products indexed under this heading.

Halazepam (Bupropion is contraindicated in patients undergoing abrupt discontinuation of sedatives (including benzodiazepines). Excessive use of sedatives (including benzodiazepines) is associated with an increased seizure risk).
No products indexed under this heading.

Haloperidol (Concurrent administration of bupropion and agents such as antipsychotics that lower seizure threshold should be undertaken only with extreme caution. Co-administration of bupropion with drugs that are metabolized by CYP2D6 isoenzyme, including antipsychotics (eg, haloperidol), should be approached with caution and should be initiated at the lower end of the dose range of the concomitant medication. If bupropion is added to the treatment regimen of a patient already receiving a drug metabolized by CYP2D6, the need to decrease the dose of the original medication should be considered, particularly for those concomitant medications with a narrow therapeutic index).
No products indexed under this heading.

Haloperidol Decanoate (Concurrent administration of bupropion and agents such as antipsychotics that lower seizure threshold should be undertaken only with extreme caution. Co-administration of bupropion with drugs that are metabolized by CYP2D6 isoenzyme, including antipsychotics (eg, haloperidol), should be approached with caution and should be initiated at the lower end of the dose range of the concomitant medication. If bupropion is added to the treatment regimen of a patient already receiving a drug metabolized by CYP2D6, the need to decrease the dose of the original medication should be considered, particularly for those concomitant medications with a narrow therapeutic index).
No products indexed under this heading.

Haloperidol Lactate (Concurrent administration of bupropion and agents such as antipsychotics that lower seizure threshold should be undertaken only with extreme caution. Co-administration of bupropion with drugs that are metabolized by CYP2D6 isoenzyme, including antipsychotics (eg, haloperidol), should be approached with caution and should be initiated at the lower end of the dose range of the concomitant medication. If bupropion is added to the treatment regimen of a patient already receiving a drug metabolized by CYP2D6, the need to decrease the dose of the original medi-

olized by CYP2D6, the need to decrease the dose of the original medication should be considered, particularly for those concomitant medications with a narrow therapeutic index).

No products indexed under this heading.

Levobunolol Hydrochloride (Co-administration of bupropion with drugs that are metabolized by the CYP2D6 isoenzyme, including beta blockers (eg, metoprolol) should be approached with caution and should be initiated at the lower end of the dose range of the concomitant medication. If bupropion is added to the treatment regimen of a patient already receiving a drug metabolized by CYP2D6, the need to decrease the dose of the original medication should be considered, particularly for those concomitant medications with a narrow therapeutic index).

No products indexed under this heading.

Levodopa (Limited clinical data suggest a higher incidence of adverse experiences in patients receiving bupropion concurrently with levodopa. Administration of bupropion to patients receiving levodopa concurrently should be undertaken with caution, using small initial doses and gradual dose increases). Products include:
Stalevo 2526

Levorphanol Tartrate (An addiction to opiates and concomitant use of opiates is associated with an increased seizure risk).

No products indexed under this heading.

Lidocaine (Co-administration of bupropion with drugs that are metabolized by the CYP2D6 isoenzyme should be approached with caution and should be initiated at the lower end of the dose range of the concomitant medication. If bupropion is added to the treatment regimen of a patient already receiving a drug metabolized by CYP2D6, the need to decrease the dose of the original medication should be considered, particularly for those concomitant medications with a narrow therapeutic index). Products include:
Lidoderm 1107

Lidocaine Base (*In vitro* studies indicate that bupropion is primarily metabolized to hydroxybupropion by the CYP2B6 isoenzyme. Therefore, the potential exists for a drug interaction between bupropion hydrochloride and drugs that are substrates or inhibitors of the CYP2B6 isoenzyme (eg, orphenadrine, thiotepa, cyclophosphamide)).

No products indexed under this heading.

Lidocaine Hydrochloride (Co-administration of bupropion with drugs that are metabolized by the CYP2D6 isoenzyme should be approached with caution and should be initiated at the lower end of the dose range of the concomitant medication. If bupropion is added to the treatment regimen of a patient already receiving a drug metabolized by CYP2D6, the need to decrease the dose of the original medication should be considered, particularly for those concomitant medications with a narrow therapeutic index).

No products indexed under this heading.

Lisdexamfetamine Dimesylate (An addiction to stimulants or use of over-the-counter stimulants with bupropion is associated with an increased seizure risk). Products include:
Vyvanse 3298

Lithium (Concurrent administration of bupropion and agents such as antipsychotics that lower seizure threshold should be undertaken with extreme caution. Co-administration of bupropion with drugs that are metabolized by CYP2D6 isoenzyme, including antipsychotics (eg, haloperidol, risperidone, thioridazine), should be approached

with caution and should be initiated at the lower end of the dose range of the concomitant medication. If bupropion is added to the treatment regimen of a patient already receiving a drug metabolized by CYP2D6, the need to decrease the dose of the original medication should be considered, particularly for those concomitant medications with a narrow therapeutic index).

No products indexed under this heading.

Lithium Carbonate (Concurrent administration of bupropion and agents such as antipsychotics that lower seizure threshold should be undertaken with extreme caution. Co-administration of bupropion with drugs that are metabolized by CYP2D6 isoenzyme, including antipsychotics (eg, haloperidol, risperidone, thioridazine), should be approached with caution and should be initiated at the lower end of the dose range of the concomitant medication. If bupropion is added to the treatment regimen of a patient already receiving a drug metabolized by CYP2D6, the need to decrease the dose of the original medication should be considered, particularly for those concomitant medications with a narrow therapeutic index).

No products indexed under this heading.

Lithium Citrate (Concurrent administration of bupropion and agents such as antipsychotics that lower seizure threshold should be undertaken with extreme caution. Co-administration of bupropion with drugs that are metabolized by CYP2D6 isoenzyme, including antipsychotics (eg, haloperidol, risperidone, thioridazine), should be approached with caution and should be initiated at the lower end of the dose range of the concomitant medication. If bupropion is added to the treatment regimen of a patient already receiving a drug metabolized by CYP2D6, the need to decrease the dose of the original medication should be considered, particularly for those concomitant medications with a narrow therapeutic index).

No products indexed under this heading.

Lorazepam (Bupropion is contraindicated in patients undergoing abrupt discontinuation of sedatives (including benzodiazepines). Excessive use of sedatives (including benzodiazepines) is associated with an increased seizure risk).

No products indexed under this heading.

Loxapine Hydrochloride (Concurrent administration of bupropion and agents such as antipsychotics that lower seizure threshold should be undertaken with extreme caution. Co-administration of bupropion with drugs that are metabolized by CYP2D6 isoenzyme, including antipsychotics (eg, haloperidol, risperidone, thioridazine), should be approached with caution and should be initiated at the lower end of the dose range of the concomitant medication. If bupropion is added to the treatment regimen of a patient already receiving a drug metabolized by CYP2D6, the need to decrease the dose of the original medication should be considered, particularly for those concomitant medications with a narrow therapeutic index).

No products indexed under this heading.

Loxapine Succinate (Concurrent administration of bupropion and agents such as antipsychotics that lower seizure threshold should be undertaken with extreme caution. Co-administration of bupropion with drugs that are metabolized by CYP2D6 isoenzyme, including antipsychotics (eg, haloperidol, risperidone, thioridazine), should be approached with caution and should be initiated at the lower end of the dose range of the concomitant medication. If bupropion is added to the treatment

regimen of a patient already receiving a drug metabolized by CYP2D6, the need to decrease the dose of the original medication should be considered, particularly for those concomitant medications with a narrow therapeutic index).

No products indexed under this heading.

Maprotiline Hydrochloride (Concurrent administration of bupropion and agents (eg, antidepressants) that lower seizure threshold should be undertaken only with extreme caution. Many drugs, including certain antidepressants (many tricyclics), are metabolized by the CYP2D6 isoenzyme. Co-administration of bupropion with drugs that are metabolized by CYP2D6 isoenzyme should be approached with caution and should be initiated at the lower end of the dose range of the concomitant medication. If bupropion is added to the treatment regimen of a patient already receiving a drug metabolized by CYP2D6, the need to decrease the dose of the original medication should be considered, particularly for those concomitant medications with a narrow therapeutic index).

No products indexed under this heading.

Mazindol (Concomitant use of anorectics with bupropion is associated with an increased seizure risk).

No products indexed under this heading.

Meperidine Hydrochloride (An addiction to opiates and concomitant use of opiates is associated with an increased seizure risk).

No products indexed under this heading.

Mephenytoin (*In vitro* studies indicate that bupropion is primarily metabolized to hydroxybupropion by the CYP2B6 isoenzyme. Therefore, the potential exists for a drug interaction between bupropion hydrochloride and drugs that are substrates or inhibitors of the CYP2B6 isoenzyme (eg, orphenadrine, thiotepa, cyclophosphamide)).

No products indexed under this heading.

Mephobarbital (*In vitro* studies indicate that bupropion is primarily metabolized to hydroxybupropion by the CYP2B6 isoenzyme. Therefore, the potential exists for a drug interaction between bupropion hydrochloride and drugs that are substrates or inhibitors of the CYP2B6 isoenzyme (eg, orphenadrine, thiotepa, cyclophosphamide)).

No products indexed under this heading.

Mesoridazine Besylate (Concurrent administration of bupropion and agents such as antipsychotics that lower seizure threshold should be undertaken with extreme caution. Co-administration of bupropion with drugs that are metabolized by CYP2D6 isoenzyme, including antipsychotics (eg, haloperidol, risperidone, thioridazine), should be approached with caution and should be initiated at the lower end of the dose range of the concomitant medication. If bupropion is added to the treatment regimen of a patient already receiving a drug metabolized by CYP2D6, the need to decrease the dose of the original medication should be considered, particularly for those concomitant medications with a narrow therapeutic index).

No products indexed under this heading.

Metformin Hydrochloride (Concomitant use of oral hypoglycemics with bupropion is associated with an increased seizure risk). Products include:
ActoPlus 3338
Avandamet 1345
Janumet 2188

Methadone Hydrochloride (An addiction to opiates and concomitant use of opiates is associated with an increased seizure risk).

No products indexed under this heading.

Methamphetamine Hydrochloride (Concomitant use of anorectics with bupropion is associated with an increased seizure risk).

No products indexed under this heading.

Methimazole (*In vitro* studies indicate that bupropion is primarily metabolized to hydroxybupropion by the CYP2B6 isoenzyme. Therefore, the potential exists for a drug interaction between bupropion hydrochloride and drugs that are substrates or inhibitors of the CYP2B6 isoenzyme (eg, orphenadrine, thiotepa, cyclophosphamide)).

No products indexed under this heading.

Methotrimeprazine (Concurrent administration of bupropion and agents such as antipsychotics that lower seizure threshold should be undertaken with extreme caution. Co-administration of bupropion with drugs that are metabolized by CYP2D6 isoenzyme, including antipsychotics (eg, haloperidol, risperidone, thioridazine), should be approached with caution and should be initiated at the lower end of the dose range of the concomitant medication. If bupropion is added to the treatment regimen of a patient already receiving a drug metabolized by CYP2D6, the need to decrease the dose of the original medication should be considered, particularly for those concomitant medications with a narrow therapeutic index).

No products indexed under this heading.

Methoxyphenamine (Co-administration of bupropion with drugs that are metabolized by the CYP2D6 isoenzyme should be approached with caution and should be initiated at the lower end of the dose range of the concomitant medication. If bupropion is added to the treatment regimen of a patient already receiving a drug metabolized by CYP2D6, the need to decrease the dose of the original medication should be considered, particularly for those concomitant medications with a narrow therapeutic index).

No products indexed under this heading.

Methylphenidate (An addiction to stimulants or use of over-the-counter stimulants with bupropion is associated with an increased seizure risk). Products include:
Daytrana 3283

Methylphenidate Hydrochloride (An addiction to stimulants or use of over-the-counter stimulants with bupropion is associated with an increased seizure risk). Products include:
Concerta 2598
Metadate CD 3439

Methylprednisolone (Concurrent administration of bupropion and agents (eg, systemic steroids) that lower seizure threshold should be undertaken only with extreme caution).

No products indexed under this heading.

Methylprednisolone Acetate (Concurrent administration of bupropion and agents (eg, systemic steroids) that lower seizure threshold should be undertaken only with extreme caution).

No products indexed under this heading.

Methylprednisolone Sodium Succinate (Concurrent administration of bupropion and agents (eg, systemic steroids) that lower seizure threshold should be undertaken only with extreme caution).

No products indexed under this heading.

Methyltestosterone (*In vitro* studies indicate that bupropion is primarily metabolized to hydroxybupropion by the CYP2B6 isoenzyme. Therefore, the potential exists for a drug interaction between bupropion hydrochloride and drugs that are substrates or inhibitors of the CYP2B6 isoenzyme (eg, orphenadrine, thiotepa, cyclophosphamide)).

No products indexed under this heading.

IMPORTANT NOTE: Always consult each drug listing in the patient's regimen for possible interactions.

Zyban Interactions Index 2198

Metipranolol Hydrochloride (Co-administration of bupropion with drugs that are metabolized by the CYP2D6 isoenzyme, including beta blockers (eg, metoprolol) should be approached with caution and should be initiated at the lower end of the dose range of the concomitant medication. If bupropion is added to the treatment regimen of a patient already receiving a drug metabolized by CYP2D6, the need to decrease the dose of the original medication should be considered, particularly for those concomitant medications with a narrow therapeutic index).
No products indexed under this heading.

Metoprolol Succinate (Co-administration of bupropion with drugs that are metabolized by the CYP2D6 isoenzyme, including β-blockers (eg, metoprolol) should be approached with caution and should be initiated at the lower end of the dose range of the concomitant medication. If bupropion is added to the treatment regimen of a patient already receiving a drug metabolized by CYP2D6, the need to decrease the dose of the original medication should be considered, particularly for those concomitant medications with a narrow therapeutic index).
Products include:
Toprol XL 732

Metoprolol Tartrate (Co-administration of bupropion with drugs that are metabolized by the CYP2D6 isoenzyme, including β-blockers (eg, metoprolol) should be approached with caution and should be initiated at the lower end of the dose range of the concomitant medication. If bupropion is added to the treatment regimen of a patient already receiving a drug metabolized by CYP2D6, the need to decrease the dose of the original medication should be considered, particularly for those concomitant medications with a narrow therapeutic index).
No products indexed under this heading.

Mexiletine Hydrochloride (Co-administration of bupropion with drugs that are metabolized by the CYP2D6 isoenzyme should be approached with caution and should be initiated at the lower end of the dose range of the concomitant medication. If bupropion is added to the treatment regimen of a patient already receiving a drug metabolized by CYP2D6, the need to decrease the dose of the original medication should be considered, particularly for those concomitant medications with a narrow therapeutic index).
No products indexed under this heading.

Miconazole (*In vitro* studies indicate that bupropion is primarily metabolized to hydroxybupropion by the CYP2B6 isoenzyme. Therefore, the potential exists for a drug interaction between bupropion hydrochloride and drugs that are substrates or inhibitors of the CYP2B6 isoenzyme (eg, orphenadrine, thiotepa, cyclophosphamide)).
No products indexed under this heading.

Miconazole Nitrate (*In vitro* studies indicate that bupropion is primarily metabolized to hydroxybupropion by the CYP2B6 isoenzyme. Therefore, the potential exists for a drug interaction between bupropion hydrochloride and drugs that are substrates or inhibitors of the CYP2B6 isoenzyme (eg, orphenadrine, thiotepa, cyclophosphamide)).
Products include:
Vusion Ointment 3335

Midazolam Hydrochloride (Bupropion is contraindicated in patients undergoing abrupt discontinuation of sedatives (including benzodiazepines). Excessive use of sedatives (including benzodiazepines) is associated with an increased seizure risk).
No products indexed under this heading.

Miglitol (Concomitant use of oral hypoglycemics with bupropion is associated with an increased seizure risk).
No products indexed under this heading.

Mirtazapine (Concurrent administration of bupropion and agents that lower seizure threshold (eg, antidepressants) should be undertaken with extreme caution. Co-administration of bupropion with drugs that are metabolized by CYP2D6 isoenzyme, including certain antidepressants (eg, nortriptyline, imipramine, desipramine, paroxetine, fluoxetine, sertraline), should be approached with caution and should be initiated at the lower end of the dose range of the concomitant medication. If bupropion is added to the treatment regimen of a patient already receiving a drug metabolized by CYP2D6, the need to decrease the dose of the original medication should be considered, particularly for those concomitant medications with a narrow therapeutic index).
Products include:
Remeron Tablets 3214
RemeronSolTab Tablets 3219

Moclobemide (Concurrent administration of bupropion and a monoamine oxidase (MAO) inhibitor is contraindicated. At least 14 days should elapse between discontinuation of an MAO inhibitor and initiation of treatment with bupropion).
No products indexed under this heading.

Molindone Hydrochloride (Concurrent administration of bupropion and agents such as antipsychotics that lower seizure threshold should be undertaken with extreme caution. Co-administration of bupropion with drugs that are metabolized by CYP2D6 isoenzyme, including antipsychotics (eg, haloperidol, risperidone, thioridazine), should be approached with caution and should be initiated at the lower end of the dose range of the concomitant medication. If bupropion is added to the treatment regimen of a patient already receiving a drug metabolized by CYP2D6, the need to decrease the dose of the original medication should be considered, particularly for those concomitant medications with a narrow therapeutic index). Products include:
Moban 1108

Mometasone Furoate (Concurrent administration of bupropion and agents (eg, systemic steroids) that lower seizure threshold should be undertaken only with extreme caution). Products include:
Asmanex 3058
Elocon Cream 3111
Elocon Lotion 3112
Elocon Ointment 3114

Mometasone Furoate Monohydrate (Concurrent administration of bupropion and agents (eg, systemic steroids) that lower seizure threshold should be undertaken only with extreme caution). Products include:
Nasonex 3166

Moricizine Hydrochloride (Co-administration of bupropion with drugs that are metabolized by the CYP2D6 isoenzyme, including antiarrhythmics, should be approached with caution and should be initiated at the lower end of the dose range of the concomitant medication. If bupropion is added to the treatment regimen of a patient already receiving a drug metabolized by CYP2D6, the need to decrease the dose of the original medication should be considered, particularly for those concomitant medications with a narrow therapeutic index).
No products indexed under this heading.

Morphine Sulfate (An addiction to opiates and concomitant use of opiates is associated with an increased seizure risk). Products include:
Avinza 1822
Embeda 1831
MS Contin 2803

Morphine Sulfate, Liposomal (An addiction to opiates and concomitant use of opiates is associated with an increased seizure risk).
No products indexed under this heading.

Nadolol (Co-administration of bupropion with drugs that are metabolized by the CYP2D6 isoenzyme, including beta blockers (eg, metoprolol) should be approached with caution and should be initiated at the lower end of the dose range of the concomitant medication. If bupropion is added to the treatment regimen of a patient already receiving a drug metabolized by CYP2D6, the need to decrease the dose of the original medication should be considered, particularly for those concomitant medications with a narrow therapeutic index).
Products include:
Nadolol 2359

Nateglinide (Concomitant use of oral hypoglycemics with bupropion is associated with an increased seizure risk).
No products indexed under this heading.

Nebivolol (Co-administration of bupropion with drugs that are metabolized by the CYP2D6 isoenzyme, including beta blockers (eg, metoprolol) should be approached with caution and should be initiated at the lower end of the dose range of the concomitant medication. If bupropion is added to the treatment regimen of a patient already receiving a drug metabolized by CYP2D6, the need to decrease the dose of the original medication should be considered, particularly for those concomitant medications with a narrow therapeutic index).
Products include:
Bystolic 1147

Nefazodone Hydrochloride (Concurrent administration of bupropion and agents that lower seizure threshold (eg, antidepressants) should be undertaken with extreme caution. Co-administration of bupropion with drugs that are metabolized by CYP2D6 isoenzyme, including certain antidepressants (eg, nortriptyline, imipramine, desipramine, paroxetine, fluoxetine, sertraline), should be approached with caution and should be initiated at the lower end of the dose range of the concomitant medication. If bupropion is added to the treatment regimen of a patient already receiving a drug metabolized by CYP2D6, the need to decrease the dose of the original medication should be considered, particularly for those concomitant medications with a narrow therapeutic index).
No products indexed under this heading.

Nelfinavir Mesylate (*In vitro* studies suggest that nelfinavir inhibits the hydroxylation of bupropion).
No products indexed under this heading.

Nevirapine (*In vitro* studies indicate that bupropion is primarily metabolized to hydroxybupropion by the CYP2B6 isoenzyme. Therefore, the potential exists for a drug interaction between bupropion hydrochloride and drugs that are substrates or inhibitors of the CYP2B6 isoenzyme (eg, orphenadrine, thiotepa, cyclophosphamide)). Products include:
Viramune Oral Suspension 897
Viramune Tablets 897

Nicotine (Data from a comparative study of bupropion, nicotine transdermal system (NTS), the combination of sustained-release bupropion plus NTS, and placebo as an aid to smoking cessation suggest a higher incidence of treatment-emergent hypertension in patients treated with the combination of bupropion and NTS. Monitoring of blood pressure is recommended in patients who receive the combination of bupropion and nicotine replacement).
No products indexed under this heading.

Nicotine Polacrilex (Data from a comparative study of bupropion, nicotine transdermal system (NTS), the combination of sustained-release bupropion plus NTS, and placebo as an aid to smoking cessation suggest a higher incidence of treatment-emergent hypertension in patients treated with the combination of bupropion and NTS. Monitoring of blood pressure is recommended in patients who receive the combination of bupropion and nicotine replacement).
No products indexed under this heading.

Nicotine Salicylate (Data from a comparative study of bupropion, nicotine transdermal system (NTS), the combination of sustained-release bupropion plus NTS, and placebo as an aid to smoking cessation suggest a higher incidence of treatment-emergent hypertension in patients treated with the combination of bupropion and NTS. Monitoring of blood pressure is recommended in patients who receive the combination of bupropion and nicotine replacement).
No products indexed under this heading.

Nicotine Sulfate (Data from a comparative study of bupropion, nicotine transdermal system (NTS), the combination of sustained-release bupropion plus NTS, and placebo as an aid to smoking cessation suggest a higher incidence of treatment-emergent hypertension in patients treated with the combination of bupropion and NTS. Monitoring of blood pressure is recommended in patients who receive the combination of bupropion and nicotine replacement).
No products indexed under this heading.

Norfluoxetine (In addition, *in vitro* studies suggest that norfluoxetine inhibits the hydroxylation of bupropion. No clinical studies have been performed to evaluate this finding).
No products indexed under this heading.

Nortriptyline Hydrochloride (Concurrent administration of bupropion and agents that lower seizure threshold (eg, antidepressants) should be undertaken with extreme caution. Co-administration of bupropion with drugs that are metabolized by CYP2D6 isoenzyme, including certain antidepressants (eg, nortriptyline), should be approached with caution and should be initiated at the lower end of the dose range of the concomitant medication. If bupropion is added to the treatment regimen of a patient already receiving a drug metabolized by CYP2D6, the need to decrease the dose of the original medication should be considered, particularly for those concomitant medications with a narrow therapeutic index).
No products indexed under this heading.

Olanzapine (Concurrent administration of bupropion and agents such as antipsychotics that lower seizure threshold should be undertaken with extreme caution. Co-administration of bupropion with drugs that are metabolized by CYP2D6 isoenzyme, including antipsychotics (eg, haloperidol, risperidone, thioridazine), should be approached with caution and should be initiated at the lower end of the dose range of the concomitant medication. If bupropion is added to the treatment regimen of a patient already receiving a drug metabolized by CYP2D6, the need to decrease the dose of the original medication should be considered, particularly for those concomitant medications with a narrow therapeutic index).
Products include:
Symbyax 1965
Zyprexa 1984
Zyprexa IntraMuscular 1984

Zyprexa ZYDIS **1984**

Omeprazole (Co-administration of bupropion with drugs that are metabolized by the CYP2D6 isoenzyme should be approached with caution and should be initiated at the lower end of the dose range of the concomitant medication. If bupropion is added to the treatment regimen of a patient already receiving a drug metabolized by CYP2D6, the need to decrease the dose of the original medication should be considered, particularly for those concomitant medications with a narrow therapeutic index).
No products indexed under this heading.

Ondansetron (Co-administration of bupropion with drugs that are metabolized by the CYP2D6 isoenzyme should be approached with caution and should be initiated at the lower end of the dose range of the concomitant medication. If bupropion is added to the treatment regimen of a patient already receiving a drug metabolized by CYP2D6, the need to decrease the dose of the original medication should be considered, particularly for those concomitant medications with a narrow therapeutic index).
No products indexed under this heading.

Ondansetron Hydrochloride (Co-administration of bupropion with drugs that are metabolized by the CYP2D6 isoenzyme should be approached with caution and should be initiated at the lower end of the dose range of the concomitant medication. If bupropion is added to the treatment regimen of a patient already receiving a drug metabolized by CYP2D6, the need to decrease the dose of the original medication should be considered, particularly for those concomitant medications with a narrow therapeutic index).
Products include:
Zofran Injection **1750**
Zofran **1756**
Zofran ODT **1756**

Orphenadrine Citrate (*In vitro* studies indicate that bupropion is primarily metabolized to hydroxybupropion by the CYP2B6 isoenzyme. Therefore, the potential exists for a drug interaction between bupropion hydrochloride and drugs that are substrates or inhibitors of the CYP2B6 isoenzyme (eg, orphenadrine, thiotepa, cyclophosphamide)).
No products indexed under this heading.

Orphenadrine Hydrochloride (*In vitro* studies indicate that bupropion is primarily metabolized to hydroxybupropion by the CYP2B6 isoenzyme. Therefore, the potential exists for a drug interaction between bupropion hydrochloride and drugs that are substrates or inhibitors of the CYP2B6 isoenzyme (eg, orphenadrine, thiotepa, cyclophosphamide)).
No products indexed under this heading.

Oxazepam (Bupropion is contraindicated in patients undergoing abrupt discontinuation of sedatives (including benzodiazepines). Excessive use of sedatives (including benzodiazepines) is associated with an increased seizure risk).
No products indexed under this heading.

Oxycodone Hydrochloride (An addiction to opiates and concomitant use of opiates is associated with an increased seizure risk). Products include:
OxyContin **2807**
Percocet **1121**
Percodan **1124**

Oxycodone Terephthalate (An addiction to opiates and concomitant use of opiates is associated with an increased seizure risk).
No products indexed under this heading.

Oxymorphone Hydrochloride (An addiction to opiates and concomitant use of opiates is associated with an increased seizure risk). Products include:
Opana **1110**
Opana ER **1114**

Paclitaxel (Co-administration of bupropion with drugs that are metabolized by the CYP2D6 isoenzyme should be approached with caution and should be initiated at the lower end of the dose range of the concomitant medication. If bupropion is added to the treatment regimen of a patient already receiving a drug metabolized by CYP2D6, the need to decrease the dose of the original medication should be considered, particularly for those concomitant medications with a narrow therapeutic index).
No products indexed under this heading.

Paliperidone (Concurrent administration of bupropion and agents such as antipsychotics that lower seizure threshold should be undertaken with extreme caution. Co-administration of bupropion with drugs that are metabolized by CYP2D6 isoenzyme, including antipsychotics (eg, haloperidol, risperidone, thioridazine), should be approached with caution and should be initiated at the lower end of the dose range of the concomitant medication. If bupropion is added to the treatment regimen of a patient already receiving a drug metabolized by CYP2D6, the need to decrease the dose of the original medication should be considered, particularly for those concomitant medications with a narrow therapeutic index).
Products include:
Invega **2613**
Invega Sustenna **2621**

Pargyline Hydrochloride (Concurrent administration of bupropion and a monoamine oxidase (MAO) inhibitor is contraindicated. At least 14 days should elapse between discontinuation of an MAO inhibitor and initiation of treatment with bupropion).
No products indexed under this heading.

Paroxetine (Concurrent administration of bupropion and agents that lower seizure threshold (eg, antidepressants) should be approached with caution. Co-administration of bupropion with drugs that are metabolized by CYP2D6 isoenzyme, including certain antidepressants (eg, paroxetine) should be approached with caution and should be initiated at the lower end of the dose range of the concomitant medication. If bupropion is added to the treatment regimen of a patient already receiving a drug metabolized by CYP2D6, the need to decrease the dose of the original medication should be considered, particularly for those concomitant medications with a narrow therapeutic index).
No products indexed under this heading.

Paroxetine Hydrochloride (Concurrent administration of bupropion and agents that lower seizure threshold (eg, antidepressants) should be approached with caution. Co-administration of bupropion with drugs that are metabolized by CYP2D6 isoenzyme, including certain antidepressants (eg, paroxetine) should be approached with caution and should be initiated at the lower end of the dose range of the concomitant medication. If bupropion is added to the treatment regimen of a patient already receiving a drug metabolized by CYP2D6, the need to decrease the dose of the original medication should be considered, particularly for those concomitant medications with a narrow therapeutic index).
Products include:
Paroxetine CR **2361**
Paroxetine ER **2371**
Paxil **1586**
Paxil CR **1596**

Paroxetine Mesylate (Concurrent administration of bupropion and agents that lower seizure threshold (eg, antidepressants) should be approached with caution. Co-administration of bupropion with drugs that are metabolized by CYP2D6 isoenzyme, including certain antidepressants (eg, paroxetine) should be approached with caution and should be initiated at the lower end of the dose range of the concomitant medication. If bupropion is added to the treatment regimen of a patient already receiving a drug metabolized by CYP2D6, the need to decrease the dose of the original medication should be considered, particularly for those concomitant medications with a narrow therapeutic index).
No products indexed under this heading.

Pemoline (An addiction to stimulants or use of over-the-counter stimulants with bupropion is associated with an increased seizure risk).
No products indexed under this heading.

Penbutolol Sulfate (Co-administration of bupropion with drugs that are metabolized by the CYP2D6 isoenzyme, including beta blockers (eg, metoprolol) should be approached with caution and should be initiated at the lower end of the dose range of the concomitant medication. If bupropion is added to the treatment regimen of a patient already receiving a drug metabolized by CYP2D6, the need to decrease the dose of the original medication should be considered, particularly for those concomitant medications with a narrow therapeutic index).
No products indexed under this heading.

Perphenazine (Concurrent administration of bupropion and agents such as antipsychotics that lower seizure threshold should be undertaken with extreme caution. Co-administration of bupropion with drugs that are metabolized by CYP2D6 isoenzyme, including antipsychotics (eg, haloperidol, risperidone, thioridazine), should be approached with caution and should be initiated at the lower end of the dose range of the concomitant medication. If bupropion is added to the treatment regimen of a patient already receiving a drug metabolized by CYP2D6, the need to decrease the dose of the original medication should be considered, particularly for those concomitant medications with a narrow therapeutic index).
No products indexed under this heading.

Phendimetrazine Tartrate (Concomitant use of anorectics with bupropion is associated with an increased seizure risk).
No products indexed under this heading.

Phenelzine Sulfate (Acute toxicity of bupropion is enhanced by phenelzine).
No products indexed under this heading.

Phenmetrazine Hydrochloride (Concomitant use of anorectics with bupropion is associated with an increased seizure risk).
No products indexed under this heading.

Phenobarbital (Phenobarbital may induce the metabolism of bupropion). Products include:
Donnatal **2711**

Phenobarbital Sodium (Phenobarbital may induce the metabolism of bupropion).
No products indexed under this heading.

Phenytoin (Because bupropion is extensively metabolized, the co-administration of other drugs may affect its clinical activity. In particular, certain drugs may induce the metabolism of bupropion including phenytoin).
No products indexed under this heading.

Phenytoin Sodium (Because bupropion is extensively metabolized, the co-administration of other drugs may affect its clinical activity. In particular, certain drugs may induce the metabolism of bupropion including phenytoin).
Products include:
Phenytek Capsules **2380**

Pimozide (Concurrent administration of bupropion and agents such as antipsychotics that lower seizure threshold should be undertaken with extreme caution. Co-administration of bupropion with drugs that are metabolized by CYP2D6 isoenzyme, including antipsychotics (eg, haloperidol, risperidone, thioridazine), should be approached with caution and should be initiated at the lower end of the dose range of the concomitant medication. If bupropion is added to the treatment regimen of a patient already receiving a drug metabolized by CYP2D6, the need to decrease the dose of the original medication should be considered, particularly for those concomitant medications with a narrow therapeutic index).
No products indexed under this heading.

Pindolol (Co-administration of bupropion with drugs that are metabolized by the CYP2D6 isoenzyme, including beta blockers (eg, metoprolol) should be approached with caution and should be initiated at the lower end of the dose range of the concomitant medication. If bupropion is added to the treatment regimen of a patient already receiving a drug metabolized by CYP2D6, the need to decrease the dose of the original medication should be considered, particularly for those concomitant medications with a narrow therapeutic index).
No products indexed under this heading.

Pioglitazone Hydrochloride (Concomitant use of oral hypoglycemics with bupropion is associated with an increased seizure risk). Products include:
ActoPlus **3338**
Actos **3345**
Duetact **3354**

Polyestradiol Phosphate (*In vitro* studies indicate that bupropion is primarily metabolized to hydroxybupropion by the CYP2B6 isoenzyme. Therefore, the potential exists for a drug interaction between bupropion hydrochloride and drugs that are substrates or inhibitors of the CYP2B6 isoenzyme (eg, orphenadrine, thiotepa, cyclophosphamide)).
No products indexed under this heading.

Prazepam (Bupropion is contraindicated in patients undergoing abrupt discontinuation of sedatives (including benzodiazepines). Excessive use of sedatives (including benzodiazepines) is associated with an increased seizure risk).
No products indexed under this heading.

Prednisolone (Concurrent administration of bupropion and agents (eg, systemic steroids) that lower seizure threshold should be undertaken only with extreme caution).
No products indexed under this heading.

Prednisolone Acetate (Concurrent administration of bupropion and agents (eg, systemic steroids) that lower seizure threshold should be undertaken only with extreme caution). Products include:
Blephamide .... ⊙**212**, ⊙**214**
Pred Forte .... ⊙**225**
Pred Mild .... ⊙**230**
Pred-G .... ⊙**226**, ⊙**227**

Prednisolone Sodium Phosphate (Concurrent administration of bupropion and agents (eg, systemic steroids) that lower seizure threshold should be undertaken only with extreme caution).
No products indexed under this heading.

Zyban Interactions Index 2200

Prednisolone Tebutate (Concurrent administration of bupropion and agents (eg, systemic steroids) that lower seizure threshold should be undertaken only with extreme caution).
No products indexed under this heading.

Prednisone (Concurrent administration of bupropion and agents (eg, systemic steroids) that lower seizure threshold should be undertaken only with extreme caution).
No products indexed under this heading.

Prednisone sodium phosphate (Concurrent administration of bupropion and agents (eg, systemic steroids) that lower seizure threshold should be undertaken only with extreme caution).
No products indexed under this heading.

Procainamide Hydrochloride (Co-administration of bupropion with drugs that are metabolized by the CYP2D6 isoenzyme, including antiarrhythmics, should be approached with caution and should be initiated at the lower end of the dose range of the concomitant medication. If bupropion is added to the treatment regimen of a patient already receiving a drug metabolized by CYP2D6, the need to decrease the dose of the original medication should be considered, particularly for those concomitant medications with a narrow therapeutic index).
No products indexed under this heading.

Procarbazine Hydrochloride (Concurrent administration of bupropion and a monoamine oxidase (MAO) inhibitor is contraindicated. At least 14 days should elapse between discontinuation of an MAO inhibitor and initiation of treatment with bupropion).
No products indexed under this heading.

Prochlorperazine (Concurrent administration of bupropion and agents such as antipsychotics that lower seizure threshold should be undertaken with extreme caution. Co-administration of bupropion with drugs that are metabolized by CYP2D6 isoenzyme, including antipsychotics (eg, haloperidol, risperidone, thioridazine), should be approached with caution and should be initiated at the lower end of the dose range of the concomitant medication. If bupropion is added to the treatment regimen of a patient already receiving a drug metabolized by CYP2D6, the need to decrease the dose of the original medication should be considered, particularly for those concomitant medications with a narrow therapeutic index).
No products indexed under this heading.

Promethazine (*In vitro* studies indicate that bupropion is primarily metabolized to hydroxybupropion by the CYP2B6 isoenzyme. Therefore, the potential exists for a drug interaction between bupropion hydrochloride and drugs that are substrates or inhibitors of the CYP2B6 isoenzyme (eg, orphenadrine, thiotepa, cyclophosphamide)).
No products indexed under this heading.

Promethazine Hydrochloride (Concurrent administration of bupropion and agents that lower seizure threshold should be undertaken only with extreme caution).
No products indexed under this heading.

Propafenone Hydrochloride (Co-administration of bupropion with drugs that are metabolized by the CYP2D6 isoenzyme, including Type 1C antiarrhythmics (eg, propafenone), should be approached with caution and should be initiated at the lower end of the dose range of the concomitant medication. If bupropion is added to the treatment regimen of a patient already receiving a drug metabolized by CYP2D6, the need to decrease the dose of the original medication should be considered, particularly for those concomitant medications with a narrow therapeutic index). Products include:
Rythmol 1648
Rythmol SR 1652

Propofol (Bupropion is contraindicated in patients undergoing abrupt discontinuation of sedatives (including benzodiazepines). Excessive use of sedatives (including benzodiazepines) is associated with an increased seizure risk).
No products indexed under this heading.

Propoxyphene Hydrochloride (An addiction to opiates and concomitant use of opiates is associated with an increased seizure risk).
No products indexed under this heading.

Propoxyphene Napsylate (An addiction to opiates and concomitant use of opiates is associated with an increased seizure risk).
No products indexed under this heading.

Propranolol Hydrochloride (Co-administration of bupropion with drugs that are metabolized by the CYP2D6 isoenzyme, including beta blockers (eg, metoprolol) should be approached with caution and should be initiated at the lower end of the dose range of the concomitant medication. If bupropion is added to the treatment regimen of a patient already receiving a drug metabolized by CYP2D6, the need to decrease the dose of the original medication should be considered, particularly for those concomitant medications with a narrow therapeutic index). Products include:
InnoPran XL 1517

Protriptyline Hydrochloride (Concurrent administration of bupropion and agents (eg, antidepressants) that lower seizure threshold should be undertaken only with extreme caution. Many drugs, including certain antidepressants (many tricyclics), are metabolized by the CYP2D6 isoenzyme. Co-administration of bupropion with drugs that are metabolized by CYP2D6 isoenzyme should be approached with caution and should be initiated at the lower end of the dose range of the concomitant medication. If bupropion is added to the treatment regimen of a patient already receiving a drug metabolized by CYP2D6, the need to decrease the dose of the original medication should be considered, particularly for those concomitant medications with a narrow therapeutic index).
No products indexed under this heading.

Quazepam (Bupropion is contraindicated in patients undergoing abrupt discontinuation of sedatives (including benzodiazepines). Excessive use of sedatives (including benzodiazepines) is associated with an increased seizure risk).
No products indexed under this heading.

Quetiapine Fumarate (Concurrent administration of bupropion and agents such as antipsychotics that lower seizure threshold should be undertaken with extreme caution. Co-administration of bupropion with drugs that are metabolized by CYP2D6 isoenzyme, including antipsychotics (eg, haloperidol, risperidone, thioridazine), should be approached with caution and should be initiated at the lower end of the dose range of the concomitant medication. If bupropion is added to the treatment regimen of a patient already receiving a drug metabolized by CYP2D6, the need to decrease the dose of the original medication should be considered, particularly for those concomitant medications with a narrow therapeutic index). Products include:
Seroquel 750
Seroquel XR 759

Quinidine Gluconate (Co-administration of bupropion with drugs that are metabolized by the CYP2D6 isoenzyme should be approached with caution and should be initiated at the lower end of the dose range of the concomitant medication. If bupropion is added to the treatment regimen of a patient already receiving a drug metabolized by CYP2D6, the need to decrease the dose of the original medication should be considered, particularly for those concomitant medications with a narrow therapeutic index).
No products indexed under this heading.

Quinidine Hydrochloride (Co-administration of bupropion with drugs that are metabolized by the CYP2D6 isoenzyme should be approached with caution and should be initiated at the lower end of the dose range of the concomitant medication. If bupropion is added to the treatment regimen of a patient already receiving a drug metabolized by CYP2D6, the need to decrease the dose of the original medication should be considered, particularly for those concomitant medications with a narrow therapeutic index).
No products indexed under this heading.

Quinidine Polygalacturonate (Co-administration of bupropion with drugs that are metabolized by the CYP2D6 isoenzyme should be approached with caution and should be initiated at the lower end of the dose range of the concomitant medication. If bupropion is added to the treatment regimen of a patient already receiving a drug metabolized by CYP2D6, the need to decrease the dose of the original medication should be considered, particularly for those concomitant medications with a narrow therapeutic index).
No products indexed under this heading.

Quinidine Sulfate (Co-administration of bupropion with drugs that are metabolized by the CYP2D6 isoenzyme should be approached with caution and should be initiated at the lower end of the dose range of the concomitant medication. If bupropion is added to the treatment regimen of a patient already receiving a drug metabolized by CYP2D6, the need to decrease the dose of the original medication should be considered, particularly for those concomitant medications with a narrow therapeutic index).
No products indexed under this heading.

Ramelteon (Bupropion is contraindicated in patients undergoing abrupt discontinuation of sedatives (including benzodiazepines). Excessive use of sedatives (including benzodiazepines) is associated with an increased seizure risk). Products include:
Rozerem 3366

Rasagiline Mesylate (Concurrent administration of bupropion and a monoamine oxidase (MAO) inhibitor is contraindicated. At least 14 days should elapse between discontinuation of an MAO inhibitor and initiation of treatment with bupropion). Products include:
Azilect 3383

Remifentanil Hydrochloride (An addiction to opiates and concomitant use of opiates is associated with an increased seizure risk).
No products indexed under this heading.

Repaglinide (Concomitant use of oral hypoglycemics with bupropion is associated with an increased seizure risk).
No products indexed under this heading.

Risperidone (Concurrent administration of bupropion and agents such as antipsychotics that lower seizure threshold should be undertaken only with extreme caution. Co-administration of bupropion with drugs that are metabolized by CYP2D6 isoenzyme, including antipsychotics (eg, risperidone), should be approached with caution and should be initiated at the lower end of the dose range of the concomitant medication. If bupropion is added to the treatment regimen of a patient already receiving a drug metabolized by CYP2D6, the need to decrease the dose of the original medication should be considered, particularly for those concomitant medications with a narrow therapeutic index). Products include:
Risperdal Consta 2682

Ritonavir (*In vitro* studies suggest that ritonavir inhibits the hydroxylation of bupropion). Products include:
Kaletra 458
Norvir 509

Ropivacaine Hydrochloride (*In vitro* studies indicate that bupropion is primarily metabolized to hydroxybupropion by the CYP2B6 isoenzyme. Therefore, the potential exists for a drug interaction between bupropion hydrochloride and drugs that are substrates or inhibitors of the CYP2B6 isoenzyme (eg, orphenadrine, thiotepa, cyclophosphamide)).
No products indexed under this heading.

Rosiglitazone Maleate (Concomitant use of oral hypoglycemics with bupropion is associated with an increased seizure risk). Products include:
Avandamet 1345
Avandaryl 1356
Avandia 1366

Secobarbital Sodium (Bupropion is contraindicated in patients undergoing abrupt discontinuation of sedatives (including benzodiazepines). Excessive use of sedatives (including benzodiazepines) is associated with an increased seizure risk).
No products indexed under this heading.

Selegiline (Concurrent administration of bupropion and a monoamine oxidase (MAO) inhibitor is contraindicated. At least 14 days should elapse between discontinuation of an MAO inhibitor and initiation of treatment with bupropion). Products include:
Emsam 3623

Selegiline Hydrochloride (Concurrent administration of bupropion and a monoamine oxidase (MAO) inhibitor is contraindicated. At least 14 days should elapse between discontinuation of an MAO inhibitor and initiation of treatment with bupropion). Products include:
Eldepryl 3312

Sertraline Hydrochloride (Concurrent administration of bupropion and agents that lower seizure threshold (eg, antidepressants) should be approached with caution. Co-administration of bupropion with drugs that are metabolized by CYP2D6 isoenzyme, including certain antidepressants (eg, sertraline), should be approached with caution and should be initiated at the lower end of the dose range of the concomitant medication. If bupropion is added to the treatment regimen of a patient already receiving a drug metabolized by CYP2D6, the need to decrease the dose of the original medication should be considered, particularly for those concomitant medications with a narrow therapeutic index).
No products indexed under this heading.

Sevoflurane (*In vitro* studies indicate that bupropion is primarily metabolized to hydroxybupropion by the CYP2B6 isoenzyme. Therefore, the potential exists for a drug interaction between bupropion hydrochloride and drugs that are substrates or inhibitors of the CYP2B6 isoenzyme (eg, orphenadrine, thiotepa, cyclophosphamide)). Products include:
Ultane 554

Sibutramine Hydrochloride Monohydrate (Concomitant use of anorec-

2201 Interactions Index Zyban

tics with bupropion is associated with an increased seizure risk). Products include:

Meridia 492

Sitagliptin Phosphate (Concomitant use of oral hypoglycemics with bupropion is associated with an increased seizure risk). Products include:

Janumet 2188
Januvia 2196

Sodium Butabarbital (Bupropion is contraindicated in patients undergoing abrupt discontinuation of sedatives (including benzodiazepines). Excessive use of sedatives (including benzodiazepines) is associated with an increased seizure risk).

No products indexed under this heading.

Sotalol Hydrochloride (Co-administration of bupropion with drugs that are metabolized by the CYP2D6 isoenzyme, including beta blockers (eg, metoprolol) should be approached with caution and should be initiated at the lower end of the dose range of the concomitant medication. If bupropion is added to the treatment regimen of a patient already receiving a drug metabolized by CYP2D6, the need to decrease the dose of the original medication should be considered, particularly for those concomitant medications with a narrow therapeutic index).

No products indexed under this heading.

Sufentanil Citrate (An addiction to opiates and concomitant use of opiates is associated with an increased seizure risk).

No products indexed under this heading.

Tamoxifen Citrate (Co-administration of bupropion with drugs that are metabolized by the CYP2D6 isoenzyme should be approached with caution and should be initiated at the lower end of the dose range of the concomitant medication. If bupropion is added to the treatment regimen of a patient already receiving a drug metabolized by CYP2D6, the need to decrease the dose of the original medication should be considered, particularly for those concomitant medications with a narrow therapeutic index).

No products indexed under this heading.

Temazepam (Bupropion is contraindicated in patients undergoing abrupt discontinuation of sedatives (including benzodiazepines). Excessive use of sedatives (including benzodiazepines) is associated with an increased seizure risk).

No products indexed under this heading.

Teniposide (Co-administration of bupropion with drugs that are metabolized by the CYP2D6 isoenzyme should be approached with caution and should be initiated at the lower end of the dose range of the concomitant medication. If bupropion is added to the treatment regimen of a patient already receiving a drug metabolized by CYP2D6, the need to decrease the dose of the original medication should be considered, particularly for those concomitant medications with a narrow therapeutic index).

No products indexed under this heading.

Testosterone (Co-administration of bupropion with drugs that are metabolized by the CYP2D6 isoenzyme should be approached with caution and should be initiated at the lower end of the dose range of the concomitant medication. If bupropion is added to the treatment regimen of a patient already receiving a drug metabolized by CYP2D6, the need to decrease the dose of the original medication should be considered, particularly for those concomitant medications with a narrow therapeutic index). Products include:

AndroGel 3456

Testosterone Cypionate (Co-administration of bupropion with drugs that are metabolized by the CYP2D6 isoenzyme should be approached with caution and should be initiated at the lower end of the dose range of the concomitant medication. If bupropion is added to the treatment regimen of a patient already receiving a drug metabolized by CYP2D6, the need to decrease the dose of the original medication should be considered, particularly for those concomitant medications with a narrow therapeutic index).

No products indexed under this heading.

Testosterone Enanthate (Co-administration of bupropion with drugs that are metabolized by the CYP2D6 isoenzyme should be approached with caution and should be initiated at the lower end of the dose range of the concomitant medication. If bupropion is added to the treatment regimen of a patient already receiving a drug metabolized by CYP2D6, the need to decrease the dose of the original medication should be considered, particularly for those concomitant medications with a narrow therapeutic index). Products include:

Delatestryl 1102

Testosterone Propionate (Co-administration of bupropion with drugs that are metabolized by the CYP2D6 isoenzyme should be approached with caution and should be initiated at the lower end of the dose range of the concomitant medication. If bupropion is added to the treatment regimen of a patient already receiving a drug metabolized by CYP2D6, the need to decrease the dose of the original medication should be considered, particularly for those concomitant medications with a narrow therapeutic index).

No products indexed under this heading.

Theophylline (Concurrent administration of bupropion and agents (eg, theophylline) that lower seizure threshold should be undertaken only with extreme caution. In addition, physiological changes resulting from smoking cessation itself, with or without treatment with bupropion, may alter the pharmacokinetics of some concomitant medications, which may require dosage adjustment. Blood concentrations of concomitant medications that are extensively metabolized, such as theophylline, may be expected to increase following smoking cessation due to de-induction of hepatic enzymes).

No products indexed under this heading.

Theophylline Anhydrous (Concurrent administration of bupropion and agents (eg, theophylline) that lower seizure threshold should be undertaken only with extreme caution. In addition, physiological changes resulting from smoking cessation itself, with or without treatment with bupropion, may alter the pharmacokinetics of some concomitant medications, which may require dosage adjustment. Blood concentrations of concomitant medications that are extensively metabolized, such as theophylline, may be expected to increase following smoking cessation due to de-induction of hepatic enzymes). Products include:

Uniphyl 2817

Theophylline Calcium Salicylate (Concurrent administration of bupropion and agents (eg, theophylline) that lower seizure threshold should be undertaken only with extreme caution. In addition, physiological changes resulting from smoking cessation itself, with or without treatment with bupropion, may alter the pharmacokinetics of some concomitant medications, which may require dosage adjustment. Blood concentrations of concomitant medications that are extensively metabolized, such as theophylline, may be expected to increase following smoking cessation due to de-induction of hepatic enzymes).

No products indexed under this heading.

Theophylline Dihydroxypropyl (Glyceryl) (Concurrent administration of bupropion and agents (eg, theophylline) that lower seizure threshold should be undertaken only with extreme caution. In addition, physiological changes resulting from smoking cessation itself, with or without treatment with bupropion, may alter the pharmacokinetics of some concomitant medications, which may require dosage adjustment. Blood concentrations of concomitant medications that are extensively metabolized, such as theophylline, may be expected to increase following smoking cessation due to de-induction of hepatic enzymes).

No products indexed under this heading.

Theophylline Ethylenediamine (Concurrent administration of bupropion and agents (eg, theophylline) that lower seizure threshold should be undertaken only with extreme caution. In addition, physiological changes resulting from smoking cessation itself, with or without treatment with bupropion, may alter the pharmacokinetics of some concomitant medications, which may require dosage adjustment. Blood concentrations of concomitant medications that are extensively metabolized, such as theophylline, may be expected to increase following smoking cessation due to de-induction of hepatic enzymes).

No products indexed under this heading.

Theophylline Sodium Glycinate (Concurrent administration of bupropion and agents (eg, theophylline) that lower seizure threshold should be undertaken only with extreme caution. In addition, physiological changes resulting from smoking cessation itself, with or without treatment with bupropion, may alter the pharmacokinetics of some concomitant medications, which may require dosage adjustment. Blood concentrations of concomitant medications that are extensively metabolized, such as theophylline, may be expected to increase following smoking cessation due to de-induction of hepatic enzymes).

No products indexed under this heading.

Thioridazine (Concurrent administration of bupropion and agents such as antipsychotics that lower seizure threshold should be undertaken only with extreme caution. Co-administration of bupropion with drugs that are metabolized by CYP2D6 isoenzyme, including antipsychotics (eg, thioridazine), should be approached with caution and should be initiated at the lower end of the dose range of the concomitant medication. If bupropion is added to the treatment regimen of a patient already receiving a drug metabolized by CYP2D6, the need to decrease the dose of the original medication should be considered, particularly for those concomitant medications with a narrow therapeutic index).

No products indexed under this heading.

Thioridazine Hydrochloride (Concurrent administration of bupropion and agents such as antipsychotics that lower seizure threshold should be undertaken only with extreme caution. Co-administration of bupropion with drugs that are metabolized by CYP2D6 isoenzyme, including antipsychotics (eg, thioridazine), should be approached with caution and should be initiated at the lower end of the dose range of the concomitant medication. If bupropion is added to the treatment regimen of a patient already receiving a drug metabolized by CYP2D6, the need to decrease the dose of the original medication should be considered, particularly for those concomitant medications with a narrow therapeutic index). Products include:

Thioridazine Hydrochloride 2384

Thiotepa (*In vitro* studies indicate that bupropion is primarily metabolized to hydroxybupropion by the CYP2B6 isoenzyme. Therefore, the potential exists for a drug interaction between bupropion hydrochloride and drugs that are substrates or inhibitors of the CYP2B6 isoenzyme (eg, orphenadrine, thiotepa, cyclophosphamide)).

No products indexed under this heading.

Thiothixene (Concurrent administration of bupropion and agents such as antipsychotics that lower seizure threshold should be undertaken with extreme caution. Co-administration of bupropion with drugs that are metabolized by CYP2D6 isoenzyme, including antipsychotics (eg, haloperidol, risperidone, thioridazine), should be approached with caution and should be initiated at the lower end of the dose range of the concomitant medication. If bupropion is added to the treatment regimen of a patient already receiving a drug metabolized by CYP2D6, the need to decrease the dose of the original medication should be considered, particularly for those concomitant medications with a narrow therapeutic index). Products include:

Thiothixene 2386

Timolol Hemihydrate (Co-administration of bupropion with drugs that are metabolized by the CYP2D6 isoenzyme, including beta blockers (eg, metoprolol) should be approached with caution and should be initiated at the lower end of the dose range of the concomitant medication. If bupropion is added to the treatment regimen of a patient already receiving a drug metabolized by CYP2D6, the need to decrease the dose of the original medication should be considered, particularly for those concomitant medications with a narrow therapeutic index). Products include:

Betimol 3490

Timolol Maleate (Co-administration of bupropion with drugs that are metabolized by the CYP2D6 isoenzyme, including beta blockers (eg, metoprolol) should be approached with caution and should be initiated at the lower end of the dose range of the concomitant medication. If bupropion is added to the treatment regimen of a patient already receiving a drug metabolized by CYP2D6, the need to decrease the dose of the original medication should be considered, particularly for those concomitant medications with a narrow therapeutic index). Products include:

Combigan 601
Dorzolamide Hydrochloride/Timolol Maleate Ophthalmic Solution .... ⊙243
Timoptic in Ocudose .... ⊙231

Tocainide Hydrochloride (Co-administration of bupropion with drugs that are metabolized by the CYP2D6 isoenzyme, including antiarrhythmics, should be approached with caution and should be initiated at the lower end of the dose range of the concomitant medication. If bupropion is added to the treatment regimen of a patient already receiving a drug metabolized by CYP2D6, the need to decrease the dose of the original medication should be considered, particularly for those concomitant medications with a narrow therapeutic index).

No products indexed under this heading.

Tolazamide (Concomitant use of oral hypoglycemics with bupropion is associated with an increased seizure risk).

No products indexed under this heading.

IMPORTANT NOTE: Always consult each drug listing in the patient's regimen for possible interactions.

Tolbutamide (Concomitant use of oral hypoglycemics with bupropion is associated with an increased seizure risk).
No products indexed under this heading.

Tolterodine Tartrate (Co-administration of bupropion with drugs that are metabolized by the CYP2D6 isoenzyme should be approached with caution and should be initiated at the lower end of the dose range of the concomitant medication. If bupropion is added to the treatment regimen of a patient already receiving a drug metabolized by CYP2D6, the need to decrease the dose of the original medication should be considered, particularly for those concomitant medications with a narrow therapeutic index).
No products indexed under this heading.

Tramadol Hydrochloride (Co-administration of bupropion with drugs that are metabolized by the CYP2D6 isoenzyme should be approached with caution and should be initiated at the lower end of the dose range of the concomitant medication. If bupropion is added to the treatment regimen of a patient already receiving a drug metabolized by CYP2D6, the need to decrease the dose of the original medication should be considered, particularly for those concomitant medications with a narrow therapeutic index). Products include:
Ryzolt 2813
Ultram ER 2693

Tranylcypromine Sulfate (Concurrent administration of bupropion and a monoamine oxidase (MAO) inhibitor is contraindicated. At least 14 days should elapse between discontinuation of an MAO inhibitor and initiation of treatment with bupropion). Products include:
Parnate 1584

Trazodone Hydrochloride (Concurrent administration of bupropion and agents that lower seizure threshold (eg, antidepressants) should be undertaken with extreme caution. Co-administration of bupropion with drugs that are metabolized by CYP2D6 isoenzyme, including certain antidepressants (eg, nortriptyline, imipramine, desipramine, paroxetine, fluoxetine, sertraline), should be approached with caution and should be initiated at the lower end of the dose range of the concomitant medication. If bupropion is added to the treatment regimen of a patient already receiving a drug metabolized by CYP2D6, the need to decrease the dose of the original medication should be considered, particularly for those concomitant medications with a narrow therapeutic index).
No products indexed under this heading.

Tretinoin (*In vitro* studies indicate that bupropion is primarily metabolized to hydroxybupropion by the CYP2B6 isoenzyme. Therefore, the potential exists for a drug interaction between bupropion hydrochloride and drugs that are substrates or inhibitors of the CYP2B6 isoenzyme (eg, orphenadrine, thiotepa, cyclophosphamide)).
No products indexed under this heading.

Triamcinolone (Concurrent administration of bupropion and agents (eg, systemic steroids) that lower seizure threshold should be undertaken only with extreme caution).
No products indexed under this heading.

Triamcinolone Acetonide (Concurrent administration of bupropion and agents (eg, systemic steroids) that lower seizure threshold should be undertaken only with extreme caution). Products include:
Azmacort 408
Nasacort AQ 3019

Triamcinolone Diacetate (Concurrent administration of bupropion and agents (eg, systemic steroids) that lower seizure threshold should be undertaken only with extreme caution).
No products indexed under this heading.

Triamcinolone Hexacetonide (Concurrent administration of bupropion and agents (eg, systemic steroids) that lower seizure threshold should be undertaken only with extreme caution).
No products indexed under this heading.

Triazolam (Bupropion is contraindicated in patients undergoing abrupt discontinuation of sedatives (including benzodiazepines). Excessive use of sedatives (including benzodiazepines) is associated with an increased seizure risk).
No products indexed under this heading.

Trifluoperazine Hydrochloride (Concurrent administration of bupropion and agents such as antipsychotics that lower seizure threshold should be undertaken with extreme caution. Co-administration of bupropion with drugs that are metabolized by CYP2D6 isoenzyme, including antipsychotics (eg, haloperidol, risperidone, thioridazine), should be approached with caution and should be initiated at the lower end of the dose range of the concomitant medication. If bupropion is added to the treatment regimen of a patient already receiving a drug metabolized by CYP2D6, the need to decrease the dose of the original medication should be considered, particularly for those concomitant medications with a narrow therapeutic index).
No products indexed under this heading.

Trimipramine Maleate (Concurrent administration of bupropion and agents (eg, antidepressants) that lower seizure threshold should be undertaken only with extreme caution. Many drugs, including certain antidepressants (many tricyclics), are metabolized by the CYP2D6 isoenzyme. Co-administration of bupropion with drugs that are metabolized by CYP2D6 isoenzyme should be approached with caution and should be initiated at the lower end of the dose range of the concomitant medication. If bupropion is added to the treatment regimen of a patient already receiving a drug metabolized by CYP2D6, the need to decrease the dose of the original medication should be considered, particularly for those concomitant medications with a narrow therapeutic index).
No products indexed under this heading.

Troglitazone (Concomitant use of oral hypoglycemics with bupropion is associated with an increased seizure risk).
No products indexed under this heading.

Valproate Sodium (*In vitro* studies indicate that bupropion is primarily metabolized to hydroxybupropion by the CYP2B6 isoenzyme. Therefore, the potential exists for a drug interaction between bupropion hydrochloride and drugs that are substrates or inhibitors of the CYP2B6 isoenzyme (eg, orphenadrine, thiotepa, cyclophosphamide)).
No products indexed under this heading.

Valproic Acid (*In vitro* studies indicate that bupropion is primarily metabolized to hydroxybupropion by the CYP2B6 isoenzyme. Therefore, the potential exists for a drug interaction between bupropion hydrochloride and drugs that are substrates or inhibitors of the CYP2B6 isoenzyme (eg, orphenadrine, thiotepa, cyclophosphamide)).
No products indexed under this heading.

Venlafaxine Hydrochloride (Concurrent administration of bupropion and agents that lower seizure threshold (eg, antidepressants) should be undertaken with extreme caution. Co-administration of bupropion with drugs that are metabolized by CYP2D6 isoenzyme, including certain antidepressants (eg, nortriptyline, imipramine, desipramine, paroxetine, fluoxetine, sertraline), should be approached with caution and should be initiated at the lower end of the dose range of the concomitant medication. If bupropion is added to the treatment regimen of a patient already receiving a drug metabolized by CYP2D6, the need to decrease the dose of the original medication should be considered, particularly for those concomitant medications with a narrow therapeutic index). Products include:
Effexor XR 3504
Venlafaxine Hydrochloride Tablets 2388

Verapamil Hydrochloride (*In vitro* studies indicate that bupropion is primarily metabolized to hydroxybupropion by the CYP2B6 isoenzyme. Therefore, the potential exists for a drug interaction between bupropion hydrochloride and drugs that are substrates or inhibitors of the CYP2B6 isoenzyme (eg, orphenadrine, thiotepa, cyclophosphamide)). Products include:
Tarka 534

Vinblastine Sulfate (Co-administration of bupropion with drugs that are metabolized by the CYP2D6 isoenzyme should be approached with caution and should be initiated at the lower end of the dose range of the concomitant medication. If bupropion is added to the treatment regimen of a patient already receiving a drug metabolized by CYP2D6, the need to decrease the dose of the original medication should be considered, particularly for those concomitant medications with a narrow therapeutic index).
No products indexed under this heading.

Warfarin Sodium (Altered PT and/or INR infrequently associated with hemorrhagic or thrombotic complications were observed when bupropion was co-administered with warfarin. In addition, physiological changes resulting from smoking cessation itself, with or without treatment with bupropion, may alter the pharmacokinetics of some concomitant medications, which may require dosage adjustment. Blood concentrations of concomitant medications that are extensively metabolized, such as warfarin, may be expected to increase following smoking cessation due to de-induction of hepatic enzymes).
No products indexed under this heading.

Zaleplon (Bupropion is contraindicated in patients undergoing abrupt discontinuation of sedatives (including benzodiazepines). Excessive use of sedatives (including benzodiazepines) is associated with an increased seizure risk).
No products indexed under this heading.

Ziprasidone Hydrochloride (Concurrent administration of bupropion and agents such as antipsychotics that lower seizure threshold should be undertaken with extreme caution. Co-administration of bupropion with drugs that are metabolized by CYP2D6 isoenzyme, including antipsychotics (eg, haloperidol, risperidone, thioridazine), should be approached with caution and should be initiated at the lower end of the dose range of the concomitant medication. If bupropion is added to the treatment regimen of a patient already receiving a drug metabolized by CYP2D6, the need to decrease the dose of the original medication should be considered, particularly for those concomitant medications with a narrow therapeutic index). Products include:
Geodon 2723

Zolpidem Tartrate (Bupropion is contraindicated in patients undergoing abrupt discontinuation of sedatives (including benzodiazepines). Excessive use of sedatives (including benzodiazepines) is associated with an increased seizure risk). Products include:
Ambien 2920
Ambien CR 2925

Zonisamide (Co-administration of bupropion with drugs that are metabolized by the CYP2D6 isoenzyme should be approached with caution and should be initiated at the lower end of the dose range of the concomitant medication. If bupropion is added to the treatment regimen of a patient already receiving a drug metabolized by CYP2D6, the need to decrease the dose of the original medication should be considered, particularly for those concomitant medications with a narrow therapeutic index). Products include:
Zonegran 1081

Food Interactions

Alcohol (Bupropion is contraindicated in patients undergoing abrupt discontinuation of alcohol. In post-marketing experience, there have been rare reports of adverse neuropsychiatric events or reduced alcohol tolerance in patients who were drinking alcohol during treatment with bupropion. The consumption of alcohol during treatment with bupropion should be minimized or avoided).

Beer, reduced-alcohol (Bupropion is contraindicated in patients undergoing abrupt discontinuation of alcohol. In post-marketing experience, there have been rare reports of adverse neuropsychiatric events or reduced alcohol tolerance in patients who were drinking alcohol during treatment with bupropion. The consumption of alcohol during treatment with bupropion should be minimized or avoided).

Beer, unspecified (Bupropion is contraindicated in patients undergoing abrupt discontinuation of alcohol. In post-marketing experience, there have been rare reports of adverse neuropsychiatric events or reduced alcohol tolerance in patients who were drinking alcohol during treatment with bupropion. The consumption of alcohol during treatment with bupropion should be minimized or avoided).

Food, unspecified (In a single-dose study, food increased the C_{max} of bupropion by 11% and the extent of absorption as defined by area under the plasma concentration-time curve (AUC) by 17%. The mean time to peak concentration (T_{max}) was prolonged by 1 hour. This effect was of no clinical significance).

Meal, unspecified (In a single-dose study, food increased the C_{max} of bupropion by 11% and the extent of absorption as defined by area under the plasma concentration-time curve (AUC) by 17%. The mean time to peak concentration (T_{max}) was prolonged by 1 hour. This effect was of no clinical significance).

Wine, Chianti (Bupropion is contraindicated in patients undergoing abrupt discontinuation of alcohol. In post-marketing experience, there have been rare reports of adverse neuropsychiatric events or reduced alcohol tolerance in patients who were drinking alcohol during treatment with bupropion. The consumption of alcohol during treatment with bupropion should be minimized or avoided).

Wine, Red (Bupropion is contraindicated in patients undergoing abrupt discontinuation of alcohol. In post-marketing experience, there have been rare reports of adverse neuropsychiatric events or reduced alcohol tolerance in patients who were drinking alcohol during treatment with bupropion. The con-

2203 Interactions Index Zydone

sumption of alcohol during treatment with bupropion should be minimized or avoided).

Wine, unspecified (Bupropion is contraindicated in patients undergoing abrupt discontinuation of alcohol. In post-marketing experience, there have been rare reports of adverse neuropsychiatric events or reduced alcohol tolerance in patients who were drinking alcohol during treatment with bupropion. The consumption of alcohol during treatment with bupropion should be minimized or avoided).

Wine products (Bupropion is contraindicated in patients undergoing abrupt discontinuation of alcohol. In post-marketing experience, there have been rare reports of adverse neuropsychiatric events or reduced alcohol tolerance in patients who were drinking alcohol during treatment with bupropion. The consumption of alcohol during treatment with bupropion should be minimized or avoided).

ZYDONE TABLETS

(Acetaminophen, Hydrocodone Bitartrate) 1138

May interact with alcohols, anticholinergics, central nervous system depressants, monoamine oxidase inhibitors, narcotic analgesics, tricyclic antidepressants, and certain other agents. Compounds in these categories include:

Alfentanil Hydrochloride (Co-administration may exhibit additive CNS depression).
No products indexed under this heading.

Alprazolam (Co-administration may exhibit additive CNS depression).
No products indexed under this heading.

Amitriptyline Hydrochloride (Co-administration of tricyclic antidepressants with hydrocodone may increase the effect of either hydrocodone or antidepressant).
No products indexed under this heading.

Amobarbital (Co-administration may exhibit additive CNS depression).
No products indexed under this heading.

Amobarbital Sodium (Co-administration may exhibit additive CNS depression).
No products indexed under this heading.

Amoxapine (Co-administration of tricyclic antidepressants with hydrocodone may increase the effect of either hydrocodone or antidepressant).
No products indexed under this heading.

Apomorphine (Co-administration may exhibit additive CNS depression).
No products indexed under this heading.

Apomorphine Hydrochloride (Co-administration may exhibit additive CNS depression).
No products indexed under this heading.

Aprobarbital (Co-administration may exhibit additive CNS depression).
No products indexed under this heading.

Atropine Sulfate (Co-administration may produce paralytic ileus). Products include:
Donnatal 2711

Belladonna Alkaloids (Co-administration may produce paralytic ileus). Products include:
Hyland's Teething Tablets 3316

Benztropine Mesylate (Co-administration may produce paralytic ileus).
No products indexed under this heading.

Biperiden Hydrochloride (Co-administration may produce paralytic ileus).
No products indexed under this heading.

Buprenorphine Hydrochloride (Co-administration may exhibit additive CNS depression).
No products indexed under this heading.

Buspirone Hydrochloride (Co-administration may exhibit additive CNS depression).
No products indexed under this heading.

Butabarbital (Co-administration may exhibit additive CNS depression).
No products indexed under this heading.

Butabarbital Sodium (Co-administration may exhibit additive CNS depression).
No products indexed under this heading.

Butalbital (Co-administration may exhibit additive CNS depression).
No products indexed under this heading.

Chlordiazepoxide (Co-administration may exhibit additive CNS depression).
No products indexed under this heading.

Chlordiazepoxide Hydrochloride (Co-administration may exhibit additive CNS depression).
No products indexed under this heading.

Chlorpromazine (Co-administration may exhibit additive CNS depression).
No products indexed under this heading.

Chlorpromazine Hydrochloride (Co-administration may exhibit additive CNS depression).
No products indexed under this heading.

Chlorprothixene (Co-administration may exhibit additive CNS depression).
No products indexed under this heading.

Chlorprothixene Hydrochloride (Co-administration may exhibit additive CNS depression).
No products indexed under this heading.

Chlorprothixene Lactate (Co-administration may exhibit additive CNS depression).
No products indexed under this heading.

Clidinium Bromide (Co-administration may produce paralytic ileus).
No products indexed under this heading.

Clomipramine Hydrochloride (Co-administration of tricyclic antidepressants with hydrocodone may increase the effect of either hydrocodone or antidepressant).
No products indexed under this heading.

Clonazepam (Co-administration may exhibit additive CNS depression). Products include:
Klonopin 2855

Clorazepate Dipotassium (Co-administration may exhibit additive CNS depression).
No products indexed under this heading.

Clozapine (Co-administration may exhibit additive CNS depression).
No products indexed under this heading.

Codeine Phosphate (Co-administration may exhibit additive CNS depression). Products include:
Tylenol with Codeine 2691

Codeine Sulfate (Co-administration may exhibit additive CNS depression).
No products indexed under this heading.

Desflurane (Co-administration may exhibit additive CNS depression).
No products indexed under this heading.

Desipramine Hydrochloride (Co-administration of tricyclic antidepressants with hydrocodone may increase the effect of either hydrocodone or antidepressant).
No products indexed under this heading.

Dezocine (Co-administration may exhibit additive CNS depression).
No products indexed under this heading.

Diazepam (Co-administration may exhibit additive CNS depression). Products include:
Valium Tablets 2880

Dicyclomine Hydrochloride (Co-administration may produce paralytic ileus). Products include:
Bentyl Capsules 780
Bentyl Injection 780
Bentyl Syrup 780
Bentyl Tablets 780

Dihydrocodeine Bitartrate (Co-administration may exhibit additive CNS depression).
No products indexed under this heading.

Dihydrocodeinone Bitartrate (Co-administration may exhibit additive CNS depression).
No products indexed under this heading.

Doxepin Hydrochloride (Co-administration of tricyclic antidepressants with hydrocodone may increase the effect of either hydrocodone or antidepressant).
No products indexed under this heading.

Droperidol (Co-administration may exhibit additive CNS depression).
No products indexed under this heading.

Enflurane (Co-administration may exhibit additive CNS depression).
No products indexed under this heading.

Estazolam (Co-administration may exhibit additive CNS depression).
No products indexed under this heading.

Ethanol (Co-administration may exhibit additive CNS depression).
No products indexed under this heading.

Ethchlorvynol (Co-administration may exhibit additive CNS depression).
No products indexed under this heading.

Ethinamate (Co-administration may exhibit additive CNS depression).
No products indexed under this heading.

Ethyl Alcohol (Co-administration may exhibit additive CNS depression).
No products indexed under this heading.

Fentanyl (Co-administration may exhibit additive CNS depression). Products include:
Duragesic 2604
Fentanyl Transdermal System 2346
Onsolis 2054

Fentanyl Citrate (Co-administration may exhibit additive CNS depression). Products include:
Fentora 966

Fluphenazine Decanoate (Co-administration may exhibit additive CNS depression).
No products indexed under this heading.

Fluphenazine Enanthate (Co-administration may exhibit additive CNS depression).
No products indexed under this heading.

Fluphenazine Hydrochloride (Co-administration may exhibit additive CNS depression).
No products indexed under this heading.

Flurazepam Hydrochloride (Co-administration may exhibit additive CNS depression).
No products indexed under this heading.

Glutethimide (Co-administration may exhibit additive CNS depression).
No products indexed under this heading.

Glycopyrrolate (Co-administration may produce paralytic ileus).
No products indexed under this heading.

Halazepam (Co-administration may exhibit additive CNS depression).
No products indexed under this heading.

Haloperidol (Co-administration may exhibit additive CNS depression).
No products indexed under this heading.

Haloperidol Decanoate (Co-administration may exhibit additive CNS depression).
No products indexed under this heading.

Haloperidol Lactate (Co-administration may exhibit additive CNS depression).
No products indexed under this heading.

Hexobarbital (Co-administration may exhibit additive CNS depression).
No products indexed under this heading.

Hydrocodone Polistirex (Co-administration may exhibit additive CNS depression). Products include:
Tussionex 3443

Hydromorphone (Co-administration may exhibit additive CNS depression).
No products indexed under this heading.

Hydromorphone Hydrochloride (Co-administration may exhibit additive CNS depression). Products include:
Dilaudid Injection 2800
Dilaudid Oral 2797
Dilaudid Tablets 2797
Dilaudid-HP 2800

Hydroxyzine Hydrochloride (Co-administration may exhibit additive CNS depression).
No products indexed under this heading.

Hyoscyamine (Co-administration may produce paralytic ileus).
No products indexed under this heading.

Hyoscyamine Sulfate (Co-administration may produce paralytic ileus). Products include:
Donnatal 2711

Imipramine Hydrochloride (Co-administration of tricyclic antidepressants with hydrocodone may increase the effect of either hydrocodone or antidepressant).
No products indexed under this heading.

Imipramine Pamoate (Co-administration of tricyclic antidepressants with hydrocodone may increase the effect of either hydrocodone or antidepressant).
No products indexed under this heading.

Ipratropium Bromide (Co-administration may produce paralytic ileus).
No products indexed under this heading.

Isocarboxazid (Co-administration of MAO inhibitors with hydrocodone may increase the effect of either hydrocodone or MAO inhibitor). Products include:
Marplan 3481

Isoflurane (Co-administration may exhibit additive CNS depression).
No products indexed under this heading.

Ketamine Hydrochloride (Co-administration may exhibit additive CNS depression).
No products indexed under this heading.

Levomethadyl Acetate Hydrochloride (Co-administration may exhibit additive CNS depression).
No products indexed under this heading.

Levorphanol Tartrate (Co-administration may exhibit additive CNS depression).
No products indexed under this heading.

Lorazepam (Co-administration may exhibit additive CNS depression).
No products indexed under this heading.

Loxapine Hydrochloride (Co-administration may exhibit additive CNS depression).
No products indexed under this heading.

Loxapine Succinate (Co-administration may exhibit additive CNS depression).
No products indexed under this heading.

Maprotiline Hydrochloride (Co-administration of tricyclic antidepressants with hydrocodone may increase the effect of either hydrocodone or antidepressant).
No products indexed under this heading.

IMPORTANT NOTE: Always consult each drug listing in the patient's regimen for possible interactions.

Mepenzolate Bromide (Co-administration may produce paralytic ileus).
No products indexed under this heading.

Meperidine Hydrochloride (Co-administration may exhibit additive CNS depression).
No products indexed under this heading.

Mephobarbital (Co-administration may exhibit additive CNS depression).
No products indexed under this heading.

Meprobamate (Co-administration may exhibit additive CNS depression).
No products indexed under this heading.

Mesoridazine Besylate (Co-administration may exhibit additive CNS depression).
No products indexed under this heading.

Methadone Hydrochloride (Co-administration may exhibit additive CNS depression).
No products indexed under this heading.

Methohexital Sodium (Co-administration may exhibit additive CNS depression).
No products indexed under this heading.

Methotrimeprazine (Co-administration may exhibit additive CNS depression).
No products indexed under this heading.

Methoxyflurane (Co-administration may exhibit additive CNS depression).
No products indexed under this heading.

Midazolam Hydrochloride (Co-administration may exhibit additive CNS depression).
No products indexed under this heading.

Moclobemide (Co-administration of MAO inhibitors with hydrocodone may increase the effect of either hydrocodone or MAO inhibitor).
No products indexed under this heading.

Molindone Hydrochloride (Co-administration may exhibit additive CNS depression). Products include:
Moban 1108

Morphine Sulfate (Co-administration may exhibit additive CNS depression). Products include:
Avinza 1822
Embeda 1831
MS Contin 2803

Morphine Sulfate, Liposomal (Co-administration may exhibit additive CNS depression).
No products indexed under this heading.

Nortriptyline Hydrochloride (Co-administration of tricyclic antidepressants with hydrocodone may increase the effect of either hydrocodone or anti-depressant).
No products indexed under this heading.

Olanzapine (Co-administration may exhibit additive CNS depression). Products include:
Symbyax 1965
Zyprexa 1984
Zyprexa IntraMuscular 1984
Zyprexa ZYDIS 1984

Oxazepam (Co-administration may exhibit additive CNS depression).
No products indexed under this heading.

Oxybutynin Chloride (Co-administration may produce paralytic ileus).
No products indexed under this heading.

Oxycodone Hydrochloride (Co-administration may exhibit additive CNS depression). Products include:
OxyContin 2807
Percocet 1121
Percodan 1124

Oxycodone Terephthalate (Co-administration may exhibit additive CNS depression).
No products indexed under this heading.

Oxymorphone Hydrochloride (Co-administration may exhibit additive CNS depression). Products include:
Opana 1110
Opana ER 1114

Pargyline Hydrochloride (Co-administration of MAO inhibitors with hydrocodone may increase the effect of either hydrocodone or MAO inhibitor).
No products indexed under this heading.

Pentobarbital (Co-administration may exhibit additive CNS depression).
No products indexed under this heading.

Pentobarbital Sodium (Co-administration may exhibit additive CNS depression). Products include:
Nembutal 2012

Perphenazine (Co-administration may exhibit additive CNS depression).
No products indexed under this heading.

Phenelzine Sulfate (Co-administration of MAO inhibitors with hydrocodone may increase the effect of either hydrocodone or MAO inhibitor).
No products indexed under this heading.

Phenobarbital (Co-administration may exhibit additive CNS depression). Products include:
Donnatal 2711

Phenobarbital Sodium (Co-administration may exhibit additive CNS depression).
No products indexed under this heading.

Prazepam (Co-administration may exhibit additive CNS depression).
No products indexed under this heading.

Procarbazine Hydrochloride (Co-administration of MAO inhibitors with hydrocodone may increase the effect of either hydrocodone or MAO inhibitor).
No products indexed under this heading.

Prochlorperazine (Co-administration may exhibit additive CNS depression).
No products indexed under this heading.

Prochlorperazine Edisylate (Co-administration may exhibit additive CNS depression).
No products indexed under this heading.

Prochlorperazine Maleate (Co-administration may exhibit additive CNS depression).
No products indexed under this heading.

Procyclidine Hydrochloride (Co-administration may produce paralytic ileus).
No products indexed under this heading.

Promethazine (Co-administration may exhibit additive CNS depression).
No products indexed under this heading.

Promethazine Hydrochloride (Co-administration may exhibit additive CNS depression).
No products indexed under this heading.

Propantheline Bromide (Co-administration may produce paralytic ileus).
No products indexed under this heading.

Propofol (Co-administration may exhibit additive CNS depression).
No products indexed under this heading.

Propoxyphene Hydrochloride (Co-administration may exhibit additive CNS depression).
No products indexed under this heading.

Propoxyphene Napsylate (Co-administration may exhibit additive CNS depression).
No products indexed under this heading.

Protriptyline Hydrochloride (Co-administration of tricyclic antidepressants with hydrocodone may increase the effect of either hydrocodone or anti-depressant).
No products indexed under this heading.

Quazepam (Co-administration may exhibit additive CNS depression).
No products indexed under this heading.

Quetiapine Fumarate (Co-administration may exhibit additive CNS depression). Products include:
Seroquel 750
Seroquel XR 759

Rasagiline Mesylate (Co-administration of MAO inhibitors with hydrocodone may increase the effect of either hydrocodone or MAO inhibitor). Products include:
Azilect 3383

Remifentanil Hydrochloride (Co-administration may exhibit additive CNS depression).
No products indexed under this heading.

Risperidone (Co-administration may exhibit additive CNS depression). Products include:
Risperdal Consta 2682

Scopolamine (Co-administration may produce paralytic ileus). Products include:
Transderm Scōp 2397

Scopolamine Hydrobromide (Co-administration may produce paralytic ileus). Products include:
Donnatal 2711

Secobarbital Sodium (Co-administration may exhibit additive CNS depression).
No products indexed under this heading.

Selegiline (Co-administration of MAO inhibitors with hydrocodone may increase the effect of either hydrocodone or MAO inhibitor). Products include:
Emsam 3623

Selegiline Hydrochloride (Co-administration of MAO inhibitors with hydrocodone may increase the effect of either hydrocodone or MAO inhibitor). Products include:
Eldepryl 3312

Sevoflurane (Co-administration may exhibit additive CNS depression). Products include:
Ultane 554

Sodium Butabarbital (Co-administration may exhibit additive CNS depression).
No products indexed under this heading.

Sodium Oxybate (Co-administration may exhibit additive CNS depression).
No products indexed under this heading.

Sodium Pentobarbital (Co-administration may exhibit additive CNS depression).
No products indexed under this heading.

Sufentanil Citrate (Co-administration may exhibit additive CNS depression).
No products indexed under this heading.

Talbutal (Co-administration may exhibit additive CNS depression).
No products indexed under this heading.

Temazepam (Co-administration may exhibit additive CNS depression).
No products indexed under this heading.

Thiamylal Sodium (Co-administration may exhibit additive CNS depression).
No products indexed under this heading.

Thioridazine (Co-administration may exhibit additive CNS depression).
No products indexed under this heading.

Thioridazine Hydrochloride (Co-administration may exhibit additive CNS depression). Products include:
Thioridazine Hydrochloride 2384

Thiothixene (Co-administration may exhibit additive CNS depression). Products include:
Thiothixene 2386

Thiothixene Hydrochloride (Co-administration may exhibit additive CNS depression).
No products indexed under this heading.

Tolterodine Tartrate (Co-administration may produce paralytic ileus).
No products indexed under this heading.

Tranylcypromine Sulfate (Co-administration of MAO inhibitors with hydrocodone may increase the effect of either hydrocodone or MAO inhibitor). Products include:
Parnate 1584

Triazolam (Co-administration may exhibit additive CNS depression).
No products indexed under this heading.

Tridihexethyl Chloride (Co-administration may produce paralytic ileus).
No products indexed under this heading.

Trifluoperazine Hydrochloride (Co-administration may exhibit additive CNS depression).
No products indexed under this heading.

Trihexyphenidyl Hydrochloride (Co-administration may produce paralytic ileus).
No products indexed under this heading.

Trimipramine Maleate (Co-administration of tricyclic antidepressants with hydrocodone may increase the effect of either hydrocodone or anti-depressant).
No products indexed under this heading.

Zaleplon (Co-administration may exhibit additive CNS depression).
No products indexed under this heading.

Ziprasidone Hydrochloride (Co-administration may exhibit additive CNS depression). Products include:
Geodon 2723

Zolpidem Tartrate (Co-administration may exhibit additive CNS depression). Products include:
Ambien 2920
Ambien CR 2925

Food Interactions

Alcohol (Co-administration may exhibit additive CNS depression).

Beer, reduced-alcohol (Co-administration may exhibit additive CNS depression).

Beer, unspecified (Co-administration may exhibit additive CNS depression).

Wine, Chianti (Co-administration may exhibit additive CNS depression).

Wine, Red (Co-administration may exhibit additive CNS depression).

Wine, unspecified (Co-administration may exhibit additive CNS depression).

Wine products (Co-administration may exhibit additive CNS depression).

ZYLET OPHTHALMIC SUSPENSION

(Loteprednol Etabonate, Tobramycin) .... ⊙252
None cited in PDR database.

ZYPREXA TABLETS

(Olanzapine) 1984
May interact with alcohols, antihypertensives, central nervous system depressants, central nervous system stimulants, cytochrome p450 1a2 inducers (selected), cytochrome p450 1a2 inhibitors (selected), dopamine agonists, drugs that elevate levels of glucuronosyl transferase, and certain other agents. Compounds in these categories include:

Acebutolol Hydrochloride (Olanzapine, because of its potential for inducing hypotension, may enhance the effects of certain antihypertensive agents).
No products indexed under this heading.

Alatrofloxacin Mesylate (Concomitant use may potentially inhibit olanzapine clearance; therefore, a dosage decrease may need to be considered).
No products indexed under this heading.

Alfentanil Hydrochloride (Given the primary CNS effects of olanzapine, caution should be used when olanzapine is taken in combination with other centrally-acting drugs).
No products indexed under this heading.

Aliskiren (Olanzapine, because of its potential for inducing hypotension, may enhance the effects of certain antihypertensive agents). Products include:
Tekturna 2538
Tekturna HCT 2541
Valturna 3637

Alprazolam (Given the primary CNS effects of olanzapine, caution should be used when olanzapine is taken in combination with other centrally-acting drugs).
No products indexed under this heading.

Amiodarone Hydrochloride (Concomitant use may potentially inhibit olanzapine clearance; therefore, a dosage decrease may need to be considered).
No products indexed under this heading.

Amlodipine Besylate (Olanzapine, because of its potential for inducing hypotension, may enhance the effects of certain antihypertensive agents). Products include:
Azor 1010
Exforge 2443
Exforge HCT 2449

Amobarbital (Given the primary CNS effects of olanzapine, caution should be used when olanzapine is taken in combination with other centrally-acting drugs).
No products indexed under this heading.

Amobarbital Sodium (Given the primary CNS effects of olanzapine, caution should be used when olanzapine is taken in combination with other centrally-acting drugs).
No products indexed under this heading.

Amphetamine Aspartate (Given the primary CNS effects of olanzapine, caution should be used when olanzapine is taken in combination with other centrally-acting drugs).
No products indexed under this heading.

Amphetamine Aspartate Monohydrate (Given the primary CNS effects of olanzapine, caution should be used when olanzapine is taken in combination with other centrally-acting drugs).
No products indexed under this heading.

Amphetamine Resins (Given the primary CNS effects of olanzapine, caution should be used when olanzapine is taken in combination with other centrally-acting drugs).
No products indexed under this heading.

Amphetamine Sulfate (Given the primary CNS effects of olanzapine, caution should be used when olanzapine is taken in combination with other centrally-acting drugs).
No products indexed under this heading.

Anastrozole (Concomitant use may potentially inhibit olanzapine clearance; therefore, a dosage decrease may need to be considered).
No products indexed under this heading.

Aprobarbital (Given the primary CNS effects of olanzapine, caution should be used when olanzapine is taken in combination with other centrally-acting drugs).
No products indexed under this heading.

Atenolol (Olanzapine, because of its potential for inducing hypotension, may enhance the effects of certain antihypertensive agents).
No products indexed under this heading.

Benazepril Hydrochloride (Olanzapine, because of its potential for inducing hypotension, may enhance the effects of certain antihypertensive agents).
No products indexed under this heading.

Bendroflumethiazide (Olanzapine, because of its potential for inducing hypotension, may enhance the effects of certain antihypertensive agents).
No products indexed under this heading.

Betaxolol Hydrochloride (Olanzapine, because of its potential for inducing hypotension, may enhance the effects of certain antihypertensive agents).
No products indexed under this heading.

Bisoprolol Fumarate (Olanzapine, because of its potential for inducing hypotension, may enhance the effects of certain antihypertensive agents).
No products indexed under this heading.

Bromocriptine Mesylate (Olanzapine may antagonize the effects of dopamine agonists).
No products indexed under this heading.

Buprenorphine Hydrochloride (Given the primary CNS effects of olanzapine, caution should be used when olanzapine is taken in combination with other centrally-acting drugs).
No products indexed under this heading.

Buspirone Hydrochloride (Given the primary CNS effects of olanzapine, caution should be used when olanzapine is taken in combination with other centrally-acting drugs).
No products indexed under this heading.

Butabarbital (Given the primary CNS effects of olanzapine, caution should be used when olanzapine is taken in combination with other centrally-acting drugs).
No products indexed under this heading.

Butabarbital Sodium (Given the primary CNS effects of olanzapine, caution should be used when olanzapine is taken in combination with other centrally-acting drugs).
No products indexed under this heading.

Butalbital (Given the primary CNS effects of olanzapine, caution should be used when olanzapine is taken in combination with other centrally-acting drugs).
No products indexed under this heading.

Candesartan Cilexetil (Olanzapine, because of its potential for inducing hypotension, may enhance the effects of certain antihypertensive agents). Products include:
Atacand 697
Atacand HCT 700

Captopril (Olanzapine, because of its potential for inducing hypotension, may enhance the effects of certain antihypertensive agents). Products include:
Captopril 2341

Carbamazepine (Carbamazepine therapy (200 mg bid) causes an approximately 50% increase in the clearance of olanzapine. This increase is likely due to the fact that carbamazepine is a potent inducer of CYP1A2 activity. Higher daily doses of carbamazepine may cause an even greater increase in olanzapine clearance). Products include:
Carbatrol 3280
Equetro 3477

Carteolol Hydrochloride (Olanzapine, because of its potential for inducing hypotension, may enhance the effects of certain antihypertensive agents).
No products indexed under this heading.

Carvedilol (Olanzapine, because of its potential for inducing hypotension, may enhance the effects of certain antihypertensive agents). Products include:
Coreg 1409

Carvedilol Phosphate (Olanzapine, because of its potential for inducing

hypotension, may enhance the effects of certain antihypertensive agents). Products include:
Coreg CR 1416

Charcoal, Activated (Co-administration with activated charcoal (1 g) reduced the C_{max} and AUC of oral olanzapine by about 60%. As peak olanzapine levels are not typically obtained until about 6 hours after dosing, charcoal may be a useful treatment for olanzapine overdose).
No products indexed under this heading.

Chlordiazepoxide (Given the primary CNS effects of olanzapine, caution should be used when olanzapine is taken in combination with other centrally-acting drugs).
No products indexed under this heading.

Chlordiazepoxide Hydrochloride (Given the primary CNS effects of olanzapine, caution should be used when olanzapine is taken in combination with other centrally-acting drugs).
No products indexed under this heading.

Chlorothiazide (Olanzapine, because of its potential for inducing hypotension, may enhance the effects of certain antihypertensive agents).
No products indexed under this heading.

Chlorothiazide Sodium (Olanzapine, because of its potential for inducing hypotension, may enhance the effects of certain antihypertensive agents). Products include:
Diuril Intravenous 2009

Chlorpromazine (Given the primary CNS effects of olanzapine, caution should be used when olanzapine is taken in combination with other centrally-acting drugs).
No products indexed under this heading.

Chlorpromazine Hydrochloride (Given the primary CNS effects of olanzapine, caution should be used when olanzapine is taken in combination with other centrally-acting drugs).
No products indexed under this heading.

Chlorprothixene (Given the primary CNS effects of olanzapine, caution should be used when olanzapine is taken in combination with other centrally-acting drugs).
No products indexed under this heading.

Chlorprothixene Hydrochloride (Given the primary CNS effects of olanzapine, caution should be used when olanzapine is taken in combination with other centrally-acting drugs).
No products indexed under this heading.

Chlorprothixene Lactate (Given the primary CNS effects of olanzapine, caution should be used when olanzapine is taken in combination with other centrally-acting drugs).
No products indexed under this heading.

Chlorthalidone (Olanzapine, because of its potential for inducing hypotension, may enhance the effects of certain antihypertensive agents). Products include:
Clorpres 2344

Cimetidine (Concomitant use may potentially inhibit olanzapine clearance; therefore, a dosage decrease may need to be considered).
No products indexed under this heading.

Cimetidine Hydrochloride (Concomitant use may potentially inhibit olanzapine clearance; therefore, a dosage decrease may need to be considered).
No products indexed under this heading.

Ciprofloxacin (Concomitant use may potentially inhibit olanzapine clearance; therefore, a dosage decrease may need to be considered). Products include:
Cipro I.V. 3082
Cipro 3073
Cipro XR 3091
Ciprodex 583

Ciprofloxacin Hydrochloride (Concomitant use may potentially inhibit olanzapine clearance; therefore, a dosage decrease may need to be considered). Products include:
Cipro 3073

Citalopram Hydrobromide (Concomitant use may cause an increase in olanzapine clearance). Products include:
Celexa 1153

Clarithromycin (Concomitant use may potentially inhibit olanzapine clearance; therefore, a dosage decrease may need to be considered). Products include:
Biaxin/Biaxin XL 412

Clonazepam (Given the primary CNS effects of olanzapine, caution should be used when olanzapine is taken in combination with other centrally-acting drugs). Products include:
Klonopin 2855

Clonidine (Olanzapine, because of its potential for inducing hypotension, may enhance the effects of certain antihypertensive agents). Products include:
Catapres-TTS 884

Clonidine Hydrochloride (Olanzapine, because of its potential for inducing hypotension, may enhance the effects of certain antihypertensive agents). Products include:
Clorpres 2344

Clorazepate Dipotassium (Given the primary CNS effects of olanzapine, caution should be used when olanzapine is taken in combination with other centrally-acting drugs).
No products indexed under this heading.

Clozapine (Given the primary CNS effects of olanzapine, caution should be used when olanzapine is taken in combination with other centrally-acting drugs).
No products indexed under this heading.

Codeine Phosphate (Given the primary CNS effects of olanzapine, caution should be used when olanzapine is taken in combination with other centrally-acting drugs). Products include:
Tylenol with Codeine 2691

Codeine Sulfate (Given the primary CNS effects of olanzapine, caution should be used when olanzapine is taken in combination with other centrally-acting drugs).
No products indexed under this heading.

Deserpidine (Olanzapine, because of its potential for inducing hypotension, may enhance the effects of certain antihypertensive agents).
No products indexed under this heading.

Desflurane (Given the primary CNS effects of olanzapine, caution should be used when olanzapine is taken in combination with other centrally-acting drugs).
No products indexed under this heading.

Desogestrel (Concomitant use may potentially inhibit olanzapine clearance; therefore, a dosage decrease may need to be considered).
No products indexed under this heading.

Dexmethylphenidate Hydrochloride (Given the primary CNS effects of olanzapine, caution should be used when olanzapine is taken in combination with other centrally-acting drugs). Products include:
Focalin XR 2472

Dextroamphetamine (Given the primary CNS effects of olanzapine, caution should be used when olanzapine is taken in combination with other centrally-acting drugs).
No products indexed under this heading.

IMPORTANT NOTE: Always consult each drug listing in the patient's regimen for possible interactions.

Dextroamphetamine Saccharate (Given the primary CNS effects of olanzapine, caution should be used when olanzapine is taken in combination with other centrally-acting drugs).
No products indexed under this heading.

Dextroamphetamine Sulfate (Given the primary CNS effects of olanzapine, caution should be used when olanzapine is taken in combination with other centrally-acting drugs). Products include:
Dexedrine 1425

Dezocine (Given the primary CNS effects of olanzapine, caution should be used when olanzapine is taken in combination with other centrally-acting drugs).
No products indexed under this heading.

Diazepam (Co-administration of diazepam with olanzapine may potentiate orthostatic hypotension). Products include:
Valium Tablets 2880

Diazoxide (Olanzapine, because of its potential for inducing hypotension, may enhance the effects of certain antihypertensive agents). Products include:
Proglycem 1179
Proglycem Suspension 1179

Diltiazem Hydrochloride (Olanzapine, because of its potential for inducing hypotension, may enhance the effects of certain antihypertensive agents). Products include:
Cardizem LA 423

Diltiazem Maleate (Olanzapine, because of its potential for inducing hypotension, may enhance the effects of certain antihypertensive agents).
No products indexed under this heading.

Dopamine Hydrochloride (Olanzapine may antagonize the effects of dopamine agonists).
No products indexed under this heading.

Doxazosin Mesylate (Olanzapine, because of its potential for inducing hypotension, may enhance the effects of certain antihypertensive agents).
No products indexed under this heading.

Droperidol (Given the primary CNS effects of olanzapine, caution should be used when olanzapine is taken in combination with other centrally-acting drugs).
No products indexed under this heading.

Enalapril Maleate (Olanzapine, because of its potential for inducing hypotension, may enhance the effects of certain antihypertensive agents).
No products indexed under this heading.

Enalaprilat (Olanzapine, because of its potential for inducing hypotension, may enhance the effects of certain antihypertensive agents).
No products indexed under this heading.

Enflurane (Given the primary CNS effects of olanzapine, caution should be used when olanzapine is taken in combination with other centrally-acting drugs).
No products indexed under this heading.

Enoxacin (Concomitant use may potentially inhibit olanzapine clearance; therefore, a dosage decrease may need to be considered).
No products indexed under this heading.

Eprosartan Mesylate (Olanzapine, because of its potential for inducing hypotension, may enhance the effects of certain antihypertensive agents). Products include:
Teveten 538
Teveten HCT 541

Erythromycin (Concomitant use may cause an increase in olanzapine clearance).
No products indexed under this heading.

Erythromycin, Topical (Concomitant use may cause an increase in olanzapine clearance).
No products indexed under this heading.

Erythromycin Estolate (Concomitant use may cause an increase in olanzapine clearance).
No products indexed under this heading.

Erythromycin Ethylsuccinate (Concomitant use may cause an increase in olanzapine clearance). Products include:
E.E.S. 437
EryPed 435

Erythromycin Gluceptate (Concomitant use may cause an increase in olanzapine clearance).
No products indexed under this heading.

Erythromycin Lactobionate (Concomitant use may cause an increase in olanzapine clearance).
No products indexed under this heading.

Erythromycin Stearate (Concomitant use may cause an increase in olanzapine clearance).
No products indexed under this heading.

Escitalopram Oxalate (Concomitant use may cause an increase in olanzapine clearance). Products include:
Lexapro Oral Suspension 1160
Lexapro Tablets 1160

Esmolol Hydrochloride (Olanzapine, because of its potential for inducing hypotension, may enhance the effects of certain antihypertensive agents).
No products indexed under this heading.

Esomeprazole Magnesium (Concomitant use may potentially inhibit olanzapine clearance; therefore, a dosage decrease may need to be considered). Products include:
Nexium Capsules 704
Nexium Oral Suspension 704

Esomeprazole Sodium (Concomitant use may potentially inhibit olanzapine clearance; therefore, a dosage decrease may need to be considered). Products include:
Nexium I.V. 712

Estazolam (Given the primary CNS effects of olanzapine, caution should be used when olanzapine is taken in combination with other centrally-acting drugs).
No products indexed under this heading.

Ethanol (Co-administration of alcohol with olanzapine potentiates orthostatic hypotension; concurrent use should be avoided. Given the primary CNS effects of olanzapine, caution should be used when olanzapine is taken in combination with other centrally-acting drugs and alcohol).
No products indexed under this heading.

Ethchlorvynol (Given the primary CNS effects of olanzapine, caution should be used when olanzapine is taken in combination with other centrally-acting drugs).
No products indexed under this heading.

Ethinamate (Given the primary CNS effects of olanzapine, caution should be used when olanzapine is taken in combination with other centrally-acting drugs).
No products indexed under this heading.

Ethinyl Estradiol (Concomitant use may potentially inhibit olanzapine clearance; therefore, a dosage decrease may need to be considered). Products include:
LoSeasonique 3407
Lybrel 3514
NuvaRing 3181
Ortho Evra 2648
Ortho-Cyclen/Ortho Tri-Cyclen 2663
Ortho Tri-Cyclen Lo Tablets 2673
Seasonique 3418
Yaz 864

Ethyl Alcohol (Co-administration of alcohol with olanzapine potentiates orthostatic hypotension; concurrent use should be avoided. Given the primary CNS effects of olanzapine, caution should be used when olanzapine is taken in combination with other centrally-acting drugs and alcohol).
No products indexed under this heading.

Felodipine (Olanzapine, because of its potential for inducing hypotension, may enhance the effects of certain antihypertensive agents).
No products indexed under this heading.

Fentanyl (Given the primary CNS effects of olanzapine, caution should be used when olanzapine is taken in combination with other centrally-acting drugs). Products include:
Duragesic 2604
Fentanyl Transdermal System 2346
Onsolis 2054

Fentanyl Citrate (Given the primary CNS effects of olanzapine, caution should be used when olanzapine is taken in combination with other centrally-acting drugs). Products include:
Fentora 966

Fluoxetine (Fluoxetine (60 mg single dose or 60 mg daily dose for 8 days) causes a small (mean 16%) increase in the maximum concentration of olanzapine and a small (mean 16%) decrease in olanzapine clearance. The magnitude of the impact of this factor is small in comparison to the overall variability between individuals, and therefore, dose modification is not routinely recommended).
No products indexed under this heading.

Fluoxetine Hydrochloride (Fluoxetine (60 mg single dose or 60 mg daily dose for 8 days) causes a small (mean 16%) increase in the maximum concentration of olanzapine and a small (mean 16%) decrease in olanzapine clearance. The magnitude of the impact of this factor is small in comparison to the overall variability between individuals, and therefore, dose modification is not routinely recommended). Products include:
Prozac Weekly 1941
Prozac Pulvules 1941
Symbyax 1965

Fluphenazine Decanoate (Given the primary CNS effects of olanzapine, caution should be used when olanzapine is taken in combination with other centrally-acting drugs).
No products indexed under this heading.

Fluphenazine Enanthate (Given the primary CNS effects of olanzapine, caution should be used when olanzapine is taken in combination with other centrally-acting drugs).
No products indexed under this heading.

Fluphenazine Hydrochloride (Given the primary CNS effects of olanzapine, caution should be used when olanzapine is taken in combination with other centrally-acting drugs).
No products indexed under this heading.

Flurazepam Hydrochloride (Given the primary CNS effects of olanzapine, caution should be used when olanzapine is taken in combination with other centrally-acting drugs).
No products indexed under this heading.

Fluvoxamine (Fluvoxamine, a CYP1A2 inhibitor, decreases the clearance of olanzapine. This results in a mean increase in olanzapine C_{max} and AUC. Lower doses of olanzapine should be considered in patients receiving concomitant treatment with fluvoxamine).
No products indexed under this heading.

Fluvoxamine Maleate (Fluvoxamine, a CYP1A2 inhibitor, decreases the clearance of olanzapine. This results in a mean increase in olanzapine C_{max} and AUC. Lower doses of olanzapine should be considered in patients receiving concomitant treatment with fluvoxamine).
No products indexed under this heading.

Fosinopril Sodium (Olanzapine, because of its potential for inducing hypotension, may enhance the effects of certain antihypertensive agents).
No products indexed under this heading.

Furosemide (Olanzapine, because of its potential for inducing hypotension, may enhance the effects of certain antihypertensive agents). Products include:
Furosemide 2354

Gatifloxacin (Concomitant use may potentially inhibit olanzapine clearance; therefore, a dosage decrease may need to be considered).
No products indexed under this heading.

Gemifloxacin Mesylate (Concomitant use may potentially inhibit olanzapine clearance; therefore, a dosage decrease may need to be considered).
No products indexed under this heading.

Glutethimide (Given the primary CNS effects of olanzapine, caution should be used when olanzapine is taken in combination with other centrally-acting drugs).
No products indexed under this heading.

Grepafloxacin Hydrochloride (Concomitant use may potentially inhibit olanzapine clearance; therefore, a dosage decrease may need to be considered).
No products indexed under this heading.

Guanabenz Acetate (Olanzapine, because of its potential for inducing hypotension, may enhance the effects of certain antihypertensive agents).
No products indexed under this heading.

Guanethidine (Olanzapine, because of its potential for inducing hypotension, may enhance the effects of certain antihypertensive agents).
No products indexed under this heading.

Guanethidine Monosulfate (Olanzapine, because of its potential for inducing hypotension, may enhance the effects of certain antihypertensive agents).
No products indexed under this heading.

Guanethidine Sulfate (Olanzapine, because of its potential for inducing hypotension, may enhance the effects of certain antihypertensive agents).
No products indexed under this heading.

Halazepam (Given the primary CNS effects of olanzapine, caution should be used when olanzapine is taken in combination with other centrally-acting drugs).
No products indexed under this heading.

Haloperidol (Given the primary CNS effects of olanzapine, caution should be used when olanzapine is taken in combination with other centrally-acting drugs).
No products indexed under this heading.

Haloperidol Decanoate (Given the primary CNS effects of olanzapine, caution should be used when olanzapine is taken in combination with other centrally-acting drugs).
No products indexed under this heading.

Haloperidol Lactate (Given the primary CNS effects of olanzapine, caution should be used when olanzapine is taken in combination with other centrally-acting drugs).
No products indexed under this heading.

Hexobarbital (Given the primary CNS effects of olanzapine, caution should be used when olanzapine is taken in combination with other centrally-acting drugs).
No products indexed under this heading.

IMPORTANT NOTE: Always consult each drug listing in the patient's regimen for possible interactions.

(⊙ Described in PDR® for Ophthalmic Medicines)

IMPORTANT NOTE: Always consult each drug listing in the patient's regimen for possible interactions.

Ambien CR 2925

Food Interactions

Alcohol (Co-administration of alcohol with olanzapine potentiates orthostatic hypotension; concurrent use should be avoided. Given the primary CNS effects of olanzapine, caution should be used when olanzapine is taken in combination with other centrally-acting drugs and alcohol).

Beer, reduced-alcohol (Co-administration of alcohol with olanzapine potentiates orthostatic hypotension; concurrent use should be avoided. Given the primary CNS effects of olanzapine, caution should be used when olanzapine is taken in combination with other centrally-acting drugs and alcohol).

Beer, unspecified (Co-administration of alcohol with olanzapine potentiates orthostatic hypotension; concurrent use should be avoided. Given the primary CNS effects of olanzapine, caution should be used when olanzapine is taken in combination with other centrally-acting drugs and alcohol).

Broccoli (Concomitant use may cause an increase in olanzapine clearance).

Brussel Sprouts (Concomitant use may cause an increase in olanzapine clearance).

Charbroiled Food (Concomitant use may cause an increase in olanzapine clearance).

Grapefruit (Concomitant use may potentially inhibit olanzapine clearance; therefore, a dosage decrease may need to be considered).

Grapefruit Juice (Concomitant use may potentially inhibit olanzapine clearance; therefore, a dosage decrease may need to be considered).

Wine, Chianti (Co-administration of alcohol with olanzapine potentiates orthostatic hypotension; concurrent use should be avoided. Given the primary CNS effects of olanzapine, caution should be used when olanzapine is taken in combination with other centrally-acting drugs and alcohol).

Wine, Red (Co-administration of alcohol with olanzapine potentiates orthostatic hypotension; concurrent use should be avoided. Given the primary CNS effects of olanzapine, caution should be used when olanzapine is taken in combination with other centrally-acting drugs and alcohol).

Wine, unspecified (Co-administration of alcohol with olanzapine potentiates orthostatic hypotension; concurrent use should be avoided. Given the primary CNS effects of olanzapine, caution should be used when olanzapine is taken in combination with other centrally-acting drugs and alcohol).

Wine products (Co-administration of alcohol with olanzapine potentiates orthostatic hypotension; concurrent use should be avoided. Given the primary CNS effects of olanzapine, caution should be used when olanzapine is taken in combination with other centrally-acting drugs and alcohol).

ZYPREXA INTRAMUSCULAR

(Olanzapine) 1984

May interact with alcohols, antihypertensives, benzodiazepines, central nervous system depressants, central nervous system stimulants, cytochrome p450 1a2 inducers (selected), cytochrome p450 1a2 inhibitors (selected), dopamine agonists, drugs that elevate levels of glucuronosyl transferase, and certain other agents. Compounds in these categories include:

Acebutolol Hydrochloride (Olanzapine, because of its potential for inducing hypotension, may enhance the effects of certain antihypertensive agents).
No products indexed under this heading.

Alatrofloxacin Mesylate (Concomitant use may potentially inhibit olanzapine clearance; therefore, a dosage decrease may need to be considered).
No products indexed under this heading.

Alfentanil Hydrochloride (Given the primary CNS effects of olanzapine, caution should be used when olanzapine is taken in combination with other centrally-acting drugs).
No products indexed under this heading.

Aliskiren (Olanzapine, because of its potential for inducing hypotension, may enhance the effects of certain antihypertensive agents). Products include:
Tekturna 2538
Tekturna HCT 2541
Valturna 3637

Alprazolam (Concomitant administration of intramuscular olanzapine and parenteral benzodiazepine has not been studied and is, therefore, not recommended. If use of intramuscular olanzapine in combination with parenteral benzodiazepines is considered, careful evaluation of clinical status for excessive sedation and cardiorespiratory depression is recommended).
No products indexed under this heading.

Amiodarone Hydrochloride (Concomitant use may potentially inhibit olanzapine clearance; therefore, a dosage decrease may need to be considered).
No products indexed under this heading.

Amlodipine Besylate (Olanzapine, because of its potential for inducing hypotension, may enhance the effects of certain antihypertensive agents). Products include:
Azor 1010
Exforge 2443
Exforge HCT 2449

Amobarbital (Given the primary CNS effects of olanzapine, caution should be used when olanzapine is taken in combination with other centrally-acting drugs).
No products indexed under this heading.

Amobarbital Sodium (Given the primary CNS effects of olanzapine, caution should be used when olanzapine is taken in combination with other centrally-acting drugs).
No products indexed under this heading.

Amphetamine Aspartate (Given the primary CNS effects of olanzapine, caution should be used when olanzapine is taken in combination with other centrally-acting drugs).
No products indexed under this heading.

Amphetamine Aspartate Monohydrate (Given the primary CNS effects of olanzapine, caution should be used when olanzapine is taken in combination with other centrally-acting drugs).
No products indexed under this heading.

Amphetamine Resins (Given the primary CNS effects of olanzapine, caution should be used when olanzapine is taken in combination with other centrally-acting drugs).
No products indexed under this heading.

Amphetamine Sulfate (Given the primary CNS effects of olanzapine, caution should be used when olanzapine is taken in combination with other centrally-acting drugs).
No products indexed under this heading.

Anastrozole (Concomitant use may potentially inhibit olanzapine clearance; therefore, a dosage decrease may need to be considered).
No products indexed under this heading.

Aprobarbital (Given the primary CNS effects of olanzapine, caution should be used when olanzapine is taken in combination with other centrally-acting drugs).
No products indexed under this heading.

Atenolol (Olanzapine, because of its potential for inducing hypotension, may enhance the effects of certain antihypertensive agents).
No products indexed under this heading.

Benazepril Hydrochloride (Olanzapine, because of its potential for inducing hypotension, may enhance the effects of certain antihypertensive agents).
No products indexed under this heading.

Bendroflumethiazide (Olanzapine, because of its potential for inducing hypotension, may enhance the effects of certain antihypertensive agents).
No products indexed under this heading.

Betaxolol Hydrochloride (Olanzapine, because of its potential for inducing hypotension, may enhance the effects of certain antihypertensive agents).
No products indexed under this heading.

Bisoprolol Fumarate (Olanzapine, because of its potential for inducing hypotension, may enhance the effects of certain antihypertensive agents).
No products indexed under this heading.

Bromocriptine Mesylate (Olanzapine may antagonize the effects of dopamine agonists).
No products indexed under this heading.

Buprenorphine Hydrochloride (Given the primary CNS effects of olanzapine, caution should be used when olanzapine is taken in combination with other centrally-acting drugs).
No products indexed under this heading.

Buspirone Hydrochloride (Given the primary CNS effects of olanzapine, caution should be used when olanzapine is taken in combination with other centrally-acting drugs).
No products indexed under this heading.

Butabarbital (Given the primary CNS effects of olanzapine, caution should be used when olanzapine is taken in combination with other centrally-acting drugs).
No products indexed under this heading.

Butabarbital Sodium (Given the primary CNS effects of olanzapine, caution should be used when olanzapine is taken in combination with other centrally-acting drugs).
No products indexed under this heading.

Butalbital (Given the primary CNS effects of olanzapine, caution should be used when olanzapine is taken in combination with other centrally-acting drugs).
No products indexed under this heading.

Candesartan Cilexetil (Olanzapine, because of its potential for inducing hypotension, may enhance the effects of certain antihypertensive agents). Products include:
Atacand 697
Atacand HCT 700

Captopril (Olanzapine, because of its potential for inducing hypotension, may enhance the effects of certain antihypertensive agents). Products include:
Captopril 2341

Carbamazepine (Carbamazepine therapy (200 mg bid) causes an approximately 50% increase in the clearance of olanzapine. This increase is likely due to the fact that carbamazepine is a potent inducer of CYP1A2 activity. Higher daily doses of carbamazepine may cause an even greater increase in olanzapine clearance). Products include:
Carbatrol 3280
Equetro 3477

Carteolol Hydrochloride (Olanzapine, because of its potential for inducing hypotension, may enhance the effects of certain antihypertensive agents).
No products indexed under this heading.

Carvedilol (Olanzapine, because of its potential for inducing hypotension, may enhance the effects of certain antihypertensive agents). Products include:
Coreg 1409

Carvedilol Phosphate (Olanzapine, because of its potential for inducing hypotension, may enhance the effects of certain antihypertensive agents). Products include:
Coreg CR 1416

Charcoal, Activated (Co-administration with activated charcoal (1 g) reduced the C_{max} and AUC of oral olanzapine by about 60%. As peak olanzapine levels are not typically obtained until about 6 hours after dosing, charcoal may be a useful treatment for olanzapine overdose).
No products indexed under this heading.

Chlordiazepoxide (Concomitant administration of intramuscular olanzapine and parenteral benzodiazepine has not been studied and is, therefore, not recommended. If use of intramuscular olanzapine in combination with parenteral benzodiazepines is considered, careful evaluation of clinical status for excessive sedation and cardiorespiratory depression is recommended).
No products indexed under this heading.

Chlordiazepoxide Hydrochloride (Concomitant administration of intramuscular olanzapine and parenteral benzodiazepine has not been studied and is, therefore, not recommended. If use of intramuscular olanzapine in combination with parenteral benzodiazepines is considered, careful evaluation of clinical status for excessive sedation and cardiorespiratory depression is recommended).
No products indexed under this heading.

Chlorothiazide (Olanzapine, because of its potential for inducing hypotension, may enhance the effects of certain antihypertensive agents).
No products indexed under this heading.

Chlorothiazide Sodium (Olanzapine, because of its potential for inducing hypotension, may enhance the effects of certain antihypertensive agents). Products include:
Diuril Intravenous 2009

Chlorpromazine (Given the primary CNS effects of olanzapine, caution should be used when olanzapine is taken in combination with other centrally-acting drugs).
No products indexed under this heading.

Chlorpromazine Hydrochloride (Given the primary CNS effects of olanzapine, caution should be used when olanzapine is taken in combination with other centrally-acting drugs).
No products indexed under this heading.

Chlorprothixene (Given the primary CNS effects of olanzapine, caution should be used when olanzapine is taken in combination with other centrally-acting drugs).
No products indexed under this heading.

Chlorprothixene Hydrochloride (Given the primary CNS effects of olanzapine, caution should be used when olanzapine is taken in combination with other centrally-acting drugs).
No products indexed under this heading.

Chlorprothixene Lactate (Given the primary CNS effects of olanzapine, caution should be used when olanzapine is taken in combination with other centrally-acting drugs).
No products indexed under this heading.

Chlorthalidone (Olanzapine, because of its potential for inducing hypotension,

2211 Interactions Index Zyprexa Intramuscular

may enhance the effects of certain antihypertensive agents). Products include:
Clorpres 2344

Cimetidine (Concomitant use may potentially inhibit olanzapine clearance; therefore, a dosage decrease may need to be considered).
No products indexed under this heading.

Cimetidine Hydrochloride (Concomitant use may potentially inhibit olanzapine clearance; therefore, a dosage decrease may need to be considered).
No products indexed under this heading.

Ciprofloxacin (Concomitant use may potentially inhibit olanzapine clearance; therefore, a dosage decrease may need to be considered). Products include:
Cipro I.V. 3082
Cipro 3073
Cipro XR 3091
Ciprodex 583

Ciprofloxacin Hydrochloride (Concomitant use may potentially inhibit olanzapine clearance; therefore, a dosage decrease may need to be considered). Products include:
Cipro 3073

Citalopram Hydrobromide (Concomitant use may cause an increase in olanzapine clearance). Products include:
Celexa 1153

Clarithromycin (Concomitant use may potentially inhibit olanzapine clearance; therefore, a dosage decrease may need to be considered). Products include:
Biaxin/Biaxin XL 412

Clonazepam (Given the primary CNS effects of olanzapine, caution should be used when olanzapine is taken in combination with other centrally-acting drugs). Products include:
Klonopin 2855

Clonidine (Olanzapine, because of its potential for inducing hypotension, may enhance the effects of certain antihypertensive agents). Products include:
Catapres-TTS 884

Clonidine Hydrochloride (Olanzapine, because of its potential for inducing hypotension, may enhance the effects of certain antihypertensive agents). Products include:
Clorpres 2344

Clorazepate Dipotassium (Concomitant administration of intramuscular olanzapine and parenteral benzodiazepine has not been studied and is, therefore, not recommended. If use of intramuscular olanzapine in combination with parenteral benzodiazepines is considered, careful evaluation of clinical status for excessive sedation and cardiorespiratory depression is recommended).
No products indexed under this heading.

Clozapine (Given the primary CNS effects of olanzapine, caution should be used when olanzapine is taken in combination with other centrally-acting drugs).
No products indexed under this heading.

Codeine Phosphate (Given the primary CNS effects of olanzapine, caution should be used when olanzapine is taken in combination with other centrally-acting drugs). Products include:
Tylenol with Codeine 2691

Codeine Sulfate (Given the primary CNS effects of olanzapine, caution should be used when olanzapine is taken in combination with other centrally-acting drugs).
No products indexed under this heading.

Deserpidine (Olanzapine, because of its potential for inducing hypotension, may enhance the effects of certain antihypertensive agents).
No products indexed under this heading.

Desflurane (Given the primary CNS effects of olanzapine, caution should be used when olanzapine is taken in combination with other centrally-acting drugs).
No products indexed under this heading.

Desogestrel (Concomitant use may potentially inhibit olanzapine clearance; therefore, a dosage decrease may need to be considered).
No products indexed under this heading.

Dexmethylphenidate Hydrochloride (Given the primary CNS effects of olanzapine, caution should be used when olanzapine is taken in combination with other centrally-acting drugs). Products include:
Focalin XR 2472

Dextroamphetamine (Given the primary CNS effects of olanzapine, caution should be used when olanzapine is taken in combination with other centrally-acting drugs).
No products indexed under this heading.

Dextroamphetamine Saccharate (Given the primary CNS effects of olanzapine, caution should be used when olanzapine is taken in combination with other centrally-acting drugs).
No products indexed under this heading.

Dextroamphetamine Sulfate (Given the primary CNS effects of olanzapine, caution should be used when olanzapine is taken in combination with other centrally-acting drugs). Products include:
Dexedrine 1425

Dezocine (Given the primary CNS effects of olanzapine, caution should be used when olanzapine is taken in combination with other centrally-acting drugs).
No products indexed under this heading.

Diazepam (Co-administration of diazepam with olanzapine may potentiate orthostatic hypotension). Products include:
Valium Tablets 2880

Diazoxide (Olanzapine, because of its potential for inducing hypotension, may enhance the effects of certain antihypertensive agents). Products include:
Proglycem 1179
Proglycem Suspension 1179

Diltiazem Hydrochloride (Olanzapine, because of its potential for inducing hypotension, may enhance the effects of certain antihypertensive agents). Products include:
Cardizem LA 423

Diltiazem Maleate (Olanzapine, because of its potential for inducing hypotension, may enhance the effects of certain antihypertensive agents).
No products indexed under this heading.

Dopamine Hydrochloride (Olanzapine may antagonize the effects of dopamine agonists).
No products indexed under this heading.

Doxazosin Mesylate (Olanzapine, because of its potential for inducing hypotension, may enhance the effects of certain antihypertensive agents).
No products indexed under this heading.

Droperidol (Given the primary CNS effects of olanzapine, caution should be used when olanzapine is taken in combination with other centrally-acting drugs).
No products indexed under this heading.

Enalapril Maleate (Olanzapine, because of its potential for inducing hypotension, may enhance the effects of certain antihypertensive agents).
No products indexed under this heading.

Enalaprilat (Olanzapine, because of its potential for inducing hypotension, may enhance the effects of certain antihypertensive agents).
No products indexed under this heading.

Enflurane (Given the primary CNS effects of olanzapine, caution should be used when olanzapine is taken in combination with other centrally-acting drugs).
No products indexed under this heading.

Enoxacin (Concomitant use may potentially inhibit olanzapine clearance; therefore, a dosage decrease may need to be considered).
No products indexed under this heading.

Eprosartan Mesylate (Olanzapine, because of its potential for inducing hypotension, may enhance the effects of certain antihypertensive agents). Products include:
Teveten 538
Teveten HCT 541

Erythromycin (Concomitant use may cause an increase in olanzapine clearance).
No products indexed under this heading.

Erythromycin, Topical (Concomitant use may cause an increase in olanzapine clearance).
No products indexed under this heading.

Erythromycin Estolate (Concomitant use may cause an increase in olanzapine clearance).
No products indexed under this heading.

Erythromycin Ethylsuccinate (Concomitant use may cause an increase in olanzapine clearance). Products include:
E.E.S. 437
EryPed 435

Erythromycin Gluceptate (Concomitant use may cause an increase in olanzapine clearance).
No products indexed under this heading.

Erythromycin Lactobionate (Concomitant use may cause an increase in olanzapine clearance).
No products indexed under this heading.

Erythromycin Stearate (Concomitant use may cause an increase in olanzapine clearance).
No products indexed under this heading.

Escitalopram Oxalate (Concomitant use may cause an increase in olanzapine clearance). Products include:
Lexapro Oral Suspension 1160
Lexapro Tablets 1160

Esmolol Hydrochloride (Olanzapine, because of its potential for inducing hypotension, may enhance the effects of certain antihypertensive agents).
No products indexed under this heading.

Esomeprazole Magnesium (Concomitant use may potentially inhibit olanzapine clearance; therefore, a dosage decrease may need to be considered). Products include:
Nexium Capsules 704
Nexium Oral Suspension 704

Esomeprazole Sodium (Concomitant use may potentially inhibit olanzapine clearance; therefore, a dosage decrease may need to be considered). Products include:
Nexium I.V. 712

Estazolam (Concomitant administration of intramuscular olanzapine and parenteral benzodiazepine has not been studied and is, therefore, not recommended. If use of intramuscular olanzapine in combination with parenteral benzodiazepines is considered, careful evaluation of clinical status for excessive sedation and cardiorespiratory depression is recommended).
No products indexed under this heading.

Ethanol (Co-administration of alcohol with olanzapine potentiates orthostatic hypotension; concurrent use should be avoided. Given the primary CNS effects of olanzapine, caution should be used when olanzapine is taken in combination with other centrally-acting drugs and alcohol).
No products indexed under this heading.

Ethchlorvynol (Given the primary CNS effects of olanzapine, caution should be used when olanzapine is taken in combination with other centrally-acting drugs).
No products indexed under this heading.

Ethinamate (Given the primary CNS effects of olanzapine, caution should be used when olanzapine is taken in combination with other centrally-acting drugs).
No products indexed under this heading.

Ethinyl Estradiol (Concomitant use may potentially inhibit olanzapine clearance; therefore, a dosage decrease may need to be considered). Products include:
LoSeasonique 3407
Lybrel 3514
NuvaRing 3181
Ortho Evra 2648
Ortho-Cyclen/Ortho Tri-Cyclen 2663
Ortho Tri-Cyclen Lo Tablets 2673
Seasonique 3418
Yaz 864

Ethyl Alcohol (Co-administration of alcohol with olanzapine potentiates orthostatic hypotension; concurrent use should be avoided. Given the primary CNS effects of olanzapine, caution should be used when olanzapine is taken in combination with other centrally-acting drugs and alcohol).
No products indexed under this heading.

Felodipine (Olanzapine, because of its potential for inducing hypotension, may enhance the effects of certain antihypertensive agents).
No products indexed under this heading.

Fentanyl (Given the primary CNS effects of olanzapine, caution should be used when olanzapine is taken in combination with other centrally-acting drugs). Products include:
Duragesic 2604
Fentanyl Transdermal System 2346
Onsolis 2054

Fentanyl Citrate (Given the primary CNS effects of olanzapine, caution should be used when olanzapine is taken in combination with other centrally-acting drugs). Products include:
Fentora 966

Fluoxetine (Fluoxetine (60 mg single dose or 60 mg daily dose for 8 days) causes a small (mean 16%) increase in the maximum concentration of olanzapine and a small (mean 16%) decrease in olanzapine clearance. The magnitude of the impact of this factor is small in comparison to the overall variability between individuals, and, therefore, dose modification is not routinely recommended).
No products indexed under this heading.

Fluoxetine Hydrochloride (Fluoxetine (60 mg single dose or 60 mg daily dose for 8 days) causes a small (mean 16%) increase in the maximum concentration of olanzapine and a small (mean 16%) decrease in olanzapine clearance. The magnitude of the impact of this factor is small in comparison to the overall variability between individuals, and, therefore, dose modification is not routinely recommended). Products include:
Prozac Weekly 1941
Prozac Pulvules 1941
Symbyax 1965

Fluphenazine Decanoate (Given the primary CNS effects of olanzapine, caution should be used when olanzapine is taken in combination with other centrally-acting drugs).
No products indexed under this heading.

Fluphenazine Enanthate (Given the primary CNS effects of olanzapine, caution should be used when olanzapine is taken in combination with other centrally-acting drugs).
No products indexed under this heading.

IMPORTANT NOTE: Always consult each drug listing in the patient's regimen for possible interactions.

Zyprexa Intramuscular — Interactions Index — 2212

Fluphenazine Hydrochloride (Given the primary CNS effects of olanzapine, caution should be used when olanzapine is taken in combination with other centrally-acting drugs).
No products indexed under this heading.

Flurazepam Hydrochloride (Concomitant administration of intramuscular olanzapine and parenteral benzodiazepine has not been studied and is, therefore, not recommended. If use of intramuscular olanzapine in combination with parenteral benzodiazepines is considered, careful evaluation of clinical status for excessive sedation and cardiorespiratory depression is recommended).
No products indexed under this heading.

Fluvoxamine (Fluvoxamine, a CYP1A2 inhibitor, decreases the clearance of olanzapine. This results in a mean increase in olanzapine C_{max} and AUC. Lower doses of olanzapine should be considered in patients receiving concomitant treatment with fluvoxamine).
No products indexed under this heading.

Fluvoxamine Maleate (Fluvoxamine, a CYP1A2 inhibitor, decreases the clearance of olanzapine. This results in a mean increase in olanzapine C_{max} and AUC. Lower doses of olanzapine should be considered in patients receiving concomitant treatment with fluvoxamine).
No products indexed under this heading.

Fosinopril Sodium (Olanzapine, because of its potential for inducing hypotension, may enhance the effects of certain antihypertensive agents).
No products indexed under this heading.

Furosemide (Olanzapine, because of its potential for inducing hypotension, may enhance the effects of certain antihypertensive agents). Products include:
Furosemide 2354

Gatifloxacin (Concomitant use may potentially inhibit olanzapine clearance; therefore, a dosage decrease may need to be considered).
No products indexed under this heading.

Gemifloxacin Mesylate (Concomitant use may potentially inhibit olanzapine clearance; therefore, a dosage decrease may need to be considered).
No products indexed under this heading.

Glutethimide (Given the primary CNS effects of olanzapine, caution should be used when olanzapine is taken in combination with other centrally-acting drugs).
No products indexed under this heading.

Grepafloxacin Hydrochloride (Concomitant use may potentially inhibit olanzapine clearance; therefore, a dosage decrease may need to be considered).
No products indexed under this heading.

Guanabenz Acetate (Olanzapine, because of its potential for inducing hypotension, may enhance the effects of certain antihypertensive agents).
No products indexed under this heading.

Guanethidine (Olanzapine, because of its potential for inducing hypotension, may enhance the effects of certain antihypertensive agents).
No products indexed under this heading.

Guanethidine Monosulfate (Olanzapine, because of its potential for inducing hypotension, may enhance the effects of certain antihypertensive agents).
No products indexed under this heading.

Guanethidine Sulfate (Olanzapine, because of its potential for inducing hypotension, may enhance the effects of certain antihypertensive agents).
No products indexed under this heading.

Halazepam (Concomitant administration of intramuscular olanzapine and parenteral benzodiazepine has not been studied and is, therefore, not recommended. If use of intramuscular olanzapine in combination with parenteral benzodiazepines is considered, careful evaluation of clinical status for excessive sedation and cardiorespiratory depression is recommended).
No products indexed under this heading.

Haloperidol (Given the primary CNS effects of olanzapine, caution should be used when olanzapine is taken in combination with other centrally-acting drugs).
No products indexed under this heading.

Haloperidol Decanoate (Given the primary CNS effects of olanzapine, caution should be used when olanzapine is taken in combination with other centrally-acting drugs).
No products indexed under this heading.

Haloperidol Lactate (Given the primary CNS effects of olanzapine, caution should be used when olanzapine is taken in combination with other centrally-acting drugs).
No products indexed under this heading.

Hexobarbital (Given the primary CNS effects of olanzapine, caution should be used when olanzapine is taken in combination with other centrally-acting drugs).
No products indexed under this heading.

Hydralazine Hydrochloride (Olanzapine, because of its potential for inducing hypotension, may enhance the effects of certain antihypertensive agents).
No products indexed under this heading.

Hydrochlorothiazide (Olanzapine, because of its potential for inducing hypotension, may enhance the effects of certain antihypertensive agents). Products include:
Atacand HCT 700
Avalide 2956
Benicar HCT 1017
Diovan HCT 2419
Dyazide 1429
Exforge HCT 2449
Hyzaar 2162
Hyzaar 100-12.5 2162
Micardis HCT 889
Prinzide 2246
Tekturna HCT 2541
Teveten HCT 541

Hydrocodone Bitartrate (Given the primary CNS effects of olanzapine, caution should be used when olanzapine is taken in combination with other centrally-acting drugs). Products include:
Vicodin 560
Vicodin ES 561
Vicodin HP 563
Vicoprofen 564
Zydone 1138

Hydrocodone Polistirex (Given the primary CNS effects of olanzapine, caution should be used when olanzapine is taken in combination with other centrally-acting drugs). Products include:
Tussionex 3443

Hydroflumethiazide (Olanzapine, because of its potential for inducing hypotension, may enhance the effects of certain antihypertensive agents).
No products indexed under this heading.

Hydromorphone (Given the primary CNS effects of olanzapine, caution should be used when olanzapine is taken in combination with other centrally-acting drugs).
No products indexed under this heading.

Hydromorphone Hydrochloride (Given the primary CNS effects of olanzapine, caution should be used when olanzapine is taken in combination with other centrally-acting drugs). Products include:
Dilaudid Injection 2800
Dilaudid Oral 2797
Dilaudid Tablets 2797
Dilaudid-HP 2800

Hydroxyamphetamine Hydrobromide (Given the primary CNS effects of olanzapine, caution should be used when olanzapine is taken in combination with other centrally-acting drugs).
No products indexed under this heading.

Hydroxyzine Hydrochloride (Given the primary CNS effects of olanzapine, caution should be used when olanzapine is taken in combination with other centrally-acting drugs).
No products indexed under this heading.

Hypericum (Concomitant use may cause an increase in olanzapine clearance).
No products indexed under this heading.

Hypericum Perforatum (Concomitant use may cause an increase in olanzapine clearance). Products include:
Traumeel 1800

Indapamide (Olanzapine, because of its potential for inducing hypotension, may enhance the effects of certain antihypertensive agents). Products include:
Indapamide 2356

Insulin (Concomitant use may cause an increase in olanzapine clearance).
No products indexed under this heading.

Insulin, Human, Zinc Suspension (Concomitant use may cause an increase in olanzapine clearance).
No products indexed under this heading.

Insulin, Human (rDNA origin) (Concomitant use may cause an increase in olanzapine clearance). Products include:
Exubera 2717

Insulin, Human NPH (Concomitant use may cause an increase in olanzapine clearance). Products include:
Humulin N Vial 1934

Insulin, Human Regular (Concomitant use may cause an increase in olanzapine clearance). Products include:
Humulin R 1937
Humulin R (U-500) 1939

Insulin, Human Regular and Human NPH Mixture (Concomitant use may cause an increase in olanzapine clearance). Products include:
Humulin 50/50 1930
Humulin 70/30 Vial 1931

Insulin, NPH (Concomitant use may cause an increase in olanzapine clearance).
No products indexed under this heading.

Insulin, Regular (Concomitant use may cause an increase in olanzapine clearance).
No products indexed under this heading.

Insulin, Regular and NPH mixture (Concomitant use may cause an increase in olanzapine clearance).
No products indexed under this heading.

Insulin, Zinc Crystals (Concomitant use may cause an increase in olanzapine clearance).
No products indexed under this heading.

Insulin, Zinc Suspension (Concomitant use may cause an increase in olanzapine clearance).
No products indexed under this heading.

Insulin Aspart (Concomitant use may cause an increase in olanzapine clearance).
No products indexed under this heading.

Insulin Aspart, Human (Concomitant use may cause an increase in olanzapine clearance). Products include:
NovoLog Mix 70/30 2581

Insulin Aspart, Human Regular (Concomitant use may cause an increase in olanzapine clearance). Products include:
NovoLog 2575

Insulin Aspart Protamine, Human (Concomitant use may cause an increase in olanzapine clearance). Products include:
NovoLog Mix 70/30 2581

Insulin Detemir (rDNA Origin) (Concomitant use may cause an increase in olanzapine clearance). Products include:
Levemir 2566

Insulin Glargine (Concomitant use may cause an increase in olanzapine clearance). Products include:
Lantus 2996

Insulin Glulisine (Concomitant use may cause an increase in olanzapine clearance). Products include:
Apidra 2937
Apidra SoloStar 2937

Insulin Lispro, Human (Concomitant use may cause an increase in olanzapine clearance). Products include:
Humalog 1910
Humalog Mix 1914
Humalog Mix75/25 1917

Insulin Lispro Protamine, Human (Concomitant use may cause an increase in olanzapine clearance). Products include:
Humalog Mix 1914
Humalog Mix75/25 1917

Irbesartan (Olanzapine, because of its potential for inducing hypotension, may enhance the effects of certain antihypertensive agents). Products include:
Avalide 2956
Avapro 2962

Isoflurane (Given the primary CNS effects of olanzapine, caution should be used when olanzapine is taken in combination with other centrally-acting drugs).
No products indexed under this heading.

Isoniazid (Concomitant use may potentially inhibit olanzapine clearance; therefore, a dosage decrease may need to be considered).
No products indexed under this heading.

Isradipine (Olanzapine, because of its potential for inducing hypotension, may enhance the effects of certain antihypertensive agents). Products include:
DynaCirc CR 1432

Ketamine Hydrochloride (Given the primary CNS effects of olanzapine, caution should be used when olanzapine is taken in combination with other centrally-acting drugs).
No products indexed under this heading.

Ketoconazole (Concomitant use may potentially inhibit olanzapine clearance; therefore, a dosage decrease may need to be considered). Products include:
Extina 3319
Xolegel 3337

Labetalol Hydrochloride (Olanzapine, because of its potential for inducing hypotension, may enhance the effects of certain antihypertensive agents).
No products indexed under this heading.

Lansoprazole (Concomitant use may cause an increase in olanzapine clearance).
No products indexed under this heading.

Levodopa (Olanzapine may antagonize the effects of levodopa). Products include:
Stalevo 2526

Levofloxacin (Concomitant use may potentially inhibit olanzapine clearance; therefore, a dosage decrease may need to be considered). Products include:
Iquix 3492
Levaquin 2629
Levaquin in 5% Dextrose 2629
Quixin 3493

2213 Interactions Index Zyprexa Intramuscular

Levomethadyl Acetate Hydrochloride (Given the primary CNS effects of olanzapine, caution should be used when olanzapine is taken in combination with other centrally-acting drugs).
No products indexed under this heading.

Levonorgestrel (Concomitant use may potentially inhibit olanzapine clearance; therefore, a dosage decrease may need to be considered). Products include:
Climara Pro 847
LoSeasonique 3407
Lybrel 3514
Mirena 854
Plan B 3416
Seasonique 3418

Levorphanol Tartrate (Given the primary CNS effects of olanzapine, caution should be used when olanzapine is taken in combination with other centrally-acting drugs).
No products indexed under this heading.

Lisdexamfetamine Dimesylate (Given the primary CNS effects of olanzapine, caution should be used when olanzapine is taken in combination with other centrally-acting drugs). Products include:
Vyvanse 3298

Lisinopril (Olanzapine, because of its potential for inducing hypotension, may enhance the effects of certain antihypertensive agents). Products include:
Prinivil 2241
Prinzide 2246

Lomefloxacin Hydrochloride (Concomitant use may potentially inhibit olanzapine clearance; therefore, a dosage decrease may need to be considered).
No products indexed under this heading.

Lorazepam (Administration of intramuscular lorazepam (2 mg) 1 hour after intramuscular olanzapine for injection (5 mg) did not significantly affect the pharmacokinetics of olanzapine, unconjugated lorazepam, or total lorazepam. However, this co-administration of intramuscular lorazepam and intramuscular olanzapine for injection added to the somnolence observed with either drug alone).
No products indexed under this heading.

Losartan Potassium (Olanzapine, because of its potential for inducing hypotension, may enhance the effects of certain antihypertensive agents). Products include:
Cozaar 2106
Hyzaar 2162
Hyzaar 100-12.5 2162

Loxapine Hydrochloride (Given the primary CNS effects of olanzapine, caution should be used when olanzapine is taken in combination with other centrally-acting drugs).
No products indexed under this heading.

Loxapine Succinate (Given the primary CNS effects of olanzapine, caution should be used when olanzapine is taken in combination with other centrally-acting drugs).
No products indexed under this heading.

Mecamylamine Hydrochloride (Olanzapine, because of its potential for inducing hypotension, may enhance the effects of certain antihypertensive agents).
No products indexed under this heading.

Meperidine Hydrochloride (Given the primary CNS effects of olanzapine, caution should be used when olanzapine is taken in combination with other centrally-acting drugs).
No products indexed under this heading.

Mephobarbital (Given the primary CNS effects of olanzapine, caution should be used when olanzapine is taken in combination with other centrally-acting drugs).
No products indexed under this heading.

Meprobamate (Given the primary CNS effects of olanzapine, caution should be used when olanzapine is taken in combination with other centrally-acting drugs).
No products indexed under this heading.

Mesoridazine Besylate (Given the primary CNS effects of olanzapine, caution should be used when olanzapine is taken in combination with other centrally-acting drugs).
No products indexed under this heading.

Mestranol (Concomitant use may potentially inhibit olanzapine clearance; therefore, a dosage decrease may need to be considered).
No products indexed under this heading.

Methadone Hydrochloride (Given the primary CNS effects of olanzapine, caution should be used when olanzapine is taken in combination with other centrally-acting drugs).
No products indexed under this heading.

Methamphetamine Hydrochloride (Given the primary CNS effects of olanzapine, caution should be used when olanzapine is taken in combination with other centrally-acting drugs).
No products indexed under this heading.

Methohexital Sodium (Given the primary CNS effects of olanzapine, caution should be used when olanzapine is taken in combination with other centrally-acting drugs).
No products indexed under this heading.

Methotrimeprazine (Given the primary CNS effects of olanzapine, caution should be used when olanzapine is taken in combination with other centrally-acting drugs).
No products indexed under this heading.

Methoxsalen (Concomitant use may potentially inhibit olanzapine clearance; therefore, a dosage decrease may need to be considered).
No products indexed under this heading.

Methoxyflurane (Given the primary CNS effects of olanzapine, caution should be used when olanzapine is taken in combination with other centrally-acting drugs).
No products indexed under this heading.

Methyclothiazide (Olanzapine, because of its potential for inducing hypotension, may enhance the effects of certain antihypertensive agents).
No products indexed under this heading.

Methyldopa (Olanzapine, because of its potential for inducing hypotension, may enhance the effects of certain antihypertensive agents).
No products indexed under this heading.

Methyldopate Hydrochloride (Olanzapine, because of its potential for inducing hypotension, may enhance the effects of certain antihypertensive agents).
No products indexed under this heading.

Methylphenidate (Given the primary CNS effects of olanzapine, caution should be used when olanzapine is taken in combination with other centrally-acting drugs). Products include:
Daytrana 3283

Methylphenidate Hydrochloride (Given the primary CNS effects of olanzapine, caution should be used when olanzapine is taken in combination with other centrally-acting drugs). Products include:
Concerta 2598
Metadate CD 3439

Metolazone (Olanzapine, because of its potential for inducing hypotension, may enhance the effects of certain antihypertensive agents).
No products indexed under this heading.

Metoprolol Succinate (Olanzapine, because of its potential for inducing hypotension, may enhance the effects of certain antihypertensive agents). Products include:
Toprol XL 732

Metoprolol Tartrate (Olanzapine, because of its potential for inducing hypotension, may enhance the effects of certain antihypertensive agents).
No products indexed under this heading.

Metyrosine (Olanzapine, because of its potential for inducing hypotension, may enhance the effects of certain antihypertensive agents).
No products indexed under this heading.

Mexiletine Hydrochloride (Concomitant use may potentially inhibit olanzapine clearance; therefore, a dosage decrease may need to be considered).
No products indexed under this heading.

Mibefradil Dihydrochloride (Olanzapine, because of its potential for inducing hypotension, may enhance the effects of certain antihypertensive agents).
No products indexed under this heading.

Midazolam Hydrochloride (Concomitant administration of intramuscular olanzapine and parenteral benzodiazepine has not been studied and is, therefore, not recommended. If use of intramuscular olanzapine in combination with parenteral benzodiazepines is considered, careful evaluation of clinical status for excessive sedation and cardiorespiratory depression is recommended).
No products indexed under this heading.

Minoxidil (Olanzapine, because of its potential for inducing hypotension, may enhance the effects of certain antihypertensive agents).
No products indexed under this heading.

Moexipril Hydrochloride (Olanzapine, because of its potential for inducing hypotension, may enhance the effects of certain antihypertensive agents).
No products indexed under this heading.

Molindone Hydrochloride (Given the primary CNS effects of olanzapine, caution should be used when olanzapine is taken in combination with other centrally-acting drugs). Products include:
Moban 1108

Morphine Sulfate (Given the primary CNS effects of olanzapine, caution should be used when olanzapine is taken in combination with other centrally-acting drugs). Products include:
Avinza 1822
Embeda 1831
MS Contin 2803

Morphine Sulfate, Liposomal (Given the primary CNS effects of olanzapine, caution should be used when olanzapine is taken in combination with other centrally-acting drugs).
No products indexed under this heading.

Moxifloxacin Hydrochloride (Concomitant use may potentially inhibit olanzapine clearance; therefore, a dosage decrease may need to be considered). Products include:
Avelox 3064
Vigamox 589

Nadolol (Olanzapine, because of its potential for inducing hypotension, may enhance the effects of certain antihypertensive agents). Products include:
Nadolol 2359

Nafcillin Sodium (Concomitant use may cause an increase in olanzapine clearance).
No products indexed under this heading.

Nalidixic Acid (Concomitant use may potentially inhibit olanzapine clearance; therefore, a dosage decrease may need to be considered).
No products indexed under this heading.

Nebivolol (Olanzapine, because of its potential for inducing hypotension, may enhance the effects of certain antihypertensive agents). Products include:
Bystolic 1147

Nicardipine Hydrochloride (Olanzapine, because of its potential for inducing hypotension, may enhance the effects of certain antihypertensive agents).
No products indexed under this heading.

Nicotine (Concomitant use may cause an increase in olanzapine clearance).
No products indexed under this heading.

Nicotine Polacrilex (Concomitant use may cause an increase in olanzapine clearance).
No products indexed under this heading.

Nicotine Salicylate (Concomitant use may cause an increase in olanzapine clearance).
No products indexed under this heading.

Nicotine Sulfate (Concomitant use may cause an increase in olanzapine clearance).
No products indexed under this heading.

Nifedipine (Olanzapine, because of its potential for inducing hypotension, may enhance the effects of certain antihypertensive agents).
No products indexed under this heading.

Nisoldipine (Olanzapine, because of its potential for inducing hypotension, may enhance the effects of certain antihypertensive agents).
No products indexed under this heading.

Nitroglycerin (Olanzapine, because of its potential for inducing hypotension, may enhance the effects of certain antihypertensive agents). Products include:
Nitro-Dur 3170
Nitrolingual 3266

Norethindrone (Concomitant use may potentially inhibit olanzapine clearance; therefore, a dosage decrease may need to be considered). Products include:
Ortho Micronor 2660

Norethindrone Acetate (Concomitant use may potentially inhibit olanzapine clearance; therefore, a dosage decrease may need to be considered). Products include:
Activella 2561

Norfloxacin (Concomitant use may potentially inhibit olanzapine clearance; therefore, a dosage decrease may need to be considered). Products include:
Noroxin 2220

Norgestrel (Concomitant use may potentially inhibit olanzapine clearance; therefore, a dosage decrease may need to be considered).
No products indexed under this heading.

Ofloxacin (Concomitant use may potentially inhibit olanzapine clearance; therefore, a dosage decrease may need to be considered).
No products indexed under this heading.

Omeprazole (Concomitant use may cause an increase in olanzapine clearance by inducing CYP1A2 or glucuronyl transferase).
No products indexed under this heading.

Omeprazole Magnesium (Concomitant use may cause an increase in olanzapine clearance by inducing CYP1A2 or glucuronyl transferase).
No products indexed under this heading.

IMPORTANT NOTE: Always consult each drug listing in the patient's regimen for possible interactions.

2215 Interactions Index Zyrtec

Sufentanil Citrate (Given the primary CNS effects of olanzapine, caution should be used when olanzapine is taken in combination with other centrally-acting drugs).
No products indexed under this heading.

Tacrine Hydrochloride (Concomitant use may potentially inhibit olanzapine clearance; therefore, a dosage decrease may need to be considered).
No products indexed under this heading.

Talbutal (Given the primary CNS effects of olanzapine, caution should be used when olanzapine is taken in combination with other centrally-acting drugs).
No products indexed under this heading.

Telmisartan (Olanzapine, because of its potential for inducing hypotension, may enhance the effects of certain antihypertensive agents). Products include:
Micardis 887
Micardis HCT 889

Temazepam (Concomitant administration of intramuscular olanzapine and parenteral benzodiazepine has not been studied and is, therefore, not recommended. If use of intramuscular olanzapine in combination with parenteral benzodiazepines is considered, careful evaluation of clinical status for excessive sedation and cardiorespiratory depression is recommended).
No products indexed under this heading.

Terazosin Hydrochloride (Olanzapine, because of its potential for inducing hypotension, may enhance the effects of certain antihypertensive agents).
No products indexed under this heading.

Thiamylal Sodium (Given the primary CNS effects of olanzapine, caution should be used when olanzapine is taken in combination with other centrally-acting drugs).
No products indexed under this heading.

Thioridazine (Given the primary CNS effects of olanzapine, caution should be used when olanzapine is taken in combination with other centrally-acting drugs).
No products indexed under this heading.

Thioridazine Hydrochloride (Given the primary CNS effects of olanzapine, caution should be used when olanzapine is taken in combination with other centrally-acting drugs). Products include:
Thioridazine Hydrochloride 2384

Thiothixene (Given the primary CNS effects of olanzapine, caution should be used when olanzapine is taken in combination with other centrally-acting drugs). Products include:
Thiothixene 2386

Thiothixene Hydrochloride (Given the primary CNS effects of olanzapine, caution should be used when olanzapine is taken in combination with other centrally-acting drugs).
No products indexed under this heading.

Ticlopidine Hydrochloride (Concomitant use may potentially inhibit olanzapine clearance; therefore, a dosage decrease may need to be considered).
No products indexed under this heading.

Timolol Maleate (Olanzapine, because of its potential for inducing hypotension, may enhance the effects of certain antihypertensive agents). Products include:
Combigan 601
Dorzolamide Hydrochloride/Timolol Maleate Ophthalmic Solution .... ⊙ 243
Timoptic in Ocudose .... ⊙ 231

Tobacco (Concomitant use may cause an increase in olanzapine clearance).
No products indexed under this heading.

Torsemide (Olanzapine, because of its potential for inducing hypotension, may enhance the effects of certain antihypertensive agents).
No products indexed under this heading.

Trandolapril (Olanzapine, because of its potential for inducing hypotension, may enhance the effects of certain antihypertensive agents). Products include:
Mavik 489
Tarka 534

Triazolam (Concomitant administration of intramuscular olanzapine and parenteral benzodiazepine has not been studied and is, therefore, not recommended. If use of intramuscular olanzapine in combination with parenteral benzodiazepines is considered, careful evaluation of clinical status for excessive sedation and cardiorespiratory depression is recommended).
No products indexed under this heading.

Trifluoperazine Hydrochloride (Given the primary CNS effects of olanzapine, caution should be used when olanzapine is taken in combination with other centrally-acting drugs).
No products indexed under this heading.

Trimethaphan Camsylate (Olanzapine, because of its potential for inducing hypotension, may enhance the effects of certain antihypertensive agents).
No products indexed under this heading.

Troleandomycin (Concomitant use may potentially inhibit olanzapine clearance; therefore, a dosage decrease may need to be considered).
No products indexed under this heading.

Trovafloxacin Mesylate (Concomitant use may potentially inhibit olanzapine clearance; therefore, a dosage decrease may need to be considered).
No products indexed under this heading.

Valsartan (Olanzapine, because of its potential for inducing hypotension, may enhance the effects of certain antihypertensive agents). Products include:
Diovan 2413
Diovan HCT 2419
Exforge 2443
Exforge HCT 2449
Valturna 3637

Vardenafil Hydrochloride (Concomitant use may potentially inhibit olanzapine clearance; therefore, a dosage decrease may need to be considered). Products include:
Levitra 3157

Verapamil Hydrochloride (Olanzapine, because of its potential for inducing hypotension, may enhance the effects of certain antihypertensive agents). Products include:
Tarka 534

Zaleplon (Given the primary CNS effects of olanzapine, caution should be used when olanzapine is taken in combination with other centrally-acting drugs).
No products indexed under this heading.

Zileuton (Concomitant use may potentially inhibit olanzapine clearance; therefore, a dosage decrease may need to be considered).
No products indexed under this heading.

Ziprasidone Hydrochloride (Given the primary CNS effects of olanzapine, caution should be used when olanzapine is taken in combination with other centrally-acting drugs). Products include:
Geodon 2723

Zolpidem Tartrate (Given the primary CNS effects of olanzapine, caution should be used when olanzapine is taken in combination with other centrally-acting drugs). Products include:
Ambien 2920
Ambien CR 2925

Food Interactions

Alcohol (Co-administration of alcohol with olanzapine potentiates orthostatic hypotension; concurrent use should be avoided. Given the primary CNS effects of olanzapine, caution should be used when olanzapine is taken in combination with other centrally-acting drugs and alcohol).

Beer, reduced-alcohol (Co-administration of alcohol with olanzapine potentiates orthostatic hypotension; concurrent use should be avoided. Given the primary CNS effects of olanzapine, caution should be used when olanzapine is taken in combination with other centrally-acting drugs and alcohol).

Beer, unspecified (Co-administration of alcohol with olanzapine potentiates orthostatic hypotension; concurrent use should be avoided. Given the primary CNS effects of olanzapine, caution should be used when olanzapine is taken in combination with other centrally-acting drugs and alcohol).

Broccoli (Concomitant use may cause an increase in olanzapine clearance).

Brussel Sprouts (Concomitant use may cause an increase in olanzapine clearance).

Charbroiled Food (Concomitant use may cause an increase in olanzapine clearance).

Grapefruit (Concomitant use may potentially inhibit olanzapine clearance; therefore, a dosage decrease may need to be considered).

Grapefruit Juice (Concomitant use may potentially inhibit olanzapine clearance; therefore, a dosage decrease may need to be considered).

Wine, Chianti (Co-administration of alcohol with olanzapine potentiates orthostatic hypotension; concurrent use should be avoided. Given the primary CNS effects of olanzapine, caution should be used when olanzapine is taken in combination with other centrally-acting drugs and alcohol).

Wine, Red (Co-administration of alcohol with olanzapine potentiates orthostatic hypotension; concurrent use should be avoided. Given the primary CNS effects of olanzapine, caution should be used when olanzapine is taken in combination with other centrally-acting drugs and alcohol).

Wine, unspecified (Co-administration of alcohol with olanzapine potentiates orthostatic hypotension; concurrent use should be avoided. Given the primary CNS effects of olanzapine, caution should be used when olanzapine is taken in combination with other centrally-acting drugs and alcohol).

Wine products (Co-administration of alcohol with olanzapine potentiates orthostatic hypotension; concurrent use should be avoided. Given the primary CNS effects of olanzapine, caution should be used when olanzapine is taken in combination with other centrally-acting drugs and alcohol).

ZYPREXA ZYDIS ORALLY DISINTEGRATING TABLETS

(Olanzapine) 1984
See Zyprexa Tablets

ZYRTEC ALLERGY TABLETS

(Cetirizine Hydrochloride) 2052
May interact with alcohols, hypnotics and sedatives, tranquilizers. Compounds in these categories include:

Alprazolam (Concomitant use may increase drowsiness).
No products indexed under this heading.

Buspirone Hydrochloride (Concomitant use may increase drowsiness).
No products indexed under this heading.

Butabarbital (Concomitant use may increase drowsiness).
No products indexed under this heading.

Butabarbital Sodium (Concomitant use may increase drowsiness).
No products indexed under this heading.

Butalbital (Concomitant use may increase drowsiness).
No products indexed under this heading.

Chloral Hydrate (Concomitant use may increase drowsiness).
No products indexed under this heading.

Chlordiazepoxide (Concomitant use may increase drowsiness).
No products indexed under this heading.

Chlordiazepoxide Hydrochloride (Concomitant use may increase drowsiness).
No products indexed under this heading.

Chlorpromazine (Concomitant use may increase drowsiness).
No products indexed under this heading.

Chlorpromazine Hydrochloride (Concomitant use may increase drowsiness).
No products indexed under this heading.

Chlorprothixene (Concomitant use may increase drowsiness).
No products indexed under this heading.

Chlorprothixene Hydrochloride (Concomitant use may increase drowsiness).
No products indexed under this heading.

Chlorprothixene Lactate (Concomitant use may increase drowsiness).
No products indexed under this heading.

Clorazepate Dipotassium (Concomitant use may increase drowsiness).
No products indexed under this heading.

Diazepam (Concomitant use may increase drowsiness). Products include:
Valium Tablets 2880

Droperidol (Concomitant use may increase drowsiness).
No products indexed under this heading.

Estazolam (Concomitant use may increase drowsiness).
No products indexed under this heading.

Ethanol (Alcohol may increase drowsiness. Avoid alcoholic drinks).
No products indexed under this heading.

Ethchlorvynol (Concomitant use may increase drowsiness).
No products indexed under this heading.

Ethinamate (Concomitant use may increase drowsiness).
No products indexed under this heading.

Ethyl Alcohol (Alcohol may increase drowsiness. Avoid alcoholic drinks).
No products indexed under this heading.

Fluphenazine Decanoate (Concomitant use may increase drowsiness).
No products indexed under this heading.

Fluphenazine Enanthate (Concomitant use may increase drowsiness).
No products indexed under this heading.

Fluphenazine Hydrochloride (Concomitant use may increase drowsiness).
No products indexed under this heading.

Flurazepam Hydrochloride (Concomitant use may increase drowsiness).
No products indexed under this heading.

Glutethimide (Concomitant use may increase drowsiness).
No products indexed under this heading.

Haloperidol (Concomitant use may increase drowsiness).
No products indexed under this heading.

IMPORTANT NOTE: Always consult each drug listing in the patient's regimen for possible interactions.

Haloperidol Decanoate (Concomitant use may increase drowsiness).
No products indexed under this heading.

Hydroxyzine Hydrochloride (Concomitant use may increase drowsiness).
No products indexed under this heading.

Lorazepam (Concomitant use may increase drowsiness).
No products indexed under this heading.

Loxapine Hydrochloride (Concomitant use may increase drowsiness).
No products indexed under this heading.

Loxapine Succinate (Concomitant use may increase drowsiness).
No products indexed under this heading.

Meprobamate (Concomitant use may increase drowsiness).
No products indexed under this heading.

Mesoridazine Besylate (Concomitant use may increase drowsiness).
No products indexed under this heading.

Midazolam Hydrochloride (Concomitant use may increase drowsiness).
No products indexed under this heading.

Molindone Hydrochloride (Concomitant use may increase drowsiness).
Products include:
Moban 1108

Oxazepam (Concomitant use may increase drowsiness).
No products indexed under this heading.

Perphenazine (Concomitant use may increase drowsiness).
No products indexed under this heading.

Prazepam (Concomitant use may increase drowsiness).
No products indexed under this heading.

Prochlorperazine (Concomitant use may increase drowsiness).
No products indexed under this heading.

Promethazine Hydrochloride (Concomitant use may increase drowsiness).
No products indexed under this heading.

Propofol (Concomitant use may increase drowsiness).
No products indexed under this heading.

Quazepam (Concomitant use may increase drowsiness).
No products indexed under this heading.

Ramelteon (Concomitant use may increase drowsiness). Products include:
Rozerem 3366

Secobarbital Sodium (Concomitant use may increase drowsiness).
No products indexed under this heading.

Sodium Butabarbital (Concomitant use may increase drowsiness).
No products indexed under this heading.

Temazepam (Concomitant use may increase drowsiness).
No products indexed under this heading.

Thioridazine Hydrochloride (Concomitant use may increase drowsiness).
Products include:
Thioridazine Hydrochloride 2384

Thiothixene (Concomitant use may increase drowsiness). Products include:
Thiothixene 2386

Triazolam (Concomitant use may increase drowsiness).
No products indexed under this heading.

Trifluoperazine Hydrochloride (Concomitant use may increase drowsiness).
No products indexed under this heading.

Zaleplon (Concomitant use may increase drowsiness).
No products indexed under this heading.

Zolpidem Tartrate (Concomitant use may increase drowsiness). Products include:
Ambien 2920
Ambien CR 2925

Food Interactions
Alcohol (Alcohol may increase drowsiness. Avoid alcoholic drinks).

Beer, reduced-alcohol (Alcohol may increase drowsiness. Avoid alcoholic drinks).

Beer, unspecified (Alcohol may increase drowsiness. Avoid alcoholic drinks).

Wine, Chianti (Alcohol may increase drowsiness. Avoid alcoholic drinks).

Wine, Red (Alcohol may increase drowsiness. Avoid alcoholic drinks).

Wine, unspecified (Alcohol may increase drowsiness. Avoid alcoholic drinks).

Wine products (Alcohol may increase drowsiness. Avoid alcoholic drinks).

CHILDREN'S ZYRTEC ALLERGY CHEWABLE TABLETS
(Cetirizine Hydrochloride) 2053
May interact with alcohols, hypnotics and sedatives, tranquilizers. Compounds in these categories include:

Alprazolam (Concomitant use may increase drowsiness).
No products indexed under this heading.

Buspirone Hydrochloride (Concomitant use may increase drowsiness).
No products indexed under this heading.

Butabarbital (Concomitant use may increase drowsiness).
No products indexed under this heading.

Butabarbital Sodium (Concomitant use may increase drowsiness).
No products indexed under this heading.

Butalbital (Concomitant use may increase drowsiness).
No products indexed under this heading.

Chloral Hydrate (Concomitant use may increase drowsiness).
No products indexed under this heading.

Chlordiazepoxide (Concomitant use may increase drowsiness).
No products indexed under this heading.

Chlordiazepoxide Hydrochloride (Concomitant use may increase drowsiness).
No products indexed under this heading.

Chlorpromazine (Concomitant use may increase drowsiness).
No products indexed under this heading.

Chlorpromazine Hydrochloride (Concomitant use may increase drowsiness).
No products indexed under this heading.

Chlorprothixene (Concomitant use may increase drowsiness).
No products indexed under this heading.

Chlorprothixene Hydrochloride (Concomitant use may increase drowsiness).
No products indexed under this heading.

Chlorprothixene Lactate (Concomitant use may increase drowsiness).
No products indexed under this heading.

Clorazepate Dipotassium (Concomitant use may increase drowsiness).
No products indexed under this heading.

Diazepam (Concomitant use may increase drowsiness). Products include:
Valium Tablets 2880

Droperidol (Concomitant use may increase drowsiness).
No products indexed under this heading.

Estazolam (Concomitant use may increase drowsiness).
No products indexed under this heading.

Ethanol (Alcohol may increase drowsiness. Avoid alcoholic drinks).

Ethchlorvynol (Concomitant use may increase drowsiness).
No products indexed under this heading.

Ethinamate (Concomitant use may increase drowsiness).
No products indexed under this heading.

Ethyl Alcohol (Alcohol may increase drowsiness. Avoid alcoholic drinks).
No products indexed under this heading.

Fluphenazine Decanoate (Concomitant use may increase drowsiness).
No products indexed under this heading.

Fluphenazine Enanthate (Concomitant use may increase drowsiness).
No products indexed under this heading.

Fluphenazine Hydrochloride (Concomitant use may increase drowsiness).
No products indexed under this heading.

Flurazepam Hydrochloride (Concomitant use may increase drowsiness).
No products indexed under this heading.

Glutethimide (Concomitant use may increase drowsiness).
No products indexed under this heading.

Haloperidol (Concomitant use may increase drowsiness).
No products indexed under this heading.

Haloperidol Decanoate (Concomitant use may increase drowsiness).
No products indexed under this heading.

Hydroxyzine Hydrochloride (Concomitant use may increase drowsiness).
No products indexed under this heading.

Lorazepam (Concomitant use may increase drowsiness).
No products indexed under this heading.

Loxapine Hydrochloride (Concomitant use may increase drowsiness).
No products indexed under this heading.

Loxapine Succinate (Concomitant use may increase drowsiness).
No products indexed under this heading.

Meprobamate (Concomitant use may increase drowsiness).
No products indexed under this heading.

Mesoridazine Besylate (Concomitant use may increase drowsiness).
No products indexed under this heading.

Midazolam Hydrochloride (Concomitant use may increase drowsiness).
No products indexed under this heading.

Molindone Hydrochloride (Concomitant use may increase drowsiness).
Products include:
Moban 1108

Oxazepam (Concomitant use may increase drowsiness).
No products indexed under this heading.

Perphenazine (Concomitant use may increase drowsiness).
No products indexed under this heading.

Prazepam (Concomitant use may increase drowsiness).
No products indexed under this heading.

Prochlorperazine (Concomitant use may increase drowsiness).
No products indexed under this heading.

Promethazine Hydrochloride (Concomitant use may increase drowsiness).
No products indexed under this heading.

Propofol (Concomitant use may increase drowsiness).
No products indexed under this heading.

Quazepam (Concomitant use may increase drowsiness).
No products indexed under this heading.

Ramelteon (Concomitant use may increase drowsiness). Products include:
Rozerem 3366

Secobarbital Sodium (Concomitant use may increase drowsiness).
No products indexed under this heading.

Sodium Butabarbital (Concomitant use may increase drowsiness).
No products indexed under this heading.

Temazepam (Concomitant use may increase drowsiness).
No products indexed under this heading.

Thioridazine Hydrochloride (Concomitant use may increase drowsiness).
Products include:
Thioridazine Hydrochloride 2384

Thiothixene (Concomitant use may increase drowsiness). Products include:
Thiothixene 2386

Triazolam (Concomitant use may increase drowsiness).
No products indexed under this heading.

Trifluoperazine Hydrochloride (Concomitant use may increase drowsiness).
No products indexed under this heading.

Zaleplon (Concomitant use may increase drowsiness).
No products indexed under this heading.

Zolpidem Tartrate (Concomitant use may increase drowsiness). Products include:
Ambien 2920
Ambien CR 2925

Food Interactions
Alcohol (Alcohol may increase drowsiness. Avoid alcoholic drinks).

Beer, reduced-alcohol (Alcohol may increase drowsiness. Avoid alcoholic drinks).

Beer, unspecified (Alcohol may increase drowsiness. Avoid alcoholic drinks).

Wine, Chianti (Alcohol may increase drowsiness. Avoid alcoholic drinks).

Wine, Red (Alcohol may increase drowsiness. Avoid alcoholic drinks).

Wine, unspecified (Alcohol may increase drowsiness. Avoid alcoholic drinks).

Wine products (Alcohol may increase drowsiness. Avoid alcoholic drinks).

CHILDREN'S ZYRTEC ALLERGY SYRUP
(Cetirizine Hydrochloride) 2053
May interact with alcohols, hypnotics and sedatives, tranquilizers. Compounds in these categories include:

Alprazolam (Concomitant use may increase drowsiness).
No products indexed under this heading.

Buspirone Hydrochloride (Concomitant use may increase drowsiness).
No products indexed under this heading.

Butabarbital (Concomitant use may increase drowsiness).
No products indexed under this heading.

Butabarbital Sodium (Concomitant use may increase drowsiness).
No products indexed under this heading.

Butalbital (Concomitant use may increase drowsiness).
No products indexed under this heading.

Chloral Hydrate (Concomitant use may increase drowsiness).
No products indexed under this heading.

Chlordiazepoxide (Concomitant use may increase drowsiness).
No products indexed under this heading.

Chlordiazepoxide Hydrochloride (Concomitant use may increase drowsiness).
No products indexed under this heading.

Chlorpromazine (Concomitant use may increase drowsiness).
No products indexed under this heading.

Chlorpromazine Hydrochloride (Concomitant use may increase drowsiness).
No products indexed under this heading.

Chlorprothixene (Concomitant use may increase drowsiness).
No products indexed under this heading.

Chlorprothixene Hydrochloride (Concomitant use may increase drowsiness).
No products indexed under this heading.

Chlorprothixene Lactate (Concomitant use may increase drowsiness).
No products indexed under this heading.

Clorazepate Dipotassium (Concomitant use may increase drowsiness).
No products indexed under this heading.

Diazepam (Concomitant use may increase drowsiness). Products include:
Valium Tablets 2880

Droperidol (Concomitant use may increase drowsiness).
No products indexed under this heading.

Estazolam (Concomitant use may increase drowsiness).
No products indexed under this heading.

Ethanol (Concomitant use may increase drowsiness).
No products indexed under this heading.

Ethchlorvynol (Concomitant use may increase drowsiness).
No products indexed under this heading.

Ethinamate (Concomitant use may increase drowsiness).
No products indexed under this heading.

Ethyl Alcohol (Concomitant use may increase drowsiness).
No products indexed under this heading.

Fluphenazine Decanoate (Concomitant use may increase drowsiness).
No products indexed under this heading.

Fluphenazine Enanthate (Concomitant use may increase drowsiness).
No products indexed under this heading.

Fluphenazine Hydrochloride (Concomitant use may increase drowsiness).
No products indexed under this heading.

Flurazepam Hydrochloride (Concomitant use may increase drowsiness).
No products indexed under this heading.

Glutethimide (Concomitant use may increase drowsiness).
No products indexed under this heading.

Haloperidol (Concomitant use may increase drowsiness).
No products indexed under this heading.

Haloperidol Decanoate (Concomitant use may increase drowsiness).
No products indexed under this heading.

Hydroxyzine Hydrochloride (Concomitant use may increase drowsiness).
No products indexed under this heading.

Lorazepam (Concomitant use may increase drowsiness).
No products indexed under this heading.

Loxapine Hydrochloride (Concomitant use may increase drowsiness).
No products indexed under this heading.

Loxapine Succinate (Concomitant use may increase drowsiness).
No products indexed under this heading.

Meprobamate (Concomitant use may increase drowsiness).
No products indexed under this heading.

Mesoridazine Besylate (Concomitant use may increase drowsiness).
No products indexed under this heading.

Midazolam Hydrochloride (Concomitant use may increase drowsiness).
No products indexed under this heading.

Molindone Hydrochloride (Concomitant use may increase drowsiness).
Products include:
Moban 1108

Oxazepam (Concomitant use may increase drowsiness).
No products indexed under this heading.

Perphenazine (Concomitant use may increase drowsiness).
No products indexed under this heading.

Prazepam (Concomitant use may increase drowsiness).
No products indexed under this heading.

Prochlorperazine (Concomitant use may increase drowsiness).
No products indexed under this heading.

Promethazine Hydrochloride (Concomitant use may increase drowsiness).
No products indexed under this heading.

Propofol (Concomitant use may increase drowsiness).
No products indexed under this heading.

Quazepam (Concomitant use may increase drowsiness).
No products indexed under this heading.

Ramelteon (Concomitant use may increase drowsiness). Products include:
Rozerem 3366

Secobarbital Sodium (Concomitant use may increase drowsiness).
No products indexed under this heading.

Sodium Butabarbital (Concomitant use may increase drowsiness).
No products indexed under this heading.

Temazepam (Concomitant use may increase drowsiness).
No products indexed under this heading.

Thioridazine Hydrochloride (Concomitant use may increase drowsiness). Products include:
Thioridazine Hydrochloride 2384

Thiothixene (Concomitant use may increase drowsiness). Products include:
Thiothixene 2386

Triazolam (Concomitant use may increase drowsiness).
No products indexed under this heading.

Trifluoperazine Hydrochloride (Concomitant use may increase drowsiness).
No products indexed under this heading.

Zaleplon (Concomitant use may increase drowsiness).
No products indexed under this heading.

Zolpidem Tartrate (Concomitant use may increase drowsiness). Products include:
Ambien 2920
Ambien CR 2925

Food Interactions

Alcohol (Concomitant use may increase drowsiness).

Beer, reduced-alcohol (Concomitant use may increase drowsiness).

Beer, unspecified (Concomitant use may increase drowsiness).

Wine, Chianti (Concomitant use may increase drowsiness).

Wine, Red (Concomitant use may increase drowsiness).

Wine, unspecified (Concomitant use may increase drowsiness).

Wine products (Concomitant use may increase drowsiness).

CHILDREN'S ZYRTEC HIVES RELIEF SYRUP

(Cetirizine Hydrochloride) 2053
May interact with alcohols, hypnotics and sedatives, tranquilizers. Compounds in these categories include:

Alprazolam (Concomitant use may increase drowsiness).
No products indexed under this heading.

Buspirone Hydrochloride (Concomitant use may increase drowsiness).
No products indexed under this heading.

Butabarbital (Concomitant use may increase drowsiness).
No products indexed under this heading.

Butabarbital Sodium (Concomitant use may increase drowsiness).
No products indexed under this heading.

Butalbital (Concomitant use may increase drowsiness).
No products indexed under this heading.

Chloral Hydrate (Concomitant use may increase drowsiness).
No products indexed under this heading.

Chlordiazepoxide (Concomitant use may increase drowsiness).
No products indexed under this heading.

Chlordiazepoxide Hydrochloride (Concomitant use may increase drowsiness).
No products indexed under this heading.

Chlorpromazine (Concomitant use may increase drowsiness).
No products indexed under this heading.

Chlorpromazine Hydrochloride (Concomitant use may increase drowsiness).
No products indexed under this heading.

Chlorprothixene (Concomitant use may increase drowsiness).
No products indexed under this heading.

Chlorprothixene Hydrochloride (Concomitant use may increase drowsiness).
No products indexed under this heading.

Chlorprothixene Lactate (Concomitant use may increase drowsiness).
No products indexed under this heading.

Clorazepate Dipotassium (Concomitant use may increase drowsiness).
No products indexed under this heading.

Diazepam (Concomitant use may increase drowsiness). Products include:
Valium Tablets 2880

Droperidol (Concomitant use may increase drowsiness).
No products indexed under this heading.

Estazolam (Concomitant use may increase drowsiness).
No products indexed under this heading.

Ethanol (Concomitant use may increase drowsiness).
No products indexed under this heading.

Ethchlorvynol (Concomitant use may increase drowsiness).
No products indexed under this heading.

Ethinamate (Concomitant use may increase drowsiness).
No products indexed under this heading.

Ethyl Alcohol (Concomitant use may increase drowsiness).
No products indexed under this heading.

Fluphenazine Decanoate (Concomitant use may increase drowsiness).
No products indexed under this heading.

Fluphenazine Enanthate (Concomitant use may increase drowsiness).
No products indexed under this heading.

Fluphenazine Hydrochloride (Concomitant use may increase drowsiness).
No products indexed under this heading.

Flurazepam Hydrochloride (Concomitant use may increase drowsiness).
No products indexed under this heading.

Glutethimide (Concomitant use may increase drowsiness).
No products indexed under this heading.

Haloperidol (Concomitant use may increase drowsiness).
No products indexed under this heading.

Haloperidol Decanoate (Concomitant use may increase drowsiness).
No products indexed under this heading.

Hydroxyzine Hydrochloride (Concomitant use may increase drowsiness).
No products indexed under this heading.

Lorazepam (Concomitant use may increase drowsiness).
No products indexed under this heading.

Loxapine Hydrochloride (Concomitant use may increase drowsiness).
No products indexed under this heading.

Loxapine Succinate (Concomitant use may increase drowsiness).
No products indexed under this heading.

Meprobamate (Concomitant use may increase drowsiness).
No products indexed under this heading.

Mesoridazine Besylate (Concomitant use may increase drowsiness).
No products indexed under this heading.

Midazolam Hydrochloride (Concomitant use may increase drowsiness).
No products indexed under this heading.

Molindone Hydrochloride (Concomitant use may increase drowsiness).
Products include:
Moban 1108

Oxazepam (Concomitant use may increase drowsiness).
No products indexed under this heading.

Perphenazine (Concomitant use may increase drowsiness).
No products indexed under this heading.

Prazepam (Concomitant use may increase drowsiness).
No products indexed under this heading.

Prochlorperazine (Concomitant use may increase drowsiness).
No products indexed under this heading.

Promethazine Hydrochloride (Concomitant use may increase drowsiness).
No products indexed under this heading.

Propofol (Concomitant use may increase drowsiness).
No products indexed under this heading.

Quazepam (Concomitant use may increase drowsiness).
No products indexed under this heading.

Ramelteon (Concomitant use may increase drowsiness). Products include:
Rozerem 3366

Secobarbital Sodium (Concomitant use may increase drowsiness).
No products indexed under this heading.

Sodium Butabarbital (Concomitant use may increase drowsiness).
No products indexed under this heading.

Temazepam (Concomitant use may increase drowsiness).
No products indexed under this heading.

Thioridazine Hydrochloride (Concomitant use may increase drowsiness).
Products include:
Thioridazine Hydrochloride 2384

Thiothixene (Concomitant use may increase drowsiness). Products include:
Thiothixene 2386

Triazolam (Concomitant use may increase drowsiness).
No products indexed under this heading.

Trifluoperazine Hydrochloride (Concomitant use may increase drowsiness).
No products indexed under this heading.

Zaleplon (Concomitant use may increase drowsiness).
No products indexed under this heading.

Zolpidem Tartrate (Concomitant use may increase drowsiness). Products include:
Ambien 2920
Ambien CR 2925

Food Interactions

Alcohol (Concomitant use may increase drowsiness).

Beer, reduced-alcohol (Concomitant use may increase drowsiness).

Beer, unspecified (Concomitant use may increase drowsiness).

Wine, Chianti (Concomitant use may increase drowsiness).

Wine, Red (Concomitant use may increase drowsiness).

Wine, unspecified (Concomitant use may increase drowsiness).

IMPORTANT NOTE: Always consult each drug listing in the patient's regimen for possible interactions.

Wine products (Concomitant use may increase drowsiness).

ZYRTEC ITCHY EYE DROPS
(Ketotifen Fumarate) 2053
None cited in PDR database.

ZYRTEC-D ALLERGY & CONGESTION EXTENDED-RELEASE TABLETS
(Cetirizine Hydrochloride, Pseudoephedrine Hydrochloride).......... 2054
May interact with alcohols, hypnotics and sedatives, monoamine oxidase inhibitors, tranquilizers. Compounds in these categories include:

Alprazolam (Concurrent use with tranquilizers may increase drowsiness).
No products indexed under this heading.

Buspirone Hydrochloride (Concurrent use with tranquilizers may increase drowsiness).
No products indexed under this heading.

Butabarbital (Concurrent use with sedatives may increase drowsiness).
No products indexed under this heading.

Butabarbital Sodium (Concurrent use with sedatives may increase drowsiness).
No products indexed under this heading.

Butalbital (Concurrent use with sedatives may increase drowsiness).
No products indexed under this heading.

Chloral Hydrate (Concurrent use with sedatives may increase drowsiness).
No products indexed under this heading.

Chlordiazepoxide (Concurrent use with tranquilizers may increase drowsiness).
No products indexed under this heading.

Chlordiazepoxide Hydrochloride (Concurrent use with tranquilizers may increase drowsiness).
No products indexed under this heading.

Chlorpromazine (Concurrent use with tranquilizers may increase drowsiness).
No products indexed under this heading.

Chlorpromazine Hydrochloride (Concurrent use with tranquilizers may increase drowsiness).
No products indexed under this heading.

Chlorprothixene (Concurrent use with tranquilizers may increase drowsiness).
No products indexed under this heading.

Chlorprothixene Hydrochloride (Concurrent use with tranquilizers may increase drowsiness).
No products indexed under this heading.

Chlorprothixene Lactate (Concurrent use with tranquilizers may increase drowsiness).
No products indexed under this heading.

Clorazepate Dipotassium (Concurrent use with tranquilizers may increase drowsiness).
No products indexed under this heading.

Diazepam (Concurrent use with tranquilizers may increase drowsiness). Products include:
Valium Tablets 2880

Droperidol (Concurrent use with tranquilizers may increase drowsiness).
No products indexed under this heading.

Estazolam (Concurrent use with sedatives may increase drowsiness).
No products indexed under this heading.

Ethanol (Concurrent use with alcohol may increase drowsiness; avoid alcohol).
No products indexed under this heading.

Ethchlorvynol (Concurrent use with sedatives may increase drowsiness).
No products indexed under this heading.

Ethinamate (Concurrent use with sedatives may increase drowsiness).
No products indexed under this heading.

Ethyl Alcohol (Concurrent use with alcohol may increase drowsiness; avoid alcohol).
No products indexed under this heading.

Fluphenazine Decanoate (Concurrent use with tranquilizers may increase drowsiness).
No products indexed under this heading.

Fluphenazine Enanthate (Concurrent use with tranquilizers may increase drowsiness).
No products indexed under this heading.

Fluphenazine Hydrochloride (Concurrent use with tranquilizers may increase drowsiness).
No products indexed under this heading.

Flurazepam Hydrochloride (Concurrent use with sedatives may increase drowsiness).
No products indexed under this heading.

Glutethimide (Concurrent use with sedatives may increase drowsiness).
No products indexed under this heading.

Haloperidol (Concurrent use with tranquilizers may increase drowsiness).
No products indexed under this heading.

Haloperidol Decanoate (Concurrent use with tranquilizers may increase drowsiness).
No products indexed under this heading.

Hydroxyzine Hydrochloride (Concurrent use with tranquilizers may increase drowsiness).
No products indexed under this heading.

Isocarboxazid (Avoid concurrent use with MAO inhibitors. Also, Zyrtec-D should not be used for two weeks after stopping an MAO inhibitor). Products include:
Marplan 3481

Lorazepam (Concurrent use with sedatives may increase drowsiness).
No products indexed under this heading.

Loxapine Hydrochloride (Concurrent use with tranquilizers may increase drowsiness).
No products indexed under this heading.

Loxapine Succinate (Concurrent use with tranquilizers may increase drowsiness).
No products indexed under this heading.

Meprobamate (Concurrent use with tranquilizers may increase drowsiness).
No products indexed under this heading.

Mesoridazine Besylate (Concurrent use with tranquilizers may increase drowsiness).
No products indexed under this heading.

Midazolam Hydrochloride (Concurrent use with sedatives may increase drowsiness).
No products indexed under this heading.

Moclobemide (Avoid concurrent use with MAO inhibitors. Also, Zyrtec-D should not be used for two weeks after stopping an MAO inhibitor).
No products indexed under this heading.

Molindone Hydrochloride (Concurrent use with tranquilizers may increase drowsiness). Products include:
Moban 1108

Oxazepam (Concurrent use with tranquilizers may increase drowsiness).
No products indexed under this heading.

Pargyline Hydrochloride (Avoid concurrent use with MAO inhibitors. Also, Zyrtec-D should not be used for two weeks after stopping an MAO inhibitor).
No products indexed under this heading.

Perphenazine (Concurrent use with tranquilizers may increase drowsiness).
No products indexed under this heading.

Phenelzine Sulfate (Avoid concurrent use with MAO inhibitors. Also, Zyrtec-D should not be used for two weeks after stopping an MAO inhibitor).
No products indexed under this heading.

Prazepam (Concurrent use with tranquilizers may increase drowsiness).
No products indexed under this heading.

Procarbazine Hydrochloride (Avoid concurrent use with MAO inhibitors. Also, Zyrtec-D should not be used for two weeks after stopping an MAO inhibitor).
No products indexed under this heading.

Prochlorperazine (Concurrent use with tranquilizers may increase drowsiness).
No products indexed under this heading.

Promethazine Hydrochloride (Concurrent use with tranquilizers may increase drowsiness).
No products indexed under this heading.

Propofol (Concurrent use with sedatives may increase drowsiness).
No products indexed under this heading.

Quazepam (Concurrent use with sedatives may increase drowsiness).
No products indexed under this heading.

Ramelteon (Concurrent use with sedatives may increase drowsiness). Products include:
Rozerem 3366

Rasagiline Mesylate (Avoid concurrent use with MAO inhibitors. Also, Zyrtec-D should not be used for two weeks after stopping an MAO inhibitor). Products include:
Azilect 3383

Secobarbital Sodium (Concurrent use with sedatives may increase drowsiness).
No products indexed under this heading.

Selegiline (Avoid concurrent use with MAO inhibitors. Also, Zyrtec-D should not be used for two weeks after stopping an MAO inhibitor). Products include:
Emsam 3623

Selegiline Hydrochloride (Avoid concurrent use with MAO inhibitors. Also, Zyrtec-D should not be used for two weeks after stopping an MAO inhibitor). Products include:
Eldepryl 3312

Sodium Butabarbital (Concurrent use with sedatives may increase drowsiness).
No products indexed under this heading.

Temazepam (Concurrent use with sedatives may increase drowsiness).
No products indexed under this heading.

Thioridazine Hydrochloride (Concurrent use with tranquilizers may increase drowsiness). Products include:
Thioridazine Hydrochloride 2384

Thiothixene (Concurrent use with tranquilizers may increase drowsiness). Products include:
Thiothixene 2386

Tranylcypromine Sulfate (Avoid concurrent use with MAO inhibitors. Also, Zyrtec-D should not be used for two weeks after stopping an MAO inhibitor). Products include:
Parnate 1584

Triazolam (Concurrent use with sedatives may increase drowsiness).
No products indexed under this heading.

Trifluoperazine Hydrochloride (Concurrent use with tranquilizers may increase drowsiness).
No products indexed under this heading.

Zaleplon (Concurrent use with sedatives may increase drowsiness).
No products indexed under this heading.

Zolpidem Tartrate (Concurrent use with sedatives may increase drowsiness). Products include:

Ambien 2920
Ambien CR 2925

Food Interactions
Alcohol (Concurrent use with alcohol may increase drowsiness; avoid alcohol).

Beer, reduced-alcohol (Concurrent use with alcohol may increase drowsiness; avoid alcohol).

Beer, unspecified (Concurrent use with alcohol may increase drowsiness; avoid alcohol).

Wine, Chianti (Concurrent use with alcohol may increase drowsiness; avoid alcohol).

Wine, Red (Concurrent use with alcohol may increase drowsiness; avoid alcohol).

Wine, unspecified (Concurrent use with alcohol may increase drowsiness; avoid alcohol).

Wine products (Concurrent use with alcohol may increase drowsiness; avoid alcohol).

ZYVOX FOR ORAL SUSPENSION
(Linezolid) 2769
See Zyvox Tablets

ZYVOX INJECTION
(Linezolid) 2769
See Zyvox Tablets

ZYVOX TABLETS
(Linezolid) 2769
May interact with 5HT1-receptor agonists, dopamine agonists, monoamine oxidase inhibitors, selective serotonin reuptake inhibitors, serotoninergic agents, sympathomimetics, tricyclic antidepressants, vasopressors, and certain other agents. Compounds in these categories include:

Albuterol (Unless patients are monitored for potential increases in BP, linezolid should not be administered to patients taking directly and indirectly acting sympathomimetic agents (eg, pseudoephedrine)).
No products indexed under this heading.

Albuterol Sulfate (Unless patients are monitored for potential increases in BP, linezolid should not be administered to patients taking directly and indirectly acting sympathomimetic agents (eg, pseudoephedrine)). Products include:
ProAir HFA 3393
Proventil HFA 3204
Ventolin HFA 1708

Almotriptan Malate (Unless patients are carefully observed for signs and/or symptoms of serotonin syndrome, linezolid should not be administered to patients taking 5-HT1 receptor agonists (triptans)). Products include:
Axert 2593

Amitriptyline Hydrochloride (Unless patients are carefully observed for signs and/or symptoms of serotonin syndrome, linezolid should not be administered to patients taking tricyclic antidepressants).
No products indexed under this heading.

Amoxapine (Unless patients are carefully observed for signs and/or symptoms of serotonin syndrome, linezolid should not be administered to patients taking tricyclic antidepressants).
No products indexed under this heading.

Bromocriptine Mesylate (Unless patients are monitored for potential increases in BP, linezolid should not be administered to patients taking dopaminergic agents (eg, dopamine, dobutamine)).
No products indexed under this heading.

Buspirone Hydrochloride (Unless patients are carefully observed for signs and/or symptoms of serotonin syndrome, linezolid should not be administered to patients taking buspirone).

No products indexed under this heading.

Citalopram Hydrobromide (Spontaneous reports of serotonin syndrome associated with the co-administration of linezolid and serotonergic agents, including antidepressants such as selective serotonin reuptake inhibitors (SSRIs), have been reported. Unless patients are carefully observed for signs and/or symptoms of serotonin syndrome, linezolid should not be administered to patients taking serotonin re-uptake inhibitors. Where administration of linezolid and concomitant serotonergic agents is clinically appropriate, patients should be closely observed for signs/symptoms of serotonin syndrome. If signs/symptoms occur, discontinuation of either one or both agents should be considered. If the concomitant serotonergic agent is withdrawn, discontinuation symptoms can be observed). Products include:
Celexa 1153

Clomipramine Hydrochloride (Unless patients are carefully observed for signs and/or symptoms of serotonin syndrome, linezolid should not be administered to patients taking tricyclic antidepressants).

No products indexed under this heading.

Desipramine Hydrochloride (Unless patients are carefully observed for signs and/or symptoms of serotonin syndrome, linezolid should not be administered to patients taking tricyclic antidepressants).

No products indexed under this heading.

Dobutamine (Unless patients are monitored for potential increases in BP, linezolid should not be administered to patients taking dopaminergic agents (eg, dopamine, dobutamine)).

No products indexed under this heading.

Dobutamine Hydrochloride (Unless patients are monitored for potential increases in BP, linezolid should not be administered to patients taking dopaminergic agents (eg, dopamine, dobutamine)).

No products indexed under this heading.

Dopamine Hydrochloride (Unless patients are monitored for potential increases in BP, linezolid should not be administered to patients taking directly and indirectly acting sympathomimetic agents (eg, pseudoephedrine)).

No products indexed under this heading.

Doxepin Hydrochloride (Unless patients are carefully observed for signs and/or symptoms of serotonin syndrome, linezolid should not be administered to patients taking tricyclic antidepressants).

No products indexed under this heading.

Eletriptan Hydrobromide (Unless patients are carefully observed for signs and/or symptoms of serotonin syndrome, linezolid should not be administered to patients taking 5-HT1 receptor agonists (triptans)).

No products indexed under this heading.

Ephedrine Hydrochloride (Unless patients are monitored for potential increases in BP, linezolid should not be administered to patients taking directly and indirectly acting sympathomimetic agents (eg, pseudoephedrine)).

No products indexed under this heading.

Ephedrine Sulfate (Unless patients are monitored for potential increases in BP, linezolid should not be administered to patients taking directly and indirectly acting sympathomimetic agents (eg, pseudoephedrine)).

No products indexed under this heading.

Ephedrine Tannate (Unless patients are monitored for potential increases in BP, linezolid should not be administered to patients taking directly and indirectly acting sympathomimetic agents (eg, pseudoephedrine)).

No products indexed under this heading.

Epinephrine (Unless patients are monitored for potential increases in BP, linezolid should not be administered to patients taking directly and indirectly acting sympathomimetic agents (eg, pseudoephedrine)). Products include:
EpiPen 3631
Twinject 3268

Epinephrine Bitartrate (Unless patients are monitored for potential increases in BP, linezolid should not be administered to patients taking directly and indirectly acting sympathomimetic agents (eg, pseudoephedrine)).

No products indexed under this heading.

Epinephrine Hydrochloride (Unless patients are monitored for potential increases in BP, linezolid should not be administered to patients taking directly and indirectly acting sympathomimetic agents (eg, pseudoephedrine)).

No products indexed under this heading.

Escitalopram Oxalate (Spontaneous reports of serotonin syndrome associated with the co-administration of linezolid and serotonergic agents, including antidepressants such as selective serotonin reuptake inhibitors (SSRIs), have been reported. Unless patients are carefully observed for signs and/or symptoms of serotonin syndrome, linezolid should not be administered to patients taking serotonin re-uptake inhibitors. Where administration of linezolid and concomitant serotonergic agents is clinically appropriate, patients should be closely observed for signs/symptoms of serotonin syndrome. If signs/symptoms occur, discontinuation of either one or both agents should be considered. If the concomitant serotonergic agent is withdrawn, discontinuation symptoms can be observed). Products include:
Lexapro Oral Suspension 1160
Lexapro Tablets 1160

Fluoxetine (Spontaneous reports of serotonin syndrome associated with the co-administration of linezolid and serotonergic agents, including antidepressants such as selective serotonin reuptake inhibitors (SSRIs), have been reported. Unless patients are carefully observed for signs and/or symptoms of serotonin syndrome, linezolid should not be administered to patients taking serotonin re-uptake inhibitors. Where administration of linezolid and concomitant serotonergic agents is clinically appropriate, patients should be closely observed for signs/symptoms of serotonin syndrome. If signs/symptoms occur, discontinuation of either one or both agents should be considered. If the concomitant serotonergic agent is withdrawn, discontinuation symptoms can be observed).

No products indexed under this heading.

Fluoxetine Hydrochloride (Spontaneous reports of serotonin syndrome associated with the co-administration of linezolid and serotonergic agents, including antidepressants such as selective serotonin reuptake inhibitors (SSRIs), have been reported. Unless patients are carefully observed for signs and/or symptoms of serotonin syndrome, linezolid should not be administered to patients taking serotonin re-uptake inhibitors. Where administration of linezolid and concomitant serotonergic agents is clinically appropriate, patients should be closely observed for signs/symptoms of serotonin syndrome. If signs/symptoms occur, discontinuation of either one or both agents should be considered. If

the concomitant serotonergic agent is withdrawn, discontinuation symptoms can be observed). Products include:
Prozac Weekly 1941
Prozac Pulvules 1941
Symbyax 1965

Fluvoxamine (Spontaneous reports of serotonin syndrome associated with the co-administration of linezolid and serotonergic agents, including antidepressants such as selective serotonin reuptake inhibitors (SSRIs), have been reported. Unless patients are carefully observed for signs and/or symptoms of serotonin syndrome, linezolid should not be administered to patients taking serotonin re-uptake inhibitors. Where administration of linezolid and concomitant serotonergic agents is clinically appropriate, patients should be closely observed for signs/symptoms of serotonin syndrome. If signs/symptoms occur, discontinuation of either one or both agents should be considered. If the concomitant serotonergic agent is withdrawn, discontinuation symptoms can be observed).

No products indexed under this heading.

Fluvoxamine Maleate (Spontaneous reports of serotonin syndrome associated with the co-administration of linezolid and serotonergic agents, including antidepressants such as selective serotonin reuptake inhibitors (SSRIs), have been reported. Unless patients are carefully observed for signs and/or symptoms of serotonin syndrome, linezolid should not be administered to patients taking serotonin re-uptake inhibitors. Where administration of linezolid and concomitant serotonergic agents is clinically appropriate, patients should be closely observed for signs/symptoms of serotonin syndrome. If signs/symptoms occur, discontinuation of either one or both agents should be considered. If the concomitant serotonergic agent is withdrawn, discontinuation symptoms can be observed).

No products indexed under this heading.

Frovatriptan Succinate (Unless patients are carefully observed for signs and/or symptoms of serotonin syndrome, linezolid should not be administered to patients taking 5-HT1 receptor agonists (triptans)). Products include:
Frova 1103

Imipramine Hydrochloride (Unless patients are carefully observed for signs and/or symptoms of serotonin syndrome, linezolid should not be administered to patients taking tricyclic antidepressants).

No products indexed under this heading.

Imipramine Pamoate (Unless patients are carefully observed for signs and/or symptoms of serotonin syndrome, linezolid should not be administered to patients taking tricyclic antidepressants).

No products indexed under this heading.

Isocarboxazid (Linezolid should not be used in patients taking any medicinal product which inhibits monoamine oxidases A or B (eg, phenelzine, isocarboxazid) or within 2 weeks of taking such medicinal product). Products include:
Marplan 3481

Isoproterenol Hydrochloride (Unless patients are monitored for potential increases in BP, linezolid should not be administered to patients taking directly and indirectly acting sympathomimetic agents (eg, pseudoephedrine)).

No products indexed under this heading.

Isoproterenol Sulfate (Unless patients are monitored for potential increases in BP, linezolid should not be administered to patients taking directly and indirectly acting sympathomimetic agents (eg, pseudoephedrine)).

No products indexed under this heading.

Levalbuterol Hydrochloride (Unless patients are monitored for potential increases in BP, linezolid should not be administered to patients taking directly and indirectly acting sympathomimetic agents (eg, pseudoephedrine)).

No products indexed under this heading.

Levodopa (Unless patients are monitored for potential increases in BP, linezolid should not be administered to patients taking dopaminergic agents (eg, dopamine, dobutamine)). Products include:
Stalevo 2526

Maprotiline Hydrochloride (Unless patients are carefully observed for signs and/or symptoms of serotonin syndrome, linezolid should not be administered to patients taking tricyclic antidepressants).

No products indexed under this heading.

Meperidine Hydrochloride (Unless patients are carefully observed for signs and/or symptoms of serotonin syndrome, linezolid should not be administered to patients taking meperidine).

No products indexed under this heading.

Mephentermine Sulfate (Unless patients are monitored for potential increases in BP, linezolid should not be administered to patients taking vasopressive agents (eg, epinephrine, norepinephrine)).

No products indexed under this heading.

Metaproterenol Sulfate (Unless patients are monitored for potential increases in BP, linezolid should not be administered to patients taking directly and indirectly acting sympathomimetic agents (eg, pseudoephedrine)).

No products indexed under this heading.

Metaraminol Bitartrate (Unless patients are monitored for potential increases in BP, linezolid should not be administered to patients taking directly and indirectly acting sympathomimetic agents (eg, pseudoephedrine)).

No products indexed under this heading.

Methoxamine Hydrochloride (Unless patients are monitored for potential increases in BP, linezolid should not be administered to patients taking directly and indirectly acting sympathomimetic agents (eg, pseudoephedrine)).

No products indexed under this heading.

Moclobemide (Linezolid should not be used in patients taking any medicinal product which inhibits monoamine oxidases A or B (eg, phenelzine, isocarboxazid) or within 2 weeks of taking such medicinal product).

No products indexed under this heading.

Naratriptan Hydrochloride (Unless patients are carefully observed for signs and/or symptoms of serotonin syndrome, linezolid should not be administered to patients taking 5-HT1 receptor agonists (triptans)). Products include:
Amerge 1306

Norepinephrine Bitartrate (Unless patients are monitored for potential increases in BP, linezolid should not be administered to patients taking directly and indirectly acting sympathomimetic agents (eg, pseudoephedrine)).

No products indexed under this heading.

IMPORTANT NOTE: Always consult each drug listing in the patient's regimen for possible interactions.

Nortriptyline Hydrochloride (Unless patients are carefully observed for signs and/or symptoms of serotonin syndrome, linezolid should not be administered to patients taking tricyclic antidepressants).

No products indexed under this heading.

Pargyline Hydrochloride (Linezolid should not be used in patients taking any medicinal product which inhibits monoamine oxidases A or B (eg, phenelzine, isocarboxazid) or within 2 weeks of taking such medicinal product).

No products indexed under this heading.

Paroxetine (Spontaneous reports of serotonin syndrome associated with the co-administration of linezolid and serotonergic agents, including antidepressants such as selective serotonin reuptake inhibitors (SSRIs), have been reported. Unless patients are carefully observed for signs and/or symptoms of serotonin syndrome, linezolid should not be administered to patients taking serotonin re-uptake inhibitors. Where administration of linezolid and concomitant serotonergic agents is clinically appropriate, patients should be closely observed for signs/symptoms of serotonin syndrome. If signs/symptoms occur, discontinuation of either one or both agents should be considered. If the concomitant serotonergic agent is withdrawn, discontinuation symptoms can be observed).

No products indexed under this heading.

Paroxetine Hydrochloride (Spontaneous reports of serotonin syndrome associated with the co-administration of linezolid and serotonergic agents, including antidepressants such as selective serotonin reuptake inhibitors (SSRIs), have been reported. Unless patients are carefully observed for signs and/or symptoms of serotonin syndrome, linezolid should not be administered to patients taking serotonin re-uptake inhibitors. Where administration of linezolid and concomitant serotonergic agents is clinically appropriate, patients should be closely observed for signs/symptoms of serotonin syndrome. If signs/symptoms occur, discontinuation of either one or both agents should be considered. If the concomitant serotonergic agent is withdrawn, discontinuation symptoms can be observed). Products include:

Paroxetine Mesylate (Spontaneous reports of serotonin syndrome associated with the co-administration of linezolid and serotonergic agents, including antidepressants such as selective serotonin reuptake inhibitors (SSRIs), have been reported. Unless patients are carefully observed for signs and/or symptoms of serotonin syndrome, linezolid should not be administered to patients taking serotonin re-uptake inhibitors. Where administration of linezolid and concomitant serotonergic agents is clinically appropriate, patients should be closely observed for signs/symptoms of serotonin syndrome. If signs/symptoms occur, discontinuation of either one or both agents should be considered. If the concomitant serotonergic agent is withdrawn, discontinuation symptoms can be observed).

No products indexed under this heading.

Pergolide Mesylate (Unless patients are monitored for potential increases in BP, linezolid should not be administered to patients taking dopaminergic agents (eg, dopamine, dobutamine)).

No products indexed under this heading.

Phenelzine Sulfate (Linezolid should not be used in patients taking any medicinal product which inhibits monoamine oxidases A or B (eg, phenelzine, isocarboxazid) or within 2 weeks of taking such medicinal product).

No products indexed under this heading.

Phenylephrine Bitartrate (Unless patients are monitored for potential increases in BP, linezolid should not be administered to patients taking directly and indirectly acting sympathomimetic agents (eg, pseudoephedrine)).

No products indexed under this heading.

Phenylephrine Hydrochloride (Unless patients are monitored for potential increases in BP, linezolid should not be administered to patients taking directly and indirectly acting sympathomimetic agents (eg, pseudoephedrine)). Products include:

Phenylephrine Tannate (Unless patients are monitored for potential increases in BP, linezolid should not be administered to patients taking directly and indirectly acting sympathomimetic agents (eg, pseudoephedrine)).

No products indexed under this heading.

Phenylpropanolamine Hydrochloride (Unless patients are monitored for potential increases in BP, linezolid should not be administered to patients taking directly and indirectly acting sympathomimetic agents (eg, pseudoephedrine)).

No products indexed under this heading.

Pirbuterol Acetate (Unless patients are monitored for potential increases in BP, linezolid should not be administered to patients taking directly and indirectly acting sympathomimetic agents (eg, pseudoephedrine)). Products include:

Pramipexole Dihydrochloride (Unless patients are monitored for potential increases in BP, linezolid should not be administered to patients taking dopaminergic agents (eg, dopamine, dobutamine)).

No products indexed under this heading.

Procarbazine Hydrochloride (Linezolid should not be used in patients taking any medicinal product which inhibits monoamine oxidases A or B (eg, phenelzine, isocarboxazid) or within 2 weeks of taking such medicinal product).

No products indexed under this heading.

Protriptyline Hydrochloride (Unless patients are carefully observed for signs and/or symptoms of serotonin syndrome, linezolid should not be administered to patients taking tricyclic antidepressants).

No products indexed under this heading.

Pseudoephedrine Hydrochloride (Unless patients are monitored for potential increases in BP, linezolid should not be administered to patients taking directly and indirectly acting sympathomimetic agents (eg, pseudoephedrine)). Products include:

Pseudoephedrine Sulfate (Unless patients are monitored for potential increases in BP, linezolid should not be administered to patients taking directly and indirectly acting sympathomimetic agents (eg, pseudoephedrine)). Products include:

Clarinex-D 12-Hour 3101
Clarinex-D 3104

Rasagiline Mesylate (Linezolid should not be used in patients taking any medicinal product which inhibits monoamine oxidases A or B (eg, phenelzine, isocarboxazid) or within 2 weeks of taking such medicinal product). Products include:

Rifampin (In health volunteers, co-administration of rifampin with linezolid resulted in a 21% decrease in linezolid C_{max} and a 32% decrease in linezolid AUC. The clinical significance of this interaction is unknown).

No products indexed under this heading.

Rizatriptan Benzoate (Unless patients are carefully observed for signs and/or symptoms of serotonin syndrome, linezolid should not be administered to patients taking 5-HT1 receptor agonists (triptans)). Products include:

Ropinirole Hydrochloride (Unless patients are monitored for potential increases in BP, linezolid should not be administered to patients taking dopaminergic agents (eg, dopamine, dobutamine)). Products include:

Salmeterol Xinafoate (Unless patients are monitored for potential increases in BP, linezolid should not be administered to patients taking directly and indirectly acting sympathomimetic agents (eg, pseudoephedrine)). Products include:

Selegiline (Linezolid should not be used in patients taking any medicinal product which inhibits monoamine oxidases A or B (eg, phenelzine, isocarboxazid) or within 2 weeks of taking such medicinal product). Products include:

Selegiline Hydrochloride (Linezolid should not be used in patients taking any medicinal product which inhibits monoamine oxidases A or B (eg, phenelzine, isocarboxazid) or within 2 weeks of taking such medicinal product). Products include:

Sertraline Hydrochloride (Spontaneous reports of serotonin syndrome associated with the co-administration of linezolid and serotonergic agents, including antidepressants such as selective serotonin reuptake inhibitors (SSRIs), have been reported. Unless patients are carefully observed for signs and/or symptoms of serotonin syndrome, linezolid should not be administered to patients taking serotonin re-uptake inhibitors. Where administration of linezolid and concomitant serotonergic agents is clinically appropriate, patients should be closely observed for signs/symptoms of serotonin syndrome. If signs/symptoms occur, discontinuation of either one or both agents should be considered. If the concomitant serotonergic agent is withdrawn, discontinuation symptoms can be observed).

No products indexed under this heading.

Sumatriptan (Unless patients are carefully observed for signs and/or symptoms of serotonin syndrome, lin-

ezolid should not be administered to patients taking 5-HT1 receptor agonists (triptans)). Products include:

Sumatriptan Succinate (Unless patients are carefully observed for signs and/or symptoms of serotonin syndrome, linezolid should not be administered to patients taking 5-HT1 receptor agonists (triptans)). Products include:

Terbutaline Sulfate (Unless patients are monitored for potential increases in BP, linezolid should not be administered to patients taking directly and indirectly acting sympathomimetic agents (eg, pseudoephedrine)).

No products indexed under this heading.

Tranylcypromine Sulfate (Linezolid should not be used in patients taking any medicinal product which inhibits monoamine oxidases A or B (eg, phenelzine, isocarboxazid) or within 2 weeks of taking such medicinal product). Products include:

Trimipramine Maleate (Unless patients are carefully observed for signs and/or symptoms of serotonin syndrome, linezolid should not be administered to patients taking tricyclic antidepressants).

No products indexed under this heading.

Tyramine (A significant pressor response has been observed in normal adult subjects receiving linezolid and tyramine doses of more than 100 mg. Therefore, patients receiving linezolid need to avoid consuming large amounts of foods or beverages with high tyramine content).

No products indexed under this heading.

Venlafaxine Hydrochloride (Spontaneous reports of serotonin syndrome associated with the co-administration of linezolid and serotonergic agents, including antidepressants such as selective serotonin reuptake inhibitors (SSRIs), have been reported. Where administration of linezolid and concomitant serotonergic agents is clinically appropriate, patients should be closely observed for signs/symptoms of serotonin syndrome. If signs/symptoms occur, discontinuation of either one or both agents. If the concomitant serotonergic agent is withdrawn, discontinuation symptoms can be observed). Products include:

Zolmitriptan (Unless patients are carefully observed for signs and/or symptoms of serotonin syndrome, linezolid should not be administered to patients taking 5-HT1 receptor agonists (triptans)). Products include:

Food Interactions

Food, unspecified (Linezolid may be administered without regard to the timing of meals. The time to reach maximum concentration is delayed from 1.5 hours to 2.2 hours and C_{max} is decreased by about 17% when high fat food is given with linezolid. However, the total exposure measured as AUC values is similar under both conditions).

Food high in tyramine (A significant pressor response has been observed in normal adult subjects receiving linezolid and tyramine doses of more than 100 mg. Therefore, patients receiving linezolid need to avoid consuming large amounts of foods or beverages with high tyramine content).

SECTION 2

FOOD INTERACTIONS CROSS-REFERENCE

In this section, drug/food and drug/alcohol interactions listed in the preceding index are cross-referenced by dietary item. Under each entry is an alphabetical list, by brand name, of drugs said to interact with the item. A brief description of the interaction follows each brand, along with the page number of the underlying text. Page numbers refer to the 2010 editions of *Physicians' Desk Reference®*

or *PDR®* *for Ophthalmic Medicines* (denoted with the ⊙ symbol).

Entries in this section are limited to drug/food and drug/alcohol interactions listed in FDA-regulated prescribing information as published by *Physicians' Desk Reference®* or supplied by the manufacturer since the printing of the 2010 *PDR*.

Alcohol

ActoPlus Met Tablets (Alcohol is known to potentiate the effect of metformin on lactate metabolism. Patients, therefore, should be warned against excessive alcohol intake, acute or chronic, while receiving ActoPlus Met. In addition, hypoglycemia does not occur in patients receiving metformin alone under usual circumstances of use, but could occur when during concomitant use with ethanol) **3338**

Adcirca Tablets (Both alcohol and tadalafil, a PDE5 inhibitor, act as mild vasodilators. When mild vasodilators are taken in combination, blood pressure–lowering effects of each individual compound may be increased. Substantial consumption of alcohol (eg, 5 units or greater) in combination with tadalafil can increase the potential for orthostatic signs and symptoms, including increase in heart rate, decrease in standing blood pressure, dizziness, and headache).............**3461**

Adipex-P Tablets (May result in adverse drug interaction) **1178**

Advicor Tablets (Concomitant alcohol may increase the flushing and its use should be avoided around the time of Advicor administration).................. **402**

Aggrenox Capsules (Patients who consume three or more alcoholic drinks every day should be counseled about the bleeding risks involved with chronic, heavy alcohol use while taking aspirin)................................ **880**

Alphagan P Ophthalmic Solution (Possible additive or potentiating effect with CNS depressants) **596**

Ambien Tablets (Since the systematic evaluations of zolpidem in combination with other CNS-active drugs have been limited, careful consideration should be given to the pharmacology of any CNS-active drug to be used with zolpidem. Any drug with CNS-depressant effects could potentially enhance the CNS depressant effects of zolpidem. Dosage adjustments may be necessary when zolpidem is combined with other CNS depressant drugs) **2920**

Ambien CR Tablets (Any drug with CNS-depressant effects could potentially enhance the CNS-depressant effects of zolpidem tartrate. Dosage adjustments may be necessary when zolpidem tartrate is combined with other CNS depressant drugs) **2925**

Amrix Capsules (Concomitant use with cyclobenzaprine HCl may enhance the effects of CNS depressants) **964**

Apidra Injection (Alcohol may either potentiate or weaken the blood glucose-lowering effect of insulin) **2937**

Aplenzin Extended-Release Tablets (Bupropion is contraindicated in patients undergoing abrupt discontinuation of alcohol. Concomitant use of alcohol with bupropion is associated with an increased seizure risk. There

have been rare reports of adverse neuropsychiatric events or reduced alcohol tolerance in patients who were drinking alcohol during treatment with bupropion. The consumption of alcohol during treatment with bupropion should be minimized or avoided) **2948**

Atacand HCT 16-12.5 Tablets (May aggravate orthostatic hypotension produced by hydrochlorothiazide)...................... **700**

Avalide Tablets (Potentiation of orthostatic hypertension may occur during concomitant administration of hydrochlorothiazide with alcohol) **2956**

Avandamet Tablets (Alcohol potentiates the effect of metformin on lactate metabolism; patients should be warned against excessive alcohol intake, acute or chronic).....**1345**

Avinza Capsules (Patients must not consume alcoholic beverages, prescription or non-prescription medications containing alcohol while on morphine sulfate therapy. Consumption of alcohol while taking morphine sulfate may result in the rapid release and absorption of a potentially fatal dose of morphine)........................**1822**

Benadryl Allergy Ultratab Tablets (Increases drowsiness effect; avoid concomitant use) **2042**

Benicar HCT Tablets (Concurrent administration could cause potentiation of orthostatic hypotension)................................**1017**

Captopril Tablets (Drugs having vasodilator activity should, if possible, be discontinued before starting captopril)................**2341**

Carbatrol Capsules (Because of its primary CNS effect, caution should be used when carbamazepine is taken with alcohol) **3280**

Catapres-TTS (Clonidine may potentiate the CNS-depressive effects of alcohol, barbiturates or other sedating drugs)................ **884**

Celebrex Capsules (Other factors that increase the risk of GI bleeding in patients treated with NSAIDs include concomitant use of alcohol. Most spontaneous reports of fatal GI events are in elderly or debilitated patients and therefore special care should be taken in treating this population) **3272**

Celexa Tablets (Although citalopram did not potentiate cognitive and motor effects of alcohol, as with other psychotropic medications, the use of alcohol by depressed patients taking citalopram is not recommended) **1153**

Cialis Tablets (Both alcohol and tadalafil act as mild vasodilators. When mild vasodilators are taken in combination, blood-pressure-lowering effects of each individual compound may be increased. Substantial consumption of alcohol (eg, 5 units or greater) in combination with tadalafil can increase the potential for orthostatic signs and symptoms, including increase in heart rate, decrease in standing blood pressure, dizziness, and headache)..............**1861**

Clinoril Tablets (Concomitant use of alcohol may increase the risk of GI bleeding) **2098**

Alcohol Food Interactions Cross-Reference 2222

Clorpres Tablets (Clonidine may enhance the CNS-depressive effects of alcohol; orthostatic hypotension may be aggravated by alcohol) 2344
Combigan Ophthalmic Solution (Although specific drug interaction studies have not been conducted with Combigan, the possibility of an additive or potentiating effect with CNS depressants (alcohol, barbiturates, opiates, sedatives or anesthetics) should be considered) 601
Comtan Tablets (Due to the possible additive sedative effects, caution should be used when concomitantly taking other CNS depressants in combination with entacapone) 2409
Crestor Tablets (Rosuvastatin calcium should be used with caution in patients who consume substantial quantities of alcohol) 736
Cymbalta Delayed-Release Capsules (Use of duloxetine concomitantly with heavy alcohol intake may be associated with severe liver injury. For this reason, duloxetine should ordinarily not be prescribed for patients with substantial alcohol use) 1871
Depakote ER Extended Release Tablets (Since valproate products may produce CNS depression, especially when combined with another CNS depressant (eg, alcohol), patients should be advised not to engage in hazardous activities, such as driving an automobile or operating dangerous machinery, until it is known that they do not become drowsy from the drug) 426
Dilaudid Oral Liquid (Hydromorphone may be expected to have additive effects when used in conjunction with alcohol. Alcohol potentiates the respiratory depressant effects of hydromorphone, increasing the risk of respiratory depression that might result in death) 2797
Dilaudid-HP Injection (Hydromorphone may be expected to have additive effects when used in conjunction with alcohol. Alcohol potentiates the respiratory depressant effects of hydromorphone, increasing the risk of respiratory depression that might result in death) 2800
Diovan HCT Tablets (Concurrent use of thiazide diuretics with alcohol may result in potentiation of orthostatic hypotension) 2419
Duetact Tablets (All sulfonylurea drugs are capable of producing hypoglycemia; hypoglycemia is more likely to occur when alcohol is ingested) 3354
Duragesic Transdermal System (The comcomitant use of fentanyl with other CNS depressants may cause respiratory depression, hypotension, and profound sedation or potentially result in coma. When such combined therapy is contemplated, the dose of one or both agents should be significantly reduced. The use of concomitant CNS active drugs requires special patient care and observation) 2604
Effexor XR Extended-Release Capsules (Although venlafaxine has not been shown to increase the impairment of mental and motor skills caused by alcohol, patients should be advised to avoid alcohol while taking venlafaxine) 3504
Elidel Cream 1% (Skin flushing due to pimecrolimus is associated with alcohol use) 2424
Embeda Extended Release Capsules (Embeda should be used with great caution and in reduced dosage in patients who are concurrently receiving other central nervous system (CNS) depressants including alcohol because of the risk of respiratory depression, hypotension, and profound sedation or coma. When such combined therapy is contemplated, the initial dose of one or both agents should be reduced by at least 50%) 1831
Emsam Transdermal System (The use of alcohol is not recommended while using selegiline transdermal system) 3623
Equetro Extended-Release Capsules (Because of its primary CNS effect, caution should be used when carbamazepine is taken with alcohol) 3477
Exforge HCT Tablets (Potentiation of orthostatic hypotension may occur when alcohol and thiazide diuretics are administered concurrently) 2449
Exubera Inhalation Powder (Alcohol may either increase or reduce the blood glucose-lowering effect of insulin. Co-administration may require insulin dose adjustment and particularly close monitoring) 2717
Fanapt Tablets (Given the primary CNS effects of iloperidone, caution should be used when it is taken in combination with alcohol) 3484
Fentanyl Transdermal System Patches (Fentanyl may be expected to have additive CNS depressant effects when used in conjunction with alcohol. The concomitant use of fentanyl with alcohol may cause respiratory depression, hypotension, and profound sedation, or potentially result in coma or death) 2346
Fentora Tablets (The concomitant use of other CNS depressants, including other opioids, sedatives or hypnotics, general anesthetics, phenothiazines, tranquilizers, skeletal muscle relaxants, sedating antihistamines, potent inhibitors of cytochrome P450 3A4 isoform (eg, erythromycin, ketoconazole, and certain protease inhibitors), and alcoholic beverages may produce increased depressant effects. Hypoventilation, hypotension, and profound sedation may occur) 966
Finacea Gel (Concomitant use with any foods and beverages that might provoke erythema, flushing, and blushing (including spicy food, alcoholic beverages, and thermally hot drinks, including hot coffee and tea) should be avoided) 1808
Flolan for Injection (Additional reductions in blood pressure may occur) 1453
Focalin XR Capsules (Dexmethylphenidate hydrochloride should be given cautiously to patients with a history of drug dependence or alcoholism) 2472
Furosemide Tablets (Aggravates orthostatic hypotension) 2354
Gabitril Tablets (Because of the possible additive effects of drugs that may depress the nervous system, ethanol should be used cautiously in combination with tiagabine) 972
Geodon Capsules (Caution should be used when ziprasidone is taken in combination with other centrally acting drugs, given the primary CNS effects of ziprasidone) 2723
Humalog-Pen and KwikPen (Co-administration with drugs with hypoglycemic activity may result in decreased insulin requirements) 1910
Humalog Mix 50/50-Pen and KwikPen (Insulin requirements may be decreased in the presence of drugs with hypoglycemic activity, such as alcohol) 1914
Humulin N Vial (Insulin requirements may be reduced in the presence of drugs that lower blood glucose or affect how the body responds to insulin) 1934
Humulin R (U-500) (Insulin requirements may be decreased in the presence of drugs that increase insulin sensitivity or have hypoglycemic activity, such as alcohol) 1939
Hyzaar 50-12.5 Tablets (Potentiation of orthostatic hypotension may occur) 2162
Indapamide Tablets (Aggravates orthostatic hypotension) 2356
Intravenous Sodium Diuril (Hypotension including orthostatic hypotension may be aggravated or potentiated by alcohol when co-administered with chlorothiazide) 2009
Intuniv Extended-Release Tablets (Caution should be exercised when guanfacine is administered concomitantly with alcohol due to the potential for additive pharmacodynamic effects) 3291
Invega Extended-Release Tablets (Given the primary CNS effects of paliperidone, paliperidone should be used with caution in combination with other centrally acting drugs and alcohol) 2613
Invega Sustenna Extended-Release Injectable Suspension (Given the primary CNS effects paliperidone should be used with caution in combination with other centrally acting drugs and alcohol. Paliperidone may antagonize the effect of levodopa and other dopamine antagonists) 2621
Janumet Tablets (Alcohol is known to potentiate the effect of metformin on lactate metabolism. Patients, therefore, should be warned against excessive alcohol intake, acute or chronic, while receiving Janumet) 2188
Klonopin Tablets (The CNS-depressant action of the benzodiazepine class of drugs may be potentiated by alcohol. Patients should be advised to avoid alcohol while taking clonazepam) 2855
Lantus Injection (May either potentiate or weaken the blood-glucose-lowering effect of insulin) 2996
Levemir Injection (Co-administration may either potentiate or weaken the blood-glucose lowering effect of insulin) 2566
Lexapro Tablets (Although escitalopram did not potentiate the cognitive and motor effects of alcohol in a clinical trial, as with other psychotropic medications, the use of alcohol by patients taking escitalopram is not recommended) 1160
Lupron Depot 3.75 mg (In patients with major risk factors for decreased bone mineral content such as chronic alcohol use, leuprolide acetate depot may pose an additional risk. In these patients, the risks and benefits must be weighed carefully before therapy with leuprolide acetate depot alone is instituted, and concomitant treatment with norethindrone acetate 5 mg daily should be considered. Retreatment with gonadotropin-releasing hormone analogs, including leuprolide acetate, is not advisable in patients with major risk factors for loss of bone mineral content) 472
Lyrica Capsules (Patients who are taking other drugs associated with angioedema (eg, angiotensin converting enzyme inhibitors [ACE inhibitors]) may be at increased risk of developing angioedema) 2731
Marplan Tablets (Isocarboxazid should not be administered in combination with central nervous system depressants) 3481
Meridia Capsules (In a double-blind, placebo-controlled, crossover study in 19 volunteers, administration of a single dose of ethanol (0.5 mL/kg) together with 20 mg of sibutramine resulted in no psychomotor interactions of clinical significance between alcohol and sibutramine. However, the concomitant use of sibutramine and excess alcohol is not recommended) 492
Metozolv ODT Orally Disintegrating Tablets (Additive sedative effects can occur when metoclopramide is given with alcohol, sedatives, hypnotics, narcotics, or tranquilizers) 2901
Mevacor Tablets (Lovastatin should be used with caution in patients who have consumed substantial quantity of alcohol and have a past history of liver disease; active liver disease and unexplained elevation in transaminase are contraindications to the use of lovastatin) 2212
Micardis HCT Tablets (Potentiation of orthostatic hypotension may occur with alcohol, barbiturates, or narcotics when administered concurrently with thiazide diuretics) 889
Moban Tablets (Concomitant use of molindone with alcohol is contraindicated) 1108
MS Contin Tablets (Profound sedation, coma, severe hypotension, respiratory depression) 2803
Nascobal Nasal Spray (Heavy alcohol intake for longer than 2 weeks may produce malabsorption of vitamin B12) 2700
Nembutal Sodium Solution (Concurrent use of barbiturates with other CNS depressants (eg, alcohol) may result in additional CNS depressant effects. Alcohol should not be consumed while taking barbiturates) 2012
Niaspan Extended-Release Tablets (Concomitant alcohol may increase the side effects of flushing and pruritus and should be avoided around the time of Niaspan ingestion) 497

(⊙ Described in PDR® for Ophthalmic Medicines)

Nitro-Dur Transdermal Infusion System (Vasodilating effects of nitroglycerin may be additive with those of other vasodilators).....**3170**

Nitrolingual Pumpspray (Alcohol may enhance sensitivity to hypotensive effects of nitrates) **3266**

NovoLog Injection (A number of substances affect glucose metabolism and may require insulin dose adjustment and particularly close monitoring. Examples of substances that may either potentiate or weaken the blood-glucose-lowering effect of insulin include alcohol) **2575**

Nucynta Tablets (Patients receiving other opioid agonist analgesics, general anesthetics, phenothiazines, antiemetics, other tranquilizers, sedatives, hypnotics, or other CNS depressants (including alcohol) concomitantly with tapentadol hydrochloride may exhibit an additive CNS depression. Interactive effects resulting in respiratory depression, hypotension, profound sedation, or coma may result if these drugs are taken in combination with tapentadol hydrochloride. When such combined therapy is contemplated, a dose reduction of one or both agents should be considered) **2643**

Nuvigil Tablets (Patients should be advised that the use of armodafinil in combination with alcohol has not been studied. Patients should be advised that it is prudent to avoid alcohol while taking armodafinil) **978**

Onsolis Film (The concomitant use of fentanyl with other CNS depressants, including other opioids, sedatives or hypnotics, general anesthetics, phenothizines, tranquilizers, skeletal muscle relaxants, sedating antihistamines, and alcoholic beverages may produce increased depressant effects. Patients on concomitant CNS depressants must be monitored for a change in opioid effects. Consideration should be given to adjusting the dose of fentanyl if warranted) **2054**

Opana Tablets (The concomitant use of other CNS depressants including sedatives, hypnotics, tranquilizers, general anesthetics, phenothiazines, other opioids, and alcohol may produce additive CNS depressant effects. Additive effects resulting in respiratory depression, hypotension, profound sedation or coma may result if these drugs are taken in combination with the usual dose of oxymorphone hydrochloride) **1110**

OsmoPrep Tablets (There have been rare reports of generalized tonic-clonic seizures and/or loss of consciousness associated with use of sodium phosphate products in patients with no prior history of seizures. Sodium phosphate should be used with caution in patients at higher risk of seizure, such as those withdrawing from alcohol) **2907**

OxyContin Tablets (Oxycodone, like all opioid analgesics, should be started at 1/3 to 1/2 of the usual dosage in patients who are concurrently receiving other central nervous system depressants including alcohol because respiratory depression, hypotension, and profound sedation or coma may result) **2807**

Parnate Tablets (Concomitant use with some central nervous system depressants, such as alcohol, is contraindicated. A marked potentiating effect on alcohol has been reported) **1584**

Paroxetine Hydrochloride Controlled-release Tablets (Avoid alcohol while taking paroxetine hydrochloride controlled-release tablets).....**2361**

Paroxetine Hydrochloride Extended-release Tablets (Avoid alcohol while taking paroxetine hydrochloride controlled-release tablets)......**2371**

Patanase Nasal Spray (Concurrent use of olopatadine nasal spray with other central nervous system depressants should be avoided because additional reductions in alertness and additional impairment of central nervous system performance may occur) **585**

Paxil Tablets (Although paroxetine has not been shown to increase the impairment of mental and motor skills caused by alcohol, patients should be advised to avoid alcohol while taking paroxetine) **1586**

Paxil CR Controlled-Release Tablets (Although paroxetine has not been shown to increase the impairment of mental and motor skills caused by alcohol, patients should be advised to avoid alcohol while taking paroxetine) **1596**

Percocet Tablets (Additive CNS depression; dose of one or both agents should be reduced) **1121**

Percodan Tablets (Additive CNS depression) **1124**

Phenytek Capsules (Acute alcohol intake with phenytoin may increase phenytoin serum levels; chronic alcohol abuse with phenytoin may decrease phenytoin serum levels) **2380**

Photofrin for Injection (Drugs that decrease vasoconstriction could decrease the efficacy of photodynamic therapy (PDT)) **786**

Prinzide Tablets (Co-administration of thiazide and alcohol may potentiate orthostatic hypotension) **2246**

Pristiq Extended-Release Tablets (Caution is advised when desvenlafaxine is taken in combination with other CNS-active drugs) **3564**

Provigil Tablets (The use of modafinil in combination with alcohol has not been studied. It is advisable to avoid alcohol while taking modafinil)......**983**

Prozac Weekly Capsules (Caution is advised if the concomitant administration of fluoxetine and CNS-acting drugs is required. In evaluating individual cases, consideration should be given to using lower initial doses of the concomitantly administered drugs, using conservative titration schedules, and monitoring of clinical status) **1941**

Pylera Capsules (Alcoholic beverages should not be consumed during Pylera therapy and for at least 1 day afterward. Psychotic reactions have been reported in alcoholic patients who are using Pylera and disulfiram concurrently. Pylera should not be given to patients who have taken disulfiram within the last 2 weeks)......**793**

Remeron Tablets (Concomitant administration of alcohol (equivalent to 60 g) had a minimal effect on plasma levels of mirtazapine (15 mg) in healthy male subjects. However, the impairment of cognitive and motor skills produced by mirtazapine were shown to be additive with those produced by alcohol. Accordingly, patients should be advised to avoid alcohol while taking mirtazapine) **3214**

Requip Tablets (Sedating medications (such as alcohol or CNS depressants), the presence of sleeping disorders, or other medications that increase plasma levels of ropinirole, may increase the risk of somnolence or falling asleep while engaged in activities of daily living. Because of possible additive effects, caution should be advised when patients are taking other sedating medications, alcohol, or other CNS depressants (eg, benzodiazepines, antipsychotics, antidepressants) in combination with ropinirole) **1620**

Requip XL Tablets (Sedating medications (such as alcohol or CNS depressants), the presence of sleeping disorders, or other medications that increase plasma levels of ropinirole, may increase the risk of somnolence or falling asleep while engaged in activities of daily living. Because of possible additive effects, caution should be advised when patients are taking other sedating medications, alcohol, or other CNS depressants (eg, benzodiazepines, antipsychotics, antidepressants) in combination with ropinirole) **1628**

Rilutek Tablets (Whether alcohol increases the risk of serious hepatotoxicity with riluzole is unknown; therefore, patients being treated with riluzole should be discouraged from drinking excessive amounts of alcohol) **3032**

Risperdal Consta Long-Acting Injection (Given the primary CNS effects of risperidone, caution should be used if taken in combination with alcohol) **2682**

Rozerem Tablets (Complex behaviors, such as "sleep driving" (eg, driving while not fully awake after ingestion of hypnotic) and other complex behaviors (eg, preparing and eating food, making phone calls, or having sex), with amnesia for the event, have been reported in association with hypnotic use. The use of alcohol and other CNS depressants may increase the risk of such behaviors) **3366**

Ryzolt Extended-Release Tablets (Tramadol hydrochloride should be used with caution and in reduced dosages when administered to patients receiving CNS depressants, such as alcohol, opioids, anesthetic agents, narcotics, phenothiazines, tranquilizers, or sedative hypnotics. Tramadol hydrochloride increases the risk of CNS and respiratory depression) **2813**

St. Joseph 81 mg Aspirin Chewable and Enteric Coated Tablets (Chronic heavy alcohol users, 3 or more drinks per day, in combination with analgesic/antipyretic drug products containing aspirin increases the risk of adverse GI events, including stomach bleeding) **2045**

Salonpas Arthritis Pain (Having 3 or more alcoholic drinks everyday may increase the chance of stomach bleeding)......**1805**

Salonpas Pain Relief Patch (Having 3 or more alcoholic drinks everyday may increase the chance of stomach bleeding) **1805**

Saphris Tablets (Given the primary CNS effects of asenapine, caution should be used when it is taken in combination with other centrally-acting drugs or alcohol) **3223**

Savella Tablets (Milnacipran hydrochloride should not be prescribed to patients with substantial alcohol use or evidence of chronic liver disease because it is possible that milnacipran hydrochloride may aggravate pre-existing liver disease) **1172**

Seromycin Capsules (Concurrent use increases the possibility and risk of epileptic episodes)......**1956**

Seroquel Tablets (The cognitive and motor effect of alcohol is potentiated; alcohol use should be avoided) **750**

Seroquel XR Extended-Release Tablets (Given the primary CNS effects of quetiapine, caution should be used when it is taken in combination with other centrally acting drugs. Quetiapine potentiated the cognitive and motor effects of alcohol in a clinical trial in subjects with selected psychotic disorders, and alcoholic beverages should be limited while taking quetiapine) **759**

Skelaxin Tablets (The sedative effects of metaxalone and other CNS depressants (eg, alcohol) may be additive. Therefore, caution should be exercised with patients who take more than one of these CNS depressants simultaneously) **1848**

Soriatane Capsules (Clinical evidence has shown that etretinate can be formed with concurrent ingestion of acitretin and ethanol) **3326**

Symbyax Capsules (The co-administration of ethanol with Symbyax may potentiate sedation and orthostatic hypotension. Patients should be advised to avoid alcohol while taking Symbyax)......**1965**

Tekturna HCT Tablets (Potentiation of orthostatic hypotension may occur with concurrent use) **2541**

Teveten HCT Tablets (May potentiate orthostatic hypotension) **541**

Thioridazine Hydrochloride Tablets (Thioridazine is capable of potentiating CNS depressants)......**2384**

Thiothixene Capsules (Patients receiving thiothixene should be cautioned about the possible additive effects (which may include hypotension) with CNS depressants and with alcohol. Extreme caution should be used in patients with a history of convulsive disorders or those in a state of alcohol withdrawal, since it may lower the convulsive threshold) **2386**

Toviaz Extended-Release Tablets (Concomitant use with alcohol may enhance the drowsiness caused by fesoterodine)......**2753**

Transderm Scōp Transdermal Therapeutic System (Scopolamine is an anticholinergic agent and causes certain CNS effects, such as drowsiness and dizziness, and hence it should be used with care in patients on concomitant therapy) **2397**

Treximet Tablets (Other factors that increase the risk for gastrointestinal bleeding in patients treated with NSAIDs include concomitant use of alcohol) **1681**

Trilipix Delayed Release Capsules (Excessive alcohol intake should be addressed before triglyceride-lowering drug therapy, such as fenofibric acid, is considered. If the decision is

made to use lipid-altering drugs, the patient should be instructed that this does not reduce the importance of adhering to diet) 548

Trizivir Tablets (Concurrent use with ethanol decreases the elimination of abacavir causing an increase in overall exposure) 1688

Tussionex Pennkinetic Extended-Release Suspension (Combined therapy may result in additive CNS depression) 3443

Regular Strength Tylenol Tablets (Severe liver damage may occur if an adult has 3 or more alcoholic drinks every day while using this product) 2049

Tylenol with Codeine Tablets (Concomitant use with other CNS depressants may produce an additive CNS depression and should be avoided) 2691

Ultram ER Extended-Release Tablets (Tramadol hydrochloride should be used with caution and in reduced dosages when administered to patients receiving CNS depressants, such as alcohol, opioids, anesthetic agents, narcotics, phenothiazines, tranquilizers, or sedative hypnotics. Tramadol hydrochloride increases the risk of CNS and respiratory depression) 2693

Uniphyl Tablets (Concurrent use with a single dose of alcohol (3mL/kg of whiskey) decreases theophylline clearance for up to 24 hours) 2817

Valium Tablets (Concomitant use with alcohol is not recommended due to enhancement of the sedative effect) 2880

Venlafaxine Hydrochloride Tablets (Although venlafaxine has not been shown to increase the impairment of mental and motor skills caused by alcohol, patients should be advised to avoid alcohol while taking venlafaxine) 2388

Vicodin Tablets (May exhibit an additive CNS depression) 560

Vicodin ES Tablets (Additive CNS depression; the dose of one or both agents should be reduced) 561

Vicodin HP Tablets (Co-administration may result in an additive CNS depression) 563

Vicoprofen Tablets (May exhibit additive CNS depression) 564

Visudyne for Injection (Co-administration with compounds that quench active oxygen species or scavenge radicals, such as ethanol, would be expected to decrease verteporfin activity) 2549

Vytorin 10/10 Tablets (Vytorin should be used with caution in patients who consume substantial quantities of alcohol and/or have a past history of liver disease) 2303

Vytorin 10/10 Tablets (Vytorin should be used with caution in patients who consume substantial quantities of alcohol and/or have a past history of liver disease) 3240

Wellbutrin Tablets (Bupropion is contraindicated in patients undergoing abrupt discontinuation of alcohol. In post-marketing experience, there have been rare reports of adverse neuropsychiatric events or reduced alcohol tolerance in patients who were drinking during treatment with bupropion. The consumption of alcohol should be minimized or avoided) 1719

Xenazine Tablets (Patients should be advised that the concomitant use of alcohol or other sedating drugs with tetrabenazine may have additive effects and

worsen sedation and somnolence) 2033

Xyzal Oral Solution (Concurrent use of levocetirizine dihydrochloride with other central nervous system depressants should be avoided because additional reductions in alertness and additional impairment of central nervous system performance may occur) 3449

Xyzal Oral Solution (Concurrent use of levocetirizine dihydrochloride with other central nervous system depressants should be avoided because additional reductions in alertness and additional impairment of central nervous system performance may occur) 3053

Ziagen Tablets (Ethanol decreases the elimination of abacavir, causing an increase in overall exposure. Co-administration of ethanol and abacavir resulted in a 41% increase in abacavir AUC and a 26% increase in abacavir $t_{1/2}$) 1740

Zocor Tablets (Simvastatin should be used with caution in patients who consume substantial quantities of alcohol) 2289

Zonegran Capsules (Concomitant administration of zonisamide and alcohol or other CNS depressants has not been evaluated in clinical studies. Because of the potential of zonisamide to cause CNS depression, as well as other cognitive and/or neuropsychiatric adverse events, zonisamide should be used with caution if used in combination with alcohol or other CNS depressants) 1081

Zyban Sustained-Release Tablets (Bupropion is contraindicated in patients undergoing abrupt discontinuation of alcohol. In post-marketing experience, there have been rare reports of adverse neuropsychiatric events or reduced alcohol tolerance in patients who were drinking alcohol during treatment with bupropion. The consumption of alcohol during treatment with bupropion should be minimized or avoided) 1762

Zydone Tablets (Co-administration may exhibit additive CNS depression) 1138

Zyprexa Tablets (Co-administration of alcohol with olanzapine potentiates orthostatic hypotension; concurrent use should be avoided. Given the primary CNS effects of olanzapine, caution should be used when olanzapine is taken in combination with other centrally-acting drugs and alcohol) 1984

Zyprexa IntraMuscular (Co-administration of alcohol with olanzapine potentiates orthostatic hypotension; concurrent use should be avoided. Given the primary CNS effects of olanzapine, caution should be used when olanzapine is taken in combination with other centrally-acting drugs and alcohol) 1984

Zyrtec Allergy Tablets (Alcohol may increase drowsiness. Avoid alcoholic drinks) 2052

Children's Zyrtec Allergy Chewable Tablets (Alcohol may increase drowsiness. Avoid alcoholic drinks) 2053

Children's Zyrtec Allergy Syrup (Concomitant use may increase drowsiness) 2053

Children's Zyrtec Hives Relief Syrup (Concomitant use may increase drowsiness) 2053

Zyrtec-D Allergy & Congestion Extended-Release Tablets (Concurrent use with alcohol may increase drowsiness; avoid alcohol) 2054

Anchovies
Parnate Tablets (Tranylcypromine is contraindicated in combination with foods with a high tyramine content. Hypertensive crises have sometimes occurred during therapy with tranylcypromine after ingestion of foods with a high tyramine content. In particular, patients should be instructed not to take foods, such as anchovies) 1584

Apple Juice
Allegra ODT Orally Disintegrating Tablets (Fruit juices such as grapefruit, orange and apple may reduce the bioavailability and exposure of fexofenadine) 2911

Allegra-D 12 Hour Extended-Release Tablets (Co-administration with grapefruit, orange or apple juice will reduce the bioavailability and exposure or fexofenadine) 2915

Avocados
Parnate Tablets (Tranylcypromine is contraindicated in combination with foods with a high tyramine content. Hypertensive crises have sometimes occurred during therapy with tranylcypromine after ingestion of foods with a high tyramine content. In particular, patients should be instructed not to take foods, such as avocados) 1584

Bananas
Parnate Tablets (Tranylcypromine is contraindicated in combination with foods with a high tyramine content. Hypertensive crises have sometimes occurred during therapy with tranylcypromine after ingestion of foods with a high tyramine content. In particular, patients should be instructed not to take foods, such as bananas) 1584

Beans, broad
Parnate Tablets (Tranylcypromine is contraindicated in combination with foods with a high tyramine content. Hypertensive crises have sometimes occurred during therapy with tranylcypromine after ingestion of food with a high tyramine content. In particular, patients should be instructed not to take foods, such as the pods of broad beans) 1584

Beans, Fava
Parnate Tablets (Tranylcypromine is contraindicated in combination with foods with a high tyramine content. Hypertensive crises have sometimes occurred during therapy with tranylcypromine after ingestion of food with a high tyramine content. In particular, patients should be instructed not to take foods, such as the pods of broad beans (fava beans)) 1584

Beer, alcohol-free
Parnate Tablets (Tranylcypromine is contraindicated in combination with foods with a high tyramine content. Hypertensive crises have sometimes occurred during therapy with tranylcypromine after ingestion of foods with a high tyramine content. In particular, patients should be instructed not to take foods,

such as beer (including non-alcoholic beer)) 1584

Beer, reduced-alcohol
ActoPlus Met Tablets (Alcohol is known to potentiate the effect of metformin on lactate metabolism. Patients, therefore, should be warned against excessive alcohol intake, acute or chronic, while receiving ActoPlus Met. In addition, hypoglycemia does not occur in patients receiving metformin alone under usual circumstances of use, but could occur when during concomitant use with ethanol) 3338

Adcirca Tablets (Both alcohol and tadalafil, a PDE5 inhibitor, act as mild vasodilators. When mild vasodilators are taken in combination, blood pressure–lowering effects of each individual compound may be increased. Substantial consumption of alcohol (eg, 5 units or greater) in combination with tadalafil can increase the potential for orthostatic signs and symptoms, including increase in heart rate, decrease in standing blood pressure, dizziness, and headache) 3461

Adipex-P Tablets (May result in adverse drug interaction) 1178

Advicor Tablets (Concomitant alcohol may increase the flushing and its use should be avoided around the time of Advicor administration)................. 402

Aggrenox Capsules (Patients who consume three or more alcoholic drinks every day should be counseled about the bleeding risks involved with chronic, heavy alcohol use while taking aspirin)................................ 880

Alphagan P Ophthalmic Solution (Possible additive or potentiating effect with CNS depressants) 596

Ambien Tablets (An additive effect on psychomotor performance between alcohol and zolpidem was demonstrated. Zolpidem should not be taken with alcohol) 2920

Ambien CR Tablets (Zolpidem tartrate has shown additive effects when combined with alcohol and should not be taken with alcohol) 2925

Amrix Capsules (Concomitant use with cyclobenzaprine HCl may enhance the effects of alcohol) 964

Apidra Injection (Alcohol may either potentiate or weaken the blood glucose-lowering effect of insulin) 2937

Aplenzin Extended-Release Tablets (Bupropion is contraindicated in patients undergoing abrupt discontinuation of alcohol. Concomitant use of alcohol with bupropion is associated with an increased seizure risk. There have been rare reports of adverse neuropsychiatric events or reduced alcohol tolerance in patients who were drinking alcohol during treatment with bupropion. The consumption of alcohol during treatment with bupropion should be minimized or avoided) 2948

Atacand HCT 16-12.5 Tablets (May aggravate orthostatic hypotension produced by hydrochlorothiazide)..................... 700

Avalide Tablets (Potentiation of orthostatic hypertension may occur during concomitant administration of hydrochlorothiazide with alcohol) 2956

Avandamet Tablets (Alcohol potentiates the effect of metformin on lactate metabolism; patients should be

and have a past history of liver disease; active liver disease and unexplained elevation in transaminase are contraindications to the use of lovastatin) 2212
Micardis HCT Tablets (Potentiation of orthostatic hypotension may occur with alcohol, barbiturates, or narcotics when administered concurrently with thiazide diuretics) 889
Moban Tablets (Concomitant use of molindone with alcohol is contraindicated) 1108
MS Contin Tablets (Respiratory depression, hypotension and profound sedation or coma may result) 2803
Nascobal Nasal Spray (Heavy alcohol intake for longer than 2 weeks may produce malabsorption of vitamin B12) 2700
Nembutal Sodium Solution (Concurrent use of barbiturates with other CNS depressants (eg, alcohol) may result in additional CNS depressant effects. Alcohol should not be consumed while taking barbiturates) 2012
Niaspan Extended-Release Tablets (Concomitant alcohol may increase the side effects of flushing and pruritus and should be avoided around the time of Niaspan ingestion) 497
Nitro-Dur Transdermal Infusion System (Enhances sensitivity to the hypotensive effects) 3170
Nitrolingual Pumpspray (Alcohol may enhance sensitivity to hypotensive effects of nitrates) 3266
NovoLog Injection (A number of substances affect glucose metabolism and may require insulin dose adjustment and particularly close monitoring. Examples of substances that may either potentiate or weaken the blood-glucose-lowering effect of insulin include alcohol) 2575
Nucynta Tablets (Due to its mu-opioid agonist activity, tapentadol hydrochloride may be expected to have additive effects when used in conjunction with alcohol, opioids, or illicit drugs that cause central nervous system depression, respiratory depression, hypotension, and profound sedation, coma or death) 2643
Nuvigil Tablets (Patients should be advised that the use of armodafinil in combination with alcohol has not been studied. Patients should be advised that it is prudent to avoid alcohol while taking armodafinil) 978
Onsolis Film (The concomitant use of fentanyl with other CNS depressants, including other opioids, sedatives or hypnotics, general anesthetics, phenothiazines, tranquilizers, skeletal muscle relaxants, sedating antihistamines, and alcoholic beverages may produce increased depressant effects) 2054
Opana Tablets (The concomitant use of other CNS depressants including sedatives, hypnotics, tranquilizers, general anesthetics, phenothiazines, other opioids, and alcohol may produce additive CNS depressant effects. Additive effects resulting in respiratory depression, hypotension, profound sedation or coma may result if these drugs are taken in combination with the usual doses of oxymorphone hydrochloride) 1110
OsmoPrep Tablets (There have been rare reports of generalized tonic-clonic seizures and/or loss of consciousness associated with use of sodium phosphate products in patients with no prior history of seizures. Sodium phosphate should be used with caution in patients at higher risk of seizure, such as those withdrawing from alcohol) 2907
OxyContin Tablets (Oxycodone, like all opioid analgesics, should be started at 1/3 to 1/2 of the usual dosage in patients who are concurrently receiving other central nervous system depressants including alcohol because respiratory depression, hypotension, and profound sedation or coma may result) 2807
Parnate Tablets (Tranylcypromine is contraindicated in combination with foods with a high tyramine content. Hypertensive crises have sometimes occurred during therapy with tranylcypromine after ingestion of foods with a high tyramine content. In particular, patients should be instructed not to take foods, such as beer (including non-alcoholic beer)) 1584
Paroxetine Hydrochloride Controlled-release Tablets (Avoid alcohol while taking paroxetine hydrochloride controlled-release tablets) 2361
Paroxetine Hydrochloride Extended-release Tablets (Avoid alcohol while taking paroxetine hydrochloride controlled-release tablets) 2371
Patanase Nasal Spray (Concurrent use of olopatadine nasal spray with alcohol should be avoided because additional reductions in alertness and additional impairment of central nervous system performance may occur) 585
Paxil Tablets (Although paroxetine has not been shown to increase the impairment of mental and motor skills caused by alcohol, patients should be advised to avoid alcohol while taking paroxetine) 1586
Paxil CR Controlled-Release Tablets (Although paroxetine has not been shown to increase the impairment of mental and motor skills caused by alcohol, patients should be advised to avoid alcohol while taking paroxetine) 1596
Percocet Tablets (Additive CNS depression) 1121
Percodan Tablets (Additive CNS depression) 1124
Phenytek Capsules (Acute alcohol intake with phenytoin may increase phenytoin serum levels; chronic alcohol abuse with phenytoin may decrease phenytoin serum levels) 2380
Photofrin for Injection (Compounds that quench active oxygen species or scavenge radicals, such as ethanol would be expected to decrease photodynamic therapy (PDT) activity) 786
Prinzide Tablets (Co-administration of thiazide and alcohol may potentiate orthostatic hypotension) 2246
Pristiq Extended-Release Tablets (A clinical study has shown that desvenlafaxine does not increase the impairment of mental and motor skills caused by ethanol. However, patients should be advised to avoid alcohol consumption while taking desvenlafaxine) 3564
Provigil Tablets (The use of modafinil in combination with alcohol has not been studied. It is advisable to avoid alcohol while taking modafinil) 983
Prozac Weekly Capsules (Concurrent use with alcohol requires caution) 1941
Pylera Capsules (Alcoholic beverages should not be consumed during Pylera therapy and for at least 1 day afterward. Psychotic reactions have been reported in alcoholic patients who are using Pylera and disulfiram concurrently. Pylera should not be given to patients who have taken disulfiram within the last 2 weeks) 793
Remeron Tablets (Concomitant administration of alcohol (equivalent to 60 g) had a minimal effect on plasma levels of mirtazapine (15 mg) in healthy male subjects. However, the impairment of cognitive and motor skills produced by mirtazapine were shown to be additive with those produced by alcohol. Accordingly, patients should be advised to avoid alcohol while taking mirtazapine) 3214
Requip Tablets (Sedating medications (such as alcohol or CNS depressants), may increase the risk of somnolence or falling asleep while engaged in activities of daily living. Because of possible additive effects, caution should be advised when patients are taking other sedating medications, alcohol, or other CNS depressants in combination with ropinirole) 1620
Requip XL Tablets (Sedating medications (such as alcohol or CNS depressants), may increase the risk of somnolence or falling asleep while engaged in activities of daily living. Because of possible additive effects, caution should be advised when patients are taking other sedating medications, alcohol, or other CNS depressants in combination with ropinirole) 1628
Rilutek Tablets (Whether alcohol increases the risk of serious hepatotoxicity with riluzole is unknown; therefore, patients being treated with riluzole should be discouraged from drinking excessive amounts of alcohol) 3032
Risperdal Consta Long-Acting Injection (Given the primary CNS effects of risperidone, caution should be used if taken in combination with alcohol) 2682
Rozerem Tablets (Complex behaviors, such as "sleep driving" (eg, driving while not fully awake after ingestion of hypnotic) and other complex behaviors (eg, preparing and eating food, making phone calls, or having sex), with amnesia for the event, have been reported in association with hypnotic use. The use of alcohol and other CNS depressants may increase the risk of such behaviors) 3366
Ryzolt Extended-Release Tablets (Patients should be cautioned about the concomitant use of tramadol products and alcohol because of potentially serious CNS-additive effects of these agents. When large doses of tramadol are administered with alcohol, respiratory depression may result. Prescribe tramadol with caution for patients who use alcohol in excess) 2813
St. Joseph 81 mg Aspirin Chewable and Enteric Coated Tablets (Chronic heavy alcohol users, 3 or more drinks per day, in combination with analgesic/antipyretic drug products containing aspirin increases the risk of adverse GI events, including stomach bleeding) 2045
Salonpas Arthritis Pain (Having 3 or more alcoholic drinks everyday may increase the chance of stomach bleeding) 1805
Salonpas Pain Relief Patch (Having 3 or more alcoholic drinks everyday may increase the chance of stomach bleeding) 1805
Saphris Tablets (Given the primary CNS effects of asenapine, caution should be used when it is taken in combination with other centrally-acting drugs or alcohol) 3223
Savella Tablets (Milnacipran hydrochloride should not be prescribed to patients with substantial alcohol use or evidence of chronic liver disease because it is possible that milnacipran hydrochloride may aggravate pre-existing liver disease) 1172
Seromycin Capsules (Concurrent use increases the possibility and risk of epileptic episodes) 1956
Seroquel Tablets (Quetiapine potentiated the cognitive and motor effects of alcohol in a clinical trial in subjects with selected psychotic disorders. Alcoholic beverages should be avoided while taking quetiapine) 750
Seroquel XR Extended-Release Tablets (Given the primary CNS effects of quetiapine, caution should be used when it is taken in combination with other centrally acting drugs. Quetiapine potentiated the cognitive and motor effects of alcohol in a clinical trial in subjects with selected psychotic disorders, and alcoholic beverages should be limited while taking quetiapine) 759
Skelaxin Tablets (The sedative effects of metaxalone and other CNS depressants (eg, alcohol) may be additive. Therefore, caution should be exercised with patients who take more than one of these CNS depressants simultaneously) 1848
Soriatane Capsules (Clinical evidence has shown that etretinate can be formed with concurrent ingestion of acitretin and ethanol) 3326
Symbyax Capsules (The co-administration of ethanol with Symbyax may potentiate sedation and orthostatic hypotension. Patients should be advised to avoid alcohol while taking Symbyax) 1965
Tekturna HCT Tablets (Potentiation of orthostatic hypotension may occur with concurrent use) 2541
Teveten HCT Tablets (May potentiate orthostatic hypotension) 541
Thioridazine Hydrochloride Tablets (Thioridazine is capable of potentiating CNS depressants) 2384
Thiothixene Capsules (Patients receiving thiothixene should be cautioned about the possible additive effects (which may include hypotension) with CNS depressants and with alcohol. Extreme caution should be used in patients with a history of convulsive disorders or those in a state of alcohol withdrawal, since it may lower the convulsive threshold) 2386
Toviaz Extended-Release Tablets (Concomitant use with alcohol may enhance the drowsiness caused by fesoterodine) 2753
Transderm Scōp Transdermal Therapeutic System (Scopolamine is an anticholinergic agent and

(☉ Described in PDR® for Ophthalmic Medicines)

causes certain CNS effects, such as drowsiness and dizziness, and hence it should be used with care in patients on concomitant therapy) **2397**

Treximet Tablets (Other factors that increase the risk for gastrointestinal bleeding in patients treated with NSAIDs include concomitant use of alcohol) **1681**

Trilipix Delayed Release Capsules (Excessive alcohol intake should be addressed before triglyceride-lowering drug therapy, such as fenofibric acid, is considered. If the decision is made to use lipid-altering drugs, the patient should be instructed that this does not reduce the importance of adhering to diet) **548**

Trizivir Tablets (Concurrent use with ethanol decreases the elimination of abacavir causing an increase in overall exposure) **1688**

Tussionex Pennkinetic Extended-Release Suspension (Combined use may result in additive CNS depression) **3443**

Regular Strength Tylenol Tablets (Severe liver damage may occur if an adult has 3 or more alcoholic drinks every day while using this product) **2049**

Tylenol with Codeine Tablets (Concomitant use with alcohol may produce an additive CNS depression and should be avoided) **2691**

Ultram ER Extended-Release Tablets (Tramadol hydrochloride is contraindicated in acute intoxication with alcohol. Tramadol hydrochloride should be used with caution and in reduced dosages when administered to patients receiving CNS depressants, such as alcohol. Tramadol may be expected to have additive effects when used in conjunction with alcohol) **2693**

Uniphyl Tablets (Concurrent use with a single dose of alcohol (3mL/kg of whiskey) decreases theophylline clearance for up to 24 hours).....................................**2817**

Valium Tablets (Concomitant use with alcohol is not recommended due to enhancement of the sedative effect) **2880**

Venlafaxine Hydrochloride Tablets (Although venlafaxine has not been shown to increase the impairment of mental and motor skills caused by alcohol, patients should be advised to avoid alcohol while taking venlafaxine) **2388**

Vicodin Tablets (May exhibit an additive CNS depression) **560**

Vicodin ES Tablets (Additive CNS depression) **561**

Vicodin HP Tablets (Concurrent use results in an additive CNS depression) **563**

Vicoprofen Tablets (May exhibit additive CNS depression) **564**

Visudyne for Injection (Co-administration with compounds that quench active oxygen species or scavenge radicals, such as ethanol, would be expected to decrease verteporfin activity) **2549**

Vytorin 10/10 Tablets (Vytorin should be used with caution in patients who consume substantial quantities of alcohol and/or have a past history of liver disease) **2303**

Vytorin 10/10 Tablets (Vytorin should be used with caution in patients who consume substantial quantities of alcohol and/or have a past history of liver disease) **3240**

Wellbutrin Tablets (Bupropion is contraindicated in patients undergoing abrupt discontinuation of alcohol. In post-marketing experience, there have been rare reports of adverse neuropsychiatric events or reduced alcohol tolerance in patients who were drinking during treatment with bupropion. The consumption of alcohol should be minimized or avoided) **1719**

Xenazine Tablets (Patients should be advised that the concomitant use of alcohol or other sedating drugs with tetrabenazine may have additive effects and worsen sedation and somnolence)................................**2033**

Xyzal Oral Solution (Concurrent use of levocetirizine dihydrochloride with alcohol should be avoided because additional reductions in alertness and additional impairment of central nervous system performance may occur) **3449**

Xyzal Oral Solution (Concurrent use of levocetirizine dihydrochloride with alcohol should be avoided because additional reductions in alertness and additional impairment of central nervous system performance may occur) **3053**

Ziagen Tablets (Ethanol decreases the elimination of abacavir, causing an increase in overall exposure. Co-administration of ethanol and abacavir resulted in a 41% increase in abacavir AUC and a 26% increase in abacavir $t_{1/2}$)........**1740**

Zocor Tablets (Simvastatin should be used with caution in patients who consume substantial quantities of alcohol) **2289**

Zonegran Capsules (Concomitant administration of zonisamide and alcohol or other CNS depressants has not been evaluated in clinical studies. Because of the potential of zonisamide to cause CNS depression, as well as other cognitive and/or neuropsychiatric adverse events, zonisamide should be used with caution if used in combination with alcohol or other CNS depressants) **1081**

Zyban Sustained-Release Tablets (Bupropion is contraindicated in patients undergoing abrupt discontinuation of alcohol. In post-marketing experience, there have been rare reports of adverse neuropsychiatric events or reduced alcohol tolerance in patients who were drinking alcohol during treatment with bupropion. The consumption of alcohol during treatment with bupropion should be minimized or avoided) **1762**

Zydone Tablets (Co-administration may exhibit additive CNS depression) **1138**

Zyprexa Tablets (Co-administration of alcohol with olanzapine potentiates orthostatic hypotension; concurrent use should be avoided. Given the primary CNS effects of olanzapine, caution should be used when olanzapine is taken in combination with other centrally-acting drugs and alcohol) **1984**

Zyprexa IntraMuscular (Co-administration of alcohol with olanzapine potentiates orthostatic hypotension; concurrent use should be avoided. Given the primary CNS effects of olanzapine, caution should be used when olanzapine is taken in combination with other centrally-acting drugs and alcohol) **1984**

Zyrtec Allergy Tablets (Alcohol may increase drowsiness. Avoid alcoholic drinks)........................**2052**

Children's Zyrtec Allergy Chewable Tablets (Alcohol may increase drowsiness. Avoid alcoholic drinks)........................**2053**

Children's Zyrtec Allergy Syrup (Concomitant use may increase drowsiness)..............................**2053**

Children's Zyrtec Hives Relief Syrup (Concomitant use may increase drowsiness)..................**2053**

Zyrtec-D Allergy & Congestion Extended-Release Tablets (Concurrent use with alcohol may increase drowsiness; avoid alcohol) **2054**

Beer, unspecified

ActoPlus Met Tablets (Alcohol is known to potentiate the effect of metformin on lactate metabolism. Patients, therefore, should be warned against excessive alcohol intake, acute or chronic, while receiving ActoPlus Met. In addition, hypoglycemia does not occur in patients receiving metformin alone under usual circumstances of use, but could occur when during concomitant use with ethanol) **3338**

Adcirca Tablets (Both alcohol and tadalafil, a PDE5 inhibitor, act as mild vasodilators. When mild vasodilators are taken in combination, blood pressure–lowering effects of each individual compound may be increased. Substantial consumption of alcohol (eg, 5 units or greater) in combination with tadalafil can increase the potential for orthostatic signs and symptoms, including increase in heart rate, decrease in standing blood pressure, dizziness, and headache)..............**3461**

Adipex-P Tablets (May result in adverse drug interaction) **1178**

Advicor Tablets (Concomitant alcohol may increase the flushing and its use should be avoided around the time of Advicor administration)..................**402**

Aggrenox Capsules (Patients who consume three or more alcoholic drinks every day should be counseled about the bleeding risks involved with chronic, heavy alcohol use while taking aspirin)..............................**880**

Alphagan P Ophthalmic Solution (Possible additive or potentiating effect with CNS depressants) **596**

Ambien Tablets (An additive effect on psychomotor performance between alcohol and zolpidem was demonstrated. Zolpidem should not be taken with alcohol) **2920**

Ambien CR Tablets (Zolpidem tartrate has shown additive effects when combined with alcohol and should not be taken with alcohol) **2925**

Amrix Capsules (Concomitant use with cyclobenzaprine HCl may enhance the effects of alcohol) **964**

Apidra Injection (Alcohol may either potentiate or weaken the blood glucose-lowering effect of insulin) **2937**

Aplenzin Extended-Release Tablets (Bupropion is contraindicated in patients undergoing abrupt discontinuation of alcohol. Concomitant use of alcohol with bupropion is associated with an increased seizure risk. There have been rare reports of adverse neuropsychiatric events or reduced alcohol tolerance in patients who were

drinking alcohol during treatment with bupropion. The consumption of alcohol during treatment with bupropion should be minimized or avoided) **2948**

Atacand HCT 16-12.5 Tablets (May aggravate orthostatic hypotension produced by hydrochlorothiazide)......................**700**

Avalide Tablets (Potentiation of orthostatic hypertension may occur during concomitant administration of hydrochlorothiazide with alcohol) **2956**

Avandamet Tablets (Alcohol potentiates the effect of metformin on lactate metabolism; patients should be warned against excessive alcohol intake, acute or chronic).....**1345**

Avinza Capsules (Patients must not consume alcoholic beverages, prescription or non-prescription medications containing alcohol while on morphine sulfate therapy. Consumption of alcohol while taking morphine sulfate may result in the rapid release and absorption of a potentially fatal dose of morphine)....................**1822**

Benadryl Allergy Ultratab Tablets (Increases drowsiness effect; avoid concomitant use) **2042**

Benicar HCT Tablets (Concurrent administration could cause potentiation of orthostatic hypotension)..............................**1017**

Carbatrol Capsules (Because of its primary CNS effect, caution should be used when carbamazepine is taken with alcohol) **3280**

Catapres-TTS (Clonidine may potentiate the CNS-depressive effects of alcohol, barbiturates or other sedating drugs) **884**

Celebrex Capsules (Other factors that increase the risk of GI bleeding in patients treated with NSAIDs include concomitant use of alcohol. Most spontaneous reports of fatal GI events are in elderly or debilitated patients and therefore special care should be taken in treating this population) **3272**

Celexa Tablets (Although citalopram did not potentiate cognitive and motor effects of alcohol, as with other psychotropic medications, the use of alcohol by depressed patients taking citalopram is not recommended)...........................**1153**

Cialis Tablets (Both alcohol and tadalafil act as mild vasodilators. When mild vasodilators are taken in combination, blood-pressure-lowering effects of each individual compound may be increased. Substantial consumption of alcohol (eg, 5 units or greater) in combination with tadalafil can increase the potential for orthostatic signs and symptoms, including increase in heart rate, decrease in standing blood pressure, dizziness, and headache)..............**1861**

Clinoril Tablets (Concomitant use of alcohol may increase the risk of GI bleeding) **2098**

Clorpres Tablets (Clonidine may enhance the CNS-depressive effects of alcohol; orthostatic hypotension may be aggravated by alcohol) **2344**

Combigan Ophthalmic Solution (Although specific drug interaction studies have not been conducted with Combigan, the possibility of an additive or potentiating effect with CNS depressants (alcohol, barbiturates, opiates, sedatives

alcoholic beverages may produce increased depressant effects) **2054**

Opana Tablets (The concomitant use of other CNS depressants including sedatives, hypnotics, tranquilizers, general anesthetics, phenothiazines, other opioids, and alcohol may produce additive CNS depressant effects. Additive effects resulting in respiratory depression, hypotension, profound sedation or coma may result if these drugs are taken in combination with the usual doses of oxymorphone hydrochloride) **1110**

OsmoPrep Tablets (There have been rare reports of generalized tonic-clonic seizures and/or loss of consciousness associated with use of sodium phosphate products in patients with no prior history of seizures. Sodium phosphate should be used with caution in patients at higher risk of seizure, such as those withdrawing from alcohol) **2907**

OxyContin Tablets (Oxycodone, like all opioid analgesics, should be started at 1/3 to 1/2 of the usual dosage in patients who are concurrently receiving other central nervous system depressants including alcohol because respiratory depression, hypotension, and profound sedation or coma may result) **2807**

Parnate Tablets (Tranylcypromine is contraindicated in combination with foods with a high tyramine content. Hypertensive crises have sometimes occurred during therapy with tranylcypromine after ingestion of foods with a high tyramine content. In particular, patients should be instructed not to take foods, such as beer (including non-alcoholic beer)).....................**1584**

Paroxetine Hydrochloride Controlled-release Tablets (Avoid alcohol while taking paroxetine hydrochloride controlled-release tablets)..............**2361**

Paroxetine Hydrochloride Extended-release Tablets (Avoid alcohol while taking paroxetine hydrochloride controlled-release tablets)...........................**2371**

Patanase Nasal Spray (Concurrent use of olopatadine nasal spray with alcohol should be avoided because additional reductions in alertness and additional impairment of central nervous system performance may occur)........................... **585**

Paxil Tablets (Although paroxetine has not been shown to increase the impairment of mental and motor skills caused by alcohol, patients should be advised to avoid alcohol while taking paroxetine) **1586**

Paxil CR Controlled-Release Tablets (Although paroxetine has not been shown to increase the impairment of mental and motor skills caused by alcohol, patients should be advised to avoid alcohol while taking paroxetine) **1596**

Percocet Tablets (Additive CNS depression) **1121**

Percodan Tablets (Additive CNS depression) **1124**

Phenytek Capsules (Acute alcohol intake with phenytoin may increase phenytoin serum levels; chronic alcohol abuse with phenytoin may decrease phenytoin serum levels) **2380**

Photofrin for Injection (Compounds that quench active oxygen species or scavenge radicals, such as ethanol would

be expected to decrease photodynamic therapy (PDT) activity).. **786**

Prinzide Tablets (Co-administration of thiazide and alcohol may potentiate orthostatic hypotension) **2246**

Pristiq Extended-Release Tablets (A clinical study has shown that desvenlafaxine does not increase the impairment of mental and motor skills caused by ethanol. However, patients should be advised to avoid alcohol consumption while taking desvenlafaxine) **3564**

Provigil Tablets (The use of modafinil in combination with alcohol has not been studied. It is advisable to avoid alcohol while taking modafinil)..................... **983**

Prozac Weekly Capsules (Concurrent use with alcohol requires caution)............................**1941**

Pylera Capsules (Alcoholic beverages should not be consumed during Pylera therapy and for at least 1 day afterward. Psychotic reactions have been reported in alcoholic patients who are using Pylera and disulfiram concurrently. Pylera should not be given to patients who have taken disulfiram within the last 2 weeks).................. **793**

Remeron Tablets (Concomitant administration of alcohol (equivalent to 60 g) had a minimal effect on plasma levels of mirtazapine (15 mg) in healthy male subjects. However, the impairment of cognitive and motor skills produced by mirtazapine were shown to be additive with those produced by alcohol. Accordingly, patients should be advised to avoid alcohol while taking mirtazapine) **3214**

Requip Tablets (Sedating medications (such as alcohol or CNS depressants), may increase the risk of somnolence or falling asleep while engaged in activities of daily living. Because of possible additive effects, caution should be advised when patients are taking other sedating medications, alcohol, or other CNS depressants in combination with ropinirole) **1620**

Requip XL Tablets (Sedating medications (such as alcohol or CNS depressants), may increase the risk of somnolence or falling asleep while engaged in activities of daily living. Because of possible additive effects, caution should be advised when patients are taking other sedating medications, alcohol, or other CNS depressants in combination with ropinirole) **1628**

Rilutek Tablets (Whether alcohol increases the risk of serious hepatotoxicity with riluzole is unknown; therefore, patients being treated with riluzole should be discouraged from drinking excessive amounts of alcohol) **3032**

Risperdal Consta Long-Acting Injection (Given the primary CNS effects of risperidone, caution should be used if taken in combination with alcohol)...........**2682**

Rozerem Tablets (Complex behaviors, such as "sleep driving" (eg, driving while not fully awake after ingestion of hypnotic) and other complex behaviors (eg, preparing and eating food, making phone calls, or having sex), with amnesia for the event, have been reported in association with hypnotic use. The use of alcohol and other CNS

depressants may increase the risk of such behaviors) **3366**

Ryzolt Extended-Release Tablets (Patients should be cautioned about the concomitant use of tramadol products and alcohol because of potentially serious CNS-additive effects of these agents. When large doses of tramadol are administered with alcohol, respiratory depression may result. Prescribe tramadol with caution for patients who use alcohol in excess)....................**2813**

St. Joseph 81 mg Aspirin Chewable and Enteric Coated Tablets (Chronic heavy alcohol users, 3 or more drinks per day, in combination with analgesic/antipyretic drug products containing aspirin increases the risk of adverse GI events, including stomach bleeding) **2045**

Salonpas Arthritis Pain (Having 3 or more alcoholic drinks everyday may increase the chance of stomach bleeding)..........**1805**

Salonpas Pain Relief Patch (Having 3 or more alcoholic drinks everyday may increase the chance of stomach bleeding) **1805**

Saphris Tablets (Given the primary CNS effects of asenapine, caution should be used when it is taken in combination with other centrally-acting drugs or alcohol) **3223**

Savella Tablets (Milnacipran hydrochloride should not be prescribed to patients with substantial alcohol use or evidence of chronic liver disease because it is possible that milnacipran hydrochloride may aggravate pre-existing liver disease)................................**1172**

Seromycin Capsules (Concurrent use increases the possibility and risk of epileptic episodes)........**1956**

Seroquel Tablets (Quetiapine potentiated the cognitive and motor effects of alcohol in a clinical trial in subjects with selected psychotic disorders. Alcoholic beverages should be avoided while taking quetiapine)..... **750**

Seroquel XR Extended-Release Tablets (Given the primary CNS effects of quetiapine, caution should be used when it is taken in combination with other centrally acting drugs. Quetiapine potentiated the cognitive and motor effects of alcohol in a clinical trial in subjects with selected psychotic disorders, and alcoholic beverages should be limited while taking quetiapine) **759**

Skelaxin Tablets (The sedative effects of metaxalone and other CNS depressants (eg, alcohol) may be additive. Therefore, caution should be exercised with patients who take more than one of these CNS depressants simultaneously) **1848**

Soriatane Capsules (Clinical evidence has shown that etretinate can be formed with concurrent ingestion of acitretin and ethanol) **3326**

Symbyax Capsules (The co-administration of ethanol with Symbyax may potentiate sedation and orthostatic hypotension. Patients should be advised to avoid alcohol while taking Symbyax)...........................**1965**

Tekturna HCT Tablets (Potentiation of orthostatic hypotension may occur with concurrent use) **2541**

Teveten HCT Tablets (May potentiate orthostatic hypotension)............................ **541**

Thioridazine Hydrochloride Tablets (Thioridazine is capable of potentiating CNS depressants).......**2384**

Thiothixene Capsules (Patients receiving thiothixene should be cautioned about the possible additive effects (which may include hypotension) with CNS depressants and with alcohol. Extreme caution should be used in patients with a history of convulsive disorders or those in a state of alcohol withdrawal, since it may lower the convulsive threshold) **2386**

Toviaz Extended-Release Tablets (Concomitant use with alcohol may enhance the drowsiness caused by fesoterodine)................**2753**

Transderm Scōp Transdermal Therapeutic System (Scopolamine is an anticholinergic agent and causes certain CNS effects, such as drowsiness and dizziness, and hence it should be used with care in patients on concomitant therapy) **2397**

Treximet Tablets (Other factors that increase the risk for gastrointestinal bleeding in patients treated with NSAIDs include concomitant use of alcohol) **1681**

Trilipix Delayed Release Capsules (Excessive alcohol intake should be addressed before triglyceride-lowering drug therapy, such as fenofibric acid, is considered. If the decision is made to use lipid-altering drugs, the patient should be instructed that this does not reduce the importance of adhering to diet) **548**

Trizivir Tablets (Concurrent use with ethanol decreases the elimination of abacavir causing an increase in overall exposure) **1688**

Tussionex Pennkinetic Extended-Release Suspension (Combined use may result in additive CNS depression)..............**3443**

Regular Strength Tylenol Tablets (Severe liver damage may occur if an adult has 3 or more alcoholic drinks every day while using this product)......................**2049**

Tylenol with Codeine Tablets (Concomitant use with alcohol may produce an additive CNS depression and should be avoided) **2691**

Ultram ER Extended-Release Tablets (Tramadol hydrochloride is contraindicated in acute intoxication with alcohol. Tramadol hydrochloride should be used with caution and in reduced dosages when administered to patients receiving CNS depressants, such as alcohol. Tramadol may be expected to have additive effects when used in conjunction with alcohol)...............**2693**

Uniphyl Tablets (Concurrent use with a single dose of alcohol (3mL/kg of whiskey) decreases theophylline clearance for up to 24 hours)................................**2817**

Valium Tablets (Concomitant use with alcohol is not recommended due to enhancement of the sedative effect) **2880**

Venlafaxine Hydrochloride Tablets (Although venlafaxine has not been shown to increase the impairment of mental and motor skills caused by alcohol, patients should be advised to avoid alcohol while taking venlafaxine) **2388**

Vicodin Tablets (May exhibit an additive CNS depression)..............**560**

Vicodin ES Tablets (Additive CNS depression) **561**

Vicodin HP Tablets (Concurrent use results in an additive CNS depression) **563**

Vicoprofen Tablets (May exhibit additive CNS depression) 564

Visudyne for Injection (Co-administration with compounds that quench active oxygen species or scavenge radicals, such as ethanol, would be expected to decrease verteporfin activity) 2549

Vytorin 10/10 Tablets (Vytorin should be used with caution in patients who consume substantial quantities of alcohol and/or have a past history of liver disease) 2303

Vytorin 10/10 Tablets (Vytorin should be used with caution in patients who consume substantial quantities of alcohol and/or have a past history of liver disease) 3240

Wellbutrin Tablets (Bupropion is contraindicated in patients undergoing abrupt discontinuation of alcohol. In post-marketing experience, there have been rare reports of adverse neuropsychiatric events or reduced alcohol tolerance in patients who were drinking during treatment with bupropion. The consumption of alcohol should be minimized or avoided) 1719

Xenazine Tablets (Patients should be advised that the concomitant use of alcohol or other sedating drugs with tetrabenazine may have additive effects and worsen sedation and somnolence) 2033

Xyzal Oral Solution (Concurrent use of levocetirizine dihydrochloride with alcohol should be avoided because additional reductions in alertness and additional impairment of central nervous system performance may occur) 3449

Xyzal Oral Solution (Concurrent use of levocetirizine dihydrochloride with alcohol should be avoided because additional reductions in alertness and additional impairment of central nervous system performance may occur) 3053

Ziagen Tablets (Ethanol decreases the elimination of abacavir, causing an increase in overall exposure. Co-administration of ethanol and abacavir resulted in a 41% increase in abacavir AUC and a 26% increase in abacavir $t_{1/2}$) 1740

Zocor Tablets (Simvastatin should be used with caution in patients who consume substantial quantities of alcohol) 2289

Zonegran Capsules (Concomitant administration of zonisamide and alcohol or other CNS depressants has not been evaluated in clinical studies. Because of the potential of zonisamide to cause CNS depression, as well as other cognitive and/or neuropsychiatric adverse events, zonisamide should be used with caution if used in combination with alcohol or other CNS depressants) 1081

Zyban Sustained-Release Tablets (Bupropion is contraindicated in patients undergoing abrupt discontinuation of alcohol. In post-marketing experience, there have been rare reports of adverse neuropsychiatric events or reduced alcohol tolerance in patients who were drinking alcohol during treatment with bupropion. The consumption of alcohol during treatment with bupropion should be minimized or avoided) ...1762

Zydone Tablets (Co-administration may exhibit additive CNS depression) 1138

Zyprexa Tablets (Co-administration of alcohol with olanzapine potentiates orthostatic hypotension; concurrent use should be avoided. Given the primary CNS effects of olanzapine, caution should be used when olanzapine is taken in combination with other centrally-acting drugs and alcohol) 1984

Zyprexa IntraMuscular (Co-administration of alcohol with olanzapine potentiates orthostatic hypotension; concurrent use should be avoided. Given the primary CNS effects of olanzapine, caution should be used when olanzapine is taken in combination with other centrally-acting drugs and alcohol) 1984

Zyrtec Allergy Tablets (Alcohol may increase drowsiness. Avoid alcoholic drinks) 2052

Children's Zyrtec Allergy Chewable Tablets (Alcohol may increase drowsiness. Avoid alcoholic drinks) 2053

Children's Zyrtec Allergy Syrup (Concomitant use may increase drowsiness) 2053

Children's Zyrtec Hives Relief Syrup (Concomitant use may increase drowsiness) 2053

Zyrtec-D Allergy & Congestion Extended-Release Tablets (Concurrent use with alcohol may increase drowsiness; avoid alcohol) 2054

Beverages, caffeine-containing

Actimmune (Preclinical studies have demonstrated a decrease in hepatic microsomal cytochrome P-450 concentrations. This could potentially lead to a depression of the hepatic metabolism of certain drugs that utilize this degradative pathway) 1810

Arcalyst for Subcutaneous Injection (This is clinically relevant for CYP450 substrates with a narrow therapeutic index, where the dose is individually adjusted (eg, warfarin). Upon initiation of rilonacept, in patients being treated with these types of medicinal products, therapeutic monitoring of the effect or drug concentration should be performed and the individual dose of the medicinal product may need to be adjusted as needed) 2824

Cipro I.V. (Ciprofloxacin has been shown to interfere with the metabolism of caffeine. This may lead to reduced clearance of caffeine and a prolongation of its serum half-life and inhibits the formation of paraxanthine after caffeine administration) 3082

Cipro Tablets (Ciprofloxacin has been shown to interfere with the metabolism of caffeine. This may lead to reduced clearance of caffeine and a prolongation of its serum half-life and inhibits the formation of paraxanthine after caffeine administration) 3073

Cipro XR Tablets (Ciprofloxacin has been shown to interfere with the metabolism of caffeine. This may lead to reduced clearance of caffeine and a prolongation of its serum half-life and inhibit the formation of paraxanthine after caffeine administration) 3091

Fosamax Tablets (Concomitant administration of alendronate with coffee reduces bioavailability by approximately 60%) 2138

Fosamax Plus D Tablets (Concomitant administration of alendronate with coffee reduces bioavailability by approximately 60%) 2147

Genotropin Lyophilized Powder (Limited published data indicates that somatropin treatment increases cytochrome P450 (CYP450)-mediated antipyrine clearance in man. These data suggest that somatropin administration may alter the clearance of compounds metabolized by CYP450 liver enzymes. Careful monitoring is advisable when somatropin is administered in combination with other drugs known to be metabolized by CYP450 liver enzymes) 2763

Humatrope Vials and Cartridges (Limited published data indicates that somatropin treatment increases cytochrome P450 (CP450)-mediated antipyrine clearance in man. These data suggest that somatropin administration may alter the clearance of compounds metabolized by CP450 liver enzymes. Therefore, careful monitoring is advised when somatropin is administered in combination with drugs metabolized by CP450 liver enzymes) 1920

Ilaris Injection (The formation of CYP450 enzymes is suppressed by increased levels of cytokines (eg, IL-1) during chronic inflammation. Thus it is expected that for a molecule that binds to IL-1, such as canakinumab, the formation of CYP450 enzymes could be normalized. This is clinically relevant for CYP450 substrates with a narrow therapeutic index, where the dose is individually adjusted (eg, warfarin). Upon initiation of canakinumab, in patients being treated with these types of medicinal products, therapeutic monitoring of the effect or drug concentration should be performed and the individual dose of the medicinal product may need to be adjusted as needed) 2488

Iquix Ophthalmic Solution (Systemic administration of some quinolones has been shown to interfere with the metabolism of caffeine) 3492

Ketek Tablets (Elevated levels of drugs metabolized by the CYP450 system may be observed when co-administered with telithromycin; therefore, increases or prolongation of the therapeutic and/or adverse effects of the concomitant drug may be observed) 2991

Lexiscan Injection (Methylxanthines (eg, caffeine) are non-specific adenosine receptor antagonists and may interfere with the vasodilation activity of regadenoson. Patients should avoid consumption of any products containing methylxanthines as well as any drugs containing theophylline for at least 12 hours before regadenoson administration) 668

Lybrel Tablets (Contraceptive effectiveness may be reduced when hormonal contraceptives are co-administered with antibiotics, anticonvulsants, and other drugs that increase the metabolism of contraceptive steroids. This could result in unintended pregnancy or unscheduled bleeding. In such cases a nonhormonal back-up method of birth control should be considered) 3514

Mylotarg for Injection (Potential for drug-drug interaction with drugs affected by CYP450 enzymes) 3524

Norditropin Cartridges (Limited published data indicate that somatropin treatment increases cytochrome P450 (CYP450)- mediated antipyrine clearance in man. These data suggest that somatropin administration may alter the clearance of compounds known to be metabolized by CYP450 liver enzymes (eg, corticosteroids, sex steroids, anticonvulsants, cyclosporine). Careful monitoring is advisable when somatropin is administered in combination with other drugs known to be metabolized by CYP450 liver enzymes) 2569

Ortho Evra Transdermal System (Although norelgestromin and its metabolites inhibit a variety of P450 enzymes in human liver microsomes, the clinical consequence of such an interaction on the levels of other concomitant medications is likely to be insignificant. Under the recommended dosing regimen, the *in vivo* concentrations of norelgestromin and its metabolites, even at the peak serum levels, are relatively low compared to the inhibitory constant (Ki) (based on results of *in vitro* studies)) 2648

Parnate Tablets (Concomitant use with excessive use of caffeine in any form is contraindicated) 1584

Rilutek Tablets (Potential inhibitors of CYP1A2, such as caffeine, could decrease the rate of riluzole elimination. CYP1A2 is the principal isoenzyme involved in the initial oxidative metabolism of riluzole; potential interactions may occur when riluzole is given concurrently with other agents which are also metabolized primarily by CYP1A2 (eg, caffeine)) 3032

Sandostatin LAR Depot (Limited published data indicate that somatostatin analogs may decrease the metabolic clearance of compounds known to be metabolized by cytochrome P450 enzymes, which may be due to the suppression of growth hormone) 2519

Simponi Injection (The formation of CYP450 enzymes may be suppressed by increased levels of cytokines (eg, TNFα) during chronic inflammation. Therefore, it is expected that for a molecule that antagonizes cytokine activity, such as golimumab, the formation of CYP450 enzymes could be normalized. Upon initiation or discontinuation of golimumab in patients being treated with CYP450 substrates with a narrow therapeutic index, monitoring of the effect (eg, warfarin) or drug concentration (eg, cyclosporine or theophylline) is recommended and the individual dose of the drug product may be adjusted as needed) 930

Tev-Tropin for Injection (Somatropin administration may alter the clearance of compounds known to be metabolized by CYP450) 1181

Zantac Injection (Ranitidine has been reported to affect the bioavailability of other drugs through several different mechanisms, such as competition for renal tubular secretion, alteration of gastric pH, and inhibition of cytochrome P450 enzymes).............................1732

Beverages, hot

Finacea Gel (Concomitant use with any foods and beverages that might provoke erythema, flushing, and blushing (including spicy food, alcoholic beverages, and thermally hot drinks, including hot coffee and tea) should be avoided).........................1808

Nascobal Nasal Spray (Hot foods may cause nasal secretions and a resulting loss of medication; therefore, patients should be told to administer cyanocobalamin nasal spray at least one hour before or one hour after ingestion of hot foods or liquids) 2700

Beverages, unspecified

Finacea Gel (Concomitant use with any foods and beverages that might provoke erythema, flushing, and blushing (including spicy food, alcoholic beverages, and thermally hot drinks, including hot coffee and tea) should be avoided).........................1808

Beverages with high tyramine

Azilect Tablets (Severe hypertensive reactions have followed the administration of tyramine rich beverages and non-selective MAO inhibitors) 3383

Eldepryl Capsules (Rare cases of hypertensive reactions associated with ingestion of tyramine-containing foods have been reported in patients taking the recommended daily dose of selegiline hydrochloride)..................3312

Emsam Transdermal System (As a class, MAO inhibitors have been associated with hypertensive crises caused by the ingestion of foods with a high concentration of tyramine) 3623

Broccoli

Aplenzin Extended-Release Tablets (Bupropion may be an inducer of drug-metabolizing enzymes in humans. In one study, following chronic administration of bupropion hydrochloride, 100 mg 3 times daily to 8 healthy male volunteers for 14 days, there was no evidence of induction of its own metabolism. Nevertheless, there may be the potential for clinically important alterations of blood levels of co-administered drugs) 2948

Biaxin Filmtab Tablets (Strong inducers of the cytochrome P450 metabolism system such as efavirenz, nevirapine, rifampicin, rifabutin, and rifapentine may accelerate the metabolism of clarithromycin and thus lower the plasma levels of clarithromycin, while increasing those of 14-OH-clarithromycin, a metabolite that is also microbiologically active. Since the microbiological activities of clarithromycin and 14-OH-clarithromycin are different for different bacteria, the intended therapeutic effect could be impaired during concomitant administration of clarithromycin and enzyme inducers) 412

Gabitril Tablets (Because of the potential for pharmacokinetic interactions between tiagabine hydrochloride and drugs that induce hepatic metabolizing

enzymes, it may be useful to obtain plasma levels of tiagabine before and after changes are made in the therapeutic regimen).....................972

Implanon Implant (Etonogestrel implant is not recommended for women who require chronic use of drugs that are potent inducers of hepatic enzymes because etonogestrel implant is likely to be less effective for these women) 3128

InnoPran XL Extended Release Capsules (Blood levels of propranolol may be decreased by administration of propranolol with inducers of hepatic drug metabolism) 1517

Klonopin Tablets (Cytochrome P-450 inducers, such as phenytoin, carbamazepine and phenobarbital induce clonazepam metabolism, causing an approximately 30% decrease in plasma clonazepam levels) 2855

Letairis Tablets (Use caution when ambrisentan is co-administered with inducers of CYPs)..................1250

Mirena Intrauterine System (The metabolism of progestogens may be increased by concomitant use of substances known to induce drug-metabolizing liver enzymes, specifically cytochrome P450 enzymes) 854

NuvaRing (Contraceptive effectiveness may be reduced when hormonal contraceptives are co-administered with some antifungals, anticonvulsants, and other drugs that increase the metabolism of contraceptive steroids. This could result in unintended pregnancy or breakthrough bleeding. Women may need to use an additional contraceptive method when taking such medications) 3181

Ortho Evra Transdermal System (If a woman on hormonal contraceptives takes a drug or herbal product that induces enzymes, including CYP3A4, that metabolize contraceptive hormones, counsel her to use additional contraception or a different method of contraception. Drugs or herbal products that induce such enzymes may decrease the plasma concentrations of contraceptive hormones, and may decrease the effectiveness of hormonal contraceptives or increase breakthrough bleeding) 2648

Ortho Micronor Tablets (The effectiveness of progestin-only pills is reduced by hepatic enzyme-inducing drugs such as the anticonvulsants phenytoin, carbamazepine, and barbiturates, and the antituberculosis drug rifampin).......2660

Ortho Tri-Cyclen Lo Tablets (Contraceptive effectiveness may be reduced when hormonal contraceptives are co-administered with antibiotics, anticonvulsants, and other drugs that increase the metabolism of contraceptive steroids. This could result in unintended pregnancy or breakthrough bleeding) 2673

Ortho-Cyclen Tablets (Contraceptive effectiveness may be reduced when hormonal contraceptives are co-administered with antibiotics, anticonvulsants, and other drugs that increase the metabolism of contraceptive steroids. This could result in unintended pregnancy or breakthrough bleeding) 2663

Plan B One-Step Tablets (Drugs or herbal products that induce enzymes, including CYP3A4,

that metabolize progestins may decrease the plasma concentrations of progestins, and may decrease the effectiveness of progestin-only pills. Some drugs or herbal products that may decrease the effectiveness of progestin-only pills include barbiturates, bosentan, carbamazepine, felbamate, griseofulvin, oxcarbazepine, phenytoin, rifampin, St. John's wort, topiramate)...........................3416

Promacta Tablets (In vitro studies demonstrate that CYP1A2 and CYP2C8 are involved in the oxidative metabolism of eltrombopag. The significance of co-administration of eltrombopag with inducers of CYP 1A2 (eg, tobacco, omeprazole) and CYP 2C8 (eg, rifampin) on the systemic exposure of eltrombopag has not been established in clinical studies. Monitor patients for signs and symptoms of excessive eltrombopag exposure when eltrombopag is administered concomitantly with these drugs) 1610

Requip Tablets (In vitro metabolism studies showed that CYP1A2 is the major enzyme responsible for the metabolism of ropinirole. There is thus the potential for inducers or inhibitors of this enzyme to alter the clearance of ropinirole. Therefore, if therapy with a drug known to be a potent inducer or inhibitor of CYP1A2 is stopped or started during treatment with ropinirole, adjustment of the dose of ropinirole may be required)............1620

Requip XL Tablets (In vitro metabolism studies showed that CYP1A2 is the major enzyme responsible for the metabolism of ropinirole. There is thus the potential for inducers or inhibitors of this enzyme to alter the clearance of ropinirole. Therefore, if therapy with a drug known to be a potent inducer or inhibitor of CYP1A2 is stopped or started during treatment with ropinirole, adjustment of the dose of ropinirole may be required)............1628

Rilutek Tablets (Potential inducers of CYP 1A2 (eg, cigarette smoke, charcoal-broiled food, rifampicin, and omeprazole) could increase the rate of riluzole elimination)........................3032

Rozerem Tablets (Efficacy may be reduced when ramelteon is used in combination with strong CYP enzyme inducers)....................3366

Seroquel XR Extended-Release Tablets (Co-administration of quetiapine with hepatic enzyme inducers may increase the clearance of quetiapine. Higher doses of quetiapine may be required when co-administered with hepatic enzyme inducers)........ 759

Symbyax Capsules (Agents that induce CYP1A2 or glucuronyl transferase enzymes may cause an increase in olanzapine concentration) 1965

Synthroid Tablets (Alters thyroid hormone or TSH levels) 529

Tarceva Tablets (CYP1A2 inducers may decrease erlotinib plasma concentrations)..............................1222

Thiothixene Capsules (Co-administration of thiothixene with hepatic microsomal enzyme inducing agents such as carbamazepine may increase the clearance of thiothixene. Patients receiving these drugs should be observed for signs of reduced thiothixene effectiveness)............2386

Treanda for Injection (Inducers of CYP1A2 (eg, omeprazole, smoking) have the potential to decrease plasma concentrations of bendamustine and increase plasma concentrations of its active metabolites. Caution should be used, or alternative treatments considered, if concomitant treatment with CYP1A2 inducers is needed) 989

Zofran Tablets (Ondansetron does not itself appear to induce or inhibit the cytochrome P-450 drug metabolizing enzyme system of the liver. Because ondansetron is metabolized by hepatic cytochrome P-450 drug-metabolizing enzymes (CYP3A4, CYP2D6, CYP1A2), inducers or inhibitors of these enzymes may change the clearance and, hence, the half-life of ondansetron. On the basis of available data, no dosage adjustment is recommended for patients on these drugs) 1756

Zonegran Capsules (Drugs that induce liver enzymes increase the metabolism and clearance of zonisamide and decrease its half-life) 1081

Zyprexa Tablets (Concomitant use may cause an increase in olanzapine clearance) 1984

Zyprexa IntraMuscular (Concomitant use may cause an increase in olanzapine clearance) 1984

Brussel Sprouts

Aplenzin Extended-Release Tablets (Bupropion may be an inducer of drug-metabolizing enzymes in humans. In one study, following chronic administration of bupropion hydrochloride, 100 mg 3 times daily to 8 healthy male volunteers for 14 days, there was no evidence of induction of its own metabolism. Nevertheless, there may be the potential for clinically important alterations of blood levels of co-administered drugs) 2948

Biaxin Filmtab Tablets (Strong inducers of the cytochrome P450 metabolism system such as efavirenz, nevirapine, rifampicin, rifabutin, and rifapentine may accelerate the metabolism of clarithromycin and thus lower the plasma levels of clarithromycin, while increasing those of 14-OH-clarithromycin, a metabolite that is also microbiologically active. Since the microbiological activities of clarithromycin and 14-OH-clarithromycin are different for different bacteria, the intended therapeutic effect could be impaired during concomitant administration of clarithromycin and enzyme inducers) 412

Gabitril Tablets (Because of the potential for pharmacokinetic interactions between tiagabine hydrochloride and drugs that induce hepatic metabolizing enzymes, it may be useful to obtain plasma levels of tiagabine before and after changes are made in the therapeutic regimen)....................... 972

Implanon Implant (Etonogestrel implant is not recommended for women who require chronic use of drugs that are potent inducers of hepatic enzymes because etonogestrel implant is likely to be less effective for these women)..............................3128

InnoPran XL Extended Release Capsules (Blood levels of propranolol may be decreased

by administration of propranolol with inducers of hepatic drug metabolism) **1517**

Klonopin Tablets (Cytochrome P-450 inducers, such as phenytoin, carbamazepine and phenobarbital induce clonazepam metabolism, causing an approximately 30% decrease in plasma clonazepam levels) **2855**

Letairis Tablets (Use caution when ambrisentan is co-administered with inducers of CYPs)....................**1250**

Mirena Intrauterine System (The metabolism of progestogens may be increased by concomitant use of substances known to induce drug-metabolizing liver enzymes, specifically cytochrome P450 enzymes) **854**

NuvaRing (Contraceptive effectiveness may be reduced when hormonal contraceptives are co-administered with some antifungals, anticonvulsants, and other drugs that increase the metabolism of contraceptive steroids. This could result in unintended pregnancy or breakthrough bleeding. Women may need to use an additional contraceptive method when taking such medications) **3181**

Ortho Evra Transdermal System (If a woman on hormonal contraceptives takes a drug or herbal product that induces enzymes, including CYP3A4, that metabolize contraceptive hormones, counsel her to use additional contraception or a different method of contraception. Drugs or herbal products that induce such enzymes may decrease the plasma concentrations of contraceptive hormones, and may decrease the effectiveness of hormonal contraceptives or increase breakthrough bleeding) **2648**

Ortho Micronor Tablets (The effectiveness of progestin-only pills is reduced by hepatic enzyme-inducing drugs such as the anticonvulsants phenytoin, carbamazepine, and barbiturates, and the antituberculosis drug rifampin).......**2660**

Ortho Tri-Cyclen Lo Tablets (Contraceptive effectiveness may be reduced when hormonal contraceptives are co-administered with antibiotics, anticonvulsants, and other drugs that increase the metabolism of contraceptive steroids. This could result in unintended pregnancy or breakthrough bleeding) **2673**

Ortho-Cyclen Tablets (Contraceptive effectiveness may be reduced when hormonal contraceptives are co-administered with antibiotics, anticonvulsants, and other drugs that increase the metabolism of contraceptive steroids. This could result in unintended pregnancy or breakthrough bleeding) **2663**

Plan B One-Step Tablets (Drugs or herbal products that induce enzymes, including CYP3A4, that metabolize progestins may decrease the plasma concentrations of progestins, and may decrease the effectiveness of progestin-only pills. Some drugs or herbal products that may decrease the effectiveness of progestin-only pills include barbiturates, bosentan, carbamazepine, felbamate, griseofulvin, oxcarbazepine, phenytoin, rifampin, St. John's wort, topiramate)..................................**3416**

Promacta Tablets (*In vitro* studies demonstrate that CYP1A2 and CYP2C8 are involved in the oxidative metabolism of eltrombopag. The significance of co-administration of eltrombopag with inducers of CYP 1A2 (eg, tobacco, omeprazole) and CYP 2C8 (eg, rifampin) on the systemic exposure of eltrombopag has not been established in clinical studies. Monitor patients for signs and symptoms of excessive eltrombopag exposure when eltrombopag is administered concomitantly with these drugs) **1610**

Requip Tablets (*In vitro* metabolism studies showed that CYP1A2 is the major enzyme responsible for the metabolism of ropinirole. There is thus the potential for inducers or inhibitors of this enzyme to alter the clearance of ropinirole. Therefore, if therapy with a drug known to be a potent inducer or inhibitor of CYP1A2 is stopped or started during treatment with ropinirole, adjustment of the dose of ropinirole may be required)............**1620**

Requip XL Tablets (*In vitro* metabolism studies showed that CYP1A2 is the major enzyme responsible for the metabolism of ropinirole. There is thus the potential for inducers or inhibitors of this enzyme to alter the clearance of ropinirole. Therefore, if therapy with a drug known to be a potent inducer or inhibitor of CYP1A2 is stopped or started during treatment with ropinirole, adjustment of the dose of ropinirole may be required)............**1628**

Rilutek Tablets (Potential inducers of CYP 1A2 (eg, cigarette smoke, charcoal-broiled food, rifampicin, and omeprazole) could increase the rate of riluzole elimination)........................**3032**

Rozerem Tablets (Efficacy may be reduced when ramelteon is used in combination with strong CYP enzyme inducers) **3366**

Seroquel XR Extended-Release Tablets (Co-administration of quetiapine with hepatic enzyme inducers may increase the clearance of quetiapine. Higher doses of quetiapine may be required when co-administered with hepatic enzyme inducers)........ **759**

Symbyax Capsules (Agents that induce CYP1A2 or glucuronyl transferase enzymes may cause an increase in olanzapine concentration) **1965**

Synthroid Tablets (Alters thyroid hormone or TSH levels) **529**

Tarceva Tablets (CYP1A2 inducers may decrease erlotinib plasma concentrations)...............................**1222**

Thiothixene Capsules (Co-administration of thiothixene with hepatic microsomal enzyme inducing agents such as carbamazepine may increase the clearance of thiothixene. Patients receiving these drugs should be observed for signs of reduced thiothixene effectiveness)..............**2386**

Treanda for Injection (Inducers of CYP1A2 (eg, omeprazole, smoking) have the potential to decrease plasma concentrations of bendamustine and increase plasma concentrations of its active metabolites. Caution should be used, or alternative treatments considered, if concomitant treatment with CYP1A2 inducers is needed) **989**

Zofran Tablets (Ondansetron does not itself appear to induce or inhibit the cytochrome P-450 drug metabolizing enzyme system of the liver. Because ondansetron is metabolized by hepatic cytochrome P-450 drug-metabolizing enzymes (CYP3A4, CYP2D6, CYP1A2), inducers or inhibitors of these enzymes may change the clearance and, hence, the half-life of ondansetron. On the basis of available data, no dosage adjustment is recommended for patients on these drugs) **1756**

Zonegran Capsules (Drugs that induce liver enzymes increase the metabolism and clearance of zonisamide and decrease its half-life) **1081**

Zyprexa Tablets (Concomitant use may cause an increase in olanzapine clearance) **1984**

Zyprexa IntraMuscular (Concomitant use may cause an increase in olanzapine clearance) **1984**

Caviar

Parnate Tablets (Tranylcypromine is contraindicated in combination with foods with a high tyramine content. Hypertensive crises have sometimes occurred during therapy with tranylcypromine after ingestion of foods with a high tyramine content. In particular, patients should be instructed not to take foods, such as caviar)..............................**1584**

Charbroiled Food

Aplenzin Extended-Release Tablets (Bupropion may be an inducer of drug-metabolizing enzymes in humans. In one study, following chronic administration of bupropion hydrochloride, 100 mg 3 times daily to 8 healthy male volunteers for 14 days, there was no evidence of induction of its own metabolism. Nevertheless, there may be the potential for clinically important alterations of blood levels of co-administered drugs) **2948**

Biaxin Filmtab Tablets (Strong inducers of the cytochrome P450 metabolism system such as efavirenz, nevirapine, rifampicin, rifabutin, and rifapentine may accelerate the metabolism of clarithromycin and thus lower the plasma levels of clarithromycin, while increasing those of 14-OH-clarithromycin, a metabolite that is also microbiologically active. Since the microbiological activities of clarithromycin and 14-OH-clarithromycin are different for different bacteria, the intended therapeutic effect could be impaired during concomitant administration of clarithromycin and enzyme inducers) **412**

Gabitril Tablets (Because of the potential for pharmacokinetic interactions between tiagabine hydrochloride and drugs that induce hepatic metabolizing enzymes, it may be useful to obtain plasma levels of tiagabine before and after changes are made in the therapeutic regimen)......................**972**

Implanon Implant (Etonogestrel implant is not recommended for women who require chronic use of drugs that are potent inducers of hepatic enzymes because etonogestrel implant is likely to be less effective for these women)...............................**3128**

InnoPran XL Extended Release Capsules (Blood levels of propranolol may be decreased by administration of propranolol

with inducers of hepatic drug metabolism) **1517**

Klonopin Tablets (Cytochrome P-450 inducers, such as phenytoin, carbamazepine and phenobarbital induce clonazepam metabolism, causing an approximately 30% decrease in plasma clonazepam levels) **2855**

Letairis Tablets (Use caution when ambrisentan is co-administered with inducers of CYPs)....................**1250**

Mirena Intrauterine System (The metabolism of progestogens may be increased by concomitant use of substances known to induce drug-metabolizing liver enzymes, specifically cytochrome P450 enzymes) **854**

NuvaRing (Contraceptive effectiveness may be reduced when hormonal contraceptives are co-administered with some antifungals, anticonvulsants, and other drugs that increase the metabolism of contraceptive steroids. This could result in unintended pregnancy or breakthrough bleeding. Women may need to use an additional contraceptive method when taking such medications) **3181**

Ortho Evra Transdermal System (If a woman on hormonal contraceptives takes a drug or herbal product that induces enzymes, including CYP3A4, that metabolize contraceptive hormones, counsel her to use additional contraception or a different method of contraception. Drugs or herbal products that induce such enzymes may decrease the plasma concentrations of contraceptive hormones, and may decrease the effectiveness of hormonal contraceptives or increase breakthrough bleeding) **2648**

Ortho Micronor Tablets (The effectiveness of progestin-only pills is reduced by hepatic enzyme-inducing drugs such as the anticonvulsants phenytoin, carbamazepine, and barbiturates, and the antituberculosis drug rifampin).......**2660**

Ortho Tri-Cyclen Lo Tablets (Contraceptive effectiveness may be reduced when hormonal contraceptives are co-administered with antibiotics, anticonvulsants, and other drugs that increase the metabolism of contraceptive steroids. This could result in unintended pregnancy or breakthrough bleeding) **2673**

Ortho-Cyclen Tablets (Contraceptive effectiveness may be reduced when hormonal contraceptives are co-administered with antibiotics, anticonvulsants, and other drugs that increase the metabolism of contraceptive steroids. This could result in unintended pregnancy or breakthrough bleeding) **2663**

Plan B One-Step Tablets (Drugs or herbal products that induce enzymes, including CYP3A4, that metabolize progestins may decrease the plasma concentrations of progestins, and may decrease the effectiveness of progestin-only pills. Some drugs or herbal products that may decrease the effectiveness of progestin-only pills include barbiturates, bosentan, carbamazepine, felbamate, griseofulvin, oxcarbazepine, phenytoin, rifampin, St. John's wort, topiramate)..................................**3416**

Promacta Tablets (*In vitro* studies demonstrate that CYP1A2 and CYP2C8 are involved in the

oxidative metabolism of eltrombopag. The significance of co-administration of eltrombopag with inducers of CYP 1A2 (eg, tobacco, omeprazole) and CYP 2C8 (eg, rifampin) on the systemic exposure of eltrombopag has not been established in clinical studies. Monitor patients for signs and symptoms of excessive eltrombopag exposure when eltrombopag is administered concomitantly with these drugs) **1610**

Requip Tablets (*In vitro* metabolism studies showed that CYP1A2 is the major enzyme responsible for the metabolism of ropinirole. There is thus the potential for inducers or inhibitors of this enzyme to alter the clearance of ropinirole. Therefore, if therapy with a drug known to be a potent inducer or inhibitor of CYP1A2 is stopped or started during treatment with ropinirole, adjustment of the dose of ropinirole may be required).............**1620**

Requip XL Tablets (*In vitro* metabolism studies showed that CYP1A2 is the major enzyme responsible for the metabolism of ropinirole. There is thus the potential for inducers or inhibitors of this enzyme to alter the clearance of ropinirole. Therefore, if therapy with a drug known to be a potent inducer or inhibitor of CYP1A2 is stopped or started during treatment with ropinirole, adjustment of the dose of ropinirole may be required).............**1628**

Rilutek Tablets (Potential inducers of CYP 1A2 (eg, cigarette smoke, charcoal-broiled food, rifampicin, and omeprazole) could increase the rate of riluzole elimination)........................**3032**

Rozerem Tablets (Efficacy may be reduced when ramelteon is used in combination with strong CYP enzyme inducers)....................**3366**

Seroquel XR Extended-Release Tablets (Co-administration of quetiapine with hepatic enzyme inducers may increase the clearance of quetiapine. Higher doses of quetiapine may be required when co-administered with hepatic enzyme inducers)........ **759**

Symbyax Capsules (Agents that induce CYP1A2 or glucuronyl transferase enzymes may cause an increase in olanzapine concentration) **1965**

Synthroid Tablets (Alters thyroid hormone or TSH levels) **529**

Tarceva Tablets (CYP1A2 inducers may decrease erlotinib plasma concentrations)..............................**1222**

Thiothixene Capsules (Co-administration of thiothixene with hepatic microsomal enzyme inducing agents such as carbamazepine may increase the clearance of thiothixene. Patients receiving these drugs should be observed for signs of reduced thiothixene effectiveness).............**2386**

Treanda for Injection (Inducers of CYP1A2 (eg, omeprazole, smoking) have the potential to decrease plasma concentrations of bendamustine and increase plasma concentrations of its active metabolites. Caution should be used, or alternative treatments considered, if concomitant treatment with CYP1A2 inducers is needed) **989**

Zofran Tablets (Ondansetron does not itself appear to induce or inhibit the cytochrome P-450 drug metabolizing enzyme system of the liver. Because

ondansetron is metabolized by hepatic cytochrome P-450 drug-metabolizing enzymes (CYP3A4, CYP2D6, CYP1A2), inducers or inhibitors of these enzymes may change the clearance and, hence, the half-life of ondansetron. On the basis of available data, no dosage adjustment is recommended for patients on these drugs) **1756**

Zonegran Capsules (Drugs that induce liver enzymes increase the metabolism and clearance of zonisamide and decrease its half-life)....................................**1081**

Zyprexa Tablets (Concomitant use may cause an increase in olanzapine clearance)....................**1984**

Zyprexa IntraMuscular (Concomitant use may cause an increase in olanzapine clearance)..................................**1984**

Cheese, aged
Parnate Tablets (Tranylcypromine is contraindicated in combination with cheese with a high tyramine content. Hypertensive crises have sometimes occurred during therapy with tranylcypromine after ingestion of foods with a high tyramine content. In particular, patients should be instructed not to take foods, such as cheese (particularly strong or aged varieties))...............**1584**

Cheese, strong, unpasteurized
Parnate Tablets (Tranylcypromine is contraindicated in combination with cheese with a high tyramine content. Hypertensive crises have sometimes occurred during therapy with tranylcypromine after ingestion of foods with a high tyramine content. In particular, patients should be instructed not to take foods, such as cheese (particularly strong or aged varieties))...............**1584**

Cheese, unspecified
Parnate Tablets (Tranylcypromine is contraindicated in combination with cheese with a high tyramine content. Hypertensive crises have sometimes occurred during therapy with tranylcypromine after ingestion of foods with a high tyramine content. In particular, patients should be instructed not to take foods, such as cheese (particularly strong or aged varieties))...............**1584**

Chocolate
Parnate Tablets (Tranylcypromine is contraindicated in combination with foods with a high tyramine content. Hypertensive crises have sometimes occurred during therapy with tranylcypromine after ingestion of foods with a high tyramine content. In particular, patients should be instructed not to take foods, such as chocolate)........................**1584**

Cotton seed meal
Levoxyl Tablets (Concurrent use of cotton seed meal may bind and decrease the absorption of levothyroxine sodium from GI tract) **1843**

Cream, sour
Parnate Tablets (Tranylcypromine is contraindicated in combination with foods with a high tyramine content. Hypertensive crises have sometimes occurred during therapy with tranylcypromine after ingestion of foods with a high tyramine content. In particular, patients should be

instructed not to take foods, such as sour cream) **1584**

Dairy products
Boniva Tablets (Milk is likely to interfere with absorption of ibandronate. Ibandronate should be taken at least 60 minutes before the first food or drink (other than water) of the day) **2844**

Cipro I.V. (Ciprofloxacin should not be taken with dairy products (like milk or yogurt) alone since absorption of ciprofloxacin may be significantly reduced; however, ciprofloxacin may be taken with a meal that contains these products) **3082**

Cipro Tablets (Ciprofloxacin should not be taken with dairy products (like milk or yogurt) alone since absorption of ciprofloxacin may be significantly reduced; however, ciprofloxacin may be taken with a meal that contains these products)...............................**3073**

Correctol Delayed-Release Tablets, USP (Patients should not take bisacodyl within 1 hour after taking an antacid or milk) **3263**

Fleet Prep Kit 3 (Concurrent use of milk or milk products with Fleet Prep Kit 3 within one hour should be avoided)........................**1145**

Noroxin Tablets (Avoid simultaneous ingestion; administer norfloxacin at least one hour before or two hours after ingestion of milk and/or other dairy products)....................**2220**

Promacta Tablets (Eltrombopag chelates polyvalent cations (such as iron, calcium, aluminum, magnesium, selenium, and zinc) in foods, mineral supplements, and antacids. In a clinical study, administration of eltrombopag with a polyvalent cation-containing antacid (1,524 mg aluminum hydroxide, 1,425 mg magnesium carbonate, and sodium alginate) decreased plasma eltrombopag systemic exposure by approximately 70%. Eltrombopag must not be taken within 4 hours of any medications or products containing polyvalent cations such as antacids, dairy products, and mineral supplements to avoid significant reduction in eltrombopag absorption due to chelation) **1610**

Pylera Capsules (Absorption of Pylera is impaired by milk or dairy products) **793**

Diet, high-lipid
Allegra-D 12 Hour Extended-Release Tablets (Co-administration with a high-fat meal decreased fexofenadine plasma concentrations C_{max} and AUC, and T_{max} was delayed by 50%; the rate of extent of pseudoephedrine absorption was not affected by food; administration of Allegra-D with food should be avoided) **2915**

Gengraf Capsules (A high fat meal within one-half hour before cyclosporine administration decreases the AUC by 13% and C_{max} by 33%) **440**

Neoral Soft Gelatin Capsules (A high-fat meal consumed within one-half hour before Neoral administration decreased the AUC by 13% and C_{max} by 33%)........**2496**

Rilutek Tablets (Co-administration with high-fat meal decreases absorption, reduces AUC by about 20% and peak blood levels by about 45%) **3032**

Uniphyl Tablets (Co-administration with a standardized high-fat meal results in increased peak plasma concentration and bioavailability; however, a precipitous increase in the rate and extent of absorption was not evident; the dosing should be ideally administered consistently either with or without food)............................**2817**

Dietary Fiber
Levoxyl Tablets (Concurrent use of dietary fiber may bind and decrease the absorption of levothyroxine sodium from GI tract) **1843**

Drinks, hot, unspecified
Advicor Tablets (Concomitant hot drinks may increase the flushing and its use should be avoided around the time of Advicor administration) **402**

Finacea Gel (Concomitant use with any foods and beverages that might provoke erythema, flushing, and blushing (including spicy food, alcoholic beverages, and thermally hot drinks, including hot coffee and tea) should be avoided)........................**1808**

Niaspan Extended-Release Tablets (Concomitant administration of hot drinks may increase the side effects of flushing and pruritus and should be avoided around the time of niacin ingestion) **497**

Egg Product
FluMist Vaccine (FluMist is contraindicated in individuals with history of hypersensitivity, especially anaphylactic reactions, to eggs and egg proteins)....................................**2078**

Hyalgan Solution (Use caution when injecting sodium hyaluronate into patients who are allergic to avian proteins, feathers, and egg products) **2988**

Eggs
Divista Softgel Capsules (Egg whites contain avidin substance that binds to biotin and block absorption resulting to altered levels of biotin) **3474**

FluMist Vaccine (FluMist is contraindicated in individuals with history of hypersensitivity, especially anaphylactic reactions, to eggs and egg proteins).....................................**2078**

Figs, canned
Parnate Tablets (Tranylcypromine is contradindicated in combination with foods with a high tyramine content. Hypertensive crises have sometimes occurred during therapy with tranylcypromine after ingestion of foods with a high tyramine content. In particular, patients should be instructed not to take foods, such as canned figs) **1584**

Food, caffeine-containing
Actimmune (Preclinical studies have demonstrated a decrease in hepatic microsomal cytochrome P-450 concentrations. This could potentially lead to a depression of the hepatic metabolism of certain drugs that utilize this degradative pathway) **1810**

Arcalyst for Subcutaneous Injection (This is clinically relevant for CYP450 substrates with a narrow therapeutic index, where the dose is individually adjusted (eg, warfarin). Upon initiation of rilonacept, in patients being treated with these types of medicinal products, therapeutic monitoring of the effect or drug concentration should be

performed and the individual dose of the medicinal product may need to be adjusted as needed) 2824

Carbatrol Capsules (Carbamazepine is known to induce CYP1A2 and CYP3A4. Therefore, the potential exists for interaction between carbamazepine and any agent metabolized by one (or more) of these enzymes. Agents that are metabolized by CYP1A2 and CYP3A4 may have decreased plasma levels when administered concomitantly with carbamazepine. Thus, if a patient has been titrated to a stable dosage on one of the agents in these categories, and then begins a course of treatment with carbamazepine, it is reasonable to expect that a dose increase for the concomitant agent may be necessary) 3280

Cipro I.V. (Ciprofloxacin is an inhibitor of the hepatic CYP1A2 enzyme pathway. Co-administration of ciprofloxacin and other drugs primarily metabolized by CYP1A2 results in increased plasma concentrations of the co-administered drug and could lead to clinically significant pharmacodynamic side effects of the co-administered drug)...........3082

Cipro Tablets (Ciprofloxacin is an inhibitor of the hepatic CYP1A2 enzyme pathway. Co-administration of ciprofloxacin and other drugs primarily metabolized by CYP1A2 results in increased plasma concentrations of the co-administered drug and could lead to clinically significant pharmacodynamic side effects of the co-administered drug)...........3073

Cipro XR Tablets (Ciprofloxacin has been shown to interfere with the metabolism of caffeine. This may lead to reduced clearance of caffeine and a prolongation of its serum half-life and inhibit the formation of paraxanthine after caffeine administration) 3091

Equetro Extended-Release Capsules (Carbamazepine is known to induce CYP1A2 and CYP3A4. Therefore, the potential exists for interaction between carbamazepine and any agent metabolized by one (or more) of these enzymes. Agents that are metabolized by CYP1A2 and CYP3A4 may have decreased plasma levels when administered concomitantly with carbamazepine) 3477

Exjade Tablets (Deferasirox inhibits human CYP1A2 *in vitro*)......2456

Genotropin Lyophilized Powder (Limited published data indicates that somatropin treatment increases cytochrome P450 (CYP450)-mediated antipyrine clearance in man. These data suggest that somatropin administration may alter the clearance of compounds metabolized by CYP450 liver enzymes. Careful monitoring is advisable when somatropin is administered in combination with other drugs known to be metabolized by CYP450 liver enzymes) 2763

Humatrope Vials and Cartridges (Limited published data indicates that somatropin treatment increases cytochrome P450 (CP450)-mediated antipyrine clearance in man. These data suggest that somatropin administration may alter the clearance of compounds

metabolized by CP450 liver enzymes. Therefore, careful monitoring is advised when somatropin is administered in combination with drugs metabolized by CP450 liver enzymes) 1920

Ilaris Injection (The formation of CYP450 enzymes is suppressed by increased levels of cytokines (eg, IL-1) during chronic inflammation. Thus it is expected that for a molecule that binds to IL-1, such as canakinumab, the formation of CYP450 enzymes could be normalized. This is clinically relevant for CYP450 substrates with a narrow therapeutic index, where the dose is individually adjusted (eg, warfarin). Upon initiation of canakinumab, in patients being treated with these types of medicinal products, therapeutic monitoring of the effect or drug concentration should be performed and the individual dose of the medicinal product may need to be adjusted as needed) 2488

InnoPran XL Extended Release Capsules (Blood levels and/or toxicity of propranolol may be increased by administration of propranolol with substrates of CYP1A2) 1517

Iquix Ophthalmic Solution ⊙ (Systemic administration of some quinolones has been shown to interfere with the metabolism of caffeine) 3492

Ketek Tablets (Elevated levels of drugs metabolized by the CYP450 system may be observed when co-administered with telithromycin; therefore, increases or prolongation of the therapeutic and/or adverse effects of the concomitant drug may be observed) 2991

Lexiscan Injection (Methylxanthines (eg, caffeine) are non-specific adenosine receptor antagonists and may interfere with the vasodilation activity of regadenoson. Patients should avoid consumption of any products containing methylxanthines as well as any drugs containing theophylline for at least 12 hours before regadenoson administration) 668

Lybrel Tablets (Contraceptive effectiveness may be reduced when hormonal contraceptives are co-administered with antibiotics, anticonvulsants, and other drugs that increase the metabolism of contraceptive steroids. This could result in unintended pregnancy or unscheduled bleeding. In such cases a nonhormonal back-up method of birth control should be considered)................................3514

Mylotarg for Injection (Potential for drug-drug interaction with drugs affected by CYP450 enzymes)....................................3524

Norditropin Cartridges (Limited published data indicate that somatropin treatment increases cytochrome P450 (CYP450)- mediated antipyrine clearance in man. These data suggest that somatropin administration may alter the clearance of compounds known to be metabolized by CYP450 liver enzymes (eg, corticosteroids, sex steroids, anticonvulsants, cyclosporine). Careful monitoring is advisable when somatropin is

administered in combination with other drugs known to be metabolized by CYP450 liver enzymes)..2569

Nuvigil Tablets (*In vitro* data demonstrated that armodafinil shows a weak inductive response for CYP1A2 and possibly CYP3A activities in a concentration related manner and demonstrated that CYP2C19 activity is reversibly inhibited by armodafinil. However, the effect on CYP1A2 activity was not observed clinically in an interaction study performed with caffeine) 978

Ortho Evra Transdermal System (Although norelgestromin and its metabolites inhibit a variety of P450 enzymes in human liver microsomes, the clinical consequence of such an interaction on the levels of other concomitant medications is likely to be insignificant. Under the recommended dosing regimen, the *in vivo* concentrations of norelgestromin and its metabolites, even at the peak serum levels, are relatively low compared to the inhibitory constant (Ki) (based on results of *in vitro* studies)) 2648

Promacta Tablets (*In vitro* studies demonstrate that CYP1A2 and CYP2C8 are involved in the oxidative metabolism of eltrombopag. The significance of co-administration of eltrombopag with other substrates of these CYP enzymes on the systemic exposure of eltrombopag has not been established in clinical studies. Monitor patients for signs and symptoms of excessive eltrombopag exposure when eltrombopag is administered concomitantly with these drugs) 1610

Requip Tablets (*In vitro* metabolism studies showed that CYP1A2 is the major enzyme responsible for the metabolism of ropinirole. There is thus the potential for inducers or inhibitors of this enzyme to alter the clearance of ropinirole. Therefore, if therapy with a drug known to be a potent inducer or inhibitor of CYP1A2 is stopped or started during treatment with ropinirole, adjustment of the dose of ropinirole may be required)..............1620

Requip XL Tablets (*In vitro* metabolism studies showed that CYP1A2 is the major enzyme responsible for the metabolism of ropinirole. There is thus the potential for inducers or inhibitors of this enzyme to alter the clearance of ropinirole. Therefore, if therapy with a drug known to be a potent inducer or inhibitor of CYP1A2 is stopped or started during treatment with ropinirole, adjustment of the dose of ropinirole may be required)..............1628

Rilutek Tablets (Potential inhibitors of CYP1A2, such as caffeine, could decrease the rate of riluzole elimination. CYP1A2 is the principal isoenzyme involved in the initial oxidative metabolism of riluzole; potential interactions may occur when riluzole is given concurrently with other agents which are also metabolized primarily by CYP1A2 (eg, caffeine))......................................3032

Risperdal Consta Long-Acting Injection (*In vitro* studies showed that drugs metabolized by other CYP isozymes, including 1A1, 1A2, 2C9, 2C19, and 3A4, are only weak

inhibitors of risperidone metabolism)..............................2682

Sandostatin LAR Depot (Limited published data indicate that somatostatin analogs may decrease the metabolic clearance of compounds known to be metabolized by cytochrome P450 enzymes, which may be due to the suppression of growth hormone)..............................2519

Simponi Injection (The formation of CYP450 enzymes may be suppressed by increased levels of cytokines (eg, TNFα) during chronic inflammation. Therefore, it is expected that for a molecule that antagonizes cytokine activity, such as golimumab, the formation of CYP450 enzymes could be normalized. Upon initiation or discontinuation of golimumab in patients being treated with CYP450 substrates with a narrow therapeutic index, monitoring of the effect (eg, warfarin) or drug concentration (eg, cyclosporine or theophylline) is recommended and the individual dose of the drug product may be adjusted as needed) 930

Tev-Tropin for Injection (Somatropin administration may alter the clearance of compounds known to be metabolized by CYP450) 1181

Zantac Injection (Ranitidine has been reported to affect the bioavailability of other drugs through several different mechanisms, such as competition for renal tubular secretion, alteration of gastric pH, and inhibition of cytochrome P450 enzymes)...............................1732

Food, calcium-rich

Cipro XR Tablets (Concomitant administration of ciprofloxacin with milk products (dairy products) or calcium-fortified juices alone should be avoided since decreased absorption is possible) 3091

Food, charcoal-broiled

Rilutek Tablets (Potential inducers of CYP1A2, such as charcoal-broiled food, could increase the rate of riluzole elimination) 3032

Food, hot

Nascobal Nasal Spray (Hot foods may cause nasal secretions and a resulting loss of medication; therefore, patients should be told to administer cyanocobalamin nasal spray at least one hour before or one hour after ingestion of hot foods or liquids) 2700

Food, unspecified

Accolate Tablets (The bioavailability of zafirlukast may be decreased when taken with food. Patients should be instructed to take zafirlukast at least 1 hour before or 2 hours after meals)................................3612

Actonel Tablets (The extent of absorption of a 30 mg dose (three 10 mg tablets) when administered 0.5 hours before breakfast is reduced by 55% compared to dosing in the fasting state (no food or drink for 10 hours prior to or 4 hours after dosing). Dosing 1 hour prior to breakfast reduces the extent of absorption by 30% compared to dosing in the fasting state. Dosing either 0.5 hours prior to breakfast or 2 hours after dinner (evening meal) results in a similar extent of absorption. Residronate is effective when administered at

2235 Food Interactions Cross-Reference Food, unspecified

least 30 minutes before breakfast)....2779
ActoPlus Met Tablets (Administration of ActoPlus Met 15 mg/850 mg with food resulted in no change in overall exposure of pioglitazone. With metformin there was no change in AUC; however, mean peak serum concentration of metformin was decreased by 28% when administered with food. A delayed time to peak serum concentration was observed for both components (1.9 hours for pioglitazone and 0.8 hours for metformin) under fed conditions. These changes are not likely to be clinically significant)....3338
Actos Tablets (Food slightly delays the time to peak serum concentration of pioglitazone to 3 to 4 hours, but does not alter the extent of absorption)....3345
Afinitor Tablets (Based on data in healthy subjects taking 1 mg everolimus tablets, a high-fat meal reduced C_{max} and AUC by 60% and 16%, respectively. No data are available with everolimus 5 mg and 10 mg tablets)....2398
Albenza Tablets (Oral bioavailability appears to be enhanced when albendazole is co-administered with a fatty meal (estimated fat content 40 g) as evidenced by higher (up to 5-fold on average) plasma concentrations of albendazole sulfoxide as compared to the fasted state)....1298
Allegra ODT Orally Disintegrating Tablets (Administration of fexofenadine hydrochloride 30 mg with a high-fat meal decreased the AUC and C_{max} by approximately 40% and 60%, respectively, and a 2-hour delay in the time to peak exposure (T_{max}) was observed)....2911
Apriso Capsules (A high fat meal did not affect C_{max} for 5-ASA, but a 27% increase in the cumulative urinary excretion of 5-ASA was observed with a high fat meal. The overall extent of absorption of N-Ac-5-ASA was not affected by a high fat meal. As mesalamine and mesalamine granules in sachet were bioequivalent, mesalamine can be taken without regard to food)....2899
Aromasin Tablets (Exemestane plasma levels increased by approximately 40% after a high-fat breakfast)....2758
Asacol HD Delayed-Release Tablets (A high fat meal does not affect the extent of systemic exposure to mesalamine after single-dose administration of mesalamine, but mesalamine C_{max} decreases by 47% and t_{max} is delayed by 14 hours under fed conditions)....2787
Avandamet Tablets (Food decreases the extent and slightly delays the absorption of metformin)....1345
Avodart Soft Gelatin Capsules (When the drug is administered with food, the maximum serum concentrations were reduced by 10% to 15%. This reduction is of no clinical significance)....1375
Banzel Tablets (Food increased the extent of absorption of rufinamide in healthy volunteers by 34% and increased peak exposure by 56% after a single dose of 400 mg, although the T_{max} was not elevated. Clinical trials were performed under fed conditions and dosing is recommended with food)....1050
Biaxin Filmtab Tablets (For a single 500 mg dose of clarithromycin, food slightly delays the onset of clarithromycin absorption, increasing the peak time from approximately 2 to 2.5 hours. Food also increases the clarithromycin peak plasma concentration by about 24%, but does not affect the extent of clarithromycin bioavailability)....412
Boniva Tablets (The oral bioavailability of ibandronate is reduced by about 90% when ibandronate is administered concomitantly with a standard breakfast in comparison with bioavailability observed in fasted subjects. There is no meaningful reduction in bioavailability when ibandronate is taken at least 60 minutes before a meal. However, both bioavailability and the effect on bone mineral density (BMD) are reduced when food or beverages are taken less than 60 minutes following an ibandronate dose)....2844
Captopril Tablets (Reduces absorption by about 30% to 40%; should be given one hour before meals)....2341
Carbatrol Capsules (A high fat meal diet increased the rate of absorption of a single 400 mg dose (mean T_{max} was reduced from 24 hours, in the fasting state, to 14 hours and C_{max} increased from 3.2 to 4.3 µg/mL) but not the extent (AUC) of absorption. The elimination half-life remains unchanged between fed and fasting state. The multiple dose study conducted in the fed state showed that the steady-state C_{max} values were within the therapeutic concentration range. The pharmacokinetic profile of extended-release carbamazepine was similar when given by sprinkling the beads over applesauce compared to the intact capsule administered in the fasted state)....3280
Ceftin Tablets (Absorption is greater when taken after food)....1399
Celebrex Capsules (When celecoxib capsules were taken with a high fat meal, peak plasma levels were delayed for about 1 to 2 hours with an increase in total absorption (AUC) of 10% to 20%. Under fasting conditions, at doses above 200 mg, there is less than a proportional increase in C_{max} and AUC, which is thought to be due to the low solubility of the drug in aqueous media. Celecoxib, at doses up to 200 mg twice daily, can be administered without regard to timing of meals. Higher doses (400 mg twice daily) should be administered with food to improve absorption)....3272
Cipro I.V. (When ciprofloxacin tablets are given concomitantly with food, there is a delay in the absorption of the drug, resulting in peak concentrations that occur closer to 2 hours after dosing rather than 1 hour, whereas there is no delay observed when ciprofloxacin suspension is given with food. The overall absorption of ciprofloxacin tablets or ciprofloxacin suspension, however, is not substantially affected. The pharmacokinetics of ciprofloxacin given as the suspension are also not affected by food)....3082
Cipro Tablets (When ciprofloxacin tablets are given concomitantly with food, there is a delay in the absorption of the drug, resulting in peak concentrations that occur closer to 2 hours after dosing rather than 1 hour, whereas there is no delay observed when ciprofloxacin suspension is given with food. The overall absorption of ciprofloxacin tablets or ciprofloxacin suspension, however, is not substantially affected. The pharmacokinetics of ciprofloxacin given as the suspension are also not affected by food)....3073
Coartem Tablets (Food enhances absorption of artemether and lumefantrine following administration of Coartem Tablets. Patients who remain averse to food during treatment should be closely monitored, as the risk of recrudescence may be greater)....2403
Coreg CR Extended-Release Capsules (Administration of carvedilol with a high-fat meal resulted in increases (~20%) in AUC and C_{max} compared to carvedilol administered with a standard meal. Decreases in AUC (27%) and C_{max} (43%) were observed when carvedilol was administered in the fasted state compared to administration after a standard meal. Carvedilol should be taken with food)....1416
Crixivan Capsules (Co-administration of indinavir with a meal high in calories, fat, and protein, may reduce the absorption of indinavir; administer without food but with water one hour before or 2 hours after a meal)....2113
Dilaudid Oral Liquid (In a study conducted with a single 8 mg dose of hydromorphone (2 mg tablets), food lowered C_{max} by 25%, prolonged T_{max} by 0.8 hour, and increased AUC by 35%. The effects may not be clinically relevant)....2797
Diovan Tablets (Food decreases the exposure (as measured by AUC) to valsartan about 40% and peak plasma concentration (C_{max}) by about 50%; valsartan may be administered with or without food)....2413
Divista Softgel Capsules (Diets high in simple sugars (eg, sucrose), compared to diets high in complex carbohydrates (eg, whole grains) increase urinary chromium excretion in adults. This effect may be related to increase insulin secretion response to the consumption of simple sugars compared to complex carbohydrates)....3474
Duetact Tablets (Food did not change the systemic exposures of glimepiride or pioglitazone. However, for glimepiride, there was a 22% increase in C_{max} when Duetact was administered with food)....3354
DynaCirc CR Controlled Release Tablets (Food has been shown to decrease the extent of bioavailability of isradipine by up to 25%)....1432
EC-Naprosyn Delayed-Release Tablets (The presence of food prolonged the time the EC-Naprosyn remained in the stomach, time to first detectable serum naproxen levels, and time to maximal naproxen levels (T_{max}), but did not affect peak naproxen levels (C_{max}))....2850
Effient Tablets (In a study of healthy subjects given a single 15 mg dose, the AUC of the active metabolite was unaffected by a high fat, high calorie meal, but C_{max} was decreased by 49% and T_{max} was increased from 0.5 to 1.5 hours. Prasugrel hydrochloride can be administered without regard to food. The active metabolite is bound about 98% to human serum albumin)....1021
Effient Tablets (In a study of healthy subjects given a single 15 mg dose, the AUC of the active metabolite was unaffected by a high fat, high calorie meal, but C_{max} was decreased by 49% and T_{max} was increased from 0.5 to 1.5 hours. Prasugrel hydrochloride can be administered without regard to food. The active metabolite is bound about 98% to human serum albumin)....1881
Eldepryl Capsules (The bioavailability of selegiline is increased 3 to 4 fold when it is taken with food)....3312
Emtriva Capsules (Emtricitabine capsules and oral solution may be taken with or without food. Emtricitabine systemic exposure (AUC) was unaffected, while C_{max} decreased by 29% when emtricitabine capsules were administered with food (an approximately 1000 kcal high-fat meal). Emtricitabine systemic exposure (AUC) and C_{max} were unaffected when 200 mg emtricitabine oral solution was administered with either a high-fat or low-fat meal)....1238
Epivir Tablets (Absorption of lamivudine was slower in the fed state (T_{max}: 3.2 ± 1.3 hours) compared with the fasted state (T_{max}: 0.9 ± 0.3 hours); C_{max} in the fed state was 40% ± 23% (mean ± SD) lower than in the fasted state. There was no significant difference in systemic exposure ($AUC_{infinity}$) in the fed and fasted states; therefore, lamivudine may be administered with or without food)....1437
Evista Tablets (Administration of raloxifene with a standardized, high fat meal increases the absorption of raloxifene, but does not lead to clinically meaningful changes in systemic exposure; Evista can be administered without regard to meals)....1887
Evoxac Capsules (When administered with food, there is a decrease in the rate of absorption of cevimeline, with a fasting T_{Max} of 1.53 hours and a T_{Max} of 2.86 hours after a meal; the peak concentration is reduced by 17.3%)....1027
Exelon Capsules (Co-administration with food delays absorption (T_{max}) by 90 minutes, lowers C_{max} by approximately 30% and increases AUC by approximately 30%)....2432
Finacea Gel (Concomitant use with any foods and beverages that might provoke erythema, flushing, and blushing (including spicy food, alcoholic beverages, and thermally hot drinks, including hot coffee and tea) should be avoided)....1808
Fleet Prep Kit 3 (Use Fleet Prep Kit 3 with caution in patients who are on a low-salt diet)....1145
Focalin XR Capsules (No food effect study was performed with Focalin XR. However, the effect of food has been studied in adults with racemic methylphenidate in the same type of extended-release formulation. The findings of that study are considered applicable to Focalin XR. After a high fat breakfast, there was a longer lag time until absorption began and variable delays in the time until the first peak concentration, the time until the interpeak minimum, and the

Food, unspecified **Food Interactions Cross-Reference** 2236

time until the second peak. The first peak concentration and the extent of absorption were unchanged after food relative to the fasting state, although the second peak was approximately 25% lower) 2472

Fosamax Plus D Tablets (Other beverages (including mineral water) and food are likely to reduce the absorption of alendronate) 2147

Gabitril Tablets (Absorption of tiagabine is rapid, with peak plasma concentrations occurring at approximately 45 minutes following an oral dose in the fasting state. Tiagabine is nearly completely absorbed (>95%), with an absolute oral bioavailability of about 90%. A high fat meal decreases the rate (mean T_{max} was prolonged to 2.5 hours, and mean C_{max} was reduced by about 40%) but not the extent (AUC) of tiagabine absorption) 972

Gengraf Capsules (The administration of food with Gengraf decreases the cyclosporine AUC and C_{max}) 440

Geodon Capsules (The absorption of oral ziprasidone is increased up to two-fold in the presence of food) 2723

Imitrex Tablets (Delays the T_{max} slightly by about 0.5 hour with no significant effect on the bioavailability) 1508

Intuniv Extended-Release Tablets (High-fat meals increase exposure of guanfacine) 3291

Invega Extended-Release Tablets (Administration of a 12 mg paliperidone extended-release tablet to healthy ambulatory subjects with a standard high-fat/high-caloric meal gave mean C_{max} and AUC values of paliperidone that were increased by 60% and 54%, respectively, compared with administration under fasting conditions. Clinical trials establishing the safety and efficacy of paliperidone were carried out in subjects without regard to the timing of meals. While paliperidone can be taken without regard to food, the presence of food at the time of paliperidone administration may increase exposure to paliperidone) 2613

Isentress Tablets (Raltegravir may be administered with or without food. Administration of multiple doses of raltegravir following a moderate-fat meal (600 Kcal, 21 g fat) did not affect raltegravir AUC to a clinically meaningful degree with an increase of 13% relative to fasting. Raltegravir C_{12hr} was 66% higher and C_{max} was 5% higher following a moderate-fat meal compared to fasting. Administration of raltegravir following a high-fat meal (825 Kcal, 52 g fat) increased AUC and C_{max} by approximately 2-fold and increased C_{12hr} by 4.1-fold. Administration of raltegravir following a low-fat meal (300 Kcal, 2.5 g fat) decreased AUC and C_{max} by 46% and 52%, respectively; C_{12hr} was essentially unchanged. Food appears to increase pharmacokinetic variability relative to fasting) 2180

Kaletra Tablets (Relative to fasting, administration of Kaletra tablets with a moderate fat meal (500 - 682 Kcal, 23 to 25% calories from fat) increased lopinavir AUC and C_{max} by 26.9% and 17.6%, respectively. Relative to fasting, administration of KALETRA tablets with a high fat meal (872 Kcal, 56% from fat) increased lopinavir AUC by 18.9% but not C_{max}. Therefore, KALETRA tablets may be taken with or without food) 458

Kapidex Delayed Release Capsules (In food-effect studies in healthy subjects receiving dexlansoprazole under various fed conditions compared to fasting, increases in C_{max} ranged from 12% to 55%, increases in AUC ranged from 9% to 37%, and T_{max} varied (ranging from a decrease of 0.7 hours to an increase of 3 hours). No significant differences in mean intragastric pH were observed between fasted and various fed conditions. However, the percentage of time intragastric pH exceeded 4 over the 24-hour dosing interval decreased slightly when dexlansoprazole was administered after a meal (57%) relative to fasting (64%), primarily due to a decreased response in intragastric pH during the first 4 hours after dosing. Because of this, while dexlansoprazole can be taken without regard to food, some patients may benefit from administering the dose prior to a meal if post-meal symptoms do not resolve under post-fed conditions) 3362

Keppra XR Extended-Release Tablets (Intake of a high fat, high calorie breakfast before the administration of extended-release levetiracetam tablets resulted in a higher peak concentration, and longer median time to peak. The median time to peak (T_{max}) was 2 hours longer in the fed state) 3434

Lanoxin Tablets (When digoxin tablets are taken after meals, the rate of absorption is slowed, but the total amount of digoxin absorbed is usually unchanged. When taken with meals high in bran fiber, however, the amount absorbed from an oral dose may be reduced) 1553

Levaquin Oral Solution (Oral administration of a 500 mg dose of levofloxacin with food prolongs the time to peak concentration by approximately 1 hour and decreases the peak concentration by approximately 25% (following oral solution administration). It is recommended that levofloxacin oral solution be taken 1 hour before, or 2 hours after eating) 2629

Levaquin Tablets (Oral administration of a 500 mg dose of levofloxacin with food prolongs the time to peak concentration by approximately 1 hour and decreases the peak concentration by approximately 14% (following tablet administration). Therefore, levofloxacin can be administered without regard to food) 2629

Levitra Tablets (Two food-effect studies were conducted which showed that high-fat meals caused a reduction in C_{max} by 18%-50%) 3157

Malarone Tablets (Dietary fat intake with atovaquone increases the rate and extent of absorption; Malarone should be taken with food or milky drink) 1572

Mavik Tablets (Slows absorption of trandolapril but does not affect AUC or C_{max}) 489

Maxalt Tablets (Delays the time to reach peak concentration by an hour; no significant effect on the bioavailability) 2206

Mepron Suspension (Food enhances absorption by approximately two-fold) 1576

Meridia Capsules (Administration of a single 20 mg dose of sibutramine with a standard breakfast resulted in reduced peak M_1 and M_2 concentrations (by 27% and 32%, respectively) and delayed the time to peak by approximately three hours. However, the AUCs of M_1 and M_2 were not significantly altered) 492

Metozolv ODT Orally Disintegrating Tablets (In a food-effect study with 28 subjects, metoclopramide taken immediately after a high-fat meal had a 17% lower peak blood level than when taken after an overnight fast. The time to peak blood levels increased from about 1.75 hours under fasted conditions to 3 hours when taken immediately after a high-fat meal. The extent of metoclopramide absorbed (area under the curve) was comparable whether metoclopramide was administered with or without food. The clinical effect of the decrease in peak plasma level if metoclopramide is inadvertently taken with food is unknown) 2901

Micardis Tablets (Food slightly reduces the bioavailability of telmisartan, with a reduction in the area under the plasma concentration-time curve (AUC) of about 6% with the 40 mg tablet and about 20% after a 160 mg dose. The absolute bioavailability of telmisartan is dose dependent. At 40 and 160 mg the bioavailability was 42% and 58%, respectively) 887

Micardis HCT Tablets (Food slightly reduces the bioavailability of telmisartan, with a reduction in the area under the plasma concentration-time curve (AUC) of about 6% with the 40 mg tablet and about 20% after a 160 mg dose. The absolute bioavailability of telmisartan is dose dependent. At 40 mg and 160 mg the bioavailability was 42% and 58%, respectively) 889

Myfortic Tablets (Co-administration of mycophenolic acid with a high fat meal decreased C_{max} by 33%, a 3.5-hour delay in the T_{lag} (range, -6 to 18 hours), and 5.0-hour delay in the T_{max} (range, -9 to 20 hours) of MPA. To avoid the variability in MPA absorption between doses, mycophenolic acid should be taken on an empty stomach) 2491

Nascobal Nasal Spray (A vegetarian diet which contains no animal products (including milk products or eggs) does not supply any vitamin B12. Therefore, patients following such a diet should be advised to take cyanocobalamin nasal spray weekly) 2700

Neoral Soft Gelatin Capsules (Administration of food with Neoral decreases the AUC and C_{max}) 2496

Nexium Delayed-Release Capsules (The AUC after administration of a single 40 mg dose of esomeprazole is decreased by 43%-53% after food intake compared to fasting conditions. Esomeprazole should be taken at least one hour before meals) 704

Niaspan Extended-Release Tablets (Concomitant administration of spicy foods may increase the side effects of flushing and pruritus and should be avoided around the time of niacin ingestion) 497

Noroxin Tablets (Co-administration may decrease the absorption of norfloxacin; administer at least one hour before or two hours after a meal) 2220

Norvir Soft Gelatin Capsules (When the oral solution was given under non-fasting conditions, peak ritonavir concentrations decreased 23% and the extent of absorption decreased 7% relative to fasting conditions. Relative to fasting conditions, the extent of absorption of ritonavir from the soft gelatin capsule formulation was 13% higher when administered with a meal) 509

NovoLog Injection (The timing of hypoglycemia usually reflects the time-action profile of the administered insulin formulations. Other factors such as changes in food intake (eg, amount of food or timing of meals) may also alter the risk of hypoglycemia. As with all insulins, use caution in patients with hypoglycemia unawareness and in patients who may be predisposed to hypoglycemia (eg, patients who are fasting or have erratic food intake)) 2575

Nucynta Tablets (The AUC and C_{max} increased by 25% and 16%, respectively, when tapentadol hydrochloride was administered after a high-fat, high-calorie breakfast. Tapentadol hydrochloride may be given with or without food) 2643

Nuvigil Tablets (Although food effect on the bioavailability of armodafinil is considered minimal, food can potentially affect the onset and time course of pharmacologic action of armodafinil. The time to reach peak concentration (T_{max}) may be delayed by approximately 2-4 hours in the fed state) 978

Omnicef Capsules (Although C_{max} and AUC of cefdinir absorption from capsules are reduced by 44% and 33%, respectively, when given with a high-fat meal, the magnitude of these reductions is not likely to be clinically significant; therefore, cefdinir may be taken without regard to food) 518

OxyContin Tablets (The peak plasma concentration of oxycodone increased by 25% when oxycodone was administered with a high-fat meal) 2807

Paxil Tablets (The effects of food on the bioavailability of paroxetine were studied in subjects administered a single dose with and without food. AUC was only slightly increased (6%) when drug was administered with food but the C_{max} was 29% greater, while the time to reach peak plasma concentration decreased from 6.4 hours post-dosing to 4.9 hours; paroxetine may be administered with or without food) 1586

Pepcid Tablets (Bioavailability may be slightly increased by antacids) 2227

Premphase Tablets (Single dose studies in healthy, postmenopausal women were conducted to investigate any potential drug interaction when PREMPHASE is administered with a high fat breakfast. Administration with food decreased the C_{max} of total estrone by 18% to 34% and increased total equilin C_{max} by 38% compared to the fasting state, with no other effect on the rate or extent of absorption of other conjugated or unconjugated estrogens. Administration with food

approximately doubles MPA C_{max} and increases MPA AUC by approximately 20% to 30%) **3549**

Prempro Tablets (Single dose studies in healthy, postmenopausal women were conducted to investigate any potential drug interaction when PREMPRO is administered with a high fat breakfast. Administration with food decreased the C_{max} of total estrone by 18% to 34% and increased total equilin C_{max} by 38% compared to the fasting state, with no other effect on the rate or extent of absorption of other conjugated or unconjugated estrogens. Administration with food approximately doubles MPA C_{max} and increases MPA AUC by approximately 20% to 30%) **3549**

Prograf Capsules (The rate and extent of tacrolimus absorption were greatest under fasted conditions. The presence and composition of food decreased both the rate and extent of tacrolimus absorption. The effect was most pronounced with a high-fat meal (848 kcal, 46% fat): mean AUC and C_{max} were decreased 37% and 77%, respectively; T_{max} was lengthened 5-fold. A high-carbohydrate meal (668 kcal, 85% carbohydrate) decreased mean AUC and mean C_{max} by 28% and 65%, respectively. The time of the meal also affected tacrolimus bioavailability. When given immediately following the meal, mean C_{max} was reduced 71%, and mean AUC was reduced 39%, relative to the fasted condition. When administered 1.5 hours following the meal, mean C_{max} was reduced 63%, and mean AUC was reduced 39%, relative to the fasted condition) **677**

Promacta Tablets (Eltrombopag chelates polyvalent cations (such as iron, calcium, aluminum, magnesium, selenium, and zinc) in foods, mineral supplements, and antacids. In a clinical study, administration of eltrombopag with a polyvalent cation-containing antacid (1,524 mg aluminum hydroxide, 1,425 mg magnesium carbonate, and sodium alginate) decreased plasma eltrombopag systemic exposure by approximately 70%. Eltrombopag must not be taken within 4 hours of any medications or products containing polyvalent cations such as antacids, dairy products, and mineral supplements to avoid significant reduction in eltrombopag absorption due to chelation) **1610**

Prometrium Capsules (100 mg, 200 mg) (Concomitant food ingestion increased the bioavailability of progesterone relative to a fasting state when administered to post-menopausal women at a dose of 200 mg) **3307**

Provigil Tablets (Delays the absorption (t_{max}) by approximately one hour; no effect on overall bioavailability) **983**

Rapamune Tablets (In healthy subjects, a high-fat meal (861.8 kcal, 54.9% kcal from fat) increased the mean total exposure (AUC) of sirolimus by 23% to 35% compared with fasting. The effect of food on the mean sirolimus C_{max} was inconsistent depending on the sirolimus dosage form evaluated) **3579**

Requip Tablets (Food does not affect the extent of absorption of ropinirole, although its T_{max} is increased by 2.5 hours and its C_{max} is decreased by approximately 25% when the drug is taken with a high-fat meal) **1620**

Requip XL Tablets (In a single-dose study, administration of ropinirole to healthy volunteers with food (eg, high-fat meal) increased AUC by approximately 30% and C_{max} by approximately 44%, compared with dosing under fasted conditions. In a repeat-dose study in patients with Parkinson's disease, food (eg, high-fat meal) increased AUC by approximately 20% and C_{max} by approximately 44%; T_{max} was prolonged by 3 hours (median prolongation) compared with dosing under fasted conditions) **1628**

Romazicon Injection (Ingestion of food during an IV infusion results in a 50% increase in clearance) **2863**

Rozerem Tablets (When administered with a high-fat meal, the AUC_{0-inf} for a single 16 mg dose of ramelteon was 31% higher and the C_{max} was 22% lower than when given in a fasted state. Median T_{max} was delayed by approximately 45 minutes when ramelteon was administered with food. Effects of food on the AUC values for M-II were similar. It is, therefore, recommended that ramelteon not be taken with or immediately after a high-fat meal) **3366**

Rythmol SR Extended Release Capsules (Increased peak blood level and bioavailability in a single dose study) **1652**

Ryzolt Extended-Release Tablets (Co-administration with a high fat meal did not significantly affect AUC (overall exposure to tramadol); however, C_{max} (peak plasma concentration) increased 67% following a single 300 mg tablet administration and 54% following a single 200 mg tablet administration. Tramadol hydrochloride was administered without regard to food in all clinical trials) **2813**

Saphris Tablets (A crossover study in 26 healthy male subjects was performed to evaluate the effect of food on the pharmacokinetics of a single 5 mg dose of asenapine. Consumption of food immediately prior to sublingual administration decreased asenapine exposure by 20%; consumption of food 4 hours after sublingual administration decreased asenapine exposure by about 10%. These effects are probably due to increased hepatic blood flow. Patients should be instructed to not eat or drink for 10 minutes after administration of asenapine) **3223**

Selzentry Tablets (Co-administration of a 300 mg tablet with a high fat breakfast reduced maraviroc C_{max} and AUC by 33% in healthy volunteers. There were no food restrictions in the studies that demonstrated the efficacy and safety of maraviroc. Therefore, maraviroc can be taken with or without food at the recommended dose) **2740**

Sensipar Tablets (A food-effect study in healthy volunteers indicated that the C_{max} and area under the curve (AUC_{0-inf}) were increased 82% and 68%, respectively, when cinacalcet

was administered with a high-fat meal compared to fasting. C_{max} and $AUC_{(0-inf)}$ of cinacalcet were increased 65% and 50%, respectively, when cinacalcet was administered with a low-fat meal compared to fasting) **640**

Seroquel Tablets (The bioavailability of quetiapine is marginally affected by administration with food, with C_{max} and AUC values increased by 25% and 15%, respectively) **750**

Seroquel XR Extended-Release Tablets (A high fat meal (approximately 800 to 1000 calories) was found to produce statistically significant increases in the quetiapine C_{max} and AUC of 44% to 52% and 20% to 22%, respectively, for the 50 mg and 300 mg tablets. In comparison, a light meal (approximately 300 calories) had no significant effect on the C_{max} or AUC of quetiapine. It is recommended that quetiapine be taken without food or with a light meal) **759**

Skelaxin Tablets (Taking metaxalone with food may enhance general CNS depression. The presence of a high fat meal at the time of drug administration increased C_{max} and AUC. T_{max} was also delayed and terminal half-life was decreased under fed conditions compared to fasted conditions) **1848**

Strattera Capsules (Atomoxetine hydrochloride can be administered with or without food. Administration of atomoxetine with a standard high–fat meal in adults did not affect the extent of oral absorption of atomoxetine (AUC), but did decrease the rate of absorption, resulting in a 37% lower C_{max}, and delayed T_{max} by 3 hours. In clinical trials with children and adolescents, administration of atomoxetine with food resulted in a 9% lower C_{max}) **1957**

Suprax for Oral Suspension (Cefixime, given orally, is about 40% to 50% absorbed whether administered with or without food; however, time to maximal absorption is increased approximately 0.8 hours when administered with food) **2038**

Tarceva Tablets (Erlotinib is about 60% absorbed after oral administration and its bioavailability is substantially increased by food to almost 100%) **1222**

Targretin Capsules (Co-administration with a fat-containing meal has resulted in higher plasma bexarotene AUC and C_{max} values; because safety and efficacy data are based upon administration with food, it is recommended that Targretin capsules be administered with or immediately following a meal)........ **1074**

Tarka Tablets (Co-administration with food decreases verapamil bioavailability and the time to peak plasma concentration is delayed; bioavailability of trandolapril is not altered; Tarka should be administered with food) **534**

Tasigna Capsules (The bioavailability of nilotinib is increased with food. Nilotinib should not be taken with food. No food should be taken at least 2 hours before and at least one hour after the dose is taken) **2533**

Temodar Capsules (Temozolomide is rapidly and completely absorbed after oral administration with a peak

plasma concentration (C_{max}) achieved in a median T_{max} of 1 hour. Food reduces the rate and extent of temozolomide absorption. Mean peak plasma concentration and AUC decreased by 32% and 9%, respectively, and median T_{max} increased by 2-fold (from 1 to 2.25 hours) when temozolomide was administered after a modified high-fat breakfast)........................ **3230**

Teveten Tablets (Co-administration with food delays absorption and causes variable changes in C_{max} and AUC values which do not appear clinically important)........................ **538**

Tricor Tablets (The absorption of fenofibrate is increased when administered with food; Tricor should be given with meals) **544**

Truvada Tablets (Truvada may be administered with or without food. Administration of Truvada following a high fat meal or a light meal delayed the time of tenofovir C_{max} by approximately 0.75 hour. The mean increases in tenofovir AUC and C_{max} were approximately 35% and 15%, respectively, when administered with a high fat or light meal, compared to administration in the fasted state. In previous safety and efficacy studies, tenofovir was taken under fed conditions. Emtricitabine systemic exposures (AUC and C_{max}) were unaffected when Truvada was administered with either a high fat or a light meal) **1258**

Uloric Tablets (Following multiple 80 mg once daily doses with a high fat meal, there was a 49% decrease in C_{max} and an 18% decrease in AUC, respectively. However, no clinically significant change in the percent decrease in serum uric acid concentration was observed (58% fed vs. 51% fasting). Thus, febuxostat may be taken without regard to food) **3370**

Urocit-K Tablets (A dose of potassium citrate taken with meals or snacks may alleviate minor gastrointestinal complaints such as abdominal discomfort, vomiting, diarrhea, loose bowel movements or nausea in some patients)............... **2333**

Uroxatral Tablets (The extent of absorption of alfuzosin is 50% lower under fasting conditions. Therefore, alfuzosin should be taken immediately following a meal)........................ **3050**

Valcyte Tablets (Co-administration with high fat meals has resulted in increased steady-state ganciclovir AUC and C_{max} without any prolongation in time to peak plasma concentrations; Valcyte should be administered with food) **2872**

Valturna Tablets (When taken with food, mean AUC and C_{max} of aliskiren are decreased by 76% and 88%, respectively; mean AUC and C_{max} of valsartan were not significantly affected. In clinical trials of Valturna, it was administered without requiring a fixed relation of administration to meals. High-fat meals decrease absorption of Valturna substantially)........................ **3637**

Vytorin 10/10 Tablets (Concomitant food administration (high-fat or non-fat meals) had no effect on the extent of absorption of ezetimibe when administered as 10-mg tablets. The C_{max} value of ezetimibe was increased by 38% with consumption of high-fat meals) **2303**

Vytorin 10/10 Tablets (Concomitant food administration (high-fat or

non-fat meals) had no effect on the extent of absorption of ezetimibe when administered as 10-mg tablets. The C_{max} value of ezetimibe was increased by 38% with consumption of high-fat meals) 3240
Xeloda Tablets (Reduces both rate and extent of absorption of capecitabine and delays T_{max} of both parent and 5-FU) 2882
Xenical Capsules (Gastrointestinal events may increase when orlistat is taken with a diet high in fat)....................2893
Zetia Tablets (The C_{max} value of ezetimibe was increased by 38% with consumption of high-fat meals. Ezetimibe can be administered with or without food) 3256
Zetia Tablets (Concomitant food administration (non-fat meals) had no effect on the extent of absorption of ezetimibe when administered as ezetimibe 10-mg tablets. The C_{max} value of ezetimibe was increased by 38% with consumption of high-fat meals. Ezetimibe can be administered with or without food) 2312
Zofran Tablets (Bioavailability is slightly enhanced by food) 1756
Zonegran Capsules (Following a 200–400 mg oral zonisamide dose, peak plasma concentrations (range: 2–5 μg/mL) in normal volunteers occur within 2–6 hours. In the presence of food, the time to maximum concentration is delayed, occurring at 4–6 hours, but food has no effect on the bioavailability of zonisamide. Zonisamide can be taken with or without food) 1081
Zyban Sustained-Release Tablets (In a single-dose study, food increased the C_{max} of bupropion by 11% and the extent of absorption as defined by area under the plasma concentration-time curve (AUC) by 17%. The mean time to peak concentration (T_{max}) was prolonged by 1 hour. This effect was of no clinical significance)........1762
Zyvox Tablets (Linezolid may be administered without regard to the timing of meals. The time to reach maximum concentration is delayed from 1.5 hours to 2.2 hours and C_{max} is decreased by about 17% when high fat food is given with linezolid. However, the total exposure measured as AUC values is similar under both conditions)............................2769

Food having a pH greater than 5.5

Creon Delayed-Release Capsules (Pancrelipase should not be crushed or chewed or mixed in foods having a pH greater than 4. These actions can disrupt the protective enteric coating, resulting in early release of enzymes, irritation of oral mucosa, and/or loss or enzyme activity)..3304
Ultrase Capsules (Can dissolve the protective coating resulting in early release of enzymes, irritation of oral mucosa, and/or loss of enzyme activity) 797
Ultrase MT Capsules (Can dissolve the protective enteric shell)... 798

Food high in tyramine

Azilect Tablets (Severe hypertensive reactions have followed the administration of tyramine rich foods and non-selective MAO inhibitors) 3383
Eldepryl Capsules (Rare cases of hypertensive reactions associated with ingestion of tyramine-containing foods have been reported in patients taking the recommended daily dose of selegiline)....................................3312
Emsam Transdermal System (As a class, MAO inhibitors have been associated with hypertensive crises caused by the ingestion of foods with a high concentration of tyramine) 3623
Marplan Tablets (Isocarboxazid should not be administered in combination with cheese or other foods with a high tyramine content. Hypertensive crises have sometimes occurred during isocarboxazid therapy after ingestion of foods with a high tyramine content. In general, patients should avoid protein foods in which aging or protein breakdown is used to increase flavor. In particular, patients should be instructed not to take foods such as cheese, sour cream, Chianti wine, sherry, beer (including non-alcoholic beer), liqueurs, pickled herring, anchovies, caviar, liver, canned figs, raisins, bananas or avocados, chocolate, soy sauce, sauerkraut, the pods of broad beans (fava beans), yeast extracts, yogurt, meat extracts, meat prepared with tenderizers, or dry sausage).................................3481
Zyvox Tablets (A significant pressor response has been observed in normal adult subjects receiving linezolid and tyramine doses of more than 100 mg. Therefore, patients receiving linezolid need to avoid consuming large amounts of foods or beverages with high tyramine content)..........................2769

Food with high concentration of tyramine

Eldepryl Capsules (Rare cases of hypertensive reactions associated with ingestion of tyramine-containing foods have been reported in patients taking the recommended daily dose of selegiline hydrochloride)................3312
Emsam Transdermal System (As a class, MAO inhibitors have been associated with hypertensive crises caused by the ingestion of foods with a high concentration of tyramine) 3623
Parnate Tablets (Tranylcypromine is contraindicated in foods with a high tyramine content. Hypertensive crises have sometimes occurred during therapy with tranylcypromine after ingestion of foods with a high tyramine content)...................1584

Fruit juices, unspecified

Allegra ODT Orally Disintegrating Tablets (Fruit juices such as grapefruit, orange and apple may reduce the bioavailability and exposure of fexofenadine) 2911
Allegra Tablets (Grapefruit, orange and apple may reduce the bioavailability and exposure of fexofenadine; it is recommended that fexofenadine should be taken with water)...................................2911
Cipro I.V. (Ciprofloxacin should not be taken with calcium-fortified juices alone since absorption of ciprofloxacin may be significantly reduced; however, ciprofloxacin may be taken with a meal that contains these products)....................................3082
Cipro Tablets (Ciprofloxacin should not be taken with calcium-fortified juices alone since absorption of ciprofloxacin may be significantly reduced; however, ciprofloxacin may be taken with a meal that contains these products)....................................3073
Dexedrine Spansule Sustained-Release Capsules (Gastrointestinal acidifying agents (eg, fruit juices) lower the absorption of amphetamines. Gastrointestinal acidifying agents lower blood levels and efficacy of amphetamines) 1425

Fruits, dried

Parnate Tablets (Tranylcypromine is contraindicated in combination with foods with a high tyramine content. Hypertensive crises have sometimes occurred during therapy with tranylcypromine after ingestion of foods with a high tyramine content. In particular, patients should be instructed not to take foods, such as dried fruits) 1584

Fruits, overripe

Parnate Tablets (Tranylcypromine is contraindicated in combination with foods with a high tyramine content. Hypertensive crises have sometimes occurred during therapy with tranylcypromine after ingestion of foods with a high tyramine content. In particular, patients should be instructed not to take foods, such as overripe fruit) 1584

Grapefruit

Adcirca Tablets (Tadalafil is metabolized predominantly by CYP3A in the liver. In patients taking potent inhibitors of CYP3A, avoid use of tadalafil. Ketoconazole (400 mg qd), a selective and potent inhibitor of CYP3A, increased tadalafil 20 mg single dose exposure (AUC) by 312% and C_{max} by 22%. Ketoconazole (200 mg qd) increased tadalafil 10 mg single dose exposure (AUC) by 107% and C_{max} by 15%. Although specific interactions have not been studied, other CYP3A inhibitors would likely increase tadalafil exposure) 3461
Advair Diskus 100/50 (Fluticasone propionate and salmeterol, the individual components of Advair Diskus, are substrates of CYP3A4. The use of strong CYP3A4 inhibitors with Advair Diskus is not recommended because increased corticosteroid and increased cardiovascular adverse effects may occur) 1275
Advair HFA 45/21 Inhalation Aerosol (Both fluticasone propionate and salmeterol are substrates of CYP 3A4. There is a potential drug interaction with CYP 3A4 inhibitors) 1288
Advicor Tablets (The risk of myopathy appears to be increased by high levels of HMG-CoA reductase inhibitory activity in plasma. Lovastatin is metabolized by the cytochrome P450 isoform 3A4. Certain drugs which share this metabolic pathway can raise the plasma levels of lovastatin and may increase the risk of myopathy).................................... 402
Afinitor Tablets (Co-administration of everolimus with strong or moderate inhibitors of CYP3A4 (eg, ketoconazole, itraconazole, clarithromycin, atazanavir, nefazodone, saquinavir, telithromycin, ritonavir, amprenavir, indinavir, nelfinavir, delavirdine, fosamprenavir, voriconazole, aprepitant, erythromycin, fluconazole, grapefruit juice, verapamil or diltazem) should be avoided due to significant increase in exposure of everolimus)................2398
Ambien Tablets (Some compounds known to inhibit CYP3A may increase exposure to zolpidem).................................2920
Ambien CR Tablets (Some compounds known to inhibit CYP3A4 may increase exposure to zolpidem tartrate) 2925
Angeliq Tablets (Inhibitors of CYP3A4 such as erythromycin, clarithromycin, ketoconazole, itraconazole, ritonavir and grapefruit juice may increase plasma concentrations of estrogens and may result in side effects) 831
Avodart Soft Gelatin Capsules (Based on *in vitro* data, blood concentrations of dutasteride may increase in the presence of inhibitors of CYP3A4/5) 1375
Azilect Tablets (Rasagiline plasma concentrations may increase up to 2 fold in patients using concomitant CYP1A2 inhibitors) 3383
Carbatrol Capsules (Carbamazepine is metabolized mainly by CYP3A4, the active carbamazepine 10,11-epoxide, which is futher metabolized to the trans-diol by epoxide hydrolase. Therefore, the potential exists for interaction between carbamazepine and any agent that inhibits CYP3A4 and/or epoxide hydrolase. Agents that are CYP3A4 inhibitors may increase the plasma levels of carbamazepine. Thus, if a patient has been titrated to a stable dosage of carbamazepine, and then begins a course of treatment with a CYP3A4 or epoxide hydrolase inhibitor, it is reasonable to expect that a dose reduction for carbamazepine may be necessary) 3280
Cardizem LA Extended Release Tablets (Diltiazem is both a substrate and an inhibitor of the CYP3A4 enzyme system. Other drugs that are specific substrates, inhibitors, or inducers of this enzyme system may have a significant impact on the efficacy and side effect profile of diltiazem) 423
Celexa Tablets (*In vitro* studies indicated that CYP3A4 and CYP2C19 are the primary enzymes involved in the metabolism of citalopram. However, co-administration of citalopram (40 mg) and ketoconazole (200 mg), a potent inhibitor of CYP3A4, did not significantly affect the pharmacokinetics of citalopram. Because citalopram is metabolized by multiple enzyme systems, inhibition of a single enzyme may not appreciably decrease citalopram clearance)......1153
Cialis Tablets (Tadalafil is a substrate of and predominantly metabolized by CYP3A4. Studies have shown that drugs that inhibit CYP3A4 can increase tadalafil exposure. When tadalafil is used on an as-needed basis, patients taking concomitant potent inhibitors of CYP3A4, such as ketoconazole or ritonavir, the maximum recommended dose of tadalafil is 10 mg, not to exceed once every 72 hours. When tadalafil is used in a once-daily regimen, patients taking concomitant potent inhibitors of CYP3A4, such as ketoconazole or ritonavir, the dose should not exceed 2.5 mg).....1861
Climara Transdermal System (Inhibitors of CYP3A4 may increase plasma concentrations of estrogens and may result in side effects) 841

Climara Pro Transdermal System (Inhibitors of CYP3A4 such as erythromycin, clarithromycin, ketoconazole, itraconazole, ritonavir and grapefruit juice may increase plasma concentrations of estrogens and may result in side effects) **847**

Coartem Tablets (When Coartem Tablets are co-administered with an inhibitor of CYP3A4, including grapefruit juice, it may result in increased concentrations of artemether and/or lumefantrine and potentiate QT prolongation) **2403**

Crixivan Capsules (Indinavir is metabolized by CYP3A4. Co-administration of indinavir and other drugs that inhibit CYP3A4 may decrease the clearance of indinavir and may result in increased plasma concentrations of indinavir) **2113**

Cymbalta Delayed-Release Capsules (Both CYP1A2 and CYP2D6 are responsible for duloxetine metabolism. When duloxetine 60 mg was co-administered with fluvoxamine 100 mg, a potent CYP1A2 inhibitor to male subjects, duloxetine AUC was increased approximately 6-fold, the C_{max} was increased approximately 2.5-fold and duloxetine $t_{1/2}$ was increased approximately 3-fold. Co-administration of duloxetine with potent CYP1A2 inhibitors should be avoided)........................**1871**

Divigel (Inhibitors of CYP3A4, such as erythromycin, clarithromycin, ketoconazole, itraconazole, ritonavir, and grapefruit juice, may increase plasma concentrations of estrogens and result in side effects) **3467**

Duragesic Transdermal System (The concomitant use of fentanyl with all CYP3A4 inhibitors may result in an increase in fentanyl plasma concentrations, which could increase or prolong adverse drug effects and may cause potentially fatal respiratory depression. Patients receiving fentanyl and any CYP3A4 inhibitor should be monitored for an extended period of time and dosage adjustments should be made if warranted) **2604**

Effexor XR Extended-Release Capsules (Concomitant use of CYP3A4 inhibitors and venlafaxine may increase levels of venlafaxine and ODV. Therefore, caution is advised if a patient's therapy includes a CYP3A4 inhibitor and venlafaxine concomitantly. The concomitant use of venlafaxine with a drug treatment(s) that potently inhibits both CYP2D6 and CYP3A4, the primary metabolizing enzymes for venlafaxine, has not been studied. Therefore, caution is advised should a patient's therapy include venlafaxine and any agent(s) that produce potent simultaneous inhibition of these two enzyme systems)........**3504**

Elidel Cream 1% (The concomitant administration of known CYP3A family of inhibitors in patients with widespread and/or erythrodermic disease should be done with caution. Some examples of such drugs are erythromycin, itraconazole, ketoconazole, fluconazole, calcium channel blockers and cimetidine)........................**2424**

Emend Capsules (Aprepitant is a substrate for CYP3A4; therefore, co-administration of fosaprepitant or aprepitant with drugs that inhibit CYP3A4

activity may result in increased plasma concentrations of aprepitant. Consequently, concomitant administration of fosaprepitant or aprepitant with strong CYP3A4 inhibitors (eg, ketoconazole, itraconazole, nefazodone, troleandomycin, clarithromycin, ritonavir, nelfinavir) should be approached with caution. Because moderate CYP3A4 inhibitors (eg, diltiazem) result in a 2-fold increase in plasma concentrations of aprepitant, concomitant administration should also be approached with caution)........................**2124**

Enjuvia Tablets (Inhibitors of CYP3A4 such as erythromycin, clarithromycin, ketoconazole, itraconazole, ritonavir and grapefruit juice may increase plasma concentrations of estrogens and may result in side effects) **3401**

Equetro Extended-Release Capsules (Carbamazepine is metabolized mainly by CYP3A4 the active carbamazepine 10,11-epoxide, which is further metabolized to the trans-diol by epoxide hydrolase. Therefore, the potential exists for interaction between carbamazepine and any agent that inhibits CYP3A4 and/or epoxide hydrolase. Agents that are CYP3A4 inhibitors may increase the plasma levels of carbamazepine) **3477**

Estrasorb Topical Emulsion (*In vitro* and *in vivo* studies have shown that estrogens are metabolized partially by cytochrome P450 3A4 (CYP3A4). Therefore, inhibitors of CYP3A4 may affect estrogen drug metabolism. Inhibitors of CYP3A4, such as erythromycin, clarithromycin, ketoconazole, itraconazole, ritonavir and grapefruit juice may increase plasma concentrations of estrogens and may result in side effects) **1777**

Evoxac Capsules (Drugs which inhibit CYP3A3/4 also inhibit the metabolism of cevimeline)........**1027**

Fentanyl Transdermal System Patches (The concomitant use of fentanyl with all CYP3A4 inhibitors (eg, grapefruit juice) may result in an increase in fentanyl plasma concentrations, which could increase or prolong adverse drug effects and may cause potentially fatal respiratory depression. Patients receiving fentanyl and any CYP3A4 inhibitor should be carefully monitored for an extended period of time and dosage adjustments should be made if warranted)........................**2346**

Fentora Tablets (The concomitant use of moderate CYP3A4 inhibitors such as amprenavir, aprepitant, diltiazem, erythromycin, fluconazole, fosamprenavir, grapefruit juice, and verapamil with fentanyl citrate may result in an increase in fentanyl plasma concentrations, which could increase or prolong adverse drug effects and may cause potentially fatal respiratory depression. Patients receiving fentanyl citrate and moderate CYP3A4 inhibitors should be carefully monitored for an extended period of time and dosage increase should be done conservatively) **966**

Flonase Nasal Spray (Caution should be exercised when potent cytochrome P450 3A4 inhibitors are co-administered with fluticasone propionate) **1459**

Gabitril Tablets (Because of the potential for pharmacokinetic interactions between tiagabine

hydrochloride and drugs that inhibit hepatic metabolizing enzymes, it may be useful to obtain plasma levels of tiagabine before and after changes are made in the therapeutic regimen) **972**

Gengraf Capsules (Affects the metabolism of cyclosporine increasing blood concentration of cyclosporine; concurrent use should be avoided)....................**440**

Geodon Capsules (Ketoconazole, a potent inhibitor of CYP3A4, at a dose of 400 mg QD for 5 days, increased the AUC and C_{max} of ziprasidone by about 35-40%. Other inhibitors of CYP3A4 would be expected to have similar effects) **2723**

Gleevec Tablets (Grapefruit juice may increase plasma concentrations of imatinib and should be avoided)........................**2477**

Implanon Implant (Inhibitors of hepatic enzymes may increase plasma hormone levels)................**3128**

InnoPran XL Extended Release Capsules (Blood levels and/or toxicity of propranolol may be increased by administration of propranolol with inhibitors of CYP1A2) **1517**

Kaletra Tablets (Although not noted with concurrent ketoconazole, co-administration of Kaletra and other drugs that inhibit CYP3A may increase lopinavir plasma concentrations)............................**458**

Klonopin Tablets (Although clinical studies have not been performed, based on the involvement of the cytochrome P-450 3A family in clonazepam metabolism, inhibitors of this enzyme system, notably oral antifungal agents, should be used cautiously in patients receiving clonazepam)....................**2855**

Letairis Tablets (Use caution when ambrisentan is co-administered with strong CYP3A-inhibitors)..........**1250**

Levitra Tablets (Although specific interactions have not been studied, other CYP3A4 inhibitors, including grapefruit juice, would likely increase vardenafil exposure)....................**3157**

Lexapro Tablets (*In vitro* studies indicated that CYP3A4 and -2C19 are the primary enzymes involved in the metabolism of escitalopram. However, co-administration of escitalopram (20 mg) and ritonavir (600 mg), a potent inhibitor of CYP3A4, did not significantly affect the pharmacokinetics of escitalopram oxalate. Because escitalopram oxalate is metabolized by multiple enzyme systems, inhibition of a single enzyme may not appreciably decrease escitalopram clearance)........................**1160**

Lexiva Tablets (Amprenavir is metabolized by CYP3A4. Co-administration of fosamprenavir calcium and drugs that inhibit CYP3A4 may increase amprenavir concentrations and increase the incidence of adverse effects) **1558**

Lipitor Tablets (Grapefruit juice contains one or more components that inhibit CYP 3A4 and can increase plasma concentrations of atorvastatin, especially with excessive grapefruit juice consumption (>1.2 liters per day)) **2703**

LoSeasonique Tablets (CYP3A4 inhibitors may increase plasma hormone levels) **3407**

Lybrel Tablets (CYP 3A4 inhibitors such as indinavir, itraconazole, ketoconazole, fluconazole, and

troleandomycin may increase plasma hormone levels)...............**3514**

Mevacor Tablets (The risk of myopathy/rhabdomyolysis is increased by concomitant use of lovastatin with potent inhibitors of CYP3A4, particularly with higher doses of lovastatin; concomitant use should be avoided unless the benefits of combined therapy outweigh the increased risk)...........**2212**

Multaq Tablets (Dronedarone is metabolized primarily by CYP 3A and is a moderate inhibitor of CYP 3A and CYP 2D6. Dronedarone's blood levels can therefore be affected by inhibitors and inducers of CYP 3A, and dronedarone can interact with drugs that are substrates of CYP 3A and CYP 2D6. Concomitant use of other potent CYP 3A inhibitors such as itraconazole, voriconazole, ritonavir, clarithromycin, and nefazodone is contraindicated).......**3015**

Neoral Soft Gelatin Capsules (Affects the metabolism of cyclosporine and should be avoided) **2496**

Nexium Delayed-Release Capsules (Concomitant administration of esomeprazole and a combined inhibitor of CYP 2C19 and CYP 3A4, such as voriconazole, may result in more than doubling of the esomeprazole exposure. Dose adjustment of esomeprazole is not normally required. However, in patients with Zollinger-Ellison's Syndrome, who may require higher doses up to 240 mg/day, dose adjustment may be considered)...... **704**

Nexium I.V. (Concomitant administration of esomeprazole and a combined inhibitor of CYP2C19 and CYP3A4, such as voriconazole, may result in more than doubling of the esomeprazole exposure. Dose adjustment of esomeprazole is not normally required for the recommended doses. However, in patients who may require higher doses, dose adjustment may be considered)...................... **712**

NuvaRing (CYP3A4 inhibitors may increase plasma hormone levels) **3181**

Onglyza Tablets (Co-administration of saxagliptin with other moderate CYP3A4/5 inhibitors (eg, amprenavir, aprepitant, erythromycin, fluconazole, fosamprenavir, grapefruit juice, verapamil) may increase plasma concentrations of saxagliptin; however, dosage adjustment is not recommended) **3615**

Onsolis Film (The concomitant use of fentanyl with CYP3A4 inhibitors (eg, indinavir, nelfinavir, ritonavir, clarithromycin, itraconazole, ketoconazole, nefazodone, saquinavir, telithromycin, aprepitant, diltiazem, erythromycin, fluconazole, grapefruit juice, verapamil, or cimetidine) may result in a potentially dangerous increase in fentanyl plasma concentrations)............................**2054**

Ortho Evra Transdermal System (CYP3A4 inhibitors, such as itraconazole or ketoconazole, may increase plasma hormone levels) **2648**

Ortho Tri-Cyclen Lo Tablets (CYP3A4 inhibitors such as itraconazole or ketoconazole may increase plasma hormone levels) **2673**

Ortho-Cyclen Tablets (CYP3A4 inhibitors, such as itraconazole or ketoconazole, may increase plasma hormone levels)................**2663**

Ultram ER Extended-Release Tablets (Administration of CYP3A4 inhibitors, such as ketoconazole and erythromycin, with tramadol hydrochloride may effect the metabolism of tramadol leading to altered tramadol exposure)........................2693
Valium Tablets (There is a potentially relevant interaction between diazepam and certain hepatic enzyme inhibitors such as CYP450 3A4. It has been shown that these compounds influence the pharmacokinetics of diazepam and may lead to increased and prolonged sedation).....................................2880
Vaprisol (The co-administration of conivaptan with potent CYP3A4 inhibitors, such as ketoconazole, itraconazole, clarithromycin, ritonavir and indinavir, is contraindicated. Conivaptan is a substrate of CYP3A4. Co-administration of conivaptan with CYP3A4 inhibitors could lead to an increase in conivaptan concentrations)............................. 689
Velcade for Injection (Patients who are concomitantly receiving bortezomib and drugs that are inhibitors or inducers of cytochrome P450 3A4 should be closely monitored for either toxicities or reduced efficacy) 2324
Venlafaxine Hydrochloride Tablets (Concomitant use of CYP3A4 inhibitors and venlafaxine may increase levels of venlafaxine and ODV. Therefore, caution is advised if a patient's therapy includes a CYP3A4 inhibitor and venlafaxine concomitantly. The concomitant use of venlafaxine with a drug treatment(s) that potently inhibits both CYP2D6 and CYP3A4, the primary metabolizing enzymes for venlafaxine, has not been studied. Therefore, caution is advised should a patient's therapy include venlafaxine and any agent(s) that produce potent simultaneous inhibition of these two enzyme systems)........2388
VESIcare Tablets (Inhibitors of CYP3A4 may alter solifenacin pharmacokinetics. Following the administration of 10 mg of solifenacin in the presence of 400 mg of ketoconazole, a potent inhibitor of CYP3A4, the mean C_{max} and AUC of solifenacin increased by 1.5 and 2.7-fold, respectively. Therefore, it is recommended not to exceed a 5 mg daily dose of solifenacin when administered with therapeutic doses of ketoconazole or other potent CYP3A4 inhibitors) 694
Vytorin 10/10 Tablets (Simvastatin is metabolized by the cytochrome P450 isoform 3A4. Certain agents that inhibit this metabolic pathway can raise plasma levels of simvastatin and may increase the risk of myopathy. These agents include large quantities of grapefruit juice (greater than 1 quart daily). The use of Vytorin concomitantly with this CYP3A4 inhibitor should be avoided).....................................2303
Vytorin 10/10 Tablets (Simvastatin is metabolized by the cytochrome P450 isoform 3A4. The risk of myopathy is increased by reducing the elimination of the simvastatin component of Vytorin. Hence when Vytorin is used with an inhibitor of CYP3A4 (eg, grapefruit juice), elevated plasma levels of HMG-CoA reductase inhibitory activity can increase the risk of myopathy and rhabdomyolysis, particularly with higher doses of Vytorin. Avoid large quantities of grapefruit juice (>1 quart daily))......3240
Zemplar Injection (A multiple dose drug-drug interaction study with ketoconazole and paricalcitol capsule demonstrated that ketoconazole approximately doubled paricalcitol AUC since paricalcitol is partially metabolized by CYP3A and ketoconazole is known to be a strong inhibitor of cytochrome P450 3A enzyme. Care should be taken while dosing paricalcitol with ketoconazole and other strong P450 3A inhibitors including atazanavir, clarithromycin, indinavir, itraconazole, nefazodone, nelfinavir, ritonavir, saquinavir, telithromycin or voriconazole) 571
Zocor Tablets (The risk of myopathy and rhabdomyolysis is increased by high level of statin activity in plasma. Simvastatin is metabolized by the cytochrome P450 isoform 3A4. Certain drugs, including the large quantities of grapefruit juice (greater than 1 quart daily), which inhibit this metabolic pathway can raise the plasma levels of simvastatin and may increase the risk of myopathy. The use of simvastatin concomitantly with this CYP3A4 inhibitor should be avoided) 2289
Zofran Tablets (Ondansetron does not itself appear to induce or inhibit the cytochrome P-450 drug metabolizing enzyme system of the liver. Because ondansetron is metabolized by hepatic cytochrome P-450 drug-metabolizing enzymes (CYP3A4, CYP2D6, CYP1A2), inducers or inhibitors of these enzymes may change the clearance and, hence, the half-life of ondansetron. On the basis of available data, no dosage adjustment is recommended for patients on these drugs) 1756
Zonegran Capsules (Concurrent use with drugs that inhibit CYP3A4 may alter serum concentrations of zonisamide)........1081
Zyprexa Tablets (Concomitant use may potentially inhibit olanzapine clearance; therefore, a dosage decrease may need to be considered) 1984
Zyprexa IntraMuscular (Concomitant use may potentially inhibit olanzapine clearance; therefore, a dosage decrease may need to be considered) 1984

Grapefruit Juice

Adcirca Tablets (Tadalafil is metabolized predominantly by CYP3A in the liver. In patients taking potent inhibitors of CYP3A, avoid use of tadalafil. Ketoconazole (400 mg qd), a selective and potent inhibitor of CYP3A, increased tadalafil 20 mg single dose exposure (AUC) by 312% and C_{max} by 22%. Ketoconazole (200 mg qd) increased tadalafil 10 mg single dose exposure (AUC) by 107% and C_{max} by 15%. Although specific interactions have not been studied, other CYP3A inhibitors, such as grapefruit juice, would likely increase tadalafil exposure) 3461
Advair Diskus 100/50 (Fluticasone propionate and salmeterol, the individual components of Advair Diskus, are substrates of CYP3A4. The use of strong CYP3A4 inhibitors with Advair Diskus is not recommended because increased corticosteroid and increased cardiovascular adverse effects may occur) 1275
Advair HFA 45/21 Inhalation Aerosol (Both fluticasone propionate and salmeterol are substrates of CYP 3A4. There is a potential drug interaction with CYP 3A4 inhibitors) 1288
Advicor Tablets (Inhibits CYP3A4 and can increase the plasma concentration of lovastatin; concurrent use should be avoided) 402
Afinitor Tablets (Co-administration of everolimus with strong or moderate inhibitors of CYP3A4 (eg, ketoconazole, itraconazole, clarithromycin, atazanavir, nefazodone, saquinavir, telithromycin, ritonavir, amprenavir, indinavir, nelfinavir, delavirdine, fosamprenavir, voriconazole, aprepitant, erythromycin, fluconazole, grapefruit juice, verapamil or diltazem) should be avoided due to significant increase in exposure of everolimus)................2398
Allegra ODT Orally Disintegrating Tablets (Fruit juices such as grapefruit, orange and apple may reduce the bioavailability and exposure of fexofenadine) 2911
Allegra-D 12 Hour Extended-Release Tablets (Co-administration with grapefruit, orange or apple juice will reduce the bioavailability and exposure or fexofenadine) 2915
Ambien Tablets (Some compounds known to inhibit CYP3A may increase exposure to zolpidem).................................2920
Ambien CR Tablets (Some compounds known to inhibit CYP3A4 may increase exposure to zolpidem tartrate) 2925
Angeliq Tablets (Inhibitors of CYP3A4 such as erythromycin, clarithromycin, ketoconazole, itraconazole, ritonavir and grapefruit juice may increase plasma concentrations of estrogens and may result in side effects) 831
Avodart Soft Gelatin Capsules (Based on *in vitro* data, blood concentrations of dutasteride may increase in the presence of inhibitors of CYP3A4/5) 1375
Azilect Tablets (Rasagiline plasma concentrations may increase up to 2 fold in patients using concomitant CYP1A2 inhibitors) 3383
Carbatrol Capsules (Carbamazepine is metabolized mainly by CYP3A4, the active carbamazepine 10,11-epoxide, which is futher metabolized to the trans-diol by epoxide hydrolase. Therefore, the potential exists for interaction between carbamazepine and any agent that inhibits CYP3A4 and/or epoxide hydrolase. Agents that are CYP3A4 inhibitors may increase the plasma levels of carbamazepine. Thus, if a patient has been titrated to a stable dosage of carbamazepine, and then begins a course of treatment with a CYP3A4 or epoxide hydrolase inhibitor, it is reasonable to expect that a dose reduction for carbamazepine may be necessary)..................................3280
Cardizem LA Extended Release Tablets (Diltiazem is both a substrate and an inhibitor of the CYP3A4 enzyme system. Other drugs that are specific substrates, inhibitors, or inducers of this enzyme system may have a significant impact on the efficacy and side effect profile of diltiazem) 423
Celexa Tablets (*In vitro* studies indicated that CYP3A4 and CYP2C19 are the primary enzymes involved in the metabolism of citalopram. However, co-administration of citalopram (40 mg) and ketoconazole (200 mg), a potent inhibitor of CYP3A4, did not significantly affect the pharmacokinetics of citalopram. Because citalopram is metabolized by multiple enzyme systems, inhibition of a single enzyme may not appreciably decrease citalopram clearance)......1153
Cialis Tablets (CYP3A4 inhibitors, such as grapefruit juice, may likely increase tadalafil exposure) 1861
Climara Transdermal System (Inhibitors of CYP3A4, such as grapefruit juice, may increase plasma concentrations of estrogens and may result in side effects) 841
Climara Pro Transdermal System (Inhibitors of CYP3A4 such as erythromycin, clarithromycin, ketoconazole, itraconazole, ritonavir and grapefruit juice may increase plasma concentrations of estrogens and may result in side effects) 847
Coartem Tablets (When Coartem Tablets are co-administered with an inhibitor of CYP3A4, including grapefruit juice, it may result in increased concentrations of artemether and/or lumefantrine and potentiate QT prolongation)...........2403
Crixivan Capsules (Indinavir is metabolized by CYP3A4. Co-administration of indinavir and other drugs that inhibit CYP3A4 may decrease the clearance of indinavir and may result in increased plasma concentrations of indinavir) 2113
Cymbalta Delayed-Release Capsules (Both CYP1A2 and CYP2D6 are responsible for duloxetine metabolism. When duloxetine 60 mg was co-administered with fluvoxamine 100 mg, a potent CYP1A2 inhibitor to male subjects, duloxetine AUC was increased approximately 6-fold, the C_{max} was increased approximately 2.5-fold and duloxetine $t_{1/2}$ was increased approximately 3-fold. Co-administration of duloxetine with potent CYP1A2 inhibitors should be avoided).......................1871
Divigel (Inhibitors of CYP3A4, such as erythromycin, clarithromycin, ketoconazole, itraconazole, ritonavir, and grapefruit juice, may increase plasma concentrations of estrogens and result in side effects) 3467
Duragesic Transdermal System (The concomitant use of fentanyl with all CYP3A4 inhibitors (eg, grapefruit juice) may result in an increase in fentanyl plasma concentrations, which could increase or prolong adverse drug effects and may cause potentially fatal respiratory depression. Patients receiving fentanyl and any CYP3A4 inhibitor should be monitored for an extended period of time and dosage adjustments should be made if warranted).................................2604
Effexor XR Extended-Release Capsules (Concomitant use of CYP3A4 inhibitors and venlafaxine may increase levels of venlafaxine and ODV. Therefore, caution is advised if a patient's therapy includes a CYP3A4 inhibitor and venlafaxine concomitantly. The concomitant use of venlafaxine with a drug treatment(s) that potently inhibits both CYP2D6 and CYP3A4, the primary

Grapefruit Juice — Food Interactions Cross-Reference — 2242

metabolizing enzymes for venlafaxine, has not been studied. Therefore, caution is advised should a patient's therapy include venlafaxine and any agent(s) that produce potent simultaneous inhibition of these two enzyme systems)........3504

Elidel Cream 1% (The concomitant administration of known CYP3A family of inhibitors in patients with widespread and/or erythrodermic disease should be done with caution. Some examples of such drugs are erythromycin, itraconazole, ketoconazole, fluconazole, calcium channel blockers and cimetidine) 2424

Emend Capsules (Aprepitant is a substrate for CYP3A4; therefore, co-administration of fosaprepitant or aprepitant with drugs that inhibit CYP3A4 activity may result in increased plasma concentrations of aprepitant. Consequently, concomitant administration of fosaprepitant or aprepitant with strong CYP3A4 inhibitors (eg, ketoconazole, itraconazole, nefazodone, troleandomycin, clarithromycin, ritonavir, nelfinavir) should be approached with caution. Because moderate CYP3A4 inhibitors (eg, diltiazem) result in a 2-fold increase in plasma concentrations of aprepitant, concomitant administration should also be approached with caution) 2124

Enjuvia Tablets (Inhibitors of CYP3A4 such as erythromycin, clarithromycin, ketoconazole, itraconazole, ritonavir and grapefruit juice may increase plasma concentrations of estrogens and may result in side effects) 3401

Equetro Extended-Release Capsules (Carbamazepine is metabolized mainly by CYP3A4 the active carbamazepine 10,11-epoxide, which is further metabolized to the trans-diol by epoxide hydrolase. Therefore, the potential exists for interaction between carbamazepine and any agent that inhibits CYP3A4 and/or epoxide hydrolase. Agents that are CYP3A4 inhibitors may increase the plasma levels of carbamazepine) 3477

Estrasorb Topical Emulsion (*In vitro* and *in vivo* studies have shown that estrogens are metabolized partially by cytochrome P450 3A4 (CYP3A4). Therefore, inhibitors of CYP3A4 may affect estrogen drug metabolism. Inhibitors of CYP3A4, such as grapefruit juice, may increase plasma concentrations of estrogens and may result in side effects) 1777

Evoxac Capsules (Drugs which inhibit CYP3A3/4 also inhibit the metabolism of cevimeline)........1027

Fentanyl Transdermal System Patches (The concomitant use of fentanyl with all CYP3A4 inhibitors (eg, grapefruit juice) may result in an increase in fentanyl plasma concentrations, which could increase or prolong adverse drug effects and may cause potentially fatal respiratory depression. Patients receiving fentanyl and any CYP3A4 inhibitor should be carefully monitored for an extended period of time and dosage adjustments should be made if warranted).........................2346

Fentora Tablets (The concomitant use of moderate CYP3A4 inhibitors such as amprenavir, aprepitant, diltiazem, erythromycin, fluconazole, fosamprenavir, grapefruit juice, and verapamil with fentanyl citrate may result in an increase in fentanyl plasma concentrations, which could increase or prolong adverse drug effects and may cause potentially fatal respiratory depression. Patients receiving fentanyl citrate and moderate CYP3A4 inhibitors should be carefully monitored for an extended period of time and dosage increase should be done conservatively) 966

Flonase Nasal Spray (Caution should be exercised when potent cytochrome P450 3A4 inhibitors are co-administered with fluticasone propionate) 1459

Gabitril Tablets (Because of the potential for pharmacokinetic interactions between tiagabine hydrochloride and drugs that inhibit hepatic metabolizing enzymes, it may be useful to obtain plasma levels of tiagabine before and after changes are made in the therapeutic regimen)...................... 972

Gengraf Capsules (Affects the metabolism of cyclosporine increasing blood concentration of cyclosporine; concurrent use should be avoided)......................... 440

Geodon Capsules (Ketoconazole, a potent inhibitor of CYP3A4, at a dose of 400 mg QD for 5 days, increased the AUC and C_{max} of ziprasidone by about 35-40%. Other inhibitors of CYP3A4 would be expected to have similar effects) 2723

Gleevec Tablets (Grapefruit juice may increase plasma concentrations of imatinib and should be avoided).........................2477

Implanon Implant (Inhibitors of hepatic enzymes may increase plasma hormone levels)................3128

InnoPran XL Extended Release Capsules (Blood levels and/or toxicity of propranolol may be increased by administration of propranolol with inhibitors of CYP1A2) 1517

Kaletra Tablets (Although not noted with concurrent ketoconazole, co-administration of Kaletra and other drugs that inhibit CYP3A may increase lopinavir plasma concentrations)............................. 458

Klonopin Tablets (Although clinical studies have not been performed, based on the involvement of the cytochrome P-450 3A family in clonazepam metabolism, inhibitors of this enzyme system, notably oral antifungal agents, should be used cautiously in patients receiving clonazepam)...................2855

Letairis Tablets (Use caution when ambrisentan is co-administered with strong CYP3A-inhibitors)..........1250

Levitra Tablets (Although specific interactions have not been studied, other CYP3A4 inhibitors, including grapefruit juice, would likely increase vardenafil exposure)......................3157

Lexapro Tablets (*In vitro* studies indicated that CYP3A4 and -2C19 are the primary enzymes involved in the metabolism of escitalopram. However, co-administration of escitalopram (20 mg) and ritonavir (600 mg), a potent inhibitor of CYP3A4, did not significantly affect the pharmacokinetics of escitalopram oxalate. Because escitalopram oxalate is metabolized by multiple enzyme systems, inhibition of a single enzyme may not appreciably decrease escitalopram clearance) 1160

Lexiva Tablets (Amprenavir is metabolized by CYP3A4. Co-administration of fosamprenavir calcium and drugs that inhibit CYP3A4 may increase amprenavir concentrations and increase the incidence of adverse effects) 1558

Lipitor Tablets (Grapefruit juice contains one or more components that inhibit CYP 3A4 and can increase plasma concentrations of atorvastatin, especially with excessive grapefruit juice consumption (>1.2 liters per day)) 2703

LoSeasonique Tablets (CYP3A4 inhibitors may increase plasma hormone levels) 3407

Lybrel Tablets (CYP 3A4 inhibitors such as indinavir, itraconazole, ketoconazole, fluconazole, and troleandomycin may increase plasma hormone levels)................3514

Mevacor Tablets (The risk of myopathy/rhabdomyolysis is increased by concomitant use of lovastatin with potent inhibitors of CYP3A4, particularly with higher doses of lovastatin; concomitant use should be avoided unless the benefits of combined therapy outweigh the increased risk)...........2212

Multaq Tablets (Grapefruit juice, a moderate inhibitor of CYP 3A, resulted in a 3-fold increase in dronedarone exposure and a 2.5-fold increase in C_{max}. Therefore, patients should avoid grapefruit juice beverages while taking dronedarone) 3015

Neoral Soft Gelatin Capsules (Affects the metabolism of cyclosporine and should be avoided) 2496

Nexium Delayed-Release Capsules (Concomitant administration of esomeprazole and a combined inhibitor of CYP 2C19 and CYP 3A4, such as voriconazole, may result in more than doubling of the esomeprazole exposure. Dose adjustment of esomeprazole is not normally required. However, in patients with Zollinger-Ellison's Syndrome, who may require higher doses up to 240 mg/day, dose adjustment may be considered)...... 704

Nexium I.V. (Concomitant administration of esomeprazole and a combined inhibitor of CYP2C19 and CYP3A4, such as voriconazole, may result in more than doubling of the esomeprazole exposure. Dose adjustment of esomeprazole is not normally required for the recommended doses. However, in patients who may require higher doses, dose adjustment may be considered)....................... 712

NuvaRing (CYP3A4 inhibitors may increase plasma hormone levels) 3181

Onglyza Tablets (Co-administration of saxagliptin with other moderate CYP3A4/5 inhibitors (eg, amprenavir, aprepitant, erythromycin, fluconazole, fosamprenavir, grapefruit juice, verapamil) may increase plasma concentrations of saxagliptin; however, dosage adjustment is not recommended) 3615

Onsolis Film (The concomitant use of fentanyl with CYP3A4 inhibitors (eg, indinavir, nelfinavir, ritonavir, clarithromycin, itraconazole, ketoconazole, nefazodone, saquinavir, telithromycin, aprepitant, diltiazem, erythromycin, fluconazole, grapefruit juice, verapamil, or cimetidine) may result in a potentially dangerous increase in fentanyl plasma concentrations)............................2054

Ortho Evra Transdermal System (CYP3A4 inhibitors, such as itraconazole or ketoconazole, may increase plasma hormone levels) 2648

Ortho Tri-Cyclen Lo Tablets (CYP3A4 inhibitors such as itraconazole or ketoconazole may increase plasma hormone levels) 2673

Ortho-Cyclen Tablets (CYP3A4 inhibitors, such as itraconazole or ketoconazole, may increase plasma hormone levels)................2663

Premarin Tablets (Co-administration of grapefruit juice with estrogens may increase plasma concentrations of estrogens and may result in side effects) 3533

Premarin Vaginal Cream (Inhibitors of CYP3A4 may affect estrogen drug metabolism. Inhibitors of CYP3A4, such as grapefruit juice, may increase plasma concentrations of estrogens and may result in side effects) 3540

Premphase Tablets (Inhibitors of CYP3A4, such as grapefruit juice, may increase plasma concentrations of estrogens and may result in side effects) 3549

Prempro Tablets (Inhibitors of CYP3A4, such as grapefruit juice, may increase plasma concentrations of estrogens and may result in side effects) 3549

Pristiq Extended-Release Tablets (CYP3A4 is a minor pathway for the metabolism of desvenlafaxine. In a clinical study, ketoconazole (200 mg b.i.d.) increased the area under the concentration vs. time curve AUC of desvenlafaxine (400 mg single dose) by about 43% and C_{max} by about 8%. Concomitant use of desvenlafaxine with potent inhibitors of CYP3A4 may result in higher concentrations of desvenlafaxine) 3564

Prograf Capsules (Grapefruit juice affects CYP3A-mediated metabolism and should be avoided during therapy with tacrolimus. Co-administered grapefruit juice has been reported to increase tacrolimus blood trough concentrations in liver transplant patients) 677

Promacta Tablets (*In vitro* studies demonstrate that CYP1A2 and CYP2C8 are involved in the oxidative metabolism of eltrombopag. The significance of co-administration of eltrombopag with moderate or strong inhibitors of CYP 1A2 (eg, ciprofloxacin, fluvoxamine) and CYP 2C8 (eg, gemfibrozil, trimethoprim) on the systemic exposure of eltrombopag has not been established in clinical studies. Monitor patients for signs and symptoms of excessive eltrombopag exposure when eltrombopag is administered concomitantly with these moderate or strong inhibitors of CYP1A2 or CYP2C8)...1610

Prometrium Capsules (100 mg, 200 mg) (The metabolism of progesterone by human liver microsomes was inhibited by ketoconazole. Ketoconazole is a known inhibitor of cytochrome P450 3A4, hence these data suggest that ketoconazole or other known inhibitors of this enzyme may increase the bioavailability of progesterone. The clinical relevance of the *in vitro* findings is unknown) 3307

2243 **Food Interactions Cross-Reference** **Grapefruit Juice**

Provigil Tablets (Co-administration of potent inhibitors of CYP3A4 could alter the plasma levels of modafinil) 983

Pulmicort Flexhaler (Concomitant administration of budesonide with known inhibitors of CYP3A4 may inhibit the metabolism of, and increase the systemic exposure to, budesonide; care should be exercised) 714

Ranexa Extended-Release Tablets (Concomitant use is contraindicated. Ranolazine is primarily metabolized by CYP3A. Use of ranolazine with potent or moderately potent inhibitors of CYP3A should be avoided because concomitant administration will increase ranolazine plasma levels and QTc prolongation) 1255

Rapamune Tablets (Because grapefruit juice inhibits the CYP3A4-mediated metabolism of sirolimus, it must not be taken with or be used for dilution of sirolimus) 3579

Requip Tablets (*In vitro* metabolism studies showed that CYP1A2 is the major enzyme responsible for the metabolism of ropinirole. There is thus the potential for inducers or inhibitors of this enzyme to alter the clearance of ropinirole. Therefore, if therapy with a drug known to be a potent inducer or inhibitor of CYP1A2 is stopped or started during treatment with ropinirole, adjustment of the dose of ropinirole may be required) 1620

Requip XL Tablets (*In vitro* metabolism studies showed that CYP1A2 is the major enzyme responsible for the metabolism of ropinirole. There is thus the potential for inducers or inhibitors of this enzyme to alter the clearance of ropinirole. Therefore, if therapy with a drug known to be a potent inducer or inhibitor of CYP1A2 is stopped or started during treatment with ropinirole, adjustment of the dose of ropinirole may be required) 1628

Rilutek Tablets (Potential inhibitors of CYP 1A2 (eg, caffeine, phenacetin, theophylline, amitriptyline, and quinolones) could decrease the rate of riluzole elimination) 3032

Rozerem Tablets (Ramelteon should be administered with caution to patients taking less strong CYP1A2 inhibitors) 3366

Rythmol Tablets (Propafenone is metabolized by CYP3A4. Agents that inhibit CYP3A4 (such as grapefruit juice), can be expected to cause increased plasma levels of propafenone. Appropriate monitoring is recommended when propafenone is used together with such agents) 1648

Rythmol SR Extended Release Capsules (Drugs that inhibit CYP1A2 might lead to increased plasma levels of propafenone; patients should be closely monitored and the propafenone dose adjusted accordingly) 1652

Ryzolt Extended-Release Tablets (Concomitant administration of CYP3A4 inhibitors, such as ketoconazole and erythromycin, may reduce metabolic clearance of tramadol increasing the risk for serious adverse events including seizures and serotonin syndrome) 2813

Seasonique Tablets (CYP3A4 inhibitors may increase plasma ethinyl estradiol levels) 3418

Selzentry Tablets (Maraviroc is a substrate of CYP3A and Pgp and hence its pharmacokinetics are likely to be modulated by inhibitors and inducers of these enzymes/transporters. The CYP3A/Pgp inhibitors ketoconazole, lopinavir/ritonavir, ritonavir, saquinavir and atazanavir all increased the C_{max} and AUC of maraviroc) 2740

Sensipar Tablets (Co-administration of ketoconazole, a strong inhibitor of CYP3A4, increased cinacalcet exposure following a single 90 mg dose of cinacalcet by 2.3-fold. Dose adjustment of cinacalcet may be required and PTH and serum calcium concentrations should be closely monitored if a patient initiates or discontinues therapy with a strong CYP3A4 inhibitor (eg, ketoconazole, erythromycin, itraconazole)) 640

Serevent Diskus (Co-administration of salmeterol and a strong CYP3A4 inhibitor ketoconazole resulted in a significant increase in plasma salmeterol exposure as determined by a 16-fold increase in AUC mainly due to increased bioavailability of swallowed portion of the dose. Although there was no statistical effect on the mean QTc, co-administration of salmeterol and ketoconazole was associated with more frequent increases in QTc duration compared with salmeterol and placebo administration. Due to the potential increased risk of cardiovascular adverse events, the concomitant use of salmeterol with strong CYP3A4 inhibitors, (eg, ketoconazole, ritonavir, atazanavir, clarithromycin, indinavir, itraconazole, nefazodone, nelfinavir, saquinavir, telithromycin) is not recommended) 1656

Seroquel Tablets (Co-administration with an inhibitor of CYP4503A may reduce oral clearance of quetiapine, resulting in an increase in maximum plasma concentration of quetiapine; dose adjustment of quetiapine will be necessary) 750

Seroquel XR Extended-Release Tablets (Co-administration of quetiapine with cytochrome P450 3A inhibitors may decrease the clearance of quetiapine. Caution (reduced dosage) of quetiapine may be necessary when co-administered with other cytochrome P450 3A inhibitors) 759

Simcor Tablets (Potent inhibitors of CYP3A4 increase the risk of myopathy by reducing the elimination of simvastatin. Hence when simvastatin is used with a potent inhibitor of CYP3A4, elevated plasma levels of HMG-CoA reductase inhibitory activity can increase the risk of myopathy and rhabdomyolysis, particularly with higher doses of simvastatin. Concomitant use of drugs labeled as potent inhibitors of CYP3A4 should be avoided unless the benefits of combined therapy outweigh the increased risk. If treatment with itraconazole, ketoconazole, erythromycin, clarithromycin or telithromycin is unavoidable, therapy with Simcor should be suspended during the course of treatment) 524

Sutent Capsules (Grapefruit may increase plasma concentrations of sunitinib malate) 2747

Symbicort 80/4.5 Inhalation Aerosol (The main route of metabolism of corticosteroids, including budesonide, a component of Symbicort, is via cytochrome P450 (CYP) isoenzyme 3A4 (CYP3A4). After oral administration of ketoconazole, a strong inhibitor of CYP3A4, the mean plasma concentration of orally administered budesonide increased. Concomitant administration of CYP3A4 inhibitors may inhibit the metabolism of, and increase the systemic exposure to, budesonide. Caution should be exercised when considering the co-administration of Symbicort with long-term ketoconazole and other known strong CYP3A4 inhibitors (eg, ritonavir, atazanavir, clarithromycin, indinavir, itraconazole, nefazodone, nelfinavir, saquinavir, telithromycin)) 720

Tarceva Tablets (Erlotinib is metabolized predominantly by CYP3A4. Inhibitors of CYP3A4 would be expected to increase exposure. Caution should be used when co-administering erlotinib with a strong CYP3A4 inhibitor, such as grapefruit juice; consider a dose reduction if severe adverse reactions occur) 1222

Targretin Capsules (Bexarotene is metabolized by CYP403A4; co-administration with inhibitors of CYP4503A4, such as grapefruit juice, would be expected to lead to an increase in plasma bexarotene concentrations) 1074

Targretin Gel 1% (Bexarotene is metabolized by CYP4503A4; co-administration with inhibitors of CYP4503A4, such as grapefruit juice, could lead to an increase in plasma bexarotene concentrations) 1079

Tasigna Capsules (Concomitant use with grapefruit products may increase serum concentrations of nilotinib and should be avoided) 2533

Taxotere Injection Concentrate (*In vitro* studies have shown that the metabolism of docetaxel may be modified by the concomitant administration of compounds that induce, inhibit, or are metabolized by cytochrome P450 3A4, such as cyclosporine, terfenadine, ketoconazole, erythromycin, and troleandomycin. Caution should be exercised with these drugs when treating patients receiving docetaxel as there is a potential for a significant interaction) 3035

Torisel Injection (Grapefruit juice may increase plasma concentrations of sirolimus (a major metabolite of temsirolimus) and should be avoided) 3592

Toviaz Extended-Release Tablets (In patients taking weak or moderate CYP3A4 inhibitors, careful assessment of tolerability at the 4 mg daily dose is advised prior to increasing the daily dose to 8 mg. While this specific interaction potential was not examined by clinical study, some pharmacokinetic interaction is expected) 2753

Tracleer Tablets (Bosentan is metabolized by CYP2C9 and CYP3A. Inhibition of these enzymes may increase the plasma concentration of bosentan. Concomitant administration of both a CYP2C9 inhibitor (such as fluconazole or amiodarone) and a strong CYP3A inhibitor (eg, ketoconazole, itraconazole) or a moderate CYP3A inhibitor (eg, amprenavir, erythromycin, fluconazole, diltiazem) with bosentan will likely lead to large increases in plasma concentrations of bosentan. Co-administration of such combinations of a CYP2C9 inhibitor plus a strong or moderate CYP3A inhibitor with bosentan is not recommended) 573

Treanda for Injection (Inhibitors of CYP1A2 (eg, fluvoxamine, ciprofloxacin) have the potential to increase plasma concentrations of bendamustine and decrease plasma concentrations of active metabolites. Caution should be used, or alternative treatments considered, if concomitant treatment with CYP1A2 inhibitors is needed) 989

Tykerb Tablets (Grapefruit may also increase plasma concentrations of lapatinib and should be avoided) 1698

Ultram ER Extended-Release Tablets (Administration of CYP3A4 inhibitors, such as ketoconazole and erythromycin, with tramadol hydrochloride may effect the metabolism of tramadol leading to altered tramadol exposure) 2693

Valium Tablets (There is a potentially relevant interaction between diazepam and certain hepatic enzyme inhibitors such as CYP450 3A4. It has been shown that these compounds influence the pharmacokinetics of diazepam and may lead to increased and prolonged sedation) 2880

Vaprisol (The co-administration of conivaptan with potent CYP3A4 inhibitors, such as ketoconazole, itraconazole, clarithromycin, ritonavir and indinavir, is contraindicated. Conivaptan is a substrate of CYP3A4. Co-administration of conivaptan with CYP3A4 inhibitors could lead to an increase in conivaptan concentrations) 689

Velcade for Injection (Patients who are concomitantly receiving bortezomib and drugs that are inhibitors or inducers of cytochrome P450 3A4 should be closely monitored for either toxicities or reduced efficacy) 2324

Venlafaxine Hydrochloride Tablets (Concomitant use of CYP3A4 inhibitors and venlafaxine may increase levels of venlafaxine and ODV. Therefore, caution is advised if a patient's therapy includes a CYP3A4 inhibitor and venlafaxine concomitantly. The concomitant use of venlafaxine with a drug treatment(s) that potently inhibits both CYP2D6 and CYP3A4, the primary metabolizing enzymes for venlafaxine, has not been studied. Therefore, caution is advised should a patient's therapy include venlafaxine and any agent(s) that produce potent simultaneous inhibition of these two enzyme systems) 2388

VESIcare Tablets (Inhibitors of CYP3A4 may alter solifenacin pharmacokinetics. Following the administration of 10 mg of solifenacin in the presence of 400 mg of ketoconazole, a potent inhibitor of CYP3A4, the mean C_{max} and AUC of solifenacin increased by 1.5 and 2.7-fold, respectively. Therefore, it is recommended not to exceed a 5 mg daily dose of solifenacin when administered with therapeutic doses of ketoconazole or other potent CYP3A4 inhibitors) 694

Vytorin 10/10 Tablets (Simvastatin is metabolized by the cytochrome P450 isoform

3A4. Certain agents that inhibit this metabolic pathway can raise plasma levels of simvastatin and may increase the risk of myopathy. These agents include large quantities of grapefruit juice (greater than 1 quart daily). The use of Vytorin concomitantly with this CYP3A4 inhibitor should be avoided) 2303

Vytorin 10/10 Tablets (Simvastatin is metabolized by the cytochrome P450 isoform 3A4. The risk of myopathy is increased by reducing the elimination of the simvastatin component of Vytorin. Hence when Vytorin is used with an inhibitor of CYP3A4 (eg, grapefruit juice), elevated plasma levels of HMG-CoA reductase inhibitory activity can increase the risk of myopathy and rhabdomyolysis, particularly with higher doses of Vytorin. Avoid large quantities of grapefruit juice (>1 quart daily))......3240

Zemplar Injection (A multiple dose drug-drug interaction study with ketoconazole and paricalcitol capsule demonstrated that ketoconazole approximately doubled paricalcitol AUC since paricalcitol is partially metabolized by CYP3A and ketoconazole is known to be a strong inhibitor of cytochrome P450 3A enzyme. Care should be taken while dosing paricalcitol with ketoconazole and other strong P450 3A inhibitors including atazanavir, clarithromycin, indinavir, itraconazole, nefazodone, nelfinavir, ritonavir, saquinavir, telithromycin or voriconazole) 571

Zocor Tablets (The risk of myopathy and rhabdomyolysis is increased by high level of statin activity in plasma. Simvastatin is metabolized by the cytochrome P450 isoform 3A4. Certain drugs, including the large quantities of grapefruit juice (greater than 1 quart daily), which inhibit this metabolic pathway can raise the plasma levels of simvastatin and may increase the risk of myopathy. The use of simvastatin concomitantly with this CYP3A4 inhibitor should be avoided) 2289

Zofran Tablets (Ondansetron does not itself appear to induce or inhibit the cytochrome P-450 drug metabolizing enzyme system of the liver. Because ondansetron is metabolized by hepatic cytochrome P-450 drug-metabolizing enzymes (CYP3A4, CYP2D6, CYP1A2), inducers or inhibitors of these enzymes may change the clearance and, hence, the half-life of ondansetron. On the basis of available data, no dosage adjustment is recommended for patients on these drugs) 1756

Zonegran Capsules (Concurrent use with drugs that inhibit CYP3A4 may alter serum concentrations of zonisamide)........1081

Zyprexa Tablets (Concomitant use may potentially inhibit olanzapine clearance; therefore, a dosage decrease may need to be considered) 1984

Zyprexa IntraMuscular (Concomitant use may potentially inhibit olanzapine clearance; therefore, a dosage decrease may need to be considered) 1984

Herring, pickled

Parnate Tablets (Tranylcypromine is contraindicated in combination with foods with a high tyramine content. Hypertensive crises have sometimes occurred during therapy with tranylcypromine after ingestion of foods with a high tyramine content. In particular, patients should be instructed not to take foods, such as pickled herring) 1584

Iron Amino Acid Chelate

Actonel Tablets (Co-administration of risedronate and calcium, antacids, or oral medications containing divalent cations will interfere with the absorption of risedronate)...................................2779

Avelox Tablets (When moxifloxacin (single 400 mg tablet dose) was administered two hours before, concomitantly, or 4 hours after an aluminum/magnesium-containing antacid (900 mg aluminum hydroxide and 600 mg magnesium hydroxide as a single oral dose) to 12 healthy volunteers there, was a 26%, 60% and 23% reduction in the mean AUC of moxifloxacin, respectively. Moxifloxacin should be taken at least 4 hours before or 8 hours after metal cations)................................3064

Boniva Tablets (Products containing calcium and other multivalent cations (such as aluminum, magnesium, iron) are likely to interfere with absorption of ibandronate sodium. Ibandronate sodium should be taken at least 60 minutes before any oral medications, including medications containing multivalent cations (such as antacids, supplements or vitamins))..............................2844

Cipro I.V. (Concurrent administration of ciprofloxacin with multivalent cation-containing products may substantially decrease its absorption, resulting in serum and urine levels considerably lower than desired) 3082

Cipro Tablets (Concurrent administration of ciprofloxacin with multivalent cation-containing products may substantially decrease its absorption, resulting in serum and urine levels considerably lower than desired) 3073

Cipro XR Tablets (Concurrent administration of ciprofloxacin with multivalent cation-containing products may substantially interfere with the absorption of ciprofloxacin, resulting in serum and urine levels considerably lower than desired. Ciprofloxacin extended release tablets should be administered at least 2 hours before or 6 hours after metal cations) 3091

Fosamax Tablets (Products containing calcium and other multivalent cations are likely to interfere with absorption of alendronate; patients must wait at least one-half hour after taking alendronate before taking any other oral medications)...............................2138

Levaquin Injection (Levaquin Injection should not be co-administered with any solution containing multivalent cations, such as magnesium, through the same intravenous line)..2629

Levaquin Oral Solution (Concurrent administration of levofloxacin tablets/oral solution with metal cations such as iron may interfere with the gastrointestinal absorption of levofloxacin, resulting in systemic levels considerably lower than desired. These agents should be taken at least two hours before or two hours after levofloxacin administration) 2629

Levaquin Tablets (Concurrent administration of levofloxacin tablets/oral solution with metal cations such as iron may interfere with the gastrointestinal absorption of levofloxacin, resulting in systemic levels considerably lower than desired. These agents should be taken at least two hours before or two hours after levofloxacin administration) 2629

Promacta Tablets (Eltrombopag chelates polyvalent cations (such as iron, calcium, aluminum, magnesium, selenium, and zinc) in foods, mineral supplements, and antacids. In a clinical study, administration of eltrombopag with a polyvalent cation-containing antacid (1,524 mg aluminum hydroxide, 1,425 mg magnesium carbonate, and sodium alginate) decreased plasma eltrombopag systemic exposure by approximately 70%. Eltrombopag must not be taken within 4 hours of any medications or products containing polyvalent cations such as antacids, dairy products, and mineral supplements to avoid significant reduction in eltrombopag absorption due to chelation) 1610

Liqueurs

Parnate Tablets (Tranylcypromine is contraindicated in combination with cheese with a high tyramine content. Hypertensive crises have sometimes occurred during therapy with tranylcypromine after ingestion of foods with a high tyramine content. In particular, patients should be instructed not to take foods, such as liqueurs) 1584

Liver

Parnate Tablets (Tranylcypromine is contraindicated in combination with foods with a high tyramine content. Hypertensive crises have sometimes occurred during therapy with tranylcypromine after ingestion of foods with a high tyramine content. In particular, patients should be instructed not to take foods, such as liver) 1584

Meal, high in bran fiber

Lanoxin Tablets (When digoxin tablets are taken after meals, the rate of absorption is slowed, but the total amount of digoxin absorbed is usually unchanged. When taken with meals high in bran fiber, however, the amount absorbed from an oral dose may be reduced) 1553

Meal, unspecified

Accolate Tablets (The bioavailability of zafirlukast may be decreased when taken with food. Patients should be instructed to take zafirlukast at least 1 hour before or 2 hours after meals) 3612

Actonel Tablets (The extent of absorption of a 30 mg dose (three 10 mg tablets) when administered 0.5 hours before breakfast is reduced by 55% compared to dosing in the fasting state (no food or drink for 10 hours prior to or 4 hours after dosing). Dosing 1 hour prior to breakfast reduces the extent of absorption by 30% compared to dosing in the fasting state. Dosing either 0.5 hours prior to breakfast or 2 hours after dinner (evening meal) results in a similar extent of absorption. Residronate is effective when administered at least 30 minutes before breakfast)....................................2779

ActoPlus Met Tablets (Administration of ActoPlus Met 15 mg/850 mg with food resulted in no change in overall exposure of pioglitazone. With metformin there was no change in AUC; however, mean peak serum concentration of metformin was decreased by 28% when administered with food. A delayed time to peak serum concentration was observed for both components (1.9 hours for pioglitazone and 0.8 hours for metformin) under fed conditions. These changes are not likely to be clinically significant)...............................3338

Actos Tablets (Food slightly delays the time to peak serum concentration of pioglitazone to 3 to 4 hours, but does not alter the extent of absorption)...............3345

Afinitor Tablets (Based on data in healthy subjects taking 1 mg everolimus tablets, a high-fat meal reduced C_{max} and AUC by 60% and 16%, respectively. No data are available with everolimus 5 mg and 10 mg tablets)..................................2398

Albenza Tablets (Oral bioavailability appears to be enhanced when albendazole is co-administered with a fatty meal (estimated fat content 40 g) as evidenced by higher (up to 5-fold on average) plasma concentrations of albendazole sulfoxide as compared to the fasted state)..............................1298

Allegra ODT Orally Disintegrating Tablets (Administration of fexofenadine hydrochloride 30 mg with a high-fat meal decreased the AUC and C_{max} by approximately 40% and 60%, respectively, and a 2-hour delay in the time to peak exposure (T_{max}) was observed) 2911

Ambien Tablets (The effect of zolpidem may be slowed by ingestion with or immediately after a meal) 2920

Apriso Capsules (A high fat meal did not affect C_{max} for 5-ASA, but a 27% increase in the cumulative urinary excretion of 5-ASA was observed with a high fat meal. The overall extent of absorption of N-Ac-5-ASA was not affected by a high fat meal. As mesalamine and mesalamine granules in sachet were bioequivalent, mesalamine can be taken without regard to food) 2899

Aromasin Tablets (Exemestane plasma levels increased by approximately 40% after a high-fat breakfast) 2758

Asacol HD Delayed-Release Tablets (A high fat meal does not affect the extent of systemic exposure to mesalamine after single-dose administration of mesalamine, but mesalamine C_{max} decreases by 47% and t_{max} is delayed by 14 hours under fed conditions) 2787

Avodart Soft Gelatin Capsules (When the drug is administered with food, the maximum serum concentrations were reduced by 10% to 15%. This reduction is of no clinical significance) 1375

Biaxin Filmtab Tablets (For a single 500 mg dose of clarithromycin, food slightly

delays the onset of clarithromycin absorption, increasing the peak time from approximately 2 to 2.5 hours. Food also increases the clarithromycin peak plasma concentration by about 24%, but does not affect the extent of clarithromycin bioavailability).......... 412

Boniva Tablets (The oral bioavailability of ibandronate is reduced by about 90% when ibandronate is administered concomitantly with a standard breakfast in comparison with bioavailability observed in fasted subjects. There is no meaningful reduction in bioavailability when ibandronate is taken at least 60 minutes before a meal. However, both bioavailability and the effect on bone mineral density (BMD) are reduced when food or beverages are taken less than 60 minutes following an ibandronate dose).........................**2844**

Carbatrol Capsules (A high fat meal diet increased the rate of absorption of a single 400 mg dose (mean T_{max} was reduced from 24 hours, in the fasting state, to 14 hours and C_{max} increased from 3.2 to 4.3 µg/mL) but not the extent (AUC) of absorption. The elimination half-life remains unchanged between fed and fasting state. The multiple dose study conducted in the fed state showed that the steady-state C_{max} values were within the therapeutic concentration range. The pharmacokinetic profile of extended-release carbamazepine was similar when given by sprinkling the beads over applesauce compared to the intact capsule administered in the fasted state) **3280**

Celebrex Capsules (When celecoxib capsules were taken with a high fat meal, peak plasma levels were delayed for about 1 to 2 hours with an increase in total absorption (AUC) of 10% to 20%. Under fasting conditions, at doses above 200 mg, there is less than a proportional increase in C_{max} and AUC, which is thought to be due to the low solubility of the drug in aqueous media. Celecoxib, at doses up to 200 mg twice daily, can be administered without regard to timing of meals. Higher doses (400 mg twice daily) should be administered with food to improve absorption).......................**3272**

Cipro I.V. (When ciprofloxacin tablets are given concomitantly with food, there is a delay in the absorption of the drug, resulting in peak concentrations that occur closer to 2 hours after dosing rather than 1 hour, whereas there is no delay observed when ciprofloxacin suspension is given with food. The overall absorption of ciprofloxacin tablets or ciprofloxacin suspension, however, is not substantially affected. The pharmacokinetics of ciprofloxacin given as the suspension are also not affected by food)...........................**3082**

Cipro Tablets (When ciprofloxacin tablets are given concomitantly with food, there is a delay in the absorption of the drug, resulting in peak concentrations that occur closer to 2 hours after dosing rather than 1 hour, whereas there is no delay observed when ciprofloxacin suspension is given with food. The overall absorption of ciprofloxacin tablets or ciprofloxacin suspension, however, is not substantially affected. The pharmacokinetics of ciprofloxacin given as the suspension are also not affected by food)...........................**3073**

Coreg CR Extended-Release Capsules (Administration of carvedilol with a high-fat meal resulted in increases (~20%) in AUC and C_{max} compared to carvedilol administered with a standard meal. Decreases in AUC (27%) and C_{max} (43%) were observed when carvedilol was administered in the fasted state compared to administration after a standard meal. Carvedilol should be taken with food) **1416**

Dilaudid Oral Liquid (In a study conducted with a single 8 mg dose of hydromorphone (2 mg tablets), food lowered C_{max} by 25%, prolonged T_{max} by 0.8 hour, and increased AUC by 35%. The effects may not be clinically relevant) **2797**

Diovan Tablets (Food decreases the exposure (as measured by AUC) to valsartan about 40% and peak plasma concentration (C_{max}) by about 50%; valsartan may be administered with or without food)...................................**2413**

Divista Softgel Capsules (Diets high in simple sugars (eg, sucrose), compared to diets high in complex carbohydrates (eg, whole grains) increase urinary chromium excretion in adults. This effect may be related to increase insulin secretion response to the consumption of simple sugars compared to complex carbohydrates).............................**3474**

Duetact Tablets (Food did not change the systemic exposures of glimepiride or pioglitazone. However, for glimepiride, there was a 22% increase in C_{max} when Duetact was administered with food) **3354**

DynaCirc CR Controlled Release Tablets (Food has been shown to decrease the extent of bioavailability of isradipine by up to 25%)...................................**1432**

Effient Tablets (In a study of healthy subjects given a single 15 mg dose, the AUC of the active metabolite was unaffected by a high fat, high calorie meal, but C_{max} was decreased by 49% and T_{max} was increased from 0.5 to 1.5 hours. Prasugrel hydrochloride can be administered without regard to food. The active metabolite is bound about 98% to human serum albumin) **1021**

Effient Tablets (In a study of healthy subjects given a single 15 mg dose, the AUC of the active metabolite was unaffected by a high fat, high calorie meal, but C_{max} was decreased by 49% and T_{max} was increased from 0.5 to 1.5 hours. Prasugrel hydrochloride can be administered without regard to food. The active metabolite is bound about 98% to human serum albumin) **1881**

Eldepryl Capsules (The bioavailability of selegiline is increased 3 to 4 fold when it is taken with food) **3312**

Emtriva Capsules (Emtricitabine capsules and oral solution may be taken with or without food. Emtricitabine systemic exposure (AUC) was unaffected, while C_{max} decreased by 29% when entricitabine capsules were administered with food (an approximately 1000 kcal high-fat meal). Emtricitabine systemic exposure (AUC) and C_{max} were unaffected when 200 mg emtricitabine oral solution was administered with either a high-fat or low-fat meal)......**1238**

Epivir Tablets (Absorption of lamivudine was slower in the fed state (T_{max}: 3.2 ± 1.3 hours) compared with the fasted state (T_{max}: 0.9 ± 0.3 hours); C_{max} in the fed state was 40% ± 23% (mean ± SD) lower than in the fasted state. There was no significant difference in systemic exposure ($AUC_{infinity}$) in the fed and fasted states; therefore, lamivudine may be administered with or without food).................................**1437**

Evoxac Capsules (When administered with food, there is a decrease in the rate of absorption of cevimeline, with a fasting T_{Max} of 1.53 hours and a T_{Max} of 2.86 hours after a meal; the peak concentration is reduced by 17.3%).........................**1027**

Finacea Gel (Concomitant use with any foods and beverages that might provoke erythema, flushing, and blushing (including spicy food, alcoholic beverages, and thermally hot drinks, including hot coffee and tea) should be avoided)........................**1808**

Fleet Prep Kit 3 (Use Fleet Prep Kit 3 with caution in patients who are on a low-salt diet).............**1145**

Focalin XR Capsules (No food effect study was performed with Focalin XR. However, the effect of food has been studied in adults with racemic methylphenidate in the same type of extended-release formulation. The findings of that study are considered applicable to Focalin XR. After a high fat breakfast, there was a longer lag time until absorption began and variable delays in the time until the first peak concentration, the time until the interpeak minimum, and the time until the second peak. The first peak concentration and the extent of absorption were unchanged after food relative to the fasting state, although the second peak was approximately 25% lower)...................................**2472**

Fosamax Tablets (Standardized breakfast decreases bioavailability by approximately 40% when alendronate is administered either one-half or 1 hour before breakfast) **2138**

Fosamax Plus D Tablets (Bioavailability was decreased (by approximately 40%) when 10 mg alendronate was administered either 0.5 or 1 hour before a standardized breakfast, when compared to dosing 2 hours before eating).........**2147**

Gabitril Tablets (Absorption of tiagabine is rapid, with peak plasma concentrations occurring at approximately 45 minutes following an oral dose in the fasting state. Tiagabine is nearly completely absorbed (>95%), with an absolute oral bioavailability of about 90%. A high fat meal decreases the rate (mean T_{max} was prolonged to 2.5 hours, and mean C_{max} was reduced by about 40%) but not the extent (AUC) of tiagabine absorption) 972

Geodon Capsules (The absorption of oral ziprasidone is increased up to two-fold in the presence of food) **2723**

Hyzaar 50-12.5 Tablets (Meal slows absorption and decreases C_{max}, but has minor effects on losartan AUC or on the AUC of the metabolite) **2162**

Intuniv Extended-Release Tablets (High-fat meals increase exposure of guanfacine)................**3291**

Invega Extended-Release Tablets (Administration of a 12 mg paliperidone extended-release tablet to healthy ambulatory subjects with a standard high-fat/high-caloric meal gave mean C_{max} and AUC values of paliperidone that were increased by 60% and 54%, respectively, compared with administration under fasting conditions. Clinical trials establishing the safety and efficacy of paliperidone were carried out in subjects without regard to the timing of meals. While paliperidone can be taken without regard to food, the presence of food at the time of paliperidone administration may increase exposure to paliperidone) **2613**

Isentress Tablets (Raltegravir may be administered with or without food. Administration of multiple doses of raltegravir following a moderate-fat meal (600 Kcal, 21 g fat) did not affect raltegravir AUC to a clinically meaningful degree with an increase of 13% relative to fasting. Raltegravir C_{12hr} was 66% higher and C_{max} was 5% higher following a moderate-fat meal compared to fasting. Administration of raltegravir following a high-fat meal (825 Kcal, 52 g fat) increased AUC and C_{max} by approximately 2-fold and increased C_{12hr} by 4.1-fold. Administration of raltegravir following a low-fat meal (300 Kcal, 2.5 g fat) decreased AUC and C_{max} by 46% and 52%, respectively; C_{12hr} was essentially unchanged. Food appears to increase pharmacokinetic variability relative to fasting)..........**2180**

Kaletra Tablets (Relative to fasting, administration of Kaletra tablets with a moderate fat meal (500 - 682 Kcal, 23 to 25% calories from fat) increased lopinavir AUC and C_{max} by 26.9% and 17.6%, respectively. Relative to fasting, administration of Kaletra tablets with a high fat meal (872 Kcal, 56% from fat) increased lopinavir AUC by 18.9% but not C_{max}. Therefore, Kaletra tablets may be taken with or without food)...................... **458**

Kapidex Delayed Release Capsules (In food-effect studies in healthy subjects receiving dexlansoprazole under various fed conditions compared to fasting, increases in C_{max} ranged from 12% to 55%, increases in AUC ranged from 9% to 37%, and T_{max} varied (ranging from a decrease of 0.7 hours to an increase of 3 hours). No significant differences in mean intragastric pH were observed between fasted and various fed conditions. However, the percentage of time intragastric pH exceeded 4 over the 24-hour dosing interval decreased slightly when dexlansoprazole was administered after a meal (57%) relative to fasting (64%), primarily due to a decreased response in intragastric pH during the first 4 hours after dosing. Because of this, while dexlansoprazole can be taken without regard to food, some patients may benefit from administering the dose prior to a meal if post-meal symptoms do not resolve under post-fed conditions) **3362**

Keppra XR Extended-Release Tablets (Intake of a high fat, high calorie breakfast before the administration of

extended-release levetiracetam tablets resulted in a higher peak concentration, and longer median time to peak. The median time to peak (T_{max}) was 2 hours longer in the fed state).......**3434**

Lanoxin Tablets (When digoxin tablets are taken after meals, the rate of absorption is slowed, but the total amount of digoxin absorbed is usually unchanged. When taken with meals high in bran fiber, however, the amount absorbed from an oral dose may be reduced) **1553**

Levaquin Oral Solution (Oral administration of a 500 mg dose of levofloxacin with food prolongs the time to peak concentration by approximately 1 hour and decreases the peak concentration by approximately 25% (following oral solution administration). It is recommended that levofloxacin oral solution be taken 1 hour before, or 2 hours after eating).......**2629**

Levaquin Tablets (Oral administration of a 500 mg dose of levofloxacin with food prolongs the time to peak concentration by approximately 1 hour and decreases the peak concentration by approximately 14% (following tablet administration). Therefore, levofloxacin can be administered without regard to food) **2629**

Levitra Tablets (Two food-effect studies were conducted which showed that high-fat meals caused a reduction in C_{max} by 18%-50%) **3157**

Meridia Capsules (Administration of a single 20 mg dose of sibutramine with a standard breakfast resulted in reduced peak M_1 and M_2 concentrations (by 27% and 32%, respectively) and delayed the time to peak by approximately three hours. However, the AUCs of M_1 and M_2 were not significantly altered)................................. **492**

Metozolv ODT Orally Disintegrating Tablets (In a food-effect study with 28 subjects, metoclopramide taken immediately after a high-fat meal had a 17% lower peak blood level than when taken after an overnight fast. The time to peak blood levels increased from about 1.75 hours under fasted conditions to 3 hours when taken immediately after a high-fat meal. The extent of metoclopramide absorbed (area under the curve) was comparable whether metoclopramide was administered with or without food. The clinical effect of the decrease in peak plasma level if metoclopramide is inadvertently taken with food is unknown) **2901**

Mevacor Tablets (When lovastatin was given under fasting conditions, plasma concentrations of total inhibitors were on average about two-thirds those found when lovastatin was administered immediately after a standard meal)...........................**2212**

Micardis Tablets (Food slightly reduces the bioavailability of telmisartan, with a reduction in the area under the plasma concentration-time curve (AUC) of about 6% with the 40 mg tablet and about 20% after a 160 mg dose. The absolute bioavailability of telmisartan is dose dependent. At 40 and 160 mg the bioavailability was 42% and 58%, respectively)........... **887**

Micardis HCT Tablets (Food slightly reduces the bioavailability of telmisartan, with a reduction in the area

under the plasma concentration-time curve (AUC) of about 6% with the 40 mg tablet and about 20% after a 160 mg dose. The absolute bioavailability of telmisartan is dose dependent. At 40 mg and 160 mg the bioavailability was 42% and 58%, respectively)........... **889**

Myfortic Tablets (Co-administration of mycophenolic acid with a high fat meal decreased C_{max} by 33%, a 3.5-hour delay in the T_{lag} (range, -6 to 18 hours), and 5.0-hour delay in the T_{max} (range, -9 to 20 hours) of MPA. To avoid the variability in MPA absorption between doses, mycophenolic acid should be taken on an empty stomach) **2491**

Nexium Delayed-Release Capsules (The AUC after administration of a single 40 mg dose of esomeprazole is decreased by 43%-53% after food intake compared to fasting conditions. Esomeprazole should be taken at least one hour before meals)........................ **704**

Niaspan Extended-Release Tablets (Concomitant administration of spicy foods may increase the side effects of flushing and pruritus and should be avoided around the time of niacin ingestion) **497**

Norvir Soft Gelatin Capsules (When the oral solution was given under non-fasting conditions, peak ritonavir concentrations decreased 23% and the extent of absorption decreased 7% relative to fasting conditions. Relative to fasting conditions, the extent of absorption of ritonavir from the soft gelatin capsule formulation was 13% higher when administered with a meal) **509**

NovoLog Injection (The timing of hypoglycemia usually reflects the time-action profile of the administered insulin formulations. Other factors such as changes in food intake (eg, amount of food or timing of meals) may also alter the risk of hypoglycemia. As with all insulins, use caution in patients with hypoglycemia unawareness and in patients who may be predisposed to hypoglycemia (eg, patients who are fasting or have erratic food intake)) **2575**

Nucynta Tablets (The AUC and C_{max} increased by 25% and 16%, respectively, when tapentadol hydrochloride was administered after a high-fat, high-calorie breakfast. Tapentadol hydrochloride may be given with or without food) **2643**

Nuvigil Tablets (Although food effect on the bioavailability of armodafinil is considered minimal, food can potentially affect the onset and time course of pharmacologic action of armodafinil. The time to reach peak concentration (T_{max}) may be delayed by approximately 2-4 hours in the fed state).. **978**

OxyContin Tablets (The peak plasma concentration of oxycodone increased by 25% when oxycodone was administered with a high-fat meal).....................................**2807**

Paxil Tablets (The effects of food on the bioavailability of paroxetine were studied in subjects administered a single dose with and without food. AUC was only slightly increased (6%) when drug was administered with food but the C_{max} was 29% greater, while the time to reach peak plasma concentration decreased from

6.4 hours post-dosing to 4.9 hours; paroxetine may be administered with or without food) **1586**

Premphase Tablets (Single dose studies in healthy, postmenopausal women were conducted to investigate any potential drug interaction when PREMPHASE is administered with a high fat breakfast. Administration with food decreased the C_{max} of total estrone by 18% to 34% and increased total equilin C_{max} by 38% compared to the fasting state, with no other effect on the rate or extent of absorption of other conjugated or unconjugated estrogens. Administration with food approximately doubles MPA C_{max} and increases MPA AUC by approximately 20% to 30%) **3549**

Prempro Tablets (Single dose studies in healthy, postmenopausal women were conducted to investigate any potential drug interaction when PREMPRO is administered with a high fat breakfast. Administration with food decreased the C_{max} of total estrone by 18% to 34% and increased total equilin C_{max} by 38% compared to the fasting state, with no other effect on the rate or extent of absorption of other conjugated or unconjugated estrogens. Administration with food approximately doubles MPA C_{max} and increases MPA AUC by approximately 20% to 30%) **3549**

Prograf Capsules (The rate and extent of tacrolimus absorption were greatest under fasted conditions. The presence and composition of food decreased both the rate and extent of tacrolimus absorption. The effect was most pronounced with a high-fat meal (848 kcal, 46% fat): mean AUC and C_{max} were decreased 37% and 77%, respectively; T_{max} was lengthened 5-fold. A high-carbohydrate meal (668 kcal, 85% carbohydrate) decreased mean AUC and mean C_{max} by 28% and 65%, respectively. The time of the meal also affected tacrolimus bioavailability. When given immediately following the meal, mean C_{max} was reduced 71%, and mean AUC was reduced 39%, relative to the fasted condition. When administered 1.5 hours following the meal, mean C_{max} was reduced 63%, and mean AUC was reduced 39%, relative to the fasted condition) **677**

Promacta Tablets (Eltrombopag chelates polyvalent cations (such as iron, calcium, aluminum, magnesium, selenium, and zinc) in foods, mineral supplements, and antacids. In a clinical study, administration of eltrombopag with a polyvalent cation-containing antacid (1,524 mg aluminum hydroxide, 1,425 mg magnesium carbonate, and sodium alginate) decreased plasma eltrombopag systemic exposure by approximately 70%. Eltrombopag must not be taken within 4 hours of any medications or products containing polyvalent cations such as antacids, dairy products, and mineral supplements to avoid significant reduction in eltrombopag absorption due to chelation) **1610**

Prometrium Capsules (100 mg, 200 mg) (Concomitant food ingestion increased the

bioavailability of progesterone relative to a fasting state when administered to post-menopausal women at a dose of 200 mg) **3307**

Requip Tablets (Food does not affect the extent of absorption of ropinirole, although its T_{max} is increased by 2.5 hours and its C_{max} is decreased by approximately 25% when the drug is taken with a high-fat meal)................................**1620**

Requip XL Tablets (In a single-dose study, administration of ropinirole to healthy volunteers with food (eg, high-fat meal) increased AUC by approximately 30% and C_{max} by approximately 44%, compared with dosing under fasted conditions. In a repeat-dose study in patients with Parkinson's disease, food (eg, high-fat meal) increased AUC by approximately 20% and C_{max} by approximately 44%; T_{max} was prolonged by 3 hours (median prolongation) compared with dosing under fasted conditions)..........................**1628**

Rozerem Tablets (When administered with a high-fat meal, the AUC_{0-inf} for a single 16 mg dose of ramelteon was 31% higher and the C_{max} was 22% lower than when given in a fasted state. Median T_{max} was delayed by approximately 45 minutes when ramelteon was administered with food. Effects of food on the AUC values for M-II were similar. It is, therefore, recommended that ramelteon not be taken with or immediately after a high-fat meal)................................**3366**

Ryzolt Extended-Release Tablets (Co-administration with a high fat meal did not significantly affect AUC (overall exposure to tramadol); however, C_{max} (peak plasma concentration) increased 67% following a single 300 mg tablet administration and 54% following a single 200 mg tablet administration. Tramadol hydrochloride was administered without regard to food in all clinical trials) **2813**

Saphris Tablets (A crossover study in 26 healthy male subjects was performed to evaluate the effect of food on the pharmacokinetics of a single 5 mg dose of asenapine. Consumption of food immediately prior to sublingual administration decreased asenapine exposure by 20%; consumption of food 4 hours after sublingual administration decreased asenapine exposure by about 10%. These effects are probably due to increased hepatic blood flow. Patients should be instructed to not eat or drink for 10 minutes after administration of asenapine).........**3223**

Selzentry Tablets (Co-administration of a 300 mg tablet with a high fat breakfast reduced maraviroc C_{max} and AUC by 33% in healthy volunteers. There were no food restrictions in the studies that demonstrated the efficacy and safety of maraviroc. Therefore, maraviroc can be taken with or without food at the recommended dose) **2740**

Sensipar Tablets (A food-effect study in healthy volunteers indicated that the C_{max} and area under the curve ($AUC_{(0-inf)}$) were increased 82% and 68%, respectively, when cinacalcet was administered with a high-fat meal compared to fasting. C_{max} and $AUC_{(0-inf)}$ of cinacalcet were

increased 65% and 50%, respectively, when cinacalcet was administered with a low-fat meal compared to fasting).............. 640

Seroquel XR Extended-Release Tablets (A high fat meal (approximately 800 to 1000 calories) was found to produce statistically significant increases in the quetiapine C_{max} and AUC of 44% to 52% and 20% to 22%, respectively, for the 50 mg and 300 mg tablets. In comparison, a light meal (approximately 300 calories) had no significant effect on the C_{max} or AUC of quetiapine. It is recommended that quetiapine be taken without food or with a light meal)............................. 759

Skelaxin Tablets (Taking metaxalone with food may enhance general CNS depression. The presence of a high fat meal at the time of drug administration increased C_{max} and AUC, T_{max} was also delayed and terminal half-life was decreased under fed conditions compared to fasted conditions)......1848

Strattera Capsules (Atomoxetine hydrochloride can be administered with or without food. Administration of atomoxetine with a standard high–fat meal in adults did not affect the extent of oral absorption of atomoxetine (AUC), but did decrease the rate of absorption, resulting in a 37% lower C_{max}, and delayed T_{max} by 3 hours. In clinical trials with children and adolescents, administration of atomoxetine with food resulted in a 9% lower C_{max}).............................1957

Tarceva Tablets (Erlotinib is about 60% absorbed after oral administration and its bioavailability is substantially increased by food to almost 100%) 1222

Tasigna Capsules (The bioavailability of nilotinib is increased with food. Nilotinib should not be taken with food. No food should be taken at least 2 hours before and at least one hour after the dose is taken)............................2533

Temodar Capsules (Temozolomide is rapidly and completely absorbed after oral administration with a peak plasma concentration (C_{max}) achieved in a median T_{max} of 1 hour. Food reduces the rate and extent of temozolomide absorption. Mean peak plasma concentration and AUC decreased by 32% and 9%, respectively, and median T_{max} increased by 2-fold (from 1 to 2.25 hours) when temozolomide was administered after a modified high-fat breakfast).........................3230

Truvada Tablets (Truvada may be administered with or without food. Administration of Truvada following a high fat meal or a light meal delayed the time of tenofovir C_{max} by approximately 0.75 hour. The mean increases in tenofovir AUC and C_{max} were approximately 35% and 15%, respectively, when administered with a high fat or light meal, compared to administration in the fasted state. In previous safety and efficacy studies, tenofovir was taken under fed conditions. Emtricitabine systemic exposures (AUC and C_{max}) were unaffected when Truvada was administered with either a high fat or a light meal) 1258

Uloric Tablets (Following multiple 80 mg once daily doses with a high fat meal, there was a 49% decrease in C_{max} and an 18% decrease in AUC, respectively. However, no clinically significant change in the percent decrease in serum uric acid concentration was observed (58% fed vs. 51% fasting). Thus, febuxostat may be taken without regard to food) 3370

Urocit-K Tablets (A dose of potassium citrate taken with meals or snacks may alleviate minor gastrointestinal complaints such as abdominal discomfort, vomiting, diarrhea, loose bowel movements or nausea in some patients)..............2333

Uroxatral Tablets (The extent of absorption of alfuzosin is 50% lower under fasting conditions. Therefore, alfuzosin should be taken immediately following a meal)............................3050

Valcyte Tablets (Co-administration with high fat meals has resulted in increased steady-state ganciclovir AUC and C_{max} without any prolongation in time to peak plasma concentrations; Valcyte should be administered with food) 2872

Valturna Tablets (When taken with food, mean AUC and C_{max} of aliskiren are decreased by 76% and 88%, respectively; mean AUC and C_{max} of valsartan were not significantly affected. In clinical trials of Valturna, it was administered without requiring a fixed relation of administration to meals. High-fat meals decrease absorption of Valturna substantially)..................3637

Vytorin 10/10 Tablets (Concomitant food administration (high-fat or non-fat meals) had no effect on the extent of absorption of ezetimibe when administered as 10-mg tablets. The C_{max} value of ezetimibe was increased by 38% with consumption of high-fat meals) 2303

Vytorin 10/10 Tablets (Concomitant food administration (high-fat or non-fat meals) had no effect on the extent of absorption of ezetimibe when administered as 10-mg tablets. The C_{max} value of ezetimibe was increased by 38% with consumption of high-fat meals) 3240

Zetia Tablets (The C_{max} value of ezetimibe was increased by 38% with consumption of high-fat meals. Ezetimibe can be administered with or without food) 3256

Zetia Tablets (Concomitant food administration (non-fat meals) had no effect on the extent of absorption of ezetimibe when administered as ezetimibe 10-mg tablets. The C_{max} value of ezetimibe was increased by 38% with consumption of high-fat meals. Ezetimibe can be administered with or without food) 2312

Zofran Tablets (Bioavailability is slightly enhanced by food) 1756

Zonegran Capsules (Following a 200–400 mg oral zonisamide dose, peak plasma concentrations (range: 2–5 μg/mL) in normal volunteers occur within 2–6 hours. In the presence of food, the time to maximum concentration is delayed, occurring at 4–6 hours, but food has no effect on the bioavailability of zonisamide. Zonisamide can be taken with or without food) 1081

Zyban Sustained-Release Tablets (In a single-dose study, food increased the C_{max} of bupropion by 11% and the extent of absorption as defined by area under the plasma concentration-time curve (AUC) by 17%. The mean time to peak concentration (T_{max}) was prolonged by 1 hour. This effect was of no clinical significance)........1762

Meat extracts

Parnate Tablets (Tranylcypromine is contraindicated in combination with foods with a high tyramine content. Hypertensive crises have sometimes occurred during therapy with tranylcypromine after ingestion of food with a high tyramine content. In particular, patients should be instructed not to take foods, such as meat extracts).................1584

Meat prepared with tenderizers

Parnate Tablets (Tranylcypromine is contraindicated in combination with foods with a high tyramine content. Hypertensive crises have sometimes occurred during therapy with tranylcypromine after ingestion of food with a high tyramine content. In particular, patients should be instructed not to take foods, such as meat prepared with tenderizers) 1584

Milk, low salt

Dyazide Capsules (Concurrent use of low-salt milk with triamterene may result in hyperkalemia, especially in patients with renal insufficiency).....1429

Dyrenium Capsules (Co-administration of triamterene with low-salt milk (may contain up to 60 mEq of potassium per liter) may promote serum potassium accumulation and possibly result in hyperkalemia because of the potassium-sparing nature of triamterene, especially in patients with renal insufficiency).....3495

Orange Juice

Allegra ODT Orally Disintegrating Tablets (Fruit juices such as grapefruit, orange and apple may reduce the bioavailability and exposure of fexofenadine) 2911

Allegra-D 12 Hour Extended-Release Tablets (Co-administration with grapefruit, orange or apple juice will reduce the bioavailability and exposure or fexofenadine) 2915

Fosamax Tablets (Concomitant administration of alendronate with orange juice reduces bioavailability by approximately 60%)............................2138

Fosamax Plus D Tablets (Concomitant administration of alendronate with orange juice reduces bioavailability by approximately 60%) 2147

Prunes

Parnate Tablets (Tranylcypromine is contraindicated in combination with foods with a high tyramine content. Hypertensive crises have sometimes occurred during therapy with tranylcypromine after ingestion of foods with a high tyramine content. In particular, patients should be instructed not to take foods, such as dried fruits (eg, prunes))........................1584

Raisins

Parnate Tablets (Tranylcypromine is contraindicated in combination with foods with a high tyramine content. Hypertensive crises have sometimes occurred during therapy with tranylcypromine after ingestion of foods with a high tyramine content. In particular, patients should be instructed not to take foods, such as fruits (eg, raisins)).............1584

Raspberries

Parnate Tablets (Tranylcypromine is contraindicated in combination with foods with a high tyramine content. Hypertensive crises have sometimes occurred during therapy with tranylcypromine after ingestion of foods with a high tyramine content. In particular, patients should be instructed not to take foods, such as raspberries) 1584

Salt Substitutes, Potassium-Containing

Cozaar Tablets (Concomitant use with salt substitutes containing potassium may lead to hyperkalemia) 2106

Dyrenium Capsules (Co-administration of triamterene with dietary potassium supplements, potassium salts, or potassium containing salt substitutes is contraindicated. Concomitant use may promote serum potassium accumulation and possibly result in hyperkalemia because of the potassium-sparing nature of triamterene, especially in patients with renal insufficiency).....3495

Prinivil Tablets (Use of lisinopril with potassium-sparing diuretics (such as spironolactone, triamterene or amiloride), potassium supplements or potassium-containing salt substitutes may lead to significant increases in serum potassium. Therefore, if concomitant use of these agents is indicated because of demonstrated hypokalemia, they should be used with caution and with frequent monitoring of serum potassium. Potassium-sparing agents should generally not be used in patients with heart failure who are receiving lisinopril) 2241

Prinzide Tablets (Risk factors for the development of hyperkalemia include the concomitant use of potassium-sparing diuretics, potassium supplements and/or potassium-containing salt substitutes. Hyperkalemia can cause serious, sometimes, fatal, arrhythmias. Prinzide should be used cautiously, if at all, with these agents and with frequent monitoring of serum potassium) 2246

Tarka Tablets (Use of potassium-sparing diuretics (spironolactone, triamterene, or amiloride), potassium supplements, or potassium-containing salt substitutes concomitantly with ACE inhibitors can increase the risk of hyperkalemia. If concomitant use of such agents is indicated, they should be used with caution and with appropriate monitoring of serum potassium)........................... 534

Valturna Tablets (Caution is advised when concomitant use of Valturna with salt substitute containing potassium may lead to increases in serum potassium and in heart failure patients to increases in serum creatinine) 3637

Sauerkraut

Parnate Tablets (Tranylcypromine is contraindicated in combination with foods with a high tyramine content. Hypertensive crises have sometimes occurred during therapy with tranylcypromine

after ingestion of food with a high tyramine content. In particular, patients should be instructed not to take foods, such as sauerkraut) **1584**

Sherry
Parnate Tablets (Tranylcypromine is contradicated in combination with foods with a high tyramine content. Hypertensive crises have sometimes occurred during therapy with tranylcypromine after ingestion of foods with a high tyramine content. In particular, patients should be instructed not to take foods, such as sherry)..............................**1584**

Soy Sauce
Parnate Tablets (Tranylcypromine is contraindicated in combination with foods with a high tyramine content. Hypertensive crises have sometimes occurred during therapy with tranylcypromine after ingestion of food with a high tyramine content. In particular, patients should be instructed not to take foods, such as soy sauce) **1584**

Soybean Formula, Children's
Levoxyl Tablets (Concurrent use of soybean flour may bind and decrease the absorption of levothyroxine sodium from GI tract) **1843**
Synthroid Tablets (Binds and decreases absorption of levothyroxine sodium from the gastrointestinal tract)....................**529**

Tannins
Finacea Gel (Avoid concurrent use with alcoholic cleansers, tinctures and astringents, abrasives and peeling agents)........**1808**

Walnuts
Levoxyl Tablets (Concurrent use of walnuts may bind and decrease the absorption of levothyroxine sodium from GI tract) **1843**

Wine, Chianti
ActoPlus Met Tablets (Alcohol is known to potentiate the effect of metformin on lactate metabolism. Patients, therefore, should be warned against excessive alcohol intake, acute or chronic, while receiving ActoPlus Met. In addition, hypoglycemia does not occur in patients receiving metformin alone under usual circumstances of use, but could occur when during concomitant use with ethanol) **3338**
Adcirca Tablets (Both alcohol and tadalafil, a PDE5 inhibitor, act as mild vasodilators. When mild vasodilators are taken in combination, blood pressure–lowering effects of each individual compound may be increased. Substantial consumption of alcohol (eg, 5 units or greater) in combination with tadalafil can increase the potential for orthostatic signs and symptoms, including increase in heart rate, decrease in standing blood pressure, dizziness, and headache)...............**3461**
Adipex-P Tablets (May result in adverse drug interaction) **1178**
Advicor Tablets (Concomitant alcohol may increase the flushing and its use should be avoided around the time of Advicor administration)..................**402**
Aggrenox Capsules (Patients who consume three or more alcoholic drinks every day should be counseled about the bleeding risks involved with chronic, heavy alcohol use while taking aspirin)...............................**880**

Alphagan P Ophthalmic Solution (Possible additive or potentiating effect with CNS depressants) **596**
Ambien Tablets (An additive effect on psychomotor performance between alcohol and zolpidem was demonstrated. Zolpidem should not be taken with alcohol) **2920**
Ambien CR Tablets (Zolpidem tartrate has shown additive effects when combined with alcohol and should not be taken with alcohol) **2925**
Amrix Capsules (Concomitant use with cyclobenzaprine HCl may enhance the effects of alcohol) **964**
Apidra Injection (Alcohol may either potentiate or weaken the blood glucose-lowering effect of insulin) **2937**
Aplenzin Extended-Release Tablets (Bupropion is contraindicated in patients undergoing abrupt discontinuation of alcohol. Concomitant use of alcohol with bupropion is associated with an increased seizure risk. There have been rare reports of adverse neuropsychiatric events or reduced alcohol tolerance in patients who were drinking alcohol during treatment with bupropion. The consumption of alcohol during treatment with bupropion should be minimized or avoided) **2948**
Atacand HCT 16-12.5 Tablets (May aggravate orthostatic hypotension produced by hydrochlorothiazide)......................**700**
Avalide Tablets (Potentiation of orthostatic hypertension may occur during concomitant administration of hydrochlorothiazide with alcohol) **2956**
Avandamet Tablets (Alcohol potentiates the effect of metformin on lactate metabolism; patients should be warned against excessive alcohol intake, acute or chronic).....**1345**
Avinza Capsules (Patients must not consume alcoholic beverages, prescription or non-prescription medications containing alcohol while on morphine sulfate therapy. Consumption of alcohol while taking morphine sulfate may result in the rapid release and absorption of a potentially fatal dose of morphine)..........................**1822**
Benadryl Allergy Ultratab Tablets (Increases drowsiness effect; avoid concomitant use) **2042**
Benicar HCT Tablets (Concurrent administration could cause potentiation of orthostatic hypotension)..............................**1017**
Carbatrol Capsules (Because of its primary CNS effect, caution should be used when carbamazepine is taken with alcohol) **3280**
Catapres-TTS (Clonidine may potentiate the CNS-depressive effects of alcohol, barbiturates or other sedating drugs) **884**
Celebrex Capsules (Other factors that increase the risk of GI bleeding in patients treated with NSAIDs include concomitant use of alcohol. Most spontaneous reports of fatal GI events are in elderly or debilitated patients and therefore special care should be taken in treating this population) **3272**
Celexa Tablets (Although citalopram did not potentiate

cognitive and motor effects of alcohol, as with other psychotropic medications, the use of alcohol by depressed patients taking citalopram is not recommended) **1153**
Cialis Tablets (Both alcohol and tadalafil act as mild vasodilators. When mild vasodilators are taken in combination, blood-pressure-lowering effects of each individual compound may be increased. Substantial consumption of alcohol (eg, 5 units or greater) in combination with tadalafil can increase the potential for orthostatic signs and symptoms, including increase in heart rate, decrease in standing blood pressure, dizziness, and headache)...............**1861**
Clinoril Tablets (Concomitant use of alcohol may increase the risk of GI bleeding) **2098**
Clorpres Tablets (Clonidine may enhance the CNS-depressive effects of alcohol; orthostatic hypotension may be aggravated by alcohol) **2344**
Combigan Ophthalmic Solution (Although specific drug interaction studies have not been conducted with Combigan, the possibility of an additive or potentiating effect with CNS depressants (alcohol, barbiturates, opiates, sedatives or anesthetics) should be considered) **601**
Crestor Tablets (Rosuvastatin calcium should be used with caution in patients who consume substantial quantities of alcohol) **736**
Cymbalta Delayed-Release Capsules (Use of duloxetine concomitantly with heavy alcohol intake may be associated with severe liver injury. For this reason, duloxetine should ordinarily not be prescribed for patients with substantial alcohol use) **1871**
Depakote ER Extended Release Tablets (Since valproate products may produce CNS depression, especially when combined with another CNS depressant (eg, alcohol), patients should be advised not to engage in hazardous activities, such as driving an automobile or operating dangerous machinery, until it is known that they do not become drowsy from the drug) **426**
Dilaudid Oral Liquid (Hydromorphone may be expected to have additive effects when used in conjunction with alcohol. Alcohol potentiates the respiratory depressant effects of hydromorphone, increasing the risk of respiratory depression that might result in death).............................**2797**
Dilaudid-HP Injection (Hydromorphone may be expected to have additive effects when used in conjunction with alcohol. Alcohol potentiates the respiratory depressant effects of hydromorphone, increasing the risk of respiratory depression that might result in death).............................**2800**
Diovan HCT Tablets (Concurrent use of thiazide diuretics with alcohol may result in potentiation of orthostatic hypotension) **2419**
Duetact Tablets (All sulfonylurea drugs are capable of producing

hypoglycemia; hypoglycemia is more likely to occur when alcohol is ingested) **3354**
Duragesic Transdermal System (Fentanyl may be expected to have additive CNS depressant effects when used in conjunction with alcohol. The concomitant use of fentanyl with alcohol may cause respiratory depression, hypotension, and profound sedation or potentially result in coma) **2604**
Effexor XR Extended-Release Capsules (Although venlafaxine has not been shown to increase the impairment of mental and motor skills caused by alcohol, patients should be advised to avoid alcohol while taking venlafaxine) **3504**
Elidel Cream 1% (Skin flushing due to pimecrolimus is associated with alcohol use) **2424**
Embeda Extended Release Capsules (Embeda should be used with great caution and in reduced dosage in patients who are concurrently receiving other central nervous system (CNS) depressants including alcohol because of the risk of respiratory depression, hypotension, and profound sedation or coma. When such combined therapy is contemplated, the initial dose of one or both agents should be reduced by at least 50%)...............**1831**
Emsam Transdermal System (The use of alcohol is not recommended while using selegiline transdermal system).......**3623**
Equetro Extended-Release Capsules (Because of its primary CNS effect, caution should be used when carbamazepine is taken with alcohol) **3477**
Exforge HCT Tablets (Potentiation of orthostatic hypotension may occur when alcohol and thiazide diuretics are administered concurrently)..................................**2449**
Exubera Inhalation Powder (Alcohol may either increase or reduce the blood glucose-lowering effect of insulin. Co-administration may require insulin dose adjustment and particularly close monitoring) **2717**
Fanapt Tablets (Given the primary CNS effects of iloperidone, caution should be used when it is taken in combination with alcohol) **3484**
Fentanyl Transdermal System Patches (Fentanyl may be expected to have additive CNS depressant effects when used in conjunction with alcohol. The concomitant use of fentanyl with alcohol may cause respiratory depression, hypotension, and profound sedation, or potentially result in coma or death) **2346**
Fentora Tablets (The concomitant use of other CNS depressants, including alcoholic beverages, may produce increased depressant effects. Hypoventilation, hypotension, and profound sedation may occur) **966**
Finacea Gel (Concomitant use with any foods and beverages that might provoke erythema, flushing, and blushing (including spicy food, alcoholic beverages, and thermally hot drinks, including hot coffee and tea) should be avoided).........................**1808**
Focalin XR Capsules (Dexmethylphenidate hydrochloride should be given

cautiously to patients with a history of drug dependence or alcoholism)........................**2472**

Furosemide Tablets (Aggravates orthostatic hypotension) **2354**

Gabitril Tablets (Because of the possible additive effects of drugs that may depress the nervous system, ethanol should be used cautiously in combination with tiagabine)............ **972**

Humalog-Pen and KwikPen (Co-administration with drugs with hypoglycemic activity may result in decreased insulin requirements)...........................**1910**

Humalog Mix 50/50-Pen and KwikPen (Insulin requirements may be decreased in the presence of drugs with hypoglycemic activity, such as alcohol) **1914**

Humulin N Vial (Insulin requirements may be reduced in the presence of drugs that lower blood glucose or affect how the body responds to insulin) **1934**

Humulin R (U-500) (Insulin requirements may be decreased in the presence of drugs that increase insulin sensitivity or have hypoglycemic activity, such as alcohol) **1939**

Hyzaar 50-12.5 Tablets (Potentiation of orthostatic hypotension may occur)..................**2162**

Indapamide Tablets (Aggravates orthostatic hypotension) **2356**

Intravenous Sodium Diuril (Hypotension including orthostatic hypotension may be aggravated or potentiated by alcohol when co-administered with chlorothiazide) **2009**

Intuniv Extended-Release Tablets (Caution should be exercised when guanfacine is administered concomitantly with alcohol due to the potential for additive pharmacodynamic effects) **3291**

Invega Extended-Release Tablets (Given the primary CNS effects of paliperidone, paliperidone should be used with caution in combination with other centrally acting drugs and alcohol) **2613**

Invega Sustenna Extended-Release Injectable Suspension (Given the primary CNS effects paliperidone should be used with caution in combination with other centrally acting drugs and alcohol. Paliperidone may antagonize the effect of levodopa and other dopamine antagonists) **2621**

Janumet Tablets (Alcohol is known to potentiate the effect of metformin on lactate metabolism. Patients, therefore, should be warned against excessive alcohol intake, acute or chronic, while receiving Janumet).........................**2188**

Klonopin Tablets (The CNS-depressant action of the benzodiazepine class of drugs may be potentiated by alcohol. Patients should be advised to avoid alcohol while taking clonazepam) **2855**

Lantus Injection (May either potentiate or weaken the blood-glucose-lowering effect of insulin) **2996**

Levemir Injection (Co-administration may either potentiate or weaken the blood-glucose lowering effect of insulin) **2566**

Lexapro Tablets (Although escitalopram did not potentiate the cognitive and motor effects of alcohol in a clinical trial, as with other psychotropic medications, the use of alcohol by patients taking escitalopram is not recommended) **1160**

Lupron Depot 3.75 mg (In patients with major risk factors for decreased bone mineral content such as chronic alcohol use, leuprolide acetate depot may pose an additional risk. In these patients, the risks and benefits must be weighed carefully before therapy with leuprolide acetate depot alone is instituted, and concomitant treatment with norethindrone acetate 5 mg daily should be considered. Retreatment with gonadotropin-releasing hormone analogs, including leuprolide acetate, is not advisable in patients with major risk factors for loss of bone mineral content)......................... **472**

Lyrica Capsules (Patients who are taking other drugs associated with angioedema (eg, angiotensin converting enzyme inhibitors [ACE inhibitors]) may be at increased risk of developing angioedema) **2731**

Marplan Tablets (Isocarboxazid should not be administered in combination with some central nervous systems depressants including alcohol) **3481**

Meridia Capsules (In a double-blind, placebo-controlled, crossover study in 19 volunteers, administration of a single dose of ethanol (0.5 mL/kg) together with 20 mg of sibutramine resulted in no psychomotor interactions of clinical significance between alcohol and sibutramine. However, the concomitant use of sibutramine and excess alcohol is not recommended) **492**

Metozolv ODT Orally Disintegrating Tablets (Additive sedative effects can occur when metoclopramide is given with alcohol, sedatives, hypnotics, narcotics, or tranquilizers)............**2901**

Mevacor Tablets (Lovastatin should be used with caution in patients who have consumed substantial quantity of alcohol and have a past history of liver disease; active liver disease and unexplained elevation in transaminase are contraindications to the use of lovastatin) **2212**

Micardis HCT Tablets (Potentiation of orthostatic hypotension may occur with alcohol, barbiturates, or narcotics when administered concurrently with thiazide diuretics) **889**

Moban Tablets (Concomitant use of molindone with alcohol is contraindicated).............................**1108**

MS Contin Tablets (Respiratory depression, hypotension and profound sedation or coma may result) **2803**

Nascobal Nasal Spray (Heavy alcohol intake for longer than 2 weeks may produce malabsorption of vitamin B12) **2700**

Nembutal Sodium Solution (Concurrent use of barbiturates with other CNS depressants (eg, alcohol) may result in additional CNS depressant effects. Alcohol should not be consumed while taking barbiturates)..........................**2012**

Niaspan Extended-Release Tablets (Concomitant alcohol may increase the side effects of flushing and pruritus and should be avoided around the time of Niaspan ingestion)........................ **497**

Nitro-Dur Transdermal Infusion System (Enhances sensitivity to the hypotensive effects)................**3170**

Nitrolingual Pumpspray (Alcohol may enhance sensitivity to hypotensive effects of nitrates) **3266**

NovoLog Injection (A number of substances affect glucose metabolism and may require insulin dose adjustment and particularly close monitoring. Examples of substances that may either potentiate or weaken the blood-glucose-lowering effect of insulin include alcohol) **2575**

Nucynta Tablets (Due to its mu-opioid agonist activity, tapentadol hydrochloride may be expected to have additive effects when used in conjunction with alcohol, opioids, or illicit drugs that cause central nervous system depression, respiratory depression, hypotension, and profound sedation, coma or death)..........................**2643**

Nuvigil Tablets (Patients should be advised that the use of armodafinil in combination with alcohol has not been studied. Patients should be advised that it is prudent to avoid alcohol while taking armodafinil) **978**

Onsolis Film (The concomitant use of fentanyl with other CNS depressants, including other opioids, sedatives or hypnotics, general anesthetics, phenothiazines, tranquilizers, skeletal muscle relaxants, sedating antihistamines, and alcoholic beverages may produce increased depressant effects) **2054**

Opana Tablets (The concomitant use of other CNS depressants including sedatives, hypnotics, tranquilizers, general anesthetics, phenothiazines, other opioids, and alcohol may produce additive CNS depressant effects. Additive effects resulting in respiratory depression, hypotension, profound sedation or coma may result if these drugs are taken in combination with the usual doses of oxymorphone hydrochloride)..............................**1110**

OsmoPrep Tablets (There have been rare reports of generalized tonic-clonic seizures and/or loss of consciousness associated with use of sodium phosphate products in patients with no prior history of seizures. Sodium phosphate should be used with caution in patients at higher risk of seizure, such as those withdrawing from alcohol) **2907**

OxyContin Tablets (Oxycodone, like all opioid analgesics, should be started at 1/3 to 1/2 of the usual dosage in patients who are concurrently receiving other central nervous system depressants including alcohol because respiratory depression, hypotension, and profound sedation or coma may result) **2807**

Parnate Tablets (Tranylcypromine is contraindicated in combination with foods with a high tyramine content. Hypertensive crises have sometimes occurred during therapy with tranylcypromine after ingestion of foods with a high tyramine content. In particular, patients should be instructed not to take foods, such as Chianti wine) **1584**

Paroxetine Hydrochloride Controlled-release Tablets (Avoid alcohol while taking paroxetine hydrochloride controlled-release tablets).............**2361**

Paroxetine Hydrochloride Extended-release Tablets (Avoid alcohol while taking paroxetine hydrochloride controlled-release tablets)..............................**2371**

Patanase Nasal Spray (Concurrent use of olopatadine nasal spray with alcohol should

be avoided because additional reductions in alertness and additional impairment of central nervous system performance may occur)................................... **585**

Paxil Tablets (Although paroxetine has not been shown to increase the impairment of mental and motor skills caused by alcohol, patients should be advised to avoid alcohol while taking paroxetine) **1586**

Paxil CR Controlled-Release Tablets (Although paroxetine has not been shown to increase the impairment of mental and motor skills caused by alcohol, patients should be advised to avoid alcohol while taking paroxetine) **1596**

Percocet Tablets (Additive CNS depression) **1121**

Percodan Tablets (Additive CNS depression) **1124**

Phenytek Capsules (Acute alcohol intake with phenytoin may increase phenytoin serum levels; chronic alcohol abuse with phenytoin may decrease phenytoin serum levels) **2380**

Photofrin for Injection (Compounds that quench active oxygen species or scavenge radicals, such as ethanol would be expected to decrease photodynamic therapy (PDT) activity)................................. **786**

Prinzide Tablets (Co-administration of thiazide and alcohol may potentiate orthostatic hypotension) **2246**

Pristiq Extended-Release Tablets (A clinical study has shown that desvenlafaxine does not increase the impairment of mental and motor skills caused by ethanol. However, patients should be advised to avoid alcohol consumption while taking desvenlafaxine) **3564**

Provigil Tablets (The use of modafinil in combination with alcohol has not been studied. It is advisable to avoid alcohol while taking modafinil).................... **983**

Prozac Weekly Capsules (Concurrent use with alcohol requires caution)....................**1941**

Pylera Capsules (Alcoholic beverages should not be consumed during Pylera therapy and for at least 1 day afterward. Psychotic reactions have been reported in alcoholic patients who are using Pylera and disulfiram concurrently. Pylera should not be given to patients who have taken disulfiram within the last 2 weeks)................. **793**

Remeron Tablets (Concomitant administration of alcohol (equivalent to 60 g) had a minimal effect on plasma levels of mirtazapine (15 mg) in healthy male subjects. However, the impairment of cognitive and motor skills produced by mirtazapine were shown to be additive with those produced by alcohol. Accordingly, patients should be advised to avoid alcohol while taking mirtazapine) **3214**

Requip Tablets (Sedating medications (such as alcohol or CNS depressants), may increase the risk of somnolence or falling asleep while engaged in activities of daily living. Because of possible additive effects, caution should be advised when patients are taking other sedating medications, alcohol, or other CNS depressants in combination with ropinirole) **1620**

Requip XL Tablets (Sedating medications (such as alcohol or CNS depressants), may increase the risk of somnolence

or falling asleep while engaged in activities of daily living. Because of possible additive effects, caution should be advised when patients are taking other sedating medications, alcohol, or other CNS depressants in combination with ropinirole) ... 1628

Rilutek Tablets (Whether alcohol increases the risk of serious hepatotoxicity with riluzole is unknown; therefore, patients being treated with riluzole should be discouraged from drinking excessive amounts of alcohol) ... 3032

Risperdal Consta Long-Acting Injection (Given the primary CNS effects of risperidone, caution should be used if taken in combination with alcohol) ... 2682

Rozerem Tablets (Complex behaviors, such as "sleep driving" (eg, driving while not fully awake after ingestion of hypnotic) and other complex behaviors (eg, preparing and eating food, making phone calls, or having sex), with amnesia for the event, have been reported in association with hypnotic use. The use of alcohol and other CNS depressants may increase the risk of such behaviors) ... 3366

Ryzolt Extended-Release Tablets (Patients should be cautioned about the concomitant use of tramadol products and alcohol because of potentially serious CNS-additive effects of these agents. When large doses of tramadol are administered with alcohol, respiratory depression may result. Prescribe tramadol with caution for patients who use alcohol in excess) ... 2813

St. Joseph 81 mg Aspirin Chewable and Enteric Coated Tablets (Chronic heavy alcohol users, 3 or more drinks per day, in combination with analgesic/antipyretic drug products containing aspirin increases the risk of adverse GI events, including stomach bleeding) ... 2045

Salonpas Arthritis Pain (Having 3 or more alcoholic drinks everyday may increase the chance of stomach bleeding) ... 1805

Salonpas Pain Relief Patch (Having 3 or more alcoholic drinks everyday may increase the chance of stomach bleeding) ... 1805

Saphris Tablets (Given the primary CNS effects of asenapine, caution should be used when it is taken in combination with other centrally-acting drugs or alcohol) ... 3223

Savella Tablets (Milnacipran hydrochloride should not be prescribed to patients with substantial alcohol use or evidence of chronic liver disease because it is possible that milnacipran hydrochloride may aggravate pre-existing liver disease) ... 1172

Seromycin Capsules (Concurrent use increases the possibility and risk of epileptic episodes) ... 1956

Seroquel Tablets (Quetiapine potentiated the cognitive and motor effects of alcohol in a clinical trial in subjects with selected psychotic disorders. Alcoholic beverages should be avoided while taking quetiapine) ... 750

Seroquel XR Extended-Release Tablets (Given the primary CNS effects of quetiapine, caution should be used when it is taken in combination with other centrally acting drugs. Quetiapine potentiated the cognitive and motor effects of alcohol in a clinical trial in subjects with selected psychotic disorders, and alcoholic beverages should be limited while taking quetiapine) ... 759

Skelaxin Tablets (The sedative effects of metaxalone and other CNS depressants (eg, alcohol) may be additive. Therefore, caution should be exercised with patients who take more than one of these CNS depressants simultaneously) ... 1848

Soriatane Capsules (Clinical evidence has shown that etretinate can be formed with concurrent ingestion of acitretin and ethanol) ... 3326

Symbyax Capsules (The co-administration of ethanol with Symbyax may potentiate sedation and orthostatic hypotension. Patients should be advised to avoid alcohol while taking Symbyax) ... 1965

Tekturna HCT Tablets (Potentiation of orthostatic hypotension may occur with concurrent use) ... 2541

Teveten HCT Tablets (May potentiate orthostatic hypotension) ... 541

Thioridazine Hydrochloride Tablets (Thioridazine is capable of potentiating CNS depressants) ... 2384

Thiothixene Capsules (Patients receiving thiothixene should be cautioned about the possible additive effects (which may include hypotension) with CNS depressants and with alcohol. Extreme caution should be used in patients with a history of convulsive disorders or those in a state of alcohol withdrawal, since it may lower the convulsive threshold) ... 2386

Toviaz Extended-Release Tablets (Concomitant use with alcohol may enhance the drowsiness caused by fesoterodine) ... 2753

Transderm Scōp Transdermal Therapeutic System (Scopolamine is an anticholinergic agent and causes certain CNS effects, such as drowsiness and dizziness, and hence it should be used with care in patients on concomitant therapy) ... 2397

Treximet Tablets (Other factors that increase the risk for gastrointestinal bleeding in patients treated with NSAIDs include concomitant use of alcohol) ... 1681

Trilipix Delayed Release Capsules (Excessive alcohol intake should be addressed before triglyceride-lowering drug therapy, such as fenofibric acid, is considered. If the decision is made to use lipid-altering drugs, the patient should be instructed that this does not reduce the importance of adhering to diet) ... 548

Trizivir Tablets (Concurrent use with ethanol decreases the elimination of abacavir causing an increase in overall exposure) ... 1688

Tussionex Pennkinetic Extended-Release Suspension (Combined use may result in additive CNS depression) ... 3443

Regular Strength Tylenol Tablets (Severe liver damage may occur if an adult has 3 or more alcoholic drinks every day while using this product) ... 2049

Tylenol with Codeine Tablets (Concomitant use with alcohol may produce an additive CNS depression and should be avoided) ... 2691

Ultram ER Extended-Release Tablets (Tramadol hydrochloride is contraindicated in acute intoxication with alcohol. Tramadol hydrochloride should be used with caution and in reduced dosages when administered to patients receiving CNS depressants, such as alcohol. Tramadol may be expected to have additive effects when used in conjunction with alcohol) ... 2693

Uniphyl Tablets (Concurrent use with a single dose of alcohol (3mL/kg of whiskey) decreases theophylline clearance for up to 24 hours) ... 2817

Valium Tablets (Concomitant use with alcohol is not recommended due to enhancement of the sedative effect) ... 2880

Venlafaxine Hydrochloride Tablets (Although venlafaxine has not been shown to increase the impairment of mental and motor skills caused by alcohol, patients should be advised to avoid alcohol while taking venlafaxine) ... 2388

Vicodin Tablets (May exhibit an additive CNS depression) ... 560

Vicodin ES Tablets (Additive CNS depression) ... 561

Vicodin HP Tablets (Concurrent use results in an additive CNS depression) ... 563

Vicoprofen Tablets (May exhibit additive CNS depression) ... 564

Visudyne for Injection (Co-administration with compounds that quench active oxygen species or scavenge radicals, such as ethanol, would be expected to decrease verteporfin activity) ... 2549

Vytorin 10/10 Tablets (Vytorin should be used with caution in patients who consume substantial quantities of alcohol and/or have a past history of liver disease) ... 2303

Vytorin 10/10 Tablets (Vytorin should be used with caution in patients who consume substantial quantities of alcohol and/or have a past history of liver disease) ... 3240

Wellbutrin Tablets (Bupropion is contraindicated in patients undergoing abrupt discontinuation of alcohol. In post-marketing experience, there have been rare reports of adverse neuropsychiatric events or reduced alcohol tolerance in patients who were drinking during treatment with bupropion. The consumption of alcohol should be minimized or avoided) ... 1719

Xenazine Tablets (Patients should be advised that the concomitant use of alcohol or other sedating drugs with tetrabenazine may have additive effects and worsen sedation and somnolence) ... 2033

Xyzal Oral Solution (Concurrent use of levocetirizine dihydrochloride with alcohol should be avoided because additional reductions in alertness and additional impairment of central nervous system performance may occur) ... 3449

Xyzal Oral Solution (Concurrent use of levocetirizine dihydrochloride with alcohol should be avoided because additional reductions in alertness and additional impairment of central nervous system performance may occur) ... 3053

Ziagen Tablets (Ethanol decreases the elimination of abacavir, causing an increase in overall exposure. Co-administration of ethanol and abacavir resulted in a 41% increase in abacavir AUC and a 26% increase in abacavir $t_{1/2}$) ... 1740

Zocor Tablets (Simvastatin should be used with caution in patients who consume substantial quantities of alcohol) ... 2289

Zonegran Capsules (Concomitant administration of zonisamide and alcohol or other CNS depressants has not been evaluated in clinical studies. Because of the potential of zonisamide to cause CNS depression, as well as other cognitive and/or neuropsychiatric adverse events, zonisamide should be used with caution if used in combination with alcohol or other CNS depressants) ... 1081

Zyban Sustained-Release Tablets (Bupropion is contraindicated in patients undergoing abrupt discontinuation of alcohol. In post-marketing experience, there have been rare reports of adverse neuropsychiatric events or reduced alcohol tolerance in patients who were drinking alcohol during treatment with bupropion. The consumption of alcohol during treatment with bupropion should be minimized or avoided) ... 1762

Zydone Tablets (Co-administration may exhibit additive CNS depression) ... 1138

Zyprexa Tablets (Co-administration of alcohol with olanzapine potentiates orthostatic hypotension; concurrent use should be avoided. Given the primary CNS effects of olanzapine, caution should be used when olanzapine is taken in combination with other centrally-acting drugs and alcohol) ... 1984

Zyprexa IntraMuscular (Co-administration of alcohol with olanzapine potentiates orthostatic hypotension; concurrent use should be avoided. Given the primary CNS effects of olanzapine, caution should be used when olanzapine is taken in combination with other centrally-acting drugs and alcohol) ... 1984

Zyrtec Allergy Tablets (Alcohol may increase drowsiness. Avoid alcoholic drinks) ... 2052

Children's Zyrtec Allergy Chewable Tablets (Alcohol may increase drowsiness. Avoid alcoholic drinks) ... 2053

Children's Zyrtec Allergy Syrup (Concomitant use may increase drowsiness) ... 2053

Children's Zyrtec Hives Relief Syrup (Concomitant use may increase drowsiness) ... 2053

Zyrtec-D Allergy & Congestion Extended-Release Tablets (Concurrent use with alcohol may increase drowsiness; avoid alcohol) ... 2054

Wine, Red

ActoPlus Met Tablets (Alcohol is known to potentiate the effect of metformin on lactate metabolism. Patients, therefore, should be warned against excessive alcohol intake, acute or chronic, while receiving ActoPlus Met. In addition, hypoglycemia does not occur in patients receiving metformin alone under usual circumstances of use, but could occur when during concomitant use with ethanol) ... 3338

Adcirca Tablets (Both alcohol and tadalafil, a PDE5 inhibitor, act as mild vasodilators. When mild vasodilators are taken in combination, blood pressure–lowering effects of each individual compound may be increased. Substantial consumption of alcohol (eg, 5 units or greater) in combination with tadalafil can increase the potential for orthostatic signs

and symptoms, including increase in heart rate, decrease in standing blood pressure, dizziness, and headache)..............3461
Adipex-P Tablets (May result in adverse drug interaction) 1178
Advicor Tablets (Concomitant alcohol may increase the flushing and its use should be avoided around the time of Advicor administration).................. 402
Aggrenox Capsules (Patients who consume three or more alcoholic drinks every day should be counseled about the bleeding risks involved with chronic, heavy alcohol use while taking aspirin).............................. 880
Alphagan P Ophthalmic Solution (Possible additive or potentiating effect with CNS depressants) 596
Ambien Tablets (An additive effect on psychomotor performance between alcohol and zolpidem was demonstrated. Zolpidem should not be taken with alcohol) 2920
Ambien CR Tablets (Zolpidem tartrate has shown additive effects when combined with alcohol and should not be taken with alcohol) 2925
Amrix Capsules (Concomitant use with cyclobenzaprine HCl may enhance the effects of alcohol) 964
Apidra Injection (Alcohol may either potentiate or weaken the blood glucose-lowering effect of insulin) 2937
Aplenzin Extended-Release Tablets (Bupropion is contraindicated in patients undergoing abrupt discontinuation of alcohol. Concomitant use of alcohol with bupropion is associated with an increased seizure risk. There have been rare reports of adverse neuropsychiatric events or reduced alcohol tolerance in patients who were drinking alcohol during treatment with bupropion. The consumption of alcohol during treatment with bupropion should be minimized or avoided) 2948
Atacand HCT 16-12.5 Tablets (May aggravate orthostatic hypotension produced by hydrochlorothiazide)...................... 700
Avalide Tablets (Potentiation of orthostatic hypertension may occur during concomitant administration of hydrochlorothiazide with alcohol) 2956
Avandamet Tablets (Alcohol potentiates the effect of metformin on lactate metabolism; patients should be warned against excessive alcohol intake, acute or chronic).....1345
Avinza Capsules (Patients must not consume alcoholic beverages, prescription or non-prescription medications containing alcohol while on morphine sulfate therapy. Consumption of alcohol while taking morphine sulfate may result in the rapid release and absorption of a potentially fatal dose of morphine).........................1822
Benadryl Allergy Ultratab Tablets (Increases drowsiness effect; avoid concomitant use)...................2042
Benicar HCT Tablets (Concurrent administration could cause potentiation of orthostatic hypotension).................................1017
Carbatrol Capsules (Because of its primary CNS effect, caution should be used when carbamazepine is taken with alcohol) 3280
Catapres-TTS (Clonidine may potentiate the CNS-depressive effects of alcohol, barbiturates or other sedating drugs) 884
Celebrex Capsules (Other factors that increase the risk of GI bleeding in patients treated with NSAIDs include concomitant use of alcohol. Most spontaneous reports of fatal GI events are in elderly or debilitated patients and therefore special care should be taken in treating this population) 3272
Celexa Tablets (Although citalopram did not potentiate cognitive and motor effects of alcohol, as with other psychotropic medications, the use of alcohol by depressed patients taking citalopram is not recommended) 1153
Cialis Tablets (Both alcohol and tadalafil act as mild vasodilators. When mild vasodilators are taken in combination, blood-pressure-lowering effects of each individual compound may be increased. Substantial consumption of alcohol (eg, 5 units or greater) in combination with tadalafil can increase the potential for orthostatic signs and symptoms, including increase in heart rate, decrease in standing blood pressure, dizziness, and headache)..............1861
Clinoril Tablets (Concomitant use of alcohol may increase the risk of GI bleeding) 2098
Clorpres Tablets (Clonidine may enhance the CNS-depressive effects of alcohol; orthostatic hypotension may be aggravated by alcohol)....................................2344
Combigan Ophthalmic Solution (Although specific drug interaction studies have not been conducted with Combigan, the possibility of an additive or potentiating effect with CNS depressants (alcohol, barbiturates, opiates, sedatives or anesthetics) should be considered) 601
Crestor Tablets (Rosuvastatin calcium should be used with caution in patients who consume substantial quantities of alcohol) 736
Cymbalta Delayed-Release Capsules (Use of duloxetine concomitantly with heavy alcohol intake may be associated with severe liver injury. For this reason, duloxetine should ordinarily not be prescribed for patients with substantial alcohol use)................1871
Depakote ER Extended Release Tablets (Since valproate products may produce CNS depression, especially when combined with another CNS depressant (eg, alcohol), patients should be advised not to engage in hazardous activities, such as driving an automobile or operating dangerous machinery, until it is known that they do not become drowsy from the drug) 426
Dilaudid Oral Liquid (Hydromorphone may be expected to have additive effects when used in conjunction with alcohol. Alcohol potentiates the respiratory depressant effects of hydromorphone, increasing the risk of respiratory depression that might result in death)..2797
Dilaudid-HP Injection (Hydromorphone may be expected to have additive effects when used in conjunction with alcohol. Alcohol potentiates the respiratory depressant effects of hydromorphone, increasing the risk of respiratory depression that might result in death)..2800
Diovan HCT Tablets (Concurrent use of thiazide diuretics with alcohol may result in potentiation of orthostatic hypotension)................................2419
Duetact Tablets (All sulfonylurea drugs are capable of producing hypoglycemia; hypoglycemia is more likely to occur when alcohol is ingested).......................3354
Duragesic Transdermal System (Fentanyl may be expected to have additive CNS depressant effects when used in conjunction with alcohol. The concomitant use of fentanyl with alcohol may cause respiratory depression, hypotension, and profound sedation or potentially result in coma)..2604
Effexor XR Extended-Release Capsules (Although venlafaxine has not been shown to increase the impairment of mental and motor skills caused by alcohol, patients should be advised to avoid alcohol while taking venlafaxine) 3504
Elidel Cream 1% (Skin flushing due to pimecrolimus is associated with alcohol use) 2424
Embeda Extended Release Capsules (Embeda should be used with great caution and in reduced dosage in patients who are concurrently receiving other central nervous system (CNS) depressants including alcohol because of the risk of respiratory depression, hypotension, and profound sedation or coma. When such combined therapy is contemplated, the initial dose of one or both agents should be reduced by at least 50%)...............1831
Emsam Transdermal System (The use of alcohol is not recommended while using selegiline transdermal system).......3623
Equetro Extended-Release Capsules (Because of its primary CNS effect, caution should be used when carbamazepine is taken with alcohol) 3477
Exforge HCT Tablets (Potentiation of orthostatic hypotension may occur when alcohol and thiazide diuretics are administered concurrently)................................2449
Exubera Inhalation Powder (Alcohol may either increase or reduce the blood glucose-lowering effect of insulin. Co-administration may require insulin dose adjustment and particularly close monitoring) 2717
Fanapt Tablets (Given the primary CNS effects of iloperidone, caution should be used when it is taken in combination with alcohol) 3484
Fentanyl Transdermal System Patches (Fentanyl may be expected to have additive CNS depressant effects when used in conjunction with alcohol. The concomitant use of fentanyl with alcohol may cause respiratory depression, hypotension, and profound sedation, or potentially result in coma or death) 2346
Fentora Tablets (The concomitant use of other CNS depressants, including alcoholic beverages, may produce increased depressant effects. Hypoventilation, hypotension, and profound sedation may occur) 966
Finacea Gel (Concomitant use with any foods and beverages that might provoke erythema, flushing, and blushing (including spicy food, alcoholic beverages, and thermally hot drinks, including hot coffee and tea) should be avoided).......................1808
Focalin XR Capsules (Dexmethylphenidate hydrochloride should be given cautiously to patients with a history of drug dependence or alcoholism).................................2472
Furosemide Tablets (Aggravates orthostatic hypotension) 2354
Gabitril Tablets (Because of the possible additive effects of drugs that may depress the nervous system, ethanol should be used cautiously in combination with tiagabine)........... 972
Humalog-Pen and KwikPen (Co-administration with drugs with hypoglycemic activity may result in decreased insulin requirements).............................1910
Humalog Mix 50/50-Pen and KwikPen (Insulin requirements may be decreased in the presence of drugs with hypoglycemic activity, such as alcohol) 1914
Humulin N Vial (Insulin requirements may be reduced in the presence of drugs that lower blood glucose or affect how the body responds to insulin) 1934
Humulin R (U-500) (Insulin requirements may be decreased in the presence of drugs that increase insulin sensitivity or have hypoglycemic activity, such as alcohol) 1939
Hyzaar 50-12.5 Tablets (Potentiation of orthostatic hypotension may occur).................2162
Indapamide Tablets (Aggravates orthostatic hypotension) 2356
Intravenous Sodium Diuril (Hypotension including orthostatic hypotension may be aggravated or potentiated by alcohol when co-administered with chlorothiazide).......................2009
Intuniv Extended-Release Tablets (Caution should be exercised when guanfacine is administered concomitantly with alcohol due to the potential for additive pharmacodynamic effects) 3291
Invega Extended-Release Tablets (Given the primary CNS effects of paliperidone, paliperidone should be used with caution in combination with other centrally acting drugs and alcohol) 2613
Invega Sustenna Extended-Release Injectable Suspension (Given the primary CNS effects paliperidone should be used with caution in combination with other centrally acting drugs and alcohol. Paliperidone may antagonize the effect of levodopa and other dopamine antagonists) 2621
Janumet Tablets (Alcohol is known to potentiate the effect of metformin on lactate metabolism. Patients, therefore, should be warned against excessive alcohol intake, acute or chronic, while receiving Janumet).......................2188
Klonopin Tablets (The CNS-depressant action of the benzodiazepine class of drugs may be potentiated by alcohol. Patients should be advised to avoid alcohol while taking clonazepam)...............................2855

(⊙ Described in PDR® for Ophthalmic Medicines)

selected psychotic disorders. Alcoholic beverages should be avoided while taking quetiapine)..... **750**

Seroquel XR Extended-Release Tablets (Given the primary CNS effects of quetiapine, caution should be used when it is taken in combination with other centrally acting drugs. Quetiapine potentiated the cognitive and motor effects of alcohol in a clinical trial in subjects with selected psychotic disorders, and alcoholic beverages should be limited while taking quetiapine) **759**

Skelaxin Tablets (The sedative effects of metaxalone and other CNS depressants (eg, alcohol) may be additive. Therefore, caution should be exercised with patients who take more than one of these CNS depressants simultaneously) **1848**

Soriatane Capsules (Clinical evidence has shown that etretinate can be formed with concurrent ingestion of acitretin and ethanol) **3326**

Symbyax Capsules (The co-administration of ethanol with Symbyax may potentiate sedation and orthostatic hypotension. Patients should be advised to avoid alcohol while taking Symbyax)................................**1965**

Tekturna HCT Tablets (Potentiation of orthostatic hypotension may occur with concurrent use) **2541**

Teveten HCT Tablets (May potentiate orthostatic hypotension)................................ **541**

Thioridazine Hydrochloride Tablets (Thioridazine is capable of potentiating CNS depressants).......**2384**

Thiothixene Capsules (Patients receiving thiothixene should be cautioned about the possible additive effects (which may include hypotension) with CNS depressants and with alcohol. Extreme caution should be used in patients with a history of convulsive disorders or those in a state of alcohol withdrawal, since it may lower the convulsive threshold) **2386**

Toviaz Extended-Release Tablets (Concomitant use with alcohol may enhance the drowsiness caused by fesoterodine).................**2753**

Transderm Scōp Transdermal Therapeutic System (Scopolamine is an anticholinergic agent and causes certain CNS effects, such as drowsiness and dizziness, and hence it should be used with care in patients on concomitant therapy) **2397**

Treximet Tablets (Other factors that increase the risk for gastrointestinal bleeding in patients treated with NSAIDs include concomitant use of alcohol) **1681**

Trilipix Delayed Release Capsules (Excessive alcohol intake should be addressed before triglyceride-lowering drug therapy, such as fenofibric acid, is considered. If the decision is made to use lipid-altering drugs, the patient should be instructed that this does not reduce the importance of adhering to diet) **548**

Trizivir Tablets (Concurrent use with ethanol decreases the elimination of abacavir causing an increase in overall exposure) **1688**

Tussionex Pennkinetic Extended-Release Suspension (Combined use may result in additive CNS depression) **3443**

Regular Strength Tylenol Tablets (Severe liver damage may occur if an adult has 3 or more alcoholic drinks every day while using this product) **2049**

Tylenol with Codeine Tablets (Concomitant use with alcohol may produce an additive CNS depression and should be avoided) **2691**

Ultram ER Extended-Release Tablets (Tramadol hydrochloride is contraindicated in acute intoxication with alcohol. Tramadol hydrochloride should be used with caution and in reduced dosages when administered to patients receiving CNS depressants, such as alcohol. Tramadol may be expected to have additive effects when used in conjunction with alcohol) **2693**

Uniphyl Tablets (Concurrent use with a single dose of alcohol (3mL/kg of whiskey) decreases theophylline clearance for up to 24 hours)..**2817**

Valium Tablets (Concomitant use with alcohol is not recommended due to enhancement of the sedative effect) **2880**

Venlafaxine Hydrochloride Tablets (Although venlafaxine has not been shown to increase the impairment of mental and motor skills caused by alcohol, patients should be advised to avoid alcohol while taking venlafaxine)................................**2388**

Vicodin Tablets (May exhibit an additive CNS depression) **560**

Vicodin ES Tablets (Additive CNS depression)................................ **561**

Vicodin HP Tablets (Concurrent use results in an additive CNS depression)................................ **563**

Vicoprofen Tablets (May exhibit additive CNS depression) **564**

Visudyne for Injection (Co-administration with compounds that quench active oxygen species or scavenge radicals, such as ethanol, would be expected to decrease verteporfin activity) **2549**

Vytorin 10/10 Tablets (Vytorin should be used with caution in patients who consume substantial quantities of alcohol and/or have a past history of liver disease) **2303**

Vytorin 10/10 Tablets (Vytorin should be used with caution in patients who consume substantial quantities of alcohol and/or have a past history of liver disease) **3240**

Wellbutrin Tablets (Bupropion is contraindicated in patients undergoing abrupt discontinuation of alcohol. In post-marketing experience, there have been rare reports of adverse neuropsychiatric events or reduced alcohol tolerance in patients who were drinking during treatment with bupropion. The consumption of alcohol should be minimized or avoided) **1719**

Xenazine Tablets (Patients should be advised that the concomitant use of alcohol or other sedating drugs with tetrabenazine may have additive effects and worsen sedation and somnolence)................................**2033**

Xyzal Oral Solution (Concurrent use of levocetirizine dihydrochloride with alcohol should be avoided because additional reductions in alertness and additional impairment of central nervous system performance may occur) **3449**

Xyzal Oral Solution (Concurrent use of levocetirizine dihydrochloride with alcohol should be avoided because additional reductions in alertness and additional impairment of central nervous system performance may occur) **3053**

Ziagen Tablets (Ethanol decreases the elimination of abacavir, causing an increase in overall exposure. Co-administration of ethanol and abacavir resulted in a 41% increase in abacavir AUC and a 26% increase in abacavir $t_{1/2}$)........**1740**

Zocor Tablets (Simvastatin should be used with caution in patients who consume substantial quantities of alcohol) **2289**

Zonegran Capsules (Concomitant administration of zonisamide and alcohol or other CNS depressants has not been evaluated in clinical studies. Because of the potential of zonisamide to cause CNS depression, as well as other cognitive and/or neuropsychiatric adverse events, zonisamide should be used with caution if used in combination with alcohol or other CNS depressants).................**1081**

Zyban Sustained-Release Tablets (Bupropion is contraindicated in patients undergoing abrupt discontinuation of alcohol. In post-marketing experience, there have been rare reports of adverse neuropsychiatric events or reduced alcohol tolerance in patients who were drinking alcohol during treatment with bupropion. The consumption of alcohol during treatment with bupropion should be minimized or avoided) **1762**

Zydone Tablets (Co-administration may exhibit additive CNS depression) **1138**

Zyprexa Tablets (Co-administration of alcohol with olanzapine potentiates orthostatic hypotension; concurrent use should be avoided. Given the primary CNS effects of olanzapine, caution should be used when olanzapine is taken in combination with other centrally-acting drugs and alcohol) **1984**

Zyprexa IntraMuscular (Co-administration of alcohol with olanzapine potentiates orthostatic hypotension; concurrent use should be avoided. Given the primary CNS effects of olanzapine, caution should be used when olanzapine is taken in combination with other centrally-acting drugs and alcohol) **1984**

Zyrtec Allergy Tablets (Alcohol may increase drowsiness. Avoid alcoholic drinks)............................**2052**

Children's Zyrtec Allergy Chewable Tablets (Alcohol may increase drowsiness. Avoid alcoholic drinks)............................**2053**

Children's Zyrtec Allergy Syrup (Concomitant use may increase drowsiness)....................................**2053**

Children's Zyrtec Hives Relief Syrup (Concomitant use may increase drowsiness)....................**2053**

Zyrtec-D Allergy & Congestion Extended-Release Tablets (Concurrent use with alcohol may increase drowsiness; avoid alcohol) **2054**

Wine, unspecified

ActoPlus Met Tablets (Alcohol is known to potentiate the effect of metformin on lactate metabolism. Patients, therefore, should be warned against excessive alcohol intake, acute or chronic, while receiving ActoPlus Met. In addition, hypoglycemia does not occur in patients receiving metformin alone under usual circumstances of use, but could occur when during concomitant use with ethanol) **3338**

Adcirca Tablets (Both alcohol and tadalafil, a PDE5 inhibitor, act as mild vasodilators. When mild vasodilators are taken in combination, blood pressure–lowering effects of each individual compound may be increased. Substantial consumption of alcohol (eg, 5 units or greater) in combination with tadalafil can increase the potential for orthostatic signs and symptoms, including increase in heart rate, decrease in standing blood pressure, dizziness, and headache)...............**3461**

Adipex-P Tablets (May result in adverse drug interaction) **1178**

Advicor Tablets (Concomitant alcohol may increase the flushing and its use should be avoided around the time of Advicor administration)................... **402**

Aggrenox Capsules (Patients who consume three or more alcoholic drinks every day should be counseled about the bleeding risks involved with chronic, heavy alcohol use while taking aspirin) **880**

Alphagan P Ophthalmic Solution (Possible additive or potentiating effect with CNS depressants) **596**

Ambien Tablets (An additive effect on psychomotor performance between alcohol and zolpidem was demonstrated. Zolpidem should not be taken with alcohol) **2920**

Ambien CR Tablets (Zolpidem tartrate has shown additive effects when combined with alcohol and should not be taken with alcohol) **2925**

Amrix Capsules (Concomitant use with cyclobenzaprine HCl may enhance the effects of alcohol) **964**

Apidra Injection (Alcohol may either potentiate or weaken the blood glucose-lowering effect of insulin) **2937**

Aplenzin Extended-Release Tablets (Bupropion is contraindicated in patients undergoing abrupt discontinuation of alcohol. Concomitant use of alcohol with bupropion is associated with an increased seizure risk. There have been rare reports of adverse neuropsychiatric events or reduced alcohol tolerance in patients who were drinking alcohol during treatment with bupropion. The consumption of alcohol during treatment with bupropion should be minimized or avoided) **2948**

Atacand HCT 16-12.5 Tablets (May aggravate orthostatic hypotension produced by hydrochlorothiazide)...................... **700**

Avalide Tablets (Potentiation of orthostatic hypertension may occur during concomitant administration of hydrochlorothiazide with alcohol) **2956**

Avandamet Tablets (Alcohol potentiates the effect of metformin on lactate metabolism; patients should be warned against excessive alcohol intake, acute or chronic).....**1345**

Avinza Capsules (Patients must not consume alcoholic beverages, prescription or non-prescription medications containing alcohol while on morphine sulfate therapy. Consumption of alcohol while taking morphine sulfate may result in the rapid release and absorption of a potentially fatal dose of morphine)......................**1822**

Benadryl Allergy Ultratab Tablets (Increases drowsiness effect; avoid concomitant use) **2042**

Benicar HCT Tablets (Concurrent administration could cause potentiation of orthostatic hypotension)................................1017

Carbatrol Capsules (Because of its primary CNS effect, caution should be used when carbamazepine is taken with alcohol)...................................3280

Catapres-TTS (Clonidine may potentiate the CNS-depressive effects of alcohol, barbiturates or other sedating drugs)................884

Celebrex Capsules (Other factors that increase the risk of GI bleeding in patients treated with NSAIDs include concomitant use of alcohol. Most spontaneous reports of fatal GI events are in elderly or debilitated patients and therefore special care should be taken in treating this population)................................3272

Celexa Tablets (Although citalopram did not potentiate cognitive and motor effects of alcohol, as with other psychotropic medications, the use of alcohol by depressed patients taking citalopram is not recommended)........................1153

Cialis Tablets (Both alcohol and tadalafil act as mild vasodilators. When mild vasodilators are taken in combination, blood-pressure-lowering effects of each individual compound may be increased. Substantial consumption of alcohol (eg, 5 units or greater) in combination with tadalafil can increase the potential for orthostatic signs and symptoms, including increase in heart rate, decrease in standing blood pressure, dizziness, and headache)..............1861

Clinoril Tablets (Concomitant use of alcohol may increase the risk of GI bleeding)................................2098

Clorpres Tablets (Clonidine may enhance the CNS-depressive effects of alcohol; orthostatic hypotension may be aggravated by alcohol)...............................2344

Combigan Ophthalmic Solution (Although specific drug interaction studies have not been conducted with Combigan, the possibility of an additive or potentiating effect with CNS depressants (alcohol, barbiturates, opiates, sedatives or anesthetics) should be considered)..................................601

Crestor Tablets (Rosuvastatin calcium should be used with caution in patients who consume substantial quantities of alcohol).............................736

Cymbalta Delayed-Release Capsules (Use of duloxetine concomitantly with heavy alcohol intake may be associated with severe liver injury. For this reason, duloxetine should ordinarily not be prescribed for patients with substantial alcohol use)................1871

Depakote ER Extended Release Tablets (Since valproate products may produce CNS depression, especially when combined with another CNS depressant (eg, alcohol), patients should be advised not to engage in hazardous activities, such as driving an automobile or operating dangerous machinery, until it is known that they do not become drowsy from the drug)...................426

Dilaudid Oral Liquid (Hydromorphone may be

expected to have additive effects when used in conjunction with alcohol. Alcohol potentiates the respiratory depressant effects of hydromorphone, increasing the risk of respiratory depression that might result in death)......................................2797

Dilaudid-HP Injection (Hydromorphone may be expected to have additive effects when used in conjunction with alcohol. Alcohol potentiates the respiratory depressant effects of hydromorphone, increasing the risk of respiratory depression that might result in death)......................................2800

Diovan HCT Tablets (Concurrent use of thiazide diuretics with alcohol may result in potentiation of orthostatic hypotension)...........................2419

Duetact Tablets (All sulfonylurea drugs are capable of producing hypoglycemia; hypoglycemia is more likely to occur when alcohol is ingested)......................3354

Duragesic Transdermal System (Fentanyl may be expected to have additive CNS depressant effects when used in conjunction with alcohol. The concomitant use of fentanyl with alcohol may cause respiratory depression, hypotension, and profound sedation or potentially result in coma)..................................2604

Effexor XR Extended-Release Capsules (Although venlafaxine has not been shown to increase the impairment of mental and motor skills caused by alcohol, patients should be advised to avoid alcohol while taking venlafaxine)............................3504

Elidel Cream 1% (Skin flushing due to pimecrolimus is associated with alcohol use).........2424

Embeda Extended Release Capsules (Embeda should be used with great caution and in reduced dosage in patients who are concurrently receiving other central nervous system (CNS) depressants including alcohol because of the risk of respiratory depression, hypotension, and profound sedation or coma. When such combined therapy is contemplated, the initial dose of one or both agents should be reduced by at least 50%)...............1831

Emsam Transdermal System (The use of alcohol is not recommended while using selegiline transdermal system).......3623

Equetro Extended-Release Capsules (Because of its primary CNS effect, caution should be used when carbamazepine is taken with alcohol)...................................3477

Exforge HCT Tablets (Potentiation of orthostatic hypotension may occur when alcohol and thiazide diuretics are administered concurrently)..........................2449

Exubera Inhalation Powder (Alcohol may either increase or reduce the blood glucose-lowering effect of insulin. Co-administration may require insulin dose adjustment and particularly close monitoring).............................2717

Fanapt Tablets (Given the primary CNS effects of iloperidone, caution should be used when it is taken in combination with alcohol)............................3484

Fentanyl Transdermal System Patches (Fentanyl may be expected to have additive CNS depressant effects when used in conjunction with alcohol. The concomitant use of fentanyl with alcohol may cause respiratory depression, hypotension, and profound sedation, or potentially result in coma or death)..................2346

Fentora Tablets (The concomitant use of other CNS depressants, including alcoholic beverages, may produce increased depressant effects. Hypoventilation, hypotension, and profound sedation may occur)......................................966

Finacea Gel (Concomitant use with any foods and beverages that might provoke erythema, flushing, and blushing (including spicy food, alcoholic beverages, and thermally hot drinks, including hot coffee and tea) should be avoided).....................1808

Focalin XR Capsules (Dexmethylphenidate hydrochloride should be given cautiously to patients with a history of drug dependence or alcoholism)..........................2472

Furosemide Tablets (Aggravates orthostatic hypotension)................2354

Gabitril Tablets (Because of the possible additive effects of drugs that may depress the nervous system, ethanol should be used cautiously in combination with tiagabine)............972

Humalog-Pen and KwikPen (Co-administration with drugs with hypoglycemic activity may result in decreased insulin requirements)................................1910

Humalog Mix 50/50-Pen and KwikPen (Insulin requirements may be decreased in the presence of drugs with hypoglycemic activity, such as alcohol).............................1914

Humulin N Vial (Insulin requirements may be reduced in the presence of drugs that lower blood glucose or affect how the body responds to insulin).................................1934

Humulin R (U-500) (Insulin requirements may be decreased in the presence of drugs that increase insulin sensitivity or have hypoglycemic activity, such as alcohol)...............1939

Hyzaar 50-12.5 Tablets (Potentiation of orthostatic hypotension may occur)..................2162

Indapamide Tablets (Aggravates orthostatic hypotension)................2356

Intravenous Sodium Diuril (Hypotension including orthostatic hypotension may be aggravated or potentiated by alcohol when co-administered with chlorothiazide).......................2009

Intuniv Extended-Release Tablets (Caution should be exercised when guanfacine is administered concomitantly with alcohol due to the potential for additive pharmacodynamic effects)...............................3291

Invega Extended-Release Tablets (Given the primary CNS effects of paliperidone, paliperidone should be used with caution in combination with other centrally acting drugs and alcohol)............2613

Invega Sustenna Extended-Release Injectable Suspension (Given the primary CNS effects paliperidone should be used with caution in combination with other centrally acting drugs and alcohol. Paliperidone may antagonize the effect of levodopa and other dopamine antagonists)................2621

Janumet Tablets (Alcohol is known to potentiate the effect of metformin on lactate

metabolism. Patients, therefore, should be warned against excessive alcohol intake, acute or chronic, while receiving Janumet)..................2188

Klonopin Tablets (The CNS-depressant action of the benzodiazepine class of drugs may be potentiated by alcohol. Patients should be advised to avoid alcohol while taking clonazepam)............................2855

Lantus Injection (May either potentiate or weaken the blood-glucose-lowering effect of insulin)...........................2996

Levemir Injection (Co-administration may either potentiate or weaken the blood-glucose lowering effect of insulin)...........................2566

Lexapro Tablets (Although escitalopram did not potentiate the cognitive and motor effects of alcohol in a clinical trial, as with other psychotropic medications, the use of alcohol by patients taking escitalopram is not recommended)...................1160

Lupron Depot 3.75 mg (In patients with major risk factors for decreased bone mineral content such as chronic alcohol use, leuprolide acetate depot may pose an additional risk. In these patients, the risks and benefits must be weighed carefully before therapy with leuprolide acetate depot alone is instituted, and concomitant treatment with norethindrone acetate 5 mg daily should be considered. Retreatment with gonadotropin-releasing hormone analogs, including leuprolide acetate, is not advisable in patients with major risk factors for loss of bone mineral content)...........................472

Lyrica Capsules (Patients who are taking other drugs associated with angioedema (eg, angiotensin converting enzyme inhibitors [ACE inhibitors]) may be at increased risk of developing angioedema)...............2731

Marplan Tablets (Isocarboxazid should not be administered in combination with some central nervous systems depressants including alcohol)....................3481

Meridia Capsules (In a double-blind, placebo-controlled, crossover study in 19 volunteers, administration of a single dose of ethanol (0.5 mL/kg) together with 20 mg of sibutramine resulted in no psychomotor interactions of clinical significance between alcohol and sibutramine. However, the concomitant use of sibutramine and excess alcohol is not recommended)............................492

Metozolv ODT Orally Disintegrating Tablets (Additive sedative effects can occur when metoclopramide is given with alcohol, sedatives, hypnotics, narcotics, or tranquilizers).............2901

Mevacor Tablets (Lovastatin should be used with caution in patients who have consumed substantial quantity of alcohol and have a past history of liver disease; active liver disease and unexplained elevation in transaminase are contraindications to the use of lovastatin)..............................2212

Micardis HCT Tablets (Potentiation of orthostatic hypotension may occur with alcohol, barbiturates, or narcotics when administered concurrently with thiazide diuretics)...............................889

Moban Tablets (Concomitant use of molindone with alcohol is contraindicated)..................1108

MS Contin Tablets (Respiratory depression, hypotension and profound sedation or coma may result) 2803

Nascobal Nasal Spray (Heavy alcohol intake for longer than 2 weeks may produce malabsorption of vitamin B12) 2700

Nembutal Sodium Solution (Concurrent use of barbiturates with other CNS depressants (eg, alcohol) may result in additional CNS depressant effects. Alcohol should not be consumed while taking barbiturates) 2012

Niaspan Extended-Release Tablets (Concomitant alcohol may increase the side effects of flushing and pruritus and should be avoided around the time of Niaspan ingestion) 497

Nitro-Dur Transdermal Infusion System (Enhances sensitivity to the hypotensive effects) 3170

Nitrolingual Pumpspray (Alcohol may enhance sensitivity to hypotensive effects of nitrates) 3266

NovoLog Injection (A number of substances affect glucose metabolism and may require insulin dose adjustment and particularly close monitoring. Examples of substances that may either potentiate or weaken the blood-glucose-lowering effect of insulin include alcohol) 2575

Nucynta Tablets (Due to its mu-opioid agonist activity, tapentadol hydrochloride may be expected to have additive effects when used in conjunction with alcohol, opioids, or illicit drugs that cause central nervous system depression, respiratory depression, hypotension, and profound sedation, coma or death) 2643

Nuvigil Tablets (Patients should be advised that the use of armodafinil in combination with alcohol has not been studied. Patients should be advised that it is prudent to avoid alcohol while taking armodafinil) 978

Onsolis Film (The concomitant use of fentanyl with other CNS depressants, including other opioids, sedatives or hypnotics, general anesthetics, phenothiazines, tranquilizers, skeletal muscle relaxants, sedating antihistamines, and alcoholic beverages may produce increased depressant effects) 2054

Opana Tablets (The concomitant use of other CNS depressants including sedatives, hypnotics, tranquilizers, general anesthetics, phenothiazines, other opioids, and alcohol may produce additive CNS depressant effects. Additive effects resulting in respiratory depression, hypotension, profound sedation or coma may result if these drugs are taken in combination with the usual doses of oxymorphone hydrochloride) 1110

OsmoPrep Tablets (There have been rare reports of generalized tonic-clonic seizures and/or loss of consciousness associated with use of sodium phosphate products in patients with no prior history of seizures. Sodium phosphate should be used with caution in patients at higher risk of seizure, such as those withdrawing from alcohol) 2907

OxyContin Tablets (Oxycodone, like all opioid analgesics, should be started at 1/3 to 1/2 of the usual dosage in patients who are concurrently receiving other central nervous system depressants including alcohol because respiratory depression, hypotension, and profound sedation or coma may result) 2807

Parnate Tablets (Concomitant use with some central nervous system depressants, such as alcohol, is contraindicated. A marked potentiating effect on alcohol has been reported) 1584

Paroxetine Hydrochloride Controlled-release Tablets (Avoid alcohol while taking paroxetine hydrochloride controlled-release tablets) 2361

Paroxetine Hydrochloride Extended-release Tablets (Avoid alcohol while taking paroxetine hydrochloride controlled-release tablets) 2371

Patanase Nasal Spray (Concurrent use of olopatadine nasal spray with alcohol should be avoided because additional reductions in alertness and additional impairment of central nervous system performance may occur) 585

Paxil Tablets (Although paroxetine has not been shown to increase the impairment of mental and motor skills caused by alcohol, patients should be advised to avoid alcohol while taking paroxetine) 1586

Paxil CR Controlled-Release Tablets (Although paroxetine has not been shown to increase the impairment of mental and motor skills caused by alcohol, patients should be advised to avoid alcohol while taking paroxetine) 1596

Percocet Tablets (Additive CNS depression) 1121

Percodan Tablets (Additive CNS depression) 1124

Phenytek Capsules (Acute alcohol intake with phenytoin may increase phenytoin serum levels; chronic alcohol abuse with phenytoin may decrease phenytoin serum levels) 2380

Photofrin for Injection (Compounds that quench active oxygen species or scavenge radicals, such as ethanol would be expected to decrease photodynamic therapy (PDT) activity) 786

Prinzide Tablets (Co-administration of thiazide and alcohol may potentiate orthostatic hypotension) 2246

Pristiq Extended-Release Tablets (A clinical study has shown that desvenlafaxine does not increase the impairment of mental and motor skills caused by ethanol. However, patients should be advised to avoid alcohol consumption while taking desvenlafaxine) 3564

Provigil Tablets (The use of modafinil in combination with alcohol has not been studied. It is advisable to avoid alcohol while taking modafinil) 983

Prozac Weekly Capsules (Concurrent use with alcohol requires caution) 1941

Pylera Capsules (Alcoholic beverages should not be consumed during Pylera therapy and for at least 1 day afterward. Psychotic reactions have been reported in alcoholic patients who are using Pylera and disulfiram concurrently. Pylera should not be given to patients who have taken disulfiram within the last 2 weeks) 793

Remeron Tablets (Concomitant administration of alcohol (equivalent to 60 g) had a minimal effect on plasma levels of mirtazapine (15 mg) in healthy male subjects. However, the impairment of cognitive and motor skills produced by mirtazapine were shown to be additive with those produced by alcohol. Accordingly, patients should be advised to avoid alcohol while taking mirtazapine) 3214

Requip Tablets (Sedating medications (such as alcohol or CNS depressants), may increase the risk of somnolence or falling asleep while engaged in activities of daily living. Because of possible additive effects, caution should be advised when patients are taking other sedating medications, alcohol, or other CNS depressants in combination with ropinirole) 1620

Requip XL Tablets (Sedating medications (such as alcohol or CNS depressants), may increase the risk of somnolence or falling asleep while engaged in activities of daily living. Because of possible additive effects, caution should be advised when patients are taking other sedating medications, alcohol, or other CNS depressants in combination with ropinirole) 1628

Rilutek Tablets (Whether alcohol increases the risk of serious hepatotoxicity with riluzole is unknown; therefore, patients being treated with riluzole should be discouraged from drinking excessive amounts of alcohol) 3032

Risperdal Consta Long-Acting Injection (Given the primary CNS effects of risperidone, caution should be used if taken in combination with alcohol) 2682

Rozerem Tablets (Complex behaviors, such as "sleep driving" (eg, driving while not fully awake after ingestion of hypnotic) and other complex behaviors (eg, preparing and eating food, making phone calls, or having sex), with amnesia for the event, have been reported in association with hypnotic use. The use of alcohol and other CNS depressants may increase the risk of such behaviors) 3366

Ryzolt Extended-Release Tablets (Patients should be cautioned about the concomitant use of tramadol products and alcohol because of potentially serious CNS-additive effects of these agents. When large doses of tramadol are administered with alcohol, respiratory depression may result. Prescribe tramadol with caution for patients who use alcohol in excess) 2813

St. Joseph 81 mg Aspirin Chewable and Enteric Coated Tablets (Chronic heavy alcohol users, 3 or more drinks per day, in combination with analgesic/antipyretic drug products containing aspirin increases the risk of adverse GI events, including stomach bleeding) 2045

Salonpas Arthritis Pain (Having 3 or more alcoholic drinks everyday may increase the chance of stomach bleeding) 1805

Salonpas Pain Relief Patch (Having 3 or more alcoholic drinks everyday may increase the chance of stomach bleeding) 1805

Saphris Tablets (Given the primary CNS effects of asenapine, caution should be used when it is taken in combination with other centrally-acting drugs or alcohol) 3223

Savella Tablets (Milnacipran hydrochloride should not be prescribed to patients with substantial alcohol use or evidence of chronic liver disease because it is possible that milnacipran hydrochloride may aggravate pre-existing liver disease) 1172

Seromycin Capsules (Concurrent use increases the possibility and risk of epileptic episodes) 1956

Seroquel Tablets (Quetiapine potentiated the cognitive and motor effects of alcohol in a clinical trial in subjects with selected psychotic disorders. Alcoholic beverages should be avoided while taking quetiapine) 750

Seroquel XR Extended-Release Tablets (Given the primary CNS effects of quetiapine, caution should be used when it is taken in combination with other centrally acting drugs. Quetiapine potentiated the cognitive and motor effects of alcohol in a clinical trial in subjects with selected psychotic disorders, and alcoholic beverages should be limited while taking quetiapine) 759

Skelaxin Tablets (The sedative effects of metaxalone and other CNS depressants (eg, alcohol) may be additive. Therefore, caution should be exercised with patients who take more than one of these CNS depressants simultaneously) 1848

Soriatane Capsules (Clinical evidence has shown that etretinate can be formed with concurrent ingestion of acitretin and ethanol) 3326

Symbyax Capsules (The co-administration of ethanol with Symbyax may potentiate sedation and orthostatic hypotension. Patients should be advised to avoid alcohol while taking Symbyax) 1965

Tekturna HCT Tablets (Potentiation of orthostatic hypotension may occur with concurrent use) 2541

Teveten HCT Tablets (May potentiate orthostatic hypotension) 541

Thioridazine Hydrochloride Tablets (Thioridazine is capable of potentiating CNS depressants) 2384

Thiothixene Capsules (Patients receiving thiothixene should be cautioned about the possible additive effects (which may include hypotension) with CNS depressants and with alcohol. Extreme caution should be used in patients with a history of convulsive disorders or those in a state of alcohol withdrawal, since it may lower the convulsive threshold) 2386

Toviaz Extended-Release Tablets (Concomitant use with alcohol may enhance the drowsiness caused by fesoterodine) 2753

Transderm Scōp Transdermal Therapeutic System (Scopolamine is an anticholinergic agent and causes certain CNS effects, such as drowsiness and dizziness, and hence it should be used with care in patients on concomitant therapy) 2397

Treximet Tablets (Other factors that increase the risk for gastrointestinal bleeding in patients treated with NSAIDs include concomitant use of alcohol) 1681

Trilipix Delayed Release Capsules (Excessive alcohol intake should be addressed before triglyceride-lowering drug therapy, such as fenofibric acid, is considered. If the decision is made to use lipid-altering drugs, the patient should be instructed that this does not reduce the importance of adhering to diet) 548

Wine, unspecified Food Interactions Cross-Reference 2256

Trizivir Tablets (Concurrent use with ethanol decreases the elimination of abacavir causing an increase in overall exposure) 1688
Tussionex Pennkinetic Extended-Release Suspension (Combined use may result in additive CNS depression) 3443
Regular Strength Tylenol Tablets (Severe liver damage may occur if an adult has 3 or more alcoholic drinks every day while using this product) 2049
Tylenol with Codeine Tablets (Concomitant use with alcohol may produce an additive CNS depression and should be avoided) 2691
Ultram ER Extended-Release Tablets (Tramadol hydrochloride is contraindicated in acute intoxication with alcohol. Tramadol hydrochloride should be used with caution and in reduced dosages when administered to patients receiving CNS depressants, such as alcohol. Tramadol may be expected to have additive effects when used in conjunction with alcohol) 2693
Uniphyl Tablets (Concurrent use with a single dose of alcohol (3mL/kg of whiskey) decreases theophylline clearance for up to 24 hours) 2817
Valium Tablets (Concomitant use with alcohol is not recommended due to enhancement of the sedative effect) 2880
Venlafaxine Hydrochloride Tablets (Although venlafaxine has not been shown to increase the impairment of mental and motor skills caused by alcohol, patients should be advised to avoid alcohol while taking venlafaxine) 2388
Vicodin Tablets (May exhibit an additive CNS depression) 560
Vicodin ES Tablets (Additive CNS depression) 561
Vicodin HP Tablets (Concurrent use results in an additive CNS depression) 563
Vicoprofen Tablets (May exhibit additive CNS depression) 564
Visudyne for Injection (Co-administration with compounds that quench active oxygen species or scavenge radicals, such as ethanol, would be expected to decrease verteporfin activity) 2549
Vytorin 10/10 Tablets (Vytorin should be used with caution in patients who consume substantial quantities of alcohol and/or have a past history of liver disease) 2303
Vytorin 10/10 Tablets (Vytorin should be used with caution in patients who consume substantial quantities of alcohol and/or have a past history of liver disease) 3240
Wellbutrin Tablets (Bupropion is contraindicated in patients undergoing abrupt discontinuation of alcohol. In post-marketing experience, there have been rare reports of adverse neuropsychiatric events or reduced alcohol tolerance in patients who were drinking during treatment with bupropion. The consumption of alcohol should be minimized or avoided) 1719
Xenazine Tablets (Patients should be advised that the concomitant use of alcohol or other sedating drugs with tetrabenazine may have additive effects and worsen sedation and somnolence) 2033
Xyzal Oral Solution (Concurrent use of levocetirizine dihydrochloride with alcohol should be avoided because additional reductions in alertness and additional impairment of central nervous system performance may occur) 3449
Xyzal Oral Solution (Concurrent use of levocetirizine dihydrochloride with alcohol should be avoided because additional reductions in alertness and additional impairment of central nervous system performance may occur) 3053
Ziagen Tablets (Ethanol decreases the elimination of abacavir, causing an increase in overall exposure. Co-administration of ethanol and abacavir resulted in a 41% increase in abacavir AUC and a 26% increase in abacavir $t_{1/2}$)........ 1740
Zocor Tablets (Simvastatin should be used with caution in patients who consume substantial quantities of alcohol) 2289
Zonegran Capsules (Concomitant administration of zonisamide and alcohol or other CNS depressants has not been evaluated in clinical studies. Because of the potential of zonisamide to cause CNS depression, as well as other cognitive and/or neuropsychiatric adverse events, zonisamide should be used with caution if used in combination with alcohol or other CNS depressants) 1081
Zyban Sustained-Release Tablets (Bupropion is contraindicated in patients undergoing abrupt discontinuation of alcohol. In post-marketing experience, there have been rare reports of adverse neuropsychiatric events or reduced alcohol tolerance in patients who were drinking alcohol during treatment with bupropion. The consumption of alcohol during treatment with bupropion should be minimized or avoided) 1762
Zydone Tablets (Co-administration may exhibit additive CNS depression) 1138
Zyprexa Tablets (Co-administration of alcohol with olanzapine potentiates orthostatic hypotension; concurrent use should be avoided. Given the primary CNS effects of olanzapine, caution should be used when olanzapine is taken in combination with other centrally-acting drugs and alcohol) 1984
Zyprexa IntraMuscular (Co-administration of alcohol with olanzapine potentiates orthostatic hypotension; concurrent use should be avoided. Given the primary CNS effects of olanzapine, caution should be used when olanzapine is taken in combination with other centrally-acting drugs and alcohol) 1984
Zyrtec Allergy Tablets (Alcohol may increase drowsiness. Avoid alcoholic drinks)........................... 2052
Children's Zyrtec Allergy Chewable Tablets (Alcohol may increase drowsiness. Avoid alcoholic drinks)........................... 2053
Children's Zyrtec Allergy Syrup (Concomitant use may increase drowsiness)............................... 2053
Children's Zyrtec Hives Relief Syrup (Concomitant use may increase drowsiness).................... 2053
Zyrtec-D Allergy & Congestion Extended-Release Tablets (Concurrent use with alcohol may increase drowsiness; avoid alcohol) 2054

Wine products

ActoPlus Met Tablets (Alcohol is known to potentiate the effect of metformin on lactate metabolism. Patients, therefore, should be warned against excessive alcohol intake, acute or chronic, while receiving ActoPlus Met. In addition, hypoglycemia does not occur in patients receiving metformin alone under usual circumstances of use, but could occur when during concomitant use with ethanol) 3338
Adcirca Tablets (Both alcohol and tadalafil, a PDE5 inhibitor, act as mild vasodilators. When mild vasodilators are taken in combination, blood pressure–lowering effects of each individual compound may be increased. Substantial consumption of alcohol (eg, 5 units or greater) in combination with tadalafil can increase the potential for orthostatic signs and symptoms, including increase in heart rate, decrease in standing blood pressure, dizziness, and headache).............. 3461
Adipex-P Tablets (May result in adverse drug interaction) 1178
Advicor Tablets (Concomitant alcohol may increase the flushing and its use should be avoided around the time of Advicor administration).................. 402
Aggrenox Capsules (Patients who consume three or more alcoholic drinks every day should be counseled about the bleeding risks involved with chronic, heavy alcohol use while taking aspirin).............................. 880
Alphagan P Ophthalmic Solution (Possible additive or potentiating effect with CNS depressants) 596
Ambien Tablets (An additive effect on psychomotor performance between alcohol and zolpidem was demonstrated. Zolpidem should not be taken with alcohol) 2920
Ambien CR Tablets (Zolpidem tartrate has shown additive effects when combined with alcohol and should not be taken with alcohol) 2925
Amrix Capsules (Concomitant use with cyclobenzaprine HCl may enhance the effects of alcohol) 964
Apidra Injection (Alcohol may either potentiate or weaken the blood glucose-lowering effect of insulin) 2937
Aplenzin Extended-Release Tablets (Bupropion is contraindicated in patients undergoing abrupt discontinuation of alcohol. Concomitant use of alcohol with bupropion is associated with an increased seizure risk. There have been rare reports of adverse neuropsychiatric events or reduced alcohol tolerance in patients who were drinking alcohol during treatment with bupropion. The consumption of alcohol during treatment with bupropion should be minimized or avoided) 2948
Atacand HCT 16-12.5 Tablets (May aggravate orthostatic hypotension produced by hydrochlorothiazide).......................... 700
Avalide Tablets (Potentiation of orthostatic hypertension may occur during concomitant administration of hydrochlorothiazide with alcohol) 2956
Avandamet Tablets (Alcohol potentiates the effect of metformin on lactate metabolism; patients should be warned against excessive alcohol intake, acute or chronic)..... 1345
Avinza Capsules (Patients must not consume alcoholic beverages, prescription or non-prescription medications containing alcohol while on morphine sulfate therapy. Consumption of alcohol while taking morphine sulfate may result in the rapid release and absorption of a potentially fatal dose of morphine)...................... 1822
Benadryl Allergy Ultratab Tablets (Increases drowsiness effect; avoid concomitant use) 2042
Benicar HCT Tablets (Concurrent administration could cause potentiation of orthostatic hypotension)................................ 1017
Carbatrol Capsules (Because of its primary CNS effect, caution should be used when carbamazepine is taken with alcohol) 3280
Catapres-TTS (Clonidine may potentiate the CNS-depressive effects of alcohol, barbiturates or other sedating drugs)................ 884
Celebrex Capsules (Other factors that increase the risk of GI bleeding in patients treated with NSAIDs include concomitant use of alcohol. Most spontaneous reports of fatal GI events are in elderly or debilitated patients and therefore special care should be taken in treating this population) 3272
Celexa Tablets (Although citalopram did not potentiate cognitive and motor effects of alcohol, as with other psychotropic medications, the use of alcohol by depressed patients taking citalopram is not recommended) 1153
Cialis Tablets (Both alcohol and tadalafil act as mild vasodilators. When mild vasodilators are taken in combination, blood-pressure-lowering effects of each individual compound may be increased. Substantial consumption of alcohol (eg, 5 units or greater) in combination with tadalafil can increase the potential for orthostatic signs and symptoms, including increase in heart rate, decrease in standing blood pressure, dizziness, and headache).............. 1861
Clinoril Tablets (Concomitant use of alcohol may increase the risk of GI bleeding) 2098
Clorpres Tablets (Clonidine may enhance the CNS-depressive effects of alcohol; orthostatic hypotension may be aggravated by alcohol) 2344
Combigan Ophthalmic Solution (Although specific drug interaction studies have not been conducted with Combigan, the possibility of an additive or potentiating effect with CNS depressants (alcohol, barbiturates, opiates, sedatives or anesthetics) should be considered).................. 601
Crestor Tablets (Rosuvastatin calcium should be used with caution in patients who consume substantial quantities of alcohol) 736
Cymbalta Delayed-Release Capsules (Use of duloxetine concomitantly with heavy alcohol intake may be associated with severe liver injury. For this reason, duloxetine should ordinarily not be prescribed for patients with substantial alcohol use)................ 1871

(⊙ Described in PDR® for Ophthalmic Medicines)

Depakote ER Extended Release Tablets (Since valproate products may produce CNS depression, especially when combined with another CNS depressant (eg, alcohol), patients should be advised not to engage in hazardous activities, such as driving an automobile or operating dangerous machinery, until it is known that they do not become drowsy from the drug) 426

Dilaudid Oral Liquid (Hydromorphone may be expected to have additive effects when used in conjunction with alcohol. Alcohol potentiates the respiratory depressant effects of hydromorphone, increasing the risk of respiratory depression that might result in death) 2797

Dilaudid-HP Injection (Hydromorphone may be expected to have additive effects when used in conjunction with alcohol. Alcohol potentiates the respiratory depressant effects of hydromorphone, increasing the risk of respiratory depression that might result in death) 2800

Diovan HCT Tablets (Concurrent use of thiazide diuretics with alcohol may result in potentiation of orthostatic hypotension) 2419

Duetact Tablets (All sulfonylurea drugs are capable of producing hypoglycemia; hypoglycemia is more likely to occur when alcohol is ingested) 3354

Duragesic Transdermal System (Fentanyl may be expected to have additive CNS depressant effects when used in conjunction with alcohol. The concomitant use of fentanyl with alcohol may cause respiratory depression, hypotension, and profound sedation or potentially result in coma) 2604

Effexor XR Extended-Release Capsules (Although venlafaxine has not been shown to increase the impairment of mental and motor skills caused by alcohol, patients should be advised to avoid alcohol while taking venlafaxine) 3504

Elidel Cream 1% (Skin flushing due to pimecrolimus is associated with alcohol use) 2424

Embeda Extended Release Capsules (Embeda should be used with great caution and in reduced dosage in patients who are concurrently receiving other central nervous system (CNS) depressants including alcohol because of the risk of respiratory depression, hypotension, and profound sedation or coma. When such combined therapy is contemplated, the initial dose of one or both agents should be reduced by at least 50%) 1831

Emsam Transdermal System (The use of alcohol is not recommended while using selegiline transdermal system) 3623

Equetro Extended-Release Capsules (Because of its primary CNS effect, caution should be used when carbamazepine is taken with alcohol) 3477

Exforge HCT Tablets (Potentiation of orthostatic hypotension may occur when alcohol and thiazide diuretics are administered concurrently) 2449

Exubera Inhalation Powder (Alcohol may either increase or reduce the blood

glucose-lowering effect of insulin. Co-administration may require insulin dose adjustment and particularly close monitoring) 2717

Fanapt Tablets (Given the primary CNS effects of iloperidone, caution should be used when it is taken in combination with alcohol) 3484

Fentanyl Transdermal System Patches (Fentanyl may be expected to have additive CNS depressant effects when used in conjunction with alcohol. The concomitant use of fentanyl with alcohol may cause respiratory depression, hypotension, and profound sedation, or potentially result in coma or death) 2346

Fentora Tablets (The concomitant use of other CNS depressants, including alcoholic beverages, may produce increased depressant effects. Hypoventilation, hypotension, and profound sedation may occur) 966

Finacea Gel (Concomitant use with any foods and beverages that might provoke erythema, flushing, and blushing (including spicy food, alcoholic beverages, and thermally hot drinks, including hot coffee and tea) should be avoided) 1808

Focalin XR Capsules (Dexmethylphenidate hydrochloride should be given cautiously to patients with a history of drug dependence or alcoholism) 2472

Furosemide Tablets (Aggravates orthostatic hypotension) 2354

Gabitril Tablets (Because of the possible additive effects of drugs that may depress the nervous system, ethanol should be used cautiously in combination with tiagabine) 972

Humalog-Pen and KwikPen (Co-administration with drugs with hypoglycemic activity may result in decreased insulin requirements) 1910

Humalog Mix 50/50-Pen and KwikPen (Insulin requirements may be decreased in the presence of drugs with hypoglycemic activity, such as alcohol) 1914

Humulin N Vial (Insulin requirements may be reduced in the presence of drugs that lower blood glucose or affect how the body responds to insulin) 1934

Humulin R (U-500) (Insulin requirements may be decreased in the presence of drugs that increase insulin sensitivity or have hypoglycemic activity, such as alcohol) 1939

Hyzaar 50-12.5 Tablets (Potentiation of orthostatic hypotension may occur) 2162

Indapamide Tablets (Aggravates orthostatic hypotension) 2356

Intravenous Sodium Diuril (Hypotension including orthostatic hypotension may be aggravated or potentiated by alcohol when co-administered with chlorothiazide) 2009

Intuniv Extended-Release Tablets (Caution should be exercised when guanfacine is administered concomitantly with alcohol due to the potential for additive pharmacodynamic effects) 3291

Invega Extended-Release Tablets (Given the primary CNS effects of paliperidone, paliperidone should be used with caution in combination with other centrally acting drugs and alcohol) 2613

Invega Sustenna Extended-Release Injectable Suspension (Given the primary

CNS effects paliperidone should be used with caution in combination with other centrally acting drugs and alcohol. Paliperidone may antagonize the effect of levodopa and other dopamine antagonists) 2621

Janumet Tablets (Alcohol is known to potentiate the effect of metformin on lactate metabolism. Patients, therefore, should be warned against excessive alcohol intake, acute or chronic, while receiving Janumet) 2188

Klonopin Tablets (The CNS-depressant action of the benzodiazepine class of drugs may be potentiated by alcohol. Patients should be advised to avoid alcohol while taking clonazepam) 2855

Lantus Injection (May either potentiate or weaken the blood-glucose-lowering effect of insulin) 2996

Levemir Injection (Co-administration may either potentiate or weaken the blood-glucose lowering effect of insulin) 2566

Lexapro Tablets (Although escitalopram did not potentiate the cognitive and motor effects of alcohol in a clinical trial, as with other psychotropic medications, the use of alcohol by patients taking escitalopram is not recommended) 1160

Lupron Depot 3.75 mg (In patients with major risk factors for decreased bone mineral content such as chronic alcohol use, leuprolide acetate depot may pose an additional risk. In these patients, the risks and benefits must be weighed carefully before therapy with leuprolide acetate depot alone is instituted, and concomitant treatment with norethindrone acetate 5 mg daily should be considered. Retreatment with gonadotropin-releasing hormone analogs, including leuprolide acetate, is not advisable in patients with major risk factors for loss of bone mineral content) 472

Lyrica Capsules (Patients who are taking other drugs associated with angioedema (eg, angiotensin converting enzyme inhibitors [ACE inhibitors]) may be at increased risk of developing angioedema) 2731

Marplan Tablets (Isocarboxazid should not be administered in combination with some central nervous systems depressants including alcohol) 3481

Meridia Capsules (In a double-blind, placebo-controlled, crossover study in 19 volunteers, administration of a single dose of ethanol (0.5 mL/kg) together with 20 mg of sibutramine resulted in no psychomotor interactions of clinical significance between alcohol and sibutramine. However, the concomitant use of sibutramine and excess alcohol is not recommended) 492

Metozolv ODT Orally Disintegrating Tablets (Additive sedative effects can occur when metoclopramide is given with alcohol, sedatives, hypnotics, narcotics, or tranquilizers) 2901

Mevacor Tablets (Lovastatin should be used with caution in patients who have consumed substantial quantity of alcohol and have a past history of liver disease; active liver disease and unexplained elevation in transaminase are contraindications to the use of lovastatin) 2212

Micardis HCT Tablets (Potentiation of orthostatic hypotension may occur with alcohol, barbiturates, or narcotics when administered concurrently with thiazide diuretics) 889

Moban Tablets (Concomitant use of molindone with alcohol is contraindicated) 1108

MS Contin Tablets (Respiratory depression, hypotension and profound sedation or coma may result) 2803

Nascobal Nasal Spray (Heavy alcohol intake for longer than 2 weeks may produce malabsorption of vitamin B12) 2700

Nembutal Sodium Solution (Concurrent use of barbiturates with other CNS depressants (eg, alcohol) may result in additional CNS depressant effects. Alcohol should not be consumed while taking barbiturates) 2012

Niaspan Extended-Release Tablets (Concomitant alcohol may increase the side effects of flushing and pruritus and should be avoided around the time of Niaspan ingestion) 497

Nitro-Dur Transdermal Infusion System (Enhances sensitivity to the hypotensive effects) 3170

Nitrolingual Pumpspray (Alcohol may enhance sensitivity to hypotensive effects of nitrates) 3266

NovoLog Injection (A number of substances affect glucose metabolism and may require insulin dose adjustment and particularly close monitoring. Examples of substances that may either potentiate or weaken the blood-glucose-lowering effect of insulin include alcohol) 2575

Nucynta Tablets (Due to its mu-opioid agonist activity, tapentadol hydrochloride may be expected to have additive effects when used in conjunction with alcohol, opioids, or illicit drugs that cause central nervous system depression, respiratory depression, hypotension, and profound sedation, coma or death) 2643

Nuvigil Tablets (Patients should be advised that the use of armodafinil in combination with alcohol has not been studied. Patients should be advised that it is prudent to avoid alcohol while taking armodafinil) 978

Onsolis Film (The concomitant use of fentanyl with other CNS depressants, including other opioids, sedatives or hypnotics, general anesthetics, phenothiazines, tranquilizers, skeletal muscle relaxants, sedating antihistamines, and alcoholic beverages may produce increased depressant effects) 2054

Opana Tablets (The concomitant use of other CNS depressants including sedatives, hypnotics, tranquilizers, general anesthetics, phenothiazines, other opioids, and alcohol may produce additive CNS depressant effects. Additive effects resulting in respiratory depression, hypotension, profound sedation or coma may result if these drugs are taken in combination with the usual doses of oxymorphone hydrochloride) 1110

OsmoPrep Tablets (There have been rare reports of generalized tonic-clonic seizures and/or loss of consciousness associated with use of sodium phosphate products in patients with no prior history of seizures. Sodium phosphate should be

used with caution in patients at higher risk of seizure, such as those withdrawing from alcohol) **2907**

OxyContin Tablets (Oxycodone, like all opioid analgesics, should be started at 1/3 to 1/2 of the usual dosage in patients who are concurrently receiving other central nervous system depressants including alcohol because respiratory depression, hypotension, and profound sedation or coma may result) **2807**

Parnate Tablets (Concomitant use with some central nervous system depressants, such as alcohol, is contraindicated. A marked potentiating effect on alcohol has been reported) **1584**

Paroxetine Hydrochloride Controlled-release Tablets (Avoid alcohol while taking paroxetine hydrochloride controlled-release tablets).............**2361**

Paroxetine Hydrochloride Extended-release Tablets (Avoid alcohol while taking paroxetine hydrochloride controlled-release tablets)...............................**2371**

Patanase Nasal Spray (Concurrent use of olopatadine nasal spray with alcohol should be avoided because additional reductions in alertness and additional impairment of central nervous system performance may occur) **585**

Paxil Tablets (Although paroxetine has not been shown to increase the impairment of mental and motor skills caused by alcohol, patients should be advised to avoid alcohol while taking paroxetine) **1586**

Paxil CR Controlled-Release Tablets (Although paroxetine has not been shown to increase the impairment of mental and motor skills caused by alcohol, patients should be advised to avoid alcohol while taking paroxetine) **1596**

Percocet Tablets (Additive CNS depression) **1121**

Percodan Tablets (Additive CNS depression) **1124**

Phenytek Capsules (Acute alcohol intake with phenytoin may increase phenytoin serum levels; chronic alcohol abuse with phenytoin may decrease phenytoin serum levels) **2380**

Photofrin for Injection (Compounds that quench active oxygen species or scavenge radicals, such as ethanol would be expected to decrease photodynamic therapy (PDT) activity).............................**786**

Prinzide Tablets (Co-administration of thiazide and alcohol may potentiate orthostatic hypotension) **2246**

Pristiq Extended-Release Tablets (A clinical study has shown that desvenlafaxine does not increase the impairment of mental and motor skills caused by ethanol. However, patients should be advised to avoid alcohol consumption while taking desvenlafaxine) **3564**

Provigil Tablets (The use of modafinil in combination with alcohol has not been studied. It is advisable to avoid alcohol while taking modafinil)...................**983**

Prozac Weekly Capsules (Concurrent use with alcohol requires caution)...........................**1941**

Pylera Capsules (Alcoholic beverages should not be consumed during Pylera therapy and for at least 1 day afterward. Psychotic reactions have been reported in alcoholic patients who are using Pylera and disulfiram concurrently. Pylera should not be given to patients

who have taken disulfiram within the last 2 weeks)................. **793**

Remeron Tablets (Concomitant administration of alcohol (equivalent to 60 g) had a minimal effect on plasma levels of mirtazapine (15 mg) in healthy male subjects. However, the impairment of cognitive and motor skills produced by mirtazapine were shown to be additive with those produced by alcohol. Accordingly, patients should be advised to avoid alcohol while taking mirtazapine) **3214**

Requip Tablets (Sedating medications (such as alcohol or CNS depressants), may increase the risk of somnolence or falling asleep while engaged in activities of daily living. Because of possible additive effects, caution should be advised when patients are taking other sedating medications, alcohol, or other CNS depressants in combination with ropinirole) **1620**

Requip XL Tablets (Sedating medications (such as alcohol or CNS depressants), may increase the risk of somnolence or falling asleep while engaged in activities of daily living. Because of possible additive effects, caution should be advised when patients are taking other sedating medications, alcohol, or other CNS depressants in combination with ropinirole) **1628**

Rilutek Tablets (Whether alcohol increases the risk of serious hepatotoxicity with riluzole is unknown; therefore, patients being treated with riluzole should be discouraged from drinking excessive amounts of alcohol) **3032**

Risperdal Consta Long-Acting Injection (Given the primary CNS effects of risperidone, caution should be used if taken in combination with alcohol) **2682**

Rozerem Tablets (Complex behaviors, such as "sleep driving" (eg, driving while not fully awake after ingestion of hypnotic) and other complex behaviors (eg, preparing and eating food, making phone calls, or having sex), with amnesia for the event, have been reported in association with hypnotic use. The use of alcohol and other CNS depressants may increase the risk of such behaviors) **3366**

Ryzolt Extended-Release Tablets (Patients should be cautioned about the concomitant use of tramadol products and alcohol because of potentially serious CNS-additive effects of these agents. When large doses of tramadol are administered with alcohol, respiratory depression may result. Prescribe tramadol with caution for patients who use alcohol in excess)...................**2813**

St. Joseph 81 mg Aspirin Chewable and Enteric Coated Tablets (Chronic heavy alcohol users, 3 or more drinks per day, in combination with analgesic/antipyretic drug products containing aspirin increases the risk of adverse GI events, including stomach bleeding) **2045**

Salonpas Arthritis Pain (Having 3 or more alcoholic drinks everyday may increase the chance of stomach bleeding)..........**1805**

Salonpas Pain Relief Patch (Having 3 or more alcoholic drinks everyday may increase the chance of stomach bleeding)........................**1805**

Saphris Tablets (Given the primary CNS effects of asenapine, caution should be used when it is taken in combination with other centrally-acting drugs or alcohol) **3223**

Savella Tablets (Milnacipran hydrochloride should not be prescribed to patients with substantial alcohol use or evidence of chronic liver disease because it is possible that milnacipran hydrochloride may aggravate pre-existing liver disease) **1172**

Seromycin Capsules (Concurrent use increases the possibility and risk of epileptic episodes)........**1956**

Seroquel Tablets (Quetiapine potentiated the cognitive and motor effects of alcohol in a clinical trial in subjects with selected psychotic disorders. Alcoholic beverages should be avoided while taking quetiapine).....**750**

Seroquel XR Extended-Release Tablets (Given the primary CNS effects of quetiapine, caution should be used when it is taken in combination with other centrally acting drugs. Quetiapine potentiated the cognitive and motor effects of alcohol in a clinical trial in subjects with selected psychotic disorders, and alcoholic beverages should be limited while taking quetiapine) **759**

Skelaxin Tablets (The sedative effects of metaxalone and other CNS depressants (eg, alcohol) may be additive. Therefore, caution should be exercised with patients who take more than one of these CNS depressants simultaneously) **1848**

Soriatane Capsules (Clinical evidence has shown that etretinate can be formed with concurrent ingestion of acitretin and ethanol) **3326**

Symbyax Capsules (The co-administration of ethanol with Symbyax may potentiate sedation and orthostatic hypotension. Patients should be advised to avoid alcohol while taking Symbyax)...........................**1965**

Tekturna HCT Tablets (Potentiation of orthostatic hypotension may occur with concurrent use) **2541**

Teveten HCT Tablets (May potentiate orthostatic hypotension)............................ **541**

Thioridazine Hydrochloride Tablets (Thioridazine is capable of potentiating CNS depressants)........**2384**

Thiothixene Capsules (Patients receiving thiothixene should be cautioned about the possible additive effects (which may include hypotension) with CNS depressants and with alcohol. Extreme caution should be used in patients with a history of convulsive disorders or those in a state of alcohol withdrawal, since it may lower the convulsive threshold) **2386**

Toviaz Extended-Release Tablets (Concomitant use with alcohol may enhance the drowsiness caused by fesoterodine)................**2753**

Transderm Scōp Transdermal Therapeutic System (Scopolamine is an anticholinergic agent and causes certain CNS effects, such as drowsiness and dizziness, and hence it should be used with care in patients on concomitant therapy) **2397**

Treximet Tablets (Other factors that increase the risk for gastrointestinal bleeding in patients treated with NSAIDs include concomitant use of alcohol) **1681**

Trilipix Delayed Release Capsules (Excessive alcohol intake should be addressed before triglyceride-lowering drug therapy, such as fenofibric acid, is considered. If the decision is made to use lipid-altering drugs, the patient should be instructed that this does not reduce the importance of adhering to diet) **548**

Trizivir Tablets (Concurrent use with ethanol decreases the elimination of abacavir causing an increase in overall exposure) **1688**

Tussionex Pennkinetic Extended-Release Suspension (Combined use may result in additive CNS depression)...............**3443**

Regular Strength Tylenol Tablets (Severe liver damage may occur if an adult has 3 or more alcoholic drinks every day while using this product) **2049**

Tylenol with Codeine Tablets (Concomitant use with alcohol may produce an additive CNS depression and should be avoided) **2691**

Ultram ER Extended-Release Tablets (Tramadol hydrochloride is contraindicated in acute intoxication with alcohol. Tramadol hydrochloride should be used with caution and in reduced dosages when administered to patients receiving CNS depressants, such as alcohol. Tramadol may be expected to have additive effects when used in conjunction with alcohol) **2693**

Uniphyl Tablets (Concurrent use with a single dose of alcohol (3mL/kg of whiskey) decreases theophylline clearance for up to 24 hours)...............................**2817**

Valium Tablets (Concomitant use with alcohol is not recommended due to enhancement of the sedative effect) **2880**

Venlafaxine Hydrochloride Tablets (Although venlafaxine has not been shown to increase the impairment of mental and motor skills caused by alcohol, patients should be advised to avoid alcohol while taking venlafaxine) **2388**

Vicodin Tablets (May exhibit an additive CNS depression)..............**560**

Vicodin ES Tablets (Additive CNS depression) **561**

Vicodin HP Tablets (Concurrent use results in an additive CNS depression) **563**

Vicoprofen Tablets (May exhibit additive CNS depression)..............**564**

Visudyne for Injection (Co-administration with compounds that quench active oxygen species or scavenge radicals, such as ethanol, would be expected to decrease verteporfin activity) **2549**

Vytorin 10/10 Tablets (Vytorin should be used with caution in patients who consume substantial quantities of alcohol and/or have a past history of liver disease) **2303**

Vytorin 10/10 Tablets (Vytorin should be used with caution in patients who consume substantial quantities of alcohol and/or have a past history of liver disease) **3240**

Wellbutrin Tablets (Bupropion is contraindicated in patients undergoing abrupt discontinuation of alcohol. In post-marketing experience, there have been rare reports of adverse neuropsychiatric events or reduced alcohol tolerance in patients who were drinking during treatment with bupropion. The consumption of alcohol should be minimized or avoided) **1719**

SECTION 3

SIDE EFFECTS INDEX

Presented in this section is an alphabetical list of every side effect reported in the "Adverse Reactions" section of the product labeling as published by *Physicians' Desk Reference*® or supplied by the manufacturer since the printing of the 2010 *PDR*. Under each side effect is an alphabetical list of brands associated with the reaction.

If noted in the underlying text, incidence is shown in parentheses immediately after the brand name. Products reporting an incidence rate of 3% or more are marked with a ▲ symbol at their left. Because incidence data are sometimes drawn from controlled clinical trials, the rates seen in actual clinical practice may vary from those found in published reports.

This index lists only side effects noted in FDA-regulated prescribing information as published by *PDR* or supplied by the manufacturer since the printing of the 2010 *PDR*. To alert you to the full range of possibilities, the entries include adverse effects shared by an entire class of drugs, but not necessarily reported for the specific drug in question. The index is restricted to reactions that may be expected to occur at recommended dosages in the general patient population. Precautions to be taken under special circumstances are not listed, nor are the effects of overdosage.

The page numbers shown for the products refer to the 2010 editions of *Physicians' Desk Reference*® or *PDR*® for *Ophthalmic Medicines* (denoted with the ⊙ symbol).

A

Abdomen, enlarged
▲ Angeliq Tablets (7%) 831
Asacol HD Delayed-Release
   Tablets 2787
Campral Tablets (Rare).................... 1150
Copaxone for Injection..................... 3388
▲ Eloxatin for Injection (2% - < 5%) 2975
Evoxac Capsules 1027
▲ Follistim AQ Cartridge (8%) 3115
Lovaza Capsules (≥ 1 patient)......... 1569
▲ Lupron Depot– 3 Month 22.5 mg
   (< 5%) 483
Nexium Delayed-Release Capsules
   (<1%)... 704
Nexium Delayed-Release Oral
   Suspension (<1%)........................... 704
Nexium I.V. (<1%)............................. 712
Norvir Oral Solution (< 2%) 509
Norvir Soft Gelatin Capsules (<
   2%)... 509
Prograf Capsules (Less frequent)..... 677
Prograf Injection (Less frequent)..... 677
▲ Proleukin for Injection (10%) 2504
Remeron Tablets (Infrequent)........... 3214
RemeronSolTab Tablets
   (Infrequent).................................... 3219
Requip Tablets (Infrequent).............. 1620
Sandostatin LAR Depot..................... 2519
Yaz Tablets.. 864

Abdomen, redistribution/accumulation of body fat
Atripla Tablets................................... 906
Kaletra Oral Solution........................ 458
Kaletra Tablets.................................. 458

Abdominal adhesion
Mirena Intrauterine System 854
Requip Tablets (Infrequent).............. 1620

Abdominal bloating
Activella Tablets................................ 2561
Angeliq Tablets................................. 831

Aralast NP Solvent (≥ 0.2% - <
   0.6%)... 806
Aricept Tablets (Frequent)................ 1045
Aricept ODT Tablets (Frequent)........ 1045
Asacol Delayed-Release Tablets
   (2% or greater)............................... 2786
Bentyl Capsules................................. 780
Bentyl Injection................................. 780
Bentyl Syrup...................................... 780
Bentyl Tablets.................................... 780
Climara Transdermal System........... 841
Climara Pro Transdermal System..... 847
▲ Crinone 4% Gel (13%) 996
▲ Crinone 8% Gel (7% to 12%) 996
Divigel.. 3467
Donnatal Extentabs.......................... 2711
Enjuvia Tablets.................................. 3401
Estrasorb Topical Emulsion.............. 1777
Fleet Prep Kit 3................................. 1145
Imitrex Nasal Spray.......................... 1503
Immunocal Powder Sachets............. 1805
Indocin Capsules (Less than 1%)...... 2167
Indocin I.V. (Less than 1%)............... 2007
Indocin Oral Suspension (Less
   than 1%).. 2167
Indocin Suppositories (Less than
   1%).. 2167
Lexapro Oral Suspension
   (Infrequent).................................... 1160
Lexapro Tablets (Infrequent)............. 1160
Lybrel Tablets................................... 3514
Nadolol Tablets (1 to 5 of 1000
   patients).. 2359
NuvaRing.. 3181
Ortho Evra Transdermal System...... 2648
Ortho Tri-Cyclen Tablets.................. 2663
Ortho Tri-Cyclen Lo Tablets............. 2673
Ortho-Cyclen Tablets........................ 2663
▲ OsmoPrep Tablets (31% - 39%) 2907
Premarin Intravenous....................... 3528
Premarin Tablets............................... 3533
Premarin Vaginal Cream 3540
Premphase Tablets............................ 3549
Prempro Tablets................................ 3549
▲ Prometrium Capsules (100 mg,
   200 mg) (8% - 12%) 3307

Seasonique Tablets 3418
Yaz Tablets....................................... 864

Abdominal conditions, acute, diagnosis or clinical course obscured
Dilaudid Injection............................. 2800
Dilaudid Oral Liquid......................... 2797
Dilaudid Tablets................................ 2797
Dilaudid-HP Injection....................... 2800
Dilaudid-HP Lyophilized Powder
   250 mg.. 2800
Embeda Extended Release
   Capsules.. 1831
Moban Tablets................................... 1108
OxyContin Tablets............................. 2807
Ryzolt Extended-Release Tablets...... 2813

Abdominal discomfort
(*see also under* Distress, abdominal; Distress, gastrointestinal)
▲ Advair HFA 45/21 Inhalation
   Aerosol (1% - 3%).......................... 1288
▲ Advair HFA 115/21 Inhalation
   Aerosol (1% - 3%).......................... 1288
▲ Advair HFA 230/21 Inhalation
   Aerosol (1% - 3%).......................... 1288
Ambien CR Tablets (1%).................... 2925
▲ Amitiza Capsules (2% to 3%) 3351
Axert Tablets..................................... 2593
Biaxin Filmtab Tablets (2%).............. 412
Biaxin Granules (2%)......................... 412
Biaxin XL Filmtab Tablets (2%)......... 412
Carafate Tablets (Less than 0.5%).... 785
Chantix Tablets................................. 2712
Cipro I.V. (≤ 1.7%)............................ 3082
Cipro Oral Suspension (<1%)............ 3073
Cipro Tablets (<1%)........................... 3073
Concerta Extended-Release
   Tablets.. 2598
▲ Cymbalta Delayed-Release
   Capsules (4%).................................. 1871
▲ DynaCirc CR Controlled Release
   Tablets (1.3% - 5.1%)..................... 1432

Embeda Extended Release
   Capsules (<1%)............................... 1831
▲ Epivir-HBV Oral Solution (16%) 1443
▲ Epivir-HBV Tablets (16%) 1443
Exforge Tablets (≥ 0.2%)................... 2443
▲ Fanapt Tablets (1% - 3%) 3484
Fleet Bisacodyl Laxatives................. 1142
Fleet Prep Kit 3................................. 1145
▲ Flovent Diskus 50 mcg (1% to
   3%).. 1463
▲ Flovent Diskus 100 mcg (1% to
   3%).. 1463
▲ Flovent Diskus 250 mcg (1% to
   3%).. 1463
Fluarix Vaccine................................. 1476
▲ Gengraf Capsules (Up to 7%) 440
Imitrex Injection (Frequent)............. 1497
Imitrex Nasal Spray (Infrequent)....... 1503
Imitrex Tablets.................................. 1508
▲ Invega Sustenna
   Extended-Release Injectable
   Suspension (0% - 3%)..................... 2621
▲ Janumet Tablets (2.2% - >5%) 2188
Kapidex Delayed Release
   Capsules (< 2%)............................... 3362
Klonopin Tablets (Infrequent)........... 2855
Klonopin Wafers (Infrequent)............ 2855
▲ Lamictal XR Extended-Release
   Tablets (6%)..................................... 1536
Letairis Tablets................................. 1250
Lexapro Oral Suspension
   (Infrequent).................................... 1160
Lexapro Tablets (Infrequent)............. 1160
▲ Lexiscan Injection (5%) 668
Lipitor Tablets................................... 2703
Nadolol Tablets (1 to 5 of 1000
   patients).. 2359
▲ Neoral Oral Solution (Up to 7%) 2496
▲ Neoral Soft Gelatin Capsules (Up
   to 7%).. 2496
Nucynta Tablets (< 1%)..................... 2643
Pepcid Tablets (Infrequent).............. 2227
Reclast Injection (1.1% - 2%)........... 2509
Requip Tablets (Infrequent).............. 1620
Ryzolt Extended-Release Tablets
   (< 1%).. 2813

▲ Sandostatin Injection (34% to 61%) 2517
▲ Sandostatin LAR Depot (29.1%) 2519
Strattera Capsules 1957
▲ Tasigna Capsules (1% to 10%) 2533
Urocit-K Tablets 2333
Vantas Implant (Less than 2%) 1133
▲ Xenical Capsules (25.5%) 2893
Zantac 25 EFFERdose Tablets 1737
Zantac 150 Tablets 1737
Zantac 300 Tablets 1737
Zantac Injection 1732
Zantac Injection Pharmacy Bulk Package 1735
Zantac Injection Premixed 1732
Zantac Syrup 1737

Abdominal distention
AmBisome for Injection (Less common) 659
▲ Amitiza Capsules (0% to 6%) 3351
▲ Arranon Injection (0% to 6%) 1327
Avalide Film-Coated Tablets 2956
Avalide Tablets 2956
Avapro Tablets (Less than 1%) 2962
Byetta Injection 648
▲ Cancidas for Injection (< 5%) 2088
Chantix Tablets 2712
Crixivan Capsules 2113
Cubicin for Injection (< 1%) 999
▲ Dacogen Injection (5%) 1054
▲ Doxil Injection (1% to 10%) 939
Duragesic Transdermal System (< 1%) 2604
DynaCirc CR Controlled Release Tablets (1.2%) 1432
Effexor XR Extended-Release Capsules (Rare) 3504
Embeda Extended Release Capsules (<1%) 1831
Exforge Tablets (≥ 0.2%) 2443
Fentanyl Transdermal System Patches (< 1%) 2346
Fentora Tablets (Greater than 1%) 966
▲ Flolan for Injection (4%) 1453
Follistim AQ Cartridge 3115
Fosamax Oral Solution (0% - 1.4%) 2138
Fosamax Tablets (0% - 1.4%) 2138
Fosamax Plus D Tablets (0% - 1.4%) 2147
Gengraf Capsules (1% to less than 3%) 440
▲ Gleevec Tablets (1% - 10%) 2477
Imitrex Injection 1497
Imitrex Nasal Spray 1503
▲ Indocin I.V. (1% to 3%) 2007
▲ Intron A for Injection (Less than 5%) 3140
Invanz for Injection (> 0.1%) 2172
Kaletra Oral Solution (< 2%) 458
Kaletra Tablets (< 2%) 458
Ketek Tablets (≥ 0.2% - < 2%) 2991
Lialda Tablets (< 1%) 3295
Lyrica Capsules (2%) 2731
Mavik Tablets (0.3% to 1%) 489
Merrem I.V. (Greater than 0.1% to 1%) 745
▲ Mirena Intrauterine System (< 5%) 854
▲ MoviPrep Oral Solution (59.8%) 2905
▲ Myfortic Tablets (3% - < 20%) 2491
NeoProfen Injection 2015
Neoral Oral Solution (1% to less than 3%) 2496
Neoral Soft Gelatin Capsules (1% to less than 3%) 2496
Noroxin Tablets (0.1% - 0.2%) 2220
Onsolis Film (≥ 1%) 2054
▲ Opana Tablets (1% to less than 10%) 1110
▲ Opana ER Tablets (1% to less than 10%) 1114
Ortho Evra Transdermal System (< 2.5%) 2648
Pentasa Capsules (Less than 1%) 3297
Percocet Tablets 1121
▲ Prometrium Capsules (100 mg, 200 mg) (8%) 3307
Reclast Injection (0.6% - 2%) 2509
ReoPro Vials (0.1%) 1952
Requip Tablets (Infrequent) 1620
Rilutek Tablets (Infrequent) 3032
Rythmol SR Extended Release Capsules 1652
Ryzolt Extended-Release Tablets (< 1%) 2813
Sabril Tablets (0% - 2%) 2025
▲ Sandostatin Injection (Less than 10% to 35%) 2517
Sandostatin LAR Depot 2519
Savella Tablets 1172
Seroquel Tablets (Rare) 750
▲ Simulect for Injection (3% to 10%) 2524
Stromectol Tablets 2277
Symbyax Capsules (2%) 1965
Tasigna Capsules (0.1% to 1%) 2533
▲ Treanda for Injection (5%) 989
Treximet Tablets (Infrequent) 1681
▲ Trisenox Injection (8%) 994
Uloric Tablets (< 1%) 3370
▲ Valcyte Tablets (< 5%) 2872
Valcyte for Oral Solution 2872
Venlafaxine Hydrochloride Tablets (Infrequent) 2388
▲ Xeloda Tablets (Less than 5%) 2882
Xifaxan Tablets (Less than 2%) 2909

Abdominal guarding
Sandostatin Injection (Rare) 2517
Sandostatin LAR Depot 2519

Abdominal pain, gynecological
▲ Follistim AQ Cartridge (25%) 3115
Ortho Micronor Tablets 2660

Abdominal pain, lower
Apriso Capsules (< 3%) 2899
Chantix Tablets 2712
▲ Cymbalta Delayed-Release Capsules (4%) 1871
Embeda Extended Release Capsules (<1%) 1831
Exjade Tablets 2456
▲ Myfortic Tablets (3% - < 20%) 2491
▲ Plan B One-Step Tablets (13.3%) 3416
Reclast Injection 2509
Requip Tablets (Infrequent) 1620
Ryzolt Extended-Release Tablets (< 1%) 2813
Zyprexa Tablets 1984
Zyprexa ZYDIS Orally Disintegrating Tablets 1984

Abdominal pain, upper
Actonel Tablets 2779
Advate (1 event) 801
▲ Apriso Capsules (5%) 2899
Arcalyst for Subcutaneous Injection 2824
Axert Tablets 2593
▲ Banzel Tablets (3%) 1050
Boniva Tablets 2844
▲ Cancidas for Injection (< 5%) 2088
▲ Celebrex Capsules (6% to 8%) 3272
Chantix Tablets 2712
Cialis Tablets (< 2%) 1861
▲ Clolar for Intravenous Infusion (7.8%) 1234
▲ Concerta Extended-Release Tablets (5.9%) 2598
Creon Delayed-Release Capsules 3304
▲ Cymbalta Delayed-Release Capsules (4%) 1871
▲ Dacogen Injection (5%) 1054
▲ Depakote ER Extended Release Tablets (8%) 426
Diovan Tablets (> 1%) 2413
Diovan HCT Tablets (> 0.2%) 2419
▲ Elidel Cream 1% (0.3% - 5.5%) 2424
Emend for Injection (Greater than 0.5%) 2132
▲ Exelon Patch (1% to 3%) 2437
Exforge Tablets (≥ 0.2%) 2443
Exforge HCT Tablets (> 0.2%) 2449
Exjade Tablets 2456
▲ Gleevec Tablets (6.2%) 2477
▲ Intuniv Extended-Release Tablets (10% - 11%) 3291
Invanz for Injection (1%) 2172
▲ Invega Extended-Release Tablets (0% - 3%) 2613
▲ Invega Sustenna Extended-Release Injectable Suspension (0% - 3%) 2621
Ketek Tablets (≥ 0.2% - < 2%) 2991
▲ MoviPrep Oral Solution (5.8%) 2905
Mycamine for Injection 670
▲ Myfortic Tablets (3% - < 20%) 2491
Nuvigil Tablets (2%) 978
▲ PegIntron Powder for Injection (12%) 3188
▲ Reclast Injection (0.9% - 4.6%) 2509
▲ Requip Tablets (3%) 1620
Rituxan I.V. (2%) 1216
▲ Ryzolt Extended-Release Tablets (1% - < 5%) 2813
▲ Sabril for Oral Solution (2% - 5%) 2017
▲ Sabril Tablets (5%) 2025
▲ Sandostatin LAR Depot (10.5%) 2519
Strattera Capsules 1957
Toviaz Extended-Release Tablets (0.5% - 1.1%) 2753
▲ Treanda for Injection (5%) 989
▲ Ultram ER Extended-Release Tablets (1% to less than 5%) 2693
▲ Velcade for Injection (12%) 2324
VESIcare Tablets (1.2% - 1.9%) 694
Zyprexa Tablets 1984
Zyprexa ZYDIS Orally Disintegrating Tablets 1984

Abdominal pain/cramps
(*see also under* Abdominal pain, lower; Abdominal pain, upper)
Accolate Tablets (1.8% to 2.8%) 3612
▲ Aciphex Tablets (3.6%) 1035
▲ Actimmune (8%) 1810
Activella Tablets 2561
▲ Actonel Tablets (7.3% to 12.2%) 2779
ActoPlus Met Tablets 3338
Actos Tablets 3345
Aczone Gel 5% 593
Advair Diskus 100/50 1275
Advair Diskus 250/50 1275
Advair Diskus 500/50 1275
▲ Advair HFA 45/21 Inhalation Aerosol (1% - 3%) 1288
▲ Advair HFA 115/21 Inhalation Aerosol (1% - 3%) 1288
▲ Advair HFA 230/21 Inhalation Aerosol (1% - 3%) 1288
▲ Advicor Tablets (4%) 402
▲ Afinitor Tablets (3% - 9%) 2398
▲ Aggrenox Capsules (17.5%) 880
▲ Albenza Tablets (0% - 6%) 1298
Aldara Cream, 5% 1771
▲ Alimta for Injection (1% - 5%) 1850
Allegra-D 12 Hour Extended-Release Tablets (1.4%) 2915
Allegra-D 24 Hour Extended-Release Tablets (1.4%) 2918
Aloxi Injection (Less than 1%) 1042
Ambien Tablets (2%) 2920
▲ AmBisome for Injection (9.9% to 19.8%) 659
Amerge Tablets (Infrequent) 1306
Aminohippurate Sodium "PAH" Injection 2084
▲ Amitiza Capsules (3% to 8%) 3351
Amoxil Capsules 1311
Amoxil Chewable Tablets 1311
Amoxil Pediatric Drops for Oral Suspension 1311
Amoxil Powder for Oral Suspension 1311
Amoxil Tablets 1311
▲ Anaprox Tablets (3% to 9%) 2850
▲ Anaprox DS Tablets (3% to 9%) 2850
▲ Angeliq Tablets (11%) 831
▲ Angiomax for Injection (5%) 2061
▲ Anzemet Injection (3.2%) 2931
Anzemet Tablets 2934
▲ Aplenzin Extended-Release Tablets (3% - 9%) 2948
Apriso Capsules 2899
▲ Aranesp for Injection (10%) 607
▲ Argatroban Injection (2.6% to 3.6%) 1314
Aricept Tablets (Frequent) 1045
Aricept ODT Tablets (Frequent) 1045
▲ Aromasin Tablets (6% - 11%) 2758
▲ Arranon Injection (0% to 9%) 1327
▲ Asacol Delayed-Release Tablets (18%) 2786
Asacol HD Delayed-Release Tablets (2.3%) 2787
▲ Asmanex Twisthaler (2% to 6%) 3058
Atacand Tablets (More than 1%) 697
Atacand HCT 16-12.5 Tablets (0.5% or greater) 700
Atacand HCT 32-12.5 Tablets (0.5% or greater) 700
▲ Atripla Tablets (Greater than or equal to 2%) 906
Augmentin Tablets 1335
Augmentin ES-600 Powder for Oral Suspension 1338
Augmentin XR Extended Release Tablets (1.6%) 1342
Avalide Film-Coated Tablets (2%) 2956
Avalide Tablets (2%) 2956
▲ Avandamet Tablets (5%) 1345
Avandaryl Tablets 1356
Avapro Tablets (1% or greater) 2962
▲ Avastin IV (8% - 61%) 1187
Avelox I.V. (≥0.1% to < 2%) 3064
Avelox Tablets (≥0.1% to < 2%) 3064
▲ Avinza Capsules (5% - 10%) 1822
Axert Tablets (Infrequent) 2593
▲ Axid Capsules (7.5%) 1381
▲ Azilect Tablets (5%) 3383
▲ Azmacort Inhalation Aerosol (1% to 3%) 408
Bactroban Cream (Less than 1%) 1383
Benicar Tablets (Greater than 0.5%) 1015
Benicar HCT Tablets (Greater than 1%) 1017
Bentyl Capsules 780
Bentyl Injection 780
Bentyl Syrup 780
Bentyl Tablets 780
Benzaclin Topical Gel 2965
▲ Betaseron for SC Injection (16%) 836
▲ Bexxar (3% to 15%) 1388
▲ Biaxin Filmtab Tablets (2% - 3%) 412
▲ Biaxin Granules (2% - 3%) 412
▲ Biaxin XL Filmtab Tablets (2% - 3%) 412
Bicillin C-R Injectable Suspension 1826
▲ Boniva Injection (5.3% to 7.8%) 2840
▲ Boniva Tablets (5% - 8%) 2844
▲ Boostrix Vaccine (1.2% to 26%) 1395
Byetta Injection 648
Bystolic Tablets (Greater than or equal to 1%) 1147
Campral Tablets (Frequent) 1150
▲ Canasa Rectal Suppositories (5.2%) 782
▲ Cancidas for Injection (4% - 9%) 2088
Captopril Tablets (About 0.5% to 2%) 2341
Carbatrol Capsules 3280
Catapres-TTS (Less frequent) 884
Ceftin for Oral Suspension (0.1% to 1%) 1399
Ceftin Tablets (0.1% to 1%) 1399
▲ Celebrex Capsules (4% to 7%) 3272
▲ Celexa Oral Solution (3%) 1153
▲ Celexa Tablets (3%) 1153
Cervidil Vaginal Insert (< 1%) 1159
▲ Chantix Tablets (5% - 7%) 2712
▲ Chemet Capsules (5.2% - 15.7%) 2001
Cialis Tablets (1% - 2%) 1861
Cimzia 3426
▲ Cipro I.V. (≤ 3.3%) 3082
▲ Cipro Oral Suspension (<1% to 3.3%) 3073
▲ Cipro Tablets (<1% to 3.3%) 3073
Cipro XR Tablets (<1%) 3091
▲ Climara Transdermal System (0% - 16%) 841
▲ Climara Pro Transdermal System (4.2%) 847
▲ Clinoril Tablets (10%) 2098
▲ Clolar for Intravenous Infusion (34.8%) 1234
Clorpres Tablets 2344
▲ Coartem Tablets (8% - 17%) 2403
▲ Combivir Tablets (6% - 9%) 1404
▲ Comtan Tablets (8%) 2409
▲ Concerta Extended-Release Tablets (Greater than 5%) 2598
Correctol Delayed-Release Tablets, USP 3263
Cosmegen for Injection 2003
Cozaar Tablets (1% or greater) 2106
▲ Creon Delayed-Release Capsules (Most common - 9%) 3304
Crestor Tablets (2.4%) 736
▲ Crinone 4% Gel (5%) 996
▲ Crinone 8% Gel (9% to 12%) 996
▲ Crixivan Capsules (16.6%) 2113
▲ Cubicin for Injection (0.2% - 5.8%) 999
▲ Cymbalta Delayed-Release Capsules (4%) 1871
▲ Dacogen Injection (14%) 1054
Dapsone Tablets USP 1819
Daytrana Transdermal Patch 3283
▲ Depakote ER Extended Release Tablets (7% - 23%) 426
Dilaudid Injection (Less frequent) 2800
Dilaudid Oral Liquid (Less frequent) 2797
Dilaudid Tablets (Less frequent) 2797
Dilaudid-HP Injection (Less frequent) 2800
Dilaudid-HP Lyophilized Powder 250 mg (Less frequent) 2800
Diovan Tablets (2%) 2413
Diovan HCT Tablets (> 0.2%) 2419
Divigel 3467
▲ Dorzolamide Hydrochloride/Timolol Maleate Ophthalmic Solution (1% - 5%) ⊙243
▲ Doxil Injection (1% to 33.5%) 939
Duac Topical Gel 3317
Duetact Tablets 3354
▲ Duragesic Transdermal System (≥ 1% to 10%) 2604
Dyazide Capsules 1429
▲ EC-Naprosyn Delayed-Release Tablets (3% to 9%) 2850
E.E.S. 200 Liquid (Most frequent) 437
E.E.S. 400 Liquid (Most frequent) 437
E.E.S. 400 Filmtab Tablets (Most frequent) 437
E.E.S. Granules (Most frequent) 437
▲ Effexor XR Extended-Release Capsules (6%) 3504
▲ Eldepryl Capsules (4 of 49 patients) 3312
▲ Elidel Cream 1% (0.3% - 4.4%) 2424
▲ Elitek (20%) 2973
Elmiron Capsules (2%) 2611
▲ Eloxatin for Injection (18% - 33%) 2975
Elspar for Injection 2122
▲ Embeda Extended Release Capsules (≥1% - <10%) 1831
▲ Emend Capsules (4.6%) 2124
▲ Emend for Injection (Greater than 0.5% - 4.6%) 2132

Incidence data in parenthesis; ▲ 3% or more   (☉ Described in PDR® for Ophthalmic Medicines)

Alopecia, reversible

Alopecia hereditaria

ALT elevation

(*see under* Alanine aminotransferase levels, elevation of)

Altered saliva

Alveolar proteinosis

Alveolitis

Alveolitis, allergic

Alveolitis, fibrosing

Alzheimer's type dementia

Amaurosis

Amblyopia

Amblyopia, toxic

Amenorrhea

Amnesia

Incidence data in parenthesis; ▲ 3% or more   (⊙ Described in PDR® for Ophthalmic Medicines)

Incidence data in parenthesis; ▲ 3% or more   (⊙ Described in PDR® for Ophthalmic Medicines)

Incidence data in parenthesis; ▲ 3% or more   (⊙ Described in PDR® for Ophthalmic Medicines)

Angioedema, cutaneous

Angioedema, extremities

Angioedema, eyes

Angioedema, face

Angioedema, glottis

Angioedema, intestinal

Angioedema, larynx

Angioedema, lips

Angioedema, mucous membranes of the mouth

Angioedema, oropharyngeal

Angioedema, throat

Angioedema, tongue

Incidence data in parenthesis; ▲ 3% or more   (⊙ Described in PDR® for Ophthalmic Medicines)

Incidence data in parenthesis; ▲ 3% or more   (⊙ Described in PDR® for Ophthalmic Medicines)

Aspartate transaminase, increased

Aspergillosis, bronchopulmonary

Asphyxia

Aspiration

AST elevation
(see under Aspartate aminotransferase levels, elevation of)

Asterixis

Asthenia

Incidence data in parenthesis; ▲ 3% or more   (⊙ Described in PDR® for Ophthalmic Medicines)

Asthenopia

Asthma, allergic

Asthma, bronchial

Asthma, worsening of

Asthmatic episodes

Behavioral deterioration

Behavioral disturbances, exacerbation of

Belching

Bell's palsy

Benign prostatic hyperplasia

Benzyl alcohol, sensitivity to

Bezoar

Bigeminy

Bile duct obstruction

Bile duct sludge, presence of metabolites

Biliary duct dilation

Biliary lithiasis

Biliary secretions, decrease in

Biliary sludge

Biliary stasis

Biliary tract abnormalities

Biliary tract spasm

Bilirubin, conjugated, increased

Bilirubin, indirect, changes

Bilirubin, total, decrease

Bilirubin, total, increase

Bilirubinemia

Bilirubinuria

Binge eating, unspecified

Bipolar illness

Birth, premature

Birth defects, increased risk of

Birth weight, low

Births, multiple

Black stools

Bladder, contracted

Bladder, hypertonic

Bladder, irritability

Bladder, neurogenic

Bladder, spasms

Bladder disorders

Bladder dysfunction

Incidence data in parenthesis; ▲ 3% or more   (⊙ Described in PDR® for Ophthalmic Medicines)

Incidence data in parenthesis; ▲ 3% or more   (☉ Described in PDR® for Ophthalmic Medicines)

Incidence data in parenthesis; ▲ 3% or more   (⊙ Described in PDR® for Ophthalmic Medicines)

Incidence data in parenthesis; ▲ 3% or more   (☉ Described in PDR® for Ophthalmic Medicines)

Incidence data in parenthesis; ▲ 3% or more   (☉ Described in PDR® for Ophthalmic Medicines)

Incidence data in parenthesis; ▲ 3% or more

(⊙ Described in PDR® for Ophthalmic Medicines)

Incidence data in parenthesis; ▲ 3% or more   (⊙ Described in PDR® for Ophthalmic Medicines)

Incidence data in parenthesis; ▲ 3% or more   (☉ Described in PDR® for Ophthalmic Medicines)

Incidence data in parenthesis; ▲ 3% or more   (⊙ Described in PDR® for Ophthalmic Medicines)

Incidence data in parenthesis; ▲ 3% or more   (⊙ Described in PDR® for Ophthalmic Medicines)

Incidence data in parenthesis; ▲ 3% or more   (☉ Described in PDR® for Ophthalmic Medicines)

E

Incidence data in parenthesis; ▲ 3% or more   (⊙ Described in PDR® for Ophthalmic Medicines)

Emesis
(*see under* Vomiting)

Emotional disturbances

Emotional lability

Emphysema

Enanthema

Encephalitis

Encephalitis, measles inclusion body

Encephalomyelitis

Encephalomyopathy, mitochondrial, exacerbation of

Encephalopathy

Encephalopathy, hepatic

Encephalopathy, hypertensive

Encephalopathy, post-viral

Endocardial fibrosis

Endocarditis

Endocarditis, infectious

Endocrine disturbances

Endometrial carcinoma
(*see under* Carcinoma, endometrial)

Endometrial disorder, unspecified

Incidence data in parenthesis; ▲ 3% or more   (⊙ Described in PDR® for Ophthalmic Medicines)

Incidence data in parenthesis; ▲ 3% or more   (⊙ Described in PDR® for Ophthalmic Medicines)

Incidence data in parenthesis; ▲ 3% or more

(☉ Described in PDR® for Ophthalmic Medicines)

Hepatic enzymes, elevation

(see also under Serum transaminase, elevation; SGPT elevation)

Hepatic enzymes, increased

Hepatic eosinophilic infiltration

Hepatic failure

Incidence data in parenthesis; ▲ 3% or more   (⊙ Described in PDR® for Ophthalmic Medicines)

Incidence data in parenthesis; ▲ 3% or more   (☉ Described in PDR® for Ophthalmic Medicines)

Incidence data in parenthesis; ▲ 3% or more   (⊙ Described in PDR® for Ophthalmic Medicines)

Incidence data in parenthesis; ▲ 3% or more   (⊙ Described in PDR® for Ophthalmic Medicines)

Incidence data in parenthesis; ▲ 3% or more   (☉ Described in PDR® for Ophthalmic Medicines)

Incidence data in parenthesis; ▲ 3% or more

(⊙ Described in PDR® for Ophthalmic Medicines)

Incidence data in parenthesis; ▲ 3% or more   (⊙ Described in PDR® for Ophthalmic Medicines)

Incidence data in parenthesis; ▲ 3% or more   (☉ Described in PDR® for Ophthalmic Medicines)

Incidence data in parenthesis; ▲ 3% or more   (⊙ Described in PDR® for Ophthalmic Medicines)

Infection, upper respiratory tract

Infection, upper respiratory tract, viral

Infection, urinary tract

Incidence data in parenthesis; ▲ 3% or more   (⊙ Described in PDR® for Ophthalmic Medicines)

Incidence data in parentheses; ▲ 3% or more   (⊙ Described in PDR® for Ophthalmic Medicines)

Incidence data in parenthesis; ▲ 3% or more

(⊙ Described in PDR® for Ophthalmic Medicines)

Incidence data in parenthesis; ▲ 3% or more   (⊙ Described in PDR® for Ophthalmic Medicines)

Incidence data in parenthesis; ▲ 3% or more   (⊙ Described in PDR® for Ophthalmic Medicines)

Incidence data in parenthesis; ▲ 3% or more   (⊙ Described in PDR® for Ophthalmic Medicines)

Incidence data in parenthesis; ▲ 3% or more   (⊙ Described in PDR® for Ophthalmic Medicines)

Incidence data in parenthesis; ▲ 3% or more   (☉ Described in PDR® for Ophthalmic Medicines)

Incidence data in parenthesis; ▲ 3% or more   (⊙ Described in PDR® for Ophthalmic Medicines)

Incidence data in parenthesis; ▲ 3% or more   (☉ Described in PDR® for Ophthalmic Medicines)

Neck, rigidity of

Necrolysis, epidermal, toxic (right column header)

Neck, spasms of

Neck, stiffness of

Neck, redistribution/accumulation of body fat

Neck tightness

Necrolysis, epidermal

Necrolysis, epidermal, toxic

Incidence data in parenthesis; ▲ 3% or more (⊙ Described in PDR® for Ophthalmic Medicines)

Incidence data in parenthesis; ▲ 3% or more   (☉ Described in PDR® for Ophthalmic Medicines)

Incidence data in parenthesis; ▲ 3% or more   (☉ Described in PDR® for Ophthalmic Medicines)

▲ Tice BCG (4% - 17%) 3238
▲ Tobi Nebulizer Solution for Inhalation (8.1%) 2546
▲ Torisel Injection (28%) 3592
▲ Travatan Z Ophthalmic Solution (1% to 5%) 587
▲ Treanda for Injection (6%) 989
Tricor Tablets 544
▲ Trilipix Delayed Release Capsules (1.4% - 3.5%) 548
▲ Trisenox Injection (15%) 994
Trizivir Tablets (<1%) 1688
▲ Truvada Tablets (≥ 5%) 1258
Uloric Tablets (< 1%) 3370
Ultane Liquid for Inhalation (Less than 1%) 554
▲ Ultram ER Extended-Release Tablets (1% to less than 5%) 2693
Uroxatral Tablets (1% - 2%) 3050
▲ Vagifem Tablets (3% to 5%) 2589
▲ Valcyte Tablets (< 5%) 2872
Valcyte for Oral Solution 2872
Vantas Implant (Less than 2%) 1133
Venlafaxine Hydrochloride Tablets 2388
Vicoprofen Tablets (Less than 3%) 564
▲ Viread Tablets (7% to 13%) 1266
▲ Welchol Tablets (6.7%) 1029
Wellbutrin Tablets (Infrequent) 1719
▲ Wellbutrin SR Sustained-Release Tablets (2% - 3%) 1725
▲ Xeloda Tablets (Less than 5%) 2882
Xifaxan Tablets (Less than 2%) 2909
▲ Xolair (7%) 1230
▲ Xolair (7%) 2551
Yaz Tablets (Greater than 1%) 864
Ziagen Oral Solution (< 1%) 1740
Ziagen Tablets (< 1%) 1740
▲ Zomig Tablets (13% - 22%) 773
▲ Zomig-ZMT Tablets (13% - 22%) 773
▲ Zosyn for Injection (1.7% to 3.2%) 3607
Zovirax Capsules 1760
Zovirax Suspension 1760
Zovirax Tablets 1760
Zyban Sustained-Release Tablets (Infrequent) 1762

Pain, upper extremities

Cipro I.V. (<= 1%) 3082
Engerix-B Vaccine (< 1%) 1434
Prinivil Tablets (0.3% to 1%) 2241
Timoptic in Ocudose ⊙ 231

Pain, urethral

Ceftin Tablets (0.1% to 1%) 1399
Protonix for Delayed-Release Oral Suspension (Less than 1%) 3571
Protonix Delayed-Release Tablets (Less than 1%) 3571
Protonix I.V. (Less than 1%) 3575
Salagen Tablets (Less than 1%) 1072
Savella Tablets (≥2%) 1172
▲ Valstar Sterile Solution for Intravesical Instillation (3%) 1131

Pain, urinary bladder

Duragesic Transdermal System (< 1%) 2604
Effexor XR Extended-Release Capsules (Infrequent) 3504
Fentanyl Transdermal System Patches (< 1%) 2346
ReoPro Vials (0.1%) 1952
▲ Valstar Sterile Solution for Intravesical Instillation (28%) 1131
Venlafaxine Hydrochloride Tablets (Infrequent) 2388
Zonegran Capsules (Rare) 1081

Pain, wrist

Cipro Oral Suspension 3073
Cipro Tablets 3073

Pain at injection site

▲ Alferon N Injection (12%) 1801
Aloxi Injection (Very rare) 1042
▲ Amevive (7% to common) 665
▲ Angiomax for Injection (2.7% to 8%) 2061
Anzemet Injection 2931
▲ Aranesp for Injection (6%) 607
Arcalyst for Subcutaneous Injection 2824
Attenuvax 2086
▲ BeneFIX Vials (6.2%) 3497
▲ Betaseron for SC Injection (16% - 78%) 836
Bicillin C-R Injectable Suspension 1826
Bicillin L-A Injection 1828
▲ Boostrix Vaccine (1.6% to 75.3%) 1395
▲ BOTOX for Injection (3% - 10%) 596
Calcijex Injection (Occasional) 422
Capastat Sulfate for Injection 1860
Cimzia 3426
Cipro I.V. (<= 1%) 3082
▲ Comvax (23.9% to 34.5%) 2103
▲ Copaxone for Injection (40%) 3388
Delatestryl Injection 1102
Dilaudid Injection (Rare) 2800
Dilaudid-HP Injection (Rare) 2800
Dilaudid-HP Lyophilized Powder 250 mg (Rare) 2800
Doxil Injection (Less than 1%) 939
▲ Dysport for Injection (3% - 5%) 1813
▲ Dysport for Injection (3% - 5%) 2067
▲ Eligard 7.5 mg (4.3%) 2968
▲ Eligard 22.5 mg (3.5%) 2968
Eligard 30 mg (2.3%) 2968
▲ Eligard 45 mg (4.6%) 2968
Eloxatin for Injection 2975
Enbrel for Subcutaneous Injection 613
Engerix-B Vaccine (< 1%) 1434
▲ Extavia Kit (16%) 2459
▲ Faslodex Injection (10.9%) 741
▲ Flolan for Injection (13%) 1453
▲ Fluarix Vaccine (12.2% - 54.7%) 1476
▲ Flulaval Injection Vaccine (21% - 24%) 1479
Fortaz Injection 1481
Fortaz for Injection 1481
Forteo for Injection 1895
▲ Fragmin Injection (2% to 12%) 1058
▲ Gardasil Injection (60.7% - 83.9%) 2154
Genotropin Lyophilized Powder (Infrequent) 2763
▲ Geodon for Injection (7% - 9%) 2723
▲ Havrix Injection Vaccine (9.5% - 21%) 1485
Humatrope Vials and Cartridges (Infrequent) 1920
▲ Humira Injection Syringe and Pen (12% - 19%) 448
▲ Hyalgan Solution (23%) 2988
Imitrex Injection 1497
▲ Infanrix Injection Vaccine (31.9% - 53.3%) 1513
▲ Intron A for Injection (Less than 5%) 3140
▲ Invega Sustenna Extended-Release Injectable Suspension (69% - 100%) 2621
Kineret Injection 877
▲ Kinrix Injection Vaccine (57%) 1519
Lantus Injection (2.7%) 2996
▲ Leustatin Injection (9% to 19%) 946
Lovenox Injection (2%) 3005
Merrem I.V. (0.4%) 745
Meruvax II 2210
Nembutal Sodium Solution 2012
Neulasta 629
Novantrone for Injection Concentrate 1088
Nutropin for Injection (Infrequent) 1204
▲ Pediarix Vaccine (31.2% - 36.1%) 1606
Liquid PedvaxHIB 2225
▲ PegIntron Powder for Injection (1% - 3%) 3188
Pneumovax 23 2230
Premarin Intravenous 3528
Prevnar 3557
Primaxin I.M. (1.2%) 2232
Primaxin I.V. (0.7%) 2235
▲ ProQuad (22%) 2254
Protonix I.V. (Greater than 1%) 3575
Reclast Injection 2509
Recombivax HB (Equal to or greater than 1%) 2262
ReoPro Vials (0.1%) 1952
Retrovir IV Infusion (Infrequent) 1640
▲ Risperdal Consta Long-Acting Injection (< 4%) 2682
Rocephin Injectable Vials (1%) 2859
▲ Romazicon Injection (3% to 9%) 2863
▲ Sandostatin Injection (7.7%) 2517
▲ Sandostatin LAR Depot (2% to 50%) 2519
Temodar Injection 3230
Timentin ADD-Vantage 1670
Timentin Injection Galaxy Container 1674
Timentin IV Infusion 1666
Timentin Pharmacy Bulk Package 1678
▲ Trisenox Injection (20%) 994
Tygacil for Injection (< 2%) 3596
▲ Vaqta (1.2% to 51.1%) 2281
▲ Varivax (19.3% to 32.5%) 2285
Velcade for Injection 2324
Vimpat Injection (2.5%) 3444
Xolair 2551
Xolair 1230
Zantac Injection 1732
Zantac Injection Pharmacy Bulk Package 1735
Zantac Injection Premixed 1732
Zeel Injection Solution 1801
▲ Zofran Injection (4%) 1750
▲ Zofran Injection Premixed (4%) 1750
▲ Zostavax Injection (33.4%) 2299
Zosyn for Injection (0.2%) 3607
Zyprexa IntraMuscular (Frequent) 1984

Pain at insertion site

▲ Implanon Implant (2.9% - 5.2%) 3128
▲ Supprelin LA Implant (4.3% to 51.1%) 1127
▲ Vantas Implant (3.6%) 1133

Pain secondary to eczema

Bactroban Cream (One report) 1383

Pain, procedural

Exforge HCT Tablets (> 0.2%) 2449
Kapidex Delayed Release Capsules (< 2%) 3362
▲ Risperdal Consta Long-Acting Injection (< 4%) 2682

Pallor

Advair Diskus 100/50 1275
Advair Diskus 250/50 1275
Advair Diskus 500/50 1275
Advair HFA 45/21 Inhalation Aerosol 1288
Advair HFA 115/21 Inhalation Aerosol 1288
Advair HFA 230/21 Inhalation Aerosol 1288
Allegra-D 12 Hour Extended-Release Tablets 2915
Allegra-D 24 Hour Extended-Release Tablets 2918
Ambien Tablets (Infrequent) 2920
Ambien CR Tablets (Infrequent) 2925
Bicillin C-R Injectable Suspension 1826
Bicillin L-A Injection 1828
Captopril Tablets (2 to 5 of 1000 patients) 2341
Catapres-TTS (Less frequent) 884
Cimzia 3426
Clorpres Tablets 2344
▲ Dacogen Injection (23%) 1054
Dapsone Tablets USP 1819
▲ Doxil Injection (1% to 10%) 939
Effexor XR Extended-Release Capsules (Rare) 3504
Enbrel for Subcutaneous Injection 613
EpiPen Auto-Injector 3631
EpiPen Jr. Auto-Injector 3631
Evoxac Capsules (< 1%) 1027
Fentora Tablets (Greater than 1%) 966
▲ Flolan for Injection (21% to 32%) 1453
Flulaval Injection Vaccine 1479
Gabitril Tablets (Infrequent) 972
Humira Injection Syringe and Pen 448
Imitrex Injection (Rare) 1497
Imitrex Nasal Spray (Rare) 1503
Imitrex Tablets (Infrequent) 1508
Intuniv Extended-Release Tablets (< 2%) 3291
Mirena Intrauterine System 854
Nitrolingual Pumpspray (Occasional) 3266
Paroxetine Hydrochloride Controlled-release Tablets 2361
Paroxetine Hydrochloride Extended-release Tablets 2371
Paxil Oral Suspension (Rare) 1586
Paxil Tablets (Rare) 1586
Paxil CR Controlled-Release Tablets (Rare) 1596
Pediarix Vaccine 1606
ReoPro Vials (0.1%) 1952
Rythmol SR Extended Release Capsules 1652
Ryzolt Extended-Release Tablets (< 1%) 2813
▲ Serevent Diskus (9%) 1656
Thioridazine Hydrochloride Tablets 2384
▲ Trisenox Injection (10%) 994
Twinject Auto-Injector 3268
Venlafaxine Hydrochloride Tablets (Rare) 2388
Wellbutrin Tablets (Rare) 1719
WinRho SDF 824

Palmar-plantar erythrodysesthesia syndrome

▲ Afinitor Tablets (5%) 2398
▲ Clolar for Intravenous Infusion (15.7%) 1234
▲ Doxil Injection (3.4% to 50.6%) 939
▲ Eloxatin for Injection (1% - 11%) 2975
Kepivance 875
▲ Sutent Capsules (3% to 14%) 2747
Taxotere Injection Concentrate 3035
▲ Tykerb Tablets (53%) 1698
▲ Xeloda Tablets (17% to 54%) 2882

Palpitations

Accutane Capsules 2832
Adcirca Tablets 3461
Adenocard IV Injection (Less than 1%) 656
Adenoscan (< 1%) 657
Adipex-P Capsules 1178
Adipex-P Tablets 1178
Advair Diskus 100/50 1275
Advair Diskus 250/50 1275
Advair Diskus 500/50 1275
Advicor Tablets 402
Aggrenox Capsules (Less than 1%) 880
Aldara Cream, 5% 1771
Allegra-D 12 Hour Extended-Release Tablets (1.9%) 2915
Allegra-D 24 Hour Extended-Release Tablets (1.9%) 2918
Ambien Tablets (2%) 2920
Ambien CR Tablets (1%) 2925
Amerge Tablets (Infrequent) 1306
Amitiza Capsules (Less than 1%) 3351
Amrix Capsules 964
Anaprox Tablets (Less than 3%) 2850
Anaprox DS Tablets (Less than 3%) 2850
Anzemet Injection (Rare) 2931
Anzemet Tablets (Rare) 2934
▲ Aplenzin Extended-Release Tablets (2% - 6%) 2948
Atacand Tablets (0.5% or greater) 697
Atacand HCT 16-12.5 Tablets (0.5% or greater) 700
Atacand HCT 32-12.5 Tablets (0.5% or greater) 700
Atripla Tablets 906
Avelox I.V. (≥0.1% to < 2%) 3064
Avelox Tablets (≥0.1% to < 2%) 3064
▲ Avinza Capsules (< 5%) 1822
Axert Tablets (Infrequent) 2593
▲ Azor Tablets (0.7% - 4.5%) 1010
Bentyl Capsules 780
Bentyl Injection 780
Bentyl Syrup 780
Bentyl Tablets 780
▲ Betaseron for SC Injection (4%) 836
Betimol Ophthalmic Solution 3490
Bicillin C-R Injectable Suspension 1826
Bicillin L-A Injection 1828
Campral Tablets (Frequent) 1150
Captopril Tablets (Approximately 1 of 100 patients) 2341
Cardizem LA Extended Release Tablets (Less than 2%) 423
Catapres-TTS (Less frequent) 884
Celebrex Capsules (0.1% to 1.9%) 3272
Celexa Oral Solution 1153
Celexa Tablets 1153
Chantix Tablets (Infrequent) 2712
Cialis Tablets (< 2%) 1861
Cipro I.V. (<= 1%) 3082
Cipro Oral Suspension (<1%) 3073
Cipro Tablets (<1%) 3073
Cipro XR Tablets 3091
Clarinex Syrup 3098
Clarinex Tablets 3098
Clarinex Reditabs Tablets 3098
Clarinex-D 12-Hour Extended-Release Tablets 3101
Clarinex-D 24-Hour Extended-Release Tablets 3104
Clinoril Tablets (Less than 1 in 100) 2098
Clorpres Tablets (5/1,000 patients) 2344
▲ Coartem Tablets (18%) 2403
Combigan Ophthalmic Solution 601
▲ Concerta Extended-Release Tablets (3.1%) 2598
▲ Copaxone for Injection (9%) 3388
▲ Coreg Tablets (> 1% - < = 3%) 1409
▲ Coreg CR Extended-Release Capsules (> 1% - < = 3%) 1416
Cozaar Tablets (Less than 1%) 2106
Cymbalta Delayed-Release Capsules (Frequent to 2%) 1871
Daytrana Transdermal Patch 3283
▲ Depakote ER Extended Release Tablets (>1% - <5%) 426
Dexedrine Spansule Sustained-Release Capsules 1425
Dilaudid Injection (Less frequent) 2800
Dilaudid Oral Liquid (Less frequent) 2797
Dilaudid Tablets (Less frequent) 2797
Dilaudid-HP Injection (Less frequent) 2800
Dilaudid-HP Lyophilized Powder 250 mg (Less frequent) 2800
Diovan Tablets (> 0.2%) 2413
Diovan HCT Tablets (> 0.2%) 2419
Donnatal Extentabs 2711
Dorzolamide Hydrochloride/Timolol Maleate Ophthalmic Solution ⊙ 243
Doxil Injection (Less than 1%) 939
▲ DynaCirc CR Controlled Release Tablets (1.2% - 4%) 1432

Paresthesia, application site

Paresthesia, circumoral

Incidence data in parenthesis; ▲ 3% or more   (⊙ Described in PDR® for Ophthalmic Medicines)

Incidence data in parenthesis; ▲ 3% or more   (⊙ Described in PDR® for Ophthalmic Medicines)

Incidence data in parenthesis; ▲ 3% or more   (⊙ Described in PDR® for Ophthalmic Medicines)

Incidence data in parenthesis; ▲ 3% or more   (⊙ Described in PDR® for Ophthalmic Medicines)

Rheumatism, articular

Rheumatoid arthritis

Rheumatoid arthritis, worsening of

Rhinitis

Serum triglyceride, elevation
(see under Hypertriglyceridemia)

Serum vitamin B12 levels, subnormal

Sex hormone binding globulin, decreased

Sex hormone binding globulin, elevated

Sex steroids, elevation of

Sexual activity, decrease

Sexual dysfunction

Sexual maturity, accelerated

SGOT changes
(see under Aspartate
aminotransferase levels,
changes in)

SGOT elevation
(see also under Aspartate
aminotransferase levels,
elevation of)

SGPT changes
(see under Alanine
aminotransferase levels,
changes in)

SGPT elevation
(see also under Alanine
aminotransferase levels,
elevation of)

Shaking
(see under Tremors)

Shininess, skin

Shivering
(see also under Tremors)

Shock

Shock, anaphylactic
(see under Anaphylactic shock)

Shock, cardiogenic

Shock, hemorrhagic

Shortness of breath

SIADH secretion syndrome
(see under ADH syndrome,
inappropriate)

Sialadenitis

Incidence data in parenthesis; ▲ 3% or more   (⊙ Described in PDR® for Ophthalmic Medicines)

Incidence data in parenthesis; ▲ 3% or more   (⊙ Described in PDR® for Ophthalmic Medicines)

Incidence data in parenthesis; ▲ 3% or more   (⊙ Described in PDR® for Ophthalmic Medicines)

Incidence data in parenthesis; ▲ 3% or more   (⊙ Described in PDR® for Ophthalmic Medicines)

Incidence data in parenthesis; ▲ 3% or more   (☉ Described in PDR® for Ophthalmic Medicines)

2501 Side Effects Index Tinnitus

Estrasorb Topical Emulsion 1777
Femara Tablets 2466
Lybrel Tablets 3514
NuvaRing 3181
Ortho Evra Transdermal System 2648
Ortho Tri-Cyclen Tablets 2663
Ortho Tri-Cyclen Lo Tablets 2673
Orthoclone OKT3 Sterile Solution 949
Ortho-Cyclen Tablets 2663
Premarin Intravenous 3528
Premarin Tablets 3533
Premarin Vaginal Cream 3540
Premphase Tablets 3549
Prempro Tablets 3549
▲ Procrit for Injection (Up to 10%) 954
Prograf Capsules 677
Prograf Injection 677
Seasonique Tablets 3418
▲ Taxotere Injection Concentrate (3.4% - 3.6%) 3035
▲ Xeloda Tablets (Less than 1% to 8%) 2882

Thrombosis at injection site
Mycamine for Injection 670

Thrombosis of vascular access
▲ Aranesp for Injection (6%) 607
▲ Epogen for Injection (39%) 621
Furosemide Tablets 2354
Procrit for Injection 954

Thrombotic events, cardiovascular
Celebrex Capsules 3272
Clinoril Tablets 2098
Flector Patch 1839
Treximet Tablets 1681
Vicoprofen Tablets 564

Thrombotic events, unspecified
▲ Aranesp for Injection (6.2%) 607
BeneFIX Vials 3497
▲ Epogen for Injection (3.2% - 10.8%) 621
Gammagard S/D 815
Gamunex 3374
Herceptin I.V. 1194
LoSeasonique Tablets 3407
Lybrel Tablets 3514
NovoSeven RT 2584
NuvaRing 3181
Ortho Tri-Cyclen Tablets 2663
Ortho Tri-Cyclen Lo Tablets 2673
Ortho-Cyclen Tablets 2663
Procrit for Injection 954
Promacta Tablets (7 patients) 1610
▲ Tarceva Tablets (11%) 1222
Treximet Tablets 1681
Wellbutrin Tablets (Infrequent) 1719
Wellbutrin SR Sustained-Release Tablets (Infrequent) 1725
Zyban Sustained-Release Tablets (Infrequent) 1762

Thrombotic events, venous
LoSeasonique Tablets 3407
Lybrel Tablets 3514
NuvaRing 3181
Symbyax Capsules 1965
Yaz Tablets 864
Zyprexa IntraMuscular 1984

Thrombotic microangiopathy
Avastin IV 1187
Epogen for Injection 621
Rapamune Oral Solution 3579
Rapamune Tablets 3579
Sutent Capsules 2747

Thrombotic vascular disease
Accutane Capsules 2832
Aranesp for Injection 607
Epogen for Injection 621
Nascobal Nasal Spray 2700
NuvaRing 3181
Ortho Evra Transdermal System 2648
Ortho Tri-Cyclen Tablets 2663
Ortho Tri-Cyclen Lo Tablets 2673
Ortho-Cyclen Tablets 2663

Thrombus formation, increased risk of
Angiomax for Injection 2061

Thrush, oral
(*see under* Candidiasis, oral)

Thymus gland abnormalities, fetal
Accutane Capsules 2832

Thyroid binding globulin, increase
(*see under* T4, increase)

Thyroid disease, exacerbation
Genotropin Lyophilized Powder 2763
Humatrope Vials and Cartridges 1920
Proleukin for Injection 2504

Thyroid disorder, unspecified
Betaseron for SC Injection 836
Chantix Tablets (Infrequent) 2712
Extavia Kit 2459
Genotropin Lyophilized Powder 2763
Humatrope Vials and Cartridges 1920
Moban Tablets 1108
PegIntron Powder for Injection 3188
Premphase Tablets 3549
Prempro Tablets 3549
▲ Rebif Prefilled Syringe for Injection (4% - 6%) 1096
Solodyn Extended Release Tablets 2073
Sutent Capsules 2747
Zomig Nasal Spray (Rare) 768

Thyroid disorders
(*see under* T3, decrease; T4, decrease; T4, increase)

Thyroid function test, abnormal
Carbatrol Capsules 3280
Crestor Tablets 736
Depakote ER Extended Release Tablets 426
InnoPran XL Extended Release Capsules 1517
Mevacor Tablets 2212

Thyroid gland discoloration
Solodyn Extended Release Tablets 2073

Thyroid hormone, changes
(*see under* T3, decrease; T4, decrease; T4, increase)

Thyroid hormone, increased
Climara Transdermal System 841
NuvaRing 3181
Ortho Evra Transdermal System 2648
Ortho Tri-Cyclen Tablets 2663
Ortho Tri-Cyclen Lo Tablets 2673
Ortho-Cyclen Tablets 2663
Premarin Vaginal Cream 3540
Premphase Tablets 3549
Prempro Tablets 3549

Thyroid nodule
Effexor XR Extended-Release Capsules (Rare) 3504
Venlafaxine Hydrochloride Tablets (Rare) 2388

Thyroid stimulating hormone elevation
Avodart Soft Gelatin Capsules 1375
Nexium Delayed-Release Capsules (≤ 1%) 704
Nexium Delayed-Release Oral Suspension (≤ 1%) 704
Nexium I.V. (≤1%) 712
PegIntron Powder for Injection 3188
Welchol Tablets (Rare) 1029

Thyroiditis
Aldara Cream, 5% 1771
Effexor XR Extended-Release Capsules (Rare) 3504
Gardasil Injection (4 patients/10,706 patients) 2154
Geodon Capsules (Rare) 2723
Paroxetine Hydrochloride Controlled-release Tablets 2361
Paroxetine Hydrochloride Extended-release Tablets 2371
Paxil Oral Suspension (Rare) 1586
Paxil Tablets (Rare) 1586
Paxil CR Controlled-Release Tablets (Rare) 1596
PegIntron Powder for Injection 3188
Tasigna Capsules 2533
Venlafaxine Hydrochloride Tablets (Rare) 2388

Thyrotoxicosis
Synthroid Tablets 529

Thyroxin-binding globulin, decrease
AndroGel 3456
Ortho Micronor Tablets 2660

Tics
Concerta Extended-Release Tablets 2598
▲ Daytrana Transdermal Patch (7%) 3283
Focalin XR Capsules 2472
Lamictal Chewable Dispersible Tablets 1522
Lamictal ODT Orally Disintegrating Tablets 1522
Lamictal Tablets 1522
Lamictal XR Extended-Release Tablets 1536
Lexapro Oral Suspension (Infrequent) 1160
Lexapro Tablets (Infrequent) 1160
▲ Vyvanse Capsules (2%) 3298

Tightness, feeling of
Axert Tablets 2593
Dysport for Injection 2067
▲ Rocephin Injectable Vials (5% - 17%) 2859

Tinea cruris
Aldara Cream, 5% (> 1%) 1771

Tingling
Alkeran for Injection 1300
Avelox I.V. 3064
Avelox Tablets 3064
Bentyl Capsules 780
Bentyl Injection 780
Bentyl Syrup 780
Bentyl Tablets 780
Cimzia 3426
Cipro I.V. 3082
Cipro Oral Suspension 3073
Cipro Tablets 3073
Cipro XR Tablets 3091
DynaCirc CR Controlled Release Tablets (≤ 0.5% - 1%) 1432
Dysport for Injection 2067
Dysport for Injection (Most frequent) 1813
▲ Elocon Ointment 0.1% (4.8%) 3114
Engerix-B Vaccine (< 1%) 1434
Gengraf Capsules (Rare) 440
Humulin 50/50, 100 Units 1930
Humulin 70/30 Vial 1931
Humulin N Vial 1934
Humulin R 1937
▲ Imitrex Injection (14%) 1497
Imitrex Nasal Spray (Infrequent) 1503
▲ Imitrex Tablets (4% to 8%) 1508
K-Phos Original (Sodium Free) Tablets (Less frequent) 874
K-Phos Neutral Tablets 873
Levaquin Injection 2629
Levaquin Oral Solution 2629
Levaquin Tablets 2629
Levaquin in 5% Dextrose Injection 2629
Neoral Oral Solution (Rare) 2496
Neoral Soft Gelatin Capsules (Rare) 2496
Niaspan Extended-Release Tablets (Most common) 497
Noroxin Tablets 2220
▲ Panretin Gel 0.1% (3% to 22%) 1070
Profilnine SD 1797
▲ Protopic Ointment (1% to 8%) 685
Twinrix Vaccine (<1%) 1694
Visine-A Eye Allergy Relief Eye Drops ⊙257

Tingling, ears
Ciprodex Otic Suspension (1 patient) 583

Tingling, extremities
Humulin R 1937
▲ Indapamide Tablets (Less than 5%) 2356

Tingling, feet
Alferon N Injection (1%) 1801
Humulin 50/50, 100 Units 1930
Humulin 70/30 Vial 1931
Humulin N Vial 1934
Humulin R 1937
Sabril for Oral Solution 2017
Sabril Tablets 2025
Uroqid-Acid No. 2 Tablets 874

Tingling, fingers
Noroxin Tablets (0.3% - 1%) 2220

Tingling, hands
Adenocard IV Injection (1%) 656
Humulin 50/50, 100 Units 1930
Humulin 70/30 Vial 1931
Humulin N Vial 1934
Humulin R 1937
Uroqid-Acid No. 2 Tablets 874

Tingling, legs
Alferon N Injection (1%) 1801

Tingling, lips
Humulin 50/50, 100 Units 1930
Humulin 70/30 Vial 1931
Humulin N Vial 1934
Humulin R 1937
K-Phos Original (Sodium Free) Tablets (Less frequent) 874
K-Phos Neutral Tablets 873
Uroqid-Acid No. 2 Tablets 874

Tingling, skin
Aldara Cream, 5% 1771
▲ Finacea Gel (4% - 16%) 1808

Tingling, toes
Sabril for Oral Solution 2017
Sabril Tablets 2025

Tingling, tongue
Humulin 50/50, 100 Units 1930
Humulin 70/30 Vial 1931
Humulin N Vial 1934
Humulin R 1937

Tinnitus
Accutane Capsules 2832
Adcirca Tablets 3461
Aggrenox Capsules (Less than 1%) 880
Alferon N Injection (One patient) 1801
Aloxi Injection (Less than 1%) 1042
Ambien Tablets (Infrequent) 2920
Ambien CR Tablets (1%) 2925
Amerge Tablets (Infrequent) 1306
▲ Anaprox Tablets (3% to 9%) 2850
▲ Anaprox DS Tablets (3% to 9%) 2850
Anzemet Injection (Rare) 2931
Anzemet Tablets (Rare) 2934
▲ Aplenzin Extended-Release Tablets (3% - 6%) 2948
Apriso Capsules (< 3%) 2899
Aricept Tablets (Infrequent) 1045
Aricept ODT Tablets (Infrequent) 1045
Asacol Delayed-Release Tablets 2786
Asacol HD Delayed-Release Tablets 2787
Atacand HCT 16-12.5 Tablets (0.5% or greater) 700
Atacand HCT 32-12.5 Tablets (0.5% or greater) 700
Atripla Tablets 906
Avelox I.V. (< 0.1%) 3064
Avelox Tablets (< 0.1%) 3064
Axert Tablets (Infrequent) 2593
Bayer Aspirin 829
Biaxin Filmtab Tablets 412
Biaxin Granules 412
Biaxin XL Filmtab Tablets 412
Bicillin C-R Injectable Suspension 1826
Bicillin L-A Injection 1828
Campral Tablets (Infrequent) 1150
Capastat Sulfate for Injection 1860
Carbatrol Capsules 3280
Cardizem LA Extended Release Tablets (Less than 2%) 423
Celebrex Capsules (0.1% to 1.9%) 3272
Celexa Oral Solution (Infrequent) 1153
Celexa Tablets (Infrequent) 1153
Chantix Tablets (Infrequent) 2712
Cialis Tablets (< 2%) 1861
Cipro I.V. (<= 1%) 3082
Cipro Oral Suspension (<1%) 3073
Cipro Tablets (<1%) 3073
Cipro XR Tablets 3091
Clinoril Tablets (Greater than 1%) 2098
Coartem Tablets (< 3%) 2403
Combigan Ophthalmic Solution 601
Coreg Tablets (> 0.1% - < = 1%) 1409
Coreg CR Extended-Release Capsules (> 0.1% - < = 1%) 1416
Cozaar Tablets (Less than 1%) 2106
Cubicin for Injection (< 1%) 999
Cymbalta Delayed-Release Capsules (Infrequent) 1871
Dapsone Tablets USP 1819
▲ Depakote ER Extended Release Tablets (>1% - 7%) 426
Diovan HCT Tablets (> 0.2%) 2419
Dorzolamide Hydrochloride/Timolol Maleate Ophthalmic Solution ⊙243
Doxil Injection (Less than 1%) 939
▲ EC-Naprosyn Delayed-Release Tablets (3% to 9%) 2850
Effexor XR Extended-Release Capsules (2%) 3504
Eldepryl Capsules 3312
Elmiron Capsules (≤ 1%) 2611
▲ Emend Capsules (3.7%) 2124
▲ Emend for Injection (3.7%) 2132
Emsam Transdermal System (Frequent) 3623
Engerix-B Vaccine 1434

Incidence data in parenthesis; ▲ 3% or more   (⊙ Described in PDR® for Ophthalmic Medicines)

Incidence data in parenthesis; ▲ 3% or more   (☉ Described in PDR® for Ophthalmic Medicines)

Visual disturbances, flashing lights

Visual field defect

Visual impairment

Vital signs, fluctuations of

Vitamin B12 deficiency

Vitiligo

Vitreous detachment

Vitreous disorder, unspecified

Vitreous floaters

Incidence data in parenthesis; ▲ 3% or more   (☉ Described in PDR® for Ophthalmic Medicines)

Vulva, dryness
(see under Vagina, dryness)

Vulvovaginal disorder, unspecified

Vulvovaginitis

W

Walking disorders

Wandering

Warm sensation

Warm to touch

Warmth

Warmth at injection site

Warts
(see under Verruca)

Water excretion, impaired

Water intoxication

Water retention
(see under Edema)

WBC, abnormal

WBC, immature

WBC counts, fluctuation

WBC counts, increase

Weakness
(see under Asthenia)

Weakness, feet

Weakness, hands

Weakness, legs

Weakness, local

Weakness, musculoskeletal

Weeping, skin

Weight change, unspecified

Weight changes, increase or decrease

Weight decrease
(see under Weight loss)

Weight gain

Incidence data in parenthesis; ▲ 3% or more   (☉ Described in PDR® for Ophthalmic Medicines)

Incidence data in parenthesis; ▲ 3% or more

(⊙ Described in PDR® for Ophthalmic Medicines)

SECTION 4

INDICATIONS INDEX

This section lists in alphabetical order every indication cited in the product labeling as published by *Physicians' Desk Reference*® or supplied by the manufacturer since the printing of the 2010 *PDR*, with cross-references to each product entry in which the indication is found. For easy comparison, each listing includes the product's brand name, generic ingredients, and manufacturer. Page numbers refer to the 2010 editions of *Physicians' Desk Reference*® or *PDR*® for Ophthalmic Medicines (denoted with the ⊙ symbol).

Because *PDR* publishes only FDA-regulated prescribing information, only approved indications are cited here. No unapproved uses are listed.

This index is intended to assist you in identifying the extent and nature of prescribing alternatives as quickly and easily as possible. However, it is only an extract of the product labeling. For more definitive information, consult the *PDR* or manufacturer.

(⊙ Described in PDR® for Ophthalmic Medicines)

(⊙ Described in PDR® for Ophthalmic Medicines)

(☉ Described in PDR® for Ophthalmic Medicines)

(⊙ Described in PDR® for Ophthalmic Medicines)

(⊙ Described in PDR® for Ophthalmic Medicines)

(⊙ Described in PDR® for Ophthalmic Medicines)

(⊙ Described in PDR® for Ophthalmic Medicines)

(⊙ Described in PDR® for Ophthalmic Medicines)

(⊙ Described in PDR® for Ophthalmic Medicines)

(⊙ Described in PDR® for Ophthalmic Medicines)

(⊙ Described in PDR® for Ophthalmic Medicines)

(⊙ Described in PDR® for Ophthalmic Medicines)

(⊙ Described in PDR® for Ophthalmic Medicines)

(⊙ Described in PDR® for Ophthalmic Medicines)

(⊙ Described in PDR® for Ophthalmic Medicines)

(⊙ Described in PDR® for Ophthalmic Medicines)

(⊙ Described in PDR® for Ophthalmic Medicines)

(⊙ Described in PDR® for Ophthalmic Medicines)

(⊙ Described in PDR® for Ophthalmic Medicines)

(⊙ Described in PDR® for Ophthalmic Medicines)

(⊙ Described in PDR® for Ophthalmic Medicines)

(☉ Described in PDR® for Ophthalmic Medicines)

SECTION 5

CONTRAINDICATIONS INDEX

This section lists in alphabetical order every medical condition cited as a contraindication in the product labeling as published by *Physicians' Desk Reference®* or supplied by the manufacturer since the printing of the 2010 *PDR*, with cross-references to all product entries in which the contraindication is found. Page numbers refer to the 2010 editions of *Physicians' Desk Reference®* or *PDR®* for *Ophthalmic Medicines* (denoted with the ⊙ symbol).

These listings help you to quickly identify drugs that generally threaten to be inappropriate in the presence of a given complication. However, a drug's suitability is sometimes affected by the severity of the complicating condition,

the age or gender of the patient, and the drug's route of administration. In ambiguous situations, consult the *PDR* or manufacturer.

Note, too, that the index does not list other drugs and dietary items whose use would present a contraindication. Contraindicated combinations can be found in the Interactions Index and the Food Interactions Cross-Reference. Hypersensitivity to the product's ingredients—an almost universal contraindication—also has not been indexed here. If the clinical picture includes the risk of allergic reaction, check individual product labeling for additional information.

(⊙ Described in PDR® for Ophthalmic Medicines)

(⊙ Described in PDR® for Ophthalmic Medicines)

(☉ Described in PDR® for Ophthalmic Medicines)

(⊙ Described in PDR® for Ophthalmic Medicines)

(⊙ Described in PDR® for Ophthalmic Medicines)

Key to Controlled Substances Categories

Products listed with the symbols shown below are subject to the Controlled Substances Act of 1970. These drugs are categorized according to their potential for abuse. The greater the potential, the more severe the limitations on their prescription.

CATEGORY	INTERPRETATION
ℂ II	**HIGH POTENTIAL FOR ABUSE.** Use may lead to severe physical or psychological dependence. Prescriptions must be written in ink, or typewritten and signed by the practitioner. Verbal prescriptions must be confirmed in writing within 72 hours, and may be given only in a genuine emergency. No renewals are permitted.
ℂ III	**SOME POTENTIAL FOR ABUSE.** Use may lead to low-to-moderate physical dependence or high psychological dependence. Prescriptions may be oral or written. Up to 5 renewals are permitted within 6 months.
ℂ IV	**LOW POTENTIAL FOR ABUSE.** Use may lead to limited physical or psychological dependence. Prescriptions may be oral or written. Up to 5 renewals are permitted within 6 months.
ℂ V	**SUBJECT TO STATE AND LOCAL REGULATION.** Abuse potential is low; a prescription may not be required.

Key to FDA Use-in-Pregnancy Ratings

The U.S. Food and Drug Administration's use-in-pregnancy rating system weighs the degree to which available information has ruled out risk to the fetus against the drug's potential benefit to the patient. The ratings, and their interpretation, are as follows:

CATEGORY	INTERPRETATION
A	**CONTROLLED STUDIES SHOW NO RISK.** Adequate, well-controlled studies in pregnant women have failed to demonstrate a risk to the fetus in any trimester of pregnancy.
B	**NO EVIDENCE OF RISK IN HUMANS.** Adequate, well-controlled studies in pregnant women have not shown increased risk of fetal abnormalities despite adverse findings in animals, or, in the absence of adequate human studies, animal studies show no fetal risk. The chance of fetal harm is remote, but remains a possibility.
C	**RISK CANNOT BE RULED OUT.** Adequate, well-controlled human studies are lacking, and animal studies have shown a risk to the fetus or are lacking as well. There is a chance of fetal harm if the drug is administered during pregnancy; but the potential benefits may outweigh the potential risk.
D	**POSITIVE EVIDENCE OF RISK.** Studies in humans, or investigational or post-marketing data, have demonstrated fetal risk. Nevertheless, potential benefits from the use of the drug may outweigh the potential risk. For example, the drug may be acceptable if needed in a life-threatening situation or serious disease for which safer drugs cannot be used or are ineffective.
X	**CONTRAINDICATED IN PREGNANCY.** Studies in animals or humans, or investigational or post-marketing reports, have demonstrated positive evidence of fetal abnormalities or risk which clearly outweighs any possible benefit to the patient.

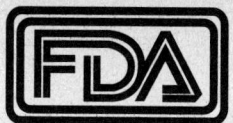

U.S. FOOD AND DRUG ADMINISTRATION

Medical Product Reporting Programs

MedWatch (24-hour service) **800-332-1088**
Reporting of problems with drugs, devices, biologics (except vaccines), medical foods, and dietary supplements.

Vaccine Adverse Event Reporting System (24-hour service) **800-822-7967**
Reporting of vaccine-related problems.

Mandatory Medical Device Reporting **240-276-1673**
Reporting required from user facilities regarding device-related deaths and serious injuries.

Veterinary Adverse Drug Reaction Program **888-332-8387**
Reporting of adverse drug events in animals.

Division of Drug Marketing, Advertising, and Communication (DDMAC) ...**301-796-1200**
Inquiries from health professionals regarding product promotion.

Information for Health Professionals

Center for Drug Evaluation and Research Drug Information Hotline **301-827-4573**
Information on human drugs including hormones.

Center for Biologics Office of Communications **301-827-2000**
Information on biological products including vaccines and blood.

Center for Devices and Radiological Health **800-638-2041**
Automated request for information on medical devices and radiation-emitting products.

Emergency Operations **301-443-1240**
Emergencies involving FDA-regulated products, tampering reports, and emergency Investigational New Drug requests.

Office of Orphan Products Development **301-827-3666**
Information on products for rare diseases.

General Information

General Consumer Inquiries **888-463-6332**
Consumer information on regulated products/issues.

Freedom of Information **301-827-6500**
Requests for publicly available FDA documents.

Office of Public Affairs **301-827-6250**
Interviews/press inquiries on FDA activities.

Center for Food Safety and Applied Nutrition **888-723-3366**
Information on food safety, seafood, dietary supplements, women's nutrition, and cosmetics.

Consumer Information Service, Center for Devices and Radiological Health ...**800-638-2041**
Information on medical devices, mammography facilities, and radiation-emitting products.

POISON CONTROL CENTERS

The American Association of Poison Control Centers (AAPCC) uses a single, nationwide emergency number to automatically link callers with their regional poison center. This toll-free number, **800-222-1222**, also works for **teletype lines (TTY)** for the hearing-impaired and **telecommunication devices (TTD)** for individuals who are deaf. However, a few local poison centers and the ASPCA/Animal Poison Control Center are not part of this nationwide system and continue to use separate numbers.

Most of the centers listed below are accredited by the AAPCC. **Certified centers are marked by an asterisk after the name.** Each has to meet certain criteria. It must, for example, serve a large geographic area; it must be open 24 hours a day and provide direct-dial or toll-free access; it must be supervised by a medical director; and it must have registered pharmacists or nurses available to answer questions from the public.

Within each state, centers are listed alphabetically by city. Some state poison centers also list their original emergency numbers (including TTY/TDD) that only work within that state. For these listings, callers may use either the state number or the nationwide 800 number.

ALABAMA

BIRMINGHAM

Regional Poison Control Center (*)
Children's Hospital of Alabama

1600 7th Ave. South
Birmingham, AL 35233
Business: 205-939-6334
Emergency: 800-222-1222
www.chsys.org

TUSCALOOSA

Alabama Poison Center (*)

2503 Phoenix Dr.
Tuscaloosa, AL 35405
Business: 800-462-0609
Emergency: 800-222-1222
             800-462-0800 (AL)
www.alapoisoncenter.org

ALASKA

JUNEAU

Alaska Poison Control System
Section of Injury Prevention and EMS

410 Willoughby Ave., Room 103
Box 110616
Juneau, AK 99811-0616
Business: 907-465-3027
Emergency: 800-222-1222
www.chems.alaska.gov

(PORTLAND, OR)

Oregon Poison Center (*)
Oregon Health and Science University

3181 SW Sam Jackson Park Rd.
CB550
Portland, OR 97239
Business: 503-494-8600
Emergency: 800-222-1222
www.oregonpoison.com

ARIZONA

PHOENIX

Banner Poison Control Center (*)
Banner Good Samaritan Medical Center

1111 E. McDowell
Phoenix, AZ 85006
Business: 602-495-4884
Emergency: 800-222-1222
www.bannerpoisoncontrol.com

TUCSON

Arizona Poison and Drug Information Center (*)
Arizona Health Sciences Center

1295 N. Martin Ave., Room B308
Tucson, AZ 85721
Business: 520-626-7899
Emergency: 800-222-1222
www.pharmacy.arizona.edu/outreach/poison

ARKANSAS

LITTLE ROCK

Arkansas Poison and Drug Information Center (*)
College of Pharmacy - UAMS

4301 West Markham St.
Mail Slot 522-2
Little Rock, AR 72205
Business: 501-686-6161
Emergency: 800-222-1222
             800-376-4766 (AR)
TDD/TTY: 800-641-3805

ASPCA/ ANIMAL POISON CONTROL CENTER

1717 South Philo Rd.
Suite 36
Urbana, IL 61802
Business: 217-337-5030
Emergency: 888-426-4435
             800-548-2423
www.aspca.org/apcc

CALIFORNIA

FRESNO/MADERA

California Poison Control System-Fresno/Madera Div. (*)
Children's Hospital Central California

9300 Valley Children's Place, MB 15
Madera, CA 93638-8762
Business: 559-622-2300
Emergency: 800-222-1222
             800-876-4766 (CA)
TDD/TTY: 800-972-3323
www.calpoison.org

SACRAMENTO

California Poison Control System-Sacramento Div. (*)
UC Davis Medical Center

2315 Stockton Blvd.
Sacramento, CA 95817
Business: 916-227-1400
Emergency: 800-222-1222
             800-876-4766 (CA)
TDD/TTY: 800-972-3323
www.calpoison.org

SAN DIEGO

California Poison Control System-San Diego Div. (*)
UC San Diego Medical Center

200 West Arbor Dr.
San Diego, CA 92103-8925
Business: 858-715-6300
Emergency: 800-222-1222
             800-876-4766 (CA)
TDD/TTY: 800-972-3323
www.calpoison.org

SAN FRANCISCO

California Poison Control System-San Francisco Div. (*)
University of California San Francisco

Box 1369
San Francisco, CA 94143-1369
Business: 415-502-6000
Emergency: 800-222-1222
             800-876-4766 (CA)
TDD/TTY: 800-972-3323
www.calpoison.org

COLORADO

DENVER

Rocky Mountain Poison and Drug Center (*)

777 Bannock St., Mail Code 0180
Denver, CO 80204
Business: 303-739-1100
Emergency: 800-222-1222
TDD/TTY: 303-739-1127 (CO)
www.RMPDC.org

CONNECTICUT

FARMINGTON

Connecticut Poison Control Center (*)
University of Connecticut Health Center

263 Farmington Ave.
Farmington, CT 06030-5365
Business: 860-679-4540
Emergency: 800-222-1222
TDD/TTY: 866-218-5372
http://poisoncontrol.uchc.edu

DELAWARE

(PHILADELPHIA, PA)

The Poison Control Center (*)
Children's Hospital of Philadelphia

34th St. & Civic Center Blvd.
Philadelphia, PA 19104-4399
Business: 215-590-2003
Emergency: 800-222-1222
TDD/TTY: 215-590-8789
www.poisoncontrol.chop.edu

DISTRICT OF COLUMBIA

WASHINGTON, DC

National Capital Poison Center (*)

3201 New Mexico Ave., NW
Suite 310
Washington, DC 20016
Business: 202-362-3867
Emergency: 800-222-1222
www.poison.org

FLORIDA

JACKSONVILLE

Florida Poison Information Center-Jacksonville (*)

655 West 8th St.
Box C23
Jacksonville, FL 32209
Business: 904-244-4465
Emergency: 800-222-1222
http://fpicjax.org

MIAMI

Florida Poison Information Center (*)
University of Miami, Dept. of Pediatrics

P.O. Box 016960 (R-131)
Miami, FL 33101
Business: 305-585-5250
Emergency: 800-222-1222
www.med.miami.edu/poisoncontrol

TAMPA

Florida Poison Information Center (*)
Tampa General Hospital

P.O. Box 1289
Tampa, FL 33601-1289
Business: 813-844-7044
Emergency: 800-222-1222
www.poisoncentertampa.org

GEORGIA

ATLANTA

Georgia Poison Center (*)
Hughes Spalding Children's Hospital, Grady Health System

80 Jesse Hill Jr. Dr., SE
P.O. Box 26066
Atlanta, GA 30303-3050
Business: 404-616-9237
Emergency: 800-222-1222
              404-616-9000 (Atlanta)
TDD: 404-616-9287
www.georgiapoisoncenter.org

HAWAII

(DENVER, CO)

Rocky Mountain Poison and Drug Center (*)

777 Bannock St., Mail Code 0180
Denver, CO 80204
Business: 303-739-1100
Emergency: 800-222-1222
TDD/TTY: 303-739-1127 (CO)
www.RMPDC.org

IDAHO

(DENVER, CO)

Rocky Mountain Poison and Drug Center (*)

777 Bannock St., Mail Code 0180
Denver, CO 80204
Business: 303-739-1100
Emergency: 800-222-1222
TDD/TTY: 303-739-1127 (CO)
www.RMPDC.org

ILLINOIS

CHICAGO

Illinois Poison Center (*)

222 South Riverside Plaza
Suite 1900
Chicago, IL 60606
Business: 312-906-6136
Emergency: 800-222-1222
TDD/TTY: 312-906-6185
www.mchc.org/ipc

INDIANA

INDIANAPOLIS

Indiana Poison Control Center (*)
Methodist Hospital, Clarian Health Partners

I-65 at 21st St.
P.O. Box 1367
Indianapolis, IN 46206-1367
Business: 317-962-2335
Emergency: 800-222-1222
              800-382-9097
              317-962-2323
              (Indianapolis)
www.clarian.org/poisoncontrol

IOWA

SIOUX CITY

Iowa Statewide Poison Control Center (*)
Iowa Health System and the University of Iowa Hospitals and Clinics

401 Douglas St., Suite 402
Sioux City, IA 51101
Business: 712-279-3710
Emergency: 800-222-1222
              712-277-2222 (IA)
www.iowapoison.org

KANSAS

KANSAS CITY

University of Kansas Poison Control Hospital Center

3901 Rainbow Blvd.
Delp - Room 4043
Kansas City, KS 66160-7231
Business: 913-588-6638
Emergency: 800-222-1222
              800-332-6633 (KS)
www.kumed.com/poison

KENTUCKY

LOUISVILLE

Kentucky Regional Poison Center (*)
Medical Towers South

234 E Gray St, Suite 847
Louisville, KY 40202
Business: 502-629-7264
Emergency: 800-222-1222
www.krpc.com

LOUISIANA

SHREVEPORT

Louisiana Poison Center (*)
LSUHSC - Shreveport
Dept. of Emergency Medicine Section of Clinical Toxology

1455 Wilkinson St
Shreveport, LA 71130
Business: 318-813-3314
Emergency: 800-222-1222

MAINE

PORTLAND

Northern New England Poison Center (*)

22 Bramhall St.
Portland, ME 04102
Business: 207-662-7042
Emergency: 800-222-1222
              800-442-6035
              207-871-2879 (ME)
TDD/TTY: 207-662-2879 (ME)
www.nnepc.org

MARYLAND

BALTIMORE

Maryland Poison Center (*)
University of Maryland at Baltimore School of Pharmacy

220 Arch St.
Office Level 01
Baltimore, MD 21201
Business: 410-706-7604
Emergency: 800-222-1222
TDD: 410-528-7530
www.mdpoison.com

(WASHINGTON, DC)

National Capital Poison Center (*)

3201 New Mexico Ave., NW
Suite 310
Washington, DC 20016
Business: 202-362-3867
Emergency: 800-222-1222
www.poison.org

MASSACHUSETTS

BOSTON

Regional Center for Poison Control and Prevention (*)
(Serving Massachusetts and Rhode Island)

300 Longwood Ave.
Boston, MA 02115
Business: 617-355-6609
Emergency: 800-222-1222
TDD/TTY: 888-244-5313
www.maripoisoncenter.com

MICHIGAN

DETROIT

Regional Poison Control Center (*)
Children's Hospital of Michigan

4160 John R. Harper Professional Office Bldg.
Suite 616
Detroit, MI 48201
Business: 313-745-5335
Emergency: 800-222-1222
www.mitoxic.org/pcc

MINNESOTA

MINNEAPOLIS

Hennepin Regional Poison Center (*)
Hennepin County Medical Center

701 Park Ave.
Mail Code RL
Minneapolis, MN 55415
Business: 612-873-3144
Emergency: 800-222-1222
www.mnpoison.org

MISSISSIPPI

JACKSON

Mississippi Regional Poison Control Center
University of Mississippi Medical Center

2500 North State St.
Jackson, MS 39216
Business: 601-984-1680
Emergency: 800-222-1222
http://poisoncontrol.umc.edu

MISSOURI

ST. LOUIS

Missouri Regional Poison Center (*)

7980 Clayton Rd. Suite 200
St. Louis, MO 63117
Business: 314-772-8300
Emergency: 800-222-1222
www.cardinalglennon.com

MONTANA

(DENVER, CO)

Rocky Mountain Poison and Drug Center (*)

777 Bannock St., Mail Code 0180
Denver, CO 80204
Business: 303-739-1100
Emergency: 800-222-1222
TDD/TTY: 303-739-1127 (CO)
www.RMPDC.org

NEBRASKA

OMAHA

Nebraska Regional Poison Center (*)

8401 W. Dodge Rd., Suite 115
Omaha, NE 68114
Business: 402-390-5555
Emergency: 800-222-1222
www.nebraskapoison.com

NEVADA

(DENVER, CO)

Rocky Mountain Poison and Drug Center (*)

777 Bannock St., Mail Code 0180
Denver, CO 80204
Business: 303-739-1100
Emergency: 800-222-1222
TDD/TTY: 303-739-1127 (CO)
www.RMPDC.org

NEW HAMPSHIRE

(PORTLAND, ME)

Northern New England Poison Center
Maine Medical Center

22 Bramhall St.
Portland, ME 04102
Business: 207-662-0111
Emergency: 800-222-1222
www.nnepc.org

NEW JERSEY

NEWARK

New Jersey Poison Information and Education System (*)
UMDNJ

140 Bergen St. PO Box 1709
Newark, NJ 07101
Business: 973-972-9280
Emergency: 800-222-1222
TDD/TTY: 973-926-8008
www.njpies.org

NEW MEXICO

ALBUQUERQUE

New Mexico Poison and Drug Information Center (*)

MSC09/5080
1 University of New Mexico
Albuquerque, NM 87131-0001
Business: 505-272-4261
Emergency: 800-222-1222
http://hsc.unm.edu/pharmacy/poison

NEW YORK

MINEOLA

Long Island Regional Poison and Drug Information Center (*)
Winthrop University Hospital

259 First St.
Mineola, NY 11501
Business: 516-663-4574
Emergency: 800-222-1222
www.lirpdic.org

NEW YORK CITY

New York City Poison Control Center (*)
NYC Bureau of Public Health

455 First Ave., Room 123, Box 81
New York, NY 10016
Business: 212-447-8152
Emergency: 800-222-1222
(English)   212-340-4494
               212-POISONS
               (212-764-7667)
Emergency: 212-venenos
(Spanish)   (212-836-3667)
TDD: 212-689-9014
www.nyc.gov/html/doh/html/poison/poison.shtml

ROCHESTER

The Ruth A. Lawrence Regional Poison and Drug Information Center (*)
University of Rochester Medical Center

601 Elmwood Ave.
Box 321
Rochester, NY 14642
Business: 585-273-4155
Emergency: 800-222-1222
TTY: 585-273-3854
www.fingerlakespoison.org

SYRACUSE

Upstate New York Poison Center (*)
SUNY Upstate Medical University

750 East Adams St.
Syracuse, NY 13210
Business: 315-464-7078
Emergency: 800-222-1222
TTY: 315-464-5424
www.upstatepoison.org

NORTH CAROLINA

CHARLOTTE

Carolinas Poison Center (*)
Carolinas Medical Center

PO Box 32861
Charlotte, NC 28232-2861
Business: 704-512-3795
Emergency: 800-222-1222
www.ncpoisoncenter.org

NORTH DAKOTA

(MINNEAPOLIS, MN)

Hennepin Regional Poison Center (*)
Hennepin County Medical Center

701 Park Ave., Mail Code RL
Minneapolis, MN 55415
Business: 612-873-3144
Emergency: 800-222-1222
www.mnpoison.org

OHIO

CINCINNATI

Cincinnati Drug and Poison Information Center (*)

3333 Burnet Ave., MLC 9004
Cincinnati, OH 45229
Business: 513-636-5063
Emergency: 800-222-1222
www.cincinnatichildrens.org/dpic

CLEVELAND

Northern Ohio Poison Center
Rainbow Babies and Children's Hospital

11100 Euclid Ave.
B261 MP 6007
Cleveland, OH 44106-6010
Business: 216-844-1573
Emergency: 800-222-1222
www.uhhospitals.org/rainbowchildren/tabid/195/Default.aspx

COLUMBUS

Central Ohio Poison Center (*)

700 Children's Dr.
Columbus, OH 43205
Business: 614-355-0435
Emergency: 800-222-1222
TTY: 866-688-0088
www.bepoisonsmart.com

OKLAHOMA

OKLAHOMA CITY

Oklahoma Poison Control Center (*)
OU Health Sciences Center

940 Northeast 13th St.
Room 3N3510
Oklahoma City, OK 73104
Business: 405-271-5062
Emergency: 800-222-1222
www.oklahomapoison.org

OREGON

PORTLAND

Oregon Poison Center (*)
Oregon Health and Science University

3181 S.W. Sam Jackson Park Rd.
CB550
Portland, OR 97239
Business: 503-494-8600
Emergency: 800-222-1222
www.ohsu.edu/poison

PENNSYLVANIA

PHILADELPHIA

The Poison Control Center (*)
Children's Hospital of Philadelphia

34th Street & Civic Center Blvd.
Philadelphia, PA 19104
Business: 215-590-2003
Emergency: 800-222-1222
               215-386-2100 (PA)
TDD/TTY: 215-590-8789
www.poisoncontrol.chop.edu

PITTSBURGH

Pittsburgh Poison Center (*)
University of Pittsburgh

200 Lothrop Street
Pittsburgh, PA 15213
Business: 412-390-3300
Emergency: 800-222-1222
               412-681-6669
www.upmc.com/services/poisoncenter

RHODE ISLAND

(BOSTON, MA)

Regional Center for Poison Control and Prevention (*)
(Serving Massachusetts and Rhode Island)

300 Longwood Ave.
Boston, MA 02115
Business: 617-355-6609
Emergency: 800-222-1222
TDD/TTY: 888-244-5313
www.maripoisoncenter.com

SOUTH CAROLINA

COLUMBIA

Palmetto Poison Center (*)
South Carolina College of Pharmacy
University of South Carolina

Columbia, SC 29208
Business: 803-777-7909
Emergency: 800-222-1222
http://poison.sc.edu

SOUTH DAKOTA

(MINNEAPOLIS, MN)

Hennepin Regional Poison Center (*)
Hennepin County Medical Center

701 Park Ave., Mail Code RL
Minneapolis, MN 55415
Business: 612-873-3144
Emergency: 800-222-1222
www.mnpoison.org

TENNESSEE

NASHVILLE

Tennessee Poison Center (*)

1161 21st Ave. South
501 Oxford House
Nashville, TN 37232-4632
Business: 615-936-0760
Emergency: 800-222-1222
www.tnpoisoncenter.org

TEXAS

AMARILLO

Texas Panhandle Poison Center (*)

1501 S. Coulter Dr.
Amarillo, TX 79106
Business: 806-354-1630
Emergency: 800-222-1222
wwww.poisoncontrol.org

DALLAS

North Texas Poison Center (*)
Texas Poison Center Network
Parkland Memorial Hospital

5201 Harry Hines Blvd.
Dallas, TX 75235
Business: 214-589-0911
Emergency: 800-222-1222
www.poisoncontrol.org

EL PASO

West Texas Regional Poison
Center (*)
At University Medical Center of
El Paso

4815 Alameda Ave.
El Paso, TX 79905
Business   915-534-3800
Emergency: 800-222-1222
www.poisoncontrol.org

GALVESTON

Southeast Texas Poison Center (*)
The University of Texas
Medical Branch

3.112 Trauma Center
Galveston, TX 77555-1175
Business: 409-772-3332
Emergency: 800-222-1222
www.utmb.edu/setpc

SAN ANTONIO

South Texas Poison Center (*)
The University of Texas Health
Science Center–San Antonio
Dept. of Surgery

7703 Floyd Curl Dr., MSC 7849
San Antonio, TX 78229-3900
Business: 210-567-5762
Emergency: 800-222-1222
www.texaspoison.com

TEMPLE

Central Texas Poison Center (*)
Scott & White Memorial Hospital

2401 South 31st St.
Temple, TX 76508
Business: 254-724-7405
Emergency: 800-222-1222
http://www.sw.org/web/
patientsAndVisitors/iwcontent/
public/poison/en_us/html/poison.jsp

UTAH

SALT LAKE CITY

Utah Poison Control Center (*)
University of Utah

585 Komas Dr. Suite #200
Salt Lake City, UT 84108-1234
Business: 801-587-0600
Emergency: 800-222-1222
http://uuhsc.utah.edu/poison

VERMONT

(PORTLAND, ME)

Northern New England
Poison Center (*)
Maine Medical Center

22 Bramhall St.
Portland, ME 04102
Business: 207-662-0111
Emergency: 800-222-1222
www.nnepc.org

VIRGINIA

CHARLOTTESVILLE

Blue Ridge Poison Center (*)
Jefferson Park Place

1222 Jefferson Park Ave.
Charlottesville, VA 22908-0774
Business: 434-924-0347
Emergency: 800-222-1222
www.healthsystem.virginia.edu/brpc

RICHMOND

Virginia Poison Center (*)
Medical College of Virginia
Hospitals
Virginia Commonwealth University
Health System

P.O. Box 980522
Richmond, VA 23298-0522
Business: 804-828-4780
Emergency: 800-222-1222
www.poison.vcu.edu

WASHINGTON

SEATTLE

Washington Poison Center (*)

155 NE 100th St.
Seattle, WA 98125-8007
Business: 206-517-2350
Emergency: 800-222-1222
www.wapc.org

WEST VIRGINIA

CHARLESTON

West Virginia Poison Center (*)
WVU Charleston Division

3110 MacCorkle Ave. SE
Charleston, WV 25314
Business: 304-347-1212
Emergency: 800-222-1222
www.wvpoisoncenter.org

WISCONSIN

MILWAUKEE

Wisconsin Poison Center

Mail Station 660
P.O. Box 1997
Milwaukee, WI 53201-1997
Business: 414-266-6973
Emergency: 800-222-1222
www.wisconsinpoison.org

WYOMING

(OMAHA, NE)

Nebraska Regional Poison
Center (*)

8401 W. Dodge St., Suite 115
Omaha, NE 68114
Business: 402-390-5555
Emergency: 800-222-1222
www.nebraskapoison.com

Designed for practicing nurses, nursing students, and other healthcare professionals...from PDR!

NEW from PDR!

2010 PDR® NURSE'S DRUG HANDBOOK
Combining effectiveness and efficiency to maintain superior patient care!

Aiming to prevent medication errors and foster clinical accountability like no other drug resource, the *2010 PDR® Nurse's Drug Handbook* places up-to-the-minute, FDA-regulated prescribing information at the reader's fingertips.

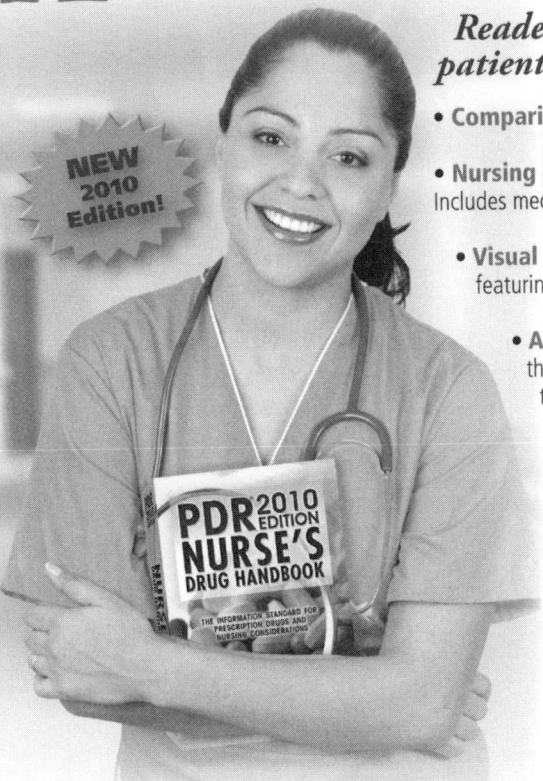

NEW 2010 Edition!

Readers can quickly and easily reference critical data on patient medications. This new edition features:

- **Comparison charts:** Scores of Rx and OTC comparison charts

- **Nursing considerations:** Considerations for monitoring disease progression and efficacy of therapy. Includes mechanism of action, pharmacokinetics, patient counseling, administration/storage, and assessment

- **Visual Identification Guide:** A color insert of drug products organized alphabetically by brand name, featuring more than 300 photographs of tablets, capsules, and other solid dosage forms

- **Appendices:** Annually revised information to assist in administering drugs and monitoring drug therapy. Key tables and charts of therapy-specific drugs, plus valuable lists of drugs, including drugs that are excreted in breast milk, drugs that should not be crushed, and drugs that may cause photosensitivity. Also included are helpful lists of associations and other nursing-specific professional resources

- **Single-column format:** Allows for quick point-of-care referencing capability

- **Expanded reference section:** Covers dosing comparisons within drug classes; OTC medications; antibiotic sensitivity and more

- **Guidelines for drug administration:** Includes changes in dosing and use recommendations

ISBN: 9781563637469 • ~~$41.95~~ • **YOUR PRICE: $37.75**

Brand & generic name

Drug's indications

Detailed dosing information

Nursing considerations

Full-color product images

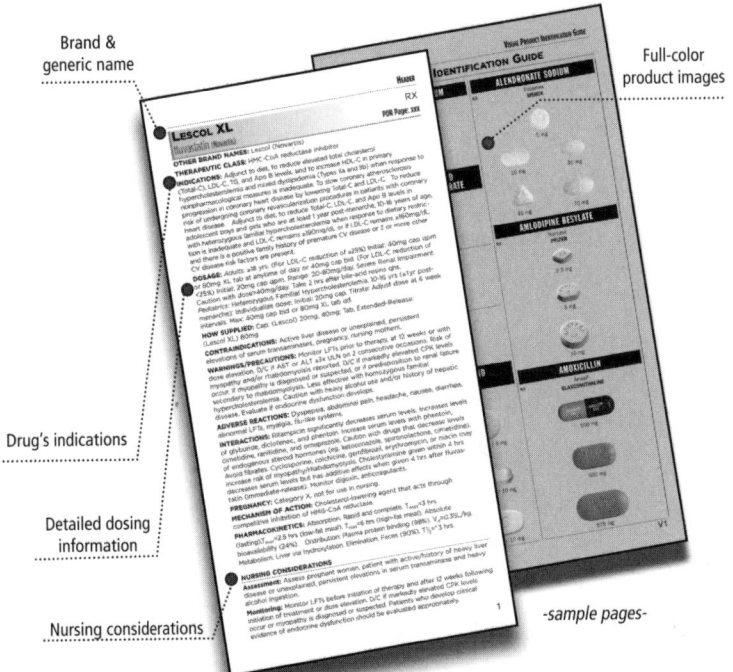

-sample pages-

Here's what the experts are saying:

*"The **PDR Nurse's Drug Handbook** provides easily accessible, critical information that will inform nursing practice and patient education efforts. With its convenient size and clear layout that aids swift access to concise, evidence-based information, this book will quickly become a useful and trusted source for medication information among nurses."*

Ivy M. Alexander, PhD, C-ANP
Associate Professor
Director—Adult, Family, Gerontological, and Women's Health Primary Care Specialty, Yale University School of Nursing

*Order online at www.PDRbookstore.com and enter promo code F9008NH07 for 10% savings!
Any questions—call toll-free 1-800-678-5689.

✔ **PDR**® Network
Safety Communication Compliance

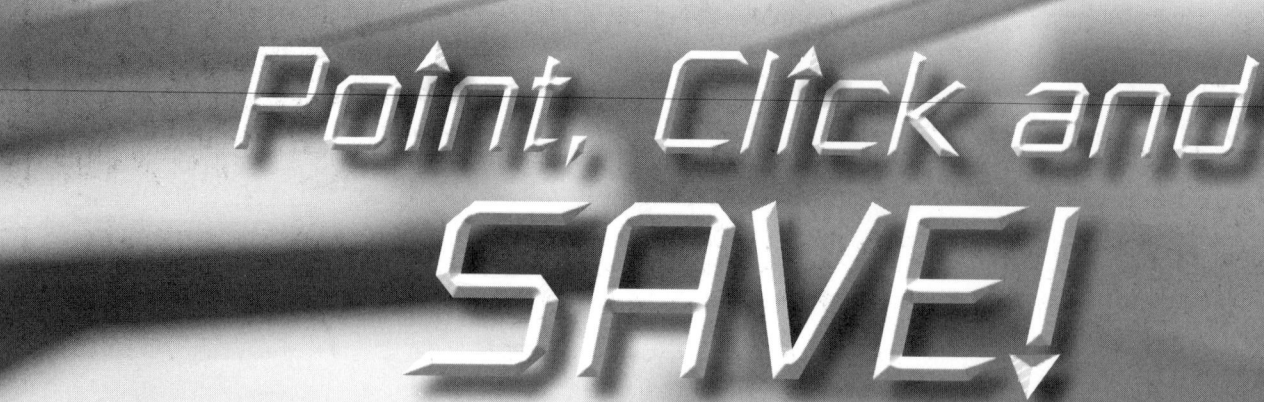
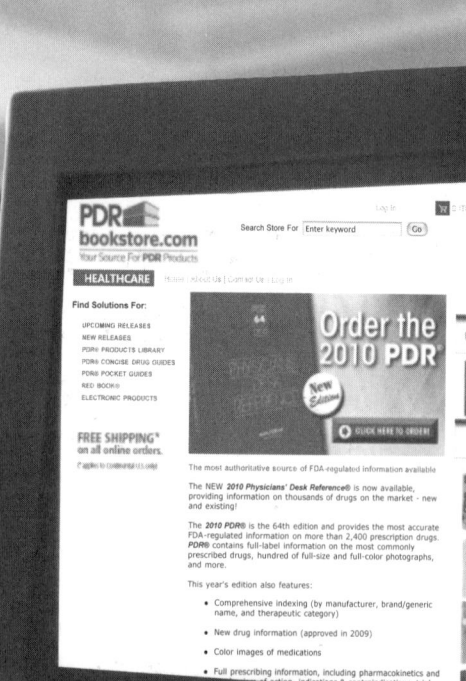